ICD-10-CM Code Book

2018

Anne B. Casto, RHIA, CCS
Consulting Editor

AHIMA
American Health Information Management Association®

ISBN: 978-1-58426-589-4
AHIMA Product No.: AC221017

AHIMA Staff:
Chelsea Brotherton, Assistant Editor
Megan Grennan, Senior Production Development Editor
Elizabeth Ranno, Vice President of Product and Planning
Caitlin Wilson, Project Editor
Pamela Woolf, Director of Publications

Cover image: © Apola, iStockphoto.com

The Centers for Medicare and Medicaid Services (CMS) and the National Center for Health Statistics (NCHS), two departments within the US Federal Government's Department of Health and Human Services (HHS) provide the *International Classification of Diseases, Tenth Revision, Clinical Modification* (ICD-10-CM) for coding and reporting. ICD-10-CM is the US modification to the World Health Organization's (WHO) International Classification of Diseases, Tenth Revision (ICD-10).

Coding Clinic for ICD-10-CM and ICD-10-PCS is a publication of the American Hospital Association (AHA).

The websites listed in this book were current and valid as of the date of publication. However, webpage addresses and the information on them may change at any time. The user is encouraged to perform his or her own general web searches to locate any site addresses listed here that are no longer valid.

For more information about AHIMA Press publications, including updates, visit http://www.ahima.org/publications/updates.aspx

American Health Information Management Association
233 North Michigan Avenue, 21st Floor
Chicago, Illinois 60601-5809
ahima.org

Contents

About the Consulting Editor iv
Acknowledgments iv

Introduction v

Index to Diseases and Injuries 1

Table of Neoplasms 324

Table of Drugs and Chemicals 346

External Cause of Injuries Index 426

Tabular List of Diseases and Injuries 459

Chapter 1 Certain Infectious and Parasitic Diseases (A00-B99) 460
Chapter 2 Neoplasms (C00-D49) 485
Chapter 3 Diseases of the Blood and Blood-forming Organs and Certain Disorders Involving the Immune Mechanism (D50-D89) 523
Chapter 4 Endocrine, Nutritional and Metabolic Diseases (E00-E89) 531
Chapter 5 Mental, Behavioral and Neurodevelopmental Disorders (F01-F99) 552
Chapter 6 Diseases of the Nervous System (G00-G99) 577
Chapter 7 Diseases of the Eye and Adnexa (H00-H59) 598
Chapter 8 Diseases of the Ear and Mastoid Process (H60-H95) 633
Chapter 9 Diseases of the Circulatory System (I00-I99) 644
Chapter 10 Diseases of the Respiratory System (J00-J99) 689
Chapter 11 Diseases of the Digestive System (K00-K95) 704
Chapter 12 Diseases of the Skin and Subcutaneous Tissue (L00-L99) 728
Chapter 13 Diseases of the Musculoskeletal System and Connective Tissue (M00-M99) 750
Chapter 14 Diseases of the Genitourinary System (N00-N99) 838
Chapter 15 Pregnancy, Childbirth and the Puerperium (O00-O9A) 858
Chapter 16 Certain Conditions Originating in the Perinatal Period (P00-P96) 894
Chapter 17 Congenital Malformations, Deformations and Chromosomal Abnormalities (Q00-Q99) 905
Chapter 18 Symptoms, Signs and Abnormal Clinical and Laboratory Findings, Not Elsewhere Classified (R00-R99) 921
Chapter 19 Injury, Poisoning and Certain Other Consequences of External Causes (S00-T88) 938
Chapter 20 External Causes of Morbidity (V00-Y99) 1233
Chapter 21 Factors Influencing Health Status and Contact with Health Services (Z00-Z99) 1300

Online Appendices:

Appendix A: CC/MCC Exclusion Lists 1330

Appendix B: Hospital-Acquired Conditions (HAC) List 1330

About the Consulting Editor

Anne B. Casto, RHIA, CCS, is the president of Casto Consulting, LLC. Casto Consulting, LLC is a consulting firm that provides services to hospitals and other healthcare stakeholders primarily in the areas of reimbursement and coding. Casto Consulting, LLC specializes in linking coding and billing practices to positive revenue cycle outcomes. Additionally, the firm provides guidance to consulting firms, healthcare organizations and healthcare insurers regarding reimbursement methodologies and Medicare regulations.

Prior to founding the firm Anne was the program manager of the HIMS Division at The Ohio State University School of Allied Medical Professions. Ms. Casto taught healthcare reimbursement, ICD-9-CM coding and CPT coding courses for several years. Additionally, Ms. Casto was responsible for curriculum revisions in the areas of chargemaster management, clinical data management and healthcare reimbursement.

Additionally, Ms. Casto was the vice president of clinical information for Cleverley & Associates where she worked very closely with APC regulations and guidelines, preparing hospitals for the implementation of the Medicare OPPS. Ms. Casto was also the clinical information product manager for CHIPS/Ingenix. She joined CHIPS/Ingenix in 1998 and spent the majority of her time developing coding compliance products for the inpatient and outpatient settings.

Ms. Casto has been responsible for inpatient and outpatient coding activities in several large hospitals including Mt. Sinai Medical Center (NYC), Beth Israel Medical Center (NYC), and The Ohio State University. She has worked extensively with CMI, quality measures, physician documentation, and coding accuracy efforts at these facilities.

Ms. Casto received her degree in Health Information Management at The Ohio State University in 1995. She received her Certified Coding Specialist credential in 1998 from the American Health Information Management Association. In 2009 Ms. Casto received her ICD-10-CM/PCS Trainer certificate from AHIMA. Ms. Casto is the co-author of an AHIMA published text book entitled *Principles of Healthcare Reimbursement*. Additionally, Ms. Casto was a contributing author to the published AHIMA books: *Severity DRGs and Reimbursement; A MS-DRG Primer* and *Effective Management of Coding Services*.

Ms. Casto received the AHIMA Legacy Award, part of the FORE Triumph Awards, in 2007 which honors a significant contribution to the knowledge base of the HIM field through an insightful publication. Additionally, Ms. Casto was honored with the Ohio Health Information Management Association's Distinguished Member Award in 2008 and the Ohio Health Information Management Association's Professional Achievement Award in 2011.

Acknowledgments

Many thanks to my family for their support during this project. Thanks to Dr. Susan White, The Ohio State University; your data manipulation skills are second to none. Thanks to Drew Beverick for providing valuable insight from the student perspective. Many thanks to Linda Hyde, RHIA and Tina L. Cressman, CCS, CCS-P, CPC CPC-H CPC-P CEMC for their very thorough technical review of the book. I thank the reviewers for their thoughtful comments and suggestions.

ICD-10-CM History and Background

The International Classification of Diseases, Tenth Revision, Clinical Modification (ICD-10-CM) is the United Stated modification to the World Health Organization's (WHO) International Classification of Diseases, Tenth Revision (ICD-10). The WHO adopted the tenth revision in 1990. Since that time, several countries, including Australia and Canada, have developed their own modification to ICD-10 and have implemented it for use.

In 1994, the National Center for Health Statistics (NCHS) began the process of determining the viability of ICD-10 and the applicability of a clinical modification of the code set for the United States. The NCHS has made draft versions of ICD-10-CM available since 2002. NCHS continued to refine and update the code set for use in the United States while the healthcare community waited for adoption of the code set by Congress. On August 22, 2008, the long-awaited official Notice of Proposed Rule Making (NPRM) regarding the adopting of the ICD-10-CM and ICD-10-PCS classifications was published in the *Federal Register*. On January 16, 2009, the Centers for Medicare and Medicaid Services (CMS) published the Final Rule for adoption of the ICD-10-CM and ICD-10-PCS code sets udders rules, 45 CFR Parts 160 and 162 of the Health Insurance Portability and Accountability Act of 1996 (HIPAA). Within this rule, a compliance (implementation) date of October 1, 2013 was released. The compliance date was revised and ICD-10-CM was successfully implemented on October 1, 2015.

Characteristics of ICD-10-CM

ICD-10-CM far exceeds its predecessors in the number of codes provided. The disease classification has been expanded to include health-related conditions and to provide greater specificity at the seventh-character level of detail. When available, these seventh characters are not optional; they are intended for use in recording the information substantiated in the clinical record.

The ICD-10-CM/PCS Coordination and Maintenance Committee

Annual modifications are made to ICD-10-CM through the ICD-10-CM Coordination and Maintenance Committee (C&M). The Committee is made up of representatives from two US federal government agencies, the National Center for Health Statistics, and the Centers for Medicare and Medicaid Services (CMS). C&M holds meetings twice a year, which are open to the public. Modification proposals submitted to C&M for consideration are presented at the meetings for public discussion. An open comment period follows each of these meetings. Those modification proposals which are approved are incorporated into the official government version of ICD-10-CM and become effective for use on October 1 of each year.

Guidance in the Use of ICD10-CM

To code accurately, it is necessary to have a working knowledge of medical terminology and to understand the characteristics, code book terminology, and conventions of ICD-10-CM. Transforming verbal descriptions of diseases, injuries, and conditions into numerical designations (coding) is a complex activity and should not be undertaken without proper training.

Originally, coding was accomplished to provide access to health records by diagnoses and operations through retrieval for medical research education and administration. Today, medical codes are utilized to facilitate payment of health services, evaluate utilization patterns, and study the appropriateness of healthcare costs. Coding also provides the basis for epidemiological studies and research into the quality of healthcare.

Coding must be performed correctly and consistently to produce meaningful statics to aid in planning for the health needs of the nation.

Official Conventions

ICD-10-CM Official Guidelines for Coding and Reporting 2018

(October 1, 2017 - September 30, 2018)

Narrative changes appear in bold text

Items <u>underlined</u> have been moved within the guidelines since the 2017 version

***Italics* are used to indicate revisions to heading changes**

The Centers for Medicare and Medicaid Services (CMS) and the National Center for Health Statistics (NCHS), two departments within the US Federal Government's Department of Health and Human Services (HHS) provide the following guidelines for coding and reporting using the International Classification of Diseases, Tenth Revision, Clinical Modification (ICD-10-CM). These guidelines should be used as a companion document to the official version of the ICD-10-CM as published on the NCHS website. The ICD-10-CM is a morbidity classification published by the United

States for classifying diagnoses and reason for visits in all healthcare settings. The ICD-10-CM is based on the ICD-10, the statistical classification of disease published by the World Health Organization (WHO).

These guidelines have been approved by the four organizations that make up the Cooperating Parties for the ICD-10-CM: the American Hospital Association (AHA), the American Health Information Management Association (AHIMA), CMS, and NCHS.

These guidelines are a set of rules that have been developed to accompany and complement the official conventions and instructions provided within the ICD-10-CM itself. The instructions and conventions of the classification take precedence over guidelines. These guidelines are based on the coding and sequencing instructions in the Tabular List and Alphabetic Index of ICD-10-CM, but provide additional instruction. Adherence to these guidelines when assigning ICD-10-CM diagnosis codes is required under the Health Insurance Portability and Accountability Act (HIPAA). The diagnosis codes (Tabular List and Alphabetic Index) have been adopted under HIPAA for all healthcare settings. A joint effort between the healthcare provider and the coder is essential to achieve complete and accurate documentation, code assignment, and reporting of diagnoses and procedures. These guidelines have been developed to assist both the healthcare provider and the coder in identifying those diagnoses that are to be reported. The importance of consistent, complete documentation in the medical record cannot be overemphasized. Without such documentation accurate coding cannot be achieved. The entire record should be reviewed to determine the specific reason for the encounter and the conditions treated.

The term encounter is used for all settings, including hospital admissions. In the context of these guidelines, the term provider is used throughout the guidelines to mean physician or any qualified healthcare practitioner who is legally accountable for establishing the patient's diagnosis. Only this set of guidelines, approved by the Cooperating Parties, is official.

The guidelines are organized into sections. Section I includes the structure and conventions of the classification and general guidelines that apply to the entire classification, and chapter-specific guidelines that correspond to the chapters as they are arranged in the classification. Section II includes guidelines for selection of principal diagnosis for non-outpatient settings. Section III includes guidelines for reporting additional diagnoses in non-outpatient settings. Section IV is for outpatient coding and reporting. It is necessary to review all sections of the guidelines to fully understand all of the rules and instructions needed to code properly.

Section I. Conventions, General Coding Guidelines and Chapter Specific Guidelines

The conventions, general guidelines and chapter-specific guidelines are applicable to all healthcare settings unless otherwise indicated. The conventions and instructions of the classification take precedence over guidelines.

A. Conventions for the ICD-10-CM

The conventions for the ICD-10-CM are the general rules for use of the classification independent of the guidelines. These conventions are incorporated within the Alphabetic Index and Tabular List of the ICD-10-CM as instructional notes.

1. The Alphabetic Index and Tabular List

The ICD-10-CM is divided into the Alphabetic Index, an alphabetical list of terms and their corresponding code, and the Tabular List, a structured list of codes divided into chapters based on body system or condition. The Alphabetic Index consists of the following parts: the Index of Diseases and Injury, the Index of External Causes of Injury, the Table of Neoplasms, and the Table of Drugs and Chemicals.

See Section I.C2. General guidelines

See Section I.C.19. Adverse effects, poisoning, underdosing and toxic effects

2. Format and Structure

The ICD-10-CM Tabular List contains categories, subcategories and codes. Characters for categories, subcategories and codes may be either a letter or a number. All categories are 3 characters. A three-character category that has no further subdivision is equivalent to a code. Subcategories are either 4 or 5 characters. Codes may be 3, 4, 5, 6, or 7 characters. That is, each level of subdivision after a category is a subcategory. The final level of subdivision is a code. Codes that have applicable 7th characters are still referred to as codes, not subcategories. A code that has an applicable 7th character is considered invalid without the 7th character.

The ICD-10-CM uses an indented format for ease in reference.

3. Use of Codes for Reporting Purposes

For reporting purposes only codes are permissible, not categories or subcategories, and any applicable 7th character is required.

4. Placeholder Character

The ICD-10-CM utilizes a placeholder character X. The X is used as a placeholder at certain codes to allow for future expansion. An example of this is at the poisoning, adverse effect and underdosing codes, categories T36–T50.

Where a placeholder exists, the X must be used in order for the code to be considered a valid code.

5. 7th Characters

Certain ICD-10-CM categories have applicable 7th characters. The applicable 7th character is required for all codes within the category, or as the notes in the Tabular List instruct. The 7th character must always be the 7th character in the data field. If a code that requires a 7th character is not 6 characters, a placeholder X must be used to fill in the empty characters.

6. Abbreviations

a. Alphabetic Index Abbreviations

NEC "Not elsewhere classifiable"
This abbreviation in the Alphabetic Index represents "other specified". When a specific code is not available for a condition, the Alphabetic Index directs the coder to the "other specified" code in the Tabular List.

NOS "Not otherwise specified"
This abbreviation is the equivalent of unspecified.

b. Tabular List Abbreviations

NEC "Not elsewhere classifiable"
This abbreviation in the Tabular List represents "other specified". When a specific code is not available for a condition the Tabular List includes an NEC entry under a code to identify the code as the "other specified" code.

NOS "Not otherwise specified"
This abbreviation is the equivalent of unspecified.

7. Punctuation

[ ] Brackets are used in the Tabular List to enclose synonyms, alternative wording or explanatory phrases. Brackets are used in the Alphabetic Index to identify manifestation codes.

( ) Parentheses are used in both the Alphabetic Index and Tabular List to enclose supplementary words that may be present or absent in the statement of a disease or procedure without affecting the code number to which it is assigned. The terms within the parentheses are referred to as nonessential modifiers. The nonessential modifiers in the Alphabetic Index to Diseases apply to subterms following a main term except when a nonessential modifier and a subentry are mutually exclusive, the subentry takes precedence. For example, in the ICD-10-CM Alphabetic Index under the main term Enteritis, "acute" is a nonessential modifier and "chronic" is a subentry. In this case, the nonessential modifier "acute" does not apply to the subentry "chronic".

: Colons are used in the Tabular List after an incomplete term which needs one or more of the modifiers following the colon to make it assignable to a given category.

8. Use of "and"

See Section I.A.14. Use of the term "And"

9. Other and Unspecified Codes

a. "Other" Codes

Codes titled "other" or "other specified" are for use when the information in the medical record provides detail for which a specific code does not exist. Alphabetic Index entries with NEC in the line designate "other" codes in the Tabular List. These Alphabetic Index entries represent specific disease entities for which no specific code exists so the term is included within an "other" code.

b. "Unspecified" Codes

Codes titled "unspecified" are for use when the information in the medical record is insufficient to assign a more specific code. For those categories for which an unspecified code is not provided, the "other specified" code may represent both other and unspecified.

See Section I.B.18 Use of Signs/Symptom/Unspecified Codes

10. Includes Notes

This note appears immediately under a three character code title to further define, or give examples of, the content of the category.

11. Inclusion Terms

List of terms is included under some codes. These terms are the conditions for which that code is to be used. The terms may be synonyms of the code title, or, in the case of "other specified" codes, the terms are a list of the various conditions assigned to that code. The inclusion terms are not necessarily exhaustive. Additional terms found only in the Alphabetic Index may also be assigned to a code.

12. Excludes Notes

The ICD-10-CM has two types of excludes notes. Each type of note has a different definition for use but they are all similar in that they indicate that codes excluded from each other are independent of each other.

a. Excludes1

A type 1 Excludes note is a pure excludes note. It means "NOT CODED HERE!" An Excludes1 note indicates that the code excluded should never be used at the same time as the code above the Excludes1 note. An Excludes1 is used when two conditions cannot occur together, such as a congenital form versus an acquired form of the same condition.

An exception to the Excludes1 definition is the circumstance when the two conditions are unrelated to each other. If it is not clear whether the two conditions involving an Excludes1 note are related or not, query the provider. For example, code F45.8, Other somatoform disorders, has an Exlcudes1 note for "sleep related teeth grinding (G47.63)," because "teeth grinding" is an inclusion term under F45.8. Only one of these two codes should be assigned for teeth grinding. However, psychogenic dysmenorrhea is also an inclusion term under F45.8, and a patient could have both this conditions and sleep related teeth grinding. In this case, the two conditions are clearly unrelated to each other, and do it would be appropriate to report F45.8 and G47.63 together.

b. Excludes2

A type 2 Excludes note represents "Not included here". An Excludes2 note indicates that the condition excluded is not part of the condition represented by the code, but a patient may have both conditions at the same time. When an Excludes2 note appears under a code, it is acceptable to use both the code and the excluded code together, when appropriate.

13. Etiology/Manifestation Convention ("Code first", "Use additional code" and "In Diseases Classified Elsewhere" Notes)

Certain conditions have both an underlying etiology and multiple body system manifestations due to the underlying etiology. For such conditions, the ICD-10-CM has a coding convention that requires the underlying condition be sequenced first, if applicable, followed by the manifestation. Wherever such a combination exists, there is a "use additional code" note at the etiology code, and a "code first" note at the manifestation code. These instructional notes indicate the proper sequencing order of the codes, etiology followed by manifestation.

In most cases the manifestation codes will have in the code title, "in diseases classified elsewhere." Codes with this title are a component of the etiology/manifestation convention. The code title indicates that it is a manifestation code. "In diseases classified elsewhere" codes are never permitted to be used as first-listed or principal diagnosis codes. They must be used in conjunction with an underlying condition code and they must be listed following the underlying condition. See category F02, Dementia in other diseases classified elsewhere, for an example of this convention.

There are manifestation codes that do not have "in diseases classified elsewhere" in the title. For such codes, there is a "use additional code" note at the etiology code and a "code first" note at the manifestation code and the rules for sequencing apply.

In addition to the notes in the Tabular List, these conditions also have a specific Alphabetic Index entry structure. In the Alphabetic Index both conditions are listed together with the etiology code first followed by the manifestation codes in brackets. The code in brackets is always to be sequenced second.

An example of the etiology/manifestation convention is dementia in Parkinson's disease. In the Alphabetic Index, code G20 is listed first, followed by code F02.80 or F02.81 in brackets. Code G20 represents the underlying etiology, Parkinson's disease, and must be sequenced first, whereas codes F02.80 and F02.81 represent the manifestation of dementia in diseases classified elsewhere, with or without behavioral disturbance.

"Code first" and "Use additional code" notes are also used as sequencing rules in the classification for certain codes that are not part of an etiology/ manifestation combination.

See Section I.B. 7. Multiple coding for a single condition.

14. "And"

The word "and" should be interpreted to mean either "and" or "or" when it appears in a title.

For example, cases of "tuberculosis of bones", "tuberculosis of joints" and "tuberculosis of bones and joints" are classified to subcategory A18.0, Tuberculosis of bones and joints.

15. **"With"**
The word "with" **or "in"** should be interpreted to mean "associated with" or "due to" when it appears in a code title, the Alphabetic Index, or an instructional note in the Tabular List. The classification presumes a causal relationship between the two conditions linked by these terms in the Alphabetic Index or Tabular List. These conditions should be coded as related even in the absence of provider documentation explicitly linking them, unless the documentation clearly states the conditions are unrelated **or when another guideline exists that specifically requires a documented linkage between two conditions (e.g., sepsis guideline for "acute organ dysfunction that is not clearly associated with the sepsis").** For conditions not specifically linked by these relational terms in the classification **or when a guideline requires that a linkage between two conditions be explicitly documented,** provider documentation must link the conditions in order to code them as related.

The word "with" in the Alphabetic Index is sequenced immediately following the main term, not in alphabetical order.

16. **"See" and "See Also"**
The "see" instruction following a main term in the Alphabetic Index indicates that another term should be referenced. It is necessary to go to the main term referenced with the "see" note to locate the correct code.

A "see also" instruction following a main term in the Alphabetic Index instructs that there is another main term that may also be referenced that may provide additional Alphabetic Index entries that may be useful. It is not necessary to follow the "see also" note when the original main term provides the necessary code.

17. **"Code Also Note"**
A "code also" note instructs that two codes may be required to fully describe a condition, but this note does not provide sequencing direction. **The sequencing depends on the circumstances of the encounter.**

18. **Default Codes**
A code listed next to a main term in the ICD-10-CM Alphabetic Index is referred to as a default code. The default code represents that condition that is most commonly associated with the main term, or is the unspecified code for the condition. If a condition is documented in a medical record (for example, appendicitis) without any additional information, such as acute or chronic, the default code should be assigned.

19. **Code Assignment and Clinical Criteria**
The assignment of a diagnosis code is based on the provider's diagnostic statement that the condition exists. The provider's statement that the patient has a particular condition is sufficient. Code assignment is not based on clinical criteria used by the provider to establish the diagnosis.

B. General Coding Guidelines

1. **Locating a Code in the ICD-10-CM**
To select a code in the classification that corresponds to a diagnosis or reason for visit documented in a medical record, first locate the term in the Alphabetic Index, and then verify the code in the Tabular List. Read and be guided by instructional notations that appear in both the Alphabetic Index and the Tabular List.

It is essential to use both the Alphabetic Index and Tabular List when locating and assigning a code. The Alphabetic Index does not always provide the full code. Selection of the full code, including laterality and any applicable 7th character can only be done in the Tabular List. A dash (-) at the end of an Alphabetic Index entry indicates that additional characters are required. Even if a dash is not included at the Alphabetic Index entry, it is necessary to refer to the Tabular List to verify that no 7th character is required.

2. **Level of Detail in Coding**
Diagnosis codes are to be used and reported at their highest number of characters available.

ICD-10-CM diagnosis codes are composed of codes with 3, 4, 5, 6, or 7 characters. Codes with three characters are included in ICD-10-CM as the heading of a category of codes that may be further subdivided by the use of fourth and/or fifth characters and/or sixth characters, which provide greater detail.

A three-character code is to be used only if it is not further subdivided. A code is invalid if it has not been coded to the full number of characters required for that code, including the 7th character, if applicable.

3. **Code or Codes from A00.0–T88.9, Z00–Z99.8**
The appropriate code or codes from A00.0–T88.9, Z00–Z99.8 must be used to identify diagnoses, symptoms, conditions, problems, complaints or other reason(s) for the encounter/visit.

4. Signs and Symptoms

Codes that describe symptoms and signs, as opposed to diagnoses, are acceptable for reporting purposes when a related definitive diagnosis has not been established (confirmed) by the provider. Chapter 18 of ICD-10-CM, Symptoms, Signs, and Abnormal Clinical and Laboratory Findings, Not Elsewhere Classified (codes R00.0–R99) contains many, but not all codes for symptoms.

See Section I.B.18 Use of Signs/Symptom/Unspecified Codes

5. Conditions that are an Integral Part of a Disease Process

Signs and symptoms that are associated routinely with a disease process should not be assigned as additional codes, unless otherwise instructed by the classification.

6. Conditions that are not an Integral Part of a Disease Process

Additional signs and symptoms that may not be associated routinely with a disease process should be coded when present.

7. Multiple Coding for a Single Condition

In addition to the etiology/manifestation convention that requires two codes to fully describe a single condition that affects multiple body systems, there are other single conditions that also require more than one code. "Use additional code" notes are found in the Tabular List at codes that are not part of an etiology/manifestation pair where a secondary code is useful to fully describe a condition. The sequencing rule is the same as the etiology/manifestation pair, "use additional code" indicates that a secondary code should be added**, if known.**

For example, for bacterial infections that are not included in chapter 1, a secondary code from category B95, Streptococcus, Staphylococcus, and Enterococcus, as the cause of diseases classified elsewhere, or B96, Other bacterial agents as the cause of diseases classified elsewhere, may be required to identify the bacterial organism causing the infection. A "use additional code" note will normally be found at the infectious disease code, indicating a need for the organism code to be added as a secondary code.

"Code first" notes are also under certain codes that are not specifically manifestation codes but may be due to an underlying cause. When there is a "code first" note and an underlying condition is present, the underlying condition should be sequenced first**, if known.**

"Code, if applicable, any causal condition first", notes indicate that this code may be assigned as a principal diagnosis when the causal condition is unknown or not applicable. If a causal condition is known, the code for that condition should be sequenced as the principal or first-listed diagnosis.

Multiple codes may be needed for sequela, complication codes and obstetric codes to more fully describe a condition. See the specific guidelines for these conditions for further instruction.

8. Acute and Chronic Conditions

If the same condition is described as both acute (subacute) and chronic, and separate subentries exist in the Alphabetic Index at the same indentation level, code both and sequence the acute (subacute) code first.

9. Combination Code

A combination code is a single code used to classify:

- Two diagnoses, or
- A diagnosis with an associated secondary process (manifestation)
- A diagnosis with an associated complication

Combination codes are identified by referring to subterm entries in the Alphabetic Index and by reading the inclusion and exclusion notes in the Tabular List.

Assign only the combination code when that code fully identifies the diagnostic conditions involved or when the Alphabetic Index so directs. Multiple coding should not be used when the classification provides a combination code that clearly identifies all of the elements documented in the diagnosis. When the combination code lacks necessary specificity in describing the manifestation or complication, an additional code should be used as a secondary code.

10. Sequela (Late Effects)

A sequela is the residual effect (condition produced) after the acute phase of an illness or injury has terminated. There is no time limit on when a sequela code can be used. The residual may be apparent early, such as in cerebral infarction, or it may occur months or years later, such as that due to a previous injury. Examples of sequela include: scar formation resulting from a burn, deviated septum due to a nasal fracture, and infertility due to tubal occlusion from old tuberculosis. Coding of sequela generally requires two codes sequenced in the following order: The condition or nature of the sequela is sequenced first. The sequela code is sequenced second.

An exception to the above guidelines are those instances where the code for the sequela is followed by a manifestation code identified in the Tabular List and title, or the sequela code has been expanded (at the fourth, fifth or sixth, character levels) to include the manifestation(s). The code for the acute phase of an illness or injury that led to the sequela is never used with a code for the late effect.

- *See Section I.C.9. Sequelae of cerebrovascular disease*
- *See Section I.C.15. Sequelae of complication of pregnancy, childbirth and the puerperium*
- *See Section I.C.19. Application of 7th characters for Chapter 19*

11. Impending or Threatened Condition

Code any condition described at the time of discharge as "impending" or "threatened" as follows:

- If it did occur, code as confirmed diagnosis.
- If it did not occur, reference the Alphabetic Index to determine if the condition has a subentry term for "impending" or "threatened" and also reference main term entries for "Impending" and for "Threatened."
- If the subterms are listed, assign the given code.
- If the subterms are not listed, code the existing underlying condition(s) and not the condition described as impending or threatened.

12. Reporting Same Diagnosis Code More than Once

Each unique ICD-10-CM diagnosis code may be reported only once for an encounter. This applies to bilateral conditions when there are no distinct codes identifying laterality or two different conditions classified to the same ICD-10-CM diagnosis code.

13. Laterality

Some ICD-10-CM codes indicate laterality, specifying whether the condition occurs on the left, right or is bilateral. If no bilateral code is provided and the condition is bilateral, assign separate codes for both the left and right side. If the side is not identified in the medical record, assign the code for the unspecified side.

When a patient has a bilateral condition and each side is treated during separate encounters, assign the "bilateral" code (as the conditions still exists on both sides), including for the encounter to treat the first side. For the second encounter for treatment after one side has previously been treated and the condition no longer exists on that side, assign the appropriate unilateral code for the side where the conditions still exists (e.g., cataract surgery performed on each eye in separate encounters). The bilateral code would not be assigned for the subsequent encounter, as the patient no longer has the condition in the previously-treated site. If the treatment on the first side did not completely resolve the condition, then the bilateral code would still be appropriate.

14. Documentation for BMI, Depth of Non-Pressure Ulcers, Pressure Ulcer Stages, Coma Scale, and NIH Stroke Scale

For the body mass index (BMI), depth of non-pressure chronic ulcers, pressure ulcer stage, coma scale, and NIH stroke scale (NIHSS) codes, code assignment may be based on medical record documentation from clinicians who are not the patient's provider (i.e., physician or other qualified healthcare practitioner legally accountable for establishing the patient's diagnosis), since this information is typically documented by other clinicians involved in the care of the patient (e.g., a dietitian often documents the BMI, a nurse often documents the pressure ulcer stages, and an emergency medical technician often documents the coma scale). However, the associated diagnosis (such as overweight, obesity, acute stroke or pressure ulcer) must be documented by the patient's provider. If there is conflicting medical record documentation, either from the same clinician or different clinicians, the patient's attending provider should be queried for clarification.

The BMI, coma scale, and NIHSS codes should only be reported as secondary diagnoses.

15. Syndromes

Follow the Alphabetic Index guidance when coding syndromes. In the absence of Alphabetic Index guidance, assign codes for the documented manifestations of the syndrome. Additional codes for manifestations that are not an integral part of the disease process may also be assigned when the condition does not have a unique code.

16. Documentation of Complications of Care

Code assignment is based on the provider's documentation of the relationship between the condition and the care or procedure, unless otherwise instructed by the classification. The guideline extends to any complications of care, regardless of the chapter the code is located in. It is important to note that not all conditions that occur during or following medical care or surgery are classified as complications. There must be a cause-and-effect relationship between the care provided and the condition, and an indication in the documentation that it is a complication. Query the provider for clarification, if the complication is not clearly documented.

17. Borderline Diagnosis

If the provider documents a "borderline" diagnosis at the time of discharge, the diagnosis is coded as confirmed, unless the classification provides a specific entry (e.g., borderline diabetes). If a borderline condition has a specific index entry in ICD-10-CM, it should be coded as such. Since borderline conditions are not uncertain diagnoses, no distinction is made between the care setting (inpatient versus outpatient). Whenever the documentation is unclear regarding a borderline condition, coders are encouraged to query for clarification.

18. Use of Sign/Symptom/Unspecified Codes

Sign/symptom and "unspecified" codes have acceptable, even necessary, uses. While specific diagnosis codes should be reported when they are supported by the available medical record documentation and clinical knowledge of the patient's health condition, there are instances when signs/symptoms or unspecified codes are the best choices for accurately reflecting the healthcare encounter. Each healthcare encounter should be coded to the level of certainty known for that encounter.

If a definitive diagnosis has not been established by the end of the encounter, it is appropriate to report codes for sign(s) and/or symptom(s) in lieu of a definitive diagnosis. When sufficient clinical information isn't known or available about a particular health condition to assign a more specific code, it is acceptable to report the appropriate "unspecified" code (e.g., a diagnosis of pneumonia has been determined, but not the specific type). Unspecified codes should be reported when they are the codes that most accurately reflects what is known about the patient's condition at the time of that particular encounter. It would be inappropriate to select a specific code that is not supported by the medical record documentation or conduct medically unnecessary diagnostic testing in order to determine a more specific code.

C. Chapter-Specific Coding Guidelines

Consulting Editor Note

In this book the Chapter-Specific Coding Guidelines are included here and in the Tabular List of Diseases and Injuries at the beginning of the chapter for which they are applicable.

Additionally, notes have been added throughout the Diagnosis and Procedure Tabular to alert the coder when the code under review is included in a chapter specific coding guideline. The user can then reference the coding guideline prior to making their final code selection. For example:

A41 Other sepsis

Review coding guideline C.1.d

This note alerts the coder to reference the chapter specific coding guidelines (C), chapter 1, guideline d, before making the final code selection. The guidelines for chapter 1, Certain Infectious and Parasitic Diseases, is located at the beginning of Chapter 1 in the Diagnosis Tabular. Please note that the coding guideline notes may be provided at the category, sub-category, or sub-classification level, whichever is applicable to the coding guidance.

In addition to general coding guidelines, there are guidelines for specific diagnoses and/or conditions in the classification. Unless otherwise indicated, these guidelines apply to all health care settings. Please refer to Section II for guidelines on the selection of principal diagnosis.

1. Chapter 1: Certain Infectious and Parasitic Diseases (A00-B99)

a. Human Immunodeficiency Virus (HIV) Infections

1) Code only confirmed cases

Code only confirmed cases of HIV infection/illness. This is an exception to the hospital inpatient guideline Section II, H.

In this context, "confirmation" does not require documentation of positive serology or culture for HIV; the provider's diagnostic statement that the patient is HIV positive, or has an HIV-related illness is sufficient.

2) Selection and sequencing of HIV codes

(a) Patient admitted for HIV-related condition

If a patient is admitted for an HIV-related condition, the principal diagnosis should be B20, Human immunodeficiency virus [HIV] disease followed by additional diagnosis codes for all reported HIV-related conditions.

(b) Patient with HIV disease admitted for unrelated condition

If a patient with HIV disease is admitted for an unrelated condition (such as a traumatic injury), the code for the unrelated condition (e.g., the nature of injury code) should be the principal diagnosis. Other diagnoses would be B20 followed by additional diagnosis codes for all reported HIV-related conditions.

(c) **Whether the patient is newly diagnosed**

Whether the patient is newly diagnosed or has had previous admissions/encounters for HIV conditions is irrelevant to the sequencing decision.

(d) **Asymptomatic human immunodeficiency virus**

Z21, Asymptomatic human immunodeficiency virus [HIV] infection status, is to be applied when the patient without any documentation of symptoms is listed as being "HIV positive," "known HIV," "HIV test positive," or similar terminology. Do not use this code if the term "AIDS" is used or if the patient is treated for any HIV-related illness or is described as having any condition(s) resulting from his/her HIV positive status; use B20 in these cases.

(e) **Patients with inconclusive HIV serology**

Patients with inconclusive HIV serology, but no definitive diagnosis or manifestations of the illness, may be assigned code R75, Inconclusive laboratory evidence of human immunodeficiency virus [HIV].

(f) **Previously diagnosed HIV-related illness**

Patients with any known prior diagnosis of an HIV-related illness should be coded to B20. Once a patient has developed an HIV-related illness, the patient should always be assigned code B20 on every subsequent admission/encounter. Patients previously diagnosed with any HIV illness (B20) should never be assigned to R75 or Z21, Asymptomatic human immunodeficiency virus [HIV] infection status.

(g) **HIV Infection in Pregnancy, Childbirth and the Puerperium**

During pregnancy, childbirth or the puerperium, a patient admitted (or presenting for a health care encounter) because of an HIV-related illness should receive a principal diagnosis code of O98.7-, Human immunodeficiency [HIV] disease complicating pregnancy, childbirth and the puerperium, followed by B20 and the code(s) for the HIV-related illness(es). Codes from Chapter 15 always take sequencing priority.

Patients with asymptomatic HIV infection status admitted (or presenting for a health care encounter) during pregnancy, childbirth, or the puerperium should receive codes of O98.7- and Z21.

(h) **Encounters for testing for HIV**

If a patient is being seen to determine his/her HIV status, use code Z11.4, Encounter for screening for human immunodeficiency virus [HIV]. Use additional codes for any associated high risk behavior.

If a patient with signs or symptoms is being seen for HIV testing, code the signs and symptoms. An additional counseling code Z71.7, Human immunodeficiency virus [HIV] counseling, may be used if counseling is provided during the encounter for the test.

When a patient returns to be informed of his/her HIV test results and the test result is negative, use code Z71.7, Human immunodeficiency virus [HIV] counseling.

If the results are positive, see previous guidelines and assign codes as appropriate.

b. Infectious agents as the cause of diseases classified to other chapters

Certain infections are classified in chapters other than Chapter 1 and no organism is identified as part of the infection code. In these instances, it is necessary to use an additional code from Chapter 1 to identify the organism. A code from category B95, Streptococcus, Staphylococcus, and Enterococcus as the cause of diseases classified to other chapters, B96, Other bacterial agents as the cause of diseases classified to other chapters, or B97, Viral agents as the cause of diseases classified to other chapters, is to be used as an additional code to identify the organism. An instructional note will be found at the infection code advising that an additional organism code is required.

c. Infections resistant to antibiotics

Many bacterial infections are resistant to current antibiotics. It is necessary to identify all infections documented as antibiotic resistant. Assign a code from category Z16, Resistance to antimicrobial drugs, following the infection code only if the infection code does not identify drug resistance.

d. Sepsis, Severe Sepsis, and Septic Shock

1) Coding of Sepsis and Severe Sepsis

(a) **Sepsis**

For a diagnosis of sepsis, assign the appropriate code for the underlying systemic infection. If the type of infection or causal organism is not further specified, assign code A41.9, Sepsis, unspecified organism.

A code from subcategory R65.2, Severe sepsis, should not be assigned unless severe sepsis or an associated acute organ dysfunction is documented.

(i) **Negative or inconclusive blood cultures and sepsis**

Negative or inconclusive blood cultures do not preclude a diagnosis of sepsis in patients with clinical evidence of the condition, however, the provider should be queried.

(ii) Urosepsis

The term urosepsis is a nonspecific term. It is not to be considered synonymous with sepsis. It has no default code in the Alphabetic Index. Should a provider use this term, he/she must be queried for clarification.

(iii) Sepsis with organ dysfunction

If a patient has sepsis and associated acute organ dysfunction or multiple organ dysfunction (MOD), follow the instructions for coding severe sepsis.

(iv) Acute organ dysfunction that is not clearly associated with the sepsis

If a patient has sepsis and an acute organ dysfunction, but the medical record documentation indicates that the acute organ dysfunction is related to a medical condition other than the sepsis, do not assign a code from subcategory R65.2, Severe sepsis. An acute organ dysfunction must be associated with the sepsis in order to assign the severe sepsis code. If the documentation is not clear as to whether an acute organ dysfunction is related to the sepsis or another medical condition, query the provider.

(b) Severe sepsis

The coding of severe sepsis requires a minimum of 2 codes: first a code for the underlying systemic infection, followed by a code from subcategory R65.2, Severe sepsis. If the causal organism is not documented, assign code A41.9, Sepsis, unspecified organism, for the infection. Additional code(s) for the associated acute organ dysfunction are also required.

Due to the complex nature of severe sepsis, some cases may require querying the provider prior to assignment of the codes.

2) Septic shock

(a) Septic shock generally refers to circulatory failure associated with severe sepsis, and therefore, it represents a type of acute organ dysfunction.

For cases of septic shock, the code for the systemic infection should be sequenced first, followed by code R65.21, Severe sepsis with septic shock or code T81.12, Postprocedural septic shock. Any additional codes for the other acute organ dysfunctions should also be assigned. As noted in the sequencing instructions in the Tabular List, the code for septic shock cannot be assigned as a principal diagnosis.

3) Sequencing of severe sepsis

If severe sepsis is present on admission, and meets the definition of principal diagnosis, the underlying systemic infection should be assigned as principal diagnosis followed by the appropriate code from subcategory R65.2 as required by the sequencing rules in the Tabular List. A code from subcategory R65.2 can never be assigned as a principal diagnosis.

When severe sepsis develops during an encounter (it was not present on admission) the underlying systemic infection and the appropriate code from subcategory R65.2 should be assigned as secondary diagnoses.

Severe sepsis may be present on admission but the diagnosis may not be confirmed until sometime after admission. If the documentation is not clear whether severe sepsis was present on admission, the provider should be queried.

4) Sepsis and severe sepsis with a localized infection

If the reason for admission is both sepsis or severe sepsis and a localized infection, such as pneumonia or cellulitis, a code(s) for the underlying systemic infection should be assigned first and the code for the localized infection should be assigned as a secondary diagnosis. If the patient has severe sepsis, a code from subcategory R65.2 should also be assigned as a secondary diagnosis. If the patient is admitted with a localized infection, such as pneumonia, and sepsis/severe sepsis doesn't develop until after admission, the localized infection should be assigned first, followed by the appropriate sepsis/severe sepsis codes.

5) Sepsis due to a postprocedural infection

(a) Documentation of causal relationship

As with all postprocedural complications, code assignment is based on the provider's documentation of the relationship between the infection and the procedure.

(b) Sepsis due to a postprocedural infection

For such cases, the postprocedural infection code, such as, T80.2, Infections following infusion, transfusion, and therapeutic injection, T81.4, Infection following a procedure, T88.0, Infection following immunization, or O86.0, Infection of obstetric surgical wound, should be coded first, followed by the code for the specific infection. If the patient has severe sepsis the appropriate code from subcategory R65.2 should also be assigned with the additional code(s) for any acute organ dysfunction.

(c) Postprocedural infection and postprocedural septic shock

In cases where a postprocedural infection has occurred and has resulted in severe sepsis and postprocedural septic shock, the code for the precipitating complication such as code T81.4, Infection following a procedure, or O86.0, Infection of obstetrical surgical wound should be coded first followed by code R65.20, Severe sepsis without septic shock. A code for the systemic infection should also be assigned.

If a postprocedural infection has resulted in postprocedural septic shock, the code for the precipitating complication such as code T81.4, Infection following a procedure, or O86.0, Infection of obstetrical surgical wound should be coded first followed by code T81.12-, Postprocedural septic shock. A code for the systemic infection should also be assigned.

6) Sepsis and severe sepsis associated with a noninfectious process (condition)

In some cases a noninfectious process (condition), such as trauma, may lead to an infection which can result in sepsis or severe sepsis. If sepsis or severe sepsis is documented as associated with a noninfectious condition, such as a burn or serious injury, and this condition meets the definition for principal diagnosis, the code for the noninfectious condition should be sequenced first, followed by the code for the resulting infection. If severe sepsis, is present a code from subcategory R65.2 should also be assigned with any associated organ dysfunction(s) codes. It is not necessary to assign a code from subcategory R65.1, Systemic inflammatory response syndrome (SIRS) of non-infectious origin, for these cases.

If the infection meets the definition of principal diagnosis it should be sequenced before the non-infectious condition. When both the associated non-infectious condition and the infection meet the definition of principal diagnosis either may be assigned as principal diagnosis.

Only one code from category R65, Symptoms and signs specifically associated with systemic inflammation and infection, should be assigned. Therefore, when a non-infectious condition leads to an infection resulting in severe sepsis, assign the appropriate code from subcategory R65.2, Severe sepsis. Do not additionally assign a code from subcategory R65.1, Systemic inflammatory response syndrome (SIRS) of non-infectious origin.

See Section I.C.18. SIRS due to non-infectious process

7) Sepsis and septic shock complicating abortion, pregnancy, childbirth, and the puerperium

See Section I.C.15. Sepsis and septic shock complicating abortion, pregnancy, childbirth and the puerperium

8) Newborn sepsis

See Section I.C.16. f. Bacterial sepsis of Newborn

e. Methicillin Resistant Staphylococcus aureus (MRSA) Conditions

1) Selection and sequencing of MRSA codes

(a) Combination codes for MRSA infection

When a patient is diagnosed with an infection that is due to methicillin resistant Staphylococcus aureus (MRSA), and that infection has a combination code that includes the causal organism (e.g., sepsis, pneumonia) assign the appropriate combination code for the condition (e.g., code A41.02, Sepsis due to Methicillin resistant Staphylococcus aureus or code J15.212, Pneumonia due to Methicillin resistant Staphylococcus aureus). Do not assign code B95.62, Methicillin resistant Staphylococcus aureus infection as the cause of diseases classified elsewhere, as an additional code because the combination code includes the type of infection and the MRSA organism. Do not assign a code from subcategory Z16.11, Resistance to penicillins, as an additional diagnosis.

See Section C.1. for instructions on coding and sequencing of sepsis and severe sepsis.

(b) Other codes for MRSA infection

When there is documentation of a current infection (e.g., wound infection, stitch abscess, urinary tract infection) due to MRSA, and that infection does not have a combination code that includes the causal organism, assign the appropriate code to identify the condition along with code B95.62, Methicillin resistant Staphylococcus aureus infection as the cause of diseases classified elsewhere for the MRSA infection. Do not assign a code from subcategory Z16.11, Resistance to penicillins.

(c) Methicillin susceptible Staphylococcus aureus (MSSA) and MRSA colonization

The condition or state of being colonized or carrying MSSA or MRSA is called colonization or carriage, while an individual person is described as being colonized or being a carrier. Colonization means that MSSA or MSRA is present on or in the body without necessarily causing illness. A positive MRSA colonization test might be documented by the provider as "MRSA screen positive" or "MRSA nasal swab positive".

Assign code Z22.322, Carrier or suspected carrier of Methicillin resistant Staphylococcus aureus, for patients documented as having MRSA colonization. Assign code Z22.321, Carrier or suspected carrier of Methicillin susceptible Staphylococcus aureus, for patient documented as having MSSA colonization. Colonization is not necessarily indicative of a disease process or as the cause of a specific condition the patient may have unless documented as such by the provider.

(d) MRSA colonization and infection

If a patient is documented as having both MRSA colonization and infection during a hospital admission, code Z22.322, Carrier or suspected carrier of Methicillin resistant Staphylococcus aureus, and a code for the MRSA infection may both be assigned.

f. Zika virus infections

1) Code only confirmed cases

Code only a confirmed diagnosis of Zika virus (A92.5, Zika virus disease) as documented by the provider. This is an exception to the hospital inpatient guideline Section II, H.

In this context, "confirmation" does not require documentation of the type of test performed; the physician's diagnostic statement that the condition is confirmed is sufficient. This code should be assigned regardless of the stated mode of transmission.

If the provider documents "suspected", "possible" or "provable" Zika, do not assign code A92.5. Assign a code(s) explaining the reason for encounter (such as fever, rash, or joint pain) or Z20.828, Contact with and (suspected) exposure to other viral communicable diseases.

2. Chapter 2: Neoplasms (C00-D49)

General guidelines

Chapter 2 of the ICD-10-CM contains the codes for most benign and all malignant neoplasms. Certain benign neoplasms, such as prostatic adenomas, may be found in the specific body system chapters. To properly code a neoplasm it is necessary to determine from the record if the neoplasm is benign, in-situ, malignant, or of uncertain histologic behavior. If malignant, any secondary (metastatic) sites should also be determined.

Primary malignant neoplasms overlapping site boundaries

A primary malignant neoplasm that overlaps two or more contiguous (next to each other) sites should be classified to the subcategory/code .8 ('overlapping lesion'), unless the combination is specifically indexed elsewhere. For multiple neoplasms of the same site that are not contiguous such as tumors in different quadrants of the same breast, codes for each site should be assigned.

Malignant neoplasm of ectopic tissue

Malignant neoplasms of ectopic tissue are to be coded to the site of origin mentioned, e.g., ectopic pancreatic malignant neoplasms involving the stomach are coded to **malignant neoplasm of** pancreas, unspecified (C25.9).

The neoplasm table in the Alphabetic Index should be referenced first. However, if the histological term is documented, that term should be referenced first, rather than going immediately to the Neoplasm Table, in order to determine which column in the Neoplasm Table is appropriate. For example, if the documentation indicates "adenoma," refer to the term in the Alphabetic Index to review the entries under this term and the instructional note to "see also neoplasm, by site, benign." The table provides the proper code based on the type of neoplasm and the site. It is important to select the proper column in the table that corresponds to the type of neoplasm. The Tabular List should then be referenced to verify that the correct code has been selected from the table and that a more specific site code does not exist.

See Section I.C.21. Factors influencing health status and contact with health services, Status, for information regarding Z15.0, codes for genetic susceptibility to cancer.

a. Treatment directed at the malignancy

If the treatment is directed at the malignancy, designate the malignancy as the principal diagnosis.

The only exception to this guideline is if a patient admission/encounter is solely for the administration of chemotherapy, immunotherapy or **external beam** radiation therapy, assign the appropriate Z51.-- code as the first-listed or principal diagnosis, and the diagnosis or problem for which the service is being performed as a secondary diagnosis.

b. Treatment of secondary site

When a patient is admitted because of a primary neoplasm with metastasis and treatment is directed toward the secondary site only, the secondary neoplasm is designated as the principal diagnosis even though the primary malignancy is still present.

c. Coding and sequencing of complications

Coding and sequencing of complications associated with the malignancies or with the therapy thereof are subject to the following guidelines:

1) Anemia associated with malignancy

When admission/encounter is for management of an anemia associated with the malignancy, and the treatment is only for anemia, the appropriate code for the malignancy is sequenced as the principal or first-listed diagnosis followed by the appropriate code for the anemia (such as code D63.0, Anemia in neoplastic disease).

2) Anemia associated with chemotherapy, immunotherapy and radiation therapy

When the admission/encounter is for management of an anemia associated with an adverse effect of the administration of chemotherapy or immunotherapy and the only treatment is for the anemia, the anemia code is sequenced first followed by the appropriate codes for the neoplasm and the adverse effect (T45.1X5, Adverse effect of antineoplastic and immunosuppressive drugs).

When the admission/encounter is for management of an anemia associated with an adverse effect of radiotherapy, the anemia code should be sequenced first, followed by the appropriate neoplasm code and code Y84.2, Radiological procedure and radiotherapy as the cause of abnormal reaction of the patient, or of later complication, without mention of misadventure at the time of the procedure.

3) Management of dehydration due to the malignancy

When the admission/encounter is for management of dehydration due to the malignancy and only the dehydration is being treated (intravenous rehydration), the dehydration is sequenced first, followed by the code(s) for the malignancy.

4) Treatment of a complication resulting from a surgical procedure

When the admission/encounter is for treatment of a complication resulting from a surgical procedure, designate the complication as the principal or first-listed diagnosis if treatment is directed at resolving the complication.

d. Primary malignancy previously excised

When a primary malignancy has been previously excised or eradicated from its site and there is no further treatment directed to that site and there is no evidence of any existing primary malignancy, a code from category Z85, Personal history of malignant neoplasm, should be used to indicate the former site of the malignancy. Any mention of extension, invasion, or metastasis to another site is coded as a secondary malignant neoplasm to that site. The secondary site may be the principal or first-listed with the Z85 code used as a secondary code.

e. Admissions/Encounters involving chemotherapy, immunotherapy and radiation therapy

1) Episode of care involves surgical removal of neoplasm

When an episode of care involves the surgical removal of a neoplasm, primary or secondary site, followed by adjunct chemotherapy or radiation treatment during the same episode of care, the code for the neoplasm should be assigned as principal or first-listed diagnosis.

2) Patient admission/encounter solely for administration of chemotherapy, immunotherapy and radiation therapy

If a patient admission/encounter is solely for the administration of chemotherapy, immunotherapy or **external beam** radiation therapy assign code Z51.0, Encounter for antineoplastic radiation therapy, or Z51.11, Encounter for antineoplastic chemotherapy, or Z51.12, Encounter for antineoplastic immunotherapy as the first-listed or principal diagnosis. If a patient receives more than one of these therapies during the same admission more than one of these codes may be assigned, in any sequence.

The malignancy for which the therapy is being administered should be assigned as a secondary diagnosis.

If a patient admission/encounter is for the insertion or implantation of radioactive elements (e.g., brachytherapy) the appropriate code for the malignancy is sequenced as the principal or first-listed diagnosis. Code Z51.0 should not be assigned.

3) Patient admitted for radiation therapy, chemotherapy or immunotherapy and develops complications

When a patient is admitted for the purpose of **external beam** radiotherapy, immunotherapy or chemotherapy and develops complications such as uncontrolled nausea and vomiting or dehydration, the principal or first-listed diagnosis is Z51.0, Encounter for antineoplastic radiation therapy, or Z51.11, Encounter for antineoplastic chemotherapy, or Z51.12, Encounter for antineoplastic immunotherapy followed by any codes for the complications.

When a patient is admitted for the purpose of insertion or implantation of radioactive elements (e.g., brachytherapy) and develops complications such as uncontrolled nausea and vomiting or dehydration, the principal or first-listed diagnosis is the appropriate code for the malignancy followed by any codes for the complications.

f. Admission/encounter to determine extent of malignancy

When the reason for admission/encounter is to determine the extent of the malignancy, or for a procedure such as paracentesis or thoracentesis, the primary malignancy or appropriate metastatic site is designated as the principal or first-listed diagnosis, even though chemotherapy or radiotherapy is administered.

g. Symptoms, signs, and abnormal findings listed in Chapter 18 associated with neoplasms

Symptoms, signs, and ill-defined conditions listed in Chapter 18 characteristic of, or associated with, an existing primary or secondary site malignancy cannot be used to replace the malignancy as principal or first-listed diagnosis, regardless of the number of admissions or encounters for treatment and care of the neoplasm.

See section I.C.21. Factors influencing health status and contact with health services, Encounter for prophylactic organ removal.

h. Admission/encounter for pain control/management

See Section I.C.6. for information on coding admission/encounter for pain control/management.

i. Malignancy in two or more noncontiguous sites

A patient may have more than one malignant tumor in the same organ. These tumors may represent different primaries or metastatic disease, depending on the site. Should the documentation be unclear, the provider should be queried as to the status of each tumor so that the correct codes can be assigned.

j. Disseminated malignant neoplasm, unspecified

Code C80.0, Disseminated malignant neoplasm, unspecified, is for use only in those cases where the patient has advanced metastatic disease and no known primary or secondary sites are specified. It should not be used in place of assigning codes for the primary site and all known secondary sites.

k. Malignant neoplasm without specification of site

Code C80.1, Malignant (primary) neoplasm, unspecified, equates to Cancer, unspecified. This code should only be used when no determination can be made as to the primary site of a malignancy. This code should rarely be used in the inpatient setting.

l. Sequencing of neoplasm codes

1) Encounter for treatment of primary malignancy

If the reason for the encounter is for treatment of a primary malignancy, assign the malignancy as the principal/first-listed diagnosis. The primary site is to be sequenced first, followed by any metastatic sites.

2) Encounter for treatment of secondary malignancy

When an encounter is for a primary malignancy with metastasis and treatment is directed toward the metastatic (secondary) site(s) only, the metastatic site(s) is designated as the principal/first-listed diagnosis. The primary malignancy is coded as an additional code.

3) Malignant neoplasm in a pregnant patient

When a pregnant woman has a malignant neoplasm, a code from subcategory O9A.1-, Malignant neoplasm complicating pregnancy, childbirth, and the puerperium, should be sequenced first, followed by the appropriate code from Chapter 2 to indicate the type of neoplasm.

4) Encounter for complication associated with a neoplasm

When an encounter is for management of a complication associated with a neoplasm, such as dehydration, and the treatment is only for the complication, the complication is coded first, followed by the appropriate code(s) for the neoplasm.

The exception to this guideline is anemia. When the admission/encounter is for management of an anemia associated with the malignancy, and the treatment is only for anemia, the appropriate code for the malignancy is sequenced as the principal or first-listed diagnosis followed by code D63.0, Anemia in neoplastic disease.

5) Complication from surgical procedure for treatment of a neoplasm

When an encounter is for treatment of a complication resulting from a surgical procedure performed for the treatment of the neoplasm, designate the complication as the principal/first- listed diagnosis. See guideline regarding the coding of a current malignancy versus personal history to determine if the code for the neoplasm should also be assigned.

6) Pathologic fracture due to a neoplasm

When an encounter is for a pathological fracture due to a neoplasm, and the focus of treatment is the fracture, a code from subcategory M84.5, Pathological fracture in neoplastic disease, should be sequenced first, followed by the code for the neoplasm.

If the focus of treatment is the neoplasm with an associated pathological fracture, the neoplasm code should be sequenced first, followed by a code from M84.5 for the pathological fracture.

m. **Current malignancy versus personal history of malignancy**

When a primary malignancy has been excised but further treatment, such as an additional surgery for the malignancy, radiation therapy or chemotherapy is directed to that site, the primary malignancy code should be used until treatment is completed.

When a primary malignancy has been previously excised or eradicated from its site, there is no further treatment (of the malignancy) directed to that site, and there is no evidence of any existing primary malignancy, a code from category Z85, Personal history of malignant neoplasm, should be used to indicate the former site of the malignancy.

See Section I.C.21. Factors influencing health status and contact with health services, History (of)

n. **Leukemia, Multiple Myeloma, and Malignant Plasma Cell Neoplasms in remission versus personal history**

The categories for leukemia, and category C90, Multiple myeloma and malignant plasma cell neoplasms, have codes indicating whether or not the leukemia has achieved remission. There are also codes Z85.6, Personal history of leukemia, and Z85.79, Personal history of other malignant neoplasms of lymphoid, hematopoietic and related tissues. If the documentation is unclear, as to whether the leukemia has achieved remission, the provider should be queried.

See Section I.C.21. Factors influencing health status and contact with health services, History (of)

o. **Aftercare following surgery for neoplasm**

See Section I.C.21. Factors influencing health status and contact with health services, Aftercare

p. **Follow-up care for completed treatment of a malignancy**

See Section I.C.21. Factors influencing health status and contact with health services, Follow-up

q. **Prophylactic organ removal for prevention of malignancy**

See Section I.C. 21, Factors influencing health status and contact with health services, Prophylactic organ removal

r. **Malignant neoplasm associated with transplanted organ**

A malignant neoplasm of a transplanted organ should be coded as a transplant complication. Assign first the appropriate code from category T86.-, Complications of transplanted organs and tissue, followed by code C80.2, Malignant neoplasm associated with transplanted organ. Use an additional code for the specific malignancy.

3. Chapter 3: Diseases of the Blood and Blood-Forming Organs and Certain Disorders Involving the Immune Mechanism (D50-D89)

Reserved for future guideline expansion

4. Chapter 4: Endocrine, Nutritional and Metabolic Diseases (E00-E89)

a. **Diabetes mellitus**

The diabetes mellitus codes are combination codes that include the type of diabetes mellitus, the body system affected, and the complications affecting that body system. As many codes within a particular category as are necessary to describe all of the complications of the disease may be used. They should be sequenced based on the reason for a particular encounter. Assign as many codes from categories E08 – E13 as needed to identify all of the associated conditions that the patient has.

1) **Type of diabetes**

The age of a patient is not the sole determining factor, though most type 1 diabetics develop the condition before reaching puberty. For this reason type 1 diabetes mellitus is also referred to as juvenile diabetes.

2) **Type of diabetes mellitus not documented**

If the type of diabetes mellitus is not documented in the medical record the default is E11.-, Type 2 diabetes mellitus.

3) **Diabetes mellitus and the use of insulin and oral hypoglycemics**

If the documentation in a medical record does not indicate the type of diabetes but does indicate that the patient uses insulin, code E11, Type 2 diabetes mellitus, should be assigned. **An additional code should be assigned from category Z79 to identify the long-term (current) use of insulin or oral hypoglycemic drugs. If the patient is treated with both oral medications and insulin, only the code for long-term (current) use of insulin should be assigned. Code Z79.4 should not be assigned if insulin is given temporarily to bring a type 2 patient's blood sugar under control during an encounter.**

4) **Diabetes mellitus in pregnancy and gestational diabetes**

See Section I.C.15. Diabetes mellitus in pregnancy.

See Section I.C.15. Gestational (pregnancy induced) diabetes

5) **Complications due to insulin pump malfunction**

(a) **Underdose of insulin due to insulin pump failure**

An underdose of insulin due to an insulin pump failure should be assigned to a code from subcategory T85.6, Mechanical complication of other specified internal and external prosthetic devices, implants and grafts, that specifies the type of pump malfunction, as the principal or first-listed code, followed by code T38.3x6-, Underdosing of insulin and oral hypoglycemic [antidiabetic] drugs. Additional codes for the type of diabetes mellitus and any associated complications due to the underdosing should also be assigned.

(b) **Overdose of insulin due to insulin pump failure**

The principal or first-listed code for an encounter due to an insulin pump malfunction resulting in an overdose of insulin, should also be T85.6-, Mechanical complication of other specified internal and external prosthetic devices, implants and grafts, followed by code T38.3x1-, Poisoning by insulin and oral hypoglycemic [antidiabetic] drugs, accidental (unintentional).

6) **Secondary diabetes mellitus**

Codes under categories E08, Diabetes mellitus due to underlying condition, E09, Drug or chemical induced diabetes mellitus, and E13, Other specified diabetes mellitus, identify complications/manifestations associated with secondary diabetes mellitus. Secondary diabetes is always caused by another condition or event (e.g., cystic fibrosis, malignant neoplasm of pancreas, pancreatectomy, adverse effect of drug, or poisoning).

(a) **Secondary diabetes mellitus and the use of insulin or *oral* hypoglycemic drugs**

For patients with secondary diabetes mellitus who routinely use insulin or oral hypoglycemic drugs, and additional code from category Z79 should be assigned to identify the long-term (current) use of insulin or oral hypoglycemic drugs. If the patient is treated with both oral medications and insulin, only the code for long-term (current) use of insulin should be assigned. Code Z79.4 should not be assigned if insulin is given temporarily to bring a type 2 patient's blood sugar under control during an encounter.

(b) **Assigning and sequencing secondary diabetes codes and its causes**

The sequencing of the secondary diabetes codes in relationship to codes for the cause of the diabetes is based on the Tabular List instructions for categories E08, E09 and E13.

(i) **Secondary diabetes mellitus due to pancreatectomy**

For postpancreatectomy diabetes mellitus (lack of insulin due to the surgical removal of all or part of the pancreas), assign code E89.1, Postprocedural hypoinsulinemia. Assign a code from category E13 and a code from subcategory Z90.41-, Acquired absence of pancreas, as additional codes.

(ii) **Secondary diabetes due to drugs**

Secondary diabetes may be caused by an adverse effect of correctly administered medications, poisoning or sequela of poisoning.

See section I.C.19.e for coding of adverse effects and poisoning, and section I.C.20 for external cause code reporting.

5. Chapter 5: Mental, Behavioral and Neurodevelopmental Disorders (F01-F99)

a. Pain disorders related to psychological factors

Assign code F45.41, for pain that is exclusively related to psychological disorders. As indicated by the Excludes 1 note under category G89, a code from category G89 should not be assigned with code F45.41

Code F45.42, Pain disorders with related psychological factors, should be used with a code from category G89, Pain, not elsewhere classified, if there is documentation of a psychological component for a patient with acute or chronic pain.

See Section I.C.6. Pain

b. Mental and behavioral disorders due to psychoactive substance use

1) **In Remission**

Selection of codes for "in remission" for categories F10-F19, Mental and behavioral disorders due to psychoactive substance use (categories F10-F19 with **-.11**, -.21) requires the provider's clinical judgment. The appropriate codes for "in remission" are assigned only on the basis of provider documentation (as defined in the Official Guidelines for Coding and Reporting)**, unless otherwise instructed by the classification.**

Mild substance use disorders in early or sustained remission are classified to the appropriate codes for substance abuse in remission, and moderate or severe substance use disorders in early or sustained remission are classified to the appropriate codes for substance dependence in remission.

2) Psychoactive Substance Use, Abuse And Dependence

When the provider documentation refers to use, abuse and dependence of the same substance (e.g. alcohol, opioid, cannabis, etc.), only one code should be assigned to identify the pattern of use based on the following hierarchy:

- If both use and abuse are documented, assign only the code for abuse
- If both abuse and dependence are documented, assign only the code for dependence
- If use, abuse and dependence are all documented, assign only the code for dependence
- If both use and dependence are documented, assign only the code for dependence.

3) Psychoactive Substance Use *Disorders*

As with all other diagnoses, the codes for psychoactive substance use **disorders** (F10.9-, F11.9-, F12.9-, F13.9-, F14.9-, F15.9-, F16.9-) should only be assigned based on provider documentation and when they meet the definition of a reportable diagnosis (see Section III, Reporting Additional Diagnoses). The codes are to be used only when the psychoactive substance use is associated with a **physical,** mental or behavioral disorder, and such a relationship is documented by the provider.

6. Chapter 6: Diseases of the Nervous System (G00-G99)

a. Dominant/nondominant side

Codes from category G81, Hemiplegia and hemiparesis, and subcategories, G83.1, Monoplegia of lower limb, G83.2, Monoplegia of upper limb, and G83.3, Monoplegia, unspecified, identify whether the dominant or nondominant side is affected. Should the affected side be documented, but not specified as dominant or nondominant, and the classification system does not indicate a default, code selection is as follows:

- For ambidextrous patients, the default should be dominant.
- If the left side is affected, the default is non-dominant.
- If the right side is affected, the default is dominant.

b. Pain-Category G89

1) General coding information

Codes in category G89, Pain, not elsewhere classified, may be used in conjunction with codes from other categories and chapters to provide more detail about acute or chronic pain and neoplasm-related pain, unless otherwise indicated below.

If the pain is not specified as acute or chronic, post- thoracotomy, post procedural, or neoplasm-related, do not assign codes from category G89.

A code from category G89 should not be assigned if the underlying (definitive) diagnosis is known, unless the reason for the encounter is pain control/management and not management of the underlying condition.

When an admission or encounter is for a procedure aimed at treating the underlying condition (e.g., spinal fusion, kyphoplasty), a code for the underlying condition (e.g., vertebral fracture, spinal stenosis) should be assigned as the principal diagnosis. No code from category G89 should be assigned.

(a) Category G89 Codes as Principal or First-Listed Diagnosis

Category G89 codes are acceptable as principal diagnosis or the first-listed code:

- When pain control or pain management is the reason for the admission/encounter (e.g., a patient with displaced intervertebral disc, nerve impingement and severe back pain presents for injection of steroid into the spinal canal). The underlying cause of the pain should be reported as an additional diagnosis, if known.
- When a patient is admitted for the insertion of a neurostimulator for pain control, assign the appropriate pain code as the principal or first-listed diagnosis. When an admission or encounter is for a procedure aimed at treating the underlying condition and a neurostimulator is inserted for pain control during the same admission/encounter, a code for the underlying condition should be assigned as the principal diagnosis and the appropriate pain code should be assigned as a secondary diagnosis.

(b) Use of Category G89 Codes in Conjunction with Site Specific Pain Codes

(i) Assigning Category G89 and Site-Specific Pain Codes

Codes from category G89 may be used in conjunction with codes that identify the site of pain (including codes from chapter 18) if the category G89 code provides additional information. For example, if the code describes the site of the pain, but does not fully describe whether the pain is acute or chronic, then both codes should be assigned.

(ii) Sequencing of Category G89 Codes with Site- Specific Pain Codes

The sequencing of category G89 codes with site-specific pain codes (including chapter 18 codes), is dependent on the circumstances of the encounter/admission as follows:

- If the encounter is for pain control or pain management, assign the code from category G89 followed by the code identifying the specific site of pain (e.g., encounter for pain management for acute neck pain from trauma is assigned code G89.11, Acute pain due to trauma, followed by code M54.2, Cervicalgia, to identify the site of pain).
- If the encounter is for any other reason except pain control or pain management, and a related definitive diagnosis has not been established (confirmed) by the provider, assign the code for the specific site of pain first, followed by the appropriate code from category G89.

2) Pain due to devices, implants and grafts

See Section I.C.19. Pain due to medical devices

3) Postoperative Pain

The provider's documentation should be used to guide the coding of postoperative pain, as well *as Section III. Reporting Additional Diagnoses and Section IV. Diagnostic Coding* and *Reporting in the Outpatient Setting.*

The default for post-thoracotomy and other postoperative pain not specified as acute or chronic is the code for the acute form.

Routine or expected postoperative pain immediately after surgery should not be coded.

(a) Postoperative pain not associated with specific postoperative complication

Postoperative pain not associated with a specific postoperative complication is assigned to the appropriate postoperative pain code in category G89.

(b) Postoperative pain associated with specific postoperative complication

Postoperative pain associated with a specific postoperative complication (such as painful wire sutures) is assigned to the appropriate code(s) found in Chapter 19, Injury, poisoning, and certain other consequences of external causes. If appropriate, use additional code(s) from category G89 to identify acute or chronic pain (G89.18 or G89.28).

4) Chronic pain

Chronic pain is classified to subcategory G89.2. There is no time frame defining when pain becomes chronic pain. The provider's documentation should be used to guide use of these codes.

5) Neoplasm Related Pain

Code G89.3 is assigned to pain documented as being related, associated or due to cancer, primary or secondary malignancy, or tumor. This code is assigned regardless of whether the pain is acute or chronic.

This code may be assigned as the principal or first- listed code when the stated reason for the admission/encounter is documented as pain control/pain management. The underlying neoplasm should be reported as an additional diagnosis.

When the reason for the admission/encounter is management of the neoplasm and the pain associated with the neoplasm is also documented, code G89.3 may be assigned as an additional diagnosis. It is not necessary to assign an additional code for the site of the pain.

See Section I.C.2 for instructions on the sequencing of neoplasms for all other stated reasons for the admission/encounter (except for pain control/pain management).

6) Chronic pain syndrome

Central pain syndrome (G89.0) and chronic pain syndrome (G89.4) are different than the term "chronic pain," and therefore codes should only be used when the provider has specifically documented this condition.

See Section I.C.5. Pain disorders related to psychological factors

7. Chapter 7: Diseases of the Eye and Adnexa (H00-H59)

a. Glaucoma

1) Assigning Glaucoma Codes

Assign as many codes from category H40, Glaucoma, as needed to identify the type of glaucoma, the affected eye, and the glaucoma stage.

2) Bilateral glaucoma with same type and stage

When a patient has bilateral glaucoma and both eyes are documented as being the same type and stage, and there is a code for bilateral glaucoma, report only the code for the type of glaucoma, bilateral, with the seventh character for the stage.

When a patient has bilateral glaucoma and both eyes are documented as being the same type and stage, and the classification does not provide a code for bilateral glaucoma (i.e. subcategories H40.10, H40.11 and H40.20) report only one code for the type of glaucoma with the appropriate seventh character for the stage.

3) Bilateral glaucoma stage with different types or stages

When a patient has bilateral glaucoma and each eye is documented as having a different type or stage, and the classification distinguishes laterality, assign the appropriatecode for each eye rather than the code for bilateral glaucoma.

When a patient has bilateral glaucoma and each eye is documented as having a different type, and the classification does not distinguish laterality (i.e. subcategories H40.10, H40.11 and H40.20), assign one code for each type of glaucoma with the appropriate seventh character for the stage.

When a patient has bilateral glaucoma and each eye is documented as having the same type, but different stage, and the classification does not distinguish laterality (i.e. subcategories H40.10, H40.11 and H40.20), assign a code for the type of glaucoma for each eye with the seventh character for the specific glaucoma stage documented for each eye.

4) Patient admitted with glaucoma and stage evolves during the admission

If a patient is admitted with glaucoma and the stage progresses during the admission, assign the code for highest stage documented.

5) Indeterminate stage glaucoma

Assignment of the seventh character "4" for "indeterminate stage" should be based on the clinical documentation. The seventh character "4" is used for glaucomas whose stage cannot be clinically determined. This seventh character should not be confused with the seventh character "0", unspecified, which should be assigned when there is no documentation regarding the stage of the glaucoma.

b. Blindness

If "blindness" or "low vision" of both eyes is documented but the visual impairment category is not documented, assign code H54.3, Unqualified visual loss, both eyes. If "blindness" or "low vision" in one eye is documented but the visual impairment category is not documented, assign a code from H54.6-, Unqualified visual loss, one eye. If "blindness" or "visual loss" is documented without any information about whether one or both eyes are affected, assign code H54.7, Unspecified visual loss.

8. Chapter 8: Diseases of the Ear and Mastoid Process (H60-H95)

Reserved for future guideline expansion

9. Chapter 9: Diseases of the Circulatory System (I00-I99)

a. Hypertension

The classification presumes a causal relationship between hypertension and heart involvement and between hypertension and kidney involvement, as the two conditions are linked by the term "with" in the Alphabetic Index. These conditions should be coded as related even in the absence of provider documentation explicitly linking them, unless the documentation clearly states the conditions are unrelated.

For hypertension and conditions not specifically linked by relational terms such as "with," "associated with" or "due to" in the classification, provider documentation must link the conditions in order to code them as related.

1) Hypertension with Heart Disease

Hypertension with heart conditions classified to I50.- or I51.4-I51.9, are assigned to, a code from category I11, Hypertensive heart disease. Use an additional code(**s**) from category I50, Heart failure, to identify the type(**s**) of heart failure in those patients with heart failure.

The same heart conditions (I50.-, I51.4-I51.9) with hypertension are coded separately if the provider has specifically documented a different cause. Sequence according to the circumstances of the admission/encounter.

2) Hypertensive Chronic Kidney Disease

Assign codes from category I12, Hypertensive chronic kidney disease, when both hypertension and a condition classifiable to category N18, Chronic kidney disease (CKD), are present. CKD should not be coded as hypertensive if the physician has specifically documented a different cause.

The appropriate code from category N18 should be used as a secondary code with a code from category I12 to identify the stage of chronic kidney disease.

See Section I.C.14. Chronic kidney disease.

If a patient has hypertensive chronic kidney disease and acute renal failure, an additional code for the acute renal failure is required.

3) **Hypertensive Heart and Chronic Kidney Disease**

Assign codes from combination category I13, Hypertensive heart and chronic kidney disease, when there is hypertension with both heart and kidney involvement. If heart failure is present, assign an additional code from category I50 to identify the type of heart failure.

The appropriate code from category N18, Chronic kidney disease, should be used as a secondary code with a code from category I13 to identify the stage of chronic kidney disease.

See Section I.C.14. Chronic kidney disease.

The codes in category I13, Hypertensive heart and chronic kidney disease, are combination codes that include hypertension, heart disease and chronic kidney disease. The Includes note at I13 specifies that the conditions included at I11 and I12 are included together in I13. If a patient has hypertension, heart disease and chronic kidney disease then a code from I13 should be used, not individual codes for hypertension, heart disease and chronic kidney disease, or codes from I11 or I12.

For patients with both acute renal failure and chronic kidney disease an additional code for acute renal failure is required.

4) **Hypertensive Cerebrovascular Disease**

For hypertensive cerebrovascular disease, first assign the appropriate code from categories I60-I69, followed by the appropriate hypertension code.

5) **Hypertensive Retinopathy**

Subcategory H35.0, Background retinopathy and retinal vascular changes, should be used with a code from category I10 – I15, Hypertensive disease to include the systemic hypertension. The sequencing is based on the reason for the encounter.

6) **Hypertension, Secondary**

Secondary hypertension is due to an underlying condition. Two codes are required: one to identify the underlying etiology and one from category I15 to identify the hypertension. Sequencing of codes is determined by the reason for admission/encounter.

7) **Hypertension, Transient**

Assign code R03.0, Elevated blood pressure reading without diagnosis of hypertension, unless patient has an established diagnosis of hypertension. Assign code O13.-, Gestational [pregnancy-induced] hypertension without significant proteinuria, or O14.-, Pre-eclampsia, for transient hypertension of pregnancy.

8) **Hypertension, Controlled**

This diagnostic statement usually refers to an existing state of hypertension under control by therapy. Assign the appropriate code from categories I10-I15, Hypertensive diseases.

9) **Hypertension, Uncontrolled**

Uncontrolled hypertension may refer to untreated hypertension or hypertension not responding to current therapeutic regimen. In either case, assign the appropriate code from categories I10-I15, Hypertensive diseases.

10) **Hypertensive Crisis**

Assign a code from category I16, Hypertensive crisis, for documented hypertensive urgency, hypertensive emergency or unspecified hypertensive crisis. Code also any identified hypertensive disease (I10-I15). The sequencing is based on the reason for the encounter.

11) **Pulmonary Hypertension**

Pulmonary hypertension is classified to category I27, Other pulmonary heart diseases. For secondary pulmonary hypertension (I27.1, I27.2-), code also any associated conditions or adverse effects of drugs or toxins. The sequencing is based on the reason for the encounter.

b. Atherosclerotic Coronary Artery Disease and Angina

ICD-10-CM has combination codes for atherosclerotic heart disease with angina pectoris. The subcategories for these codes are I25.11, Atherosclerotic heart disease of native coronary artery with angina pectoris and I25.7, Atherosclerosis of coronary artery bypass graft(s) and coronary artery of transplanted heart with angina pectoris.

When using one of these combination codes it is not necessary to use an additional code for angina pectoris. A causal relationship can be assumed in a patient with both atherosclerosis and angina pectoris, unless the documentation indicates the angina is due to something other than the atherosclerosis.

If a patient with coronary artery disease is admitted due to an acute myocardial infarction (AMI), the AMI should be sequenced before the coronary artery disease.

See Section I.C.9. Acute myocardial infarction (AMI)

c. Intraoperative and Postprocedural Cerebrovascular Accident

Medical record documentation should clearly specify the cause- and-effect relationship between the medical intervention and the cerebrovascular accident in order to assign a code for intraoperative or postprocedural cerebrovascular accident.

Proper code assignment depends on whether it was an infarction or hemorrhage and whether it occurred intraoperatively or postoperatively. If it was a cerebral hemorrhage, code assignment depends on the type of procedure performed.

d. Sequelae of Cerebrovascular Disease

1) Category I69, Sequelae of Cerebrovascular disease

Category I69 is used to indicate conditions classifiable to categories I60-I67 as the causes of sequela (neurologic deficits), themselves classified elsewhere. These "late effects" include neurologic deficits that persist after initial onset of conditions classifiable to categories I60-I67. The neurologic deficits caused by cerebrovascular disease may be present from the onset or may arise at any time after the onset of the condition classifiable to categories I60-I67.

Codes from category I69, Sequelae of cerebrovascular disease, that specify hemiplegia, hemiparesis and monoplegia identify whether the dominant or nondominant side is affected. Should the affected side be documented, but not specified as dominant or nondominant, and the classification system does not indicate a default, code selection is as follows:

- For ambidextrous patients, the default should be dominant.
- If the left side is affected, the default is non-dominant.
- If the right side is affected, the default is dominant.

2) Codes from category I69 with codes from I60-I67

Codes from category I69 may be assigned on a health care record with codes from I60-I67, if the patient has a current cerebrovascular disease and deficits from an old cerebrovascular disease.

3) Codes from category I69 and Personal history of transient ischemic attack (TIA) and cerebral infarction (Z86.73)

Codes from category I69 should not be assigned if the patient does not have neurologic deficits.

See Section I.C.21. 4. History (of) for use of personal history codes

e. Acute myocardial infarction (AMI)

1) ST elevation myocardial infarction (STEMI) and non ST elevation myocardial infarction (NSTEMI)

The ICD-10-CM codes for **type 1** acute myocardial infarction (AMI) identify the site, such as anterolateral wall or true posterior wall. Subcategories I21.0-I21.2 and code I21.3 are used for **type 1** ST elevation myocardial infarction (STEMI). Code I21.4, Non-ST elevation (NSTEMI) myocardial infarction, is used for **type 1** non ST elevation myocardial infarction (NSTEMI) and nontransmural MIs.

If **a type 1** NSTEMI evolves to STEMI, assign the STEMI code. If **a type 1** STEMI converts to NSTEMI due to thrombolytic therapy, it is still coded as STEMI.

For encounters occurring while the myocardial infarction is equal to, or less than, four weeks old, including transfers to another acute setting or a postacute setting, and the myocardial infarction meets the definition for "other diagnoses" (see Section III, Reporting Additional Diagnoses), codes from category I21 may continue to be reported. For encounters after the 4 week time frame and the patient is still receiving care related to the myocardial infarction, the appropriate aftercare code should be assigned, rather than a code from category I21. For old or healed myocardial infarctions not requiring further care, code I25.2, Old myocardial infarction, may be assigned.

2) Acute myocardial infarction, unspecified

Code **I21.9, Acute myocardial infarction, unspecified**, is the default for unspecified acute myocardial infarction **or unspecified type**. If only **type 1** STEMI or transmural MI without the site is documented, assign code I21.3, **ST elevation (STEMI) myocardial infarction of unspecified site.**

3) AMI documented as nontransmural or subendocardial but site provided

If an AMI is documented as nontransmural or subendocardial, but the site is provided, it is still coded as a subendocardial AMI.

See Section I.C.21.3 for information on coding status post administration of tPA in a different facility within the last 24 hours.

4) Subsequent acute myocardial infarction

A code from category I22, Subsequent ST elevation (STEMI) and non ST elevation (NSTEMI) myocardial infarction, is to be used when a patient who has suffered **a type 1 or unspecified** AMI has a new AMI within the 4 week time frame of the initial AMI. A code from category I22 must be used in conjunction with a code from category I21. The sequencing of the I22 and I21 codes depends on the circumstances of the encounter.

Do not assign code I22 for subsequent myocardial infarctions other than type 1 or unspecified. For subsequent type 2 AMI assign only code I21.A1. For subsequent type 4 or type 5 AMI, assign only code I21.A9.

5) **Other Types of Myocardial Infarction**

The ICD-10-CM provides codes for different types of myocardial infarction. Type 1 myocardial infarctions are assigned to codes I21.0-I21.4.

Type 2 myocardial infarctions, and myocardial infarction due to demand ischemia or secondary to ischemic balance, is assigned to code I21.A1, Myocardial infarction type 2 with a code for the underlying cause. Do not assign code I24.8, Other forms of acute ischemic heart disease for the demand ischemia. Sequencing of type 2 AMI or the underlying cause is dependent on the circumstances of admission. When a type 2 AMI code is described as NSTEMI or STEMI, only assign code I21.A1. Codes I21.0-I21.4 should only be assigned for type 1 AMIs.

Acute myocardial infarctions type 3, 4a, 4b, 4c and 5 are assigned to code I21.A9, Other myocardial infarction type.

The "Code also" and "Code first" notes should be followed related to complications, and for coding of postprocedural myocardial infarctions during or following cardiac surgery.

10. Chapter 10: Diseases of the Respiratory System (J00-J99)

a. Chronic Obstructive Pulmonary Disease [COPD] and Asthma

1) Acute exacerbation of chronic obstructive bronchitis and asthma

The codes in categories J44 and J45 distinguish between uncomplicated cases and those in acute exacerbation. An acute exacerbation is a worsening or a decompensation of a chronic condition. An acute exacerbation is not equivalent to an infection superimposed on a chronic condition, though an exacerbation may be triggered by an infection.

b. Acute Respiratory Failure

1) Acute respiratory failure as principal diagnosis

A code from subcategory J96.0, Acute respiratory failure, or subcategory J96.2, Acute and chronic respiratory failure, may be assigned as a principal diagnosis when it is the condition established after study to be chiefly responsible for occasioning the admission to the hospital, and the selection is supported by the Alphabetic Index and Tabular List. However, chapter- specific coding guidelines (such as obstetrics, poisoning, HIV, newborn) that provide sequencing direction take precedence.

2) Acute respiratory failure as secondary diagnosis

Respiratory failure may be listed as a secondary diagnosis if it occurs after admission, or if it is present on admission, but does not meet the definition of principal diagnosis.

3) Sequencing of acute respiratory failure and another acute condition

When a patient is admitted with respiratory failure and another acute condition, (e.g., myocardial infarction, cerebrovascular accident, aspiration pneumonia), the principal diagnosis will not be the same in every situation. This applies whether the other acute condition is a respiratory or nonrespiratory condition. Selection of the principal diagnosis will be dependent on the circumstances of admission. If both the respiratory failure and the other acute condition are equally responsible for occasioning the admission to the hospital, and there are no chapter-specific sequencing rules, the guideline regarding two or more diagnoses that equally meet the definition for principal diagnosis *(Section II, C.)* may be applied in these situations.

If the documentation is not clear as to whether acute respiratory failure and another condition are equally responsible for occasioning the admission, query the provider for clarification.

c. Influenza due to certain identified influenza viruses

Code only confirmed cases of influenza due to certain identified influenza viruses (category J09), and due to other identified influenza virus (category J10). This is an exception to the hospital inpatient guideline Section II, H. (Uncertain Diagnosis).

In this context, "confirmation" does not require documentation of positive laboratory testing specific for avian or other novel influenza A or other identified influenza virus. However, coding should be based on the provider's diagnostic statement that the patient has avian influenza, or other novel influenza A, for category J09, or has another particular identified strain of influenza, such as H1N1 or H3N2, but not identified as novel or variant, for category J10.

If the provider records "suspected" or "possible" or "probable" avian influenza, or novel influenza, or other identified influenza, then the appropriate influenza code from category J11, Influenza due to unidentified influenza virus, should be assigned. A code from category J09, Influenza due to certain identified influenza viruses, should not be assigned nor should a code from category J10, Influenza due to other identified influenza virus.

d. Ventilator associated Pneumonia

1) Documentation of Ventilator associated Pneumonia

As with all procedural or postprocedural complications, code assignment is based on the provider's documentation of the relationship between the condition and the procedure.

Code J95.851, Ventilator associated pneumonia, should be assigned only when the provider has documented ventilator associated pneumonia (VAP). An additional code to identify the organism (e.g., Pseudomonas aeruginosa, code B96.5) should also be assigned. Do not assign an additional code from categories J12-J18 to identify the type of pneumonia.

Code J95.851 should not be assigned for cases where the patient has pneumonia and is on a mechanical ventilator and the provider has not specifically stated that the pneumonia is ventilator-associated pneumonia. If the documentation is unclear as to whether the patient has a pneumonia that is a complication attributable to the mechanical ventilator, query the provider.

2) Ventilator associated Pneumonia Develops after Admission

A patient may be admitted with one type of pneumonia (e.g., code J13, Pneumonia due to Streptococcus pneumonia) and subsequently develop VAP. In this instance, the principal diagnosis would be the appropriate code from categories J12- J18 for the pneumonia diagnosed at the time of admission. Code J95.851, Ventilator associated pneumonia, would be assigned as an additional diagnosis when the provider has also documented the presence of ventilator associated pneumonia.

11. Chapter 11: Diseases of the Digestive System (K00-K95)

Reserved for future guideline expansion

12. Chapter 12: Diseases of the Skin and Subcutaneous Tissue (L00-L99)

a. Pressure ulcer stage codes

1) Pressure ulcer stages

Codes from category L89, Pressure ulcer, are combination codes that identify the site of the pressure ulcer as well as the stage of the ulcer.

The ICD-10-CM classifies pressure ulcer stages based on severity, which is designated by stages 1-4, unspecified stage and unstageable.

Assign as many codes from category L89 as needed to identify all the pressure ulcers the patient has, if applicable.

2) Unstageable pressure ulcers

Assignment of the code for unstageable pressure ulcer (L89.--0) should be based on the clinical documentation. These codes are used for pressure ulcers whose stage cannot be clinically determined (e.g., the ulcer is covered by eschar or has been treated with a skin or muscle graft) and pressure ulcers that are documented as deep tissue injury but not documented as due to trauma. This code should not be confused with the codes for unspecified stage (L89.--9). When there is no documentation regarding the stage of the pressure ulcer, assign the appropriate code for unspecified stage (L89.--9).

3) Documented pressure ulcer stage

Assignment of the pressure ulcer stage code should be guided by clinical documentation of the stage or documentation of the terms found in the Alphabetic Index. For clinical terms describing the stage that are not found in the Alphabetic Index, and there is no documentation of the stage, the provider should be queried.

4) Patients admitted with pressure ulcers documented as healed

No code is assigned if the documentation states that the pressure ulcer is completely healed.

5) Patients admitted with pressure ulcers documented as healing

Pressure ulcers described as healing should be assigned the appropriate pressure ulcer stage code based on the documentation in the medical record. If the documentation does not provide information about the stage of the healing pressure ulcer, assign the appropriate code for unspecified stage.

If the documentation is unclear as to whether the patient has a current (new) pressure ulcer or if the patient is being treated for a healing pressure ulcer, query the provider.

For ulcers that were present on admission but healed at the time of discharge, assign the code for the site and stage of the pressure ulcer at the time of admission.

6) Patient admitted with pressure ulcer evolving into another stage during the admission

If a patient is admitted **to an inpatient hospital** with a pressure ulcer at one stage and it progresses to a higher stage, two separate codes should be assigned: one code for the site and stage of the ulcer on admission and a second code for the same ulcer site and the highest stage reported during the stay.

b. **Non-Pressure Chronic Ulcers**

1) **Patients admitted with non-pressure ulcers documented as healed**

No code is assigned if the documentation states that the non-pressure ulcer is completely healed.

2) **Patients admitted with non-pressure ulcers documented as healing**

Non-pressure ulcers described as healing should be assigned the appropriate non-pressure ulcer code based on the documentation in the medical record. If the documentation does not provide information about the severity of the healing non-pressure ulcer, assign the appropriate code unspecified severity.

If the documentation is unclear as to whether the patient has a current (new) non-pressure ulcer or if the patient is being treated for a healing non-pressure ulcer, query the provider.

For ulcers that were present on admission but healed at the time of discharge, assign the code for the site and severity of the non-pressure ulcer at the time of admission.

3) **Patient admitted with non-pressure ulcer that progresses to another severity level during the admission**

If a patient is admitted to an inpatient hospital with a non-pressure ulcer at one severity level and it progresses to a higher severity level, two separate codes should be assigned; one code for the site and severity level of the ulcer on admission and a second code for the same ulcer site and the highest severity level reported during the stay.

13. Chapter 13: Diseases of the Musculoskeletal System and Connective Tissue (M00-M99)

a. Site and laterality

Most of the codes within Chapter 13 have site and laterality designations. The site represents the bone, joint or the muscle involved. For some conditions where more than one bone, joint or muscle is usually involved, such as osteoarthritis, there is a "multiple sites" code available. For categories where no multiple site code is provided and more than one bone, joint or muscle is involved, multiple codes should be used to indicate the different sites involved.

1) Bone versus joint

For certain conditions, the bone may be affected at the upper or lower end, (e.g., avascular necrosis of bone, M87, Osteoporosis, M80, M81). Though the portion of the bone affected may be at the joint, the site designation will be the bone, not the joint.

b. Acute traumatic versus chronic or recurrent musculoskeletal conditions

Many musculoskeletal conditions are a result of previous injury or trauma to a site, or are recurrent conditions. Bone, joint or muscle conditions that are the result of a healed injury are usually found in chapter 13. Recurrent bone, joint or muscle conditions are also usually found in chapter 13. Any current, acute injury should be coded to the appropriate injury code from chapter 19. Chronic or recurrent conditions should generally be coded with a code from chapter 13. If it is difficult to determine from the documentation in the record which code is best to describe a condition, query the provider.

c. Coding of Pathologic Fractures

7th character A is for use as long as the patient is receiving active treatment for the fracture. While the patient may be seen by a new or different provider over the course of treatment for a pathological fracture, assignment of the 7th character is based on whether the patient is undergoing active treatment and not whether the provider is seeing the patient for the first time.

7th character, D is to be used for encounters after the patient has completed active treatment **for the fracture and is receiving routine care for the fracture during the healing or recovery phase**. The other 7th characters, listed under each subcategory in the Tabular List, are to be used for subsequent encounters for routine care of fractures during the healing and recovery phase as well as treatment of problems associated with the healing, such as malunions, nonunions, and sequelae.

Care for complications of surgical treatment for fracture repairs during the healing or recovery phase should be coded with the appropriate complication codes.

See Section I.C.19. Coding of traumatic fractures.

d. Osteoporosis

Osteoporosis is a systemic condition, meaning that all bones of the musculoskeletal system are affected. Therefore, site is not a component of the codes under category M81, Osteoporosis without current pathological fracture. The site codes under category M80, Osteoporosis with current pathological fracture, identify the site of the fracture, not the osteoporosis.

1) Osteoporosis without pathological fracture

Category M81, Osteoporosis without current pathological fracture, is for use for patients with osteoporosis who do not currently have a pathologic fracture due to the osteoporosis, even if they have had a fracture in the past. For patients with a history of osteoporosis fractures, status code Z87.310, Personal history of (healed) osteoporosis fracture, should follow the code from M81.

2) Osteoporosis with current pathological fracture

Category M80, Osteoporosis with current pathological fracture, is for patients who have a current pathologic fracture at the time of an encounter. The codes under M80 identify the site of the fracture. A code from category M80, not a traumatic fracture code, should be used for any patient with known osteoporosis who suffers a fracture, even if the patient had a minor fall or trauma, if that fall or trauma would not usually break a normal, healthy bone.

14. Chapter 14: Diseases of the Genitourinary System (N00-N99)

a. Chronic kidney disease

1) Stages of chronic kidney disease (CKD)

The ICD-10-CM classifies CKD based on severity. The severity of CKD is designated by stages 1-5. Stage 2, code N18.2, equates to mild CKD; stage 3, code N18.3, equates to moderate CKD; and stage 4, code N18.4, equates to severe CKD. Code N18.6, End stage renal disease (ESRD), is assigned when the provider has documented end-stage-renal disease (ESRD).

If both a stage of CKD and ESRD are documented, assign code N18.6 only.

2) Chronic kidney disease and kidney transplant status

Patients who have undergone kidney transplant may still have some form of chronic kidney disease (CKD) because the kidney transplant may not fully restore kidney function. Therefore, the presence of CKD alone does not constitute a transplant complication. Assign the appropriate N18 code for the patient's stage of CKD and code Z94.0, Kidney transplant status. If a transplant complication such as failure or rejection or other transplant complication is documented, see section I.C.19.g for information on coding complications of a kidney transplant. If the documentation is unclear as to whether the patient has a complication of the transplant, query the provider.

3) Chronic kidney disease with other conditions

Patients with CKD may also suffer from other serious conditions, most commonly diabetes mellitus and hypertension. The sequencing of the CKD code in relationship to codes for other contributing conditions is based on the conventions in the Tabular List.

See I.C.9. Hypertensive chronic kidney disease.

See I.C.19. Chronic kidney disease and kidney transplant complications.

15. Chapter 15: Pregnancy, Childbirth and the Puerperium (O00-O9A)

a. General Rules for Obstetric Cases

1) Codes from chapter 15 and sequencing priority

Obstetric cases require codes from chapter 15, codes in the range O00-O9A, Pregnancy, Childbirth, and the Puerperium. Chapter 15 codes have sequencing priority over codes from other chapters. Additional codes from other chapters may be used in conjunction with chapter 15 codes to further specify conditions. Should the provider document that the pregnancy is incidental to the encounter, then code Z33.1, Pregnant state, incidental, should be used in place of any chapter 15 codes. It is the provider's responsibility to state that the condition being treated is not affecting the pregnancy.

2) Chapter 15 codes used only on the maternal record

Chapter 15 codes are to be used only on the maternal record, never on the record of the newborn.

3) Final character for trimester

The majority of codes in Chapter 15 have a final character indicating the trimester of pregnancy. The timeframes for the trimesters are indicated at the beginning of the chapter. If trimester is not a component of a code it is because the condition always occurs in a specific trimester, or the concept of trimester of pregnancy is not applicable. Certain codes have characters for only certain trimesters because the condition does not occur in all trimesters, but it may occur in more than just one.

Assignment of the final character for trimester should be based on the provider's documentation of the trimester (or number of weeks) for the current admission/encounter. This applies to the assignment of trimester for pre-existing conditions as well as those that develop during or are due to the pregnancy. The provider's documentation of the number of weeks may be used to assign the appropriate code identifying the trimester.

Whenever delivery occurs during the current admission, and there is an "in childbirth" option for the obstetric complication being coded, the "in childbirth" code should be assigned.

4) Selection of trimester for inpatient admissions that encompass more than one trimester

In instances when a patient is admitted to a hospital for complications of pregnancy during one trimester and remains in the hospital into a subsequent trimester, the trimester character for the antepartum complication code should be assigned on the basis of the trimester when the complication developed, not the trimester of the discharge. If the condition developed prior to the current admission/encounter or represents a pre-existing condition, the trimester character for the trimester at the time of the admission/encounter should be assigned.

5) Unspecified trimester

Each category that includes codes for trimester has a code for "unspecified trimester." The "unspecified trimester" code should rarely be used, such as when the documentation in the record is insufficient to determine the trimester and it is not possible to obtain clarification.

6) 7th character for Fetus Identification

Where applicable, a 7th character is to be assigned for certain categories (O31, O32, O33.3 - O33.6, O35, O36, O40, O41, O60.1, O60.2, O64, and O69) to identify the fetus for which the complication code applies.

Assign 7th character "0":

- For single gestations
- When the documentation in the record is insufficient to determine the fetus affected and it is not possible to obtain clarification.
- When it is not possible to clinically determine which fetus is affected.

b. Selection of OB Principal or First-listed Diagnosis

1) Routine outpatient prenatal visits

For routine outpatient prenatal visits when no complications are present, a code from category Z34, Encounter for supervision of normal pregnancy, should be used as the first-listed diagnosis. These codes should not be used in conjunction with chapter 15 codes.

2) Supervision of High-Risk Pregnancy

Codes from category O09, Supervision of high-risk pregnancy, are intended for use only during the prenatal period. For complications during the labor or delivery episode as a result of a high-risk pregnancy, assign the applicable complication codes from Chapter 15. If there are no complications during the labor or delivery episode, assign code O80, Encounter for full-term uncomplicated delivery.

For routine prenatal outpatient visits for patients with high-risk pregnancies, a code from category O09, Supervision of high-risk pregnancy, should be used as the first-listed diagnosis. Secondary chapter 15 codes may be used in conjunction with these codes if appropriate.

3) Episodes when no delivery occurs

In episodes when no delivery occurs, the principal diagnosis should correspond to the principal complication of the pregnancy which necessitated the encounter. Should more than one complication exist, all of which are treated or monitored, any of the complications codes may be sequenced first.

4) When a delivery occurs

When an obstetric patient is admitted and delivers during that admission, the condition that prompted the admission should be sequenced as the principal diagnosis. If multiple conditions prompted the admission, sequence the one most related to the delivery as the principal diagnosis. A code for any complication of the delivery should be assigned as an additional diagnosis. In cases of cesarean delivery, if the patient was admitted with a condition that resulted in the performance of a cesarean procedure, that condition should be selected as the principal diagnosis. If the reason for the admission was unrelated to the condition resulting in the cesarean delivery, the condition related to the reason for the admission should be selected as the principal diagnosis.

5) Outcome of delivery

A code from category Z37, Outcome of delivery, should be included on every maternal record when a delivery has occurred. These codes are not to be used on subsequent records or on the newborn record.

c. Pre-existing conditions versus conditions due to the pregnancy

Certain categories in Chapter 15 distinguish between conditions of the mother that existed prior to pregnancy (pre-existing) and those that are a direct result of pregnancy. When assigning codes from Chapter 15, it is important to assess if a condition was pre-existing prior to pregnancy or developed during or due to the pregnancy in order to assign the correct code.

Categories that do not distinguish between pre-existing and pregnancy- related conditions may be used for either. It is acceptable to use codes specifically for the puerperium with codes complicating pregnancy and childbirth if a condition arises postpartum during the delivery encounter.

d. Pre-existing hypertension in pregnancy

Category O10, Pre-existing hypertension complicating pregnancy, childbirth and the puerperium, includes codes for hypertensive heart and hypertensive chronic kidney disease. When assigning one of the O10 codes that includes hypertensive heart disease or hypertensive chronic kidney disease, it is necessary to add a secondary code from the appropriate hypertension category to specify the type of heart failure or chronic kidney disease.

See Section I.C.9. Hypertension.

e. Fetal Conditions Affecting the Management of the Mother

1) Codes from categories O35 and O36

Codes from categories O35, Maternal care for known or suspected fetal abnormality and damage, and O36, Maternal care for other fetal problems, are assigned only when the fetal condition is actually responsible for modifying the management of the mother, i.e., by requiring diagnostic studies, additional observation, special care, or termination of pregnancy. The fact that the fetal condition exists does not justify assigning a code from this series to the mother's record.

2) In utero surgery

In cases when surgery is performed on the fetus, a diagnosis code from category O35, Maternal care for known or suspected fetal abnormality and damage, should be assigned identifying the fetal condition. Assign the appropriate procedure code for the procedure performed.

No code from Chapter 16, the perinatal codes, should be used on the mother's record to identify fetal conditions. Surgery performed in utero on a fetus is still to be coded as an obstetric encounter.

f. HIV Infection in Pregnancy, Childbirth and the Puerperium

During pregnancy, childbirth or the puerperium, a patient admitted because of an HIV-related illness should receive a principal diagnosis from subcategory O98.7-, Human immunodeficiency [HIV] disease complicating pregnancy, childbirth and the puerperium, followed by the code(s) for the HIV-related illness(es).

Patients with asymptomatic HIV infection status admitted during pregnancy, childbirth, or the puerperium should receive codes of O98.7- and Z21, Asymptomatic human immunodeficiency virus [HIV] infection status.

g. Diabetes mellitus in pregnancy

Diabetes mellitus is a significant complicating factor in pregnancy. Pregnant women who are diabetic should be assigned a code from category O24, Diabetes mellitus in pregnancy, childbirth, and the puerperium, first, followed by the appropriate diabetes code(s) (E08- E13) from Chapter 4.

h. Long term use of insulin and oral hypoglycemics

See section I.C.4.a.3 for information on the long term use of insulin and oral hypoglycemic.

i. Gestational (pregnancy induced) diabetes

Gestational (pregnancy induced) diabetes can occur during the second and third trimester of pregnancy in women who were not diabetic prior to pregnancy. Gestational diabetes can cause complications in the pregnancy similar to those of pre-existing diabetes mellitus. It also puts the woman at greater risk of developing diabetes after the pregnancy. Codes for gestational diabetes are in subcategory O24.4, Gestational diabetes mellitus. No other code from category O24, Diabetes mellitus in pregnancy, childbirth, and the puerperium, should be used with a code from O24.4

The codes under subcategory O24.4 include diet controlled, insulin controlled, and controlled by oral hypoglycemic drugs. If a patient with gestational diabetes is treated with both diet and insulin, only the code for insulin-controlled is required. If a patient with gestational diabetes is treated with both diet and oral hypoglycemic medications, only the code for "controlled by oral hypoglycemic drugs" is required.

Code Z79.4, Long-term (current) use of insulin or code Z79.84, Long-term (current) use of oral hypoglycemic drugs, should not be assigned with codes from subcategory O24.4.

An abnormal glucose tolerance in pregnancy is assigned a code from subcategory O99.81, Abnormal glucose complicating pregnancy, childbirth, and the puerperium.

j. Sepsis and septic shock complicating abortion, pregnancy, childbirth and the puerperium

When assigning a chapter 15 code for sepsis complicating abortion, pregnancy, childbirth, and the puerperium, a code for the specific type of infection should be assigned as an additional diagnosis. If severe sepsis is present, a code from subcategory R65.2, Severe sepsis, and code(s) for associated organ dysfunction(s) should also be assigned as additional diagnoses.

k. Puerperal sepsis

Code O85, Puerperal sepsis, should be assigned with a secondary code to identify the causal organism (e.g., for a bacterial infection, assign a code from category B95-B96, Bacterial infections in conditions classified elsewhere). A code from category A40, Streptococcal sepsis, or A41, Other sepsis, should not be used for puerperal sepsis. If applicable, use additional codes to identify severe sepsis (R65.2-) and any associated acute organ dysfunction.

l. Alcohol and tobacco use during pregnancy, childbirth and the puerperium

1) Alcohol use during pregnancy, childbirth and the puerperium

Codes under subcategory O99.31, Alcohol use complicating pregnancy, childbirth, and the puerperium, should be assigned for any pregnancy case when a mother uses alcohol during the pregnancy or postpartum. A secondary code from category F10, Alcohol related disorders, should also be assigned to identify manifestations of the alcohol use.

2) Tobacco use during pregnancy, childbirth and the puerperium

Codes under subcategory O99.33, Smoking (tobacco) complicating pregnancy, childbirth, and the puerperium, should be assigned for any pregnancy case when a mother uses any type of tobacco product during the pregnancy or postpartum. A secondary code from category F17, Nicotine dependence, should also be assigned to identify the type of nicotine dependence.

m. Poisoning, toxic effects, adverse effects and underdosing in a pregnant patient

A code from subcategory O9A.2, Injury, poisoning and certain other consequences of external causes complicating pregnancy, childbirth, and the puerperium, should be sequenced first, followed by the appropriate injury, poisoning, toxic effect, adverse effect or underdosing code, and then the additional code(s) that specifies the condition caused by the poisoning, toxic effect, adverse effect or underdosing.

See Section I.C.19. Adverse effects, poisoning, underdosing and toxic effects.

n. Normal Delivery, Code O80

1) Encounter for full term uncomplicated delivery

Code O80 should be assigned when a woman is admitted for a full-term normal delivery and delivers a single, healthy infant without any complications antepartum, during the delivery, or postpartum during the delivery episode. Code O80 is always a principal diagnosis. It is not to be used if any other code from chapter 15 is needed to describe a current complication of the antenatal, delivery, or perinatal period. Additional codes from other chapters may be used with code O80 if they are not related to or are in any way complicating the pregnancy.

2) Uncomplicated delivery with resolved antepartum complication

Code O80 may be used if the patient had a complication at some point during the pregnancy, but the complication is not present at the time of the admission for delivery.

3) Outcome of delivery for O80

Z37.0, Single live birth, is the only outcome of delivery code appropriate for use with O80.

o. The Peripartum and Postpartum Periods

1) Peripartum and Postpartum periods

The postpartum period begins immediately after delivery and continues for six weeks following delivery. The peripartum period is defined as the last month of pregnancy to five months postpartum.

2) Peripartum and postpartum complication

A postpartum complication is any complication occurring within the six-week period.

3) Pregnancy-related complications after 6 week period

Chapter 15 codes may also be used to describe pregnancy-related complications after the peripartum or postpartum period if the provider documents that a condition is pregnancy related.

4) Admission for routine postpartum care following delivery outside hospital

When the mother delivers outside the hospital prior to admission and is admitted for routine postpartum care and no complications are noted, code Z39.0, Encounter for care and examination of mother immediately after delivery, should be assigned as the principal diagnosis.

5) Pregnancy associated cardiomyopathy

Pregnancy associated cardiomyopathy, code O90.3, is unique in that it may be diagnosed in the third trimester of pregnancy but may continue to progress months after delivery. For this reason, it is referred to as peripartum cardiomyopathy. Code O90.3 is only for use when the cardiomyopathy develops as a result of pregnancy in a woman who did not have pre-existing heart disease.

p. Code O94, Sequelae of complication of pregnancy, childbirth, and the puerperium

1) Code O94

Code O94, Sequelae of complication of pregnancy, childbirth, and the puerperium, is for use in those cases when an initial complication of a pregnancy develops a sequelae requiring care or treatment at a future date.

2) After the initial postpartum period

This code may be used at any time after the initial postpartum period.

3) Sequencing of Code O94

This code, like all sequela codes, is to be sequenced following the code describing the sequelae of the complication.

q. Termination of Pregnancy and Spontaneous abortions

1) Abortion with Liveborn Fetus

When an attempted termination of pregnancy results in a liveborn fetus, assign code Z33.2, Encounter for elective termination of pregnancy and a code from category Z37, Outcome of Delivery.

2) Retained Products of Conception following an abortion

Subsequent encounters for retained products of conception following a spontaneous abortion or elective termination of pregnancy**, without complications** are assigned O03**.4, Incomplete spontaneous,** abortion **without complication,** or codes O07.4, Failed attempted termination of pregnancy without complication. This advice is appropriate even when the patient was discharged previously with a discharge diagnosis of complete abortion. **If the patient has a specific complication associated with the spontaneous abortion or elective termination of pregnancy in addition to retained products of conception, assign the appropriate complication in category O03 or O07 instead of code O03.4 or O07.4.**

3) Complications leading to abortion

Codes from Chapter 15 may be used as additional codes to identify any documented complications of the pregnancy in conjunction with codes in categories in **O04**, O07 and O08.

r. Abuse in a pregnant patient

For suspected or confirmed cases of abuse of a pregnant patient, a code(s) from subcategories O9A.3, Physical abuse complicating pregnancy, childbirth, and the puerperium, O9A.4, Sexual abuse complicating pregnancy, childbirth, and the puerperium, and O9A.5, Psychological abuse complicating pregnancy, childbirth, and the puerperium, should be sequenced first, followed by the appropriate codes (if applicable) to identify any associated current injury due to physical abuse, sexual abuse, and the perpetrator of abuse.

See Section I.C.19. Adult and child abuse, neglect and other maltreatment.

16. Chapter 16: Certain Conditions Originating in the Perinatal Period (P00-P96)

For coding and reporting purposes the perinatal period is defined as before birth through the 28th day following birth. The following guidelines are provided for reporting purposes

a. General Perinatal Rules

1) Use of Chapter 16 Codes

Codes in this chapter are <u>never</u> for use on the maternal record. Codes from Chapter 15, the obstetric chapter, are never permitted on the newborn record. Chapter 16 codes may be used throughout the life of the patient if the condition is still present.

2) Principal Diagnosis for Birth Record

When coding the birth episode in a newborn record, assign a code from category Z38, Liveborn infants according to place of birth and type of delivery, as the principal diagnosis. A code from category Z38 is assigned only once, to a newborn at the time of birth. If a newborn is transferred to another institution, a code from category Z38 should not be used at the receiving hospital.

A code from category Z38 is used only on the newborn record, not on the mother's record.

3) Use of Codes from other Chapters with Codes from Chapter 16

Codes from other chapters may be used with codes from chapter 16 if the codes from the other chapters provide more specific detail. Codes for signs and symptoms may be assigned when a definitive diagnosis has not been established. If the reason for the encounter is a perinatal condition, the code from chapter 16 should be sequenced first.

4) Use of Chapter 16 Codes after the Perinatal Period

Should a condition originate in the perinatal period, and continue throughout the life of the patient, the perinatal code should continue to be used regardless of the patient's age.

5) **Birth process or community acquired conditions**

If a newborn has a condition that may be either due to the birth process or community acquired and the documentation does not indicate which it is, the default is due to the birth process and the code from Chapter 16 should be used. If the condition is community-acquired, a code from Chapter 16 should not be assigned.

6) **Code all clinically significant conditions**

All clinically significant conditions noted on routine newborn examination should be coded. A condition is clinically significant if it requires:

- clinical evaluation; or
- therapeutic treatment; or
- diagnostic procedures; or
- extended length of hospital stay; or
- increased nursing care and/or monitoring; or
- has implications for future health care needs

Note: The perinatal guidelines listed above are the same as the general coding guidelines for "additional diagnoses", except for the final point regarding implications for future health care needs. Codes should be assigned for conditions that have been specified by the provider as having implications for future health care needs.

b. Observation and Evaluation of Newborns for Suspected Conditions not Found

1) ***Use of Z05 codes***

Assign a code from category Z05, Observation and evaluation of newborns and infants for suspected conditions ruled out, to identify those instances when a healthy newborn is evaluated for a suspected condition that is determined after study not to be present. Do not use a code from category Z05 when the patient has identified signs or symptoms of a suspected problem; in such cases code the sign or symptom.

2) ***Z05 on Other than the Birth Record***

A code from category Z05 may also be assigned as a principal or first-listed code for readmissions or encounters when the code from category Z38 code no longer applies. Codes from category Z05 are fur use only for healthy newborns and infants for which no condition after study is found to be present.

3) **Z05 on a birth record**

A code from category Z05 is to be used as a secondary code after the code from category Z38, Liveborn infants according to place of birth and type of delivery.

c. Coding Additional Perinatal Diagnoses

1) **Assigning codes for conditions that require treatment**

Assign codes for conditions that require treatment or further investigation, prolong the length of stay, or require resource utilization.

2) **Codes for conditions specified as having implications for future health care needs**

Assign codes for conditions that have been specified by the provider as having implications for future health care needs.

Note: This guideline should not be used for adult patients.

d. Prematurity and Fetal Growth Retardation

Providers utilize different criteria in determining prematurity. A code for prematurity should not be assigned unless it is documented. Assignment of codes in categories P05, Disorders of newborn related to slow fetal growth and fetal malnutrition, and P07, Disorders of newborn related to short gestation and low birth weight, not elsewhere classified, should be based on the recorded birth weight and estimated gestational age.

When both birth weight and gestational age are available, two codes from category P07 should be assigned, with the code for birth weight sequenced before the code for gestational age.

e. Low birth weight and immaturity status

Codes from category P07, Disorders of newborn related to short gestation and low birth weight, not elsewhere classified, are for use for a child or adult who was premature or had a low birth weight as a newborn and this is affecting the patient's current health status.

See Section I.C.21. Factors influencing health status and contact with health services, Status.

f. Bacterial Sepsis of Newborn

Category P36, Bacterial sepsis of newborn, includes congenital sepsis. If a perinate is documented as having sepsis without documentation of congenital or community acquired, the default is congenital and a code from category

P36 should be assigned. If the P36 code includes the causal organism, an additional code from category B95, Streptococcus, Staphylococcus, and Enterococcus as the cause of diseases classified elsewhere, or B96, Other bacterial agents as the cause of diseases classified elsewhere, should not be assigned. If the P36 code does not include the causal organism, assign an additional code from category B96. If applicable, use additional codes to identify severe sepsis (R65.2-) and any associated acute organ dysfunction.

g. Stillbirth

Code P95, Stillbirth, is only for use in institutions that maintain separate records for stillbirths. No other code should be used with P95. Code P95 should not be used on the mother's record.

17. Chapter 17: Congenital Malformations, Deformations and Chromosomal Abnormalities (Q00-Q99)

Assign an appropriate code(s) from categories Q00-Q99, Congenital malformations, deformations, and chromosomal abnormalities when a malformation/deformation or chromosomal abnormality is documented. A malformation/deformation or chromosomal abnormality may be the principal/first-listed diagnosis on a record or a secondary diagnosis.

When a malformation/deformation or chromosomal abnormality does not have a unique code assignment, assign additional code(s) for any manifestations that may be present.

When the code assignment specifically identifies the malformation/deformation or chromosomal abnormality, manifestations that are an inherent component of the anomaly should not be coded separately. Additional codes should be assigned for manifestations that are not an inherent component.

Codes from Chapter 17 may be used throughout the life of the patient. If a congenital malformation or deformity has been corrected, a personal history code should be used to identify the history of the malformation or deformity. Although present at birth, malformation/deformation or chromosomal abnormality may not be identified until later in life. Whenever the condition is diagnosed by the physician, it is appropriate to assign a code from codes Q00-Q99. For the birth admission, the appropriate code from category Z38, Liveborn infants, according to place of birth and type of delivery, should be sequenced as the principal diagnosis, followed by any congenital anomaly codes, Q00-Q99.

18. Chapter 18: Symptoms, Signs, and Abnormal Clinical and Laboratory Findings, Not Elsewhere Classified (R00-R99)

Chapter 18 includes symptoms, signs, abnormal results of clinical or other investigative procedures, and ill-defined conditions regarding which no diagnosis classifiable elsewhere is recorded. Signs and symptoms that point to a specific diagnosis have been assigned to a category in other chapters of the classification.

a. Use of symptom codes

Codes that describe symptoms and signs are acceptable for reporting purposes when a related definitive diagnosis has not been established (confirmed) by the provider.

b. Use of a symptom code with a definitive diagnosis code

Codes for signs and symptoms may be reported in addition to a related definitive diagnosis when the sign or symptom is not routinely associated with that diagnosis, such as the various signs and symptoms associated with complex syndromes. The definitive diagnosis code should be sequenced before the symptom code.

Signs or symptoms that are associated routinely with a disease process should not be assigned as additional codes, unless otherwise instructed by the classification.

c. Combination codes that include symptoms

ICD-10-CM contains a number of combination codes that identify both the definitive diagnosis and common symptoms of that diagnosis. When using one of these combination codes, an additional code should not be assigned for the symptom.

d. Repeated falls

Code R29.6, Repeated falls, is for use for encounters when a patient has recently fallen and the reason for the fall is being investigated.

Code Z91.81, History of falling, is for use when a patient has fallen in the past and is at risk for future falls. When appropriate, both codes R29.6 and Z91.81 may be assigned together.

e. Coma scale

The coma scale codes (R40.2-) can be used in conjunction with traumatic brain injury codes, acute cerebrovascular disease or sequelae of cerebrovascular disease codes. These codes are primarily for use by trauma registries, but they may be used in any setting where this information is collected. The coma scale may also be used to assess the status of the central nervous system for other non-trauma conditions, such as monitoring patients in the intensive care unit regardless of medical conditions. The coma scale codes should be sequenced after the diagnosis code(s).

These codes, one from each subcategory, are needed to complete the scale. The 7th character indicates when the scale was recorded. The 7th character should match for all three codes.

At a minimum, report the initial score documented on presentation at your facility. This may be a score from the emergency medicine technician (EMT) or in the emergency department. If desired, a facility may choose to capture multiple coma scale scores.

Assign code R40.24, Glasgow coma scale, total score, when only the total score is documented in the medical record and not the individual score(s).

f. Functional quadriplegia

GUIDELINE HAS BEEN DELETED EFFECTIVE OCTOBER 1, 2017

g. SIRS due to Non-Infectious Process

The systemic inflammatory response syndrome (SIRS) can develop as a result of certain non-infectious disease processes, such as trauma, malignant neoplasm, or pancreatitis. When SIRS is documented with a noninfectious condition, and no subsequent infection is documented, the code for the underlying condition, such as an injury, should be assigned, followed by code R65.10, Systemic inflammatory response syndrome (SIRS) of non-infectious origin without acute organ dysfunction, or code R65.11, Systemic inflammatory response syndrome (SIRS) of non-infectious origin with acute organ dysfunction. If an associated acute organ dysfunction is documented, the appropriate code(s) for the specific type of organ dysfunction(s) should be assigned in addition to code R65.11. If acute organ dysfunction is documented, but it cannot be determined if the acute organ dysfunction is associated with SIRS or due to another condition (e.g., directly due to the trauma), the provider should be queried.

h. Death NOS

Code R99, Ill-defined and unknown cause of mortality, is only for use in the very limited circumstance when a patient who has already died is brought into an emergency department or other healthcare facility and is pronounced dead upon arrival. It does not represent the discharge disposition of death.

i. NIHSS Stroke Scale

The NIH stroke scale (NIHSS) codes (R29.7--) can be used in conjunction with acute stroke codes (I63) to identify the patient's neurological status and the severity of the stroke. The stroke scale codes should be sequenced after the acute stroke diagnosis code(s).

At a minimum, report the initial score documented. If desired, a facility may choose to capture multiple stroke scale scores.

See Section I.B.14 for information concerning the medical record documentations that may be used for assignment of the NIHSS codes.

19. Chapter 19: Injury, Poisoning and Certain Other Consequences of External Causes (S00-T88)

a. Application of 7th Characters in Chapter 19

Most categories in chapter 19 have a 7th character requirement for each applicable code. Most categories in this chapter have three 7th character values (with the exception of fractures): A, initial encounter, D, subsequent encounter and S, sequela. Categories for traumatic fractures have additional 7th character values. While the patient may be seen by a new or different provider over the course of treatment for an injury, assignment of the 7th character is based on whether the patient is undergoing active treatment and not whether the provider is seeing the patient for the first time.

For complication codes, active treatment refers to treatment for the condition described by the code, even though it may be related to an earlier precipitating problem. For example, code T84.50XA, Infection and inflammatory reaction due to unspecified internal joint prosthesis, initial encounter, is used when active treatment is provided for the infection, even though the condition relates to the prosthetic device, implant or graft that was placed at a previous encounter.

7th character "A", initial encounter is used for each encounter where the patient is receiving active treatment for the condition.

7th character "D" subsequent encounter is used for encounters after the patient has completed active treatment of the condition and is receiving routine care for the condition during the healing or recovery phase.

The aftercare Z codes should not be used for aftercare for conditions such as injuries or poisonings, where 7th characters are provided to identify subsequent care. For example, for aftercare of an injury, assign the acute injury code with the 7th character "D" (subsequent encounter).

7th character "S", sequela, is for use for complications or conditions that arise as a direct result of a condition, such as scar formation after a burn. The scars are sequelae of the burn. When using 7th character "S", it is necessary to use both the injury code that precipitated the sequela and the code for the sequela itself. The "S" is added only to the injury code, not the sequela code. The 7th character "S" identifies the injury responsible for the sequela. The specific type of sequela (e.g. scar) is sequenced first, followed by the injury code.

See Section I.B.10 Sequela (Late Effects)

b. Coding of Injuries

When coding injuries, assign separate codes for each injury unless a combination code is provided, in which case the combination code is assigned. **Codes from category** T07, Unspecified multiple injuries should not be assigned in the inpatient setting unless information for a more specific code is not available. Traumatic injury codes (S00-T14.9) are not to be used for normal, healing surgical wounds or to identify complications of surgical wounds.

The code for the most serious injury, as determined by the provider and the focus of treatment, is sequenced first.

1) Superficial injuries

Superficial injuries such as abrasions or contusions are not coded when associated with more severe injuries of the same site.

2) Primary injury with damage to nerves/blood vessels

When a primary injury results in minor damage to peripheral nerves or blood vessels, the primary injury is sequenced first with additional code(s) for injuries to nerves and spinal cord (such as category S04), and/or injury to blood vessels (such as category S15). When the primary injury is to the blood vessels or nerves, that injury should be sequenced first.

c. Coding of Traumatic Fractures

The principles of multiple coding of injuries should be followed in coding fractures. Fractures of specified sites are coded individually by site in accordance with both the provisions within categories S02, S12, S22, S32, S42, S49, S52, S59, S62, S72, S79, S82, S89, S92 and the level of detail furnished by medical record content.

A fracture not indicated as open or closed should be coded to closed. A fracture not indicated whether displaced or not displaced should be coded to displaced.

More specific guidelines are as follows:

1) Initial vs. Subsequent Encounter for Fractures

Traumatic fractures are coded using the appropriate 7th character for initial encounter (A, B, C) for each encounter where the patient is receiving active treatment for the fracture. The appropriate 7th character for initial encounter should also be assigned for a patient who delayed seeking treatment for the fracture or nonunion.

Fractures are coded using the appropriate 7th character for subsequent care for encounters after the patient has completed active treatment of the fracture and is receiving routine care for the fracture during the healing or recovery phase.

Care for complications of surgical treatment for fracture repairs during the healing or recovery phase should be coded with the appropriate complication codes.

Care of complications of fractures, such as malunion and nonunion, should be reported with the appropriate 7th character for subsequent care with nonunion (K, M, N,) or subsequent care with malunion (P, Q, R).

Malunion/nonunion: The appropriate 7th character for initial encounter should also be assigned for a patient who delayed seeking treatment for the fracture or nonunion.

The open fracture designations in the assignment of the 7th character for fractures of the forearm, femur and lower leg, including ankle are based on the Gustilo open fracture classification. When the Gustilo classification type is not specified for an open fracture, the 7th character for open fracture type I or II should be assigned (B, E, H, M, Q).

A code from category M80, not a traumatic fracture code, should be used for any patient with known osteoporosis who suffers a fracture, even if the patient had a minor fall or trauma, if that fall or trauma would not usually break a normal, healthy bone.

See Section I.C.13. Osteoporosis.

The aftercare Z codes should not be used for aftercare for traumatic fractures. For aftercare of a traumatic fracture, assign the acute fracture code with the appropriate 7th character.

2) Multiple fractures sequencing

Multiple fractures are sequenced in accordance with the severity of the fracture.

d. Coding of Burns and Corrosions

The ICD-10-CM makes a distinction between burns and corrosions. The burn codes are for thermal burns, except sunburns, that come from a heat source, such as a fire or hot appliance. The burn codes are also for burns resulting from electricity and radiation. Corrosions are burns due to chemicals. The guidelines are the same for burns and corrosions.

Current burns (T20-T25) are classified by depth, extent and by agent (X code). Burns are classified by depth as first degree (erythema), second degree (blistering), and third degree (full-thickness involvement). Burns of the eye and internal organs (T26-T28) are classified by site, but not by degree.

1) Sequencing of burn and related condition codes

Sequence first the code that reflects the highest degree of burn when more than one burn is present.

a. When the reason for the admission or encounter is for treatment of external multiple burns, sequence first the code that reflects the burn of the highest degree.

b. When a patient has both internal and external burns, the circumstances of admission govern the selection of the principal diagnosis or first-listed diagnosis.

c. When a patient is admitted for burn injuries and other related conditions such as smoke inhalation and/or respiratory failure, the circumstances of admission govern the selection of the principal or first-listed diagnosis.

2) Burns of the same local site

Classify burns of the same local site (three-character category level, T20-T28) but of different degrees to the subcategory identifying the highest degree recorded in the diagnosis.

3) Non-healing burns

Non-healing burns are coded as acute burns.

Necrosis of burned skin should be coded as a non-healed burn.

4) Infected Burn

For any documented infected burn site, use an additional code for the infection.

5) Assign separate codes for each burn site

When coding burns, assign separate codes for each burn site. Category T30, Burn and corrosion, body region unspecified is extremely vague and should rarely be used.

6) Burns and Corrosions Classified According to Extent of Body Surface Involved

Assign codes from category T31, Burns classified according to extent of body surface involved, or T32, Corrosions classified according to extent of body surface involved, when the site of the burn is not specified or when there is a need for additional data. It is advisable to use category T31 as additional coding when needed to provide data for evaluating burn mortality, such as that needed by burn units. It is also advisable to use category T31 as an additional code for reporting purposes when there is mention of a third-degree burn involving 20 percent or more of the body surface.

Categories T31 and T32 are based on the classic "rule of nines" in estimating body surface involved: head and neck are assigned nine percent, each arm nine percent, each leg 18 percent, the anterior trunk 18 percent, posterior trunk 18 percent, and genitalia one percent. Providers may change these percentage assignments where necessary to accommodate infants and children who have proportionately larger heads than adults, and patients who have large buttocks, thighs, or abdomen that involve burns.

7) Encounters for treatment of sequela of burns

Encounters for the treatment of the late effects of burns or corrosions (i.e., scars or joint contractures) should be coded with a burn or corrosion code with the 7th character "S" for sequela.

8) Sequelae with a late effect code and current burn

When appropriate, both a code for a current burn or corrosion with 7th character "A" or "D" and a burn or corrosion code with 7th character "S" may be assigned on the same record (when both a current burn and sequelae of an old burn exist). Burns and corrosions do not heal at the same rate and a current healing wound may still exist with sequela of a healed burn or corrosion.

See Section I.B.10 Sequela (Late Effects)

9) Use of an external cause code with burns and corrosions

An external cause code should be used with burns and corrosions to identify the source and intent of the burn, as well as the place where it occurred.

e. Adverse Effects, Poisoning, Underdosing and Toxic Effects

Codes in categories T36-T65 are combination codes that include the substance that was taken as well as the intent. No additional external cause code is required for poisonings, toxic effects, adverse effects and underdosing codes.

1) Do not code directly from the Table of Drugs

Do not code directly from the Table of Drugs and Chemicals. Always refer back to the Tabular List.

2) Use as many codes as necessary to describe

Use as many codes as necessary to describe completely all drugs, medicinal or biological substances.

3) If the same code would describe the causative agent

If the same code would describe the causative agent for more than one adverse reaction, poisoning, toxic effect or underdosing, assign the code only once.

4) If two or more drugs, medicinal or biological substances

If two or more drugs, medicinal or biological substances are reported, code each individually unless a combination code is listed in the Table of Drugs and Chemicals.

5) The occurrence of drug toxicity is classified in ICD-10-CM as follows:

(a) Adverse Effect

When coding an adverse effect of a drug that has been correctly prescribed and properly administered, assign the appropriate code for the nature of the adverse effect followed by the appropriate code for the adverse effect of the drug (T36-T50). The code for the drug should have a 5th or 6th character "5" (for example T36.0X5-) Examples of the nature of an adverse effect are tachycardia, delirium, gastrointestinal hemorrhaging, vomiting, hypokalemia, hepatitis, renal failure, or respiratory failure.

(b) Poisoning

When coding a poisoning or reaction to the improper use of a medication (e.g., overdose, wrong substance given or taken in error, wrong route of administration), first assign the appropriate code from categories T36-T50. The poisoning codes have an associated intent as their 5th or 6th character (accidental, intentional self-harm, assault and undetermined.) If the intent of the poisoning is unknown or unspecified, code the intent as accidental intent. The undetermined intent is only for use if the documentation in the record specifies that the intent cannot be determined. Use additional code(s) for all manifestations of poisonings.

If there is also a diagnosis of abuse or dependence of the substance, the abuse or dependence is assigned as an additional code.

Examples of poisoning include:

(i) Error was made in drug prescription

Errors made in drug prescription or in the administration of the drug by provider, nurse, patient, or other person.

(ii) Overdose of a drug intentionally taken

If an overdose of a drug was intentionally taken or administered and resulted in drug toxicity, it would be coded as a poisoning.

(iii) Nonprescribed drug taken with correctly prescribed and properly administered drug

If a nonprescribed drug or medicinal agent was taken in combination with a correctly prescribed and properly administered drug, any drug toxicity or other reaction resulting from the interaction of the two drugs would be classified as a poisoning.

(iv) Interaction of drug(s) and alcohol

When a reaction results from the interaction of a drug(s) and alcohol, this would be classified as poisoning.

See Section I.C.4. if poisoning is the result of insulin pump malfunctions.

(c) Underdosing

Underdosing refers to taking less of a medication than is prescribed by a provider or a manufacturer's instruction. For underdosing, assign the code from categories T36-T50 (fifth or sixth character "6").

Codes for underdosing should never be assigned as principal or first-listed codes. If a patient has a relapse or exacerbation of the medical condition for which the drug is prescribed because of the reduction in dose, then the medical condition itself should be coded.

Noncompliance (Z91.12-, Z91.13-) or complication of care (Y63.6-Y63.9) codes are to be used with an underdosing code to indicate intent, if known.

(d) Toxic Effects

When a harmful substance is ingested or comes in contact with a person, this is classified as a toxic effect. The toxic effect codes are in categories T51-T65.

Toxic effect codes have an associated intent: accidental, intentional self-harm, assault and undetermined.

f. Adult and child abuse, neglect and other maltreatment

Sequence first the appropriate code from categories T74.- (Adult and child abuse, neglect and other maltreatment, confirmed) or T76.- (Adult and child abuse, neglect and other maltreatment, suspected) for abuse, neglect and other maltreatment, followed by any accompanying mental health or injury code(s).

If the documentation in the medical record states abuse or neglect it is coded as confirmed (T74.-). It is coded as suspected if it is documented as suspected (T76.-).

For cases of confirmed abuse or neglect an external cause code from the assault section (X92-Y09) should be added to identify the cause of any physical injuries. A perpetrator code (Y07) should be added when the perpetrator of the abuse is known. For suspected cases of abuse or neglect, do not report external cause or perpetrator code.

If a suspected case of abuse, neglect or mistreatment is ruled out during an encounter code Z04.71, Encounter for examination and observation following alleged physical adult abuse, ruled out, or code Z04.72, Encounter for examination and observation following alleged child physical abuse, ruled out, should be used, not a code from T76.

If a suspected case of alleged rape or sexual abuse is ruled out during an encounter code Z04.41, Encounter for examination and observation following alleged adult rape or code Z04.42, Encounter for examination and observation following alleged child rape, should be used, not a code from T76.

See Section I.C.15. Abuse in a pregnant patient.

g. Complications of care

1) General guidelines for complications of care

(a) Documentation of complications of care

See Section I.B.16. for information on documentation of complications of care.

2) Pain due to medical devices

Pain associated with devices, implants or grafts left in a surgical site (for example painful hip prosthesis) is assigned to the appropriate code(s) found in Chapter 19, Injury, poisoning, and certain other consequences of external causes. Specific codes for pain due to medical devices are found in the T code section of the ICD-10-CM. Use additional code(s) from category G89 to identify acute or chronic pain due to presence of the device, implant or graft (G89.18 or G89.28).

3) Transplant complications

(a) Transplant complications other than kidney

Codes under category T86, Complications of transplanted organs and tissues, are for use for both complications and rejection of transplanted organs. A transplant complication code is only assigned if the complication affects the function of the transplanted organ. Two codes are required to fully describe a transplant complication: the appropriate code from category T86 and a secondary code that identifies the complication.

Pre-existing conditions or conditions that develop after the transplant are not coded as complications unless they affect the function of the transplanted organs.

See I.C.21. for transplant organ removal status.

See I.C.2. for malignant neoplasm associated with transplanted organ.

(b) Kidney transplant complications

Patients who have undergone kidney transplant may still have some form of chronic kidney disease (CKD) because the kidney transplant may not fully restore kidney function. Code T86.1- should be assigned for documented complications of a kidney transplant, such as transplant failure or rejection or other transplant complication. Code T86.1- should not be assigned for post kidney transplant patients who have chronic kidney (CKD) unless a transplant complication such as transplant failure or rejection is documented. If the documentation is unclear as to whether the patient has a complication of the transplant, query the provider.

Conditions that affect the function of the transplanted kidney, other than CKD, should be assigned a code from subcategory T86.1, Complications of transplanted organ, Kidney, and a secondary code that identifies the complication.

For patients with CKD following a kidney transplant, but who do not have a complication such as failure or rejection, *see section I.C.14. Chronic kidney disease and kidney transplant status.*

4) Complication codes that include the external cause

As with certain other T codes, some of the complications of care codes have the external cause included in the code. The code includes the nature of the complication as well as the type of procedure that caused the complication. No external cause code indicating the type of procedure is necessary for these codes.

5) Complications of care codes within the body system chapters

Intraoperative and postprocedural complication codes are found within the body system chapters with codes specific to the organs and structures of that body system. These codes should be sequenced first, followed by a code(s) for the specific complication, if applicable.

20. Chapter 20: External Causes of Morbidity (V00-Y99)

The external causes of morbidity codes should never be sequenced as the first-listed or principal diagnosis.

External cause codes are intended to provide data for injury research and evaluation of injury prevention strategies. These codes capture how the injury or health condition happened (cause), the intent (unintentional or accidental; or intentional, such as suicide or assault), the place where the event occurred the activity of the patient at the time of the event, and the person's status (e.g., civilian, military).

There is no national requirement for mandatory ICD-10-CM external cause code reporting. Unless a provider is subject to a state-based external cause code reporting mandate or these codes are required by a particular payer, reporting of ICD-10-CM codes in Chapter 20, External Causes of Morbidity, is not required. In the absence of a mandatory reporting requirement, providers are encouraged to voluntarily report external cause codes, as they provide valuable data for injury research and evaluation of injury prevention strategies.

a. General External Cause Coding Guidelines

1) Used with any code in the range of A00.0-T88.9, Z00-Z99

An external cause code may be used with any code in the range of A00.0-T88.9, Z00-Z99, classification that **represents** a health condition due to an external cause. Though they are most applicable to injuries, they are also valid for use with such things as infections or diseases due to an external source, and other health conditions, such as a heart attack that occurs during strenuous physical activity.

2) External cause code used for length of treatment

Assign the external cause code, with the appropriate 7th character (initial encounter, subsequent encounter or sequela) for each encounter for which the injury or condition is being treated. Most categories in chapter 20 have a 7th character requirement for each applicable code.

Most categories in this chapter have three 7th character values: A, initial encounter, D, subsequent encounter and S, sequela. While the patient may be seen by a new or different provider over the course of treatment for an injury or condition, assignment of the 7th character for external cause should match the 7th character of the code assigned for the associated injury or condition for the encounter.

3) Use the full range of external cause codes

Use the full range of external cause codes to completely describe the cause, the intent, the place of occurrence, and if applicable, the activity of the patient at the time of the event, and the patient's status, for all injuries, and other health conditions due to an external cause.

4) Assign as many external cause codes as necessary

Assign as many external cause codes as necessary to fully explain each cause. If only one external code can be recorded, assign the code most related to the principal diagnosis.

5) The selection of the appropriate external cause code

The selection of the appropriate external cause code is guided by the Alphabetic Index of External Causes and by Inclusion and Exclusion notes in the Tabular List.

6) External cause code can never be a principal diagnosis

An external cause code can never be a principal (first-listed) diagnosis.

7) Combination external cause codes

Certain of the external cause codes are combination codes that identify sequential events that result in an injury, such as a fall which results in striking against an object. The injury may be due to either event or both. The combination external cause code used should correspond to the sequence of events regardless of which caused the most serious injury.

8) No external cause code needed in certain circumstances

No external cause code from Chapter 20 is needed if the external cause and intent are included in a code from another chapter (e.g. T36.0X1- Poisoning by penicillins, accidental (unintentional)).

b. Place of Occurrence Guideline

Codes from category Y92, Place of occurrence of the external cause, are secondary codes for use after other external cause codes to identify the location of the patient at the time of injury or other condition.

Generally, a place of occurrent code is assigned only once, at the initial encounter for treatment. However, in the rare instance that a new injury occurs during hospitalization, an additional place of occurrence code may be assigned. No 7th characters are used for Y92.

Do not use place of occurrence code Y92.9 if the place is not stated or is not applicable.

c. Activity Code

Assign a code from category Y93, Activity code, to describe the activity of the patient at the time the injury or other health condition occurred.

An activity code is used only once, at the initial encounter for treatment. Only one code from Y93 should be recorded on a medical record.

The activity codes are not applicable to poisonings, adverse effects, misadventures or sequela.

Do not assign Y93.9, Unspecified activity, if the activity is not stated.

A code from category Y93 is appropriate for use with external cause and intent codes if identifying the activity provides additional information about the event.

d. Place of Occurrence, Activity, and Status Codes Used with other External Cause Code

When applicable, place of occurrence, activity, and external cause status codes are sequenced after the main external cause code(s). Regardless of the number of external cause codes assigned, there should be only one place of occurrence code, one activity code, and one external cause status code assigned to an encounter. However, in the rare instance that a new injury occurs during hospitalization, an additional place of occurrence code may be assigned.

e. If the Reporting Format Limits the Number of External Cause Codes

If the reporting format limits the number of external cause codes that can be used in reporting clinical data, report the code for the cause/intent most related to the principal diagnosis. If the format permits capture of additional external cause codes, the cause/intent, including medical misadventures, of the additional events should be reported rather than the codes for place, activity, or external status.

f. Multiple External Cause Coding Guidelines

More than one external cause code is required to fully describe the external cause of an illness or injury. The assignment of external cause codes should be sequenced in the following priority:

If two or more events cause separate injuries, an external cause code should be assigned for each cause. The first-listed external cause code will be selected in the following order:

External codes for child and adult abuse take priority over all other external cause codes.

See Section I.C.19., Child and Adult abuse guidelines.

External cause codes for terrorism events take priority over all other external cause codes except child and adult abuse.

External cause codes for cataclysmic events take priority over all other external cause codes except child and adult abuse and terrorism.

External cause codes for transport accidents take priority over all other external cause codes except cataclysmic events, child and adult abuse and terrorism.

Activity and external cause status codes are assigned following all causal (intent) external cause codes.

The first-listed external cause code should correspond to the cause of the most serious diagnosis due to an assault, accident, or self-harm, following the order of hierarchy listed above.

g. Child and Adult Abuse Guideline

Adult and child abuse, neglect and maltreatment are classified as assault. Any of the assault codes may be used to indicate the external cause of any injury resulting from the confirmed abuse.

For confirmed cases of abuse, neglect and maltreatment, when the perpetrator is known, a code from Y07, Perpetrator of maltreatment and neglect, should accompany any other assault codes.

See Section I.C.19. Adult and child abuse, neglect and other maltreatment

h. Unknown or Undetermined Intent Guideline

If the intent (accident, self-harm, assault) of the cause of an injury or other condition is unknown or unspecified, code the intent as accidental intent. All transport accident categories assume accidental intent.

1) Use of undetermined intent

External cause codes for events of undetermined intent are only for use if the documentation in the record specifies that the intent cannot be determined.

i. Sequelae (Late Effects) of External Cause Guidelines

1) Sequelae external cause codes

Sequela are reported using the external cause code with the 7th character "S" for sequela. These codes should be used with any report of a late effect or sequela resulting from a previous injury.

See Section I.B.10 Sequela (Late Effects)

2) Sequela external cause code with a related current injury

A sequela external cause code should never be used with a related current nature of injury code.

3) Use of sequela external cause codes for subsequent visits

Use a late effect external cause code for subsequent visits when a late effect of the initial injury is being treated. Do not use a late effect external cause code for subsequent visits for follow- up care (e.g., to assess healing, to receive rehabilitative therapy) of the injury when no late effect of the injury has been documented.

j. Terrorism Guidelines

1) Cause of injury identified by the Federal Government (FBI) as terrorism

When the cause of an injury is identified by the Federal Government (FBI) as terrorism, the first-listed external cause code should be a code from category Y38, Terrorism. The definition of terrorism employed by the FBI is found at the inclusion note at the beginning of category Y38. Use additional code for place of occurrence (Y92.-). More than one Y38 code may be assigned if the injury is the result of more than one mechanism of terrorism.

2) Cause of an injury is suspected to be the result of terrorism

When the cause of an injury is suspected to be the result of terrorism a code from category Y38 should not be assigned. Suspected cases should be classified as assault.

3) Code Y38.9, Terrorism, secondary effects

Assign code Y38.9, Terrorism, secondary effects, for conditions occurring subsequent to the terrorist event. This code should not be assigned for conditions that are due to the initial terrorist act.

It is acceptable to assign code Y38.9 with another code from Y38 if there is an injury due to the initial terrorist event and an injury that is a subsequent result of the terrorist event.

k. External cause status

A code from category Y99, External cause status, should be assigned whenever any other external cause code is assigned for an encounter, including an Activity code, except for the events noted below. Assign a code from category Y99, External cause status, to indicate the work status of the person at the time the event occurred. The status code indicates whether the event occurred during military activity, whether a non-military person was at work, whether an individual including a student or volunteer was involved in a non-work activity at the time of the causal event.

A code from Y99, External cause status, should be assigned, when applicable, with other external cause codes, such as transport accidents and falls. The external cause status codes are not applicable to poisonings, adverse effects, misadventures or late effects. Do not assign a code from category Y99 if no other external cause codes (cause, activity) are applicable for the encounter.

An external cause status code is used only once, at the initial encounter for treatment. Only one code from Y99 should be recorded on a medical record.

Do not assign code Y99.9, Unspecified external cause status, if the status is not stated.

21. Chapter 21: Factors Influencing Health Status and Contact with Health Services (Z00-Z99)

NOTE The chapter specific guidelines provide additional information about the use of Z codes for specified encounters.

a. Use of Z codes in any healthcare setting

Z codes are for use in any healthcare setting. Z codes may be used as either a first-listed (principal diagnosis code in the inpatient setting) or secondary code, depending on the circumstances of the encounter. Certain Z codes may only be used as first-listed or principal diagnosis.

b. Z Codes indicate a reason for an encounter

Z codes are not procedure codes. A corresponding procedure code must accompany a Z code to describe any procedure performed.

c. Categories of Z Codes

1) Contact/Exposure

Category Z20 indicates contact with, and suspected exposure to, communicable diseases. These codes are for patients who do not show any sign or symptom of a disease but are suspected to have been exposed to it by close personal contact with an infected individual or are in an area where a disease is epidemic.

Category Z77, Other contact with and (suspected) exposures hazardous to health, indicates contact with and suspected exposures hazardous to health.

Contact/exposure codes may be used as a first-listed code to explain an encounter for testing, or, more commonly, as a secondary code to identify a potential risk.

2) Inoculations and vaccinations

Code Z23 is for encounters for inoculations and vaccinations. It indicates that a patient is being seen to receive a prophylactic inoculation against a disease. Procedure codes are required to identify the actual administration of the injection and the type(s) of immunizations given. Code Z23 may be used as a secondary code if the inoculation is given as a routine part of preventive health care, such as a well-baby visit.

3) Status

Status codes indicate that a patient is either a carrier of a disease or has the sequelae or residual of a past disease or condition. This includes such things as the presence of prosthetic or mechanical devices resulting from past treatment. A status code is informative, because the status may affect the course of treatment and its outcome. A status code is distinct from a history code. The history code indicates that the patient no longer has the condition.

A status code should not be used with a diagnosis code from one of the body system chapters, if the diagnosis code includes the information provided by the status code. For example, code Z94.1, Heart transplant status, should not be used with a code from subcategory T86.2, Complications of heart transplant. The status code does not provide additional information. The complication code indicates that the patient is a heart transplant patient.

For encounters for weaning from a mechanical ventilator, assign a code from subcategory J96.1, Chronic respiratory failure, followed by code Z99.11, Dependence on respirator [ventilator] status.

The status Z codes/categories are:

Z14 Genetic carrier

Genetic carrier status indicates that a person carries a gene, associated with a particular disease, which may be passed to offspring who may develop that disease. The person does not have the disease and is not at risk of developing the disease.

Z15 Genetic susceptibility to disease

Genetic susceptibility indicates that a person has a gene that increases the risk of that person developing the disease.

Codes from category Z15 should not be used as principal or first-listed codes. If the patient has the condition to which he/she is susceptible, and that condition is the reason for the encounter, the code for the current condition should be sequenced first. If the patient is being seen for follow-up after completed treatment for this condition, and the condition no longer exists, a follow-up code should be sequenced first, followed by the appropriate personal history and genetic susceptibility codes. If the purpose of the encounter is genetic counseling associated with procreative management, code Z31.5, Encounter for genetic counseling, should be assigned as the first-listed code, followed by a code from category Z15. Additional codes should be assigned for any applicable family or personal history.

Z16 Resistance to antimicrobial drugs

This code indicates that a patient has a condition that is resistant to antimicrobial drug treatment. Sequence the infection code first.

Z17 Estrogen receptor status

Z18 Retained foreign body fragments

Z19 Hormone sensitivity malignancy status

Z21 Asymptomatic HIV infection status

This code indicates that a patient has tested positive for HIV but has manifested no signs or symptoms of the disease.

Z22 Carrier of infectious disease

Carrier status indicates that a person harbors the specific organisms of a disease without manifest symptoms and is capable of transmitting the infection.

Z28.3 Underimmunization status

Z33.1 Pregnant state, incidental

This code is a secondary code only for use when the pregnancy is in no way complicating the reason for visit. Otherwise, a code from the obstetric chapter is required.

Z66 Do not resuscitate

This code may be used when it is documented by the provider that a patient is on do not resuscitate status at any time during the stay.

Z67 Blood type

Z68 Body mass index (BMI)

As with all other secondary diagnosis codes, the BMI codes should only be assigned when they meet the definition of a reportable diagnosis (see Section III, Reporting Additional Diagnoses).

Z74.01 Bed confinement status

Z76.82 Awaiting organ transplant status

Z78 Other specified health status

Code Z78.1, Physical restraint status, may be used when it is documented by the provider that a patient has been put in restraints during the current encounter. Please note that this code should not be reported when it is documented by the provider that a patient is temporarily restrained during a procedure.

Z79 Long-term (current) drug therapy

Codes from this category indicate a patient's continuous use of a prescribed drug (including such things as aspirin therapy) for the long-term treatment of a condition or for prophylactic use. It is not for use for patients who have addictions to drugs. This subcategory is not for use of medications for detoxification or maintenance programs to prevent withdrawal symptoms in patients with drug dependence (e.g., methadone maintenance for opiate dependence). Assign the appropriate code for the drug dependence instead.

Assign a code from Z79 if the patient is receiving a medication for an extended period as a prophylactic measure (such as for the prevention of deep vein thrombosis) or as treatment of a chronic condition (such as arthritis) or a disease requiring a lengthy course of treatment (such as cancer). Do not assign a code from category Z79 for medication being administered for a brief period of time to treat an acute illness or injury (such as a course of antibiotics to treat acute bronchitis).

Z88 Allergy status to drugs, medicaments and biological substances

Except: Z88.9, Allergy status to unspecified drugs, medicaments and biological substances status

Z89 Acquired absence of limb

Z90 Acquired absence of organs, not elsewhere classified

Z91.0- Allergy status, other than to drugs and biological substances

Z92.82 Status post administration of tPA (rtPA) in a different facility within the last 24 hours prior to admission to a current facility

Assign code Z92.82, Status post administration of tPA (rtPA) in a different facility within the last 24 hours prior to admission to current facility, as a secondary diagnosis when a patient is received by transfer into a facility and documentation indicates they were administered tissue plasminogen activator (tPA) within the last 24 hours prior to admission to the current facility.

This guideline applies even if the patient is still receiving the tPA at the time they are received into the current facility.

The appropriate code for the condition for which the tPA was administered (such as cerebrovascular disease or myocardial infarction) should be assigned first.

Code Z92.82 is only applicable to the receiving facility record and not to the transferring facility record.

Z93 Artificial opening status

Z94 Transplanted organ and tissue status

Z95 Presence of cardiac and vascular implants and grafts

Z96 Presence of other functional implants

Z97 Presence of other devices

Z98 Other postprocedural states

Assign code Z98.85, Transplanted organ removal status, to indicate that a transplanted organ has been previously removed. This code should not be assigned for the encounter in which the transplanted organ is removed. The complication necessitating removal of the transplant organ should be assigned for that encounter.

See section I.C19. for information on the coding of organ transplant complications.

Z99 Dependence on enabling machines and devices, not elsewhere classified

NOTE Categories Z89-Z90 and Z93-Z99 are for use only if there are no complications or malfunctions of the organ or tissue replaced, the amputation site or the equipment on which the patient is dependent.

4) History (of)

There are two types of history Z codes, personal and family. Personal history codes explain a patient's past medical condition that no longer exists and is not receiving any treatment, but that has the potential for recurrence, and therefore may require continued monitoring.

Family history codes are for use when a patient has a family member(s) who has had a particular disease that causes the patient to be at higher risk of also contracting the disease.

Personal history codes may be used in conjunction with follow- up codes and family history codes may be used in conjunction with screening codes to explain the need for a test or procedure. History codes are also acceptable on any medical record regardless of the reason for visit. A history of an illness, even if no longer present, is important information that may alter the type of treatment ordered.

The history Z code categories are:

Z80 Family history of primary malignant neoplasm

Z81 Family history of mental and behavioral disorders

Z82 Family history of certain disabilities and chronic diseases (leading to disablement)

Z83 Family history of other specific disorders

Z84 Family history of other conditions

Z85 Personal history of malignant neoplasm

Z86 Personal history of certain other diseases

Z87 Personal history of other diseases and conditions

Z91.4- Personal history of psychological trauma, not elsewhere classified

Z91.5 Personal history of self-harm

Z91.81 History of falling

Z91.82 Personal history of military deployment

Z92 Personal history of medical treatment

Except: Z92.0, Personal history of contraception Except: Z92.82, Status post administration of tPA (rtPA) in a different facility within the last 24 hours prior to admission to a current facility

5) Screening

Screening is the testing for disease or disease precursors in seemingly well individuals so that early detection and treatment can be provided for those who test positive for the disease (e.g., screening mammogram).

The testing of a person to rule out or confirm a suspected diagnosis because the patient has some sign or symptom is a diagnostic examination, not a screening. In these cases, the sign or symptom is used to explain the reason for the test.

A screening code may be a first-listed code if the reason for the visit is specifically the screening exam. It may also be used as an additional code if the screening is done during an office visit for other health problems. A screening code is not necessary if the screening is inherent to a routine examination, such as a pap smear done during a routine pelvic examination.

Should a condition be discovered during the screening then the code for the condition may be assigned as an additional diagnosis.

The Z code indicates that a screening exam is planned. A procedure code is required to confirm that the screening was performed.

The screening Z codes/categories:

Z11 Encounter for screening for infectious and parasitic diseases

Z12 Encounter for screening for malignant neoplasms

Z13 Encounter for screening for other diseases and disorders

Except: Z13.9, Encounter for screening, unspecified

Z36 Encounter for antenatal screening for mother

6) **Observation**

There are three observation Z code categories. They are for use in very limited circumstances when a person is being observed for a suspected condition that is ruled out. The observation codes are not for use if an injury or illness or any signs or symptoms related to the suspected condition are present. In such cases the diagnosis/symptom code is used with the corresponding external cause code.

The observation codes are to be used as principal diagnosis only. The only exception to this is when the principal diagnosis is required to be a code from category Z38, Liveborn infants according to place of birth and type of delivery. Then a code form category Z05, Encounter for observation and evaluation of newborn for suspected diseases and conditions ruled out, is sequenced after the Z38 code. Additional codes may be used in addition to the observation code but only if they are unrelated to the suspected condition being observed.

Codes from subcategory Z03.7, Encounter for suspected maternal and fetal conditions ruled out, may either be used as a first-listed or as an additional code assignment depending on the case. They are for use in very limited circumstances on a maternal record when an encounter is for a suspected maternal or fetal condition that is ruled out during that encounter (for example, a maternal or fetal condition may be suspected due to an abnormal test result). These codes should not be used when the condition is confirmed. In those cases, the confirmed condition should be coded. In addition, these codes are not for use if an illness or any signs or symptoms related to the suspected condition or problem are present. In such cases the diagnosis/symptom code is used.

Additional codes may be used in addition to the code from subcategory Z03.7, but only if they are unrelated to the suspected condition being evaluated.

Codes from subcategory Z03.7 may not be used for encounters for antenatal screening of mother. *See Section I.C.21. Screening.*

For encounters for suspected fetal condition that are inconclusive following testing and evaluation, assign the appropriate code from category O35, O36, O40 or O41.

The observation Z code categories:

Z03	Encounter for medical observation for suspected diseases and conditions ruled out
Z04	Encounter for examination and observation for other reasons
	Except: Z04.9, Encounter for examination and observation for unspecified reason
Z05	Encounter for observation and evaluation of newborn for suspected diseases and conditions ruled out

7) **Aftercare**

Aftercare visit codes cover situations when the initial treatment of a disease has been performed and the patient requires continued care during the healing or recovery phase, or for the long-term consequences of the disease. The aftercare Z code should not be used if treatment is directed at a current, acute disease. The diagnosis code is to be used in these cases. Exceptions to this rule are codes Z51.0, Encounter for antineoplastic radiation therapy, and codes from subcategory Z51.1, Encounter for antineoplastic chemotherapy and immunotherapy. These codes are to be first-listed, followed by the diagnosis code when a patient's encounter is solely to receive radiation therapy, chemotherapy, or immunotherapy for the treatment of a neoplasm. If the reason for the encounter is more than one type of antineoplastic therapy, code Z51.0 and a code from subcategory Z51.1 may be assigned together, in which case one of these codes would be reported as a secondary diagnosis.

The aftercare Z codes should also not be used for aftercare for injuries. For aftercare of an injury, assign the acute injury code with the appropriate 7th character (for subsequent encounter).

The aftercare codes are generally first-listed to explain the specific reason for the encounter. An aftercare code may be used as an additional code when some type of aftercare is provided in addition to the reason for admission and no diagnosis code is applicable. An example of this would be the closure of a colostomy during an encounter for treatment of another condition.

Aftercare codes should be used in conjunction with other aftercare codes or diagnosis codes to provide better detail on the specifics of an aftercare encounter visit, unless otherwise directed by the classification. Should a patient receive multiple types of antineoplastic therapy during the same encounter, code Z51.0, Encounter for antineoplastic radiation therapy, and codes from subcategory Z51.1, Encounter for antineoplastic chemotherapy and immunotherapy, may be used together on a record. The sequencing of multiple aftercare codes depends on the circumstances of the encounter.

Certain aftercare Z code categories need a secondary diagnosis code to describe the resolving condition or sequelae. For others, the condition is included in the code title.

Additional Z code aftercare category terms include fitting and adjustment, and attention to artificial openings.

Status Z codes may be used with aftercare Z codes to indicate the nature of the aftercare. For example code Z95.1, Presence of aortocoronary bypass graft, may be used with code Z48.812, Encounter for surgical aftercare following surgery on the circulatory system, to indicate the surgery for which the aftercare is being performed. A status code should not be used when the aftercare code indicates the type of status, such as using Z43.0, Encounter for attention to tracheostomy, with Z93.0, Tracheostomy status.

The aftercare Z category/codes:

Z42	Encounter for plastic and reconstructive surgery following medical procedure or healed injury
Z43	Encounter for attention to artificial openings
Z44	Encounter for fitting and adjustment of external prosthetic device
Z45	Encounter for adjustment and management of implanted device
Z46	Encounter for fitting and adjustment of other devices
Z47	Orthopedic aftercare
Z48	Encounter for other postprocedural aftercare
Z49	Encounter for care involving renal dialysis
Z51	Encounter for other aftercare and medical care

8) Follow-up

The follow-up codes are used to explain continuing surveillance following completed treatment of a disease, condition, or injury. They imply that the condition has been fully treated and no longer exists. They should not be confused with aftercare codes, or injury codes with a 7th character for subsequent encounter, that explain ongoing care of a healing condition or its sequelae. Follow-up codes may be used in conjunction with history codes to provide the full picture of the healed condition and its treatment. The follow-up code is sequenced first, followed by the history code.

A follow-up code may be used to explain multiple visits. Should a condition be found to have recurred on the follow-up visit, then the diagnosis code for the condition should be assigned in place of the follow-up code.

The follow-up Z code categories:

Z08	Encounter for follow-up examination after completed treatment for malignant neoplasm
Z09	Encounter for follow-up examination after completed treatment for conditions other than malignant neoplasm
Z39	Encounter for maternal postpartum care and examination

9) Donor

Codes in category Z52, Donors of organs and tissues, are used for living individuals who are donating blood or other body tissue. These codes are only for individuals donating for others, not for self-donations. They are not used to identify cadaveric donations.

10) Counseling

Counseling Z codes are used when a patient or family member receives assistance in the aftermath of an illness or injury, or when support is required in coping with family or social problems.

The counseling Z codes/categories:

Z30.0-	Encounter for general counseling and advice on contraception
Z31.5	Encounter for **procreative** genetic counseling
Z31.6-	Encounter for general counseling and advice on procreation
Z32.2	Encounter for childbirth instruction
Z32.3	Encounter for childcare instruction
Z69	Encounter for mental health services for victim and perpetrator of abuse
Z70	Counseling related to sexual attitude, behavior and orientation
Z71	Persons encountering health services for other counseling and medical advice, not elsewhere classified
Z76.81	Expectant mother prebirth pediatrician visit

11) Encounters for Obstetrical and Reproductive Services

See Section I.C.15. Pregnancy, Childbirth, and the Puerperium, for further instruction on the use of these codes.

Z codes for pregnancy are for use in those circumstances when none of the problems or complications included in the codes from the Obstetrics chapter exist (a routine prenatal visit or postpartum care). Codes in category Z34, Encounter for supervision of normal pregnancy, are always first-listed and are not to be used with any other code from the OB chapter.

Codes in category Z3A, Weeks of gestation, may be assigned to provide additional information about the pregnancy. Category Z3A codes should not be assigned for pregnancies with abortive outcomes (categories O00-O08), elective termination of pregnancy (code **Z33.2**), nor for postpartum conditions, as category Z3A is not applicable to these conditions. The date of the admission should be used to determine weeks of gestation for inpatient admissions that encompass more than one gestational week.

The outcome of delivery, category Z37, should be included on all maternal delivery records. It is always a secondary code. Codes in category Z37 should not be used on the newborn record.

Z codes for family planning (contraceptive) or procreative management and counseling should be included on an obstetric record either during the pregnancy or the postpartum stage, if applicable.

Z codes/categories for obstetrical and reproductive services:

Z30	Encounter for contraceptive management
Z31	Encounter for procreative management
Z32.2	Encounter for childbirth instruction
Z32.3	Encounter for childcare instruction
Z33	Pregnant state
Z34	Encounter for supervision of normal pregnancy
Z36	Encounter for antenatal screening of mother
Z3A	Weeks of gestation
Z37	Outcome of delivery
Z39	Encounter for maternal postpartum care and examination
Z76.81	Expectant mother prebirth pediatrician visit

12) Newborns and Infants

See Section I.C.16. Newborn (Perinatal) Guidelines, for further instruction on the use of these codes.

Newborn Z codes/categories:

Z76.1	Encounter for health supervision and care of foundling
Z00.1-	Encounter for routine child health examination
Z38	Liveborn infants according to place of birth and type of delivery

13) Routine and administrative examinations

The Z codes allow for the description of encounters for routine examinations, such as, a general check-up, or, examinations for administrative purposes, such as, a pre-employment physical. The codes are not to be used if the examination is for diagnosis of a suspected condition or for treatment purposes. In such cases the diagnosis code is used. During a routine exam, should a diagnosis or condition be discovered, it should be coded as an additional code. Pre-existing and chronic conditions and history codes may also be included as additional codes as long as the examination is for administrative purposes and not focused on any particular condition.

Some of the codes for routine health examinations distinguish between "with" and "without" abnormal findings. Code assignment depends on the information that is known at the time the encounter is being coded. For example, if no abnormal findings were found during the examination, but the encounter is being coded before test results are back, it is acceptable to assign the code for "without abnormal findings." When assigning a code for "with abnormal findings," additional code(s) should be assigned to identify the specific abnormal finding(s).

Pre-operative examination and pre-procedural laboratory examination Z codes are for use only in those situations when a patient is being cleared for a procedure or surgery and no treatment is given.

The Z codes/categories for routine and administrative examinations:

Z00	Encounter for general examination without complaint, suspected or reported diagnosis
Z01	Encounter for other special examination without complaint, suspected or reported diagnosis
Z02	Encounter for administrative examination
	Except: Z02.9, Encounter for administrative examinations, unspecified
Z32.0-	Encounter for pregnancy test

14) Miscellaneous Z codes

The miscellaneous Z codes capture a number of other health care encounters that do not fall into one of the other categories. Certain of these codes identify the reason for the encounter; others are for use as additional codes that provide useful information on circumstances that may affect a patient's care and treatment.

Prophylactic Organ Removal

For encounters specifically for prophylactic removal of an organ (such as prophylactic removal of breasts due to a genetic susceptibility to cancer or a family history of cancer), the principal or first-listed code should be a code from category Z40, Encounter for prophylactic surgery, followed by the appropriate codes to identify the associated risk factor (such as genetic susceptibility or family history).

If the patient has a malignancy of one site and is having prophylactic removal at another site to prevent either a new primary malignancy or metastatic disease, a code for the malignancy should also be assigned in addition to a code from subcategory Z40.0, Encounter for prophylactic surgery for risk factors related to malignant neoplasms. A Z40.0 code should not be assigned if the patient is having organ removal for treatment of a malignancy, such as the removal of the testes for the treatment of prostate cancer.

Miscellaneous Z codes/categories:

Z28	Immunization not carried out
	Except: Z28.3, Underimmunization status
Z29	Encounter for other prophylactic measures
Z40	Encounter for prophylactic surgery
Z41	Encounter for procedures for purposes other than remedying health state
	Except: Z41.9, Encounter for procedure for purposes other than remedying health state, unspecified
Z53	Persons encountering health services for specific procedures and treatment, not carried out
Z55	Problems related to education and literacy
Z56	Problems related to employment and unemployment
Z57	Occupational exposure to risk factors
Z58	Problems related to physical environment
Z59	Problems related to housing and economic circumstances
Z60	Problems related to social environment
Z62	Problems related to upbringing
Z63	Other problems related to primary support group, including family circumstances
Z64	Problems related to certain psychosocial circumstances
Z65	Problems related to other psychosocial circumstances
Z72	Problems related to lifestyle
	Note: These codes should be assigned only when the documentation specifies that the patient has an associated problem.
Z73	Problems related to life management difficulty
Z74	Problems related to care provider dependency
	Except: Z74.01, Bed confinement status
Z75	Problems related to medical facilities and other health care
Z76.0	Encounter for issue of repeat prescription
Z76.3	Healthy person accompanying sick person
Z76.4	Other boarder to healthcare facility
Z76.5	Malingerer [conscious simulation]
Z91.1-	Patient's noncompliance with medical treatment and regimen
Z91.83	Wandering in diseases classified elsewhere
Z91.84-	**Oral health risk factors**
Z91.89	Other specified personal risk factors, not elsewhere classified

15) Nonspecific Z codes

Certain Z codes are so non-specific, or potentially redundant with other codes in the classification, that there can be little justification for their use in the inpatient setting. Their use in the outpatient setting should be limited to those instances when there is no further documentation to permit more precise coding. Otherwise, any sign or symptom or any other reason for visit that is captured in another code should be used.

Nonspecific Z codes/categories:

Z02.9	Encounter for administrative examinations, unspecified
Z04.9	Encounter for examination and observation for unspecified reason

Z13.9	Encounter for screening, unspecified
Z41.9	Encounter for procedure for purposes other than remedying health state, unspecified
Z52.9	Donor of unspecified organ or tissue
Z86.59	Personal history of other mental and behavioral disorders
Z88.9	Allergy status to unspecified drugs, medicaments and biological substances status
Z92.0	Personal history of contraception

16) Z Codes That May Only be Principal/First-Listed Diagnosis

The following Z codes/categories may only be reported as the principal/first-listed diagnosis, except when there are multiple encounters on the same day and the medical records for the encounters are combined:

Z00	Encounter for general examination without complaint, suspected or reported diagnosis Except: Z00.6
Z01	Encounter for other special examination without complaint, suspected or reported diagnosis
Z02	Encounter for administrative examination
Z03	Encounter for medical observation for suspected diseases and conditions ruled out
Z04	Encounter for examination and observation for other reasons
Z33.2	Encounter for elective termination of pregnancy
Z31.81	Encounter for male factor infertility in female patient
Z31.83	Encounter for assisted reproductive fertility procedure cycle
Z31.84	Encounter for fertility preservation procedure
Z34	Encounter for supervision of normal pregnancy
Z39	Encounter for maternal postpartum care and examination
Z38	Liveborn infants according to place of birth and type of delivery
Z40	**Encounter for prophylactic surgery**
Z42	Encounter for plastic and reconstructive surgery following medical procedure or healed injury
Z51.0	Encounter for antineoplastic radiation therapy
Z51.1-	Encounter for antineoplastic chemotherapy and immunotherapy
Z52	Donors of organs and tissues Except: Z52.9, Donor of unspecified organ or tissue
Z76.1	Encounter for health supervision and care of foundling
Z76.2	Encounter for health supervision and care of other healthy infant and child
Z99.12	Encounter for respirator [ventilator] dependence during power failure

Section II. Selection of Principal Diagnosis

The circumstances of inpatient admission always govern the selection of principal diagnosis. The principal diagnosis is defined in the Uniform Hospital Discharge Data Set (UHDDS) as "that condition established after study to be chiefly responsible for occasioning the admission of the patient to the hospital for care."

The UHDDS definitions are used by hospitals to report inpatient data elements in a standardized manner. These data elements and their definitions can be found in the July 31, 1985, Federal Register (Vol. 50, No, 147), pp. 31038–40.

Since that time the application of the UHDDS definitions has been expanded to include all non-outpatient settings (acute care, short term, long term care and psychiatric hospitals; home health agencies; rehab facilities; nursing homes, etc). The UHDDS definitions also apply to hospice services (all levels of care).

In determining principal diagnosis, coding conventions in the ICD-10-CM, the Tabular List and Alphabetic Index take precedence over these official coding guidelines.

(See Section I.A., Conventions for the ICD-10-CM)

The importance of consistent, complete documentation in the medical record cannot be overemphasized. Without such documentation the application of all coding guidelines is a difficult, if not impossible, task.

A. Codes for Symptoms, Signs, and Ill-Defined Conditions

Codes for symptoms, signs, and ill-defined conditions from Chapter 18 are not to be used as principal diagnosis when a related definitive diagnosis has been established.

B. Two or More Interrelated Conditions, Each Potentially Meeting the Definition for Principal Diagnosis

When there are two or more interrelated conditions (such as diseases in the same ICD-10-CM chapter or manifestations characteristically associated with a certain disease) potentially meeting the definition of principal diagnosis, either condition may be sequenced first, unless the circumstances of the admission, the therapy provided, the Tabular List, or the Alphabetic Index indicate otherwise.

C. Two or More Diagnoses that Equally Meet the Definition for Principal Diagnosis

In the unusual instance when two or more diagnoses equally meet the criteria for principal diagnosis as determined by the circumstances of admission, diagnostic workup and/or therapy provided, and the Alphabetic Index, Tabular List, or another coding guidelines does not provide sequencing direction, any one of the diagnoses may be sequenced first.

D. Two or More Comparative or Contrasting Conditions

In those rare instances when two or more contrasting or comparative diagnoses are documented as "either/or" (or similar terminology), they are coded as if the diagnoses were confirmed and the diagnoses are sequenced according to the circumstances of the admission. If no further determination can be made as to which diagnosis should be principal, either diagnosis may be sequenced first.

E. A Symptom(s) Followed by Contrasting/Comparative Diagnoses

GUIDELINE HAS BEEN DELETED EFFECTIVE OCTOBER 1, 2014.

F. Original Treatment Plan not Carried out

Sequence as the principal diagnosis the condition, which after study occasioned the admission to the hospital, even though treatment may not have been carried out due to unforeseen circumstances.

G. Complications of Surgery and Other Medical Care

When the admission is for treatment of a complication resulting from surgery or other medical care, the complication code is sequenced as the principal diagnosis. If the complication is classified to the T80–T88 series and the code lacks the necessary specificity in describing the complication, an additional code for the specific complication should be assigned.

H. Uncertain Diagnosis

If the diagnosis documented at the time of discharge is qualified as "probable", "suspected", "likely", "questionable", "possible", or "still to be ruled out", or other similar terms indicating uncertainty, code the condition as if it existed or was established. The bases for these guidelines are the diagnostic workup, arrangements for further workup or observation, and initial therapeutic approach that correspond most closely with the established diagnosis.

Note: This guideline is applicable only to inpatient admissions to short-term, acute, long-term care and psychiatric hospitals.

I. Admission from Observation Unit

1. Admission Following Medical Observation

When a patient is admitted to an observation unit for a medical condition, which either worsens or does not improve, and is subsequently admitted as an inpatient of the same hospital for this same medical condition, the principal diagnosis would be the medical condition which led to the hospital admission.

2. Admission Following Post-Operative Observation

When a patient is admitted to an observation unit to monitor a condition (or complication) that develops following outpatient surgery, and then is subsequently admitted as an inpatient of the same hospital, hospitals should apply the Uniform Hospital Discharge Data Set (UHDDS) definition of principal diagnosis as "that condition established after study to be chiefly responsible for occasioning the admission of the patient to the hospital for care."

J. Admission from Outpatient Surgery

When a patient receives surgery in the hospital's outpatient surgery department and is subsequently admitted for continuing inpatient care at the same hospital, the following guidelines should be followed in selecting the principal diagnosis for the inpatient admission:

- If the reason for the inpatient admission is a complication, assign the complication as the principal diagnosis.
- If no complication, or other condition, is documented as the reason for the inpatient admission, assign the reason for the outpatient surgery as the principal diagnosis.
- If the reason for the inpatient admission is another condition unrelated to the surgery, assign the unrelated condition as the principal diagnosis.

K. Admissions/Encounters for Rehabilitation

When the purpose for the admission/encounter is rehabilitation, sequence first the code for the condition for which the service is being performed. For example, for an admission/encounter for rehabilitation for rightsided dominant hemiplegia following a cerebrovascular infarction, report code I69.351, Hemiplegia and hemiparesis following cerebral infarction affecting right dominant side, as the first-listed or principal diagnosis.

If the condition for which the rehabilitation service **is being provided** is no longer present, report the appropriate aftercare code **as the first-listed or principal diagnosis, unless the rehabilitation service is being provided following an injury. For rehabilitation services following active treatment of an injury, assign the injury code with the appropriate seventh character for subsequent encounter** as the first-listed or principal diagnosis. For example, if a patient with severe degenerative osteoarthritis of the hip, underwent hip replacement and the current encounter/admission is for rehabilitation, report code Z47.1, Aftercare following joint replacement surgery, as the first-listed or principal diagnosis. **If the patient requires rehabilitation post hip replacement for right intertrochanteric femur fracture, report code S72.141D, Displaced intertrochanteric fracture of right femur, subsequent encounter for closed fracture with routine healing, as the first-listed or principal diagnosis.**

See Section I.C.21.c.7, Factors influencing health states and contact with health services, Aftercare.
See Section I.C.19.a for additional information about the use of 7th characters for injury codes.

Section III. Reporting Additional Diagnoses

GENERAL RULES FOR OTHER (ADDITIONAL) DIAGNOSES

For reporting purposes the definition for "other diagnoses" is interpreted as additional conditions that affect patient care in terms of requiring:

- clinical evaluation; or
- therapeutic treatment; or
- diagnostic procedures; or
- extended length of hospital stay; or
- increased nursing care and/or
- monitoring

The UHDDS item #11-b defines Other Diagnoses as "all conditions that coexist at the time of admission, that develop subsequently, or that affect the treatment received and/or the length of stay. Diagnoses that relate to an earlier episode which have no bearing on the current hospital stay are to be excluded." UHDDS definitions apply to inpatients in acute-care, short-term, long term care and psychiatric hospital setting. The UHDDS definitions are used by acute-care shortterm hospitals to report inpatient data elements in a standardized manner. These data elements and their definitions can be found in the July 31, 1985, *Federal Register* (Vol. 50, No, 147), pp. 31038–40.

Since that time the application of the UHDDS definitions has been expanded to include all nonoutpatient settings (acute-care, short-term, long-term care and psychiatric hospitals; home health agencies; rehab facilities; nursing homes, etc). The UHDDS definitions also apply to hospice services (all levels of care).

The following guidelines are to be applied in designating "other diagnoses" when neither the Alphabetic Index nor the Tabular List in ICD-10-CM provide direction. The listing of the diagnoses in the patient record is the responsibility of the attending provider.

A. Previous Conditions

If the provider has included a diagnosis in the final diagnostic statement, such as the discharge summary or the face sheet, it should ordinarily be coded. Some providers include in the diagnostic statement resolved conditions or diagnoses and status-post procedures from previous admission that have no bearing on the current stay. Such conditions are not to be reported and are coded only if required by hospital policy.

However, history codes (categories Z80–Z87) may be used as secondary codes if the historical condition or family history has an impact on current care or influences treatment.

B. Abnormal Findings

Abnormal findings (laboratory, x-ray, pathologic, and other diagnostic results) are not coded and reported unless the provider indicates their clinical significance. If the findings are outside the normal range and the attending provider has ordered other tests to evaluate the condition or prescribed treatment, it is appropriate to ask the provider whether the abnormal finding should be added.

Note: This differs from the coding practices in the outpatient setting for coding encounters for diagnostic tests that have been interpreted by a provider.

C. Uncertain Diagnosis

If the diagnosis documented at the time of discharge is qualified as "probable", "suspected", "likely", "questionable", "possible", or "still to be ruled out" or other similar terms indicating uncertainty, code the condition as if it existed or was established. The bases for these guidelines are the diagnostic workup, arrangements for further workup or observation, and initial therapeutic approach that correspond most closely with the established diagnosis.

Note: This guideline is applicable only to inpatient admissions to short-term, acute-care, long-term care and psychiatric hospitals.

Section IV. Diagnostic Coding and Reporting Guidelines for Outpatient Services

These coding guidelines for outpatient diagnoses have been approved for use by hospitals/ providers in coding and reporting hospital-based outpatient services and provider-based office visits. Guidelines in Section I, Conventions, general coding guidelines and chapter-specific guidelines, should also be applied for outpatient services and office visits.

Information about the use of certain abbreviations, punctuation, symbols, and other conventions used in the ICD-10-CM Tabular List (code numbers and titles), can be found in Section IA of these guidelines, under "Conventions Used in the Tabular List." Section I.B. contains general guidelines that apply to the entire classification. Section I.C. contains chapter-specific guidelines that correspond to the chapters as they are arranged in the classification. Information about the correct sequence to use in finding a code is also described in Section I.

The terms encounter and visit are often used interchangeably in describing outpatient service contacts and, therefore, appear together in these guidelines without distinguishing one from the other.

Though the conventions and general guidelines apply to all settings, coding guidelines for outpatient and provider reporting of diagnoses will vary in a number of instances from those for inpatient diagnoses, recognizing that:

The Uniform Hospital Discharge Data Set (UHDDS) definition of principal diagnosis does not apply to hospital-based outpatient services and provider-based office visits.

Coding guidelines for inconclusive diagnoses (probable, suspected, rule out, etc.) were developed for inpatient reporting and do not apply to outpatients.

A. Selection of First-Listed Condition

In the outpatient setting, the term first-listed diagnosis is used in lieu of principal diagnosis.

In determining the first-listed diagnosis the coding conventions of ICD-10-CM, as well as the general and disease specific guidelines take precedence over the outpatient guidelines.

Diagnoses often are not established at the time of the initial encounter/visit. It may take two or more visits before the diagnosis is confirmed.

The most critical rule involves beginning the search for the correct code assignment through the Alphabetic Index. Never begin searching initially in the Tabular List as this will lead to coding errors.

1. Outpatient Surgery

When a patient presents for outpatient surgery (same day surgery), code the reason for the surgery as the first-listed diagnosis (reason for the encounter), even if the surgery is not performed due to a contraindication.

2. Observation Stay

When a patient is admitted for observation for a medical condition, assign a code for the medical condition as the first-listed diagnosis.

When a patient presents for outpatient surgery and develops complications requiring admission to observation, code the reason for the surgery as the first reported diagnosis (reason for the encounter), followed by codes for the complications as secondary diagnoses.

B. Codes from A00.0–T88.9, Z00–Z99

The appropriate code(s) from A00.0–T88.9, Z00–Z99 must be used to identify diagnoses, symptoms, conditions, problems, complaints, or other reason(s) for the encounter/visit.

C. Accurate Reporting of ICD-10-CM Diagnosis Codes

For accurate reporting of ICD-10-CM diagnosis codes, the documentation should describe the patient's condition, using terminology which includes specific diagnoses as well as symptoms, problems, or reasons for the encounter. There are ICD-10-CM codes to describe all of these.

D. Codes that Describe Symptoms and Signs

Codes that describe symptoms and signs, as opposed to diagnoses, are acceptable for reporting purposes when a diagnosis has not been established (confirmed) by the provider. Chapter 18 of ICD-10-CM, Symptoms, Signs, and Abnormal Clinical, and Laboratory Findings Not Elsewhere Classified (codes R00–R99) contain many, but not all codes for symptoms.

E. Encounters for Circumstances Other than a Disease or Injury

ICD-10-CM provides codes to deal with encounters for circumstances other than a disease or injury. The Factors Influencing Health Status and Contact with Health Services codes (Z00–Z99) are provided to deal with occasions when circumstances other than a disease or injury are recorded as diagnosis or problems.

See Section I.C.21. Factors influencing health status and contact with health services.

F. Level of Detail in Coding

1. ICD-10-CM Codes with 3, 4, 5, 6, Or 7 Characters

ICD-10-CM is composed of codes with 3, 4, 5, 6, or 7 characters. Codes with three characters are included in ICD-10-CM as the heading of a category of codes that may be further subdivided by the use of fourth**,** fifth, sixth, or seventh characters to provide greater specificity.

2. Use of Full Number of Characters Required for a Code

A three-character code is to be used only if it is not further subdivided. A code is invalid if it has not been coded to the full number of characters required for that code, including the 7th character, if applicable.

G. ICD-10-CM Code for the Diagnosis, Condition, Problem, or Other Reason for Encounter/Visit

List first the ICD-10-CM code for the diagnosis, condition, problem, or other reason for encounter/visit shown in the medical record to be chiefly responsible for the services provided. List additional codes that describe any coexisting conditions. In some cases the first-listed diagnosis may be a symptom when a diagnosis has not been established (confirmed) by the physician.

H. Uncertain Diagnosis

Do not code diagnoses documented as "probable", "suspected," "questionable," "rule out," or "working diagnosis" or other similar terms indicating uncertainty. Rather, code the condition(s) to the highest degree of certainty for that encounter/visit, such as symptoms, signs, abnormal test results, or other reason for the visit.

Note: This differs from the coding practices used by short-term, acute-care, long-term care and psychiatric hospitals.

I. Chronic Diseases

Chronic diseases treated on an ongoing basis may be coded and reported as many times as the patient receives treatment and care for the condition(s).

J. Code All Documented Conditions that Coexist

Code all documented conditions that coexist at the time of the encounter/visit, and require or affect patient care treatment or management. Do not code conditions that were previously treated and no longer exist. However, history codes (categories Z80–Z87) may be used as secondary codes if the historical condition or family history has an impact on current care or influences treatment.

K. Patients Receiving Diagnostic Services Only

For patients receiving diagnostic services only during an encounter/visit, sequence first the diagnosis, condition, problem, or other reason for encounter/visit shown in the medical record to be chiefly responsible for the outpatient services provided during the encounter/visit. Codes for other diagnoses (e.g., chronic conditions) may be sequenced as additional diagnoses.

For encounters for routine laboratory/radiology testing in the absence of any signs, symptoms, or associated diagnosis, assign Z01.89, Encounter for other specified special examinations. If routine testing is performed during the same encounter as a test to evaluate a sign, symptom, or diagnosis, it is appropriate to assign both the Z code and the code describing the reason for the non-routine test.

For outpatient encounters for diagnostic tests that have been interpreted by a physician, and the final report is available at the time of coding, code any confirmed or definitive diagnosis(es) documented in the interpretation. Do not code related signs and symptoms as additional diagnoses.

Note: This differs from the coding practice in the hospital inpatient setting regarding abnormal findings on test results.

L. Patients Receiving Therapeutic Services Only

For patients receiving therapeutic services only during an encounter/visit, sequence first the diagnosis, condition, problem, or other reason for encounter/visit shown in the medical record to be chiefly responsible for the outpatient services provided during the encounter/visit. Codes for other diagnoses (e.g., chronic conditions) may be sequenced as additional diagnoses.

The only exception to this rule is that when the primary reason for the admission/encounter is chemotherapy or radiation therapy, the appropriate Z code for the service is listed first, and the diagnosis or problem for which the service is being performed listed second.

M. Patients Receiving Preoperative Evaluations Only

For patients receiving preoperative evaluations only, sequence first a code from subcategory Z01.81, Encounter for pre-procedural examinations, to describe the pre-op consultations. Assign a code for the condition to describe the reason for the surgery as an additional diagnosis. Code also any findings related to the pre-op evaluation.

N. Ambulatory Surgery

For ambulatory surgery, code the diagnosis for which the surgery was performed. If the postoperative diagnosis is known to be different from the preoperative diagnosis at the time the diagnosis is confirmed, select the postoperative diagnosis for coding, since it is the most definitive.

O. Routine Outpatient Prenatal Visits

See Section I.C.15. Routine outpatient prenatal visits.

P. Encounters for General Medical Examinations with Abnormal Findings

The subcategories for encounters for general medical examinations, Z00.0- **and encounter for routine child health examination, Z00.12-,** provide codes for with and without abnormal findings. Should a general medical examination result in an abnormal finding, the code for general medical examination with abnormal finding should be assigned as the first-listed diagnosis. An examination with abnormal findings refers to a condition/diagnosis that is newly identified or a change in severity of a chronic condition (such as uncontrolled hypertension, or an acute exacerbation of chronic obstructive pulmonary disease) during a routine physical examination. A secondary code for the abnormal finding should also be coded.

Q. Encounters for Routine Health Screenings

See Section I.C.21. Factors influencing health status and contact with health services, Screening

Appendix I. Present on Admission Reporting Guidelines

Introduction

These guidelines are to be used as a supplement to the *ICD-10-CM Official Guidelines for Coding and Reporting* to facilitate the assignment of the Present on Admission (POA) indicator for each diagnosis and external cause of injury code reported on claim forms (UB-04 and 837 Institutional).

These guidelines are not intended to replace any guidelines in the main body of the *ICD-10-CM Official Guidelines for Coding and Reporting.* The POA guidelines are not intended to provide guidance on when a condition should be coded, but rather, how to apply the POA indicator to the final set of diagnosis codes that have been assigned in accordance with Sections I, II, and III of the official coding guidelines. Subsequent to the assignment of the ICD-10-CM codes, the POA indicator should then be assigned to those conditions that have been coded.

As stated in the Introduction to the ICD-10-CM Official Guidelines for Coding and Reporting, a joint effort between the healthcare provider and the coder is essential to achieve complete and accurate documentation, code assignment, and reporting of diagnoses and procedures. The importance of consistent, complete documentation in the medical record cannot be overemphasized. Medical record documentation from any provider involved in the care and treatment of the patient may be used to support the determination of whether a condition was present on admission or not. In the context of the official coding guidelines, the term "provider" means a physician or any qualified healthcare practitioner who is legally accountable for establishing the patient's diagnosis.

These guidelines are not a substitute for the provider's clinical judgment as to the determination of whether a condition was or was not present on admission. The provider should be queried regarding issues related to the linking of signs/symptoms, timing of test results, and the timing of findings.

Please see the CDC website for the detailed list of ICD-10-CM codes that do not require the use of a POA indicator (https://www.cdc.gov/nchs/icd/icd10cm.htm) (https://www.cms.gov/Medicare/Coding/ICD10/2018-ICD-10-CM-and-GEMs.html).

The **codes and categories** on this exempt list **are** for circumstances regarding the healthcare encounter or factors influencing health status that do not represent a current disease or injury or **that describe conditions that** are always present on admission.

General Reporting Requirements

All claims involving inpatient admissions to general acute-care hospitals or other facilities that are subject to a law or regulation mandating collection of present on admission information.

Present on admission is defined as present at the time the order for inpatient admission occurs—conditions that develop during an outpatient encounter, including emergency department, observation, or outpatient surgery, are considered as present on admission.

POA indicator is assigned to principal and secondary diagnoses (as defined in Section II of the Official Guidelines for Coding and Reporting) and the external cause of injury codes.

Issues related to inconsistent, missing, conflicting or unclear documentation must still be resolved by the provider.

If a condition would not be coded and reported based on UHDDS definitions and current official coding guidelines, then the POA indicator would not be reported.

Reporting Options

Y—Yes
N—No
U—Unknown
W—Clinically undetermined
Unreported/Not used—(Exempt from POA reporting)

Reporting Definitions

Y = present at the time of inpatient admission
N = not present at the time of inpatient admission
U = documentation is insufficient to determine if condition is present on admission
W = provider is unable to clinically determine whether condition was present on admission or not

Timeframe for POA Identification and Documentation

There is no required timeframe as to when a provider (per the definition of "provider" used in these guidelines) must identify or document a condition to be present on admission. In some clinical situations, it may not be possible for a provider to make a definitive diagnosis (or a condition may not be recognized or reported by the patient) for a period of time after admission. In some cases it may be several days before the provider arrives at a definitive diagnosis. This does not mean that the condition was not present on admission. Determination of whether the condition was present on admission or not will be based on the applicable POA guideline as identified in this document, or on the provider's best clinical judgment.

If at the time of code assignment the documentation is unclear as to whether a condition was present on admission or not, it is appropriate to query the provider for clarification.

Assigning the POA Indicator

Condition is on the "Exempt from Reporting" list

Leave the "present on admission" field blank if the condition is on the list of ICD-10-CM codes for which this field is not applicable. This is the only circumstance in which the field may be left blank.

POA Explicitly Documented

Assign "Y" for any condition the provider explicitly documents as being present on admission.

Assign "N" for any condition the provider explicitly documents as not present at the time of admission.

Conditions diagnosed prior to inpatient admission

Assign "Y" for conditions that were diagnosed prior to admission (example: hypertension, diabetes mellitus, asthma)

Conditions diagnosed during the admission but clearly present before admission

Assign "Y" for conditions diagnosed during the admission that were clearly present but not diagnosed until after admission occurred.

Diagnoses subsequently confirmed after admission are considered present on admission if at the time of admission they are documented as suspected, possible, rule out, differential diagnosis, or constitute an underlying cause of a symptom that is present at the time of admission.

Condition develops during outpatient encounter prior to inpatient admission

Assign "Y" for any condition that develops during an outpatient encounter prior to a written order for inpatient admission.

Documentation does not indicate whether condition was present on admission

Assign “U” when the medical record documentation is unclear as to whether the condition was present on admission. “U” should not be routinely assigned and used only in very limited circumstances. Coders are encouraged to query the providers when the documentation is unclear.

Documentation states that it cannot be determined whether the condition was or was not present on admission

Assign “W” when the medical record documentation indicates that it cannot be clinically determined whether or not the condition was present on admission.

Chronic condition with acute exacerbation during the admission

If a single code identifies both the chronic condition and the acute exacerbation, see POA guidelines pertaining to codes that contain multiple clinical concepts.

If a single code only identifies the chronic condition and not the acute exacerbation (e.g., acute exacerbation of chronic leukemia), assign “Y.”

Conditions documented as possible, probable, suspected, or rule out at the time of discharge

If the final diagnosis contains a possible, probable, suspected, or rule out diagnosis, and this diagnosis was based on signs, symptoms or clinical findings suspected at the time of inpatient admission, assign “Y.”

If the final diagnosis contains a possible, probable, suspected, or rule out diagnosis, and this diagnosis was based on signs, symptoms or clinical findings that were not present on admission, assign “N”.

Conditions documented as impending or threatened at the time of discharge

If the final diagnosis contains an impending or threatened diagnosis, and this diagnosis is based on symptoms or clinical findings that were present on admission, assign “Y”.

If the final diagnosis contains an impending or threatened diagnosis, and this diagnosis is based on symptoms or clinical findings that were not present on admission, assign “N”.

Acute and Chronic Conditions

Assign “Y” for acute conditions that are present at time of admission and N for acute conditions that are not present at time of admission.

Assign “Y” for chronic conditions, even though the condition may not be diagnosed until after admission.

If a single code identifies both an acute and chronic condition, see the POA guidelines for codes that contain multiple clinical concepts.

Codes That Contain Multiple Clinical Concepts

Assign “N” if at least one of the clinical concepts included in the code was not present on admission (e.g., COPD with acute exacerbation and the exacerbation was not present on admission; gastric ulcer that does not start bleeding until after admission; asthma patient develops status asthmaticus after admission)

Assign “Y” if all parts of the clinical concepts included in the code were present on admission (e.g., duodenal ulcer that perforates prior to admission)

For infection codes that include the causal organism, assign “Y” if the infection (or signs of the infection) were present on admission, even though the culture results may not be known until after admission (e.g., patient is admitted with pneumonia and the provider documents pseudomonas as the causal organism a few days later).

Same Diagnosis Code for Two or More Conditions

When the same ICD-10-CM diagnosis code applies to two or more conditions during the same encounter (e.g. two separate conditions classified to the same ICD-10-CM diagnosis code):

Assign “Y” if all conditions represented by the single ICD-10-CM code were present on admission (e.g. bilateral unspecified age-related cataracts).

Assign “N” if any of the conditions represented by the single ICD-10-CM code was not present on admission (e.g. traumatic secondary and recurrent hemorrhage and seroma is assigned to a single code T79.2, but only one of the conditions was present on admission).

Obstetrical Conditions

Whether or not the patient delivers during the current hospitalization does not affect assignment of the POA indicator. The determining factor for POA assignment is whether the pregnancy complication or obstetrical condition described by the code was present at the time of admission or not.

If the pregnancy complication or obstetrical condition was present on admission (e.g., patient admitted in preterm labor), assign “Y”.

If the pregnancy complication or obstetrical condition was not present on admission (e.g., 2nd degree laceration during delivery, postpartum hemorrhage that occurred during current hospitalization, fetal distress develops after admission), assign “N”.

If the obstetrical code includes more than one diagnosis and any of the diagnoses identified by the code were not present on admission assign “N” (e.g., Category O11, Pre-existing hypertension with pre-eclampsia).

Perinatal Conditions

Newborns are not considered to be admitted until after birth. Therefore, any condition present at birth or that developed in utero is considered present at admission and should be assigned "Y". This includes conditions that occur during delivery (e.g., injury during delivery, meconium aspiration, exposure to streptococcus B in the vaginal canal).

Congenital Conditions and Anomalies

Assign "Y" for congenital conditions and anomalies except for categories Q00–Q99, Congenital anomalies, which are on the exempt list. Congenital conditions are always considered present on admission.

External Cause of Injury Codes

Assign "Y" for any external cause code representing an external cause of morbidity that occurred prior to inpatient admission (e.g., patient fell out of bed at home, patient fell out of bed in emergency room prior to admission).

Assign "N" for any external cause code representing an external cause of morbidity that occurred during inpatient hospitalization (e.g., patient fell out of hospital bed during hospital stay, patient experienced an adverse reaction to a medication administered after inpatient admission).

Consulting Editor's Note

The Official Coding Guidelines Appendix I, Present on Admission Reporting Guidelines, no longer provides a listing of Present on Admission (POA) exempt codes by category/sub-category. Instead interested parties can view a full list of the POA exempt code list via the National Center for Health Statistics webpage.

Here we are providing an updated 2018 POA exempt code list by category/sub-category to be used as a reference guide for the users of this code book. Users, including educators, can use this list to provide examples of the types of codes included on the POA exempt code list.

B90–B94	Sequelae of infectious and parasitic diseases
E64	Sequelae of malnutrition and other nutritional deficiencies
I25.2	Old myocardial infarction
I69	Sequelae of cerebrovascular disease
M84.7	Nontraumatic fracture, NEC (excluding codes ending in 7th character A)
M97	Periprosthetic fracture around internal prosthetic joint (excluding codes ending in 7th character A)
O09	Supervision of high risk pregnancy
O66.5	Attempted application of vacuum extractor and forceps
O80	Encounter for full-term uncomplicated delivery
O94	Sequelae of complication of pregnancy, childbirth, and the puerperium
P00	Newborn affected by maternal conditions that may be unrelated to present pregnancy
P29.3	Persistent fetal circulation
P78.84	Gestational alloimmune liver disease
P83.8	Other specified conditions of integument specific to newborn
P91.81	Neonatal encephalopathy
P91.88	Other specified disturbances of cerebral status of newborn
Q00–Q99	Congenital malformations, deformations and chromosomal abnormalities
S00–T88.9	Injury, poisoning and certain other consequences of external causes with 7th character representing subsequent encounter or sequela
V00–V09	Pedestrian injured in transport accident
	Except V00.81-, Accident with wheelchair (powered)
	V00.83-, Accident with motorized mobility scooter
V10–V19	Pedal cycle rider injured in transport accident
V20–V29	Motorcycle rider injured in transport accident
V30–V39	Occupant of three-wheeled motor vehicle injured in transport accident
V40–V49	Car occupant injured in transport accident

V50–V59	Occupant of pick-up truck or van injured in transport accident
V60–V69	Occupant of heavy transport vehicle injured in transport accident
V70–V79	Bus occupant injured in transport accident
V80–V89	Other land transport accidents
V90–V94	Water transport accidents
V95–V97	Air and space transport accidents
V98–V99	Other and unspecified transport accidents
W09	Fall on and from playground equipment (except codes ending in 7th character A)
W14	Fall from tree
W15	Fall from cliff
W16	Fall, jump or diving into water (excluding codes that end in 7th character A)
W17.0	Fall into well
W17.1	Fall into storm drain or manhole
W17.3	Fall into empty swimming pool
W17.4	Fall from dock
W17.8	Other fall from one level to another
W18.00	Striking against unspecified object with subsequent fall (excluding codes ending in 7th character A)
W18.01	Striking against sports equipment with subsequent fall
W18.02	Striking against glass with subsequent fall (except codes ending in 7th character A)
W18.09	Striking against other object with subsequent fall (except codes ending in 7th character A)
W18.1	Fall from or off toilet (except codes ending in 7th character A)
W18.2	Fall in (into) shower or empty bathtub (except codes ending in 7th character A)
W18.3	Other and unspecified fall on same level (except codes ending in 7th character A)
W18.4	Slipping, tripping and stumbling without falling (except codes ending in 7th character A)
W21	Striking against or struck by sports equipment
W22.01	Walked into wall (except codes ending in 7th character A)
W22.02	Walked into lamppost
W22.03	Walked into furniture (except codes ending in 7th character A)
W22.04	Striking against wall of swimming pool (except codes ending in 7th character A)
W22.09	Striking against other stationary object (except codes ending in 7th character A)
W22.1	Striking against or struck by automobile airbag
W22.8	Striking against or struck by other objects
W24.0	Contact with lifting devices, not elsewhere classified (except codes ending in 7th character A)
W24.1	Contact with transmission devices, NEC
W26.1–W26.9	Contact with knife, sword or dagger
W27.0	Contact with workbench
W27.1	Contact with garden tool
W27.2	Contact with scissors (except codes ending in 7th character A)
W27.3	Contact with needle (except codes ending in 7th character A)
W27.4	Contact with kitchen utensil (except codes ending in 7th character A)
W27.5	Contact with paper-cutter (except codes ending in 7th character A)
W27.8	Contact with other nonpowered hand tool
W28	Contact with powered lawn mower
W29	Contact with other powered hand tools and household machinery
W30	Contact with agricultural machinery
W31	Contact with other and unspecified machinery

W32–W34	Accidental handgun discharge and malfunction
W35–W40	Exposure to inanimate mechanical forces
W42.0	Exposure to supersonic waves
W42.9	Exposure to other noise (except codes ending in 7th character A)
W45.0	Nail entering through skin
W49	Exposure to other inanimate mechanical forces (except codes ending in 7th character A)
W52	Crushed, pushed or stepped on by crowd or human stampede
W53	Contact with rodent
W54	Contact with dog
W55	Contact with other mammals
W56	Contact with nonvenomous marine animal
W57	Bitten or stung by nonvenomous insect and other nonvenomous arthropods (except codes ending in 7th character A)
W58	Contact with crocodile or alligator
W59.01	Bitten by nonvenomous lizards (except codes ending in 7th character A)
W59.02–W59.8	Contact with other nonvenomous reptiles
W60	Contact with nonvenomous plant thorns and spines and sharp leaves
W61	Contact with birds (domestic) (wild)
W62	Contact with nonvenomous amphibians
W64	Exposure to other animate mechanical forces
W65	Accidental drowning and submersion while in bath-tub (except codes ending in 7th character A)
W67	Accidental drowning and submersion while in swimming pool (except codes ending in 7th character A)
W69	Accidental drowning and submersion while in natural water
W73	Other specified cause of accidental non-transport drowning and submersion
W74	Unspecified cause of accidental drowning and submersion
W85	Exposure to electric transmission lines (except codes ending in 7th character A)
W86	Exposure to other specified electric current (except codes ending in 7th character A)
W88	Exposure to ionizing radiation (except codes ending in 7th character A)
W89	Exposure to man-made visible and ultraviolet light
W90	Exposure to other nonionizing radiation (except codes ending in 7th character A)
W92	Exposure to excessive heat of man-made origin
W93	Exposure to excessive cold of man-made origin
W94	Exposure to high and low air pressure and changes in air pressure
W99	Exposure to other man-made environmental factors
X02	Exposure to controlled fire in building or structure (except codes ending in 7th character A)
X03	Exposure to controlled fire, not in building or structure (except codes ending in 7th character A)
X04	Exposure to ignition of highly flammable material
X30	Exposure to excessive natural heat
X31	Exposure to excessive natural cold
X32	Exposure to sunlight
X34	Earthquake (except codes ending in 7th character A)
X35	Volcanic eruption
X36	Avalanche, landslide and other earth movements (except codes ending in 7th character A)
X37	Cataclysmic storm (except codes ending in 7th character A)
X38	Flood (except codes ending in 7th character A)
X39	Exposure to other forces of nature

X50	Overexertion and strenuous or repetitive movements
X52	Prolonged stay in weightless environment
X71	Intentional self-harm by drowning and submersion (except codes ending in 7th character A) Except X71.0-, Intentional self-harm by drowning and submersion while in bath tub
X72	Intentional self-harm by handgun discharge
X73	Intentional self-harm by rifle, shotgun and larger firearm discharge
X74	Intentional self-harm by other and unspecified firearm and gun discharge
X75	Intentional self-harm by explosive material
X76	Intentional self-harm by smoke, fire and flames
X77	Intentional self-harm by steam, hot vapors and hot objects
X81	Intentional self-harm by jumping or lying in front of moving object
X82	Intentional self-harm by crashing of motor vehicle
X83	Intentional self-harm by other specified means
X92	Assault by drowning and submersion (except codes ending in 7th character A)
X93	Assault by handgun discharge (except codes ending in 7th character A)
X94	Assault by rifle, shotgun and larger firearm discharge (except codes ending in 7th character A)
X95	Assault by other and unspecified firearm and gun discharge (except codes ending in 7th character A)
X96	Assault by explosive material (except codes ending in 7th character A)
X97	Assault by smoke, fire and flames (except codes ending in 7th character A)
X98	Assault by steam, hot vapors and hot objects (except codes ending in 7th character A)
X99	Assault by sharp object (except codes ending in 7th character A)
Y00	Assault by blunt object (except codes ending in 7th character A)
Y01	Assault by pushing from high place (except codes ending in 7th character A)
Y02	Assault by pushing or placing victim in front of moving object
Y03	Assault by crashing of motor vehicle
Y04	Assault by bodily force (except codes ending in 7th character A)
Y07	Perpetrator of assault, maltreatment and neglect
Y08	Assault by other specified means
Y21	Drowning and submersion, undetermined intent
Y22	Handgun discharge, undetermined intent (except codes ending in 7th character A)
Y23	Rifle, shotgun and larger firearm discharge, undetermined intent (except codes ending in 7th character A)
Y24	Other and unspecified firearm discharge, undetermined intent (except Y24.9, Unspecified firearm discharge, undetermined intent, initial encounter)
Y30	Falling, jumping or pushed from a high place, undetermined intent
Y32	Assault by crashing of motor vehicle, undetermined intent
Y35	Legal intervention (except codes ending in 7th character A)
Y36	Operations of war
Y37	Military operations
Y38	Terrorism (except codes ending in 7th character A)
Y92	Place of occurrence of the external cause (except Y92.23-, Y92.530 and Y92.538)
Y93.12–Y93.9	Activity code
Y99	External cause status
Z00	Encounter for general examination without complaint, suspected or reported diagnosis
Z01	Encounter for other special examination without complaint, suspected or reported diagnosis
Z02	Encounter for administrative examination
Z03	Encounter for medical observation for suspected diseases and conditions ruled out
Z05	Encounter for observation and evaluation of newborn for suspected diseases and conditions ruled out

Z08	Encounter for follow-up examination following completed treatment for malignant neoplasm
Z09	Encounter for follow-up examination after completed treatment for conditions other than malignant neoplasm
Z11	Encounter for screening for infectious and parasitic diseases
Z11.8	Encounter for screening for other infectious and parasitic diseases
Z12	Encounter for screening for malignant neoplasms
Z13	Encounter for screening for other diseases and disorders
Z13.4	Encounter for screening for certain developmental disorders in childhood
Z13.5	Encounter for screening for eye and ear disorders
Z13.6	Encounter for screening for cardiovascular disorders
Z13.83	Encounter for screening for respiratory disorder NEC
Z13.89	Encounter for screening for other disorder
Z13.89	Encounter for screening for other disorder
Z14	Genetic carrier
Z15	Genetic susceptibility to disease
Z17	Estrogen receptor status
Z18	Retained foreign body fragments
Z19	Hormone sensitivity malignancy status
Z22	Carrier of infectious disease
Z23	Encounter for immunization
Z28	Immunization not carried out and underimmunization status
Z29	Encounter for prophylactic measures
Z30	Encounter for contraceptive management
Z31	Encounter for procreative management
Z34	Encounter for supervision of normal pregnancy
Z3A	Weeks of gestation
Z36	Encounter for antenatal screening of mother
Z37	Outcome of delivery
Z38	Liveborn infants according to place of birth and type of delivery
Z39	Encounter for maternal postpartum care and examination
Z40.3	Encounter for prophylactic removal of fallopian tube(s)
Z41	Encounter for procedures for purposes other than remedying health state
Z42	Encounter for plastic and reconstructive surgery following medical procedure or healed injury
Z43	Encounter for attention to artificial openings
Z44	Encounter for fitting and adjustment of external prosthetic device
Z45	Encounter for adjustment and management of implanted device
Z46	Encounter for fitting and adjustment of other devices
Z47	Orthopedic aftercare
Z48	Encounter for other postprocedural aftercare
Z49	Encounter for care involving renal dialysis
Z51	Encounter for other aftercare (except Z51.5, Encounter for palliative care)
Z52	Donors of organs and tissues
Z53.3	Procedure converted to open procedure
Z55	Problems related to education and literacy
Z56	Problems related to employment and unemployment
Z57	Occupational exposure to risk factors
Z59	Problems related to housing and economic circumstances
Z63	Other problems related to primary support group, including family circumstances

Z64	Problems related to certain psychosocial circumstances
Z65	Problems related to other psychosocial circumstances
Z65.8	Other specified problems related to psychosocial circumstances
Z67.1–Z67.9	Blood type
Z68	Body mass index (BMI)
Z69	Encounter for mental health services for victim and perpetrator of abuse
Z70	Counseling related to sexual attitude, behavior and orientation
Z71	Persons encountering health services for other counseling and medical advice, NEC
Z72	Problems related to lifestyle
Z73	Problems related to life management difficulty
Z74.01	Bed confinement status
Z75	Problems related to medical facilities and other health care
Z76	Persons encountering health services in other circumstances
Z77.110–Z77.128	Environmental pollution and hazards in the physical environment
Z78	Other specified health status
Z79	Long-term (current) drug therapy
Z80	Family history of primary malignant neoplasm
Z81	Family history of mental and behavioral disorders
Z82	Family history of certain disabilities and chronic diseases (leading to disablement)
Z83	Family history of other specific disorders
Z84	Family history of other conditions
Z85	Personal history of primary malignant neoplasm
Z86	Personal history of certain other diseases
Z87	Personal history of other diseases and conditions
Z87.828	Personal history of other (healed) physical injury and trauma
Z87.891	Personal history of nicotine dependence
Z88	Allergy status to drugs, medicaments and biological substances
Z89	Acquired absence of limb
Z90	Acquired absence of organs, NEC
Z91	Personal risk factors, NEC
Z92	Personal history of medical treatment
Z93	Artificial opening status
Z94	Transplanted organ and tissue status
Z95	Presence of cardiac and vascular implants and grafts
Z97	Presence of other devices
Z98	Other postprocedural states
Z99	Dependence on enabling machines and devices, not elsewhere classified

Additional Conventions

The use of symbols and color-coding has been added to this code book to alert the user to Medicare reimbursement logic and edits that are impacted by diagnosis coding. Although some third-party payers have adopted Medicare's reimbursement methodology, others have not. Therefore, it is important to review your facilities payer reporting requirements for non-Medicare payers prior to diagnosis coding.

Some codes may be included in multiple reimbursement issues and, therefore, may have more than one symbol or color-coding feature. For a quick reference review, the legend at the bottom of each page of the Tabular as well as the inside cover of the code book. The symbols and color-coding features are described in detail here.

Tabular Enhancements

In an effort to make the Tabular more user-friendly, the following symbols and color-coding features have been added. These features are indented to help the user in selecting a complete and accurate diagnosis code.

Final Character Indicator

ICD-10-CM codes range in length from 3 to 7 characters. In order for a code to be "valid" it must be listed to the fullest character length available. For example, if a fourth character is available, a three-character code is considered invalid.

To help users comply with this convention, a red plus sign (+) is listed to the left of any subcategory or subclassification code that requires an additional character. For example:

+ **J45.2 Mild intermittent asthma**

The assignment of the seventh character can, at times, be tricky. There are designated categories of codes that require a seventh character even though the code may not already have six characters present. For these codes, the user must insert the placeholder character of X after the code to fill any open characters prior to the seventh character.

To help users comply with this convention, in this book, the phrase X+7th is in red and is located to the left of the code that requires the placeholder of X and/or the seventh character. For example:

X+7th **M80.00 Age-related osteoporosis with current pathological fracture**

Additionally, there are six character codes that require the application of a seventh character. For these codes a placeholder X is not required. To help users differentiate these codes, in this book, the phrase +7th is in red and is located to the left of the code that requires the seventh character. For example:

+7th **S72.021 Displaced fracture of epiphysis (separation) (upper) of right femur**

Lastly, there are some codes that have only three characters. They require no further specification with additional characters and are therefore valid codes. The following note: Valid 3-character code, no further characters required is located below the code description in this book. This note alerts the coder that the three-character code is valid and can be used for reporting.

Color Identification

The Tabular section of this code book contains many instructional notes for the user. In order to help navigate the various types of instructional notes, a color-coding system has been applied:

- Category block headers are presented in dark green font.
- Category codes (three characters) are presented in blue font.
- Includes notes have a gray color bar over the **Includes**
- Excludes1 notes have a yellow color bar over the ***Excludes1***
- Excludes2 notes have a bright green color bar over the ***Excludes2***
- Notes have a maroon color bar over the **NOTE**
- *Use additional code* notes are presented in orange font
- *Code also* notes are presented in orange font
- *Code first* notes are presented in orange font
- Seventh character options are presented in a box and are highlighted in gray

The following excerpt from the Tabular illustrates the color-coding applied in this code book.

Disorders of bone density and structure (M80–M85)

M80 Osteoporosis with current pathological fracture

Includes: osteoporosis with current fragility fracture

Use additional code to identify major osseous defect, if applicable (M89.7-)

Excludes1: *collapsed vertebra NOS (M48.5)*
pathological fracture NOS (M84.4)
wedging of vertebra NOS (M48.5)

Excludes2: *personal history of (healed) osteoporosis fracture (Z87.310)*

The appropriate 7th character is to be added to each code from category M80:
A initial encounter for fracture
D subsequent encounter for fracture with routine healing
G subsequent encounter for fracture with delayed healing
K subsequent encounter for fracture with nonunion
P subsequent encounter for fracture with malunion
S sequela

Medicare Code Edits

Hospital inpatient Medicare claims paid under the Inpatient Prospective payment System (IPPS) are processed through the Medicare Code Editor (MCE) prior to payment by the Medicare administrative contractor (MAC). The code edits are intended to ensure that all claims processed by the MAC are accurate and complete. The information in this manual is based on the MCE v35.

Several of the MCE edits pertain to diagnoses. We have identified the codes included in these edits throughout the Tabular section this manual to assist users with preparing accurate and complete claims. The MCE edits included in this manual:

- Age conflict
- Sex Conflict Edit
- Manifestation codes not allowed as principal diagnosis
- Unacceptable principal diagnoses

Note: It is important to remember these edits are Medicare edits and may not apply to other third-party payers claim processing.

Age Conflict

The age conflict edit is activated when the age of the patient and the type diagnosis code reported does not match. The following symbols are used to identify the four age conflict categories.

- Newborn diagnosis age 0: This symbol appears to the left of the applicable code in the Tabular.
- Pediatric diagnosis age 0–17: This symbol appears to the left of the applicable code in the Tabular.
- Maternity diagnosis age 12–55: This symbol appears to the left of the applicable code in the Tabular.
- Adult diagnosis age 15–124: This symbol appears to the left of the applicable code in the Tabular.

Sex Conflict Edit

The sex conflict edit is activated when the sex of the patient and the diagnosis reported does not match. The following symbols are used to identify female-only and male-only diagnoses.

♀ Female-only diagnosis: This symbol appears to the left of the applicable code in the Tabular.

♂ Male-only diagnosis: This symbol appears to the left of the applicable code in the Tabular.

Manifestation Code Not Allowed as Principal Diagnosis

Manifestation codes are used to report the manifestation of an underlying disease, not to report the disease itself. Therefore, within ICD-10-CM the manifestation should not be reported as the principal diagnosis; rather it should always be reported as a secondary diagnosis.

Manifestation codes are identified with a light green color bar over the code in the Tabular. For example:

D63.0 Anemia in neoplastic disease

Unacceptable Principal Diagnosis

There are specified codes that describe a circumstance which influences an individual's health status but not a current illness or injury, or codes that are not specific manifestations but may be due to an underlying cause. These codes are considered unacceptable as a principal diagnosis.

Unacceptable principal diagnosis codes are identified with a light blue color bar over the code in the Tabular:

B60.13 Keratoconjunctivitis due to Acanthamoeba

MS-DRG Diagnosis Designations

The MS-DRG system is utilized within the IPPS to determine the unadjusted reimbursement amount for Medicare hospital inpatient claims. The MS-DRG Definitions Manual includes the logic for MS-DRG refinement and selection as well as logic based on the IPPS final rules released each August. The information in this book is based on the MS-DRG v35. *Note:* It is important to remember that these edits are Medicare edits and may not apply to other third-party payers claim processing.

CC and MCC Codes

Within the MS-DRG system, one of the refinement pathways is whether there is a complication/comorbidity (CC) or major complication/comorbidity (MCC) code reported as a secondary diagnosis. For some of the MS-DRG families, the presence of a CC or MCC allows for an MS-DRG assignment that has a higher relative weight and, therefore, a higher reimbursement amount. There are exceptions to the application of the CC or MCC codes and the exceptions are referred to as *CC Exclusions* or *MCC Exclusions*. If exclusions apply, the CC/MCC code is assigned a principal diagnosis collection. Within this collection are the codes that, when reported as principal diagnosis, excludes the CC/MCC status from the secondary diagnosis code under review. Essentially, it takes away the CC/MCC code's ability to influence the MS-DRG assignment.

Codes that are considered CC codes have a purple CC to the left of the code in the Tabular. Below the code description, the phrase ***CC Exclusion see Appendix A PDX collection xxxx*** appears, alerting the coder to review the principal diagnosis collection identified if required for the task at hand. If the code requires a seventh character, the characters that are eligible for CC status are included within the CC Exclusion note.

Codes that are considered MCC codes have a purple MCC to the left of the code in the Tabular. Below the code description, the phrase ***MCC Exclusion see Appendix A PDX collection xxxx*** appears, alerting the coder to review the principal diagnosis collection identified if required for the task at hand. If the code requires a seventh character, the characters that are eligible for MCC status are included within the MCC Exclusion note.

Hospital-Acquired Conditions Related Diagnoses

As part of the Medicare Value-Based Purchasing program, CMS has implemented a Paying for Value program entitled Hospital-Acquired Conditions (HACs) Reduction Program. This program is designed to reduce reimbursements to facilities where the value of the medical or surgical services have been comprised due to preventable conditions. Reimbursement for facilities with HAC scores in the lowest-performance quartile will be reduced. In this manual, the HAC-associated procedures are identified with an orange rectangle HAC with HAC. The orange rectangle is located below the code description in the code listing. If there is conditional logic for the diagnosis code, it is included in Appendix B.

AHA *Coding Clinic for ICD-10-CM and ICD-10-PCS*

The American Hospital Association began publishing coding guidance for ICD-10-CM and ICD-10-PCS in the fourth quarter of 2012. In this code book we identify diagnosis codes that are discussed in the *Coding Clinic* guidance fourth quarter 2012 through second quarter 2017. Within the Tabular the following sky-blue note alerts the coder to review the AHA *Coding Clinic* prior to assignment of the code to ensure appropriate and accurate reporting. The quarter of publication, year, and page number(s) are provided in the note.

AHA CC: 4Q; 2012; pg#-pg#

CMS Hierarchical Condition Categories Risk Adjustment System

Since 2004, Medicare has utilized the CMS Hierarchical Condition Categories (HCC) model to risk adjust within the Medicare Advantage capitation payment system. Using the CMS HCC model Medicare uses large pools of data to predict costs on average for a predetermined set of factors; one of the factors is individual disease groups. The HCC diagnosis code listing is utilized to determine the individual disease groups from Medicare claims data. Additionally, CMS HCCs are utilized in accountable care organizations payment methodologies (inpatient and outpatient settings) and in Medicare's inpatient acute care (IPPS) value-based purchasing program. The use of HCCs for risk adjustment within payment systems continues to grow. Therefore, it is imperative that coding professionals in all settings are familiar with the reporting of HCC diagnosis codes. The most current list of ICD-10-CM HCC diagnosis codes are identified in this code book. HCC codes are updated each year with an effective date of January 1.

ICD-10-CM HCC diagnosis codes are identified with a lavender color bar over the code in the Tabular:

E11.21 Type 2 diabetes mellitus with diabetic nephropathy

Basic Steps in ICD-10-CM Coding

To code each disease or condition completely and accurately, the coder should:

1. Identify all main terms included in the diagnostic statement.
2. Locate each main term in the Alphabetic Index.
3. Refer to any subterms indented under the main term. The subterms form individual line entries and describe essential differences by site, etiology, or clinical type.
4. Follow the instructions (see, see also) provided in the Alphabetic Index if the needed code is not located under the first main entry consulted.
5. Verify the code selected in the Tabular List.
6. Read and be guided by any instructional terms in the Tabular List.
7. Assign codes to their highest level of specificity, up to a total of seven characters if applicable.
8. Continue coding the diagnostic statement until all the component elements are fully identified.

(*Source:* Schraffenberger, L.A. *Basic ICD-10-CM/PCS Coding*, 2016 Edition, pg. 34. AHIMA.)

Index to Diseases and Injuries

A

- **Aarskog's syndrome** Q87.1
- **Abandonment** *—see* Maltreatment
- **Abasia** (-astasia) (hysterical) F44.4
- **Abderhalden-Kaufmann-Lignac syndrome** (cystinosis) E72.04
- **Abdomen, abdominal** *—see also* condition
  - acute R10.0
  - angina K55.1
  - muscle deficiency syndrome Q79.4
- **Abdominalgia** *—see* Pain, abdominal
- **Abduction contracture, hip or other joint** *—see* Contraction, joint
- **Aberrant** (congenital) *—see also* Malposition, congenital
  - adrenal gland Q89.1
  - artery (peripheral) Q27.8
    - basilar NEC Q28.1
    - cerebral Q28.3
    - coronary Q24.5
    - digestive system Q27.8
    - eye Q15.8
    - lower limb Q27.8
    - precerebral Q28.1
    - pulmonary Q25.79
    - renal Q27.2
    - retina Q14.1
    - specified site NEC Q27.8
    - subclavian Q27.8
    - upper limb Q27.8
    - vertebral Q28.1
  - breast Q83.8
  - endocrine gland NEC Q89.2
  - hepatic duct Q44.5
  - pancreas Q45.3
  - parathyroid gland Q89.2
  - pituitary gland Q89.2
  - sebaceous glands, mucous membrane, mouth, congenital Q38.6
  - spleen Q89.09
  - subclavian artery Q27.8
  - thymus (gland) Q89.2
  - thyroid gland Q89.2
  - vein (peripheral) NEC Q27.8
    - cerebral Q28.3
    - digestive system Q27.8
    - lower limb Q27.8
    - precerebral Q28.1
    - specified site NEC Q27.8
    - upper limb Q27.8
- **Aberration**
  - distantial *—see* Disturbance, visual
  - mental F99
- **Abetalipoproteinemia** E78.6
- **Abiotrophy** R68.89
- **Ablatio, ablation**
  - retinae *—see* Detachment, retina
- **Ablepharia, ablepharon** Q10.3
- **Abnormal, abnormality, abnormalities** *—see also* Anomaly
  - acid-base balance (mixed) E87.4
  - albumin R77.0
  - alphafetoprotein R77.2
  - alveolar ridge K08.9
  - anatomical relationship Q89.9
  - apertures, congenital, diaphragm Q79.1
  - auditory perception H93.29-
    - diplacusis *—see* Diplacusis
    - hyperacusis *—see* Hyperacusis

Abnormal, abnormality, abnormalities *(continued)*

  - auditory perception *(continued)*
    - recruitment *—see* Recruitment, auditory
    - threshold shift *—see* Shift, auditory threshold
  - autosomes Q99.9
    - fragile site Q95.5
  - basal metabolic rate R94.8
  - biosynthesis, testicular androgen E29.1
  - bleeding time R79.1
  - blood-gas level R79.81
  - blood level (of)
    - cobalt R79.0
    - copper R79.0
    - iron R79.0
    - lithium R78.89
    - magnesium R79.0
    - mineral NEC R79.0
    - zinc R79.0
  - blood pressure
    - elevated R03.0
    - low reading (nonspecific) R03.1
  - blood sugar R73.09
  - bowel sounds R19.15
    - absent R19.11
    - hyperactive R19.12
  - brain scan R94.02
  - breathing R06.9
  - caloric test R94.138
  - cerebrospinal fluid R83.9
    - cytology R83.6
    - drug level R83.2
    - enzyme level R83.0
    - hormones R83.1
    - immunology R83.4
    - microbiology R83.5
    - nonmedicinal level R83.3
    - specified type NEC R83.8
  - chemistry, blood R79.9
    - C-reactive protein R79.82
    - drugs *—see* Findings, abnormal, in blood
    - gas level R79.81
    - minerals R79.0
    - pancytopenia D61.818
    - PTT R79.1
    - specified NEC R79.89
    - toxins *—see* Findings, abnormal, in blood
  - chest sounds (friction) (rales) R09.89
  - chromosome, chromosomal Q99.9
    - with more than three X chromosomes, female Q97.1
    - analysis result R89.8
      - bronchial washings R84.8
      - cerebrospinal fluid R83.8
      - cervix uteri NEC R87.89
      - nasal secretions R84.8
      - nipple discharge R89.8
      - peritoneal fluid R85.89
      - pleural fluid R84.8
      - prostatic secretions R86.8
      - saliva R85.89
      - seminal fluid R86.8
      - sputum R84.8
      - synovial fluid R89.8
      - throat scrapings R84.8
      - vagina R87.89
      - vulva R87.89
      - wound secretions R89.8
    - dicentric replacement Q93.2
    - ring replacement Q93.2

Abnormal, abnormality, abnormalities *(continued)*

  - chromosome *(continued)*
    - sex Q99.8
      - female phenotype Q97.9
        - specified NEC Q97.8
      - male phenotype Q98.9
        - specified NEC Q98.8
      - structural male Q98.6
    - specified NEC Q99.8
  - clinical findings NEC R68.89
  - coagulation D68.9
    - newborn, transient P61.6
    - profile R79.1
    - time R79.1
  - communication *—see* Fistula
  - conjunctiva, vascular H11.41-
  - coronary artery Q24.5
  - cortisol-binding globulin E27.8
  - course, eustachian tube Q17.8
  - creatinine clearance R94.4
  - cytology
    - anus R85.619
      - atypical squamous cells cannot exclude high grade squamous intraepithelial lesion (ASC-H) R85.611
      - atypical squamous cells of undetermined significance (ASC-US) R85.610
      - cytologic evidence of malignancy R85.614
      - high grade squamous intraepithelial lesion (HGSIL) R85.613
      - human papillomavirus (HPV) DNA test
        - high risk positive R85.81
        - low risk postive R85.82
      - inadequate smear R85.615
      - low grade squamous intraepithelial lesion (LGSIL) R85.612
      - satisfactory anal smear but lacking transformation zone R85.616
      - specified NEC R85.618
      - unsatisfactory smear R85.615
    - female genital organs *—see* Abnormal, Papanicolaou (smear)
  - dark adaptation curve H53.61
  - dentofacial NEC *—see* Anomaly, dentofacial
  - development, developmental Q89.9
    - central nervous system Q07.9
  - diagnostic imaging
    - abdomen, abdominal region NEC R93.5
    - biliary tract R93.2
    - bladder R93.41
    - breast R92.8
    - central nervous system NEC R90.89
    - cerebrovascular NEC R90.89
    - coronary circulation R93.1
    - digestive tract NEC R93.3
    - gastrointestinal (tract) R93.3
    - genitourinary organs R93.8
    - head R93.0
    - heart R93.1
    - intrathoracic organ NEC R93.8
    - kidney R93.42-
    - limbs R93.6
    - liver R93.2
    - lung (field) R91.8
    - musculoskeletal system NEC R93.7

Abnormal, abnormality, abnormalities *(continued)*

  - diagnostic imaging *(continued)*
    - renal pelvis R93.41
    - retroperitoneum R93.5
    - site specified NEC R93.8
    - skin and subcutaneous tissue R93.8
    - skull R93.0
    - urinary organs specified NEC R93.49
    - ureter R93.41
  - direction, teeth, fully erupted M26.30
  - ear ossicles, acquired NEC H74.39-
    - ankylosis *—see* Ankylosis, ear ossicles
    - discontinuity *—see* Discontinuity, ossicles, ear
    - partial loss *—see* Loss, ossicles, ear (partial)
  - Ebstein Q22.5
  - echocardiogram R93.1
  - echoencephalogram R90.81
  - echogram *—see* Abnormal, diagnostic imaging
  - electrocardiogram [ECG] [EKG] R94.31
  - electroencephalogram [EEG] R94.01
  - electrolyte *—see* Imbalance, electrolyte
  - electromyogram [EMG] R94.131
  - electro-oculogram [EOG] R94.110
  - electrophysiological intracardiac studies R94.39
  - electroretinogram [ERG] R94.111
  - erythrocytes
    - congenital, with perinatal jaundice D58.9
  - feces (color) (contents) (mucus) R19.5
  - finding *—see* Findings, abnormal, without diagnosis
  - fluid
    - amniotic *—see* Abnormal, specimen, specified
    - cerebrospinal *—see* Abnormal, cerebrospinal fluid
    - peritoneal *—see* Abnormal, specimen, digestive organs
    - pleural *—see* Abnormal, specimen, respiratory organs
    - synovial *—see* Abnormal, specimen, specified
    - thorax (bronchial washings) (pleural fluid) *—see* Abnormal, specimen, respiratory organs
    - vaginal *—see* Abnormal, specimen, female genital organs
  - form
    - teeth K00.2
    - uterus *—see* Anomaly, uterus
  - function studies
    - auditory R94.120
    - bladder R94.8
    - brain R94.09
    - cardiovascular R94.30
    - ear R94.128
    - endocrine NEC R94.7
    - eye NEC R94.118
    - kidney R94.4
    - liver R94.5
    - nervous system
      - central NEC R94.09
      - peripheral NEC R94.138
    - pancreas R94.8
    - placenta R94.8
    - pulmonary R94.2
    - special senses NEC R94.128
    - spleen R94.8

Abnormal, abnormality, abnormalities *(continued)*
- function studies *(continued)*
  - thyroid R94.6
  - vestibular R94.121
- gait —*see* Gait
  - hysterical F44.4
- gastrin secretion E16.4
- globulin R77.1
  - cortisol-binding E27.8
  - thyroid-binding E07.89
- glomerular, minor (*see also* N00-N07 with fourth character .0) N05.0
- glucagon secretion E16.3
- glucose tolerance (test) (non-fasting) R73.09
- gravitational (G) forces or states (effect of) T75.81
- hair (color) (shaft) L67.9
  - specified NEC L67.8
- hard tissue formation in pulp (dental) K04.3
- head movement R25.0
- heart
  - rate R00.9
    - specified NEC R00.8
  - shadow R93.1
  - sounds NEC R01.2
- hemoglobin (disease) —*see also* Disease, hemoglobin D58.2
  - trait —*see* Trait, hemoglobin, abnormal
- histology NEC R89.7
- immunological findings R89.4
  - in serum R76.9
    - specified NEC R76.8
- increase in appetite R63.2
- involuntary movement —*see* Abnormal, movement, involuntary
- jaw closure M26.51
- karyotype R89.8
- kidney function test R94.4
- knee jerk R29.2
- leukocyte (cell) (differential) NEC D72.9
- liver function test R94.5
- loss of
  - height R29.890
  - weight R63.4
- mammogram NEC R92.8
  - calcification (calculus) R92.1
  - microcalcification R92.0
- Mantoux test R76.11
- movement (disorder) —*see also* Disorder, movement
  - head R25.0
  - involuntary R25.9
    - fasciculation R25.3
    - of head R25.0
    - spasm R25.2
    - specified type NEC R25.8
    - tremor R25.1
- myoglobin (Aberdeen) (Annapolis) R89.7
- neonatal screening P09
- oculomotor study R94.113
- palmar creases Q82.8
- Papanicolaou (smear)
  - anus R85.619
    - atypical squamous cells cannot exclude high grade squamous intraepithelial lesion (ASC-H) R85.611
    - atypical squamous cells of undetermined significance (ASC-US) R85.610
    - cytologic evidence of malignancy R85.614
    - high grade squamous intraepithelial lesion (HGSIL) R85.613

Abnormal, abnormality, abnormalities *(continued)*
- Papanicolaou *(continued)*
  - anus *(continued)*
    - human papillomavirus (HPV) DNA test
      - high risk positive R85.81
      - low risk postive R85.82
    - inadequate smear R85.615
    - low grade squamous intraepithelial lesion (LGSIL) R85.612
    - satisfactory anal smear but lacking transformation zone R85.616
    - specified NEC R85.618
    - unsatisfactory smear R85.615
  - bronchial washings R84.6
  - cerebrospinal fluid R83.6
  - cervix R87.619
    - atypical squamous cells cannot exclude high grade squamous intraepithelial lesion (ASC-H) R87.611
    - atypical squamous cells of undetermined significance (ASC-US) R87.610
    - cytologic evidence of malignancy R87.614
    - high grade squamous intraepithelial lesion (HGSIL) R87.613
    - inadequate smear R87.615
    - low grade squamous intraepithelial lesion (LGSIL) R87.612
    - non-atypical endometrial cells R87.618
    - satisfactory cervical smear but lacking transformation zone R87.616
    - specified NEC R87.618
    - thin preparaton R87.619
    - unsatisfactory smear R87.615
  - nasal secretions R84.6
  - nipple discharge R89.6
  - peritoneal fluid R85.69
  - pleural fluid R84.6
  - prostatic secretions R86.6
  - saliva R85.69
  - seminal fluid R86.6
  - sites NEC R89.6
  - sputum R84.6
  - synovial fluid R89.6
  - throat scrapings R84.6
  - vagina R87.629
    - atypical squamous cells cannot exclude high grade squamous intraepithelial lesion (ASC-H) R87.621
    - atypical squamous cells of undetermined significance (ASC-US) R87.620
    - cytologic evidence of malignancy R87.624
    - high grade squamous intraepithelial lesion (HGSIL) R87.623
    - inadequate smear R87.625
    - low grade squamous intraepithelial lesion (LGSIL) R87.622
    - specified NEC R87.628
    - thin preparation R87.629
    - unsatisfactory smear R87.625
  - vulva R87.69
  - wound secretions R89.6
- partial thromboplastin time (PTT) R79.1
- pelvis (bony) —*see* Deformity, pelvis

Abnormal, abnormality, abnormalities *(continued)*
- percussion, chest (tympany) R09.89
- periods (grossly) —*see* Menstruation
- phonocardiogram R94.39
- plantar reflex R29.2
- plasma
  - protein R77.9
    - specified NEC R77.8
  - viscosity R70.1
- pleural (folds) Q34.0
- posture R29.3
- product of conception O02.9
  - specified type NEC O02.89
- prothrombin time (PT) R79.1
- pulmonary
  - artery, congenital Q25.79
  - function, newborn P28.89
  - test results R94.2
- pulsations in neck R00.2
- pupillary H21.56-
  - function (reaction) (reflex) —*see* Anomaly, pupil, function
- radiological examination —*see* Abnormal, diagnostic imaging
- red blood cell(s) (morphology) (volume) R71.8
- reflex —*see* Reflex
- renal function test R94.4
- response to nerve stimulation R94.130
- retinal correspondence H53.31
- retinal function study R94.111
- rhythm, heart —*see also* Arrhythmia
- saliva —*see* Abnormal, specimen, digestive organs
- scan
  - kidney R94.4
  - liver R93.2
  - thyroid R94.6
- secretion
  - gastrin E16.4
  - glucagon E16.3
- semen, seminal fluid —*see* Abnormal, specimen, male genital organs
- serum level (of)
  - acid phosphatase R74.8
  - alkaline phosphatase R74.8
  - amylase R74.8
  - enzymes R74.9
    - specified NEC R74.8
  - lipase R74.8
  - triacylglycerol lipase R74.8
- shape
  - gravid uterus —*see* Anomaly, uterus
- sinus venosus Q21.1
- size, tooth, teeth K00.2
- spacing, tooth, teeth, fully erupted M26.30
- specimen
  - digestive organs (peritoneal fluid) (saliva) R85.9
    - cytology R85.69
    - drug level R85.2
    - enzyme level R85.0
    - histology R85.7
    - hormones R85.1
    - immunology R85.4
    - microbiology R85.5
    - nonmedicinal level R85.3
    - specified type NEC R85.89
  - female genital organs (secretions) (smears) R87.9
    - cytology R87.69
      - cervix R87.619
        - human papillomavirus (HPV) DNA test
          - high risk positive R87.810
          - low risk positive R87.820

Abnormal, abnormality, abnormalities *(continued)*
- specimen *(continued)*
  - female genital organs *(continued)*
    - cytology *(continued)*
      - cervix *(continued)*
        - inadequate (unsatisfactory) smear R87.615
        - non-atypical endometrial cells R87.618
        - specified NEC R87.618
      - vagina R87.629
        - human papillomavirus (HPV) DNA test
          - high risk positive R87.811
          - low risk positive R87.821
        - inadequate (unsatisfactory) smear R87.625
      - vulva R87.69
    - drug level R87.2
    - enzyme level R87.0
    - histological R87.7
    - hormones R87.1
    - immunology R87.4
    - microbiology R87.5
    - nonmedicinal level R87.3
    - specified type NEC R87.89
  - male genital organs (prostatic secretions) (semen) R86.9
    - cytology R86.6
    - drug level R86.2
    - enzyme level R86.0
    - histological R86.7
    - hormones R86.1
    - immunology R86.4
    - microbiology R86.5
    - nonmedicinal level R86.3
    - specified type NEC R86.8
  - nipple discharge —*see* Abnormal, specimen, specified
  - respiratory organs (bronchial washings) (nasal secretions) (pleural fluid) (sputum) R84.9
    - cytology R84.6
    - drug level R84.2
    - enzyme level R84.0
    - histology R84.7
    - hormones R84.1
    - immunology R84.4
    - microbiology R84.5
    - nonmedicinal level R84.3
    - specified type NEC R84.8
  - specified organ, system and tissue NOS R89.9
    - cytology R89.6
    - drug level R89.2
    - enzyme level R89.0
    - histology R89.7
    - hormones R89.1
    - immunology R89.4
    - microbiology R89.5
    - nonmedicinal level R89.3
    - specified type NEC R89.8
  - synovial fluid —*see* Abnormal, specimen, specified
  - thorax (bronchial washings) (pleural fluids) —*see* Abnormal, specimen, respiratory organs
  - vagina (secretion) (smear) R87.629
  - vulva (secretion) (smear) R87.69
  - wound secretion —*see* Abnormal, specimen, specified
- spermatozoa —*see* Abnormal, specimen, male genital organs
- sputum (amount) (color) (odor) R09.3
- stool (color) (contents) (mucus) R19.5
  - bloody K92.1
  - guaiac positive R19.5
- synchondrosis Q78.8

Abnormal, abnormality, abnormalities *(continued)*
thermography —*see also* Abnormal, diagnostic imaging R93.8
thyroid-binding globulin E07.89
tooth, teeth (form) (size) K00.2
toxicology (findings) R78.9
transport protein E88.09
tumor marker NEC R97.8
ultrasound results —*see* Abnormal, diagnostic imaging
umbilical cord complicating delivery O69.9
urination NEC R39.198
urine (constituents) R82.90
bile R82.2
cytological examination R82.8
drugs R82.5
fat R82.0
glucose R81
heavy metals R82.6
hemoglobin R82.3
histological examination R82.8
ketones R82.4
microbiological examination (culture) R82.79
myoglobin R82.1
positive culture R82.79
protein —*see* Proteinuria
specified substance NEC R82.99
chromoabnormality NEC R82.91
substances nonmedical R82.6
uterine hemorrhage —*see* Hemorrhage, uterus
vectorcardiogram R94.39
visually evoked potential (VEP) R94.112
white blood cells D72.9
specified NEC D72.89
X-ray examination —*see* Abnormal, diagnostic imaging

Abnormity (any organ or part) —*see* Anomaly

Abocclusion M26.29
hemolytic disease (newborn) P55.1
incompatibility reaction ABO —*see* Complication(s), transfusion, incompatibility reaction, ABO

Abolition, language R48.8

Aborter, habitual or recurrent —*see* Loss (of), pregnancy, recurrent

Abortion (complete) (spontaneous) O03.9
with
retained products of conception —*see* Abortion, incomplete
attempted (elective) (failed) O07.4
complicated by O07.30
afibrinogenemia O07.1
cardiac arrest O07.36
chemical damage of pelvic organ(s) O07.34
circulatory collapse O07.31
cystitis O07.38
defibrination syndrome O07.1
electrolyte imbalance O07.33
embolism (air) (amniotic fluid) (blood clot) (fat) (pulmonary) (septic) (soap) O07.2
endometritis O07.0
genital tract and pelvic infection O07.0
hemolysis O07.1
hemorrhage (delayed) (excessive) O07.1
infection
genital tract or pelvic O07.0
urinary tract tract O07.38
intravascular coagulation O07.1

Abortion *(continued)*
attempted *(continued)*
complicated by *(continued)*
laceration of pelvic organ(s) O07.34
metabolic disorder O07.33
oliguria O07.32
oophoritis O07.0
parametritis O07.0
pelvic peritonitis O07.0
perforation of pelvic organ(s) O07.34
renal failure or shutdown O07.32
salpingitis or salpingo-oophoritis O07.0
sepsis O07.37
shock O07.31
specified condition NEC O07.39
tubular necrosis (renal) O07.32
uremia O07.32
urinary tract infection O07.38
venous complication NEC O07.35
embolism (air) (amniotic fluid) (blood clot) (fat) (pulmonary) (septic) (soap) O07.2
complicated (by) (following) O03.80
afibrinogenemia O03.6
cardiac arrest O03.86
chemical damage of pelvic organ(s) O03.84
circulatory collapse O03.81
cystitis O03.88
defibrination syndrome O03.6
electrolyte imbalance O03.83
embolism (air) (amniotic fluid) (blood clot) (fat) (pulmonary) (septic) (soap) O03.7
endometritis O03.5
genital tract and pelvic infection O03.5
hemolysis O03.6
hemorrhage (delayed) (excessive) O03.6
infection
genital tract or pelvic O03.5
urinary tract O03.88
intravascular coagulation O03.6
laceration of pelvic organ(s) O03.84
metabolic disorder O03.83
oliguria O03.82
oophoritis O03.5
parametritis O03.5
pelvic peritonitis O03.5
perforation of pelvic organ(s) O03.84
renal failure or shutdown O03.82
salpingitis or salpingo-oophoritis O03.5
sepsis O03.87
shock O03.81
specified condition NEC O03.89
tubular necrosis (renal) O03.82
uremia O03.82
urinary tract infection O03.88
venous complication NEC O03.85
embolism (air) (amniotic fluid) (blood clot) (fat) (pulmonary) (septic) (soap) O03.7
failed —*see* Abortion, attempted
habitual or recurrent N96
with current abortion —*see* categories O03-O04
without current pregnancy N96
care in current pregnancy O26.2-
incomplete (spontaneous) O03.4
complicated (by) (following) O03.30

Abortion *(continued)*
incomplete *(continued)*
complicated *(continued)*
afibrinogenemia O03.1
cardiac arrest O03.36
chemical damage of pelvic organ(s) O03.34
circulatory collapse O03.31
cystitis O03.38
defibrination syndrome O03.1
electrolyte imbalance O03.33
embolism (air) (amniotic fluid) (blood clot) (fat) (pulmonary) (septic) (soap) O03.2
endometritis O03.0
genital tract and pelvic infection O03.0
hemolysis O03.1
hemorrhage (delayed) (excessive) O03.1
infection
genital tract or pelvic O03.0
urinary tract O03.38
intravascular coagulation O03.1
laceration of pelvic organ(s) O03.34
metabolic disorder O03.33
oliguria O03.32
oophoritis O03.0
parametritis O03.0
pelvic peritonitis O03.0
perforation of pelvic organ(s) O03.34
renal failure or shutdown O03.32
salpingitis or salpingo-oophoritis O03.0
sepsis O03.37
shock O03.31
specified condition NEC O03.39
tubular necrosis (renal) O03.32
uremia O03.32
urinary infection O03.38
venous complication NEC O03.35
embolism (air) (amniotic fluid) (blood clot) (fat) (pulmonary) (septic) (soap) O03.2
induced (encounter for) Z33.2
complicated by O04.80
afibrinogenemia O04.6
cardiac arrest O04.86
chemical damage of pelvic organ(s) O04.84
circulatory collapse O04.81
cystitis O04.88
defibrination syndrome O04.6
electrolyte imbalance O04.83
embolism (air) (amniotic fluid) (blood clot) (fat) (pulmonary) (septic) (soap) O04.7
endometritis O04.5
genital tract and pelvic infection O04.5
hemolysis O04.6
hemorrhage (delayed) (excessive) O04.6
infection
genital tract or pelvic O04.5
urinary tract O04.88
intravascular coagulation O04.6
laceration of pelvic organ(s) O04.84
metabolic disorder O04.83
oliguria O04.82
oophoritis O04.5
parametritis O04.5
pelvic peritonitis O04.5

Abortion *(continued)*
induced *(continued)*
complicated by *(continued)*
perforation of pelvic organ(s) O04.84
renal failure or shutdown O04.82
salpingitis or salpingo-oophoritis O04.5
sepsis O04.87
shock O04.81
specified condition NEC O04.89
tubular necrosis (renal) O04.82
uremia O04.82
urinary tract infection O04.88
venous complication NEC O04.85
embolism (air) (amniotic fluid) (blood clot) (fat) (pulmonary) (septic) (soap) O04.7
missed O02.1
spontaneous —*see* Abortion (complete) (spontaneous)
threatened O20.0
threatened (spontaneous) O20.0
tubal O00.10-
with intrauterine pregnancy O00.11-

Abortus fever A23.1

Aboulomania F60.7

Abrami's disease D59.8

Abramov-Fiedler myocarditis (acute isolated myocarditis) I40.1

Abrasion T14.8
abdomen, abdominal (wall) S30.811
alveolar process S00.512
ankle S90.51-
antecubital space —*see* Abrasion, elbow
anus S30.817
arm (upper) S40.81-
auditory canal —*see* Abrasion, ear
auricle —*see* Abrasion, ear
axilla —*see* Abrasion, arm
back, lower S30.810
breast S20.11-
brow S00.81
buttock S30.810
calf —*see* Abrasion, leg
canthus —*see* Abrasion, eyelid
cheek S00.81
internal S00.512
chest wall —*see* Abrasion, thorax
chin S00.81
clitoris S30.814
cornea S05.0-
costal region —*see* Abrasion, thorax
dental K03.1
digit(s)
foot —*see* Abrasion, toe
hand —*see* Abrasion, finger
ear S00.41-
elbow S50.31-
epididymis S30.813
epigastric region S30.811
epiglottis S10.11
esophagus (thoracic) S27.818
cervical S10.11
eyebrow —*see* Abrasion, eyelid
eyelid S00.21-
face S00.81
finger(s) S60.41-
index S60.41-
little S60.41-
middle S60.41-
ring S60.41-
flank S30.811
foot (except toe(s) alone) S90.81-
toe —*see* Abrasion, toe

Abrasion *(continued)*
- forearm S50.81-
  - elbow only *—see* Abrasion, elbow
- forehead S00.81
- genital organs, external
  - female S30.816
  - male S30.815
- groin S30.811
- gum S00.512
- hand S60.51-
- head S00.91
  - ear *—see* Abrasion, ear
  - eyelid *—see* Abrasion, eyelid
  - lip S00.511
  - nose S00.31
  - oral cavity S00.512
  - scalp S00.01
  - specified site NEC S00.81
- heel *—see* Abrasion, foot
- hip S70.21-
- inguinal region S30.811
- interscapular region S20.419
- jaw S00.81
- knee S80.21-
- labium (majus) (minus) S30.814
- larynx S10.11
- leg (lower) S80.81-
  - knee *—see* Abrasion, knee
  - upper *—see* Abrasion, thigh
- lip S00.511
- lower back S30.810
- lumbar region S30.810
- malar region S00.81
- mammary *—see* Abrasion, breast
- mastoid region S00.81
- mouth S00.512
- nail
  - finger *—see* Abrasion, finger
  - toe *—see* Abrasion, toe
- nape S10.81
- nasal S00.31
- neck S10.91
  - specified site NEC S10.81
  - throat S10.11
- nose S00.31
- occipital region S00.01
- oral cavity S00.512
- orbital region *—see* Abrasion, eyelid
- palate S00.512
- palm *—see* Abrasion, hand
- parietal region S00.01
- pelvis S30.810
- penis S30.812
- perineum
  - female S30.814
  - male S30.810
- periocular area *—see* Abrasion, eyelid
- phalanges
  - finger *—see* Abrasion, finger
  - toe *—see* Abrasion, toe
- pharynx S10.11
- pinna *—see* Abrasion, ear
- popliteal space *—see* Abrasion, knee
- prepuce S30.812
- pubic region S30.810
- pudendum
  - female S30.816
  - male S30.815
- sacral region S30.810
- scalp S00.01
- scapular region *—see* Abrasion, shoulder
- scrotum S30.813
- shin *—see* Abrasion, leg
- shoulder S40.21-
- skin NEC T14.8
- sternal region S20.319
- submaxillary region S00.81
- submental region S00.81
- subungual
  - finger(s) *—see* Abrasion, finger
  - toe(s) *—see* Abrasion, toe
- supraclavicular fossa S10.81
- supraorbital S00.81
- temple S00.81
- temporal region S00.81
- testis S30.813
- thigh S70.31-
- thorax, thoracic (wall) S20.91
  - back S20.41-
  - front S20.31-
- throat S10.11
- thumb S60.31-
- toe(s) (lesser) S90.416
  - great S90.41-
- tongue S00.512
- tooth, teeth (dentifrice) (habitual) (hard tissues) (occupational) (ritual) (traditional) K03.1
- trachea S10.11
- tunica vaginalis S30.813
- tympanum, tympanic membrane *—see* Abrasion, ear
- uvula S00.512
- vagina S30.814
- vocal cords S10.11
- vulva S30.814
- wrist S60.81-

Abrism *—see* Poisoning, food, noxious, plant

Abruptio placentae O45.9-
- with
  - afibrinogenemia O45.01-
  - coagulation defect O45.00-
    - specified NEC O45.09-
  - disseminated intravascular coagulation O45.02-
  - hypofibrinogenemia O45.01-
- specified NEC O45.8-

Abruption, placenta *—see* Abruptio placentae

Abscess (connective tissue) (embolic) (fistulous) (infective) (metastatic) (multiple) (pernicious) (pyogenic) (septic) L02.91
- with
  - diverticular disease (intestine) K57.80
    - with bleeding K57.81
    - large intestine K57.20
      - with
        - bleeding K57.21
        - small intestine K57.40
          - with bleeding K57.41
    - small intestine K57.00
      - with
        - bleeding K57.01
        - large intestine K57.40
          - with bleeding K57.41
  - lymphangitis - code by site under Abscess
- abdomen, abdominal
  - cavity K65.1
  - wall L02.211
- abdominopelvic K65.1
- accessory sinus *—see* Sinusitis
- adrenal (capsule) (gland) E27.8
- alveolar K04.7
  - with sinus K04.6
- amebic A06.4
  - brain (and liver or lung abscess) A06.6
  - genitourinary tract A06.82
  - liver (without mention of brain or lung abscess) A06.4
  - lung (and liver) (without mention of brain abscess) A06.5
  - specified site NEC A06.89
  - spleen A06.89

Abscess *(continued)*
- anerobic A48.0
- ankle *—see* Abscess, lower limb
- anorectal K61.2
- antecubital space *—see* Abscess, upper limb
- antrum (chronic) (Highmore) *—see* Sinusitis, maxillary
- anus K61.0
- apical (tooth) K04.7
  - with sinus (alveolar) K04.6
- appendix K35.3
- areola (acute) (chronic) (nonpuerperal) N61.1
  - puerperal, postpartum or gestational *—see* Infection, nipple
- arm (any part) *—see* Abscess, upper limb
- artery (wall) I77.89
- atheromatous I77.2
- auricle, ear *—see* Abscess, ear, external
- axilla (region) L02.41-
  - lymph gland or node L04.2
- back (any part, except buttock) L02.212
- Bartholin's gland N75.1
  - with
    - abortion *—see* Abortion, by type complicated by, sepsis
    - ectopic or molar pregnancy O08.0
  - following ectopic or molar pregnancy O08.0
- Bezold's *—see* Mastoiditis, acute
- bilharziasis B65.1
- bladder (wall) *—see* Cystitis, specified type NEC
- bone (subperiosteal) *—see also* Osteomyelitis, specified type NEC
  - accessory sinus (chronic) *—see* Sinusitis
  - chronic or old *—see* Osteomyelitis, chronic
  - jaw (lower) (upper) M27.2
  - mastoid *—see* Mastoiditis, acute, subperiosteal
  - petrous *—see* Petrositis
  - spinal (tuberculous) A18.01
    - nontuberculous *—see* Osteomyelitis, vertebra
- bowel K63.0
- brain (any part) (cystic) (otogenic) G06.0
  - amebic (with abscess of any other site) A06.6
  - gonococcal A54.82
  - pheomycotic (chromomycotic) B43.1
  - tuberculous A17.81
- breast (acute) (chronic) (nonpuerperal) N61.1
  - newborn P39.0
  - puerperal, postpartum, gestational *—see* Mastitis, obstetric, purulent
- broad ligament N73.2
  - acute N73.0
  - chronic N73.1
- Brodie's (localized) (chronic) M86.8X-
- bronchi J98.09
- buccal cavity K12.2
- bulbourethral gland N34.0
- bursa M71.00
  - ankle M71.07-
  - elbow M71.02-
  - foot M71.07-
  - hand M71.04-
  - hip M71.05-

Abscess *(continued)*
- bursa *(continued)*
  - knee M71.06-
  - multiple sites M71.09
  - pharyngeal J39.1
  - shoulder M71.01-
  - specified site NEC M71.08
  - wrist M71.03-
- buttock L02.31
- canthus *—see* Blepharoconjunctivitis
- cartilage *—see* Disorder, cartilage, specified type NEC
- cecum K35.3
- cerebellum, cerebellar G06.0
  - sequelae G09
- cerebral (embolic) G06.0
  - sequelae G09
- cervical (meaning neck) L02.11
  - lymph gland or node L04.0
- cervix (stump) (uteri) *—see* Cervicitis
- cheek (external) L02.01
  - inner K12.2
- chest J86.9
  - with fistula J86.0
  - wall L02.213
- chin L02.01
- choroid *—see* Inflammation, chorioretinal
- circumtonsillar J36
- cold (lung) (tuberculous) *—see also* Tuberculosis, abscess, lung
  - articular *—see* Tuberculosis, joint
- colon (wall) K63.0
- colostomy K94.02
- conjunctiva *—see* Conjunctivitis, acute
- cornea H16.31-
- corpus
  - cavernosum N48.21
  - luteum *—see* Oophoritis
- Cowper's gland N34.0
- cranium G06.0
- cul-de-sac (Douglas') (posterior) *—see* Peritonitis, pelvic, female
- cutaneous *—see* Abscess, by site
- dental K04.7
  - with sinus (alveolar) K04.6
- dentoalveolar K04.7
  - with sinus K04.6
- diaphragm, diaphragmatic K65.1
- Douglas' cul-de-sac or pouch *—see* Peritonitis, pelvic, female
- Dubois A50.59
- ear (middle) *—see also* Otitis, media, suppurative
  - acute *—see* Otitis, media, suppurative, acute
  - external H60.0-
- entamebic *—see* Abscess, amebic
- enterostomy K94.12
- epididymis N45.4
- epidural G06.2
  - brain G06.0
  - spinal cord G06.1
- epiglottis J38.7
- epiploon, epiploic K65.1
- erysipelatous *—see* Erysipelas
- esophagus K20.8
- ethmoid (bone) (chronic) (sinus) J32.2
- external auditory canal *—see* Abscess, ear, external
- extradural G06.2
  - brain G06.0
    - sequelae G09
  - spinal cord G06.1
- extraperitoneal K68.19
- eye *—see* Endophthalmitis, purulent
- eyelid H00.03-

Abscess *(continued)*
- face (any part, except ear, eye and nose) L02.01
- fallopian tube —*see* Salpingitis
- fascia M72.8
- fauces J39.1
- fecal K63.0
- femoral (region) —*see* Abscess, lower limb
- filaria, filarial —*see* Infestation, filarial
- finger (any) —*see also* Abscess, hand
  - nail —*see* Cellulitis, finger
- foot L02.61-
- forehead L02.01
- frontal sinus (chronic) J32.1
- gallbladder K81.0
- genital organ or tract
  - female (external) N76.4
  - male N49.9
    - multiple sites N49.8
    - specified NEC N49.8
- gestational mammary O91.11-
- gestational subareolar O91.11-
- gingival — *see* Peridontitis, aggressive, localized
- gland, glandular (lymph) (acute) —*see* Lymphadenitis, acute
- gluteal (region) L02.31
- gonorrheal —*see* Gonococcus
- groin L02.214
- gum — *see* Peridontitis, aggressive, localized
- hand L02.51-
- head NEC L02.811
  - face (any part, except ear, eye and nose) L02.01
- heart —*see* Carditis
- heel —*see* Abscess, foot
- helminthic —*see* Infestation, helminth
- hepatic (cholangitic) (hematogenic) (lymphogenic) (pylephlebitic) K75.0
  - amebic A06.4
- hip (region) —*see* Abscess, lower limb
- ileocecal K35.3
- ileostomy (bud) K94.12
- iliac (region) L02.214
  - fossa K35.3
- infraclavicular (fossa) —*see* Abscess, upper limb
- inguinal (region) L02.214
  - lymph gland or node L04.1
- intestine, intestinal NEC K63.0
  - rectal K61.1
- intra-abdominal (*see also* Abscess, peritoneum) K65.1
  - postprocedural T81.4
    - retroperitoneal K68.11
- intracranial G06.0
- intramammary —*see* Abscess, breast
- intraorbital —*see* Abscess, orbit
- intraperitoneal K65.1
- intrasphincteric (anus) K61.4
- intraspinal G06.1
- intratonsillar J36
- ischiorectal (fossa) K61.3
- jaw (bone) (lower) (upper) M27.2
- joint —*see* Arthritis, pyogenic or pyemic
  - spine (tuberculous) A18.01
    - nontuberculous —*see* Spondylopathy, infective
- kidney N15.1
  - with calculus N20.0
    - with hydronephrosis N13.6
  - puerperal (postpartum) O86.21
- knee —*see also* Abscess, lower limb
  - joint M00.9

Abscess *(continued)*
- labium (majus) (minus) N76.4
- lacrimal
  - caruncle —*see* Inflammation, lacrimal, passages, acute
  - gland —*see* Dacryoadenitis
  - passages (duct) (sac) —*see* Inflammation, lacrimal, passages, acute
- lacunar N34.0
- larynx J38.7
- lateral (alveolar) K04.7
  - with sinus K04.6
- leg (any part) —*see* Abscess, lower limb
- lens H27.8
- lingual K14.0
  - tonsil J36
- lip K13.0
- Littre's gland N34.0
- liver (cholangitic) (hematogenic) (lymphogenic) (pylephlebitic) (pyogenic) K75.0
  - amebic (due to Entamoeba histolytica) (dysenteric) (tropical) A06.4
    - with
      - brain abscess (and liver or lung abscess) A06.6
      - lung abscess A06.5
- loin (region) L02.211
- lower limb L02.41-
- lumbar (tuberculous) A18.01
  - nontuberculous L02.212
- lung (miliary) (putrid) J85.2
  - with pneumonia J85.1
    - due to specified organism (*see* Pneumonia, in (due to))
  - amebic (with liver abscess) A06.5
    - with
      - brain abscess A06.6
      - pneumonia A06.5
- lymph, lymphatic, gland or node (acute) —*see also* Lymphadenitis, acute
  - mesentery I88.0
- malar M27.2
- mammary gland —*see* Abscess, breast
- marginal, anus K61.0
- mastoid —*see* Mastoiditis, acute
- maxilla, maxillary M27.2
  - molar (tooth) K04.7
    - with sinus K04.6
  - premolar K04.7
  - sinus (chronic) J32.0
- mediastinum J85.3
- meibomian gland —*see* Hordeolum
- meninges G06.2
- mesentery, mesenteric K65.1
- mesosalpinx —*see* Salpingitis
- mons pubis L02.215
- mouth (floor) K12.2
- muscle —*see* Myositis, infective
- myocardium I40.0
- nabothian (follicle) —*see* Cervicitis
- nasal J32.9
- nasopharyngeal J39.1
- navel L02.216
  - newborn P38.9
    - with mild hemorrhage P38.1
    - without hemorrhage P38.9
- neck (region) L02.11
  - lymph gland or node L04.0
- nephritic —*see* Abscess, kidney
- nipple N61.1
  - associated with
    - lactation —*see* Pregnancy, complicated by

Abscess *(continued)*
- nipple *(continued)*
  - associated with *(continued)*
    - pregnancy —*see* Pregnancy, complicated by
- nose (external) (fossa) (septum) J34.0
  - sinus (chronic) —*see* Sinusitis
- omentum K65.1
- operative wound T81.4
- orbit, orbital —*see* Cellulitis, orbit
- otogenic G06.0
- ovary, ovarian (corpus luteum) —*see* Oophoritis
- oviduct —*see* Oophoritis
- palate (soft) K12.2
  - hard M27.2
- palmar (space) —*see* Abscess, hand
- pancreas (duct) —*see* Pancreatitis, acute
- parafrenal N48.21
- parametric, parametrium N73.2
  - acute N73.0
  - chronic N73.1
- paranephric N15.1
- parapancreatic —*see* Pancreatitis, acute
- parapharyngeal J39.0
- pararectal K61.1
- parasinus —*see* Sinusitis
- parauterine —*see also* Disease, pelvis, inflammatory N73.2
- paravaginal —*see* Vaginitis
- parietal region (scalp) L02.811
- parodontal —*see* Peridontitis, aggressive, localized
- parotid (duct) (gland) K11.3
  - region K12.2
- pectoral (region) L02.213
- pelvis, pelvic
  - female —*see* Disease, pelvis, inflammatory
  - male, peritoneal K65.1
- penis N48.21
  - gonococcal (accessory gland) (periurethral) A54.1
- perianal K61.0
- periapical K04.7
  - with sinus (alveolar) K04.6
- periappendicular K35.3
- pericardial I30.1
- pericecal K35.3
- pericemental —*see* Peridontitis, aggressive, localized
- pericholecystic —*see* Cholecystitis, acute
- pericoronal —*see* Peridontitis, aggressive, localized
- peridental —*see* Peridontitis, aggressive, localized
- perimetric —*see also* Disease, pelvis, inflammatory N73.2
- perinephric, perinephritic —*see* Abscess, kidney
- perineum, perineal (superficial) L02.215
  - urethra N34.0
- periodontal (parietal) —*see* Peridontitis, aggressive, localized
  - apical K04.7
- periosteum, periosteal —*see also* Osteomyelitis, specified type NEC
  - with osteomyelitis —*see also* Osteomyelitis, specified type NEC
    - acute —*see* Osteomyelitis, acute
    - chronic —*see* Osteomyelitis, chronic
- peripharyngeal J39.0
- peripleuritic J86.9
  - with fistula J86.0

Abscess *(continued)*
- periprostatic N41.2
- perirectal K61.1
- perirenal (tissue) —*see* Abscess, kidney
- perisinuous (nose) —*see* Sinusitis
- peritoneum, peritoneal (perforated) (ruptured) K65.1
  - with appendicitis K35.3
  - pelvic
    - female —*see* Peritonitis, pelvic, female
    - male K65.1
  - postoperative T81.4
  - puerperal, postpartum, childbirth O85
  - tuberculous A18.31
- peritonsillar J36
- perityphlic K35.3
- periureteral N28.89
- periurethral N34.0
  - gonococcal (accessory gland) (periurethral) A54.1
- periuterine —*see also* Disease, pelvis, inflammatory N73.2
- perivesical —*see* Cystitis, specified type NEC
- petrous bone —*see* Petrositis
- phagedenic NOS L02.91
  - chancroid A57
- pharynx, pharyngeal (lateral) J39.1
- pilonidal L05.01
- pituitary (gland) E23.6
- pleura J86.9
  - with fistula J86.0
- popliteal —*see* Abscess, lower limb
- postcecal K35.3
- postlaryngeal J38.7
- postnasal J34.0
- postoperative (any site) T81.4
  - retroperitoneal K68.11
- postpharyngeal J39.0
- posttonsillar J36
- post-typhoid A01.09
- pouch of Douglas —*see* Peritonitis, pelvic, female
- premammary —*see* Abscess, breast
- prepatellar —*see* Abscess, lower limb
- prostate N41.2
  - gonococcal (acute) (chronic) A54.22
- psoas muscle K68.12
- puerperal - code by site under Puerperal, abscess
- pulmonary —*see* Abscess, lung
- pulp, pulpal (dental) K04.01
  - irreversible K04.02
  - reversible K04.01
- rectovaginal septum K63.0
- rectovesical —*see* Cystitis, specified type NEC
- rectum K61.1
- renal —*see* Abscess, kidney
- retina —*see* Inflammation, chorioretinal
- retrobulbar —*see* Abscess, orbit
- retrocecal K65.1
- retrolaryngeal J38.7
- retromammary —*see* Abscess, breast
- retroperitoneal NEC K68.19
  - postprocedural K68.11
- retropharyngeal J39.0
- retrouterine —*see* Peritonitis, pelvic, female
- retrovesical —*see* Cystitis, specified type NEC
- root, tooth K04.7
  - with sinus (alveolar) K04.6
- round ligament —*see also* Disease, pelvis, inflammatory N73.2

Abscess *(continued)*
- rupture (spontaneous) NOS L02.91
- sacrum (tuberculous) A18.01
  - nontuberculous M46.28
- salivary (duct) (gland) K11.3
- scalp (any part) L02.811
- scapular *—see* Osteomyelitis, specified type NEC
- sclera *—see* Scleritis
- scrofulous (tuberculous) A18.2
- scrotum N49.2
- seminal vesicle N49.0
- septal, dental K04.7
  - with sinus (alveolar) K04.6
- serous *—see* Periostitis
- shoulder (region) *—see* Abscess, upper limb
- sigmoid K63.0
- sinus (accessory) (chronic) (nasal) *—see also* Sinusitis
  - intracranial venous (any) G06.0
- Skene's duct or gland N34.0
- skin *—see* Abscess, by site
- specified site NEC L02.818
- spermatic cord N49.1
- sphenoidal (sinus) (chronic) J32.3
- spinal cord (any part) (staphylococcal) G06.1
  - tuberculous A17.81
- spine (column) (tuberculous) A18.01
  - epidural G06.1
  - nontuberculous *—see* Osteomyelitis, vertebra
- spleen D73.3
  - amebic A06.89
- stitch T81.4
- subarachnoid G06.2
  - brain G06.0
  - spinal cord G06.1
- subareolar *—see* Abscess, breast
- subcecal K35.3
- subcutaneous *—see also* Abscess, by site
  - pheomycotic (chromomycotic) B43.2
- subdiaphragmatic K65.1
- subdural G06.2
  - brain G06.0
    - sequelae G09
  - spinal cord G06.1
- subgaleal L02.811
- subhepatic K65.1
- sublingual K12.2
  - gland K11.3
- submammary *—see* Abscess, breast
- submandibular (region) (space) (triangle) K12.2
  - gland K11.3
- submaxillary (region) L02.01
  - gland K11.3
- submental L02.01
  - gland K11.3
- subperiosteal *—see* Osteomyelitis, specified type NEC
- subphrenic K65.1
  - postoperative T81.4
- suburethral N34.0
- sudoriparous L75.8
- supraclavicular (fossa) *—see* Abscess, upper limb
- suprapelvic, acute N73.0
- suprarenal (capsule) (gland) E27.8
- sweat gland L74.8
- tear duct *—see* Inflammation, lacrimal, passages, acute
- temple L02.01
- temporal region L02.01
- temporosphenoidal G06.0
- tendon (sheath) M65.00
  - ankle M65.07-
  - foot M65.07-

Abscess *(continued)*
- tendon *(continued)*
  - forearm M65.03-
  - hand M65.04-
  - lower leg M65.06-
  - pelvic region M65.05-
  - shoulder region M65.01-
  - specified site NEC M65.08
  - thigh M65.05-
  - upper arm M65.02-
- testis N45.4
- thigh *—see* Abscess, lower limb
- thorax J86.9
  - with fistula J86.0
- throat J39.1
- thumb *—see also* Abscess, hand
  - nail *—see* Cellulitis, finger
- thymus (gland) E32.1
- thyroid (gland) E06.0
- toe (any) *—see also* Abscess, foot
  - nail *—see* Cellulitis, toe
- tongue (staphylococcal) K14.0
- tonsil(s) (lingual) J36
- tonsillopharyngeal J36
- tooth, teeth (root) K04.7
  - with sinus (alveolar) K04.6
  - supporting structures NEC *— see* Peridontitis, aggressive, localized
- trachea J39.8
- trunk L02.219
  - abdominal wall L02.211
  - back L02.212
  - chest wall L02.213
  - groin L02.214
  - perineum L02.215
  - umbilicus L02.216
- tubal *—see* Salpingitis
- tuberculous *—see* Tuberculosis, abscess
- tubo-ovarian *—see* Salpingo-oophoritis
- tunica vaginalis N49.1
- umbilicus L02.216
- upper
  - limb L02.41-
  - respiratory J39.8
- urethral (gland) N34.0
- urinary N34.0
- uterus, uterine (wall) *—see also* Endometritis
  - ligament *—see also* Disease, pelvis, inflammatory N73.2
  - neck *—see* Cervicitis
- uvula K12.2
- vagina (wall) *—see* Vaginitis
- vaginorectal *—see* Vaginitis
- vas deferens N49.1
- vermiform appendix K35.3
- vertebra (column) (tuberculous) A18.01
  - nontuberculous *—see* Osteomyelitis, vertebra
- vesical *—see* Cystitis, specified type NEC
- vesico-uterine pouch *—see* Peritonitis, pelvic, female
- vitreous (humor) *—see* Endophthalmitis, purulent
- vocal cord J38.3
- von Bezold's *—see* Mastoiditis, acute
- vulva N76.4
- vulvovaginal gland N75.1
- web space *—see* Abscess, hand
- wound T81.4
- wrist *—see* Abscess, upper limb

Absence (of) (organ or part) (complete or partial)
- adrenal (gland) (congenital) Q89.1
  - acquired E89.6
- albumin in blood E88.09

Absence *(continued)*
- alimentary tract (congenital) Q45.8
  - upper Q40.8
- alveolar process (acquired) *—see* Anomaly, alveolar
- ankle (acquired) Z89.44-
- anus (congenital) Q42.3
  - with fistula Q42.2
- aorta (congenital) Q25.41
- appendix, congenital Q42.8
- arm (acquired) Z89.20-
  - above elbow Z89.22-
    - congenital (with hand present) *—see* Agenesis, arm, with hand present
      - and hand *—see* Agenesis, forearm, and hand
  - below elbow Z89.21-
    - congenital (with hand present) *—see* Agenesis, arm, with hand present
      - and hand *—see* Agenesis, forearm, and hand
  - congenital *—see* Defect, reduction, upper limb
  - shoulder (following explantation of shoulder joint prosthesis) (joint) (with or without presence of antibiotic-impregnated cement spacer) Z89.23-
    - congenital (with hand present) *—see* Agenesis, arm, with hand present
- artery (congenital) (peripheral) Q27.8
  - brain Q28.3
  - coronary Q24.5
  - pulmonary Q25.79
  - specified NEC Q27.8
  - umbilical Q27.0
- atrial septum (congenital) Q21.1
- auditory canal (congenital) (external) Q16.1
- auricle (ear), congenital Q16.0
- bile, biliary duct, congenital Q44.5
- bladder (acquired) Z90.6
  - congenital Q64.5
- bowel sounds R19.11
- brain Q00.0
  - part of Q04.3
- breast(s) (and nipple(s)) (acquired) Z90.1-
  - congenital Q83.8
- broad ligament Q50.6
- bronchus (congenital) Q32.4
- canaliculus lacrimalis, congenital Q10.4
- cerebellum (vermis) Q04.3
- cervix (acquired) (with uterus) Z90.710
  - with remaining uterus Z90.712
  - congenital Q51.5
- chin, congenital Q18.8
- cilia (congenital) Q10.3
  - acquired *—see* Madarosis
- clitoris (congenital) Q52.6
- coccyx, congenital Q76.49
- cold sense R20.8
- congenital
  - lumen *—see* Atresia
  - organ or site NEC *—see* Agenesis
  - septum *—see* Imperfect, closure
- corpus callosum Q04.0
- cricoid cartilage, congenital Q31,8
- diaphragm (with hernia), congenital Q79.1
- digestive organ(s) or tract, congenital Q45.8
  - acquired NEC Z90.49
  - upper Q40.8
- ductus arteriosus Q28.8

Absence *(continued)*
- duodenum (acquired) Z90.49
  - congenital Q41.0
- ear, congenital Q16.9
  - acquired H93.8-
  - auricle Q16.0
  - external Q16.0
  - inner Q16.5
  - lobe, lobule Q17.8
  - middle, except ossicles Q16.4
    - ossicles Q16.3
  - ossicles Q16.3
- ejaculatory duct (congenital) Q55.4
- endocrine gland (congenital) NEC Q89.2
  - acquired E89.89
- epididymis (congenital) Q55.4
  - acquired Z90.79
- epiglottis, congenital Q31.8
- esophagus (congenital) Q39.8
  - acquired (partial) Z90.49
- eustachian tube (congenital) Q16.2
- extremity (acquired) Z89.9
  - congenital Q73.0
  - knee (following explantation of knee joint prosthesis) (joint) (with or without presence of antibiotic-impregnated cement spacer) Z89.52-
  - lower (above knee) Z89.619
    - below knee Z89.51-
  - upper *—see* Absence, arm
- eye (acquired) Z90.01
  - congenital Q11.1
  - muscle (congenital) Q10.3
- eyeball (acquired) Z90.01
- eyelid (fold) (congenital) Q10.3
  - acquired Z90.01
- face, specified part NEC Q18.8
- fallopian tube(s) (acquired) Z90.79
  - congenital Q50.6
- family member (causing problem in home) NEC *—see also* Disruption, family Z63.32
- femur, congenital *—see* Defect, reduction, lower limb, longitudinal, femur
- fibrinogen (congenital) D68.2
  - acquired D65
- finger(s) (acquired) Z89.02-
  - congenital *—see* Agenesis, hand
- foot (acquired) Z89.43-
  - congenital *—see* Agenesis, foot
- forearm (acquired) *—see* Absence, arm, below elbow
- gallbladder (acquired) Z90.49
  - congenital Q44.0
- gamma globulin in blood D80.1
  - hereditary D80.0
- genital organs
  - acquired (female) (male) Z90.79
  - female, congenital Q52.8
    - external Q52.71
    - internal NEC Q52.8
  - male, congenital Q55.8
- genitourinary organs, congenital NEC
  - female Q52.8
  - male Q55.8
- globe (acquired) Z90.01
  - congenital Q11.1
- glottis, congenital Q31.8
- hand and wrist (acquired) Z89.11-
  - congenital *—see* Agenesis, hand
- head, part (acquired) NEC Z90.09
- heat sense R20.8
- hip (following explantation of hip joint prosthesis) (joint) (with or without presence of antibiotic-impregnated cement spacer) Z89.62-
- hymen (congenital) Q52.4

Absence *(continued)*
- ileum (acquired) Z90.49
  - congenital Q41.2
- immunoglobulin, isolated NEC D80.3
  - IgA D80.2
  - IgG D80.3
  - IgM D80.4
- incus (acquired) *—see* Loss, ossicles, ear
  - congenital Q16.3
- inner ear, congenital Q16.5
- intestine (acquired) (small) Z90.49
  - congenital Q41.9
    - specified NEC Q41.8
  - large Z90.49
    - congenital Q42.9
      - specified NEC Q42.8
- iris, congenital Q13.1
- jejunum (acquired) Z90.49
  - congenital Q41.1
- joint
  - acquired
    - hip (following explantation of hip joint prosthesis) (with or without presence of antibiotic-impregnated cement spacer) Z89.62-
    - knee (following explantation of knee joint prosthesis) (with or without presence of antibiotic-impregnated cement spacer) Z89.52-
    - shoulder (following explantation of shoulder joint prosthesis) (with or without presence of antibiotic-impregnated cement spacer) Z89.23-
  - congenital NEC Q74.8
- kidney(s) (acquired) Z90.5
  - congenital Q60.2
    - bilateral Q60.1
    - unilateral Q60.0
- knee (following explantation of knee joint prosthesis) (joint) (with or without presence of antibiotic-impregnated cement spacer) Z89.52-
- labyrinth, membranous Q16.5
- larynx (congenital) Q31.8
  - acquired Z90.02
- leg (acquired) (above knee) Z89.61-
  - below knee (acquired) Z89.51-
  - congenital *—see* Defect, reduction, lower limb
- lens (acquired) *—see also* Aphakia
  - congenital Q12.3
  - post cataract extraction Z98.4-
- limb (acquired) *—see* Absence, extremity
- lip Q38.6
- liver (congenital) Q44.7
- lung (fissure) (lobe) (bilateral) (unilateral) (congenital) Q33.3
  - acquired (any part) Z90.2
- menstruation *—see* Amenorrhea
- muscle (congenital) (pectoral) Q79.8
  - ocular Q10.3
- neck, part Q18.8
- neutrophil *—see* Agranulocytosis
- nipple(s) (with breast(s)) (acquired) Z90.1-
  - congenital Q83.2
- nose (congenital) Q30.1
  - acquired Z90.09
- organ
  - of Corti, congenital Q16.5
  - or site, congenital NEC Q89.8
    - acquired NEC Z90.89

Absence *(continued)*
- osseous meatus (ear) Q16.4
- ovary (acquired)
  - bilateral Z90.722
  - congenital
    - bilateral Q50.02
    - unilateral Q50.01
  - unilateral Z90.721
- oviduct (acquired)
  - bilateral Z90.722
  - congenital Q50.6
  - unilateral Z90.721
- pancreas (congenital) Q45.0
  - acquired Z90.410
    - complete Z90.410
    - partial Z90.411
    - total Z90.410
- parathyroid gland (acquired) E89.2
  - congenital Q89.2
- patella, congenital Q74.1
- penis (congenital) Q55.5
  - acquired Z90.79
- pericardium (congenital) Q24.8
- pituitary gland (congenital) Q89.2
  - acquired E89.3
- prostate (acquired) Z90.79
  - congenital Q55.4
- pulmonary valve Q22.0
- punctum lacrimale (congenital) Q10.4
- radius, congenital *—see* Defect, reduction, upper limb, longitudinal, radius
- rectum (congenital) Q42.1
  - with fistula Q42.0
  - acquired Z90.49
- respiratory organ NOS Q34.9
- rib (acquired) Z90.89
  - congenital Q76.6
- sacrum, congenital Q76.49
- salivary gland(s), congenital Q38.4
- scrotum, congenital Q55.29
- seminal vesicles (congenital) Q55.4
  - acquired Z90.79
- septum
  - atrial (congenital) Q21.1
  - between aorta and pulmonary artery Q21.4
  - ventricular (congenital) Q20.4
- sex chromosome
  - female phenotype Q97.8
  - male phenotype Q98.8
- skull bone (congenital) Q75.8
  - with
    - anencephaly Q00.0
    - encephalocele *—see* Encephalocele
    - hydrocephalus Q03.9
      - with spina bifida *—see* Spina bifida, by site, with hydrocephalus
    - microcephaly Q02
- spermatic cord, congenital Q55.4
- spine, congenital Q76.49
- spleen (congenital) Q89.01
  - acquired Z90.81
- sternum, congenital Q76.7
- stomach (acquired) (partial) Z90.3
  - congenital Q40.2
- superior vena cava, congenital Q26.8
- teeth, tooth (congenital) K00.0
  - acquired (complete) K08.109
    - class I K08.101
    - class II K08.102
    - class III K08.103
    - class IV K08.104
    - due to
      - caries K08.139
        - class I K08.131
        - class II K08.132
        - class III K08.133
        - class IV K08.134

Absence *(continued)*
- teeth, tooth *(continued)*
  - acquired *(continued)*
    - due to *(continued)*
      - periodontal disease K08.129
        - class I K08.121
        - class II K08.122
        - class III K08.123
        - class IV K08.124
      - specified NEC K08.199
        - class I K08.191
        - class II K08.192
        - class III K08.193
        - class IV K08.194
      - trauma K08.119
        - class I K08.111
        - class II K08.112
        - class III K08.113
        - class IV K08.114
    - partial K08.409
      - class I K08.401
      - class II K08.402
      - class III K08.403
      - class IV K08.404
      - due to
        - caries K08.439
          - class I K08.431
          - class II K08.432
          - class III K08.433
          - class IV K08.434
        - periodontal disease K08.429
          - class I K08.421
          - class II K08.422
          - class III K08.423
          - class IV K08.424
        - specified NEC K08.499
          - class I K08.491
          - class II K08.492
          - class III K08.493
          - class IV K08.494
        - trauma K08.419
          - class I K08.411
          - class II K08.412
          - class III K08.413
          - class IV K08.414
- tendon (congenital) Q79.8
- testis (congenital) Q55.0
  - acquired Z90.79
- thumb (acquired) Z89.01-
  - congenital *—see* Agenesis, hand
- thymus gland Q89.2
- thyroid (gland) (acquired) E89.0
  - cartilage, congenital Q31.8
  - congenital E03.1
- toe(s) (acquired) Z89.42-
  - with foot *—see* Absence, foot and ankle
  - congenital *—see* Agenesis, foot
  - great Z89.41-
- tongue, congenital Q38.3
- trachea (cartilage), congenital Q32.1
- transverse aortic arch, congenital Q25.49
- tricuspid valve Q22.4
- umbilical artery, congenital Q27.0
- upper arm and forearm with hand present, congenital *—see* Agenesis, arm, with hand present
- ureter (congenital) Q62.4
  - acquired Z90.6
- urethra, congenital Q64.5
- uterus (acquired) Z90.710
  - with cervix Z90.710
  - with remaining cervical stump Z90.711
  - congenital Q51.0
- uvula, congenital Q38.5
- vagina, congenital Q52.0
- vas deferens (congenital) Q55.4
  - acquired Z90.79

Absence *(continued)*
- vein (peripheral) congenital NEC Q27.8
  - cerebral Q28.3
  - digestive system Q27.8
  - great Q26.8
  - lower limb Q27.8
  - portal Q26.5
  - precerebral Q28.1
  - specified site NEC Q27.8
  - upper limb Q27.8
- vena cava (inferior) (superior), congenital Q26.8
- ventricular septum Q20.4
- vertebra, congenital Q76.49
- vulva, congenital Q52.71
- wrist (acquired) Z89.12-

Absorbent system disease I87.8

Absorption
- carbohydrate, disturbance K90.49
- chemical *—see* Table of Drugs and Chemicals
  - through placenta (newborn) P04.9
    - environmental substance P04.6
    - nutritional substance P04.5
    - obstetric anesthetic or analgesic drug P04.0
- drug NEC *—see* Table of Drugs and Chemicals
  - addictive
    - through placenta (newborn) P04.49
      - cocaine P04.41
  - medicinal
    - through placenta (newborn) P04.1
  - through placenta (newborn) P04.1
    - obstetric anesthetic or analgesic drug P04.0
- fat, disturbance K90.49
  - pancreatic K90.3
- noxious substance *—see* Table of Drugs and Chemicals
- protein, disturbance K90.49
- starch, disturbance K90.49
- toxic substance *—see* Table of Drugs and Chemicals
- uremic *—see* Uremia

Abstinence symptoms, syndrome
- alcohol F10.239
  - with delirium F10.231
- cocaine F14.23
- neonatal P96.1
- nicotine *—see* Dependence, drug, nicotine, with, withdrawal
- opioid F11.93
  - with dependence F11.23
- psychoactive NEC F19.939
  - with
    - delirium F19.931
    - dependence F19.239
      - with
        - delirium F19.231
        - perceptual disturbance F19.232
      - uncomplicated F19.230
    - perceptual disturbance F19.932
  - uncomplicated F19.930
- sedative F13.939
  - with
    - delirium F13.931
    - dependence F13.239
      - with
        - delirium F13.231
        - perceptual disturbance F13.232
      - uncomplicated F13.230
    - perceptual disturbance F13.932
  - uncomplicated F13.930
- stimulant NEC F15.93
  - with dependence F15.23

- **Abulia** R68.89
- **Abulomania** F60.7
- **Abuse**
  - adult —*see* Maltreatment, adult
    - as reason for
      - couple see king advice (including offender) Z63.0
  - alcohol (non-dependent) F10.10
    - with
      - anxiety disorder F10.180
      - intoxication F10.129
        - with delirium F10.121
        - uncomplicated F10.120
      - mood disorder F10.14
      - other specified disorder F10.188
      - psychosis F10.159
        - delusions F10.150
        - hallucinations F10.151
      - sexual dysfunction F10.181
      - sleep disorder F10.182
      - unspecified disorder F10.19
    - counseling and surveillance Z71.41
    - in remission (early) (sustained) F10.11
  - amphetamine (or related substance) —*see* Abuse, drug, stimulant NEC
  - analgesics (non-prescribed) (over the counter) F55.8
  - antacids F55.0
  - antidepressants —*see* Abuse, drug, psychoactive NEC
  - anxiolytic —*see* Abuse, drug, sedative
  - barbiturates —*see* Abuse, drug, sedative
  - caffeine —*see* Abuse, drug, stimulant NEC
  - cannabis, cannabinoids —*see* Abuse, drug, cannabis
  - child —*see* Maltreatment, child
  - cocaine —*see* Abuse, drug, cocaine
  - drug NEC (non-dependent) F19.10
    - with sleep disorder F19.182
    - amphetamine type —*see* Abuse, drug, stimulant NEC
    - analgesics (non-prescribed) (over the counter) F55.8
    - antacids F55.0
    - antidepressants —*see* Abuse, drug, psychoactive NEC
    - anxiolytics —*see* Abuse, drug, sedative
    - barbiturates —*see* Abuse, drug, sedative
    - caffeine —*see* Abuse, drug, stimulant NEC
    - cannabis F12.10
      - with
        - anxiety disorder F12.180
        - intoxication F12.129
          - with
            - delirium F12.121
            - perceptual disturbance F12.122
          - uncomplicated F12.120
        - other specified disorder F12.188
        - psychosis F12.159
          - delusions F12.150
          - hallucinations F12.151
        - unspecified disorder F12.19
      - in remission (early) (sustained) F12.11
    - cocaine F14.10
      - with
        - anxiety disorder F14.180
        - intoxication F14.129
          - with
            - delirium F14.121
            - perceptual disturbance F14.122
          - uncomplicated F14.120

Abuse *(continued)*
  - drug NEC *(continued)*
    - cocaine *(continued)*
      - with *(continued)*
        - mood disorder F14.14
        - other specified disorder F14.188
        - psychosis F14.159
          - delusions F14.150
          - hallucinations F14.151
        - sexual dysfunction F14.181
        - sleep disorder F14.182
        - unspecified disorder F14.19
      - in remission (early) (sustained) F14.11
    - counseling and surveillance Z71.51
    - hallucinogen F16.10
      - with
        - anxiety disorder F16.180
        - flashbacks F16.183
        - intoxication F16.129
          - with
            - delirium F16.121
            - perceptual disturbance F16.122
          - uncomplicated F16.120
        - mood disorder F16.14
        - other specified disorder F16.188
        - perception disorder, persisting F16.183
        - psychosis F16.159
          - delusions F16.150
          - hallucinations F16.151
        - unspecified disorder F16.19
      - in remission (early) (sustained) F16.11
    - hashish —*see* Abuse, drug, cannabis
    - herbal or folk remedies F55.1
    - hormones F55.3
    - hypnotics —*see* Abuse, drug, sedative
    - inhalant F18.10
      - with
        - anxiety disorder F18.180
        - dementia, persisting F18.17
        - intoxication F18.129
          - with delirium F18.121
          - uncomplicated F18.120
        - mood disorder F18.14
        - other specified disorder F18.188
        - psychosis F18.159
          - delusions F18.150
          - hallucinations F18.151
        - unspecified disorder F18.19
      - in remission (early) (sustained) F18.11
    - laxatives F55.2
    - in remission (early) (sustained) F19.11
    - LSD —*see* Abuse, drug, hallucinogen
    - marihuana —*see* Abuse, drug, cannabis
    - morphine type (opioids) —*see* Abuse, drug, opioid
    - opioid F11.10
      - with
        - intoxication F11.129
          - with
            - delirium F11.121
            - perceptual disturbance F11.122
          - uncomplicated F11.120
        - mood disorder F11.14
        - other specified disorder F11.188
        - psychosis F11.159
          - delusions F11.150
          - hallucinations F11.151
        - sexual dysfunction F11.181

Abuse *(continued)*
  - drug NEC *(continued)*
    - opioid *(continued)*
      - with *(continued)*
        - sleep disorder F11.182
        - unspecified disorder F11.19
      - in remission (early) (sustained) F11.11
    - PCP (phencyclidine) (or related substance) —*see* Abuse, drug, hallucinogen
    - psychoactive NEC F19.10
      - with
        - amnestic disorder F19.16
        - anxiety disorder F19.180
        - dementia F19.17
        - intoxication F19.129
          - with
            - delirium F19.121
            - perceptual disturbance F19.122
          - uncomplicated F19.120
        - mood disorder F19.14
        - other specified disorder F19.188
        - psychosis F19.159
          - delusions F19.150
          - hallucinations F19.151
        - sexual dysfunction F19.181
        - sleep disorder F19.182
        - unspecified disorder F19.19
    - sedative, hypnotic or anxiolytic F13.10
      - with
        - anxiety disorder F13.180
        - intoxication F13.129
          - with delirium F13.121
          - uncomplicated F13.120
        - mood disorder F13.14
        - other specified disorder F13.188
        - psychosis F13.159
          - delusions F13.150
          - hallucinations F13.151
        - sexual dysfunction F13.181
        - sleep disorder F13.182
        - unspecified disorder F13.19
      - in remission (early) (sustained) F13.11
    - solvent —*see* Abuse, drug, inhalant
    - steroids F55.3
    - stimulant NEC F15.10
      - with
        - anxiety disorder F15.180
        - intoxication F15.129
          - with
            - delirium F15.121
            - perceptual disturbance F15.122
          - uncomplicated F15.120
        - mood disorder F15.14
        - other specified disorder F15.188
        - psychosis F15.159
          - delusions F15.150
          - hallucinations F15.151
        - sexual dysfunction F15.181
        - sleep disorder F15.182
        - unspecified disorder F15.19
      - in remission (early) (sustained) F15.11
    - tranquilizers —*see* Abuse, drug, sedative
    - vitamins F55.4
  - hallucinogens —*see* Abuse, drug, hallucinogen
  - hashish —*see* Abuse, drug, cannabis
  - herbal or folk remedies F55.1
  - hormones F55.3
  - hypnotic —*see* Abuse, drug, sedative
  - inhalant —*see* Abuse, drug, inhalant

Abuse *(continued)*
  - laxatives F55.2
  - LSD —*see* Abuse, drug, hallucinogen
  - marihuana —*see* Abuse, drug, cannabis
  - morphine type (opioids) —*see* Abuse, drug, opioid
  - non-psychoactive substance NEC F55.8
    - antacids F55.0
    - folk remedies F55.1
    - herbal remedies F55.1
    - hormones F55.3
    - laxatives F55.2
    - steroids F55.3
    - vitamins F55.4
  - opioids —*see* Abuse, drug, opioid
  - PCP (phencyclidine) (or related substance) —*see* Abuse, drug, hallucinogen
  - physical (adult) (child) —*see* Maltreatment
  - psychoactive substance —*see* Abuse, drug, psychoactive NEC
  - psychological (adult) (child) —*see* Maltreatment
  - sedative —*see* Abuse, drug, sedative
  - sexual —*see* Maltreatment
  - solvent —*see* Abuse, drug, inhalant
  - steroids F55.3
  - vitamins F55.4
- **Acalculia** R48.8
  - developmental F81.2
- **Acanthamebiasis** (with) B60.10
  - conjunctiva B60.12
  - keratoconjunctivitis B60.13
  - meningoencephalitis B60.11
  - other specified B60.19
- **Acanthocephaliasis** B83.8
- **Acanthocheilonemiasis** B74.4
- **Acanthocytosis** E78.6
- **Acantholysis** L11.9
- **Acanthosis** (acquired) (nigricans) L83
  - benign Q82.8
  - congenital Q82.8
  - seborrheic L82.1
    - inflamed L82.0
  - tongue K14.3
- **Acapnia** E87.3
- **Acarbia** E87.2
- **Acardia, acardius** Q89.8
- **Acardiacus amorphus** Q89.8
- **Acardiotrophia** I51.4
- **Acariasis** B88.0
  - scabies B86
- **Acarodermatitis** (urticarioides) B88.0
- **Acarophobia** F40.218
- **Acatalasemia, acatalasia** E80.3
- **Acathisia** (drug induced) G25.71
- **Accelerated atrioventricular conduction** I45.6
- **Accentuation of personality traits** (type A) Z73.1
- **Accessory** (congenital)
  - adrenal gland Q89.1
  - anus Q43.4
  - appendix Q43.4
  - atrioventricular conduction I45.6
  - auditory ossicles Q16.3
  - auricle (ear) Q17.0
  - biliary duct or passage Q44.5
  - bladder Q64.79
  - blood vessels NEC Q27.9
    - coronary Q24.5
  - bone NEC Q79.8
  - breast tissue, axilla Q83.1

- **Accessory** *(continued)*
  - carpal bones Q74.0
  - cecum Q43.4
  - chromosome(s) NEC (nonsex) Q92.9
    - with complex rearrangements NEC Q92.5
      - seen only at prometaphase Q92.8
    - partial Q92.9
    - sex
      - female phenotype Q97.8
    - 13 *—see* Trisomy, 13
    - 18 *—see* Trisomy, 18
    - 21 *—see* Trisomy, 21
  - coronary artery Q24.5
  - cusp(s), heart valve NEC Q24.8
    - pulmonary Q22.3
  - cystic duct Q44.5
  - digit(s) Q69.9
  - ear (auricle) (lobe) Q17.0
  - endocrine gland NEC Q89.2
  - eye muscle Q10.3
  - eyelid Q10.3
  - face bone(s) Q75.8
  - fallopian tube (fimbria) (ostium) Q50.6
  - finger(s) Q69.0
  - foreskin N47.8
  - frontonasal process Q75.8
  - gallbladder Q44.1
  - genital organ(s)
    - female Q52.8
      - external Q52.79
      - internal NEC Q52.8
    - male Q55.8
  - genitourinary organs NEC Q89.8
    - female Q52.8
    - male Q55.8
  - hallux Q69.2
  - heart Q24.8
    - valve NEC Q24.8
      - pulmonary Q22.3
  - hepatic ducts Q44.5
  - hymen Q52.4
  - intestine (large) (small) Q43.4
  - kidney Q63.0
  - lacrimal canal Q10.6
  - leaflet, heart valve NEC Q24.8
  - ligament, broad Q50.6
  - liver Q44.7
    - duct Q44.5
  - lobule (ear) Q17.0
  - lung (lobe) Q33.1
  - muscle Q79.8
  - navicular of carpus Q74.0
  - nervous system, part NEC Q07.8
  - nipple Q83.3
  - nose Q30.8
  - organ or site not listed *—see* Anomaly, by site
  - ovary Q50.31
  - oviduct Q50.6
  - pancreas Q45.3
  - parathyroid gland Q89.2
  - parotid gland (and duct) Q38.4
  - pituitary gland Q89.2
  - preauricular appendage Q17.0
  - prepuce N47.8
  - renal arteries (multiple) Q27.2
  - rib Q76.6
    - cervical Q76.5
  - roots (teeth) K00.2
  - salivary gland Q38.4
  - sesamoid bones Q74.8
    - foot Q74.2
    - hand Q74.0
  - skin tags Q82.8
  - spleen Q89.09
  - sternum Q76.7
  - submaxillary gland Q38.4
  - tarsal bones Q74.2
  - teeth, tooth K00.1
  - tendon Q79.8
  - thumb Q69.1
  - thymus gland Q89.2
  - thyroid gland Q89.2
  - toes Q69.2
  - tongue Q38.3
  - tooth, teeth K00.1
  - tragus Q17.0
  - ureter Q62.5
  - urethra Q64.79
  - urinary organ or tract NEC Q64.8
  - uterus Q51.2
  - vagina Q52.10
  - valve, heart NEC Q24.8
    - pulmonary Q22.3
  - vertebra Q76.49
  - vocal cords Q31.8
  - vulva Q52.79
- **Accident**
  - birth *—see* Birth, injury
  - cardiac *—see* Infarct, myocardium
  - cerebral I63.9
  - cerebrovascular (embolic) (ischemic) (thrombotic) I63.9
    - aborted I63.9
    - hemorrhagic *—see* Hemorrhage, intracranial, intracerebral
    - old (without sequelae) Z86.73
      - with sequelae (of) *—see* Sequelae, infarction, cerebral
  - coronary *—see* Infarct, myocardium
  - craniovascular I63.9
  - vascular, brain I63.9
- **Accidental** *—see* condition
- **Accommodation** (disorder) *—see also* condition
  - hysterical paralysis of F44.89
  - insufficiency of H52.4
  - paresis *—see* Paresis, of accommodation
  - spasm *—see* Spasm, of accommodation
- **Accouchement** *—see* Delivery
- **Accreta placenta** O43.21-
- **Accretio cordis** (nonrheumatic) I31.0
- **Accretions, tooth, teeth** K03.6
- **Acculturation difficulty** Z60.3
- **Accumulation secretion, prostate** N42.89
- **Acephalia, acephalism, acephalus, acephaly** Q00.0
- **Acephalobrachia monster** Q89.8
- **Acephalochirus monster** Q89.8
- **Acephalogaster** Q89.8
- **Acephalostomus monster** Q89.8
- **Acephalothorax** Q89.8
- **Acerophobia** F40.298
- **Acetonemia** R79.89
  - in Type 1 diabetes E10.10
    - with coma E10.11
- **Acetonuria** R82.4
- **Achalasia** (cardia) (esophagus) K22.0
  - congenital Q39.5
  - pylorus Q40.0
  - sphincteral NEC K59.8
- **Ache**(s) *—see* Pain
- **Acheilia** Q38.6
- **Achillobursitis** *—see* Tendinitis, Achilles
- **Achillodynia** *—see* Tendinitis, Achilles
- **Achlorhydria, achlorhydric** (neurogenic) K31.83
  - anemia D50.8
  - diarrhea K31.83
  - psychogenic F45.8
  - secondary to vagotomy K91.1
- **Achluophobia** F40.228
- **Acholia** K82.8
- **Acholuric jaundice** (familial) (splenomegalic) *—see also* Spherocytosis
  - acquired D59.8
- **Achondrogenesis** Q77.0
- **Achondroplasia** (osteosclerosis congenita) Q77.4
- **Achroma, cutis** L80
- **Achromat** (ism), achromatopsia (acquired) (congenital) H53.51
- **Achromia, congenital** *—see* Albinism
- **Achromia parasitica** B36.0
- **Achylia gastrica** K31.89
  - psychogenic F45.8
- **Acid**
  - burn *—see* Corrosion
  - deficiency
    - amide nicotinic E52
    - ascorbic E54
    - folic E53.8
    - nicotinic E52
    - pantothenic E53.8
  - intoxication E87.2
  - peptic disease K30
  - phosphatase deficiency E83.39
  - stomach K30
    - psychogenic F45.8
- **Acidemia** E87.2
  - argininosuccinic E72.22
  - isovaleric E71.110
  - metabolic (newborn) P19.9
    - first noted before onset of labor P19.0
    - first noted during labor P19.1
    - noted at birth P19.2
  - methylmalonic E71.120
  - pipecolic E72.3
  - propionic E71.121
- **Acidity, gastric** (high) K30
  - psychogenic F45.8
- **Acidocytopenia** *—see* Agranulocytosis
- **Acidocytosis** D72.1
- **Acidopenia** *—see* Agranulocytosis
- **Acidosis** (lactic) (respiratory) E87.2
  - in Type 1 diabetes E10.10
    - with coma E10.11
  - kidney, tubular N25.89
  - lactic E87.2
  - metabolic NEC E87.2
    - with respiratory acidosis E87.4
    - late, of newborn P74.0
  - mixed metabolic and respiratory, newborn P84
  - newborn P84
  - renal (hyperchloremic) (tubular) N25.89
  - respiratory E87.2
    - complicated by
      - metabolic
        - acidosis E87.4
        - alkalosis E87.4
- **Aciduria**
  - argininosuccinic E72.22
  - glutaric (type I) E72.3
    - type II E71.313
    - type III E71.5-
  - orotic (congenital) (hereditary) (pyrimidine deficiency) E79.8
    - anemia D53.0
- **Acladiosis** (skin) B36.0
- **Aclasis, diaphyseal** Q78.6
- **Acleistocardia** Q21.1
- **Aclusion** *—see* Anomaly, dentofacial, malocclusion
- **Acne** L70.9
  - artificialis L70.8
  - atrophica L70.2
  - cachecticorum (Hebra) L70.8
  - conglobata L70.1
  - cystic L70.0
  - decalvans L66.2
  - excoriée (des jeunes filles) L70.5
  - frontalis L70.2
  - indurata L70.0
  - infantile L70.4
  - keloid L73.0
  - lupoid L70.2
  - necrotic, necrotica (miliaris) L70.2
  - neonatal L70.4
  - nodular L70.0
  - occupational L70.8
  - picker's L70.5
  - pustular L70.0
  - rodens L70.2
  - rosacea L71.9
  - specified NEC L70.8
  - tropica L70.3
  - varioliformis L70.2
  - vulgaris L70.0
- **Acnitis** (primary) A18.4
- **Acosta's disease** T70.29
- **Acoustic** *—see* condition
- **Acousticophobia** F40.298
- **Acquired** *—see also* condition
  - immunodeficiency syndrome (AIDS) B20
- **Acrania** Q00.0
- **Acroangiodermatitis** I78.9
- **Acroasphyxia, chronic** I73.89
- **Acrobystitis** N47.7
- **Acrocephalopolysyndactyly** Q87.0
- **Acrocephalosyndactyly** Q87.0
- **Acrocephaly** Q75.0
- **Acrochondrohyperplasia** *—see* Syndrome, Marfan's
- **Acrocyanosis** I73.8
  - newborn P28.2
    - meaning transient blue hands and feet - omit code
- **Acrodermatitis** L30.8
  - atrophicans (chronica) L90.4
  - continua (Hallopeau) L40.2
  - enteropathica (hereditary) E83.2
  - Hallopeau's L40.2
  - infantile papular L44.4
  - perstans L40.2
  - pustulosa continua L40.2
  - recalcitrant pustular L40.2
- **Acrodynia** *—see* Poisoning, mercury
- **Acromegaly, acromegalia** E22.0
- **Acromelalgia** I73.81
- **Acromicria, acromikria** Q79.8
- **Acronyx** L60.0
- **Acropachy, thyroid** *—see* Thyrotoxicosis
- **Acroparesthesia** (simple) (vasomotor) I73.89
- **Acropathy, thyroid** *—see* Thyrotoxicosis
- **Acrophobia** F40.241
- **Acroposthitis** N47.7
- **Acroscleriasis, acroscleroderma, acrosclerosis** *—see* Sclerosis, systemic
- **Acrosphacelus** I96
- **Acrospiroma, eccrine** *—see* Neoplasm, skin, benign

Acrostealgia —*see* Osteochondropathy

Acrotrophodynia —*see* Immersion

ACTH ectopic syndrome E24.3

Actinic —*see* condition

Actinobacillosis, actinobacillus A28.8
- mallei A24.0
- muris A25.1

Actinomyces israelii (infection) —*see* Actinomycosis

Actinomycetoma (foot) B47.1

Actinomycosis, actinomycotic A42.9
- with pneumonia A42.0
- abdominal A42.1
- cervicofacial A42.2
- cutaneous A42.89
- gastrointestinal A42.1
- pulmonary A42.0
- sepsis A42.7
- specified site NEC A42.89

Actinoneuritis G62.82

Action, heart
- disorder I49.9
- irregular I49.9
  - psychogenic F45.8

Activated protein C resistance D68.51

Activation
- mast cell (disorder) (syndrom) D89.40
  - idiopathic D89.42
  - monoclonal D89.41
  - secondary D89.43
  - specified type NEC D89.49

Active —*see* condition

Acute —*see also* condition
- abdomen R10.0
- gallbladder —*see* Cholecystitis, acute

Acyanotic heart disease (congenital) Q24.9

Acystia Q64.5

Adair-Dighton syndrome (brittle bones and blue sclera, deafness) Q78.0

Adamantinoblastoma —*see* Ameloblastoma

Adamantinoma —*see also* Cyst, calcifying odontogenic
- long bones C40.90
  - lower limb C40.2-
  - upper limb C40.0-
- malignant C41.1
  - jaw (bone) (lower) C41.1
    - upper C41.0
- tibial C40.2-

Adamantoblastoma —*see* Ameloblastoma

Adams-Stokes (-Morgagni) **disease or syndrome** I45.9

Adaption reaction —*see* Disorder, adjustment

Addiction —*see also* Dependence F19.20
- alcohol, alcoholic (ethyl) (methyl) (wood) (without remission) F10.20
  - with remission F10.21
- drug —*see* Dependence, drug
- ethyl alcohol (without remission) F10.20
  - with remission F10.21
- heroin —*see* Dependence, drug, opioid
- methyl alcohol (without remission) F10.20
  - with remission F10.21

Addiction *(continued)*
- methylated spirit (without remission) F10.20
  - with remission F10.21
- morphine(-like substances) —*see* Dependence, drug, opioid
- nicotine —*see* Dependence, drug, nicotine
- opium and opioids —*see* Dependence, drug, opioid
- tobacco —*see* Dependence, drug, nicotine

Addisonian crisis E27.2

Addison's
- anemia (pernicious) D51.0
- disease (bronze) or syndrome E27.1
  - tuberculous A18.7
- keloid L94.0

Addison-Biermer anemia (pernicious) D51.0

Addison-Schilder complex E71.528

Additional —*see also* Accessory
- chromosome(s) Q99.8
  - sex —*see* Abnormal, chromosome, sex
  - 21 —*see* Trisomy, 21

Adduction contracture, hip or other joint —*see* Contraction, joint

Adenitis —*see also* Lymphadenitis
- acute, unspecified site L04.9
- axillary I88.9
  - acute L04.2
  - chronic or subacute I88.1
- Bartholin's gland N75.8
- bulbourethral gland —*see* Urethritis
- cervical I88.9
  - acute L04.0
  - chronic or subacute I88.1
- chancroid (Hemophilus ducreyi) A57
- chronic, unspecified site I88.1
- Cowper's gland —*see* Urethritis
- due to Pasteurella multocida (P. septica) A28.0
- epidemic, acute B27.09
- gangrenous L04.9
- gonorrheal NEC A54.89
- groin I88.9
  - acute L04.1
  - chronic or subacute I88.1
- infectious (acute) (epidemic) B27.09
- inguinal I88.9
  - acute L04.1
  - chronic or subacute I88.1
- lymph gland or node, except mesenteric I88.9
  - acute —*see* Lymphadenitis, acute
  - chronic or subacute I88.1
- mesenteric (acute) (chronic) (nonspecific) (subacute) I88.0
- parotid gland (suppurative) —*see* Sialoadenitis
- salivary gland (any) (suppurative) —*see* Sialoadenitis
- scrofulous (tuberculous) A18.2
- Skene's duct or gland —*see* Urethritis
- strumous, tuberculous A18.2
- subacute, unspecified site I88.1
- sublingual gland (suppurative) —*see* Sialoadenitis
- submandibular gland (suppurative) —*see* Sialoadenitis
- submaxillary gland (suppurative) —*see* Sialoadenitis
- tuberculous —*see* Tuberculosis, lymph gland
- urethral gland —*see* Urethritis
- Wharton's duct (suppurative) —*see* Sialoadenitis

Adenoacanthoma —*see* Neoplasm, malignant, by site

Adenoameloblastoma —*see* Cyst, calcifying odontogenic

Adenocarcinoid (tumor) —*see* Neoplasm, malignant, by site

Adenocarcinoma —*see also* Neoplasm, malignant, by site
- acidophil
  - specified site —*see* Neoplasm, malignant, by site
  - unspecified site C75.1
- adrenal cortical C74.0-
- alveolar —*see* Neoplasm, lung, malignant
- apocrine
  - breast —*see* Neoplasm, breast, malignant
  - in situ
    - breast D05.8-
    - specified site NEC —*see* Neoplasm, skin, in situ
    - unspecified site D04.9
  - specified site NEC —*see* Neoplasm, skin, malignant
  - unspecified site C44.99
- basal cell
  - specified site —*see* Neoplasm, skin, malignant
  - unspecified site C08.9
- basophil
  - specified site —*see* Neoplasm, malignant, by site
  - unspecified site C75.1
- bile duct type C22.1
  - liver C22.1
  - specified site NEC —*see* Neoplasm, malignant, by site
  - unspecified site C22.1
- bronchiolar —*see* Neoplasm, lung, malignant
- bronchioloalveolar —*see* Neoplasm, lung, malignant
- ceruminous C44.29-
- cervix, in situ —*see also* Carcinoma, cervix uteri, in situ D06.9
- chromophobe
  - specified site —*see* Neoplasm, malignant, by site
  - unspecified site C75.1
- diffuse type
  - specified site —*see* Neoplasm, malignant, by site
  - unspecified site C16.9
- duct
  - infiltrating
    - with Paget's disease —*see* Neoplasm, breast, malignant
    - specified site —*see* Neoplasm, malignant, by site
    - unspecified site (female) 50.91-
      - male C50.92-
  - specified site —*see* Neoplasm, malignant, by site
  - unspecified site
    - female C56.9
    - male C61
- eosinophil
  - specified site —*see* Neoplasm, malignant, by site
  - unspecified site C75.1
- follicular
  - with papillary C73
  - moderately differentiated C73
  - specified site —*see* Neoplasm, malignant, by site
  - trabecular C73
  - unspecified site C73
  - well differentiated C73

Adenocarcinoma *(continued)*
- Hurthle cell C73
- in
  - adenomatous
    - polyposis coli C18.9
- infiltrating duct
  - with Paget's disease —*see* Neoplasm, breast, malignant
  - specified site —*see* Neoplasm, by site, malignant
  - unspecified site (female) C50.91-
    - male C50.92-
- inflammatory
  - specified site —*see* Neoplasm, by site, malignant
  - unspecified site (female) C50.91-
    - male C50.92-
- intestinal type
  - specified site —*see* Neoplasm, by site, malignant
  - unspecified site C16.9
- intracystic papillary
- intraductal
  - breast D05.1-
  - noninfiltrating
    - breast D05.1-
    - papillary
      - with invasion
        - specified site —*see* Neoplasm, by site, malignant
        - unspecified site (female) C50.91-
          - male C50.92-
      - breast D05.1-
      - specified site NEC —*see* Neoplasm, in situ, by site
      - unspecified site D05.1-
    - specified site NEC —*see* Neoplasm, in situ, by site
    - unspecified site D05.1-
  - papillary
    - with invasion
      - specified site —*see* Neoplasm, malignant, by site
      - unspecified site (female) C50.91-
        - male C50.92-
    - breast D05.1-
    - specified site —*see* Neoplasm, in situ, by site
    - unspecified site D05.1-
  - specified site NEC —*see* Neoplasm, in situ, by site
  - unspecified site D05.1-
- islet cell
  - with exocrine, mixed
    - specified site —*see* Neoplasm, malignant, by site
    - unspecified site C25.9
  - pancreas C25.4
  - specified site NEC —*see* Neoplasm, malignant, by site
  - unspecified site C25.4
- lobular
  - in situ
    - breast D05.0-
    - specified site NEC —*see* Neoplasm, in situ, by site
    - unspecified site D05.0-
  - specified site —*see* Neoplasm, malignant, by site
  - unspecified site (female) C50.91-
    - male C50.92-
- mucoid —*see also* Neoplasm, malignant, by site
  - cell
    - specified site —*see* Neoplasm, malignant, by site
    - unspecified site C75.1

Adenocarcinoma *(continued)*
- nonencapsulated sclerosing C73
- papillary
  - with follicular C73
  - follicular variant C73
  - intraductal (noninfiltrating)
    - with invasion
      - specified site *—see* Neoplasm, malignant, by site
      - unspecified site (female) C50.91-
        - male C50.92-
    - breast D05.1-
    - specified site NEC *—see* Neoplasm, in situ, by site
    - unspecified site D05.1-
  - serous
    - specified site *—see* Neoplasm, malignant, by site
    - unspecified site C56.9
- papillocystic
  - specified site *—see* Neoplasm, malignant, by site
  - unspecified site C56.9
- pseudomucinous
  - specified site *—see* Neoplasm, malignant, by site
  - unspecified site C56.9
- renal cell C64-
- sebaceous *—see* Neoplasm, skin, malignant
- serous *—see also* Neoplasm, malignant, by site
  - papillary
    - specified site *—see* Neoplasm, malignant, by site
    - unspecified site C56.9
- sweat gland *—see* Neoplasm, skin, malignant
- water-clear cell C75.0

Adenocarcinoma-in-situ *—see also* Neoplasm, in situ, by site
- breast D05.9-

Adenofibroma
- clear cell *—see* Neoplasm, benign, by site
- endometrioid D27.9
  - borderline malignancy D39.10
  - malignant C56-
- mucinous
  - specified site *—see* Neoplasm, benign, by site
  - unspecified site D27.9
- papillary
  - specified site *—see* Neoplasm, benign, by site
  - unspecified site D27.9
- prostate *—see* Enlargement, enlarged, prostate
- serous
  - specified site *—see* Neoplasm, benign, by site
  - unspecified site D27.9
- specified site *—see* Neoplasm, benign, by site
- unspecified site D27.9

Adenofibrosis
- breast *—see* Fibroadenosis, breast
- endometrioid N80.0

Adenoiditis (chronic) J35.02
- with tonsillitis J35.03
- acute J03.90
  - recurrent J03.91
  - specified organism NEC J03.80
    - recurrent J03.81
  - staphylococcal J03.80
    - recurrent J03.81
  - streptococcal J03.00
    - recurrent J03.01

Adenoids *—see* condition

Adenolipoma *—see* Neoplasm, benign, by site

Adenolipomatosis, Launois-Bensaude E88.89

Adenolymphoma
- specified site *—see* Neoplasm, benign, by site
- unspecified site D11.9

Adenoma *—see also* Neoplasm, benign, by site
- acidophil
  - specified site *—see* Neoplasm, benign, by site
  - unspecified site D35.2
- acidophil-basophil, mixed
  - specified site *—see* Neoplasm, benign, by site
  - unspecified site D35.2
- adrenal (cortical) D35.00
  - clear cell D35.00
  - compact cell D35.00
  - glomerulosa cell D35.00
  - heavily pigmented variant D35.00
  - mixed cell D35.00
- alpha-cell
  - pancreas D13.7
  - specified site NEC *—see* Neoplasm, benign, by site
  - unspecified site D13.7
- alveolar D14.30
- apocrine
  - breast D24-
  - specified site NEC *—see* Neoplasm, skin, benign, by site
  - unspecified site D23.9
- basal cell D11.9
- basophil
  - specified site *—see* Neoplasm, benign, by site
  - unspecified site D35.2
- basophil-acidophil, mixed
  - specified site *—see* Neoplasm, benign, by site
  - unspecified site D35.2
- beta-cell
  - pancreas D13.7
  - specified site NEC *—see* Neoplasm, benign, by site
  - unspecified site D13.7
- bile duct D13.4
  - common D13.5
  - extrahepatic D13.5
  - intrahepatic D13.4
  - specified site NEC *—see* Neoplasm, benign, by site
  - unspecified site D13.4
- black D35.00
- bronchial D38.1
  - cylindroid type *—see* Neoplasm, lung, malignant
- ceruminous D23.2-
- chief cell D35.1
- chromophobe
  - specified site *—see* Neoplasm, benign, by site
  - unspecified site D35.2
- colloid
  - specified site *—see* Neoplasm, benign, by site
  - unspecified site D34
- duct
- eccrine, papillary *—see* Neoplasm, skin, benign
- endocrine, multiple
  - single specified site *—see* Neoplasm, uncertain behavior, by site
  - two or more specified sites D44-
  - unspecified site D44.9

Adenoma *(continued)*
- endometrioid *—see also* Neoplasm, benign
  - borderline malignancy *—see* Neoplasm, uncertain behavior, by site
- eosinophil
  - specified site *—see* Neoplasm, benign, by site
  - unspecified site D35.2
- fetal
  - specified site *—see* Neoplasm, benign, by site
  - unspecified site D34
- follicular
  - specified site *—see* Neoplasm, benign, by site
  - unspecified site D34
- hepatocellular D13.4
- Hurthle cell D34
- islet cell
  - pancreas D13.7
  - specified site NEC *—see* Neoplasm, benign, by site
  - unspecified site D13.7
- liver cell D13.4
- macrofollicular
  - specified site *—see* Neoplasm, benign, by site
  - unspecified site D34
- malignant, malignum *—see* Neoplasm, malignant, by site
- microcystic
  - pancreas D13.6
  - specified site NEC *—see* Neoplasm, benign, by site
  - unspecified site D13.6
- microfollicular
  - specified site *—see* Neoplasm, benign, by site
  - unspecified site D34
- mucoid cell
  - specified site *—see* Neoplasm, benign, by site
  - unspecified site D35.2
- multiple endocrine
  - single specified site *—see* Neoplasm, uncertain behavior, by site
  - two or more specified sites D44-
  - unspecified site D44.9
- nipple D24-
- papillary *—see also* Neoplasm, benign, by site
  - eccrine *—see* Neoplasm, skin, benign, by site
- Pick's tubular
  - specified site *—see* Neoplasm, benign, by site
  - unspecified site
    - female D27.9
    - male D29.20
- pleomorphic
  - carcinoma in *—see* Neoplasm, salivary gland, malignant
    - specified site *—see* Neoplasm, malignant, by site
    - unspecified site C08.9
- polypoid *—see also* Neoplasm, benign
  - adenocarcinoma in *—see* Neoplasm, malignant, by site
  - adenocarcinoma in situ *—see* Neoplasm, in situ, by site
- prostate *—see* Neoplasm, benign, prostate
- rete cell D29.20
- sebaceous *—see* Neoplasm, skin, benign

Adenoma *(continued)*
- Sertoli cell
  - specified site *—see* Neoplasm, benign, by site
  - unspecified site
    - female D27.9
    - male D29.20
- skin appendage *—see* Neoplasm, skin, benign
- sudoriferous gland *—see* Neoplasm, skin, benign
- sweat gland *—see* Neoplasm, skin, benign
- testicular
  - specified site *—see* Neoplasm, benign, by site
  - unspecified site
    - female D27.9
    - male D29.20
- tubular *—see also* Neoplasm, benign, by site
  - adenocarcinoma in *—see* Neoplasm, malignant, by site
  - adenocarcinoma in situ *—see* Neoplasm, in situ, by site
  - Pick's
    - specified site *—see* Neoplasm, benign, by site
    - unspecified site
      - female D27.9
      - male D29.20
- tubulovillous *—see also* Neoplasm, benign, by site
  - adenocarcinoma in *—see* Neoplasm, malignant, by site
  - adenocarcinoma in situ *—see* Neoplasm, in situ, by site
- villous *—see* Neoplasm, uncertain behavior, by site
  - adenocarcinoma in *—see* Neoplasm, malignant, by site
  - adenocarcinoma in situ *—see* Neoplasm, in situ, by site
- water-clear cell D35.1

Adenomatosis
- endocrine (multiple) E31.20
  - single specified site *—see* Neoplasm, uncertain behavior, by site
- erosive of nipple D24-
- pluriendocrine *—see* Adenomatosis, endocrine
- pulmonary D38.1
  - malignant *—see* Neoplasm, lung, malignant
- specified site *—see* Neoplasm, benign, by site
- unspecified site D12.6

Adenomatous
- goiter (nontoxic) E04.9
  - with hyperthyroidism *—see* Hyperthyroidism, with, goiter, nodular
  - toxic *—see* Hyperthyroidism, with, goiter, nodular

Adenomyoma *—see also* Neoplasm, benign, by site
- prostate *—see* Enlarged, prostate

Adenomyometritis N80.0

Adenomyosis N80.0

Adenopathy (lymph gland) R59.9
- generalized R59.1
- inguinal R59.0
- localized R59.0
- mediastinal R59.0
- mesentery R59.0
- syphilitic (secondary) A51.49
- tracheobronchial R59.0
  - tuberculous A15.4
    - primary (progressive) A15.7

Adenopathy *(continued)*
- tuberculous —*see also* Tuberculosis, lymph gland
  - tracheobronchial A15.4
    - primary (progressive) A15.7

Adenosalpingitis —*see* Salpingitis

Adenosarcoma —*see* Neoplasm, malignant, by site

Adenosclerosis I88.8

Adenosis (sclerosing) breast —*see* Fibroadenosis, breast

Adenovirus, as cause of disease classified elsewhere B97.0

Adentia (complete) (partial) —*see* Absence, teeth

Adherent —*see also* Adhesions
- labia (minora) N90.89
- pericardium (nonrheumatic) I31.0
  - rheumatic I09.2
- placenta (with hemorrhage) O72.0
  - without hemorrhage O73.0
- prepuce, newborn N47.0
- scar (skin) L90.5
- tendon in scar L90.5

Adhesions, adhesive (postinfective) K66.0
- with intestinal obstruction K56.50
  - complete K56.52
  - incomplete K56.51
  - partial K56.51
- abdominal (wall) —*see* Adhesions, peritoneum
- appendix K38.8
- bile duct (common) (hepatic) K83.8
- bladder (sphincter) N32.89
- bowel —*see* Adhesions, peritoneum
- cardiac I31.0
  - rheumatic I09.2
- cecum —*see* Adhesions, peritoneum
- cervicovaginal N88.1
  - congenital Q52.8
  - postpartal O90.89
    - old N88.1
- cervix N88.1
- ciliary body NEC —*see* Adhesions, iris
- clitoris N90.89
- colon —*see* Adhesions, peritoneum
- common duct K83.8
- congenital —*see also* Anomaly, by site
  - fingers —*see* Syndactylism, complex, fingers
  - omental, anomalous Q43.3
  - peritoneal Q43.3
  - tongue (to gum or roof of mouth) Q38.3
- conjunctiva (acquired) H11.21-
  - congenital Q15.8
- cystic duct K82.8
- diaphragm —*see* Adhesions, peritoneum
- due to foreign body —*see* Foreign body
- duodenum —*see* Adhesions, peritoneum
- ear
  - middle H74.1-
- epididymis N50.89
- epidural —*see* Adhesions, meninges
- epiglottis J38.7
- eyelid H02.59
- female pelvis N73.6
- gallbladder K82.8
- globe H44.89
- heart I31.0
  - rheumatic I09.2
- ileocecal (coil) —*see* Adhesions, peritoneum
- ileum —*see* Adhesions, peritoneum

Adhesions, adhesive *(continued)*
- intestine —*see also* Adhesions, peritoneum
  - with obstruction K56.50
    - complete K56.52
    - incomplete K56.51
    - partial K56.51
- intra-abdominal —*see* Adhesions, peritoneum
- iris H21.50-
  - anterior H21.51-
  - goniosynechiae H21.52-
  - posterior H21.54-
  - to corneal graft T85.898
- joint —*see* Ankylosis
  - knee M23.8X
  - temporomandibular M26.61-
- labium (majus) (minus), congenital Q52.5
- liver —*see* Adhesions, peritoneum
- lung J98.4
- mediastinum J98.59
- meninges (cerebral) (spinal) G96.12
  - congenital Q07.8
  - tuberculous (cerebral) (spinal) A17.0
- mesenteric —*see* Adhesions, peritoneum
- nasal (septum) (to turbinates) J34.89
- ocular muscle —*see* Strabismus, mechanical
- omentum —*see* Adhesions, peritoneum
- ovary N73.6
  - congenital (to cecum, kidney or omentum) Q50.39
- paraovarian N73.6
- pelvic (peritoneal)
  - female N73.6
    - postprocedural N99.4
  - male —*see* Adhesions, peritoneum
  - postpartal (old) N73.6
  - tuberculous A18.17
- penis to scrotum (congenital) Q55.8
- periappendiceal —*see also* Adhesions, peritoneum
- pericardium (nonrheumatic) I31.0
  - focal I31.8
  - rheumatic I09.2
  - tuberculous A18.84
- pericholecystic K82.8
- perigastric —*see* Adhesions, peritoneum
- periovarian N73.6
- periprostatic N42.89
- perirectal —*see* Adhesions, peritoneum
- perirenal N28.89
- peritoneum, peritoneal (postinfective)
  - with obstruction (intestinal) K56.50
    - complete K56.52
    - incomplete K56.51
    - partial K56.51
  - congenital Q43.3
  - pelvic, female N73.6
    - postprocedural N99.4
  - postpartal, pelvic N73.6
  - postprocedural K66.0
  - to uterus N73.6
- peritubal N73.6
- periureteral N28.89
- periuterine N73.6
- perivesical N32.89
- perivesicular (seminal vesicle) N50.89
- pleura, pleuritic J94.8
  - tuberculous NEC A15.6
- pleuropericardial J94.8
- postoperative (gastrointestinal tract) K66.0
  - with obstruction (*see also* Obstruction, intestine, postoperative) K91.30

Adhesions, adhesive *(continued)*
- postoperative *(continued)*
  - due to foreign body accidentally left in wound —*see* Foreign body, accidentally left during a procedure
  - pelvic peritoneal N99.4
  - urethra —*see* Stricture, urethra, postprocedural
  - vagina N99.2
- postpartal, old (vulva or perineum) N90.89
- preputial, prepuce N47.5
- pulmonary J98.4
- pylorus —*see* Adhesions, peritoneum
- sciatic nerve —*see* Lesion, nerve, sciatic
- seminal vesicle N50.89
- shoulder (joint) —*see* Capsulitis, adhesive
- sigmoid flexure —*see* Adhesions, peritoneum
- spermatic cord (acquired) N50.89
  - congenital Q55.4
- spinal canal G96.12
- stomach —*see* Adhesions, peritoneum
- subscapular —*see* Capsulitis, adhesive
- temporomandibular M26.61-
- tendinitis —*see also* Tenosynovitis, specified type NEC
  - shoulder —*see* Capsulitis, adhesive
- testis N44.8
- tongue, congenital (to gum or roof of mouth) Q38.3
  - acquired K14.8
- trachea J39.8
- tubo-ovarian N73.6
- tunica vaginalis N44.8
- uterus N73.6
  - internal N85.6
  - to abdominal wall N73.6
- vagina (chronic) N89.5
  - postoperative N99.2
- vitreomacular H43.82-
- vitreous H43.89
- vulva N90.89

Adiaspiromycosis B48.88

Adie (-Holmes) **pupil or syndrome** —*see* Anomaly, pupil, function, tonic pupil

Adiponecrosis neonatorum P83.88

Adiposis —*see also* Obesity
- cerebralis E23.6
- dolorosa E88.2

Adiposity —*see also* Obesity
- heart —*see* Degeneration, myocardial
- localized E65

Adiposogenital dystrophy E23.6

Adjustment
- disorder —*see* Disorder, adjustment
- implanted device —*see* Encounter (for), adjustment (of)
- prosthesis, external —*see* Fitting
- reaction —*see* Disorder, adjustment

Administration of tPA (rtPA) **in a different facility within the last 24 hours prior to admission to current facility** Z92.82

Admission (for) —*see also* Encounter (for)
- adjustment (of)
  - artificial
    - arm Z44.00-
      - complete Z44.01-
      - partial Z44.02-
    - eye Z44.2
    - leg Z44.10-
      - complete Z44.11-
      - partial Z44.12-

Admission *(continued)*
- adjustment *(continued)*
  - brain neuropacemaker Z46.2
    - implanted Z45.42
  - breast
    - implant Z45.81
    - prosthesis (external) Z44.3
  - colostomy belt Z46.89
  - contact lenses Z46.0
  - cystostomy device Z46.6
  - dental prosthesis Z46.3
  - device NEC
    - abdominal Z46.89
    - implanted Z45.89
      - cardiac Z45.09
        - defibrillator (with synchronous cardiace pacemaker) Z45.02
        - pacemaker (cardiac resynchronization therapy (CRT-P)) Z45.018
          - pulse generator Z45.010
        - resynchronization therapy defibrillator (CRT-D) Z45.02
      - hearing device Z45.328
        - bone conduction Z45.320
        - cochlear Z45.321
      - infusion pump Z45.1
      - nervous system Z45.49
        - CSF drainage Z45.41
        - hearing device —*see* Admission, adjustment, device, implanted, hearing device
        - neuropacemaker Z45.42
        - visual substitution Z45.31
      - specified NEC Z45.89
      - vascular access Z45.2
      - visual substitution Z45.31
    - nervous system Z46.2
      - implanted —*see* Admission, adjustment, device, implanted, nervous system
    - orthodontic Z46.4
    - prosthetic Z44.9
      - arm —*see* Admission, adjustment, artificial, arm
      - breast Z44.3
      - dental Z46.3
      - eye Z44.2
      - leg —*see* Admission, adjustment, artificial, leg
      - specified type NEC Z44.8
    - substitution
      - auditory Z46.2
        - implanted —*see* Admission, adjustment, device, implanted, hearing device
      - nervous system Z46.2
        - implanted —*see* Admission, adjustment, device, implanted, nervous system
      - visual Z46.2
        - implanted Z45.31
    - urinary Z46.6
  - hearing aid Z46.1
    - implanted —*see* Admission, adjustment, device, implanted, hearing device
  - ileostomy device Z46.89
  - intestinal appliance or device NEC Z46.89
  - neuropacemaker (brain) (peripheral nerve) (spinal cord) Z46.2
    - implanted Z45.42

Admission *(continued)*
- adjustment *(continued)*
  - orthodontic device Z46.4
  - orthopedic (brace) (cast) (device) (shoes) Z46.89
  - pacemaker (cardiac resynchronization therapy (CRT-P))
    - cardiac Z45.018
      - pulse generator Z45.010
    - nervous system Z46.2
      - implanted Z45.42
  - portacath (port-a-cath) Z45.2
  - prosthesis Z44.9
    - arm *—see* Admission, adjustment, artificial, arm
    - breast Z44.3
    - dental Z46.3
    - eye Z44.2
    - leg *—see* Admission, adjustment, artificial, leg
    - specified NEC Z44.8
  - spectacles Z46.0
- aftercare *—see also* Aftercare Z51.89
  - postpartum
    - immediately after delivery Z39.0
    - routine follow-up Z39.2
  - radiation therapy (antineoplastic) Z51.0
- attention to artificial opening (of) Z43.9
  - artificial vagina Z43.7
  - colostomy Z43.3
  - cystostomy Z43.5
  - enterostomy Z43.4
  - gastrostomy Z43.1
  - ileostomy Z43.2
  - jejunostomy Z43.4
  - nephrostomy Z43.6
  - specified site NEC Z43.8
    - intestinal tract Z43.4
    - urinary tract Z43.6
  - tracheostomy Z43.0
  - ureterostomy Z43.6
  - urethrostomy Z43.6
- breast augmentation or reduction Z41.1
- breast reconstruction following mastectomy Z42.1
- change of
  - dressing (nonsurgical) Z48.00
  - neuropacemaker device (brain) (peripheral nerve) (spinal cord) Z46.2
    - implanted Z45.42
  - surgical dressing Z48.01
- circumcision, ritual or routine (in absence of diagnosis) Z41.2
- clinical research investigation (control) (normal comparison) (participant) Z00.6
- contraceptive management Z30.9
- cosmetic surgery NEC Z41.1
- counseling *—see also* Counseling
  - dietary Z71.3
  - gestational carrier Z31.7
  - HIV Z71.7
  - human immunodeficiency virus Z71.7
  - nonattending third party Z71.0
  - procreative management NEC Z31.69
- delivery, full-term, uncomplicated O80
  - cesarean, without indication O82
- desensitization to allergens Z51.6

Admission *(continued)*
- dietary surveillance and counseling Z71.3
- ear piercing Z41.3
- examination at health care facility (adult) (*see also* Examination) Z00.00
  - with abnormal findings Z00.01
  - clinical research investigation (control) (normal comparison) (participant) Z00.6
  - dental Z01.20
    - with abnormal findings Z01.21
  - donor (potential) Z00.5
  - ear Z01.10
    - with abnormal findings NEC Z01.118
  - eye Z01.00
    - with abnormal findings Z01.01
  - general, specified reason NEC Z00.8
  - hearing Z01.10
    - with abnormal findings NEC Z01.118
  - postpartum checkup Z39.2
  - psychiatric (general) Z00.8
    - requested by authority Z04.6
  - vision Z01.00
    - with abnormal findings Z01.01
- fitting (of)
  - artificial
    - arm *—see* Admission, adjustment, artificial, arm
    - eye Z44.2
    - leg *—see* Admission, adjustment, artificial, leg
  - brain neuropacemaker Z46.2
    - implanted Z45.42
  - breast prosthesis (external) Z44.3
  - colostomy belt Z46.89
  - contact lenses Z46.0
  - cystostomy device Z46.6
  - dental prosthesis Z46.3
  - dentures Z46.3
  - device NEC
    - abdominal Z46.89
    - nervous system Z46.2
      - implanted *—see* Admission, adjustment, device, implanted, nervous system
    - orthodontic Z46.4
    - prosthetic Z44.9
      - breast Z44.3
      - dental Z46.3
      - eye Z44.2
    - substitution
      - auditory Z46.2
        - implanted *—see* Admission, adjustment, device, implanted, hearing device
      - nervous system Z46.2
        - implanted *—see* Admission, adjustment, device, implanted, nervous system
      - visual Z46.2
        - implanted Z45.31
  - hearing aid Z46.1
  - ileostomy device Z46.89
  - intestinal appliance or device NEC Z46.89
  - neuropacemaker (brain) (peripheral nerve) (spinal cord) Z46.2
    - implanted Z45.42
  - orthodontic device Z46.4

Admission *(continued)*
- fitting (of) *(continued)*
  - orthopedic device (brace) (cast) (shoes) Z46.89
  - prosthesis Z44.9
    - arm *—see* Admission, adjustment, artificial, arm
    - breast Z44.3
    - dental Z46.3
    - eye Z44.2
    - leg *—see* Admission, adjustment, artificial, leg
    - specified type NEC Z44.8
  - spectacles Z46.0
- follow-up examination Z09
- intrauterine device management Z30.431
  - initial prescription Z30.014
- mental health evaluation Z00.8
  - requested by authority Z04.6
- observation *—see* Observation
- Papanicolaou smear, cervix Z12.4
  - for suspected malignant neoplasm Z12.4
- plastic and reconstructive surgery following medical procedure or healed injury NEC Z42.8
- plastic surgery, cosmetic NEC Z41.1
- postpartum observation
  - immediately after delivery Z39.0
  - routine follow-up Z39.2
- poststerilization (for restoration) Z31.0
  - aftercare Z31.42
- procreative management Z31.9
- prophylactic (measure) - *see also* Encounter, prophylactic measures
  - organ removal Z40.00
    - breast Z40.01
    - fallopian tube(s) Z40.03
      - with ovary(s) Z40.02
    - ovary(s) Z40.02
    - specified organ NEC Z40.09
    - testes Z40.09
  - vaccination Z23
- psychiatric examination (general) Z00.8
  - requested by authority Z04.6
- radiation therapy (antineoplastic) Z51.0
- reconstructive surgery following medical procedure or healed injury NEC Z42.8
- removal of
  - cystostomy catheter Z43.5
  - drains Z48.03
  - dressing (nonsurgical) Z48.00
  - implantable subdermal contraceptive Z30.46
  - intrauterine contraceptive device Z30.432
  - neuropacemaker (brain) (peripheral nerve) (spinal cord) Z46.2
    - implanted Z45.42
  - staples Z48.02
  - surgical dressing Z48.01
  - sutures Z48.02
  - ureteral stent Z46.6
- respirator [ventilator] use during power failure Z99.12
- restoration of organ continuity (poststerilization) Z31.0
  - aftercare Z31.42
- sensitivity test *—see also* Test, skin
  - allergy NEC Z01.82
  - Mantoux Z11.1
- tuboplasty following previous sterilization Z31.0
  - aftercare Z31.42
- vasoplasty following previous sterilization Z31.0
  - aftercare Z31.42

Admission *(continued)*
- vision examination Z01.00
  - with abnormal findings Z01.01
- waiting period for admission to other facility Z75.1

Adnexitis (suppurative) *—see* Salpingo-oophoritis

Adolescent X-linked adrenoleukodystrophy E71.521

Adrenal (gland) *—see* condition

Adrenalism, tuberculous A18.7

Adrenalitis, adrenitis E27.8
- autoimmune E27.1
- meningococcal, hemorrhagic A39.1

Adrenarche, premature E27.0

Adrenocortical syndrome *—see* Cushing's, syndrome

Adrenogenital syndrome E25.9
- acquired E25.8
- congenital E25.0
- salt loss E25.0

Adrenogenitalism, congenital E25.0

Adrenoleukodystrophy E71.529
- neonatal E71.511
- X-linked E71.529
  - Addison only phenotype E71.528
  - Addison-Schilder E71.528
  - adolescent E71.521
  - adrenomyeloneuropathy E71.522
  - childhood cerebral E71.520
  - other specified E71.528

Adrenomyeloneuropathy E71.522

Adventitious bursa *—see* Bursopathy, specified type NEC

Adverse effect *—see* Table of Drugs and Chemicals, categories T36-T50, with 6th character 5

Advice *—see* Counseling

Adynamia (episodica) (hereditary) (periodic) G72.3

Aeration lung imperfect, newborn *—see* Atelectasis

Aerobullosis T70.3

Aerocele *—see* Embolism, air

Aerodermectasia
- subcutaneous (traumatic) T79.7

Aerodontalgia T70.29

Aeroembolism T70.3

Aerogenes capsulatus infection A48.0

Aero-otitis media T70.0

Aerophagy, aerophagia (psychogenic) F45.8

Aerophobia F40.228

Aerosinusitis T70.1

Aerotitis T70.0

Affection *—see* Disease

Afibrinogenemia (*see also* Defect, coagulation) D68.8
- acquired D65
- congenital D68.2
- following ectopic or molar pregnancy O08.1
- in abortion *—see* Abortion, by type, complicated by, afibrinogenemia
- puerperal O72.3

African
- sleeping sickness B56.9
- tick fever A68.1
- trypanosomiasis B56.9
  - gambian B56.0
  - rhodesian B56.1

Aftercare (*see also* Care) Z51.89
  following surgery (for) (on)
    amputation Z47.81
    attention to
      drains Z48.03
      dressings (nonsurgical) Z48.00
        surgical Z48.01
      sutures Z48.02
    circulatory system Z48.812
    delayed (planned) wound closure Z48.1
    digestive system Z48.815
    explantation of joint prosthesis (staged procedure)
      hip Z47.32
      knee Z47.33
      shoulder Z47.31
    genitourinary system Z48.816
    joint replacement Z47.1
    neoplasm Z48.3
    nervous system Z48.811
    oral cavity Z48.814
    organ transplant
      bone marrow Z48.290
      heart Z48.21
      heart-lung Z48.280
      kidney Z48.22
      liver Z48.23
      lung Z48.24
      multiple organs NEC Z48.288
      specified NEC Z48.298
    orthopedic NEC Z47.89
    planned wound closure Z48.1
    removal of internal fixation device Z47.2
    respiratory system Z48.813
    scoliosis Z47.82
    sense organs Z48.810
    skin and subcutaneous tissue Z48.817
    specified body system
      circulatory Z48.812
      digestive Z48.815
      genitourinary Z48.816
      nervous Z48.811
      oral cavity Z48.814
      respiratory Z48.813
      sense organs Z48.810
      skin and subcutaneous tissue Z48.817
      teeth Z48.814
    specified NEC Z48.89
    spinal Z47.89
    teeth Z48.814
  fracture - code to fracture with seventh character D
  involving
    removal of
      drains Z48.03
      dressings (nonsurgical) Z48.00
      staples Z48.02
      surgical dressings Z48.01
      sutures Z48.02
  neuropacemaker (brain) (peripheral nerve) (spinal cord) Z46.2
    implanted Z45.42
  orthopedic NEC Z47.89
  postprocedural —*see* Aftercare, following surgery

After-cataract —*see* Cataract, secondary

Agalactia (primary) O92.3
  elective, secondary or therapeutic O92.5

Agammaglobulinemia (acquired (secondary)) (nonfamilial) D80.1
  with
    immunoglobulin-bearing B-lymphocytes D80.1
    lymphopenia D81.9

Agammaglobulinemia *(continued)*
  autosomal recessive (Swiss type) D80.0
  Bruton's X-linked D80.0
  common variable (CVAgamma) D80.1
  congenital sex-linked D80.0
  hereditary D80.0
  lymphopenic D81.9
  Swiss type (autosomal recessive) D80.0
  X-linked (with growth hormone deficiency) (Bruton) D80.0

Aganglionosis (bowel) (colon) Q43.1

Age (old) —*see* Senility

Agenesis
  adrenal (gland) Q89.1
  alimentary tract (complete) (partial) NEC Q45.8
    upper Q40.8
  anus, anal (canal) Q42.3
    with fistula Q42.2
  aorta Q25.41
  appendix Q42.8
  arm (complete) Q71.0-
    with hand present Q71.1-
  artery (peripheral) Q27.9
    brain Q28.3
    coronary Q24.5
    pulmonary Q25.79
    specified NEC Q27.8
    umbilical Q27.0
  auditory (canal) (external) Q16.1
  auricle (ear) Q16.0
  bile duct or passage Q44.5
  bladder Q64.5
  bone Q79.9
  brain Q00.0
    part of Q04.3
  breast (with nipple present) Q83.8
    with absent nipple Q83.0
  bronchus Q32.4
  canaliculus lacrimalis Q10.4
  carpus —*see* Agenesis, hand
  cartilage Q79.9
  cecum Q42.8
  cerebellum Q04.3
  cervix Q51.5
  chin Q18.8
  cilia Q10.3
  circulatory system, part NOS Q28.9
  clavicle Q74.0
  clitoris Q52.6
  coccyx Q76.49
  colon Q42.9
    specified NEC Q42.8
  corpus callosum Q04.0
  cricoid cartilage Q31.8
  diaphragm (with hernia) Q79.1
  digestive organ(s) or tract (complete) (partial) NEC Q45.8
    upper Q40.8
  ductus arteriosus Q28.8
  duodenum Q41.0
  ear Q16.9
    auricle Q16.0
    lobe Q17.8
  ejaculatory duct Q55.4
  endocrine (gland) NEC Q89.2
  epiglottis Q31.8
  esophagus Q39.8
  eustachian tube Q16.2
  eye Q11.1
    adnexa Q15.8
  eyelid (fold) Q10.3
  face
    bones NEC Q75.8
    specified part NEC Q18.8
  fallopian tube Q50.6

Agenesis *(continued)*
  femur —*see* Defect, reduction, lower limb, longitudinal, femur
  fibula —*see* Defect, reduction, lower limb, longitudinal, fibula
  finger (complete) (partial) —*see* Agenesis, hand
  foot (and toes) (complete) (partial) Q72.3-
  forearm (with hand present) —*see* Agenesis, arm, with hand present
    and hand Q71.2-
  gallbladder Q44.0
  gastric Q40.2
  genitalia, genital (organ(s))
    female Q52.8
      external Q52.71
      internal NEC Q52.8
    male Q55.8
  glottis Q31.8
  hair Q84.0
  hand(and fingers) (complete) (partial) Q71.3-
  heart Q24.8
    valve NEC Q24.8
      pulmonary Q22.0
  hepatic Q44.7
  humerus —*see* Defect, reduction, upper limb
  hymen Q52.4
  ileum Q41.2
  incus Q16.3
  intestine (small) Q41.9
    large Q42.9
      specified NEC Q42.8
  iris (dilator fibers) Q13.1
  jaw M26.09
  jejunum Q41.1
  kidney(s) (partial) Q60.2
    bilateral Q60.1
    unilateral Q60.0
  labium (majus) (minus) Q52.71
  labyrinth, membranous Q16.5
  lacrimal apparatus Q10.4
  larynx Q31.8
  leg (complete) Q72.0-
    with foot present Q72.1-
    lower leg (with foot present) —*see* Agenesis, leg, with foot present and foot Q72.2-
  lens Q12.3
  limb (complete) Q73.0
    lower —*see* Agenesis, leg
    upper —*see* Agenesis, arm
  lip Q38.0
  liver Q44.7
  lung (fissure) (lobe) (bilateral) (unilateral) Q33.3
  mandible, maxilla M26.09
  metacarpus —*see* Agenesis, hand
  metatarsus —*see* Agenesis, foot
  muscle Q79.8
    eyelid Q10.3
    ocular Q15.8
  musculoskeletal system NEC Q79.8
  nail(s) Q84.3
  neck, part Q18.8
  nerve Q07.8
  nervous system, part NEC Q07.8
  nipple Q83.2
  nose Q30.1
  nuclear Q07.8
  organ
    of Corti Q16.5
    or site not listed —*see* Anomaly, by site
  osseous meatus (ear) Q16.1
  ovary
    bilateral Q50.02
    unilateral Q50.01

Agenesis *(continued)*
  oviduct Q50.6
  pancreas Q45.0
  parathyroid (gland) Q89.2
  parotid gland(s) Q38.4
  patella Q74.1
  pelvic girdle (complete) (partial) Q74.2
  penis Q55.5
  pericardium Q24.8
  pituitary (gland) Q89.2
  prostate Q55.4
  punctum lacrimale Q10.4
  radioulnar —*see* Defect, reduction, upper limb
  radius —*see* Defect, reduction, upper limb, longitudinal, radius
  rectum Q42.1
    with fistula Q42.0
  renal Q60.2
    bilateral Q60.1
    unilateral Q60.0
  respiratory organ NEC Q34.8
  rib Q76.6
  roof of orbit Q75.8
  round ligament Q52.8
  sacrum Q76.49
  salivary gland Q38.4
  scapula Q74.0
  scrotum Q55.29
  seminal vesicles Q55.4
  septum
    atrial Q21.1
    between aorta and pulmonary artery Q21.4
    ventricular Q20.4
  shoulder girdle (complete) (partial) Q74.0
  skull (bone) Q75.8
    with
      anencephaly Q00.0
      encephalocele —*see* Encephalocele
      hydrocephalus Q03.9
        with spina bifida —*see* Spina bifida, by site, with hydrocephalus
      microcephaly Q02
  spermatic cord Q55.4
  spinal cord Q06.0
  spine Q76.49
  spleen Q89.01
  sternum Q76.7
  stomach Q40.2
  submaxillary gland(s) (congenital) Q38.4
  tarsus —*see* Agenesis, foot
  tendon Q79.8
  testicle Q55.0
  thymus (gland) Q89.2
  thyroid (gland) E03.1
    cartilage Q31.8
  tibia —*see* Defect, reduction, lower limb, longitudinal, tibia
  tibiofibular —*see* Defect, reduction, lower limb, specified type NEC
  toe (and foot) (complete) (partial) —*see* Agenesis, foot
  tongue Q38.3
  trachea (cartilage) Q32.1
  ulna —*see* Defect, reduction, upper limb, longitudinal, ulna
  upper limb —*see* Agenesis, arm
  ureter Q62.4
  urethra Q64.5
  urinary tract NEC Q64.8
  uterus Q51.0
  uvula Q38.5
  vagina Q52.0
  vas deferens Q55.4

Agenesis *(continued)*
- vein(s) (peripheral) Q27.9
  - brain Q28.3
  - great NEC Q26.8
  - portal Q26.5
- vena cava (inferior) (superior) Q26.8
- vermis of cerebellum Q04.3
- vertebra Q76.49
- vulva Q52.71

Ageusia R43.2

Agitated *—see* condition

Agitation R45.1

Aglossia (congenital) Q38.3

Aglossia-adactylia syndrome Q87.0

Aglycogenosis E74.00

Agnosia (body image) (other senses) (tactile) R48.1
- developmental F88
- verbal R48.1
  - auditory R48.1
    - developmental F80.2
  - developmental F80.2
- visual (object) R48.3

Agoraphobia F40.00
- with panic disorder F40.01
- without panic disorder F40.02

Agrammatism R48.8

Agranulocytopenia *—see* Agranulocytosis

Agranulocytosis (chronic) (cyclical) (genetic) (infantile) (periodic) (pernicious) *—see also* Neutropenia D70.9
- congenital D70.0
- cytoreductive cancer chemotherapy sequela D70.1
- drug-induced D70.2
  - due to cytoreductive cancer chemotherapy D70.1
- due to infection D70.3
- secondary D70.4
  - drug-induced D70.2
    - due to cytoreductive cancer chemotherapy D70.1

Agraphia (absolute) R48.8
- with alexia R48.0
- developmental F81.81

Ague (dumb) *—see* Malaria

Agyria Q04.3

Ahumada-del Castillo syndrome E23.0

Aichomophobia F40.298

AIDS (related complex) B20

Ailment heart *—see* Disease, heart

Ailurophobia F40.218

AIN *—see* Neoplasia, intraepithelial, anal

Ainhum (disease) L94.6

AIPHI (acute idiopathic pulmonary hemorrhage in infants (over 28 days old)) R04.81

Air
- anterior mediastinum J98.2
- compressed, disease T70.3
- conditioner lung or pneumonitis J67.7
- embolism (artery) (cerebral) (any site) T79.0
  - with ectopic or molar pregnancy O08.2
  - due to implanted device NEC *—see* Complications, by site and type, specified NEC

Air *(continued)*
- embolism *(continued)*
  - following
    - abortion *—see* Abortion by type, complicated by, embolism
    - ectopic or molar pregnancy O08.2
    - infusion, therapeutic injection or transfusion T80.0
  - in pregnancy, childbirth or puerperium *—see* Embolism, obstetric
  - traumatic T79.0
- hunger, psychogenic F45.8
- rarefied, effects of *—see* Effect, adverse, high altitude
- sickness T75.3

Airplane sickness T75.3

Akathisia (drug-induced) (treatment-induced) G25.71
- neuroleptic induced (acute) G25.71
- tardive G25.71

Akinesia R29.898

Akinetic mutism R41.89

Akureyri's disease G93.3

Alactasia, congenital E73.0

Alagille's syndrome Q44.7

Alastrim B03

Albers-Schönberg syndrome Q78.2

Albert's syndrome *—see* Tendinitis, Achilles

Albinism, albino E70.30
- with hematologic abnormality E70.339
  - Chédiak-Higashi syndrome E70.330
  - Hermansky-Pudlak syndrome E70.331
  - other specified E70.338
- I E70.320
- II E70.321
- ocular E70.319
  - autosomal recessive E70.311
  - other specified E70.318
  - X-linked E70.310
- oculocutaneous E70.329
  - other specified E70.328
  - tyrosinase (ty) negative E70.320
  - tyrosinase (ty) positive E70.321
- other specified E70.39

Albinismus E70.30

Albright (-McCune) (-Sternberg) syndrome Q78.1

Albuminous *—see* condition

Albuminuria, albuminuric (acute) (chronic) (subacute) (*see also* Proteinuria) R80.9
- complicating pregnancy *—see* Proteinuria, gestational
  - with
    - gestational hypertension *—see* Pre-eclampsia
    - pre-existing hypertension *—see* Hypertension, complicating pregnancy, pre-existing, with, pre-eclampsia
- gestational *—see* Proteinuria, gestational
  - with
    - gestational hypertension *—see* Pre-eclampsia
    - pre-existing hypertension *—see* Hypertension, complicating pregnancy, pre-existing, with, pre-eclampsia
- orthostatic R80.2
- postural R80.2
- pre-eclamptic *—see* Pre-eclampsia
- scarlatinal A38.8

Albuminurophobia F40.298

Alcaptonuria E70.29

Alcohol, alcoholic, alcohol-induced
- addiction (without remission) F10.20
  - with remission F10.21
- amnestic disorder, persisting F10.96
  - with dependence F10.26
- anxiety disorder F10.980
- bipolar and related disorder F10.94
- brain syndrome, chronic F10.97
  - with dependence F10.27
- cardiopathy I42.6
- counseling and surveillance Z71.41
  - family member Z71.42
- delirium (acute) (tremens) (withdrawal) F10.231
  - with intoxication F10.921
    - in
      - abuse F10.121
      - dependence F10.221
- dementia F10.97
  - with dependence F10.27
- depressive disorder F10.94
  - with dependence F10.27
- deterioration F10.97
- hallucinosis (acute) F10.951
  - in
    - abuse F10.151
    - dependence F10.251
- insanity F10.959
- intoxication (acute) (without dependence) F10.129
  - with
    - delirium F10.121
    - dependence F10.229
      - with delirium F10.221
      - uncomplicated F10.220
  - uncomplicated F10.120
- jealousy F10.988
- Korsakoff's, Korsakov's, Korsakow's F10.26
- liver K70.9
  - acute *—see* Disease, liver, alcoholic, hepatitis
- major neurocognitive disorder, amnestic-confabulatory type F10.96
- major neurocognitive disorder, nonamnestic-confabulatory type F10.97
- mania (acute) (chronic) F10.959
- mild neurocognitive disorder F10.988
- paranoia, paranoid (type) psychosis F10.950
- pellagra E52
- poisoning, accidental (acute)
  - NEC *—see* Table of Drugs and Chemicals, alcohol, poisoning
- psychosis *—see* Psychosis, alcoholic
- psychotic disorder F10.959
- sexual dysfunction F10.981
- sleep disorder F10.982
- withdrawal (without convulsions) F10.239
  - with delirium F10.231

Alcoholism (chronic) (without remission) F10.20
- with
  - psychosis *—see* Psychosis, alcoholic
  - remission F10.21
- Korsakov's F10.96
  - with dependence F10.26

Alder (-Reilly) anomaly or syndrome (leukocyte granulation) D72.0

Aldosteronism E26.9
- familial (type I) E26.02
- glucocorticoid-remediable E26.02
- primary (due to (bilateral) adrenal hyperplasia) E26.09
- primary NEC E26.09
- secondary E26.1
- specified NEC E26.89

Aldosteronoma D44.10

Aldrich (-Wiskott) syndrome (eczema-thrombocytopenia) D82.0

Alektorophobia F40.218

Aleppo boil B55.1

Aleukemic *—see* condition

Aleukia
- congenital D70.0
- hemorrhagica D61.9
  - congenital D61.09
- splenica D73.1

Alexia R48.0
- developmental F81.0
- secondary to organic lesion R48.0

Algoneurodystrophy M89.00
- ankle M89.07-
- foot M89.07-
- forearm M89.03-
- hand M89.04-
- lower leg M89.06-
- multiple sites M89.0-
- shoulder M89.01-
- specified site NEC M89.08
- thigh M89.05-
- upper arm M89.02-

Algophobia F40.298

Alienation, mental *—see* Psychosis

Alkalemia E87.3

Alkalosis E87.3
- metabolic E87.3
  - with respiratory acidosis E87.4
- respiratory E87.3

Alkaptonuria E70.29

Allen-Masters syndrome N83.8

Allergy, allergic (reaction) (to) T78.40
- air-borne substance NEC (rhinitis) J30.89
- alveolitis (extrinsic) J67.9
  - due to
    - Aspergillus clavatus J67.4
    - Cryptostroma corticale J67.6
    - organisms (fungal, thermophilic actinomycete) growing in ventilation (air conditioning) systems J67.7
  - specified type NEC J67.8
- anaphylactic reaction or shock T78.2
- angioneurotic edema T78.3
- animal (dander) (epidermal) (hair) (rhinitis) J30.81
- bee sting (anaphylactic shock) *—see* Toxicity, venom, arthropod, bee
- biological *—see* Allergy, drug
- colitis (*see also* Colitis, allergic) K52.29
- dander (animal) (rhinitis) J30.81
- dandruff (rhinitis) J30.81
- dental restorative material (existing) K08.55
- dermatitis *—see* Dermatitis, contact, allergic
- diathesis *—see* History, allergy
- drug, medicament & biological (any) (external) (internal) T78.40
  - correct substance properly administered *—see* Table of Drugs and Chemicals, by drug, adverse effect

Allergy, allergic *(continued)*
- drug, medicament *(continued)*
  - wrong substance given or taken NEC (by accident) —*see* Table of Drugs and Chemicals, by drug, poisoning
- due to pollen J30.1
- dust (house) (stock) (rhinitis) J30.89
  - with asthma —*see* Asthma, allergic extrinsic
- eczema —*see* Dermatitis, contact, allergic
- epidermal (animal) (rhinitis) J30.81
- feathers (rhinitis) J30.89
- food (any) (ingested) NEC T78.1
  - anaphylactic shock —*see* Shock, anaphylactic, due to food
  - dermatitis —*see* Dermatitis, due to, food
  - dietary counseling and surveillance Z71.3
  - in contact with skin L23.6
  - rhinitis J30.5
  - status (without reaction) Z91.018
    - eggs Z91.012
    - milk products Z91.011
    - peanuts Z91.010
    - seafood Z91.013
    - specified NEC Z91.018
- gastrointestinal —*see also* specific type of allergic reaction
  - meaning colitis (*see also* Colitis, allergic) K52.29
  - meaning gastroenteritis (*see also* Gastroenteritis, allergic) K52.29
  - meaning other adverse food reaction not elsewhere classified T78.1
- grain J30.1
- grass (hay fever) (pollen) J30.1
  - asthma —*see* Asthma, allergic extrinsic
- hair (animal) (rhinitis) J30.81
- history (of) —*see* History, allergy
- horse serum —*see* Allergy, serum
- inhalant (rhinitis) J30.89
  - pollen J30.1
- kapok (rhinitis) J30.89
- medicine —*see* Allergy, drug
- milk protein (*see also* Allergy, food) Z91.011
  - anaphylactic reaction T78.07
  - dematitis L27.2
  - entercolitis syndrome K52.21
  - enteropathy K52.22
  - gastroenteritis K52.29
  - gastroesophageal reflux (*see also* Reaction, adverse, food) K21.9
    - with esophagitis K21.0
  - proctocolitis K52.82
- nasal, seasonal due to pollen J30.1
- pneumonia J82
- pollen (any) (hay fever) J30.1
  - asthma —*see* Asthma, allergic extrinsic
- primrose J30.1
- primula J30.1
- proctocolitis K52.82
- purpura D69.0
- ragweed (hay fever) (pollen) J30.1
  - asthma —*see* Asthma, allergic extrinsic
- rose (pollen) J30.1
- seasonal NEC J30.2
- Senecio jacobae (pollen) J30.1
- serum (*see also* Reaction, serum) T80.69
  - anaphylactic shock T80.59
- shock (anaphylactic) T78.2

Allergy, allergic *(continued)*
- shock *(continued)*
  - due to
    - administration of blood and blood products T80.51
    - adverse effect of correct medicinal substance properly administered T88.6
    - immunization T80.52
    - serum NEC T80.59
    - vaccination T80.52
- specific NEC T78.49
- tree (any) (hay fever) (pollen) J30.1
  - asthma —*see* Asthma, allergic extrinsic
- upper respiratory J30.9
- urticaria L50.0
- vaccine —*see* Allergy, serum
- wheat —*see* Allergy, food

Allescheriasis B48.2

Alligator skin disease Q80.9

Allocheiria, allochiria R20.8

Almeida's disease —*see* Paracoccidioidomycosis

Alopecia (hereditaria) (seborrheica) L65.9
- androgenic L64.9
  - drug-induced L64.0
  - specified NEC L64.8
- areata L63.9
  - ophiasis L63.2
  - specified NEC L63.8
  - totalis L63.0
  - universalis L63.1
- cicatricial L66.9
  - specified NEC L66.8
- circumscripta L63.9
- congenital, congenitalis Q84.0
- due to cytotoxic drugs NEC L65.8
- mucinosa L65.2
- postinfective NEC L65.8
- postpartum L65.0
- premature L64.8
- specific (syphilitic) A51.32
- specified NEC L65.8
- syphilitic (secondary) A51.32
- totalis (capitis) L63.0
- universalis (entire body) L63.1
- X-ray L58.1

Alpers' disease G31.81

Alpine sickness T70.29

Alport syndrome Q87.81

ALTE (apparent life threatening event) in newborn and infant R68.13

Alteration (of), **Altered**
- awareness
  - transient R40.4
  - unintended under general anesthesia, during procedure T88.53
- mental status R41.82
- pattern of family relationships affecting child Z62.898
- sensation
  - following
    - cerebrovascular disease I69.998
      - cerebral infarction I69.398
      - intracerebral hemorrhage I69.198
      - nontraumatic intracranial hemorrhage NEC I69.298
      - specified disease NEC I69.898
      - subarachnoid hemorrhage I69.098

Alternating —*see* condition

Altitude, high (effects) —*see* Effect, adverse, high altitude

Aluminosis (of lung) J63.0

Alveolitis
- allergic (extrinsic) —*see* Pneumonitis, hypersensitivity
- due to
  - Aspergillus clavatus J67.4
  - Cryptostroma corticale J67.6
- fibrosing (cryptogenic) (idiopathic) J84.112
- jaw M27.3
- sicca dolorosa M27.3

Alveolus, alveolar —*see* condition

Alymphocytosis D72.810
- thymic (with immunodeficiency) D82.1

Alymphoplasia, thymic D82.1

Alzheimer's disease or sclerosis —*see* Disease, Alzheimer's

Amastia (with nipple present) Q83.8
- with absent nipple Q83.0

Amathophobia F40.228

Amaurosis (acquired) (congenital) —*see also* Blindness
- fugax G45.3
- hysterical F44.6
- Leber's congenital H35.50
- uremic —*see* Uremia

Amaurotic idiocy (infantile) (juvenile) (late) E75.4

Amaxophobia F40.248

Ambiguous genitalia Q56.4

Amblyopia (congenital) (ex anopsia) (partial) (suppression) H53.00-
- anisometropic —*see* Amblyopia, refractive
- deprivation H53.01-
- hysterical F44.6
- nocturnal —*see also* Blindness, night
  - vitamin A deficiency E50.5
- refractive H53.02-
- strabismic H53.03-
- suspect H53.04-
- tobacco H53.8
- toxic NEC H53.8
- uremic —*see* Uremia

Ameba, amebic (histolytica) —*see also* Amebiasis
- abscess (liver) A06.4

Amebiasis A06.9
- with abscess —*see* Abscess, amebic
- acute A06.0
- chronic (intestine) A06.1
  - with abscess —*see* Abscess, amebic
- cutaneous A06.7
- cutis A06.7
- cystitis A06.81
- genitourinary tract NEC A06.82
- hepatic —*see* Abscess, liver, amebic
- intestine A06.0
- nondysenteric colitis A06.2
- skin A06.7
- specified site NEC A06.89

Ameboma (of intestine) A06.3

Amelia Q73.0
- lower limb —*see* Agenesis, leg
- upper limb —*see* Agenesis, arm

Ameloblastoma —*see also* Cyst, calcifying odontogenic
- long bones C40.9-
  - lower limb C40.2-
  - upper limb C40.0-
- malignant C41.1
  - jaw (bone) (lower) C41.1
    - upper C41.0
- tibial C40.2-

Amelogenesis imperfecta K00.5
- nonhereditaria (segmentalis) K00.4

Amenorrhea N91.2
- hyperhormonal E28.8
- primary N91.0
- secondary N91.1

Amentia —*see* Disability, intellectual
- Meynert's (nonalcoholic) F04

American
- leishmaniasis B55.2
- mountain tick fever A93.2

Ametropia —*see* Disorder, refraction

AMH (asymptomatic microscopic hematuria) R31.21

Amianthosis J61

Amimia R48.8

Amino-acid disorder E72.9
- anemia D53.0

Aminoacidopathy E72.9

Aminoaciduria E72.9

Amnes(t)**ic syndrome** (post-traumatic) F04
- induced by
  - alcohol F10.96
    - with dependence F10.26
  - psychoactive NEC F19.96
    - with
      - abuse F19.16
      - dependence F19.26
  - sedative F13.96
    - with dependence F13.26

Amnesia R41.3
- anterograde R41.1
- auditory R48.8
- dissociative F44.0
  - with dissociative fugue F44.1
- hysterical F44.0
- postictal in epilepsy —*see* Epilepsy
- psychogenic F44.0
- retrograde R41.2
- transient global G45.4

Amnion, amniotic —*see* condition

Amnionitis —*see* Pregnancy, complicated by

Amok F68.8

Amoral traits F60.89

Amphetamine (or other stimulant) -induced
- anxiety disorder F15.980
- bipolar and related disorder F15.94
- delirium F15.921
- depressive disorder F15.94
- obsessive-compulsive and related disorder F15.988
- psychotic disorder F15.959
- sexual dysfunction F15.981
- sleep disorder F15.982
- stimulant withdrawal F15.23

Ampulla
- lower esophagus K22.8
- phrenic K22.8

Amputation —*see also* Absence, by site, acquired
- neuroma (postoperative) (traumatic) —*see* Complications, amputation stump, neuroma
- stump (surgical)
  - abnormal, painful, or with complication (late) —*see* Complications, amputation stump
  - healed or old NOS Z89.9

Amputation *(continued)*
- traumatic (complete) (partial)
  - arm (upper) (complete) S48.91-
    - at
      - elbow S58.01-
        - partial S58.02-
      - shoulder joint (complete) S48.01-
        - partial S48.02-
    - between
      - elbow and wrist (complete) S58.11-
        - partial S58.12-
      - shoulder and elbow (complete) S48.11-
        - partial S48.12-
    - partial S48.92-
  - breast (complete) S28.21-
    - partial S28.22-
  - clitoris (complete) S38.211
    - partial S38.212
  - ear (complete) S08.11-
    - partial S08.12-
  - finger (complete) (metacarpophalangeal) S68.11-
    - index S68.11-
    - little S68.11-
    - middle S68.11-
    - partial S68.12-
      - index S68.12-
      - little S68.12-
      - middle S68.12-
      - ring S68.12-
    - ring S68.11-
    - thumb *—see* Amputation, traumatic, thumb
    - transphalangeal (complete) S68.61-
      - index S68.61-
      - little S68.61-
      - middle S68.61-
      - partial S68.62-
        - index S68.62-
        - little S68.62-
        - middle S68.62-
        - ring S68.62-
      - ring S68.61-
  - foot (complete) S98.91-
    - at ankle level S98.01-
      - partial S98.02-
    - midfoot S98.31-
      - partial S98.32-
    - partial S98.92-
  - forearm (complete) S58.91-
    - at elbow level (complete) S58.01-
      - partial S58.02-
    - between elbow and wrist (complete) S58.11-
      - partial S58.12-
    - partial S58.92-
  - genital organ(s) (external)
    - female (complete) S38.211
      - partial S38.212
    - male
      - penis (complete) S38.221
        - partial S38.222
      - scrotum (complete) S38.231
        - partial S38.232
      - testes (complete) S38.231
        - partial S38.232
  - hand (complete) (wrist level) S68.41-
    - finger(s) alone *—see* Amputation, traumatic, finger
    - partial S68.42-
    - thumb alone *—see* Amputation, traumatic, thumb
    - transmetacarpal (complete) S68.71-
      - partial S68.72-

Amputation *(continued)*
- traumatic *(continued)*
  - head
    - ear *—see* Amputation, traumatic, ear
    - nose (partial) S08.812
      - complete S08.811
    - part S08.89
      - scalp S08.0
  - hip (and thigh) (complete) S78.91-
    - at hip joint (complete) S78.01-
      - partial S78.02-
    - between hip and knee (complete) S78.11-
      - partial S78.12-
    - partial S78.92-
  - labium (majus) (minus) (complete) S38.21-
    - partial S38.21-
  - leg (lower) S88.91-
    - at knee level S88.01-
      - partial S88.02-
    - between knee and ankle S88.11-
      - partial S88.12-
    - partial S88.92-
  - nose (partial) S08.812
    - complete S08.811
  - penis (complete) S38.221
    - partial S38.222
  - scrotum (complete) S38.231
    - partial S38.232
  - shoulder *—see* Amputation, traumatic, arm
    - at shoulder joint *—see* Amputation, traumatic, arm, at shoulder joint
  - testes (complete) S38.231
    - partial S38.232
  - thigh *—see* Amputation, traumatic, hip
  - thorax, part of S28.1
    - breast *—see* Amputation, traumatic, breast
  - thumb (complete) (metacarpophalangeal) S68.01-
    - partial S68.02-
    - transphalangeal (complete) S68.51-
      - partial S68.52-
  - toe (lesser) S98.13-
    - great S98.11-
      - partial S98.12-
    - more than one S98.21-
      - partial S98.22-
    - partial S98.14-
  - vulva (complete) S38.211
    - partial S38.212

Amputee (bilateral) (old) Z89.9

Amsterdam dwarfism Q87.1

Amusia R48.8
- developmental F80.89

Amyelencephalus, amyelencephaly Q00.0

Amyelia Q06.0

Amygdalitis *—see* Tonsillitis

Amygdalolith J35.8

Amyloid heart (disease) E85.4 *[I43]*

Amyloidosis (generalized) (primary) E85.9
- with lung involvement E85.4 *[J99]*
- familial E85.2
- genetic E85.2
- heart E85.4 *[I43]*
- hemodialysis-associated E85.3
- liver E85.4 *[K77]*
- light chain (AL) E85.81
- localized E85.4

Amyloidosis *(continued)*
- neuropathic heredofamilial E85.1
- non-neuropathic heredofamilial E85.0
- organ limited E85.4
- Portuguese E85.1
- pulmonary E85.4 *[J99]*
- secondary systemic E85.3
- senile systemic (SSA) E85.82
- skin (lichen) (macular) E85.4 *[L99]*
- specified NEC E85.89
- subglottic E85.4 *[J99]*
- wild-type transthyretin-related (ATTR) E85.82

Amylopectinosis (brancher enzyme deficiency) E74.03

Amylophagia *—see* Pica

Amyoplasia congenita Q79.8

Amyotonia M62.89
- congenita G70.2

Amyotrophia, amyotrophy, amyotrophic G71.8
- congenita Q79.8
- diabetic *—see* Diabetes, amyotrophy
- lateral sclerosis G12.21
- neuralgic G54.5
- spinal progressive G12.25

Anacidity, gastric K31.83
- psychogenic F45.8

Anaerosis of newborn P28.89

Analbuminemia E88.09

Analgesia *—see* Anesthesia

Analphalipoproteinemia E78.6

Anaphylactic
- purpura D69.0
- shock or reaction *—see* Shock, anaphylactic

Anaphylactoid shock or reaction *—see* Shock, anaphylactic

Anaphylactoid syndrome of pregnancy O88.01-

Anaphylaxis *—see* Shock, anaphylactic

Anaplasia cervix *—see also* Dysplasia, cervix N87.9

Anaplasmosis, human A77.49

Anarthria R47.1

Anasarca R60.1
- cardiac *—see* Failure, heart, congestive
- lung J18.2
- newborn P83.2
- nutritional E43
- pulmonary J18.2
- renal N04.9

Anastomosis
- aneurysmal *—see* Aneurysm
- arteriovenous ruptured brain I60.8
- intestinal K63.89
  - complicated NEC K91.89
    - involving urinary tract N99.89
- retinal and choroidal vessels (congenital) Q14.8

Anatomical narrow angle H40.03-

Ancylostoma, ancylostomiasis (braziliense) (caninum) (ceylanicum) (duodenale) B76.0
- Necator americanus B76.1

Andersen's disease (glycogen storage) E74.09

Anderson-Fabry disease E75.21

Andes disease T70.29

Andrews' disease (bacterid) L08.89

Androblastoma
- benign
  - specified site *—see* Neoplasm, benign, by site
  - unspecified site
    - female D27.9
    - male D29.20
- malignant
  - specified site *—see* Neoplasm, malignant, by site
  - unspecified site
    - female C56.9
    - male C62.90
- specified site *—see* Neoplasm, uncertain behavior, by site
- tubular
  - with lipid storage
    - specified site *—see* Neoplasm, benign, by site
    - unspecified site
      - female D27.9
      - male D29.20
  - specified site *—see* Neoplasm, benign, by site
  - unspecified site
    - female D27.9
    - male D29.20
- unspecified site
  - female D39.10
  - male D40.10

Androgen insensitivity syndrome *—see also* Syndrome, androgen insensitivity E34.50

Androgen resistance syndrome *—see also* Syndrome, androgen insensitivity E34.50

Android pelvis Q74.2
- with disproportion (fetopelvic) O33.3
  - causing obstructed labor O65.3

Androphobia F40.290

Anectasis, pulmonary (newborn) *—see* Atelectasis

Anemia (essential) (general) (hemoglobin deficiency) (infantile) (primary) (profound) D64.9
- with (due to) (in)
  - disorder of
    - anaerobic glycolysis D55.2
    - pentose phosphate pathway D55.1
  - koilonychia D50.9
- achlorhydric D50.8
- achrestic D53.1
- Addison (-Biermer) (pernicious) D51.0
- agranulocytic *—see* Agranulocytosis
- amino-acid-deficiency D53.0
- aplastic D61.9
  - congenital D61.09
  - drug-induced D61.1
  - due to
    - drugs D61.1
    - external agents NEC D61.2
    - infection D61.2
    - radiation D61.2
  - idiopathic D61.3
  - red cell (pure) D60.9
    - chronic D60.0
    - congenital D61.01
    - specified type NEC D60.8
    - transient D60.1
  - specified type NEC D61.89
  - toxic D61.2
- aregenerative
  - congenital D61.09
- asiderotic D50.9
- atypical (primary) D64.9

Anemia *(continued)*
- Baghdad spring D55.0
- Balantidium coli A07.0
- Biermer's (pernicious) D51.0
- blood loss (chronic) D50.0
  - acute D62
- bothriocephalus B70.0 *[D63.8]*
- brickmaker's B76.9 *[D63.8]*
- cerebral I67.89
- childhood D58.9
- chlorotic D50.8
- chronic
  - blood loss D50.0
  - hemolytic D58.9
    - idiopathic D59.9
  - simple D53.9
- chronica congenita aregenerativa D61.09
- combined system disease NEC D51.0 *[G32.0]*
  - due to dietary vitamin B12 deficiency D51.3 *[G32.0]*
- complicating pregnancy, childbirth or puerperium *—see* Pregnancy, complicated by (management affected by), anemia
- congenital P61.4
  - aplastic D61.09
  - due to isoimmunization NOS P55.9
  - dyserythropoietic, dyshematopoietic D64.4
  - following fetal blood loss P61.3
  - Heinz body D58.2
  - hereditary hemolytic NOS D58.9
  - pernicious D51.0
  - spherocytic D58.0
- Cooley's (erythroblastic) D56.1
- cytogenic D51.0
- deficiency D53.9
  - 2, 3 diphosphoglycurate mutase D55.2
  - 2, 3 PG D55.2
  - 6 phosphogluconate dehydrogenase D55.1
  - 6-PGD D55.1
  - amino-acid D53.0
  - combined B12 and folate D53.1
  - enzyme D55.9
    - drug-induced (hemolytic) D59.2
    - glucose-6-phosphate dehydrogenase (G6PD) D55.0
    - glycolytic D55.2
    - nucleotide metabolism D55.3
    - related to hexose monophosphate (HMP) shunt pathway NEC D55.1
    - specified type NEC D55.8
  - erythrocytic glutathione D55.1
  - folate D52.9
    - dietary D52.0
    - drug-induced D52.1
  - folic acid D52.9
    - dietary D52.0
    - drug-induced D52.1
  - G SH D55.1
  - GGS-R D55.1
  - glucose-6-phosphate dehydrogenase D55.0
  - glutathione reductase D55.1
  - glyceraldehyde phosphate dehydrogenase D55.2
  - G6PD D55.0
  - hexokinase D55.2
  - iron D50.9
    - secondary to blood loss (chronic) D50.0

Anemia *(continued)*
- deficiency *(continued)*
  - nutritional D53.9
    - with
      - poor iron absorption D50.8
      - specified deficiency NEC D53.8
  - phosphofructo-aldolase D55.2
  - phosphoglycerate kinase D55.2
  - PK D55.2
  - protein D53.0
  - pyruvate kinase D55.2
  - transcobalamin II D51.2
  - triose-phosphate isomerase D55.2
  - vitamin B12 NOS D51.9
    - dietary D51.3
    - due to
      - intrinsic factor deficiency D51.0
      - selective vitamin B12 malabsorption with proteinuria D51.1
    - pernicious D51.0
    - specified type NEC D51.8
- Diamond-Blackfan (congenital hypoplastic) D61.01
- dibothriocephalus B70.0 *[D63.8]*
- dimorphic D53.1
- diphasic D53.1
- Diphyllobothrium (Dibothriocephalus) B70.0 *[D63.8]*
- due to (in) (with)
  - antineoplastic chemotherapy D64.81
  - blood loss (chronic) D50.0
    - acute D62
  - chemotherapy, antineoplastic D64.81
  - chronic disease classified elsewhere NEC D63.8
  - chronic kidney disease D63.1
  - deficiency
    - amino-acid D53.0
    - copper D53.8
    - folate (folic acid) D52.9
      - dietary D52.0
      - drug-induced D52.1
    - molybdenum D53.8
    - protein D53.0
    - zinc D53.8
  - dietary vitamin B12 deficiency D51.3
  - disorder of
    - glutathione metabolism D55.1
    - nucleotide metabolism D55.3
  - drug *—see* Anemia, by type *— see also* Table of Drugs and Chemicals
  - end stage renal disease D63.1
  - enzyme disorder D55.9
  - fetal blood loss P61.3
  - fish tapeworm (D.latum) infestation B70.0 *[D63.8]*
  - hemorrhage (chronic) D50.0
    - acute D62
  - impaired absorption D50.9
  - loss of blood (chronic) D50.0
    - acute D62
  - myxedema E03.9 *[D63.8]*
  - Necator americanus B76.1 *[D63.8]*
  - prematurity P61.2
  - selective vitamin B12 malabsorption with proteinuria D51.1
  - transcobalamin II deficiency D51.2
- Dyke-Young type (secondary) (symptomatic) D59.1
- dyserythropoietic (congenital) D64.4
- dyshematopoietic (congenital) D64.4

Anemia *(continued)*
- Egyptian B76.9 *[D63.8]*
- elliptocytosis *—see* Elliptocytosis
- enzyme-deficiency, drug-induced D59.2
- epidemic *—see also* Ancylostomiasis B76.9 *[D63.8]*
- erythroblastic
  - familial D56.1
  - newborn (*see also* Disease, hemolytic) P55.9
  - of childhood D56.1
- erythrocytic glutathione deficiency D55.1
- erythropoietin-resistant anemia (EPO resistant anemia) D63.1
- Faber's (achlorhydric anemia) D50.9
- factitious (self-induced blood letting) D50.0
- familial erythroblastic D56.1
- Fanconi's (congenital pancytopenia) D61.09
- favism D55.0
- fish tapeworm (D. latum) infestation B70.0 *[D63.8]*
- folate (folic acid) deficiency D52.9
- glucose-6-phosphate dehydrogenase (G6PD) deficiency D55.0
- glutathione-reductase deficiency D55.1
- goat's milk D52.0
- granulocytic *—see* Agranulocytosis
- Heinz body, congenital D58.2
- hemolytic D58.9
  - acquired D59.9
    - with hemoglobinuria NEC D59.6
    - autoimmune NEC D59.1
    - infectious D59.4
    - specified type NEC D59.8
    - toxic D59.4
  - acute D59.9
    - due to enzyme deficiency specified type NEC D55.8
    - Lederer's D59.1
  - autoimmune D59.1
    - drug-induced D59.0
  - chronic D58.9
    - idiopathic D59.9
  - cold type (secondary) (symptomatic) D59.1
  - congenital (spherocytic) *—see* Spherocytosis
  - due to
    - cardiac conditions D59.4
    - drugs (nonautoimmune) D59.2
      - autoimmune D59.0
    - enzyme disorder D55.9
      - drug-induced D59.2
    - presence of shunt or other internal prosthetic device D59.4
  - familial D58.9
  - hereditary D58.9
    - due to enzyme disorder D55.9
      - specified type NEC D55.8
    - specified type NEC D58.8
  - idiopathic (chronic) D59.9
  - mechanical D59.4
  - microangiopathic D59.4
  - nonautoimmune D59.4
    - drug-induced D59.2
  - nonspherocytic
    - congenital or hereditary NEC D55.8
      - glucose-6-phosphate dehydrogenase deficiency D55.0
      - pyruvate kinase deficiency D55.2

Anemia *(continued)*
- hemolytic *(continued)*
  - nonspherocytic *(continued)*
    - congenital or hereditary NEC *(continued)*
      - type
        - I D55.1
        - II D55.2
    - type
      - I D55.1
      - II D55.2
  - secondary D59.4
    - autoimmune D59.1
  - specified (hereditary) type NEC D58.8
  - Stransky-Regala type (*see also* Hemoglobinopathy) D58.8
  - symptomatic D59.4
    - autoimmune D59.1
  - toxic D59.4
  - warm type (secondary) (symptomatic) D59.1
- hemorrhagic (chronic) D50.0
  - acute D62
- Herrick's D57.1
- hexokinase deficiency D55.2
- hookworm B76.9 *[D63.8]*
- hypochromic (idiopathic) (microcytic) (normoblastic) D50.9
  - due to blood loss (chronic) D50.0
    - acute D62
  - familial sex-linked D64.0
  - pyridoxine-responsive D64.3
  - sideroblastic, sex-linked D64.0
- hypoplasia, red blood cells D61.9
  - congenital or familial D61.01
- hypoplastic (idiopathic) D61.9
  - congenital or familial (of childhood) D61.01
- hypoproliferative (refractive) D61.9
- idiopathic D64.9
  - aplastic D61.3
  - hemolytic, chronic D59.9
- in (due to) (with)
  - chronic kidney disease D63.1
  - end stage renal disease D63.1
  - failure, kidney (renal) D63.1
  - neoplastic disease (*see also* Neoplasm) D63.0
- intertropical *—see also* Ancylostomiasis D63.8
- iron deficiency D50.9
  - secondary to blood loss (chronic) D50.0
    - acute D62
  - specified type NEC D50.8
- Joseph-Diamond-Blackfan (congenital hypoplastic) D61.01
- Lederer's (hemolytic) D59.1
- leukoerythroblastic D61.82
- macrocytic D53.9
  - nutritional D52.0
  - tropical D52.8
- malarial (*see also* Malaria) B54 *[D63.8]*
- malignant (progressive) D51.0
- malnutrition D53.9
- marsh (*see also* Malaria) B54 *[D63.8]*
- Mediterranean (with other hemoglobinopathy) D56.9
- megaloblastic D53.1
  - combined B12 and folate deficiency D53.1
  - hereditary D51.1
  - nutritional D52.0
  - orotic aciduria D53.0
  - refractory D53.1
  - specified type NEC D53.1
- megalocytic D53.1

Anemia *(continued)*
- microcytic (hypochromic) D50.9
  - due to blood loss (chronic) D50.0
    - acute D62
  - familial D56.8
- microdrepanocytosis D57.40
- microelliptopoikilocytic (Rietti-Greppi- Micheli) D56.9
- miner's B76.9 *[D63.8]*
- myelodysplastic D46.9
- myelofibrosis D75.81
- myelogenous D64.89
- myelopathic D64.89
- myelophthisic D61.82
- myeloproliferative D47.Z9
- newborn P61.4
  - due to
    - ABO (antibodies, isoimmunization, maternal/fetal incompatibility) P55.1
    - Rh (antibodies, isoimmunization, maternal/fetal incompatibility) P55.0
  - following fetal blood loss P61.3
  - posthemorrhagic (fetal) P61.3
- nonspherocytic hemolytic —*see* Anemia, hemolytic, nonspherocytic
- normocytic (infectional) D64.9
  - due to blood loss (chronic) D50.0
    - acute D62
  - myelophthisic D61.82
- nutritional (deficiency) D53.9
  - with
    - poor iron absorption D50.8
    - specified deficiency NEC D53.8
  - megaloblastic D52.0
- of prematurity P61.2
- orotaciduric (congenital) (hereditary) D53.0
- osteosclerotic D64.89
- ovalocytosis (hereditary) —*see* Elliptocytosis
- paludal (*see also* Malaria) B54 *[D63.8]*
- pernicious (congenital) (malignant) (progressive) D51.0
- pleochromic D64.89
  - of sprue D52.8
- posthemorrhagic (chronic) D50.0
  - acute D62
  - newborn P61.3
- postoperative (postprocedural)
  - due to (acute) blood loss D62
    - chronic blood loss D50.0
  - specified NEC D64.9
- postpartum O90.81
- pressure D64.89
- progressive D64.9
  - malignant D51.0
  - pernicious D51.0
- protein-deficiency D53.0
- pseudoleukemica infantum D64.89
- pure red cell D60.9
  - congenital D61.01
- pyridoxine-responsive D64.3
- pyruvate kinase deficiency D55.2
- refractory D46.4
  - with
    - excess of blasts D46.20
      - 1(RAEB 1) D46.21
      - 2(RAEB 2) D46.22
      - in transformation (RAEB T) —*see* Leukemia, acute myeloblastic
    - hemochromatosis D46.1
    - sideroblasts (ring) (RARS) D46.1
  - megaloblastic D53.1
  - sideroblastic D46.1

Anemia *(continued)*
- refractory *(continued)*
  - sideropenic D50.9
  - without ring sideroblasts, so stated D46.0
  - without sideroblasts without excess of blasts D46.0
- Rietti-Greppi-Micheli D56.9
- scorbutic D53.2
- secondary to
  - blood loss (chronic) D50.0
    - acute D62
  - hemorrhage (chronic) D50.0
    - acute D62
- semiplastic D61.89
- sickle-cell —*see* Disease, sickle-cell
- sideroblastic D64.3
  - hereditary D64.0
  - hypochromic, sex-linked D64.0
  - pyridoxine-responsive NEC D64.3
  - refractory D46.1
  - secondary (due to)
    - disease D64.1
    - drugs and toxins D64.2
  - specified type NEC D64.3
- sideropenic (refractory) D50.9
  - due to blood loss (chronic) D50.0
    - acute D62
- simple chronic D53.9
- specified type NEC D64.89
- spherocytic (hereditary) —*see* Spherocytosis
- splenic D64.89
- splenomegalic D64.89
- stomatocytosis D58.8
- syphilitic (acquired) (late) A52.79 *[D63.8]*
- target cell D64.89
- thalassemia D56.9
- thrombocytopenic —*see* Thrombocytopenia
- toxic D61.2
- tropical B76.9 *[D63.8]*
  - macrocytic D52.8
- tuberculous A18.89 *[D63.8]*
- vegan D51.3
- vitamin
  - B6-responsive D64.3
  - B12 deficiency (dietary)
    - pernicious D51.0
- von Jaksch's D64.89
- Witts'(achlorhydric anemia) D50.8

Anemophobia F40.228

Anencephalus, anencephaly Q00.0

Anergasia —*see* Psychosis, organic

Anesthesia, anesthetic R20.0
- complication or reaction NEC (*see also* Complications, anesthesia) T88.59
  - due to
    - correct substance properly administered —*see* Table of Drugs and Chemicals, by drug, adverse effect
    - overdose or wrong substance given —*see* Table of Drugs and Chemicals, by drug, poisoning
  - unintended awareness under general anesthesia during procedure T88.53
    - personal history of Z92.84
- cornea H18.81-
- dissociative F44.6
- functional (hysterical) F44.6
- hyperesthetic, thalamic G89.0
- hysterical F44.6
- local skin lesion R20.0
- sexual (psychogenic) F52.1
- shock (due to) T88.2
- skin R20.0
- testicular N50.9

Anetoderma (maculosum) (of) L90.8
- Jadassohn-Pellizzari L90.2
- Schweniger-Buzzi L90.1

Aneurin deficiency E51.9

Aneurysm (anastomotic) (artery) (cirsoid) (diffuse) (false) (fusiform) (multiple) (saccular) I72.9
- abdominal (aorta) I71.4
  - ruptured I71.3
  - syphilitic A52.01
- aorta, aortic (nonsyphilitic) I71.9
  - abdominal I71.4
    - ruptured I71.3
  - arch I71.2
    - ruptured I71.1
  - arteriosclerotic I71.9
    - ruptured I71.8
  - ascending I71.2
    - ruptured I71.1
  - congenital Q25.43
  - descending I71.9
    - abdominal I71.4
      - ruptured I71.3
    - ruptured I71.8
    - thoracic I71.2
      - ruptured I71.1
  - root Q25.43
  - ruptured I71.8
  - sinus, congenital Q25.43
  - syphilitic A52.01
  - thoracic I71.2
    - ruptured I71.1
  - thoracoabdominal I71.6
    - ruptured I71.5
  - thorax, thoracic (arch) I71.2
    - ruptured I71.1
    - root Q25.43
  - transverse I71.2
    - ruptured I71.1
  - valve (heart) (*see also* Endocarditis, aortic) I35.8
- arteriosclerotic I72.9
  - cerebral I67.1
    - ruptured —*see* Hemorrhage, intracranial, subarachnoid
- arteriovenous (congenital) —*see also* Malformation, arteriovenous
  - acquired I77.0
    - brain I67.1
    - coronary I25.41
    - pulmonary I28.0
  - brain Q28.2
    - ruptured I60.8
  - peripheral —*see* Malformation, arteriovenous, peripheral
  - precerebral vessels Q28.0
  - specified site NEC —*see also* Malformation, arteriovenous
    - acquired I77.0
- basal —*see* Aneurysm, brain
- basilar (trunk) I72.5
- berry (congenital) (nonruptured) I67.1
  - ruptured I60.7
- brain I67.1
  - arteriosclerotic I67.1
    - ruptured —*see* Hemorrhage, intracranial, subarachnoid
  - arteriovenous (congenital) (nonruptured) Q28.2
    - acquired I67.1
      - ruptured I60.8
    - ruptured I60.8
  - berry (congenital) (nonruptured) I67.1
    - ruptured (*see also* Hemorrhage, intracranial, subarachnoid) I60.7
  - congenital Q28.3
    - ruptured I60.7
  - meninges I67.1
    - ruptured I60.8

Aneurysm *(continued)*
- brain *(continued)*
  - miliary (congenital) (nonruptured) I67.1
    - ruptured (*see also* Hemorrhage, intracranial, subarachnoid) I60.7
  - mycotic I33.0
  - ruptured —*see* Hemorrhage, intracranial, subarachnoid
  - syphilitic (hemorrhage) A52.05
- cardiac (false) (*see also* Aneurysm, heart) I25.3
- carotid artery (common) (external) I72.0
  - internal (intracranial) I67.1
    - extracranial portion I72.0
  - ruptured into brain I60.0-
  - syphilitic A52.09
    - intracranial A52.05
- cavernous sinus I67.1
  - arteriovenous (congenital) (nonruptured) Q28.3
    - ruptured I60.8
- celiac I72.8
- central nervous system, syphilitic A52.05
- cerebral —*see* Aneurysm, brain
- chest —*see* Aneurysm, thorax
- circle of Willis I67.1
  - congenital Q28.3
    - ruptured I60.6
  - ruptured I60.6
- common iliac artery I72.3
- congenital (peripheral) Q27.8
  - aorta (root) (sinus) Q25.43
  - brain Q28.3
    - ruptured I60.7
  - coronary Q24.5
  - digestive system Q27.8
  - lower limb Q27.8
  - pulmonary Q25.79
  - retina Q14.1
  - specified site NEC Q27.8
  - upper limb Q27.8
- conjunctiva —*see* Abnormality, conjunctiva, vascular
- conus arteriosus —*see* Aneurysm, heart
- coronary (arteriosclerotic) (artery) I25.41
  - arteriovenous, congenital Q24.5
  - congenital Q24.5
  - ruptured —*see* Infarct, myocardium
  - syphilitic A52.06
  - vein I25.89
- cylindroid (aorta) I71.9
  - ruptured I71.8
  - syphilitic A52.01
- ductus arteriosus Q25.0
- endocardial, infective (any valve) I33.0
- femoral (artery) (ruptured) I72.4
- gastroduodenal I72.8
- gastroepiploic I72.8
- heart (wall) (chronic or with a stated duration of over 4 weeks) I25.3
  - valve —*see* Endocarditis
- hepatic I72.8
- iliac (common) (artery) (ruptured) I72.3
- infective I72.9
  - endocardial (any valve) I33.0
- innominate (nonsyphilitic) I72.8
  - syphilitic A52.09
- interauricular septum —*see* Aneurysm, heart
- interventricular septum —*see* Aneurysm, heart
- intrathoracic (nonsyphilitic) I71.2
  - ruptured I71.1
  - syphilitic A52.01

Aneurysm *(continued)*
- lower limb I72.4
- lung (pulmonary artery) I28.1
- mediastinal (nonsyphilitic) I72.8
  - syphilitic A52.09
- miliary (congenital) I67.1
  - ruptured —*see* Hemorrhage, intracerebral, subarachnoid, intracranial
- mitral (heart) (valve) I34.8
- mural —*see* Aneurysm, heart
- mycotic I72.9
  - endocardial (any valve) I33.0
  - ruptured, brain —*see* Hemorrhage, intracerebral, subarachnoid
- myocardium —*see* Aneurysm, heart
- neck I72.0
- pancreaticoduodenal I72.8
- patent ductus arteriosus Q25.0
- peripheral NEC I72.8
  - congenital Q27.8
    - digestive system Q27.8
    - lower limb Q27.8
    - specified site NEC Q27.8
    - upper limb Q27.8
- popliteal (artery) (ruptured) I72.4
- precerebral
  - congenital (nonruptured) Q28.1
  - specified site, NEC I72.5
- pulmonary I28.1
  - arteriovenous Q25.72
    - acquired I28.0
  - syphilitic A52.09
  - valve (heart) —*see* Endocarditis, pulmonary
- racemose (peripheral) I72.9
  - congenital —*see* Aneurysm, congenital
- radial I72.1
- Rasmussen NEC A15.0
- renal (artery) I72.2
- retina —*see also* Disorder, retina, microaneurysms
  - congenital Q14.1
  - diabetic —*see* Diabetes, microaneurysms, retinal
- sinus of Valsalva Q25.49
- specified NEC I72.8
- spinal (cord) I72.8
  - syphilitic (hemorrhage) A52.09
- splenic I72.8
- subclavian (artery) (ruptured) I72.8
  - syphilitic A52.09
- superior mesenteric I72.8
- syphilitic (aorta) A52.01
  - central nervous system A52.05
  - congenital (late) A50.54 *[I79.0]*
  - spine, spinal A52.09
- thoracoabdominal (aorta) I71.6
  - ruptured I71.5
  - syphilitic A52.01
- thorax, thoracic (aorta) (arch) (nonsyphilitic) I71.2
  - ruptured I71.1
  - syphilitic A52.01
- traumatic (complication) (early), specified site —*see* Injury, blood vessel
- tricuspid (heart) (valve) I07.8
- ulnar I72.1
- upper limb (ruptured) I72.1
- valve, valvular —*see* Endocarditis
- venous (*see also* Varix) I86.8
  - congenital Q27.8
    - digestive system Q27.8
    - lower limb Q27.8
    - specified site NEC Q27.8
    - upper limb Q27.8
- ventricle —*see* Aneurysm, heart
- vertebral artery I72.6
- visceral NEC I72.8

Angelman syndrome Q93.5

Anger R45.4

Angiectasis, angiectopia I99.8

Angiitis I77.6
- allergic granulomatous M30.1
- hypersensitivity M31.0
- necrotizing M31.9
  - specified NEC M31.8
- nervous system, granulomatous I67.7

Angina (attack) (cardiac) (chest) (heart) (pectoris) (syndrome) (vasomotor) I20.9
- with
  - atherosclerotic heart disease —*see* Arteriosclerosis, coronary (artery),
  - documented spasm I20.1
- abdominal K55.1
- accelerated —*see* Angina, unstable
- agranulocytic —*see* Agranulocytosis
- angiospastic —*see* Angina, with documented spasm
- aphthous B08.5
- crescendo —*see* Angina, unstable
- croupous J05.0
- cruris I73.9
- de novo effort —*see* Angina, unstable
- diphtheritic, membranous A36.0
- equivalent I20.8
- exudative, chronic J37.0
- following acute myocardial infarction I23.7
- gangrenous diphtheritic A36.0
- intestinal K55.1
- Ludovici K12.2
- Ludwig's K12.2
- malignant diphtheritic A36.0
- membranous J05.0
  - diphtheritic A36.0
  - Vincent's A69.1
- mesenteric K55.1
- monocytic —*see* Mononucleosis, infectious
- of effort —*see* Angina, specified NEC
- phlegmonous J36
  - diphtheritic A36.0
- post-infarctional I23.7
- pre-infarctional —*see* Angina, unstable
- Prinzmetal —*see* Angina, with documented spasm
- progressive —*see* Angina, unstable
- pseudomembranous A69.1
- pultaceous, diphtheritic A36.0
- spasm-induced —*see* Angina, with documented spasm
- specified NEC I20.8
- stable I20.8
- stenocardia —*see* Angina, specified NEC
- stridulous, diphtheritic A36.2
- tonsil J36
- trachealis J05.0
- unstable I20.0
- variant —*see* Angina, with documented spasm
- Vincent's A69.1
- worsening effort —*see* Angina, unstable

Angioblastoma —*see* Neoplasm, connective tissue, uncertain behavior

Angiocholecystitis —*see* Cholecystitis, acute

Angiocholitis —*see also* Cholecystitis, acute K83.0

Angiodysgenesis spinalis G95.19

Angiodysplasia (cecum) (colon) K55.20
- with bleeding K55.21
- duodenum (and stomach) K31.819
  - with bleeding K31.811
- stomach (and duodenum) K31.819
  - with bleeding K31.811

Angioedema (allergic) (any site) (with urticaria) T78.3
- hereditary D84.1

Angioendothelioma —*see* Neoplasm, uncertain behavior, by site
- benign D18.00
  - intra-abdominal D18.03
  - intracranial D18.02
  - skin D18.01
  - specified site NEC D18.09
- bone —*see* Neoplasm, bone, malignant
- Ewing's —*see* Neoplasm, bone, malignant

Angioendotheliomatosis C85.8-

Angiofibroma —*see also* Neoplasm, benign, by site
- juvenile
  - specified site —*see* Neoplasm, benign, by site
  - unspecified site D10.6

Angiohemophilia (A) (B) D68.0

Angioid streaks (choroid) (macula) (retina) H35.33

Angiokeratoma —*see* Neoplasm, skin, benign
- corporis diffusum E75.21

Angioleiomyoma —*see* Neoplasm, connective tissue, benign

Angiolipoma —*see also* Lipoma
- infiltrating —*see* Lipoma

Angioma —*see also* Hemangioma, by site
- capillary I78.1
- hemorrhagicum hereditaria I78.0
- intra-abdominal D18.03
- intracranial D18.02
- malignant —*see* Neoplasm, connective tissue, malignant
- plexiform D18.00
  - intra-abdominal D18.03
  - intracranial D18.02
  - skin D18.01
  - specified site NEC D18.09
- senile I78.1
- serpiginosum L81.7
- skin D18.01
- specified site NEC D18.09
- spider I78.1
- stellate I78.1
- venous Q28.3

Angiomatosis Q82.8
- bacillary A79.89
- encephalotrigeminal Q85.8
- hemorrhagic familial I78.0
- hereditary familial I78.0
- liver K76.4

Angiomyolipoma —*see* Lipoma

Angiomyoliposarcoma —*see* Neoplasm, connective tissue, malignant

Angiomyoma —*see* Neoplasm, connective tissue, benign

Angiomyosarcoma —*see* Neoplasm, connective tissue, malignant

Angiomyxoma —*see* Neoplasm, connective tissue, uncertain behavior

Angioneurosis F45.8

Angioneurotic edema (allergic) (any site) (with urticaria) T78.3
- hereditary D84.1

Angiopathia, angiopathy I99.9
- cerebral I67.9
  - amyloid E85.4 *[I68.0]*
- diabetic (peripheral) —*see* Diabetes, angiopathy
- peripheral I73.9
  - diabetic —*see* Diabetes, angiopathy
  - specified type NEC I73.89
- retinae syphilitica A52.05
- retinalis (juvenilis)
  - diabetic —*see* Diabetes, retinopathy
  - proliferative —*see* Retinopathy, proliferative

Angiosarcoma —*see also* Neoplasm, connective tissue, malignant
- liver C22.3

Angiosclerosis —*see* Arteriosclerosis

Angiospasm (peripheral) (traumatic) (vessel) I73.9
- brachial plexus G54.0
- cerebral G45.9
- cervical plexus G54.2
- nerve
  - arm —*see* Mononeuropathy, upper limb
    - axillary G54.0
    - median —*see* Lesion, nerve, median
    - ulnar —*see* Lesion, nerve, ulnar
  - axillary G54.0
  - leg —*see* Mononeuropathy, lower limb
  - median —*see* Lesion, nerve, median
  - plantar —*see* Lesion, nerve, plantar
  - ulnar —*see* Lesion, nerve, ulnar

Angiospastic disease or edema I73.9

Angiostrongyliasis
- due to
  - Parastrongylus
    - cantonensis B83.2
    - costaricensis B81.3
- intestinal B81.3

Anguillulosis —*see* Strongyloidiasis

Angulation
- cecum —*see* Obstruction, intestine
- coccyx (acquired) (*see also* subcategory) M43.8
  - congenital NEC Q76.49
- femur (acquired) —*see also* Deformity, limb, specified type NEC, thigh
  - congenital Q74.2
- intestine (large) (small) —*see* Obstruction, intestine
- sacrum (acquired) (*see also* subcategory) M43.8
  - congenital NEC Q76.49
- sigmoid (flexure) —*see* Obstruction, intestine
- spine —*see* Dorsopathy, deforming, specified NEC
- tibia (acquired) —*see also* Deformity, limb, specified type NEC, lower leg
  - congenital Q74.2
- ureter N13.5
  - with infection N13.6
- wrist (acquired) —*see also* Deformity, limb, specified type NEC, forearm
  - congenital Q74.0

Angulus infectiosus (lips) K13.0
Anhedonia R45.84
  sexual F52.0
Anhidrosis L74.4
Anhydration E86.0
Anhydremia E86.0
Anidrosis L74.4
Aniridia (congenital) Q13.1
Anisakiasis (infection) (infestation) B81.0
Anisakis larvae infestation B81.0
Aniseikonia H52.32
Anisocoria (pupil) H57.02
  congenital Q13.2
Anisocytosis R71.8
Anisometropia (congenital) H52.31
Ankle —*see* condition
Ankyloblepharon (eyelid) (acquired) —*see also* Blepharophimosis
  filiforme (adnatum) (congenital) Q10.3
  total Q10.3
Ankyloglossia Q38.1
Ankylosis (fibrous) (osseous) (joint) M24.60
  ankle M24.67-
  arthrodesis status Z98.1
  cricoarytenoid (cartilage) (joint) (larynx) J38.7
  dental K03.5
  ear ossicles H74.31-
  elbow M24.62-
  foot M24.67-
  hand M24.64-
  hip M24.65-
  incostapedial joint (infectional) —*see* Ankylosis, ear ossicles
  jaw (temporomandibular) M26.61-
  knee M24.66-
  lumbosacral (joint) M43.27
  postoperative (status) Z98.1
  produced by surgical fusion, status Z98.1
  sacro-iliac (joint) M43.28
  shoulder M24.61-
  spine (joint) —*see also* Fusion, spine
    spondylitic —*see* Spondylitis, ankylosing
  surgical Z98.1
  temporomandibular M26.61-
  tooth, teeth (hard tissues) K03.5
  wrist M24.63-
Ankylostoma —*see* Ancylostoma
Ankylostomiasis —*see* Ancylostomiasis
Ankylurethria —*see* Stricture, urethra
Annular —*see also* condition
  detachment, cervix N88.8
  organ or site, congenital NEC —*see* Distortion
  pancreas (congenital) Q45.1
Anodontia (complete) (partial) (vera) K00.0
  acquired K08.10
Anomaly, anomalous (congenital) (unspecified type) Q89.9
  abdominal wall NEC Q79.59
  acoustic nerve Q07.8
  adrenal (gland) Q89.1
  Alder (-Reilly) (leukocyte granulation) D72.0
  alimentary tract Q45.9
    upper Q40.9

Anomaly, anomalous *(continued)*
  alveolar M26.70
    hyperplasia M26.79
      mandibular M26.72
      maxillary M26.71
    hypoplasia M26.79
      mandibular M26.74
      maxillary M26.73
    ridge (process) M26.79
    specified NEC M26.79
  ankle (joint) Q74.2
  anus Q43.9
  aorta (arch) NEC Q25.40
    coarctation (preductal) (postductal) Q25.1
  aortic cusp or valve Q23.9
  appendix Q43.8
  apple peel syndrome Q41.1
  aqueduct of Sylvius Q03.0
    with spina bifida —*see* Spina bifida, with hydrocephalus
  arm Q74.0
  arteriovenous NEC
    coronary Q24.5
    gastrointestinal Q27.33
      acquired —*see* Angiodysplasia
  artery (peripheral) Q27.9
    basilar NEC Q28.1
    cerebral Q28.3
    coronary Q24.5
    digestive system Q27.8
    eye Q15.8
    great Q25.9
      specified NEC Q25.8
    lower limb Q27.8
    peripheral Q27.9
      specified NEC Q27.8
    pulmonary NEC Q25.79
    renal Q27.2
    retina Q14.1
    specified site NEC Q27.8
    subclavian Q27.8
      origin Q25.48
    umbilical Q27.0
    upper limb Q27.8
    vertebral NEC Q28.1
  aryteno-epiglottic folds Q31.8
  atrial
    bands or folds Q20.8
    septa Q21.1
  atrioventricular
    excitation I45.6
    septum Q21.0
  auditory canal Q17.8
  auricle
    ear Q17.8
      causing impairment of hearing Q16.9
    heart Q20.8
  Axenfeld's Q15.0
  back Q89.9
  band
    atrial Q20.8
    heart Q24.8
    ventricular Q24.8
  Bartholin's duct Q38.4
  biliary duct or passage Q44.5
  bladder Q64.70
    absence Q64.5
    diverticulum Q64.6
    exstrophy Q64.10
      cloacal Q64.12
      extroversion Q64.19
      specified type NEC Q64.19
      supravesical fissure Q64.11
    neck obstruction Q64.31
    specified type NEC Q64.79
  bone Q79.9
    arm Q74.0
    face Q75.9

Anomaly, anomalous *(continued)*
  bone *(continued)*
    leg Q74.2
    pelvic girdle Q74.2
    shoulder girdle Q74.0
    skull Q75.9
      with
        anencephaly Q00.0
        encephalocele —*see* Encephalocele
        hydrocephalus Q03.9
          with spina bifida —*see* Spina bifida, by site, with hydrocephalus
        microcephaly Q02
  brain (multiple) Q04.9
    vessel Q28.3
  breast Q83.9
  broad ligament Q50.6
  bronchus Q32.4
  bulbus cordis Q21.9
  bursa Q79.9
  canal of Nuck Q52.4
  canthus Q10.3
  capillary Q27.9
  cardiac Q24.9
    chambers Q20.9
      specified NEC Q20.8
    septal closure Q21.9
      specified NEC Q21.8
    valve NEC Q24.8
      pulmonary Q22.3
  cardiovascular system Q28.8
  carpus Q74.0
  caruncle, lacrimal Q10.6
  cascade stomach Q40.2
  cauda equina Q06.3
  cecum Q43.9
  cerebral Q04.9
    vessels Q28.3
  cervix Q51.9
  Chédiak-Higashi (-Steinbrinck) (congenital gigantism of peroxidase granules) E70.330
  cheek Q18.9
  chest wall Q67.8
    bones Q76.9
  chin Q18.9
  chordae tendineae Q24.8
  choroid Q14.3
    plexus Q07.8
  chromosomes, chromosomal Q99.9
    D (1) —*see* condition, chromosome 13
    E (3) —*see* condition, chromosome 18
    G —*see* condition, chromosome 21
    sex
      female phenotype Q97.8
      gonadal dysgenesis (pure) Q99.1
      Klinefelter's Q98.4
      male phenotype Q98.9
      Turner's Q96.9
    specified NEC Q99.8
  cilia Q10.3
  circulatory system Q28.9
  clavicle Q74.0
  clitoris Q52.6
  coccyx Q76.49
  colon Q43.9
  common duct Q44.5
  communication
    coronary artery Q24.5
    left ventricle with right atrium Q21.0
  concha (ear) Q17.3
  connection
    portal vein Q26.5
    pulmonary venous Q26.4
      partial Q26.3

Anomaly, anomalous *(continued)*
  connection *(continued)*
    pulmonary venous *(continued)*
      total Q26.2
    renal artery with kidney Q27.2
  cornea (shape) Q13.4
  coronary artery or vein Q24.5
  cranium —*see* Anomaly, skull
  cricoid cartilage Q31.8
  cystic duct Q44.5
  dental
    alveolar —*see* Anomaly, alveolar
    arch relationship M26.20
      specified NEC M26.29
  dentofacial M26.9
    alveolar —*see* Anomaly, alveolar
    dental arch relationship M26.20
      specified NEC M26.29
    functional M26.50
      specified NEC M26.59
    jaw-cranial base relationship M26.10
      asymmetry M26.12
        maxillary M26.11
      specified type NEC M26.19
    jaw size M26.00
      macrogenia M26.05
      mandibular
        hyperplasia M26.03
        hypoplasia M26.04
      maxillary
        hyperplasia M26.01
        hypoplasia M26.02
      microgenia M26.06
      specified type NEC M26.09
    malocclusion M26.4
      dental arch relationship NEC M26.29
      jaw-cranial base relationship —*see* Anomaly, dentofacial, jaw-cranial base relationship
      jaw size —*see* Anomaly, dentofacial, jaw size
    specified type NEC M26.89
    temporomandibular joint M26.60 -
      adhesions M26.61 -
      ankylosis M26.61 -
      arthralgia M26.62 -
      articular disc M26.63 -
      specified type NEC M26.69
    tooth position, fully erupted M26.30
      specified NEC M26.39
  dermatoglyphic Q82.8
  diaphragm (apertures) NEC Q79.1
  digestive organ(s) or tract Q45.9
    lower Q43.9
    upper Q40.9
  distance, interarch (excessive) (inadequate) M26.25
  distribution, coronary artery Q24.5
  ductus
    arteriosus Q25.0
    botalli Q25.0
  duodenum Q43.9
  dura (brain) Q04.9
    spinal cord Q06.9
  ear (external) Q17.9
    causing impairment of hearing Q16.9
    inner Q16.5
    middle (causing impairment of hearing) Q16.4
    ossicles Q16.3
  Ebstein's (heart) (tricuspid valve) Q22.5
  ectodermal Q82.9
  Eisenmenger's (ventricular septal defect) Q21.8
  ejaculatory duct Q55.4

Anomaly, anomalous *(continued)*
- elbow Q74.0
- endocrine gland NEC Q89.2
- epididymis Q55.4
- epiglottis Q31.8
- esophagus Q39.9
- eustachian tube Q17.8
- eye Q15.9
  - anterior segment Q13.9
    - specified NEC Q13.89
  - posterior segment Q14.9
    - specified NEC Q14.8
  - ptosis (eyelid) Q10.0
  - specified NEC Q15.8
- eyebrow Q18.8
- eyelid Q10.3
  - ptosis Q10.0
- face Q18.9
  - bone(s) Q75.9
- fallopian tube Q50.6
- fascia Q79.9
- femur NEC Q74.2
- fibula NEC Q74.2
- finger Q74.0
- fixation, intestine Q43.3
- flexion (joint) NOS Q74.9
  - hip or thigh Q65.89
- foot NEC Q74.2
  - varus (congenital) Q66.3
- foramen
  - Botalli Q21.1
  - ovale Q21.1
- forearm Q74.0
- forehead Q75.8
- form, teeth K00.2
- fovea centralis Q14.1
- frontal bone —*see* Anomaly, skull
- gallbladder (position) (shape) (size) Q44.1
- Gartner's duct Q52.4
- gastrointestinal tract Q45.9
- genitalia, genital organ(s) or system
  - female Q52.9
    - external Q52.70
    - internal NOS Q52.9
  - male Q55.9
    - hydrocele P83.5
    - specified NEC Q55.8
- genitourinary NEC
  - female Q52.9
  - male Q55.9
- Gerbode Q21.0
- glottis Q31.8
- granulation or granulocyte, genetic (constitutional) (leukocyte) D72.0
- gum Q38.6
- gyri Q07.9
- hair Q84.2
- hand Q74.0
- hard tissue formation in pulp K04.3
- head —*see* Anomaly, skull
- heart Q24.9
  - auricle Q20.8
  - bands or folds Q24.8
  - fibroelastosis cordis I42.4
  - obstructive NEC Q22.6
  - patent ductus arteriosus (Botalli) Q25.0
  - septum Q21.9
    - auricular Q21.1
    - interatrial Q21.1
    - interventricular Q21.0
      - with pulmonary stenosis or atresia, dextraposition of aorta and hypertrophy of right ventricle Q21.3
    - specified NEC Q21.8

Anomaly, anomalous *(continued)*
- heart *(continued)*
  - septum *(continued)*
    - ventricular Q21.0
      - with pulmonary stenosis or atresia, dextraposition of aorta and hypertrophy of right ventricle Q21.3
  - tetralogy of Fallot Q21.3
  - valve NEC Q24.8
    - aortic
      - bicuspid valve Q23.1
      - insufficiency Q23.1
      - stenosis Q23.0
        - subaortic Q24.4
    - mitral
      - insufficiency Q23.3
      - stenosis Q23.2
    - pulmonary Q22.3
      - atresia Q22.0
      - insufficiency Q22.2
      - stenosis Q22.1
        - infundibular Q24.3
        - subvalvular Q24.3
    - tricuspid
      - atresia Q22.4
      - stenosis Q22.4
  - ventricle Q20.8
- heel NEC Q74.2
- Hegglin's D72.0
- hemianencephaly Q00.0
- hemicephaly Q00.0
- hemicrania Q00.0
- hepatic duct Q44.5
- hip NEC Q74.2
- hourglass stomach Q40.2
- humerus Q74.0
- hydatid of Morgagni
  - female Q50.5
  - male (epididymal) Q55.4
    - testicular Q55.29
- hymen Q52.4
- hypersegmentation of neutrophils, hereditary D72.0
- hypophyseal Q89.2
- ileocecal (coil) (valve) Q43.9
- ileum Q43.9
- ilium NEC Q74.2
- integument Q84.9
  - specified NEC Q84.8
- interarch distance (excessive) (inadequate) M26.25
- intervertebral cartilage or disc Q76.49
- intestine (large) (small) Q43.9
  - with anomalous adhesions, fixation or malrotation Q43.3
- iris Q13.2
- ischium NEC Q74.2
- jaw —*see* Anomaly, dentofacial
  - alveolar —*see* Anomaly, alveolar
- jaw-cranial base relationship —*see* Anomaly, dentofacial, jaw-cranial base relationship
- jejunum Q43.8
- joint Q74.9
  - specified NEC Q74.8
- Jordan's D72.0
- kidney(s) (calyx) (pelvis) Q63.9
  - artery Q27.2
  - specified NEC Q63.8
- Klippel-Feil (brevicollis) Q76.1
- knee Q74.1
- labium (majus) (minus) Q52.70
- labyrinth, membranous Q16.5
- lacrimal apparatus or duct Q10.6
- larynx, laryngeal (muscle) Q31.9
  - web (bed) Q31.0
- lens Q12.9
- leukocytes, genetic D72.0
  - granulation (constitutional) D72.0

Anomaly, anomalous *(continued)*
- lid (fold) Q10.3
- ligament Q79.9
  - broad Q50.6
  - round Q52.8
- limb Q74.9
  - lower NEC Q74.2
    - reduction deformity —*see* Defect, reduction, lower limb
  - upper Q74.0
- lip Q38.0
- liver Q44.7
  - duct Q44.5
- lower limb NEC Q74.2
- lumbosacral (joint) (region) Q76.49
  - kyphosis —*see* Kyphosis, congenital
  - lordosis —*see* Lordosis, congenital
- lung (fissure) (lobe) Q33.9
- mandible —*see* Anomaly, dentofacial
- maxilla —*see* Anomaly, dentofacial
- May (-Hegglin) D72.0
- meatus urinarius NEC Q64.79
- meningeal bands or folds Q07.9
  - constriction of Q07.8
  - spinal Q06.9
- meninges Q07.9
  - cerebral Q04.8
  - spinal Q06.9
- meningocele Q05.9
- mesentery Q45.9
- metacarpus Q74.0
- metatarsus NEC Q74.2
- middle ear Q16.4
  - ossicles Q16.3
- mitral (leaflets) (valve) Q23.9
  - insufficiency Q23.3
  - specified NEC Q23.8
  - stenosis Q23.2
- mouth Q38.6
- Müllerian —*see also* Anomaly, by site
  - uterus NEC Q51.818
- multiple NEC Q89.7
- muscle Q79.9
  - eyelid Q10.3
- musculoskeletal system, except limbs Q79.9
- myocardium Q24.8
- nail Q84.6
- narrowness, eyelid Q10.3
- nasal sinus (wall) Q30.8
- neck (any part) Q18.9
- nerve Q07.9
  - acoustic Q07.8
  - optic Q07.8
- nervous system (central) Q07.9
- nipple Q83.9
- nose, nasal (bones) (cartilage) (septum) (sinus) Q30.9
  - specified NEC Q30.8
- ocular muscle Q15.8
- omphalomesenteric duct Q43.0
- opening, pulmonary veins Q26.4
- optic
  - disc Q14.2
  - nerve Q07.8
- opticociliary vessels Q13.2
- orbit (eye) Q10.7
- organ Q89.9
  - of Corti Q16.5
- origin
  - artery
    - innominate Q25.48
    - pulmonary Q25.79
    - renal Q27.2
    - subclavian Q25.48
- osseous meatus (ear) Q16.1

Anomaly, anomalous *(continued)*
- ovary Q50.39
- oviduct Q50.6
- palate (hard) (soft) NEC Q38.5
- pancreas or pancreatic duct Q45.3
- papillary muscles Q24.8
- parathyroid gland Q89.2
- paraurethral ducts Q64.79
- parotid (gland) Q38.4
- patella Q74.1
- Pelger-Huët (hereditary hyposegmentation) D72.0
- pelvic girdle NEC Q74.2
- pelvis (bony) NEC Q74.2
  - rachitic E64.3
- penis (glans) Q55.69
- pericardium Q24.8
- peripheral vascular system Q27.9
- Peter's Q13.4
- pharynx Q38.8
- pigmentation L81.9
  - congenital Q82.8
- pituitary (gland) Q89.2
- pleural (folds) Q34.0
- portal vein Q26.5
  - connection Q26.5
- position, tooth, teeth, fully erupted M26.30
  - specified NEC M26.39
- precerebral vessel Q28.1
- prepuce Q55.69
- prostate Q55.4
- pulmonary Q33.9
  - artery NEC Q25.79
  - valve Q22.3
    - atresia Q22.0
    - insufficiency Q22.2
    - specified type NEC Q22.3
    - stenosis Q22.1
      - infundibular Q24.3
      - subvalvular Q24.3
  - venous connection Q26.4
    - partial Q26.3
    - total Q26.2
- pupil Q13.2
  - function H57.00
    - anisocoria H57.02
    - Argyll Robertson pupil H57.01
    - miosis H57.03
    - mydriasis H57.04
    - specified type NEC H57.09
    - tonic pupil H57.05-
- pylorus Q40.3
- radius Q74.0
- rectum Q43.9
- reduction (extremity) (limb)
  - femur (longitudinal) —*see* Defect, reduction, lower limb, longitudinal, femur
  - fibula (longitudinal) —*see* Defect, reduction, lower limb, longitudinal, fibula
  - lower limb —*see* Defect, reduction, lower limb
  - radius (longitudinal) —*see* Defect, reduction, upper limb, longitudinal, radius
  - tibia (longitudinal) —*see* Defect, reduction, lower limb, longitudinal, tibia
  - ulna (longitudinal) —*see* Defect, reduction, upper limb, longitudinal, ulna
  - upper limb —*see* Defect, reduction, upper limb
- refraction —*see* Disorder, refraction
- renal Q63.9
  - artery Q27.2
  - pelvis Q63.9
    - specified NEC Q63.8

Anomaly, anomalous *(continued)*
respiratory system Q34.9
specified NEC Q34.8
retina Q14.1
rib Q76.6
cervical Q76.5
Rieger's Q13.81
rotation *—see* Malrotation
hip or thigh Q65.89
round ligament Q52.8
sacroiliac (joint) NEC Q74.2
sacrum NEC Q76.49
kyphosis *—see* Kyphosis, congenital
lordosis *—see* Lordosis, congenital
saddle nose, syphilitic A50.57
salivary duct or gland Q38.4
scapula Q74.0
scrotum *—see* Malformation, testis and scrotum
sebaceous gland Q82.9
seminal vesicles Q55.4
sense organs NEC Q07.8
sex chromosomes NEC *—see also* Anomaly, chromosomes
female phenotype Q97.8
male phenotype Q98.9
shoulder (girdle) (joint) Q74.0
sigmoid (flexure) Q43.9
simian crease Q82.8
sinus of Valsalva Q25.49
skeleton generalized Q78.9
skin (appendage) Q82.9
skull Q75.9
with
anencephaly Q00.0
encephalocele *—see* Encephalocele
hydrocephalus Q03.9
with spina bifida *—see* Spina bifida, by site, with hydrocephalus
microcephaly Q02
specified organ or site NEC Q89.8
spermatic cord Q55.4
spine, spinal NEC Q76.49
column NEC Q76.49
kyphosis *—see* Kyphosis, congenital
lordosis *—see* Lordosis, congenital
cord Q06.9
nerve root Q07.8
spleen Q89.09
agenesis Q89.01
stenonian duct Q38.4
sternum NEC Q76.7
stomach Q40.3
submaxillary gland Q38.4
tarsus NEC Q74.2
tendon Q79.9
testis *—see* Malformation, testis and scrotum
thigh NEC Q74.2
thorax (wall) Q67.8
bony Q76.9
throat Q38.8
thumb Q74.0
thymus gland Q89.2
thyroid (gland) Q89.2
cartilage Q31.8
tibia NEC Q74.2
saber A50.56
toe Q74.2
tongue Q38.3
tooth, teeth K00.9
eruption K00.6
position, fully erupted M26.30
spacing, fully erupted M26.30

Anomaly, anomalous *(continued)*
trachea (cartilage) Q32.1
tragus Q17.9
tricuspid (leaflet) (valve) Q22.9
atresia or stenosis Q22.4
Ebstein's Q22.5
Uhl's (hypoplasia of myocardium, right ventricle) Q24.8
ulna Q74.0
umbilical artery Q27.0
union
cricoid cartilage and thyroid cartilage Q31.8
thyroid cartilage and hyoid bone Q31.8
trachea with larynx Q31.8
upper limb Q74.0
urachus Q64.4
ureter Q62.8
obstructive NEC Q62.39
cecoureterocele Q62.32
orthotopic ureterocele Q62.31
urethra Q64.70
absence Q64.5
double Q64.74
fistula to rectum Q64.73
obstructive Q64.39
stricture Q64.32
prolapse Q64.71
specified type NEC Q64.79
urinary tract Q64.9
uterus Q51.9
with only one functioning horn Q51.4
uvula Q38.5
vagina Q52.4
valleculae Q31.8
valve (heart) NEC Q24.8
coronary sinus Q24.5
inferior vena cava Q24.8
pulmonary Q22.3
sinus coronario Q24.5
venae cavae inferioris Q24.8
vas deferens Q55.4
vascular Q27.9
brain Q28.3
ring Q25.45
vein(s) (peripheral) Q27.9
brain Q28.3
cerebral Q28.3
coronary Q24.5
developmental Q28.3
great Q26.9
specified NEC Q26.8
vena cava (inferior) (superior) Q26.9
venous *—see* Anomaly, vein(s)
venous return Q26.8
ventricular
bands or folds Q24.8
septa Q21.0
vertebra Q76.49
kyphosis *—see* Kyphosis, congenital
lordosis *—see* Lordosis, congenital
vesicourethral orifice Q64.79
vessel(s) Q27.9
optic papilla Q14.2
precerebral Q28.1
vitelline duct Q43.0
vitreous body or humor Q14.0
vulva Q52.70
wrist (joint) Q74.0

Anomia R48.8

Anonychia (congenital) Q84.3
acquired L60.8

Anophthalmos, anophthalmus (congenital) (globe) Q11.1
acquired Z90.01

Anopia, anopsia H53.46-
quadrant H53.46-

Anorchia, anorchism, anorchidism Q55.0

Anorexia R63.0
hysterical F44.89
nervosa F50.00
atypical F50.9
binge-eating type F50.2
with purging F50.02
restricting type F50.01

Anorgasmy, psychogenic (female) F52.31
male F52.32

Anosmia R43.0
hysterical F44.6
postinfectional J39.8

Anosognosia R41.89

Anosteoplasia Q78.9

Anovulatory cycle N97.0

Anoxemia R09.02
newborn P84

Anoxia (pathological) R09.02
altitude T70.29
cerebral G93.1
complicating
anesthesia (general) (local) or other sedation T88.59
in labor and delivery O74.3
in pregnancy O29.21-
postpartum, puerperal O89.2
delivery (cesarean) (instrumental) O75.4
during a procedure G97.81
newborn P84
resulting from a procedure G97.82
due to
drowning T75.1
high altitude T70.29
heart *—see* Insufficiency, coronary
intrauterine P84
myocardial *—see* Insufficiency, coronary
newborn P84
spinal cord G95.11
systemic (by suffocation) (low content in atmosphere) *—see* Asphyxia, traumatic

Anteflexion *—see* Anteversion

Antenatal
care (normal pregnancy) Z34.90
screening (encounter for) of mother (*see also* Encounter, antenatal screening) Z36.9

Antepartum *—see* condition

Anterior *—see* condition

Antero-occlusion M26.220

Anteversion
cervix *—see* Anteversion, uterus
femur (neck), congenital Q65.89
uterus, uterine (cervix) (postinfectional) (postpartal, old) N85.4
congenital Q51.818
in pregnancy or childbirth *—see* Pregnancy, complicated by

Anthophobia F40.228

Anthracosilicosis J60

Anthracosis (lung) (occupational) J60
lingua K14.3

Anthrax A22.9
with pneumonia A22.1
cerebral A22.8
colitis A22.2
cutaneous A22.0

Anthrax *(continued)*
gastrointestinal A22.2
inhalation A22.1
intestinal A22.2
meningitis A22.8
pulmonary A22.1
respiratory A22.1
sepsis A22.7
specified manifestation NEC A22.8

Anthropoid pelvis Q74.2
with disproportion (fetopelvic) O33.0

Anthropophobia F40.10
generalized F40.11

Antibodies, maternal (blood group) *—see* Isoimmunization, affecting management of pregnancy
anti-D *—see* Isoimmunization, affecting management of pregnancy, Rh
newborn P55.0

Antibody
anticardiolipin R76.0
with
hemorrhagic disorder D68.312
hypercoagulable state D68.61
antiphosphatidylglycerol R76.0
with
hemorrhagic disorder D68.312
hypercoagulable state D68.61
antiphosphatidylinositol R76.0
with
hemorrhagic disorder D68.312
hypercoagulable state D68.61
antiphosphatidylserine R76.0
with
hemorrhagic disorder D68.312
hypercoagulable state D68.61
antiphospholipid R76.0
with
hemorrhagic disorder D68.312
hypercoagulable state D68.61

Anticardiolipin syndrome D68.61

Anticoagulant, circulating (intrinsic) (*see also* Disorder, hemorrhagic) D68.318
drug-induced (extrinsic) (*see also* Disorder, hemorrhagic) D68.32
iatrogenic D68.32

Antidiuretic hormone syndrome E22.2

Antimonial cholera *—see* Poisoning, antimony

Antiphospholipid
antibody
with hemorrhagic disorder D68.312
syndrome D68.61

Antisocial personality F60.2

Antithrombinemia *—see* Circulating anticoagulants

Antithromboplastinemia D68.318

Antithromboplastinogenemia D68.318

Antitoxin complication or reaction *—see* Complications, vaccination

Antlophobia F40.228

Antritis J32.0
maxilla J32.0
acute J01.00
recurrent J01.01
stomach K29.60
with bleeding K29.61

Antrum, antral *—see* condition

Anuria R34
calculous (impacted) (recurrent) (*see also* Calculus, urinary) N20.9

Anuria *(continued)*
- following
  - abortion —*see* Abortion by type complicated by, renal failure
  - ectopic or molar pregnancy O08.4
- newborn P96.0
- postprocedural N99.0
- postrenal N13.8
- traumatic (following crushing) T79.5

Anus, anal —*see* condition

Anusitis K62.89

Anxiety F41.9
- depression F41.8
- episodic paroxysmal F41.0
- generalized F41.1
- hysteria F41.8
- neurosis F41.1
- panic type F41.0
- reaction F41.1
- separation, abnormal (of childhood) F93.0
- specified NEC F41.8
- state F41.1

Aorta, aortic —*see* condition

Aortectasia —*see* Ectasia, aorta
- with aneurysm —*see* Aneurysm, aorta

Aortitis (nonsyphilitic) (calcific) I77.6
- arteriosclerotic I70.0
- Doehle-Heller A52.02
- luetic A52.02
- rheumatic —*see* Endocarditis, acute, rheumatic
- specific (syphilitic) A52.02
- syphilitic A52.02
  - congenital A50.54 *[I79.1]*

Apathetic thyroid storm —*see* Thyrotoxicosis

Apathy R45.3

Apeirophobia F40.228

Apepsia K30
- psychogenic F45.8

Aperistalsis, esophagus K22.0

Apertognathia M26.29

Apert's syndrome Q87.0

Aphagia R13.0
- psychogenic F50.9

Aphakia (acquired) (postoperative) H27.0-
- congenital Q12.3

Aphasia (amnestic) (global) (nominal) (semantic) (syntactic) R47.01
- acquired, with epilepsy (Landau-Kleffner syndrome) —*see* Epilepsy, specified NEC
- auditory (developmental) F80.2
- developmental (receptive type) F80.2
  - expressive type F80.1
  - Wernicke's F80.2
- following
  - cerebrovascular disease I69.920
    - cerebral infarction I69.320
    - intracerebral hemorrhage I69.120
    - nontraumatic intracranial hemorrhage NEC I69.220
    - specified disease NEC I69.820
    - subarachnoid hemorrhage I69.020
- primary progressive G31.01 *[F02.80]*
  - with behavioral disturbance G31.01 *[F02.81]*

Aphasia *(continued)*
- progressive isolated G31.01 *[F02.80]*
  - with behavioral disturbance G31.01 *[F02.81]*
- sensory F80.2
- syphilis, tertiary A52.19
- Wernicke's (developmental) F80.2

Aphonia (organic) R49.1
- hysterical F44.4
- psychogenic F44.4

Aphthae, aphthous —*see also* condition
- Bednar's K12.0
- cachectic K14.0
- epizootic B08.8
- fever B08.8
- oral (recurrent) K12.0
- stomatitis (major) (minor) K12.0
- thrush B37.0
- ulcer (oral) (recurrent) K12.0
  - genital organ(s) NEC
    - female N76.6
    - male N50.89
  - larynx J38.7

Apical —*see* condition

Apiphobia F40.218

Aplasia —*see also* Agenesis
- abdominal muscle syndrome Q79.4
- alveolar process (acquired) —*see* Anomaly, alveolar
  - congenital Q38.6
- aorta (congenital) Q25.41
- axialis extracorticalis (congenita) E75.29
- bone marrow (myeloid) D61.9
  - congenital D61.01
- brain Q00.0
  - part of Q04.3
- bronchus Q32.4
- cementum K00.4
- cerebellum Q04.3
- cervix (congenital) Q51.5
- congenital pure red cell D61.01
- corpus callosum Q04.0
- cutis congenita Q84.8
- erythrocyte congenital D61.01
- extracortical axial E75.29
- eye Q11.1
- fovea centralis (congenital) Q14.1
- gallbladder, congenital Q44.0
- iris Q13.1
- labyrinth, membranous Q16.5
- limb (congenital) Q73.8
  - lower —*see* Defect, reduction, lower limb
  - upper —*see* Agenesis, arm
- lung, congenital (bilateral) (unilateral) Q33.3
- pancreas Q45.0
- parathyroid-thymic D82.1
- Pelizaeus-Merzbacher E75.29
- penis Q55.5
- prostate Q55.4
- red cell (with thymoma) D60.9
  - acquired D60.9
    - due to drugs D60.9
  - adult D60.9
  - chronic D60.0
  - congenital D61.01
  - constitutional D61.01
  - due to drugs D60.9
  - hereditary D61.01
  - of infants D61.01
  - primary D61.01
  - pure D61.01
    - due to drugs D60.9
  - specified type NEC D60.8
  - transient D60.1

Aplasia *(continued)*
- round ligament Q52.8
- skin Q84.8
- spermatic cord Q55.4
- spleen Q89.01
- testicle Q55.0
- thymic, with immunodeficiency D82.1
- thyroid (congenital) (with myxedema) E03.1
- uterus Q51.0
- ventral horn cell Q06.1

Apnea, apneic (of) (spells) R06.81
- newborn NEC P28.4
  - obstructive P28.4
  - sleep (central) (obstructive) (primary) P28.3
- prematurity P28.4
- sleep G47.30
  - central (primary) G47.31
    - idiopathic G47.31
    - in conditions classified elsewhere G47.37
  - obstructive (adult) (pediatric) G47.33
    - hypopnea G47.33
  - primary central G47.31
  - specified NEC G47.39

Apneumatosis, newborn P28.0

Apocrine metaplasia (breast) —*see* Dysplasia, mammary, specified type NEC

Apophysitis (bone) —*see also* Osteochondropathy
- calcaneus M92.8
- juvenile M92.9

Apoplectiform convulsions (cerebral ischemia) I67.82

Apoplexia, apoplexy, apoplectic
- adrenal A39.1
- heart (auricle) (ventricle) —*see* Infarct, myocardium
- heat T67.0
- hemorrhagic (stroke) —*see* Hemorrhage, intracranial
- meninges, hemorrhagic —*see* Hemorrhage, intracranial, subarachnoid
- uremic N18.9 *[I68.8]*

Appearance
- bizarre R46.1
- specified NEC R46.89
- very low level of personal hygiene R46.0

Appendage
- epididymal (organ of Morgagni) Q55.4
- intestine (epiploic) Q43.8
- preauricular Q17.0
- testicular (organ of Morgagni) Q55.29

Appendicitis (pneumococcal) (retrocecal) K37
- with
  - perforation or rupture K35.2
  - peritoneal abscess K35.3
  - peritonitis NEC K35.3
    - generalized (with perforation or rupture) K35.2
    - localized (with perforation or rupture) K35.3
- acute (catarrhal) (fulminating) (gangrenous) (obstructive) (retrocecal) (suppurative) K35.80
  - with
    - peritoneal abscess K35.3
    - peritonitis NEC K35.3
      - generalized (with perforation or rupture) K35.2
      - localized (with perforation or rupture) K35.3
  - specified NEC K35.89

Appendicitis *(continued)*
- amebic A06.89
- chronic (recurrent) K36
- exacerbation —*see* Appendicitis, acute
- gangrenous —*see* Appendicitis, acute
- healed (obliterative) K36
- interval K36
- neurogenic K36
- obstructive K36
- recurrent K36
- relapsing K36
- subacute (adhesive) K36
- subsiding K36
- suppurative —*see* Appendicitis, acute
- tuberculous A18.32

Appendicopathia oxyurica B80

Appendix, appendicular —*see also* condition
- epididymis Q55.4
- Morgagni
  - female Q50.5
  - male (epididymal) Q55.4
    - testicular Q55.29
- testis Q55.29

Appetite
- depraved —*see* Pica
- excessive R63.2
- lack or loss (*see also* Anorexia) R63.0
  - nonorganic origin F50.89
  - psychogenic F50.89
- perverted (hysterical) —*see* Pica

Apple peel syndrome Q41.1

Apprehension state F41.1

Apprehensiveness, abnormal F41.9

Approximal wear K03.0

Apraxia (classic) (ideational) (ideokinetic) (ideomotor) (motor) (verbal) R48.2
- following
  - cerebrovascular disease I69.990
    - cerebral infarction I69.390
    - intracerebral hemorrhage I69.190
    - nontraumatic intracranial hemorrhage NEC I69.290
    - specified disease NEC I69.890
    - subarachnoid hemorrhage I69.090
- oculomotor, congenital H51.8

Aptyalism K11.7

Apudoma —*see* Neoplasm, uncertain behavior, by site

Aqueous misdirection H40.83-

Arabicum elephantiasis —*see* Infestation, filarial

Arachnitis —*see* Meningitis

Arachnodactyly —*see* Syndrome, Marfan's

Arachnoiditis (acute) (adhesive) (basal) (brain) (cerebrospinal) —*see* Meningitis

Arachnophobia F40.210

Arboencephalitis, Australian A83.4

Arborization block (heart) I45.5

ARC (AIDS-related complex) B20

Arch
- aortic Q25.49
- bovine Q25.49

Arches —*see* condition

Arcuate uterus Q51.810

Arcuatus uterus Q51.810

Arcus (cornea) **senilis** —*see* Degeneration, cornea, senile

Arc-welder's lung J63.4

Areflexia R29.2

Areola —*see* condition

Argentaffinoma —*see also* Neoplasm, uncertain behavior, by site
- malignant —*see* Neoplasm, malignant, by site
- syndrome E34.0

Argininemia E72.21

Arginosuccinic aciduria E72.22

Argyll Robertson phenomenon, pupil or syndrome (syphilitic) A52.19
- atypical H57.09
- nonsyphilitic H57.09

Argyria, argyriasis
- conjunctival H11.13-
- from drug or medicament —*see* Table of Drugs and Chemicals, by substance

Argyrosis, conjunctival H11.13-

Arhinencephaly Q04.1

Ariboflavinosis E53.0

Arm —*see* condition

Arnold-Chiari disease, obstruction or syndrome (type II) Q07.00
- with
  - hydrocephalus Q07.02
    - with spina bifida Q07.03
  - spina bifida Q07.01
    - with hydrocephalus Q07.03
- type III —*see* Encephalocele
- type IV Q04.8

Aromatic amino-acid metabolism disorder E70.9
- specified NEC E70.8

Arousals, confusional G47.51

Arrest, arrested
- cardiac I46.9
  - complicating
    - abortion —*see* Abortion, by type, complicated by, cardiac arrest
    - anesthesia (general) (local) or other sedation —*see* Table of Drugs and Chemicals, by drug,
      - in labor and delivery O74.2
      - in pregnancy O29.11-
      - postpartum, puerperal O89.1
    - delivery (cesarean) (instrumental) O75.4
  - due to
    - cardiac condition I46.2
    - specified condition NEC I46.8
  - intraoperative I97.71-
  - newborn P29.81
  - personal history, successfully resuscitated Z86.74
  - postprocedural I97.12-
    - obstetric procedure O75.4
- cardiorespiratory —*see* Arrest, cardiac
- circulatory —*see* Arrest, cardiac
- deep transverse O64.0
- development or growth
  - bone —*see* Disorder, bone, development or growth
  - child R62.50
  - tracheal rings Q32.1
- epiphyseal
  - complete
    - femur M89.15-
    - humerus M89.12-
    - tibia M89.16-
    - ulna M89.13-
  - forearm M89.13-
    - specified NEC M89.13-

Arrest, arrested *(continued)*
- epiphyseal *(continued)*
  - forearm *(continued)*
    - ulna —*see* Arrest, epiphyseal, by type, ulna
  - lower leg M89.16-
    - specified NEC M89.168
    - tibia —*see* Arrest, epiphyseal, by type, tibia
  - partial
    - femur M89.15-
    - humerus M89.12-
    - tibia M89.16-
    - ulna M89.13-
  - specified NEC M89.18
- granulopoiesis —*see* Agranulocytosis
- growth plate —*see* Arrest, epiphyseal
- heart —*see* Arrest, cardiac
- legal, anxiety concerning Z65.3
- physeal —*see* Arrest, epiphyseal
- respiratory R09.2
  - newborn P28.81
- sinus I45.5
- spermatogenesis (complete) —*see* Azoospermia
  - incomplete —*see* Oligospermia
- transverse (deep) O64.0

Arrhenoblastoma
- benign
  - specified site —*see* Neoplasm, benign, by site
  - unspecified site
    - female D27.9
    - male D29.20
- malignant
  - specified site —*see* Neoplasm, malignant, by site
  - unspecified site
    - female C56.9
    - male C62.90
- specified site —*see* Neoplasm, uncertain behavior, by site
- unspecified site
  - female D39.10
  - male D40.10

Arrhythmia (auricle)(cardiac) (juvenile)(nodal) (reflex)(sinus) (supraventricular)(transitory) (ventricle) I49.9
- block I45.9
- extrasystolic I49.49
- newborn
  - bradycardia P29.12
  - occurring before birth P03.819
    - before onset of labor P03.810
    - during labor P03.811
  - tachycardia P29.11
- psychogenic F45.8
- specified NEC I49.8
- vagal R55
- ventricular re-entry I47.0

Arrillaga-Ayerza syndrome (pulmonary sclerosis with pulmonary hypertension) I27.0

Arsenical pigmentation L81.8
- from drug or medicament —*see* Table of Drugs and Chemicals

Arsenism —*see* Poisoning, arsenic

Arterial —*see* condition

Arteriofibrosis —*see* Arteriosclerosis

Arteriolar sclerosis —*see* Arteriosclerosis

Arteriolith —*see* Arteriosclerosis

Arteriolitis I77.6
- necrotizing, kidney I77.5
- renal —*see* Hypertension, kidney

Arteriolosclerosis —*see* Arteriosclerosis

Arterionephrosclerosis —*see* Hypertension, kidney

Arteriopathy I77.9

Arteriosclerosis, arteriosclerotic (diffuse) (obliterans) (of) (senile) (with calcification) I70.90
- aorta I70.0
- arteries of extremities —*see* Arteriosclerosis, extremities
- brain I67.2
- bypass graft
  - coronary —*see* Arteriosclerosis, coronary, bypass graft
  - extremities —*see* Arteriosclerosis, extremities, bypass graft
- cardiac —*see* Disease, heart, ischemic, atherosclerotic
- cardiopathy —*see* Disease, heart, ischemic, atherosclerotic
- cardiorenal —*see* Hypertension, cardiorenal
- cardiovascular —*see* Disease, heart, ischemic, atherosclerotic
- carotid (*see also* Occlusion, artery, carotid) I65.2-
- central nervous system I67.2
- cerebral I67.2
- cerebrovascular I67.2
- coronary (artery) I25.10
  - due to
    - calcified coronary lesion (severely) I25.84
    - lipid rich plaque I25.83
  - bypass graft I25.810
    - with
      - angina pectoris I25.709
        - with documented spasm I25.701
        - specified type NEC I25.708
        - unstable I25.700
      - ischemic chest pain I25.709
    - autologous artery I25.810
      - with
        - angina pectoris I25.729
          - with documented spasm I25.721
          - specified type I25.728
          - unstable I25.720
        - ischemic chest pain I25.729
    - autologous vein I25.810
      - with
        - angina pectoris I25.719
          - with documented spasm I25.711
          - specified type I25.718
          - unstable I25.710
        - ischemic chest pain I25.719
    - nonautologous biological I25.810
      - with
        - angina pectoris I25.739
          - with documented spasm I25.731
          - specified type I25.738
          - unstable I25.730
        - ischemic chest pain I25.739
    - specified type NEC I25.810
      - with
        - angina pectoris I25.799
          - with documented spasm I25.791
          - specified type I25.798
          - unstable I25.790
        - ischemic chest pain I25.799

Arteriosclerosis, arteriosclerotic *(continued)*
- coronary *(continued)*
  - native vessel
    - with
      - angina pectoris I25.119
        - with documented spasm I25.111
        - specified type NEC I25.118
        - unstable I25.110
      - ischemic chest pain I25.119
  - transplanted heart I25.811
    - bypass graft I25.812
      - with
        - angina pectoris I25.769
          - with documented spasm I25.761
          - specified type I25.768
          - unstable I25.760
        - ischemic chest pain I25.769
    - native coronary artery I25.811
      - with
        - angina pectoris I25.759
          - with documented spasm I25.751
          - specified type I25.758
          - unstable I25.750
        - ischemic chest pain I25.759
- extremities (native arteries) I70.209
  - bypass graft I70.309
    - autologous vein graft I70.409
      - leg I70.409
        - with
          - gangrene (and intermittent claudication, rest pain and ulcer) I70.469
          - intermittent claudication I70.419
          - rest pain (and intermittent claudication) I70.429
        - bilateral I70.403
          - with
            - gangrene (and intermittent claudication, rest pain and ulcer) I70.463
            - intermittent claudication I70.413
            - rest pain (and intermittent claudication) I70.423
          - specified type NEC I70.493
        - left I70.402
          - with
            - gangrene (and intermittent claudication, rest pain and ulcer) I70.462
            - intermittent claudication I70.412
            - rest pain (and intermittent claudication) I70.422
            - ulceration (and intermittent claudication and rest pain) I70.449
              - ankle I70.443

Arteriosclerosis, arteriosclerotic *(continued)*

- extremities *(continued)*
  - bypass graft *(continued)*
    - autologous vein graft *(continued)*
      - leg *(continued)*
        - left *(continued)*
          - with *(continued)*
            - ulceration *(continued)*
              - calf I70.442
              - foot site NEC I70.445
              - heel I70.444
              - lower leg NEC I70.448
              - midfoot I70.444
              - thigh I70.441
          - specified type NEC I70.492
        - right I70.401
          - with
            - gangrene (and intermittent claudication, rest pain and ulcer) I70.461
            - intermittent claudication I70.411
            - rest pain (and intermittent claudication) I70.421
            - ulceration (and intermittent claudication and rest pain) I70.439
              - ankle I70.433
              - calf I70.432
              - foot site NEC I70.435
              - heel I70.434
              - lower leg NEC I70.438
              - midfoot I70.434
              - thigh I70.431
          - specified type NEC I70.491
        - specified type NEC I70.499
      - specified NEC I70.408
        - with
          - gangrene (and intermittent claudication, rest pain and ulcer) I70.468
          - intermittent claudication I70.418
          - rest pain (and intermittent claudication) I70.428
          - ulceration (and intermittent claudication and rest pain) I70.45
        - specified type NEC I70.498
    - leg I70.309
      - with
        - gangrene (and intermittent claudication, rest pain and ulcer) I70.369
        - intermittent claudication I70.319
        - rest pain (and intermittent claudication) I70.329
      - bilateral I70.303
        - with
          - gangrene (and intermittent claudication, rest pain and ulcer) I70.363
          - intermittent claudication I70.313
          - rest pain (and intermittent claudication) I70.323
        - specified type NEC I70.393
      - left I70.302
        - with
          - gangrene (and intermittent claudication, rest pain and ulcer) I70.362
          - intermittent claudication I70.312
          - rest pain (and intermittent claudication) I70.322
          - ulceration (and intermittent claudication and rest pain) I70.349
            - ankle I70.343
            - calf I70.342
            - foot site NEC I70.345
            - heel I70.344
            - lower leg NEC I70.348
            - midfoot I70.344
            - thigh I70.341
        - specified type NEC I70.392
      - right I70.301
        - with
          - gangrene (and intermittent claudication, rest pain and ulcer) I70.361
          - intermittent claudication I70.311
          - rest pain (and intermittent claudication) I70.321
          - ulceration (and intermittent claudication and rest pain) I70.339
            - ankle I70.333
            - calf I70.332
            - foot site NEC I70.335
            - heel I70.334
            - lower leg NEC I70.338
            - midfoot I70.334
            - thigh I70.331
        - specified type NEC I70.391
      - specified type NEC I70.399
    - nonautologous biological graft I70.509
      - leg I70.509
        - with
          - gangrene (and intermittent claudication, rest pain and ulcer) I70.569
          - intermittent claudication I70.519
          - rest pain (and intermittent claudication) I70.529
        - bilateral I70.503
          - with
            - gangrene (and intermittent claudication, rest pain and ulcer) I70.563
            - intermittent claudication I70.513
            - rest pain (and intermittent claudication) I70.523
          - specified type NEC I70.593
        - left I70.502
          - with
            - gangrene (and intermittent claudication, rest pain and ulcer) I70.562
            - intermittent claudication I70.512
            - rest pain (and intermittent claudication) I70.522
            - ulceration (and intermittent claudication and rest pain) I70.549
              - ankle I70.543
              - calf I70.542
              - foot site NEC I70.545
              - heel I70.544
              - lower leg NEC I70.548
              - midfoot I70.544
              - thigh I70.541
          - specified type NEC I70.592
        - right I70.501
          - with
            - gangrene (and intermittent claudication, rest pain and ulcer) I70.561
            - intermittent claudication I70.511
            - rest pain (and intermittent claudication) I70.521
            - ulceration (and intermittent claudication and rest pain) I70.539
              - ankle I70.533
              - calf I70.532
              - foot site NEC I70.535
              - heel I70.534
              - lower leg NEC I70.538
              - midfoot I70.534
              - thigh I70.531
          - specified type NEC I70.591
        - specified type NEC I70.599
      - specified NEC I70.508
        - with
          - gangrene (and intermittent claudication, rest pain and ulcer) I70.568
          - intermittent claudication I70.518
          - rest pain (and intermittent claudication) I70.528
          - ulceration (and intermittent claudication and rest pain) I70.55
        - specified type NEC I70.598
    - nonbiological graft I70.609
      - leg I70.609
        - with
          - gangrene (and intermittent claudication, rest pain and ulcer) I70.669
          - intermittent claudication I70.619
          - rest pain (and intermittent claudication) I70.629
        - bilateral I70.603
          - with
            - gangrene (and intermittent claudication, rest pain and ulcer) I70.663
            - intermittent claudication I70.613
            - rest pain(and intermittent claudication) I70.623
          - specified type NEC I70.693
        - left I70.602
          - with
            - gangrene (and intermittent claudication, rest pain and ulcer) I70.662
            - intermittent claudication I70.612
            - rest pain (and intermittent claudication) I70.622
            - ulceration (and intermittent claudication and rest pain) I70.649
              - ankle I70.643
              - calf I70.642
              - foot site NEC I70.645
              - heel I70.644
              - lower leg NEC I70.648
              - midfoot I70.644
              - thigh I70.641
          - specified type NEC I70.692

Arteriosclerosis, arteriosclerotic *(continued)*
- extremities *(continued)*
  - bypass graft *(continued)*
    - nonbiological graft *(continued)*
      - leg *(continued)*
        - right I70.601
          - with
            - gangrene (and intermittent claudication, rest pain and ulcer) I70.661
            - intermittent claudication I70.611
            - rest pain (and intermittent claudication) I70.621
            - ulceration (and intermittent claudication and rest pain) I70.639
              - ankle I70.633
              - calf I70.632
              - foot site NEC I70.635
              - heel I70.634
              - lower leg NEC I70.638
              - midfoot I70.634
              - thigh I70.631
          - specified type NEC I70.691
        - specified type NEC I70.699
      - specified NEC I70.608
        - with
          - gangrene (and intermittent claudication, rest pain and ulcer) I70.668
          - intermittent claudication I70.618
          - rest pain (and intermittent claudication) I70.628
          - ulceration (and intermittent claudication and rest pain) I70.65
        - specified type NEC I70.698
    - specified graft NEC I70.709
      - leg I70.709
        - with
          - gangrene (and intermittent claudication, rest pain and ulcer) I70.769
          - intermittent claudication I70.719
          - rest pain (and intermittent claudication) I70.729
        - bilateral I70.703
          - with
            - gangrene (and intermittent claudication, rest pain and ulcer) I70.763
            - intermittent claudication I70.713
            - rest pain (and intermittent claudication) I70.723

Arteriosclerosis, arteriosclerotic *(continued)*
- extremities *(continued)*
  - bypass graft *(continued)*
    - specified graft NEC *(continued)*
      - leg *(continued)*
        - bilateral *(continued)*
          - specified type NEC I70.793
        - left I70.702
          - with
            - gangrene (and intermittent claudication, rest pain and ulcer) I70.762
            - intermittent claudication I70.712
            - rest pain (and intermittent claudication) I70.722
            - ulceration (and intermittent claudication and rest pain) I70.749
              - ankle I70.743
              - calf I70.742
              - foot site NEC I70.745
              - heel I70.744
              - lower leg NEC I70.748
              - midfoot I70.744
              - thigh I70.741
          - specified type NEC I70.792
        - right I70.701
          - with
            - gangrene (and intermittent claudication, rest pain and ulcer) I70.761
            - intermittent claudication I70.711
            - rest pain (and intermittent claudication) I70.721
            - ulceration (and intermittent claudication and rest pain) I70.739
              - ankle I70.733
              - calf I70.732
              - foot site NEC I70.735
              - heel I70.734
              - lower leg NEC I70.738
              - midfoot I70.734
              - thigh I70.731
          - specified type NEC I70.791
        - specified type NEC I70.799
      - specified NEC I70.708
        - with
          - gangrene (and intermittent claudication, rest pain and ulcer) I70.768
          - intermittent claudication I70.718
          - rest pain (and intermittent claudication) I70.728

Arteriosclerosis, arteriosclerotic *(continued)*
- extremities *(continued)*
  - bypass graft *(continued)*
    - specified graft NEC *(continued)*
      - specified NEC *(continued)*
        - with *(continued)*
          - ulceration (and intermittent claudication and rest pain) I70.75
        - specified type NEC I70.798
    - specified NEC I70.308
      - with
        - gangrene (and intermittent claudication, rest pain and ulcer) I70.368
        - intermittent claudication I70.318
        - rest pain (and intermittent claudication) I70.328
        - ulceration (and intermittent claudication and rest pain) I70.35
      - specified type NEC I70.398
  - leg I70.209
    - with
      - gangrene (and intermittent claudication, rest pain and ulcer) I70.269
      - intermittent claudication I70.219
      - rest pain (and intermittent claudication) I70.229
    - bilateral I70.203
      - with
        - gangrene (and intermittent claudication, rest pain and ulcer) I70.263
        - intermittent claudication I70.213
        - rest pain (and intermittent claudication) I70.223
      - specified type NEC I70.293
    - left I70.202
      - with
        - gangrene (and intermittent claudication, rest pain and ulcer) I70.262
        - intermittent claudication I70.212
        - rest pain (and intermittent claudication) I70.222
        - ulceration (and intermittent claudication and rest pain) I70.249
          - ankle I70.243
          - calf I70.242
          - foot site NEC I70.245
          - heel I70.244
          - lower leg NEC I70.248
          - midfoot I70.244
          - thigh I70.241
      - specified type NEC I70.292
    - right I70.201
      - with
        - gangrene (and intermittent claudication, rest pain and ulcer) I70.261
        - intermittent claudication I70.211
        - rest pain (and intermittent claudication) I70.221
        - ulceration (and intermittent claudication and rest pain) I70.239
          - ankle I70.233
          - calf I70.232
          - foot site NEC I70.235

Arteriosclerosis, arteriosclerotic *(continued)*
- extremities *(continued)*
  - leg *(continued)*
    - right *(continued)*
      - with *(continued)*
        - ulceration *(continued)*
          - heel I70.234
          - lower leg NEC I70.238
          - midfoot I70.234
          - thigh I70.231
      - specified type NEC I70.291
    - specified type NEC I70.299
  - specified site NEC I70.208
    - with
      - gangrene (and intermittent claudication, rest pain and ulcer) I70.268
      - intermittent claudication I70.218
      - rest pain (and intermittent claudication) I70.228
      - ulceration (and intermittent claudication and rest pain) I70.25
    - specified type NEC I70.298
- generalized I70.91
- heart (disease) *—see* Arteriosclerosis, coronary (artery),
- kidney *—see* Hypertension, kidney
- medial *—see* Arteriosclerosis, extremities
- mesenteric (artery) K55.1
- Mönckeberg's *—see* Arteriosclerosis, extremities
- myocarditis I51.4
- peripheral (of extremities) *—see* Arteriosclerosis, extremities
- pulmonary (idiopathic) I27.0
- renal (arterioles) *—see also* Hypertension, kidney
  - artery I70.1
- retina (vascular) I70.8 *[H35.0]-*
- specified artery NEC I70.8
- spinal (cord) G95.19
- vertebral (artery) I67.2

Arteriospasm I73.9

Arteriovenous *—see* condition

Arteritis I77.6
- allergic M31.0
- aorta (nonsyphilitic) I77.6
  - syphilitic A52.02
- aortic arch M31.4
- brachiocephalic M31.4
- brain I67.7
  - syphilitic A52.04
- cerebral I67.7
  - in
    - diseases classified elsewhere I68.2
    - systemic lupus erythematosus M32.19
  - listerial A32.89
  - syphilitic A52.04
  - tuberculous A18.89
- coronary (artery) I25.89
  - rheumatic I01.8
    - chronic I09.89
  - syphilitic A52.06
- cranial (left) (right), giant cell M31.6
- deformans *—see* Arteriosclerosis
- giant cell NEC M31.6
  - with polymyalgia rheumatica M31.5
- necrosing or necrotizing M31.9
  - specified NEC M31.8
- nodosa M30.0
- obliterans *—see* Arteriosclerosis

Arteritis *(continued)*
- pulmonary I28.8
- rheumatic *—see* Fever, rheumatic
- senile *—see* Arteriosclerosis
- suppurative I77.2
- syphilitic (general) A52.09
  - brain A52.04
  - coronary A52.06
  - spinal A52.09
- temporal, giant cell M31.6
- young female aortic arch syndrome M31.4

Artery, arterial *—see also* condition
- abscess I77.89
- single umbilical Q27.0

Arthralgia (allergic) *—see also* Pain, joint
- in caisson disease T70.3
- temporomandibular M26.62-

Arthritis, arthritic (acute) (chronic) (nonpyogenic) (subacute) M19.90
- allergic *—see* Arthritis, specified form NEC
- ankylosing (crippling) (spine) *—see also* Spondylitis, ankylosing
  - sites other than spine *—see* Arthritis, specified form NEC
- atrophic *—see* Osteoarthritis
  - spine *—see* Spondylitis, ankylosing
- back *—see* Spondylopathy, inflammatory
- blennorrhagic (gonococcal) A54.42
- Charcot's *—see* Arthropathy, neuropathic
  - diabetic *—see* Diabetes, arthropathy, neuropathic
  - syringomyelic G95.0
- chylous (filarial) (*see also* category M01) B74.9
- climacteric (any site) NEC *—see* Arthritis, specified form NEC
- crystal (-induced) *—see* Arthritis, in, crystals
- deformans *—see* Osteoarthritis
- degenerative *—see* Osteoarthritis
- due to or associated with
  - acromegaly E22.0
  - brucellosis *—see* Brucellosis
  - caisson disease T70.3
  - diabetes *—see* Diabetes, arthropathy
  - dracontiasis (*see also* category M01) B72
  - enteritis NEC
    - regional *—see* Enteritis, regional
  - erysipelas (*see also* category M01) A46
  - erythema
    - epidemic A25.1
    - nodosum L52
  - filariasis NOS B74.9
  - glanders A24.0
  - helminthiasis (*see also* category M01) B83.9
  - hemophilia D66 *[M36.2]*
  - Henoch-(Schönlein) purpura D69.0 *[M36.4]*
  - human parvovirus (*see also* category M01) B97.6
  - infectious disease NEC M01
  - leprosy (*see also* category M01) *—see also* Leprosy A30.9
  - Lyme disease A69.23
  - mycobacteria (*see also* category M01) A31.8

Arthritis, arthritic *(continued)*
- due to or associated *(continued)*
  - parasitic disease NEC (*see also* category M01) B89
  - paratyphoid fever (*see also* category M01) (*see also* Fever, paratyphoid) A01.4
  - rat bite fever (*see also* category M01) A25.1
  - regional enteritis *—see* Enteritis, regional
  - respiratory disorder NOS J98.9
  - serum sickness (*see also* Reaction, serum) T80.69
  - syringomyelia G95.0
  - typhoid fever A01.04
- epidemic erythema A25.1
- febrile *—see* Fever, rheumatic
- gonococcal A54.42
- gouty (acute) *—see* Gout
- in (due to)
  - acromegaly (*see also* subcategory M14.8-) E22.0
  - amyloidosis (*see also* subcategory M14.8-) E85.4
  - bacterial disease (*see also* subcategory M01) A49.9
  - Behçet's syndrome M35.2
  - caisson disease (*see also* subcategory M14.8-) T70.3
  - coliform bacilli (Escherichia coli) *—see* Arthritis, in, pyogenic organism NEC
  - crystals M11.9
    - dicalcium phosphate *—see* Arthritis, in, crystals, specified type NEC
    - hydroxyapatite M11.0-
    - pyrophosphate *—see* Arthritis, in, crystals, specified type NEC
    - specified type NEC M11.80
      - ankle M11.87-
      - elbow M11.82-
      - foot joint M11.87-
      - hand joint M11.84-
      - hip M11.85-
      - knee M11.86-
      - multiple sites M11.8-
      - shoulder M11.81-
      - vertebrae M11.88
      - wrist M11.83-
  - dermatoarthritis, lipoid E78.81
  - dracontiasis (dracunculiasis) (*see also* category M01) B72
  - endocrine disorder NEC (*see also* subcategory M14.8-) E34.9
  - enteritis, infectious NEC (*see also* category M01) A09
    - specified organism NEC (*see also* category M01) A08.8
  - erythema
    - multiforme (*see also* subcategory M14.8-) L51.9
    - nodosum (*see also* subcategory M14.8-) L52
  - gout *—see* Gout
  - helminthiasis NEC (*see also* category M01) B83.9
  - hemochromatosis (*see also* subcategory M14.8-) E83.118
  - hemoglobinopathy NEC D58.2 *[M36.3]*
  - hemophilia NEC D66 *[M36.2]*
  - Hemophilus influenzae M00.8- *[B96.2]*
  - Henoch (-Schönlein) purpura D69.0 *[M36.4]*
  - hyperparathyroidism NEC (*see also* subcategory M14.8-) E21.3

Arthritis, arthritic *(continued)*
- in *(continued)*
  - hypersensitivity reaction NEC T78.49 *[M36.4]*
  - hypogammaglobulinemia (*see also* subcategory M14.8-) D80.1
  - hypothyroidism NEC (*see also* subcategory M14.8-) E03.9
  - infection *—see* Arthritis, pyogenic or pyemic
    - spine *—see* Spondylopathy, infective
  - infectious disease NEC M01
  - leprosy (*see also* category M01) A30.9
  - leukemia NEC C95.9- *[M36.1]*
  - lipoid dermatoarthritis E78.81
  - Lyme disease A69.23
  - Mediterranean fever, familial (*see also* subcategory M14.8-) M04.1
  - Meningococcus A39.83
  - metabolic disorder NEC (*see also* subcategory M14.8-) E88.9
  - multiple myelomatosis C90.0- *[M36.1]*
  - mumps B26.85
  - mycosis NEC (*see also* category M01) B49
  - myelomatosis (multiple) C90.0- *[M36.1]*
  - neurological disorder NEC G98.0
  - ochronosis (*see also* subcategory M14.8-) E70.29
  - O'nyong-nyong (*see also* category M01) A92.1
  - parasitic disease NEC (*see also* category M01) B89
  - paratyphoid fever (*see also* category M01) A01.4
  - Pseudomonas *—see* Arthritis, pyogenic, bacterial NEC
  - psoriasis L40.50
  - pyogenic organism NEC *—see* Arthritis, pyogenic, bacterial NEC
  - Reiter's disease *—see* Reiter's disease
  - respiratory disorder NEC (*see also* subcategory M14.8-) J98.9
  - reticulosis, malignant (*see also* subcategory M14.8-) C86.0
  - rubella B06.82
  - Salmonella (arizonae) (cholerae-suis) (enteritidis) (typhimurium) A02.23
  - sarcoidosis D86.86
  - specified bacteria NEC *—see* Arthritis, pyogenic, bacterial NEC
  - sporotrichosis B42.82
  - syringomyelia G95.0
  - thalassemia NEC D56.9 *[M36.3]*
  - tuberculosis *—see* Tuberculosis, arthritis
  - typhoid fever A01.04
  - urethritis, Reiter's *—see* Reiter's disease
  - viral disease NEC (*see also* category M01) B34.9
- infectious or infective *—see also* Arthritis, pyogenic or pyemic
  - spine *—see* Spondylopathy, infective
- juvenile M08.90
  - with systemic onset *—see* Still's disease
  - ankle M08.97-
  - elbow M08.92-
  - foot joint M08.97-

Arthritis, arthritic *(continued)*
- juvenile *(continued)*
  - hand joint M08.94-
  - hip M08.95-
  - knee M08.96-
  - multiple site M08.99
  - pauciarticular M08.40
    - ankle M08.47-
    - elbow M08.42-
    - foot joint M08.47-
    - hand joint M08.44-
    - hip M08.45-
    - knee M08.46-
    - shoulder M08.41-
    - vertebrae M08.48
    - wrist M08.43-
  - psoriatic L40.54
  - rheumatoid *—see* Arthritis, rheumatoid, juvenile
  - shoulder M08.91-
  - vertebra M08.98
  - specified type NEC M08.80
    - ankle M08.87-
    - elbow M08.82-
    - foot joint M08.87-
    - hand joint M08.84-
    - hip M08.85-
    - knee M08.86-
    - multiple site M08.89
    - shoulder M08.81-
    - specified joint NEC M08.88
    - vertebrae M08.88
    - wrist M08.83-
  - wrist M08.93-
- meaning osteoarthritis *—see* Osteoarthritis
- meningococcal A39.83
- menopausal (any site) NEC *—see* Arthritis, specified form NEC
- mutilans (psoriatic) L40.52
- mycotic NEC (*see also* category M01) B49
- neuropathic (Charcot) *—see* Arthropathy, neuropathic
  - diabetic *—see* Diabetes, arthropathy, neuropathic
  - nonsyphilitic NEC G98.0
  - syringomyelic G95.0
- ochronotic (*see also* subcategory M14.8-) E70.29
- palindromic (any site) *—see* Rheumatism, palindromic
- pneumococcal M00.10
  - ankle M00.17-
  - elbow M00.12-
  - foot joint *—see* Arthritis, pneumococcal, ankle
  - hand joint M00.14-
  - hip M00.15-
  - knee M00.16-
  - multiple site M00.19
  - shoulder M00.11-
  - vertebra M00.18
  - wrist M00.13-
- postdysenteric *—see* Arthropathy, postdysenteric
- postmeningococcal A39.84
- postrheumatic, chronic *—see* Arthropathy, postrheumatic, chronic
- primary progressive *—see also* Arthritis, specified form NEC
  - spine *—see* Spondylitis, ankylosing
- psoriatic L40.50
- purulent (any site except spine) *—see* Arthritis, pyogenic or pyemic
  - spine *—see* Spondylopathy, infective

Arthritis, arthritic *(continued)*
- pyogenic or pyemic (any site except spine) M00.9
  - bacterial NEC M00.80
    - ankle M00.87-
    - elbow M00.82-
    - foot joint *—see* Arthritis, pyogenic, bacterial NEC, ankle
    - hand joint M00.84-
    - hip M00.85-
    - knee M00.86-
    - multiple site M00.89
    - shoulder M00.81-
    - vertebra M00.88
    - wrist M00.83-
  - pneumococcal *—see* Arthritis, pneumococcal
  - spine *—see* Spondylopathy, infective
  - staphylococcal *—see* Arthritis, staphylococcal
  - streptococcal *—see* Arthritis, streptococcal NEC
    - pneumococcal *—see* Arthritis, pneumococcal
- reactive *—see* Reiter's disease
- rheumatic *—see also* Arthritis, rheumatoid
  - acute or subacute *—see* Fever, rheumatic
- rheumatoid M06.9
  - with
    - carditis *—see* Rheumatoid, carditis
    - endocarditis *—see* Rheumatoid, carditis
    - heart involvement NEC *—see* Rheumatoid, carditis
    - lung involvement *—see* Rheumatoid, lung
    - myocarditis *—see* Rheumatoid, carditis
    - myopathy *—see* Rheumatoid, myopathy
    - pericarditis *—see* Rheumatoid, carditis
    - polyneuropathy *—see* Rheumatoid, polyneuropathy
    - rheumatoid factor *—see* Arthritis, rheumatoid, seropositive
    - splenoadenomegaly and leukopenia *—see* Felty's syndrome
    - vasculitis *—see* Rheumatoid, vasculitis
    - visceral involvement NEC *— see* Rheumatoid, arthritis, with involvement of organs NEC
  - juvenile (with or without rheumatoid factor) M08.00
    - ankle M08.07-
    - elbow M08.02-
    - foot joint M08.07-
    - hand joint M08.04-
    - hip M08.05-
    - knee M08.06-
    - multiple site M08.09
    - shoulder M08.01-
    - vertebra M08.08
    - wrist M08.03-
  - seronegative M06.00
    - ankle M06.07-
    - elbow M06.02-
    - foot joint M06.07-
    - hand joint M06.04-
    - hip M06.05-
    - knee M06.06-

Arthritis, arthritic *(continued)*
- rheumatoid *(continued)*
  - seronegative *(continued)*
    - multiple site M06.09
    - shoulder M06.01-
    - vertebra M06.08
    - wrist M06.03-
  - seropositive M05.9
    - specified NEC M05.80
      - ankle M05.87-
      - elbow M05.82-
      - foot joint M05.87-
      - hand joint M05.84-
      - hip M05.85-
      - knee M05.86-
      - multiple sites M05.89
      - shoulder M05.81-
      - vertebra *—see* Spondylitis, ankylosing
      - wrist M05.83-
    - without organ involvement M05.70
      - ankle M05.77-
      - elbow M05.72-
      - foot joint M05.77-
      - hand joint M05.74-
      - hip M05.75-
      - knee M05.76-
      - multiple sites M05.79
      - shoulder M05.71-
      - vertebra *—see* Spondylitis, ankylosing
      - wrist M05.73-
  - specified type NEC M06.80
    - ankle M06.87-
    - elbow M06.82-
    - foot joint M06.87-
    - hand joint M06.84-
    - hip M06.85-
    - knee M06.86-
    - multiple site M06.89
    - shoulder M06.81-
    - vertebra M06.88
    - wrist M06.83-
  - spine *—see* Spondylitis, ankylosing
- rubella B06.82
- scorbutic (*see also* subcategory M14.8-) E54
- senile or senescent *—see* Osteoarthritis
- septic (any site except spine) *—see* Arthritis, pyogenic or pyemic
  - spine *—see* Spondylopathy, infective
- serum (nontherapeutic) (therapeutic) *—see* Arthropathy, postimmunization
- specified form NEC M13.80
  - ankle M13.87-
  - elbow M13.82-
  - foot joint M13.87-
  - hand joint M13.84-
  - hip M13.85-
  - knee M13.86-
  - multiple site M13.89
  - shoulder M13.81-
  - specified joint NEC M13.88
  - wrist M13.83-
- spine *—see also* Spondylopathy, inflammatory
  - infectious or infective NEC *—see* Spondylopathy, infective
  - Marie-Strümpell *—see* Spondylitis, ankylosing
  - pyogenic *—see* Spondylopathy, infective
  - rheumatoid *—see* Spondylitis, ankylosing
  - traumatic (old) *—see* Spondylopathy, traumatic
  - tuberculous A18.01

Arthritis, arthritic *(continued)*
- staphylococcal M00.00
  - ankle M00.07-
  - elbow M00.02-
  - foot joint *—see* Arthritis, staphylococcal, ankle
  - hand joint M00.04-
  - hip M00.05-
  - knee M00.06-
  - multiple site M00.09
  - shoulder M00.01-
  - vertebra M00.08
  - wrist M00.03-
- streptococcal NEC M00.20
  - ankle M00.27-
  - elbow M00.22-
  - foot joint *—see* Arthritis, streptococcal, ankle
  - hand joint M00.24-
  - hip M00.25-
  - knee M00.26-
  - multiple site M00.29
  - shoulder M00.21-
  - vertebra M00.28
  - wrist M00.23-
- suppurative *—see* Arthritis, pyogenic or pyemic
- syphilitic (late) A52.16
  - congenital A50.55 *[M12.80]*
- syphilitica deformans (Charcot) A52.16
- temporomandibular M26.69
- toxic of menopause (any site) *—see* Arthritis, specified form NEC
- transient *—see* Arthropathy, specified form NEC
- traumatic (chronic) *—see* Arthropathy, traumatic
- tuberculous A18.02
  - spine A18.01
- uratic *—see* Gout
- urethritica (Reiter's) *—see* Reiter's disease
- vertebral *—see* Spondylopathy, inflammatory
- villous (any site) *—see* Arthropathy, specified form NEC

Arthrocele *—see* Effusion, joint

Arthrodesis status Z98.1

Arthrodynia *—see also* Pain, joint

Arthrodysplasia Q74.9

Arthrofibrosis, joint *—see* Ankylosis

Arthrogryposis (congenital) Q68.8
- multiplex congenita Q74.3

Arthrokatadysis M24.7

Arthropathy *—see also* Arthritis M12.9
- Charcot's *—see* Arthropathy, neuropathic
  - diabetic *—see* Diabetes, arthropathy, neuropathic
  - syringomyelic G95.0
- cricoarytenoid J38.7
- crystal (-induced) *—see* Arthritis, in, crystals
- diabetic NEC *—see* Diabetes, arthropathy
- distal interphalangeal, psoriatic L40.51
- enteropathic M07.60
  - ankle M07.67-
  - elbow M07.62-
  - foot joint M07.67-
  - hand joint M07.64-
  - hip M07.65-
  - knee M07.66-
  - multiple site M07.69
  - shoulder M07.61-
  - vertebra M07.68
  - wrist M07.63-

Arthropathy *(continued)*
- following intestinal bypass M02.00
  - ankle M02.07-
  - elbow M02.02-
  - foot joint M02.07-
  - hand joint M02.04-
  - hip M02.05-
  - knee M02.06-
  - multiple site M02.09
  - shoulder M02.01-
  - vertebra M02.08
  - wrist M02.03-
- gouty *—see also* Gout
  - in (due to)
    - Lesch-Nyhan syndrome E79.1 *[M14.8-]*
    - sickle-cell disorders D57- *[M14.8-]*
- hemophilic NEC D66 *[M36.2]*
  - in (due to)
    - hyperparathyroidism NEC E21.3 *[M14.8-]*
    - metabolic disease NOS E88.9 *[M14.8-]*
- in (due to)
  - acromegaly E22.0 *[M14.8-]*
  - amyloidosis E85.4 *[M14.8-]*
  - blood disorder NOS D75.9 *[M36.3]*
  - diabetes *—see* Diabetes, arthropathy
  - endocrine disease NOS E34.9 *[M14.8-]*
  - erythema
    - multiforme L51.9 *[M14.8-]*
    - nodosum L52 *[M14.8-]*
  - hemochromatosis E83.118 *[M14.8-]*
  - hemoglobinopathy NEC D58.2 *[M36.3]*
  - hemophilia NEC D66 *[M36.2]*
  - Henoch-Schönlein purpura D69.0 *[M36.4]*
  - hyperthyroidism E05.90 *[M14.8-]*
  - hypothyroidism E03.9 *[M14.8-]*
  - infective endocarditis I33.0 *[M12.80]*
  - leukemia NEC C95.9- *[M36.1]*
  - malignant histiocytosis C96.A *[M36.1]*
  - metabolic disease NOS E88.9 *[M14.8-]*
  - multiple myeloma C90.0- *[M36.1]*
  - neoplastic disease NOS (*see also* Neoplasm) D49.9 *[M36.1]*
  - nutritional deficiency (*see also* subcategory M14.8-) E63.9
  - psoriasis NOS L40.50
  - sarcoidosis D86.86
  - syphilis (late) A52.77
    - congenital A50.55 *[M12.80]*
  - thyrotoxicosis (*see also* subcategory M14.8-) E05.90
  - ulcerative colitis K51.90 *[M07.60]*
  - viral hepatitis (postinfectious) NEC B19.9 *[M12.80]*
  - Whipple's disease (*see also* subcategory M14.8-) K90.81
- Jaccoud *—see* Arthropathy, postrheumatic, chronic
- juvenile *—see* Arthritis, juvenile
  - psoriatic L40.54
- mutilans (psoriatic) L40.52
- neuropathic (Charcot) M14.60
  - ankle M14.67-
  - diabetic *—see* Diabetes, arthropathy, neuropathic
  - elbow M14.62-
  - foot joint M14.67-
  - hand joint M14.64-
  - hip M14.65-

Arthropathy *(continued)*
neuropathic *(continued)*
knee M14.66-
multiple site M14.69
nonsyphilitic NEC G98.0
shoulder M14.61-
syringomyelic G95.0
vertebra M14.68
wrist M14.63-
osteopulmonary *—see* Osteoarthropathy, hypertrophic, specified NEC
postdysenteric M02.10
ankle M02.17-
elbow M02.12-
foot joint M02.17-
hand joint M02.14-
hip M02.15-
knee M02.16-
multiple site M02.19
shoulder M02.11-
vertebra M02.18
wrist M02.13-
postimmunization M02.20
ankle M02.27-
elbow M02.22-
foot joint M02.27-
hand joint M02.24-
hip M02.25-
knee M02.26-
multiple site M02.29
shoulder M02.21-
vertebra M02.28
wrist M02.23-
postinfectious NEC B99 *[M12.80]*
in (due to)
enteritis due to Yersinia enterocolitica A04.6 *[M12.80]*
syphilis A52.77
viral hepatitis NEC B19.9 *[M12.80]*
postrheumatic, chronic (Jaccoud) M12.00
ankle M12.07-
elbow M12.02-
foot joint M12.07-
hand joint M12.04-
hip M12.05-
knee M12.06-
multiple site M12.09
shoulder M12.01-
specified joint NEC M12.08
vertebrae M12.08
wrist M12.03-
psoriatic NEC L40.59
interphalangeal, distal L40.51
reactive M02.9
in (due to)
infective endocarditis I33.0 *[M02.9]*
specified type NEC M02.80
ankle M02.87-
elbow M02.82-
foot joint M02.87-
hand joint M02.84-
hip M02.85-
knee M02.86-
multiple site M02.89
shoulder M02.81-
vertebra M02.88
wrist M02.83-
specified form NEC M12.80
ankle M12.87-
elbow M12.82-
foot joint M12.87-
hand joint M12.84-
hip M12.85-
knee M12.86-
multiple site M12.89
shoulder M12.81-

Arthropathy *(continued)*
specified form *(continued)*
specified joint NEC M12.88
vertebrae M12.88
wrist M12.83-
syringomyelic G95.0
tabes dorsalis A52.16
tabetic A52.16
transient *—see* Arthropathy, specified form NEC
traumatic M12.50
ankle M12.57-
elbow M12.52-
foot joint M12.57-
hand joint M12.54-
hip M12.55-
knee M12.56-
multiple site M12.59
shoulder M12.51-
specified joint NEC M12.58
vertebrae M12.58
wrist M12.53-

Arthropyosis *—see* Arthritis, pyogenic or pyemic

Arthrosis (deformans) (degenerative) (localized) *—see also* Osteoarthritis M19.90
spine *—see* Spondylosis

Arthus' phenomenon or reaction T78.41
due to
drug *—see* Table of Drugs and Chemicals, by drug

Articular *—see* condition

Articulation, reverse (teeth) M26.24

Artificial
insemination complication *— see* Complications, artificial, fertilization
opening status (functioning) (without complication) Z93.9
anus (colostomy) Z93.3
colostomy Z93.3
cystostomy Z93.50
appendico-vesicostomy Z93.52
cutaneous Z93.51
specified NEC Z93.59
enterostomy Z93.4
gastrostomy Z93.1
ileostomy Z93.2
intestinal tract NEC Z93.4
jejunostomy Z93.4
nephrostomy Z93.6
specified site NEC Z93.8
tracheostomy Z93.0
ureterostomy Z93.6
urethrostomy Z93.6
urinary tract NEC Z93.6
vagina Z93.8
vagina status Z93.8

Arytenoid *—see* condition

Asbestosis (occupational) J61

ASC-H (atypical squamous cells cannot exclude high grade squamous intraepithelial lesion on cytologic smear)
anus R85.611
cervix R87.611
vagina R87.621

ASC-US (atypical squamous cells of undetermined significance on cytologic smear)
anus R85.610
cervix R87.610
vagina R87.620

Ascariasis B77.9
with
complications NEC B77.89
intestinal complications B77.0
pneumonia, pneumonitis B77.81

Ascaridosis, ascaridiasis *—see* Ascariasis

Ascaris (infection) (infestation) (lumbricoides) *—see* Ascariasis

Ascending *—see* condition

Aschoff's bodies *—see* Myocarditis, rheumatic

Ascites (abdominal) R18.8
cardiac (*see also* Failure, heart, right) I50.810
chylous (nonfilarial) I89.8
filarial *—see* Infestation, filarial
due to
cirrhosis, alcoholic K70.31
hepatitis
alcoholic K70.11
chronic active K71.51
S. japonicum B65.2
heart (*see also* Failure, heart, right) I50.810
malignant R18.0
pseudochylous R18.8
syphilitic A52.74
tuberculous A18.31

Aseptic *—see* condition

Asherman's syndrome N85.6

Asialia K11.7

Asiatic cholera *—see* Cholera

Asimultagnosia (simultanagnosia) R48.3

Askin's tumor *—see* Neoplasm, connective tissue, malignant

Asocial personality F60.2

Asomatognosia R41.4

Aspartylglucosaminuria E77.1

Asperger's disease or syndrome F84.5

Aspergilloma *—see* Aspergillosis

Aspergillosis (with pneumonia) B44.9
bronchopulmonary, allergic B44.81
disseminated B44.7
generalized B44.7
pulmonary NEC B44.1
allergic B44.81
invasive B44.0
specified NEC B44.89
tonsillar B44.2

Aspergillus (flavus) (fumigatus) (infection) (terreus) *—see* Aspergillosis

Aspermatogenesis *—see* Azoospermia

Aspermia (testis) *—see* Azoospermia

Asphyxia, asphyxiation (by) R09.01
antenatal P84
birth P84
bunny bag *—see* Asphyxia, due to, mechanical threat to breathing, trapped in bed clothes
crushing S28.0
drowning T75.1
gas, fumes, or vapor *—see* Table of Drugs and Chemicals
inhalation *—see* Inhalation
intrauterine P84
local I73.00
with gangrene I73.01
mucus *—see also* Foreign body, respiratory tract, causing asphyxia
newborn P84
pathological R09.01

Asphyxia, asphyxiation *(continued)*
postnatal P84
mechanical *—see* Asphyxia, due to, mechanical threat to breathing
prenatal P84
reticularis R23.1
strangulation *—see* Asphyxia, due to, mechanical threat to breathing
submersion T75.1
traumatic T71.9
due to
crushed chest S28.0
foreign body (in) *—see* Foreign body, respiratory tract, causing asphyxia
low oxygen content of ambient air T71.20
due to
being trapped in
low oxygen environment T71.29
in car trunk T71.221
circumstances undetermined T71.224
done with intent to harm by
another person T71.223
self T71.222
in refrigerator T71.231
circumstances undetermined T71.234
done with intent to harm by
another person T71.233
self T71.232
cave-in T71.21
mechanical threat to breathing (accidental) T71.191
circumstances undetermined T71.194
done with intent to harm by
another person T71.193
self T71.192
hanging T71.161
circumstances undetermined T71.164
done with intent to harm by
another person T71.163
self T71.162
plastic bag T71.121
circumstances undetermined T71.124
done with intent to harm by
another person T71.123
self T71.122
smothering
in furniture T71.151
circumstances undetermined T71.154
done with intent to harm by
another person T71.153
self T71.152
under
another person's body T71.141
circumstances undetermined T71.144
done with intent to harm T71.143

Asphyxia, asphyxiation *(continued)*
- traumatic *(continued)*
  - due to *(continued)*
    - mechanical *(continued)*
      - smothering *(continued)*
        - under *(continued)*
          - pillow T71.111
            - circumstances undetermined T71.114
            - done with intent to harm by
              - another person T71.113
              - self T71.112
      - trapped in bed clothes T71.131
        - circumstances undetermined T71.134
        - done with intent to harm by
          - another person T71.133
          - self T71.132
- vomiting, vomitus *—see* Foreign body, respiratory tract, causing asphyxia

Aspiration
- amniotic (clear) fluid (newborn) P24.10
  - with
    - pneumonia (pneumonitis) P24.11
    - respiratory symptoms P24.11
- blood
  - newborn (without respiratory symptoms) P24.20
    - with
      - pneumonia (pneumonitis) P24.21
      - respiratory symptoms P24.21
  - specified age NEC *—see* Foreign body, respiratory tract
- bronchitis J69.0
- food or foreign body (with asphyxiation) *—see* Asphyxia, food
- liquor (amnii) (newborn) P24.10
  - with
    - pneumonia (pneumonitis) P24.11
    - respiratory symptoms P24.11
- meconium (newborn) (without respiratory symptoms) P24.00
  - with
    - pneumonitis (pneumonitis) P24.01
    - respiratory symptoms P24.01
- milk (newborn) (without respiratory symptoms) P24.30
  - with
    - pneumonia (pneumonitis) P24.31
    - respiratory symptoms P24.31
  - specified age NEC *—see* Foreign body, respiratory tract
- mucus *—see also* Foreign body, by site, causing asphyxia
  - newborn P24.10
    - with
      - pneumonia (pneumonitis) P24.11
      - respiratory symptoms P24.11
- neonatal P24.9
  - specific NEC (without respiratory symptoms) P24.80
    - with
      - pneumonia (pneumonitis) P24.81
      - respiratory symptoms P24.81
- newborn P24.9
  - specific NEC (without respiratory symptoms) P24.80
    - with
      - pneumonia (pneumonitis) P24.81
      - respiratory symptoms P24.81
- pneumonia J69.0
- pneumonitis J69.0
- syndrome of newborn *—see* Aspiration, by substance, with pneumonia
- vernix caseosa (newborn) P24.80
  - with
    - pneumonia (pneumonitis) P24.81
    - respiratory symptoms P24.81
- vomitus *—see also* Foreign body, respiratory tract
  - newborn (without respiratory symptoms) P24.30
    - with
      - pneumonia (pneumonitis) P24.31
      - respiratory symptoms P24.31

Asplenia (congenital) Q89.01
- postsurgical Z90.81

Assam fever B55.0

Assault, sexual *—see* Maltreatment

Assmann's focus NEC A15.0

Astasia(-abasia) (hysterical) F44.4

Asteatosis cutis L85.3

Astereognosia, astereognosis R48.1

Asterixis R27.8
- in liver disease K71.3

Asteroid hyalitis *—see* Deposit, crystalline

Asthenia, asthenic R53.1
- cardiac (*see also* Failure, heart) I50.9
  - psychogenic F45.8
- cardiovascular (*see also* Failure, heart) I50.9
  - psychogenic F45.8
- heart (*see also* Failure, heart) I50.9
  - psychogenic F45.8
- hysterical F44.4
- myocardial (*see also* Failure, heart) I50.9
  - psychogenic F45.8
- nervous F48.8
- neurocirculatory F45.8
- neurotic F48.8
- psychogenic F48.8
- psychoneurotic F48.8
- psychophysiologic F48.8
- reaction (psychophysiologic) F48.8
- senile R54

Asthenopia *—see also* Discomfort, visual
- hysterical F44.6
- psychogenic F44.6

Asthenospermia *—see* Abnormal, specimen, male genital organs

Asthma, asthmatic (bronchial) (catarrh) (spasmodic) J45.909
- with
  - chronic obstructive bronchitis J44.9
    - with
      - acute lower respiratory infection J44.0
      - exacerbation (acute) J44.1
  - chronic obstructive pulmonary disease J44.9
    - with
      - acute lower respiratory infection J44.0
      - exacerbation (acute) J44.1
  - exacerbation (acute) J45.901
  - hay fever *—see* Asthma, allergic extrinsic
  - rhinitis, allergic *—see* Asthma, allergic extrinsic
  - status asthmaticus J45.902
- allergic extrinsic J45.909
  - with
    - exacerbation (acute) J45.901
    - status asthmaticus J45.902
- atopic *—see* Asthma, allergic extrinsic
- cardiac *—see* Failure, ventricular, left
- cardiobronchial I50.1
- childhood J45.909
  - with
    - exacerbation (acute) J45.901
    - status asthmaticus J45.902
- chronic obstructive J44.9
  - with
    - acute lower respiratory infection J44.0
    - exacerbation (acute) J44.1
- collier's J60
- cough variant J45.991
- detergent J69.8
- due to
  - detergent J69.8
  - inhalation of fumes J68.3
- eosinophilic J82
- extrinsic, allergic *—see* Asthma, allergic extrinsic
- grinder's J62.8
- hay *—see* Asthma, allergic extrinsic
- heart I50.1
- idiosyncratic *—see* Asthma, nonallergic
- intermittent (mild) J45.20
  - with
    - exacerbation (acute) J45.21
    - status asthmaticus J45.22
- intrinsic, nonallergic *—see* Asthma, nonallergic
- Kopp's E32.8
- late-onset J45.909
  - with
    - exacerbation (acute) J45.901
    - status asthmaticus J45.902
- mild intermittent J45.20
  - with
    - exacerbation (acute) J45.21
    - status asthmaticus J45.22
- mild persistent J45.30
  - with
    - exacerbation (acute) J45.31
    - status asthmaticus J45.32
- Millar's (laryngismus stridulus) J38.5
- miner's J60
- mixed J45.909
  - with
    - exacerbation (acute) J45.901
    - status asthmaticus J45.902
- moderate persistent J45.40
  - with
    - exacerbation (acute) J45.41
    - status asthmaticus J45.42
- nervous *—see* Asthma, nonallergic
- nonallergic (intrinsic) J45.909
  - with
    - exacerbation (acute) J45.901
    - status asthmaticus J45.902
- persistent
  - mild J45.30
    - with
      - exacerbation (acute) J45.31
      - status asthmaticus J45.32
  - moderate J45.40
    - with
      - exacerbation (acute) J45.41
      - status asthmaticus J45.42
  - severe J45.50
    - with
      - exacerbation (acute) J45.51
      - status asthmaticus J45.52
- platinum J45.998
- pneumoconiotic NEC J64
- potter's J62.8
- predominantly allergic J45.909
- psychogenic F54
- pulmonary eosinophilic J82
- red cedar J67.8
- Rostan's I50.1
- sandblaster's J62.8
- sequoiosis J67.8
- severe persistent J45.50
  - with
    - exacerbation (acute) J45.51
    - status asthmaticus J45.52
- specified NEC J45.998
- stonemason's J62.8
- thymic E32.8
- tuberculous *—see* Tuberculosis, pulmonary
- Wichmann's (laryngismus stridulus) J38.5
- wood J67.8

Astigmatism (compound) (congenital) H52.20-
- irregular H52.21-
- regular H52.22-

Astraphobia F40.220

Astroblastoma
- specified site *—see* Neoplasm, malignant, by site
- unspecified site C71.9

Astrocytoma (cystic)
- anaplastic
  - specified site *—see* Neoplasm, malignant, by site
  - unspecified site C71.9
- fibrillary
  - specified site *—see* Neoplasm, malignant, by site
  - unspecified site C71.9
- fibrous
  - specified site *—see* Neoplasm, malignant, by site
  - unspecified site C71.9
- gemistocytic
  - specified site *—see* Neoplasm, malignant, by site
  - unspecified site C71.9
- juvenile
  - specified site *—see* Neoplasm, malignant, by site
  - unspecified site C71.9
- pilocytic
  - specified site *—see* Neoplasm, malignant, by site
  - unspecified site C71.9
- piloid
  - specified site *—see* Neoplasm, malignant, by site
  - unspecified site C71.9
- protoplasmic
  - specified site *—see* Neoplasm, malignant, by site
  - unspecified site C71.9
- specified site NEC *—see* Neoplasm, malignant, by site
- subependymal D43.2

Astrocytoma *(continued)*
- subependymal *(continued)*
  - giant cell
    - specified site —*see* Neoplasm, uncertain behavior, by site
    - unspecified site D43.2
  - specified site —*see* Neoplasm, uncertain behavior, by site
  - unspecified site D43.2
- unspecified site C71.9

Astroglioma
- specified site —*see* Neoplasm, malignant, by site
- unspecified site C71.9

Asymbolia R48.8

Asymmetry —*see also* Distortion
- between native and reconstructed breast N65.1
- face Q67.0
- jaw (lower) —*see* Anomaly, dentofacial, jaw-cranial base relationship, asymmetry

Asynergia, asynergy R27.8
- ventricular I51.89

Asystole (heart) —*see* Arrest, cardiac

At risk
- for
  - dental caries Z91.849
    - high Z91.843
    - low Z91.841
    - moderate Z91.842
- falling Z91.81

Ataxia, ataxy, ataxic R27.0
- acute R27.8
- brain (hereditary) G11.9
- cerebellar (hereditary) G11.9
  - with defective DNA repair G11.3
  - alcoholic G31.2
  - early-onset G11.1
  - in
    - alcoholism G31.2
    - myxedema E03.9 *[G13.2]*
    - neoplastic disease (*see also* Neoplasm) D49.9 *[G32.81]*
    - specified disease NEC G32.81
  - late-onset (Marie's) G11.2
- cerebral (hereditary) G11.9
- congenital nonprogressive G11.0
- family, familial —*see* Ataxia, hereditary
- following
  - cerebrovascular disease I69.993
    - cerebral infarction I69.393
    - intracerebral hemorrhage I69.193
    - nontraumatic intracranial hemorrhage NEC I69.293
    - specified disease NEC I69.893
    - subarachnoid hemorrhage I69.093
- Friedreich's (heredofamilial) (cerebellar) (spinal) G11.1
- gait R26.0
  - hysterical F44.4
- general R27.8
- gluten M35.9 *[G32.81]*
  - with celiac disease K90.0 *[G32.81]*
- hereditary G11.9
  - with neuropathy G60.2
  - cerebellar —*see* Ataxia, cerebellar
  - spastic G11.4
  - specified NEC G11.8
  - spinal (Friedreich's) G11.1
- heredofamilial —*see* Ataxia, hereditary
- Hunt's G11.1
- hysterical F44.4
- locomotor (progressive) (syphilitic) (partial) (spastic) A52.11
  - diabetic —*see* Diabetes, ataxia

Ataxia, ataxy, ataxic *(continued)*
- Marie's (cerebellar) (heredofamilial) (late- onset) G11.2
- nonorganic origin F44.4
- nonprogressive, congenital G11.0
- psychogenic F44.4
- Roussy-Lévy G60.0
- Sanger-Brown's (hereditary) G11.2
- spastic hereditary G11.4
- spinal
  - hereditary (Friedreich's) G11.1
  - progressive (syphilitic) A52.11
- spinocerebellar, X-linked recessive G11.1
- telangiectasia (Louis-Bar) G11.3

Ataxia-telangiectasia (Louis-Bar) G11.3

Atelectasis (massive) (partial) (pressure) (pulmonary) J98.11
- newborn P28.10
  - due to resorption P28.11
  - partial P28.19
  - primary P28.0
  - secondary P28.19
- primary (newborn) P28.0
- tuberculous —*see* Tuberculosis, pulmonary

Atelocardia Q24.9

Atelomyelia Q06.1

Atheroembolism
- of
  - extremities
    - lower I75.02-
    - upper I75.01-
  - kidney I75.81
  - specified NEC I75.89

Atheroma, atheromatous —*see also* Arteriosclerosis I70.90
- aorta, aortic I70.0
  - valve —*see also* Endocarditis, aortic I35.8
- aorto-iliac I70.0
- artery —*see* Arteriosclerosis
- basilar (artery) I67.2
- carotid (artery) (common) (internal) I67.2
- cerebral (arteries) I67.2
- coronary (artery) I25.10
  - with angina pectoris —*see* Arteriosclerosis, coronary (artery),
- degeneration —*see* Arteriosclerosis
- heart, cardiac —*see* Disease, heart, ischemic, atherosclerotic
- mitral (valve) I34.8
- myocardium, myocardial —*see* Disease, heart, ischemic, atherosclerotic
- pulmonary valve (heart) (*see also* Endocarditis, pulmonary) I37.8
- tricuspid (heart) (valve) I36.8
- valve, valvular —*see* Endocarditis
- vertebral (artery) I67.2

Atheromatosis —*see* Arteriosclerosis

Atherosclerosis —*see also* Arteriosclerosis
- coronary
  - artery I25.10
    - with angina pectoris —*see* Arteriosclerosis, coronary (artery),
    - due to
      - calcified coronary lesion (severely) I25.84
      - lipid rich plaque I25.83
- transplanted heart I25.811
  - bypass graft I25.812

Atherosclerosis *(continued)*
- transplanted heart *(continued)*
  - bypass graft *(continued)*
    - with angina pectoris —*see* Arteriosclerosis, coronary (artery),
  - native coronary artery I25.811
    - with angina pectoris —*see* Arteriosclerosis, coronary (artery),

Athetosis (acquired) R25.8
- bilateral (congenital) G80.3
- congenital (bilateral) (double) G80.3
- double (congenital) G80.3
- unilateral R25.8

Athlete's
- foot B35.3
- heart I51.7

Athrepsia E41

Athyrea (acquired) —*see also* Hypothyroidism
- congenital E03.1

Atonia, atony, atonic
- bladder (sphincter) (neurogenic) N31.2
- capillary I78.8
- cecum K59.8
  - psychogenic F45.8
- colon —*see* Atony, intestine
- congenital P94.2
- esophagus K22.8
- intestine K59.8
  - psychogenic F45.8
- stomach K31.89
  - neurotic or psychogenic F45.8
- uterus (during labor) O62.2
  - with hemorrhage (postpartum) O72.1
  - postpartum (with hemorrhage) O72.1
    - without hemorrhage O75.89

Atopy —*see* History, allergy

Atransferrinemia, congenital E88.09

Atresia, atretic
- alimentary organ or tract NEC Q45.8
  - upper Q40.8
- ani, anus, anal (canal) Q42.3
  - with fistula Q42.2
- aorta (ring) Q25.29
- aortic (orifice) (valve) Q23.0
  - arch Q25.21
  - congenital with hypoplasia of ascending aorta and defective development of left ventricle (with mitral stenosis) Q23.4
  - in hypoplastic left heart syndrome Q23.4
- aqueduct of Sylvius Q03.0
  - with spina bifida —*see* Spina bifida, with hydrocephalus
- artery NEC Q27.8
  - cerebral Q28.3
  - coronary Q24.5
  - digestive system Q27.8
  - eye Q15.8
  - lower limb Q27.8
  - pulmonary Q25.5
  - specified site NEC Q27.8
  - umbilical Q27.0
  - upper limb Q27.8
- auditory canal (external) Q16.1
- bile duct (common) (congenital) (hepatic) Q44.2
  - acquired —*see* Obstruction, bile duct
- bladder (neck) Q64.39
  - obstruction Q64.31
- bronchus Q32.4

Atresia, atretic *(continued)*
- cecum Q42.8
- cervix (acquired) N88.2
  - congenital Q51.828
  - in pregnancy or childbirth —*see* Anomaly, cervix, in pregnancy or childbirth
    - causing obstructed labor O65.5
- choana Q30.0
- colon Q42.9
  - specified NEC Q42.8
- common duct Q44.2
- cricoid cartilage Q31.8
- cystic duct Q44.2
  - acquired K82.8
    - with obstruction K82.0
- digestive organs NEC Q45.8
- duodenum Q41.0
- ear canal Q16.1
- ejaculatory duct Q55.4
- epiglottis Q31.8
- esophagus Q39.0
  - with tracheoesophageal fistula Q39.1
- eustachian tube Q17.8
- fallopian tube (congenital) Q50.6
  - acquired N97.1
- follicular cyst N83.0-
- foramen of
  - Luschka Q03.1
    - with spina bifida —*see* Spina bifida, with hydrocephalus
  - Magendie Q03.1
    - with spina bifida —*see* Spina bifida, with hydrocephalus
- gallbladder Q44.1
- genital organ
  - external
    - female Q52.79
    - male Q55.8
  - internal
    - female Q52.8
    - male Q55.8
- glottis Q31.8
- gullet Q39.0
  - with tracheoesophageal fistula Q39.1
- heart valve NEC Q24.8
  - pulmonary Q22.0
  - tricuspid Q22.4
- hymen Q52.3
  - acquired (postinfective) N89.6
- ileum Q41.2
- intestine (small) Q41.9
  - large Q42.9
    - specified NEC Q42.8
- iris, filtration angle Q15.0
- jejunum Q41.1
- lacrimal apparatus Q10.4
- larynx Q31.8
- meatus urinarius Q64.33
- mitral valve Q23.2
  - in hypoplastic left heart syndrome Q23.4
- nares (anterior) (posterior) Q30.0
- nasopharynx Q34.8
- nose, nostril Q30.0
  - acquired J34.89
- organ or site NEC Q89.8
- osseous meatus (ear) Q16.1
- oviduct (congenital) Q50.6
  - acquired N97.1
- parotid duct Q38.4
  - acquired K11.8
- pulmonary (artery) Q25.5
  - valve Q22.0
- pulmonic Q22.0
- pupil Q13.2
- rectum Q42.1
  - with fistula Q42.0

Atresia, atretic *(continued)*
salivary duct Q38.4
acquired K11.8
sublingual duct Q38.4
acquired K11.8
submandibular duct Q38.4
acquired K11.8
submaxillary duct Q38.4
acquired K11.8
thyroid cartilage Q31.8
trachea Q32.1
tricuspid valve Q22.4
ureter Q62.10
pelvic junction Q62.11
vesical orifice Q62.12
ureteropelvic junction Q62.11
ureterovesical orifice Q62.12
urethra (valvular) Q64.39
stricture Q64.32
urinary tract NEC Q64.8
uterus Q51.818
acquired N85.8
vagina (congenital) Q52.4
acquired (postinfectional) (senile) N89.5
vas deferens Q55.3
vascular NEC Q27.8
cerebral Q28.3
digestive system Q27.8
lower limb Q27.8
specified site NEC Q27.8
upper limb Q27.8
vein NEC Q27.8
digestive system Q27.8
great Q26.8
lower limb Q27.8
portal Q26.5
pulmonary Q26.4
partial Q26.3
total Q26.2
specified site NEC Q27.8
upper limb Q27.8
vena cava (inferior) (superior) Q26.8
vesicourethral orifice Q64.31
vulva Q52.79
acquired N90.5

Atrichia, atrichosis *—see* Alopecia

Atrophia *—see also* Atrophy
cutis senilis L90.8
due to radiation L57.8
gyrata of choroid and retina H31.23
senilis R54
dermatological L90.8
due to radiation (nonionizing) (solar) L57.8
unguium L60.3
congenita Q84.6

Atrophie blanche (en plaque) (de Milian) L95.0

Atrophoderma, atrophodermia (of) L90.9
diffusum (idiopathic) L90.4
maculatum L90.8
et striatum L90.8
due to syphilis A52.79
syphilitic A51.39
neuriticum L90.8
Pasini and Pierini L90.3
pigmentosum Q82.1
reticulatum symmetricum faciei L66.4
senile L90.8
due to radiation (nonionizing) (solar) L57.8
vermiculata (cheeks) L66.4

Atrophy, atrophic (of)
adrenal (capsule) (gland) E27.49
primary (autoimmune) E27.1
alveolar process or ridge (edentulous) K08.20

Atrophy, atrophic *(continued)*
anal sphincter (disuse) N81.84
appendix K38.8
arteriosclerotic *—see* Arteriosclerosis
bile duct (common) (hepatic) K83.8
bladder N32.89
neurogenic N31.8
blanche (en plaque) (of Milian) L95.0
bone (senile) NEC *—see also* Disorder, bone, specified type NEC
due to
tabes dorsalis (neurogenic) A52.11
brain (cortex) (progressive) G31.9
frontotemporal circumscribed G31.01 *[F02.80]*
with behavioral disturbance G31.01 *[F02.81]*
senile NEC G31.1
breast N64.2
obstetric *—see* Disorder, breast, specified type NEC
buccal cavity K13.79
cardiac *—see* Degeneration, myocardial
cartilage (infectional) (joint) *—see* Disorder, cartilage, specified NEC
cerebellar *—see* Atrophy, brain
cerebral *—see* Atrophy, brain
cervix (mucosa) (senile) (uteri) N88.8
menopausal N95.8
Charcot-Marie-Tooth G60.0
choroid (central) (macular) (myopic) (retina) H31.10-
diffuse secondary H31.12-
gyrate H31.23
senile H31.11-
ciliary body *—see* Atrophy, iris
conjunctiva (senile) H11.89
corpus cavernosum N48.89
cortical *—see* Atrophy, brain
cystic duct K82.8
Déjérine-Thomas G23.8
disuse NEC *—see* Atrophy, muscle
Duchenne-Aran G12.21
ear H93.8-
edentulous alveolar ridge K08.20
endometrium (senile) N85.8
cervix N88.8
enteric K63.89
epididymis N50.89
eyeball *—see* Disorder, globe, degenerated condition, atrophy
eyelid (senile) *—see* Disorder, eyelid, degenerative
facial (skin) L90.9
fallopian tube (senile) N83.32-
with ovary N83.33-
fascioscapulohumeral (Landouzy-Déjérine) G71.0
fatty, thymus (gland) E32.8
gallbladder K82.8
gastric K29.40
with bleeding K29.41
gastrointestinal K63.89
glandular I89.8
globe H44.52-
gum *-see* Recession, gingival
hair L67.8
heart (brown) *—see* Degeneration, myocardial
hemifacial Q67.4
Romberg G51.8
infantile E41
paralysis, acute *—see* Poliomyelitis, paralytic

Atrophy, atrophic *(continued)*
intestine K63.89
iris (essential) (progressive) H21.26-
specified NEC H21.29
kidney (senile) (terminal) (*see also* Sclerosis, renal) N26.1
congenital or infantile Q60.5
bilateral Q60.4
unilateral Q60.3
hydronephrotic *—see* Hydronephrosis
lacrimal gland (primary) H04.14-
secondary H04.15-
Landouzy-Déjérine G71.0
laryngitis, infective J37.0
larynx J38.7
Leber's optic (hereditary) H47.22
lip K13.0
liver (yellow) K72.90
with coma K72.91
acute, subacute K72.00
with coma K72.01
chronic K72.10
with coma K72.11
lung (senile) J98.4
macular (dermatological) L90.8
syphilitic, skin A51.39
striated A52.79
mandible (edentulous) K08.20
minimal K08.21
moderate K08.22
severe K08.23
maxilla K08.20
minimal K08.24
moderate K08.25
severe K08.26
muscle, muscular (diffuse) (general) (idiopathic) (primary) M62.50
ankle M62.57-
Duchenne-Aran G12.21
foot M62.57-
forearm M62.53-
hand M62.54-
infantile spinal G12.0
lower leg M62.56-
multiple sites M62.59
myelopathic *—see* Atrophy, muscle, spinal
myotonic G71.11
neuritic G58.9
neuropathic (peroneal) (progressive) G60.0
pelvic (disuse) N81.84
peroneal G60.0
progressive (bulbar) G12.21
adult G12.1
infantile (spinal) G12.0
spinal G12.25
adult G12.1
infantile G12.0
pseudohypertrophic G71.0
shoulder region M62.51-
specified site NEC M62.58
spinal G12.9
adult form G12.1
Aran-Duchenne G12.21
childhood form, type II G12.1
distal G12.1
hereditary NEC G12.1
infantile, type I (Werdnig-Hoffmann) G12.0
juvenile form, type III (Kugelberg- Welander) G12.1
progressive G12.25
scapuloperoneal form G12.1
specified NEC G12.8
syphilitic A52.78
thigh M62.55-
upper arm M62.52-
myocardium *—see* Degeneration, myocardial

Atrophy, atrophic *(continued)*
myometrium (senile) N85.8
cervix N88.8
myopathic NEC *—see* Atrophy, muscle
myotonia G71.11
nail L60.3
nasopharynx J31.1
nerve *—see also* Disorder, nerve
abducens *—see* Strabismus, paralytic, sixth nerve
accessory G52.8
acoustic or auditory H93.3
cranial G52.9
eighth (auditory) H93.3
eleventh (accessory) G52.8
fifth (trigeminal) G50.8
first (olfactory) G52.0
fourth (trochlear) *—see* Strabismus, paralytic, fourth nerve
second (optic) H47.20
sixth (abducens) *—see* Strabismus, paralytic, sixth nerve
tenth (pneumogastric) (vagus) G52.2
third (oculomotor) *—see* Strabismus, paralytic, third nerve
twelfth (hypoglossal) G52.3
hypoglossal G52.3
oculomotor *—see* Strabismus, paralytic, third nerve
olfactory G52.0
optic (papillomacular bundle)
syphilitic (late) A52.15
congenital A50.44
pneumogastric G52.2
trigeminal G50.8
trochlear *—see* Strabismus, paralytic, fourth nerve
vagus (pneumogastric) G52.2
neurogenic, bone, tabetic A52.11
nutritional E41
old age R54
olivopontocerebellar G23.8
optic (nerve) H47.20
glaucomatous H47.23-
hereditary H47.22
primary H47.21-
specified type NEC H47.29-
syphilitic (late) A52.15
congenital A50.44
orbit H05.31-
ovary (senile) N83.31-
with fallopian tube N83.33-
oviduct (senile) *—see* Atrophy, fallopian tube
palsy, diffuse (progressive) G12.22
pancreas (duct) (senile) K86.89
parotid gland K11.0
pelvic muscle N81.84
penis N48.89
pharynx J39.2
pluriglandular E31.8
autoimmune E31.0
polyarthritis M15.9
prostate N42.89
pseudohypertrophic (muscle) G71.0
renal (*see also* Sclerosis, renal) N26.1
retina, retinal (postinfectional) H35.89
rhinitis J31.0
salivary gland K11.0
scar L90.5
sclerosis, lobar (of brain) G31.09 *[F02.80]*
with behavioral disturbance G31.09 *[F02.81]*

Atrophy, atrophic *(continued)*
scrotum N50.89
seminal vesicle N50.89
senile R54
due to radiation (nonionizing) (solar) L57.8
skin (patches) (spots) L90.9
degenerative (senile) L90.8
due to radiation (nonionizing) (solar) L57.8
senile L90.8
spermatic cord N50.89
spinal (acute) (cord) G95.89
muscular *—see* Atrophy, muscle, spinal
paralysis G12.20
acute *—see* Poliomyelitis, paralytic
meaning progressive muscular atrophy G12.21
spine (column) *—see* Spondylopathy, specified NEC
spleen (senile) D73.0
stomach K29.40
with bleeding K29.41
striate (skin) L90.6
syphilitic A52.79
subcutaneous L90.9
sublingual gland K11.0
submandibular gland K11.0
submaxillary gland K11.0
Sudeck's *—see* Algoneurodystrophy
suprarenal (capsule) (gland) E27.49
primary E27.1
systemic affecting central nervous system
in
myxedema E03.9 *[G13.2]*
neoplastic disease (*see also* Neoplasm) D49.9 *[G13.1]*
specified disease NEC G13.8
tarso-orbital fascia, congenital Q10.3
testis N50.0
thenar, partial *—see* Syndrome, carpal tunnel
thymus (fatty) E32.8
thyroid (gland) (acquired) E03.4
with cretinism E03.1
congenital (with myxedema) E03.1
tongue (senile) K14.8
papillae K14.4
trachea J39.8
tunica vaginalis N50.89
turbinate J34.89
tympanic membrane (nonflaccid) H73.82-
flaccid H73.81-
upper respiratory tract J39.8
uterus, uterine (senile) N85.8
cervix N88.8
due to radiation (intended effect) N85.8
adverse effect or misadventure N99.89
vagina (senile) N95.2
vas deferens N50.89
vascular I99.8
vertebra (senile) *—see* Spondylopathy, specified NEC
vulva (senile) N90.5
Werdnig-Hoffmann G12.0
yellow *—see* Failure, hepatic

Attack, attacks
with alteration of consciousness (with automatisms) *—see* Epilepsy, localization-related, symptomatic, with complex partial seizures
Adams-Stokes I45.9

Attack, attacks *(continued)*
akinetic *—see* Epilepsy, generalized, specified NEC
angina *—see* Angina
atonic *—see* Epilepsy, generalized, specified NEC
benign shuddering G25.83
cataleptic *—see* Catalepsy
coronary *—see* Infarct, myocardium
cyanotic, newborn P28.2
drop NEC R55
epileptic *—see* Epilepsy
heart *—see* infarct, myocardium
hysterical F44.9
jacksonian *—see* Epilepsy, localization-related, symptomatic, with simple partial seizures
myocardium, myocardial *—see* Infarct, myocardium
myoclonic *—see* Epilepsy, generalized, specified NEC
panic F41.0
psychomotor *—see* Epilepsy, localization-related, symptomatic, with complex partial seizures
salaam *—see* Epilepsy, spasms
schizophreniform, brief F23
shuddering, benign G25.83
Stokes-Adams I45.9
syncope R55
transient ischemic (TIA) G45.9
specified NEC G45.8
unconsciousness R55
hysterical F44.89
vasomotor R55
vasovagal (paroxysmal) (idiopathic) R55
without alteration of consciousness *—see* Epilepsy, localization-related, symptomatic, with simple partial seizures

Attention (to)
artificial
opening (of) Z43.9
digestive tract NEC Z43.4
colon Z43.3
ilium Z43.2
stomach Z43.1
specified NEC Z43.8
trachea Z43.0
urinary tract NEC Z43.6
cystostomy Z43.5
nephrostomy Z43.6
ureterostomy Z43.6
urethrostomy Z43.6
vagina Z43.7
colostomy Z43.3
cystostomy Z43.5
deficit disorder or syndrome F98.8
with hyperactivity *—see* Disorder, attention-deficit hyperactivity
gastrostomy Z43.1
ileostomy Z43.2
jejunostomy Z43.4
nephrostomy Z43.6
surgical dressings Z48.01
sutures Z48.02
tracheostomy Z43.0
ureterostomy Z43.6
urethrostomy Z43.6

Attrition
gum *-see* Recession, gingival
tooth, teeth (excessive) (hard tissues) K03.0

Atypical, atypism *—see also* condition
cells (on cytological smear) (endocervical) (endometrial) (glandular)
cervix R87.619
vagina R87.629

Atypical, atypism *(continued)*
cervical N87.9
endometrium N85.9
hyperplasia N85.00
parenting situation Z62.9

Auditory *—see* condition

Aujeszky's disease B33.8

Aurantiasis, cutis E67.1

Auricle, auricular *—see also* condition
cervical Q18.2

Auriculotemporal syndrome G50.8

Austin Flint murmur (aortic insufficiency) I35.1

Australian
Q fever A78
X disease A83.4

Autism, autistic (childhood) (infantile) F84.0
atypical F84.9
spectrum disorder F84.0

Autodigestion R68.89

Autoerythrocyte sensitization (syndrome) D69.2

Autographism L50.3

Autoimmune
disease (systemic) M35.9
inhibitors to clotting factors D68.311
lymphoproliferative syndrome [ALPS] D89.82
thyroiditis E06.3

Autointoxication R68.89

Automatism G93.89
with temporal sclerosis G93.81
epileptic *—see* Epilepsy, localization-related, symptomatic, with complex partial seizures
paroxysmal, idiopathic *—see* Epilepsy, localization-related, symptomatic, with complex partial seizures

Autonomic, autonomous
bladder (neurogenic) N31.2
hysteria seizure F44.5

Autosensitivity, erythrocyte D69.2

Autosensitization, cutaneous L30.2

Autosome *—see* condition by chromosome involved

Autotopagnosia R48.1

Autotoxemia R68.89

Autumn *—see* condition

Avellis' syndrome G46.8

Aversion
oral R63.3
newborn P92.-
nonorganic origin F98.2
sexual F52.1

Aviator's
disease or sickness *—see* Effect, adverse, high altitude
ear T70.0

Avitaminosis (multiple) (*see also* Deficiency, vitamin) E56.9
B E53.9
with
beriberi E51.11
pellagra E52
B2 E53.0
B6 E53.1
B12 E53.8
D E55.9
with rickets E55.0

Avitaminosis *(continued)*
G E53.0
K E56.1
nicotinic acid E52

AVNRT (atrioventricular nodal re-entrant tachycardia) I47.1

AVRT (atrioventricular nodal re-entrant tachycardia) I47.1

Avulsion (traumatic)
blood vessel *—see* Injury, blood vessel
bone *—see* Fracture, by site
cartilage *—see also* Dislocation, by site
symphyseal (inner), complicating delivery O71.6
external site other than limb *—see* Wound, open, by site
eye S05.7-
head (intracranial)
external site NEC S08.89
scalp S08.0
internal organ or site *—see* Injury, by site
joint *—see also* Dislocation, by site
capsule *—see* Sprain, by site
kidney S37.06-
ligament *—see* Sprain, by site
limb *—see also* Amputation, traumatic, by site
skin and subcutaneous tissue *— see* Wound, open, by site
muscle *—see* Injury, muscle
nerve (root) *—see* Injury, nerve
scalp S08.0
skin and subcutaneous tissue *—see* Wound, open, by site
spleen S36.032
symphyseal cartilage (inner), complicating delivery O71.6
tendon *—see* Injury, muscle
tooth S03.2

Awareness of heart beat R00.2

Axenfeld's
anomaly or syndrome Q15.0
degeneration (calcareous) Q13.4

Axilla, axillary *—see also* condition
breast Q83.1

Axonotmesis *—see* Injury, nerve

Ayerza's disease or syndrome (pulmonary artery sclerosis with pulmonary hypertension) I27.0

Azoospermia (organic) N46.01
due to
drug therapy N46.021
efferent duct obstruction N46.023
infection N46.022
radiation N46.024
specified cause NEC N46.029
systemic disease N46.025

Azotemia R79.89
meaning uremia N19

Aztec ear Q17.3

Azygos
continuation inferior vena cava Q26.8
lobe (lung) Q33.1

B

Baastrup's disease *—see* Kissing spine

Babesiosis B60.0

Babington's disease (familial hemorrhagic telangiectasia) I78.0

Babinski's syndrome A52.79
Baby
  crying constantly R68.11
  floppy (syndrome) P94.2
Bacillary *—see* condition
Bacilluria R82.71
Bacillus *—see also* Infection, bacillus
  abortus infection A23.1
  anthracis infection A22.9
  coli infection *—see also* Escherichia coli B96.20
  Flexner's A03.1
  mallei infection A24.0
  Shiga's A03.0
  suipestifer infection *—see* Infection, salmonella
Back *—see* condition
Backache (postural) M54.9
  sacroiliac M53.3
  specified NEC M54.89
Backflow *—see* Reflux
Backward reading (dyslexia) F81.0
Bacteremia R78.81
  with sepsis *—see* Sepsis
Bactericholia *—see* Cholecystitis, acute
Bacterid, bacteride (pustular) L40.3
Bacterium, bacteria, bacterial
  agent NEC, as cause of disease classified elsewhere B96.89
  in blood *—see* Bacteremia
  in urine *—see* Bacteriuria
Bacteriuria, bacteruria R82.71
  asymptomatic R82.71
Bacteroides
  fragilis, as cause of disease classified elsewhere B96.6
Bad
  heart *—see* Disease, heart
  trip
    due to drug abuse *—see* Abuse, drug, hallucinogen
    due to drug dependence *—see* Dependence, drug, hallucinogen
Baelz's disease (cheilitis glandularis apostematosa) K13.0
Baerensprung's disease (eczema marginatum) B35.6
Bagasse disease or pneumonitis J67.1
Bagassosis J67.1
Baker's cyst *—see* Cyst, Baker's
Bakwin-Krida syndrome (metaphyseal dysplasia) Q78.5
Balancing side interference M26.56
Balanitis (circinata) (erosiva) (gangrenosa) (phagedenic) (vulgaris) N48.1
  amebic A06.82
  candidal B37.42
  due to Haemophilus ducreyi A57
  gonococcal (acute) (chronic) A54.09
  xerotica obliterans N48.0
Balanoposthitis N47.6
  gonococcal (acute) (chronic) A54.09
  ulcerative (specific) A63.8
Balanorrhagia *—see* Balanitis
Balantidiasis, balantidiosis A07.0
Bald tongue K14.4
Baldness *—see also* Alopecia
  male-pattern *—see* Alopecia, androgenic
Balkan grippe A78
Balloon disease *—see* Effect, adverse, high altitude
Balo's disease (concentric sclerosis) G37.5
Bamberger-Marie disease *—see* Osteoarthropathy, hypertrophic, specified type NEC
Bancroft's filariasis B74.0
Band(s)
  adhesive *—see* Adhesions, peritoneum
  anomalous or congenital *—see also* Anomaly, by site
    heart (atrial) (ventricular) Q24.8
    intestine Q43.3
    omentum Q43.3
  cervix N88.1
  constricting, congenital Q79.8
  gallbladder (congenital) Q44.1
  intestinal (adhesive) *—see* Adhesions, peritoneum
  obstructive
    intestine K56.50
      complete K56.52
      incomplete K56.51
      partial K56.51
    peritoneum K56.50
      complete K56.52
      incomplete K56.51
      partial K56.51
  periappendiceal, congenital Q43.3
  peritoneal (adhesive) *—see* Adhesions, peritoneum
  uterus N73.6
    internal N85.6
  vagina N89.5
Bandemia D72.825
Bandl's ring (contraction), **complicating delivery** O62.4
Bangkok hemorrhagic fever A91
Bang's disease (brucella abortus) A23.1
Bankruptcy, anxiety concerning Z59.8
Bannister's disease T78.3
  hereditary D84.1
Banti's disease or syndrome (with cirrhosis) (with portal hypertension) K76.6
Bar, median, prostate *—see* Enlargement, enlarged, prostate
Barcoo disease or rot *—see* Ulcer, skin
Barlow's disease E54
Barodontalgia T70.29
Baron Münchausen syndrome *—see* Disorder, factitious
Barosinusitis T70.1
Barotitis T70.0
Barotrauma T70.29
  odontalgia T70.29
  otitic T70.0
  sinus T70.1
Barraquer (-Simons) **disease or syndrome** (progressive lipodystrophy) E88.1
Barré-Guillain disease or syndrome G61.0
Barré-Liéou syndrome (posterior cervical sympathetic) M53.0
Barrel chest M95.4
Barrett's
  disease *—see* Barrett's, esophagus
  esophagus K22.70
    with dysplasia K22.719
      high grade K22.711
      low grade K22.710
    without dysplasia K22.70
  syndrome *—see* Barrett's, esophagus
  ulcer K22.10
    with bleeding K22.11
    without bleeding K22.10
Bársony (-Polgár) (-Teschendorf) syndrome (corkscrew esophagus) K22.4
Bartholinitis (suppurating) N75.8
  gonococcal (acute) (chronic) (with abscess) A54.1
Barth syndrome E78.71
Bartonellosis A44.9
  cutaneous A44.1
  mucocutaneous A44.1
  specified NEC A44.8
  systemic A44.0
Barton's fracture S52.56-
Bartter's syndrome E26.81
Basal *—see* condition
Basan's (hidrotic) **ectodermal dysplasia** Q82.4
Baseball finger *—see* Dislocation, finger
Basedow's disease (exophthalmic goiter) *—see* Hyperthyroidism, with, goiter
Basic *—see* condition
Basilar *—see* condition
Bason's (hidrotic) **ectodermal dysplasia** Q82.4
Basopenia *—see* Agranulocytosis
Basophilia D72.824
Basophilism (cortico-adrenal) (Cushing's) (pituitary) E24.0
Bassen-Kornzweig disease or syndrome E78.6
Bat ear Q17.5
Bateman's
  disease B08.1
  purpura (senile) D69.2
Bathing cramp T75.1
Bathophobia F40.248
Batten (-Mayou) **disease** E75.4
  retina E75.4 *[H36]*
Batten-Steinert syndrome G71.11
Battered *—see* Maltreatment
Battey Mycobacterium infection A31.0
Battle exhaustion F43.0
Battledore placenta O43.19-
Baumgarten-Cruveilhier cirrhosis, disease or syndrome K74.69
Bauxite fibrosis (of lung) J63.1
Bayle's disease (general paresis) A52.17
Bazin's disease (primary) (tuberculous) A18.4
Beach ear *—see* Swimmer's, ear
Beaded hair (congenital) Q84.1
Béal conjunctivitis or syndrome B30.2
Beard's disease (neurasthenia) F48.8
Beat(s)
  atrial, premature I49.1
  ectopic I49.49
  elbow *—see* Bursitis, elbow
  escaped, heart I49.49
  hand *—see* Bursitis, hand
  knee *—see* Bursitis, knee
  premature I49.40
    atrial I49.1
    auricular I49.1
    supraventricular I49.1
Beau's
  disease or syndrome *—see* Degeneration, myocardial
  lines (transverse furrows on fingernails) L60.4
Bechterev's syndrome *—see* Spondylitis, ankylosing
Beck's syndrome (anterior spinal artery occlusion) I65.8
Becker's
  cardiomyopathy I42.8
  disease
    idiopathic mural endomyocardial disease I42.3
    myotonia congenita, recessive form G71.12
  dystrophy G71.0
  pigmented hairy nevus D22.5
Beckwith-Wiedemann syndrome Q87.3
Bed confinement status Z74.01
Bed sore *—see* Ulcer, pressure, by site
Bedbug bite(s) *—see* Bite(s), by site, superficial, insect
Bedclothes, asphyxiation or suffocation by *—see* Asphyxia, traumatic, due to, mechanical, trapped
Bednar's
  aphthae K12.0
  tumor *—see* Neoplasm, malignant, by site
Bedridden Z74.01
Bedsore *—see* Ulcer, pressure, by site
Bedwetting *—see* Enuresis
Bee sting (with allergic or anaphylactic shock) *—see* Toxicity, venom, arthropod, bee
Beer drinker's heart (disease) I42.6
Begbie's disease (exophthalmic goiter) *—see* Hyperthyroidism, with, goiter
Behavior
  antisocial
    adult Z72.811
    child or adolescent Z72.810
  disorder, disturbance *—see* Disorder, conduct
  disruptive *—see* Disorder, conduct
  drug seeking Z76.5
  inexplicable R46.2
  marked evasiveness R46.5
  obsessive-compulsive R46.81
  overactivity R46.3
  poor responsiveness R46.4
  self-damaging(life-style) Z72.89
  sleep-incompatible Z72.821
  slowness R46.4
  specified NEC R46.89
  strange (and inexplicable) R46.2
  suspiciousness R46.5
  type A pattern Z73.1
  undue concern or preoccupation with stressful events R46.6
  verbosity and circumstantial detail obscuring reason for contact R46.7
Behçet's disease or syndrome M35.2

- **Behr's disease** *—see* Degeneration, macula
- **Beigel's disease or morbus** (white piedra) B36.2
- **Bejel** A65
- **Bekhterev's syndrome** *—see* Spondylitis, ankylosing
- **Belching** *—see* Eructation
- **Bell's**
  - mania F30.8
  - palsy, paralysis G51.0
    - infant or newborn P11.3
  - spasm G51.3
- **Bence Jones albuminuria or proteinuria NEC** R80.3
- **Bends** T70.3
- **Benedikt's paralysis or syndrome** G46.3
- **Benign** *—see also* condition
  - prostatic hyperplasia *—see* Hyperplasia, prostate
- **Bennett's fracture** (displaced) S62.21-
- **Benson's disease** *—see* Deposit, crystalline
- **Bent**
  - back (hysterical) F44.4
  - nose M95.0
    - congenital Q67.4
- **Bereavement** (uncomplicated) Z63.4
- **Bergeron's disease** (hysterical chorea) F44.4
- **Berger's disease** *—see* Nephropathy, IgA
- **Beriberi** (dry) E51.11
  - heart (disease) E51.12
  - polyneuropathy E51.11
  - wet E51.12
    - involving circulatory system E51.11
- **Berlin's disease or edema** (traumatic) S05.8X-
- **Berlock** (berloque) **dermatitis** L56.2
- **Bernard-Horner syndrome** G90.2
- **Bernard-Soulier disease or thrombopathia** D69.1
- **Bernhardt** (-Roth) **disease** *—see* Mononeuropathy, lower limb, meralgia paresthetica
- **Bernheim's syndrome** *—see* Failure, heart, right
- **Bertielliasis** B71.8
- **Berylliosis** (lung) J63.2
- **Besnier-Boeck** (-Schaumann) **disease** *—see* Sarcoidosis
- **Besnier's**
  - lupus pernio D86.3
  - prurigo L20.0
- **Bestiality** F65.89
- **Best's disease** H35.50
- **Beta-mercaptolactate-cysteine disulfiduria** E72.09
- **Betalipoproteinemia, broad or floating** E78.2
- **Betting and gambling** Z72.6
  - pathological (compulsive) F63.0
- **Bezoar** T18.9
  - intestine T18.3
  - stomach T18.2
- **Bezold's abscess** *—see* Mastoiditis, acute
- **Bianchi's syndrome** R48.8
- **Bicornate or bicornis uterus** Q51.3
  - in pregnancy or childbirth O34.00
    - causing obstructed labor O65.5
- **Bicuspid aortic valve** Q23.1
- **Biedl-Bardet syndrome** Q87.89
- **Bielschowsky** (-Jansky) **disease** E75.4
- **Biermer's** (pernicious) **anemia or disease** D51.0
- **Biett's disease** L93.0
- **Bifid** (congenital)
  - apex, heart Q24.8
  - clitoris Q52.6
  - kidney Q63.8
  - nose Q30.2
  - patella Q74.1
  - scrotum Q55.29
  - toe NEC Q74.2
  - tongue Q38.3
  - ureter Q62.8
  - uterus Q51.3
  - uvula Q35.7
- **Biforis uterus** (suprasimplex) Q51.3
- **Bifurcation** (congenital)
  - gallbladder Q44.1
  - kidney pelvis Q63.8
  - renal pelvis Q63.8
  - rib Q76.6
  - tongue, congenital Q38.3
  - trachea Q32.1
  - ureter Q62.8
  - urethra Q64.74
  - vertebra Q76.49
- **Big spleen syndrome** D73.1
- **Bigeminal pulse** R00.8
- **Bilateral** *—see* condition
- **Bile**
  - duct *—see* condition
  - pigments in urine R82.2
- **Bilharziasis** *—see also* Schistosomiasis
  - chyluria B65.0
  - cutaneous B65.3
  - galacturia B65.0
  - hematochyluria B65.0
  - intestinal B65.1
  - lipemia B65.9
  - lipuria B65.0
  - oriental B65.2
  - piarhemia B65.9
  - pulmonary NOS B65.9 *[J99]*
    - pneumonia B65.9 *[J17]*
  - tropical hematuria B65.0
  - vesical B65.0
- **Biliary** *—see* condition
- **Bilirubin metabolism disorder** E80.7
  - specified NEC E80.6
- **Bilirubinemia, familial nonhemolytic** E80.4
- **Bilirubinuria** R82.2
- **Biliuria** R82.2
- **Bilocular stomach** K31.2
- **Binswanger's disease** I67.3
- **Biparta, bipartite**
  - carpal scaphoid Q74.0
  - patella Q74.1
  - vagina Q52.10
- **Bird**
  - face Q75.8
  - fancier's disease or lung J67.2
- **Birt-Hogg-Dube syndrome** Q87.89
- **Birth**
  - complications in mother *—see* Delivery, complicated
  - compression during NOS P15.9
  - defect *—see* Anomaly
  - immature (less than 37 completed weeks) *—see* Preterm, newborn
    - extremely (less than 28 completed weeks) *—see* Immaturity, extreme
  - inattention, at or after *—see* Maltreatment, child, neglect
  - injury NOS P15.9
    - basal ganglia P11.1
    - brachial plexus NEC P14.3
    - brain (compression) (pressure) P11.2
    - central nervous system NOS P11.9
    - cerebellum P11.1
    - cerebral hemorrhage P10.1
    - external genitalia P15.5
    - eye P15.3
    - face P15.4
    - fracture
      - bone P13.9
        - specified NEC P13.8
      - clavicle P13.4
      - femur P13.2
      - humerus P13.3
      - long bone, except femur P13.3
      - radius and ulna P13.3
      - skull P13.0
      - spine P11.5
      - tibia and fibula P13.3
    - intracranial P11.2
      - laceration or hemorrhage P10.9
        - specified NEC P10.8
    - intraventricular hemorrhage P10.2
    - laceration
      - brain P10.1
      - by scalpel P15.8
      - peripheral nerve P14.9
    - liver P15.0
    - meninges
      - brain P11.1
      - spinal cord P11.5
    - nerve
      - brachial plexus P14.3
      - cranial NEC (except facial) P11.4
      - facial P11.3
      - peripheral P14.9
      - phrenic (paralysis) P14.2
    - paralysis
      - facial nerve P11.3
      - spinal P11.5
    - penis P15.5
    - rupture
      - spinal cord P11.5
    - scalp P12.9
    - scalpel wound P15.8
    - scrotum P15.5
    - skull NEC P13.1
      - fracture P13.0
    - specified type NEC P15.8
    - spinal cord P11.5
    - spine P11.5
    - spleen P15.1
    - sternomastoid (hematoma) P15.2
    - subarachnoid hemorrhage P10.3
    - subcutaneous fat necrosis P15.6
    - subdural hemorrhage P10.0
    - tentorial tear P10.4
    - testes P15.5
    - vulva P15.5
  - lack of care, at or after *—see* Maltreatment, child, neglect
  - neglect, at or after *—see* Maltreatment, child, neglect
  - palsy or paralysis, newborn, NOS (birth injury) P14.9

Birth *(continued)*

  - premature (infant) *—see* Preterm, newborn
  - shock, newborn P96.89
  - trauma *—see* Birth, injury
  - weight
    - low (2499 grams or less) *—see* Low, birthweight
      - extremely (999 grams or less) *—see* Low, birthweight, extreme
    - 4000 grams to 4499 grams P08.1
    - 4500 grams or more P08.0
- **Birthmark** Q82.5
- **Bisalbuminemia** E88.09
- **Biskra's button** B55.1
- **Bite**(s) (animal) (human)
  - abdomen, abdominal
    - wall S31.159
      - with penetration into peritoneal cavity S31.659
      - epigastric region S31.152
        - with penetration into peritoneal cavity S31.652
      - left
        - lower quadrant S31.154
          - with penetration into peritoneal cavity S31.654
        - upper quadrant S31.151
          - with penetration into peritoneal cavity S31.651
      - periumbilic region S31.155
        - with penetration into peritoneal cavity S31.655
      - right
        - lower quadrant S31.153
          - with penetration into peritoneal cavity S31.653
        - upper quadrant S31.150
          - with penetration into peritoneal cavity S31.650
      - superficial NEC S30.871
        - insect S30.861
  - alveolar (process) *—see* Bite, oral cavity
  - amphibian (venomous) *—see* Venom, bite, amphibian
  - animal *—see also* Bite, by site
    - venomous *—see* Venom
  - ankle S91.05-
    - superficial NEC S90.57-
      - insect S90.56-
  - antecubital space *—see* Bite, elbow
  - anus S31.835
    - superficial NEC S30.877
      - insect S30.867
  - arm (upper) S41.15-
    - lower *—see* Bite, forearm
    - superficial NEC S40.87-
      - insect S40.86-
  - arthropod NEC *—see* Venom, bite, arthropod
  - auditory canal (external) (meatus) *—see* Bite, ear
  - auricle, ear *—see* Bite, ear
  - axilla *—see* Bite, arm
  - back *—see also* Bite, thorax, back
    - lower S31.050
      - with penetration into retroperitoneal space S31.051
      - superficial NEC S30.870
        - insect S30.860
  - bedbug *—see* Bite(s), by site, superficial, insect

Bite *(continued)*
- breast S21.05-
  - superficial NEC S20.17-
    - insect S20.16-
- brow *—see* Bite, head, specified site NEC
- buttock S31.805
  - left S31.825
  - right S31.815
  - superficial NEC S30.870
    - insect S30.860
- calf *—see* Bite, leg
- canaliculus lacrimalis *—see* Bite, eyelid
- canthus, eye *—see* Bite, eyelid
- centipede *—see* Toxicity, venom, arthropod, centipede
- cheek (external) S01.45-
  - superficial NEC S00.87
    - insect S00.86
  - internal *—see* Bite, oral cavity
- chest wall *—see* Bite, thorax
- chigger B88.0
- chin *—see* Bite, head, specified site NEC
- clitoris *—see* Bite, vulva
- costal region *—see* Bite, thorax
- digit(s)
  - hand *—see* Bite, finger
  - toe *—see* Bite, toe
- ear (canal) (external) S01.35-
  - superficial NEC S00.47-
    - insect S00.46-
- elbow S51.05-
  - superficial NEC S50.37-
    - insect S50.36-
- epididymis *—see* Bite, testis
- epigastric region *—see* Bite, abdomen
- epiglottis *—see* Bite, neck, specified site NEC
- esophagus, cervical S11.25
  - superficial NEC S10.17
    - insect S10.16
- eyebrow *—see* Bite, eyelid
- eyelid S01.15-
  - superficial NEC S00.27-
    - insect S00.26-
- face NEC *—see* Bite, head, specified site NEC
- finger(s) S61.259
  - with
    - damage to nail S61.359
  - index S61.258
    - with
      - damage to nail S61.358
    - left S61.251
      - with
        - damage to nail S61.351
    - right S61.250
      - with
        - damage to nail S61.350
    - superficial NEC S60.478
      - insect S60.46-
  - little S61.25-
    - with
      - damage to nail S61.35-
    - superficial NEC S60.47-
      - insect S60.46-
  - middle S61.25-
    - with
      - damage to nail S61.35-
    - superficial NEC S60.47-
      - insect S60.46-
  - ring S61.25-
    - with
      - damage to nail S61.35-
    - superficial NEC S60.47-
      - insect S60.46-
  - superficial NEC S60.479
    - insect S60.469
  - thumb *—see* Bite, thumb

Bite *(continued)*
- flank *—see* Bite, abdomen, wall
- flea *—see* Bite, by site, superficial, insect
- foot (except toe(s) alone) S91.35-
  - superficial NEC S90.87-
    - insect S90.86-
  - toe *—see* Bite, toe
- forearm S51.85-
  - elbow only *—see* Bite, elbow
  - superficial NEC S50.87-
    - insect S50.86-
- forehead *—see* Bite, head, specified site NEC
- genital organs, external
  - female S31.552
    - superficial NEC S30.876
      - insect S30.866
    - vagina and vulva *—see* Bite, vulva
  - male S31.551
    - penis *—see* Bite, penis
    - scrotum *—see* Bite, scrotum
    - superficial NEC S30.875
      - insect S30.865
    - testes *—see* Bite, testis
- groin *—see* Bite, abdomen, wall
- gum *—see* Bite, oral cavity
- hand S61.45-
  - finger *—see* Bite, finger
  - superficial NEC S60.57-
    - insect S60.56-
  - thumb *—see* Bite, thumb
- head S01.95
  - cheek *—see* Bite, cheek
  - ear *—see* Bite, ear
  - eyelid *—see* Bite, eyelid
  - lip *—see* Bite, lip
  - nose *—see* Bite, nose
  - oral cavity *—see* Bite, oral cavity
  - scalp *—see* Bite, scalp
  - specified site NEC S01.85
    - superficial NEC S00.87
      - insect S00.86
  - superficial NEC S00.97
    - insect S00.96
  - temporomandibular area *—see* Bite, cheek
- heel *—see* Bite, foot
- hip S71.05-
  - superficial NEC S70.27-
    - insect S70.26-
- hymen S31.45
- hypochondrium *—see* Bite, abdomen, wall
- hypogastric region *—see* Bite, abdomen, wall
- inguinal region *—see* Bite, abdomen, wall
- insect *—see* Bite, by site, superficial, insect
- instep *—see* Bite, foot
- interscapular region *—see* Bite, thorax, back
- jaw *—see* Bite, head, specified site NEC
- knee S81.05-
  - superficial NEC S80.27-
    - insect S80.26-
- labium (majus) (minus) *—see* Bite, vulva
- lacrimal duct *—see* Bite, eyelid
- larynx S11.015
  - superficial NEC S10.17
    - insect S10.16
- leg (lower) S81.85-
  - ankle *—see* Bite, ankle
  - foot *—see* Bite, foot
  - knee *—see* Bite, knee
  - superficial NEC S80.87-
    - insect S80.86-

Bite *(continued)*
- leg *(continued)*
  - toe *—see* Bite, toe
  - upper *—see* Bite, thigh
- lip S01.551
  - superficial NEC S00.571
    - insect S00.561
- lizard (venomous) *—see* Venom, bite, reptile
- loin *—see* Bite, abdomen, wall
- lower back *—see* Bite, back, lower
- lumbar region *—see* Bite, back, lower
- malar region *—see* Bite, head, specified site NEC
- mammary *—see* Bite, breast
- marine animals (venomous) *—see* Toxicity, venom, marine animal
- mastoid region *—see* Bite, head, specified site NEC
- mouth *—see* Bite, oral cavity
- nail
  - finger *—see* Bite, finger
  - toe *—see* Bite, toe
- nape *—see* Bite, neck, specified site NEC
- nasal (septum) (sinus) *—see* Bite, nose
- nasopharynx *—see* Bite, head, specified site NEC
- neck S11.95
  - involving
    - cervical esophagus *—see* Bite, esophagus, cervical
    - larynx *—see* Bite, larynx
    - pharynx *—see* Bite, pharynx
    - thyroid gland S11.15
    - trachea *—see* Bite, trachea
  - specified site NEC S11.85
    - superficial NEC S10.87
      - insect S10.86
  - superficial NEC S10.97
    - insect S10.96
  - throat S11.85
    - superficial NEC S10.17
      - insect S10.16
- nose (septum) (sinus) S01.25
  - superficial NEC S00.37
    - insect S00.36
- occipital region *—see* Bite, scalp
- oral cavity S01.552
  - superficial NEC S00.572
    - insect S00.562
- orbital region *—see* Bite, eyelid
- palate *—see* Bite, oral cavity
- palm *—see* Bite, hand
- parietal region *—see* Bite, scalp
- pelvis S31.050
  - with penetration into retroperitoneal space S31.051
  - superficial NEC S30.870
    - insect S30.860
- penis S31.25
  - superficial NEC S30.872
    - insect S30.862
- perineum
  - female *—see* Bite, vulva
  - male *—see* Bite, pelvis
- periocular area (with or without lacrimal passages) *—see* Bite, eyelid
- phalanges
  - finger *—see* Bite, finger
  - toe *—see* Bite, toe
- pharynx S11.25
  - superficial NEC S10.17
    - insect S10.16
- pinna *—see* Bite, ear
- poisonous *—see* Venom
- popliteal space *—see* Bite, knee
- prepuce *—see* Bite, penis

Bite *(continued)*
- pubic region *—see* Bite, abdomen, wall
- rectovaginal septum *—see* Bite, vulva
- red bug B88.0
- reptile NEC *—see also* Venom, bite, reptile
  - nonvenomous *—see* Bite, by site
  - snake *—see* Venom, bite, snake
- sacral region *—see* Bite, back, lower
- sacroiliac region *—see* Bite, back, lower
- salivary gland *—see* Bite, oral cavity
- scalp S01.05
  - superficial NEC S00.07
    - insect S00.06
- scapular region *—see* Bite, shoulder
- scrotum S31.35
  - superficial NEC S30.873
    - insect S30.863
- sea-snake (venomous) *—see* Toxicity, venom, snake, sea snake
- shin *—see* Bite, leg
- shoulder S41.05-
  - superficial NEC S40.27-
    - insect S40.26-
- snake *—see also* Venom, bite, snake
  - nonvenomous *—see* Bite, by site
- spermatic cord *—see* Bite, testis
- spider (venomous) *—see* Toxicity, venom, spider
  - nonvenomous *—see* Bite, by site, superficial, insect
- sternal region *—see* Bite, thorax, front
- submaxillary region *—see* Bite, head, specified site NEC
- submental region *—see* Bite, head, specified site NEC
- subungual
  - finger(s) *—see* Bite, finger
  - toe *—see* Bite, toe
- superficial *—see* Bite, by site, superficial
- supraclavicular fossa S11.85
- supraorbital *—see* Bite, head, specified site NEC
- temple, temporal region *—see* Bite, head, specified site NEC
- temporomandibular area *—see* Bite, cheek
- testis S31.35
  - superficial NEC S30.873
    - insect S30.863
- thigh S71.15-
  - superficial NEC S70.37-
    - insect S70.36-
- thorax, thoracic (wall) S21.95
  - back S21.25-
    - with penetration into thoracic cavity S21.45-
  - breast *—see* Bite, breast
  - front S21.15-
    - with penetration into thoracic cavity S21.35-
  - superficial NEC S20.97
    - back S20.47-
    - front S20.37-
    - insect S20.96
      - back S20.46-
      - front S20.36-
- throat *—see* Bite, neck, throat
- thumb S61.05-
  - with
    - damage to nail S61.15-
  - superficial NEC S60.37-
    - insect S60.36-
- thyroid S11.15
  - superficial NEC S10.87
    - insect S10.86

Bite *(continued)*
- toe(s) S91.15-
  - with
    - damage to nail S91.25-
  - great S91.15-
    - with
      - damage to nail S91.25-
  - lesser S91.15-
    - with
      - damage to nail S91.25-
  - superficial NEC S90.47-
    - great S90.47-
    - insect S90.46-
      - great S90.46-
- tongue S01.552
- trachea S11.025
  - superficial NEC S10.17
    - insect S10.16
- tunica vaginalis *—see* Bite, testis
- tympanum, tympanic membrane *—see* Bite, ear
- umbilical region S31.155
- uvula *—see* Bite, oral cavity
- vagina *—see* Bite, vulva
- venomous *—see* Venom
- vocal cords S11.035
  - superficial NEC S10.17
    - insect S10.16
- vulva S31.45
  - superficial NEC S30.874
    - insect S30.864
- wrist S61.55-
  - superficial NEC S60.87-
    - insect S60.86-

Biting, cheek or lip K13.1

Biventricular failure (heart) I50.82

Björck (-Thorson) **syndrome** (malignant carcinoid) E34.0

Black
- death A20.9
- eye S00.1-
- hairy tongue K14.3
- heel (foot) S90.3-
- lung (disease) J60
- palm (hand) S60.22-

Blackfan-Diamond anemia or syndrome (congenital hypoplastic anemia) D61.01

Blackhead L70.0

Blackout R55

Bladder *—see* condition

Blast (air) (hydraulic) (immersion) (underwater)
- blindness S05.8X-
- injury
  - abdomen or thorax *—see* Injury, by site
  - ear (acoustic nerve trauma) *—see* Injury, nerve, acoustic, specified type NEC
  - syndrome NEC T70.8

Blastoma *—see* Neoplasm, malignant, by site
- pulmonary *—see* Neoplasm, lung, malignant

Blastomycosis, blastomycotic B40.9
- Brazilian *—see* Paracoccidioidomycosis
- cutaneous B40.3
- disseminated B40.7
- European *—see* Cryptococcosis
- generalized B40.7
- keloidal B48.0
- North American B40.9
- primary pulmonary B40.0

Blastomycosis, blastomycotic *(continued)*
- pulmonary B40.2
  - acute B40.0
  - chronic B40.1
- skin B40.3
- South American *—see* Paracoccidioidomycosis
- specified NEC B40.89

Bleb(s) R23.8
- emphysematous (lung) (solitary) J43.9
- endophthalmitis H59.43
- filtering (vitreous), after glaucoma surgery Z98.83
- inflammed (infected), postprocedural H59.40
  - stage 1 H59.41
  - stage 2 H59.42
  - stage 3 H59.43
- lung (ruptured) J43.9
  - congenital *—see* Atelectasis
  - newborn P25.8
- subpleural (emphysematous) J43.9

Blebitis, postprocedural H59.40
- stage 1 H59.41
- stage 2 H59.42
- stage 3 H59.43

Bleeder (familial) (hereditary) *—see* Hemophilia

Bleeding *—see also* Hemorrhage
- anal K62.5
- anovulatory N97.0
- atonic, following delivery O72.1
- capillary I78.8
  - puerperal O72.2
- contact (postcoital) N93.0
- due to uterine subinvolution N85.3
- ear *—see* Otorrhagia
- excessive, associated with menopausal onset N92.4
- familial *—see* Defect, coagulation
- following intercourse N93.0
- gastrointestinal K92.2
- hemorrhoids *—see* Hemorrhoids
- intermenstrual (regular) N92.3
  - irregular N92.1
- intraoperative *—see* Complication, intraoperative, hemorrhage
- irregular N92.6
- menopausal N92.4
- newborn, intraventricular *—see* Newborn, affected by, hemorrhage, intraventricular
- nipple N64.59
- nose R04.0
- ovulation N92.3
- pre-pubertal vaginal N93.1
- postclimacteric N95.0
- postcoital N93.0
- postmenopausal N95.0
- postoperative *—see* Complication, postprocedural, hemorrhage
- preclimacteric N92.4
- puberty (excessive, with onset of menstrual periods) N92.2
- rectum, rectal K62.5
  - newborn P54.2
- tendencies *—see* Defect, coagulation
- throat R04.1
- tooth socket (post-extraction) K91.840
- umbilical stump P51.9
- uterus, uterine NEC N93.9
  - climacteric N92.4
  - dysfunctional or functional N93.8
  - menopausal N92.4
  - preclimacteric or premenopausal N92.4
  - unrelated to menstrual cycle N93.9

Bleeding *(continued)*
- vagina, vaginal (abnormal) N93.9
  - dysfunctional or functional N93.8
  - newborn P54.6
  - pre-pubertal N93.1
- vicarious N94.89

Blennorrhagia, blennorrhagic *—see* Gonorrhea

Blennorrhea (acute) (chronic) *—see also* Gonorrhea
- inclusion (neonatal) (newborn) P39.1
- lower genitourinary tract (gonococcal) A54.00
- neonatorum (gonococcal ophthalmia) A54.31

Blepharelosis *—see* Entropion

Blepharitis (angularis) (ciliaris) (eyelid) (marginal) (nonulcerative) H01.009
- herpes zoster B02.39
- left H01.006
  - lower H01.005
  - upper H01.004
- right H01.003
  - lower H01.002
  - upper H01.001
- squamous H01.029
  - left H01.026
    - lower H01.025
    - upper H01.024
  - right H01.023
    - lower H01.022
    - upper H01.021
- ulcerative H01.019
  - left H01.016
    - lower H01.015
    - upper H01.014
  - right H01.013
    - lower H01.012
    - upper H01.011

Blepharochalasis H02.30
- congenital Q10.0
- left H02.36
  - lower H02.35
  - upper H02.34
- right H02.33
  - lower H02.32
  - upper H02.31

Blepharoclonus H02.59

Blepharoconjunctivitis H10.50-
- angular H10.52-
- contact H10.53-
- ligneous H10.51-

Blepharophimosis (eyelid) H02.529
- congenital Q10.3
- left H02.526
  - lower H02.525
  - upper H02.524
- right H02.523
  - lower H02.522
  - upper H02.521

Blepharoptosis H02.40-
- congenital Q10.0
- mechanical H02.41-
- myogenic H02.42-
- neurogenic H02.43-
- paralytic H02.43-

Blepharopyorrhea, gonococcal A54.39

Blepharospasm G24.5
- drug induced G24.01

Blighted ovum O02.0

Blind *—see also* Blindness
- bronchus (congenital) Q32.4
- loop syndrome K90.2
  - congenital Q43.8
- sac, fallopian tube (congenital) Q50.6

Blind *(continued)*
- spot, enlarged *—see* Defect, visual field, localized, scotoma, blind spot area
- tract or tube, congenital NEC *—see* Atresia, by site

Blindness (acquired) (congenital) (both eyes) H54.0X-
- blast S05.8X-
- color *—see* Deficiency, color vision
- concussion S05.8X-
- cortical H47.619
  - left brain H47.612
  - right brain H47.611
- day H53.11
- due to injury (current episode) S05.9-
  - sequelae -- code to injury with seventh character S
- eclipse (total) *—see* Retinopathy, solar
- emotional (hysterical) F44.6
- face H53.16
- hysterical F44.6
- legal (both eyes) (USA definition) H54.8
- mind R48.8
- night H53.60
  - abnormal dark adaptation curve H53.61
  - acquired H53.62
  - congenital H53.63
  - specified type NEC H53.69
  - vitamin A deficiency E50.5
- one eye (other eye normal) H54.40
  - left (normal vision on right) H54.42-
    - low vision on right H54.12-
  - low vision, other eye H54.10
  - right (normal vision on left) H54.41-
    - low vision on left H54.11-
- psychic R48.8
- river B73.01
- snow *—see* Photokeratitis
- sun, solar *—see* Retinopathy, solar
- transient *—see* Disturbance, vision, subjective, loss, transient
- traumatic (current episode) S05.9-
- word (developmental) F81.0
  - acquired R48.0
  - secondary to organic lesion R48.0

Blister (nonthermal)
- abdominal wall S30.821
- alveolar process S00.522
- ankle S90.52-
- antecubital space *—see* Blister, elbow
- anus S30.827
- arm (upper) S40.82-
- auditory canal *—see* Blister, ear
- auricle *—see* Blister, ear
- axilla *—see* Blister, arm
- back, lower S30.820
- beetle dermatitis L24.89
- breast S20.12-
- brow S00.82
- calf *—see* Blister, leg
- canthus *—see* Blister, eyelid
- cheek S00.82
  - internal S00.522
- chest wall *—see* Blister, thorax
- chin S00.82
- costal region *—see* Blister, thorax
- digit(s)
  - foot *—see* Blister, toe
  - hand *—see* Blister, finger
- due to burn *—see* Burn, by site, second degree
- ear S00.42-

Blister *(continued)*
  elbow S50.32-
  epiglottis S10.12
  esophagus, cervical S10.12
  eyebrow *—see* Blister, eyelid
  eyelid S00.22-
  face S00.82
  fever B00.1
  finger(s) S60.429
    index S60.42-
    little S60.42-
    middle S60.42-
    ring S60.42-
  foot (except toe(s) alone) S90.82-
    toe *—see* Blister, toe
  forearm S50.82-
    elbow only *—see* Blister, elbow
  forehead S00.82
  fracture - omit code
  genital organ
    female S30.826
    male S30.825
  gum S00.522
  hand S60.52-
  head S00.92
    ear *—see* Blister, ear
    eyelid *—see* Blister, eyelid
    lip S00.521
    nose S00.32
    oral cavity S00.522
    scalp S00.02
    specified site NEC S00.82
  heel *—see* Blister, foot
  hip S70.22-
  interscapular region S20.429
  jaw S00.82
  knee S80.22-
  larynx S10.12
  leg (lower) S80.82-
    knee *—see* Blister, knee
    upper *—see* Blister, thigh
  lip S00.521
  malar region S00.82
  mammary *—see* Blister, breast
  mastoid region S00.82
  mouth S00.522
  multiple, skin, nontraumatic R23.8
  nail
    finger *—see* Blister, finger
    toe *—see* Blister, toe
  nasal S00.32
  neck S10.92
    specified site NEC S10.82
    throat S10.12
  nose S00.32
  occipital region S00.02
  oral cavity S00.522
  orbital region *—see* Blister, eyelid
  palate S00.522
  palm *—see* Blister, hand
  parietal region S00.02
  pelvis S30.820
  penis S30.822
  periocular area *—see* Blister, eyelid
  phalanges
    finger *—see* Blister, finger
    toe *—see* Blister, toe
  pharynx S10.12
  pinna *—see* Blister, ear
  popliteal space *—see* Blister, knee
  scalp S00.02
  scapular region *—see* Blister, shoulder
  scrotum S30.823
  shin *—see* Blister, leg
  shoulder S40.22-
  sternal region S20.329
  submaxillary region S00.82
  submental region S00.82
  subungual
    finger(s) *—see* Blister, finger
    toe(s) *—see* Blister, toe

Blister *(continued)*
  supraclavicular fossa S10.82
  supraorbital S00.82
  temple S00.82
  temporal region S00.82
  testis S30.823
  thermal *—see* Burn, second degree, by site
  thigh S70.32-
  thorax, thoracic (wall) S20.92
    back S20.42-
    front S20.32-
  throat S10.12
  thumb S60.32-
  toe(s) S90.42-
    great S90.42-
  tongue S00.522
  trachea S10.12
  tympanum, tympanic membrane *—see* Blister, ear
  upper arm *—see* Blister, arm (upper)
  uvula S00.522
  vagina S30.824
  vocal cords S10.12
  vulva S30.824
  wrist S60.82-

Bloating R14.0

Bloch-Sulzberger disease or syndrome Q82.3

Block, blocked
  alveolocapillary J84.10
  arborization (heart) I45.5
  arrhythmic I45.9
  atrioventricular (incomplete) (partial) I44.30
    with atrioventricular dissociation I44.2
    complete I44.2
      congenital Q24.6
    congenital Q24.6
    first degree I44.0
    second degree (types I and II) I44.1
    specified NEC I44.39
    third degree I44.2
    types I and II I44.1
  auriculoventricular *—see* Block, atrioventricular
  bifascicular (cardiac) I45.2
  bundle-branch (complete) (false) (incomplete) I45.4
    bilateral I45.2
    left I44.7
      with right bundle branch block I45.2
      hemiblock I44.60
        anterior I44.4
        posterior I44.5
      incomplete I44.7
        with right bundle branch block I45.2
    right I45.10
      with
        left bundle branch block I45.2
        left fascicular block I45.2
      specified NEC I45.19
    Wilson's type I45.19
  cardiac I45.9
  conduction I45.9
    complete I44.2
  fascicular (left) I44.60
    anterior I44.4
    posterior I44.5
    right I45.0
    specified NEC I44.69
  foramen Magendie (acquired) G91.1
    congenital Q03.1
      with spina bifida *—see* Spina bifida, by site, with hydrocephalus

Block, blocked *(continued)*
  heart I45.9
    bundle branch I45.4
      bilateral I45.2
    complete (atrioventricular) I44.2
    congenital Q24.6
    first degree (atrioventricular) I44.0
    second degree (atrioventricular) I44.1
    specified type NEC I45.5
    third degree (atrioventricular) I44.2
  hepatic vein I82.0
  intraventricular (nonspecific) I45.4
    bundle branch
      bilateral I45.2
  kidney N28.9
    postcystoscopic or postprocedural N99.0
  Mobitz (types I and II) I44.1
  myocardial *—see* Block, heart
  nodal I45.5
  organ or site, congenital NEC *—see* Atresia, by site
  portal (vein) I81
  second degree (types I and II) I44.1
  sinoatrial I45.5
  sinoauricular I45.5
  third degree I44.2
  trifascicular I45.3
  tubal N97.1
  vein NOS I82.90
  Wenckebach (types I and II) I44.1

Blockage *—see* Obstruction

Blocq's disease F44.4

Blood
  constituents, abnormal R78.9
  disease D75.9
  donor *—see* Donor, blood
  dyscrasia D75.9
    with
      abortion *—see* Abortion, by type, complicated by, hemorrhage
      ectopic pregnancy O08.1
      molar pregnancy O08.1
    following ectopic or molar pregnancy O08.1
    newborn P61.9
    puerperal, postpartum O72.3
  flukes NEC *—see* Schistosomiasis
  in
    feces K92.1
      occult R19.5
    urine *—see* Hematuria
  mole O02.0
  occult in feces R19.5
  pressure
    decreased, due to shock following injury T79.4
    examination only Z01.30
    fluctuating I99.8
    high *—see* Hypertension
      borderline R03.0
      incidental reading, without diagnosis of hypertension R03.0
    low *—see also* Hypotension
      incidental reading, without diagnosis of hypotension R03.1
  spitting *—see* Hemoptysis
  staining cornea *—see* Pigmentation, cornea, stromal
  transfusion
    reaction or complication *—see* Complications, transfusion
  type
    A (Rh positive) Z67.10
      Rh negative Z67.11

Blood *(continued)*
  type *(continued)*
    AB (Rh positive) Z67.30
      Rh negative Z67.31
    B (Rh positive) Z67.20
      Rh negative Z67.21
    O (Rh positive) Z67.40
      Rh negative Z67.41
    Rh (positive) Z67.90
      negative Z67.91
  vessel rupture *—see* Hemorrhage
  vomiting *—see* Hematemesis

Blood-forming organs, disease D75.9

Bloodgood's disease *—see* Mastopathy, cystic

Bloom (-Machacek) (-Torre) syndrome Q82.8

Blount's disease or osteochondrosis *—see* Osteochondrosis, juvenile, tibia

Blue
  baby Q24.9
  diaper syndrome E72.09
  dome cyst (breast) *—see* Cyst, breast
  dot cataract Q12.0
  nevus D22.9
  sclera Q13.5
    with fragility of bone and deafness Q78.0
  toe syndrome I75.02-

Blueness *—see* Cyanosis

Blues, postpartal O90.6
  baby O90.6

Blurring, visual H53.8

Blushing (abnormal) (excessive) R23.2

BMI *—see* Body, mass index

Boarder, hospital NEC Z76.4
  accompanying sick person Z76.3
  healthy infant or child Z76.2
    foundling Z76.1

Bockhart's impetigo L01.02

Bodechtel-Guttman disease (subacute sclerosing panencephalitis) A81.1

Boder-Sedgwick syndrome (ataxia-telangiectasia) G11.3

Body, bodies
  Aschoff's *—see* Myocarditis, rheumatic
  asteroid, vitreous *—see* Deposit, crystalline
  cytoid (retina) *—see* Occlusion, artery, retina
  drusen (degenerative) (macula) (retinal) *—see also* Degeneration, macula, drusen
    optic disc *—see* Drusen, optic disc
  foreign *—see* Foreign body
  loose
    joint, except knee *—see* Loose, body, joint
      knee M23.4-
    sheath, tendon *—see* Disorder, tendon, specified type NEC
  mass index (BMI)
    adult
      19.9 or less Z68.1
      20.0-20.9 Z68.20
      21.0-21.9 Z68.21
      22.0-22.9 Z68.22
      23.0-23.9 Z68.23
      24.0-24.9 Z68.24
      25.0-25.9 Z68.25
      26.0-26.9 Z68.26
      27.0-27.9 Z68.27
      28.0-28.9 Z68.28
      29.0-29.9 Z68.29

Body, bodies *(continued)*
- mass index *(continued)*
  - adult *(continued)*
    - 30.0-30.9 Z68.30
    - 31.0-31.9 Z68.31
    - 32.0-32.9 Z68.32
    - 33.0-33.9 Z68.33
    - 34.0-34.9 Z68.34
    - 35.0-35.9 Z68.35
    - 36.0-36.9 Z68.36
    - 37.0-37.9 Z68.37
    - 38.0-38.9 Z68.38
    - 39.0-39.9 Z68.39
    - 40.0-44.9 Z68.41
    - 45.0-49.9 Z68.42
    - 50.0-59.9 Z68.43
    - 60.0-69.9 Z68.44
    - 70 and over Z68.45
  - pediatric
    - 5th percentile to less than 85th percentile for age Z68.52
    - 85th percentile to less than 95th percentile for age Z68.53
    - greater than or equal to ninety-fifth percentile for age Z68.54
    - less than fifth percentile for age Z68.51
- Mooser's A75.2
- rice —*see also* Loose, body, joint
  - knee M23.4-
- rocking F98.4

Boeck's
- disease or sarcoid —*see* Sarcoidosis
- lupoid (miliary) D86.3

Boerhaave's syndrome (spontaneous esophageal rupture) K22.3

Boggy
- cervix N88.8
- uterus N85.8

Boil —*see also* Furuncle, by site
- Aleppo B55.1
- Baghdad B55.1
- Delhi B55.1
- lacrimal
  - gland —*see* Dacryoadenitis
  - passages (duct) (sac) —*see* Inflammation, lacrimal, passages, acute
- Natal B55.1
- orbit, orbital —*see* Abscess, orbit
- tropical B55.1

Bold hives —*see* Urticaria

Bombé, iris —*see* Membrane, pupillary

Bone —*see* condition

Bonnevie-Ullrich syndrome (*see also* Turner's syndrome) Q87.1

Bonnier's syndrome —*see* subcategory H81.8

Bonvale dam fever T73.3

Bony block of joint —*see* Ankylosis

BOOP (bronchiolitis obliterans organized pneumonia) J84.89

Borderline
- diabetes mellitus R73.03
- hypertension R03.0
- osteopenia M85.8-
- pelvis, with obstruction during labor O65.1
- personality F60.3

Borna disease A83.9

Bornholm disease B33.0

Boston exanthem A88.0

Botalli, ductus (patent) (persistent) Q25.0

Bothriocephalus latus infestation B70.0

Botulism (foodborne intoxication) A05.1
- infant A48.51
- non-foodborne A48.52
- wound A48.52

Bouba —*see* Yaws

Bouchard's nodes (with arthropathy) M15.2

Bouffée délirante F23

Bouillaud's disease or syndrome (rheumatic heart disease) I01.9

Bourneville's disease Q85.1

Boutonniere deformity (finger) —*see* Deformity, finger, boutonniere

Bouveret (-Hoffmann) syndrome (paroxysmal tachycardia) I47.9

Bovine heart —*see* Hypertrophy, cardiac

Bowel —*see* condition

Bowen's
- dermatosis (precancerous) —*see* Neoplasm, skin, in situ
- disease —*see* Neoplasm, skin, in situ
- epithelioma —*see* Neoplasm, skin, in situ
- type
  - epidermoid carcinoma-in-situ —*see* Neoplasm, skin, in situ
  - intraepidermal squamous cell carcinoma —*see* Neoplasm, skin, in situ

Bowing
- femur —*see also* Deformity, limb, specified type NEC, thigh
  - congenital Q68.3
- fibula —*see also* Deformity, limb, specified type NEC, lower leg
  - congenital Q68.4
- forearm —*see* Deformity, limb, specified type NEC, forearm
- leg(s), long bones, congenital Q68.5
- radius —*see* Deformity, limb, specified type NEC, forearm
- tibia —*see also* Deformity, limb, specified type NEC, lower leg
  - congenital Q68.4

Bowleg(s) (acquired) M21.16-
- congenital Q68.5
- rachitic E64.3

Boyd's dysentery A03.2

Brachial —*see* condition

Brachycardia R00.1

Brachycephaly Q75.0

Bradley's disease A08.19

Bradyarrhythmia, cardiac I49.8

Bradycardia (sinoatrial) (sinus) (vagal) R00.1
- neonatal P29.12
- reflex G90.09
- tachycardia syndrome I49.5

Bradykinesia R25.8

Bradypnea R06.89

Bradytachycardia I49.5

Brailsford's disease or osteochondrosis —*see* Osteochondrosis, juvenile, radius

Brain —*see also* condition
- death G93.82
- syndrome —*see* Syndrome, brain

Branched-chain amino-acid disorder E71.2

Branchial —*see* condition
- cartilage, congenital Q18.2

Branchiogenic remnant (in neck) Q18.0

Brandt's syndrome (acrodermatitis enteropathica) E83.2

Brash (water) R12

Bravais-jacksonian epilepsy —*see* Epilepsy, localization-related, symptomatic, with simple partial seizures

Braxton Hicks contractions —*see* False, labor

Brazilian leishmaniasis B55.2

BRBPR K62.5

Break, retina (without detachment) H33.30-
- with retinal detachment —*see* Detachment, retina
- horseshoe tear H33.31-
- multiple H33.33-
- round hole H33.32-

Breakdown
- device, graft or implant —*see also* Complications, by site and type, mechanical T85.618
  - arterial graft NEC —*see* Complication, cardiovascular device, mechanical, vascular
  - breast (implant) T85.41
  - catheter NEC T85.618
    - cystostomy T83.010
    - dialysis (renal) T82.41
      - intraperitoneal T85.611
    - Hopkins T83.018
    - ileostomy T83.018
    - infusion NEC T82.514
      - cranial T85.610
      - epidural T85.610
      - intrathecal T85.610
      - spinal T85.610
      - subarachnoid T85.610
      - subdural T85.610
    - nephrostomy T83.012
    - urethral indwelling T83.011
    - urinary NEC T83.018
    - urostomy T83.018
  - electronic (electrode) (pulse generator) (stimulator)
    - bone T84.310
    - cardiac T82.119
      - electrode T82.110
      - pulse generator T82.111
      - specified type NEC T82.118
    - nervous system —*see* Complication, prosthetic device, mechanical, electronic nervous system stimulator
    - urinary —*see* Complication, genitourinary, device, urinary, mechanical
  - fixation, internal (orthopedic) NEC —*see* Complication, fixation device, mechanical
  - gastrointestinal —*see* Complications, prosthetic device, mechanical, gastrointestinal device
  - genital NEC T83.418
    - intrauterine contraceptive device T83.31
    - penile prosthesis (cylinder) (implanted) (pump) (resevoir) T83.410
    - testicular prosthesis T83.411
  - heart NEC —*see* Complication, cardiovascular device, mechanical

Breakdown *(continued)*
- device, graft or implant *(continued)*
  - intrathecal infusion pump T85.615
  - joint prosthesis —*see* Complications..., joint prosthesis,internal, mechanical, by site
  - nervous system, specified device NEC T85.615
  - ocular NEC —*see* Complications, prosthetic device, mechanical, ocular device
  - orthopedic NEC —*see* Complication, orthopedic, device, mechanical
  - specified NEC T85.618
  - subcutaneous device pocket
    - nervous system prosthetic device, implant, or graft T85.890
    - other internal prosthetic device, implant or graft T85.898
  - sutures, permanent T85.612
    - used in bone repair —*see* Complications, fixation device, internal (orthopedic), mechanical
  - urinary NEC T83.118
    - graft T83.21
    - sphincter, implanted T83.111
    - stent (ileal conduit) (nephroureteral) T83.113
      - ureteral indwelling T83.112
  - vascular NEC —*see* Complication, cardiovascular device, mechanical
  - ventricular intracranial shunt T85.01
- nervous F48.8
- perineum O90.1
- respirator J95.850
  - specified NEC J95.859
- ventilator J95.850
  - specified NEC J95.859

Breast —*see also* condition
- buds E30.1
  - in newborn P96.89
- dense R92.2
- nodule (*see also* Lump, breast) N63.0

Breath
- foul R19.6
- holder, child R06.89
- holding spell R06.89
- shortness R06.02

Breathing
- labored —*see* Hyperventilation
- mouth R06.5
  - causing malocclusion M26.5
- periodic R06.3
  - high altitude G47.32

Breathlessness R06.81

Breda's disease —*see* Yaws

Breech presentation (mother) O32.1
- causing obstructed labor O64.1
- footling O32.8
  - causing obstructed labor O64.8
- incomplete O32.8
  - causing obstructed labor O64.8

Breisky's disease N90.4

Brennemann's syndrome I88.0

Brenner
- tumor (benign) D27.9
  - borderline malignancy D39.1-
  - malignant C56
  - proliferating D39.1-

Bretonneau's disease or angina A36.0

Breus' mole O02.0

Brevicollis Q76.49

Brickmakers' anemia B76.9 *[D63.8]*

Bridge, myocardial Q24.5

Bright red blood per rectum (BRBPR) K62.5

Bright's disease *—see also* Nephritis
- arteriosclerotic *—see* Hypertension, kidney

Brill (-Zinsser) disease (recrudescent typhus) A75.1
- flea-borne A75.2
- louse-borne A75.1

Brill-Symmers' disease C82.90

Brion-Kayser disease *—see* Fever, parathyroid

Briquet's disorder or syndrome F45.0

Brissaud's
- infantilism or dwarfism E23.0
- motor-verbal tic F95.2

Brittle
- bones disease Q78.0
- nails L60.3
  - congenital Q84.6

Broad *—see also* condition
- beta disease E78.2
- ligament laceration syndrome N83.8

Broad- or floating-betalipoproteinemia E78.2

Brock's syndrome (atelectasis due to enlarged lymph nodes) J98.19

Brocq-Duhring disease (dermatitis herpetiformis) L13.0

Brodie's abscess or disease M86.8X-

Broken
- arches *—see also* Deformity, limb, flat foot
- arm (meaning upper limb) *—see* Fracture, arm
- back *—see* Fracture, vertebra
- bone *—see* Fracture
- implant or internal device *—see* Complications, by site and type, mechanical
- leg (meaning lower limb) *—see* Fracture, leg
- nose S02.2
- tooth, teeth *—see* Fracture, tooth

Bromhidrosis, bromidrosis L75.0

Bromidism, bromism G92
- due to
  - correct substance properly administered *—see* Table of Drugs and Chemicals, by drug, adverse effect
  - overdose or wrong substance given or taken *—see* Table of Drugs and Chemicals, by drug, poisoning
- chronic (dependence) F13.20

Bromidrosiphobia F40.298

Bronchi, bronchial *—see* condition

Bronchiectasis (cylindrical) (diffuse) (fusiform) (localized) (saccular) J47.9
- with
  - acute
    - bronchitis J47.0
    - lower respiratory infection J47.0
  - exacerbation (acute) J47.1
- congenital Q33.4
- tuberculous NEC *—see* Tuberculosis, pulmonary

Bronchiolectasis *—see* Bronchiectasis

Bronchiolitis (acute) (infective) (subacute) J21.9
- with
  - bronchospasm or obstruction J21.9
  - influenza, flu or grippe *—see* Influenza, with, respiratory manifestations NEC
- chemical (chronic) J68.4
  - acute J68.0
- chronic (fibrosing) (obliterative) J44.9
- due to
  - external agent *—see* Bronchitis, acute, due to
  - human metapneumovirus J21.1
  - respiratory syncytial virus J21.0
  - specified organism NEC J21.8
- fibrosa obliterans J44.9
- influenzal *—see* Influenza, with, respiratory manifestations NEC
- obliterans J42
  - with organizing pneumonia (BOOP) J84.89
- obliterative (chronic) (subacute) J44.9
  - due to fumes or vapors J68.4
  - due to chemicals, gases, fumes or vapors (inhalation) J68.4
- respiratory, interstitial lung disease J84.115

Bronchitis (diffuse) (fibrinous) (hypostatic) (infective) (membranous) J40
- with
  - influenza, flu or grippe *—see* Influenza, with, respiratory manifestations NEC
  - obstruction (airway) (lung) J44.9
  - tracheitis (15 years of age and above) J40
    - acute or subacute J20.9
    - chronic J42
    - under 15 years of age J20.9
- acute or subacute (with bronchospasm or obstruction) J20.9
  - with
    - bronchiectasis J47.0
    - chronic obstructive pulmonary disease J44.0
  - chemical (due to gases, fumes or vapors) J68.0
  - due to
    - fumes or vapors J68.0
    - Haemophilus influenzae J20.1
    - Mycoplasma pneumoniae J20.0
    - radiation J70.0
    - specified organism NEC J20.8
    - Streptococcus J20.2
    - virus
      - coxsackie J20.3
      - echovirus J20.7
      - parainfluenzae J20.4
      - respiratory syncytial J20.5
      - rhinovirus J20.6
  - viral NEC J20.8
- allergic (acute) J45.909
  - with
    - exacerbation (acute) J45.901
    - status asthmaticus J45.902
- arachidic T17.528
- aspiration (due to fumes or vapors) J68.0
- asthmatic J45.9
  - chronic J44.9
    - with
      - acute lower respiratory infection J44.0
      - exacerbation (acute) J44.1

Bronchitis *(continued)*
- capillary *—see* Pneumonia, broncho
- caseous (tuberculous) A15.5
- Castellani's A69.8
- catarrhal (15 years of age and above) J40
  - acute *—see* Bronchitis, acute
  - chronic J41.0
  - under 15 years of age J20.9
- chemical (acute) (subacute) J68.0
  - chronic J68.4
  - due to fumes or vapors J68.0
    - chronic J68.4
- chronic J42
  - with
    - airways obstruction J44.9
    - tracheitis (chronic) J42
  - asthmatic (obstructive) J44.9
  - catarrhal J41.0
  - chemical (due to fumes or vapors) J68.4
  - due to
    - chemicals, gases, fumes or vapors (inhalation) J68.4
    - radiation J70.1
    - tobacco smoking J41.0
  - emphysematous J44.9
  - mucopurulent J41.1
  - non-obstructive J41.0
  - obliterans J44.9
  - obstructive J44.9
  - purulent J41.1
  - simple J41.0
- croupous *—see* Bronchitis, acute
- due to gases, fumes or vapors (chemical) J68.0
- emphysematous (obstructive) J44.9
- exudative *—see* Bronchitis, acute
- fetid J41.1
- grippal *—see* Influenza, with, respiratory manifestations NEC
- in those under 15 years age *—see* Bronchitis, acute
  - chronic *—see* Bronchitis, chronic
- influenzal *—see* Influenza, with, respiratory manifestations NEC
- mixed simple and mucopurulent J41.8
- moulder's J62.8
- mucopurulent (chronic) (recurrent) J41.1
  - acute or subacute J20.9
  - simple (mixed) J41.8
- obliterans (chronic) J44.9
- obstructive (chronic) (diffuse) J44.9
- pituitous J41.1
- pneumococcal, acute or subacute J20.2
- pseudomembranous, acute or subacute *—see* Bronchitis, acute
- purulent (chronic) (recurrent) J41.1
  - acute or subacute *—see* Bronchitis, acute
- putrid J41.1
- senile (chronic) J42
- simple and mucopurulent (mixed) J41.8
- smokers' J41.0
- spirochetal NEC A69.8
- subacute *—see* Bronchitis, acute
- suppurative (chronic) J41.1
  - acute or subacute *—see* Bronchitis, acute
- tuberculous A15.5
- under 15 years of age *—see* Bronchitis, acute
  - chronic *—see* Bronchitis, chronic
- viral NEC, acute or subacute *—see also* Bronchitis, acute J20.8

Bronchoalveolitis J18.0

Bronchoaspergillosis B44.1

Bronchocele meaning goiter E04.0

Broncholithiasis J98.09
- tuberculous NEC A15.5

Bronchomalacia J98.09
- congenital Q32.2

Bronchomycosis NOS B49 *[J99]*
- candidal B37.1

Bronchopleuropneumonia *—see* Pneumonia, broncho

Bronchopneumonia *—see* Pneumonia, broncho

Bronchopneumonitis *—see* Pneumonia, broncho

Bronchopulmonary *—see* condition

Bronchopulmonitis *—see* Pneumonia, broncho

Bronchorrhagia (*see* Hemoptysis)

Bronchorrhea J98.09
- acute J20.9
- chronic (infective) (purulent) J42

Bronchospasm (acute) J98.01
- with
  - bronchiolitis, acute J21.9
  - bronchitis, acute (conditions in J20) *—see* Bronchitis, acute
- due to external agent *—see* condition, respiratory, acute, due to
- exercise induced J45.990

Bronchospirochetosis A69.8
- Castellani A69.8

Bronchostenosis J98.09

Bronchus *—see* condition

Brontophobia F40.220

Bronze baby syndrome P83.88

Brooke's tumor *—see* Neoplasm, skin, benign

Brown enamel of teeth (hereditary) K00.5

Brown's sheath syndrome H50.61-

Brown-Séquard disease, paralysis or syndrome G83.81

Bruce sepsis A23.0

Brucellosis (infection) A23.9
- abortus A23.1
- canis A23.3
- dermatitis A23.9
- melitensis A23.0
- mixed A23.8
- sepsis A23.9
  - melitensis A23.0
  - specified NEC A23.8
- suis A23.2

Bruck-de Lange disease Q87.1

Bruck's disease *—see* Deformity, limb

BRUE (brief resolved unexplained event) R68.13

Brugsch's syndrome Q82.8

Bruise (skin surface intact) *—see also* Contusion
- with
  - open wound *—see* Wound, open
- internal organ *—see* Injury, by site
- newborn P54.5
- scalp, due to birth injury, newborn P12.3
- umbilical cord O69.5

Bruit (arterial) R09.89
- cardiac R01.1

Brush burn *—see* Abrasion, by site

Bruton's X-linked agammaglobulinemia D80.0

Bruxism
- psychogenic F45.8
- sleep related G47.63

Bubbly lung syndrome P27.0

Bubo I88.8
- blennorrhagic (gonococcal) A54.89
- chancroidal A57
- climatic A55
- due to Haemophilus ducreyi A57
- gonococcal A54.89
- indolent (nonspecific) I88.8
- inguinal (nonspecific) I88.8
  - chancroidal A57
  - climatic A55
  - due to H. ducreyi A57
  - infective I88.8
- scrofulous (tuberculous) A18.2
- soft chancre A57
- suppurating —*see* Lymphadenitis, acute
- syphilitic (primary) A51.0
  - congenital A50.07
- tropical A55
- virulent (chancroidal) A57

Bubonic plague A20.0

Bubonocele —*see* Hernia, inguinal

Buccal —*see* condition

Buchanan's disease or osteochondrosis M91.0

Buchem's syndrome (hyperostosis corticalis) M85.2

Bucket-handle fracture or tear (semilunar cartilage) —*see* Tear, meniscus

Budd-Chiari syndrome (hepatic vein thrombosis) I82.0

Budgerigar fancier's disease or lung J67.2

Buds
- breast E30.1
  - in newborn P96.89

Buerger's disease (thromboangiitis obliterans) I73.1

Bulbar —*see* condition

Bulbus cordis (left ventricle) (persistent) Q21.8

Bulimia (nervosa) F50.2
- atypical F50.9
- normal weight F50.9

Bulky
- stools R19.5
- uterus N85.2

Bulla (e) R23.8
- lung (emphysematous) (solitary) J43.9
  - newborn P25.8

Bullet wound —*see also* Wound, open
- fracture - code as Fracture, by site
- internal organ —*see* Injury, by site

Bundle
- branch block (complete) (false) (incomplete) —*see* Block, bundle-branch
- of His —*see* condition

Bunion M21.61-
- tailor's M21.62-

Bunionette M21.62-

Buphthalmia, buphthalmos (congenital) Q15.0

Burdwan fever B55.0

Bürger-Grütz disease or syndrome E78.3

Buried
- penis (congenital) Q55.64
  - acquired N48.83
- roots K08.3

Burke's syndrome K86.89

Burkitt
- cell leukemia C91.0-
- lymphoma (malignant) C83.7-
  - small noncleaved, diffuse C83.7-
  - spleen C83.77
  - undifferentiated C83.7-
- tumor C83.7-
- type
  - acute lymphoblastic leukemia C91.0-
  - undifferentiated C83.7-

Burn (electricity) (flame) (hot gas, liquid or hot object) (radiation) (steam) (thermal) T30.0
- abdomen, abdominal (muscle) (wall) T21.02
  - first degree T21.12
  - second degree T21.22
  - third degree T21.32
- above elbow T22.039
  - first degree T22.139
  - left T22.032
    - first degree T22.132
    - second degree T22.232
    - third degree T22.332
  - right T22.031
    - first degree T22.131
    - second degree T22.231
    - third degree T22.331
  - second degree T22.239
  - third degree T22.339
- acid (caustic) (external) (internal) —*see* Corrosion, by site
- alimentary tract NEC T28.2
  - esophagus T28.1
  - mouth T28.0
  - pharynx T28.0
- alkaline (caustic) (external) (internal) —*see* Corrosion, by site
- ankle T25.019
  - first degree T25.119
  - left T25.012
    - first degree T25.112
    - second degree T25.212
    - third degree T25.312
  - multiple with foot —*see* Burn, lower, limb, multiple, ankle and foot
  - right T25.011
    - first degree T25.111
    - second degree T25.211
    - third degree T25.311
  - second degree T25.219
  - third degree T25.319
- anus —*see* Burn, buttock
- arm (lower) (upper) —*see* Burn, upper, limb
- axilla T22.049
  - first degree T22.149
  - left T22.042
    - first degree T22.142
    - second degree T22.242
    - third degree T22.342
  - right T22.041
    - first degree T22.141
    - second degree T22.241
    - third degree T22.341
  - second degree T22.249
  - third degree T22.349
- back (lower) T21.04
  - first degree T21.14
  - second degree T21.24
  - third degree T21.34
  - upper T21.03
    - first degree T21.13
    - second degree T21.23
    - third degree T21.33
- blisters - code as Burn, second degree, by site

Burn *(continued)*
- breast(s) —*see* Burn, chest wall
- buttock(s) T21.05
  - first degree T21.15
  - second degree T21.25
  - third degree T21.35
- calf T24.039
  - first degree T24.139
  - left T24.032
    - first degree T24.132
    - second degree T24.232
    - third degree T24.332
  - right T24.031
    - first degree T24.131
    - second degree T24.231
    - third degree T24.331
  - second degree T24.239
  - third degree T24.339
- canthus (eye) —*see* Burn, eyelid
- caustic acid or alkaline —*see* Corrosion, by site
- cervix T28.3
- cheek T20.06
  - first degree T20.16
  - second degree T20.26
  - third degree T20.36
- chemical (acids) (alkalines) (caustics) (external) (internal) —*see* Corrosion, by site
- chest wall T21.01
  - first degree T21.11
  - second degree T21.21
  - third degree T21.31
- chin T20.03
  - first degree T20.13
  - second degree T20.23
  - third degree T20.33
- colon T28.2
- conjunctiva (and cornea) —*see* Burn, cornea
- cornea (and conjunctiva) T26.1-
  - chemical —*see* Corrosion, cornea
- corrosion (external) (internal) —*see* Corrosion, by site
- deep necrosis of underlying tissue - code as Burn, third degree, by site
- dorsum of hand T23.069
  - first degree T23.169
  - left T23.062
    - first degree T23.162
    - second degree T23.262
    - third degree T23.362
  - right T23.061
    - first degree T23.161
    - second degree T23.261
    - third degree T23.361
  - second degree T23.269
  - third degree T23.369
- due to ingested chemical agent —*see* Corrosion, by site
- ear (auricle) (external) (canal) T20.01
  - first degree T20.11
  - second degree T20.21
  - third degree T20.31
- elbow T22.029
  - first degree T22.129
  - left T22.022
    - first degree T22.122
    - second degree T22.222
    - third degree T22.322
  - right T22.021
    - first degree T22.121
    - second degree T22.221
    - third degree T22.321
  - second degree T22.229
  - third degree T22.329
- epidermal loss - code as Burn, second degree, by site

Burn *(continued)*
- erythema, erythematous - code as Burn, first degree, by site
- esophagus T28.1
- extent (percentage of body surface)
  - less than 10 percent T31.0
  - 10-19 percent T31.10
    - with 0-9 percent third degree burns T31.10
    - with 10-19 percent third degree burns T31.11
  - 20-29 percent T31.20
    - with 0-9 percent third degree burns T31.20
    - with 10-19 percent third degree burns T31.21
    - with 20-29 percent third degree burns T31.22
  - 30-39 percent T31.30
    - with 0-9 percent third degree burns T31.30
    - with 10-19 percent third degree burns T31.31
    - with 20-29 percent third degree burns T31.32
    - with 30-39 percent third degree burns T31.33
  - 40-49 percent T31.40
    - with 0-9 percent third degree burns T31.40
    - with 10-19 percent third degree burns T31.41
    - with 20-29 percent third degree burns T31.42
    - with 30-39 percent third degree burns T31.43
    - with 40-49 percent third degree burns T31.44
  - 50-59 percent T31.50
    - with 0-9 percent third degree burns T31.50
    - with 10-19 percent third degree burns T31.51
    - with 20-29 percent third degree burns T31.52
    - with 30-39 percent third degree burns T31.53
    - with 40-49 percent third degree burns T31.54
    - with 50-59 percent third degree burns T31.55
  - 60-69 percent T31.60
    - with 0-9 percent third degree burns T31.60
    - with 10-19 percent third degree burns T31.61
    - with 20-29 percent third degree burns T31.62
    - with 30-39 percent third degree burns T31.63
    - with 40-49 percent third degree burns T31.64
    - with 50-59 percent third degree burns T31.65
    - with 60-69 percent third degree burns T31.66
  - 70-79 percent T31.70
    - with 0-9 percent third degree burns T31.70
    - with 10-19 percent third degree burns T31.71
    - with 20-29 percent third degree burns T31.72
    - with 30-39 percent third degree burns T31.73
    - with 40-49 percent third degree burns T31.74
    - with 50-59 percent third degree burns T31.75
    - with 60-69 percent third degree burns T31.76

Burn *(continued)*
- extent *(continued)*
  - 70-79 percent T31.70 *(continued)*
    - with 70-79 percent third degree burns T31.77
  - 80-89 percent T31.80
    - with 0-9 percent third degree burns T31.80
    - with 10-19 percent third degree burns T31.81
    - with 20-29 percent third degree burns T31.82
    - with 30-39 percent third degree burns T31.83
    - with 40-49 percent third degree burns T31.84
    - with 50-59 percent third degree burns T31.85
    - with 60-69 percent third degree burns T31.86
    - with 70-79 percent third degree burns T31.87
    - with 80-89 percent third degree burns T31.88
  - 90 percent or more T31.90
    - with 0-9 percent third degree burns T31.90
    - with 10-19 percent third degree burns T31.91
    - with 20-29 percent third degree burns T31.92
    - with 30-39 percent third degree burns T31.93
    - with 40-49 percent third degree burns T31.94
    - with 50-59 percent third degree burns T31.95
    - with 60-69 percent third degree burns T31.96
    - with 70-79 percent third degree burns T31.97
    - with 80-89 percent third degree burns T31.98
    - with 90 percent or more third degree burns T31.99
- extremity *—see* Burn, limb
- eye(s) and adnexa T26.4-
  - with resulting rupture and destruction of eyeball T26.2-
  - conjunctival sac *—see* Burn, cornea
  - cornea *—see* Burn, cornea
  - lid *—see* Burn, eyelid
  - periocular area *—see* Burn, eyelid
  - specified site NEC T26.3-
- eyeball *—see* Burn, eye
- eyelid(s) T26.0-
  - chemical *—see* Corrosion, eyelid
- face *—see* Burn, head
- finger T23.029
  - first degree T23.129
  - left T23.022
    - first degree T23.122
    - second degree T23.222
    - third degree T23.322
  - multiple sites (without thumb) T23.039
    - with thumb T23.049
      - first degree T23.149
      - left T23.042
        - first degree T23.142
        - second degree T23.242
        - third degree T23.342
      - right T23.041
        - first degree T23.141
        - second degree T23.241
        - third degree T23.341
      - second degree T23.249
      - third degree T23.349
    - first degree T23.139

Burn *(continued)*
- finger *(continued)*
  - multiple sites *(continued)*
    - left T23.032
      - first degree T23.132
      - second degree T23.232
      - third degree T23.332
    - right T23.031
      - first degree T23.131
      - second degree T23.231
      - third degree T23.331
    - second degree T23.239
    - third degree T23.339
  - right T23.021
    - first degree T23.121
    - second degree T23.221
    - third degree T23.321
  - second degree T23.229
  - third degree T23.329
- flank *—see* Burn, abdominal wall
- foot T25.029
  - first degree T25.129
  - left T25.022
    - first degree T25.122
    - second degree T25.222
    - third degree T25.322
    - multiple with ankle *—see* Burn, lower, limb, multiple, ankle and foot
  - right T25.021
    - first degree T25.121
    - second degree T25.221
    - third degree T25.321
  - second degree T25.229
  - third degree T25.329
- forearm T22.019
  - first degree T22.119
  - left T22.012
    - first degree T22.112
    - second degree T22.212
    - third degree T22.312
  - right T22.011
    - first degree T22.111
    - second degree T22.211
    - third degree T22.311
  - second degree T22.219
  - third degree T22.319
- forehead T20.06
  - first degree T20.16
  - second degree T20.26
  - third degree T20.36
- fourth degree - code as Burn, third degree, by site
- friction *—see* Burn, by site
- from swallowing caustic or corrosive substance NEC *—see* Corrosion, by site
- full thickness skin loss - code as Burn, third degree, by site
- gastrointestinal tract NEC T28.2
  - from swallowing caustic or corrosive substance T28.7
- genital organs
  - external
    - female T21.07
      - first degree T21.17
      - second degree T21.27
      - third degree T21.37
    - male T21.06
      - first degree T21.16
      - second degree T21.26
      - third degree T21.36
  - internal T28.3
    - from caustic or corrosive substance T28.8
- groin *—see* Burn, abdominal wall
- hand(s) T23.009
  - back *—see* Burn, dorsum of hand
  - finger *—see* Burn, finger
  - first degree T23.109
  - left T23.002

Burn *(continued)*
- hand *(continued)*
  - left *(continued)*
    - first degree T23.102
    - second degree T23.202
    - third degree T23.302
  - multiple sites with wrist T23.099
    - first degree T23.199
    - left T23.092
      - first degree T23.192
      - second degree T23.292
      - third degree T23.392
    - right T23.091
      - first degree T23.191
      - second degree T23.291
      - third degree T23.391
    - second degree T23.299
    - third degree T23.399
  - palm *—see* Burn, palm
  - right T23.001
    - first degree T23.101
    - second degree T23.201
    - third degree T23.301
  - second degree T23.209
  - third degree T23.309
  - thumb *—see* Burn, thumb
- head (and face) (and neck) T20.00
  - cheek *—see* Burn, cheek
  - chin *—see* Burn, chin
  - ear *—see* Burn, ear
  - eye(s) only *—see* Burn, eye
  - first degree T20.10
  - forehead *—see* Burn, forehead
  - lip *—see* Burn, lip
  - multiple sites T20.09
    - first degree T20.19
    - second degree T20.29
    - third degree T20.39
  - neck *—see* Burn, neck
  - nose *—see* Burn, nose
  - scalp *—see* Burn, scalp
  - second degree T20.20
  - third degree T20.30
- hip(s) *—see* Burn, thigh
- inhalation *—see* Burn, respiratory tract
  - caustic or corrosive substance (fumes) *—see* Corrosion, respiratory tract
- internal organ(s) T28.40
  - alimentary tract T28.2
    - esophagus T28.1
  - eardrum T28.41
  - esophagus T28.1
  - from caustic or corrosive substance (swallowing) NEC *— see* Corrosion, by site
  - genitourinary T28.3
  - mouth T28.0
  - pharynx T28.0
  - respiratory tract *—see* Burn, respiratory tract
  - specified organ NEC T28.49
- interscapular region *—see* Burn, back, upper
- intestine (large) (small) T28.2
- knee T24.029
  - first degree T24.129
  - left T24.022
    - first degree T24.122
    - second degree T24.222
    - third degree T24.322
  - right T24.021
    - first degree T24.121
    - second degree T24.221
    - third degree T24.321
  - second degree T24.229
  - third degree T24.329
- labium (majus) (minus) *—see* Burn, genital organs, external, female
- lacrimal apparatus, duct, gland or sac *—see* Burn, eye, specified site NEC

Burn *(continued)*
- larynx T27.0
  - with lung T27.1
- leg(s) (lower) (upper) *—see* Burn, lower, limb
- lightning *—see* Burn, by site
- limb(s)
  - lower (except ankle or foot alone) *—see* Burn, lower, limb
  - upper *—see* Burn, upper limb
- lip(s) T20.02
  - first degree T20.12
  - second degree T20.22
  - third degree T20.32
- lower
  - back *—see* Burn, back
  - limb T24.009
    - ankle *—see* Burn, ankle
    - calf *—see* Burn, calf
    - first degree T24.109
    - foot *—see* Burn, foot
    - hip *—see* Burn, thigh
    - knee *—see* Burn, knee
    - left T24.002
      - first degree T24.102
      - second degree T24.202
      - third degree T24.302
    - multiple sites, except ankle and foot T24.099
      - ankle and foot T25.099
        - first degree T25.199
        - left T25.092
          - first degree T25.192
          - second degree T25.292
          - third degree T25.392
        - right T25.091
          - first degree T25.191
          - second degree T25.291
          - third degree T25.391
        - second degree T25.299
        - third degree T25.399
      - first degree T24.199
      - left T24.092
        - first degree T24.192
        - second degree T24.292
        - third degree T24.392
      - right T24.091
        - first degree T24.191
        - second degree T24.291
        - third degree T24.391
      - second degree T24.299
      - third degree T24.399
    - right T24.001
      - first degree T24.101
      - second degree T24.201
      - third degree T24.301
    - second degree T24.209
    - thigh *—see* Burn, thigh
    - third degree T24.309
    - toe *—see* Burn, toe
- lung (with larynx and trachea) T27.1
- mouth T28.0
- neck T20.07
  - first degree T20.17
  - second degree T20.27
  - third degree T20.37
- nose (septum) T20.04
  - first degree T20.14
  - second degree T20.24
  - third degree T20.34
- ocular adnexa *—see* Burn, eye
- orbit region *—see* Burn, eyelid
- palm T23.059
  - first degree T23.159
  - left T23.052
    - first degree T23.152
    - second degree T23.252
    - third degree T23.352
  - right T23.051
    - first degree T23.151

Burn *(continued)*
palm *(continued)*
right *(continued)*
second degree T23.251
third degree T23.351
second degree T23.259
third degree T23.359
partial thickness - code as Burn, unspecified degree, by site
pelvis —*see* Burn, trunk
penis —*see* Burn, genital organs, external, male
perineum
female —*see* Burn, genital organs, external, female
male —*see* Burn, genital organs, external, male
periocular area —*see* Burn, eyelid
pharynx T28.0
rectum T28.2
respiratory tract T27.3
larynx —*see* Burn, larynx
specified part NEC T27.2
trachea —*see* Burn, trachea
sac, lacrimal —*see* Burn, eye, specified site NEC
scalp T20.05
first degree T20.15
second degree T20.25
third degree T20.35
scapular region T22.069
first degree T22.169
left T22.062
first degree T22.162
second degree T22.262
third degree T22.362
right T22.061
first degree T22.161
second degree T22.261
third degree T22.361
second degree T22.269
third degree T22.369
sclera —*see* Burn, eye, specified site NEC
scrotum —*see* Burn, genital organs, external, male
shoulder T22.059
first degree T22.159
left T22.052
first degree T22.152
second degree T22.252
third degree T22.352
right T22.051
first degree T22.151
second degree T22.251
third degree T22.351
second degree T22.259
third degree T22.359
stomach T28.2
temple —*see* Burn, head
testis —*see* Burn, genital organs, external, male
thigh T24.019
first degree T24.119
left T24.012
first degree T24.112
second degree T24.212
third degree T24.312
right T24.011
first degree T24.111
second degree T24.211
third degree T24.311
second degree T24.219
third degree T24.319
thorax (external) —*see* Burn, trunk
throat (meaning pharynx) T28.0
thumb(s) T23.019
first degree T23.119
left T23.012
first degree T23.112
second degree T23.212

Burn *(continued)*
thumb *(continued)*
left *(continued)*
third degree T23.312
multiple sites with fingers T23.049
first degree T23.149
left T23.042
first degree T23.142
second degree T23.242
third degree T23.342
right T23.041
first degree T23.141
second degree T23.241
third degree T23.341
second degree T23.249
third degree T23.349
right T23.011
first degree T23.111
second degree T23.211
third degree T23.311
second degree T23.219
third degree T23.319
toe T25.039
first degree T25.139
left T25.032
first degree T25.132
second degree T25.232
third degree T25.332
right T25.031
first degree T25.131
second degree T25.231
third degree T25.331
second degree T25.239
third degree T25.339
tongue T28.0
tonsil(s) T28.0
trachea T27.0
with lung T27.1
trunk T21.00
abdominal wall —*see* Burn, abdominal wall
anus —*see* Burn, buttock
axilla —*see* Burn, upper limb
back —*see* Burn, back
breast —*see* Burn, chest wall
buttock —*see* Burn, buttock
chest wall —*see* Burn, chest wall
first degree T21.10
flank —*see* Burn, abdominal wall
genital
female —*see* Burn, genital organs, external, female
male —*see* Burn, genital organs, external, male
groin —*see* Burn, abdominal wall
interscapular region —*see* Burn, back, upper
labia —*see* Burn, genital organs, external, female
lower back —*see* Burn, back
penis —*see* Burn, genital organs, external, male
perineum
female —*see* Burn, genital organs, external, female
male —*see* Burn, genital organs, external, male
scapula region —*see* Burn, scapular region
scrotum —*see* Burn, genital organs, external, male
second degree T21.20
specified site NEC T21.09
first degree T21.19
second degree T21.29
third degree T21.39
testes —*see* Burn, genital organs, external, male
third degree T21.30
upper back —*see* Burn, back, upper

Burn *(continued)*
trunk *(continued)*
vulva —*see* Burn, genital organs, external, female
unspecified site with extent of body surface involved specified
less than 10 percent T31.0
10-19 percent (0-9 percent third degree) T31.10
with 10-19 percent third degree T31.11
20-29 percent (0-9 percent third degree) T31.20
with
10-19 percent third degree T31.21
20-29 percent third degree T31.22
30-39 percent (0-9 percent third degree) T31.30
with
10-19 percent third degree T31.31
20-29 percent third degree T31.32
30-39 percent third degree T31.33
40-49 percent (0-9 percent third degree) T31.40
with
10-19 percent third degree T31.41
20-29 percent third degree T31.42
30-39 percent third degree T31.43
40-49 percent third degree T31.44
50-59 percent (0-9 percent third degree) T31.50
with
10-19 percent third degree T31.51
20-29 percent third degree T31.52
30-39 percent third degree T31.53
40-49 percent third degree T31.54
50-59 percent third degree T31.55
60-69 percent (0-9 percent third degree) T31.60
with
10-19 percent third degree T31.61
20-29 percent third degree T31.62
30-39 percent third degree T31.63
40-49 percent third degree T31.64
50-59 percent third degree T31.65
60-69 percent third degree T31.66
70-79 percent (0-9 percent third degree) T31.70
with
10-19 percent third degree T31.71
20-29 percent third degree T31.72
30-39 percent third degree T31.73
40-49 percent third degree T31.74
50-59 percent third degree T31.75
60-69 percent third degree T31.76

Burn *(continued)*
unspecified site with extent of body surface involved specified *(continued)*
70-79 percent (0-9 percent third degree) *(continued)*
70-79 percent third degree T31.77
80-89 percent (0-9 percent third degree) T31.80
with
10-19 percent third degree T31.81
20-29 percent third degree T31.82
30-39 percent third degree T31.83
40-49 percent third degree T31.84
50-59 percent third degree T31.85
60-69 percent third degree T31.86
70-79 percent third degree T31.87
80-89 percent third degree T31.88
90 percent or more (0-9 percent third degree) T31.90
with
10-19 percent third degree T31.91
20-29 percent third degree T31.92
30-39 percent third degree T31.93
40-49 percent third degree T31.94
50-59 percent third degree T31.95
60-69 percent third degree T31.96
70-79 percent third degree T31.97
80-89 percent third degree T31.98
90-99 percent third degree T31.99
upper limb T22.00
above elbow —*see* Burn, above elbow
axilla —*see* Burn, axilla
elbow —*see* Burn, elbow
first degree T22.10
forearm —*see* Burn, forearm
hand —*see* Burn, hand
interscapular region —*see* Burn, back, upper
multiple sites T22.099
first degree T22.199
left T22.092
first degree T22.192
second degree T22.292
third degree T22.392
right T22.091
first degree T22.191
second degree T22.291
third degree T22.391
second degree T22.299
third degree T22.399
scapular region —*see* Burn, scapular region
second degree T22.20
shoulder —*see* Burn, shoulder
third degree T22.30
wrist —*see* Burn, wrist
uterus T28.3
vagina T28.3
vulva —*see* Burn, genital organs, external, female
wrist T23.079
first degree T23.179

Burn *(continued)*
- wrist *(continued)*
  - left T23.072
    - first degree T23.172
    - second degree T23.272
    - third degree T23.372
  - multiple sites with hand T23.099
    - first degree T23.199
    - left T23.092
      - first degree T23.192
      - second degree T23.292
      - third degree T23.392
    - right T23.091
      - first degree T23.191
      - second degree T23.291
      - third degree T23.391
    - second degree T23.299
    - third degree T23.399
  - right T23.071
    - first degree T23.171
    - second degree T23.271
    - third degree T23.371
  - second degree T23.279
  - third degree T23.379

Burnett's syndrome E83.52

Burning
- feet syndrome E53.9
- sensation R20.8
- tongue K14.6

Burn-out (state) Z73.0

Burns' disease or osteochondrosis —*see* Osteochondrosis, juvenile, ulna

Bursa —*see* condition

Bursitis M71.9
- Achilles —*see* Tendinitis, Achilles
- adhesive —*see* Bursitis, specified NEC
- ankle —*see* Enthesopathy, lower limb, ankle, specified type NEC
- calcaneal —*see* Enthesopathy, foot, specified type NEC
- collateral ligament, tibial —*see* Bursitis, tibial collateral
- due to use, overuse, pressure —*see also* Disorder, soft tissue, due to use, specified type NEC
  - specified NEC —*see* Disorder, soft tissue, due to use, specified NEC
- Duplay's M75.0
- elbow NEC M70.3-
  - olecranon M70.2-
- finger —*see* Disorder, soft tissue, due to use, specified type NEC, hand
- foot —*see* Enthesopathy, foot, specified type NEC
- gonococcal A54.49
- gouty —*see* Gout
- hand M70.1-
- hip NEC M70.7-
  - trochanteric M70.6-
- infective NEC M71.10
  - abscess —*see* Abscess, bursa
  - ankle M71.17-
  - elbow M71.12-
  - foot M71.17-
  - hand M71.14-
  - hip M71.15-
  - knee M71.16-
  - multiple sites M71.19
  - shoulder M71.11-
  - specified site NEC M71.18
  - wrist M71.13-
- ischial —*see* Bursitis, hip
- knee NEC M70.5-
  - prepatellar M70.4-
- occupational NEC —*see also* Disorder, soft tissue, due to, use

Bursitis *(continued)*
- olecranon —*see* Bursitis, elbow, olecranon
- pharyngeal J39.1
- popliteal —*see* Bursitis, knee
- prepatellar M70.4-
- radiohumeral M77.8
- rheumatoid M06.20
  - ankle M06.27-
  - elbow M06.22-
  - foot joint M06.27-
  - hand joint M06.24-
  - hip M06.25-
  - knee M06.26-
  - multiple site M06.29
  - shoulder M06.21-
  - vertebra M06.28
  - wrist M06.23-
- scapulohumeral —*see* Bursitis, shoulder
- semimembranous muscle (knee) —*see* Bursitis, knee
- shoulder M75.5-
  - adhesive —*see* Capsulitis, adhesive
- specified NEC M71.50
  - ankle M71.57-
  - due to use, overuse or pressure —*see* Disorder, soft tissue, due to, use
  - elbow M71.52-
  - foot M71.57-
  - hand M71.54-
  - hip M71.55-
  - knee M71.56-
  - shoulder —*see* Bursitis, shoulder
  - specified site NEC M71.58
  - tibial collateral M76.4-
  - wrist M71.53-
- subacromial —*see* Bursitis, shoulder
- subcoracoid —*see* Bursitis, shoulder
- subdeltoid —*see* Bursitis, shoulder
- syphilitic A52.78
- Thornwaldt, Tornwaldt J39.2
- tibial collateral M76.4-
- toe —*see* Enthesopathy, foot, specified type NEC
- trochanteric (area) —*see* Bursitis, hip, trochanteric
- wrist —*see* Bursitis, hand

Bursopathy M71.9
- specified type NEC M71.80
  - ankle M71.87-
  - elbow M71.82-
  - foot M71.87-
  - hand M71.84-
  - hip M71.85-
  - knee M71.86-
  - multiple sites M71.89
  - shoulder M71.81-
  - specified site NEC M71.88
  - wrist M71.83-

Burst stitches or sutures (complication of surgery) T81.31
- external operation wound T81.31
- internal operation wound T81.32

Buruli ulcer A31.1

Bury's disease L95.1

Buschke's
- disease B45.3
- scleredema —*see* Sclerosis, systemic

Busse-Buschke disease B45.3

Buttock —*see* condition

Button
- Biskra B55.1
- Delhi B55.1
- oriental B55.1

Buttonhole deformity (finger) —*see* Deformity, finger, boutonniere

Bwamba fever A92.8

Byssinosis J66.0

Bywaters' syndrome T79.5

C

Cachexia R64
- cancerous R64
- cardiac —*see* Disease, heart
- dehydration E86.0
- due to malnutrition R64
- exophthalmic —*see* Hyperthyroidism
- heart —*see* Disease, heart
- hypophyseal E23.0
- hypopituitary E23.0
- lead —*see* Poisoning, lead
- malignant R64
- marsh —*see* Malaria
- nervous F48.8
- old age R54
- paludal —*see* Malaria
- pituitary E23.0
- renal N28.9
- saturnine —*see* Poisoning, lead
- senile R54
- Simmonds' E23.0
- splenica D73.0
- strumipriva E03.4
- tuberculous NEC —*see* Tuberculosis

Café, au lait spots L81.3

Caffeine-induced
- anxiety disorder F15.980
- sleep disorder F15.982

Caffey's syndrome Q78.8

Caisson disease T70.3

Cake kidney Q63.1

Caked breast (puerperal, postpartum) O92.79

Calabar swelling B74.3

Calcaneal spur —*see* Spur, bone, calcaneal

Calcaneo-apophysitis M92.8

Calcareous —*see* condition

Calcicosis J62.8

Calciferol (vitamin D) **deficiency** E55.9
- with rickets E55.0

Calcification
- adrenal (capsule) (gland) E27.49
  - tuberculous E35 *[B90.8]*
- aorta I70.0
- artery (annular) —*see* Arteriosclerosis
- auricle (ear) —*see* Disorder, pinna, specified type NEC
- basal ganglia G23.8
- bladder N32.89
  - due to Schistosoma hematobium B65.0
- brain (cortex) —*see* Calcification, cerebral
- bronchus J98.09
- bursa M71.40
  - ankle M71.47-
  - elbow M71.42-
  - foot M71.47-
  - hand M71.44-
  - hip M71.45-
  - knee M71.46-
  - multiple sites M71.49
  - shoulder M75.3-
  - specified site NEC M71.48
  - wrist M71.43-

Calcification *(continued)*
- cardiac —*see* Degeneration, myocardial
- cerebral (cortex) G93.89
  - artery I67.2
- cervix (uteri) N88.8
- choroid plexus G93.89
- conjunctiva —*see* Concretion, conjunctiva
- corpora cavernosa (penis) N48.89
- cortex (brain) —*see* Calcification, cerebral
- dental pulp (nodular) K04.2
- dentinal papilla K00.4
- fallopian tube N83.8
- falx cerebri G96.19
- gallbladder K82.8
- general E83.59
- heart —*see also* Degeneration, myocardial
  - valve —*see* Endocarditis
- idiopathic infantile arterial (IIAC) Q28.8
- intervertebral cartilage or disc (postinfective) —*see* Disorder, disc, specified NEC
- intracranial —*see* Calcification, cerebral
- joint —*see* Disorder, joint, specified type NEC
- kidney N28.89
  - tuberculous N29 *[B90.1]*
- larynx (senile) J38.7
- lens —*see* Cataract, specified NEC
- lung (active) (postinfectional) J98.4
  - tuberculous B90.9
- lymph gland or node (postinfectional) I89.8
  - tuberculous (*see also* Tuberculosis, lymph gland) B90.8
- mammographic R92.1
- massive (paraplegic) —*see* Myositis, ossificans, in, quadriplegia
- medial —*see* Arteriosclerosis, extremities
- meninges (cerebral) (spinal) G96.19
- metastatic E83.59
- Mönckeberg's —*see* Arteriosclerosis, extremities
- muscle M61.9
  - due to burns —*see* Myositis, ossificans, in, burns
  - paralytic —*see* Myositis, ossificans, in, quadriplegia
  - specified type NEC M61.40
    - ankle M61.47-
    - foot M61.47-
    - forearm M61.43-
    - hand M61.44-
    - lower leg M61.46-
    - multiple sites M61.49
    - pelvic region M61.45-
    - shoulder region M61.41-
    - specified site NEC M61.48
    - thigh M61.45-
    - upper arm M61.42-
- myocardium, myocardial —*see* Degeneration, myocardial
- ovary N83.8
- pancreas K86.89
- penis N48.89
- periarticular —*see* Disorder, joint, specified type NEC
- pericardium —*see also* Pericarditis I31.1
- pineal gland E34.8
- pleura J94.8
  - postinfectional J94.8
  - tuberculous NEC B90.9
- pulpal (dental) (nodular) K04.2
- sclera H15.89

Calcification *(continued)*
spleen D73.89
subcutaneous L94.2
suprarenal (capsule) (gland) E27.49
tendon (sheath) *—see also* Tenosynovitis, specified type NEC
with bursitis, synovitis or tenosynovitis *—see* Tendinitis, calcific
trachea J39.8
ureter N28.89
uterus N85.8
vitreous *—see* Deposit, crystalline

Calcified *—see* Calcification

Calcinosis (interstitial) (tumoral) (universalis) E83.59
with Raynaud's phenomenon, esophageal dysfunction, sclerodactyly, telangiectasia (CREST syndrome) M34.1
circumscripta (skin) L94.2
cutis L94.2

Calciphylaxis *—see also* Calcification, by site E83.59

Calcium
deposits *—see* Calcification, by site
metabolism disorder E83.50
salts or soaps in vitreous *—see* Deposit, crystalline

Calciuria R82.99

Calculi *—see* Calculus

Calculosis, intrahepatic *—see* Calculus, bile duct

Calculus, calculi, calculous
ampulla of Vater *—see* Calculus, bile duct
anuria (impacted) (recurrent) *—see also* Calculus, urinary N20.9
appendix K38.1
bile duct (common) (hepatic) K80.50
with
calculus of gallbladder *—see* Calculus, gallbladder and bile duct
cholangitis K80.30
with
cholecystitis *—see* Calculus, bile duct, with cholecystitis
obstruction K80.31
acute K80.32
with
chronic cholangitis K80.36
with obstruction K80.37
obstruction K80.33
chronic K80.34
with
acute cholangitis K80.36
with obstruction K80.37
obstruction K80.35
cholecystitis (with cholangitis) K80.40
with obstruction K80.41
acute K80.42
with
chronic cholecystitis K80.46
with obstruction K80.47
obstruction K80.43
chronic K80.44
with
acute cholecystitis K80.46

Calculus, calculi, calculous *(continued)*
bile duct *(continued)*
with *(continued)*
cholecystitis *(continued)*
chronic *(continued)*
with obstruction K80.47
obstruction K80.45
obstruction K80.51
biliary *—see also* Calculus, gallbladder
specified NEC K80.80
with obstruction K80.81
bilirubin, multiple *—see* Calculus, gallbladder
bladder (encysted) (impacted) (urinary) (diverticulum) N21.0
bronchus J98.09
calyx (kidney) (renal) *—see* Calculus, kidney
cholesterol (pure) (solitary) *—see* Calculus, gallbladder
common duct (bile) *—see* Calculus, bile duct
conjunctiva *—see* Concretion, conjunctiva
cystic N21.0
duct *—see* Calculus, gallbladder
dental (subgingival) (supragingival) K03.6
diverticulum
bladder N21.0
kidney N20.0
epididymis N50.89
gallbladder K80.20
with
bile duct calculus *—see* Calculus, gallbladder and bile duct
cholecystitis K80.10
with obstruction K80.11
acute K80.00
with
chronic cholecystitis K80.12
with obstruction K80.13
obstruction K80.01
chronic K80.10
with
acute cholecystitis K80.12
with obstruction K80.13
obstruction K80.11
specified NEC K80.18
with obstruction K80.19
obstruction K80.21
gallbladder and bile duct K80.70
with
cholecystitis K80.60
with obstruction K80.61
acute K80.62
with
chronic cholecystitis K80.66
with obstruction K80.67
obstruction K80.63
chronic K80.64
with
acute cholecystitis K80.66
with obstruction K80.67
obstruction K80.65
obstruction K80.71
hepatic (duct) *—see* Calculus, bile duct
hepatobiliary K80.80
with obstruction K80.81

Calculus, calculi, calculous *(continued)*
ileal conduit N21.8
intestinal (impaction) (obstruction) K56.49
kidney (impacted) (multiple) (pelvis) (recurrent) (staghorn) N20.0
with calculus, ureter N20.2
congenital Q63.8
lacrimal passages *—see* Dacryolith
liver (impacted) *—see* Calculus, bile duct
lung J98.4
mammographic R92.1
nephritic (impacted) (recurrent) *—see* Calculus, kidney
nose J34.89
pancreas (duct) K86.89
parotid duct or gland K11.5
pelvis, encysted *—see* Calculus, kidney
prostate N42.0
pulmonary J98.4
pyelitis (impacted) (recurrent) N20.0
with hydronephrosis N13.2
pyelonephritis (impacted) (recurrent) N20
with hydronephrosis N13.2
renal (impacted) (recurrent) *—see* Calculus, kidney
salivary (duct) (gland) K11.5
seminal vesicle N50.89
staghorn *—see* Calculus, kidney
Stensen's duct K11.5
stomach K31.89
sublingual duct or gland K11.5
congenital Q38.4
submandibular duct, gland or region K11.5
submaxillary duct, gland or region K11.5
suburethral N21.8
tonsil J35.8
tooth, teeth (subgingival) (supragingival) K03.6
tunica vaginalis N50.89
ureter (impacted) (recurrent) N20.1
with calculus, kidney N20.2
with hydronephrosis N13.2
with infection N13.6
urethra (impacted) N21.1
urinary (duct) (impacted) (passage) (tract) N20.9
with hydronephrosis N13.2
with infection N13.6
in (due to)
lower N21.9
specified NEC N21.8
vagina N89.8
vesical (impacted) N21.0
Wharton's duct K11.5
xanthine E79.8 *[N22]*

Calicectasis N28.89

Caliectasis N28.89

California
disease B38.9
encephalitis A83.5

Caligo cornea *—see* Opacity, cornea, central

Callositas, callosity (infected) L84

Callus (infected) L84
bone *—see* Osteophyte
excessive, following fracture - code as Sequelae of fracture

CALME (childhood asymmetric labium majus enlargement) N90.61

Calorie deficiency or malnutrition (*see also* Malnutrition) E46

Calvé-Perthes disease *—see* Legg-Calvé-Perthes disease

Calvé's disease *—see* Osteochondrosis, juvenile, spine

Calvities *—see* Alopecia, androgenic

Cameroon fever *—see* Malaria

Camptocormia (hysterical) F44.4

Camurati-Engelmann syndrome Q78.3

Canal *—see also* condition
atrioventricular common Q21.2

Canaliculitis (lacrimal) (acute) (subacute) H04.33-
Actinomyces A42.89
chronic H04.42-

Canavan's disease E75.29

Canceled procedure (surgical) Z53.9
because of
contraindication Z53.09
smoking Z53.01
left against medical advice (AMA) Z53.21
patient's decision Z53.20
for reasons of belief or group pressure Z53.1
specified reason NEC Z53.29
specified reason NEC Z53.8

Cancer *—see also* Neoplasm, by site, malignant
bile duct type liver C22.1
blood *—see* Leukemia
breast (*see also* Neoplasm, breast, malignant) C50.91-
hepatocellular C22.0
lung (*see also* Neoplasm, lung, malignant) C34.90-
ovarian (*see also* Neoplasm, ovary, malignant) C56.9-
unspecified site (primary) C80.1

Cancer (o)phobia F45.29

Cancerous *—see* Neoplasm, malignant, by site

Cancrum oris A69.0

Candidiasis, candidal B37.9
balanitis B37.42
bronchitis B37.1
cheilitis B37.83
congenital P37.5
cystitis B37.41
disseminated B37.7
endocarditis B37.6
enteritis B37.82
esophagitis B37.81
intertrigo B37.2
lung B37.1
meningitis B37.5
mouth B37.0
nails B37.2
neonatal P37.5
onychia B37.2
oral B37.0
osteomyelitis B37.89
otitis externa B37.84
paronychia B37.2
perionyxis B37.2
pneumonia B37.1
proctitis B37.82
pulmonary B37.1
pyelonephritis B37.49
sepsis B37.7
skin B37.2
specified site NEC B37.89
stomatitis B37.0
systemic B37.7
urethritis B37.41
urogenital site NEC B37.49
vagina B37.3

Candidiasis, candidal *(continued)*
- vulva B37.3
- vulvovaginitis B37.3

Candidid L30.2

Candidosis *—see* Candidiasis

Candiru infection or infestation B88.8

Canities (premature) L67.1
- congenital Q84.2

Canker (mouth) (sore) K12.0
- rash A38.9

Cannabinosis J66.2

Cannabis induced
- anxiety disorder F12.980
- psychotic disorder F12.959
- sleep disorder F12.988

Canton fever A75.9

Cantrell's syndrome Q87.89

Capillariasis (intestinal) B81.1
- hepatic B83.8

Capillary *—see* condition

Caplan's syndrome *—see* Rheumatoid, lung

Capsule *—see* condition

Capsulitis (joint) *—see also* Enthesopathy
- adhesive (shoulder) M75.0-
- hepatic K65.8
- labyrinthine *—see* Otosclerosis, specified NEC
- thyroid E06.9

Caput
- crepitus Q75.8
- medusae I86.8
- succedaneum P12.81

Car sickness T75.3

Carapata (disease) A68.0

Carate *—see* Pinta

Carbon lung J60

Carbuncle L02.93
- abdominal wall L02.231
- anus K61.0
- auditory canal, external *—see* Abscess, ear, external
- auricle ear *—see* Abscess, ear, external
- axilla L02.43-
- back (any part) L02.232
- breast N61.1
- buttock L02.33
- cheek (external) L02.03
- chest wall L02.233
- chin L02.03
- corpus cavernosum N48.21
- ear (any part) (external) (middle) *—see* Abscess, ear, external
- external auditory canal *—see* Abscess, ear, external
- eyelid *—see* Abscess, eyelid
- face NEC L02.03
- femoral (region) *—see* Carbuncle, lower limb
- finger *—see* Carbuncle, hand
- flank L02.231
- foot L02.63-
- forehead L02.03
- genital *—see* Abscess, genital
- gluteal (region) L02.33
- groin L02.234
- hand L02.53-
- head NEC L02.831
- heel *—see* Carbuncle, foot
- hip *—see* Carbuncle, lower limb
- kidney *—see* Abscess, kidney

Carbuncle *(continued)*
- knee *—see* Carbuncle, lower limb
- labium (majus) (minus) N76.4
- lacrimal
  - gland *—see* Dacryoadenitis
  - passages (duct) (sac) *—see* Inflammation, lacrimal, passages, acute
- leg *—see* Carbuncle, lower limb
- lower limb L02.43-
- malignant A22.0
- navel L02.236
- neck L02.13
- nose (external) (septum) J34.0
- orbit, orbital *—see* Abscess, orbit
- palmar (space) *—see* Carbuncle, hand
- partes posteriores L02.33
- pectoral region L02.233
- penis N48.21
- perineum L02.235
- pinna *—see* Abscess, ear, external
- popliteal *—see* Carbuncle, lower limb
- scalp L02.831
- seminal vesicle N49.0
- shoulder *—see* Carbuncle, upper limb
- specified site NEC L02.838
- temple (region) L02.03
- thumb *—see* Carbuncle, hand
- toe *—see* Carbuncle, foot
- trunk L02.239
  - abdominal wall L02.231
  - back L02.232
  - chest wall L02.233
  - groin L02.234
  - perineum L02.235
  - umbilicus L02.236
- umbilicus L02.236
- upper limb L02.43-
- urethra N34.0
- vulva N76.4

Carbunculus *—see* Carbuncle

Carcinoid (tumor) *—see* Tumor, carcinoid

Carcinoidosis E34.0

Carcinoma (malignant) *—see also* Neoplasm, by site, malignant
- acidophil
  - specified site *—see* Neoplasm, malignant, by site
  - unspecified site C75.1
- acidophil-basophil, mixed
  - specified site *—see* Neoplasm, malignant, by site
  - unspecified site C75.1
- adnexal (skin) *—see* Neoplasm, skin, malignant
- adrenal cortical C74.0-
- alveolar *—see* Neoplasm, lung, malignant
  - cell *—see* Neoplasm, lung, malignant
- ameloblastic C41.1
  - upper jaw (bone) C41.0
- apocrine
  - breast *—see* Neoplasm, breast, malignant
  - specified site NEC *—see* Neoplasm, skin, malignant
  - unspecified site C44.99
- basal cell (pigmented) (*see also* Neoplasm, skin, malignant) C44.91
  - fibro-epithelial *—see* Neoplasm, skin, malignant
  - morphea *—see* Neoplasm, skin, malignant
  - multicentric *—see* Neoplasm, skin, malignant

Carcinoma *(continued)*
- basaloid
- basal-squamous cell, mixed *—see* Neoplasm, skin, malignant
- basophil
  - specified site *—see* Neoplasm, malignant, by site
  - unspecified site C75.1
- basophil-acidophil, mixed
  - specified site *—see* Neoplasm, malignant, by site
  - unspecified site C75.1
- basosquamous *—see* Neoplasm, skin, malignant
- bile duct
  - with hepatocellular, mixed C22.0
  - liver C22.1
  - specified site NEC *—see* Neoplasm, malignant, by site
  - unspecified site C22.1
- branchial or branchiogenic C10.4
- bronchial or bronchogenic *—see* Neoplasm, lung, malignant
- bronchiolar *—see* Neoplasm, lung, malignant
- bronchioloalveolar *—see* Neoplasm, lung, malignant
- C cell
  - specified site *—see* Neoplasm, malignant, by site
  - unspecified site C73
- ceruminous C44.29-
- cervix uteri
  - in situ D06.9
    - endocervix D06.0
    - exocervix D06.1
    - specified site NEC D06.7
- chorionic
  - specified site *—see* Neoplasm, malignant, by site
  - unspecified site
    - female C58
    - male C62.90
- chromophobe
  - specified site *—see* Neoplasm, malignant, by site
  - unspecified site C75.1
- cloacogenic
  - specified site *—see* Neoplasm, malignant, by site
  - unspecified site C21.2
- diffuse type
  - specified site *—see* Neoplasm, malignant, by site
  - unspecified site C16.9
- duct (cell)
  - with Paget's disease *—see* Neoplasm, breast, malignant
  - infiltrating
    - with lobular carcinoma (in situ)
      - specified site *—see* Neoplasm, malignant, by site
      - unspecified site (female) C50.91-
        - male C50.92-
    - specified site *—see* Neoplasm, malignant, by site
    - unspecified site (female) C50.91-
      - male C50.92-
- ductal
  - with lobular
    - specified site *—see* Neoplasm, malignant, by site
    - unspecified site (female) C50.91-
      - male C50.92-
- ductular, infiltrating
  - specified site *—see* Neoplasm, malignant, by site

Carcinoma *(continued)*
- ductular, infiltrating *(continued)*
  - unspecified site (female) C50.91-
    - male C50.92-
- embryonal
  - liver C22.7
- endometrioid
  - specified site *—see* Neoplasm, malignant, by site
  - unspecified site
    - female C56.9
    - male C61
- eosinophil
  - specified site *—see* Neoplasm, malignant, by site
  - unspecified site C75.1
- epidermoid *—see also* Neoplasm, skin malignant
  - in situ, Bowen's type *—see* Neoplasm, skin, in situ
- fibroepithelial, basal cell *—see* Neoplasm, skin, malignant
- follicular
  - with papillary (mixed) C73
  - moderately differentiated C73
  - pure follicle C73
  - specified site *—see* Neoplasm, malignant, by site
  - trabecular C73
  - unspecified site C73
  - well differentiated C73
- generalized, with unspecified primary site C80.0
- glycogen-rich *—see* Neoplasm, breast, malignant
- granulosa cell C56-
- hepatic cell C22.0
- hepatocellular C22.0
  - with bile duct, mixed C22.0
  - fibrolamellar C22.0
- hepatocholangiolitic C22.0
- Hurthle cell C73
- in
  - adenomatous
    - polyposis coli C18.9
  - pleomorphic adenoma *—see* Neoplasm, salivary glands, malignant
  - situ *—see* Carcinoma-in-situ
- infiltrating
  - duct
    - with lobular
      - specified site *—see* Neoplasm, malignant, by site
      - unspecified site (female) C50.91-
        - male C50.92-
    - with Paget's disease *—see* Neoplasm, breast, malignant
    - specified site *—see* Neoplasm, malignant
    - unspecified site (female) C50.91-
      - male C50.92-
  - ductular
    - specified site *—see* Neoplasm, malignant
    - unspecified site (female) C50.91-
      - male C50.92-
  - lobular
    - specified site *—see* Neoplasm, malignant
    - unspecified site (female) C50.91-
      - male C50.92-
- inflammatory
  - specified site *—see* Neoplasm, malignant
  - unspecified site (female) C50.91-
    - male C50.92-

Carcinoma *(continued)*
- intestinal type
  - specified site *—see* Neoplasm, malignant, by site
  - unspecified site C16.9
- intracystic
  - noninfiltrating *—see* Neoplasm, in situ, by site
- intraductal (noninfiltrating)
  - with Paget's disease *—see* Neoplasm, breast, malignant
  - breast D05.1-
  - papillary
    - with invasion
      - specified site *—see* Neoplasm, malignant, by site
      - unspecified site (female) C50.91-
        - male C50.92-
    - breast D05.1-
    - specified site NEC *—see* Neoplasm, in situ, by site
    - unspecified site (female) D05.1-
  - specified site NEC *—see* Neoplasm, in situ, by site
  - unspecified site (female) D05.1-
- intraepidermal *—see* Neoplasm, in situ
  - squamous cell, Bowen's type *—see* Neoplasm, skin, in situ
- intraepithelial *—see* Neoplasm, in situ, by site
  - squamous cell *—see* Neoplasm, in situ, by site
- intraosseous C41.1
  - upper jaw (bone) C41.0
- islet cell
  - with exocrine, mixed
    - specified site *—see* Neoplasm, malignant, by site
    - unspecified site C25.9
  - pancreas C25.4
  - specified site NEC *—see* Neoplasm, malignant, by site
  - unspecified site C25.4
- juvenile, breast *—see* Neoplasm, breast, malignant
- large cell
  - small cell
    - specified site *—see* Neoplasm, malignant, by site
    - unspecified site C34.90
- Leydig cell (testis)
  - specified site *—see* Neoplasm, malignant, by site
  - unspecified site
    - female C56.9
    - male C62.90
- lipid-rich (female) C50.91-
  - male C50.92-
- liver cell C22.0
- liver NEC C22.7
- lobular (infiltrating)
  - with intraductal
    - specified site *—see* Neoplasm, malignant, by site
    - unspecified site (female) C50.91-
      - male C50.92-
  - noninfiltrating
    - breast D05.0-
    - specified site NEC *—see* Neoplasm, in situ, by site
    - unspecified site D05.0-
  - specified site *—see* Neoplasm, malignant, by site
  - unspecified site (female) C50.91-
    - male C50.92-

Carcinoma *(continued)*
- medullary
  - with
    - amyloid stroma
      - specified site *—see* Neoplasm, malignant, by site
      - unspecified site C73
    - lymphoid stroma
      - specified site *—see* Neoplasm, malignant, by site
      - unspecified site (female) C50.91-
        - male C50.92-
- Merkel cell C4A.9
  - anal margin C4A.51
  - anal skin C4A.51
  - canthus C4A.1-
  - ear and external auricular canal C4A.2-
  - external auricular canal C4A.2-
  - eyelid, including canthus C4A.1-
  - face C4A.30
    - specified NEC C4A.39
  - hip C4A.7-
  - lip C4A.0
  - lower limb, including hip C4A.7-
  - neck C4A.4
  - nodal presentation C7B.1
  - nose C4A.31
  - overlapping sites C4A.8
  - perianal skin C4A.51
  - scalp C4A.4
  - secondary C7B.1
  - shoulder C4A.6-
  - skin of breast C4A.52
  - trunk NEC C4A.59
  - upper limb, including shoulder C4A.6-
  - visceral metastatic C7B.1
- metastatic *—see* Neoplasm, secondary, by site
- metatypical *—see* Neoplasm, skin, malignant
- morphea, basal cell *—see* Neoplasm, skin, malignant
- mucoid
  - cell
    - specified site *—see* Neoplasm, malignant, by site
    - unspecified site C75.1
- neuroendocrine *—see also* Tumor, neuroendocrine
  - high grade, any site C7A.1
  - poorly differentiated, any site C7A.1
- nonencapsulated sclerosing C73
- noninfiltrating
  - intracystic *—see* Neoplasm, in situ, by site
  - intraductal
    - breast D05.1-
    - papillary
      - breast D05.1-
      - specified site NEC *—see* Neoplasm, in situ, by site
      - unspecified site D05.1-
    - specified site *—see* Neoplasm, in situ, by site
    - unspecified site D05.1-
  - lobular
    - breast D05.0-
    - specified site NEC *—see* Neoplasm, in situ, by site
    - unspecified site (female) D05.0-
- oat cell
  - specified site *—see* Neoplasm, malignant, by site
  - unspecified site C34.90

Carcinoma *(continued)*
- odontogenic C41.1
  - upper jaw (bone) C41.0
- papillary
  - with follicular (mixed) C73
  - follicular variant C73
  - intraductal (noninfiltrating)
    - with invasion
      - specified site *—see* Neoplasm, malignant, by site
      - unspecified site (female) C50.91-
        - male C50.92-
    - breast D05.1-
    - specified site NEC *—see* Neoplasm, in situ, by site
    - unspecified site D05.1-
  - serous
    - specified site *—see* Neoplasm, malignant, by site
    - surface
      - specified site *—see* Neoplasm, malignant, by site
      - unspecified site C56.9
    - unspecified site C56.9
- papillocystic
  - specified site *—see* Neoplasm, malignant, by site
  - unspecified site C56.9
- parafollicular cell
  - specified site *—see* Neoplasm, malignant, by site
  - unspecified site C73
- pilomatrix *—see* Neoplasm, skin, malignant
- pseudomucinous
  - specified site *—see* Neoplasm, malignant, by site
  - unspecified site C56.9
- renal cell C64-
- Schmincke *—see* Neoplasm, nasopharynx, malignant
- Schneiderian
  - specified site *—see* Neoplasm, malignant, by site
  - unspecified site C30.0
- sebaceous *—see* Neoplasm, skin, malignant
- secondary *—see also* Neoplasm, secondary, by site
  - Merkel cell C7B.1
- secretory, breast *—see* Neoplasm, breast, malignant
- serous
  - papillary
    - specified site *—see* Neoplasm, malignant, by site
    - unspecified site C56.9
  - surface, papillary
    - specified site *—see* Neoplasm, malignant, by site
    - unspecified site C56.9
- Sertoli cell
  - specified site *—see* Neoplasm, malignant, by site
  - unspecified site C62.90
    - female C56.9
    - male C62.90
- skin appendage *—see* Neoplasm, skin, malignant
- small cell
  - fusiform cell
    - specified site *—see* Neoplasm, malignant, by site
    - unspecified site C34.90
  - intermediate cell
    - specified site *—see* Neoplasm, malignant, by site
    - unspecified site C34.90

Carcinoma *(continued)*
- small cell *(continued)*
  - large cell
    - specified site *—see* Neoplasm, malignant, by site
    - unspecified site C34.90
- solid
  - with amyloid stroma
    - specified site *—see* Neoplasm, malignant, by site
    - unspecified site C73
  - microinvasive
    - specified site *—see* Neoplasm, malignant, by site
    - unspecified site C53.9
- sweat gland *—see* Neoplasm, skin, malignant
- theca cell C56.-
- thymic C37
- unspecified site (primary) C80.1
- water-clear cell C75.0

Carcinoma-in-situ *—see also* Neoplasm, in situ, by site
- breast NOS D05.9-
  - specified type NEC D05.8-
- epidermoid *—see also* Neoplasm, in situ, by site
  - with questionable stromal invasion
    - cervix D06.9
    - specified site NEC *—see* Neoplasm, in situ, by site
    - unspecified site D06.9
  - Bowen's type *—see* Neoplasm, skin, in situ
- intraductal
  - breast D05.1-
  - specified site NEC *—see* Neoplasm, in situ, by site
  - unspecified site D05.1-
- lobular
  - with
    - infiltrating duct
      - breast (female) C50.91-
        - male C50.92-
      - specified site NEC *—see* Neoplasm, malignant
      - unspecified site (female) C50.91-
        - male C50.92-
    - intraductal
      - breast D05.8-
      - specified site NEC *—see* Neoplasm, in situ, by site
      - unspecified site (female) D05.8-
  - breast D05.0-
  - specified site NEC *—see* Neoplasm, in situ, by site
  - unspecified site D05.0-
- squamous cell *—see also* Neoplasm, in situ, by site
  - with questionable stromal invasion
    - cervix D06.9
    - specified site NEC *—see* Neoplasm, in situ, by site
    - unspecified site D06.9

Carcinomaphobia F45.29

Carcinomatosis C80.0
- peritonei C78.6
- unspecified site (primary) (secondary) C80.0

Carcinosarcoma *—see* Neoplasm, malignant, by site
- embryonal *—see* Neoplasm, malignant, by site

Cardia, cardial *—see* condition

Cardiac *—see also* condition
- death, sudden *—see* Arrest, cardiac

Cardiac *(continued)*
- pacemaker
  - in situ Z95.0
  - management or adjustment Z45.018
- tamponade I31.4

Cardialgia *—see* Pain, precordial

Cardiectasis *—see* Hypertrophy, cardiac

Cardiochalasia K21.9

Cardiomalacia I51.5

Cardiomegalia glycogenica diffusa E74.02 *[I43]*

Cardiomegaly *—see also* Hypertrophy, cardiac
- congenital Q24.8
- glycogen E74.02 *[I43]*
- idiopathic I51.7

Cardiomyoliposis I51.5

Cardiomyopathy (familial) (idiopathic) I42.9
- alcoholic I42.6
- amyloid E85.4 *[I43]*
  - transthyretin-related (ATTR) familial E85.4
- arteriosclerotic *—see* Disease, heart, ischemic, atherosclerotic
- beriberi E51.12
- cobalt-beer I42.6
- congenital I42.4
- congestive I42.0
- constrictive NOS I42.5
- dilated I42.0
- due to
  - alcohol I42.6
  - beriberi E51.12
  - cardiac glycogenosis E74.02 *[I43]*
  - drugs I42.7
  - external agents NEC I42.7
  - Friedreich's ataxia G11.1
  - myotonia atrophica G71.11 *[I43]*
  - progressive muscular dystrophy G71.0 *[I43]*
- glycogen storage E74.02 *[I43]*
- hypertensive *—see* Hypertension, heart
- hypertrophic (nonobstructive) I42.2
  - obstructive I42.1
    - congenital Q24.8
- in
  - Chagas' disease (chronic) B57.2
    - acute B57.0
  - sarcoidosis D86.85
- ischemic I25.5
- metabolic E88.9 *[I43]*
  - thyrotoxic E05.90 *[I43]*
    - with thyroid storm E05.91 *[I43]*
- newborn I42.8
  - congenital I42.4
- nutritional E63.9 *[I43]*
  - beriberi E51.12
- obscure of Africa I42.8
- peripartum O90.3
- postpartum O90.3
- restrictive NEC I42.5
- rheumatic I09.0
- secondary I42.9
- stress induced I51.81
- takotsubo I51.81
- thyrotoxic E05.90 *[I43]*
  - with thyroid storm E05.91 *[I43]*
- toxic NEC I42.7
- transthyretin-related (ATTR) familial amyloid E85.4
- tuberculous A18.84
- viral B33.24

Cardionephritis *—see* Hypertension, cardiorenal

Cardionephropathy *—see* Hypertension, cardiorenal

Cardionephrosis *—see* Hypertension, cardiorenal

Cardiopathia nigra I27.0

Cardiopathy *—see also* Disease, heart I51.9
- idiopathic I42.9
- mucopolysaccharidosis E76.3 *[I52]*

Cardiopericarditis *—see* Pericarditis

Cardiophobia F45.29

Cardiorenal *—see* condition

Cardiorrhexis *—see* Infarct, myocardium

Cardiosclerosis *—see* Disease, heart, ischemic, atherosclerotic

Cardiosis *—see* Disease, heart

Cardiospasm (esophagus) (reflex) (stomach) K22.0
- congenital Q39.5
  - with megaesophagus Q39.5

Cardiostenosis *—see* Disease, heart

Cardiosymphysis I31.0

Cardiovascular *—see* condition

Carditis (acute) (bacterial) (chronic) (subacute) I51.89
- meningococcal A39.50
- rheumatic *—see* Disease, heart, rheumatic
- rheumatoid *—see* Rheumatoid, carditis
- viral B33.20

Care (of) (for) (following)
- child (routine) Z76.2
- family member (handicapped) (sick)
  - creating problem for family Z63.6
  - provided away from home for holiday relief Z75.5
  - unavailable, due to
    - absence (person rendering care) (sufferer) Z74.2
    - inability (any reason) of person rendering care Z74.2
- foundling Z76.1
- holiday relief Z75.5
- improper *—see* Maltreatment
- lack of (at or after birth) (infant) *—see* Maltreatment, child, neglect
- lactating mother Z39.1
- palliative Z51.5
- postpartum
  - immediately after delivery Z39.0
  - routine follow-up Z39.2
- respite Z75.5
- unavailable, due to
  - absence of person rendering care Z74.2
  - inability (any reason) of person rendering care Z74.2
- well-baby Z76.2

Caries
- bone NEC A18.03
- dental (dentino enamel junction) (early in childhood) (of dentine) (pre-eruptive) (recurrent) (to the pulp) K02.9
  - arrested (coronal) (root) K02.3
  - chewing surface
    - limited to enamel K02.51
    - penetrating into dentin K02.52
    - penetrating into pulp K02.53
  - coronal surface
    - chewing surface
      - limited to enamel K02.51
      - penetrating into dentin K02.52
      - penetrating into pulp K02.53
    - pit and fissure surface
      - limited to enamel K02.51
      - penetrating into dentin K02.52
      - penetrating into pulp K02.53
    - smooth surface
      - limited to enamel K02.61
      - penetrating into dentin K02.62
      - penetrating into pulp K02.63
  - pit and fissure surface
    - limited to enamel K02.51
    - penetrating into dentin K02.52
    - penetrating into pulp K02.53
  - primary, cervical origin K02.52
  - root K02.7
  - smooth surface
    - limited to enamel K02.61
    - penetrating into dentin K02.62
    - penetrating into pulp K02.63
- external meatus *—see* Disorder, ear, external, specified type NEC
- hip (tuberculous) A18.02
- initial (tooth)
  - chewing surface K02.51
  - pit and fissure surface K02.51
  - smooth surface K02.61
- knee (tuberculous) A18.02
- labyrinth *—see* subcategory H83.8
- limb NEC (tuberculous) A18.03
- mastoid process (chronic) *—see* Mastoiditis, chronic
  - tuberculous A18.03
- middle ear *—see* subcategory H74.8
- nose (tuberculous) A18.03
- orbit (tuberculous) A18.03
- ossicles, ear *—see* Abnormal, ear ossicles
- petrous bone *—see* Petrositis
- root (dental) (tooth) K02.7
- sacrum (tuberculous) A18.01
- spine, spinal (column) (tuberculous) A18.01
- syphilitic A52.77
  - congenital (early) A50.02 *[M90.80]*
- tooth, teeth *—see* Caries, dental
- tuberculous A18.03
- vertebra (column) (tuberculous) A18.01

Carious teeth *—see* Caries, dental

Carneous mole O02.0

Carnitine insufficiency E71.40

Carotid body or sinus syndrome G90.01

Carotidynia G90.01

Carotinemia (dietary) E67.1

Carotinosis (cutis) (skin) E67.1

Carpal tunnel syndrome *—see* Syndrome, carpal tunnel

Carpenter's syndrome Q87.0

Carpopedal spasm *—see* Tetany

Carr-Barr-Plunkett syndrome Q97.1

Carrier (suspected) **of**
- amebiasis Z22.1
- bacterial disease NEC Z22.39
  - diphtheria Z22.2
  - intestinal infectious NEC Z22.1
    - typhoid Z22.0
  - meningococcal Z22.31
  - sexually transmitted Z22.4
  - specified NEC Z22.39
  - staphylococcal (Methicillin susceptible) Z22.321
    - Methicillin resistant Z22.322
  - streptococcal Z22.338
    - group B Z22.330
      - complicating pregnancy or delivery O99.82-
  - typhoid Z22.0
- cholera Z22.1
- diphtheria Z22.2
- gastrointestinal pathogens NEC Z22.1
- genetic Z14.8
  - cystic fibrosis Z14.1
  - hemophilia A (asymptomatic) Z14.01
    - symptomatic Z14.02
- gestational, pregnant Z33.1
- gonorrhea Z22.4
- HAA (hepatitis Australian-antigen) B18.8
- HB (c)(s)-AG B18.1
- hepatitis (viral) B18.9
  - Australia-antigen (HAA) B18.8
  - B surface antigen (HBsAg) B18.1
    - with acute delta-(super) infection B17.0
  - C B18.2
  - specified NEC B18.8
- human T-cell lymphotropic virus type-1(HTLV-1) infection Z22.6
- infectious organism Z22.9
  - specified NEC Z22.8
- meningococci Z22.31
- Salmonella typhosa Z22.0
- serum hepatitis *—see* Carrier, hepatitis
- staphylococci (Methicillin susceptible) Z22.321
  - Methicillin resistant Z22.322
- streptococci Z22.338
  - group B Z22.330
    - complicating pregnancy or delivery O99.82-
- syphilis Z22.4
- typhoid Z22.0
- venereal disease NEC Z22.4

Carrion's disease A44.0

Carter's relapsing fever (Asiatic) A68.1

Cartilage *—see* condition

Caruncle (inflamed)
- conjunctiva (acute) *—see* Conjunctivitis, acute
- labium (majus) (minus) N90.89
- lacrimal *—see* Inflammation, lacrimal, passages
- myrtiform N89.8
- urethral (benign) N36.2

Cascade stomach K31.2

Caseation lymphatic gland (tuberculous) A18.2

Cassidy (-Scholte) **syndrome** (malignant carcinoid) E34.0

Castellani's disease A69.8

Castration, traumatic, male S38.231

Casts in urine R82.99

Cat
- cry syndrome Q93.4
- ear Q17.3
- eye syndrome Q92.8

Catabolism, senile R54

Catalepsy (hysterical) F44.2
- schizophrenic F20.2

Cataplexy (idiopathic) *—see* - Narcolepsy

Cataract (cortical) (immature) (incipient) H26.9
- with
  - neovascularization —*see* Cataract, complicated
- age-related —*see* Cataract, senile
- anterior
  - and posterior axial embryonal Q12.0
  - pyramidal Q12.0
- associated with
  - galactosemia E74.21 *[H28]*
  - myotonic disorders G71.19 *[H28]*
- blue Q12.0
- central Q12.0
- cerulean Q12.0
- complicated H26.20
  - with
    - neovascularization H26.21-
    - ocular disorder H26.22-
  - glaucomatous flecks H26.23-
- congenital Q12.0
- coraliform Q12.0
- coronary Q12.0
- crystalline Q12.0
- diabetic —*see* Diabetes, cataract
- drug-induced H26.3-
- due to
  - ocular disorder —*see* Cataract, complicated
  - radiation H26.8
- electric H26.8
- extraction status Z98.4-
- glass-blower's H26.8
- heat ray H26.8
- heterochromic —*see* Cataract, complicated
- hypermature —*see* Cataract, senile, morgagnian type
- in (due to)
  - chronic iridocyclitis —*see* Cataract, complicated
  - diabetes —*see* Diabetes, cataract
  - endocrine disease E34.9 *[H28]*
  - eye disease —*see* Cataract, complicated
  - hypoparathyroidism E20.9 *[H28]*
  - malnutrition-dehydration E46 *[H28]*
  - metabolic disease E88.9 *[H28]*
  - myotonic disorders G71.19 *[H28]*
  - nutritional disease E63.9 *[H28]*
- infantile —*see* Cataract, presenile
- irradiational —*see* Cataract, specified NEC
- juvenile —*see* Cataract, presenile
- malnutrition-dehydration E46 *[H28]*
- morgagnian —*see* Cataract, senile, morgagnian type
- myotonic G71.19 *[H28]*
- myxedema E03.9 *[H28]*
- nuclear
  - embryonal Q12.0
  - sclerosis —*see* Cataract, senile, nuclear
- presenile H26.00-
  - combined forms H26.06-
  - cortical H26.01-
  - lamellar —*see* Cataract, presenile, cortical
  - nuclear H26.03-
  - specified NEC H26.09
  - subcapsular polar (anterior) H26.04-
    - posterior H26.05-
  - zonular —*see* Cataract, presenile, cortical
- secondary H26.40
  - Soemmering's ring H26.41-

Cataract *(continued)*
- secondary *(continued)*
  - specified NEC H26.49-
  - to eye disease —*see* Cataract, complicated
- senile H25.9
  - brunescens —*see* Cataract, senile, nuclear
  - combined forms H25.81-
  - coronary —*see* Cataract, senile, incipient
  - cortical H25.01-
  - hypermature —*see* Cataract, senile, morgagnian type
  - incipient (mature) (total) H25.09-
    - cortical —*see* Cataract, senile, cortical
    - subcapsular —*see* Cataract, senile, subcapsular
  - morgagnian type (hypermature) H25.2-
  - nuclear (sclerosis) H25.1-
  - polar subcapsular (anterior) (posterior) —*see* Cataract, senile, incipient
  - punctate —*see* Cataract, senile, incipient
  - specified NEC H25.89
  - subcapsular polar (anterior) H25.03-
    - posterior H25.04-
- snowflake —*see* Diabetes, cataract
- specified NEC H26.8
- toxic —*see* Cataract, drug-induced
- traumatic H26.10-
  - localized H26.11-
  - partially resolved H26.12-
  - total H26.13-
- zonular (perinuclear) Q12.0

Cataracta —*see also* Cataract
- brunescens —*see* Cataract, senile, nuclear
- centralis pulverulenta Q12.0
- cerulea Q12.0
- complicata —*see* Cataract, complicated
- congenita Q12.0
- coralliformis Q12.0
- coronaria Q12.0
- diabetic —*see* Diabetes, cataract
- membranacea
  - accreta —*see* Cataract, secondary
  - congenita Q12.0
- nigra —*see* Cataract, senile, nuclear
- sunflower —*see* Cataract, complicated

Catarrh, catarrhal (acute) (febrile) (infectious) (inflammation) —*see also* condition J00
- bronchial —*see* Bronchitis
- chest —*see* Bronchitis
- chronic J31.0
- due to congenital syphilis A50.03
- enteric —*see* Enteritis
- eustachian H68.009
- fauces —*see* Pharyngitis
- gastrointestinal —*see* Enteritis
- gingivitis K05.00
  - nonplaque induced K05.01
  - plaque induced K05.00
- hay —*see* Fever, hay
- intestinal —*see* Enteritis
- larynx, chronic J37.0
- liver B15.9
  - with hepatic coma B15.0
- lung —*see* Bronchitis
- middle ear, chronic —*see* Otitis, media, nonsuppurative, chronic, serous
- mouth K12.1

Catarrh, catarrhal *(continued)*
- nasal (chronic) —*see* Rhinitis
- nasobronchial J31.1
- nasopharyngeal (chronic) J31.1
  - acute J00
- pulmonary —*see* Bronchitis
- spring (eye) (vernal) —*see* Conjunctivitis, acute, atopic
- summer (hay) —*see* Fever, hay
- throat J31.2
- tubotympanal —*see also* Otitis, media, nonsuppurative
  - chronic —*see* Otitis, media, nonsuppurative, chronic, serous

Catatonia (schizophrenic) F20.2

Catatonic
- disorder due to known physiologic condition F06.1
- schizophrenia F20.2
- stupor R40.1

Cat-scratch —*see also* Abrasion
- disease or fever A28.1

Cauda equina —*see* condition

Cauliflower ear M95.1-

Causalgia (upper limb) G56.4-
- lower limb G57.7-

Cause
- external, general effects T75.89

Caustic burn —*see* Corrosion, by site

Cavare's disease (familial periodic paralysis) G72.3

Cave-in, injury
- crushing (severe) —*see* Crush
- suffocation —*see* Asphyxia, traumatic, due to low oxygen, due to cave-in

Cavernitis (penis) N48.29

Cavernositis N48.29

Cavernous —*see* condition

Cavitation of lung —*see also* Tuberculosis, pulmonary
- nontuberculous J98.4

Cavities, dental —*see* Caries, dental

Cavity
- lung —*see* Cavitation of lung
- optic papilla Q14.2
- pulmonary —*see* Cavitation of lung

Cavovarus foot, congenital Q66.1

Cavus foot (congenital) Q66.7
- acquired —*see* Deformity, limb, foot, specified NEC

Cazenave's disease L10.2

Cecitis K52.9
- with perforation, peritonitis, or rupture K65.8

Cecum —*see* condition

Celiac
- artery compression syndrome I77.4
- disease (with steatorrhea) K90.0
- infantilism K90.0

Cell(s), cellular —*see also* condition
- in urine R82.99

Cellulitis (diffuse) (phlegmonous) (septic) (suppurative) L03.90
- abdominal wall L03.311
- anaerobic A48.0
- ankle —*see* Cellulitis, lower limb
- anus K61.0
- arm —*see* Cellulitis, upper limb
- auricle (ear) —*see* Cellulitis, ear
- axilla L03.11-

Cellulitis *(continued)*
- back (any part) L03.312
- breast (acute) (nonpuerperal) (subacute) N61.0
  - nipple N61.0
- broad ligament
  - acute N73.0
- buttock L03.317
- cervical (meaning neck) L03.221
- cervix (uteri) —*see* Cervicitis
- cheek (external) L03.211
  - internal K12.2
- chest wall L03.313
- chronic L03.90
- clostridial A48.0
- corpus cavernosum N48.22
- digit
  - finger —*see* Cellulitis, finger
  - toe —*see* Cellulitis, toe
- Douglas' cul-de-sac or pouch
  - acute N73.0
- drainage site (following operation) T81.4
- ear (external) H60.1-
- eosinophilic (granulomatous) L98.3
- erysipelatous —*see* Erysipelas
- external auditory canal —*see* Cellulitis, ear
- eyelid —*see* Abscess, eyelid
- face NEC L03.211
- finger (intrathecal) (periosteal) (subcutaneous) (subcuticular) L03.01-
- foot —*see* Cellulitis, lower limb
- gangrenous —*see* Gangrene
- genital organ NEC
  - female (external) N76.4
  - male N49.9
    - multiple sites N49.8
    - specified NEC N49.8
- gluteal (region) L03.317
- gonococcal A54.89
- groin L03.314
- hand —*see* Cellulitis, upper limb
- head NEC L03.811
  - face (any part, except ear, eye and nose) L03.211
- heel —*see* Cellulitis, lower limb
- hip —*see* Cellulitis, lower limb
- jaw (region) L03.211
- knee —*see* Cellulitis, lower limb
- labium (majus) (minus) —*see* Vulvitis
- lacrimal passages —*see* Inflammation, lacrimal, passages
- larynx J38.7
- leg —*see* Cellulitis, lower limb
- lip K13.0
- lower limb L03.11-
  - toe —*see* Cellulitis, toe
- mouth (floor) K12.2
- multiple sites, so stated L03.90
- nasopharynx J39.1
- navel L03.316
  - newborn P38.9
    - with mild hemorrhage P38.1
    - without hemorrhage P38.9
- neck (region) L03.221
- nipple (acute) (nonpuerperal) (subacute) N61.0
- nose (septum) (external) J34.0
- orbit, orbital H05.01-
- palate (soft) K12.2
- pectoral (region) L03.313
- pelvis, pelvic (chronic)
  - female —*see also* Disease, pelvis, inflammatory N73.2
    - acute N73.0
  - following ectopic or molar pregnancy O08.0
  - male K65.0

Cellulitis *(continued)*
- penis N48.22
- perineal, perineum L03.315
- periorbital L03.213
- perirectal K61.1
- peritonsillar J36
- periurethral N34.0
- periuterine (*see also* Disease pelvis, inflammatory) N73.2
  - acute N73.0
- pharynx J39.1
- preseptal L03.213
- rectum K61.1
- retroperitoneal K68.9
- round ligament
  - acute N73.0
- scalp (any part) L03.811
- scrotum N49.2
- seminal vesicle N49.0
- shoulder *—see* Cellulitis, upper limb
- specified site NEC L03.818
- submandibular (region) (space) (triangle) K12.2
  - gland K11.3
- submaxillary (region) K12.2
  - gland K11.3
- thigh *—see* Cellulitis, lower limb
- thumb (intrathecal) (periosteal) (subcutaneous) (subcuticular) *— see* Cellulitis, finger
- toe (intrathecal) (periosteal) (subcutaneous) (subcuticular) L03.03-
- tonsil J36
- trunk L03.319
  - abdominal wall L03.311
  - back (any part) L03.312
  - buttock L03.317
  - chest wall L03.313
  - groin L03.314
  - perineal, perineum L03.315
  - umbilicus L03.316
- tuberculous (primary) A18.4
- umbilicus L03.316
- upper limb L03.11-
  - axilla *—see* Cellulitis, axilla
  - finger *—see* Cellulitis, finger
  - thumb *—see* Cellulitis, finger
- vaccinal T88.0
- vocal cord J38.3
- vulva *—see* Vulvitis
- wrist *—see* Cellulitis, upper limb

Cementoblastoma, benign *—see* Cyst, calcifying odontogenic

Cementoma *—see* Cyst, calcifying odontogenic

Cementoperiostitis *—see* Periodontitis

Cementosis K03.4

Central auditory processing disorder H93.25

Central pain syndrome G89.0

Cephalematocele, cephalhematocele
- newborn P52.8
  - birth injury P10.8
- traumatic *—see* Hematoma, brain

Cephalematoma, cephalhematoma (calcified)
- newborn (birth injury) P12.0
- traumatic *—see* Hematoma, brain

Cephalgia, cephalalgia *—see also* Headache
- histamine G44.009
  - intractable G44.001
  - not intractable G44.009
- trigeminal autonomic (TAC) NEC G44.099
  - intractable G44.091
  - not intractable G44.099

Cephalic *—see* condition

Cephalitis *—see* Encephalitis

Cephalocele *—see* Encephalocele

Cephalomenia N94.89

Cephalopelvic *—see* condition

Cerclage (with cervical incompetence) **in pregnancy** *—see* Incompetence, cervix, in pregnancy

Cerebellitis *—see* Encephalitis

Cerebellum, cerebellar *—see* condition

Cerebral *—see* condition

Cerebritis *—see* Encephalitis

Cerebro-hepato-renal syndrome Q87.89

Cerebromalacia *—see* Softening, brain
- sequelae of cerebrovascular disease I69.398

Cerebroside lipidosis E75.22

Cerebrospasticity (congenital) G80.1

Cerebrospinal *—see* condition

Cerebrum *—see* condition

Ceroid-lipofuscinosis, neuronal E75.4

Cerumen (accumulation) (impacted) H61.2-

Cervical *—see also* condition
- auricle Q18.2
- dysplasia in pregnancy *—see* Abnormal, cervix, in pregnancy or childbirth
- erosion in pregnancy *—see* Abnormal, cervix, in pregnancy or childbirth
- fibrosis in pregnancy *—see* Abnormal, cervix, in pregnancy or childbirth
- fusion syndrome Q76.1
- rib Q76.5
- shortening (complicating pregnancy) O26.87-

Cervicalgia M54.2

Cervicitis (acute) (chronic) (nonvenereal) (senile (atrophic)) (subacute) (with ulceration) N72
- with
  - abortion *—see* Abortion, by type complicated by genital tract and pelvic infection
  - ectopic pregnancy O08.0
  - molar pregnancy O08.0
- chlamydial A56.09
- gonococcal A54.03
- herpesviral A60.03
- puerperal (postpartum) O86.11
- syphilitic A52.76
- trichomonal A59.09
- tuberculous A18.16

Cervicocolpitis (emphysematosa) (*see also* Cervicitis) N72

Cervix *—see* condition

Cesarean delivery, previous, affecting management of pregnancy O34.219
- classical (vertical) scar O34.212
- low transverse scar O34.211

Céstan (-Chenais) **paralysis or syndrome** G46.3

Céstan-Raymond syndrome I65.8

Cestode infestation B71.9
- specified type NEC B71.8

Cestodiasis B71.9

Chabert's disease A22.9

Chacaleh E53.8

Chafing L30.4

Chagas' (-Mazza) **disease** (chronic) B57.2
- with
  - cardiovascular involvement NEC B57.2
  - digestive system involvement B57.30
    - megacolon B57.32
    - megaesophagus B57.31
    - other specified B57.39
  - megacolon B57.32
  - megaesophagus B57.31
  - myocarditis B57.2
  - nervous system involvement B57.40
    - meningitis B57.41
    - meningoencephalitis B57.42
    - other specified B57.49
  - specified organ involvement NEC B57.5
- acute (with) B57.1
  - cardiovascular NEC B57.0
  - myocarditis B57.0

Chagres fever B50.9

Chairridden Z74.09

Chalasia (cardiac sphincter) K21.9

Chalazion H00.19
- left H00.16
  - lower H00.15
  - upper H00.14
- right H00.13
  - lower H00.12
  - upper H00.11

Chalcosis *—see also* Disorder, globe, degenerative, chalcosis
- cornea *—see* Deposit, cornea
- crystalline lens *—see* Cataract, complicated
- retina H35.89

Chalicosis (pulmonum) J62.8

Chancre (any genital site) (hard) (hunterian) (mixed) (primary) (seronegative) (seropositive) (syphilitic) A51.0
- congenital A50.07
- conjunctiva NEC A51.2
- Ducrey's A57
- extragenital A51.2
- eyelid A51.2
- lip A51.2
- nipple A51.2
- Nisbet's A57
- of
  - carate A67.0
  - pinta A67.0
  - yaws A66.0
- palate, soft A51.2
- phagedenic A57
- simple A57
- soft A57
  - bubo A57
  - palate A51.2
- urethra A51.0
- yaws A66.0

Chancroid (anus) (genital) (penis) (perineum) (rectum) (urethra) (vulva) A57

Chandler's disease (osteochondritis dissecans, hip) *—see* Osteochondritis, dissecans, hip

Change(s) (in) (of) *—see also* Removal

Change *(continued)*
- arteriosclerotic *—see* Arteriosclerosis
- bone *—see also* Disorder, bone
  - diabetic *—see* Diabetes, bone change
- bowel habit R19.4
- cardiorenal (vascular) *—see* Hypertension, cardiorenal
- cardiovascular *—see* Disease, cardiovascular
- circulatory I99.9
- cognitive (mild) (organic) R41.89
- color, tooth, teeth
  - during formation K00.8
  - posteruptive K03.7
- contraceptive device Z30.433
- corneal membrane H18.30
  - Bowman's membrane fold or rupture H18.31-
  - Descemet's membrane
    - fold H18.32-
    - rupture H18.33-
- coronary *—see* Disease, heart, ischemic
- degenerative, spine or vertebra *—see* Spondylosis
- dental pulp, regressive K04.2
- dressing (nonsurgical) Z48.00
  - surgical Z48.01
- heart *—see* Disease, heart
- hip joint *—see* Derangement, joint, hip
- hyperplastic larynx J38.7
- hypertrophic
  - nasal sinus J34.89
  - turbinate, nasal J34.3
  - upper respiratory tract J39.8
- indwelling catheter Z46.6
- inflammatory *—see also* Inflammation
  - sacroiliac M46.1
- job, anxiety concerning Z56.1
- joint *—see* Derangement, joint
- life *—see* Menopause
- mental status R41.82
- minimal (glomerular) (*see also* N00-N07 with fourth character .0) N05.0
- myocardium, myocardial *—see* Degeneration, myocardial
- of life *—see* Menopause
- pacemaker Z45.018
  - pulse generator Z45.010
- personality (enduring) F68.8
  - due to (secondary to)
    - general medical condition F07.0
  - secondary (nonspecific) F60.89
- regressive, dental pulp K04.2
- renal *—see* Disease, renal
- retina H35.9
  - myopic (*see also* Myopia, degenerative) H44.2-
- sacroiliac joint M53.3
- senile (*see also* condition) R54
- sensory R20.8
- skin R23.9
  - acute, due to ultraviolet radiation L56.9
    - specified NEC L56.8
  - chronic, due to nonionizing radiation L57.9
    - specified NEC L57.8
  - cyanosis R23.0
  - flushing R23.2
  - pallor R23.1
  - petechiae R23.3
  - specified change NEC R23.8
  - swelling *—see* Mass, localized
  - texture R23.4

Change *(continued)*
- trophic
  - arm *—see* Mononeuropathy, upper limb
  - leg *—see* Mononeuropathy, lower limb
- vascular I99.9
- vasomotor I73.9
- voice R49.9
  - psychogenic F44.4
  - specified NEC R49.8

Changing sleep-work schedule, affecting sleep G47.26

Changuinola fever A93.1

Chapping skin T69.8

Charcot-Marie-Tooth disease, paralysis or syndrome G60.0

Charcot's
- arthropathy *—see* Arthropathy, neuropathic
- cirrhosis K74.3
- disease (tabetic arthropathy) A52.16
- joint (disease) (tabetic) A52.16
  - diabetic *—see* Diabetes, with, arthropathy
  - syringomyelic G95.0
- syndrome (intermittent claudication) I73.9

CHARGE association Q89.8

Charley-horse (quadriceps) M62.831
- traumatic (quadriceps) S76.11-

Charlouis' disease *—see* Yaws

Cheadle's disease E54

Checking (of)
- cardiac pacemaker (battery) (electrode(s)) Z45.018
  - pulse generator Z45.010
- implantable subdermal contraceptive Z30.46
- intrauterine contraceptive device Z30.431
- wound Z48.0-
  - due to injury - code to Injury, by site, using appropriate seventh character for subsequent encounter

Check-up *—see* Examination

Chédiak-Higashi (-Steinbrinck) **syndrome** (congenital gigantism of peroxidase granules) E70.330

Cheek *—see* condition

Cheese itch B88.0

Cheese-washer's lung J67.8

Cheese-worker's lung J67.8

Cheilitis (acute) (angular) (catarrhal) (chronic) (exfoliative) (gangrenous) (glandular) (infectional) (suppurative) (ulcerative) (vesicular) K13.0
- actinic (due to sun) L56.8
  - other than from sun L59.8
- candidal B37.83

Cheilodynia K13.0

Cheiloschisis *—see* Cleft, lip

Cheilosis (angular) K13.0
- with pellagra E52
- due to
  - vitamin B2(riboflavin) deficiency E53.0

Cheiromegaly M79.89

Cheiropompholyx L30.1

Cheloid *—see* Keloid

Chemical burn *—see* Corrosion, by site

Chemodectoma *—see* Paraganglioma, nonchromaffin

Chemosis, conjunctiva *—see* Edema, conjunctiva

Chemotherapy (session) (for)
- cancer Z51.11
- neoplasm Z51.11

Cherubism M27.8

Chest *—see* condition

Cheyne-Stokes breathing (respiration) R06.3

Chiari's
- disease or syndrome (hepatic vein thrombosis) I82.0
- malformation
  - type I G93.5
  - type II *—see* Spina bifida
- net Q24.8

Chicago disease B40.9

Chickenpox *—see* Varicella

Chiclero ulcer or sore B55.1

Chigger (infestation) B88.0

Chignon (disease) B36.8
- newborn (from vacuum extraction) (birth injury) P12.1

Chilaiditi's syndrome (subphrenic displacement, colon) Q43.3

Chilblain(s) (lupus) T69.1

Child
- custody dispute Z65.3

Childbirth *—see* Delivery

Childhood
- cerebral X-linked adrenoleukodystrophy E71.520
- period of rapid growth Z00.2

Chill(s) R68.83
- with fever R50.9
- congestive in malarial regions B54
- without fever R68.83

Chilomastigiasis A07.8

Chimera 46,XX/46,XY Q99.0

Chin *—see* condition

Chinese dysentery A03.9

Chionophobia F40.228

Chitral fever A93.1

Chlamydia, chlamydial A74.9
- cervicitis A56.09
- conjunctivitis A74.0
- cystitis A56.01
- endometritis A56.11
- epididymitis A56.19
- female
  - pelvic inflammatory disease A56.11
  - pelviperitonitis A56.11
- orchitis A56.19
- peritonitis A74.81
- pharyngitis A56.4
- proctitis A56.3
- psittaci (infection) A70
- salpingitis A56.11
- sexually-transmitted infection NEC A56.8
- specified NEC A74.89
- urethritis A56.01
- vulvovaginitis A56.02

Chlamydiosis *—see* Chlamydia

Chloasma (skin) (idiopathic) (symptomatic) L81.1
- eyelid H02.719
  - hyperthyroid E05.90 *[H02.719]*
    - with thyroid storm E05.91 *[H02.719]*
  - left H02.716
    - lower H02.715
    - upper H02.714
  - right H02.713
    - lower H02.712
    - upper H02.711

Chloroma C92.3-

Chlorosis D50.9
- Egyptian B76.9 *[D63.8]*
- miner's B76.9 *[D63.8]*

Chlorotic anemia D50.8

Chocolate cyst (ovary) N80.1

Choked
- disc or disk *—see* Papilledema
- on food, phlegm, or vomitus NOS *—see* Foreign body, by site
- while vomiting NOS *—see* Foreign body, by site

Chokes (resulting from bends) T70.3

Choking sensation R09.89

Cholangiectasis K83.8

Cholangiocarcinoma
- with hepatocellular carcinoma, combined C22.0
- liver C22.1
- specified site NEC *—see* Neoplasm, malignant, by site
- unspecified site C22.1

Cholangiohepatitis K83.8
- due to fluke infestation B66.1

Cholangiohepatoma C22.0

Cholangiolitis (acute) (chronic) (extrahepatic) (gangrenous) (intrahepatic) K83.0
- paratyphoidal *—see* Fever, paratyphoid
- typhoidal A01.09

Cholangioma D13.4
- malignant *—see* Cholangiocarcinoma

Cholangitis (ascending) (primary) (recurrent) (sclerosing) (secondary) (stenosing) (suppurative) K83.0
- with calculus, bile duct *—see* Calculus, bile duct, with cholangitis
- chronic nonsuppurative destructive K74.3

Cholecystectasia K82.8

Cholecystitis K81.9
- with
  - calculus, stones in
    - bile duct (common) (hepatic) *—see* Calculus, bile duct, with cholecystitis
    - cystic duct *—see* Calculus, gallbladder, with cholecystitis
    - gallbladder *—see* Calculus, gallbladder, with cholecystitis
  - choledocholithiasis *—see* Calculus, bile duct, with cholecystitis
  - cholelithiasis *—see* Calculus, gallbladder, with cholecystitis
- acute (emphysematous) (gangrenous) (suppurative) K81.0
  - with
    - calculus, stones in
      - cystic duct *—see* Calculus, gallbladder, with cholecystitis, acute
      - gallbladder *—see* Calculus, gallbladder, with cholecystitis, acute
    - choledocholithiasis *—see* Calculus, bile duct, with cholecystitis, acute
    - cholelithiasis *—see* Calculus, gallbladder, with cholecystitis, acute
    - chronic cholecystitis K81.2
      - with gallbladder calculus K80.12
        - with obstruction K80.13
- chronic K81.1
  - with acute cholecystitis K81.2
    - with gallbladder calculus K80.12
      - with obstruction K80.13
- emphysematous (acute) *—see* Cholecystitis, acute
- gangrenous *—see* Cholecystitis, acute
- paratyphoidal, current A01.4
- suppurative *—see* Cholecystitis, acute
- typhoidal A01.09

Cholecystolithiasis *—see* Calculus, gallbladder

Choledochitis (suppurative) K83.0

Choledocholith *—see* Calculus, bile duct

Choledocholithiasis (common duct) (hepatic duct) *—see* Calculus, bile duct
- cystic *—see* Calculus, gallbladder
- typhoidal A01.09

Cholelithiasis (cystic duct) (gallbladder) (impacted) (multiple) *—see* Calculus, gallbladder
- bile duct (common) (hepatic) *—see* Calculus, bile duct
- hepatic duct *—see* Calculus, bile duct
- specified NEC K80.80
  - with obstruction K80.81

Cholemia *—see also* Jaundice
- familial (simple) (congenital) E80.4
- Gilbert's E80.4

Choleperitoneum, choleperitonitis K65.3

Cholera (Asiatic) (epidemic) (malignant) A00.9
- antimonial *—see* Poisoning, antimony
- classical A00.0
- due to Vibrio cholerae 01 A00.9
  - biovar cholerae A00.0
  - biovar eltor A00.1
  - el tor A00.1
- el tor A00.1

Cholerine *—see* Cholera

Cholestasis NEC K83.1
- with hepatocyte injury K71.0
- due to total parenteral nutrition (TPN) K76.89
- pure K71.0

Cholesteatoma (ear) (middle) (with reaction) H71.9-
- attic H71.0-
- external ear (canal) H60.4-
- mastoid H71.2-
- postmastoidectomy cavity (recurrent) *—see* Complications, postmastoidectomy, recurrent cholesteatoma

Cholesteatoma *(continued)*
- recurrent (postmastoidectomy) *—see* Complications, postmastoidectomy, recurrent cholesteatoma
- tympanum H71.1-

Cholesteatosis, diffuse H71.3-

Cholesteremia E78.00

Cholesterin in vitreous *—see* Deposit, crystalline

Cholesterol
- deposit
  - retina H35.89
  - vitreous *—see* Deposit, crystalline
- elevated (high) E78.00
  - with elevated (high) triglycerides E78.2
  - screening for Z13.220
- imbibition of gallbladder K82.4

Cholesterolemia (essential) (pure) E78.00
- familial E78.01
- hereditary E78.01

Cholesterolosis, cholesterosis (gallbladder) K82.4
- cerebrotendinous E75.5

Cholocolic fistula K82.3

Choluria R82.2

Chondritis M94.8X9
- aurical H61.03-
- costal (Tietze's) M94.0
- external ear H61.03-
- patella, posttraumatic *—see* Chondromalacia, patella
- pinna H61.03-
- purulent M94.8X-
- tuberculous NEC A18.02
  - intervertebral A18.01

Chondroblastoma *—see also* Neoplasm, bone, benign
- malignant *—see* Neoplasm, bone, malignant

Chondrocalcinosis M11.20
- ankle M11.27-
- elbow M11.22-
- familial M11.10
  - ankle M11.17-
  - elbow M11.12-
  - foot joint M11.17-
  - hand joint M11.14-
  - hip M11.15-
  - knee M11.16-
  - multiple site M11.19
  - shoulder M11.11-
  - vertebrae M11.18
  - wrist M11.13-
- foot joint M11.27-
- hand joint M11.24-
- hip M11.25-
- knee M11.26-
- multiple site M11.29
- shoulder M11.21-
- vertebrae M11.28
- specified type NEC M11.20
  - ankle M11.27-
  - elbow M11.22-
  - foot joint M11.27-
  - hand joint M11.24-
  - hip M11.25-
  - knee M11.26-
  - multiple site M11.29
  - shoulder M11.21-
  - vertebrae M11.28
  - wrist M11.23-
- wrist M11.23-

Chondrodermatitis nodularis helicis or anthelicis *—see* Perichondritis, ear

Chondrodysplasia Q78.9
- with hemangioma Q78.4
- calcificans congenita Q77.3
- fetalis Q77.4
- metaphyseal (Jansen's) (McKusick's) (Schmid's) Q78.8
- punctata Q77.3

Chondrodystrophy, chondrodystrophia (familial) (fetalis) (hypoplastic) Q78.9
- calcificans congenita Q77.3
- myotonic (congenital) G71.13
- punctata Q77.3

Chondroectodermal dysplasia Q77.6

Chondrogenesis imperfecta Q77.4

Chondrolysis M94.35-

Chondroma *—see also* Neoplasm, cartilage, benign
- juxtacortical *—see* Neoplasm, bone, benign
- periosteal *—see* Neoplasm, bone, benign

Chondromalacia (systemic) M94.20
- acromioclavicular joint M94.21-
- ankle M94.27-
- elbow M94.22-
- foot joint M94.27-
- glenohumeral joint M94.21-
- hand joint M94.24-
- hip M94.25-
- knee M94.26-
  - patella M22.4-
- multiple sites M94.29
- patella M22.4-
- rib M94.28
- sacroiliac joint M94.259
- shoulder M94.21-
- sternoclavicular joint M94.21-
- vertebral joint M94.28
- wrist M94.23-

Chondromatosis *—see also* Neoplasm, cartilage, uncertain behavior
- internal Q78.4

Chondromyxosarcoma *—see* Neoplasm, cartilage, malignant

Chondro-osteodysplasia (Morquio-Brailsford type) E76.219

Chondro-osteodystrophy E76.29

Chondro-osteoma *—see* Neoplasm, bone, benign

Chondropathia tuberosa M94.0

Chondrosarcoma *—see* Neoplasm, cartilage, malignant
- juxtacortical *—see* Neoplasm, bone, malignant
- mesenchymal *—see* Neoplasm, connective tissue, malignant
- myxoid *—see* Neoplasm, cartilage, malignant

Chordee (nonvenereal) N48.89
- congenital Q54.4
- gonococcal A54.09

Chorditis (fibrinous) (nodosa) (tuberosa) J38.2

Chordoma *—see* Neoplasm, vertebral (column), malignant

Chorea (chronic) (gravis) (posthemiplegic) (senile) (spasmodic) G25.5
- with
  - heart involvement I02.0
    - active or acute (conditions in I01-) I02.0
    - rheumatic I02.9
      - with valvular disorder I02.0
  - rheumatic heart disease (chronic) (inactive) (quiescent) - code to rheumatic heart condition involved
- drug-induced G25.4
- habit F95.8
- hereditary G10
- Huntington's G10
- hysterical F44.4
- minor I02.9
  - with heart involvement I02.0
- progressive G25.5
  - hereditary G10
- rheumatic (chronic) I02.9
  - with heart involvement I02.0
- Sydenham's I02.9
  - with heart involvement *—see* Chorea, with rheumatic heart disease
  - nonrheumatic G25.5

Choreoathetosis (paroxysmal) G25.5

Chorioadenoma (destruens) D39.2

Chorioamnionitis O41.12-

Chorioangioma D26.7

Choriocarcinoma *—see* Neoplasm, malignant, by site
- combined with
  - embryonal carcinoma *—see* Neoplasm, malignant, by site
  - other germ cell elements *—see* Neoplasm, malignant, by site
  - teratoma *—see* Neoplasm, malignant, by site
- specified site *—see* Neoplasm, malignant, by site
- unspecified site
  - female C58
  - male C62.90

Chorioencephalitis (acute) (lymphocytic) (serous) A87.2

Chorioepithelioma *—see* Choriocarcinoma

Choriomeningitis (acute) (lymphocytic) (serous) A87.2

Chorionepithelioma *—see* Choriocarcinoma

Chorioretinitis *—see also* Inflammation, chorioretinal
- disseminated *—see also* Inflammation, chorioretinal, disseminated
  - in neurosyphilis A52.19
- Egyptian B76.9 *[D63.8]*
- focal *—see also* Inflammation, chorioretinal, focal
- histoplasmic B39.9 *[H32]*
- in (due to)
  - histoplasmosis B39.9 *[H32]*
  - syphilis (secondary) A51.43
    - late A52.71
  - toxoplasmosis (acquired) B58.01
    - congenital (active) P37.1 *[H32]*
  - tuberculosis A18.53
- juxtapapillary, juxtapapillaris *—see* Inflammation, chorioretinal, focal, juxtapapillary
- leprous A30.9 *[H32]*
- miner's B76.9 *[D63.8]*
- progressive myopia (degeneration) (*see also* Myopia, degenerative) H44.2-

Chorioretinitis *(continued)*
- syphilitic (secondary) A51.43
  - congenital (early) A50.01 *[H32]*
    - late A50.32
  - late A52.71
- tuberculous A18.53

Chorioretinopathy, central serous H35.71-

Choroid *—see* condition

Choroideremia H31.21

Choroiditis *—see* Chorioretinitis

Choroidopathy *—see* Disorder, choroid

Choroidoretinitis *—see* Chorioretinitis

Choroidoretinopathy, central serous *—see* Chorioretinopathy, central serous

Christian-Weber disease M35.6

Christmas disease D67

Chromaffinoma *—see also* Neoplasm, benign, by site
- malignant *—see* Neoplasm, malignant, by site

Chromatopsia *—see* Deficiency, color vision

Chromhidrosis, chromidrosis L75.1

Chromoblastomycosis *—see* Chromomycosis

Chromoconversion R82.91

Chromomycosis B43.9
- brain abscess B43.1
- cerebral B43.1
- cutaneous B43.0
- skin B43.0
- specified NEC B43.8
- subcutaneous abscess or cyst B43.2

Chromophytosis B36.0

Chromosome *—see* condition by chromosome involved
- D (1) *—see* condition, chromosome 13
- E (3) *—see* condition, chromosome 18
- G *—see* condition, chromosome 21

Chromotrichomycosis B36.8

Chronic *—see* condition
- fracture *—see* Fracture, pathological

Churg-Strauss syndrome M30.1

Chyle cyst, mesentery I89.8

Chylocele (nonfilarial) I89.8
- filarial (*see also* Infestation, filarial) B74.9 *[N51]*
- tunica vaginalis N50.89
  - filarial (*see also* Infestation, filarial) B74.9 *[N51]*

Chylomicronemia (fasting) (with hyperprebetalipoproteinemia) E78.3

Chylopericardium I31.3
- acute I30.9

Chylothorax (nonfilarial) I89.8
- filarial (*see also* Infestation, filarial) B74.9 *[J91.8]*

Chylous *—see* condition

Chyluria (nonfilarial) R82.0
- due to
  - bilharziasis B65.0
  - Brugia (malayi) B74.1
    - timori B74.2
  - schistosomiasis (bilharziasis) B65.0
  - Wuchereria (bancrofti) B74.0
- filarial *—see* Infestation, filarial

- **Cicatricial** (deformity) *—see* Cicatrix
- **Cicatrix** (adherent) (contracted) (painful) (vicious) (*see also* Scar) L90.5
  - adenoid (and tonsil) J35.8
  - alveolar process M26.79
  - anus K62.89
  - auricle *—see* Disorder, pinna, specified type NEC
  - bile duct (common) (hepatic) K83.8
  - bladder N32.89
  - bone *—see* Disorder, bone, specified type NEC
  - brain G93.89
  - cervix (postoperative) (postpartal) N88.1
  - common duct K83.8
  - cornea H17.9
    - tuberculous A18.59
  - duodenum (bulb), obstructive K31.5
  - esophagus K22.2
  - eyelid *—see* Disorder, eyelid function
  - hypopharynx J39.2
  - lacrimal passages *—see* Obstruction, lacrimal
  - larynx J38.7
  - lung J98.4
  - middle ear H74.8
  - mouth K13.79
  - muscle M62.89
    - with contracture *—see* Contraction, muscle NEC
  - nasopharynx J39.2
  - palate (soft) K13.79
  - penis N48.89
  - pharynx J39.2
  - prostate N42.89
  - rectum K62.89
  - retina *—see* Scar, chorioretinal
  - semilunar cartilage *—see* Derangement, meniscus
  - seminal vesicle N50.89
  - skin L90.5
    - infected L08.89
    - postinfective L90.5
    - tuberculous B90.8
  - specified site NEC L90.5
  - throat J39.2
  - tongue K14.8
  - tonsil (and adenoid) J35.8
  - trachea J39.8
  - tuberculous NEC B90.9
  - urethra N36.8
  - uterus N85.8
  - vagina N89.8
    - postoperative N99.2
  - vocal cord J38.3
  - wrist, constricting (annular) L90.5
- **CIDP** (chronic inflammatory demyelinating polyneuropathy) G61.81
- **CIN** *—see* Neoplasia, intraepithelial, cervix
- **CINCA (chronic infantile neurological, cutaneous and articular syndrome)** M04.2
- **Cinchonism** *—see* Deafness, ototoxic
  - correct substance properly administered *—see* Table of Drugs and Chemicals, by drug, adverse effect
  - overdose or wrong substance given or taken *—see* Table of Drugs and Chemicals, by drug, poisoning
- **Circle of Willis** *—see* condition
- **Circular** *—see* condition
- **Circulating anticoagulants** (*see also* Disorder, hemorrhagic) D68.318
  - due to drugs (*see also* Disorder, hemorrhagic) D68.32
  - following childbirth O72.3
- **Circulation**
  - collateral, any site I99.8
  - defective (lower extremity) I99.9
    - congenital Q28.9
  - embryonic Q28.9
  - failure (peripheral) R57.9
    - newborn P29.89
  - fetal, persistent P29.38
  - heart, incomplete Q28.9
- **Circulatory system** *—see* condition
- **Circulus senilis** (cornea) *—see* Degeneration, cornea, senile
- **Circumcision** (in absence of medical indication) (ritual) (routine) Z41.2
- **Circumscribed** *—see* condition
- **Circumvallate placenta** O43.11-
- **Cirrhosis, cirrhotic** (hepatic) (liver) K74.60
  - alcoholic K70.30
    - with ascites K70.31
  - atrophic *—see* Cirrhosis, liver
  - Baumgarten-Cruveilhier K74.69
  - biliary (cholangiolitic) (cholangitic) (hypertrophic) (obstructive) (pericholangiolitic) K74.5
    - due to
      - Clonorchiasis B66.1
      - flukes B66.3
    - primary K74.3
    - secondary K74.4
  - cardiac (of liver) K76.1
  - Charcot's K74.3
  - cholangiolitic, cholangitic, cholostatic (primary) K74.3
  - congestive K76.1
  - Cruveilhier-Baumgarten K74.69
  - cryptogenic (liver) K74.69
  - due to
    - hepatolenticular degeneration E83.01
    - Wilson's disease E83.01
    - xanthomatosis E78.2
  - fatty K76.0
    - alcoholic K70.0
  - Hanot's (hypertrophic) K74.3
  - hepatic *—see* Cirrhosis, liver
  - hypertrophic K74.3
  - Indian childhood K74.69
  - kidney *—see* Sclerosis, renal
  - Laennec's K70.30
    - with ascites K70.31
    - alcoholic K70.30
      - with ascites K70.31
    - nonalcoholic K74.69
  - liver K74.60
    - alcoholic K70.30
      - with ascites K70.31
      - fatty K70.0
    - congenital P78.81
    - syphilitic A52.74
  - lung (chronic) J84.10
  - macronodular K74.69
    - alcoholic K70.30
      - with ascites K70.31
  - micronodular K74.69
    - alcoholic K70.30
      - with ascites K70.31
  - mixed type K74.69
  - monolobular K74.3
  - nephritis *—see* Sclerosis, renal
  - nutritional K74.69
    - alcoholic K70.30
      - with ascites K70.31
  - obstructive *—see* Cirrhosis, biliary
- **Cirrhosis, cirrhotic** *(continued)*
  - ovarian N83.8
  - pancreas (duct) K86.89
  - pigmentary E83.110
  - portal K74.69
    - alcoholic K70.30
      - with ascites K70.31
  - postnecrotic K74.69
    - alcoholic K70.30
      - with ascites K70.31
  - pulmonary J84.10
  - renal *—see* Sclerosis, renal
  - spleen D73.2
  - stasis K76.1
  - Todd's K74.3
  - unilobar K74.3
  - xanthomatous (biliary) K74.5
    - due to xanthomatosis (familial) (metabolic) (primary) E78.2
- **Cistern, subarachnoid** R93.0
- **Citrullinemia** E72.23
- **Citrullinuria** E72.23
- **Civatte's disease or poikiloderma** L57.3
- **Clam digger's itch** B65.3
- **Clammy skin** R23.1
- **Clap** *—see* Gonorrhea
- **Clarke-Hadfield syndrome** (pancreatic infantilism) K86.89
- **Clark's paralysis** G80.9
- **Clastothrix** L67.8
- **Claude Bernard-Horner syndrome** G90.2
  - traumatic *—see* Injury, nerve, cervical sympathetic
- **Claude's disease or syndrome** G46.3
- **Claudication (intermittent)** I73.9
  - cerebral (artery) G45.9
  - spinal cord (arteriosclerotic) G95.19
    - syphilitic A52.09
  - venous (axillary) I87.8
- **Claudicatio venosa intermittens** I87.8
- **Claustrophobia** F40.240
- **Clavus** (infected) L84
- **Clawfoot** (congenital) Q66.89
  - acquired *—see* Deformity, limb, clawfoot
- **Clawhand** (acquired) *—see also* Deformity, limb, clawhand
  - congenital Q68.1
- **Clawtoe** (congenital) Q66.89
  - acquired *—see* Deformity, toe, specified NEC
- **Clay eating** *—see* Pica
- **Cleansing of artificial opening** *—see* Attention to, artificial, opening
- **Cleft** (congenital) *—see also* Imperfect, closure
  - alveolar process M26.79
  - branchial (persistent) Q18.2
    - cyst Q18.0
      - fistula Q18.0
      - sinus Q18.0
  - cricoid cartilage, posterior Q31.8
  - foot Q72.7
  - hand Q71.6
  - lip (unilateral) Q36.9
    - with cleft palate Q37.9
      - hard Q37.1
        - with soft Q37.5
      - soft Q37.3
        - with hard Q37.5
    - bilateral Q36.0
      - with cleft palate Q37.8
        - hard Q37.0
          - with soft Q37.4
        - soft Q37.2
          - with hard Q37.4
- **Cleft** *(continued)*
  - lip *(continued)*
    - median Q36.1
  - nose Q30.2
  - palate Q35.9
    - with cleft lip (unilateral) Q37.9
      - bilateral Q37.8
    - hard Q35.1
      - with
        - cleft lip (unilateral) Q37.1
          - bilateral Q37.0
        - soft Q35.5
          - with cleft lip (unilateral) Q37.5
            - bilateral Q37.4
    - medial Q35.5
    - soft Q35.3
      - with
        - cleft lip (unilateral) Q37.3
          - bilateral Q37.2
        - hard Q35.5
          - with cleft lip (unilateral) Q37.5
            - bilateral Q37.4
  - penis Q55.69
  - scrotum Q55.29
  - thyroid cartilage Q31.8
  - uvula Q35.7
- **Cleidocranial dysostosis** Q74.0
- **Cleptomania** F63.2
- **Clicking hip** (newborn) R29.4
- **Climacteric** (female) *—see also* Menopause
  - arthritis (any site) NEC *—see* Arthritis, specified form NEC
  - depression (single episode) F32.89
    - recurrent episode F33.8
  - melancholia (single episodie) F32.89
    - recurrent episode F33.8
  - male (symptoms) (syndrome) NEC N50.89
  - paranoid state F22
  - polyarthritis NEC *—see* Arthritis, specified form NEC
  - symptoms (female) N95.1
- **Clinical research investigation** (clinical trial) (control subject) (normal comparison) (participant) Z00.6
- **Clitoris** *—see* condition
- **Cloaca** (persistent) Q43.7
- **Clonorchiasis, clonorchis infection** (liver) B66.1
- **Clonus** R25.8
- **Closed bite** M26.29
- **Clostridium** (C.) **perfringens, as cause of disease classified elsewhere** B96.7
- **Closure**
  - congenital, nose Q30.0
  - cranial sutures, premature Q75.0
  - defective or imperfect NEC *—see* Imperfect, closure
  - fistula, delayed *—see* Fistula
  - foramen ovale, imperfect Q21.1
  - hymen N89.6
  - interauricular septum, defective Q21.1
  - interventricular septum, defective Q21.0
  - lacrimal duct *—see also* Stenosis, lacrimal, duct
    - congenital Q10.5
  - nose (congenital) Q30.0
    - acquired M95.0
  - of artificial opening *—see* Attention to, artificial, opening
  - primary angle, without glaucoma damage H40.06-

Closure *(continued)*
- vagina N89.5
- valve *—see* Endocarditis
- vulva N90.5

Clot (blood) *—see also* Embolism
- artery (obstruction) (occlusion) *—see* Embolism
- bladder N32.89
- brain (intradural or extradural) *—see* Occlusion, artery, cerebral
- circulation I74.9
- heart *—see also* Infarct, myocardium
  - not resulting in infarction I51.3
- vein *—see* Thrombosis

Clouded state R40.1
- epileptic *—see* Epilepsy, specified NEC
- paroxysmal *—see* Epilepsy, specified NEC

Cloudy antrum, antra J32.0

Clouston's (hidrotic) **ectodermal dysplasia** Q82.4

Clubbed nail pachydermoperiostosis M89.40 *[L62]*

Clubbing of finger(s) (nails) R68.3

Clubfinger R68.3
- congenital Q68.1

Clubfoot (congenital) Q66.89
- acquired *—see* Deformity, limb, clubfoot
- equinovarus Q66.0
- paralytic *—see* Deformity, limb, clubfoot

Clubhand (congenital) (radial) Q71.4-
- acquired *—see* Deformity, limb, clubhand

Clubnail R68.3
- congenital Q84.6

Clump, kidney Q63.1

Clumsiness, clumsy child syndrome F82

Cluttering F80.81

Clutton's joints A50.51 *[M12.80]*

Coagulation, intravascular (diffuse) (disseminated) *—see also* Defibrination syndrome
- complicating abortion *—see* Abortion, by type, complicated by, intravascular coagulation
- following ectopic or molar pregnancy O08.1

Coagulopathy *—see also* Defect, coagulation
- consumption D65
- intravascular D65
  - newborn P60

Coalition
- calcaneo-scaphoid Q66.89
- tarsal Q66.89

Coalminer's
- elbow *—see* Bursitis, elbow, olecranon
- lung or pneumoconiosis J60

Coalworker's lung or pneumoconiosis J60

Coarctation
- aorta (preductal) (postductal) Q25.1
- pulmonary artery Q25.71

Coated tongue K14.3

Coats' disease (exudative retinopathy) *—see* Retinopathy, exudative

Cocaine-induced
- anxiety disorder F14.980
- bipolar and related disorder F14.94
- depressive disorder F14.94

Cocaine-induced *(continued)*
- obsessive-compulsive and related disorder F14.988
- psychotic disorder F14.959
- sleep disorder F14.982
- sexual dysfunction F14.981

Cocainism *—see* Disorder, cocaine use

Coccidioidomycosis B38.9
- cutaneous B38.3
- disseminated B38.7
- generalized B38.7
- meninges B38.4
- prostate B38.81
- pulmonary B38.2
  - acute B38.0
  - chronic B38.1
- skin B38.3
- specified NEC B38.89

Coccidioidosis *—see* Coccidioidomycosis

Coccidiosis (intestinal) A07.3

Coccydynia, coccygodynia M53.3

Coccyx *—see* condition

Cochin-China diarrhea K90.1

Cockayne's syndrome Q87.1

Cocked up toe *—see* Deformity, toe, specified NEC

Cock's peculiar tumor L72.3

Codman's tumor *—see* Neoplasm, bone, benign

Coenurosis B71.8

Coffee-worker's lung J67.8

Cogan's syndrome H16.32-
- oculomotor apraxia H51.8

Coitus, painful (female) N94.10
- male N53.12
- psychogenic F52.6

Cold J00
- with influenza, flu, or grippe *—see* Influenza, with, respiratory manifestations NEC
- agglutinin disease or hemoglobinuria (chronic) D59.1
- bronchial *—see* Bronchitis
- chest *—see* Bronchitis
- common (head) J00
- effects of T69.9
  - specified effect NEC T69.8
- excessive, effects of T69.9
  - specified effect NEC T69.8
- exhaustion from T69.8
- exposure to T69.9
  - specified effect NEC T69.8
- head J00
- injury syndrome (newborn) P80.0
- on lung *—see* Bronchitis
- rose J30.1
- sensitivity, auto-immune D59.1
- symptoms J00
- virus J00

Coldsore B00.1

Colibacillosis A49.8
- as the cause of other disease (*see also* Escherichia coli) B96.20
- generalized A41.50

Colic (bilious) (infantile) (intestinal) (recurrent) (spasmodic) R10.83
- abdomen R10.83
  - psychogenic F45.8
- appendix, appendicular K38.8
- bile duct *—see* Calculus, bile duct
- biliary *—see* Calculus, bile duct
- common duct *—see* Calculus, bile duct

Colic *(continued)*
- cystic duct *—see* Calculus, gallbladder
- Devonshire NEC *—see* Poisoning, lead
- gallbladder *—see* Calculus, gallbladder
- gallstone *—see* Calculus, gallbladder
  - gallbladder or cystic duct *—see* Calculus, gallbladder
- hepatic (duct) *—see* Calculus, bile duct
- hysterical F45.8
- kidney N23
- lead NEC *—see* Poisoning, lead
- mucous K58.9
  - with diarrhea K58.0
  - psychogenic F54
- nephritic N23
- painter's NEC *—see* Poisoning, lead
- pancreas K86.89
- psychogenic F45.8
- renal N23
- saturnine NEC *—see* Poisoning, lead
- ureter N23
- urethral N36.8
  - due to calculus N21.1
- uterus NEC N94.89
  - menstrual *—see* Dysmenorrhea
- worm NOS B83.9

Colicystitis *—see* Cystitis

Colitis (acute) (catarrhal) (chronic) (noninfective) (hemorrhagic) (*see also* Enteritis) K52.9
- allergic K52.29
  - with
    - food protein-induced enterocolitis syndrome K52.21
    - proctocolitis K52.82
- amebic (acute) (*see also* Amebiasis) A06.0
  - nondysenteric A06.2
- anthrax A22.2
- bacillary *—see* Infection, Shigella
- balantidial A07.0
- Clostridium difficile
  - not specified as recurrent A04.72
  - recurrent A04.71
- coccidial A07.3
- collagenous K52.831
- cystica superficialis K52.89
- dietary counseling and surveillance (for) Z71.3
- dietetic (*see also* Colitis, allergic) K52.29
- drug-induced K52.1
- due to radiation K52.0
- eosinophilic K52.82
- food hypersensitivity (*see also* Colitis, allergic) K52.29
- giardial A07.1
- granulomatous *—see* Enteritis, regional, large intestine
- indeterminate, so stated K52.3
- infectious *—see* Enteritis, infectious
- ischemic K55.9
  - acute (subacute) (*see also* Ischemia, intestine, acute) K55.039
  - chronic K55.1
  - due to mesenteric artery insufficiency K55.1
  - fulminant (acute) (*see also* Ischemia, intestine, acute) K55.039
- left sided K51.50
  - with
    - abscess K51.514
    - complication K51.519
      - specified NEC K51.518
    - fistula K51.513
    - obstruction K51.512
    - rectal bleeding K51.511
- lymphocytic K52.832

Colitis *(continued)*
- membranous
  - psychogenic F54
- microscopic K52.839
  - specified NEC K52.838
- mucous *—see* Syndrome, irritable, bowel
  - psychogenic F54
- noninfective K52.9
  - specified NEC K52.89
- polyposa *—see* Polyp, colon, inflammatory
- protozoal A07.9
- pseudomembranous
  - not specified as recurrent A04.72
  - recurrent A04.71
- pseudomucinous *—see* Syndrome, irritable, bowel
- regional *—see* Enteritis, regional, large intestine
  - infectious A09
- segmental *—see* Enteritis, regional, large intestine
- septic *—see* Enteritis, infectious
- spastic K58.9
  - with diarrhea K58.0
  - psychogenic F54
- staphylococcal A04.8
  - foodborne A05.0
- subacute ischemic (*see also* Ischemia, intestine, acute) K55.039
- thromboulcerative (*see also* Ischemia, intestine, acute) K55.039
- toxic NEC K52.1
  - due to Clostridium difficile
    - not specified as recurrent A04.72
    - recurrent A04.71
- transmural *—see* Enteritis, regional, large intestine
- trichomonal A07.8
- tuberculous (ulcerative) A18.32
- ulcerative (chronic) K51.90
  - with
    - complication K51.919
      - abscess K51.914
      - fistula K51.913
      - obstruction K51.912
      - rectal bleeding K51.911
      - specified complication NEC K51.918
  - enterocolitis *—see* Enterocolitis, ulcerative
  - ileocolitis *—see* Ileocolitis, ulcerative
  - mucosal proctocolitis *—see* Proctocolitis, mucosal
  - proctitis *—see* Proctitis, ulcerative
  - pseudopolyposis *—see* Polyp, colon, inflammatory
  - psychogenic F54
  - rectosigmoiditis *—see* Rectosigmoiditis, ulcerative
  - specified type NEC K51.80
    - with
      - complication K51.819
        - abscess K51.814
        - fistula K51.813
        - obstruction K51.812
        - rectal bleeding K51.811
        - specified complication NEC K51.818

Collagenosis, collagen disease (nonvascular) (vascular) M35.9
- cardiovascular I42.8
- reactive perforating L87.1
- specified NEC M35.8

Collapse R55
- adrenal E27.2
- cardiorespiratory R57.0
- cardiovascular R57.0
  - newborn P29.89

Collapse *(continued)*
- circulatory (peripheral) R57.9
  - during or after labor and delivery O75.1
  - following ectopic or molar pregnancy O08.3
  - newborn P29.89
- during or
  - after labor and delivery O75.1
  - resulting from a procedure, not elsewhere classified T81.10
- external ear canal *—see* Stenosis, external ear canal
- general R55
- heart *—see* Disease, heart
- heat T67.1
- hysterical F44.89
- labyrinth, membranous (congenital) Q16.5
- lung (massive) (*see also* Atelectasis) J98.19
  - pressure due to anesthesia (general) (local) or other sedation T88.2
    - during labor and delivery O74.1
    - in pregnancy O29.02-
    - postpartum, puerperal O89.09
- myocardial *—see* Disease, heart
- nervous F48.8
- neurocirculatory F45.8
- nose M95.0
- postoperative T81.10
- pulmonary (*see also* Atelectasis) J98.19
  - newborn *—see* Atelectasis
- trachea J39.8
- tracheobronchial J98.09
- valvular *—see* Endocarditis
- vascular (peripheral) R57.9
  - during or after labor and delivery O75.1
  - following ectopic or molar pregnancy O08.3
  - newborn P29.89
- vertebra M48.50-
  - cervical region M48.52-
  - cervicothoracic region M48.53-
  - in (due to)
    - metastasis *—see* Collapse, vertebra, in, specified disease NEC
    - osteoporosis (*see also* Osteoporosis) M80.88
      - cervical region M80.88
      - cervicothoracic region M80.88
      - lumbar region M80.88
      - lumbosacral region M80.88
      - multiple sites M80.88
      - occipito-atlanto-axial region M80.88
      - sacrococcygeal region M80.88
      - thoracic region M80.88
      - thoracolumbar region M80.88
    - specified disease NEC M48.50-
      - cervical region M48.52-
      - cervicothoracic region M48.53-
      - lumbar region M48.56-
      - lumbosacral region M48.57-
      - occipito-atlanto-axial region M48.51-
      - sacrococcygeal region M48.58-
      - thoracic region M48.54-
      - thoracolumbar region M48.55-
  - lumbar region M48.56-
  - lumbosacral region M48.57-
  - occipito-atlanto-axial region M48.51-
  - sacrococcygeal region M48.58-

Collapse *(continued)*
- vertebra *(continued)*
  - thoracic region M48.54-
  - thoracolumbar region M48.55-

Collateral *—see also* condition
- circulation (venous) I87.8
- dilation, veins I87.8

Colles' fracture S52.53-

Collet (-Sicard) **syndrome** G52.7

Collier's asthma or lung J60

Collodion baby Q80.2

Colloid nodule (of thyroid) (cystic) E04.1

Coloboma (iris) Q13.0
- eyelid Q10.3
- fundus Q14.8
- lens Q12.2
- optic disc (congenital) Q14.2
  - acquired H47.31-

Coloenteritis *—see* Enteritis

Colon *—see* condition

Colonization
- MRSA (Methicillin resistant Staphylococcus aureus) Z22.322
- MSSA (Methicillin susceptible Staphylococcus aureus) Z22.321
- status *—see* Carrier (suspected) of

Coloptosis K63.4

Color blindness *—see* Deficiency, color vision

Colostomy
- attention to Z43.3
- fitting or adjustment Z46.89
- malfunctioning K94.03
- status Z93.3

Colpitis (acute) *—see* Vaginitis

Colpocele N81.5

Colpocystitis *—see* Vaginitis

Colpospasm N94.2

Column, spinal, vertebral *—see* condition

Coma R40.20
- with
  - motor response (none) R40.231
    - abnormal R40.233
    - abnormal extensor posturing to pain or noxious stimuli (<2 years of age) R40.232
    - abnormal flexure posturing to pain or noxious stimuli (0-5 years of age) R40.233
    - extension R40.232
    - extensor posturing to pain or noxious stimuli (2-5 years of age) R40.232
    - flexion/decorticate posturing (<2 years of age) R40.233
    - flexion withdrawal R40.234
    - localizes pain (2-5 years of age) R40.235
    - normal or spontaneous movement (<2 years of age) R40.236
    - abnormal flexure posturing to pain or noxious stimuli (0-5 years of age) R40.233
    - obeys commands (2-5 years of age) R40.236
    - withdraws from pain or noxious stimuli (0-5 years of age) R40.234
    - withdraws to touch (<2 years of age) R40.235
  - opening of eyes (never) R40.211
    - in response to
      - pain R40.212
      - sound R40.213
    - spontaneous R40.214

Coma *(continued)*
- with *(continued)*
  - verbal response (none) R40.221
    - confused conversation R40.224
    - cooing or babbling or crying appropriately (<2 years of age) R40.225
    - inappropriate crying or screaming (<2 years of age) R40.223
    - inappropriate words (2-5 years of age) R40.224
    - incomprehensible sounds (2-5 years of age) R40.222
    - incomprehensible words R40.222
    - irritable cries (<2 years of age) R40.224
    - moans/grunts to pain; restless (<2 years of age) R40.222
    - oriented R40.225
    - screaming (2-5 years of age) R40.223
    - uses appropriate words (2-5 years of age) R40.225
- eclamptic *—see* Eclampsia
- epileptic *—see* Epilepsy
- Glasgow, scale score *—see* Glasgow coma scale
- hepatic *—see* Failure, hepatic, by type, with coma
- hyperglycemic (diabetic) *—see* Diabetes, by type, with hyperosmolarity, with coma
- hyperosmolar (diabetic) *—see* Diabetes, by type, with hyperosmolarity, with coma
- hypoglycemic (diabetic) *—see* Diabetes, by type, with hypoglycemia, with coma
  - nondiabetic E15
- in diabetes *—see* Diabetes, coma
- insulin-induced *—see* Coma, hypoglycemic
- ketoacidotic (diabetic) - *see* Diabetes, by type, with ketoacidosis, with coma
- myxedematous E03.5
- newborn P91.5
- persistent vegetative state R40.3
- specified NEC, without documented Glasgow coma scale score, or with partial Glasgow coma scale score reported R40.244

Comatose *—see* Coma

Combat fatigue F43.0

Combined *—see* condition

Comedo, comedones (giant) L70.0

Comedocarcinoma *—see also* Neoplasm, breast, malignant
- noninfiltrating
  - breast D05.8-
  - specified site *—see* Neoplasm, in situ, by site
  - unspecified site D05.8-

Comedomastitis *—see* Ectasia, mammary duct

Comminuted fracture - code as Fracture, closed

Common
- arterial trunk Q20.0
- atrioventricular canal Q21.2
- atrium Q21.1
- cold (head) J00
- truncus (arteriosus) Q20.0
- variable immunodeficiency *—see* Immunodeficiency, common variable
- ventricle Q20.4

Commotio, commotion (current)
- brain *—see* Injury, intracranial, concussion
- cerebri *—see* Injury, intracranial, concussion
- retinae S05.8X-
- spinal cord *—see* Injury, spinal cord, by region
- spinalis *—see* Injury, spinal cord, by region

Communication
- between
  - base of aorta and pulmonary artery Q21.4
  - left ventricle and right atrium Q20.5
  - pericardial sac and pleural sac Q34.8
  - pulmonary artery and pulmonary vein, congenital Q25.72
- congenital between uterus and digestive or urinary tract Q51.7

Compartment syndrome (deep) (posterior) (traumatic) T79.A0
- abdomen T79.A3
- lower extremity (hip, buttock, thigh, leg, foot, toes) T79.A2
- nontraumatic
  - abdomen M79.A3
  - lower extremity (hip, buttock, thigh, leg, foot, toes) M79.A2-
  - specified site NEC M79.A9
  - upper extremity (shoulder, arm, forearm, wrist, hand, fingers) M79.A1-
- specified site NEC T79.A9
- upper extremity (shoulder, arm, forearm, wrist, hand, fingers) T79.A1

Compensation
- failure *—see* Disease, heart
- neurosis, psychoneurosis *—see* Disorder, factitious

Complaint *—see also* Disease
- bowel, functional K59.9
  - psychogenic F45.8
- intestine, functional K59.9
  - psychogenic F45.8
- kidney *—see* Disease, renal
- miners' J60

Complete *—see* condition

Complex
- Addison-Schilder E71.528
- cardiorenal *—see* Hypertension, cardiorenal
- Costen's M26.69
- disseminated mycobacterium avium-intracellulare (DMAC) A31.2
- Eisenmenger's (ventricular septal defect) I27.83
- hypersexual F52.8
- jumped process, spine *—see* Dislocation, vertebra
- primary, tuberculous A15.7
- Schilder-Addison E71.528
- subluxation (vertebral) M99.19
  - abdomen M99.19
  - acromioclavicular M99.17
  - cervical region M99.11
  - cervicothoracic M99.11
  - costochondral M99.18
  - costovertebral M99.18
  - head region M99.10
  - hip M99.15
  - lower extremity M99.16
  - lumbar region M99.13
  - lumbosacral M99.13
  - occipitocervical M99.10
  - pelvic region M99.15
  - pubic M99.15

Complex *(continued)*
subluxation *(continued)*
rib cage M99.18
sacral region M99.14
sacrococcygeal M99.14
sacroiliac M99.14
specified NEC M99.19
sternochondral M99.18
sternoclavicular M99.17
thoracic region M99.12
thoracolumbar M99.12
upper extremity M99.17
Taussig-Bing (transposition, aorta and overriding pulmonary artery) Q20.1

Complication(s) (from) (of)
accidental puncture or laceration during a procedure (of) *—see* Complications, intraoperative (intraprocedural), puncture or laceration
amputation stump (surgical) (late) NEC T87.9
dehiscence T87.81
infection or inflammation T87.40
lower limb T87.4-
upper limb T87.4-
necrosis T87.50
lower limb T87.5-
upper limb T87.5-
neuroma T87.30
lower limb T87.3-
upper limb T87.3-
specified type NEC T87.89
anastomosis (and bypass) *—see also* Complications, prosthetic device or implant
intestinal (internal) NEC K91.89
involving urinary tract N99.89
urinary tract (involving intestinal tract) N99.89
vascular *—see* Complications, cardiovascular device or implant
anesthesia, anesthetic (*see also* Anesthesia, complication) T88.59
general, unintended awareness during procedure T88.53
unintended awareness under general anesthesia during procedure T88.53
brain, postpartum, puerperal O89.2
cardiac
in
labor and delivery O74.2
pregnancy O29.19-
postpartum, puerperal O89.1
central nervous system
in
labor and delivery O74.3
pregnancy O29.29-
postpartum, puerperal O89.2
difficult or failed intubation T88.4
in pregnancy O29.6-
failed sedation (conscious) (moderate) during procedure T88.52
hyperthermia, malignant T88.3
hypothermia T88.51
intubation failure T88.4
malignant hyperthermia T88.3
pulmonary
in
labor and delivery O74.1
pregnancy NEC O29.09-
postpartum, puerperal O89.09
shock T88.2

Complication *(continued)*
anesthesia, anesthetic *(continued)*
spinal and epidural
in
labor and delivery NEC O74.6
headache O74.5
pregnancy NEC O29.5X-
postpartum, puerperal NEC O89.5
headache O89.4
anti-reflux device *—see* Complications, esophageal anti-reflux device
aortic (bifurcation) graft *—see* Complications, graft, vascular
aortocoronary (bypass) graft *—see* Complications, coronary artery (bypass) graft
aortofemoral (bypass) graft *—see* Complications, extremity artery (bypass) graft
arteriovenous
fistula, surgically created T82.9
embolism T82.818
fibrosis T82.828
hemorrhage T82.838
infection or inflammation T82.7
mechanical
breakdown T82.510
displacement T82.520
leakage T82.530
malposition T82.520
obstruction T82.590
perforation T82.590
protrusion T82.590
pain T82.848
specified type NEC T82.898
stenosis T82.858
thrombosis T82.868
shunt, surgically created T82.9
embolism T82.818
fibrosis T82.828
hemorrhage T82.838
infection or inflammation T82.7
mechanical
breakdown T82.511
displacement T82.521
leakage T82.531
malposition T82.521
obstruction T82.591
perforation T82.591
protrusion T82.591
pain T82.848
specified type NEC T82.898
stenosis T82.858
thrombosis T82.868
arthroplasty *—see* Complications, joint prosthesis
artificial
fertilization or insemination N98.9
attempted introduction (of)
embryo in embryo transfer N98.3
ovum following in vitro fertilization N98.2
hyperstimulation of ovaries N98.1
infection N98.0
specified NEC N98.8
heart T82.9
embolism T82.817
fibrosis T82.827
hemorrhage T82.837
infection or inflammation T82.7
mechanical
breakdown T82.512
displacement T82.522
leakage T82.532
malposition T82.522
obstruction T82.592
perforation T82.592
protrusion T82.592

Complication *(continued)*
artificial *(continued)*
heart *(continued)*
pain T82.847
specified type NEC T82.897
stenosis T82.857
thrombosis T82.867
opening
cecostomy *—see* Complications, colostomy
colostomy *—see* Complications, colostomy
cystostomy *—see* Complications, cystostomy
enterostomy *—see* Complications, enterostomy
gastrostomy *—see* Complications, gastrostomy
ileostomy *—see* Complications, enterostomy
jejunostomy *—see* Complications, enterostomy
nephrostomy *—see* Complications, stoma, urinary tract
tracheostomy *—see* Complications, tracheostomy
ureterostomy *—see* Complications, stoma, urinary tract
urethrostomy *—see* Complications, stoma, urinary tract
balloon implant or device
gastrointestinal T85.9
embolism T85.818
fibrosis T85.828
hemorrhage T85.838
infection and inflammation T85.79
pain T85.848
specified type NEC T85.898
stenosis T85.858
thrombosis T85.868
vascular (counterpulsation) T82.9
embolism T82.818
fibrosis T82.828
hemorrhage T82.838
infection or inflammation T82.7
mechanical
breakdown T82.513
displacement T82.523
leakage T82.533
malposition T82.523
obstruction T82.593
perforation T82.593
protrusion T82.593
pain T82.848
specified type NEC T82.898
stenosis T82.858
thrombosis T82.868
bariatric procedure
gastric band procedure K95.09
infection K95.01
specified procedure NEC K95.89
infection K95.81
bile duct implant (prosthetic) T85.9
embolism T85.818
fibrosis T85.828
hemorrhage T85.838
infection and inflammation T85.79
mechanical
breakdown T85.510
displacement T85.520
malfunction T85.510
malposition T85.520
obstruction T85.590
perforation T85.590
protrusion T85.590
specified NEC T85.590
pain T85.848
specified type NEC T85.898

Complication *(continued)*
bile duct implant *(continued)*
stenosis T85.858
thrombosis T85.868
bladder device (auxiliary) *—see* Complications, genitourinary, device or implant, urinary system
bleeding (postoperative) *—see* Complication, postoperative, hemorrhage
intraoperative *—see* Complication, intraoperative, hemorrhage
blood vessel graft *—see* Complications, graft, vascular
bone
device NEC T84.9
embolism T84.81
fibrosis T84.82
hemorrhage T84.83
infection or inflammation T84.7
mechanical
breakdown T84.318
displacement T84.328
malposition T84.328
obstruction T84.398
perforation T84.398
protrusion T84.398
pain T84.84
specified type NEC T84.89
stenosis T84.85
thrombosis T84.86
graft *—see* Complications, graft, bone
growth stimulator (electrode) *—see* Complications, electronic stimulator device, bone
marrow transplant *—see* Complications, transplant, bone, marrow
brain neurostimulator (electrode) *—see* Complications, electronic stimulator device, brain
breast implant (prosthetic) T85.9
capsular contracture T85.44
embolism T85.818
fibrosis T85.828
hemorrhage T85.838
infection and inflammation T85.79
mechanical
breakdown T85.41
displacement T85.42
leakage T85.43
malposition T85.42
obstruction T85.49
perforation T85.49
protrusion T85.49
specified NEC T85.49
pain T85.848
specified type NEC T85.898
stenosis T85.858
thrombosis T85.868
bypass *—see also* Complications, prosthetic device or implant
aortocoronary *—see* Complications, coronary artery (bypass) graft
arterial *—see also* Complications, graft, vascular
extremity *—see* Complications, extremity artery (bypass) graft
cardiac *—see also* Disease, heart
device, implant or graft T82.9
embolism T82.817
fibrosis T82.827
hemorrhage T82.837
infection or inflammation T82.7
valve prosthesis T82.6
mechanical
breakdown T82.519
specified device NEC T82.518

Complication *(continued)*
cardiac *(continued)*
device, implant or graft *(continued)*
mechanical *(continued)*
displacement T82.529
specified device NEC T82.528
leakage T82.539
specified device NEC T82.538
malposition T82.529
specified device NEC T82.528
obstruction T82.599
specified device NEC T82.598
perforation T82.599
specified device NEC T82.598
protrusion T82.599
specified device NEC T82.598
pain T82.847
specified type NEC T82.897
stenosis T82.857
thrombosis T82.867
cardiovascular device, graft or implant T82.9
aortic graft *—see* Complications, graft, vascular
arteriovenous
fistula, artificial *—see* Complication, arteriovenous, fistula, surgically created
shunt *—see* Complication, arteriovenous, shunt, surgically created
artificial heart *—see* Complication, artificial, heart
balloon (counterpulsation) device *—see* Complication, balloon implant, vascular
carotid artery graft *—see* Complications, graft, vascular
coronary bypass graft *—see* Complication, coronary artery (bypass) graft
dialysis catheter (vascular) *—see* Complication, catheter, dialysis
electronic T82.9
electrode T82.9
embolism T82.817
fibrosis T82.827
hemorrhage T82.837
infection T82.7
mechanical
breakdown T82.110
displacement T82.120
leakage T82.190
obstruction T82.190
perforation T82.190
protrusion T82.190
specified type NEC T82.190
pain T82.847
specified NEC T82.897
stenosis T82.857
thrombosis T82.867
embolism T82.817
fibrosis T82.827
hemorrhage T82.837
infection T82.7
mechanical
breakdown T82.119
displacement T82.129
leakage T82.199
obstruction T82.199
perforation T82.199
protrusion T82.199
specified type NEC T82.199

Complication *(continued)*
cardiovascular device, graft or implant *(continued)*
electronic *(continued)*
pain T82.847
pulse generator T82.9
embolism T82.817
fibrosis T82.827
hemorrhage T82.837
infection T82.7
mechanical
breakdown T82.111
displacement T82.121
leakage T82.191
obstruction T82.191
perforation T82.191
protrusion T82.191
specified type NEC T82.191
pain T82.847
specified NEC T82.897
stenosis T82.857
thrombosis T82.867
specified condition NEC T82.897
specified device NEC T82.9
embolism T82.817
fibrosis T82.827
hemorrhage T82.837
infection T82.7
mechanical
breakdown T82.118
displacement T82.128
leakage T82.198
obstruction T82.198
perforation T82.198
protrusion T82.198
specified type NEC T82.198
pain T82.847
specified NEC T82.897
stenosis T82.857
thrombosis T82.867
stenosis T82.857
thrombosis T82.867
extremity artery graft *—see* Complication, extremity artery (bypass) graft
femoral artery graft *—see* Complication, extremity artery (bypass) graft
heart-lung transplant *—see* Complication, transplant, heart, with lung
heart
transplant *—see* Complication, transplant, heart
valve *—see* Complication, prosthetic device, heart valve
graft *—see* Complication, heart, valve, graft
infection or inflammation T82.7
umbrella device *—see* Complication, umbrella device, vascular
vascular graft (or anastomosis) *—see* Complication, graft, vascular
carotid artery (bypass) graft *—see* Complications, graft, vascular
catheter (device) NEC *—see also* Complications, prosthetic device or implant
cranial infusion
infection and inflammation T85.735
mechanical
breakdown T85.610
displacement T85.620
leakage T85.630
malfunction T85.690
malposition T85.620
obstruction T85.690
perforation T85.690
protrusion T85.690
specified NEC T85.690

Complication *(continued)*
catheter *(continued)*
cystostomy T83.9
embolism T83.81
fibrosis T83.82
hemorrhage T83.83
infection and inflammation T83.510
mechanical
breakdown T83.010
displacement T83.020
leakage T83.030
malposition T83.020
obstruction T83.090
perforation T83.090
protrusion T83.090
specified NEC T83.090
pain T83.84
specified type NEC T83.89
stenosis T83.85
thrombosis T83.86
dialysis (vascular) T82.9
embolism T82.818
fibrosis T82.828
hemorrhage T82.838
infection and inflammation T82.7
intraperitoneal *—see* Complications, catheter, intraperitoneal
mechanical
breakdown T82.41
displacement T82.42
leakage T82.43
malposition T82.42
obstruction T82.49
perforation T82.49
protrusion T82.49
pain T82.848
specified type NEC T82.898
stenosis T82.858
thrombosis T82.868
epidural infusion T85.9
embolism T85.810
fibrosis T85.820
hemorrhage T85.830
infection and inflammation T85.735
mechanical
breakdown T85.610
displacement T85.620
leakage T85.630
malfunction T85.610
malposition T85.620
obstruction T85.690
perforation T85.690
protrusion T85.690
specified NEC T85.690
pain T85.840
specified type NEC T85.890
stenosis T85.850
thrombosis T85.860
intraperitoneal dialysis T85.9
embolism T85.818
fibrosis T85.828
hemorrhage T85.838
infection and inflammation T85.735
mechanical
breakdown T85.611
displacement T85.621
leakage T85.631
malfunction T85.611
malposition T85.621
obstruction T85.691
perforation T85.691
protrusion T85.691
specified NEC T85.691
pain T85.848
specified type NEC T85.898
stenosis T85.858
thrombosis T85.868

Complication *(continued)*
catheter *(continued)*
intrathecal infusion
infection and inflammation T85.735
mechanical
breakdown T85.610
displacement T85.620
leakage T85.630
malfunction T85.690
malposition T85.620
obstruction T85.690
perforation T85.690
protrusion T85.690
specified NEC T85.690
intravenous infusion T82.9
embolism T82.818
fibrosis T82.828
hemorrhage T82.838
infection or inflammation T82.7
mechanical
breakdown T82.514
displacement T82.524
leakage T82.534
malposition T82.524
obstruction T82.594
perforation T82.594
protrusion T82.594
pain T82.848
specified type NEC T82.898
stenosis T82.858
thrombosis T82.868
spinal infusion
infection and inflammation T85.735
mechanical
breakdown T85.610
displacement T85.620
leakage T85.630
malfunction T85.690
malposition T85.620
obstruction T85.690
perforation T85.690
protrusion T85.690
specified NEC T85.690
subarachnoid infusion
infection and inflammation T85.735
mechanical
breakdown T85.610
displacement T85.620
leakage T85.630
malfunction T85.690
malposition T85.620
obstruction T85.690
perforation T85.690
protrusion T85.690
specified NEC T85.690
subdural infusion T85.9
embolism T85.810
fibrosis T85.820
hemorrhage T85.830
infection and inflammation T85.735
mechanical
breakdown T85.610
displacement T85.620
leakage T85.630
malfunction T85.610
malposition T85.620
obstruction T85.690
perforation T85.690
protrusion T85.690
specified NEC T85.690
pain T85.840
specified type NEC T85.890
stenosis T85.850
thrombosis T85.860
urethral T83.9
displacement T83.028
embolism T83.81

catheter (continued)
urethral (continued)
fibrosis T83.82
hemorrhage T83.83
indwelling
breakdown T83.011
displacement T83.021
infection and inflammation T83.511
leakage T83.031
specified complication NEC T83.091
infection and inflammation T83.511
leakage T83.038
malposition T83.028
mechanical
breakdown T83.011
obstruction (mechanical) T83.091
pain T83.84
perforation T83.091
protrusion T83.091
specified type NEC T83.091
stenosis T83.85
thrombosis T83.86
urinary NEC
breakdown T83.018
displacement T83.028
infection and inflammation T83.518
leakage T83.038
specified complication NEC T83.098
cecostomy (stoma) *—see* Complications, colostomy
cesarean delivery wound NEC O90.89
disruption O90.0
hematoma O90.2
infection (following delivery) O86.0
chemotherapy (antineoplastic) NEC T88.7
chin implant (prosthetic) *—see* Complication, prosthetic device or implant, specified NEC
circulatory system I99.8
intraoperative I97.88
postprocedural I97.89
following cardiac surgery (*see also* Infarct, myocardium, associated with revascularization procedure) I97.19-
postcardiotomy syndrome I97.0
hypertension I97.3
lymphedema after mastectomy I97.2
postcardiotomy syndrome I97.0
seroma - *see* Complications, postprocedural, seroma (of), mastoid process
specified NEC I97.89
colostomy (stoma) K94.00
hemorrhage K94.01
infection K94.02
malfunction K94.03
mechanical K94.03
specified complication NEC K94.09
contraceptive device, intrauterine *—see* Complications, intrauterine, contraceptive device
cord (umbilical) *—see* Complications, umbilical cord
corneal graft *—see* Complications, graft, cornea
coronary artery (bypass) graft T82.9
atherosclerosis *—see* Arteriosclerosis, coronary (artery),
embolism T82.818

coronary artery (bypass) graft *(continued)*
fibrosis T82.828
hemorrhage T82.838
infection and inflammation T82.7
mechanical
breakdown T82.211
displacement T82.212
leakage T82.213
malposition T82.212
obstruction T82.218
perforation T82.218
protrusion T82.218
specified NEC T82.218
pain T82.848
specified type NEC T82.898
stenosis T82.858
thrombosis T82.868
counterpulsation device (balloon), intra- aortic *—see* Complications, balloon implant, vascular
cystostomy (stoma) N99.518
catheter *—see* Complications, catheter, cystostomy
hemorrhage N99.510
infection N99.511
malfunction N99.512
specified type NEC N99.518
delivery (*see also* Complications, obstetric) O75.9
procedure (instrumental) (manual) (surgical) O75.4
specified NEC O75.89
dialysis (peritoneal) (renal) *—see also* Complications, infusion
catheter (vascular) *—see* Complication, catheter, dialysis
peritoneal, intraperitoneal *—see* Complications, catheter, intraperitoneal
dorsal column (spinal)
neurostimulator *—see* Complications, electronic stimulator device, spinal cord
drug NEC T88.7
ear procedure *—see also* Disorder, ear
intraoperative H95.88
hematoma *—see* Complications, intraoperative, hemorrhage (hematoma) (of), ear
hemorrhage *—see* Complications, intraoperative, hemorrhage (hematoma) (of), ear
laceration *—see* Complications, intraoperative, puncture or laceration..., ear
specified NEC H95.88
postoperative H95.89
external ear canal stenosis H95.81-
hematoma *—see* Complications, postprocedural, hematoma (of), ear
hemorrhage *—see* Complications, postprocedural, hemorrhage (of), ear
postmastoidectomy *— see* Complications, postmastoidectomy
specified NEC H95.89
seroma *— see* Complications, postprocedural, seroma (of), mastoid process
ectopic pregnancy O08.9
damage to pelvic organs O08.6
embolism O08.2
genital infection O08.0
hemorrhage (delayed) (excessive) O08.1
metabolic disorder O08.5
renal failure O08.4

ectopic pregnancy *(continued)*
shock O08.3
specified type NEC O08.0
venous complication NEC O08.7
electronic stimulator device
bladder (urinary) *—see* Complications, electronic stimulator device, urinary
bone T84.9
breakdown T84.310
displacement T84.320
embolism T84.81
fibrosis T84.82
hemorrhage T84.83
infection or inflammation T84.7
malfunction T84.310
malposition T84.320
mechanical NEC T84.390
obstruction T84.390
pain T84.84
perforation T84.390
protrusion T84.390
specified type NEC T84.89
stenosis T84.85
thrombosis T84.86
brain T85.9
embolism T85.810
fibrosis T85.820
hemorrhage T85.830
infection and inflammation T85.731
mechanical
breakdown T85.110
displacement T85.120
leakage T85.190
malposition T85.120
obstruction T85.190
perforation T85.190
protrusion T85.190
specified NEC T85.190
pain T85.840
specified type NEC T85.890
stenosis T85.850
thrombosis T85.860
cardiac (defibrillator) (pacemaker) *—see* Complications, cardiovascular device or implant, electronic
generator (brain) (gastric) (peripheral) (sacral) (spinal)
breakdown T85.113
displacement T85.123
leakage T85.193
malposition T85.123
obstruction T85.193
perforation T85.193
protrusion T85.193
specified NEC T85.193
muscle T84.9
breakdown T84.418
displacement T84.428
embolism T84.81
fibrosis T84.82
hemorrhage T84.83
infection or inflammation T84.7
mechanical NEC T84.498
pain T84.84
specified type NEC T84.89
stenosis T84.85
thrombosis T84.86
nervous system T85.9
brain *—see* Complications, electronic stimulator device, brain
cranial nerve - *see* Complications, electronic stimulator device, peripheral nerve
embolism T85.810
fibrosis T85.820

electronic stimulator device *(continued)*
nervous system *(continued)*
gastric nerve - *see* Complications, electronic stimulator device, peripheral nerve
hemorrhage T85.830
infection and inflammation T85.738
mechanical
breakdown T85.118
displacement T85.128
leakage T85.199
malposition T85.128
obstruction T85.199
perforation T85.199
protrusion T85.199
specified NEC T85.199
pain T85.840
peripheral nerve *—see* Complications, electronic stimulator device, peripheral nerve
sacral nerve - *see* Complications, electronic stimulator device, peripheral nerve
specified type NEC T85.890
spinal cord *—see* Complications, electronic stimulator device, spinal cord
stenosis T85.850
thrombosis T85.860
vagal nerve - *see* Complications, electronic stimulator device, peripheral nerve
peripheral nerve T85.9
embolism T85.810
fibrosis T85.820
hemorrhage T85.830
infection and inflammation T85.732
mechanical
breakdown T85.111
displacement T85.121
leakage T85.191
malposition T85.121
obstruction T85.191
perforation T85.191
protrusion T85.191
specified NEC T85.191
pain T85.840
specified type NEC T85.890
stenosis T85.850
thrombosis T85.860
spinal cord T85.9
embolism T85.810
fibrosis T85.820
hemorrhage T85.830
infection and inflammation T85.733
mechanical
breakdown T85.112
displacement T85.122
leakage T85.192
malposition T85.122
obstruction T85.192
perforation T85.192
protrusion T85.192
specified NEC T85.192
pain T85.840
specified type NEC T85.890
stenosis T85.850
thrombosis T85.860
urinary T83.9
embolism T83.81
fibrosis T83.82
hemorrhage T83.83

Complication *(continued)*
electronic stimulator device *(continued)*
urinary T83.9 *(continued)*
infection and inflammation T83.598
mechanical
breakdown T83.110
displacement T83.120
malposition T83.120
perforation T83.190
protrusion T83.190
specified NEC T83.190
pain T83.84
specified type NEC T83.89
stenosis T83.85
thrombosis T83.86
electroshock therapy T88.9
specified NEC T88.8
endocrine E34.9
postprocedural
adrenal hypofunction E89.6
hypoinsulinemia E89.1
hypoparathyroidism E89.2
hypopituitarism E89.3
hypothyroidism E89.0
ovarian failure E89.40
asymptomatic E89.40
symptomatic E89.41
specified NEC E89.89
testicular hypofunction E89.5
endodontic treatment NEC M27.59
enterostomy (stoma) K94.10
hemorrhage K94.11
infection K94.12
malfunction K94.13
mechanical K94.13
specified complication NEC K94.19
episiotomy, disruption O90.1
esophageal anti-reflux device T85.9
embolism T85.818
fibrosis T85.828
hemorrhage T85.838
infection and inflammation T85.79
mechanical
breakdown T85.511
displacement T85.521
malfunction T85.511
malposition T85.521
obstruction T85.591
perforation T85.591
protrusion T85.591
specified NEC T85.591
pain T85.848
specified type NEC T85.898
stenosis T85.858
thrombosis T85.868
esophagostomy K94.30
hemorrhage K94.31
infection K94.32
malfunction K94.33
mechanical K94.33
specified complication NEC K94.39
extracorporeal circulation T80.90
extremity artery (bypass) graft T82.9
arteriosclerosis —*see* Arteriosclerosis, extremities, bypass graft
embolism T82.818
fibrosis T82.828
hemorrhage T82.838
infection and inflammation T82.7
mechanical
breakdown T82.318
femoral artery T82.312
displacement T82.328
femoral artery T82.322
leakage T82.338
femoral artery T82.332

Complication *(continued)*
extremity artery *(continued)*
mechanical *(continued)*
malposition T82.328
femoral artery T82.322
obstruction T82.398
femoral artery T82.392
perforation T82.398
femoral artery T82.392
protrusion T82.398
femoral artery T82.392
pain T82.848
specified type NEC T82.898
stenosis T82.858
thrombosis T82.868
eye H57.9
corneal graft —*see* Complications, graft, cornea
implant (prosthetic) T85.9
embolism T85.818
fibrosis T85.828
hemorrhage T85.838
infection and inflammation T85.79
mechanical
breakdown T85.318
displacement T85.328
leakage T85.398
malposition T85.328
obstruction T85.398
perforation T85.398
protrusion T85.398
specified NEC T85.398
pain T85.848
specified type NEC T85.898
stenosis T85.858
thrombosis T85.868
intraocular lens —*see* Complications, intraocular lens
orbital prosthesis —*see* Complications, orbital prosthesis
female genital N94.9
device, implant or graft NEC —*see* Complications, genitourinary, device or implant, genital tract
femoral artery (bypass) graft —*see* Complication, extremity artery (bypass) graft
fixation device, internal (orthopedic) T84.9
infection and inflammation T84.60
arm T84.61-
humerus T84.61-
radius T84.61-
ulna T84.61-
leg T84.629
femur T84.62-
fibula T84.62-
tibia T84.62-
specified site NEC T84.69
spine T84.63
mechanical
breakdown
limb T84.119
carpal T84.210
femur T84.11-
fibula T84.11-
humerus T84.11-
metacarpal T84.210
metatarsal T84.213
phalanx
foot T84.213
hand T84.210
radius T84.11-
tarsal T84.213
tibia T84.11-
ulna T84.11-
specified bone NEC T84.218
spine T84.216

Complication *(continued)*
fixation device, internal *(continued)*
mechanical *(continued)*
displacement
limb T84.129
carpal T84.220
femur T84.12-
fibula T84.12-
humerus T84.12-
metacarpal T84.220
metatarsal T84.223
phalanx
foot T84.223
hand T84.220
radius T84.12-
tarsal T84.223
tibia T84.12-
ulna T84.12-
specified bone NEC T84.228
spine T84.226
malposition —*see* Complications, fixation device, internal, mechanical, displacement
obstruction —*see* Complications, fixation device, internal, mechanical, specified type NEC
perforation —*see* Complications, fixation device, internal, mechanical, specified type NEC
protrusion —*see* Complications, fixation device, internal, mechanical, specified type NEC
specified type NEC
limb T84.199
carpal T84.290
femur T84.19-
fibula T84.19-
humerus T84.19-
metacarpal T84.290
metatarsal T84.293
phalanx
foot T84.293
hand T84.290
radius T84.19-
tarsal T84.293
tibia T84.19-
ulna T84.19-
specified bone NEC T84.298
vertebra T84.296
specified type NEC T84.89
embolism T84.81
fibrosis T84.82
hemorrhage T84.83
pain T84.84
specified complication NEC T84.89
stenosis T84.85
thrombosis T84.86
following
acute myocardial infarction NEC I23.8
aneurysm (false) (of cardiac wall) (of heart wall) (ruptured) I23.3
angina I23.7
atrial
septal defect I23.1
thrombosis I23.6
cardiac wall rupture I23.3
chordae tendinae rupture I23.4
defect
septal
atrial (heart) I23.1
ventricular (heart) I23.2
hemopericardium I23.0
papillary muscle rupture I23.5

Complication *(continued)*
following *(continued)*
acute myocardial infarction *(continued)*
rupture
cardiac wall I23.3
with hemopericardium I23.0
chordae tendineae I23.4
papillary muscle I23.5
specified NEC I23.8
thrombosis
atrium I23.6
auricular appendage I23.6
ventricle (heart) I23.6
ventricular
septal defect I23.2
thrombosis I23.6
ectopic or molar pregnancy O08.9
cardiac arrest O08.81
sepsis O08.82
specified type NEC O08.89
urinary tract infection O08.83
termination of pregnancy —*see* Abortion
gastrointestinal K92.9
bile duct prosthesis —*see* Complications, bile duct implant
esophageal anti-reflux device —*see* Complications, esophageal anti-reflux device
postoperative
colostomy —*see* Complications, colostomy
dumping syndrome K91.1
enterostomy —*see* Complications, enterostomy
gastrostomy —*see* Complications, gastrostomy
malabsorption NEC K91.2
obstruction (*see also* Obstruction, intestine, postoperative) K91.30
postcholecystectomy syndrome K91.5
specified NEC K91.89
vomiting after GI surgery K91.0
prosthetic device or implant
bile duct prosthesis —*see* Complications, bile duct implant
esophageal anti-reflux device —*see* Complications, esophageal anti-reflux device
specified type NEC
embolism T85.818
fibrosis T85.828
hemorrhage T85.838
mechanical
breakdown T85.518
displacement T85.528
malfunction T85.518
malposition T85.528
obstruction T85.598
perforation T85.598
protrusion T85.598
specified NEC T85.598
pain T85.848
specified complication NEC T85.898
stenosis T85.858
thrombosis T85.868
gastrostomy (stoma) K94.20
hemorrhage K94.21
infection K94.22
malfunction K94.23
mechanical K94.23
specified complication NEC K94.29

Complication *(continued)*
genitourinary
device or implant T83.9
genital tract T83.9
infection or inflammation T83.69
intrauterine contraceptive device —*see* Complications, intrauterine, contraceptive device
mechanical —*see* Complications, by device, mechanical
mesh —*see* Complications, mesh
penile prosthesis —*see* Complications, prosthetic device, penile
specified type NEC T83.89
embolism T83.81
fibrosis T83.82
hemorrhage T83.83
pain T83.84
specified complication NEC T83.89
stenosis T83.85
thrombosis T83.86
vaginal mesh —*see* Complications, mesh
urinary system T83.9
cystostomy catheter —*see* Complication, catheter, cystostomy
electronic stimulator —*see* Complications, electronic stimulator device, urinary
indwelling urethral catheter —*see* Complications, catheter, urethral, indwelling
infection or inflammation T83.598
indwelling urethral catheter T83.511
kidney transplant —*see* Complication, transplant, kidney
organ graft —*see* Complication, graft, urinary organ
specified type NEC T83.89
embolism T83.81
fibrosis T83.82
hemorrhage T83.83
mechanical T83.198
breakdown T83.118
displacement T83.128
malfunction T83.118
malposition T83.128
obstruction T83.198
perforation T83.198
protrusion T83.198
specified NEC T83.198
sphincter implant —*see* Complications, implant, urinary sphincter
sphincter, implanted T83.191
stent (ileal conduit) (nephroureteral) T83.193
pain T83.84
specified complication NEC T83.89
stenosis T83.85
thrombosis T83.86
ureteral indwelling T83.192
postprocedural
pelvic peritoneal adhesions N99.4
renal failure N99.0
specified NEC N99.89

Complication *(continued)*
genitourinary *(continued)*
postprocedural *(continued)*
stoma —*see* Complications, stoma, urinary tract
urethral stricture —*see* Stricture, urethra, postprocedural
vaginal
adhesions N99.2
vault prolapse N99.3
graft (bypass) (patch) —*see also* Complications, prosthetic device or implant
aorta —*see* Complications, graft, vascular
arterial —*see* Complication, graft, vascular
bone T86.839
failure T86.831
infection T86.832
mechanical T84.318
breakdown T84.318
displacement T84.328
protrusion T84.398
specified type NEC T84.398
rejection T86.830
specified type NEC T86.838
carotid artery —*see* Complications, graft, vascular
cornea T86.849
failure T86.841
infection T86.842
mechanical T85.398
breakdown T85.318
displacement T85.328
protrusion T85.398
specified type NEC T85.398
rejection T86.840
retroprosthetic membrane T85.398
specified type NEC T86.848
femoral artery (bypass) —*see* Complication, extremity artery (bypass) graft
genital organ or tract —*see* Complications, genitourinary, device or implant, genital tract
muscle T84.9
breakdown T84.410
displacement T84.420
embolism T84.81
fibrosis T84.82
hemorrhage T84.83
infection and inflammation T84.7
mechanical NEC T84.490
pain T84.84
specified type NEC T84.89
stenosis T84.85
thrombosis T84.86
nerve —*see* Complication, prosthetic device or implant, specified NEC
skin —*see* Complications, prosthetic device or implant, skin graft
tendon T84.9
breakdown T84.410
displacement T84.420
embolism T84.81
fibrosis T84.82
hemorrhage T84.83
infection and inflammation T84.7
mechanical NEC T84.490
pain T84.84
specified type NEC T84.89
stenosis T84.85
thrombosis T84.86

Complication *(continued)*
graft *(continued)*
urinary organ T83.9
embolism T83.81
fibrosis T83.82
hemorrhage T83.83
infection and inflammation T83.598
indwelling urethral catheter T83.511
mechanical
breakdown T83.21
displacement T83.22
erosion T83.24
exposure T83.25
leakage T83.23
malposition T83.22
obstruction T83.29
perforation T83.29
protrusion T83.29
specified NEC T83.29
pain T83.84
specified type NEC T83.89
stenosis T83.85
thrombosis T83.86
vascular T82.9
embolism T82.818
femoral artery —*see* Complication, extremity artery (bypass) graft
fibrosis T82.828
hemorrhage T82.838
mechanical
breakdown T82.319
aorta (bifurcation) T82.310
carotid artery T82.311
specified vessel NEC T82.318
displacement T82.329
aorta (bifurcation) T82.320
carotid artery T82.321
specified vessel NEC T82.328
leakage T82.339
aorta (bifurcation) T82.330
carotid artery T82.331
specified vessel NEC T82.338
malposition T82.329
aorta (bifurcation) T82.320
carotid artery T82.321
specified vessel NEC T82.328
obstruction T82.399
aorta (bifurcation) T82.390
carotid artery T82.391
specified vessel NEC T82.398
perforation T82.399
aorta (bifurcation) T82.390
carotid artery T82.391
specified vessel NEC T82.398
protrusion T82.399
aorta (bifurcation) T82.390
carotid artery T82.391
specified vessel NEC T82.398
pain T82.848
specified complication NEC T82.898
stenosis T82.858
thrombosis T82.868
heart I51.9
assist device
infection and inflammation T82.7
following acute myocardial infarction —*see* Complications, following, acute myocardial infarction

Complication *(continued)*
heart *(continued)*
postoperative —*see* Complications, circulatory system
transplant —*see* Complication, transplant, heart
and lung(s) —*see* Complications, transplant, heart, with lung
valve
graft (biological) T82.9
embolism T82.817
fibrosis T82.827
hemorrhage T82.837
infection and inflammation T82.7
mechanical T82.228
breakdown T82.221
displacement T82.222
leakage T82.223
malposition T82.222
obstruction T82.228
perforation T82.228
protrusion T82.228
pain T82.847
specified type NEC T82.897
stenosis T82.857
thrombosis T82.867
prosthesis T82.9
embolism T82.817
fibrosis T82.827
hemorrhage T82.837
infection or inflammation T82.6
mechanical T82.09
breakdown T82.01
displacement T82.02
leakage T82.03
malposition T82.02
obstruction T82.09
perforation T82.09
protrusion T82.09
pain T82.847
specified type NEC T82.897
mechanical T82.09
stenosis T82.857
thrombosis T82.867
hematoma
intraoperative —*see* Complication, intraoperative, hemorrhage
postprocedural —*see* Complication, postprocedural, hematoma
hemodialysis —*see* Complications, dialysis
hemorrhage
intraoperative —*see* Complication, intraoperative, hemorrhage
postprocedural —*see* Complication, postprocedural, hemorrhage
ileostomy (stoma) —*see* Complications, enterostomy
immunization (procedure) —*see* Complications, vaccination
implant —*see also* Complications, by site and type
urinary sphincter T83.9
embolism T83.81
fibrosis T83.82
hemorrhage T83.83
infection and inflammation T83.591
mechanical
breakdown T83.111
displacement T83.121
leakage T83.191
malposition T83.121
obstruction T83.191
perforation T83.191

- **Complication** *(continued)*
  - implant *(continued)*
    - urinary sphincter *(continued)*
      - mechanical *(continued)*
        - protrusion T83.191
        - specified NEC T83.191
      - pain T83.84
      - specified type NEC T83.89
      - stenosis T83.85
      - thrombosis T83.86
  - infusion (procedure) T80.90
    - air embolism T80.0
    - blood —*see* Complications, transfusion
    - catheter —*see* Complications, catheter
    - infection T80.29
    - pump —*see* Complications, cardiovascular, device or implant
    - sepsis T80.29
    - serum reaction (*see also* Reaction, serum) T80.69
      - anaphylactic shock (*see also* Shock, anaphylactic) T80.59
    - specified type NEC T80.89
  - inhalation therapy NEC T81.81
  - injection (procedure) T80.90
    - drug reaction —*see* Reaction, drug
    - infection T80.29
    - sepsis T80.29
    - serum (prophylactic) (therapeutic) —*see* Complications, vaccination
    - specified type NEC T80.89
    - vaccine (any) —*see* Complications, vaccination
  - inoculation (any) —*see* Complications, vaccination
  - insulin pump
    - infection and inflammation T85.72
    - mechanical
      - breakdown T85.614
      - displacement T85.624
      - leakage T85.633
      - malposition T85.624
      - obstruction T85.694
      - perforation T85.694
      - protrusion T85.694
      - specified NEC T85.694
  - intestinal pouch NEC K91.858
  - intraocular lens (prosthetic) T85.9
    - embolism T85.818
    - fibrosis T85.828
    - hemorrhage T85.838
    - infection and inflammation T85.79
    - mechanical
      - breakdown T85.21
      - displacement T85.22
      - malposition T85.22
      - obstruction T85.29
      - perforation T85.29
      - protrusion T85.29
      - specified NEC T85.29
    - pain T85.848
    - specified type NEC T85.898
    - stenosis T85.858
    - thrombosis T85.868
  - intraoperative (intraprocedural)
    - cardiac arrest - *see also* Infarct, myocardium, associated with revascularization procedure
      - during cardiac surgery I97.710
      - during other surgery I97.711
    - cardiac functional disturbance NEC - *see also* Infarct, myocardium, associated with revascularization procedure
      - during cardiac surgery I97.790
      - during other surgery I97.791
    - hemorrhage (hematoma) (of)

- **Complication** *(continued)*
  - intraoperative *(continued)*
    - hemorrhage *(continued)*
      - circulatory system organ or structure
        - during cardiac bypass I97.411
        - during cardiac catheterization I97.410
        - during other circulatory system procedure I97.418
        - during other procedure I97.42
      - digestive system organ
        - during procedure on digestive system K91.61
        - during procedure on other organ K91.62
      - ear
        - during procedure on ear and mastoid process H95.21
        - during procedure on other organ H95.22
      - endocrine system organ or structure
        - during procedure on endocrine system organ or structure E36.01
        - during procedure on other organ E36.02
      - eye and adnexa
        - during ophthalmic procedure H59.11-
        - during other procedure H59.12-
      - genitourinary organ or structure
        - during procedure on genitourinary organ or structure N99.61
        - during procedure on other organ N99.62
      - mastoid process
        - during procedure on ear and mastoid process H95.21
        - during procedure on other organ H95.22
      - musculoskeletal structure
        - during musculoskeletal surgery M96.810
        - during non-orthopedic surgery M96.811
        - during orthopedic surgery M96.810
      - nervous system
        - during a nervous system procedure G97.31
        - during other procedure G97.32
      - respiratory system
        - during other procedure J95.62
        - during procedure on respiratory system organ or structure J95.61
      - skin and subcutaneous tissue
        - during a dermatologic procedure L76.01
        - during a procedure on other organ L76.02
      - spleen
        - during a procedure on other organ D78.02
        - during a procedure on the spleen D78.01
    - puncture or laceration (accidental) (unintentional) (of)
      - brain
        - during a nervous system procedure G97.48
        - during other procedure G97.49
      - circulatory system organ or structure
        - during circulatory system procedure I97.51
        - during other procedure I97.52

- **Complication** *(continued)*
  - intraoperative *(continued)*
    - puncture or laceration *(continued)*
      - digestive system
        - during procedure on digestive system K91.71
        - during procedure on other organ K91.72
      - ear
        - during procedure on ear and mastoid process H95.31
        - during procedure on other organ H95.32
      - endocrine system organ or structure
        - during procedure on endocrine system organ or structure E36.11
        - during procedure on other organ E36.12
      - eye and adnexa
        - during ophthalmic procedure H59.21-
        - during other procedure H59.22-
      - genitourinary organ or structure
        - during procedure on genitourinary organ or structure N99.71
        - during procedure on other organ N99.72
      - mastoid process
        - during procedure on ear and mastoid process H95.31
        - during procedure on other organ H95.32
      - musculoskeletal structure
        - during musculoskeletal surgery M96.820
        - during non-orthopedic surgery M96.821
        - during orthopedic surgery M96.820
      - nervous system
        - during a nervous system procedure G97.48
        - during other procedure G97.49
      - respiratory system
        - during other procedure J95.72
        - during procedure on respiratory system organ or structure J95.71
      - skin and subcutaneous tissue
        - during a dermatologic procedure L76.11
        - during a procedure on other organ L76.12
      - spleen
        - during a procedure on other organ D78.12
        - during a procedure on the spleen D78.11
    - specified NEC
      - circulatory system I97.88
      - digestive system K91.81
      - ear H95.88
      - endocrine system E36.8
      - eye and adnexa H59.88
      - genitourinary system N99.81
      - mastoid process H95.88
      - musculoskeletal structure M96.89
      - nervous system G97.81
      - respiratory system J95.88
      - skin and subcutaneous tissue L76.81
      - spleen D78.81
  - intraperitoneal catheter (dialysis) (infusion) —*see* Complications, catheter, intraperitoneal
  - intrathecal infusion pump
    - infection and inflammation T85.738

- **Complication** *(continued)*
  - intrathecal infusion pump *(continued)*
    - mechanical
      - breakdown T85.615
      - displacement T85.625
      - leakage T85.635
      - malfunction T85.695
      - malposition T85.625
      - obstruction T85.695
      - perforation T85.695
      - protrusion T85.695
      - specified NEC T85.695
  - intrauterine
    - contraceptive device
      - embolism T83.81
      - fibrosis T83.82
      - hemorrhage T83.83
      - infection and inflammation T83.69
      - mechanical
        - breakdown T83.31
        - displacement T83.32
        - malposition T83.32
        - obstruction T83.39
        - perforation T83.39
        - protrusion T83.39
        - specified NEC T83.39
      - pain T83.84
      - specified type NEC T83.89
      - stenosis T83.85
      - thrombosis T83.86
    - procedure (fetal), to newborn P96.5
  - jejunostomy (stoma) —*see* Complications, enterostomy
  - joint prosthesis, internal T84.9
    - breakage (fracture) T84.01-
    - dislocation T84.02-
    - fracture T84.01-
    - infection or inflammation T84.50
      - hip T84.5-
      - knee T84.5-
      - specified joint NEC T84.59
    - instability T84.02-
    - malposition —*see* Complications, joint prosthesis, mechanical, displacement
    - mechanical
      - breakage, broken T84.01-
      - dislocation T84.02-
      - fracture T84.01-
      - instability T84.02-
      - leakage —*see* Complications, joint prosthesis, mechanical, specified NEC
      - loosening T84.039
        - hip T84.03-
        - knee T84.03-
        - specified joint NEC T84.038
      - obstruction —*see* Complications, joint prosthesis, mechanical, specified NEC
      - perforation —*see* Complications, joint prosthesis, mechanical, specified NEC
        - osteolysis T84.059
          - hip T84.05-
          - knee T84.05-
          - other specified joint T84.058
      - protrusion —*see* Complications, joint prosthesis, mechanical, specified NEC
      - specified complication NEC T84.099
        - hip T84.09-
        - knee T84.09-
        - other specified joint T84.098
      - subluxation T84.02-
      - wear of articular bearing surface T84.069
        - hip T84.06-
        - knee T84.06-
        - other specified joint T84.068

Complication *(continued)*

- joint prosthesis, internal *(continued)*
  - specified joint NEC T84.89
    - embolism T84.81
    - fibrosis T84.82
    - hemorrhage T84.83
    - pain T84.84
    - specified complication NEC T84.89
    - stenosis T84.85
    - thrombosis T84.86
  - subluxation T84.02-
- kidney transplant *—see* Complications, transplant, kidney
- labor O75.9
  - specified NEC O75.89
- liver transplant (immune or nonimmune) *—see* Complications, transplant, liver
- lumbar puncture G97.1
  - cerebrospinal fluid leak G97.0
  - headache or reaction G97.1
- lung transplant *—see* Complications, transplant, lung
  - and heart *—see* Complications, transplant, lung, with heart
- male genital N50.9
  - device, implant or graft *—see* Complications, genitourinary, device or implant, genital tract
  - postprocedural or postoperative *—see* Complications, genitourinary, postprocedural
    - specified NEC N99.89
- mastoid (process) procedure
  - intraoperative H95.88
    - hematoma *—see* Complications, intraoperative, hemorrhage (hematoma) (of), mastoid process
    - hemorrhage *—see* Complications, intraoperative, hemorrhage (hematoma) (of), mastoid process
    - laceration *—see* Complications, intraoperative, puncture or laceration..., mastoid process
    - specified NEC H95.88
  - postmastoidectomy *—see* Complications, postmastoidectomy
  - postoperative H95.89
    - external ear canal stenosis H95.81-
    - hematoma *—see* Complications..., postprocedural, hematoma (of), mastoid process
    - hemorrhage *—see* Complications..., postprocedural, hemorrhage (of), mastoid process
    - postmastoidectomy *—see* Complications, postmastoidectomy
    - seroma - *see* Complications, postprocedureal, seroma (of), mastoid process
    - specified NEC H95.89
- mastoidectomy cavity *—see* Complications, postmastoidectomy
- mechanical *—see* Complications, by site and type, mechanical
- medical procedures (*see also* Complication(s), intraoperative) T88.9
- metabolic E88.9
  - postoperative E89.89
    - specified NEC E89.89
- molar pregnancy NOS O08.9
  - damage to pelvic organs O08.6

Complication *(continued)*

- molar pregnancy NOS *(continued)*
  - embolism O08.2
  - genital infection O08.0
  - hemorrhage (delayed) (excessive) O08.1
  - metabolic disorder O08.5
  - renal failure O08.4
  - shock O08.3
  - specified type NEC O08.0
  - venous complication NEC O08.7
- musculoskeletal system *—see also* Complication, intraoperative (intraprocedural), by site
  - device, implant or graft NEC *—see* Complications, orthopedic, device or implant
  - internal fixation (nail) (plate) (rod) *—see* Complications, fixation device, internal
  - joint prosthesis *—see* Complications, joint prosthesis
  - postoperative (postprocedural) M96.89
    - with osteoporosis *—see* Osteoporosis
    - fracture following insertion of device *—see* Fracture, following insertion of orthopedic implant, joint prosthesis or bone plate
    - joint instability after prosthesis removal M96.89
    - lordosis M96.4
    - postlaminectomy syndrome NEC M96.1
      - kyphosis M96.3
    - pseudarthrosis M96.0
    - specified complication NEC M96.89
  - post radiation M96.89
    - kyphosis M96.2
    - scoliosis M96.5
    - specified complication NEC M96.89
- nephrostomy (stoma) *—see* Complications, stoma, urinary tract, external NEC
- nervous system G98.8
  - central G96.9
  - device, implant or graft *—see also* Complication, prosthetic device or implant, specified NEC
    - electronic stimulator (electrode(s)) *—see* Complications, electronic stimulator device
    - specified NEC
      - infection and inflammation T85.738
      - mechanical T85.695
        - breakdown T85.615
        - displacement T85.625
        - leakage T85.635
        - malfunction T85.695
        - malposition T85.625
        - obstruction T85.695
        - perforation T85.695
        - protrusion T85.695
        - specified NEC T85.695
    - ventricular shunt *—see* Complications, ventricular shunt
  - electronic stimulator (electrode(s)) *—see* Complications, electronic stimulator device
  - postprocedural G97.82
    - intracranial hypotension G97.2
    - specified NEC G97.82
    - spinal fluid leak G97.0
- newborn, due to intrauterine (fetal) procedure P96.5

Complication *(continued)*

- nonabsorbable (permanent) sutures *—see* Complication, sutures, permanent
- obstetric O75.9
  - procedure (instrumental) (manual) (surgical) specified NEC O75.4
  - specified NEC O75.89
  - surgical wound NEC O90.89
    - hematoma O90.2
    - infection O86.0
- ocular lens implant *—see* Complications, intraocular lens
- ophthalmologic
  - postprocedural bleb *—see* Blebitis
- orbital prosthesis T85.9
  - embolism T85.818
  - fibrosis T85.828
  - hemorrhage T85.838
  - infection and inflammation T85.79
  - mechanical
    - breakdown T85.31-
    - displacement T85.32-
    - malposition T85.32-
    - obstruction T85.39-
    - perforation T85.39-
    - protrusion T85.39-
    - specified NEC T85.39-
  - pain T85.848
  - specified type NEC T85.898
  - stenosis T85.858
  - thrombosis T85.868
- organ or tissue transplant (partial) (total) *—see* Complications, transplant
- orthopedic *—see also* Disorder, soft tissue
  - device or implant T84.9
    - bone
      - device or implant *—see* Complication, bone, device NEC
      - graft *—see* Complication, graft, bone
    - breakdown T84.418
    - displacement T84.428
    - electronic bone stimulator *—see* Complications, electronic stimulator device, bone
    - embolism T84.81
    - fibrosis T84.82
    - fixation device *—see* Complication, fixation device, internal
    - hemorrhage T84.83
    - infection or inflammation T84.7
    - joint prosthesis *—see* Complication, joint prosthesis, internal
    - malfunction T84.418
    - malposition T84.428
    - mechanical NEC T84.498
    - muscle graft *—see* Complications, graft, muscle
    - obstruction T84.498
    - pain T84.84
    - perforation T84.498
    - protrusion T84.498
    - specified complication NEC T84.89
    - stenosis T84.85
    - tendon graft *—see* Complications, graft, tendon
    - thrombosis T84.86
  - fracture (following insertion of device) *—see* Fracture, following insertion of orthopedic implant, joint prosthesis or bone plate

Complication *(continued)*

- orthopedic *(continued)*
  - postprocedural M96.89
    - fracture *—see* Fracture, following insertion of orthopedic implant, joint prosthesis or bone plate
    - postlaminectomy syndrome NEC M96.1
      - kyphosis M96.3
      - lordosis M96.4
    - postradiation
      - kyphosis M96.2
      - scoliosis M96.5
    - pseudarthrosis post-fusion M96.0
    - specified type NEC M96.89
- pacemaker (cardiac) *—see* Complications, cardiovascular device or implant, electronic
- pancreas transplant *—see* Complications, transplant, pancreas
- penile prosthesis (implant) *—see* Complications, prosthetic device, penile
- perfusion NEC T80.90
- perineal repair (obstetrical) NEC O90.89
  - disruption O90.1
  - hematoma O90.2
  - infection (following delivery) O86.0
- phototherapy T88.9
  - specified NEC T88.8
- postmastoidectomy NEC H95.19-
  - cyst, mucosal H95.13-
  - granulation H95.12-
  - inflammation, chronic H95.11-
  - recurrent cholesteatoma H95.0-
- postoperative *—see* Complications, postprocedural
  - circulatory *—see* Complications, circulatory system
  - ear *—see* Complications, ear
  - endocrine *—see* Complications, endocrine
  - eye *—see* Complications, eye
  - lumbar puncture G97.1
    - cerebrospinal fluid leak G97.0
  - nervous system (central) (peripheral) *—see* Complications, nervous system
  - respiratory system *—see* Complications, respiratory system
- postprocedural *—see also* Complications, surgical procedure
  - cardiac arrest - *see also* Infarct, myocardium, associated with revascularization procedure
    - following cardiac surgery I97.120
    - following other surgery I97.121
  - cardiac functional disturbance NEC - *see also* Infarct, myocardium, associated with revascularization procedure
    - following cardiac surgery I97.190
    - following other surgery I97.191
  - cardiac insufficiency
    - following cardiac surgery I97.110
    - following other surgery I97.111
  - chorioretinal scars following retinal surgery H59.81-
  - following cataract surgery
    - cataract (lens) fragments H59.02-
    - cystoid macular edema H59.03-
    - specified NEC H59.09-
    - vitreous (touch) syndrome H59.01-
  - heart failure
    - following cardiac surgery I97.130
    - following other surgery I97.131

Complication *(continued)*
postprocedural *(continued)*
hematoma (of)
circulatory system organ or structure
following cardiac bypass I97.631
following cardiac catheterization I97.630
following other circulatory system procedure I97.638
following other procedure I97.621
digestive system
following procedure on digestive system K91.870
following procedure on other organ K91.871
ear
following other procedure H95.52
following procedure on ear and mastoid process H95.51
endocrine system
following endocrine system procedure E89.820
following other procedure E89.821
eye and adnexa
following ophthalmic procedure H59.33-
following other procedure H59.34-
genitourinary organ or structure
following procedure on genitourinary organ or structure N99.840
following procedure on other organ N99.841
mastoid process
following other procedure H95.52
following procedure on ear and mastoid process H95.51
musculoskeletal structure
following musculoskeletal surgery M96.840
following non-orthopedic surgery M96.841
following orthopedic surgery M96.840
nervous system
following nervous system procedure G97.61
following other procedure G97.62
respiratory system
following other procedure J95.861
following procedure on respiratory system organ or structure J95.860
skin and subcutaneous tissue
following dematologic procedure L76.31
following procedure on other organ L76.32
spleen
following procedure on other organ D78.32
following procedure on the spleen D78.31
hemorrhage (of)
circulatory system organ or structure
following cardiac bypass I97.611
following cardiac catheterization I97.610

Complication *(continued)*
postprocedural *(continued)*
hemorrhage *(continued)*
circulatory system organ or structure *(continued)*
following other circulatory system procedure I97.618
following other procedure I97.620
digestive system
following procedure on digestive system K91.840
following procedure on other organ K91.841
ear
following other procedure H95.42
following procedure on ear and mastoid process H95.41
endocrine system
following endocrine system procedure E89.810
following other procedure E89.811
eye and adnexa
following ophthalmic procedure H59.31-
following other procedure H59.32-
genitourinary organ or structure
following procedure on genitourinary organ or structure N99.820
following procedure on other organ N99.821
mastoid process
following other procedure H95.42
following procedure on ear and mastoid process H95.41
musculoskeletal structure
following musculoskeletal surgery M96.830
following non-orthopedic surgery M96.831
following orthopedic surgery M96.830
nervous system
following nervous system procedure G97.51
following other procedure G97.52
respiratory system
following other procedure J95.831
following procedure on respiratory system organ or structure J95.830
skin and subcutaneous tissue
following dermatologic procedure L76.21
following a procedure on other organ L76.22
spleen
following procedure on other organ D78.22
following procedure on the spleen D78.21
seroma (of)
circulatory system organ or structure
following cardiac bypass I97.641
following cardiac catheterization I97.640
following other circulatory system procedure I97.648
following other procedure I97.622

Complication *(continued)*
postprocedural *(continued)*
seroma (of) *(continued)*
digestive system
following procedure on digestive system K91.872
following procedure on other organ K91.873
ear
following other procedure H95.54
following procedure on ear and mastoid process H95.53
endocrine system
following endocrine system procedure E89.822
following other procedure E89.823
eye and adnexa
following ophthalmic procedure H59.35-
following other procedure H59.36-
genitourinary organ or structure
following procedure on genitourinary organ or structure N99.842
following procedure on other organ N99.843
mastoid process
following other procedure H95.54
following procedure on ear and mastoid process H95.53
musculoskeletal structure
following musculoskeletal surgery M96.842
following non-orthopedic surgery M96.843
following orthopedic surgery M96.842
nervous system
following nervous system procedure G97.63
following other procedure G97.64
respiratory system
following other procedure J95.863
following procedure on respiratory system organ or structure J95.862
skin and subcutaneous tissue
following dematologic procedure L76.33
following procedure on other organ L76.34
spleen
following procedure on other organ D78.34
following procedure on the spleen D78.33
specified NEC
circulatory system I97.89
digestive K91.89
ear H95.89
endocrine E89.89
eye and adnexa H59.89
genitourinary N99.89
mastoid process H95.89
metabolic E89.89
musculoskeletal structure M96.89
nervous system G97.82
respiratory system J95.89
skin and subcutaneous tissue L76.82
spleen D78.89
pregnancy NEC —*see* Pregnancy, complicated by

Complication *(continued)*
prosthetic device or implant T85.9
bile duct —*see* Complications, bile duct implant
breast —*see* Complications, breast implant
bulking agent
ureteral
erosion T83.714
exposure T83.724
urethral
erosion T83.713
exposure T83.723
cardiac and vascular NEC —*see* Complications, cardiovascular device or implant
corneal transplant —*see* Complications, graft, cornea
electronic nervous system stimulator —*see* Complications, electronic stimulator device
epidural infusion catheter —*see* Complications, catheter, epidural
esophageal anti-reflux device —*see* Complications, esophageal anti-reflux device
genital organ or tract —*see* Complications, genitourinary, device or implant, genital tract
specified NEC T83.79
heart valve —*see* Complications, heart, valve, prosthesis
infection or inflammation T85.79
intestine transplant T86.892
liver transplant T86.43
lung transplant T86.812
pancreas transplant T86.892
skin graft T86.822
intraocular lens —*see* Complications, intraocular lens
intraperitoneal (dialysis) catheter —*see* Complications, catheter, intraperitoneal
joint —*see* Complications, joint prosthesis, internal
mechanical NEC T85.698
dialysis catheter (vascular) —*see also* Complication, catheter, dialysis, mechanical
peritoneal —*see* Complication, catheter, intraperitoneal, mechanical
gastrointestinal device T85.598
ocular device T85.398
subdural (infusion) catheter T85.690
suture, permanent T85.692
that for bone repair —*see* Complications, fixation device, internal (orthopedic), mechanical
ventricular shunt
breakdown T85.01
displacement T85.02
leakage T85.03
malposition T85.02
obstruction T85.09
perforation T85.09
protrusion T85.09
specified NEC T85.09
mesh
erosion (to surrounding organ or tissue) T83.718
vaginal (into pelvic floor muscles) T83.711
urethral (into pelvic floor muscles) T83.712
exposure (into surrounding organ or tissue) T83.728
vaginal (into vagina) (through vaginal wall) T83.721

Complication *(continued)*
- prosthetic device or implant *(continued)*
  - mesh *(continued)*
    - exposure *(continued)*
      - urethral (through urethral wall) T83.722
  - orbital *—see* Complications, orbital prosthesis
  - penile T83.9
    - embolism T83.81
    - fibrosis T83.82
    - hemorrhage T83.83
    - infection and inflammation T83.61
    - mechanical
      - breakdown T83.410
      - displacement T83.420
      - leakage T83.490
      - malposition T83.420
      - obstruction T83.490
      - perforation T83.490
      - protrusion T83.490
      - specified NEC T83.490
    - pain T83.848
    - specified type NEC T83.89
    - stenosis T83.85
    - thrombosis T83.86
  - prosthetic materials NEC
    - erosion (to surrounding organ or tissue) T83.718
    - exposure (into surrounding organ or tissue) T83.728
  - skin graft T86.829
    - artificial skin or decellularized allodermis
      - embolism T85.818
      - fibrosis T85.828
      - hemorrhage T85.838
      - infection and inflammation T85.79
      - mechanical
        - breakdown T85.613
        - displacement T85.623
      - malfunction T85.613
        - malposition T85.623
        - obstruction T85.693
        - perforation T85.693
        - protrusion T85.693
        - specified NEC T85.693
      - pain T85.848
      - specified type NEC T85.898
      - stenosis T85.858
      - thrombosis T85.868
    - failure T86.821
    - infection T86.822
    - rejection T86.820
    - specified NEC T86.828
  - sling
    - urethral (female) (male)
      - erosion T83.712
      - exposure T83.722
  - specified NEC T85.9
    - embolism T85.818
    - fibrosis T85.828
    - hemorrhage T85.838
    - infection and inflammation T85.79
    - mechanical
      - breakdown T85.618
      - displacement T85.628
      - leakage T85.638
      - malfunction T85.618
      - malposition T85.628
      - obstruction T85.698
      - perforation T85.698
      - protrusion T85.698
      - specified NEC T85.698
    - pain T85.848
    - specified type NEC T85.898
    - stenosis T85.858
    - thrombosis T85.868

Complication *(continued)*
- prosthetic device or implant *(continued)*
  - subdural infusion catheter *—see* Complications, catheter, subdural
  - sutures *—see* Complications, sutures
  - urinary organ or tract NEC *—see* Complications, genitourinary, device or implant, urinary system
  - vascular *—see* Complications, cardiovascular device or implant
  - ventricular shunt *—see* Complications, ventricular shunt (device)
- puerperium *—see* Puerperal
- puncture, spinal G97.1
  - cerebrospinal fluid leak G97.0
  - headache or reaction G97.1
- pyelogram N99.89
- radiation
  - kyphosis M96.2
  - scoliosis M96.5
- reattached
  - extremity (infection) (rejection)
    - lower T87.1X-
    - upper T87.0X-
  - specified body part NEC T87.2
- reconstructed breast
  - asymmetry between native and reconstructed breast N65.1
  - deformity N65.0
  - disproportion between native and reconstructed breast N65.1
  - excess tissue N65.0
  - misshappen N65.0
- reimplant NEC *—see also* Complications, prosthetic device or implant
  - limb (infection) (rejection) *—see* Complications, reattached, extremity
  - organ (partial) (total) *—see* Complications, transplant
  - prosthetic device NEC *—see* Complications, prosthetic device
- renal N28.9
  - allograft *—see* Complications, transplant, kidney
  - dialysis *—see* Complications, dialysis
- respirator
  - mechancial J95.850
    - specified NEC J95.859
- respiratory system J98.9
  - device, implant or graft *—see* Complication, prosthetic device or implant, specified NEC
  - lung transplant *—see* Complications, prosthetic device or implant, lung transplant
  - postoperative J95.89
    - air leak J95.812
    - Mendelson's syndrome (chemical pneumonitis) J95.4
    - pneumothorax J95.811
    - pulmonary insufficiency (acute) (after nonthoracic surgery) J95.2
      - chronic J95.3
      - following thoracic surgery J95.1
    - respiratory failure (acute) J95.821
      - acute and chronic J95.822
    - specified NEC J95.89
    - subglottic stenosis J95.5
    - tracheostomy complication *—see* Complications, tracheostomy
  - therapy T81.89

Complication *(continued)*
- sedation during labor and delivery O74.9
  - cardiac O74.2
  - central nervous system O74.3
  - pulmonary NEC O74.1
- shunt *—see also* Complications, prosthetic device or implant
  - arteriovenous *—see* Complications, arteriovenous, shunt
  - ventricular (communicating) *— see* Complications, ventricular shunt
- skin
  - graft T86.829
    - failure T86.821
    - infection T86.822
    - rejection T86.820
    - specified type NEC T86.828
- spinal
  - anesthesia *—see* Complications, anesthesia, spinal
  - catheter (epidural) (subdural) *— see* Complications, catheter
  - puncture or tap G97.1
    - cerebrospinal fluid leak G97.0
    - headache or reaction G97.1
- stent
  - bile duct *—see* Complications, bile duct prosthesis
  - ureteral indwelling
    - breakdown T83.112
    - displacement T83.122
    - leakage T83.192
    - malposition T83.122
    - obstruction T83.192
    - perforation T83.192
    - protrusion T83.192
    - specified NEC T83.192
  - urinary NEC (ileal conduit) (nephroureteral) T83.193
    - embolism T83.81
    - fibrosis T83.82
    - hemorrhage T83.83
    - infection and inflammation T83.593
    - mechanical
      - breakdown T83.113
      - displacement T83.123
      - leakage T83.193
      - malposition T83.123
      - obstruction T83.193
      - perforation T83.193
      - protrusion T83.193
      - specified NEC T83.193
    - pain T83.84
    - specified type NEC T83.89
    - stenosis T83.85
    - thrombosis T83.86
  - vascular
    - end stent stenosis - *see* Restenosis, stent
    - in stent stenosis - *see* Restenosis, stent
- stoma
  - digestive tract
    - colostomy *—see* Complications, colostomy
    - enterostomy *—see* Complications, enterostomy
    - esophagostomy *—see* Complications, esophagostomy
    - gastrostomy *—see* Complications, gastrostomy
  - urinary tract N99.528
    - continent N99.538
      - hemorrhage N99.530
      - herniation N99.533
      - infection N99.531
      - malfunction N99.532
      - specified type NEC N99.538

Complication *(continued)*
- stoma *(continued)*
  - urinary tract *(continued)*
    - continent *(continued)*
      - stenosis N99.534
    - cystostomy *—see* Complications, cystostomy
    - external NOS N99.528
    - hemorrhage N99.520
    - herniation N99.523
    - incontinent N99.528
      - hemorrhage N99.520
      - herniation N99.523
      - infection N99.521
      - malfunction N99.522
      - specified type NEC N99.528
      - stenosis N99.524
    - infection N99.521
    - malfunction N99.522
    - specified type NEC N99.528
  - stenosis N99.524
- stomach banding *—see* Complication(s), bariatric procedure
- stomach stapling *—see* Complication(s), bariatric procedure
- surgical material, nonabsorbable *—see* Complication, suture, permanent
- surgical procedure (on) T81.9
  - amputation stump (late) *—see* Complications, amputation stump
  - cardiac *—see* Complications, circulatory system
  - cholesteatoma, recurrent *—see* Complications, postmastoidectomy, recurrent cholesteatoma
  - circulatory (early) *—see* Complications, circulatory system
  - digestive system *—see* Complications, gastrointestinal
  - dumping syndrome (postgastrectomy) K91.1
  - ear *—see* Complications, ear
  - elephantiasis or lymphedema I97.89
    - postmastectomy I97.2
  - emphysema (surgical) T81.82
  - endocrine *—see* Complications, endocrine
  - eye *—see* Complications, eye
  - fistula (persistent postoperative) T81.83
  - foreign body inadvertently left in wound (sponge) (suture) (swab) *—see* Foreign body, accidentally left during a procedure
  - gastrointestinal *—see* Complications, gastrointestinal
  - genitourinary NEC N99.89
  - hematoma
    - intraoperative *—see* Complication, intraoperative, hemorrhage
    - postprocedural *— see* Complication, postprocedural, hematoma
  - hemorrhage
    - intraoperative *—see* Complication, intraoperative, hemorrhage
    - postprocedural *— see* Complication, postprocedural, hemorrhage
  - hepatic failure K91.82
  - hyperglycemia (postpancreatectomy) E89.1
  - hypoinsulinemia (postpancreatectomy) E89.1
  - hypoparathyroidism (postparathyroidectomy) E89.2

Complication *(continued)*
- surgical procedure *(continued)*
  - hypopituitarism (posthypophysectomy) E89.3
  - hypothyroidism (post-thyroidectomy) E89.0
  - intestinal obstruction (*see also* Obstruction, intestine, postoperative) K91.30
  - intracranial hypotension following ventricular shunting (ventriculostomy) G97.2
  - lymphedema I97.89
    - postmastectomy I97.2
  - malabsorption (postsurgical) NEC K91.2
    - osteoporosis *—see* Osteoporosis, postsurgical malabsorption
  - mastoidectomy cavity NEC *—see* Complications, postmastoidectomy
  - metabolic E89.89
    - specified NEC E89.89
  - musculoskeletal *—see* Complications, musculoskeletal system
  - nervous system (central) (peripheral) *—see* Complications, nervous system
  - ovarian failure E89.40
    - asymptomatic E89.40
    - symptomatic E89.41
  - peripheral vascular *—see* Complications, surgical procedure, vascular
  - postcardiotomy syndrome I97.0
  - postcholecystectomy syndrome K91.5
  - postcommissurotomy syndrome I97.0
  - postgastrectomy dumping syndrome K91.1
  - postlaminectomy syndrome NEC M96.1
    - kyphosis M96.3
  - postmastectomy lymphedema syndrome I97.2
  - postmastoidectomy cholesteatoma *—see* Complications, postmastoidectomy, recurrent cholesteatoma
  - postvagotomy syndrome K91.1
  - postvalvulotomy syndrome I97.0
  - pulmonary insufficiency (acute) J95.2
    - chronic J95.3
    - following thoracic surgery J95.1
  - reattached body part *—see* Complications, reattached
  - respiratory *—see* Complications, respiratory system
  - shock (hypovolemic) T81.19
  - spleen (postoperative) D78.89
    - intraoperative D78.81
  - stitch abscess T81.4
  - subglottic stenosis (postsurgical) J95.5
  - testicular hypofunction E89.5
  - transplant *—see* Complications, organ or tissue transplant
  - urinary NEC N99.89
  - vaginal vault prolapse (posthysterectomy) N99.3
  - vascular (peripheral)
    - artery T81.719
      - mesenteric T81.710
      - renal T81.711
      - specified NEC T81.718
    - vein T81.72
  - wound infection T81.4

Complication *(continued)*
- suture, permanent (wire) NEC T85.9
  - with repair of bone *—see* Complications, fixation device, internal
  - embolism T85.818
  - fibrosis T85.828
  - hemorrhage T85.838
  - infection and inflammation T85.79
  - mechanical
    - breakdown T85.612
    - displacement T85.622
    - malfunction T85.612
    - malposition T85.622
    - obstruction T85.692
    - perforation T85.692
    - protrusion T85.692
    - specified NEC T85.692
  - pain T85.848
  - specified type NEC T85.898
  - stenosis T85.858
  - thrombosis T85.868
- tracheostomy J95.00
  - granuloma J95.09
  - hemorrhage J95.01
  - infection J95.02
  - malfunction J95.03
  - mechanical J95.03
  - obstruction J95.03
  - specified type NEC J95.09
  - tracheo-esophageal fistula J95.04
- transfusion (blood) (lymphocytes) (plasma) T80.92
  - air emblism T80.0
  - circulatory overload E87.71
  - febrile nonhemolytic transfusion reaction R50.84
  - hemolysis T80.89
  - hemochromatosis E83.111
  - hemolytic reaction (antigen unspecified) T80.919
  - incompatibility reaction (antigen unspecified) T80.919
    - ABO T80.30
      - delayed serologic (DSTR) T80.39
      - hemolytic transfusion reaction (HTR) (unspecified time after transfusion) T80.319
        - acute (AHTR) (less than 24 hours after transfusion) T80.310
        - delayed (DHTR) (24 hours or more after transfusion) T80.311
      - specified NEC T80.39
    - acute (antigen unspecified) T80.910
    - delayed (antigen unspecified) T80.911
    - delayed serologic (DSTR) T80.89
    - Non-ABO (minor antigens (Duffy) (Kell) (Kidd) (Lewis) (M) (N) (P) (S)) T80.A0
      - delayed serologic (DSTR) T80.A9
      - hemolytic transfusion reaction (HTR) (unspecified time after transfusion) T80.A19
        - acute (AHTR) (less than 24 hours after transfusion) T80.A10
        - delayed (DHTR) (24 hours or more after transfusion) T80.A11
      - specified NEC T80.A9
    - Rh (antigens (C) (c) (D) (E) (e)) (factor) T80.40
      - delayed serologic (DSTR) T80.49

Complication *(continued)*
- transfusion *(continued)*
  - incompatibility reaction *(continued)*
    - Rh *(continued)*
      - hemolytic transfusion reaction (HTR) (unspecified time after transfusion) T80.419
        - acute (AHTR) (less than 24 hours after transfusion) T80.410
        - delayed (DHTR) (24 hours or more after transfusion) T80.411
      - specified NEC T80.49
  - infection T80.29
    - acute T80.22
  - reaction NEC T80.89
  - sepsis T80.29
  - shock T80.89
- transplant T86.90
  - bone T86.839
    - failure T86.831
    - infection T86.832
    - rejection T86.830
    - specified type NEC T86.838
  - bone marrow T86.00
    - failure T86.02
    - infection T86.03
    - rejection T86.01
    - specified type NEC T86.09
  - cornea T86.849
    - failure T86.841
    - infection T86.842
    - rejection T86.840
    - specified type NEC T86.848
  - failure T86.92
  - heart T86.20
    - with lung T86.30
    - cardiac allograft vasculopathy T86.290
      - failure T86.32
      - infection T86.33
      - rejection T86.31
      - specified type NEC T86.39
    - failure T86.22
    - infection T86.23
    - rejection T86.21
    - specified type NEC T86.298
  - infection T86.93
  - intestine T86.859
    - failure T86.851
    - infection T86.852
    - rejection T86.850
    - specified type NEC T86.858
  - kidney T86.10
    - failure T86.12
    - infection T86.13
    - rejection T86.11
    - specified type NEC T86.19
  - liver T86.40
    - failure T86.42
    - infection T86.43
    - rejection T86.41
    - specified type NEC T86.49
  - lung T86.819
    - with heart T86.30
      - failure T86.32
      - infection T86.33
      - rejection T86.31
      - specified type NEC T86.39
    - failure T86.811
    - infection T86.812
    - rejection T86.810
    - specified type NEC T86.818
  - malignant neoplasm C80.2
  - pancreas T86.899
    - failure T86.891
    - infection T86.892
    - rejection T86.890
    - specified type NEC T86.898

Complication *(continued)*
- transplant *(continued)*
  - peripheral blood stem cells T86.5
  - post-transplant lymphoproliferative disorder (PTLD) D47.Z1
  - rejection T86.91
  - skin T86.829
    - failure T86.821
    - infection T86.822
    - rejection T86.820
    - specified type NEC T86.828
  - specified
    - tissue T86.899
      - failure T86.891
      - infection T86.892
      - rejection T86.890
      - specified type NEC T86.898
    - type NEC T86.99
  - stem cell (from peripheral blood) (from umbilical cord) T86.5
  - umbilical cord stem cells T86.5
- trauma (early) T79.9
  - specified NEC T79.8
- ultrasound therapy NEC T88.9
- umbilical cord NEC
  - complicating delivery O69.9
    - specified NEC O69.89
- umbrella device, vascular T82.9
  - embolism T82.818
  - fibrosis T82.828
  - hemorrhage T82.838
  - infection or inflammation T82.7
  - mechanical
    - breakdown T82.515
    - displacement T82.525
    - leakage T82.535
    - malposition T82.525
    - obstruction T82.595
    - perforation T82.595
    - protrusion T82.595
  - pain T82.848
  - specified type NEC T82.898
  - stenosis T82.858
  - thrombosis T82.868
- urethral catheter *—see* Complications, catheter, urethral, indwelling
- vaccination T88.1
  - anaphylaxis NEC T80.52
  - arthropathy *—see* Arthropathy, postimmunization
  - cellulitis T88.0
  - encephalitis or encephalomyelitis G04.02
  - infection (general) (local) NEC T88.0
  - meningitis G03.8
  - myelitis G04.02
  - protein sickness T80.62
  - rash T88.1
  - reaction (allergic) T88.1
    - serum T80.62
  - sepsis T88.0
  - serum intoxication, sickness, rash, or other serum reaction NEC T80.62
    - anaphylactic shock T80.52
  - shock (allergic) (anaphylactic) T80.52
  - vaccinia (generalized) (localized) T88.1
- vas deferens device or implant *—see* Complications, genitourinary, device or implant, genital tract
- vascular I99.9
  - device or implant T82.9
    - embolism T82.818
    - fibrosis T82.828
    - hemorrhage T82.838
    - infection or inflammation T82.7

Complication *(continued)*
vascular *(continued)*
device or implant *(continued)*
mechanical
breakdown T82.519
specified device NEC T82.518
displacement T82.529
specified device NEC T82.528
leakage T82.539
specified device NEC T82.538
malposition T82.529
specified device NEC T82.528
obstruction T82.599
specified device NEC T82.598
perforation T82.599
specified device NEC T82.598
protrusion T82.599
specified device NEC T82.598
pain T82.848
specified type NEC T82.898
stenosis T82.858
thrombosis T82.868
dialysis catheter *—see* Complication, catheter, dialysis
following infusion, therapeutic injection or transfusion T80.1
graft T82.9
embolism T82.818
fibrosis T82.828
hemorrhage T82.838
mechanical
breakdown T82.319
aorta (bifurcation) T82.310
carotid artery T82.311
specified vessel NEC T82.318
displacement T82.329
aorta (bifurcation) T82.320
carotid artery T82.321
specified vessel NEC T82.328
leakage T82.339
aorta (bifurcation) T82.330
carotid artery T82.331
specified vessel NEC T82.338
malposition T82.329
aorta (bifurcation) T82.320
carotid artery T82.321
specified vessel NEC T82.328
obstruction T82.399
aorta (bifurcation) T82.390
carotid artery T82.391
specified vessel NEC T82.398
perforation T82.399
aorta (bifurcation) T82.390
carotid artery T82.391
specified vessel NEC T82.398
protrusion T82.399
aorta (bifurcation) T82.390
carotid artery T82.391
specified vessel NEC T82.398
pain T82.848
specified complication NEC T82.898
stenosis T82.858
thrombosis T82.868
postoperative *—see* Complications, postoperative, circulatory

Complication *(continued)*
vena cava device (filter) (sieve) (umbrella) *—see* Complications, umbrella device, vascular
ventilation therapy NEC T81.81
ventilator
mechanical J95.850
specified NEC J95.859
ventricular (communicating) shunt (device) T85.9
embolism T85.810
fibrosis T85.820
hemorrhage T85.830
infection and inflammation T85.730
mechanical
breakdown T85.01
displacement T85.02
leakage T85.03
malposition T85.02
obstruction T85.09
perforation T85.09
protrusion T85.09
specified NEC T85.09
pain T85.840
specified type NEC T85.890
stenosis T85.850
thrombosis T85.860
wire suture, permanent (implanted) *—see* Complications, suture, permanent

Compressed air disease T70.3

Compression
with injury - code by Nature of injury
artery I77.1
celiac, syndrome I77.4
brachial plexus G54.0
brain (stem) G93.5
due to
contusion (diffuse) *—see* Injury, intracranial, diffuse
focal *—see* Injury, intracranial, focal
injury NEC *—see* Injury, intracranial, diffuse
traumatic *—see* Injury, intracranial, diffuse
bronchus J98.09
cauda equina G83.4
celiac (artery) (axis) I77.4
cerebral *—see* Compression, brain
cervical plexus G54.2
cord
spinal *—see* Compression, spinal
umbilical *—see* Compression, umbilical cord
cranial nerve G52.9
eighth H93.3
eleventh G52.8
fifth G50.8
first G52.0
fourth *—see* Strabismus, paralytic, fourth nerve
ninth G52.1
second *—see* Disorder, nerve, optic
seventh G51.8
sixth *—see* Strabismus, paralytic, sixth nerve
tenth G52.2
third *—see* Strabismus, paralytic, third nerve
twelfth G52.3
diver's squeeze T70.3
during birth (newborn) P15.9
esophagus K22.2
eustachian tube *—see* Obstruction, eustachian tube, cartilaginous
facies Q67.1
fracture
nontraumatic NOS *—see* Collapse, vertebra

Compression *(continued)*
fracture *(continued)*
pathological *—see* Fracture, pathological
traumatic *—see* Fracture, traumatic
heart *—see* Disease, heart
intestine *—see* Obstruction, intestine
laryngeal nerve, recurrent G52.2
with paralysis of vocal cords and larynx J38.00
bilateral J38.02
unilateral J38.01
lumbosacral plexus G54.1
lung J98.4
lymphatic vessel I89.0
medulla *—see* Compression, brain
nerve (*see also* Disorder, nerve) G58.9
arm NEC *—see* Mononeuropathy, upper limb
axillary G54.0
cranial *—see* Compression, cranial nerve
leg NEC *—see* Mononeuropathy, lower limb
median (in carpal tunnel) *—see* Syndrome, carpal tunnel
optic *—see* Disorder, nerve, optic
plantar *—see* Lesion, nerve, plantar
posterior tibial (in tarsal tunnel) *—see* Syndrome, tarsal tunnel
root or plexus NOS (in) G54.9
intervertebral disc disorder NEC *—see* Disorder, disc, with, radiculopathy
with myelopathy *—see* Disorder, disc, with, myelopathy
neoplastic disease *—see also* Neoplasm D49.9 *[G55]*
spondylosis *—see* Spondylosis, with radiculopathy
sciatic (acute) *—see* Lesion, nerve, sciatic
sympathetic G90.8
traumatic *—see* Injury, nerve
ulnar *—see* Lesion, nerve, ulnar
upper extremity NEC *—see* Mononeuropathy, upper limb
spinal (cord) G95.20
by displacement of intervertebral disc NEC *—see also* Disorder, disc, with, myelopathy
nerve root NOS G54.9
due to displacement of intervertebral disc NEC *—see* Disorder, disc, with, radiculopathy
with myelopathy *—see* Disorder, disc, with, myelopathy
specified NEC G95.29
spondylogenic (cervical) (lumbar, lumbosacral) (thoracic) *—see* Spondylosis, with myelopathy NEC
anterior *—see* Syndrome, anterior, spinal artery, compression
traumatic *—see* Injury, spinal cord, by region
subcostal nerve (syndrome) *—see* Mononeuropathy, upper limb, specified NEC
sympathetic nerve NEC G90.8
syndrome T79.5
trachea J39.8
ulnar nerve (by scar tissue) *—see* Lesion, nerve, ulnar
umbilical cord
complicating delivery O69.2
cord around neck O69.1
prolapse O69.0
specified NEC O69.2

Compression *(continued)*
ureter N13.5
vein I87.1
vena cava (inferior) (superior) I87.1

Compulsion, compulsive
gambling F63.0
neurosis F42.8
personality F60.5
states F42.8
swearing F42.8
in Gilles de la Tourette's syndrome F95.2
tics and spasms F95.9

Concato's disease (pericardial polyserositis) A19.9
nontubercular I31.1
pleural *—see* Pleurisy, with effusion

Concavity chest wall M95.4

Concealed penis Q55.69

Concern (normal) about sick person in family Z63.6

Concrescence (teeth) K00.2

Concretio cordis I31.1
rheumatic I09.2

Concretion *—see also* Calculus
appendicular K38.1
canaliculus *—see* Dacryolith
clitoris N90.89
conjunctiva H11.12-
eyelid *—see* Disorder, eyelid, specified type NEC
lacrimal passages *—see* Dacryolith
prepuce (male) N47.8
salivary gland (any) K11.5
seminal vesicle N50.89
tonsil J35.8

Concussion (brain) (cerebral) (current) S06.0X9
with
loss of consciousness of 30 minutes or less S06.0X1
loss of consciousness of unspecified duration S06.0X9
blast (air) (hydraulic) (immersion) (underwater)
abdomen or thorax *—see* Injury, blast, by site
ear with acoustic nerve injury *—see* Injury, nerve, acoustic, specified type NEC
cauda equina S34.3
conus medullaris S34.02
ocular S05.8X-
spinal (cord)
cervical S14.0
lumbar S34.01
sacral S34.02
thoracic S24.0
syndrome F07.81
without loss of consciousness S06.0X0

Condition *—see* Disease

Conditions arising in the perinatal period *—see* Newborn, affected by

Conduct disorder *—see* Disorder, conduct

Condyloma A63.0
acuminatum A63.0
gonorrheal A54.09
latum A51.31
syphilitic A51.31
congenital A50.07
venereal, syphilitic A51.31

Conflagration *—see also* Burn
asphyxia (by inhalation of gases, fumes or vapors) (*see also* Table of Drugs and Chemicals) T59.9-

Conflict (with) *—see also* Discord
- family Z73.9
- marital Z63.0
  - involving divorce or estrangement Z63.5
- parent-child Z62.820
  - parent-adopted child Z62.821
  - parent-biological child Z62.820
  - parent-foster child Z62.822
- social role NEC Z73.5

Confluent *—see* condition

Confusion, confused R41.0
- epileptic F05
- mental state (psychogenic) F44.89
- psychogenic F44.89
- reactive (from emotional stress, psychological trauma) F44.89

Confusional arousals G47.51

Congelation T69.9

Congenital *—see also* condition
- aortic septum Q25.49
- intrinsic factor deficiency D51.0
- malformation *—see* Anomaly

Congestion, congestive
- bladder N32.89
- bowel K63.89
- brain G93.89
- breast N64.59
- bronchial J98.09
- catarrhal J31.0
- chest R09.89
- chill, malarial *—see* Malaria
- circulatory NEC I99.8
- duodenum K31.89
- eye *—see* Hyperemia, conjunctiva
- facial, due to birth injury P15.4
- general R68.89
- glottis J37.0
- heart *—see* Failure, heart, congestive
- hepatic K76.1
- hypostatic (lung) *—see* Edema, lung
- intestine K63.89
- kidney N28.89
- labyrinth *—see* subcategory H83.8
- larynx J37.0
- liver K76.1
- lung R09.89
  - active or acute *—see* Pneumonia
- malaria, malarial *—see* Malaria
- nasal R09.81
- nose R09.81
- orbit, orbital *—see also* Exophthalmos
  - inflammatory (chronic) *—see* Inflammation, orbit
- ovary N83.8
- pancreas K86.89
- pelvic, female N94.89
- pleural J94.8
- prostate (active) N42.1
- pulmonary *—see* Congestion, lung
- renal N28.89
- retina H35.81
- seminal vesicle N50.1
- spinal cord G95.19
- spleen (chronic) D73.2
- stomach K31.89
- trachea *—see* Tracheitis
- urethra N36.8
- uterus N85.8
  - with subinvolution N85.3
- venous (passive) I87.8
- viscera R68.89

Congestive *—see* Congestion

Conical
- cervix (hypertrophic elongation) N88.4
- cornea *—see* Keratoconus
- teeth K00.2

Conjoined twins Q89.4

Conjugal maladjustment Z63.0
- involving divorce or estrangement Z63.5

Conjunctiva *—see* condition

Conjunctivitis (staphylococcal) (streptococcal) **NOS** H10.9
- Acanthamoeba B60.12
- acute H10.3-
  - atopic H10.1-
  - mucopurulent H10.02-
    - follicular H10.01-
  - chemical (*see also* Corrosion, cornea) H10.21-
  - pseudomembranous H10.22-
  - serous except viral H10.23-
    - viral *—see* Conjunctivitis, viral
  - toxic H10.21-
- adenoviral (acute) (follicular) B30.1
- allergic (acute) *—see* Conjunctivitis, acute, atopic
  - chronic H10.45
    - vernal H10.44
- anaphylactic *—see* Conjunctivitis, acute, atopic
- Apollo B30.3
- atopic (acute) *—see* Conjunctivitis, acute, atopic
- Béal's B30.2
- blennorrhagic (gonococcal) (neonatorum) A54.31
- chemical (acute) (*see also* Corrosion, cornea) H10.21-
- chlamydial A74.0
  - due to trachoma A71.1
  - neonatal P39.1
- chronic (nodosa) (petrificans) (phlyctenular) H10.40-
  - allergic H10.45
    - vernal H10.44
  - follicular H10.43-
  - giant papillary H10.41-
  - simple H10.42-
  - vernal H10.44
- coxsackievirus 24 B30.3
- diphtheritic A36.86
- due to
  - dust *—see* Conjunctivitis, acute, atopic
  - filariasis B74.9
  - mucocutaneous leishmaniasis B55.2
- enterovirus type 70 (hemorrhagic) B30.3
- epidemic (viral) B30.9
  - hemorrhagic B30.3
- gonococcal (neonatorum) A54.31
- granular (trachomatous) A71.1
  - sequelae (late effect) B94.0
- hemorrhagic (acute) (epidemic) B30.3
- herpes zoster B02.31
- in (due to)
  - Acanthamoeba B60.12
  - adenovirus (acute) (follicular) B30.1
  - Chlamydia A74.0
  - coxsackievirus 24 B30.3
  - diphtheria A36.86
  - enterovirus type 70 (hemorrhagic) B30.3
  - filariasis B74.9
  - gonococci A54.31
  - herpes (simplex) virus B00.53
    - zoster B02.31
  - infectious disease NEC B99
  - meningococci A39.89
  - mucocutaneous leishmaniasis B55.2
  - rosacea L71.9
  - syphilis (late) A52.71
  - zoster B02.31
- inclusion A74.0

Conjunctivitis *(continued)*
- infantile P39.1
  - gonococcal A54.31
- Koch-Weeks' *—see* Conjunctivitis, acute, mucopurulent
- light *—see* Conjunctivitis, acute, atopic
- ligneous *—see* Blepharoconjunctivitis, ligneous
- meningococcal A39.89
- mucopurulent *—see* Conjunctivitis, acute, mucopurulent
- neonatal P39.1
  - gonococcal A54.31
- Newcastle B30.8
- of Béal B30.2
- parasitic
  - filariasis B74.9
  - mucocutaneous leishmaniasis B55.2
- Parinaud's H10.89
- petrificans H10.89
- rosacea L71.9
- specified NEC H10.89
- swimming-pool B30.1
- trachomatous A71.1
  - acute A71.0
  - sequelae (late effect) B94.0
- traumatic NEC H10.89
- tuberculous A18.59
- tularemic A21.1
- tularensis A21.1
- viral B30.9
  - due to
    - adenovirus B30.1
    - enterovirus B30.3
  - specified NEC B30.8

Conjunctivochalasis H11.82-

Connective tissue *—see* condition

Conn's syndrome E26.01

Conradi (-Hunermann) **disease** Q77.3

Consanguinity Z84.3
- counseling Z71.89

Conscious simulation (of illness) Z76.5

Consecutive *—see* condition

Consolidation lung (base) *—see* Pneumonia, lobar

Constipation (atonic) (neurogenic) (simple) (spastic) K59.00
- chronic K59.09
  - idiopathic K59.04
- drug-induced K59.03
- functional K59.04
- outlet dysfunction K59.02
- psychogenic F45.8
- slow transit K59.01
- specified NEC K59.09

Constitutional *—see also* condition
- substandard F60.7

Constitutionally substandard F60.7

Constriction *—see also* Stricture
- auditory canal *—see* Stenosis, external ear canal
- bronchial J98.09
- duodenum K31.5
- esophagus K22.2
- external
  - abdomen, abdominal (wall) S30.841
  - alveolar process S00.542
  - ankle S90.54-
  - antecubital space *—see* Constriction, external, forearm
  - arm (upper) S40.84-
  - auricle *—see* Constriction, external, ear
  - axilla *—see* Constriction, external, arm
  - back, lower S30.840

Constriction *(continued)*
- external *(continued)*
  - breast S20.14-
  - brow S00.84
  - buttock S30.840
  - calf *—see* Constriction, external, leg
  - canthus *—see* Constriction, external, eyelid
  - cheek S00.84
    - internal S00.542
  - chest wall *—see* Constriction, external, thorax
  - chin S00.84
  - clitoris S30.844
  - costal region *—see* Constriction, external, thorax
  - digit(s)
    - foot *—see* Constriction, external, toe
    - hand *—see* Constriction, external, finger
  - ear S00.44-
  - elbow S50.34-
  - epididymis S30.843
  - epigastric region S30.841
  - esophagus, cervical S10.14
  - eyebrow *—see* Constriction, external, eyelid
  - eyelid S00.24-
  - face S00.84
  - finger(s) S60.44-
    - index S60.44-
    - little S60.44-
    - middle S60.44-
    - ring S60.44-
  - flank S30.841
  - foot (except toe(s) alone) S90.84-
    - toe *—see* Constriction, external, toe
  - forearm S50.84-
    - elbow only *—see* Constriction, external, elbow
  - forehead S00.84
  - genital organs, external
    - female S30.846
    - male S30.845
  - groin S30.841
  - gum S00.542
  - hand S60.54-
  - head S00.94
    - ear *—see* Constriction, external, ear
    - eyelid *—see* Constriction, external, eyelid
    - lip S00.541
    - nose S00.34
    - oral cavity S00.542
    - scalp S00.04
    - specified site NEC S00.84
  - heel *—see* Constriction, external, foot
  - hip S70.24-
  - inguinal region S30.841
  - interscapular region S20.449
  - jaw S00.84
  - knee S80.24-
  - labium (majus) (minus) S30.844
  - larynx S10.14
  - leg (lower) S80.84-
    - knee *—see* Constriction, external, knee
    - upper *—see* Constriction, external, thigh
  - lip S00.541
  - lower back S30.840
  - lumbar region S30.840
  - malar region S00.84
  - mammary *—see* Constriction, external, breast

Constriction *(continued)*
external *(continued)*
mastoid region S00.84
mouth S00.542
nail
finger *—see* Constriction, external, finger
toe *—see* Constriction, external, toe
nasal S00.34
neck S10.94
specified site NEC S10.84
throat S10.14
nose S00.34
occipital region S00.04
oral cavity S00.542
orbital region *—see* Constriction, external, eyelid
palate S00.542
palm *—see* Constriction, external, hand
parietal region S00.04
pelvis S30.840
penis S30.842
perineum
female S30.844
male S30.840
periocular area *—see* Constriction, external, eyelid
phalanges
finger *—see* Constriction, external, finger
toe *—see* Constriction, external, toe
pharynx S10.14
pinna *—see* Constriction, external, ear
popliteal space *—see* Constriction, external, knee
prepuce S30.842
pubic region S30.840
pudendum
female S30.846
male S30.845
sacral region S30.840
scalp S00.04
scapular region *—see* Constriction, external, shoulder
scrotum S30.843
shin *—see* Constriction, external, leg
shoulder S40.24-
sternal region S20.349
submaxillary region S00.84
submental region S00.84
subungual
finger(s) *—see* Constriction, external, finger
toe(s) *—see* Constriction, external, toe
supraclavicular fossa S10.84
supraorbital S00.84
temple S00.84
temporal region S00.84
testis S30.843
thigh S70.34-
thorax, thoracic (wall) S20.94
back S20.44-
front S20.34-
throat S10.14
thumb S60.34-
toe(s) (lesser) S90.44-
great S90.44-
tongue S00.542
trachea S10.14
tunica vaginalis S30.843
uvula S00.542
vagina S30.844
vulva S30.844
wrist S60.84-
gallbladder *—see* Obstruction, gallbladder

Constriction *(continued)*
intestine *—see* Obstruction, intestine
larynx J38.6
congenital Q31.8
specified NEC Q31.8
subglottic Q31.1
organ or site, congenital NEC *—see* Atresia, by site
prepuce (acquired) (congenital) N47.1
pylorus (adult hypertrophic) K31.1
congenital or infantile Q40.0
newborn Q40.0
ring dystocia (uterus) O62.4
spastic *—see also* Spasm
ureter N13.5
ureter N13.5
with infection N13.6
urethra *—see* Stricture, urethra
visual field (peripheral) (functional) *—see* Defect, visual field

Constrictive *—see* condition

Consultation
medical *—see* Counseling, medical
religious Z71.81
specified reason NEC Z71.89
spiritual Z71.81
without complaint or sickness Z71.9
feared complaint unfounded Z71.1
specified reason NEC Z71.89

Consumption *—see* Tuberculosis

Contact (with) *—see also* Exposure (to)
acariasis Z20.7
AIDS virus Z20.6
air pollution Z77.110
algae and algae toxins Z77.121
algae bloom Z77.121
anthrax Z20.810
aromatic amines Z77.020
aromatic (hazardous) compounds NEC Z77.028
aromatic dyes NOS Z77.028
arsenic Z77.010
asbestos Z77.090
bacterial disease NEC Z20.818
benzene Z77.021
blue-green algae bloom Z77.121
body fluids (potentially hazardous) Z77.21
brown tide Z77.121
chemicals (chiefly nonmedicinal) (hazardous) NEC Z77.098
cholera Z20.09
chromium compounds Z77.018
communicable disease Z20.9
bacterial NEC Z20.818
specified NEC Z20.89
viral NEC Z20.828
cyanobacteria bloom Z77.121
dyes Z77.098
Escherichia coli (E. coli) Z20.01
fiberglass *—see* Table of Drugs and Chemicals, fiberglass
German measles Z20.4
gonorrhea Z20.2
hazardous metals NEC Z77.018
hazardous substances NEC Z77.29
hazards in the physical environment NEC Z77.128
hazards to health NEC Z77.9
HIV Z20.6
HTLV-III/LAV Z20.6
human immunodeficiency virus (HIV) Z20.6
infection Z20.9
specified NEC Z20.89
infestation (parasitic) NEC Z20.7
intestinal infectious disease NEC Z20.09
Escherichia coli (E. coli) Z20.01

Contact *(continued)*
lead Z77.011
meningococcus Z20.811
mold (toxic) Z77.120
nickel dust Z77.018
noise Z77.122
parasitic disease Z20.7
pediculosis Z20.7
pfiesteria piscicida Z77.121
poliomyelitis Z20.89
pollution
air Z77.110
environmental NEC Z77.118
soil Z77.112
water Z77.111
polycyclic aromatic hydrocarbons Z77.028
rabies Z20.3
radiation, naturally occurring NEC Z77.123
radon Z77.123
red tide (Florida) Z77.121
rubella Z20.4
sexually-transmitted disease Z20.2
smallpox (laboratory) Z20.89
syphilis Z20.2
tuberculosis Z20.1
uranium Z77.012
varicella Z20.820
venereal disease Z20.2
viral disease NEC Z20.828
viral hepatitis Z20.5
water pollution Z77.111

Contamination, food *—see* Intoxication, foodborne

Contraception, contraceptive
advice Z30.09
counseling Z30.09
device (intrauterine) (in situ) Z97.5
causing menorrhagia T83.83
checking Z30.431
complications *—see* Complications, intrauterine, contraceptive device
in place Z97.5
initial prescription Z30.014
reinsertion Z30.433
removal Z30.432
replacement Z30.433
emergency (postcoital) Z30.012
initial prescription Z30.019
barrier Z30.018
diaphragm Z30.018
injectable Z30.013
intrauterine device Z30.014
pills Z30.011
postcoital (emergency) Z30.012
specified type NEC Z30.018
subdermal implantable Z30.017
transdermal patch hormonal Z30.016
vaginal ring hormonal Z30.015
maintenance Z30.40
barrier Z30.49
diaphragm Z30.49
examination Z30.8
injectable Z30.42
intrauterine device Z30.431
pills Z30.41
specified type NEC Z30.49
subdermal implantable Z30.46
transdermal patch hormonal Z30.45
vaginal ring hormonal Z30.44
management Z30.9
specified NEC Z30.8
postcoital (emergency) Z30.012
prescription Z30.019
repeat Z30.40
sterilization Z30.2
surveillance (drug) *—see* Contraception, maintenance

Contraction(s), contracture, contracted
Achilles tendon *—see also* Short, tendon, Achilles
congenital Q66.89
amputation stump (surgical) (flexion) (late) (next proximal joint) T87.89
anus K59.8
bile duct (common) (hepatic) K83.8
bladder N32.89
neck or sphincter N32.0
bowel, cecum, colon or intestine, any part *—see* Obstruction, intestine
Braxton Hicks *—see* False, labor
breast implant, capsular T85.44
bronchial J98.09
burn (old) *—see* Cicatrix
cervix *—see* Stricture, cervix
cicatricial *—see* Cicatrix
conjunctiva, trachomatous, active A71.1
sequelae (late effect) B94.0
Dupuytren's M72.0
eyelid *—see* Disorder, eyelid function
fascia (lata) (postural) M72.8
Dupuytren's M72.0
palmar M72.0
plantar M72.2
finger NEC *—see also* Deformity, finger
congenital Q68.1
joint *—see* Contraction, joint, hand
flaccid *—see* Contraction, paralytic
gallbladder K82.0
heart valve *—see* Endocarditis
hip *—see* Contraction, joint, hip
hourglass
bladder N32.89
congenital Q64.79
gallbladder K82.0
congenital Q44.1
stomach K31.89
congenital Q40.2
psychogenic F45.8
uterus (complicating delivery) O62.4
hysterical F44.4
internal os *—see* Stricture, cervix
joint (abduction) (acquired) (adduction) (flexion) (rotation) M24.50
ankle M24.57-
congenital NEC Q68.8
hip Q65.89
elbow M24.52-
foot joint M24.57-
hand joint M24.54-
hip M24.55-
congenital Q65.89
hysterical F44.4
knee M24.56-
shoulder M24.51-
wrist M24.53-
kidney (granular) (secondary) N26.9
congenital Q63.8
hydronephritic *—see* Hydronephrosis
Page N26.2
pyelonephritic *—see* Pyelitis, chronic
tuberculous A18.11
ligament *—see also* Disorder, ligament
congenital Q79.8
muscle (postinfective) (postural) NEC M62.40
with contracture of joint *—see* Contraction, joint
ankle M62.47-
congenital Q79.8
sternocleidomastoid Q68.0
extraocular *—see* Strabismus

Contraction(s), contracture, contracted *(continued)*
- muscle *(continued)*
  - eye (extrinsic) —*see* Strabismus
  - foot M62.47-
  - forearm M62.43-
  - hand M62.44-
  - hysterical F44.4
  - ischemic (Volkmann's) T79.6
  - lower leg M62.46-
  - multiple sites M62.49
  - pelvic region M62.45-
  - posttraumatic —*see* Strabismus, paralytic
  - psychogenic F45.8
    - conversion reaction F44.4
  - shoulder region M62.41-
  - specified site NEC M62.48
  - thigh M62.45-
  - upper arm M62.42-
- neck —*see* Torticollis
- ocular muscle —*see* Strabismus
- organ or site, congenital NEC —*see* Atresia, by site
- outlet (pelvis) —*see* Contraction, pelvis
- palmar fascia M72.0
- paralytic
  - joint —*see* Contraction, joint
  - muscle —*see also* Contraction, muscle NEC
    - ocular —*see* Strabismus, paralytic
- pelvis (acquired) (general) M95.5
  - with disproportion (fetopelvic) O33.1
    - causing obstructed labor O65.1
    - inlet O33.2
    - mid-cavity O33.3
    - outlet O33.3
- plantar fascia M72.2
- premature
  - atrium I49.1
  - auriculoventricular I49.49
  - heart I49.49
  - junctional I49.2
  - supraventricular I49.1
  - ventricular I49.3
- prostate N42.89
- pylorus NEC —*see also* Pylorospasm
  - psychogenic F45.8
- rectum, rectal (sphincter) K59.8
- ring (Bandl's) (complicating delivery) O62.4
- scar —*see* Cicatrix
- spine —*see* Dorsopathy, deforming
- sternocleidomastoid (muscle), congenital Q68.0
- stomach K31.89
  - hourglass K31.89
    - congenital Q40.2
    - psychogenic F45.8
  - psychogenic F45.8
- tendon (sheath) M62.40
  - with contracture of joint —*see* Contraction, joint
  - Achilles —*see* Short, tendon, Achilles
  - ankle M62.47-
    - Achilles —*see* Short, tendon, Achilles
  - foot M62.47-
  - forearm M62.43-
  - hand M62.44-
  - lower leg M62.46-
  - multiple sites M62.49
  - neck M62.48
  - pelvic region M62.45-
  - shoulder region M62.41-
  - specified site NEC M62.48
  - thigh M62.45-
  - thorax M62.48

Contraction(s), contracture, contracted *(continued)*
- tendon *(continued)*
  - trunk M62.48
  - upper arm M62.42-
- toe —*see* Deformity, toe, specified NEC
- ureterovesical orifice (postinfectional) N13.5
  - with infection N13.6
- urethra —*see also* Stricture, urethra orifice N32.0
- uterus N85.8
  - abnormal NEC O62.9
  - clonic (complicating delivery) O62.4
  - dyscoordinate (complicating delivery) O62.4
  - hourglass (complicating delivery) O62.4
  - hypertonic O62.4
  - hypotonic NEC O62.2
  - inadequate
    - primary O62.0
    - secondary O62.1
  - incoordinate (complicating delivery) O62.4
  - poor O62.2
  - tetanic (complicating delivery) O62.4
- vagina (outlet) N89.5
- vesical N32.89
  - neck or urethral orifice N32.0
- visual field —*see* Defect, visual field, generalized
- Volkmann's (ischemic) T79.6

Contusion (skin surface intact) T14.8
- abdomen, abdominal (muscle) (wall) S30.1
- adnexa, eye NEC S05.8X-
- adrenal gland S37.812
- alveolar process S00.532
- ankle S90.0-
- antecubital space —*see* Contusion, forearm
- anus S30.3
- arm (upper) S40.02-
  - lower (with elbow) —*see* Contusion, forearm
- auditory canal —*see* Contusion, ear
- auricle —*see* Contusion, ear
- axilla —*see* Contusion, arm, upper
- back —*see also* Contusion, thorax, back
  - lower S30.0
- bile duct S36.13
- bladder S37.22
- bone NEC T14.8
- brain (diffuse) —*see* Injury, intracranial, diffuse
  - focal —*see* Injury, intracranial, focal
- brainstem S06.38-
- breast S20.0-
- broad ligament S37.892
- brow S00.83
- buttock S30.0
- canthus, eye S00.1-
- cauda equina S34.3
- cerebellar, traumatic S06.37-
- cerebral S06.33-
  - left side S06.32-
  - right side S06.31-
- cheek S00.83
  - internal S00.532
- chest (wall) —*see* Contusion, thorax
- chin S00.83
- clitoris S30.23
- colon —*see* Injury, intestine, large, contusion
- common bile duct S36.13
- conjunctiva S05.1-

Contusion *(continued)*
- conjunctiva *(continued)*
  - with foreign body (in conjunctival sac) —*see* Foreign body, conjunctival sac
- conus medullaris (spine) S34.139
- cornea —*see* Contusion, eyeball
  - with foreign body —*see* Foreign body, cornea
- corpus cavernosum S30.21
- cortex (brain) (cerebral) —*see* Injury, intracranial, diffuse
  - focal —*see* Injury, intracranial, focal
- costal region —*see* Contusion, thorax
- cystic duct S36.13
- diaphragm S27.802
- duodenum S36.420
- ear S00.43-
- elbow S50.0-
  - with forearm —*see* Contusion, forearm
- epididymis S30.22
- epigastric region S30.1
- epiglottis S10.0
- esophagus (thoracic) S27.812
  - cervical S10.0
- eyeball S05.1-
- eyebrow S00.1-
- eyelid (and periocular area) S00.1-
- face NEC S00.83
- fallopian tube S37.529
  - bilateral S37.522
  - unilateral S37.521
- femoral triangle S30.1
- finger(s) S60.00
  - with damage to nail (matrix) S60.10
  - index S60.02-
    - with damage to nail S60.12-
  - little S60.05-
    - with damage to nail S60.15-
  - middle S60.03-
    - with damage to nail S60.13-
  - ring S60.04-
    - with damage to nail S60.14-
  - thumb —*see* Contusion, thumb
- flank S30.1
- foot (except toe(s) alone) S90.3-
  - toe —*see* Contusion, toe
- forearm S50.1-
  - elbow only —*see* Contusion, elbow
- forehead S00.83
- gallbladder S36.122
- genital organs, external
  - female S30.202
  - male S30.201
- globe (eye) —*see* Contusion, eyeball
- groin S30.1
- gum S00.532
- hand S60.22-
  - finger(s) —*see* Contusion, finger
  - wrist —*see* Contusion, wrist
- head S00.93
  - ear —*see* Contusion, ear
  - eyelid —*see* Contusion, eyelid
  - lip S00.531
  - nose S00.33
  - oral cavity S00.532
  - scalp S00.03
  - specified part NEC S00.83
- heart (*see also* Injury, heart) S26.91
- heel —*see* Contusion, foot
- hepatic duct S36.13
- hip S70.0-
- ileum S36.428
- iliac region S30.1
- inguinal region S30.1
- interscapular region S20.229
- intra-abdominal organ S36.92
  - colon —*see* Injury, intestine, large, contusion
  - liver S36.112

Contusion *(continued)*
- intra-abdominal organ *(continued)*
  - pancreas —*see* Contusion, pancreas
  - rectum S36.62
  - small intestine —*see* Injury, intestine, small, contusion
  - specified organ NEC S36.892
  - spleen —*see* Contusion, spleen
  - stomach S36.32
- iris (eye) —*see* Contusion, eyeball
- jaw S00.83
- jejunum S36.428
- kidney S37.01-
  - major (greater than 2 cm) S37.02-
  - minor (less than 2 cm) S37.01-
- knee S80.0-
- labium (majus) (minus) S30.23
- lacrimal apparatus, gland or sac S05.8X-
- larynx S10.0
- leg (lower) S80.1-
  - knee —*see* Contusion, knee
- lens —*see* Contusion, eyeball
- lip S00.531
- liver S36.112
- lower back S30.0
- lumbar region S30.0
- lung S27.329
  - bilateral S27.322
  - unilateral S27.321
- malar region S00.83
- mastoid region S00.83
- membrane, brain —*see* Injury, intracranial, diffuse
  - focal —*see* Injury, intracranial, focal
- mesentery S36.892
- mesosalpinx S37.892
- mouth S00.532
- muscle —*see* Contusion, by site
- nail
  - finger —*see* Contusion, finger, with damage to nail
  - toe —*see* Contusion, toe, with damage to nail
- nasal S00.33
- neck S10.93
  - specified site NEC S10.83
  - throat S10.0
- nerve —*see* Injury, nerve
- newborn P54.5
- nose S00.33
- occipital
  - lobe (brain) —*see* Injury, intracranial, diffuse
    - focal —*see* Injury, intracranial, focal
  - region (scalp) S00.03
- orbit (region) (tissues) S05.1-
- ovary S37.429
  - bilateral S37.422
  - unilateral S37.421
- palate S00.532
- pancreas S36.229
  - body S36.221
  - head S36.220
  - tail S36.222
- parietal
  - lobe (brain) —*see* Injury, intracranial, diffuse
    - focal —*see* Injury, intracranial, focal
  - region (scalp) S00.03
- pelvic organ S37.92
  - adrenal gland S37.812
  - bladder S37.22
  - fallopian tube —*see* Contusion, fallopian tube
  - kidney —*see* Contusion, kidney
  - ovary —*see* Contusion, ovary
  - prostate S37.822

Contusion *(continued)*
- pelvic organ *(continued)*
  - specified organ NEC S37.892
  - ureter S37.12
  - urethra S37.32
  - uterus S37.62
- pelvis S30.0
- penis S30.21
- perineum
  - female S30.23
  - male S30.0
- periocular area S00.1-
- peritoneum S36.81
- periurethral tissue —*see* Contusion, urethra
- pharynx S10.0
- pinna —*see* Contusion, ear
- popliteal space —*see* Contusion, knee
- prepuce S30.21
- prostate S37.822
- pubic region S30.1
- pudendum
  - female S30.202
  - male S30.201
- quadriceps femoris —*see* Contusion, thigh
- rectum S36.62
- retroperitoneum S36.892
- round ligament S37.892
- sacral region S30.0
- scalp S00.03
  - due to birth injury P12.3
- scapular region —*see* Contusion, shoulder
- sclera —*see* Contusion, eyeball
- scrotum S30.22
- seminal vesicle S37.892
- shoulder S40.01-
- skin NEC T14.8
- small intestine —*see* Injury, intestine, small, contusion
- spermatic cord S30.22
- spinal cord —*see* Injury, spinal cord, by region
  - cauda equina S34.3
  - conus medullaris S34.139
- spleen S36.029
  - major S36.021
  - minor S36.020
- sternal region S20.219
- stomach S36.32
- subconjunctival S05.1-
- subcutaneous NEC T14.8
- submaxillary region S00.83
- submental region S00.83
- subperiosteal NEC T14.8
- subungual
  - finger —*see* Contusion, finger, with damage to nail
  - toe —*see* Contusion, toe, with damage to nail
- supraclavicular fossa S10.83
- supraorbital S00.83
- suprarenal gland S37.812
- temple (region) S00.83
- temporal
  - lobe (brain) —*see* Injury, intracranial, diffuse
    - focal —*see* Injury, intracranial, focal
  - region S00.83
- testis S30.22
- thigh S70.1-
- thorax (wall) S20.20
  - back S20.22-
  - front S20.21-
- throat S10.0
- thumb S60.01-
  - with damage to nail S60.11-

Contusion *(continued)*
- toe(s) (lesser) S90.12-
  - with damage to nail S90.22-
  - great S90.11-
    - with damage to nail S90.21-
- tongue S00.532
- trachea (cervical) S10.0
  - thoracic S27.52
- tunica vaginalis S30.22
- tympanum, tympanic membrane —*see* Contusion, ear
- ureter S37.12
- urethra S37.32
- urinary organ NEC S37.892
- uterus S37.62
- uvula S00.532
- vagina S30.23
- vas deferens S37.892
- vesical S37.22
- vocal cord(s) S10.0
- vulva S30.23
- wrist S60.21-

Conus (congenital) (any type) Q14.8
- cornea —*see* Keratoconus
- medullaris syndrome G95.81

Conversion hysteria, neurosis or reaction F44.9

Converter, tuberculosis (test reaction) R76.11

Conviction (legal)**, anxiety concerning** Z65.0
- with imprisonment Z65.1

Convulsions (idiopathic) (*see also* Seizure(s)) R56.9
- apoplectiform (cerebral ischemia) I67.82
- dissociative F44.5
- epileptic —*see* Epilepsy
- epileptiform, epileptoid —*see* Seizure, epileptiform
- ether (anesthetic) —*see* Table of Drugs and Chemicals, by drug
- febrile R56.00
  - with status epilepticus G40.901
  - complex R56.01
    - with status epilepticus G40.901
  - simple R56.00
- hysterical F44.5
- infantile P90
  - epilepsy —*see* Epilepsy
- jacksonian —*see* Epilepsy, localization-related, symptomatic, with simple partial seizures
- myoclonic G25.3
- newborn P90
- obstetrical (nephritic) (uremic) —*see* Eclampsia
- paretic A52.17
- post traumatic R56.1
- psychomotor —*see* Epilepsy, localization-related, symptomatic, with complex partial seizures
- recurrent R56.9
- reflex R25.8
- scarlatinal A38.8
- tetanus, tetanic —*see* Tetanus
- thymic E32.8

Convulsive —*see also* Convulsions

Cooley's anemia D56.1

Coolie itch B76.9

Cooper's
- disease —*see* Mastopathy, cystic
- hernia —*see* Hernia, abdomen, specified site NEC

Copra itch B88.0

Coprophagy F50.89

Coprophobia F40.298

Coproporphyria, hereditary E80.29

Cor
- biloculare Q20.8
- bovis, bovinum —*see* Hypertrophy, cardiac
- pulmonale (chronic) I27.81
  - acute I26.09
- triatriatum, triatrium Q24.2
- triloculare Q20.8
  - biatrium Q20.4
  - biventriculare Q21.1

Corbus' disease (gangrenous balanitis) N48.1

Cord —*see also* condition
- around neck
  - complicating delivery O69.81
    - with compression O69.1
- bladder G95.89
  - tabetic A52.19

Cordis ectopia Q24.8

Corditis (spermatic) N49.1

Corectopia Q13.2

Cori's disease (glycogen storage) E74.03

Corkhandler's disease or lung J67.3

Corkscrew esophagus K22.4

Corkworker's disease or lung J67.3

Corn (infected) L84

Cornea —*see also* condition
- donor Z52.5
- plana Q13.4

Cornelia de Lange syndrome Q87.1

Cornu cutaneum L85.8

Cornual gestation or pregnancy O00.80
- with intrauterine pregnancy O00.81

Coronary (artery) —*see* condition

Coronavirus, as cause of disease classified elsewhere B97.29
- SARS-associated B97.21

Corpora —*see also* condition
- amylacea, prostate N42.89
- cavernosa —*see* condition

Corpulence —*see* Obesity

Corpus —*see* condition

Corrected transposition Q20.5

Corrosion (injury) (acid) (caustic) (chemical) (lime) (external) (internal) T30.4
- abdomen, abdominal (muscle) (wall) T21.42
  - first degree T21.52
  - second degree T21.62
  - third degree T21.72
- above elbow T22.439
  - first degree T22.539
  - left T22.432
    - first degree T22.532
    - second degree T22.632
    - third degree T22.732
  - right T22.431
    - first degree T22.531
    - second degree T22.631
    - third degree T22.731
  - second degree T22.639
  - third degree T22.739
- alimentary tract NEC T28.7
- ankle T25.419
  - first degree T25.519
  - left T25.412
    - first degree T25.512
    - second degree T25.612
    - third degree T25.712
  - multiple with foot —*see* Corrosion, lower, limb, multiple, ankle and foot

Corrosion *(continued)*
- ankle *(continued)*
  - right T25.411
    - first degree T25.511
    - second degree T25.611
    - third degree T25.711
  - second degree T25.619
  - third degree T25.719
- anus —*see* Corrosion, buttock
- arm(s) (meaning upper limb(s)) —*see* Corrosion, upper limb
- axilla T22.449
  - first degree T22.549
  - left T22.442
    - first degree T22.542
    - second degree T22.642
    - third degree T22.742
  - right T22.441
    - first degree T22.541
    - second degree T22.641
    - third degree T22.741
  - second degree T22.649
  - third degree T22.749
- back (lower) T21.44
  - first degree T21.54
  - second degree T21.64
  - third degree T21.74
  - upper T21.43
    - first degree T21.53
    - second degree T21.63
    - third degree T21.73
- blisters - code as Corrosion, second degree, by site
- breast(s) —*see* Corrosion, chest wall
- buttock(s) T21.45
  - first degree T21.55
  - second degree T21.65
  - third degree T21.75
- calf T24.439
  - first degree T24.539
  - left T24.432
    - first degree T24.532
    - second degree T24.632
    - third degree T24.732
  - right T24.431
    - first degree T24.531
    - second degree T24.631
    - third degree T24.731
  - second degree T24.639
  - third degree T24.739
- canthus (eye) —*see* Corrosion, eyelid
- cervix T28.8
- cheek T20.46
  - first degree T20.56
  - second degree T20.66
  - third degree T20.76
- chest wall T21.41
  - first degree T21.51
  - second degree T21.61
  - third degree T21.71
- chin T20.43
  - first degree T20.53
  - second degree T20.63
  - third degree T20.73
- colon T28.7
- conjunctiva (and cornea) —*see* Corrosion, cornea
- cornea (and conjunctiva) T26.6-
- deep necrosis of underlying tissue - code as Corrosion, third degree, by site
- dorsum of hand T23.469
  - first degree T23.569
  - left T23.462
    - first degree T23.562
    - second degree T23.662
    - third degree T23.762

Corrosion *(continued)*
dorsum of hand *(continued)*
right T23.461
first degree T23.561
second degree T23.661
third degree T23.761
second degree T23.669
third degree T23.769
ear (auricle) (external) (canal) T20.41
drum T28.91
first degree T20.51
second degree T20.61
third degree T20.71
elbow T22.429
first degree T22.529
left T22.422
first degree T22.522
second degree T22.622
third degree T22.722
right T22.421
first degree T22.521
second degree T22.621
third degree T22.721
second degree T22.629
third degree T22.729
entire body —*see* Corrosion, multiple body regions
epidermal loss - code as Corrosion, second degree, by site
epiglottis T27.4
erythema, erythematous - code as Corrosion, first degree, by site
esophagus T28.6
extent (percentage of body surface)
less than 10 percent T32.0
10-19 percent (0-9 percent third degree) T32.10
with 10-19 percent third degree T32.11
20-29 percent (0-9 percent third degree) T32.20
with
10-19 percent third degree T32.21
20-29 percent third degree T32.22
30-39 percent (0-9 percent third degree) T32.30
with
10-19 percent third degree T32.31
20-29 percent third degree T32.32
30-39 percent third degree T32.33
40-49 percent (0-9 percent third degree) T32.40
with
10-19 percent third degree T32.41
20-29 percent third degree T32.42
30-39 percent third degree T32.43
40-49 percent third degree T32.44
50-59 percent (0-9 percent third degree) T32.50
with
10-19 percent third degree T32.51
20-29 percent third degree T32.52
30-39 percent third degree T32.53
40-49 percent third degree T32.54
50-59 percent third degree T32.55

Corrosion *(continued)*
extent *(continued)*
60-69 percent (0-9 percent third degree) T32.60
with
10-19 percent third degree T32.61
20-29 percent third degree T32.62
30-39 percent third degree T32.63
40-49 percent third degree T32.64
50-59 percent third degree T32.65
60-69 percent third degree T32.66
70-79 percent (0-9 percent third degree) T32.70
with
10-19 percent third degree T32.71
20-29 percent third degree T32.72
30-39 percent third degree T32.73
40-49 percent third degree T32.74
50-59 percent third degree T32.75
60-69 percent third degree T32.76
70-79 percent third degree T32.77
80-89 percent (0-9 percent third degree) T32.80
with
10-19 percent third degree T32.81
20-29 percent third degree T32.82
30-39 percent third degree T32.83
40-49 percent third degree T32.84
50-59 percent third degree T32.85
60-69 percent third degree T32.86
70-79 percent third degree T32.87
80-89 percent third degree T32.88
90 percent or more (0-9 percent third degree) T32.90
with
10-19 percent third degree T32.91
20-29 percent third degree T32.92
30-39 percent third degree T32.93
40-49 percent third degree T32.94
50-59 percent third degree T32.95
60-69 percent third degree T32.96
70-79 percent third degree T32.97
80-89 percent third degree T32.98
90-99 percent third degree T32.99
extremity —*see* Corrosion, limb
eye(s) and adnexa T26.9-
with resulting rupture and destruction of eyeball T26.7-
conjunctival sac —*see* Corrosion, cornea

Corrosion *(continued)*
eye(s) and adnexa *(continued)*
cornea —*see* Corrosion, cornea
lid —*see* Corrosion, eyelid
periocular area —*see* Corrosion eyelid
specified site NEC T26.8-
eyeball —*see* Corrosion, eye
eyelid(s) T26.5-
face —*see* Corrosion, head
finger T23.429
first degree T23.529
left T23.422
first degree T23.522
second degree T23.622
third degree T23.722
multiple sites (without thumb) T23.439
with thumb T23.449
first degree T23.549
left T23.442
first degree T23.542
second degree T23.642
third degree T23.742
right T23.441
first degree T23.541
second degree T23.641
third degree T23.741
second degree T23.649
third degree T23.749
first degree T23.539
left T23.432
first degree T23.532
second degree T23.632
third degree T23.732
right T23.431
first degree T23.531
second degree T23.631
third degree T23.731
second degree T23.639
third degree T23.739
right T23.421
first degree T23.521
second degree T23.621
third degree T23.721
second degree T23.629
third degree T23.729
flank —*see* Corrosion, abdomen
foot T25.429
first degree T25.529
left T25.422
first degree T25.522
second degree T25.622
third degree T25.722
multiple with ankle —*see* Corrosion, lower, limb, multiple, ankle and foot
right T25.421
first degree T25.521
second degree T25.621
third degree T25.721
second degree T25.629
third degree T25.729
forearm T22.419
first degree T22.519
left T22.412
first degree T22.512
second degree T22.612
third degree T22.712
right T22.411
first degree T22.511
second degree T22.611
third degree T22.711
second degree T22.619
third degree T22.719
forehead T20.46
first degree T20.56
second degree T20.66
third degree T20.76

Corrosion *(continued)*
fourth degree - code as Corrosion, third degree, by site
full thickness skin loss - code as Corrosion, third degree, by site
gastrointestinal tract NEC T28.7
genital organs
external
female T21.47
first degree T21.57
second degree T21.67
third degree T21.77
male T21.46
first degree T21.56
second degree T21.66
third degree T21.76
internal T28.8
groin —*see* Corrosion, abdominal wall
hand(s) T23.409
back —*see* Corrosion, dorsum of hand
finger —*see* Corrosion, finger
first degree T23.509
left T23.402
first degree T23.502
second degree T23.602
third degree T23.702
multiple sites with wrist T23.499
first degree T23.599
left T23.492
first degree T23.592
second degree T23.692
third degree T23.792
right T23.491
first degree T23.591
second degree T23.691
third degree T23.791
second degree T23.699
third degree T23.799
palm —*see* Corrosion, palm
right T23.401
first degree T23.501
second degree T23.601
third degree T23.701
second degree T23.609
third degree T23.709
thumb —*see* Corrosion, thumb
head (and face) (and neck) T20.40
cheek —*see* Corrosion, cheek
chin —*see* Corrosion, chin
ear —*see* Corrosion, ear
eye(s) only —*see* Corrosion, eye
first degree T20.50
forehead —*see* Corrosion, forehead
lip —*see* Corrosion, lip
multiple sites T20.49
first degree T20.59
second degree T20.69
third degree T20.79
neck —*see* Corrosion, neck
nose —*see* Corrosion, nose
scalp —*see* Corrosion, scalp
second degree T20.60
third degree T20.70
hip(s) —*see* Corrosion, lower, limb
inhalation —*see* Corrosion, respiratory tract
internal organ(s) (*see also* Corrosion, by site) T28.90
alimentary tract T28.7
esophagus T28.6
esophagus T28.6
genitourinary T28.8
mouth T28.5
pharynx T28.5
specified organ NEC T28.99
interscapular region —*see* Corrosion, back, upper
intestine (large) (small) T28.7
knee T24.429

Corrosion *(continued)*
- knee *(continued)*
  - first degree T24.529
  - left T24.422
    - first degree T24.522
    - second degree T24.622
    - third degree T24.722
  - right T24.421
    - first degree T24.521
    - second degree T24.621
    - third degree T24.721
  - second degree T24.629
  - third degree T24.729
- labium (majus) (minus) —*see* Corrosion, genital organs, external, female
- lacrimal apparatus, duct, gland or sac —*see* Corrosion, eye, specified site NEC
- larynx T27.4
  - with lung T27.5
- leg(s) (meaning lower limb(s)) —*see* Corrosion, lower limb
- limb(s)
  - lower —*see* Corrosion, lower, limb
  - upper —*see* Corrosion, upper limb
- lip(s) T20.42
  - first degree T20.52
  - second degree T20.62
  - third degree T20.72
- lower
  - back —*see* Corrosion, back
  - limb T24.409
    - ankle —*see* Corrosion, ankle
    - calf —*see* Corrosion, calf
    - first degree T24.509
    - foot —*see* Corrosion, foot
    - knee —*see* Corrosion, knee
    - left T24.402
      - first degree T24.502
      - second degree T24.602
      - third degree T24.702
    - multiple sites, except ankle and foot T24.499
      - ankle and foot T25.499
        - first degree T25.599
        - left T25.492
          - first degree T25.592
          - second degree T25.692
          - third degree T25.792
        - right T25.491
          - first degree T25.591
          - second degree T25.691
          - third degree T25.791
        - second degree T25.699
        - third degree T25.799
      - first degree T24.599
      - left T24.492
        - first degree T24.592
        - second degree T24.692
        - third degree T24.792
      - right T24.491
        - first degree T24.591
        - second degree T24.691
        - third degree T24.791
      - second degree T24.699
      - third degree T24.799
    - right T24.401
      - first degree T24.501
      - second degree T24.601
      - third degree T24.701
    - second degree T24.609
    - hip —*see* Corrosion, thigh
    - thigh —*see* Corrosion, thigh
    - third degree T24.709
- lung (with larynx and trachea) T27.5
- mouth T28.5
- neck T20.47
  - first degree T20.57
  - second degree T20.67
  - third degree T20.77
- nose (septum) T20.44
  - first degree T20.54
  - second degree T20.64
  - third degree T20.74
- ocular adnexa —*see* Corrosion, eye
- orbit region —*see* Corrosion, eyelid
- palm T23.459
  - first degree T23.559
  - left T23.452
    - first degree T23.552
    - second degree T23.652
    - third degree T23.752
  - right T23.451
    - first degree T23.551
    - second degree T23.651
    - third degree T23.751
  - second degree T23.659
  - third degree T23.759
- partial thickness - code as Corrosion, unspecified degree, by site
- pelvis —*see* Corrosion, trunk
- penis —*see* Corrosion, genital organs, external, male
- perineum
  - female —*see* Corrosion, genital organs, external, female
  - male —*see* Corrosion, genital organs, external, male
- periocular area —*see* Corrosion, eyelid
- pharynx T28.5
- rectum T28.7
- respiratory tract T27.7
  - larynx —*see* Corrosion, larynx
  - specified part NEC T27.6
  - trachea —*see* Corrosion, larynx
- sac, lacrimal —*see* Corrosion, eye, specified site NEC
- scalp T20.45
  - first degree T20.55
  - second degree T20.65
  - third degree T20.75
- scapular region T22.469
  - first degree T22.569
  - left T22.462
    - first degree T22.562
    - second degree T22.662
    - third degree T22.762
  - right T22.461
    - first degree T22.561
    - second degree T22.661
    - third degree T22.761
  - second degree T22.669
  - third degree T22.769
- sclera —*see* Corrosion, eye, specified site NEC
- scrotum —*see* Corrosion, genital organs, external, male
- shoulder T22.459
  - first degree T22.559
  - left T22.452
    - first degree T22.552
    - second degree T22.652
    - third degree T22.752
  - right T22.451
    - first degree T22.551
    - second degree T22.651
    - third degree T22.751
  - second degree T22.659
  - third degree T22.759
- stomach T28.7
- temple —*see* Corrosion, head
- testis —*see* Corrosion, genital organs, external, male
- thigh T24.419
  - first degree T24.519
  - left T24.412
    - first degree T24.512
    - second degree T24.612
    - third degree T24.712

Corrosion *(continued)*
- thigh *(continued)*
  - right T24.411
    - first degree T24.511
    - second degree T24.611
    - third degree T24.711
  - second degree T24.619
  - third degree T24.719
- thorax (external) —*see* Corrosion, trunk
- throat (meaning pharynx) T28.5
- thumb(s) T23.419
  - first degree T23.519
  - left T23.412
    - first degree T23.512
    - second degree T23.612
    - third degree T23.712
  - multiple sites with fingers T23.449
    - first degree T23.549
    - left T23.442
      - first degree T23.542
      - second degree T23.642
      - third degree T23.742
    - right T23.441
      - first degree T23.541
      - second degree T23.641
      - third degree T23.741
    - second degree T23.649
    - third degree T23.749
  - right T23.411
    - first degree T23.511
    - second degree T23.611
    - third degree T23.711
  - second degree T23.619
  - third degree T23.719
- toe T25.439
  - first degree T25.539
  - left T25.432
    - first degree T25.532
    - second degree T25.632
    - third degree T25.732
  - right T25.431
    - first degree T25.531
    - second degree T25.631
    - third degree T25.731
  - second degree T25.639
  - third degree T25.739
- tongue T28.5
- tonsil(s) T28.5
- total body —*see* Corrosion, multiple body regions
- trachea T27.4
  - with lung T27.5
- trunk T21.40
  - abdominal wall —*see* Corrosion, abdominal wall
  - anus —*see* Corrosion, buttock
  - axilla —*see* Corrosion, upper limb
  - back —*see* Corrosion, back
  - breast —*see* Corrosion, chest wall
  - buttock —*see* Corrosion, buttock
  - chest wall —*see* Corrosion, chest wall
  - first degree T21.50
  - flank —*see* Corrosion, abdominal wall
  - genital
    - female —*see* Corrosion, genital organs, external, female
    - male —*see* Corrosion, genital organs, external, male
  - groin —*see* Corrosion, abdominal wall
  - interscapular region —*see* Corrosion, back, upper
  - labia —*see* Corrosion, genital organs, external, female
  - lower back —*see* Corrosion, back
  - penis —*see* Corrosion, genital organs, external, male

Corrosion *(continued)*
- trunk *(continued)*
  - perineum
    - female —*see* Corrosion, genital organs, external, female
    - male —*see* Corrosion, genital organs, external, male
  - scapular region —*see* Corrosion, upper limb
  - scrotum —*see* Corrosion, genital organs, external, male
  - second degree T21.60
  - shoulder —*see* Corrosion, upper limb
  - specified site NEC T21.49
    - first degree T21.59
    - second degree T21.69
    - third degree T21.79
  - testes —*see* Corrosion, genital organs, external, male
  - third degree T21.70
  - upper back —*see* Corrosion, back, upper
  - vagina T28.8
  - vulva —*see* Corrosion, genital organs, external, female
- unspecified site with extent of body surface involved specified
  - less than 10 percent T32.0
  - 10-19 percent (0-9 percent third degree) T32.10
    - with 10-19 percent third degree T32.11
  - 20-29 percent (0-9 percent third degree) T32.20
    - with
      - 10-19 percent third degree T32.21
      - 20-29 percent third degree T32.22
  - 30-39 percent (0-9 percent third degree) T32.30
    - with
      - 10-19 percent third degree T32.31
      - 20-29 percent third degree T32.32
      - 30-39 percent third degree T32.33
  - 40-49 percent (0-9 percent third degree) T32.40
    - with
      - 10-19 percent third degree T32.41
      - 20-29 percent third degree T32.42
      - 30-39 percent third degree T32.43
      - 40-49 percent third degree T32.44
  - 50-59 percent (0-9 percent third degree) T32.50
    - with
      - 10-19 percent third degree T32.51
      - 20-29 percent third degree T32.52
      - 30-39 percent third degree T32.53
      - 40-49 percent third degree T32.54
      - 50-59 percent third degree T32.55
  - 60-69 percent (0-9 percent third degree) T32.60
    - with
      - 10-19 percent third degree T32.61
      - 20-29 percent third degree T32.62

Corrosion *(continued)*
- unspecified site with extent of body surface involved specified *(continued)*
  - 60-69 percent *(continued)*
    - with *(continued)*
      - 30-39 percent third degree T32.63
      - 40-49 percent third degree T32.64
      - 50-59 percent third degree T32.65
      - 60-69 percent third degree T32.66
  - 70-79 percent (0-9 percent third degree) T32.70
    - with
      - 10-19 percent third degree T32.71
      - 20-29 percent third degree T32.72
      - 30-39 percent third degree T32.73
      - 40-49 percent third degree T32.74
      - 50-59 percent third degree T32.75
      - 60-69 percent third degree T32.76
      - 70-79 percent third degree T32.77
  - 80-89 percent (0-9 percent third degree) T32.80
    - with
      - 10-19 percent third degree T32.81
      - 20-29 percent third degree T32.82
      - 30-39 percent third degree T32.83
      - 40-49 percent third degree T32.84
      - 50-59 percent third degree T32.85
      - 60-69 percent third degree T32.86
      - 70-79 percent third degree T32.87
      - 80-89 percent third degree T32.88
  - 90 percent or more (0-9 percent third degree) T32.90
    - with
      - 10-19 percent third degree T32.91
      - 20-29 percent third degree T32.92
      - 30-39 percent third degree T32.93
      - 40-49 percent third degree T32.94
      - 50-59 percent third degree T32.95
      - 60-69 percent third degree T32.96
      - 70-79 percent third degree T32.97
      - 80-89 percent third degree T32.98
      - 90-99 percent third degree T32.99
- upper limb (axilla) (scapular region) T22.40
  - above elbow —*see* Corrosion, above elbow
  - axilla —*see* Corrosion, axilla
  - elbow —*see* Corrosion, elbow
  - first degree T22.50
  - forearm —*see* Corrosion, forearm
  - hand —*see* Corrosion, hand

Corrosion *(continued)*
- upper limb *(continued)*
  - interscapular region —*see* Corrosion, back, upper
  - multiple sites T22.499
    - first degree T22.599
    - left T22.492
      - first degree T22.592
      - second degree T22.692
      - third degree T22.792
    - right T22.491
      - first degree T22.591
      - second degree T22.691
      - third degree T22.791
    - second degree T22.699
    - third degree T22.799
  - scapular region —*see* Corrosion, scapular region
  - second degree T22.60
  - shoulder —*see* Corrosion, shoulder
  - third degree T22.70
  - wrist —*see* Corrosion, hand
- uterus T28.8
- vagina T28.8
- vulva —*see* Corrosion, genital organs, external, female
- wrist T23.479
  - first degree T23.579
  - left T23.472
    - first degree T23.572
    - second degree T23.672
    - third degree T23.772
  - multiple sites with hand T23.499
    - first degree T23.599
    - left T23.492
      - first degree T23.592
      - second degree T23.692
      - third degree T23.792
    - right T23.491
      - first degree T23.591
      - second degree T23.691
      - third degree T23.791
    - second degree T23.699
    - third degree T23.799
  - right T23.471
    - first degree T23.571
    - second degree T23.671
    - third degree T23.771
  - second degree T23.679
  - third degree T23.779

Corrosive burn —*see* Corrosion

Corsican fever —*see* Malaria

Cortical —*see* condition

Cortico-adrenal —*see* condition

Coryza (acute) J00
- with grippe or influenza —*see* Influenza, with, respiratory manifestations NEC
- syphilitic
  - congenital (chronic) A50.05

Costen's syndrome or complex M26.69

Costiveness —*see* Constipation

Costochondritis M94.0

Cotard's syndrome F22

Cot death R99

Cotia virus B08.8

Cotton wool spots (retinal) H35.81

Cotungo's disease —*see* Sciatica

Cough (affected) (chronic) (epidemic) (nervous) R05
- with hemorrhage —*see* Hemoptysis
- bronchial R05
  - with grippe or influenza —*see* Influenza, with, respiratory manifestations NEC
- functional F45.8

Cough *(continued)*
- hysterical F45.8
- laryngeal, spasmodic R05
- psychogenic F45.8
- smokers' J41.0
- tea taster's B49

Counseling (for) Z71.9
- abuse NEC
  - perpetrator Z69.82
  - victim Z69.81
- alcohol abuser Z71.41
  - family Z71.42
- child abuse
  - nonparental
    - perpetrator Z69.021
    - victim Z69.020
  - parental
    - perpetrator Z69.011
    - victim Z69.010
- consanguinity Z71.89
- contraceptive Z30.09
- dietary Z71.3
- drug abuser Z71.51
  - family member Z71.52
- exercise Z71.82
- family Z71.89
- fertility preservation (prior to cancer therapy) (prior to removal of gonads) Z31.62
- for non-attending third party Z71.0
  - related to sexual behavior or orientation Z70.2
- genetic
  - nonprocreative Z71.83
  - procreative NEC Z31.5
- gestational carrier Z31.7
- health (advice) (education) (instruction) —*see* Counseling, medical
- human immunodeficiency virus (HIV) Z71.7
- impotence Z70.1
- insulin pump use Z46.81
- medical (for) Z71.9
  - boarding school resident Z59.3
  - consanguinity Z71.89
  - feared complaint and no disease found Z71.1
  - human immunodeficiency virus (HIV) Z71.7
  - institutional resident Z59.3
  - on behalf of another Z71.0
    - related to sexual behavior or orientation Z70.2
  - person living alone Z60.2
  - specified reason NEC Z71.89
- natural family planning
  - procreative Z31.61
  - to avoid pregnancy Z30.02
- perpetrator (of)
  - abuse NEC Z69.82
  - child abuse
    - non-parental Z69.021
    - parental Z69.011
  - rape NEC Z69.82
  - spousal abuse Z69.12
- procreative NEC Z31.69
  - fertility preservation (prior to cancer therapy) (prior to removal of gonads) Z31.62
  - using natural family planning Z31.61
- promiscuity Z70.1
- rape victim Z69.81
- religious Z71.81
- sex, sexual (related to) Z70.9
  - attitude(s) Z70.0
  - behavior or orientation Z70.1
  - combined concerns Z70.3
  - non-responsiveness Z70.1
  - on behalf of third party Z70.2
  - specified reason NEC Z70.8

Counseling *(continued)*
- specified reason NEC Z71.89
- spiritual Z71.81
- spousal abuse (perpetrator) Z69.12
  - victim Z69.11
- substance abuse Z71.89
  - alcohol Z71.41
  - drug Z71.51
  - tobacco Z71.6
- tobacco use Z71.6
- use (of)
  - insulin pump Z46.81
- victim (of)
  - abuse Z69.81
  - child abuse
    - by parent Z69.010
    - non-parental Z69.020
  - rape NEC Z69.81

Coupled rhythm R00.8

Couvelaire syndrome or uterus (complicating delivery) O45.8X-

Cowperitis —*see* Urethritis

Cowper's gland —*see* condition

Cowpox B08.010
- due to vaccination T88.1

Coxa
- magna M91.4-
- plana M91.2-
- valga (acquired) —*see also* Deformity, limb, specified type NEC, thigh
  - congenital Q65.81
  - sequelae (late effect) of rickets E64.3
- vara (acquired) —*see also* Deformity, limb, specified type NEC, thigh
  - congenital Q65.82
  - sequelae (late effect) of rickets E64.3

Coxalgia, coxalgic (nontuberculous) —*see also* Pain, joint, hip
- tuberculous A18.02

Coxitis —*see* Monoarthritis, hip

Coxsackie (virus) (infection) B34.1
- as cause of disease classified elsewhere B97.11
- carditis B33.20
- central nervous system NEC A88.8
- endocarditis B33.21
- enteritis A08.39
- meningitis (aseptic) A87.0
- myocarditis B33.22
- pericarditis B33.23
- pharyngitis B08.5
- pleurodynia B33.0
- specific disease NEC B33.8

Crabs, meaning pubic lice B85.3

Crack baby P04.41

Cracked nipple N64.0
- associated with
  - lactation O92.13
  - pregnancy O92.11-
  - puerperium O92.12

Cracked tooth K03.81

Cradle cap L21.0

Craft neurosis F48.8

Cramp(s) R25.2
- abdominal —*see* Pain, abdominal
- bathing T75.1
- colic R10.83
  - psychogenic F45.8
- due to immersion T75.1
- fireman T67.2
- heat T67.2
- immersion T75.1
- intestinal —*see* Pain, abdominal
  - psychogenic F45.8

Cramp(s) *(continued)*
leg, sleep related G47.62
limb (lower) (upper) NEC R25.2
sleep related G47.62
linotypist's F48.8
organic G25.89
muscle (limb) (general) R25.2
due to immersion T75.1
psychogenic F45.8
occupational (hand) F48.8
organic G25.89
salt-depletion E87.1
sleep related, leg G47.62
stoker's T67.2
swimmer's T75.1
telegrapher's F48.8
organic G25.89
typist's F48.8
organic G25.89
uterus N94.89
menstrual —*see* Dysmenorrhea
writer's F48.8
organic G25.89

Cranial —*see* condition

Craniocleidodysostosis Q74.0

Craniofenestria (skull) Q75.8

Craniolacunia (skull) Q75.8

Craniopagus Q89.4

Craniopathy, metabolic M85.2

Craniopharyngeal —*see* condition

Craniopharyngioma D44.4

Craniorachischisis (totalis) Q00.1

Cranioschisis Q75.8

Craniostenosis Q75.0

Craniosynostosis Q75.0

Craniotabes (cause unknown) M83.8
neonatal P96.3
rachitic E64.3
syphilitic A50.56

Cranium —*see* condition

Craw-craw —*see* Onchocerciasis

Creaking joint —*see* Derangement, joint, specified type NEC

Creeping
eruption B76.9
palsy or paralysis G12.22

Crenated tongue K14.8

Creotoxism A05.9

Crepitus
caput Q75.8
joint —*see* Derangement, joint, specified type NEC

Crescent or conus choroid, congenital Q14.3

CREST syndrome M34.1

Cretin, cretinism (congenital) (endemic) (nongoitrous) (sporadic) E00.9
pelvis
with disproportion (fetopelvic) O33.0
causing obstructed labor O65.0
type
hypothyroid E00.1
mixed E00.2
myxedematous E00.1
neurological E00.0

Creutzfeldt-Jakob disease or syndrome (with dementia) A81.00
familial A81.09
iatrogenic A81.09
specified NEC A81.09
sporadic A81.09
variant (vCJD) A81.01

Crib death R99

Cribriform hymen Q52.3

Cri-du-chat syndrome Q93.4

Crigler-Najjar disease or syndrome E80.5

Crime, victim of Z65.4

Crimean hemorrhagic fever A98.0

Criminalism F60.2

Crisis
abdomen R10.0
acute reaction F43.0
addisonian E27.2
adrenal (cortical) E27.2
celiac K90.0
Dietl's N13.8
emotional —*see also* Disorder, adjustment
acute reaction to stress F43.0
specific to childhood and adolescence F93.8
glaucomatocyclitic —*see* Glaucoma, secondary, inflammation
heart —*see* Failure, heart
nitritoid I95.2
correct substance properly administered —*see* Table of Drugs and Chemicals, by drug, adverse effect
overdose or wrong substance given or taken —*see* Table of Drugs and Chemicals, by drug, poisoning
oculogyric H51.8
psychogenic F45.8
Pel's (tabetic) A52.11
psychosexual identity F64.2
renal N28.0
sickle-cell D57.00
with
acute chest syndrome D57.01
splenic sequestration D57.02
state (acute reaction) F43.0
tabetic A52.11
thyroid —*see* Thyrotoxicosis with thyroid storm
thyrotoxic —*see* Thyrotoxicosis with thyroid storm

Crocq's disease (acrocyanosis) I73.89

Crohn's disease —*see* Enteritis, regional

Crooked septum, nasal J34.2

Cross syndrome E70.328

Crossbite (anterior) (posterior) M26.24

Cross-eye —*see* Strabismus, convergent concomitant

Croup, croupous (catarrhal) (infectious) (inflammatory) (nondiphtheritic) J05.0
bronchial J20.9
diphtheritic A36.2
false J38.5
spasmodic J38.5
diphtheritic A36.2
stridulous J38.5
diphtheritic A36.2

Crouzon's disease Q75.1

Crowding, tooth, teeth, fully erupted M26.31

CRST syndrome M34.1

Cruchet's disease A85.8

Cruelty in children —*see also* Disorder, conduct

Crural ulcer —*see* Ulcer, lower limb

Crush, crushed, crushing T14.8

Crush, crushed, crushing *(continued)*
abdomen S38.1
ankle S97.0-
arm (upper) (and shoulder) S47.-
axilla —*see* Crush, arm
back, lower S38.1
buttock S38.1
cheek S07.0
chest S28.0
cranium S07.1
ear S07.0
elbow S57.0-
extremity
lower
ankle —*see* Crush, ankle
below knee —*see* Crush, leg
foot —*see* Crush, foot
hip —*see* Crush, hip
knee —*see* Crush, knee
thigh —*see* Crush, thigh
toe —*see* Crush, toe
upper
below elbow S67.9-
elbow —*see* Crush, elbow
finger —*see* Crush, finger
forearm —*see* Crush, forearm
hand —*see* Crush, hand
thumb —*see* Crush, thumb
upper arm —*see* Crush, arm
wrist —*see* Crush, wrist
face S07.0
finger(s) S67.1-
with hand (and wrist) —*see* Crush, hand, specified site NEC
index S67.19-
little S67.19-
middle S67.19-
ring S67.19-
thumb —*see* Crush, thumb
foot S97.8-
toe —*see* Crush, toe
forearm S57.8-
genitalia, external
female S38.002
vagina S38.03
vulva S38.03
male S38.001
penis S38.01
scrotum S38.02
testis S38.02
hand (except fingers alone) S67.2-
with wrist S67.4-
head S07.9
specified NEC S07.8
heel —*see* Crush, foot
hip S77.0-
with thigh S77.2-
internal organ (abdomen, chest, or pelvis) NEC T14.8
knee S87.0-
labium (majus) (minus) S38.03
larynx S17.0
leg (lower) S87.8-
knee —*see* Crush, knee
lip S07.0
lower
back S38.1
leg —*see* Crush, leg
neck S17.9
nerve —*see* Injury, nerve
nose S07.0
pelvis S38.1
penis S38.01
scalp S07.8
scapular region —*see* Crush, arm
scrotum S38.02
severe, unspecified site T14.8
shoulder (and upper arm) —*see* Crush, arm
skull S07.1

Crush, crushed, crushing *(continued)*
syndrome (complication of trauma) T79.5
testis S38.02
thigh S77.1-
with hip S77.2-
throat S17.8
thumb S67.0-
with hand (and wrist) —*see* Crush, hand, specified site NEC
toe(s) S97.10-
great S97.11-
lesser S97.12-
trachea S17.0
vagina S38.03
vulva S38.03
wrist S67.3-
with hand S67.4-

Crusta lactea L21.0

Crusts R23.4

Crutch paralysis —*see* Injury, brachial plexus

Cruveilhier-Baumgarten cirrhosis, disease or syndrome K74.69

Cruveilhier's atrophy or disease G12.8

Crying (constant) (continuous) (excessive)
child, adolescent, or adult R45.83
infant (baby) (newborn) R68.11

Cryofibrinogenemia D89.2

Cryoglobulinemia (essential) (idiopathic) (mixed) (primary) (purpura) (secondary) (vasculitis) D89.1
with lung involvement D89.1 *[J99]*

Cryptitis (anal) (rectal) K62.89

Cryptococcosis, cryptococcus (infection) (neoformans) B45.9
bone B45.3
cerebral B45.1
cutaneous B45.2
disseminated B45.7
generalized B45.7
meningitis B45.1
meningocerebralis B45.1
osseous B45.3
pulmonary B45.0
skin B45.2
specified NEC B45.8

Cryptopapillitis (anus) K62.89

Cryptophthalmos Q11.2
syndrome Q87.0

Cryptorchid, cryptorchism, cryptorchidism Q53.9
bilateral Q53.20
abdominal Q53.211
perineal Q53.22
unilateral Q53.10
abdominal Q53.111
perineal Q53.12

Cryptosporidiosis A07.2
hepatobiliary B88.8
respiratory B88.8

Cryptostromosis J67.6

Crystalluria R82.99

Cubitus
congenital Q68.8
valgus (acquired) M21.0-
congenital Q68.8
sequelae (late effect) of rickets E64.3
varus (acquired) M21.1-
congenital Q68.8
sequelae (late effect) of rickets E64.3

Cultural deprivation or shock Z60.3

Curling esophagus K22.4

Curling's ulcer *—see* Ulcer, peptic, acute

Curschmann (-Batten) (-Steinert) disease or syndrome G71.11

Curse, Ondine's *—see* Apnea, sleep

Curvature
- organ or site, congenital NEC *—see* Distortion
- penis (lateral) Q55.61
- Pott's (spinal) A18.01
- radius, idiopathic, progressive (congenital) Q74.0
- spine (acquired) (angular) (idiopathic) (incorrect) (postural) *—see* Dorsopathy, deforming
  - congenital Q67.5
  - due to or associated with
    - Charcot-Marie-Tooth disease (*see also* subcategory M49.8) G60.0
    - osteitis
      - deformans M88.88
      - fibrosa cystica (*see also* subcategory M49.8) E21.0
    - tuberculosis (Pott's curvature) A18.01
  - sequelae (late effect) of rickets E64.3
  - tuberculous A18.01

Cushingoid due to steroid therapy E24.2
- correct substance properly administered *—see* Table of Drugs and Chemicals, by drug, adverse effect
- overdose or wrong substance given or taken *—see* Table of Drugs and Chemicals, by drug, poisoning

Cushing's
- syndrome or disease E24.9
  - drug-induced E24.2
  - iatrogenic E24.2
  - pituitary-dependent E24.0
  - specified NEC E24.8
- ulcer *—see* Ulcer, peptic, acute

Cusp, Carabelli - omit code

Cut (external) *—see also* Laceration
- muscle *—see* Injury, muscle

Cutaneous *—see also* condition
- hemorrhage R23.3
- larva migrans B76.9

Cutis *—see also* condition
- hyperelastica Q82.8
  - acquired L57.4
- laxa (hyperelastica) *—see* Dermatolysis
- marmorata R23.8
- osteosis L94.2
- pendula *—see* Dermatolysis
- rhomboidalis nuchae L57.2
- verticis gyrata Q82.8
  - acquired L91.8

Cyanosis R23.0
- due to
  - patent foramen botalli Q21.1
  - persistent foramen ovale Q21.1
- enterogenous D74.8
- paroxysmal digital *—see* Raynaud's disease
  - with gangrene I73.01
- retina, retinal H35.89

Cyanotic heart disease I24.9
- congenital Q24.9

Cycle
- anovulatory N97.0
- menstrual, irregular N92.6

Cyclencephaly Q04.9

Cyclical vomiting (*see also* Vomiting, cyclica) G43.A0
- psychogenic F50.89

Cyclitis (*see also* Iridocyclitis) H20.9
- chronic *—see* Iridocyclitis, chronic
- Fuchs' heterochromic H20.81-

Cyclitis
- granulomatous *—see* Iridocyclitis, chronic
- lens-induced *—see* Iridocyclitis, lens-induced
- posterior H30.2-

Cycloid personality F34.0

Cyclophoria H50.54

Cyclopia, cyclops Q87.0

Cyclopism Q87.0

Cyclosporiasis A07.4

Cyclothymia F34.0

Cyclothymic personality F34.0

Cyclotropia H50.41-

Cylindroma *—see also* Neoplasm, malignant, by site
- eccrine dermal *—see* Neoplasm, skin, benign
- skin *—see* Neoplasm, skin, benign

Cylindruria R82.99

Cynanche
- diphtheritic A36.2
- tonsillaris J36

Cynophobia F40.218

Cynorexia R63.2

Cyphosis *—see* Kyphosis

Cyprus fever *—see* Brucellosis

Cyst (colloid) (mucous) (simple) (retention)
- adenoid (infected) J35.8
- aneurysmal M27.49
- adrenal gland E27.8
  - congenital Q89.1
- air, lung J98.4
- allantoic Q64.4
- alveolar process (jaw bone) M27.40
- amnion, amniotic O41.8X-
- anterior
  - chamber (eye) *—see* Cyst, iris
  - nasopalatine K09.1
- antrum J34.1
- anus K62.89
- apical (tooth) (periodontal) K04.8
- appendix K38.8
- arachnoid, brain (acquired) G93.0
  - congenital Q04.6
- arytenoid J38.7
- Baker's M71.2-
  - ruptured M66.0
  - tuberculous A18.02
- Bartholin's gland N75.0
- bile duct (common) (hepatic) K83.5
- bladder (multiple) (trigone) N32.89
- blue dome (breast) *—see* Cyst, breast
- bone (local) NEC M85.60
  - aneurysmal M85.50
    - ankle M85.57-
    - foot M85.57-
    - forearm M85.53-
    - hand M85.54-
    - jaw M27.49
    - lower leg M85.56-
    - multiple site M85.59
    - neck M85.58
    - rib M85.58
    - shoulder M85.51-
    - skull M85.58

Cyst *(continued)*
- bone *(continued)*
  - aneurysmal *(continued)*
    - specified site NEC M85.58
    - thigh M85.55-
    - toe M85.57-
    - upper arm M85.52-
    - vertebra M85.58
  - solitary M85.40
    - ankle M85.47-
    - fibula M85.46-
    - foot M85.47-
    - hand M85.44-
    - humerus M85.42-
    - jaw M27.49
    - neck M85.48
    - pelvis M85.45-
    - radius M85.43-
    - rib M85.48
    - shoulder M85.41-
    - skull M85.48
    - specified site NEC M85.48
    - tibia M85.46-
    - toe M85.47-
    - ulna M85.43-
    - vertebra M85.48
  - specified type NEC M85.60
    - ankle M85.67-
    - foot M85.67-
    - forearm M85.63-
    - hand M85.64-
    - jaw M27.40
      - developmental (nonodontogenic) K09.1
        - odontogenic K09.0
      - latent M27.0
    - lower leg M85.66-
    - multiple site M85.69
    - neck M85.68
    - rib M85.68
    - shoulder M85.61-
    - skull M85.68
    - specified site NEC M85.68
    - thigh M85.65-
    - toe M85.67-
    - upper arm M85.62-
    - vertebra M85.68
- brain (acquired) G93.0
  - congenital Q04.6
  - hydatid B67.99 *[G94]*
  - third ventricle (colloid), congenital Q04.6
- branchial (cleft) Q18.0
- branchiogenic Q18.0
- breast (benign) (blue dome) (pedunculated) (solitary) N60.0-
  - involution *—see* Dysplasia, mammary, specified type NEC
  - sebaceous *—see* Dysplasia, mammary, specified type NEC
- broad ligament (benign) N83.8
- bronchogenic (mediastinal) (sequestration) J98.4
  - congenital Q33.0
- buccal K09.8
- bulbourethral gland N36.8
- bursa, bursal NEC M71.30
  - with rupture *—see* Rupture, synovium
  - ankle M71.37-
  - elbow M71.32-
  - foot M71.37-
  - hand M71.34-
  - hip M71.35-
  - multiple sites M71.39
  - pharyngeal J39.2
  - popliteal space *—see* Cyst, Baker's
  - shoulder M71.31-
  - specified site NEC M71.38
  - wrist M71.33-

Cyst *(continued)*
- calcifying odontogenic D16.5
  - upper jaw (bone) (maxilla) D16.4
- canal of Nuck (female) N94.89
  - congenital Q52.4
- canthus *—see* Cyst, conjunctiva
- carcinomatous *—see* Neoplasm, malignant, by site
- cauda equina G95.89
- cavum septi pellucidi *—see* Cyst, brain
- celomic (pericardium) Q24.8
- cerebellopontine (angle) *—see* Cyst, brain
- cerebellum *—see* Cyst, brain
- cerebral *—see* Cyst, brain
- cervical lateral Q18.0
- cervix NEC N88.8
  - embryonic Q51.6
  - nabothian N88.8
- chiasmal optic NEC *—see* Disorder, optic, chiasm
- chocolate (ovary) N80.1
- choledochus, congenital Q44.4
- chorion O41.8X-
- choroid plexus G93.0
- ciliary body *—see* Cyst, iris
- clitoris N90.7
- colon K63.89
- common (bile) duct K83.5
- congenital NEC Q89.8
  - adrenal gland Q89.1
  - epiglottis Q31.8
  - esophagus Q39.8
  - fallopian tube Q50.4
  - kidney Q61.00
    - more than one (multiple) Q61.02
      - specified as polycystic Q61.3
        - adult type Q61.2
        - infantile type NEC Q61.19
          - collecting duct dilation Q61.11
    - solitary Q61.01
  - larynx Q31.8
  - liver Q44.6
  - lung Q33.0
  - mediastinum Q34.1
  - ovary Q50.1
  - oviduct Q50.4
  - periurethral (tissue) Q64.79
  - prepuce Q55.69
  - salivary gland (any) Q38.4
  - sublingual Q38.6
  - submaxillary gland Q38.6
  - thymus (gland) Q89.2
  - tongue Q38.3
  - ureterovesical orifice Q62.8
  - vulva Q52.79
- conjunctiva H11.44-
- cornea H18.89-
- corpora quadrigemina G93.0
- corpus
  - albicans N83.29-
  - luteum (hemorrhagic) (ruptured) N83.1-
- Cowper's gland (benign) (infected) N36.8
- cranial meninges G93.0
- craniobuccal pouch E23.6
- craniopharyngeal pouch E23.6
- cystic duct K82.8
- Cysticercus *—see* Cysticercosis
- Dandy-Walker Q03.1
  - with spina bifida *—see* Spina bifida
- dental (root) K04.8
  - developmental K09.0
  - eruption K09.0
  - primordial K09.0

Cyst *(continued)*
- dentigerous (mandible) (maxilla) K09.0
- dermoid *—see* Neoplasm, benign, by site
  - with malignant transformation C56.-
  - implantation
    - external area or site (skin) NEC L72.0
    - iris *—see* Cyst, iris, implantation
    - vagina N89.8
    - vulva N90.7
  - mouth K09.8
  - oral soft tissue K09.8
  - sacrococcygeal *—see* Cyst, pilonidal
- developmental K09.1
  - odontogenic K09.0
  - oral region (nonodontogenic) K09.1
  - ovary, ovarian Q50.1
- dura (cerebral) G93.0
  - spinal G96.19
- ear (external) Q18.1
- echinococcal *—see* Echinococcus
- embryonic
  - cervix uteri Q51.6
  - fallopian tube Q50.4
  - vagina Q52.4
- endometrium, endometrial (uterus) N85.8
  - ectopic *—see* Endometriosis
- enterogenous Q43.8
- epidermal, epidermoid (inclusion) (*see also* Cyst, skin) L72.0
  - mouth K09.8
  - oral soft tissue K09.8
- epididymis N50.3
- epiglottis J38.7
- epiphysis cerebri E34.8
- epithelial (inclusion) L72.0
- epoophoron Q50.5
- eruption K09.0
- esophagus K22.8
- ethmoid sinus J34.1
- external female genital organs NEC N90.7
- eye NEC H57.8
  - congenital Q15.8
- eyelid (sebaceous) H02.829
  - infected *—see* Hordeolum
  - left H02.826
    - lower H02.825
    - upper H02.824
  - right H02.823
    - lower H02.822
    - upper H02.821
- fallopian tube N83.8
  - congenital Q50.4
- fimbrial (twisted) Q50.4
- fissural (oral region) K09.1
- follicle (graafian) (hemorrhagic) N83.0-
  - nabothian N88.8
- follicular (atretic) (hemorrhagic) (ovarian) N83.0-
  - dentigerous K09.0
  - odontogenic K09.0
  - skin L72.9
    - specified NEC L72.8
- frontal sinus J34.1
- gallbladder K82.8
- ganglion *—see* Ganglion
- Gartner's duct Q52.4
- gingiva K09.0
- gland of Moll *—see* Cyst, eyelid
- globulomaxillary K09.1
- graafian follicle (hemorrhagic) N83.0-
- granulosal lutein (hemorrhagic) N83.1-
- hemangiomatous D18.00
  - intra-abdominal D18.03
  - intracranial D18.02
  - skin D18.01
- hemangiomatous *(continued)*
  - specified site NEC D18.09
- hemorrhagic M27.49
- hydatid (*see also* Echinococcus) B67.90
  - brain B67.99 *[G94]*
  - liver (*see also* Cyst, liver, hydatid) B67.8
  - lung NEC B67.99 *[J99]*
  - Morgagni
    - female Q50.5
    - male (epididymal) Q55.4
      - testicular Q55.29
  - specified site NEC B67.99
- hymen N89.8
  - embryonic Q52.4
- hypopharynx J39.2
- hypophysis, hypophyseal (duct) (recurrent) E23.6
  - cerebri E23.6
- implantation (dermoid)
  - external area or site (skin) NEC L72.0
  - iris *—see* Cyst, iris, implantation
  - vagina N89.8
  - vulva N90.7
- incisive canal K09.1
- inclusion (epidermal) (epithelial) (epidermoid) (squamous) L72.0
  - not of skin - code under Cyst, by site
- intestine (large) (small) K63.89
- intracranial *—see* Cyst, brain
- intraligamentous *—see also* Disorder, ligament
  - knee *—see* Derangement, knee
- intrasellar E23.6
- iris H21.309
  - exudative H21.31-
  - idiopathic H21.30-
  - implantation H21.32-
  - parasitic H21.33-
  - pars plana (primary) H21.34-
    - exudative H21.35-
- jaw (bone) M27.40
  - aneurysmal M27.49
  - developmental (odontogenic) K09.0
  - fissural K09.1
  - hemorrhagic M27.49
  - traumatic M27.49
- joint NEC *—see* Disorder, joint, specified type NEC
- kidney (acquired) N28.1
  - calyceal *—see* Hydronephrosis
  - congenital Q61.00
  - more than one (multiple) Q61.02
    - specified as polycystic Q61.3
      - adult type (autosomal dominant) Q61.2
      - infantile type (autosomal recessive) NEC Q61.19
        - collecting duct dilation Q61.11
  - pyelogenic *—see* Hydronephrosis
  - simple N28.1
  - solitary (single) Q61.01
    - acquired N28.1
- labium (majus) (minus) N90.7
  - sebaceous N90.7
- lacrimal *—see also* Disorder, lacrimal system, specified NEC
  - gland H04.13-
  - passages or sac *—see* Disorder, lacrimal system, specified NEC
- larynx J38.7
- lateral periodontal K09.0
- lens H27.8
  - congenital Q12.8
- lip (gland) K13.0
- liver (idiopathic) (simple) K76.89
  - congenital Q44.6
- liver *(continued)*
  - hydatid B67.8
    - granulosus B67.0
    - multilocularis B67.5
- lung J98.4
  - congenital Q33.0
  - giant bullous J43.9
- lutein N83.1-
- lymphangiomatous D18.1
- lymphoepithelial, oral soft tissue K09.8
- macula *—see* Degeneration, macula, hole
- malignant *—see* Neoplasm, malignant, by site
- mammary gland *—see* Cyst, breast
- mandible M27.40
  - dentigerous K09.0
  - radicular K04.8
- maxilla M27.40
  - dentigerous K09.0
  - radicular K04.8
- medial, face and neck Q18.8
- median
  - anterior maxillary K09.1
  - palatal K09.1
- mediastinum, congenital Q34.1
- meibomian (gland) *—see* Chalazion
  - infected *—see* Hordeolum
- membrane, brain G93.0
- meninges (cerebral) G93.0
  - spinal G96.19
- meniscus, knee *—see* Derangement, knee, meniscus, cystic
- mesentery, mesenteric K66.8
  - chyle I89.8
- mesonephric duct
  - female Q50.5
  - male Q55.4
- milk N64.89
- Morgagni (hydatid)
  - female Q50.5
  - male (epididymal) Q55.4
    - testicular Q55.29
- mouth K09.8
- Müllerian duct Q50.4
  - appendix testis Q55.29
  - cervix Q51.6
  - fallopian tube Q50.4
  - female Q50.4
  - male Q55.29
  - prostatic utricle Q55.4
  - vagina (embryonal) Q52.4
- multilocular (ovary) D39.10
  - benign *—see* Neoplasm, benign, by site
- myometrium N85.8
- nabothian (follicle) (ruptured) N88.8
- nasoalveolar K09.1
- nasolabial K09.1
- nasopalatine (anterior) (duct) K09.1
- nasopharynx J39.2
- neoplastic *—see* Neoplasm, uncertain behavior, by site
  - benign *—see* Neoplasm, benign, by site
- nervous system NEC G96.8
- neuroenteric (congenital) Q06.8
- nipple *—see* Cyst, breast
- nose (turbinates) J34.1
  - sinus J34.1
- odontogenic, developmental K09.0
- omentum (lesser) K66.8
  - congenital Q45.8
- ora serrata *—see* Cyst, retina, ora serrata
- oral
  - region K09.9
    - developmental (nonodontogenic) K09.1
- oral *(continued)*
  - region *(continued)*
    - specified NEC K09.8
  - soft tissue K09.9
    - specified NEC K09.8
- orbit H05.81-
- ovary, ovarian (twisted) N83.20-
  - adherent N83.20-
  - chocolate N80.1
  - corpus
    - albicans N83.29-
    - luteum (hemorrhagic) N83.1-
  - dermoid D27.9
  - developmental Q50.1
  - due to failure of involution NEC N83.20-
  - endometrial N80.1
  - follicular (graafian) (hemorrhagic) N83.0-
  - hemorrhagic N83.20-
  - in pregnancy or childbirth O34.8-
    - with obstructed labor O65.5
  - multilocular D39.10
  - pseudomucinous D27.9
  - retention N83.29-
  - serous N83.20-
  - specified NEC N83.29-
  - theca lutein (hemorrhagic) N83.1-
  - tuberculous A18.18
- oviduct N83.8
- palate (median) (fissural) K09.1
- palatine papilla (jaw) K09.1
- pancreas, pancreatic (hemorrhagic) (true) K86.2
  - congenital Q45.2
  - false K86.3
- paralabral
  - hip M24.85-
  - shoulder S43.43-
- paramesonephric duct Q50.4
  - female Q50.4
  - male Q55.29
- paranephric N28.1
- paraphysis, cerebri, congenital Q04.6
- parasitic B89
- parathyroid (gland) E21.4
- paratubal N83.8
- paraurethral duct N36.8
- paroophoron Q50.5
- parotid gland K11.6
- parovarian Q50.5
- pelvis, female N94.89
  - in pregnancy or childbirth O34.8-
    - causing obstructed labor O65.5
- penis (sebaceous) N48.89
- periapical K04.8
- pericardial (congenital) Q24.8
  - acquired (secondary) I31.8
- pericoronal K09.0
- periodontal K04.8
  - lateral K09.0
- peripelvic (lymphatic) N28.1
- peritoneum K66.8
  - chylous I89.8
- periventricular, acquired, newborn P91.1
- pharynx (wall) J39.2
- pilar L72.11
- pilonidal (infected) (rectum) L05.91
  - with abscess L05.01
  - malignant C44.59-
- pituitary (duct) (gland) E23.6
- placenta O43.19-
- pleura J94.8
- popliteal *—see* Cyst, Baker's
- porencephalic Q04.6
  - acquired G93.0
- postanal (infected) *—see* Cyst, pilonidal
- postmastoidectomy cavity (mucosal) *—see* Complications, postmastoidectomy, cyst

Cyst *(continued)*
- preauricular Q18.1
- prepuce N47.4
  - congenital Q55.69
- primordial (jaw) K09.0
- prostate N42.83
- pseudomucinous (ovary) D27.9
- pupillary, miotic H21.27-
- radicular (residual) K04.8
- radiculodental K04.8
- ranular K11.8
- Rathke's pouch E23.6
- rectum (epithelium) (mucous) K62.89
- renal *—see* Cyst, kidney
- residual (radicular) K04.8
- retention (ovary) N83.29-
  - salivary gland K11.6
- retina H33.19-
  - ora serrata H33.11-
  - parasitic H33.12-
- retroperitoneal K68.9
- sacrococcygeal (dermoid) *—see* Cyst, pilonidal
- salivary gland or duct (mucous extravasation or retention) K11.6
- Sampson's N80.1
- sclera H15.89
- scrotum L72.9
  - sebaceous L72.3
- sebaceous (duct) (gland) L72.3
  - breast *—see* Dysplasia, mammary, specified type NEC
  - eyelid *—see* Cyst, eyelid
  - genital organ NEC
    - female N94.89
    - male N50.89
  - scrotum L72.3
- semilunar cartilage (knee) (multiple) *—see* Derangement, knee, meniscus, cystic
- seminal vesicle N50.89
- serous (ovary) N83.20-
- sinus (accessory) (nasal) J34.1
- Skene's gland N36.8
- skin L72.9
  - breast *—see* Dysplasia, mammary, specified type NEC
  - epidermal, epidermoid L72.0
  - epithelial L72.0
  - eyelid *—see* Cyst, eyelid
  - genital organ NEC
    - female N90.7
    - male N50.89
  - inclusion L72.0
  - scrotum L72.9
  - sebaceous L72.3
  - sweat gland or duct L74.8
- solitary
  - bone *—see* Cyst, bone, solitary
  - jaw M27.40
  - kidney N28.1
- spermatic cord N50.89
- sphenoid sinus J34.1
- spinal meninges G96.19
- spleen NEC D73.4
  - congenital Q89.09
  - hydatid (*see also* Echinococcus) B67.99 *[D77]*
- Stafne's M27.0
- subarachnoid intrasellar R93.0
- subcutaneous, pheomycotic (chromomycotic) B43.2
- subdural (cerebral) G93.0
  - spinal cord G96.19
- sublingual gland K11.6
- submandibular gland K11.6
- submaxillary gland K11.6
- suburethral N36.8
- suprarenal gland E27.8
- suprasellar *—see* Cyst, brain
- sweat gland or duct L74.8

Cyst *(continued)*
- synovial *—see also* Cyst, bursa
  - ruptured *—see* Rupture, synovium
- tarsal *—see* Chalazion
- tendon (sheath) *—see* Disorder, tendon, specified type NEC
- testis N44.2
  - tunica albuginea N44.1
- theca lutein (ovary) N83.1-
- Thornwaldt's J39.2
- thymus (gland) E32.8
- thyroglossal duct (infected) (persistent) Q89.2
- thyrolingual duct (infected) (persistent) Q89.2
- thyroid (gland) E04.1
- tongue K14.8
- tonsil J35.8
- tooth *—see* Cyst, dental
- Tornwaldt's J39.2
- trichilemmal (proliferating) L72.12
- trichodermal L72.12
- tubal (fallopian) N83.8
  - inflammatory *—see* Salpingitis, chronic
- tubo-ovarian N83.8
  - inflammatory N70.13
- tunica
  - albuginea testis N44.1
  - vaginalis N50.89
- turbinate (nose) J34.1
- Tyson's gland N48.89
- urachus, congenital Q64.4
- ureter N28.89
- ureterovesical orifice N28.89
- urethra, urethral (gland) N36.8
- uterine ligament N83.8
- uterus (body) (corpus) (recurrent) N85.8
  - embryonic Q51.818
    - cervix Q51.6
- vagina, vaginal (implantation) (inclusion) (squamous cell) (wall) N89.8
  - embryonic Q52.4
- vallecula, vallecular (epiglottis) J38.7
- vesical (orifice) N32.89
- vitreous body H43.89
- vulva (implantation) (inclusion) N90.7
  - congenital Q52.79
  - sebaceous gland N90.7
- vulvovaginal gland N90.7
- wolffian
  - female Q50.5
  - male Q55.4

Cystadenocarcinoma *—see* Neoplasm, malignant, by site
- bile duct C22.1
- endometrioid *—see* Neoplasm, malignant, by site
  - specified site *—see* Neoplasm, malignant, by site
  - unspecified site
    - female C56.9
    - male C61
- mucinous
  - papillary
    - specified site *—see* Neoplasm, malignant, by site
    - unspecified site C56.9
  - specified site *—see* Neoplasm, malignant, by site
  - unspecified site C56.9
- papillary
  - mucinous
    - specified site *—see* Neoplasm, malignant, by site
    - unspecified site C56.9
  - pseudomucinous
    - specified site *—see* Neoplasm, malignant, by site
    - unspecified site C56.9

Cystadenocarcinoma *(continued)*
- papillary *(continued)*
  - serous
    - specified site *—see* Neoplasm, malignant, by site
    - unspecified site C56.9
  - specified site *—see* Neoplasm, malignant, by site
  - unspecified site C56.9
- pseudomucinous
  - papillary
    - specified site *—see* Neoplasm, malignant, by site
    - unspecified site C56.9
  - specified site *—see* Neoplasm, malignant, by site
  - unspecified site C56.9
- serous
  - papillary
    - specified site *—see* Neoplasm, malignant, by site
    - unspecified site C56.9
  - specified site *—see* Neoplasm, malignant, by site
  - unspecified site C56.9

Cystadenofibroma
- clear cell *—see* Neoplasm, benign, by site
- endometrioid D27.9
  - borderline malignancy D39.1-
  - malignant C56.-
- mucinous
  - specified site *—see* Neoplasm, benign, by site
  - unspecified site D27.9
- serous
  - specified site *—see* Neoplasm, benign, by site
  - unspecified site D27.9
- specified site *—see* Neoplasm, benign, by site
- unspecified site D27.9

Cystadenoma *—see also* Neoplasm, benign, by site
- bile duct D13.4
- endometrioid *—see* Neoplasm, benign, by site
  - borderline malignancy *—see* Neoplasm, uncertain behavior, by site
- malignant *—see* Neoplasm, malignant, by site
- mucinous
  - borderline malignancy
    - ovary C56.-
    - specified site NEC *—see* Neoplasm, uncertain behavior, by site
    - unspecified site C56.9
  - papillary
    - borderline malignancy
      - ovary C56.-
      - specified site NEC *—see* Neoplasm, uncertain behavior, by site
      - unspecified site C56.9
    - specified site *—see* Neoplasm, benign, by site
    - unspecified site D27.9
  - specified site *—see* Neoplasm, benign, by site
  - unspecified site D27.9
- papillary
  - borderline malignancy
    - ovary C56.-
    - specified site NEC *—see* Neoplasm, uncertain behavior, by site
    - unspecified site C56.9

Cystadenoma *(continued)*
- papillary *(continued)*
  - lymphomatosum
    - specified site *—see* Neoplasm, benign, by site
    - unspecified site D11.9
  - mucinous
    - borderline malignancy
      - ovary C56.-
      - specified site NEC *—see* Neoplasm, uncertain behavior, by site
      - unspecified site C56.9
    - specified site *—see* Neoplasm, benign, by site
    - unspecified site D27.9
  - pseudomucinous
    - borderline malignancy
      - ovary C56.-
      - specified site NEC *—see* Neoplasm, uncertain behavior, by site
      - unspecified site C56.9
    - specified site *—see* Neoplasm, benign, by site
    - unspecified site D27.9
  - serous
    - borderline malignancy
      - ovary C56.-
      - specified site NEC *—see* Neoplasm, uncertain behavior, by site
      - unspecified site C56.9
    - specified site *—see* Neoplasm, benign, by site
    - unspecified site D27.9
  - specified site *—see* Neoplasm, benign, by site
  - unspecified site D27.9
- pseudomucinous
  - borderline malignancy
    - ovary C56.-
    - specified site NEC *—see* Neoplasm, uncertain behavior, by site
    - unspecified site C56.9
  - papillary
    - borderline malignancy
      - ovary C56.-
      - specified site NEC *—see* Neoplasm, uncertain behavior, by site
      - unspecified site C56.9
    - specified site *—see* Neoplasm, benign, by site
    - unspecified site D27.9
  - specified site *—see* Neoplasm, benign, by site
  - unspecified site D27.9
- serous
  - borderline malignancy
    - ovary C56.-
    - specified site NEC *—see* Neoplasm, uncertain behavior, by site
    - unspecified site C56.9
  - papillary
    - borderline malignancy
      - ovary C56.-
      - specified site NEC *—see* Neoplasm, uncertain behavior, by site
      - unspecified site C56.9
    - specified site *—see* Neoplasm, benign, by site
    - unspecified site D27.9
  - specified site *—see* Neoplasm, benign, by site
  - unspecified site D27.9

Cystathionine synthase deficiency E72.11

- **Cystathioninemia** E72.19
- **Cystathioninuria** E72.19
- **Cystic** —*see also* condition
  - breast (chronic) —*see* Mastopathy, cystic
  - corpora lutea (hemorrhagic) N83.1-
  - duct —*see* condition
  - eyeball (congenital) Q11.0
  - fibrosis —*see* Fibrosis, cystic
  - kidney (congenital) Q61.9
    - adult type Q61.2
    - infantile type NEC Q61.19
      - collecting duct dilatation Q61.11
    - medullary Q61.5
  - liver, congenital Q44.6
  - lung disease J98.4
    - congenital Q33.0
  - mastitis, chronic —*see* Mastopathy, cystic
  - medullary, kidney Q61.5
  - meniscus —*see* Derangement, knee, meniscus, cystic
  - ovary N83.20-
- **Cysticercosis, cysticerciasis** B69.9
  - with
    - epileptiform fits B69.0
    - myositis B69.81
  - brain B69.0
  - central nervous system B69.0
  - cerebral B69.0
  - ocular B69.1
  - specified NEC B69.89
- **Cysticercus cellulose infestation** —*see* Cysticercosis
- **Cystinosis** (malignant) E72.04
- **Cystinuria** E72.01
- **Cystitis** (exudative) (hemorrhagic) (septic) (suppurative) N30.90
  - with
    - fibrosis —*see* Cystitis, chronic, interstitial
    - hematuria N30.91
    - leukoplakia —*see* Cystitis, chronic, interstitial
    - malakoplakia —*see* Cystitis, chronic, interstitial
    - metaplasia —*see* Cystitis, chronic, interstitial
    - prostatitis N41.3
  - acute N30.00
    - with hematuria N30.01
    - of trigone N30.30
      - with hematuria N30.31
  - allergic —*see* Cystitis, specified type NEC
  - amebic A06.81
  - bilharzial B65.9 *[N33]*
  - blennorrhagic (gonococcal) A54.01
  - bullous —*see* Cystitis, specified type NEC
  - calculous N21.0
  - chlamydial A56.01
  - chronic N30.20
    - with hematuria N30.21
    - interstitial N30.10
      - with hematuria N30.11
    - of trigone N30.30
      - with hematuria N30.31
    - specified NEC N30.20
      - with hematuria N30.21
  - cystic (a) —*see* Cystitis, specified type NEC
  - diphtheritic A36.85
  - echinococcal
    - granulosus B67.39
    - multilocularis B67.69
  - emphysematous —*see* Cystitis, specified type NEC
  - encysted —*see* Cystitis, specified type NEC

Cystitis *(continued)*

  - eosinophilic —*see* Cystitis, specified type NEC
  - follicular —*see* Cystitis, of trigone
  - gangrenous —*see* Cystitis, specified type NEC
  - glandularis —*see* Cystitis, specified type NEC
  - gonococcal A54.01
  - incrusted —*see* Cystitis, specified type NEC
  - interstitial (chronic) —*see* Cystitis, chronic, interstitial
  - irradiation N30.40
    - with hematuria N30.41
  - irritation —*see* Cystitis, specified type NEC
  - malignant —*see* Cystitis, specified type NEC
  - of trigone N30.30
    - with hematuria N30.31
  - panmural —*see* Cystitis, chronic, interstitial
  - polyposa —*see* Cystitis, specified type NEC
  - prostatic N41.3
  - puerperal (postpartum) O86.22
  - radiation —*see* Cystitis, irradiation
  - specified type NEC N30.80
    - with hematuria N30.81
  - subacute —*see* Cystitis, chronic
  - submucous —*see* Cystitis, chronic, interstitial
  - syphilitic (late) A52.76
  - trichomonal A59.03
  - tuberculous A18.12
  - ulcerative —*see* Cystitis, chronic, interstitial
- **Cystocele** (-urethrocele)
  - female N81.10
    - with prolapse of uterus —*see* Prolapse, uterus
    - lateral N81.12
    - midline N81.11
    - paravaginal N81.12
  - in pregnancy or childbirth O34.8-
    - causing obstructed labor O65.5
  - male N32.89
- **Cystolithiasis** N21.0
- **Cystoma** —*see also* Neoplasm, benign, by site
  - endometrial, ovary N80.1
  - mucinous
    - specified site —*see* Neoplasm, benign, by site
    - unspecified site D27.9
  - serous
    - specified site —*see* Neoplasm, benign, by site
    - unspecified site D27.9
  - simple (ovary) N83.29-
- **Cystoplegia** N31.2
- **Cystoptosis** N32.89
- **Cystopyelitis** —*see* Pyelonephritis
- **Cystorrhagia** N32.89
- **Cystosarcoma phyllodes** D48.6-
  - benign D24-
  - malignant —*see* Neoplasm, breast, malignant
- **Cystostomy**
  - attention to Z43.5
  - complication —*see* Complications, cystostomy
  - status Z93.50
    - appendico-vesicostomy Z93.52
    - cutaneous Z93.51
    - specified NEC Z93.59
- **Cystourethritis** —*see* Urethritis
- **Cystourethrocele** —*see also* Cystocele
  - female N81.10
    - with uterine prolapse —*see* Prolapse, uterus
    - lateral N81.12
    - midline N81.11
    - paravaginal N81.12
  - male N32.89
- **Cytomegalic inclusion disease**
  - congenital P35.1
- **Cytomegalovirus infection** B25.9
- **Cytomycosis** (reticuloendothelial) B39.4
- **Cytopenia** D75.9
  - refractory
    - with multilineage dysplasia D46.A
      - and ring sideroblasts (RCMD RS) D46.B
- **Czerny's disease** (periodic hydrarthrosis of the knee) —*see* Effusion, joint, knee

D

- **Daae** (-Finsen) **disease** (epidemic pleurodynia) B33.0
- **Da Costa's syndrome** F45.8
- **Dabney's grip** B33.0
- **Dacryoadenitis, dacryadenitis** H04.00-
  - acute H04.01-
  - chronic H04.02-
- **Dacryocystitis** H04.30-
  - acute H04.32-
  - chronic H04.41-
  - neonatal P39.1
  - phlegmonous H04.31-
  - syphilitic A52.71
    - congenital (early) A50.01
  - trachomatous, active A71.1
    - sequelae (late effect) B94.0
- **Dacryocystoblenorrhea** —*see* Inflammation, lacrimal, passages, chronic
- **Dacryocystocele** —*see* Disorder, lacrimal system, changes
- **Dacryolith, dacryolithiasis** H04.51-
- **Dacryoma** —*see* Disorder, lacrimal system, changes
- **Dacryopericystitis** —*see* Dacryocystitis
- **Dacryops** H04.11-
- **Dacryostenosis** —*see also* Stenosis, lacrimal
  - congenital Q10.5
- **Dactylitis**
  - bone —*see* Osteomyelitis
  - sickle-cell D57.00
    - Hb C D57.219
    - Hb SS D57.00
    - specified NEC D57.819
  - skin L08.9
  - syphilitic A52.77
  - tuberculous A18.03
- **Dactylolysis spontanea** (ainhum) L94.6
- **Dactylosymphysis** Q70.9
  - fingers —*see* Syndactylism, complex, fingers
  - toes —*see* Syndactylism, complex, toes
- **Damage**
  - arteriosclerotic —*see* Arteriosclerosis
  - brain (nontraumatic) G93.9
    - anoxic, hypoxic G93.1
      - resulting from a procedure G97.82
    - child NEC G80.9
    - due to birth injury P11.2
  - cardiorenal (vascular) —*see* Hypertension, cardiorenal
  - cerebral NEC —*see* Damage, brain
  - coccyx, complicating delivery O71.6
  - coronary —*see* Disease, heart, ischemic
  - eye, birth injury P15.3
  - liver (nontraumatic) K76.9
    - alcoholic K70.9
    - due to drugs —*see* Disease, liver, toxic
    - toxic —*see* Disease, liver, toxic
  - medication T88.7
  - pelvic
    - joint or ligament, during delivery O71.6
    - organ NEC
      - during delivery O71.5
      - following ectopic or molar pregnancy O08.6
  - renal —*see* Disease, renal
  - subendocardium, subendocardial —*see* Degeneration, myocardial
  - vascular I99.9
- **Dana-Putnam syndrome** (subacute combined sclerosis with pernicious anemia) —*see* Degeneration, combined
- **Danbolt** (-Cross) **syndrome** (acrodermatitis enteropathica) E83.2
- **Dandruff** L21.0
- **Dandy-Walker syndrome** Q03.1
  - with spina bifida —*see* Spina bifida
- **Danlos' syndrome** Q79.6
- **Darier** (-White) disease (congenital) Q82.8
  - meaning erythema annulare centrifugum L53.1
- **Darier-Roussy sarcoid** D86.3
- **Darling's disease or histoplasmosis** B39.4
- **Darwin's tubercle** Q17.8
- **Dawson's** (inclusion body) **encephalitis** A81.1
- **De Beurmann** (-Gougerot) **disease** B42.1
- **De la Tourette's syndrome** F95.2
- **De Lange's syndrome** Q87.1
- **De Morgan's spots** (senile angiomas) I78.1
- **De Quervain's**
  - disease (tendon sheath) M65.4
  - syndrome E34.51
  - thyroiditis (subacute granulomatous thyroiditis) E06.1
- **De Toni-Fanconi** (-Debré) **syndrome** E72.09
  - with cystinosis E72.04
- **Dead**
  - fetus, retained (mother) O36.4
    - early pregnancy O02.1
  - labyrinth H83.2
  - ovum, retained O02.0
- **Deaf nonspeaking NEC** H91.3
- **Deafmutism** (acquired) (congenital) **NEC** H91.3
  - hysterical F44.6
  - syphilitic, congenital (*see also* subcategory H94.8) A50.09

Deafness (acquired) (complete) (hereditary) (partial) H91.9-
- with blue sclera and fragility of bone Q78.0
- auditory fatigue —*see* Deafness, specified type NEC
- aviation T70.0
  - nerve injury —*see* Injury, nerve, acoustic, specified type NEC
- boilermaker's —*see* subcategory H83.3
- central —*see* Deafness, sensorineural
- conductive H90.2
  - and sensorineural
    - mixed H90.8
      - bilateral H90.6
  - bilateral H90.0
  - unilateral H90.1-
    - with restricted hearing on the contralateral side H90.A-
- congenital H90.5
  - with blue sclera and fragility of bone Q78.0
- due to toxic agents —*see* Deafness, ototoxic
- emotional (hysterical) F44.6
- functional (hysterical) F44.6
- high frequency H91.9-
- hysterical F44.6
- low frequency H91.9-
- mental R48.8
- mixed conductive and sensorineural H90.8
  - bilateral H90.6
  - unilateral H90.7-
- nerve —*see* Deafness, sensorineural
- neural —*see* Deafness, sensorineural
- noise-induced —*see also* subcategory H83.3
  - nerve injury —*see* Injury, nerve, acoustic, specified type NEC
- nonspeaking H91.3
- ototoxic H91.0
- perceptive —*see* Deafness, sensorineural
- psychogenic (hysterical) F44.6
- sensorineural H90.5
  - and conductive
    - mixed H90.8
      - bilateral H90.6
  - bilateral H90.3
  - unilateral H90.4-
    - with restricted hearing on the contralateral side H90.A-
- sensory —*see* Deafness, sensorineural
- specified type NEC H91.8
- sudden (idiopathic) H91.2-
- syphilitic A52.15
- transient ischemic H93.01-
- traumatic —*see* Injury, nerve, acoustic, specified type NEC
- word (developmental) H93.25

Death (cause unknown) (of) (unexplained) (unspecified cause) R99
- brain G93.82
- cardiac (sudden) (with successful resuscitation) - code to underlying disease
  - family history of Z82.41
  - personal history of Z86.74
- family member (assumed) Z63.4

Debility (chronic) (general) (nervous) R53.81
- congenital or neonatal NOS P96.9
- nervous R53.81
- old age R54
- senile R54

Débove's disease (splenomegaly) R16.1

Decalcification
- bone —*see* Osteoporosis
- teeth K03.89

Decapsulation, kidney N28.89

Decay
- dental —*see* Caries, dental
- senile R54
- tooth, teeth —*see* Caries, dental

Deciduitis (acute)
- following ectopic or molar pregnancy O08.0

Decline (general) —*see* Debility
- cognitive, age-associated R41.81

Decompensation
- cardiac (acute) (chronic) —*see* Disease, heart
- cardiovascular —*see* Disease, cardiovascular
- heart —*see* Disease, heart
- hepatic —*see* Failure, hepatic
- myocardial (acute) (chronic) —*see* Disease, heart
- respiratory J98.8

Decompression sickness T70.3

Decrease (d)
- absolute neutrophile count —*see* Neutropenia
- blood
  - platelets —*see* Thrombocytopenia
  - pressure R03.1
    - due to shock following
      - injury T79.4
      - operation T81.19
- estrogen E28.39
  - postablative E89.40
    - asymptomatic E89.40
    - symptomatic E89.41
- fragility of erythrocytes D58.8
- function
  - lipase (pancreatic) K90.3
  - ovary in hypopituitarism E23.0
  - parenchyma of pancreas K86.89
  - pituitary (gland) (anterior) (lobe) E23.0
    - posterior (lobe) E23.0
- functional activity R68.89
- glucose R73.09
- hematocrit R71.0
- hemoglobin R71.0
- leukocytes D72.819
  - specified NEC D72.818
- libido R68.82
- lymphocytes D72.810
- platelets D69.6
- respiration, due to shock following injury T79.4
- sexual desire R68.82
- tear secretion NEC —*see* Syndrome, dry eye
- tolerance
  - fat K90.49
  - glucose R73.09
  - pancreatic K90.3
  - salt and water E87.8
- vision NEC H54.7
- white blood cell count D72.819
  - specified NEC D72.818

Decubitus (ulcer) —*see* Ulcer, pressure, by site
- cervix N86

Deepening acetabulum —*see* Derangement, joint, specified type NEC, hip

Defect, defective Q89.9
- 3-beta-hydroxysteroid dehydrogenase E25.0
- 11-hydroxylase E25.0
- 21-hydroxylase E25.0
- abdominal wall, congenital Q79.59
- antibody immunodeficiency D80.9
- aorticopulmonary septum Q21.4
- atrial septal (ostium secundum type) Q21.1
  - following acute myocardial infarction (current complication) I23.1
  - ostium primum type Q21.2
- atrioventricular
  - canal Q21.2
  - septum Q21.2
- auricular septal Q21.1
- bilirubin excretion NEC E80.6
- biosynthesis, androgen (testicular) E29.1
- bulbar septum Q21.0
- catalase E80.3
- cell membrane receptor complex (CR3) D71
- circulation I99.9
  - congenital Q28.9
  - newborn Q28.9
- coagulation (factor) (*see also* Deficiency, factor) D68.9
  - with
    - ectopic pregnancy O08.1
    - molar pregnancy O08.1
  - acquired D68.4
  - antepartum with hemorrhage —*see* Hemorrhage, antepartum, with coagulation defect
  - due to
    - liver disease D68.4
    - vitamin K deficiency D68.4
  - hereditary NEC D68.2
  - intrapartum O67.0
  - newborn, transient P61.6
  - postpartum O99.13
    - with hemorrhage O72.3
  - specified type NEC D68.8
- complement system D84.1
- conduction (heart) I45.9
  - bone —*see* Deafness, conductive
- congenital, organ or site not listed —*see* Anomaly, by site
- coronary sinus Q21.1
- cushion, endocardial Q21.2
- degradation, glycoprotein E77.1
- dental bridge, crown, fillings —*see* Defect, dental restoration
- dental restoration K08.50
  - specified NEC K08.59
- dentin (hereditary) K00.5
- Descemet's membrane, congenital Q13.89
- developmental —*see also* Anomaly
  - cauda equina Q06.3
- diaphragm
  - with elevation, eventration or hernia —*see* Hernia, diaphragm
  - congenital Q79.1
    - with hernia Q79.0
    - gross (with hernia) Q79.0
- ectodermal, congenital Q82.9
- Eisenmenger's Q21.8
- enzyme
  - catalase E80.3
  - peroxidase E80.3
- esophagus, congenital Q39.9
- extensor retinaculum M62.89
- fibrin polymerization D68.2
- filling
  - bladder R93.41
  - kidney R93.42-
  - renal pelvis R93.41
  - stomach R93.3
  - ureter R93.41

Defect, defective *(continued)*
- filling *(continued)*
  - urinary organs, specified NEC R93.49
- Gerbode Q21.0
- glycoprotein degradation E77.1
- Hageman (factor) D68.2
- hearing —*see* Deafness
- high grade F70
- interatrial septal Q21.1
- interauricular septal Q21.1
- interventricular septal Q21.0
  - with dextroposition of aorta, pulmonary stenosis and hypertrophy of right ventricle Q21.3
  - in tetralogy of Fallot Q21.3
- learning (specific) —*see* Disorder, learning
- lymphocyte function antigen-1(LFA-1) D84.0
- lysosomal enzyme, post-translational modification E77.0
- major osseous M89.70
  - ankle M89.77-
  - carpus M89.74-
  - clavicle M89.71-
  - femur M89.75-
  - fibula M89.76-
  - fingers M89.74-
  - foot M89.77-
  - forearm M89.73-
  - hand M89.74-
  - humerus M89.72-
  - lower leg M89.76-
  - metacarpus M89.74-
  - metatarsus M89.77-
  - multiple sites M89.79
  - pelvic region M89.75-
  - pelvis M89.75-
  - radius M89.73-
  - scapula M89.71-
  - shoulder region M89.71-
  - specified NEC M89.78
  - tarsus M89.77-
  - thigh M89.75-
  - tibia M89.76-
  - toes M89.77-
  - ulna M89.73-
- mental —*see* Disability, intellectual
- modification, lysosomal enzymes, post-translational E77.0
- obstructive, congenital
  - renal pelvis Q62.39
  - ureter Q62.39
    - atresia —*see* Atresia, ureter
    - cecoureterocele Q62.32
    - megaureter Q62.2
    - orthotopic ureterocele Q62.31
- osseous, major M89.70
  - ankle M89.77-
  - carpus M89.74-
  - clavicle M89.71-
  - femur M89.75-
  - fibula M89.76-
  - fingers M89.74-
  - foot M89.77-
  - forearm M89.73-
  - hand M89.74-
  - humerus M89.72-
  - lower leg M89.76-
  - metacarpus M89.74-
  - metatarsus M89.77-
  - multiple sites M89.9
  - pelvic region M89.75-
  - pelvis M89.75-
  - radius M89.73-
  - scapula M89.71-
  - shoulder region M89.71-
  - specified NEC M89.78

Defect, defective *(continued)*
osseous, major *(continued)*
tarsus M89.77-
thigh M89.75-
tibia M89.76-
toes M89.77-
ulna M89.73-
osteochondral NEC *(see also* Deformity) M95.8
ostium
primum Q21.2
secundum Q21.1
peroxidase E80.3
placental blood supply *—see* Insufficiency, placental
platelets, qualitative D69.1
constitutional D68.0
postural NEC, spine *—see* Dorsopathy, deforming
reduction
limb Q73.8
lower Q72.9-
absence *—see* Agenesis, leg
foot *—see* Agenesis, foot
longitudinal
femur Q72.4-
fibula Q72.6-
tibia Q72.5-
specified type NEC Q72.89-
split foot Q72.7-
specified type NEC Q73.8
upper Q71.9-
absence *—see* Agenesis, arm
forearm *—see* Agenesis, forearm
hand *—see* Agenesis, hand
lobster-claw hand Q71.6-
longitudinal
radius Q71.4-
ulna Q71.5-
specified type NEC Q71.89-
renal pelvis Q63.8
obstructive Q62.39
respiratory system, congenital Q34.9
restoration, dental K08.50
specified NEC K08.59
retinal nerve bundle fibers H35.89
septal (heart) NOS Q21.9
acquired (atrial) (auricular) (ventricular) (old) I51.0
atrial Q21.1
concurrent with acute myocardial infarction *—see* Infarct, myocardium
following acute myocardial infarction (current complication) I23.1
ventricular *(see also* Defect, ventricular septal) Q21.0
sinus venosus Q21.1
speech R47.9
developmental F80.9
specified NEC R47.89
Taussig-Bing (aortic transposition and overriding pulmonary artery) Q20.1
teeth, wedge K03.1
vascular (local) I99.9
congenital Q27.9
ventricular septal Q21.0
concurrent with acute myocardial infarction *—see* Infarct, myocardium
following acute myocardial infarction (current complication) I23.2
in tetralogy of Fallot Q21.3
vision NEC H54.7

Defect, defective *(continued)*
visual field H53.40
bilateral
heteronymous H53.47
homonymous H53.46-
generalized contraction H53.48-
localized
arcuate H53.43-
scotoma (central area) H53.41-
blind spot area H53.42-
sector H53.43-
specified type NEC H53.45-
voice R49.9
specified NEC R49.8
wedge, tooth, teeth (abrasion) K03.1

Deferentitis N49.1
gonorrheal (acute) (chronic) A54.23

Defibrination (syndrome) D65
antepartum *—see* Hemorrhage, antepartum, with coagulation defect, disseminated intravascular coagulation
following ectopic or molar pregnancy O08.1
intrapartum O67.0
newborn P60
postpartum O72.3

Deficiency, deficient
3-beta hydroxysteroid dehydrogenase E25.0
5-alpha reductase (with male pseudohermaphroditism) E29.1
11-hydroxylase E25.0
21-hydroxylase E25.0
abdominal muscle syndrome Q79.4
accelerator globulin (Ac G) (blood) D68.2
AC globulin (congenital) (hereditary) D68.2
acquired D68.4
acid phosphatase E83.39
activating factor (blood) D68.2
adenosine deaminase (ADA) D81.3
aldolase (hereditary) E74.19
alpha-1-antitrypsin E88.01
amino-acids E72.9
anemia *—see* Anemia
aneurin E51.9
antibody with
hyperimmunoglobulinemia D80.6
near-normal immunoglobins D80.6
antidiuretic hormone E23.2
anti-hemophilic
factor (A) D66
B D67
C D68.1
globulin (AHG) NEC D66
antithrombin (antithrombin III) D68.59
ascorbic acid E54
attention (disorder) (syndrome) F98.8
with hyperactivity *—see* Disorder, attention-deficit hyperactivity
autoprothrombin
I D68.2
II D67
C D68.2
beta-glucuronidase E76.29
biotin E53.8
biotin-dependent carboxylase D81.819
biotinidase D81.810
brancher enzyme (amylopectinosis) E74.03
calciferol E55.9
with
adult osteomalacia M83.8
rickets *—see* Rickets

Deficiency, deficient *(continued)*
calcium (dietary) E58
calorie, severe E43
with marasmus E41
and kwashiorkor E42
cardiac *—see* Insufficiency, myocardial
carnitine E71.40
due to
hemodialysis E71.43
inborn errors of metabolism E71.42
Valproic acid therapy E71.43
iatrogenic E71.43
muscle palmityltransferase E71.314
primary E71.41
secondary E71.448
carotene E50.9
central nervous system G96.8
ceruloplasmin (Wilson) E83.01
choline E53.8
Christmas factor D67
chromium E61.4
clotting (blood) *(see also* Deficiency, coagulation factor) D68.9
clotting factor NEC (hereditary) *(see also* Deficiency, factor) D68.2
coagulation NOS D68.9
with
ectopic pregnancy O08.1
molar pregnancy O08.1
acquired (any) D68.4
antepartum hemorrhage *—see* Hemorrhage, antepartum, with coagulation defect
clotting factor NEC *(see also* Deficiency, factor) D68.2
due to
hyperprothrombinemia D68.4
liver disease D68.4
vitamin K deficiency D68.4
newborn, transient P61.6
postpartum O72.3
specified NEC D68.8
cognitive F09
color vision H53.50
achromatopsia H53.51
acquired H53.52
deuteranomaly H53.53
protanomaly H53.54
specified type NEC H53.59
tritanomaly H53.55
combined glucocorticoid and mineralocorticoid E27.49
contact factor D68.2
copper (nutritional) E61.0
corticoadrenal E27.40
primary E27.1
craniofacial axis Q75.0
cyanocobalamin E53.8
C1 esterase inhibitor (C1-INH) D84.1
debrancher enzyme (limit dextrinosis) E74.03
dehydrogenase
long chain/very long chain acyl CoA E71.310
medium chain acyl CoA E71.311
short chain acyl CoA E71.312
diet E63.9
dihydropyrimidine dehydrogenase (DPD) E88.89
disaccharidase E73.9
edema *—see* Malnutrition, severe
endocrine E34.9
energy-supply *—see* Malnutrition
enzymes, circulating NEC E88.09
ergosterol E55.9
with
adult osteomalacia M83.8
rickets *—see* Rickets
essential fatty acid (EFA) E63.0

Deficiency, deficient *(continued)*
factor *—see also* Deficiency, coagulation
Hageman D68.2
I (congenital) (hereditary) D68.2
II (congenital) (hereditary) D68.2
IX (congenital) (functional) (hereditary) (with functional defect) D67
multiple (congenital) D68.8
acquired D68.4
V (congenital) (hereditary) D68.2
VII (congenital) (hereditary) D68.2
VIII (congenital) (functional) (hereditary) (with functional defect) D66
with vascular defect D68.0
X (congenital) (hereditary) D68.2
XI (congenital) (hereditary) D68.1
XII (congenital) (hereditary) D68.2
XIII (congenital) (hereditary) D68.2
femoral, proximal focal (congenital) *—see* Defect, reduction, lower limb, longitudinal, femur
fibrin-stabilizing factor (congenital) (hereditary) D68.2
acquired D68.4
fibrinase D68.2
fibrinogen (congenital) (hereditary) D68.2
acquired D65
folate E53.8
folic acid E53.8
foreskin N47.3
fructokinase E74.11
fructose 1,6-diphosphatase E74.19
fructose-1-phosphate aldolase E74.19
galactokinase E74.29
galactose-1-phosphate uridyl transferase E74.29
gammaglobulin in blood D80.1
hereditary D80.0
glass factor D68.2
glucocorticoid E27.49
mineralocorticoid E27.49
glucose-6-phosphatase E74.01
glucose-6-phosphate dehydrogenase anemia D55.0
glucuronyl transferase E80.5
glycogen synthetase E74.09
gonadotropin (isolated) E23.0
growth hormone (idiopathic) (isolated) E23.0
Hageman factor D68.2
hemoglobin D64.9
hepatophosphorylase E74.09
homogentisate 1,2-dioxygenase E70.29
hormone
anterior pituitary (partial) NEC E23.0
growth E23.0
growth (isolated) E23.0
pituitary E23.0
testicular E29.1
hypoxanthine-(guanine)-phosphoribosyltransferase (HG-PRT) (total H-PRT) E79.1
immunity D84.9
cell-mediated D84.8
with thrombocytopenia and eczema D82.0
combined D81.9
humoral D80.9
IgA (secretory) D80.2
IgG D80.3
IgM D80.4
immuno *—see* Immunodeficiency
immunoglobulin, selective
A (IgA) D80.2

Deficiency, deficient *(continued)*
- immunoglobulin, selective *(continued)*
  - G (IgG) (subclasses) D80.3
  - M (IgM) D80.4
- inositol (B complex) E53.8
- intrinsic
  - factor (congenital) D51.0
  - sphincter N36.42
    - with urethral hypermobility N36.43
- iodine E61.8
  - congenital syndrome *—see* Syndrome, iodine-deficiency, congenital
- iron E61.1
  - anemia D50.9
- kalium E87.6
- kappa-light chain D80.8
- labile factor (congenital) (hereditary) D68.2
  - acquired D68.4
- lacrimal fluid (acquired) *—see also* Syndrome, dry eye
  - congenital Q10.6
- lactase
  - congenital E73.0
  - secondary E73.1
- Laki-Lorand factor D68.2
- lecithin cholesterol acyltransferase E78.6
- lipocaic K86.89
- lipoprotein (familial) (high density) E78.6
- liver phosphorylase E74.09
- lysosomal alpha-1, 4 glucosidase E74.02
- magnesium E61.2
- major histocompatibility complex
  - class I D81.6
  - class II D81.7
- manganese E61.3
- menadione (vitamin K) E56.1
  - newborn P53
- mental (familial) (hereditary) *—see* Disability, intellectual
- methylenetetrahydrofolate reductase (MTHFR) E72.12
- mevalonate kinase M04.1
- mineral NEC E61.8
- mineralocorticoid E27.49
  - with glucocorticoid E27.49
- molybdenum (nutritional) E61.5
- moral F60.2
- multiple nutrient elements E61.7
- muscle
  - carnitine (palmityltransferase) E71.314
  - phosphofructokinase E74.09
- myoadenylate deaminase E79.2
- myocardial *—see* Insufficiency, myocardial
- myophosphorylase E74.04
- NADH diaphorase or reductase (congenital) D74.0
- NADH-methemoglobin reductase (congenital) D74.0
- natrium E87.1
- niacin (amide) (-tryptophan) E52
- nicotinamide E52
- nicotinic acid E52
- number of teeth *—see* Anodontia
- nutrient element E61.9
  - multiple E61.7
  - specified NEC E61.8
- nutrition, nutritional E63.9
  - sequelae *—see* Sequelae, nutritional deficiency
  - specified NEC E63.8
- of interleukin 1 receptor antagonist [DIRA] M04.8
- ornithine transcarbamylase E72.4

Deficiency, deficient *(continued)*
- ovarian E28.39
- oxygen *—see* Anoxia
- pantothenic acid E53.8
- parathyroid (gland) E20.9
- perineum (female) N81.89
- phenylalanine hydroxylase E70.1
- phosphoenolpyruvate carboxykinase E74.4
- phosphofructokinase E74.19
- phosphomannomutuse E74.8
- phosphomannose isomerase E74.8
- phosphomannosyl mutase E74.8
- phosphorylase kinase, liver E74.09
- pituitary hormone (isolated) E23.0
- plasma thromboplastin
  - antecedent (PTA) D68.1
  - component (PTC) D67
- platelet NEC D69.1
  - constitutional D68.0
- polyglandular E31.8
  - autoimmune E31.0
- potassium (K) E87.6
- prepuce N47.3
- proaccelerin (congenital) (hereditary) D68.2
  - acquired D68.4
- proconvertin factor (congenital) (hereditary) D68.2
  - acquired D68.4
- protein (*see also* Malnutrition) E46
  - anemia D53.0
  - C D68.59
  - S D68.59
- prothrombin (congenital) (hereditary) D68.2
  - acquired D68.4
- Prower factor D68.2
- pseudocholinesterase E88.09
- PTA (plasma thromboplastin antecedent) D68.1
- PTC (plasma thromboplastin component) D67
- purine nucleoside phosphorylase (PNP) D81.5
- pyracin (alpha) (beta) E53.1
- pyridoxal E53.1
- pyridoxamine E53.1
- pyridoxine (derivatives) E53.1
- pyruvate
  - carboxylase E74.4
  - dehydrogenase E74.4
- riboflavin (vitamin B2) E53.0
- salt E87.1
- secretion
  - ovary E28.39
  - salivary gland (any) K11.7
  - urine R34
- selenium (dietary) E59
- serum antitrypsin, familial E88.01
- short stature homeobox gene (SHOX)
  - with
    - dyschondrosteosis Q78.8
    - short stature (idiopathic) E34.3
    - Turner's syndrome Q96.9
- sodium (Na) E87.1
- SPCA(factor VII) D68.2
- sphincter, intrinsic N36.42
  - with urethral hypermobility N36.43
- stable factor (congenital) (hereditary) D68.2
  - acquired D68.4
- Stuart-Prower (factor X) D68.2
- sucrase E74.39
- sulfatase E75.29
- sulfite oxidase E72.19
- thiamin, thiaminic (chloride) E51.9
  - beriberi (dry) E51.11
    - wet E51.12
- thrombokinase D68.2
  - newborn P53

Deficiency, deficient *(continued)*
- thyroid (gland) *—see* Hypothyroidism
- tocopherol E56.0
- tooth bud K00.0
- transcobalamine II (anemia) D51.2
- vanadium E61.6
- vascular I99.9
- vasopressin E23.2
- vertical ridge K06.8
- viosterol *—see* Deficiency, calciferol
- vitamin (multiple) NOS E56.9
  - A E50.9
    - with
      - Bitot's spot (corneal) E50.1
      - follicular keratosis E50.8
      - keratomalacia E50.4
      - manifestations NEC E50.8
      - night blindness E50.5
      - scar of cornea, xerophthalmic E50.6
      - xeroderma E50.8
      - xerophthalmia E50.7
      - xerosis
        - conjunctival E50.0
          - and Bitot's spot E50.1
        - cornea E50.2
          - and ulceration E50.3
    - sequelae E64.1
  - B (complex) NOS E53.9
    - with
      - beriberi (dry) E51.11
        - wet E51.12
      - pellagra E52
  - B1 NOS E51.9
    - beriberi (dry) E51.11
      - with circulatory system manifestations E51.11
      - wet E51.12
  - B12 E53.8
  - B2 (riboflavin) E53.0
  - B6 E53.1
  - C E54
    - sequelae E64.2
  - D E55.9
    - with
      - adult osteomalacia M83.8
      - rickets *—see* Rickets
    - 25-hydroxylase E83.32
  - E E56.0
  - folic acid E53.8
  - G E53.0
  - group B E53.9
    - specified NEC E53.8
  - H (biotin) E53.8
  - K E56.1
    - of newborn P53
  - nicotinic E52
  - P E56.8
  - PP (pellagra-preventing) E52
  - specified NEC E56.8
  - thiamin E51.9
    - beriberi *—see* Beriberi
- zinc, dietary E60

Deficit *—see also* Deficiency
- attention and concentration R41.840
  - disorder *—see* Attention, deficit
  - following
    - cerebral infarction I69.310
    - cerebrovascular disease I69.910
      - specified disease NEC I69.810
    - nontraumatic
      - intracerebral hemorrhage I69.110
      - specified intracranial hemorrhage NEC I69.210
      - subarachnoid hemorrhage I69.010
- cognitive
  - communication R41.841
  - emotional
    - following

Deficit *(continued)*
- cognitive *(continued)*
  - emotional *(continued)*
    - following *(continued)*
      - cerebral infarction I69.315
      - cerebrovascular disease I69.915
        - specified disease NEC I69.815
      - nontraumantic
        - intracerebral hemorrhage I69.115
        - specified intracranial hemorrhage NEC I69.215
        - subarachnoid hemorrhage I69.015
  - following
    - cerebral infarction I69.319
    - cerebrovascular disease I69.919
      - specified disease NEC I69.819
    - nontraumatic
      - intracerebral hemorrhage I69.119
      - specified intracranial hemorrhage NEC I69.219
      - subarachnoid hemorrhage I69.019
  - social
    - following
      - cerebral infarction I69.315
      - cerebrovascular disease I69.915
        - specified disease NEC I69.815
      - nontraumatic
        - intracerebral hemorrhage I69.115
        - specified intracranial hemorrhage NEC I69.215
        - subarachnoid hemorrhage I69.015
- cognitive NEC R41.89
  - following
    - cerebral infarction I69.318
    - cerebrovascular disease I69.918
      - specified disease NEC I69.818
    - nontraumatic
      - intracerebral hemorrhage I69.118
      - specified intracaranial hemorrhage NEC I69.218
      - subarachnoid hemorrhage I69.018
- concentration R41.840
- executive function R41.844
  - following
    - cerebral infarction I69.314
    - cerebrovascular disease I69.914
      - specified disease NEC I69.814
    - nontraumatic
      - intracerebral hemorrhage I69.114
      - specified intracranial hemorrhage NEC I69.214
      - subarachnoid hemorrhage I69.014
- frontal lobe R41.844
  - following
    - cerebral infarction I69.314
    - cerebrovascular disease I69.914
      - specified disease NEC I69.814
    - nontraumatic
      - intracerebral hemorrhage I69.114
      - specified intracranial hemorrhage NEC I69.214
      - subarachnoid hemorrhage I69.014
- memory
  - following
    - cerebral infarction I69.311
    - cerebrovascular disease I69.911
      - specified disease NEC I69.811

Deficit *(continued)*
memory *(continued)*
following *(continued)*
nontraumatic
intracerebral hemorrhage I69.111
specified intracranial hemorrhage NEC I69.211
subarachnoid hemorrhage I69.011
neurologic NEC R29.818
ischemic
reversible (RIND) I63.9
prolonged (PRIND) I63.9
oxygen R09.02
prolonged reversible ischemic neurologic (PRIND) I63.9
psychomotor R41.843
following
cerebral infarction I69.313
cerebrovascular disease I69.913
specified disease NEC I69.813
nontraumatic
intracerebral hemorrhage I69.113
specified intracranial hemorrhage NEC I69.213
subarachnoid hemorrhage I69.013
visuospatial R41.842
following
cerebral infarction I69.312
cerebrovascular disease I69.912
specified disease NEC I69.812
nontraumatic
intracerebral hemorrhage I69.112
specified intracranial hemorrhage NEC I69.212
subarachnoid hemorrhage I69.012

Deflection
radius *—see* Deformity, limb, specified type NEC, forearm
septum (acquired) (nasal) (nose) J34.2
spine *—see* Curvature, spine
turbinate (nose) J34.2

Defluvium
capillorum *—see* Alopecia
ciliorum *—see* Madarosis
unguium L60.8

Deformity Q89.9
abdomen, congenital Q89.9
abdominal wall
acquired M95.8
congenital Q79.59
acquired (unspecified site) M95.9
adrenal gland Q89.1
alimentary tract, congenital Q45.9
upper Q40.9
ankle (joint) (acquired) *—see also* Deformity, limb, lower leg
abduction *—see* Contraction, joint, ankle
congenital Q68.8
contraction *—see* Contraction, joint, ankle
specified type NEC *—see* Deformity, limb, foot, specified NEC
anus (acquired) K62.89
congenital Q43.9
aorta (arch) (congenital) Q25.40
acquired I77.89
aortic
arch, acquired I77.89
cusp or valve (congenital) Q23.8
acquired (*see also* Endocarditis, aortic) I35.8

Deformity *(continued)*
arm (acquired) (upper) *—see also* Deformity, limb, upper arm
congenital Q68.8
forearm *—see* Deformity, limb, forearm
artery (congenital) (peripheral) NOS Q27.9
acquired I77.89
coronary (acquired) I25.9
congenital Q24.5
umbilical Q27.0
atrial septal Q21.1
auditory canal (external) (congenital) *—see also* Malformation, ear, external
acquired *—see* Disorder, ear, external, specified type NEC
auricle
ear (congenital) *—see also* Malformation, ear, external
acquired *—see* Disorder, pinna, deformity
back *—see* Dorsopathy, deforming
bile duct (common) (congenital) (hepatic) Q44.5
acquired K83.8
biliary duct or passage (congenital) Q44.5
acquired K83.8
bladder (neck) (trigone) (sphincter) (acquired) N32.89
congenital Q64.79
bone (acquired) NOS M95.9
congenital Q79.9
turbinate M95.0
brain (congenital) Q04.9
acquired G93.89
reduction Q04.3
breast (acquired) N64.89
congenital Q83.9
reconstructed N65.0
bronchus (congenital) Q32.4
acquired NEC J98.09
bursa, congenital Q79.9
canaliculi (lacrimalis) (acquired) *—see also* Disorder, lacrimal system, changes
congenital Q10.6
canthus, acquired *—see* Disorder, eyelid, specified type NEC
capillary (acquired) I78.8
cardiovascular system, congenital Q28.9
caruncle, lacrimal (acquired) *—see also* Disorder, lacrimal system, changes
congenital Q10.6
cascade, stomach K31.2
cecum (congenital) Q43.9
acquired K63.89
cerebral, acquired G93.89
congenital Q04.9
cervix (uterus) (acquired) NEC N88.8
congenital Q51.9
cheek (acquired) M95.2
congenital Q18.9
chest (acquired) (wall) M95.4
congenital Q67.8
sequelae (late effect) of rickets E64.3
chin (acquired) M95.2
congenital Q18.9
choroid (congenital) Q14.3
acquired H31.8
plexus Q07.8
acquired G96.19
cicatricial *—see* Cicatrix
cilia, acquired *—see* Disorder, eyelid, specified type NEC
clavicle (acquired) M95.8
congenital Q68.8

Deformity *(continued)*
clitoris (congenital) Q52.6
acquired N90.89
clubfoot *—see* Clubfoot
coccyx (acquired) M43.8
colon (congenital) Q43.9
acquired K63.89
concha (ear), congenital *—see also* Malformation, ear, external
acquired *—see* Disorder, pinna, deformity
cornea (acquired) H18.70
congenital Q13.4
descemetocele *—see* Descemetocele
ectasia *—see* Ectasia, cornea
specified NEC H18.79-
staphyloma *—see* Staphyloma, cornea
coronary artery (acquired) I25.9
congenital Q24.5
cranium (acquired) *—see* Deformity, skull
cricoid cartilage (congenital) Q31.8
acquired J38.7
cystic duct (congenital) Q44.5
acquired K82.8
Dandy-Walker Q03.1
with spina bifida *—see* Spina bifida
diaphragm (congenital) Q79.1
acquired J98.6
digestive organ NOS Q45.9
ductus arteriosus Q25.0
duodenal bulb K31.89
duodenum (congenital) Q43.9
acquired K31.89
dura *—see* Deformity, meninges
ear (acquired) *—see also* Disorder, pinna, deformity
congenital (external) Q17.9
internal Q16.5
middle Q16.4
ossicles Q16.3
ossicles Q16.3
ectodermal (congenital) NEC Q84.9
ejaculatory duct (congenital) Q55.4
acquired N50.89
elbow (joint) (acquired) *—see also* Deformity, limb, upper arm
congenital Q68.8
contraction *—see* Contraction, joint, elbow
endocrine gland NEC Q89.2
epididymis (congenital) Q55.4
acquired N50.89
epiglottis (congenital) Q31.8
acquired J38.7
esophagus (congenital) Q39.9
acquired K22.8
eustachian tube (congenital) NEC Q17.8
eye, congenital Q15.9
eyebrow (congenital) Q18.8
eyelid (acquired) *—see also* Disorder, eyelid, specified type NEC
congenital Q10.3
face (acquired) M95.2
congenital Q18.9
fallopian tube, acquired N83.8
femur (acquired) *—see* Deformity, limb, specified type NEC, thigh
fetal
with fetopelvic disproportion O33.7
causing obstructed labor O66.3
finger (acquired) M20.00-
boutonniere M20.02-
congenital Q68.1
flexion contracture *—see* Contraction, joint, hand
mallet finger M20.01-
specified NEC M20.09-
swan-neck M20.03-

Deformity *(continued)*
flexion (joint) (acquired) (*see also* Deformity, limb, flexion) M21.20
congenital NOS Q74.9
hip Q65.89
foot (acquired) *—see also* Deformity, limb, lower leg
cavovarus (congenital) Q66.1
congenital NOS Q66.9
specified type NEC Q66.89
specified type NEC *—see* Deformity, limb, foot, specified NEC
valgus (congenital) Q66.6
acquired *—see* Deformity, valgus, ankle
varus (congenital) NEC Q66.3
acquired *—see* Deformity, varus, ankle
forearm (acquired) *—see also* Deformity, limb, forearm
congenital Q68.8
forehead (acquired) M95.2
congenital Q75.8
frontal bone (acquired) M95.2
congenital Q75.8
gallbladder (congenital) Q44.1
acquired K82.8
gastrointestinal tract (congenital) NOS Q45.9
acquired K63.89
genitalia, genital organ(s) or system NEC
female (congenital) Q52.9
acquired N94.89
external Q52.70
male (congenital) Q55.9
acquired N50.89
globe (eye) (congenital) Q15.8
acquired H44.89
gum, acquired NEC K06.8
hand (acquired) *—see* Deformity, limb, hand
congenital Q68.1
head (acquired) M95.2
congenital Q75.8
heart (congenital) Q24.9
septum Q21.9
auricular Q21.1
ventricular Q21.0
valve (congenital) NEC Q24.8
acquired *—see* Endocarditis
heel (acquired) *—see* Deformity, foot
hepatic duct (congenital) Q44.5
acquired K83.8
hip (joint) (acquired) *—see also* Deformity, limb, thigh
congenital Q65.9
due to (previous) juvenile osteochondrosis *—see* Coxa, plana
flexion *—see* Contraction, joint, hip
hourglass *—see* Contraction, hourglass
humerus (acquired) M21.82-
congenital Q74.0
hypophyseal (congenital) Q89.2
ileocecal (coil) (valve) (acquired) K63.89
congenital Q43.9
ileum (congenital) Q43.9
acquired K63.89
ilium (acquired) M95.5
congenital Q74.2
integument (congenital) Q84.9
intervertebral cartilage or disc (acquired) *—see* Disorder, disc, specified NEC
intestine (large) (small) (congenital) NOS Q43.9
acquired K63.89

Deformity *(continued)*
- intrinsic minus or plus (hand) *—see* Deformity, limb, specified type NEC, forearm
- iris (acquired) H21.89
  - congenital Q13.2
- ischium (acquired) M95.5
  - congenital Q74.2
- jaw (acquired) (congenital) M26.9
- joint (acquired) NEC M21.90
  - congenital Q68.8
  - elbow M21.92-
  - hand M21.94-
  - hip M21.95-
  - knee M21.96-
  - shoulder M21.92-
  - wrist M21.93-
- kidney(s) (calyx) (pelvis) (congenital) Q63.9
  - acquired N28.89
  - artery (congenital) Q27.2
    - acquired I77.89
- Klippel-Feil (brevicollis) Q76.1
- knee (acquired) NEC *—see also* Deformity, limb, lower leg
  - congenital Q68.2
- labium (majus) (minus) (congenital) Q52.79
  - acquired N90.89
- lacrimal passages or duct (congenital) NEC Q10.6
  - acquired *—see* Disorder, lacrimal system, changes
- larynx (muscle) (congenital) Q31.8
  - acquired J38.7
  - web (glottic) Q31.0
- leg (upper) (acquired) NEC *—see also* Deformity, limb, thigh
  - congenital Q68.8
  - lower leg *—see* Deformity, limb, lower leg
- lens (acquired) H27.8
  - congenital Q12.9
- lid (fold) (acquired) *—see also* Disorder, eyelid, specified type NEC
  - congenital Q10.3
- ligament (acquired) *—see* Disorder, ligament
  - congenital Q79.9
- limb (acquired) M21.90
  - clawfoot M21.53-
  - clawhand M21.51-
  - clubfoot M21.54-
  - clubhand M21.52-
  - congenital, except reduction deformity Q74.9
  - flat foot M21.4-
  - flexion M21.20
    - ankle M21.27-
    - elbow M21.22-
    - finger M21.24-
    - hip M21.25-
    - knee M21.26-
    - shoulder M21.21-
    - toe M21.27-
    - wrist M21.23-
  - foot
    - claw *—see* Deformity, limb, clawfoot
    - club *—see* Deformity, limb, clubfoot
    - drop M21.37-
    - flat *—see* Deformity, limb, flat foot
    - specified NEC M21.6X-
  - forearm M21.93-
  - hand M21.94-
  - lower leg M21.96-
  - specified type NEC M21.80
    - forearm M21.83-
    - lower leg M21.86-

Deformity *(continued)*
- limb (acquired) *(continued)*
  - specified type *(continued)*
    - thigh M21.85-
    - upper arm M21.82-
  - thigh M21.95-
  - unequal length M21.70
    - short site is
      - femur M21.75-
      - fibula M21.76-
      - humerus M21.72-
      - radius M21.73-
      - tibia M21.76-
      - ulna M21.73-
  - upper arm M21.92-
  - valgus *—see* Deformity, valgus
  - varus *—see* Deformity, varus
  - wrist drop M21.33-
- lip (acquired) NEC K13.0
  - congenital Q38.0
- liver (congenital) Q44.7
  - acquired K76.89
- lumbosacral (congenital) (joint) (region) Q76.49
  - acquired M43.8
  - kyphosis *—see* Kyphosis, congenital
  - lordosis *—see* Lordosis, congenital
- lung (congenital) Q33.9
  - acquired J98.4
- lymphatic system, congenital Q89.9
- Madelung's (radius) Q74.0
- mandible (acquired) (congenital) M26.9
- maxilla (acquired) (congenital) M26.9
- meninges or membrane (congenital) Q07.9
  - cerebral Q04.8
    - acquired G96.19
  - spinal cord (congenital) G96.19
    - acquired G96.19
- metacarpus (acquired) *—see* Deformity, limb, forearm
  - congenital Q74.0
- metatarsus (acquired) *—see* Deformity, foot
  - congenital Q66.9
- middle ear (congenital) Q16.4
  - ossicles Q16.3
- mitral (leaflets) (valve) I05.8
  - parachute Q23.2
  - stenosis, congenital Q23.2
- mouth (acquired) K13.79
  - congenital Q38.6
- multiple, congenital NEC Q89.7
- muscle (acquired) M62.89
  - congenital Q79.9
    - sternocleidomastoid Q68.0
- musculoskeletal system (acquired) M95.9
  - congenital Q79.9
  - specified NEC M95.8
- nail (acquired) L60.8
  - congenital Q84.6
- nasal *—see* Deformity, nose
- neck (acquired) M95.3
  - congenital Q18.9
    - sternocleidomastoid Q68.0
- nervous system (congenital) Q07.9
- nipple (congenital) Q83.9
  - acquired N64.89
- nose (acquired) (cartilage) M95.0
  - bone (turbinate) M95.0
  - congenital Q30.9
    - bent or squashed Q67.4
  - saddle M95.0
    - syphilitic A50.57
  - septum (acquired) J34.2
    - congenital Q30.8
  - sinus (wall) (congenital) Q30.8
    - acquired M95.0
  - syphilitic (congenital) A50.57
    - late A52.73

Deformity *(continued)*
- ocular muscle (congenital) Q10.3
  - acquired *—see* Strabismus, mechanical
- opticociliary vessels (congenital) Q13.2
- orbit (eye) (acquired) H05.30
  - atrophy *—see* Atrophy, orbit
  - congenital Q10.7
  - due to
    - bone disease NEC H05.32-
    - trauma or surgery H05.33-
  - enlargement *—see* Enlargement, orbit
  - exostosis *—see* Exostosis, orbit
- organ of Corti (congenital) Q16.5
- ovary (congenital) Q50.39
  - acquired N83.8
- oviduct, acquired N83.8
- palate (congenital) Q38.5
  - acquired M27.8
  - cleft (congenital) *—see* Cleft, palate
- pancreas (congenital) Q45.3
  - acquired K86.89
- parathyroid (gland) Q89.2
- parotid (gland) (congenital) Q38.4
  - acquired K11.8
- patella (acquired) *—see* Disorder, patella, specified NEC
- pelvis, pelvic (acquired) (bony) M95.5
  - with disproportion (fetopelvic) O33.0
    - causing obstructed labor O65.0
  - congenital Q74.2
  - rachitic sequelae (late effect) E64.3
- penis (glans) (congenital) Q55.69
  - acquired N48.89
- pericardium (congenital) Q24.8
  - acquired *—see* Pericarditis
- pharynx (congenital) Q38.8
  - acquired J39.2
- pinna, acquired *—see also* Disorder, pinna, deformity
  - congenital Q17.9
- pituitary (congenital) Q89.2
- posture *—see* Dorsopathy, deforming
- prepuce (congenital) Q55.69
  - acquired N47.8
- prostate (congenital) Q55.4
  - acquired N42.89
- pupil (congenital) Q13.2
  - acquired *—see* Abnormality, pupillary
- pylorus (congenital) Q40.3
  - acquired K31.89
- rachitic (acquired), old or healed E64.3
- radius (acquired) *—see also* Deformity, limb, forearm
  - congenital Q68.8
- rectum (congenital) Q43.9
  - acquired K62.89
- reduction (extremity) (limb), congenital (*see also* condition and site) Q73.8
  - brain Q04.3
  - lower *—see* Defect, reduction, lower limb
  - upper *—see* Defect, reduction, upper limb
- renal *—see* Deformity, kidney
- respiratory system (congenital) Q34.9
- rib (acquired) M95.4
  - congenital Q76.6
    - cervical Q76.5
- rotation (joint) (acquired) *—see* Deformity, limb, specified site NEC
  - congenital Q74.9
  - hip *—see* Deformity, limb, specified type NEC, thigh
    - congenital Q65.89
- sacroiliac joint (congenital) Q74.2
  - acquired *—see* subcategory M43.8

Deformity *(continued)*
- sacrum (acquired) *—see* subcategory M43.8
- saddle
  - back *—see* Lordosis
  - nose M95.0
    - syphilitic A50.57
- salivary gland or duct (congenital) Q38.4
  - acquired K11.8
- scapula (acquired) M95.8
  - congenital Q68.8
- scrotum (congenital) *—see also* Malformation, testis and scrotum
  - acquired N50.89
- seminal vesicles (congenital) Q55.4
  - acquired N50.89
- septum, nasal (acquired) J34.2
- shoulder (joint) (acquired) *—see* Deformity, limb, upper arm
  - congenital Q74.0
  - contraction *—see* Contraction, joint, shoulder
- sigmoid (flexure) (congenital) Q43.9
  - acquired K63.89
- skin (congenital) Q82.9
- skull (acquired) M95.2
  - congenital Q75.8
    - with
      - anencephaly Q00.0
      - encephalocele *—see* Encephalocele
      - hydrocephalus Q03.9
        - with spina bifida *—see* Spina bifida, by site, with hydrocephalus
      - microcephaly Q02
- soft parts, organs or tissues (of pelvis)
  - in pregnancy or childbirth NEC O34.8-
    - causing obstructed labor O65.5
- spermatic cord (congenital) Q55.4
  - acquired N50.89
    - torsion *—see* Torsion, spermatic cord
- spinal *—see* Dorsopathy, deforming
  - column (acquired) *—see* Dorsopathy, deforming
  - congenital Q67.5
  - cord (congenital) Q06.9
    - acquired G95.89
  - nerve root (congenital) Q07.9
- spine (acquired) *—see also* Dorsopathy, deforming
  - congenital Q67.5
  - rachitic E64.3
  - specified NEC *—see* Dorsopathy, deforming, specified NEC
- spleen
  - acquired D73.89
  - congenital Q89.09
- Sprengel's (congenital) Q74.0
- sternocleidomastoid (muscle), congenital Q68.0
- sternum (acquired) M95.4
  - congenital NEC Q76.7
- stomach (congenital) Q40.3
  - acquired K31.89
- submandibular gland (congenital) Q38.4
- submaxillary gland (congenital) Q38.4
  - acquired K11.8
- talipes *—see* Talipes
- testis (congenital) *—see also* Malformation, testis and scrotum
  - acquired N44.8
    - torsion *—see* Torsion, testis
- thigh (acquired) *—see also* Deformity, limb, thigh
  - congenital NEC Q68.8

Deformity *(continued)*
thorax (acquired) (wall) M95.4
congenital Q67.8
sequelae of rickets E64.3
thumb (acquired) *—see also* Deformity, finger
congenital NEC Q68.1
thymus (tissue) (congenital) Q89.2
thyroid (gland) (congenital) Q89.2
cartilage Q31.8
acquired J38.7
tibia (acquired) *—see also* Deformity, limb, specified type NEC, lower leg
congenital NEC Q68.8
saber (syphilitic) A50.56
toe (acquired) M20.6-
congenital Q66.9
hallux rigidus M20.2-
hallux valgus M20.1-
hallux varus M20.3-
hammer toe M20.4-
specified NEC M20.5X-
tongue (congenital) Q38.3
acquired K14.8
tooth, teeth K00.2
trachea (rings) (congenital) Q32.1
acquired J39.8
transverse aortic arch (congenital) Q25.49
tricuspid (leaflets) (valve) I07.8
atresia or stenosis Q22.4
Ebstein's Q22.5
trunk (acquired) M95.8
congenital Q89.9
ulna (acquired) *—see also* Deformity, limb, forearm
congenital NEC Q68.8
urachus, congenital Q64.4
ureter (opening) (congenital) Q62.8
acquired N28.89
urethra (congenital) Q64.79
acquired N36.8
urinary tract (congenital) Q64.9
urachus Q64.4
uterus (congenital) Q51.9
acquired N85.8
uvula (congenital) Q38.5
vagina (acquired) N89.8
congenital Q52.4
valgus NEC M21.00
ankle M21.07-
elbow M21.02-
hip M21.05-
knee M21.06-
valve, valvular (congenital) (heart) Q24.8
acquired *—see* Endocarditis
varus NEC M21.10
ankle M21.17-
elbow M21.12-
hip M21.15
knee M21.16-
tibia *—see* Osteochondrosis, juvenile, tibia
vas deferens (congenital) Q55.4
acquired N50.89
vein (congenital) Q27.9
great Q26.9
vertebra *—see* Dorsopathy, deforming
vertical talus (congenital) Q66.80
left foot Q66.82
right foot Q66.81
vesicourethral orifice (acquired) N32.89
congenital NEC Q64.79
vessels of optic papilla (congenital) Q14.2
visual field (contraction) *—see* Defect, visual field
vitreous body, acquired H43.89

Deformity *(continued)*
vulva (congenital) Q52.79
acquired N90.89
wrist (joint) (acquired) *—see also* Deformity, limb, forearm
congenital Q68.8
contraction *—see* Contraction, joint, wrist

Degeneration, degenerative
adrenal (capsule) (fatty) (gland) (hyaline) (infectional) E27.8
amyloid (*see also* Amyloidosis) E85.9
anterior cornua, spinal cord G12.29
anterior labral S43.49-
aorta, aortic I70.0
fatty I77.89
aortic valve (heart) *—see* Endocarditis, aortic
arteriovascular *—see* Arteriosclerosis
artery, arterial (atheromatous) (calcareous) *—see also* Arteriosclerosis
cerebral, amyloid E85.4 *[I68.0]*
medial *—see* Arteriosclerosis, extremities
articular cartilage NEC *—see* Derangement, joint, articular cartilage, by site
atheromatous *—see* Arteriosclerosis
basal nuclei or ganglia G23.9
specified NEC G23.8
bone NEC *—see* Disorder, bone, specified type NEC
brachial plexus G54.0
brain (cortical) (progressive) G31.9
alcoholic G31.2
arteriosclerotic I67.2
childhood G31.9
specified NEC G31.89
cystic G31.89
congenital Q04.6
in
alcoholism G31.2
beriberi E51.2
cerebrovascular disease I67.9
congenital hydrocephalus Q03.9
with spina bifida *—see also* Spina bifida
Fabry-Anderson disease E75.21
Gaucher's disease E75.22
Hunter's syndrome E76.1
lipidosis
cerebral E75.4
generalized E75.6
mucopolysaccharidosis *—see* Mucopolysaccharidosis
myxedema E03.9 *[G32.89]*
neoplastic disease (*see also* Neoplasm) D49.6 *[G32.89]*
Niemann-Pick disease E75.249 *[G32.89]*
sphingolipidosis E75.3 *[G32.89]*
vitamin B12 deficiency E53.8 *[G32.89]*
senile NEC G31.1
breast N64.89
Bruch's membrane *—see* Degeneration, choroid
capillaries (fatty) I78.8
amyloid E85.89 *[I79.8]*
cardiac *—see also* Degeneration, myocardial
valve, valvular *—see* Endocarditis
cardiorenal *—see* Hypertension, cardiorenal
cardiovascular *—see also* Disease, cardiovascular
renal *—see* Hypertension, cardiorenal
cerebellar NOS G31.9
alcoholic G31.2
primary (hereditary) (sporadic) G11.9

Degeneration, degenerative *(continued)*
cerebral *—see* Degeneration, brain
cerebrovascular I67.9
due to hypertension I67.4
cervical plexus G54.2
cervix N88.8
due to radiation (intended effect) N88.8
adverse effect or misadventure N99.89
chamber angle H21.21-
changes, spine or vertebra *—see* Spondylosis
chorioretinal *—see also* Degeneration, choroid
hereditary H31.20
choroid (colloid) (drusen) H31.10-
atrophy *—see* Atrophy, choroidal
hereditary *—see* Dystrophy, choroidal, hereditary
ciliary body H21.22-
cochlear H83.8
combined (spinal cord) (subacute) E53.8 *[G32.0]*
with anemia (pernicious) D51.0 *[G32.0]*
due to dietary vitamin B12 deficiency D51.3 *[G32.0]*
in (due to)
vitamin B12 deficiency E53.8 *[G32.0]*
anemia D51.9 *[G32.0]*
conjunctiva H11.10
concretions *—see* Concretion, conjunctiva
deposits *—see* Deposit, conjunctiva
pigmentations *—see* Pigmentation, conjunctiva
pinguecula *—see* Pinguecula
xerosis *—see* Xerosis, conjunctiva
cornea H18.40
calcerous H18.43
band keratopathy H18.42-
familial, hereditary *—see* Dystrophy, cornea
hyaline (of old scars) H18.49
keratomalacia *—see* Keratomalacia
nodular H18.45-
peripheral H18.46-
senile H18.41-
specified type NEC H18.49
cortical (cerebellar) (parenchymatous) G31.89
alcoholic G31.2
diffuse, due to arteriopathy I67.2
corticobasal G31.85
cutis L98.8
amyloid E85.4 *[L99]*
dental pulp K04.2
disc disease *—see* Degeneration, intervertebral disc NEC
dorsolateral (spinal cord) *—see* Degeneration, combined
extrapyramidal G25.9
eye, macular *—see also* Degeneration, macula
congenital or hereditary *—see* Dystrophy, retina
facet joints *—see* Spondylosis
fatty
liver NEC K76.0
alcoholic K70.0
grey matter (brain) (Alpers') G31.81
heart *—see also* Degeneration, myocardial
amyloid E85.4 *[I43]*
atheromatous *—see* Disease, heart, ischemic, atherosclerotic
ischemic *—see* Disease, heart, ischemic

Degeneration, degenerative *(continued)*
hepatolenticular (Wilson's) E83.01
hepatorenal K76.7
hyaline (diffuse) (generalized)
localized *—see* Degeneration, by site
infrapatellar fat pad M79.4
intervertebral disc NOS
with
myelopathy *—see* Disorder, disc, with, myelopathy
radiculitis or radiculopathy *—see* Disorder, disc, with, radiculopathy
cervical, cervicothoracic *—see* Disorder, disc, cervical, degeneration
with
myelopathy *—see* Disorder, disc, cervical, with myelopathy
neuritis, radiculitis or radiculopathy *—see* Disorder, disc, cervical, with neuritis
lumbar region M51.36
with
myelopathy M51.06
neuritis, radiculitis, radiculopathy or sciatica M51.16
lumbosacral region M51.37
with
neuritis, radiculitis, radiculopathy or sciatica M51.17
sacrococcygeal region M53.3
thoracic region M51.34
with
myelopathy M51.04
neuritis, radiculitis, radiculopathy M51.14
thoracolumbar region M51.35
with
myelopathy M51.05
neuritis, radiculitis, radiculopathy M51.15
intestine, amyloid E85.4
iris (pigmentary) H21.23-
ischemic *—see* Ischemia
joint disease *—see* Osteoarthritis
kidney N28.89
amyloid E85.4 *[N29]*
cystic, congenital Q61.9
fatty N28.89
polycystic Q61.3
adult type (autosomal dominant) Q61.2
infantile type (autosomal recessive) NEC Q61.19
collecting duct dilatation Q61.11
Kuhnt-Junius (*see also* Degeneration, macula) H35.32-
lens *—see* Cataract
lenticular (familial) (progressive) (Wilson's) (with cirrhosis of liver) E83.01
liver (diffuse) NEC K76.89
amyloid E85.4 *[K77]*
cystic K76.89
congenital Q44.6
fatty NEC K76.0
alcoholic K70.0
hypertrophic K76.89
parenchymatous, acute or subacute K72.00
with coma K72.01
pigmentary K76.89
toxic (acute) K71.9
lung J98.4

Degeneration, degenerative *(continued)*
lymph gland I89.8
hyaline I89.8
macula, macular (acquired) (age-related) (senile) H35.30
angioid streaks H35.33
atrophic age-related H35.31-
congenital or hereditary *—see* Dystrophy, retina
cystoid H35.35-
dry age-related H35.31-
drusen H35.36-
exudative H35.32-
hole H35.34-
nonexudative H35.31-
puckering H35.37-
toxic H35.38-
wet age-related H35.32-
membranous labyrinth, congenital (causing impairment of hearing) Q16.5
meniscus *—see* Derangement, meniscus
mitral *—see* Insufficiency, mitral
Mönckeberg's *—see* Arteriosclerosis, extremities
motor centers, senile G31.1
multi-system G90.3
mural *—see* Degeneration, myocardial
muscle (fatty) (fibrous) (hyaline) (progressive) M62.89
heart *—see* Degeneration, myocardial
myelin, central nervous system G37.9
myocardial, myocardium (fatty) (hyaline) (senile) I51.5
with rheumatic fever (conditions in I00) I09.0
active, acute or subacute I01.2
with chorea I02.0
inactive or quiescent (with chorea) I09.0
hypertensive *—see* Hypertension, heart
rheumatic *—see* Degeneration, myocardial, with rheumatic fever
syphilitic A52.06
nasal sinus (mucosa) J32.9
frontal J32.1
maxillary J32.0
nerve *—see* Disorder, nerve
nervous system G31.9
alcoholic G31.2
amyloid E85.4 *[G99.8]*
autonomic G90.9
fatty G31.89
specified NEC G31.89
nipple N64.89
olivopontocerebellar (hereditary) (familial) G23.8
osseous labyrinth *—see* subcategory H83.8
ovary N83.8
cystic N83.20-
microcystic N83.20-
pallidal pigmentary (progressive) G23.0
pancreas K86.89
tuberculous A18.83
penis N48.89
pigmentary (diffuse) (general)
localized *—see* Degeneration, by site
pallidal (progressive) G23.0
pineal gland E34.8
pituitary (gland) E23.6
popliteal fat pad M79.4
posterolateral (spinal cord) *—see* Degeneration, combined
pulmonary valve (heart) I37.8
pulp (tooth) K04.2

Degeneration, degenerative *(continued)*
pupillary margin H21.24-
renal *—see* Degeneration, kidney
retina H35.9
hereditary (cerebroretinal) (congenital) (juvenile) (macula) (peripheral) (pigmentary) *—see* Dystrophy, retina
Kuhnt-Junius *(see also* Degeneration, macula) H35.32-
macula (cystic) (exudative) (hole) (nonexudative) (pseudohole) (senile) (toxic) *—see* Degeneration, macula
peripheral H35.40
lattice H35.41-
microcystoid H35.42-
paving stone H35.43-
secondary
pigmentary H35.45-
vitreoretinal H35.46-
senile reticular H35.44-
pigmentary (primary) *—see also* Dystrophy, retina
secondary *—see* Degeneration, retina, peripheral, secondary
posterior pole *—see* Degeneration, macula
saccule, congenital (causing impairment of hearing) Q16.5
senile R54
brain G31.1
cardiac, heart or myocardium *—see* Degeneration, myocardial
motor centers G31.1
vascular *—see* Arteriosclerosis
sinus (cystic) *—see also* Sinusitis
polypoid J33.1
skin L98.8
amyloid E85.4 *[L99]*
colloid L98.8
spinal (cord) G31.89
amyloid E85.4 *[G32.89]*
combined (subacute) *—see* Degeneration, combined
dorsolateral *—see* Degeneration, combined
familial NEC G31.89
fatty G31.89
funicular *—see* Degeneration, combined
posterolateral *—see* Degeneration, combined
subacute combined *—see* Degeneration, combined
tuberculous A17.81
spleen D73.0
amyloid E85.4 *[D77]*
stomach K31.89
striatonigral G23.2
suprarenal (capsule) (gland) E27.8
synovial membrane (pulpy) *—see* Disorder, synovium, specified type NEC
tapetoretinal *—see* Dystrophy, retina
thymus (gland) E32.8
fatty E32.8
thyroid (gland) E07.89
tricuspid (heart) (valve) I07.9
tuberculous NEC *—see* Tuberculosis
turbinate J34.89
uterus (cystic) N85.8
vascular (senile) *—see* Arteriosclerosis
hypertensive *—see* Hypertension
vitreoretinal, secondary *—see* Degeneration, retina, peripheral, secondary, vitreoretinal
vitreous (body) H43.81-
Wallerian *—see* Disorder, nerve
Wilson's hepatolenticular E83.01

Deglutition
paralysis R13.0
hysterical F44.4
pneumonia J69.0

Degos' disease I77.89

Dehiscence (of)
amputation stump T87.81
cesarean wound O90.0
closure of
cornea T81.31
craniotomy T81.32
fascia (muscular) (superficial) T81.32
internal organ or tissue T81.32
laceration (external) (internal) T81.33
ligament T81.32
mucosa T81.31
muscle or muscle flap T81.32
ribs or rib cage T81.32
skin and subcutaneous tissue (full-thickness) (superficial) T81.31
skull T81.32
sternum (sternotomy) T81.32
tendon T81.32
traumatic laceration (external) (internal) T81.33
episiotomy O90.1
operation wound NEC T81.31
external operation wound (superficial) T81.31
internal operation wound (deep) T81.32
perineal wound (postpartum) O90.1
traumatic injury wound repair T81.33
wound T81.30
traumatic repair T81.33

Dehydration E86.0
newborn P74.1

Déjérine-Roussy syndrome G89.0

Déjérine-Sottas disease or neuropathy (hypertrophic) G60.0

Déjérine-Thomas atrophy G23.8

Delay, delayed
any plane in pelvis
complicating delivery O66.9
birth or delivery NOS O63.9
closure, ductus arteriosus (Botalli) P29.38
coagulation *—see* Defect, coagulation
conduction (cardiac) (ventricular) I45.9
delivery, second twin, triplet, etc O63.2
development R62.50
global F88
intellectual (specific) F81.9
language F80.9
due to hearing loss F80.4
learning F81.9
pervasive F84.9
physiological R62.50
specified stage NEC R62.0
reading F81.0
sexual E30.0
speech F80.9
due to hearing loss F80.4
spelling F81.81
ejaculation F52.32
gastric emptying K30
menarche E30.0
menstruation (cause unknown) N91.0
milestone R62.0
passage of meconium (newborn) P76.0
primary respiration P28.9

Delay, delayed *(continued)*
puberty (constitutional) E30.0
separation of umbilical cord P96.82
sexual maturation, female E30.0
sleep phase syndrome G47.21
union, fracture *—see* Fracture, by site
vaccination Z28.9

Deletion(s)
autosome Q93.9
identified by fluorescence in situ hybridization (FISH) Q93.89
identified by in situ hybridization (ISH) Q93.89
chromosome
with complex rearrangements NEC Q93.7
part of NEC Q93.5
seen only at prometaphase Q93.89
short arm
4 Q93.3
5p Q93.4
22q11.2 Q93.81
specified NEC Q93.89
long arm chromosome 18 or 21 Q93.89
with complex rearrangements NEC Q93.7
microdeletions NEC Q93.88

Delhi boil or button B55.1

Delinquency (juvenile) (neurotic) F91.8
group Z72.810

Delinquent immunization status Z28.3

Delirium, delirious (acute or subacute) (not alcohol- or drug-induced) (with dementia) R41.0
alcoholic (acute) (tremens) (withdrawal) F10.921
with intoxication F10.921
in
abuse F10.121
dependence F10.221
due to (secondary to)
alcohol
intoxication F10.921
in
abuse F10.121
dependence F10.221
withdrawal F10.231
amphetamine intoxication F15.921
in
abuse F15.121
dependence F15.221
anxiolytic
intoxication F13.921
in
abuse F13.121
dependence F13.221
withdrawal F13.231
cannabis intoxication (acute) F12.921
in
abuse F12.121
dependence F12.221
cocaine intoxication (acute) F14.921
in
abuse F14.121
dependence F14.221
general medical condition F05
hallucinogen intoxication F16.921
in
abuse F16.121
dependence F16.221
hypnotic
intoxication F13.921
in
abuse F13.121
dependence F13.221
withdrawal F13.231

Delirium, delirious *(continued)*
due to (secondary to) *(continued)*
inhalant intoxication (acute) F18.921
in
abuse F18.121
dependence F18.221
multiple etiologies F05
opioid intoxication (acute) F11.921
in
abuse F11.121
dependence F11.221
other (or unknown) substance F19.921
phencyclidine intoxication (acute) F16.921
in
abuse F16.121
dependence F16.221
psychoactive substance NEC
intoxication (acute) F19.921
in
abuse F19.121
dependence F19.221
sedative
intoxication F13.921
in
abuse F13.121
dependence F13.221
withdrawal F13.231
unknown etiology F05
exhaustion F43.0
hysterical F44.89
postprocedural (postoperative) F05
puerperal F05
thyroid *—see* Thyrotoxicosis with thyroid storm
traumatic *—see* Injury, intracranial
tremens (alcohol-induced) F10.231
sedative-induced F13.231

Delivery (childbirth) (labor)
arrested active phase O62.1
cesarean (for)
abnormal
pelvis (bony) (deformity) (major) NEC with disproportion (fetopelvic) O33.0
with obstructed labor O65.0
presentation or position O32.9
abruptio placentae (*see also* Abruptio placentae) O45.9-
acromion presentation O32.2
atony, uterus O62.2
breech presentation O32.1
incomplete O32.8
brow presentation O32.3
cephalopelvic disproportion O33.9
cerclage O34.3-
chin presentation O32.3
cicatrix of cervix O34.4-
contracted pelvis (general)
inlet O33.2
outlet O33.3
cord presentation or prolapse O69.0
cystocele O34.8-
deformity (acquired) (congenital)
pelvic organs or tissues NEC O34.8-
pelvis (bony) NEC O33.0
disproportion NOS O33.9
eclampsia *—see* Eclampsia
face presentation O32.3
failed
forceps O66.5
induction of labor O61.9
instrumental O61.1
mechanical O61.1
medical O61.0
specified NEC O61.8
surgical O61.1

Delivery *(continued)*
cesarean *(continued)*
failed *(continued)*
trial of labor NOS O66.40
following previous cesarean delivery O66.41
vacuum extraction O66.5
ventouse O66.5
fetal-maternal hemorrhage O43.01-
hemorrhage (intrapartum) O67.9
with coagulation defect O67.0
specified cause NEC O67.8
high head at term O32.4
hydrocephalic fetus O33.6
incarceration of uterus O34.51-
incoordinate uterine action O62.4
increased size, fetus O33.5
inertia, uterus O62.2
primary O62.0
secondary O62.1
lateroversion, uterus O34.59-
mal lie O32.9
malposition
fetus O32.9
pelvic organs or tissues NEC O34.8-
uterus NEC O34.59-
malpresentation NOS O32.9
oblique presentation O32.2
occurring after 37 completed weeks of gestation but before 39 completed weeks gestation due to (spontaneous) onset of labor O75.82
oversize fetus O33.5
pelvic tumor NEC O34.8-
placenta previa O44.0-
complete O44.0-
with hemorrhage O44.1-
placental insufficiency O36.51-
planned, occurring after 37 completed weeks of gestation but before 39 completed weeks gestation due to (spontaneous) onset of labor O75.82
polyp, cervix O34.4-
causing obstructed labor O65.5
poor dilatation, cervix O62.0
pre-eclampsia O14.94
mild O14.04
moderate O14.04
severe O14.14
with hemolysis, elevated liver enzymes and low platelet count (HELLP) O14.24
previous
cesarean delivery O34.219
classical (vertical) O34.212
low transverse scar O34.211
surgery (to)
cervix O34.4-
gynecological NEC O34.8-
rectum O34.7-
uterus O34.29
vagina O34.6-
prolapse
arm or hand O32.2
uterus O34.52-
prolonged labor NOS O63.9
rectocele O34.8-
retroversion
uterus O34.53-
rigid
cervix O34.4-
pelvic floor O34.8-
perineum O34.7-
vagina O34.6-
vulva O34.7-
sacculation, pregnant uterus O34.59-

Delivery *(continued)*
cesarean *(continued)*
scar(s)
cervix O34.4-
cesarean delivery O34.219
classical (vertical) O34.212
low transverse O34.211
transmural uterine O34.29
uterus O34.29
Shirodkar suture in situ O34.3-
shoulder presentation O32.2
stenosis or stricture, cervix O34.4-
streptococcus group B (GBS) carrier state O99.824
transmural uterine scar O34.29
transverse presentation or lie O32.2
tumor, pelvic organs or tissues NEC O34.8-
cervix O34.4-
umbilical cord presentation or prolapse O69.0
without indication O82
completely normal case O80
complicated O75.9
by
abnormal, abnormality (of)
forces of labor O62.9
specified type NEC O62.8
glucose O99.814
uterine contractions NOS O62.9
abruptio placentae (*see also* Abruptio placentae) O45.9-
abuse
physical O9A.32
psychological O9A.52
sexual O9A.42
adherent placenta O72.0
without hemorrhage O73.0
alcohol use O99.314
anemia (pre-existing) O99.02
anesthetic death O74.8
annular detachment of cervix O71.3
atony, uterus O62.2
attempted vacuum extraction and forceps O66.5
Bandl's ring O62.4
bariatric surgery status O99.844
biliary tract disorder O26.62
bleeding *—see* Delivery, complicated by, hemorrhage
blood disorder NEC O99.12
cervical dystocia (hypotonic) O62.2
primary O62.0
secondary O62.1
circulatory system disorder O99.42
compression of cord (umbilical) NEC O69.2
condition NEC O99.89
contraction, contracted ring O62.4
cord (umbilical)
around neck
with compression O69.1
without compression O69.81
bruising O69.5
complication O69.9
specified NEC O69.89
compression NEC O69.2
entanglement O69.2
without compression O69.82
hematoma O69.5
presentation O69.0
prolapse O69.0
short O69.3
thrombosis (vessels) O69.5
vascular lesion O69.5

Delivery *(continued)*
complicated *(continued)*
by *(continued)*
Couvelaire uterus O45.8X-
damage to (injury to) NEC
perineum O71.82
periurethral tissue O71.82
vulva O71.82
delay following rupture of membranes (spontaneous) — *see* Pregnancy, complicated by, premature rupture of membranes
depressed fetal heart tones O76
diabetes O24.92
gestational
diabetes O24.429
diet controlled O24.420
insulin (and diet) controlled O24.424
oral drug controlled (antidiabetic) (hypoglycemic) O24.425
edema O12.04
with proteinuria O12.24
proteinuria O12.14
pre-existing O24.32
specified NEC O24.82
type 1 O24.02
type 2 O24.12
diastasis recti (abdominis) O71.89
dilatation
bladder O66.8
cervix incomplete, poor or slow O62.0
disease NEC O99.89
disruptio uteri *—see* Delivery, complicated by, rupture, uterus
drug use O99.324
dysfunction, uterus NOS O62.9
hypertonic O62.4
hypotonic O62.2
primary O62.0
secondary O62.1
incoordinate O62.4
eclampsia O15.1
embolism (pulmonary) *—see* Embolism, obstetric
endocrine, nutritional or metabolic disease NEC O99.284
failed
attempted vaginal birth after previous cesarean delivery O66.41
induction of labor O61.9
instrumental O61.1
mechanical O61.1
medical O61.0
specified NEC O61.8
surgical O61.1
trial of labor O66.40
female genital mutilation O65.5
fetal
abnormal acid-base balance O68
acidemia O68
acidosis O68
alkalosis O68
death, early O02.1
deformity O66.3
heart rate or rhythm (abnormal) (non-reassuring) O76
hypoxia O77.8
stress O77.9
due to drug administration O77.1

Delivery *(continued)*
 complicated *(continued)*
  by *(continued)*
   fetal *(continued)*
    stress *(continued)*
     electrocardiographic evidence of O77.8
     specified NEC O77.8
     ultrasound evidence of O77.8
   fever during labor O75.2
   gastric banding status O99.844
   gastric bypass status O99.844
   gastrointestinal disease NEC O99.62
   gestational
    diabetes O24.429
     diet controlled O24.420
     insulin (and diet) controlled O24.424
     oral drug controlled (antidiabetic) (hypoglycemic) O24.425
    edema O12.04
     with proteinuria O12.14
    proteinuria O12.14
   gonorrhea O98.22
   hematoma O71.7
    ischial spine O71.7
    pelvic O71.7
    vagina O71.7
    vulva or perineum O71.7
   hemorrhage (uterine) O67.9
    associated with
     afibrinogenemia O67.0
     coagulation defect O67.0
     hyperfibrinolysis O67.0
     hypofibrinogenemia O67.0
    due to
     low implantation of placenta O44.5-
     low-lying placenta O44.5-
     placenta previa O44.1-
      marginal O44.3-
      partial O44.3-
     premature separation of placenta (normally implanted) (*see also* Abruptio placentae) O45.9-
     retained placenta O72.0
     uterine leiomyoma O67.8
    placenta NEC O67.8
    postpartum NEC (atonic) (immediate) O72.1
     with retained or trapped placenta O72.0
     delayed O72.2
     secondary O72.2
     third stage O72.0
   hourglass contraction, uterus O62.4
   hypertension, hypertensive (pre-existing) *—see* Hypertension, complicated by, childbirth (labor)
   hypotension O26.5-
   incomplete dilatation (cervix) O62.0
   incoordinate uterus contractions O62.4
   inertia, uterus O62.2
    during latent phase of labor O62.0
    primary O62.0
    secondary O62.1
   infection (maternal) O98.92
    carrier state NEC O99.834
    gonorrhea O98.22
    human immunodeficiency virus (HIV) O98.72

Delivery *(continued)*
 complicated *(continued)*
  by *(continued)*
   infection (maternal) *(continued)*
    sexually transmitted NEC O98.32
    specified NEC O98.82
    syphilis O98.12
    tuberculosis O98.02
    viral hepatitis O98.42
    viral NEC O98.52
   injury (to mother) (*see also* Delivery, complicated by, damage to) O71.9
    nonobstetric O9A.22
     caused by abuse *—see* Delivery, complicated by, abuse
   intrauterine fetal death, early O02.1
   inversion, uterus O71.2
   laceration (perineal) O70.9
    anus (sphincter) O70.4
     with third degree laceration (*see also* Delivery, complicated, by, laceration, perineum, third degree) O70.20
      with mucosa O70.3
     without third degree laceration O70.4
    bladder (urinary) O71.5
    bowel O71.5
    cervix (uteri) O71.3
    fourchette O70.0
    hymen O70.0
    labia O70.0
    pelvic
     floor O70.1
     organ NEC O71.5
    perineum, perineal O70.9
     first degree O70.0
     fourth degree O70.3
     muscles O70.1
     second degree O70.1
     skin O70.0
     slight O70.0
     third degree O70.20
      with
       both external anal sphincter (EAS) and internal anal sphincter (IAS) torm (IIIc) O70.23
       less than 50% of external anal sphincter (EAS) thickness torn (IIIa) O70.21
       more than 50% of external anal sphincter (EAS) thickness torn (IIIb) O70.22
      IIIa O70.21
      IIIb O70.22
      IIIc O70.23
    peritoneum (pelvic) O71.5
    rectovaginal (septum) (without perineal laceration) O71.4
     with perineum (*see also* Delivery, complicated, by, laceration, perineum, third degree) O70.20
      with anal or rectal mucosa O70.3
    specified NEC O71.89
    sphincter ani *—see* Delivery, complicated, by, laceration, anus (sphincter)
    urethra O71.5

Delivery *(continued)*
 complicated *(continued)*
  by *(continued)*
   laceration (perineal) *(continued)*
    uterus O71.81
     before labor O71.81
    vagina, vaginal (deep) (high) (without perineal laceration) O71.4
     with perineum O70.0
     muscles, with perineum O70.1
    vulva O70.0
   liver disorder O26.62
   malignancy O9A.12
   malnutrition O25.2
   malposition, malpresentation
    placenta O44.0-
     with hemorrhage O44.1-
    uterus or cervix O65.5
    without obstruction (*see also* Delivery, complicated by, obstruction) O32.9
     breech O32.1
     compound O32.6
     face (brow) (chin) O32.3
     footling O32.8
     high head O32.4
     oblique O32.2
     specified NEC O32.8
     transverse O32.2
     unstable lie O32.0
   meconium in amniotic fluid O77.0
   mental disorder NEC O99.344
   metrorrhexis *—see* Delivery, complicated by, rupture, uterus
   nervous system disorder O99.354
   obesity (pre-existing) O99.214
   obesity surgery status O99.844
   obstetric trauma O71.9
    specified NEC O71.89
   obstructed labor
    due to
     breech (complete) (frank) presentation O64.1
      incomplete O64.8
     brow presenation O64.3
     buttock presentation O64.1
     chin presentation O64.2
     compound presentation O64.5
     contracted pelvis O65.1
     deep transverse arrest O64.0
     deformed pelvis O65.0
     dystocia (fetal) O66.9
      due to
       conjoined twins O66.3
       fetal
        abnormality NEC O66.3
        ascites O66.3
        hydrops O66.3
        meningomyelocele O66.3
        sacral teratoma O66.3
        tumor O66.3
       hydrocephalic fetus O66.3
      shoulder O66.0
     face presentation O64.2
     fetopelvic disproportion O65.4
     footling presentation O64.8
     impacted shoulders O66.0
     incomplete rotation of fetal head O64.0
     large fetus O66.2
     locked twins O66.1
     malposition O64.9
      specified NEC O64.8

Delivery *(continued)*
 complicated *(continued)*
  by *(continued)*
   obstructed labor *(continued)*
    due to *(continued)*
     malpresentation O64.9
      specified NEC O64.8
     multiple fetuses NEC O66.6
     pelvic
      abnormality (maternal) O65.9
       organ O65.5
       specified NEC O65.8
      contraction
       inlet O65.2
       mid-cavity O65.3
       outlet O65.3
     persistent (position)
      occipitoiliac O64.0
      occipitoposterior O64.0
      occipitosacral O64.0
      occipitotransverse O64.0
     prolapsed arm O64.4
     shoulder presentation O64.4
    specified NEC O66.8
   pathological retraction ring, uterus O62.4
   penetration, pregnant uterus by instrument O71.1
   perforation *—see* Delivery, complicated by, laceration
   placenta, placental
    ablatio (*see also* Abruptio placentae) O45.9-
    abnormality O43.9-
     specified NEC O43.89-
    abruptio (*see also* Abruptio placentae) O45.9-
    accreta O43.21-
    adherent (with hemorrhage) O72.0
     without hemorrhage O73.0
    detachment (premature) (*see also* Abruptio placentae) O45.9-
    disorder O43.9-
     specified NEC O43.89-
    hemorrhage NEC O67.8
    increta O43.22-
    low (implantation) (lying) O44.4-
     with hemorrhage O44.5-
    malformation O43.10-
    malposition O44.0-
     with hemorrhage O44.1-
    percreta O43.23-
    previa (central) (complete) (lateral) (total) O44.0-
     with hemorrhage O44.1-
     marginal O44.2-
      with hemorrhage O44.3-
     partial O44.2-
      with hemorrhage O44.3-
     with hemorrhage O44.1-
    retained (with hemorrhage) O72.0
     without hemorrhage O73.0
    separation (premature) O45.9-
     specified NEC O45.8X-
    vicious insertion O44.1-
   precipitate labor O62.3
   premature rupture, membranes (*see also* Pregnancy, complicated by, premature rupture of membranes) O42.90
   prolapse
    arm or hand O32.2
    cord (umbilical) O69.0
    foot or leg O32.8
    uterus O34.52-

Delivery *(continued)*
complicated *(continued)*
by *(continued)*
prolonged labor O63.9
first stage O63.0
second stage O63.1
protozoal disease (maternal) O98.62
respiratory disease NEC O99.52
retained membranes or portions of placenta O72.2
without hemorrhage O73.1
retarded birth O63.9
retention of secundines (with hemorrhage) O72.0
without hemorrhage O73.0
partial O72.2
without hemorrhage O73.1
rupture
bladder (urinary) O71.5
cervix O71.3
pelvic organ NEC O71.5
urethra O71.5
uterus (during or after labor) O71.1
before labor O71.0-
separation, pubic bone (symphysis pubis) O71.6
shock O75.1
shoulder presentation O64.4
skin disorder NEC O99.72
spasm, cervix O62.4
stenosis or stricture, cervix O65.5
streptococcus group B (GBS) carrier state O99.824
subluxation of symphysis (pubis) O26.72
syphilis (maternal) O98.12
tear *—see* Delivery, complicated by, laceration
tetanic uterus O62.4
trauma (obstetrical) (*see also* Delivery, complicated by, damage to) O71.9
non-obstetric O9A.22
periurethral O71.82
specified NEC O71.89
tuberculosis (maternal) O98.02
tumor, pelvic organs or tissues NEC O65.5
umbilical cord around neck
with compression O69.1
without compression O69.81
uterine inertia O62.2
during latent phase of labor O62.0
primary O62.0
secondary O62.1
vasa previa O69.4
velamentous insertion of cord O43.12-
specified complication NEC O75.89
delayed NOS O63.9
following rupture of membranes
artificial O75.5
second twin, triplet, etc. O63.2
forceps, low following failed vacuum extraction O66.5
missed (at or near term) O36.4
normal O80
obstructed *—see* Delivery, complicated by, obstructed labor
precipitate O62.3
preterm (*see also* Pregnancy, complicated by, preterm labor) O60.10
spontaneous O80
term pregnancy NOS O80
uncomplicated O80

Delivery *(continued)*
vaginal, following previous cesarean delivery O34.219
classical (vertical) scar O34.212
low transverse scar O34.211

Delusions (paranoid) *—see* Disorder, delusional

Dementia (degenerative (primary)) (old age) (persisting) F03.90
with
aggressive behavior F03.91
behavioral disturbance F03.91
combative behavior F03.91
Lewy bodies G31.83 *[F02.80]*
with behavioral disturbance G31.83 *[F02.81]*
Parkinsonism G31.83 *[F02.80]*
with behavioral disturbance G31.83 *[F02.81]*
Parkinson's disease G20 *[F02.80]*
with behavioral disturbance G20 *[F02.81]*
violent behavior F03.91
alcoholic F10.97
with dependence F10.27
Alzheimer's type *—see* Disease, Alzheimer's
arteriosclerotic *—see* Dementia, vascular
atypical, Alzheimer's type *—see* Disease, Alzheimer's, specified NEC
congenital *—see* Disability, intellectual
frontal (lobe) G31.09 *[F02.80]*
with behavioral disturbance G31.09 *[F02.81]*
frontotemporal G31.09 *[F02.80]*
with behavioral disturbance G31.09 *[F02.81]*
specified NEC G31.09 *[F02.80]*
with behavioral disturbance G31.09 *[F02.81]*
in (due to)
alcohol F10.97
with dependence F10.27
Alzheimer's disease *—see* Disease, Alzheimer's
arteriosclerotic brain disease *— see* Dementia, vascular
cerebral lipidoses E75.- *[F02.80]*
with behavioral disturbance E75.- *[F02.81]*
Creutzfeldt-Jakob disease *—see also* Creutzfeldt-Jakob disease or syndrome (with dementia) A81.00
epilepsy G40.- *[F02.80]*
with behavioral disturbance G40.- *[F02.81]*
hepatolenticular degeneration E83.01 *[F02.80]*
with behavioral disturbance E83.01 *[F02.81]*
human immunodeficiency virus (HIV) disease B20 *[F02.80]*
with behavioral disturbance B20 *[F02.81]*
Huntington's disease or chorea G10 *[F02.80]*
with behavioral disturbance G10 *[F02.81]*
hypercalcemia E83.52 *[F02.80]*
with behavioral disturbance E83.52 *[F02.81]*
hypothyroidism, acquired E03.9 *[F02.80]*
with behavioral disturbance E03.9 *[F02.81]*
due to iodine deficiency E01.8 *[F02.80]*
with behavioral disturbance E01.8 *[F02.81]*

Dementia *(continued)*
in *(continued)*
inhalants F18.97
with dependence F18.27
multiple
etiologies F03
sclerosis G35 *[F02.80]*
with behavioral disturbance G35 *[F02.81]*
neurosyphilis A52.17 *[F02.80]*
with behavioral disturbance A52.17 *[F02.81]*
juvenile A50.49 *[F02.80]*
with behavioral disturbance A50.49 *[F02.81]*
niacin deficiency E52 *[F02.80]*
with behavioral disturbance E52 *[F02.81]*
paralysis agitans G20 *[F02.80]*
with behavioral disturbance G20 *[F02.81]*
Parkinson's disease G20 *[F02.80]*
pellagra E52 *[F02.80]*
with behavioral disturbance E52 *[F02.81]*
Pick's G31.01 *[F02.80]*
with behavioral disturbance G31.01 *[F02.81]*
polyarteritis nodosa M30.0 *[F02.80]*
with behavioral disturbance M30.0 *[F02.81]*
psychoactive drug F19.97
with dependence F19.27
inhalants F18.97
with dependence F18.27
sedatives, hypnotics or anxiolytics F13.97
with dependence F13.27
sedatives, hypnotics or anxiolytics F13.97
with dependence F13.27
systemic lupus erythematosus M32.- *[F02.80]*
with behavioral disturbance M32.- *[F02.81]*
trypanosomiasis
African B56.9 *[F02.80]*
with behavioral disturbance B56.9 *[F02.81]*
unknown etiology F03
vitamin B12 deficiency E53.8 *[F02.80]*
with behavioral disturbance E53.8 *[F02.81]*
volatile solvents F18.97
with dependence F18.27
with behavioral disturbance G31.83 *[F02.81]*
infantile, infantilis F84.3
Lewy body G31.83 *[F02.80]*
with behavioral disturbance G31.83 *[F02.81]*
multi-infarct *—see* Dementia, vascular
paralytica, paralytic (syphilitic) A52.17 *[F02.80]*
with behavioral disturbance A52.17 *[F02.81]*
juvenilis A50.45
paretic A52.17
praecox *—see* Schizophrenia
presenile F03
Alzheimer's type *—see* Disease, Alzheimer's, early onset
primary degenerative F03
progressive, syphilitic A52.17
senile F03
with acute confusional state F05
Alzheimer's type *—see* Disease, Alzheimer's, late onset
depressed or paranoid type F03

Dementia *(continued)*
vascular (acute onset) (mixed) (multi-infarct) (subcortical) F01.50
with behavioral disturbance F01.51

Demineralization, bone *—see* Osteoporosis

Demodex folliculorum (infestation) B88.0

Demophobia F40.248

Demoralization R45.3

Demyelination, demyelinization
central nervous system G37.9
specified NEC G37.8
corpus callosum (central) G37.1
disseminated, acute G36.9
specified NEC G36.8
global G35
in optic neuritis G36.0

Dengue (classical) (fever) A90
hemorrhagic A91
sandfly A93.1

Dennie-Marfan syphilitic syndrome A50.45

Dens evaginatus, in dente or invaginatus K00.2

Dense breasts R92.2

Density
increased, bone (disseminated) (generalized) (spotted) *—see* Disorder, bone, density and structure, specified type NEC
lung (nodular) J98.4

Dental *—see also* condition
examination Z01.20
with abnormal findings Z01.21
restoration
aesthetically inadequate or displeasing K08.56
defective K08.50
specified NEC K08.59
failure of marginal integrity K08.51
failure of periodontal anatomical integrity K08.54

Dentia praecox K00.6

Denticles (pulp) K04.2

Dentigerous cyst K09.0

Dentin
irregular (in pulp) K04.3
opalescent K00.5
secondary (in pulp) K04.3
sensitive K03.89

Dentinogenesis imperfecta K00.5

Dentinoma *—see* Cyst, calcifying odontogenic

Dentition (syndrome) K00.7
delayed K00.6
difficult K00.7
precocious K00.6
premature K00.6
retarded K00.6

Dependence (on) (syndrome) F19.20
with remission F19.21
alcohol (ethyl) (methyl) (without remission) F10.20
with
amnestic disorder, persisting F10.26
anxiety disorder F10.280
dementia, persisting F10.27
intoxication F10.229
with delirium F10.221
uncomplicated F10.220
mood disorder F10.24
psychotic disorder F10.259
with
delusions F10.250
hallucinations F10.251

Dependence *(continued)*
  alcohol *(continued)*
    with *(continued)*
      remission F10.21
      sexual dysfunction F10.281
      sleep disorder F10.282
      specified disorder NEC F10.288
      withdrawal F10.239
        with
          delirium F10.231
          perceptual disturbance F10.232
        uncomplicated F10.230
    counseling and surveillance Z71.41
  amobarbital —*see* Dependence, drug, sedative
  amphetamine(s) (type) —*see* Dependence, drug, stimulant NEC
  amytal (sodium) —*see* Dependence, drug, sedative
  analgesic NEC F55.8
  anesthetic (agent) (gas) (general) (local) NEC —*see* Dependence, drug, psychoactive NEC
  anxiolytic NEC —*see* Dependence, drug, sedative
  barbital(s) —*see* Dependence, drug, sedative
  barbiturate(s) (compounds) (drugs classifiable to T42) —*see* Dependence, drug, sedative
  benzedrine —*see* Dependence, drug, stimulant NEC
  bhang —*see* Dependence, drug, cannabis
  bromide(s) NEC —*see* Dependence, drug, sedative
  caffeine —*see* Dependence, drug, stimulant NEC
  cannabis (sativa) (indica) (resin) (derivatives) (type) —*see* Dependence, drug, cannabis
  chloral (betaine) (hydrate) —*see* Dependence, drug, sedative
  chlordiazepoxide —*see* Dependence, drug, sedative
  coca (leaf) (derivatives) —*see* Dependence, drug, cocaine
  cocaine —*see* Dependence, drug, cocaine
  codeine —*see* Dependence, drug, opioid
  combinations of drugs F19.20
  dagga —*see* Dependence, drug, cannabis
  demerol —*see* Dependence, drug, opioid
  dexamphetamine —*see* Dependence, drug, stimulant NEC
  dexedrine —*see* Dependence, drug, stimulant NEC
  dextromethorphan —*see* Dependence, drug, opioid
  dextromoramide —*see* Dependence, drug, opioid
  dextro-nor-pseudo-ephedrine —*see* Dependence, drug, stimulant NEC
  dextrorphan —*see* Dependence, drug, opioid
  diazepam —*see* Dependence, drug, sedative
  dilaudid —*see* Dependence, drug, opioid
  D-lysergic acid diethylamide —*see* Dependence, drug, hallucinogen
  drug NEC F19.20
    with sleep disorder F19.282
    cannabis F12.20
      with
        anxiety disorder F12.280
        intoxication F12.229
          with
            delirium F12.221
            perceptual disturbance F12.222
          uncomplicated F12.220
        other specified disorder F12.288
        psychosis F12.259
          delusions F12.250
          hallucinations F12.251
        unspecified disorder F12.29
      in remission F12.21
    cocaine F14.20
      with
        anxiety disorder F14.280
        intoxication F14.229
          with
            delirium F14.221
            perceptual disturbance F14.222
          uncomplicated F14.220
        mood disorder F14.24
        other specified disorder F14.288
        psychosis F14.259
          delusions F14.250
          hallucinations F14.251
        sexual dysfunction F14.281
        sleep disorder F14.282
        unspecified disorder F14.29
        withdrawal F14.23
      in remission F14.21
      withdrawal symptoms in newborn P96.1
    counseling and surveillance Z71.51
    hallucinogen F16.20
      with
        anxiety disorder F16.280
        flashbacks F16.283
        intoxication F16.229
          with delirium F16.221
          uncomplicated F16.220
        mood disorder F16.24
        other specified disorder F16.288
        perception disorder, persisting F16.283
        psychosis F16.259
          delusions F16.250
          hallucinations F16.251
        unspecified disorder F16.29
      in remission F16.21
    in remission F19.21
    inhalant F18.20
      with
        anxiety disorder F18.280
        dementia, persisting F18.27
        intoxication F18.229
          with delirium F18.221
          uncomplicated F18.220
        mood disorder F18.24
        other specified disorder F18.288
        psychosis F18.259
          delusions F18.250
          hallucinations F18.251
        unspecified disorder F18.29
      in remission F18.21
    nicotine F17.200
      with disorder F17.209
        in remission F17.201
        specified disorder NEC F17.208
        withdrawal F17.203
      chewing tobacco F17.220
        with disorder F17.229
          in remission F17.221
          specified disorder NEC F17.228
          withdrawal F17.223
      cigarettes F17.210
        with disorder F17.219
          in remission F17.211
          specified disorder NEC F17.218
          withdrawal F17.213
      specified product NEC F17.290
        with disorder F17.299
          remission F17.291
          specified disorder NEC F17.298
          withdrawal F17.293
    opioid F11.20
      with
        intoxication F11.229
          with
            delirium F11.221
            perceptual disturbance F11.222
          uncomplicated F11.220
        mood disorder F11.24
        other specified disorder F11.288
        psychosis F11.259
          delusions F11.250
          hallucinations F11.251
        sexual dysfunction F11.281
        sleep disorder F11.282
        unspecified disorder F11.29
        withdrawal F11.23
      in remission F11.21
    psychoactive NEC F19.20
      with
        amnestic disorder F19.26
        anxiety disorder F19.280
        dementia F19.27
        intoxication F19.229
          with
            delirium F19.221
            perceptual disturbance F19.222
          uncomplicated F19.220
        mood disorder F19.24
        other specified disorder F19.288
        psychosis F19.259
          delusions F19.250
          hallucinations F19.251
        sexual dysfunction F19.281
        sleep disorder F19.282
        unspecified disorder F19.29
        withdrawal F19.239
          with
            delirium F19.231
            perceptual disturbance F19.232
          uncomplicated F19.230
    sedative, hypnotic or anxiolytic F13.20
      with
        amnestic disorder F13.26
        anxiety disorder F13.280
        dementia, persisting F13.27
        intoxication F13.229
          with delirium F13.221
          uncomplicated F13.220
        mood disorder F13.24
        other specified disorder F13.288
        psychosis F13.259
          delusions F13.250
          hallucinations F13.251
        sexual dysfunction F13.281
        sleep disorder F13.282
        unspecified disorder F13.29
        withdrawal F13.239
          with
            delirium F13.231
            perceptual disturbance F13.232
          uncomplicated F13.230
      in remission F13.21
    stimulant NEC F15.20
      with
        anxiety disorder F15.280
        intoxication F15.229
          with
            delirium F15.221
            perceptual disturbance F15.222
          uncomplicated F15.220
        mood disorder F15.24
        other specified disorder F15.288
        psychosis F15.259
          delusions F15.250
          hallucinations F15.251
        sexual dysfunction F15.281
        sleep disorder F15.282
        unspecified disorder F15.29
        withdrawal F15.23
      in remission F15.21
  ethyl
    alcohol (without remission) F10.20
      with remission F10.21
    bromide —*see* Dependence, drug, sedative
    carbamate F19.20
    chloride F19.20
    morphine —*see* Dependence, drug, opioid
  ganja —*see* Dependence, drug, cannabis
  glue (airplane) (sniffing) —*see* Dependence, drug, inhalant
  glutethimide —*see* Dependence, drug, sedative
  hallucinogenics —*see* Dependence, drug, hallucinogen
  hashish —*see* Dependence, drug, cannabis
  hemp —*see* Dependence, drug, cannabis
  heroin (salt) (any) —*see* Dependence, drug, opioid
  hypnotic NEC —*see* Dependence, drug, sedative
  Indian hemp —*see* Dependence, drug, cannabis
  inhalants —*see* Dependence, drug, inhalant
  khat —*see* Dependence, drug, stimulant NEC
  laudanum —*see* Dependence, drug, opioid
  LSD(-25) (derivatives) —*see* Dependence, drug, hallucinogen
  luminal —*see* Dependence, drug, sedative
  lysergic acid —*see* Dependence, drug, hallucinogen
  maconha —*see* Dependence, drug, cannabis

Dependence *(continued)*
marihuana *—see* Dependence, drug, cannabis
meprobamate *—see* Dependence, drug, sedative
mescaline *—see* Dependence, drug, hallucinogen
methadone *—see* Dependence, drug, opioid
methamphetamine(s) *—see* Dependence, drug, stimulant NEC
methaqualone *—see* Dependence, drug, sedative
methyl
alcohol (without remission) F10.20
with remission F10.21
bromide *—see* Dependence, drug, sedative
morphine *—see* Dependence, drug, opioid
phenidate *—see* Dependence, drug, stimulant NEC
sulfonal *—see* Dependence, drug, sedative
morphine (sulfate) (sulfite) (type) *—see* Dependence, drug, opioid
narcotic (drug) NEC *—see* Dependence, drug, opioid
nembutal *—see* Dependence, drug, sedative
neraval *—see* Dependence, drug, sedative
neravan *—see* Dependence, drug, sedative
neurobarb *—see* Dependence, drug, sedative
nicotine *—see* Dependence, drug, nicotine
nitrous oxide F19.20
nonbarbiturate sedatives and tranquilizers with similar effect *—see* Dependence, drug, sedative
on
artificial heart (fully implantable) (mechanical) Z95.812
aspirator Z99.0
care provider (because of) Z74.9
impaired mobility Z74.09
need for
assistance with personal care Z74.1
continuous supervision Z74.3
no other household member able to render care Z74.2
specified reason NEC Z74.8
machine Z99.89
enabling NEC Z99.89
specified type NEC Z99.89
renal dialysis (hemodialysis) (peritoneal) Z99.2
respirator Z99.11
ventilator Z99.11
wheelchair Z99.3
opiate *—see* Dependence, drug, opioid
opioids *—see* Dependence, drug, opioid
opium (alkaloids) (derivatives) (tincture) *—see* Dependence, drug, opioid
oxygen (long-term) (supplemental) Z99.81
paraldehyde *—see* Dependence, drug, sedative
paregoric *—see* Dependence, drug, opioid
PCP (phencyclidine) (or related substance) - *see* Dependence, drug, hallucinogen

Dependence *(continued)*
pentobarbital *—see* Dependence, drug, sedative
pentobarbitone (sodium) *—see* Dependence, drug, sedative
pentothal *—see* Dependence, drug, sedative
peyote *—see* Dependence, drug, hallucinogen
phencyclidine (PCP) (or related substance) - *see* Dependence, drug, hallucinogen
phenmetrazine *—see* Dependence, drug, stimulant NEC
phenobarbital *—see* Dependence, drug, sedative
polysubstance F19.20
psilocibin, psilocin, psilocyn, psilocyline *—see* Dependence, drug, hallucinogen
psychostimulant NEC *—see* Dependence, drug, stimulant NEC
secobarbital *—see* Dependence, drug, sedative
seconal *—see* Dependence, drug, sedative
sedative NEC *—see* Dependence, drug, sedative
specified drug NEC *—see* Dependence, drug
stimulant NEC *—see* Dependence, drug, stimulant NEC
substance NEC *—see* Dependence, drug
supplemental oxygen Z99.81
tobacco *—see* Dependence, drug, nicotine
counseling and surveillance Z71.6
tranquilizer NEC *—see* Dependence, drug, sedative
vitamin B6 E53.1
volatile solvents *—see* Dependence, drug, inhalant

Dependency
care-provider Z74.9
passive F60.7
reactions (persistent) F60.7

Depersonalization (in neurotic state) (neurotic) (syndrome) F48.1

Depletion
extracellular fluid E86.9
plasma E86.1
potassium E87.6
nephropathy N25.89
salt or sodium E87.1
causing heat exhaustion or prostration T67.4
nephropathy N28.9
volume NOS E86.9

Deployment (current) (military) **status** Z56.82
in theater or in support of military war, peacekeeping and humanitarian operations Z56.82
personal history of Z91.82
military war, peacekeeping and humanitarian deployment (current or past conflict) Z91.82
returned from Z91.82

Depolarization, premature I49.40
atrial I49.1
junctional I49.2
specified NEC I49.49
ventricular I49.3

Deposit
bone in Boeck's sarcoid D86.89
calcareous, calcium *—see* Calcification

Deposit *(continued)*
cholesterol
retina H35.89
vitreous (body) (humor) *—see* Deposit, crystalline
conjunctiva H11.11-
cornea H18.00-
argentous H18.02-
due to metabolic disorder H18.03-
Kayser-Fleischer ring H18.04-
pigmentation *—see* Pigmentation, cornea
crystalline, vitreous (body) (humor) H43.2-
hemosiderin in old scars of cornea *—see* Pigmentation, cornea, stromal
metallic in lens *—see* Cataract, specified NEC
skin R23.8
tooth, teeth (betel) (black) (green) (materia alba) (orange) (tobacco) K03.6
urate, kidney *—see* Calculus, kidney

Depraved appetite *—see* Pica

Depressed
HDL cholesterol E78.6

Depression (acute) (mental) F32.9
agitated (single episode) F32.2
anaclitic *—see* Disorder, adjustment
anxiety F41.8
persistent F34.1
arches *—see also* Deformity, limb, flat foot
atypical (single episode) F32.89
recurrent episode F33.8
basal metabolic rate R94.8
bone marrow D75.89
central nervous system R09.2
cerebral R29.818
newborn P91.4
cerebrovascular I67.9
chest wall M95.4
climacteric (single episode) F32.89
recurrent episode F33.8
endogenous (without psychotic symptoms) F33.2
with psychotic symptoms F33.3
functional activity R68.89
hysterical F44.89
involutional (single episode) F32.89
recurrent episode F33.8
major F32.9
with psychotic symptoms F32.3
recurrent *—see* Disorder, depressive, recurrent
manic-depressive *—see* Disorder, depressive, recurrent
masked (single episode) F32.89
medullary G93.89
menopausal (single episode) F32.89
recurrent episode F33.8
metatarsus *—see* Depression, arches
monopolar F33.9
nervous F34.1
neurotic F34.1
nose M95.0
postnatal F53
postpartum F53
post-psychotic of schizophrenia F32.89
post-schizophrenic F32.89
psychogenic (reactive) (single episode) F32.9
psychoneurotic F34.1
psychotic (single episode) F32.3
recurrent F33.3
reactive (psychogenic) (single episode) F32.9
psychotic (single episode) F32.3

Depression *(continued)*
recurrent *—see* Disorder, depressive, recurrent
respiratory center G93.89
seasonal *—see* Disorder, depressive, recurrent
senile F03
severe, single episode F32.2
situational F43.21
skull Q67.4
specified NEC (single episode) F32.89
sternum M95.4
visual field *—see* Defect, visual field
vital (recurrent) (without psychotic symptoms) F33.2
with psychotic symptoms F33.3
single episode F32.2

Deprivation
cultural Z60.3
effects NOS T73.9
specified NEC T73.8
emotional NEC Z65.8
affecting infant or child *—see* Maltreatment, child, psychological
food T73.0
protein *—see* Malnutrition
sleep Z72.820
social Z60.4
affecting infant or child *—see* Maltreatment, child, psychological
specified NEC T73.8
vitamins *—see* Deficiency, vitamin
water T73.1

Derangement
ankle (internal) *—see* Derangement, joint, ankle
cartilage (articular) NEC *—see* Derangement, joint, articular cartilage, by site
recurrent *—see* Dislocation, recurrent
cruciate ligament, anterior, current injury *—see* Sprain, knee, cruciate, anterior
elbow (internal) *—see* Derangement, joint, elbow
hip (joint) (internal) (old) *—see* Derangement, joint, hip
joint (internal) M24.9
ankylosis *—see* Ankylosis
articular cartilage M24.10
ankle M24.17-
elbow M24.12-
foot M24.17-
hand M24.14-
hip M24.15-
knee NEC M23.9-
loose body *—see* Loose, body
shoulder M24.11-
wrist M24.13-
contracture *—see* Contraction, joint
current injury *—see also* Dislocation
knee, meniscus or cartilage *—see* Tear, meniscus
dislocation
pathological *—see* Dislocation, pathological
recurrent *—see* Dislocation, recurrent
knee *—see* Derangement, knee
ligament *—see* Disorder, ligament
loose body *—see* Loose, body
recurrent *—see* Dislocation, recurrent

- **Derangement** *(continued)*
  - joint *(continued)*
    - specified type NEC M24.80
      - ankle M24.87-
      - elbow M24.82-
      - foot joint M24.87-
      - hand joint M24.84-
      - hip M24.85-
      - shoulder M24.81-
      - wrist M24.83-
    - temporomandibular M26.69
  - knee (recurrent) M23.9-
    - ligament disruption, spontaneous M23.60-
      - anterior cruciate M23.61-
      - capsular M23.67-
      - instability, chronic M23.5-
      - lateral collateral M23.64-
      - medial collateral M23.63-
      - posterior cruciate M23.62-
    - loose body M23.4-
    - meniscus M23.30-
      - cystic M23.00-
        - lateral M23.002
          - anterior horn M23.04-
          - posterior horn M23.05-
          - specified NEC M23.06-
        - medial M23.005
          - anterior horn M23.01-
          - posterior horn M23.02-
          - specified NEC M23.03-
      - degenerate *—see* Derangement, knee, meniscus, specified NEC
      - detached *—see* Derangement, knee, meniscus, specified NEC
      - due to old tear or injury M23.20-
        - lateral M23.20-
          - anterior horn M23.24-
          - posterior horn M23.25-
          - specified NEC M23.26-
        - medial M23.20-
          - anterior horn M23.21-
          - posterior horn M23.22-
          - specified NEC M23.23-
      - retained *—see* Derangement, knee, meniscus, specified NEC
      - specified NEC M23.30-
        - lateral M23.30-
          - anterior horn M23.34-
          - posterior horn M23.35-
          - specified NEC M23.36-
        - medial M23.30-
          - anterior horn M23.31-
          - posterior horn M23.32-
          - specified NEC M23.33-
    - old M23.8X-
    - specified NEC *—see* subcategory M23.8
  - low back NEC *—see* Dorsopathy, specified NEC
  - meniscus *—see* Derangement, knee, meniscus
  - mental *—see* Psychosis
  - patella, specified NEC *—see* Disorder, patella, derangement NEC
  - semilunar cartilage (knee) *—see* Derangement, knee, meniscus, specified NEC
  - shoulder (internal) *—see* Derangement, joint, shoulder
- **Dercum's disease** E88.2
- **Derealization** (neurotic) F48.1
- **Dermal** *—see* condition
- **Dermaphytid** *—see* Dermatophytosis
- **Dermatitis** (eczematous) L30.9
  - ab igne L59.0
  - acarine B88.0
  - actinic (due to sun) L57.8
    - other than from sun L59.8
  - allergic *—see* Dermatitis, contact, allergic
  - ambustionis, due to burn or scald *—see* Burn
  - amebic A06.7
  - ammonia L22
  - arsenical (ingested) L27.8
  - artefacta L98.1
    - psychogenic F54
  - atopic L20.9
    - psychogenic F54
    - specified NEC L20.89
  - autoimmune progesterone L30.8
  - berlock, berloque L56.2
  - blastomycotic B40.3
  - blister beetle L24.89
  - bullous, bullosa L13.9
    - mucosynechial, atrophic L12.1
    - seasonal L30.8
    - specified NEC L13.8
  - calorica L59.0
    - due to burn or scald *—see* Burn
  - caterpillar L24.89
  - cercarial B65.3
  - combustionis L59.0
    - due to burn or scald *—see* Burn
  - congelationis T69.1
  - contact (occupational) L25.9
    - allergic L23.9
      - due to
        - adhesives L23.1
        - cement L23.5
        - chemical products NEC L23.5
        - chromium L23.0
        - cosmetics L23.2
        - dander (cat) (dog) L23.81
        - drugs in contact with skin L23.3
        - dyes L23.4
        - food in contact with skin L23.6
        - hair (cat) (dog) L23.81
        - insecticide L23.5
        - metals L23.0
        - nickel L23.0
        - plants, non-food L23.7
        - plastic L23.5
        - rubber L23.5
        - specified agent NEC L23.89
    - due to
      - cement L25.3
      - chemical products NEC L25.3
      - cosmetics L25.0
      - dander (cat) (dog) L23.81
      - drugs in contact with skin L25.1
      - dyes L25.2
      - food in contact with skin L25.4
      - hair (cat) (dog) L23.81
      - plants, non-food L25.5
      - specified agent NEC L25.8
    - irritant L24.9
      - due to
        - cement L24.5
        - chemical products NEC L24.5
        - cosmetics L24.3
        - detergents L24.0
        - drugs in contact with skin L24.4
        - food in contact with skin L24.6
        - oils and greases L24.1
        - plants, non-food L24.7
        - solvents L24.2
        - specified agent NEC L24.89
- **Dermatitis** *(continued)*
  - contusiformis L52
  - diabetic *—see* E08-E13 with .620
  - diaper L22
  - diphtheritica A36.3
  - dry skin L85.3
  - due to
    - acetone (contact) (irritant) L24.2
    - acids (contact) (irritant) L24.5
    - adhesive(s) (allergic) (contact) (plaster) L23.1
      - irritant L24.5
    - alcohol (irritant) (skin contact) (substances in category T51) L24.2
      - taken internally L27.8
    - alkalis (contact) (irritant) L24.5
    - arsenic (ingested) L27.8
    - carbon disulfide (contact) (irritant) L24.2
    - caustics (contact) (irritant) L24.5
    - cement (contact) L25.3
    - cereal (ingested) L27.2
    - chemical(s) NEC L25.3
      - taken internally L27.8
    - chlorocompounds L24.2
    - chromium (contact) (irritant) L24.81
    - coffee (ingested) L27.2
    - cold weather L30.8
    - cosmetics (contact) L25.0
      - allergic L23.2
      - irritant L24.3
    - cyclohexanes L24.2
    - dander (cat) (dog) L23.81
    - Demodex species B88.0
    - Dermanyssus gallinae B88.0
    - detergents (contact) (irritant) L24.0
    - dichromate L24.81
    - drugs and medicaments (generalized) (internal use) L27.0
      - external *—see* Dermatitis, due to, drugs, in contact with skin
      - in contact with skin L25.1
        - allergic L23.3
        - irritant L24.4
      - localized skin eruption L27.1
      - specified substance *—see* Table of Drugs and Chemicals
    - dyes (contact) L25.2
      - allergic L23.4
      - irritant L24.89
    - epidermophytosis *—see* Dermatophytosis
    - esters L24.2
    - external irritant NEC L24.9
    - fish (ingested) L27.2
    - flour (ingested) L27.2
    - food (ingested) L27.2
      - in contact with skin L25.4
    - fruit (ingested) L27.2
    - furs (allergic) (contact) L23.81
    - glues *—see* Dermatitis, due to, adhesives
    - glycols L24.2
    - greases NEC (contact) (irritant) L24.1
    - hair (cat) (dog) L23.81
    - hot
      - objects and materials *—see* Burn
      - weather or places L59.0
    - hydrocarbons L24.2
    - infrared rays L59.8
    - ingestion, ingested substance L27.9
      - chemical NEC L27.8
      - drugs and medicaments *—see* Dermatitis, due to, drugs
      - food L27.2
      - specified NEC L27.8
- **Dermatitis** *(continued)*
  - due to *(continued)*
    - insecticide in contact with skin L24.5
    - internal agent L27.9
      - drugs and medicaments (generalized) *—see* Dermatitis, due to, drugs
      - food L27.2
    - irradiation *—see* Dermatitis, due to, radioactive substance
    - ketones L24.2
    - lacquer tree (allergic) (contact) L23.7
    - light (sun) NEC L57.8
      - acute L56.8
      - other L59.8
    - Liponyssoides sanguineus B88.0
    - low temperature L30.8
    - meat (ingested) L27.2
    - metals, metal salts (contact) (irritant) L24.81
    - milk (ingested) L27.2
    - nickel (contact) (irritant) L24.81
    - nylon (contact) (irritant) L24.5
    - oils NEC (contact) (irritant) L24.1
    - paint solvent (contact) (irritant) L24.2
    - petroleum products (contact) (irritant) (substances in T52.0) L24.2
    - plants NEC (contact) L25.5
      - allergic L23.7
      - irritant L24.7
    - plasters (adhesive) (any) (allergic) (contact) L23.1
      - irritant L24.5
    - plastic (contact) L25.3
    - preservatives (contact) *—see* Dermatitis, due to, chemical, in contact with skin
    - primrose (allergic) (contact) L23.7
    - primula (allergic) (contact) L23.7
    - radiation L59.8
      - nonionizing (chronic exposure) L57.8
      - sun NEC L57.8
        - acute L56.8
    - radioactive substance L58.9
      - acute L58.0
      - chronic L58.1
    - radium L58.9
      - acute L58.0
      - chronic L58.1
    - ragweed (allergic) (contact) L23.7
    - Rhus (allergic) (contact) (diversiloba) (radicans) (toxicodendron) (venenata) (verniciflua) L23.7
    - rubber (contact) L24.5
    - Senecio jacobaea (allergic) (contact) L23.7
    - solvents (contact) (irritant) (substances in categories T52) L24.2
    - specified agent NEC (contact) L25.8
      - allergic L23.89
      - irritant L24.89
    - sunshine NEC L57.8
      - acute L56.8
    - tetrachlorethylene (contact) (irritant) L24.2
    - toluene (contact) (irritant) L24.2
    - turpentine (contact) L24.2
    - ultraviolet rays (sun NEC) (chronic exposure) L57.8
      - acute L56.8
    - vaccine or vaccination L27.0
      - specified substance *—see* Table of Drugs and Chemicals

Dermatitis *(continued)*
due to *(continued)*
varicose veins *—see* Varix, leg, with, inflammation
X-rays L58.9
acute L58.0
chronic L58.1
dyshydrotic L30.1
dysmenorrheica N94.6
escharotica *—see* Burn
exfoliative, exfoliativa (generalized) L26
neonatorum L00
eyelid *—see also* Dermatosis, eyelid
allergic H01.119
left H01.116
lower H01.115
upper H01.114
right H01.113
lower H01.112
upper H01.111
contact *—see* Dermatitis, eyelid, allergic
due to
Demodex species B88.0
herpes (zoster) B02.39
simplex B00.59
eczematous H01.139
left H01.136
lower H01.135
upper H01.134
right H01.133
lower H01.132
upper H01.131
facta, factitia, factitial L98.1
psychogenic F54
flexural NEC L20.82
friction L30.4
fungus B36.9
specified type NEC B36.8
gangrenosa, gangrenous infantum L08.0
harvest mite B88.0
heat L59.0
herpesviral, vesicular (ear) (lip) B00.1
herpetiformis (bullous) (erythematous) (pustular) (vesicular) L13.0
juvenile L12.2
senile L12.0
hiemalis L30.8
hypostatic, hypostatica *—see* Varix, leg, with, inflammation
infectious eczematoid L30.3
infective L30.3
irritant *—see* Dermatitis, contact, irritant
Jacquet's (diaper dermatitis) L22
Leptus B88.0
lichenified NEC L28.0
medicamentosa (generalized) (internal use) *—see* Dermatitis, due to drugs
mite B88.0
multiformis L13.0
juvenile L12.2
napkin L22
neurotica L13.0
nummular L30.0
papillaris capillitii L73.0
pellagrous E52
perioral L71.0
photocontact L56.2
polymorpha dolorosa L13.0
pruriginosa L13.0
pruritic NEC L30.8
psychogenic F54
purulent L08.0
pustular
contagious B08.02
subcorneal L13.1

Dermatitis *(continued)*
pyococcal L08.0
pyogenica L08.0
repens L40.2
Ritter's (exfoliativa) L00
Schamberg's L81.7
schistosome B65.3
seasonal bullous L30.8
seborrheic L21.9
infantile L21.1
specified NEC L21.8
sensitization NOS L23.9
septic L08.0
solare L57.8
specified NEC L30.8
stasis I87.2
with
varicose ulcer - *see* Varix, leg, with ulcer, with inflammation
Varicose veins - *see* Varix, leg, with, inflammation
due to postthrombotic syndrome *—see* Syndrome, postthrombotic
suppurative L08.0
traumatic NEC L30.4
trophoneurotica L13.0
ultraviolet (sun) (chronic exposure) L57.8
acute L56.8
varicose *—see* Varix, leg, with, inflammation
vegetans L10.1
verrucosa B43.0
vesicular, herpesviral B00.1

Dermatoarthritis, lipoid E78.81

Dermatochalasis, eyelid H02.839
left H02.836
lower H02.835
upper H02.834
right H02.833
lower H02.832
upper H02.831

Dermatofibroma (lenticulare) *—see* Neoplasm, skin, benign
protuberans *—see* Neoplasm, skin, uncertain behavior

Dermatofibrosarcoma (pigmented) (protuberans) *—see* Neoplasm, skin, malignant

Dermatographia L50.3

Dermatolysis (exfoliativa) (congenital) Q82.8
acquired L57.4
eyelids *—see* Blepharochalasis
palpebrarum *—see* Blepharochalasis
senile L57.4

Dermatomegaly NEC Q82.8

Dermatomucosomyositis M33.10
with
myopathy M33.12
respiratory involvement M33.11
specified organ involvement NEC M33.19

Dermatomycosis B36.9
furfuracea B36.0
specified type NEC B36.8

Dermatomyositis (acute) (chronic) *—see also* Dermatopolymyositis
adult (*see also* Dematomyositis, specified NEC) M33.10
in (due to) neoplastic disease (*see also* Neoplasm) D49.9 *[M36.0]*
juvenile M33.00
with
myopathy M33.02
respiratory involvement M33.01
specified organ involvement NEC M33.09

Dermatomyositis *(continued)*
juvenile *(continued)*
without myopathy M33.03
specified NEC M33.10
with
myopathy M33.12
respiratory involvement M33.11
specified organ involvement NEC M33.19
without myopathy M33.13

Dermatoneuritis of children *—see* Poisoning, mercury

Dermatophilosis A48.8

Dermatophytid L30.2

Dermatophytide *—see* Dermatophytosis

Dermatophytosis (epidermophyton) (infection) (Microsporum) (tinea) (Trichophyton) B35.9
beard B35.0
body B35.4
capitis B35.0
corporis B35.4
deep-seated B35.8
disseminated B35.8
foot B35.3
granulomatous B35.8
groin B35.6
hand B35.2
nail B35.1
perianal (area) B35.6
scalp B35.0
specified NEC B35.8

Dermatopolymyositis M33.90
with
myopathy M33.92
respiratory involvement M33.91
specified organ involvement NEC M33.99
without myopathy M33.93
in neoplastic disease (*see also* Neoplasm) D49.9 *[M36.0]*
juvenile M33.00
with
myopathy M33.02
respiratory involvement M33.01
specified organ involvement NEC M33.09
specified NEC M33.10
myopathy M33.12
respiratory involvement M33.11
specified organ involvement NEC M33.19

Dermatopolyneuritis *—see* Poisoning, mercury

Dermatorrhexis Q79.6
acquired L57.4

Dermatosclerosis *—see also* Scleroderma
localized L94.0

Dermatosis L98.9
Andrews' L08.89
Bowen's *—see* Neoplasm, skin, in situ
bullous L13.9
specified NEC L13.8
exfoliativa L26
eyelid (noninfectious)
dermatitis *—see* Dermatitis, eyelid
discoid lupus erythematosus *—see* Lupus, erythematosus, eyelid
xeroderma *—see* Xeroderma, acquired, eyelid
factitial L98.1
febrile neutrophilic L98.2
gonococcal A54.89
herpetiformis L13.0
juvenile L12.2
linear IgA L13.8
menstrual NEC L98.8
neutrophilic, febrile L98.2

Dermatosis *(continued)*
occupational *—see* Dermatitis, contact
papulosa nigra L82.1
pigmentary L81.9
progressive L81.7
Schamberg's L81.7
psychogenic F54
purpuric, pigmented L81.7
pustular, subcorneal L13.1
transient acantholytic L11.1

Dermographia, dermographism L50.3

Dermoid (cyst) *—see also* Neoplasm, benign, by site
with malignant transformation C56-
due to radiation (nonionizing) L57.8

Dermopathy
infiltrative with thyrotoxicosis *—see* Thyrotoxicosis
nephrogenic fibrosing L90.8

Dermophytosis *—see* Dermatophytosis

Descemetocele H18.73-

Descemet's membrane *—see* condition

Descending *—see* condition

Descensus uteri *—see* Prolapse, uterus

Desert
rheumatism B38.0
sore *—see* Ulcer, skin

Desertion (newborn) *—see* Maltreatment

Desmoid (extra-abdominal) (tumor) *—see* Neoplasm, connective tissue, uncertain behavior
abdominal D48.1

Despondency F32.9

Desquamation, skin R23.4

Destruction, destructive *—see also* Damage
articular facet *—see also* Derangement, joint, specified type NEC
knee M23.8X-
vertebra *—see* Spondylosis
bone *—see also* Disorder, bone, specified type NEC
syphilitic A52.77
joint *—see also* Derangement, joint, specified type NEC
sacroiliac M53.3
rectal sphincter K62.89
septum (nasal) J34.89
tuberculous NEC *—see* Tuberculosis
tympanum, tympanic membrane (nontraumatic) *—see* Disorder, tympanic membrane, specified NEC
vertebral disc *—see* Degeneration, intervertebral disc

Destructiveness *—see also* Disorder, conduct
adjustment reaction *—see* Disorder, adjustment

Desultory labor O62.2

Detachment
cartilage *—see* Sprain
cervix, annular N88.8
complicating delivery O71.3
choroid (old) (postinfectional) (simple) (spontaneous) H31.40-
hemorrhagic H31.41-
serous H31.42-
ligament *—see* Sprain
meniscus (knee) *—see also* Derangement, knee, meniscus, specified NEC
current injury *—see* Tear, meniscus
due to old tear or injury *—see* Derangement, knee, meniscus, due to old tear

Detachment *(continued)*
- retina (without retinal break) (serous) H33.2-
  - with retinal:
    - break H33.00-
      - giant H33.03-
      - multiple H33.02-
      - single H33.01-
    - dialysis H33.04-
  - pigment epithelium *—see* Degeneration, retina, separation of layers, pigment epithelium detachment
  - rhegmatogenous *—see* Detachment, retina, with retinal, break
  - specified NEC H33.8
  - total H33.05-
  - traction H33.4-
- vitreous (body) H43.81

Detergent asthma J69.8

Deterioration
- epileptic F06.8
- general physical R53.81
- heart, cardiac *—see* Degeneration, myocardial
- mental *—see* Psychosis
- myocardial, myocardium *—see* Degeneration, myocardial
- senile (simple) R54

Deuteranomaly (anomalous trichromat) H53.53

Deuteranopia (complete) (incomplete) H53.53

Development
- abnormal, bone Q79.9
- arrested R62.50
  - bone *—see* Arrest, development or growth, bone
  - child R62.50
  - due to malnutrition E45
- defective, congenital *—see also* Anomaly, by site
  - cauda equina Q06.3
  - left ventricle Q24.8
    - in hypoplastic left heart syndrome Q23.4
  - valve Q24.8
    - pulmonary Q22.3
- delayed *—see also* Delay, development R62.50
  - arithmetical skills F81.2
  - language (skills) (expressive) F80.1
  - learning skill F81.9
  - mixed skills F88
  - motor coordination F82
  - reading F81.0
  - specified learning skill NEC F81.89
  - speech F80.9
  - spelling F81.81
  - written expression F81.81
- imperfect, congenital *—see also* Anomaly, by site
  - heart Q24.9
  - lungs Q33.6
- incomplete
  - bronchial tree Q32.4
  - organ or site not listed *—see* Hypoplasia, by site
  - respiratory system Q34.9
- sexual, precocious NEC E30.1
- tardy, mental (*see also* Disability, intellectual) F79

Developmental *—see* condition
- testing, infant or child - *see* Examination, child

Devergie's disease (pityriasis rubra pilaris) L44.0

Deviation (in)
- conjugate palsy (eye) (spastic) H51.0
- esophagus (acquired) K22.8
- eye, skew H51.8
- midline (jaw) (teeth) (dental arch) M26.29
  - specified site NEC *—see* Malposition
- nasal septum J34.2
  - congenital Q67.4
- opening and closing of the mandible M26.53
- organ or site, congenital NEC *—see* Malposition, congenital
- septum (nasal) (acquired) J34.2
  - congenital Q67.4
- sexual F65.9
  - bestiality F65.89
  - erotomania F52.8
  - exhibitionism F65.2
  - fetishism, fetishistic F65.0
    - transvestism F65.1
  - frotteurism F65.81
  - masochism F65.51
  - multiple F65.89
  - necrophilia F65.89
  - nymphomania F52.8
  - pederosis F65.4
  - pedophilia F65.4
  - sadism, sadomasochism F65.52
  - satyriasis F52.8
  - specified type NEC F65.89
  - transvestism F64.1
  - voyeurism F65.3
- teeth, midline M26.29
- trachea J39.8
- ureter, congenital Q62.61

Device
- cerebral ventricle (communicating) in situ Z98.2
- contraceptive *—see* Contraceptive, device
- drainage, cerebrospinal fluid, in situ Z98.2

Devic's disease G36.0

Devil's
- grip B33.0
- pinches (purpura simplex) D69.2

Devitalized tooth K04.99

Devonshire colic *—see* Poisoning, lead

Dextraposition, aorta Q20.3
- in tetralogy of Fallot Q21.3

Dextrinosis, limit (debrancher enzyme deficiency) E74.03

Dextrocardia (true) Q24.0
- with
  - complete transposition of viscera Q89.3
  - situs inversus Q89.3

Dextrotransposition, aorta Q20.3

d-glycericacidemia E72.59

Dhat syndrome F48.8

Dhobi itch B35.6

Di George's syndrome D82.1

Di Guglielmo's disease C94.0-

Diabetes, diabetic (mellitus) (sugar) E11.9
- with
  - amyotrophy E11.44
  - arthropathy NEC E11.618
  - autonomic (poly)neuropathy E11.43
  - cataract E11.36
  - Charcot's joints E11.610
  - chronic kidney disease E11.22

Diabetes, diabetic *(continued)*
- with *(continued)*
  - circulatory complication NEC E11.59
  - complication E11.8
    - specified NEC E11.69
  - dermatitis E11.620
  - foot ulcer E11.621
  - gangrene E11.52
  - gastroparalysis E11.43
  - gastroparesis E11.43
  - glomerulonephrosis, intracapillary E11.21
  - glomerulosclerosis, intercapillary E11.21
  - hyperglycemia E11.65
  - hyperosmolarity E11.00
    - with coma E11.01
  - hypoglycemia E11.649
    - with coma E11.641
  - ketoacidosis E11.10
    - with coma E11.11
  - kidney complications NEC E11.29
  - Kimmelsteil-Wilson disease E11.21
  - loss of protective sensation (LOPS) *—see* Diabetes, by type, with neuropathy
  - mononeuropathy E11.41
  - myasthenia E11.44
  - necrobiosis lipoidica E11.620
  - nephropathy E11.21
  - neuralgia E11.42
  - neurologic complication NEC E11.49
  - neuropathic arthropathy E11.610
  - neuropathy E11.40
  - ophthalmic complication NEC E11.39
  - oral complication NEC E11.638
  - osteomyelitis E11.69
  - periodontal disease E11.630
  - peripheral angiopathy E11.51
    - with gangrene E11.52
  - polyneuropathy E11.42
  - renal complication NEC E11.29
  - renal tubular degeneration E11.29
  - retinopathy E11.319
    - with macular edema E11.311
      - resolved following treatment E11.37
    - nonproliferative E11.329
      - with macular edema E11.321
      - mild E11.329
        - with macular edema E11.321
      - moderate E11.339
        - with macular edema E11.331
      - severe E11.349
        - with macular edema E11.341
        - with
          - combined traction retinal detachment and rhegmatogenous retinal detachment E11.354
          - macular edema E11.351
          - stable proliferative diabetic retinopathy E11.355
          - traction retinal detachment involving the macula E11.352
          - traction retinal detachment no involving the macula E11.353
    - proliferative E11.359
      - with
        - combined traction retinal detachment and rhegmatogenous retinal detachment E11.354
        - macular edema E11.351

Diabetes, diabetic *(continued)*
- with *(continued)*
  - retinopathy *(continued)*
    - proliferative *(continued)*
      - with *(continued)*
        - stable proliferative diabetic retinopathy E11.355
        - traction retinal detachment involving the macula E11.352
        - traction retinal detachement not involving the macula E11.353
  - skin complication NEC E11.628
  - skin ulcer NEC E11.622
- brittle - *see* Diabetes, type 1
- bronzed E83.110
- complicating pregnancy *—see* Pregnancy, complicated by, diabetes
- dietary counseling and surveillance Z71.3
- due to
  - autoimmune process *—see* Diabetes, type 1
  - immune mediated pancreatic islet beta-cell destruction *—see* Diabetes, type 1
- due to drug or chemical E09.9
  - with
    - amyotrophy E09.44
    - arthropathy NEC E09.618
    - autonomic (poly)neuropathy E09.43
    - cataract E09.36
    - Charcot's joints E09.610
    - chronic kidney disease E09.22
    - circulatory complication NEC E09.59
    - complication E09.8
      - specified NEC E09.69
    - dermatitis E09.620
    - foot ulcer E09.621
    - gangrene E09.52
    - gastroparalysis E09.43
    - gastroparesis E09.43
    - glomerulonephrosis, intracapillary E09.21
    - glomerulosclerosis, intercapillary E09.21
    - hyperglycemia E09.65
    - hyperosmolarity E09.00
      - with coma E09.01
    - hypoglycemia E09.649
      - with coma E09.641
    - ketoacidosis E09.10
      - with coma E09.11
    - kidney complications NEC E09.29
    - Kimmelsteil-Wilson disease E09.21
    - mononeuropathy E09.41
    - myasthenia E09.44
    - necrobiosis lipoidica E09.620
    - nephropathy E09.21
    - neuralgia E09.42
    - neurologic complication NEC E09.49
    - neuropathic arthropathy E09.610
    - neuropathy E09.40
    - ophthalmic complication NEC E09.39
    - oral complication NEC E09.638
    - periodontal disease E09.630
    - peripheral angiopathy E09.51
      - with gangrene E09.52
    - polyneuropathy E09.42
    - renal complication NEC E09.29
    - renal tubular degeneration E09.29
    - retinopathy E09.319
      - with macular edema E09.311
        - resolved following treatment E09.37

Diabetes, diabetic *(continued)*
- due to drug or chemical *(continued)*
  - with *(continued)*
    - retinopathy *(continued)*
      - nonproliferative E09.329
        - with macular edema E09.321
        - mild E09.329
          - with macular edema E09.321
        - moderate E09.339
          - with macular edema E09.331
        - severe E09.349
          - with macular edema E09.341
      - proliferative E09.359
        - with
          - combined traction retinal detachment and rhegmatogenous retinal detachment E09.354
          - macular edema E09.351
          - stable proliferative diabetic retinopathy E09.355
          - traction retinal detachment involving the macula E09.352
          - traction retinal detachment not involving the macula E09.353
    - skin complication NEC E09.628
    - skin ulcer NEC E09.622
- due to underlying condition E08.9
  - with
    - amyotrophy E08.44
    - arthropathy NEC E08.618
    - autonomic (poly)neuropathy E08.43
    - cataract E08.36
    - Charcot's joints E08.610
    - chronic kidney disease E08.22
    - circulatory complication NEC E08.59
    - complication E08.8
      - specified NEC E08.69
    - dermatitis E08.620
    - foot ulcer E08.621
    - gangrene E08.52
    - gastroparalysis E08.43
    - gastroparesis E08.43
    - glomerulonephrosis, intracapillary E08.21
    - glomerulosclerosis, intercapillary E08.21
    - hyperglycemia E08.65
    - hyperosmolarity E08.00
      - with coma E08.01
    - hypoglycemia E08.649
      - with coma E08.641
    - ketoacidosis E08.10
      - with coma E08.11
    - kidney complications NEC E08.29
    - Kimmelsteil-WIlson disease E08.21
    - mononeuropathy E08.41
    - myasthenia E08.44
    - necrobiosis lipoidica E08.620
    - nephropathy E08.21
    - neuralgia E08.42
    - neurologic complication NEC E08.49
    - neuropathic arthropathy E08.610
    - neuropathy E08.40
    - ophthalmic complication NEC E08.39
    - oral complication NEC E08.638
    - periodontal disease E08.630
    - peripheral angiopathy E08.51
      - with gangrene E08.52
    - polyneuropathy E08.42

Diabetes, diabetic *(continued)*
- due to underlying condition *(continued)*
  - with *(continued)*
    - renal complication NEC E08.29
    - renal tubular degeneration E08.29
    - retinopathy E08.319
      - with macular edema E08.311
      - resolved following treatment E08.37
      - nonproliferative E08.329
        - with macular edema E08.321
        - mild E08.329
          - with macular edema E08.321
        - moderate E08.339
          - with macular edema E08.331
        - severe E08.349
          - with macular edema E08.341
      - proliferative E08.359
        - with
          - combined traction retinal detachment and rhegmatogenous retinal detachment E08.354
          - macular edema E08.351
          - stable proliferative diabetic retinopathy E08.355
          - traction retinal detachment involving the macula E08.352
          - traction retinal detachment not involving the macula E08.353
    - skin complication NEC E08.628
    - skin ulcer NEC E08.622
- gestational (in pregnancy) O24.419
  - affecting newborn P70.0
  - diet controlled O24.410
  - in childbirth O24.429
    - diet controlled O24.420
    - insulin (and diet) controlled O24.424
    - oral drug controlled (antidiabetic) (hypoglycemic) O24.425
  - oral drug controlled (antidiabetic) (hypoglycemic) O24.415
  - insulin (and diet) controlled O24.414
  - puerperal O24.439
    - diet controlled O24.430
    - insulin (and diet) controlled O24.434
    - oral drug controlled (antidiabetic) (hypoglycemic) O24.435
- hepatogenous E13.9
- idiopathic - *see* Diabetes, type 1
- inadequately controlled - code to Diabetes, by type, with hyperglycemia
- insipidus E23.2
  - nephrogenic N25.1
  - pituitary E23.2
  - vasopressin resistant N25.1
- insulin dependent - code to type of diabetes
- juvenile-onset —*see* Diabetes, type 1
- ketosis-prone —*see* Diabetes, type 1
- latent R73.03
- neonatal (transient) P70.2
- non-insulin dependent - code to type of diabetes

Diabetes, diabetic *(continued)*
- out of control - code to Diabetes, by type, with hyperglycemia
- phosphate E83.39
- poorly controlled - code to Diabetes, by type, with hyperglycemia
- postpancreatectomy —*see* Diabetes, specified type NEC
- postprocedural —*see* Diabetes, specified type NEC
- secondary diabetes mellitus NEC —*see* Diabetes, specified type NEC
- specified type NEC E13.9
  - with
    - amyotrophy E13.44
    - arthropathy NEC E13.618
    - autonomic (poly)neuropathy E13.43
    - cataract E13.36
    - Charcot's joints E13.610
    - chronic kidney disease E13.22
    - circulatory complication NEC E13.59
    - complication E13.8
      - specified NEC E13.69
    - dermatitis E13.620
    - foot ulcer E13.621
    - gangrene E13.52
    - gastroparalysis E13.43
    - gastroparesis E13.43
    - glomerulonephrosis, intracapillary E13.21
    - glomerulosclerosis, intercapillary E13.21
    - hyperglycemia E13.65
    - hyperosmolarity E13.00
      - with coma E13.01
    - hypoglycemia E13.649
      - with coma E13.641
    - ketoacidosis E13.10
      - with coma E13.11
    - kidney complications NEC E13.29
    - Kimmelsteil-Wilson disease E13.21
    - mononeuropathy E13.41
    - myasthenia E13.44
    - necrobiosis lipoidica E13.620
    - nephropathy E13.21
    - neuralgia E13.42
    - neurologic complication NEC E13.49
    - neuropathic arthropathy E13.610
    - neuropathy E13.40
    - ophthalmic complication NEC E13.39
    - oral complication NEC E13.638
    - periodontal disease E13.630
    - peripheral angiopathy E13.51
      - with gangrene E13.52
    - polyneuropathy E13.42
    - renal complication NEC E13.29
    - renal tubular degeneration E13.29
    - retinopathy E13.319
      - with macular edema E13.311
      - resolved following treatment E13.37
      - nonproliferative E13.329
        - with macular edema E13.321
        - mild E13.329
          - with macular edema E13.321
        - moderate E13.339
          - with macular edema E13.331
        - severe E13.349
          - with macular edema E13.341

Diabetes, diabetic *(continued)*
- specified type *(continued)*
  - with *(continued)*
    - retinopathy *(continued)*
      - proliferative E13.359
        - with
          - combined traction retinal detachment and rhegmatogenous retinal detachment E13.354
          - macular edema E13.351
          - stable proliferative diabetic retinopathy E13.355
          - traction retinal detachment involving the macula E13.352
          - traction retinal detachment not involving the macula E13.353
    - skin complication NEC E13.628
    - skin ulcer NEC E13.622
- steroid-induced —*see* Diabetes, due to, drug or chemical
- type 1 E10.9
  - with
    - amyotrophy E10.44
    - arthropathy NEC E10.618
    - autonomic (poly)neuropathy E10.43
    - cataract E10.36
    - Charcot's joints E10.610
    - chronic kidney disease E10.22
    - circulatory complication NEC E10.59
    - complication E10.8
      - specified NEC E10.69
    - dermatitis E10.620
    - foot ulcer E10.621
    - gangrene E10.52
    - gastroparalysis E10.43
    - gastroparesis E10.43
    - glomerulonephrosis, intracapillary E10.21
    - glomerulosclerosis, intercapillary E10.21
    - hyperglycemia E10.65
    - hypoglycemia E10.649
      - with coma E10.641
    - ketoacidosis E10.10
      - with coma E10.11
    - kidney complications NEC E10.29
    - Kimmelsteil-Wilson disease E10.21
    - mononeuropathy E10.41
    - myasthenia E10.44
    - necrobiosis lipoidica E10.620
    - nephropathy E10.21
    - neuralgia E10.42
    - neurologic complication NEC E10.49
    - neuropathic arthropathy E10.610
    - neuropathy E10.40
    - ophthalmic complication NEC E10.39
    - oral complication NEC E10.638
    - osteomyelitis E10.69
    - periodontal disease E10.630
    - peripheral angiopathy E10.51
      - with gangrene E10.52
    - polyneuropathy E10.42
    - renal complication NEC E10.29
    - renal tubular degeneration E10.29
    - retinopathy E10.319
      - with macular edema E10.311
      - resolved following treatment E10.37
      - nonproliferative E10.329

- **Diabetes, diabetic** *(continued)*
  - type 1 *(continued)*
    - with *(continued)*
      - retinopathy *(continued)*
        - nonproliferative *(continued)*
          - with macular edema E10.321
          - mild E10.329
            - with macular edema E10.321
          - moderate E10.339
            - with macular edema E10.331
          - severe E10.349
            - with macular edema E10.341
        - proliferative E10.359
          - with
            - combined traction retinal detachment and rhegmatogenous retinal detachment E10.354
          - with
            - macular edema E10.351
            - stable proliferative diabetic retinopathy E10.355
            - traction retinal detachment involving the macula E10.352
            - traction retinal detachment not involving the macula E10.353
      - skin complication NEC E10.628
      - skin ulcer NEC E10.622
  - type 2 E11.9
    - with
      - amyotrophy E11.44
      - arthropathy NEC E11.618
      - autonomic (poly)neuropathy E11.43
      - cataract E11.36
      - Charcot's joints E11.610
      - chronic kidney disease E11.22
      - circulatory complication NEC E11.59
      - complication E11.8
        - specified NEC E11.69
      - dermatitis E11.620
      - foot ulcer E11.621
      - gangrene E11.52
      - gastroparalysis E11.43
      - gastroparesis E11.43
      - glomerulonephrosis, intracapillary E11.21
      - glomerulosclerosis, intercapillary E11.21
      - hyperglycemia E11.65
      - hyperosmolarity E11.00
        - with coma E11.01
      - hypoglycemia E11.649
        - with coma E11.641
      - ketoacidosis E11.10
        - with coma E11.11
      - kidney complications NEC E11.29
      - Kimmelsteil-Wilson disease E11.21
      - mononeuropathy E11.41
      - myasthenia E11.44
      - necrobiosis lipoidica E11.620
      - nephropathy E11.21
      - neuralgia E11.42
      - neurologic complication NEC E11.49
      - neuropathic arthropathy E11.610
      - neuropathy E11.40
      - ophthalmic complication NEC E11.39
      - oral complication NEC E11.638
      - osteomyelitis E11.69
      - periodontal disease E11.630

- **Diabetes, diabetic** *(continued)*
  - type 2 *(continued)*
    - with *(continued)*
      - peripheral angiopathy E11.51
        - with gangrene E11.52
      - polyneuropathy E11.42
      - renal complication NEC E11.29
      - renal tubular degeneration E11.29
      - retinopathy E11.319
        - with macular edema E11.311
        - resolved following treatment E11.37
        - nonproliferative E11.329
          - with macular edema E11.321
          - mild E11.329
            - with macular edema E11.321
          - moderate E11.339
            - with macular edema E11.331
          - severe E11.349
            - with macular edema E11.341
        - proliferative E11.359
          - with
            - combined traction retinal detachment and rhegmatogenous retinal detachment E11.354
            - macular edema E11.351
            - stable proliferative diabetic retinopathy E11.355
            - traction retinal detachment involving the macula E11.352
            - traction retinal detachment not involving the macula E11.353
      - skin complication NEC E11.628
      - skin ulcer NEC E11.622
  - uncontrolled
  - meaning
  - hyperglycemia *—see* Diabetes, by type, with, hyperglycemia
  - hypoglycemia *—see* Diabetes, by type, with, hypoglycemia

- **Diacyclothrombopathia** D69.1
- **Diagnosis deferred** R69
- **Dialysis** (intermittent) (treatment)
  - noncompliance (with) Z91.15
  - renal (hemodialysis) (peritoneal), status Z99.2
  - retina, retinal *—see* Detachment, retina, with retinal, dialysis
- **Diamond-Blackfan anemia** (congenital hypoplastic) D61.01
- **Diamond-Gardener syndrome** (autoerythrocyte sensitization) D69.2
- **Diaper rash** L22
- **Diaphoresis** (excessive) R61
- **Diaphragm** *—see* condition
- **Diaphragmalgia** R07.1
- **Diaphragmatitis, diaphragmitis** J98.6
- **Diaphysial aclasis** Q78.6
- **Diaphysitis** *—see* Osteomyelitis, specified type NEC
- **Diarrhea, diarrheal** (disease) (infantile) (inflammatory) R19.7
  - achlorhydric K31.83
  - allergic K52.29
    - due to
      - colitis *—see* Colitis, allergic
      - enteritis *—see* Enteritis, allergic

- **Diarrhea, diarrheal** *(continued)*
  - amebic (*see also* Amebiasis) A06.0
    - with abscess *—see* Abscess, amebic
    - acute A06.0
    - chronic A06.1
    - nondysenteric A06.2
  - bacillary *—see* Dysentery, bacillary
  - balantidial A07.0
  - cachectic NEC K52.89
  - Chilomastix A07.8
  - choleriformis A00.1
  - chronic (noninfectious) K52.9
  - coccidial A07.3
  - Cochin-China K90.1
    - strongyloidiasis B78.0
  - Dientamoeba A07.8
  - dietetic (*see also* Diarrhea, allergic) K52.29
  - drug-induced K52.1
  - due to
    - bacteria A04.9
      - specified NEC A04.8
    - Campylobacter A04.5
    - Capillaria philippinensis B81.1
    - Clostridium difficile
      - not specified as recurrent A04.72
      - recurrent A04.71
    - Clostridium perfringens (C) (F) A04.8
    - Cryptosporidium A07.2
    - drugs K52.1
    - Escherichia coli A04.4
      - enteroaggregative A04.4
      - enterohemorrhagic A04.3
      - enteroinvasive A04.2
      - enteropathogenic A04.0
      - enterotoxigenic A04.1
      - specified NEC A04.4
    - food hypersensitivity (*see also* Diarrhea, allergic) K52.29
    - Necator americanus B76.1
    - S. japonicum B65.2
    - specified organism NEC A08.8
      - bacterial A04.8
      - viral A08.39
    - Staphylococcus A04.8
    - Trichuris trichiuria B79
    - virus *—see* Enteritis, viral
    - Yersinia enterocolitica A04.6
  - dysenteric A09
  - endemic A09
  - epidemic A09
  - flagellate A07.9
  - Flexner's (ulcerative) A03.1
  - functional K59.1
    - following gastrointestinal surgery K91.89
    - psychogenic F45.8
  - Giardia lamblia A07.1
  - giardial A07.1
  - hill K90.1
  - infectious A09
  - malarial *—see* Malaria
  - mite B88.0
  - mycotic NEC B49
  - neonatal (noninfectious) P78.3
  - nervous F45.8
  - neurogenic K59.1
  - noninfectious K52.9
  - postgastrectomy K91.1
  - postvagotomy K91.1
  - protozoal A07.9
    - specified NEC A07.8
  - psychogenic F45.8
  - specified
    - bacterium NEC A04.8
    - virus NEC A08.39
  - strongyloidiasis B78.0
  - toxic K52.1
  - trichomonal A07.8

- **Diarrhea, diarrheal** *(continued)*
  - tropical K90.1
  - tuberculous A18.32
  - viral *—see* Enteritis, viral
- **Diastasis**
  - cranial bones M84.88
    - congenital NEC Q75.8
  - joint (traumatic) *—see* Dislocation
  - muscle M62.00
    - ankle M62.07-
    - congenital Q79.8
    - foot M62.07-
    - forearm M62.03-
    - hand M62.04-
    - lower leg M62.06-
    - pelvic region M62.05-
    - shoulder region M62.01-
    - specified site NEC M62.08
    - thigh M62.05-
    - upper arm M62.02-
  - recti (abdomen)
    - complicating delivery O71.89
    - congenital Q79.59
- **Diastema, tooth, teeth, fully erupted** M26.32
- **Diastematomyelia** Q06.2
- **Diataxia, cerebral** G80.4
- **Diathesis**
  - allergic *—see* History, allergy
  - bleeding (familial) D69.9
  - cystine (familial) E72.00
  - gouty *—see* Gout
  - hemorrhagic (familial) D69.9
    - newborn NEC P53
  - spasmophilic R29.0
- **Diaz's disease or osteochondrosis** (juvenile) (talus) *—see* Osteochondrosis, juvenile, tarsus
- **Dibothriocephalus, dibothriocephaliasis** (latus) (infection) (infestation) B70.0
  - larval B70.1
- **Dicephalus, dicephaly** Q89.4
- **Dichotomy, teeth** K00.2
- **Dichromat, dichromatopsia** (congenital) *—see* Deficiency, color vision
- **Dichuchwa** A65
- **Dicroceliasis** B66.2
- **Didelphia, didelphys** *—see* Double uterus
- **Didymytis** N45.1
  - with orchitis N45.3
- **Dietary**
  - inadequacy or deficiency E63.9
  - surveillance and counseling Z71.3
- **Dietl's crisis** N13.8
- **Dieulafoy lesion** (hemorrhagic)
  - duodenum K31.82
  - esophagus K22.8
  - intestine (colon) K63.81
  - stomach K31.82
- **Difficult, difficulty** (in)
  - acculturation Z60.3
  - feeding R63.3
    - newborn P92.9
      - breast P92.5
      - specified NEC P92.8
    - nonorganic (infant or child) F98.29
  - intubation, in anesthesia T88.4
  - mechanical, gastroduodenal stoma K91.89
    - causing obstruction (*see also* Obstruction, intestine, postoperative) K91.30

Difficult, difficulty *(continued)*
micturition
need to immediately re-void R39.191
position dependent R39.192
specified NEC R39.198
reading (developmental) F81.0
secondary to emotional disorders F93.9
spelling (specific) F81.81
with reading disorder F81.89
due to inadequate teaching Z55.8
swallowing —*see* Dysphagia
walking R26.2
work
conditions NEC Z56.5
schedule Z56.3

Diffuse —*see* condition

DiGeorge's syndrome (thymic hypoplasia) D82.1

Digestive —*see* condition

Dihydropyrimidine dehydrogenase disease (DPD) E88.89

Diktyoma —*see* Neoplasm, malignant, by site

Dilaceration, tooth K00.4

Dilatation
anus K59.8
venule —*see* Hemorrhoids
aorta (focal) (general) —*see* Ectasia, aorta
with aneuysm —*see* Aneurysm, aorta
congenital Q25.44
artery —*see* Aneurysm
bladder (sphincter) N32.89
congenital Q64.79
blood vessel I99.8
bronchial J47.9
with
exacerbation (acute) J47.1
lower respiratory infection J47.0
calyx (due to obstruction) —*see* Hydronephrosis
capillaries I78.8
cardiac (acute) (chronic) —*see also* Hypertrophy, cardiac
congenital Q24.8
valve NEC Q24.8
pulmonary Q22.3
valve —*see* Endocarditis
cavum septi pellucidi Q06.8
cervix (uteri) —*see also* Incompetency, cervix
incomplete, poor, slow
complicating delivery O62.0
colon K59.39
congenital Q43.1
psychogenic F45.8
toxic K59.31
common duct (acquired) K83.8
congenital Q44.5
cystic duct (acquired) K82.8
congenital Q44.5
duct, mammary —*see* Ectasia, mammary duct
duodenum K59.8
esophagus K22.8
congenital Q39.5
due to achalasia K22.0
eustachian tube, congenital Q17.8
gallbladder K82.8
gastric —*see* Dilatation, stomach
heart (acute) (chronic) —*see also* Hypertrophy, cardiac
congenital Q24.8
valve —*see* Endocarditis
ileum K59.8
psychogenic F45.8

Dilatation *(continued)*
jejunum K59.8
psychogenic F45.8
kidney (calyx) (collecting structures) (cystic) (parenchyma) (pelvis) (idiopathic) N28.89
lacrimal passages or duct —*see* Disorder, lacrimal system, changes
lymphatic vessel I89.0
mammary duct —*see* Ectasia, mammary duct
Meckel's diverticulum (congenital) Q43.0
malignant —*see* Table of Neoplasms, small intestine, malignant
myocardium (acute) (chronic) —*see* Hypertrophy, cardiac
organ or site, congenital NEC —*see* Distortion
pancreatic duct K86.89
pericardium —*see* Pericarditis
pharynx J39.2
prostate N42.89
pulmonary
artery (idiopathic) I28.8
valve, congenital Q22.3
pupil H57.04
rectum K59.39
saccule, congenital Q16.5
salivary gland (duct) K11.8
sphincter ani K62.89
stomach K31.89
acute K31.0
psychogenic F45.8
submaxillary duct K11.8
trachea, congenital Q32.1
ureter (idiopathic) N28.82
congenital Q62.2
due to obstruction N13.4
urethra (acquired) N36.8
vasomotor I73.9
vein I86.8
ventricular, ventricle (acute) (chronic) —*see also* Hypertrophy, cardiac
cerebral, congenital Q04.8
venule NEC I86.8
vesical orifice N32.89

Dilated, dilation —*see* Dilatation

Diminished, diminution
hearing (acuity) —*see* Deafness
sense or sensation (cold) (heat) (tactile) (vibratory) R20.8
vision NEC H54.7
vital capacity R94.2

Diminuta taenia B71.0

Dimitri-Sturge-Weber disease Q85.8

Dimple
congenital sacral Q82.6
parasacral Q82.6
pilonidal or postanal - *see* Cyst, pilonidal

Dioctophyme renalis (infection) (infestation) B83.8

Dipetalonemiasis B74.4

Diphallus Q55.69

Diphtheria, diphtheritic (gangrenous) (hemorrhagic) A36.9
carrier (suspected) Z22.2
cutaneous A36.3
faucial A36.0
infection of wound A36.3
laryngeal A36.2
myocarditis A36.81
nasal, anterior A36.89
nasopharyngeal A36.1
neurological complication A36.89
pharyngeal A36.0
specified site NEC A36.89
tonsillar A36.0

Diphyllobothriasis (intestine) B70.0
larval B70.1

Diplacusis H93.22-

Diplegia (upper limbs) G83.0
congenital (cerebral) G80.8
facial G51.0
lower limbs G82.20
spastic G80.1

Diplococcus, diplococcal —*see* condition

Diplopia H53.2

Dipsomania F10.20
with
psychosis —*see* Psychosis, alcoholic
remission F10.21

Dipylidiasis B71.1

DIRA (deficiency of interleukin 1 receptor antagonist) M04.8

Direction, teeth, abnormal, fully erupted M26.30

Dirofilariasis B74.8

Dirt-eating child F98.3

Disability, disabilities
heart —*see* Disease, heart
intellectual F79
with
autistic features F84.9
mild (I.Q.50-69) F70
moderate (I.Q.35-49) F71
profound (I.Q. under 20) F73
severe (I.Q.20-34) F72
specified level NEC F78
knowledge acquisition F81.9
learning F81.9
limiting activities Z73.6
spelling, specific F81.81

Disappearance of family member Z63.4

Disarticulation —*see* Amputation
meaning traumatic amputation —*see* Amputation, traumatic

Discharge (from)
abnormal finding in —*see* Abnormal, specimen
breast (female) (male) N64.52
diencephalic autonomic idiopathic —*see* Epilepsy, specified NEC
ear —*see also* Otorrhea
blood —*see* Otorrhagia
excessive urine R35.8
nipple N64.52
penile R36.9
postnasal R09.82
prison, anxiety concerning Z65.2
urethral R36.9
without blood R36.0
hematospermia R36.1
vaginal N89.8

Discitis, diskitis M46.40
cervical region M46.42
cervicothoracic region M46.43
lumbar region M46.46
lumbosacral region M46.47
multiple sites M46.49
occipito-atlanto-axial region M46.41
pyogenic —*see* Infection, intervertebral disc, pyogenic
sacrococcygeal region M46.48
thoracic region M46.44
thoracolumbar region M46.45

Discoid
meniscus (congenital) Q68.6
semilunar cartilage (congenital) —*see* Derangement, knee, meniscus, specified NEC

Discoloration
nails L60.8
teeth (posteruptive) K03.7
during formation K00.8

Discomfort
chest R07.89
visual H53.14-

Discontinuity, ossicles, ear H74.2-

Discord (with)
boss Z56.4
classmates Z55.4
counselor Z64.4
employer Z56.4
family Z63.8
fellow employees Z56.4
in-laws Z63.1
landlord Z59.2
lodgers Z59.2
neighbors Z59.2
probation officer Z64.4
social worker Z64.4
teachers Z55.4
workmates Z56.4

Discordant connection
atrioventricular (congenital) Q20.5
ventriculoarterial Q20.3

Discrepancy
centric occlusion maximum intercuspation M26.55
leg length (acquired) —*see* Deformity, limb, unequal length
congenital —*see* Defect, reduction, lower limb
uterine size date O26.84-

Discrimination
ethnic Z60.5
political Z60.5
racial Z60.5
religious Z60.5
sex Z60.5

Disease, diseased —*see also* Syndrome
absorbent system I87.8
acid-peptic K30
Acosta's T70.29
Adams-Stokes (-Morgagni) (syncope with heart block) I45.9
Addison's anemia (pernicious) D51.0
adenoids (and tonsils) J35.9
adrenal (capsule) (cortex) (gland) (medullary) E27.9
hyperfunction E27.0
specified NEC E27.8
ainhum L94.6
airway
obstructive, chronic J44.9
due to
cotton dust J66.0
specific organic dusts NEC J66.8
reactive —*see* Asthma
akamushi (scrub typhus) A75.3
Albers-Schönberg (marble bones) Q78.2
Albert's —*see* Tendinitis, Achilles
alimentary canal K63.9
alligator-skin Q80.9
acquired L85.0
alpha heavy chain C88.3
alpine T70.29
altitude T70.20
alveolar ridge
edentulous K06.9
specified NEC K06.8
alveoli, teeth K08.9
Alzheimer's G30.9 *[F02.80]*
with behavioral disturbance G30.9 *[F02.81]*

Disease, diseased *(continued)*

- Alzheimer's *(continued)*
  - early onset G30.0 *[F02.80]*
    - with behavioral disturbance G30.0 *[F02.81]*
  - late onset G30.1 *[F02.80]*
    - with behavioral disturbance G30.1 *[F02.81]*
  - specified NEC G30.8 *[F02.80]*
    - with behavioral disturbance G30.8 *[F02.81]*
- amyloid —*see* Amyloidosis
- Andersen's (glycogenosis IV) E74.09
- Andes T70.29
- Andrews'(bacterid) L08.89
- angiospastic I73.9
  - cerebral G45.9
  - vein I87.8
- anterior
  - chamber H21.9
  - horn cell G12.29
- antiglomerular basement membrane (anti- GBM) antibody M31.0
  - tubulo-interstitial nephritis N12
- antral —*see* Sinusitis, maxillary
- anus K62.9
  - specified NEC K62.89
- aorta (nonsyphilitic) I77.9
  - syphilitic NEC A52.02
- aortic (heart) (valve) I35.9
  - rheumatic I06.9
- Apollo B30.3
- aponeuroses —*see* Enthesopathy
- appendix K38.9
  - specified NEC K38.8
- aqueous (chamber) H21.9
- Arnold-Chiari —*see* Arnold-Chiari disease
- arterial I77.9
  - occlusive —*see* Occlusion, by site
    - due to stricture or stenosis I77.1
- arteriocardiorenal —*see* Hypertension, cardiorenal
- arteriolar (generalized) (obliterative) I77.9
- arteriorenal —*see* Hypertension, kidney
- arteriosclerotic —*see also* Arteriosclerosis
  - cardiovascular —*see* Disease, heart, ischemic, atherosclerotic
  - coronary (artery) —*see* Disease, heart, ischemic, atherosclerotic
  - heart —*see* Disease, heart, ischemic, atherosclerotic
- artery I77.9
  - cerebral I67.9
  - coronary I25.10
    - with angina pectoris —*see* Arteriosclerosis, coronary (artery),
- arthropod-borne NOS (viral) A94
  - specified type NEC A93.8
- atticoantral, chronic H66.20
  - left H66.22
    - with right H66.23
  - right H66.21
    - with left H66.23
- auditory canal —*see* Disorder, ear, external
- auricle, ear NEC —*see* Disorder, pinna
- Australian X A83.4
- autoimmune (systemic) NOS M35.9
  - hemolytic (cold type) (warm type) D59.1
    - drug-induced D59.0
  - thyroid E06.3
- aviator's —*see* Effect, adverse, high altitude
- Ayerza's (pulmonary artery sclerosis with pulmonary hypertension) I27.0

Disease, diseased *(continued)*

- Babington's (familial hemorrhagic telangiectasia) I78.0
- bacterial A49.9
  - specified NEC A48.8
  - zoonotic A28.9
    - specified type NEC A28.8
- Baelz's (cheilitis glandularis apostematosa) K13.0
- bagasse J67.1
- balloon —*see* Effect, adverse, high altitude
- Bang's (brucella abortus) A23.1
- Bannister's T78.3
- barometer makers' —*see* Poisoning, mercury
- Barraquer (-Simons') (progressive lipodystrophy) E88.1
- Barrett's —*see* Barrett's, esophagus
- Bartholin's gland N75.9
- basal ganglia G25.9
  - degenerative G23.9
    - specified NEC G23.8
  - specified NEC G25.89
- Basedow's (exophthalmic goiter) —*see* Hyperthyroidism, with, goiter (diffuse)
- Bateman's B08.1
- Batten-Steinert G71.11
- Battey A31.0
- Beard's (neurasthenia) F48.8
- Becker
  - idiopathic mural endomyocardial I42.3
  - myotonia congenita G71.12
- Begbie's (exophthalmic goiter) —*see* Hyperthyroidism, with, goiter (diffuse)
- behavioral, organic F07.9
- Beigel's (white piedra) B36.2
- Benson's —*see* Deposit, crystalline
- Bernard-Soulier (thrombopathy) D69.1
- Bernhardt (-Roth) —*see* Mononeuropathy, lower limb, meralgia paresthetica
- Biermer's (pernicious anemia) D51.0
- bile duct (common) (hepatic) K83.9
  - with calculus, stones —*see* Calculus, bile duct
  - specified NEC K83.8
- biliary (tract) K83.9
  - specified NEC K83.8
- Billroth's —*see* Spina bifida
- bird fancier's J67.2
- black lung J60
- bladder N32.9
  - in (due to)
    - schistosomiasis (bilharziasis) B65.0 *[N33]*
  - specified NEC N32.89
- bleeder's D66
- blood D75.9
  - forming organs D75.9
  - vessel I99.9
- Bloodgood's —*see* Mastopathy, cystic
- Bodechtel-Guttmann (subacute sclerosing panencephalitis) A81.1
- bone —*see also* Disorder, bone
  - aluminum M83.4
  - fibrocystic NEC
    - jaw M27.49
- bone-marrow D75.9
- Borna A83.9
- Bornholm (epidemic pleurodynia) B33.0
- Bouchard's (myopathic dilatation of the stomach) K31.0
- Bouillaud's (rheumatic heart disease) I01.9

Disease, diseased *(continued)*

- Bourneville (-Brissaud) (tuberous sclerosis) Q85.1
- Bouveret (-Hoffmann) (paroxysmal tachycardia) I47.9
- bowel K63.9
  - functional K59.9
    - psychogenic F45.8
- brain G93.9
  - arterial, artery I67.9
  - arteriosclerotic I67.2
  - congenital Q04.9
  - degenerative —*see* Degeneration, brain
  - inflammatory —*see* Encephalitis
  - organic G93.9
    - arteriosclerotic I67.2
  - parasitic NEC B71.9 *[G94]*
  - senile NEC G31.1
  - specified NEC G93.89
- breast —*see also* Disorder, breast N64.9
  - cystic (chronic) —*see* Mastopathy, cystic
  - fibrocystic —*see* Mastopathy, cystic
  - Paget's
    - female, unspecified side C50.91-
    - male, unspecified side C50.92-
  - specified NEC N64.89
- Breda's —*see* Yaws
- Bretonneau's (diphtheritic malignant angina) A36.0
- Bright's —*see* Nephritis
  - arteriosclerotic —*see* Hypertension, kidney
- Brill's (recrudescent typhus) A75.1
- Brill-Zinsser (recrudescent typhus) A75.1
- Brion-Kayser —*see* Fever, paratyphoid
- broad
  - beta E78.2
  - ligament (noninflammatory) N83.9
    - inflammatory —*see* Disease, pelvis, inflammatory
    - specified NEC N83.8
- Brocq-Duhring (dermatitis herpetiformis) L13.0
- Brocq's
  - meaning
    - dermatitis herpetiformis L13.0
    - prurigo L28.2
- bronchopulmonary J98.4
- bronchus NEC J98.09
- bronze Addison's E27.1
  - tuberculous A18.7
- budgerigar fancier's J67.2
- bullous L13.9
  - chronic of childhood L12.2
  - specified NEC L13.8
- Buerger's (thromboangiitis obliterans) I73.1
- Bürger-Grütz (essential familial hyperlipemia) E78.3
- bursa —*see* Bursopathy
- caisson T70.3
- California —*see* Coccidioidomycosis
- capillaries I78.9
  - specified NEC I78.8
- Carapata A68.0
- cardiac —*see* Disease, heart
- cardiopulmonary, chronic I27.9
- cardiorenal (hepatic) (hypertensive) (vascular) —*see* Hypertension, cardiorenal
- cardiovascular (atherosclerotic) I25.10
  - with angina pectoris —*see* Arteriosclerosis, coronary (artery),

Disease, diseased *(continued)*

- cardiovascular *(continued)*
  - congenital Q28.9
  - newborn P29.9
    - specified NEC P29.89
  - hypertensive —*see* Hypertension, heart
  - renal (hypertensive) —*see* Hypertension, cardiorenal
  - syphilitic (asymptomatic) A52.00
- cartilage —*see* Disorder, cartilage
- Castellani's A69.8
- Castleman (unicentric) (multicentric) D47.Z2
  - HHV-8-associated (*see also* Herpesvirus, human, 8) D47.Z2
- cat-scratch A28.1
- Cavare's (familial periodic paralysis) G72.3
- cecum K63.9
- celiac (adult) (infantile) (with steatorrhea) K90.0
- cellular tissue L98.9
- central core G71.2
- cerebellar, cerebellum —*see* Disease, brain
- cerebral —*see also* Disease, brain
  - degenerative —*see* Degeneration, brain
- cerebrospinal G96.9
- cerebrovascular I67.9
  - acute I67.89
    - embolic I63.4-
    - thrombotic I63.3-
  - arteriosclerotic I67.2
  - specified NEC I67.89
- cervix (uteri) (noninflammatory) N88.9
  - inflammatory —*see* Cervicitis
  - specified NEC N88.8
- Chabert's A22.9
- Chandler's (osteochondritis dissecans, hip) —*see* Osteochondritis, dissecans, hip
- Charlouis —*see* Yaws
- Chédiak-Steinbrinck (-Higashi) (congenital gigantism of peroxidase granules) E70.330
- chest J98.9
- Chiari's (hepatic vein thrombosis) I82.0
- Chicago B40.9
- Chignon B36.8
- chigo, chigoe B88.1
- childhood granulomatous D71
- Chinese liver fluke B66.1
- chlamydial A74.9
  - specified NEC A74.89
- cholecystic K82.9
- choroid H31.9
  - specified NEC H31.8
- Christmas D67
- chronic bullous of childhood L12.2
- chylomicron retention E78.3
- ciliary body H21.9
  - specified NEC H21.89
- circulatory (system) NEC I99.8
  - newborn P29.9
  - syphilitic A52.00
    - congenital A50.54
- coagulation factor deficiency (congenital) —*see* Defect, coagulation
- coccidioidal —*see* Coccidioidomycosis
- cold
  - agglutinin or hemoglobinuria D59.1
    - paroxysmal D59.6
  - hemagglutinin (chronic) D59.1

Disease, diseased *(continued)*
- collagen NOS (nonvascular) (vascular) M35.9
  - specified NEC M35.8
- colon K63.9
  - functional K59.9
    - congenital Q43.2
  - ischemic (*see also* Ischemia, intestine, acute) K55.039
- colonic inflammatory bowel, unclassified (IBDU) K52.3
- combined system *—see* Degeneration, combined
- compressed air T70.3
- Concato's (pericardial polyserositis) A19.9
  - nontubercular I31.1
  - pleural *—see* Pleurisy, with effusion
- conjunctiva H11.9
  - chlamydial A74.0
  - specified NEC H11.89
  - viral B30.9
    - specified NEC B30.8
- connective tissue, systemic (diffuse) M35.9
  - in (due to)
    - hypogammaglobulinemia D80.1 *[M36.8]*
    - ochronosis E70.29 *[M36.8]*
  - specified NEC M35.8
- Conor and Bruch's (boutonneuse fever) A77.1
- Cooper's *—see* Mastopathy, cystic
- Cori's (glycogenosis III) E74.03
- corkhandler's or corkworker's J67.3
- cornea H18.9
  - specified NEC H18.89-
- coronary (artery) *—see* Disease, heart, ischemic, atherosclerotic
  - congenital Q24.5
  - ostial, syphilitic (aortic) (mitral) (pulmonary) A52.03
- corpus cavernosum N48.9
  - specified NEC N48.89
- Cotugno's *—see* Sciatica
- coxsackie (virus) NEC B34.1
- cranial nerve NOS G52.9
- Creutzfeldt-Jakob *—see* Creutzfeldt-Jakob disease or syndrome
- Crocq's (acrocyanosis) I73.89
- Crohn's *—see* Enteritis, regional
- Curschmann G71.11
- cystic
  - breast (chronic) *—see* Mastopathy, cystic
  - kidney, congenital Q61.9
  - liver, congenital Q44.6
  - lung J98.4
    - congenital Q33.0
- cytomegalic inclusion (generalized) B25.9
  - with pneumonia B25.0
  - congenital P35.1
- cytomegaloviral B25.9
  - specified NEC B25.8
- Czerny's (periodic hydrarthrosis of the knee) *—see* Effusion, joint, knee
- Daae (-Finsen) (epidemic pleurodynia) B33.0
- Darling's *—see* Histoplasmosis capsulati
- Débove's (splenomegaly) R16.1
- deer fly *—see* Tularemia
- Degos' I77.89
- demyelinating, demyelinizating (nervous system) G37.9
  - multiple sclerosis G35
  - specified NEC G37.8
- dense deposit (*see also* N00-N07 with fourth character .6) N05.6

Disease, diseased *(continued)*
- deposition, hydroxyapatite *—see* Disease, hydroxyapatite deposition
- de Quervain's (tendon sheath) M65.4
  - thyroid (subacute granulomatous thyroiditis) E06.1
- Devergie's (pityriasis rubra pilaris) L44.0
- Devic's G36.0
- diaphorase deficiency D74.0
- diaphragm J98.6
- diarrheal, infectious NEC A09
- digestive system K92.9
  - specified NEC K92.89
- disc, degenerative *—see* Degeneration, intervertebral disc
- discogenic *—see also* Displacement, intervertebral disc NEC
  - with myelopathy *—see* Disorder, disc, with, myelopathy
- diverticular *—see* Diverticula
- Dubois (thymus) A50.59 *[E35]*
- Duchenne-Griesinger G71.0
- Duchenne's
  - muscular dystrophy G71.0
  - pseudohypertrophy, muscles G71.0
- ductless glands E34.9
- Duhring's (dermatitis herpetiformis) L13.0
- duodenum K31.9
  - specified NEC K31.89
- Dupré's (meningism) R29.1
- Dupuytren's (muscle contracture) M72.0
- Durand-Nicholas-Favre (climatic bubo) A55
- Duroziez's (congenital mitral stenosis) Q23.2
- ear *—see* Disorder, ear
- Eberth's *—see* Fever, typhoid
- Ebola (virus) A98.4
- Ebstein's heart Q22.5
- Echinococcus *—see* Echinococcus
- echovirus NEC B34.1
- Eddowes'(brittle bones and blue sclera) Q78.0
- edentulous (alveolar) ridge K06.9
  - specified NEC K06.8
- Edsall's T67.2
- Eichstedt's (pityriasis versicolor) B36.0
- Eisenmenger's (irreversible) I27.83
- Ellis-van Creveld (chondroectodermal dysplasia) Q77.6
- end stage renal (ESRD) N18.6
  - due to hypertension I12.0
- endocrine glands or system NEC E34.9
- endomyocardial (eosinophilic) I42.3
- English (rickets) E55.0
- enteroviral, enterovirus NEC B34.1
  - central nervous system NEC A88.8
- epidemic B99.9
  - specified NEC B99.8
- epididymis N50.9
- Erb (-Landouzy) G71.0
- Erdheim-Chester (ECD) E88.89
- esophagus K22.9
  - functional K22.4
  - psychogenic F45.8
  - specified NEC K22.8
- Eulenburg's (congenital paramyotonia) G71.19
- eustachian tube *—see* Disorder, eustachian tube
- external
  - auditory canal *—see* Disorder, ear, external
  - ear *—see* Disorder, ear, external
- extrapyramidal G25.9
  - specified NEC G25.89

Disease, diseased *(continued)*
- eye H57.9
  - anterior chamber H21.9
  - inflammatory NEC H57.8
  - muscle (external) *—see* Strabismus
  - specified NEC H57.8
  - syphilitic *—see* Oculopathy, syphilitic
- eyeball H44.9
  - specified NEC H44.89
- eyelid *—see* Disorder, eyelid
  - specified NEC *—see* Disorder, eyelid, specified type NEC
- eyeworm of Africa B74.3
- facial nerve (seventh) G51.9
  - newborn (birth injury) P11.3
- Fahr (of brain) G23.8
- Fahr Volhard (of kidney) I12.-
- fallopian tube (noninflammatory) N83.9
  - inflammatory *—see* Salpingo-oophoritis
  - specified NEC N83.8
- familial periodic paralysis G72.3
- Fanconi's (congenital pancytopenia) D61.09
- fascia NEC *—see also* Disorder, muscle
  - inflammatory *—see* Myositis
  - specified NEC M62.89
- Fauchard's (periodontitis) *—see* Periodontitis
- Favre-Durand-Nicolas (climatic bubo) A55
- Fede's K14.0
- Feer's *—see* Poisoning, mercury
- female pelvic inflammatory *—see also* Disease, pelvis, inflammatory N73.9
  - syphilitic (secondary) A51.42
  - tuberculous A18.17
- Fernels'(aortic aneurysm) I71.9
- fibrocaseous of lung *—see* Tuberculosis, pulmonary
- fibrocystic *—see* Fibrocystic disease
- Fiedler's (leptospiral jaundice) A27.0
- fifth B08.3
- file-cutter's *—see* Poisoning, lead
- fish-skin Q80.9
  - acquired L85.0
- Flajani (-Basedow) (exophthalmic goiter) *—see* Hyperthyroidism, with, goiter (diffuse)
- flax-dresser's J66.1
- fluke *—see* Infestation, fluke
- foot and mouth B08.8
- foot process N04.9
- Forbes'(glycogenosis III) E74.03
- Fordyce-Fox (apocrine miliaria) L75.2
- Fordyce's (ectopic sebaceous glands) (mouth) Q38.6
- Forestier's (rhizomelic pseudopolyarthritis) M35.3
  - meaning ankylosing hyperostosis *—see* Hyperostosis, ankylosing
- Fothergill's
  - neuralgia *—see* Neuralgia, trigeminal
  - scarlatina anginosa A38.9
- Fournier (gangrene) N49.3
  - female N76.89
- fourth B08.8
- Fox (-Fordyce) (apocrine miliaria) L75.2
- Francis' *—see* Tularemia
- Franklin C88.2
- Frei's (climatic bubo) A55
- Friedreich's
  - combined systemic or ataxia G11.1
  - myoclonia G25.3

Disease, diseased *(continued)*
- frontal sinus *—see* Sinusitis, frontal
- fungus NEC B49
- Gaisböck's (polycythemia hypertonica) D75.1
- gallbladder K82.9
  - calculus *—see* Calculus, gallbladder
  - cholecystitis *—see* Cholecystitis
  - cholesterolosis K82.4
  - fistula *—see* Fistula, gallbladder
  - hydrops K82.1
  - obstruction *—see* Obstruction, gallbladder
  - perforation K82.2
  - specified NEC K82.8
- gamma heavy chain C88.2
- Gamna's (siderotic splenomegaly) D73.2
- Gamstorp's (adynamia episodica hereditaria) G72.3
- Gandy-Nanta (siderotic splenomegaly) D73.2
- ganister J62.8
- gastric *—see* Disease, stomach
- gastroesophageal reflux (GERD) K21.9
  - with esophagitis K21.0
- gastrointestinal (tract) K92.9
  - amyloid E85.4
  - functional K59.9
    - psychogenic F45.8
  - specified NEC K92.89
- Gee (-Herter) (-Heubner) (-Thaysen) (nontropical sprue) K90.0
- genital organs
  - female N94.9
  - male N50.9
- Gerhardt's (erythromelalgia) I73.81
- Gibert's (pityriasis rosea) L42
- Gierke's (glycogenosis I) E74.01
- Gilles de la Tourette's (motor-verbal tic) F95.2
- gingiva K06.9
  - plaque induced K05.00
  - specified NEC K06.8
- gland (lymph) I89.9
- Glanzmann's (hereditary hemorrhagic thrombasthenia) D69.1
- glass-blower's (cataract) *—see* Cataract, specified NEC
  - salivary gland hypertrophy K11.1
- Glisson's *—see* Rickets
- globe H44.9
  - specified NEC H44.89
- glomerular *—see also* Glomerulonephritis
  - with edema *—see* Nephrosis
  - acute *—see* Nephritis, acute
  - chronic *—see* Nephritis, chronic
  - minimal change N05.0
  - rapidly progressive N01.9
- glycogen storage E74.00
  - Andersen's E74.09
  - Cori's E74.03
  - Forbes' E74.03
  - generalized E74.00
  - glucose-6-phosphatase deficiency E74.01
  - heart E74.02 *[I43]*
  - hepatorenal E74.09
  - Hers' E74.09
  - liver and kidney E74.09
  - McArdle's E74.04
  - muscle phosphofructokinase E74.09
  - myocardium E74.02 *[I43]*
  - Pompe's E74.02
  - Tauri's E74.09

Disease, diseased *(continued)*
glycogen storage *(continued)*
type 0 E74.09
type I E74.01
type II E74.02
type III E74.03
type IV E74.09
type V E74.04
type VI-XI E74.09
Von Gierke's E74.01
Goldstein's (familial hemorrhagic telangiectasia) I78.0
gonococcal NOS A54.9
graft-versus-host (GVH) D89.813
acute D89.810
acute on chronic D89.812
chronic D89.811
grainhandler's J67.8
granulomatous (childhood) (chronic) D71
Graves' (exophthalmic goiter) —*see* Hyperthyroidism, with, goiter (diffuse)
Griesinger's —*see* Ancylostomiasis
Grisel's M43.6
Gruby's (tinea tonsurans) B35.0
Guillain-Barré G61.0
Guinon's (motor-verbal tic) F95.2
gum K06.9
gynecological N94.9
H (Hartnup's) E72.02
Haff —*see* Poisoning, mercury
Hageman (congenital factor XII deficiency) D68.2
hair (color) (shaft) L67.9
follicles L73.9
specified NEC L73.8
Hamman's (spontaneous mediastinal emphysema) J98.2
hand, foot and mouth B08.4
Hansen's —*see* Leprosy
Hantavirus, with pulmonary manifestations B33.4
with renal manifestations A98.5
Harada's H30.81-
Hartnup (pellagra-cerebellar ataxia-renal aminoaciduria) E72.02
Hart's (pellagra-cerebellar ataxia-renal aminoaciduria) E72.02
Hashimoto's (struma lymphomatosa) E06.3
Hb —*see* Disease, hemoglobin
heart (organic) I51.9
with
pulmonary edema (acute) —*see also* Failure, ventricular, left I50.1
rheumatic fever (conditions in I00)
active I01.9
with chorea I02.0
specified NEC I01.8
inactive or quiescent (with chorea) I09.9
specified NEC I09.89
amyloid E85.4 *[I43]*
aortic (valve) I35.9
arteriosclerotic or sclerotic (senile) —*see* Disease, heart, ischemic, atherosclerotic
artery, arterial —*see* Disease, heart, ischemic, atherosclerotic
beer drinkers' I42.6
beriberi (wet) E51.12
black I27.0
congenital Q24.9
cyanotic Q24.9
specified NEC Q24.8
coronary —*see* Disease, heart, ischemic
cryptogenic I51.9

Disease, diseased *(continued)*
heart *(continued)*
fibroid —*see* Myocarditis
functional I51.89
psychogenic F45.8
glycogen storage E74.02 *[I43]*
gonococcal A54.83
hypertensive —*see* Hypertension, heart
hyperthyroid —*see also* Hyperthyroidism E05.90 *[I43]*
with thyroid storm E05.91 *[I43]*
ischemic (chronic or with a stated duration of over 4 weeks) I25.9
atherosclerotic (of) I25.10
with angina pectoris —*see* Arteriosclerosis, coronary (artery)
coronary artery bypass graft —*see* Arteriosclerosis, coronary (artery),
cardiomyopathy I25.5
diagnosed on ECG or other special investigation, but currently presenting no symptoms I25.6
silent I25.6
specified form NEC I25.89
kyphoscoliotic I27.1
meningococcal A39.50
endocarditis A39.51
myocarditis A39.52
pericarditis A39.53
mitral I05.9
specified NEC I05.8
muscular —*see* Degeneration, myocardial
psychogenic (functional) F45.8
pulmonary (chronic) I27.9
in schistosomiasis B65.9 *[I52]*
specified NEC I27.89
rheumatic (chronic) (inactive) (old) (quiescent) (with chorea) I09.9
active or acute I01.9
with chorea (acute) (rheumatic) (Sydenham's) I02.0
specified NEC I09.89
senile —*see* Myocarditis
syphilitic A52.06
aortic A52.03
aneurysm A52.01
congenital A50.54 *[I52]*
thyrotoxic (*see also* Thyrotoxicosis) E05.90 *[I43]*
with thyroid storm E05.91 *[I43]*
valve, valvular (obstructive) (regurgitant) —*see also* Endocarditis
congenital NEC Q24.8
pulmonary Q22.3
vascular —*see* Disease, cardiovascular
heavy chain NEC C88.2
alpha C88.3
gamma C88.2
mu C88.2
Hebra's
pityriasis
maculata et circinata L42
rubra pilaris L44.0
prurigo L28.2
hematopoietic organs D75.9
hemoglobin or Hb
abnormal (mixed) NEC D58.2
with thalassemia D56.9
AS genotype D57.3
Bart's D56.0
C (Hb-C) D58.2
with other abnormal hemoglobin NEC D58.2

Disease, diseased *(continued)*
hemoglobin or Hb *(continued)*
C *(continued)*
elliptocytosis D58.1
Hb-S D57.2-
sickle-cell D57.2-
thalassemia D56.8
Constant Spring D58.2
D(Hb-D) D58.2
E(Hb-E) D58.2
E-beta thalassemia D56.5
elliptocytosis D58.1
H(Hb-H) (thalassemia) D56.0
with other abnormal hemoglobin NEC D56.9
Constant Spring D56.0
I thalassemia D56.9
M D74.0
S or SS D57.1
SC D57.2-
SD D57.8-
SE D57.8-
spherocytosis D58.0
unstable, hemolytic D58.2
hemolytic (newborn) P55.9
autoimmune (cold type) (warm type) D59.1
drug-induced D59.0
due to or with
incompatibility
ABO (blood group) P55.1
blood (group) (Duffy) (K (ell)) (Kidd) (Lewis) (M) (S) NEC P55.8
Rh (blood group) (factor) P55.0
Rh negative mother P55.0
specified type NEC P55.8
unstable hemoglobin D58.2
hemorrhagic D69.9
newborn P53
Henoch (-Schönlein) (purpura nervosa) D69.0
hepatic —*see* Disease, liver
hepatobiliary K83.9
toxic K71.9
hepatolenticular E83.01
heredodegenerative NEC
spinal cord G95.89
herpesviral, disseminated B00.7
Hers' (glycogenosis VI) E74.09
Herter (-Gee) (-Heubner) (nontropical sprue) K90.0
Heubner-Herter (nontropical sprue) K90.0
high fetal gene or hemoglobin thalassemia D56.9
Hildenbrand's —*see* Typhus
hip (joint) M25.9
congenital Q65.89
suppurative M00.9
tuberculous A18.02
His (-Werner) (trench fever) A79.0
Hodgson's I71.2
ruptured I71.1
Holla —*see* Spherocytosis
hookworm B76.9
specified NEC B76.8
host-versus-graft D89.813
acute D89.810
acute on chronic D89.812
chronic D89.811
human immunodeficiency virus (HIV) B20
Huntington's G10
with dementia G10 *[F02.80]*
Hutchinson's (cheiropompholyx) —*see* Hutchinson's disease
hyaline (diffuse) (generalized)
membrane (lung) (newborn) P22.0
adult J80

Disease, diseased *(continued)*
hydatid —*see* Echinococcus
hydroxyapatite deposition M11.00
ankle M11.07-
elbow M11.02-
foot joint M11.07-
hand joint M11.04-
hip M11.05-
knee M11.06-
multiple site M11.09
shoulder M11.01-
vertebra M11.08
wrist M11.03-
hyperkinetic —*see* Hyperkinesia
hypertensive —*see* Hypertension
hypophysis E23.7
Iceland G93.3
I-cell E77.0
immune D89.9
immunoproliferative (malignant) C88.9
small intestinal C88.3
specified NEC C88.8
inclusion B25.9
salivary gland B25.9
infectious, infective B99.9
congenital P37.9
specified NEC P37.8
viral P35.9
specified type NEC P35.8
specified NEC B99.8
inflammatory
penis N48.29
abscess N48.21
cellulitis N48.22
prepuce N47.7
balanoposthitis N47.6
tubo-ovarian —*see* Salpingo-oophoritis
intervertebral disc —*see also* Disorder, disc
with myelopathy —*see* Disorder, disc, with, myelopathy
cervical, cervicothoracic —*see* Disorder, disc, cervical
with
myelopathy —*see* Disorder, disc, cervical, with myelopathy
neuritis, radiculitis or radiculopathy —*see* Disorder, disc, cervical, with neuritis
specified NEC —*see* Disorder, disc, cervical, specified type NEC
lumbar (with)
myelopathy M51.06
neuritis, radiculitis, radiculopathy or sciatica M51.16
specified NEC M51.86
lumbosacral (with)
neuritis, radiculitis, radiculopathy or sciatica M51.17
specified NEC M51.87
specified NEC —*see* Disorder, disc, specified NEC
thoracic (with)
myelopathy M51.04
neuritis, radiculitis or radiculopathy M51.14
specified NEC M51.84
thoracolumbar (with)
myelopathy M51.05
neuritis, radiculitis or radiculopathy M51.15
specified NEC M51.85
intestine K63.9
functional K59.9
psychogenic F45.8
specified NEC K59.8

- intestine *(continued)*
  - organic K63.9
  - protozoal A07.9
  - specified NEC K63.89
- iris H21.9
  - specified NEC H21.89
- iron metabolism or storage E83.10
- island (scrub typhus) A75.3
- itai-itai *—see* Poisoning, cadmium
- Jakob-Creutzfeldt *—see* Creutzfeldt-Jakob disease or syndrome
- jaw M27.9
  - fibrocystic M27.49
  - specified NEC M27.8
- jigger B88.1
- joint *—see also* Disorder, joint
  - Charcot's *—see* Arthropathy, neuropathic (Charcot)
  - degenerative *—see* Osteoarthritis
    - multiple M15.9
    - spine *—see* Spondylosis
  - hypertrophic *—see* Osteoarthritis
  - sacroiliac M53.3
  - specified NEC *—see* Disorder, joint, specified type NEC
  - spine NEC *—see* Dorsopathy
  - suppurative *—see* Arthritis, pyogenic or pyemic
- Jourdain's (acute gingivitis) K05.00
  - nonplaque induced K05.01
  - plaque induced K05.00
- Kaschin-Beck (endemic polyarthritis) M12.10
  - ankle M12.17-
  - elbow M12.12-
  - foot joint M12.17-
  - hand joint M12.14-
  - hip M12.15-
  - knee M12.16-
  - multiple site M12.19
  - shoulder M12.11-
  - vertebra M12.18
  - wrist M12.13-
- Katayama B65.2
- Kedani (scrub typhus) A75.3
- Keshan E59
- kidney (functional) (pelvis) N28.9
  - chronic N18.9
    - hypertensive *—see* Hypertension, kidney
    - stage 1 N18.1
    - stage 2(mild) N18.2
    - stage 3(moderate) N18.3
    - stage 4(severe) N18.4
    - stage 5 N18.5
  - complicating pregnancy *—see* Pregnancy, complicated by, renal disease
  - cystic (congenital) Q61.9
  - diabetic *—see* E08-E13 with .22
  - fibrocystic (congenital) Q61.8
  - hypertensive *—see* Hypertension, kidney
  - in (due to)
    - schistosomiasis (bilharziasis) B65.9 *[N29]*
  - multicystic Q61.4
  - polycystic Q61.3
    - adult type Q61.2
    - childhood type NEC Q61.19
      - collecting duct dilatation Q61.11
- Kimmelstiel (-Wilson) (intercapillary polycystic (congenital) glomerulosclerosis) *—see* E08-E13 with .21
- Kimura D21.9
  - specified site (*see* Neoplasm, connective tissue benign)

Disease, diseased *(continued)*

- Kinnier Wilson's (hepatolenticular degeneration) E83.01
- kissing *—see* Mononucleosis, infectious
- Klebs' (*see also* Glomerulonephritis) N05.-
- Klippel-Feil (brevicollis) Q76.1
- Köhler-Pellegrini-Stieda (calcification, knee joint) *—see* Bursitis, tibial collateral
- Kok Q89.8
- König's (osteochondritis dissecans) *—see* Osteochondritis, dissecans
- Korsakoff's (nonalcoholic) F04
  - alcoholic F10.96
    - with dependence F10.26
- Kostmann's (infantile genetic agranulocytosis) D70.0
- kuru A81.81
- Kyasanur Forest A98.2
- labyrinth, ear *—see* Disorder, ear, inner
- lacrimal system *—see* Disorder, lacrimal system
- Lafora's *—see* Epilepsy, generalized, idiopathic
- Lancereaux-Mathieu (leptospiral jaundice) A27.0
- Landry's G61.0
- Larrey-Weil (leptospiral jaundice) A27.0
- larynx J38.7
- legionnaires' A48.1
  - nonpneumonic A48.2
- Lenegre's I44.2
- lens H27.9
  - specified NEC H27.8
- Lev's (acquired complete heart block) I44.2
- Lewy body (dementia) G31.83 *[F02.80]*
  - with behavioral disturbance G31.83 *[F02.81]*
- Lichtheim's (subacute combined sclerosis with pernicious anemia) D51.0
- Lightwood's (renal tubular acidosis) N25.89
- Lignac's (cystinosis) E72.04
- lip K13.0
- lipid-storage E75.6
  - specified NEC E75.5
- Lipschütz's N76.6
- liver (chronic) (organic) K76.9
  - alcoholic (chronic) K70.9
    - acute *—see* Disease, liver, alcoholic, hepatitis
    - cirrhosis K70.30
      - with ascites K70.31
    - failure K70.40
      - with coma K70.41
    - fatty liver K70.0
    - fibrosis K70.2
    - hepatitis K70.10
      - with ascites K70.11
    - sclerosis K70.2
  - cystic, congenital Q44.6
  - drug-induced (idiosyncratic) (toxic) (predictable) (unpredictable) *—see* Disease, liver, toxic
  - end stage K72.90
    - due to hepatitis *—see* Hepatitis
  - fatty, nonalcoholic (NAFLD) K76.0
    - alcoholic K70.0
  - fibrocystic (congenital) Q44.6
  - fluke
    - Chinese B66.1
    - oriental B66.1
    - sheep B66.3

Disease, diseased *(continued)*

- liver *(continued)*
  - gestational alloimmune (GALD) P78.84
  - glycogen storage E74.09 *[K77]*
  - in (due to)
    - schistosomiasis (bilharziasis) B65.9 *[K77]*
  - inflammatory K75.9
    - alcoholic K70.1
    - specified NEC K75.89
  - polycystic (congenital) Q44.6
  - toxic K71.9
    - with
      - cholestasis K71.0
      - cirrhosis (liver) K71.7
      - fibrosis (liver) K71.7
      - focal nodular hyperplasia K71.8
      - hepatic granuloma K71.8
      - hepatic necrosis K71.10
        - with coma K71.11
      - hepatitis NEC K71.6
        - acute K71.2
        - chronic
          - active K71.50
            - with ascites K71.51
          - lobular K71.4
          - persistent K71.3
        - lupoid K71.50
          - with ascites K71.51
      - peliosis hepatis K71.8
      - veno-occlusive disease (VOD) of liver K71.8
  - veno-occlusive K76.5
- Lobo's (keloid blastomycosis) B48.0
- Lobstein's (brittle bones and blue sclera) Q78.0
- Ludwig's (submaxillary cellulitis) K12.2
- lumbosacral region M53.87
- lung J98.4
  - black J60
  - congenital Q33.9
  - cystic J98.4
    - congenital Q33.0
  - fibroid (chronic) *—see* Fibrosis, lung
  - fluke B66.4
    - oriental B66.4
  - in
    - amyloidosis E85.4 *[J99]*
    - sarcoidosis D86.0
    - Sjögren's syndrome M35.02
    - systemic
      - lupus erythematosus M32.13
      - sclerosis M34.81
  - interstitial J84.9
    - of childhood, specified NEC J84.848
    - respiratory bronchiolitis J84.115
    - specified NEC J84.89
  - obstructive (chronic) J44.9
    - with
      - acute
        - bronchitis J44.0
        - exacerbation NEC J44.1
        - lower respiratory infection J44.0
      - alveolitis, allergic J67.9
      - asthma J44.9
      - bronchiectasis J47.9
        - with
          - exacerbation (acute) J47.1
          - lower respiratory infection J47.0
      - bronchitis J44.9
        - with
          - exacerbation (acute) J44.1

Disease, diseased *(continued)*

- lung *(continued)*
  - obstructive *(continued)*
    - with *(continued)*
      - bronchitis *(continued)*
        - with *(continued)*
          - lower respiratory infection J44.0
      - emphysema J43.9
      - hypersensitivity pneumonitis J67.9
    - decompensated J44.1
      - with
        - exacerbation (acute) J44.1
  - polycystic J98.4
    - congenital Q33.0
  - rheumatoid (diffuse) (interstitial) *—see* Rheumatoid, lung
- Lutembacher's (atrial septal defect with mitral stenosis) Q21.1
- Lyme A69.20
- lymphatic (gland) (system) (channel) (vessel) I89.9
- lymphoproliferative D47.9
  - specified NEC D47.Z9
  - T-gamma D47.Z9
  - X-linked D82.3
- Magitot's M27.2
- malarial *—see* Malaria
- malignant *—see also* Neoplasm, malignant, by site
- Manson's B65.1
- maple bark J67.6
- maple-syrup-urine E71.0
- Marburg (virus) A98.3
- Marion's (bladder neck obstruction) N32.0
- Marsh's (exophthalmic goiter) *—see* Hyperthyroidism, with, goiter (diffuse)
- mastoid (process) *—see* Disorder, ear, middle
- Mathieu's (leptospiral jaundice) A27.0
- Maxcy's A75.2
- McArdle (-Schmid-Pearson) (glycogenosis V) E74.04
- mediastinum J98.59
- medullary center (idiopathic) (respiratory) G93.89
- Meige's (chronic hereditary edema) Q82.0
- meningococcal *—see* Infection, meningococcal
- mental F99
  - organic F09
- mesenchymal M35.9
- mesenteric embolic (*see also* Ischemia, intestine, acute) K55.039
- metabolic, metabolism E88.9
  - bilirubin E80.7
- metal-polisher's J62.8
- metastatic (*see also* Neoplasm, secondary, by site) C79.9
- microvascular - code to condition
- microvillus
  - atrophy Q43.8
  - inclusion (MVD) Q43.8
- middle ear *—see* Disorder, ear, middle
- Mikulicz'(dryness of mouth, absent or decreased lacrimation) K11.8
- Milroy's (chronic hereditary edema) Q82.0
- Minamata *—see* Poisoning, mercury
- minicore G71.2
- Minor's G95.19
- Minot's (hemorrhagic disease, newborn) P53
- Minot-von Willebrand-Jürgens (angiohemophilia) D68.0

Disease, diseased *(continued)*

- Mitchell's (erythromelalgia) I73.81
- mitral (valve) I05.9
  - nonrheumatic I34.9
- mixed connective tissue M35.1
- moldy hay J67.0
- Monge's T70.29
- Morgagni-Adams-Stokes (syncope with heart block) I45.9
- Morgagni's (syndrome) (hyperostosis frontalis interna) M85.2
- Morton's (with metatarsalgia) —*see* Lesion, nerve, plantar
- Morvan's G60.8
- motor neuron (bulbar) (mixed type) (spinal) G12.20
  - amyotrophic lateral sclerosis G12.21
  - familial G12.24
  - progressive bulbar palsy G12.22
  - specified NEC G12.29
- moyamoya I67.5
- mu heavy chain disease C88.2
- multicore G71.2
- muscle —*see also* Disorder, muscle
  - inflammatory —*see* Myositis
  - ocular (external) —*see* Strabismus
- musculoskeletal system, soft tissue —*see also* Disorder, soft tissue
  - specified NEC —*see* Disorder, soft tissue, specified type NEC
- mushroom workers' J67.5
- mycotic B49
- myelodysplastic, not classified C94.6
- myeloproliferative, not classified C94.6
  - chronic D47.1
- myocardium, myocardial (*see also* Degeneration, myocardial) I51.5
  - primary (idiopathic) I42.9
- myoneural G70.9
- Naegeli's D69.1
- nails L60.9
  - specified NEC L60.8
- Nairobi (sheep virus) A93.8
- nasal J34.9
- nemaline body G71.2
- nerve —*see* Disorder, nerve
- nervous system G98.8
  - autonomic G90.9
  - central G96.9
    - specified NEC G96.8
  - congenital Q07.9
  - parasympathetic G90.9
  - specified NEC G98.8
  - sympathetic G90.9
  - vegetative G90.9
- neuromuscular system G70.9
- Newcastle B30.8
- Nicolas (-Durand)-Favre (climatic bubo) A55
- nipple N64.9
  - Paget's C50.01-
    - female C50.01-
    - male C50.02-
- Nishimoto (-Takeuchi) I67.5
- nonarthropod-borne NOS (viral) B34.9
  - enterovirus NEC B34.1
- nonautoimmune hemolytic D59.4
  - drug-induced D59.2
- Nonne-Milroy-Meige (chronic hereditary edema) Q82.0
- nose J34.9
- nucleus pulposus —*see* Disorder, disc
- nutritional E63.9
- oast-house-urine E72.19
  - ocular
    - herpesviral B00.50
    - zoster B02.30
- obliterative vascular I77.1
- Ohara's —*see* Tularemia
- Opitz's (congestive splenomegaly) D73.2
- Oppenheim-Urbach (necrobiosis lipoidica diabeticorum) —*see* E08-E13 with .620
- optic nerve NEC —*see* Disorder, nerve, optic
- orbit —*see* Disorder, orbit
- Oriental liver fluke B66.1
- Oriental lung fluke B66.4
- Ormond's N13.5
- Oropouche virus A93.0
- Osler-Rendu (familial hemorrhagic telangiectasia) I78.0
- osteofibrocystic E21.0
- Otto's M24.7
- outer ear —*see* Disorder, ear, external
- ovary (noninflammatory) N83.9
  - cystic N83.20-
  - inflammatory —*see* Salpingo-oophoritis
  - polycystic E28.2
  - specified NEC N83.8
- Owren's (congenital) —*see* Defect, coagulation
- pancreas K86.9
  - cystic K86.2
  - fibrocystic E84.9
  - specified NEC K86.89
- panvalvular I08.9
  - specified NEC I08.8
- parametrium (noninflammatory) N83.9
- parasitic B89
  - cerebral NEC B71.9 *[G94]*
  - intestinal NOS B82.9
  - mouth B37.0
  - skin NOS B88.9
  - specified type —*see* Infestation
  - tongue B37.0
- parathyroid (gland) E21.5
  - specified NEC E21.4
- Parkinson's G20
- parodontal K05.6
- Parrot's (syphilitic osteochondritis) A50.02
- Parry's (exophthalmic goiter) —*see* Hyperthyroidism, with, goiter (diffuse)
- Parson's (exophthalmic goiter) —*see* Hyperthyroidism, with, goiter (diffuse)
- Paxton's (white piedra) B36.2
- pearl-worker's —*see* Osteomyelitis, specified type NEC
- Pellegrini-Stieda (calcification, knee joint) —*see* Bursitis, tibial collateral
- pelvis, pelvic
  - female NOS N94.9
    - specified NEC N94.89
  - gonococcal (acute) (chronic) A54.24
  - inflammatory (female) N73.9
    - acute N73.0
    - chlamydial A56.11
    - chronic N73.1
    - specified NEC N73.8
    - syphilitic (secondary) A51.42
      - late A52.76
    - tuberculous A18.17
  - organ, female N94.9
  - peritoneum, female NEC N94.89
- penis N48.9
  - inflammatory N48.29
    - abscess N48.21
    - cellulitis N48.22
  - specified NEC N48.89
- periapical tissues NOS K04.90
- periodontal K05.6
  - specified NEC K05.5
- periosteum —*see* Disorder, bone, specified type NEC
- peripheral
  - arterial I73.9
  - autonomic nervous system G90.9
  - nerves —*see* Polyneuropathy
  - vascular NOS I73.9
- peritoneum K66.9
  - pelvic, female NEC N94.89
  - specified NEC K66.8
- persistent mucosal (middle ear) H66.20
  - left H66.22
    - with right H66.23
  - right H66.21
    - with left H66.23
- Petit's —*see* Hernia, abdomen, specified site NEC
- pharynx J39.2
  - specified NEC J39.2
- Phocas' —*see* Mastopathy, cystic
- photochromogenic (acid-fast bacilli) (pulmonary) A31.0
  - nonpulmonary A31.9
- Pick's G31.01 *[F02.80]*
  - with behavioral disturbance G31.01 *[F02.81]*
  - brain G31.01 *[F02.80]*
    - with behavioral disturbance G31.01 *[F02.81]*
  - of pericardium (pericardial pseudocirrhosis of liver) I31.1
- pigeon fancier's J67.2
- pineal gland E34.8
- pink —*see* Poisoning, mercury
- Pinkus'(lichen nitidus) L44.1
- pinworm B80
- Piry virus A93.8
- pituitary (gland) E23.7
- pituitary-snuff-taker's J67.8
- pleura (cavity) J94.9
  - specified NEC J94.8
- pneumatic drill (hammer) T75.21
- Pollitzer's (hidradenitis suppurativa) L73.2
- polycystic
  - kidney or renal Q61.3
    - adult type Q61.2
    - childhood type NEC Q61.19
      - collecting duct dilatation Q61.11
  - liver or hepatic Q44.6
  - lung or pulmonary J98.4
    - congenital Q33.0
  - ovary, ovaries E28.2
  - spleen Q89.09
- polyethylene T84.05-
- Pompe's (glycogenosis II) E74.02
- Posadas-Wernicke B38.9
- Potain's (pulmonary edema) —*see* Edema, lung
- prepuce N47.8
  - inflammatory N47.7
    - balanoposthitis N47.6
- Pringle's (tuberous sclerosis) Q85.1
- prion, central nervous system A81.9
  - specified NEC A81.89
- prostate N42.9
  - specified NEC N42.89
- protozoal B64
  - acanthamebiasis —*see* Acanthamebiasis
  - African trypanosomiasis —*see* African trypanosomiasis
  - babesiosis B60.0
  - Chagas disease —*see* Chagas disease
  - intestine, intestinal A07.9
  - leishmaniasis —*see* Leishmaniasis
  - malaria —*see* Malaria
  - naegleriasis B60.2
  - pneumocystosis B59
  - specified organism NEC B60.8
  - toxoplasmosis —*see* Toxoplasmosis
- pseudo-Hurler's E77.0
- psychiatric F99
- psychotic —*see* Psychosis
- Puente's (simple glandular cheilitis) K13.0
- puerperal (*see also* Puerperal) O90.89
- pulmonary —*see also* Disease, lung
  - artery I28.9
  - chronic obstructive J44.9
    - with
      - acute bronchitis J44.0
      - exacerbation (acute) J44.1
      - lower respiratory infection (acute) J44.0
    - decompensated J44.1
      - with
        - exacerbation (acute) J44.1
  - heart I27.9
    - specified NEC I27.89
  - hypertensive (vascular) (*see also* Hypertension, pulmonary) I27.20
    - primary (idiopathic) I27.0
  - valve I37.9
    - rheumatic I09.89
- pulp (dental) NOS K04.90
- pulseless M31.4
- Putnam's (subacute combined sclerosis with pernicious anemia) D51.0
- Pyle (-Cohn) (metaphyseal dysplasia) Q78.5
- ragpicker's or ragsorter's A22.1
- Raynaud's —*see* Raynaud's disease
- reactive airway —*see* Asthma
- Reclus'(cystic) —*see* Mastopathy, cystic
- rectum K62.9
  - specified NEC K62.89
- Refsum's (heredopathia atactica polyneuritiformis) G60.1
- renal (functional) (pelvis) (*see also* Disease, kidney) N28.9
  - with
    - edema —*see* Nephrosis
    - glomerular lesion —*see* Glomerulonephritis
      - with edema —*see* Nephrosis
    - interstitial nephritis N12
  - acute N28.9
  - chronic (*see also* Disease, kidney, chronic) N18.9
  - cystic, congenital Q61.9
  - diabetic —*see* E08-E13 with .22
  - end-stage (failure) N18.6
    - due to hypertension I12.0
  - fibrocystic (congenital) Q61.8
  - hypertensive —*see* Hypertension, kidney
  - lupus M32.14
  - phosphate-losing (tubular) N25.0
  - polycystic (congenital) Q61.3
    - adult type Q61.2
    - childhood type NEC Q61.19
      - collecting duct dilatation Q61.11
  - rapidly progressive N01.9
  - subacute N01.9
- Rendu-Osler-Weber (familial hemorrhagic telangiectasia) I78.0
- renovascular (arteriosclerotic) —*see* Hypertension, kidney

Disease, diseased *(continued)*
- respiratory (tract) J98.9
  - acute or subacute NOS J06.9
    - due to
      - chemicals, gases, fumes or vapors (inhalation) J68.3
      - external agent J70.9
        - specified NEC J70.8
      - radiation J70.0
      - smoke inhalation J70.5
    - noninfectious J39.8
  - chronic NOS J98.9
    - due to
      - chemicals, gases, fumes or vapors J68.4
      - external agent J70.9
        - specified NEC J70.8
      - radiation J70.1
    - newborn P27.9
      - specified NEC P27.8
  - due to
    - chemicals, gases, fumes or vapors J68.9
      - acute or subacute NEC J68.3
      - chronic J68.4
    - external agent J70.9
      - specified NEC J70.8
  - newborn P28.9
    - specified type NEC P28.89
  - upper J39.9
    - acute or subacute J06.9
    - noninfectious NEC J39.8
    - specified NEC J39.8
    - streptococcal J06.9
- retina, retinal H35.9
  - Batten's or Batten-Mayou E75.4 *[H36]*
  - specified NEC H35.89
- rheumatoid *—see* Arthritis, rheumatoid
- rickettsial NOS A79.9
  - specified type NEC A79.89
- Riga (-Fede) (cachectic aphthae) K14.0
- Riggs'(compound periodontitis) *—see* Periodontitis
- Ritter's L00
- Rivalta's (cervicofacial actinomycosis) A42.2
- Robles'(onchocerciasis) B73.01
- Roger's (congenital interventricular septal defect) Q21.0
- Rosenthal's (factor XI deficiency) D68.1
- Rossbach's (hyperchlorhydria) K30
- Ross River B33.1
- Rotes Quérol *—see* Hyperostosis, ankylosing
- Roth (-Bernhardt) *—see* Mononeuropathy, lower limb, meralgia paresthetica
- Runeberg's (progressive pernicious anemia) D51.0
- sacroiliac NEC M53.3
- salivary gland or duct K11.9
  - inclusion B25.9
  - specified NEC K11.8
  - virus B25.9
- sandworm B76.9
- Schimmelbusch's *—see* Mastopathy, cystic
- Schmorl's *—see* Schmorl's disease or nodes
- Schönlein (-Henoch) (purpura rheumatica) D69.0
- Schottmüller's *—see* Fever, paratyphoid

Disease, diseased *(continued)*
- Schultz's (agranulocytosis) *—see* Agranulocytosis
- Schwalbe-Ziehen-Oppenheim G24.1
- Schwartz-Jampel G71.13
- sclera H15.9
  - specified NEC H15.89
- scrofulous (tuberculous) A18.2
- scrotum N50.9
- sebaceous glands L73.9
- semilunar cartilage, cystic *—see also* Derangement, knee, meniscus, cystic
- seminal vesicle N50.9
- serum NEC (*see also* Reaction, serum) T80.69
- sexually transmitted A64
  - anogenital
    - herpesviral infection *—see* Herpes, anogenital
    - warts A63.0
  - chancroid A57
  - chlamydial infection *—see* Chlamydia
  - gonorrhea *—see* Gonorrhea
  - granuloma inguinale A58
  - specified organism NEC A63.8
  - syphilis *—see* Syphilis
  - trichomoniasis *—see* Trichomoniasis
- Sézary C84.1-
- shimamushi (scrub typhus) A75.3
- shipyard B30.0
- sickle-cell D57.1
  - with crisis (vasoocclusive pain) D57.00
    - with
      - acute chest syndrome D57.01
      - splenic sequestration D57.02
  - elliptocytosis D57.8-
  - Hb-C D57.20
    - with crisis (vasoocclusive pain) D57.219
      - with
        - acute chest syndrome D57.211
        - splenic sequestration D57.212
    - without crisis D57.20
  - Hb-SD D57.80
    - with crisis D57.819
      - with
        - acute chest syndrome D57.811
        - splenic sequestration D57.812
  - Hb-SE D57.80
    - with crisis D57.819
      - with
        - acute chest syndrome D57.811
        - splenic sequestration D57.812
  - specified NEC D57.80
    - with crisis D57.819
      - with
        - acute chest syndrome D57.811
        - splenic sequestration D57.812
  - spherocytosis D57.80
    - with crisis D57.819
      - with
        - acute chest syndrome D57.811
        - splenic sequestration D57.812

Disease, diseased *(continued)*
- sickle-cell *(continued)*
  - thalassemia D57.40
    - with crisis (vasoocclusive pain) D57.419
      - with
        - acute chest syndrome D57.411
        - splenic sequestration D57.412
    - without crisis D57.40
- silo-filler's J68.8
  - bronchitis J68.0
  - pneumonitis J68.0
  - pulmonary edema J68.1
- simian B B00.4
- Simons'(progressive lipodystrophy) E88.1
- sin nombre virus B33.4
- sinus *—see* Sinusitis
- Sirkari's B55.0
- sixth B08.20
  - due to human herpesvirus 6 B08.21
  - due to human herpesvirus 7 B08.22
- skin L98.9
  - due to metabolic disorder NEC E88.9 *[L99]*
  - specified NEC L98.8
- slim (HIV) B20
- small vessel I73.9
- Sneddon-Wilkinson (subcorneal pustular dermatosis) L13.1
- South African creeping B88.0
- spinal (cord) G95.9
  - congenital Q06.9
  - specified NEC G95.89
- spine *—see also* Spondylopathy
  - joint *—see* Dorsopathy
  - tuberculous A18.01
- spinocerebellar (hereditary) G11.9
  - specified NEC G11.8
- spleen D73.9
  - amyloid E85.4 *[D77]*
  - organic D73.9
  - polycystic Q89.09
  - postinfectional D73.89
- sponge-diver's *—see* Toxicity, venom, marine animal, sea anemone
- Startle Q89.8
- Steinert's G71.11
- Sticker's (erythema infectiosum) B08.3
- Stieda's (calcification, knee joint) *—see* Bursitis, tibial collateral
- Stokes'(exophthalmic goiter) *—see* Hyperthyroidism, with, goiter (diffuse)
- Stokes-Adams (syncope with heart block) I45.9
- stomach K31.9
  - functional, psychogenic F45.8
  - specified NEC K31.89
- stonemason's J62.8
- storage
  - glycogen *—see* Disease, glycogen storage
  - mucopolysaccharide *—see* Mucopolysaccharidosis
- striatopallidal system NEC G25.89
- Stuart-Prower (congenital factor X deficiency) D68.2
- Stuart's (congenital factor X deficiency) D68.2
- subcutaneous tissue *—see* Disease, skin
- supporting structures of teeth K08.9
  - specified NEC K08.89

Disease, diseased *(continued)*
- suprarenal (capsule) (gland) E27.9
  - hyperfunction E27.0
  - specified NEC E27.8
- sweat glands L74.9
  - specified NEC L74.8
- Sweeley-Klionsky E75.21
- Swift (-Feer) *—see* Poisoning, mercury
- swimming-pool granuloma A31.1
- Sylvest's (epidemic pleurodynia) B33.0
- sympathetic nervous system G90.9
- synovium *—see* Disorder, synovium
- syphilitic *—see* Syphilis
- systemic tissue mast cell C96.20
- tanapox (virus) B08.71
- Tangier E78.6
- Tarral-Besnier (pityriasis rubra pilaris) L44.0
- Tauri's E74.09
- tear duct *—see* Disorder, lacrimal system
- tendon, tendinous *—see also* Disorder, tendon
  - nodular *—see* Trigger finger
- terminal vessel I73.9
- testis N50.9
- thalassemia Hb-S *—see* Disease, sickle-cell, thalassemia
- Thaysen-Gee (nontropical sprue) K90.0
- Thomsen G71.12
- throat J39.2
  - septic J02.0
- thromboembolic *—see* Embolism
- thymus (gland) E32.9
  - specified NEC E32.8
- thyroid (gland) E07.9
  - heart (*see also* Hyperthyroidism) E05.90 *[I43]*
    - with thyroid storm E05.91 *[I43]*
  - specified NEC E07.89
- Tietze's M94.0
- tongue K14.9
  - specified NEC K14.8
- tonsils, tonsillar (and adenoids) J35.9
- tooth, teeth K08.9
  - hard tissues K03.9
    - specified NEC K03.89
  - pulp NEC K04.99
  - specified NEC K08.89
- Tourette's F95.2
- trachea NEC J39.8
- tricuspid I07.9
  - nonrheumatic I36.9
- triglyceride-storage E75.5
- trophoblastic *—see* Mole, hydatidiform
- tsutsugamushi A75.3
- tube (fallopian) (noninflammatory) N83.9
  - inflammatory *—see* Salpingitis
  - specified NEC N83.8
- tuberculous NEC *—see* Tuberculosis
- tubo-ovarian (noninflammatory) N83.9
  - inflammatory *—see* Salpingo-oophoritis
  - specified NEC N83.8
- tubotympanic, chronic *—see* Otitis, media, suppurative, chronic, tubotympanic
- tubulo-interstitial N15.9
  - specified NEC N15.8
- tympanum *—see* Disorder, tympanic membrane
- Uhl's Q24.8
- Underwood's (sclerema neonatorum) P83.0
- Unverricht (-Lundborg) *—see* Epilepsy, generalized, idiopathic

Disease, diseased *(continued)*
- Urbach-Oppenheim (necrobiosis lipoidica diabeticorum) *—see* E08-E13 with .620
- ureter N28.9
  - in (due to)
    - schistosomiasis (bilharziasis) B65.0 *[N29]*
- urethra N36.9
  - specified NEC N36.8
- urinary (tract) N39.9
  - bladder N32.9
    - specified NEC N32.89
  - specified NEC N39.8
- uterus (noninflammatory) N85.9
  - infective *—see* Endometritis
  - inflammatory *—see* Endometritis
  - specified NEC N85.8
- uveal tract (anterior) H21.9
  - posterior H31.9
- vagabond's B85.1
- vagina, vaginal (noninflammatory) N89.9
  - inflammatory NEC N76.89
  - specified NEC N89.8
- valve, valvular I38
  - multiple I08.9
    - specified NEC I08.8
- van Creveld-von Gierke (glycogenosis I) E74.01
- vas deferens N50.9
- vascular I99.9
  - arteriosclerotic *—see* Arteriosclerosis
  - ciliary body NEC *—see* Disorder, iris, vascular
  - hypertensive *—see* Hypertension
  - iris NEC *—see* Disorder, iris, vascular
  - obliterative I77.1
    - peripheral I73.9
  - occlusive I99.8
  - peripheral (occlusive) I73.9
    - in diabetes mellitus *—see* E08-E13 with .51
- vasomotor I73.9
- vasospastic I73.9
- vein I87.9
- venereal (*see also* Disease, sexually transmitted) A64
  - chlamydial NEC A56.8
    - anus A56.3
    - genitourinary NOS A56.2
    - pharynx A56.4
    - rectum A56.3
  - fifth A55
  - sixth A55
  - specified nature or type NEC A63.8
- vertebra, vertebral *—see also* Spondylopathy
  - disc *—see* Disorder, disc
- vibration *—see* Vibration, adverse effects
- viral, virus (*see also* Disease, by type of virus) B34.9
  - arbovirus NOS A94
  - arthropod-borne NOS A94
  - congenital P35.9
    - specified NEC P35.8
  - Hanta (with renal manifestations) (Dobrava) (Puumala) (Seoul) A98.5
    - with pulmonary manifestations (Andes) (Bayou) (Bermejo) (Black Creek Canal) (Choclo) (Juquitiba) (Laguna negra) (Lechiguanas) (New York) (Oran) (Sin nombre) B33.4

Disease, diseased *(continued)*
- viral, virus *(continued)*
  - Hantaan (Korean hemorrhagic fever) A98.5
  - human immunodeficiency (HIV) B20
  - Kunjin A83.4
  - nonarthropod-borne NOS B34.9
  - Powassan A84.8
  - Rocio (encephalitis) A83.6
  - Sin nombre (Hantavirus) (cardio)-pulmonary syndrome) B33.4
  - Tahyna B33.8
  - vesicular stomatitis A93.8
- vitreous H43.9
  - specified NEC H43.89
- vocal cord J38.3
- Volkmann's, acquired T79.6
- von Eulenburg's (congenital paramyotonia) G71.19
- von Gierke's (glycogenosis I) E74.01
- von Graefe's *—see* Strabismus, paralytic, ophthalmoplegia, progressive
- von Willebrand (-Jürgens) (angiohemophilia) D68.0
- Vrolik's (osteogenesis imperfecta) Q78.0
- vulva (noninflammatory) N90.9
  - inflammatory NEC N76.89
  - specified NEC N90.89
- Wallgren's (obstruction of splenic vein with collateral circulation) I87.8
- Wassilieff's (leptospiral jaundice) A27.0
- wasting NEC R64
  - due to malnutrition E41
- Waterhouse-Friderichsen A39.1
- Wegner's (syphilitic osteochondritis) A50.02
- Weil's (leptospiral jaundice of lung) A27.0
- Weir Mitchell's (erythromelalgia) I73.81
- Werdnig-Hoffmann G12.0
- Wermer's E31.21
- Werner-His (trench fever) A79.0
- Werner-Schultz (neutropenic splenomegaly) D73.81
- Wernicke-Posadas B38.9
- whipworm B79
- white blood cells D72.9
  - specified NEC D72.89
- white matter R90.82
- white-spot, meaning lichen sclerosus et atrophicus L90.0
  - penis N48.0
  - vulva N90.4
- Wilkie's K55.1
- Wilkinson-Sneddon (subcorneal pustular dermatosis) L13.1
- Willis' *—see* Diabetes
- Wilson's (hepatolenticular degeneration) E83.01
- woolsorter's A22.1
- yaba monkey tumor B08.72
- yaba pox (virus) B08.72
- Zika virus A92.5
- zoonotic, bacterial A28.9
  - specified type NEC A28.8

Disfigurement (due to scar) L90.5

Disgerminoma *—see* Dysgerminoma

DISH (diffuse idiopathic skeletal hyperostosis) *—see* Hyperostosis, ankylosing

Disinsertion, retina *—see* Detachment, retina

Dislocatable hip, congenital Q65.6

Dislocation (articular)
- with fracture *—see* Fracture
- acromioclavicular (joint) S43.10-
  - with displacement
    - 100%-200% S43.12-
    - more than 200% S43.13-
  - inferior S43.14-
  - posterior S43.15-
- ankle S93.0-
- astragalus *—see* Dislocation, ankle
- atlantoaxial S13.121
- atlantooccipital S13.111
- atloidooccipital S13.111
- breast bone S23.29
- capsule, joint - code by site under Dislocation
- carpal (bone) *—see* Dislocation, wrist
- carpometacarpal (joint) NEC S63.05-
  - thumb S63.04-
- cartilage (joint) - code by site under Dislocation
- cervical spine (vertebra) *—see* Dislocation, vertebra, cervical
- chronic *—see* Dislocation, recurrent
- clavicle *—see* Dislocation, acromioclavicular joint
- coccyx S33.2
- congenital NEC Q68.8
- coracoid *—see* Dislocation, shoulder
- costal cartilage S23.29
- costochondral S23.29
- cricoarytenoid articulation S13.29
- cricothyroid articulation S13.29
- dorsal vertebra *—see* Dislocation, vertebra, thoracic
- ear ossicle *—see* Discontinuity, ossicles, ear
- elbow S53.10-
  - congenital Q68.8
  - pathological *—see* Dislocation, pathological NEC, elbow
  - radial head alone *—see* Dislocation, radial head
  - recurrent *—see* Dislocation, recurrent, elbow
  - traumatic S53.10-
    - anterior S53.11-
    - lateral S53.14-
    - medial S53.13-
    - posterior S53.12-
    - specified type NEC S53.19-
- eye, nontraumatic *—see* Luxation, globe
- eyeball, nontraumatic *—see* Luxation, globe
- femur
  - distal end *—see* Dislocation, knee
  - proximal end *—see* Dislocation, hip
- fibula
  - distal end *—see* Dislocation, ankle
  - proximal end *—see* Dislocation, knee
- finger S63.25-
  - index S63.25-
  - interphalangeal S63.27-
    - distal S63.29-
      - index S63.29-
      - little S63.29-
      - middle S63.29-
      - ring S63.29-
    - index S63.27-
    - little S63.27-

Dislocation *(continued)*
- finger *(continued)*
  - interphalangeal *(continued)*
    - middle S63.27-
    - proximal S63.28-
      - index S63.28-
      - little S63.28-
      - middle S63.28-
      - ring S63.28-
    - ring S63.27-
  - little S63.25-
  - metacarpophalangeal S63.26-
    - index S63.26-
    - little S63.26-
    - middle S63.26-
    - ring S63.26-
  - middle S63.25-
  - recurrent *—see* Dislocation, recurrent, finger
  - ring S63.25-
  - thumb *—see* Dislocation, thumb
- foot S93.30-
  - recurrent *—see* Dislocation, recurrent, foot
  - specified site NEC S93.33-
  - tarsal joint S93.31-
  - tarsometatarsal joint S93.32-
  - toe *—see* Dislocation, toe
- fracture *—see* Fracture
- glenohumeral (joint) *—see* Dislocation, shoulder
- glenoid *—see* Dislocation, shoulder
- habitual *—see* Dislocation, recurrent
- hip S73.00-
  - anterior S73.03-
    - obturator S73.02-
  - central S73.04-
  - congenital (total) Q65.2
    - bilateral Q65.1
    - partial Q65.5
      - bilateral Q65.4
      - unilateral Q65.3-
    - unilateral Q65.0-
  - developmental M24.85-
  - pathological *—see* Dislocation, pathological NEC, hip
  - posterior S73.01-
  - recurrent *—see* Dislocation, recurrent, hip
- humerus, proximal end *—see* Dislocation, shoulder
- incomplete *—see* Subluxation, by site
- incus *—see* Discontinuity, ossicles, ear
- infracoracoid *—see* Dislocation, shoulder
- innominate (pubic junction) (sacral junction) S33.39
  - acetabulum *—see* Dislocation, hip
- interphalangeal (joint(s))
  - finger S63.279
    - distal S63.29-
      - index S63.29-
      - little S63.29-
      - middle S63.29-
      - ring S63.29-
    - index S63.27-
    - little S63.27-
    - middle S63.27-
    - proximal S63.28-
      - index S63.28-
      - little S63.28-
      - middle S63.28-
      - ring S63.28-
    - ring S63.27-
  - foot or toe *—see* Dislocation, toe
  - thumb S63.12-
    - distal joint S63.14-
    - proximal joint S63.13-

Dislocation *(continued)*

- jaw (cartilage) (meniscus) S03.0-
- joint prosthesis —*see* Complications, joint prosthesis, mechanical, displacement, by site
- knee S83.106
  - cap —*see* Dislocation, patella
  - congenital Q68.2
  - old M23.8X-
  - patella —*see* Dislocation, patella
  - pathological —*see* Dislocation, pathological NEC, knee
  - proximal tibia
    - anteriorly S83.11-
    - laterally S83.14-
    - medially S83.13-
    - posteriorly S83.12-
  - recurrent —*see also* Derangement, knee, specified NEC
  - specified type NEC S83.19-
- lacrimal gland H04.16-
- lens (complete) H27.10
  - anterior H27.12-
  - congenital Q12.1
  - ocular implant —*see* Complications, intraocular lens
  - partial H27.11-
  - posterior H27.13-
  - traumatic S05.8X-
- ligament - code by site under Dislocation
- lumbar (vertebra) —*see* Dislocation, vertebra, lumbar
- lumbosacral (vertebra) —*see also* Dislocation, vertebra, lumbar
  - congenital Q76.49
- mandible S03.0-
- meniscus (knee) —*see* Tear, meniscus
  - other sites - code by site under Dislocation
- metacarpal (bone)
  - distal end —*see* Dislocation, finger
  - proximal end S63.06-
- metacarpophalangeal (joint)
  - finger S63.26-
    - index S63.26-
    - little S63.26-
    - middle S63.26-
    - ring S63.26-
  - thumb S63.11-
- metatarsal (bone) —*see* Dislocation, foot
- metatarsophalangeal (joint(s)) —*see* Dislocation, toe
- midcarpal (joint) S63.03-
- midtarsal (joint) —*see* Dislocation, foot
- neck S13.20
  - specified site NEC S13.29
  - vertebra —*see* Dislocation, vertebra, cervical
- nose (septal cartilage) S03.1
- occipitoatloid S13.111
- old —*see* Derangement, joint, specified type NEC
- ossicles, ear —*see* Discontinuity, ossicles, ear
- partial —*see* Subluxation, by site
- patella S83.006
  - congenital Q74.1
  - lateral S83.01-
  - recurrent (nontraumatic) M22.0-
    - incomplete M22.1-
  - specified type NEC S83.09-
- pathological NEC M24.30
  - ankle M24.37-
  - elbow M24.32-
  - foot joint M24.37-

Dislocation *(continued)*

- pathological *(continued)*
  - hand joint M24.34-
  - hip M24.35-
  - knee M24.36-
  - lumbosacral joint —*see* subcategory M53.2
  - pelvic region —*see* Dislocation, pathological, hip
  - sacroiliac —*see* subcategory M53.2
  - shoulder M24.31-
  - wrist M24.33-
- pelvis NEC S33.30
  - specified NEC S33.39
- phalanx
  - finger or hand —*see* Dislocation, finger
  - foot or toe —*see* Dislocation, toe
- prosthesis, internal —*see* Complications, prosthetic device, by site, mechanical
- radial head S53.006
  - anterior S53.01-
  - posterior S53.02-
  - specified type NEC S53.09-
- radiocarpal (joint) S63.02-
- radiohumeral (joint) —*see* Dislocation, radial head
- radioulnar (joint)
  - distal S63.01-
  - proximal —*see* Dislocation, elbow
- radius
  - distal end —*see* Dislocation, wrist
  - proximal end —*see* Dislocation, radial head
- recurrent M24.40
  - ankle M24.47-
  - elbow M24.42-
  - finger M24.44-
  - foot joint M24.47-
  - hand joint M24.44-
  - hip M24.45-
  - knee M24.46-
    - patella —*see* Dislocation, patella, recurrent
  - patella —*see* Dislocation, patella, recurrent
  - sacroiliac —*see* subcategory M53.2
  - shoulder M24.41-
  - toe M24.47-
  - vertebra (*see also* subcategory) M43.5
    - atlantoaxial M43.4
      - with myelopathy M43.3
  - wrist M24.43-
- rib (cartilage) S23.29
- sacrococcygeal S33.2
- sacroiliac (joint) (ligament) S33.2
  - congenital Q74.2
  - recurrent M53.2
- sacrum S33.2
- scaphoid (bone) (hand) (wrist) —*see* Dislocation, wrist
  - foot —*see* Dislocation, foot
- scapula —*see* Dislocation, shoulder, girdle, scapula
- semilunar cartilage, knee —*see* Tear, meniscus
- septal cartilage (nose) S03.1
- septum (nasal) (old) J34.2
- sesamoid bone - code by site under Dislocation
- shoulder (blade) (ligament) (joint) (traumatic) S43.006
  - acromioclavicular —*see* Dislocation, acromioclavicular
  - chronic —*see* Dislocation, recurrent, shoulder
  - congenital Q68.8

Dislocation *(continued)*

- shoulder *(continued)*
  - girdle S43.30-
    - scapula S43.31-
    - specified site NEC S43.39-
  - humerus S43.00-
    - anterior S43.01-
    - inferior S43.03-
    - posterior S43.02-
  - pathological —*see* Dislocation, pathological NEC, shoulder
  - recurrent —*see* Dislocation, recurrent, shoulder
  - specified type NEC S43.08-
- spine
  - cervical —*see* Dislocation, vertebra, cervical
  - congenital Q76.49
  - due to birth trauma P11.5
  - lumbar —*see* Dislocation, vertebra, lumbar
  - thoracic —*see* Dislocation, vertebra, thoracic
- spontaneous —*see* Dislocation, pathological
- sternoclavicular (joint) S43.206
  - anterior S43.21-
  - posterior S43.22-
- sternum S23.29
- subglenoid —*see* Dislocation, shoulder
- symphysis pubis S33.4
- talus —*see* Dislocation, ankle
- tarsal (bone(s)) (joint(s)) —*see* Dislocation, foot
- tarsometatarsal (joint(s)) —*see* Dislocation, foot
- temporomandibular (joint) S03.0-
- thigh, proximal end —*see* Dislocation, hip
- thorax S23.20
  - specified site NEC S23.29
  - vertebra —*see* Dislocation, vertebra
- thumb S63.10-
  - interphalangeal joint —*see* Dislocation, interphalangeal (joint), thumb
  - metacarpophalangeal joint —*see* Dislocation, metacarpophalangeal (joint), thumb
- thyroid cartilage S13.29
- tibia
  - distal end —*see* Dislocation, ankle
  - proximal end —*see* Dislocation, knee
- tibiofibular (joint)
  - distal —*see* Dislocation, ankle
  - superior —*see* Dislocation, knee
- toe(s) S93.106
  - great S93.10-
    - interphalangeal joint S93.11-
    - metatarsophalangeal joint S93.12-
  - interphalangeal joint S93.119
  - lesser S93.106
    - interphalangeal joint S93.11-
    - metatarsophalangeal joint S93.12-
  - metatarsophalangeal joint S93.12-
- tooth S03.2
- trachea S23.29
- ulna
  - distal end S63.07-
  - proximal end —*see* Dislocation, elbow
- ulnohumeral (joint) —*see* Dislocation, elbow

Dislocation *(continued)*

- vertebra (articular process) (body) (traumatic)
  - cervical S13.101
    - atlantoaxial joint S13.121
    - atlantooccipital joint S13.111
    - atloidooccipital joint S13.111
    - joint between
      - C0 and C1 S13.111
      - C1 and C2 S13.121
      - C2 and C3 S13.131
      - C3 and C4 S13.141
      - C4 and C5 S13.151
      - C5and C6 S13.161
      - C6and C7 S13.171
      - C7and T1 S13.181
    - occipitoatloid joint S13.111
  - congenital Q76.49
  - lumbar S33.101
    - joint between
      - L1and L2 S33.111
      - L2and L3 S33.121
      - L3 and L4 S33.131
      - L4and L5 S33.141
  - nontraumatic —*see* Displacement, intervertebral disc
  - partial —*see* Subluxation, by site
  - recurrent NEC —*see* subcategory M43.5
  - thoracic S23.101
    - joint between
      - T1 and T2 S23.111
      - T2 and T3 S23.121
      - T3 and T4 S23.123
      - T4 and T5 S23.131
      - T5 and T6 S23.133
      - T6 and T7 S23.141
      - T7 and T8 S23.143
      - T8 and T9 S23.151
      - T9 and T10 S23.153
      - T10 and T11 S23.161
      - T11 and T12 S23.163
      - T12 and L1 S23.171
- wrist (carpal bone) S63.006
  - carpometacarpal joint —*see* Dislocation, carpometacarpal (joint)
  - distal radioulnar joint —*see* Dislocation, radioulnar (joint), distal
  - metacarpal bone, proximal —*see* Dislocation, metacarpal (bone), proximal end
  - midcarpal —*see* Dislocation, midcarpal (joint)
  - radiocarpal joint —*see* Dislocation, radiocarpal (joint)
  - recurrent —*see* Dislocation, recurrent, wrist
  - specified site NEC S63.09-
  - ulna —*see* Dislocation, ulna, distal end
- xiphoid cartilage S23.29

Disorder (of) —*see also* Disease

- acantholytic L11.9
  - specified NEC L11.8
- acute
  - psychotic —*see* Psychosis, acute
  - stress F43.0
- adjustment (grief) F43.20
  - with
    - anxiety F43.22
      - with depressed mood F43.23
    - conduct disturbance F43.24
      - with emotional disturbance F43.25
    - depressed mood F43.21
      - with anxiety F43.23
    - other specified symptom F43.29

Disorder *(continued)*
  adrenal (capsule) (gland) (medullary) E27.9
    specified NEC E27.8
  adrenogenital E25.9
    drug-induced E25.8
    iatrogenic E25.8
    idiopathic E25.8
  adult personality (and behavior) F69
    specified NEC F68.8
  affective (mood) —*see* Disorder, mood
  aggressive, unsocialized F91.1
  alcohol-related F10.99
    with
      amnestic disorder, persisting F10.96
      anxiety disorder F10.980
      dementia, persisting F10.97
      intoxication F10.929
        with delirium F10.921
        uncomplicated F10.920
      mood disorder F10.94
      other specified F10.988
      psychotic disorder F10.959
        with
          delusions F10.950
          hallucinations F10.951
      sexual dysfunction F10.981
      sleep disorder F10.982
  alcohol use
    mild F10.10
      with
        alcohol-induced
          anxiety disorder F10.180
          bipolar and related disorder F10.14
          depressive disorder F10.14
          psychotic disorder F10.159
          sexual dysfunction F10.181
          sleep disorder F10.182
        alcohol intoxication F10.129
          delirium F10.121
      in remission (early) (sustained) F10.11
    moderate or severe F10.20
      with
        alcohol-induced
          anxiety disorder F10.280
          bipolar and related disorder F10.24
          depressive disorder F10.24
          major neurocognitive disorder, amnestic-confabulatory type F10.26
          major neurocognitive disorder, nonamnestic-confabulatory type F10.27
          mild neurocognitive disorder F10.288
          psychotic disorder F10.259
          sexual dysfunction F10.281
          sleep disorder F10.282
        alcohol intoxication F10.229
          delirium F10.221
      in remission (early) (sustained) F10.21
  allergic —*see* Allergy
  alveolar NEC J84.09
  amino-acid
    cystathioninuria E72.19
    cystinosis E72.04
    cystinuria E72.01
    glycinuria E72.09
    homocystinuria E72.11
    metabolism —*see* Disturbance, metabolism, amino-acid
      specified NEC E72.8
    neonatal, transitory P74.8

Disorder *(continued)*
  amino-acid *(continued)*
    renal transport NEC E72.09
    transport NEC E72.09
  amnesic, amnestic
    alcohol-induced F10.96
      with dependence F10.26
    due to (secondary to) general medical condition F04
    psychoactive NEC-induced F19.96
      with
        abuse F19.16
        dependence F19.26
    sedative, hypnotic or anxiolytic-induced F13.96
      with dependence F13.26
  amphetamine-type substance use
    mild F15.10
      in remission (early) (sustained) F15.11
    moderate F15.20
      in remission (early) (sustained) F15.21
    severe 15.20
      in remission (early) (sustained) F15.21
  amphetamine (or other stimulant) use
    mild F15.10
      with
        amphetamine (or other stimulant) -induced
          anxiety disorder F15.180
          bipolar and related disorder F15.14
          depressive disorder F15.14
          obsessive-compulsive and related disorder F15.188
          psychotic disorder F15.159
          sexual dysfunction F15.181
        amphetamine, cocaine, or other stimulant intoxication
          with perceptual disturbances F15.122
          without perceptual disturbances F15.129
        intoxication delirium F15.121
      in remission (early) (sustained) F15.11
    moderate or severe
      with
        amphetamine (or other stimulant) -induced
          anxiety disorder F15.280
          bipolar and related disorder F15.14
          depressive disorder F15.24
          obsessive-compulsive and related disorder F15.288
          psychotic disorder F15.259
          sexual dysfunction F15.281
        amphetamine, cocaine, or other stimulant intoxication
          with perceptual disturbances F15.222
          without perceptual disturbances F15.229
        intoxication delirium F15.221
  anaerobic glycolysis with anemia D55.2
  anxiety F41.9
    due to (secondary to)
      alcohol F10.980
        in
          abuse F10.980
          dependence F10.280
      amphetamine F15.980
        in
          abuse F15.180
          dependence F15.280
      anxiolytic F13.980

Disorder *(continued)*
  anxiety *(continued)*
    due to *(continued)*
      anxiolytic *(continued)*
        in
          abuse F13.180
          dependence F13.280
      caffeine F15.980
        in
          abuse F15.180
          dependence F15.280
      cannabis F12.980
        in
          abuse F12.180
          dependence F12.280
      cocaine F14.980
        in
          abuse F14.180
          dependence F14.180
      general medical condition F06.4
      hallucinogen F16.980
        in
          abuse F16.180
          dependence F16.280
      hypnotic F13.980
        in
          abuse F13.180
          dependence F13.280
      inhalant F18.980
        in
          abuse F18.180
          dependence F18.280
      phencyclidine F16.980
        in
          abuse F16.180
          dependence F16.280
      psychoactive substance NEC F19.980
        in
          abuse F19.180
          dependence F19.280
      sedative F13.980
        in
          abuse F13.180
          dependence F13.280
      volatile solvents F18.980
        in
          abuse F18.180
          dependence F18.280
    generalized F41.1
    illness F45.21
    mixed
      with depression (mild) F41.8
      specified NEC F41.3
    organic F06.4
    phobic F40.9
      of childhood F40.8
    specified NEC F41.8
  aortic valve —*see* Endocarditis, aortic
  aromatic amino-acid metabolism E70.9
    specified NEC E70.8
  arteriole NEC I77.89
  artery NEC I77.89
  articulation —*see* Disorder, joint
  attachment (childhood)
    disinhibited F94.2
    reactive F94.1
  attention-deficit hyperactivity (adolescent) (adult) (child) F90.0
    combined
      presentation F90.2
      type F90.2
    hyperactive
      impulsive presentation F90.1
      type F90.1
    inattentive
      presentation F90.0
      type F90.0
    specified type NEC F90.8

Disorder *(continued)*
  attention-deficit without hyperactivity (adolescent) (adult) (child) F98.8
  auditory processing (central) H93.25
  autistic F84.0
  autoimmune D89.89
  autonomic nervous system G90.9
    specified NEC G90.8
  autism spectrum F84.0
  avoidant
    child or adolescent F40.10
    restrictive food intake F50.82
  balance
    acid-base E87.8
      mixed E87.4
    electrolyte E87.8
    fluid NEC E87.8
  behavioral (disruptive) —*see* Disorder, conduct
  beta-amino-acid metabolism E72.8
  bile acid and cholesterol metabolism E78.70
    Barth syndrome E78.71
    other specified E78.79
    Smith-Lemli-Opitz syndrome E78.72
  bilirubin excretion E80.6
  binge eating F50.81
  binocular
    movement H51.9
      convergence
        excess H51.12
        insufficiency H51.11
      internuclear ophthalmoplegia —*see* Ophthalmoplegia, internuclear
      palsy of conjugate gaze H51.0
      specified type NEC H51.8
    vision NEC —*see* Disorder, vision, binocular
  bipolar (I) (type 1) F31.9
    and related due to a known physiological condition
      with
        manic features F06.33
        manic- or hypomanic-like episodes F06.33
        mixed features F06.34
    current (or most recent) episode
      depressed F31.9
        with psychotic features F31.5
        without psychotic features F31.30
          mild F31.31
          moderate F31.32
          severe (without psychotic features) F31.4
            with psychotic features F31.5
      hypomanic F31.0
      manic F31.9
        with psychotic features F31.2
        without psychotic features F31.10
          mild F31.11
          moderate F31.12
          severe (without psychotic features) F31.13
            with psychotic features F31.2
      mixed F31.60
        mild F31.61
        moderate F31.62
        severe (without psychotic features) F31.63
          with psychotic features F31.64
      severe depression (without psychotic features) F31.4
        with psychotic features F31.5

Disorder *(continued)*
- bipolar (I) (type 1) *(continued)*
  - in remission (currently) F31.70
    - in full remission
      - most recent episode
        - depressed F31.76
        - hypomanic F31.72
        - manic F31.74
        - mixed F31.78
    - in partial remission
      - most recent episode
        - depressed F31.75
        - hypomanic F31.71
        - manic F31.73
        - mixed F31.77
  - specified NEC F31.89
  - II (type 2) F31.81
  - organic F06.30
  - single manic episode F30.9
    - mild F30.11
    - moderate F30.12
    - severe (without psychotic symptoms) F30.13
      - with psychotic symptoms F30.2
- bladder N32.9
  - functional NEC N31.9
  - in schistosomiasis B65.0 *[N33]*
  - specified NEC N32.89
- bleeding D68.9
- blood D75.9
  - in congenital early syphilis A50.09 *[D77]*
- body dysmorphic F45.22
- bone M89.9
  - continuity M84.9
    - specified type NEC M84.80
      - ankle M84.87-
      - fibula M84.86-
      - foot M84.87-
      - hand M84.84-
      - humerus M84.82-
      - neck M84.88
      - pelvis M84.859
      - radius M84.83-
      - rib M84.88
      - shoulder M84.81-
      - skull M84.88
      - thigh M84.85-
      - tibia M84.86-
      - ulna M84.83-
      - vertebra M84.88
  - density and structure M85.9
    - cyst *—see also* Cyst, bone, specified type NEC
      - aneurysmal *—see* Cyst, bone, aneurysmal
      - solitary *—see* Cyst, bone, solitary
    - diffuse idiopathic skeletal hyperostosis *—see* Hyperostosis, ankylosing
    - fibrous dysplasia (monostotic) *—see* Dysplasia, fibrous, bone
    - fluorosis *—see* Fluorosis, skeletal
    - hyperostosis of skull M85.2
    - osteitis condensans *—see* Osteitis, condensans
    - specified type NEC M85.8-
      - ankle M85.87-
      - foot M85.87-
      - forearm M85.83-
      - hand M85.84-
      - lower leg M85.86-
      - multiple sites M85.89
      - neck M85.88

Disorder *(continued)*
- bone *(continued)*
  - density and structure *(continued)*
    - specified type *(continued)*
      - rib M85.88
      - shoulder M85.81-
      - skull M85.88
      - thigh M85.85-
      - upper arm M85.82-
      - vertebra M85.88
  - development and growth NEC M89.20
    - carpus M89.24-
    - clavicle M89.21-
    - femur M89.25-
    - fibula M89.26-
    - finger M89.24-
    - humerus M89.22-
    - ilium M89.259
    - ischium M89.259
    - metacarpus M89.24-
    - metatarsus M89.27-
    - multiple sites M89.29
    - neck M89.28
    - radius M89.23-
    - rib M89.28
    - scapula M89.21-
    - skull M89.28
    - tarsus M89.27-
    - tibia M89.26-
    - toe M89.27-
    - ulna M89.23-
    - vertebra M89.28
  - specified type NEC M89.8X-
- brachial plexus G54.0
- branched-chain amino-acid metabolism E71.2
  - specified NEC E71.19
- breast N64.9
  - agalactia *—see* Agalactia
  - associated with
    - lactation O92.70
      - specified NEC O92.79
    - pregnancy O92.20
      - specified NEC O92.29
    - puerperium O92.20
      - specified NEC O92.29
  - cracked nipple *—see* Cracked nipple
  - galactorrhea *—see* Galactorrhea
  - hypogalactia O92.4
  - lactation disorder NEC O92.79
  - mastitis *—see* Mastitis
  - nipple infection *—see* Infection, nipple
  - retracted nipple *—see* Retraction, nipple
  - specified type NEC N64.89
- Briquet's F45.0
- bullous, in diseases classified elsewhere L14
- caffeine use
  - mild
    - with
      - caffeine-induced
        - anxiety disorder F15.180
        - sleep disorder F15.182
  - moderate or severe
    - with
      - caffeine-induced
        - anxiety disorder F15.280
        - sleep disorder F15.282
- cannabis use
  - mild F12.10
    - with
      - cannabis-induced
        - anxiety disorder F12.180
        - psychotic disorder F12.159
        - sleep disorder F12.188

Disorder *(continued)*
- cannabis *(continued)*
  - mild *(continued)*
    - with *(continued)*
      - cannabis intoxication
        - delirium F12.121
        - with perceptual disturbances F12.122
        - without perceptual disturbances F12.129
    - in remission (early) (sustained) F12.11
  - moderate or severe F12.20
    - with
      - cannabis-induced
        - anxiety disorder F12.280
        - psychotic disorder F12.259
        - sleep disorder F12.288
      - cannabis intoxication
        - with perceptual disturbances F12.222
        - without perceptual disturbances F12.229
      - delirium F12.221
    - in remission (early) (sustained) F12.21
- carbohydrate
  - absorption, intestinal NEC E74.39
  - metabolism (congenital) E74.9
    - specified NEC E74.8
- cardiac, functional I51.89
- carnitine metabolism E71.40
- cartilage M94.9
  - articular NEC *—see* Derangement, joint, articular cartilage
    - chondrocalcinosis *—see* Chondrocalcinosis
  - specified type NEC M94.8X-
    - articular *—see* Derangement, joint, articular cartilage
    - multiple sites M94.8X0
- catatonia (due to known physiological condition) (with another mental disorder) F06.1
- catatonic
  - due to (secondary to) known physiological condition F06.1
  - organic F06.1
- central auditory processing H93.25
- cervical
  - region NEC M53.82
  - root (nerve) NEC G54.2
- character NOS F60.9
- childhood disintegrative NEC F84.3
- cholesterol and bile acid metabolism E78.70
  - Barth syndrome E78.71
  - other specified E78.79
  - Smith-Lemli-Opitz syndrome E78.72
- choroid H31.9
  - atrophy *—see* Atrophy, choroid
  - degeneration *—see* Degeneration, choroid
  - detachment *—see* Detachment, choroid
  - dystrophy *—see* Dystrophy, choroid
  - hemorrhage *—see* Hemorrhage, choroid
  - rupture *—see* Rupture, choroid
  - scar *—see* Scar, chorioretinal
  - solar retinopathy *—see* Retinopathy, solar
  - specified type NEC H31.8
- ciliary body *—see* Disorder, iris
  - degeneration *—see* Degeneration, ciliary body
- coagulation (factor) (*see also* Defect, coagulation) D68.9
  - newborn, transient P61.6

Disorder *(continued)*
- cocaine use
  - mild F14.10
    - with
      - amphetamine, cocaine, or other stimulant intoxication
        - with perceptual disturbances F14.122
        - without perceptual disturbances F14.129
      - cocaine-induced
        - anxiety disorder F14.180
        - bipolar and related disorder F14.14
        - depressive disorder F14.14
        - obsessive-compulsive and related disorder F14.188
        - psychotic disorder F14.159
        - sexual dysfunction F14.181
        - sleep disorder F14.182
      - cocaine intoxication delirium F14.121
    - in remission (early) (sustained) F14.11
  - moderate or severe
    - with
      - amphetamine, cocaine, or other stimulant intoxication
        - with perceptual disturbances F14.222
        - without perceptual disturbances F14.229
      - cocaine-induced
        - anxiety disorder F14.280
        - bipolar and related disorder F14.24
        - depressive disorder F14.24
        - obsessive-compulsive and related disorder F14.288
        - psychotic disorder F14.259
        - sexual dysfunction F14.281
        - sleep disorder F14.282
      - cocaine intoxication delirium F14.221
    - in remission (early) (sustained) F14.21
- coccyx NEC M53.3
- cognitive F09
  - due to (secondary to) general medical condition F09
  - persisting R41.89
    - due to
      - alcohol F10.97
        - with dependence F10.27
      - anxiolytics F13.97
        - with dependence F13.27
      - hypnotics F13.97
        - with dependence F13.27
      - sedatives F13.97
        - with dependence F13.27
      - specified substance NEC F19.97
        - with
          - abuse F19.17
          - dependence F19.27
- communication F80.9
  - social pragmatic F80.82
- conduct (childhood) F91.9
  - adjustment reaction *—see* Disorder, adjustment
  - adolescent onset type F91.2
  - childhood onset type F91.1
  - compulsive F63.9
  - confined to family context F91.0
  - depressive F91.8
  - group type F91.2
  - hyperkinetic *—see* Disorder, attention-deficit hyperactivity
  - oppositional defiance F91.3

Disorder *(continued)*
- conduct *(continued)*
  - socialized F91.2
  - solitary aggressive type F91.1
  - specified NEC F91.8
  - unsocialized (aggressive) F91.1
- conduction, heart I45.9
- congenital glycosylation (CDG) E74.8
- conjunctiva H11.9
  - infection —*see* Conjunctivitis
- connective tissue, localized L94.9
  - specified NEC L94.8
- conversion (functional neurological symptom disorder)
  - with
    - abnormal movement F44.4
    - anesthesia or sensory loss F44.6
    - attacks or seizures F44.5
    - mixed symptoms F44.7
    - special sensory symptoms F44.6
    - speech symptoms F44.4
    - swallowing symptoms F44.4
    - weakness or paralysis F44.4
- convulsive (secondary) —*see* Convulsions
- cornea H18.9
  - deformity —*see* Deformity, cornea
  - degeneration —*see* Degeneration, cornea
  - deposits —*see* Deposit, cornea
  - due to contact lens H18.82-
    - specified as edema —*see* Edema, cornea
  - edema —*see* Edema, cornea
  - keratitis —*see* Keratitis
  - keratoconjunctivitis —*see* Keratoconjunctivitis
  - membrane change —*see* Change, corneal membrane
  - neovascularization —*see* Neovascularization, cornea
  - scar —*see* Opacity, cornea
  - specified type NEC H18.89-
  - ulcer —*see* Ulcer, cornea
- corpus cavernosum N48.9
- cranial nerve —*see* Disorder, nerve, cranial
- cyclothymic F34.0
- defiant oppositional F91.3
- delusional (persistent) (systematized) F22
  - induced F24
- depersonalization F48.1
- depressive F32.9
  - due to known physiological condition
    - with
      - depressive features F06.31
      - major depressive-like episode F06.32
      - mixed features F06.34
  - major F32.9
    - with psychotic symptoms F32.3
    - in remission (full) F32.5
      - partial F32.4
    - recurrent F33.9
      - with psychotic features F33.3
    - single episode F32.9
      - mild F32.0
      - moderate F32.1
      - severe (without psychotic symptoms) F32.2
        - with psychotic symptoms F32.3
  - organic F06.31
  - persistent F34.1
  - recurrent F33.9
    - current episode
      - mild F33.0
      - moderate F33.1

Disorder *(continued)*
- depressive *(continued)*
  - recurrent *(continued)*
    - current episode *(continued)*
      - severe (without psychotic symptoms) F33.2
        - with psychotic symptoms F33.3
    - in remission F33.40
      - full F33.42
      - partial F33.41
    - specified NEC F33.8
  - single episode —*see* Episode, depressive
  - specified NEC F32.89
- developmental F89
  - arithmetical skills F81.2
  - coordination (motor) F82
  - expressive writing F81.81
  - language F80.9
    - expressive F80.1
    - mixed receptive and expressive F80.2
    - receptive type F80.2
    - specified NEC F80.89
  - learning F81.9
    - arithmetical F81.2
    - reading F81.0
  - mixed F88
  - motor coordination or function F82
  - pervasive F84.9
    - specified NEC F84.8
  - phonological F80.0
  - reading F81.0
  - scholastic skills —*see also* Disorder, learning
    - mixed F81.89
  - specified NEC F88
  - speech F80.9
    - articulation F80.0
    - specified NEC F80.89
  - written expression F81.81
- diaphragm J98.6
- digestive (system) K92.9
  - newborn P78.9
    - specified NEC P78.89
  - postprocedural —*see* Complication, gastrointestinal
  - psychogenic F45.8
- disc (intervertebral) M51.9
  - with
    - myelopathy
      - cervical region M50.00
      - cervicothoracic region M50.03
      - high cervical region M50.01
      - lumbar region M51.06
      - mid-cervical region M50.020
      - sacrococcygeal region M53.3
      - thoracic region M51.04
      - thoracolumbar region M51.05
    - radiculopathy
      - cervical region M50.10
      - cervicothoracic region M50.13
      - high cervical region M50.11
      - lumbar region M51.16
      - lumbosacral region M51.17
      - mid-cervical region M50.120
      - sacrococcygeal region M53.3
      - thoracic region M51.14
      - thoracolumbar region M51.15
  - cervical M50.90
    - with
      - myelopathy M50.00
        - C2-C3 M50.01
        - C3-C4 M50.01
        - C4-C5 M50.021
        - C5-C6 M50.022

Disorder *(continued)*
- disc *(continued)*
  - cervical *(continued)*
    - with *(continued)*
      - myelopathy *(continued)*
        - C6-C7 M50.023
        - C7-T1 M50.03
        - cervicothoracic region M50.03
        - high cervical region M50.01
        - mid-cervical region M50.020
      - neuritis, radiculitis or radiculopathy M50.10
        - C2-C3 M50.11
        - C3-C4 M50.11
        - C4-C5 M50.121
        - C5-C6 M50.122
        - C6-C7 M50.123
        - C7-T1 M50.13
        - cervicothoracic region M50.13
        - high cervical region M50.11
        - mid-cervical region M50.120
    - C2-C3 M50.91
    - C3-C4 M50.91
    - C4-C5 M50.921
    - C5-C6 M50.922
    - C6-C7 M50.923
    - C7-T1 M50.93
    - cervicothoracic region M50.93
    - degeneration M50.30
      - C2-C3 M50.31
      - C3-C4 M50.31
      - C4-C5 M50.321
      - C5-C6 M50.322
      - C6-C7 M50.323
      - C7-T1 M50.33
      - cervicothoracic region M50.33
      - high cervical region M50.31
      - mid-cervical region M50.320
    - displacement M50.20
      - C2-C3 M50.21
      - C3-C4 M50.21
      - C4-C5 M50.221
      - C5-C6 M50.222
      - C6-C7 M50.223
      - C7-T1 M50.23
      - cervicothoracic region M50.23
      - high cervical region M50.21
      - mid-cervical region M50.220
    - high cervical region M50.91
    - mid-cervical region M50.920
    - specified type NEC M50.80
      - C2-C3 M50.81
      - C3-C4 M50.81
      - C4-C5 M50.821
      - C5-C6 M50.822
      - C6-C7 M50.823
      - C7-T1 M50.83
      - cervicothoracic region M50.83
      - high cervical region M50.81
      - mid-cervical region M50.820
  - specified NEC
    - lumbar region M51.86
    - lumbosacral region M51.87
    - sacrococcygeal region M53.3
    - thoracic region M51.84
    - thoracolumbar region M51.85
- disinhibited attachment (childhood) F94.2
- disintegrative, childhood NEC F84.3
- disruptive F91.9
  - mood dysregulation F34.81
  - specified NEC F91.8

Disorder *(continued)*
- disruptive behavior - *see* Disorder, conduct
- dissocial personality F60.2
- dissociative F44.9
  - affecting
    - motor function F44.4
      - and sensation F44.7
    - sensation F44.6
      - and motor function F44.7
  - brief reactive F43.0
  - due to (secondary to) general medical condition F06.8
  - mixed F44.7
  - organic F06.8
  - other specified NEC F44.89
- double heterozygous sickling —*see* Disease, sickle-cell
- dream anxiety F51.5
- drug induced hemorrhagic D68.32
- drug related F19.99
  - abuse —*see* Abuse, drug
  - dependence —*see* Dependence, drug
- dysmorphic body F45.22
- dysthymic F34.1
- ear H93.9-
  - bleeding —*see* Otorrhagia
  - deafness —*see* Deafness
  - degenerative H93.09-
  - discharge —*see* Otorrhea
  - external H61.9-
    - auditory canal stenosis —*see* Stenosis, external ear canal
    - exostosis —*see* Exostosis, external ear canal
    - impacted cerumen —*see* Impaction, cerumen
    - otitis —*see* Otitis, externa
    - perichondritis —*see* Perichondritis, ear
    - pinna —*see* Disorder, pinna
    - specified type NEC H61.89-
      - in diseases classified elsewhere H62.8X-
  - inner H83.9-
    - vestibular dysfunction —*see* Disorder, vestibular function
  - middle H74.9-
    - adhesive H74.1-
    - ossicle —*see* Abnormal, ear ossicles
    - polyp —*see* Polyp, ear (middle)
    - specified NEC, in diseases classified elsewhere H75.8-
  - postprocedural —*see* Complications, ear, procedure
  - specified NEC, in diseases classified elsewhere H94.8-
- eating (adult) (psychogenic) F50.9
  - anorexia —*see* Anorexia
  - binge F50.81
  - bulimia F50.2
  - child F98.29
    - pica F98.3
    - rumination disorder F98.21
  - pica F50.89
    - childhood F98.3
- electrolyte (balance) NEC E87.8
  - with
    - abortion —*see* Abortion by type complicated by specified condition NEC
    - ectopic pregnancy O08.5
    - molar pregnancy O08.5
  - acidosis (metabolic) (respiratory) E87.2
  - alkalosis (metabolic) (respiratory) E87.3
- elimination, transepidermal L87.9
  - specified NEC L87.8

Disorder *(continued)*
  emotional (persistent) F34.9
    of childhood F93.9
      specified NEC F93.8
  endocrine E34.9
    postprocedural E89.89
      specified NEC E89.89
  erectile (male) (organic) (*see also* Dysfunction, sexual, male, erectile) N52.9
    nonorganic F52.21
  erythematous —*see* Erythema
  esophagus K22.9
    functional K22.4
    psychogenic F45.8
  eustachian tube H69.9-
    infection —*see* Salpingitis, eustachian
    obstruction —*see* Obstruction, eustachian tube
    patulous —*see* Patulous, eustachian tube
    specified NEC H69.8-
  exhibitionistic F65.2
  extrapyramidal G25.9
    in diseases classified elsewhere —*see* category G26
    specified type NEC G25.89
  eye H57.9
    postprocedural —*see* Complication, postprocedural, eye
  eyelid H02.9
    cyst —*see* Cyst, eyelid
    degenerative H02.70
      chloasma —*see* Chloasma, eyelid
      madarosis —*see* Madarosis
      specified type NEC H02.79
      vitiligo —*see* Vitiligo, eyelid
      xanthelasma —*see* Xanthelasma
    dermatochalasis —*see* Dermatochalasis
    edema —*see* Edema, eyelid
    elephantiasis —*see* Elephantiasis, eyelid
    foreign body, retained —*see* Foreign body, retained, eyelid
    function H02.59
      abnormal innervation syndrome —*see* Syndrome, abnormal innervation
      blepharochalasis —*see* Blepharochalasis
      blepharoclonus —*see* Blepharoclonus
      blepharophimosis —*see* Blepharophimosis
      blepharoptosis —*see* Blepharoptosis
      lagophthalmos —*see* Lagophthalmos
      lid retraction —*see* Retraction, lid
    hypertrichosis —*see* Hypertrichosis, eyelid
    specified type NEC H02.89
    vascular H02.879
      left H02.876
        lower H02.875
        upper H02.874
      right H02.873
        lower H02.872
        upper H02.871
  factitious F68.10
    with predominantly
      psychological symptoms F68.11
        with physical symptoms F68.13
      physical symptoms F68.12
        with psychological symptoms F68.13

Disorder *(continued)*
  factor, coagulation —*see* Defect, coagulation
  fatty acid
    metabolism E71.30
      specified NEC E71.39
    oxidation
      LCAD E71.310
      MCAD E71.311
      SCAD E71.312
      specified deficiency NEC E71.318
  feeding (infant or child) (*see also* Disorder, eating) R63.3
    or eating disorder F50.9
    specified NEC F50.9
  feigned (with obvious motivation) Z76.5
    without obvious motivation —*see* Disorder, factitious
  female
    hypoactive sexual desire F52.0
    orgasmic F52.31
    sexual interest/arousal F52.22
  fetishistic F65.0
  fibroblastic M72.9
    specified NEC M72.8
  fluency
    adult onset F98.5
    childhood onset F80.81
    following
      cerebral infarction I69.323
      cerebrovascular disease I69.923
        specified disease NEC I69.823
      intracerebral hemorrhage I69.123
      nontraumatic intracranial hemorrhage NEC I69.223
      subarachnoid hemorrhage I69.023
    in conditions classified elsewhere R47.82
  fluid balance E87.8
  follicular (skin) L73.9
    specified NEC L73.8
  frotteuristic F65.81
  fructose metabolism E74.10
    essential fructosuria E74.11
    fructokinase deficiency E74.11
    fructose-1, 6-diphosphatase deficiency E74.19
    hereditary fructose intolerance E74.12
    other specified E74.19
  functional polymorphonuclear neutrophils D71
  gallbladder, biliary tract and pancreas in diseases classified elsewhere K87
  gambling F63.0
  gamma-glutamyl cycle E72.8
  gastric (functional) K31.9
    motility K30
    psychogenic F45.8
    secretion K30
  gastrointestinal (functional) NOS K92.9
    newborn P78.9
    psychogenic F45.8
  gender-identity or -role F64.9
    childhood F64.2
    effect on relationship F66
    of adolescence or adulthood F64.0
      nontranssexual F64.8
    specified NEC F64.8
    uncertainty F66
  genito-pelvic pain penetration F52.6
  genitourinary system
    female N94.9
    male N50.9
    psychogenic F45.8

Disorder *(continued)*
  globe H44.9
    degenerated condition H44.50
      absolute glaucoma H44.51-
      atrophy H44.52-
      leucocoria H44.53-
    degenerative H44.30
      chalcosis H44.31-
      myopia (*see also* Myopia, degenerative) H44.2-
      siderosis H44.32-
      specified type NEC H44.39-
    endophthalmitis —*see* Endophthalmitis
    foreign body, retained —*see* Foreign body, intraocular, old, retained
    hemophthalmos —*see* Hemophthalmos
    hypotony H44.40
      due to
        ocular fistula H44.42-
        specified disorder NEC H44.43-
      flat anterior chamber H44.41-
      primary H44.44-
    luxation —*see* Luxation, globe
    specified type NEC H44.89
  glomerular (in) N05.9
    amyloidosis E85.4 *[N08]*
    cryoglobulinemia D89.1 *[N08]*
    disseminated intravascular coagulation D65 *[N08]*
    Fabry's disease E75.21 *[N08]*
    familial lecithin cholesterol acyltransferase deficiency E78.6 *[N08]*
    Goodpasture's syndrome M31.0
    hemolytic-uremic syndrome D59.3
    Henoch (-Schönlein) purpura D69.0 *[N08]*
    malariae malaria B52.0
    microscopic polyangiitis M31.7 *[N08]*
    multiple myeloma C90.0- *[N08]*
    mumps B26.83
    schistosomiasis B65.9 *[N08]*
    sepsis NEC A41.- *[N08]*
      streptococcal A40.- [*N08]*
    sickle-cell disorders D57.- *[N08]*
    strongyloidiasis B78.9 *[N08]*
    subacute bacterial endocarditis I33.0 *[N08]*
    syphilis A52.75
    systemic lupus erythematosus M32.14
    thrombotic thrombocytopenic purpura M31.1 *[N08]*
    Waldenström macroglobulinemia C88.0 *[N08]*
    Wegener's granulomatosis M31.31
  gluconeogenesis E74.4
  glucosaminoglycan metabolism —*see* Disorder, metabolism, glucosaminoglycan
  glycine metabolism E72.50
    d-glycericacidemia E72.59
    hyperhydroxyprolinemia E72.59
    hyperoxaluria E72.53
    hyperprolinemia E72.59
    non-ketotic hyperglycinemia E72.51
    oxalosis E72.53
    oxaluria E72.53
    sarcosinemia E72.59
    trimethylaminuria E72.52
  glycoprotein metabolism E77.9
    specified NEC E77.8
  habit (and impulse) F63.9
    involving sexual behavior NEC F65.9
    specified NEC F63.89

Disorder *(continued)*
  hallucinogen use
    mild F16.10
      with
        hallucinogen-induced
          anxiety disorder F16.180
          bipolar and related disorder F16.14
          depressive disorder F16.14
          psychotic disorder F16.159
        hallucinogen intoxication delirium F16.121
        other hallucinogen intoxication F16.129
      in remission (early) (sustained) F16.11
    moderate or severe F16.20
      with
        hallucinogen-induced
          anxiety disorder F16.280
          bipolar and related disorder F16.24
          depressive disorder F16.24
          psychotic disorder F16.259
        hallucinogen intoxication delirium F16.221
        other hallucinogen intoxication F16.229
      in remission (early) (sustained) F16.21
  heart action I49.9
  hematological D75.9
    newborn (transient) P61.9
      specified NEC P61.8
  hematopoietic organs D75.9
  hemorrhagic NEC D69.9
    drug-induced D68.32
    due to
      extrinsic circulating anticoagulants D68.32
      increase in
        anti-IIa D68.32
        anti-Xa D68.32
      intrinsic
        circulating anticoagulants D68.318
        increase in
          antithrombin D68.318
          anti-VIIIa D68.318
          anti-IXa D68.318
          anti-XIa D68.318
    following childbirth O72.3
  hemostasis —*see* Defect, coagulation
  histidine metabolism E70.40
    histidinemia E70.41
    other specified E70.49
  hoarding F42.3
  hyperkinetic —*see* Disorder, attention-deficit hyperactivity
  hyperleucine-isoleucinemia E71.19
  hypervalinemia E71.19
  hypoactive sexual desire F52.0
  hypochondriacal F45.20
    body dysmorphic F45.22
    neurosis F45.21
    other specified F45.29
  identity
    dissociative F44.81
    illness anxiety F45.21
    of childhood F93.8
  immune mechanism (immunity) D89.9
    specified type NEC D89.89
  impaired renal tubular function N25.9
    specified NEC N25.89
  impulse (control) F63.9

Disorder *(continued)*
- inflammatory
  - pelvic, in diseases classified elsewhere *—see* category N74
  - penis N48.29
    - abscess N48.21
    - cellulitis N48.22
- inhalant use
  - mild F18.10
    - with
      - inhalant-induced
        - anxiety disorder F18.180
        - depressive disorder F18.14
        - major neurocognitive disorder F18.17
        - mild neurocognitive disorder F18.188
        - psychotic disorder F18.159
      - inhalant intoxication F18.129
      - inhalant intoxication delirium F18.121
    - in remission (early) (sustained) F18.11
  - moderate or severe F18.20
    - with
      - inhalant-induced
        - anxiety disorder F18.280
        - depressive disorder F18.24
        - major neurocognitive disorder F18.27
        - mild neurocognitive disorder F18.288
        - psychotic disorder F18.259
      - inhalant intoxication F18.229
      - inhalant intoxication delirium F18.221
    - in remission (early) (sustained) F18.21
- integument, newborn P83.9
  - specified NEC P83.88
- intermittent explosive F63.81
- internal secretion pancreas *—see* Increased, secretion, pancreas, endocrine
- intestine, intestinal
  - carbohydrate absorption NEC E74.39
    - postoperative K91.2
  - functional NEC K59.9
    - postoperative K91.89
  - psychogenic F45.8
  - vascular K55.9
    - chronic K55.1
    - specified NEC K55.8
- intraoperative (intraprocedural) *—see* Complications, intraoperative
- involuntary emotional expression (IEED) F48.2
- iris H21.9
  - adhesions *—see* Adhesions, iris
  - atrophy *—see* Atrophy, iris
  - chamber angle recession *—see* Recession, chamber angle
  - cyst *—see* Cyst, iris
  - degeneration *—see* Degeneration, iris
  - in diseases classified elsewhere H22
  - iridodialysis *—see* Iridodialysis
  - iridoschisis *—see* Iridoschisis
  - miotic pupillary cyst *—see* Cyst, pupillary
  - pupillary
    - abnormality *—see* Abnormality, pupillary
    - membrane *—see* Membrane, pupillary
  - specified type NEC H21.89
  - vascular NEC H21.1X-
- iron metabolism E83.10
  - specified NEC E83.19

Disorder *(continued)*
- isovaleric acidemia E71.110
- jaw, developmental M27.0
  - temporomandibular (*see* Anomaly, dentofacial, temporomandibular joint) M26.60-
- joint M25.9
  - derangement *—see* Derangement, joint
  - effusion *—see* Effusion, joint
  - fistula *—see* Fistula, joint
  - hemarthrosis *—see* Hemarthrosis
  - instability *—see* Instability, joint
  - osteophyte *—see* Osteophyte
  - pain *—see* Pain, joint
  - psychogenic F45.8
  - specified type NEC M25.80
    - ankle M25.87-
    - elbow M25.82-
    - foot joint M25.87-
    - hand joint M25.84-
    - hip M25.85-
    - knee M25.86-
    - shoulder M25.81-
    - wrist M25.83-
  - stiffness *—see* Stiffness, joint
- ketone metabolism E71.32
- kidney N28.9
  - functional (tubular) N25.9
  - in
    - schistosomiasis B65.9 *[N29]*
  - tubular function N25.9
    - specified NEC N25.89
- lacrimal system H04.9
  - changes H04.69
    - fistula *—see* Fistula, lacrimal
  - gland H04.19
    - atrophy *—see* Atrophy, lacrimal gland
    - cyst *—see* Cyst, lacrimal, gland
    - dacryops *—see* Dacryops
    - dislocation *—see* Dislocation, lacrimal gland
    - dry eye syndrome *—see* Syndrome, dry eye
    - infection *—see* Dacryoadenitis
  - granuloma *—see* Granuloma, lacrimal
  - inflammation *—see* Inflammation, lacrimal
  - obstruction *—see* Obstruction, lacrimal
  - specified NEC H04.89
- lactation NEC O92.79
- language (developmental) F80.9
  - expressive F80.1
  - mixed receptive and expressive F80.2
  - receptive F80.2
- late luteal phase dysphoric N94.89
- learning (specific) F81.9
  - acalculia R48.8
  - alexia R48.0
  - mathematics F81.2
  - reading F81.0
  - specified
    - with impairment in
      - mathematics F81.2
      - reading F81.0
      - written expression F81.81
  - specified NEC F81.89
  - spelling F81.81
  - written expression F81.81
- lens H27.9
  - aphakia *—see* Aphakia
  - cataract *—see* Cataract
  - dislocation *—see* Dislocation, lens
  - specified type NEC H27.8
- ligament M24.20
  - ankle M24.27-
  - attachment, spine *—see* Enthesopathy, spinal

Disorder *(continued)*
- ligament *(continued)*
  - elbow M24.22-
  - foot joint M24.27-
  - hand joint M24.24-
  - hip M24.25-
  - knee *—see* Derangement, knee, specified NEC
  - shoulder M24.21-
  - vertebra M24.28
  - wrist M24.23-
- ligamentous attachments *—see also* Enthesopathy
  - spine *—see* Enthesopathy, spinal
- lipid
  - metabolism, congenital E78.9
  - storage E75.6
    - specified NEC E75.5
- lipoprotein
  - deficiency (familial) E78.6
  - metabolism E78.9
    - specified NEC E78.89
- liver K76.9
  - malarial B54 *[K77]*
- low back *—see also* Dorsopathy, specified NEC
- lumbosacral
  - plexus G54.1
  - root (nerve) NEC G54.4
- lung, interstitial, drug-induced J70.4
  - acute J70.2
  - chronic J70.3
- lymphoproliferative, post-transplant (PTLD) D47.Z1
- lysine and hydroxylysine metabolism E72.3
- male
  - erectile (organic) (*see also* Dysfunction, sexual, male, erectile) N52.9
    - nonorganic F52.21
  - hypoactive sexual desire F52.0
  - orgasmic F52.32
- major neurocognitive *—see* Dementia, in (due to)
- manic F30.9
  - organic F06.33
- mast cell activation *—see* Activation, mast cell
- mastoid *—see also* Disorder, ear, middle
  - postprocedural *—see* Complications, ear, procedure
- meniscus *—see* Derangement, knee, meniscus
- menopausal N95.9
  - specified NEC N95.8
- menstrual N92.6
  - psychogenic F45.8
  - specified NEC N92.5
- mental (or behavioral) (nonpsychotic) F99
  - due to (secondary to)
    - amphetamine
      - due to drug abuse *—see* Abuse, drug, stimulant
      - due to drug dependence *—see* Dependence, drug, stimulant
    - brain disease, damage and dysfunction F09
    - caffeine use
      - due to drug abuse *—see* Abuse, drug, stimulant
      - due to drug dependence *—see* Dependence, drug, stimulant
    - cannabis use
      - due to drug abuse *—see* Abuse, drug, cannabis

Disorder *(continued)*
- mental *(continued)*
  - due to *(continued)*
    - cannabis use *(continued)*
      - due to drug dependence *—see* Dependence, drug, cannabis
    - general medical condition F09
    - sedative or hypnotic use
      - due to drug abuse *—see* Abuse, drug, sedative
      - due to drug dependence *—see* Dependence, drug, sedative
    - tobacco (nicotine) use *—see* Dependence, drug, nicotine
  - following organic brain damage F07.9
    - frontal lobe syndrome F07.0
    - personality change F07.0
    - postconcussional syndrome F07.81
    - specified NEC F07.89
  - infancy, childhood or adolescence F98.9
  - neurotic *—see* Neurosis
  - organic or symptomatic F09
  - presenile, psychotic F03
  - problem NEC
  - psychoneurotic *—see* Neurosis
  - psychotic *—see* Psychosis
  - puerperal F53
  - senile, psychotic NEC F03
- metabolic, amino acid, transitory, newborn P74.8
- metabolism NOS E88.9
  - amino-acid E72.9
    - aromatic E70.9
      - albinism *—see* Albinism
      - histidine E70.40
        - histidinemia E70.41
        - other specified E70.49
      - hyperphenylalaninemia E70.1
        - classical phenylketonuria E70.0
      - other specified E70.8
      - tryptophan E70.5
      - tyrosine E70.20
        - hypertyrosinemia E70.21
        - other specified E70.29
    - branched chain E71.2
      - 3-methylglutaconic aciduria E71.111
      - hyperleucine-isoleucinemia E71.19
      - hypervalinemia E71.19
      - isovaleric acidemia E71.110
      - maple syrup urine disease E71.0
      - methylmalonic acidemia E71.120
      - organic aciduria NEC E71.118
      - other specified E71.19
      - proprionate NEC E71.128
      - proprionic acidemia E71.121
    - glycine E72.50
      - d-glycericacidemia E72.59
      - hyperhydroxyprolinemia E72.59
      - hyperoxaluria E72.53
      - hyperprolinemia E72.59
      - non-ketotic hyperglycinemia E72.51
      - other specified E72.59
      - sarcosinemia E72.59
      - trimethylaminuria E72.52
    - hydroxylysine E72.3
    - lysine E72.3
    - ornithine E72.4

- **Disorder** *(continued)*
  - metabolism *(continued)*
    - amino-acid *(continued)*
      - other specified E72.8
        - beta-amino acid E72.8
        - gamma-glutamyl cycle E72.8
      - straight-chain E72.8
      - sulfur-bearing E72.10
        - homocystinuria E72.11
        - methylenetetrahydrofolate reductase deficiency E72.12
        - other specified E72.19
    - bile acid and cholesterol metabolism E78.70
    - bilirubin E80.7
      - specified NEC E80.6
    - calcium E83.50
      - hypercalcemia E83.52
      - hypocalcemia E83.51
      - other specified E83.59
    - carbohydrate E74.9
      - specified NEC E74.8
    - cholesterol and bile acid metabolism E78.70
    - congenital E88.9
    - copper E83.00
      - Wilson's disease E83.01
      - specified type NEC E83.09
    - cystinuria E72.01
    - fructose E74.10
    - galactose E74.20
    - glucosaminoglycan E76.9
      - mucopolysaccharidosis *—see* Mucopolysaccharidosis
      - specified NEC E76.8
    - glutamine E72.8
    - glycine E72.50
    - glycogen storage (hepatorenal) E74.09
    - glycoprotein E77.9
      - specified NEC E77.8
    - glycosaminoglycan E76.9
      - specified NEC E76.8
    - in labor and delivery O75.89
    - iron E83.10
    - isoleucine E71.19
    - leucine E71.19
    - lipoid E78.9
    - lipoprotein E78.9
      - specified NEC E78.89
    - magnesium E83.40
      - hypermagnesemia E83.41
      - hypomagnesemia E83.42
      - other specified E83.49
    - mineral E83.9
      - specified NEC E83.89
    - mitochondrial E88.40
      - MELAS syndrome E88.41
      - MERRF syndrome (myoclonic epilepsy associated with ragged-red fibers) E88.42
      - other specified E88.49
    - ornithine E72.4
    - phosphatases E83.30
    - phosphorus E83.30
      - acid phosphatase deficiency E83.39
      - hypophosphatasia E83.39
      - hypophosphatemia E83.39
        - familial E83.31
      - other specified E83.39
      - pseudovitamin D deficiency E83.32
    - plasma protein NEC E88.09
    - porphyrin *—see* Porphyria
    - postprocedural E89.89
      - specified NEC E89.89
    - purine E79.9
      - specified NEC E79.8
    - pyrimidine E79.9
      - specified NEC E79.8
    - pyruvate E74.4
    - serine E72.8
    - sodium E87.8
    - specified NEC E88.89
    - threonine E72.8
    - valine E71.19
    - zinc E83.2
  - methylmalonic acidemia E71.120
  - micturition NEC (*see also* Difficulty, micturition) R39.198
    - feeling of incomplete emptying R39.14
    - hesitancy R39.11
    - poor stream R39.12
    - psychogenic F45.8
    - split stream R39.13
    - straining R39.16
    - urgency R39.15
  - mild neurocognitive G31.84
  - mitochondrial metabolism E88.40
  - mitral (valve) *—see* Endocarditis, mitral
  - mixed
    - anxiety and depressive F41.8
    - of scholastic skills (developmental) F81.89
    - receptive expressive language F80.2
  - mood F39
    - bipolar *—see* Disorder, bipolar
    - depressive *—see* Disorder, depressive
    - due to (secondary to)
      - alcohol F10.94
      - amphetamine F15.94
        - in
          - abuse F15.14
          - dependence F15.24
      - anxiolytic F13.94
        - in
          - abuse F13.14
          - dependence F13.24
      - cocaine F14.94
        - in
          - abuse F14.14
          - dependence F14.24
      - general medical condition F06.30
      - hallucinogen F16.94
        - in
          - abuse F16.14
          - dependence F16.24
      - hypnotic F13.94
        - in
          - abuse F13.14
          - dependence F13.24
      - inhalant F18.94
        - in
          - abuse F18.14
          - dependence F18.24
      - opioid F11.94
        - in
          - abuse F11.14
          - dependence F11.24
      - phencyclidine (PCP) F16.94
        - in
          - abuse F16.14
          - dependence F16.24
      - physiological condition F06.30
        - with
          - depressive features F06.31
          - major depressive-like episode F06.32
          - manic features F06.33
          - mixed features F06.34
      - psychoactive substance NEC F19.94
        - in
          - abuse F19.14
          - dependence F19.24
      - sedative F13.94
        - in
          - abuse F13.14
          - dependence F13.24
      - volatile solvents F18.94
        - in
          - abuse F18.14
          - dependence F18.24
    - manic episode F30.9
      - with psychotic symptoms F30.2
      - in remission (full) F30.4
        - partial F30.3
      - specified type NEC F30.8
      - without psychotic symptoms F30.10
        - mild F30.11
        - moderate F30.12
        - severe F30.13
    - organic F06.30
      - right hemisphere F07.89
    - persistent F34.9
      - cyclothymia F34.0
      - dysthymia F34.1
      - specified type NEC F34.89
    - recurrent F39
    - right hemisphere organic F07.89
  - movement G25.9
    - drug-induced G25.70
      - akathisia G25.71
      - specified NEC G25.79
    - hysterical F44.4
    - in diseases classified elsewhere *—see* category G26
    - periodic limb G47.61
      - sleep related G47.61
    - specified NEC G25.89
    - sleep related NEC G47.69
    - stereotyped F98.4
    - treatment-induced G25.9
  - multiple personality F44.81
  - muscle M62.9
    - attachment, spine *—see* Enthesopathy, spinal
    - in trichinellosis *—see* Trichinellosis, with muscle disorder
    - psychogenic F45.8
    - specified type NEC M62.89
    - tone, newborn P94.9
      - specified NEC P94.8
  - muscular
    - attachments *—see also* Enthesopathy
      - spine *—see* Enthesopathy, spinal
    - urethra N36.44
  - musculoskeletal system, soft tissue *—see* Disorder, soft tissue
    - postprocedural M96.89
    - psychogenic F45.8
  - myoneural G70.9
    - due to lead G70.1
    - specified NEC G70.89
    - toxic G70.1
  - myotonic NEC G71.19
  - nail, in diseases classified elsewhere L62
  - neck region NEC *—see* Dorsopathy, specified NEC
  - neonatal onset multisystemic inflammatory (NOMID) M04.2
  - nerve G58.9
    - abducent NEC *—see* Strabismus, paralytic, sixth nerve
    - accessory G52.8
    - acoustic *—see* subcategory H93.3
    - auditory *—see* subcategory H93.3
    - auriculotemporal G50.8
    - axillary G54.0
    - cerebral *—see* Disorder, nerve, cranial
    - cranial G52.9
      - eighth *—see* subcategory H93.3
      - eleventh G52.8
      - fifth G50.9
      - first G52.0
      - fourth NEC *—see* Strabismus, paralytic, fourth nerve
      - multiple G52.7
      - ninth G52.1
      - second NEC *—see* Disorder, nerve, optic
      - seventh NEC G51.8
      - sixth NEC *—see* Strabismus, paralytic, sixth nerve
      - specified NEC G52.8
      - tenth G52.2
      - third NEC *—see* Strabismus, paralytic, third nerve
      - twelfth G52.3
    - entrapment *—see* Neuropathy, entrapment
    - facial G51.9
      - specified NEC G51.8
    - femoral *—see* Lesion, nerve, femoral
    - glossopharyngeal NEC G52.1
    - hypoglossal G52.3
    - intercostal G58.0
    - lateral
      - cutaneous of thigh *—see* Mononeuropathy, lower limb, meralgia paresthetica
      - popliteal *—see* Lesion, nerve, popliteal
    - lower limb *—see* Mononeuropathy, lower limb
    - medial popliteal *—see* Lesion, nerve, popliteal, medial
    - median NEC *—see* Lesion, nerve, median
    - multiple G58.7
    - oculomotor NEC *—see* Strabismus, paralytic, third nerve
    - olfactory G52.0
    - optic NEC H47.09-
      - hemorrhage into sheath *—see* Hemorrhage, optic nerve
      - ischemic H47.01-
    - peroneal *—see* Lesion, nerve, popliteal
    - phrenic G58.8
    - plantar *—see* Lesion, nerve, plantar
    - pneumogastric G52.2
    - posterior tibial *—see* Syndrome, tarsal tunnel
    - radial *—see* Lesion, nerve, radial
    - recurrent laryngeal G52.2
    - root G54.9
      - cervical G54.2
      - lumbosacral G54.1
      - specified NEC G54.8
      - thoracic G54.3
    - sciatic NEC *—see* Lesion, nerve, sciatic
    - specified NEC G58.8
      - lower limb *—see* Mononeuropathy, lower limb, specified NEC
      - upper limb *—see* Mononeuropathy, upper limb, specified NEC
    - sympathetic G90.9

Disorder *(continued)*
- nerve *(continued)*
  - tibial *—see* Lesion, nerve, popliteal, medial
  - trigeminal G50.9
    - specified NEC G50.8
  - trochlear NEC *—see* Strabismus, paralytic, fourth nerve
  - ulnar *—see* Lesion, nerve, ulnar
  - upper limb *—see* Mononeuropathy, upper limb
  - vagus G52.2
- nervous system G98.8
  - autonomic (peripheral) G90.9
    - specified NEC G90.8
  - central G96.9
    - specified NEC G96.8
  - parasympathetic G90.9
  - specified NEC G98.8
  - sympathetic G90.9
  - vegetative G90.9
- neurocognitive R41.9
  - major
    - with
      - aggressive behavior F01.51
      - combative behavior F01.51
      - violent behavior F01.51
    - due to vascular disease, with behavioral disturbance F01.51
    - in (due to) (other diseases classified elsewhere) (*see also* Dementia, in (due to)) F02.80
      - with
        - aggressive behavior F02.81
        - combative behavior F02.81
        - violent behavior F02.81
      - without behavioral disturbance F01.50
  - mild G31.84
- neurodevelopment F89
  - specified NEC F88
- neurohypophysis NEC E23.3
- neurological NEC R29.818
- neuromuscular G70.9
  - hereditary NEC G71.9
  - specified NEC G70.89
  - toxic G70.1
- neurotic F48.9
  - specified NEC F48.8
- neutrophil, polymorphonuclear D71
- nicotine use *—see* Dependence, drug, nicotine
- nightmare F51.5
- non-rapid eye movement sleep arousal
  - sleep terror type F51.4
  - sleepwalking type F51.3
- nose J34.9
  - specified NEC J34.89
- obsessive-compulsive F42.9
  - and related disorder due to a known physiological condition F06.8
- odontogenesis NOS K00.9
- opioid use
  - with
    - opioid-induced psychotic disorder F11.959
      - with
        - delusions F11.950
        - hallucinations F11.951
  - due to drug abuse *—see* Abuse, drug, opioid
  - due to drug dependence *—see* Dependence, drug, opioid
  - mild F11.10
    - with
      - opioid-induced
        - anxiety disorder F11.188

Disorder *(continued)*
- opioid use *(continued)*
  - mild *(continued)*
    - with *(continued)*
      - opioid-induced *(continued)*
        - depressive disorder F11.14
        - sexual dysfunction F11.181
      - opioid intoxication
        - with perceptual disturbances F11.122
        - delirium F11.121
        - without perceptual disturbances F11.129
    - in remission (early) (sustained) F11.11
  - moderate or severe F11.20
    - with
      - opioid-induced
        - anxiety disorder F11.288
        - anxiety disorder F11.988
        - depressive disorder F11.24
        - depressive disorder F11.94
        - sexual dysfunction F11.281
        - sexual dysfunction F11.981
      - opioid intoxication
        - with perceptual disturbances F11.222
        - delirium F11.221
        - without perceptual disturbances F11.229
    - in remission (early) (sustained) F11.21
- oppositional defiant F91.3
- optic
  - chiasm H47.49
    - due to
      - inflammatory disorder H47.41
      - neoplasm H47.42
      - vascular disorder H47.43
  - disc H47.39-
    - coloboma *—see* Coloboma, optic disc
    - drusen *—see* Drusen, optic disc
    - pseudopapilledema *—see* Pseudopapilledema
  - radiations *—see* Disorder, visual, pathway
  - tracts *—see* Disorder, visual, pathway
- orbit H05.9
  - cyst *—see* Cyst, orbit
  - deformity *—see* Deformity, orbit
  - edema *—see* Edema, orbit
  - enophthalmos *—see* Enophthalmos
  - exophthalmos *—see* Exophthalmos
  - hemorrhage *—see* Hemorrhage, orbit
  - inflammation *—see* Inflammation, orbit
  - myopathy *—see* Myopathy, extraocular muscles
  - retained foreign body *—see* Foreign body, orbit, old
  - specified type NEC H05.89
- organic
  - anxiety F06.4
  - catatonic F06.1
  - delusional F06.2
  - dissociative F06.8
  - emotionally labile (asthenic) F06.8
  - mood (affective) F06.30
  - schizophrenia-like F06.2
- orgasmic (female) F52.31
  - male F52.32
- ornithine metabolism E72.4
- overanxious F41.1
  - of childhood F93.8

Disorder *(continued)*
- pain
  - with related psychological factors F45.42
  - exclusively related to psychological factors F45.41
  - genito-pelvic penetration disorder F52.6
- pancreatic internal secretion E16.9
  - specified NEC E16.8
- panic F41.0
  - with agoraphobia F40.01
- papulosquamous L44.9
  - in diseases classified elsewhere L45
  - specified NEC L44.8
- paranoid F22
  - induced F24
  - shared F24
- paraphilic F65.9
  - specified NEC F65.89
- parathyroid (gland) E21.5
  - specified NEC E21.4
- parietoalveolar NEC J84.09
- paroxysmal, mixed R56.9
- patella M22.9-
  - chondromalacia *—see* Chondromalacia, patella
  - derangement NEC M22.3X-
  - recurrent
    - dislocation *—see* Dislocation, patella, recurrent
    - subluxation *—see* Dislocation, patella, recurrent, incomplete
  - specified NEC M22.8X-
- patellofemoral M22.2X-
- pedophilic F65.4
- pentose phosphate pathway with anemia D55.1
- perception, due to hallucinogens F16.983
  - in
    - abuse F16.183
    - dependence F16.283
- peripheral nervous system NEC G64
- peroxisomal E71.50
  - biogenesis
    - neonatal adrenoleukodystrophy E71.511
    - specified disorder NEC E71.518
    - Zellweger syndrome E71.510
  - rhizomelic chondrodysplasia punctata E71.540
  - specified form NEC E71.548
    - group 1 E71.518
    - group 2 E71.53
    - group 3 E71.542
  - X-linked adrenoleukodystrophy E71.529
    - adolescent E71.521
    - adrenomyeloneuropathy E71.522
    - childhood E71.520
    - specified form NEC E71.528
  - Zellweger-like syndrome E71.541
- persistent
  - (somatoform) pain F45.41
  - affective (mood) F34.9
- personality *—see also* Personality F60.9
  - affective F34.0
  - aggressive F60.3
  - amoral F60.2
  - anankastic F60.5
  - antisocial F60.2
  - anxious F60.6
  - asocial F60.2
  - asthenic F60.7
  - avoidant F60.6
  - borderline F60.3
  - change (secondary) due to general medical condition F07.0
  - compulsive F60.5

Disorder *(continued)*
- personality *(continued)*
  - cyclothymic F34.0
  - dependent (passive) F60.7
  - depressive F34.1
  - dissocial F60.2
  - emotional instability F60.3
  - expansive paranoid F60.0
  - explosive F60.3
  - following organic brain damage F07.9
  - histrionic F60.4
  - hyperthymic F34.0
  - hypothymic F34.1
  - hysterical F60.4
  - immature F60.89
  - inadequate F60.7
  - labile F60.3
  - mixed (nonspecific) F60.89
  - moral deficiency F60.2
  - narcissistic F60.81
  - negativistic F60.89
  - obsessional F60.5
  - obsessive (-compulsive) F60.5
  - organic F07.9
  - overconscientious F60.5
  - paranoid F60.0
  - passive (-dependent) F60.7
  - passive-aggressive F60.89
  - pathological NEC F60.9
  - pseudosocial F60.2
  - psychopathic F60.2
  - schizoid F60.1
  - schizotypal F21
  - self-defeating F60.7
  - specified NEC F60.89
  - type A F60.5
  - unstable (emotional) F60.3
- pervasive, developmental F84.9
- phencyclidine use
  - mild F16.10
    - with
      - phencyclidine-induced
        - anxiety disorder F16.180
        - bipolar and related disorder F16.14
        - depressive disorder F16.14
        - psychotic disorder F16.159
      - phencyclidine intoxication F16.129
      - phencyclidine intoxication delirium F16.121
    - in remission (early) (sustained) F16.11
  - moderate or severe F16.20
    - with
      - phencyclidine-induced
        - anxiety disorder F16.280
        - bipolar and related disorder F16.24
        - depressive disorder F16.24
        - psychotic disorder F16.259
      - phencyclidine intoxication F16.229
      - phencyclidine intoxication delirium F16.221
    - in remission (early) (sustained) F16.21
- phobic anxiety, childhood F40.8
- phosphate-losing tubular N25.0
- pigmentation L81.9
  - choroid, congenital Q14.3
  - diminished melanin formation L81.6
  - iron L81.8
  - specified NEC L81.8
- pinna (noninfective) H61.10-
  - deformity, acquired H61.11-
  - hematoma H61.12-
  - perichondritis *—see* Perichondritis, ear
  - specified type NEC H61.19-

Disorder *(continued)*
  pituitary gland E23.7
    iatrogenic (postprocedural) E89.3
    specified NEC E23.6
  platelets D69.1
  plexus G54.9
    specified NEC G54.8
  polymorphonuclear neutrophils D71
  porphyrin metabolism *—see* Porphyria
  postconcussional F07.81
  posthallucinogen perception F16.983
    in
      abuse F16.183
      dependence F16.283
  postmenopausal N95.9
    specified NEC N95.8
  postprocedural (postoperative) *—see* Complications, postprocedural
  post-transplant lymphoproliferative D47.Z1
  post-traumatic stress (PTSD) F43.10
    acute F43.11
    chronic F43.12
  premenstrual dysphoric (PMDD) F32.81
  prepuce N47.8
  propionic acidemia E71.121
  prostate N42.9
    specified NEC N42.89
  psychogenic NOS (*see also* condition) F45.9
    anxiety F41.8
    appetite F50.9
    asthenic F48.8
    cardiovascular (system) F45.8
    compulsive F42.8
    cutaneous F54
    depressive F32.9
    digestive (system) F45.8
    dysmenorrheic F45.8
    dyspneic F45.8
    endocrine (system) F54
    eye NEC F45.8
    feeding *—see* Disorder, eating
    functional NEC F45.8
    gastric F45.8
    gastrointestinal (system) F45.8
    genitourinary (system) F45.8
    heart (function) (rhythm) F45.8
    hyperventilatory F45.8
    hypochondriacal *—see* Disorder, hypochondriacal
    intestinal F45.8
    joint F45.8
    learning F81.9
    limb F45.8
    lymphatic (system) F45.8
    menstrual F45.8
    micturition F45.8
    monoplegic NEC F44.4
    motor F44.4
    muscle F45.8
    musculoskeletal F45.8
    neurocirculatory F45.8
    obsessive F42.8
    occupational F48.8
    organ or part of body NEC F45.8
    paralytic NEC F44.4
    phobic F40.9
    physical NEC F45.8
    rectal F45.8
    respiratory (system) F45.8
    rheumatic F45.8
    sexual (function) F52.9
    skin (allergic) (eczematous) F54
    sleep F51.9
    specified part of body NEC F45.8
    stomach F45.8
  psychological F99
    associated with
      disease classified elsewhere F54
      sexual
        development F66
        relationship F66
      uncertainty about gender identity F64.9
  psychomotor NEC F44.4
    hysterical F44.4
  psychoneurotic *—see also* Neurosis
    mixed NEC F48.8
  psychophysiologic *—see* Disorder, somatoform
  psychosexual F65.9
    development F66
    identity of childhood F64.2
  psychosomatic NOS *—see* Disorder, somatoform
    multiple F45.0
    undifferentiated F45.1
  psychotic *—see* Psychosis
    transient (acute) F23
  puberty E30.9
    specified NEC E30.8
  pulmonary (valve) *—see* Endocarditis, pulmonary
  purine metabolism E79.9
  pyrimidine metabolism E79.9
  pyruvate metabolism E74.4
  reactive attachment (childhood) F94.1
  reading R48.0
    developmental (specific) F81.0
  receptive language F80.2
  receptor, hormonal, peripheral (*see also* Syndrome, androgen insensitivity) E34.50
  recurrent brief depressive F33.8
  reflex R29.2
  refraction H52.7
    aniseikonia H52.32
    anisometropia H52.31
    astigmatism *—see* Astigmatism
    hypermetropia *—see* Hypermetropia
    myopia *—see* Myopia
    presbyopia H52.4
    specified NEC H52.6
  relationship F68.8
    due to sexual orientation F66
  REM sleep behavior G47.52
  renal function, impaired (tubular) N25.9
  resonance R49.9
    specified NEC R49.8
  respiratory function, impaired *—see also* Failure, respiration
    postprocedural *—see* Complication, postoperative, respiratory system
    psychogenic F45.8
  retina H35.9
    angioid streaks H35.33
    changes in vascular appearance H35.01-
    degeneration *—see* Degeneration, retina
    dystrophy (hereditary) *—see* Dystrophy, retina
    edema H35.81
    hemorrhage *—see* Hemorrhage, retina
    ischemia H35.82
    macular degeneration *—see* Degeneration, macula
    microaneurysms H35.04-
    microvascular abnormality NEC H35.09
    neovascularization *—see* Neovascularization, retina
    retinopathy *—see* Retinopathy

Disorder *(continued)*
  retina *(continued)*
    separation of layers H35.70
      central serous chorioretinopathy H35.71-
      pigment epithelium detachment (serous) H35.72-
        hemorrhagic H35.73-
    specified type NEC H35.89
    telangiectasis *—see* Telangiectasis, retina
    vasculitis *—see* Vasculitis, retina
  retroperitoneal K68.9
  right hemisphere organic affective F07.89
  rumination (infant or child) F98.21
  sacrum, sacrococcygeal NEC M53.3
  schizoaffective F25.9
    bipolar type F25.0
    depressive type F25.1
    manic type F25.0
    mixed type F25.0
    specified NEC F25.8
  schizoid of childhood F84.5
  schizophrenia spectrum and other psychotic disorder F29
    specified NEC F28
  schizophreniform F20.81
    brief F23
  schizotypal (personality) F21
  secretion, thyrocalcitonin E07.0
  sedative, hypnotic, or anxiolytic-induced
    mild F13.10
      with
        sedative, hypnotic, or anxiolytic-induced
          anxiety disorder F13.180
          bipolar and related disorder F13.14
          depressive disorder F13.14
          psychotic disorder F13.159
          sexual dysfunction F13.181
        sedative, hypnotic, or anxiolytic intoxication F13.129
        sedative, hypnotic, or anxiolytic intoxication delirium F13.121
      in remission (early) (sustained) F13.11
    moderate or severe F13.20
      with
        sedative, hypnotic, or anxiolytic-induced
          anxiety disorder F13.280
          bipolar and related disorder F13.24
          depressive disorder F13.24
          major neurocognitive disorder F13.27
          mild neurocognitive disorder F13.288
          psychotic disorder F13.259
          sexual dysfunction F13.281
        sedative, hypnotic, or anxiolytic intoxication F13.229
        sedative, hypnotic, or anxiolytic intoxication delirium F13.221
      in remission (early) (sustained) F13.21
  seizure (*see also* Epilepsy) G40.909
    intractable G40.919
      with status epilepticus G40.911
  semantic pragmatic F80.89
    with autism F84.0
  sense of smell R43.1
    psychogenic F45.8
  separation anxiety, of childhood F93.0

Disorder *(continued)*
  sexual
    arousal, female F52.22
    aversion F52.1
    function, psychogenic F52.9
    interest/arousal, female F52.22
    masochism F65.51
    maturation F66
    nonorganic F52.9
    preference (*see also* Deviation, sexual) F65.9
      fetishistic transvestism F65.1
    relationship F66
    sadism F65.52
  shyness, of childhood and adolescence F40.10
  sibling rivalry F93.8
  sickle-cell (sickling) (homozygous) *—see* Disease, sickle-cell
    heterozygous D57.3
    specified type NEC D57.8-
    trait D57.3
  sinus (nasal) J34.9
    specified NEC J34.89
  skin L98.9
    atrophic L90.9
      specified NEC L90.8
    granulomatous L92.9
      specified NEC L92.8
    hypertrophic L91.9
      specified NEC L91.8
    infiltrative NEC L98.6
    newborn P83.9
      specified NEC P83.88
    picking F42.4
    psychogenic (allergic) (eczematous) F54
  sleep G47.9
    breathing-related *—see* Apnea, sleep
    circadian rhythm G47.20
      advance sleep phase type G47.22
      delayed sleep phase type G47.21
      due to
        alcohol
          abuse F10.182
          dependence F10.282
          use F10.982
        amphetamines
          abuse F15.182
          dependence F15.282
          use F15.982
        caffeine
          abuse F15.182
          dependence F15.282
          use F15.982
        cocaine
          abuse F14.182
          dependence F14.282
          use F14.982
        drug NEC
          abuse F19.182
          dependence F19.282
          use F19.982
        opioid
          abuse F11.182
          dependence F11.282
          use F11.982
        psychoactive substance NEC
          abuse F19.182
          dependence F19.282
          use F19.982
        sedative, hypnotic, or anxiolytic
          abuse F13.182
          dependence F13.282
          use F13.982
        stimulant NEC
          abuse F15.182
          dependence F15.282
          use F15.982

Disorder *(continued)*
- sleep *(continued)*
  - circadian rhythm (continued)
    - due to *(continued)*
      - free running type G47.24
      - in conditions classified elsewhere G47.27
      - irregular sleep wake type G47.23
      - jet lag type G47.25
      - non-24-hour sleep-wake type G47.24
      - shift work type G47.26
      - specified NEC G47.29
  - due to
    - alcohol
      - abuse F10.182
      - dependence F10.282
      - use F10.982
    - amphetamine
      - abuse F15.182
      - dependence F15.282
      - use F15.982
    - anxiolytic
      - abuse F13.182
      - dependence F13.282
      - use F13.982
    - caffeine
      - abuse F15.182
      - dependence F15.282
      - use F15.982
    - cocaine
      - abuse F14.182
      - dependence F14.282
      - use F14.982
    - drug NEC
      - abuse F19.182
      - dependence F19.282
      - use F19.982
    - hypnotic
      - abuse F13.182
      - dependence F13.282
      - use F13.982
    - opioid
      - abuse F11.182
      - dependence F11.282
      - use F11.982
    - psychoactive substance NEC
      - abuse F19.182
      - dependence F19.282
      - use F19.982
    - sedative
      - abuse F13.182
      - dependence F13.282
      - use F13.982
    - stimulant NEC
      - abuse F15.182
      - dependence F15.282
      - use F15.982
  - emotional F51.9
  - excessive somnolence —*see* Hypersomnia
  - hypersomnia type —*see* Hypersomnia
  - initiating or maintaining —*see* Insomnia
  - nightmares F51.5
  - nonorganic F51.9
    - specified NEC F51.8
  - parasomnia type G47.50
  - specified NEC G47.8
  - terrors F51.4
  - walking F51.3
- sleep-wake pattern or schedule —(*see also* Disorder, sleep, circadian rhythm) G47.9
  - specified NEC G47.8
- social
  - anxiety (of childhood) F40.10
    - generalized F40.11
  - functioning in childhood F94.9
    - specified NEC F94.8

Disorder *(continued)*
- social *(continued)*
  - pragmatic F80.82
- soft tissue M79.9
  - ankle M79.9
  - due to use, overuse and pressure M70.90
    - ankle M70.97-
    - bursitis —*see* Bursitis
    - foot M70.97-
    - forearm M70.93-
    - hand M70.94-
    - lower leg M70.96-
    - multiple sites M70.99
    - pelvic region M70.95-
    - shoulder region M70.91-
    - specified site NEC M70.98
    - specified type NEC M70.80
      - ankle M70.87-
      - foot M70.87-
      - forearm M70.83-
      - hand M70.84-
      - lower leg M70.86-
      - multiple sites M70.89
      - pelvic region M70.85-
      - shoulder region M70.81-
      - specified site NEC M70.88
      - thigh M70.85-
      - upper arm M70.82-
    - thigh M70.95-
    - upper arm M70.92-
  - foot M79.9
  - forearm M79.9
  - hand M79.9
  - lower leg M79.9
  - multiple sites M79.9
  - occupational —*see* Disorder, soft tissue, due to use, overuse and pressure
  - pelvic region M79.9
  - shoulder region M79.9
  - specified type NEC M79.89
  - thigh M79.9
  - upper arm M79.9
- somatic symptom F45.1
- somatization F45.0
- somatoform F45.9
  - pain (persistent) F45.41
  - somatization (multiple) (long-lasting) F45.0
  - specified NEC F45.8
  - undifferentiated F45.1
- somnolence, excessive —*see* Hypersomnia
- specific
  - arithmetical F81.2
  - developmental, of motor F82
  - reading F81.0
  - speech and language F80.9
  - spelling F81.81
  - written expression F81.81
- speech R47.9
  - articulation (functional) (specific) F80.0
  - developmental F80.9
  - specified NEC R47.89
- speech-sound F80.0
- spelling (specific) F81.81
- spine —*see also* Dorsopathy
  - ligamentous or muscular attachments, peripheral —*see* Enthesopathy, spinal
  - specified NEC —*see* Dorsopathy, specified NEC
- stereotyped, habit or movement F98.4
- stimulant use (other) (unspecified)
  - mild F15.10
    - in remission (early) (sustained) F15.11
  - moderate or severe F15.20
    - in remission (early) (sustained) F15.21

Disorder *(continued)*
- stomach (functional) —*see* Disorder, gastric
- stress F43.9
  - acute F43.0
  - post-traumatic F43.10
    - acute F43.11
    - chronic F43.12
- substance use (other) (unknown)
  - mild F19.10
    - with substance-induced
      - anxiety disorder F19.180
      - bipolar and related disorder F19.14
      - depressive disorder F19.14
      - major neurocognitive disorder F19.17
      - mild neurocognitive disorder F19.188
      - obsessive-compulsive and related disorder F19.188
      - sexual dysfunction F19.181
    - substance intoxication F19.129
    - substance intoxication delirium F19.121
  - moderate or severe F19.20
    - with substance-induced
      - anxiety disorder F19.280
      - bipolar and related disorder F19.24
      - depressive disorder F19.24
      - major neurocognitive disorder F19.27
      - mild neurocognitive disorder F19.288
      - obsessive-compulsive and related disorder F19.288
      - sexual dysfunction F19.281
    - in remission (early) (sustained) F19.21
    - substance intoxication F19.229
    - substance intoxication delirium F19.221
- sulfur-bearing amino-acid metabolism E72.10
- sweat gland (eccrine) L74.9
  - apocrine L75.9
    - specified NEC L75.8
  - specified NEC L74.8
- synovium M67.90
  - acromioclavicular M67.91-
  - ankle M67.97-
  - elbow M67.92-
  - foot M67.97-
  - forearm M67.93-
  - hand M67.94-
  - hip M67.95-
  - knee M67.96-
  - multiple sites M67.99
  - rupture —*see* Rupture, synovium
  - shoulder M67.91-
  - specified type NEC M67.80
    - acromioclavicular M67.81-
    - ankle M67.87-
    - elbow M67.82-
    - foot M67.87-
    - hand M67.84-
    - hip M67.85-
    - knee M67.86-
    - multiple sites M67.89
    - wrist M67.83-
  - synovitis —*see* Synovitis
  - upper arm M67.92-
  - wrist M67.93-
- temperature regulation, newborn P81.9
  - specified NEC P81.8
- temporomandibular joint M26.60-
- tendon M67.90
  - acromioclavicular M67.91-
  - ankle M67.97-
  - contracture —*see* Contracture, tendon

Disorder *(continued)*
- tendon *(continued)*
  - elbow M67.92-
  - foot M67.97-
  - forearm M67.93-
  - hand M67.94-
  - hip M67.95-
  - knee M67.96-
  - multiple sites M67.99
  - rupture —*see* Rupture, tendon
  - shoulder M67.91-
  - specified type NEC M67.80
    - acromioclavicular M67.81-
    - ankle M67.87-
    - elbow M67.82-
    - foot M67.87-
    - hand M67.84-
    - hip M67.85-
    - knee M67.86-
    - multiple sites M67.89
    - trunk M67.88
    - wrist M67.83-
  - synovitis —*see* Synovitis
  - tendinitis —*see* Tendinitis
  - tenosynovitis —*see* Tenosynovitis
  - trunk M67.98
  - upper arm M67.92-
  - wrist M67.93-
- thoracic root (nerve) NEC G54.3
- thyrocalcitonin hypersecretion E07.0
- thyroid (gland) E07.9
  - function NEC, neonatal, transitory P72.2
  - iodine-deficiency related E01.8
  - specified NEC E07.89
- tic —*see* Tic
- tobacco use
  - chewing tobacco (mild) (moderate) (severe)
    - in remission (early) (sustained) F17.221
  - cigarettes (mild) (moderate) (severe)
    - in remission (early) (sustained) F17.211
  - mild Z72.0
    - in remission (early) (sustained) F17.201
  - moderate F17.200
    - in remission (early) (sustained) F17.201
  - severe F17.200
    - in remission (early) (sustained) F17.201
  - specified product NEC (mild) (moderate) (severe)
    - in remission (early) (sustained) F17.291
- tooth K08.9
  - development K00.9
    - specified NEC K00.8
  - eruption K00.6
- Tourette's F95.2
- trance and possession F44.89
- transvestic F65.1
- trauma and stressor-related F43.9
  - other specified F43.8
- tricuspid (valve) —*see* Endocarditis, tricuspid
- tryptophan metabolism E70.5
- tubular, phosphate-losing N25.0
- tubulo-interstitial (in)
  - brucellosis A23.9 *[N16]*
  - cystinosis E72.04
  - diphtheria A36.84
  - glycogen storage disease E74.00 *[N16]*
  - leukemia NEC C95.9- *[N16]*
  - lymphoma NEC C85.9- *[N16]*
  - mixed cryoglobulinemia D89.1 *[N16]*
  - multiple myeloma C90.0- *[N16]*

Disorder *(continued)*
- tubulo-interstitial *(continued)*
  - Salmonella infection A02.25
  - sarcoidosis D86.84
  - sepsis A41.9 *[N16]*
    - streptococcal A40.9 *[N16]*
  - systemic lupus erythematosus M32.15
  - toxoplasmosis B58.83
  - transplant rejection T86.91 *[N16]*
  - Wilson's disease E83.01 *[N16]*
- tubulo-renal function, impaired N25.9
  - specified NEC N25.89
- tympanic membrane H73.9-
  - atrophy —*see* Atrophy, tympanic membrane
  - infection —*see* Myringitis
  - perforation —*see* Perforation, tympanum
  - specified NEC H73.89-
- unsocialized aggressive F91.1
- urea cycle metabolism E72.20
  - argininemia E72.21
  - arginosuccinic aciduria E72.22
  - citrullinemia E72.23
  - ornithine transcarbamylase deficiency E72.4
  - other specified E72.29
- ureter (in) N28.9
  - schistosomiasis B65.0 *[N29]*
  - tuberculosis A18.11
- urethra N36.9
  - specified NEC N36.8
- urinary system N39.9
  - specified NEC N39.8
- valve, heart
  - aortic —*see* Endocarditis, aortic
  - mitral —*see* Endocarditis, mitral
  - pulmonary —*see* Endocarditis, pulmonary
  - rheumatic
    - aortic —*see* Endocarditis, aortic, rheumatic
    - mitral —*see* Endocarditis, mitral
    - pulmonary —*see* Endocarditis, pulmonary, rheumatic
    - tricuspid —*see* Endocarditis, tricuspid
  - tricuspid —*see* Endocarditis, tricuspid
- vestibular function H81.9-
  - specified NEC —*see* subcategory H81.8
    - in diseases classified elsewhere H82.-
  - vertigo —*see* Vertigo
- vision, binocular H53.30
  - abnormal retinal correspondence H53.31
  - diplopia H53.2
  - fusion with defective stereopsis H53.32
  - simultaneous perception H53.33
  - suppression H53.34
- visual
  - cortex
    - blindness H47.619
      - left brain H47.612
      - right brain H47.611
    - due to
      - inflammatory disorder H47.629
        - left brain H47.622
        - right brain H47.621
      - neoplasm H47.639
        - left brain H47.632
        - right brain H47.631
      - vascular disorder H47.649
        - left brain H47.642
        - right brain H47.641

Disorder *(continued)*
- visual *(continued)*
  - pathway H47.9
    - due to
      - inflammatory disorder H47.51-
      - neoplasm H47.52-
      - vascular disorder H47.53-
    - optic chiasm —*see* Disorder, optic, chiasm
- vitreous body H43.9
  - crystalline deposits —*see* Deposit, crystalline
  - degeneration —*see* Degeneration, vitreous
  - hemorrhage —*see* Hemorrhage, vitreous
  - opacities —*see* Opacity, vitreous
  - prolapse —*see* Prolapse, vitreous
  - specified type NEC H43.89
- voice R49.9
  - specified type NEC R49.8
- volatile solvent use
  - due to drug abuse —*see* Abuse, drug, inhalant
  - due to drug dependence —*see* Dependence, drug, inhalant
- voyeuristic F65.3
- white blood cells D72.9
  - specified NEC D72.89
- withdrawing, child or adolescent F40.10

Disorientation R41.0

Displacement, displaced
- acquired traumatic of bone, cartilage, joint, tendon NEC —*see* Dislocation
- adrenal gland (congenital) Q89.1
- appendix, retrocecal (congenital) Q43.8
- auricle (congenital) Q17.4
- bladder (acquired) N32.89
  - congenital Q64.19
- brachial plexus (congenital) Q07.8
- brain stem, caudal (congenital) Q04.8
- canaliculus (lacrimalis), congenital Q10.6
- cardia through esophageal hiatus (congenital) Q40.1
- cerebellum, caudal (congenital) Q04.8
- cervix —*see* Malposition, uterus
- colon (congenital) Q43.3
- device, implant or graft (*see also* Complications, by site and type, mechanical) T85.628
  - arterial graft NEC —*see* Complication, cardiovascular device, mechanical, vascular
  - breast (implant) T85.42
  - catheter NEC T85.628
    - dialysis (renal) T82.42
      - intraperitoneal T85.621
    - infusion NEC T82.524
      - spinal (epidural) (subdural) T85.620
    - urinary
      - cystostomy T83.020
      - Hopkins T83.028
      - ileostomy T83.028
      - indwelling T83.021
      - nephrostomy T83.022
      - specified NEC T83.028
      - urostomy T83.028
  - electronic (electrode) (pulse generator) (stimulator) —*see* Complication, electronic stimulator
  - fixation, internal (orthopedic) NEC —*see* Complication, fixation device, mechanical

Displacement, displaced *(continued)*
- device, implant or graft *(continued)*
  - gastrointestinal —*see* Complications, prosthetic device, mechanical, gastrointestinal device
  - genital NEC T83.428
    - intrauterine contraceptive device (string) T83.32
    - penile prosthesis (cylinder) (implanted) (pump) (resevoir) T83.420
    - testicular prosthesis T83.421
  - heart NEC —*see* Complication, cardiovascular device, mechanical
  - joint prosthesis —*see* Complications, joint prosthesis, mechanical
  - ocular —*see* Complications, prosthetic device, mechanical, ocular device
  - orthopedic NEC —*see* Complication, orthopedic, device or graft, mechanical
  - specified NEC T85.628
  - urinary NEC T83.128
    - graft T83.22
    - sphincter, implanted T83.121
    - stent (ileal conduit) (nephroureteral) T83.123
      - ureteral indwelling T83.122
  - vascular NEC —*see* Complication, cardiovascular device, mechanical
  - ventricular intracranial shunt T85.02
- electronic stimulator
  - bone T84.320
  - cardiac —*see* Complications, cardiac device, electronic
  - nervous system —*see* Complication, prosthetic device, mechanical, electronic nervous system stimulator
  - urinary —*see* Complications, electronic stimulator, urinary
- esophageal mucosa into cardia of stomach, congenital Q39.8
- esophagus (acquired) K22.8
  - congenital Q39.8
- eyeball (acquired) (lateral) (old) —*see* Displacement, globe
  - congenital Q15.8
  - current —*see* Avulsion, eye
- fallopian tube (acquired) N83.4-
  - congenital Q50.6
  - opening (congenital) Q50.6
- gallbladder (congenital) Q44.1
- gastric mucosa (congenital) Q40.2
- globe (acquired) (old) (lateral) H05.21-
  - current —*see* Avulsion, eye
- heart (congenital) Q24.8
  - acquired I51.89
- hymen (upward) (congenital) Q52.4
- intervertebral disc NEC
  - with myelopathy —*see* Disorder, disc, with, myelopathy
  - cervical, cervicothoracic (with) M50.20
    - myelopathy —*see* Disorder, disc, cervical, with myelopathy
    - neuritis, radiculitis or radiculopathy —*see* Disorder, disc, cervical, with neuritis
  - due to trauma —*see* Dislocation, vertebra

Displacement, displaced *(continued)*
- intervertebral disc NEC *(continued)*
  - lumbar region M51.26
    - with
      - myelopathy M51.06
      - neuritis, radiculitis, radiculopathy or sciatica M51.16
  - lumbosacral region M51.27
    - with
      - neuritis, radiculitis, radiculopathy or sciatica M51.17
  - sacrococcygeal region M53.3
  - thoracic region M51.24
    - with
      - myelopathy M51.04
      - neuritis, radiculitis, radiculopathy M51.14
  - thoracolumbar region M51.25
    - with
      - myelopathy M51.05
      - neuritis, radiculitis, radiculopathy M51.15
- intrauterine device (string) T83.32
- kidney (acquired) N28.83
  - congenital Q63.2
- lachrymal, lacrimal apparatus or duct (congenital) Q10.6
- lens, congenital Q12.1
- macula (congenital) Q14.1
- Meckel's diverticulum Q43.0
  - malignant —*see* Table of Neoplasms, small intestine, malignant
- nail (congenital) Q84.6
  - acquired L60.8
- opening of Wharton's duct in mouth Q38.4
- organ or site, congenital NEC —*see* Malposition, congenital
- ovary (acquired) N83.4-
  - congenital Q50.39
  - free in peritoneal cavity (congenital) Q50.39
  - into hernial sac N83.4-
- oviduct (acquired) N83.4-
  - congenital Q50.6
- parathyroid (gland) E21.4
- parotid gland (congenital) Q38.4
- punctum lacrimale (congenital) Q10.6
- sacro-iliac (joint) (congenital) Q74.2
  - current injury S33.2
  - old —*see* subcategory M53.2
- salivary gland (any) (congenital) Q38.4
- spleen (congenital) Q89.09
- stomach, congenital Q40.2
- sublingual duct Q38.4
- tongue (downward) (congenital) Q38.3
- tooth, teeth, fully erupted M26.30
  - horizontal M26.33
  - vertical M26.34
- trachea (congenital) Q32.1
- ureter or ureteric opening or orifice (congenital) Q62.62
- uterine opening of oviducts or fallopian tubes Q50.6
- uterus, uterine —*see* Malposition, uterus
- ventricular septum Q21.0
  - with rudimentary ventricle Q20.4

Disproportion
- between native and reconstructed breast N65.1
- fiber-type G71.2

Disruptio uteri —*see* Rupture, uterus

Disruption (of)
- ciliary body NEC H21.89
- closure of
  - cornea T81.31
  - craniotomy T81.32
  - fascia (muscular) (superficial) T81.32
  - internal organ or tissue T81.32
  - laceration (external) (internal) T81.33
  - ligament T81.32
  - mucosa T81.31
  - muscle or muscle flap T81.32
  - ribs or rib cage T81.32
  - skin and subcutaneous tissue (full-thickness) (superficial) T81.31
  - skull T81.32
  - sternum (sternotomy) T81.32
  - tendon T81.32
  - traumatic laceration (external) (internal) T81.33
- family Z63.8
  - due to
    - absence of family member due to military deployment Z63.31
    - absence of family member NEC Z63.32
    - alcoholism and drug addiction in family Z63.72
    - bereavement Z63.4
    - death (assumed) or disappearance of family member Z63.4
    - divorce or separation Z63.5
    - drug addiction in family Z63.72
    - return of family member from military deployment (current or past conflict) Z63.71
    - stressful life events NEC Z63.79
- iris NEC H21.89
- ligament(s) —*see also* Sprain
  - knee
    - current injury —*see* Dislocation, knee
    - old (chronic) —*see* Derangement, knee, ligament, instability, chronic
    - spontaneous NEC —*see* Derangement, knee, disruption ligament
- ossicular chain —*see* Discontinuity, ossicles, ear
- pelvic ring (stable) S32.810
  - unstable S32.811
- wound T81.30
  - episiotomy O90.1
  - operation T81.31
    - cesarean O90.0
    - external operation wound (superficial) T81.31
    - internal operation wound (deep) T81.32
  - perineal (obstetric) O90.1
  - traumatic injury repair T81.33
- traumatic injury wound repair T81.33

Dissatisfaction with
- employment Z56.9
- school environment Z55.4

Dissecting —*see* condition

Dissection
- aorta I71.00
  - abdominal I71.02
  - thoracic I71.01
  - thoracoabdominal I71.03
- artery I77.70
  - basilar (trunk) I77.75
  - carotid I77.71
  - cerebral (nonruptured) I67.0
    - ruptured —*see* Hemorrhage, intracranial, subarachnoid
  - coronary I25.42
  - extremity
    - lower I77.77
    - upper I77.76
  - iliac I77.72
  - precerebral
    - congenital (nonruptured) Q28.1
    - specified site NEC I77.75
  - renal I77.73
  - specified NEC I77.79
  - vertebral I77.74
- precerebral artery, congential (nonruptured) Q28.1
  - Heartland A93.8
- traumatic —*see* Wound, open, by site
- vascular I99.8
- wound —*see* Wound, open

Disseminated —*see* condition

Dissociation
- auriculoventricular or atrioventricular (AV) (any degree) (isorhythmic) I45.89
  - with heart block I44.2
- interference I45.89

Dissociative reaction, state F44.9

Dissolution, vertebra —*see* Osteoporosis

Distension, distention
- abdomen R14.0
- bladder N32.89
- cecum K63.89
- colon K63.89
- gallbladder K82.8
- intestine K63.89
- kidney N28.89
- liver K76.89
- seminal vesicle N50.89
- stomach K31.89
  - acute K31.0
  - psychogenic F45.8
- ureter —*see* Dilatation, ureter
- uterus N85.8

Distoma hepaticum infestation B66.3

Distomiasis B66.9
- bile passages B66.3
- hemic B65.9
- hepatic B66.3
  - due to Clonorchis sinensis B66.1
- intestinal B66.5
- liver B66.3
  - due to Clonorchis sinensis B66.1
- lung B66.4
- pulmonary B66.4

Distomolar (fourth molar) K00.1

Disto-occlusion (Division I) (Division II) M26.212

Distortion(s) (congenital)
- adrenal (gland) Q89.1
- arm NEC Q68.8
- bile duct or passage Q44.5
- bladder Q64.79
- brain Q04.9
- cervix (uteri) Q51.9
- chest (wall) Q67.8
  - bones Q76.8
- clavicle Q74.0
- clitoris Q52.6
- coccyx Q76.49
- common duct Q44.5
- coronary Q24.5
- cystic duct Q44.5
- ear (auricle) (external) Q17.3
  - inner Q16.5
  - middle Q16.4
    - ossicles Q16.3
- endocrine NEC Q89.2
- eustachian tube Q17.8
- eye (adnexa) Q15.8
- face bone(s) NEC Q75.8
- fallopian tube Q50.6
- femur NEC Q68.8
- fibula NEC Q68.8
- finger(s) Q68.1
- foot Q66.9
- genitalia, genital organ(s)
  - female Q52.8
    - external Q52.79
    - internal NEC Q52.8
- gyri Q04.8
- hand bone(s) Q68.1
- heart (auricle) (ventricle) Q24.8
  - valve (cusp) Q24.8
- hepatic duct Q44.5
- humerus NEC Q68.8
- hymen Q52.4
- intrafamilial communications Z63.8
- jaw NEC M26.89
- labium (majus) (minus) Q52.79
- leg NEC Q68.8
- lens Q12.8
- liver Q44.7
- lumbar spine Q76.49
  - with disproportion O33.8
    - causing obstructed labor O65.0
- lumbosacral (joint) (region) Q76.49
  - kyphosis —*see* Kyphosis, congenital
  - lordosis —*see* Lordosis, congenital
- nerve Q07.8
- nose Q30.8
- organ
  - of Corti Q16.5
  - or site not listed —*see* Anomaly, by site
- ossicles, ear Q16.3
- oviduct Q50.6
- pancreas Q45.3
- parathyroid (gland) Q89.2
- pituitary (gland) Q89.2
- radius NEC Q68.8
- sacroiliac joint Q74.2
- sacrum Q76.49
- scapula Q74.0
- shoulder girdle Q74.0
- skull bone(s) NEC Q75.8
  - with
    - anencephalus Q00.0
    - encephalocele —*see* Encephalocele
    - hydrocephalus Q03.9
      - with spina bifida —*see* Spina bifida, with hydrocephalus
    - microcephaly Q02
- spinal cord Q06.8
- spine Q76.49
  - kyphosis —*see* Kyphosis, congenital
  - lordosis —*see* Lordosis, congenital
- spleen Q89.09
- sternum NEC Q76.7
- thorax (wall) Q67.8
  - bony Q76.8
- thymus (gland) Q89.2
- thyroid (gland) Q89.2
- tibia NEC Q68.8
- toe(s) Q66.9
- tongue Q38.3
- trachea (cartilage) Q32.1
- ulna NEC Q68.8
- ureter Q62.8
- urethra Q64.79
  - causing obstruction Q64.39
- uterus Q51.9
- vagina Q52.4
- vertebra Q76.49
  - kyphosis —*see* Kyphosis, congenital
  - lordosis —*see* Lordosis, congenital
- visual —*see also* Disturbance, vision
  - shape and size H53.15
- vulva Q52.79
- wrist (bones) (joint) Q68.8

Distress
- abdomen —*see* Pain, abdominal
- acute respiratory R06.03
  - syndrome (adult) (child) J80
- epigastric R10.13
- fetal P84
  - complicating pregnancy —*see* Stress, fetal
- gastrointestinal (functional) K30
  - psychogenic F45.8
- intestinal (functional) NOS K59.9
  - psychogenic F45.8
- maternal, during labor and delivery O75.0
- relationship, with spouse or intimate partner Z63.0
- respiratory (adult) (child) R06.03
  - newborn P22.9
    - specified NEC P22.8
  - orthopnea R06.01
  - psychogenic F45.8
  - shortness of breath R06.02
  - specified type NEC R06.09

Distribution vessel, atypical Q27.9
- coronary artery Q24.5
- precerebral Q28.1

Districhiasis L68.8

Disturbance(s) —*see also* Disease
- absorption K90.9
  - calcium E58
  - carbohydrate K90.49
  - fat K90.49
    - pancreatic K90.3
  - protein K90.49
  - starch K90.49
  - vitamin —*see* Deficiency, vitamin
- acid-base equilibrium E87.8
  - mixed E87.4
- activity and attention (with hyperkinesis) —*see* Disorder, attention-deficit hyperactivity
- amino acid transport E72.00
- assimilation, food K90.9
- auditory nerve, except deafness —*see* subcategory H93.3
- behavior —*see* Disorder, conduct
- blood clotting (mechanism) (*see also* Defect, coagulation) D68.9
- cerebral
  - nerve —*see* Disorder, nerve, cranial
  - status, newborn P91.9
    - specified NEC P91.88
- circulatory I99.9
- conduct (*see also* Disorder, conduct) F91.9
  - adjustment reaction —*see* Disorder, adjustment
  - compulsive F63.9
  - disruptive F91.9
  - hyperkinetic —*see* Disorder, attention-deficit hyperactivity
  - socialized F91.2
  - specified NEC F91.8
  - unsocialized F91.1
- coordination R27.8
- cranial nerve —*see* Disorder, nerve, cranial

Disturbance *(continued)*
- deep sensibility *—see* Disturbance, sensation
- digestive K30
  - psychogenic F45.8
- electrolyte *—see also* Imbalance, electrolyte
  - newborn, transitory P74.4
    - hyperammonemia P74.6
    - potassium balance P74.3
    - sodium balance P74.2
    - specified type NEC P74.4
- emotions specific to childhood and adolescence F93.9
  - with
    - anxiety and fearfulness NEC F93.8
    - elective mutism F94.0
    - oppositional disorder F91.3
    - sensitivity (withdrawal) F40.10
    - shyness F40.10
    - social withdrawal F40.10
  - involving relationship problems F93.8
  - mixed F93.8
  - specified NEC F93.8
- endocrine (gland) E34.9
  - neonatal, transitory P72.9
    - specified NEC P72.8
- equilibrium R42
- fructose metabolism E74.10
- gait *—see* Gait
  - hysterical F44.4
  - psychogenic F44.4
- gastrointestinal (functional) K30
  - psychogenic F45.8
- habit, child F98.9
- hearing, except deafness and tinnitus *—see* Abnormal, auditory perception
- heart, functional (conditions in I44-I50)
  - due to presence of (cardiac) prosthesis I97.19-
  - postoperative I97.89
    - cardiac surgery (*see also* Infarct, myocardium, associated with revascularization procedure) I97.19-
- hormones E34.9
- innervation uterus (parasympathetic) (sympathetic) N85.8
- keratinization NEC
  - gingiva K05.10
    - nonplaque induced K05.11
    - plaque induced K05.10
  - lip K13.0
  - oral (mucosa) (soft tissue) K13.29
  - tongue K13.29
- learning (specific) *—see* Disorder, learning
- memory *—see* Amnesia
  - mild, following organic brain damage F06.8
- mental F99
  - associated with diseases classified elsewhere F54
- metabolism E88.9
  - with
    - abortion *—see* Abortion, by type with other specified complication
    - ectopic pregnancy O08.5
    - molar pregnancy O08.5
  - amino-acid E72.9
    - aromatic E70.9
    - branched-chain E71.2
    - straight-chain E72.8
    - sulfur-bearing E72.10

Disturbance *(continued)*
- metabolism *(continued)*
  - ammonia E72.20
  - arginine E72.21
  - arginosuccinic acid E72.22
  - carbohydrate E74.9
  - cholesterol E78.9
  - citrulline E72.23
  - cystathionine E72.19
  - general E88.9
  - glutamine E72.8
  - histidine E70.40
  - homocystine E72.19
  - hydroxylysine E72.3
  - in labor or delivery O75.89
  - iron E83.10
  - lipoid E78.9
  - lysine E72.3
  - methionine E72.19
  - neonatal, transitory P74.9
    - calcium and magnesium P71.9
      - specified type NEC P71.8
    - carbohydrate metabolism P70.9
      - specified type NEC P70.8
    - specified NEC P74.8
  - ornithine E72.4
  - phosphate E83.39
  - sodium NEC E87.8
  - threonine E72.8
  - tryptophan E70.5
  - tyrosine E70.20
  - urea cycle E72.20
- motor R29.2
- nervous, functional R45.0
- neuromuscular mechanism (eye), due to syphilis A52.15
- nutritional E63.9
  - nail L60.3
- ocular motion H51.9
  - psychogenic F45.8
- oculogyric H51.8
  - psychogenic F45.8
- oculomotor H51.9
  - psychogenic F45.8
- olfactory nerve R43.1
- optic nerve NEC *—see* Disorder, nerve, optic
- oral epithelium, including tongue NEC K13.29
- perceptual due to
  - alcohol withdrawal F10.232
  - amphetamine intoxication F15.922
    - in
      - abuse F15.122
      - dependence F15.222
  - anxiolytic withdrawal F13.232
  - cannabis intoxication (acute) F12.922
    - in
      - abuse F12.122
      - dependence F12.222
  - cocaine intoxication (acute) F14.922
    - in
      - abuse F14.122
      - dependence F14.222
  - hypnotic withdrawal F13.232
  - opioid intoxication (acute) F19.122
  - phencyclidine intoxication (acute) F16.122
  - sedative withdrawal F13.232
- personality (pattern) (trait) *—see also* Disorder, personality F60.9
  - following organic brain damage F07.9
- polyglandular E31.9
  - specified NEC E31.8
- potassium balance, newborn P74.3
- psychogenic F45.9
- psychomotor F44.4

Disturbance *(continued)*
- psychophysical visual H53.16
- pupillary *—see* Anomaly, pupil, function
- reflex R29.2
- rhythm, heart I49.9
- salivary secretion K11.7
- sensation (cold) (heat) (localization) (tactile discrimination) (texture) (vibratory) NEC R20.9
  - hysterical F44.6
  - skin R20.9
    - anesthesia R20.0
    - hyperesthesia R20.3
    - hypoesthesia R20.1
    - paresthesia R20.2
    - specified type NEC R20.8
  - smell R43.9
    - and taste (mixed) R43.8
    - anosmia R43.0
    - parosmia R43.1
    - specified NEC R43.8
  - taste R43.9
    - and smell (mixed) R43.8
    - parageusia R43.2
    - specified NEC R43.8
- sensory *—see* Disturbance, sensation
- situational (transient) *—see also* Disorder, adjustment
  - acute F43.0
- sleep G47.9
  - nonorganic origin F51.9
- smell *—see* Disturbance, sensation, smell
- sociopathic F60.2
- sodium balance, newborn P74.2
- speech R47.9
  - developmental F80.9
  - specified NEC R47.89
- stomach (functional) K31.9
- sympathetic (nerve) G90.9
- taste *—see* Disturbance, sensation, taste
- temperature
  - regulation, newborn P81.9
    - specified NEC P81.8
  - sense R20.8
    - hysterical F44.6
- tooth
  - eruption K00.6
  - formation K00.4
  - structure, hereditary NEC K00.5
- touch *—see* Disturbance, sensation
- vascular I99.9
  - arteriosclerotic *—see* Arteriosclerosis
- vasomotor I73.9
- vasospastic I73.9
- vision, visual H53.9
  - following
    - cerebral infarction I69.398
    - cerebrovascular disease I69.998
      - specified NEC I69.898
    - intracerebral hemorrhage I69.198
    - nontraumatic intracranial hemorrhage NEC I69.298
    - specified disease NEC I69.898
    - subarachnoid hemorrhage I69.098
  - psychophysical H53.16
  - specified NEC H53.8
  - subjective H53.10
    - day blindness H53.11
    - discomfort H53.14-
    - distortions of shape and size H53.15
    - loss
      - sudden H53.13-
      - transient H53.12-
    - specified type NEC H53.19

Disturbance *(continued)*
- voice R49.9
  - psychogenic F44.4
  - specified NEC R49.8

Diuresis R35.8

Diver's palsy, paralysis or squeeze T70.3

Diverticulitis (acute) K57.92
- bladder *—see* Cystitis
- ileum *—see* Diverticulitis, intestine, small
- intestine K57.92
  - with
    - abscess, perforation or peritonitis K57.80
      - with bleeding K57.81
    - bleeding K57.93
  - congenital Q43.8
  - large K57.32
    - with
      - abscess, perforation or peritonitis K57.20
        - with bleeding K57.21
      - bleeding K57.33
      - small intestine K57.52
        - with
          - abscess, perforation or peritonitis K57.40
            - with bleeding K57.41
          - bleeding K57.53
  - small K57.12
    - with
      - abscess, perforation or peritonitis K57.00
        - with bleeding K57.01
      - bleeding K57.13
      - large intestine K57.52
        - with
          - abscess, perforation or peritonitis K57.40
            - with bleeding K57.41
          - bleeding K57.53

Diverticulosis K57.90
- with bleeding K57.91
- large intestine K57.30
  - with
    - bleeding K57.31
    - small intestine K57.50
      - with bleeding K57.51
- small intestine K57.10
  - with
    - bleeding K57.11
    - large intestine K57.50
      - with bleeding K57.51

Diverticulum, diverticula (multiple) K57.90
- appendix (noninflammatory) K38.2
- bladder (sphincter) N32.3
  - congenital Q64.6
- bronchus (congenital) Q32.4
  - acquired J98.09
- calyx, calyceal (kidney) N28.89
- cardia (stomach) K31.4
- cecum *—see* Diverticulosis, intestine, large
  - congenital Q43.8
- colon *—see* Diverticulosis, intestine, large
  - congenital Q43.8
- duodenum *—see* Diverticulosis, intestine, small
  - congenital Q43.8
- epiphrenic (esophagus) K22.5
- esophagus (congenital) Q39.6
  - acquired (epiphrenic) (pulsion) (traction) K22.5
- eustachian tube *—see* Disorder, eustachian tube, specified NEC
- fallopian tube N83.8

Diverticulum, diverticula *(continued)*
- gastric K31.4
- heart (congenital) Q24.8
- ileum *—see* Diverticulosis, intestine, small
- jejunum *—see* Diverticulosis, intestine, small
- kidney (pelvis) (calyces) N28.89
  - with calculus *—see* Calculus, kidney
- Meckel's (displaced) (hypertrophic) Q43.0
  - malignant *—see* Table of Neoplasms, small intestine, malignant
- midthoracic K22.5
- organ or site, congenital NEC *—see* Distortion
- pericardium (congenital) (cyst) Q24.8
  - acquired I31.8
- pharyngoesophageal (congenital) Q39.6
  - acquired K22.5
- pharynx (congenital) Q38.7
- rectosigmoid *—see* Diverticulosis, intestine, large
  - congenital Q43.8
- rectum *—see* Diverticulosis, intestine, large
- Rokitansky's K22.5
- seminal vesicle N50.89
- sigmoid *—see* Diverticulosis, intestine, large
  - congenital Q43.8
- stomach (acquired) K31.4
  - congenital Q40.2
- trachea (acquired) J39.8
- ureter (acquired) N28.89
  - congenital Q62.8
- ureterovesical orifice N28.89
- urethra (acquired) N36.1
  - congenital Q64.79
- ventricle, left (congenital) Q24.8
- vesical N32.3
  - congenital Q64.6
- Zenker's (esophagus) K22.5

Division
- cervix uteri (acquired) N88.8
- glans penis Q55.69
- labia minora (congenital) Q52.79
- ligament (partial or complete) (current) *—see also* Sprain
  - with open wound *—see* Wound, open
- muscle (partial or complete) (current) *—see also* Injury, muscle
  - with open wound *—see* Wound, open
- nerve (traumatic) *—see* Injury, nerve
- spinal cord *—see* Injury, spinal cord, by region
- vein I87.8

Divorce, causing family disruption Z63.5

Dix-Hallpike neurolabyrinthitis *—see* Neuronitis, vestibular

Dizziness R42
- hysterical F44.89
- psychogenic F45.8

DMAC (disseminated mycobacterium avium- intracellulare complex) A31.2

DNR (do not resuscitate) Z66

Doan-Wiseman syndrome (primary splenic neutropenia) *—see* Agranulocytosis

Doehle-Heller aortitis A52.02

Dog bite *—see* Bite

Dohle body panmyelopathic syndrome D72.0

Dolichocephaly Q67.2

Dolichocolon Q43.8

Dolichostenomelia *—see* Syndrome, Marfan's

Donohue's syndrome E34.8

Donor (organ or tissue) Z52.9
- blood (whole) Z52.000
  - autologous Z52.010
  - specified component (lymphocytes) (platelets) NEC Z52.008
    - autologous Z52.018
    - specified donor NEC Z52.098
  - specified donor NEC Z52.090
  - stem cells Z52.001
    - autologous Z52.011
    - specified donor NEC Z52.091
- bone Z52.20
  - autologous Z52.21
  - marrow Z52.3
  - specified type NEC Z52.29
- cornea Z52.5
- egg (Oocyte) Z52.819
  - age 35 and over Z52.812
    - anonymous recipient Z52.812
    - designated recipient Z52.813
  - under age 35 Z52.810
    - anonymous recipient Z52.810
    - designated recipient Z52.811
- kidney Z52.4
- liver Z52.6
- lung Z52.89
- lymphocyte *—see* Donor, blood, specified components NEC
- Oocyte *—see* Donor, egg
- platelets Z52.008
- potential, examination of Z00.5
- semen Z52.89
- skin Z52.10
  - autologous Z52.11
  - specified type NEC Z52.19
- specified organ or tissue NEC Z52.89
- sperm Z52.89

Donovanosis A58

Dorsalgia M54.9
- psychogenic F45.41
- specified NEC M54.89

Dorsopathy M53.9
- deforming M43.9
  - specified NEC *—see* subcategory M43.8
- specified NEC M53.80
  - cervical region M53.82
  - cervicothoracic region M53.83
  - lumbar region M53.86
  - lumbosacral region M53.87
  - occipito-atlanto-axial region M53.81
  - sacrococcygeal region M53.88
  - thoracic region M53.84
  - thoracolumbar region M53.85

Double
- albumin E88.09
- aortic arch Q25.45
- auditory canal Q17.8
- auricle (heart) Q20.8
- bladder Q64.79
- cervix Q51.820
  - with doubling of uterus (and vagina) Q51.10
    - with obstruction Q51.11
- inlet ventricle Q20.4
- kidney with double pelvis (renal) Q63.0
- meatus urinarius Q64.75

Double *(continued)*
- monster Q89.4
- outlet
  - left ventricle Q20.2
  - right ventricle Q20.1
- pelvis (renal) with double ureter Q62.5
- tongue Q38.3
- ureter (one or both sides) Q62.5
  - with double pelvis (renal) Q62.5
- urethra Q64.74
- urinary meatus Q64.75
- uterus Q51.2
  - with
    - doubling of cervix (and vagina) Q51.10
      - with obstruction Q51.11
  - in pregnancy or childbirth O34.59-
    - causing obstructed labor O65.5
- vagina Q52.10
  - with doubling of uterus (and cervix) Q51.10
    - with obstruction Q51.11
- vision H53.2
- vulva Q52.79

Douglas' pouch, cul-de-sac *—see* condition

Down syndrome Q90.9
- meiotic nondisjunction Q90.0
- mitotic nondisjunction Q90.1
- mosaicism Q90.1
- translocation Q90.2

DPD (dihydropyrimidine dehydrogenase deficiency) E88.89

Dracontiasis B72

Dracunculiasis, dracunculosis B72

Dream state, hysterical F44.89

Dreschlera (hawaiiensis) (infection) B43.8

Drepanocytic anemia *—see* Disease, sickle-cell

Dresbach's syndrome (elliptocytosis) D58.1

Dressler's syndrome I24.1

Drift, ulnar *—see* Deformity, limb, specified type NEC, forearm

Drinking (alcohol)
- excessive, to excess NEC (without dependence) F10.10
  - habitual (continual) (without remission) F10.20
    - with remission F10.21

Drip, postnasal (chronic) R09.82
- due to
  - allergic rhinitis *—see* Rhinitis, allergic
  - common cold J00
  - gastroesophageal reflux *—see* Reflux, gastroesophageal
  - nasopharyngitis *—see* Nasopharyngitis
  - other know condition - code to condition
  - sinusitis *—see* Sinusitis

Droop
- facial R29.810
  - cerebrovascular disease I69.992
    - cerebral infarction I69.392
    - intracerebral hemorrhage I69.192
    - nontraumatic intracranial hemorrhage NEC I69.292
    - specified disease NEC I69.892
    - subarachnoid hemorrhage I69.092

Drop (in)
- attack NEC R55
- finger *—see* Deformity, finger
- foot *—see* Deformity, limb, foot, drop
- hematocrit (precipitous) R71.0
- hemoglobin R71.0
- toe *—see* Deformity, toe, specified NEC
- wrist *—see* Deformity, limb, wrist drop

Dropped heart beats I45.9

Dropsy, dropsical *—see also* Hydrops
- abdomen R18.8
- brain *—see* Hydrocephalus
- cardiac, heart *—see* Failure, heart, congestive
- gangrenous *—see* Gangrene
- heart *—see* Failure, heart, congestive
- kidney *—see* Nephrosis
- lung *—see* Edema, lung
- newborn due to isoimmunization P56.0
- pericardium *—see* Pericarditis

Drowned, drowning (near) T75.1

Drowsiness R40.0

Drug
- abuse counseling and surveillance Z71.51
- addiction *—see* Dependence
- dependence *—see* Dependence
- habit *—see* Dependence
- harmful use *—see* Abuse, drug
- induced fever R50.2
- overdose *—see* Table of Drugs and Chemicals, by drug, poisoning
- poisoning *—see* Table of Drugs and Chemicals, by drug, poisoning
- resistant organism infection (*see also* Resistant, organism, to, drug) Z16.30
- therapy
  - long term (current) (prophylactic) *—see* Therapy, drug long-term (current) (prophylactic)
  - short term - omit code
- wrong substance given or taken in error *—see* Table of Drugs and Chemicals, by drug, poisoning

Drunkenness (without dependence) F10.129
- acute in alcoholism F10.229
- chronic (without remission) F10.20
  - with remission F10.21
- pathological (without dependence) F10.129
  - with dependence F10.229
- sleep F51.9

Drusen
- macula (degenerative) (retina) *—see* Degeneration, macula, drusen
- optic disc H47.32-

Dry, dryness *—see also* condition
- larynx J38.7
- mouth R68.2
  - due to dehydration E86.0
- nose J34.89
- socket (teeth) M27.3
- throat J39.2

DSAP L56.5

Duane's syndrome H50.81-

Dubin-Johnson disease or syndrome E80.6

Dubois' disease (thymus gland) A50.59 *[E35]*

Dubowitz' syndrome Q87.1

Duchenne-Aran muscular atrophy G12.21
Duchenne-Griesinger disease G71.0
Duchenne's
disease or syndrome
motor neuron disease G12.22
muscular dystrophy G71.0
locomotor ataxia (syphilitic) A52.11
paralysis
birth injury P14.0
due to or associated with
motor neuron disease G12.22
muscular dystrophy G71.0
Ducrey's chancre A57
Duct, ductus *—see* condition
Duhring's disease (dermatitis herpetiformis) L13.0
Dullness, cardiac (decreased) (increased) R01.2
Dumb ague *—see* Malaria
Dumbness *—see* Aphasia
Dumdum fever B55.0
Dumping syndrome (postgastrectomy) K91.1
Duodenitis (nonspecific) (peptic) K29.80
with bleeding K29.81
Duodenocholangitis *—see* Cholangitis
Duodenum, duodenal *—see* condition
Duplay's bursitis or periarthritis *— see* Tendinitis, calcific, shoulder
Duplication, duplex *—see also* Accessory
alimentary tract Q45.8
anus Q43.4
appendix (and cecum) Q43.4
biliary duct (any) Q44.5
bladder Q64.79
cecum (and appendix) Q43.4
cervix Q51.820
chromosome NEC
with complex rearrangements NEC Q92.5
seen only at prometaphase Q92.8
cystic duct Q44.5
digestive organs Q45.8
esophagus Q39.8
frontonasal process Q75.8
intestine (large) (small) Q43.4
kidney Q63.0
liver Q44.7
pancreas Q45.3
penis Q55.69
respiratory organs NEC Q34.8
salivary duct Q38.4
spinal cord (incomplete) Q06.2
stomach Q40.2
Dupré's disease (meningism) R29.1
Dupuytren's contraction or disease M72.0
Durand-Nicolas-Favre disease A55
Durotomy (inadvertent) (incidental) G97.41
Duroziez's disease (congenital mitral stenosis) Q23.2
Dutton's relapsing fever (West African) A68.1
Dwarfism E34.3
achondroplastic Q77.4
congenital E34.3
constitutional E34.3
hypochondroplastic Q77.4
hypophyseal E23.0
Dwarfism *(continued)*
infantile E34.3
Laron-type E34.3
Lorain (-Levi) type E23.0
metatropic Q77.8
nephrotic-glycosuric (with hypophosphatemic rickets) E72.09
nutritional E45
pancreatic K86.89
pituitary E23.0
renal N25.0
thanatophoric Q77.1
Dyke-Young anemia (secondary) (symptomatic) D59.1
Dysacusis *—see* Abnormal, auditory perception
Dysadrenocortism E27.9
hyperfunction E27.0
Dysarthria R47.1
following
cerebral infarction I69.322
cerebrovascular disease I69.922
specified disease NEC I69.822
intracerebral hemorrhage I69.122
nontraumatic intracranial hemorrhage NEC I69.222
subarachnoid hemorrhage I69.022
Dysautonomia (familial) G90.1
Dysbarism T70.3
Dysbasia R26.2
angiosclerotica intermittens I73.9
hysterical F44.4
lordotica (progressiva) G24.1
nonorganic origin F44.4
psychogenic F44.4
Dysbetalipoproteinemia (familial) E78.2
Dyscalculia R48.8
developmental F81.2
Dyschezia K59.00
Dyschondroplasia (with hemangiomata) Q78.4
Dyschromia (skin) L81.9
Dyscollagenosis M35.9
Dyscranio-pygo-phalangy Q87.0
Dyscrasia
blood (with) D75.9
antepartum hemorrhage *—see* Hemorrhage, antepartum, with coagulation defect
newborn P61.9
specified type NEC P61.8
intrapartum hemorrhage O67.0
puerperal, postpartum O72.3
polyglandular, pluriglandular E31.9
Dysendocrinism E34.9
Dysentery, dysenteric (catarrhal) (diarrhea) (epidemic) (hemorrhagic) (infectious) (sporadic) (tropical) A09
abscess, liver A06.4
amebic (*see also* Amebiasis) A06.0
with abscess *—see* Abscess, amebic
acute A06.0
chronic A06.1
arthritis (*see also* category M01) A09
bacillary (*see also* category M01) A03.9
bacillary A03.9
arthritis (*see also* category M01) A03.9
Boyd A03.2
Flexner A03.1
Schmitz (-Stutzer) A03.0
Shiga (-Kruse) A03.0
Dysentery, dysenteric *(continued)*
bacillary *(continued)*
Shigella A03.9
boydii A03.2
dysenteriae A03.0
flexneri A03.1
group A A03.0
group B A03.1
group C A03.2
group D A03.3
sonnei A03.3
specified type NEC A03.8
Sonne A03.3
specified type NEC A03.8
balantidial A07.0
Balantidium coli A07.0
Boyd's A03.2
candidal B37.82
Chilomastix A07.8
Chinese A03.9
coccidial A07.3
Dientamoeba (fragilis) A07.8
Embadomonas A07.8
Entamoeba, entamebic *—see* Dysentery, amebic
Flexner-Boyd A03.2
Flexner's A03.1
Giardia lamblia A07.1
Hiss-Russell A03.1
Lamblia A07.1
leishmanial B55.0
malarial *—see* Malaria
metazoal B82.0
monilial B37.82
protozoal A07.9
Salmonella A02.0
schistosomal B65.1
Schmitz (-Stutzer) A03.0
Shiga (-Kruse) A03.0
Shigella NOS *—see* Dysentery, bacillary
Sonne A03.3
strongyloidiasis B78.0
trichomonal A07.8
viral *—see also* Enteritis, viral A08.4
Dysequilibrium R42
Dysesthesia R20.8
hysterical F44.6
Dysfibrinogenemia (congenital) D68.2
Dysfunction
adrenal E27.9
hyperfunction E27.0
autonomic
due to alcohol G31.2
somatoform F45.8
bladder N31.9
neurogenic NOS *—see* Dysfunction, bladder, neuromuscular
neuromuscular NOS N31.9
atonic (motor) (sensory) N31.2
autonomous N31.2
flaccid N31.2
nonreflex N31.2
reflex N31.1
specified NEC N31.8
uninhibited N31.0
bleeding, uterus N93.8
cerebral G93.89
colon K59.9
psychogenic F45.8
colostomy K94.03
cystic duct K82.8
cystostomy (stoma) *—see* Complications, cystostomy
ejaculatory N53.19
anejaculatory orgasm N53.13
painful N53.12
premature F52.4
retarded N53.11
Dysfunction *(continued)*
endocrine NOS E34.9
endometrium N85.8
enterostomy K94.13
erectile - *see* Dysfunction, sexual, male, erectile
gallbladder K82.8
gastrostomy (stoma) K94.23
gland, glandular NOS E34.9
heart I51.89
hemoglobin D75.89
hepatic K76.89
hypophysis E23.7
hypothalamic NEC E23.3
ileostomy (stoma) K94.13
jejunostomy (stoma) K94.13
kidney *—see* Disease, renal
labyrinthine *—see* subcategory H83.2
left ventricular, following sudden emotional stress I51.81
liver K76.89
male *—see* Dysfunction, sexual, male
orgasmic (female) F52.31
male F52.32
ovary E28.9
specified NEC E28.8
papillary muscle I51.89
parathyroid E21.4
physiological NEC R68.89
psychogenic F59
pineal gland E34.8
pituitary (gland) E23.3
platelets D69.1
polyglandular E31.9
specified NEC E31.8
psychophysiologic F59
psychosexual F52.9
with
dyspareunia F52.6
premature ejaculation F52.4
vaginismus F52.5
pylorus K31.9
rectum K59.9
psychogenic F45.8
reflex (sympathetic) *—see* Syndrome, pain, complex regional I
segmental *—see* Dysfunction, somatic
senile R54
sexual (due to) R37
alcohol F10.981
amphetamine F15.981
in
abuse F15.181
dependence F15.281
anxiolytic F13.981
in
abuse F13.181
dependence F13.281
cocaine F14.981
in
abuse F14.181
dependence F14.281
excessive sexual drive F52.8
failure of genital response (male) F52.21
female F52.22
female N94.9
aversion F52.1
dyspareunia N94.10
psychogenic F52.6
frigidity F52.22
nymphomania F52.8
orgasmic F52.31
psychogenic F52.9
aversion F52.1
dyspareunia F52.6
frigidity F52.22
nymphomania F52.8

Dysfunction *(continued)*
- sexual *(continued)*
  - female *(continued)*
    - psychogenic *(continued)*
      - orgasmic F52.31
      - vaginismus F52.5
    - vaginismus N94.2
      - psychogenic F52.5
  - hypnotic F13.981
    - in
      - abuse F13.181
      - dependence F13.281
  - inhibited orgasm (female) F52.31
    - male F52.32
  - lack
    - of sexual enjoyment F52.1
    - or loss of sexual desire F52.0
  - male N53.9
    - anejaculatory orgasm N53.13
    - ejaculatory N53.19
      - painful N53.12
      - premature F52.4
      - retarded N53.11
    - erectile N52.9
      - drug induced N52.2
      - due to
        - disease classified elsewhere N52.1
        - drug N52.2
      - postoperative (postprocedural) N52.39
        - following
          - cryotherapy N52.37
          - interstitial *see*d therapy N52.36
          - prostate ablative therapy N52.37
          - prostatectomy N52.34
            - radical N52.31
          - radical cystectomy N52.32
          - radiation therapy N52.35
          - ultrasound ablative therapy N52.37
          - urethral surgery N52.33
      - psychogenic F52.21
      - specified cause NEC N52.8
      - vasculogenic
        - arterial insufficiency N52.01
          - with corporo-venous occlusive N52.03
        - corporo-venous occlusive N52.02
          - with arterial insufficiency N52.03
    - impotence *—see* Dysfunction, sexual, male, erectile
    - psychogenic F52.9
      - aversion F52.1
      - erectile F52.21
      - orgasmic F52.32
      - premature ejaculation F52.4
      - satyriasis F52.8
      - specified type NEC F52.8
    - specified type NEC N53.8
  - nonorganic F52.9
    - specified NEC F52.8
  - opioid F11.981
    - in
      - abuse F11.181
      - dependence F11.281
  - orgasmic dysfunction (female) F52.31
    - male F52.32
  - premature ejaculation F52.4
  - psychoactive substances NEC F19.981
    - in
      - abuse F19.181
      - dependence F19.281

Dysfunction *(continued)*
- sexual *(continued)*
  - psychogenic F52.9
  - sedative F13.981
    - in
      - abuse F13.181
      - dependence F13.281
  - sexual aversion F52.1
  - vaginismus (nonorganic) (psychogenic) F52.5
- sinoatrial node I49.5
- somatic M99.09
  - abdomen M99.09
  - acromioclavicular M99.07
  - cervical region M99.01
  - cervicothoracic M99.01
  - costochondral M99.08
  - costovertebral M99.08
  - head region M99.00
  - hip M99.05
  - lower extremity M99.06
  - lumbar region M99.03
  - lumbosacral M99.03
  - occipitocervical M99.00
  - pelvic region M99.05
  - pubic M99.05
  - rib cage M99.08
  - sacral region M99.04
  - sacrococcygeal M99.04
  - sacroiliac M99.04
  - specified NEC M99.09
  - sternochondral M99.08
  - sternoclavicular M99.07
  - thoracic region M99.02
  - thoracolumbar M99.02
  - upper extremity M99.07
- somatoform autonomic F45.8
- stomach K31.89
  - psychogenic F45.8
- suprarenal E27.9
  - hyperfunction E27.0
- symbolic R48.9
  - specified type NEC R48.8
- temporomandibular (joint) M26.69
  - joint-pain syndrome M26.62-
- testicular (endocrine) E29.9
  - specified NEC E29.8
- thymus E32.9
- thyroid E07.9
- ureterostomy (stoma) *—see* Complications, stoma, urinary tract
- urethrostomy (stoma) *—see* Complications, stoma, urinary tract
- uterus, complicating delivery O62.9
  - hypertonic O62.4
  - hypotonic O62.2
    - primary O62.0
    - secondary O62.1
- ventricular I51.9
  - with congestive heart failure (*see also* Failure, heart) I50.9
  - left, reversible, following sudden emotional stress I51.81

Dysgenesis
- gonadal (due to chromosomal anomaly) Q96.9
  - pure Q99.1
- renal Q60.5
  - bilateral Q60.4
  - unilateral Q60.3
- reticular D72.0
- tidal platelet D69.3

Dysgerminoma
- specified site *—see* Neoplasm, malignant, by site
- unspecified site
  - female C56.9
  - male C62.90

Dysgeusia R43.2

Dysgraphia R27.8

Dyshidrosis, dysidrosis L30.1

Dyskaryotic cervical smear R87.619

Dyskeratosis L85.8
- cervix *—see* Dysplasia, cervix
- congenital Q82.8
- uterus NEC N85.8

Dyskinesia G24.9
- biliary (cystic duct or gallbladder) K82.8
- drug induced
  - orofacial G24.01
- esophagus K22.4
- hysterical F44.4
- intestinal K59.8
- nonorganic origin F44.4
- orofacial (idiopathic) G24.4
  - drug induced G24.01
- psychogenic F44.4
- subacute, drug induced G24.01
- tardive G24.01
  - neuroleptic induced G24.01
- trachea J39.8
- tracheobronchial J98.09

Dyslalia (developmental) F80.0

Dyslexia R48.0
- developmental F81.0

Dyslipidemia E78.5
- depressed HDL cholesterol E78.6
- elevated fasting triglycerides E78.1

Dysmaturity *—see also* Light for dates
- pulmonary (newborn) (Wilson-Mikity) P27.0

Dysmenorrhea (essential) (exfoliative) N94.6
- congestive (syndrome) N94.6
- primary N94.4
- psychogenic F45.8
- secondary N94.5

Dysmetabolic syndrome X E88.81

Dysmetria R27.8

Dysmorphism (due to)
- alcohol Q86.0
- exogenous cause NEC Q86.8
- hydantoin Q86.1
- warfarin Q86.2

Dysmorphophobia (nondelusional) F45.22
- delusional F22

Dysnomia R47.01

Dysorexia R63.0
- psychogenic F50.89

Dysostosis
- cleidocranial, cleidocranialis Q74.0
- craniofacial Q75.1
- Fairbank's (idiopathic familial generalized osteophytosis) Q78.9
- mandibulofacial (incomplete) Q75.4
- multiplex E76.01
- oculomandibular Q75.5

Dyspareunia (female) N94.10
- deep N94.12
- male N53.12
- nonorganic F52.6
- psychogenic F52.6
- secondary N94.19
- specified NEC N94.19
- superficial (introital) N94.11

Dyspepsia R10.13
- atonic K30
- functional (allergic) (congenital) (gastrointestinal) (occupational) (reflex) K30
- intestinal K59.8
- nervous F45.8

Dyspepsia *(continued)*
- neurotic F45.8
- psychogenic F45.8

Dysphagia R13.10
- cervical R13.19
- following
  - cerebral infarction I69.391
  - cerebrovascular disease I69.991
    - specified NEC I69.891
  - intracerebral hemorrhage I69.191
  - nontraumatic intracranial hemorrhage NEC I69.291
  - specified disease NEC I69.891
  - subarachnoid hemorrhage I69.091
- functional (hysterical) F45.8
- hysterical F45.8
- nervous (hysterical) F45.8
- neurogenic R13.19
- oral phase R13.11
- oropharyngeal phase R13.12
- pharyngeal phase R13.13
- pharyngoesophageal phase R13.14
- psychogenic F45.8
- sideropenic D50.1
- spastica K22.4
- specified NEC R13.19

Dysphagocytosis, congenital D71

Dysphasia R47.02
- developmental
  - expressive type F80.1
  - receptive type F80.2
- following
  - cerebrovascular disease I69.921
    - cerebral infarction I69.321
    - intracerebral hemorrhage I69.121
    - nontraumatic intracranial hemorrhage NEC I69.221
    - specified disease NEC I69.821
    - subarachnoid hemorrhage I69.021

Dysphonia R49.0
- functional F44.4
- hysterical F44.4
- psychogenic F44.4
- spastica J38.3

Dysphoria
- gender F64.9
  - in
    - adolescence and adulthood F64.0
    - children F64.2
  - postpartal O90.6
  - specified NEC F64.8

Dyspituitarism E23.3

Dysplasia *—see also* Anomaly
- acetabular, congenital Q65.89
- alveolar capillary, with vein misalignment J84.843
- anus (histologically confirmed) (mild) (moderate) K62.82
  - severe D01.3
- arrhythmogenic right ventricular I42.8
- arterial, fibromuscular I77.3
- asphyxiating thoracic (congenital) Q77.2
- brain Q07.9
- bronchopulmonary, perinatal P27.1
- cervix (uteri) N87.9
  - mild N87.0
  - moderate N87.1
  - severe D06.9
- chondroectodermal Q77.6
- colon D12.6
- craniometaphyseal Q78.8
- dentinal K00.5
- diaphyseal, progressive Q78.3
- dystrophic Q77.5

Dysplasia *(continued)*
- ectodermal (anhidrotic) (congenital) (hereditary) Q82.4
  - hydrotic Q82.8
- epithelial, uterine cervix *—see* Dysplasia, cervix
- eye (congenital) Q11.2
- fibrous
  - bone NEC (monostotic) M85.00
    - ankle M85.07-
    - foot M85.07-
    - forearm M85.03-
    - hand M85.04-
    - lower leg M85.06-
    - multiple site M85.09
    - neck M85.08
    - rib M85.08
    - shoulder M85.01-
    - skull M85.08
    - specified site NEC M85.08
    - thigh M85.05-
    - toe M85.07-
    - upper arm M85.02-
    - vertebra M85.08
  - diaphyseal, progressive Q78.3
  - jaw M27.8
  - polyostotic Q78.1
- florid osseous *—see also* Cyst, calcifying odontogenic
- high grade, focal D12.6
- hip, congenital Q65.89
- joint, congenital Q74.8
- kidney Q61.4
  - multicystic Q61.4
- leg Q74.2
- lung, congenital (not associated with short gestation) Q33.6
- mammary (gland) (benign) N60.9-
  - cyst (solitary) *—see* Cyst, breast
  - cystic *—see* Mastopathy, cystic
  - duct ectasia *—see* Ectasia, mammary duct
  - fibroadenosis *—see* Fibroadenosis, breast
  - fibrosclerosis *—see* Fibrosclerosis, breast
  - specified type NEC N60.8-
- metaphyseal Q78.5
  - specified NEC N42.39
- muscle Q79.8
- oculodentodigital Q87.0
- periapical (cemental) (cemento-osseous) *—see* Cyst, calcifying odontogenic
- periosteum *—see* Disorder, bone, specified type NEC
- polyostotic fibrous Q78.1
- prostate (*see also* Neoplasia, intraepithelial, prostate) N42.30
  - severe D07.5
  - specified NEC N42.39
- renal Q61.4
  - multicystic Q61.4
- retinal, congenital Q14.1
- right ventricular, arrhythmogenic I42.8
- septo-optic Q04.4
- skin L98.8
- spinal cord Q06.1
- spondyloepiphyseal Q77.7
- thymic, with immunodeficiency D82.1
- vagina N89.3
  - mild N89.0
  - moderate N89.1
  - severe NEC D07.2
- vulva N90.3
  - mild N90.0
  - moderate N90.1
  - severe NEC D07.1

Dyspnea (nocturnal) (paroxysmal) R06.00
- asthmatic (bronchial) J45.909
  - with
    - exacerbation (acute) J45.901
    - bronchitis J45.909
      - with
        - exacerbation (acute) J45.901
        - status asthmaticus J45.902
      - chronic J44.9
    - status asthmaticus J45.902
  - cardiac *—see* Failure, ventricular, left
- cardiac *—see* Failure, ventricular, left
- functional F45.8
- hyperventilation R06.4
- hysterical F45.8
- newborn P28.89
- orthopnea R06.01
- psychogenic F45.8
- shortness of breath R06.02
- specified type NEC R06.09

Dyspraxia R27.8
- developmental (syndrome) F82

Dysproteinemia E88.09

Dysreflexia, autonomic G90.4

Dysrhythmia
- cardiac I49.9
  - newborn
    - bradycardia P29.12
    - occurring before birth P03.819
      - before onset of labor P03.810
      - during labor P03.811
    - tachycardia P29.11
  - postoperative I97.89
- cerebral or cortical *—see* Epilepsy

Dyssomnia *—see* Disorder, sleep

Dyssynergia
- biliary K83.8
- bladder sphincter N36.44
- cerebellaris myoclonica (Hunt's ataxia) G11.1

Dysthymia F34.1

Dysthyroidism E07.9

Dystocia O66.9
- affecting newborn P03.1
- cervical (hypotonic) O62.2
  - affecting newborn P03.6
  - primary O62.0
  - secondary O62.1
- contraction ring O62.4
- fetal O66.9
  - abnormality NEC O66.3
  - conjoined twins O66.3
  - oversize O66.2
- maternal O66.9
- positional O64.9
- shoulder (girdle) O66.0
  - causing obstructed labor O66.0
- uterine NEC O62.4

Dystonia G24.9
- deformans progressiva G24.1
- drug induced NEC G24.09
  - acute G24.02
  - specified NEC G24.09
- familial G24.1
- idiopathic G24.1
  - familial G24.1
  - nonfamilial G24.2
  - orofacial G24.4
- lenticularis G24.8
- musculorum deformans G24.1
- neuroleptic induced (acute) G24.02
- orofacial (idiopathic) G24.4
- oromandibular G24.4
  - due to drug G24.01

Dystonia *(continued)*
- specified NEC G24.8
- torsion (familial) (idiopathic) G24.1
  - acquired G24.8
  - genetic G24.1
  - symptomatic (nonfamilial) G24.2

Dystonic movements R25.8

Dystrophy, dystrophia
- adiposogenital E23.6
- Becker's type G71.0
- cervical sympathetic G90.2
- choroid (hereditary) H31.20
  - central areolar H31.22
  - choroideremia H31.21
  - gyrate atrophy H31.23
  - specified type NEC H31.29
- cornea (hereditary) H18.50
  - endothelial H18.51
  - epithelial H18.52
  - granular H18.53
  - lattice H18.54
  - macular H18.55
  - specified type NEC H18.59
- Duchenne's type G71.0
- due to malnutrition E45
- Erb's G71.0
- Fuchs' H18.51
- Gower's muscular G71.0
- hair L67.8
- infantile neuraxonal G31.89
- Landouzy-Déjérine G71.0
- Leyden-Möbius G71.0
- muscular G71.0
  - benign (Becker type) G71.0
  - congenital (hereditary) (progressive) (with specific morphological abnormalities of the muscle fiber) G71.0
    - myotonic G71.11
  - distal G71.0
  - Duchenne type G71.0
  - Emery-Dreifuss G71.0
  - Erb type G71.0
  - facioscapulohumeral G71.0
  - Gower's G71.0
  - hereditary (progressive) G71.0
  - Landouzy-Déjérine type G71.0
  - limb-girdle G71.0
  - myotonic G71.11
  - progressive (hereditary) G71.0
    - Charcot-Marie (-Tooth) type G60.0
  - pseudohypertrophic (infantile) G71.0
  - severe (Duchenne type) G71.0
- myocardium, myocardial *—see* Degeneration, myocardial
- nail L60.3
  - congenital Q84.6
- nutritional E45
- ocular G71.0
- oculocerebrorenal E72.03
- oculopharyngeal G71.0
- ovarian N83.8
- polyglandular E31.8
- reflex (neuromuscular) (sympathetic) *—see* Syndrome, pain, complex regional I
- retinal (hereditary) H35.50
  - in
    - lipid storage disorders E75.6 *[H36]*
    - systemic lipidoses E75.6 *[H36]*
  - involving
    - pigment epithelium H35.54
    - sensory area H35.53
  - pigmentary H35.52
  - vitreoretinal H35.51
- Salzmann's nodular *—see* Degeneration, cornea, nodular

Dystrophy, dystrophia *(continued)*
- scapuloperoneal G71.0
- skin NEC L98.8
- sympathetic (reflex) *—see* Syndrome, pain, complex regional I
  - cervical G90.2
- tapetoretinal H35.54
- thoracic, asphyxiating Q77.2
- unguium L60.3
  - congenital Q84.6
- vitreoretinal H35.51
- vulva N90.4
- yellow (liver) *—see* Failure, hepatic

Dysuria R30.0
- psychogenic F45.8

E

Eales' disease H35.06-

Ear *—see also* condition
- piercing Z41.3
- tropical NEC B36.9 *[H62.40]*
  - in
    - aspergillosis B44.89
    - candidiasis B37.84
    - moniliasis B37.84
- wax (impacted) H61.20
  - left H61.22
    - with right H61.23
  - right H61.21
    - with left H61.23

Earache *—see* subcategory H92.0

Early satiety R68.81

Eaton-Lambert syndrome *—see* Syndrome, Lambert-Eaton

Eberth's disease (typhoid fever) A01.00

Ebola virus disease A98.4

Ebstein's anomaly or syndrome (heart) Q22.5

Eccentro-osteochondrodysplasia E76.29

Ecchondroma *—see* Neoplasm, bone, benign

Ecchondrosis D48.0

Ecchymosis R58
- conjunctiva *—see* Hemorrhage, conjunctiva
- eye (traumatic) *—see* Contusion, eyeball
- eyelid (traumatic) *—see* Contusion, eyelid
- newborn P54.5
- spontaneous R23.3
- traumatic *—see* Contusion

Echinococciasis *—see* Echinococcus

Echinococcosis *—see* Echinococcus

Echinococcus (infection) B67.90
- granulosus B67.4
  - bone B67.2
  - liver B67.0
  - lung B67.1
  - multiple sites B67.32
  - specified site NEC B67.39
  - thyroid B67.31
- liver NOS B67.8
  - granulosus B67.0
  - multilocularis B67.5
- lung NEC B67.99
  - granulosus B67.1
  - multilocularis B67.69
- multilocularis B67.7
  - liver B67.5
  - multiple sites B67.61
  - specified site NEC B67.69

Echinococcus *(continued)*
- specified site NEC B67.99
  - granulosus B67.39
  - multilocularis B67.69
- thyroid NEC B67.99
  - granulosus B67.31
  - multilocularis B67.69 *[E35]*

Echinorhynchiasis B83.8

Echinostomiasis B66.8

Echolalia R48.8

Echovirus, as cause of disease classified elsewhere B97.12

Eclampsia, eclamptic (coma) (convulsions) (delirium) (with hypertension) **NEC** O15.9
- complicating
  - labor and delivery O15.1
  - postpartum O15.2
  - pregnancy O15.0-
  - puerperal O15.2

Economic circumstances affecting care Z59.9

Economo's disease A85.8

Ectasia, ectasis
- annuloaortic I35.8
- aorta I77.819
  - with aneurysm —*see* Aneurysm, aorta
  - abdominal I77.811
  - thoracic I77.810
  - thoracoabdominal I77.812
- breast —*see* Ectasia, mammary duct
- capillary I78.8
- cornea H18.71-
- gastric antral vascular (GAVE) K31.819
  - with hemorrhage K31.811
  - without hemorrhage K31.819
- mammary duct N60.4-
- salivary gland (duct) K11.8
- sclera —*see* Sclerectasia

Ecthyma L08.0
- contagiosum B08.02
- gangrenosum L08.0
- infectiosum B08.02

Ectocardia Q24.8

Ectodermal dysplasia (anhidrotic) Q82.4

Ectodermosis erosiva pluriorificialis L51.1

Ectopic, ectopia (congenital)
- abdominal viscera Q45.8
  - due to defect in anterior abdominal wall Q79.59
- ACTH syndrome E24.3
- adrenal gland Q89.1
- anus Q43.5
- atrial beats I49.1
- beats I49.49
  - atrial I49.1
  - ventricular I49.3
- bladder Q64.10
- bone and cartilage in lung Q33.5
- brain Q04.8
- breast tissue Q83.8
- cardiac Q24.8
- cerebral Q04.8
- cordis Q24.8
- endometrium —*see* Endometriosis
- gastric mucosa Q40.2
- gestation —*see* Pregnancy, by site
- heart Q24.8
- hormone secretion NEC E34.2
- kidney (crossed) (pelvis) Q63.2
- lens, lentis Q12.1
- mole —*see* Pregnancy, by site

Ectopic, ectopia *(continued)*
- organ or site NEC —*see* Malposition, congenital
- pancreas Q45.3
- pregnancy —*see* Pregnancy, ectopic
- pupil —*see* Abnormality, pupillary
- renal Q63.2
- sebaceous glands of mouth Q38.6
- spleen Q89.09
- testis Q53.00
  - bilateral Q53.02
  - unilateral Q53.01
- thyroid Q89.2
- tissue in lung Q33.5
- ureter Q62.63
- ventricular beats I49.3
- vesicae Q64.10

Ectromelia Q73.8
- lower limb —*see* Defect, reduction, limb, lower, specified type NEC
- upper limb —*see* Defect, reduction, limb, upper, specified type NEC

Ectropion H02.109
- cervix N86
  - with cervicitis N72
- congenital Q10.1
- eyelid (paralytic) H02.109
  - cicatricial H02.119
    - left H02.116
      - lower H02.115
      - upper H02.114
    - right H02.113
      - lower H02.112
      - upper H02.111
  - congenital Q10.1
  - left H02.106
    - lower H02.105
    - upper H02.104
  - mechanical H02.129
    - left H02.126
      - lower H02.125
      - upper H02.124
    - right H02.123
      - lower H02.122
      - upper H02.121
  - right H02.103
    - lower H02.102
    - upper H02.101
  - senile H02.139
    - left H02.136
      - lower H02.135
      - upper H02.134
    - right H02.133
      - lower H02.132
      - upper H02.131
  - spastic H02.149
    - left H02.146
      - lower H02.145
      - upper H02.144
    - right H02.143
      - lower H02.142
      - upper H02.141
- iris H21.89
- lip (acquired) K13.0
  - congenital Q38.0
- urethra N36.8
- uvea H21.89

Eczema (acute) (chronic) (erythematous) (fissum) (rubrum) (squamous) —*see also* Dermatitis L30.9
- contact —*see* Dermatitis, contact
- dyshydrotic L30.1
- external ear —*see* Otitis, externa, acute, eczematoid
- flexural L20.82
- herpeticum B00.0
- hypertrophicum L28.0
- hypostatic —*see* Varix, leg, with, inflammation

Eczema *(continued)*
- impetiginous L01.1
- infantile (due to any substance) L20.83
  - intertriginous L21.1
  - seborrheic L21.1
- intertriginous NEC L30.4
  - infantile L21.1
- intrinsic (allergic) L20.84
- lichenified NEC L28.0
- marginatum (hebrae) B35.6
- pustular L30.3
- stasis I87.2
  - with varicose veins - *see* Varix, leg, with, inflammation
- vaccination, vaccinatum T88.1
- varicose —*see* Varix, leg, with, inflammation

Eczematid L30.2

Eddowes (-Spurway) **syndrome** Q78.0

Edema, edematous (infectious) (pitting) (toxic) R60.9
- with nephritis —*see* Nephrosis
- allergic T78.3
- amputation stump (surgical) (sequelae (late effect)) T87.89
- angioneurotic (allergic) (any site) (with urticaria) T78.3
  - hereditary D84.1
- angiospastic I73.9
- Berlin's (traumatic) S05.8X-
- brain (cytotoxic) (vasogenic) G93.6
  - due to birth injury P11.0
  - newborn (anoxia or hypoxia) P52.4
    - birth injury P11.0
  - traumatic —*see* Injury, intracranial, cerebral edema
- cardiac —*see* Failure, heart, congestive
- cardiovascular —*see* Failure, heart, congestive
- cerebral —*see* Edema, brain
- cerebrospinal —*see* Edema, brain
- cervix (uteri) (acute) N88.8
  - puerperal, postpartum O90.89
- chronic hereditary Q82.0
- circumscribed, acute T78.3
  - hereditary D84.1
- conjunctiva H11.42-
- cornea H18.2-
  - idiopathic H18.22-
  - secondary H18.23-
    - due to contact lens H18.21-
- due to
  - lymphatic obstruction I89.0
  - salt retention E87.0
- epiglottis —*see* Edema, glottis
- essential, acute T78.3
  - hereditary D84.1
- extremities, lower —*see* Edema, legs
- eyelid NEC H02.849
  - left H02.846
    - lower H02.845
    - upper H02.844
  - right H02.843
    - lower H02.842
    - upper H02.841
- familial, hereditary Q82.0
- famine —*see* Malnutrition, severe
- generalized R60.1
- glottis, glottic, glottidis (obstructive) (passive) J38.4
  - allergic T78.3
    - hereditary D84.1
- heart —*see* Failure, heart, congestive
- heat T67.7
- hereditary Q82.0
- inanition —*see* Malnutrition, severe
- intracranial G93.6

Edema, edematous *(continued)*
- iris H21.89
- joint —*see* Effusion, joint
- larynx —*see* Edema, glottis
- legs R60.0
  - due to venous obstruction I87.1
  - hereditary Q82.0
- localized R60.0
  - due to venous obstruction I87.1
- lower limbs —*see* Edema, legs
- lung J81.1
  - with heart condition or failure —*see* Failure, ventricular, left
  - acute J81.0
  - chemical (acute) J68.1
    - chronic J68.1
  - chronic J81.1
    - due to
      - chemicals, gases, fumes or vapors (inhalation) J68.1
      - external agent J70.9
        - specified NEC J70.8
      - radiation J70.1
  - due to
    - chemicals, fumes or vapors (inhalation) J68.1
    - external agent J70.9
      - specified NEC J70.8
    - high altitude T70.29
    - near drowning T75.1
    - radiation J70.0
  - meaning failure, left ventricle I50.1
- lymphatic I89.0
  - due to mastectomy I97.2
- macula H35.81
  - cystoid, following cataract surgery —*see* Complications, postprocedural, following cataract surgery
  - diabetic —*see* Diabetes, by type, with, retinopathy, with macular edema
- malignant —*see* Gangrene, gas
- Milroy's Q82.0
- nasopharynx J39.2
- newborn P83.30
  - hydrops fetalis —*see* Hydrops, fetalis
  - specified NEC P83.39
- nutritional —*see also* Malnutrition, severe
  - with dyspigmentation, skin and hair E40
- optic disc or nerve —*see* Papilledema
- orbit H05.22-
- pancreas K86.89
- papilla, optic —*see* Papilledema
- penis N48.89
- periodic T78.3
  - hereditary D84.1
- pharynx J39.2
- pulmonary —*see* Edema, lung
- Quincke's T78.3
  - hereditary D84.1
- renal —*see* Nephrosis
- retina H35.81
  - diabetic —*see* Diabetes, by type, with, retinopathy, with macular edema
- salt E87.0
- scrotum N50.89
- seminal vesicle N50.89
- spermatic cord N50.89
- spinal (cord) (vascular) (nontraumatic) G95.19
- starvation —*see* Malnutrition, severe
- stasis —*see* Hypertension, venous, (chronic)
- subglottic —*see* Edema, glottis
- supraglottic —*see* Edema, glottis

Edema, edematous *(continued)*
  testis N44.8
  tunica vaginalis N50.89
  vas deferens N50.89
  vulva (acute) N90.89

Edentulism *—see* Absence, teeth, acquired

Edsall's disease T67.2

Educational handicap Z55.9
  specified NEC Z55.8

Edward's syndrome *—see* Trisomy, 18

Effect, adverse
  abnormal gravitational (G) forces or states T75.81
  abuse *—see* Maltreatment
  air pressure T70.9
    specified NEC T70.8
  altitude (high) *—see* Effect, adverse, high altitude
  anesthesia (*see also* Anesthesia) T88.59
    in labor and delivery O74.9
    local, toxic
      in labor and delivery O74.4
      in pregnancy NEC O29.3-
      postpartum, puerperal O89.3
    postpartum, puerperal O89.9
    specified NEC T88.59
      in labor and delivery O74.8
      postpartum, puerperal O89.8
    spinal and epidural T88.59
      headache T88.59
        in labor and delivery O74.5
        postpartum, puerperal O89.4
      specified NEC
        in labor and delivery O74.6
        postpartum, puerperal O89.5
  antitoxin *—see* Complications, vaccination
  atmospheric pressure T70.9
    due to explosion T70.8
    high T70.3
    low *—see* Effect, adverse, high altitude
    specified effect NEC T70.8
  biological, correct substance properly administered *—see* Effect, adverse, drug
  blood (derivatives) (serum) (transfusion) *—see* Complications, transfusion
  chemical substance *—see* Table of Drugs and Chemicals
  cold (temperature) (weather) T69.9
    chilblains T69.1
    frostbite *—see* Frostbite
    specified effect NEC T69.8
  drugs and medicaments T88.7
    specified drug *—see* Table of Drugs and Chemicals, by drug, adverse effect
    specified effect - code to condition
  electric current, electricity (shock) T75.4
    burn *—see* Burn
  exertion (excessive) T73.3
  exposure *—see* Exposure
  external cause NEC T75.89
  foodstuffs T78.1
    allergic reaction *—see* Allergy, food
      causing anaphylaxis *—see* Shock, anaphylactic, due to food
    noxious *—see* Poisoning, food, noxious
  gases, fumes, or vapors T59.9-
    specified agent *—see* Table of Drugs and Chemicals

Effect, adverse *(continued)*
  glue (airplane) sniffing
    due to drug abuse *—see* Abuse, drug, inhalant
    due to drug dependence *—see* Dependence, drug, inhalant
  heat *—see* Heat
  high altitude NEC T70.29
    anoxia T70.29
    on
      ears T70.0
      sinuses T70.1
    polycythemia D75.1
  high pressure fluids T70.4
  hot weather *—see* Heat
  hunger T73.0
  immersion, foot *—see* Immersion
  immunization *—see* Complications, vaccination
  immunological agents *—see* Complications, vaccination
  infrared (radiation) (rays) NOS T66
    dermatitis or eczema L59.8
  infusion *—see* Complications, infusion
  lack of care of infants *—see* Maltreatment, child
  lightning *—see* Lightning
  medical care T88.9
    specified NEC T88.8
  medicinal substance, correct, properly administered *—see* Effect, adverse, drug
  motion T75.3
  noise, on inner ear *—see* subcategory H83.3
  overheated places *—see* Heat
  psychosocial, of work environment Z56.5
  radiation (diagnostic) (infrared) (natural source) (therapeutic) (ultraviolet) (X-ray) NOS T66
    dermatitis or eczema *—see* Dermatitis, due to, radiation
    fibrosis of lung J70.1
    pneumonitis J70.0
    pulmonary manifestations
      acute J70.0
      chronic J70.1
    skin L59.9
  radioactive substance NOS
    dermatitis or eczema *—see* Radiodermatitis
  reduced temperature T69.9
    immersion foot or hand *—see* Immersion
    specified effect NEC T69.8
  serum NEC (*see also* Reaction, serum) T80.69
  specified NEC T78.8
    external cause NEC T75.89
  strangulation *—see* Asphyxia, traumatic
  submersion T75.1
  thirst T73.1
  toxic *—see* Toxicity
  transfusion *—see* Complications, transfusion
  ultraviolet (radiation) (rays) NOS T66
    burn *—see* Burn
    dermatitis or eczema *—see* Dermatitis, due to, ultraviolet rays
      acute L56.8
  vaccine (any) *—see* Complications, vaccination
  vibration *—see* Vibration, adverse effects
  water pressure NEC T70.9
    specified NEC T70.8

Effect, adverse *(continued)*
  weightlessness T75.82
  whole blood *—see* Complications, transfusion
  work environment Z56.5

Effect(s) (of) (from) *—see* Effect, adverse NEC

Effects, late *—see* Sequelae

Effluvium
  anagen L65.1
  telogen L65.0

Effort syndrome (psychogenic) F45.8

Effusion
  amniotic fluid *—see* Pregnancy, complicated by, prematue rupture of membranes
  brain (serous) G93.6
  bronchial *—see* Bronchitis
  cerebral G93.6
  cerebrospinal *—see also* Meningitis
    vessel G93.6
  chest *—see* Effusion, pleura
  chylous, chyliform (pleura) J94.0
  intracranial G93.6
  joint M25.40
    ankle M25.47-
    elbow M25.42-
    foot joint M25.47-
    hand joint M25.44-
    hip M25.45-
    knee M25.46-
    shoulder M25.41-
    specified joint NEC M25.48
    wrist M25.43-
  malignant pleural J91.0
  meninges *—see* Meningitis
  pericardium, pericardial (noninflammatory) I31.3
    acute *—see* Pericarditis, acute
  peritoneal (chronic) R18.8
  pleura, pleurisy, pleuritic, pleuropericardial J90
    chylous, chyliform J94.0
    due to systemic lupus erythematosis M32.13
    in conditions classified elsewhere J91.8
    influenzal *—see* Influenza, with, respiratory manifestations NEC
    malignant J91.0
    newborn P28.89
    tuberculous NEC A15.6
      primary (progressive) A15.7
  spinal *—see* Meningitis
  thorax, thoracic *—see* Effusion, pleura

Egg shell nails L60.3
  congenital Q84.6

Egyptian splenomegaly B65.1

Ehrlichiosis A77.40
  due to
    E. chafeensis A77.41
    E. sennetsu A79.81
    specified organism NEC A77.49

Ehlers-Danlos syndrome Q79.6

Eichstedt's disease B36.0

Eisenmenger's
  complex or syndrome I27.83
  defect Q21.8

Ejaculation
  delayed F52.32
  painful N53.12
  premature F52.4
  retarded N53.11
  retrograde N53.14
  semen, painful N53.12
    psychogenic F52.6

Ekbom's syndrome (restless legs) G25.81

Ekman's syndrome (brittle bones and blue sclera) Q78.0

Elastic skin Q82.8
  acquired L57.4

Elastofibroma *—see* Neoplasm, connective tissue, benign

Elastoma (juvenile) Q82.8
  Miescher's L87.2

Elastomyofibrosis I42.4

Elastosis
  actinic, solar L57.8
  atrophicans (senile) L57.4
  perforans serpiginosa L87.2
  senilis L57.4

Elbow *—see* condition

Electric current, electricity, effects (concussion) (fatal) (nonfatal) (shock) T75.4
  burn *—see* Burn

Electric feet syndrome E53.8

Electrocution T75.4
  from electroshock gun (taser) T75.4

Electrolyte imbalance E87.8
  with
    abortion *—see* Abortion by type, complicated by, electrolyte imbalance
    ectopic pregnancy O08.5
    molar pregnancy O08.5

Elephantiasis (nonfilarial) I89.0
  arabicum *—see* Infestation, filarial
  bancroftian B74.0
  congenital (any site) (hereditary) Q82.0
  due to
    Brugia (malayi) B74.1
      timori B74.2
    mastectomy I97.2
    Wuchereria (bancrofti) B74.0
  eyelid H02.859
    left H02.856
      lower H02.855
      upper H02.854
    right H02.853
      lower H02.852
      upper H02.851
  filarial, filariensis *—see* Infestation, filarial
  glandular I89.0
  graecorum A30.9
  lymphangiectatic I89.0
  lymphatic vessel I89.0
    due to mastectomy I97.2
  scrotum (nonfilarial) I89.0
  streptococcal I89.0
  surgical I97.89
    postmastectomy I97.2
  telangiectodes I89.0
  vulva (nonfilarial) N90.89

Elevated, elevation
  antibody titer R76.0
  basal metabolic rate R94.8
  blood pressure *—see also* Hypertension
    reading (incidental) (isolated) (nonspecific), no diagnosis of hypertension R03.0
  blood sugar R73.9
  body temperature (of unknown origin) R50.9
  C-reactive protein (CRP) R79.82
  cancer antigen 125 [CA 125] R97.1
  carcinoembryonic antigen [CEA] R97.0

Elevated, elevation *(continued)*
- cholesterol E78.00
  - with high triglycerides E78.2
- conjugate, eye H51.0
- diaphragm, congenital Q79.1
- erythrocyte sedimentation rate R70.0
- fasting glucose R73.01
- fasting triglycerides E78.1
- finding on laboratory examination —*see* Findings, abnormal, inconclusive, without diagnosis, by type of exam
- GFR (glomerular filtration rate) —*see* Findings, abnormal, inconclusive, without diagnosis, by type of exam
- glucose tolerance (oral) R73.02
- immunoglobulin level R76.8
- indoleacetic acid R82.5
- lactic acid dehydrogenase (LDH) level R74.0
- leukocytes D72.829
- lipoprotein a level E78.8
- liver function
  - study R94.5
  - test R79.89
    - alkaline phosphatase R74.8
    - aminotransferase R74.0
    - bilirubin R17
    - hepatic enzyme R74.8
    - lactate dehydrogenase R74.0
- lymphocytes D72.820
- prostate specific antigen [PSA] R97.20
- Rh titer —*see* Complication(s), transfusion, incompatibility reaction, Rh (factor)
- scapula, congenital Q74.0
- sedimentation rate R70.0
- SGOT R74.0
- SGPT R74.0
- transaminase level R74.0
- triglycerides E78.1
  - with high cholesterol E78.2
- tumor associated antigens [TAA] NEC R97.8
- tumor specific antigens [TSA] NEC R97.8
- urine level of
  - catecholamine R82.5
  - indoleacetic acid R82.5
  - 17-ketosteroids R82.5
  - steroids R82.5
  - vanillylmandelic acid (VMA) R82.5
- venous pressure I87.8
- white blood cell count D72.829
  - specified NEC D72.828

Elliptocytosis (congenital) (hereditary) D58.1
- Hb C (disease) D58.1
- hemoglobin disease D58.1
- sickle-cell (disease) D57.8-
  - trait D57.3

Ellison-Zollinger syndrome E16.4

Ellis-van Creveld syndrome (chondroectodermal dysplasia) Q77.6

Elongated, elongation (congenital) —*see also* Distortion
- bone Q79.9
- cervix (uteri) Q51.828
  - acquired N88.4
  - hypertrophic N88.4
- colon Q43.8
- common bile duct Q44.5
- cystic duct Q44.5
- frenulum, penis Q55.69
- labia minora (acquired) N90.69

Elongated, elongation *(continued)*
- ligamentum patellae Q74.1
- petiolus (epiglottidis) Q31.8
- tooth, teeth K00.2
- uvula Q38.6

Eltor cholera A00.1

Emaciation (due to malnutrition) E41

Embadomoniasis A07.8

Embedded tooth, teeth K01.0
- root only K08.3

Embolic —*see* condition

Embolism (multiple) (paradoxical) I74.9
- air (any site) (traumatic) T79.0
  - following
    - abortion —*see* Abortion by type complicated by embolism
    - ectopic pregnancy O08.2
    - infusion, therapeutic injection or transfusion T80.0
    - molar pregnancy O08.2
    - procedure NEC
      - artery T81.719
        - mesenteric T81.710
        - renal T81.711
        - specified NEC T81.718
      - vein T81.72
  - in pregnancy, childbirth or puerperium —*see* Embolism, obstetric
- amniotic fluid (pulmonary) —*see also* Embolism, obstetric
  - following
    - abortion —*see* Abortion by type complicated by embolism
    - ectopic pregnancy O08.2
    - molar pregnancy O08.2
- aorta, aortic I74.10
  - abdominal I74.09
    - saddle I74.01
  - bifurcation I74.09
  - saddle I74.01
  - thoracic I74.11
- artery I74.9
  - auditory, internal I65.8
  - basilar —*see* Occlusion, artery, basilar
  - carotid (common) (internal) —*see* Occlusion, artery, carotid
  - cerebellar (anterior inferior) (posterior inferior) (superior) I66.3
  - cerebral —*see* Occlusion, artery, cerebral
  - choroidal (anterior) I65.8
  - communicating posterior I65.8
  - coronary —*see also* Infarct, myocardium
    - not resulting in infarction I24.0
  - extremity I74.4
    - lower I74.3
    - upper I74.2
  - hypophyseal I65.8
  - iliac I74.5
  - limb I74.4
    - lower I74.3
    - upper I74.2
  - mesenteric (with gangrene) (*see also* Ischemia, intestine, acute) K55.059
  - ophthalmic —*see* Occlusion, artery, retina
  - peripheral I74.4
  - pontine I65.8
  - precerebral —*see* Occlusion, artery, precerebral
  - pulmonary —*see* Embolism, pulmonary

Embolism *(continued)*
- artery *(continued)*
  - renal N28.0
  - retinal —*see* Occlusion, artery, retina
  - septic I76
  - specified NEC I74.8
  - vertebral —*see* Occlusion, artery, vertebral
- basilar (artery) I65.1
- blood clot
  - following
    - abortion —*see* Abortion by type complicated by embolism
    - ectopic or molar pregnancy O08.2
  - in pregnancy, childbirth or puerperium —*see* Embolism, obstetric
- brain —*see also* Occlusion, artery, cerebral
  - following
    - abortion —*see* Abortion by type complicated by embolism
    - ectopic or molar pregnancy O08.2
  - puerperal, postpartum, childbirth —*see* Embolism, obstetric
- capillary I78.8
- cardiac —*see also* Infarct, myocardium
  - not resulting in infarction I51.3
- carotid (artery) (common) (internal) —*see* Occlusion, artery, carotid
- cavernous sinus (venous) —*see* Embolism, intracranial venous sinus
- cerebral —*see* Occlusion, artery, cerebral
- cholesterol —*see* Atheroembolism
- coronary (artery or vein) (systemic) —*see* Occlusion, coronary
- due to device, implant or graft —*see also* Complications, by site and type, specified NEC
  - arterial graft NEC T82.818
  - breast (implant) T85.818
  - catheter NEC T85.818
    - dialysis (renal) T82.818
      - intraperitoneal T85.818
    - infusion NEC T82.818
      - spinal (epidural) (subdural) T85.810
    - urinary (indwelling) T83.81
  - electronic (electrode) (pulse generator) (stimulator)
    - bone T84.81
    - cardiac T82.817
    - nervous system (brain) (peripheral nerve) (spinal) T85.810
    - urinary T83.81
  - fixation, internal (orthopedic) NEC T84.81
  - gastrointestinal (bile duct) (esophagus) T85.818
  - genital NEC T83.81
  - heart (graft) (valve) T82.817
  - joint prosthesis T84.81
  - ocular (corneal graft) (orbital implant) T85.818
  - orthopedic (bone graft) NEC T86.838
  - specified NEC T85.818
  - urinary (graft) NEC T83.81
  - vascular NEC T82.818
  - ventricular intracranial shunt T85.810
- extremities
  - lower —*see* Embolism, vein, lower extremity
    - arterial I74.3
  - upper I74.2

Embolism *(continued)*
- eye H34.9
- fat (cerebral) (pulmonary) (systemic) T79.1
  - following
    - abortion —*see* Abortion by type complicated by embolism
    - ectopic or molar pregnancy O08.2
  - complicating delivery —*see* Embolism, obstetric
- following
  - abortion —*see* Abortion by type complicated by embolism
  - ectopic or molar pregnancy O08.2
  - infusion, therapeutic injection or transfusion
    - air T80.0
- heart (fatty) —*see also* Infarct, myocardium
  - not resulting in infarction I51.3
- hepatic (vein) I82.0
- in pregnancy, childbirth or puerperium —*see* Embolism, obstetric
- intestine (artery) (vein) (with gangrene) (*see also* Ischemia, intestine, acute) K55.039
- intracranial —*see also* Occlusion, artery, cerebral
  - venous sinus (any) G08
    - nonpyogenic I67.6
- intraspinal venous sinuses or veins G08
  - nonpyogenic G95.19
- kidney (artery) N28.0
- lateral sinus (venous) —*see* Embolism, intracranial, venous sinus
- leg —*see* Embolism, vein, lower extremity
  - arterial I74.3
- longitudinal sinus (venous) —*see* Embolism, intracranial, venous sinus
- lung (massive) —*see* Embolism, pulmonary
- meninges I66.8
- mesenteric (artery) (vein) (with gangrene) (*see also* Ischemia, intestine, acute) K55.059
- obstetric (in) (pulmonary)
  - childbirth O88.22
    - air O88.02
    - amniotic fluid O88.12
    - blood clot O88.22
    - fat O88.82
    - pyemic O88.32
    - septic O88.32
    - specified type NEC O88.82
  - pregnancy O88.21-
    - air O88.01-
    - amniotic fluid O88.11-
    - blood clot O88.21-
    - fat O88.81-
    - pyemic O88.31-
    - septic O88.31-
    - specified type NEC O88.81-
  - puerperal O88.23
    - air O88.03
    - amniotic fluid O88.13
    - blood clot O88.23
    - fat O88.83
    - pyemic O88.33
    - septic O88.33
    - specified type NEC O88.83
- ophthalmic —*see* Occlusion, artery, retina
- penis N48.81
- peripheral artery NOS I74.4

Embolism *(continued)*
pituitary E23.6
popliteal (artery) I74.3
portal (vein) I81
postoperative, postrprocedural
artery T81.719
mesenteric T81.710
renal T81.711
specified NEC T81.718
vein T81.72
precerebral artery —*see* Occlusion, artery, precerebral
puerperal —*see* Embolism, obstetric
pulmonary (acute) (artery) (vein) I26.99
with acute cor pulmonale I26.09
chronic I27.82
following
abortion —*see* Abortion by type complicated by embolism
ectopic or molar pregnancy O08.2
healed or old Z86.711
in pregnancy, childbirth or puerperium —*see* Embolism, obstetric
personal history of Z86.711
saddle I26.92
with acute cor pulmonale I26.02
septic I26.90
with acute cor pulmonale I26.01
pyemic (multiple) I76
following
abortion —*see* Abortion by type complicated by embolism
ectopic or molar pregnancy O08.2
Hemophilus influenzae A41.3
pneumococcal A40.3
with pneumonia J13
puerperal, postpartum, childbirth (any organism) —*see* Embolism, obstetric
specified organism NEC A41.89
staphylococcal A41.2
streptococcal A40.9
renal (artery) N28.0
vein I82.3
retina, retinal —*see* Occlusion, artery, retina
saddle
abdominal aorta I74.01
pulmonary artery I26.92
with acute cor pulmonale I26.02
septic (arterial) I76
complicating abortion —*see* Abortion, by type, complicated by, embolism
sinus —*see* Embolism, intracranial, venous sinus
soap complicating abortion —*see* Abortion, by type, complicated by, embolism
spinal cord G95.19
pyogenic origin G06.1
spleen, splenic (artery) I74.8
upper extremity I74.2
vein (acute) I82.90
antecubital I82.61-
chronic I82.71-
axillary I82.A1-
chronic I82.A2-
basilic I82.61-
chronic I82.71-
brachial I82.62-
chronic I82.72-
brachiocephalic (innominate) I82.290
chronic I82.291

Embolism *(continued)*
vein *(continued)*
cephalic I82.61-
chronic I82.71-
chronic I82.91
deep (DVT) I82.40-
calf I82.4Z-
chronic I82.5Z-
lower leg I82.4Z-
chronic I82.5Z-
thigh I82.4Y-
chronic I82.5Y-
upper leg I82.4Y
chronic I82.5y-
femoral I82.41-
chronic I82.51-
iliac (iliofemoral) I82.42-
chronic I82.52-
innominate I82.290
chronic I82.291
internal jugular I82.C1-
chronic I82.C2-
lower extremity
deep I82.40-
chronic I82.50-
specified NEC I82.49-
chronic NEC I82.59-
distal
deep I82.4Z-
proximal
deep I82.4Y-
chronic I82.5Y-
superficial I82.81-
popliteal I82.43-
chronic I82.53-
radial I82.62-
chronic I82.72-
renal I82.3
saphenous (greater) (lesser) I82.81-
specified NEC I82.890
chronic NEC I82.891
subclavian I82.B1-
chronic I82.B2-
thoracic NEC I82.290
chronic I82.291
tibial I82.44-
chronic I82.54-
ulnar I82.62-
chronic I82.72-
upper extremity I82.60-
chronic I82.70-
deep I82.62-
chronic I82.72-
superficial I82.61-
chronic I82.71-
vena cava
inferior (acute) I82.220
chronic I82.221
superior (acute) I82.210
chronic I82.211
venous sinus G08
vessels of brain —*see* Occlusion, artery, cerebral

Embolus —*see* Embolism

Embryoma —*see also* Neoplasm, uncertain behavior, by site
benign —*see* Neoplasm, benign, by site
kidney C64.-
liver C22.0
malignant —*see also* Neoplasm, malignant, by site
kidney C64.-
liver C22.0
testis C62.9-
descended (scrotal) C62.1-
undescended C62.0-
testis C62.9-
descended (scrotal) C62.1-
undescended C62.0-

Embryonic
circulation Q28.9
heart Q28.9
vas deferens Q55.4

Embryopathia NOS Q89.9

Embryotoxon Q13.4

Emesis —*see* Vomiting

Emotional lability R45.86

Emotionality, pathological F60.3

Emotogenic disease —*see* Disorder, psychogenic

Emphysema (atrophic) (bullous) (chronic) (interlobular) (lung) (obstructive) (pulmonary) (senile) (vesicular) J43.9
cellular tissue (traumatic) T79.7
surgical T81.82
centrilobular J43.2
compensatory J98.3
congenital (interstitial) P25.0
conjunctiva H11.89
connective tissue (traumatic) T79.7
surgical T81.82
due to chemicals, gases, fumes or vapors J68.4
eyelid(s) —*see* Disorder, eyelid, specified type NEC
surgical T81.82
traumatic T79.7
interstitial J98.2
congenital P25.0
perinatal period P25.0
laminated tissue T79.7
surgical T81.82
mediastinal J98.2
newborn P25.2
orbit, orbital —*see* Disorder, orbit, specified type NEC
panacinar J43.1
panlobular J43.1
specified NEC J43.8
subcutaneous (traumatic) T79.7
nontraumatic J98.2
postprocedural T81.82
surgical T81.82
surgical T81.82
thymus (gland) (congenital) E32.8
traumatic (subcutaneous) T79.7
unilateral J43.0

Empty nest syndrome Z60.0

Empyema (acute) (chest) (double) (pleura) (supradiaphragmatic) (thorax) J86.9
with fistula J86.0
accessory sinus (chronic) —*see* Sinusitis
antrum (chronic) —*see* Sinusitis, maxillary
brain (any part) —*see* Abscess, brain
ethmoidal (chronic) (sinus) —*see* Sinusitis, ethmoidal
extradural —*see* Abscess, extradural
frontal (chronic) (sinus) —*see* Sinusitis, frontal
gallbladder K81.0
mastoid (process) (acute) —*see* Mastoiditis, acute
maxilla, maxillary M27.2
sinus (chronic) —*see* Sinusitis, maxillary
nasal sinus (chronic) —*see* Sinusitis
sinus (accessory) (chronic) (nasal) —*see* Sinusitis
sphenoidal (sinus) (chronic) —*see* Sinusitis, sphenoidal
subarachnoid —*see* Abscess, extradural

Empyema *(continued)*
subdural —*see* Abscess, subdural
tuberculous A15.6
ureter —*see* Ureteritis
ventricular —*see* Abscess, brain

En coup de sabre lesion L94.1

Enamel pearls K00.2

Enameloma K00.2

Enanthema, viral B09

Encephalitis (chronic) (hemorrhagic) (idiopathic) (nonepidemic) (spurious) (subacute) G04.90
acute (*see also* Encephalitis, viral) A86
disseminated G04.00
infectious G04.01
noninfectious G04.81
postimmunization (postvaccination) G04.02
postinfectious G04.01
inclusion body A85.8
necrotizing hemorrhagic G04.30
postimmunization G04.32
postinfectious G04.31
specified NEC G04.39
arboviral, arbovirus NEC A85.2
arthropod-borne NEC (viral) A85.2
Australian A83.4
California (virus) A83.5
Central European (tick-borne) A84.1
Czechoslovakian A84.1
Dawson's (inclusion body) A81.1
diffuse sclerosing A81.1
disseminated, acute G04.00
due to
cat scratch disease A28.1
human immunodeficiency virus (HIV) disease B20 *[G05.3]*
malaria —*see* Malaria
rickettsiosis —*see* Rickettsiosis
smallpox inoculation G04.02
typhus —*see* Typhus
Eastern equine A83.2
endemic (viral) A86
epidemic NEC (viral) A86
equine (acute) (infectious) (viral) A83.9
Eastern A83.2
Venezuelan A92.2
Western A83.1
Far Eastern (tick-borne) A84.0
following vaccination or other immunization procedure G04.02
herpes zoster B02.0
herpesviral B00.4
due to herpesvirus 6 B10.01
due to herpesvirus 7 B10.09
specified NEC B10.09
Ilheus (virus) A83.8
inclusion body A81.1
in (due to)
actinomycosis A42.82
adenovirus A85.1
African trypanosomiasis B56.9 *[G05.3]*
Chagas' disease (chronic) B57.42
cytomegalovirus B25.8
enterovirus A85.0
herpes (simplex) virus B00.4
due to herpesvirus 6 B10.01
due to herpesvirus 7 B10.09
specified NEC B10.09
infectious disease NEC B99 *[G05.3]*
influenza —*see* Influenza, with, encephalopathy
listeriosis A32.12
measles B05.0

Encephalitis *(continued)*
- in *(continued)*
  - mumps B26.2
  - naegleriasis B60.2
  - parasitic disease NEC B89 *[G05.3]*
  - poliovirus A80.9 *[G05.3]*
  - rubella B06.01
  - syphilis
    - congenital A50.42
    - late A52.14
  - systemic lupus erythematosus M32.19
  - toxoplasmosis (acquired) B58.2
    - congenital P37.1
  - tuberculosis A17.82
  - zoster B02.0
- infectious (acute) (virus) NEC A86
- Japanese (B type) A83.0
- La Crosse A83.5
- lead *—see* Poisoning, lead
- lethargica (acute) (infectious) A85.8
- louping ill A84.8
- lupus erythematosus, systemic M32.19
- lymphatica A87.2
- Mengo A85.8
- meningococcal A39.81
- Murray Valley A83.4
- otitic NEC H66.40 *[G05.3]*
- parasitic NOS B71.9
- periaxial G37.0
- periaxialis (concentrica) (diffuse) G37.5
- postchickenpox B01.11
- postexanthematous NEC B09
- postimmunization G04.02
- postinfectious NEC G04.01
- postmeasles B05.0
- postvaccinal G04.02
- postvaricella B01.11
- postviral NEC A86
- Powassan A84.8
- Rasmussen G04.81
- Rio Bravo A85.8
- Russian
  - autumnal A83.0
  - spring-summer (taiga) A84.0
- saturnine *—see* Poisoning, lead
- specified NEC G04.81
- St. Louis A83.3
- subacute sclerosing A81.1
- summer A83.0
- suppurative G04.81
- tick-borne A84.9
- Torula, torular (cryptococcal) B45.1
- toxic NEC G92
- trichinosis B75 *[G05.3]*
- type
  - B A83.0
  - C A83.3
- van Bogaert's A81.1
- Venezuelan equine A92.2
- Vienna A85.8
- viral, virus A86
  - arthropod-borne NEC A85.2
    - mosquito-borne A83.9
      - Australian X disease A83.4
      - California virus A83.5
      - Eastern equine A83.2
      - Japanese (B type) A83.0
      - Murray Valley A83.4
      - specified NEC A83.8
      - St. Louis A83.3
      - type B A83.0
      - type C A83.3
      - Western equine A83.1
    - tick-borne A84.9
      - biundulant A84.1
      - central European A84.1
      - Czechoslovakian A84.1

Encephalitis *(continued)*
- viral, virus *(continued)*
  - arthropod-borne *(continued)*
    - tick-borne *(continued)*
      - diphasic meningoencephalitis A84.1
      - Far Eastern A84.0
      - Russian spring-summer (taiga) A84.0
      - specified NEC A84.8
    - specified type NEC A85.8
  - Western equine A83.1

Encephalocele Q01.9
- frontal Q01.0
- nasofrontal Q01.1
- occipital Q01.2
- specified NEC Q01.8

Encephalocystocele *—see* Encephalocele

Encephaloduroarteriomyosynangiosis (EDAMS) I67.5

Encephalomalacia (brain) (cerebellar) (cerebral) *—see* Softening, brain

Encephalomeningitis *—see* Meningoencephalitis

Encephalomeningocele *—see* Encephalocele

Encephalomeningomyelitis *—see* Meningoencephalitis

Encephalomyelitis *—see also* Encephalitis G04.90
- acute disseminated G04.00
  - infectious G04.01
  - noninfectious G04.81
  - postimmunization G04.02
  - postinfectious G04.01
- acute necrotizing hemorrhagic G04.30
  - postimmunization G04.32
  - postinfectious G04.31
  - specified NEC G04.39
- benign myalgic G93.3
- equine A83.9
  - Eastern A83.2
  - Venezuelan A92.2
  - Western A83.1
- in diseases classified elsewhere G05.3
- myalgic, benign G93.3
- postchickenpox B01.11
- postinfectious NEC G04.01
- postmeasles B05.0
- postvaccinal G04.02
- postvaricella B01.11
- rubella B06.01
- specified NEC G04.81
- Venezuelan equine A92.2

Encephalomyelocele *—see* Encephalocele

Encephalomyelomeningitis *—see* Meningoencephalitis

Encephalomyelopathy G96.9

Encephalomyeloradiculitis (acute) G61.0

Encephalomyeloradiculoneuritis (acute) (Guillain-Barré) G61.0

Encephalomyeloradiculopathy G96.9

Encephalopathia hyperbilirubinemica, newborn P57.9
- due to isoimmunization (conditions in P55) P57.0

Encephalopathy (acute) G93.40
- acute necrotizing hemorrhagic G04.30
  - postimmunization G04.32
  - postinfectious G04.31
  - specified NEC G04.39
- alcoholic G31.2
- anoxic *—see* Damage, brain, anoxic
- arteriosclerotic I67.2
- centrolobar progressive (Schilder) G37.0
- congenital Q07.9
- degenerative, in specified disease NEC G32.89
- demyelinating callosal G37.1
- due to
  - drugs (*see also* Table of Drugs and Chemicals) G92
- hepatic *—see* Failure, hepatic
- hyperbilirubinemic, newborn P57.9
  - due to isoimmunization (conditions in P55) P57.0
- hypertensive I67.4
- hypoglycemic E16.2
- hypoxic *—see* Damage, brain, anoxic
- hypoxic ischemic P91.60
  - mild P91.61
  - moderate P91.62
  - severe P91.63
- in (due to) (with)
  - birth injury P11.1
  - hyperinsulinism E16.1 *[G94]*
  - influenza *—see* Influenza, with, encephalopathy
  - lack of vitamin (*see also* Deficiency, vitamin) E56.9 *[G32.89]*
  - neoplastic disease (*see also* Neoplasm) D49.9 *[G13.1]*
  - serum (*see also* Reaction, serum) T80.69
  - syphilis A52.17
  - trauma (postconcussional) F07.81
    - current injury *—see* Injury, intracranial
  - vaccination G04.02
- lead *—see* Poisoning, lead
- metabolic G93.41
  - drug induced G92
  - toxic G92
- myoclonic, early, symptomatic *—see* Epilepsy, generalized, specified NEC
- necrotizing, subacute (Leigh) G31.82
- neonatal P91.819
  - in diseases classified elsewhere P91.811
- pellagrous E52 *[G32.89]*
- portosystemic *—see* Failure, hepatic
- postcontusional F07.81
  - current injury *—see* Injury, intracranial, diffuse
- posthypoglycemic (coma) E16.1 *[G94]*
- postradiation G93.89
- saturnine *—see* Poisoning, lead
- septic G93.41
- specified NEC G93.49
- spongioform, subacute (viral) A81.09
- toxic G92
  - metabolic G92
- traumatic (postconcussional) F07.81
  - current injury *—see* Injury, intracranial
- vitamin B deficiency NEC E53.9 *[G32.89]*
  - vitamin B1 E51.2
- Wernicke's E51.2

Encephalorrhagia *—see* Hemorrhage, intracranial, intracerebral

Encephalosis, posttraumatic F07.81

Enchondroma *—see also* Neoplasm, bone, benign

Enchondromatosis (cartilaginous) (multiple) Q78.4

Encopresis R15.9
- functional F98.1
- nonorganic origin F98.1
- psychogenic F98.1

Encounter (with health service) (for) Z76.89
- adjustment and management (of)
  - breast implant Z45.81
  - implanted device NEC Z45.89
  - myringotomy device (stent) (tube) Z45.82
- administrative purpose only Z02.9
  - examination for
    - adoption Z02.82
    - armed forces Z02.3
    - disability determination Z02.71
    - driving license Z02.4
    - employment Z02.1
    - insurance Z02.6
    - medical certificate NEC Z02.79
    - paternity testing Z02.81
    - residential institution admission Z02.2
    - school admission Z02.0
    - sports Z02.5
  - specified reason NEC Z02.89
- aftercare *—see* Aftercare
- antenatal screening Z36.9
  - cervical length Z36.86
  - chromosomal anomalies Z36.0
  - congenital cardiac abnormalities Z36.83
  - elevated maternal serum alphafetoprotein level Z36.1
  - fetal growth retardation Z36.4
  - fetal lung maturity Z36.84
  - fetal macrosomia Z36.88
  - hydrops fetalis Z36.81
  - intrauterine growth restriction (IUGR)/small-for-dates Z36.4
  - isoimmunization Z36.5
  - large-for-dates Z36.88
  - malformations Z36.3
  - non-visualized anatomy on a previous scan Z36.2
  - nuchal translucency Z36.82
  - raised alphafetoprotein level Z36.1
  - risk of pre-term labor Z36.86
  - specified type NEC Z36.89
  - specified follow-up NEC Z36.2
  - specified genetic defects NEC Z36.8A
  - Streptococcus B Z36.85
  - suspected anomaly Z36.3
  - uncertain dates Z36.87
- assisted reproductive fertility procedure cycle Z31.83
- blood typing Z01.83
  - Rh typing Z01.83
- breast augmentation or reduction Z41.1
- breast implant exchange (different material) (different size) Z45.81
- breast reconstruction following mastectomy Z42.1
- check-up *—see* Examination
- chemotherapy for neoplasm Z51.11
- colonoscopy, screening Z12.11
- counseling *—see* Counseling
- delivery, full-term, uncomplicated O80
  - cesarean, without indication O82
- desensitization to allergens Z51.6
- ear piercing Z41.3

Encounter *(continued)*
examination —*see* Examination
expectant parent(s) (adoptive)
pre-birth pediatrician visit Z76.81
fertility preservation procedure (prior to cancer therapy) (prior to removal of gonads) Z31.84
fitting (of) —*see* Fitting (and adjustment) (of)
genetic
counseling
nonprocreative Z71.83
procreative Z31.5
testing —*see* Test, genetic
hearing conservation and treatment Z01.12
immunotherapy for neoplasm Z51.12
in vitro fertilization cycle Z31.83
instruction (in)
childbirth Z32.2
child care (postpartal) (prenatal) Z32.3
natural family planning
procreative Z31.61
to avoid pregnancy Z30.02
insulin pump titration Z46.81
joint prosthesis insertion following prior explantation of joint prosthesis (staged procedure)
hip Z47.32
knee Z47.33
shoulder Z47.31
laboratory (as part of a general medical examination) Z00.00
with abnormal findings Z00.01
mental health services (for)
abuse NEC
perpetrator Z69.82
victim Z69.81
child abuse
nonparental
perpetrator Z69.021
victim Z69.020
parental
perpetrator Z69.011
victim Z69.010
child neglect
nonparental
perpetrator Z69.021
victim Z69.020
parental
perpetrator Z69.011
victim Z69.010
child psychological abuse
nonparental
perpetrator Z69.021
victim Z69.020
parental
perpetrator Z69.011
victim Z69.010
child sexual abuse
nonparental
perpetrator Z69.021
victim Z69.020
parental
perpetrator Z69.011
victim Z69.010
non-spousal adult abuse (perpetrator) (victim) Z69.81
spousal or parter
abuse
perpetrator Z69.12
victim Z69.11
neglect
perpetrator Z69.12
victim Z69.11
psychological abuse
perpetrator Z69.12
victim Z69.11

Encounter *(continued)*
mental health services *(continued)*
spousal or parter *(continued)*
violence
perpetrator (physical) (sexual) Z69.12
victim (physical) Z69.11
sexual Z69.81
observation (for) (ruled out)
exposure to (suspected)
anthrax Z03.810
biological agent NEC Z03.818
pediatrician visit, by expectant parent(s) (adoptive) Z76.81
placental sample (taken vaginally) (*see also* Encounter, antenatal screening) Z36.9
plastic and reconstructive surgery following medical procedure or healed injury NEC Z42.8
pregnancy
supervision of —*see* Pregnancy, supervision of
test Z32.00
result negative Z32.02
result positive Z32.01
procreative management and counseling for gestational carrier Z31.7
prophylactic measures Z29.9
antivenin Z29.12
fluoride administration Z29.3
immunotherapy for respiratory syncytial virus (RSV) Z29.11
rabies immune globulin Z29.14
Rho (D) immune globulin Z29.13
specified NEC Z29.8
radiation therapy (antineoplastic) Z51.0
radiological (as part of a general medical examination) Z00.00
with abnormal findings Z00.01
reconstructive surgery following medical procedure or healed injury NEC Z42.8
removal (of) —*see also* Removal
artificial
arm Z44.00-
complete Z44.01-
partial Z44.02-
eye Z44.2-
leg Z44.10-
complete Z44.11-
partial Z44.12-
breast implant Z45.81
tissue expander (without synchronous insertion of permanent implant) Z45.81
device Z46.9
specified NEC Z46.89
external
fixation device - code to fracture with seventh character D
prosthesis, prosthetic device Z44.9
breast Z44.3-
specified NEC Z44.8
implanted device NEC Z45.89
insulin pump Z46.81
internal fixation device Z47.2
myringotomy device (stent) (tube) Z45.82
nervous system device NEC Z46.2
brain neuropacemaker Z46.2
visual substitution device Z46.2
implanted Z45.31
non-vascular catheter Z46.82
orthodontic device Z46.4
stent
ureteral Z46.6
urinary device Z46.6

Encounter *(continued)*
repeat cervical smear to confirm findings of recent normal smear following initial abnormal smear Z01.42
respirator [ventilator] use during power failure Z99.12
Rh typing Z01.83
screening —*see* Screening
specified NEC Z76.89
sterilization Z30.2
suspected condition, ruled out
amniotic cavity and membrane Z03.71
cervical shortening Z03.75
fetal anomaly Z03.73
fetal growth Z03.74
maternal and fetal conditions NEC Z03.79
oligohydramnios Z03.71
placental problem Z03.72
polyhydramnios Z03.71
suspected exposure (to), ruled out
anthrax Z03.810
biological agents NEC Z03.818
termination of pregnancy, elective Z33.2
testing —*see* Test
therapeutic drug level monitoring Z51.81
titration, insulin pump Z46.81
to determine fetal viability of pregnancy O36.80
training
insulin pump Z46.81
X-ray of chest (as part of a general medical examination) Z00.00
with abnormal findings Z00.01

Encystment —*see* Cyst

Endarteritis (bacterial, subacute) (infective) I77.6
brain I67.7
cerebral or cerebrospinal I67.7
deformans —*see* Arteriosclerosis
embolic —*see* Embolism
obliterans —*see also* Arteriosclerosis
pulmonary I28.8
pulmonary I28.8
retina —*see* Vasculitis, retina
senile —*see* Arteriosclerosis
syphilitic A52.09
brain or cerebral A52.04
congenital A50.54 *[I79.8]*
tuberculous A18.89

Endemic —*see* condition

Endocarditis (chronic) (marantic) (nonbacterial) (thrombotic) (valvular) I38
with rheumatic fever (conditions in I00)
active —*see* Endocarditis, acute, rheumatic
inactive or quiescent (with chorea) I09.1
acute or subacute I33.9
infective I33.0
rheumatic (aortic) (mitral) (pulmonary) (tricuspid) I01.1
with chorea (acute) (rheumatic) (Sydenham's) I02.0
aortic (heart) (nonrheumatic) (valve) I35.8
with
mitral disease I08.0
with tricuspid (valve) disease I08.3
active or acute I01.1
with chorea (acute) (rheumatic) (Sydenham's) I02.0

Endocarditis *(continued)*
aortic *(continued)*
with *(continued)*
rheumatic fever (conditions in I00)
active —*see* Endocarditis, acute, rheumatic
inactive or quiescent (with chorea) I06.9
tricuspid (valve) disease I08.2
with mitral (valve) disease I08.3
acute or subacute I33.9
arteriosclerotic I35.8
rheumatic I06.9
with mitral disease I08.0
with tricuspid (valve) disease I08.3
active or acute I01.1
with chorea (acute) (rheumatic) (Sydenham's) I02.0
active or acute I01.1
with chorea (acute) (rheumatic) (Sydenham's) I02.0
specified NEC I06.8
specified cause NEC I35.8
syphilitic A52.03
arteriosclerotic I38
atypical verrucous (Libman-Sacks) M32.11
bacterial (acute) (any valve) (subacute) I33.0
candidal B37.6
congenital Q24.8
constrictive I33.0
Coxiella burnetii A78 *[I39]*
Coxsackie B33.21
due to
prosthetic cardiac valve T82.6
Q fever A78 *[I39]*
Serratia marcescens I33.0
typhoid (fever) A01.02
gonococcal A54.83
infectious or infective (acute) (any valve) (subacute) I33.0
lenta (acute) (any valve) (subacute) I33.0
Libman-Sacks M32.11
listerial A32.82
Löffler's I42.3
malignant (acute) (any valve) (subacute) I33.0
meningococcal A39.51
mitral (chronic) (double) (fibroid) (heart) (inactive) (valve) (with chorea) I05.9
with
aortic (valve) disease I08.0
with tricuspid (valve) disease I08.3
active or acute I01.1
with chorea (acute) (rheumatic) (Sydenham's) I02.0
rheumatic fever (conditions in I00)
active —*see* Endocarditis, acute, rheumatic
inactive or quiescent (with chorea) I05.9
tricuspid (valve) disease I08.1
with aortic (valve) disease I08.3
active or acute I01.1
with chorea (acute) (rheumatic) (Sydenham's) I02.0
bacterial I33.0
arteriosclerotic I34.8
nonrheumatic I34.8
acute or subacute I33.9
specified NEC I05.8

Endocarditis *(continued)*
- monilial B37.6
- multiple valves I08.9
  - specified disorders I08.8
- mycotic (acute) (any valve) (subacute) I33.0
- pneumococcal (acute) (any valve) (subacute) I33.0
- pulmonary (chronic) (heart) (valve) I37.8
  - with rheumatic fever (conditions in I00)
    - active —*see* Endocarditis, acute, rheumatic
    - inactive or quiescent (with chorea) I09.89
      - with aortic, mitral or tricuspid disease I08.8
  - acute or subacute I33.9
    - rheumatic I01.1
      - with chorea (acute) (rheumatic) (Sydenham's) I02.0
  - arteriosclerotic I37.8
  - congenital Q22.2
  - rheumatic (chronic) (inactive) (with chorea) I09.89
    - active or acute I01.1
      - with chorea (acute) (rheumatic) (Sydenham's) I02.0
  - syphilitic A52.03
- purulent (acute) (any valve) (subacute) I33.0
- Q fever A78 *[I39]*
- rheumatic (chronic) (inactive) (with chorea) I09.1
  - active or acute (aortic) (mitral) (pulmonary) (tricuspid) I01.1
    - with chorea (acute) (rheumatic) (Sydenham's) I02.0
- rheumatoid —*see* Rheumatoid, carditis
- septic (acute) (any valve) (subacute) I33.0
- streptococcal (acute) (any valve) (subacute) I33.0
- subacute —*see* Endocarditis, acute
- suppurative (acute) (any valve) (subacute) I33.0
- syphilitic A52.03
- toxic I33.9
- tricuspid (chronic) (heart) (inactive) (rheumatic) (valve) (with chorea) I07.9
  - with
    - aortic (valve) disease I08.2
      - mitral (valve) disease I08.3
    - mitral (valve) disease I08.1
      - aortic (valve) disease I08.3
    - rheumatic fever (conditions in I00)
      - active —*see* Endocarditis, acute, rheumatic
      - inactive or quiescent (with chorea) I07.8
  - active or acute I01.1
    - with chorea (acute) (rheumatic) (Sydenham's) I02.0
  - arteriosclerotic I36.8
  - nonrheumatic I36.8
    - acute or subacute I33.9
  - specified cause, except rheumatic I36.8
- tuberculous —*see* Tuberculosis, endocarditis
- typhoid A01.02
- ulcerative (acute) (any valve) (subacute) I33.0
- vegetative (acute) (any valve) (subacute) I33.0

Endocarditis *(continued)*
- verrucous (atypical) (nonbacterial) (nonrheumatic) M32.11

Endocardium, endocardial —*see also* condition
- cushion defect Q21.2

Endocervicitis —*see also* Cervicitis
- due to intrauterine (contraceptive) device T83.69
- hyperplastic N72

Endocrine —*see* condition

Endocrinopathy, pluriglandular E31.9

Endodontic
- overfill M27.52
- underfill M27.53

Endodontitis K04.01
- irreversible K04.02
- reversible K04.01

Endomastoiditis —*see* Mastoiditis

Endometrioma N80.9

Endometriosis N80.9
- appendix N80.5
- bladder N80.8
- bowel N80.5
- broad ligament N80.3
- cervix N80.0
- colon N80.5
- cul-de-sac (Douglas') N80.3
- exocervix N80.0
- fallopian tube N80.2
- female genital organ NEC N80.8
- gallbladder N80.8
- in scar of skin N80.6
- internal N80.0
- intestine N80.5
- lung N80.8
- myometrium N80.0
- ovary N80.1
- parametrium N80.3
- pelvic peritoneum N80.3
- peritoneal (pelvic) N80.3
- rectovaginal septum N80.4
- rectum N80.5
- round ligament N80.3
- skin (scar) N80.6
- specified site NEC N80.8
- stromal D39.0
- thorax N80.8
- umbilicus N80.8
- uterus (internal) N80.0
- vagina N80.4
- vulva N80.8

Endometritis (decidual) (nonspecific) (purulent) (senile) (atrophic) (suppurative) N71.9
- with ectopic pregnancy O08.0
- acute N71.0
- blenorrhagic (gonococcal) (acute) (chronic) A54.24
- cervix, cervical (with erosion or ectropion) —*see also* Cervicitis
  - hyperplastic N72
- chlamydial A56.11
- chronic N71.1
- following
  - abortion —*see* Abortion by type complicated by genital infection
  - ectopic or molar pregnancy O08.0
- gonococcal, gonorrheal (acute) (chronic) A54.24
- hyperplastic (*see also* Hyperplasia, endometrial) N85.00-
  - cervix N72
- puerperal, postpartum, childbirth O86.12

Endometritis *(continued)*
- subacute N71.0
- tuberculous A18.17

Endometrium —*see* condition

Endomyocardiopathy, South African I42.3

Endomyocarditis —*see* Endocarditis

Endomyofibrosis I42.3

Endomyometritis —*see* Endometritis

Endopericarditis —*see* Endocarditis

Endoperineuritis —*see* Disorder, nerve

Endophlebitis —*see* Phlebitis

Endophthalmia —*see* Endophthalmitis, purulent

Endophthalmitis (acute) (infective) (metastatic) (subacute) H44.009
- bleb associated H59.4 —*see also* Bleb, inflammed (infected), postprocedural
- gonorrheal A54.39
- in (due to)
  - cysticercosis B69.1
  - onchocerciasis B73.01
  - toxocariasis B83.0
- panuveitis —*see* Panuveitis
- parasitic H44.12-
- purulent H44.00-
  - panophthalmitis —*see* Panophthalmitis
  - vitreous abscess H44.02-
- specified NEC H44.19
- sympathetic —*see* Uveitis, sympathetic

Endosalpingioma D28.2

Endosalpingiosis N94.89

Endosteitis —*see* Osteomyelitis

Endothelioma, bone —*see* Neoplasm, bone, malignant

Endotheliosis (hemorrhagic infectional) D69.8

Endotoxemia - code to condition

Endotrachelitis —*see* Cervicitis

Engelmann (-Camurati) **syndrome** Q78.3

English disease —*see* Rickets

Engman's disease L30.3

Engorgement
- breast N64.59
  - newborn P83.4
  - puerperal, postpartum O92.79
- lung (passive) —*see* Edema, lung
- pulmonary (passive) —*see* Edema, lung
- stomach K31.89
- venous, retina —*see* Occlusion, retina, vein, engorgement

Enlargement, enlarged —*see also* Hypertrophy
- adenoids J35.2
  - with tonsils J35.3
- alveolar ridge K08.89
  - congenital —*see* Anomaly, alveolar
- apertures of diaphragm (congenital) Q79.1
- gingival K06.1
- heart, cardiac —*see* Hypertrophy, cardiac
- labium majus, childhood asymmetric (CALME) N90.61
- lacrimal gland, chronic H04.03-
- liver —*see* Hypertrophy, liver
- lymph gland or node R59.9
  - generalized R59.1
  - localized R59.0

Enlargement, enlarged *(continued)*
- orbit H05.34-
- organ or site, congenital NEC —*see* Anomaly, by site
- parathyroid (gland) E21.0
- pituitary fossa R93.0
- prostate N40.0
  - with lower urinary tract symptoms (LUTS) N40.1
  - without lower urinary tract symtpoms (LUTS) N40.0
- sella turcica R93.0
- spleen —*see* Splenomegaly
- thymus (gland) (congenital) E32.0
- thyroid (gland) —*see* Goiter
- tongue K14.8
- tonsils J35.1
  - with adenoids J35.3
- uterus N85.2
- vestibular aqueduct A16.5

Enophthalmos H05.40-
- due to
  - orbital tissue atrophy H05.41-
  - trauma or surgery H05.42-

Enostosis M27.8

Entamebic, entamebiasis —*see* Amebiasis

Entanglement
- umbilical cord(s) O69.82
  - with compression O69.2
  - around neck (with compression) O69.81
    - with compression O69.1
    - without compression O69.81
  - of twins in monoamniotic sac O69.2
  - without compression O69.82

Enteralgia —*see* Pain, abdominal

Enteric —*see* condition

Enteritis (acute) (diarrheal) (hemorrhagic) (noninfective) K52.9
- adenovirus A08.2
- aertrycke infection A02.0
- allergic K52.29
  - with
    - eosinophilic gastritis or gastroenteritis K52.81
    - food protein-induced entercolitis syndrome K52.21
    - food protein-induced enteropathy K52.22
- amebic (acute) A06.0
  - with abscess —*see* Abscess, amebic
  - chronic A06.1
    - with abscess —*see* Abscess, amebic
    - nondysenteric A06.2
  - nondysenteric A06.2
- astrovirus A08.32
- bacillary NOS A03.9
- bacterial A04.9
  - specified NEC A04.8
- calicivirus A08.31
- candidal B37.82
- Chilomastix A07.8
- choleriformis A00.1
- chronic (noninfectious) K52.9
  - ulcerative —*see* Colitis, ulcerative
- cicatrizing (chronic) —*see* Enteritis, regional, small intestine
- Clostridium
  - botulinum (food poisoning) A05.1
  - difficile
    - not specified as recurrent A04.72
    - recurrent A04.71
- coccidial A07.3

Enteritis *(continued)*
coxsackie virus A08.39
dietetic (*see also* Enteritis, allergic) K52.29
drug-induced K52.1
due to
astrovirus A08.32
calicivirus A08.31
coxsackie virus A08.39
drugs K52.1
echovirus A08.39
enterovirus NEC A08.39
food hypersensitivity (*see also* Enteritis, allergic) K52.29
infectious organism (bacterial) (viral) —*see* Enteritis, infectious
torovirus A08.39
Yersinia enterocolitica A04.6
echovirus A08.39
eltor A00.1
enterovirus NEC A08.39
eosinophilic K52.81
epidemic (infectious) A09
fulminant (*see also* Ischemia, intestine acute) K55.019
gangrenous —*see* Enteritis, infectious
giardial A07.1
infectious NOS A09
due to
adenovirus A08.2
Aerobacter aerogenes A04.8
Arizona (bacillus) A02.0
bacteria NOS A04.9
specified NEC A04.8
Campylobacter A04.5
Clostridium difficile
not specified as recurrent A04.72
recurrent A04.71
Clostridium perfringens A04.8
Enterobacter aerogenes A04.8
enterovirus A08.39
Escherichia coli A04.4
enteroaggregative A04.4
enterohemorrhagic A04.3
enteroinvasive A04.2
enteropathogenic A04.0
enterotoxigenic A04.1
specified NEC A04.4
specified
bacteria NEC A04.8
virus NEC A08.39
Staphylococcus A04.8
virus NEC A08.4
specified type NEC A08.39
Yersinia enterocolitica A04.6
specified organism NEC A08.8
influenzal —*see* Influenza, with, digestive manifestations
ischemic K55.9
acute (*see also* Ischemia, intestine acute) K55.019
chronic K55.1
microsporidial A07.8
mucomembranous, myxomembranous —*see* Syndrome, irritable bowel
mucous —*see* Syndrome, irritable bowel
necroticans A05.2
necrotizing of newborn —*see* Enterocolitis, necrotizing, in newborn
neurogenic —*see* Syndrome, irritable bowel
newborn necrotizing —*see* Enterocolitis, necrotizing, in newborn
noninfectious K52.9

Enteritis *(continued)*
norovirus A08.11
parasitic NEC B82.9
paratyphoid (fever) —*see* Fever, paratyphoid
protozoal A07.9
specified NEC A07.8
radiation K52.0
regional (of) K50.90
with
complication K50.919
abscess K50.914
fistula K50.913
intestinal obstruction K50.912
rectal bleeding K50.911
specified complication NEC K50.918
colon —*see* Enteritis, regional, large intestine
duodenum —*see* Enteritis, regional, small intestine
ileum —*see* Enteritis, regional, small intestine
jejunum —*see* Enteritis, regional, small intestine
large bowel —*see* Enteritis, regional, large intestine
large intestine (colon) (rectum) K50.10
with
complication K50.119
abscess K50.114
fistula K50.113
intestinal obstruction K50.112
rectal bleeding K50.111
small intestine (duodenum) (ileum) (jejunum) involvement K50.80
with
complication K50.819
abscess K50.814
fistula K50.813
intestinal obstruction K50.812
rectal bleeding K50.811
specified complication NEC K50.818
specified complication NEC K50.118
rectum —*see* Enteritis, regional, large intestine
small intestine (duodenum) (ileum) (jejunum) K50.00
with
complication K50.019
abscess K50.014
fistula K50.013
intestinal obstruction K50.012
large intestine (colon) (rectum) involvement K50.80
with
complication K50.819
abscess K50.814
fistula K50.813
intestinal obstruction K50.812
rectal bleeding K50.811
specified complication NEC K50.818
rectal bleeding K50.011
specified complication NEC K50.018

Enteritis *(continued)*
rotaviral A08.0
Salmonella, salmonellosis (arizonae) (cholerae-suis) (enteritidis) (typhimurium) A02.0
segmental —*see* Enteritis, regional
septic A09
Shigella —*see* Infection, Shigella
small round structured NEC A08.19
spasmodic, spastic —*see* Syndrome, irritable bowel
staphylococcal A04.8
due to food A05.0
torovirus A08.39
toxic NEC K52.1
due to Clostridium difficile
not specified as recurrent A04.72
recurrent A04.71
trichomonal A07.8
tuberculous A18.32
typhosa A01.00
ulcerative (chronic) —*see* Colitis, ulcerative
viral A08.4
adenovirus A08.2
enterovirus A08.39
Rotavirus A08.0
small round structured NEC A08.19
specified NEC A08.39
virus specified NEC A08.39

Enterobiasis B80

Enterobius vermicularis (infection) (infestation) B80

Enterocele —*see also* Hernia, abdomen
pelvic, pelvis (acquired) (congenital) N81.5
vagina, vaginal (acquired) (congenital) NEC N81.5

Enterocolitis (*see also* Enteritis) K52.9
due to Clostridium difficile
not specified as recurrent A04.72
recurrent A04.71
fulminant ischemic (*see also* Ischemia, intestine acute) K55.059
granulomatous —*see* Enteritis, regional
hemorrhagic (acute) (*see also* Ischemia, intestine acute) K55.059
chronic K55.1
infectious NEC A09
ischemic K55.9
necrotizing K55.30
with
perforation K55.33
pneumatosis K55.32
and perforation K55.33
due to Clostridium difficile
not specified as recurrent A04.72
recurrent A04.71
in newborn P77.9
stage 1 (without pneumatosis, without perforation) P77.1
stage 2 (with pneumatosis, without perforation) P77.2
stage 3 (with pneumatosis, with perforation) P77.3
in non-newborn K55.30
stage 1 (without pneumatosis, without perforation) K55.31
stage 2 (with pneumatosis, without perforation) K55.32
stage 3 (with pneumatosis, with perforation) K55.33
without pneumatosis or perforation K55.31

Enterocolitis *(continued)*
noninfectious K52.9
newborn —*see* Enterocolitis, necrotizing, in newborn
pseudomembranous (newborn)
not specified as recurrent A04.72
recurrent A04.71
radiation K52.0
newborn —*see* Enterocolitis, necrotizing, in newborn
ulcerative (chronic) —*see* Pancolitis, ulcerative (chronic)

Enterogastritis —*see* Enteritis

Enteropathy K63.9
celiac-gluten-sensitive K90.0
non-celiac K90.41
food protein-induced enterocolitis K52.22
hemorrhagic, terminal (*see also* Ischemia, intestine, acute) K55.059
protein-losing K90.49

Enteroperitonitis —*see* Peritonitis

Enteroptosis K63.4

Enterorrhagia K92.2

Enterospasm —*see also* Syndrome, irritable, bowel
psychogenic F45.8

Enterostenosis (*see also* Obstruction, intestine specified NEC) K56.699

Enterostomy
complication —*see* Complication, enterostomy
status Z93.4

Enterovirus, as cause of disease classified elsewhere B97.10
coxsackievirus B97.11
echovirus B97.12
other specified B97.19

Enthesopathy (peripheral) M77.9
Achilles tendinitis —*see* Tendinitis, Achilles
ankle and tarsus M77.9
specified type NEC —*see* Enthesopathy, foot, specified type NEC
anterior tibial syndrome M76.81-
calcaneal spur —*see* Spur, bone, calcaneal
elbow region M77.8
lateral epicondylitis —*see* Epicondylitis, lateral
medial epicondylitis —*see* Epicondylitis, medial
foot NEC M77.9
metatarsalgia —*see* Metatarsalgia
specified type NEC M77.5-
forearm M77.9
gluteal tendinitis —*see* Tendinitis, gluteal
hand M77.9
hip —*see* Enthesopathy, lower limb, specified type NEC
iliac crest spur —*see* Spur, bone, iliac crest
iliotibial band syndrome —*see* Syndrome, iliotibial band
knee —*see* Enthesopathy, lower limb, lower leg, specified type NEC
lateral epicondylitis —*see* Epicondylitis, lateral
lower limb (excluding foot) M76.9
Achilles tendinitis —*see* Tendinitis, Achilles
anterior tibial syndrome M76.81-

Enthesopathy *(continued)*
- lower limb *(continued)*
  - gluteal tendinitis —*see* Tendinitis, gluteal
  - iliac crest spur —*see* Spur, bone, iliac crest
  - iliotibial band syndrome —*see* Syndrome, iliotibial band
  - patellar tendinitis —*see* Tendinitis, patellar
  - pelvic region —*see* Enthesopathy, lower limb, specified type NEC
  - peroneal tendinitis —*see* Tendinitis, peroneal
  - posterior tibial syndrome M76.82-
  - psoas tendinitis —*see* Tendinitis, psoas
  - shoulder M77.9
  - specified type NEC M76.89-
  - tibial collateral bursitis —*see* Bursitis, tibial collateral
- medial epicondylitis —*see* Epicondylitis, medial
- metatarsalgia —*see* Metatarsalgia
- multiple sites M77.9
- patellar tendinitis —*see* Tendinitis, patellar
- pelvis M77.9
- periarthritis of wrist —*see* Periarthritis, wrist
- peroneal tendinitis —*see* Tendinitis, peroneal
- posterior tibial syndrome M76.82-
- psoas tendinitis —*see* Tendinitis, psoas
- shoulder region —*see* Lesion, shoulder
- specified site NEC M77.9
- specified type NEC M77.8
- spinal M46.00
  - cervical region M46.02
  - cervicothoracic region M46.03
  - lumbar region M46.06
  - lumbosacral region M46.07
  - multiple sites M46.09
  - occipito-atlanto-axial region M46.01
  - sacrococcygeal region M46.08
  - thoracic region M46.04
  - thoracolumbar region M46.05
- tibial collateral bursitis —*see* Bursitis, tibial collateral
- upper arm M77.9
- wrist and carpus NEC M77.8
  - calcaneal spur —*see* Spur, bone, calcaneal
  - periarthritis of wrist —*see* Periarthritis, wrist

Entomophobia F40.218

Entomophthoromycosis B46.8

Entrance, air into vein —*see* Embolism, air

Entrapment, nerve —*see* Neuropathy, entrapment

Entropion (eyelid) (paralytic) H02.009
- cicatricial H02.019
  - left H02.016
    - lower H02.015
    - upper H02.014
  - right H02.013
    - lower H02.012
    - upper H02.011
- congenital Q10.2
- left H02.006
  - lower H02.005
  - upper H02.004
- mechanical H02.029
  - left H02.026
    - lower H02.025
    - upper H02.024

Entropion *(continued)*
- mechanical *(continued)*
  - right H02.023
    - lower H02.022
    - upper H02.021
- right H02.003
  - lower H02.002
  - upper H02.001
- senile H02.039
  - left H02.036
    - lower H02.035
    - upper H02.034
  - right H02.033
    - lower H02.032
    - upper H02.031
- spastic H02.049
  - left H02.046
    - lower H02.045
    - upper H02.044
  - right H02.043
    - lower H02.042
    - upper H02.041

Enucleated eye (traumatic, current) S05.7-

Enuresis R32
- functional F98.0
- habit disturbance F98.0
- nocturnal N39.44
  - psychogenic F98.0
- nonorganic origin F98.0
- psychogenic F98.0

Eosinopenia —*see* Agranulocytosis

Eosinophilia (allergic) (hereditary) (idiopathic) (secondary) D72.1
- with
  - angiolymphoid hyperplasia (ALHE) D18.01
- infiltrative J82
- Löffler's J82
- peritoneal —*see* Peritonitis, eosinophilic
- pulmonary NEC J82
- tropical (pulmonary) J82

Eosinophilia-myalgia syndrome M35.8

Ependymitis (acute) (cerebral) (chronic) (granular) —*see* Encephalomyelitis

Ependymoblastoma
- specified site —*see* Neoplasm, malignant, by site
- unspecified site C71.9

Ependymoma (epithelial) (malignant)
- anaplastic
  - specified site —*see* Neoplasm, malignant, by site
  - unspecified site C71.9
- benign
  - specified site —*see* Neoplasm, benign, by site
  - unspecified site D33.2
- myxopapillary D43.2
  - specified site —*see* Neoplasm, uncertain behavior, by site
  - unspecified site D43.2
- papillary D43.2
  - specified site —*see* Neoplasm, uncertain behavior, by site
  - unspecified site D43.2
- specified site —*see* Neoplasm, malignant, by site
- unspecified site C71.9

Ependymopathy G93.89

Ephelis, ephelides L81.2

Epiblepharon (congenital) Q10.3

Epicanthus, epicanthic fold (eyelid) (congenital) Q10.3

Epicondylitis (elbow)
- lateral M77.1-
- medial M77.0-

Epicystitis —*see* Cystitis

Epidemic —*see* condition

Epidermidalization, cervix —*see* Dysplasia, cervix

Epidermis, epidermal —*see* condition

Epidermodysplasia verruciformis B07.8

Epidermolysis
- bullosa (congenital) Q81.9
  - acquired L12.30
    - drug-induced L12.31
    - specified cause NEC L12.35
  - dystrophica Q81.2
  - letalis Q81.1
  - simplex Q81.0
  - specified NEC Q81.8
- necroticans combustiformis L51.2
  - due to drug —*see* Table of Drugs and Chemicals, by drug

Epidermophytid —*see* Dermatophytosis

Epidermophytosis (infected) —*see* Dermatophytosis

Epididymis —*see* condition

Epididymitis (acute) (nonvenereal) (recurrent) (residual) N45.1
- with orchitis N45.3
- blennorrhagic (gonococcal) A54.23
- caseous (tuberculous) A18.15
- chlamydial A56.19
- filarial (*see also* Infestation, filarial) B74.9 *[N51]*
- gonococcal A54.23
- syphilitic A52.76
- tuberculous A18.15

Epididymo-orchitis (*see also* Epididymitis) N45.3

Epidural —*see* condition

Epigastrium, epigastric —*see* condition

Epigastrocele —*see* Hernia, ventral

Epiglottis —*see* condition

Epiglottitis, epiglottiditis (acute) J05.10
- with obstruction J05.11
- chronic J37.0

Epignathus Q89.4

Epilepsia partialis continua (*see also* Kozhevnikof's epilepsy) G40.1-

Epilepsy, epileptic, epilepsia (attack) (cerebral) (convulsion) (fit) (seizure) G40.909

> Note: the following terms are to be considered equivalent to intractable: pharmacoresistant (pharmacologically resistant), treatment resistant, refractory (medically) and poorly controlled

- with
  - complex partial seizures —*see* Epilepsy, localization-related, symptomatic, with complex partial seizures
  - grand mal seizures on awakening —*see* Epilepsy, generalized, specified NEC
  - myoclonic absences —*see* Epilepsy, generalized, specified NEC
  - myoclonic-astatic seizures —*see* Epilepsy, generalized, specified NEC
  - simple partial seizures —*see* Epilepsy, localization-related, symptomatic, with simple partial seizures

Epilepsy, epileptic, epilepsia *(continued)*
- akinetic —*see* Epilepsy, generalized, specified NEC
- benign childhood with centrotemporal EEG spikes —*see* Epilepsy, localization-related, idiopathic
- benign myoclonic in infancy G40.80-
- Bravais-jacksonian —*see* Epilepsy, localization-related, symptomatic, with simple partial seizures
- childhood
  - with occipital EEG paroxysms —*see* Epilepsy, localization-related, idiopathic
  - absence G40.A09
    - intractable G40.A19
      - with status epilepticus G40.A11
      - without status epilepticus G40.A19
    - not intractable G40.A09
      - with status epilepticus G40.A01
      - without status epilepticus G40.A09
- climacteric —*see* Epilepsy, specified NEC
- cysticercosis B69.0
- deterioration (mental) F06.8
- due to syphilis A52.19
- focal —*see* Epilepsy, localization-related, symptomatic, with simple partial seizures
- generalized
  - idiopathic G40.309
    - intractable G40.319
      - with status epilepticus G40.311
      - without status epilepticus G40.319
    - not intractable G40.309
      - with status epilepticus G40.301
      - without status epilepticus G40.309
  - specified NEC G40.409
    - intractable G40.419
      - with status epilepticus G40.411
      - without status epilepticus G40.419
    - not intractable G40.409
      - with status epilepticus G40.401
      - without status epilepticus G40.409
- impulsive petit mal —*see* Epilepsy, juvenile myoclonic
- intractable G40.919
  - with status epilepticus G40.911
  - without status epilepticus G40.919
- juvenile absence G40.A09
  - intractable G40.A19
    - with status epilepticus G40.A11
    - without status epilepticus G40.A19
  - not intractable G40.A09
    - with status epilepticus G40.A01
    - without status epilepticus G40.A09
- juvenile myoclonic G40.B09
  - intractable G40.B19
    - with status epilepticus G40.B11
    - without status epilepticus G40.B19
  - not intractable G40.B09
    - with status epilepticus G40.B01
    - without status epilepticus G40.B09

Epilepsy, epileptic, epilepsia *(continued)*
- localization-related (focal) (partial)
  - idiopathic G40.009
    - with seizures of localized onset G40.009
      - intractable G40.019
        - with status epilepticus G40.011
        - without status epilepticus G40.019
      - not intractable G40.009
        - with status epilepticus G40.001
        - without status epilepticus G40.009
  - symptomatic
    - with complex partial seizures G40.209
      - intractable G40.219
        - with status epilepticus G40.211
        - without status epilepticus G40.219
      - not intractable G40.209
        - with status epilepticus G40.201
        - without status epilepticus G40.209
    - with simple partial seizures G40.109
      - intractable G40.119
        - with status epilepticus G40.111
        - without status epilepticus G40.119
      - not intractable G40.109
        - with status epilepticus G40.101
        - without status epilepticus G40.109
- myoclonus, myoclonic —*see* Epilepsy, generalized, specified NEC
  - progressive —*see* Epilepsy, generalized, idiopathic
- not intractable G40.909
  - with status epilepticus G40.901
  - without status epilepticus G40.909
- on awakening —*see* Epilepsy, generalized, specified NEC
- parasitic NOS B71.9 *[G94]*
- partialis continua (*see also* Kozhevnikof's epilepsy) G40.1-
- peripheral —*see* Epilepsy, specified NEC
- procursiva —*see* Epilepsy, localization-related, symptomatic, with simple partial seizures
- progressive (familial) myoclonic —*see* Epilepsy, generalized, idiopathic
- reflex —*see* Epilepsy, specified NEC
- related to
  - alcohol G40.509
    - not intractable G40.509
      - with status epilepticus G40.501
      - without status eplipticus G40.509
  - drugs G40.509
    - not intractable G40.509
      - with status epilepticus G40.501
      - without status eplipticus G40.509
  - external causes G40.509
    - not intractable G40.509
      - with status epilepticus G40.501
      - without status eplipticus G40.509

Epilepsy, epileptic, epilepsia *(continued)*
- related to *(continued)*
  - hormonal changes G40.509
    - not intractable G40.509
      - with status epilepticus G40.501
      - without status eplipticus G40.509
  - sleep deprivation G40.509
    - not intractable G40.509
      - with status epilepticus G40.501
      - without status eplipticus G40.509
  - stress G40.509
    - not intractable G40.509
      - with status epilepticus G40.501
      - without status eplipticus G40.509
- somatomotor —*see* Epilepsy, localization-related, symptomatic, with simple partial seizures
- somatosensory —*see* Epilepsy, localization-related, symptomatic, with simple partial seizures
- spasms G40.822
  - intractable G40.824
    - with status epilepticus G40.823
    - without status epilepticus G40.824
  - not intractable G40.822
    - with status epilepticus G40.821
    - without status epilepticus G40.822
- specified NEC G40.802
  - intractable G40.804
    - with status epilepticus G40.803
    - without status epilepticus G40.804
  - not intractable G40.802
    - with status epilepticus G40.801
    - without status epilepticus G40.802
- syndromes
  - generalized
    - idiopathic G40.309
      - intractable G40.319
        - with status epilepticus G40.311
        - without status epilepticus G40.319
      - not intractable G40.309
        - with status epilepticus G40.301
        - without status epilepticus G40.309
    - specified NEC G40.409
      - intractable G40.419
        - with status epilepticus G40.411
        - without status epilepticus G40.419
      - not intractable G40.409
        - with status epilepticus G40.401
        - without status epilepticus G40.409
  - localization-related (focal) (partial)
    - idiopathic G40.009
      - with seizures of localized onset G40.009
        - intractable G40.019
          - with status epilepticus G40.011
          - without status epilepticus G40.019

Epilepsy, epileptic, epilepsia *(continued)*
- syndromes *(continued)*
  - localization-related *(continued)*
    - idiopathic *(continued)*
      - with seizures of localized onset *(continued)*
        - not intractable G40.009
          - with status epilepticus G40.001
          - without status epilepticus G40.009
    - symptomatic
      - with complex partial seizures G40.209
        - intractable G40.219
          - with status epilepticus G40.211
          - without status epilepticus G40.219
        - not intractable G40.209
          - with status epilepticus G40.201
          - without status epilepticus G40.209
      - with simple partial seizures G40.109
        - intractable G40.119
          - with status epilepticus G40.111
          - without status epilepticus G40.119
        - not intractable G40.109
          - with status epilepticus G40.101
          - without status epilepticus G40.109
  - specified NEC G40.802
    - intractable G40.804
      - with status epilepticus G40.803
      - without status epilepticus G40.804
    - not intractable G40.802
      - with status epilepticus G40.801
      - without status epilepticus G40.802
- tonic (-clonic) —*see* Epilepsy, generalized, specified NEC
- twilight F05
- uncinate (gyrus) —*see* Epilepsy, localization-related, symptomatic, with complex partial seizures
- Unverricht (-Lundborg) (familial myoclonic) —*see* Epilepsy, generalized, idiopathic
- visceral —*see* Epilepsy, specified NEC
- visual —*see* Epilepsy, specified NEC

Epiloia Q85.1

Epimenorrhea N92.0

Epipharyngitis —*see* Nasopharyngitis

Epiphora H04.20-
- due to
  - excess lacrimation H04.21-
  - insufficient drainage H04.22-

Epiphyseal arrest —*see* Arrest, epiphyseal

Epiphyseolysis, epiphysiolysis —*see* Osteochondropathy

Epiphysitis —*see also* Osteochondropathy
- juvenile M92.9
- syphilitic (congenital) A50.02

Epiplocele —*see* Hernia, abdomen

Epiploitis —*see* Peritonitis

Epiplosarcomphalocele —*see* Hernia, umbilicus

Episcleritis (suppurative) H15.10-
- in (due to)
  - syphilis A52.71
  - tuberculosis A18.51
- nodular H15.12-
- periodica fugax H15.11-
  - angioneurotic —*see* Edema, angioneurotic
- syphilitic (late) A52.71
- tuberculous A18.51

Episode
- affective, mixed F39
- depersonalization (in neurotic state) F48.1
- depressive F32.9
  - major F32.9
    - mild F32.0
    - moderate F32.1
    - severe (without psychotic symptoms) F32.2
      - with psychotic symptoms F32.3
  - recurrent F33.9
    - brief F33.8
  - specified NEC F32.89
- hypomanic F30.8
- manic F30.9
  - with
    - psychotic symptoms F30.2
    - remission (full) F30.4
      - partial F30.3
  - other specified F30.8
  - recurrent F31.89
  - without psychotic symptoms F30.10
    - mild F30.11
    - moderate F30.12
    - severe (without psychotic symptoms) F30.13
      - with psychotic symptoms F30.2
- psychotic F23
  - organic F06.8
- schizophrenic (acute) NEC, brief F23

Epispadias (female) (male) Q64.0

Episplenitis D73.89

Epistaxis (multiple) R04.0
- hereditary I78.0
- vicarious menstruation N94.89

Epithelioma (malignant) —*see also* Neoplasm, malignant, by site
- adenoides cysticum —*see* Neoplasm, skin, benign
- basal cell —*see* Neoplasm, skin, malignant
- benign —*see* Neoplasm, benign, by site
- Bowen's —*see* Neoplasm, skin, in situ
- calcifying, of Malherbe —*see* Neoplasm, skin, benign
- external site —*see* Neoplasm, skin, malignant
- intraepidermal, Jadassohn —*see* Neoplasm, skin, benign
- squamous cell —*see* Neoplasm, malignant, by site

Epitheliomatosis pigmented Q82.1

Epitheliopathy, multifocal placoid pigment H30.14-

Epithelium, epithelial —*see* condition

Epituberculosis (with atelectasis) (allergic) A15.7

Eponychia Q84.6

Epstein's
- nephrosis or syndrome *—see* Nephrosis
- pearl K09.8

Epulis (gingiva) (fibrous) (giant cell) K06.8

Equinia A24.0

Equinovarus (congenital) (talipes) Q66.0
- acquired *—see* Deformity, limb, clubfoot

Equivalent
- convulsive (abdominal) *—see* Epilepsy, specified NEC
- epileptic (psychic) *—see* Epilepsy, localization-related, symptomatic, with complex partial seizures

Erb (-Duchenne) **paralysis** (birth injury) (newborn) P14.0

Erb-Goldflam disease or syndrome G70.00
- with exacerbation (acute) G70.01
- in crisis G70.01

Erb's
- disease G71.0
- palsy, paralysis (brachial) (birth) (newborn) P14.0
  - spinal (spastic) syphilitic A52.17
- pseudohypertrophic muscular dystrophy G71.0

Erdheim's syndrome (acromegalic macrospondylitis) E22.0

Erection, painful (persistent) *—see* Priapism

Ergosterol deficiency (vitamin D) E55.9
- with
  - adult osteomalacia M83.8
  - rickets *—see* Rickets

Ergotism *—see also* Poisoning, food, noxious, plant
- from ergot used as drug (migraine therapy) *—see* Table of Drugs and Chemicals

Erosio interdigitalis blastomycetica B37.2

Erosion
- artery I77.2
  - without rupture I77.89
- bone *—see* Disorder, bone, density and structure, specified NEC
- bronchus J98.09
- cartilage (joint) *—see* Disorder, cartilage, specified type NEC
- cervix (uteri) (acquired) (chronic) (congenital) N86
  - with cervicitis N72
- cornea (nontraumatic) *—see* Ulcer, cornea
  - recurrent H18.83-
  - traumatic *—see* Abrasion, cornea
- dental (idiopathic) (occupational) (due to diet, drugs or vomiting) K03.2
- duodenum, postpyloric *—see* Ulcer, duodenum
- esophagus K22.10
  - with bleeding K22.11
- gastric *—see* Ulcer, stomach
- gastrojejunal *—see* Ulcer, gastrojejunal
- implanted mesh *—see* Complications, mesh
- intestine K63.3
- lymphatic vessel I89.8

Erosion *(continued)*
- pylorus, pyloric (ulcer) *—see* Ulcer, stomach
- spine, aneurysmal A52.09
- stomach *—see* Ulcer, stomach
- subcutaneous device pocket
  - nervous system prosthetic device, implant, or graft T85.890
  - other internal prosthetic device, implant, or graft T85.898
- teeth (idiopathic) (occupational) (due to diet, drugs or vomiting) K03.2
- urethra N36.8
- uterus N85.8

Erotomania F52.8

Error
- metabolism, inborn -- se Disorder, metabolism
- refractive *—see* Disorder, refraction

Eructation R14.2
- nervous or psychogenic F45.8

Eruption
- creeping B76.9
- drug (generalized) (taken internally) L27.0
  - fixed L27.1
  - in contact with skin *—see* Dermatitis, due to drugs
  - localized L27.1
- Hutchinson, summer L56.4
- Kaposi's varicelliform B00.0
- napkin L22
- polymorphous light (sun) L56.4
- recalcitrant pustular L13.8
- ringed R23.8
- skin (nonspecific) R21
  - creeping (meaning hookworm) B76.9
  - due to inoculation/vaccination (generalized) (*see also* Dermatitis, due to, vaccine) L27.0
    - localized L27.1
  - erysipeloid A26.0
  - feigned L98.1
  - Kaposi's varicelliform B00.0
  - lichenoid L28.0
  - meaning dermatitis *—see* Dermatitis
  - toxic NEC L53.0
- tooth, teeth, abnormal (incomplete) (late) (premature) (sequence) K00.6
- vesicular R23.8

Erysipelas (gangrenous) (infantile) (newborn) (phlegmonous) (suppurative) A46
- external ear A46 *[H62.40]*
- puerperal, postpartum O86.89

Erysipeloid A26.9
- cutaneous (Rosenbach's) A26.0
- disseminated A26.8
- sepsis A26.7
- specified NEC A26.8

Erythema, erythematous (infectional) (inflammation) L53.9
- ab igne L59.0
- annulare (centrifugum) (rheumaticum) L53.1
- arthriticum epidemicum A25.1
- brucellum *—see* Brucellosis
- chronic figurate NEC L53.3
- chronicum migrans (Borrelia burgdorferi) A69.20
- diaper L22
- due to
  - chemical NEC L53.0
    - in contact with skin L24.5
  - drug (internal use) *—see* Dermatitis, due to, drugs

Erythema, erythematous *(continued)*
- elevatum diutinum L95.1
- endemic E52
- epidemic, arthritic A25.1
- figuratum perstans L53.3
- gluteal L22
- heat - code by site under Burn, first degree
- ichthyosiforme congenitum bullous Q80.3
- in diseases classified elsewhere L54
- induratum (nontuberculous) L52
  - tuberculous A18.4
- infectiosum B08.3
- intertrigo L30.4
- iris L51.9
- marginatum L53.2
  - in (due to) acute rheumatic fever I00
- medicamentosum *—see* Dermatitis, due to, drugs
- migrans A26.0
  - chronicum A69.20
  - tongue K14.1
- multiforme (major) (minor) L51.9
  - bullous, bullosum L51.1
  - conjunctiva L51.1
  - nonbullous L51.0
  - pemphigoides L12.0
  - specified NEC L51.8
- napkin L22
- neonatorum P83.88
  - toxic P83.1
- nodosum L52
  - tuberculous A18.4
- palmar L53.8
- pernio T69.1
- rash, newborn P83.88
- scarlatiniform (recurrent) (exfoliative) L53.8
- solare L55.0
- specified NEC L53.8
- toxic, toxicum NEC L53.0
  - newborn P83.1
- tuberculous (primary) A18.4

Erythematous, erythematosus *—see* condition

Erythermalgia (primary) I73.81

Erythralgia I73.81

Erythrasma L08.1

Erythredema (polyneuropathy) *—see* Poisoning, mercury

Erythremia (acute) C94.0-
- chronic D45
- secondary D75.1

Erythroblastopenia *—see also* Aplasia, red cell D60.9
- congenital D61.01

Erythroblastophthisis D61.09

Erythroblastosis (fetalis) (newborn) P55.9
- due to
  - ABO (antibodies) (incompatibility) (isoimmunization) P55.1
  - Rh (antibodies) (incompatibility) (isoimmunization) P55.0

Erythrocyanosis (crurum) I73.89

Erythrocythemia *—see* Erythremia

Erythrocytosis (megalosplenic) (secondary) D75.1
- familial D75.0
- oval, hereditary *—see* Elliptocytosis
- secondary D75.1
- stress D75.1

Erythroderma (secondary) (*see also* Erythema) L53.9
- bullous ichthyosiform, congenital Q80.3
- desquamativum L21.1
- ichthyosiform, congenital (bullous) Q80.3
- neonatorum P83.88
- psoriaticum L40.8

Erythrodysesthesia, palmar plantar (PPE) L27.1

Erythrogenesis imperfecta D61.09

Erythroleukemia C94.0-

Erythromelalgia I73.81

Erythrophagocytosis D75.89

Erythrophobia F40.298

Erythroplakia, oral epithelium, and tongue K13.29

Erythroplasia (Queyrat) D07.4
- specified site *—see* Neoplasm, skin, in situ
- unspecified site D07.4

Escherichia coli (E. coli)**, as cause of disease classified elsewhere** B96.20
- non-O157 Shiga toxin-producing (with known O group) B96.22
- non-Shiga toxin-producing B96.29
- O157 with confirmation of Shiga toxin when H antigen is unknown, or is not H7 B96.21
- O157:H-(nonmotile) with confirmation of Shiga toxin B96.21
- Shiga toxin-producing (with unspecified O group) (STEC) B96.23
- O157 B96.21
- O157:H7 with or without confirmation of Shiga toxin-production B96.21
- specified NEC B96.29

Esophagismus K22.4

Esophagitis (acute) (alkaline) (chemical) (chronic) (infectional) (necrotic) (peptic) (postoperative) K20.9
- candidal B37.81
- due to gastrointestinal reflux disease K21.0
- eosinophilic K20.0
- reflux K21.0
- specified NEC K20.8
- tuberculous A18.83
- ulcerative K22.10
  - with bleeding K22.11

Esophagocele K22.5

Esophagomalacia K22.8

Esophagospasm K22.4

Esophagostenosis K22.2

Esophagostomiasis B81.8

Esophagotracheal *—see* condition

Esophagus *—see* condition

Esophoria H50.51
- convergence, excess H51.12
- divergence, insufficiency H51.8

Esotropia *—see* Strabismus, convergent concomitant

Espundia B55.2

Essential *—see* condition

Esthesioneuroblastoma C30.0

Esthesioneurocytoma C30.0

Esthesioneuroepithelioma C30.0

Esthiomene A55

Estivo-autumnal malaria (fever) B50.9

Estrangement (marital) Z63.5
- parent-child NEC Z62.890

Estriasis —*see* Myiasis

Ethanolism —*see* Alcoholism

Etherism —*see* Dependence, drug, inhalant

Ethmoid, ethmoidal —*see* condition

Ethmoiditis (chronic) (nonpurulent) (purulent) —*see also* Sinusitis, ethmoidal
- influenzal —*see* Influenza, with, respiratory manifestations NEC
- Woakes' J33.1

Ethylism —*see* Alcoholism

Eulenburg's disease (congenital paramyotonia) G71.19

Eumycetoma B47.0

Eunuchoidism E29.1
- hypogonadotropic E23.0

European blastomycosis —*see* Cryptococcosis

Eustachian —*see* condition

Evaluation (for) (of)
- development state
  - adolescent Z00.3
  - period of
    - delayed growth in childhood Z00.70
      - with abnormal findings Z00.71
    - rapid growth in childhood Z00.2
  - puberty Z00.3
- growth and developmental state (period of rapid growth) Z00.2
  - delayed growth Z00.70
    - with abnormal findings Z00.71
- mental health (status) Z00.8
  - requested by authority Z04.6
- period of
  - delayed growth in childhood Z00.70
    - with abnormal findings Z00.71
  - rapid growth in childhood Z00.2
- suspected condition —*see* Observation

Evans syndrome D69.41

Event
- apparent life threatening in newborn and infact (ALTE) R68.13
- brief resolved unexplained event (BRUE) R68.13

Eventration —*see also* Hernia, ventral
- colon into chest —*see* Hernia, diaphragm
- diaphragm (congenital) Q79.1

Eversion
- bladder N32.89
- cervix (uteri) N86
  - with cervicitis N72
- foot NEC —*see also* Deformity, valgus, ankle
  - congenital Q66.6
- punctum lacrimale (postinfectional) (senile) H04.52-
- ureter (meatus) N28.89
- urethra (meatus) N36.8
- uterus N81.4

Evidence
- cytologic
  - of malignancy on anal smear R85.614
  - of malignancy on cervical smear R87.614
  - of malignancy on vaginal smear R87.624

Evisceration
- birth injury P15.8
- traumatic NEC
  - eye —*see* Enucleated eye

Evulsion —*see* Avulsion

Ewing's sarcoma or tumor - —*see* Neoplasm, bone, malignant

Examination (for) (following) (general) (of) (routine) Z00.00
- with abnormal findings Z00.01
- abuse, physical (alleged), ruled out
  - adult Z04.71
  - child Z04.72
- adolescent (development state) Z00.3
- alleged rape or sexual assault (victim), ruled out
  - adult Z04.41
  - child Z04.42
- allergy Z01.82
- annual (adult) (periodic) (physical) Z00.00
  - with abnormal findings Z00.01
  - gynecological Z01.419
    - with abnormal findings Z01.411
- antibody response Z01.84
- blood —*see* Examination, laboratory
- blood pressure Z01.30
  - with abnormal findings Z01.31
- cancer staging —*see* Neoplasm, malignant, by site
- cervical Papanicolaou smear Z12.4
  - as part of routine gynecological examination Z01.419
    - with abnormal findings Z01.411
- child (over 28 days old) Z00.129
  - with abnormal findings Z00.121
  - under 28 days old —*see* Newborn, examination
- clinical research control or normal comparison (control) (participant) Z00.6
- contraceptive (drug) maintenance (routine) Z30.8
  - device (intrauterine) Z30.431
- dental Z01.20
  - with abnormal findings Z01.21
- developmental —*see* Examination, child
- donor (potential) Z00.5
- ear Z01.10
  - with abnormal findings NEC Z01.118
- eye Z01.00
  - with abnormal findings Z01.01
- following
  - accident NEC Z04.3
    - transport Z04.1
    - work Z04.2
  - assault, alleged, ruled out
    - adult Z04.71
    - child Z04.72
  - motor vehicle accident Z04.1
  - treatment (for) Z09
    - combined NEC Z09
      - fracture Z09
      - malignant neoplasm Z08
    - malignant neoplasm Z08
    - mental disorder Z09
    - specified condition NEC Z09
- follow-up (routine) (following) Z09
  - chemotherapy NEC Z09
    - malignant neoplasm Z08
  - fracture Z09
  - malignant neoplasm Z08
  - postpartum Z39.2
  - psychotherapy Z09
  - radiotherapy NEC Z09
    - malignant neoplasm Z08
  - surgery NEC Z09
    - malignant neoplasm Z08

Examination *(continued)*
- gynecological Z01.419
  - with abnormal findings Z01.411
  - for contraceptive maintenance Z30.8
- health —*see* Examination, medical
- hearing Z01.10
  - with abnormal findings NEC Z01.118
  - following failed hearing screening Z01.110
- immunity status testing Z01.84
- laboratory (as part of a general medical examination) Z00.00
  - with abnormal findings Z00.01
  - preprocedural Z01.812
- lactating mother Z39.1
- medical (adult) (for) (of) Z00.00
  - with abnormal findings Z00.01
  - administrative purpose only Z02.9
    - specified NEC Z02.89
  - admission to
    - armed forces Z02.3
    - old age home Z02.2
    - prison Z02.89
    - residential institution Z02.2
    - school Z02.0
      - following illness or medical treatment Z02.0
    - summer camp Z02.89
  - adoption Z02.82
  - blood alcohol or drug level Z02.83
  - camp (summer) Z02.89
  - clinical research, normal subject (control) (participant) Z00.6
  - control subject in clinical research (normal comparison) (participant) Z00.6
  - donor (potential) Z00.5
  - driving license Z02.4
  - general (adult) Z00.00
    - with abnormal findings Z00.01
  - immigration Z02.89
  - insurance purposes Z02.6
  - marriage Z02.89
  - medicolegal reasons NEC Z04.8
  - naturalization Z02.89
  - participation in sport Z02.5
  - paternity testing Z02.81
  - population survey Z00.8
  - pre-employment Z02.1
  - pre-operative —*see* Examination, pre-procedural
  - pre-procedural
    - cardiovascular Z01.810
    - respiratory Z01.811
    - specified NEC Z01.818
  - preschool children
    - for admission to school Z02.0
  - prisoners
    - for entrance into prison Z02.89
  - recruitment for armed forces Z02.3
  - specified NEC Z00.8
  - sport competition Z02.5
- medicolegal reason NEC Z04.8
- newborn —*see* Newborn, examination
- pelvic (annual) (periodic) Z01.419
  - with abnormal findings Z01.411
- period of rapid growth in childhood Z00.2
- periodic (adult) (annual) (routine) Z00.00
  - with abnormal findings Z00.01
- physical (adult) (*see also* Examination, medical) Z00.00
  - sports Z02.5
- postpartum
  - immediately after delivery Z39.0
  - routine follow-up Z39.2

Examination *(continued)*
- prenatal (normal pregnancy) (*see also* Pregnancy, normal) Z34.9-
- pre-chemotherapy (antineoplastic) Z01.818
- pre-procedural (pre-operative)
  - cardiovascular Z01.810
  - laboratory Z01.812
  - respiratory Z01.811
  - specified NEC Z01.818
- prior to chemotherapy (antineoplastic) Z01.818
- psychiatric NEC Z00.8
  - follow-up not needing further care Z09
  - requested by authority Z04.6
- radiological (as part of a general medical examination) Z00.00
  - with abnormal findings Z00.01
- repeat cervical smear to confirm findings of recent normal smear following initial abnormal smear Z01.42
- skin (hypersensitivity) Z01.82
- special (*see also* Examination, by type) Z01.89
  - specified type NEC Z01.89
- specified type or reason NEC Z04.8
- teeth Z01.20
  - with abnormal findings Z01.21
- urine —*see* Examination, laboratory
- vision Z01.00
  - with abnormal findings Z01.01

Exanthem, exanthema —*see also* Rash
- with enteroviral vesicular stomatitis B08.4
- Boston A88.0
- epidemic with meningitis A88.0 *[G02]*
- subitum B08.20
  - due to human herpesvirus 6 B08.21
  - due to human herpesvirus 7 B08.22
- viral, virus B09
  - specified type NEC B08.8

Excess, excessive, excessively
- alcohol level in blood R78.0
- androgen (ovarian) E28.1
- attrition, tooth, teeth K03.0
- carotene, carotin (dietary) E67.1
- cold, effects of T69.9
  - specified effect NEC T69.8
- convergence H51.12
- crying
  - in child, adolescent, or adult R45.83
  - in infant R68.11
- development, breast N62
- divergence H51.8
- drinking (alcohol) NEC (without dependence) F10.10
  - habitual (continual) (without remission) F10.20
- eating R63.2
- estrogen E28.0
- fat —*see also* Obesity
  - in heart —*see* Degeneration, myocardial
  - localized E65
- foreskin N47.8
- gas R14.0
- glucagon E16.3
- heat —*see* Heat
- intermaxillary vertical dimension of fully erupted teeth M26.37
- interocclusal distance of fully erupted teeth M26.37
- kalium E87.5

Excess, excessive, excessively *(continued)*
- large
  - colon K59.39
    - congenital Q43.8
  - infant P08.0
  - organ or site, congenital NEC —*see* Anomaly, by site
- long
  - organ or site, congenital NEC —*see* Anomaly, by site
- menstruation (with regular cycle) N92.0
  - with irregular cycle N92.1
- napping Z72.821
- natrium E87.0
- number of teeth K00.1
- nutrient (dietary) NEC R63.2
- potassium (K) E87.5
- salivation K11.7
- secretion —*see also* Hypersecretion
  - milk O92.6
  - sputum R09.3
  - sweat R61
- sexual drive F52.8
- short
  - organ or site, congenital NEC —*see* Anomaly, by site
  - umbilical cord in labor or delivery O69.3
- skin L98.7
  - and subcutaneous tissue L98.7
  - eyelid (acquired) —*see* Blepharochalasis
    - congenital Q10.3
- sodium (Na) E87.0
- spacing of fully erupted teeth M26.32
- sputum R09.3
- sweating R61
- thirst R63.1
  - due to deprivation of water T73.1
- tuberosity of jaw M26.07
- vitamin
  - A (dietary) E67.0
    - administered as drug (prolonged intake) —*see* Table of Drugs and Chemicals, vitamins, adverse effect
    - overdose or wrong substance given or taken —*see* Table of Drugs and Chemicals, vitamins, poisoning
  - D (dietary) E67.3
    - administered as drug (prolonged intake) —*see* Table of Drugs and Chemicals, vitamins, adverse effect
    - overdose or wrong substance given or taken —*see* Table of Drugs and Chemicals, vitamins, poisoning
- weight
  - gain R63.5
  - loss R63.4

Excitability, abnormal, under minor stress (personality disorder) F60.3

Excitation
- anomalous atrioventricular I45.6
- psychogenic F30.8
- reactive (from emotional stress, psychological trauma) F30.8

Excitement
- hypomanic F30.8
- manic F30.9
- mental, reactive (from emotional stress, psychological trauma) F30.8
- state, reactive (from emotional stress, psychological trauma) F30.8

Excoriation (traumatic) —*see also* Abrasion
- neurotic L98.1
- skin picking disorder F42.4

Exfoliation
- due to erythematous conditions according to extent of body surface involved L49.0
  - 10-19 percent of body surface L49.1
  - 20-29 percent of body surface L49.2
  - 30-39 percent of body surface L49.3
  - 40-49 percent of body surface L49.4
  - 50-59 percent of body surface L49.5
  - 60-69 percent of body surface L49.6
  - 70-79 percent of body surface L49.7
  - 80-89 percent of body surface L49.8
  - 90-99 percent of body surface L49.9
  - less than 10 percent of body surface L49.0
- teeth, due to systemic causes K08.0

Exfoliative —*see* condition

Exhaustion, exhaustive (physical NEC) R53.83
- battle F43.0
- cardiac —*see* Failure, heart
- delirium F43.0
- due to
  - cold T69.8
  - excessive exertion T73.3
  - exposure T73.2
  - neurasthenia F48.8
- heart —*see* Failure, heart
- heat (*see also* Heat, exhaustion) T67.5
  - due to
    - salt depletion T67.4
    - water depletion T67.3
- maternal, complicating delivery O75.81
- mental F48.8
- myocardium, myocardial —*see* Failure, heart
- nervous F48.8
- old age R54
- psychogenic F48.8
- psychosis F43.0
- senile R54
- vital NEC Z73.0

Exhibitionism F65.2

Exocervicitis —*see* Cervicitis

Exomphalos Q79.2
- meaning hernia —*see* Hernia, umbilicus

Exophoria H50.52
- convergence, insufficiency H51.11
- divergence, excess H51.8

Exophthalmos H05.2-
- congenital Q15.8
- constant NEC H05.24-
- displacement, globe —*see* Displacement, globe
- due to thyrotoxicosis (hyperthyroidism) —*see* Hyperthyroidism, with, goiter (diffuse)
- dysthyroid —*see* Hyperthyroidism, with, goiter (diffuse)
- goiter —*see* Hyperthyroidism, with, goiter (diffuse)
- intermittent NEC H05.25-

Exophthalmos *(continued)*
- malignant —*see* Hyperthyroidism, with, goiter (diffuse)
- orbital
  - edema —*see* Edema, orbit
  - hemorrhage —*see* Hemorrhage, orbit
- pulsating NEC H05.26-
- thyrotoxic, thyrotropic —*see* Hyperthyroidism, with, goiter (diffuse)

Exostosis —*see also* Disorder, bone
- cartilaginous —*see* Neoplasm, bone, benign
- congenital (multiple) Q78.6
- external ear canal H61.81-
- gonococcal A54.49
- jaw (bone) M27.8
- multiple, congenital Q78.6
- orbit H05.35-
- osteocartilaginous —*see* Neoplasm, bone, benign
- syphilitic A52.77

Exotropia —*see* Strabismus, divergent concomitant

Explanation of
- investigation finding Z71.2
- medication Z71.89

Exposure (to) (*see also* Contact, with) T75.89
- acariasis Z20.7
- AIDS virus Z20.6
- air pollution Z77.110
- algae and algae toxins Z77.121
- algae bloom Z77.121
- anthrax Z20.810
- aromatic amines Z77.020
- aromatic (hazardous) compounds NEC Z77.028
- aromatic dyes NOS Z77.028
- arsenic Z77.010
- asbestos Z77.090
- bacterial disease NEC Z20.818
- benzene Z77.021
- blue-green algae bloom Z77.121
- body fluids (potentially hazardous) Z77.21
- brown tide Z77.121
- chemicals (chiefly nonmedicinal) (hazardous) NEC Z77.098
- cholera Z20.09
- chromium compounds Z77.018
- cold, effects of T69.9
  - specified effect NEC T69.8
- communicable disease Z20.9
  - bacterial NEC Z20.818
  - specified NEC Z20.89
  - viral NEC Z20.828
- cyanobacteria bloom Z77.121
- disaster Z65.5
- discrimination Z60.5
- dyes Z77.098
- effects of T73.9
- environmental tobacco smoke (acute) (chronic) Z77.22
- Escherichia coli (E. coli) Z20.01
- exhaustion due to T73.2
- fiberglass —*see* Table of Drugs and Chemicals, fiberglass
- German measles Z20.4
- gonorrhea Z20.2
- hazardous metals NEC Z77.018
- hazardous substances NEC Z77.29
- hazards in the physical environment NEC Z77.128
- hazards to health NEC Z77.9
- human immunodeficiency virus (HIV) Z20.6
- human T-lymphotropic virus type-1 (HTLV-1) Z20.89

Exposure *(continued)*
- implanted
  - mesh —*see* Complications, mesh
  - prosthetic materials NEC —*see* Complications, prosthetic materials NEC
- infestation (parasitic) NEC Z20.7
- intestinal infectious disease NEC Z20.09
  - Escherichia coli (E. coli) Z20.01
- lead Z77.011
- meningococcus Z20.811
- mold (toxic) Z77.120
- nickel dust Z77.018
- noise Z77.122
- occupational
  - air contaminants NEC Z57.39
  - dust Z57.2
  - environmental tobacco smoke Z57.31
  - extreme temperature Z57.6
  - noise Z57.0
  - radiation Z57.1
  - risk factors Z57.9
    - specified NEC Z57.8
  - toxic agents (gases) (liquids) (solids) (vapors) in agriculture Z57.4
  - toxic agents (gases) (liquids) (solids) (vapors) in industry NEC Z57.5
  - vibration Z57.7
- parasitic disease NEC Z20.7
- pediculosis Z20.7
- persecution Z60.5
- pfiesteria piscicida Z77.121
- poliomyelitis Z20.89
- polycyclic aromatic hydrocarbons Z77.028
- pollution
  - air Z77.110
  - environmental NEC Z77.118
  - soil Z77.112
  - water Z77.111
- prenatal (drugs) (toxic chemicals) —*see* Newborn, affected by, noxious substances transmitted via placenta or breast milk
- rabies Z20.3
- radiation, naturally occurring NEC Z77.123
- radon Z77.123
- red tide (Florida) Z77.121
- rubella Z20.4
- second hand tobacco smoke (acute) (chronic) Z77.22
  - in the perinatal period P96.81
- sexually-transmitted disease Z20.2
- smallpox (laboratory) Z20.89
- syphilis Z20.2
- terrorism Z65.4
- torture Z65.4
- tuberculosis Z20.1
- uranium Z77.012
- varicella Z20.820
- venereal disease Z20.2
- viral disease NEC Z20.828
- war Z65.5
- water pollution Z77.111

Exsanguination —*see* Hemorrhage

Exstrophy
- abdominal contents Q45.8
- bladder Q64.10
  - cloacal Q64.12
  - specified type NEC Q64.19
  - supravesical fissure Q64.11

Extensive —*see* condition

Extra (*see also* Accessory marker chromosomes) (normal individual) Q92.61
- in abnormal individual Q92.62
- rib Q76.6
  - cervical Q76.5

Extrasystoles (supraventricular) I49.49
- atrial I49.1
- auricular I49.1
- junctional I49.2
- ventricular I49.3

Extrauterine gestation or pregnancy —*see* Pregnancy, by site

Extravasation
- blood R58
- chyle into mesentery I89.8
- pelvicalyceal N13.8
- pyelosinus N13.8
- urine (from ureter) R39.0
- vesicant agent
  - antineoplastic chemotherapy T80.810
  - other agent NEC T80.818

Extremity —*see* condition, limb

Extrophy —*see* Exstrophy

Extroversion
- bladder Q64.19
- uterus N81.4
  - complicating delivery O71.2
  - postpartal (old) N81.4

Extruded tooth (teeth) M26.34

Extrusion
- breast implant (prosthetic) T85.42
- eye implant (globe) (ball) T85.328
- intervertebral disc —*see* Displacement, intervertebral disc
- ocular lens implant (prosthetic) —*see* Complications, intraocular lens
- vitreous —*see* Prolapse, vitreous

Exudate
- pleural —*see* Effusion, pleura
- retina H35.89

Exudative —*see* condition

Eye, eyeball, eyelid —*see* condition

Eyestrain —*see* Disturbance, vision, subjective

Eyeworm disease of Africa B74.3

F

Faber's syndrome (achlorhydric anemia) D50.9

Fabry (-Anderson) **disease** E75.21

Faciocephalalgia, autonomic (*see also* Neuropathy, peripheral, autonomic) G90.09

Factor(s)
- psychic, associated with diseases classified elsewhere F54
- psychological
  - affecting physical conditions F54
  - or behavioral
    - affecting general medical condition F54
    - associated with disorders or diseases classified elsewhere F54

Fahr disease (of brain) G23.8

Fahr Volhard disease (of kidney) I12.-

Failure, failed
- abortion —*see* Abortion, attempted
- aortic (valve) I35.8
  - rheumatic I06.8

Failure, failed *(continued)*
- attempted abortion —*see* Abortion, attempted
- biventricular I50.82
  - due to left heart failure I50.814
- bone marrow —*see* Anemia, aplastic
- cardiac —*see* Failure, heart
- cardiorenal (chronic) (*see also* Failure, renal, and Failure, heart) I50.9
  - hypertensive I13.2
- cardiorespiratory (*see also* Failure, heart) R09.2
- cardiovascular (chronic) —*see* Failure, heart
- cerebrovascular I67.9
- cervical dilatation in labor O62.0
- circulation, circulatory (peripheral) R57.9
  - newborn P29.89
- compensation —*see* Disease, heart
- compliance with medical treatment or regimen —*see* Noncompliance
- congestive —*see* Failure, heart, congestive
- dental implant (endosseous) M27.69
  - due to
    - failure of dental prosthesis M27.63
    - lack of attached gingiva M27.62
    - occlusal trauma (poor prosthetic design) M27.62
    - parafunctional habits M27.62
    - periodontal infection (peri-implantitis) M27.62
    - poor oral hygiene M27.62
  - osseointegration M27.61
    - due to
      - complications of systemic disease M27.61
      - poor bone quality M27.61
    - iatrogenic M27.61
  - post-osseointegration
    - biological M27.62
    - due to complications of systemic disease M27.62
    - iatrogenic M27.62
    - mechanical M27.63
  - pre-integration M27.61
  - pre-osseointegration M27.61
  - specified NEC M27.69
- descent of head (at term) of pregnancy (mother) O32.4
- endosseous dental implant —*see* Failure, dental implant
- engagement of head (term of pregnancy) (mother) O32.4
- erection (penile) (*see also* Dysfunction, sexual, male, erectile) N52.9
  - nonorganic F52.21
- examination(s), anxiety concerning Z55.2
- expansion terminal respiratory units (newborn) (primary) P28.0
- forceps NOS (with subsequent cesarean delivery) O66.5
- gain weight (child over 28 days old) R62.51
  - adult R62.7
  - newborn P92.6
- genital response (male) F52.21
  - female F52.22
- heart (acute) (senile) (sudden) I50.9
  - with
    - acute pulmonary edema —*see* Failure, ventricular, left
    - decompensation —*see also* Failure, heart, by type as diastolic or systolic, acute and chronic I50.9

Failure, failed *(continued)*
- heart *(continued)*
  - with *(continued)*
    - dilatation —*see* Disease, heart
    - normal ejection fraction —*see* Failure, heart diastolic
    - preserved ejection fraction —*see* Failure, heart diastolic
    - reduced ejection fraction - *see* Failure, heart systolic
  - arteriosclerotic I70.90
  - biventricular I50.82
    - due to left heart failure I50.814
  - combined left-right sided I50.82
    - due to left heart failure I50.814
  - compensated (*see also* Failure, heart, by type as diastolic or systolic, chronic) I50.9
  - complicating
    - anesthesia (general) (local) or other sedation
      - in labor and delivery O74.2
      - in pregnancy O29.12-
      - postpartum, puerperal O89.1
    - delivery (cesarean) (instrumental) O75.4
  - congestive I50.9
    - with rheumatic fever (conditions in I00)
      - active I01.8
      - inactive or quiescent (with chorea) I09.81
    - newborn P29.0
    - rheumatic (chronic) (inactive) (with chorea) I09.81
      - active or acute I01.8
        - with chorea I02.0
  - decompensated (*see also* Failure, heart, by type as diastolic or systolic, acute and chronic) I50.9
  - degenerative —*see* Degeneration, myocardial
  - diastolic (congestive) (left ventricular) I50.30
    - acute (congestive) I50.31
      - and (on) chronic (congestive) I50.33
    - chronic (congestive) I50.32
      - and (on) acute (congestive) I50.33
    - combined with systolic (congestive) I50.40
      - acute (congestive) I50.41
        - and (on) chronic (congestive) I50.43
      - chronic (congestive) I50.42
        - and (on) acute (congestive) I50.43
  - due to presence of cardiac prosthesis I97.13-
  - end stage (*see also* Failure, heart, by type as diastolic or systolic, chronic) I50.84
  - following cardiac surgery I97.13-
  - high output NOS I50.83
  - hypertensive —*see* Hypertension, heart
  - left (ventricular) —*see also* Failure, ventricular, left
    - combined diastolic and systolic —*see* Failure, heart, diastolic, combined with systolic
    - diastolic —*see* Failure, heart, diastolic
    - systolic —*see* Failure, heart, systolic
  - low output (syndrome) NOS I50.9
  - newborn P29.0
  - organic —*see* Disease, heart
  - peripartum O90.3

Failure, failed *(continued)*
- heart *(continued)*
  - postprocedural I97.13-
  - rheumatic (chronic) (inactive) I09.9
  - right (isolated) I50.810
    - acute I50.811
      - and (on) chronic I50.813
    - chronic I50.812
      - and acute I50.813
    - secondary to left heart failure I50.814
  - specified NEC I50.89

  Note: heart failure stages A, B, C and D are based on the American College of Cardiology and American Heart Association stages of heart failure, which complement and should not be confused with the New York Heart Association Classification of Heart Failure, into Class I, Class II, Class III and Class IV

  - stage A Z91.89
  - stage B (*see also* Failure, heart, by type as diastolic or systolic) I50.9
  - stage C (*see also* Failure, heart, by type as diastolic or systolic) I50.9
  - stage D (*see also* Failure, heart, by type as diastolic or systolic, chronic) I50.84
  - systolic (congestive) (left ventricular) I50.20
    - acute (congestive) I50.21
      - and (on) chronic (congestive) I50.23
    - chronic (congestive) I50.22
      - and (on) acute (congestive) I50.23
    - combined with diastolic (congestive) I50.40
      - acute (congestive) I50.41
        - and (on) chronic (congestive) I50.43
      - chronic (congestive) I50.42
        - and (on) acute (congestive) I50.43
  - thyrotoxic (*see also* Thyrotoxicosis) E05.90 *[I43]*
    - with
      - high output (*see also* Thyrotoxicosis) I50.83
      - thyroid storm E05.91 *[I43]*
        - high output (*see also* Thyrotoxicosis) I50.83
  - valvular —*see* Endocarditis
- hepatic K72.90
  - with coma K72.91
  - acute or subacute K72.00
    - with coma K72.01
    - due to drugs K71.10
      - with coma K71.11
  - alcoholic (acute) (chronic) (subacute) K70.40
    - with coma K70.41
  - chronic K72.10
    - with coma K72.11
    - due to drugs (acute) (subacute) (chronic) K71.10
      - with coma K71.11
  - due to drugs (acute) (subacute) (chronic) K71.10
    - with coma K71.11
  - postprocedural K91.82
- hepatorenal K76.7
- induction (of labor) O61.9
  - abortion —*see* Abortion, attempted

Failure, failed *(continued)*
induction *(continued)*
by
oxytocic drugs O61.0
prostaglandins O61.0
instrumental O61.1
mechanical O61.1
medical O61.0
specified NEC O61.8
surgical O61.1
intubation during anesthesia T88.4
in pregnancy O29.6-
labor and delivery O74.7
postpartum, puerperal O89.6
involution, thymus (gland) E32.0
kidney (*see also* Disease, kidney, chronic) N19
acute (*see also* Failure, renal, acute) N17.9-
diabetic *—see* E08-E13 with .22
lactation (complete) O92.3
partial O92.4
Leydig's cell, adult E29.1
liver *—see* Failure, hepatic
menstruation at puberty N91.0
mitral I05.8
myocardial, myocardium (*see also* Failure, heart) I50.9
chronic (*see also* Failure, heart, congestive) I50.9
congestive (*see also* Failure, heart, congestive) I50.9
orgasm (female) (psychogenic) F52.31
male F52.32
ovarian (primary) E28.39
iatrogenic E89.40
asymptomatic E89.40
symptomatic E89.41
postprocedural (postablative) (postirradiation) (postsurgical) E89.40
asymptomatic E89.40
symptomatic E89.41
ovulation causing infertility N97.0
polyglandular, autoimmune E31.0
prosthetic joint implant *—see* Complications, joint prosthesis, mechanical, breakdown, by site
renal N19
with
tubular necrosis (acute) N17.0
acute N17.9
with
cortical necrosis N17.1
medullary necrosis N17.2
tubular necrosis N17.0
specified NEC N17.8
chronic N18.9
hypertensive *—see* Hypertension, kidney
congenital P96.0
end stage (chronic) N18.6
due to hypertension I12.0
following
abortion *—see* Abortion by type complicated by specified condition NEC
crushing T79.5
ectopic or molar pregnancy O08.4
labor and delivery (acute) O90.4
hypertensive *—see* Hypertension, kidney
postprocedural N99.0
respiration, respiratory J96.90
with
hypercarbia J96.02
hypercapnia J96.92
hypoxia J96.91

Failure, failed *(continued)*
respiration, respiratory *(continued)*
acute J96.00
with
hypercarbia J96.02
hypercapnia J96.02
hypoxia J96.01
center G93.89
acute and (on) chronic J96.20
with
hypercarbia J96.22
hypercapnia J96.22
hypoxia J96.21
chronic J96.10
with
hypercarbia J96.12
hypercapnia J96.12
hypoxia J96.11
newborn P28.5
postprocedural (acute) J95.821
acute and chronic J95.822
rotation
cecum Q43.3
colon Q43.3
intestine Q43.3
kidney Q63.2
sedation (conscious) (moderate) during procedure T88.52
history of Z92.83
segmentation *—see also* Fusion
fingers *—see* Syndactylism, complex, fingers
vertebra Q76.49
with scoliosis Q76.3
seminiferous tubule, adult E29.1
senile (general) R54
sexual arousal (male) F52.21
female F52.22
testicular endocrine function E29.1
to thrive (child over 28 days old) R62.51
adult R62.7
newborn P92.6
transplant T86.92
bone T86.831
marrow T86.02
cornea T86.841
heart T86.22
with lung(s) T86.32
intestine T86.851
kidney T86.12
liver T86.42
lung(s) T86.811
with heart T86.32
pancreas T86.891
skin (allograft) (autograft) T86.821
specified organ or tissue NEC T86.891
stem cell (peripheral blood) (umbilical cord) T86.5
trial of labor (with subsequent cesarean delivery) O66.40
following previous cesarean delivery O66.41
tubal ligation N99.89
urinary *—see* Disease, kidney, chronic
vacuum extraction NOS (with subsequent cesarean delivery) O66.5
vasectomy N99.89
ventouse NOS (with subsequent cesarean delivery) O66.5
ventricular (*see also* Failure, heart) I50.9

Failure, failed *(continued)*
ventricular *(continued)*
left (*see also* Failure, heart) I50.1
with rheumatic fever (conditions in I00)
active I01.8
with chorea I02.0
inactive or quiescent (with chorea) I09.81
rheumatic (chronic) (inactive) (with chorea) I09.81
active or acute I01.8
with chorea I02.0
right *—see* Failure, heart, right
vital centers, newborn P91.88

Fainting (fit) R55

Fallen arches *—see* Deformity, limb, flat foot

Falling, falls (repeated) R29.6
any organ or part *—see* Prolapse

Fallopian
insufflation Z31.41
tube *—see* condition

Fallot's
pentalogy Q21.8
tetrad or tetralogy Q21.3
triad or trilogy Q22.3

False *—see also* condition
croup J38.5
joint *—see* Nonunion, fracture
labor (pains) O47.9
at or after 37 completed weeks of gestation O47.1
before 37 completed weeks of gestation O47.0-
passage, urethra (prostatic) N36.5
pregnancy F45.8

Family, familial *—see also* condition
disruption Z63.8
involving divorce or separation Z63.5
Li-Fraumeni (syndrome) Z15.01
planning advice Z30.09
problem Z63.9
specified NEC Z63.8
retinoblastoma C69.2-

Famine (effects of) T73.0
edema *—see* Malnutrition, severe

Fanconi (-de Toni) (-Debré) **syndrome** E72.09
with cystinosis E72.04

Fanconi's anemia (congenital pancytopenia) D61.09

Farber's disease or syndrome E75.29

Farcy A24.0

Farmer's
lung J67.0
skin L57.8

Farsightedness *—see* Hypermetropia

Fascia *—see* condition

Fasciculation R25.3

Fasciitis M72.9
diffuse (eosinophilic) M35.4
infective M72.8
necrotizing M72.6
necrotizing M72.6
nodular M72.4
perirenal (with ureteral obstruction) N13.5
with infection N13.6
plantar M72.2
specified NEC M72.8
traumatic (old) M72.8
current - code by site under Sprain

Fascioliasis B66.3

Fasciolopsis, fasciolopsiasis (intestinal) B66.5

Fascioscapulohumeral myopathy G71.0

Fast pulse R00.0

Fat
embolism *—see* Embolism, fat
excessive *—see also* Obesity
in heart *—see* Degeneration, myocardial
in stool R19.5
localized (pad) E65
heart *—see* Degeneration, myocardial
knee M79.4
retropatellar M79.4
necrosis
breast N64.1
mesentery K65.4
omentum K65.4
pad E65
knee M79.4

Fatigue R53.83
auditory deafness *—see* Deafness
chronic R53.82
combat F43.0
general R53.83
psychogenic F48.8
heat (transient) T67.6
muscle M62.89
myocardium *—see* Failure, heart
neoplasm-related R53.0
nervous, neurosis F48.8
operational F48.8
psychogenic (general) F48.8
senile R54
voice R49.8

Fatness *—see* Obesity

Fatty *—see also* condition
apron E65
degeneration *—see* Degeneration, fatty
heart (enlarged) *—see* Degeneration, myocardial
liver NEC K76.0
alcoholic K70.0
nonalcoholic K76.0
necrosis *—see* Degeneration, fatty

Fauces *—see* condition

Fauchard's disease (periodontitis) *—see* Periodontitis

Faucitis J02.9

Favism (anemia) D55.0

Favus *—see* Dermatophytosis

Fazio-Londe disease or syndrome G12.1

Fear complex or reaction F40.9

Fear of *—see* Phobia

Feared complaint unfounded Z71.1

Febris, febrile *—see also* Fever
flava (*see also* Fever, yellow) A95.9
melitensis A23.0
pestis *—see* Plague
recurrens *—see* Fever, relapsing
rubra A38.9

Fecal
incontinence R15.9
smearing R15.1
soiling R15.1
urgency R15.2

Fecalith (impaction) K56.41
appendix K38.1
congenital P76.8

- **Fede's disease** K14.0
- **Feeble rapid pulse due to shock following injury** T79.4
- **Feeble-minded** F70
- **Feeding**
  - difficulties R63.3
  - problem R63.3
    - newborn P92.9
      - specified NEC P92.8
    - nonorganic (adult) *—see* Disorder, eating
- **Feeling** (of)
  - foreign body in throat R09.89
- **Feer's disease** *—see* Poisoning, mercury
- **Feet** *—see* condition
- **Feigned illness** Z76.5
- **Feil-Klippel syndrome** (brevicollis) Q76.1
- **Feinmesser's** (hidrotic) **ectodermal dysplasia** Q82.4
- **Felinophobia** F40.218
- **Felon** *—see also* Cellulitis, digit
  - with lymphangitis *—see* Lymphangitis, acute, digit
- **Felty's syndrome** M05.00
  - ankle M05.07-
  - elbow M05.02-
  - foot joint M05.07-
  - hand joint M05.04-
  - hip M05.05-
  - knee M05.06-
  - multiple site M05.09
  - shoulder M05.01-
  - vertebra *—see* Spondylitis, ankylosing
  - wrist M05.03-
- **Female genital cutting status** *—see* Female genital mutilation status (FGM)
- **Female genital mutilation status** (FGM) N90.810
  - specified NEC N90.818
  - type I (clitorectomy status) N90.811
  - type II (clitorectomy with excision of labia minora status) N90.812
  - type III (infibulation status) N90.813
  - type IV N90.818
- **Femur, femoral** *—see* condition
- **Fenestration, fenestrated** *—see also* Imperfect, closure
  - aortico-pulmonary Q21.4
  - cusps, heart valve NEC Q24.8
    - pulmonary Q22.3
  - pulmonic cusps Q22.3
- **Fernell's disease** (aortic aneurysm) I71.9
- **Fertile eunuch syndrome** E23.0
- **Fetid**
  - breath R19.6
  - sweat L75.0
- **Fetishism** F65.0
  - transvestic F65.1
- **Fetus, fetal** *—see also* condition
  - alcohol syndrome (dysmorphic) Q86.0
  - compressus O31.0-
  - hydantoin syndrome Q86.1
  - lung tissue P28.0
  - papyraceous O31.0-
- **Fever** (inanition) (of unknown origin) (persistent) (with chills) (with rigor) R50.9

Fever *(continued)*

- abortus A23.1
- Aden (dengue) A90
- African tick-borne A68.1
- American
  - mountain (tick) A93.2
  - spotted A77.0
- aphthous B08.8
- arbovirus, arboviral A94
  - hemorrhagic A94
  - specified NEC A93.8
- Argentinian hemorrhagic A96.0
- Assam B55.0
- Australian Q A78
- Bangkok hemorrhagic A91
- Barmah forest A92.8
- Bartonella A44.0
- bilious, hemoglobinuric B50.8
- blackwater B50.8
- blister B00.1
- Bolivian hemorrhagic A96.1
- Bonvale dam T73.3
- boutonneuse A77.1
- brain *—see* Encephalitis
- Brazilian purpuric A48.4
- breakbone A90
- Bullis A77.0
- Bunyamwera A92.8
- Burdwan B55.0
- Bwamba A92.8
- Cameroon *—see* Malaria
- Canton A75.9
- catarrhal (acute) J00
  - chronic J31.0
- cat-scratch A28.1
- Central Asian hemorrhagic A98.0
- cerebral *—see* Encephalitis
- cerebrospinal meningococcal A39.0
- Chagres B50.9
- Chandipura A92.8
- Changuinola A93.1
- Charcot's (biliary) (hepatic) (intermittent) *—see* Calculus, bile duct
- Chikungunya (viral) (hemorrhagic) A92.0
- Chitral A93.1
- Colombo *—see* Fever, paratyphoid
- Colorado tick (virus) A93.2
- congestive (remittent) *—see* Malaria
- Congo virus A98.0
- continued malarial B50.9
- Corsican *—see* Malaria
- Crimean-Congo hemorrhagic A98.0
- Cyprus *—see* Brucellosis
- dandy A90
- deer fly *—see* Tularemia
- dengue (virus) A90
  - hemorrhagic A91
  - sandfly A93.1
- desert B38.0
- drug induced R50.2
- due to
  - conditions classified elsewhere R50.81
  - heat T67.0
- enteric A01.00
- enteroviral exanthematous (Boston exanthem) A88.0
- ephemeral (of unknown origin) R50.9
- epidemic hemorrhagic A98.5
- erysipelatous *—see* Erysipelas
- estivo-autumnal (malarial) B50.9
- famine A75.0
- five day A79.0
- following delivery O86.4
- Fort Bragg A27.89
- gastroenteric A01.00
- gastromalarial *—see* Malaria
- Gibraltar *—see* Brucellosis

Fever *(continued)*

- glandular *—see* Mononucleosis, infectious
- Guama (viral) A92.8
- Haverhill A25.1
- hay (allergic) J30.1
  - with asthma (bronchial) J45.909
    - with
      - exacerbation (acute) J45.901
      - status asthmaticus J45.902
  - due to
    - allergen other than pollen J30.89
    - pollen, any plant or tree J30.1
- heat (effects) T67.0
- hematuric, bilious B50.8
- hemoglobinuric (malarial) (bilious) B50.8
- hemorrhagic (arthropod-borne) NOS A94
  - with renal syndrome A98.5
  - arenaviral A96.9
    - specified NEC A96.8
  - Argentinian A96.0
  - Bangkok A91
  - Bolivian A96.1
  - Central Asian A98.0
  - Chikungunya A92.0
  - Crimean-Congo A98.0
  - dengue (virus) A91
  - epidemic A98.5
  - Junin (virus) A96.0
  - Korean A98.5
  - Kyasanur forest A98.2
  - Machupo (virus) A96.1
  - mite-borne A93.8
  - mosquito-borne A92.8
  - Omsk A98.1
  - Philippine A91
  - Russian A98.5
  - Singapore A91
  - Southeast Asia A91
  - Thailand A91
  - tick-borne NEC A93.8
  - viral A99
    - specified NEC A98.8
- hepatic *—see* Cholecystitis
- herpetic *—see* Herpes
- icterohemorrhagic A27.0
- Indiana A93.8
- infective B99.9
  - specified NEC B99.8
- intermittent (bilious) *—see also* Malaria
  - of unknown origin R50.9
  - pernicious B50.9
- iodide R50.2
- Japanese river A75.3
- jungle *—see also* Malaria
  - yellow A95.0
- Junin (virus) hemorrhagic A96.0
- Katayama B65.2
- kedani A75.3
- Kenya (tick) A77.1
- Kew Garden A79.1
- Korean hemorrhagic A98.5
- Lassa A96.2
- Lone Star A77.0
- Machupo (virus) hemorrhagic A96.1
- malaria, malarial *—see* Malaria
- Malta A23.9
- Marseilles A77.1
- marsh *—see* Malaria
- Mayaro (viral) A92.8
- Mediterranean (*see also* Brucellosis) A23.9
  - familial M04.1
  - tick A77.1
- meningeal *—see* Meningitis
- Meuse A79.0
- Mexican A75.2
- mianeh A68.1

Fever *(continued)*

- miasmatic *—see* Malaria
- mosquito-borne (viral) A92.9
  - hemorrhagic A92.8
- mountain (*see also* Brucellosis)
  - meaning Rocky Mountain spotted fever A77.0
  - tick (American) (Colorado) (viral) A93.2
- Mucambo (viral) A92.8
- mud A27.9
- Neapolitan *—see* Brucellosis
- neutropenic D70.9
- newborn P81.9
  - environmental P81.0
- Nine-Mile A78
- non-exanthematous tick A93.2
- North Asian tick-borne A77.2
- Omsk hemorrhagic A98.1
- O'nyong-nyong (viral) A92.1
- Oropouche (viral) A93.0
- Oroya A44.0
- paludal *—see* Malaria
- Panama (malarial) B50.9
- Pappataci A93.1
- paratyphoid A01.4
  - A A01.1
  - B A01.2
  - C A01.3
- parrot A70
- periodic (Mediterranean) M04.1
- persistent (of unknown origin) R50.9
- petechial A39.0
- pharyngoconjunctival B30.2
- Philippine hemorrhagic A91
- phlebotomus A93.1
- Piry (virus) A93.8
- Pixuna (viral) A92.8
- Plasmodium ovale B53.0
- polioviral (nonparalytic) A80.4
- Pontiac A48.2
- postimmunization R50.83
- postoperative R50.82
  - due to infection T81.4
- posttransfusion R50.84
- postvaccination R50.83
- presenting with conditions classified elsewhere R50.81
- pretibial A27.89
- puerperal O86.4
- Q A78
- quadrilateral A78
- quartan (malaria) B52.9
- Queensland (coastal) (tick) A77.3
- quintan A79.0
- rabbit *—see* Tularemia
- rat-bite A25.9
  - due to
    - Spirillum A25.0
    - Streptobacillus moniliformis A25.1
- recurrent *—see* Fever, relapsing
- relapsing (Borrelia) A68.9
  - Carter's (Asiatic) A68.1
  - Dutton's (West African) A68.1
  - Koch's A68.9
  - louse-borne A68.0
  - Novy's
    - louse-borne A68.0
    - tick-borne A68.1
  - Obermeyer's (European) A68.0
  - tick-borne A68.1
- remittent (bilious) (congestive) (gastric) *—see* Malaria
- rheumatic (active) (acute) (chronic) (subacute) I00
  - with central nervous system involvement I02.9
  - active with heart involvement *— see* category I01

Fever *(continued)*
- rheumatic *(continued)*
  - inactive or quiescent with
    - cardiac hypertrophy I09.89
    - carditis I09.9
    - endocarditis I09.1
      - aortic (valve) I06.9
        - with mitral (valve) disease I08.0
      - mitral (valve) I05.9
        - with aortic (valve) disease I08.0
      - pulmonary (valve) I09.89
      - tricuspid (valve) I07.8
    - heart disease NEC I09.89
    - heart failure (congestive) (conditions in I50.-) I09.81
    - left ventricular failure (conditions in I50.1-I50.4-) I09.81
    - myocarditis, myocardial degeneration (conditions in I51.4) I09.0
    - pancarditis I09.9
    - pericarditis I09.2
- Rift Valley (viral) A92.4
- Rocky Mountain spotted A77.0
- rose J30.1
- Ross River B33.1
- Russian hemorrhagic A98.5
- San Joaquin (Valley) B38.0
- sandfly A93.1
- Sao Paulo A77.0
- scarlet A38.9
- seven day (leptospirosis) (autumnal) (Japanese) A27.89
  - dengue A90
- shin-bone A79.0
- Singapore hemorrhagic A91
- solar A90
- Songo A98.5
- sore B00.1
- South African tick-bite A68.1
- Southeast Asia hemorrhagic A91
- spinal *—see* Meningitis
- spirillary A25.0
- splenic *—see* Anthrax
- spotted A77.9
  - American A77.0
  - Brazilian A77.0
  - cerebrospinal meningitis A39.0
  - Colombian A77.0
  - due to Rickettsia
    - australis A77.3
    - conorii A77.1
    - rickettsii A77.0
    - sibirica A77.2
    - specified type NEC A77.8
  - Ehrlichiosis A77.40
    - due to
      - E. chafeensis A77.41
      - specified organism NEC A77.49
  - Rocky Mountain A77.0
- steroid R50.2
- streptobacillary A25.1
- subtertian B50.9
- Sumatran mite A75.3
- sun A90
- swamp A27.9
- swine A02.8
- sylvatic, yellow A95.0
- Tahyna B33.8
- tertian *—see* Malaria, tertian
- Thailand hemorrhagic A91
- thermic T67.0
- three-day A93.1
- tick
  - American mountain A93.2
  - Colorado A93.2

Fever *(continued)*
- tick *(continued)*
  - Kemerovo A93.8
  - Mediterranean A77.1
  - mountain A93.2
  - nonexanthematous A93.2
  - Quaranfil A93.8
- tick-bite NEC A93.8
- tick-borne (hemorrhagic) NEC A93.8
- trench A79.0
- tsutsugamushi A75.3
- typhogastric A01.00
- typhoid (abortive) (hemorrhagic) (intermittent) (malignant) A01.00
  - complicated by
    - arthritis A01.04
    - heart involvement A01.02
    - meningitis A01.01
    - osteomyelitis A01.05
    - pneumonia A01.03
    - specified NEC A01.09
- typhomalarial *—see* Malaria
- typhus *—see* Typhus (fever)
- undulant *—see* Brucellosis
- unknown origin R50.9
- uveoparotid D86.89
- valley B38.0
- Venezuelan equine A92.2
- vesicular stomatitis A93.8
- viral hemorrhagic *—see* Fever, hemorrhagic, by type of virus
- Volhynian A79.0
- Wesselsbron (viral) A92.8
- West
  - African B50.8
  - Nile (viral) A92.30
    - with
      - complications NEC A92.39
      - cranial nerve disorders A92.32
      - encephalitis A92.31
      - encephalomyelitis A92.31
      - neurologic manifestation NEC A92.32
      - optic neuritis A92.32
      - polyradiculitis A92.32
- Whitmore's *—see* Melioidosis
- Wolhynian A79.0
- worm B83.9
- yellow A95.9
  - jungle A95.0
  - sylvatic A95.0
  - urban A95.1
- Zika virus A92.5

Fibrillation
- atrial or auricular (established) I48.91
  - chronic I48.2
  - paroxysmal I48.0
  - permanent I48.2
  - persistent I48.1
- cardiac I49.8
- heart I49.8
- muscular M62.89
- ventricular I49.01

Fibrin
- ball or bodies, pleural (sac) J94.1
- chamber, anterior (eye) (gelatinous exudate) *—see* Iridocyclitis, acute

Fibrinogenolysis *—see* Fibrinolysis

Fibrinogenopenia D68.8
- acquired D65
- congenital D68.2

Fibrinolysis (hemorrhagic) (acquired) D65
- antepartum hemorrhage *—see* Hemorrhage, antepartum, with coagulation defect

Fibrinolysis *(continued)*
- following
  - abortion *—see* Abortion by type complicated by hemorrhage
  - ectopic or molar pregnancy O08.1
- intrapartum O67.0
- newborn, transient P60
- postpartum O72.3

Fibrinopenia (hereditary) D68.2
- acquired D68.4

Fibrinopurulent *—see* condition

Fibrinous *—see* condition

Fibroadenoma
- cellular intracanalicular D24-
- giant D24-
- intracanalicular
  - cellular D24-
  - giant D24-
  - specified site *—see* Neoplasm, benign, by site
  - unspecified site D24-
- juvenile D24-
- pericanalicular
  - specified site *—see* Neoplasm, benign, by site
  - unspecified site D24-
- phyllodes D24-
- prostate D29.1
- specified site NEC *—see* Neoplasm, benign, by site
- unspecified site D24-

Fibroadenosis, breast (chronic) (cystic) (diffuse) (periodic) (segmental) N60.2-

Fibroangioma *—see also* Neoplasm, benign, by site
- juvenile
  - specified site *—see* Neoplasm, benign, by site
  - unspecified site D10.6

Fibrochondrosarcoma *—see* Neoplasm, cartilage, malignant

Fibrocystic
- disease *—see also* Fibrosis, cystic
  - breast *—see* Mastopathy, cystic
  - jaw M27.49
  - kidney (congenital) Q61.8
  - liver Q44.6
  - pancreas E84.9
- kidney (congenital) Q61.8

Fibrodysplasia ossificans progressiva *—see* Myositis, ossificans, progressiva

Fibroelastosis (cordis) (endocardial) (endomyocardial) I42.4

Fibroid (tumor) *—see also* Neoplasm, connective tissue, benign
- disease, lung (chronic) *—see* Fibrosis, lung
- heart (disease) *—see* Myocarditis
- in pregnancy or childbirth O34.1-
  - causing obstructed labor O65.5
- induration, lung (chronic) *—see* Fibrosis, lung
- lung *—see* Fibrosis, lung
- pneumonia (chronic) *—see* Fibrosis, lung
- uterus (*see also* Leiomyoma, uterus) D25.9

Fibrolipoma *—see* Lipoma

Fibroliposarcoma *—see* Neoplasm, connective tissue, malignant

Fibroma *—see also* Neoplasm, connective tissue, benign
- ameloblastic *—see* Cyst, calcifying odontogenic

Fibroma *(continued)*
- bone (nonossifying) *—see* Disorder, bone, specified type NEC
  - ossifying *—see* Neoplasm, bone, benign
- cementifying *—see* Neoplasm, bone, benign
- chondromyxoid *—see* Neoplasm, bone, benign
- desmoplastic *—see* Neoplasm, connective tissue, uncertain behavior
- durum *—see* Neoplasm, connective tissue, benign
- fascial *—see* Neoplasm, connective tissue, benign
- invasive *—see* Neoplasm, connective tissue, uncertain behavior
- molle *—see* Lipoma
- myxoid *—see* Neoplasm, connective tissue, benign
- nasopharynx, nasopharyngeal (juvenile) D10.6
- nonosteogenic (nonossifying) *—see* Dysplasia, fibrous
- odontogenic (central) *—see* Cyst, calcifying odontogenic
- ossifying *—see* Neoplasm, bone, benign
- periosteal *—see* Neoplasm, bone, benign
- soft *—see* Lipoma

Fibromatosis M72.9
- abdominal *—see* Neoplasm, connective tissue, uncertain behavior
- aggressive *—see* Neoplasm, connective tissue, uncertain behavior
- congenital generalized *—see* Neoplasm, connective tissue, uncertain behavior
- Dupuytren's M72.0
- gingival K06.1
- palmar (fascial) M72.0
- plantar (fascial) M72.2
- pseudosarcomatous (proliferative) (subcutaneous) M72.4
- retroperitoneal D48.3
- specified NEC M72.8

Fibromyalgia M79.7

Fibromyoma *—see also* Neoplasm, connective tissue, benign
- uterus (corpus) *—see also* Leiomyoma, uterus
  - in pregnancy or childbirth *—see* Fibroid, in pregnancy or childbirth
    - causing obstructed labor O65.5

Fibromyositis M79.7

Fibromyxolipoma D17.9

Fibromyxoma *—see* Neoplasm, connective tissue, benign

Fibromyxosarcoma *—see* Neoplasm, connective tissue, malignant

Fibro-odontoma, ameloblastic *—see* Cyst, calcifying odontogenic

Fibro-osteoma *—see* Neoplasm, bone, benign

Fibroplasia, retrolental H35.17-

Fibropurulent *—see* condition

Fibrosarcoma *—see also* Neoplasm, connective tissue, malignant
- ameloblastic C41.1
  - upper jaw (bone) C41.0

Fibrosarcoma *(continued)*
- congenital —*see* Neoplasm, connective tissue, malignant
- fascial —*see* Neoplasm, connective tissue, malignant
- infantile —*see* Neoplasm, connective tissue, malignant
- odontogenic C41.1
  - upper jaw (bone) C41.0
- periosteal —*see* Neoplasm, bone, malignant

Fibrosclerosis
- breast N60.3-
- multifocal M35.5
- penis (corpora cavernosa) N48.6

Fibrosis, fibrotic
- adrenal (gland) E27.8
- amnion O41.8X-
- anal papillae K62.89
- arteriocapillary —*see* Arteriosclerosis
- bladder N32.89
  - interstitial —*see* Cystitis, chronic, interstitial
  - localized submucosal —*see* Cystitis, chronic, interstitial
  - panmural —*see* Cystitis, chronic, interstitial
- breast —*see* Fibrosclerosis, breast
- capillary (*see also* Arteriosclerosis) I70.90
  - lung (chronic) —*see* Fibrosis, lung
- cardiac —*see* Myocarditis
- cervix N88.8
- chorion O41.8X-
- corpus cavernosum (sclerosing) N48.6
- cystic (of pancreas) E84.9
  - with
    - distal intestinal obstruction syndrome E84.19
    - fecal impaction E84.19
    - intestinal manifestations NEC E84.19
    - pulmonary manifestations E84.0
    - specified manifestations NEC E84.8
- due to device, implant or graft (*see also* Complications, by site and type, specified) NEC T85.828
  - arterial graft NEC T82.828
  - breast (implant) T85.828
  - catheter NEC T85.828
    - dialysis (renal) T82.828
      - intraperitoneal T85.828
    - infusion NEC T82.828
      - spinal (epidural) (subdural) T85.820
    - urinary (indwelling) T83.82
  - electronic (electrode) (pulse generator) (stimulator)
    - bone T84.82
    - cardiac T82.827
    - nervous system (brain) (peripheral nerve) (spinal) T85.820
    - urinary T83.82
  - fixation, internal (orthopedic) NEC T84.82
  - gastrointestinal (bile duct) (esophagus) T85.828
  - genital NEC T83.82
  - heart NEC T82.827
  - joint prosthesis T84.82
  - ocular (corneal graft) (orbital implant) NEC T85.828
  - orthopedic NEC T84.82
  - specified NEC T85.828
  - urinary NEC T83.82
  - vascular NEC T82.828
  - ventricular intracranial shunt T85.820

Fibrosis, fibrotic *(continued)*
- ejaculatory duct N50.89
- endocardium —*see* Endocarditis
- endomyocardial (tropical) I42.3
- epididymis N50.89
- eye muscle —*see* Strabismus, mechanical
- heart —*see* Myocarditis
- hepatic —*see* Fibrosis, liver
- hepatolienal (portal hypertension) K76.6
- hepatosplenic (portal hypertension) K76.6
- infrapatellar fat pad M79.4
- intrascrotal N50.89
- kidney N26.9
- liver K74.0
  - with sclerosis K74.2
  - alcoholic K70.2
- lung (atrophic) (chronic) (confluent) (massive) (perialveolar) (peribronchial) J84.10
  - with
    - anthracosilicosis J60
    - anthracosis J60
    - asbestosis J61
    - bagassosis J67.1
    - bauxite J63.1
    - berylliosis J63.2
    - byssinosis J66.0
    - calcicosis J62.8
    - chalicosis J62.8
    - dust reticulation J64
    - farmer's lung J67.0
    - ganister disease J62.8
    - graphite J63.3
    - pneumoconiosis NOS J64
    - siderosis J63.4
    - silicosis J62.8
  - capillary J84.10
  - congenital P27.8
  - diffuse (idiopathic) J84.10
    - chemicals, gases, fumes or vapors (inhalation) J68.4
    - interstitial J84.10
      - acute J84.114
    - talc J62.0
  - following radiation J70.1
  - idiopathic J84.112
  - postinflammatory J84.10
  - silicotic J62.8
  - tuberculous —*see* Tuberculosis, pulmonary
- lymphatic gland I89.8
- median bar —*see* Hyperplasia, prostate
- mediastinum (idiopathic) J98.59
- meninges G96.19
- myocardium, myocardial —*see* Myocarditis
- ovary N83.8
- oviduct N83.8
- pancreas K86.89
- penis NEC N48.6
- pericardium I31.0
- perineum, in pregnancy or childbirth O34.7-
  - causing obstructed labor O65.5
- pleura J94.1
- popliteal fat pad M79.4
- prostate (chronic) —*see* Hyperplasia, prostate
- pulmonary (*see also* Fibrosis, lung) J84.10
  - congenital P27.8
  - idiopathic J84.112
- rectal sphincter K62.89
- retroperitoneal, idiopathic (with ureteral obstruction) N13.5
  - with infection N13.6

Fibrosis, fibrotic *(continued)*
- sclerosing mesenteric (idiopathic) K65.4
- scrotum N50.89
- seminal vesicle N50.89
- senile R54
- skin L90.5
- spermatic cord N50.89
- spleen D73.89
  - in schistosomiasis (bilharziasis) B65.9 *[D77]*
- subepidermal nodular —*see* Neoplasm, skin, benign
- submucous (oral) (tongue) K13.5
- testis N44.8
  - chronic, due to syphilis A52.76
- thymus (gland) E32.8
- tongue, submucous K13.5
- tunica vaginalis N50.89
- uterus (non-neoplastic) N85.8
- vagina N89.8
- valve, heart —*see* Endocarditis
- vas deferens N50.89
- vein I87.8

Fibrositis (periarticular) M79.7
- nodular, chronic (Jaccoud's) (rheumatoid) —*see* Arthropathy, postrheumatic, chronic

Fibrothorax J94.1

Fibrotic —*see* Fibrosis

Fibrous —*see* condition

Fibroxanthoma —*see also* Neoplasm, connective tissue, benign
- atypical —*see* Neoplasm, connective tissue, uncertain behavior
- malignant —*see* Neoplasm, connective tissue, malignant

Fibroxanthosarcoma —*see* Neoplasm, connective tissue, malignant

Fiedler's
- disease (icterohemorrhagic leptospirosis) A27.0
- myocarditis (acute) I40.1

Fifth disease B08.3
- venereal A55

Filaria, filarial, filariasis —*see* Infestation, filarial

Filatov's disease —*see* Mononucleosis, infectious

File-cutter's disease —*see* Poisoning, lead

Filling defect
- biliary tract R93.2
- bladder R93.41
- duodenum R93.3
- gallbladder R93.2
- gastrointestinal tract R93.3
- intestine R93.3
- kidney R93.42-
- stomach R93.3
- ureter R93.41
- urinary organs, specified NEC R93.49

Fimbrial cyst Q50.4

Financial problem affecting care NOS Z59.9
- bankruptcy Z59.8
- foreclosure on loan Z59.8

Findings, abnormal, inconclusive, without diagnosis —*see also* Abnormal
- 17-ketosteroids, elevated R82.5
- acetonuria R82.4
- alcohol in blood R78.0
- anisocytosis R71.8

Findings, abnormal, inconclusive, without diagnosis *(continued)*
- antenatal screening of mother O28.9
  - biochemical O28.1
  - chromosomal O28.5
  - cytological O28.2
  - genetic O28.5
  - hematological O28.0
  - radiological O28.4
  - specified NEC O28.8
  - ultrasonic O28.3
- antibody titer, elevated R76.0
- anticardiolipin antibody R76.0
- antiphosphatidylglycerol antibody R76.0
- antiphosphatidylinositol antibody R76.0
- antiphosphatidylserine antibody R76.0
- antiphospholipid antibody R76.0
- bacteriuria R82.71
- bicarbonate E87.8
- bile in urine R82.2
- blood sugar R73.09
  - high R73.9
  - low (transient) E16.2
- body fluid or substance, specified NEC R88.8
- casts, urine R82.99
- catecholamines R82.5
- cells, urine R82.99
- chloride E87.8
- cholesterol E78.9
  - high E78.00
    - with high triglycerides E78.2
- chyluria R82.0
- cloudy
  - dialysis effluent R88.0
  - urine R82.90
- creatinine clearance R94.4
- crystals, urine R82.99
- culture
  - blood R78.81
  - positive —*see* Positive, culture
- echocardiogram R93.1
- electrolyte level, urinary R82.99
- function study NEC R94.8
  - bladder R94.8
  - endocrine NEC R94.7
    - thyroid R94.6
  - kidney R94.4
  - liver R94.5
  - pancreas R94.8
  - placenta R94.8
  - pulmonary R94.2
  - spleen R94.8
- gallbladder, nonvisualization R93.2
- glucose (tolerance test) (non-fasting) R73.09
- glycosuria R81
- heart
  - shadow R93.1
  - sounds R01.2
- hematinuria R82.3
- hematocrit drop (precipitous) R71.0
- hemoglobinuria R82.3
- human papillomavirus (HPV) DNA test positive
  - cervix
    - high risk R87.810
    - low risk R87.820
  - vagina
    - high risk R87.811
    - low risk R87.821
- in blood (of substance not normally found in blood) R78.9
  - addictive drug NEC R78.4
  - alcohol (excessive level) R78.0
  - cocaine R78.2
  - hallucinogen R78.3

Findings, abnormal, inconclusive, without diagnosis *(continued)*
- in blood (continued)
  - heavy metals (abnormal level) R78.79
  - lead R78.71
  - lithium (abnormal level) R78.89
  - opiate drug R78.1
  - psychotropic drug R78.5
  - specified substance NEC R78.89
  - steroid agent R78.6
- indoleacetic acid, elevated R82.5
- ketonuria R82.4
- lactic acid dehydrogenase (LDH) R74.0
- liver function test R79.89
- mammogram NEC R92.8
  - calcification (calculus) R92.1
  - inconclusive result (due to dense breasts) R92.2
  - microcalcification R92.0
- mediastinal shift R93.8
- melanin, urine R82.99
- myoglobinuria R82.1
- neonatal screening P09
- nonvisualization of gallbladder R93.2
- odor of urine NOS R82.90
- Papanicolaou cervix R87.619
  - non-atypical endometrial cells R87.618
- pneumoencephalogram R93.0
- poikilocytosis R71.8
- potassium (deficiency) E87.6
  - excess E87.5
- PPD R76.11
- radiologic (X-ray) R93.8
  - abdomen R93.5
  - biliary tract R93.2
  - breast R92.8
  - gastrointestinal tract R93.3
  - genitourinary organs R93.8
  - head R93.0
  - inconclusive due to excess body fat of patient R93.9
  - intrathoracic organs NEC R93.1
  - placenta R93.8
  - retroperitoneum R93.5
  - skin R93.8
  - skull R93.0
  - subcutaneous tissue R93.8
- red blood cell (count) (morphology) (sickling) (volume) R71.8
- scan NEC R94.8
  - bladder R94.8
  - bone R94.8
  - kidney R94.4
  - liver R93.2
  - lung R94.2
  - pancreas R94.8
  - placental R94.8
  - spleen R94.8
  - thyroid R94.6
- sedimentation rate, elevated R70.0
- SGOT R74.0
- SGPT R74.0
- sodium (deficiency) E87.1
  - excess E87.0
- specified body fluid NEC R88.8
- stress test R94.39
- thyroid (function) (metabolic rate) (scan) (uptake) R94.6
- transaminase (level) R74.0
- triglycerides E78.9
  - high E78.1
    - with high cholesterol E78.2
- tuberculin skin test (without active tuberculosis) R76.11
- urine R82.90
  - acetone R82.4
  - bacteria R82.71
  - bile R82.2

Findings, abnormal, inconclusive, without diagnosis *(continued)*
- urine *(continued)*
  - casts or cells R82.99
  - chyle R82.0
  - culture positive R82.79
  - glucose R81
  - hemoglobin R82.3
  - ketone R82.4
  - sugar R81
- vanillylmandelic acid (VMA), elevated R82.5
- vectorcardiogram (VCG) R94.39
- ventriculogram R93.0
- white blood cell (count) (differential) (morphology) D72.9
- xerography R92.8

Finger —*see* condition

Fire, Saint Anthony's —*see* Erysipelas

Fire-setting
- pathological (compulsive) F63.1

Fish hook stomach K31.89

Fishmeal-worker's lung J67.8

Fissure, fissured
- anus, anal K60.2
  - acute K60.0
  - chronic K60.1
  - congenital Q43.8
- ear, lobule, congenital Q17.8
- epiglottis (congenital) Q31.8
- larynx J38.7
  - congenital Q31.8
- lip K13.0
  - congenital —*see* Cleft, lip
- nipple N64.0
  - associated with
    - lactation O92.13
    - pregnancy O92.11-
    - puerperium O92.12
- nose Q30.2
- palate (congenital) —*see* Cleft, palate
- skin R23.4
- spine (congenital) —*see also* Spina bifida
  - with hydrocephalus —*see* Spina bifida, by site, with hydrocephalus
- tongue (acquired) K14.5
  - congenital Q38.3

Fistula (cutaneous) L98.8
- abdomen (wall) K63.2
  - bladder N32.2
  - intestine NEC K63.2
  - ureter N28.89
  - uterus N82.5
- abdominorectal K63.2
- abdominosigmoidal K63.2
- abdominothoracic J86.0
- abdominouterine N82.5
  - congenital Q51.7
- abdominovesical N32.2
- accessory sinuses —*see* Sinusitis
- actinomycotic —*see* Actinomycosis
- alveolar antrum —*see* Sinusitis, maxillary
- alveolar process K04.6
- anorectal K60.5
- antrobuccal —*see* Sinusitis, maxillary
- antrum —*see* Sinusitis, maxillary
- anus, anal (recurrent) (infectional) K60.3
  - congenital Q43.6
    - with absence, atresia and stenosis Q42.2
  - tuberculous A18.32
- aorta-duodenal I77.2
- appendix, appendicular K38.3

Fistula *(continued)*
- arteriovenous (acquired) (nonruptured) I77.0
  - brain I67.1
    - congenital Q28.2
      - ruptured I60.8
    - ruptured I60.8
  - cerebral —*see* Fistula, arteriovenous, brain
  - congenital (peripheral) —*see also* Malformation, arteriovenous
    - brain Q28.2
      - ruptured I60.8
    - coronary Q24.5
    - pulmonary Q25.72
  - coronary I25.41
    - congenital Q24.5
  - pulmonary I28.0
    - congenital Q25.72
  - surgically created (for dialysis) Z99.2
    - complication —*see* Complication, arteriovenous, fistula, surgically created
  - traumatic —*see* Injury, blood vessel
- artery I77.2
- aural (mastoid) —*see* Mastoiditis, chronic
- auricle —*see also* Disorder, pinna, specified type NEC
  - congenital Q18.1
- Bartholin's gland N82.8
- bile duct (common) (hepatic) K83.3
  - with calculus, stones —*see* Calculus, bile duct
- biliary (tract) —*see* Fistula, bile duct
- bladder (sphincter) NEC (*see also* Fistula, vesico-) N32.2
  - into seminal vesicle N32.2
- bone —*see also* Disorder, bone, specified type NEC
  - with osteomyelitis, chronic —*see* Osteomyelitis, chronic, with draining sinus
- brain G93.89
  - arteriovenous (acquired) I67.1
    - congenital Q28.2
- branchial (cleft) Q18.0
- branchiogenous Q18.0
- breast N61.0
  - puerperal, postpartum or gestational, due to mastitis (purulent) —*see* Mastitis, obstetric, purulent
- bronchial J86.0
- bronchocutaneous, bronchomediastinal, bronchopleural, bronchopleuromediastinal (infective) J86.0
  - tuberculous NEC A15.5
- bronchoesophageal J86.0
  - congenital Q39.2
    - with atresia of esophagus Q39.1
- bronchovisceral J86.0
- buccal cavity (infective) K12.2
- cecosigmoidal K63.2
- cecum K63.2
- cerebrospinal (fluid) G96.0
- cervical, lateral Q18.1
- cervicoaural Q18.1
- cervicosigmoidal N82.4
- cervicovesical N82.1
- cervix N82.8
- chest (wall) J86.0
- cholecystenteric —*see* Fistula, gallbladder
- cholecystocolic —*see* Fistula, gallbladder
- cholecystocolonic —*see* Fistula, gallbladder

Fistula *(continued)*
- cholecystoduodenal —*see* Fistula, gallbladder
- cholecystogastric —*see* Fistula, gallbladder
- cholecystointestinal —*see* Fistula, gallbladder
- choledochoduodenal —*see* Fistula, bile duct
- cholocolic K82.3
- coccyx —*see* Sinus, pilonidal
- colon K63.2
- colostomy K94.09
- common duct —*see* Fistula, bile duct
- congenital, site not listed —*see* Anomaly, by site
- coronary, arteriovenous I25.41
  - congenital Q24.5
- costal region J86.0
- cul-de-sac, Douglas' N82.8
- cystic duct —*see also* Fistula, gallbladder
  - congenital Q44.5
- dental K04.6
- diaphragm J86.0
- duodenum K31.6
- ear (external) (canal) —*see* Disorder, ear, external, specified type NEC
- enterocolic K63.2
- enterocutaneous K63.2
- enterouterine N82.4
  - congenital Q51.7
- enterovaginal N82.4
  - congenital Q52.2
  - large intestine N82.3
  - small intestine N82.2
- enterovesical N32.1
- epididymis N50.89
  - tuberculous A18.15
- esophagobronchial J86.0
  - congenital Q39.2
    - with atresia of esophagus Q39.1
- esophagocutaneous K22.8
- esophagopleural-cutaneous J86.0
- esophagotracheal J86.0
  - congenital Q39.2
    - with atresia of esophagus Q39.1
- esophagus K22.8
  - congenital Q39.2
    - with atresia of esophagus Q39.1
- ethmoid —*see* Sinusitis, ethmoidal
- eyeball (cornea) (sclera) —*see* Disorder, globe, hypotony
- eyelid H01.8
- fallopian tube, external N82.5
- fecal K63.2
  - congenital Q43.6
- from periapical abscess K04.6
- frontal sinus —*see* Sinusitis, frontal
- gallbladder K82.3
  - with calculus, cholelithiasis, stones —*see* Calculus, gallbladder
- gastric K31.6
- gastrocolic K31.6
  - congenital Q40.2
  - tuberculous A18.32
- gastroenterocolic K31.6
- gastroesophageal K31.6
- gastrojejunal K31.6
- gastrojejunocolic K31.6
- genital tract (female) N82.9
  - specified NEC N82.8
  - to intestine NEC N82.4
  - to skin N82.5
- hepatic artery-portal vein, congenital Q26.6
- hepatopleural J86.0
- hepatopulmonary J86.0
- ileorectal or ileosigmoidal K63.2
- ileovaginal N82.2

Fistula *(continued)*
- ileovesical N32.1
- ileum K63.2
- in ano K60.3
  - tuberculous A18.32
- inner ear (labyrinth) H83.1
- intestine NEC K63.2
- intestinocolonic (abdominal) K63.2
- intestinoureteral N28.89
- intestinouterine N82.4
- intestinovaginal N82.4
  - large intestine N82.3
  - small intestine N82.2
- intestinovesical N32.1
- ischiorectal (fossa) K61.3
- jejunum K63.2
- joint M25.10
  - ankle M25.17-
  - elbow M25.12-
  - foot joint M25.17-
  - hand joint M25.14-
  - hip M25.15-
  - knee M25.16-
  - shoulder M25.11-
  - specified joint NEC M25.18
  - tuberculous *—see* Tuberculosis, joint
  - vertebrae M25.18
  - wrist M25.13-
- kidney N28.89
- labium (majus) (minus) N82.8
- labyrinth H83.1
- lacrimal (gland) (sac) H04.61-
- lacrimonasal duct *—see* Fistula, lacrimal
- laryngotracheal, congenital Q34.8
- larynx J38.7
- lip K13.0
  - congenital Q38.0
- lumbar, tuberculous A18.01
- lung J86.0
- lymphatic I89.8
- mammary (gland) N61.0
- mastoid (process) (region) *—see* Mastoiditis, chronic
- maxillary J32.0
- medial, face and neck Q18.8
- mediastinal J86.0
- mediastinobronchial J86.0
- mediastinocutaneous J86.0
- middle ear H74.8
- mouth K12.2
- nasal J34.89
  - sinus *—see* Sinusitis
- nasopharynx J39.2
- nipple N64.0
- nose J34.89
- oral (cutaneous) K12.2
  - maxillary J32.0
  - nasal (with cleft palate) *—see* Cleft, palate
- orbit, orbital *—see* Disorder, orbit, specified type NEC
- oroantral J32.0
- oviduct, external N82.5
- palate (hard) M27.8
- pancreatic K86.89
- pancreaticoduodenal K86.89
- parotid (gland) K11.4
  - region K12.2
- penis N48.89
- perianal K60.3
- pericardium (pleura) (sac) *—see* Pericarditis
- pericecal K63.2
- perineorectal K60.4
- perineosigmoidal K63.2
- perineum, perineal (with urethral involvement) NEC N36.0
  - tuberculous A18.13
  - ureter N28.89

Fistula *(continued)*
- perirectal K60.4
  - tuberculous A18.32
- peritoneum K65.9
- pharyngoesophageal J39.2
- pharynx J39.2
  - branchial cleft (congenital) Q18.0
- pilonidal (infected) (rectum) *—see* Sinus, pilonidal
- pleura, pleural, pleurocutaneous, pleuroperitoneal J86.0
  - tuberculous NEC A15.6
- pleuropericardial I31.8
- portal vein-hepatic artery, congenital Q26.6
- postauricular H70.81-
- postoperative, persistent T81.83
  - specified site *—see* Fistula, by site
- preauricular (congenital) Q18.1
- prostate N42.89
- pulmonary J86.0
  - arteriovenous I28.0
    - congenital Q25.72
  - tuberculous *—see* Tuberculosis, pulmonary
- pulmonoperitoneal J86.0
- rectolabial N82.4
- rectosigmoid (intercommunicating) K63.2
- rectoureteral N28.89
- rectourethral N36.0
  - congenital Q64.73
- rectouterine N82.4
  - congenital Q51.7
- rectovaginal N82.3
  - congenital Q52.2
  - tuberculous A18.18
- rectovesical N32.1
  - congenital Q64.79
- rectovesicovaginal N82.3
- rectovulval N82.4
  - congenital Q52.79
- rectum (to skin) K60.4
  - congenital Q43.6
    - with absence, atresia and stenosis Q42.0
  - tuberculous A18.32
- renal N28.89
- retroauricular *—see* Fistula, postauricular
- salivary duct or gland (any) K11.4
  - congenital Q38.4
- scrotum (urinary) N50.89
  - tuberculous A18.15
- semicircular canals H83.1
- sigmoid K63.2
  - to bladder N32.1
- sinus *—see* Sinusitis
- skin L98.8
  - to genital tract (female) N82.5
- splenocolic D73.89
- stercoral K63.2
- stomach K31.6
- sublingual gland K11.4
- submandibular gland K11.4
- submaxillary (gland) K11.4
  - region K12.2
- thoracic J86.0
  - duct I89.8
- thoracoabdominal J86.0
- thoracogastric J86.0
- thoracointestinal J86.0
- thorax J86.0
- thyroglossal duct Q89.2
- thyroid E07.89
- trachea, congenital (external) (internal) Q32.1
- tracheoesophageal J86.0
  - congenital Q39.2
    - with atresia of esophagus Q39.1
  - following tracheostomy J95.04

Fistula *(continued)*
- traumatic arteriovenous *—see* Injury, blood vessel, by site
- tuberculous - code by site under Tuberculosis
- typhoid A01.09
- umbilicourinary Q64.8
- urachus, congenital Q64.4
- ureter (persistent) N28.89
- ureteroabdominal N28.89
- ureterorectal N28.89
- ureterosigmoido-abdominal N28.89
- ureterovaginal N82.1
- ureterovesical N32.2
- urethra N36.0
  - congenital Q64.79
  - tuberculous A18.13
- urethroperineal N36.0
- urethroperineovesical N32.2
- urethrorectal N36.0
  - congenital Q64.73
- urethroscrotal N50.89
- urethrovaginal N82.1
- urethrovesical N32.2
- urinary (tract) (persistent) (recurrent) N36.0
- uteroabdominal N82.5
  - congenital Q51.7
- uteroenteric, uterointestinal N82.4
  - congenital Q51.7
- uterorectal N82.4
  - congenital Q51.7
- uteroureteric N82.1
- uterourethral Q51.7
- uterovaginal N82.8
- uterovesical N82.1
  - congenital Q51.7
- uterus N82.8
- vagina (postpartal) (wall) N82.8
- vaginocutaneous (postpartal) N82.5
- vaginointestinal NEC N82.4
  - large intestine N82.3
  - small intestine N82.2
- vaginoperineal N82.5
- vasocutaneous, congenital Q55.7
- vesical NEC N32.2
- vesicoabdominal N32.2
- vesicocervicovaginal N82.1
- vesicocolic N32.1
- vesicocutaneous N32.2
- vesicoenteric N32.1
- vesicointestinal N32.1
- vesicometrorectal N82.4
- vesicoperineal N32.2
- vesicorectal N32.1
  - congenital Q64.79
- vesicosigmoidal N32.1
- vesicosigmoidovaginal N82.3
- vesicoureteral N32.2
- vesicoureterovaginal N82.1
- vesicourethral N32.2
- vesicourethrorectal N32.1
- vesicouterine N82.1
  - congenital Q51.7
- vesicovaginal N82.0
- vulvorectal N82.4
  - congenital Q52.79

Fit R56.9
- epileptic *—see* Epilepsy
- fainting R55
- hysterical F44.5
- newborn P90

Fitting (and adjustment) (of)
- artificial
  - arm *—see* Admission, adjustment, artificial, arm
  - breast Z44.3
  - eye Z44.2
  - leg *—see* Admission, adjustment, artificial, leg

Fitting *(continued)*
- automatic implantable cardiac defibrillator (with synchronous cardiac pacemaker) Z45.02
- brain neuropacemaker Z46.2
  - implanted Z45.42
- cardiac defibrillator *—see* Fitting (and adjustment) (of), automatic implantable cardiac defibrillator
- catheter, non-vascular Z46.82
- colostomy belt Z46.89
- contact lenses Z46.0
- CRT-D (resynchronization therapy defibrillator) Z45.02
- CRT-P (cardiac resynchronization therapy pacemaker) Z45.018
  - pulse generator Z45.010
- cystostomy device Z46.6
- defibrillator, cardiac *—see* Fitting (and adjustment) (of), automatic implantable cardiac defibrillator
- dentures Z46.3
- device NOS Z46.9
  - abdominal Z46.89
  - gastrointestinal NEC Z46.59
  - implanted NEC Z45.89
  - nervous system Z46.2
    - implanted *—see* Admission, adjustment, device, implanted, nervous system
  - orthodontic Z46.4
  - orthoptic Z46.0
  - orthotic Z46.89
  - prosthetic (external) Z44.9
    - breast Z44.3
    - dental Z46.3
    - eye Z44.2
    - specified NEC Z44.8
  - specified NEC Z46.89
  - substitution
    - auditory Z46.2
      - implanted *—see* Admission, adjustment, device, implanted, hearing device
    - nervous system Z46.2
      - implanted *—see* Admission, adjustment, device, implanted, nervous system
    - visual Z46.2
      - implanted Z45.31
  - urinary Z46.6
- gastric lap band Z46.51
- gastrointestinal appliance NEC Z46.59
- glasses (reading) Z46.0
- hearing aid Z46.1
- ileostomy device Z46.89
- insulin pump Z46.81
- intestinal appliance NEC Z46.89
- myringotomy device (stent) (tube) Z45.82
- neuropacemaker Z46.2
  - implanted Z45.42
- non-vascular catheter Z46.82
- orthodontic device Z46.4
- orthopedic device (brace) (cast) (corset) (shoes) Z46.89
- pacemaker (cardiac) (cardiac resynchronization therapy (CRT-P)) Z45.018
  - nervous system (brain) (peripheral nerve) (spinal cord) Z46.2
    - implanted Z45.42
  - pulse generator Z45.010
- portacath (port-a-cath) Z45.2
- prosthesis (external) Z44.9
  - arm *—see* Admission, adjustment, artificial, arm
  - breast Z44.3
  - dental Z46.3
  - eye Z44.2

Fitting *(continued)*
prosthesis *(continued)*
leg *—see* Admission, adjustment, artificial, leg
specified NEC Z44.8
spectacles Z46.0
wheelchair Z46.89
Fitzhugh-Curtis syndrome
due to
Chlamydia trachomatis A74.81
Neisseria gonorrhorea (gonococcal peritonitis) A54.85
Fitz's syndrome (acute hemorrhagic pancreatitis) (*see also* Pancreatitis, acute) K85.80
Fixation
joint *—see* Ankylosis
larynx J38.7
stapes *—see* Ankylosis, ear ossicles
deafness *—see* Deafness, conductive
uterus (acquired) *—see* Malposition, uterus
vocal cord J38.3
Flabby ridge K06.8
Flaccid *—see also* condition
palate, congenital Q38.5
Flail
chest S22.5
newborn (birth injury) P13.8
joint (paralytic) M25.20
ankle M25.27-
elbow M25.22-
foot joint M25.27-
hand joint M25.24-
hip M25.25-
knee M25.26-
shoulder M25.21-
specified joint NEC M25.28
wrist M25.23-
Flajani's disease *—see* Hyperthyroidism, with, goiter (diffuse)
Flap, liver K71.3
Flashbacks (residual to hallucinogen use) F16.283
Flat
chamber (eye) *—see* Disorder, globe, hypotony, flat anterior chamber
chest, congenital Q67.8
foot (acquired) (fixed type) (painful) (postural) *—see also* Deformity, limb, flat foot
congenital (rigid) (spastic (everted)) Q66.5-
rachitic sequelae (late effect) E64.3
organ or site, congenital NEC *—see* Anomaly, by site
pelvis M95.5
with disproportion (fetopelvic) O33.0
causing obstructed labor O65.0
congenital Q74.2
Flatau-Schilder disease G37.0
Flatback syndrome M40.30
lumbar region M40.36
lumbosacral region M40.37
thoracolumbar region M40.35
Flattening
head, femur M89.8X5
hip *—see* Coxa, plana
lip (congenital) Q18.8
nose (congenital) Q67.4
acquired M95.0
Flatulence R14.3
psychogenic F45.8
Flatus R14.3
vaginalis N89.8
Flax-dresser's disease J66.1
Flea bite *—see* Injury, bite, by site, superficial, insect
Flecks, glaucomatous (subcapsular) *—see* Cataract, complicated
Fleischer (-Kayser) **ring** (cornea) H18.04-
Fleshy mole O02.0
Flexibilitas cerea *—see* Catalepsy
Flexion
amputation stump (surgical) T87.89
cervix *—see* Malposition, uterus
contracture, joint *—see* Contraction, joint
deformity, joint (*see also* Deformity, limb, flexion) M21.20
hip, congenital Q65.89
uterus *—see also* Malposition, uterus
lateral *—see* Lateroversion, uterus
Flexner-Boyd dysentery A03.2
Flexner's dysentery A03.1
Flexure *—see* Flexion
Flint murmur (aortic insufficiency) I35.1
Floater, vitreous *—see* Opacity, vitreous
Floating
cartilage (joint) *—see also* Loose, body, joint
knee *—see* Derangement, knee, loose body
gallbladder, congenital Q44.1
kidney N28.89
congenital Q63.8
spleen D73.89
Flooding N92.0
Floor *—see* condition
Floppy
baby syndrome (nonspecific) P94.2
iris syndrome (intraoperative) (IFIS) H21.81
nonrheumatic mitral valve syndrome I34.1
Flu *—see also* Influenza
avian (*see also* Influenza, due to, identified novel influenza A virus) J09.X2
bird (*see also* Influenza, due to, identified novel influenza A virus) J09.X2
intestinal NEC A08.4
swine (viruses that normally cause infections in pigs) (*see also* Influenza, due to, identified novel influenza A virus) J09.X2
Fluctuating blood pressure I99.8
Fluid
abdomen R18.8
chest J94.8
heart *—see* Failure, heart, congestive
joint *—see* Effusion, joint
loss (acute) E86.9
lung *—see* Edema, lung
overload E87.70
specified NEC E87.79
peritoneal cavity R18.8
pleural cavity J94.8
retention R60.9
Flukes NEC *—see also* Infestation, fluke
blood NEC *—see* Schistosomiasis
liver B66.3
Fluor (vaginalis) N89.8
trichomonal or due to Trichomonas (vaginalis) A59.00
Fluorosis
dental K00.3
skeletal M85.10
ankle M85.17-
foot M85.17-
forearm M85.13-
hand M85.14-
lower leg M85.16-
multiple site M85.19
neck M85.18
rib M85.18
shoulder M85.11-
skull M85.18
specified site NEC M85.18
thigh M85.15-
toe M85.17-
upper arm M85.12-
vertebra M85.18
Flush syndrome E34.0
Flushing R23.2
menopausal N95.1
Flutter
atrial or auricular I48.92
atypical I48.4
type I I48.3
type II I48.4
typical I48.3
heart I49.8
atrial or auricular I48.92
atypical I48.4
type I I48.3
type II I48.4
typical I48.3
ventricular I49.02
ventricular I49.02
FNHTR (febrile nonhemolytic transfusion reaction) R50.84
Fochier's abscess - code by site under Abscess
Focus, Assmann's *—see* Tuberculosis, pulmonary
Fogo selvagem L10.3
Foix-Alajouanine syndrome G95.19
Fold, folds (anomalous) *—see also* Anomaly, by site
Descemet's membrane *—see* Change, corneal membrane, Descemet's, fold
epicanthic Q10.3
heart Q24.8
Folie à deux F24
Follicle
cervix (nabothian) (ruptured) N88.8
graafian, ruptured, with hemorrhage N83.0-
nabothian N88.8
Follicular *—see* condition
Folliculitis (superficial) L73.9
abscedens et suffodiens L66.3
cyst N83.0-
decalvans L66.2
deep *—see* Furuncle, by site
gonococcal (acute) (chronic) A54.01
keloid, keloidalis L73.0
pustular L01.02
ulerythematosa reticulata L66.4
Folliculome lipidique
specified site *—see* Neoplasm, benign, by site
unspecified site
female D27.9
male D29.20
Følling's disease E70.0
Follow-up *—see* Examination, follow-up
Fong's syndrome (hereditary osteo-onychodysplasia) Q87.2
Food
allergy L27.2
asphyxia (from aspiration or inhalation) *—see* Foreign body, by site
choked on *—see* Foreign body, by site
deprivation T73.0
specified kind of food NEC E63.8
intoxication *—see* Poisoning, food
lack of T73.0
poisoning *—see* Poisoning, food
rejection NEC *—see* Disorder, eating
strangulation or suffocation *—see* Foreign body, by site
toxemia *—see* Poisoning, food
Foot *—see* condition
Foramen ovale (nonclosure) (patent) (persistent) Q21.1
Forbes' glycogen storage disease E74.03
Fordyce-Fox disease L75.2
Fordyce's disease (mouth) Q38.6
Forearm *—see* condition
Foreign body
with
laceration *—see* Laceration, by site, with foreign body
puncture wound *—see* Puncture, by site, with foreign body
accidentally left following a procedure T81.509
aspiration T81.506
resulting in
adhesions T81.516
obstruction T81.526
perforation T81.536
specified complication NEC T81.596
cardiac catheterization T81.505
resulting in
acute reaction T81.60
aseptic peritonitis T81.61
specified NEC T81.69
accidentally left following a
adhesions T81.515
obstruction T81.525
perforation T81.535
specified complication NEC T81.595
causing
acute reaction T81.60
aseptic peritonitis T81.61
specified complication NEC T81.69
adhesions T81.519
aseptic peritonitis T81.61
obstruction T81.529
perforation T81.539
specified complication NEC T81.599

Foreign body *(continued)*
accidentally left following a *(continued)*
endoscopy T81.504
resulting in
adhesions T81.514
obstruction T81.524
perforation T81.534
specified complication NEC T81.594
immunization T81.503
resulting in
adhesions T81.513
obstruction T81.523
perforation T81.533
specified complication NEC T81.593
infusion T81.501
resulting in
adhesions T81.511
obstruction T81.521
perforation T81.531
specified complication NEC T81.591
injection T81.503
resulting in
adhesions T81.513
obstruction T81.523
perforation T81.533
specified complication NEC T81.593
kidney dialysis T81.502
resulting in
adhesions T81.512
obstruction T81.522
perforation T81.532
specified complication NEC T81.592
packing removal T81.507
resulting in
acute reaction T81.60
aseptic peritonitis T81.61
specified NEC T81.69
adhesions T81.517
obstruction T81.527
perforation T81.537
specified complication NEC T81.597
puncture T81.506
resulting in
adhesions T81.516
obstruction T81.526
perforation T81.536
specified complication NEC T81.596
specified procedure NEC T81.508
resulting in
acute reaction T81.60
aseptic peritonitis T81.61
specified NEC T81.69
adhesions T81.518
obstruction T81.528
perforation T81.538
specified complication NEC T81.598
surgical operation T81.500
resulting in
acute reaction T81.60
aseptic peritonitis T81.61
specified NEC T81.69
adhesions T81.510
obstruction T81.520
perforation T81.530
specified complication NEC T81.590
transfusion T81.501
resulting in
adhesions T81.511
obstruction T81.521
perforation T81.531

Foreign body *(continued)*
accidentally left following a *(continued)*
transfusion *(continued)*
resulting in *(continued)*
specified complication NEC T81.591
alimentary tract T18.9
anus T18.5
colon T18.4
esophagus *—see* Foreign body, esophagus
mouth T18.0
multiple sites T18.8
rectosigmoid (junction) T18.5
rectum T18.5
small intestine T18.3
specified site NEC T18.8
stomach T18.2
anterior chamber (eye) S05.5-
auditory canal *—see* Foreign body, entering through orifice, ear
bronchus T17.508
causing
asphyxiation T17.500
food (bone) (seed) T17.520
gastric contents (vomitus) T17.510
specified type NEC T17.590
injury NEC T17.508
food (bone) (seed) T17.528
gastric contents (vomitus) T17.518
specified type NEC T17.598
canthus *—see* Foreign body, conjunctival sac
ciliary body (eye) S05.5-
conjunctival sac T15.1-
cornea T15.0-
entering through orifice
accessory sinus T17.0
alimentary canal T18.9
multiple parts T18.8
specified part NEC T18.8
alveolar process T18.0
antrum (Highmore's) T17.0
anus T18.5
appendix T18.4
auditory canal *—see* Foreign body, entering through orifice, ear
auricle *—see* Foreign body, entering through orifice, ear
bladder T19.1
bronchioles *—see* Foreign body, respiratory tract, specified site NEC
bronchus (main) *—see* Foreign body, bronchus
buccal cavity T18.0
canthus (inner) *—see* Foreign body, conjunctival sac
cecum T18.4
cervix (canal) (uteri) T19.3
colon T18.4
conjunctival sac *—see* Foreign body, conjunctival sac
cornea *—see* Foreign body, cornea
digestive organ or tract NOS T18.9
multiple parts T18.8
specified part NEC T18.8
duodenum T18.3
ear (external) T16.-
esophagus *—see* Foreign body, esophagus
eye (external) NOS T15.9-
conjunctival sac *—see* Foreign body, conjunctival sac
cornea *—see* Foreign body, cornea
specified part NEC T15.8-

Foreign body *(continued)*
entering through orifice *(continued)*
eyeball *—see also* Foreign body, entering through orifice, eye, specified part NEC
with penetrating wound *—see* Puncture, eyeball
eyelid *—see also* Foreign body, conjunctival sac
with
laceration *—see* Laceration, eyelid, with foreign body
puncture *—see* Puncture, eyelid, with foreign body
superficial injury *—see* Foreign body, superficial, eyelid
gastrointestinal tract T18.9
multiple parts T18.8
specified part NEC T18.8
genitourinary tract T19.9
multiple parts T19.8
specified part NEC T19.8
globe *—see* Foreign body, entering through orifice, eyeball
gum T18.0
Highmore's antrum T17.0
hypopharynx *—see* Foreign body, pharynx
ileum T18.3
intestine (small) T18.3
large T18.4
lacrimal apparatus (punctum) *—see* Foreign body, entering through orifice, eye, specified part NEC
large intestine T18.4
larynx *—see* Foreign body, larynx
lung *—see* Foreign body, respiratory tract, specified site NEC
maxillary sinus T17.0
mouth T18.0
nasal sinus T17.0
nasopharynx *—see* Foreign body, pharynx
nose (passage) T17.1
nostril T17.1
oral cavity T18.0
palate T18.0
penis T19.4
pharynx *—see* Foreign body, pharynx
piriform sinus *—see* Foreign body, pharynx
rectosigmoid (junction) T18.5
rectum T18.5
respiratory tract *—see* Foreign body, respiratory tract
sinus (accessory) (frontal) (maxillary) (nasal) T17.0
piriform *—see* Foreign body, pharynx
small intestine T18.3
stomach T18.2
suffocation by *—see* Foreign body, by site
tear ducts or glands *—see* Foreign body, entering through orifice, eye, specified part NEC
throat *—see* Foreign body, pharynx
tongue T18.0
tonsil, tonsillar (fossa) *—see* Foreign body, pharynx
trachea *—see* Foreign body, trachea
ureter T19.8
urethra T19.0
uterus (any part) T19.3
vagina T19.2
vulva T19.2

Foreign body *(continued)*
esophagus T18.108
causing
injury NEC T18.108
food (bone) (seed) T18.128
gastric contents (vomitus) T18.118
specified type NEC T18.198
tracheal compression T18.100
food (bone) (seed) T18.120
gastric contents (vomitus) T18.110
specified type NEC T18.190
feeling of, in throat R09.89
fragment *—see* Retained, foreign body fragments (type of)
genitourinary tract T19.9
bladder T19.1
multiple parts T19.8
penis T19.4
specified site NEC T19.8
urethra T19.0
uterus T19.3
IUD Z97.5
vagina T19.2
contraceptive device Z97.5
vulva T19.2
granuloma (old) (soft tissue) *—see also* Granuloma, foreign body
skin L92.3
in
laceration *—see* Laceration, by site, with foreign body
puncture wound *—see* Puncture, by site, with foreign body
soft tissue (residual) M79.5
inadvertently left in operation wound *—see* Foreign body, accidentally left during a procedure
ingestion, ingested NOS T18.9
inhalation or inspiration *—see* Foreign body, by site
internal organ, not entering through a natural orifice - code as specific injury with foreign body
intraocular S05.5-
old, retained (nonmagnetic) H44.70-
anterior chamber H44.71-
ciliary body H44.72-
iris H44.72-
lens H44.73-
magnetic H44.60-
anterior chamber H44.61-
ciliary body H44.62-
iris H44.62-
lens H44.63-
posterior wall H44.64-
specified site NEC H44.69-
vitreous body H44.65-
posterior wall H44.74-
specified site NEC H44.79-
vitreous body H44.75-
iris *—see* Foreign body, intraocular
lacrimal punctum *—see* Foreign body, entering through orifice, eye, specified part NEC
larynx T17.308
causing
asphyxiation T17.300
food (bone) (seed) T17.320
gastric contents (vomitus) T17.310
specified type NEC T17.390
injury NEC T17.308
food (bone) (seed) T17.328
gastric contents (vomitus) T17.318
specified type NEC T17.398
lens *—see* Foreign body, intraocular

Foreign body *(continued)*
  ocular muscle S05.4-
    old, retained —*see* Foreign body, orbit, old
  old or residual
    soft tissue (residual) M79.5
  operation wound, left accidentally —*see* Foreign body, accidentally left during a procedure
  orbit S05.4-
    old, retained H05.5-
  pharynx T17.208
    causing
      asphyxiation T17.200
        food (bone) (seed) T17.220
        gastric contents (vomitus) T17.210
        specified type NEC T17.290
      injury NEC T17.208
        food (bone) (seed) T17.228
        gastric contents (vomitus) T17.218
        specified type NEC T17.298
  respiratory tract T17.908
    bronchioles —*see* Foreign body, respiratory tract, specified site NEC
    bronchus —*see* Foreign body, bronchus
    causing
      asphyxiation T17.900
        food (bone) (seed) T17.920
        gastric contents (vomitus) T17.910
        specified type NEC T17.990
      injury NEC T17.908
        food (bone) (seed) T17.928
        gastric contents (vomitus) T17.918
        specified type NEC T17.998
    larynx —*see* Foreign body, larynx
    lung —*see* Foreign body, respiratory tract, specified site NEC
    multiple parts —*see* Foreign body, respiratory tract, specified site NEC
    nasal sinus T17.0
    nasopharynx —*see* Foreign body, pharynx
    nose T17.1
    nostril T17.1
    pharynx —*see* Foreign body, pharynx
    specified site NEC T17.808
      causing
        asphyxiation T17.800
          food (bone) (seed) T17.820
          gastric contents (vomitus) T17.810
          specified type NEC T17.890
        injury NEC T17.808
          food (bone) (seed) T17.828
          gastric contents (vomitus) T17.818
          specified type NEC T17.898
    throat —*see* Foreign body, pharynx
    trachea —*see* Foreign body, trachea
  retained (old) (nonmagnetic) (in)
    anterior chamber (eye) —*see* Foreign body, intraocular, old, retained, anterior chamber
      magnetic —*see* Foreign body, intraocular, old, retained, magnetic, anterior chamber

Foreign body *(continued)*
  retained *(continued)*
    ciliary body —*see* Foreign body, intraocular, old, retained, ciliary body
      magnetic —*see* Foreign body, intraocular, old, retained, magnetic, ciliary body
    eyelid H02.819
      left H02.816
        lower H02.815
        upper H02.814
      right H02.813
        lower H02.812
        upper H02.811
    fragments —*see* Retained, foreign body fragments (type of)
    globe —*see* Foreign body, intraocular, old, retained
      magnetic —*see* Foreign body, intraocular, old, retained, magnetic
    intraocular —*see* Foreign body, intraocular, old, retained
      magnetic —*see* Foreign body, intraocular, old, retained, magnetic
    iris —*see* Foreign body, intraocular, old, retained, iris
      magnetic —*see* Foreign body, intraocular, old, retained, magnetic, iris
    lens —*see* Foreign body, intraocular, old, retained, lens
      magnetic —*see* Foreign body, intraocular, old, retained, magnetic, lens
    muscle —*see* Foreign body, retained, soft tissue
    orbit —*see* Foreign body, orbit, old
    posterior wall of globe —*see* Foreign body, intraocular, old, retained, posterior wall
      magnetic —*see* Foreign body, intraocular, old, retained, magnetic, posterior wall
    retrobulbar —*see* Foreign body, orbit, old, retrobulbar
    soft tissue M79.5
    vitreous —*see* Foreign body, intraocular, old, retained, vitreous body
      magnetic —*see* Foreign body, intraocular, old, retained, magnetic, vitreous body
  retina S05.5-
  superficial, without open wound
    abdomen, abdominal (wall) S30.851
    alveolar process S00.552
    ankle S90.55-
    antecubital space —*see* Foreign body, superficial, forearm
    anus S30.857
    arm (upper) S40.85-
    auditory canal —*see* Foreign body, superficial, ear
    auricle —*see* Foreign body, superficial, ear
    axilla —*see* Foreign body, superficial, arm
    back, lower S30.850
    breast S20.15-
    brow S00.85
    buttock S30.850
    calf —*see* Foreign body, superficial, leg
    canthus —*see* Foreign body, superficial, eyelid

Foreign body *(continued)*
  superficial, without open wound *(continued)*
    cheek S00.85
      internal S00.552
    chest wall —*see* Foreign body, superficial, thorax
    chin S00.85
    clitoris S30.854
    costal region —*see* Foreign body, superficial, thorax
    digit(s)
      hand —*see* Foreign body, superficial, finger
      foot —*see* Foreign body, superficial, toe
    ear S00.45-
    elbow S50.35-
    epididymis S30.853
    epigastric region S30.851
    epiglottis S10.15
    esophagus, cervical S10.15
    eyebrow —*see* Foreign body, superficial, eyelid
    eyelid S00.25-
    face S00.85
    finger(s) S60.459
      index S60.45-
      little S60.45-
      middle S60.45-
      ring S60.45-
    flank S30.851
    foot (except toe(s) alone) S90.85-
      toe —*see* Foreign body, superficial, toe
    forearm S50.85-
      elbow only —*see* Foreign body, superficial, elbow
    forehead S00.85
    genital organs, external
      female S30.856
      male S30.855
    groin S30.851
    gum S00.552
    hand S60.55-
    head S00.95
      ear —*see* Foreign body, superficial, ear
      eyelid —*see* Foreign body, superficial, eyelid
      lip S00.551
      nose S00.35
      oral cavity S00.552
      scalp S00.05
      specified site NEC S00.85
    heel —*see* Foreign body, superficial, foot
    hip S70.25-
    inguinal region S30.851
    interscapular region S20.459
    jaw S00.85
    knee S80.25-
    labium (majus) (minus) S30.854
    larynx S10.15
    leg (lower) S80.85-
      knee —*see* Foreign body, superficial, knee
      upper —*see* Foreign body, superficial, thigh
    lip S00.551
    lower back S30.850
    lumbar region S30.850
    malar region S00.85
    mammary —*see* Foreign body, superficial, breast
    mastoid region S00.85
    mouth S00.552
    nail
      finger —*see* Foreign body, superficial, finger

Foreign body *(continued)*
  superficial, without open wound *(continued)*
    nail *(continued)*
      toe —*see* Foreign body, superficial, toe
    nape S10.85
    nasal S00.35
    neck S10.95
      specified site NEC S10.85
      throat S10.15
    nose S00.35
    occipital region S00.05
    oral cavity S00.552
    orbital region —*see* Foreign body, superficial, eyelid
    palate S00.552
    palm —*see* Foreign body, superficial, hand
    parietal region S00.05
    pelvis S30.850
    penis S30.852
    perineum
      female S30.854
      male S30.850
    periocular area —*see* Foreign body, superficial, eyelid
    phalanges
      finger —*see* Foreign body, superficial, finger
      toe —*see* Foreign body, superficial, toe
    pharynx S10.15
    pinna —*see* Foreign body, superficial, ear
    popliteal space —*see* Foreign body, superficial, knee
    prepuce S30.852
    pubic region S30.850
    pudendum
      female S30.856
      male S30.855
    sacral region S30.850
    scalp S00.05
    scapular region —*see* Foreign body, superficial, shoulder
    scrotum S30.853
    shin —*see* Foreign body, superficial, leg
    shoulder S40.25-
    sternal region S20.359
    submaxillary region S00.85
    submental region S00.85
    subungual
      finger(s) —*see* Foreign body, superficial, finger
      toe(s) —*see* Foreign body, superficial, toe
    supraclavicular fossa S10.85
    supraorbital S00.85
    temple S00.85
    temporal region S00.85
    testis S30.853
    thigh S70.35-
    thorax, thoracic (wall) S20.95
      back S20.45-
      front S20.35-
    throat S10.15
    thumb S60.35-
    toe(s) (lesser) S90.456
      great S90.45-
    tongue S00.552
    trachea S10.15
    tunica vaginalis S30.853
    tympanum, tympanic membrane —*see* Foreign body, superficial, ear
    uvula S00.552
    vagina S30.854
    vocal cords S10.15

Foreign body *(continued)*
- superficial, without open wound *(continued)*
  - vulva S30.854
  - wrist S60.85-
- swallowed T18.9
- trachea T17.408
  - causing
    - asphyxiation T17.400
      - food (bone) (seed) T17.420
      - gastric contents (vomitus) T17.410
      - specified type NEC T17.490
    - injury NEC T17.408
      - food (bone) (seed) T17.428
      - gastric contents (vomitus) T17.418
      - specified type NEC T17.498
- type of fragment *—see* Retained, foreign body fragments (type of)
- vitreous (humor) S05.5-

Forestier's disease (rhizomelic pseudopolyarthritis) M35.3
- meaning ankylosing hyperostosis *—see* Hyperostosis, ankylosing

Formation
- hyalin in cornea *—see* Degeneration, cornea
- sequestrum in bone (due to infection) *—see* Osteomyelitis, chronic
- valve
  - colon, congenital Q43.8
  - ureter (congenital) Q62.39

Formication R20.2

Fort Bragg fever A27.89

Fossa *—see also* condition
- pyriform *—see* condition

Foster-Kennedy syndrome H47.14-

Fothergill's
- disease (trigeminal neuralgia) *—see also* Neuralgia, trigeminal
  - scarlatina anginosa A38.9

Foul breath R19.6

Foundling Z76.1

Fournier disease or gangrene N49.3
- female N76.89

Fourth
- cranial nerve *—see* condition
- molar K00.1

Foville's (peduncular) **disease or syndrome** G46.3

Fox (-Fordyce) disease (apocrine miliaria) L75.2

Fracture, burst *—see* Fracture, traumatic, by site

Fracture, chronic *—see* Fracture, pathological, by site

Fracture, insufficiency *—see* Fracture, pathologic, by site

Fracture, nontraumatic, NEC
- atypical
  - femur M84.750-
    - complete
      - oblique M84.759
        - left side M84.758
        - right side M84.757
      - transverse M84.756
        - left side M84.755
        - right side M84.754
    - incomplete M84.753
      - left side M84.752
      - right side M84.751

Fracture, pathological (pathologic) *—see also* Fracture, traumatic M84.40
- ankle M84.47-
- carpus M84.44-
- clavicle M84.41-
- compression (not due to trauma) (*see also* Collapse, vertebra) M48.50-
- dental implant M27.63
- dental restorative material K08.539
  - with loss of material K08.531
  - without loss of material K08.530
- due to
  - neoplastic disease NEC (*see also* Neoplasm) M84.50
    - ankle M84.57-
    - carpus M84.54-
    - clavicle M84.51-
    - femur M84.55-
    - fibula M84.56-
    - finger M84.54-
    - hip M84.559
    - humerus M84.52-
    - ilium M84.550
    - ischium M84.550
    - metacarpus M84.54-
    - metatarsus M84.57-
    - neck M84.58
    - pelvis M84.550
    - radius M84.53-
    - rib M84.58
    - scapula M84.51-
    - skull M84.58
    - specified site NEC M84.58
    - tarsus M84.57-
    - tibia M84.56-
    - toe M84.57-
    - ulna M84.53-
    - vertebra M84.58
  - osteoporosis M80.00
    - disuse *—see* Osteoporosis, specified type NEC, with pathological fracture
    - drug-induced *—see* Osteoporosis, drug induced, with pathological fracture
    - idiopathic *—see* Osteoporosis, specified type NEC, with pathological fracture
    - postmenopausal *—see* Osteoporosis, postmenopausal, with pathological fracture
    - postoophorectomy *—see* Osteoporosis, postoophorectomy, with pathological fracture
    - postsurgical malabsorption *—see* Osteoporosis, specified type NEC, with pathological fracture
    - specified cause NEC *—see* Osteoporosis, specified type NEC, with pathological fracture
  - specified disease NEC M84.60
    - ankle M84.67-
    - carpus M84.64-
    - clavicle M84.61-
    - femur M84.65-
    - fibula M84.66-
    - finger M84.64-
    - hip M84.65-
    - humerus M84.62-
    - ilium M84.650
    - ischium M84.650
    - metacarpus M84.64-
    - metatarsus M84.67-
    - neck M84.68
    - radius M84.63-
    - rib M84.68

Fracture, pathological *(continued)*
- due to *(continued)*
  - specified disease NEC *(continued)*
    - scapula M84.61-
    - skull M84.68
    - tarsus M84.67-
    - tibia M84.66-
    - toe M84.67-
    - ulna M84.63-
    - vertebra M84.68
- femur M84.45-
- fibula M84.46-
- finger M84.44-
- hip M84.459
- humerus M84.42-
- ilium M84.454
- ischium M84.454
- joint prosthesis *—see* Complications, joint prosthesis, mechanical, breakdown, by site
  - periprosthetic *—see* Fracture, pathological, periprosthetic
- metacarpus M84.44-
- metatarsus M84.47-
- neck M84.48
- pelvis M84.454
- periprosthetic M97.9
  - ankle M97.2-
  - elbow M97.4-
  - finger M97.8
  - hip M97.0-
  - knee M97.1-
  - other specified joint M97.8
  - shoulder M97.3-
  - spinal joint M97.8
  - toe joint M97.8
  - wrist joint M97.8
- radius M84.43-
- restorative material (dental) K08.539
  - with loss of material K08.531
  - without loss of material K08.530
- rib M84.48
- scapula M84.41-
- skull M84.48
- tarsus M84.47-
- tibia M84.46-
- toe M84.47-
- ulna M84.43-
- vertebra M84.48

Fracture, traumatic (abduction) (adduction) (separation) (*see also* Fracture, pathological) T14.8
- acetabulum S32.40-
  - column
    - anterior (displaced) (iliopubic) S32.43-
      - nondisplaced S32.436
    - posterior (displaced) (ilioischial) S32.443
      - nondisplaced S32.44-
  - dome (displaced) S32.48-
    - nondisplaced S32.48
  - specified NEC S32.49-
  - transverse (displaced) S32.45-
    - with associated posterior wall fracture (displaced) S32.46-
      - nondisplaced S32.46-
    - nondisplaced S32.45-
  - wall
    - anterior (displaced) S32.41-
      - nondisplaced S32.41-
    - medial (displaced) S32.47-
      - nondisplaced S32.47-
    - posterior (displaced) S32.42-
      - with associated transverse fracture (displaced) S32.46-
        - nondisplaced S32.46-
      - nondisplaced S32.42-
- acromion *—see* Fracture, scapula, acromial process

Fracture, traumatic *(continued)*
- ankle S82.899
  - bimalleolar (displaced) S82.84-
    - nondisplaced S82.84-
  - lateral malleolus only (displaced) S82.6-
    - nondisplaced S82.6-
  - medial malleolus (displaced) S82.5-
    - associated with Maisonneuve's fracture *—see* Fracture, Maisonneuve's
    - nondisplaced S82.5-
  - talus *—see* Fracture, tarsal, talus
  - trimalleolar (displaced) S82.85-
    - nondisplaced S82.85-
- arm (upper) *—see also* Fracture, humerus, shaft
  - humerus *—see* Fracture, humerus
  - radius *—see* Fracture, radius
  - ulna *—see* Fracture, ulna
- astragalus *—see* Fracture, tarsal, talus
- atlas *—see* Fracture, neck, cervical vertebra, first
- axis *—see* Fracture, neck, cervical vertebra, second
- back *—see* Fracture, vertebra
- Barton's *—see* Barton's fracture
- base of skull *—see* Fracture, skull, base
- basicervical (basal) (femoral) S72.0
- Bennett's *—see* Bennett's fracture
- bimalleolar *—see* Fracture, ankle, bimalleolar
- blow-out S02.3-
- bone NEC T14.8
  - birth injury P13.9
  - following insertion of orthopedic implant, joint prosthesis or bone plate *—see* Fracture, following insertion of orthopedic implant, joint prosthesis or bone plate
  - in (due to) neoplastic disease NEC *—see* Fracture, pathological, due to, neoplastic disease
  - pathological (cause unknown) *—see* Fracture, pathological
- breast bone *—see* Fracture, sternum
- bucket handle (semilunar cartilage) *—see* Tear, meniscus
- burst *—see* Fracture, traumatic, by site
- calcaneus *—see* Fracture, tarsal, calcaneus
- carpal bone(s) S62.10-
  - capitate (displaced) S62.13-
    - nondisplaced S62.13-
  - cuneiform *—see* Fracture, carpal bone, triquetrum
  - hamate (body) (displaced) S62.143
    - hook process (displaced) S62.15-
      - nondisplaced S62.15-
    - nondisplaced S62.14-
  - larger multangular *—see* Fracture, carpal bones, trapezium
  - lunate (displaced) S62.12-
    - nondisplaced S62.12-
  - navicular S62.00-
    - distal pole (displaced) S62.01-
      - nondisplaced S62.01-
    - middle third (displaced) S62.02-
      - nondisplaced S62.02-
    - proximal third (displaced) S62.03-
      - nondisplaced S62.03-

Fracture, traumatic *(continued)*
- carpal bone(s) *(continued)*
  - navicular *(continued)*
    - volar tuberosity —*see* Fracture, carpal bones, navicular, distal pole
  - os magnum —*see* Fracture, carpal bones, capitate
  - pisiform (displaced) S62.16-
    - nondisplaced S62.16-
  - semilunar —*see* Fracture, carpal bones, lunate
  - smaller multangular —*see* Fracture, carpal bones, trapezoid
  - trapezium (displaced) S62.17-
    - nondisplaced S62.17-
  - trapezoid (displaced) S62.18-
    - nondisplaced S62.18-
  - triquetrum (displaced) S62.11-
    - nondisplaced S62.11-
  - unciform —*see* Fracture, carpal bones, hamate
- cervical —*see* Fracture, vertebra, cervical
- clavicle S42.00-
  - acromial end (displaced) S42.03-
    - nondisplaced S42.03-
  - birth injury P13.4
  - lateral end —*see* Fracture, clavicle, acromial end
  - shaft (displaced) S42.02-
    - nondisplaced S42.02-
  - sternal end (anterior) (displaced) S42.01-
    - nondisplaced S42.01-
    - posterior S42.01-
- coccyx S32.2
- collapsed —*see* Collapse, vertebra
- collar bone —*see* Fracture, clavicle
- Colles' —*see* Colles' fracture
- coronoid process —*see* Fracture, ulna, upper end, coronoid process
- corpus cavernosum penis S39.840
- costochondral cartilage S23.41
- costochondral, costosternal junction —*see* Fracture, rib
- cranium —*see* Fracture, skull
- cricoid cartilage S12.8
- cuboid (ankle) —*see* Fracture, tarsal, cuboid
- cuneiform
  - foot —*see* Fracture, tarsal, cuneiform
  - wrist —*see* Fracture, carpal, triquetrum
- delayed union —*see* Delay, union, fracture
- dental restorative material K08.539
  - with loss of material K08.531
  - without loss of material K08.530
- due to
  - birth injury —*see* Birth, injury, fracture
  - osteoporosis —*see* Osteoporosis, with fracture
- Dupuytren's —*see* Fracture, ankle, lateral malleolus
- elbow S42.40-
- ethmoid (bone) (sinus) —*see* Fracture, skull, base
- face bone S02.92
- fatigue —*see also* Fracture, stress
  - vertebra M48.40
    - cervical region M48.42
    - cervicothoracic region M48.43
    - lumbar region M48.46
    - lumbosacral region M48.47

Fracture, traumatic *(continued)*
- fatigue *(continued)*
  - vertebra *(continued)*
    - occipito-atlanto-axial region M48.41
    - sacrococcygeal region M48.48
    - thoracic region M48.44
    - thoracolumbar region M48.45
- femur, femoral S72.9-
  - basicervical (basal) S72.0
  - birth injury P13.2
  - capital epiphyseal S79.01-
  - condyles, epicondyles —*see* Fracture, femur, lower end
  - distal end —*see* Fracture, femur, lower end
  - epiphysis
    - head —*see* Fracture, femur, upper end, epiphysis
    - lower —*see* Fracture, femur, lower end, epiphysis
    - upper —*see* Fracture, femur, upper end, epiphysis
  - following insertion of implant, prosthesis or plate M96.66-
  - head —*see* Fracture, femur, upper end, head
  - intertrochanteric —*see* Fracture, femur, trochanteric
  - intratrochanteric —*see* Fracture, femur, trochanteric
  - lower end S72.40-
    - condyle (displaced) S72.41-
      - lateral (displaced) S72.42-
        - nondisplaced S72.42-
      - medial (displaced) S72.43-
        - nondisplaced S72.43-
      - nondisplaced S72.41-
    - epiphysis (displaced) S72.44-
      - nondisplaced S72.44-
    - physeal S79.10-
      - Salter-Harris
        - Type I S79.11-
        - Type II S79.12-
        - Type III S79.13-
        - Type IV S79.14-
      - specified NEC S79.19-
    - specified NEC S72.49-
    - supracondylar (displaced) S72.45-
      - with intracondylar extension (displaced) S72.46-
        - nondisplaced S72.46-
      - nondisplaced S72.45-
    - torus S72.47-
  - neck —*see* Fracture, femur, upper end, neck
  - pertrochanteric —*see* Fracture, femur, trochanteric
  - shaft (lower third) (middle third) (upper third) S72.30-
    - comminuted (displaced) S72.35-
      - nondisplaced S72.35-
    - oblique (displaced) S72.33-
      - nondisplaced S72.33-
    - segmental (displaced) S72.36-
      - nondisplaced S72.36-
    - specified NEC S72.39-
    - spiral (displaced) S72.34-
      - nondisplaced S72.34-
    - transverse (displaced) S72.32-
      - nondisplaced S72.32-
  - specified site NEC S72.8
  - subcapital (displaced) S72.01-
  - subtrochanteric (region) (section) (displaced) S72.2-
    - nondisplaced S72.2-
  - transcervical —*see* Fracture, femur, upper end, neck

Fracture, traumatic *(continued)*
- femur, femoral *(continued)*
  - transtrochanteric —*see* Fracture, femur, trochanteric
  - trochanteric S72.10-
    - apophyseal (displaced) S72.13-
      - nondisplaced S72.13-
    - greater trochanter (displaced) S72.11-
      - nondisplaced S72.11-
    - intertrochanteric (displaced) S72.14-
      - nondisplaced S72.14-
    - lesser trochanter (displaced) S72.12-
      - nondisplaced S72.12-
  - upper end S72.00-
    - apophyseal (displaced) S72.13-
      - nondisplaced S72.13-
    - cervicotrochanteric —*see* Fracture, femur, upper end, neck, base
    - epiphysis (displaced) S72.02-
      - nondisplaced S72.02-
    - head S72.05-
      - articular (displaced) S72.06-
        - nondisplaced S72.06-
      - specified NEC S72.09-
    - intertrochanteric (displaced) S72.14-
      - nondisplaced S72.14-
    - intracapsular S72.01-
    - midcervical (displaced) S72.03-
      - nondisplaced S72.03-
    - neck S72.00-
      - base (displaced) S72.04-
        - nondisplaced S72.04-
      - specified NEC S72.09-
    - pertrochanteric —*see* Fracture, femur, upper end, trochanteric
    - physeal S79.00-
      - Salter-Harris type I S79.01-
      - specified NEC S79.09-
    - subcapital (displaced) S72.01-
    - subtrochanteric (displaced) S72.2-
      - nondisplaced S72.2-
    - transcervical —*see* Fracture, femur, upper end, midcervical
    - trochanteric S72.10-
      - greater (displaced) S72.11-
        - nondisplaced S72.11-
      - lesser (displaced) S72.12-
        - nondisplaced S72.12-
- fibula (shaft) (styloid) S82.40-
  - comminuted (displaced) S82.45-
    - nondisplaced S82.45-
  - following insertion of implant, prosthesis or plate M96.67-
  - involving ankle or malleolus —*see* Fracture, fibula, lateral malleolus
  - lateral malleolus (displaced) S82.6-
    - nondisplaced S82.6-
  - lower end
    - physeal S89.30-
      - Salter-Harris
        - Type I S89.31-
        - Type II S89.32-
      - specified NEC S89.39-
    - specified NEC S82.83-
    - torus S82.82-
  - oblique (displaced) S82.43-
    - nondisplaced S82.43-
  - segmental (displaced) S82.46-
    - nondisplaced S82.46-
  - specified NEC S82.49-

Fracture, traumatic *(continued)*
- fibula *(continued)*
  - spiral (displaced) S82.44-
    - nondisplaced S82.44-
  - transverse (displaced) S82.42-
    - nondisplaced S82.42-
  - upper end
    - physeal S89.20-
      - Salter-Harris
        - Type I S89.21-
        - Type II S89.22-
      - specified NEC S89.29-
    - specified NEC S82.83-
    - torus S82.81-
- finger (except thumb) S62.60-
  - distal phalanx (displaced) S62.63-
    - nondisplaced S62.66-
  - index S62.60-
    - distal phalanx (displaced) S62.63-
      - nondisplaced S62.66-
    - medial phalanx (displaced) S62.62-
      - nondisplaced S62.65-
    - proximal phalanx (displaced) S62.61-
      - nondisplaced S62.64-
  - little S62.60-
    - distal phalanx (displaced) S62.63-
      - nondisplaced S62.66-
    - medial phalanx (displaced) S62.62-
      - nondisplaced S62.65-
    - proximal phalanx (displaced) S62.61-
      - nondisplaced S62.64-
  - medial phalanx (displaced) S62.62-
    - nondisplaced S62.65-
  - middle S62.60-
    - distal phalanx (displaced) S62.63-
      - nondisplaced S62.66-
    - medial phalanx (displaced) S62.62-
      - nondisplaced S62.65-
    - proximal phalanx (displaced) S62.61-
      - nondisplaced S62.64-
  - proximal phalanx (displaced) S62.61-
    - nondisplaced S62.64-
  - ring S62.60-
    - distal phalanx (displaced) S62.63-
      - nondisplaced S62.66-
    - medial phalanx (displaced) S62.62-
      - nondisplaced S62.65-
    - proximal phalanx (displaced) S62.61-
      - nondisplaced S62.64-
  - thumb —*see* Fracture, thumb
- following insertion (intraoperative) (postoperative) of orthopedic implant, joint prosthesis or bone plate M96.69
  - femur M96.66-
  - fibula M96.67-
  - humerus M96.62-
  - pelvis M96.65
  - radius M96.63-
  - specified bone NEC M96.69
  - tibia M96.67-
  - ulna M96.63-
- foot S92.90-
  - astragalus —*see* Fracture, tarsal, talus

- foot *(continued)*
  - calcaneus *—see* Fracture, tarsal, calcaneus
  - cuboid *—see* Fracture, tarsal, cuboid
  - cuneiform *—see* Fracture, tarsal, cuneiform
  - metatarsal *—see* Fracture, metatarsal
  - navicular *—see* Fracture, tarsal, navicular
  - sesamoid S92.81-
  - specified NEC S92.81-
  - talus *—see* Fracture, tarsal, talus
  - tarsal *—see* Fracture, tarsal
  - toe *—see* Fracture, toe
- forearm S52.9-
  - radius *—see* Fracture, radius
  - ulna *—see* Fracture, ulna
- fossa (anterior) (middle) (posterior) S02.19
- frontal (bone) (skull) S02.0
  - sinus S02.19
- glenoid (cavity) (scapula) *—see* Fracture, scapula, glenoid cavity
- greenstick *—see* Fracture, by site
- hallux *—see* Fracture, toe, great
- hand S62.9-
  - carpal *—see* Fracture, carpal bone
  - finger (except thumb) *—see* Fracture, finger
  - metacarpal *—see* Fracture, metacarpal
  - navicular (scaphoid) (hand) *—see* Fracture, carpal bone, navicular
  - thumb *—see* Fracture, thumb
- healed or old
  - with complications - code by Nature of the complication
- heel bone *—see* Fracture, tarsal, calcaneus
- Hill-Sachs S42.29-
- hip *—see* Fracture, femur, neck
- humerus S42.30-
  - anatomical neck *—see* Fracture, humerus, upper end
  - articular process *—see* Fracture, humerus, lower end
  - capitellum *—see* Fracture, humerus, lower end, condyle, lateral
  - distal end *—see* Fracture, humerus, lower end
  - epiphysis
    - lower *—see* Fracture, humerus, lower end, physeal
    - upper *—see* Fracture, humerus, upper end, physeal
  - external condyle *—see* Fracture, humerus, lower end, condyle, lateral
  - following insertion of implant, prosthesis or plate M96.62-
  - great tuberosity *—see* Fracture, humerus, upper end, greater tuberosity
  - intercondylar *—see* Fracture, humerus, lower end
  - internal epicondyle *—see* Fracture, humerus, lower end, epicondyle, medial
  - lesser tuberosity *—see* Fracture, humerus, upper end, lesser tuberosity
  - lower end S42.40-
    - condyle
      - lateral (displaced) S42.45-
        - nondisplaced S42.45-
      - medial (displaced) S42.46-
        - nondisplaced S42.46-

- humerus *(continued)*
  - lower end *(continued)*
    - epicondyle
      - lateral (displaced) S42.43-
        - nondisplaced S42.43-
      - medial (displaced) S42.44-
        - incarcerated S42.44-
        - nondisplaced S42.44-
    - physeal S49.10-
      - Salter-Harris
        - Type I S49.11-
        - Type II S49.12-
        - Type III S49.13-
        - Type IV S49.14-
      - specified NEC S49.19-
    - specified NEC (displaced) S42.49-
      - nondisplaced S42.49-
    - supracondylar (simple) (displaced) S42.41-
      - with intercondylar fracture - *see* Fracture, humerus, lower end
      - comminuted (displaced) S42.42-
        - nondisplaced S42.42-
      - nondisplaced S42.41-
    - torus S42.48-
    - transcondylar (displaced) S42.47-
      - nondisplaced S42.47-
  - proximal end *—see* Fracture, humerus, upper end
  - shaft S42.30-
    - comminuted (displaced) S42.35-
      - nondisplaced S42.35-
    - greenstick S42.31-
    - oblique (displaced) S42.33-
      - nondisplaced S42.33-
    - segmental (displaced) S42.36-
      - nondisplaced S42.36-
    - specified NEC S42.39-
    - spiral (displaced) S42.34-
      - nondisplaced S42.34-
    - transverse (displaced) S42.32-
      - nondisplaced S42.32-
  - supracondylar *—see* Fracture, humerus, lower end
  - surgical neck *—see* Fracture, humerus, upper end, surgical neck
  - trochlea *—see* Fracture, humerus, lower end, condyle, medial
  - tuberosity *—see* Fracture, humerus, upper end
  - upper end S42.20-
    - anatomical neck *—see* Fracture, humerus, upper end, specified NEC
    - articular head *—see* Fracture, humerus, upper end, specified NEC
    - epiphysis *—see* Fracture, humerus, upper end, physeal
    - greater tuberosity (displaced) S42.25-
      - nondisplaced S42.25-
    - lesser tuberosity (displaced) S42.26-
      - nondisplaced S42.26-
    - physeal S49.00-
      - Salter-Harris
        - Type I S49.01-
        - Type II S49.02-
        - Type III S49.03-
        - Type IV S49.04-
      - specified NEC S49.09-
    - specified NEC (displaced) S42.29-
      - nondisplaced S42.29-

- humerus *(continued)*
  - upper end *(continued)*
    - surgical neck (displaced) S42.21-
      - four-part S42.24-
      - nondisplaced S42.21-
      - three-part S42.23-
      - two-part (displaced) S42.22-
        - nondisplaced S42.22-
    - torus S42.27-
    - transepiphyseal *—see* Fracture, humerus, upper end, physeal
- hyoid bone S12.8
- ilium S32.30-
  - with disruption of pelvic ring *— see* Disruption, pelvic ring
  - avulsion (displaced) S32.31-
    - nondisplaced S32.31-
  - specified NEC S32.39-
- impaction, impacted - code as Fracture, by site
- innominate bone *—see* Fracture, ilium
- instep *—see* Fracture, foot
- ischium S32.60-
  - with disruption of pelvic ring *— see* Disruption, pelvic ring
  - avulsion (displaced) S32.61-
    - nondisplaced S32.61-
  - specified NEC S32.69-
- jaw (bone) (lower) *—see* Fracture, mandible
  - upper *—see* Fracture, maxilla
- joint prosthesis *—see* Complications, joint prosthesis, mechanical, breakdown, by site
  - periprosthetic *—see* Fracture, traumatic, periprosthetic
- knee cap *—see* Fracture, patella
- larynx S12.8
- late effects *—see* Sequelae, fracture
- leg (lower) S82.9-
  - ankle *—see* Fracture, ankle
  - femur *—see* Fracture, femur
  - fibula *—see* Fracture, fibula
  - malleolus *—see* Fracture, ankle
  - patella *—see* Fracture, patella
  - specified site NEC S82.89-
  - tibia *—see* Fracture, tibia
- lumbar spine *—see* Fracture, vertebra, lumbar
- lumbosacral spine S32.9
- Maisonneuve's (displaced) S82.86-
  - nondisplaced S82.86-
- malar bone *—see also* Fracture, maxilla S02.400
  - left side S02.40B
  - right side S02.40A
- malleolus *—see* Fracture, ankle
- malunion *—see* Fracture, by site
- mandible (lower jaw (bone)) S02.609
  - alveolus S02.67-
  - angle (of jaw) S02.65-
  - body, unspecified S02.600
    - left side S02.602
    - right side S02.601
  - condylar process S02.61-
  - coronoid process S02.63-
  - ramus, unspecified S02.64-
  - specified site NEC S02.69
  - subcondylar process S02.62-
  - symphysis S02.66
- manubrium (sterni) S22.21
  - dissociation from sternum S22.23
- march *—see* Fracture, traumatic, stress, by site
- maxilla, maxillary (bone) (sinus) (superior) (upper jaw) S02.401
  - alveolus S02.42

- maxilla, maxillary *(continued)*
  - inferior *—see* Fracture, mandible
  - LeFort I S02.411
  - LeFort II S02.412
  - LeFort III S02.413
  - left side S02.40D
  - right side S02.40C
- metacarpal S62.309
  - base (displaced) S62.319
    - nondisplaced S62.349
  - fifth S62.30-
    - base (displaced) S62.31-
      - nondisplaced S62.34-
    - neck (displaced) S62.33-
      - nondisplaced S62.36-
    - shaft (displaced) S62.32-
      - nondisplaced S62.35-
    - specified NEC S62.398
  - first S62.20-
    - base NEC (displaced) S62.23-
      - nondisplaced S62.23-
    - Bennett's *—see* Bennett's fracture
    - neck (displaced) S62.25-
      - nondisplaced S62.25-
    - shaft (displaced) S62.24-
      - nondisplaced S62.24-
    - specified NEC S62.29-
  - fourth S62.30-
    - base (displaced) S62.31-
      - nondisplaced S62.34-
    - neck (displaced) S62.33-
      - nondisplaced S62.36-
    - shaft (displaced) S62.32-
      - nondisplaced S62.35-
    - specified NEC S62.39-
  - neck (displaced) S62.33-
    - nondisplaced S62.36-
  - Rolando's *—see* Rolando's fracture
  - second S62.30-
    - base (displaced) S62.31-
      - nondisplaced S62.34-
    - neck (displaced) S62.33-
      - nondisplaced S62.36-
    - shaft (displaced) S62.32-
      - nondisplaced S62.35-
    - specified NEC S62.39-
  - shaft (displaced) S62.32-
    - nondisplaced S62.35-
  - third S62.30-
    - base (displaced) S62.31-
      - nondisplaced S62.34-
    - neck (displaced) S62.33-
      - nondisplaced S62.36-
    - shaft (displaced) S62.32-
      - nondisplaced S62.35-
    - specified NEC S62.39-
  - specified NEC S62.399
- metastatic *—see* Fracture, pathological, due to, neoplastic disease *—see also* Neoplasm
- metatarsal bone S92.30-
  - fifth (displaced) S92.35-
    - nondisplaced S92.35-
  - first (displaced) S92.31-
    - nondisplaced S92.31-
  - fourth (displaced) S92.34-
    - nondisplaced S92.34-
  - physeal S99.10-
    - Salter-Harris
      - Type I S99.11-
      - Type II S99.12-
      - Type III S99.13-
      - Type IV S99.14-
    - specified NEC S99.19-
  - second (displaced) S92.32-
    - nondisplaced S92.32-
  - third (displaced) S92.33-
    - nondisplaced S92.33-

Fracture, traumatic *(continued)*
Monteggia's —*see* Monteggia's fracture
multiple
hand (and wrist) NEC —*see* Fracture, by site
ribs —*see* Fracture, rib, multiple
nasal (bone(s)) S02.2
navicular (scaphoid) (foot) —*see also* Fracture, tarsal, navicular
hand —*see* Fracture, carpal, navicular
neck S12.9
cervical vertebra S12.9
fifth (displaced) S12.400
nondisplaced S12.401
specified type NEC (displaced) S12.490
nondisplaced S12.491
first (displaced) S12.000
burst (stable) S12.01
unstable S12.02
lateral mass (displaced) S12.040
nondisplaced S12.041
nondisplaced S12.001
posterior arch (displaced) S12.030
nondisplaced S12.031
specified type NEC (displaced) S12.090
nondisplaced S12.091
fourth (displaced) S12.300
nondisplaced S12.301
specified type NEC (displaced) S12.390
nondisplaced S12.391
second (displaced) S12.100
nondisplaced S12.101
dens (anterior) (displaced) (type II) S12.110
nondisplaced S12.112
posterior S12.111
specified type NEC (displaced) S12.120
nondisplaced S12.121
specified type NEC (displaced) S12.190
nondisplaced S12.191
seventh (displaced) S12.600
nondisplaced S12.601
specified type NEC (displaced) S12.690
non displaced S12.691
sixth (displaced) S12.500
nondisplaced S12.501
specified type NEC (displaced) S12.590
non displaced S12.591
third (displaced) S12.200
nondisplaced S12.201
specified type NEC (displaced) S12.290
non displaced S12.291
hyoid bone S12.8
larynx S12.8
specified site NEC S12.8
thyroid cartilage S12.8
trachea S12.8
neoplastic NEC —*see* Fracture, pathological, due to, neoplastic disease
neural arch —*see* Fracture, vertebra
newborn —*see* Birth, injury, fracture
nontraumatic —*see* Fracture, pathological
nonunion —*see* Nonunion, fracture
nose, nasal (bone) (septum) S02.2
occiput —*see* Fracture, skull, base, occiput

Fracture, traumatic *(continued)*
odontoid process —*see* Fracture, neck, cervical vertebra, second
olecranon (process) (ulna) —*see* Fracture, ulna, upper end, olecranon process
orbit, orbital (bone) (region) S02.8-
floor (blow-out) S02.3-
roof S02.19
os
calcis —*see* Fracture, tarsal, calcaneus
magnum —*see* Fracture, carpal, capitate
pubis —*see* Fracture, pubis
palate S02.8-
parietal bone (skull) S02.0
patella S82.00-
comminuted (displaced) S82.04-
nondisplaced S82.04-
longitudinal (displaced) S82.02-
nondisplaced S82.02-
osteochondral (displaced) S82.01-
nondisplaced S82.01-
specified NEC S82.09-
transverse (displaced) S82.03-
nondisplaced S82.03-
pedicle (of vertebral arch) —*see* Fracture, vertebra
pelvis, pelvic (bone) S32.9
acetabulum —*see* Fracture, acetabulum
circle —*see* Disruption, pelvic ring
following insertion of implant, prosthesis or plate M96.65
ilium —*see* Fracture, ilium
ischium —*see* Fracture, ischium
multiple
with disruption of pelvic ring (circle) —*see* Disruption, pelvic ring
without disruption of pelvic ring (circle) S32.82
pubis —*see* Fracture, pubis
specified site NEC S32.89
sacrum —*see* Fracture, sacrum
periprosthetic, around internal prosthetic joint M97.9
ankle M97.2-
elbow M97.4-
finger M97.8
hip M97.0-
knee M97.1-
shoulder M97.3-
specified joint NEC M97.8
spine M97.8
toe M97.8
wrist M97.8
phalanx
foot —*see* Fracture, toe
hand —*see* Fracture, finger
pisiform —*see* Fracture, carpal, pisiform
pond —*see* Fracture, skull
prosthetic device, internal —*see* Complications, prosthetic device, by site, mechanical
pubis S32.50-
with disruption of pelvic ring —*see* Disruption, pelvic ring
specified site NEC S32.59-
superior rim S32.51-
radius S52.9-
distal end —*see* Fracture, radius, lower end
following insertion of implant, prosthesis or plate M96.63-
head —*see* Fracture, radius, upper end, head
lower end S52.50-

Fracture, traumatic *(continued)*
radius *(continued)*
lower end *(continued)*
Barton's —*see* Barton's fracture
Colles' —*see* Colles' fracture
extraarticular NEC S52.55-
intraarticular NEC S52.57-
physeal S59.20-
Salter-Harris
Type I S59.21-
Type II S59.22-
Type III S59.23-
Type IV S59.24-
specified NEC S59.29-
Smith's —*see* Smith's fracture
specified NEC S52.59-
styloid process (displaced) S52.51-
nondisplaced S52.51-
torus S52.52-
neck —*see* Fracture, radius, upper end
proximal end —*see* Fracture, radius, upper end
shaft S52.30-
bent bone S52.38-
comminuted (displaced) S52.35-
nondisplaced S52.35-
Galeazzi's —*see* Galeazzi's fracture
greenstick S52.31-
oblique (displaced) S52.33-
nondisplaced S52.33-
segmental (displaced) S52.36-
nondisplaced S52.36-
specified NEC S52.39-
spiral (displaced) S52.34-
nondisplaced S52.34-
transverse (displaced) S52.32-
nondisplaced S52.32-
upper end S52.10-
head (displaced) S52.12-
nondisplaced S52.12-
neck (displaced) S52.13-
nondisplaced S52.13-
specified NEC S52.18-
physeal S59.10-
Salter-Harris
Type I S59.11-
Type II S59.12-
Type III S59.13-
Type IV S59.14-
specified NEC S59.19-
torus S52.11-
ramus
inferior or superior, pubis —*see* Fracture, pubis
mandible —*see* Fracture, mandible
restorative material (dental) K08.539
with loss of material K08.531
without loss of material K08.530
rib S22.3-
with flail chest —*see* Flail, chest
multiple S22.4-
with flail chest —*see* Flail, chest
root, tooth —*see* Fracture, tooth
sacrum S32.10
specified NEC S32.19
Type
1 S32.14
2 S32.15
3 S32.16
4 S32.17
Zone
I S32.119
displaced (minimally) S32.111
severely S32.112
nondisplaced S32.110

Fracture, traumatic *(continued)*
sacrum *(continued)*
Zone *(continued)*
II S32.129
displaced (minimally) S32.121
severely S32.122
nondisplaced S32.120
III S32.139
displaced (minimally) S32.131
severely S32.132
nondisplaced S32.130
scaphoid (hand) —*see also* Fracture, carpal, navicular
foot —*see* Fracture, tarsal, navicular
scapula S42.10-
acromial process (displaced) S42.12-
nondisplaced S42.12-
body (displaced) S42.11-
nondisplaced S42.11-
coracoid process (displaced) S42.13-
nondisplaced S42.13-
glenoid cavity (displaced) S42.14-
nondisplaced S42.14-
neck (displaced) S42.15-
nondisplaced S42.15-
specified NEC S42.19-
semilunar bone, wrist —*see* Fracture, carpal, lunate
sequelae —*see* Sequelae, fracture
sesamoid bone
hand —*see* Fracture, carpal
foot S92.81-
other —*see* Fracture, traumatic, by site
shepherd's —*see* Fracture, tarsal, talus
shoulder (girdle) S42.9-
blade —*see* Fracture, scapula
sinus (ethmoid) (frontal) S02.19
skull S02.91
base S02.10-
occiput S02.119
condyle S02.113
type I S02.110
left side S02.11B
right side S02.11A
type II S02.111
left side S02.11D
right side S02.11C
type III S02.112
left side S02.11F
right side S02.11E
specified NEC S02.118
left side S02.11H
right side S02.11G
specified NEC S02.19
birth injury P13.0
frontal bone S02.0
parietal bone S02.0
specified site NEC S02.8-
temporal bone S02.19
vault S02.0
Smith's —*see* Smith's fracture
sphenoid (bone) (sinus) S02.19
spine —*see* Fracture, vertebra
spinous process —*see* Fracture, vertebra
spontaneous (cause unknown) —*see* Fracture, pathological
stave (of thumb) —*see* Fracture, metacarpal, first
sternum S22.20
with flail chest —*see* Flail, chest
body S22.22
manubrium S22.21
xiphoid (process) S22.24

Fracture, traumatic *(continued)*
stress M84.30
ankle M84.37-
carpus M84.34-
clavicle M84.31-
femoral neck M84.359
femur M84.35-
fibula M84.36-
finger M84.34-
hip M84.359
humerus M84.32-
ilium M84.350
ischium M84.350
metacarpus M84.34-
metatarsus M84.37-
neck *—see* Fracture, fatigue, vertebra
pelvis M84.350
radius M84.33-
rib M84.38
scapula M84.31-
skull M84.38
tarsus M84.37-
tibia M84.36-
toe M84.37-
ulna M84.33-
vertebra *—see* Fracture, fatigue, vertebra
supracondylar, elbow *—see* Fracture, humerus, lower end, supracondylar
symphysis pubis *—see* Fracture, pubis
talus (ankle bone) *—see* Fracture, tarsal, talus
tarsal bone(s) S92.20-
astragalus *—see* Fracture, tarsal, talus
calcaneus S92.00-
anterior process (displaced) S92.02-
nondisplaced S92.02-
body (displaced) S92.01-
nondisplaced S92.01-
extraarticular NEC (displaced) S92.05-
nondisplaced S92.05-
intraarticular (displaced) S92.06-
nondisplaced S92.06-
physeal S99.00-
Salter-Harris
Type I S99.01-
Type II S99.02-
Type III S99.03-
Type IV S99.04-
specified NEC S99.09-
tuberosity (displaced) S92.04-
avulsion (displaced) S92.03-
nondisplaced S92.03-
nondisplaced S92.04-
cuboid (displaced) S92.21-
nondisplaced S92.21-
cuneiform
intermediate (displaced) S92.23-
nondisplaced S92.23-
lateral (displaced) S92.22-
nondisplaced S92.22-
medial (displaced) S92.24-
nondisplaced S92.24-
navicular (displaced) S92.25-
nondisplaced S92.25-
scaphoid *—see* Fracture, tarsal, navicular
talus S92.10-
avulsion (displaced) S92.15-
nondisplaced S92.15-
body (displaced) S92.12-
nondisplaced S92.12-
dome (displaced) S92.14-

Fracture, traumatic *(continued)*
tarsal bone(s) *(continued)*
talus *(continued)*
dome (displaced) *(continued)*
nondisplaced S92.14-
head (displaced) S92.12-
nondisplaced S92.12-
lateral process (displaced) S92.14-
nondisplaced S92.14-
neck (displaced) S92.11-
nondisplaced S92.11-
posterior process (displaced) S92.13-
nondisplaced S92.13-
specified NEC S92.19-
temporal bone (styloid) S02.19
thorax (bony) S22.9
with flail chest *—see* Flail, chest
rib S22.3-
multiple S22.4-
with flail chest *—see* Flail, chest
sternum S22.20
body S22.22
manubrium S22.21
xiphoid process S22.24
vertebra (displaced) S22.009
burst (stable) S22.001
unstable S22.002
eighth S22.069
burst (stable) S22.061
unstable S22.062
specified type NEC S22.068
wedge compression S22.060
eleventh S22.089
burst (stable) S22.081
unstable S22.082
specified type NEC S22.088
wedge compression S22.080
fifth S22.059
burst (stable) S22.051
unstable S22.052
specified type NEC S22.058
wedge compression S22.050
first S22.019
burst (stable) S22.011
unstable S22.012
specified type NEC S22.018
wedge compression S22.010
fourth S22.049
burst (stable) S22.041
unstable S22.042
specified type NEC S22.048
wedge compression S22.040
ninth S22.079
burst (stable) S22.071
unstable S22.072
specified type NEC S22.078
wedge compression S22.070
nondisplaced S22.001
second S22.029
burst (stable) S22.021
unstable S22.022
specified type NEC S22.028
wedge compression S22.020
seventh S22.069
burst (stable) S22.061
unstable S22.062
specified type NEC S22.068
wedge compression S22.060
sixth S22.059
burst (stable) S22.051
unstable S22.052
specified type NEC S22.058
wedge compression S22.050
specified type NEC S22.008
tenth S22.079
burst (stable) S22.071
unstable S22.072
specified type NEC S22.078
wedge compression S22.070

Fracture, traumatic *(continued)*
thorax *(continued)*
vertebra *(continued)*
third S22.039
burst (stable) S22.031
unstable S22.032
specified type NEC S22.038
wedge compression S22.030
twelfth S22.089
burst (stable) S22.081
unstable S22.082
specified type NEC S22.088
wedge compression S22.080
wedge compression S22.000
thumb S62.50-
distal phalanx (displaced) S62.52-
nondisplaced S62.52-
proximal phalanx (displaced) S62.51-
nondisplaced S62.51-
thyroid cartilage S12.8
tibia (shaft) S82.20-
comminuted (displaced) S82.25-
nondisplaced S82.25-
condyles *—see* Fracture, tibia, upper end
distal end *—see* Fracture, tibia, lower end
epiphysis
lower *—see* Fracture, tibia, lower end
upper *—see* Fracture, tibia, upper end
following insertion of implant, prosthesis or plate M96.67-
head (involving knee joint) *—see* Fracture, tibia, upper end
intercondyloid eminence *—see* Fracture, tibia, upper end
involving ankle or malleolus *—see* Fracture, ankle, medial malleolus
lower end S82.30-
physeal S89.10-
Salter-Harris
Type I S89.11-
Type II S89.12-
Type III S89.13-
Type IV S89.14-
specified NEC S89.19-
pilon (displaced) S82.87-
nondisplaced S82.87-
specified NEC S82.39-
torus S82.31-
malleolus *—see* Fracture, ankle, medial malleolus
oblique (displaced) S82.23-
nondisplaced S82.23-
pilon *—see* Fracture, tibia, lower end, pilon
proximal end *—see* Fracture, tibia, upper end
segmental (displaced) S82.26-
nondisplaced S82.26-
specified NEC S82.29-
spine *—see* Fracture, tibia, upper end, spine
spiral (displaced) S82.24-
nondisplaced S82.24-
transverse (displaced) S82.22-
nondisplaced S82.22-
tuberosity *—see* Fracture, tibia, upper end, tuberosity
upper end S82.10-
bicondylar (displaced) S82.14-
nondisplaced S82.14-
lateral condyle (displaced) S82.12-
nondisplaced S82.12-

Fracture, traumatic *(continued)*
tibia *(continued)*
upper end *(continued)*
medial condyle (displaced) S82.13-
nondisplaced S82.13-
physeal S89.00-
Salter-Harris
Type I S89.01-
Type II S89.02-
Type III S89.03-
Type IV S89.04-
specified NEC S89.09-
plateau *—see* Fracture, tibia, upper end, bicondylar
spine (displaced) S82.11-
nondisplaced S82.11-
torus S82.16-
specified NEC S82.19-
tuberosity (displaced) S82.15-
nondisplaced S82.15-
toe S92.91-
great (displaced) S92.40-
distal phalanx (displaced) S92.42-
nondisplaced S92.42-
nondisplaced S92.40-
proximal phalanx (displaced) S92.41-
nondisplaced S92.41-
specified NEC S92.49-
lesser (displaced) S92.50-
distal phalanx (displaced) S92.53-
nondisplaced S92.53-
medial phalanx (displaced) S92.52-
nondisplaced S92.52-
nondisplaced S92.50-
proximal phalanx (displaced) S92.51-
nondisplaced S92.51-
specified NEC S92.59-
physeal
phalanx S99.20-
Salter-Harris
Type I S99.21-
Type II S99.22-
Type III S99.23-
Type IV S99.24-
specified NEC S99.29-
tooth (root) S02.5
trachea (cartilage) S12.8
transverse process *—see* Fracture, vertebra
trapezium or trapezoid bone *—see* Fracture, carpal
trimalleolar *—see* Fracture, ankle, trimalleolar
triquetrum (cuneiform of carpus) *—see* Fracture, carpal, triquetrum
trochanter *—see* Fracture, femur, trochanteric
tuberosity (external) *-see* Fracture, traumatic, by site
ulna (shaft) S52.20-
bent bone S52.28-
coronoid process *—see* Fracture, ulna, upper end, coronoid process
distal end *—see* Fracture, ulna, lower end
following insertion of implant, prosthesis or plate M96.63-
head S52.60-
lower end S52.60-
physeal S59.00-
Salter-Harris
Type I S59.01-
Type II S59.02-
Type III S59.03-
Type IV S59.04-
specified NEC S59.09-

Fracture, traumatic *(continued)*
ulna *(continued)*
lower end *(continued)*
specified NEC S52.69-
styloid process (displaced) S52.61-
nondisplaced S52.61-
torus S52.62-
proximal end *—see* Fracture, ulna, upper end
shaft S52.20-
comminuted (displaced) S52.25-
nondisplaced S52.25-
greenstick S52.21-
Monteggia's *—see* Monteggia's fracture
oblique (displaced) S52.23-
nondisplaced S52.23-
segmental (displaced) S52.26-
nondisplaced S52.26-
specified NEC S52.29-
spiral (displaced) S52.24-
nondisplaced S52.24-
transverse (displaced) S52.22-
nondisplaced S52.22-
upper end S52.00-
coronoid process (displaced) S52.04-
nondisplaced S52.04-
olecranon process (displaced) S52.02-
with intraarticular extension S52.03-
nondisplaced S52.02-
with intraarticular extension S52.03-
specified NEC S52.09-
torus S52.01-
unciform *—see* Fracture, carpal, hamate
vault of skull S02.0
vertebra, vertebral (arch) (body) (column) (neural arch) (pedicle) (spinous process) (transverse process)
atlas *—see* Fracture, neck, cervical vertebra, first
axis *—see* Fracture, neck, cervical vertebra, second
cervical (teardrop) S12.9
axis *—see* Fracture, neck, cervical vertebra, second
first (atlas) *—see* Fracture, neck, cervical vertebra, first
second (axis) *—see* Fracture, neck, cervical vertebra, second
chronic M84.48
coccyx S32.2
dorsal *—see* Fracture, thorax, vertebra
lumbar S32.009
burst (stable) S32.001
unstable S32.002
fifth S32.059
burst (stable) S32.051
unstable S32.052
specified type NEC S32.058
wedge compression S32.050
first S32.019
burst (stable) S32.011
unstable S32.012
specified type NEC S32.018
wedge compression S32.010
fourth S32.049
burst (stable) S32.041
unstable S32.042
specified type NEC S32.048
wedge compression S32.040
second S32.029
burst (stable) S32.021
unstable S32.022

Fracture, traumatic *(continued)*
vertebra, vertebral *(continued)*
lumbar *(continued)*
second *(continued)*
specified type NEC S32.028
wedge compression S32.020
specified type NEC S32.008
third S32.039
burst (stable) S32.031
unstable S32.032
specified type NEC S32.038
wedge compression S32.030
wedge compression S32.000
metastatic *—see* Collapse, vertebra, in, specified disease NEC *—see also* Neoplasm
newborn (birth injury) P11.5
sacrum S32.10
specified NEC S32.19
Type
1 S32.14
2 S32.15
3 S32.16
4 S32.17
Zone
I S32.119
displaced (minimally) S32.111
severely S32.112
nondisplaced S32.110
II S32.129
displaced (minimally) S32.121
severely S32.122
nondisplaced S32.120
III S32.139
displaced (minimally) S32.131
severely S32.132
nondisplaced S32.130
thoracic *—see* Fracture, thorax, vertebra
vertex S02.0
vomer (bone) S02.2
wrist S62.10-
carpal *—see* Fracture, carpal bone
navicular (scaphoid) (hand) *—see* Fracture, carpal, navicular
xiphisternum, xiphoid (process) S22.24
zygoma S02.402
left side S02.40F
right side S02.40E

Fragile, fragility
autosomal site Q95.5
bone, congenital (with blue sclera) Q78.0
capillary (hereditary) D69.8
hair L67.8
nails L60.3
non-sex chromosome site Q95.5
X chromosome Q99.2

Fragilitas
crinium L67.8
ossium (with blue sclerae) (hereditary) Q78.0
unguium L60.3
congenital Q84.6

Fragments, cataract (lens)**, following cataract surgery** H59.02-
retained foreign body *—see* Retained, foreign body fragments (type of)

Frailty (frail) R54
mental R41.81

Frambesia, frambesial (tropica) *—see also* Yaws
initial lesion or ulcer A66.0
primary A66.0

Frambeside
gummatous A66.4
of early yaws A66.2

Frambesioma A66.1

Franceschetti-Klein (-Wildervanck) **disease or syndrome** Q75.4

Francis' disease *—see* Tularemia

Franklin disease C88.2

Frank's essential thrombocytopenia D69.3

Fraser's syndrome Q87.0

Freckle(s) L81.2
malignant melanoma in *—see* Melanoma
melanotic (Hutchinson's) *—see* Melanoma, in situ
retinal D49.81

Frederickson's hyperlipoproteinemia, type
I and V E78.3
IIA E78.00
IIB and III E78.2
IV E78.1

Freeman Sheldon syndrome Q87.0

Freezing (*see also* Effect, adverse, cold) T69.9

Freiberg's disease (infraction of metatarsal head or osteochondrosis) *—see* Osteochondrosis, juvenile, metatarsus

Frei's disease A55

Fremitus, friction, cardiac R01.2

Frenum, frenulum
external os Q51.828
tongue (shortening) (congenital) Q38.1

Frequency micturition (nocturnal) R35.0
psychogenic F45.8

Frey's syndrome
auriculotemporal G50.8
hyperhidrosis L74.52

Friction
burn *—see* Burn, by site
fremitus, cardiac R01.2
precordial R01.2
sounds, chest R09.89

Friderichsen-Waterhouse syndrome or disease A39.1

Friedländer's B (bacillus) **NEC** (*see also* condition) A49.8

Friedreich's
ataxia G11.1
combined systemic disease G11.1
facial hemihypertrophy Q67.4
sclerosis (cerebellum) (spinal cord) G11.1

Frigidity F52.22

Fröhlich's syndrome E23.6

Frontal *—see also* condition
lobe syndrome F07.0

Frostbite (superficial) T33.90
with
partial thickness skin loss *—see* Frostbite (superficial), by site
tissue necrosis T34.90
abdominal wall T33.3
with tissue necrosis T34.3
ankle T33.81-
with tissue necrosis T34.81-
arm T33.4-
with tissue necrosis T34.4-
finger(s) *—see* Frostbite, finger
hand *—see* Frostbite, hand
wrist *—see* Frostbite, wrist

Frostbite *(continued)*
ear T33.01-
with tissue necrosis T34.01-
face T33.09
with tissue necrosis T34.09
finger T33.53-
with tissue necrosis T34.53-
foot T33.82-
with tissue necrosis T34.82-
hand T33.52-
with tissue necrosis T34.52-
head T33.09
with tissue necrosis T34.09
ear *—see* Frostbite, ear
nose *—see* Frostbite, nose
hip (and thigh) T33.6-
with tissue necrosis T34.6-
knee T33.7-
with tissue necrosis T34.7-
leg T33.9-
with tissue necrosis T34.9-
ankle *—see* Frostbite, ankle
foot *—see* Frostbite, foot
knee *—see* Frostbite, knee
lower T33.7-
with tissue necrosis T34.7-
thigh *—see* Frostbite, hip
toe *—see* Frostbite, toe
limb
lower T33.99
with tissue necrosis T34.99
upper *—see* Frostbite, arm
neck T33.1
with tissue necrosis T34.1
nose T33.02
with tissue necrosis T34.02
pelvis T33.3
with tissue necrosis T34.3
specified site NEC T33.99
with tissue necrosis T34.99
thigh *—see* Frostbite, hip
thorax T33.2
with tissue necrosis T34.2
toes T33.83-
with tissue necrosis T34.83-
trunk T33.99
with tissue necrosis T34.99
wrist T33.51-
with tissue necrosis T34.51-

Frotteurism F65.81

Frozen *—see also* Effect, adverse, col T69.9
pelvis (female) N94.89
male K66.8
shoulder *—see* Capsulitis, adhesive

Fructokinase deficiency E74.11

Fructose 1,6 diphosphatase deficiency E74.19

Fructosemia (benign) (essential) E74.12

Fructosuria (benign) (essential) E74.11

Fuchs'
black spot (myopic) (*see also* Myopia, degenerative) H44.2-
dystrophy (corneal endothelium) H18.51
heterochromic cyclitis *—see* Cyclitis, Fuchs' heterochromic

Fucosidosis E77.1

Fugue R68.89
dissociative F44.1
hysterical (dissociative) F44.1
postictal in epilepsy *—see* Epilepsy
reaction to exceptional stress (transient) F43.0

Fulminant, fulminating *—see* conditio

Functional *—see also* condition
bleeding (uterus) N93.8

Functioning, intellectual, borderline R41.83

Fundus *—see* condition

Fungemia NOS B49

Fungus, fungous
- cerebral G93.89
- disease NOS B49
- infection *—see* Infection, fungus

Funiculitis (acute) (chronic) (endemic) N49.1
- gonococcal (acute) (chronic) A54.23
- tuberculous A18.15

Funnel
- breast (acquired) M95.4
  - congenital Q67.6
  - sequelae (late effect) of rickets E64.3
- chest (acquired) M95.4
  - congenital Q67.6
  - sequelae (late effect) of rickets E64.3
- pelvis (acquired) M95.5
  - with disproportion (fetopelvic) O33.3
    - causing obstructed labor O65.3
  - congenital Q74.2

FUO (fever of unknown origin) R50.9

Furfur L21.0
- microsporon B36.0

Furrier's lung J67.8

Furrowed K14.5
- nail(s) (transverse) L60.4
  - congenital Q84.6
- tongue K14.5
  - congenital Q38.3

Furuncle L02.92
- abdominal wall L02.221
- ankle *—see* Furuncle, lower limb
- anus K61.0
- antecubital space *—see* Furuncle, upper limb
- arm *—see* Furuncle, upper limb
- auditory canal, external *—see* Abscess, ear, external
- auricle (ear) *—see* Abscess, ear, external
- axilla (region) L02.42-
- back (any part) L02.222
- breast N61.1
- buttock L02.32
- cheek (external) L02.02
- chest wall L02.223
- chin L02.02
- corpus cavernosum N48.21
- ear, external *—see* Abscess, ear, external
- external auditory canal *—see* Abscess, ear, external
- eyelid *—see* Abscess, eyelid
- face L02.02
- femoral (region) *—see* Furuncle, lower limb
- finger *—see* Furuncle, hand
- flank L02.221
- foot L02.62-
- forehead L02.02
- gluteal (region) L02.32
- groin L02.224
- hand L02.52-
- head L02.821
  - face L02.02
- hip *—see* Furuncle, lower limb
- kidney *—see* Abscess, kidney
- knee *—see* Furuncle, lower limb
- labium (majus) (minus) N76.4
- lacrimal
  - gland *—see* Dacryoadenitis
  - passages (duct) (sac) *—see* Inflammation, lacrimal, passages, acute
- leg (any part) *—see* Furuncle, lower limb
- lower limb L02.42-
- malignant A22.0
- mouth K12.2
- navel L02.226
- neck L02.12
- nose J34.0
- orbit, orbital *—see* Abscess, orbit
- palmar (space) *—see* Furuncle, hand
- partes posteriores L02.32
- pectoral region L02.223
- penis N48.21
- perineum L02.225
- pinna *—see* Abscess, ear, external
- popliteal *—see* Furuncle, lower limb
- prepatellar *—see* Furuncle, lower limb
- scalp L02.821
- seminal vesicle N49.0
- shoulder *—see* Furuncle, upper limb
- specified site NEC L02.828
- submandibular K12.2
- temple (region) L02.02
- thumb *—see* Furuncle, hand
- toe *—see* Furuncle, foot
- trunk L02.229
  - abdominal wall L02.221
  - back L02.222
  - chest wall L02.223
  - groin L02.224
  - perineum L02.225
  - umbilicus L02.226
- umbilicus L02.226
- upper limb L02.42-
- vulva N76.4

Furunculosis *—see* Furuncle

Fused *—see* Fusion, fused

Fusion, fused (congenital)
- astragaloscaphoid Q74.2
- atria Q21.1
- auditory canal Q16.1
- auricles, heart Q21.1
- binocular with defective stereopsis H53.32
- bone Q79.8
- cervical spine M43.22
- choanal Q30.0
- commissure, mitral valve Q23.2
- cusps, heart valve NEC Q24.8
  - mitral Q23.2
  - pulmonary Q22.1
  - tricuspid Q22.4
- ear ossicles Q16.3
- fingers Q70.0-
- hymen Q52.3
- joint (acquired) *—see also* Ankylosis
  - congenital Q74.8
- kidneys (incomplete) Q63.1
- labium (majus) (minus) Q52.5
- larynx and trachea Q34.8
- limb, congenital Q74.8
  - lower Q74.2
  - upper Q74.0
- lobes, lung Q33.8
- lumbosacral (acquired) M43.27
  - arthrodesis status Z98.1
  - congenital Q76.49
  - postprocedural status Z98.1
- nares, nose, nasal, nostril(s) Q30.0
- organ or site not listed *—see* Anomaly, by site
- ossicles Q79.9
  - auditory Q16.3
- pulmonic cusps Q22.1
- ribs Q76.6
- sacroiliac (joint) (acquired) M43.28
  - arthrodesis status Z98.1
  - congenital Q74.2
  - postprocedural status Z98.1
- spine (acquired) NEC M43.20
  - arthrodesis status Z98.1
  - cervical region M43.22
  - cervicothoracic region M43.23
  - congenital Q76.49
  - lumbar M43.26
  - lumbosacral region M43.27
  - occipito-atlanto-axial region M43.21
  - postoperative status Z98.1
  - sacrococcygeal region M43.28
  - thoracic region M43.24
  - thoracolumbar region M43.25
- sublingual duct with submaxillary duct at opening in mouth Q38.4
- testes Q55.1
- toes Q70.2-
- tooth, teeth K00.2
- trachea and esophagus Q39.8
- twins Q89.4
- vagina Q52.4
- ventricles, heart Q21.0
- vertebra (arch) *—see* Fusion, spine
- vulva Q52.5

Fusospirillosis (mouth) (tongue) (tonsil) A69.1

Fussy baby R68.12

G

Gain in weight (abnormal) (excessive) *—see also* Weight, gain

Gaisböck's disease (polycythemia hypertonica) D75.1

Gait abnormality R26.9
- ataxic R26.0
- falling R29.6
- hysterical (ataxic) (staggering) F44.4
- paralytic R26.1
- spastic R26.1
- specified type NEC R26.89
- staggering R26.0
- unsteadiness R26.81
- walking difficulty NEC R26.2

Galactocele (breast) N64.89
- puerperal, postpartum O92.79

Galactokinase deficiency E74.29

Galactophoritis N61.0
- gestational, puerperal, postpartum O91.2-

Galactorrhea O92.6
- not associated with childbirth N64.3

Galactosemia (classic) (congenital) E74.21

Galactosuria E74.29

Galacturia R82.0
- schistosomiasis (bilharziasis) B65.0

GALD (gestational alloimmune liver disease) P78.84

Galeazzi's fracture S52.37-

Galen's vein *—see* condition

Galeophobia F40.218

Gall duct *—see* condition

Gallbladder *—see also* condition
- acute K81.0

Gallop rhythm R00.8

Gallstone (colic) (cystic duct) (gallbladder) (impacted) (multiple) *—see also* Calculus, gallbladder
- with
  - cholecystitis *—see* Calculus, gallbladder, with cholecystitis
- bile duct (common) (hepatic) *—see* Calculus, bile duct
- causing intestinal obstruction K56.3
- specified NEC K80.80
  - with obstruction K80.81

Gambling Z72.6
- pathological (compulsive) F63.0

Gammopathy (of undetermined significance [MGUS]) D47.2
- associated with lymphoplasmacytic dyscrasia D47.2
- monoclonal D47.2
- polyclonal D89.0

Gamna's disease (siderotic splenomegaly) D73.1

Gamophobia F40.298

Gampsodactylia (congenital) Q66.7

Gamstorp's disease (adynamia episodica hereditaria) G72.3

Gandy-Nanta disease (siderotic splenomegaly) D73.1

Gang
- membership offenses Z72.810

Gangliocytoma D36.10

Ganglioglioma *—see* Neoplasm, uncertain behavior, by site

Ganglion (compound) (diffuse) (joint) (tendon (sheath)) M67.40
- ankle M67.47-
- foot M67.47-
- forearm M67.43-
- hand M67.44-
- lower leg M67.46-
- multiple sites M67.49
- of yaws (early) (late) A66.6
- pelvic region M67.45-
- periosteal *—see* Periostitis
- shoulder region M67.41-
- specified site NEC M67.48
- thigh region M67.45-
- tuberculous A18.09
- upper arm M67.42-
- wrist M67.43-

Ganglioneuroblastoma *—see* Neoplasm, nerve, malignant

Ganglioneuroma D36.10
- malignant *—see* Neoplasm, nerve, malignant

Ganglioneuromatosis D36.10

Ganglionitis
- fifth nerve *—see* Neuralgia, trigeminal
- gasserian (postherpetic) (postzoster) B02.21
- geniculate G51.1
  - newborn (birth injury) P11.3
  - postherpetic, postzoster B02.21
- herpes zoster B02.21
- postherpetic geniculate B02.21

Gangliosidosis E75.10
- GM1 E75.19
- GM2 E75.00
  - other specified E75.09
  - Sandhoff disease E75.01
  - Tay-Sachs disease E75.02
- GM3 E75.19
- mucolipidosis IV E75.11

Gangosa A66.5

Gangrene, gangrenous (connective tissue) (dropsical) (dry) (moist) (skin) (ulcer) *—see also* Necrosis I96

Gangrene, gangrenous *(continued)*
with diabetes (mellitus) *—see* Diabetes, gangrene
abdomen (wall) I96
alveolar M27.3
appendix K35.80
with
perforation or rupture K35.2
peritoneal abscess K35.3
peritonitis NEC K35.3
generalized (with perforation or rupture) K35.2
localized (with perforation or rupture) K35.3
arteriosclerotic (general) (senile) *—see* Arteriosclerosis, extremities, with, gangrene
auricle I96
Bacillus welchii A48.0
bladder (infectious) *—see* Cystitis, specified type NEC
bowel, cecum, or colon *—see* Gangrene, intestine
Clostridium perfringens or welchii A48.0
cornea H18.89-
corpora cavernosa N48.29
noninfective N48.89
cutaneous, spreading I96
decubital *—see* Ulcer, pressure, by site
diabetic (any site) *—see* Diabetes, gangrene
epidemic *—see* Poisoning, food, noxious, plant
epididymis (infectional) N45.1
erysipelas *—see* Erysipelas
emphysematous *—see* Gangrene, gas
extremity (lower) (upper) I96
Fournier N49.3
female N76.89
fusospirochetal A69.0
gallbladder *—see* Cholecystitis, acute
gas (bacillus) A48.0
following
abortion *—see* Abortion by type complicated by infection
ectopic or molar pregnancy O08.0
glossitis K14.0
hernia *—see* Hernia, by site, with gangrene
intestine, intestinal (hemorrhagic) (massive) (*see also* Infarct, intestine) K55.069
with
mesenteric embolism (*see also* Infarct, intestine) K55.069
obstruction *—see* Obstruction, intestine
laryngitis J04.0
limb (lower) (upper) I96
lung J85.0
spirochetal A69.8
lymphangitis I89.1
Meleney's (synergistic) *—see* Ulcer, skin
mesentery (*see also* Infarct, intestine) K55.069
with
embolism (*see also* Infarct, intestine) K55.069
intestinal obstruction *—see* Obstruction, intestine
mouth A69.0
ovary *—see* Oophoritis
pancreas - *see* Pancreatitis, acute
penis N48.29
noninfective N48.89

Gangrene, gangrenous *(continued)*
perineum I96
pharynx *—see also* Pharyngitis
Vincent's A69.1
presenile I73.1
progressive synergistic *—see* Ulcer, skin
pulmonary J85.0
pulpal (dental) K04.1
quinsy J36
Raynaud's (symmetric gangrene) I73.01
retropharyngeal J39.2
scrotum N49.3
noninfective N50.89
senile (atherosclerotic) *—see* Arteriosclerosis, extremities, with, gangrene
spermatic cord N49.1
noninfective N50.89
spine I96
spirochetal NEC A69.8
spreading cutaneous I96
stomatitis A69.0
symmetrical I73.01
testis (infectional) N45.2
noninfective N44.8
throat *—see also* Pharyngitis
diphtheritic A36.0
Vincent's A69.1
thyroid (gland) E07.89
tooth (pulp) K04.1
tuberculous NEC *—see* Tuberculosis
tunica vaginalis N49.1
noninfective N50.89
umbilicus I96
uterus *—see* Endometritis
uvulitis K12.2
vas deferens N49.1
noninfective N50.89
vulva N76.89

Ganister disease J62.8

Ganser's syndrome (hysterical) F44.89

Gardner-Diamond syndrome (autoerythrocyte sensitization) D69.2

Gargoylism E76.01

Garré's disease, osteitis (sclerosing), **osteomyelitis** *—see* Osteomyelitis, specified type NEC

Garrod's pad, knuckle M72.1

Gartner's duct
cyst Q52.4
persistent Q50.6

Gas R14.3
asphyxiation, inhalation, poisoning, suffocation NEC *—see* Table of Drugs and Chemicals
excessive R14.0
gangrene A48.0
following
abortion *—see* Abortion by type complicated by infection
ectopic or molar pregnancy O08.0
on stomach R14.0
pains R14.1

Gastralgia *—see also* Pain, abdominal

Gastrectasis K31.0
psychogenic F45.8

Gastric *—see* condition

Gastrinoma
malignant
pancreas C25.4
specified site NEC *—see* Neoplasm, malignant, by site
unspecified site C25.4
specified site *—see* Neoplasm, uncertain behavior
unspecified site D37.9

Gastritis (simple) K29.70
with bleeding K29.71
acute (erosive) K29.00
with bleeding K29.01
alcoholic K29.20
with bleeding K29.21
allergic K29.60
with bleeding K29.61
atrophic (chronic) K29.40
with bleeding K29.41
chronic (antral) (fundal) K29.50
with bleeding K29.51
atrophic K29.40
with bleeding K29.41
superficial K29.30
with bleeding K29.31
dietary counseling and surveillance Z71.3
due to diet deficiency E63.9
eosinophilic K52.81
giant hypertrophic K29.60
with bleeding K29.61
granulomatous K29.60
with bleeding K29.61
hypertrophic (mucosa) K29.60
with bleeding K29.61
nervous F54
spastic K29.60
with bleeding K29.61
specified NEC K29.60
with bleeding K29.61
superficial chronic K29.30
with bleeding K29.31
tuberculous A18.83
viral NEC A08.4

Gastrocarcinoma *—see* Neoplasm, malignant, stomach

Gastrocolic *—see* condition

Gastrodisciasis, gastrodiscoidiasis B66.8

Gastroduodenitis K29.90
with bleeding K29.91
virus, viral A08.4
specified type NEC A08.39

Gastrodynia *—see* Pain, abdominal

Gastroenteritis (acute) (chronic) (noninfectious) (*see also* Enteritis) K52.9
allergic K52.29
with
eosinophilic gastritis or gastroenteritis K52.81
food protein-induced enterocolitis syndrome K52.21
food protein-induced enteropathy K52.22
dietetic (*see also* Gastroenteritis, allergic) K52.29
drug-induced K52.1
due to
Cryptosporidium A07.2
drugs K52.1
food poisoning *—see* Intoxication, foodborne
radiation K52.0
eosinophilic K52.81
epidemic (infectious) A09
food hypersensitivity (*see also* Gastroenteritis, allergic) K52.29
infectious *—see* Enteritis, infectious
influenzal *—see* Influenza, with gastroenteritis
noninfectious K52.9
specified NEC K52.89
rotaviral A08.0
Salmonella A02.0
toxic K52.1
viral NEC A08.4

Gastroenteritis *(continued)*
viral NEC *(continued)*
acute infectious A08.39
type Norwalk A08.11
infantile (acute) A08.39
Norwalk agent A08.11
rotaviral A08.0
severe of infants A08.39
specified type NEC A08.39

Gastroenteropathy (*see also* Gastroenteritis) K52.9
acute, due to Norwalk agent A08.11
acute, due to Norovirus A08.11
infectious A09

Gastroenteroptosis K63.4

Gastroesophageal laceration-hemorrhage syndrome K22.6

Gastrointestinal *—see* condition

Gastrojejunal *—see* condition

Gastrojejunitis (*see also* Enteritis) K52.9

Gastrojejunocolic *—see* condition

Gastroliths K31.89

Gastromalacia K31.89

Gastroparalysis K31.84
diabetic *—see* Diabetes, gastroparalysis

Gastroparesis K31.84
diabetic *—see* Diabetes, by type, with gastroparesis

Gastropathy K31.9
congestive portal K31.89
erythematous K29.70
exudative K90.89
portal hypertensive K31.89

Gastroptosis K31.89

Gastrorrhagia K92.2
psychogenic F45.8

Gastroschisis (congenital) Q79.3

Gastrospasm (neurogenic) (reflex) K31.89
neurotic F45.8
psychogenic F45.8

Gastrostaxis *—see* Gastritis, with bleeding

Gastrostenosis K31.89

Gastrostomy
attention to Z43.1
status Z93.1

Gastrosuccorrhea (continuous) (intermittent) K31.89
neurotic F45.8
psychogenic F45.8

Gatophobia F40.218

Gaucher's disease or splenomegaly (adult) (infantile) E75.22

Gee (-Herter) (-Thaysen) **disease** (nontropical sprue) K90.0

Gélineau's syndrome G47.419
with cataplexy G47.411

Gemination, tooth, teeth K00.2

Gemistocytoma
specified site *—see* Neoplasm, malignant, by site
unspecified site C71.9

General, generalized *—see* condition

Genetic
carrier (status)
cystic fibrosis Z14.1

Genetic *(continued)*
- carrier (status) *(continued)*
  - hemophilia A (asymptomatic) Z14.01
    - symptomatic Z14.02
  - specified NEC Z14.8
- susceptibility to disease NEC Z15.89
  - malignant neoplasm Z15.09
    - breast Z15.01
    - endometrium Z15.04
    - ovary Z15.02
    - prostate Z15.03
    - specified NEC Z15.09
  - multiple endocrine neoplasia Z15.81

Genital *—see* condition

Genito-anorectal syndrome A55

Genitourinary system *—see* condition

Genu
- congenital Q74.1
- extrorsum (acquired) *—see also* Deformity, varus, knee
  - congenital Q74.1
  - sequelae (late effect) of rickets E64.3
- introrsum (acquired) *—see also* Deformity, valgus, knee
  - congenital Q74.1
  - sequelae (late effect) of rickets E64.3
- rachitic (old) E64.3
- recurvatum (acquired) *—see also* Deformity, limb, specified type NEC, lower leg
  - congenital Q68.2
  - sequelae (late effect) of rickets E64.3
- valgum (acquired) (knock-knee) M21.06-
  - congenital Q74.1
  - sequelae (late effect) of rickets E64.3
- varum (acquired) (bowleg) M21.16-
  - congenital Q74.1
  - sequelae (late effect) of rickets E64.3

Geographic tongue K14.1

Geophagia *—see* Pica

Geotrichosis B48.3
- stomatitis B48.3

Gephyrophobia F40.242

Gerbode defect Q21.0

GERD (gastroesophageal reflux disease) K21.9

Gerhardt's
- disease (erythromelalgia) I73.81
- syndrome (vocal cord paralysis) J38.00
  - bilateral J38.02
  - unilateral J38.01

German measles *—see also* Rubella
- exposure to Z20.4

Germinoblastoma (diffuse) C85.9-
- follicular C82.9-

Germinoma *—see* Neoplasm, malignant, by site

Gerontoxon *—see* Degeneration, cornea, senile

Gerstmann-Sträussler-Scheinker syndrome (GSS) A81.82

Gerstmann's syndrome R48.8
- developmental F81.2

Gestation (period) *—see also* Pregnancy
- ectopic *—see* Pregnancy, by site
- multiple O30.9-
  - greater than quadruplets *—see* Pregnancy, multiple (gestation), specified NEC
  - specified NEC *—see* Pregnancy, multiple (gestation), specified NEC

Gestational
- mammary abscess O91.11-
- purulent mastitis O91.11-
- subareolar abscess O91.11-

Ghon tubercle, primary infection A15.7

Ghost
- teeth K00.4
- vessels (cornea) H16.41-

Ghoul hand A66.3

Gianotti-Crosti disease L44.4

Giant
- cell
  - epulis K06.8
  - peripheral granuloma K06.8
- esophagus, congenital Q39.5
- kidney, congenital Q63.3
- urticaria T78.3
  - hereditary D84.1

Giardiasis A07.1

Gibert's disease or pityriasis L42

Giddiness R42
- hysterical F44.89
- psychogenic F45.8

Gierke's disease (glycogenosis I) E74.01

Gigantism (cerebral) (hypophyseal) (pituitary) E22.0
- constitutional E34.4

Gilbert's disease or syndrome E80.4

Gilchrist's disease B40.9

Gilford-Hutchinson disease E34.8

Gilles de la Tourette's disease or syndrome (motor-verbal tic) F95.2

Gingivitis K05.10
- acute (catarrhal) K05.00
  - necrotizing A69.1
  - nonplaque induced K05.01
  - plaque induced K05.00
- chronic (desquamative) (hyperplastic) (simple marginal) (pregnancy associated) (ulcerative) K05.10
  - nonplaque induced K05.11
  - plaque induced K05.10
- expulsiva *—see* Periodontitis
- necrotizing ulcerative (acute) A69.1
- pellagrous E52
  - acute necrotizing A69.1
- Vincent's A69.1

Gingivoglossitis K14.0

Gingivopericementitis *—see* Periodontitis

Gingivosis *—see* Gingivitis, chronic

Gingivostomatitis K05.10
- herpesviral B00.2
- necrotizing ulcerative (acute) A69.1

Gland, glandular *—see* condition

Glanders A24.0

Glanzmann (-Naegeli) **disease or thrombasthenia** D69.1

Glasgow coma scale
- total score
  - 3-8 R40.243
  - 9-12 R40.242
  - 13-15 R40.241

Glass-blower's disease (cataract) *—see* Cataract, specified NEC

Glaucoma H40.9
- with
  - increased episcleral venous pressure H40.81-
  - pseudoexfoliation of lens *—see* Glaucoma, open angle, primary, capsular
- absolute H44.51-
- angle-closure (primary) H40.20-
  - acute (attack) (crisis) H40.21-
  - chronic H40.22-
  - intermittent H40.23-
  - residual stage H40.24-
- borderline H40.00-
- capsular (with pseudoexfoliation of lens) *—see* Glaucoma, open angle, primary, capsular
- childhood Q15.0
- closed angle *—see* Glaucoma, angle-closure
- congenital Q15.0
- corticosteroid-induced *—see* Glaucoma, secondary, drugs
- hypersecretion H40.82-
- in (due to)
  - amyloidosis E85.4 *[H42]*
  - aniridia Q13.1 *[H42]*
  - concussion of globe *—see* Glaucoma, secondary, trauma
  - dislocation of lens *—see* Glaucoma, secondary
  - disorder of lens NEC *—see* Glaucoma, secondary
  - drugs *—see* Glaucoma, secondary, drugs
  - endocrine disease NOS E34.9 *[H42]*
  - eye
    - inflammation *—see* Glaucoma, secondary, inflammation
    - trauma *—see* Glaucoma, secondary, trauma
  - hypermature cataract *—see* Glaucoma, secondary
  - iridocyclitis *—see* Glaucoma, secondary, inflammation
  - lens disorder *—see* Glaucoma, secondary,
  - Lowe's syndrome E72.03 *[H42]*
  - metabolic disease NOS E88.9 *[H42]*
  - ocular disorders NEC *—see* Glaucoma, secondary
  - onchocerciasis B73.02
  - pupillary block *—see* Glaucoma, secondary
  - retinal vein occlusion *—see* Glaucoma, secondary
  - Rieger's anomaly Q13.81 *[H42]*
  - rubeosis of iris *—see* Glaucoma, secondary
  - tumor of globe *—see* Glaucoma, secondary
- infantile Q15.0
- low tension *—see* Glaucoma, open angle, primary, low-tension
- malignant H40.83-
- narrow angle *—see* Glaucoma, angle-closure
- newborn Q15.0
- noncongestive (chronic) *—see* Glaucoma, open angle
- nonobstructive *—see* Glaucoma, open angle
- obstructive *—see also* Glaucoma, angle-closure
  - due to lens changes *—see* Glaucoma, secondary
- open angle H40.10-
  - primary H40.11-
    - capsular (with pseudoexfoliation of lens) H40.14-
    - low-tension H40.12-
    - pigmentary H40.13-
    - residual stage H40.15-
- phacolytic *—see* Glaucoma, secondary
- pigmentary *—see* Glaucoma, open angle, primary, pigmentary
- postinfectious *—see* Glaucoma, secondary, inflammation
- secondary (to) H40.5-
  - drugs H40.6-
  - inflammation H40.4-
  - trauma H40.3-
- simple (chronic) H40.11-
- simplex H40.11-
- specified type NEC H40.89
- suspect H40.00-
- syphilitic A52.71
- traumatic *—see also* Glaucoma, secondary, trauma
  - newborn (birth injury) P15.3
- tuberculous A18.59

Glaucomatous flecks (subcapsular) *—see* Cataract, complicated

Glazed tongue K14.4

Gleet (gonococcal) A54.01

Glénard's disease K63.4

Glioblastoma (multiforme)
- with sarcomatous component
  - specified site *—see* Neoplasm, malignant, by site
  - unspecified site C71.9
- giant cell
  - specified site *—see* Neoplasm, malignant, by site
  - unspecified site C71.9
- specified site *—see* Neoplasm, malignant, by site
- unspecified site C71.9

Glioma (malignant)
- astrocytic
  - specified site *—see* Neoplasm, malignant, by site
  - unspecified site C71.9
- mixed
  - specified site *—see* Neoplasm, malignant, by site
  - unspecified site C71.9
- nose Q30.8
- specified site NEC *—see* Neoplasm, malignant, by site
- subependymal D43.2
  - specified site *—see* Neoplasm, uncertain behavior, by site
  - unspecified site D43.2
- unspecified site C71.9

Gliomatosis cerebri C71.0

Glioneuroma *—see* Neoplasm, uncertain behavior, by site

Gliosarcoma
- specified site *—see* Neoplasm, malignant, by site
- unspecified site C71.9

Gliosis (cerebral) G93.89
- spinal G95.89

Glisson's disease *—see* Rickets

Globinuria R82.3

Globus (hystericus) F45.8

Glomangioma D18.00
- intra-abdominal D18.03
- intracranial D18.02
- skin D18.01
- specified site NEC D18.09

Glomangiomyoma D18.00
- intra-abdominal D18.03
- intracranial D18.02
- skin D18.01
- specified site NEC D18.09

Glomangiosarcoma *—see* Neoplasm, connective tissue, malignant

Glomerular
- disease in syphilis A52.75
- nephritis *—see* Glomerulonephritis

Glomerulitis *—see* Glomerulonephritis

Glomerulonephritis (*see also* Nephritis) N05.9
- with
  - edema *—see* Nephrosis
  - minimal change N05.0
  - minor glomerular abnormality N05.0
- acute N00.9
- chronic N03.9
- crescentic (diffuse) NEC (*see also* N00-N07 with fourth character .7) N05.7
- dense deposit (*see also* N00-N07 with fourth character .6) N05.6
- diffuse
  - crescentic (*see also* N00-N07 with fourth character .7) N05.7
  - endocapillary proliferative (*see also* N00-N07 with fourth character .4) N05.4
  - membranous (*see also* N00-N07 with fourth character .2) N05.2
  - mesangial proliferative (*see also* N00-N07 with fourth character .3) N05.3
  - mesangiocapillary (*see also* N00-N07 with fourth character .5) N05.5
  - sclerosing N18.9
- endocapillary proliferative (diffuse) NEC (*see also* N00-N07 with fourth character .4) N05.4
- extracapillary NEC (*see also* N00-N07 with fourth character .7) N05.7
- focal (and segmental) (*see also* N00-N07 with fourth character .1) N05.1
- hypocomplementemic *—see* Glomerulonephritis, membranoproliferative
- IgA *—see* Nephropathy, IgA
- immune complex (circulating) NEC N05.8
- in (due to)
  - amyloidosis E85.4 *[N08]*
  - bilharziasis B65.9 *[N08]*
  - cryoglobulinemia D89.1 *[N08]*
  - defibrination syndrome D65 *[N08]*
  - diabetes mellitus *—see* Diabetes, glomerulosclerosis
  - disseminated intravascular coagulation D65 *[N08]*
  - Fabry (-Anderson) disease E75.21 *[N08]*
  - Goodpasture's syndrome M31.0

Glomerulonephritis *(continued)*
- in *(continued)*
  - hemolytic-uremic syndrome D59.3
  - Henoch (-Schönlein) purpura D69.0 *[N08]*
  - lecithin cholesterol acyltransferase deficiency E78.6 *[N08]*
  - microscopic polyangiitis M31.7 *[N08]*
  - multiple myeloma C90.0- *[N08]*
  - Plasmodium malariae B52.0
  - schistosomiasis B65.9 *[N08]*
  - sepsis A41.9 *[N08]*
    - streptococcal A40- *[N08]*
  - sickle-cell disorders D57.- *[N08]*
  - strongyloidiasis B78.9 *[N08]*
  - subacute bacterial endocarditis I33.0 *[N08]*
  - syphilis (late) congenital A50.59 *[N08]*
  - systemic lupus erythematosus M32.14
  - thrombotic thrombocytopenic purpura M31.1 *[N08]*
  - typhoid fever A01.09
  - Waldenström macroglobulinemia C88.0 *[N08]*
  - Wegener's granulomatosis M31.31
- latent or quiescent N03.9
- lobular, lobulonodular *—see* Glomerulonephritis, membranoproliferative
- membranoproliferative (diffuse) (type 1 or 3) (*see also* N00-N07 with fourth character .5) N05.5
  - dense deposit (type 2) NEC (*see also* N00-N07 with fourth character .6) N05.6
- membranous (diffuse) NEC (*see also* N00-N07 with fourth character .2) N05.2
- mesangial
  - IgA/IgG *—see* Nephropathy, IgA
  - proliferative (diffuse) NEC (*see also* N00-N07 with fourth character .3) N05.3
- mesangiocapillary (diffuse) NEC (*see also* N00-N07 with fourth character .5) N05.5
- necrotic, necrotizing NEC (*see also* N00-N07 with fourth character .8) N05.8
- nodular *—see* Glomerulonephritis, membranoproliferative
- poststreptococcal NEC N05.9
  - acute N00.9
  - chronic N03.9
  - rapidly progressive N01.9
- proliferative NEC (*see also* N00-N07 with fourth character .8) N05.8
  - diffuse (lupus) M32.14
- rapidly progressive N01.9
- sclerosing, diffuse N18.9
- specified pathology NEC (*see also* N00-N07 with fourth character .8) N05.8
- subacute N01.9

Glomerulopathy *—see* Glomerulonephritis

Glomerulosclerosis *—see also* Sclerosis, renal
- intercapillary (nodular) (with diabetes) *—see* Diabetes, glomerulosclerosis
- intracapillary *—see* Diabetes, glomerulosclerosis

Glossagra K14.6

Glossalgia K14.6

Glossitis (chronic superficial) (gangrenous) (Moeller's) K14.0
- areata exfoliativa K14.1
- atrophic K14.4
- benign migratory K14.1
- cortical superficial, sclerotic K14.0
- Hunter's D51.0
- interstitial, sclerous K14.0
- median rhomboid K14.2
- pellagrous E52
- superficial, chronic K14.0

Glossocele K14.8

Glossodynia K14.6
- exfoliativa K14.4

Glossoncus K14.8

Glossopathy K14.9

Glossophytia K14.3

Glossoplegia K14.8

Glossoptosis K14.8

Glossopyrosis K14.6

Glossotrichia K14.3

Glossy skin L90.8

Glottis *—see* condition

Glottitis *—see also* Laryngitis J04.0

Glucagonoma
- pancreas
  - benign D13.7
  - malignant C25.4
  - uncertain behavior D37.8
- specified site NEC
  - benign *—see* Neoplasm, benign, by site
  - malignant *—see* Neoplasm, malignant, by site
  - uncertain behavior *—see* Neoplasm, uncertain behavior, by site
- unspecified site
  - benign D13.7
  - malignant C25.4
  - uncertain behavior D37.8

Glucoglycinuria E72.51

Glucose-galactose malabsorption E74.39

Glue
- ear *—see* Otitis, media, nonsuppurative, chronic, mucoid
- sniffing (airplane) *—see* Abuse, drug, inhalant
  - dependence *—see* Dependence, drug, inhalant

Glutaric aciduria E72.3

Glycinemia E72.51

Glycinuria (renal) (with ketosis) E72.09

Glycogen
- infiltration *—see* Disease, glycogen storage
- storage disease *—see* Disease, glycogen storage

Glycogenosis (diffuse) (generalized) *—see also* Disease, glycogen storage
- cardiac E74.02 *[I43]*
- diabetic, secondary *—see* Diabetes, glycogenosis, secondary
- pulmonary interstitial J84.842

Glycopenia E16.2

Glycosuria R81
- renal E74.8

Gnathostoma spinigerum (infection) (infestation), gnathostomiasis (wandering swelling) B83.1

Goiter (plunging) (substernal) E04.9
- with
  - hyperthyroidism (recurrent) *—see* Hyperthyroidism, with, goiter
  - thyrotoxicosis *—see* Hyperthyroidism, with, goiter
- adenomatous *—see* Goiter, nodular
- cancerous C73
- congenital (nontoxic) E03.0
  - diffuse E03.0
  - parenchymatous E03.0
  - transitory, with normal functioning P72.0
- cystic E04.2
  - due to iodine-deficiency E01.1
- due to
  - enzyme defect in synthesis of thyroid hormone E07.1
  - iodine-deficiency (endemic) E01.2
- dyshormonogenetic (familial) E07.1
- endemic (iodine-deficiency) E01.2
  - diffuse E01.0
  - multinodular E01.1
- exophthalmic *—see* Hyperthyroidism, with, goiter
- iodine-deficiency (endemic) E01.2
  - diffuse E01.0
  - multinodular E01.1
  - nodular E01.1
- lingual Q89.2
- lymphadenoid E06.3
- malignant C73
- multinodular (cystic) (nontoxic) E04.2
  - toxic or with hyperthyroidism E05.20
    - with thyroid storm E05.21
- neonatal NEC P72.0
- nodular (nontoxic) (due to) E04.9
  - with
    - hyperthyroidism E05.20
      - with thyroid storm E05.21
    - thyrotoxicosis E05.20
      - with thyroid storm E05.21
  - endemic E01.1
  - iodine-deficiency E01.1
  - sporadic E04.9
  - toxic E05.20
    - with thyroid storm E05.21
- nontoxic E04.9
  - diffuse (colloid) E04.0
  - multinodular E04.2
  - simple E04.0
  - specified NEC E04.8
  - uninodular E04.1
- simple E04.0
- toxic *—see* Hyperthyroidism, with, goiter
- uninodular (nontoxic) E04.1
  - toxic or with hyperthyroidism E05.10
    - with thyroid storm E05.11

Goiter-deafness syndrome E07.1

Goldberg syndrome Q89.8

Goldberg-Maxwell syndrome E34.51

Goldblatt's hypertension or kidney I70.1

Goldenhar (-Gorlin) **syndrome** Q87.0

Goldflam-Erb disease or syndrome G70.00
- with exacerbation (acute) G70.01
- in crisis G70.01

Goldscheider's disease Q81.8

Goldstein's disease (familial hemorrhagic telangiectasia) I78.0

Golfer's elbow *—see* Epicondylitis, medial

Gonadoblastoma
- specified site —*see* Neoplasm, uncertain behavior, by site
- unspecified site
  - female D39.10
  - male D40.10

Gonecystitis —*see* Vesiculitis

Gongylonemiasis B83.8

Goniosynechiae —*see* Adhesions, iris, goniosynechiae

Gonococcemia A54.86

Gonococcus, gonococcal (disease) (infection) (*see also* condition) A54.9
- anus A54.6
- bursa, bursitis A54.49
- conjunctiva, conjunctivitis (neonatorum) A54.31
- endocardium A54.83
- eye A54.30
  - conjunctivitis A54.31
  - iridocyclitis A54.32
  - keratitis A54.33
  - newborn A54.31
  - other specified A54.39
- fallopian tubes (acute) (chronic) A54.24
- genitourinary (organ) (system) (tract) (acute)
  - lower A54.00
    - with abscess (accessory gland) (periurethral) A54.1
  - upper (*see also* condition) A54.29
- heart A54.83
- iridocyclitis A54.32
- joint A54.42
- lymphatic (gland) (node) A54.89
- meninges, meningitis A54.81
- musculoskeletal A54.40
  - arthritis A54.42
  - osteomyelitis A54.43
  - other specified A54.49
  - spondylopathy A54.41
- pelviperitonitis A54.24
- pelvis (acute) (chronic) A54.24
- pharynx A54.5
- proctitis A54.6
- pyosalpinx (acute) (chronic) A54.24
- rectum A54.6
- skin A54.89
- specified site NEC A54.89
- tendon sheath A54.49
- throat A54.5
- urethra (acute) (chronic) A54.01
  - with abscess (accessory gland) (periurethral) A54.1
- vulva (acute) (chronic) A54.02

Gonocytoma
- specified site —*see* Neoplasm, uncertain behavior, by site
- unspecified site
  - female D39.10
  - male D40.10

Gonorrhea (acute) (chronic) A54.9
- Bartholin's gland (acute) (chronic) (purulent) A54.02
  - with abscess (accessory gland) (periurethral) A54.1
- bladder A54.01
- cervix A54.03
- conjunctiva, conjunctivitis (neonatorum) A54.31
- contact Z20.2
- Cowper's gland (with abscess) A54.1
- exposure to Z20.2
- fallopian tube (acute) (chronic) A54.24
- kidney (acute) (chronic) A54.21

Gonorrhea *(continued)*
- lower genitourinary tract A54.00
  - with abscess (accessory gland) (periurethral) A54.1
- ovary (acute) (chronic) A54.24
- pelvis (acute) (chronic) A54.24
  - female pelvic inflammatory disease A54.24
- penis A54.09
- prostate (acute) (chronic) A54.22
- seminal vesicle (acute) (chronic) A54.23
- specified site not listed (*see also* Gonococcus) A54.89
- spermatic cord (acute) (chronic) A54.23
- urethra A54.01
  - with abscess (accessory gland) (periurethral) A54.1
- vagina A54.02
- vas deferens (acute) (chronic) A54.23
- vulva A54.02

Goodall's disease A08.19

Goodpasture's syndrome M31.0

Gopalan's syndrome (burning feet) E53.0

Gorlin-Chaudry-Moss syndrome Q87.0

Gottron's papules L94.4

Gougerot's syndrome (trisymptomatic) L81.7

Gougerot-Blum syndrome (pigmented purpuric lichenoid dermatitis) L81.7

Gougerot-Carteaud disease or syndrome (confluent reticulate papillomatosis) L83

Gouley's syndrome (constrictive pericarditis) I31.1

Goundou A66.6

Gout, gouty (acute) (attack) (flare) (*see also* Gout, chronic) M10.9
- drug-induced M10.20
  - ankle M10.27-
  - elbow M10.22-
  - foot joint M10.27-
  - hand joint M10.24-
  - hip M10.25-
  - knee M10.26-
  - multiple site M10.29
  - shoulder M10.21-
  - vertebrae M10.28
  - wrist M10.23-
- idiopathic M10.00
  - ankle M10.07-
  - elbow M10.02-
  - foot joint M10.07-
  - hand joint M10.04-
  - hip M10.05-
  - knee M10.06-
  - multiple site M10.09
  - shoulder M10.01-
  - vertebrae M10.08
  - wrist M10.03-
- in (due to) renal impairment M10.30
  - ankle M10.37-
  - elbow M10.32-
  - foot joint M10.37-
  - hand joint M10.34-
  - hip M10.35-
  - knee M10.36-
  - multiple site M10.39
  - shoulder M10.31-
  - vertebrae M10.38
  - wrist M10.33-
- lead-induced M10.10
  - ankle M10.17-

Gout, gouty *(continued)*
- lead-induced *(continued)*
  - elbow M10.12-
  - foot joint M10.17-
  - hand joint M10.14-
  - hip M10.15-
  - knee M10.16-
  - multiple site M10.19
  - shoulder M10.11-
  - vertebrae M10.18
  - wrist M10.13-
- primary —*see* Gout, idiopathic
- saturnine —*see* Gout, lead-induced
- secondary NEC M10.40
  - ankle M10.47-
  - elbow M10.42-
  - foot joint M10.47-
  - hand joint M10.44-
  - hip M10.45-
  - knee M10.46-
  - multiple site M10.49
  - shoulder M10.41-
  - vertebrae M10.48
  - wrist M10.43-
- syphilitic (*see also* subcategory M14.8-) A52.77
- tophi —*see* Gout, chronic

Gout, chronic (*see also* Gout, gouty) M1A.9
- drug-induced M1A.20
  - ankle M1A.27-
  - elbow M1A.22-
  - foot joint M1A.27-
  - hand joint M1A.24-
  - hip M1A.25-
  - knee M1A.26-
  - multiple site M1A.29-
  - shoulder M1A.21-
  - vertebrae M1A.28
  - wrist M1A.23-
- idiopathic M1A.00
  - ankle M1A.07-
  - elbow M1A.02-
  - foot joint M1A.07-
  - hand joint M1A.04-
  - hip M1A.05-
  - knee M1A.06-
  - multiple site M1A.09
  - shoulder M1A.01-
  - vertebrae M1A.08
  - wrist M1A.03-
- in (due to) renal impairment M1A.30
  - ankle M1A.37-
  - elbow M1A.32-
  - foot joint M1A.37-
  - hand joint M1A.34-
  - hip M1A.35-
  - knee M1A.36-
  - multiple site M1A.39
  - shoulder M1A.31-
  - vertebrae M1A.38
  - wrist M1A.33-
- lead-induced M1A.10
  - ankle M1A.17-
  - elbow M1A.12-
  - foot joint M1A.17-
  - hand joint M1A.14-
  - hip M1A.15-
  - knee M1A.16-
  - multiple site M1A.19
  - shoulder M1A.11-
  - vertebrae M1A.18
  - wrist M1A.13-
- primary —*see* Gout, chronic, idiopathic
- saturnine —*see* Gout, chronic, lead-induced
- secondary NEC M1A.40
  - ankle M1A.47-
  - elbow M1A.42-

Gout, chronic *(continued)*
- secondary NEC *(continued)*
  - foot joint M1A.47-
  - hand joint M1A.44-
  - hip M1A.45-
  - knee M1A.46-
  - multiple site M1A.49
  - shoulder M1A.41-
  - vertebrae M1A.48
  - wrist M1A.43-
- syphilitic (*see also* subcategory M14.8-) A52.77
- tophi M1A.9

Gower's
- muscular dystrophy G71.0
- syndrome (vasovagal attack) R55

Gradenigo's syndrome —*see* Otitis, media, suppurative, acute

Graefe's disease —*see* Strabismus, paralytic, ophthalmoplegia, progressive

Graft-versus-host disease D89.813
- acute D89.810
- acute on chronic D89.812
- chronic D89.811

Grainhandler's disease or lung J67.8

Grain mite (itch) B88.0

Grand mal —*see* Epilepsy, generalized, specified NEC

Grand multipara status only (not pregnant) Z64.1
- pregnant —*see* Pregnancy, complicated by, grand multiparity

Granite worker's lung J62.8

Granular —*see also* condition
- inflammation, pharynx J31.2
- kidney (contracting) —*see* Sclerosis, renal
- liver K74.69

Granulation tissue (abnormal) (excessive) L92.9
- postmastoidectomy cavity —*see* Complications, postmastoidectomy, granulation

Granulocytopenia (primary) (malignant) —*see* Agranulocytosis

Granuloma L92.9
- abdomen K66.8
  - from residual foreign body L92.3
  - pyogenicum L98.0
- actinic L57.5
- annulare (perforating) L92.0
- apical K04.5
- aural —*see* Otitis, externa, specified NEC
- beryllium (skin) L92.3
- bone
  - eosinophilic C96.6
  - from residual foreign body —*see* Osteomyelitis, specified type NEC
  - lung C96.6
- brain (any site) G06.0
  - schistosomiasis B65.9 *[G07]*
- canaliculus lacrimalis —*see* Granuloma, lacrimal
- candidal (cutaneous) B37.2
- cerebral (any site) G06.0
- coccidioidal (primary) (progressive) B38.7
  - lung B38.1
  - meninges B38.4
- colon K63.89
- conjunctiva H11.22-
- dental K04.5
- ear, middle —*see* Cholesteatoma

- **Granuloma** *(continued)*
  - eosinophilic C96.6
    - bone C96.6
    - lung C96.6
    - oral mucosa K13.4
    - skin L92.2
  - eyelid H01.8
  - facial (e) L92.2
  - foreign body (in soft tissue) NEC M60.20
    - ankle M60.27-
    - foot M60.27-
    - forearm M60.23-
    - hand M60.24-
    - in operation wound *—see* Foreign body, accidentally left during a procedure
    - lower leg M60.26-
    - pelvic region M60.25-
    - shoulder region M60.21-
    - skin L92.3
    - specified site NEC M60.28
    - subcutaneous tissue L92.3
    - thigh M60.25-
    - upper arm M60.22-
  - gangraenescens M31.2
  - genito-inguinale A58
  - giant cell (central) (reparative) (jaw) M27.1
    - gingiva (peripheral) K06.8
  - gland (lymph) I88.8
  - hepatic NEC K75.3
    - in (due to)
      - berylliosis J63.2 *[K77]*
      - sarcoidosis D86.89
  - Hodgkin C81.9
  - ileum K63.89
  - infectious B99.9
    - specified NEC B99.8
  - inguinale (Donovan) (venereal) A58
  - intestine NEC K63.89
  - intracranial (any site) G06.0
  - intraspinal (any part) G06.1
  - iridocyclitis *—see* Iridocyclitis, chronic
  - jaw (bone) (central) M27.1
    - reparative giant cell M27.1
  - kidney (*see also* Infection, kidney) N15.8
  - lacrimal H04.81-
  - larynx J38.7
  - lethal midline (faciale(e)) M31.2
  - liver NEC *—see* Granuloma, hepatic
  - lung (infectious) *—see also* Fibrosis, lung
    - coccidioidal B38.1
    - eosinophilic C96.6
  - Majocchi's B35.8
  - malignant (facial(e)) M31.2
  - mandible (central) M27.1
  - midline (lethal) M31.2
  - monilial (cutaneous) B37.2
  - nasal sinus *—see* Sinusitis
  - operation wound T81.89
    - foreign body *—see* Foreign body, accidentally left during a procedure
    - stitch T81.89
    - talc *—see* Foreign body, accidentally left during a procedure
  - oral mucosa K13.4
  - orbit, orbital H05.11-
  - paracoccidioidal B41.8
  - penis, venereal A58
  - periapical K04.5
  - peritoneum K66.8
    - due to ova of helminths NOS (*see also* Helminthiasis) B83.9 *[K67]*

- **Granuloma** *(continued)*
  - postmastoidectomy cavity *—see* Complications, postmastoidectomy, recurrent cholesteatoma
  - prostate N42.89
  - pudendi (ulcerating) A58
  - pulp, internal (tooth) K03.3
  - pyogenic, pyogenicum (of) (skin) L98.0
    - gingiva K06.8
    - maxillary alveolar ridge K04.5
    - oral mucosa K13.4
  - rectum K62.89
  - reticulohistiocytic D76.3
  - rubrum nasi L74.8
  - Schistosoma *—see* Schistosomiasis
  - septic (skin) L98.0
  - silica (skin) L92.3
  - sinus (accessory) (infective) (nasal) *—see* Sinusitis
  - skin L92.9
    - from residual foreign body L92.3
    - pyogenicum L98.0
  - spine
    - syphilitic (epidural) A52.19
    - tuberculous A18.01
  - stitch (postoperative) T81.89
  - suppurative (skin) L98.0
  - swimming pool A31.1
  - talc *—see also* Granuloma, foreign body
    - in operation wound *—see* Foreign body, accidentally left during a procedure
  - telangiectaticum (skin) L98.0
  - tracheostomy J95.09
  - trichophyticum B35.8
  - tropicum A66.4
  - umbilical P83.81
  - umbilicus P83.81
  - urethra N36.8
  - uveitis *—see* Iridocyclitis, chronic
  - vagina A58
  - venereum A58
  - vocal cord J38.3
- **Granulomatosis** L92.9
  - lymphoid C83.8-
  - miliary (listerial) A32.89
  - necrotizing, respiratory M31.30
  - progressive septic D71
  - specified NEC L92.8
  - Wegener's M31.30
    - with renal involvement M31.31
- **Granulomatous tissue** (abnormal) (excessive) L92.9
- **Granulosis rubra nasi** L74.8
- **Graphite fibrosis** (of lung) J63.3
- **Graphospasm** F48.8
  - organic G25.89
- **Grating scapula** M89.8X1
- **Gravel** (urinary) *—see* Calculus, urinary
- **Graves' disease** *—see* Hyperthyroidism, with, goiter
- **Gravis** *—see* condition
- **Grawitz tumor** C64.-
- **Gray syndrome** (newborn) P93.0
- **Grayness, hair** (premature) L67.1
  - congenital Q84.2
- **Green sickness** D50.8
- **Greenfield's disease**
  - meaning
    - concentric sclerosis (encephalitis periaxialis concentrica) G37.5
    - metachromatic leukodystrophy E75.25

- **Greenstick fracture** - code as Fracture, by site
- **Grey syndrome** (newborn) P93.0
- **Grief** F43.21
  - prolonged F43.29
  - reaction (*see also* Disorder, adjustment) F43.20
- **Griesinger's disease** B76.9
- **Grinder's lung or pneumoconiosis** J62.8
- **Grinding, teeth**
  - psychogenic F45.8
  - sleep related G47.63
- **Grip**
  - Dabney's B33.0
  - devil's B33.0
- **Grippe, grippal** *—see also* Influenza
  - Balkan A78
  - summer, of Italy A93.1
- **Grisel's disease** M43.6
- **Groin** *—see* condition
- **Grooved tongue** K14.5
- **Ground itch** B76.9
- **Grover's disease or syndrome** L11.1
- **Growing pains, children** R29.898
- **Growth** (fungoid) (neoplastic) (new) *—see also* Neoplasm
  - adenoid (vegetative) J35.8
  - benign *—see* Neoplasm, benign, by site
  - malignant *—see* Neoplasm, malignant, by site
  - rapid, childhood Z00.2
  - secondary *—see* Neoplasm, secondary, by site
- **Gruby's disease** B35.0
- **Gubler-Millard paralysis or syndrome** G46.3
- **Guerin-Stern syndrome** Q74.3
- **Guidance, insufficient anterior** (occlusal) M26.54
- **Guillain-Barré disease or syndrome** G61.0
  - sequelae G65.0
- **Guinea worms** (infection) (infestation) B72
- **Guinon's disease** (motor-verbal tic) F95.2
- **Gull's disease** E03.4
- **Gum** *—see* condition
- **Gumboil** K04.7
  - with sinus K04.6
- **Gumma** (syphilitic) A52.79
  - artery A52.09
    - cerebral A52.04
  - bone A52.77
    - of yaws (late) A66.6
  - brain A52.19
  - cauda equina A52.19
  - central nervous system A52.3
  - ciliary body A52.71
  - congenital A50.59
  - eyelid A52.71
  - heart A52.06
  - intracranial A52.19
  - iris A52.71
  - kidney A52.75
  - larynx A52.73
  - leptomeninges A52.19
  - liver A52.74
  - meninges A52.19
  - myocardium A52.06

- **Gumma** *(continued)*
  - nasopharynx A52.73
  - neurosyphilitic A52.3
  - nose A52.73
  - orbit A52.71
  - palate (soft) A52.79
  - penis A52.76
  - pericardium A52.06
  - pharynx A52.73
  - pituitary A52.79
  - scrofulous (tuberculous) A18.4
  - skin A52.79
  - specified site NEC A52.79
  - spinal cord A52.19
  - tongue A52.79
  - tonsil A52.73
  - trachea A52.73
  - tuberculous A18.4
  - ulcerative due to yaws A66.4
  - ureter A52.75
  - yaws A66.4
    - bone A66.6
- **Gunn's syndrome** Q07.8
- **Gunshot wound** *—see also* Wound, open
  - fracture - code as Fracture, by site
  - internal organs *—see* Injury, by site
- **Gynandrism** Q56.0
- **Gynandroblastoma**
  - specified site *—see* Neoplasm, uncertain behavior, by site
  - unspecified site
    - female D39.10
    - male D40.10
- **Gynecological examination** (periodic) (routine) Z01.419
  - with abnormal findings Z01.411
- **Gynecomastia** N62
- **Gynephobia** F40.291
- **Gyrate scalp** Q82.8

H

- **H** (Hartnup's) **disease** E72.02
- **Haas' disease or osteochondrosis** (juvenile) (head of humerus) *—see* Osteochondrosis, juvenile, humerus
- **Habit, habituation**
  - bad sleep Z72.821
  - chorea F95.8
  - disturbance, child F98.9
  - drug *—see* Dependence, drug
  - irregular sleep Z72.821
  - laxative F55.2
  - spasm *—see* Tic
  - tic *—see* Tic
- **Haemophilus** (H.) **influenzae, as cause of disease classified elsewhere** B96.3
- **Haff disease** *—see* Poisoning, mercury
- **Hageman's factor defect, deficiency or disease** D68.2
- **Haglund's disease or osteochondrosis** (juvenile) (os tibiale externum) *—see* Osteochondrosis, juvenile, tarsus
- **Hailey-Hailey disease** Q82.8
- **Hair** *—see also* condition
  - plucking F63.3
    - in stereotyped movement disorder F98.4
  - tourniquet syndrome *—see also* Constriction, external, by site
    - finger S60.44-
    - penis S30.842
    - thumb S60.34-
    - toe S90.44-

Hairball in stomach T18.2

Hair-pulling, pathological (compulsive) F63.3

Hairy black tongue K14.3

Half vertebra Q76.49

Halitosis R19.6

Hallerman-Streiff syndrome Q87.0

Hallervorden-Spatz disease G23.0

Hallopeau's acrodermatitis or disease L40.2

Hallucination R44.3
- auditory R44.0
- gustatory R44.2
- olfactory R44.2
- specified NEC R44.2
- tactile R44.2
- visual R44.1

Hallucinosis (chronic) F28
- alcoholic (acute) F10.951
  - in
    - abuse F10.151
    - dependence F10.251
- drug-induced F19.951
  - cannabis F12.951
  - cocaine F14.951
  - hallucinogen F16.151
  - in
    - abuse F19.151
      - cannabis F12.151
      - cocaine F14.151
      - hallucinogen F16.151
      - inhalant F18.151
      - opioid F11.151
      - sedative, anxiolytic or hypnotic F13.151
      - stimulant NEC F15.151
    - dependence F19.251
      - cannabis F12.251
      - cocaine F14.251
      - hallucinogen F16.251
      - inhalant F18.251
      - opioid F11.251
      - sedative, anxiolytic or hypnotic F13.251
      - stimulant NEC F15.251
  - inhalant F18.951
  - opioid F11.951
  - sedative, anxiolytic or hypnotic F13.951
  - stimulant NEC F15.951
- organic F06.0

Hallux
- deformity (acquired) NEC M20.5X-
- limitus M20.5X-
- malleus (acquired) NEC M20.3-
- rigidus (acquired) M20.2-
  - congenital Q74.2
  - sequelae (late effect) of rickets E64.3
- valgus (acquired) M20.1-
  - congenital Q66.6
- varus (acquired) M20.3-
  - congenital Q66.3

Halo, visual H53.19

Hamartoma, hamartoblastoma Q85.9
- epithelial (gingival), odontogenic, central or peripheral *—see* Cyst, calcifying odontogenic

Hamartosis Q85.9

Hamman-Rich syndrome J84.114

Hammer toe (acquired) **NEC** *—see also* Deformity, toe, hammer toe
- congenital Q66.89
- sequelae (late effect) of rickets E64.3

Hand *—see* condition

Hand-foot syndrome L27.1

Handicap, handicapped
- educational Z55.9
  - specified NEC Z55.8

Hand-Schüller-Christian disease or syndrome C96.5

Hanging (asphyxia) (strangulation) (suffocation) *—see* Asphyxia, traumatic, due to mechanical threat

Hangnail *—see also* Cellulitis, digit
- with lymphangitis *—see* Lymphangitis, acute, digit

Hangover (alcohol) F10.129

Hanhart's syndrome Q87.0

Hanot-Chauffard (-Troisier) **syndrome** E83.19

Hanot's cirrhosis or disease K74.3

Hansen's disease *—see* Leprosy

Hantaan virus disease (Korean hemorrhagic fever) A98.5

Hantavirus disease (with renal manifestations) (Dobrava) (Puumala) (Seoul) A98.5
- with pulmonary manifestations (Andes) (Bayou) (Bermejo) (Black Creek Canal) (Choclo) (Juquitiba) (Laguna negra) (Lechiguanas) (New York) (Oran) (Sin nombre) B33.4

Happy puppet syndrome Q93.5

Harada's disease or syndrome H30.81-

Hardening
- artery *—see* Arteriosclerosis
- brain G93.89

Harelip (complete) (incomplete) *—see* Cleft, lip

Harlequin (newborn) Q80.4

Harley's disease D59.6

Harmful use (of)
- alcohol F10.10
- anxiolytics *—see* Abuse, drug, sedative
- cannabinoids *—see* Abuse, drug, cannabis
- cocaine *—see* Abuse, drug, cocaine
- drug *—see* Abuse, drug
- hallucinogens *—see* Abuse, drug, hallucinogen
- hypnotics *—see* Abuse, drug, sedative
- opioids *—see* Abuse, drug, opioid
- PCP (phencyclidine) *—see* Abuse, drug, hallucinogen
- sedatives *—see* Abuse, drug, sedative
- stimulants NEC *—see* Abuse, drug, stimulant

Harris' lines *—see* Arrest, epiphyseal

Hartnup's disease E72.02

Harvester's lung J67.0

Harvesting ovum for in vitro fertilization Z31.83

Hashimoto's disease or thyroiditis E06.3

Hashitoxicosis (transient) E06.3

Hassal-Henle bodies or warts (cornea) H18.49

Haut mal *—see* Epilepsy, generalized, specified NEC

Haverhill fever A25.1

Hay fever (*see also* Fever, hay) J30.1

Hayem-Widal syndrome D59.8

Haygarth's nodes M15.8

Haymaker's lung J67.0

Hb (abnormal)
- Bart's disease D56.0
- disease *—see* Disease, hemoglobin
- trait *—see* Trait

Head *—see* condition

Headache R51
- allergic NEC G44.89
- associated with sexual activity G44.82
- chronic daily R51
- cluster G44.009
  - chronic G44.029
    - intractable G44.021
    - not intractable G44.029
  - episodic G44.019
    - intractable G44.011
    - not intractable G44.019
  - intractable G44.001
  - not intractable G44.009
- cough (primary) G44.83
- daily chronic R51
- drug-induced NEC G44.40
  - intractable G44.41
  - not intractable G44.40
- exertional (primary) G44.84
- histamine G44.009
  - intractable G44.001
  - not intractable G44.009
- hypnic G44.81
- lumbar puncture G97.1
- medication overuse G44.40
  - intractable G44.41
  - not intractable G44.40
- menstrual *—see* Migraine, menstrual
- migraine (type) (*see also* Migraine) G43.909
- nasal septum R51
- neuralgiform, short lasting unilateral, with conjunctival injection and tearing (SUNCT) G44.059
  - intractable G44.051
  - not intractable G44.059
- new daily persistent (NDPH) G44.52
- orgasmic G44.82
- periodic syndromes in adults and children G43.C0
  - with refractory migraine G43.C1
  - intractable G43.C1
  - not intractable G43.C0
  - without refractory migraine G43.C0
- postspinal puncture G97.1
- post-traumatic G44.309
  - acute G44.319
    - intractable G44.311
    - not intractable G44.319
  - chronic G44.329
    - intractable G44.321
    - not intractable G44.329
  - intractable G44.301
  - not intractable G44.309
- pre-menstrual *—see* Migraine, menstrual
- preorgasmic G44.82
- primary
  - cough G44.83
  - exertional G44.84
  - stabbing G44.85
  - thunderclap G44.53
- rebound G44.40
  - intractable G44.41
  - not intractable G44.40

Headache
- short lasting unilateral neuralgiform, with conjunctival injection and tearing (SUNCT) G44.059
  - intractable G44.051
  - not intractable G44.059
- specified syndrome NEC G44.89
- spinal and epidural anesthesia - induced T88.59
  - in labor and delivery O74.5
  - in pregnancy O29.4-
  - postpartum, puerperal O89.4
- spinal fluid loss (from puncture) G97.1
- stabbing (primary) G44.85
- tension (-type) G44.209
  - chronic G44.229
    - intractable G44.221
    - not intractable G44.229
  - episodic G44.219
    - intractable G44.211
    - not intractable G44.219
  - intractable G44.201
  - not intractable G44.209
- thunderclap (primary) G44.53
- vascular NEC G44.1

Healthy
- infant
  - accompanying sick mother Z76.3
  - receiving care Z76.2
- person accompanying sick person Z76.3

Hearing examination Z01.10
- with abnormal findings NEC Z01.118
- following failed hearing screening Z01.110
- for hearing conservation and treatment Z01.12

Heart *—see* condition

Heart beat
- abnormality R00.9
  - specified NEC R00.8
- awareness R00.2
- rapid R00.0
- slow R00.1

Heartburn R12
- psychogenic F45.8

Heartland virus disease A93.8

Heat (effects) T67.9
- apoplexy T67.0
- burn (*see also* Burn) L55.9
- collapse T67.1
- cramps T67.2
- dermatitis or eczema L59.0
- edema T67.7
- erythema - code by site under Burn, first degree
- excessive T67.9
  - specified effect NEC T67.8
- exhaustion T67.5
  - anhydrotic T67.3
  - due to
    - salt (and water) depletion T67.4
    - water depletion T67.3
      - with salt depletion T67.4
- fatigue (transient) T67.6
- fever T67.0
- hyperpyrexia T67.0
- prickly L74.0
- prostration *—see* Heat, exhaustion
- pyrexia T67.0
- rash L74.0
- specified effect NEC T67.8
- stroke T67.0
- sunburn *—see* Sunburn
- syncope T67.1

Heavy-for-dates NEC (infant) (4000g to 4499g) P08.1
exceptionally (4500g or more) P08.0

Hebephrenia, hebephrenic (schizophrenia) F20.1

Heberden's disease or nodes (with arthropathy) M15.1

Hebra's
pityriasis L26
prurigo L28.2

Heel —*see* condition

Heerfordt's disease D86.89

Hegglin's anomaly or syndrome D72.0

Heilmeyer-Schoner disease D45

Heine-Medin disease A80.9

Heinz body anemia, congenital D58.2

Heliophobia F40.228

Heller's disease or syndrome F84.3

HELLP syndrome (hemolysis, elevated liver enzymes and low platelet count) O14.2-
complicating
childbirth O14.24
puerperium O14.25

Helminthiasis —*see also* Infestation, helminth
Ancylostoma B76.0
intestinal B82.0
mixed types (types classifiable to more than one of the titles B65.0-B81.3 and B81.8) B81.4
specified type NEC B81.8
mixed types (intestinal) (types classifiable to more than one of the titles B65.0-B81.3 and B81.8) B81.4
Necator (americanus) B76.1
specified type NEC B83.8

Heloma L84

Hemangioblastoma —*see* Neoplasm, connective tissue, uncertain behavior
malignant —*see* Neoplasm, connective tissue, malignant

Hemangioendothelioma —*see also* Neoplasm, uncertain behavior, by site
benign D18.00
intra-abdominal D18.03
intracranial D18.02
skin D18.01
specified site NEC D18.09
bone (diffuse) —*see* Neoplasm, bone, malignant
epithelioid —*see also* Neoplasm, uncertain behavior, by site
malignant —*see* Neoplasm, malignant, by site
malignant —*see* Neoplasm, connective tissue, malignant

Hemangiofibroma —*see* Neoplasm, benign, by site

Hemangiolipoma —*see* Lipoma

Hemangioma D18.00
arteriovenous D18.00
intra-abdominal D18.03
intracranial D18.02
skin D18.01
specified site NEC D18.09

Hemangioma *(continued)*
capillary D18.00
intra-abdominal D18.03
intracranial D18.02
skin D18.01
specified site NEC D18.09
cavernous D18.00
intra-abdominal D18.03
intracranial D18.02
skin D18.01
specified site NEC D18.09
epithelioid D18.00
intra-abdominal D18.03
intracranial D18.02
skin D18.01
specified site NEC D18.09
histiocytoid D18.00
intra-abdominal D18.03
intracranial D18.02
skin D18.01
specified site NEC D18.09
infantile D18.00
intra-abdominal D18.03
intracranial D18.02
skin D18.01
specified site NEC D18.09
intra-abdominal D18.03
intracranial D18.02
intramuscular D18.00
intra-abdominal D18.03
intracranial D18.02
skin D18.01
specified site NEC D18.09
intrathoracic structures D18.09
juvenile D18.00
malignant —*see* Neoplasm,connective tissue, malignant
plexiform D18.00
intra-abdominal D18.03
intracranial D18.02
skin D18.01
specified site NEC D18.09
racemose D18.00
intra-abdominal D18.03
intracranial D18.02
skin D18.01
specified site NEC D18.09
sclerosing —*see* Neoplasm,skin, benign
simplex D18.00
intra-abdominal D18.03
intracranial D18.02
skin D18.01
specified site NEC D18.09
skin D18.01
specified site NEC D18.09
venous D18.00
intra-abdominal D18.03
intracranial D18.02
skin D18.01
specified site NEC D18.09
verrucous keratotic D18.00
intra-abdominal D18.03
intracranial D18.02
skin D18.01
specified site NEC D18.09

Hemangiomatosis (systemic) I78.8
involving single site —*see* Hemangioma

Hemangiopericytoma —*see also* Neoplasm, connective tissue, uncertain behavior
benign —*see* Neoplasm, connective tissue, benign
malignant —*see* Neoplasm, connective tissue, malignant

Hemangiosarcoma —*see* Neoplasm, connective tissue, malignant

Hemarthrosis (nontraumatic) M25.00
ankle M25.07-
elbow M25.02-
foot joint M25.07-
hand joint M25.04-
hip M25.05-
in hemophilic arthropathy —*see* Arthropathy, hemophilic
knee M25.06-
shoulder M25.01-
specified joint NEC M25.08
traumatic —*see* Sprain, by site
vertebrae M25.08
wrist M25.03-

Hematemesis K92.0
with ulcer - code by site under Ulcer, with hemorrhage K27.4
newborn, neonatal P54.0
due to swallowed maternal blood P78.2

Hematidrosis L74.8

Hematinuria —*see also* Hemoglobinuria
malarial B50.8

Hematobilia K83.8

Hematocele
female NEC N94.89
with ectopic pregnancy O00.90
with intrauterine pregnancy O00.91
ovary N83.8
male N50.1

Hematochezia (*see also* Melena) K92.1

Hematochyluria —*see also* Infestation, filarial
schistosomiasis (bilharziasis) B65.0

Hematocolpos (with hematometra or hematosalpinx) N89.7

Hematocornea —*see* Pigmentation, cornea, stromal

Hematogenous —*see* condition

Hematoma (traumatic) (skin surface intact) —*see also* Contusion
with
injury of internal organs —*see* Injury, by site
open wound —*see* Wound, open
amputation stump (surgical) (late) T87.89
aorta, dissecting I71.00
abdominal I71.02
thoracic I71.01
thoracoabdominal I71.03
aortic intramural —*see* Dissection, aorta
arterial (complicating trauma) —*see* Injury, blood vessel, by site
auricle —*see* Contusion, ear
nontraumatic —*see* Disorder, pinna, hematoma
birth injury NEC P15.8
brain (traumatic)
with
cerebral laceration or contusion (diffuse) —*see* Injury, intracranial, diffuse
focal —*see* Injury, intracranial, focal
cerebellar, traumatic S06.37-
newborn NEC P52.4
birth injury P10.1
intracerebral, traumatic —*see* Injury, intracranial, intracerebral hemorrhage

Hematoma *(continued)*
brain *(continued)*
nontraumatic —*see* Hemorrhage, intracranial
subarachnoid, arachnoid, traumatic —*see* Injury, intracranial, subarachnoid hemorrhage
subdural, traumatic —*see* Injury, intracranial, subdural hemorrhage
breast (nontraumatic) N64.89
broad ligament (nontraumatic) N83.
traumatic S37.892
cerebellar, traumatic S06.37-
cerebral —*see* Hematoma, brain
cerebrum S06.36-
left S06.35-
right S06.34-
cesarean delivery wound O90.2
complicating delivery (perineal) (pelvic) (vagina) (vulva) O71.7
corpus cavernosum (nontraumatic) N48.89
epididymis (nontraumatic) N50.1
epidural (traumatic) —*see* Injury, intracranial, epidural hemorrhage
spinal —*see* Injury, spinal cord, by region
episiotomy O90.2
face, birth injury P15.4
genital organ NEC (nontraumatic)
female (nonobstetric) N94.89
traumatic S30.202
male N50.1
traumatic S30.201
internal organs —*see* Injury, by site
intracerebral, traumatic —*see* Injury, intracranial, intracerebral hemorrhage
intraoperative —*see* Complications, intraoperative, hemorrhage
labia (nontraumatic) (nonobstetric) N90.89
liver (subcapsular) (nontraumatic) K76.89
birth injury P15.0
mediastinum —*see* Injury, intrathoracic
mesosalpinx (nontraumatic) N83.7
traumatic S37.898
muscle - code by site under Contusion
nontraumatic
muscle M79.81
soft tissue M79.81
obstetrical surgical wound O90.2
orbit, orbital (nontraumatic) —*see also* Hemorrhage, orbit
traumatic —*see* Contusion, orbit
pelvis (female) (nontraumatic) (nonobstetric) N94.89
obstetric O71.7
traumatic —*see* Injury, by site
penis (nontraumatic) N48.89
birth injury P15.5
perianal (nontraumatic) K64.5
perineal S30.23
complicating delivery O71.7
perirenal —*see* Injury, kidney
pinna —*see* Contusion, ear
nontraumatic —*see* Disorder, pinna, hematoma
placenta O43.89-
postoperative (postprocedural) —*see* Complication, postprocedural, hematoma
retroperitoneal (nontraumatic) K66.1
traumatic S36.892
scrotum, superficial S30.22
birth injury P15.5

Hematoma *(continued)*
seminal vesicle (nontraumatic) N50.1
traumatic S37.892
spermatic cord (traumatic) S37.892
nontraumatic N50.1
spinal (cord) (meninges) *—see also* Injury, spinal cord, by region
newborn (birth injury) P11.5
spleen D73.5
intraoperative *—see* Complications, intraoperative, hemorrhage, spleen
postprocedural (postoperative) *—see* Complications, postprocedural, hemorrhage, spleen
sternocleidomastoid, birth injury P15.2
sternomastoid, birth injury P15.2
subarachnoid (traumatic) *—see* Injury, intracranial, subarachnoid hemorrhage
newborn (nontraumatic) P52.5
due to birth injury P10.3
nontraumatic *—see* Hemorrhage, intracranial, subarachnoid
subdural (traumatic) *—see* Injury, intracranial, subdural hemorrhage
newborn (localized) P52.8
birth injury P10.0
nontraumatic *—see* Hemorrhage, intracranial, subdural
superficial, newborn P54.5
testis (nontraumatic) N50.1
birth injury P15.5
tunica vaginalis (nontraumatic) N50.1
umbilical cord, complicating delivery O69.5
uterine ligament (broad) (nontraumatic) N83.7
traumatic S37.892
vagina (ruptured) (nontraumatic) N89.8
complicating delivery O71.7
vas deferens (nontraumatic) N50.1
traumatic S37.892
vitreous *—see* Hemorrhage, vitreous
vulva (nontraumatic) (nonobstetric) N90.89
complicating delivery O71.7
newborn (birth injury) P15.5

Hematometra N85.7
with hematocolpos N89.7

Hematomyelia (central) G95.19
newborn (birth injury) P11.5
traumatic T14.8

Hematomyelitis G04.90

Hematoperitoneum *—see* Hemoperitoneum

Hematophobia F40.230

Hematopneumothorax (*see* Hemothorax)

Hematopoiesis, cyclic D70.4

Hematoporphyria *—see* Porphyria

Hematorachis, hematorrhachis G95.19
newborn (birth injury) P11.5

Hematosalpinx N83.6
with
hematocolpos N89.7
hematometra N85.7
with hematocolpos N89.7
infectional *—see* Salpingitis

Hematospermia R36.1

Hematothorax (see Hemothorax)

Hematuria R31.9
due to sulphonamide, sulfonamide *—see* Table of Drugs and Chemicals, by drug
benign (familial) (of childhood) *— see also* Hematuria, idiopathic
essential microscopic R31.1
endemic (*see also* Schistosomiasis) B65.0
gross R31.0
idiopathic N02.9
with glomerular lesion
crescentic (diffuse) glomerulonephritis N02.7
dense deposit disease N02.6
endocapillary proliferative glomerulonephritis N02.4
focal and segmental hyalinosis or sclerosis N02.1
membranoproliferative (diffuse) N02.5
membranous (diffuse) N02.2
mesangial proliferative (diffuse) N02.3
mesangiocapillary (diffuse) N02.5
minor abnormality N02.0
proliferative NEC N02.8
specified pathology NEC N02.8
intermittent *—see* Hematuria, idiopathic
malarial B50.8
microscopic NEC (with symptoms) R31.29
asymptomatic R31.21
benign essential R31.1
paroxysmal *—see also* Hematuria, idiopathic
nocturnal D59.5
persistent *—see* Hematuria, idiopathic
recurrent *—see* Hematuria, idiopathic
tropical (*see also* Schistosomiasis) B65.0
tuberculous A18.13

Hemeralopia (day blindness) H53.11
vitamin A deficiency E50.5

Hemi-akinesia R41.4

Hemianalgesia R20.0

Hemianencephaly Q00.0

Hemianesthesia R20.0

Hemianopia, hemianopsia (heteronymous) H53.47
homonymous H53.46-
syphilitic A52.71

Hemiathetosis R25.8

Hemiatrophy R68.89
cerebellar G31.9
face, facial, progressive (Romberg) G51.8
tongue K14.8

Hemiballism (us) G25.5

Hemicardia Q24.8

Hemicephalus, hemicephaly Q00.0

Hemichorea G25.5

Hemicolitis, left *—see* Colitis, left sided

Hemicrania
congenital malformation Q00.0
continua G44.51
meaning migraine (*see also* Migraine) G43.909
paroxysmal G44.039
chronic G44.049
intractable G44.041
not intractable G44.049

Hemicrania *(continued)*
paroxysmal *(continued)*
episodic G44.039
intractable G44.031
not intractable G44.039
intractable G44.031
not intractable G44.039

Hemidystrophy *—see* Hemiatrophy

Hemiectromelia Q73.8

Hemihypalgesia R20.8

Hemihypesthesia R20.1

Hemi-inattention R41.4

Hemimelia Q73.8
lower limb *—see* Defect, reduction, lower limb, specified type NEC
upper limb *—see* Defect, reduction, upper limb, specified type NEC

Hemiparalysis *—see* Hemiplegia

Hemiparesis *—see* Hemiplegia

Hemiparesthesia R20.2

Hemiparkinsonism G20

Hemiplegia G81.9-
alternans facialis G83.89
ascending NEC G81.90
spinal G95.89
congenital (cerebral) G80.8
spastic G80.2
embolic (current episode) I63.4-
flaccid G81.0-
following
cerebrovascular disease I69.959
cerebral infarction I69.35-
intracerebral hemorrhage I69.15-
nontraumatic intracranial hemorrhage NEC I69.25-
specified disease NEC I69.85-
stroke NOS I69.35-
subarachnoid hemorrhage I69.05-
hysterical F44.4
newborn NEC P91.88
birth injury P11.9
spastic G81.1-
congenital G80.2
thrombotic (current episode) I63.3-

Hemisection, spinal cord *—see* Injury, spinal cord, by region

Hemispasm (facial) R25.2

Hemisporosis B48.8

Hemitremor R25.1

Hemivertebra Q76.49
failure of segmentation with scoliosis Q76.3
fusion with scoliosis Q76.3

Hemochromatosis E83.119
with refractory anemia D46.1
due to repeated red blood cell transfusion E83.111
hereditary (primary) E83.110
neonatal P78.84
primary E83.110
specified NEC E83.118

Hemoglobin *—see also* condition
abnormal (disease) *—see* Disease, hemoglobin
AS genotype D57.3
Constant Spring D58.2
E-beta thalassemia D56.5
fetal, hereditary persistence (HPFH) D56.4
H Constant Spring D56.0
low NOS D64.9
S (Hb S), heterozygous D57.3

Hemoglobinemia D59.9
due to blood transfusion T80.89
paroxysmal D59.6
nocturnal D59.5

Hemoglobinopathy (mixed) D58.2
with thalassemia D56.8
sickle-cell D57.1
with thalassemia D57.40
with crisis (vasoocclusive pain) D57.419
with
acute chest syndrome D57.411
splenic sequestration D57.412
without crisis D57.40

Hemoglobinuria R82.3
with anemia, hemolytic, acquired (chronic) NEC D59.6
cold (agglutinin) (paroxysmal) (with Raynaud's syndrome) D59.6
due to exertion or hemolysis NEC D59.6
intermittent D59.6
malarial B50.8
march D59.6
nocturnal (paroxysmal) D59.5
paroxysmal (cold) D59.6
nocturnal D59.5

Hemolymphangioma D18.1

Hemolysis
intravascular
with
abortion *—see* Abortion, by type, complicated by, hemorrhage
ectopic or molar pregnancy O08.1
hemorrhage
antepartum *—see* Hemorrhage, antepartum, with coagulation defect
intrapartum (*see also* Hemorrhage, complicating, delivery) O67.0
postpartum O72.3
neonatal (excessive) P58.9
specified NEC P58.8

Hemolytic *—see* condition

Hemopericardium I31.2
following acute myocardial infarction (current complication) I23.0
newborn P54.8
traumatic *—see* Injury, heart, with hemopericardium

Hemoperitoneum K66.1
infectional K65.9
traumatic S36.899
with open wound *—see* Wound, open, with penetration into peritoneal cavity

Hemophilia (classical) (familial) (hereditary) D66
A D66
B D67
C D68.1
acquired D68.311
autoimmune D68.311

Hemophilia
calcipriva (*see also* Defect, coagulation) D68.4
nonfamilial (*see also* Defect, coagulation) D68.4
secondary D68.311
vascular D68.0

- **Hemophthalmos** H44.81-
- **Hemopneumothorax** —*see also* Hemothorax
  - traumatic S27.2
- **Hemoptysis** R04.2
  - newborn P26.9
  - tuberculous —*see* Tuberculosis, pulmonary
- **Hemorrhage, hemorrhagic** (concealed) R58
  - abdomen R58
  - accidental antepartum —*see* Hemorrhage, antepartum
  - acute idiopathic pulmonary, in infants R04.81
  - adenoid J35.8
  - adrenal (capsule) (gland) E27.49
    - medulla E27.8
    - newborn P54.4
  - after delivery —*see* Hemorrhage, postpartum
  - alveolar
    - lung, newborn P26.8
    - process K08.89
  - alveolus K08.89
  - amputation stump (surgical) T87.89
  - anemia (chronic) D50.0
    - acute D62
  - antepartum (with) O46.90
    - with coagulation defect O46.00-
      - afibrinogenemia O46.01-
      - disseminated intravascular coagulation O46.02-
      - hypofibrinogenemia O46.01-
      - specified defect NEC O46.09-
    - before 20 weeks gestation O20.9
      - specified type NEC O20.8
      - threatened abortion O20.0
    - due to
      - abruptio placenta (*see also* Abuptio placentae) O45.9-
      - leiomyoma, uterus —*see* Hemorrhage, antepartum, specified cause NEC
      - placenta previa O44.1-
    - specified cause NEC O46.8X-
  - anus (sphincter) K62.5
  - apoplexy (stroke) —*see* Hemorrhage, intracranial, intracerebral
  - arachnoid —*see* Hemorrhage, intracranial, subarachnoid
  - artery R58
    - brain —*see* Hemorrhage, intracranial, intracerebral
  - basilar (ganglion) I61.0
  - bladder N32.89
  - bowel K92.2
    - newborn P54.3
  - brain (miliary) (nontraumatic) —*see* Hemorrhage, intracranial, intracerebral
    - due to
      - birth injury P10.1
      - syphilis A52.05
    - epidural or extradural (traumatic) —*see* Injury, intracranial, epidural hemorrhage
    - newborn P52.4
      - birth injury P10.1
    - subarachnoid —*see* Hemorrhage, intracranial, subarachnoid
    - subdural —*see* Hemorrhage, intracranial, subdural
  - brainstem (nontraumatic) I61.3
    - traumatic S06.38-
  - breast N64.59
  - bronchial tube —*see* Hemorrhage, lung

Hemorrhage, hemorrhagic *(continued)*

  - bronchopulmonary —*see* Hemorrhage, lung
  - bronchus —*see* Hemorrhage, lung
  - bulbar I61.5
  - capillary I78.8
    - primary D69.8
  - cecum K92.2
  - cerebellar, cerebellum (nontraumatic) I61.4
    - newborn P52.6
    - traumatic S06.37-
  - cerebral, cerebrum —*see also* Hemorrhage, intracranial, intracerebral
    - newborn (anoxic) P52.4
      - birth injury P10.1
    - lobe I61.1
  - cerebromeningeal I61.8
  - cerebrospinal —*see* Hemorrhage, intracranial, intracerebral
  - cervix (uteri) (stump) NEC N88.8
  - chamber, anterior (eye) —*see* Hyphema
  - childbirth —*see* Hemorrhage, complicating, delivery
  - choroid H31.30-
    - expulsive H31.31-
  - ciliary body —*see* Hyphema
  - cochlea —*see* subcategory H83.8
  - colon K92.2
  - complicating
    - abortion —*see* Abortion, by type, complicated by, hemorrhage
    - delivery O67.9
      - associated with coagulation defect (afibrinogenemia) (DIC) (hyperfibrinolysis) O67.0
      - specified cause NEC O67.8
    - surgical procedure —*see* Hemorrhage, intraoperative
  - conjunctiva H11.3-
    - newborn P54.8
  - cord, newborn (stump) P51.9
  - corpus luteum (ruptured) cyst N83.1-
  - cortical (brain) I61.1
  - cranial —*see* Hemorrhage, intracranial
  - cutaneous R23.3
    - due to autosensitivity, erythrocyte D69.2
    - newborn P54.5
  - delayed
    - following ectopic or molar pregnancy O08.1
    - postpartum O72.2
  - diathesis (familial) D69.9
  - disease D69.9
    - newborn P53
    - specified type NEC D69.8
  - due to or associated with
    - afibrinogenemia or other coagulation defect (conditions in categories D65-D69)
      - antepartum —*see* Hemorrhage, antepartum, with coagulation defect
      - intrapartum O67.0
    - dental implant M27.61
    - device, implant or graft (*see also* Complications, by site and type, specified NEC) T85.838
      - arterial graft NEC T82.838
      - breast T85.838
      - catheter NEC T85.838
        - dialysis (renal) T82.838
          - intraperitoneal T85.838

Hemorrhage, hemorrhagic *(continued)*

  - due to or associated with *(continued)*
    - device, implant or graft *(continued)*
      - catheter *(continued)*
        - infusion NEC T82.838
          - spinal (epidural) (subdural) T85.830
        - urinary (indwelling) T83.83
      - electronic (electrode) (pulse generator) (stimulator)
        - bone T84.83
        - cardiac T82.837
        - nervous system (brain) (peripheral nerve) (spinal) T85.830
        - urinary T83.83
      - fixation, internal (orthopedic) NEC T84.83
      - gastrointestinal (bile duct) (esophagus) T85.838
      - genital NEC T83.83
      - heart NEC T82.837
      - joint prosthesis T84.83
      - ocular (corneal graft) (orbital implant) NEC T85.838
      - orthopedic NEC T84.83
        - bone graft T86.838
      - specified NEC T85.838
      - urinary NEC T83.83
      - vascular NEC T82.838
      - ventricular intracranial shunt T85.830
  - duodenum, duodenal K92.2
    - ulcer —*see* Ulcer, duodenum, with hemorrhage
  - dura mater —*see* Hemorrhage, intracranial, subdural
  - endotracheal —*see* Hemorrhage, lung
  - epicranial subaponeurotic (massive), birth injury P12.2
  - epidural (traumatic) —*see also* Injury, intracranial, epidural hemorrhage
    - nontraumatic I62.1
  - esophagus K22.8
    - varix I85.01
      - secondary I85.11
  - excessive, following ectopic gestation (subsequent episode) O08.1
  - extradural (traumatic) —*see* Injury, intracranial, epidural hemorrhage
    - birth injury P10.8
    - newborn (anoxic) (nontraumatic) P52.8
    - nontraumatic I62.1
  - eye NEC H57.8
    - fundus —*see* Hemorrhage, retina
    - lid —*see* Disorder, eyelid, specified type NEC
  - fallopian tube N83.6
  - fibrinogenolysis —*see* Fibrinolysis
  - fibrinolytic (acquired) —*see* Fibrinolysis
  - from
    - ear (nontraumatic) —*see* Otorrhagia
    - tracheostomy stoma J95.01
  - fundus, eye —*see* Hemorrhage, retina
  - funis —*see* Hemorrhage, umbilicus, cord
  - gastric —*see* Hemorrhage, stomach
  - gastroenteric K92.2
    - newborn P54.3
  - gastrointestinal (tract) K92.2
    - newborn P54.3

Hemorrhage, hemorrhagic *(continued)*

  - genital organ, male N50.1
  - genitourinary (tract) NOS R31.9
  - gingiva K06.8
  - globe (eye) —*see* Hemophthalmos
  - graafian follicle cyst (ruptured) N83.0-
  - gum K06.8
  - heart I51.89
  - hypopharyngeal (throat) R04.1
  - intermenstrual (regular) N92.3
    - irregular N92.1
  - internal (organs) NEC R58
    - capsule I61.0
    - ear H83.8
    - newborn P54.8
  - intestine K92.2
    - newborn P54.3
  - intra-abdominal R58
  - intra-alveolar (lung), newborn P26.8
  - intracerebral (nontraumatic) —*see* Hemorrhage, intracranial, intracerebral
  - intracranial (nontraumatic) I62.9
    - birth injury P10.9
    - epidural, nontraumatic I62.1
    - extradural, nontraumatic I62.1
    - newborn P52.9
      - specified NEC P52.8
    - intracerebral (nontraumatic) (in) I61.9
      - brain stem I61.3
      - cerebellum I61.4
      - newborn P52.4
        - birth injury P10.1
      - hemisphere I61.2
        - cortical (superficial) I61.1
        - subcortical (deep) I61.0
      - intraoperative
        - during a nervous system procedure G97.31
        - during other procedure G97.32
      - intraventricular I61.5
      - multiple localized I61.6
      - postprocedural
        - following a nervous system procedure G97.51
        - following other procedure G97.52
      - specified NEC I61.8
      - superficial I61.1
      - traumatic (diffuse) —*see* Injury, intracranial, diffuse
        - focal —*see* Injury, intracranial, focal
    - subarachnoid (nontraumatic) (from) I60.9
      - newborn P52.5
        - birth injury P10.3
      - intracranial (cerebral) artery I60.7
        - anterior communicating I60.2
        - basilar I60.4
        - carotid siphon and bifurcation I60.0-
        - communicating I60.7
          - anterior I60.2
          - posterior I60.3-
        - middle cerebral I60.1-
        - posterior communicating I60.3-
        - specified artery NEC I60.6
        - vertebral I60.5-
      - specified NEC I60.8
      - traumatic S06.6X-
    - subdural (nontraumatic) I62.00
      - acute I62.01
      - birth injury P10.0
      - chronic I62.03

Hemorrhage, hemorrhagic *(continued)*
- intracranial *(continued)*
  - subdural *(continued)*
    - newborn (anoxic) (hypoxic) P52.8
      - birth injury P10.0
    - spinal G95.19
    - subacute I62.02
    - traumatic *—see* Injury, intracranial, subdural hemorrhage
  - traumatic *—see* Injury, intracranial, focal brain injury
- intramedullary NEC G95.19
- intraocular *—see* Hemophthalmos
- intraoperative, intraprocedural *—see* Complication, hemorrhage (hematoma), intraoperative (intraprocedural), by site
- intrapartum *—see* Hemorrhage, complicating, delivery
- intrapelvic
  - female N94.89
  - male K66.1
- intraperitoneal K66.1
- intrapontine I61.3
- intraprocedural *—see* Complication, hemorrhage (hematoma), intraoperative (intraprocedural), by site
- intrauterine N85.7
  - complicating delivery (*see also* Hemorrhage, complicating, delivery) O67.9
  - postpartum *—see* Hemorrhage, postpartum
- intraventricular I61.5
  - newborn (nontraumatic) (*see also* Newborn, affected by, hemorrhage) P52.3
    - due to birth injury P10.2
    - grade
      - 1 P52.0
      - 2 P52.1
      - 3 P52.21
      - 4 P52.22
- intravesical N32.89
- iris (postinfectional) (postinflammatory) (toxic) *—see* Hyphema
- joint (nontraumatic) *—see* Hemarthrosis
- kidney N28.89
- knee (joint) (nontraumatic) *—see* Hemarthrosis, knee
- labyrinth *—see* subcategory H83.8
- lenticular striate artery I61.0
- ligature, vessel *—see* Hemorrhage, postoperative
- liver K76.89
- lung R04.89
  - newborn P26.9
    - massive P26.1
    - specified NEC P26.8
  - tuberculous *—see* Tuberculosis, pulmonary
- massive umbilical, newborn P51.0
- mediastinum *—see* Hemorrhage, lung
- medulla I61.3
- membrane (brain) I60.8
  - spinal cord *—see* Hemorrhage, spinal cord
- meninges, meningeal (brain) (middle) I60.8
  - spinal cord *—see* Hemorrhage, spinal cord
- mesentery K66.1

Hemorrhage, hemorrhagic *(continued)*
- metritis *—see* Endometritis
- mouth K13.79
- mucous membrane NEC R58
  - newborn P54.8
- muscle M62.89
- nail (subungual) L60.8
- nasal turbinate R04.0
  - newborn P54.8
- navel, newborn P51.9
- newborn P54.9
  - specified NEC P54.8
- nipple N64.59
- nose R04.0
  - newborn P54.8
- omentum K66.1
- optic nerve (sheath) H47.02-
- orbit, orbital H05.23-
- ovary NEC N83.8
- oviduct N83.6
- pancreas K86.89
- parathyroid (gland) (spontaneous) E21.4
- parturition *—see* Hemorrhage, complicating, delivery
- penis N48.89
- pericardium, pericarditis I31.2
- peritoneum, peritoneal K66.1
- peritonsillar tissue J35.8
  - due to infection J36
- petechial R23.3
  - due to autosensitivity, erythrocyte D69.2
- pituitary (gland) E23.6
- pleura *—see* Hemorrhage, lung
- polioencephalitis, superior E51.2
- polymyositis *—see* Polymyositis
- pons, pontine I61.3
- posterior fossa (nontraumatic) I61.8
  - newborn P52.6
- postmenopausal N95.0
- postnasal R04.0
- postoperative *—see* Complications, postprocedural, hemorrhage, by site
- postpartum NEC (following delivery of placenta) O72.1
  - delayed or secondary O72.2
  - retained placenta O72.0
  - third stage O72.0
- pregnancy *—see* Hemorrhage, antepartum
- preretinal *—see* Hemorrhage, retina
- prostate N42.1
- puerperal *—see* Hemorrhage, postpartum
  - delayed or secondary O72.2
- pulmonary R04.89
  - newborn P26.9
    - massive P26.1
    - specified NEC P26.8
  - tuberculous *—see* Tuberculosis, pulmonary
- purpura (primary) D69.3
- rectum (sphincter) K62.5
  - newborn P54.2
- recurring, following initial hemorrhage at time of injury T79.2
- renal N28.89
- respiratory passage or tract R04.9
  - specified NEC R04.89
- retina, retinal (vessels) H35.6-
  - diabetic *—see* Diabetes, retinal, hemorrhage
- retroperitoneal R58
- scalp R58
- scrotum N50.1
- secondary (nontraumatic) R58

Hemorrhage, hemorrhagic *(continued)*
- secondary *(continued)*
  - following initial hemorrhage at time of injury T79.2
- seminal vesicle N50.1
- skin R23.3
  - newborn P54.5
- slipped umbilical ligature P51.8
- spermatic cord N50.1
- spinal (cord) G95.19
  - newborn (birth injury) P11.5
- spleen D73.5
  - intraoperative *—see* Complications, intraoperative, hemorrhage, spleen
  - postprocedural *—see* Complications, postprocedural, hemorrhage, spleen
- stomach K92.2
  - newborn P54.3
  - ulcer *—see* Ulcer, stomach, with hemorrhage
- subarachnoid (nontraumatic) *—see* Hemorrhage, intracranial, subarachnoid
- subconjunctival *—see also* Hemorrhage, conjunctiva
  - birth injury P15.3
- subcortical (brain) I61.0
- subcutaneous R23.3
- subdiaphragmatic R58
- subdural (acute) (nontraumatic) *—see* Hemorrhage, intracranial, subdural
- subependymal
  - newborn P52.0
    - with intraventricular extension P52.1
      - and intracerebral extension P52.22
- subgaleal P12.2
- subhyaloid *—see* Hemorrhage, retina
- subperiosteal *—see* Disorder, bone, specified type NEC
- subretinal *—see* Hemorrhage, retina
- subtentorial *—see* Hemorrhage, intracranial, subdural
- subungual L60.8
- suprarenal (capsule) (gland) E27.49
  - newborn P54.4
- tentorium (traumatic) NEC *—see* Hemorrhage, brain
  - newborn (birth injury) P10.4
- testis N50.1
- third stage (postpartum) O72.0
- thorax *—see* Hemorrhage, lung
- throat R04.1
- thymus (gland) E32.8
- thyroid (cyst) (gland) E07.89
- tongue K14.8
- tonsil J35.8
- trachea *—see* Hemorrhage, lung
- tracheobronchial R04.89
  - newborn P26.0
- traumatic - code to specific injury
  - cerebellar *—see* Hemorrhage, brain
  - intracranial *—see* Hemorrhage, brain
  - recurring or secondary (following initial hemorrhage at time of injury) T79.2
- tuberculous NEC (*see also* Tuberculosis, pulmonary) A15.0
- tunica vaginalis N50.1
- ulcer - code by site under Ulcer, with hemorrhage K27.4

Hemorrhage, hemorrhagic *(continued)*
- umbilicus, umbilical
  - cord
    - after birth, newborn P51.9
    - complicating delivery O69.5
  - newborn P51.9
    - massive P51.0
    - slipped ligature P51.8
  - stump P51.9
- urethra (idiopathic) N36.8
- uterus, uterine (abnormal) N93.9
  - climacteric N92.4
  - complicating delivery *—see* Hemorrhage, complicating, delivery
  - dysfunctional or functional N93.8
  - intermenstrual (regular) N92.3
    - irregular N92.1
  - postmenopausal N95.0
  - postpartum *—see* Hemorrhage, postpartum
  - preclimacteric or premenopausal N92.4
  - prepubertal N93.8
  - pubertal N92.2
- vagina (abnormal) N93.9
  - newborn P54.6
- vas deferens N50.1
- vasa previa O69.4
- ventricular I61.5
- vesical N32.89
- viscera NEC R58
  - newborn P54.8
- vitreous (humor) (intraocular) H43.1-
- vulva N90.89

Hemorrhoids (bleeding) (without mention of degree) K64.9
- 1st degree (grade/stage I) (without prolapse outside of anal canal) K64.0
- 2nd degree (grade/stage II) (that prolapse with straining but retract spontaneously) K64.1
- 3rd degree (grade/stage III) (that prolapse with straining and require manual replacement back inside anal canal) K64.2
- 4th degree (grade/stage IV) (with prolapsed tissue that cannot be manually replaced) K64.3
- complicating
  - pregnancy O22.4
  - puerperium O87.2
- external K64.4
  - with
    - thrombosis K64.5
- internal (without mention of degree) K64.8
- prolapsed K64.8
- skin tags
  - anus K64.4
  - residual K64.4
- specified NEC K64.8
- strangulated (*see also* Hemorrhoids, by degree) K64.8
- thrombosed (*see also* Hemorrhoids, by degree) K64.5
- ulcerated (*see also* Hemorrhoids, by degree) K64.8

Hemosalpinx N83.6
- with
  - hematocolpos N89.7
  - hematometra N85.7
    - with hematocolpos N89.7

Hemosiderosis (dietary) E83.19
- pulmonary, idiopathic E83.1- *[J84.03]*
- transfusion T80.89

Hemothorax (bacterial) (nontuberculous) J94.2
- newborn P54.8
- traumatic S27.1
  - with pneumothorax S27.2
- tuberculous NEC A15.6

Henoch (-Schönlein) **disease or syndrome** (purpura) D69.0

Henpue, henpuye A66.6

Hepar lobatum (syphilitic) A52.74

Hepatalgia K76.89

Hepatitis K75.9
- acute B17.9
  - with coma K72.01
  - with hepatic failure *—see* Failure, hepatic
  - alcoholic *—see* Hepatitis, alcoholic
  - infectious B17.9
  - non-viral K72.0
  - viral B17.9
- alcoholic (acute) (chronic) K70.10
  - with ascites K70.11
- amebic *—see* Abscess, liver, amebic
- anicteric,(viral) *—see* Hepatitis, viral
- antigen-associated (HAA) *—see* Hepatitis, B
- Australia-antigen (positive) *—see* Hepatitis, B
- autoimmune K75.4
- B B19.10
  - with hepatic coma B19.11
  - acute B16.9
    - with
      - delta-agent (coinfection) (without hepatic coma) B16.1
        - with hepatic coma B16.0
      - hepatic coma (without delta-agent coinfection) B16.2
  - chronic B18.1
    - with delta-agent B18.0
- bacterial NEC K75.89
- C (viral) B19.20
  - with hepatic coma B19.21
  - acute B17.10
    - with hepatic coma B17.11
  - chronic B18.2
- catarrhal (acute) B15.9
  - with hepatic coma B15.0
- cholangiolitic K75.89
- cholestatic K75.89
- chronic K73.9
  - active NEC K73.2
  - lobular NEC K73.1
  - persistent NEC K73.0
  - specified NEC K73.8
- cytomegaloviral B25.1
- due to ethanol (acute) (chronic) *—see* Hepatitis, alcoholic
- epidemic B15.9
  - with hepatic coma B15.0
- fulminant NEC (viral) *—see* Hepatitis, viral
- neonatal giant cell P59.29
- granulomatous NEC K75.3
- herpesviral B00.81
- history of
  - B Z86.19
  - C Z86.19
- homologous serum *—see* Hepatitis, viral, type B
- in (due to)
  - mumps B26.81
  - toxoplasmosis (acquired) B58.1
    - congenital (active) P37.1 *[K77]*

Hepatitis *(continued)*
- infectious, infective B15.9
  - acute (subacute) B17.9
  - chronic B18.9
- inoculation *—see* Hepatitis, viral, type B
- interstitial (chronic) K74.69
- lupoid NEC K75.4
- malignant NEC (with hepatic failure) K72.90
  - with coma K72.91
- neonatal (idiopathic) (toxic) P59.29
- newborn P59.29
- postimmunization *—see* Hepatitis, viral, type B
- post-transfusion *—see* Hepatitis, viral, type B
- reactive, nonspecific K75.2
- serum *—see* Hepatitis, viral, type B
- specified type NEC
  - with hepatic failure *—see* Failure, hepatic
- syphilitic (late) A52.74
  - congenital (early) A50.08 *[K77]*
    - late A50.59 *[K77]*
  - secondary A51.45
- toxic (*see also* Disease, liver, toxic) K71.6
- tuberculous A18.83
- viral, virus B19.9
  - with hepatic coma B19.0
  - acute B17.9
  - chronic B18.9
    - specified NEC B18.8
    - type
      - B B18.1
        - with delta-agent B18.0
      - C B18.2
  - congenital P35.3
  - coxsackie B33.8 *[K77]*
  - cytomegalic inclusion B25.1
  - in remission, any type - code to Hepatitis, chronic, by type
  - non-A, non-B B17.8
  - specified type NEC (with or without coma) B17.8
  - type
    - A B15.9
      - with hepatic coma B15.0
    - B B19.10
      - with hepatic coma B19.11
      - acute B16.9
        - with
          - delta-agent (coinfection) (without hepatic coma) B16.1
            - with hepatic coma B16.0
          - hepatic coma (without delta-agent coinfection) B16.2
      - chronic B18.1
        - with delta-agent B18.0
    - C B19.20
      - with hepatic coma B19.21
      - acute B17.10
        - with hepatic coma B17.11
      - chronic B18.2
    - E B17.2
    - non-A, non-B B17.8

Hepatization lung (acute) *—see* Pneumonia, lobar

Hepatoblastoma C22.2

Hepatocarcinoma C22.0

Hepatocholangiocarcinoma C22.0

Hepatocholangioma, benign D13.4

Hepatocholangitis K75.89

Hepatolenticular degeneration E83.01

Hepatoma (malignant) C22.0
- benign D13.4
- embryonal C22.0

Hepatomegaly *—see also* Hypertrophy, liver
- with splenomegaly R16.2
- congenital Q44.7
- in mononucleosis
  - gammaherpesviral B27.09
  - infectious specified NEC B27.89

Hepatoptosis K76.89

Hepatorenal syndrome following labor and delivery O90.4

Hepatosis K76.89

Hepatosplenomegaly R16.2
- hyperlipemic (Bürger-Grütz type) E78.3 *[K77]*

Hereditary *—see* condition

Heredodegeneration, macular *—see* Dystrophy, retina

Heredopathia atactica polyneuritiformis G60.1

Heredosyphilis *—see* Syphilis, congenital

Herlitz' syndrome Q81.1

Hermansky-Pudlak syndrome E70.331

Hermaphrodite, hermaphroditism (true) Q56.0
- 46,XX with streak gonads Q99.1
- 46,XX/46,XY Q99.0
- 46,XY with streak gonads Q99.1
- chimera 46,XX/46,XY Q99.0

Hernia, hernial (acquired) (recurrent) K46.9
- with
  - gangrene *—see* Hernia, by site, with, gangrene
  - incarceration *—see* Hernia, by site, with, obstruction
  - irreducible *—see* Hernia, by site, with, obstruction
  - obstruction *—see* Hernia, by site, with, obstruction
  - strangulation *—see* Hernia, by site, with, obstruction
- abdomen, abdominal K46.9
  - with
    - gangrene (and obstruction) K46.1
    - obstruction K46.0
  - femoral *—see* Hernia, femoral
  - incisional *—see* Hernia, incisional
  - inguinal *—see* Hernia, inguinal
  - specified site NEC K45.8
    - with
      - gangrene (and obstruction) K45.1
      - obstruction K45.0
  - umbilical *—see* Hernia, umbilical
  - wall *—see* Hernia, ventral
- appendix *—see* Hernia, abdomen
- bladder (mucosa) (sphincter)
  - congenital (female) (male) Q79.51
  - female *—see* Cystocele
  - male N32.89
- brain, congenital *—see* Encephalocele
- cartilage, vertebra *—see* Displacement, intervertebral disc
- cerebral, congenital *—see also* Encephalocele
  - endaural Q01.8
- ciliary body (traumatic) S05.2-

Hernia, hernial *(continued)*
- colon *—see* Hernia, abdomen
- Cooper's *—see* Hernia, abdomen, specified site NEC
- crural *—see* Hernia, femoral
- diaphragm, diaphragmatic K44.9
  - with
    - gangrene (and obstruction) K44.1
    - obstruction K44.0
  - congenital Q79.0
- direct (inguinal) *—see* Hernia, inguinal
- diverticulum, intestine *—see* Hernia, abdomen
- double (inguinal) *—see* Hernia, inguinal, bilateral
- due to adhesions (with obstruction) K56.50
- epigastric (*see also* Hernia, ventral) K43.9
- esophageal hiatus *—see* Hernia, hiatal
- external (inguinal) *—see* Hernia, inguinal
- fallopian tube N83.4-
- fascia M62.89
- femoral K41.90
  - with
    - gangrene (and obstruction) K41.40
      - not specified as recurrent K41.40
      - recurrent K41.41
    - obstruction K41.30
      - not specified as recurrent K41.30
      - recurrent K41.31
  - bilateral K41.20
    - with
      - gangrene (and obstruction) K41.10
        - not specified as recurrent K41.10
        - recurrent K41.11
      - obstruction K41.00
        - not specified as recurrent K41.00
        - recurrent K41.01
    - not specified as recurrent K41.20
    - recurrent K41.21
  - unilateral K41.90
    - with
      - gangrene (and obstruction) K41.40
        - not specified as recurrent K41.40
        - recurrent K41.41
      - obstruction K41.30
        - not specified as recurrent K41.30
        - recurrent K41.31
    - not specified as recurrent K41.90
    - recurrent K41.91
  - not specified as recurrent K41.90
  - recurrent K41.91
- foramen magnum G93.5
  - congenital Q01.8
- funicular (umbilical) *—see also* Hernia, umbilicus
  - spermatic (cord) *—see* Hernia, inguinal
- gastrointestinal tract *—see* Hernia, abdomen
- Hesselbach's *—see* Hernia, femoral, specified site NEC
- hiatal (esophageal) (sliding) K44.9

Hernia, hernial *(continued)*
hiatal *(continued)*
with
gangrene (and obstruction) K44.1
obstruction K44.0
congenital Q40.1
hypogastric *—see* Hernia, ventral
incarcerated *—see also* Hernia, by site, with obstruction
with gangrene *—see* Hernia, by site, with gangrene
incisional K43.2
with
gangrene (and obstruction) K43.1
obstruction K43.0
indirect (inguinal) *—see* Hernia, inguinal
inguinal (direct) (external) (funicular) (indirect) (internal) (oblique) (scrotal) (sliding) K40.90
with
gangrene (and obstruction) K40.40
not specified as recurrent K40.40
recurrent K40.41
obstruction K40.30
not specified as recurrent K40.30
recurrent K40.31
not specified as recurrent K40.90
recurrent K40.91
bilateral K40.20
with
gangrene (and obstruction) K40.10
not specified as recurrent K40.10
recurrent K40.11
obstruction K40.00
not specified as recurrent K40.00
recurrent K40.01
not specified as recurrent K40.20
recurrent K40.21
unilateral K40.90
with
gangrene (and obstruction) K40.40
not specified as recurrent K40.40
recurrent K40.41
obstruction K40.30
not specified as recurrent K40.30
recurrent K40.31
not specified as recurrent K40.90
recurrent K40.91
internal *—see also* Hernia, abdomen
inguinal *—see* Hernia, inguinal
interstitial *—see* Hernia, abdomen
intervertebral cartilage or disc *—see* Displacement, intervertebral disc
intestine, intestinal *—see* Hernia, by site
intra-abdominal *—see* Hernia, abdomen
iris (traumatic) S05.2-
irreducible *—see also* Hernia, by site, with obstruction
with gangrene *—see* Hernia, by site, with gangrene
ischiatic *—see* Hernia, abdomen, specified site NEC
ischiorectal *—see* Hernia, abdomen, specified site NEC

Hernia, hernial *(continued)*
lens (traumatic) S05.2-
linea (alba) (semilunaris) *—see* Hernia, ventral
Littre's *—see* Hernia, abdomen
lumbar *—see* Hernia, abdomen, specified site NEC
lung (subcutaneous) J98.4
mediastinum J98.59
mesenteric (internal) *—see* Hernia, abdomen
midline *—see* Hernia, ventral
muscle (sheath) M62.89
nucleus pulposus *—see* Displacement, intervertebral disc
oblique (inguinal) *—see* Hernia, inguinal
obstructive *—see also* Hernia, by site, with obstruction
with gangrene *—see* Hernia, by site, with gangrene
obturator *—see* Hernia, abdomen, specified site NEC
omental *—see* Hernia, abdomen
ovary N83.4-
oviduct N83.4-
paraesophageal *—see also* Hernia, diaphragm
congenital Q40.1
parastomal K43.5
with
gangrene (and obstruction) K43.4
obstruction K43.3
paraumbilical *—see* Hernia, umbilicus
perineal *—see* Hernia, abdomen, specified site NEC
Petit's *—see* Hernia, abdomen, specified site NEC
postoperative *—see* Hernia, incisional
pregnant uterus *—see* Abnormal, uterus in pregnancy or childbirth
prevesical N32.89
properitoneal *—see* Hernia, abdomen, specified site NEC
pudendal *—see* Hernia, abdomen, specified site NEC
rectovaginal N81.6
retroperitoneal *—see* Hernia, abdomen, specified site NEC
Richter's *—see* Hernia, abdomen, with obstruction
Rieux's, Riex's *—see* Hernia, abdomen, specified site NEC
sac condition (adhesion) (dropsy) (inflammation) (laceration) (suppuration) - code by site under Hernia
sciatic *—see* Hernia, abdomen, specified site NEC
scrotum, scrotal *—see* Hernia, inguinal
sliding (inguinal) *—see also* Hernia, inguinal
hiatus *—see* Hernia, hiatal
spigelian *—see* Hernia, ventral
spinal *—see* Spina bifida
strangulated *—see also* Hernia, by site, with obstruction
with gangrene *—see* Hernia, by site, with gangrene
subxiphoid *—see* Hernia, ventral
supra-umbilicus *—see* Hernia, ventral
tendon *—see* Disorder, tendon, specified type NEC

Hernia, hernial *(continued)*
Treitz's (fossa) *—see* Hernia, abdomen, specified site NEC
tunica vaginalis Q55.29
umbilicus, umbilical K42.9
with
gangrene (and obstruction) K42.1
obstruction K42.0
ureter N28.89
urethra, congenital Q64.79
urinary meatus, congenital Q64.79
uterus N81.4
pregnant *—see* Abnormal, uterus in pregnancy or childbirth
vaginal (anterior) (wall) *—see* Cystocele
Velpeau's *—see* Hernia, femoral
ventral K43.9
with
gangrene (and obstruction) K43.7
obstruction K43.6
recurrent *—see* Hernia, incisional
incisional K43.2
with
gangrene (and obstruction) K43.1
obstruction K43.0
specified NEC K43.9
with
gangrene (and obstruction) K43.7
obstruction K43.6
vesical
congenital (female) (male) Q79.51
female *—see* Cystocele
male N32.89
vitreous (into wound) S05.2-
into anterior chamber *—see* Prolapse, vitreous

Herniation *—see also* Hernia
brain (stem) G93.5
cerebral G93.5
mediastinum J98.59
nucleus pulposus *—see* Displacement, intervertebral disc

Herpangina B08.5

Herpes, herpesvirus, herpetic B00.9
anogenital A60.9
perianal skin A60.1
rectum A60.1
urogenital tract A60.00
cervix A60.03
male genital organ NEC A60.02
penis A60.01
specified site NEC A60.09
vagina A60.04
vulva A60.04
blepharitis (zoster) B02.39
simplex B00.59
circinatus B35.4
bullosus L12.0
conjunctivitis (simplex) B00.53
zoster B02.31
cornea B02.33
encephalitis B00.4
due to herpesvirus 6 B10.01
due to herpesvirus 7 B10.09
specified NEC B10.09
eye (zoster) B02.30
simplex B00.50
eyelid (zoster) B02.39
simplex B00.59
facialis B00.1
febrilis B00.1
geniculate ganglionitis B02.21
genital, genitalis A60.00

Herpes, herpesvirus, herpetic *(continued)*
genital, genitalis *(continued)*
female A60.09
male A60.02
gestational, gestationis O26.4-
gingivostomatitis B00.2
human B00.9
1 *—see* Herpes, simplex
2 *—see* Herpes, simplex
3 *—see* Varicella
4 *—see* Mononucleosis, Epstein-Barr (virus)
5 *—see* Disease, cytomegalic inclusion (generalized)
6
encephalitis B10.01
specified NEC B10.81
7
encephalitis B10.09
specified NEC B10.82
8 B10.89
infection NEC B10.89
Kaposi's sarcoma associated B10.89
iridocyclitis (simplex) B00.51
zoster B02.32
iris (vesicular erythema multiforme) L51.9
iritis (simplex) B00.51
Kaposi's sarcoma associated B10.89
keratitis (simplex) (dendritic) (disciform) (interstitial) B00.52
zoster (interstitial) B02.33
keratoconjunctivitis (simplex) B00.52
zoster B02.33
labialis B00.1
lip B00.1
meningitis (simplex) B00.3
zoster B02.1
ophthalmicus (zoster) NEC B02.30
simplex B00.50
penis A60.01
perianal skin A60.1
pharyngitis, pharyngotonsillitis B00.2
rectum A60.1
scrotum A60.02
sepsis B00.7
simplex B00.9
complicated NEC B00.89
congenital P35.2
conjunctivitis B00.53
external ear B00.1
eyelid B00.59
hepatitis B00.81
keratitis (interstitial) B00.52
myleitis B00.82
specified complication NEC B00.89
visceral B00.89
stomatitis B00.2
tonsurans B35.0
visceral B00.89
vulva A60.04
whitlow B00.89
zoster (*see also* condition) B02.9
auricularis B02.21
complicated NEC B02.8
conjunctivitis B02.31
disseminated B02.7
encephalitis B02.0
eye (lid) B02.39
geniculate ganglionitis B02.21
keratitis (interstitial) B02.33
meningitis B02.1
myelitis B02.24
neuritis, neuralgia B02.29
ophthalmicus NEC B02.30

Herpes, herpesvirus, herpetic *(continued)*
- zoster *(continued)*
  - oticus B02.21
  - polyneuropathy B02.23
  - specified complication NEC B02.8
  - trigeminal neuralgia B02.22

Herpesvirus (human) *—see* Herpes

Herpetophobia F40.218

Herrick's anemia *—see* Disease, sickle-cell

Hers' disease E74.09

Herter-Gee syndrome K90.0

Herxheimer's reaction R68.89

Hesitancy
- of micturition R39.11
- urinary R39.11

Hesselbach's hernia *—see* Hernia, femoral, specified site NEC

Heterochromia (congenital) Q13.2
- cataract *—see* Cataract, complicated
- cyclitis (Fuchs) *—see* Cyclitis, Fuchs' heterochromic
- hair L67.1
- iritis *—see* Cyclitis, Fuchs' heterochromic
- retained metallic foreign body (nonmagnetic) *—see* Foreign body, intraocular, old, retained
  - magnetic *—see* Foreign body, intraocular, old, retained, magnetic
- uveitis *—see* Cyclitis, Fuchs' heterochromic

Heterophoria *—see* Strabismus, heterophoria

Heterophyes, heterophyiasis (small intestine) B66.8

Heterotopia, heterotopic *—see also* Malposition, congenital
- cerebralis Q04.8

Heterotropia *—see* Strabismus

Heubner-Herter disease K90.0

Hexadactylism Q69.9

HGSIL (cytology finding) (high grade squamous intraepithelial lesion on cytologic smear) (Pap smear finding)
- anus R85.613
- cervix R87.613
  - biopsy (histology) finding *—see* Neoplasia, intraepithelial, cervix, grade II or grade III
- vagina R87.623
  - biopsy (histology) finding *—see* Neoplasia, intraepithelial, vagina, grade II or grade III

Hibernoma *—see* Lipoma

Hiccup, hiccough R06.6
- epidemic B33.0
- psychogenic F45.8

Hidden penis (congenital) Q55.64
- acquired N48.83

Hidradenitis (axillaris) (suppurative) L73.2

Hidradenoma (nodular) *—see also* Neoplasm, skin, benign
- clear cell *—see* Neoplasm, skin, benign
- papillary *—see* Neoplasm, skin, benign

Hidrocystoma *—see* Neoplasm, skin, benign

High
- altitude effects T70.20
  - anoxia T70.29
  - on
    - ears T70.0
    - sinuses T70.1
  - polycythemia D75.1
- arch
  - foot Q66.7
  - palate, congenital Q38.5
- arterial tension *—see* Hypertension
- basal metabolic rate R94.8
- blood pressure *—see also* Hypertension
  - borderline R03.0
  - reading (incidental) (isolated) (nonspecific), without diagnosis of hypertension R03.0
- cholesterol E78.00
  - with high triglycerides E78.2
- diaphragm (congenital) Q79.1
- expressed emotional level within family Z63.8
- head at term O32.4
- palate, congenital Q38.5
- risk
  - infant NEC Z76.2
  - sexual behavior (heterosexual) Z72.51
    - bisexual Z72.53
    - homosexual Z72.52
- scrotal testis, testes
  - bilateral Q53.23
  - unilateral Q53.13
- temperature (of unknown origin) R50.9
- thoracic rib Q76.6
- triglycerides E78.1
  - with high cholesterol E78.2

Hildenbrand's disease A75.0

Hilum *—see* condition

Hip *—see* condition

Hippel's disease Q85.8

Hippophobia F40.218

Hippus H57.09

Hirschsprung's disease or megacolon Q43.1

Hirsutism, hirsuties L68.0

Hirudiniasis
- external B88.3
- internal B83.4

Hiss-Russell dysentery A03.1

Histidinemia, histidinuria E70.41

Histiocytoma *—see also* Neoplasm, skin, benign
- fibrous *—see also* Neoplasm, skin, benign
  - atypical *—see* Neoplasm, connective tissue, uncertain behavior
  - malignant *—see* Neoplasm, connective tissue, malignant

Histiocytosis D76.3
- acute differentiated progressive C96.0
- Langerhans' cell NEC C96.6
  - multifocal X
    - multisystemic (disseminated) C96.0
    - unisystemic C96.5
  - pulmonary, adult (adult PLCH) J84.82
  - unifocal (X) C96.6
- lipid, lipoid D76.3
  - essential E75.29
- malignant C96.A
- mononuclear phagocytes NEC D76.1
  - Langerhans' cells C96.6
- non-Langerhans cell D76.3
- polyostotic sclerosing D76.3
- sinus, with massive lymphadenopathy D76.3
- syndrome NEC D76.3
- X NEC C96.6
  - acute (progressive) C96.0
  - chronic C96.6
  - multifocal C96.5
  - multisystemic C96.0
  - unifocal C96.6

Histoplasmosis B39.9
- with pneumonia NEC B39.2
- African B39.5
- American *—see* Histoplasmosis, capsulati
- capsulati B39.4
  - disseminated B39.3
  - generalized B39.3
  - pulmonary B39.2
    - acute B39.0
    - chronic B39.1
- Darling's B39.4
- duboisii B39.5
- lung NEC B39.2

History
- family (of) *—see also* History, personal (of)
  - alcohol abuse Z81.1
  - allergy NEC Z84.89
  - anemia Z83.2
  - arthritis Z82.61
  - asthma Z82.5
  - blindness Z82.1
  - cardiac death (sudden) Z82.41
  - carrier of genetic disease Z84.81
  - chromosomal anomaly Z82.79
  - chronic
    - disabling disease NEC Z82.8
    - lower respiratory disease Z82.5
  - colonic polyps Z83.71
  - congenital malformations and deformations Z82.79
    - polycystic kidney Z82.71
  - consanguinity Z84.3
  - deafness Z82.2
  - diabetes mellitus Z83.3
  - disability NEC Z82.8
  - disease or disorder (of)
    - allergic NEC Z84.89
    - behavioral NEC Z81.8
    - blood and blood-forming organs Z83.2
    - cardiovascular NEC Z82.49
    - chronic disabling NEC Z82.8
    - digestive Z83.79
    - ear NEC Z83.52
    - endocrine NEC Z83.49
    - eye NEC Z83.518
      - glaucoma Z83.511
    - familial hypercholesterolemia Z83.42
    - genitourinary NEC Z84.2
    - glaucoma Z83.511
    - hematological Z83.2
    - immune mechanism Z83.2
    - infectious NEC Z83.1
    - ischemic heart Z82.49
    - kidney Z84.1
    - mental NEC Z81.8
    - metabolic Z83.49
    - musculoskeletal NEC Z82.69
    - neurological NEC Z82.0
    - nutritional Z83.49
    - parasitic NEC Z83.1
    - psychiatric NEC Z81.8
    - respiratory NEC Z83.6
    - skin and subcutaneous tissue NEC Z84.0
    - specified NEC Z84.89
  - drug abuse NEC Z81.3
  - epilepsy Z82.0
  - familial hypercholesterolemia Z83.42
  - genetic disease carrier Z84.81
  - glaucoma Z83.511
  - hearing loss Z82.2
  - human immunodeficiency virus (HIV) infection Z83.0
  - Huntington's chorea Z82.0
  - intellectual disability Z81.0
  - leukemia Z80.6
  - malignant neoplasm (of) NOS Z80.9
    - bladder Z80.52
    - breast Z80.3
    - bronchus Z80.1
    - digestive organ Z80.0
    - gastrointestinal tract Z80.0
    - genital organ Z80.49
      - ovary Z80.41
      - prostate Z80.42
      - specified organ NEC Z80.49
      - testis Z80.43
    - hematopoietic NEC Z80.7
    - intrathoracic organ NEC Z80.2
    - kidney Z80.51
    - lung Z80.1
    - lymphatic NEC Z80.7
    - ovary Z80.41
    - prostate Z80.42
    - respiratory organ NEC Z80.2
    - specified site NEC Z80.8
    - testis Z80.43
    - trachea Z80.1
    - urinary organ or tract Z80.59
      - bladder Z80.52
      - kidney Z80.51
  - mental
    - disorder NEC Z81.8
  - multiple endocrine neoplasia (MEN) syndrome Z83.41
  - osteoporosis Z82.62
  - polycystic kidney Z82.71
  - polyps (colon) Z83.71
  - psychiatric disorder Z81.8
  - psychoactive substance abuse NEC Z81.3
  - respiratory condition NEC Z83.6
    - asthma and other lower respiratory conditions Z82.5
  - self-harmful behavior Z81.8
  - SIDS (sudden infant death syndrome) Z84.82
  - skin condition Z84.0
  - specified condition NEC Z84.89
  - stroke (cerebrovascular) Z82.3
  - substance abuse NEC Z81.4
    - alcohol Z81.1
    - drug NEC Z81.3
    - psychoactive NEC Z81.3
    - tobacco Z81.2
  - sudden
    - cardiac death Z82.41
    - infant death syndrome (SIDS) Z84.82
  - tobacco abuse Z81.2
  - violence, violent behavior Z81.8
  - visual loss Z82.1
- personal (of) *—see also* History, family (of)
  - abuse

History *(continued)*

- personal (of) *(continued)*
  - abuse *(continued)*
    - childhood Z62.819
      - physical Z62.810
      - psychological Z62.811
      - sexual Z62.810
    - adult Z91.419
      - physical and sexual Z91.410
      - psychological Z91.411
  - alcohol dependence F10.21
  - allergy (to) Z88.9
    - analgesic agent NEC Z88.6
    - anesthetic Z88.4
    - antibiotic agent NEC Z88.1
    - anti-infective agent NEC Z88.3
    - contrast media Z91.041
    - drugs, medicaments and biological substances Z88.9
      - specified NEC Z88.8
    - food Z91.018
      - additives Z91.02
      - eggs Z91.012
      - milk products Z91.011
      - peanuts Z91.010
      - seafood Z91.013
      - specified food NEC Z91.018
    - insect Z91.038
      - bee Z91.030
    - latex Z91.040
    - medicinal agents Z88.9
      - specified NEC Z88.8
    - narcotic agent NEC Z88.5
    - nonmedicinal agents Z91.048
    - penicillin Z88.0
    - serum Z88.7
    - specified NEC Z91.09
    - sulfonamides Z88.2
    - vaccine Z88.7
  - anaphylactic shock Z87.892
  - anaphylaxis Z87.892
  - behavioral disorders Z86.59
  - benign carcinoid tumor Z86.012
  - benign neoplasm Z86.018
    - carcinoid Z86.012
    - brain Z86.011
    - colonic polyps Z86.010
  - brain injury (traumatic) Z87.820
  - breast implant removal Z98.86
  - calculi, renal Z87.442
  - cancer *—see* History, personal (of), malignant neoplasm (of)
  - cardiac arrest (death), successfully resuscitated Z86.74
  - cerebral infarction without residual deficit Z86.73
  - cervical dysplasia Z87.410
  - chemotherapy for neoplastic condition Z92.21
  - childhood abuse *—see* History, personal (of), abuse
  - cleft lip (corrected) Z87.730
  - cleft palate (corrected) Z87.730
  - collapsed vertebra (healed) Z87.311
    - due to osteoporosis Z87.310
  - combat and operational stress reaction Z86.51
  - congenital malformation (corrected) Z87.798
    - circulatory system (corrected) Z87.74
    - digestive system (corrected) NEC Z87.738
    - ear (corrected) Z87.721
    - eye (corrected) Z87.720
    - face and neck (corrected) Z87.790

History *(continued)*
personal *(continued)*
congenital malformation *(continued)*

- personal *(continued)*
  - congenital malformation *(continued)*
    - genitourinary system (corrected) NEC Z87.718
    - heart (corrected) Z87.74
    - integument (corrected) Z87.76
    - limb(s) (corrected) Z87.76
    - musculoskeletal system (corrected) Z87.76
    - neck (corrected) Z87.790
    - nervous system (corrected) NEC Z87.728
    - respiratory system (corrected) Z87.75
    - sense organs (corrected) NEC Z87.728
    - specified NEC Z87.798
  - contraception Z92.0
  - deployment (military) Z91.82
  - diabetic foot ulcer Z86.31
  - disease or disorder (of) Z87.898
    - blood and blood-forming organs Z86.2
    - circulatory system Z86.79
      - specified condition NEC Z86.79
    - connective tissue NEC Z87.39
    - digestive system Z87.19
      - colonic polyp Z86.010
      - peptic ulcer disease Z87.11
      - specified condition NEC Z87.19
    - ear Z86.69
    - endocrine Z86.39
      - diabetic foot ulcer Z86.31
      - gestational diabetes Z86.32
      - specified type NEC Z86.39
    - eye Z86.69
    - genital (track) system NEC
      - female Z87.42
      - male Z87.438
    - hematological Z86.2
    - Hodgkin Z85.71
    - immune mechanism Z86.2
    - infectious Z86.19
      - malaria Z86.13
      - Methicillin resistant Staphylococcus aureus (MRSA) Z86.14
      - poliomyelitis Z86.12
      - specified NEC Z86.19
      - tuberculosis Z86.11
    - mental NEC Z86.59
    - metabolic Z86.39
      - diabetic foot ulcer Z86.31
      - gestational diabetes Z86.32
      - specified type NEC Z86.39
    - musculoskeletal NEC Z87.39
    - nervous system Z86.69
    - nutritional Z86.39
    - parasitic Z86.19
    - respiratory system NEC Z87.09
    - sense organs Z86.69
    - skin Z87.2
    - specified site or type NEC Z87.898
    - subcutaneous tissue Z87.2
    - trophoblastic Z87.59
    - urinary system NEC Z87.448
  - drug dependence *—see* Dependence, drug, by type, in remission
  - drug therapy
    - antineoplastic chemotherapy Z92.21
    - estrogen Z92.23
    - immunosupression Z92.25

History *(continued)*
personal *(continued)*
drug therapy *(continued)*

- personal *(continued)*
  - drug therapy *(continued)*
    - inhaled steroids Z92.240
    - monoclonal drug Z92.22
    - specified NEC Z92.29
    - steroid Z92.241
    - systemic steroids Z92.241
  - dysplasia
    - cervical (mild) (moderate) Z87.410
      - severe (grade III) Z86.001
    - prostatic Z87.430
    - vaginal (mild) (moderate) Z87.411 severe (grade III) Z86.008
    - vulvar (mild) (moderate) Z87.412
      - severe (grade III) Z86.008
  - embolism (venous) Z86.718
    - pulmonary Z86.711
  - encephalitis Z86.61
  - estrogen therapy Z92.23
  - extracorporeal membrane oxygenation (ECMO) Z92.81
  - failed moderate sedation Z92.83
  - failed conscious sedation Z92.83
  - fall, falling Z91.81
  - fracture (healed)
    - fatigue Z87.312
    - fragility Z87.310
    - osteoporosis Z87.310
    - pathological NEC Z87.311
    - stress Z87.312
    - traumatic Z87.81
  - gestational diabetes Z86.32
  - hepatitis
    - B Z86.19
    - C Z86.19
  - Hodgkin disease Z85.71
  - hyperthermia, malignant Z88.4
  - hypospadias (corrected) Z87.710
  - hysterectomy Z90.710
  - immunosupression therapy Z92.25
  - in situ neoplasm
    - breast Z86.000
    - cervix uteri Z86.001
    - specified NEC Z86.008
  - infection NEC Z86.19
    - central nervous system Z86.61
    - Methicillin resistant Staphylococcus aureus (MRSA) Z86.14
    - urinary (recurrent) (tract) Z87.440
  - injury NEC Z87.828
  - in utero procedure during pregnancy Z98.870
  - in utero procedure while a fetus Z98.871
  - irradiation Z92.3
  - kidney stones Z87.442
  - leukemia Z85.6
  - lymphoma (non-Hodgkin) Z85.72
  - malignant melanoma (skin) Z85.820
  - malignant neoplasm (of) Z85.9
    - accessory sinuses Z85.22
    - anus NEC Z85.048
      - carcinoid Z85.040
    - bladder Z85.51
    - bone Z85.830
    - brain Z85.841
    - breast Z85.3
    - bronchus NEC Z85.118
      - carcinoid Z85.110
    - carcinoid *—see* History, personal (of), malignant neoplasm, by site, carcinioid

History *(continued)*
personal *(continued)*
malignant neoplasm *(continued)*

- personal *(continued)*
  - malignant neoplasm *(continued)*
    - cervix Z85.41
    - colon NEC Z85.038
      - carcinoid Z85.030
    - digestive organ Z85.00
      - specified NEC Z85.09
    - endocrine gland NEC Z85.858
    - epididymis Z85.48
    - esophagus Z85.01
    - eye Z85.840
    - gastrointestinal tract *—see* History, malignant neoplasm, digestive organ
    - genital organ
      - female Z85.40
        - specified NEC Z85.44
      - male Z85.45
        - specified NEC Z85.49
    - hematopoietic NEC Z85.79
    - intrathoracic organ Z85.20
    - kidney NEC Z85.528
      - carcinoid Z85.520
    - large intestine NEC Z85.038
      - carcinoid Z85.030
    - larynx Z85.21
    - liver Z85.05
    - lung NEC Z85.118
      - carcinoid Z85.110
    - mediastinum Z85.29
    - Merkel cell Z85.821
    - middle ear Z85.22
    - nasal cavities Z85.22
    - nervous system NEC Z85.848
    - oral cavity Z85.819
      - specified site NEC Z85.818
    - ovary Z85.43
    - pancreas Z85.07
    - pharynx Z85.819
      - specified site NEC Z85.818
    - pelvis Z85.53
    - pleura Z85.29
    - prostate Z85.46
    - rectosigmoid junction NEC Z85.048
      - carcinoid Z85.040
    - rectum NEC Z85.048
      - carcinoid Z85.040
    - respiratory organ Z85.20
    - sinuses, accessory Z85.22
    - skin NEC Z85.828
      - melanoma Z85.820
      - Merkel cell Z85.821
    - small intestine NEC Z85.068
      - carcinoid Z85.060
    - soft tissue Z85.831
    - specified site NEC Z85.89
    - stomach NEC Z85.028
      - carcinoid Z85.020
    - testis Z85.47
    - thymus NEC Z85.238
      - carcinoid Z85.230
    - thyroid Z85.850
    - tongue Z85.810
    - trachea Z85.12
    - ureter Z85.54
    - urinary organ or tract Z85.50
      - specified NEC Z85.59
    - uterus Z85.42
  - maltreatment Z91.89
  - medical treatment NEC Z92.89
  - melanoma (malignant) (skin) Z85.820
  - meningitis Z86.61
  - mental disorder Z86.59
  - Merkel cell carcinoma (skin) Z85.821
  - Methicillin resistant Staphylococcus aureus (MRSA) Z86.14

History *(continued)*
- personal *(continued)*
  - military deployment Z91.82
  - military war, peacekeeping and humanitarian deployment (current or past conflict) Z91.82
  - myocardial infarction (old) I25.2
  - neglect (in)
    - adult Z91.412
    - childhood Z62.812
  - neoplasm
    - benign Z86.018
      - brain Z86.011
      - colon polyp Z86.010
    - in situ
      - breast Z86.000
      - cervix uteri Z86.001
      - specified NEC Z86.008
    - malignant *—see* History of, malignant neoplasm
    - uncertain behavior Z86.03
  - nephrotic syndrome Z87.441
  - nicotine dependence Z87.891
  - noncompliance with medical treatment or regimen *—see* Noncompliance
  - nutritional deficiency Z86.39
  - obstetric complications Z87.59
    - childbirth Z87.59
    - pregnancy Z87.59
    - pre-term labor Z87.51
    - puerperium Z87.59
  - osteoporosis fractures Z87.31
  - parasuicide (attempt) Z91.5
  - physical trauma NEC Z87.828
    - self-harm or suicide attempt Z91.5
  - poisoning NEC Z91.89
    - self-harm or suicide attempt Z91.5
  - poor personal hygiene Z91.89
  - pneumonia (recurrent) Z87.01
  - preterm labor Z87.51
  - prolonged reversible ischemic neurologic deficit (PRIND) Z86.73
  - procedure during pregnancy Z98.870
  - procedure while a fetus Z98.871
  - prostatic dysplasia Z87.430
  - psychological
    - abuse
      - adult Z91.411
      - child Z62.811
    - trauma, specified NEC Z91.49
  - radiation therapy Z92.3
  - removal
    - implant
      - breast Z98.86
  - renal calculi Z87.442
  - respiratory condition NEC Z87.09
  - retained foreign body fully removed Z87.821
  - risk factors NEC Z91.89
  - self-harm Z91.5
  - self-poisoning attempt Z91.5
  - sex reassignment Z87.890
  - sleep-wake cycle problem Z72.821
  - specified NEC Z87.898
  - steroid therapy (systemic) Z92.241
    - inhaled Z92.240
  - stroke without residual deficits Z86.73
  - substance abuse NEC F10-F19
  - sudden cardiac arrest Z86.74
  - sudden cardiac death successfully resuscitated Z86.74

History *(continued)*
- personal *(continued)*
  - suicide attempt Z91.5
  - surgery NEC Z98.890
    - with uterine scar Z98.891
    - sex reassignment Z87.890
    - transplant *—see* Transplant
  - thrombophlebitis Z86.72
  - thrombosis (venous) Z86.718
    - pulmonary Z86.711
  - tobacco dependence Z87.891
  - transient ischemic attack (TIA)
    - without residual deficits Z86.73
  - trauma (physical) NEC Z87.828
    - psychological NEC Z91.49
    - self-harm Z91.5
  - traumatic brain injury Z87.820
  - unhealthy sleep-wake cycle Z72.821
  - unintended awareness under general anesthesia Z92.84
  - urinary calculi Z87.442
  - urinary (recurrent) (tract) infection(s) Z87.440
  - uterine scar from previous surgery Z98.891
  - vaginal dysplasia Z87.411
  - venous thrombosis or embolism Z86.718
    - pulmonary Z86.711
  - vulvar dysplasia Z87.412

His-Werner disease A79.0

HIV (*see also* Human, immunodeficiency virus) B20
- laboratory evidence (nonconclusive) R75
- positive, seropositive Z21
- nonconclusive test (in infants) R75

Hives (bold) *—see* Urticaria

Hoarseness R49.0

Hobo Z59.0

Hodgkin disease *—see* Lymphoma, Hodgkin

Hodgson's disease I71.2
- ruptured I71.1

Hoffa-Kastert disease E88.89

Hoffa's disease E88.89

Hoffmann-Bouveret syndrome I47.9

Hoffmann's syndrome E03.9 *[G73.7]*

Hole (round)
- macula H35.34-
- retina (without detachment) *—see* Break, retina, round hole
  - with detachment *—see* Detachment, retina, with retinal, break

Holiday relief care Z75.5

Hollenhorst's plaque *—see* Occlusion, artery, retina

Hollow foot (congenital) Q66.7
- acquired *—see* Deformity, limb, foot, specified NEC

Holoprosencephaly Q04.2

Holt-Oram syndrome Q87.2

Homelessness Z59.0

Homesickness *—see* Disorder, adjustment

Homocystinemia, homocystinuria E72.11

Homogentisate 1,2-dioxygenase deficiency E70.29

Homologous serum hepatitis (prophylactic) (therapeutic) *—see* Hepatitis, viral, type B

Honeycomb lung J98.4
- congenital Q33.0

Hooded
- clitoris Q52.6
- penis Q55.69

Hookworm (anemia) (disease) (infection) (infestation) B76.9
- specified NEC B76.8

Hordeolum (eyelid) (externum) (recurrent) H00.019
- internum H00.029
  - left H00.026
    - lower H00.025
    - upper H00.024
  - right H00.023
    - lower H00.022
    - upper H00.021
- left H00.016
  - lower H00.015
  - upper H00.014
- right H00.013
  - lower H00.012
  - upper H00.011

Horn
- cutaneous L85.8
- nail L60.2
  - congenital Q84.6

Horner (-Claude Bernard) **syndrome** G90.2
- traumatic *—see* Injury, nerve, cervical sympathetic

Horseshoe kidney (congenital) Q63.1

Horton's headache or neuralgia G44.099
- intractable G44.091
- not intractable G44.099

Hospital hopper syndrome *—see* Disorder, factitious

Hospitalism in children *—see* Disorder, adjustment

Hostility R45.5
- towards child Z62.3

Hot flashes
- menopausal N95.1

Hourglass (contracture) *—see also* Contraction, hourglass
- stomach K31.89
  - congenital Q40.2
  - stricture K31.2

Household, housing circumstance affecting care Z59.9
- specified NEC Z59.8

Housemaid's knee *—see* Bursitis, prepatellar

Hudson (-Stähli) **line** (cornea) *—see* Pigmentation, cornea, anterior

Human
- bite (open wound) *—see also* Bite
  - intact skin surface *—see* Bite, superficial
- herpesvirus *—see* Herpes
- immunodeficiency virus (HIV) disease (infection) B20
  - asymptomatic status Z21
  - contact Z20.6
  - counseling Z71.7
  - dementia B20 *[F02.80]*
    - with behavioral disturbance B20 *[F02.81]*
  - exposure to Z20.6
  - laboratory evidence R75
  - type-2(HIV 2) as cause of disease classified elsewhere B97.35
- papillomavirus (HPV)
  - DNA test positive

Human *(continued)*
- papillomavirus *(continued)*
  - DNA test positive *(continued)*
    - high risk
      - cervix R87.810
      - vagina R87.811
    - low risk
      - cervix R87.820
      - vagina R87.821
  - screening for Z11.51
- T-cell lymphotropic virus
  - type-1(HTLV-I) infection B33.3
    - as cause of disease classified elsewhere B97.33
    - carrier Z22.6
  - type-2(HTLV-II) as cause of disease classified elsewhere B97.34

Humidifier lung or pneumonitis J67.7

Humiliation (experience) **in childhood** Z62.898

Humpback (acquired) *—see* Kyphosis

Hunchback (acquired) *—see* Kyphosis

Hunger T73.0
- air, psychogenic F45.8

Hungry bone syndrome E83.81

Hunner's ulcer *—see* Cystitis, chronic, interstitial

Hunter's
- glossitis D51.0
- syndrome E76.1

Huntington's disease or chorea G10
- with dementia G10 *[F02.80]*
  - with behavioral disturbance G10 *[F02.81]*

Hunt's
- disease or syndrome (herpetic geniculate ganglionitis) B02.21
  - dyssynergia cerebellaris myoclonica G11.1
- neuralgia B02.21

Hurler (-Scheie) **disease or syndrome** E76.02

Hurst's disease G36.1

Hurthle cell
- adenocarcinoma C73
- adenoma D34
- carcinoma C73
- tumor D34

Hutchinson-Boeck disease or syndrome *—see* Sarcoidosis

Hutchinson-Gilford disease or syndrome E34.8

Hutchinson's
- disease, meaning
  - angioma serpiginosum L81.7
  - pompholyx (cheiropompholyx) L30.1
  - prurigo estivalis L56.4
  - summer eruption or summer prurigo L56.4
- melanotic freckle *—see* Melanoma, in situ
  - malignant melanoma in *—see* Melanoma
- teeth or incisors (congenital syphilis) A50.52
- triad (congenital syphilis) A50.53

Hyalin plaque, sclera, senile H15.89

Hyaline membrane (disease) (lung) (pulmonary) (newborn) P22.0

Hyalinosis
- cutis (et mucosae) E78.89

Hyalinosis *(continued)*
focal and segmental (glomerular) (*see also* N00-N07 with fourth character .1) N05.1

Hyalitis, hyalosis, asteroid *—see also* Deposit, crystalline
syphilitic (late) A52.71

Hydatid
cyst or tumor *—see* Echinococcus
mole *—see* Hydatidiform mole
Morgagni
female Q50.5
male (epididymal) Q55.4
testicular Q55.29

Hydatidiform mole (benign) (complicating pregnancy) (delivered) (undelivered) O01.9
classical O01.0
complete O01.0
incomplete O01.1
invasive D39.2
malignant D39.2
partial O01.1

Hydatidosis *—see* Echinococcus

Hydradenitis (axillaris) (suppurative) L73.2

Hydradenoma *—see* Hidradenoma

Hydramnios O40.-

Hydrancephaly, hydranencephaly Q04.3
with spina bifida *—see* Spina bifida, with hydrocephalus

Hydrargyrism NEC *—see* Poisoning, mercury

Hydrarthrosis *—see also* Effusion, joint
gonococcal A54.42
intermittent M12.40
ankle M12.47-
elbow M12.42-
foot joint M12.47-
hand joint M12.44-
hip M12.45-
knee M12.46-
multiple site M12.49
shoulder M12.41-
specified joint NEC M12.48
wrist M12.43-
of yaws (early) (late) (*see also* subcategory M14.8-) A66.6
syphilitic (late) A52.77
congenital A50.55 *[M12.80]*

Hydremia D64.89

Hydrencephalocele (congenital) *—see* Encephalocele

Hydrencephalomeningocele (congenital) *—see* Encephalocele

Hydroa R23.8
aestivale L56.4
vacciniforme L56.4

Hydroadenitis (axillaris) (suppurative) L73.2

Hydrocalycosis *—see* Hydronephrosis

Hydrocele (spermatic cord) (testis) (tunica vaginalis) N43.3
canal of Nuck N94.89
communicating N43.2
congenital P83.5
congenital P83.5
encysted N43.0
female NEC N94.89
infected N43.1
newborn P83.5
round ligament N94.89
specified NEC N43.2

Hydrocele *(continued)*
spinalis *—see* Spina bifida
vulva N90.89

Hydrocephalus (acquired) (external) (internal) (malignant) (recurrent) G91.9
aqueduct Sylvius stricture Q03.0
causing disproportion O33.6
with obstructed labor O66.3
communicating G91.0
congenital (external) (internal) Q03.9
with spina bifida Q05.4
cervical Q05.0
dorsal Q05.1
lumbar Q05.2
lumbosacral Q05.2
sacral Q05.3
thoracic Q05.1
thoracolumbar Q05.1
specified NEC Q03.8
due to toxoplasmosis (congenital) P37.1
foramen Magendie block (acquired) G91.1
congenital (*see also* Hydrocephalus, congenital) Q03.1
in (due to)
infectious disease NEC B89 *[G91.4]*
neoplastic disease NEC (*see also* Neoplasm) G91.4
parasitic disease B89 *[G91.4]*
newborn Q03.9
with spina bifida *—see* Spina bifida, with hydrocephalus
noncommunicating G91.1
normal pressure G91.2
secondary G91.0
obstructive G91.1
otitic G93.2
post-traumatic NEC G91.3
secondary G91.4
post-traumatic G91.3
specified NEC G91.8
syphilitic, congenital A50.49

Hydrocolpos (congenital) N89.8

Hydrocystoma *—see* Neoplasm, skin, benign

Hydroencephalocele (congenital) *—see* Encephalocele

Hydroencephalomeningocele (congenital) *—see* Encephalocele

Hydrohematopneumothorax *—see* Hemothorax

Hydromeningitis *—see* Meningitis

Hydromeningocele (spinal) *—see also* Spina bifida
cranial *—see* Encephalocele

Hydrometra N85.8

Hydrometrocolpos N89.8

Hydromicrocephaly Q02

Hydromphalos (since birth) Q45.8

Hydromyelia Q06.4

Hydromyelocele *—see* Spina bifida

Hydronephrosis (atrophic) (early) (functionless) (intermittent) (primary) (secondary) **NEC** N13.30
with
infection N13.6
obstruction (by) (of)
renal calculus N13.2
with infection N13.6
ureteral NEC N13.1
with infection N13.6
calculus N13.2
with infection N13.6

Hydronephrosis *(continued)*
with *(continued)*
obstruction *(continued)*
ureteropelvic junction (congenital) Q62.11
acquired N13.0
with infection N13.6
ureteral stricture NEC N13.1
with infection N13.6
congenital Q62.0
due to acquired occlusion of ureteropelvic junction N13.0
specified type NEC N13.39
tuberculous A18.11

Hydropericarditis *—see* Pericarditis

Hydropericardium *—see* Pericarditis

Hydroperitoneum R18.8

Hydrophobia *—see* Rabies

Hydrophthalmos Q15.0

Hydropneumohemothorax *—see* Hemothorax

Hydropneumopericarditis *—see* Pericarditis

Hydropneumopericardium *—see* Pericarditis

Hydropneumothorax J94.8
traumatic *—see* Injury, intrathoracic, lung
tuberculous NEC A15.6

Hydrops R60.9
abdominis R18.8
articulorum intermittens *—see* Hydrarthrosis, intermittent
cardiac *—see* Failure, heart, congestive
causing obstructed labor (mother) O66.3
endolymphatic H81.0-
fetal *—see* Pregnancy, complicated by, hydrops, fetalis
fetalis P83.2
due to
ABO isoimmunization P56.0
alpha thalassemia D56.0
hemolytic disease P56.90
specified NEC P56.99
isoimmunization (ABO) (Rh) P56.0
other specified nonhemolytic disease NEC P83.2
Rh incompatibility P56.0
during pregnancy *—see* Pregnancy, complicated by, hydrops, fetalis
gallbladder K82.1
joint *—see* Effusion, joint
labyrinth H81.0-
newborn (idiopathic) P83.2
due to
ABO isoimmunization P56.0
alpha thalassemia D56.0
hemolytic disease P56.90
specified NEC P56.99
isoimmunization (ABO) (Rh) P56.0
Rh incompatibility P56.0
nutritional *—see* Malnutrition, severe
pericardium *—see* Pericarditis
pleura *—see* Hydrothorax
spermatic cord *—see* Hydrocele

Hydropyonephrosis N13.6

Hydrorachis Q06.4

Hydrorrhea (nasal) J34.89
pregnancy *—see* Rupture, membranes, premature

Hydrosadenitis (axillaris) (suppurative) L73.2

Hydrosalpinx (fallopian tube) (follicularis) N70.11

Hydrothorax (double) (pleura) J94.8
chylous (nonfilarial) I89.8
filarial (*see also* Infestation, filarial) B74.9 *[J91.8]*
traumatic *—see* Injury, intrathoracic
tuberculous NEC (non primary) A15.6

Hydroureter (*see also* Hydronephrosis) N13.4
with infection N13.6
congenital Q62.39

Hydroureteronephrosis *—see* Hydronephrosis

Hydrourethra N36.8

Hydroxykynureninuria E70.8

Hydroxylysinemia E72.3

Hydroxyprolinemia E72.59

Hygiene, sleep
abuse Z72.821
inadequate Z72.821
poor Z72.821

Hygroma (congenital) (cystic) D18.1
praepatellare, prepatellar *—see* Bursitis, prepatellar

Hymen *—see* condition

Hymenolepis, hymenolepiasis (diminuta) (infection) (infestation) (nana) B71.0

Hypalgesia R20.8

Hyperacidity (gastric) K31.89
psychogenic F45.8

Hyperactive, hyperactivity F90.9
basal cell, uterine cervix *—see* Dysplasia, cervix
bowel sounds R19.12
cervix epithelial (basal) *—see* Dysplasia, cervix
child F90.9
attention deficit *—see* Disorder, attention-deficit hyperactivity
detrusor muscle N32.81
gastrointestinal K31.89
psychogenic F45.8
nasal mucous membrane J34.3
stomach K31.89
thyroid (gland) *—see* Hyperthyroidism

Hyperacusis H93.23-

Hyperadrenalism E27.5

Hyperadrenocorticism E24.9
congenital E25.0
iatrogenic E24.2
correct substance properly administered *—see* Table of Drugs and Chemicals, by drug, adverse effect
overdose or wrong substance given or taken *—see* Table of Drugs and Chemicals, by drug, poisoning
not associated with Cushing's syndrome E27.0
pituitary-dependent E24.0

Hyperaldosteronism E26.9
familial (type I) E26.02
glucocorticoid-remediable E26.02

Hyperaldosteronism *(continued)*
- primary (due to (bilateral) adrenal hyperplasia) E26.09
- primary NEC E26.09
- secondary E26.1
- specified NEC E26.89

Hyperalgesia R20.8

Hyperalimentation R63.2
- carotene, carotin E67.1
- specified NEC E67.8
- vitamin
  - A E67.0
  - D E67.3

Hyperaminoaciduria
- arginine E72.21
- cystine E72.01
- lysine E72.3
- ornithine E72.4

Hyperammonemia (congenital) E72.20

Hyperazotemia —*see* Uremia

Hyperbetalipoproteinemia (familial) E78.00
- with prebetalipoproteinemia E78.2

Hyperbilirubinemia
- constitutional E80.6
- familial conjugated E80.6
- neonatal (transient) —*see* Jaundice, newborn

Hypercalcemia, hypocalciuric, familial E83.52

Hypercalciuria, idiopathic E83.52

Hypercapnia R06.89
- newborn P84

Hypercarotenemia, hypercarotinemia (dietary) E67.1

Hypercementosis K03.4

Hyperchloremia E87.8

Hyperchlorhydria K31.89
- neurotic F45.8
- psychogenic F45.8

Hypercholesterinemia —*see* Hypercholesterolemia

Hypercholesterolemia (essential) (primary) (pure) E78.00
- with hyperglyceridemia, endogenous E78.2
- dietary counseling and surveillance Z71.3
- familial E78.01
- hereditary E78.01

Hyperchylia gastrica, psychogenic F45.8

Hyperchylomicronemia (familial) (primary) E78.3
- with hyperbetalipoproteinemia E78.3

Hypercoagulable (state) D68.59
- activated protein C resistance D68.51
- antithrombin (III) deficiency D68.59
- factor V Leiden mutation D68.51
- primary NEC D68.59
- protein C deficiency D68.59
- protein S deficiency D68.59
- prothrombin gene mutation D68.52
- secondary D68.69
- specified NEC D68.69

Hypercoagulation (state) D68.59

Hypercorticalism, pituitary-dependent E24.0

Hypercorticosolism —*see* Cushing's, syndrome

Hypercorticosteronism E24.2
- correct substance properly administered —*see* Table of Drugs and Chemicals, by drug, adverse effect
- overdose or wrong substance given or taken —*see* Table of Drugs and Chemicals, by drug, poisoning

Hypercortisonism E24.2
- correct substance properly administered —*see* Table of Drugs and Chemicals, by drug, adverse effect
- overdose or wrong substance given or taken —*see* Table of Drugs and Chemicals, by drug, poisoning

Hyperekplexia Q89.8

Hyperelectrolytemia E87.8

Hyperemesis R11.10
- with nausea R11.2
- gravidarum (mild) O21.0
  - with
    - carbohydrate depletion O21.1
    - dehydration O21.1
    - electrolyte imbalance O21.1
    - metabolic disturbance O21.1
  - severe (with metabolic disturbance) O21.1
- projectile R11.12
- psychogenic F45.8

Hyperemia (acute) (passive) R68.89
- anal mucosa K62.89
- bladder N32.89
- cerebral I67.89
- conjunctiva H11.43-
- ear internal, acute H83.0
- enteric K59.8
- eye —*see* Hyperemia, conjunctiva
- eyelid (active) (passive) —*see* Disorder, eyelid, specified type NEC
- intestine K59.8
- iris —*see* Disorder, iris, vascular
- kidney N28.89
- labyrinth H83.0
- liver (active) K76.89
- lung (passive) —*see* Edema, lung
- pulmonary (passive) —*see* Edema, lung
- renal N28.89
- retina H35.89
- stomach K31.89

Hyperesthesia (body surface) R20.3
- larynx (reflex) J38.7
  - hysterical F44.89
- pharynx (reflex) J39.2
  - hysterical F44.89

Hyperestrogenism (drug-induced) (iatrogenic) E28.0

Hyperexplexia Q89.8

Hyperfibrinolysis —*see* Fibrinolysis

Hyperfructosemia E74.19

Hyperfunction
- adrenal cortex, not associated with Cushing's syndrome E27.0
  - medulla E27.5
    - adrenomedullary E27.5
  - virilism E25.9
    - congenital E25.0
- ovarian E28.8
- pancreas K86.89
- parathyroid (gland) E21.3
- pituitary (gland) (anterior) E22.9
  - specified NEC E22.8
- polyglandular E31.1
- testicular E29.0

Hypergammaglobulinemia D89.2
- polyclonal D89.0
- Waldenström D89.0

Hypergastrinemia E16.4

Hyperglobulinemia R77.1

Hyperglycemia, hyperglycemic (transient) R73.9
- coma —*see* Diabetes, by type, with coma
- postpancreatectomy E89.1

Hyperglyceridemia (endogenous) (essential) (familial) (hereditary) (pure) E78.1
- mixed E78.3

Hyperglycinemia (non-ketotic) E72.51

Hypergonadism
- ovarian E28.8
- testicular (primary) (infantile) E29.0

Hyperheparinemia D68.32

Hyperhidrosis, hyperidrosis R61
- focal
  - primary L74.519
    - axilla L74.510
    - face L74.511
    - palms L74.512
    - soles L74.513
  - secondary L74.52
- generalized R61
- localized
  - primary L74.519
    - axilla L74.510
    - face L74.511
    - palms L74.512
    - soles L74.513
  - secondary L74.52
- psychogenic F45.8
- secondary R61
  - focal L74.52

Hyperhistidinemia E70.41

Hyperhomocysteinemia E72.11

Hyperhydroxyprolinemia E72.59

Hyperinsulinism (functional) E16.1
- with
  - coma (hypoglycemic) E15
  - encephalopathy E16.1 *[G94]*
- ectopic E16.1
- therapeutic misadventure (from administration of insulin) T38.3

Hyperkalemia E87.5

Hyperkeratosis (*see also* Keratosis) L85.9
- cervix N88.0
- due to yaws (early) (late) (palmar or plantar) A66.3
- follicularis Q82.8
  - penetrans (in cutem) L87.0
- palmoplantaris climacterica L85.1
- pinta A67.1
- senile (with pruritus) L57.0
- universalis congenita Q80.8
- vocal cord J38.3
- vulva N90.4

Hyperkinesia, hyperkinetic (disease) (reaction) (syndrome) (childhood) (adolescence) —*see also* Disorder, attention-deficit hyperactivity
- heart I51.89

Hyperleucine-isoleucinemia E71.19

Hyperlipemia, hyperlipidemia E78.5
- combined E78.2
  - familial E78.4
- group
  - A E78.00
  - B E78.1

Hyperlipemia, hyperlipidemia *(continued)*
- group *(continued)*
  - C E78.2
  - D E78.3
- mixed E78.2
- specified NEC E78.4

Hyperlipidosis E75.6
- hereditary NEC E75.5

Hyperlipoproteinemia E78.5
- Fredrickson's type
  - I E78.3
  - IIa E78.00
  - IIb E78.2
  - III E78.2
  - IV E78.1
  - V E78.3
- low-density-lipoprotein-type (LDL) E78.00
- very-low-density-lipoprotein-type (VLDL) E78.1

Hyperlucent lung, unilateral J43.0

Hyperlysinemia E72.3

Hypermagnesemia E83.41
- neonatal P71.8

Hypermenorrhea N92.0

Hypermethioninemia E72.19

Hypermetropia (congenital) H52.0-

Hypermobility, hypermotility
- cecum —*see* Syndrome, irritable bowel
- coccyx —*see* subcategory M53.2
- colon —*see* Syndrome, irritable bowel
  - psychogenic F45.8
- ileum K58.9
- intestine (*see also* Syndrome, irritable bowel) K58.9
  - psychogenic F45.8
- meniscus (knee) —*see* Derangement, knee, meniscus
- scapula —*see* Instability, joint, shoulder
- stomach K31.89
  - psychogenic F45.8
- syndrome M35.7
- urethra N36.41
  - with intrinsic sphincter deficiency N36.43

Hypernasality R49.21

Hypernatremia E87.0

Hypernephroma C64.-

Hyperopia —*see* Hypermetropia

Hyperorexia nervosa F50.2

Hyperornithinemia E72.4

Hyperosmia R43.1

Hyperosmolality E87.0

Hyperostosis (monomelic) —*see also* Disorder, bone, density and structure, specified NEC
- ankylosing (spine) M48.10
  - cervical region M48.12
  - cervicothoracic region M48.13
  - lumbar region M48.16
  - lumbosacral region M48.17
  - multiple sites M48.19
  - occipito-atlanto-axial region M48.11
  - sacrococcygeal region M48.18
  - thoracic region M48.14
  - thoracolumbar region M48.15
- cortical (skull) M85.2
  - infantile M89.8X-
- frontal, internal of skull M85.2

Hyperostosis *(continued)*
- interna frontalis M85.2
- skeletal, diffuse idiopathic *—see* Hyperostosis, ankylosing
- skull M85.2
  - congenital Q75.8
- vertebral, ankylosing *—see* Hyperostosis, ankylosing

Hyperovarism E28.8

Hyperoxaluria (primary) E72.53

Hyperparathyroidism E21.3
- primary E21.0
- secondary (renal) N25.81
  - non-renal E21.1
- specified NEC E21.2
- tertiary E21.2

Hyperpathia R20.8

Hyperperistalsis R19.2
- psychogenic F45.8

Hyperpermeability, capillary I78.8

Hyperphagia R63.2

Hyperphenylalaninemia NEC E70.1

Hyperphoria (alternating) H50.53

Hyperphosphatemia E83.39

Hyperpiesis, hyperpiesia *—see* Hypertension

Hyperpigmentation *—see also* Pigmentation
- melanin NEC L81.4
- postinflammatory L81.0

Hyperpinealism E34.8

Hyperpituitarism E22.9

Hyperplasia, hyperplastic
- adenoids J35.2
- adrenal (capsule) (cortex) (gland) E27.8
  - with
    - sexual precocity (male) E25.9
      - congenital E25.0
    - virilism, adrenal E25.9
      - congenital E25.0
    - virilization (female) E25.9
      - congenital E25.0
  - congenital E25.0
    - salt-losing E25.0
- adrenomedullary E27.5
- angiolymphoid, eosinophilia (ALHE) D18.01
- appendix (lymphoid) K38.0
- artery, fibromuscular I77.3
- bone *—see also* Hypertrophy, bone
  - marrow D75.89
- breast *—see also* Hypertrophy, breast
  - ductal (atypical) N60.9-
- C-cell, thyroid E07.0
- cementation (tooth) (teeth) K03.4
- cervical gland R59.0
- cervix (uteri) (basal cell) (endometrium) (polypoid) *—see also* Dysplasia, cervix
  - congenital Q51.828
- clitoris, congenital Q52.6
- denture K06.2
- endocervicitis N72
- endometrium, endometrial (adenomatous) (benign) (cystic) (glandular) (glandular-cystic) (polypoid) N85.00
  - with atypia N85.02
  - cervix *—see* Dysplasia, cervix
  - complex (without atypia) N85.01
  - simple (without atypia) N85.01
- epithelial L85.9
  - focal, oral, including tongue K13.29
  - nipple N62

Hyperplasia, hyperplastic *(continued)*
- epithelial *(continued)*
  - skin L85.9
  - tongue K13.29
  - vaginal wall N89.3
- erythroid D75.89
- fibromuscular of artery (carotid) (renal) I77.3
- genital
  - female NEC N94.89
  - male N50.89
- gingiva K06.1
- glandularis cystica uteri (interstitialis) *(see also* Hyperplasia, endometrial) N85.00-
- gum K06.1
- hymen, congenital Q52.4
- irritative, edentulous (alveolar) K06.2
- jaw M26.09
  - alveolar M26.79
  - lower M26.03
    - alveolar M26.72
  - upper M26.01
    - alveolar M26.71
- kidney (congenital) Q63.3
- labia N90.69
  - epithelial N90.3
- liver (congenital) Q44.7
  - nodular, focal K76.89
- lymph gland or node R59.9
- mandible, mandibular M26.03
  - alveolar M26.72
  - unilateral condylar M27.8
- maxilla, maxillary M26.01
  - alveolar M26.71
- myometrium, myometrial N85.2
- neuroendocrine cell, of infancy J84.841
- nose
  - lymphoid J34.89
  - polypoid J33.9
- oral mucosa (irritative) K13.6
- organ or site, congenital NEC *—see* Anomaly, by site
- ovary N83.8
- palate, papillary (irritative) K13.6
- pancreatic islet cells E16.9
  - alpha E16.8
    - with excess
      - gastrin E16.4
      - glucagon E16.3
  - beta E16.1
- parathyroid (gland) E21.0
- pharynx (lymphoid) J39.2
- prostate (adenofibromatous) (nodular) N40.0
  - with lower urinary tract symptoms (LUTS) N40.1
  - without lower urinary tract symtpoms (LUTS) N40.0
- renal artery I77.89
- reticulo-endothelial (cell) D75.89
- salivary gland (any) K11.1
- Schimmelbusch's *—see* Mastopathy, cystic
- suprarenal capsule (gland) E27.8
- thymus (gland) (persistent) E32.0
- thyroid (gland) *—see* Goiter
- tonsils (faucial) (infective) (lingual) (lymphoid) J35.1
  - with adenoids J35.3
- unilateral condylar M27.8
- uterus, uterine N85.2
  - endometrium (glandular) *(see also* Hyperplasia, endometrial) N85.00-
- vulva N90.69
  - epithelial N90.3

Hyperpnea *—see* Hyperventilation

Hyperpotassemia E87.5

Hyperprebetalipoproteinemia (familial) E78.1

Hyperprolactinemia E22.1

Hyperprolinemia (type I) (type II) E72.59

Hyperproteinemia E88.09

Hyperprothrombinemia, causing coagulation factor deficiency D68.4

Hyperpyrexia R50.9
- heat (effects) T67.0
- malignant, due to anesthetic T88.3
- rheumatic *—see* Fever, rheumatic
- unknown origin R50.9

Hyper-reflexia R29.2

Hypersalivation K11.7

Hypersecretion
- ACTH (not associated with Cushing's syndrome) E27.0
  - pituitary E24.0
- adrenaline E27.5
- adrenomedullary E27.5
- androgen (testicular) E29.0
  - ovarian (drug-induced) (iatrogenic) E28.1
- calcitonin E07.0
- catecholamine E27.5
- corticoadrenal E24.9
- cortisol E24.9
- epinephrine E27.5
- estrogen E28.0
- gastric K31.89
  - psychogenic F45.8
- gastrin E16.4
- glucagon E16.3
- hormone(s)
  - ACTH (not associated with Cushing's syndrome) E27.0
    - pituitary E24.0
  - antidiuretic E22.2
  - growth E22.0
  - intestinal NEC E34.1
  - ovarian androgen E28.1
  - pituitary E22.9
  - testicular E29.0
  - thyroid stimulating E05.80
    - with thyroid storm E05.81
- insulin *—see* Hyperinsulinism
- lacrimal glands *—see* Epiphora
- medulloadrenal E27.5
- milk O92.6
- ovarian androgens E28.1
- salivary gland (any) K11.7
- thyrocalcitonin E07.0
- upper respiratory J39.8

Hypersegmentation, leukocytic, hereditary D72.0

Hypersensitive, hypersensitiveness, hypersensitivity *—see also* Allergy
- carotid sinus G90.01
- colon *—see* Irritable, colon
- drug T88.7
- gastrointestinal K52.29
  - immediate K52.29
  - psychogenic F45.8
- labyrinth H83.2
- pain R20.8
- pneumonitis *—see* Pneumonitis, allergic
- reaction T78.40
  - upper respiratory tract NEC J39.3

Hypersomnia (organic) G47.10
- due to
  - alcohol
    - abuse F10.182

Hypersomnia *(continued)*
- due to *(continued)*
  - alcohol *(continued)*
    - dependence F10.282
    - use F10.982
  - amphetamines
    - abuse F15.182
    - dependence F15.282
    - use F15.982
  - caffeine
    - abuse F15.182
    - dependence F15.282
    - use F15.982
  - cocaine
    - abuse F14.182
    - dependence F14.282
    - use F14.982
  - drug NEC
    - abuse F19.182
    - dependence F19.282
    - use F19.982
  - medical condition G47.14
  - mental disorder F51.13
  - opioid
    - abuse F11.182
    - dependence F11.282
    - use F11.982
  - psychoactive substance NEC
    - abuse F19.182
    - dependence F19.282
    - use F19.982
  - sedative, hypnotic, or anxiolytic
    - abuse F13.182
    - dependence F13.282
    - use F13.982
  - stimulant NEC
    - abuse F15.182
    - dependence F15.282
    - use F15.982
- idiopathic G47.11
  - with long sleep time G47.11
  - without long sleep time G47.12
- menstrual related G47.13
- nonorganic origin F51.11
  - specified NEC F51.19
- not due to a substance or known physiological condition F51.11
  - specified NEC F51.19
- primary F51.11
- recurrent G47.13
- specified NEC G47.19

Hypersplenia, hypersplenism D73.1

Hyperstimulation, ovaries (associated with induced ovulation) N98.1

Hypersusceptibility *—see* Allergy

Hypertelorism (ocular) (orbital) Q75.2

Hypertension, hypertensive (accelerated) (benign) (essential) (idiopathic) (malignant) (systemic) I10
- with
  - heart failure (congestive) I11.0
  - heart involvement (conditions in I50.-, I51.4- I51.9 due to hypertension) *—see* Hypertension, heart
  - kidney involvement *—see* Hypertension, kidney
- benign, intracranial G93.2
- borderline R03.0
- cardiorenal (disease) I13.10
  - with heart failure I13.0
    - with stage 1 through stage 4 chronic kidney disease I13.0
    - with stage 5 or end stage renal disease I13.2

Hypertension, hypertensive *(continued)*
cardiorenal *(continued)*
without heart failure I13.10
with stage 1 through stage 4 chronic kidney disease I13.10
with stage 5 or end stage renal disease I13.11
cardiovascular
disease (arteriosclerotic) (sclerotic) —*see* Hypertension, heart
renal (disease) —*see* Hypertension, cardiorenal
chronic venous —*see* Hypertension, venous (chronic)
complicating
childbirth (labor) O16.4
pre-existing O10.92
with
heart disease O12.12
with renal disease O10.32
pre-eclampsia O11.4
renal disease O10.22
with heart disease O10.32
essential O10.02
secondary O10.42
pregnancy O16.-
with edema (*see also* Pre-eclampsia) O14.9-
gestational (pregnancy induced) (without proteinuria) O13.-
with proteinuria O14.9-
mild pre-eclampsia O14.0-
moderate pre-eclampsia O14.0-
severe pre-eclampsia O14.1-
with hemolysis, elevated liver enzymes and low platelet count (HELLP) O14.2-
pre-existing O10.91-
with
heart disease O10.11-
with renal disease O10.31-
pre-eclampsia - *see* category O11
renal disease O10.21-
with heart disease O10.31-
essential O10.01-
secondary O10.41-
transient O13.-
puerperium, pre-existing O16.5
pre-existing
with
heart disease O10.13
with renal disease O10.33
pre-eclampsia O11.5
renal disease O10.23
with heart disease O10.33
essential O10.03
pregnancy-induced O13.9
secondary O10.43
crisis I16.9
due to
endocrine disorders I15.2
pheochromocytoma I15.2
renal disorders NEC I15.1
arterial I15.0
renovascular disorders I15.0
specified disease NEC I15.8
emergency I16.1
encephalopathy I67.4
gestational (without significant proteinuria) (pregnancy-induced) (transient) O13.-
with significant proteinuria —*see* Pre-eclampsia

Hypertension, hypertensive *(continued)*
gestational *(continued)*
complicating
delivery O13.4
puerperium O13.5
Goldblatt's I70.1
heart (disease) (conditions in I51.4-I51.9 due to hypertension) I11.9
with
heart failure (congestive) I11.0
kidney disease (chronic) —*see* Hypertension, cardiorenal
intracranial (benign) G93.2
kidney I12.9
with
heart disease —*see* Hypertension, cardiorenal
stage 5 chronic kidney disease (CKD) or end stage renal disease (ESRD) I12.0
stage 1 through stage 4 chronic kidney disease I12.9
lesser circulation I27.0
maternal O16.-
newborn P29.2
pulmonary (persistent) P29.30
ocular H40.05-
pancreatic duct - code to underlying condition
with chronic pancreatitis K86.1
portal (due to chronic liver disease) (idiopathic) K76.6
gastropathy K31.89
in (due to) schistosomiasis (bilharziasis) B65.9 *[K77]*
postoperative I97.3
psychogenic F45.8
pulmonary I27.20
with
cor pulmonale (chronic) I27.29
acute I26.09
right heart ventricular strain/failure I27.29
acute I26.09
right to left shunt related to congenital heart disease I27.83
unclear multifactorial mechanisms I27.29
arterial (associated) (drug-induced) (toxin-induced) I27.21
chronic thromboembolic I27.24
due to
hematologic disorders I27.29
left heart disease I27.22
lung diseases and hypoxia I27.23
metabolic disorders I27.29
specified systemic disorders NEC I27.29
group 1 (associated) (drug-induced) (toxin-induced) I27.21
group 2 I27.22
group 3 I27.23
group 4 I27.24
group 5 I27.29
of newborn (persistent) P29.30
secondary
arterial I27.21
specified NEC I27.29
primary (idiopathic) I27.0
renal —*see* Hypertension, kidney
renovascular I15.0
secondary NEC I15.9
due to
endocrine disorders I15.2
pheochromocytoma I15.2
renal disorders NEC I15.1
arterial I15.0

Hypertension, hypertensive *(continued)*
secondary *(continued)*
due to *(continued)*
renovascular disorders I15.0
specified NEC I15.8
transient, of pregnancy O13.-
urgency I16.0
venous (chronic)
due to
deep vein thrombosis —*see* Syndrome, postthrombotic
idiopathic I87.309
with
inflammation I87.32-
with ulcer I87.33-
specified complication NEC I87.39-
ulcer I87.31-
with inflammation I87.33-
asymptomatic I87.30-

Hypertensive urgency —*see* Hypertension

Hyperthecosis ovary E28.8

Hyperthermia (of unknown origin) —*see also* Hyperpyrexia
malignant, due to anesthesia T88.3
newborn P81.9
environmental P81.0

Hyperthyroid (recurrent) —*see* Hyperthyroidism

Hyperthyroidism (latent) (pre-adult) (recurrent) E05.90
with
goiter (diffuse) E05.00
with thyroid storm E05.01
nodular (multinodular) E05.20
with thyroid storm E05.21
uninodular E05.10
with thyroid storm E05.11
storm E05.91
due to ectopic thyroid tissue E05.30
with thyroid storm E05.31
neonatal, transitory P72.1
specified NEC E05.80
with thyroid storm E05.81

Hypertony, hypertonia, hypertonicity
bladder N31.8
congenital P94.1
stomach K31.89
psychogenic F45.8
uterus, uterine (contractions) (complicating delivery) O62.4

Hypertrichosis L68.9
congenital Q84.2
eyelid H02.869
left H02.866
lower H02.865
upper H02.864
right H02.863
lower H02.862
upper H02.861
lanuginosa Q84.2
acquired L68.1
localized L68.2
specified NEC L68.8

Hypertriglyceridemia, essential E78.1

Hypertrophy, hypertrophic
adenofibromatous, prostate —*see* Enlargement, enlarged, prostate
adenoids (infective) J35.2
with tonsils J35.3
adrenal cortex E27.8
alveolar process or ridge —*see* Anomaly, alveolar

Hypertrophy, hypertrophic *(continued)*
anal papillae K62.89
artery I77.89
congenital NEC Q27.8
digestive system Q27.8
lower limb Q27.8
specified site NEC Q27.8
upper limb Q27.8
auricular —*see* Hypertrophy, cardiac
Bartholin's gland N75.8
bile duct (common) (hepatic) K83.8
bladder (sphincter) (trigone) N32.89
bone M89.30
carpus M89.34-
clavicle M89.31-
femur M89.35-
fibula M89.36-
finger M89.34-
humerus M89.32-
ilium M89.359
ischium M89.359
metacarpus M89.34-
metatarsus M89.37-
multiple sites M89.39
neck M89.38
radius M89.33-
rib M89.38
scapula M89.31-
skull M89.38
tarsus M89.37-
tibia M89.36-
toe M89.37-
ulna M89.33-
vertebra M89.38
brain G93.89
breast N62
cystic —*see* Mastopathy, cystic
newborn P83.4
pubertal, massive N62
puerperal, postpartum —*see* Disorder, breast, specified type NEC
senile (parenchymatous) N62
cardiac (chronic) (idiopathic) I51.7
with rheumatic fever (conditions in I00)
active I01.8
inactive or quiescent (with chorea) I09.89
congenital NEC Q24.8
fatty —*see* Degeneration, myocardial
hypertensive —*see* Hypertension, heart
rheumatic (with chorea) I09.89
active or acute I01.8
with chorea I02.0
valve —*see* Endocarditis
cartilage —*see* Disorder, cartilage, specified type NEC
cecum —*see* Megacolon
cervix (uteri) N88.8
congenital Q51.828
elongation N88.4
clitoris (cirrhotic) N90.89
congenital Q52.6
colon —*see also* Megacolon
congenital Q43.2
conjunctiva, lymphoid H11.89
corpora cavernosa N48.89
cystic duct K82.8
duodenum K31.89
endometrium (glandular) (*see also* Hyperplasia, endometrial) N85.00-
cervix N88.8
epididymis N50.89
esophageal hiatus (congenital) Q79.1
with hernia —*see* Hernia, hiatal
eyelid —*see* Disorder, eyelid, specified type NEC

Hypertrophy, hypertrophic *(continued)*
- fat pad E65
  - knee (infrapatellar) (popliteal) (prepatellar) (retropatellar) M79.4
- foot (congenital) Q74.2
- frenulum, frenum (tongue) K14.8
  - lip K13.0
- gallbladder K82.8
- gastric mucosa K29.60
  - with bleeding K29.61
- gland, glandular R59.9
  - generalized R59.1
  - localized R59.0
- gum (mucous membrane) K06.1
- heart (idiopathic) —*see also* Hypertrophy, cardiac
  - valve (*see also* Endocarditis) I38
- hemifacial Q67.4
- hepatic —*see* Hypertrophy, liver
- hiatus (esophageal) Q79.1
- hilus gland R59.0
- hymen, congenital Q52.4
- ileum K63.89
- intestine NEC K63.89
- jejunum K63.89
- kidney (compensatory) N28.81
  - congenital Q63.3
- labium (majus) (minus) N90.60
- ligament —*see* Disorder, ligament
- lingual tonsil (infective) J35.1
  - with adenoids J35.3
- lip K13.0
  - congenital Q18.6
- liver R16.0
  - acute K76.89
  - congenital Q44.7
  - cirrhotic —*see* Cirrhosis, liver
  - fatty —*see* Fatty, liver
- lymph, lymphatic gland R59.9
  - generalized R59.1
  - localized R59.0
  - tuberculous —*see* Tuberculosis, lymph gland
- mammary gland —*see* Hypertrophy, breast
- Meckel's diverticulum (congenital) Q43.0
  - malignant —*see* Table of Neoplasms, small intestine, malignant
- median bar —*see* Hyperplasia, prostate
- meibomian gland —*see* Chalazion
- meniscus, knee, congenital Q74.1
- metatarsal head —*see* Hypertrophy, bone, metatarsus
- metatarsus —*see* Hypertrophy, bone, metatarsus
- mucous membrane
  - alveolar ridge K06.2
  - gum K06.1
  - nose (turbinate) J34.3
- muscle M62.89
- muscular coat, artery I77.89
- myocardium —*see also* Hypertrophy, cardiac
  - idiopathic I42.2
- myometrium N85.2
- nail L60.2
  - congenital Q84.5
- nasal J34.89
  - alae J34.89
  - bone J34.89
  - cartilage J34.89
  - mucous membrane (septum) J34.3
  - sinus J34.89
  - turbinate J34.3
- nasopharynx, lymphoid (infectional) (tissue) (wall) J35.2
- nipple N62

Hypertrophy, hypertrophic *(continued)*
- organ or site, congenital NEC —*see* Anomaly, by site
- ovary N83.8
- palate (hard) M27.8
  - soft K13.79
- pancreas, congenital Q45.3
- parathyroid (gland) E21.0
- parotid gland K11.1
- penis N48.89
- pharyngeal tonsil J35.2
- pharynx J39.2
  - lymphoid (infectional) (tissue) (wall) J35.2
- pituitary (anterior) (fossa) (gland) E23.6
- prepuce (congenital) N47.8
  - female N90.89
- prostate —*see* Enlargement, enlarged, prostate
  - congenital Q55.4
- pseudomuscular G71.0
- pylorus (adult) (muscle) (sphincter) K31.1
  - congenital or infantile Q40.0
- rectal, rectum (sphincter) K62.89
- rhinitis (turbinate) J31.0
- salivary gland (any) K11.1
  - congenital Q38.4
- scaphoid (tarsal) —*see* Hypertrophy, bone, tarsus
- scar L91.0
- scrotum N50.89
- seminal vesicle N50.89
- sigmoid —*see* Megacolon
- skin L91.9
  - specified NEC L91.8
- spermatic cord N50.89
- spleen —*see* Splenomegaly
- spondylitis —*see* Spondylosis
- stomach K31.89
- sublingual gland K11.1
- submandibular gland K11.1
- suprarenal cortex (gland) E27.8
- synovial NEC M67.20
  - acromioclavicular M67.21-
  - ankle M67.27-
  - elbow M67.22-
  - foot M67.27-
  - hand M67.24-
  - hip M67.25-
  - knee M67.26-
  - multiple sites M67.29
  - specified site NEC M67.28
  - wrist M67.23-
- tendon —*see* Disorder, tendon, specified type NEC
- testis N44.8
  - congenital Q55.29
- thymic, thymus (gland) (congenital) E32.0
- thyroid (gland) —*see* Goiter
- toe (congenital) Q74.2
  - acquired —*see also* Deformity, toe, specified NEC
- tongue K14.8
  - congenital Q38.2
  - papillae (foliate) K14.3
- tonsils (faucial) (infective) (lingual) (lymphoid) J35.1
  - with adenoids J35.3
- tunica vaginalis N50.89
- ureter N28.89
- urethra N36.8
- uterus N85.2
  - neck (with elongation) N88.4
  - puerperal O90.89
- uvula K13.79
- vagina N89.8
- vas deferens N50.89

Hypertrophy, hypertrophic *(continued)*
- vein I87.8
- ventricle, ventricular (heart) —*see also* Hypertrophy, cardiac
  - congenital Q24.8
  - in tetralogy of Fallot Q21.3
- verumontanum N36.8
- vocal cord J38.3
- vulva N90.60
  - stasis (nonfilarial) N90.69

Hypertropia H50.2-

Hypertyrosinemia E70.21

Hyperuricemia (asymptomatic) E79.0

Hypervalinemia E71.19

Hyperventilation (tetany) R06.4
- hysterical F45.8
- psychogenic F45.8
- syndrome F45.8

Hypervitaminosis (dietary) **NEC** E67.8
- A E67.0
  - administered as drug (prolonged intake) —*see* Table of Drugs and Chemicals, vitamins, adverse effect
  - overdose or wrong substance given or taken —*see* Table of Drugs and Chemicals, vitamins, poisoning
- B6 E67.2
- D E67.3
  - administered as drug (prolonged intake) —*see* Table of Drugs and Chemicals, vitamins, adverse effect
  - overdose or wrong substance given or taken —*see* Table of Drugs and Chemicals, vitamins, poisoning
- K E67.8
  - administered as drug (prolonged intake) —*see* Table of Drugs and Chemicals, vitamins, adverse effect
  - overdose or wrong substance given or taken —*see* Table of Drugs and Chemicals, vitamins, poisoning

Hypervolemia E87.70
- specified NEC E87.79

Hypesthesia R20.1
- cornea —*see* Anesthesia, cornea

Hyphema H21.0-
- traumatic S05.1-

Hypoacidity, gastric K31.89
- psychogenic F45.8

Hypoadrenalism, hypoadrenia E27.40
- primary E27.1
- tuberculous A18.7

Hypoadrenocorticism E27.40
- pituitary E23.0
- primary E27.1

Hypoalbuminemia E88.09

Hypoaldosteronism E27.40

Hypoalphalipoproteinemia E78.6

Hypobarism T70.29

Hypobaropathy T70.29

Hypobetalipoproteinemia (familial) E78.6

Hypocalcemia E83.51
- dietary E58
- neonatal P71.1
  - due to cow's milk P71.0
- phosphate-loading (newborn) P71.1

Hypochloremia E87.8

Hypochlorhydria K31.89
- neurotic F45.8
- psychogenic F45.8

Hypochondria, hypochondriac, hypochondriasis (reaction) F45.21
- sleep F51.03

Hypochondrogenesis Q77.0

Hypochondroplasia Q77.4

Hypochromasia, blood cells D50.8

Hypodontia —*see* Anodontia

Hypoeosinophilia D72.89

Hypoesthesia R20.1

Hypofibrinogenemia D68.8
- acquired D65
- congenital (hereditary) D68.2

Hypofunction
- adrenocortical E27.40
  - drug-induced E27.3
  - postprocedural E89.6
  - primary E27.1
- adrenomedullary, postprocedural E89.6
- cerebral R29.818
- corticoadrenal NEC E27.40
- intestinal K59.8
- labyrinth H83.2
- ovary E28.39
- pituitary (gland) (anterior) E23.0
- testicular E29.1
  - postprocedural (postsurgical) (postirradiation) (iatrogenic) E89.5

Hypogalactia O92.4

Hypogammaglobulinemia (*see also* Agammaglobulinemia) D80.1
- hereditary D80.0
- nonfamilial D80.1
- transient, of infancy D80.7

Hypogenitalism (congenital) —*see* Hypogonadism

Hypoglossia Q38.3

Hypoglycemia (spontaneous) E16.2
- coma E15
  - diabetic —*see* Diabetes, by type, with hypoglycemia, with coma
- diabetic —*see* Diabetes, hypoglycemia
- dietary counseling and surveillance Z71.3
- drug-induced E16.0
  - with coma (nondiabetic) E15
- due to insulin E16.0
  - with coma (nondiabetic) E15
  - therapeutic misadventure —*see* subcategory T38.3
- functional, nonhyperinsulinemic E16.1
- iatrogenic E16.0
  - with coma (nondiabetic) E15
- in infant of diabetic mother P70.1
  - gestational diabetes P70.0
- infantile E16.1
- leucine-induced E71.19
- neonatal (transitory) P70.4
  - iatrogenic P70.3
- reactive (not drug-induced) E16.1
- transitory neonatal P70.4

Hypogonadism
- female E28.39
- hypogonadotropic E23.0
- male E29.1
- ovarian (primary) E28.39
- pituitary E23.0
- testicular (primary) E29.1

Hypohidrosis, hypoidrosis L74.4

Hypoinsulinemia, postprocedural E89.1

Hypokalemia E87.6

Hypoleukocytosis *—see* Agranulocytosis

Hypolipoproteinemia (alpha) (beta) E78.6

Hypomagnesemia E83.42
- neonatal P71.2

Hypomania, hypomanic reaction F30.8

Hypomenorrhea *—see* Oligomenorrhea

Hypometabolism R63.8

Hypomotility
- gastrointestinal (tract) K31.89
  - psychogenic F45.8
- intestine K59.8
  - psychogenic F45.8
- stomach K31.89
  - psychogenic F45.8

Hyponasality R49.22

Hyponatremia E87.1

Hypo-osmolality E87.1

Hypo-ovarianism, hypo-ovarism E28.39

Hypoparathyroidism E20.9
- familial E20.8
- idiopathic E20.0
- neonatal, transitory P71.4
- postprocedural E89.2
- specified NEC E20.8

Hypoperfusion (in)
- newborn P96.89

Hypopharyngitis *—see* Laryngopharyngitis

Hypophoria H50.53

Hypophosphatemia, hypophosphatasia (acquired) (congenital) (renal) E83.39
- familial E83.31

Hypophyseal, hypophysis *—see also* condition
- dwarfism E23.0
- gigantism E22.0

Hypopiesis *—see* Hypotension

Hypopinealism E34.8

Hypopituitarism (juvenile) E23.0
- drug-induced E23.1
- due to
  - hypophysectomy E89.3
  - radiotherapy E89.3
- iatrogenic NEC E23.1
- postirradiation E89.3
- postpartum O99.285
- postprocedural E89.3

Hypoplasia, hypoplastic
- adrenal (gland), congenital Q89.1
- alimentary tract, congenital Q45.8
  - upper Q40.8
- anus, anal (canal) Q42.3
  - with fistula Q42.2
- aorta, aortic Q25.42
  - ascending, in hypoplastic left heart syndrome Q23.4
  - valve Q23.1
    - in hypoplastic left heart syndrome Q23.4
- areola, congenital Q83.8
- arm (congenital) *—see* Defect, reduction, upper limb

Hypoplasia, hypoplastic *(continued)*
- artery (peripheral) Q27.8
  - brain (congenital) Q28.3
  - coronary Q24.5
  - digestive system Q27.8
  - lower limb Q27.8
  - pulmonary Q25.79
    - functional, unilateral J43.0
  - retinal (congenital) Q14.1
  - specified site NEC Q27.8
  - umbilical Q27.0
  - upper limb Q27.8
- auditory canal Q17.8
  - causing impairment of hearing Q16.9
- biliary duct or passage Q44.5
- bone NOS Q79.9
  - face Q75.8
  - marrow D61.9
    - megakaryocytic D69.49
  - skull *—see* Hypoplasia, skull
- brain Q02
  - gyri Q04.3
  - part of Q04.3
- breast (areola) N64.82
- bronchus Q32.4
- cardiac Q24.8
- carpus *—see* Defect, reduction, upper limb, specified type NEC
- cartilage hair Q78.8
- cecum Q42.8
- cementum K00.4
- cephalic Q02
- cerebellum Q04.3
- cervix (uteri), congenital Q51.821
- clavicle (congenital) Q74.0
- coccyx Q76.49
- colon Q42.9
  - specified NEC Q42.8
- corpus callosum Q04.0
- cricoid cartilage Q31.2
- digestive organ(s) or tract NEC Q45.8
  - upper (congenital) Q40.8
- ear (auricle) (lobe) Q17.2
  - middle Q16.4
- enamel of teeth (neonatal) (postnatal) (prenatal) K00.4
- endocrine (gland) NEC Q89.2
- endometrium N85.8
- epididymis (congenital) Q55.4
- epiglottis Q31.2
- erythroid, congenital D61.01
- esophagus (congenital) Q39.8
- eustachian tube Q17.8
- eye Q11.2
- eyelid (congenital) Q10.3
- face Q18.8
  - bone(s) Q75.8
- femur (congenital) *—see* Defect, reduction, lower limb, specified type NEC
- fibula (congenital) *—see* Defect, reduction, lower limb, specified type NEC
- finger (congenital) *—see* Defect, reduction, upper limb, specified type NEC
- focal dermal Q82.8
- foot *—see* Defect, reduction, lower limb, specified type NEC
- gallbladder Q44.0
- genitalia, genital organ(s)
  - female, congenital Q52.8
    - external Q52.79
    - internal NEC Q52.8
  - in adiposogenital dystrophy E23.6
- glottis Q31.2
- hair Q84.2

Hypoplasia, hypoplastic *(continued)*
- hand (congenital) *—see* Defect, reduction, upper limb, specified type NEC
- heart Q24.8
- humerus (congenital) *—see* Defect, reduction, upper limb, specified type NEC
- intestine (small) Q41.9
  - large Q42.9
    - specified NEC Q42.8
- jaw M26.09
  - alveolar M26.79
  - lower M26.04
    - alveolar M26.74
  - upper M26.02
    - alveolar M26.73
- kidney(s) Q60.5
  - bilateral Q60.4
  - unilateral Q60.3
- labium (majus) (minus), congenital Q52.79
- larynx Q31.2
- left heart syndrome Q23.4
- leg (congenital) *—see* Defect, reduction, lower limb
- limb Q73.8
  - lower (congenital) *—see* Defect, reduction, lower limb
  - upper (congenital) *—see* Defect, reduction, upper limb
- liver Q44.7
- lung (lobe) (not associated with short gestation) Q33.6
  - associated with immaturity, low birth weight, prematurity, or short gestation P28.0
- mammary (areola), congenital Q83.8
- mandible, mandibular M26.04
  - alveolar M26.74
  - unilateral condylar M27.8
- maxillary M26.02
  - alveolar M26.73
- medullary D61.9
- megakaryocytic D69.49
- metacarpus *—see* Defect, reduction, upper limb, specified type NEC
- metatarsus *—see* Defect, reduction, lower limb, specified type NEC
- muscle Q79.8
- nail(s) Q84.6
- nose, nasal Q30.1
- optic nerve H47.03-
- osseous meatus (ear) Q17.8
- ovary, congenital Q50.39
- pancreas Q45.0
- parathyroid (gland) Q89.2
- parotid gland Q38.4
- patella Q74.1
- pelvis, pelvic girdle Q74.2
- penis (congenital) Q55.62
- peripheral vascular system Q27.8
  - digestive system Q27.8
  - lower limb Q27.8
  - specified site NEC Q27.8
  - upper limb Q27.8
- pituitary (gland) (congenital) Q89.2
- pulmonary (not associated with short gestation) Q33.6
  - artery, functional J43.0
  - associated with short gestation P28.0
- radioulnar *—see* Defect, reduction, upper limb, specified type NEC
- radius *—see* Defect, reduction, upper limb
- rectum Q42.1
  - with fistula Q42.0
- respiratory system NEC Q34.8
- rib Q76.6

Hypoplasia, hypoplastic *(continued)*
- right heart syndrome Q22.6
- sacrum Q76.49
- scapula Q74.0
- scrotum Q55.1
- shoulder girdle Q74.0
- skin Q82.8
- skull (bone) Q75.8
  - with
    - anencephaly Q00.0
    - encephalocele *—see* Encephalocele
    - hydrocephalus Q03.9
      - with spina bifida *—see* Spina bifida, by site, with hydrocephalus
    - microcephaly Q02
- spinal (cord) (ventral horn cell) Q06.1
- spine Q76.49
- sternum Q76.7
- tarsus *—see* Defect, reduction, lower limb, specified type NEC
- testis Q55.1
- thymic, with immunodeficiency D82.1
- thymus (gland) Q89.2
  - with immunodeficiency D82.1
- thyroid (gland) E03.1
  - cartilage Q31.2
- tibiofibular (congenital) *—see* Defect, reduction, lower limb, specified type NEC
- toe *—see* Defect, reduction, lower limb, specified type NEC
- tongue Q38.3
- Turner's K00.4
- ulna (congenital) *—see* Defect, reduction, upper limb
- umbilical artery Q27.0
- unilateral condylar M27.8
- ureter Q62.8
- uterus, congenital Q51.811
- vagina Q52.4
- vascular NEC peripheral Q27.8
  - brain Q28.3
  - digestive system Q27.8
  - lower limb Q27.8
  - specified site NEC Q27.8
  - upper limb Q27.8
- vein(s) (peripheral) Q27.8
  - brain Q28.3
  - digestive system Q27.8
  - great Q26.8
  - lower limb Q27.8
  - specified site NEC Q27.8
  - upper limb Q27.8
- vena cava (inferior) (superior) Q26.8
- vertebra Q76.49
- vulva, congenital Q52.79
- zonule (ciliary) Q12.8

Hypopnea, obstructive sleep apnea G47.33

Hypopotassemia E87.6

Hypoproconvertinemia, congenital (hereditary) D68.2

Hypoproteinemia E77.8

Hypoprothrombinemia (congenital) (hereditary) (idiopathic) D68.2
- acquired D68.4
- newborn, transient P61.6

Hypoptyalism K11.7

Hypopyon (eye) (anterior chamber) *—see* Iridocyclitis, acute, hypopyon

Hypopyrexia R68.0

Hyporeflexia R29.2

Hyposecretion
- ACTH E23.0
- antidiuretic hormone E23.2

Hyposecretion *(continued)*
- ovary E28.39
- salivary gland (any) K11.7
- vasopressin E23.2

Hyposegmentation, leukocytic, hereditary D72.0

Hyposiderinemia D50.9

Hypospadias Q54.9
- balanic Q54.0
- coronal Q54.0
- glandular Q54.0
- penile Q54.1
- penoscrotal Q54.2
- perineal Q54.3
- specified NEC Q54.8

Hypospermatogenesis *—see* Oligospermia

Hyposplenism D73.0

Hypostasis pulmonary, passive *—see* Edema, lung

Hypostatic *—see* condition

Hyposthenuria N28.89

Hypotension (arterial) (constitutional) I95.9
- chronic I95.89
- due to (of) hemodialysis I95.3
- drug-induced I95.2
- iatrogenic I95.89
- idiopathic (permanent) I95.0
- intracranial, following ventricular shunting (ventriculostomy) G97.2
- intra-dialytic I95.3
- maternal, syndrome (following labor and delivery) O26.5-
- neurogenic, orthostatic G90.3
- orthostatic (chronic) I95.1
  - due to drugs I95.2
  - neurogenic G90.3
- postoperative I95.81
- postural I95.1
- specified NEC I95.89

Hypothermia (accidental) T68
- due to anesthesia, anesthetic T88.51
- low environmental temperature T68
- neonatal P80.9
  - environmental (mild) NEC P80.8
  - mild P80.8
  - severe (chronic) (cold injury syndrome) P80.0
  - specified NEC P80.8
- not associated with low environmental temperature R68.0

Hypothyroidism (acquired) E03.9
- autoimmune - *see* Thyroiditis, autoimmune
- congenital (without goiter) E03.1
  - with goiter (diffuse) E03.0
- due to
  - exogenous substance NEC E03.2
  - iodine-deficiency, acquired E01.8
    - subclinical E02
  - irradiation therapy E89.0
  - medicament NEC E03.2
  - P-aminosalicylic acid (PAS) E03.2
  - phenylbutazone E03.2
  - resorcinol E03.2
  - sulfonamide E03.2
  - surgery E89.0
  - thiourea group drugs E03.2
- iatrogenic NEC E03.2
- iodine-deficiency (acquired) E01.8
  - congenital *—see* Syndrome, iodine- deficiency, congenital
  - subclinical E02
- neonatal, transitory P72.2
- postinfectious E03.3
- postirradiation E89.0

Hypothyroidism *(continued)*
- postprocedural E89.0
- postsurgical E89.0
- specified NEC E03.8
- subclinical, iodine-deficiency related E02

Hypotonia, hypotonicity, hypotony
- bladder N31.2
- congenital (benign) P94.2
- eye *—see* Disorder, globe, hypotony

Hypotrichosis *—see* Alopecia

Hypotropia H50.2-

Hypoventilation R06.89
- congenital central alveolar G47.35
- sleep related
  - idiopathic nonobstructive alveolar G47.34
  - in conditions classified elsewhere G47.36

Hypovitaminosis *—see* Deficiency, vitamin

Hypovolemia E86.1
- surgical shock T81.19
- traumatic (shock) T79.4

Hypoxemia R09.02
- newborn P84
- sleep related, in conditions classified elsewhere G47.36

Hypoxia (*see also* Anoxia) R09.02
- cerebral, during a procedure NEC G97.81
  - postprocedural NEC G97.82
- intrauterine P84
- myocardial *—see* Insufficiency, coronary
- newborn P84
- sleep-related G47.34

Hypsarhythmia *—see* Epilepsy, generalized, specified NEC

Hysteralgia, pregnant uterus O26.89-

Hysteria, hysterical (conversion) (dissociative state) F44.9
- anxiety F41.8
- convulsions F44.5
- psychosis, acute F44.9

Hysteroepilepsy F44.5

I

IBDU (colonic inflammatory bowel disease unclassified) K52.3

Ichthyoparasitism due to Vandellia cirrhosa B88.8

Ichthyosis (congenital) Q80.9
- acquired L85.0
- fetalis Q80.4
- hystrix Q80.8
- lamellar Q80.2
- lingual K13.29
- palmaris and plantaris Q82.8
- simplex Q80.0
- vera Q80.8
- vulgaris Q80.0
- X-linked Q80.1

Ichthyotoxism *—see* Poisoning, fish
- bacterial *—see* Intoxication, foodborne

Icteroanemia, hemolytic (acquired) D59.9
- congenital *—see* Spherocytosis

Icterus *—see also* Jaundice
- conjunctiva R17
- newborn P59.9
- gravis, newborn P55.0

Icterus *(continued)*
- hematogenous (acquired) D59.9
- hemolytic (acquired) D59.9
  - congenital *—see* Spherocytosis
- hemorrhagic (acute) (leptospiral) (spirochetal) A27.0
  - newborn P53
- infectious B15.9
  - with hepatic coma B15.0
  - leptospiral A27.0
  - spirochetal A27.0
- neonatorum *—see* Jaundice, newborn
- spirochetal A27.0

Ictus solaris, solis T67.0

Ideation
- homicidal R45.850
- suicidal R45.851

Identity disorder (child) F64.9
- gender role F64.2
- psychosexual F64.2

Id reaction (due to bacteria) L30.2

Idioglossia F80.0

Idiopathic *—see* condition

Idiot, idiocy (congenital) F73
- amaurotic (Bielschowsky (-Jansky)) (family) (infantile (late)) (juvenile (late)) (Vogt-Spielmeyer) E75.4
- microcephalic Q02

IgE asthma J45.909

IIAC (idiopathic infantile arterial calcification) Q28.8

Ileitis (chronic) (noninfectious) *—see also* Enteritis K52.9
- backwash *—see* Pancolitis, ulcerative (chronic)
- infectious A09
- regional (ulcerative) *—see* Enteritis, regional, small intestine
- segmental *—see* Enteritis, regional
- terminal (ulcerative) *—see* Enteritis, regional, small intestine

Ileocolitis (*see also* Enteritis) K52.9
- regional *—see* Enteritis, regional
- infectious A09
- ulcerative K51.0-

Ileostomy
- attention to Z43.2
- malfunctioning K94.13
- status Z93.2
  - with complication *—see* Complications, enterostomy

Ileotyphus *—see* Typhoid

Ileum *—see* condition

Ileus (bowel) (colon) (inhibitory) (intestine) K56.7
- adynamic K56.0
- due to gallstone (in intestine) K56.3
- duodenal (chronic) K31.5
- gallstone K56.3
- mechanical NEC (*see also* Obstruction, intestine, specified NEC) K56.699
- meconium P76.0
  - in cystic fibrosis E84.11
  - meaning meconium plug (without cystic fibrosis) P76.0
- myxedema K59.8
- neurogenic K56.0
  - Hirschsprung's disease or megacolon Q43.1
- newborn
  - due to meconium P76.0
    - in cystic fibrosis E84.11
    - meaning meconium plug (without cystic fibrosis) P76.0
  - transitory P76.1

Ileus *(continued)*
- obstructive (*see also* Obstruction, intestine, specified NEC) K56.699
- paralytic K56.0
- postoperative K91.89

Iliac *—see* condition

Iliotibial band syndrome M76.3-

Illiteracy Z55.0

Illness (*see also* Disease) R69
- manic-depressive *—see* Disorder, bipolar

Imbalance R26.89
- autonomic G90.8
- constituents of food intake E63.1
- electrolyte E87.8
  - with
    - abortion *—see* Abortion by type, complicated by, electrolyte imbalance
    - molar pregnancy O08.5
  - due to hyperemesis gravidarum O21.1
  - following ectopic or molar pregnancy O08.5
  - neonatal, transitory NEC P74.4
    - potassium P74.3
    - sodium P74.2
- endocrine E34.9
- eye muscle NOS H50.9
- hormone E34.9
- hysterical F44.4
- labyrinth H83.2
- posture R29.3
- protein-energy *—see* Malnutrition
- sympathetic G90.8

Imbecile, imbecility (I.Q.35-49) F71

Imbedding, intrauterine device T83.39

Imbibition, cholesterol (gallbladder) K82.4

Imbrication, teeth,, fully erupted M26.30

Imerslund (-Gräsbeck) **syndrome** D51.1

Immature *—see also* Immaturity
- birth (less than 37 completed weeks) *—see* Preterm, newborn
  - extremely (less than 28 completed weeks) *—see* Immaturity, extreme
- personality F60.89

Immaturity (less than 37 completed weeks) *—see also* Preterm, newborn
- extreme of newborn (less than 28 completed weeks of gestation) (less than 196 completed days of gestation) (unspecified weeks of gestation) P07.20
  - gestational age
    - 23 completed weeks (23 weeks, 0 days through 23 weeks, 6 days) P07.22
    - 24 completed weeks (24 weeks, 0 days through 24 weeks, 6 days) P07.23
    - 25 completed weeks (25 weeks, 0 days through 25 weeks, 6 days) P07.24
    - 26 completed weeks (26 weeks, 0 days through 26 weeks, 6 days) P07.25
    - 27 completed weeks (27 weeks, 0 days through 27 weeks, 6 days) P07.26
    - less than 23 completed weeks P07.21
- fetus or infant light-for-dates *—see* Light-for-dates

Immaturity *(continued)*
- lung, newborn P28.0
- organ or site NEC *—see* Hypoplasia
- pulmonary, newborn P28.0
- reaction F60.89
- sexual (female) (male), after puberty E30.0

Immersion T75.1
- hand T69.01-
- foot T69.02-

Immobile, immobility
- complete, due to severe physical disability or frailty R53.2
- intestine K59.8
- syndrome (paraplegic) M62.3

Immune reconstitution (inflammatory) **syndrome [IRIS]** D89.3

Immunization *—see also* Vaccination
- ABO *—see* Incompatibility, ABO
  - in newborn P55.1
- complication *—see* Complications, vaccination
- encounter for Z23
- not done (not carried out) Z28.9
  - because (of)
    - acute illness of patient Z28.01
    - allergy to vaccine (or component) Z28.04
    - caregiver refusal Z28.82
    - chronic illness of patient Z28.02
    - contraindication NEC Z28.09
    - group pressure Z28.1
    - guardian refusal Z28.82
    - immune compromised state of patient Z28.03
    - parent refusal Z28.82
    - patient's belief Z28.1
    - patient had disease being vaccinated against Z28.81
    - patient refusal Z28.21
    - religious beliefs of patient Z28.1
    - specified reason NEC Z28.89
      - of patient Z28.29
    - unspecified patient reason Z28.20
- Rh factor
  - affecting management of pregnancy NEC O36.09-
    - anti-D antibody O36.01-
  - from transfusion *—see* Complication(s), transfusion, incompatibility reaction, Rh (factor)

Immunocytoma C83.0-

Immunodeficiency D84.9
- with
  - adenosine-deaminase deficiency D81.3
  - antibody defects D80.9
    - specified type NEC D80.8
  - hyperimmunoglobulinemia D80.6
  - increased immunoglobulin M (IgM) D80.5
  - major defect D82.9
    - specified type NEC D82.8
  - partial albinism D82.8
  - short-limbed stature D82.2
  - thrombocytopenia and eczema D82.0
- antibody with
  - hyperimmunoglobulinemia D80.6
  - near-normal immunoglobulins D80.6

Immunodeficiency *(continued)*
- autosomal recessive, Swiss type D80.0
- combined D81.9
  - biotin-dependent carboxylase D81.819
    - biotinidase D81.810
    - holocarboxylase synthetase D81.818
    - specified type NEC D81.818
  - severe (SCID) D81.9
    - with
      - low or normal B-cell numbers D81.2
      - low T- and B-cell numbers D81.1
      - reticular dysgenesis D81.0
  - specified type NEC D81.89
- common variable D83.9
  - with
    - abnormalities of B-cell numbers and function D83.0
    - autoantibodies to B- or T-cells D83.2
    - immunoregulatory T-cell disorders D83.1
  - specified type NEC D83.8
- following hereditary defective response to Epstein-Barr virus (EBV) D82.3
- selective, immunoglobulin
  - A (IgA) D80.2
  - G (IgG) (subclasses) D80.3
  - M (IgM) D80.4
- severe combined (SCID) D81.9
- specified type NEC D84.8
- X-linked, with increased IgM D80.5

Immunotherapy (encounter for)
- antineoplastic Z51.12

Impaction, impacted
- bowel, colon, rectum (*see also* Impaction, fecal) K56.49
  - by gallstone K56.3
- calculus *—see* Calculus
- cerumen (ear) (external) H61.2-
- cuspid *—see* Impaction, tooth
- dental (same or adjacent tooth) K01.1
- fecal, feces K56.41
- fracture *—see* Fracture, by site
- gallbladder *—see* Calculus, gallbladder
- gallstone(s) *—see* Calculus, gallbladder
  - bile duct (common) (hepatic) *—see* Calculus, bile duct
  - cystic duct *—see* Calculus, gallbladder
  - in intestine, with obstruction (any part) K56.3
- intestine (calculous) NEC *—see also* Impaction, fecal K56.49
  - gallstone, with ileus K56.3
- intrauterine device (IUD) T83.39
- molar *—see* Impaction, tooth
- shoulder, causing obstructed labor O66.0
- tooth, teeth K01.1
- turbinate J34.89

Impaired, impairment (function)
- auditory discrimination *—see* Abnormal, auditory perception
- cognitive, mild, so stated G31.84
- dual sensory Z73.82
- fasting glucose R73.01
- glucose tolerance (oral) R73.02
- hearing *—see* Deafness
- heart *—see* Disease, heart
- kidney N28.9
  - disorder resulting from N25.9
    - specified NEC N25.89

Impaired, impairment *(continued)*
- liver K72.90
  - with coma K72.91
- mastication K08.89
- mild cognitive, so stated G31.84
- mobility
  - ear ossicles *—see* Ankylosis, ear ossicles
  - requiring care provider Z74.09
- myocardium, myocardial *—see* Insufficiency, myocardial
- rectal sphincter R19.8
- renal (acute) (chronic) N28.9
  - disorder resulting from N25.9
    - specified NEC N25.89
- vision NEC H54.7
  - both eyes H54.3

Impediment, speech R47.9
- psychogenic (childhood) F98.8
- slurring R47.81
- specified NEC R47.89

Impending
- coronary syndrome I20.0
- delirium tremens F10.239
- myocardial infarction I20.0

Imperception auditory (acquired) *— see also* Deafness
- congenital H93.25

Imperfect
- aeration, lung (newborn) NEC *—see* Atelectasis
- closure (congenital)
  - alimentary tract NEC Q45.8
    - lower Q43.8
    - upper Q40.8
  - atrioventricular ostium Q21.2
  - atrium (secundum) Q21.1
  - branchial cleft NOS Q18.2
    - cyst Q18.0
    - fistula Q18.0
    - sinus Q18.0
  - choroid Q14.3
  - cricoid cartilage Q31.8
  - cusps, heart valve NEC Q24.8
    - pulmonary Q22.3
  - ductus
    - arteriosus Q25.0
    - Botalli Q25.0
  - ear drum (causing impairment of hearing) Q16.4
  - esophagus with communication to bronchus or trachea Q39.1
  - eyelid Q10.3
  - foramen
    - botalli Q21.1
    - ovale Q21.1
  - genitalia, genital organ(s) or system
    - female Q52.8
      - external Q52.79
      - internal NEC Q52.8
    - male Q55.8
  - glottis Q31.8
  - interatrial ostium or septum Q21.1
  - interauricular ostium or septum Q21.1
  - interventricular ostium or septum Q21.0
  - larynx Q31.8
  - lip *—see* Cleft, lip
  - nasal septum Q30.3
  - nose Q30.2
  - omphalomesenteric duct Q43.0
  - optic nerve entry Q14.2
  - organ or site not listed *—see* Anomaly, by site

Imperfect *(continued)*
- closure (congenital) *(continued)*
  - organ or site not listed *(continued)* Anomaly, by site *(continued)*
  - ostium
    - interatrial Q21.1
    - interauricular Q21.1
    - interventricular Q21.0
  - palate *—see* Cleft, palate
  - preauricular sinus Q18.1
  - retina Q14.1
  - roof of orbit Q75.8
  - sclera Q13.5
  - septum
    - aorticopulmonary Q21.4
    - atrial (secundum) Q21.1
    - between aorta and pulmonary artery Q21.4
    - heart Q21.9
    - interatrial (secundum) Q21.1
    - interauricular (secundum) Q21.1
    - interventricular Q21.0
      - in tetralogy of Fallot Q21.3
    - nasal Q30.3
    - ventricular Q21.0
      - with pulmonary stenosis or atresia, dextraposition of aorta, and hypertrophy of right ventricle Q21.3
      - in tetralogy of Fallot Q21.3
  - skull Q75.0
    - with
      - anencephaly Q00.0
      - encephalocele *—see* Encephalocele
      - hydrocephalus Q03.9
        - with spina bifida *—see* Spina bifida, by site, with hydrocephalus
      - microcephaly Q02
  - spine (with meningocele) *—see* Spina bifida
  - trachea Q32.1
  - tympanic membrane (causing impairment of hearing) Q16.4
  - uterus Q51.818
  - vitelline duct Q43.0
- erection *—see* Dysfunction, sexual, male, erectile
- fusion *—see* Imperfect, closure
- inflation, lung (newborn) *—see* Atelectasis
- posture R29.3
- rotation, intestine Q43.3
- septum, ventricular Q21.0

Imperfectly descended testis *—see* Cryptorchid

Imperforate (congenital) *—see also* Atresia
- anus Q42.3
  - with fistula Q42.2
- cervix (uteri) Q51.828
- esophagus Q39.0
  - with tracheoesophageal fistula Q39.1
- hymen Q52.3
- jejunum Q41.1
- pharynx Q38.8
- rectum Q42.1
  - with fistula Q42.0
- urethra Q64.39
- vagina Q52.4

Impervious (congenital) *—see also* Atresia
- anus Q42.3
  - with fistula Q42.2
- bile duct Q44.2
- esophagus Q39.0
  - with tracheoesophageal fistula Q39.1

Impervious *(continued)*
- intestine (small) Q41.9
  - large Q42.9
    - specified NEC Q42.8
- rectum Q42.1
  - with fistula Q42.0
- ureter *—see* Atresia, ureter
- urethra Q64.39

Impetiginization of dermatoses L01.1

Impetigo (any organism) (any site) (circinate) (contagiosa) (simplex) (vulgaris) L01.00
- Bockhart's L01.02
- bullous, bullosa L01.03
- external ear L01.00 *[H62.40]*
- follicularis L01.02
- furfuracea L30.5
- herpetiformis L40.1
  - nonobstetrical L40.1
- neonatorum L01.03
- nonbullous L01.01
- specified type NEC L01.09
- ulcerative L01.09

Impingement (on teeth)
- soft tissue
  - anterior M26.81
  - posterior M26.82

Implant, endometrial N80.9

Implantation
- anomalous *—see* Anomaly, by site
  - ureter Q62.63
- cyst
  - external area or site (skin) NEC L72.0
  - iris *—see* Cyst, iris, implantation
  - vagina N89.8
  - vulva N90.7
- dermoid (cyst) *—see* Implantation, cyst

Impotence (sexual) N52.9
- counseling Z70.1
- organic origin (*see also* Dysfunction, sexual, male, erectile) N52.9
- psychogenic F52.21

Impression, basilar Q75.8

Imprisonment, anxiety concerning Z65.1

Improper care (child) (newborn) — *see* Maltreatment

Improperly tied umbilical cord (causing hemorrhage) P51.8

Impulsiveness (impulsive) R45.87

Inability to swallow *—see* Aphagia

Inaccessible, inaccessibility
- health care NEC Z75.3
  - due to
    - waiting period Z75.2
      - for admission to facility elsewhere Z75.1
- other helping agencies Z75.4

Inactive *—see* condition

Inadequate, inadequacy
- aesthetics of dental restoration K08.56
- biologic, constitutional, functional, or social F60.7
- development
  - child R62.50
  - genitalia
    - after puberty NEC E30.0
    - congenital
      - female Q52.8
        - external Q52.79

Inadequate, inadequacy *(continued)*
- development *(continued)*
  - genitalia *(continued)*
    - congenital *(continued)*
      - female *(continued)*
        - internal Q52.8
      - male Q55.8
  - lungs Q33.6
    - associated with short gestation P28.0
  - organ or site not listed *—see* Anomaly, by site
- diet (causing nutritional deficiency) E63.9
- eating habits Z72.4
- environment, household Z59.1
- family support Z63.8
- food (supply) NEC Z59.4
  - hunger effects T73.0
- functional F60.7
- household care, due to
  - family member
    - handicapped or ill Z74.2
    - on vacation Z75.5
    - temporarily away from home Z74.2
  - technical defects in home Z59.1
  - temporary absence from home of person rendering care Z74.2
- housing (heating) (space) Z59.1
- income (financial) Z59.6
- intrafamilial communication Z63.8
- material resources Z59.9
- mental *—see* Disability, intellectual
- parental supervision or control of child Z62.0
- personality F60.7
- pulmonary
  - function R06.89
    - newborn P28.5
  - ventilation, newborn P28.5
- sample of cytologic smear
  - anus R85.615
  - cervix R87.615
  - vagina R87.625
- social F60.7
  - insurance Z59.7
  - skills NEC Z73.4
- supervision of child by parent Z62.0
- teaching affecting education Z55.8
- welfare support Z59.7

Inanition R64
- with edema *—see* Malnutrition, severe
- due to
  - deprivation of food T73.0
  - malnutrition *—see* Malnutrition
- fever R50.9

Inappropriate
- change in quantitative human chorionic gonadotropin (hCG) in early pregnancy O02.81
- diet or eating habits Z72.4
- level of quantitative human chorionic gonadotropin (hCG) for gestational age in early pregnancy O02.81
- secretion
  - antidiuretic hormone (ADH) (excessive) E22.2
    - deficiency E23.2
  - pituitary (posterior) E22.2

Inattention at or after birth *—see* Neglect

Incarceration, incarcerated
- enterocele K46.0
  - gangrenous K46.1
- epiplocele K46.0
  - gangrenous K46.1
- exomphalos K42.0

Incarceration, incarcerated *(continued)*
- exomphalos *(continued)*
  - gangrenous K42.1
- hernia *—see also* Hernia, by site,
  - with obstruction
  - with gangrene *—see* Hernia, by site, with gangrene
- iris, in wound *—see* Injury, eye, laceration, with prolapse
- lens, in wound *—see* Injury, eye, laceration, with prolapse
- omphalocele K42.0
- prison, anxiety concerning Z65.1
- rupture *—see* Hernia, by site
- sarcoepiplocele K46.0
  - gangrenous K46.1
- sarcoepiplomphalocele K42.0
  - with gangrene K42.1
- uterus N85.8
  - gravid O34.51-
    - causing obstructed labor O65.5

Incised wound
- external *—see* Laceration
- internal organs *—see* Injury, by site

Incision, incisional
- hernia K43.2
  - with
    - gangrene (and obstruction) K43.1
    - obstruction K43.0
- surgical, complication *—see* Complications, surgical procedure
- traumatic
  - external *—see* Laceration
  - internal organs *—see* Injury, by site

Inclusion
- azurophilic leukocytic D72.0
- blennorrhea (neonatal) (newborn) P39.1
- gallbladder in liver (congenital) Q44.1

Incompatibility
- ABO
  - affecting management of pregnancy O36.11-
    - anti-A sensitization O36.11-
    - anti-B sensitization O36.19-
    - specified NEC O36.19-
  - infusion or transfusion reaction — *see* Complication(s), transfusion, incompatibility reaction, ABO
  - newborn P55.1
- blood (group) (Duffy) (K(ell)) (Kidd) (Lewis) (M) (S) NEC
  - affecting management of pregnancy O36.11-
    - anti-A sensitization O36.11-
    - anti-B sensitization O36.19-
  - infusion or transfusion reaction T80.89
  - newborn P55.8
- divorce or estrangement Z63.5
- Rh (blood group) (factor) Z31.82
  - affecting management of pregnancy NEC O36.09-
    - anti-D antibody O36.01-
  - infusion or transfusion reaction *—see* Complication(s), transfusion, incompatibility reaction, Rh (factor)
  - newborn P55.0
- rhesus *—see* Incompatibility, Rh

Incompetency, incompetent, incompetence
- annular
  - aortic (valve) *—see* Insufficiency, aortic
  - mitral (valve) I34.0
  - pulmonary valve (heart) I37.1
- aortic (valve) *—see* Insufficiency, aortic
- cardiac valve *—see* Endocarditis
- cervix, cervical (os) N88.3
  - in pregnancy O34.3-
- chronotropic I45.89
  - with
    - autonomic dysfunction G90.8
    - ischemic heart disease I25.89
    - left ventricular dysfunction I51.89
    - sinus node dysfunction I49.8
- esophagogastric (junction) (sphincter) K22.0
- mitral (valve) *—see* Insufficiency, mitral
- pelvic fundus N81.89
- pubocervical tissue N81.82
- pulmonary valve (heart) I37.1
  - congenital Q22.3
- rectovaginal tissue N81.83
- tricuspid (annular) (valve) *—see* Insufficiency, tricuspid
- valvular *—see* Endocarditis
  - congenital Q24.8
- vein, venous (saphenous) (varicose) *—see* Varix, leg

Incomplete *—see also* condition
- bladder, emptying R33.9
- defecation R15.0
- expansion lungs (newborn) NEC — *see* Atelectasis
- rotation, intestine Q43.3

Inconclusive
- diagnostic imaging due to excess body fat of patient R93.9
- findings on diagnostic imaging of breast NEC R92.8
- mammogram (due to dense breasts) R92.2

Incontinence R32
- anal sphincter R15.9
- coital N39.491
- feces R15.9
  - nonorganic origin F98.1
- insensible (urinary) N39.42
- overflow N39.490
- postural (urinary) N39.492
- psychogenic F45.8
- rectal R15.9
- reflex N39.498
- stress (female) (male) N39.3
  - and urge N39.46
- urethral sphincter R32
- urge N39.41
  - and stress (female) (male) N39.46
- urine (urinary) R32
  - continuous N39.45
  - due to cognitive impairment, or severe physical disability or immobility R39.81
  - functional R39.81
  - insensible N39.42
  - mixed (stress and urge) N39.46
  - nocturnal N39.44
  - nonorganic origin F98.0
  - overflow N39.490
  - post dribbling N39.43
  - postural N39.492
  - reflex N39.498
  - specified NEC N39.498

Incontinence *(continued)*
- urine *(continued)*
  - stress (female) (male) N39.3
    - and urge N39.46
  - total N39.498
  - unaware N39.42
  - urge N39.41
    - and stress (female) (male) N39.46

Incontinentia pigmenti Q82.3

Incoordinate, incoordination
- esophageal-pharyngeal (newborn) —*see* Dysphagia
- muscular R27.8
- uterus (action) (contractions) (complicating delivery) O62.4

Increase, increased
- abnormal, in development R63.8
- androgens (ovarian) E28.1
- anticoagulants (antithrombin) (anti-VIIIa) (anti-IXa) (anti-Xa) (anti-XIa) —*see* Circulating anticoagulants
- cold sense R20.8
- estrogen E28.0
- function
  - adrenal
    - cortex —*see* Cushing's, syndrome
    - medulla E27.5
  - pituitary (gland) (anterior) (lobe) E22.9
    - posterior E22.2
- heat sense R20.8
- intracranial pressure (benign) G93.2
- permeability, capillaries I78.8
- pressure, intracranial G93.2
- secretion
  - gastrin E16.4
  - glucagon E16.3
  - pancreas, endocrine E16.9
    - growth hormone-releasing hormone E16.8
    - pancreatic polypeptide E16.8
    - somatostatin E16.8
    - vasoactive-intestinal polypeptide E16.8
- sphericity, lens Q12.4
- splenic activity D73.1
- venous pressure I87.8
  - portal K76.6

Increta placenta O43.22-

Incrustation, cornea, foreign body (lead) (zinc) —*see* Foreign body, cornea

Incyclophoria H50.54

Incyclotropia —*see* Cyclotropia

Indeterminate sex Q56.4

India rubber skin Q82.8

Indigestion (acid) (bilious) (functional) K30
- catarrhal K31.89
- due to decomposed food NOS A05.9
- nervous F45.8
- psychogenic F45.8

Indirect —*see* condition

Induratio penis plastica N48.6

Induration, indurated
- brain G93.89
- breast (fibrous) N64.51
  - puerperal, postpartum O92.29
- broad ligament N83.8
- chancre
  - anus A51.1
  - congenital A50.07
  - extragenital NEC A51.2

Induration, indurated *(continued)*
- corpora cavernosa (penis) (plastic) N48.6
- liver (chronic) K76.89
- lung (black) (chronic) (fibroid) —*see also* Fibrosis, lung J84.10
  - essential brown J84.03
- penile (plastic) N48.6
- phlebitic —*see* Phlebitis
- skin R23.4

Inebriety (without dependence) —*see* Alcohol, intoxication

Inefficiency, kidney N28.9

Inelasticity, skin R23.4

Inequality, leg (length) (acquired) —*see also* Deformity, limb, unequal length
- congenital —*see* Defect, reduction, lower limb
- lower leg —*see* Deformity, limb, unequal length

Inertia
- bladder (neurogenic) N31.2
- stomach K31.89
  - psychogenic F45.8
- uterus, uterine during labor O62.2
  - during latent phase of labor O62.0
  - primary O62.0
  - secondary O62.1
- vesical (neurogenic) N31.2

Infancy, infantile, infantilism —*see also* condition
- celiac K90.0
- genitalia, genitals (after puberty) E30.0
- Herter's (nontropical sprue) K90.0
- intestinal K90.0
- Lorain E23.0
- pancreatic K86.89
- pelvis M95.5
  - with disproportion (fetopelvic) O33.1
    - causing obstructed labor O65.1
- pituitary E23.0
- renal N25.0
- uterus —*see* Infantile, genitalia

Infant(s) —*see also* Infancy
- excessive crying R68.11
- irritable child R68.12
- lack of care —*see* Neglect
- liveborn (singleton) Z38.2
  - born in hospital Z38.00
    - by cesarean Z38.01
  - born outside hospital Z38.1
  - multiple NEC Z38.8
    - born in hospital Z38.68
      - by cesarean Z38.69
    - born outside hospital Z38.7
  - quadruplet Z38.8
    - born in hospital Z38.63
      - by cesarean Z38.64
    - born outside hospital Z38.7
  - quintuplet Z38.8
    - born in hospital Z38.65
      - by cesarean Z38.66
    - born outside hospital Z38.7
  - triplet Z38.8
    - born in hospital Z38.61
      - by cesarean Z38.62
    - born outside hospital Z38.7
  - twin Z38.5
    - born in hospital Z38.30
      - by cesarean Z38.31
    - born outside hospital Z38.4
- of diabetic mother (syndrome of) P70.1
  - gestational diabetes P70.0

Infantile —*see also* condition
- genitalia, genitals E30.0
- os, uterine E30.0
- penis E30.0
- testis E29.1
- uterus E30.0

Infantilism —*see* Infancy

Infarct, infarction
- adrenal (capsule) (gland) E27.49
- appendices epiploicae (*see also* Infarct, intestine) K55.069
- bowel (*see also* Infarct, intestine) K55.0 069
- brain (stem) —*see* Infarct, cerebral
- breast N64.89
- brewer's (kidney) N28.0
- cardiac —*see* Infarct, myocardium
- cerebellar —*see* Infarct, cerebral
- cerebral —*see also* Occlusion, artery
  - cerebral or precerebral, with infarction I63.9-
  - aborted I63.9
  - cortical I63.9
  - due to
    - cerebral venous thrombosis, nonpyogenic I63.6
    - embolism
      - cerebral arteries I63.4-
      - precerebral arteries I63.1-
    - occlusion NEC
      - cerebral arteries I63.5-
      - precerebral arteries I63.2-
    - stenosis NEC
      - cerebral arteries I63.5-
      - precerebral arteries I63.2-
    - thrombosis
      - cerebral artery I63.3-
      - precerebral artery I63.0-
  - intraoperative
    - during cardiac surgery I97.810
    - during other surgery I97.811
  - postprocedural
    - following cardiac surgery I97.820
    - following other surgery I97.821
  - specified NEC I63.8
- colon (acute) (agnogenic) (embolic) (hemorrhagic) (nonocclusive) (nonthrombotic) (occlusive) (segmental) (thrombotic) (with gangrene) (*see also* Infarct, intestine) K55.049
- coronary artery —*see* Infarct, myocardium
- embolic —*see* Embolism
- fallopian tube N83.8
- gallbladder K82.8
- heart —*see* Infarct, myocardium
- hepatic K76.3
- hypophysis (anterior lobe) E23.6
- impending (myocardium) I20.0
- intestine (acute) (agnogenic) (embolic) (hemorrhagic) (nonocclusive) (nonthrombotic) (occlusive) (thrombotic) (with gangrene) K55.069
  - diffuse K55.062
  - focal K55.061
  - large K55.049
    - diffuse K55.042
    - focal K55.041
  - small K55.029
    - diffuse K55.029
    - focal K55.021
- kidney N28.0
- liver K76.3
- lung (embolic) (thrombotic) —*see* Embolism, pulmonary
- lymph node I89.8

Infarct, infarction *(continued)*
- mesentery, mesenteric (embolic) (thrombotic) (with gangrene) (*see also* Infarct, intestine) K55.069
- muscle (ischemic) M62.20
  - ankle M62.27-
  - foot M62.27-
  - forearm M62.23-
  - hand M62.24-
  - lower leg M62.26-
  - pelvic region M62.25-
  - shoulder region M62.21-
  - specified site NEC M62.28
  - thigh M62.25-
  - upper arm M62.22-
- myocardium, myocardial (acute) (with stated duration of 4 weeks or less) I21.9
  - associated with revascularization procedure I21.A9
  - diagnosed on ECG, but presenting no symptoms I25.2
  - due to
    - demand ischemia I21.A1
    - ischemic imbalance I21.A1
  - healed or old I25.2
  - intraoperative —*see also* Infarct, myocardium, associated with revascularization procedure
    - during cardiac surgery I97.790
    - during other surgery I97.791
  - non-Q wave I21.4
  - non-ST elevation (NSTEMI) I21.4
    - subsequent I22.2
  - nontransmural I21.4
  - past (diagnosed on ECG or other investigation, but currently presenting no symptoms) I25.2
  - postprocedural —*see also* Infarct, myocardium, associated with revascularization procedure
    - following cardiac surgery (*see also* Infarct, myocardium, type 4 or type 5) I97.190
    - following other surgery I97.191
  - Q wave (*see also*, Infarct, myocardium, by site) I21.3
  - secondary to
    - demand ischemia I21.A1
    - ischemic imbalance I21.A1
  - ST elevation (STEMI) I21.3
    - anterior (anteroapical) (anterolateral) (anteroseptal) (Q wave) (wall) I21.09
      - subsequent I22.0
    - inferior (diaphragmatic) (inferolateral) (inferoposterior) (wall) NEC I21.19
      - subsequent I22.1
    - inferoposterior transmural (Q wave) I21.11
    - involving
      - coronary artery of anterior wall NEC I21.09
      - coronary artery of inferior wall NEC I21.19
      - diagonal coronary artery I21.02
      - left anterior descending coronary artery I21.02
      - left circumflex coronary artery I21.21
      - left main coronary artery I21.01
      - oblique marginal coronary artery I21.21
      - right coronary artery I21.11
    - lateral (apical-lateral) (basal-lateral) (high) I21.29
      - subsequent I22.8

Infarct, infarction *(continued)*
- myocardium, myocardial *(continued)*
  - ST elevation *(continued)*
    - posterior (posterobasal) (posterolateral) (posteroseptal) (true) I21.29
      - subsequent I22.8
    - septal I21.29
      - subsequent I22.8
    - specified NEC I21.29
      - subsequent I22.8
    - subsequent I22.9
  - subsequent (recurrent) (reinfarction) I22.9
    - anterior (anteroapical) (anterolateral) (anteroseptal) (wall) I22.0
    - diaphragmatic (wall) I22.1
    - inferior (diaphragmatic) (inferolateral) (inferoposterior) (wall) I22.1
    - lateral (apical-lateral) (basal-lateral) (high) I22.8
    - non-ST elevation (NSTEMI) I22.2
    - posterior (posterobasal) (posterolateral) (posteroseptal) (true) I22.8
    - septal I22.8
    - specified NEC I22.8
    - ST elevation I22.9
      - anterior (anteroapical) (anterolateral) (anteroseptal) (wall) I22.0
      - inferior (diaphragmatic) (inferolateral) (inferoposterior) (wall) I22.1
      - specified NEC I22.8
    - subendocardial I22.2
    - transmural I22.9
      - anterior (anteroapical) (anterolateral) (anteroseptal) (wall) I22.0
    - transmural
      - diaphragmatic (wall) I22.1
      - inferior (diaphragmatic) (inferolateral) (inferoposterior) (wall) I22.1
      - lateral (apical-lateral) (basal-lateral) (high) I22.8
      - posterior (posterobasal) (posterolateral) (posteroseptal) (true) I22.8
      - specified NEC I22.8
    - type 1 (*see also* Infarction, myocardial, subsequent, by site, or by ST elevation or non-ST elevation) I22.9
    - type 2 I21.A1
    - type 3 I21.A9
    - type 4 I21.A9
    - type 5 I21.A9
  - syphilitic A52.06
  - transmural I21.9
    - anterior (anteroapical) (anterolateral) (anteroseptal) (Q wave) (wall) NEC I21.09
    - inferior (diaphragmatic) (inferolateral) (inferoposterior) (Q wave) (wall) NEC I21.19
    - inferoposterior (Q wave) I21.11
    - lateral (apical-lateral) (basal-lateral) (high) NEC I21.29
    - posterior (posterobasal) (posterolateral) (posteroseptal) (true) NEC I21.29

Infarct, infarction *(continued)*
- myocardium, myocardial *(continued)*
  - transmural *(continued)*
    - septal NEC I21.29
    - specified NEC I21.29
  - type 1 (*see also* Infarction, myocardial, by site, or by ST elevation or non-ST elevation) I21.9
  - type 2 I21.A1
  - type 3 I21.A9
  - type 4 (a) (b) (c) I21.A9
  - type 5 I21.A9
- nontransmural I21.4
- omentum (*see also* Infarct, intestine) K55.069
- ovary N83.8
- pancreas K86.89
- papillary muscle *—see* Infarct, myocardium
- parathyroid gland E21.4
- pituitary (gland) E23.6
- placenta O43.81-
- prostate N42.89
- pulmonary (artery) (vein) (hemorrhagic) *—see* Embolism, pulmonary
- renal (embolic) (thrombotic) N28.0
- retina, retinal (artery) *—see* Occlusion, artery, retina
- spinal (cord) (acute) (embolic) (nonembolic) G95.11
- spleen D73.5
  - embolic or thrombotic I74.8
- subendocardial (acute) (nontransmural) I21.4
- suprarenal (capsule) (gland) E27.49
- testis N50.1
- thrombotic *—see also* Thrombosis
  - artery, arterial *—see* Embolism
- thyroid (gland) E07.89
- ventricle (heart) *—see* Infarct, myocardium

Infecting *—see* condition

Infection, infected, infective (opportunistic) B99.9
- with
  - drug resistant organism *—see* Resistance (to), drug *—see also* specific organism
  - lymphangitis *—see* Lymphangitis
  - organ dysfunction (acute) R65.20
    - with septic shock R65.21
- abscess (skin)- code by site under Abscess
- Absidia *—see* Mucormycosis
- Acanthamoeba *—see* Acanthamebiasis
- Acanthocheilonema (perstans) (streptocerca) B74.4
- accessory sinus (chronic) *—see* Sinusitis
- achorion *—see* Dermatophytosis
- Acremonium falciforme B47.0
- acromioclavicular M00.9
- Actinobacillus (actinomycetem-comitans) A28.8
  - mallei A24.0
  - muris A25.1
- Actinomadura B47.1
- Actinomyces (israelii) (*see also* Actinomycosis) A42.9
- Actinomycetales *—see* Actinomycosis
- actinomycotic NOS *—see* Actinomycosis
- adenoid (and tonsil) J03.90
  - chronic J35.02

Infection, infected, infective *(continued)*
- adenovirus NEC
  - as cause of disease classified elsewhere B97.0
  - unspecified nature or site B34.0
- aerogenes capsulatus A48.0
- aertrycke *—see* Infection, salmonella
- alimentary canal NOS *—see* Enteritis, infectious
- Allescheria boydii B48.2
- Alternaria B48.8
- alveolus, alveolar (process) K04.7
- Ameba, amebic (histolytica) *—see* Amebiasis
- amniotic fluid, sac or cavity O41.10-
  - chorioamnionitis O41.12-
  - placentitis O41.14-
- amputation stump (surgical) *—see* Complication, amputation stump, infection
- Ancylostoma (duodenalis) B76.0
- Anisakiasis, Anisakis larvae B81.0
- anthrax *—see* Anthrax
- antrum (chronic) *—see* Sinusitis, maxillary
- anus, anal (papillae) (sphincter) K62.89
- arbovirus (arbor virus) A94
  - specified type NEC A93.8
- artificial insemination N98.0
- Ascaris lumbricoides *—see* Ascariasis
- Ascomycetes B47.0
- Aspergillus (flavus) (fumigatus) (terreus) *—see* Aspergillosis
- atypical
  - acid-fast (bacilli) *—see* Mycobacterium, atypical
  - mycobacteria *—see* Mycobacterium, atypical
  - virus A81.9
    - specified type NEC A81.89
- auditory meatus (external) *—see* Otitis, externa, infective
- auricle (ear) *—see* Otitis, externa, infective
- axillary gland (lymph) L04.2
- Bacillus A49.9
  - abortus A23.1
  - anthracis *—see* Anthrax
  - Ducrey's (any location) A57
  - Flexner's A03.1
  - Friedländer's NEC A49.8
  - gas (gangrene) A48.0
  - mallei A24.0
  - melitensis A23.0
  - paratyphoid, paratyphosus A01.4
    - A A01.1
    - B A01.2
    - C A01.3
  - Shiga (-Kruse) A03.0
  - suipestifer *—see* Infection, salmonella
  - swimming pool A31.1
  - typhosa A01.00
  - welchii *—see* Gangrene, gas
- bacterial NOS A49.9
  - as cause of disease classified elsewhere B96.89
    - Clostridium perfringens [C. perfringens] B96.7
    - Bacteroides fragilis [B. fragilis] B96.6
    - Enterobacter sakazakii B96.89
    - Enterococcus B95.2
    - Escherichia coli [E. coli] *—see also* Escherichia coli B96.20

Infection, infected, infective *(continued)*
- bacterial NOS *(continued)*
  - as cause of disease classified elsewhere *(continued)*
    - Helicobacter pylori [H.pylori] B96.81
    - Hemophilus influenzae [H. influenzae] B96.3
    - Klebsiella pneumoniae [K. pneumoniae] B96.1
    - Mycoplasma pneumoniae [M. pneumoniae] B96.0
    - Proteus (mirabilis) (morganii) B96.4
    - Pseudomonas (aeruginosa) (mallei) (pseudomallei) B96.5
    - Staphylococcus B95.8
      - aureus (methicillin susceptible) (MSSA) B95.61
        - methicillin resistant (MRSA) B95.62
      - specified NEC B95.7
    - Streptococcus B95.5
      - group A B95.0
      - group B B95.1
      - pneumoniae B95.3
      - specified NEC B95.4
    - Vibrio vulnificus B96.82
  - specified NEC A48.8
- Bacterium
  - paratyphosum A01.4
    - A A01.1
    - B A01.2
    - C A01.3
  - typhosum A01.00
- Bacteroides NEC A49.8
  - fragilis, as cause of disease classified elsewhere B96.6
- Balantidium coli A07.0
- Bartholin's gland N75.8
- Basidiobolus B46.8
- bile duct (common) (hepatic) *—see* Cholangitis
- bladder *—see* Cystitis
- Blastomyces, blastomycotic *—see also* Blastomycosis
  - brasiliensis *—see* Paracoccidioidomycosis
  - dermatitidis *—see* Blastomycosis
  - European *—see* Cryptococcosis
  - Loboi B48.0
  - North American B40.9
  - South American *—see* Paracoccidioidomycosis
- bleb, postprocedure *—see* Blebitis
- bone *—see* Osteomyelitis
- Bordetella *—see* Whooping cough
- Borrelia bergdorfi A69.20
- brain (*see also* Encephalitis) G04.90
  - membranes *—see* Meningitis
  - septic G06.0
    - meninges *—see* Meningitis, bacterial
- branchial cyst Q18.0
- breast *—see* Mastitis
- bronchus *—see* Bronchitis
- Brucella A23.9
  - abortus A23.1
  - canis A23.3
  - melitensis A23.0
  - mixed A23.8
  - specified NEC A23.8
  - suis A23.2
- Brugia (malayi) B74.1
  - timori B74.2
- bursa *—see* Bursitis, infective

Infection, infected, infective *(continued)*

- buttocks (skin) L08.9
- Campylobacter, intestinal A04.5
  - as cause of disease classified elsewhere B96.81
- Candida (albicans) (tropicalis) *—see* Candidiasis
- candiru B88.8
- Capillaria (intestinal) B81.1
  - hepatica B83.8
  - philippinensis B81.1
- cartilage *—see* Disorder, cartilage, specified type NEC
- catheter-related bloodstream (CRBSI) T80.211
- cat liver fluke B66.0
- cellulitis - code by site under Cellulitis
- central line-associated T80.219
  - bloodstream (CLABSI) T80.211
  - specified NEC T80.218
- Cephalosporium falciforme B47.0
- cerebrospinal *—see* Meningitis
- cervical gland (lymph) L04.0
- cervix *—see* Cervicitis
- cesarean delivery wound (puerperal) O86.0
- cestodes *—see* Infestation, cestodes
- chest J22
- Chilomastix (intestinal) A07.8
- Chlamydia, chlamydial A74.9
  - anus A56.3
  - genitourinary tract A56.2
    - lower A56.00
    - specified NEC A56.19
  - lymphogranuloma A55
  - pharynx A56.4
  - psittaci A70
  - rectum A56.3
  - sexually transmitted NEC A56.8
- cholera *—see* Cholera
- Cladosporium
  - bantianum (brain abscess) B43.1
  - carrionii B43.0
  - castellanii B36.1
  - trichoides (brain abscess) B43.1
  - werneckii B36.1
- Clonorchis (sinensis) (liver) B66.1
- Clostridium NEC
  - bifermentans A48.0
  - botulinum (food poisoning) A05.1
    - infant A48.51
    - wound A48.52
  - difficile
    - as cause of disease classified elsewhere B96.89
    - foodborne (disease)
      - not specified as recurrent A04.72
      - recurrent A04.71
    - gas gangrene A48.0
    - necrotizing enterocolitis
      - not specified as recurrent A04.72
      - recurrent A04.71
    - sepsis A41.4
  - gas-forming NEC A48.0
  - histolyticum A48.0
  - novyi, causing gas gangrene A48.0
  - oedematiens A48.0
  - perfringens
    - as cause of disease classified elsewhere B96.7
    - due to food A05.2
    - foodborne (disease) A05.2
    - gas gangrene A48.0
    - sepsis A41.4

Infection, infected, infective *(continued)*

- Clostridium NEC *(continued)*
  - septicum, causing gas gangrene A48.0
  - sordellii, causing gas gangrene A48.0
  - welchii
    - as cause of disease classified elsewhere B96.7
    - foodborne (disease) A05.2
    - gas gangrene A48.0
    - necrotizing enteritis A05.2
    - sepsis A41.4
- Coccidioides (immitis) *—see* Coccidioidomycosis
- colon *—see* Enteritis, infectious
- colostomy K94.02
- common duct *—see* Cholangitis
- congenital P39.9
  - Candida (albicans) P37.5
  - cytomegalovirus P35.1
  - hepatitis, viral P35.3
  - herpes simplex P35.2
  - infectious or parasitic disease P37.9
    - specified NEC P37.8
  - listeriosis (disseminated) P37.2
  - malaria NEC P37.4
    - falciparum P37.3
  - Plasmodium falciparum P37.3
  - poliomyelitis P35.8
  - rubella P35.0
  - skin P39.4
  - toxoplasmosis (acute) (subacute) (chronic) P37.1
  - tuberculosis P37.0
  - urinary (tract) P39.3
  - vaccinia P35.8
  - virus P35.9
    - specified type NEC P35.8
- Conidiobolus B46.8
- coronavirus NEC B34.2
  - as cause of disease classified elsewhere B97.29
  - severe acute respiratory syndrome (SARS associated) B97.21
- corpus luteum *—see* Salpingo-oophoritis
- Corynebacterium diphtheriae *—see* Diphtheria
- cotia virus B08.8
- Coxiella burnetii A78
- coxsackie *—see* Coxsackie
- Cryptococcus neoformans *—see* Cryptococcosis
- Cryptosporidium A07.2
- Cunninghamella *—see* Mucormycosis
- cyst *—see* Cyst
- cystic duct (*see also* Cholecystitis) K81.9
- Cysticercus cellulosae *—see* Cysticercosis
- cytomegalovirus, cytomegaloviral B25.9
  - congenital P35.1
  - maternal, maternal care for (suspected) damage to fetus O35.3
  - mononucleosis B27.10
    - with
      - complication NEC B27.19
      - meningitis B27.12
      - polyneuropathy B27.11
- delta-agent (acute), in hepatitis B carrier B17.0
- dental (pulpal origin) K04.7
- Deuteromycetes B47.0
- Dicrocoelium dendriticum B66.2
- Dipetalonema (perstans) (streptocerca) B74.4

Infection, infected, infective *(continued)*

- diphtherial *—see* Diphtheria
- Diphyllobothrium (adult) (latum) (pacificum) B70.0
  - larval B70.1
- Diplogonoporus (grandis) B71.8
- Dipylidium caninum B67.4
- Dirofilaria B74.8
- Dracunculus medinensis B72
- Drechslera (hawaiiensis) B43.8
- Ducrey Haemophilus (any location) A57
- due to or resulting from
  - artificial insemination N98.0
  - central venous catheter T80.219
    - bloodstream T80.211
    - exit or insertion site T80.212
    - localized T80.212
    - port or reservoir T80.212
    - specified NEC T80.218
    - tunnel T80.212
  - device, implant or graft (*see also* Complications, by site and type, infection or inflammation) T85.79
    - arterial graft NEC T82.7
    - breast (implant) T85.79
    - catheter NEC T85.79
      - dialysis (renal) T82.7
        - intraperitoneal T85.71
      - infusion NEC T82.7
        - cranial T85.735
        - intrathecal T85.735
        - spinal (epidural) (subdural) T85.735
        - subarachnoid T85.735
      - urinary T83.518
        - cystostomy T83.510
        - Hopkins T83.518
        - ileostomy T83.518
        - nephrostomy T83.512
        - specified NEC T83.518
        - urethral indwelling T83.511
        - urostomy T83.518
    - electronic (electrode) (pulse generator) (stimulator)
      - bone T84.7
      - cardiac T82.7
      - nervous system T85.738
        - brain T85.731
        - cranial nerve T85.732
        - gastric nerve T85.732
        - generator pocket T85.734
        - neurostimulator generator T85.734
        - peripheral nerve T85.732
        - sacral nerve T85.732
        - spinal cord T85.733
        - vagal nerve T85.732
      - urinary T83.590
    - fixation, internal (orthopedic) NEC *—see* Complication, fixation device, infection
    - gastrointestinal (bile duct) (esophagus) T85.79
      - neurostimulator electrode (lead) T85.732
    - genital NEC T83.69
    - heart NEC T82.7
      - valve (prosthesis) T82.6
        - graft T82.7
    - joint prosthesis *—see* Complication, joint prosthesis, infection
    - ocular (corneal graft) (orbital implant) NEC T85.79
    - orthopedic NEC T84.7
    - penile (cylinder) (pump) (resevoir) T83.61
    - specified NEC T85.79

Infection, infected, infective *(continued)*

- due to or resulting from *(continued)*
  - device, implant or graft *(continued)*
    - testicular T83.62
    - urinary NEC T83.598
      - ileal conduit stent T83.593
      - implanted neurostimulation T83.590
      - implanted sphincter T83.591
      - indwelling ureteral stent T83.592
      - nephroureteral stent T83.593
      - specified stent NEC T83.593
    - vascular NEC T82.7
    - ventricular intracranial (communicating) shunt T85.730
  - Hickman catheter T80.219
    - bloodstream T80.211
    - localized T80.212
    - specified NEC T80.218
  - immunization or vaccination T88.0
  - infusion, injection or transfusion NEC T80.29
    - acute T80.22
  - injury NEC - code by site under Wound, open
  - peripherally inserted central catheter (PICC) T80.219
    - bloodstream T80.211
    - localized T80.212
    - specified NEC T80.218
  - portacath (port-a-cath) T80.219
    - bloodstream T80.211
    - localized T80.212
    - specified NEC T80.218
  - surgery T81.4
  - Swan Ganz catheter *—see* Infection, due to or resulting from, central venous catheter
  - triple lumen catheter T80.219
    - bloodstream T80.211
    - localized T80.212
    - specified NEC T80.218
  - umbilical venous catheter T80.219
    - bloodstream T80.211
    - localized T80.212
    - specified NEC T80.218
- during labor NEC O75.3
- ear (middle) *—see also* Otitis media
  - external *—see* Otitis, externa, infective
  - inner *—see* subcategory H83.0
- Eberthella typhosa A01.00
- Echinococcus *—see* Echinococcus
- echovirus
  - as cause of disease classified elsewhere B97.12
  - unspecified nature or site B34.1
- endocardium I33.0
- endocervix *—see* Cervicitis
- Entamoeba *—see* Amebiasis
- enteric *—see* Enteritis, infectious
- Enterobacter sakazakii B96.89
- Enterobius vermicularis B80
- enterostomy K94.12
- enterovirus B34.1
  - as cause of disease classified elsewhere B97.10
    - coxsackievirus B97.11
    - echovirus B97.12
    - specified NEC B97.19
- Entomophthora B46.8
- Epidermophyton *—see* Dermatophytosis
- epididymis *—see* Epididymitis
- episiotomy (puerperal) O86.0

Infection, infected, infective *(continued)*
Erysipelothrix (insidiosa) (rhusiopathiae) *—see* Erysipeloid
erythema infectiosum B08.3
Escherichia (E.) coli NEC A49.8
as cause of disease classified elsewhere (*see also* Escherichia coli) B96.20
congenital P39.8
sepsis P36.4
generalized A41.51
intestinal *—see* Enteritis, infectious, due to, Escherichia coli
ethmoidal (chronic) (sinus) *—see* Sinusitis, ethmoidal
eustachian tube (ear) *—see* Salpingitis, eustachian
external auditory canal (meatus) NEC *—see* Otitis, externa, infective
eye (purulent) *—see* Endophthalmitis, purulent
eyelid *—see* Inflammation, eyelid
fallopian tube *—see* Salpingo-oophoritis
Fasciola (gigantica) (hepatica) (indica) B66.3
Fasciolopsis (buski) B66.5
filarial *—see* Infestation, filarial
finger (skin) L08.9
nail L03.01-
fungus B35.1
fish tapeworm B70.0
larval B70.1
flagellate, intestinal A07.9
fluke *—see* Infestation, fluke
focal
teeth (pulpal origin) K04.7
tonsils J35.01
Fonsecaea (compactum) (pedrosoi) B43.0
food *—see* Intoxication, foodborne
foot (skin) L08.9
dermatophytic fungus B35.3
Francisella tularensis *—see* Tularemia
frontal (sinus) (chronic) *—see* Sinusitis, frontal
fungus NOS B49
beard B35.0
dermatophytic *—see* Dermatophytosis
foot B35.3
groin B35.6
hand B35.2
nail B35.1
pathogenic to compromised host only B48.8
perianal (area) B35.6
scalp B35.0
skin B36.9
foot B35.3
hand B35.2
toenails B35.1
Fusarium B48.8
gallbladder *—see* Cholecystitis
gas bacillus *—see* Gangrene, gas
gastrointestinal *—see* Enteritis, infectious
generalized NEC *—see* Sepsis
generator pocket, implanted electronic neurostimulator T85.734
genital organ or tract
female *—see* Disease, pelvis, inflammatory
male N49.9
multiple sites N49.8
specified NEC N49.8

Infection, infected, infective *(continued)*
Ghon tubercle, primary A15.7
Giardia lamblia A07.1
gingiva (chronic) K05.10
acute K05.00
nonplaque induced K05.01
plaque induced K05.00
nonplaque induced K05.11
plaque induced K05.10
glanders A24.0
glenosporopsis B48.0
Gnathostoma (spinigerum) B83.1
Gongylonema B83.8
gonococcal *—see* Gonococcus
gram-negative bacilli NOS A49.9
guinea worm B72
gum (chronic) K05.10
acute K05.00
nonplaque induced K05.01
plaque induced K05.00
nonplaque induced K05.11
plaque induced K05.10
Haemophilus *—see* Infection, Hemophilus
heart *—see* Carditis
Helicobacter pylori A04.8
as cause of disease classified elsewhere B96.81
helminths B83.9
intestinal B82.0
mixed (types classifiable to more than one of the titles B65.0-B81.3 and B81.8) B81.4
specified type NEC B81.8
specified type NEC B83.8
Hemophilus
aegyptius, systemic A48.4
ducrey (any location) A57
influenzae NEC A49.2
as cause of disease classified elsewhere B96.3
generalized A41.3
herpes (simplex) *—see also* Herpes
congenital P35.2
disseminated B00.7
zoster B02.9
herpesvirus, herpesviral *—see* Herpes
hip (joint) NEC M00.9
due to internal joint prosthesis
left T84.52
right T84.51
skin NEC L08.9
Heterophyes (heterophyes) B66.8
Histoplasma *—see* Histoplasmosis
American B39.4
capsulatum B39.4
hookworm B76.9
human
papilloma virus A63.0
T-cell lymphotropic virus type-1(HTLV-1) B33.3
hydrocele N43.0
Hymenolepis B71.0
hypopharynx *—see* Pharyngitis
inguinal (lymph) glands L04.1
due to soft chancre A57
intervertebral disc, pyogenic M46.30
cervical region M46.32
cervicothoracic region M46.33
lumbar region M46.36
lumbosacral region M46.37
multiple sites M46.39
occipito-atlanto-axial region M46.31
sacrococcygeal region M46.38
thoracic region M46.34
thoracolumbar region M46.35

Infection, infected, infective *(continued)*
intestine, intestinal *—see* Enteritis, infectious
specified NEC A08.8
intra-amniotic affecting newborn NEC P39.2
Isospora belli or hominis A07.3
Japanese B encephalitis A83.0
jaw (bone) (lower) (upper) M27.2
joint NEC M00.9
due to internal joint prosthesis T84.50
kidney (cortex) (hematogenous) N15.9
with calculus N20.0
with hydronephrosis N13.6
following ectopic gestation O08.83
pelvis and ureter (cystic) N28.85
puerperal (postpartum) O86.21
specified NEC N15.8
Klebsiella (K.) pneumoniae NEC A49.8
as cause of disease classified elsewhere B96.1
knee (joint) NEC M00.9
joint M00.9
due to internal joint prosthesis
left T84.54
right T84.53
skin L08.9
Koch's *—see* Tuberculosis
labia (majora) (minora) (acute) *—see* Vulvitis
lacrimal
gland *—see* Dacryoadenitis
passages (duct) (sac) *—see* Inflammation, lacrimal, passages
lancet fluke B66.2
larynx NEC J38.7
leg (skin) NOS L08.9
Legionella pneumophila A48.1
nonpneumonic A48.2
Leishmania *—see also* Leishmaniasis
aethiopica B55.1
braziliensis B55.2
chagasi B55.0
donovani B55.0
infantum B55.0
major B55.1
mexicana B55.1
tropica B55.1
lentivirus, as cause of disease classified elsewhere B97.31
Leptosphaeria senegalensis B47.0
Leptospira interrogans A27.9
autumnalis A27.89
canicola A27.89
hebdomadis A27.89
icterohaemorrhagiae A27.0
pomona A27.89
specified type NEC A27.89
leptospirochetal NEC *—see* Leptospirosis
Listeria monocytogenes *—see also* Listeriosis
congenital P37.2
Loa loa B74.3
with conjunctival infestation B74.3
eyelid B74.3
Loboa loboi B48.0
local, skin (staphylococcal) (streptococcal) L08.9
abscess - code by site under Abscess
cellulitis - code by site under Cellulitis

Infection, infected, infective *(continued)*
local, skin *(continued)*
specified NEC L08.89
ulcer *—see* Ulcer, skin
Loefflerella mallei A24.0
lung (*see also* Pneumonia) J18.9
atypical Mycobacterium A31.0
spirochetal A69.8
tuberculous *—see* Tuberculosis, pulmonary
virus *—see* Pneumonia, viral
lymph gland *—see also* Lymphadenitis, acute
mesenteric I88.0
lymphoid tissue, base of tongue or posterior pharynx, NEC (chronic) J35.03
Madurella (grisea) (mycetomii) B47.0
major
following ectopic or molar pregnancy O08.0
puerperal, postpartum, childbirth O85
Malassezia furfur B36.0
Malleomyces
mallei A24.0
pseudomallei (whitmori) *—see* Melioidosis
mammary gland N61.0
Mansonella (ozzardi) (perstans) (streptocerca) B74.4
mastoid *—see* Mastoiditis
maxilla, maxillary M27.2
sinus (chronic) *—see* Sinusitis, maxillary
mediastinum J98.51
Medina (worm) B72
meibomian cyst or gland *—see* Hordeolum
meninges *—see* Meningitis, bacterial
meningococcal (*see also* condition) A39.9
adrenals A39.1
brain A39.81
cerebrospinal A39.0
conjunctiva A39.89
endocardium A39.51
heart A39.50
endocardium A39.51
myocardium A39.52
pericardium A39.53
joint A39.83
meninges A39.0
meningococcemia A39.4
acute A39.2
chronic A39.3
myocardium A39.52
pericardium A39.53
retrobulbar neuritis A39.82
specified site NEC A39.89
mesenteric lymph nodes or glands NEC I88.0
Metagonimus B66.8
metatarsophalangeal M00.9
methicillin
resistant Staphylococcus aureus (MRSA) A49.02
susceptible Staphylococcus aureus (MSSA) A49.01
Microsporum, microsporic *—see* Dermatophytosis
mixed flora (bacterial) NEC A49.8
Monilia *—see* Candidiasis
Monosporium apiospermum B48.2
mouth, parasitic B37.0
Mucor *—see* Mucormycosis

Infection, infected, infective *(continued)*
muscle NEC *—see* Myositis, infective
mycelium NOS B49
mycetoma B47.9
actinomycotic NEC B47.1
mycotic NEC B47.0
Mycobacterium, mycobacterial *—see* Mycobacterium
Mycoplasma NEC A49.3
pneumoniae, as cause of disease classified elsewhere B96.0
mycotic NOS B49
pathogenic to compromised host only B48.8
skin NOS B36.9
myocardium NEC I40.0
nail (chronic)
with lymphangitis *—see* Lymphangitis, acute, digit
finger L03.01-
fungus B35.1
ingrowing L60.0
toe L03.03-
fungus B35.1
nasal sinus (chronic) *—see* Sinusitis
nasopharynx *—see* Nasopharyngitis
navel L08.82
Necator americanus B76.1
Neisseria *—see* Gonococcus
Neotestudina rosatii B47.0
newborn P39.9
vintra-amniotic NEC P39.2
skin P39.4
specified type NEC P39.8
nipple N61.0
associated with
lactation O91.03
pregnancy O91.01-
puerperium O91.02
Nocardia *—see* Nocardiosis
obstetrical surgical wound (puerperal) O86.0
Oesophagostomum (apiostomum) B81.8
Oestrus ovis *—see* Myiasis
Oidium albicans B37.9
Onchocerca (volvulus) *—see* Onchocerciasis
oncovirus, as cause of disease classified elsewhere B97.32
operation wound T81.4
Opisthorchis (felineus) (viverrini) B66.0
orbit, orbital *—see* Inflammation, orbit
orthopoxvirus NEC B08.09
ovary *—see* Salpingo-oophoritis
Oxyuris vermicularis B80
pancreas (acute) *—see* Pancreatitis, acute
abscess *—see* Pancreatitis, acute
specified NEC (*see also* Pancreatitis, acute) K85.80
papillomavirus, as cause of disease classified elsewhere B97.7
papovavirus NEC B34.4
Paracoccidioides brasiliensis *—see* Paracoccidioidomycosis
Paragonimus (westermani) B66.4
parainfluenza virus B34.8
parameningococcus NOS A39.9
parapoxvirus B08.60
specified NEC B08.69
parasitic B89
Parastrongylus
cantonensis B83.2
costaricensis B81.3
paratyphoid A01.4
Type A A01.1
Type B A01.2

Infection, infected, infective *(continued)*
Parastrongylus *(continued)*
paratyphoid *(continued)*
Type C A01.3
paraurethral ducts N34.2
parotid gland *—see* Sialoadenitis
parvovirus NEC B34.3
as cause of disease classified elsewhere B97.6
Pasteurella NEC A28.0
multocida A28.0
pestis *—see* Plague
pseudotuberculosis A28.0
septica (cat bite) (dog bite) A28.0
tularensis *—see* Tularemia
pelvic, female *—see* Disease, pelvis, inflammatory
Penicillium (marneffei) B48.4
penis (glans) (retention) NEC N48.29
periapical K04.5
peridental, periodontal K05.20
generalized *—see* Peridontitis, aggressive, generalized
localized *—see* Peridontitis, aggressive, localized
perinatal period P39.9
specified type NEC P39.8
perineal repair (puerperal) O86.0
periorbital *—see* Inflammation, orbit
perirectal K62.89
perirenal *—see* Infection, kidney
peritoneal *—see* Peritonitis
periureteral N28.89
Petriellidium boydii B48.2
pharynx *—see also* Pharyngitis
coxsackievirus B08.5
posterior, lymphoid (chronic) J35.03
Phialophora
gougerotii (subcutaneous abscess or cyst) B43.2
jeanselmei (subcutaneous abscess or cyst) B43.2
verrucosa (skin) B43.0
Piedraia hortae B36.3
pinta A67.9
intermediate A67.1
late A67.2
mixed A67.3
primary A67.0
pinworm B80
pityrosporum furfur B36.0
pleuro-pneumonia-like organism (PPLO) NEC A49.3
as cause of disease classified elsewhere B96.0
pneumococcus, pneumococcal NEC A49.1
as cause of disease classified elsewhere B95.3
generalized (purulent) A40.3
with pneumonia J13
Pneumocystis carinii (pneumonia) B59
Pneumocystis jiroveci (pneumonia) B59
port or reservoir T80.212
postoperative T81.4
postoperative wound T81.4
postprocedural T81.4
postvaccinal T88.0
prepuce NEC N47.7
with penile inflammation N47.6
prion *—see* Disease, prion, central nervous system
prostate (capsule) *—see* Prostatitis
Proteus (mirabilis) (morganii) (vulgaris) NEC A49.8

Infection, infected, infective *(continued)*
Proteus *(continued)*
as cause of disease classified elsewhere B96.4
protozoal NEC B64
intestinal A07.9
specified NEC A07.8
specified NEC B60.8
Pseudoallescheria boydii B48.2
Pseudomonas NEC A49.8
as cause of disease classified elsewhere B96.5
mallei A24.0
pneumonia J15.1
pseudomallei *—see* Melioidosis
puerperal O86.4
genitourinary tract NEC O86.89
major or generalized O85
minor O86.4
specified NEC O86.89
pulmonary *—see* Infection, lung
purulent *—see* Abscess
Pyrenochaeta romeroi B47.0
Q fever A78
rectum (sphincter) K62.89
renal *—see also* Infection, kidney
pelvis and ureter (cystic) N28.85
reovirus, as cause of disease classified elsewhere B97.5
respiratory (tract) NEC J98.8
acute J22
chronic J98.8
influenzal (upper) (acute) *—see* Influenza, with, respiratory manifestations NEC
lower (acute) J22
chronic *—see* Bronchitis, chronic
rhinovirus J00
syncytial virus, as cause of disease classified elsewhere B97.4
upper (acute) NOS J06.9
chronic J39.8
streptococcal J06.9
viral NOS J06.9
resulting from
presence of internal prosthesis, implant, graft *—see* Complications, by site and type, infection
retortamoniasis A07.8
retroperitoneal NEC K68.9
retrovirus B33.3
as cause of disease classified elsewhere B97.30
human
immunodeficiency, type 2(HIV 2) B97.35
T-cell lymphotropic
type I (HTLV-I) B97.33
type II (HTLV-II) B97.34
lentivirus B97.31
oncovirus B97.32
specified NEC B97.39
Rhinosporidium (*see*beri) B48.1
rhinovirus
as cause of disease classified elsewhere B97.89
unspecified nature or site B34.8
Rhizopus *—see* Mucormycosis
rickettsial NOS A79.9
roundworm (large) NEC B82.0
Ascariasis (*see also* Ascariasis) B77.9
rubella *—see* Rubella
Saccharomyces *—see* Candidiasis
salivary duct or gland (any) *—see* Sialoadenitis

Infection, infected, infective *(continued)*
Salmonella (aertrycke) (arizonae) (callinarum) (cholerae-suis) (enteritidis) (suipestifer) (typhimurium) A02.9
with
(gastro)enteritis A02.0
sepsis A02.1
specified manifestation NEC A02.8
due to food (poisoning) A02.9
hirschfeldii A01.3
localized A02.20
arthritis A02.23
meningitis A02.21
osteomyelitis A02.24
pneumonia A02.22
pyelonephritis A02.25
specified NEC A02.29
paratyphi A01.4
A A01.1
B A01.2
C A01.3
schottmuelleri A01.2
typhi, typhosa *—see* Typhoid
Sarcocystis A07.8
scabies B86
Schistosoma *—see* Infestation, Schistosoma
scrotum (acute) NEC N49.2
seminal vesicle *—see* Vesiculitis
septic
localized, skin *—see* Abscess
sheep liver fluke B66.3
Shigella A03.9
boydii A03.2
dysenteriae A03.0
flexneri A03.1
group
A A03.0
B A03.1
C A03.2
D A03.3
Schmitz (-Stutzer) A03.0
schmitzii A03.0
shigae A03.0
sonnei A03.3
specified NEC A03.8
shoulder (joint) NEC M00.9
due to internal joint prosthesis T84.59
skin NEC L08.9
sinus (accessory) (chronic) (nasal) *—see also* Sinusitis
pilonidal *—see* Sinus, pilonidal
skin NEC L08.89
Skene's duct or gland *—see* Urethritis
skin (local) (staphylococcal) (streptococcal) L08.9
abscess - code by site under Abscess
cellulitis - code by site under Cellulitis
due to fungus B36.9
specified type NEC B36.8
mycotic B36.9
specified type NEC B36.8
newborn P39.4
ulcer *—see* Ulcer, skin
slow virus A81.9
specified NEC A81.89
Sparganum (mansoni) (proliferum) (baxteri) B70.1
specific *—see also* Syphilis
to perinatal period *—see* Infection, congenital
specified NEC B99.8
spermatic cord NEC N49.1

Infection, infected, infective *(continued)*

- sphenoidal (sinus) *—see* Sinusitis, sphenoidal
- spinal cord NOS *—see also* Myelitis G04.91
  - abscess G06.1
  - meninges *—see* Meningitis
  - streptococcal G04.89
- Spirillum A25.0
- spirochetal NOS A69.9
  - lung A69.8
  - specified NEC A69.8
- Spirometra larvae B70.1
- spleen D73.89
- Sporotrichum, Sporothrix (schenckii) *—see* Sporotrichosis
- staphylococcal, unspecified site
  - aureus (methicillin susceptible) (MSSA) A49.01
    - methicillin resistant (MRSA) A49.02
  - as cause of disease classified elsewhere B95.8
    - aureus (methicillin susceptible) (MSSA) B95.61
      - methicillin resistant (MRSA) B95.62
    - specified NEC B95.7
  - food poisoning A05.0
  - generalized (purulent) A41.2
  - pneumonia *—see* Pneumonia, staphylococcal
- Stellantchasmus falcatus B66.8
- streptobacillus moniliformis A25.1
- streptococcal NEC A49.1
  - as cause of disease classified elsewhere B95.5
  - B genitourinary complicating
    - childbirth O98.82
    - pregnancy O98.81-
    - puerperium O98.83
  - congenital
    - sepsis P36.10
      - group B P36.0
      - specified NEC P36.19
  - generalized (purulent) A40.9
- Streptomyces B47.1
- Strongyloides (stercoralis) *—see* Strongyloidiasis
- stump (amputation) (surgical) *—see* Complication, amputation stump, infection
- subcutaneous tissue, local L08.9
- suipestifer *—see* Infection, salmonella
- swimming pool bacillus A31.1
- Taenia *—see* Infestation, Taenia
- Taeniarhynchus saginatus B68.1
- tapeworm *—see* Infestation, tapeworm
- tendon (sheath) *—see* Tenosynovitis, infective NEC
- Ternidens diminutus B81.8
- testis *—see* Orchitis
- threadworm B80
- throat *—see* Pharyngitis
- thyroglossal duct K14.8
- toe (skin) L08.9
  - cellulitis L03.03-
    - fungus B35.1
  - nail L03.03-
    - fungus B35.1
- tongue NEC K14.0
  - parasitic B37.0
- tonsil (and adenoid) (faucial) (lingual) (pharyngeal) *—see* Tonsillitis
- tooth, teeth K04.7
  - periapical K04.7

Infection, infected, infective *(continued)*

- tooth, teeth *(continued)*
  - peridental, periodontal K05.20
    - generalized - *see* Peridontitis, aggressive, generalized
    - localized - *see* Peridontitis, aggressive, localized
  - pulp K04.01
    - irreversible K04.02
    - reversible K04.01
  - socket M27.3
- TORCH *—see* Infection, congenital
  - without active infection P00.2
- Torula histolytica *—see* Cryptococcosis
- Toxocara (canis) (cati) (felis) B83.0
- Toxoplasma gondii *—see* Toxoplasma
- trachea, chronic J42
- trematode NEC *—see* Infestation, fluke
- trench fever A79.0
- Treponema pallidum *—see* Syphilis
- Trichinella (spiralis) B75
- Trichomonas A59.9
  - cervix A59.09
  - intestine A07.8
  - prostate A59.02
  - specified site NEC A59.8
  - urethra A59.03
  - urogenitalis A59.00
  - vagina A59.01
  - vulva A59.01
- Trichophyton, trichophytic *—see* Dermatophytosis
- Trichosporon (beigelii) cutaneum B36.2
- Trichostrongylus B81.2
- Trichuris (trichiura) B79
- Trombicula (irritans) B88.0
- Trypanosoma
  - brucei
    - gambiense B56.0
    - rhodesiense B56.1
  - cruzi *—see* Chagas' disease
- tubal *—see* Salpingo-oophoritis
- tuberculous NEC *—see* Tuberculosis
- tubo-ovarian *—see* Salpingo-oophoritis
- tunnel T80.212
- tunica vaginalis N49.1
- tympanic membrane NEC *—see* Myringitis
- typhoid (abortive) (ambulant) (bacillus) *—see* Typhoid
- typhus A75.9
  - flea-borne A75.2
  - mite-borne A75.3
  - recrudescent A75.1
  - tick-borne A77.9
    - African A77.1
    - North Asian A77.2
- umbilicus L08.82
- ureter N28.86
- urethra *—see* Urethritis
- urinary (tract) N39.0
  - bladder *—see* Cystitis
  - complicating
    - pregnancy O23.4-
      - specified type NEC O23.3-
  - kidney *—see* Infection, kidney
  - newborn P39.3
  - puerperal (postpartum) O86.20
  - tuberculous A18.13
  - urethra *—see* Urethritis
- uterus, uterine *—see* Endometritis
- vaccination T88.0
- vaccinia not from vaccination B08.011
- vagina (acute) *—see* Vaginitis

Infection, infected, infective *(continued)*

- varicella B01.9
- varicose veins *—see* Varix
- vas deferens NEC N49.1
- vesical *—see* Cystitis
- Vibrio
  - cholerae A00.0
    - El Tor A00.1
  - parahaemolyticus (food poisoning) A05.3
  - vulnificus
    - as cause of disease classified elsewhere B96.82
    - foodborne intoxication A05.5
- Vincent's (gum) (mouth) (tonsil) A69.1
- virus, viral NOS B34.9
  - adenovirus
    - as cause of disease classified elsewhere B97.0
    - unspecified nature or site B34.0
  - arborvirus, arbovirus arthropod-borne A94
  - as cause of disease classified elsewhere B97.89
    - adenovirus B97.0
    - coronavirus B97.29
      - SARS-associated B97.21
    - coxsackievirus B97.11
    - echovirus B97.12
    - enterovirus B97.10
      - coxsackievirus B97.11
      - echovirus B97.12
      - specified NEC B97.19
    - human
      - immunodeficiency, type 2 (HIV 2) B97.35
      - T-cell lymphotropic,
        - type I (HTLV-I) B97.33
        - type II (HTLV-II) B97.34
      - metapneumovirus B97.81
    - papillomavirus B97.7
    - parvovirus B97.6
    - reovirus B97.5
    - respiratory syncytial B97.4
    - retrovirus B97.30
      - human
        - immunodeficiency, type 2(HIV 2) B97.35
        - T-cell lymphotropic,
          - type I (HTLV-I) B97.33
          - type II (HTLV-II) B97.34
      - lentivirus B97.31
      - oncovirus B97.32
      - specified NEC B97.39
    - specified NEC B97.89
  - central nervous system A89
    - atypical A81.9
      - specified NEC A81.89
    - enterovirus NEC A88.8
      - meningitis A87.0
    - slow virus A81.9
      - specified NEC A81.89
    - specified NEC A88.8
  - chest J98.8
  - cotia B08.8
  - coxsackie (*see also* Infection, coxsackie) B34.1
    - as cause of disease classified elsewhere B97.11
  - ECHO
    - as cause of disease classified elsewhere B97.12
    - unspecified nature or site B34.1
  - encephalitis, tick-borne A84.9
  - enterovirus, as cause of disease classified elsewhere B97.10
    - coxsackievirus B97.11
    - echovirus B97.12
    - specified NEC B97.19

Infection, infected, infective *(continued)*

- virus, viral *(continued)*
  - exanthem NOS B09
  - human papilloma as cause of disease classified elsewhere B97.7
  - human metapneumovirus as cause of disease classified elsewhere B97.81
  - intestine *—see* Enteritis, viral
  - respiratory syncytial
    - as cause of disease classified elsewhere B97.4
    - bronchopneumonia J12.1
    - common cold syndrome J00
    - nasopharyngitis (acute) J00
  - rhinovirus
    - as cause of disease classified elsewhere B97.89
    - unspecified nature or site B34.8
  - slow A81.9
    - specified NEC A81.89
  - specified type NEC B33.8
    - as cause of disease classified elsewhere B97.89
    - unspecified nature or site B34.8
  - unspecified nature or site B34.9
  - West Nile *—see* Virus, West Nile
- vulva (acute) *—see* Vulvitis
- West Nile *—see* Virus, West Nile
- whipworm B79
- worms B83.9
  - specified type NEC B83.8
- Wuchereria (bancrofti) B74.0
  - malayi B74.1
- yatapoxvirus B08.70
  - specified NEC B08.79
- yeast (*see also* Candidiasis) B37.9
- yellow fever *—see* Fever, yellow
- Yersinia
  - enterocolitica (intestinal) A04.6
  - pestis *—see* Plague
  - pseudotuberculosis A28.2
- Zeis' gland *—see* Hordeolum
- Zika virus A92.5
- zoonotic bacterial NOS A28.9
- Zopfia senegalensis B47.0

Infective, infectious *—see* condition

Infertility

- female N97.9
  - age-related N97.8
  - associated with
    - anovulation N97.0
    - cervical (mucus) disease or anomaly N88.3
    - congenital anomaly
      - cervix N88.3
      - fallopian tube N97.1
      - uterus N97.2
      - vagina N97.8
    - dysmucorrhea N88.3
    - fallopian tube disease or anomaly N97.1
    - pituitary-hypothalamic origin E23.0
    - specified origin NEC N97.8
    - Stein-Leventhal syndrome E28.2
    - uterine disease or anomaly N97.2
    - vaginal disease or anomaly N97.8
  - due to
    - cervical anomaly N88.3
    - fallopian tube anomaly N97.1
    - ovarian failure E28.39
    - Stein-Leventhal syndrome E28.2
    - uterine anomaly N97.2
    - vaginal anomaly N97.8

Infertility *(continued)*
female *(continued)*
nonimplantation N97.2
origin
cervical N88.3
tubal (block) (occlusion) (stenosis) N97.1
uterine N97.2
vaginal N97.8
male N46.9
azoospermia N46.01
extratesticular cause N46.029
drug therapy N46.021
efferent duct obstruction N46.023
infection N46.022
radiation N46.024
specified cause NEC N46.029
systemic disease N46.025
oligospermia N46.11
extratesticular cause N46.129
drug therapy N46.121
efferent duct obstruction N46.123
infection N46.122
radiation N46.124
specified cause NEC N46.129
systemic disease N46.125
specified type NEC N46.8

Infestation B88.9
Acanthocheilonema (perstans) (streptocerca) B74.4
Acariasis B88.0
demodex folliculorum B88.0
sarcoptes scabiei B86
trombiculae B88.0
Agamofilaria streptocerca B74.4
Ancylostoma, ankylostoma (braziliense) (caninum) (ceylanicum) (duodenale) B76.0
americanum B76.1
new world B76.1
Anisakis larvae, anisakiasis B81.0
arthropod NEC B88.2
Ascaris lumbricoides *—see* Ascariasis
Balantidium coli A07.0
beef tapeworm B68.1
Bothriocephalus (latus) B70.0
larval B70.1
broad tapeworm B70.0
larval B70.1
Brugia (malayi) B74.1
timori B74.2
candiru B88.8
Capillaria
hepatica B83.8
philippinensis B81.1
cat liver fluke B66.0
cestodes B71.9
diphyllobothrium *—see* Infestation, diphyllobothrium
dipylidiasis B71.1
hymenolepiasis B71.0
specified type NEC B71.8
chigger B88.0
chigo, chigoe B88.1
Clonorchis (sinensis) (liver) B66.1
coccidial A07.3
crab-lice B85.3
Cysticercus cellulosae *—see* Cysticercosis
Demodex (folliculorum) B88.0
Dermanyssus gallinae B88.0
Dermatobia (hominis) *—see* Myiasis
Dibothriocephalus (latus) B70.0
larval B70.1
Dicrocoelium dendriticum B66.2

Infestation *(continued)*
Diphyllobothrium (adult) (latum) (intestinal) (pacificum) B70.0
larval B70.1
Diplogonoporus (grandis) B71.8
Dipylidium caninum B67.4
Distoma hepaticum B66.3
dog tapeworm B67.4
Dracunculus medinensis B72
dragon worm B72
dwarf tapeworm B71.0
Echinococcus *—see* Echinococcus
Echinostomum ilocanum B66.8
Entamoeba (histolytica) *—see* Infection, Ameba
Enterobius vermicularis B80
eyelid
in (due to)
leishmaniasis B55.1
loiasis B74.3
onchocerciasis B73.09
phthiriasis B85.3
parasitic NOS B89
eyeworm B74.3
Fasciola (gigantica) (hepatica) (indica) B66.3
Fasciolopsis (buski) (intestine) B66.5
filarial B74.9
bancroftian B74.0
conjunctiva B74.9
due to
Acanthocheilonema (perstans) (streptocerca) B74.4
Brugia (malayi) B74.1
timori B74.2
Dracunculus medinensis B72
guinea worm B72
loa loa B74.3
Mansonella (ozzardi) (perstans) (streptocerca) B74.4
Onchocerca volvulus B73.00
eye B73.00
eyelid B73.09
Wuchereria (bancrofti) B74.0
Malayan B74.1
ozzardi B74.4
specified type NEC B74.8
fish tapeworm B70.0
larval B70.1
fluke B66.9
blood NOS *—see* Schistosomiasis
cat liver B66.0
intestinal B66.5
liver (sheep) B66.3
cat B66.0
Chinese B66.1
due to clonorchiasis B66.1
oriental B66.1
lancet B66.2
lung (oriental) B66.4
sheep liver B66.3
specified type NEC B66.8
fly larvae *—see* Myiasis
Gasterophilus (intestinalis) *—see* Myiasis
Gastrodiscoides hominis B66.8
Giardia lamblia A07.1
Gnathostoma (spinigerum) B83.1
Gongylonema B83.8
guinea worm B72
helminth B83.9
angiostrongyliasis B83.2
intestinal B81.3
gnathostomiasis B83.1
hirudiniasis, internal B83.4
intestinal B82.0
angiostrongyliasis B81.3
anisakiasis B81.0
ascariasis *—see* Ascariasis

Infestation *(continued)*
helminth *(continued)*
intestinal *(continued)*
capillariasis B81.1
cysticercosis *—see* Cysticercosis
diphyllobothriasis *—see* Infestation, diphyllobothriasis
dracunculiasis B72
echinococcus *—see* Echinococcosis
enterobiasis B80
filariasis *—see* Infestation, filarial
fluke *—see* Infestation, fluke
hookworm *—see* Infestation, hookworm
mixed (types classifiable to more than one of the titles B65.0-B81.3 and B81.8) B81.4
onchocerciasis *—see* Onchocerciasis
schistosomiasis *—see* Infestation, schistosoma
specified
cestode NEC *—see* Infestation, cestode
type NEC B81.8
strongyloidiasis *—see* Strongyloidiasis
taenia *—see* Infestation, taenia
trichinellosis B75
trichostrongyliasis B81.2
trichuriasis B79
specified type NEC B83.8
syngamiasis B83.3
visceral larva migrans B83.0
Heterophyes (heterophyes) B66.8
hookworm B76.9
ancylostomiasis B76.0
necatoriasis B76.1
specified type NEC B76.8
Hymenolepis (diminuta) (nana) B71.0
intestinal NEC B82.9
leeches (aquatic) (land) *—see* Hirudiniasis
Leishmania *—see* Leishmaniasis
lice, louse *—see* Infestation, Pediculus
Linguatula B88.8
Liponyssoides sanguineus B88.0
Loa loa B74.3
conjunctival B74.3
eyelid B74.3
louse *—see* Infestation, Pediculus
maggots *—see* Myiasis
Mansonella (ozzardi) (perstans) (streptocerca) B74.4
Medina (worm) B72
Metagonimus (yokogawai) B66.8
microfilaria streptocerca *—see* Onchocerciasis
eye B73.00
eyelid B73.09
mites B88.9
scabic B86
Monilia (albicans) *—see* Candidiasis
mouth B37.0
Necator americanus B76.1
nematode NEC (intestinal) B82.0
Ancylostoma B76.0
conjunctiva NEC B83.9
Enterobius vermicularis B80
Gnathostoma spinigerum B83.1
physaloptera B80
specified NEC B81.8
trichostrongylus B81.2
trichuris (trichuria) B79

Infestation *(continued)*
Oesophagostomum (apiostomum) B81.8
Oestrus ovis (*see also* Myiasis) B87.9
Onchocerca (volvulus) *—see* Onchocerciasis
Opisthorchis (felineus) (viverrini) B66.0
orbit, parasitic NOS B89
Oxyuris vermicularis B80
Paragonimus (westermani) B66.4
parasite, parasitic B89
eyelid B89
intestinal NOS B82.9
mouth B37.0
skin B88.9
tongue B37.0
Parastrongylus
cantonensis B83.2
costaricensis B81.3
Pediculus B85.2
body B85.1
capitis (humanus) (any site) B85.0
corporis (humanus) (any site) B85.1
head B85.0
mixed (classifiable to more than one of the titles B85.0-B85.3) B85.4
pubis (any site) B85.3
Pentastoma B88.8
Phthirus (pubis) (any site) B85.3
with any infestation classifiable to B85.0-B85.2 B85.4
pinworm B80
pork tapeworm (adult) B68.0
protozoal NEC B64
intestinal A07.9
specified NEC A07.8
specified NEC B60.8
pubic, louse B85.3
rat tapeworm B71.0
red bug B88.0
roundworm (large) NEC B82.0
Ascariasis (*see also* Ascariasis) B77.9
sandflea B88.1
Sarcoptes scabiei B86
scabies B86
Schistosoma B65.9
bovis B65.8
cercariae B65.3
haematobium B65.0
intercalatum B65.8
japonicum B65.2
mansoni B65.1
mattheei B65.8
mekongi B65.8
specified type NEC B65.8
spindale B65.8
screw worms *—see* Myiasis
skin NOS B88.9
Sparganum (mansoni) (proliferum) (baxteri) B70.1
larval B70.1
specified type NEC B88.8
Spirometra larvae B70.1
Stellantchasmus falcatus B66.8
Strongyloides stercoralis *—see* Strongyloidiasis
Taenia B68.9
diminuta B71.0
echinococcus *—see* Echinococcus
mediocanellata B68.1
nana B71.0
saginata B68.1
solium (intestinal form) B68.0
larval form *—see* Cysticercosis

Infestation *(continued)*
- Taeniarhynchus saginatus B68.1
- tapeworm B71.9
  - beef B68.1
  - broad B70.0
    - larval B70.1
  - dog B67.4
  - dwarf B71.0
  - fish B70.0
    - larval B70.1
  - pork B68.0
  - rat B71.0
- Ternidens diminutus B81.8
- Tetranychus molestissimus B88.0
- threadworm B80
- tongue B37.0
- Toxocara (canis) (cati) (felis) B83.0
- trematode(s) NEC *—see* Infestation, fluke
- Trichinella (spiralis) B75
- Trichocephalus B79
- Trichomonas *—see* Trichomoniasis
- Trichostrongylus B81.2
- Trichuris (trichiura) B79
- Trombicula (irritans) B88.0
- Tunga penetrans B88.1
- Uncinaria americana B76.1
- Vandellia cirrhosa B88.8
- whipworm B79
- worms B83.9
  - intestinal B82.0
- Wuchereria (bancrofti) B74.0

Infiltrate, infiltration
- amyloid (generalized) (localized) *—see* Amyloidosis
- calcareous NEC R89.7
  - localized *—see* Degeneration, by site
- calcium salt R89.7
- cardiac
  - fatty *—see* Degeneration, myocardial
  - glycogenic E74.02 *[I43]*
- corneal *—see* Edema, cornea
- eyelid *—see* Inflammation, eyelid
- glycogen, glycogenic *—see* Disease, glycogen storage
- heart, cardiac
  - fatty *—see* Degeneration, myocardial
  - glycogenic E74.02 *[I43]*
- inflammatory in vitreous H43.89
- kidney N28.89
- leukemic *—see* Leukemia
- liver K76.89
  - fatty *—see* Fatty, liver NEC
  - glycogen (*see also* Disease, glycogen storage) E74.03 *[K77]*
- lung R91.8
  - eosinophilic J82
- lymphatic (*see also* Leukemia, lymphatic) C91.9-
  - gland I88.9
- muscle, fatty M62.89
- myocardium, myocardial
  - fatty *—see* Degeneration, myocardial
  - glycogenic E74.02 *[I43]*
- on chest x-ray R91.8
- pulmonary R91.8
  - with eosinophilia J82
- skin (lymphocytic) L98.6
- thymus (gland) (fatty) E32.8
- urine R39.0
- vesicant agent
  - antineoplastic chemotherapy T80.810
  - other agent NEC T80.818
- vitreous body H43.89

Infirmity R68.89
- senile R54

Inflammation, inflamed, inflammatory (with exudation)
- abducent (nerve) *—see* Strabismus, paralytic, sixth nerve
- accessory sinus (chronic) *—see* Sinusitis
- adrenal (gland) E27.8
- alveoli, teeth M27.3
  - scorbutic E54
- anal canal, anus K62.89
- antrum (chronic) *—see* Sinusitis, maxillary
- appendix *—see* Appendicitis
- arachnoid *—see* Meningitis
- areola N61.0
  - puerperal, postpartum or gestational *—see* Infection, nipple
- areolar tissue NOS L08.9
- artery *—see* Arteritis
- auditory meatus (external) *—see* Otitis, externa
- Bartholin's gland N75.8
- bile duct (common) (hepatic) or passage *—see* Cholangitis
- bladder *—see* Cystitis
- bone *—see* Osteomyelitis
- brain *—see also* Encephalitis
  - membrane *—see* Meningitis
- breast N61.0
  - puerperal, postpartum, gestational *—see* Mastitis, obstetric
- broad ligament *—see* Disease, pelvis, inflammatory
- bronchi *—see* Bronchitis
- catarrhal J00
- cecum *—see* Appendicitis
- cerebral *—see also* Encephalitis
  - membrane *—see* Meningitis
- cerebrospinal
  - meningococcal A39.0
- cervix (uteri) *—see* Cervicitis
- chest J98.8
- chorioretinal H30.9-
  - cyclitis *—see* Cyclitis
  - disseminated H30.10-
    - generalized H30.13-
    - peripheral H30.12-
    - posterior pole H30.11-
  - epitheliopathy *—see* Epitheliopathy
  - focal H30.00-
    - juxtapapillary H30.01-
    - macular H30.04-
    - paramacular *—see* Inflammation, chorioretinal, focal, macular
    - peripheral H30.03-
    - posterior pole H30.02-
  - specified type NEC H30.89-
- choroid *—see* Inflammation, chorioretinal
- chronic, postmastoidectomy cavity *—see* Complications, postmastoidectomy, inflammation
- colon *—see* Enteritis
- connective tissue (diffuse) NEC *—see* Disorder, soft tissue, specified type NEC
- cornea *—see* Keratitis
- corpora cavernosa N48.29
- cranial nerve *—see* Disorder, nerve, cranial
- Douglas' cul-de-sac or pouch (chronic) N73.0

Inflammation, inflamed, inflammatory *(continued)*
- due to device, implant or graft *—see also* Complications, by site and type, infection or inflammation
  - arterial graft T82.7
  - breast (implant) T85.79
  - catheter T85.79
    - dialysis (renal) T82.7
      - intraperitoneal T85.71
    - infusion T82.7
      - cranial T85.735
      - intrathecal T85.735
      - spinal (epidural) (subdural) T85.735
      - subarachnoid T85.735
    - urinary T83.51
      - cystostomy T83.510
      - Hopkins T83.518
      - ileostomy T83.518
      - nephrostomy T83.512
      - specified NEC T83.518
      - urethral indwelling T83.511
      - urostomy T83.518
  - electronic (electrode) (pulse generator) (stimulator)
    - bone T84.7
    - cardiac T82.7
    - nervous system T85.738
      - brain T85.731
      - cranial nerve T85.732
      - gastric nerve T85.732
      - neurostimulator generator T85.734
      - peripheral nerve T85.732
      - sacral nerve T85.732
      - spinal cord T85.733
      - vagal nerve T85.732
    - urinary T83.590
  - fixation, internal (orthopedic)
    - NEC *—see* Complication, fixation device, infection
  - gastrointestinal (bile duct) (esophagus) T85.79
    - neurostimulator electrode (lead) T85.732
  - genital NEC T83.69
  - heart NEC T82.7
    - valve (prosthesis) T82.6
      - graft T82.7
  - joint prosthesis *—see* Complication, joint prosthesis, infection
  - ocular (corneal graft) (orbital implant) NEC T85.79
  - orthopedic NEC T84.7
  - penile (cylinder) (pump) (resevoir) T83.61
  - specified NEC T85.79
  - testicular T83.62
  - urinary NEC T83.598
    - ileal conduit stent T83.593
    - implanted neurostimulation T83.590
    - implanted sphincter T83.591
    - indwelling ureteral stent T83.592
    - nephroureteral stent T83.593
    - specified stent NEC T83.593
  - vascular NEC T82.7
  - ventricular intracranial (communicating) shunt T85.730
- duodenum K29.80
  - with bleeding K29.81
- dura mater *—see* Meningitis
- ear (middle) *—see also* Otitis, media
  - external *—see* Otitis, externa
  - inner *—see* subcategory H83.0
- epididymis *—see* Epididymitis
- esophagus K20.9
- ethmoidal (sinus) (chronic) *—see* Sinusitis, ethmoidal
- eustachian tube (catarrhal) *—see* Salpingitis, eustachian
- eyelid H01.9
  - abscess *—see* Abscess, eyelid
  - blepharitis *—see* Blepharitis
  - chalazion *—see* Chalazion
  - dermatosis (noninfectious) *—see* Dermatosis, eyelid
  - hordeolum *—see* Hordeolum
  - specified NEC H01.8
- fallopian tube *—see* Salpingo-oophoritis
- fascia *—see* Myositis
- follicular, pharynx J31.2
- frontal (sinus) (chronic) *—see* Sinusitis, frontal
- gallbladder *—see* Cholecystitis
- gastric *—see* Gastritis
- gastrointestinal *—see* Enteritis
- genital organ (internal) (diffuse)
  - female *—see* Disease, pelvis, inflammatory
  - male N49.9
    - multiple sites N49.8
    - specified NEC N49.8
- gland (lymph) *—see* Lymphadenitis
- glottis *—see* Laryngitis
- granular, pharynx J31.2
- gum K05.10
  - nonplaque induced K05.11
  - plaque induced K05.10
- heart *—see* Carditis
- hepatic duct *—see* Cholangitis
- ileoanal (internal) pouch K91.850
- ileum *—see also* Enteritis
  - regional or terminal *—see* Enteritis, regional
- intestine (any part) *—see* Enteritis
- intestinal pouch K91.850
- jaw (acute) (bone) (chronic) (lower) (suppurative) (upper) M27.2
- joint NEC *—see* Arthritis
  - sacroiliac M46.1
- kidney *—see* Nephritis
- knee (joint) M13.169
  - tuberculous A18.02
- labium (majus) (minus) *—see* Vulvitis
- lacrimal
  - gland *—see* Dacryoadenitis
  - passages (duct) (sac) *—see also* Dacryocystitis
    - canaliculitis *—see* Canaliculitis, lacrimal
- larynx *—see* Laryngitis
- leg NOS L08.9
- lip K13.0
- liver (capsule) *—see also* Hepatitis
  - chronic K73.9
  - suppurative K75.0
- lung (acute) *—see also* Pneumonia
  - chronic J98.4
- lymph gland or node *—see* Lymphadenitis
- lymphatic vessel *—see* Lymphangitis
- maxilla, maxillary M27.2
  - sinus (chronic) *—see* Sinusitis, maxillary
- membranes of brain or spinal cord *—see* Meningitis
- meninges *—see* Meningitis
- mouth K12.1
- muscle *—see* Myositis
- myocardium *—see* Myocarditis

Inflammation, inflamed, inflammatory *(continued)*
- nasal sinus (chronic) —*see* Sinusitis
- nasopharynx —*see* Nasopharyngitis
- navel L08.82
- nerve NEC —*see* Neuralgia
- nipple N61.0
  - puerperal, postpartum or gestational —*see* Infection, nipple
- nose —*see* Rhinitis
- oculomotor (nerve) —*see* Strabismus, paralytic, third nerve
- optic nerve —*see* Neuritis, optic
- orbit (chronic) H05.10
  - acute H05.00
    - abscess —*see* Abscess, orbit
    - cellulitis —*see* Cellulitis, orbit
    - osteomyelitis —*see* Osteomyelitis, orbit
    - periostitis —*see* Periostitis, orbital
    - tenonitis —*see* Tenonitis, eye
  - granuloma —*see* Granuloma, orbit
  - myositis —*see* Myositis, orbital
- ovary —*see* Salpingo-oophoritis
- oviduct —*see* Salpingo-oophoritis
- pancreas (acute) —*see* Pancreatitis
- parametrium N73.0
- parotid region L08.9
- pelvis, female —*see* Disease, pelvis, inflammatory
- penis (corpora cavernosa) N48.29
- perianal K62.89
- pericardium —*see* Pericarditis
- perineum (female) (male) L08.9
- perirectal K62.89
- peritoneum —*see* Peritonitis
- periuterine —*see* Disease, pelvis, inflammatory
- perivesical —*see* Cystitis
- petrous bone (acute) (chronic) —*see* Petrositis
- pharynx (acute) —*see* Pharyngitis
- pia mater —*see* Meningitis
- pleura —*see* Pleurisy
- polyp, colon (*see also* Polyp, colon, inflammatory) K51.40
- prostate —*see also* Prostatitis
  - specified type NEC N41.8
- rectosigmoid —*see* Rectosigmoiditis
- rectum (*see also* Proctitis) K62.89
- respiratory, upper (*see also* Infection, respiratory, upper) J06.9
  - acute, due to radiation J70.0
  - chronic, due to external agent —*see* condition, respiratory, chronic, due to
  - due to
    - chemicals, gases, fumes or vapors (inhalation) J68.2
    - radiation J70.1
- retina —*see* Chorioretinitis
- retrocecal —*see* Appendicitis
- retroperitoneal —*see* Peritonitis
- salivary duct or gland (any) (suppurative) —*see* Sialoadenitis
- scorbutic, alveoli, teeth E54
- scrotum N49.2
- seminal vesicle —*see* Vesiculitis
- sigmoid —*see* Enteritis
- sinus —*see* Sinusitis
- Skene's duct or gland —*see* Urethritis
- skin L08.9
- spermatic cord N49.1
- sphenoidal (sinus) —*see* Sinusitis, sphenoidal
- spinal
  - cord —*see* Encephalitis
  - membrane —*see* Meningitis
  - nerve —*see* Disorder, nerve
- spine —*see* Spondylopathy, inflammatory
- spleen (capsule) D73.89
- stomach —*see* Gastritis
- subcutaneous tissue L08.9
- suprarenal (gland) E27.8
- synovial —*see* Tenosynovitis
- tendon (sheath) NEC —*see* Tenosynovitis
- testis —*see* Orchitis
- throat (acute) —*see* Pharyngitis
- thymus (gland) E32.8
- thyroid (gland) —*see* Thyroiditis
- tongue K14.0
- tonsil —*see* Tonsillitis
- trachea —*see* Tracheitis
- trochlear (nerve) —*see* Strabismus, paralytic, fourth nerve
- tubal —*see* Salpingo-oophoritis
- tuberculous NEC —*see* Tuberculosis
- tubo-ovarian —*see* Salpingo-oophoritis
- tunica vaginalis N49.1
- tympanic membrane —*see* Tympanitis
- umbilicus, umbilical L08.82
- uterine ligament —*see* Disease, pelvis, inflammatory
- uterus (catarrhal) —*see* Endometritis
- uveal tract (anterior) NOS —*see also* Iridocyclitis
  - posterior —*see* Chorioretinitis
- vagina —*see* Vaginitis
- vas deferens N49.1
- vein —*see also* Phlebitis
  - intracranial or intraspinal (septic) G08
  - thrombotic I80.9
    - leg —*see* Phlebitis, leg
    - lower extremity —*see* Phlebitis, leg
- vocal cord J38.3
- vulva —*see* Vulvitis
- Wharton's duct (suppurative) —*see* Sialoadenitis

Inflation, lung, imperfect (newborn) —*see* Atelectasis

Influenza (bronchial) (epidemic) (respiratory (upper)) (unidentified influenza virus) J11.1
- with
  - digestive manifestations J11.2
  - encephalopathy J11.81
  - enteritis J11.2
  - gastroenteritis J11.2
  - gastrointestinal manifestations J11.2
  - laryngitis J11.1
  - myocarditis J11.82
  - otitis media J11.83
  - pharyngitis J11.1
  - pneumonia J11.00
    - specified type J11.08
  - respiratory manifestations NEC J11.1
  - specified manifestation NEC J11.89
- A/H5N1 (*see also* Influenza, due to, identified novel influenza A virus) J09.X2
- avian (*see also* Influenza, due to, identified novel influenza A virus) J09.X2
- bird (*see also* Influenza, due to, identified novel influenza A virus) J09.X2
- novel (2009) H1N1 influenza (*see also* Influenza, due to, identified novel influenza A virus) NEC J10.1
- novel influenza A/H1N1 (*see also* Influenza, due to, identified novel influenza A virus) NEC J10.1
- due to
  - avian (*see also* Influenza, due to, identified novel influenza A virus) J09.X2
  - identified influenza virus NEC J10.1
    - with
      - digestive manifestations J10.2
      - encephalopathy J10.81
      - enteritis J10.2
      - gastroenteritis J10.2
      - gastrointestinal manifestations J10.2
      - laryngitis J10.1
      - myocarditis J10.82
      - otitis media J10.83
      - pharyngitis J10.1
      - pneumonia (unspecified type) J10.00
        - with same identified influenza virus J10.01
        - specified type NEC J10.08
      - respiratory manifestations NEC J10.1
      - specified manifestation NEC J10.89
  - identified novel influenza A virus J09.X2
    - with
      - digestive manifestations J09.X3
      - encephalopathy J09.X9
      - enteritis J09.X3
      - gastroenteritis J09.X3
      - gastrointestinal manifestations J09.X3
      - laryngitis J09.X2
      - myocarditis J09.X9
      - otitis media J09.X9
      - pharyngitis J09.X2
      - pneumonia J09.X1
      - respiratory manifestations NEC J09.X2
      - specified manifestation NEC J09.X9
      - upper respiratory symptoms J09.X2
- of other animal origin, not bird or swine (*see also* Influenza, due to, identified novel influenza A virus) J09.X2
- swine (viruses that normally cause infections in pigs) (*see also* Influenza, due to, identified novel influenza A virus) J09.X2

Influenza-like disease —*see* Influenza

Influenzal —*see* Influenza

Infraction, Freiberg's (metatarsal head) —*see* Osteochondrosis, juvenile, metatarsus

Infraeruption of tooth (teeth) M26.34

Infusion complication, misadventure, or reaction —*see* Complications, infusion

Ingestion
- chemical —*see* Table of Drugs and Chemicals, by substance, poisoning
- drug or medicament
  - correct substance properly administered —*see* Table of Drugs and Chemicals, by drug, adverse effect
  - overdose or wrong substance given or taken —*see* Table of Drugs and Chemicals, by drug, poisoning
- foreign body —*see* Foreign body, alimentary tract
- tularemia A21.3

Ingrowing
- hair (beard) L73.1
- nail (finger) (toe) L60.0

Inguinal —*see also* condition
- testicle Q53.9
  - bilateral Q53.212
  - unilateral Q53.112

Inhalant-induced
- anxiety disorder F18.980
- depressive disorder F18.94
- major neurocognitive disorder F18.97
- mild neurocognitive disorder F18.988
- psychotic disorder F18.959

Inhalation
- anthrax A22.1
- flame T27.3
- food or foreign body —*see* Foreign body, by site
- gases, fumes, or vapors NEC T59.9-
  - specified agent —*see* Table of Drugs and Chemicals, by substance
- liquid or vomitus —*see* Asphyxia
- meconium (newborn) P24.00
  - with
    - pneumonia (pneumonitis) P24.01
    - with respiratory symptoms P24.01
- mucus —*see* Asphyxia, mucus
- oil or gasoline (causing suffocation) —*see* Foreign body, by site
- smoke J70.5
  - due to chemicals, gases, fumes and vapors J68.9
- steam —*see* Toxicity, vapors
- stomach contents or secretions —*see* Foreign body, by site
  - due to anesthesia (general) (local) or other sedation T88.59
    - in labor and delivery O74.0
    - in pregnancy O29.01-
    - postpartum, puerperal O89.01

Inhibition, orgasm
- female F52.31
- male F52.32

Inhibitor, systemic lupus erythematosus (presence of) D68.62

Iniencephalus, iniencephaly Q00.2

Injection, traumatic jet (air) (industrial) (water) (paint or dye) T70.4

Injury (*see also* specified injury type) T14.90
- abdomen, abdominal S39.91
  - blood vessel —*see* Injury, blood vessel, abdomen

Injury *(continued)*
abdomen, abdominal *(continued)*
cavity —*see* Injury, intra-abdominal
contusion S30.1
internal —*see* Injury, intra-abdominal
intra-abdominal organ —*see* Injury, intra-abdominal
nerve —*see* Injury, nerve, abdomen
open —*see* Wound, open, abdomen
specified NEC S39.81
superficial —*see* Injury, superficial, abdomen
Achilles tendon S86.00-
laceration S86.02-
specified type NEC S86.09-
strain S86.01-
acoustic, resulting in deafness —*see* Injury, nerve, acoustic
adrenal (gland) S37.819
contusion S37.812
laceration S37.813
specified type NEC S37.818
alveolar (process) S09.93
ankle S99.91-
contusion —*see* Contusion, ankle
dislocation —*see* Dislocation, ankle
fracture —*see* Fracture, ankle
nerve —*see* Injury, nerve, ankle
open —*see* Wound, open, ankle
specified type NEC S99.81-
sprain —*see* Sprain, ankle
superficial —*see* Injury, superficial, ankle
anterior chamber, eye —*see* Injury, eye, specified site NEC
anus —*see* Injury, abdomen
aorta (thoracic) S25.00
abdominal S35.00
laceration (minor) (superficial) S35.01
major S35.02
specified type NEC S35.09
laceration (minor) (superficial) S25.01
major S25.02
specified type NEC S25.09
arm (upper) S49.9-
blood vessel —*see* Injury, blood vessel, arm
contusion —*see* Contusion, arm, upper
fracture —*see* Fracture, humerus
lower —*see* Injury, forearm
muscle —*see* Injury, muscle, shoulder
nerve —*see* Injury, nerve, arm
open —*see* Wound, open, arm
specified type NEC S49.8-
superficial —*see* Injury, superficial, arm
artery (complicating trauma) —*see also* Injury, blood vessel, by site
cerebral or meningeal —*see* Injury, intracranial
auditory canal (external) (meatus) S09.91
auricle, auris, ear S09.91
axilla —*see* Injury, shoulder
back —*see* Injury, back, lower
bile duct S36.13
birth —*see also* Birth, injury P15.9
bladder (sphincter) S37.20
at delivery O71.5
contusion S37.22
laceration S37.23
obstetrical trauma O71.5
specified type NEC S37.29

Injury *(continued)*
blast (air) (hydraulic) (immersion) (underwater) NEC T14.8
acoustic nerve trauma —*see* Injury, nerve, acoustic
bladder —*see* Injury, bladder
brain —*see* Concussion
colon —*see* Injury, intestine, large, blast injury
ear (primary) S09.31-
secondary S09.39-
generalized T70.8
lung —*see* Injury, intrathoracic, lung, blast injury
multiple body organs T70.8
peritoneum S36.81
rectum S36.61
retroperitoneum S36.898
small intestine S36.419
duodenum S36.410
specified site NEC S36.418
specified
intra-abdominal organ NEC S36.898
pelvic organ NEC S37.899
blood vessel NEC T14.8
abdomen S35.9-
aorta —*see* Injury, aorta, abdominal
celiac artery —*see* Injury, blood vessel, celiac artery
iliac vessel —*see* Injury, blood vessel, iliac
laceration S35.91
mesenteric vessel —*see* Injury, mesenteric
portal vein —*see* Injury, blood vessel, portal vein
renal vessel —*see* Injury, blood vessel, renal
specified vessel NEC S35.8X-
splenic vessel —*see* Injury, blood vessel, splenic
vena cava —*see* Injury, vena cava, inferior
ankle —*see* Injury, blood vessel, foot
aorta (abdominal) (thoracic) —*see* Injury, aorta
arm (upper) NEC S45.90-
forearm —*see* Injury, blood vessel, forearm
laceration S45.91-
specified
site NEC S45.80-
laceration S45.81-
specified type NEC S45.89-
type NEC S45.99-
superficial vein S45.30-
laceration S45.31-
specified type NEC S45.39-
axillary
artery S45.00-
laceration S45.01-
specified type NEC S45.09-
vein S45.20-
laceration S45.21-
specified type NEC S45.29-
azygos vein —*see* Injury, blood vessel, thoracic, specified site NEC
brachial
artery S45.10-
laceration S45.11-
specified type NEC S45.19-
vein S45.20-
laceration S45.219
specified type NEC S45.29-

Injury *(continued)*
blood vessel NEC *(continued)*
carotid artery (common) (external) (internal, extracranial) S15.00-
internal, intracranial S06.8-
laceration (minor) (superficial) S15.01-
major S15.02-
specified type NEC S15.09-
celiac artery S35.219
branch S35.299
laceration (minor) (superficial) S35.291
major S35.292
specified NEC S35.298
laceration (minor) (superficial) S35.211
major S35.212
specified type NEC S35.218
cerebral —*see* Injury, intracranial
deep plantar —*see* Injury, blood vessel, plantar artery
digital (hand) —*see* Injury, blood vessel, finger
dorsal
artery (foot) S95.00-
laceration S95.01-
specified type NEC S95.09-
vein (foot) S95.20-
laceration S95.21-
specified type NEC S95.29-
due to accidental laceration during procedure —*see* Laceration, accidental complicating surgery
extremity —*see* Injury, blood vessel, limb
femoral
artery (common) (superficial) S75.00-
laceration (minor) (superficial) S75.01-
major S75.02-
specified type NEC S75.09-
vein (hip level) (thigh level) S75.10-
laceration (minor) (superficial) S75.11-
major S75.12-
specified type NEC S75.19-
finger S65.50-
index S65.50-
laceration S65.51-
specified type NEC S65.59-
laceration S65.51-
little S65.50-
laceration S65.51-
specified type NEC S65.59-
middle S65.50-
laceration S65.51-
specified type NEC S65.59-
specified type NEC S65.59-
thumb —*see* Injury, blood vessel, thumb
foot S95.90-
dorsal
artery —*see* Injury, blood vessel, dorsal, artery
vein —*see* Injury, blood vessel, dorsal, vein
laceration S95.91-
plantar artery —*see* Injury, blood vessel, plantar artery
specified
site NEC S95.80-
laceration S95.81-
specified type NEC S95.89-
specified type NEC S95.99-

Injury *(continued)*
blood vessel NEC *(continued)*
forearm S55.90-
laceration S55.91-
radial artery —*see* Injury, blood vessel, radial artery
specified
site NEC S55.80-
laceration S55.81-
specified type NEC S55.89-
type NEC S55.99-
ulnar artery —*see* Injury, blood vessel, ulnar artery
vein S55.20-
laceration S55.21-
specified type NEC S55.29-
gastric
artery —*see* Injury, mesenteric, artery, branch
vein —*see* Injury, blood vessel, abdomen
gastroduodenal artery —*see* Injury, mesenteric, artery, branch
greater saphenous vein (lower leg level) S85.30-
hip (and thigh) level S75.20-
laceration (minor) (superficial) S75.21-
major S75.22-
specified type NEC S75.29-
laceration S85.31-
specified type NEC S85.39-
hand (level) S65.90-
finger —*see* Injury, blood vessel, finger
laceration S65.91-
palmar arch —*see* Injury, blood vessel, palmar arch
radial artery —*see* Injury, blood vessel, radial artery, hand
specified
site NEC S65.80-
laceration S65.81-
specified type NEC S65.89-
type NEC S65.99-
thumb —*see* Injury, blood vessel, thumb
ulnar artery —*see* Injury, blood vessel, ulnar artery, hand
head S09.0
intracranial —*see* Injury, intracranial
multiple S09.0
hepatic
artery —*see* Injury, mesenteric, artery
vein —*see* Injury, vena cava, inferior
hip S75.90-
femoral artery —*see* Injury, blood vessel, femoral, artery
femoral vein —*see* Injury, blood vessel, femoral, vein
greater saphenous vein —*see* Injury, blood vessel, greater saphenous, hip level
laceration S75.91-
specified
site NEC S75.80-
laceration S75.81-
specified type NEC S75.89-
type NEC S75.99-
hypogastric (artery) (vein) —*see* Injury, blood vessel, iliac

Injury *(continued)*
- blood vessel NEC *(continued)*
  - iliac S35.5-
    - artery S35.51-
    - specified vessel NEC S35.5-
    - uterine vessel *—see* Injury, blood vessel, uterine
    - vein S35.51-
  - innominate *—see* Injury, blood vessel, thoracic, innominate
  - intercostal (artery) (vein) *—see* Injury, blood vessel, thoracic, intercostal
  - jugular vein (external) S15.20-
    - internal S15.30-
      - laceration (minor) (superficial) S15.31-
        - major S15.32-
      - specified type NEC S15.39-
    - laceration (minor) (superficial) S15.21-
      - major S15.22-
    - specified type NEC S15.29-
  - leg (level) (lower) S85.90-
    - greater saphenous *—see* Injury, blood vessel, greater saphenous
    - laceration S85.91-
    - lesser saphenous *—see* Injury, blood vessel, lesser saphenous
    - peroneal artery *—see* Injury, blood vessel, peroneal artery
    - popliteal
      - artery *—see* Injury, blood vessel, popliteal, artery
      - vein *—see* Injury, blood vessel, popliteal, vein
    - specified
      - site NEC S85.80-
        - laceration S85.81-
        - specified type NEC S85.89-
      - type NEC S85.99-
    - thigh *—see* Injury, blood vessel, hip
    - tibial artery *—see* Injury, blood vessel, tibial artery
  - lesser saphenous vein (lower leg level) S85.40-
    - laceration S85.41-
    - specified type NEC S85.49-
  - limb
    - lower *—see* Injury, blood vessel, leg
    - upper *—see* Injury, blood vessel, arm
  - lower back *—see* Injury, blood vessel, abdomen
    - specified NEC *—see* Injury, blood vessel, abdomen, specified, site NEC
  - mammary (artery) (vein) *—see* Injury, blood vessel, thoracic, specified site NEC
  - mesenteric (inferior) (superior)
    - artery *—see* Injury, mesenteric, artery
    - vein *—see* Injury, mesenteric, vein
  - neck S15.9
    - specified site NEC S15.8
  - ovarian (artery) (vein) *—see* subcategory S35.8
  - palmar arch (superficial) S65.20-
    - deep S65.30-
      - laceration S65.31-
      - specified type NEC S65.39-
    - laceration S65.21-
    - specified type NEC S65.29-

Injury *(continued)*
- blood vessel NEC *(continued)*
  - pelvis *—see* Injury, blood vessel, abdomen
    - specified NEC *—see* Injury, blood vessel, abdomen, specified, site NEC
  - peroneal artery S85.20-
    - laceration S85.21-
    - specified type NEC S85.29-
  - plantar artery (deep) (foot) S95.10-
    - laceration S95.11-
    - specified type NEC S95.19-
  - popliteal
    - artery S85.00-
      - laceration S85.01-
      - specified type NEC S85.09-
    - vein S85.50-
      - laceration S85.51-
      - specified type NEC S85.59-
  - portal vein S35.319
    - laceration S35.311
    - specified type NEC S35.318
  - precerebral *—see* Injury, blood vessel, neck
  - pulmonary (artery) (vein) *—see* Injury, blood vessel, thoracic, pulmonary
  - radial artery (forearm level) S55.10-
    - hand and wrist (level) S65.10-
      - laceration S65.11-
      - specified type NEC S65.19-
    - laceration S55.11-
    - specified type NEC S55.19-
  - renal
    - artery S35.40-
      - laceration S35.41-
      - specified NEC S35.49-
    - vein S35.40-
      - laceration S35.41-
      - specified NEC S35.49-
  - saphenous vein (greater) (lower leg level) *—see* Injury, blood vessel, greater saphenous
    - hip and thigh level *—see* Injury, blood vessel, greater saphenous, hip level
    - lesser *—see* Injury, blood vessel, lesser saphenous
  - shoulder
    - specified NEC *—see* Injury, blood vessel, arm, specified site NEC
    - superficial vein *—see* Injury, blood vessel, arm, superficial vein
  - specified NEC T14.8
  - splenic
    - artery *—see* Injury, blood vessel, celiac artery, branch
    - vein S35.329
      - laceration S35.321
      - specified NEC S35.328
  - subclavian *—see* Injury, blood vessel, thoracic, innominate
  - thigh *—see* Injury, blood vessel, hip
  - thoracic S25.90
    - aorta S25.00
      - laceration (minor) (superficial) S25.01
        - major S25.02
      - specified type NEC S25.09
    - azygos vein *—see* Injury, blood vessel, thoracic, specified, site NEC

Injury *(continued)*
- blood vessel NEC *(continued)*
  - thoracic *(continued)*
    - innominate
      - artery S25.10-
        - laceration (minor) (superficial) S25.11-
          - major S25.12-
        - specified type NEC S25.19-
      - vein S25.30-
        - laceration (minor) (superficial) S25.31-
          - major S25.32-
        - specified type NEC S25.39-
    - intercostal S25.50-
      - laceration S25.51-
      - specified type NEC S25.59-
    - laceration S25.91
    - mammary vessel *—see* Injury, blood vessel, thoracic, specified, site NEC
    - pulmonary S25.40-
      - laceration (minor) (superficial) S25.41-
        - major S25.42-
      - specified type NEC S25.49-
    - specified
      - site NEC S25.80-
        - laceration S25.81-
        - specified type NEC S25.89-
      - type NEC S25.99
    - subclavian *—see* Injury, blood vessel, thoracic, innominate
    - vena cava (superior) S25.20
      - laceration (minor) (superficial) S25.21
        - major S25.22
      - specified type NEC S25.29
  - thumb S65.40-
    - laceration S65.41-
    - specified type NEC S65.49-
  - tibial artery S85.10-
    - anterior S85.13-
      - laceration S85.14-
      - specified injury NEC S85.15-
    - laceration S85.11-
    - posterior S85.16-
      - laceration S85.17-
      - specified injury NEC S85.18-
    - specified injury NEC S85.12-
  - ulnar artery (forearm level) S55.00-
    - hand and wrist (level) S65.00-
      - laceration S65.01-
      - specified type NEC S65.09-
    - laceration S55.01-
    - specified type NEC S55.09-
  - upper arm (level) *—see* Injury, blood vessel, arm
    - superficial vein *—see* Injury, blood vessel, arm, superficial vein
  - uterine S35.5-
    - artery S35.53-
    - vein S35.53-
  - vena cava *—see* Injury, vena cava
  - vertebral artery S15.10-
    - laceration (minor) (superficial) S15.11-
      - major S15.12-
    - specified type NEC S15.19-
  - wrist (level) *—see* Injury, blood vessel, hand
- brachial plexus S14.3
  - newborn P14.3

Injury *(continued)*
- brain (traumatic) S06.9-
  - diffuse (axonal) S06.2X-
  - focal S06.30-
- brainstem S06.38-
- breast NOS S29.9
- broad ligament *—see* Injury, pelvic organ, specified site NEC
- bronchus, bronchi *—see* Injury, intrathoracic, bronchus
- brow S09.90
- buttock S39.92
- canthus, eye S05.90
- cardiac plexus *—see* Injury, nerve, thorax, sympathetic
- cauda equina S34.3
- cavernous sinus *—see* Injury, intracranial
- cecum *—see* Injury, colon
- celiac ganglion or plexus *—see* Injury, nerve, lumbosacral, sympathetic
- cerebellum *—see* Injury, intracranial
- cerebral *—see* Injury, intracranial
- cervix (uteri) *—see* Injury, uterus
- cheek (wall) S09.93
- chest *—see* Injury, thorax
- childbirth (newborn) *—see also* Birth, injury
  - maternal NEC O71.9
- chin S09.93
- choroid (eye) *—see* Injury, eye, specified site NEC
- clitoris S39.94
- coccyx *—see also* Injury, back, lower
  - complicating delivery O71.6
- colon *—see* Injury, intestine, large
- common bile duct *—see* Injury, liver
- conjunctiva (superficial) *—see* Injury, eye, conjunctiva
- conus medullaris *—see* Injury, spinal, sacral
- cord
  - spermatic (pelvic region) S37.898
    - scrotal region S39.848
  - spinal *—see* Injury, spinal cord, by region
- cornea *—see* Injury, eye, specified site NEC
  - abrasion *—see* Injury, eye, cornea, abrasion
- cortex (cerebral) *—see also* Injury, intracranial
  - visual *—see* Injury, nerve, optic
- costal region NEC S29.9
- costochondral NEC S29.9
- cranial
  - cavity *—see* Injury, intracranial
  - nerve *—see* Injury, nerve, cranial
- crushing *—see* Crush
- cutaneous sensory nerve
- cystic duct *—see* Injury, liver
- deep tissue *—see* Contusion, by site
  - meaning pressure ulcer *—see* Ulcer, pressure, unstageable, by site
- delivery (newborn) P15.9
  - maternal NEC O71.9
- Descemet's membrane *—see* Injury, eyeball, penetrating
- diaphragm *—see* Injury, intrathoracic, diaphragm
- duodenum *—see* Injury, intestine, small, duodenum
- ear (auricle) (external) (canal) S09.91
  - abrasion *—see* Abrasion, ear
  - bite *—see* Bite, ear

Injury–Injury

Injury *(continued)*
- ear *(continued)*
  - blister —*see* Blister, ear
  - bruise —*see* Contusion, ear
  - contusion —*see* Contusion, ear
  - external constriction —*see* Constriction, external, ear
  - hematoma —*see* Hematoma, ear
  - inner —*see* Injury, ear, middle
  - laceration —*see* Laceration, ear
  - middle S09.30-
    - blast —*see* Injury, blast, ear
    - specified NEC S09.39-
  - puncture —*see* Puncture, ear
  - superficial —*see* Injury, superficial, ear
- eighth cranial nerve (acoustic or auditory) —*see* Injury, nerve, acoustic
- elbow S59.90-
  - contusion —*see* Contusion, elbow
  - dislocation —*see* Dislocation, elbow
  - fracture —*see* Fracture, ulna, upper end
  - open —*see* Wound, open, elbow
  - specified NEC S59.80-
  - sprain —*see* Sprain, elbow
  - superficial —*see* Injury, superficial, elbow
- eleventh cranial nerve (accessory) —*see* Injury, nerve, accessory
- epididymis S39.94
- epigastric region S39.91
- epiglottis NEC S19.89
- esophageal plexus —*see* Injury, nerve, thorax, sympathetic
- esophagus (thoracic part) —*see also* Injury, intrathoracic, esophagus
  - cervical NEC S19.85
- eustachian tube S09.30-
- eye S05.9-
  - avulsion S05.7-
  - ball —*see* Injury, eyeball
  - conjunctiva S05.0-
  - cornea
    - abrasion S05.0-
  - laceration S05.3-
    - with prolapse S05.2-
  - lacrimal apparatus S05.8X-
  - orbit penetration S05.4-
  - specified site NEC S05.8X-
- eyeball S05.8X-
  - contusion S05.1-
  - penetrating S05.6-
    - with
      - foreign body S05.5-
      - prolapse or loss of intraocular tissue S05.2-
    - without prolapse or loss of intraocular tissue S05.3-
  - specified type NEC S05.8-
- eyebrow S09.93
- eyelid S09.93
  - abrasion —*see* Abrasion, eyelid
  - contusion —*see* Contusion, eyelid
  - open —*see* Wound, open, eyelid
- face S09.93
- fallopian tube S37.509
  - bilateral S37.502
    - blast injury S37.512
    - contusion S37.522
    - laceration S37.532
    - specified type NEC S37.592
  - blast injury (primary) S37.519
    - bilateral S37.512
    - secondary —*see* Injury, fallopian tube, specified type NEC
    - unilateral S37.511

Injury *(continued)*
- fallopian tube *(continued)*
  - contusion S37.529
    - bilateral S37.522
    - unilateral S37.521
  - laceration S37.539
    - bilateral S37.532
    - unilateral S37.531
  - specified type NEC S37.599
    - bilateral S37.592
    - unilateral S37.591
  - unilateral S37.501
    - blast injury S37.511
    - contusion S37.521
    - laceration S37.531
    - specified type NEC S37.591
- fascia —*see* Injury, muscle
- fifth cranial nerve (trigeminal) —*see* Injury, nerve, trigeminal
- finger (nail) S69.9-
  - blood vessel —*see* Injury, blood vessel, finger
  - contusion —*see* Contusion, finger
  - dislocation —*see* Dislocation, finger
  - fracture —*see* Fracture, finger
  - muscle —*see* Injury, muscle, finger
  - nerve —*see* Injury, nerve, digital, finger
  - open —*see* Wound, open, finger
  - specified NEC S69.8-
  - sprain —*see* Sprain, finger
  - superficial —*see* Injury, superficial, finger
- first cranial nerve (olfactory) —*see* Injury, nerve, olfactory
- flank —*see* Injury, abdomen
- foot S99.92-
  - blood vessel —*see* Injury, blood vessel, foot
  - contusion —*see* Contusion, foot
  - dislocation —*see* Dislocation, foot
  - fracture —*see* Fracture, foot
  - muscle —*see* Injury, muscle, foot
  - open —*see* Wound, open, foot
  - specified type NEC S99.82-
  - sprain —*see* Sprain, foot
  - superficial —*see* Injury, superficial, foot
- forceps NOS P15.9
- forearm S59.91-
  - blood vessel —*see* Injury, blood vessel, forearm
  - contusion —*see* Contusion, forearm
  - fracture —*see* Fracture, forearm
  - muscle —*see* Injury, muscle, forearm
  - nerve —*see* Injury, nerve, forearm
  - open —*see* Wound, open, forearm
  - specified NEC S59.81-
  - superficial —*see* Injury, superficial, forearm
- forehead S09.90
- fourth cranial nerve (trochlear) —*see* Injury, nerve, trochlear
- gallbladder S36.129
  - contusion S36.122
  - laceration S36.123
  - specified NEC S36.128
- ganglion
  - celiac, coeliac —*see* Injury, nerve, lumbosacral, sympathetic
  - gasserian —*see* Injury, nerve, trigeminal
  - stellate —*see* Injury, nerve, thorax, sympathetic
  - thoracic sympathetic —*see* Injury, nerve, thorax, sympathetic

Injury *(continued)*
- gasserian ganglion —*see* Injury, nerve, trigeminal
- gastric artery —*see* Injury, blood vessel, celiac artery, branch
- gastroduodenal artery —*see* Injury, blood vessel, celiac artery, branch
- gastrointestinal tract —*see* Injury, intra-abdominal
  - with open wound into abdominal cavity —*see* Wound, open, with penetration into peritoneal cavity
  - colon —*see* Injury, intestine, large
  - rectum —*see* Injury, intestine, large, rectum
    - with open wound into abdominal cavity S36.61
  - specified site NEC —*see* Injury, intra-abdominal, specified, site NEC
  - stomach —*see* Injury, stomach
  - small intestine —*see* Injury, intestine, small
- genital organ(s)
  - external S39.94
    - specified NEC S39.848
  - internal S37.90
    - fallopian tube —*see* Injury, fallopian tube
    - ovary —*see* Injury, ovary
    - prostate —*see* Injury, prostate
    - seminal vesicle —*see* Injury, pelvis, organ, specified site NEC
    - uterus —*see* Injury, uterus
    - vas deferens —*see* Injury, pelvis, organ, specified site NEC
  - obstetrical trauma O71.9
- gland
  - lacrimal laceration —*see* Injury, eye, specified site NEC
  - salivary S09.93
  - thyroid NEC S19.84
- globe (eye) S05.90
  - specified NEC S05.8X-
- groin —*see* Injury, abdomen
- gum S09.90
- hand S69.9-
  - blood vessel —*see* Injury, blood vessel, hand
  - contusion —*see* Contusion, hand
  - fracture —*see* Fracture, hand
  - muscle —*see* Injury, muscle, hand
  - nerve —*see* Injury, nerve, hand
  - open —*see* Wound, open, hand
  - specified NEC S69.8-
  - sprain —*see* Sprain, hand
  - superficial —*see* Injury, superficial, hand
- head S09.90
  - with loss of consciousness S06.9-
  - specified NEC S09.8
- heart S26.90
  - with hemopericardium S26.00
    - contusion S26.01
    - laceration (mild) S26.020
      - moderate S26.021
      - major S26.022
    - specified type NEC S26.09
  - contusion S26.91
  - laceration S26.92
  - specified type NEC S26.99
  - without hemopericardium S26.10
    - contusion S26.11
    - laceration S26.12
    - specified type NEC S26.19

Injury *(continued)*
- heel —*see* Injury, foot
- hepatic
  - artery —*see* Injury, blood vessel, celiac artery, branch
  - duct —*see* Injury, liver
  - vein —*see* Injury, vena cava, inferior
- hip S79.91-
  - blood vessel —*see* Injury, blood vessel, hip
  - contusion —*see* Contusion, hip
  - dislocation —*see* Dislocation, hip
  - fracture —*see* Fracture, femur, neck
  - muscle —*see* Injury, muscle, hip
  - nerve —*see* Injury, nerve, hip
  - open —*see* Wound, open, hip
  - sprain —*see* Sprain, hip
  - superficial —*see* Injury, superficial, hip
  - specified NEC S79.81-
- hymen S39.94
- hypogastric
  - blood vessel —*see* Injury, blood vessel, iliac
  - plexus —*see* Injury, nerve, lumbosacral, sympathetic
- ileum —*see* Injury, intestine, small
- iliac region S39.91
- instrumental (during surgery) —*see* Laceration, accidental complicating surgery
  - birth injury —*see* Birth, injury
  - nonsurgical —*see* Injury, by site
  - obstetrical O71.9
    - bladder O71.5
    - cervix O71.3
    - high vaginal O71.4
    - perineal NOS O70.9
    - urethra O71.5
    - uterus O71.5
      - with rupture or perforation O71.1
- internal T14.8
  - aorta —*see* Injury, aorta
  - bladder (sphincter) —*see* Injury, bladder
    - with
      - ectopic or molar pregnancy O08.6
    - following ectopic or molar pregnancy O08.6
    - obstetrical trauma O71.5
  - bronchus, bronchi —*see* Injury, intrathoracic, bronchus
  - cecum —*see* Injury, intestine, large
  - cervix (uteri) —*see also* Injury, uterus
    - with ectopic or molar pregnancy O08.6
    - following ectopic or molar pregnancy O08.6
    - obstetrical trauma O71.3
  - chest —*see* Injury, intrathoracic
  - gastrointestinal tract —*see* Injury, intra-abdominal
  - heart —*see* Injury, heart
  - intestine NEC —*see* Injury, intestine
  - intrauterine —*see* Injury, uterus
  - mesentery —*see* Injury, intra-abdominal, specified, site NEC
  - pelvis, pelvic (organ) S37.90
    - following ectopic or molar pregnancy (subsequent episode) O08.6

- **Injury** *(continued)*
  - internal *(continued)*
    - pelvis, pelvic *(continued)*
      - obstetrical trauma NEC O71.5
        - rupture or perforation O71.1
      - specified NEC S39.83
    - rectum —*see* Injury, intestine, large, rectum
    - stomach —*see* Injury, stomach
    - ureter —*see* Injury, ureter
    - urethra (sphincter) following ectopic or molar pregnancy O08.6
    - uterus —*see* Injury, uterus
  - interscapular area —*see* Injury, thorax
  - intestine
    - large S36.509
      - ascending (right) S36.500
        - blast injury (primary) S36.510
          - secondary S36.590
        - contusion S36.520
        - laceration S36.530
        - specified type NEC S36.590
      - blast injury (primary) S36.519
        - ascending (right) S36.510
        - descending (left) S36.512
        - rectum S36.61
        - sigmoid S36.513
        - specified site NEC S36.518
        - transverse S36.511
      - contusion S36.529
        - ascending (right) S36.520
        - descending (left) S36.522
        - rectum S36.62
        - sigmoid S36.523
        - specified site NEC S36.528
        - transverse S36.521
      - descending (left) S36.502
        - blast injury (primary) S36.512
          - secondary S36.592
        - contusion S36.522
        - laceration S36.532
        - specified type NEC S36.592
      - laceration S36.539
        - ascending (right) S36.530
        - descending (left) S36.532
        - rectum S36.63
        - sigmoid S36.533
        - specified site NEC S36.538
        - transverse S36.531
      - rectum S36.60
        - blast injury (primary) S36.61
          - secondary S36.69
        - contusion S36.62
        - laceration S36.63
        - specified type NEC S36.69
      - sigmoid S36.503
        - blast injury (primary) S36.513
          - secondary S36.593
        - contusion S36.523
        - laceration S36.533
        - specified type NEC S36.593
      - specified
        - site NEC S36.508
          - blast injury (primary) S36.518
            - secondary S36.598
          - contusion S36.528
          - laceration S36.538
          - specified type NEC S36.598
        - type NEC S36.599
          - ascending (right) S36.590
          - descending (left) S36.592
          - rectum S36.69
          - sigmoid S36.593
          - specified site NEC S36.598
          - transverse S36.591

- **Injury** *(continued)*
  - intestine *(continued)*
    - large *(continued)*
      - transverse S36.501
        - blast injury (primary) S36.511
          - secondary S36.591
        - contusion S36.521
        - laceration S36.531
        - specified type NEC S36.591
    - small S36.409
      - blast injury (primary) S36.419
        - duodenum S36.410
        - secondary S36.499
          - duodenum S36.490
          - specified site NEC S36.498
        - specified site NEC S36.418
      - contusion S36.429
        - duodenum S36.420
        - specified site NEC S36.428
      - duodenum S36.400
        - blast injury (primary) S36.410
          - secondary S36.490
        - contusion S36.420
        - laceration S36.430
        - specified NEC S36.490
      - laceration S36.439
        - duodenum S36.430
        - specified site NEC S36.438
      - specified
        - type NEC S36.499
          - duodenum S36.490
          - specified site NEC S36.498
        - site NEC S36.408
  - intra-abdominal S36.90
    - adrenal gland —*see* Injury, adrenal gland
    - bladder —*see* Injury, bladder
    - colon —*see* Injury, intestine, large
    - contusion S36.92
    - fallopian tube —*see* Injury, fallopian tube
    - gallbladder —*see* Injury, gallbladder
    - intestine —*see* Injury, intestine
    - laceration S36.93
    - liver —*see* Injury, liver
    - kidney —*see* Injury, kidney
    - ovary —*see* Injury, ovary
    - pancreas —*see* Injury, pancreas
    - pelvic NOS S37.90
    - peritoneum —*see* Injury, intra-abdominal, specified, site NEC
    - prostate —*see* Injury, prostate
    - rectum —*see* Injury, intestine, large, rectum
    - retroperitoneum —*see* Injury, intra-abdominal, specified, site NEC
    - seminal vesicle —*see* Injury, pelvis, organ, specified site NEC
    - small intestine —*see* Injury, intestine, small
    - specified
      - site NEC S36.899
        - contusion S36.892
        - laceration S36.893
        - specified type NEC S36.898
      - type NEC S36.99
    - pelvic S37.90
      - specified
        - site NEC S37.899
          - specified type NEC S37.898
        - type NEC S37.99
    - spleen —*see* Injury, spleen

- **Injury** *(continued)*
  - intra-abdominal *(continued)*
    - stomach —*see* Injury, stomach
    - ureter —*see* Injury, ureter
    - urethra —*see* Injury, urethra
    - uterus —*see* Injury, uterus
    - vas deferens —*see* Injury, pelvis, organ, specified site NEC
  - intracranial (traumatic) S06.9-
    - cerebellar hemorrhage, traumatic —*see* Injury, intracranial, focal
    - cerebral edema, traumatic S06.1X-
      - diffuse S06.1X-
      - focal S06.1X-
    - diffuse (axonal) S06.2X-
    - epidural hemorrhage (traumatic) S06.4X-
    - focal brain injury S06.30-
      - contusion —*see* Contusion, cerebral
      - laceration —*see* Laceration, cerebral
    - intracerebral hemorrhage, traumatic S06.36-
      - left side S06.35-
      - right side S06.34-
    - subarachnoid hemorrhage, traumatic S06.6X-
    - subdural hemorrhage, traumatic S06.5X-
  - intraocular —*see* Injury, eyeball, penetrating
  - intrathoracic S27.9
    - bronchus S27.409
      - bilateral S27.402
      - blast injury (primary) S27.419
        - bilateral S27.412
        - secondary —*see* Injury, intrathoracic, bronchus, specified type NEC
        - unilateral S27.411
      - contusion S27.429
        - bilateral S27.422
        - unilateral S27.421
      - laceration S27.439
        - bilateral S27.432
        - unilateral S27.431
      - specified type NEC S27.499
        - bilateral S27.492
        - unilateral S27.491
      - unilateral S27.401
    - diaphragm S27.809
      - contusion S27.802
      - laceration S27.803
      - specified type NEC S27.808
    - esophagus (thoracic) S27.819
      - contusion S27.812
      - laceration S27.813
      - specified type NEC S27.818
    - heart —*see* Injury, heart
    - hemopneumothorax S27.2
    - hemothorax S27.1
    - lung S27.309
      - aspiration J69.0
      - bilateral S27.302
      - blast injury (primary) S27.319
        - bilateral S27.312
        - secondary —*see* Injury, intrathoracic, lung, specified type NEC
        - unilateral S27.311
      - contusion S27.329
        - bilateral S27.322
        - unilateral S27.321
      - laceration S27.339
        - bilateral S27.332
        - unilateral S27.331
      - specified type NEC S27.399
        - bilateral S27.392
        - unilateral S27.391

- **Injury** *(continued)*
  - intrathoracic *(continued)*
    - lung *(continued)*
      - unilateral S27.301
    - pleura S27.60
      - laceration S27.63
      - specified type NEC S27.69
    - pneumothorax S27.0
    - specified organ NEC S27.899
      - contusion S27.892
      - laceration S27.893
      - specified type NEC S27.898
    - thoracic duct —*see* Injury, intrathoracic, specified organ NEC
    - thymus gland —*see* Injury, intrathoracic, specified organ NEC
    - trachea, thoracic S27.50
      - blast (primary) S27.51
      - contusion S27.52
      - laceration S27.53
      - specified type NEC S27.59
  - iris —*see* Injury, eye, specified site NEC
    - penetrating —*see* Injury, eyeball, penetrating
  - jaw S09.93
  - jejunum —*see* Injury, intestine, small
  - joint NOS T14.8
    - old or residual —*see* Disorder, joint, specified type NEC
  - kidney S37.00-
    - acute (nontraumatic) N17.9
    - contusion —*see* Contusion, kidney
    - laceration —*see* Laceration, kidney
    - specified NEC S37.09-
  - knee S89.9-
    - contusion —*see* Contusion, knee
    - dislocation —*see* Dislocation, knee
    - meniscus (lateral) (medial) —*see* Sprain, knee, specified site NEC
      - old injury or tear —*see* Derangement, knee, meniscus, due to old injury
    - open —*see* Wound, open, knee
    - specified NEC S89.8-
    - sprain —*see* Sprain, knee
    - superficial —*see* Injury, superficial, knee
  - labium (majus) (minus) S39.94
  - labyrinth, ear S09.30-
  - lacrimal apparatus, duct, gland, or sac —*see* Injury, eye, specified site NEC
  - larynx NEC S19.81
  - leg (lower) S89.9-
    - blood vessel —*see* Injury, blood vessel, leg
    - contusion —*see* Contusion, leg
    - fracture —*see* Fracture, leg
    - muscle —*see* Injury, muscle, leg
    - nerve —*see* Injury, nerve, leg
    - open —*see* Wound, open, leg
    - specified NEC S89.8-
    - superficial —*see* Injury, superficial, leg
  - lens, eye —*see* Injury, eye, specified site NEC
    - penetrating —*see* Injury, eyeball, penetrating
  - limb NEC T14.8
  - lip S09.93
  - liver S36.119
    - contusion S36.112
    - laceration S36.113
      - major (stellate) S36.116
      - minor S36.114
      - moderate S36.115

Injury *(continued)*
- liver *(continued)*
  - specified NEC S36.118
- lower back S39.92
  - specified NEC S39.82
- lumbar, lumbosacral (region) S39.92
  - plexus —*see* Injury, lumbosacral plexus
- lumbosacral plexus S34.4
- lung —*see also* Injury, intrathoracic, lung
  - aspiration J69.0
  - transfusion-related (TRALI) J95.84
- lymphatic thoracic duct —*see* Injury, intrathoracic, specified organ NEC
- malar region S09.93
- mastoid region S09.90
- maxilla S09.93
- mediastinum —*see* Injury, intrathoracic, specified organ NEC
- membrane, brain —*see* Injury, intracranial
- meningeal artery —*see* Injury, intracranial, subdural hemorrhage
- meninges (cerebral) —*see* Injury, intracranial
- mesenteric
  - artery
    - branch S35.299
      - laceration (minor) (superficial) S35.291
        - major S35.292
      - specified NEC S35.298
    - inferior S35.239
      - laceration (minor) (superficial) S35.231
        - major S35.232
      - specified NEC S35.238
    - superior S35.229
      - laceration (minor) (superficial) S35.221
        - major S35.222
      - specified NEC S35.228
  - plexus (inferior) (superior) —*see* Injury, nerve, lumbosacral, sympathetic
  - vein
    - inferior S35.349
      - laceration S35.341
      - specified NEC S35.348
    - superior S35.339
      - laceration S35.331
      - specified NEC S35.338
- mesentery —*see* Injury, intra-abdominal, specified site NEC
- mesosalpinx —*see* Injury, pelvic organ, specified site NEC
- middle ear S09.30-
- midthoracic region NOS S29.9
- mouth S09.93
- multiple NOS T07
- muscle (and fascia) (and tendon)
  - abdomen S39.001
    - laceration S39.021
    - specified type NEC S39.091
    - strain S39.011
  - abductor
    - thumb, forearm level —*see* Injury, muscle, thumb, abductor
  - adductor
    - thigh S76.20-
      - laceration S76.22-
      - specified type NEC S76.29-
      - strain S76.21-
  - ankle —*see* Injury, muscle, foot
  - anterior muscle group, at leg level (lower) S86.20-

Injury *(continued)*
- muscle *(continued)*
  - anterior muscle group, at leg level *(continued)*
    - laceration S86.22-
    - specified type NEC S86.29-
    - strain S86.21-
  - arm (upper) —*see* Injury, muscle, shoulder
  - biceps (parts NEC) S46.20-
    - laceration S46.22-
    - long head S46.10-
      - laceration S46.12-
      - strain S46.11-
      - specified type NEC S46.19-
    - specified type NEC S46.29-
    - strain S46.21-
  - extensor
    - finger(s) (other than thumb) —*see* Injury, muscle, finger by site, extensor
    - forearm level, specified NEC —*see* Injury, muscle, forearm, extensor
    - thumb —*see* Injury, muscle, thumb, extensor
    - toe (large) (ankle level) (foot level) —*see* Injury, muscle, toe, extensor
  - finger
    - extensor (forearm level) S56.40-
      - hand level S66.309
        - laceration S66.329
        - specified type NEC S66.399
        - strain S66.319
      - laceration S56.429
      - specified type NEC S56.499
      - strain S56.419
    - flexor (forearm level) S56.10-
      - hand level S66.109
        - laceration S66.129
        - specified type NEC S66.199
        - strain S66.119
      - laceration S56.129
      - specified type NEC S56.199
      - strain S56.119
    - intrinsic S66.509
      - laceration S66.529
      - specified type NEC S66.599
      - strain S66.519
    - index
      - extensor (forearm level)
        - hand level S66.308
          - laceration S66.32-
          - specified type NEC S66.39-
          - strain S66.31-
        - specified type NEC S56.492-
      - flexor (forearm level)
        - hand level S66.108
          - laceration S66.12-
          - specified type NEC S66.19-
          - strain S66.11-
        - specified type NEC S56.19-
        - strain S56.11-
      - intrinsic S66.50-
        - laceration S66.52-
        - specified type NEC S66.59-
        - strain S66.51-
    - little
      - extensor (forearm level)
        - hand level S66.30-

Injury *(continued)*
- muscle *(continued)*
  - finger *(continued)*
    - little *(continued)*
      - extensor *(continued)*
        - hand level *(continued)*
          - laceration S66.32-
          - specified type NEC S66.39-
          - strain S66.31-
        - laceration S56.42-
        - specified type NEC S56.49-
        - strain S56.41-
      - flexor (forearm level)
        - hand level S66.10-
          - laceration S66.12-
          - specified type NEC S66.19-
          - strain S66.11-
        - laceration S56.12-
        - specified type NEC S56.19-
        - strain S56.11-
      - intrinsic S66.50-
        - laceration S66.52-
        - specified type NEC S66.59-
        - strain S66.51-
    - middle
      - extensor (forearm level)
        - hand level S66.30-
          - laceration S66.32-
          - specified type NEC S66.39-
          - strain S66.31-
        - laceration S56.42-
        - specified type NEC S56.49-
        - strain S56.41-
      - flexor (forearm level)
        - hand level S66.10-
          - laceration S66.12-
          - specified type NEC S66.19-
          - strain S66.11-
        - laceration S56.12-
        - specified type NEC S56.19-
        - strain S56.11-
      - intrinsic S66.50-
        - laceration S66.52-
        - specified type NEC S66.59-
        - strain S66.51-
    - ring
      - extensor (forearm level)
        - hand level S66.30-
          - laceration S66.32-
          - specified type NEC S66.39-
          - strain S66.31-
        - laceration S56.42-
        - specified type NEC S56.49-
        - strain S56.41-
      - flexor (forearm level)
        - hand level S66.10-
          - laceration S66.12-
          - specified type NEC S66.19-
          - strain S66.11-
        - laceration S56.12-
        - specified type NEC S56.19-
        - strain S56.11-
      - intrinsic S66.50-
        - laceration S66.52-
        - specified type NEC S66.59-
        - strain S66.51-

Injury *(continued)*
- muscle *(continued)*
  - flexor
    - finger(s) (other than thumb) —*see* Injury, muscle, finger
    - forearm level, specified NEC —*see* Injury, muscle, forearm, flexor
    - thumb —*see* Injury, muscle, thumb, flexor
    - toe (long) (ankle level) (foot level) —*see* Injury, muscle, toe, flexor
  - foot S96.90-
    - intrinsic S96.20-
      - laceration S96.22-
      - specified type NEC S96.29-
      - strain S96.21-
    - laceration S96.92-
    - long extensor, toe —*see* Injury, muscle, toe, extensor
    - long flexor, toe —*see* Injury, muscle, toe, flexor
    - specified
      - site NEC S96.80-
        - laceration S96.82-
        - specified type NEC S96.89-
        - strain S96.81-
      - type NEC S96.99-
    - strain S96.91-
  - forearm (level) S56.90-
    - extensor S56.50-
      - laceration S56.52-
      - specified type NEC S56.59-
      - strain S56.51-
    - flexor S56.20-
      - laceration S56.22-
      - specified type NEC S56.29-
      - strain S56.21-
    - laceration S56.92-
    - specified S56.99-
      - site NEC S56.80-
        - laceration S56.82-
        - strain S56.81-
      - type NEC S56.89-
    - strain S56.91-
  - hand (level) S66.90-
    - laceration S66.92-
    - specified
      - site NEC S66.80-
        - laceration S66.82-
        - specified type NEC S66.89-
        - strain S66.81-
      - type NEC S66.99-
    - strain S66.91-
  - head S09.10
    - laceration S09.12
    - specified type NEC S09.19
    - strain S09.11
  - hip NEC S76.00-
    - laceration S76.02-
    - specified type NEC S76.09-
    - strain S76.01-
  - intrinsic
    - ankle and foot level —*see* Injury, muscle, foot, intrinsic
    - finger (other than thumb) —*see* Injury, muscle, finger by site, intrinsic
    - foot (level) —*see* Injury, muscle, foot, intrinsic
    - thumb —*see* Injury, muscle, thumb, intrinsic

- **Injury** *(continued)*
  - muscle *(continued)*
    - leg (level) (lower) S86.90-
      - Achilles tendon —*see* Injury, Achilles tendon
      - anterior muscle group —*see* Injury, muscle, anterior muscle group
      - laceration S86.92-
      - peroneal muscle group —*see* Injury, muscle, peroneal muscle group
      - posterior muscle group —*see* Injury, muscle, posterior muscle group, leg level
      - specified
        - site NEC S86.80-
          - laceration S86.82-
          - specified type NEC S86.89-
          - strain S86.81-
        - type NEC S86.99-
      - strain S86.91-
    - long
      - extensor toe, at ankle and foot level —*see* Injury, muscle, toe, extensor
      - flexor, toe, at ankle and foot level —*see* Injury, muscle, toe, flexor
      - head, biceps —*see* Injury, muscle, biceps, long head
    - lower back S39.002
      - laceration S39.022
      - specified type NEC S39.092
      - strain S39.012
    - neck (level) S16.9
      - laceration S16.2
      - specified type NEC S16.8
      - strain S16.1
    - pelvis S39.003
      - laceration S39.023
      - specified type NEC S39.093
      - strain S39.013
    - peroneal muscle group, at leg level (lower) S86.30-
      - laceration S86.32-
      - specified type NEC S86.39-
      - strain S86.31-
    - posterior muscle (group)
      - leg level (lower) S86.10-
        - laceration S86.12-
        - specified type NEC S86.19-
        - strain S86.11-
      - thigh level S76.30-
        - laceration S76.32-
        - specified type NEC S76.39-
        - strain S76.31-
    - quadriceps (thigh) S76.10-
      - laceration S76.12-
      - specified type NEC S76.19-
      - strain S76.11-
    - shoulder S46.90-
      - laceration S46.92-
      - rotator cuff —*see* Injury, rotator cuff
      - specified site NEC S46.80-
        - laceration S46.82-
        - strain S46.81-
        - specified type NEC S46.89-
      - strain S46.91-
      - specified type NEC S46.99-
    - thigh NEC (level) S76.90-
      - adductor —*see* Injury, muscle, adductor, thigh
      - laceration S76.92-
      - posterior muscle (group) —*see* Injury, muscle, posterior muscle, thigh level
      - quadriceps —*see* Injury, muscle, quadriceps

- **Injury** *(continued)*
  - muscle *(continued)*
    - thigh NEC *(continued)*
      - specified
        - site NEC S76.80-
          - laceration S76.82-
          - specified type NEC S76.89-
          - strain S76.81-
        - type NEC S76.99-
      - strain S76.91-
    - thorax (level) S29.009
      - back wall S29.002
      - front wall S29.001
      - laceration S29.029
        - back wall S29.022
        - front wall S29.021
      - specified type NEC S29.099
        - back wall S29.092
        - front wall S29.091
      - strain S29.019
        - back wall S29.012
        - front wall S29.011
    - thumb
      - abductor (forearm level) S56.30-
        - laceration S56.32-
        - specified type NEC S56.39-
        - strain S56.31-
      - extensor (forearm level) S56.30-
        - hand level S66.20-
          - laceration S66.22-
          - specified type NEC S66.29-
          - strain S66.21-
        - laceration S56.32-
        - specified type NEC S56.39-
        - strain S56.31-
      - flexor (forearm level) S56.00-
        - hand level S66.00-
          - laceration S66.02-
          - specified type NEC S66.09-
          - strain S66.01-
        - laceration S56.02-
        - specified type NEC S56.09-
        - strain S56.01-
        - wrist level —*see* Injury, muscle, thumb, flexor, hand level
      - intrinsic S66.40-
        - laceration S66.42-
        - specified type NEC S66.49-
        - strain S66.41-
    - toe —*see also* Injury, muscle, foot
      - extensor, long S96.10-
        - laceration S96.12-
        - specified type NEC S96.19-
        - strain S96.11-
      - flexor, long S96.00-
        - laceration S96.02-
        - specified type NEC S96.09-
        - strain S96.01-
    - triceps S46.30-
      - laceration S46.32-
      - specified type NEC S46.39-
      - strain S46.31-
    - wrist (and hand) level —*see* Injury, muscle, hand
  - musculocutaneous nerve —*see* Injury, nerve, musculocutaneous
  - myocardium —*see* Injury, heart
  - nape —*see* Injury, neck
  - nasal (septum) (sinus) S09.92
  - nasopharynx S09.92
  - neck S19.9
    - specified NEC S19.80
      - specified site NEC S19.89

- **Injury** *(continued)*
  - nerve NEC T14.8
    - abdomen S34.9
      - peripheral S34.6
      - specified site NEC S34.8
    - abducens S04.4-
      - contusion S04.4-
      - laceration S04.4-
      - specified type NEC S04.4-
    - abducent —*see* Injury, nerve, abducens
    - accessory S04.7-
      - contusion S04.7-
      - laceration S04.7-
      - specified type NEC S04.7-
    - acoustic S04.6-
      - contusion S04.6-
      - laceration S04.6-
      - specified type NEC S04.6-
    - ankle S94.9-
      - cutaneous sensory S94.3-
      - specified site NEC —*see* subcategory S94.8
    - anterior crural, femoral —*see* Injury, nerve, femoral
    - arm (upper) S44.9-
      - axillary —*see* Injury, nerve, axillary
      - cutaneous —*see* Injury, nerve, cutaneous, arm
      - median —*see* Injury, nerve, median, upper arm
      - musculocutaneous —*see* Injury, nerve, musculocutaneous
      - radial —*see* Injury, nerve, radial, upper arm
      - specified site NEC S44.8
      - ulnar —*see* Injury, nerve, ulnar, arm
    - auditory —*see* Injury, nerve, acoustic
    - axillary S44.3-
    - brachial plexus —*see* Injury, brachial plexus
    - cervical sympathetic S14.5
    - cranial S04.9
      - contusion S04.9
      - eighth (acoustic or auditory) —*see* Injury, nerve, acoustic
      - eleventh (accessory) —*see* Injury, nerve, accessory
      - fifth (trigeminal) —*see* Injury, nerve, trigeminal
      - first (olfactory) —*see* Injury, nerve, olfactory
      - fourth (trochlear) —*see* Injury, nerve, trochlear
      - laceration S04.9
      - ninth (glossopharyngeal) —*see* Injury, nerve, glossopharyngeal
      - second (optic) —*see* Injury, nerve, optic
      - seventh (facial) —*see* Injury, nerve, facial
      - sixth (abducent) —*see* Injury, nerve, abducens
      - specified
        - nerve NEC S04.89-
          - contusion S04.89-
          - laceration S04.89-
          - specified type NEC S04.89-
        - type NEC S04.9
      - tenth (pneumogastric or vagus) —*see* Injury, nerve, vagus
      - third (oculomotor) —*see* Injury, nerve, oculomotor
      - twelfth (hypoglossal) —*see* Injury, nerve, hypoglossal

- **Injury** *(continued)*
  - nerve NEC *(continued)*
    - cutaneous sensory
      - ankle (level) S94.3-
      - arm (upper) (level) S44.5-
      - foot (level) —*see* Injury, nerve, cutaneous sensory, ankle
      - forearm (level) S54.3-
      - hip (level) S74.2-
      - leg (lower level) S84.2-
      - shoulder (level) —*see* Injury, nerve, cutaneous sensory, arm
      - thigh (level) —*see* Injury, nerve, cutaneous sensory, hip
    - deep peroneal —*see* Injury, nerve, peroneal, foot
    - digital
      - finger S64.4-
        - index S64.49-
        - little S64.49-
        - middle S64.49-
        - ring S64.49-
      - thumb S64.3-
      - toe —*see* Injury, nerve, ankle, specified site NEC
    - eighth cranial (acoustic or auditory) —*see* Injury, nerve, acoustic
    - eleventh cranial (accessory) —*see* Injury, nerve, accessory
    - facial S04.5-
      - contusion S04.5-
      - laceration S04.5-
      - newborn P11.3
      - specified type NEC S04.5-
    - femoral (hip level) (thigh level) S74.1-
    - fifth cranial (trigeminal) —*see* Injury, nerve, trigeminal
    - finger (digital) —*see* Injury, nerve, digital, finger
    - first cranial (olfactory) —*see* Injury, nerve, olfactory
    - foot S94.9-
      - cutaneous sensory S94.3-
      - deep peroneal S94.2-
      - lateral plantar S94.0-
      - medial plantar S94.1-
      - specified site NEC —*see* subcategory S94.8
    - forearm (level) S54.9-
      - cutaneous sensory —*see* Injury, nerve, cutaneous sensory, forearm
      - median —*see* Injury, nerve, median
      - radial —*see* Injury, nerve, radial
      - specified site NEC —*see* subcategory S54.8
      - ulnar —*see* Injury, nerve, ulnar
    - fourth cranial (trochlear) —*see* Injury, nerve, trochlear
    - glossopharyngeal S04.89-
      - specified type NEC S04.89-
    - hand S64.9-
      - median —*see* Injury, nerve, median, hand
      - radial —*see* Injury, nerve, radial, hand
      - specified NEC —*see* subcategory S64.8
      - ulnar —*see* Injury, nerve, ulnar, hand
    - hip (level) S74.9-
      - cutaneous sensory —*see* Injury, nerve, cutaneous sensory, hip
      - femoral —*see* Injury, nerve, femoral

Injury (continued)
- nerve NEC (continued)
  - hip (continued)
    - sciatic —*see* Injury, nerve, sciatic
    - specified site NEC S74.8
  - hypoglossal S04.89-
    - specified type NEC S04.89-
  - lateral plantar S94.0-
  - leg (lower) S84.9-
    - cutaneous sensory —*see* Injury, nerve, cutaneous sensory, leg
    - peroneal —*see* Injury, nerve, peroneal
    - specified site NEC —*see* subcategory S84.8
    - tibial —*see* Injury, nerve, tibial
    - upper —*see* Injury, nerve, thigh
  - lower
    - back —*see* Injury, nerve, abdomen, specified site NEC
      - peripheral —*see* Injury, nerve, abdomen, peripheral
    - limb —*see* Injury, nerve, leg
  - lumbar spinal —*see* Injury, nerve, spinal, lumbar
  - lumbar plexus —*see* Injury, nerve, lumbosacral, sympathetic
  - lumbosacral
    - plexus —*see* Injury, nerve, lumbosacral, sympathetic
    - sympathetic S34.5
  - medial plantar S94.1-
  - median (forearm level) S54.1-
    - hand (level) S64.1-
    - upper arm (level) S44.1-
    - wrist (level) —*see* Injury, nerve, median, hand
  - musculocutaneous S44.4-
  - musculospiral (upper arm level) —*see* Injury, nerve, radial, upper arm
  - neck S14.9
    - peripheral S14.4
    - specified site NEC S14.8
    - sympathetic S14.5
  - ninth cranial (glossopharyngeal) —*see* Injury, nerve, glossopharyngeal
  - oculomotor S04.1-
    - contusion S04.1-
    - laceration S04.1-
    - specified type NEC S04.1-
  - olfactory S04.81-
    - specified type NEC S04.81-
  - optic S04.01-
    - contusion S04.01-
    - laceration S04.01-
    - specified type NEC S04.01-
  - pelvic girdle —*see* Injury, nerve, hip
  - pelvis —*see* Injury, nerve, abdomen, specified site NEC
    - peripheral —*see* Injury, nerve, abdomen, peripheral
  - peripheral NEC T14.8
    - abdomen —*see* Injury, nerve, abdomen, peripheral
    - lower back —*see* Injury, nerve, abdomen, peripheral
    - neck —*see* Injury, nerve, neck, peripheral
    - pelvis —*see* Injury, nerve, abdomen, peripheral
    - specified NEC T14.8
  - peroneal (lower leg level) S84.1-
    - foot S94.2-

Injury (continued)
- nerve NEC (continued)
  - plexus
    - brachial —*see* Injury, brachial plexus
    - celiac, coeliac —*see* Injury, nerve, lumbosacral, sympathetic
    - mesenteric, inferior —*see* Injury, nerve, lumbosacral, sympathetic
    - sacral —*see* Injury, lumbosacral plexus
    - spinal
      - brachial —*see* Injury, brachial plexus
      - lumbosacral —*see* Injury, lumbosacral plexus
  - pneumogastric —*see* Injury, nerve, vagus
  - radial (forearm level) S54.2-
    - hand (level) S64.2-
    - upper arm (level) S44.2-
    - wrist (level) —*see* Injury, nerve, radial, hand
  - root —*see* Injury, nerve, spinal, root
  - sacral plexus —*see* Injury, lumbosacral plexus
  - sacral spinal —*see* Injury, nerve, spinal, sacral
  - sciatic (hip level) (thigh level) S74.0-
  - second cranial (optic) —*see* Injury, nerve, optic
  - seventh cranial (facial) —*see* Injury, nerve, facial
  - shoulder —*see* Injury, nerve, arm
  - sixth cranial (abducent) —*see* Injury, nerve, abducens
  - spinal
    - plexus —*see* Injury, nerve, plexus, spinal
    - root
      - cervical S14.2
      - dorsal S24.2
      - lumbar S34.21
      - sacral S34.22
      - thoracic —*see* Injury, nerve, spinal, root, dorsal
  - splanchnic —*see* Injury, nerve, lumbosacral, sympathetic
  - sympathetic NEC —*see* Injury, nerve, lumbosacral, sympathetic
    - cervical —*see* Injury, nerve, cervical sympathetic
  - tenth cranial (pneumogastric or vagus) —*see* Injury, nerve, vagus
  - thigh (level) —*see* Injury, nerve, hip
    - cutaneous sensory —*see* Injury, nerve, cutaneous sensory, hip
    - femoral —*see* Injury, nerve, femoral
    - sciatic —*see* Injury, nerve, sciatic
    - specified NEC —*see* Injury, nerve, hip
  - third cranial (oculomotor) —*see* Injury, nerve, oculomotor
  - thorax S24.9
    - peripheral S24.3
    - specified site NEC S24.8
    - sympathetic S24.4
  - thumb, digital —*see* Injury, nerve, digital, thumb
  - tibial (lower leg level) (posterior) S84.0-
  - toe —*see* Injury, nerve, ankle

Injury (continued)
- nerve NEC (continued)
  - trigeminal S04.3-
    - contusion S04.3-
    - laceration S04.3-
    - specified type NEC S04.3-
  - trochlear S04.2-
    - contusion S04.2-
    - laceration S04.2-
    - specified type NEC S04.2-
  - twelfth cranial (hypoglossal) —*see* Injury, nerve, hypoglossal
  - ulnar (forearm level) S54.0-
    - arm (upper) (level) S44.0-
    - hand (level) S64.0-
    - wrist (level) —*see* Injury, nerve, ulnar, hand
  - vagus S04.89-
    - specified type NEC S04.89-
  - wrist (level) —*see* Injury, nerve, hand
- ninth cranial nerve (glossopharyngeal) —*see* Injury, nerve, glossopharyngeal
- nose (septum) S09.92
- obstetrical O71.9
  - specified NEC O71.89
- occipital (region) (scalp) S09.90
  - lobe —*see* Injury, intracranial
- optic chiasm S04.02
- optic radiation S04.03-
- optic tract and pathways S04.03-
- orbit, orbital (region) —*see* Injury, eye
  - penetrating (with foreign body) —*see* Injury, eye, orbit, penetrating
  - specified NEC —*see* Injury, eye, specified site NEC
- ovary, ovarian S37.409
  - bilateral S37.402
    - contusion S37.422
    - laceration S37.432
    - specified type NEC S37.492
  - blood vessel —*see* Injury, blood vessel, ovarian
  - contusion S37.429
    - bilateral S37.422
    - unilateral S37.421
  - laceration S37.439
    - bilateral S37.432
    - unilateral S37.431
  - specified type NEC S37.499
    - bilateral S37.492
    - unilateral S37.491
  - unilateral S37.401
    - contusion S37.421
    - laceration S37.431
    - specified type NEC S37.491
- palate (hard) (soft) S09.93
- pancreas S36.209
  - body S36.201
    - contusion S36.221
    - laceration S36.231
      - major S36.261
      - minor S36.241
      - moderate S36.251
    - specified type NEC S36.291
  - contusion S36.229
  - head S36.200
    - contusion S36.220
    - laceration S36.230
      - major S36.260
      - minor S36.240
      - moderate S36.250
    - specified type NEC S36.290
  - laceration S36.239
    - major S36.269
    - minor S36.249
    - moderate S36.259

Injury (continued)
- pancreas (continued)
  - specified type NEC S36.299
  - tail S36.202
    - contusion S36.222
    - laceration S36.232
      - major S36.262
      - minor S36.242
      - moderate S36.252
    - specified type NEC S36.292
- parietal (region) (scalp) S09.90
  - lobe —*see* Injury, intracranial
- patellar ligament (tendon) S76.10-
  - laceration S76.12-
  - specified NEC S76.19-
  - strain S76.11-
- pelvis, pelvic (floor) S39.93
  - complicating delivery O70.1
  - joint or ligament, complicating delivery O71.6
  - organ S37.90
    - with ectopic or molar pregnancy O08.6
    - complication of abortion —*see* Abortion
    - contusion S37.92
    - following ectopic or molar pregnancy O08.6
    - laceration S37.93
    - obstetrical trauma NEC O71.5
    - specified
      - site NEC S37.899
        - contusion S37.892
        - laceration S37.893
        - specified type NEC S37.898
      - type NEC S37.99
  - specified NEC S39.83
- penis S39.94
- perineum S39.94
- peritoneum S36.81
  - laceration S36.893
- periurethral tissue —*see* Injury, urethra
  - complicating delivery O71.82
- phalanges
  - foot —*see* Injury, foot
  - hand —*see* Injury, hand
- pharynx NEC S19.85
- pleura —*see* Injury, intrathoracic, pleura
- plexus
  - brachial —*see* Injury, brachial plexus
  - cardiac —*see* Injury, nerve, thorax, sympathetic
  - celiac, coeliac —*see* Injury, nerve, lumbosacral, sympathetic
  - esophageal —*see* Injury, nerve, thorax, sympathetic
  - hypogastric —*see* Injury, nerve, lumbosacral, sympathetic
  - lumbar, lumbosacral —*see* Injury, lumbosacral plexus
  - mesenteric —*see* Injury, nerve, lumbosacral, sympathetic
  - pulmonary —*see* Injury, nerve, thorax, sympathetic
- postcardiac surgery (syndrome) I97.0
- prepuce S39.94
- prostate S37.829
  - contusion S37.822
  - laceration S37.823
  - specified type NEC S37.828
- pubic region S39.94
- pudendum S39.94
- pulmonary plexus —*see* Injury, nerve, thorax, sympathetic

Injury *(continued)*
rectovaginal septum NEC S39.83
rectum —*see* Injury, intestine, large, rectum
retina —*see* Injury, eye, specified site NEC
penetrating —*see* Injury, eyeball, penetrating
retroperitoneal —*see* Injury, intra-abdominal, specified site NEC
rotator cuff (muscle(s)) (tendon(s)) S46.00-
laceration S46.02-
specified type NEC S46.09-
strain S46.01-
round ligament —*see* Injury, pelvic organ, specified site NEC
sacral plexus —*see* Injury, lumbosacral plexus
salivary duct or gland S09.93
scalp S09.90
newborn (birth injury) P12.9
due to monitoring (electrode) (sampling incision) P12.4
specified NEC P12.89
caput succedaneum P12.81
scapular region —*see* Injury, shoulder
sclera —*see* Injury, eye, specified site NEC
penetrating —*see* Injury, eyeball, penetrating
scrotum S39.94
second cranial nerve (optic) —*see* Injury, nerve, optic
seminal vesicle —*see* Injury, pelvic organ, specified site NEC
seventh cranial nerve (facial) —*see* Injury, nerve, facial
shoulder S49.9-
blood vessel —*see* Injury, blood vessel, arm
contusion —*see* Contusion, shoulder
dislocation —*see* Dislocation, shoulder
fracture —*see* Fracture, shoulder
shoulder S49.9-
muscle —*see* Injury, muscle, shoulder
nerve —*see* Injury, nerve, shoulder
open —*see* Wound, open, shoulder
specified type NEC S49.8-
sprain —*see* Sprain, shoulder girdle
superficial —*see* Injury, superficial, shoulder
sinus
cavernous —*see* Injury, intracranial
nasal S09.92
sixth cranial nerve (abducent) —*see* Injury, nerve, abducens
skeleton, birth injury P13.9
specified part NEC P13.8
skin NEC T14.8
surface intact —*see* Injury, superficial
skull NEC S09.90
specified NEC T14.8
spermatic cord (pelvic region) S37.898
scrotal region S39.848
spinal (cord)
cervical (neck) S14.109
anterior cord syndrome S14.139
C1 level S14.131
C2 level S14.132
C3 level S14.133

Injury *(continued)*
spinal *(continued)*
cervical *(continued)*
anterior cord syndrome *(continued)*
C4 level S14.134
C5 level S14.135
C6 level S14.136
C7 level S14.137
C8 level S14.138
Brown-Séquard syndrome S14.149
C1 level S14.141
C2 level S14.142
C3 level S14.143
C4 level S14.144
C5 level S14.145
C6 level S14.146
C7 level S14.147
C8 level S14.148
C1 level S14.101
C2 level S14.102
C3 level S14.103
C4 level S14.104
C5 level S14.105
C6 level S14.106
C7 level S14.107
C8 level S14.108
central cord syndrome S14.129
C1 level S14.121
C2 level S14.122
C3 level S14.123
C4 level S14.124
C5 level S14.125
C6 level S14.126
C7 level S14.127
C8 level S14.128
complete lesion S14.119
C1 level S14.111
C2 level S14.112
C3 level S14.113
C4 level S14.114
C5 level S14.115
C6 level S14.116
C7 level S14.117
C8 level S14.118
concussion S14.0
edema S14.0
incomplete lesion specified NEC S14.159
C1 level S14.151
C2 level S14.152
C3 level S14.153
C4 level S14.154
C5 level S14.155
C6 level S14.156
C7 level S14.157
C8 level S14.158
posterior cord syndrome S14.159
C1 level S14.151
C2 level S14.152
C3 level S14.153
C4 level S14.154
C5 level S14.155
C6 level S14.156
C7 level S14.157
C8 level S14.158
dorsal —*see* Injury, spinal, thoracic
lumbar S34.109
complete lesion S34.119
L1 level S34.111
L2 level S34.112
L3 level S34.113
L4 level S34.114
L5 level S34.115
concussion S34.01
edema S34.01
incomplete lesion S34.129

Injury *(continued)*
spinal *(continued)*
lumbar *(continued)*
incomplete lesion *(continued)*
L1 level S34.121
L2 level S34.122
L3 level S34.123
L4 level S34.124
L5 level S34.125
L1 level S34.101
L2 level S34.102
L3 level S34.103
L4 level S34.104
L5 level S34.105
nerve root NEC
cervical —*see* Injury, nerve, spinal, root, cervical
dorsal —*see* Injury, nerve, spinal, root, dorsal
lumbar S34.21
sacral S34.22
thoracic —*see* Injury, nerve, spinal, root, dorsal
plexus
brachial —*see* Injury, brachial plexus
lumbosacral —*see* Injury, lumbosacral plexus
sacral S34.139
complete lesion S34.131
incomplete lesion S34.132
thoracic S24.109
anterior cord syndrome S24.139
T1 level S24.131
T2-T6 level S24.132
T7-T10 level S24.133
T11-T12 level S24.134
Brown-Séquard syndrome S24.149
T1 level S24.141
T2-T6 level S24.142
T7-T10 level S24.143
T11-T12 level S24.144
complete lesion S24.119
T1 level S24.111
T2-T6 level S24.112
T7-T10 level S24.113
T11-T12 level S24.114
concussion S24.0
edema S24.0
incomplete lesion specified NEC S24.159
T1 level S24.151
T2-T6 level S24.152
T7-T10 level S24.153
T11-T12 level S24.154
posterior cord syndrome S24.159
T1 level S24.151
T2-T6 level S24.152
T7-T10 level S24.153
T11-T12 level S24.154
T1 level S24.101
T2-T6 level S24.102
T7-T10 level S24.103
T11-T12 level S24.104
splanchnic nerve —*see* Injury, nerve, lumbosacral, sympathetic
spleen S36.00
contusion S36.029
major S36.021
minor S36.020
laceration S36.039
major (massive) (stellate) S36.032
moderate S36.031
superficial (capsular) (minor) S36.030

Injury *(continued)*
spleen *(continued)*
specified type NEC S36.09
splenic artery —*see* Injury, blood vessel, celiac artery, branch
stellate ganglion —*see* Injury, nerve thorax, sympathetic
sternal region S29.9
stomach S36.30
contusion S36.32
laceration S36.33
specified type NEC S36.39
subconjunctival —*see* Injury, eye, conjunctiva
subcutaneous NEC T14.8
submaxillary region S09.93
submental region S09.93
subungual
fingers —*see* Injury, hand
toes —*see* Injury, foot
superficial NEC T14.8
abdomen, abdominal (wall) S30.92
abrasion S30.811
bite S30.871
insect S30.861
contusion S30.1
external constriction S30.841
foreign body S30.851
abrasion —*see* Abrasion, by site
adnexa, eye NEC —*see* Injury, eye, specified site NEC
alveolar process —*see* Injury, superficial, oral cavity
ankle S90.91-
abrasion —*see* Abrasion, ankle
blister —*see* Blister, ankle
bite —*see* Bite, ankle
contusion —*see* Contusion, ankle
external constriction —*see* Constriction, external, ankle
foreign body —*see* Foreign body, superficial, ankle
anus S30.98
arm (upper) S40.92-
abrasion —*see* Abrasion, arm
bite —*see* Bite, superficial, arm
blister —*see* Blister, arm (upper)
contusion —*see* Contusion, arm
external constriction —*see* Constriction, external, arm
foreign body —*see* Foreign body, superficial, arm
auditory canal (external) (meatus) —*see* Injury, superficial, ear
auricle —*see* Injury, superficial, ear
axilla —*see* Injury, superficial, arm
back —*see also* Injury, superficial, thorax, back
lower S30.91
abrasion S30.810
contusion S30.0
external constriction S30.840
superficial
bite NEC S30.870
insect S30.860
foreign body S30.850
bite NEC —*see* Bite, superficial NEC, by site
blister —*see* Blister, by site
breast S20.10-
abrasion —*see* Abrasion, breast
bite —*see* Bite, superficial, breast

Injury *(continued)*
- superficial NEC *(continued)*
  - breast *(continued)*
    - contusion *—see* Contusion, breast
    - external constriction *—see* Constriction, external, breast
    - foreign body *—see* Foreign body, superficial, breast
  - brow *—see* Injury, superficial, head, specified NEC
  - buttock S30.91
  - calf *—see* Injury, superficial, leg
  - canthus, eye *—see* Injury, superficial, periocular area
  - cheek (external) *—see* Injury, superficial, head, specified NEC
    - internal *—see* Injury, superficial, oral cavity
  - chest wall *—see* Injury, superficial, thorax
  - chin *—see* Injury, superficial, head NEC
  - clitoris S30.95
  - conjunctiva *—see* Injury, eye, conjunctiva
    - with foreign body (in conjunctival sac) *—see* Foreign body, conjunctival sac
  - contusion *—see* Contusion, by site
  - costal region *—see* Injury, superficial, thorax
  - digit(s)
    - hand *—see* Injury, superficial, finger
  - ear (auricle) (canal) (external) S00.40-
    - abrasion *—see* Abrasion, ear
    - bite *—see* Bite, superficial, ear
    - contusion *—see* Contusion, ear
    - external constriction *—see* Constriction, external, ear
    - foreign body *—see* Foreign body, superficial, ear
  - elbow S50.90-
    - abrasion *—see* Abrasion, elbow
    - bite *—see* Bite, superficial, elbow
    - blister *—see* Blister, elbow
    - contusion *—see* Contusion, elbow
    - external constriction *—see* Constriction, external, elbow
    - foreign body *—see* Foreign body, superficial, elbow
  - epididymis S30.94
  - epigastric region S30.92
  - epiglottis *—see* Injury, superficial, throat
  - esophagus
    - cervical *—see* Injury, superficial, throat
  - external constriction *—see* Constriction, external, by site
  - extremity NEC T14.8
  - eyeball NEC *—see* Injury, eye, specified site NEC
  - eyebrow *—see* Injury, superficial, periocular area
  - eyelid S00.20-
    - abrasion *—see* Abrasion, eyelid
    - bite *—see* Bite, superficial, eyelid
    - contusion *—see* Contusion, eyelid
    - external constriction *—see* Constriction, external, eyelid

Injury *(continued)*
- superficial NEC *(continued)*
  - eyelid *(continued)*
    - foreign body *—see* Foreign body, superficial, eyelid
  - face NEC *—see* Injury, superficial, head, specified NEC
  - finger(s) S60.949
    - abrasion *—see* Abrasion, finger
    - bite *—see* Bite, superficial, finger
    - blister *—see* Blister, finger
    - contusion *—see* Contusion, finger
    - external constriction *—see* Constriction, external, finger
    - foreign body *—see* Foreign body, superficial, finger
    - insect bite *—see* Bite, by site, superficial, insect
    - index S60.94-
    - little S60.94-
    - middle S60.94-
    - ring S60.94-
  - flank S30.92
  - foot S90.92-
    - abrasion *—see* Abrasion, foot
    - bite *—see* Bite, foot
    - blister *—see* Blister, foot
    - contusion *—see* Contusion, foot
    - external constriction *—see* Constriction, external, foot
    - foreign body *—see* Foreign body, superficial, foot
  - forearm S50.91-
    - abrasion *—see* Abrasion, forearm
    - bite *—see* Bite, forearm, superficial
    - blister *—see* Blister, forearm
    - contusion *—see* Contusion, forearm
    - elbow only *—see* Injury, superficial, elbow
    - external constriction *—see* Constriction, external, forearm
    - foreign body *—see* Foreign body, superficial, forearm
  - forehead *—see* Injury, superficial, head NEC
  - foreign body *—see* Foreign body, superficial
  - genital organs, external
    - female S30.97
    - male S30.96
  - globe (eye) *—see* Injury, eye, specified site NEC
  - groin S30.92
  - gum *—see* Injury, superficial, oral cavity
  - hand S60.92-
    - abrasion *—see* Abrasion, hand
    - bite *—see* Bite, superficial, hand
    - contusion *—see* Contusion, hand
    - external constriction *—see* Constriction, external, hand
    - foreign body *—see* Foreign body, superficial, hand
  - head S00.90
    - ear *—see* Injury, superficial, ear
    - eyelid *—see* Injury, superficial, eyelid
    - nose S00.30
    - oral cavity S00.502
    - scalp S00.00
    - specified site NEC S00.80

Injury *(continued)*
- superficial NEC *(continued)*
  - heel *—see* Injury, superficial, foot
  - hip S70.91-
    - abrasion *—see* Abrasion, hip
    - bite *—see* Bite, superficial, hip
    - blister *—see* Blister, hip
    - contusion *—see* Contusion, hip
    - external constriction *—see* Constriction, external, hip
    - foreign body *—see* Foreign body, superficial, hip
  - iliac region *—see* Injury, superficial, abdomen
  - inguinal region *—see* Injury, superficial, abdomen
  - insect bite *—see* Bite, by site, superficial, insect
  - interscapular region *—see* Injury, superficial, thorax, back
  - jaw *—see* Injury, superficial, head, specified NEC
  - knee S80.91-
    - abrasion *—see* Abrasion, knee
    - bite *—see* Bite, superficial, knee
    - blister *—see* Blister, knee
    - contusion *—see* Contusion, knee
    - external constriction *—see* Constriction, external, knee
    - foreign body *—see* Foreign body, superficial, knee
  - labium (majus) (minus) S30.95
  - lacrimal (apparatus) (gland) (sac) *—see* Injury, eye, specified site NEC
  - larynx *—see* Injury, superficial, throat
  - leg (lower) S80.92-
    - abrasion *—see* Abrasion, leg
    - bite *—see* Bite, superficial, leg
    - contusion *—see* Contusion, leg
    - external constriction *—see* Constriction, external, leg
    - foreign body *—see* Foreign body, superficial, leg
    - knee *—see* Injury, superficial, knee
  - limb NEC T14.8
  - lip S00.501
  - lower back S30.91
  - lumbar region S30.91
  - malar region *—see* Injury, superficial, head, specified NEC
  - mammary *—see* Injury, superficial, breast
  - mastoid region *—see* Injury, superficial, head, specified NEC
  - mouth *—see* Injury, superficial, oral cavity
  - muscle NEC T14.8
  - nail NEC T14.8
    - finger *—see* Injury, superficial, finger
    - toe *—see* Injury, superficial, toe
  - nasal (septum) *—see* Injury, superficial, nose
  - neck S10.90
    - specified site NEC S10.80
  - nose (septum) S00.30
  - occipital region *—see* Injury, superficial, scalp
  - oral cavity S00.502
  - orbital region *—see* Injury, superficial, periocular area
  - palate *—see* Injury, superficial, oral cavity
  - palm *—see* Injury, superficial, hand

Injury *(continued)*
- superficial NEC *(continued)*
  - parietal region *—see* Injury, superficial, scalp
  - pelvis S30.91
    - girdle *—see* Injury, superficial, hip
  - penis S30.93
  - perineum
    - female S30.95
    - male S30.91
  - periocular area S00.20-
    - abrasion *—see* Abrasion, eyelid
    - bite *—see* Bite, superficial, eyelid
    - contusion *—see* Contusion, eyelid
    - external constriction *—see* Constriction, external, eyelid
    - foreign body *—see* Foreign body, superficial, eyelid
  - phalanges
    - finger *—see* Injury, superficial, finger
    - toe *—see* Injury, superficial, toe
  - pharynx *—see* Injury, superficial, throat
  - pinna *—see* Injury, superficial, ear
  - popliteal space *—see* Injury, superficial, knee
  - prepuce S30.93
  - pubic region S30.91
  - pudendum
    - female S30.97
    - male S30.96
  - sacral region S30.91
  - scalp S00.00
  - scapular region *—see* Injury, superficial, shoulder
  - sclera *—see* Injury, eye, specified site NEC
  - scrotum S30.94
  - shin *—see* Injury, superficial, leg
  - shoulder S40.91-
    - abrasion *—see* Abrasion, shoulder
    - bite *—see* Bite, superficial, shoulder
    - blister *—see* Blister, shoulder
    - contusion *—see* Contusion, shoulder
    - external constriction *—see* Constriction, external, shoulder
    - foreign body *—see* Foreign body, superficial, shoulder
  - skin NEC T14.8
  - sternal region *—see* Injury, superficial, thorax, front
  - subconjunctival *—see* Injury, eye, specified site NEC
  - subcutaneous NEC T14.8
  - submaxillary region *—see* Injury, superficial, head, specified NEC
  - submental region *—see* Injury, superficial, head, specified NEC
  - subungual
    - finger(s) *—see* Injury, superficial, finger
    - toe(s) *—see* Injury, superficial, toe
  - supraclavicular fossa *—see* Injury, superficial, neck
  - supraorbital *—see* Injury, superficial, head, specified NEC
  - temple *—see* Injury, superficial, head, specified NEC
  - temporal region *—see* Injury, superficial, head, specified NEC

Injury *(continued)*
superficial NEC *(continued)*
testis S30.94
thigh S70.92-
abrasion *—see* Abrasion, thigh
bite *—see* Bite, superficial, thigh
blister *—see* Blister, thigh
contusion *—see* Contusion, thigh
external constriction *—see* Constriction, external, thigh
foreign body *—see* Foreign body, superficial, thigh
thorax, thoracic (wall) S20.90
abrasion *—see* Abrasion, thorax
back S20.40-
bite *—see* Bite, thorax, superficial
blister *—see* Blister, thorax
contusion *—see* Contusion, thorax
external constriction *—see* Constriction, external, thorax
foreign body *—see* Foreign body, superficial, thorax
front S20.30-
throat S10.10
abrasion S10.11
bite S10.17
insect S10.16
blister S10.12
contusion S10.0
external constriction S10.14
foreign body S10.15
thumb S60.93-
abrasion *—see* Abrasion, thumb
bite *—see* Bite, superficial, thumb
blister *—see* Blister, thumb
contusion *—see* Contusion, thumb
external constriction *—see* Constriction, external, thumb
foreign body *—see* Foreign body, superficial, thumb
insect bite *—see* Bite, by site, superficial, insect
specified type NEC S60.39-
toe(s) S90.93-
abrasion *—see* Abrasion, toe
bite *—see* Bite, toe
blister *—see* Blister, toe
contusion *—see* Contusion, toe
external constriction *—see* Constriction, external, toe
foreign body *—see* Foreign body, superficial, toe
great S90.93-
tongue *—see* Injury, superficial, oral cavity
tooth, teeth *—see* Injury, superficial, oral cavity
trachea S10.10
tunica vaginalis S30.94
tympanum, tympanic membrane *—see* Injury, superficial, ear
uvula *—see* Injury, superficial, oral cavity
vagina S30.95
vocal cords *—see* Injury, superficial, throat
vulva S30.95
wrist S60.91-
supraclavicular region *—see* Injury, neck
supraorbital S09.93
suprarenal gland (multiple) *—see* Injury, adrenal

Injury *(continued)*
surgical complication (external or internal site) *—see* Laceration, accidental complicating surgery
temple S09.90
temporal region S09.90
tendon *—see also* Injury, muscle, by site
abdomen *—see* Injury, muscle, abdomen
Achilles *—see* Injury, Achilles tendon
lower back *—see* Injury, muscle, lower back
pelvic organs *—see* Injury, muscle, pelvis
tenth cranial nerve (pneumogastric or vagus) *—see* Injury, nerve, vagus
testis S39.94
thigh S79.92-
blood vessel *—see* Injury, blood vessel, hip
contusion *—see* Contusion, thigh
fracture *—see* Fracture, femur
muscle *—see* Injury, muscle, thigh
nerve *—see* Injury, nerve, thigh
open *—see* Wound, open, thigh
specified NEC S79.82-
superficial *—see* Injury, superficial, thigh
third cranial nerve (oculomotor) *—see* Injury, nerve, oculomotor
thorax, thoracic S29.9
blood vessel *—see* Injury, blood vessel, thorax
cavity *—see* Injury, intrathoracic
dislocation *—see* Dislocation, thorax
external (wall) S29.9
contusion *—see* Contusion, thorax
nerve *—see* Injury, nerve, thorax
open *—see* Wound, open, thorax
specified NEC S29.8
sprain *—see* Sprain, thorax
superficial *—see* Injury, superficial, thorax
fracture *—see* Fracture, thorax
internal *—see* Injury, intrathoracic
intrathoracic organ *—see* Injury, intrathoracic
sympathetic ganglion *—see* Injury, nerve, thorax, sympathetic
throat (*see also* Injury, neck) S19.9
thumb S69.9-
blood vessel *—see* Injury, blood vessel, thumb
contusion *—see* Contusion, thumb
dislocation *—see* Dislocation, thumb
fracture *—see* Fracture, thumb
muscle *—see* Injury, muscle, thumb
nerve *—see* Injury, nerve, digital, thumb
open *—see* Wound, open, thumb
specified NEC S69.8-
sprain *—see* Sprain, thumb
superficial *—see* Injury, superficial, thumb
thymus (gland) *—see* Injury, intrathoracic, specified organ NEC
thyroid (gland) NEC S19.84
toe S99.92-
contusion *—see* Contusion, toe
dislocation *—see* Dislocation, toe
fracture *—see* Fracture, toe
muscle *—see* Injury, muscle, toe

Injury *(continued)*
toe *(continued)*
open *—see* Wound, open, toe
specified type NEC S99.82-
sprain *—see* Sprain, toe
superficial *—see* Injury, superficial, toe
tongue S09.93
tonsil S09.93
tooth S09.93
trachea (cervical) NEC S19.82
thoracic *—see* Injury, intrathoracic, trachea, thoracic
transfusion-related acute lung (TRALI) J95.84
tunica vaginalis S39.94
twelfth cranial nerve (hypoglossal) *—see* Injury, nerve, hypoglossal
ureter S37.10
contusion S37.12
laceration S37.13
specified type NEC S37.19
urethra (sphincter) S37.30
at delivery O71.5
contusion S37.32
laceration S37.33
specified type NEC S37.39
urinary organ S37.90
contusion S37.92
laceration S37.93
specified
site NEC S37.899
contusion S37.892
laceration S37.893
specified type NEC S37.898
type NEC S37.99
uterus, uterine S37.60
with ectopic or molar pregnancy O08.6
blood vessel *—see* Injury, blood vessel, iliac
contusion S37.62
laceration S37.63
cervix at delivery O71.3
rupture associated with obstetrics *—see* Rupture, uterus
specified type NEC S37.69
uvula S09.93
vagina S39.93
abrasion S30.814
bite S31.45
insect S30.864
superficial NEC S30.874
contusion S30.23
crush S38.03
during delivery *—see* Laceration, vagina, during delivery
external constriction S30.844
insect bite S30.864
laceration S31.41
with foreign body S31.42
open wound S31.40
puncture S31.43
with foreign body S31.44
superficial S30.95
foreign body S30.854
vas deferens *—see* Injury, pelvic organ, specified site NEC
vascular NEC T14.8
vein *—see* Injury, blood vessel
vena cava (superior) S25.20
inferior S35.10
laceration (minor) (superficial) S35.11
major S35.12
specified type NEC S35.19
laceration (minor) (superficial) S25.21
major S25.22
specified type NEC S25.29

Injury *(continued)*
vesical (sphincter) *—see* Injury, bladder
visual cortex S04.04-
vitreous (humor) S05.90
specified NEC S05.8X-
vocal cord NEC S19.83
vulva S39.94
abrasion S30.814
bite S31.45
insect S30.864
superficial NEC S30.874
contusion S30.23
crush S38.03
during delivery *—see* Laceration, perineum, female, during delivery
external constriction S30.844
insect bite S30.864
laceration S31.41
with foreign body S31.42
open wound S31.40
puncture S31.43
with foreign body S31.44
superficial S30.95
foreign body S30.854
whiplash (cervical spine) S13.4
wrist S69.9-
blood vessel *—see* Injury, blood vessel, hand
contusion *—see* Contusion, wrist
dislocation *—see* Dislocation, wrist
fracture *—see* Fracture, wrist
muscle *—see* Injury, muscle, hand
nerve *—see* Injury, nerve, hand
open *—see* Wound, open, wrist
specified NEC S69.8-
sprain *—see* Sprain, wrist
superficial *—see* Injury, superficial, wrist

Inoculation *—see also* Vaccination
complication or reaction *—see* Complications, vaccination

Insanity, insane *—see also* Psychosis
adolescent *—see* Schizophrenia
confusional F28
acute or subacute F05
delusional F22
senile F03

Insect
bite *—see* Bite, by site, superficial, insect
venomous, poisoning NEC (by) *—see* Venom, arthropod

Insensitivity
adrenocorticotropin hormone (ACTH) E27.49
androgen E34.50
complete E34.51
partial E34.52

Insertion
cord (umbilical) lateral or velamentous O43.12-
intrauterine contraceptive device (encounter for) *—see* Intrauterine contraceptive device

Insolation (sunstroke) T67.0

Insomnia (organic) G47.00
adjustment F51.02
adjustment disorder F51.02
behavioral, of childhood Z73.819
combined type Z73.812
limit setting type Z73.811
sleep-onset association type Z73.810

Insomnia *(continued)*
- childhood Z73.819
- chronic F51.04
  - somatized tension F51.04
- conditioned F51.04
- due to
  - alcohol
    - abuse F10.182
    - dependence F10.282
    - use F10.982
  - amphetamines
    - abuse F15.182
    - dependence F15.282
    - use F15.982
  - anxiety disorder F51.05
  - caffeine
    - abuse F15.182
    - dependence F15.282
    - use F15.982
  - cocaine
    - abuse F14.182
    - dependence F14.282
    - use F14.982
  - depression F51.05
  - drug NEC
    - abuse F19.182
    - dependence F19.282
    - use F19.982
  - medical condition G47.01
  - mental disorder NEC F51.05
  - opioid
    - abuse F11.182
    - dependence F11.282
    - use F11.982
  - psychoactive substance NEC
    - abuse F19.182
    - dependence F19.282
    - use F19.982
  - sedative, hypnotic, or anxiolytic
    - abuse F13.182
    - dependence F13.282
    - use F13.982
  - stimulant NEC
    - abuse F15.182
    - dependence F15.282
    - use F15.982
- fatal familial (FFI) A81.83
- idiopathic F51.01
- learned F51.3
- nonorganic origin F51.01
- not due to a substance or known physiological condition F51.01
  - specified NEC F51.09
- paradoxical F51.03
- primary F51.01
- psychiatric F51.05
- psychophysiologic F51.04
- related to psychopathology F51.05
- short-term F51.02
- specified NEC G47.09
- stress-related F51.02
- transient F51.02
- without objective findings F51.02

Inspiration
- food or foreign body *—see* Foreign body, by site
- mucus *—see* Asphyxia, mucus

Inspissated bile syndrome (newborn) P59.1

Instability
- emotional (excessive) F60.3
- joint (post-traumatic) M25.30
  - ankle M25.37-
  - due to old ligament injury *—see* Disorder, ligament
  - elbow M25.32-
  - flail *—see* Flail, joint
  - foot M25.37-
  - hand M25.34-

Instability *(continued)*
- joint *(continued)*
  - hip M25.35-
  - knee M25.36-
  - lumbosacral M53.2
  - prosthesis *—see* Complications, joint prosthesis, mechanical, displacement, by site
  - sacroiliac M53.2
  - secondary to
    - old ligament injury *—see* Disorder, ligament
    - removal of joint prosthesis M96.89
  - shoulder (region) M25.31-
  - spine M53.2
  - wrist M25.33-
- knee (chronic) M23.5-
- lumbosacral M53.2
- nervous F48.8
- personality (emotional) F60.3
- spine *—see* Instability, joint, spine
- vasomotor R55

Institutional syndrome (childhood) F94.2

Institutionalization, affecting child Z62.22
- disinhibited attachment F94.2

Insufficiency, insufficient
- accommodation, old age H52.4
- adrenal (gland) E27.40
  - primary E27.1
- adrenocortical E27.40
  - drug-induced E27.3
  - iatrogenic E27.3
  - primary E27.1
- anatomic crown height K08.89
- anterior (occlusal) guidance M26.54
- anus K62.89
- aortic (valve) I35.1
  - with
    - mitral (valve) disease I08.0
      - with tricuspid (valve) disease I08.3
    - stenosis I35.2
    - tricuspid (valve) disease I08.2
      - with mitral (valve) disease I08.3
  - congenital Q23.1
  - rheumatic I06.1
    - with
      - mitral (valve) disease I08.0
        - with tricuspid (valve) disease I08.3
      - stenosis I06.2
        - with mitral (valve) disease I08.0
          - with tricuspid (valve) disease I08.3
      - tricuspid (valve) disease I08.2
        - with mitral (valve) disease I08.3
  - specified cause NEC I35.1
  - syphilitic A52.03
- arterial I77.1
  - basilar G45.0
  - carotid (hemispheric) G45.1
  - cerebral I67.81
  - coronary (acute or subacute) I24.8
  - mesenteric K55.1
  - peripheral I73.9
  - precerebral (multiple) (bilateral) G45.2
  - vertebral G45.0
- arteriovenous I99.8
- biliary K83.8
- cardiac *—see also* Insufficiency, myocardial
  - due to presence of (cardiac) prosthesis I97.11-

Insufficiency, insufficient *(continued)*
- cardiac *(continued)*
  - postprocedural I97.11-
- cardiorenal, hypertensive I13.2
- cardiovascular *—see* Disease, cardiovascular
- cerebrovascular (acute) I67.81
  - with transient focal neurological signs and symptoms G45.8
- circulatory NEC I99.8
  - newborn P29.89
- clinical crown height K08.89
- convergence H51.11
- coronary (acute or subacute) I24.8
  - chronic or with a stated duration of over 4 weeks I25.89
- corticoadrenal E27.40
  - primary E27.1
- dietary E63.9
- divergence H51.8
- food T73.0
- gastroesophageal K22.8
- gonadal
  - ovary E28.39
  - testis E29.1
- heart *—see also* Insufficiency, myocardial
  - newborn P29.0
  - valve *—see* Endocarditis
- hepatic *—see* Failure, hepatic
- idiopathic autonomic G90.09
- interocclusal distance of fully erupted teeth (ridge) M26.36
- kidney N28.9
  - acute N28.9
  - chronic N18.9
- lacrimal (secretion) H04.12-
  - passages *—see* Stenosis, lacrimal
- liver *—see* Failure, hepatic
- lung *—see* Insufficiency, pulmonary
- mental (congenital) *—see* Disability, intellectual
- mesenteric K55.1
- mitral (valve) I34.0
  - with
    - aortic valve disease I08.0
      - with tricuspid (valve) disease I08.3
    - obstruction or stenosis I05.2
      - with aortic valve disease I08.0
    - tricuspid (valve) disease I08.1
      - with aortic (valve) disease I08.3
  - congenital Q23.3
  - rheumatic I05.1
    - with
      - aortic valve disease I08.0
        - with tricuspid (valve) disease I08.3
      - obstruction or stenosis I05.2
        - with aortic valve disease I08.0
          - with tricuspid (valve) disease I08.3
      - tricuspid (valve) disease I08.1
        - with aortic (valve) disease I08.3
    - active or acute I01.1
      - with chorea, rheumatic (Sydenham's) I02.0
  - specified cause, except rheumatic I34.0
- muscle *—see also* Disease, muscle
  - heart *—see* Insufficiency, myocardial
  - ocular NEC H50.9
- myocardial, myocardium (with arteriosclerosis) (*see also* Failure, heart) I50.9

Insufficiency, insufficient *(continued)*
- myocardial, myocardium *(continued)*
  - with
    - rheumatic fever (conditions in I00) I09.0
      - active, acute or subacute I01.2
        - with chorea I02.0
      - inactive or quiescent (with chorea) I09.0
  - congenital Q24.8
  - hypertensive *—see* Hypertension, heart
  - newborn P29.0
  - rheumatic I09.0
    - active, acute, or subacute I01.2
  - syphilitic A52.06
- nourishment T73.0
- pancreatic K86.89
  - exocrine K86.81
- parathyroid (gland) E20.9
- peripheral vascular (arterial) I73.9
- pituitary E23.0
- placental (mother) O36.51-
- platelets D69.6
- prenatal care affecting management of pregnancy O09.3-
- progressive pluriglandular E31.0
- pulmonary J98.4
  - acute, following surgery (nonthoracic) J95.2
    - thoracic J95.1
  - chronic, following surgery J95.3
  - following
    - shock J98.4
    - trauma J98.4
  - newborn P28.5
  - valve I37.1
    - with stenosis I37.2
    - congenital Q22.2
    - rheumatic I09.89
      - with aortic, mitral or tricuspid (valve) disease I08.8
- pyloric K31.89
- renal (acute) N28.9
  - chronic N18.9
- respiratory R06.89
  - newborn P28.5
- rotation *—see* Malrotation
- sleep syndrome F51.12
- social insurance Z59.7
- suprarenal E27.40
  - primary E27.1
- tarso-orbital fascia, congenital Q10.3
- testis E29.1
- thyroid (gland) (acquired) E03.9
  - congenital E03.1
- tricuspid (valve) (rheumatic) I07.1
  - with
    - aortic (valve) disease I08.2
      - with mitral (valve) disease I08.3
    - mitral (valve) disease I08.1
      - with aortic (valve) disease I08.3
    - obstruction or stenosis I07.2
      - with aortic (valve) disease I08.2
        - with mitral (valve) disease I08.3
  - congenital Q22.8
  - nonrheumatic I36.1
    - with stenosis I36.2
- urethral sphincter R32
- valve, valvular (heart) I38
  - aortic *—see* Insufficiency, aortic (valve)
  - congenital Q24.8
  - mitral *—see* Insufficiency, mitral (valve)

Insufficiency, insufficient *(continued)*
- valve, valvular *(continued)*
  - pulmonary *—see* Insufficiency, pulmonary valve
  - tricuspid *—see* Insufficiency, tricuspid (valve)
- vascular I99.8
  - intestine K55.9
    - acute (*see also* Ischemia, intestine, acute) K55.059
  - mesenteric K55.1
  - peripheral I73.9
  - renal *—see* Hypertension, kidney
- velopharyngeal
  - acquired K13.79
  - congenital Q38.8
- venous (chronic) (peripheral) I87.2
- ventricular *—see* Insufficiency, myocardial
- welfare support Z59.7

Insufflation, fallopian Z31.41

Insular *—see* condition

Insulinoma
- pancreas
  - benign D13.7
  - malignant C25.4
  - uncertain behavior D37.8
- specified site
  - benign *—see* Neoplasm, by site, benign
  - malignant *—see* Neoplasm, by site, malignant
  - uncertain behavior *—see* Neoplasm, by site, uncertain behavior
- unspecified site
  - benign D13.7
  - malignant C25.4
  - uncertain behavior D37.8

Insuloma *—see* Insulinoma

Interference
- balancing side M26.56
- non-working side M26.56

Intermenstrual *—see* condition

Intermittent *—see* condition

Internal *—see* condition

Interrogation
- cardiac defibrillator (automatic) (implantable) Z45.02
- cardiac pacemaker Z45.018
- cardiac (event) (loop) recorder Z45.09
- infusion pump (implanted) (intrathecal) Z45.1
- neurostimulator Z46.2

Interruption
- aortic arch Q25.21
- bundle of His I44.30
- phase-shift, sleep cycle *—see* Disorder, sleep, circadian rhythm
- sleep phase-shift, or 24 hour sleep-wake cycle *—see* Disorder, sleep, circadian rhythm

Interstitial *—see* condition

Intertrigo L30.4
- labialis K13.0

Intervertebral disc *—see* condition

Intestine, intestinal *—see* condition

Intolerance
- carbohydrate K90.49
- disaccharide, hereditary E73.0
- fat NEC K90.49
  - pancreatic K90.3

Intolerance *(continued)*
- food K90.49
  - dietary counseling and surveillance Z71.3
- fructose E74.10
  - hereditary E74.12
- glucose (-galactose) E74.39
- gluten K90.41
- lactose E73.9
  - specified NEC E73.8
- lysine E72.3
- milk NEC K90.49
  - lactose E73.9
- protein K90.49
- starch NEC K90.49
- sucrose (-isomaltose) E74.31

Intoxicated NEC (without dependence) *—see* Alcohol, intoxication

Intoxication
- acid E87.2
- alcoholic (acute) (without dependence) *—see* Alcohol, intoxication
- alimentary canal K52.1
- amphetamine (without dependence) *—see* Abuse, drug, stimulant, with intoxication
  - with dependence *—see* Dependence, drug, stimulant, with intoxication
- anxiolytic (acute) (without dependence) *—see* Abuse, drug, sedative, with intoxication
  - with dependence *—see* Dependence, drug, sedative, with intoxication
- caffeine F15.929
  - with
    - abuse - *see* Abuse, drug, cannabis, with intoxication
    - dependence *—see* Dependence, drug, cannabis, with intoxication
- cannabinoids (acute) (without dependence) *—see* Use, cannabis, with intoxication
  - with
    - abuse - *see* Abuse, drug, cannabis, with intoxication
    - dependence - *see* Dependence, drug, cannabis, with intoxication
- chemical *—see* Table of Drugs and Chemicals
  - via placenta or breast milk *—see* - Absorption, chemical, through placenta
- cocaine (acute) (without dependence) *—see* Abuse, drug, cocaine, with intoxication
  - with dependence *—see* Dependence, drug, cocaine, with intoxication
- drug
  - acute (without dependence) *—see* Abuse, drug, by type with intoxication
    - with dependence *—see* Dependence, drug, by type with intoxication
  - addictive
    - via placenta or breast milk *—see* Absorption, drug, addictive, through placenta
  - newborn P93.8
    - gray baby syndrome P93.0
  - overdose or wrong substance given or taken *—see* Table of Drugs and Chemicals, by drug, poisoning
- enteric K52.1

Intoxication *(continued)*
- foodborne A05.9
  - bacterial A05.9
  - classical (Clostridium botulinum) A05.1
  - due to
    - Bacillus cereus A05.4
    - bacterium A05.9
      - specified NEC A05.8
    - Clostridium
      - botulinum A05.1
      - perfringens A05.2
      - welchii A05.2
    - Salmonella A02.9
      - with
        - (gastro)enteritis A02.0
        - localized infection(s) A02.20
          - arthritis A02.23
          - meningitis A02.21
          - osteomyelitis A02.24
          - pneumonia A02.22
          - pyelonephritis A02.25
          - specified NEC A02.29
        - sepsis A02.1
        - specified manifestation NEC A02.8
    - Staphylococcus A05.0
    - Vibrio
      - parahaemolyticus A05.3
      - vulnificus A05.5
  - enterotoxin, staphylococcal A05.0
  - noxious *—see* Poisoning, food, noxious
- gastrointestinal K52.1
- hallucinogenic (without dependence) *—see* Abuse, drug, hallucinogen, with intoxication
  - with dependence *—see* Dependence, drug, hallucinogen, with intoxication
- hypnotic (acute) (without dependence) *—see* Abuse, drug, sedative, with intoxication
  - with dependence *—see* Dependence, drug, sedative, with intoxication
- inhalant (acute) (without dependence) *—see* Abuse, drug, inhalant, with intoxication
  - with dependence *—see* Dependence, drug, inhalant, with intoxication
- meaning
  - inebriation F10
  - poisoning *—see* Table of Drugs and Chemicals
- methyl alcohol (acute) (without dependence) *—see* Alcohol, intoxication
- opioid (acute) (without dependence) *—see* Abuse, drug, opioid, with intoxication
  - with dependence *—see* Dependence, drug, opioid, with intoxication
- pathologic NEC (without dependence) *—see* Alcohol, intoxication
- phencyclidine (without dependence) *—see* Abuse, drug, hallucinogen, with intoxication
  - with dependence *—see* Dependence, drug, hallucinogen, with intoxication
- potassium (K) E87.5
- psychoactive substance NEC (without dependence) *—see* Abuse, drug, psychoactive NEC, with intoxication

Intoxication *(continued)*
- psychoactive substance NEC *(continued)*
  - with dependence *—see* Dependence, drug, psychoactive NEC, with intoxication
- sedative (acute) (without dependence) *—see* Abuse, drug, sedative, with intoxication
  - with dependence *—see* Dependence, drug, sedative, with intoxication
- serum (*see also* Reaction, serum) T80.69
- uremic *—see* Uremia
- volatile solvents (acute) (without dependence) *—see* Abuse, drug, inhalant, with intoxication
  - with dependence *—see* Dependence, drug, inhalant, with intoxication
- water E87.79

Intraabdominal testis, testes
- bilateral Q53.211
- unilateral Q53.111

Intracranial *—see* condition

Intrahepatic gallbladder Q44.1

Intraligamentous *—see* condition

Intrathoracic *—see also* condition
- kidney Q63.2

Intrauterine contraceptive device
- checking Z30.431
- insertion Z30.430
  - immediately following removal Z30.433
- in situ Z97.5
- management Z30.431
- reinsertion Z30.433
- removal Z30.432
- replacement Z30.433
- retention in pregnancy O26.3-

Intraventricular *—see* condition

Intrinsic deformity *—see* Deformity

Intubation, difficult or failed T88.4

Intumescence, lens (eye) (cataract) *—see* Cataract

Intussusception (bowel) (colon) (enteric) (ileocecal) (ileocolic) (intestine) (rectum) K56.1
- appendix K38.8
- congenital Q43.8
- ureter (with obstruction) N13.5

Invagination (bowel, colon, intestine or rectum) K56.1

Inversion
- albumin-globulin (A-G) ratio E88.09
- bladder N32.89
- cecum *—see* Intussusception
- cervix N88.8
- chromosome in normal individual Q95.1
- circadian rhythm *—see* Disorder, sleep, circadian rhythm
- nipple N64.59
  - congenital Q83.8
  - gestational *—see* Retraction, nipple
  - puerperal, postpartum *—see* Retraction, nipple
- nyctohemeral rhythm *—see* Disorder, sleep, circadian rhythm
- optic papilla Q14.2
- organ or site, congenital NEC *—see* Anomaly, by site

Inversion *(continued)*
- sleep rhythm *—see* Disorder, sleep, circadian rhythm
- testis (congenital) Q55.29
- uterus (chronic) (postinfectional) (postpartal, old) N85.5
  - postpartum O71.2
- vagina (posthysterectomy) N99.3
- ventricular Q20.5

Investigation (*see also* Examination) Z04.9
- clinical research subject (control) (normal comparison) (participant) Z00.6

Involuntary movement, abnormal R25.9

Involution, involutional *—see also* condition
- breast, cystic *—see* Dysplasia, mammary, specified type NEC
- depression (single episode) F32.89
  - recurrent episode F33.9
- melancholia (single episode) F32.89
  - recurrent episode F33.8
- ovary, senile *—see* Atrophy, ovary
- thymus failure E32.8

I.Q.
- under 20 F73
- 20-34 F72
- 35-49 F71
- 50-69 F70

IRDS (type I) P22.0
- type II P22.1

Irideremia Q13.1

Iridis rubeosis *—see* Disorder, iris, vascular

Iridochoroiditis (panuveitis) *—see* Panuveitis

Iridocyclitis H20.9
- acute H20.0-
  - hypopyon H20.05-
  - primary H20.01-
  - recurrent H20.02-
  - secondary (noninfectious) H20.04-
    - infectious H20.03-
- chronic H20.1-
- due to allergy *—see* Iridocyclitis, acute, secondary
- endogenous *—see* Iridocyclitis, acute, primary
- Fuchs' *—see* Cyclitis, Fuchs' heterochromic
- gonococcal A54.32
- granulomatous *—see* Iridocyclitis, chronic
- herpes, herpetic (simplex) B00.51
  - zoster B02.32
- hypopyon *—see* Iridocyclitis, acute, hypopyon
- in (due to)
  - ankylosing spondylitis M45.9
  - gonococcal infection A54.32
  - herpes (simplex) virus B00.51
    - zoster B02.32
  - infectious disease NOS B99
  - parasitic disease NOS B89 *[H22]*
  - sarcoidosis D86.83
  - syphilis A51.43
  - tuberculosis A18.54
  - zoster B02.32
- lens-induced H20.2-
- nongranulomatous *—see* Iridocyclitis, acute
- recurrent *—see* Iridocyclitis, acute, recurrent

Iridocyclitis *(continued)*
- rheumatic *—see* Iridocyclitis, chronic
- subacute *—see* Iridocyclitis, acute
- sympathetic *—see* Uveitis, sympathetic
- syphilitic (secondary) A51.43
- tuberculous (chronic) A18.54
- Vogt-Koyanagi H20.82-

Iridocyclochoroiditis (panuveitis) *— see* Panuveitis

Iridodialysis H21.53-

Iridodonesis H21.89

Iridoplegia (complete) (partial) (reflex) H57.09

Iridoschisis H21.25-

Iris *—see also* condition
- bombé *—see* Membrane, pupillary

Iritis *—see also* Iridocyclitis
- chronic *—see* Iridocyclitis, chronic
- diabetic *—see* E08-E13 with .39
- due to
  - herpes simplex B00.51
  - leprosy A30.9 *[H22]*
- gonococcal A54.32
- gouty (*see also* Gout, by type) M10.9 *[H22]*
- granulomatous *—see* Iridocyclitis, chronic
- lens induced *—see* Iridocyclitis, lens-induced
- papulosa (syphilitic) A52.71
- rheumatic *—see* Iridocyclitis, chronic
- syphilitic (secondary) A51.43
  - congenital (early) A50.01
  - late A52.71
- tuberculous A18.54

Iron *—see* condition

Iron-miner's lung J63.4

Irradiated enamel (tooth, teeth) K03.89

Irradiation effects, adverse T66

Irreducible, irreducibility *—see* condition

Irregular, irregularity
- action, heart I49.9
- alveolar process K08.89
- bleeding N92.6
- breathing R06.89
- contour of cornea (acquired) *—see* Deformity, cornea
  - congenital Q13.4
- contour, reconstructed breast N65.0
- dentin (in pulp) K04.3
- eye movements H55.89
  - nystagmus *—see* Nystagmus
  - saccadic H55.81
- labor O62.2
- menstruation (cause unknown) N92.6
- periods N92.6
- prostate N42.9
- pupil *—see* Abnormality, pupillary
- reconstructed breast N65.0
- respiratory R06.89
- septum (nasal) J34.2
- shape, organ or site, congenital NEC *—see* Distortion
- sleep-wake pattern (rhythm) G47.23

Irritable, irritability R45.4
- bladder N32.89
- bowel (syndrome) K58.9
  - with
    - constipation K58.1
    - diarrhea K58.0

Irritable, irritability *(continued)*
- bowel *(continued)*
  - mixed K58.2
  - psychogenic F45.8
  - specified NEC K58.8
- bronchial *—see* Bronchitis
- cerebral, in newborn P91.3
- colon (*see also* Irritable, bowel) K58.9
  - with diarrhea K58.0
  - psychogenic F45.8
- duodenum K59.8
- heart (psychogenic) F45.8
- hip *—see* Derangement, joint, specified type NEC, hip
- ileum K59.8
- infant R68.12
- jejunum K59.8
- rectum K59.8
- stomach K31.89
  - psychogenic F45.8
- sympathetic G90.8
- urethra N36.8

Irritation
- anus K62.89
- axillary nerve G54.0
- bladder N32.89
- brachial plexus G54.0
- bronchial *—see* Bronchitis
- cervical plexus G54.2
- cervix *—see* Cervicitis
- choroid, sympathetic *—see* Endophthalmitis
- cranial nerve *—see* Disorder, nerve, cranial
- gastric K31.89
  - psychogenic F45.8
- globe, sympathetic *—see* Uveitis, sympathetic
- labyrinth *—see* subcategory H83.2
- lumbosacral plexus G54.1
- meninges (traumatic) *—see* Injury, intracranial
  - nontraumatic *—see* Meningismus
- nerve *—see* Disorder, nerve
- nervous R45.0
- penis N48.89
- perineum NEC L29.3
- peripheral autonomic nervous system G90.8
- peritoneum *—see* Peritonitis
- pharynx J39.2
- plantar nerve *—see* Lesion, nerve, plantar
- spinal (cord) (traumatic) *—see also* Injury, spinal cord, by region
  - nerve G58.9
    - root NEC *—see* Radiculopathy
  - nontraumatic *—see* Myelopathy
- stomach K31.89
  - psychogenic F45.8
- sympathetic nerve NEC G90.8
- ulnar nerve *—see* Lesion, nerve, ulnar
- vagina N89.8

Ischemia, ischemic I99.8
- brain *—see* Ischemia, cerebral
- bowel (transient)
  - acute (*see also* Ischemia, intestine, acute) K55.019
    - diffuse K55.012
    - focal K55.011
  - chronic K55.1
  - due to mesenteric artery insufficiency K55.1
- cardiac (*see* Disease, heart, ischemic)
- cardiomyopathy I25.5
- cerebral (chronic) (generalized) I67.82
  - arteriosclerotic I67.2
  - intermittent G45.9
  - newborn P91.0

Ischemia, ischemic *(continued)*
- cerebral *(continued)*
  - recurrent focal G45.8
  - transient G45.9
- colon chronic (due to mesenteric artery insufficiency) K55.1
- coronary *—see* Disease, heart, ischemic
- demand (coronary) (*see also* Angina) I24.8
  - with myocardial infarction I21.A1
  - resulting in myocardial infarction I21.A1
- heart (chronic or with a stated duration of over 4 weeks) I25.9
  - acute or with a stated duration of 4 weeks or less I24.9
  - subacute I24.9
- infarction, muscle *—see* Infarct, muscle
- intestine (large) (small) (transient) K55.9
  - acute K55.059
  - diffuse K55.052
  - focal K55.051
  - large K55.039
    - diffuse K55.032
    - focal K55.031
  - small K55.019
    - diffuse K55.012
    - focal K55.011
  - chronic K55.1
  - due to mesenteric artery insufficiency K55.1
- kidney N28.0
- mesenteric, acute (*see also* Ischemia, intestine, acute) K55.059
- muscle, traumatic T79.6
- myocardium, myocardial (chronic or with a stated duration of over 4 weeks) I25.9
  - acute, without myocardial infarction I51.3
  - silent (asymptomatic) I25.6
  - transient of newborn P29.4
- renal N28.0
- retina, retinal *—see* Occlusion, artery, retina
- small bowel
  - acute K55.019
    - diffuse K55.012
    - focal K55.011
  - chronic K55.1
  - due to mesenteric artery insufficiency K55.1
- spinal cord G95.11
- subendocardial *—see* Insufficiency, coronary
- supply (coronary) (*see also* Angina) I25.9
  - due to vasospasm I20.1

Ischial spine *—see* condition

Ischialgia *—see* Sciatica

Ischiopagus Q89.4

Ischium, ischial *—see* condition

Ischuria R34

Iselin's disease or osteochondrosis *—see* Osteochondrosis, juvenile, metatarsus

Islands of
- parotid tissue in
  - lymph nodes Q38.6
  - neck structures Q38.6
- submaxillary glands in
  - fascia Q38.6
  - lymph nodes Q38.6
  - neck muscles Q38.6

Islet cell tumor, pancreas D13.7

Isoimmunization NEC *—see also* Incompatibility
- affecting management of pregnancy (ABO) (with hydrops fetalis) O36.11-
  - anti-A sensitization O36.11-
  - anti-B sensitization O36.19-
  - anti-c sensitization O36.09-
  - anti-C sensitization O36.09-
  - anti-e sensitization O36.09-
  - anti-E sensitization O36.09-
  - Rh NEC O36.09-
    - anti-D antibody O36.01-
  - specified NEC O36.19-
- newborn P55.9
  - with
    - hydrops fetalis P56.0
    - kernicterus P57.0
  - ABO (blood groups) P55.1
  - Rhesus (Rh) factor P55.0
  - specified type NEC P55.8

Isolation, isolated
- dwelling Z59.8
- family Z63.79
- social Z60.4

Isoleucinosis E71.19

Isomerism atrial appendages (with asplenia or polysplenia) Q20.6

Isosporiasis, isosporosis A07.3

Isovaleric acidemia E71.110

Issue of
- medical certificate Z02.79
  - for disability determination Z02.71
- repeat prescription (appliance) (glasses) (medicinal substance, medicament, medicine) Z76.0
  - contraception *—see* Contraception

Itch, itching *—see also* Pruritus
- baker's L23.6
- barber's B35.0
- bricklayer's L24.5
- cheese B88.0
- clam digger's B65.3
- coolie B76.9
- copra B88.0
- dew B76.9
- dhobi B35.6
- filarial *—see* Infestation, filarial
- grain B88.0
- grocer's B88.0
- ground B76.9
- harvest B88.0
- jock B35.6
- Malabar B35.5
  - beard B35.0
  - foot B35.3
  - scalp B35.0
- meaning scabies B86
- Norwegian B86
- perianal L29.0
- poultrymen's B88.0
- sarcoptic B86
- scabies B86
- scrub B88.0
- straw B88.0
- swimmer's B65.3
- water B76.9
- winter L29.8

Ivemark's syndrome (asplenia with congenital heart disease) Q89.01

Ivory bones Q78.2

Ixodiasis NEC B88.8

J

Jaccoud's syndrome *—see* Arthropathy, postrheumatic, chronic

Jackson's
- membrane Q43.3
- paralysis or syndrome G83.89
- veil Q43.3

Jacquet's dermatitis (diaper dermatitis) L22

Jadassohn-Pellizari's disease or anetoderma L90.2

Jadassohn's
- blue nevus *—see* Nevus
- intraepidermal epithelioma *—see* Neoplasm, skin, benign

Jaffe-Lichtenstein (-Uehlinger) **syndrome** *—see* Dysplasia, fibrous, bone NEC

Jakob-Creutzfeldt disease or syndrome *—see* Creutzfeldt-Jakob disease or syndrome

Jaksch-Luzet disease D64.89

Jamaican
- neuropathy G92
- paraplegic tropical ataxic-spastic syndrome G92

Janet's disease F48.8

Janiceps Q89.4

Jansky-Bielschowsky amaurotic idiocy E75.4

Japanese
- B-type encephalitis A83.0
- river fever A75.3

Jaundice (yellow) R17
- acholuric (familial) (splenomegalic) *—see also* Spherocytosis
  - acquired D59.8
- breast-milk (inhibitor) P59.3
- catarrhal (acute) B15.9
  - with hepatic coma B15.0
- cholestatic (benign) R17
- due to or associated with
  - delayed conjugation P59.8
    - associated with (due to) preterm delivery P59.0
  - preterm delivery P59.0
- epidemic (catarrhal) B15.9
  - with hepatic coma B15.0
  - leptospiral A27.0
  - spirochetal A27.0
- familial nonhemolytic (congenital) (Gilbert) E80.4
  - Crigler-Najjar E80.5
- febrile (acute) B15.9
  - with hepatic coma B15.0
  - leptospiral A27.0
  - spirochetal A27.0
- hematogenous D59.9
- hemolytic (acquired) D59.9
  - congenital *—see* Spherocytosis
- hemorrhagic (acute) (leptospiral) (spirochetal) A27.0
- infectious (acute) (subacute) B15.9
  - with hepatic coma B15.0
  - leptospiral A27.0
  - spirochetal A27.0
- leptospiral (hemorrhagic) A27.0
- malignant (without coma) K72.90
  - with coma K72.91
- newborn P59.9
  - due to or associated with
    - ABO
      - antibodies P55.1
      - incompatibility, maternal/fetal P55.1
      - isoimmunization P55.1
    - absence or deficiency of enzyme system for bilirubin conjugation (congenital) P59.8

Jaundice *(continued)*
- newborn *(continued)*
  - due to or associated with *(continued)*
    - bleeding P58.1
    - breast milk inhibitors to conjugation P59.3
      - associated with preterm delivery P59.0
    - bruising P58.0
    - Crigler-Najjar syndrome E80.5
    - delayed conjugation P59.8
      - associated with preterm delivery P59.0
    - drugs or toxins
      - given to newborn P58.42
      - transmitted from mother P58.41
    - excessive hemolysis P58.9
      - due to
        - bleeding P58.1
        - bruising P58.0
        - drugs or toxins
          - given to newborn P58.42
          - transmitted from mother P58.41
        - infection P58.2
        - polycythemia P58.3
        - swallowed maternal blood P58.5
      - specified type NEC P58.8
    - galactosemia E74.21
    - Gilbert syndrome E80.4
    - hemolytic disease P55.9
      - ABO isoimmunization P55.1
      - Rh isoimmunization P55.0
      - specified NEC P55.8
    - hepatocellular damage P59.20
      - specified NEC P59.29
    - hereditary hemolytic anemia P58.8
    - hypothyroidism, congenital E03.1
    - incompatibility, maternal/fetal NOS P55.9
    - infection P58.2
    - inspissated bile syndrome P59.1
    - isoimmunization NOS P55.9
    - mucoviscidosis E84.9
    - polycythemia P58.3
    - preterm delivery P59.0
    - Rh
      - antibodies P55.0
      - incompatibility, maternal/fetal P55.0
      - isoimmunization P55.0
    - specified cause NEC P59.8
    - swallowed maternal blood P58.5
  - spherocytosis (congenital) D58.0
- neonatal *—see* Jaundice, newborn
- nonhemolytic congenital familial (Gilbert) E80.4
- nuclear, newborn (*see also* Kernicterus of newborn) P57.9
- obstructive (*see also* Obstruction, bile duct) K83.1
- post-immunization *—see* Hepatitis, viral, type, B
- post-transfusion *—see* Hepatitis, viral, type, B
- regurgitation (*see also* Obstruction, bile duct) K83.1
- serum (homologous) (prophylactic) (therapeutic) *—see* Hepatitis, viral, type, B
- spirochetal (hemorrhagic) A27.0
- symptomatic R17
  - newborn P59.9

Jaw *—see* condition

Jaw-winking phenomenon or syndrome Q07.8

Jealousy
- alcoholic F10.988
- childhood F93.8
- sibling F93.8

Jejunitis *—see* Enteritis

Jejunostomy status Z93.4

Jejunum, jejunal *—see* condition

Jensen's disease *—see* Inflammation, chorioretinal, focal, juxtapapillary

Jerks, myoclonic G25.3

Jervell-Lange-Nielsen syndrome I45.81

Jeune's disease Q77.2

Jigger disease B88.1

Job's syndrome (chronic granulomatous disease) D71

Joint *—see also* condition
- mice *—see* Loose, body, joint
  - knee M23.4-

Jordan's anomaly or syndrome D72.0

Joseph-Diamond-Blackfan anemia (congenital hypoplastic) D61.01

Jungle yellow fever A95.0

Jüngling's disease *—see* Sarcoidosis

Juvenile *—see* condition

K

Kahler's disease C90.0-

Kakke E51.11

Kala-azar B55.0

Kallmann's syndrome E23.0

Kanner's syndrome (autism) *—see* Psychosis, childhood

Kaposi's
- dermatosis (xeroderma pigmentosum) Q82.1
- lichen ruber L44.0
  - acuminatus L44.0
- sarcoma
  - colon C46.4
  - connective tissue C46.1
  - gastrointestinal organ C46.4
  - lung C46.5-
  - lymph node (multiple) C46.3
  - palate (hard) (soft) C46.2
  - rectum C46.4
  - skin (multiple sites) C46.0
  - specified site NEC C46.7
  - stomach C46.4
  - unspecified site C46.9
- varicelliform eruption B00.0
  - vaccinia T88.1

Kartagener's syndrome or triad (sinusitis, bronchiectasis, situs inversus) Q89.3

Karyotype
- with abnormality except iso (Xq) Q96.2
- 45,X Q96.0
- 46,X
  - iso (Xq) Q96.1
- 46,XX Q98.3
  - with streak gonads Q50.32
  - hermaphrodite (true) Q99.1
  - male Q98.3

Karyotype *(continued)*
46,XY
with streak gonads Q56.1
female Q97.3
hermaphrodite (true) Q99.1
47,XXX Q97.0
47,XXY Q98.0
47,XYY Q98.5
Kaschin-Beck disease *—see* Disease, Kaschin-Beck
Katayama's disease or fever B65.2
Kawasaki's syndrome M30.3
Kayser-Fleischer ring (cornea) (pseudosclerosis) H18.04-
Kaznelson's syndrome (congenital hypoplastic anemia) D61.01
Kearns-Sayre syndrome H49.81-
Kedani fever A75.3
Kelis L91.0
Kelly (-Patterson) **syndrome** (sideropenic dysphagia) D50.1
Keloid, cheloid L91.0
acne L73.0
Addison's L94.0
cornea *—see* Opacity, cornea
Hawkin's L91.0
scar L91.0
Keloma L91.0
Kenya fever A77.1
Keratectasia *—see also* Ectasia, cornea
congenital Q13.4
Keratinization of alveolar ridge mucosa
excessive K13.23
minimal K13.22
Keratinized residual ridge mucosa
excessive K13.23
minimal K13.22
Keratitis (nodular) (nonulcerative) (simple) (zonular) H16.9
with ulceration (central) (marginal) (perforated) (ring) *—see* Ulcer, cornea
actinic *—see* Photokeratitis
arborescens (herpes simplex) B00.52
areolar H16.11-
bullosa H16.8
deep H16.309
specified type NEC H16.399
dendritic (a) (herpes simplex) B00.52
disciform (is) (herpes simplex) B00.52
varicella B01.81
filamentary H16.12-
gonococcal (congenital or prenatal) A54.33
herpes, herpetic (simplex) B00.52
zoster B02.33
in (due to)
acanthamebiasis B60.13
adenovirus B30.0
exanthema (*see also* Exanthem) B09
herpes (simplex) virus B00.52
measles B05.81
syphilis A50.31
tuberculosis A18.52
zoster B02.33
interstitial (nonsyphilitic) H16.30-
diffuse H16.32-
herpes, herpetic (simplex) B00.52
zoster B02.33
sclerosing H16.33-
specified type NEC H16.39-
Keratitis *(continued)*
interstitial (nonsyphilitic) *(continued)*
syphilitic (congenital) (late) A50.31
tuberculous A18.52
macular H16.11-
nummular H16.11-
oyster shuckers' H16.8
parenchymatous *—see* Keratitis, interstitial
petrificans H16.8
postmeasles B05.81
punctata
leprosa A30.9 *[H16.14-]*
syphilitic (profunda) A50.31
punctate H16.14-
purulent H16.8
rosacea L71.8
sclerosing H16.33-
specified type NEC H16.8
stellate H16.11-
striate H16.11-
superficial H16.10-
with conjunctivitis *—see* Keratoconjunctivitis
due to light *—see* Photokeratitis
suppurative H16.8
syphilitic (congenital) (prenatal) A50.31
trachomatous A71.1
sequelae B94.0
tuberculous A18.52
vesicular H16.8
xerotic (*see also* Keratomlacia) H16.8
vitamin A deficiency E50.4
Keratoacanthoma L85.8
Keratocele *—see* Descemetocele
Keratoconjunctivitis H16.20-
Acanthamoeba B60.13
adenoviral B30.0
epidemic B30.0
exposure H16.21-
herpes, herpetic (simplex) B00.52
zoster B02.33
in exanthema (*see also* Exanthem) B09
infectious B30.0
lagophthalmic *—see* Keratoconjunctivitis, specified type NEC
neurotrophic H16.23-
phlyctenular H16.25-
postmeasles B05.81
shipyard B30.0
sicca (Sjogren's) M35.0-
not Sjogren's H16.22-
specified type NEC H16.29-
tuberculous (phlyctenular) A18.52
vernal H16.26-
Keratoconus H18.60-
congenital Q13.4
stable H18.61-
unstable H18.62-
Keratocyst (dental) (odontogenic) *—see* Cyst, calcifying odontogenic
Keratoderma, keratodermia (congenital) (palmaris et plantaris) (symmetrical) Q82.8
acquired L85.1
in diseases classified elsewhere L86
climactericum L85.1
gonococcal A54.89
gonorrheal A54.89
punctata L85.2
Reiter's *—see* Reiter's disease
Keratodermatocele *—see* Descemetocele
Keratoglobus H18.79
congenital Q15.8
with glaucoma Q15.0
Keratohemia *—see* Pigmentation, cornea, stromal
Keratoiritis *—see also* Iridocyclitis
syphilitic A50.39
tuberculous A18.54
Keratoma L57.0
palmaris and plantaris hereditarium Q82.8
senile L57.0
Keratomalacia H18.44-
vitamin A deficiency E50.4
Keratomegaly Q13.4
Keratomycosis B49
nigrans, nigricans (palmaris) B36.1
Keratopathy H18.9
band H18.42-
bullous H18.1-
bullous (aphakic), following cataract surgery H59.01-
Keratoscleritis, tuberculous A18.52
Keratosis L57.0
actinic L57.0
arsenical L85.8
congenital, specified NEC Q80.8
female genital NEC N94.89
follicularis Q82.8
acquired L11.0
congenita Q82.8
et parafollicularis in cutem penetrans L87.0
spinulosa (decalvans) Q82.8
vitamin A deficiency E50.8
gonococcal A54.89
male genital (external) N50.89
nigricans L83
obturans, external ear (canal) *—see* Cholesteatoma, external ear
palmaris et plantaris (inherited) (symmetrical) Q82.8
acquired L85.1
penile N48.89
pharynx J39.2
pilaris, acquired L85.8
punctata (palmaris et plantaris) L85.2
scrotal N50.89
seborrheic L82.1
inflamed L82.0
senile L57.0
solar L57.0
tonsillaris J35.8
vagina N89.4
vegetans Q82.8
vitamin A deficiency E50.8
vocal cord J38.3
Kerato-uveitis *—see* Iridocyclitis
Kerunoparalysis T75.09
Kerion (celsi) B35.0
Kernicterus of newborn (not due to isoimmunization) P57.9
due to isoimmunization (conditions in P55.0-P55.9) P57.0
specified type NEC P57.8
Keshan disease E59
Ketoacidosis E87.2
diabetic *—see* Diabetes, by type, with ketoacidosis
Ketonuria R82.4
Ketosis NEC E88.89
diabetic *—see* Diabetes, by type, with with ketoacidosis
Kew Garden fever A79.1
Kidney *—see* condition
Kienböck's disease *—see also* Osteochondrosis, juvenile, hand, carpal lunate
adult M93.1
Kimmelstiel (-Wilson) **disease** *—see* Diabetes, Kimmelstiel (-Wilson) disease
Kimura disease D21.9
specified site *—see* Neoplasm, connective tissue benign
Kink, kinking
artery I77.1
hair (acquired) L67.8
ileum or intestine *—see* Obstruction, intestine
Lane's *—see* Obstruction, intestine
organ or site, congenital NEC *—see* Anomaly, by site
ureter (pelvic junction) N13.5
with
hydronephrosis N13.1
with infection N13.6
pyelonephritis (chronic) N11.1
congenital Q62.39
vein(s) I87.8
caval I87.1
peripheral I87.1
Kinnier Wilson's disease (hepatolenticular degeneration) E83.01
Kissing spine M48.20
cervical region M48.22
cervicothoracic region M48.23
lumbar region M48.26
lumbosacral region M48.27
occipito-atlanto-axial region M48.21
thoracic region M48.24
thoracolumbar region M48.25
Klatskin's tumor C24.0
Klauder's disease A26.8
Klebs' disease (*see also* Glomerulonephritis) N05.-
Klebsiella (K.) **pneumoniae, as cause of disease classified elsewhere** B96.1
Klein (e)**-Levin syndrome** G47.13
Kleptomania F63.2
Klinefelter's syndrome Q98.4
karyotype 47,XXY Q98.0
male with more than two X chromosomes Q98.1
Klippel-Feil deficiency, disease, or syndrome (brevicollis) Q76.1
Klippel's disease I67.2
Klippel-Trenaunay (-Weber) **syndrome** Q87.2
Klumpke (-Déjerine) palsy, paralysis (birth) (newborn) P14.1
Knee *—see* condition
Knock knee (acquired) M21.06-
congenital Q74.1
Knot(s)
intestinal, syndrome (volvulus) K56.2
surfer S89.8-
umbilical cord (true) O69.2

Knotting (of)
- hair L67.8
- intestine K56.2

Knuckle pad (Garrod's) M72.1

Koch's
- infection —*see* Tuberculosis
- relapsing fever A68.9

Koch-Weeks' conjunctivitis —*see* Conjunctivitis, acute, mucopurulent

Köebner's syndrome Q81.8

Köenig's disease (osteochondritis dissecans) —*see* Osteochondritis, dissecans

Köhler-Pellegrini-Steida disease or syndrome (calcification, knee joint) —*see* Bursitis, tibial collateral

Köhler's disease
- patellar —*see* Osteochondrosis, juvenile, patella
- tarsal navicular —*see* Osteochondrosis, juvenile, tarsus

Koilonychia L60.3
- congenital Q84.6

Kojevnikov's, epilepsy —*see* Kozhevnikof's epilepsy

Koplik's spots B05.9

Kopp's asthma E32.8

Korsakoff's (Wernicke) disease, psychosis or syndrome (alcoholic) F10.96
- with dependence F10.26
- drug-induced
  - due to drug abuse —*see* Abuse, drug, by type, with amnestic disorder
  - due to drug dependence —*see* Dependence, drug, by type, with amnestic disorder
- nonalcoholic F04

Korsakov's disease, psychosis or syndrome —*see* Korsakoff's disease

Korsakow's disease, psychosis or syndrome —*see* Korsakoff's disease

Kostmann's disease or syndrome (infantile genetic agranulocytosis) —*see* Agranulocytosis

Kozhevnikof's epilepsy G40.109
- intractable G40.119
  - with status epilepticus G40.111
  - without status epilepticus G40.119
- not intractable G40.109
  - with status epilepticus G40.101
  - without status epilepticus G40.109

Krabbe's
- disease E75.23
- syndrome, congenital muscle hypoplasia Q79.8

Kraepelin-Morel disease —*see* Schizophrenia

Kraft-Weber-Dimitri disease Q85.8

Kraurosis
- ani K62.89
- penis N48.0
- vagina N89.8
- vulva N90.4

Kreotoxism A05.9

Krukenberg's
- spindle —*see* Pigmentation, cornea, posterior
- tumor C79.6-

Kufs' disease E75.4

Kugelberg-Welander disease G12.1

Kuhnt-Junius degeneration (*see also* Degeneration, macula) H35.32 -

Kümmell's disease or spondylitis —*see* Spondylopathy, traumatic

Kupffer cell sarcoma C22.3

Kuru A81.81

Kussmaul's
- disease M30.0
- respiration E87.2
  - in diabetic acidosis —*see* Diabetes, by type, with ketoacidosis

Kwashiorkor E40
- marasmic, marasmus type E42

Kyasanur Forest disease A98.2

Kyphoscoliosis, kyphoscoliotic (acquired) (*see also* Scoliosis) M41.9
- congenital Q67.5
- heart (disease) I27.1
- sequelae of rickets E64.3
- tuberculous A18.01

Kyphosis, kyphotic (acquired) M40.209
- cervical region M40.202
- cervicothoracic region M40.203
- congenital Q76.419
  - cervical region Q76.412
  - cervicothoracic region Q76.413
  - occipito-atlanto-axial region Q76.411
  - thoracic region Q76.414
  - thoracolumbar region Q76.415
- Morquio-Brailsford type (spinal) (*see also* subcategory M49.8) E76.219
- postlaminectomy M96.3
- postradiation therapy M96.2
- postural (adolescent) M40.00
  - cervicothoracic region M40.03
  - thoracic region M40.04
  - thoracolumbar region M40.05
- secondary NEC M40.10
  - cervical region M40.12
  - cervicothoracic region M40.13
  - thoracic region M40.14
  - thoracolumbar region M40.15
- sequelae of rickets E64.3
- specified type NEC M40.299
  - cervical region M40.292
  - cervicothoracic region M40.293
  - thoracic region M40.294
  - thoracolumbar region M40.295
- syphilitic, congenital A50.56
- thoracic region M40.204
- thoracolumbar region M40.205
- tuberculous A18.01

Kyrle disease L87.0

L

Labia, labium —*see* condition

Labile
- blood pressure R09.89
- vasomotor system I73.9

Labioglossal paralysis G12.29

Labium leporinum —*see* Cleft, lip

Labor —*see* Delivery

Labored breathing —*see* Hyperventilation

Labyrinthitis (circumscribed) (destructive) (diffuse) (inner ear) (latent) (purulent) (suppurative) —*see also* subcategory H83.0
- syphilitic A52.79

Laceration
- with abortion —*see* Abortion, by type, complicated by laceration of pelvic organs
- abdomen, abdominal
  - wall S31.119
    - with
      - foreign body S31.129
      - penetration into peritoneal cavity S31.619
        - with foreign body S31.629
    - epigastric region S31.112
      - with
        - foreign body S31.122
        - penetration into peritoneal cavity S31.612
          - with foreign body S31.622
    - left
      - lower quadrant S31.114
        - with
          - foreign body S31.124
          - penetration into peritoneal cavity S31.614
            - with foreign body S31.624
      - upper quadrant S31.111
        - with
          - foreign body S31.121
          - penetration into peritoneal cavity S31.611
            - with foreign body S31.621
    - periumbilic region S31.115
      - with
        - foreign body S31.125
        - penetration into peritoneal cavity S31.615
          - with foreign body S31.625
    - right
      - lower quadrant S31.113
        - with
          - foreign body S31.123
          - penetration into peritoneal cavity S31.613
            - with foreign body S31.623
      - upper quadrant S31.110
        - with
          - foreign body S31.120
          - penetration into peritoneal cavity S31.610
            - with foreign body S31.620
- accidental, complicating surgery —*see* Complications, surgical, accidental puncture or laceration
- Achilles tendon S86.02-
- adrenal gland S37.813
- alveolar (process) —*see* Laceration, oral cavity
- ankle S91.01-
  - with
    - foreign body S91.02-
- antecubital space —*see* Laceration, elbow
- anus (sphincter) S31.831
  - with
    - ectopic or molar pregnancy O08.6
    - foreign body S31.832
  - complicating delivery —*see* Delivery, complicated, by, laceration, anus (sphincter)
  - following ectopic or molar pregnancy O08.6

Laceration *(continued)*
- anus (sphincter) *(continued)*
  - nontraumatic, nonpuerperal —*see* Fissure, anus
- arm (upper) S41.11-
  - with foreign body S41.12-
  - lower —*see* Laceration, forearm
- auditory canal (external) (meatus) —*see* Laceration, ear
- auricle, ear —*see* Laceration, ear
- axilla —*see* Laceration, arm
- back —*see also* Laceration, thorax, back
  - lower S31.010
    - with
      - foreign body S31.020
        - with penetration into retroperitoneal space S31.021
      - penetration into retroperitoneal space S31.011
- bile duct S36.13
- bladder S37.23
  - with ectopic or molar pregnancy O08.6
  - following ectopic or molar pregnancy O08.6
  - obstetrical trauma O71.5
- blood vessel —*see* Injury, blood vessel
- bowel —*see also* Laceration, intestine
  - with ectopic or molar pregnancy O08.6
  - complicating abortion —*see* Abortion, by type, complicated by, specified condition NEC
  - following ectopic or molar pregnancy O08.6
  - obstetrical trauma O71.5
- brain (any part) (cortex) (diffuse) (membrane) —*see also* Injury, intracranial, diffuse
  - during birth P10.8
    - with hemorrhage P10.1
  - focal —*see* Injury, intracranial, focal brain injury
- brainstem S06.38-
- breast S21.01-
  - with foreign body S21.02-
- broad ligament S37.893
  - with ectopic or molar pregnancy O08.6
  - following ectopic or molar pregnancy O08.6
  - laceration syndrome N83.8
  - obstetrical trauma O71.6
  - syndrome (laceration) N83.8
- buttock S31.801
  - with foreign body S31.802
  - left S31.821
    - with foreign body S31.822
  - right S31.811
    - with foreign body S31.812
- calf —*see* Laceration, leg
- canaliculus lacrimalis —*see* Laceration, eyelid
- canthus, eye —*see* Laceration, eyelid
- capsule, joint —*see* Sprain
- causing eversion of cervix uteri (old) N86
- central (perineal), complicating delivery O70.9
- cerebellum, traumatic S06.37-
- cerebral S06.33-
  - left side S06.32-
  - during birth P10.8
    - with hemorrhage P10.1
  - right side S06.31-

Laceration *(continued)*
- cervix (uteri)
  - with ectopic or molar pregnancy O08.6
  - following ectopic or molar pregnancy O08.6
  - nonpuerperal, nontraumatic N88.1
  - obstetrical trauma (current) O71.3
  - old (postpartal) N88.1
  - traumatic S37.63
- cheek (external) S01.41-
  - with foreign body S01.42-
  - internal —*see* Laceration, oral cavity
- chest wall —*see* Laceration, thorax
- chin —*see* Laceration, head, specified site NEC
- chordae tendinae NEC I51.1
  - concurrent with acute myocardial infarction —*see* Infarct, myocardium
  - following acute myocardial infarction (current complication) I23.4
- clitoris —*see* Laceration, vulva
- colon —*see* Laceration, intestine, large, colon
- common bile duct S36.13
- cortex (cerebral) —*see* Injury, intracranial, diffuse
- costal region —*see* Laceration, thorax
- cystic duct S36.13
- diaphragm S27.803
- digit(s)
  - hand —*see* Laceration, finger
  - foot —*see* Laceration, toe
- duodenum S36.430
- ear (canal) (external) S01.31-
  - with foreign body S01.32-
  - drum S09.2-
- elbow S51.01-
  - with
    - foreign body S51.02-
- epididymis —*see* Laceration, testis
- epigastric region —*see* Laceration, abdomen, wall, epigastric region
- esophagus K22.8
  - traumatic
    - cervical S11.21
      - with foreign body S11.22
    - thoracic S27.813
- eye (ball) S05.3-
  - with prolapse or loss of intraocular tissue S05.2-
  - penetrating S05.6-
- eyebrow —*see* Laceration, eyelid
- eyelid S01.11-
  - with foreign body S01.12-
- face NEC —*see* Laceration, head, specified site NEC
- fallopian tube S37.539
  - bilateral S37.532
  - unilateral S37.531
- finger(s) S61.219
  - with
    - damage to nail S61.319
      - with
        - foreign body S61.329
    - foreign body S61.229
  - index S61.218
    - with
      - damage to nail S61.318
        - with
          - foreign body S61.328
      - foreign body S61.228
    - left S61.211
      - with
        - damage to nail S61.311
          - with
            - foreign body S61.321
        - foreign body S61.221

Laceration *(continued)*
- finger *(continued)*
  - index *(continued)*
    - right S61.210
      - with
        - damage to nail S61.310
          - with
            - foreign body S61.320
        - foreign body S61.220
  - little S61.218
    - with
      - damage to nail S61.318
        - with
          - foreign body S61.328
      - foreign body S61.228
    - left S61.217
      - with
        - damage to nail S61.317
          - with
            - foreign body S61.327
        - foreign body S61.227
    - right S61.216
      - with
        - damage to nail S61.316
          - with
            - foreign body S61.326
        - foreign body S61.226
  - middle S61.218
    - with
      - damage to nail S61.318
        - with
          - foreign body S61.328
      - foreign body S61.228
    - left S61.213
      - with
        - damage to nail S61.313
          - with
            - foreign body S61.323
        - foreign body S61.223
    - right S61.212
      - with
        - damage to nail S61.312
          - with
            - foreign body S61.322
        - foreign body S61.222
  - ring S61.218
    - with
      - damage to nail S61.318
        - with
          - foreign body S61.328
      - foreign body S61.228
    - left S61.215
      - with
        - damage to nail S61.315
          - with
            - foreign body S61.325
        - foreign body S61.225
    - right S61.214
      - with
        - damage to nail S61.314
          - with
            - foreign body S61.324
        - foreign body S61.224
- flank S31.119
  - with foreign body S31.129
- foot (except toe(s) alone) S91.319
  - with foreign body S91.329
  - left S91.312
    - with foreign body S91.322
  - right S91.311
    - with foreign body S91.321
  - toe —*see* Laceration, toe
- forearm S51.819
  - with
    - foreign body S51.829
  - elbow only —*see* Laceration, elbow
  - left S51.812
    - with
      - foreign body S51.822

Laceration *(continued)*
- forearm *(continued)*
  - right S51.811
    - with
      - foreign body S51.821
- forehead S01.81
  - with foreign body S01.82
- fourchette O70.0
  - with ectopic or molar pregnancy O08.6
  - complicating delivery O70.0
  - following ectopic or molar pregnancy O08.6
- gallbladder S36.123
- genital organs, external
  - female S31.512
    - with foreign body S31.522
    - vagina —*see* Laceration, vagina
    - vulva —*see* Laceration, vulva
  - male S31.511
    - with foreign body S31.521
    - penis —*see* Laceration, penis
    - scrotum —*see* Laceration, scrotum
    - testis —*see* Laceration, testis
- groin —*see* Laceration, abdomen, wall
- gum —*see* Laceration, oral cavity
- hand S61.419
  - with
    - foreign body S61.429
  - finger —*see* Laceration, finger
  - left S61.412
    - with
      - foreign body S61.422
  - right S61.411
    - with
      - foreign body S61.421
  - thumb —*see* Laceration, thumb
- head S01.91
  - with foreign body S01.92
  - cheek —*see* Laceration, cheek
  - ear —*see* Laceration, ear
  - eyelid —*see* Laceration, eyelid
  - lip —*see* Laceration, lip
  - nose —*see* Laceration, nose
  - oral cavity —*see* Laceration, oral cavity
  - scalp S01.01
    - with foreign body S01.02
  - specified site NEC S01.81
    - with foreign body S01.82
  - temporomandibular area —*see* Laceration, cheek
- heart —*see* Injury, heart, laceration
- heel —*see* Laceration, foot
- hepatic duct S36.13
- hip S71.019
  - with foreign body S71.029
  - left S71.012
    - with foreign body S71.022
  - right S71.011
    - with foreign body S71.021
- hymen —*see* Laceration, vagina
- hypochondrium —*see* Laceration, abdomen, wall
- hypogastric region —*see* Laceration, abdomen, wall
- ileum S36.438
- inguinal region —*see* Laceration, abdomen, wall
- instep —*see* Laceration, foot
- internal organ —*see* Injury, by site
- interscapular region —*see* Laceration, thorax, back

Laceration *(continued)*
- intestine
  - large
    - colon S36.539
      - ascending S36.530
      - descending S36.532
      - sigmoid S36.533
      - specified site NEC S36.538
    - rectum S36.63
      - transverse S36.531
  - small S36.439
    - duodenum S36.430
    - specified site NEC S36.438
- intra-abdominal organ S36.93
  - intestine —*see* Laceration, intestine
  - liver —*see* Laceration, liver
  - pancreas —*see* Laceration, pancreas
  - peritoneum S36.81
  - specified site NEC S36.893
  - spleen —*see* Laceration, spleen
  - stomach —*see* Laceration, stomach
- intracranial NEC —*see also* Injury, intracranial, diffuse
  - birth injury P10.9
- jaw —*see* Laceration, head, specified site NEC
- jejunum S36.438
- joint capsule —*see* Sprain, by site
- kidney S37.03-
  - major (greater than 3 cm) (massive) (stellate) S37.06-
  - minor (less than 1 cm) S37.04-
  - moderate (1 to 3 cm) S37.05-
    - multiple S37.06-
- knee S81.01-
  - with foreign body S81.02-
- labium (majus) (minus) —*see* Laceration, vulva
- lacrimal duct —*see* Laceration, eyelid
- large intestine —*see* Laceration, intestine, large
- larynx S11.011
  - with foreign body S11.012
- leg (lower) S81.819
  - with foreign body S81.829
  - foot —*see* Laceration, foot
  - knee —*see* Laceration, knee
  - left S81.812
    - with foreign body S81.822
  - right S81.811
    - with foreign body S81.821
  - upper —*see* Laceration, thigh
- ligament —*see* Sprain
- lip S01.511
  - with foreign body S01.521
- liver S36.113
  - major (stellate) S36.116
  - minor S36.114
  - moderate S36.115
- loin —*see* Laceration, abdomen, wall
- lower back —*see* Laceration, back, lower
- lumbar region —*see* Laceration, back, lower
- lung S27.339
  - bilateral S27.332
  - unilateral S27.331
- malar region —*see* Laceration, head, specified site NEC
- mammary —*see* Laceration, breast
- mastoid region —*see* Laceration, head, specified site NEC
- meninges —*see* Injury, intracranial, diffuse
- meniscus —*see* Tear, meniscus
- mesentery S36.893

Laceration *(continued)*
- mesosalpinx S37.893
- mouth *—see* Laceration, oral cavity
- muscle *—see* Injury, muscle, by site, laceration
- nail
  - finger *—see* Laceration, finger, with damage to nail
  - toe *—see* Laceration, toe, with damage to nail
- nasal (septum) (sinus) *—see* Laceration, nose
- nasopharynx *—see* Laceration, head, specified site NEC
- neck S11.91
  - with foreign body S11.92
  - involving
    - cervical esophagus S11.21
      - with foreign body S11.22
    - larynx *—see* Laceration, larynx
    - pharynx *—see* Laceration, pharynx
    - thyroid gland *—see* Laceration, thyroid gland
    - trachea *—see* Laceration, trachea
  - specified site NEC S11.81
    - with foreign body S11.82
- nerve *—see* Injury, nerve
- nose (septum) (sinus) S01.21
  - with foreign body S01.22
- ocular NOS S05.3-
  - adnexa NOS S01.11-
- oral cavity S01.512
  - with foreign body S01.522
- orbit (eye) *—see* Wound, open, ocular, orbit
- ovary S37.439
  - bilateral S37.432
  - unilateral S37.431
- palate *—see* Laceration, oral cavity
- palm *—see* Laceration, hand
- pancreas S36.239
  - body S36.231
    - major S36.261
    - minor S36.241
    - moderate S36.251
  - head S36.230
    - major S36.260
    - minor S36.240
    - moderate S36.250
  - major S36.269
  - minor S36.249
  - moderate S36.259
  - tail S36.232
    - major S36.262
    - minor S36.242
    - moderate S36.252
- pelvic S31.010
  - with
    - foreign body S31.020
      - penetration into retroperitoneal cavity S31.021
    - penetration into retroperitoneal cavity S31.011
  - floor *—see also* Laceration, back, lower
    - with ectopic or molar pregnancy O08.6
    - complicating delivery O70.1
    - following ectopic or molar pregnancy O08.6
    - old (postpartal) N81.89
  - organ S37.93
    - with ectopic or molar pregnancy O08.6
    - adrenal gland S37.813
    - bladder S37.23
    - fallopian tube *—see* Laceration, fallopian tube

Laceration *(continued)*
- pelvic *(continued)*
  - organ *(continued)*
    - following ectopic or molar pregnancy O08.6
    - kidney *—see* Laceration, kidney
    - obstetrical trauma O71.5
    - ovary *—see* Laceration, ovary
    - prostate S37.823
    - specified site NEC S37.893
    - ureter S37.13
    - urethra S37.33
    - uterus S37.63
- penis S31.21
  - with foreign body S31.22
- perineum
  - female S31.41
    - with
      - ectopic or molar pregnancy O08.6
      - foreign body S31.42
    - during delivery O70.9
      - first degree O70.0
      - fourth degree O70.3
      - second degree O70.1
      - third degree (*see also* Delivery, complicated, by, laceraton, perineum, third degree) O70.20
    - old (postpartal) N81.89
    - postpartal N81.89
    - secondary (postpartal) O90.1
  - male S31.119
    - with foreign body S31.129
- periocular area (with or without lacrimal passages) *—see* Laceration, eyelid
- peritoneum S36.893
- periumbilic region *—see* Laceration, abdomen, wall, periumbilic
- periurethral tissue *—see* Laceration, urethra
- phalanges
  - finger *—see* Laceration, finger
  - toe *—see* Laceration, toe
- pharynx S11.21
  - with foreign body S11.22
- pinna *—see* Laceration, ear
- popliteal space *—see* Laceration, knee
- prepuce *—see* Laceration, penis
- prostate S37.823
- pubic region S31.119
  - with foreign body S31.129
- pudendum *—see* Laceration, genital organs, external
- rectovaginal septum *—see* Laceration, vagina
- rectum S36.63
- retroperitoneum S36.893
- round ligament S37.893
- sacral region *—see* Laceration, back, lower
- sacroiliac region *—see* Laceration, back, lower
- salivary gland *—see* Laceration, oral cavity
- scalp S01.01
  - with foreign body S01.02
- scapular region *—see* Laceration, shoulder
- scrotum S31.31
  - with foreign body S31.32
- seminal vesicle S37.893
- shin *—see* Laceration, leg
- shoulder S41.019
  - with foreign body S41.029
  - left S41.012
    - with foreign body S41.022
  - right S41.011
    - with foreign body S41.021

Laceration *(continued)*
- small intestine *—see* Laceration, intestine, small
- spermatic cord *—see* Laceration, testis
- spinal cord (meninges) *—see also* Injury, spinal cord, by region
  - due to injury at birth P11.5
  - newborn (birth injury) P11.5
- spleen S36.039
  - major (massive) (stellate) S36.032
  - moderate S36.031
  - superficial (minor) S36.030
- sternal region *—see* Laceration, thorax, front
- stomach S36.33
- submaxillary region *—see* Laceration, head, specified site NEC
- submental region *—see* Laceration, head, specified site NEC
- subungual
  - finger(s) *—see* Laceration, finger, with damage to nail
  - toe(s) *—see* Laceration, toe, with damage to nail
- suprarenal gland *—see* Laceration, adrenal gland
- temple, temporal region *—see* Laceration, head, specified site NEC
- temporomandibular area *—see* Laceration, cheek
- tendon *—see* Injury, muscle, by site, laceration
  - Achilles S86.02-
- tentorium cerebelli *—see* Injury, intracranial, diffuse
- testis S31.31
  - with foreign body S31.32
- thigh S71.11-
  - with foreign body S71.12-
- thorax, thoracic (wall) S21.91
  - with foreign body S21.92
    - back S21.22-
      - with penetration into thoracic cavity S21.42-
    - front S21.12-
      - with penetration into thoracic cavity S21.32-
  - back S21.21-
    - with
      - foreign body S21.22-
        - with penetration into thoracic cavity S21.42-
      - penetration into thoracic cavity S21.41-
  - breast *—see* Laceration, breast
  - front S21.11-
    - with
      - foreign body S21.12-
        - with penetration into thoracic cavity S21.32-
      - penetration into thoracic cavity S21.31-
- thumb S61.019
  - with
    - damage to nail S61.119
      - with
        - foreign body S61.129
    - foreign body S61.029
  - left S61.012
    - with
      - damage to nail S61.112
        - with
          - foreign body S61.122
      - foreign body S61.022
  - right S61.011
    - with
      - damage to nail S61.111
        - with
          - foreign body S61.121
      - foreign body S61.021

Laceration *(continued)*
- thyroid gland S11.11
  - with foreign body S11.12
- toe(s) S91.119
  - with
    - damage to nail S91.219
      - with
        - foreign body S91.229
    - foreign body S91.129
  - great S91.113
    - with
      - damage to nail S91.213
        - with
          - foreign body S91.223
      - foreign body S91.123
    - left S91.112
      - with
        - damage to nail S91.212
          - with
            - foreign body S91.222
        - foreign body S91.122
    - right S91.111
      - with
        - damage to nail S91.211
          - with
            - foreign body S91.221
        - foreign body S91.121
  - lesser S91.116
    - with
      - damage to nail S91.216
        - with
          - foreign body S91.226
      - foreign body S91.126
    - left S91.115
      - with
        - damage to nail S91.215
          - with
            - foreign body S91.225
        - foreign body S91.125
    - right S91.114
      - with
        - damage to nail S91.214
          - with
            - foreign body S91.224
        - foreign body S91.124
- tongue *—see* Laceration, oral cavity
- trachea S11.021
  - with foreign body S11.022
- tunica vaginalis *—see* Laceration, testis
- tympanum, tympanic membrane *—see* Laceration, ear, drum
- umbilical region S31.115
  - with foreign body S31.125
- ureter S37.13
- urethra S37.33
  - with or following ectopic or molar pregnancy O08.6
  - obstetrical trauma O71.5
- urinary organ NEC S37.893
- uterus S37.63
  - with ectopic or molar pregnancy O08.6
  - following ectopic or molar pregnancy O08.6
  - nonpuerperal, nontraumatic N85.8
  - obstetrical trauma NEC O71.81
  - old (postpartal) N85.8
- uvula *—see* Laceration, oral cavity
- vagina S31.41
  - with
    - ectopic or molar pregnancy O08.6
    - foreign body S31.42
  - during delivery O71.4
    - with perineal laceration *—see* Laceration, perineum, female, during delivery
  - following ectopic or molar pregnancy O08.6

Laceration *(continued)*
- vagina *(continued)*
  - nonpuerperal, nontraumatic N89.8
  - old (postpartal) N89.8
- vas deferens S37.893
- vesical *—see* Laceration, bladder
- vocal cords S11.031
  - with foreign body S11.032
- vulva S31.41
  - with
    - ectopic or molar pregnancy O08.6
    - foreign body S31.42
  - complicating delivery O70.0
  - following ectopic or molar pregnancy O08.6
  - nonpuerperal, nontraumatic N90.89
  - old (postpartal) N90.89
- wrist S61.519
  - with
    - foreign body S61.529
  - left S61.512
    - with
      - foreign body S61.522
  - right S61.511
    - with
      - foreign body S61.521

Lack of
- achievement in school Z55.3
- adequate
  - food Z59.4
  - intermaxillary vertical dimension of fully erupted teeth M26.36
  - sleep Z72.820
- appetite (*see* Anorexia) R63.0
- awareness R41.9
- care
  - in home Z74.2
  - of infant (at or after birth) T76.02
    - confirmed T74.02
- cognitive functions R41.9
- coordination R27.9
  - ataxia R27.0
  - specified type NEC R27.8
- development (physiological) R62.50
  - failure to thrive (child over 28 days old) R62.51
    - adult R62.7
    - newborn P92.6
  - short stature R62.52
  - specified type NEC R62.59
- energy R53.83
- financial resources Z59.6
- food T73.0
- growth R62.52
- heating Z59.1
- housing (permanent) (temporary) Z59.0
  - adequate Z59.1
- learning experiences in childhood Z62.898
- leisure time (affecting life-style) Z73.2
- material resources Z59.9
- memory *—see also* Amnesia
  - mild, following organic brain damage F06.8
- ovulation N97.0
- parental supervision or control of child Z62.0
- person able to render necessary care Z74.2
- physical exercise Z72.3
- play experience in childhood Z62.898
- posterior occlusal support M26.57
- relaxation (affecting life-style) Z73.2
- sexual
  - desire F52.0
  - enjoyment F52.1

Lack of *(continued)*
- shelter Z59.0
- sleep (adequate) Z72.820
- supervision of child by parent Z62.0
- support, posterior occlusal M26.57
- water T73.1

Lacrimal *—see* condition

Lacrimation, abnormal *—see* Epiphora

Lacrimonasal duct *—see* condition

Lactation, lactating (breast) (puerperal, postpartum)
- associated
  - cracked nipple O92.13
  - retracted nipple O92.03
- defective O92.4
- disorder NEC O92.79
- excessive O92.6
- failed (complete) O92.3
  - partial O92.4
- mastitis NEC *—see* Mastitis, obstetric
- mother (care and/or examination) Z39.1
- nonpuerperal N64.3

Lacticemia, excessive E87.2

Lacunar skull Q75.8

Laennec's cirrhosis K70.30
- with ascites K70.31
- nonalcoholic K74.69

Lafora's disease *—see* Epilepsy, generalized, idiopathic

Lag, lid (nervous) *—see* Retraction, lid

Lagophthalmos (eyelid) (nervous) H02.209
- cicatricial H02.219
  - left H02.216
    - lower H02.215
    - upper H02.214
  - right H02.213
    - lower H02.212
    - upper H02.211
- keratoconjunctivitis *—see* Keratoconjunctivitis
- left H02.206
  - lower H02.205
  - upper H02.204
- mechanical H02.229
  - left H02.226
    - lower H02.225
    - upper H02.224
  - right H02.223
    - lower H02.222
    - upper H02.221
- paralytic H02.239
  - left H02.236
    - lower H02.235
    - upper H02.234
  - right H02.233
    - lower H02.232
    - upper H02.231
- right H02.203
  - lower H02.202
  - upper H02.201

Laki-Lorand factor deficiency *—see* Defect, coagulation, specified type NEC

Lalling F80.0

Lambert-Eaton syndrome *—see* Syndrome, Lambert-Eaton

Lambliasis, lambliosis A07.1

Landau-Kleffner syndrome *—see* Epilepsy, specified NEC

Landouzy-Déjérine dystrophy or facioscapulohumeral atrophy G71.0

Landouzy's disease (icterohemorrhagic leptospirosis) A27.0

Landry-Guillain-Barré, syndrome or paralysis G61.0

Landry's disease or paralysis G61.0

Lane's
- band Q43.3
- kink *—see* Obstruction, intestine
- syndrome K90.2

Langdon Down syndrome *—see* Trisomy, 21

Lapsed immunization schedule status Z28.3

Large
- baby (regardless of gestational age) (4000g to 4499g) P08.1
- ear, congenital Q17.1
- physiological cup Q14.2
- stature R68.89

Large-for-dates NEC (infant) (4000g to 4499g) P08.1
- affecting management of pregnancy O36.6-
- exceptionally (4500g or more) P08.0

Larsen-Johansson disease orosteochondrosis *—see* Osteochondrosis, juvenile, patella

Larsen's syndrome (flattened facies and multiple congenital dislocations) Q74.8

Larva migrans
- cutaneous B76.9
  - Ancylostoma B76.0
- visceral B83.0

Laryngeal *—see* condition

Laryngismus (stridulus) J38.5
- congenital P28.89
- diphtheritic A36.2

Laryngitis (acute) (edematous) (fibrinous) (infective) (infiltrative) (malignant) (membranous) (phlegmonous) (pneumococcal) (pseudomembranous) (septic) (subglottic) (suppurative) (ulcerative) J04.0
- with
  - influenza, flu, or grippe *—see* Influenza, with, laryngitis
  - tracheitis (acute) *—see* Laryngotracheitis
- atrophic J37.0
- catarrhal J37.0
- chronic J37.0
  - with tracheitis (chronic) J37.1
- diphtheritic A36.2
- due to external agent *—see* Inflammation, respiratory, upper, due to
- Hemophilus influenzae J04.0
- H. influenzae J04.0
- hypertrophic J37.0
- influenzal *—see* Influenza, with, respiratory manifestations NEC
- obstructive J05.0
- sicca J37.0
- spasmodic J05.0
  - acute J04.0
- streptococcal J04.0
- stridulous J05.0
- syphilitic (late) A52.73
  - congenital A50.59 *[J99]*
    - early A50.03 *[J99]*
- tuberculous A15.5
- Vincent's A69.1

Laryngocele (congenital) (ventricular) Q31.3

Laryngofissure J38.7
- congenital Q31.8

Laryngomalacia (congenital) Q31.5

Laryngopharyngitis (acute) J06.0
- chronic J37.0
- due to external agent *—see* Inflammation, respiratory, upper, due to

Laryngoplegia J38.00
- bilateral J38.02
- unilateral J38.01

Laryngoptosis J38.7

Laryngospasm J38.5

Laryngostenosis J38.6

Laryngotracheitis (acute) (Infectional) (infective) (viral) J04.2
- atrophic J37.1
- catarrhal J37.1
- chronic J37.1
- diphtheritic A36.2
- due to external agent *—see* Inflammation, respiratory, upper, due to
- Hemophilus influenzae J04.2
- hypertrophic J37.1
- influenzal *—see* Influenza, with, respiratory manifestations NEC
- pachydermic J38.7
- sicca J37.1
- spasmodic J38.5
  - acute J05.0
- streptococcal J04.2
- stridulous J38.5
- syphilitic (late) A52.73
  - congenital A50.59 *[J99]*
    - early A50.03 *[J99]*
- tuberculous A15.5
- Vincent's A69.1

Laryngotracheobronchitis *—see* Bronchitis

Larynx, laryngeal *—see* condition

Lassa fever A96.2

Lassitude *—see* Weakness

Late
- talker R62.0
- walker R62.0

Late effect(s) *—see* Sequelae

Latent *—see* condition

Laterocession *—see* Lateroversion

Lateroflexion *—see* Lateroversion

Lateroversion
- cervix *—see* Lateroversion, uterus
- uterus, uterine (cervix) (postinfectional) (postpartal, old) N85.4
  - congenital Q51.818
  - in pregnancy or childbirth O34.59-

Lathyrism *—see* Poisoning, food, noxious, plant

Launois' syndrome (pituitary gigantism) E22.0

Launois-Bensaude adenolipomatosis E88.89

Laurence-Moon (-Bardet)-**Biedl syndrome** Q87.89

Lax, laxity *—see also* Relaxation
- ligament (ous) *—see also* Disorder, ligament
  - familial M35.7
  - knee *—see* Derangement, knee
- skin (acquired) L57.4
  - congenital Q82.8

Laxative habit F55.2

Lazy leukocyte syndrome D70.8

Lead miner's lung J63.6

Leak, leakage
- air NEC J93.82
  - postprocedural J95.812
- amniotic fluid —*see* Rupture, membranes, premature
- blood (microscopic), fetal, into maternal circulation affecting management of pregnancy —*see* Pregnancy, complicated by
- cerebrospinal fluid G96.0
  - from spinal (lumbar) puncture G97.0
- device, implant or graft —*see also* Complications, by site and type, mechanical
  - arterial graft NEC —*see* Complication, cardiovascular device, mechanical, vascular
  - breast (implant) T85.43
  - catheter NEC T85.638
    - urinary T83.038
      - cystostomy T83.030
      - Hopkins T83.038
      - ileostomy T83.038
      - indwelling T83.031
      - nephrostomy T83.032
      - specified NEC T83.038
      - urostomy T83.038
    - dialysis (renal) T82.43
      - intraperitoneal T85.631
    - infusion NEC T82.534
      - spinal (epidural) (subdural) T85.630
  - gastrointestinal —*see* Complications, prosthetic device, mechanical, gastrointestinal device
  - genital NEC T83.498
    - penile prosthesis (cylinder) (implanted) (pump) (resevoir) T83.490
    - testicular prosthesis T83.491
  - heart NEC —*see* Complication, cardiovascular device, mechanical
  - joint prosthesis —*see* Complications, joint prosthesis, mechanical, specified NEC, by site
  - ocular NEC —*see* Complications, prosthetic device, mechanical, ocular device
  - orthopedic NEC —*see* Complication, orthopedic, device, mechanical
  - persistent air J93.82
  - specified NEC T85.638
  - urinary NEC —*see also* Complication, genitourinary, device, urinary, mechanical
    - graft T83.23
  - vascular NEC —*see* Complication, cardiovascular device, mechanical
  - ventricular intracranial shunt T85.03
- urine —*see* Incontinence

Leaky heart —*see* Endocarditis

Learning defect (specific) F81.9

Leather bottle stomach C16.9

Leber's
- congenital amaurosis H35.50
- optic atrophy (hereditary) H47.22

Lederer's anemia D59.1

Leeches (external) —*see* Hirudiniasis

Leg —*see* condition

Legg (-Calvé)-Perthes disease, syndrome or osteochondrosis M91.1-

Legionellosis A48.1
- nonpneumonic A48.2

Legionnaires'
- disease A48.1
  - nonpneumonic A48.2
- pneumonia A48.1

Leigh's disease G31.82

Leiner's disease L21.1

Leiofibromyoma —*see* Leiomyoma

Leiomyoblastoma —*see* Neoplasm, connective tissue, benign

Leiomyofibroma —*see also* Neoplasm, connective tissue, benign
- uterus (cervix) (corpus) D25.9

Leiomyoma —*see also* Neoplasm, connective tissue, benign
- bizarre —*see* Neoplasm, connective tissue, benign
- cellular —*see* Neoplasm, connective tissue, benign
- epithelioid —*see* Neoplasm, connective tissue, benign
- uterus (cervix) (corpus) D25.9
  - intramural D25.1
  - submucous D25.0
  - subserosal D25.2
- vascular —*see* Neoplasm, connective tissue, benign

Leiomyoma, leiomyomatosis (intravascular) —*see* Neoplasm, connective tissue, uncertain behavior

Leiomyosarcoma —*see also* Neoplasm, connective tissue, malignant
- epithelioid —*see* Neoplasm, connective tissue, malignant
- myxoid —*see* Neoplasm, connective tissue, malignant

Leishmaniasis B55.9
- American (mucocutaneous) B55.2
  - cutaneous B55.1
- Asian Desert B55.1
- Brazilian B55.2
- cutaneous (any type) B55.1
- dermal —*see also* Leishmaniasis, cutaneous
  - post-kala-azar B55.0
- eyelid B55.1
- infantile B55.0
- Mediterranean B55.0
- mucocutaneous (American) (New World) B55.2
- naso-oral B55.2
- nasopharyngeal B55.2
- old world B55.1
- tegumentaria diffusa B55.1
- visceral B55.0

Leishmanoid, dermal —*see also* Leishmaniasis, cutaneous
- post-kala-azar B55.0

Lenegre's disease I44.2

Lengthening, leg —*see* Deformity, limb, unequal length

Lennert's lymphoma —*see* Lymphoma, Lennert's

Lennox-Gastaut syndrome G40.812
- intractable G40.814
  - with status epilepticus G40.813
  - without status epilepticus G40.814
- not intractable G40.812
  - with status epilepticus G40.811
  - without status epilepticus G40.812

Lens —*see* condition

Lenticonus (anterior) (posterior) (congenital) Q12.8

Lenticular degeneration, progressive E83.01

Lentiglobus (posterior) (congenital) Q12.8

Lentigo (congenital) L81.4
- maligna —*see also* Melanoma, in situ
  - melanoma —*see* Melanoma

Lentivirus, as cause of disease classified elsewhere B97.31

Leontiasis
- ossium M85.2
- syphilitic (late) A52.78
  - congenital A50.59

Lepothrix A48.8

Lepra —*see* Leprosy

Leprechaunism E34.8

Leprosy A30.-
- with muscle disorder A30.9 *[M63.80]*
  - ankle A30.9 *[M63.87-]*
  - foot A30.9 *[M63.87-]*
  - forearm A30.9 *[M63.83-]*
  - hand A30.9 *[M63.84-]*
  - lower leg A30.9 *[M63.86-]*
  - multiple sites A30.9 *[M63.89]*
  - pelvic region A30.9 *[M63.85-]*
  - shoulder region A30.9 *[M63.81-]*
  - specified site NEC A30.9 *[M63.88]*
  - thigh A30.9 *[M63.85-]*
  - upper arm A30.9 *[M63.82-]*
- anesthetic A30.9
- BB A30.3
- BL A30.4
- borderline (infiltrated) (neuritic) A30.3
  - lepromatous A30.4
  - tuberculoid A30.2
- BT A30.2
- dimorphous (infiltrated) (neuritic) A30.3
- I A30.0
- indeterminate (macular) (neuritic) A30.0
- lepromatous (diffuse) (infiltrated) (macular) (neuritic) (nodular) A30.5
- LL A30.5
- macular (early) (neuritic) (simple) A30.9
- maculoanesthetic A30.9
- mixed A30.3
- neural A30.9
- nodular A30.5
- primary neuritic A30.3
- specified type NEC A30.8
- TT A30.1
- tuberculoid (major) (minor) A30.1

Leptocytosis, hereditary D56.9

Leptomeningitis (chronic) (circumscribed) (hemorrhagic) (nonsuppurative) —*see* Meningitis

Leptomeningopathy G96.19

Leptospiral —*see* condition

Leptospirochetal —*see* condition

Leptospirosis A27.9
- canicola A27.89
- due to Leptospira interrogans serovar icterohaemorrhagiae A27.0
- icterohemorrhagica A27.0
- pomona A27.89
- Weil's disease A27.0

Leptus dermatitis B88.0

Leriche's syndrome (aortic bifurcation occlusion) I74.09

Leri's pleonosteosis Q78.8

Leri-Weill syndrome Q77.8

Lermoyez' syndrome —*see* Vertigo, peripheral NEC

Lesch-Nyhan syndrome E79.1

Leser-Trélat disease L82.1
- inflamed L82.0

Lesion(s) (nontraumatic)
- abducens nerve —*see* Strabismus, paralytic, sixth nerve
- alveolar process K08.9
- angiocentric immunoproliferative D47.Z9
- anorectal K62.9
- aortic (valve) I35.9
- auditory nerve —*see* subcategory H93.3
- basal ganglion G25.9
- bile duct —*see* Disease, bile duct
- biomechanical M99.9
  - specified type NEC M99.89
    - abdomen M99.89
    - acromioclavicular M99.87
    - cervical region M99.81
    - cervicothoracic M99.81
    - costochondral M99.88
    - costovertebral M99.88
    - head region M99.80
    - hip M99.85
    - lower extremity M99.86
    - lumbar region M99.83
    - lumbosacral M99.83
    - occipitocervical M99.80
    - pelvic region M99.85
    - pubic M99.85
    - rib cage M99.88
    - sacral region M99.84
    - sacrococcygeal M99.84
    - sacroiliac M99.84
    - specified NEC M99.89
    - sternochondral M99.88
    - sternoclavicular M99.87
    - thoracic region M99.82
    - thoracolumbar M99.82
    - upper extremity M99.87
- bladder N32.9
- bone —*see* Disorder, bone
- brachial plexus G54.0
- brain G93.9
  - congenital Q04.9
  - vascular I67.9
    - degenerative I67.9
    - hypertensive I67.4
- buccal cavity K13.79
- calcified —*see* Calcification
- canthus —*see* Disorder, eyelid
- carate —*see* Pinta, lesions
- cardia K31.9
- cardiac (*see also* Disease, heart) I51.9
  - congenital Q24.9
  - valvular —*see* Endocarditis
- cauda equina G83.4
- cecum K63.9
- cerebral —*see* Lesion, brain
- cerebrovascular I67.9
  - degenerative I67.9
  - hypertensive I67.4
- cervical (nerve) root NEC G54.2
- chiasmal —*see* Disorder, optic, chiasm
- chorda tympani G51.8
- coin, lung R91.1
- colon K63.9

Lesion *(continued)*
combined periodontic - endodontic K05.5
congenital *—see* Anomaly, by site
conjunctiva H11.9
conus medullaris *—see* Injury, conus medullaris
coronary artery *—see* Ischemia, heart
cranial nerve G52.9
eighth *—see* Disorder, ear
eleventh G52.9
fifth G50.9
first G52.0
fourth *—see* Strabismus, paralytic, fourth nerve
seventh G51.9
sixth *—see* Strabismus, paralytic, sixth nerve
tenth G52.2
twelfth G52.3
cystic *—see* Cyst
degenerative *—see* Degeneration
duodenum K31.9
edentulous (alveolar) ridge, associated with trauma, due to traumatic occlusion K06.2
en coup de sabre L94.1
eyelid *—see* Disorder, eyelid
gasserian ganglion G50.8
gastric K31.9
gastroduodenal K31.9
gastrointestinal K63.9
gingiva, associated with trauma K06.2
glomerular
focal and segmental (*see also* N00-N07 with fourth character .1) N05.1
minimal change (*see also* N00-N07 with fourth character .0) N05.0
heart (organic) *—see* Disease, heart
hyperchromic, due to pinta (carate) A67.1
hyperkeratotic *—see* Hyperkeratosis
hypothalamic E23.7
ileocecal K63.9
ileum K63.9
iliohypogastric nerve G57.8-
inflammatory *—see* Inflammation
intestine K63.9
intracerebral *—see* Lesion, brain
intrachiasmal (optic) *—see* Disorder, optic, chiasm
intracranial, space-occupying R90.0
joint *—see* Disorder, joint
sacroiliac (old) M53.3
keratotic *—see* Keratosis
kidney *—see* Disease, renal
laryngeal nerve (recurrent) G52.2
lip K13.0
liver K76.9
lumbosacral
plexus G54.1
root (nerve) NEC G54.4
lung (coin) R91.1
maxillary sinus J32.0
mitral I05.9
Morel-Lavallée *—see* Hematoma, by site
motor cortex NEC G93.89
mouth K13.79
nerve G58.9
femoral G57.2-
median G56.1-
carpal tunnel syndrome *—see* Syndrome, carpal tunnel
plantar G57.6-

Lesion *(continued)*
nerve *(continued)*
popliteal (lateral) G57.3-
medial G57.4-
radial G56.3-
sciatic G57.0-
spinal *—see* Injury, nerve, spinal
ulnar G56.2-
nervous system, congenital Q07.9
nonallopathic *—see* Lesion, biomechanical
nose (internal) J34.89
obstructive *—see* Obstruction
obturator nerve G57.8-
oral mucosa K13.70
organ or site NEC *—see* Disease, by site
osteolytic *—see* Osteolysis
peptic K27.9
periodontal, due to traumatic occlusion K05.5
pharynx J39.2
pigment, pigmented (skin) L81.9
pinta *—see* Pinta, lesions
polypoid *—see* Polyp
prechiasmal (optic) *—see* Disorder, optic, chiasm
primary (*see also* Syphilis, primary) A51.0
carate A67.0
pinta A67.0
yaws A66.0
pulmonary J98.4
valve I37.9
pylorus K31.9
rectosigmoid K63.9
retina, retinal H35.9
sacroiliac (joint) (old) M53.3
salivary gland K11.9
benign lymphoepithelial K11.8
saphenous nerve G57.8-
sciatic nerve G57.0-
secondary *—see* Syphilis, secondary
shoulder (region) M75.9-
specified NEC M75.8-
sigmoid K63.9
sinus (accessory) (nasal) J34.89
skin L98.9
suppurative L08.0
SLAP S43.43-
spinal cord G95.9
congenital Q06.9
spleen D73.89
stomach K31.9
superior glenoid labrum S43.43-
syphilitic *—see* Syphilis
tertiary *—see* Syphilis, tertiary
thoracic root (nerve) NEC G54.3
tonsillar fossa J35.9
tooth, teeth K08.9
white spot
chewing surface K02.51
pit and fissure surface K02.51
smooth surface K02.61
traumatic *—see* specific type of injury by site
tricuspid (valve) I07.9
nonrheumatic I36.9
trigeminal nerve G50.9
ulcerated or ulcerative *—see* Ulcer, skin
uterus N85.9
vagus nerve G52.2
valvular *—see* Endocarditis
vascular I99.9
affecting central nervous system I67.9
following trauma NEC T14.8
umbilical cord, complicating delivery O69.5

Lesion *(continued)*
warty *—see* Verruca
white spot (tooth)
chewing surface K02.51
pit and fissure surface K02.51
smooth surface K02.61

Lethargic *—see* condition

Lethargy R53.83

Letterer-Siwe's disease C96.0

Leukemia, leukemic C95.9-
acute basophilic C94.8-
acute bilineal C95.0-
acute erythroid C94.0-
acute lymphoblastic C91.0-
acute megakaryoblastic C94.2-
acute megakaryocytic C94.2-
acute mixed lineage C95.0-
acute monoblastic (monoblastic/monocytic) C93.0-
acute monocytic (monoblastic/monocytic) C93.0-
acute myeloblastic (minimal differentiation) (with maturation) C92.0-
acute myeloid
with
11q23-abnormality C92.6-
dysplasia of remaining hematopoesis and/or myelodysplastic disease in its history C92.A-
multilineage dysplasia C92.A-
variation of MLL-gene C92.6-
M6 (a)(b) C94.0-
M7 C94.2-
acute myelomonocytic C92.5-
acute promyelocytic C92.4-
adult T-cell (HTLV-1-associated) (acute variant) (chronic variant) (lymphomatoid variant) (smouldering variant) C91.5-
aggressive NK-cell C94.8-
AML (1/ETO) (M0) (M1) (M2) (without a FAB classification) C92.0-
AML M3 C92.4-
AML M4 (Eo with inv (16) or t (16;16)) C92.5-
AML M5 C93.0-
AML M5a C93.0-
AML M5b C93.0-
AML Me with t (15;17) and variants C92.4-
atypical chronic myeloid, BCR/ABL-negative C92.2-
biphenotypic acute C95.0-
blast cell C95.0-
Burkitt-type, mature B-cell C91.A-
chronic lymphocytic, of B-cell type C91.1-
chronic monocytic C93.1-
chronic myelogenous (Philadelphia chromosome (Ph1) positive) (t (9;22)) (q34;q11) (with crisis of blast cells) C92.1-
chronic myeloid, BCR/ABL-positive C92.1-
atypical, BCR/ABL-negative C92.2-
chronic myelomonocytic C93.1-
chronic neutrophilic D47.1
CMML (-1) (-2) (with eosinophilia) C93.1-
granulocytic (*see also* Category C92) C92.9-
hairy cell C91.4-
juvenile myelomonocytic C93.3-

Leukemia, leukemic *(continued)*
lymphoid C91.9-
specified NEC C91.Z-
mast cell C94.3-
mature B-cell, Burkitt-type C91.A-
monocytic (subacute) C93.9-
specified NEC C93.Z-
myelogenous (*see also* Category C92) C92.9-
myeloid C92.9-
specified NEC C92.Z-
plasma cell C90.1-
plasmacytic C90.1-
prolymphocytic
of B-cell type C91.3-
of T-cell type C91.6-
specified NEC C94.8-
stem cell, of unclear lineage C95.0-
subacute lymphocytic C91.9-
T-cell large granular lymphocytic C91.Z-
unspecified cell type C95.9-
acute C95.0-
chronic C95.1-

Leukemoid reaction (*see also* Reaction, leukemoid) D72.823-

Leukoaraiosis (hypertensive) I67.81

Leukoariosis *—see* Leukoaraiosis

Leukocoria *—see* Disorder, globe, degenerated condition, leucocoria

Leukocytopenia D72.819

Leukocytosis D72.829
eosinophilic D72.1

Leukoderma, leukodermia NEC L81.5
syphilitic A51.39
late A52.79

Leukodystrophy E75.29

Leukoedema, oral epithelium K13.29

Leukoencephalitis G04.81
acute (subacute) hemorrhagic G36.1
postimmunization or postvaccinal G04.02
postinfectious G04.01
subacute sclerosing A81.1
van Bogaert's (sclerosing) A81.1

Leukoencephalopathy (*see also* Encephalopathy) G93.49
Binswanger's I67.3
heroin vapor G92
metachromatic E75.25
multifocal (progressive) A81.2
postimmunization and postvaccinal G04.02
progressive multifocal A81.2
reversible, posterior G93.6
van Bogaert's (sclerosing) A81.1
vascular, progressive I67.3

Leukoerythroblastosis D75.9

Leukokeratosis *—see also* Leukoplakia
mouth K13.21
nicotina palati K13.24
oral mucosa K13.21
tongue K13.21
vocal cord J38.3

Leukokraurosis vulva (e) N90.4

Leukoma (cornea) *—see also* Opacity, cornea
adherent H17.0-
interfering with central vision *—see* Opacity, cornea, central

Leukomalacia, cerebral, newborn P91.2
periventricular P91.2

Leukomelanopathy, hereditary D72.0

Leukonychia (punctata) (striata) L60.8
- congenital Q84.4

Leukopathia unguium L60.8
- congenital Q84.4

Leukopenia D72.819
- basophilic D72.818
- chemotherapy (cancer) induced D70.1
- congenital D70.0
- cyclic D70.0
- drug induced NEC D70.2
  - due to cytoreductive cancer chemotherapy D70.1
- eosinophilic D72.818
- familial D70.0
- infantile genetic D70.0
- malignant D70.9
- periodic D70.0
- transitory neonatal P61.5

Leukopenic —*see* condition

Leukoplakia
- anus K62.89
- bladder (postinfectional) N32.89
- buccal K13.21
- cervix (uteri) N88.0
- esophagus K22.8
- gingiva K13.21
- hairy (oral mucosa) (tongue) K13.3
- kidney (pelvis) N28.89
- larynx J38.7
- lip K13.21
- mouth K13.21
- oral epithelium, including tongue (mucosa) K13.21
- palate K13.21
- pelvis (kidney) N28.89
- penis (infectional) N48.0
- rectum K62.89
- syphilitic (late) A52.79
- tongue K13.21
- ureter (postinfectional) N28.89
- urethra (postinfectional) N36.8
- uterus N85.8
- vagina N89.4
- vocal cord J38.3
- vulva N90.4

Leukorrhea N89.8
- due to Trichomonas (vaginalis) A59.00
- trichomonal A59.00

Leukosarcoma C85.9-

Levocardia (isolated) Q24.1
- with situs inversus Q89.3

Levotransposition Q20.5

Lev's disease or syndrome (acquired complete heart block) I44.2

Levulosuria —*see* Fructosuria

Levurid L30.2

Lewy body (ies) (dementia) (disease) G31.83

Leyden-Moebius dystrophy G71.0

Leydig cell
- carcinoma
  - specified site —*see* Neoplasm, malignant, by site
  - unspecified site
    - female C56.9
    - male C62.9-
- tumor
  - benign
    - specified site —*see* Neoplasm, benign, by site
    - unspecified site
      - female D27.-
      - male D29.2-

Leydig cell *(continued)*
- tumor *(continued)*
  - malignant
    - specified site —*see* Neoplasm, malignant, by site
    - unspecified site
      - female C56.-
      - male C62.9-
  - specified site —*see* Neoplasm, uncertain behavior, by site
  - unspecified site
    - female D39.1-
    - male D40.1-

Leydig-Sertoli cell tumor
- specified site —*see* Neoplasm, benign, by site
- unspecified site
  - female D27.-
  - male D29.2-

LGSIL (Low grade squamous intraepithelial lesion on cytologic smear of)
- anus R85.612
- cervix R87.612
- vagina R87.622

Liar, pathologic F60.2

Libido
- decreased R68.82

Libman-Sacks disease M32.11

Lice (infestation) B85.2
- body (Pediculus corporis) B85.1
- crab B85.3
- head (Pediculus capitis) B85.0
- mixed (classifiable to more than one of the titles B85.0-B85.3) B85.4
- pubic (Phthirus pubis) B85.3

Lichen L28.0
- albus L90.0
  - penis N48.0
  - vulva N90.4
- amyloidosis E85.4 *[L99]*
- atrophicus L90.0
  - penis N48.0
  - vulva N90.4
- congenital Q82.8
- myxedematosus L98.5
- nitidus L44.1
- pilaris Q82.8
  - acquired L85.8
- planopilaris L66.1
- planus (chronicus) L43.9
  - annularis L43.8
  - bullous L43.1
  - follicular L66.1
  - hypertrophic L43.0
  - moniliformis L44.3
  - of Wilson L43.9
  - specified NEC L43.8
  - subacute (active) L43.3
  - tropicus L43.3
- ruber
  - acuminatus L44.0
  - moniliformis L44.3
  - planus L43.9
- sclerosus (et atrophicus) L90.0
  - penis N48.0
  - vulva N90.4
- scrofulosus (primary) (tuberculous) A18.4
- simplex (chronicus) (circumscriptus) L28.0
- striatus L44.2
- urticatus L28.2

Lichenification L28.0

Lichenoides tuberculosis (primary) A18.4

Lichtheim's disease or syndrome —*see* Degeneration, combined

Lien migrans D73.89

Ligament —*see* condition

Light
- for gestational age —*see* Light for dates
- headedness R42

Light-for-dates (infant) P05.00
- with weight of
  - 499 grams or less P05.01
  - 500-749 grams P05.02
  - 750-999 grams P05.03
  - 1000-1249 grams P05.04
  - 1250-1499 grams P05.05
  - 1500-1749 grams P05.06
  - 1750-1999 grams P05.07
  - 2000-2499 grams P05.08
  - 2500 grams and over P05.09
- and small-for-dates —*see* Small for dates
- affecting management of pregnancy O36.59-
- specified NEC P05.09

Lightning (effects) (stroke) (struck by) T75.00
- burn —*see* Burn
- foot E53.8
- shock T75.01
- specified effect NEC T75.09

Lightwood-Albright syndrome N25.89

Lightwood's disease or syndrome (renal tubular acidosis) N25.89

Lignac (-de Toni) (-Fanconi) (-Debré) **disease or syndrome** E72.09
- with cystinosis E72.04

Ligneous thyroiditis E06.5

Likoff's syndrome I20.8

Limb —*see* condition

Limbic epilepsy personality syndrome F07.0

Limitation, limited
- activities due to disability Z73.6
- cardiac reserve —*see* Disease, heart
- eye muscle duction, traumatic —*see* Strabismus, mechanical
- mandibular range of motion M26.52

Lindau (-von Hippel) **disease** Q85.8

Line(s)
- Beau's L60.4
- Harris' —*see* Arrest, epiphyseal
- Hudson's (cornea) —*see* Pigmentation, cornea, anterior
- Stähli's (cornea) —*see* Pigmentation, cornea, anterior

Linea corneae senilis —*see* Change, cornea, senile

Lingua
- geographica K14.1
- nigra (villosa) K14.3
- plicata K14.5
- tylosis K13.29

Lingual —*see* condition

Linguatulosis B88.8

Linitis (gastric) **plastica C16.9**

Lip —*see* condition

Lipedema —*see* Edema

Lipemia —*see also* Hyperlipidemia
- retina, retinalis E78.3

Lipidosis E75.6
- cerebral (infantile) (juvenile) (late) E75.4
- cerebroretinal E75.4

Lipidosis *(continued)*
- cerebroside E75.22
- cholesterol (cerebral) E75.5
- glycolipid E75.21
- hepatosplenomegalic E78.3
- sphingomyelin —*see* Niemann-Pick disease or syndrome
- sulfatide E75.29

Lipoadenoma —*see* Neoplasm, benign, by site

Lipoblastoma —*see* Lipoma

Lipoblastomatosis —*see* Lipoma

Lipochondrodystrophy E76.01

Lipodermatosclerosis —*see* Varix, leg, with, inflammation
- ulcerated —*see* Varix, leg, with, ulcer, with inflammation by site

Lipochrome histiocytosis (familial) D71

Lipodystrophia progressiva E88.1

Lipodystrophy (progressive) E88.1
- insulin E88.1
- intestinal K90.81
- mesenteric K65.4

Lipofibroma —*see* Lipoma

Lipofuscinosis, neuronal (with ceroidosis) E75.4

Lipogranuloma, sclerosing L92.8

Lipogranulomatosis E78.89

Lipoid —*see also* condition
- histiocytosis D76.3
  - essential E75.29
- nephrosis N04.9
- proteinosis of Urbach E78.89

Lipoidemia —*see* Hyperlipidemia

Lipoidosis —*see* Lipidosis

Lipoma D17.9
- fetal D17.9
  - fat cell D17.9
- infiltrating D17.9
- intramuscular D17.9
- pleomorphic D17.9
- site classification
  - arms (skin) (subcutaneous) D17.2-
  - connective tissue D17.30
    - intra-abdominal D17.5
    - intrathoracic D17.4
    - peritoneum D17.79
    - retroperitoneum D17.79
    - specified site NEC D17.39
    - spermatic cord D17.6
  - face (skin) (subcutaneous) D17.0
  - genitourinary organ NEC D17.72
  - head (skin) (subcutaneous) D17.0
  - intra-abdominal D17.5
  - intrathoracic D17.4
  - kidney D17.71
  - legs (skin) (subcutaneous) D17.2-
  - neck (skin) (subcutaneous) D17.0
  - peritoneum D17.79
  - retroperitoneum D17.79
  - skin D17.30
    - specified site NEC D17.39
  - specified site NEC D17.79
  - spermatic cord D17.6
  - subcutaneous D17.30
    - specified site NEC D17.39
  - trunk (skin) (subcutaneous) D17.1
  - unspecified D17.9
- spindle cell D17.9

Lipomatosis E88.2
- dolorosa (Dercum) E88.2
- fetal —*see* Lipoma
- Launois-Bensaude E88.89

Lipomyoma —*see* Lipoma

Lipomyxoma *—see* Lipoma

Lipomyxosarcoma *—see* Neoplasm, connective tissue, malignant

Lipoprotein metabolism disorder E78.9

Lipoproteinemia E78.5
- broad-beta E78.2
- floating-beta E78.2
- hyper-pre-beta E78.1

Liposarcoma *—see also* Neoplasm, connective tissue, malignant
- dedifferentiated *—see* Neoplasm, connective tissue, malignant
- differentiated type *—see* Neoplasm, connective tissue, malignant
- embryonal *—see* Neoplasm, connective tissue, malignant
- mixed type *—see* Neoplasm, connective tissue, malignant
- myxoid *—see* Neoplasm, connective tissue, malignant
- pleomorphic *—see* Neoplasm, connective tissue, malignant
- round cell *—see* Neoplasm, connective tissue, malignant
- well differentiated type *—see* Neoplasm, connective tissue, malignant

Liposynovitis prepatellaris E88.89

Lipping, cervix N86

Lipschütz disease or ulcer N76.6

Lipuria R82.0
- schistosomiasis (bilharziasis) B65.0

Lisping F80.0

Lissauer's paralysis A52.17

Lissencephalia, lissencephaly Q04.3

Listeriosis, listerellosis A32.9
- congenital (disseminated) P37.2
- cutaneous A32.0
- neonatal, newborn (disseminated) P37.2
- oculoglandular A32.81
- specified NEC A32.89

Lithemia E79.0

Lithiasis *—see* Calculus

Lithosis J62.8

Lithuria R82.99

Litigation, anxiety concerning Z65.3

Little leaguer's elbow *—see* Epicondylitis, medial

Little's disease G80.9

Littre's
- gland *—see* condition
- hernia *—see* Hernia, abdomen

Littritis *—see* Urethritis

Livedo (annularis) (racemosa) (reticularis) R23.1

Liver *—see* condition

Living alone (problems with) Z60.2
- with handicapped person Z74.2

Lloyd's syndrome *—see* Adenomatosis, endocrine

Loa loa, loaiasis, loasis B74.3

Lobar *—see* condition

Lobomycosis B48.0

Lobo's disease B48.0

Lobotomy syndrome F07.0

Lobstein (-Ekman) **disease or syndrome** Q78.0

Lobster-claw hand Q71.6-

Lobulation (congenital) *—see also* Anomaly, by site
- kidney, Q63.1
- liver, abnormal Q44.7
- spleen Q89.09

Lobule, lobular *—see* condition

Local, localized *—see* condition

Locked-in state G83.5

Locked twins causing obstructed labor O66.1

Locking
- joint *—see* Derangement, joint, specified type NEC
  - knee *—see* Derangement, knee

Lockjaw *—see* Tetanus

Löffler's
- endocarditis I42.3
- eosinophilia J82
- pneumonia J82
- syndrome (eosinophilic pneumonitis) J82

Loiasis (with conjunctival infestation) (eyelid) B74.3

Lone Star fever A77.0

Long
- labor O63.9
  - first stage O63.0
  - second stage O63.1
- QT syndrome I45.81

Long-term (current) (prophylactic)
- drug therapy (use of)
- agents affecting estrogen receptors and estrogen levels NEC Z79.818
- anastrozole (Arimidex) Z79.811
- antibiotics Z79.2
  - short-term use - omit code
- anticoagulants Z79.01
- anti-inflammatory, non-steroidal (NSAID) Z79.1
- antiplatelet Z79.02
- antithrombotics Z79.02
- aromatase inhibitors Z79.811
- aspirin Z79.82
- birth control pill or patch Z79.3
- bisphosphonates Z79.83
- contraceptive, oral Z79.3
- drug, specified NEC Z79.899
- estrogen receptor downregulators Z79.818
- Evista Z79.810
- exemestane (Aromasin) Z79.811
- Fareston Z79.810
- fulvestrant (Faslodex) Z79.818
- gonadotropin-releasing hormone (GnRH) agonist Z79.818
- goserelin acetate (Zoladex) Z79.818
- hormone replacement Z79.890
- insulin Z79.4
- letrozole (Femara) Z79.811
- leuprolide acetate (leuprorelin) (Lupron) Z79.818
- megestrol acetate (Megace) Z79.818
- methadone for pain management Z79.891
- Nolvadex Z79.810
- non-steroidal anti-inflammatories (NSAID) Z79.1
- opiate analgesic Z79.891
- oral
  - antidiabetic Z79.84
  - contraceptive Z79.3
  - hypoglycemic Z79.84
- raloxifene (Evista) Z79.810
- selective estrogen receptor modulators (SERMs) Z79.810

Long-term *(continued)*
- steroids
  - inhaled Z79.51
  - systemic Z79.52
- tamoxifen (Nolvadex) Z79.810
- toremifene (Fareston) Z79.810

Longitudinal stripes or grooves, nails L60.8
- congenital Q84.6

Loop
- intestine *—see* Volvulus
- vascular on papilla (optic) Q14.2

Loose *—see also* condition
- body
  - joint M24.00
    - ankle M24.07-
    - elbow M24.02-
    - hand M24.04-
    - hip M24.05-
    - knee M23.4-
    - shoulder (region) M24.01-
    - specified site NEC M24.08
    - vertebra M24.08
    - toe M24.07-
    - wrist M24.03-
  - knee M23.4-
  - sheath, tendon *—see* Disorder, tendon, specified type NEC
- cartilage *—see* Loose, body, joint
- skin and subcutaneous tissue (following bariatric surgery weight loss) (following dietary weight loss) L98.7
- tooth, teeth K08.89

Loosening
- aseptic
  - joint prosthesis *—see* Complications, joint prosthesis, mechanical, loosening, by site
- epiphysis *—see* Osteochondropathy
- mechanical
  - joint prosthesis *—see* Complications, joint prosthesis, mechanical, loosening, by site

Looser-Milkman (-Debray) **syndrome** M83.8

Lop ear (deformity) Q17.3

Lorain (-Levi) **short stature syndrome** E23.0

Lordosis M40.50
- acquired *—see* Lordosis, specified type NEC
- congenital Q76.429
  - lumbar region Q76.426
  - lumbosacral region Q76.427
  - sacral region Q76.428
  - sacrococcygeal region Q76.428
  - thoracolumbar region Q76.425
- lumbar region M40.56
- lumbosacral region M40.57
- postsurgical M96.4
- postural *—see* Lordosis, specified type NEC
- rachitic (late effect) (sequelae) E64.3
- sequelae of rickets E64.3
- specified type NEC M40.40
  - lumbar region M40.46
  - lumbosacral region M40.47
  - thoracolumbar region M40.45
- thoracolumbar region M40.55
- tuberculous A18.01

Loss (of)
- appetite (*see* Anorexia) R63.0
  - hysterical F50.89
  - nonorganic origin F50.89
  - psychogenic F50.89
- blood *—see* Hemorrhage

Loss *(continued)*
- bone *—see* Loss, substance of, bone
- control, sphincter, rectum R15.9
  - nonorganic origin F98.1
- consciousness, transient R55
  - traumatic *—see* Injury, intracranial
- elasticity, skin R23.4
- family (member) in childhood Z62.898
- fluid (acute) E86.9
- function of labyrinth H83.2
- hair, nonscarring *—see* Alopecia
- hearing *—see also* Deafness
  - central NOS H90.5
  - conductive H90.2
    - bilateral H90.0
    - unilateral
      - with
        - restricted hearing on the contralateral side H90.A1-
        - unrestricted hearing on the contralateral side H90.1-
  - mixed conductive and sensorineural hearing loss H90.8
    - bilateral H90.6
    - unilateral
      - with
        - restricted hearing on the contralateral side H90.A3-
        - unrestricted hearing on the contralateral side H90.7-
  - neural NOS H90.5
  - perceptive NOS H90.5
  - sensorineural NOS H90.5
    - bilateral H90.3
    - unilateral
      - with
        - restricted hearing on the contralateral side H90.A2-
        - unrestricted hearing on the contralateral side H90.4-
  - sensory NOS H90.5
- height R29.890
- limb or member, traumatic, current *—see* Amputation, traumatic
- love relationship in childhood Z62.898
- memory *—see also* Amnesia
  - mild, following organic brain damage F06.8
- mind *—see* Psychosis
- occlusal vertical dimension of fully erupted teeth M26.37
- organ or part *—see* Absence, by site, acquired
- ossicles, ear (partial) H74.32-
- parent in childhood Z63.4
- pregnancy, recurrent N96
  - care in current pregnancy O26.2-
  - without current pregnancy N96
- recurrent pregnancy *—see* Loss, pregnancy, recurrent
- self-esteem, in childhood Z62.898
- sense of
  - smell *—see* Disturbance, sensation, smell
  - taste *—see* Disturbance, sensation, taste
  - touch R20.8
- sensory R44.9
  - dissociative F44.6
- sexual desire F52.0
- sight (acquired) (complete) (congenital) *—see* Blindness

- **Loss** *(continued)*
  - substance of
    - bone *—see* Disorder, bone, density and structure, specified NEC
      - horizontal alveolar K06.3
    - cartilage *—see* Disorder, cartilage, specified type NEC
      - auricle (ear) *—see* Disorder, pinna, specified type NEC
    - vitreous (humor) H15.89
  - tooth, teeth *—see* Absence, teeth, acquired
  - vision, visual H54.7
    - both eyes H54.3
    - one eye H54.60
      - left (normal vision on right) H54.62
      - right (normal vision on left) H54.61
    - specified as blindness *—see* Blindness
    - subjective
      - sudden H53.13-
      - transient H53.12-
  - vitreous *—see* Prolapse, vitreous
  - voice *—see* Aphonia
  - weight (abnormal) (cause unknown) R63.4
- **Louis-Bar syndrome** (ataxia-telangiectasia) G11.3
- **Louping ill** (encephalitis) A84.8
- **Louse, lousiness** *—see* Lice
- **Low**
  - achiever, school Z55.3
  - back syndrome M54.5
  - basal metabolic rate R94.8
  - birthweight (2499 grams or less) P07.10
    - with weight of
      - 1000-1249 grams P07.14
      - 1250-1499 grams P07.15
      - 1500-1749 grams P07.16
      - 1750-1999 grams P07.17
      - 2000-2499 grams P07.18
    - extreme (999 grams or less) P07.00
      - with weight of
        - 499 grams or less P07.01
        - 500-749 grams P07.02
        - 750-999 grams P07.03
    - for gestational age *—see* Light for dates
  - blood pressure *—see also* Hypotension
    - reading (incidental) (isolated) (nonspecific) R03.1
  - cardiac reserve *—see* Disease, heart
  - function *—see also* Hypofunction
    - kidney N28.9
  - hematocrit D64.9
  - hemoglobin D64.9
  - income Z59.6
  - level of literacy Z55.0
  - lying
    - kidney N28.89
    - organ or site, congenital *—see* Malposition, congenital
  - output syndrome (cardiac) *—see* Failure, heart
  - platelets (blood) *—see* Thrombocytopenia
  - reserve, kidney N28.89
  - salt syndrome E87.1
  - self esteem R45.81
  - set ears Q17.4
  - vision H54.2X-
    - one eye (other eye normal) H54.50
      - left (normal vision on right) H54.52A-
      - other eye blind *—see* Blindness
      - right (normal vision on left) H54.511-
- **Low-density-lipoprotein-type** (LDL) **hyperlipoproteinemia** E78.00
- **Lowe's syndrome** E72.03
- **Lown-Ganong-Levine syndrome** I45.6
- **LSD reaction** (acute) (without dependence) F16.90
  - with dependence F16.20
- **L-shaped kidney** Q63.8
- **Ludwig's angina or disease** K12.2
- **Lues** (venerea)**, luetic** *—see* Syphilis
- **Luetscher's syndrome** (dehydration) E86.0
- **Lumbago, lumbalgia** M54.5
  - with sciatica M54.4-
    - due to intervertebral disc disorder M51.17
  - due to displacement, intervertebral disc M51.27
    - with sciatica M51.17
- **Lumbar** *—see* condition
- **Lumbarization, vertebra, congenital** Q76.49
- **Lumbermen's itch** B88.0
- **Lump** *—see also* Mass
  - breast N63.0
    - axillary tail
      - left N63.32
      - right N63.31
    - left
      - lower inner quadrant N63.24
      - lower outer quadrant N63.23
      - unspecified quadrant N63.20
      - upper inner quadrant N63.22
      - upper outer quadrant N63.21
    - right
      - lower inner quadrant N63.14
      - lower outer quadrant N63.13
      - unspecified quadrant N63.10
      - upper inner quadrant N63.12
      - upper outer quadrant N63.11
    - subareolar
      - left N63.42
      - right N63.41
- **Lunacy** *—see* Psychosis
- **Lung** *—see* condition
- **Lupoid** (miliary) **of Boeck** D86.3
- **Lupus**
  - anticoagulant D68.62
    - with
      - hemorrhagic disorder D68.312
      - hypercoagulable state D68.62
    - finding without diagnosis R76.0
  - discoid (local) L93.0
  - erythematosus (discoid) (local) L93.0
    - disseminated *—see* Lupus, erythematosus, systemic
    - eyelid H01.129
      - left H01.126
        - lower H01.125
        - upper H01.124
      - right H01.123
        - lower H01.122
        - upper H01.121
    - profundus L93.2
    - specified NEC L93.2
    - subacute cutaneous L93.1
    - systemic M32.9
      - with organ or system involvement M32.10
        - endocarditis M32.11
        - lung M32.13
        - pericarditis M32.12
        - renal (glomerular) M32.14
          - tubulo-interstitial M32.15
        - specified organ or system NEC M32.19
      - drug-induced M32.0
      - inhibitor (presence of) D68.62
        - with
          - hemorrhagic disorder D68.312
          - hypercoagulable state D68.62
        - finding without diagnosis R76.0
      - specified NEC M32.8
  - exedens A18.4
  - hydralazine M32.0
    - correct substance properly administered *—see* Table of Drugs and Chemicals, by drug, adverse effect
    - overdose or wrong substance given or taken *—see* Table of Drugs and Chemicals, by drug, poisoning
  - nephritis (chronic) M32.14
  - nontuberculous, not disseminated L93.0
  - panniculitis L93.2
  - pernio (Besnier) D86.3
  - systemic *—see* Lupus, erythematosus, systemic
  - tuberculous A18.4
    - eyelid A18.4
  - vulgaris A18.4
    - eyelid A18.4
- **Luteinoma** D27.-
- **Lutembacher's disease or syndrome** (atrial septal defect with mitral stenosis) Q21.1
- **Luteoma** D27.-
- **Lutz** (-Splendore-de Almeida) **disease** *—see* Paracoccidioidomycosis
- **Luxation** *—see also* Dislocation
  - eyeball (nontraumatic) *—see* Luxation, globe
    - birth injury P15.3
  - globe, nontraumatic H44.82-
  - lacrimal gland *—see* Dislocation, lacrimal gland
  - lens (old) (partial) (spontaneous)
    - congenital Q12.1
      - syphilitic A50.39
- **Lycanthropy** F22
- **Lyell's syndrome** L51.2
  - due to drug L51.2
    - correct substance properly administered *—see* Table of Drugs and Chemicals, by drug, adverse effect
    - overdose or wrong substance given or taken *—see* Table of Drugs and Chemicals, by drug, poisoning
- **Lyme disease** A69.20
- **Lymph**
  - gland or node *—see* condition
  - scrotum *—see* Infestation, filarial
- **Lymphadenitis** I88.9
  - with ectopic or molar pregnancy O08.0
  - acute L04.9
    - axilla L04.2
    - face L04.0
    - head L04.0
    - hip L04.3
    - limb
      - lower L04.3
      - upper L04.2
    - neck L04.0
    - shoulder L04.2
    - specified site NEC L04.8
    - trunk L04.1
  - anthracosis (occupational) J60
  - any site, except mesenteric I88.9
    - chronic I88.1
    - subacute I88.1
  - breast
    - gestational *—see* Mastitis, obstetric
    - puerperal, postpartum (nonpurulent) O91.22
  - chancroidal (congenital) A57
  - chronic I88.1
    - mesenteric I88.0
  - due to
    - Brugia (malayi) B74.1
      - timori B74.2
    - chlamydial lymphogranuloma A55
    - diphtheria (toxin) A36.89
    - lymphogranuloma venereum A55
    - Wuchereria bancrofti B74.0
  - following ectopic or molar pregnancy O08.0
  - gonorrheal A54.89
  - infective *—see* Lymphadenitis, acute
  - mesenteric (acute) (chronic) (nonspecific) (subacute) I88.0
    - due to Salmonella typhi A01.09
    - tuberculous A18.39
  - mycobacterial A31.8
  - purulent *—see* Lymphadenitis, acute
  - pyogenic *—see* Lymphadenitis, acute
  - regional, nonbacterial I88.8
  - septic *—see* Lymphadenitis, acute
  - subacute, unspecified site I88.1
  - suppurative *—see* Lymphadenitis, acute
  - syphilitic (early) (secondary) A51.49
    - late A52.79
  - tuberculous *—see* Tuberculosis, lymph gland
  - venereal (chlamydial) A55
- **Lymphadenoid goiter** E06.3
- **Lymphadenopathy** (generalized) R59.1
  - angioimmunoblastic, with dysproteinemia (AILD) C86.5
  - due to toxoplasmosis (acquired) B58.89
    - congenital (acute) (subacute) (chronic) P37.1
  - localized R59.0
  - syphilitic (early) (secondary) A51.49
- **Lymphadenosis** R59.1
- **Lymphangiectasis** I89.0
  - conjunctiva H11.89
  - postinfectional I89.0
  - scrotum I89.0
- **Lymphangiectatic elephantiasis, nonfilarial** I89.0

- **Lymphangioendothelioma** D18.1
  - malignant —*see* Neoplasm, connective tissue, malignant
- **Lymphangioleiomyomatosis** J84.81
- **Lymphangioma** D18.1
  - capillary D18.1
  - cavernous D18.1
  - cystic D18.1
  - malignant —*see* Neoplasm, connective tissue, malignant
- **Lymphangiomyoma** D18.1
- **Lymphangiomyomatosis** J84.81
- **Lymphangiosarcoma** —*see* Neoplasm, connective tissue, malignant
- **Lymphangitis** I89.1
  - with
    - abscess - code by site under Abscess
    - cellulitis - code by site under Cellulitis
    - ectopic or molar pregnancy O08.0
  - acute L03.91
    - abdominal wall L03.321
    - ankle —*see* Lymphangitis, acute, lower limb
    - arm —*see* Lymphangitis, acute, upper limb
    - auricle (ear) —*see* Lymphangitis, acute, ear
    - axilla L03.12-
    - back (any part) L03.322
    - buttock L03.327
    - cervical (meaning neck) L03.222
    - cheek (external) L03.212
    - chest wall L03.323
    - digit
      - finger —*see* Lymphangitis, acute, finger
      - toe —*see* Lymphangitis, acute, toe
    - ear (external) H60.1-
    - external auditory canal —*see* Lymphangitis, acute, ear
    - eyelid —*see* Abscess, eyelid
    - face NEC L03.212
    - finger (intrathecal) (periosteal) (subcutaneous) (subcuticular) L03.02-
    - foot —*see* Lymphangitis, acute, lower limb
    - gluteal (region) L03.327
    - groin L03.324
    - hand —*see* Lymphangitis, acute, upper limb
    - head NEC L03.891
      - face (any part, except ear, eye and nose) L03.212
    - heel —*see* Lymphangitis, acute, lower limb
    - hip —*see* Lymphangitis, acute, lower limb
    - jaw (region) L03.212
    - knee —*see* Lymphangitis, acute, lower limb
    - leg —*see* Lymphangitis, acute, lower limb
    - lower limb L03.12-
      - toe —*see* Lymphangitis, acute, toe
    - navel L03.326
    - neck (region) L03.222
    - orbit, orbital —*see* Cellulitis, orbit
    - pectoral (region) L03.323
    - perineal, perineum L03.325
    - scalp (any part) L03.891
    - shoulder —*see* Lymphangitis, acute, upper limb

- **Lymphangitis** *(continued)*
  - acute *(continued)*
    - specified site NEC L03.898
    - thigh —*see* Lymphangitis, acute, lower limb
    - thumb (intrathecal) (periosteal) (subcutaneous) (subcuticular) —*see* Lymphangitis, acute, finger
    - toe (intrathecal) (periosteal) (subcutaneous) (subcuticular) L03.04-
    - trunk L03.329
      - abdominal wall L03.321
      - back (any part) L03.322
      - buttock L03.327
      - chest wall L03.323
      - groin L03.324
      - perineal, perineum L03.325
      - umbilicus L03.326
    - umbilicus L03.326
    - upper limb L03.12-
      - axilla —*see* Lymphangitis, acute, axilla
      - finger —*see* Lymphangitis, acute, finger
      - thumb —*see* Lymphangitis, acute, finger
    - wrist —*see* Lymphangitis, acute, upper limb
  - breast
    - gestational —*see* Mastitis, obstetric
  - chancroidal A57
  - chronic (any site) I89.1
  - due to
    - Brugia (malayi) B74.1
      - timori B74.2
    - Wuchereria bancrofti B74.0
  - following ectopic or molar pregnancy O08.89
  - penis
    - acute N48.29
    - gonococcal (acute) (chronic) A54.09
  - puerperal, postpartum, childbirth O86.89
  - strumous, tuberculous A18.2
  - subacute (any site) I89.1
  - tuberculous —*see* Tuberculosis, lymph gland
- **Lymphatic** (vessel) —*see* condition
- **Lymphatism** E32.8
- **Lymphectasia** I89.0
- **Lymphedema** (acquired) —*see also* Elephantiasis
  - congenital Q82.0
  - hereditary (chronic) (idiopathic) Q82.0
  - postmastectomy I97.2
  - praecox I89.0
  - secondary I89.0
  - surgical NEC I97.89
    - postmastectomy (syndrome) I97.2
- **Lymphoblastic** —*see* condition
- **Lymphoblastoma** (diffuse) —*see* Lymphoma, lymphoblastic (diffuse)
  - giant follicular —*see* Lymphoma, lymphoblastic (diffuse)
  - macrofollicular —*see* Lymphoma, lymphoblastic (diffuse)
- **Lymphocele** I89.8
- **Lymphocytic**
  - chorioencephalitis (acute) (serous) A87.2
  - choriomeningitis (acute) (serous) A87.2
  - meningoencephalitis A87.2

- **Lymphocytoma, benign cutis** L98.8
- **Lymphocytopenia** D72.810
- **Lymphocytosis** (symptomatic) D72.820
  - infectious (acute) B33.8
- **Lymphoepithelioma** —*see* Neoplasm, malignant, by site
- **Lymphogranuloma** (malignant) —*see also* Lymphoma, Hodgkin
  - chlamydial A55
  - inguinale A55
  - venereum (any site) (chlamydial) (with stricture of rectum) A55
- **Lymphogranulomatosis** (malignant) —*see also* Lymphoma, Hodgkin
  - benign (Boeck's sarcoid) (Schaumann's) D86.1
- **Lymphohistiocytosis, hemophagocytic** (familial) D76.1
- **Lymphoid** —*see* condition
- **Lymphoma** (of) (malignant) C85.90
  - adult T-cell (HTLV-1-associated) (acute variant) (chronic variant) (lymphomatoid variant) (smouldering variant) C91.5-
  - anaplastic large cell
    - ALK-negative C84.7-
    - ALK-positive C84.6-
    - CD30-positive C84.6-
    - primary cutaneous C86.6
  - angioimmunoblastic T-cell C86.5
  - BALT C88.4
  - B-cell C85.1-
  - B-precursor C83.5-
  - blastic NK-cell C86.4
  - blastic plasmacytoid dendritic cell neoplasm (BPDCN) C86.4
  - blastic plasmacytoid dendritic cell neoplasm (BPDCN) C86.4
  - bronchial-associated lymphoid tissue [BALT-lymphoma] C88.4
  - Burkitt (atypical) C83.7-
  - Burkitt-like C83.7-
  - centrocytic C83.1-
  - cutaneous follicle center C82.6-
  - cutaneous T-cell C84.A-
  - diffuse follicle center C82.5-
  - diffuse large cell C83.3-
    - anaplastic C83.3-
    - B-cell C83.3-
    - CD30-positive C83.3-
    - centroblastic C83.3-
    - immunoblastic C83.3-
    - plasmablastic C83.3-
    - subtype not specified C83.3-
    - T-cell rich C83.3-
  - enteropathy-type (associated) (intestinal) T-cell C86.2
  - extranodal NK/T-cell, nasal type C86.0
  - extranodal marginal zone B-cell lymphoma of mucosa-associated lymphoid tissue [MALT-lymphoma] C88.4
  - follicular C82.9-
    - grade
      - I C82.0-
      - II C82.1-
      - III C82.2-
      - IIIa C82.3-
      - IIIb C82.4-
    - specified NEC C82.8-
  - hepatosplenic T-cell (alpha-beta) (gamma-delta) C86.1
  - histiocytic C85.9-
    - true C96.A
  - Hodgkin C81.9
    - lymphocyte-rich (classical) C81.4-

- **Lymphoma** *(continued)*
  - Hodgkin *(continued)*
    - lymphocyte depleted (classical) C81.3-
    - mixed cellularity (classical) C81.2-
    - nodular sclerosis (classical) C81.1-
    - specified NEC (classical) C81.7-
    - nodular
      - lymphocyte predominant C81.0-
      - sclerosis (classical) C81.1-
  - intravascular large B-cell C83.8-
  - Lennert's C84.4-
  - lymphoblastic B-cell C83.5-
  - lymphoblastic (diffuse) C83.5-
  - lymphoblastic T-cell C83.5-
  - lymphoepithelioid C84.4-
  - lymphoplasmacytic C83.0-
    - with IgM-production C88.0
  - MALT C88.4
  - mantle cell C83.1-
  - mature T-cell NEC C84.4-
  - mature T/NK-cell C84.9-
    - specified NEC C84.Z-
  - mediastinal (thymic) large B-cell C85.2-
  - Mediterranean C88.3
  - mucosa-associated lymphoid tissue [MALT-lymphoma] C88.4
  - NK/T cell C84.9-
  - nodal marginal zone C83.0-
  - non-follicular (diffuse) C83.9-
    - specified NEC C83.8-
  - non-Hodgkin (*see also* Lymphoma, by type) C85.9-
    - specified NEC C85.8-
  - non-leukemic variant of B-CLL C83.0-
  - peripheral T-cell, not classified C84.4-
  - primary cutaneous
    - anaplastic large cell C86.6
    - CD30-positive large T-cell C86.6
  - primary effusion B-cell C83.8-
  - SALT C88.4
  - skin-associated lymphoid tissue [SALT-lymphoma] C88.4
  - small cell B-cell C83.0-
  - splenic marginal zone C83.0-
  - subcutaneous panniculitis-like T-cell C86.3
  - T-precursor C83.5-
  - true histiocytic C96.A
- **Lymphomatosis** —*see* Lymphoma
- **Lymphopathia venereum, veneris** A55
- **Lymphopenia** D72.810
- **Lymphoplasmacytic leukemia** —*see* Leukemia, chronic lymphocytic, B-cell type
- **Lymphoproliferation, X-linked disease** D82.3
- **Lymphoreticulosis, benign** (of inoculation) A28.1
- **Lymphorrhea** I89.8
- **Lymphosarcoma** (diffuse) (*see also* Lymphoma) C85.9-
- **Lymphostasis** I89.8
- **Lypemania** —*see* Melancholia
- **Lysine and hydroxylysine metabolism disorder** E72.3
- **Lyssa** —*see* Rabies

M

Macacus ear Q17.3

Maceration, wet feet, tropical (syndrome) T69.02-

MacLeod's syndrome J43.0

Macrocephalia, macrocephaly Q75.3

Macrocheilia, macrochilia (congenital) Q18.6

Macrocolon (*see also* Megacolon) Q43.1

Macrocornea Q15.8
- with glaucoma Q15.0

Macrocytic *—see* condition

Macrocytosis D75.89

Macrodactylia, macrodactylism (fingers) (thumbs) Q74.0
- toes Q74.2

Macrodontia K00.2

Macrogenia M26.05

Macrogenitosomia (adrenal) (male) (praecox) E25.9
- congenital E25.0

Macroglobulinemia (idiopathic) (primary) C88.0
- monoclonal (essential) D47.2
- Waldenström C88.0

Macroglossia (congenital) Q38.2
- acquired K14.8

Macrognathia, macrognathism (congenital) (mandibular) (maxillary) M26.09

Macrogyria (congenital) Q04.8

Macrohydrocephalus *—see* Hydrocephalus

Macromastia *—see* Hypertrophy, breast

Macrophthalmos Q11.3
- in congenital glaucoma Q15.0

Macropsia H53.15

Macrosigmoid K59.39
- congenital Q43.2

Macrospondylitis, acromegalic E22.0

Macrostomia (congenital) Q18.4

Macrotia (external ear) (congenital) Q17.1

Macula
- cornea, corneal *—see* Opacity, cornea
- degeneration (atrophic) (exudative) (senile) *—see also* Degeneration, macula
  - hereditary *—see* Dystrophy, retina

Maculae ceruleae B85.1

Maculopathy, toxic *—see* Degeneration, macula, toxic

Madarosis (eyelid) H02.729
- left H02.726
  - lower H02.725
  - upper H02.724
- right H02.723
  - lower H02.722
  - upper H02.721

Madelung's
- deformity (radius) Q74.0
- disease
  - radial deformity Q74.0
  - symmetrical lipomas, neck E88.89

Madness *—see* Psychosis

Madura
- foot B47.9
  - actinomycotic B47.1
  - mycotic B47.0

Maduromycosis B47.0

Maffucci's syndrome Q78.4

Magnesium metabolism disorder *—see* Disorder, metabolism, magnesium

Main en griffe (acquired) *—see also* Deformity, limb, clawhand
- congenital Q74.0

Maintenance (encounter for)
- antineoplastic chemotherapy Z51.11
- antineoplastic radiation therapy Z51.0
- methadone F11.20

Majocchi's
- disease L81.7
- granuloma B35.8

Major *—see* condition

Malabar itch (any site) B35.5

Malabsorption K90.9
- calcium K90.89
- carbohydrate K90.49
- disaccharide E73.9
- fat K90.49
- galactose E74.20
- glucose (-galactose) E74.39
- intestinal K90.9
  - specified NEC K90.89
- isomaltose E74.31
- lactose E73.9
- methionine E72.19
- monosaccharide E74.39
- postgastrectomy K91.2
- postsurgical K91.2
- protein K90.49
- starch K90.49
- sucrose E74.39
- syndrome K90.9
  - postsurgical K91.2

Malacia, bone (adult) M83.9
- juvenile *—see* Rickets

Malacoplakia
- bladder N32.89
- pelvis (kidney) N28.89
- ureter N28.89
- urethra N36.8

Malacosteon, juvenile *—see* Rickets

Maladaptation *—see* Maladjustment

Maladie de Roger Q21.0

Maladjustment
- conjugal Z63.0
  - involving divorce or estrangement Z63.5
- educational Z55.4
- family Z63.9
- marital Z63.0
  - involving divorce or estrangement Z63.5
- occupational NEC Z56.89
- simple, adult *—see* Disorder, adjustment
- situational *—see* Disorder, adjustment
- social Z60.9
  - due to
    - acculturation difficulty Z60.3
    - discrimination and persecution (perceived) Z60.5
    - exclusion and isolation Z60.4
    - life-cycle (phase of life) transition Z60.0
    - rejection Z60.4
    - specified reason NEC Z60.8

Malaise R53.81

Malakoplakia *—see* Malacoplakia

Malaria, malarial (fever) B54
- with
  - blackwater fever B50.8
    - hemoglobinuric (bilious) B50.8
  - hemoglobinuria B50.8
- accidentally induced (therapeutically) - code by type under Malaria
- algid B50.9
- cerebral B50.0 *[G94]*
- clinically diagnosed (without parasitological confirmation) B54
- congenital NEC P37.4
  - falciparum P37.3
- congestion, congestive B54
- continued (fever) B50.9
- estivo-autumnal B50.9
- falciparum B50.9
  - with complications NEC B50.8
    - cerebral B50.0 *[G94]*
  - severe B50.8
- hemorrhagic B54
- malariae B52.9
  - with
    - complications NEC B52.8
    - glomerular disorder B52.0
- malignant (tertian) *—see* Malaria, falciparum
- mixed infections - code to first listed type in B50-B53
- ovale B53.0
- parasitologically confirmed NEC B53.8
- pernicious, acute *—see* Malaria, falciparum
- Plasmodium (P.)
  - falciparum NEC *—see* Malaria, falciparum
  - malariae NEC B52.9
    - with Plasmodium
      - falciparum (and or vivax) *—see* Malaria, falciparum
      - vivax *—see also* Malaria, vivax
        - and falciparum *—see* Malaria, falciparum
  - ovale B53.0
    - with Plasmodium malariae *—see also* Malaria, malariae
      - and vivax *—see also* Malaria, vivax
        - and falciparum *—see* Malaria, falciparum
  - simian B53.1
    - with Plasmodium malariae *—see also* Malaria, malariae
      - and vivax *—see also* Malaria, vivax
        - and falciparum *—see* Malaria, falciparum
  - vivax NEC B51.9
    - with Plasmodium falciparum *—see* Malaria, falciparum
- quartan *—see* Malaria, malariae
- quotidian *—see* Malaria, falciparum
- recurrent B54
- remittent B54
- specified type NEC (parasitologically confirmed) B53.8
- spleen B54
- subtertian (fever) *—see* Malaria, falciparum
- tertian (benign) *—see also* Malaria, vivax
  - malignant B50.9
- tropical B50.9

Malaria, malarial *(continued)*
- typhoid B54
- vivax B51.9
  - with
    - complications NEC B51.8
    - ruptured spleen B51.0

Malassimilation K90.9

Malassez's disease (cystic) N50.89

Mal de los pintos *—see* Pinta

Mal de mer T75.3

Maldescent, testis Q53.9
- bilateral Q53.20
  - abdominal Q53.211
  - perineal Q53.22
- unilateral Q53.10
  - abdominal Q53.111
  - perineal Q53.12

Maldevelopment *—see also* Anomaly
- brain Q07.9
- colon Q43.9
- hip Q74.2
  - congenital dislocation Q65.2
    - bilateral Q65.1
    - unilateral Q65.0-
- mastoid process Q75.8
- middle ear Q16.4
  - except ossicles Q16.4
  - ossicles Q16.3
- ossicles Q16.3
- spine Q76.49
- toe Q74.2

Male type pelvis Q74.2
- with disproportion (fetopelvic) O33.3
  - causing obstructed labor O65.3

Malformation (congenital) *—see also* Anomaly
- adrenal gland Q89.1
- affecting multiple systems with skeletal changes NEC Q87.5
- alimentary tract Q45.9
  - specified type NEC Q45.8
  - upper Q40.9
    - specified type NEC Q40.8
- aorta Q25.40
  - absence Q25.41
  - aneurysm, congenital Q25.43
  - aplasia Q25.41
  - atresia Q25.29
    - aortic arch Q25.21
  - coarctation (preductal) (postductal) Q25.1
  - dilatation, congenital Q25.44
  - hypoplasia Q25.42
  - patent ductus arteriosus Q25.0
  - specified type NEC Q25.49
  - stenosis Q25.1
    - supravalvular Q25.3
- aortic valve Q23.9
  - specified NEC Q23.8
- arteriovenous, aneurysmatic (congenital) Q27.30
  - brain Q28.2
  - cerebral Q28.2
  - peripheral Q27.30
    - digestive system Q27.33
    - lower limb Q27.32
    - other specified site Q27.39
    - renal vessel Q27.34
    - upper limb Q27.31
  - precerebral vessels (nonruptured) Q28.0
- auricle
  - ear (congenital) Q17.3
    - acquired H61.119
      - left H61.112
        - with right H61.113
      - right H61.111
        - with left H61.113

Malformation *(continued)*
bile duct Q44.5
bladder Q64.79
aplasia Q64.5
diverticulum Q64.6
exstrophy *—see* Exstrophy, bladder
neck obstruction Q64.31
bone Q79.9
face Q75.9
specified type NEC Q75.8
skull Q75.9
specified type NEC Q75.8
brain (multiple) Q04.9
arteriovenous Q28.2
specified type NEC Q04.8
branchial cleft Q18.2
breast Q83.9
specified type NEC Q83.8
broad ligament Q50.6
bronchus Q32.4
bursa Q79.9
cardiac
chambers Q20.9
specified type NEC Q20.8
septum Q21.9
specified type NEC Q21.8
cerebral Q04.9
vessels Q28.3
cervix uteri Q51.9
specified type NEC Q51.828
Chiari
Type I G93.5
Type II Q07.01
choroid (congenital) Q14.3
plexus Q07.8
circulatory system Q28.9
cochlea Q16.5
cornea Q13.4
coronary vessels Q24.5
corpus callosum (congenital) Q04.0
diaphragm Q79.1
digestive system NEC, specified type NEC Q45.8
dura Q07.9
brain Q04.9
spinal Q06.9
ear Q17.9
causing impairment of hearing Q16.9
external Q17.9
accessory auricle Q17.0
causing impairment of hearing Q16.9
absence of
auditory canal Q16.1
auricle Q16.0
macrotia Q17.1
microtia Q17.2
misplacement Q17.4
misshapen NEC Q17.3
prominence Q17.5
specified type NEC Q17.8
inner Q16.5
middle Q16.4
absence of eustachian tube Q16.2
ossicles (fusion) Q16.3
ossicles Q16.3
specified type NEC Q17.8
epididymis Q55.4
esophagus Q39.9
specified type NEC Q39.8
eye Q15.9
lid Q10.3
specified NEC Q15.8
fallopian tube Q50.6
genital organ *—see* Anomaly, genitalia

Malformation *(continued)*
great
artery Q25.9
aorta *—see* Malformation, aorta
pulmonary artery *—see* Malformation, pulmonary, artery
specified type NEC Q25.8
vein Q26.9
anomalous
portal venous connection Q26.5
pulmonary venous connection Q26.4
partial Q26.3
total Q26.2
persistent left superior vena cava Q26.1
portal vein-hepatic artery fistula Q26.6
specified type NEC Q26.8
vena cava stenosis, congenital Q26.0
gum Q38.6
hair Q84.2
heart Q24.9
specified type NEC Q24.8
integument Q84.9
specified type NEC Q84.8
internal ear Q16.5
intestine Q43.9
specified type NEC Q43.8
iris Q13.2
joint Q74.9
ankle Q74.2
lumbosacral Q76.49
sacroiliac Q74.2
specified type NEC Q74.8
kidney Q63.9
accessory Q63.0
giant Q63.3
horseshoe Q63.1
hydronephrosis Q62.0
malposition Q63.2
specified type NEC Q63.8
lacrimal apparatus Q10.6
lip Q38.0
lingual Q38.3
liver Q44.7
lung Q33.9
meninges or membrane (congenital) Q07.9
cerebral Q04.8
spinal (cord) Q06.9
middle ear Q16.4
ossicles Q16.3
mitral valve Q23.9
specified NEC Q23.8
Mondini's (congenital) (malformation, cochlea) Q16.5
mouth (congenital) Q38.6
multiple types NEC Q89.7
musculoskeletal system Q79.9
myocardium Q24.8
nail Q84.6
nervous system (central) Q07.9
nose Q30.9
specified type NEC Q30.8
optic disc Q14.2
orbit Q10.7
ovary Q50.39
palate Q38.5
parathyroid gland Q89.2
pelvic organs or tissues NEC
in pregnancy or childbirth O34.8-
causing obstructed labor O65.5
penis Q55.69
aplasia Q55.5
curvature (lateral) Q55.61

Malformation *(continued)*
penis *(continued)*
hypoplasia Q55.62
pericardium Q24.8
peripheral vascular system Q27.9
specified type NEC Q27.8
pharynx Q38.8
precerebral vessels Q28.1
prostate Q55.4
pulmonary
arteriovenous Q25.72
artery Q25.9
atresia Q25.5
specified type NEC Q25.79
stenosis Q25.6
valve Q22.3
renal artery Q27.2
respiratory system Q34.9
retina Q14.1
scrotum *—see* Malformation, testis and scrotum
seminal vesicles Q55.4
sense organs NEC Q07.9
skin Q82.9
specified NEC Q89.8
spinal
cord Q06.9
nerve root Q07.8
spine Q76.49
kyphosis *—see* Kyphosis, congenital
lordosis *—see* Lordosis, congenital
spleen Q89.09
stomach Q40.3
specified type NEC Q40.2
teeth, tooth K00.9
tendon Q79.9
testis and scrotum Q55.20
aplasia Q55.0
hypoplasia Q55.1
polyorchism Q55.21
retractile testis Q55.22
scrotal transposition Q55.23
specified NEC Q55.29
throat Q38.8
thorax, bony Q76.9
thyroid gland Q89.2
tongue (congenital) Q38.3
hypertrophy Q38.2
tie Q38.1
trachea Q32.1
tricuspid valve Q22.9
specified type NEC Q22.8
umbilical cord NEC (complicating delivery) O69.89
umbilicus Q89.9
ureter Q62.8
agenesis Q62.4
duplication Q62.5
malposition *—see* Malposition, congenital, ureter
obstructive defect *—see* Defect, obstructive, ureter
vesico-uretero-renal reflux Q62.7
urethra Q64.79
aplasia Q64.5
duplication Q64.74
posterior valves Q64.2
prolapse Q64.71
stricture Q64.32
urinary system Q64.9
uterus Q51.9
specified type NEC Q51.818
vagina Q52.4
vascular system, peripheral Q27.9
vas deferens Q55.4
atresia Q55.3
venous *—see* Anomaly, vein(s)
vulva Q52.70

Malfunction *—see also* Dysfunction
cardiac electronic device T82.119
electrode T82.110
pulse generator T82.111
specified type NEC T82.118
catheter device NEC T85.618
cystostomy T83.010
dialysis (renal) (vascular) T82.41
intraperitoneal T85.611
infusion NEC T82.514
cranial T85.610
epidural T85.610
intrathecal T85.610
spinal T85.610
subarachnoid T85.610
subdural T85.610
urinary (*see also* Breakdown, device, catheter), T83.018
colostomy K94.03
valve K94.03
cystostomy (stoma) N99.512
catheter T83.010
enteric stoma K94.13
enterostomy K94.13
esophagostomy K94.33
gastroenteric K31.89
gastrostomy K94.23
ileostomy K94.13
valve K94.13
intrathecal infusion pump T85.615
jejunostomy K94.13
nervous system device, implant or graft, specified NEC T85.615
pacemaker *—see* Malfunction, cardiac electronic device
prosthetic device, internal *—see* Complications, prosthetic device, by site, mechanical
tracheostomy J95.03
urinary device NEC *—see* Complication, genitourinary, device, urinary, mechanical
valve
colostomy K94.03
heart T82.09
ileostomy K94.13
vascular graft or shunt NEC *—see* Complication, cardiovascular device, mechanical, vascular
ventricular (communicating shunt) T85.01

Malherbe's tumor *—see* Neoplasm, skin, benign

Malibu disease L98.8

Malignancy *—see also* Neoplasm, malignant, by site
unspecified site (primary) C80.1

Malignant *—see* condition

Malingerer, malingering Z76.5

Mallet finger (acquired) *—see* Deformity, finger, mallet finger
congenital Q74.0
sequelae of rickets E64.3

Malleus A24.0

Mallory's bodies R89.7

Mallory-Weiss syndrome K22.6

Malnutrition E46
degree
first E44.1
mild (protein) E44.1
moderate (protein) E44.0
second E44.0

Malnutrition *(continued)*
- degree *(continued)*
  - severe (protein-energy) E43
    - intermediate form E42
      - with
        - kwashiorkor (and marasmus) E42
        - marasmus E41
  - third E43
- following gastrointestinal surgery K91.2
- intrauterine
  - light-for-dates —*see* Light for dates
  - small-for-dates —*see* Small for dates
- lack of care, or neglect (child) (infant) T76.02
  - confirmed T74.02
- malignant E40
- protein E46
  - calorie E46
    - mild E44.1
    - moderate E44.0
    - severe E43
      - intermediate form E42
        - with
          - kwashiorkor (and marasmus) E42
          - marasmus E41
  - energy E46
    - mild E44.1
    - moderate E44.0
    - severe E43
      - intermediate form E42
        - with
          - kwashiorkor (and marasmus) E42
          - marasmus E41
- severe (protein-energy) E43
  - with
    - kwashiorkor (and marasmus) E42
    - marasmus E41

Malocclusion (teeth) M26.4
- Angle's M26.219
  - class I M26.211
  - class II M26.212
  - class III M26.213
- due to
  - abnormal swallowing M26.59
  - mouth breathing M26.59
  - tongue, lip or finger habits M26.59
- temporomandibular (joint) M26.69

Malposition
- cervix —*see* Malposition, uterus
- congenital
  - adrenal (gland) Q89.1
  - alimentary tract Q45.8
    - lower Q43.8
    - upper Q40.8
  - aorta Q25.49
  - appendix Q43.8
  - arterial trunk Q20.0
  - artery (peripheral) Q27.8
    - coronary Q24.5
    - digestive system Q27.8
    - lower limb Q27.8
    - pulmonary Q25.79
    - specified site NEC Q27.8
    - upper limb Q27.8
  - auditory canal Q17.8
    - causing impairment of hearing Q16.9
  - auricle (ear) Q17.4
    - causing impairment of hearing Q16.9
    - cervical Q18.2
  - biliary duct or passage Q44.5
  - bladder (mucosa) —*see* Exstrophy, bladder
  - brachial plexus Q07.8
  - brain tissue Q04.8
  - breast Q83.8
  - bronchus Q32.4
  - cecum Q43.8
  - clavicle Q74.0
  - colon Q43.8
  - digestive organ or tract NEC Q45.8
    - lower Q43.8
    - upper Q40.8
  - ear (auricle) (external) Q17.4
    - ossicles Q16.3
  - endocrine (gland) NEC Q89.2
  - epiglottis Q31.8
  - eustachian tube Q17.8
  - eye Q15.8
  - facial features Q18.8
  - fallopian tube Q50.6
  - finger(s) Q68.1
    - supernumerary Q69.0
  - foot Q66.9
  - gallbladder Q44.1
  - gastrointestinal tract Q45.8
  - genitalia, genital organ(s) or tract
    - female Q52.8
      - external Q52.79
      - internal NEC Q52.8
    - male Q55.8
  - glottis Q31.8
  - hand Q68.1
  - heart Q24.8
    - dextrocardia Q24.0
      - with complete transposition of viscera Q89.3
  - hepatic duct Q44.5
  - hip (joint) Q65.89
  - intestine (large) (small) Q43.8
    - with anomalous adhesions, fixation or malrotation Q43.3
  - joint NEC Q68.8
  - kidney Q63.2
  - larynx Q31.8
  - limb Q68.8
    - lower Q68.8
    - upper Q68.8
  - liver Q44.7
  - lung (lobe) Q33.8
  - nail(s) Q84.6
  - nerve Q07.8
  - nervous system NEC Q07.8
  - nose, nasal (septum) Q30.8
  - organ or site not listed —*see* Anomaly, by site
  - ovary Q50.39
  - pancreas Q45.3
  - parathyroid (gland) Q89.2
  - patella Q74.1
  - peripheral vascular system Q27.8
  - pituitary (gland) Q89.2
  - respiratory organ or system NEC Q34.8
  - rib (cage) Q76.6
    - supernumerary in cervical region Q76.5
  - scapula Q74.0
  - shoulder Q74.0
  - spinal cord Q06.8
  - spleen Q89.09
  - sternum NEC Q76.7
  - stomach Q40.2
  - symphysis pubis Q74.2
  - thymus (gland) Q89.2
  - thyroid (gland) (tissue) Q89.2
    - cartilage Q31.8
  - toe(s) Q66.9
    - supernumerary Q69.2
  - tongue Q38.3
  - trachea Q32.1
  - ureter Q62.60
    - deviation Q62.61
    - displacement Q62.62
    - ectopia Q62.63
    - specified type NEC Q62.69
  - uterus Q51.818
  - vein(s) (peripheral) Q27.8
    - great Q26.8
  - vena cava (inferior) (superior) Q26.8
- device, implant or graft (*see also* Complications, by site and type, mechanical) T85.628
  - arterial graft NEC —*see* Complication, cardiovascular device, mechanical, vascular
  - breast (implant) T85.42
  - catheter NEC T85.628
    - cystostomy T83.020
    - dialysis (renal) T82.42
      - intraperitoneal T85.621
    - infusion NEC T82.524
      - spinal (epidural) (subdural) T85.620
    - urinary (*see also* Displacement, device, catheter, urinary), T83.028
  - electronic (electrode) (pulse generator) (stimulator)
    - bone T84.320
    - cardiac T82.129
      - electrode T82.120
      - pulse generator T82.121
      - specified type NEC T82.128
    - nervous system —*see* Complication, prosthetic device, mechanical, electronic nervous system stimulator
    - urinary —*see* Complication, genitourinary, device, urinary, mechanical
  - fixation, internal (orthopedic) NEC —*see* Complication, fixation device, mechanical
  - gastrointestinal —*see* Complications, prosthetic device, mechanical, gastrointestinal device
  - genital NEC T83.428
    - intrauterine contraceptive device (string) T83.32
    - penile prosthesis (cylinder) (implanted) (pump) (resevoir) T83.420
    - testicular prosthesis T83.421
  - heart NEC —*see* Complication, cardiovascular device, mechanical
  - joint prosthesis —*see* Complication, joint prosthesis, mechanical
  - ocular NEC —*see* Complications, prosthetic device, mechanical, ocular device
  - orthopedic NEC —*see* Complication, orthopedic, device, mechanical
  - specified NEC T85.628
  - urinary NEC —*see also* Complication, genitourinary, device, urinary, mechanical
    - graft T83.22
  - vascular NEC —*see* Complication, cardiovascular device, mechanical
  - ventricular intracranial shunt T85.02
- fetus —*see* Pregnancy, complicated by (management affected by), presentation, fetal
- gallbladder K82.8
- gastrointestinal tract, congenital Q45.8
- heart, congenital NEC Q24.8
- joint prosthesis —*see* Complications, joint prosthesis, mechanical, displacement, by site
- stomach K31.89
  - congenital Q40.2
- tooth, teeth, fully erupted M26.30
- uterus (acute) (acquired) (adherent) (asymptomatic) (postinfectional) (postpartal, old) N85.4
  - anteflexion or anteversion N85.4
    - congenital Q51.818
  - flexion N85.4
    - lateral —*see* Lateroversion, uterus
  - inversion N85.5
  - lateral (flexion) (version) —*see* Lateroversion, uterus
    - in pregnancy or childbirth —*see* subcategory O34.5
  - retroflexion or retroversion —*see* Retroversion, uterus

Malposture R29.3

Malrotation
- cecum Q43.3
- colon Q43.3
- intestine Q43.3
- kidney Q63.2

Maltreatment
- adult
  - abandonment
    - confirmed T74.01
    - suspected T76.01
  - confirmed T74.91
  - history of Z91.419
  - neglect
    - confirmed T74.01
    - suspected T76.01
  - physical abuse
    - confirmed T74.11
    - suspected T76.11
  - psychological abuse
    - confirmed T74.31
    - suspected T76.31
    - history of Z91.411
  - sexual abuse
    - confirmed T74.21
    - suspected T76.21
  - suspected T76.91
- child
  - abandonment
    - confirmed T74.02
    - suspected T76.02
  - confirmed T74.92
  - history of —*see* History, personal (of), abuse
  - neglect
    - confirmed T74.02
    - history of —*see* History, personal (of), abuse
    - suspected T76.02
  - physical abuse
    - confirmed T74.12
    - history of —*see* History, personal (of), abuse
    - suspected T76.12

Maltreatment *(continued)*
child *(continued)*
psychological abuse
confirmed T74.32
history of *—see* History, personal (of), abuse
suspected T76.32
sexual abuse
confirmed T74.22
history of *—see* History, personal (of), abuse
suspected T76.22
suspected T76.92
personal history of Z91.89

Malta fever *—see* Brucellosis

Maltworker's lung J67.4

Malunion, fracture *—see* Fracture, by site

Mammillitis N61.0
puerperal, postpartum O91.02

Mammitis *—see* Mastitis

Mammogram (examination) Z12.39
routine Z12.31

Mammoplasia N62

Management (of)
bone conduction hearing device (implanted) Z45.320
cardiac pacemaker NEC Z45.018
cerebrospinal fluid drainage device Z45.41
cochlear device (implanted) Z45.321
contraceptive Z30.9
specified NEC Z30.8
implanted device Z45.9
specified NEC Z45.89
infusion pump Z45.1
procreative Z31.9
male factor infertility in female Z31.81
specified NEC Z31.89
prosthesis (external) (*see also* Fitting) Z44.9
implanted Z45.9
specified NEC Z45.89
renal dialysis catheter Z49.01
vascular access device Z45.2

Mangled *—see* specified injury by site

Mania (monopolar) *—see also* Disorder, mood, manic episode
with psychotic symptoms F30.2
without psychotic symptoms F30.10
mild F30.11
moderate F30.12
severe F30.13
Bell's F30.8
chronic (recurrent) F31.89
hysterical F44.89
puerperal F30.8
recurrent F31.89

Manic depression F31.9

Manic-depressive insanity, psychosis, or syndrome *—see* Disorder, bipolar

Mannosidosis E77.1

Mansonelliasis, mansonellosis B74.4

Manson's
disease B65.1
schistosomiasis B65.1

Manual *—see* condition

Maple-bark-stripper's lung (disease) J67.6

Maple-syrup-urine disease E71.0

Marable's syndrome (celiac artery compression) I77.4

Marasmus E41
due to malnutrition E41
intestinal E41
nutritional E41
senile R54
tuberculous NEC *—see* Tuberculosis

Marble
bones Q78.2
skin R23.8

Marburg virus disease A98.3

March
fracture *—see* Fracture, traumatic, stress, by site
hemoglobinuria D59.6

Marchesani (-Weill) **syndrome** Q87.0

Marchiafava (-Bignami) **syndrome or disease** G37.1

Marchiafava-Micheli syndrome D59.5

Marcus Gunn's syndrome Q07.8

Marfan's syndrome *—see* Syndrome, Marfan's

Marie-Bamberger disease *—see* Osteoarthropathy, hypertrophic, specified NEC

Marie-Charcot-Tooth neuropathic muscular atrophy G60.0

Marie's
cerebellar ataxia (late-onset) G11.2
disease or syndrome (acromegaly) E22.0

Marie-Strümpell arthritis, disease or spondylitis *—see* Spondylitis, ankylosing

Marion's disease (bladder neck obstruction) N32.0

Marital conflict Z63.0

Mark
port wine Q82.5
raspberry Q82.5
strawberry Q82.5
stretch L90.6
tattoo L81.8

Marker heterochromatin *—see* Extra, marker chromosomes

Maroteaux-Lamy syndrome (mild) (severe) E76.29

Marrow (bone)
arrest D61.9
poor function D75.89

Marseilles fever A77.1

Marsh fever *—see* Malaria

Marshall's (hidrotic) **ectodermal dysplasia** Q82.4

Marsh's disease (exophthalmic goiter) E05.00
with storm E05.01

Masculinization (female) **with adrenal hyperplasia** E25.9
congenital E25.0

Masculinovoblastoma D27.-

Masochism (sexual) F65.51

Mason's lung J62.8

Mass
abdominal R19.00
epigastric R19.06
generalized R19.07
left lower quadrant R19.04

Mass *(continued)*
abdominal *(continued)*
left upper quadrant R19.02
periumbilic R19.05
right lower quadrant R19.03
right upper quadrant R19.01
specified site NEC R19.09
breast (*see also* Lump, breast) N63.0
chest R22.2
cystic *—see* Cyst
ear H93.8-
head R22.0
intra-abdominal (diffuse) (generalized) *—see* Mass, abdominal
kidney N28.89
liver R16.0
localized (skin) R22.9
chest R22.2
head R22.0
limb
lower R22.4-
upper R22.3-
neck R22.1
trunk R22.2
lung R91.8
malignant *—see* Neoplasm, malignant, by site
neck R22.1
pelvic (diffuse) (generalized) *—see* Mass, abdominal
specified organ NEC *—see* Disease, by site
splenic R16.1
substernal thyroid *—see* Goiter
superficial (localized) R22.9
umbilical (diffuse) (generalized) R19.09

Massive *—see* condition

Mast cell
disease, systemic tissue D47.02
neoplasm
malignant C96.20
specified type NEC C96.29
of uncertain behavior NEC D47.09
leukemia C94.3-
sarcoma C96.22
tumor D47.09

Mastalgia N64.4

Masters-Allen syndrome N83.8

Mastitis (acute) (diffuse) (nonpuerperal) (subacute) N61.0
with abscess N61.1
chronic (cystic) *—see* Mastopathy, cystic
cystic (Schimmelbusch's type) *—see* Mastopathy, cystic
fibrocystic *—see* Mastopathy, cystic
infective N61.0
newborn P39.0
interstitial, gestational or puerperal *—see* Mastitis, obstetric
neonatal (noninfective) P83.4
infective P39.0
obstetric (interstitial) (nonpurulent)
associated with
lactation O91.23
pregnancy O91.21-
puerperium O91.22
purulent
associated with
lactation O91.13
pregnancy O91.11-
puerperium O91.12
periductal *—see* Ectasia, mammary duct
phlegmonous *—see* Mastopathy, cystic

Mastitis *(continued)*
plasma cell *—see* Ectasia, mammary duct
without abscess N61.0

Mastocytoma (extracutaneous) D47.09
malignant C96.29
solitary D47.01

Mastocytosis D47.09
aggressive systemic C96.21
cutaneous (diffuse) (maculopapular) D47.01
congenital Q82.2
of neonatal onset Q82.2
of newborn onset Q82.2
indolent systemic D47.02
isolated bone marrow D47.02
malignant C96.29
systemic (indolent) (smoldering)
with an associated hematological non-mast cell lineage disease (SM-AHNMD) D47.02

Mastodynia N64.4

Mastoid *—see* condition

Mastoidalgia *—see* subcategory H92.0

Mastoiditis (coalescent) (hemorrhagic) (suppurative) H70.9-
acute, subacute H70.00-
complicated NEC H70.09-
subperiosteal H70.01-
chronic (necrotic) (recurrent) H70.1-
in (due to)
infectious disease NEC B99 *[H75.0-]*
parasitic disease NEC B89 *[H75.0-]*
tuberculosis A18.03
petrositis *—see* Petrositis
postauricular fistula *—see* Fistula, postauricular
specified NEC H70.89-
tuberculous A18.03

Mastopathy, mastopathia N64.9
chronica cystica *—see* Mastopathy, cystic
cystic (chronic) (diffuse) N60.1-
with epithelial proliferation N60.3-
diffuse cystic *—see* Mastopathy, cystic
estrogenic, oestrogenica N64.89
ovarian origin N64.89

Mastoplasia, mastoplastia N62

Masturbation (excessive) F98.8

Maternal care (for) *—see* Pregnancy (complicated by) (management affected by)

Matheiu's disease (leptospiral jaundice) A27.0

Mauclaire's disease or osteochondrosis *—see* Osteochondrosis, juvenile, hand, metacarpal

Maxcy's disease A75.2

Maxilla, maxillary *—see* condition

May (-Hegglin) **anomaly or syndrome** D72.0

McArdle (-Schmid) (-Pearson) **disease** (glycogen storage) E74.04

McCune-Albright syndrome Q78.1

McQuarrie's syndrome (idiopathic familial hypoglycemia) E16.2

Meadow's syndrome Q86.1

Measles (black) (hemorrhagic) (suppressed) B05.9

Measles *(continued)*
with
complications NEC B05.89
encephalitis B05.0
intestinal complications B05.4
keratitis (keratoconjunctivitis) B05.81
meningitis B05.1
otitis media B05.3
pneumonia B05.2
French *—see* Rubella
German *—see* Rubella
Liberty *—see* Rubella

Meatitis, urethral *—see* Urethritis

Meatus, meatal *—see* condition

Meat-wrappers' asthma J68.9

Meckel-Gruber syndrome Q61.9

Meckel's diverticulitis, diverticulum (displaced) (hypertrophic) Q43.0
malignant *—see* Table of Neoplasms, small intestine, malignant

Meconium
ileus, newborn P76.0
in cystic fibrosis E84.11
meaning meconium plug (without cystic fibrosis) P76.0
obstruction, newborn P76.0
due to fecaliths P76.0
in mucoviscidosis E84.11
peritonitis P78.0
plug syndrome (newborn) NEC P76.0

Median *—see also* condition
arcuate ligament syndrome I77.4
bar (prostate) (vesical orifice) *—see* Hyperplasia, prostate
rhomboid glossitis K14.2

Mediastinal shift R93.8

Mediastinitis (acute) (chronic) J98.51
syphilitic A52.73
tuberculous A15.8

Mediastinopericarditis *—see also* Pericarditis
acute I30.9
adhesive I31.0
chronic I31.8
rheumatic I09.2

Mediastinum, mediastinal *—see* condition

Medicine poisoning *—see* Table of Drugs and Chemicals, by drug, poisoning

Mediterranean
fever *—see* Brucellosis
familial M04.1
tick A77.1
kala-azar B55.0
leishmaniasis B55.0
tick fever A77.1

Medulla *—see* condition

Medullary cystic kidney Q61.5

Medullated fibers
optic (nerve) Q14.8
retina Q14.1

Medulloblastoma
desmoplastic C71.6
specified site *—see* Neoplasm, malignant, by site
unspecified site C71.6

Medulloepithelioma *—see also* Neoplasm, malignant, by site
teratoid *—see* Neoplasm, malignant, by site

Medullomyoblastoma
specified site *—see* Neoplasm, malignant, by site
unspecified site C71.6

Meekeren-Ehlers-Danlos syndrome Q79.6

Megacolon (acquired) (functional) (not Hirschsprung's disease) (in) K59.39
Chagas' disease B57.32
congenital, congenitum (aganglionic) Q43.1
Hirschsprung's (disease) Q43.1
toxic NEC K59.31
due to Clostridium difficile
not specified as recurrent A04.72
recurrent A04.71

Megaesophagus (functional) K22.0
congenital Q39.5
in (due to) Chagas' disease B57.31

Megalencephaly Q04.5

Megalerythema (epidemic) B08.3

Megaloappendix Q43.8

Megalocephalus, megalocephaly NEC Q75.3

Megalocornea Q15.8
with glaucoma Q15.0

Megalocytic anemia D53.1

Megalodactylia (fingers) (thumbs) (congenital) Q74.0
toes Q74.2

Megaloduodenum Q43.8

Megaloesophagus (functional) K22.0
congenital Q39.5

Megalogastria (acquired) K31.89
congenital Q40.2

Megalophthalmos Q11.3

Megalopsia H53.15

Megalosplenia *—see* Splenomegaly

Megaloureter N28.82
congenital Q62.2

Megarectum K62.89

Megasigmoid K59.39
congenital Q43.2

Megaureter N28.82
congenital Q62.2

Megavitamin-B6 syndrome E67.2

Megrim *—see* Migraine

Meibomian
cyst, infected *—see* Hordeolum
gland *—see* condition
sty, stye *—see* Hordeolum

Meibomitis *—see* Hordeolum

Meige-Milroy disease (chronic hereditary edema) Q82.0

Meige's syndrome Q82.0

Melalgia, nutritional E53.8

Melancholia F32.9
climacteric (single episode) F32.89
recurrent episode F33.8
hypochondriac F45.29
intermittent (single episode) F32.89
recurrent episode F33.8
involutional (single episode) F32.89
recurrent episode F33.8
menopausal (single episode) F32.89
recurrent episode F33.8
puerperal F32.89
reactive (emotional stress or trauma) F32.3
recurrent F33.9

Melancholia *(continued)*
senile F03
stuporous (single episode) F32.89
recurrent episode F33.8

Melanemia R79.89

Melanoameloblastoma *—see* Neoplasm, bone, benign

Melanoblastoma *—see* Melanoma

Melanocarcinoma *—see* Melanoma

Melanocytoma, eyeball D31.9-

Melanocytosis, neurocutaneous Q82.8

Melanoderma, melanodermia L81.4

Melanodontia, infantile K03.89

Melanodontoclasia K03.89

Melanoepithelioma *—see* Melanoma

Melanoma (malignant) C43.9
acral lentiginous, malignant *—see* Melanoma, skin, by site
amelanotic *—see* Melanoma, skin, by site
balloon cell *—see* Melanoma, skin, by site
benign *—see* Nevus
desmoplastic, malignant *—see* Melanoma, skin, by site
epithelioid cell *—see* Melanoma, skin, by site
with spindle cell, mixed *—see* Melanoma, skin, by site
in
giant pigmented nevus *—see* Melanoma, skin, by site
Hutchinson's melanotic freckle *—see* Melanoma, skin, by site
junctional nevus *—see* Melanoma, skin, by site
precancerous melanosis *—see* Melanoma, skin, by site
in situ D03.9
abdominal wall D03.59
ala nasi D03.39
ankle D03.7-
anus, anal (margin) (skin) D03.51
arm D03.6-
auditory canal D03.2-
auricle (ear) D03.2-
auricular canal (external) D03.2-
axilla, axillary fold D03.59
back D03.59
breast D03.52
brow D03.39
buttock D03.59
canthus (eye) D03.1-
cheek (external) D03.39
chest wall D03.59
chin D03.39
choroid D03.8
conjunctiva D03.8
ear (external) D03.2-
external meatus (ear) D03.2-
eye D03.8
eyebrow D03.39
eyelid (lower) (upper) D03.1-
face D03.30
specified NEC D03.39
female genital organ (external) NEC D03.8
finger D03.6-
flank D03.59
foot D03.7-
forearm D03.6-
forehead D03.39
foreskin D03.8
gluteal region D03.59

Melanoma *(continued)*
in situ *(continued)*
groin D03.59
hand D03.6-
heel D03.7-
helix D03.2-
hip D03.7-
interscapular region D03.59
iris D03.8
jaw D03.39
knee D03.7-
labium (majus) (minus) D03.8
lacrimal gland D03.8
leg D03.7-
lip (lower) (upper) D03.0
lower limb NEC D03.7-
male genital organ (external) NEC D03.8
nail D03.9
finger D03.6-
toe D03.7-
neck D03.4
nose (external) D03.39
orbit D03.8
penis D03.8
perianal skin D03.51
perineum D03.51
pinna D03.2-
popliteal fossa or space D03.7-
prepuce D03.8
pudendum D03.8
retina D03.8
retrobulbar D03.8
scalp D03.4
scrotum D03.8
shoulder D03.6-
specified site NEC D03.8
submammary fold D03.52
temple D03.39
thigh D03.7-
toe D03.7-
trunk NEC D03.59
umbilicus D03.59
upper limb NEC D03.6-
vulva D03.8
juvenile *—see* Nevus
malignant, of soft parts except skin *—see* Neoplasm, connective tissue, malignant
metastatic
breast C79.81
genital organ C79.82
specified site NEC C79.89
neurotropic, malignant *—see* Melanoma, skin, by site
nodular *—see* Melanoma, skin, by site
regressing, malignant *—see* Melanoma, skin, by site
skin C43.9
abdominal wall C43.59
ala nasi C43.31
ankle C43.7-
anus, anal (skin) C43.51
arm C43.6-
auditory canal (external) C43.2-
auricle (ear) C43.2-
auricular canal (external) C43.2-
axilla, axillary fold C43.59
back C43.59
breast (female) (male) C43.52
brow C43.39
buttock C43.59
canthus (eye) C43.1-
cheek (external) C43.39
chest wall C43.59
chin C43.39
ear (external) C43.2-
elbow C43.6-
external meatus (ear) C43.2-

Melanoma *(continued)*
- skin *(continued)*
  - eyebrow C43.39
  - eyelid (lower) (upper) C43.1-
  - face C43.30
    - specified NEC C43.39
  - female genital organ (external) NEC C51.9
  - finger C43.6-
  - flank C43.59
  - foot C43.7-
  - forearm C43.6-
  - forehead C43.39
  - foreskin C60.0
  - glabella C43.39
  - gluteal region C43.59
  - groin C43.59
  - hand C43.6-
  - heel C43.7-
  - helix C43.2-
  - hip C43.7-
  - interscapular region C43.59
  - jaw (external) C43.39
  - knee C43.7-
  - labium C51.9
    - majus C51.0
    - minus C51.1
  - leg C43.7-
  - lip (lower) (upper) C43.0
  - lower limb NEC C43.7-
  - male genital organ (external) NEC C63.9
  - nail
    - finger C43.6-
    - toe C43.7-
  - nasolabial groove C43.39
  - nates C43.59
  - neck C43.4
  - nose (external) C43.31
  - overlapping site C43.8
  - palpebra C43.1-
  - penis C60.9
  - perianal skin C43.51
  - perineum C43.51
  - pinna C43.2-
  - popliteal fossa or space C43.7-
  - prepuce C60.0
  - pudendum C51.9
  - scalp C43.4
  - scrotum C63.2
  - shoulder C43.6-
  - skin NEC C43.9
  - submammary fold C43.52
  - temple C43.39
  - thigh C43.7-
  - toe C43.7-
  - trunk NEC C43.59
  - umbilicus C43.59
  - upper limb NEC C43.6-
  - vulva C51.9
    - overlapping sites C51.8
- spindle cell
  - with epithelioid, mixed *—see* Melanoma, skin, by site
  - type A C69.4-
  - type B C69.4-
- superficial spreading *—see* Melanoma, skin, by site

Melanosarcoma *—see also* Melanoma
- epithelioid cell *—see* Melanoma

Melanosis L81.4
- addisonian E27.1
  - tuberculous A18.7
- adrenal E27.1
- colon K63.89
- conjunctiva *—see* Pigmentation, conjunctiva
  - congenital Q13.89
- cornea (presenile) (senile) *—see also* Pigmentation, cornea
  - congenital Q13.4
- eye NEC H57.8
  - congenital Q15.8
- lenticularis progressiva Q82.1
- liver K76.89
- precancerous *—see also* Melanoma, in situ
  - malignant melanoma in *—see* Melanoma
- Riehl's L81.4
- sclera H15.89
  - congenital Q13.89
- suprarenal E27.1
- tar L81.4
- toxic L81.4

Melanuria R82.99

MELAS syndrome E88.41

Melasma L81.1
- adrenal (gland) E27.1
- suprarenal (gland) E27.1

Melena K92.1
- with ulcer - code by site under Ulcer, with hemorrhage K27.4
- due to swallowed maternal blood P78.2
- newborn, neonatal P54.1
  - due to swallowed maternal blood P78.2

Meleney's
- gangrene (cutaneous) *—see* Ulcer, skin
- ulcer (chronic undermining) *—see* Ulcer, skin

Melioidosis A24.9
- acute A24.1
- chronic A24.2
- fulminating A24.1
- pneumonia A24.1
- pulmonary (chronic) A24.2
  - acute A24.1
  - subacute A24.2
- sepsis A24.1
- specified NEC A24.3
- subacute A24.2

Melitensis, febris A23.0

Melkersson (-Rosenthal) **syndrome** G51.2

Mellitus, diabetes *—see* Diabetes

Melorheostosis (bone) *—see* Disorder, bone, density and structure, specified NEC

Meloschisis Q18.4

Melotia Q17.4

Membrana
- capsularis lentis posterior Q13.89
- epipapillaris Q14.2

Membranacea placenta O43.19-

Membranaceous uterus N85.8

Membrane(s), membranous *—see also* condition
- cyclitic *—see* Membrane, pupillary
- folds, congenital *—see* Web
- Jackson's Q43.3
- over face of newborn P28.9
- premature rupture *—see* Rupture, membranes, premature
- pupillary H21.4-
  - persistent Q13.89
- retained (with hemorrhage) (complicating delivery) O72.2
  - without hemorrhage O73.1
- secondary cataract *—see* Cataract, secondary
- unruptured (causing asphyxia) *—see* Asphyxia, newborn
- vitreous *—see* Opacity, vitreous, membranes and strands

Membranitis *—see* Chorioamnionitis

Memory disturbance, lack or loss *—see also* Amnesia
- mild, following organic brain damage F06.8

Menadione deficiency E56.1

Menarche
- delayed E30.0
- precocious E30.1

Mendacity, pathologic F60.2

Mendelson's syndrome (due to anesthesia) J95.4
- in labor and delivery O74.0
- in pregnancy O29.01-
- obstetric O74.0
- postpartum, puerperal O89.01

Ménétrier's disease or syndrome K29.60
- with bleeding K29.61

Ménière's disease, syndrome or vertigo H81.0-

Meninges, meningeal *—see* condition

Meningioma *—see also* Neoplasm, meninges, benign
- angioblastic *—see* Neoplasm, meninges, benign
- angiomatous *—see* Neoplasm, meninges, benign
- endotheliomatous *—see* Neoplasm, meninges, benign
- fibroblastic *—see* Neoplasm, meninges, benign
- fibrous *—see* Neoplasm, meninges, benign
- hemangioblastic *—see* Neoplasm, meninges, benign
- hemangiopericytic *—see* Neoplasm, meninges, benign
- malignant *—see* Neoplasm, meninges, malignant
- meningiothelial *—see* Neoplasm, meninges, benign
- meningotheliomatous *—see* Neoplasm, meninges, benign
- mixed *—see* Neoplasm, meninges, benign
- multiple *—see* Neoplasm, meninges, uncertain behavior
- papillary *—see* Neoplasm, meninges, uncertain behavior
- psammomatous *—see* Neoplasm, meninges, benign
- syncytial *—see* Neoplasm, meninges, benign
- transitional *—see* Neoplasm, meninges, benign

Meningiomatosis (diffuse) *—see* Neoplasm, meninges, uncertain behavior

Meningism *—see* Meningismus

Meningismus (infectional) (pneumococcal) R29.1
- due to serum or vaccine R29.1
- influenzal *—see* Influenza, with, manifestations NEC

Meningitis (basal) (basic) (brain) (cerebral) (cervical) (congestive) (diffuse) (hemorrhagic) (infantile) (membranous) (metastatic) (nonspecific) (pontine) (progressive) (simple) (spinal) (subacute) (sympathetic) (toxic) G03.9
- abacterial G03.0
- actinomycotic A42.81
- adenoviral A87.1
- arbovirus A87.8
- aseptic (acute) G03.0
- bacterial G00.9
  - Escherichia coli (E. coli) G00.8
  - Friedländer (bacillus) G00.8
  - gram-negative G00.9
  - H. influenzae G00.0
  - Klebsiella G00.8
  - pneumococcal G00.1
  - specified organism NEC G00.8
  - staphylococcal G00.3
  - streptococcal (acute) G00.2
- benign recurrent (Mollaret) G03.2
- candidal B37.5
- caseous (tuberculous) A17.0
- cerebrospinal A39.0
- chronic NEC G03.1
- clear cerebrospinal fluid NEC G03.0
- coxsackievirus A87.0
- cryptococcal B45.1
- diplococcal (gram positive) A39.0
- echovirus A87.0
- enteroviral A87.0
- eosinophilic B83.2
- epidemic NEC A39.0
- Escherichia coli (E. coli) G00.8
- fibrinopurulent G00.9
  - specified organism NEC G00.8
- Friedländer (bacillus) G00.8
- gonococcal A54.81
- gram-negative cocci G00.9
- gram-positive cocci G00.9
- Haemophilus (influenzae) G00.0
- H. influenzae G00.0
- in (due to)
  - adenovirus A87.1
  - African trypanosomiasis B56.9 *[G02]*
  - anthrax A22.8
  - bacterial disease NEC A48.8 *[G01]*
  - Chagas' disease (chronic) B57.41
  - chickenpox B01.0
  - coccidioidomycosis B38.4
  - Diplococcus pneumoniae G00.1
  - enterovirus A87.0
  - herpes (simplex) virus B00.3
    - zoster B02.1
  - infectious mononucleosis B27.92
  - leptospirosis A27.81
  - Listeria monocytogenes A32.11
  - Lyme disease A69.21
  - measles B05.1
  - mumps (virus) B26.1
  - neurosyphilis (late) A52.13
  - parasitic disease NEC B89 *[G02]*
  - poliovirus A80.9 *[G02]*
  - preventive immunization, inoculation or vaccination G03.8
  - rubella B06.02
  - Salmonella infection A02.21
  - specified cause NEC G03.8
  - Streptococcal pneumoniae G00.1
  - typhoid fever A01.01
  - varicella B01.0
  - viral disease NEC A87.8
  - whooping cough A37.90
  - zoster B02.1

Meningitis *(continued)*
- infectious G00.9
- influenzal (H. influenzae) G00.0
- Klebsiella G00.8
- leptospiral (aseptic) A27.81
- lymphocytic (acute) (benign) (serous) A87.2
- meningococcal A39.0
- Mima polymorpha G00.8
- Mollaret (benign recurrent) G03.2
- monilial B37.5
- mycotic NEC B49 *[G02]*
- Neisseria A39.0
- nonbacterial G03.0
- nonpyogenic NEC G03.0
- ossificans G96.19
- pneumococcal streptococcus pneumoniae G00.1
- poliovirus A80.9 *[G02]*
- postmeasles B05.1
- purulent G00.9
  - specified organism NEC G00.8
- pyogenic G00.9
  - specified organism NEC G00.8
- Salmonella (arizonae) (Cholerae-Suis) (enteritidis) (typhimurium) A02.21
- septic G00.9
  - specified organism NEC G00.8
- serosa circumscripta NEC G03.0
- serous NEC G93.2
- specified organism NEC G00.8
- sporotrichosis B42.81
- staphylococcal G00.3
- sterile G03.0
- Streptococcal (acute) G00.2
  - pneumoniae G00.1
- suppurative G00.9
  - specified organism NEC G00.8
- syphilitic (late) (tertiary) A52.13
  - acute A51.41
  - congenital A50.41
  - secondary A51.41
- Torula histolytica (cryptococcal) B45.1
- traumatic (complication of injury) T79.8
- tuberculous A17.0
- typhoid A01.01
- viral NEC A87.9
- Yersinia pestis A20.3

Meningocele (spinal) *—see also* Spina bifida
- with hydrocephalus *—see* Spina bifida, by site, with hydrocephalus
- acquired (traumatic) G96.19
- cerebral *—see* Encephalocele

Meningocerebritis *—see* Meningoencephalitis

Meningococcemia A39.4
- acute A39.2
- chronic A39.3

Meningococcus, meningococcal *—see also* condition A39.9
- adrenalitis, hemorrhagic A39.1
- carrier (suspected) of Z22.31
- meningitis (cerebrospinal) A39.0

Meningoencephalitis (*see also* Encephalitis) G04.90
- acute NEC (*see also* Encephalitis, viral) A86
- bacterial NEC G04.2
- California A83.5
- diphasic A84.1
- eosinophilic B83.2
- epidemic A39.81
- herpesviral, herpetic B00.4
  - due to herpesvirus 6 B10.01
  - due to herpesvirus 7 B10.09
  - specified NEC B10.09

Meningoencephalitis *(continued)*
- in (due to)
  - blastomycosis NEC B40.81
  - diseases classified elsewhere G05.3
  - free-living amebae B60.2
  - Hemophilus influenzae (H .influenzae) G00.0
  - herpes B00.4
    - due to herpesvirus 6 B10.01
    - due to herpesvirus 7 B10.09
    - specified NEC B10.09
  - H. influenzae G00.0
  - Lyme disease A69.22
  - mercury *—see* subcategory T56.1
  - mumps B26.2
  - Naegleria (amebae) (organisms) (fowleri) B60.2
  - Parastrongylus cantonensis B83.2
  - toxoplasmosis (acquired) B58.2
    - congenital P37.1
- infectious (acute) (viral) A86
- influenzal (H. influenzae) G00.0
- Listeria monocytogenes A32.12
- lymphocytic (serous) A87.2
- mumps B26.2
- parasitic NEC B89 *[G05.3]*
- pneumococcal G04.2
- primary amebic B60.2
- specific (syphilitic) A52.14
- specified organism NEC G04.81
- staphylococcal G04.2
- streptococcal G04.2
- syphilitic A52.14
- toxic NEC G92
  - due to mercury *—see* subcategory T56.1
- tuberculous A17.82
- virus NEC A86

Meningoencephalocele *—see also* Encephalocele
- syphilitic A52.19
  - congenital A50.49

Meningoencephalomyelitis *—see also* Meningoencephalitis
- acute NEC (viral) A86
  - disseminated G04.00
    - postimmunization or postvaccination G04.02
    - postinfectious G04.01
- due to
  - actinomycosis A42.82
  - Torula B45.1
  - Toxoplasma or toxoplasmosis (acquired) B58.2
    - congenital P37.1
- postimmunization or postvaccination G04.02

Meningoencephalomyelopathy G96.9

Meningoencephalopathy G96.9

Meningomyelitis *—see also* Meningoencephalitis
- bacterial NEC G04.2
- blastomycotic NEC B40.81
- cryptococcal B45.1
- in diseases classified elsewhere G05.4
- meningococcal A39.81
- syphilitic A52.14
- tuberculous A17.82

Meningomyelocele *—see also* Spina bifida
- syphilitic A52.19

Meningomyeloneuritis *—see* Meningoencephalitis

Meningoradiculitis *—see* Meningitis

Meningovascular *—see* condition

Menkes' disease or syndrome E83.09
- meaning maple-syrup-urine disease E71.0

Menometrorrhagia N92.1

Menopause, menopausal (asymptomatic) (state) Z78.0
- arthritis (any site) NEC *—see* Arthritis, specified form NEC
- bleeding N92.4
- depression (single episode) F32.89
  - agitated (single episode) F32.2
    - recurrent episode F33.9
  - psychotic (single episode) F32.89
    - recurrent episode F33.8
  - recurrent episode F33.9
- melancholia (single episode) F32.89
  - recurrent episode F33.8
- paranoid state F22
- premature E28.319
  - asymptomatic E28.319
    - postirradiation E89.40
    - postsurgical E89.40
  - symptomatic E28.310
    - postirradiation E89.41
    - postsurgical E89.41
- psychosis NEC F28
- symptomatic N95.1
- toxic polyarthritis NEC *—see* Arthritis, specified form NEC

Menorrhagia (primary) N92.0
- climacteric N92.4
  - menopausal N92.4
- menopausal N92.4
- postclimacteric N95.0
- postmenopausal N95.0
- preclimacteric or premenopausal N92.4
- pubertal (menses retained) N92.2

Menostaxis N92.0

Menses, retention N94.89

Menstrual *—see* Menstruation

Menstruation
- absent *—see* Amenorrhea
- anovulatory N97.0
- cycle, irregular N92.6
- delayed N91.0
- disorder N93.9
  - psychogenic F45.8
- during pregnancy O20.8
- excessive (with regular cycle) N92.0
  - with irregular cycle N92.1
  - at puberty N92.2
- frequent N92.0
- infrequent *—see* Oligomenorrhea
- irregular N92.6
  - specified NEC N92.5
- latent N92.5
- membranous N92.5
- painful (*see also* Dysmenorrhea) N94.6
  - primary N94.4
  - psychogenic F45.8
  - secondary N94.5
- passage of clots N92.0
- precocious E30.1
- protracted N92.5
- rare *—see* Oligomenorrhea
- retained N94.89
- retrograde N92.5
- scanty *—see* Oligomenorrhea
- suppression N94.89
- vicarious (nasal) N94.89

Mental *—see also* condition
- deficiency *—see* Disability, intellectual
- deterioration *—see* Psychosis
- disorder *—see* Disorder, mental
- exhaustion F48.8

Mental *(continued)*
- insufficiency (congenital) *—see* Disability, intellectual
- observation without need for further medical care Z03.89
- retardation *—see* Disability, intellectual
- subnormality *—see* Disability, intellectuall
- upset *—see* Disorder, mental

Meralgia paresthetica G57.1-

Mercurial *—see* condition

Mercurialism *—see* subcategory T56.1

MERRF syndrome (myoclonic epilepsy associated with ragged-red fiber) E88.42

Merkel cell tumor *—see* Carcinoma, Merkel cell

Merocele *—see* Hernia, femoral

Meromelia
- lower limb *—see* Defect, reduction, lower limb
  - intercalary
    - femur *—see* Defect, reduction, lower limb, specified type NEC
    - tibiofibular (complete) (incomplete) *—see* Defect, reduction, lower limb
- upper limb *—see* Defect, reduction, upper limb
  - intercalary, humeral, radioulnar *—see* Agenesis, arm, with hand present

Merzbacher-Pelizaeus disease E75.29

Mesaortitis *—see* Aortitis

Mesarteritis *—see* Arteritis

Mesencephalitis *—see* Encephalitis

Mesenchymoma *—see also* Neoplasm, connective tissue, uncertain behavior
- benign *—see* Neoplasm, connective tissue, benign
- malignant *—see* Neoplasm, connective tissue, malignant

Mesenteritis
- retractile K65.4
- sclerosing K65.4

Mesentery, mesenteric *—see* condition

Mesiodens, mesiodentes K00.1

Mesio-occlusion M26.213

Mesocolon *—see* condition

Mesonephroma (malignant) *—see* Neoplasm, malignant, by site
- benign *—see* Neoplasm, benign, by site

Mesophlebitis *—see* Phlebitis

Mesostromal dysgenesia Q13.89

Mesothelioma (malignant) C45.9
- benign
  - mesentery D19.1
  - mesocolon D19.1
  - omentum D19.1
  - peritoneum D19.1
  - pleura D19.0
  - specified site NEC D19.7
  - unspecified site D19.9

Mesothelioma *(continued)*
- biphasic C45.9
  - benign
    - mesentery D19.1
    - mesocolon D19.1
    - omentum D19.1
    - peritoneum D19.1
    - pleura D19.0
    - specified site NEC D19.7
    - unspecified site D19.9
- cystic D48.4
- epithelioid C45.9
  - benign
    - mesentery D19.1
    - mesocolon D19.1
    - omentum D19.1
    - peritoneum D19.1
    - pleura D19.0
    - specified site NEC D19.7
    - unspecified site D19.9
- fibrous C45.9
  - benign
    - mesentery D19.1
    - mesocolon D19.1
    - omentum D19.1
    - peritoneum D19.1
    - pleura D19.0
    - specified site NEC D19.7
    - unspecified site D19.9
- site classification
  - liver C45.7
  - lung C45.7
  - mediastinum C45.7
  - mesentery C45.1
  - mesocolon C45.1
  - omentum C45.1
  - pericardium C45.2
  - peritoneum C45.1
  - pleura C45.0
    - parietal C45.0
  - retroperitoneum C45.7
  - specified site NEC C45.7
  - unspecified C45.9

Metabolic syndrome E88.81

Metagonimiasis B66.8

Metagonimus infestation (intestine) B66.8

Metal
- pigmentation L81.8
- polisher's disease J62.8

Metamorphopsia H53.15

Metaplasia
- apocrine (breast) —*see* Dysplasia, mammary, specified type NEC
- cervix (squamous) —*see* Dysplasia, cervix
- endometrium (squamous) (uterus) N85.8
- esophagus K22.7-
- kidney (pelvis) (squamous) N28.89
- myelogenous D73.1
- myeloid (agnogenic) (megakaryocytic) D73.1
- spleen D73.1
- squamous cell, bladder N32.89

Metastasis, metastatic
- abscess —*see* Abscess
- calcification E83.59
- cancer
  - from specified site —*see* Neoplasm, malignant, by site
  - to specified site —*see* Neoplasm, secondary, by site
- deposits (in) —*see* Neoplasm, secondary, by site
- disease (*see also* Neoplasm, secondary, by site) C79.9

Metastasis, metastatic *(continued)*
- spread (to) —*see* Neoplasm, secondary, by site

Metastrongyliasis B83.8

Metatarsalgia M77.4-
- anterior G57.6-
- Morton's G57.6-

Metatarsus, metatarsal —*see also* condition
- adductus, congenital Q66.22
- valgus (abductus), congenital Q66.6
- varus (congenital) Q66.22
  - primus Q66.21

Methadone use —*see* Use, opioid

Methemoglobinemia D74.9
- acquired (with sulfhemoglobinemia) D74.8
- congenital D74.0
- enzymatic (congenital) D74.0
- Hb M disease D74.0
- hereditary D74.0
- toxic D74.8

Methemoglobinuria —*see* Hemoglobinuria

Methioninemia E72.19

Methylmalonic acidemia E71.120

Metritis (catarrhal) (hemorrhagic) (septic) (suppurative) —*see also* Endometritis
- cervical —*see* Cervicitis

Metropathia hemorrhagica N93.8

Metroperitonitis —*see* Peritonitis, pelvic, female

Metrorrhagia N92.1
- climacteric N92.4
- menopausal N92.4
- postpartum NEC (atonic) (following delivery of placenta) O72.1
  - delayed or secondary O72.2
- preclimacteric or premenopausal N92.4
- psychogenic F45.8

Metrorrhexis —*see* Rupture, uterus

Metrosalpingitis N70.91

Metrostaxis N93.8

Metrovaginitis —*see* Endometritis

Meyer-Schwickerath and Weyers syndrome Q87.0

Meynert's amentia (nonalcoholic) F04
- alcoholic F10.96
  - with dependence F10.26

Mibelli's disease (porokeratosis) Q82.8

Mice, joint —*see* Loose, body, joint
- knee M23.4-

Micrencephalon, micrencephaly Q02

Microalbuminuria R80.9

Microaneurysm, retinal —*see also* Disorder, retina, microaneurysms
- diabetic —*see* E08-E13 with .31

Microangiopathy (peripheral) I73.9
- thrombotic M31.1

Microcalcifications, breast R92.0

Microcephalus, microcephalic, microcephaly Q02
- due to toxoplasmosis (congenital) P37.1

Microcheilia Q18.7

Microcolon (congenital) Q43.8

Microcornea (congenital) Q13.4

Microcytic —*see* condition

Microdeletions NEC Q93.88

Microdontia K00.2

Microdrepanocytosis D57.40
- with crisis (vasoocclusive pain) D57.419
  - with
    - acute chest syndrome D57.411
    - splenic sequestration D57.412

Microembolism
- atherothrombotic —*see* Atheroembolism
- retinal —*see* Occlusion, artery, retina

Microencephalon Q02

Microfilaria streptocerca infestation —*see* Onchocerciasis

Microgastria (congenital) Q40.2

Microgenia M26.06

Microgenitalia, congenital
- female Q52.8
- male Q55.8

Microglioma —*see* Lymphoma, non-Hodgkin, specified NEC

Microglossia (congenital) Q38.3

Micrognathia, micrognathism (congenital) (mandibular) (maxillary) M26.09

Microgyria (congenital) Q04.3

Microinfarct of heart —*see* Insufficiency, coronary

Microlentia (congenital) Q12.8

Microlithiasis, alveolar, pulmonary J84.02

Micromastia N64.82

Micromyelia (congenital) Q06.8

Micropenis Q55.62

Microphakia (congenital) Q12.8

Microphthalmos, microphthalmia (congenital) Q11.2
- due to toxoplasmosis P37.1

Micropsia H53.15

Microscopic polyangiitis (polyarteritis) M31.7

Microsporidiosis B60.8
- intestinal A07.8

Microsporon furfur infestation B36.0

Microsporosis —*see also* Dermatophytosis
- nigra B36.1

Microstomia (congenital) Q18.5

Microtia (congenital) (external ear) Q17.2

Microtropia H50.40

Microvillus inclusion disease (MVD) (MVID) Q43.8

Micturition
- disorder NEC (*see also* Difficulty, micturition) R39.198
  - psychogenic F45.8
- frequency R35.0
  - psychogenic F45.8
- hesitancy R39.11
- incomplete emptying R39.14
- nocturnal R35.1
- painful R30.9
  - dysuria R30.0
  - psychogenic F45.8
  - tenesmus R30.1

Micturition *(continued)*
- poor stream R39.12
- position dependent R39.192
- split stream R39.13
- straining R39.16
- urgency R39.15

Mid plane —*see* condition

Middle
- ear —*see* condition
- lobe (right) syndrome J98.19

Miescher's elastoma L87.2

Mietens' syndrome Q87.2

Migraine (idiopathic) G43.909
- with refractory migraine G43.919
  - with status migrainosus G43.911
  - without status migrainosus G43.919
- with aura (acute-onset) (prolonged) (typical) (without headache) G43.109
  - with refractory migraine G43.119
    - with status migrainosus G43.111
    - without status migrainosus G43.119
  - intractable G43.119
    - with status migrainosus G43.111
    - without status migrainosus G43.119
  - not intractable G43.109
    - with status migrainosus G43.101
    - without status migrainosus G43.109
  - persistent G43.509
    - with cerebral infarction G43.609
      - with refractory migraine G43.619
        - with status migrainosus G43.611
        - without status migrainosus G43.619
      - intractable G43.619
        - with status migrainosus G43.611
        - without status migrainosus G43.619
      - not intractable G43.609
        - with status migrainosus G43.601
        - without status migrainosus G43.609
      - without refractory migraine G43.609
        - with status migrainosus G43.601
        - without status migrainosus G43.609
    - without cerebral infarction G43.509
      - with refractory migraine G43.519
        - with status migrainosus G43.511
        - without status migrainosus G43.519
      - intractable G43.519
        - with status migrainosus G43.511
        - without status migrainosus G43.519
      - not intractable G43.509
        - with status migrainosus G43.501

Migraine *(continued)*
with aura *(continued)*
persistent *(continued)*
without cerebral infarction *(continued)*
without status migrainosus G43.509
without refractory migraine G43.509
with status migrainosus G43.501
without status migrainosus G43.509
without mention of refractory migraine G43.109
with status migrainosus G43.101
without status migrainosus G43.109
abdominal G43.D0
with refractory migraine G43.D1
intractable G43.D1
not intractable G43.D0
without refractory migraine G43.D0
basilar *—see* Migraine, with aura
classical *—see* Migraine, with aura
common *—see* Migraine, without aura
complicated G43.109
equivalents *—see* Migraine, with aura
familiar *—see* Migraine, hemiplegic
hemiplegic G43.409
with refractory migraine G43.419
with status migrainosus G43.411
without status migrainosus G43.419
intractable G43.419
with status migrainosus G43.411
without status migrainosus G43.419
not intractable G43.409
with status migrainosus G43.401
without status migrainosus G43.409
without refractory migraine G43.409
with status migrainosus G43.401
without status migrainosus G43.409
intractable G43.919
with status migrainosus G43.911
without status migrainosus G43.919
menstrual G43.829
with refractory migraine G43.839
with status migrainosus G43.831
without status migrainosus G43.839
intractable G43.839
with status migrainosus G43.831
without status migrainosus G43.839
not intractable 4G43.829
with status migrainosus G43.821
without status migrainosus G43.829
without refractory migraine G43.829
with status migrainosus G43.821
without status migrainosus G43.829

Migraine *(continued)*
menstrually related *—see* Migraine, menstrual
not intractable G43.909
with status migrainosus G43.901
without status migrainosus G43.919
ophthalmoplegic G43.B0
with refractory migraine G43.B1
intractable G43.B1
not intractable G43.B0
without refractory migraine G43.B0
persistent aura (with, without) cerebral infarction *—see* Migraine, with aura, persistent
preceded or accompanied by transient focal neurological phenomena *—see* Migraine, with aura
pre-menstrual *—see* Migraine, menstrual
pure menstrual *—see* Migraine, menstrual
retinal *—see* Migraine, with aura
specified NEC G43.809
intractable G43.819
with status migrainosus G43.811
without status migrainosus G43.819
not intractable G43.809
with status migrainosus G43.801
without status migrainosus G43.809
sporadic *—see* Migraine, hemiplegic
transformed *—see* Migraine, without aura, chronic
triggered seizures *—see* Migraine, with aura
without aura G43.009
with refractory migraine G43.019
with status migrainosus G43.011
without status migrainosus G43.019
chronic G43.709
with refractory migraine G43.719
with status migrainosus G43.711
without status migrainosus G43.719
intractable
with status migrainosus G43.711
without status migrainosus G43.719
not intractable
with status migrainosus G43.701
without status migrainosus G43.709
without refractory migraine G43.709
with status migrainosus G43.701
without status migrainosus G43.709
intractable
with status migrainosus G43.011
without status migrainosus G43.019
not intractable
with status migrainosus G43.001
without status migrainosus G43.009

Migraine *(continued)*
without aura *(continued)*
without mention of refractory migraine G43.009
with status migrainosus G43.001
without status migrainosus G43.009
without refractory migraine G43.909
with status migrainosus G43.901
without status migrainosus G43.919

Migrant, social Z59.0

Migration, anxiety concerning Z60.3

Migratory, migrating *—see also* condition
person Z59.0
testis Q55.29

Mikity-Wilson disease or syndrome P27.0

Mikulicz' disease or syndrome K11.8

Miliaria L74.3
alba L74.1
apocrine L75.2
crystallina L74.1
profunda L74.2
rubra L74.0
tropicalis L74.2

Miliary *—see* condition

Milium L72.0
colloid L57.8

Milk
crust L21.0
excessive secretion O92.6
poisoning *—see* Poisoning, food, noxious
retention O92.79
sickness *—see* Poisoning, food, noxious
spots I31.0

Milk-alkali disease or syndrome E83.52

Milk-leg (deep vessels) (nonpuerperal) *—see* Embolism, vein, lower extremity
complicating pregnancy O22.3-
puerperal, postpartum, childbirth O87.1

Milkman's disease or syndrome M83.8

Milky urine *—see* Chyluria

Millard-Gubler (-Foville) **paralysis or syndrome** G46.3

Millar's asthma J38.5

Miller Fisher syndrome G61.0

Mills' disease *—see* Hemiplegia

Millstone maker's pneumoconiosis J62.8

Milroy's disease (chronic hereditary edema) Q82.0

Minamata disease T56.1

Miners' asthma or lung J60

Minkowski-Chauffard syndrome *—see* Spherocytosis

Minor *—see* condition

Minor's disease (hematomyelia) G95.19

Minot's disease (hemorrhagic disease), **newborn** P53

Minot-von Willebrand-Jurgens disease or syndrome (angiohemophilia) D68.0

Minus (and plus) hand (intrinsic) *—see* Deformity, limb, specified type NEC, forearm

Miosis (pupil) H57.03

Mirizzi's syndrome (hepatic duct stenosis) K83.1

Mirror writing F81.0

Misadventure (of) (prophylactic) (therapeutic) (*see also* Complications) T88.9
administration of insulin (by accident) T38.3
infusion *—see* Complications, infusion
local applications (of fomentations, plasters, etc.) T88.9
burn or scald *—see* Burn
specified NEC T88.8
medical care (early) (late) T88.9
adverse effect of drugs or chemicals *—see* Table of Drugs and Chemicals
burn or scald *—see* Burn
specified NEC T88.8
specified NEC T88.8
surgical procedure (early) (late) *—see* Complications, surgical procedure
transfusion *—see* Complications, transfusion
vaccination or other immunological procedure *—see* Complications, vaccination

Miscarriage O03.9

Misdirection, aqueous H40.83-

Misperception, sleep state F51.02

Misplaced, misplacement
ear Q17.4
kidney (acquired) N28.89
congenital Q63.2
organ or site, congenital NEC *—see* Malposition, congenital

Missed
abortion O02.1
delivery O36.4

Missing *—see also* Absence
string of intrauterine contraceptive device T83.32

Misuse of drugs F19.99

Mitchell's disease (erythromelalgia) I73.81

Mite(s) (infestation) B88.9
diarrhea B88.0
grain (itch) B88.0
hair follicle (itch) B88.0
in sputum B88.0

Mitral *—see* condition

Mittelschmerz N94.0

Mixed *—see* condition

MMN (multifocal motor neuropathy) G61.82

MNGIE (Mitochondrial Neurogastrointestinal Encephalopathy) **syndrome** E88.49

Mobile, mobility
cecum Q43.3
excessive *—see* Hypermobility
gallbladder, congenital Q44.1
kidney N28.89
organ or site, congenital NEC *—see* Malposition, congenital

Mobitz heart block (atrioventricular) I44.1

Moebius, Möbius
- disease (ophthalmoplegic migraine) —*see* Migraine, ophthalmoplegic
- syndrome Q87.0
  - congenital oculofacial paralysis (with other anomalies) Q87.0
  - ophthalmoplegic migraine —*see* Migraine, ophthalmoplegic

Moeller's glossitis K14.0

Mohr's syndrome (Types I and II) Q87.0

Mola destruens D39.2

Molar pregnancy O02.0

Molarization of premolars K00.2

Molding, head (during birth) - omit code

Mole (pigmented) —*see also* Nevus
- blood O02.0
- Breus' O02.0
- cancerous —*see* Melanoma
- carneous O02.0
- destructive D39.2
- fleshy O02.0
- hydatid, hydatidiform (benign) (complicating pregnancy) (delivered) (undelivered) O01.9
  - classical O01.0
  - complete O01.0
  - incomplete O01.1
  - invasive D39.2
  - malignant D39.2
  - partial O01.1
- intrauterine O02.0
- invasive (hydatidiform) D39.2
- malignant
  - meaning
    - malignant hydatidiform mole D39.2
    - melanoma —*see* Melanoma
- nonhydatidiform O02.0
- nonpigmented —*see* Nevus
- pregnancy NEC O02.0
- skin —*see* Nevus
- tubal O00.10-
  - with intrauterine pregnancy O00.11-
- vesicular —*see* Mole, hydatidiform

Molimen, molimina (menstrual) N94.3

Molluscum contagiosum (epitheliale) B08.1

Mönckeberg's arteriosclerosis, disease, or sclerosis —*see* Arteriosclerosis, extremities

Mondini's malformation (cochlea) Q16.5

Mondor's disease I80.8

Monge's disease T70.29

Monilethrix (congenital) Q84.1

Moniliasis (*see also* Candidiasis) B37.9
- neonatal P37.5

Monitoring (encounter for)
- therapeutic drug level Z51.81

Monkey malaria B53.1

Monkeypox B04

Monoarthritis M13.10
- ankle M13.17-
- elbow M13.12-

Monoarthritis *(continued)*
- foot joint M13.17-
- hand joint M13.14-
- hip M13.15-
- knee M13.16-
- shoulder M13.11-
- wrist M13.13-

Monoblastic —*see* condition

Monochromat (ism), monochromatopsia (acquired) (congenital) H53.51

Monocytic —*see* condition

Monocytopenia D72.818

Monocytosis (symptomatic) D72.821

Monomania —*see* Psychosis

Mononeuritis G58.9
- cranial nerve —*see* Disorder, nerve, cranial
- femoral nerve G57.2-
- lateral
  - cutaneous nerve of thigh G57.1-
  - popliteal nerve G57.3-
- lower limb G57.9-
  - specified nerve NEC G57.8-
- medial popliteal nerve G57.4-
- median nerve G56.1-
- multiplex G58.7
- plantar nerve G57.6-
- posterior tibial nerve G57.5-
- radial nerve G56.3-
- sciatic nerve G57.0-
- specified NEC G58.8
- tibial nerve G57.4-
- ulnar nerve G56.2-
- upper limb G56.9-
  - specified nerve NEC G56.8-
- vestibular —*see* subcategory H93.3

Mononeuropathy G58.9
- carpal tunnel syndrome —*see* Syndrome, carpal tunnel
- diabetic NEC —*see* E08-E13 with .41
- femoral nerve —*see* Lesion, nerve, femoral
- ilioinguinal nerve G57.8-
- in diseases classified elsewhere —*see* category G59
- intercostal G58.0
- lower limb G57.9-
  - causalgia —*see* Causalgia, lower limb
  - femoral nerve —*see* Lesion, nerve, femoral
  - meralgia paresthetica G57.1-
  - plantar nerve —*see* Lesion, nerve, plantar
  - popliteal nerve —*see* Lesion, nerve, popliteal
  - sciatic nerve —*see* Lesion, nerve, sciatic
  - specified NEC G57.8-
  - tarsal tunnel syndrome —*see* Syndrome, tarsal tunnel
- median nerve —*see* Lesion, nerve, median
- multiplex G58.7
- obturator nerve G57.8-
- popliteal nerve —*see* Lesion, nerve, popliteal
- radial nerve —*see* Lesion, nerve, radial
- saphenous nerve G57.8-
- specified NEC G58.8
- tarsal tunnel syndrome —*see* Syndrome, tarsal tunnel

Mononeuropathy *(continued)*
- tuberculous A17.83
- ulnar nerve —*see* Lesion, nerve, ulnar
- upper limb G56.9-
  - carpal tunnel syndrome —*see* Syndrome, carpal tunnel
  - causalgia —*see* Causalgia
  - median nerve —*see* Lesion, nerve, median
  - radial nerve —*see* Lesion, nerve, radial
  - specified site NEC G56.8-
  - ulnar nerve —*see* Lesion, nerve, ulnar

Mononucleosis, infectious B27.90
- with
  - complication NEC B27.99
  - meningitis B27.92
  - polyneuropathy B27.91
- cytomegaloviral B27.10
  - with
    - complication NEC B27.19
    - meningitis B27.12
    - polyneuropathy B27.11
- Epstein-Barr (virus) B27.00
  - with
    - complication NEC B27.09
    - meningitis B27.02
    - polyneuropathy B27.01
- gammaherpesviral B27.00
  - with
    - complication NEC B27.09
    - meningitis B27.02
    - polyneuropathy B27.01
- specified NEC B27.80
  - with
    - complication NEC B27.89
    - meningitis B27.82
    - polyneuropathy B27.81

Monoplegia G83.3-
- congenital (cerebral) G80.8
  - spastic G80.1
- embolic (current episode) I63.4-
- following
  - cerebrovascular disease
    - cerebral infarction
      - lower limb I69.34-
      - upper limb I69.33-
    - intracerebral hemorrhage
      - lower limb I69.14-
      - upper limb I69.13-
    - lower limb I69.94-
    - nontraumatic intracranial hemorrhage NEC
      - lower limb I69.24-
      - upper limb I69.23-
    - specified disease NEC
      - lower limb I69.84-
      - upper limb I69.83-
    - stroke NOS
      - lower limb I69.34-
      - upper limb I69.33-
    - subarachnoid hemorrhage
      - lower limb I69.04-
      - upper limb I69.03-
    - upper limb I69.93-
- hysterical (transient) F44.4
- lower limb G83.1-
- psychogenic (conversion reaction) F44.4
- thrombotic (current episode) I63.3-
- transient R29.818
- upper limb G83.2-

Monorchism, monorchidism Q55.0

Monosomy (*see also* Deletion, chromosome) Q93.9
- specified NEC Q93.89

Monosomy *(continued)*
- whole chromosome
  - meiotic nondisjunction Q93.0
  - mitotic nondisjunction Q93.1
  - mosaicism Q93.1
- X Q96.9

Monster, monstrosity (single) Q89.7
- acephalic Q00.0
- twin Q89.4

Monteggia's fracture (-dislocation) S52.27-

Mooren's ulcer (cornea) —*see* Ulcer, cornea, Mooren's

Moore's syndrome —*see* Epilepsy, specified NEC

Mooser-Neill reaction A75.2

Mooser's bodies A75.2

Morbidity not stated or unknown R69

Morbilli —*see* Measles

Morbus —*see also* Disease
- angelicus, anglorum E55.0
- Beigel B36.2
- caducus —*see* Epilepsy
- celiacus K90.0
- comitialis —*see* Epilepsy
- cordis (*see also* Disease, heart) I51.9
  - valvulorum —*see* Endocarditis
- coxae senilis M16.9
  - tuberculous A18.02
- hemorrhagicus neonatorum P53
- maculosus neonatorum P54.5

Morel (-Stewart) (-Morgagni) **syndrome** M85.2

Morel-Kraepelin disease —*see* Schizophrenia

Morel-Moore syndrome M85.2

Morgagni's
- cyst, organ, hydatid, or appendage
  - female Q50.5
  - male (epididymal) Q55.4
    - testicular Q55.29
- syndrome M85.2

Morgagni-Stokes-Adams syndrome I45.9

Morgagni-Stewart-Morel syndrome M85.2

Morgagni-Turner (-Albright) **syndrome** Q96.9

Moria F07.0

Moron (I.Q.50-69) F70

Morphea L94.0

Morphinism (without remission) F11.20
- with remission F11.21

Morphinomania (without remission) F11.20
- with remission F11.21

Morquio (-Ullrich) (-Brailsford) **disease or syndrome** —*see* Mucopolysaccharidosis

Mortification (dry) (moist) —*see* Gangrene

Morton's metatarsalgia (neuralgia) (neuroma) (syndrome) G57.6-

Morvan's disease or syndrome G60.8

Mosaicism, mosaic (autosomal) (chromosomal)
- 45,X/other cell lines NEC with abnormal sex chromosome Q96.4

Mosaicism, mosaic *(continued)*
45,X/46,XX Q96.3
sex chromosome
female Q97.8
lines with various numbers of X chromosomes Q97.2
male Q98.7
XY Q96.3
Moschowitz' disease M31.1
Mother yaw A66.0
Motion sickness (from travel, any vehicle) (from roundabouts or swings) T75.3
Mottled, mottling, teeth (enamel) (endemic) (nonendemic) K00.3
Mounier-Kuhn syndrome Q32.4
with bronchiectasis J47.9
exacerbation (acute) J47.1
lower respiratory infection J47.0
acquired J98.09
with bronchiectasis J47.9
with
exacerbation (acute) J47.1
lower respiratory infection J47.0
Mountain
sickness T70.29
with polycythemia, acquired (acute) D75.1
tick fever A93.2
Mouse, joint *—see* Loose, body, joint
knee M23.4-
Mouth *—see* condition
Movable
coccyx *—see* subcategory M53.2
kidney N28.89
congenital Q63.8
spleen D73.89
Movements, dystonic R25.8
Moyamoya disease I67.5
MRSA (Methicillin resistant Staphylococcus aureus)
infection A49.02
as the cause of diseases classified elsewhere B95.62
sepsis A41.02
MSSA (Methicillin susceptible Staphylococcus aureus)
infection A49.01
as the cause of diseases classified elsewhere B95.61
sepsis A41.01
Mucha-Habermann disease L41.0
Mucinosis (cutaneous) (focal) (papular) (reticular erythematous) (skin) L98.5
oral K13.79
Mucocele
appendix K38.8
buccal cavity K13.79
gallbladder K82.1
lacrimal sac, chronic H04.43-
nasal sinus J34.1
nose J34.1
salivary gland (any) K11.6
sinus (accessory) (nasal) J34.1
turbinate (bone) (middle) (nasal) J34.1
uterus N85.8
Mucolipidosis
I E77.1
II, III E77.0
IV E75.11
Mucopolysaccharidosis E76.3
beta-gluduronidase deficiency E76.29
cardiopathy E76.3 *[I52]*
Hunter's syndrome E76.1
Hurler's syndrome E76.01
Hurler-Scheie syndrome E76.02
Maroteaux-Lamy syndrome E76.29
Morquio syndrome E76.219
A E76.210
B E76.211
classic E76.210
Sanfilippo syndrome E76.22
Scheie's syndrome E76.03
specified NEC E76.29
type
I
Hurler's syndrome E76.01
Hurler-Scheie syndrome E76.02
Scheie's syndrome E76.03
II E76.1
III E76.22
IV E76.219
IVA E76.210
IVB E76.211
VI E76.29
VII E76.29
Mucormycosis B46.5
cutaneous B46.3
disseminated B46.4
gastrointestinal B46.2
generalized B46.4
pulmonary B46.0
rhinocerebral B46.1
skin B46.3
subcutaneous B46.3
Mucositis (ulcerative) K12.30
due to drugs NEC K12.32
gastrointestinal K92.81
mouth (oral) (oropharyngeal) K12.30
due to antineoplastic therapy K12.31
due to drugs NEC K12.32
due to radiation K12.33
specified NEC K12.39
viral K12.39
nasal J34.81
oral cavity *—see* Mucositis, mouth
oral soft tissues *—see* Mucositis, mouth
vagina and vulva N76.81
Mucositis necroticans agranulocytica *—see* Agranulocytosis
Mucous *—see also* condition
patches (syphilitic) A51.39
congenital A50.07
Mucoviscidosis E84.9
with meconium obstruction E84.11
Mucus
asphyxia or suffocation *—see* Asphyxia, mucus
in stool R19.5
plug *—see* Asphyxia, mucus
Muguet B37.0
Mulberry molars (congenital syphilis) A50.52
Müllerian mixed tumor
specified site *—see* Neoplasm, malignant, by site
unspecified site C54.9
Multicystic kidney (development) Q61.4
Multiparity (grand) Z64.1
affecting management of pregnancy, labor and delivery (supervision only) O09.4-
requiring contraceptive management *—see* Contraception
Multipartita placenta O43.19-
Multiple, multiplex *—see also* condition
digits (congenital) Q69.9
endocrine neoplasia *—see* Neoplasia, endocrine, multiple (MEN)
personality F44.81
Mumps B26.9
arthritis B26.85
complication NEC B26.89
encephalitis B26.2
hepatitis B26.81
meningitis (aseptic) B26.1
meningoencephalitis B26.2
myocarditis B26.82
oophoritis B26.89
orchitis B26.0
pancreatitis B26.3
polyneuropathy B26.84
Mumu *—see also* Infestation, filarial B74.9 *[N51]*
Münchhausen's syndrome *—see* Disorder, factitious
Münchmeyer's syndrome *—see* Myositis, ossificans, progressiva
Mural *—see* condition
Murmur (cardiac) (heart) (organic) R01.1
abdominal R19.15
aortic (valve) *—see* Endocarditis, aortic
benign R01.0
diastolic *—see* Endocarditis
Flint I35.1
functional R01.0
Graham Steell I37.1
innocent R01.0
mitral (valve) *—see* Insufficiency, mitral
nonorganic R01.0
presystolic, mitral *—see* Insufficiency, mitral
pulmonic (valve) I37.8
systolic R01.1
tricuspid (valve) I07.9
valvular *—see* Endocarditis
Murri's disease (intermittent hemoglobinuria) D59.6
Muscle, muscular *—see also* condition
carnitine (palmityltransferase) deficiency E71.314
Musculoneuralgia *—see* Neuralgia
Mushroom-workers'(pickers') **disease or lung** J67.5
Mushrooming hip *—see* Derangement, joint, specified NEC, hip
Mutation(s)
factor V Leiden D68.51
surfactant, of lung J84.83
prothrombin gene D68.52
Mutism *—see also* Aphasia
deaf (acquired) (congenital) NEC H91.3
elective (adjustment reaction) (childhood) F94.0
hysterical F44.4
selective (childhood) F94.0
MVD (microvillus inclusion disease) Q43.8
MVID (microvillus inclusion disease) Q43.8
Myalgia M79.1
epidemic (cervical) B33.0
traumatic NEC T14.8
Myasthenia G70.9
congenital G70.2
cordis *—see* Failure, heart
developmental G70.2
gravis G70.00
with exacerbation (acute) G70.01
in crisis G70.01
neonatal, transient P94.0
pseudoparalytica G70.00
with exacerbation (acute) G70.01
in crisis G70.01
stomach, psychogenic F45.8
syndrome
in
diabetes mellitus *—see* E08-E13 with .44
neoplastic disease (*see also* Neoplasm) D49.9 *[G73.3]*
pernicious anemia D51.0 *[G73.3]*
thyrotoxicosis E05.90 *[G73.3]*
with thyroid storm E05.91 *[G73.3]*
Myasthenic M62.81
Mycelium infection B49
Mycetismus *—see* Poisoning, food, noxious, mushroom
Mycetoma B47.9
actinomycotic B47.1
bone (mycotic) B47.9 *[M90.80]*
eumycotic B47.0
foot B47.9
actinomycotic B47.1
mycotic B47.0
madurae NEC B47.9
mycotic B47.0
maduromycotic B47.0
mycotic B47.0
nocardial B47.1
Mycobacteriosis *—see* Mycobacterium
Mycobacterium, mycobacterial (infection) A31.9
anonymous A31.9
atypical A31.9
cutaneous A31.1
pulmonary A31.0
tuberculous *—see* Tuberculosis, pulmonary
specified site NEC A31.8
avium (intracellulare complex) A31.0
balnei A31.1
Battey A31.0
chelonei A31.8
cutaneous A31.1
extrapulmonary systemic A31.8
fortuitum A31.8
intracellulare (Battey bacillus) A31.0
kansasii (yellow bacillus) A31.0
kakaferifu A31.8
kasongo A31.8
leprae (*see also* Leprosy) A30.9
luciflavum A31.1
marinum (M. balnei) A31.1
nonspecific *—see* Mycobacterium, atypical
pulmonary (atypical) A31.0
tuberculous *—see* Tuberculosis, pulmonary
scrofulaceum A31.8
simiae A31.8
systemic, extrapulmonary A31.8
szulgai A31.8

Mycobacterium, mycobacterial *(continued)*
terrae A31.8
triviale A31.8
tuberculosis (human, bovine) - see Tuberculosis
ulcerans A31.1
xenopi A31.8

Mycoplasma (M.) **pneumoniae, as cause of disease classified elsewhere** B96.0

Mycosis, mycotic B49
cutaneous NEC B36.9
ear B36.9
in
aspergillosis B44.89
candidiasis B37.84
moniliasis B37.84
fungoides (extranodal) (solid organ) C84.0-
mouth B37.0
nails B35.1
opportunistic B48.8
skin NEC B36.9
specified NEC B48.8
stomatitis B37.0
vagina, vaginitis (candidal) B37.3

Mydriasis (pupil) H57.04

Myelatelia Q06.1

Myelinolysis, pontine, central G37.2

Myelitis (acute) (ascending) (childhood) (chronic) (descending) (diffuse) (disseminated) (idiopathic) (pressure) (progressive) (spinal cord) (subacute) (*see also* Encephalitis) G04.91
herpes simplex B00.82
herpes zoster B02.24
in diseases classified elsewhere G05.4
necrotizing, subacute G37.4
optic neuritis in G36.0
postchickenpox B01.12
postherpetic B02.24
postimmunization G04.02
postinfectious NEC G04.89
postvaccinal G04.02
specified NEC G04.89
syphilitic (transverse) A52.14
toxic G92
transverse (in demyelinating diseases of central nervous system) G37.3
tuberculous A17.82
varicella B01.12

Myeloblastic —*see* condition

Myeloblastoma
granular cell —*see also* Neoplasm, connective tissue
malignant —*see* Neoplasm, connective tissue, malignant
tongue D10.1

Myelocele —*see* Spina bifida

Myelocystocele —*see* Spina bifida

Myelocytic —*see* condition

Myelodysplasia D46.9
specified NEC D46.Z
spinal cord (congenital) Q06.1

Myelodysplastic syndrome D46.9
with
5q deletion D46.C
isolated del (5q) chromosomal abnormality D46.C
specified NEC D46.Z

Myeloencephalitis —*see* Encephalitis

Myelofibrosis D75.81
with myeloid metaplasia D47.4
acute C94.4-
idiopathic (chronic) D47.4
primary D47.1
secondary D75.81
in myeloproliferative disease D47.4

Myelogenous —*see* condition

Myeloid —*see* condition

Myelokathexis D70.9

Myeloleukodystrophy E75.29

Myelolipoma —*see* Lipoma

Myeloma (multiple) C90.0-
monostotic C90.3
plasma cell C90.0-
plasma cell C90.0-
solitary (*see also* Plasmacytoma, solitary) C90.3-

Myelomalacia G95.89

Myelomatosis C90.0-

Myelomeningitis —*see* Meningoencephalitis

Myelomeningocele (spinal cord) —*see* Spina bifida

Myelo-osteo-musculodysplasia hereditaria Q79.8

Myelopathic
anemia D64.89
muscle atrophy —*see* Atrophy, muscle, spinal
pain syndrome G89.0

Myelopathy (spinal cord) G95.9
drug-induced G95.89
in (due to)
degeneration or displacement, intervertebral disc NEC —*see* Disorder, disc, with, myelopathy
infection —*see* Encephalitis
intervertebral disc disorder —*see also* Disorder, disc, with, myelopathy
mercury —*see* subcategory T56.1
neoplastic disease (*see also* Neoplasm) D49.9 *[G99.2]*
pernicious anemia D51.0 *[G99.2]*
spondylosis —*see* Spondylosis, with myelopathy NEC
necrotic (subacute) (vascular) G95.19
radiation-induced G95.89
spondylogenic NEC —*see* Spondylosis, with myelopathy NEC
toxic G95.89
transverse, acute G37.3
vascular G95.19
vitamin B12 E53.8 *[G32.0]*

Myelophthisis D61.82

Myeloradiculitis G04.91

Myeloradiculodysplasia (spinal) Q06.1

Myelosarcoma C92.3-

Myelosclerosis D75.89
with myeloid metaplasia D47.4
disseminated, of nervous system G35
megakaryocytic D47.4
with myeloid metaplasia D47.4

Myelosis
acute C92.0-
aleukemic C92.9-
chronic D47.1

Myelosis *(continued)*
erythremic (acute) C94.0-
megakaryocytic C94.2-
nonleukemic D72.828
subacute C92.9-

Myiasis (cavernous) B87.9
aural B87.4
creeping B87.0
cutaneous B87.0
dermal B87.0
ear (external) (middle) B87.4
eye B87.2
genitourinary B87.81
intestinal B87.82
laryngeal B87.3
nasopharyngeal B87.3
ocular B87.2
orbit B87.2
skin B87.0
specified site NEC B87.89
traumatic B87.1
wound B87.1

Myoadenoma, prostate —*see* Hyperplasia, prostate

Myoblastoma
granular cell —*see also* Neoplasm, connective tissue, benign
malignant —*see* Neoplasm, connective tissue, malignant
tongue D10.1

Myocardial —*see* condition

Myocardiopathy (congestive) (constrictive) (familial) (hypertrophic nonobstructive) (idiopathic) (infiltrative) (obstructive) (primary) (restrictive) (sporadic) (*see also* Cardiomyopathy) I42.9
alcoholic I42.6
cobalt-beer I42.6
glycogen storage E74.02 *[I43]*
hypertrophic obstructive I42.1
in (due to)
beriberi E51.12
cardiac glycogenosis E74.02 *[I43]*
Friedreich's ataxia G11.1 *[I43]*
myotonia atrophica G71.11 *[I43]*
progressive muscular dystrophy G71.0 *[I43]*
obscure (African) I42.8
secondary I42.9
thyrotoxic E05.90 *[I43]*
with storm E05.91 *[I43]*
toxic NEC I42.7

Myocarditis (with arteriosclerosis) (chronic) (fibroid) (interstitial) (old) (progressive) (senile) I51.4
with
rheumatic fever (conditions in I00) I09.0
active —*see* Myocarditis, acute, rheumatic
inactive or quiescent (with chorea) I09.0
active I40.9
rheumatic I01.2
with chorea (acute) (rheumatic) (Sydenham's) I02.0
acute or subacute (interstitial) I40.9
due to
streptococcus (beta-hemolytic) I01.2
idiopathic I40.1
rheumatic I01.2
with chorea (acute) (rheumatic) (Sydenham's) I02.0
specified NEC I40.8
aseptic of newborn B33.22

Myocarditis *(continued)*
bacterial (acute) I40.0
Coxsackie (virus) B33.22
diphtheritic A36.81
eosinophilic I40.1
epidemic of newborn (Coxsackie) B33.22
Fiedler's (acute) (isolated) I40.1
giant cell (acute) (subacute) I40.1
gonococcal A54.83
granulomatous (idiopathic) (isolated) (nonspecific) I40.1
hypertensive —*see* Hypertension, heart
idiopathic (granulomatous) I40.1
in (due to)
diphtheria A36.81
epidemic louse-borne typhus A75.0 *[I41]*
Lyme disease A69.29
sarcoidosis D86.85
scarlet fever A38.1
toxoplasmosis (acquired) B58.81
typhoid A01.02
typhus NEC A75.9 *[I41]*
infective I40.0
influenzal —*see* Influenza, with, myocarditis
isolated (acute) I40.1
meningococcal A39.52
mumps B26.82
nonrheumatic, active I40.9
parenchymatous I40.9
pneumococcal I40.0
rheumatic (chronic) (inactive) (with chorea) I09.0
active or acute I01.2
with chorea (acute) (rheumatic) (Sydenham's) I02.0
rheumatoid —*see* Rheumatoid, carditis
septic I40.0
staphylococcal I40.0
suppurative I40.0
syphilitic (chronic) A52.06
toxic I40.8
rheumatic —*see* Myocarditis, acute, rheumatic
tuberculous A18.84
typhoid A01.02
valvular —*see* Endocarditis
virus, viral I40.0
of newborn (Coxsackie) B33.22

Myocardium, myocardial —*see* condition

Myocardosis —*see* Cardiomyopathy

Myoclonus, myoclonic, myoclonia (familial) (essential) (multifocal) (simplex) G25.3
drug-induced G25.3
epilepsy (*see also* Epilepsy, generalized, specified NEC) G40.4-
familial (progressive) G25.3
epileptica G40.409
with status epilepticus G40.401
facial G51.3
familial progressive G25.3
Friedreich's G25.3
jerks G25.3
massive G25.3
palatal G25.3
pharyngeal G25.3

Myocytolysis I51.5

Myodiastasis —*see* Diastasis, muscle

Myoendocarditis —*see* Endocarditis

Myoepithelioma —*see* Neoplasm, benign, by site

Myofasciitis (acute) *—see* Myositis

Myofibroma *—see also* Neoplasm, connective tissue, benign
uterus (cervix) (corpus) *—see* Leiomyoma

Myofibromatosis D48.1
infantile Q89.8

Myofibrosis M62.89
heart *—see* Myocarditis
scapulohumeral *—see* Lesion, shoulder, specified NEC

Myofibrositis M79.7
scapulohumeral *—see* Lesion, shoulder, specified NEC

Myoglobulinuria, myoglobinuria (primary) R82.1

Myokymia, facial G51.4

Myolipoma *—see* Lipoma

Myoma *—see also* Neoplasm, connective tissue, benign
malignant *—see* Neoplasm, connective tissue, malignant
prostate D29.1
uterus (cervix) (corpus) *—see* Leiomyoma

Myomalacia M62.89

Myometritis *—see* Endometritis

Myometrium *—see* condition

Myonecrosis, clostridial A48.0

Myopathy G72.9
acute
necrotizing G72.81
quadriplegic G72.81
alcoholic G72.1
benign congenital G71.2
central core G71.2
centronuclear G71.2
congenital (benign) G71.2
critical illness G72.81
distal G71.0
drug-induced G72.0
endocrine NEC E34.9 *[G73.7]*
extraocular muscles H05.82-
facioscapulohumeral G71.0
hereditary G71.9
specified NEC G71.8
immune NEC G72.49
in (due to)
Addison's disease E27.1 *[G73.7]*
alcohol G72.1
amyloidosis E85.0 *[G73.7]*
cretinism E00.9 *[G73.7]*
Cushing's syndrome E24.9 *[G73.7]*
drugs G72.0
endocrine disease NEC E34.9 *[G73.7]*
giant cell arteritis M31.6 *[G73.7]*
glycogen storage disease E74.00 *[G73.7]*
hyperadrenocorticism E24.9 *[G73.7]*
hyperparathyroidism NEC E21.3 *[G73.7]*
hypoparathyroidism E20.9 *[G73.7]*
hypopituitarism E23.0 *[G73.7]*
hypothyroidism E03.9 *[G73.7]*
infectious disease NEC B99 *[G73.7]*
lipid storage disease E75.6 *[G73.7]*
metabolic disease NEC E88.9 *[G73.7]*
myxedema E03.9 *[G73.7]*
parasitic disease NEC B89 *[G73.7]*

Myopathy *(continued)*
in *(continued)*
polyarteritis nodosa M30.0 *[G73.7]*
rheumatoid arthritis *—see* Rheumatoid, myopathy
sarcoidosis D86.87
scleroderma M34.82
sicca syndrome M35.03
Sjögren's syndrome M35.03
systemic lupus erythematosus M32.19
thyrotoxicosis (hyperthyroidism) E05.90 *[G73.7]*
with thyroid storm E05.91 *[G73.7]*
toxic agent NEC G72.2
inflammatory NEC G72.49
intensive care (ICU) G72.81
limb-girdle G71.0
mitochondrial NEC G71.3
mytonic, proximal (PROMM) G71.11
myotubular G71.2
nemaline G71.2
ocular G71.0
oculopharyngeal G71.0
of critical illness G72.81
primary G71.9
specified NEC G71.8
progressive NEC G72.89
proximal myotonic (PROMM) G71.11
rod G71.2
scapulohumeral G71.0
specified NEC G72.89
toxic G72.2

Myopericarditis *—see also* Pericarditis
chronic rheumatic I09.2

Myopia (axial) (congenital) H52.1-
degenerative (malignant) H44.20
with
choroidal neovascularization H44.2A-
foveoschisis H44.2D-
macular hole H44.2B-
retinal detachment H44.2C-
specified maculopathy NEC H44.2E-
bilateral H44.23
left eye H44.22
right eye H44.21
malignant (*see also* Myopia, degenerative) H44.2-
pernicious (*see also* Myopia, degenerative) H44.2-
progressive high (degenerative) (*see also* Myopia, degenerative) H44.2-

Myosarcoma *—see* Neoplasm, connective tissue, malignant

Myosis (pupil) H57.03
stromal (endolymphatic) D39.0

Myositis M60.9
clostridial A48.0
due to posture *—see* Myositis, specified type NEC
epidemic B33.0
fibrosa or fibrous (chronic), Volkmann's T79.6
foreign body granuloma *—see* Granuloma, foreign body
in (due to)
bilharziasis B65.9 *[M63.8-]*
cysticercosis B69.81
leprosy A30.9 *[M63.8-]*
mycosis B49 *[M63.8-]*
sarcoidosis D86.87

Myositis *(continued)*
in *(continued)*
schistosomiasis B65.9 *[M63.8-]*
syphilis
late A52.78
secondary A51.49
toxoplasmosis (acquired) B58.82
trichinellosis B75 *[M63.8-]*
tuberculosis A18.09
inclusion body [IBM] G72.41
infective M60.009
arm M60.002
left M60.001
right M60.000
leg M60.005
left M60.004
right M60.003
lower limb M60.005
ankle M60.07-
foot M60.07-
lower leg M60.06-
thigh M60.05-
toe M60.07-
multiple sites M60.09
specified site NEC M60.08
upper limb M60.002
finger M60.04-
forearm M60.03-
hand M60.04-
shoulder region M60.01-
upper arm M60.02-
interstitial M60.10
ankle M60.17-
foot M60.17-
forearm M60.13-
hand M60.14-
lower leg M60.16-
multiple sites M60.19
shoulder region M60.11-
specified site NEC M60.18
thigh M60.15-
upper arm M60.12-
mycotic B49 *[M63.8-]*
orbital, chronic H05.12-
ossificans or ossifying (circumscripta) *—see also* Ossification, muscle, specified NEC
in (due to)
burns M61.30
ankle M61.37-
foot M61.37-
forearm M61.33-
hand M61.34-
lower leg M61.36-
multiple sites M61.39
pelvic region M61.35-
shoulder region M61.31-
specified site NEC M61.38
thigh M61.35-
upper arm M61.32-
quadriplegia or paraplegia M61.20
ankle M61.27-
foot M61.27-
forearm M61.23-
hand M61.24-
lower leg M61.26-
multiple sites M61.29
pelvic region M61.25-
shoulder region M61.21-
specified site NEC M61.28
thigh M61.25-
upper arm M61.22-
progressiva M61.10
ankle M61.17-
finger M61.14-
foot M61.17-
forearm M61.13-
hand M61.14-

Myositis *(continued)*
ossificans or ossifying *(continued)*
progressiva *(continued)*
lower leg M61.16-
multiple sites M61.19
pelvic region M61.15-
shoulder region M61.11-
specified site NEC M61.18
thigh M61.15-
toe M61.17-
upper arm M61.12-
traumatica M61.00
ankle M61.07-
foot M61.07-
forearm M61.03-
hand M61.04-
lower leg M61.06-
multiple sites M61.09
pelvic region M61.05-
shoulder region M61.01-
specified site NEC M61.08
thigh M61.05-
upper arm M61.02-
purulent *—see* Myositis, infective
specified type NEC M60.80
ankle M60.87-
foot M60.87-
forearm M60.83-
hand M60.84-
lower leg M60.86-
multiple sites M60.89
pelvic region M60.85-
shoulder region M60.81-
specified site NEC M60.88
thigh M60.85-
upper arm M60.82-
suppurative *—see* Myositis, infective
traumatic (old) *—see* Myositis, specified type NEC

Myospasia impulsiva F95.2

Myotonia (acquisita) (intermittens) M62.89
atrophica G71.11
chondrodystrophic G71.13
congenita (acetazolamide responsive) (dominant) (recessive) G71.12
drug-induced G71.14
dystrophica G71.11
fluctuans G71.19
levior G71.12
permanens G71.19
symptomatic G71.19

Myotonic pupil *—see* Anomaly, pupil, function, tonic pupil

Myriapodiasis B88.2

Myringitis H73.2-
with otitis media *—see* Otitis, media
acute H73.00-
bullous H73.01-
specified NEC H73.09-
bullous *—see* Myringitis, acute, bullous
chronic H73.1-

Mysophobia F40.228

Mytilotoxism *—see* Poisoning, fish

Myxadenitis labialis K13.0

Myxedema (adult) (idiocy) (infantile) (juvenile) (*see also* Hypothyroidism) E03.9
circumscribed E05.90
with storm E05.91
coma E03.5
congenital E00.1
cutis L98.5

Myxedema *(continued)*
localized (pretibial) E05.90
with storm E05.91
papular L98.5

Myxochondrosarcoma *—see* Neoplasm, cartilage, malignant

Myxofibroma *—see* Neoplasm, connective tissue, benign
odontogenic *—see* Cyst, calcifying odontogenic

Myxofibrosarcoma *—see* Neoplasm, connective tissue, malignant

Myxolipoma D17.9

Myxoliposarcoma *—see* Neoplasm, connective tissue, malignant

Myxoma *—see also* Neoplasm, connective tissue, benign
nerve sheath *—see* Neoplasm, nerve, benign
odontogenic *—see* Cyst, calcifying odontogenic

Myxosarcoma *—see* Neoplasm, connective tissue, malignant

N

Naegeli's
disease Q82.8
leukemia, monocytic C93.1-

Naegleriasis (with meningoencephalitis) B60.2

Naffziger's syndrome G54.0

Naga sore *—see* Ulcer, skin

Nägele's pelvis M95.5
with disproportion (fetopelvic) O33.0
causing obstructed labor O65.0

Nail *—see also* condition
biting F98.8
patella syndrome Q87.2

Nanism, nanosomia *—see* Dwarfism

Nanophyetiasis B66.8

Nanukayami A27.89

Napkin rash L22

Narcolepsy G47.419
with cataplexy G47.411
in conditions classified elsewhere G47.429
with cataplexy G47.421

Narcosis R06.89

Narcotism *—see* Dependence

NARP (Neuropathy, Ataxia and Retinitis pigmentosa) **syndrome** E88.49

Narrow
anterior chamber angle H40.03-
gingival width (of periodontal soft tissue) K05.5
pelvis *—see* Contraction, pelvis

Narrowing *—see also* Stenosis
artery I77.1
auditory, internal I65.8
basilar *—see* Occlusion, artery, basilar
carotid *—see* Occlusion, artery, carotid
cerebellar *—see* Occlusion, artery, cerebellar
cerebral *—see* Occlusion artery, cerebral
choroidal *—see* Occlusion, artery, cerebral, specified NEC

Narrowing *(continued)*
artery *(continued)*
communicating posterior *—see* Occlusion, artery, cerebral, specified NEC
coronary *—see also* Disease, heart, ischemic, atherosclerotic
congenital Q24.5
syphilitic A50.54 *[I52]*
due to syphilis NEC A52.06
hypophyseal *—see* Occlusion, artery, cerebral, specified NEC
pontine *—see* Occlusion, artery, cerebral, specified NEC
precerebral *—see* Occlusion, artery, precerebral
vertebral *—see* Occlusion, artery, vertebral
auditory canal (external) *—see* Stenosis, external ear canal
eustachian tube *—see* Obstruction, eustachian tube
eyelid *—see* Disorder, eyelid function
larynx J38.6
mesenteric artery (*see also* Ischemia, intestine, acute) K55.059
palate M26.89
palpebral fissure *—see* Disorder, eyelid function
ureter N13.5
with infection N13.6
urethra *—see* Stricture, urethra

Narrowness, abnormal, eyelid Q10.3

Nasal *—see* condition

Nasolachrymal, nasolacrimal *—see* condition

Nasopharyngeal *—see also* condition
pituitary gland Q89.2
torticollis M43.6

Nasopharyngitis (acute) (infective) (streptococcal) (subacute) J00
chronic (suppurative) (ulcerative) J31.1

Nasopharynx, nasopharyngeal *—see* condition

Natal tooth, teeth K00.6

Nausea (without vomiting) R11.0
with vomiting R11.2
gravidarum *—see* Hyperemesis, gravidarum
marina T75.3
navalis T75.3

Navel *—see* condition

Neapolitan fever *—see* Brucellosis

Near drowning T75.1

Nearsightedness *—see* Myopia

Near-syncope R55

Nebula, cornea *—see* Opacity, cornea

Necator americanus infestation B76.1

Necatoriasis B76.1

Neck *—see* condition

Necrobiosis R68.89
lipoidica NEC L92.1
with diabetes *—see* E08-E13 with .620

Necrolysis, toxic epidermal L51.2
due to drug
correct substance properly administered *—see* Table of Drugs and Chemicals, by drug, adverse effect

Necrolysis, toxic epidermal *(continued)*
due to drug *(continued)*
overdose or wrong substance given or taken *—see* Table of Drugs and Chemicals, by drug, poisoning

Necrophilia F65.89

Necrosis, necrotic (ischemic) *—see also* Gangrene
adrenal (capsule) (gland) E27.49
amputation stump (surgical) (late) T87.50
arm T87.5-
leg T87.5-
antrum J32.0
aorta (hyaline) *—see also* Aneurysm, aorta
cystic medial *—see* Dissection, aorta
artery I77.5
bladder (aseptic) (sphincter) N32.89
bone *—see also* Osteonecrosis M87.9
aseptic or avascular *—see* Osteonecrosis
idiopathic M87.00
ethmoid J32.2
jaw M27.2
tuberculous *—see* Tuberculosis, bone
brain I67.89
breast (aseptic) (fat) (segmental) N64.1
bronchus J98.09
central nervous system NEC I67.89
cerebellar I67.89
cerebral I67.89
colon (*see also* Infarct, intestine) K55.049
cornea H18.89-
cortical (acute) (renal) N17.1
cystic medial (aorta) *—see* Dissection, aorta
dental pulp K04.1
esophagus K22.8
ethmoid (bone) J32.2
eyelid *—see* Disorder, eyelid, degenerative
fat, fatty (generalized) *—see also* Disorder, soft tissue, specified type NEC
abdominal wall K65.4
breast (aseptic) (segmental) N64.1
localized *—see* Degeneration, by site, fatty
mesentery K65.4
omentum K65.4
pancreas K86.89
peritoneum K65.4
skin (subcutaneous), newborn P83.0
subcutaneous, due to birth injury P15.6
gallbladder *—see* Cholecystitis, acute
heart *—see* Infarct, myocardium
hip, aseptic or avascular *—see* Osteonecrosis, by type, femur
intestine (acute) (hemorrhagic) (massive) (*see also* Infarct, intestine) K55.069
jaw M27.2
kidney (bilateral) N28.0
acute N17.9
cortical (acute) (bilateral) N17.1
with ectopic or molar pregnancy O08.4
medullary (bilateral) (in acute renal failure) (papillary) N17.2

Necrosis, necrotic *(continued)*
kidney (bilateral) *(continued)*
papillary (bilateral) (in acute renal failure) N17.2
tubular N17.0
with ectopic or molar pregnancy O08.4
complicating
abortion *—see* Abortion, by type, complicated by, tubular necrosis
ectopic or molar pregnancy O08.4
pregnancy *—see* Pregnancy, complicated by, diseases of, specified type or system NEC
following ectopic or molar pregnancy O08.4
traumatic T79.5
larynx J38.7
liver (with hepatic failure) (cell) *—see* Failure, hepatic
hemorrhagic, central K76.2
lung J85.0
lymphatic gland *—see* Lymphadenitis, acute
mammary gland (fat) (segmental) N64.1
mastoid (chronic) *—see* Mastoiditis, chronic
medullary (acute) (renal) N17.2
mesentery (*see also* Infarct, intestine) K55.069
fat K65.4
mitral valve *—see* Insufficiency, mitral
myocardium, myocardial *—see* Infarct, myocardium
nose J34.0
omentum (with mesenteric infarction) (*see also* Infarct, intestine) K55.069
fat K65.4
orbit, orbital *—see* Osteomyelitis, orbit
ossicles, ear *—see* Abnormal, ear ossicles
ovary N70.92
pancreas (aseptic) (duct) (fat) K86.89
acute (infective) *—see* Pancreatitis, acute
infective *—see* Pancreatitis, acute
papillary (acute) (renal) N17.2
perineum N90.89
peritoneum (with mesenteric infarction) (*see also* Infarct, intestine) K55.069
fat K65.4
pharynx J02.9
in granulocytopenia *—see* Neutropenia
Vincent's A69.1
phosphorus *—see* subcategory T54.2
pituitary (gland) E23.0
postpartum O99.285
Sheehan O99.285
pressure *—see* Ulcer, pressure, by site
pulmonary J85.0
pulp (dental) K04.1
radiation *—see* Necrosis, by site
radium *—see* Necrosis, by site
renal *—see* Necrosis, kidney
sclera H15.89
scrotum N50.89
skin or subcutaneous tissue NEC I96

Necrosis, necrotic *(continued)*
spine, spinal (column) *—see also* Osteonecrosis, by type, vertebra
cord G95.19
spleen D73.5
stomach K31.89
stomatitis (ulcerative) A69.0
subcutaneous fat, newborn P83.88
subendocardial (acute) I21.4
chronic I25.89
suprarenal (capsule) (gland) E27.49
testis N50.89
thymus (gland) E32.8
tonsil J35.8
trachea J39.8
tuberculous NEC *—see* Tuberculosis
tubular (acute) (anoxic) (renal) (toxic) N17.0
postprocedural N99.0
vagina N89.8
vertebra *—see also* Osteonecrosis, by type, vertebra
tuberculous A18.01
vulva N90.89
X-ray *—see* Necrosis, by site

Necrospermia *—see* Infertility, male

Need (for)
care provider because (of)
assistance with personal care Z74.1
continuous supervision required Z74.3
impaired mobility Z74.09
no other household member able to render care Z74.2
specified reason NEC Z74.8
immunization *—see* Vaccination
vaccination *—see* Vaccination

Neglect
adult
confirmed T74.01
history of Z91.412
suspected T76.01
child (childhood)
confirmed T74.02
history of Z62.812
suspected T76.02
emotional, in childhood Z62.898
hemispatial R41.4
left-sided R41.4
sensory R41.4
visuospatial R41.4

Neisserian infection NEC *—see* Gonococcus

Nelaton's syndrome G60.8

Nelson's syndrome E24.1

Nematodiasis (intestinal) B82.0
Ancylostoma B76.0

Neonatal *—see also* Newborn
acne L70.4
bradycardia P29.12
tachycardia P29.11
screening, abnormal findings on P09
tooth, teeth K00.6

Neonatorum *—see* condition

Neoplasia
endocrine, multiple (MEN) E31.20
type I E31.21
type IIA E31.22
type IIB E31.23
intraepithelial (histologically confirmed)
anal (AIN) (histologically confirmed) K62.82

Neoplasia *(continued)*
intraepithelial *(continued)*
anal *(continued)*
grade I K62.82
grade II K62.82
severe D01.3
cervical glandular (histologically confirmed) D06.9
cervix (uteri) (CIN) (histologically confirmed) N87.9
glandular D06.9
grade I N87.0
grade II N87.1
grade III (severe dysplasia) (*see also* Carcinoma, cervix uteri, in situ) D06.9
prostate (histologically confirmed) (PIN) N42.31
grade I N42.31
grade II N42.31
grade III (severe dysplasia) D07.5
vagina (histologically confirmed) (VAIN) N89.3
grade I N89.0
grade II N89.1
grade III (severe dysplasia) D07.2
vulva (histologically confirmed) (VIN) N90.3
grade I N90.0
grade II N90.1
grade III (severe dysplasia) D07.1

Neoplasm, neoplastic *—see also* Table of Neoplasms
lipomatous, benign *—see* Lipoma
malignant mast cell C96.20
specified type NEC C96.29
mast cell, of uncertain behavior NEC D47.09

Neovascularization
ciliary body *—see* Disorder, iris, vascular
cornea H16.40-
deep H16.44-
ghost vessels *—see* Ghost, vessels
localized H16.43-
pannus *—see* Pannus
iris *—see* Disorder, iris, vascular
retina H35.05-

Nephralgia N23

Nephritis, nephritic (albuminuric) (azotemic) (congenital) (disseminated) (epithelial) (familial) (focal) (granulomatous) (hemorrhagic) (infantile) (nonsuppurative, excretory) (uremic) N05.9
with
dense deposit disease N05.6
diffuse
crescentic glomerulonephritis N05.7
endocapillary proliferative glomerulonephritis N05.4
membranous glomerulonephritis N05.2
mesangial proliferative glomerulonephritis N05.3
mesangiocapillary glomerulonephritis N05.5
edema *—see* Nephrosis
focal and segmental glomerular lesions N05.1
foot process disease N04.9
glomerular lesion
diffuse sclerosing N05.8

Nephritis, nephritic *(continued)*
with *(continued)*
glomerular lesion *(continued)*
hypocomplementemic *—see* Nephritis, membranoproliferative
IgA *—see* Nephropathy, IgA
lobular, lobulonodular *—see* Nephritis, membranoproliferative
nodular *—see* Nephritis, membranoproliferative
lesion of
glomerulonephritis, proliferative N05.8
renal necrosis N05.9
minor glomerular abnormality N05.0
specified morphological changes NEC N05.8
acute N00.9
with
dense deposit disease N00.6
diffuse
crescentic glomerulonephritis N00.7
endocapillary proliferative glomerulonephritis N00.4
membranous glomerulonephritis N00.2
mesangial proliferative glomerulonephritis N00.3
mesangiocapillary glomerulonephritis N00.5
focal and segmental glomerular lesions N00.1
minor glomerular abnormality N00.0
specified morphological changes NEC N00.8
amyloid E85.4 *[N08]*
antiglomerular basement membrane (anti-GBM) antibody NEC
in Goodpasture's syndrome M31.0
antitubular basement membrane (tubulo-interstitial) NEC N12
toxic *—see* Nephropathy, toxic
arteriolar *—see* Hypertension, kidney
arteriosclerotic *—see* Hypertension, kidney
ascending *—see* Nephritis, tubulo-interstitial
atrophic N03.9
Balkan (endemic) N15.0
calculous, calculus *—see* Calculus, kidney
cardiac *—see* Hypertension, kidney
cardiovascular *—see* Hypertension, kidney
chronic N03.9
with
dense deposit disease N03.6
diffuse
crescentic glomerulonephritis N03.7
endocapillary proliferative glomerulonephritis N03.4
membranous glomerulonephritis N03.2
mesangial proliferative glomerulonephritis N03.3
mesangiocapillary glomerulonephritis N03.5
focal and segmental glomerular lesions N03.1
minor glomerular abnormality N03.0
specified morphological changes NEC N03.8

Nephritis, nephritic *(continued)*
chronic *(continued)*
arteriosclerotic *—see* Hypertension, kidney
cirrhotic N26.9
complicating pregnancy O26.83-
croupous N00.9
degenerative *—see* Nephrosis
diffuse sclerosing N05.8
due to
diabetes mellitus *—see* E08-E13 with .21
subacute bacterial endocarditis I33.0
systemic lupus erythematosus (chronic) M32.14
typhoid fever A01.09
gonococcal (acute) (chronic) A54.21
hypocomplementemic *—see* Nephritis, membranoproliferative
IgA *—see* Nephropathy, IgA
immune complex (circulating) NEC N05.8
infective *—see* Nephritis, tubulo-interstitial
interstitial *—see* Nephritis, tubulo-interstitial
lead N14.3
membranoproliferative (diffuse) (type 1 or 3) (*see also* N00-N07 with fourth character .5) N05.5
type 2 (*see also* N00-N07 with fourth character .6) N05.6
minimal change N05.0
necrotic, necrotizing NEC (*see also* N00-N07 with fourth character .8) N05.8
nephrotic *—see* Nephrosis
nodular *—see* Nephritis, membranoproliferative
polycystic Q61.3
adult type Q61.2
autosomal
dominant Q61.2
recessive NEC Q61.19
childhood type NEC Q61.19
infantile type NEC Q61.19
poststreptococcal N05.9
acute N00.9
chronic N03.9
rapidly progressive N01.9
proliferative NEC (*see also* N00-N07 with fourth character .8) N05.8
purulent *—see* Nephritis, tubulo-interstitial
rapidly progressive N01.9
with
dense deposit disease N01.6
diffuse
crescentic glomerulonephritis N01.7
endocapillary proliferative glomerulonephritis N01.4
membranous glomerulonephritis N01.2
mesangial proliferative glomerulonephritis N01.3
mesangiocapillary glomerulonephritis N01.5
focal and segmental glomerular lesions N01.1
minor glomerular abnormality N01.0
specified morphological changes NEC N01.8
salt losing or wasting NEC N28.89
saturnine N14.3
sclerosing, diffuse N05.8

- **Nephritis, nephritic** *(continued)*
  - septic *—see* Nephritis, tubulo-interstitial
  - specified pathology NEC (*see also* N00-N07 with fourth character .8) N05.8
  - subacute N01.9
  - suppurative *—see* Nephritis, tubulo-interstitial
  - syphilitic (late) A52.75
    - congenital A50.59 *[N08]*
    - early (secondary) A51.44
  - toxic *—see* Nephropathy, toxic
  - tubal, tubular *—see* Nephritis, tubulo-interstitial
  - tuberculous A18.11
  - tubulo-interstitial (in) N12
    - acute (infectious) N10
    - chronic (infectious) N11.9
      - nonobstructive N11.8
        - reflux-associated N11.0
      - obstructive N11.1
      - specified NEC N11.8
    - due to
      - brucellosis A23.9 *[N16]*
      - cryoglobulinemia D89.1 *[N16]*
      - glycogen storage disease E74.00 *[N16]*
    - Sjögren's syndrome M35.04
  - vascular *—see* Hypertension, kidney
  - war N00.9
- **Nephroblastoma** (epithelial) (mesenchymal) C64-
- **Nephrocalcinosis** E83.59 *[N29]*
- **Nephrocystitis, pustular** *—see* Nephritis, tubulo-interstitial
- **Nephrolithiasis** (congenital) (pelvis) (recurrent) *—see also* Calculus, kidney
- **Nephroma** C64-
  - mesoblastic D41.0-
- **Nephronephritis** *—see* Nephrosis
- **Nephronophthisis** Q61.5
- **Nephropathia epidemica** A98.5
- **Nephropathy** *—see also* Nephritis N28.9
  - with
    - edema *—see* Nephrosis
    - glomerular lesion *—see* Glomerulonephritis
  - amyloid, hereditary E85.0
  - analgesic N14.0
    - with medullary necrosis, acute N17.2
  - Balkan (endemic) N15.0
  - chemical *—see* Nephropathy, toxic
  - diabetic *—see* E08-E13 with .21
  - drug-induced N14.2
    - specified NEC N14.1
  - focal and segmental hyalinosis or sclerosis N02.1
  - heavy metal-induced N14.3
  - hereditary NEC N07.9
    - with
      - dense deposit disease N07.6
      - diffuse
        - crescentic glomerulonephritis N07.7
        - endocapillary proliferative glomerulonephritis N07.4
        - membranous glomerulonephritis N07.2
        - mesangial proliferative glomerulonephritis N07.3
        - mesangiocapillary glomerulonephritis N07.5
- **Nephropathy** *(continued)*
  - hereditary NEC *(continued)*
    - with *(continued)*
      - focal and segmental glomerular lesions N07.1
      - minor glomerular abnormality N07.0
      - specified morphological changes NEC N07.8
  - hypercalcemic N25.89
  - hypertensive *—see* Hypertension, kidney
  - hypokalemic (vacuolar) N25.89
  - IgA N02.8
    - with glomerular lesion N02.9
      - focal and segmental hyalinosis or sclerosis N02.1
      - membranoproliferative (diffuse) N02.5
      - membranous (diffuse) N02.2
      - mesangial proliferative (diffuse) N02.3
      - mesangiocapillary (diffuse) N02.5
      - proliferative NEC N02.8
      - specified pathology NEC N02.8
  - lead N14.3
  - membranoproliferative (diffuse) N02.5
  - membranous (diffuse) N02.2
  - mesangial (IgA/IgG) *—see* Nephropathy, IgA
    - proliferative (diffuse) N02.3
  - mesangiocapillary (diffuse) N02.5
  - obstructive N13.8
  - phenacetin N17.2
  - phosphate-losing N25.0
  - potassium depletion N25.89
  - pregnancy-related O26.83-
  - proliferative NEC (*see also* N00-N07 with fourth character .8) N05.8
  - protein-losing N25.89
  - saturnine N14.3
  - sickle-cell D57.- *[N08]*
  - toxic NEC N14.4
    - due to
      - drugs N14.2
        - analgesic N14.0
        - specified NEC N14.1
      - heavy metals N14.3
  - vasomotor N17.0
  - water-losing N25.89
- **Nephroptosis** N28.83
- **Nephropyosis** *—see* Abscess, kidney
- **Nephrorrhagia** N28.89
- **Nephrosclerosis** (arteriolar) (arteriosclerotic) (chronic) (hyaline) *—see also* Hypertension, kidney
  - hyperplastic *—see* Hypertension, kidney
  - senile N26.9
- **Nephrosis, nephrotic** (Epstein's) (syndrome) (congenital) N04.9
  - with
    - foot process disease N04.9
    - glomerular lesion N04.1
    - hypocomplementemic N04.5
  - acute N04.9
  - anoxic *—see* Nephrosis, tubular
  - chemical *—see* Nephrosis, tubular
  - cholemic K76.7
  - diabetic *—see* E08-E13 with .21
  - Finnish type (congenital) Q89.8
  - hemoglobin N10
  - hemoglobinuric *—see* Nephrosis, tubular
- **Nephrosis, nephrotic** *(continued)*
  - in
    - amyloidosis E85.4 *[N08]*
    - diabetes mellitus *—see* E08-E13 with .21
    - epidemic hemorrhagic fever A98.5
    - malaria (malariae) B52.0
  - ischemic *—see* Nephrosis, tubular
  - lipoid N04.9
  - lower nephron *—see* Nephrosis, tubular
  - malarial (malariae) B52.0
  - minimal change N04.0
  - myoglobin N10
  - necrotizing *—see* Nephrosis, tubular
  - osmotic (sucrose) N25.89
  - radiation N04.9
  - syphilitic (late) A52.75
  - toxic *—see* Nephrosis, tubular
  - tubular (acute) N17.0
    - postprocedural N99.0
    - radiation N04.9
- **Nephrosonephritis, hemorrhagic** (endemic) A98.5
- **Nephrostomy**
  - attention to Z43.6
  - status Z93.6
- **Nerve** *—see also* condition
  - injury *—see* Injury, nerve, by body site
- **Nerves** R45.0
- **Nervous** (*see also* condition) R45.0
  - heart F45.8
  - stomach F45.8
  - tension R45.0
- **Nervousness** R45.0
- **Nesidioblastoma**
  - pancreas D13.7
  - specified site NEC *—see* Neoplasm, benign, by site
  - unspecified site D13.7
- **Nettleship's syndrome** - *see* Urticaria pigmentosa
- **Neumann's disease or syndrome** L10.1
- **Neuralgia, neuralgic** (acute) M79.2
  - accessory (nerve) G52.8
  - acoustic (nerve) H93.3
  - auditory (nerve) H93.3
  - ciliary G44.009
    - intractable G44.001
    - not intractable G44.009
  - cranial
    - nerve *—see also* Disorder, nerve, cranial
      - fifth or trigeminal *—see* Neuralgia, trigeminal
    - postherpetic, postzoster B02.29
  - ear *—see* subcategory H92.0
  - facialis vera G51.1
  - Fothergill's *—see* Neuralgia, trigeminal
  - glossopharyngeal (nerve) G52.1
  - Horton's G44.099
    - intractable G44.091
    - not intractable G44.099
  - Hunt's B02.21
  - hypoglossal (nerve) G52.3
  - infraorbital *—see* Neuralgia, trigeminal
  - malarial *—see* Malaria
  - migrainous G44.009
    - intractable G44.001
    - not intractable G44.009
  - Morton's G57.6-
- **Neuralgia, neuralgic** *(continued)*
  - nerve, cranial *—see* Disorder, nerve, cranial
  - nose G52.0
  - occipital M54.81
  - olfactory G52.0
  - penis N48.9
  - perineum R10.2
  - postherpetic NEC B02.29
    - trigeminal B02.22
  - pubic region R10.2
  - scrotum R10.2
  - Sluder's G44.89
  - specified nerve NEC G58.8
  - spermatic cord R10.2
  - sphenopalatine (ganglion) G90.09
  - trifacial *—see* Neuralgia, trigeminal
  - trigeminal G50.0
    - postherpetic, postzoster B02.22
  - vagus (nerve) G52.2
  - writer's F48.8
    - organic G25.89
- **Neurapraxia** *—see* Injury, nerve
- **Neurasthenia** F48.8
  - cardiac F45.8
  - gastric F45.8
  - heart F45.8
- **Neurilemmoma** *—see also* Neoplasm, nerve, benign
  - acoustic (nerve) D33.3
  - malignant *—see also* Neoplasm, nerve, malignant
    - acoustic (nerve) C72.4-
- **Neurilemmosarcoma** *—see* Neoplasm, nerve, malignant
- **Neurinoma** *—see* Neoplasm, nerve, benign
- **Neurinomatosis** *—see* Neoplasm, nerve, uncertain behavior
- **Neuritis** (rheumatoid) M79.2
  - abducens (nerve) *—see* Strabismus, paralytic, sixth nerve
  - accessory (nerve) G52.8
  - acoustic (nerve) (*see also* subcategory) H93.3
    - in (due to)
      - infectious disease NEC B99 *[H94.0-]*
      - parasitic disease NEC B89 *[H94.0-]*
    - syphilitic A52.15
  - alcoholic G62.1
    - with psychosis *—see* Psychosis, alcoholic
  - amyloid, any site E85.4 *[G63]*
  - auditory (nerve) *—see* subcategory H93.3
  - brachial *—see* Radiculopathy
    - due to displacement, intervertebral disc *—see* Disorder, disc, cervical, with neuritis
  - cranial nerve
    - due to Lyme disease A69.22
    - eighth or acoustic or auditory H93.3
    - eleventh or accessory G52.8
    - fifth or trigeminal G51.0
    - first or olfactory G52.0
    - fourth or trochlear *—see* Strabismus, paralytic, fourth nerve
    - second or optic *—see* Neuritis, optic
    - seventh or facial G51.8
      - newborn (birth injury) P11.3

- **Neuritis** *(continued)*
  - cranial nerve *(continued)*
    - sixth or abducent *—see* Strabismus, paralytic, sixth nerve
    - tenth or vagus G52.2
    - third or oculomotor *—see* Strabismus, paralytic, third nerve
    - twelfth or hypoglossal G52.3
  - Déjérine-Sottas G60.0
  - diabetic (mononeuropathy) *—see* E08-E13 with .41
    - polyneuropathy *—see* E08-E13 with .42
  - due to
    - beriberi E51.11
    - displacement, prolapse or rupture, intervertebral disc *—see* Disorder, disc, with, radiculopathy
    - herniation, nucleus pulposus M51.9 *[G55]*
  - endemic E51.11
  - facial G51.8
    - newborn (birth injury) P11.3
  - general *—see* Polyneuropathy
  - geniculate ganglion G51.1
    - due to herpes (zoster) B02.21
  - gouty (*see also* Gout, by type) M10.9 *[G63]*
  - hypoglossal (nerve) G52.3
  - ilioinguinal (nerve) G57.9-
  - infectious (multiple) NEC G61.0
  - interstitial hypertrophic progressive G60.0
  - lumbar M54.16
  - lumbosacral M54.17
  - multiple *—see also* Polyneuropathy
    - endemic E51.11
    - infective, acute G61.0
  - multiplex endemica E51.11
  - nerve root *—see* Radiculopathy
  - oculomotor (nerve) *—see* Strabismus, paralytic, third nerve
  - olfactory nerve G52.0
  - optic (nerve) (hereditary) (sympathetic) H46.9
    - with demyelination G36.0
    - in myelitis G36.0
    - nutritional H46.2
    - papillitis *—see* Papillitis, optic
    - retrobulbar H46.1-
    - specified type NEC H46.8
    - toxic H46.3
  - peripheral (nerve) G62.9
    - multiple *—see* Polyneuropathy
    - single *—see* Mononeuritis
  - pneumogastric (nerve) G52.2
  - postherpetic, postzoster B02.29
  - progressive hypertrophic interstitial G60.0
  - retrobulbar *—see also* Neuritis, optic, retrobulbar
    - in (due to)
      - late syphilis A52.15
      - meningococcal infection A39.82
    - meningococcal A39.82
    - syphilitic A52.15
  - sciatic (nerve) *—see also* Sciatica
    - due to displacement of intervertebral disc *—see* Disorder, disc, with, radiculopathy
  - serum (*see also* Reaction, serum) T80.69
  - shoulder-girdle G54.5
  - specified nerve NEC G58.8
  - spinal (nerve) root *—see* Radiculopathy
  - syphilitic A52.15
  - thenar (median) G56.1-
  - thoracic M54.14
  - toxic NEC G62.2
  - trochlear (nerve) *—see* Strabismus, paralytic, fourth nerve
  - vagus (nerve) G52.2
- **Neuroastrocytoma** *—see* Neoplasm, uncertain behavior, by site
- **Neuroavitaminosis** E56.9 *[G99.8]*
- **Neuroblastoma**
  - olfactory C30.0
  - specified site *—see* Neoplasm, malignant, by site
  - unspecified site C74.90
- **Neurochorioretinitis** *—see* Chorioretinitis
- **Neurocirculatory asthenia** F45.8
- **Neurocysticercosis** B69.0
- **Neurocytoma** *—see* Neoplasm, benign, by site
- **Neurodermatitis** (circumscribed) (circumscripta) (local) L28.0
  - atopic L20.81
  - diffuse (Brocq) L20.81
  - disseminated L20.81
- **Neuroencephalomyelopathy, optic** G36.0
- **Neuroepithelioma** *—see also* Neoplasm, malignant, by site
  - olfactory C30.0
- **Neurofibroma** *—see also* Neoplasm, nerve, benign
  - melanotic *—see* Neoplasm, nerve, benign
  - multiple *—see* Neurofibromatosis
  - plexiform *—see* Neoplasm, nerve, benign
- **Neurofibromatosis** (multiple) (nonmalignant) Q85.00
  - acoustic Q85.02
  - malignant *—see* Neoplasm, nerve, malignant
  - specified NEC Q85.09
  - type 1 (von Recklinghausen) Q85.01
  - type 2 Q85.02
- **Neurofibrosarcoma** *—see* Neoplasm, nerve, malignant
- **Neurogenic** *—see also* condition
  - bladder (*see also* Dysfunction bladder, neuromuscular) N31.9
    - cauda equina syndrome G83.4
  - bowel NEC K59.2
  - heart F45.8
- **Neuroglioma** *—see* Neoplasm, uncertain behavior, by site
- **Neurolabyrinthitis** (of Dix and Hallpike) *—see* Neuronitis, vestibular
- **Neurolathyrism** *—see* Poisoning, food, noxious, plant
- **Neuroleprosy** A30.9
- **Neuroma** *—see also* Neoplasm, nerve, benign
  - acoustic (nerve) D33.3
  - amputation (stump) (traumatic) (surgical complication) (late) T87.3-
    - arm T87.3-
    - leg T87.3-
  - digital (toe) G57.6-
  - interdigital G58.8
    - lower limb (toe) G57.8-
    - upper limb G56.8-
  - intermetatarsal G57.8-
  - Morton's G57.6-
  - nonneoplastic
    - arm G56.9-
    - leg G57.9-
    - lower extremity G57.9-
    - upper extremity G56.9-
  - optic (nerve) D33.3
  - plantar G57.6-
  - plexiform *—see* Neoplasm, nerve, benign
  - surgical (nonneoplastic)
    - arm G56.9-
    - leg G57.9-
    - lower extremity G57.9-
    - upper extremity G56.9-
- **Neuromyalgia** *—see* Neuralgia
- **Neuromyasthenia** (epidemic) (postinfectious) G93.3
- **Neuromyelitis** G36.9
  - ascending G61.0
  - optica G36.0
- **Neuromyopathy** G70.9
  - paraneoplastic D49.9 *[G13.0]*
- **Neuromyotonia** (Isaacs) G71.19
- **Neuronevus** *—see* Nevus
- **Neuronitis** G58.9
  - ascending (acute) G57.2-
  - vestibular H81.2-
- **Neuroparalytic** *—see* condition
- **Neuropathy, neuropathic** G62.9
  - acute motor G62.81
  - alcoholic G62.1
    - with psychosis *—see* Psychosis, alcoholic
  - arm G56.9-
  - autonomic, peripheral *—see* Neuropathy, peripheral, autonomic
  - axillary G56.9-
  - bladder N31.9
    - atonic (motor) (sensory) N31.2
    - autonomous N31.2
    - flaccid N31.2
    - nonreflex N31.2
    - reflex N31.1
    - uninhibited N31.0
  - brachial plexus G54.0
  - cervical plexus G54.2
  - chronic
    - progressive segmentally demyelinating G62.89
    - relapsing demyelinating G62.89
  - Déjérine-Sottas G60.0
  - diabetic *—see* E08-E13 with .40
    - mononeuropathy *—see* E08-E13 with .41
    - polyneuropathy *—see* E08-E13 with .42
  - entrapment G58.9
    - iliohypogastric nerve G57.8-
    - ilioinguinal nerve G57.8-
    - lateral cutaneous nerve of thigh G57.1-
    - median nerve G56.0-
    - obturator nerve G57.8-
    - peroneal nerve G57.3-
    - posterior tibial nerve G57.5-
    - saphenous nerve G57.8-
    - ulnar nerve G56.2-
  - facial nerve G51.9
  - hereditary G60.9
    - motor and sensory (types I-IV) G60.0
    - sensory G60.8
    - specified NEC G60.8
  - hypertrophic G60.0
    - Charcot-Marie-Tooth G60.0
    - Déjérine-Sottas G60.0
    - interstitial progressive G60.0
    - of infancy G60.0
    - Refsum G60.1
  - idiopathic G60.9
    - progressive G60.3
    - specified NEC G60.8
  - in association with hereditary ataxia G60.2
  - intercostal G58.0
  - ischemic *—see* Disorder, nerve
  - Jamaica (ginger) G62.2
  - leg NEC G57.9-
  - lower extremity G57.9-
  - lumbar plexus G54.1
  - median nerve G56.1-
  - motor and sensory *—see also* Polyneuropathy
    - hereditary (types I-IV) G60.0
  - multifocal motor (MMN) G61.82
  - multiple (acute) (chronic) *—see* Polyneuropathy
  - optic (nerve) *—see also* Neuritis, optic
    - ischemic H47.01-
  - paraneoplastic (sensorial) (Denny Brown) D49.9 *[G13.0]*
  - peripheral (nerve) (*see also* Polyneuropathy) G62.9
    - autonomic G90.9
      - idiopathic G90.09
      - in (due to)
        - amyloidosis E85.4 *[G99.0]*
        - diabetes mellitus *—see* E08-E13 with .43
        - endocrine disease NEC E34.9 *[G99.0]*
        - gout M10.00 *[G99.0]*
        - hyperthyroidism E05.90 *[G99.0]*
          - with thyroid storm E05.91 *[G99.0]*
        - metabolic disease NEC E88.9 *[G99.0]*
    - idiopathic G60.9
      - progressive G60.3
    - in (due to)
      - antitetanus serum G62.0
      - arsenic G62.2
      - drugs NEC G62.0
      - lead G62.2
      - organophosphate compounds G62.2
      - toxic agent NEC G62.2
  - plantar nerves G57.6-
  - progressive
    - hypertrophic interstitial G60.0
    - inflammatory G62.81
  - radicular NEC *—see* Radiculopathy
  - sacral plexus G54.1
  - sciatic G57.0-
  - serum G61.1
  - toxic NEC G62.2
  - trigeminal sensory G50.8
  - ulnar nerve G56.2-
  - uremic N18.9 *[G63]*
  - vitamin B12 E53.8 *[G63]*
    - with anemia (pernicious) D51.0 *[G63]*
      - due to dietary deficiency D51.3 *[G63]*

Neurophthisis —*see also* Disorder, nerve
- peripheral, diabetic —*see* E08-E13 with .42

Neuroretinitis —*see* Chorioretinitis

Neuroretinopathy, hereditary optic H47.22

Neurosarcoma —*see* Neoplasm, nerve, malignant

Neurosclerosis —*see* Disorder, nerve

Neurosis, neurotic F48.9
- anankastic F42.8
- anxiety (state) F41.1
  - panic type F41.0
- asthenic F48.8
- bladder F45.8
- cardiac (reflex) F45.8
- cardiovascular F45.8
- character F60.9
- colon F45.8
- compensation F68.1
- compulsive, compulsion F42.8
- conversion F44.9
- craft F48.8
- cutaneous F45.8
- depersonalization F48.1
- depressive (reaction) (type) F34.1
- environmental F48.8
- excoriation L98.1
- fatigue F48.8
- functional —*see* Disorder, somatoform
- gastric F45.8
- gastrointestinal F45.8
- heart F45.8
- hypochondriacal F45.21
- hysterical F44.9
- incoordination F45.8
  - larynx F45.8
  - vocal cord F45.8
- intestine F45.8
- larynx (sensory) F45.8
  - hysterical F44.4
- mixed NEC F48.8
- musculoskeletal F45.8
- obsessional F42.8
- obsessive-compulsive F42.8
- occupational F48.8
- ocular NEC F45.8
- organ —*see* Disorder, somatoform
- pharynx F45.8
- phobic F40.9
- posttraumatic (situational) F43.10
  - acute F43.11
  - chronic F43.12
- psychasthenic (type) F48.8
- railroad F48.8
- rectum F45.8
- respiratory F45.8
- rumination F45.8
- sexual F65.9
- situational F48.8
- social F40.10
  - generalized F40.11
- specified type NEC F48.8
- state F48.9
  - with depersonalization episode F48.1
- stomach F45.8
- traumatic F43.10
  - acute F43.11
  - chronic F43.12
- vasomotor F45.8
- visceral F45.8
- war F48.8

Neurospongioblastosis diffusa Q85.1

Neurosyphilis (arrested) (early) (gumma) (late) (latent) (recurrent) (relapse) A52.3
- with ataxia (cerebellar) (locomotor) (spastic) (spinal) A52.19
- aneurysm (cerebral) A52.05
- arachnoid (adhesive) A52.13
- arteritis (any artery) (cerebral) A52.04
- asymptomatic A52.2
- congenital A50.40
- dura (mater) A52.13
- general paresis A52.17
- hemorrhagic A52.05
- juvenile (asymptomatic) (meningeal) A50.40
- leptomeninges (aseptic) A52.13
- meningeal, meninges (adhesive) A52.13
- meningitis A52.13
- meningovascular (diffuse) A52.13
- optic atrophy A52.15
- parenchymatous (degenerative) A52.19
- paresis, paretic A52.17
  - juvenile A50.45
- remission in (sustained) A52.3
- serological (without symptoms) A52.2
- specified nature or site NEC A52.19
- tabes, tabetic (dorsalis) A52.11
  - juvenile A50.45
- taboparesis A52.17
  - juvenile A50.45
- thrombosis (cerebral) A52.05
- vascular (cerebral) NEC A52.05

Neurothekeoma —*see* Neoplasm, nerve, benign

Neurotic —*see* Neurosis

Neurotoxemia —*see* Toxemia

Neutroclusion M26.211

Neutropenia, neutropenic (chronic) (genetic) (idiopathic) (immune) (infantile) (malignant) (pernicious) (splenic) D70.9
- congenital (primary) D70.0
- cyclic D70.4
- cytoreductive cancer chemotherapy sequela D70.1
- drug-induced D70.2
  - due to cytoreductive cancer chemotherapy D70.1
- due to infection D70.3
- fever D70.9
- neonatal, transitory (isoimmune) (maternal transfer) P61.5
- periodic D70.4
- secondary (cyclic) (periodic) (splenic) D70.4
  - drug-induced D70.2
    - due to cytoreductive cancer chemotherapy D70.1
- toxic D70.8

Neutrophilia, hereditary giant D72.0

Nevocarcinoma —*see* Melanoma

Nevus D22.9
- achromic —*see* Neoplasm, skin, benign
- amelanotic —*see* Neoplasm, skin, benign
- angiomatous D18.00
  - intra-abdominal D18.03
  - intracranial D18.02
  - skin D18.01
  - specified site NEC D18.09
- araneus I78.1

Nevus *(continued)*
- balloon cell —*see* Neoplasm, skin, benign
- bathing trunk D48.5
- blue —*see* Neoplasm, skin, benign
  - cellular —*see* Neoplasm, skin, benign
  - giant —*see* Neoplasm, skin, benign
  - Jadassohn's —*see* Neoplasm, skin, benign
  - malignant —*see* Melanoma
- capillary D18.00
  - intra-abdominal D18.03
  - intracranial D18.02
  - skin D18.01
  - specified site NEC D18.09
- cavernous D18.00
  - intra-abdominal D18.03
  - intracranial D18.02
  - skin D18.01
  - specified site NEC D18.09
- cellular —*see* Neoplasm, skin, benign
  - blue —*see* Neoplasm, skin, benign
- choroid D31.3-
- comedonicus Q82.5
- conjunctiva D31.0-
- dermal —*see* Neoplasm, skin, benign
  - with epidermal nevus —*see* Neoplasm, skin, benign
- dysplastic —*see* Neoplasm, skin, benign
- eye D31.9-
- flammeus Q82.5
- hemangiomatous D18.00
  - intra-abdominal D18.03
  - intracranial D18.02
  - skin D18.01
  - specified site NEC D18.09
- iris D31.4-
- lacrimal gland D31.5-
- lymphatic D18.1
- magnocellular
  - specified site —*see* Neoplasm, benign, by site
  - unspecified site D31.40
- malignant —*see* Melanoma
- meaning hemangioma D18.00
  - intra-abdominal D18.03
  - intracranial D18.02
  - skin D18.01
  - specified site NEC D18.09
- mouth (mucosa) D10.30
  - specified site NEC D10.39
  - white sponge Q38.6
- multiplex Q85.1
- non-neoplastic I78.1
- oral mucosa D10.30
  - specified site NEC D10.39
  - white sponge Q38.6
- orbit D31.6-
- pigmented
  - giant (*see also* Neoplasm, skin, uncertain behavior) D48.5
    - malignant melanoma in —*see* Melanoma
- portwine Q82.5
- retina D31.2-
- retrobulbar D31.6-
- sanguineous Q82.5
- senile I78.1
- skin D22.9
  - abdominal wall D22.5
  - ala nasi D22.39
  - ankle D22.7-
  - anus, anal D22.5
  - arm D22.6-
  - auditory canal (external) D22.2-

Nevus *(continued)*
- skin *(continued)*
  - auricle (ear) D22.2-
  - auricular canal (external) D22.2-
  - axilla, axillary fold D22.5
  - back D22.5
  - breast D22.5
  - brow D22.39
  - buttock D22.5
  - canthus (eye) D22.1-
  - cheek (external) D22.39
  - chest wall D22.5
  - chin D22.39
  - ear (external) D22.2-
  - external meatus (ear) D22.2-
  - eyebrow D22.39
  - eyelid (lower) (upper) D22.1-
  - face D22.30
    - specified NEC D22.39
  - female genital organ (external) NEC D28.0
  - finger D22.6-
  - flank D22.5
  - foot D22.7-
  - forearm D22.6-
  - forehead D22.39
  - foreskin D29.0
  - genital organ (external) NEC
    - female D28.0
    - male D29.9
  - gluteal region D22.5
  - groin D22.5
  - hand D22.6-
  - heel D22.7-
  - helix D22.2-
  - hip D22.7-
  - interscapular region D22.5
  - jaw D22.39
  - knee D22.7-
  - labium (majus) (minus) D28.0
  - leg D22.7-
  - lip (lower) (upper) D22.0
  - lower limb D22.7-
  - male genital organ (external) D29.9
  - nail D22.9
    - finger D22.6-
    - toe D22.7-
  - nasolabial groove D22.39
  - nates D22.5
  - neck D22.4
  - nose (external) D22.39
  - palpebra D22.1-
  - penis D29.0
  - perianal skin D22.5
  - perineum D22.5
  - pinna D22.2-
  - popliteal fossa or space D22.7-
  - prepuce D29.0
  - pudendum D28.0
  - scalp D22.4
  - scrotum D29.4
  - shoulder D22.6-
  - submammary fold D22.5
  - temple D22.39
  - thigh D22.7-
  - toe D22.7-
  - trunk NEC D22.5
  - umbilicus D22.5
  - upper limb D22.6-
  - vulva D28.0
- specified site NEC —*see* Neoplasm, by site, benign
- spider I78.1
- stellar I78.1
- strawberry Q82.5
- Sutton's benign D22.9
- unius lateris Q82.5
- Unna's Q82.5
- vascular Q82.5
- verrucous Q82.5

Newborn (infant) (liveborn) (singleton) Z38.2
  acne L70.4
  abstinence syndrome P96.1
  affected by
    abnormalities of membranes P02.9
      specified NEC P02.8
    abruptio placenta P02.1
    amino-acid metabolic disorder, transitory P74.8
    amniocentesis (while in utero) P00.6
    amnionitis P02.7
    apparent life threatening event (ALTE) R68.13
    bleeding (into)
      cerebral cortex P52.22
      germinal matrix P52.0
      ventricles P52.1
    breech delivery P03.0
    cardiac arrest P29.81
    cardiomyopathy I42.8
      congenital I42.4
    cerebral ischemia P91.0
    Cesarean delivery P03.4
    chemotherapy agents P04.1
    chorioamnionitis P02.7
    cocaine (crack) P04.41
    complications of labor and delivery P03.9
      specified NEC P03.89
    compression of umbilical cord NEC P02.5
    contracted pelvis P03.1
    delivery P03.9
      Cesarean P03.4
      forceps P03.2
      vacuum extractor P03.3
    environmental chemicals P04.6
    entanglement (knot) in umbilical cord P02.5
    fetal (intrauterine)
      growth retardation P05.9
      malnutrition not light or small for gestational age P05.2
    forceps delivery P03.2
    heart rate abnormalities
      bradycardia P29.12
      intrauterine P03.819
        before onset of labor P03.810
        during labor P03.811
      tachycardia P29.11
    hemorrhage (antepartum) P02.1
      cerebellar (nontraumatic) P52.6
      intracerebral (nontraumatic) P52.4
      intracranial (nontraumatic) P52.9
        specified NEC P52.8
      intraventricular (nontraumatic) P52.3
        grade 1 P52.0
        grade 2 P52.1
        grade 3 P52.21
        grade 4 P52.22
      posterior fossa (nontraumatic) P52.6
      subarachnoid (nontraumatic) P52.5
      subependymal P52.0
        with intracerebral extension P52.22
        with intraventricular extension P52.1
          with enlargment of ventricles P52.21
        without intraventricular extension P52.0

Newborn *(continued)*
  affected by *(continued)*
    hypoxic ischemic encephalopathy [HIE] P91.60
      mild P91.61
      moderate P91.62
      severe P91.63
    induction of labor P03.89
    intestinal perforation P78.0
    intrauterine (fetal) blood loss P50.9
      due to (from)
        cut end of co-twin cord P50.5
        hemorrhage into
          co-twin P50.3
          maternal circulation P50.4
        placenta P50.2
        ruptured cord blood P50.1
        vasa previa P50.0
      specified NEC P50.8
    intrauterine (fetal) hemorrhage P50.9
    intrauterine (in utero) procedure P96.5
    malpresentation (malposition) NEC P03.1
    maternal (complication of) (use of)
      alcohol P04.3
      analgesia (maternal) P04.0
      anesthesia (maternal) P04.0
      blood loss P02.1
      circulatory disease P00.3
      condition P00.9
        specified NEC P00.89
      delivery P03.9
        Cesarean P03.4
        forceps P03.2
        vacuum extractor P03.3
      diabetes mellitus (pre-existing) P70.1
      disorder P00.9
        specified NEC P00.89
      drugs (addictive) (illegal) NEC P04.49
      ectopic pregnancy P01.4
      gestational diabetes P70.0
      hemorrhage P02.1
      hypertensive disorder P00.0
      incompetent cervix P01.0
      infectious disease P00.2
      injury P00.5
      labor and delivery P03.9
      malpresentation before labor P01.7
      maternal death P01.6
      medical procedure P00.7
      medication P04.1
      multiple pregnancy P01.5
      nutritional disorder P00.4
      oligohydramnios P01.2
      parasitic disease P00.2
      periodontal disease P00.81
      placenta previa P02.0
      polyhydramnios P01.3
      precipitate delivery P03.5
      pregnancy P01.9
        specified P01.8
      premature rupture of membranes P01.1
      renal disease P00.1
      respiratory disease P00.3
      surgical procedure P00.6
      urinary tract disease P00.1
      uterine contraction (abnormal) P03.6
    meconium peritonitis P78.0

Newborn *(continued)*
  affected by *(continued)*
    medication (legal) (maternal use) (prescribed) P04.1
    membrane abnormalities P02.9
      specified NEC P02.8
    membranitis P02.7
    methamphetamine(s) P04.49
    mixed metabolic and respiratory acidosis P84
    neonatal abstinence syndrome P96.1
    noxious substances transmitted via placenta or breast milk P04.9
      specified NEC P04.8
    nutritional supplements P04.5
    placenta previa P02.0
    placental
      abnormality (functional) (morphological) P02.20
        specified NEC P02.29
      dysfunction P02.29
      infarction P02.29
      insufficiency P02.29
      separation NEC P02.1
      transfusion syndromes P02.3
    placentitis P02.7
    precipitate delivery P03.5
    prolapsed cord P02.4
    respiratory arrest P28.81
    slow intrauterine growth P05.9
    tobacco P04.2
    twin to twin transplacental transfusion P02.3
    umbilical cord (tightly) around neck P02.5
    umbilical cord condition P02.60
      short cord P02.69
      specified NEC P02.69
    uterine contractions (abnormal) P03.6
    vasa previa P02.69
      from intrauterine blood loss P50.0
  apnea P28.4
    primary P28.3
    obstructive P28.4
    sleep (central) (obstructive) (primary) P28.3
  born in hospital Z38.00
    by cesarean Z38.01
  born outside hospital Z38.1
  breast buds P96.89
  breast engorgement P83.4
  check-up —*see* Newborn, examination
  convulsion P90
  dehydration P74.1
  examination
    8 to 28 days old Z00.111
    under 8 days old Z00.110
  fever P81.9
    environmentally-induced P81.0
  hyperbilirubinemia P59.9
    of prematurity P59.0
  hypernatremia P74.2
  hyponatremia P74.2
  infection P39.9
    candidal P37.5
    specified NEC P39.8
    urinary tract P39.3
  jaundice P59.9
    due to
      breast milk inhibitor P59.3
      hepatocellular damage P59.20
        specified NEC P59.29
      preterm delivery P59.0
    of prematurity P59.0
    specified NEC P59.8
  late metabolic acidosis P74.0

Newborn *(continued)*
  mastitis P39.0
    infective P39.0
    noninfective P83.4
  multiple born NEC Z38.8
    born in hospital Z38.68
      by cesarean Z38.69
    born outside hospital Z38.7
  omphalitis P38.9
    with mild hemorrhage P38.1
    without hemorrhage P38.9
  post-term P08.21
  prolonged gestation (over 42 completed weeks) P08.22
  quadruplet Z38.8
    born in hospital Z38.63
      by cesarean Z38.64
    born outside hospital Z38.7
  quintuplet Z38.8
    born in hospital Z38.65
      by cesarean Z38.66
    born outside hospital Z38.7
  seizure P90
  sepsis (congenital) P36.9
    due to
      anaerobes NEC P36.5
      Escherichia coli P36.4
      Staphylococcus P36.30
        aureus P36.2
        specified NEC P36.39
      Streptococcus P36.10
        group B P36.0
        specified NEC P36.19
    specified NEC P36.8
  triplet Z38.8
    born in hospital Z38.61
      by cesarean Z38.62
    born outside hospital Z38.7
  twin Z38.5
    born in hospital Z38.30
      by cesarean Z38.31
    born outside hospital Z38.4
  vomiting P92.09
    bilious P92.01
  weight check Z00.111

Newcastle conjunctivitis or disease B30.8

Nezelof's syndrome (pure alymphocytosis) D81.4

Niacin (amide) **deficiency** E52

Nicolas (-Durand)-**Favre disease** A55

Nicotine —*see* Tobacco

Nicotinic acid deficiency E52

Niemann-Pick disease or syndrome E75.249
  specified NEC E75.248
  type
    A E75.240
    B E75.241
    C E75.242
    D E75.243

Night
  blindness —*see* Blindness, night
  sweats R61
  terrors (child) F51.4

Nightmares (REM sleep type) F51.5

NIHSS (National Institutes of Health Stroke Scale) score R29.7-

Nipple —*see* condition

Nisbet's chancre A57

Nishimoto (-Takeuchi) **disease** I67.5

Nitritoid crisis or reaction —*see* Crisis, nitritoid

Nitrosohemoglobinemia D74.8

Njovera A65

Nocardiosis, nocardiasis A43.9
- cutaneous A43.1
- lung A43.0
- pneumonia A43.0
- pulmonary A43.0
- specified site NEC A43.8

Nocturia R35.1
- psychogenic F45.8

Nocturnal *—see* condition

Nodal rhythm I49.8

Node(s) *—see also* Nodule
- Bouchard's (with arthropathy) M15.2
- Haygarth's M15.8
- Heberden's (with arthropathy) M15.1
- larynx J38.7
- lymph *—see* condition
- milker's B08.03
- Osler's I33.0
- Schmorl's *—see* Schmorl's disease
- singer's J38.2
- teacher's J38.2
- tuberculous *—see* Tuberculosis, lymph gland
- vocal cord J38.2

Nodule(s), **nodular**
- actinomycotic *—see* Actinomycosis
- breast NEC (*see also* Lump, breast) N63.0
- colloid (cystic), thyroid E04.1
- cutaneous *—see* Swelling, localized
- endometrial (stromal) D26.1
- Haygarth's M15.8
- inflammatory *—see* Inflammation
- juxta-articular
  - syphilitic A52.77
  - yaws A66.7
- larynx J38.7
- lung, solitary (subsegmental branch of the bronchial tree) R91.1
  - multiple R91.8
- milker's B08.03
- prostate N40.2
  - with lower urinary tract symptoms (LUTS) N40.3
  - without lower urinary tract symtpoms (LUTS) N40.2
- pulmonary, solitary (subsegmental branch of the bronchial tree) R91.1
- retrocardiac R09.89
- rheumatoid M06.30
  - ankle M06.37-
  - elbow M06.32-
  - foot joint M06.37-
  - hand joint M06.34-
  - hip M06.35-
  - knee M06.36-
  - multiple site M06.39
  - shoulder M06.31-
  - vertebra M06.38
  - wrist M06.33-
- scrotum (inflammatory) N49.2
- singer's J38.2
- solitary, lung (subsegmental branch of the bronchial tree) R91.1
  - multiple R91.8
- subcutaneous *—see* Swelling, localized
- teacher's J38.2
- thyroid (cold) (gland) (nontoxic) E04.1
  - with thyrotoxicosis E05.20
    - with thyroid storm E05.21

Nodule(s), **nodular** *(continued)*
- thyroid *(continued)*
  - toxic or with hyperthyroidism E05.20
    - with thyroid storm E05.21
- vocal cord J38.2

Noma (gangrenous) (hospital) (infective) A69.0
- auricle I96
- mouth A69.0
- pudendi N76.89
- vulvae N76.89

Nomad, nomadism Z59.0

NOMID (neonatal onset multisystemic inflammatory disorder) M04.2

Nonadherence to medical treatment Z91.19

Nonautoimmune hemolytic anemia D59.4
- drug-induced D59.2

Nonclosure *—see also* Imperfect, closure
- ductus arteriosus (Botallo's) Q25.0
- foramen
  - botalli Q21.1
  - ovale Q21.1

Noncompliance Z91.19
- with
  - dietary regimen Z91.11
  - dialysis Z91.15
  - medical treatment Z91.19
  - medication regimen NEC Z91.14
    - underdosing (*see also* Table of Drugs and Chemicals, categories T36-T50, with final character 6) Z91.14
    - intentional NEC Z91.128
      - due to financial hardship of patient Z91.120
    - unintentional NEC Z91.138
      - due to patient's age related debility Z91.130
  - renal dialysis Z91.15

Nondescent (congenital) *—see also* Malposition, congenital
- cecum Q43.3
- colon Q43.3
- testicle Q53.9
  - bilateral Q53.20
    - abdominal Q53.211
    - perineal Q53.22
  - unilateral Q53.10
    - abdominal Q53.111
    - perineal Q53.12

Nondevelopment
- brain Q02
  - part of Q04.3
- heart Q24.8
- organ or site, congenital NEC *—see* Hypoplasia

Nonengagement
- head NEC O32.4
  - in labor, causing obstructed labor O64.8

Nonexanthematous tick fever A93.2

Nonexpansion, lung (newborn) P28.0

Nonfunctioning
- cystic duct (*see also* Disease, gallbladder) K82.8
- gallbladder (*see also* Disease, gallbladder) K82.8
- kidney N28.9
- labyrinth H83.2

Non-Hodgkin lymphoma NEC *—see* Lymphoma, non-Hodgkin

Non-working side interference M26.56

Nonimplantation, ovum N97.2

Noninsufflation, fallopian tube N97.1

Non-ketotic hyperglycinemia E72.51

Nonne-Milroy syndrome Q82.0

Nonovulation N97.0

Nonpatent fallopian tube N97.1

Non-palpable testicle(s)
- bilateral R39.84
- unilateral R39.83

Nonpneumatization, lung NEC P28.0

Nonrotation *—see* Malrotation

Nonsecretion, urine *—see* Anuria

Nonunion
- fracture *—see* Fracture, by site
- joint, following fusion or arthrodesis M96.0
- organ or site, congenital NEC *—see* Imperfect, closure
- symphysis pubis, congenital Q74.2

Nonvisualization, gallbladder R93.2

Nonvital, nonvitalized tooth K04.99

Noonan's syndrome Q87.1

Normocytic anemia (infectional) **due to blood loss** (chronic) D50.0
- acute D62

Norrie's disease (congenital) Q15.8

North American blastomycosis B40.9

Norwegian itch B86

Nose, nasal *—see* condition

Nosebleed R04.0

Nose-picking F98.8

Nosomania F45.21

Nosophobia F45.22

Nostalgia F43.20

Notch of iris Q13.2

Notching nose, congenital (tip) Q30.2

Nothnagel's
- syndrome *—see* Strabismus, paralytic, third nerve
- vasomotor acroparesthesia I73.89

Novy's relapsing fever A68.9
- louse-borne A68.0
- tick-borne A68.1

Noxious
- foodstuffs, poisoning by *—see* Poisoning, food, noxious, plant
- substances transmitted through placenta or breast milk P04.9

Nucleus pulposus *—see* condition

Numbness R20.0

Nuns' knee *—see* Bursitis, prepatellar

Nursemaid's elbow S53.03-

Nutcracker esophagus K22.4

Nutmeg liver K76.1

Nutrient element deficiency E61.9
- specified NEC E61.8

Nutrition deficient or insufficient (*see also* Malnutrition) E46
- due to
  - insufficient food T73.0
  - lack of
    - care (child) T76.02
      - adult T76.01
    - food T73.0

Nutritional stunting E45

Nyctalopia (night blindness) *—see* Blindness, night

Nycturia R35.1
- psychogenic F45.8

Nymphomania F52.8

Nystagmus H55.00
- benign paroxysmal *—see* Vertigo, benign paroxysmal
- central positional H81.4-
- congenital H55.01
- dissociated H55.04
- latent H55.02
- miners' H55.09
- positional
  - benign paroxysmal H81.4-
  - central H81.4-
- specified form NEC H55.09
- visual deprivation H55.03

O

Obermeyer's relapsing fever (European) A68.0

Obesity E66.9
- with alveolar hypoventilation E66.2
- adrenal E27.8
- complicating
  - childbirth O99.214
  - pregnancy O99.21-
  - puerperium O99.215
- constitutional E66.8
- dietary counseling and surveillance Z71.3
- drug-induced E66.1
- due to
  - drug E66.1
  - excess calories E66.09
    - morbid E66.01
    - severe E66.01
- endocrine E66.8
- endogenous E66.8
- exogenous E66.09
- familial E66.8
- glandular E66.8
- hypothyroid *—see* Hypothyroidism
- hypoventilation syndrome (OHS) E66.2
- morbid E66.01
  - with
    - alveolar hypoventilation E66.2
    - obesity hypoventilation syndrome (OHS) E66.2
  - due to excess calories E66.01
- nutritional E66.09
- pituitary E23.6
- severe E66.01
- specified type NEC E66.8

Oblique *—see* condition

Obliteration
- appendix (lumen) K38.8
- artery I77.1
- bile duct (noncalculous) K83.1
- common duct (noncalculous) K83.1
- cystic duct *—see* Obstruction, gallbladder
- disease, arteriolar I77.1
- endometrium N85.8
- eye, anterior chamber *—see* Disorder, globe, hypotony
- fallopian tube N97.1
- lymphatic vessel I89.0
  - due to mastectomy I97.2
- organ or site, congenital NEC *—see* Atresia, by site
- ureter N13.5
  - with infection N13.6

Obliteration *(continued)*
- urethra —*see* Stricture, urethra
- vein I87.8
- vestibule (oral) K08.89

Observation (following) (for) (without need for further medical care) Z04.9
- accident NEC Z04.3
  - at work Z04.2
  - transport Z04.1
- adverse effect of drug Z03.6
- alleged rape or sexual assault (victim), ruled out
  - adult Z04.41
  - child Z04.42
- criminal assault Z04.8
- development state
  - adolescent Z00.3
  - period of rapid growth in childhood Z00.2
  - puberty Z00.3
- disease, specified NEC Z03.89
- following work accident Z04.2
- growth and development state —*see* Observation, development state
- injuries (accidental) NEC —*see also* Observation, accident
- newborn (for)
  - suspected condition, related to exposure from the mother or birth process —*see* Newborn, affected by, maternal
    - ruled out Z05.9
      - cardiac Z05.0
      - connective tissue Z05.73
      - gastrointestinal Z05.5
      - genetic Z05.41
      - genitourinary Z05.6
      - immunologic Z05.43
      - infectious Z05.1
      - metabolic Z05.42
      - mesculoskeletal Z05.72
      - neurological Z05.2
      - respiratory Z05.3
      - skin and subcutaneous tissue Z05.71
      - specified condition NEC Z05.8
- postpartum
  - immediately after delivery Z39.0
  - routine follow-up Z39.2
- pregnancy (normal) (without complication) Z34.9-
  - high risk O09.9-
- suicide attempt, alleged NEC Z03.89
  - self-poisoning Z03.6
- suspected, ruled out —*see also* Suspected condition, ruled out
  - abuse, physical
    - adult Z04.71
    - child Z04.72
  - accident at work Z04.2
  - adult battering victim Z04.71
  - child battering victim Z04.72
  - condition NEC Z03.89
    - newborn (*see also* Observation, newborn (for), suspected condition, ruled out) Z05.9
  - drug poisoning or adverse effect Z03.6
  - exposure (to)
    - anthrax Z03.810
    - biological agent NEC Z03.818
  - inflicted injury NEC Z04.8
  - suicide attempt, alleged Z03.89
    - self-poisoning Z03.6
  - toxic effects from ingested substance (drug) (poison) Z03.6
- toxic effects from ingested substance (drug) (poison) Z03.6

Obsession, obsessional state F42.8
- mixed thoughts and acts F42.2

Obsessive-compulsive neurosis or reaction F42.8

Obstetric embolism, septic —*see* Embolism, obstetric, septic

Obstetrical trauma (complicating delivery) O71.9
- with or following ectopic or molar pregnancy O08.6
- specified type NEC O71.89

Obstipation —*see* Constipation

Obstruction, obstructed, obstructive
- airway J98.8
  - with
    - allergic alveolitis J67.9
    - asthma J45.909
      - with
        - exacerbation (acute) J45.901
        - status asthmaticus J45.902
    - bronchiectasis J47.9
      - with
        - exacerbation (acute) J47.1
        - lower respiratory infection J47.0
    - bronchitis (chronic) J44.9
    - emphysema J43.9
  - chronic J44.9
    - with
      - allergic alveolitis —*see* Pneumonitis, hypersensitivity
      - bronchiectasis J47.9
        - with
          - exacerbation (acute) J47.1
          - lower respiratory infection J47.0
  - due to
    - foreign body —*see* Foreign body, by site, causing asphyxia
    - inhalation of fumes or vapors J68.9
    - laryngospasm J38.5
- ampulla of Vater K83.1
- aortic (heart) (valve) —*see* Stenosis, aortic
- aortoiliac I74.09
- aqueduct of Sylvius G91.1
  - congenital Q03.0
    - with spina bifida —*see* Spina bifida, by site, with hydrocephalus
- Arnold-Chiari —*see* Arnold-Chiari disease
- artery (*see also* Atherosclerosis, artery) I70.9
  - basilar (complete) (partial) —*see* Occlusion, artery, basilar
  - carotid (complete) (partial) —*see* Occlusion, artery, carotid
  - cerebellar —*see* Occlusion, artery, cerebellar
  - cerebral (anterior) (middle) (posterior) —*see* Occlusion, artery, cerebral
  - precerebral —*see* Occlusion, artery, precerebral
  - renal N28.0
  - retinal NEC —*see* Occlusion, artery, retina
  - stent —*see* Restenosis, stent
  - vertebral (complete) (partial) —*see* Occlusion, artery, vertebral
- band (intestinal) (*see also* Obstruction, intestine, specified NEC) K56.699

Obstruction, obstructed, obstructive *(continued)*
- bile duct or passage (common) (hepatic) (noncalculous) K83.1
  - with calculus K80.51
  - congenital (causing jaundice) Q44.3
- biliary (duct) (tract) K83.1
  - gallbladder K82.0
- bladder-neck (acquired) N32.0
  - congenital Q64.31
  - due to hyperplasia (hypertrophy) of prostate —*see* Hyperplasia, prostate
- bowel —*see* Obstruction, intestine
- bronchus J98.09
- canal, ear —*see* Stenosis, external ear canal
- cardia K22.2
- caval veins (inferior) (superior) I87.1
- cecum —*see* Obstruction, intestine
- circulatory I99.8
- colon —*see* Obstruction, intestine
- common duct (noncalculous) K83.1
- coronary (artery) —*see* Occlusion, coronary
- cystic duct —*see also* Obstruction, gallbladder
  - with calculus K80.21
- device, implant or graft (*see also* Complications, by site and type, mechanical) T85.698
  - arterial graft NEC —*see* Complication, cardiovascular device, mechanical, vascular
  - catheter NEC T85.628
    - cystostomy T83.090
    - dialysis (renal) T82.49
      - intraperitoneal T85.691
    - Hopkins T83.098
    - ileostomy T83.098
    - infusion NEC T82.594
      - spinal (epidural) (subdural) T85.690
    - nephrostomy T83.092
    - urethral indwelling T83.091
    - urinary T83.098
    - urostomy T83.098
  - due to infection T85.79
  - gastrointestinal —*see* Complications, prosthetic device, mechanical, gastrointestinal device
  - genital NEC T83.498
    - intrauterine contraceptive device T83.39
    - penile prosthesis (cylinder) (implanted) (pump) (resevoir) T83.490
    - testicular prosthesis T83.491
  - heart NEC —*see* Complication, cardiovascular device, mechanical
  - joint prosthesis —*see* Complications, joint prosthesis, mechanical, specified NEC, by site
  - orthopedic NEC —*see* Complication, orthopedic, device, mechanical
  - specified NEC T85.628
  - urinary NEC —*see also* Complication, genitourinary, device, urinary, mechanical
    - graft T83.29
  - vascular NEC —*see* Complication, cardiovascular device, mechanical
  - ventricular intracranial shunt T85.09

Obstruction, obstructed, obstructive *(continued)*
- due to foreign body accidentally left in operative wound T81.529
- duodenum K31.5
- ejaculatory duct N50.89
- esophagus K22.2
- eustachian tube (complete) (partial) H68.10-
  - cartilagenous (extrinsic) H68.13-
    - intrinsic H68.12-
  - osseous H68.11-
- fallopian tube (bilateral) N97.1
- fecal K56.41
  - with hernia —*see* Hernia, by site, with obstruction
- foramen of Monro (congenital) Q03.8
  - with spina bifida —*see* Spina bifida, by site, with hydrocephalus
- foreign body —*see* Foreign body
- gallbladder K82.0
  - with calculus, stones K80.21
  - congenital Q44.1
- gastric outlet K31.1
- gastrointestinal —*see* Obstruction, intestine
- hepatic K76.89
  - duct (noncalculous) K83.1
- hepatobiliary K83.1
- ileum —*see* Obstruction, intestine
- iliofemoral (artery) I74.5
- intestine K56.609
  - complete K56.601
  - incomplete K56.600
  - partial K56.600
  - with
    - adhesions (intestinal) (peritoneal) K56.50
    - complete K56.52
    - incomplete K56.51
    - partial K56.51
  - adynamic K56.0
  - by gallstone K56.3
  - congenital (small) Q41.9
    - large Q42.9
      - specified part NEC Q42.8
  - neurogenic K56.0
    - Hirschsprung's disease or megacolon Q43.1
  - newborn P76.9
    - due to
      - fecaliths P76.8
      - inspissated milk P76.2
      - meconium (plug) P76.0
        - in mucoviscidosis E84.11
    - specified NEC P76.8
  - postoperative K91.30
    - complete K91.32
    - incomplete K91.31
    - partial K91.31
  - reflex K56.0
  - specified NEC K56.699
    - complete K56.691
    - incomplete K56.690
    - partial K56.690
  - volvulus K56.2
- intracardiac ball valve prosthesis T82.09
- jejunum —*see* Obstruction, intestine
- joint prosthesis —*see* Complications, joint prosthesis, mechanical, specified NEC, by site
- kidney (calices) N28.89
- labor —*see* Delivery
- lacrimal (passages) (duct)
  - by
    - dacryolith —*see* Dacryolith
    - stenosis —*see* Stenosis, lacrimal

Obstruction, obstructed, obstructive *(continued)*
- lacrimal *(continued)*
  - congenital Q10.5
  - neonatal H04.53-
- lacrimonasal duct —*see* Obstruction, lacrimal
- lacteal, with steatorrhea K90.2
- laryngitis —*see* Laryngitis
- larynx NEC J38.6
  - congenital Q31.8
- lung J98.4
  - disease, chronic J44.9
- lymphatic I89.0
- meconium (plug)
  - newborn P76.0
    - due to fecaliths P76.0
    - in mucoviscidosis E84.11
- mitral —*see* Stenosis, mitral
- nasal J34.89
- nasolacrimal duct —*see also* Obstruction, lacrimal
  - congenital Q10.5
- nasopharynx J39.2
- nose J34.89
- organ or site, congenital NEC —*see* Atresia, by site
- pancreatic duct K86.89
- parotid duct or gland K11.8
- pelviureteral junction N13.5
  - with hydronephrosis N13.0
  - congenital Q62.39
- pharynx J39.2
- portal (circulation) (vein) I81
- prostate —*see also* Hyperplasia, prostate
  - valve (urinary) N32.0
- pulmonary valve (heart) I37.0
- pyelonephritis (chronic) N11.1
- pylorus
  - adult K31.1
  - congenital or infantile Q40.0
- rectosigmoid —*see* Obstruction, intestine
- rectum K62.4
- renal N28.89
  - outflow N13.8
  - pelvis, congenital Q62.39
- respiratory J98.8
  - chronic J44.9
- retinal (vessels) H34.9
- salivary duct (any) K11.8
  - with calculus K11.5
- sigmoid —*see* Obstruction, intestine
- sinus (accessory) (nasal) J34.89
- Stensen's duct K11.8
- stomach NEC K31.89
  - acute K31.0
  - congenital Q40.2
  - due to pylorospasm K31.3
- submandibular duct K11.8
- submaxillary gland K11.8
  - with calculus K11.5
- thoracic duct I89.0
- thrombotic —*see* Thrombosis
- trachea J39.8
- tracheostomy airway J95.03
- tricuspid (valve) —*see* Stenosis, tricuspid
- upper respiratory, congenital Q34.8
- ureter (functional) (pelvic junction) NEC N13.5
  - with
    - hydronephrosis N13.1
      - with infection N13.6
    - pyelonephritis (chronic) N11.1
  - congenital Q62.39
  - due to calculus —*see* Calculus, ureter
- urethra NEC N36.8
  - congenital Q64.39

Obstruction, obstructed, obstructive *(continued)*
- urinary (moderate) N13.9
  - due to hyperplasia (hypertrophy) of prostate —*see* Hyperplasia, prostate
  - organ or tract (lower) N13.9
  - prostatic valve N32.0
  - specified NEC N13.8
- uropathy N13.9
- uterus N85.8
- vagina N89.5
- valvular —*see* Endocarditis
- vein, venous I87.1
  - caval (inferior) (superior) I87.1
  - thrombotic —*see* Thrombosis
- vena cava (inferior) (superior) I87.1
- vesical NEC N32.0
- vesicourethral orifice N32.0
  - congenital Q64.31
- vessel NEC I99.8
  - stent —*see* Restenosis, stent

Obturator —*see* condition

Occlusal wear, teeth K03.0

Occlusio pupillae —*see* Membrane, pupillary

Occlusion, occluded
- anus K62.4
  - congenital Q42.3
    - with fistula Q42.2
- aortoiliac (chronic) I74.09
- aqueduct of Sylvius G91.1
  - congenital Q03.0
    - with spina bifida —*see* Spina bifida, by site, with hydrocephalus
- artery (*see also* Atherosclerosis, artery) I70.9
  - auditory, internal I65.8
  - basilar I65.1
    - with
      - infarction I63.22
        - due to
          - embolism I63.12
          - thrombosis I63.02
  - brain or cerebral I66.9
    - with infarction (due to) I63.5-
      - embolism I63.4-
      - thrombosis I63.3-
  - carotid I65.2-
    - with
      - infarction I63.23-
        - due to
          - embolism I63.13-
          - thrombosis I63.03-
  - cerebellar (anterior inferior) (posterior inferior) (superior) I66.3
    - with infarction I63.54-
      - due to
        - embolism I63.44-
        - thrombosis I63.34-
  - cerebral I66.9
    - with infarction I63.50
      - due to
        - embolism I63.40
          - specified NEC I63.49
        - thrombosis I63.30
          - specified NEC I63.39
    - anterior I66.1-
      - with infarction I63.52-
        - due to
          - embolism I63.42-
          - thrombosis I63.32-
    - middle I66.0-
      - with infarction I63.51-
        - due to
          - embolism I63.41-
          - thrombosis I63.31-

Occlusion, occluded *(continued)*
- artery *(continued)*
  - cerebral *(continued)*
    - posterior I66.2-
      - with infarction I63.53-
        - due to
          - embolism I63.43-
          - thrombosis I63.33-
    - specified NEC I66.8
      - with infarction I63.59
        - due to
          - embolism I63.4-
          - thrombosis I63.3-
  - choroidal (anterior) —*see* Occlusion, artery, precerebral, specified NEC
  - communicating posterior —*see* Occlusion, artery, precerebral, specified NEC
  - complete
    - coronary I25.82
    - extremities I70.92
  - coronary (acute) (thrombotic) (without myocardial infarction) I24.0
    - with myocardial infarction —*see* Infarction, myocardium
    - chronic total I25.82
    - complete I25.82
    - healed or old I25.2
    - total (chronic) I25.82
  - hypophyseal —*see* Occlusion, artery, precerebral, specified NEC
  - iliac I74.5
  - lower extremities due to stenosis or stricture I77.1
  - mesenteric (embolic) (thrombotic) (*see also* Infarct, intestine) K55.069
  - perforating —*see* Occlusion, artery, cerebral, specified NEC
  - peripheral I77.9
    - thrombotic or embolic I74.4
  - pontine —*see* Occlusion, artery, precerebral, specified NEC
  - precerebral I65.9
    - with infarction I63.20
      - specified NEC I63.29
      - due to
        - embolism I63.10
          - specified NEC I63.19
        - thrombosis I63.09
          - specified NEC I63.09
    - basilar —*see* Occlusion, artery, basilar
    - carotid —*see* Occlusion, artery, carotid
    - puerperal O88.23
    - specified NEC I65.8
      - with infarction I63.29
        - due to
          - embolism I63.19
          - thrombosis I63.09
    - vertebral —*see* Occlusion, artery, vertebral
  - renal N28.0
  - retinal
    - central H34.1-
    - partial H34.21-
    - branch H34.23-
    - transient H34.0-
  - spinal —*see* Occlusion, artery, precerebral, vertebral
  - total (chronic)
    - coronary I25.82
    - extremities I70.92
  - vertebral I65.0-
    - with
      - infarction I63.21-
        - due to

Occlusion, occluded *(continued)*
- artery *(continued)*
  - vertebral *(continued)*
    - with *(continued)*
      - infarction *(continued)*
        - due to *(continued)*
          - embolism I63.11-
          - thrombosis I63.01-
- basilar artery —*see* Occlusion, artery, basilar
- bile duct (common) (hepatic) (noncalculous) K83.1
- bowel —*see* Obstruction, intestine
- carotid (artery) (common) (internal) —*see* Occlusion, artery, carotid
- centric (of teeth) M26.59
  - maximum intercuspation discrepancy M26.55
- cerebellar (artery) —*see* Occlusion, artery, cerebellar
- cerebral (artery) —*see* Occlusion, artery, cerebral
- cerebrovascular —*see also* Occlusion, artery, cerebral
  - with infarction I63.5-
- cervical canal —*see* Stricture, cervix
- cervix (uteri) —*see* Stricture, cervix
- choanal Q30.0
- choroidal (artery) —*see* Occlusion, artery, precerebral, specified NEC
- colon —*see* Obstruction, intestine
- communicating posterior artery —*see* Occlusion, artery, precerebral, specified NEC
- coronary (artery) (vein) (thrombotic) —*see also* Infarct, myocardium
  - chronic total I25.82
  - healed or old I25.2
  - not resulting in infarction I24.0
  - total (chronic) I25.82
- cystic duct —*see* Obstruction, gallbladder
- embolic —*see* Embolism
- fallopian tube N97.1
  - congenital Q50.6
- gallbladder —*see also* Obstruction, gallbladder
  - congenital (causing jaundice) Q44.1
- gingiva, traumatic K06.2
- hymen N89.6
  - congenital Q52.3
- hypophyseal (artery) —*see* Occlusion, artery, precerebral, specified NEC
- iliac artery I74.5
- intestine —*see* Obstruction, intestine
- lacrimal passages —*see* Obstruction, lacrimal
- lung J98.4
- lymph or lymphatic channel I89.0
- mammary duct N64.89
- mesenteric artery (embolic) (thrombotic) (*see also* Infarct, intestine) K55.069
- nose J34.89
  - congenital Q30.0
- organ or site, congenital NEC —*see* Atresia, by site
- oviduct N97.1
  - congenital Q50.6
- peripheral arteries
  - due to stricture or stenosis I77.1
  - upper extremity I74.2
- pontine (artery) —*see* Occlusion, artery, precerebral, specified NEC
- posterior lingual, of mandibular teeth M26.29
- precerebral artery —*see* Occlusion, artery, precerebral

Occlusion, occluded *(continued)*
- punctum lacrimale *—see* Obstruction, lacrimal
- pupil *—see* Membrane, pupillary
- pylorus, adult (*see also* Stricture, pylorus) K31.1
- renal artery N28.0
- retina, retinal
  - artery *—see* Occlusion, artery, retinal
  - vein (central) H34.81-
    - engorgement H34.82-
    - tributary H34.83-
  - vessels H34.9
- spinal artery *—see* Occlusion, artery, precerebral, vertebral
- teeth (mandibular) (posterior lingual) M26.29
- thoracic duct I89.0
- thrombotic *—see* Thrombosis, artery
- traumatic
  - edentulous (alveolar) ridge K06.2
  - gingiva K06.2
  - periodontal K05.5
- tubal N97.1
- ureter (complete) (partial) N13.5
  - congenital Q62.10
- ureteropelvic junction N13.5
  - congenital Q62.11
- ureterovesical orifice N13.5
  - congenital Q62.12
- urethra *—see* Stricture, urethra
- uterus N85.8
- vagina N89.5
- vascular NEC I99.8
- vein *—see* Thrombosis
  - retinal *—see* Occlusion, retinal, vein
- vena cava (inferior) (superior) *—see* Embolism, vena cava
- ventricle (brain) NEC G91.1
- vertebral (artery) *—see* Occlusion, artery, vertebral
- vessel (blood) I99.8
- vulva N90.5

Occult
- blood in feces (stools) R19.5

Occupational
- problems NEC Z56.89

Ochlophobia *—see* Agoraphobia

Ochronosis (endogenous) E70.29

Ocular muscle *—see* condition

Oculogyric crisis or disturbance H51.8
- psychogenic F45.8

Oculomotor syndrome H51.9

Oculopathy
- syphilitic NEC A52.71
  - congenital
    - early A50.01
    - late A50.30
  - early (secondary) A51.43
  - late A52.71

Oddi's sphincter spasm K83.4

Odontalgia K08.89

Odontoameloblastoma *—see* Cyst, calcifying odontogenic

Odontoclasia K03.89

Odontodysplasia, regional K00.4

Odontogenesis imperfecta K00.5

Odontoma (ameloblastic) (complex) (compound) (fibroameloblastic) *—see* Cyst, calcifying odontogenic

Odontomyelitis (closed) (open) K04.01
- irreversible K04.02
- reversible K04.01

Odontorrhagia K08.89

Odontosarcoma, ameloblastic C41.1
- upper jaw (bone) C41.0

Oestriasis *—see* Myiasis

Oguchi's disease H53.63

Ohara's disease *—see* Tularemia

OHS (obesity hypoventilation syndrome) E66.2

Oidiomycosis *—see* Candidiasis

Oidium albicans infection *—see* Candidiasis

Old age (without mention of debility) R54
- dementia F03

Old (previous) **myocardial infarction** I25.2

Olfactory *—see* condition

Oligemia *—see* Anemia

Oligoastrocytoma
- specified site *—see* Neoplasm, malignant, by site
- unspecified site C71.9

Oligocythemia D64.9

Oligodendroblastoma
- specified site *—see* Neoplasm, malignant
- unspecified site C71.9

Oligodendroglioma
- anaplastic type
  - specified site *—see* Neoplasm, malignant, by site
  - unspecified site C71.9
- specified site *—see* Neoplasm, malignant, by site
- unspecified site C71.9

Oligodontia *—see* Anodontia

Oligoencephalon Q02

Oligohidrosis L74.4

Oligohydramnios O41.0-

Oligohydrosis L74.4

Oligomenorrhea N91.5
- primary N91.3
- secondary N91.4

Oligophrenia *—see also* Disability, intellectual
- phenylpyruvic E70.0

Oligospermia N46.11
- due to
  - drug therapy N46.121
  - efferent duct obstruction N46.123
  - infection N46.122
  - radiation N46.124
  - specified cause NEC N46.129
  - systemic disease N46.125

Oligotrichia *—see* Alopecia

Oliguria R34
- with, complicating or following ectopic or molar pregnancy O08.4
- postprocedural N99.0

Ollier's disease Q78.4

Omentitis *—see* Peritonitis

Omenotocele *—see* Hernia, abdomen, specified site NEC

Omentum, omental *—see* condition

Omphalitis (congenital) (newborn) P38.9
- with mild hemorrhage P38.1
- without hemorrhage P38.9
- not of newborn L08.82
- tetanus A33

Omphalocele Q79.2

Omphalomesenteric duct, persistent Q43.0

Omphalorrhagia, newborn P51.9

Omsk hemorrhagic fever A98.1

Onanism (excessive) F98.8

Onchocerciasis, onchocercosis B73.1
- with
  - eye disease B73.00
    - endophthalmitis B73.01
    - eyelid B73.09
    - glaucoma B73.02
    - specified NEC B73.09
- eye NEC B73.00
- eyelid B73.09

Oncocytoma *—see* Neoplasm, benign, by site

Oncovirus, as cause of disease classified elsewhere B97.32

Ondine's curse *—see* Apnea, sleep

Oneirophrenia F23

Onychauxis L60.2
- congenital Q84.5

Onychia *—see also* Cellulitis, digit
- with lymphangitis *—see* Lymphangitis, acute, digit
- candidal B37.2
- dermatophytic B35.1

Onychitis *—see also* Cellulitis, digit
- with lymphangitis *—see* Lymphangitis, acute, digit

Onychocryptosis L60.0

Onychodystrophy L60.3
- congenital Q84.6

Onychogryphosis, onychogryposis L60.2

Onycholysis L60.1

Onychomadesis L60.8

Onychomalacia L60.3

Onychomycosis (finger) (toe) B35.1

Onycho-osteodysplasia Q87.2

Onychophagia F98.8

Onychophosis L60.8

Onychoptosis L60.8

Onychorrhexis L60.3
- congenital Q84.6

Onychoschizia L60.3

Onyxis (finger) (toe) L60.0

Onyxitis *—see also* Cellulitis, digit
- with lymphangitis *—see* Lymphangitis, acute, digit

Oophoritis (cystic) (infectional) (interstitial) N70.92
- with salpingitis N70.93
- acute N70.02
  - with salpingitis N70.03
- chronic N70.12
  - with salpingitis N70.13
- complicating abortion *—see* Abortion, by type, complicated by, oophoritis

Oophorocele N83.4-

Opacity, opacities
- cornea H17.-
  - central H17.1-
  - congenital Q13.3
  - degenerative *—see* Degeneration, cornea
  - hereditary *—see* Dystrophy, cornea
  - inflammatory *—see* Keratitis
  - minor H17.81-
  - peripheral H17.82-

Opacity, opacities *(continued)*
- cornea
  - sequelae of trachoma (healed) B94.0
  - specified NEC H17.89
- enamel (teeth) (fluoride) (nonfluoride) K00.3
- lens *—see* Cataract
- snowball *—see* Deposit, crystalline
- vitreous (humor) NEC H43.39-
  - congenital Q14.0
  - membranes and strands H43.31-

Opalescent dentin (hereditary) K00.5

Open, opening
- abnormal, organ or site, congenital *—see* Imperfect, closure
- angle with
  - borderline
    - findings
      - high risk H40.02-
      - low risk H40.01-
    - intraocular pressure H40.00-
  - cupping of discs H40.01-
  - glaucoma (primary) *—see* Glaucoma, open angle
- bite
  - anterior M26.220
  - posterior M26.221
- false *—see* Imperfect, closure
- margin on tooth restoration K08.51
- restoration margins of tooth K08.51
- wound *—see* Wound, open

Operational fatigue F48.8

Operative *—see* condition

Operculitis *—see* Periodontitis

Operculum *—see* Break, retina

Ophiasis L63.2

Ophthalmia (*see also* Conjunctivitis) H10.9
- actinic rays *—see* Photokeratitis
- allergic (acute) *—see* Conjunctivitis, acute, atopic
- blennorrhagic (gonococcal) (neonatorum) A54.31
- diphtheritic A36.86
- Egyptian A71.1
- electrica *—see* Photokeratitis
- gonococcal (neonatorum) A54.31
- metastatic *—see* Endophthalmitis, purulent
- migraine *—see* Migraine, ophthalmoplegic
- neonatorum, newborn P39.1
  - gonococcal A54.31
- nodosa H16.24-
- purulent *—see* Conjunctivitis, acute, mucopurulent
- spring *—see* Conjunctivitis, acute, atopic
- sympathetic *—see* Uveitis, sympathetic

Ophthalmitis *—see* Ophthalmia

Ophthalmocele (congenital) Q15.8

Ophthalmoneuromyelitis G36.0

Ophthalmoplegia *—see also* Strabismus, paralytic
- anterior internuclear *—see* Ophthalmoplegia, internuclear
- ataxia-areflexia G61.0
- diabetic *—see* E08-E13 with .39
- exophthalmic E05.00
  - with thyroid storm E05.01
- external H49.88-
  - progressive H49.4-
    - with pigmentary retinopathy *—see* Kearns-Sayre syndrome

Ophthalmoplegia *(continued)*
- external *(continued)*
  - total H49.3-
- internal (complete) (total) H52.51-
- internuclear H51.2-
- migraine —*see* Migraine, ophthalmoplegic
- Parinaud's H49.88-
- progressive external —*see* Ophthalmoplegia, external, progressive
- supranuclear, progressive G23.1
- total (external) —*see* Ophthalmoplegia, external, total

Opioid(s)
- abuse —*see* Abuse, drug, opioids
- dependence —*see* Dependence, drug, opioids
- induced, without use disorder
  - anxiety disorder F11.988
  - delirium F11.921
  - depressive disorder F11.94
  - sexual dysfunction F11.981
  - sleep disorder F11.982

Opisthognathism M26.09

Opisthorchiasis (felineus) (viverrini) B66.0

Opitz' disease D73.2

Opiumism —*see* Dependence, drug, opioid

Oppenheim's disease G70.2

Oppenheim-Urbach disease (necrobiosis lipoidica diabeticorum) —*see* E08-E13 with .620

Optic nerve —*see* condition

Orbit —*see* condition

Orchioblastoma C62.9-

Orchitis (gangrenous) (nonspecific) (septic) (suppurative) N45.2
- blennorrhagic (gonococcal) (acute) (chronic) A54.23
- chlamydial A56.19
- filarial —*see also* Infestation, filarial B74.9 *[N51]*
- gonococcal (acute) (chronic) A54.23
- mumps B26.0
- syphilitic A52.76
- tuberculous A18.15

Orf (virus disease) B08.02

Organic —*see also* condition
- brain syndrome F09
- heart —*see* Disease, heart
- mental disorder F09
- psychosis F09

Orgasm
- anejaculatory N53.13

Oriental
- bilharziasis B65.2
- schistosomiasis B65.2

Orifice —*see* condition

Origin of both great vessels from right ventricle Q20.1

Ormond's disease (with ureteral obstruction) N13.5
- with infection N13.6

Ornithine metabolism disorder E72.4

Ornithinemia (Type I) (Type II) E72.4

Ornithosis A70

Orotaciduria, oroticaciduria (congenital) (hereditary) (pyrimidine deficiency) E79.8
- anemia D53.0

Orthodontics
- adjustment Z46.4
- fitting Z46.4

Orthopnea R06.01

Orthopoxvirus B08.09
- specified NEC B08.09

Os, uterus —*see* condition

Osgood-Schlatter disease or osteochondrosis —*see* Osteochondrosis, juvenile, tibia

Osler (-Weber)-**Rendu disease** I78.0

Osler's nodes I33.0

Osmidrosis L75.0

Osseous —*see* condition

Ossification
- artery —*see* Arteriosclerosis
- auricle (ear) —*see* Disorder, pinna, specified type NEC
- bronchial J98.09
- cardiac —*see* Degeneration, myocardial
- cartilage (senile) —*see* Disorder, cartilage, specified type NEC
- coronary (artery) —*see* Disease, heart, ischemic, atherosclerotic
- diaphragm J98.6
- ear, middle —*see* Otosclerosis
- falx cerebri G96.19
- fontanel, premature Q75.0
- heart —*see also* Degeneration, myocardial
  - valve —*see* Endocarditis
- larynx J38.7
- ligament —*see* Disorder, tendon, specified type NEC
  - posterior longitudinal —*see* Spondylopathy, specified NEC
- meninges (cerebral) (spinal) G96.19
- multiple, eccentric centers —*see* Disorder, bone, development or growth
- muscle —*see also* Calcification, muscle
  - due to burns —*see* Myositis, ossificans, in, burns
  - paralytic —*see* Myositis, ossificans, in, quadriplegia
  - progressive —*see* Myositis, ossificans, progressiva
  - specified NEC M61.50
    - ankle M61.57-
    - foot M61.57-
    - forearm M61.53-
    - hand M61.54-
    - lower leg M61.56-
    - multiple sites M61.59
    - pelvic region M61.55-
    - shoulder region M61.51-
    - specified site NEC M61.58
    - thigh M61.55-
    - upper arm M61.52-
  - traumatic —*see* Myositis, ossificans, traumatica
- myocardium, myocardial —*see* Degeneration, myocardial
- penis N48.89
- periarticular —*see* Disorder, joint, specified type NEC
- pinna —*see* Disorder, pinna, specified type NEC
- rider's bone —*see* Ossification, muscle, specified NEC
- sclera H15.89
- subperiosteal, post-traumatic M89.8X-
- tendon —*see* Disorder, tendon, specified type NEC

Ossification *(continued)*
- trachea J39.8
- tympanic membrane —*see* Disorder, tympanic membrane, specified NEC
- vitreous (humor) —*see* Deposit, crystalline

Osteitis —*see also* Osteomyelitis
- alveolar M27.3
- condensans M85.30
  - ankle M85.37-
  - foot M85.37-
  - forearm M85.33-
  - hand M85.34-
  - lower leg M85.36-
  - multiple site M85.39
  - neck M85.38
  - rib M85.38
  - shoulder M85.31-
  - skull M85.38
  - specified site NEC M85.38
  - thigh M85.35-
  - toe M85.37-
  - upper arm M85.32-
  - vertebra M85.38
- deformans M88.9
  - in (due to)
    - malignant neoplasm of bone C41.9 *[M90.60]*
    - neoplastic disease (*see also* Neoplasm) D49.9 *[M90.60]*
      - carpus D49.9 *[M90.64-]*
      - clavicle D49.9 *[M90.61-]*
      - femur D49.9 *[M90.65-]*
      - fibula D49.9 *[M90.66-]*
      - finger D49.9 *[M90.64-]*
      - humerus D49.9 *[M90.62-]*
      - ilium D49.9 *[M90.65-]*
      - ischium D49.9 *[M90.65-]*
      - metacarpus D49.9 *[M90.64-]*
      - metatarsus D49.9 *[M90.67-]*
      - multiple sites D49.9 *[M90.69]*
      - neck D49.9 *[M90.68]*
      - radius D49.9 *[M90.63-]*
      - rib D49.9 *[M90.68]*
      - scapula D49.9 *[M90.61-]*
      - skull D49.9 *[M90.68]*
      - tarsus D49.9 *[M90.67-]*
      - tibia D49.9 *[M90.66-]*
      - toe D49.9 *[M90.67-]*
      - ulna D49.9 *[M90.63-]*
      - vertebra D49.9 *[M90.68]*
  - skull M88.0
  - specified NEC —*see* Paget's disease, bone, by site
  - vertebra M88.1
- due to yaws A66.6
- fibrosa NEC —*see* Cyst, bone, by site
  - circumscripta —*see* Dysplasia, fibrous, bone NEC
  - cystica (generalisata) E21.0
  - disseminata Q78.1
  - osteoplastica E21.0
- fragilitans Q78.0
- Garr's (sclerosing) —*see* Osteomyelitis, specified type NEC
- jaw (acute) (chronic) (lower) (suppurative) (upper) M27.2
- parathyroid E21.0
- petrous bone (acute) (chronic) —*see* Petrositis
- sclerotic, nonsuppurative —*see* Osteomyelitis, specified type NEC
- tuberculosa A18.09
  - cystica D86.89
  - multiplex cystoides D86.89

Osteoarthritis M19.90
- ankle M19.07-
- elbow M19.02-

Osteoarthritis *(continued)*
- foot joint M19.07-
- generalized M15.9
  - erosive M15.4
  - primary M15.0
  - specified NEC M15.8
- hand joint M19.04-
  - first carpometacarpal joint M18.9
- hip M16.1-
  - bilateral M16.0
  - due to hip dysplasia (unilateral) M16.3-
    - bilateral M16.2
- interphalangeal
  - distal (Heberden) M15.1
  - proximal (Bouchard) M15.2
- knee M17.1-
  - bilateral M17.0
- shoulder M19.01-
- spine —*see* Spondylosis
- wrist M19.03-
- post-traumatic NEC M19.92
  - ankle M19.17-
  - elbow M19.12-
  - foot joint M19.17-
  - hand joint M19.14-
    - first carpometacarpal joint M18.3-
      - bilateral M18.2
  - hip M16.5-
    - bilateral M16.4
  - knee M17.3-
    - bilateral M17.2
  - shoulder M19.11-
  - wrist M19.13-
- primary M19.91
  - ankle M19.07-
  - elbow M19.02-
  - foot joint M19.07-
  - hand joint M19.04-
    - first carpometacarpal joint M18.1-
      - bilateral M18.0
  - hip M16.1-
    - bilateral M16.0
  - knee M17.1-
    - bilateral M17.0
  - shoulder M19.01-
  - spine —*see* Spondylosis
  - wrist M19.03-
- secondary M19.93
  - ankle M19.27-
  - elbow M19.22-
  - foot joint M19.27-
  - hand joint M19.24-
    - first carpometacarpal joint M18.5-
      - bilateral M18.4
  - hip M16.7
    - bilateral M16.6
  - knee M17.5
    - bilateral M17.4
  - multiple M15.3
  - shoulder M19.21-
  - spine —*see* Spondylosis
  - wrist M19.23-

Osteoarthropathy (hypertrophic) M19.90
- ankle —*see* Osteoarthritis, primary, ankle
- elbow —*see* Osteoarthritis, primary, elbow
- foot joint —*see* Osteoarthritis, primary, foot
- hand joint —*see* Osteoarthritis, primary, hand joint
- knee joint —*see* Osteoarthritis, primary, knee
- multiple site —*see* Osteoarthritis, primary, multiple joint

Osteoarthropathy *(continued)*
  pulmonary *—see also* Osteoarthropathy, specified type NEC
    hypertrophic *—see* Osteoarthropathy, hypertrophic, specified type NEC
  secondary hypertrophic *—see* Osteoarthropathy, specified type NEC
  shoulder *—see* Osteoarthritis, primary, shoulder
  specified joint NEC *—see* Osteoarthritis, primary, specified joint NEC
  specified type NEC M89.40
    carpus M89.44-
    clavicle M89.41-
    femur M89.45-
    fibula M89.46-
    finger M89.44-
    humerus M89.42-
    ilium M89.459
    ischium M89.459
    metacarpus M89.44-
    metatarsus M89.47-
    multiple sites M89.49
    neck M89.48
    radius M89.43-
    rib M89.48
    scapula M89.41-
    skull M89.48
    tarsus M89.47-
    tibia M89.46-
    toe M89.47-
    ulna M89.43-
    vertebra M89.48
  secondary *—see* Osteoarthropathy, specified type NEC
  spine *—see* Spondylosis
  wrist *—see* Osteoarthritis, primary, wrist

Osteoarthrosis (degenerative) (hypertrophic) (joint) *—see also* Osteoarthritis
  deformans alkaptonurica E70.29 *[M36.8]*
  erosive M15.4
  generalized M15.9
    primary M15.0
  polyarticular M15.9
  spine *—see* Spondylosis

Osteoblastoma *—see* Neoplasm, bone, benign
  aggressive *—see* Neoplasm, bone, uncertain behavior

Osteochondroarthrosis deformans endemica *—see* Disease, Kaschin-Beck

Osteochondritis *—see also* Osteochondropathy, by site
  Brailsford's *—see* Osteochondrosis, juvenile, radius
  dissecans M93.20
    ankle M93.27-
    elbow M93.22-
    foot M93.27-
    hand M93.24-
    hip M93.25-
    knee M93.26-
    multiple sites M93.29
    shoulder joint M93.21-
    specified site NEC M93.28
    wrist M93.23-
  juvenile M92.9
    patellar *—see* Osteochondrosis, juvenile, patella
  syphilitic (congenital) (early) A50.02 *[M90.80]*

Osteochondritis *(continued)*
  syphilitic *(continued)*
    ankle A50.02 *[M90.87-]*
    elbow A50.02 *[M90.82-]*
    foot A50.02 *[M90.87-]*
    forearm A50.02 *[M90.83-]*
    hand A50.02 *[M90.84-]*
    hip A50.02 *[M90.85-]*
    knee A50.02 *[M90.86-]*
    multiple sites A50.02 *[M90.89]*
    shoulder joint A50.02 *[M90.81-]*
    specified site NEC A50.02 *[M90.88]*

Osteochondrodysplasia Q78.9
  with defects of growth of tubular bones and spine Q77.9
    specified NEC Q77.8
  specified NEC Q78.8

Osteochondrodystrophy E78.9

Osteochondrolysis *—see* Osteochondritis, dissecans

Osteochondroma *—see* Neoplasm, bone, benign

Osteochondromatosis D48.0
  syndrome Q78.4

Osteochondromyxosarcoma *—see* Neoplasm, bone, malignant

Osteochondropathy M93.90
  ankle M93.97-
  elbow M93.92-
  foot M93.97-
  hand M93.94-
  hip M93.95-
  Kienböck's disease of adults M93.1
  knee M93.96-
  multiple joints M93.99
  osteochondritis dissecans *—see* Osteochondritis, dissecans
  osteochondrosis *—see* Osteochondrosis
  shoulder region M93.91-
  slipped upper femoral epiphysis *—see* Slipped, epiphysis, upper femoral
  specified joint NEC M93.98
  specified type NEC M93.80
    ankle M93.87-
    elbow M93.82-
    foot M93.87-
    hand M93.84-
    hip M93.85-
    knee M93.86-
    multiple joints M93.89
    shoulder region M93.81-
    specified joint NEC M93.88
    wrist M93.83-
  syphilitic, congenital
    early A50.02 *[M90.80]*
    late A50.56 *[M90.80]*
  wrist M93.93-

Osteochondrosarcoma *—see* Neoplasm, bone, malignant

Osteochondrosis *—see also* Osteochondropathy, by site
  acetabulum (juvenile) M91.0
  adult *—see* Osteochondropathy, specified type NEC, by site
  astragalus (juvenile) *—see* Osteochondrosis, juvenile, tarsus
  Blount's *—see* Osteochondrosis, juvenile, tibia
  Buchanan's M91.0
  Burns' *—see* Osteochondrosis, juvenile, ulna
  calcaneus (juvenile) *—see* Osteochondrosis, juvenile, tarsus

Osteochondrosis *(continued)*
  capitular epiphysis (femur) (juvenile) *—see* Legg-Calvé-Perthes disease
  carpal (juvenile) (lunate) (scaphoid) *—see* Osteochondrosis, juvenile, hand, carpal lunate
    adult M93.1
  coxae juvenilis *—see* Legg-Calvé-Perthes disease
  deformans juvenilis, coxae *—see* Legg-Calvé-Perthes disease
  Diaz's *—see* Osteochondrosis, juvenile, tarsus
  dissecans (knee) (shoulder) *—see* Osteochondritis, dissecans
  femoral capital epiphysis (juvenile) *—see* Legg-Calvé-Perthes disease
  femur (head), juvenile *—see* Legg-Calvé-Perthes disease
  fibula (juvenile) *—see* Osteochondrosis, juvenile, fibula
  foot NEC (juvenile) M92.8
  Freiberg's *—see* Osteochondrosis, juvenile, metatarsus
  Haas' (juvenile) *—see* Osteochondrosis, juvenile, humerus
  Haglund's *—see* Osteochondrosis, juvenile, tarsus
  hip (juvenile) *—see* Legg-Calvé-Perthes disease
  humerus (capitulum) (head) (juvenile) *—see* Osteochondrosis, juvenile, humerus
  ilium, iliac crest (juvenile) M91.0
  ischiopubic synchondrosis M91.0
  Iselin's *—see* Osteochondrosis, juvenile, metatarsus
  juvenile, juvenilis M92.9
    after congenital dislocation of hip reduction *—see* Osteochondrosis, juvenile, hip, specified NEC
    arm *—see* Osteochondrosis, juvenile, upper limb NEC
    capitular epiphysis (femur) *—see* Legg-Calvé-Perthes disease
    clavicle, sternal epiphysis *—see* Osteochondrosis, juvenile, upper limb NEC
    coxae *—see* Legg-Calvé-Perthes disease
    deformans M92.9
    fibula M92.5-
    foot NEC M92.8
    hand M92.20-
      carpal lunate M92.21-
      metacarpal head M92.22-
      specified site NEC M92.29-
    head of femur *—see* Legg-Calvé-Perthes disease
    hip and pelvis M91.9-
      coxa plana *—see* Coxa, plana
      femoral head *—see* Legg-Calvé-Perthes disease
      pelvis M91.0
      pseudocoxalgia *—see* Pseudocoxalgia
      specified NEC M91.8-
    humerus M92.0-
    limb
      lower NEC M92.8
      upper NEC *—see* Osteochondrosis, juvenile, upper limb NEC
    medial cuneiform bone *—see* Osteochondrosis, juvenile, tarsus
    metatarsus M92.7-
    patella M92.4-

Osteochondrosis *(continued)*
  juvenile, juvenilis *(continued)*
    radius M92.1-
    specified site NEC M92.8
    spine M42.00
      cervical region M42.02
      cervicothoracic region M42.03
      lumbar region M42.06
      lumbosacral region M42.07
      multiple sites M42.09
      occipito-atlanto-axial region M42.01
      sacrococcygeal region M42.08
      thoracic region M42.04
      thoracolumbar region M42.05
    tarsus M92.6-
    tibia M92.5-
    ulna M92.1-
    upper limb NEC M92.3-
    vertebra (body) (epiphyseal plates) (Calvé's) (Scheuermann's) *—see* Osteochondrosis, juvenile, spine
  Kienböck's *—see* Osteochondrosis, juvenile, hand, carpal lunate
    adult M93.1
  Köhler's
    patellar *—see* Osteochondrosis, juvenile, patella
    tarsal navicular *—see* Osteochondrosis, juvenile, tarsus
  Legg-Perthes (-Calvé) (-Waldenström) *—see* Legg-Calvé-Perthes disease
  limb
    lower NEC (juvenile) M92.8
    upper NEC (juvenile) *—see* Osteochondrosis, juvenile, upper limb NEC
  lunate bone (carpal) (juvenile) *—see also* Osteochondrosis, juvenile, hand, carpal lunate
    adult M93.1
  Mauclaire's *—see* Osteochondrosis, juvenile, hand, metacarpal
  metacarpal (head) (juvenile) *—see* Osteochondrosis, juvenile, hand, metacarpal
  metatarsus (fifth) (head) (juvenile) (second) *—see* Osteochondrosis, juvenile, metatarsus
  navicular (juvenile) *—see* Osteochondrosis, juvenile, tarsus
  os
    calcis (juvenile) *—see* Osteochondrosis, juvenile, tarsus
    tibiale externum (juvenile) *—see* Osteochondrosis, juvenile, tarsus
  Osgood-Schlatter *—see* Osteochondrosis, juvenile, tibia
  Panner's *—see* Osteochondrosis, juvenile, humerus
  patellar center (juvenile) (primary) (secondary) *—see* Osteochondrosis, juvenile, patella
  pelvis (juvenile) M91.0
  Pierson's M91.0
  radius (head) (juvenile) *—see* Osteochondrosis, juvenile, radius
  Scheuermann's *—see* Osteochondrosis, juvenile, spine
  Sever's *—see* Osteochondrosis, juvenile, tarsus
  Sinding-Larsen *—see* Osteochondrosis, juvenile, patella

Osteochondrosis *(continued)*
spine M42.9
adult M42.10
cervical region M42.12
cervicothoracic region M42.13
lumbar region M42.16
lumbosacral region M42.17
multiple sites M42.19
occipito-atlanto-axial region M42.11
sacrococcygeal region M42.18
thoracic region M42.14
thoracolumbar region M42.15
juvenile *—see* Osteochondrosis, juvenile, spine
symphysis pubis (juvenile) M91.0
syphilitic (congenital) A50.02
talus (juvenile) *—see* Osteochondrosis, juvenile, tarsus
tarsus (navicular) (juvenile) *—see* Osteochondrosis, juvenile, tarsus
tibia (proximal) (tubercle) (juvenile) *—see* Osteochondrosis, juvenile, tibia
tuberculous *—see* Tuberculosis, bone
ulna (lower) (juvenile) *—see* Osteochondrosis, juvenile, ulna
van Neck's M91.0
vertebral *—see* Osteochondrosis, spine
Osteoclastoma D48.0
malignant *—see* Neoplasm, bone, malignant
Osteodynia *—see* Disorder, bone, specified type NEC
Osteodystrophy Q78.9
azotemic N25.0
congenital Q78.9
parathyroid, secondary E21.1
renal N25.0
Osteofibroma *—see* Neoplasm, bone, benign
Osteofibrosarcoma *—see* Neoplasm, bone, malignant
Osteogenesis imperfecta Q78.0
Osteogenic *—see* condition
Osteolysis M89.50
carpus M89.54-
clavicle M89.51-
femur M89.55-
fibula M89.56-
finger M89.54-
humerus M89.52-
ilium M89.559
ischium M89.559
joint prosthesis (periprosthetic) *—see* Complications, joint prosthesis, mechanical, periprosthetic, osteolysis, by site
metacarpus M89.54-
metatarsus M89.57-
multiple sites M89.59
neck M89.58
periprosthetic *—see* Complications, joint prosthesis, mechanical, periprosthetic, osteolysis, by site
radius M89.53-
rib M89.58
scapula M89.51-
skull M89.58
tarsus M89.57-
tibia M89.56-
toe M89.57-
ulna M89.53-
vertebra M89.58
Osteoma *—see also* Neoplasm, bone, benign
osteoid *—see also* Neoplasm, bone, benign
giant *—see* Neoplasm, bone, benign
Osteomalacia M83.9
adult M83.9
drug-induced NEC M83.5
due to
malabsorption (postsurgical) M83.2
malnutrition M83.3
specified NEC M83.8
aluminium-induced M83.4
infantile *—see* Rickets
juvenile *—see* Rickets
oncogenic E83.89
pelvis M83.8
puerperal M83.0
senile M83.1
vitamin-D-resistant in adults E83.31 *[M90.8-]*
carpus E83.31 *[M90.84-]*
clavicle E83.31 *[M90.81-]*
femur E83.31 *[M90.85-]*
fibula E83.31 *[M90.86-]*
finger E83.31 *[M90.84-]*
humerus E83.31 *[M90.82-]*
ilium E83.31 *[M90.859]*
ischium E83.31 *[M90.859]*
metacarpus E83.31 *[M90.84-]*
metatarsus E83.31 *[M90.87-]*
multiple sites E83.31 *[M90.89]*
neck E83.31 *[M90.88]*
radius E83.31 *[M90.83-]*
rib E83.31 *[M90.88]*
scapula E83.31 *[M90.819]*
skull E83.31 *[M90.88]*
tarsus E83.31 *[M90.879]*
tibia E83.31 *[M90.869]*
toe E83.31 *[M90.879]*
ulna E83.31 *[M90.839]*
vertebra E83.31 *[M90.88]*
Osteomyelitis (general) (infective) (localized) (neonatal) (purulent) (septic) (staphylococcal) (streptococcal) (suppurative) (with periostitis) M86.9
acute M86.10
carpus M86.14-
clavicle M86.11-
femur M86.15-
fibula M86.16-
finger M86.14-
hematogenous M86.00
carpus M86.04-
clavicle M86.01-
femur M86.05-
fibula M86.06-
finger M86.04-
humerus M86.02-
ilium M86.059
ischium M86.059
mandible M27.2
metacarpus M86.04-
metatarsus M86.07-
multiple sites M86.09
neck M86.08
orbit H05.02-
petrous bone *—see* Petrositis
radius M86.03-
rib M86.08
scapula M86.01-
skull M86.08
tarsus M86.07-
tibia M86.06-
toe M86.07-
ulna M86.03-
Osteomyelitis *(continued)*
acute *(continued)*
hematogenous *(continued)*
vertebra *—see* Osteomyelitis, vertebra
humerus M86.12-
ilium M86.159
ischium M86.159
mandible M27.2
metacarpus M86.14-
metatarsus M86.17-
multiple sites M86.19
neck M86.18
orbit H05.02-
petrous bone *—see* Petrositis
radius M86.13-
rib M86.18
scapula M86.11-
skull M86.18
tarsus M86.17-
tibia M86.16-
toe M86.17-
ulna M86.13-
vertebra *—see* Osteomyelitis, vertebra
chronic (or old) M86.60
with draining sinus M86.40
carpus M86.44-
clavicle M86.41-
femur M86.45-
fibula M86.46-
finger M86.44-
humerus M86.42-
ilium M86.459
ischium M86.459
mandible M27.2
metacarpus M86.44-
metatarsus M86.47-
multiple sites M86.49
neck M86.48
orbit H05.02-
petrous bone *—see* Petrositis
radius M86.43-
rib M86.48
scapula M86.41-
skull M86.48
tarsus M86.47-
tibia M86.46-
toe M86.47-
ulna M86.43-
vertebra *—see* Osteomyelitis, vertebra
carpus M86.64-
clavicle M86.61-
femur M86.65-
fibula M86.66-
finger M86.64-
hematogenous NEC M86.50
carpus M86.54-
clavicle M86.51-
femur M86.55-
fibula M86.56-
finger M86.54-
humerus M86.52-
ilium M86.559
ischium M86.559
mandible M27.2
metacarpus M86.54-
metatarsus M86.57-
multifocal M86.30
carpus M86.34-
clavicle M86.31-
femur M86.35-
fibula M86.36-
finger M86.34-
humerus M86.32-
ilium M86.359
ischium M86.359
metacarpus M86.34-
metatarsus M86.37-
Osteomyelitis *(continued)*
chronic *(continued)*
hematogenous *(continued)*
multifocal *(continued)*
multiple sites M86.39
neck M86.38
radius M86.33-
rib M86.38
scapula M86.31-
skull M86.38
tarsus M86.37-
tibia M86.36-
toe M86.37-
ulna M86.33-
vertebra *—see* Osteomyelitis, vertebra
multiple sites M86.59
neck M86.58
orbit H05.02-
petrous bone *—see* Petrositis
radius M86.53-
rib M86.58
scapula M86.51-
skull M86.58
tarsus M86.57-
tibia M86.56-
toe M86.57-
ulna M86.53-
vertebra *—see* Osteomyelitis, vertebra
humerus M86.62-
ilium M86.659
ischium M86.659
mandible M27.2
metacarpus M86.64-
metatarsus M86.67-
multifocal *—see* Osteomyelitis, chronic, hematogenous, multifocal
multiple sites M86.69
neck M86.68
orbit H05.02-
petrous bone *—see* Petrositis
radius M86.63-
rib M86.68
scapula M86.61-
skull M86.68
tarsus M86.67-
tibia M86.66-
toe M86.67-
ulna M86.63-
vertebra *—see* Osteomyelitis, vertebra
echinococcal B67.2
Garr's *—see* Osteomyelitis, specified type NEC
in diabetes mellitus *—see* E08-E13 with .69
jaw (acute) (chronic) (lower) (neonatal) (suppurative) (upper) M27.2
nonsuppurating *—see* Osteomyelitis, specified type NEC
orbit H05.02-
petrous bone *—see* Petrositis
Salmonella (arizonae) (cholerae-suis) (enteritidis) (typhimurium) A02.24
sclerosing, nonsuppurative *—see* Osteomyelitis, specified type NEC
specified type NEC (*see also* subcategory) M86.8X-
mandible M27.2
orbit H05.02-
petrous bone *—see* Petrositis
vertebra *—see* Osteomyelitis, vertebra
subacute M86.20
carpus M86.24-
clavicle M86.21-

Osteomyelitis *(continued)*
subacute *(continued)*
femur M86.25-
fibula M86.26-
finger M86.24-
humerus M86.22-
mandible M27.2
metacarpus M86.24-
metatarsus M86.27-
multiple sites M86.29
neck M86.28
orbit H05.02-
petrous bone *—see* Petrositis
radius M86.23-
rib M86.28
scapula M86.21-
skull M86.28
tarsus M86.27-
tibia M86.26-
toe M86.27-
ulna M86.23-
vertebra *—see* Osteomyelitis, vertebra
syphilitic A52.77
congenital (early) A50.02 *[M90.80]*
tuberculous *—see* Tuberculosis, bone
typhoid A01.05
vertebra M46.20
cervical region M46.22
cervicothoracic region M46.23
lumbar region M46.26
lumbosacral region M46.27
occipito-atlanto-axial region M46.21
sacrococcygeal region M46.28
thoracic region M46.24
thoracolumbar region M46.25

Osteomyelofibrosis D47.4

Osteomyelosclerosis D75.89

Osteonecrosis M87.9
due to
drugs *—see* Osteonecrosis, secondary, due to, drugs
trauma *—see* Osteonecrosis, secondary, due to, trauma
idiopathic aseptic M87.00
ankle M87.07-
carpus M87.03-
clavicle M87.01-
femur M87.05-
fibula M87.06-
finger M87.04-
humerus M87.02-
ilium M87.050
ischium M87.050
metacarpus M87.04-
metatarsus M87.07-
multiple sites M87.09
neck M87.08
pelvis M87.050
radius M87.03-
rib M87.08
scapula M87.01-
skull M87.08
tarsus M87.07-
tibia M87.06-
toe M87.07-
ulna M87.03-
vertebra M87.08
secondary NEC M87.30
carpus M87.33-
clavicle M87.31-
due to
drugs M87.10
carpus M87.13-
clavicle M87.11-
femur M87.15-

Osteonecrosis *(continued)*
secondary NEC *(continued)*
due to *(continued)*
drugs *(continued)*
fibula M87.16-
finger M87.14-
humerus M87.12-
ilium M87.159
ischium M87.159
jaw M87.180
metacarpus M87.14-
metatarsus M87.17-
multiple sites M87.19
neck M87.18
radius M87.13-
rib M87.18
scapula M87.11-
skull M87.18
tarsus M87.17-
tibia M87.16-
toe M87.17-
ulna M87.13-
vertebra M87.18
hemoglobinopathy NEC D58.2 *[M90.50]*
carpus D58.2 *[M90.54-]*
clavicle D58.2 *[M90.51-]*
femur D58.2 *[M90.55-]*
fibula D58.2 *[M90.56-]*
finger D58.2 *[M90.54-]*
humerus D58.2 *[M90.52-]*
ilium D58.2 *[M90.55-]*
ischium D58.2 *[M90.55-]*
metacarpus D58.2 *[M90.54-]*
metatarsus D58.2 *[M90.57-]*
multiple sites D58.2 *[M90.58]*
neck D58.2 *[M90.58]*
radius D58.2 *[M90.53-]*
rib D58.2 *[M90.58]*
scapula D58.2 *[M90.51-]*
skull D58.2 *[M90.58]*
tarsus D58.2 *[M90.57-]*
tibia D58.2 *[M90.56-]*
toe D58.2 *[M90.57-]*
ulna D58.2 *[M90.53-]*
vertebra D58.2 *[M90.58]*
trauma (previous) M87.20
carpus M87.23-
clavicle M87.21-
femur M87.25-
fibula M87.26-
finger M87.24-
humerus M87.22-
ilium M87.25-
ischium M87.25-
metacarpus M87.24-
metatarsus M87.27-
multiple sites M87.29
neck M87.28
radius M87.23-
rib M87.28
scapula M87.21-
skull M87.28
tarsus M87.27-
tibia M87.26-
toe M87.27-
ulna M87.23-
vertebra M87.28
femur M87.35-
fibula M87.36-
finger M87.34-
humerus M87.32-
ilium M87.350
in
caisson disease T70.3 *[M90.50]*
carpus T70.3 *[M90.54-]*
clavicle T70.3 *[M90.51-]*
femur T70.3 *[M90.55-]*

Osteonecrosis *(continued)*
secondary NEC *(continued)*
in *(continued)*
caisson disease *(continued)*
fibula T70.3 *[M90.56-]*
finger T70.3 *[M90.54-]*
humerus T70.3 *[M90.52-]*
ilium T70.3 *[M90.55-]*
ischium T70.3 *[M90.55-]*
metacarpus T70.3 *[M90.54-]*
metatarsus T70.3 *[M90.57-]*
multiple sites T70.3 *[M90.59]*
neck T70.3 *[M90.58]*
radius T70.3 *[M90.53-]*
rib T70.3 *[M90.58]*
scapula T70.3 *[M90.51-]*
skull T70.3 *[M90.58]*
tarsus T70.3 *[M90.57-]*
tibia T70.3 *[M90.56-]*
toe T70.3 *[M90.57-]*
ulna T70.3 *[M90.53-]*
vertebra T70.3 *[M90.58]*
ischium M87.350
metacarpus M87.34-
metatarsus M87.37-
multiple site M87.39
neck M87.38
radius M87.33-
rib M87.38
scapula M87.319
skull M87.38
tarsus M87.379
tibia M87.366
toe M87.379
ulna M87.33-
vertebra M87.38
specified type NEC M87.80
carpus M87.83-
clavicle M87.81-
femur M87.85-
fibula M87.86-
finger M87.84-
humerus M87.82-
ilium M87.85-
ischium M87.85-
metacarpus M87.84-
metatarsus M87.87-
multiple sites M87.89
neck M87.88
radius M87.83-
rib M87.88
scapula M87.81-
skull M87.88
tarsus M87.87-
tibia M87.86-
toe M87.87-
ulna M87.83-
vertebra M87.88

Osteo-onycho-arthro-dysplasia Q87.2

Osteo-onychodysplasia, hereditary Q87.2

Osteopathia condensans disseminata Q78.8

Osteopathy *—see also* Osteomyelitis, Osteonecrosis, Osteoporosis
after poliomyelitis M89.60
carpus M89.64-
clavicle M89.61-
femur M89.65-
fibula M89.66-
finger M89.64-
humerus M89.62-
ilium M89.659
ischium M89.659
metacarpus M89.64-
metatarsus M89.67-
multiple sites M89.69
neck M89.68

Osteopathy *(continued)*
after poliomyelitis *(continued)*
radius M89.63-
rib M89.68
scapula M89.61-
skull M89.68
tarsus M89.67-
tibia M89.66-
toe M89.67-
ulna M89.63-
vertebra M89.68
in (due to)
renal osteodystrophy N25.0
specified diseases classified elsewhere M90.8

Osteopenia M85.8-
borderline M85.8-

Osteoperiostitis *—see* Osteomyelitis, specified type NEC

Osteopetrosis (familial) Q78.2

Osteophyte M25.70
ankle M25.77-
elbow M25.72-
foot joint M25.77-
hand joint M25.74-
hip M25.75-
knee M25.76-
shoulder M25.71-
spine M25.78
vertebrae M25.78
wrist M25.73-

Osteopoikilosis Q78.8

Osteoporosis (female) (male) M81.0
with current pathological fracture M80.00
age-related M81.0
with current pathologic fracture M80.00
carpus M80.04-
clavicle M80.01-
fibula M80.06-
finger M80.04-
humerus M80.02-
ilium M80.05-
ischium M80.05-
metacarpus M80.04-
metatarsus M80.07-
pelvis M80.05-
radius M80.03-
scapula M80.01-
tarsus M80.07-
tibia M80.06-
toe M80.07-
ulna M80.03-
vertebra M80.08
disuse M81.8
with current pathological fracture M80.80
carpus M80.84-
clavicle M80.81-
fibula M80.86-
finger M80.84-
humerus M80.82-
ilium M80.85-
ischium M80.85-
metacarpus M80.84-
metatarsus M80.87-
pelvis M80.85-
radius M80.83-
scapula M80.81-
tarsus M80.87-
tibia M80.86-
toe M80.87-
ulna M80.83-
vertebra M80.88
drug-induced *—see* Osteoporosis, specified type NEC

Osteoporosis *(continued)*
- idiopathic —*see* Osteoporosis, specified type NEC
- involutional —*see* Osteoporosis, age-related
- Lequesne M81.6
- localized M81.6
- postmenopausal M81.0
  - with pathological fracture M80.00
    - carpus M80.04-
    - clavicle M80.01-
    - fibula M80.06-
    - finger M80.04-
    - humerus M80.02-
    - ilium M80.05-
    - ischium M80.05-
    - metacarpus M80.04-
    - metatarsus M80.07-
    - pelvis M80.05-
    - radius M80.03-
    - scapula M80.01-
    - tarsus M80.07-
    - tibia M80.06-
    - toe M80.07-
    - ulna M80.03-
    - vertebra M80.08
- postoophorectomy —*see* Osteoporosis, specified type NEC
- postsurgical malabsorption —*see* Osteoporosis, specified type NEC
- post-traumatic —*see* Osteoporosis, specified type NEC
- senile —*see* Osteoporosis, age-related
- specified type NEC M81.8
  - with pathological fracture M80.80
    - carpus M80.84-
    - clavicle M80.81-
    - fibula M80.86-
    - finger M80.84-
    - humerus M80.82-
    - ilium M80.85-
    - ischium M80.85-
    - metacarpus M80.84-
    - metatarsus M80.87-
    - pelvis M80.85-
    - radius M80.83-
    - scapula M80.81-
    - tarsus M80.87-
    - tibia M80.86-
    - toe M80.87-
    - ulna M80.83-
    - vertebra M80.88

Osteopsathyrosis (idiopathica) Q78.0

Osteoradionecrosis, jaw (acute) (chronic) (lower) (suppurative) (upper) M27.2

Osteosarcoma (any form) —*see* Neoplasm, bone, malignant

Osteosclerosis Q78.2
- acquired M85.8-
- congenita Q77.4
- fragilitas (generalisata) Q78.2
- myelofibrosis D75.81

Osteosclerotic anemia D64.89

Osteosis
- cutis L94.2
- renal fibrocystic N25.0

Österreicher-Turner syndrome Q87.2

Ostium
- atrioventriculare commune Q21.2
- primum (arteriosum) (defect) (persistent) Q21.2
- secundum (arteriosum) (defect) (patent) (persistent) Q21.1

Ostrum-Furst syndrome Q75.8

Otalgia —*see* subcategory H92.0

Otitis (acute) H66.90
- with effusion —*see also* Otitis, media, nonsuppurative
  - purulent —*see* Otitis, media, suppurative
- adhesive H74.1
- chronic —*see also* Otitis, media, chronic
  - with effusion —*see also* Otitis, media, nonsuppurative, chronic
- externa H60.9-
  - abscess —*see* Abscess, ear, external
  - acute (noninfective) H60.50-
    - actinic H60.51-
    - chemical H60.52-
    - contact H60.53-
    - eczematoid H60.54-
    - infective —*see* Otitis, externa, infective
    - reactive H60.55-
    - specified NEC H60.59-
  - cellulitis —*see* Cellulitis, ear
  - chronic H60.6-
  - diffuse —*see* Otitis, externa, infective, diffuse
  - hemorrhagic —*see* Otitis, externa, infective, hemorrhagic
  - in (due to)
    - aspergillosis B44.89
    - candidiasis B37.84
    - erysipelas A46 *[H62.40]*
    - herpes (simplex) virus infection B00.1
      - zoster B02.8
    - impetigo L01.00 *[H62.40]*
    - infectious disease NEC B99 *[H62.4-]*
    - mycosis NEC B36.9 *[H62.40]*
    - parasitic disease NEC B89 *[H62.40]*
    - viral disease NEC B34.9 *[H62.40]*
    - zoster B02.8
  - infective NEC H60.39-
    - abscess —*see* Abscess, ear, external
    - cellulitis —*see* Cellulitis, ear
    - diffuse H60.31-
    - hemorrhagic H60.32-
    - swimmer's ear —*see* Swimmer's, ear
  - malignant H60.2-
  - mycotic NEC B36.9 *[H62.40]*
    - in
      - aspergillosis B44.89
      - candidiasis B37.84
      - moniliasis B37.84
  - necrotizing —*see* Otitis, externa, malignant
  - Pseudomonas aeruginosa —*see* Otitis, externa, malignant
  - reactive —*see* Otitis, externa, acute, reactive
  - specified NEC —*see* subcategory H60.8
  - tropical NEC B36.9 *[H62.40]*
    - in
      - aspergillosis B44.89
      - candidiasis B37.84
      - moniliasis B37.84
- insidiosa —*see* Otosclerosis
- interna —*see* subcategory H83.0
- media (hemorrhagic) (staphylococcal) (streptococcal) H66.9-
  - with effusion (nonpurulent) —*see* Otitis, media, nonsuppurative
  - acute, subacute H66.90
    - allergic —*see* Otitis, media, nonsuppurative, acute, allergic
    - exudative —*see* Otitis, media, suppurative, acute
    - mucoid —*see* Otitis, media, nonsuppurative, acute
    - necrotizing —*see also* Otitis, media, suppurative, acute
      - in
        - measles B05.3
        - scarlet fever A38.0
    - nonsuppurative NEC —*see* Otitis, media, nonsuppurative, acute
    - purulent —*see* Otitis, media, suppurative, acute
    - sanguinous —*see* Otitis, media, nonsuppurative, acute
    - secretory —*see* Otitis, media, nonsuppurative, acute, serous
    - seromucinous —*see* Otitis, media, nonsuppurative, acute
    - serous —*see* Otitis, media, nonsuppurative, acute, serous
    - suppurative —*see* Otitis, media, suppurative, acute
  - allergic —*see* Otitis, media, nonsuppurative
  - catarrhal —*see* Otitis, media, nonsuppurative
  - chronic H66.90
    - with effusion (nonpurulent) —*see* Otitis, media, nonsuppurative, chronic
    - allergic —*see* Otitis, media, nonsuppurative, chronic, allergic
    - benign suppurative —*see* Otitis, media, suppurative, chronic, tubotympanic
    - catarrhal —*see* Otitis, media, nonsuppurative, chronic, serous
    - exudative —*see* Otitis, media, nonsuppurative, chronic
    - mucinous —*see* Otitis, media, nonsuppurative, chronic, mucoid
    - mucoid —*see* Otitis, media, nonsuppurative, chronic, mucoid
    - nonsuppurative NEC —*see* Otitis, media, nonsuppurative, chronic
    - purulent —*see* Otitis, media, suppurative, chronic
    - secretory —*see* Otitis, media, nonsuppurative, chronic, mucoid
    - seromucinous —*see* Otitis, media, nonsuppurative, chronic
    - serous —*see* Otitis, media, nonsuppurative, chronic, serous
    - suppurative —*see* Otitis, media, suppurative, chronic
    - transudative —*see* Otitis, media, nonsuppurative, chronic, mucoid
  - exudative —*see* Otitis, media, suppurative
  - in (due to) (with)
    - influenza —*see* Influenza, with, otitis media
    - measles B05.3
    - scarlet fever A38.0
    - tuberculosis A18.6
    - viral disease NEC B34.- *[H67.-]*
  - mucoid —*see* Otitis, media, nonsuppurative
  - nonsuppurative H65.9-
    - acute or subacute NEC H65.19-
      - allergic H65.11-
        - recurrent H65.11-
      - recurrent H65.19-
      - secretory —*see* Otitis, media, nonsuppurative, serous
      - serous H65.0-
        - recurrent H65.0-
    - chronic H65.49-
      - allergic H65.41-
      - mucoid H65.3-
      - serous H65.2-
  - postmeasles B05.3
  - purulent —*see* Otitis, media, suppurative
  - secretory —*see* Otitis, media, nonsuppurative
  - seromucinous —*see* Otitis, media, nonsuppurative
  - serous —*see* Otitis, media, nonsuppurative
  - suppurative H66.4-
    - acute H66.00-
      - with rupture of ear drum H66.01-
      - recurrent H66.00-
        - with rupture of ear drum H66.01-
    - chronic (*see also* subcategory) H66.3
      - atticoantral H66.2-
      - benign —*see* Otitis, media, suppurative, chronic, tubotympanic
      - tubotympanic H66.1-
  - transudative —*see* Otitis, media, nonsuppurative
  - tuberculous A18.6

Otocephaly Q18.2

Otolith syndrome —*see* subcategory H81.8

Otomycosis (diffuse) **NEC** B36.9 *[H62.40]*
- in
  - aspergillosis B44.89
  - candidiasis B37.84
  - moniliasis B37.84

Otoporosis —*see* Otosclerosis

Otorrhagia (nontraumatic) H92.2-
- traumatic - code by Type of injury

Otorrhea H92.1-
- cerebrospinal G96.0

Otosclerosis (general) H80.9-
- cochlear (endosteal) H80.2-
- involving
  - otic capsule —*see* Otosclerosis, cochlear
  - oval window
    - nonobliterative H80.0-
    - obliterative H80.1-
  - round window —*see* Otosclerosis, cochlear
- nonobliterative —*see* Otosclerosis, involving, oval window, nonobliterative

Otosclerosis *(continued)*
- obliterative *—see* Otosclerosis, involving, oval window, obliterative
- specified NEC H80.8-

Otospongiosis *—see* Otosclerosis

Otto's disease or pelvis M24.7

Outcome of delivery Z37.9
- multiple births Z37.9
  - all liveborn Z37.50
    - quadruplets Z37.52
    - quintuplets Z37.53
    - sextuplets Z37.54
    - specified number NEC Z37.59
    - triplets Z37.51
  - all stillborn Z37.7
  - some liveborn Z37.60
    - quadruplets Z37.62
    - quintuplets Z37.63
    - sextuplets Z37.64
    - specified number NEC Z37.69
    - triplets Z37.61
- single NEC Z37.9
  - liveborn Z37.0
  - stillborn Z37.1
- twins NEC Z37.9
  - both liveborn Z37.2
  - both stillborn Z37.4
  - one liveborn, one stillborn Z37.3

Outlet *—see* condition

Ovalocytosis (congenital) (hereditary) *—see* Elliptocytosis

Ovarian *—see* Condition

Ovariocele N83.4-

Ovaritis (cystic) *—see* Oophoritis

Ovary, ovarian *—see also* condition
- resistant syndrome E28.39
- vein syndrome N13.8

Overactive *—see also* Hyperfunction
- adrenal cortex NEC E27.0
- bladder N32.81
- hypothalamus E23.3
- thyroid *—see* Hyperthyroidism

Overactivity R46.3
- child *—see* Disorder, attention-deficit hyperactivity

Overbite (deep) (excessive) (horizontal) (vertical) M26.29

Overbreathing *—see* Hyperventilation

Overconscientious personality vF60.5

Overdevelopment *—see* Hypertrophy

Overdistension *—see* Distension

Overdose, overdosage (drug) *—see* Table of Drugs and Chemicals, by drug, poisoning

Overeating R63.2
- nonorganic origin F50.89
- psychogenic F50.89

Overexertion (effects) (exhaustion) T73.3

Overexposure (effects) T73.9
- exhaustion T73.2

Overfeeding *—see* Overeating
- newborn P92.4

Overfill, endodontic M27.52

Overgrowth, bone *—see* Hypertrophy, bone

Overhanging of dental restorative material (unrepairable) K08.52

Overheated (places) (effects) *—see* Heat

Overjet (excessive horizontal) M26.23

Overlaid, overlying (suffocation) *—see* Asphyxia, traumatic, due to mechanical threat

Overlap, excessive horizontal (teeth) M26.23

Overlapping toe (acquired) *—see also* Deformity, toe, specified NEC
- congenital (fifth toe) Q66.89

Overload
- circulatory, due to transfusion (blood) (blood components) (TACO) E87.71
- fluid E87.70
  - due to transfusion (blood) (blood components) E87.71
  - specified NEC E87.79
- iron, due to repeated red blood cell transfusions E83.111
- potassium (K) E87.5
- sodium (Na) E87.0

Overnutrition *—see* Hyperalimentation

Overproduction *—see also* Hypersecretion
- ACTH E27.0
- catecholamine E27.5
- growth hormone E22.0

Overprotection, child by parent Z62.1

Overriding
- aorta Q25.49
- finger (acquired) *—see* Deformity, finger
  - congenital Q68.1
- toe (acquired) *—see also* Deformity, toe, specified NEC
  - congenital Q66.89

Overstrained R53.83
- heart *—see* Hypertrophy, cardiac

Overuse, muscle NEC M70.8-

Overweight E66.3

Overworked R53.83

Oviduct *—see* condition

Ovotestis Q56.0

Ovulation (cycle)
- failure or lack of N97.0
- pain N94.0

Ovum *—see* condition

Owren's disease or syndrome (parahemophilia) D68.2

Ox heart *—see* Hypertrophy, cardiac

Oxalosis E72.53

Oxaluria E72.53

Oxycephaly, oxycephalic Q75.0
- syphilitic, congenital A50.02

Oxyuriasis B80

Oxyuris vermicularis (infestation) B80

Ozena J31.0

P

Pachyderma, pachydermia L85.9
- larynx (verrucosa) J38.7

Pachydermatocele (congenital) Q82.8

Pachydermoperiostosis *—see also* Osteoarthropathy, hypertrophic, specified type NEC
- clubbed nail M89.40 *[L62]*

Pachygyria Q04.3

Pachymeningitis (adhesive) (basal) (brain) (cervical) (chronic) (circumscribed) (external) (fibrous) (hemorrhagic) (hypertrophic) (internal) (purulent) (spinal) (suppurative) *—see* Meningitis

Pachyonychia (congenital) Q84.5

Pacinian tumor *—see* Neoplasm, skin, benign

Pad, knuckle or Garrod's M72.1

Paget-Schroetter syndrome I82.890

Paget's disease
- with infiltrating duct carcinoma *—see* Neoplasm, breast, malignant
- bone M88.9
  - carpus M88.84-
  - clavicle M88.81-
  - femur M88.85-
  - fibula M88.86-
  - finger M88.84-
  - humerus M88.82-
  - ilium M88.85-
  - in neoplastic disease *—see* Osteitis, deformans, in neoplastic disease
  - ischium M88.85-
  - metacarpus M88.84-
  - metatarsus M88.87-
  - multiple sites M88.89
  - neck M88.88
  - radius M88.83-
  - rib M88.88
  - scapula M88.81-
  - skull M88.0
  - tarsus M88.87-
  - tibia M88.86-
  - toe M88.87-
  - ulna M88.83-
  - vertebra M88.88
- breast (female) C50.01-
  - male C50.02-
- extramammary *—see also* Neoplasm, skin, malignant
  - anus C21.0
    - margin C44.590
    - skin C44.590
- intraductal carcinoma *—see* Neoplasm, breast, malignant
- malignant *—see* Neoplasm, skin, malignant
  - breast (female) C50.01-
    - male C50.02-
  - unspecified site (female) C50.01-
    - male C50.02-
- mammary *—see* Paget's disease, breast
- nipple *—see* Paget's disease, breast
- osteitis deformans *—see* Paget's disease, bone

Pain(s) (*see also* Painful) R52
- abdominal R10.9
  - colic R10.83
  - generalized R10.84
    - with acute abdomen R10.0
  - lower R10.30
    - left quadrant R10.32
    - pelvic or perineal R10.2
    - periumbilical R10.33
    - right quadrant R10.31
  - rebound *—see* Tenderness, abdominal, rebound
  - severe with abdominal rigidity R10.0
  - tenderness *—see* Tenderness, abdominal
  - upper R10.10
    - epigastric R10.13

Pain *(continued)*
- abdominal *(continued)*
  - upper *(continued)*
    - left quadrant R10.12
    - right quadrant R10.11
- acute R52
  - due to trauma G89.11
  - neoplasm related G89.3
  - postprocedural NEC G89.18
  - post-thoracotomy G89.12
  - specified by site - code to Pain, by site
- adnexa (uteri) R10.2
- anginoid *—see* Pain, precordial
- anus K62.89
- arm *—see* Pain, limb, upper
- axillary (axilla) M79.62-
- back (postural) M54.9
- bladder R39.89
  - associated with micturition *—see* Micturition, painful
  - chronic R39.82
- bone *—see* Disorder, bone, specified type NEC
- breast N64.4
- broad ligament R10.2
- cancer associated (acute) (chronic) G89.3
- cecum *—see* Pain, abdominal
- cervicobrachial M53.1
- chest (central) R07.9
  - anterior wall R07.89
  - atypical R07.89
  - ischemic I20.9
  - musculoskeletal R07.89
  - non-cardiac R07.89
  - on breathing R07.1
  - pleurodynia R07.81
  - precordial R07.2
  - wall (anterior) R07.89
- chronic G89.29
  - associated with significant psychosocial dysfunction G89.4
  - due to trauma G89.21
  - neoplasm related G89.3
  - postoperative NEC G89.28
  - postprocedural NEC G89.28
  - post-thoracotomy G89.22
  - specified NEC G89.29
- coccyx M53.3
- colon *—see* Pain, abdominal
- coronary *—see* Angina
- costochondral R07.1
- diaphragm R07.1
- due to cancer G89.3
- due to device, implant or graft (*see also* Complications, by site and type, specified NEC) T85.848
  - arterial graft NEC T82.848
  - breast (implant) T85.848
  - catheter NEC T85.848
    - dialysis (renal) T82.848
      - intraperitoneal T85.848
    - infusion NEC T82.848
      - spinal (epidural) (subdural) T85.840
    - urinary (indwelling) T83.84
  - electronic (electrode) (pulse generator) (stimulator)
    - bone T84.84
    - cardiac T82.847
    - nervous system (brain) (peripheral nerve) (spinal) T85.840
    - urinary T83.84
  - fixation, internal (orthopedic) NEC T84.84
  - gastrointestinal (bile duct) (esophagus) T85.848
  - genital NEC T83.84
  - heart NEC T82.847

Pain *(continued)*
- due to device, implant or graft *(continued)*
  - infusion NEC T85.848
  - joint prosthesis T84.84
  - ocular (corneal graft) (orbital implant) NEC T85.848
  - orthopedic NEC T84.84
  - specified NEC T85.848
  - urinary NEC T83.84
  - vascular NEC T82.848
  - ventricular intracranial shunt T85.840
- due to malignancy (primary) (secondary) G89.3
- ear —*see* subcategory H92.0
- epigastric, epigastrium R10.13
- eye —*see* Pain, ocular
- face, facial R51
  - atypical G50.1
- female genital organs NEC N94.89
- finger —*see* Pain, limb, upper
- flank —*see* Pain, abdominal
- foot —*see* Pain, limb, lower
- gallbladder K82.9
- gas (intestinal) R14.1
- gastric —*see* Pain, abdominal
- generalized NOS R52
- genital organ
  - female N94.89
  - male N50.89
- groin —*see* Pain, abdominal, lower
- hand —*see* Pain, limb, upper
- head —*see* Headache
- heart —*see* Pain, precordial
- infra-orbital —*see* Neuralgia, trigeminal
- intercostal R07.82
- intermenstrual N94.0
- jaw R68.84
- joint M25.50
  - ankle M25.57-
  - elbow M25.52-
  - finger M25.54-
  - foot M25.57-
  - hand M25.54-
  - hip M25.55-
  - knee M25.56-
  - shoulder M25.51-
  - toe M25.57-
  - wrist M25.53-
- kidney N23
- laryngeal R07.0
- leg —*see* Pain, limb, lower
- limb M79.609
  - lower M79.60-
    - foot M79.67-
    - lower leg M79.66-
    - thigh M79.65-
    - toe M79.67-
  - upper M79.60-
    - axilla M79.62-
    - finger M79.64-
    - forearm M79.63-
    - hand M79.64-
    - upper arm M79.62-
- loin M54.5
- low back M54.5
- lumbar region M54.5
- mandibular R68.84
- mastoid —*see* subcategory H92.0
- maxilla R68.84
- menstrual (*see also* Dysmenorrhea) N94.6
- metacarpophalangeal (joint) —*see* Pain, joint, hand
- metatarsophalangeal (joint) —*see* Pain, joint, foot
- mouth K13.79
- muscle —*see* Myalgia

Pain *(continued)*
- muscle *(continued)*
  - musculoskeletal (*see also* Pain, by site) M79.1
  - myofascial M79.1
- nasal J34.89
- nasopharynx J39.2
- neck NEC M54.2
- nerve NEC —*see* Neuralgia
- neuromuscular —*see* Neuralgia
- nose J34.89
- ocular H57.1-
- ophthalmic —*see* Pain, ocular
- orbital region —*see* Pain, ocular
- ovary N94.89
- over heart —*see* Pain, precordial
- ovulation N94.0
- pelvic (female) R10.2
- penis N48.89
- pericardial —*see* Pain, precordial
- perineal, perineum R10.2
- pharynx J39.2
- pleura, pleural, pleuritic R07.81
- postoperative NOS G89.18
- postprocedural NOS G89.18
- post-thoracotomy G89.12
- precordial (region) R07.2
- premenstrual N94.3
- psychogenic (persistent) (any site) F45.41
- radicular (spinal) —*see* Radiculopathy
- rectum K62.89
- respiration R07.1
- retrosternal R07.2
- rheumatoid, muscular —*see* Myalgia
- rib R07.81
- root (spinal) —*see* Radiculopathy
- round ligament (stretch) R10.2
- sacroiliac M53.3
- sciatic —*see* Sciatica
- scrotum N50.82
- seminal vesicle N50.89
- shoulder M25.51-
- spermatic cord N50.89
- spinal root —*see* Radiculopathy
- spine M54.9
  - cervical M54.2
  - low back M54.5
    - with sciatica M54.4-
  - thoracic M54.6
- stomach —*see* Pain, abdominal
- substernal R07.2
- temporomandibular (joint) M26.62-
- testis N50.81-
- thoracic spine M54.6
  - with radicular and visceral pain M54.14
- throat R07.0
- tibia —*see* Pain, limb, lower
- toe —*see* Pain, limb, lower
- tongue K14.6
- tooth K08.89
- trigeminal —*see* Neuralgia, trigeminal
- tumor associated G89.3
- ureter N23
- urinary (organ) (system) N23
- uterus NEC N94.89
- vagina R10.2
- vertebrogenic (syndrome) M54.89
- vesical R39.89
  - associated with micturition —*see* Micturition, painful
- vulva R10.2

Painful —*see also* Pain
- coitus
  - female N94.10
  - male N53.12
  - psychogenic F52.6

Painful *(continued)*
- ejaculation (semen) N53.12
  - psychogenic F52.6
- erection —*see* Priapism
- feet syndrome E53.8
- joint replacement (hip) (knee) T84.84
- menstruation —*see* Dysmenorrhea
  - psychogenic F45.8
- micturition —*see* Micturition, painful
- respiration R07.1
- scar NEC L90.5
- wire sutures T81.89

Painter's colic —*see* subcategory T56.0

Palate —*see* condition

Palatoplegia K13.79

Palatoschisis —*see* Cleft, palate

Palilalia R48.8

Palliative care Z51.5

Pallor R23.1
- optic disc, temporal —*see* Atrophy, optic

Palmar —*see also* condition
- fascia —*see* condition

Palpable
- cecum K63.89
- kidney N28.89
- ovary N83.8
- prostate N42.9
- spleen —*see* Splenomegaly

Palpitations (heart) R00.2
- psychogenic F45.8

Palsy (*see also* Paralysis) G83.9
- atrophic diffuse (progressive) G12.22
- Bell's —*see also* Palsy, facial
  - newborn P11.3
- brachial plexus NEC G54.0
  - newborn (birth injury) P14.3
- brain —*see* Palsy, cerebral
- bulbar (progressive) (chronic) G12.22
  - of childhood (Fazio-Londe) G12.1
  - pseudo NEC G12.29
  - supranuclear (progressive) G23.1
- cerebral (congenital) G80.9
  - ataxic G80.4
  - athetoid G80.3
  - choreathetoid G80.3
  - diplegic G80.8
    - spastic G80.1
  - dyskinetic G80.3
    - athetoid G80.3
    - choreathetoid G80.3
    - distonic G80.3
  - dystonic G80.3
  - hemiplegic G80.8
    - spastic G80.2
  - mixed G80.8
  - monoplegic G80.8
    - spastic G80.1
  - paraplegic G80.8
    - spastic G80.1
  - quadriplegic G80.8
    - spastic G80.0
  - spastic G80.1
    - diplegic G80.1
    - hemiplegic G80.2
    - monoplegic G80.1
    - quadriplegic G80.0
    - specified NEC G80.1
    - tetrapelgic G80.0
  - specified NEC G80.8

Palsy *(continued)*
- cerebral *(continued)*
  - syphilitic A52.12
    - congenital A50.49
  - tetraplegic G80.8
    - spastic G80.0
- cranial nerve —*see also* Disorder, nerve, cranial
  - multiple G52.7
    - in
      - infectious disease B99 *[G53]*
      - neoplastic disease (*see also* Neoplasm) D49.9 *[G53]*
      - parasitic disease B89 *[G53]*
      - sarcoidosis D86.82
- creeping G12.22
- diver's T70.3
- Erb's P14.0
- facial G51.0
  - newborn (birth injury) P11.3
- glossopharyngeal G52.1
- Klumpke (-Déjérine) P14.1
- lead —*see* subcategory T56.0
- median nerve (tardy) G56.1-
- nerve G58.9
  - specified NEC G58.8
- peroneal nerve (acute) (tardy) G57.3-
- progressive supranuclear G23.1
- pseudobulbar NEC G12.29
- radial nerve (acute) G56.3-
- seventh nerve —*see also* Palsy, facial
  - newborn P11.3
- shaking —*see* Parkinsonism
- spastic (cerebral) (spinal) G80.1
- ulnar nerve (tardy) G56.2-
- wasting G12.29

Paludism —*see* Malaria

Panangiitis M30.0

Panaris, panaritium —*see also* Cellulitis, digit
- with lymphangitis —*see* Lymphangitis, acute, digit

Panarteritis nodosa M30.0
- brain or cerebral I67.7

Pancake heart R93.1
- with cor pulmonale (chronic) I27.81

Pancarditis (acute) (chronic) I51.89
- rheumatic I09.89
  - active or acute I01.8

Pancoast's syndrome or tumor C34.1-

Pancolitis, ulcerative (chronic) K51.00
- with
  - complication K51.019
  - abscess K51.014
  - fistula K51.013
  - obstruction K51.012
  - rectal bleeding K51.011
  - specified complication NEC K51.018

Pancreas, pancreatic —*see* condition

Pancreatitis (annular) (apoplectic) (calcareous) (edematous) (hemorrhagic) (malignant) (recurrent) (subacute) (suppurative) K85.90
- with necrosis (uninfected) K85.91
  - infected K85.92
- acute (without necrosis or infection) K85.90
  - with necrosis (uninfected) K85.91
    - infected K85.92
  - alcohol induced (without necrosis or infection) K85.20

Pancreatitis *(continued)*
- acute *(continued)*
  - alcohol induced *(continued)*
    - with necrosis (uninfected) K85.21
      - infected K85.22
  - biliary (without necrosis or infection) K85.10
    - with necrosis (uninfected) K85.11
      - infected K85.12
  - drug induced (without necrosis or infection) K85.30
    - with necrosis (uninfected) K85.31
      - infected K85.32
  - gallstone (without necrosis or infection) K85.10
    - with necrosis (uninfected) K85.11
      - infected K85.12
  - idiopathic (without necrosis or infection) K85.00
    - with necrosis (uninfected) K85.01
      - infected K85.02
  - specified NEC (without necrosis or infection) K85.80
    - with necrosis (uninfected) K85.81
      - infected K85.82
- chronic (infectious) K86.1
  - alcohol-induced K86.0
  - recurrent K86.1
  - relapsing K86.1
- cystic (chronic) K86.1
- cytomegaloviral B25.2
- fibrous (chronic) K86.1
- gangrenous *—see* Pancreatitis, acute
- gallstone (without necrosis or infection) K85.10
  - with necrosis (uninfected) K85.11
  - infected K85.12
- interstitial (chronic) K86.1
  - acute (*see also* Pancreatitis, acute) K85.80
- mumps B26.3
- recurrent (chronic) K86.1
- relapsing, chronic K86.1
- syphilitic A52.74

Pancreatoblastoma *—see* Neoplasm, pancreas, malignant

Pancreolithiasis K86.89

Pancytolysis D75.89

Pancytopenia (acquired) D61.818
- with
  - malformations D61.09
  - myelodysplastic syndrome *—see* Syndrome, myelodysplastic
- antineoplastic chemotherapy induced D61.810
- congenital D61.09
- drug-induced NEC D61.811

PANDAS (pediatric autoimmune neuropsychiatric disorders associated with streptococcal infections syndrome) D89.89

Panencephalitis, subacute, sclerosing A81.1

Panhematopenia D61.9
- congenital D61.09
- constitutional D61.09
- splenic, primary D73.1

Panhemocytopenia D61.9
- congenital D61.09
- constitutional D61.09

Panhypogonadism E29.1

Panhypopituitarism E23.0
- prepubertal E23.0

Panic (attack) (state) F41.0
- reaction to exceptional stress (transient) F43.0

Panmyelopathy, familial, constitutional D61.09

Panmyelophthisis D61.82
- congenital D61.09

Panmyelosis (acute) (with myelofibrosis) C94.4-

Panner's disease *—see* Osteochondrosis, juvenile, humerus

Panneuritis endemica E51.11

Panniculitis (nodular) (nonsuppurative) M79.3
- back M54.00
  - cervical region M54.02
  - cervicothoracic region M54.03
  - lumbar region M54.06
  - lumbosacral region M54.07
  - multiple sites M54.09
  - occipito-atlanto-axial region M54.01
  - sacrococcygeal region M54.08
  - thoracic region M54.04
  - thoracolumbar region M54.05
- lupus L93.2
- mesenteric K65.4
- neck M54.02
  - cervicothoracic region M54.03
  - occipito-atlanto-axial region M54.01
- relapsing M35.6

Panniculus adiposus (abdominal) E65

Pannus (allergic) (cornea) (degenerativus) (keratic) H16.42-
- abdominal (symptomatic) E65
- trachomatosus, trachomatous (active) A71.1

Panophthalmitis H44.01-

Pansinusitis (chronic) (hyperplastic) (nonpurulent) (purulent) J32.4
- acute J01.40
  - recurrent J01.41
- tuberculous A15.8

Panuveitis (sympathetic) H44.11-

Panvalvular disease I08.9
- specified NEC I08.8

PAPA (pyogenic arthritis, pyoderma gangrenosum, and acne syndrome) M04.8

Papanicolaou smear, cervix Z12.4
- as part of routine gynecological examination Z01.419
  - with abnormal findings Z01.411
- for suspected neoplasm Z12.4
- nonspecific abnormal finding R87.619
- routine Z01.419
  - with abnormal findings Z01.411

Papilledema (choked disc) H47.10
- associated with
  - decreased ocular pressure H47.12
  - increased intracranial pressure H47.11
  - retinal disorder H47.13
- Foster-Kennedy syndrome H47.14-

Papillitis H46.00
- anus K62.89
- chronic lingual K14.4
- necrotizing, kidney N17.2
- optic H46.0-
- rectum K62.89
- renal, necrotizing N17.2
- tongue K14.0

Papilloma *—see also* Neoplasm, benign, by site
- basal cell L82.1
  - inflamed L82.0
- acuminatum (female) (male) (anogenital) A63.0
- benign pinta (primary) A67.0
- bladder (urinary) (transitional cell) D41.4
- choroid plexus (lateral ventricle) (third ventricle) D33.0
  - anaplastic C71.5
  - fourth ventricle D33.1
  - malignant C71.5
- renal pelvis (transitional cell) D41.1-
  - benign D30.1-
- Schneiderian
  - specified site *—see* Neoplasm, benign, by site
  - unspecified site D14.0
- serous surface
  - borderline malignancy
    - specified site *—see* Neoplasm, uncertain behavior, by site
    - unspecified site D39.10
  - specified site *—see* Neoplasm, benign, by site
  - unspecified site D27.9
- transitional (cell)
  - bladder (urinary) D41.4
  - inverted type *—see* Neoplasm, uncertain behavior, by site
  - renal pelvis D41.1-
  - ureter D41.2-
- ureter (transitional cell) D41.2-
  - benign D30.2-
- urothelial *—see* Neoplasm, uncertain behavior, by site
- villous *—see* Neoplasm, uncertain behavior, by site
  - adenocarcinoma in *—see* Neoplasm, malignant, by site
  - in situ *—see* Neoplasm, in situ
- yaws, plantar or palmar A66.1

Papillomata, multiple, of yaws A66.1

Papillomatosis *—see also* Neoplasm, benign, by site
- confluent and reticulated L83
- cystic, breast *—see* Mastopathy, cystic
- ductal, breast *—see* Mastopathy, cystic
- intraductal (diffuse) *—see* Neoplasm, benign, by site
- subareolar duct D24-

Papillomavirus, as cause of disease classified elsewhere B97.7

Papillon-Léage and Psaume syndrome Q87.0

Papule(s) R23.8
- carate (primary) A67.0
- fibrous, of nose D22.39
- Gottron's L94.4
- pinta (primary) A67.0

Papulosis
- lymphomatoid C86.6
- malignant I77.89

Papyraceous fetus O31.0-

Para-albuminemia E88.09

Paracephalus Q89.7

Parachute mitral valve Q23.2

Paracoccidioidomycosis B41.9
- disseminated B41.7
- generalized B41.7
- mucocutaneous-lymphangitic B41.8
- pulmonary B41.0
- specified NEC B41.8
- visceral B41.8

Paradentosis K05.4

Paraffinoma T88.8

Paraganglioma D44.7
- adrenal D35.0-
  - malignant C74.1-
- aortic body D44.7
  - malignant C75.5
- carotid body D44.6
  - malignant C75.4
- chromaffin *—see also* Neoplasm, benign, by site
  - malignant *—see* Neoplasm, malignant, by site
- extra-adrenal D44.7
  - malignant C75.5
    - specified site *—see* Neoplasm, malignant, by site
    - unspecified site C75.5
  - specified site *—see* Neoplasm, uncertain behavior, by site
  - unspecified site D44.7
- gangliocytic D13.2
  - specified site *—see* Neoplasm, benign, by site
  - unspecified site D13.2
- glomus jugulare D44.7
  - malignant C75.5
- jugular D44.7
- malignant C75.5
  - specified site *—see* Neoplasm, malignant, by site
  - unspecified site C75.5
- nonchromaffin D44.7
  - malignant C75.5
    - specified site *—see* Neoplasm, malignant, by site
    - unspecified site C75.5
  - specified site *—see* Neoplasm, uncertain behavior, by site
  - unspecified site D44.7
- parasympathetic D44.7
  - specified site *—see* Neoplasm, uncertain behavior, by site
  - unspecified site D44.7
- specified site *—see* Neoplasm, uncertain behavior, by site
- sympathetic D44.7
  - specified site *—see* Neoplasm, uncertain behavior, by site
  - unspecified site D44.7
- unspecified site D44.7

Parageusia R43.2
- psychogenic F45.8

Paragonimiasis B66.4

Paragranuloma, Hodgkin *—see* Lymphoma, Hodgkin, specified NEC

Parahemophilia (*see also* Defect, coagulation) D68.2

Parakeratosis R23.4
- variegata L41.0

Paralysis, paralytic (complete) (incomplete) G83.9
- with
  - syphilis A52.17
- abducens, abducent (nerve) *—see* Strabismus, paralytic, sixth nerve
- abductor, lower extremity G57.9-
- accessory nerve G52.8
- accommodation *—see also* Paresis, of accommodation
  - hysterical F44.89
- acoustic nerve (except Deafness) *—see* subcategory H93.3
- agitans (*see also* Parkinsonism) G20
  - arteriosclerotic G21.4

Paralysis, paralytic *(continued)*

- alternating (oculomotor) G83.89
- amyotrophic G12.21
- ankle G57.9-
- anus (sphincter) K62.89
- arm —*see* Monoplegia, upper limb
- ascending (spinal), acute G61.0
- association G12.29
- asthenic bulbar G70.00
  - with exacerbation (acute) G70.01
  - in crisis G70.01
- ataxic (hereditary) G11.9
  - general (syphilitic) A52.17
- atrophic G58.9
  - infantile, acute —*see* Poliomyelitis, paralytic
  - progressive G12.22
  - spinal (acute) —*see* Poliomyelitis, paralytic
- axillary G54.0
- Babinski-Nageotte's G83.89
- Bell's G51.0
  - newborn P11.3
- Benedikt's G46.3
- birth injury P14.9
  - spinal cord P11.5
- bladder (neurogenic) (sphincter) N31.2
- bowel, colon or intestine K56.0
- brachial plexus G54.0
  - birth injury P14.3
  - newborn (birth injury) P14.3
- brain G83.9
  - diplegia G83.0
  - triplegia G83.89
- bronchial J98.09
- Brown-Séquard G83.81
- bulbar (chronic) (progressive) G12.22
  - infantile —*see* Poliomyelitis, paralytic
  - poliomyelitic —*see* Poliomyelitis, paralytic
  - pseudo G12.29
- bulbospinal G70.00
  - with exacerbation (acute) G70.01
  - in crisis G70.01
- cardiac (*see also* Failure, heart) I50.9
- cerebrocerebellar, diplegic G80.1
- cervical
  - plexus G54.2
  - sympathetic G90.09
- Céstan-Chenais G46.3
- Charcot-Marie-Tooth type G60.0
- Clark's G80.9
- colon K56.0
- compressed air T70.3
- compression
  - arm G56.9-
  - leg G57.9-
  - lower extremity G57.9-
  - upper extremity G56.9-
- congenital (cerebral) —*see* Palsy, cerebral
- conjugate movement (gaze) (of eye) H51.0
  - cortical (nuclear) (supranuclear) H51.0
- cordis —*see* Failure, heart
- cranial or cerebral nerve G52.9
- creeping G12.22
- crossed leg G83.89
- crutch —*see* Injury, brachial plexus
- deglutition R13.0
  - hysterical F44.4
- dementia A52.17
- descending (spinal) NEC G12.29
- diaphragm (flaccid) J98.6
  - due to accidental dissection of phrenic nerve during procedure —*see* Puncture, accidental complicating surgery

Paralysis, paralytic *(continued)*

- digestive organs NEC K59.8
- diplegic —*see* Diplegia
- divergence (nuclear) H51.8
- diver's T70.3
- Duchenne's
  - birth injury P14.0
  - due to or associated with
    - motor neuron disease G12.22
    - muscular dystrophy G71.0
- due to intracranial or spinal birth injury —*see* Palsy, cerebral
- embolic (current episode) I63.4-
- Erb (-Duchenne) (birth) (newborn) P14.0
- Erb's syphilitic spastic spinal A52.17
- esophagus K22.8
- eye muscle (extrinsic) H49.9
  - intrinsic —*see also* Paresis, of accommodation
- facial (nerve) G51.0
  - birth injury P11.3
  - congenital P11.3
  - following operation NEC —*see* Puncture, accidental complicating surgery
  - newborn (birth injury) P11.3
- familial (recurrent) (periodic) G72.3
  - spastic G11.4
- fauces J39.2
- finger G56.9-
- gait R26.1
- gastric nerve (nondiabetic) G52.2
- gaze, conjugate H51.0
- general (progressive) (syphilitic) A52.17
  - juvenile A50.45
- glottis J38.00
  - bilateral J38.02
  - unilateral J38.01
- gluteal G54.1
- Gubler (-Millard) G46.3
- hand —*see* Monoplegia, upper limb
- heart —*see* Arrest, cardiac
- hemiplegic —*see* Hemiplegia
- hyperkalemic periodic (familial) G72.3
- hypoglossal (nerve) G52.3
- hypokalemic periodic G72.3
- hysterical F44.4
- ileus K56.0
- infantile (*see also* Poliomyelitis, paralytic) A80.30
  - bulbar —*see* Poliomyelitis, paralytic
  - cerebral —*see* Palsy, cerebral
  - spastic —*see* Palsy, cerebral, spastic
- infective —*see* Poliomyelitis, paralytic
- inferior nuclear G83.9
- internuclear —*see* Ophthalmoplegia, internuclear
- intestine K56.0
- iris H57.09
  - due to diphtheria (toxin) A36.89
- ischemic, Volkmann's (complicating trauma) T79.6
- Jackson's G83.89
- jake —*see* Poisoning, food, noxious, plant
- Jamaica ginger (jake) G62.2
- juvenile general A50.45
- Klumpke (-Déjérine) (birth) (newborn) P14.1
- labioglossal (laryngeal) (pharyngeal) G12.29
- Landry's G61.0
- laryngeal nerve (recurrent) (superior) (unilateral) J38.00
  - bilateral J38.02
  - unilateral J38.01

Paralysis, paralytic *(continued)*

- larynx J38.00
  - bilateral J38.02
  - due to diphtheria (toxin) A36.2
  - unilateral J38.01
- lateral G12.23
- lead —*see* subcategory T56.0
- left side —*see* Hemiplegia
- leg G83.1-
  - both —*see* Paraplegia
  - crossed G83.89
  - hysterical F44.4
  - psychogenic F44.4
  - transient or transitory R29.818
    - traumatic NEC —*see* Injury, nerve, leg
- levator palpebrae superioris —*see* Blepharoptosis, paralytic
- limb —*see* Monoplegia
- lip K13.0
- Lissauer's A52.17
- lower limb —*see* Monoplegia, lower limb
  - both —*see* Paraplegia
- lung J98.4
- median nerve G56.1-
- medullary (tegmental) G83.89
- mesencephalic NEC G83.89
  - tegmental G83.89
- middle alternating G83.89
- Millard-Gubler-Foville G46.3
- monoplegic —*see* Monoplegia
- motor G83.9
- muscle, muscular NEC G72.89
  - due to nerve lesion G58.9
  - eye (extrinsic) H49.9
    - intrinsic —*see* Paresis, of accommodation
    - oblique —*see* Strabismus, paralytic, fourth nerve
  - iris sphincter H21.9
  - ischemic (Volkmann's) (complicating trauma) T79.6
  - progressive G12.21
  - pseudohypertrophic G71.0
- musculocutaneous nerve G56.9-
- musculospiral G56.9-
- nerve —*see also* Disorder, nerve
  - abducent —*see* Strabismus, paralytic, sixth nerve
  - accessory G52.8
  - auditory (except Deafness) —*see* subcategory H93.3
  - birth injury P14.9
  - cranial or cerebral G52.9
  - facial G51.0
    - birth injury P11.3
    - congenital P11.3
    - newborn (birth injury) P11.3
  - fourth or trochlear —*see* Strabismus, paralytic, fourth nerve
  - newborn (birth injury) P14.9
  - oculomotor —*see* Strabismus, paralytic, third nerve
  - phrenic (birth injury) P14.2
  - radial G56.3-
  - seventh or facial G51.0
    - newborn (birth injury) P11.3
  - sixth or abducent —*see* Strabismus, paralytic, sixth nerve
  - syphilitic A52.15
  - third or oculomotor —*see* Strabismus, paralytic, third nerve
  - trigeminal G50.9
  - trochlear —*see* Strabismus, paralytic, fourth nerve
  - ulnar G56.2-
- normokalemic periodic G72.3

Paralysis, paralytic *(continued)*

- ocular H49.9
  - alternating G83.89
- oculofacial, congenital (Moebius) Q87.0
- oculomotor (external bilateral) (nerve) —*see* Strabismus, paralytic, third nerve
- palate (soft) K13.79
- paratrigeminal G50.9
- periodic (familial) (hyperkalemic) (hypokalemic) (myotonic) (normokalemic) (potassium sensitive) (secondary) G72.3
- peripheral autonomic nervous system —*see* Neuropathy, peripheral, autonomic
- peroneal (nerve) G57.3-
- pharynx J39.2
- phrenic nerve G56.8-
- plantar nerve(s) G57.6-
- pneumogastric nerve G52.2
- poliomyelitis (current) —*see* Poliomyelitis, paralytic
- popliteal nerve G57.3-
- postepileptic transitory G83.84
- progressive (atrophic) (bulbar) (spinal) G12.22
  - general A52.17
  - infantile acute —*see* Poliomyelitis, paralytic
  - supranuclear G23.1
- pseudobulbar G12.29
- pseudohypertrophic (muscle) G71.0
- psychogenic F44.4
- quadriceps G57.9-
- quadriplegic —*see* Tetraplegia
- radial nerve G56.3-
- rectus muscle (eye) H49.9
- recurrent isolated sleep G47.53
- respiratory (muscle) (system) (tract) R06.81
  - center NEC G93.89
  - congenital P28.89
  - newborn P28.89
- right side —*see* Hemiplegia
- saturnine —*see* subcategory T56.0
- sciatic nerve G57.0-
- senile G83.9
- shaking —*see* Parkinsonism
- shoulder G56.9-
- sleep, recurrent isolated G47.53
- spastic G83.9
  - cerebral —*see* Palsy, cerebral, spastic
  - congenital (cerebral) —*see* Palsy, cerebral, spastic
  - familial G11.4
  - hereditary G11.4
  - quadriplegic G80.0
  - syphilitic (spinal) A52.17
- sphincter, bladder —*see* Paralysis, bladder
- spinal (cord) G83.9
  - accessory nerve G52.8
  - acute —*see* Poliomyelitis, paralytic
  - ascending acute G61.0
  - atrophic (acute) —*see also* Poliomyelitis, paralytic
    - spastic, syphilitic A52.17
  - congenital NEC —*see* Palsy, cerebral
  - infantile —*see* Poliomyelitis, paralytic
  - hereditary G95.89
  - progressive G12.21
  - sequelae NEC G83.89
- sternomastoid G52.8
- stomach K31.84

Paralysis, paralytic *(continued)*
- stomach *(continued)*
  - diabetic *—see* Diabetes, by type, with gastroparesis
  - nerve G52.2
    - diabetic *—see* Diabetes, by type, with gastroparesis
- stroke *—see* Infarct, brain
- subcapsularis G56.8-
- supranuclear (progressive) G23.1
- sympathetic G90.8
  - cervical G90.09
  - nervous system *—see* Neuropathy, peripheral, autonomic
- syndrome G83.9
  - specified NEC G83.89
- syphilitic spastic spinal (Erb's) A52.17
- thigh G57.9-
- throat J39.2
  - diphtheritic A36.0
  - muscle J39.2
- thrombotic (current episode) I63.3-
- thumb G56.9-
- tick *—see* Toxicity, venom, arthropod, specified NEC
- Todd's (postepileptic transitory paralysis) G83.84
- toe G57.6-
- tongue K14.8
- transient R29.5
  - arm or leg NEC R29.818
  - traumatic NEC *—see* Injury, nerve
- trapezius G52.8
- traumatic, transient NEC *—see* Injury, nerve
- trembling *—see* Parkinsonism
- triceps brachii G56.9-
- trigeminal nerve G50.9
- trochlear (nerve) *—see* Strabismus, paralytic, fourth nerve
- ulnar nerve G56.2-
- upper limb *—see* Monoplegia, upper limb
- uremic N18.9 *[G99.8]*
- uveoparotitic D86.89
- uvula K13.79
  - postdiphtheritic A36.0
- vagus nerve G52.2
- vasomotor NEC G90.8
- velum palati K13.79
- vesical *—see* Paralysis, bladder
- vestibular nerve (except Vertigo) *—see* subcategory H93.3
- vocal cords J38.00
  - bilateral J38.02
  - unilateral J38.01
- Volkmann's (complicating trauma) T79.6
- wasting G12.29
- Weber's G46.3
- wrist G56.9-

Paramedial urethrovesical orifice Q64.79

Paramenia N92.6

Parametritis (*see also* Disease, pelvis, inflammatory) N73.2
- acute N73.0
- complicating abortion *—see* Abortion, by type, complicated by, parametritis

Parametrium, parametric *—see* condition

Paramnesia *—see* Amnesia

Paramolar K00.1

Paramyloidosis E85.89

Paramyoclonus multiplex G25.3

Paramyotonia (congenita) G71.19

Parangi *—see* Yaws

Paranoia (querulans) F22
- senile F03

Paranoid
- dementia (senile) F03
  - praecox *—see* Schizophrenia
- personality F60.0
- psychosis (climacteric) (involutional) (menopausal) F22
  - psychogenic (acute) F23
  - senile F03
- reaction (acute) F23
  - chronic F22
- schizophrenia F20.0
- state (climacteric) (involutional) (menopausal) (simple) F22
  - senile F03
- tendencies F60.0
- traits F60.0
- trends F60.0
- type, psychopathic personality F60.0

Paraparesis *—see* Paraplegia

Paraphasia R47.02

Paraphilia F65.9

Paraphimosis (congenital) N47.2
- chancroidal A57

Paraphrenia, paraphrenic (late) F22
- schizophrenia F20.0

Paraplegia (lower) G82.20
- ataxic *—see* Degeneration, combined, spinal cord
- complete G82.21
- congenital (cerebral) G80.8
  - spastic G80.1
- familial spastic G11.4
- functional (hysterical) F44.4
- hereditary, spastic G11.4
- hysterical F44.4
- incomplete G82.22
- Pott's A18.01
- psychogenic F44.4
- spastic
  - Erb's spinal, syphilitic A52.17
  - hereditary G11.4
  - tropical G04.1
- syphilitic (spastic) A52.17
- tropical spastic G04.1

Parapoxvirus B08.60
- specified NEC B08.69

Paraproteinemia D89.2
- benign (familial) D89.2
- monoclonal D47.2
- secondary to malignant disease D47.2

Parapsoriasis L41.9
- en plaques L41.4
- guttata L41.1
- large plaque L41.4
- retiform, retiformis L41.5
- small plaque L41.3
- specified NEC L41.8
- varioliformis (acuta) L41.0

Parasitic *—see also* condition
- disease NEC B89
- stomatitis B37.0
- sycosis (beard) (scalp) B35.0
- twin Q89.4

Parasitism B89
- intestinal B82.9
- skin B88.9
- specified *—see* Infestation

Parasitophobia F40.218

Parasomnia G47.50
- due to
  - alcohol
    - abuse F10.182
    - dependence F10.282
    - use F10.982
  - amphetamines
    - abuse F15.182
    - dependence F15.282
    - use F15.982
  - caffeine
    - abuse F15.182
    - dependence F15.282
    - use F15.982
  - cocaine
    - abuse F14.182
    - dependence F14.282
    - use F14.982
  - drug NEC
    - abuse F19.182
    - dependence F19.282
    - use F19.982
  - opioid
    - abuse F11.182
    - dependence F11.282
    - use F11.982
  - psychoactive substance NEC
    - abuse F19.182
    - dependence F19.282
    - use F19.982
  - sedative, hypnotic, or anxiolytic
    - abuse F13.182
    - dependence F13.282
    - use F13.982
  - stimulant NEC
    - abuse F15.182
    - dependence F15.282
    - use F15.982
- in conditions classified elsewhere G47.54
- nonorganic origin F51.8
- organic G47.50
- specified NEC G47.59

Paraspadias Q54.9

Paraspasmus facialis G51.8

Parasuicide (attempt)
- history of (personal) Z91.5
  - in family Z81.8

Parathyroid gland *—see* condition

Parathyroid tetany E20.9

Paratrachoma A74.0

Paratyphilitis *—see* Appendicitis

Paratyphoid (fever) *—see* Fever, paratyphoid

Paratyphus *—see* Fever, paratyphoid

Paraurethral duct Q64.79
- nonorganic origin F51.5

Paraurethritis *—see also* Urethritis
- gonococcal (acute) (chronic) (with abscess) A54.1

Paravaccinia NEC B08.04

Paravaginitis *—see* Vaginitis

Parencephalitis *—see also* Encephalitis
- sequelae G09

Parent-child conflict *—see* Conflict, parent-child
- estrangement NEC Z62.890

Paresis *—see also* Paralysis
- accommodation *—see* Paresis, of accommodation
- Bernhardt's G57.1-
- bladder (sphincter) *—see also* Paralysis, bladder
  - tabetic A52.17

Paresis *(continued)*
- bowel, colon or intestine K56.0
- extrinsic muscle, eye H49.9
- general (progressive) (syphilitic) A52.17
  - juvenile A50.45
- heart *—see* Failure, heart
- insane (syphilitic) A52.17
- juvenile (general) A50.45
- of accommodation H52.52-
- peripheral progressive (idiopathic) G60.3
- pseudohypertrophic G71.0
- senile G83.9
- syphilitic (general) A52.17
  - congenital A50.45
- vesical NEC N31.2

Paresthesia (*see also* Disturbance, sensation, skin) R20.2
- Bernhardt G57.1-

Paretic *—see* condition

Parinaud's
- conjunctivitis H10.89
- oculoglandular syndrome H10.89
- ophthalmoplegia H49.88-

Parkinsonism (idiopathic) (primary) G20
- with neurogenic orthostatic hypotension (symptomatic) G90.3
- arteriosclerotic G21.4
- dementia G31.83 *[F02.80]*
  - with behavioral disturbance G31.83 *[F02.81]*
- due to
  - drugs NEC G21.19
    - neuroleptic G21.11
- medication-induced NEC G21.19
- neuroleptic induced G21.11
- postencephalitic G21.3
- secondary G21.9
  - due to
    - arteriosclerosis G21.4
    - drugs NEC G21.19
      - neuroleptic G21.11
    - encephalitis G21.3
    - external agents NEC G21.2
    - syphilis A52.19
  - specified NEC G21.8
- syphilitic A52.19
- treatment-induced NEC G21.19
- vascular G21.4

Parkinson's disease, syndrome or tremor *—see* Parkinsonism

Parodontitis *—see* Periodontitis

Parodontosis K05.4

Paronychia *—see also* Cellulitis, digit
- with lymphangitis *—see* Lymphangitis, acute, digit
- candidal (chronic) B37.2
- tuberculous (primary) A18.4

Parorexia (psychogenic) F50.89

Parosmia R43.1
- psychogenic F45.8

Parotid gland *—see* condition

Parotitis, parotiditis (allergic) (nonspecific toxic) (purulent) (septic) (suppurative) *—see also* Sialoadenitis
- epidemic *—see* Mumps
- infectious *—see* Mumps
- postoperative K91.89
- surgical K91.89

Parrot fever A70

Parrot's disease (early congenital syphilitic pseudoparalysis) A50.02

Parry-Romberg syndrome G51.8

Parry's disease or syndrome E05.00
- with thyroid storm E05.01

Pars planitis —*see* Cyclitis

Parsonage (-Aldren)-**Turner syndrome** G54.5

Parson's disease (exophthalmic goiter) E05.00
- with thyroid storm E05.01

Particolored infant Q82.8

Parturition —*see* Delivery

Parulis K04.7
- with sinus K04.6

Parvovirus, as cause of disease classified elsewhere B97.6

Pasini and Pierini's atrophoderma L90.3

Passage
- false, urethra N36.5
- meconium (newborn) during delivery P03.82
- of sounds or bougies —*see* Attention to, artificial, opening

Passive —*see* condition
- smoking Z77.22

Pasteurella septica A28.0

Pasteurellosis —*see* Infection, Pasteurella

PAT (paroxysmal atrial tachycardia) I47.1

Patau's syndrome —*see* Trisomy, 13

Patches
- mucous (syphilitic) A51.39
  - congenital A50.07
- smokers' (mouth) K13.24

Patellar —*see* condition

Patent —*see also* Imperfect, closure
- canal of Nuck Q52.4
- cervix N88.3
- ductus arteriosus or Botallo's Q25.0
- foramen
  - botalli Q21.1
  - ovale Q21.1
- interauricular septum Q21.1
- interventricular septum Q21.0
- omphalomesenteric duct Q43.0
- os (uteri) —*see* Patent, cervix
- ostium secundum Q21.1
- urachus Q64.4
- vitelline duct Q43.0

Paterson (-Brown) (-Kelly) **syndrome or web** D50.1

Pathologic, pathological —*see also* condition
- asphyxia R09.01
- fire-setting F63.1
- gambling F63.0
- ovum O02.0
- resorption, tooth K03.3
- stealing F63.2

Pathology (of) —*see* Disease
- periradicular, associated with previous endodontic treatment NEC M27.59

Pattern, sleep-wake, irregular G47.23

Patulous —*see also* Imperfect, closure (congenital)
- alimentary tract Q45.8
  - lower Q43.8
  - upper Q40.8
- eustachian tube H69.0-

Pause, sinoatrial I49.5

Paxton's disease B36.2

Pearl(s)
- enamel K00.2
- Epstein's K09.8

Pearl-worker's disease —*see* Osteomyelitis, specified type NEC

Pectenosis K62.4

Pectoral —*see* condition

Pectus
- carinatum (congenital) Q67.7
  - acquired M95.4
  - rachitic sequelae (late effect) E64.3
- excavatum (congenital) Q67.6
  - acquired M95.4
  - rachitic sequelae (late effect) E64.3
- recurvatum (congenital) Q67.6

Pedatrophia E41

Pederosis F65.4

Pediculosis (infestation) B85.2
- capitis (head-louse) (any site) B85.0
- corporis (body-louse) (any site) B85.1
- eyelid B85.0
- mixed (classifiable to more than one of the titles B85.0-B85.3) B85.4
- pubis (pubic louse) (any site) B85.3
- vestimenti B85.1
- vulvae B85.3

Pediculus (infestation) —*see* Pediculosis

Pedophilia F65.4

Peg-shaped teeth K00.2

Pelade —*see* Alopecia, areata

Pelger-Huët anomaly or syndrome D72.0

Peliosis (rheumatica) D69.0
- hepatis K76.4
  - with toxic liver disease K71.8

Pelizaeus-Merzbacher disease E75.29

Pellagra (alcoholic) (with polyneuropathy) E52

Pellagra-cerebellar-ataxia-renal aminoaciduria syndrome E72.02

Pellegrini (-Stieda) **disease or syndrome** —*see* Bursitis, tibial collateral

Pellizzi's syndrome E34.8

Pel's crisis A52.11

Pelvic —*see also* condition
- examination (periodic) (routine) Z01.419
  - with abnormal findings Z01.411
- kidney, congenital Q63.2

Pelviolithiasis —*see* Calculus, kidney

Pelviperitonitis —*see also* Peritonitis, pelvic
- gonococcal A54.24
- puerperal O85

Pelvis —*see* condition or type

Pemphigoid L12.9
- benign, mucous membrane L12.1
- bullous L12.0
- cicatricial L12.1
- juvenile L12.2
- ocular L12.1
- specified NEC L12.8

Pemphigus L10.9
- benign familial (chronic) Q82.8
- Brazilian L10.3
- circinatus L13.0
- conjunctiva L12.1
- drug-induced L10.5
- erythematosus L10.4
- foliaceous L10.2
- gangrenous —*see* Gangrene
- neonatorum L01.03
- ocular L12.1
- paraneoplastic L10.81
- specified NEC L10.89
- syphilitic (congenital) A50.06
- vegetans L10.1
- vulgaris L10.0
- wildfire L10.3

Pendred's syndrome E07.1

Pendulous
- abdomen, in pregnancy —*see* Pregnancy, complicated by, abnormal, pelvic organs or tissues NEC
- breast N64.89

Penetrating wound —*see also* Puncture
- with internal injury —*see* Injury, by site
- eyeball —*see* Puncture, eyeball
- orbit (with or without foreign body) —*see* Puncture, orbit
- uterus by instrument with or following ectopic or molar pregnancy O08.6

Penicillosis B48.4

Penis —*see* condition

Penitis N48.29

Pentalogy of Fallot Q21.8

Pentasomy X syndrome Q97.1

Pentosuria (essential) E74.8

Percreta placenta O43.23-

Peregrinating patient —*see* Disorder, factitious

Perforation, perforated (nontraumatic) (of)
- accidental during procedure (blood vessel) (nerve) (organ) —*see* Complication, accidental puncture or laceration
- antrum —*see* Sinusitis, maxillary
- appendix K35.2
  - with localized peritonitis K35.3
- atrial septum, multiple Q21.1
- attic, ear —*see* Perforation, tympanum, attic
- bile duct (common) (hepatic) K83.2
  - cystic K82.2
- bladder (urinary)
  - with or following ectopic or molar pregnancy O08.6
  - obstetrical trauma O71.5
  - traumatic S37.29
    - at delivery O71.5
- bowel K63.1
  - with or following ectopic or molar pregnancy O08.6
  - newborn P78.0
  - obstetrical trauma O71.5
  - traumatic —*see* Laceration, intestine
- broad ligament N83.8
  - with or following ectopic or molar pregnancy O08.6
  - obstetrical trauma O71.6

Perforation, perforated *(continued)*
- by
  - device, implant or graft (*see also* Complications, by site and type, mechanical) T85.628
    - arterial graft NEC —*see* Complication, cardiovascular device, mechanical, vascular
    - breast (implant) T85.49
    - catheter NEC T85.698
      - cystostomy T83.090
      - dialysis (renal) T82.49
        - intraperitoneal T85.691
      - infusion NEC T82.594
        - spinal (epidural) (subdural) T85.690
      - urinary (*see also* Complications, catheter, urinary) T83.098
    - electronic (electrode) (pulse generator) (stimulator)
      - bone T84.390
      - cardiac T82.199
        - electrode T82.190
        - pulse generator T82.191
        - specified type NEC T82.198
      - nervous system —*see* Complication, prosthetic device, mechanical, electronic nervous system stimulator
      - urinary —*see* Complication, genitourinary, device, urinary, mechanical
    - fixation, internal (orthopedic) NEC —*see* Complication, fixation device, mechanical
    - gastrointestinal —*see* Complications, prosthetic device, mechanical, gastrointestinal device
    - genital NEC T83.498
      - intrauterine contraceptive device T83.39
      - penile prosthesis T83.490
    - heart NEC —*see* Complication, cardiovascular device, mechanical
    - joint prosthesis —*see* Complications, joint prosthesis, mechanical, specified NEC, by site
    - ocular NEC —*see* Complications, prosthetic device, mechanical, ocular device
    - orthopedic NEC —*see* Complication, orthopedic, device, mechanical
    - specified NEC T85.628
    - urinary NEC —*see also* Complication, genitourinary, device, urinary, mechanical
      - graft T83.29
    - vascular NEC —*see* Complication, cardiovascular device, mechanical
    - ventricular intracranial shunt T85.09
  - foreign body left accidentally in operative wound T81.539
  - instrument (any) during a procedure, accidental —*see* Puncture, accidental complicating surgery
- cecum K35.2
  - with localized peritonitis K35.3
- cervix (uteri) N88.8
  - with or following ectopic or molar pregnancy O08.6

Perforation, perforated *(continued)*
- cervix *(continued)*
  - obstetrical trauma O71.3
- colon K63.1
  - newborn P78.0
  - obstetrical trauma O71.5
  - traumatic —*see* Laceration, intestine, large
- common duct (bile) K83.2
- cornea (due to ulceration) —*see* Ulcer, cornea, perforated
- cystic duct K82.2
- diverticulum (intestine) K57.80
  - with bleeding K57.81
  - large intestine K57.20
    - with
      - bleeding K57.21
      - small intestine K57.40
        - with bleeding K57.41
  - small intestine K57.00
    - with
      - bleeding K57.01
      - large intestine K57.40
        - with bleeding K57.41
- ear drum —*see* Perforation, tympanum
- esophagus K22.3
- ethmoidal sinus —*see* Sinusitis, ethmoidal
- frontal sinus —*see* Sinusitis, frontal
- gallbladder K82.2
- heart valve —*see* Endocarditis
- ileum K63.1
  - newborn P78.0
  - obstetrical trauma O71.5
  - traumatic —*see* Laceration, intestine, small
- instrumental, surgical (accidental) (blood vessel) (nerve) (organ) —*see* Puncture, accidental complicating surgery
- intestine NEC K63.1
  - with ectopic or molar pregnancy O08.6
  - newborn P78.0
  - obstetrical trauma O71.5
  - traumatic —*see* Laceration, intestine
  - ulcerative NEC K63.1
    - newborn P78.0
- jejunum, jejunal K63.1
  - obstetrical trauma O71.5
  - traumatic —*see* Laceration, intestine, small
  - ulcer —*see* Ulcer, gastrojejunal, with perforation
- joint prosthesis —*see* Complications, joint prosthesis, mechanical, specified NEC, by site
- mastoid (antrum) (cell) —*see* Disorder, mastoid, specified NEC
- maxillary sinus —*see* Sinusitis, maxillary
- membrana tympani —*see* Perforation, tympanum
- nasal
  - septum J34.89
    - congenital Q30.3
    - syphilitic A52.73
  - sinus J34.89
    - congenital Q30.8
    - due to sinusitis —*see* Sinusitis
- palate (*see also* Cleft, palate) Q35.9
  - syphilitic A52.79
- palatine vault (*see also* Cleft, palate, hard) Q35.1
  - syphilitic A52.79
    - congenital A50.59
- pars flaccida (ear drum) —*see* Perforation, tympanum, attic

Perforation, perforated *(continued)*
- pelvic
  - floor S31.030
    - with
      - ectopic or molar pregnancy O08.6
      - penetration into retroperitoneal space S31.031
      - retained foreign body S31.040
        - with penetration into retroperitoneal space S31.041
    - following ectopic or molar pregnancy O08.6
    - obstetrical trauma O70.1
  - organ S37.99
    - adrenal gland S37.818
    - bladder —*see* Perforation, bladder
    - fallopian tube S37.599
      - bilateral S37.592
      - unilateral S37.591
    - kidney S37.09-
    - obstetrical trauma O71.5
    - ovary S37.499
      - bilateral S37.492
      - unilateral S37.491
    - prostate S37.828
    - specified organ NEC S37.898
    - ureter —*see* Perforation, ureter
    - urethra —*see* Perforation, urethra
    - uterus —*see* Perforation, uterus
- perineum —*see* Laceration, perineum
- pharynx J39.2
- rectum K63.1
  - newborn P78.0
  - obstetrical trauma O71.5
  - traumatic S36.63
- root canal space due to endodontic treatment M27.51
- sigmoid K63.1
  - newborn P78.0
  - obstetrical trauma O71.5
  - traumatic S36.533
- sinus (accessory) (chronic) (nasal) J34.89
- sphenoidal sinus —*see* Sinusitis, sphenoidal
- surgical (accidental) (by instrument) (blood vessel) (nerve) (organ) —*see* Puncture, accidental complicating surgery
- traumatic
  - external —*see* Puncture
  - eye —*see* Puncture, eyeball
  - internal organ —*see* Injury, by site
- tympanum, tympanic (membrane) (persistent post-traumatic) (postinflammatory) H72.9-
  - attic H72.1-
    - multiple —*see* Perforation, tympanum, multiple
    - total —*see* Perforation, tympanum, total
  - central H72.0-
    - multiple —*see* Perforation, tympanum, multiple
    - total —*see* Perforation, tympanum, total
  - marginal NEC —*see* subcategory H72.2
  - multiple H72.81-
  - pars flaccida —*see* Perforation, tympanum, attic
  - total H72.82-
  - traumatic, current episode S09.2-
- typhoid, gastrointestinal —*see* Typhoid

Perforation, perforated *(continued)*
- ulcer —*see* Ulcer, by site, with perforation
- ureter N28.89
  - traumatic S37.19
- urethra N36.8
  - with ectopic or molar pregnancy O08.6
  - following ectopic or molar pregnancy O08.6
  - obstetrical trauma O71.5
  - traumatic S37.39
    - at delivery O71.5
- uterus
  - with ectopic or molar pregnancy O08.6
  - by intrauterine contraceptive device T83.39
  - following ectopic or molar pregnancy O08.6
  - obstetrical trauma O71.1
  - traumatic S37.69
    - obstetric O71.1
- uvula K13.79
  - syphilitic A52.79
- vagina
  - obstetrical trauma O71.4
  - other trauma —*see* Puncture, vagina

Periadenitis mucosa necrotica recurrens K12.0

Periappendicitis (acute) —*see* Appendicitis

Periarteritis nodosa (disseminated) (infectious) (necrotizing) M30.0

Periarthritis (joint) —*see also* Enthesopathy
- Duplay's M75.0-
- gonococcal A54.42
- humeroscapularis —*see* Capsulitis, adhesive
- scapulohumeral —*see* Capsulitis, adhesive
- shoulder —*see* Capsulitis, adhesive
- wrist M77.2-

Periarthrosis (angioneural) —*see* Enthesopathy

Pericapsulitis, adhesive (shoulder) —*see* Capsulitis, adhesive

Pericarditis (with decompensation) (with effusion) I31.9
- with rheumatic fever (conditions in I00)
  - active —*see* Pericarditis, rheumatic
  - inactive or quiescent I09.2
- acute (hemorrhagic) (nonrheumatic) (Sicca) I30.9
  - with chorea (acute) (rheumatic) (Sydenham's) I02.0
  - benign I30.8
  - nonspecific I30.0
  - rheumatic I01.0
    - with chorea (acute) (Sydenham's) I02.0
- adhesive or adherent (chronic) (external) (internal) I31.0
  - acute —*see* Pericarditis, acute
  - rheumatic I09.2
- bacterial (acute) (subacute) (with serous or seropurulent effusion) I30.1
- calcareous I31.1
- cholesterol (chronic) I31.8
  - acute I30.9
- chronic (nonrheumatic) I31.9
  - rheumatic I09.2
- constrictive (chronic) I31.1
- coxsackie B33.23

Pericarditis *(continued)*
- fibrinocaseous (tuberculous) A18.84
- fibrinopurulent I30.1
- fibrinous I30.8
- fibrous I31.0
- gonococcal A54.83
- idiopathic I30.0
- in systemic lupus erythematosus M32.12
- infective I30.1
- meningococcal A39.53
- neoplastic (chronic) I31.8
  - acute I30.9
- obliterans, obliterating I31.0
- plastic I31.0
- pneumococcal I30.1
- postinfarction I24.1
- purulent I30.1
- rheumatic (active) (acute) (with effusion) (with pneumonia) I01.0
  - with chorea (acute) (rheumatic) (Sydenham's) I02.0
  - chronic or inactive (with chorea) I09.2
- rheumatoid —*see* Rheumatoid, carditis
- septic I30.1
- serofibrinous I30.8
- staphylococcal I30.1
- streptococcal I30.1
- suppurative I30.1
- syphilitic A52.06
- tuberculous A18.84
- uremic N18.9 *[I32]*
- viral I30.1

Pericardium, pericardial —*see* condition

Pericellulitis —*see* Cellulitis

Pericementitis (chronic) (suppurative) —*see also* Periodontitis
- acute K05.20
  - generalized —*see* Peridontitis, aggressive, generalized
  - localized —*see* Peridontitis, aggressive, localized

Perichondritis
- auricle —*see* Perichondritis, ear
- bronchus J98.09
- ear (external) H61.00-
  - acute H61.01-
  - chronic H61.02-
- external auditory canal —*see* Perichondritis, ear
- larynx J38.7
  - syphilitic A52.73
  - typhoid A01.09
- nose J34.89
- pinna —*see* Perichondritis, ear
- trachea J39.8

Periclasia K05.4

Pericoronitis —*see* Periodontitis

Pericystitis N30.90
- with hematuria N30.91

Peridiverticulitis (intestine) K57.92
- cecum —*see* Diverticulitis, intestine, large
- colon —*see* Diverticulitis, intestine, large
- duodenum —*see* Diverticulitis, intestine, small
- intestine —*see* Diverticulitis, intestine
- jejunum —*see* Diverticulitis, intestine, small
- rectosigmoid —*see* Diverticulitis, intestine, large
- rectum —*see* Diverticulitis, intestine, large

eridiverticulitis *(continued)*
sigmoid *—see* Diverticulitis, intestine, large
eriendocarditis *—see* Endocarditis
eriepididymitis N45.1
erifolliculitis L01.02
abscedens, caput, scalp L66.3
capitis, abscedens (et suffodiens) L66.3
superficial pustular L01.02
erihepatitis K65.8
erilabyrinthitis (acute) *—see* subcategory H83.0
erimeningitis *—see* Meningitis
erimetritis *—see* Endometritis
erimetrosalpingitis *—see* Salpingo-oophoritis
erineocele N81.81
erinephric, perinephritic *—see* condition
erinephritis *—see also* Infection, kidney
purulent *—see* Abscess, kidney
erineum, perineal *—see* condition
erineuritis NEC *—see* Neuralgia
eriodic *—see* condition
eriodontitis (chronic) (complex) (compound) (local) (simplex) K05.30
acute K05.20
generalized K05.229
moderate K05.222
severe K05.223
slight K05.221
localized K05.219
moderate K05.212
severe K05.213
slight K05.211
apical K04.5
acute (pulpal origin) K04.4
generalized K05.329
moderate K05.322
severe K05.323
slight K05.321
localized K05.319
moderate K05.312
severe K05.313
slight K05.311
eriodontoclasia K05.4
eriodontosis (juvenile) K05.4
eriods *—see also* Menstruation
heavy N92.0
irregular N92.6
shortened intervals (irregular) N92.1
erionychia *—see also* Cellulitis, digit
with lymphangitis *—see* Lymphangitis, acute, digit
erioophoritis *—see* Salpingo-oophoritis
eriorchitis N45.2
eriosteum, periosteal *—see* condition
eriostitis (albuminosa) (circumscribed) (diffuse) (infective) (monomelic) *—see also* Osteomyelitis
alveolar M27.3
alveolodental M27.3
dental M27.3
gonorrheal A54.43
jaw (lower) (upper) M27.2
orbit H05.03-
syphilitic A52.77
congenital (early) A50.02 *[M90.80]*
secondary A51.46

Periostitis *(continued)*
tuberculous *—see* Tuberculosis, bone
yaws (hypertrophic) (early) (late) A66.6 *[M90.80]*
Periostosis (hyperplastic) *—see also* Disorder, bone, specified type NEC
with osteomyelitis *—see* Osteomyelitis, specified type NEC
Peripartum
cardiomyopathy O90.3
Periphlebitis *—see* Phlebitis
Periproctitis K62.89
Periprostatitis *—see* Prostatitis
Perirectal *—see* condition
Perirenal *—see* condition
Perisalpingitis *—see* Salpingo-oophoritis
Perisplenitis (infectional) D73.89
Peristalsis, visible or reversed R19.2
Peritendinitis *—see* Enthesopathy
Peritoneum, peritoneal *—see* condition
Peritonitis (adhesive) (bacterial) (fibrinous) (hemorrhagic) (idiopathic) (localized) (perforative) (primary) (with adhesions) (with effusion) K65.9
with or following
abscess K65.1
appendicitis K35.3
with perforation or rupture K35.2
generalized K35.2
localized K35.3
diverticular disease (intestine) K57.80
with bleeding K57.81
large intestine K57.20
with
bleeding K57.21
small intestine K57.40
with bleeding K57.41
small intestine K57.00
with
bleeding K57.01
large intestine K57.40
with bleeding K57.41
ectopic or molar pregnancy O08.0
acute (generalized) K65.0
aseptic T81.61
bile, biliary K65.3
chemical T81.61
chlamydial A74.81
complicating abortion *—see* Abortion, by type, complicated by, pelvic peritonitis
congenital P78.1
chronic proliferative K65.8
diaphragmatic K65.0
diffuse K65.0
diphtheritic A36.89
disseminated K65.0
due to
bile K65.3
foreign
body or object accidentally left during a procedure (instrument) (sponge) (swab) T81.599
substance accidentally left during a procedure (chemical) (powder) (talc) T81.61
talc T81.61
urine K65.8

Peritonitis *(continued)*
eosinophilic K65.8
acute K65.0
fibrocaseous (tuberculous) A18.31
fibropurulent K65.0
following ectopic or molar pregnancy O08.0
general (ized) K65.0
gonococcal A54.85
meconium (newborn) P78.0
neonatal P78.1
meconium P78.0
pancreatic K65.0
paroxysmal, familial E85.0
benign E85.0
pelvic
female N73.5
acute N73.3
chronic N73.4
with adhesions N73.6
male K65.0
periodic, familial E85.0
proliferative, chronic K65.8
puerperal, postpartum, childbirth O85
purulent K65.0
septic K65.0
specified NEC K65.8
spontaneous bacterial K65.2
subdiaphragmatic K65.0
subphrenic K65.0
suppurative K65.0
syphilitic A52.74
congenital (early) A50.08 *[K67]*
talc T81.61
tuberculous A18.31
urine K65.8
Peritonsillar *—see* condition
Peritonsillitis J36
Perityphlitis K37
Periureteritis N28.89
Periurethral *—see* condition
Periurethritis (gangrenous) *—see* Urethritis
Periuterine *—see* condition
Perivaginitis *—see* Vaginitis
Perivasculitis, retinal H35.06-
Perivasitis (chronic) N49.1
Perivesiculitis (seminal) *—see* Vesiculitis
Perlèche NEC K13.0
due to
candidiasis B37.83
moniliasis B37.83
riboflavin deficiency E53.0
vitamin B2 (riboflavin) deficiency E53.0
Pernicious *—see* condition
Pernio, perniosis T69.1
Perpetrator (of abuse) *—see* Index to External Causes of Injury, Perpetrator
Persecution
delusion F22
social Z60.5
Perseveration (tonic) R48.8
Persistence, persistent (congenital)
anal membrane Q42.3
with fistula Q42.2
arteria stapedia Q16.3
atrioventricular canal Q21.2
branchial cleft NOS Q18.2
cyst Q18.0
fistula Q18.0
sinus Q18.0

Persistence, persistent *(continued)*
bulbus cordis in left ventricle Q21.8
canal of Cloquet Q14.0
capsule (opaque) Q12.8
cilioretinal artery or vein Q14.8
cloaca Q43.7
communication *—see* Fistula, congenital
convolutions
aortic arch Q25.46
fallopian tube Q50.6
oviduct Q50.6
uterine tube Q50.6
double aortic arch Q25.45
ductus arteriosus (Botalli) Q25.0
fetal
circulation P29.38
form of cervix (uteri) Q51.828
hemoglobin, hereditary (HPFH) D56.4
foramen
Botalli Q21.1
ovale Q21.1
Gartner's duct Q52.4
hemoglobin, fetal (hereditary) (HPFH) D56.4
hyaloid
artery (generally incomplete) Q14.0
system Q14.8
hymen, in pregnancy or childbirth *—see* Pregnancy, complicated by, abnormal, vulva
lanugo Q84.2
left
posterior cardinal vein Q26.8
root with right arch of aorta Q25.49
superior vena cava Q26.1
Meckel's diverticulum Q43.0
malignant *—see* Table of Neoplasms, small intestine, malignant
mucosal disease (middle ear) *—see* Otitis, media, suppurative, chronic, tubotympanic
nail(s), anomalous Q84.6
omphalomesenteric duct Q43.0
organ or site not listed *—see* Anomaly, by site
ostium
atrioventriculare commune Q21.2
primum Q21.2
secundum Q21.1
ovarian rests in fallopian tube Q50.6
pancreatic tissue in intestinal tract Q43.8
primary (deciduous)
teeth K00.6
vitreous hyperplasia Q14.0
pupillary membrane Q13.89
right aortic arch Q25.47
rhesus (Rh) titer *—see* Complication(s), transfusion, incompatibility reaction, Rh (factor)
sinus
urogenitalis
female Q52.8
male Q55.8
venosus with imperfect incorporation in right auricle Q26.8
thymus (gland) (hyperplasia) E32.0
thyroglossal duct Q89.2
thyrolingual duct Q89.2
truncus arteriosus or communis Q20.0
tunica vasculosa lentis Q12.2
umbilical sinus Q64.4

Persistence, persistent *(continued)*
urachus Q64.4
vitelline duct Q43.0
Person (with)
admitted for clinical research, as a control subject (normal comparison) (participant) Z00.6
awaiting admission to adequate facility elsewhere Z75.1
concern (normal) about sick person in family Z63.6
consulting on behalf of another Z71.0
feigning illness Z76.5
living (in)
alone Z60.2
boarding school Z59.3
residential institution Z59.3
without
adequate housing (heating) (space) Z59.1
housing (permanent) (temporary) Z59.0
person able to render necessary care Z74.2
shelter Z59.0
on waiting list Z75.1
sick or handicapped in family Z63.6
Personality (disorder) F60.9
accentuation of traits (type A pattern) Z73.1
affective F34.0
aggressive F60.3
amoral F60.2
anacastic, anankastic F60.5
antisocial F60.2
anxious F60.6
asocial F60.2
asthenic F60.7
avoidant F60.6
borderline F60.3
change due to organic condition (enduring) F07.0
compulsive F60.5
cycloid F34.0
cyclothymic F34.0
dependent F60.7
depressive F34.1
dissocial F60.2
dual F44.81
eccentric F60.89
emotionally unstable F60.3
expansive paranoid F60.0
explosive F60.3
fanatic F60.0
haltlose type F60.89
histrionic F60.4
hyperthymic F34.0
hypothymic F34.1
hysterical F60.4
immature F60.89
inadequate F60.7
labile (emotional) F60.3
mixed (nonspecific) F60.89
morally defective F60.2
multiple F44.81
narcissistic F60.81
obsessional F60.5
obsessive (-compulsive) F60.5
organic F07.0
overconscientious F60.5
paranoid F60.0
passive (-dependent) F60.7
passive-aggressive F60.89
pathologic F60.9
pattern defect or disturbance F60.9
pseudopsychopathic (organic) F07.0
pseudoretarded (organic) F07.0
psychoinfantile F60.4
psychoneurotic NEC F60.89
Personality *(continued)*
psychopathic F60.2
querulant F60.0
sadistic F60.89
schizoid F60.1
self-defeating F60.7
sensitive paranoid F60.0
sociopathic (amoral) (antisocial) (asocial) (dissocial) F60.2
specified NEC F60.89
type A Z73.1
unstable (emotional) F60.3
Perthes' disease *—see* Legg-Calvé-Perthes disease
Pertussis (*see also* Whooping cough) A37.90
Perversion, perverted
appetite F50.89
psychogenic F50.89
function
pituitary gland E23.2
posterior lobe E22.2
sense of smell and taste R43.8
psychogenic F45.8
sexual *—see* Deviation, sexual
Pervious, congenital *—see also* Imperfect, closure
ductus arteriosus Q25.0
Pes (congenital) *—see also* Talipes
acquired *—see also* Deformity, limb, foot, specified NEC
planus *—see* Deformity, limb, flat foot
adductus Q66.89
cavus Q66.7
deformity NEC, acquired *—see* Deformity, limb, foot, specified NEC
planus (acquired) (any degree) *—see also* Deformity, limb, flat foot
rachitic sequelae (late effect) E64.3
valgus Q66.6
Pest, pestis *—see* Plague
Petechia, petechiae R23.3
newborn P54.5
Petechial typhus A75.9
Peter's anomaly Q13.4
Petit mal seizure *—see* Epilepsy, generalized, specified NEC
Petit's hernia *—see* Hernia, abdomen, specified site NEC
Petrellidosis B48.2
Petrositis H70.20-
acute H70.21-
chronic H70.22-
Peutz-Jeghers disease or syndrome Q85.8
Peyronie's disease N48.6
PFAPA (periodic fever, aphthous stomatitis, pharyngitis, and adenopathy syndrome) M04.8
Pfeiffer's disease *—see* Mononucleosis, infectious
Phagedena (dry) (moist) (sloughing) *—see also* Gangrene
geometric L88
penis N48.29
tropical *—see* Ulcer, skin
vulva N76.6
Phagedenic *—see* condition
Phakoma H35.89
Phakomatosis (*see also* specific eponymous syndromes) Q85.9
Phakomatosis *(continued)*
Bourneville's Q85.1
specified NEC Q85.8
Phantom limb syndrome (without pain) G54.7
with pain G54.6
Pharyngeal pouch syndrome D82.1
Pharyngitis (acute) (catarrhal) (gangrenous) (infective) (malignant) (membranous) (phlegmonous) (pseudomembranous) (simple) (subacute) (suppurative) (ulcerative) (viral) J02.9
with influenza, flu, or grippe *—see* Influenza, with, pharyngitis
aphthous B08.5
atrophic J31.2
chlamydial A56.4
chronic (atrophic) (granular) (hypertrophic) J31.2
coxsackievirus B08.5
diphtheritic A36.0
enteroviral vesicular B08.5
follicular (chronic) J31.2
fusospirochetal A69.1
gonococcal A54.5
granular (chronic) J31.2
herpesviral B00.2
hypertrophic J31.2
infectional, chronic J31.2
influenzal *—see* Influenza, with, respiratory manifestations NEC
lymphonodular, acute (enteroviral) B08.8
pneumococcal J02.8
purulent J02.9
putrid J02.9
septic J02.0
sicca J31.2
specified organism NEC J02.8
staphylococcal J02.8
streptococcal J02.0
syphilitic, congenital (early) A50.03
tuberculous A15.8
vesicular, enteroviral B08.5
viral NEC J02.8
Pharyngoconjunctivitis, viral B30.2
Pharyngolaryngitis (acute) J06.0
chronic J37.0
Pharyngoplegia J39.2
Pharyngotonsillitis, herpesviral B00.2
Pharyngotracheitis, chronic J42
Pharynx, pharyngeal *—see* condition
Phencyclidine-induced
anxiety disorder F16.980
bipolar and related disorder F16.94
depressive disorder F16.94
psychotic disorder F16.959
Phenomenon
Arthus' *—see* Arthus' phenomenon
jaw-winking Q07.8
lupus erythematosus (LE) cell M32.9
Raynaud's (secondary) I73.00
with gangrene I73.01
vasomotor R55
vasospastic I73.9
vasovagal R55
Wenckebach's I44.1
Phenylketonuria E70.1
classical E70.0
maternal E70.1
Pheochromoblastoma
specified site *—see* Neoplasm, malignant, by site
unspecified site C74.10
Pheochromocytoma
malignant
specified site *—see* Neoplasm, malignant, by site
unspecified site C74.10
specified site *—see* Neoplasm, benign, by site
unspecified site D35.00
Pheohyphomycosis *—see* Chromomycosis
Pheomycosis *—see* Chromomycosis
Phimosis (congenital) (due to infection) N47.1
chancroidal A57
Phlebectasia *—see also* Varix
congenital Q27.4
Phlebitis (infective) (pyemic) (septic) (suppurative) I80.9
antepartum *—see* Thrombophlebitis, antepartum
blue *—see* Phlebitis, leg, deep
breast, superficial I80.8
cavernous (venous) sinus *—see* Phlebitis, intracranial (venous) sinus
cerebral (venous) sinus *—see* Phlebitis, intracranial (venous) sinus
chest wall, superficial I80.8
cranial (venous) sinus *—see* Phlebitis, intracranial (venous) sinus
deep (vessels) *—see* Phlebitis, leg, deep
due to implanted device *—see* Complications, by site and type, specified NEC
during or resulting from a procedure T81.72
femoral vein (superficial) I80.1-
femoropopliteal vein I80.0-
gestational *—see* Phlebopathy, gestational
hepatic veins I80.8
iliofemoral *—see* Phlebitis, femoral vein
intracranial (venous) sinus (any) G08
nonpyogenic I67.6
intraspinal venous sinuses and veins G08
nonpyogenic G95.19
lateral (venous) sinus *—see* Phlebitis, intracranial (venous) sinus
leg I80.3
antepartum *—see* Thrombophlebitis, antepartum
deep (vessels) NEC I80.20-
iliac I80.21-
popliteal vein I80.22-
specified vessel NEC I80.29-
tibial vein I80.23-
femoral vein (superficial) I80.1-
superficial (vessels) I80.0-
longitudinal sinus *—see* Phlebitis, intracranial (venous) sinus
lower limb *—see* Phlebitis, leg
migrans, migrating (superficial) I82.1
pelvic
with ectopic or molar pregnancy O08.0
following ectopic or molar pregnancy O08.0
puerperal, postpartum O87.1

Phlebitis *(continued)*
popliteal vein *—see* Phlebitis, leg, deep, popliteal
portal (vein) K75.1
postoperative T81.72
pregnancy *—see* Thrombophlebitis, antepartum
puerperal, postpartum, childbirth O87.0
deep O87.1
pelvic O87.1
superficial O87.0
retina *—see* Vasculitis, retina
saphenous (accessory) (great) (long) (small) *—see* Phlebitis, leg, superficial
sinus (meninges) *—see* Phlebitis, intracranial (venous) sinus
specified site NEC I80.8
syphilitic A52.09
tibial vein *—see* Phlebitis, leg, deep, tibial
ulcerative I80.9
leg *—see* Phlebitis, leg
umbilicus I80.8
uterus (septic) *—see* Endometritis
varicose (leg) (lower limb) *—see* Varix, leg, with, inflammation

Phlebofibrosis I87.8

Phleboliths I87.8

Phlebopathy,
gestational O22.9-
puerperal O87.9

Phlebosclerosis I87.8

Phlebothrombosis *—see also* Thrombosis
antepartum *—see* Thrombophlebitis, antepartum
pregnancy *—see* Thrombophlebitis, antepartum
puerperal *—see* Thrombophlebitis, puerperal

Phlebotomus fever A93.1

Phlegmasia
alba dolens O87.1
nonpuerperal *—see* Phlebitis, femoral vein
cerulea dolens *—see* Phlebitis, leg, deep

Phlegmon *—see* Abscess

Phlegmonous *—see* condition

Phlyctenulosis (allergic) (keratoconjunctivitis) (nontuberculous) *—see also* Keratoconjunctivitis
cornea *—see* Keratoconjunctivitis
tuberculous A18.52

Phobia, phobic F40.9
animal F40.218
spiders F40.210
examination F40.298
reaction F40.9
simple F40.298
social F40.10
generalized F40.11
specific (isolated) F40.298
animal F40.218
spiders F40.210
blood F40.230
injection F40.231
injury F40.233
men F40.290
natural environment F40.228
thunderstorms F40.220
situational F40.248
bridges F40.242
closed in spaces F40.240

Phobia, phobic *(continued)*
specific *(continued)*
situational *(continued)*
flying F40.243
heights F40.241
specified focus NEC F40.298
transfusion F40.231
women F40.291
specified NEC F40.8
medical care NEC F40.232
state F40.9

Phocas' disease *—see* Mastopathy, cystic

Phocomelia Q73.1
lower limb *—see* Agenesis, leg, with foot present
upper limb *—see* Agenesis, arm, with hand present

Phoria H50.50

Phosphate-losing tubular disorder N25.0

Phosphatemia E83.39

Phosphaturia E83.39

Photodermatitis (sun) L56.8
chronic L57.8
due to drug L56.8
light other than sun L59.8

Photokeratitis H16.13-

Photophobia H53.14-

Photophthalmia *—see* Photokeratitis

Photopsia H53.19

Photoretinitis *—see* Retinopathy, solar

Photosensitivity, photosensitization (sun) **skin** L56.8
light other than sun L59.8

Phrenitis *—see* Encephalitis

Phrynoderma (vitamin A deficiency) E50.8

Phthiriasis (pubis) B85.3
with any infestation classifiable to B85.0-B85.2 *[B85.4]*

Phthirus infestation *—see* Phthiriasis

Phthisis *—see also* Tuberculosis
bulbi (infectional) *—see* Disorder, globe, degenerated condition, atrophy
eyeball (due to infection) *—see* Disorder, globe, degenerated condition, atrophy

Phycomycosis *—see* Zygomycosis

Physalopteriasis B81.8

Physical restraint status Z78.1

Phytobezoar T18.9
intestine T18.3
stomach T18.2

Pian *—see* Yaws

Pianoma A66.1

Pica F50.89
in adults F50.89
infant or child F98.3

Picking, nose F98.8

Pick-Niemann disease *—see* Niemann-Pick disease or syndrome

Pick's
cerebral atrophy G31.01 *[F02.80]*
with behavioral disturbance G31.01 *[F02.81]*
disease or syndrome (brain) G31.01 *[F02.80]*

Pick's *(continued)*
disease or syndrome *(continued)*
with behavioral disturbance G31.01 *[F02.81]*
brain G31.01 *[F02.80]*
with behavioral disturbance G31.01 *[F02.81]*
pericardium (pericardial pseudocirrhosis of liver) I31.1
syndrome
brain G31.01 *[F02.80]*
with behavioral disturbance G31.01 *[F02.81]*
of heart (pericardial pseudocirrhosis of liver) I31.1

Pickwickian syndrome E66.2

Piebaldism E70.39

Piedra (beard) (scalp) B36.8
black B36.3
white B36.2

Pierre Robin deformity or syndrome Q87.0

Pierson's disease or osteochondrosis M91.0

Pig-bel A05.2

Pigeon
breast or chest (acquired) M95.4
congenital Q67.7
rachitic sequelae (late effect) E64.3
breeder's disease or lung J67.2
fancier's disease or lung J67.2
toe *—see* Deformity, toe, specified NEC

Pigmentation (abnormal) (anomaly) L81.9
conjunctiva H11.13-
cornea (anterior) H18.01-
posterior H18.05-
stromal H18.06-
diminished melanin formation NEC L81.6
iron L81.8
lids, congenital Q82.8
limbus corneae *—see* Pigmentation, cornea
metals L81.8
optic papilla, congenital Q14.2
retina, congenital (grouped) (nevoid) Q14.1
scrotum, congenital Q82.8
tattoo L81.8

Piles (*see also* Hemorrhoids) K64.9

Pili
annulati or torti (congenital) Q84.1
incarnati L73.1

Pill roller hand (intrinsic) *—see* Parkinsonism

Pilomatrixoma *—see* Neoplasm, skin, benign
malignant *—see* Neoplasm, skin, malignant

Pilonidal *—see* condition

Pimple R23.8

PIN - *see* Neoplasia, intraepithelial, prostate

Pinched nerve *—see* Neuropathy, entrapment

Pindborg tumor *—see* Cyst, calcifying odontogenic

Pineal body or gland *—see* condition

Pinealoblastoma C75.3

Pinealoma D44.5
malignant C75.3

Pineoblastoma C75.3

Pineocytoma D44.5

Pinguecula H11.15-

Pingueculitis H10.81-

Pinhole meatus (*see also* Stricture, urethra) N35.9

Pink
disease *—see* subcategory T56.1
eye *—see* Conjunctivitis, acute, mucopurulent

Pinkus' disease (lichen nitidus) L44.1

Pinpoint
meatus *—see* Stricture, urethra
os (uteri) *—see* Stricture, cervix

Pins and needles R20.2

Pinta A67.9
cardiovascular lesions A67.2
chancre (primary) A67.0
erythematous plaques A67.1
hyperchromic lesions A67.1
hyperkeratosis A67.1
lesions A67.9
cardiovascular A67.2
hyperchromic A67.1
intermediate A67.1
late A67.2
mixed A67.3
primary A67.0
skin (achromic) (cicatricial) (dyschromic) A67.2
hyperchromic A67.1
mixed (achromic and hyperchromic) A67.3
papule (primary) A67.0
skin lesions (achromic) (cicatricial) (dyschromic) A67.2
hyperchromic A67.1
mixed (achromic and hyperchromic) A67.3
vitiligo A67.2

Pintids A67.1

Pinworm (disease) (infection) (infestation) B80

Piroplasmosis B60.0

Pistol wound *—see* Gunshot wound

Pitchers' elbow *—see* Derangement, joint, specified type NEC, elbow

Pithecoid pelvis Q74.2
with disproportion (fetopelvic) O33.0
causing obstructed labor O65.0

Pithiatism F48.8

Pitted *—see* Pitting

Pitting (*see also* Edema) R60.9
lip R60.0
nail L60.8
teeth K00.4

Pituitary gland *—see* condition

Pituitary-snuff-taker's disease J67.8

Pityriasis (capitis) L21.0
alba L30.5
circinata (et maculata) L42
furfuracea L21.0
Hebra's L26
lichenoides L41.0
chronica L41.1
et varioliformis (acuta) L41.0
maculata (et circinata) L30.5
nigra B36.1
pilaris, Hebra's L44.0

Pityriasis *(continued)*
- rosea L42
- rotunda L44.8
- rubra (Hebra) pilaris L44.0
- simplex L30.5
- specified type NEC L30.5
- streptogenes L30.5
- versicolor (scrotal) B36.0

Placenta, placental *—see* Pregnancy, complicated by (care of) (management affected by), specified condition

Placentitis O41.14-

Plagiocephaly Q67.3

Plague A20.9
- abortive A20.8
- ambulatory A20.8
- asymptomatic A20.8
- bubonic A20.0
- cellulocutaneous A20.1
- cutaneobubonic A20.1
- lymphatic gland A20.0
- meningitis A20.3
- pharyngeal A20.8
- pneumonic (primary) (secondary) A20.2
- pulmonary, pulmonic A20.2
- septicemic A20.7
- tonsillar A20.8
  - septicemic A20.7

Planning, family
- contraception Z30.9
- procreation Z31.69

Plaque(s)
- artery, arterial *—see* Arteriosclerosis
- calcareous *—see* Calcification
- coronary, lipid rich I25.83
- epicardial I31.8
- erythematous, of pinta A67.1
- Hollenhorst's *—see* Occlusion, artery, retina
- lipid rich, coronary I25.83
- pleural (without asbestos) J92.9
  - with asbestos J92.0
- tongue K13.29

Plasmacytoma C90.3-
- extramedullary C90.2-
- medullary C90.0-
- solitary C90.3-

Plasmacytopenia D72.818

Plasmacytosis D72.822

Plaster ulcer *—see* Ulcer, pressure, by site

Plateau iris syndrome (post-iridectomy) (postprocedural) (without glaucoma) H21.82
- with glaucoma H40.22-

Platybasia Q75.8

Platyonychia (congenital) Q84.6
- acquired L60.8

Platypelloid pelvis M95.5
- with disproportion (fetopelvic) O33.0
  - causing obstructed labor O65.0
- congenital Q74.2

Platyspondylisis Q76.49

Plaut (-Vincent) **disease** (*see also* Vincent's) A69.1

Plethora R23.2
- newborn P61.1

Pleura, pleural *—see* condition

Pleuralgia R07.81

Pleurisy (acute) (adhesive) (chronic) (costal) (diaphragmatic) (double) (dry) (fibrinous) (fibrous) (interlobar) (latent) (plastic) (primary) (residual) (sicca) (sterile) (subacute) (unresolved) R09.1
- with
  - adherent pleura J86.0
  - effusion J90
    - chylous, chyliform J94.0
    - tuberculous (non primary) A15.6
      - primary (progressive) A15.7
  - tuberculosis *—see* Pleurisy, tuberculous (non primary)
- encysted *—see* Pleurisy, with effusion
- exudative *—see* Pleurisy, with effusion
- fibrinopurulent, fibropurulent *—see* Pyothorax
- hemorrhagic *—see* Hemothorax
- pneumococcal J90
- purulent *—see* Pyothorax
- septic *—see* Pyothorax
- serofibrinous *—see* Pleurisy, with effusion
- seropurulent *—see* Pyothorax
- serous *—see* Pleurisy, with effusion
- staphylococcal J86.9
- streptococcal J90
- suppurative *—see* Pyothorax
- traumatic (post) (current) *—see* Injury, intrathoracic, pleura
- tuberculous (with effusion) (non primary) A15.6
  - primary (progressive) A15.7

Pleuritis sicca *—see* Pleurisy

Pleurobronchopneumonia *—see* Pneumonia, broncho-

Pleurodynia R07.81
- epidemic B33.0
- viral B33.0

Pleuropericarditis *—see also* Pericarditis
- acute I30.9

Pleuropneumonia (acute) (bilateral) (double) (septic) (*see also* Pneumonia) J18.8
- chronic *—see* Fibrosis, lung

Pleuro-pneumonia-like-organism (PPLO)**, as cause of disease classified elsewhere** B96.0

Pleurorrhea *—see* Pleurisy, with effusion

Plexitis, brachial G54.0

Plica
- polonica B85.0
- syndrome, knee M67.5-
- tonsil J35.8

Plicated tongue K14.5

Plug
- bronchus NEC J98.09
- meconium (newborn) NEC
  - syndrome P76.0
- mucus *—see* Asphyxia, mucus

Plumbism *—see* subcategory T56.0

Plummer's disease E05.20
- with thyroid storm E05.21

Plummer-Vinson syndrome D50.1

Pluricarential syndrome of infancy E40

Plus (and minus) hand (intrinsic) *—see* Deformity, limb, specified type NEC, forearm

Pneumathemia *—see* Air, embolism

Pneumatic hammer (drill) **syndrome** T75.21

Pneumatocele (lung) J98.4
- intracranial G93.89
- tension J44.9

Pneumatosis
- cystoides intestinalis K63.89
- intestinalis K63.89
- peritonei K66.8

Pneumaturia R39.89

Pneumoblastoma *—see* Neoplasm, lung, malignant

Pneumocephalus G93.89

Pneumococcemia A40.3

Pneumococcus, pneumococcal *—see* condition

Pneumoconiosis (due to) (inhalation of) J64
- with tuberculosis (any type in A15) J65
- aluminum J63.0
- asbestos J61
- bagasse, bagassosis J67.1
- bauxite J63.1
- beryllium J63.2
- coal miners' (simple) J60
- coalworkers' (simple) J60
- collier's J60
- cotton dust J66.0
- diatomite (diatomaceous earth) J62.8
- dust
  - inorganic NEC J63.6
  - lime J62.8
  - marble J62.8
  - organic NEC J66.8
- fumes or vapors (from silo) J68.9
- graphite J63.3
- grinder's J62.8
- kaolin J62.8
- mica J62.8
- millstone maker's J62.8
- mineral fibers NEC J61
- miner's J60
- moldy hay J67.0
- potter's J62.8
- rheumatoid *—see* Rheumatoid, lung
- sandblaster's J62.8
- silica, silicate NEC J62.8
  - with carbon J60
- stonemason's J62.8
- talc (dust) J62.0

Pneumocystis carinii pneumonia B59

Pneumocystis jiroveci (pneumonia) B59

Pneumocystosis (with pneumonia) B59

Pneumohemopericardium I31.2

Pneumohemothorax J94.2
- traumatic S27.2

Pneumohydropericardium *—see* Pericarditis

Pneumohydrothorax *—see* Hydrothorax

Pneumomediastinum J98.2
- congenital or perinatal P25.2

Pneumomycosis B49 *[J99]*

Pneumonia (acute) (double) (migratory) (purulent) (septic) (unresolved) J18.9
- with
  - lung abscess J85.1
    - due to specified organism *—see* Pneumonia, in (due to)
  - influenza *—see* Influenza, with, pneumonia

Pneumonia *(continued)*
- adenoviral J12.0
- adynamic J18.2
- alba A50.04
- allergic (eosinophilic) J82
- alveolar *—see* Pneumonia, lobar
- anaerobes J15.8
- anthrax A22.1
- apex, apical *—see* Pneumonia, lo
- Ascaris B77.81
- aspiration J69.0
  - due to
    - aspiration of microorganisms
      - bacterial J15.9
      - viral J12.9
    - food (regurgitated) J69.0
    - gastric secretions J69.0
    - milk (regurgitated) J69.0
    - oils, essences J69.1
    - solids, liquids NEC J69.8
    - vomitus J69.0
  - newborn P24.81
    - amniotic fluid (clear) P24.11
    - blood P24.21
    - liquor (amnii) P24.11
    - meconium P24.01
    - milk P24.31
    - mucus P24.11
    - food (regurgitated) P24.31
    - specified NEC P24.81
    - stomach contents P24.31
  - postprocedural J95.4
- atypical NEC J18.9
- bacillus J15.9
  - specified NEC J15.8
- bacterial J15.9
  - specified NEC J15.8
- Bacteroides (fragilis) (oralis) (melaninogenicus) J15.8
- basal, basic, basilar *—see* Pneumonia, by type
- bronchiolitis obliterans organized (BOOP) J84.89
- broncho-, bronchial (confluent) (croupous) (diffuse) (disseminated) (hemorrhagic) (involving lobes) (lobar) (terminal) J18.0
  - allergic (eosinophilic) J82
  - aspiration *—see* Pneumonia, aspiration
  - bacterial J15.9
    - specified NEC J15.8
  - chronic *—see* Fibrosis, lung
  - diplococcal J13
  - Eaton's agent J15.7
  - Escherichia coli (E. coli) J15.5
  - Friedländer's bacillus J15.0
  - Hemophilus influenzae J14
  - hypostatic J18.2
  - inhalation *—see also* Pneumoni aspiration
    - due to fumes or vapors (chemical) J68.0
    - of oils or essences J69.1
  - Klebsiella (pneumoniae) J15.0
  - lipid, lipoid J69.1
    - endogenous J84.89
  - Mycoplasma (pneumoniae) J15.
  - pleuro-pneumonia-like-organism (PPLO) J15.7
  - pneumococcal J13
  - Proteus J15.6
  - Pseudomonas J15.1
  - Serratia marcescens J15.6
  - specified organism NEC J16.8
  - staphylococcal *—see* Pneumoni staphylococcal
  - streptococcal NEC J15.4
    - group B J15.3
    - pneumoniae J13

neumonia *(continued)*
- broncho-, bronchial *(continued)*
  - viral, virus —*see* Pneumonia, viral
- Butyrivibrio (fibriosolvens) J15.8
- Candida B37.1
- caseous —*see* Tuberculosis, pulmonary
- catarrhal —*see* Pneumonia, broncho
- chlamydial J16.0
  - congenital P23.1
- cholesterol J84.89
- cirrhotic (chronic) —*see* Fibrosis, lung
- Clostridium (haemolyticum) (novyi) J15.8
- confluent —*see* Pneumonia, broncho
- congenital (infective) P23.9
  - due to
    - bacterium NEC P23.6
    - Chlamydia P23.1
    - Escherichia coli P23.4
    - Haemophilus influenzae P23.6
    - infective organism NEC P23.8
    - Klebsiella pneumoniae P23.6
    - Mycoplasma P23.6
    - Pseudomonas P23.5
    - Staphylococcus P23.2
    - Streptococcus (except group B) P23.6
      - group B P23.3
    - viral agent P23.0
  - specified NEC P23.8
- croupous —*see* Pneumonia, lobar
- cryptogenic organizing J84.116
- cytomegalic inclusion B25.0
- cytomegaloviral B25.0
- deglutition —*see* Pneumonia, aspiration
- desquamative interstitial J84.117
- diffuse —*see* Pneumonia, broncho
- diplococcal, diplococcus (broncho-) (lobar) J13
- disseminated (focal) —*see* Pneumonia, broncho
- Eaton's agent J15.7
- embolic, embolism —*see* Embolism, pulmonary
- Enterobacter J15.6
- eosinophilic J82
- Escherichia coli (E. coli) J15.5
- Eubacterium J15.8
- fibrinous —*see* Pneumonia, lobar
- fibroid, fibrous (chronic) —*see* Fibrosis, lung
- Friedländer's bacillus J15.0
- Fusobacterium (nucleatum) J15.8
- gangrenous J85.0
- giant cell (measles) B05.2
- gonococcal A54.84
- gram-negative bacteria NEC J15.6
  - anaerobic J15.8
- Hemophilus influenzae (broncho) (lobar) J14
- human metapneumovirus J12.3
- hypostatic (broncho) (lobar) J18.2
- in (due to)
  - actinomycosis A42.0
  - adenovirus J12.0
  - anthrax A22.1
  - ascariasis B77.81
  - aspergillosis B44.9
  - Bacillus anthracis A22.1
  - Bacterium anitratum J15.6
  - candidiasis B37.1
  - chickenpox B01.2
  - Chlamydia J16.0
    - neonatal P23.1
  - coccidioidomycosis B38.2
    - acute B38.0

Pneumonia *(continued)*
- in *(continued)*
  - coccidioidomycosis *(continued)*
    - chronic B38.1
  - cytomegalovirus disease B25.0
  - Diplococcus (pneumoniae) J13
  - Eaton's agent J15.7
  - Enterobacter J15.6
  - Escherichia coli (E. coli) J15.5
  - Friedländer's bacillus J15.0
  - fumes and vapors (chemical) (inhalation) J68.0
  - gonorrhea A54.84
  - Hemophilus influenzae (H. influenzae) J14
  - Herellea J15.6
  - histoplasmosis B39.2
    - acute B39.0
    - chronic B39.1
  - human metapneumovirus J12.3
  - Klebsiella (pneumoniae) J15.0
  - measles B05.2
  - Mycoplasma (pneumoniae) J15.7
  - nocardiosis, nocardiasis A43.0
  - ornithosis A70
  - parainfluenza virus J12.2
  - pleuro-pneumonia-like-organism (PPLO) J15.7
  - pneumococcus J13
  - pneumocystosis (Pneumocystis carinii) (Pneumocystis jiroveci) B59
  - Proteus J15.6
  - Pseudomonas NEC J15.1
    - pseudomallei A24.1
  - psittacosis A70
  - Q fever A78
  - respiratory syncytial virus J12.1
  - rheumatic fever I00 *[J17]*
  - rubella B06.81
  - Salmonella (infection) A02.22
    - typhi A01.03
  - schistosomiasis B65.9 *[J17]*
  - Serratia marcescens J15.6
  - specified
    - bacterium NEC J15.8
    - organism NEC J16.8
  - spirochetal NEC A69.8
  - Staphylococcus J15.20
    - aureus (methicillin susceptible) (MSSA) J15.211
      - methicillin resistant (MRSA) J15.212
    - specified NEC J15.29
  - Streptococcus J15.4
    - group B J15.3
    - pneumoniae J13
    - specified NEC J15.4
  - toxoplasmosis B58.3
  - tularemia A21.2
  - typhoid (fever) A01.03
  - varicella B01.2
  - virus —*see* Pneumonia, viral
  - whooping cough A37.91
    - due to
      - Bordetella parapertussis A37.11
      - Bordetella pertussis A37.01
      - specified NEC A37.81
  - Yersinia pestis A20.2
- inhalation of food or vomit —*see* Pneumonia, aspiration
- interstitial J84.9
  - chronic J84.111
  - desquamative J84.117
  - due to
    - collagen vascular disease J84.17
    - known underlying cause J84.17
  - idiopathic NOS J84.111

Pneumonia *(continued)*
- interstitial *(continued)*
  - in disease classified elsewhere J84.17
  - lymphocytic (due to collagen vascular disease) (in diseases classified elsewhere) J84.17
  - lymphoid J84.2
  - non-specific J84.89
    - due to
      - collagen vascular disease J84.17
      - known underlying cause J84.17
    - idiopathic J84.113
    - in diseases classified elsewhere J84.17
  - plasma cell B59
  - pseudomonas J15.1
  - usual J84.112
    - due to collagen vascular disease J84.17
    - idiopathic J84.112
    - in diseases classified elsewhere J84.17
- Klebsiella (pneumoniae) J15.0
- lipid, lipoid (exogenous) J69.1
  - endogenous J84.89
- lobar (disseminated) (double) (interstitial) J18.1
  - bacterial J15.9
    - specified NEC J15.8
  - chronic —*see* Fibrosis, lung
  - Escherichia coli (E. coli) J15.5
  - Friedländer's bacillus J15.0
  - Hemophilus influenzae J14
  - hypostatic J18.2
  - Klebsiella (pneumoniae) J15.0
  - pneumococcal J13
  - Proteus J15.6
  - Pseudomonas J15.1
  - specified organism NEC J16.8
  - staphylococcal —*see* Pneumonia, staphylococcal
  - streptococcal NEC J15.4
  - Streptococcus pneumoniae J13
  - viral, virus —*see* Pneumonia, viral
- lobular —*see* Pneumonia, broncho
- Löffler's J82
- lymphoid interstitial J84.2
- massive —*see* Pneumonia, lobar
- meconium P24.01
- MRSA (Methicillin resistant Staphylococcus aureus) J15.212
- MSSA (methicillin susceptible Staphylococcus aureus) J15.211
- multilobar —*see* Pneumonia, by type
- Mycoplasma (pneumoniae) J15.7
- necrotic J85.0
- neonatal P23.9
  - aspiration —*see* Aspiration, by substance, with pneumonia
- nitrogen dioxide J68.0
- organizing J84.89
  - due to
    - collagen vascular disease J84.17
    - known underlying cause J84.17
  - in diseases classified elsewhere J84.17
- orthostatic J18.2
- parainfluenza virus J12.2
- parenchymatous —*see* Fibrosis, lung
- passive J18.2
- patchy —*see* Pneumonia, broncho
- Peptococcus J15.8
- Peptostreptococcus J15.8
- plasma cell (of infants) B59
- pleurolobar —*see* Pneumonia, lobar

Pneumonia *(continued)*
- pleuro-pneumonia-like organism (PPLO) J15.7
- pneumococcal (broncho) (lobar) J13
- Pneumocystis (carinii) (jiroveci) B59
- postinfectional NEC B99 *[J17]*
- postmeasles B05.2
- Proteus J15.6
- Pseudomonas J15.1
- psittacosis A70
- radiation J70.0
- respiratory syncytial virus J12.1
- resulting from a procedure J95.89
- rheumatic I00 *[J17]*
- Salmonella (arizonae) (cholerae-suis) (enteritidis) (typhimurium) A02.22
  - typhi A01.03
  - typhoid fever A01.03
- SARS-associated coronavirus J12.81
- segmented, segmental —*see* Pneumonia, broncho-
- Serratia marcescens J15.6
- specified NEC J18.8
  - bacterium NEC J15.8
  - organism NEC J16.8
  - virus NEC J12.89
- spirochetal NEC A69.8
- staphylococcal (broncho) (lobar) J15.20
  - aureus (methicillin susceptible) (MSSA) J15.211
    - methicillin resistant (MRSA) J15.212
  - specified NEC J15.29
- static, stasis J18.2
- streptococcal NEC (broncho) (lobar) J15.4
  - group
    - A J15.4
    - B J15.3
    - specified NEC J15.4
- Streptococcus pneumoniae J13
- syphilitic, congenital (early) A50.04
- traumatic (complication) (early) (secondary) T79.8
- tuberculous (any) —*see* Tuberculosis, pulmonary
- tularemic A21.2
- varicella B01.2
- Veillonella J15.8
- ventilator associated J95.851
- viral, virus (broncho) (interstitial) (lobar) J12.9
  - adenoviral J12.0
  - congenital P23.0
  - human metapneumovirus J12.3
  - parainfluenza J12.2
  - respiratory syncytial J12.1
  - SARS-associated coronavirus J12.81
  - specified NEC J12.89
- white (congenital) A50.04

Pneumonic —*see* condition

Pneumonitis (acute) (primary) —*see also* Pneumonia
- air-conditioner J67.7
- allergic (due to) J67.9
  - organic dust NEC J67.8
  - red cedar dust J67.8
  - sequoiosis J67.8
  - wood dust J67.8
- aspiration J69.0
  - due to
    - anesthesia J95.4
      - during
        - labor and delivery O74.0
        - pregnancy O29.01-
        - puerperium O89.01

Pneumonitis *(continued)*
aspiration *(continued)*
due to *(continued)*
fumes or gases J68.0
obstetric O74.0
chemical (due to gases, fumes or vapors) (inhalation) J68.0
due to anesthesia J95.4
cholesterol J84.89
crack (cocaine) J68.0
chronic *—see* Fibrosis, lung
congenital rubella P35.0
due to
beryllium J68.0
cadmium J68.0
crack (cocaine) J68.0
detergent J69.8
fluorocarbon-polymer J68.0
food, vomit (aspiration) J69.0
fumes or vapors J68.0
gases, fumes or vapors (inhalation) J68.0
inhalation
blood J69.8
essences J69.1
food (regurgitated), milk, vomit J69.0
oils, essences J69.1
saliva J69.0
solids, liquids NEC J69.8
manganese J68.0
nitrogen dioxide J68.0
oils, essences J69.1
solids, liquids NEC J69.8
toxoplasmosis (acquired) B58.3
congenital P37.1
vanadium J68.0
ventilator J95.851
eosinophilic J82
hypersensitivity J67.9
air conditioner lung J67.7
bagassosis J67.1
bird fancier's lung J67.2
farmer's lung J67.0
maltworker's lung J67.4
maple bark-stripper's lung J67.6
mushroom worker's lung J67.5
specified organic dust NEC J67.8
suberosis J67.3
interstitial (chronic) J84.89
acute J84.114
lymphoid J84.2
non-specific J84.89
idiopathic J84.113
lymphoid, interstitial J84.2
meconium P24.01
postanesthetic J95.4
correct substance properly administered *—see* Table of Drugs and Chemicals, by drug, adverse effect
in labor and delivery O74.0
in pregnancy O29.01-
obstetric O74.0
overdose or wrong substance given or taken (by accident) *—see* Table of Drugs and Chemicals, by drug, poisoning
postpartum, puerperal O89.01
postoperative J95.4
obstetric O74.0
radiation J70.0
rubella, congenital P35.0
ventilation (air-conditioning) J67.7
ventilator associated J95.851
wood-dust J67.8

Pneumonoconiosis *—see* Pneumoconiosis

Pneumoparotid K11.8

Pneumopathy NEC J98.4
alveolar J84.09
due to organic dust NEC J66.8
parietoalveolar J84.09

Pneumopericarditis *—see also* Pericarditis
acute I30.9

Pneumopericardium *—see also* Pericarditis
congenital P25.3
newborn P25.3
traumatic (post) *—see* Injury, heart

Pneumophagia (psychogenic) F45.8

Pneumopleurisy, pneumopleuritis (*see also* Pneumonia) J18.8

Pneumopyopericardium I30.1

Pneumopyothorax *—see* Pyopneumothorax
with fistula J86.0

Pneumorrhagia *—see also* Hemorrhage, lung
tuberculous *—see* Tuberculosis, pulmonary

Pneumothorax NOS J93.9
acute J93.83
chronic J93.81
congenital P25.1
perinatal period P25.1
postprocedural J95.811
specified NEC J93.83
spontaneous NOS J93.83
newborn P25.1
primary J93.11
secondary J93.12
tension J93.0
tense valvular, infectional J93.0
tension (spontaneous) J93.0
traumatic S27.0
with hemothorax S27.2
tuberculous *—see* Tuberculosis, pulmonary

Podagra (*see also* Gout) M10.9

Podencephalus Q01.9

Poikilocytosis R71.8

Poikiloderma L81.6
Civatte's L57.3
congenital Q82.8
vasculare atrophicans L94.5

Poikilodermatomyositis M33.10
with
myopathy M33.12
respiratory involvement M33.11
specified organ involvement NEC M33.19

Pointed ear (congenital) Q17.3

Poison ivy, oak, sumac or other plant dermatitis (allergic) (contact) L23.7

Poisoning (acute) *—see also* Table of Drugs and Chemicals
algae and toxins T65.82-
Bacillus B (aertrycke) (cholerae (suis)) (paratyphosus) (suipestifer) A02.9
botulinus A05.1
bacterial toxins A05.9
berries, noxious *—see* Poisoning, food, noxious, berries
botulism A05.1
ciguatera fish T61.0-
Clostridium botulinum A05.1
death-cap (Amanita phalloides) (Amanita verna) *—see* Poisoning, food, noxious, mushrooms

Poisoning *(continued)*
drug *—see* Table of Drugs and Chemicals, by drug, poisoning
epidemic, fish (noxious) *—see* Poisoning, seafood
bacterial A05.9
fava bean D55.0
fish (noxious) T61.9-
bacterial *—see* Intoxication, foodborne, by agent
ciguatera fish *—see* Poisoning, ciguatera fish
scombroid fish *—see* Poisoning, scombroid fish
specified type NEC T61.77-
food (acute) (diseased) (infected) (noxious) NEC T62.9-
bacterial *—see* Intoxication, foodborne, by agent
due to
Bacillus (aertrycke) (choleraesuis) (paratyphosus) (suipestifer) A02.9
botulinus A05.1
Clostridium (perfringens) (Welchii) A05.2
salmonella (aertrycke) (callinarum) (choleraesuis) (enteritidis) (paratyphi) (suipestifer) A02.9
with
gastroenteritis A02.0
sepsis A02.1
staphylococcus A05.0
Vibrio
parahaemolyticus A05.3
vulnificus A05.5
noxious or naturally toxic T62.9-
berries *—see* subcategory T62.1-
fish *—see* Poisoning, seafood
mushrooms *—see* subcategory T62.0X-
plants NEC *—see* subcategory T62.2X-
seafood *—see* Poisoning, seafood
specified NEC T62.8X-
ichthyotoxism *—see* Poisoning, seafood
kreotoxism, food A05.9
latex T65.81-
lead T56.0-
mushroom *—see* Poisoning, food, noxious, mushroom
mussels *—see also* Poisoning, shellfish
bacterial *—see* Intoxication, foodborne, by agent
nicotine (tobacco) T65.2-
noxious foodstuffs *—see* Poisoning, food, noxious
plants, noxious *—see* Poisoning, food, noxious, plants NEC
ptomaine *—see* Poisoning, food
radiation J70.0
Salmonella (arizonae) (cholerae-suis) (enteritidis) (typhimurium) A02.9
scombroid fish T61.1-
seafood (noxious) T61.9-
bacterial *—see* Intoxication, foodborne, by agent
fish *—see* Poisoning, fish
shellfish *—see* Poisoning, shellfish
specified NEC *—see* subcategory T61.8X-

Poisoning *(continued)*
shellfish (amnesic) (azaspiracid) (diarrheic) (neurotoxic) (noxious) (paralytic) T61.78-
bacterial *—see* Intoxication, foodborne, by agent
ciguatera mollusk *—see* Poisoning, ciguatera fish
specified substance NEC T65.891
Staphylococcus, food A05.0
tobacco (nicotine) T65.2-
water E87.79

Poker spine *—see* Spondylitis, ankylosing

Poland syndrome Q79.8

Polioencephalitis (acute) (bulbar) A80.9
inferior G12.22
influenzal *—see* Influenza, with, encephalopathy
superior hemorrhagic (acute) (Wernicke's) E51.2
Wernicke's E51.2

Polioencephalomyelitis (acute) (anterior) A80.9
with beriberi E51.2

Polioencephalopathy, superior hemorrhagic E51.2
with
beriberi E51.11
pellagra E52

Poliomeningoencephalitis *—see* Meningoencephalitis

Poliomyelitis (acute) (anterior) (epidemic) A80.9
with paralysis (bulbar) *—see* Poliomyelitis, paralytic
abortive A80.4
ascending (progressive) *—see* Poliomyelitis, paralytic
bulbar (paralytic) *—see* Poliomyelitis, paralytic
congenital P35.8
nonepidemic A80.9
nonparalytic A80.4
paralytic A80.30
specified NEC A80.39
vaccine-associated A80.0
wild virus
imported A80.1
indigenous A80.2
spinal, acute A80.9

Poliosis (eyebrow) (eyelashes) L67.1
circumscripta, acquired L67.1

Pollakiuria R35.0
psychogenic F45.8

Pollinosis J30.1

Pollitzer's disease L73.2

Polyadenitis *—see also* Lymphadenitis
malignant A20.0

Polyalgia M79.89

Polyangiitis M30.0
microscopic M31.7
overlap syndrome M30.8

Polyarteritis
microscopic M31.7
nodosa M30.0
with lung involvement M30.1
juvenile M30.2
related condition NEC M30.8

Polyarthralgia *—see* Pain, joint

Polyarthritis, polyarthropathy (*see also* Arthritis) M13.0

lyarthritis, polyarthropathy *(continued)*
- due to or associated with
  - other specified conditions *—see* Arthritis
- epidemic (Australian) (with exanthema) B33.1
- infective *—see* Arthritis, pyogenic or pyemic
- inflammatory M06.4
- juvenile (chronic) (seronegative) M08.3
- migratory *—see* Fever, rheumatic
- rheumatic, acute *—see* Fever, rheumatic

lyarthrosis M15.9
- post-traumatic M15.3
- primary M15.0
- specified NEC M15.8

lycarential syndrome of infancy E40

lychondritis (atrophic) (chronic) *—see also* Disorder, cartilage, specified type NEC
- relapsing M94.1

lycoria Q13.2

lycystic (disease)
- degeneration, kidney Q61.3
  - autosomal dominant (adult type) Q61.2
  - autosomal recessive (infantile type) NEC Q61.19
- kidney Q61.3
  - autosomal
    - dominant Q61.2
    - recessive NEC Q61.19
  - autosomal dominant (adult type) Q61.2
  - autosomal recessive (childhood type) NEC Q61.19
  - infantile type NEC Q61.19
- liver Q44.6
- lung J98.4
  - congenital Q33.0
- ovary, ovaries E28.2
- spleen Q89.09

olycythemia (secondary) D75.1
- acquired D75.1
- benign (familial) D75.0
- due to
  - donor twin P61.1
  - erythropoietin D75.1
  - fall in plasma volume D75.1
  - high altitude D75.1
  - maternal-fetal transfusion P61.1
  - stress D75.1
- emotional D75.1
- erythropoietin D75.1
- familial (benign) D75.0
- Gaisböck's (hypertonica) D75.1
- high altitude D75.1
- hypertonica D75.1
- hypoxemic D75.1
- neonatorum P61.1
- nephrogenous D75.1
- relative D75.1
- secondary D75.1
- spurious D75.1
- stress D75.1
- vera D45

olycytosis cryptogenica D75.1

olydactylism, polydactyly Q69.9
- toes Q69.2

olydipsia R63.1

olydystrophy, pseudo-Hurler E77.0

Polyembryoma *—see* Neoplasm, malignant, by site

Polyglandular
- deficiency E31.0
- dyscrasia E31.9
- dysfunction E31.9
- syndrome E31.8

Polyhydramnios O40.-

Polymastia Q83.1

Polymenorrhea N92.0

Polymyalgia M35.3
- arteritica, giant cell M31.5
- rheumatica M35.3
  - with giant cell arteritis M31.5

Polymyositis (acute) (chronic) (hemorrhagic) M33.20
- with
  - myopathy M33.22
  - respiratory involvement M33.21
  - skin involvement *—see* Dermatopolymyositis
  - specified organ involvement NEC M33.29
- ossificans (generalisata) (progressiva) *—see* Myositis, ossificans, progressiva

Polyneuritis, polyneuritic *—see also* Polyneuropathy
- acute (post-)infective G61.0
- alcoholic G62.1
- cranialis G52.7
- demyelinating, chronic inflammatory (CIDP) G61.81
- diabetic *—see* Diabetes, polyneuropathy
- diphtheritic A36.83
- due to lack of vitamin NEC E56.9 *[G63]*
- endemic E51.11
- erythredema *—see* subcategory T56.1
- febrile, acute G61.0
- hereditary ataxic G60.1
- idiopathic, acute G61.0
- infective (acute) G61.0
- inflammatory, chronic demyelinating (CIDP) G61.81
- nutritional E63.9 *[G63]*
- postinfective (acute) G61.0
- specified NEC G62.89

Polyneuropathy (peripheral) G62.9
- alcoholic G62.1
- amyloid (Portuguese) E85.1 *[G63]*
  - transthyretin-related (ATTR) familial E85.1
- arsenical G62.2
- critical illness G62.81
- demyelinating, chronic inflammatory (CIDP) G61.81
- diabetic *—see* Diabetes, polyneuropathy
- drug-induced G62.0
- hereditary G60.9
  - specified NEC G60.8
- idiopathic G60.9
  - progressive G60.3
- in (due to)
  - alcohol G62.1
    - sequelae G65.2
  - amyloidosis, familial (Portuguese) E85.1 *[G63]*
  - antitetanus serum G61.1
  - arsenic G62.2
    - sequelae G65.2
  - avitaminosis NEC E56.9 *[G63]*
  - beriberi E51.11
  - collagen vascular disease NEC M35.9 *[G63]*

Polyneuropathy *(continued)*
- in (due to) *(continued)*
  - deficiency (of)
    - B (-complex) vitamins E53.9 *[G63]*
    - vitamin B6 E53.1 *[G63]*
  - diabetes *—see* Diabetes, polyneuropathy
  - diphtheria A36.83
  - drug or medicament G62.0
    - correct substance properly administered *—see* Table of Drugs and Chemicals, by drug, adverse effect
    - overdose or wrong substance given or taken *—see* Table of Drugs and Chemicals, by drug, poisoning
  - endocrine disease NEC E34.9 *[G63]*
  - herpes zoster B02.23
  - hypoglycemia E16.2 *[G63]*
  - infectious
    - disease NEC B99 *[G63]*
    - mononucleosis B27.91
  - lack of vitamin NEC E56.9 *[G63]*
  - lead G62.2
    - sequelae G65.2
  - leprosy A30.9 *[G63]*
  - Lyme disease A69.22
  - metabolic disease NEC E88.9 *[G63]*
  - microscopic polyangiitis M31.7 *[G63]*
  - mumps B26.84
  - neoplastic disease (*see also* Neoplasm) D49.9 *[G63]*
  - nutritional deficiency NEC E63.9 *[G63]*
  - organophosphate compounds G62.2
    - sequelae G65.2
  - parasitic disease NEC B89 *[G63]*
  - pellagra E52 *[G63]*
  - polyarteritis nodosa M30.0
  - porphyria E80.20 *[G63]*
  - radiation G62.82
  - rheumatoid arthritis *—see* Rheumatoid, polyneuropathy
  - sarcoidosis D86.89
  - serum G61.1
  - syphilis (late) A52.15
    - congenital A50.43
  - systemic
    - connective tissue disorder M35.9 *[G63]*
    - lupus erythematosus M32.19
  - toxic agent NEC G62.2
    - sequelae G65.2
- inflammatory G61.9
  - chronic demyelinating (CIDP) G61.81
  - sequelae G65.1
  - specified NEC G61.89
- lead G62.2
  - sequelae G65.2
- nutritional NEC E63.9 *[G63]*
- postherpetic (zoster) B02.23
- progressive G60.3
- radiation-induced G62.82
- sensory (hereditary) (idiopathic) G60.8
- specified NEC G62.89
- syphilitic (late) A52.15
  - congenital A50.43
- transthyretin-related (ATTR) familial amyloid E85.1
  - triorthocresyl phosphate G62.2
    - sequelae G65.2
  - tuberculosis A17.89

Polyneuropathy *(continued)*
- transthyretin-related *(continued)*
  - uremia N18.9 *[G63]*
  - vitamin B12 deficiency E53.8 *[G63]*
    - with anemia (pernicious) D51.0 *[G63]*
      - due to dietary deficiency D51.3 *[G63]*
  - zoster B02.23

Polyopia H53.8

Polyorchism, polyorchidism Q55.21

Polyosteoarthritis (*see also* Osteoarthritis, generalized) M15.9-
- post-traumatic M15.3
- specified NEC M15.8

Polyostotic fibrous dysplasia Q78.1

Polyotia Q17.0

Polyp, polypus
- accessory sinus J33.8
- adenocarcinoma in *—see* Neoplasm, malignant, by site
- adenocarcinoma in situ in *—see* Neoplasm, in situ, by site
- adenoid tissue J33.0
- adenomatous *—see also* Neoplasm, benign, by site
  - adenocarcinoma in *—see* Neoplasm, malignant, by site
  - adenocarcinoma in situ in *—see* Neoplasm, in situ, by site
  - carcinoma in *—see* Neoplasm, malignant, by site
  - carcinoma in situ in *—see* Neoplasm, in situ, by site
  - multiple *—see* Neoplasm, benign
    - adenocarcinoma in *—see* Neoplasm, malignant, by site
    - adenocarcinoma in situ in *—see* Neoplasm, in situ, by site
- antrum J33.8
- anus, anal (canal) K62.0
- Bartholin's gland N84.3
- bladder D41.4
- carcinoma in *—see* Neoplasm, malignant, by site
- carcinoma in situ in *—see* Neoplasm, in situ, by site
- cecum D12.0
- cervix (uteri) N84.1
  - in pregnancy or childbirth *—see* Pregnancy, complicated by, abnormal, cervix
  - mucous N84.1
  - nonneoplastic N84.1
- choanal J33.0
- cholesterol K82.4
- clitoris N84.3
- colon K63.5
  - adenomatous D12.6
  - ascending D12.2
  - cecum D12.0
  - descending D12.4
  - inflammatory K51.40
    - with
      - abscess K51.414
      - complication K51.419
        - specified NEC K51.418
      - fistula K51.413
      - intestinal obstruction K51.412
      - rectal bleeding K51.411
  - sigmoid D12.5
  - transverse D12.3
- corpus uteri N84.0
- dental K04.01

Polyp, polypus *(continued)*
- dental *(continued)*
  - irreversible K04.02
  - reversible K04.01
- duodenum K31.7
- ear (middle) H74.4-
- endometrium N84.0
- ethmoidal (sinus) J33.8
- fallopian tube N84.8
- female genital tract N84.9
  - specified NEC N84.8
- frontal (sinus) J33.8
- gallbladder K82.4
- gingiva, gum K06.8
- labia, labium (majus) (minus) N84.3
- larynx (mucous) J38.1
  - adenomatous D14.1
- malignant —*see* Neoplasm, malignant, by site
- maxillary (sinus) J33.8
- middle ear —*see* Polyp, ear (middle)
- myometrium N84.0
- nares
  - anterior J33.9
  - posterior J33.0
- nasal (mucous) J33.9
  - cavity J33.0
  - septum J33.0
- nasopharyngeal J33.0
- nose (mucous) J33.9
- oviduct N84.8
- pharynx J39.2
- placenta O90.89
- prostate —*see* Enlargement, enlarged, prostate
- pudenda, pudendum N84.3
- pulpal (dental) K04.01
  - irreversible K04.02
  - reversible K04.01
- rectum (nonadenomatous) K62.1
  - adenomatous —*see* Polyp, adenomatous
- septum (nasal) J33.0
- sinus (accessory) (ethmoidal) (frontal) (maxillary) (sphenoidal) J33.8
- sphenoidal (sinus) J33.8
- stomach K31.7
  - adenomatous D13.1
- tube, fallopian N84.8
- turbinate, mucous membrane J33.8
- umbilical, newborn P83.6
- ureter N28.89
- urethra N36.2
- uterus (body) (corpus) (mucous) N84.0
  - cervix N84.1
  - in pregnancy or childbirth —*see* Pregnancy, complicated by, tumor, uterus
- vagina N84.2
- vocal cord (mucous) J38.1
- vulva N84.3

Polyphagia R63.2

Polyploidy Q92.7

Polypoid —*see* condition

Polyposis —*see also* Polyp
- coli (adenomatous) D12.6
  - adenocarcinoma in C18.9
  - adenocarcinoma in situ in —*see* Neoplasm, in situ, by site
  - carcinoma in C18.9
- colon (adenomatous) D12.6
- familial D12.6
  - adenocarcinoma in situ in —*see* Neoplasm, in situ, by site
- intestinal (adenomatous) D12.6
- malignant lymphomatous C83.1-

Polyposis *(continued)*
- multiple, adenomatous (*see also* Neoplasm, benign) D36.9

Polyradiculitis —*see* Polyneuropathy

Polyradiculoneuropathy (acute) (postinfective) (segmentally demyelinating) G61.0

Polyserositis
- due to pericarditis I31.1
- pericardial I31.1
- periodic, familial E85.0
- tuberculous A19.9
  - acute A19.1
  - chronic A19.8

Polysplenia syndrome Q89.09

Polysyndactyly (*see also* Syndactylism, syndactyly) Q70.4

Polytrichia L68.3

Polyunguia Q84.6

Polyuria R35.8
- nocturnal R35.1
- psychogenic F45.8

Pompe's disease (glycogen storage) E74.02

Pompholyx L30.1

Poncet's disease (tuberculous rheumatism) A18.09

Pond fracture —*see* Fracture, skull

Ponos B55.0

Pons, pontine —*see* condition

Poor
- aesthetic of existing restoration of tooth K08.56
- contractions, labor O62.2
- gingival margin to tooth restoration K08.51
- personal hygiene R46.0
- prenatal care, affecting management of pregnancy —*see* Pregnancy, complicated by, insufficient, prenatal care
- sucking reflex (newborn) R29.2
- urinary stream R39.12
- vision NEC H54.7

Poradenitis, nostras inguinalis or venerea A55

Porencephaly (congenital) (developmental) (true) Q04.6
- acquired G93.0
- nondevelopmental G93.0
- traumatic (post) F07.89

Porocephaliasis B88.8

Porokeratosis Q82.8

Poroma, eccrine —*see* Neoplasm, skin, benign

Porphyria (South African) E80.20
- acquired E80.20
- acute intermittent (hepatic) (Swedish) E80.21
- cutanea tarda (hereditary) (symptomatic) E80.1
- due to drugs E80.20
  - correct substance properly administered —*see* Table of Drugs and Chemicals, by drug, adverse effect
  - overdose or wrong substance given or taken —*see* Table of Drugs and Chemicals, by drug, poisoning

Porphyria *(continued)*
- erythropoietic (congenital) (hereditary) E80.0
- hepatocutaneous type E80.1
- secondary E80.20
- toxic NEC E80.20
- variegata E80.20

Porphyrinuria —*see* Porphyria

Porphyruria —*see* Porphyria

Portal —*see* condition

Port wine nevus, mark, or stain Q82.5

Posadas-Wernicke disease B38.9

Positive
- culture (nonspecific)
  - blood R78.81
  - bronchial washings R84.5
  - cerebrospinal fluid R83.5
  - cervix uteri R87.5
  - nasal secretions R84.5
  - nipple discharge R89.5
  - nose R84.5
    - staphylococcus (Methicillin susceptible) Z22.321
      - Methicillin resistant Z22.322
  - peritoneal fluid R85.5
  - pleural fluid R84.5
  - prostatic secretions R86.5
  - saliva R85.5
  - seminal fluid R86.5
  - sputum R84.5
  - synovial fluid R89.5
  - throat scrapings R84.5
  - urine R82.79
  - vagina R87.5
  - vulva R87.5
  - wound secretions R89.5
- PPD (skin test) R76.11
- serology for syphilis A53.0
  - false R76.8
  - with signs or symptoms - code as Syphilis, by site and stage
- skin test, tuberculin (without active tuberculosis) R76.11
- test, human immunodeficiency virus (HIV) R75
- VDRL A53.0
  - with signs or symptoms - code by site and stage under Syphilis A53.9
- Wassermann reaction A53.0

Postcardiotomy syndrome I97.0

Postcaval ureter Q62.62

Postcholecystectomy syndrome K91.5

Postclimacteric bleeding N95.0

Postcommissurotomy syndrome I97.0

Postconcussional syndrome F07.81

Postcontusional syndrome F07.81

Postcricoid region —*see* condition

Post-dates (40-42 weeks) (pregnancy) (mother) O48.0
- more than 42 weeks gestation O48.1

Postencephalitic syndrome F07.89

Posterior —*see* condition

Posterolateral sclerosis (spinal cord) —*see* Degeneration, combined

Postexanthematous —*see* condition

Postfebrile —*see* condition

Postgastrectomy dumping syndrome K91.1

Posthemiplegic chorea —*see* Monoplegia

Posthemorrhagic anemia (chronic) D50.0
- acute D62
- newborn P61.3

Postherpetic neuralgia (zoster) B02.
- trigeminal B02.22

Posthitis N47.7

Postimmunization complication or reaction —*see* Complications, vaccination

Postinfectious —*see* condition

Postlaminectomy syndrome NEC M96.1

Postleukotomy syndrome F07.0

Postmastectomy lymphedema (syndrome) I97.2

Postmaturity, postmature (over 42 weeks)
- maternal (over 42 weeks gestation) O48.1
- newborn P08.22

Postmeasles complication NEC —*se also* condition B05.89

Postmenopausal
- endometrium (atrophic) N95.8
  - suppurative (*see also* Endometritis) N71.9
- osteoporosis —*see* Osteoporosis, postmenopausal

Postnasal drip R09.82
- due to
  - allergic rhinitis —*see* Rhinitis, allergic
  - common cold J00
  - gastroesophageal reflux —*see* Reflux, gastroesophageal
  - nasopharyngitis —*see* Nasopharyngitis
  - other know condition - code to condition
  - sinusitis —*see* Sinusitis

Postnatal —*see* condition

Postoperative (postprocedural) —*see* Complication, postoperative
- pneumothorax, therapeutic Z98.3
- state NEC Z98.890

Postpancreatectomy hyperglycemia E89.1

Postpartum —*see* Puerperal

Postphlebitic syndrome —*see* Syndrome, postthrombotic

Postpoliomyelitic —*see also* conditic
- osteopathy —*see* Osteopathy, after poliomyelitis

Postpolio (myelitic) **syndrome** G14

Postprocedural —*see also* Postoperative
- hypoinsulinemia E89.1

Postschizophrenic depression F32.8

Postsurgery status —*see also* Status (post)
- pneumothorax, therapeutic Z98.3

Post-term (40-42 weeks) (pregnancy) (mother) O48.0
- infant P08.21
- more than 42 weeks gestation (mother) O48.1

Post-traumatic brain syndrome, nonpsychotic F07.81

ost-typhoid abscess A01.09

ostures, hysterical F44.2

ostvaccinal reaction or complication —*see* Complications, vaccination

ostvalvulotomy syndrome I97.0

otain's
- disease (pulmonary edema) —*see* Edema, lung
- syndrome (gastrectasis with dyspepsia) K31.0

otter's
- asthma J62.8
- facies Q60.6
- lung J62.8
- syndrome (with renal agenesis) Q60.6

ott's
- curvature (spinal) A18.01
- disease or paraplegia A18.01
- spinal curvature A18.01
- tumor, puffy —*see* Osteomyelitis, specified type NEC

ouch
- bronchus Q32.4
- Douglas' —*see* condition
- esophagus, esophageal, congenital Q39.6
  - acquired K22.5
- gastric K31.4
- Hartmann's K82.8
- pharynx, pharyngeal (congenital) Q38.7

ouchitis K91.850

oultrymen's itch B88.0

overty NEC Z59.6
- extreme Z59.5

oxvirus NEC B08.8

rader-Willi syndrome Q87.1

reauricular appendage or tag Q17.0

rebetalipoproteinemia (acquired) (essential) (familial) (hereditary) (primary) (secondary) E78.1
- with chylomicronemia E78.3

recipitate labor or delivery O62.3

reclimacteric bleeding (menorrhagia) N92.4

recocious
- adrenarche E30.1
- menarche E30.1
- menstruation E30.1
- pubarche E30.1
- puberty E30.1
  - central E22.8
- sexual development NEC E30.1
- thelarche E30.8

recocity, sexual (constitutional) (cryptogenic) (female) (idiopathic) (male) E30.1
- with adrenal hyperplasia E25.9
  - congenital E25.0

recordial pain R07.2

redeciduous teeth K00.2

rediabetes, prediabetic R73.03
- complicating
  - pregnancy —*see* Pregnancy, complicated by, diseases of, specified type or system NEC
  - puerperium O99.89

Predislocation status of hip at birth Q65.6

Pre-eclampsia O14.9-
- with pre-existing hypertension —*see* Hypertension, complicating pregnancy, pre-existing, with, pre-eclampsia
- complicating
  - childbirth O14.94
  - puerperium O14.95
- mild O14.0-
  - complicating
    - childbirth O14.04
    - puerperium O14.05
- moderate O14.0-
  - complicating
    - childbirth O14.04
    - puerperium O14.05
- severe O14.1-
  - with hemolysis, elevated liver enzymes and low platelet count (HELLP) O14.2-
    - complicating
      - childbirth O14.24
      - puerperium O14.25
  - complicating
    - childbirth O14.14
    - puerperium O14.15

Pre-eruptive color change, teeth, tooth K00.8

Pre-excitation atrioventricular conduction I45.6

Preglaucoma H40.00-

Pregnancy (single) (uterine) —*see also* Delivery and Puerperal

> Note: The Tabular must be reviewed for assignment of the appropriate character indicating the trimester of the pregnancy
> Note: The Tabular must be reviewed for assignment of appropriate seventh character for multiple gestation codes in Chapter 15

- abdominal (ectopic) O00.00
  - with intrauterine pregnancy O00.01
  - with viable fetus O36.7-
- ampullar O00.10-
  - with intrauterine pregnancy O00.11-
- biochemical O02.81
- broad ligament O00.80
  - with intrauterine pregnancy O00.81
- cervical O00.80
  - with intrauterine pregnancy O00.81
- chemical O02.81
- complicated NOS O26.9-
- complicated by (care of) (management affected by)
  - abnormal, abnormality
    - cervix O34.4-
      - causing obstructed labor O65.5
    - cord (umbilical) O69.9
    - fetal heart rate or rhythm O36.83-
    - findings on antenatal screening of mother O28.9
      - biochemical O28.1
      - cytological O28.2
      - chromosomal O28.5
      - genetic O28.5
      - hematological O28.0
      - radiological O28.4
      - specified NEC O28.8
      - ultrasonic O28.3

Pregnancy *(continued)*
- complicated by *(continued)*
  - findings on antenatal screening of mother *(continued)*
    - glucose (tolerance) NEC O99.810
    - pelvic organs O34.9-
      - specified NEC O34.8-
        - causing obstructed labor O65.5
    - pelvis (bony) (major) NEC O33.0
    - perineum O34.7-
    - position
      - placenta O44.0
        - with hemorrhage O44.1-
      - uterus O34.59-
    - uterus O34.59-
      - causing obstructed labor O65.5
      - congenital O34.0-
    - vagina O34.6-
      - causing obstructed labor O65.5
    - vulva O34.7-
      - causing obstructed labor O65.5
  - abruptio placentae —*see* Abruptio placentae
  - abscess or cellulitis
    - bladder O23.1-
    - breast O91.11-
    - genital organ or tract O23.9-
  - abuse
    - physical O9A.31-
    - psychological O9A.51-
    - sexual O9A.41-
  - adverse effect anesthesia O29.9-
    - aspiration pneumonitis O29.01-
    - cardiac arrest O29.11-
    - cardiac complication NEC O29.19-
    - cardiac failure O29.12-
    - central nervous system complication NEC O29.29-
    - cerebral anoxia O29.21-
    - failed or difficult intubation O29.6-
    - inhalation of stomach contents or secretions NOS O29.01-
    - local, toxic reaction O29.3X
    - Mendelson's syndrome O29.01-
    - pressure collapse of lung O29.02-
    - pulmonary complications NEC O29.09-
    - specified NEC O29.8X-
    - spinal and epidural type NEC O29.5X
      - induced headache O29.4-
  - albuminuria (*see also* Proteinuria, gestational) O12.1-
  - alcohol use O99.31-
  - amnionitis O41.12-
  - anaphylactoid syndrome of pregnancy O88.01-
  - anemia (conditions in D50-D64) (pre-existing) O99.01-
    - complicating the puerperium O99.03
  - antepartum hemorrhage O46.9-
    - with coagulation defect —*see* Hemorrhage, antepartum, with coagulation defect
    - specified NEC O46.8X-
  - appendicitis O99.61-
  - atrophy (yellow) (acute) liver (subacute) O26.61-
  - bariatric surgery status O99.84-
  - bicornis or bicornuate uterus O34.0-

Pregnancy *(continued)*
- complicated by *(continued)*
  - biliary tract problems O26.61-
  - breech presentation O32.1
  - cardiovascular diseases (conditions in I00-I09, I20-I52, I70-I99) O99.41-
  - cerebrovascular disorders (conditions in I60-I69) O99.41-
  - cervical shortening O26.87-
  - cervicitis O23.51-
  - chloasma (gravidarum) O26.89-
  - cholestasis (intrahepatic) O26.61-
  - cholecystitis O99.61-
  - chorioamnionitis O41.12-
  - circulatory system disorder (conditions in I00-I09, I20-I99, O99.41-)
  - compound presentation O32.6
  - conjoined twins O30.02-
  - connective system disorders (conditions in M00-M99) O99.89
  - contracted pelvis (general) O33.1
    - inlet O33.2
    - outlet O33.3
  - convulsions (eclamptic) (uremic) (*see also* Eclampsia) O15.9-
  - cracked nipple O92.11-
  - cystitis O23.1-
  - cystocele O34.8-
  - death of fetus (near term) O36.4
    - early pregnancy O02.1
    - of one fetus or more in multiple gestation O31.2-
  - deciduitis O41.14-
  - decreased fetal movement O36.81-
  - dental problems O99.61-
  - diabetes (mellitus) O24.91-
    - gestational (pregnancy induced) —*see* - Diabetes, gestational
    - pre-existing O24.31-
      - specified NEC O24.81-
      - type 1 O24.01-
      - type 2 O24.11-
  - digestive system disorders (conditions in K00-K93) O99.61-
  - diseases of —*see* Pregnancy, complicated by, specified body system disease
    - biliary tract O26.61-
    - blood NEC (conditions in D65-D77) O99.11-
    - liver O26.61-
    - specified NEC O99.89
  - disorders of —*see* Pregnancy, complicated by, specified body system disorder
    - amniotic fluid and membranes O41.9-
      - specified NEC O41.8X-
    - biliary tract O26.61-
    - ear and mastoid process (conditions in H60-H95) O99.89
    - eye and adnexa (conditions in H00-H59) O99.89
    - liver O26.61-
    - skin (conditions in L00-L99) O99.71-
    - specified NEC O99.89
  - displacement, uterus NEC O34.59-
    - causing obstructed labor O6
  - disproportion (due to) O33.
    - fetal (ascites) (hydrop
      (meningomyeloc
      teratoma) (tu
      NEC O33.7

Pregnancy *(continued)*
complicated by *(continued)*
disproportion *(continued)*
generally contracted pelvis O33.1
hydrocephalic fetus O33.6
inlet contraction of pelvis O33.2
mixed maternal and fetal origin O33.4
specified NEC O33.8
double uterus O34.0-
causing obstructed labor O65.5
drug use (conditions in F11-F19) O99.32-
eclampsia, eclamptic (coma) (convulsions) (delirium) (nephritis) (uremia) (*see also* Eclampsia) O15.-
ectopic pregnancy —*see* Pregnancy, ectopic
edema O12.0-
with
gestational hypertension, mild (*see also* Pre-eclampsia) O14.0-
proteinuria O12.2-
effusion, amniotic fluid —*see* Pregnancy, complicated by, premature rupture of membranes
elderly
multigravida O09.52-
primigravida O09.51-
embolism (*see also* Embolism, obstetric, pregnancy) O88.-
endocrine diseases NEC O99.28-
endometritis O86.12
excessive weight gain O26.0-
exhaustion O26.81-
during labor and delivery O75.81
face presentation O32.3
failed induction of labor O61.9
instrumental O61.1
mechanical O61.1
medical O61.0
specified NEC O61.8
surgical O61.1
failed or difficult intubation for anesthesia O29.6-
false labor (pains) O47.9
at or after 37 completed weeks of pregnancy O47.1
before 37 completed weeks of pregnancy O47.0-
fatigue O26.81-
during labor and delivery O75.81
fatty metamorphosis of liver O26.61-
female genital mutilation O34.8- *[N90.81-]*
fetal (maternal care for)
abnormality or damage O35.9
acid-base balance O68
specified type NEC O35.8
acidemia O68
acidosis O68
...penia

Pregnancy *(continued)*
complicated by *(continued)*
fetal *(continued)*
damage from *(continued)*
hematological investigation O35.7
intrauterine contraceptive device O35.7
maternal
alcohol addiction O35.4
cytomegalovirus infection O35.3
disease NEC O35.8
drug addiction O35.5
listeriosis O35.8
rubella O35.3
toxoplasmosis O35.8
viral infection O35.3
medical procedure NEC O35.7
radiation O35.6
death (near term) O36.4
early pregnancy O02.1
decreased movement O36.81-
disproportion due to deformity (fetal) O33.7
excessive growth (large for dates) O36.6-
growth retardation O36.59-
light for dates O36.59-
small for dates O36.59-
heart rate irregularity (bradycardia) (decelerations) (tachycardia) O76
hereditary disease O35.2
hydrocephalus O35.0
intrauterine death O36.4
poor growth O36.59-
light for dates O36.59-
small for dates O36.59-
problem O36.9-
specified NEC O36.89-
reduction (elective) O31.3-
selective termination O31.3-
spina bifida O35.0
thrombocytopenia O36.82-
fibroid (tumor) (uterus) O34.1-
fissure of nipple O92.11-
gallstones O99.61-
gastric banding status O99.84-
gastric bypass status O99.84-
genital herpes (asymptomatic) (history of) (inactive) O98.3-
genital tract infection O23.9-
glomerular diseases (conditions in N00-N07) O26.83-
with hypertension, pre-existing —*see* Hypertension, complicating, pregnancy, pre-existing, with, renal disease
gonorrhea O98.21-
grand multiparity O09.4
habitual aborter —*see* Pregnancy, complicated by, recurrent pregnancy loss
HELLP syndrome (hemolysis, elevated liver enzymes and low platelet count) O14.2-
hemorrhage
antepartum —*see* Hemorrhage, antepartum
before 20 completed weeks gestation O20.9
specified NEC O20.8
due to premature separation, placenta (*see also* Abruptio placentae) O45.9-
early O20.9
specified NEC O20.8
threatened abortion O20.0

Pregnancy *(continued)*
complicated by *(continued)*
hemorrhoids O22.4-
hepatitis (viral) O98.41-
herniation of uterus O34.59-
high
head at term O32.4
risk —*see* Supervision (of) (for), high-risk
history of in utero procedure during previous pregnancy O09.82-
HIV O98.71-
human immunodeficiency virus (HIV) disease O98.71-
hydatidiform mole (*see also* Mole, hydatidiform) O01.9-
hydramnios O40.-
hydrocephalic fetus (disproportion) O33.6
hydrops
amnii O40.-
fetalis O36.2-
associated with isoimmunization (*see also* Pregnancy, complicated by, isoimmunization) O36.11-
hydrorrhea O42.90
hyperemesis (gravidarum) (mild) (*see also* Hyperemesis, gravidarum) O21.0-
hypertension —*see* Hypertension, complicating pregnancy
hypertensive
heart and renal disease, pre-existing —*see* Hypertension, complicating, pregnancy, pre-existing, with, heart disease, with renal disease
heart disease, pre-existing —*see* Hypertension, complicating, pregnancy, pre-existing, with, heart disease
renal disease, pre-existing —*see* Hypertension, complicating, pregnancy, pre-existing, with, renal disease
hypotension O26.5-
immune disorders NEC (conditions in D80-D89) O99.11-
incarceration, uterus O34.51-
incompetent cervix O34.3-
inconclusive fetal viability O36.80
infection(s) O98.91-
amniotic fluid or sac O41.10-
bladder O23.1-
carrier state NEC O99.830
streptococcus B O99.820
genital organ or tract O23.9-
specified NEC O23.59-
genitourinary tract O23.9-
gonorrhea O98.21-
hepatitis (viral) O98.41-
HIV O98.71-
human immunodeficiency virus (HIV) O98.71-
kidney O23.0-
nipple O91.01-
parasitic disease O98.91-
specified NEC O98.81-
protozoal disease O98.61-
sexually transmitted NEC O98.31-
specified type NEC O98.81-
syphilis O98.11-
tuberculosis O98.01-
urethra O23.2-
urinary (tract) O23.4-
specified NEC O23.3-

Pregnancy *(continued)*
complicated by *(continued)*
infection(s) *(continued)*
viral disease O98.51-
injury or poisoning (conditions in S00-T88) O9A.21-
due to abuse
physical O9A.31-
psychological O9A.51-
sexual O9A.41-
insufficient
prenatal care O09.3-
weight gain O26.1-
insulin resistance O26.89
intrauterine fetal death (near term) O36.4
early pregnancy O02.1
multiple gestation (one fetus or more) O31.2-
isoimmunization O36.11-
anti-A sensitization O36.11-
anti-B sensitization O36.19-
Rh O36.09-
anti-D antibody O36.01-
specified NEC O36.19-
laceration of uterus NEC O71.81
malformation
placenta, placental (vessel) O43.10-
specified NEC O43.19-
uterus (congenital) O34.0-
malnutrition (conditions in E40-E46) O25.1-
maternal hypotension syndrome O26.5-
mental disorders (conditions in F01-F09, F20-F99) O99.34-
alcohol use O99.31-
drug use O99.32-
smoking O99.33-
mentum presentation O32.3
metabolic disorders O99.28-
missed
abortion O02.1
delivery O36.4
multiple gestations O30.9-
conjoined twins O30.02-
specified number of multiples NEC —*see* Pregnancy, multiple (gestation), specified NEC
quadruplet —*see* Pregnancy, quadruplet
specified complication NEC O31.8X-
triplet —*see* Pregnancy, triplet
twin —*see* Pregnancy, twin
musculoskeletal condition (conditions is M00-M99) O99.89
necrosis, liver (conditions in K72) O26.61-
neoplasm
benign
cervix O34.4-
corpus uteri O34.1-
uterus O34.1-
malignant O9A.11-
nephropathy NEC O26.83-
nervous system condition (conditions in G00-G99) O99.35-
nutritional diseases NEC O99.28-
obesity (pre-existing) O99.21-
obesity surgery status O99.84-
oblique lie or presentation O32.2
older mother —*see* Pregnancy, complicated by, elderly
oligohydramnios O41.0-

Pregnancy *(continued)*
complicated by *(continued)*
oligohydramnios *(continued)*
with premature rupture of membranes (*see also* Pregnancy, complicated by, premature rupture of membranes) O42.-
onset (spontaneous) of labor after 37 completed weeks of gestation but before 39 completed weeks gestation, with delivery by (planned) cesarean section O75.82
oophoritis O23.52-
overdose, drug (*see also* Table of Drugs and Chemicals, by drug, poisoning) O9A.21-
oversize fetus O33.5
papyraceous fetus O31.0-
pelvic inflammatory disease O99.89
periodontal disease O99.61-
peripheral neuritis O26.82-
peritoneal (pelvic) adhesions O99.89
phlebitis O22.9-
phlebopathy O22.9-
phlebothrombosis (superficial) O22.2-
deep O22.3-
placenta accreta O43.21-
placenta increta O43.22-
placenta percreta O43.23-
placenta previa O44.0-
complete O44.0-
with hemorrhage O44.1-
marginal O44.2-
with hemorrhage O44.3-
partial O44.2-
with hemorrhage O44.3-
placental disorder O43.9-
specified NEC O43.89-
placental dysfunction O43.89-
placental infarction O43.81-
placental insufficiency O36.51-
placental transfusion syndromes
fetomaternal O43.01-
fetus to fetus O43.02-
maternofetal O43.01-
placentitis O41.14-
pneumonia O99.51-
poisoning (*see also* Table of Drugs and Chemicals) O9A.21-
polyhydramnios O40-
polymorphic eruption of pregnancy O26.86
poor obstetric history NEC O09.29-
postmaturity (post-term) (40 to 42 weeks) O48.0
more than 42 completed weeks gestation (prolonged) O48.1
pre-eclampsia O14.9-
mild O14.0-
moderate O14.0-
severe O14.1-
with hemolysis, elevated liver enzymes and low platelet count (HELLP) O14.2-
premature labor *—see* Pregnancy, complicated by, preterm labor
premature rupture of membranes O42.90
full-term, unspecified as to length of time between rupture and onset of labor O42.92
with onset of labor
within 24 hours O42.00

Pregnancy *(continued)*
complicated by *(continued)*
premature rupture of membranes *(continued)*
with onset of labor *(continued)*
within 24 hours *(continued)*
at or after 37 weeks gestation, onset of labor within 24 hours of rupture O42.02
pre-term (before 37 completed weeks of gestation) O42.01-
after 24 hours O42.10
at or after 37 weeks gestation, onset of labor more than 24 hours following rupture O42.12
pre-term (before 37 completed weeks of gestation) O42.11-
at or after 37 weeks gestation, unspecified as to length of time between rupture and onset of labor O42.92
pre-term (before 37 completed weeks of gestation) O42.91-
premature separation of placenta (*see also* Abruptio placentae) O45.9-
presentation, fetal - *—see* Delivery, complicated by, malposition
preterm delivery O60.10
preterm labor
with delivery O60.10
preterm O60.10
term O60.20
second trimester
with term delivery O60.22
without delivery O60.02
with preterm delivery
second trimester O60.12
third trimester O60.13
third trimester
with term delivery O60.23
without delivery O60.03
with third trimester preterm delivery O60.14
without delivery O60.00
second trimester O60.02
third trimester O60.03
previous history of *—see* Pregnancy, supervision of, high-risk
prolapse, uterus O34.52-
proteinuria (gestational) (*see also* Proteinuria, gestational) O12.1-
with edema O12.2-
pruritic urticarial papules and plaques of pregnancy (PUPPP) O26.86
pruritus (neurogenic) O26.89-
psychosis or psychoneurosis (puerperal) F53
ptyalism O26.89-
PUPPP (pruritic urticarial papules and plaques of pregnancy) O26.86
pyelitis O23.0-
recurrent pregnancy loss O26.2-
renal disease or failure NEC O26.83-
with secondary hypertension, pre-existing *—see* Hypertension, complicating, pregnancy, pre-existing, secondary

Pregnancy *(continued)*
complicated by *(continued)*
renal disease or failure NEC *(continued)*
hypertensive, pre-existing *—see* Hypertension, complicating, pregnancy, pre-existing, with, renal disease
respiratory condition (conditions in J00-J99) O99.51-
retained, retention
dead ovum O02.0
intrauterine contraceptive device O26.3-
retroversion, uterus O34.53-
Rh immunization, incompatibility or sensitization NEC O36.09-
anti-D antibody O36.01-
rupture
amnion (premature) (*see also* Pregnancy, complicated by, premature rupture of membranes) O42-
membranes (premature) (*see also* Pregnancy, complicated by, premature rupture of membranes) O42-
uterus (during labor) O71.1
before onset of labor O71.0-
salivation (excessive) O26.89-
salpingitis O23.52-
salpingo-oophoritis O23.52-
sepsis (conditions in A40, A41) O98.81-
size date discrepancy (uterine) O26.84-
skin condition (conditions in L00-L99) O99.71-
smoking (tobacco) O99.33-
social problem O09.7-
specified condition NEC O26.89-
spotting O26.85-
streptococcus group B (GBS) carrier state O99.820
subluxation of symphysis (pubis) O26.71-
syphilis (conditions in A50-A53) O98.11-
threatened
abortion O20.0
labor O47.9
at or after 37 completed weeks of gestation O47.1
before 37 completed weeks of gestation O47.0-
thrombophlebitis (superficial) O22.2-
thrombosis O22.9-
cerebral venous O22.5-
cerebrovenous sinus O22.5-
deep O22.3-
tobacco use disorder (smoking) O99.33-
torsion of uterus O34.59-
toxemia O14.9-
transverse lie or presentation O32.2
tuberculosis (conditions in A15-A19) O98.01-
tumor (benign)
cervix O34.4-
malignant O9A.11-
uterus O34.1-
unstable lie O32.0
upper respiratory infection O99.51-
urethritis O23.2-
uterine size date discrepancy O26.84-
vaginitis or vulvitis O23.59-

Pregnancy *(continued)*
complicated by *(continued)*
varicose veins (lower extremities) O22.0-
genitals O22.1-
legs O22.0-
perineal O22.1-
vaginal or vulval O22.1-
venereal disease NEC (conditions in A63.8) O98.31-
venous disorders O22.9-
specified NEC O22.8X-
viral diseases (conditions in A80-B09, B25-B34) O98.51-
very young mother *—see* Pregnancy, complicated by, young mother
vomiting O21.9
due to diseases classified elsewhere O21.8
hyperemesis gravidarum (mild) (*see also* Hyperemesis, gravidarum) O21.0-
late (occurring after 20 weeks of gestation) O21.2
young mother
multigravida O09.62-
primigravida O09.61-
concealed O09.3-
continuing following
elective fetal reduction of one or more fetus O31.3-
intrauterine death of one or more fetus O31.2-
spontaneous abortion of one or more fetus O31.1-
cornual O00.80
with intrauterine pregnancy O00.81
ectopic (ruptured) O00.90
with intrauterine pregnancy O00.91
abdominal O00.00
with
intrauterine pregnancy O00.01
viable fetus O36.7-
cervical O00.80
with intrauterine pregnancy O00.81
complicated (by) O08.9
afibrinogenemia O08.1
cardiac arrest O08.81
chemical damage of pelvic organ(s) O08.6
circulatory collapse O08.3
defibrination syndrome O08.1
electrolyte imbalance O08.5
embolism (amniotic fluid) (blood clot) (pulmonary) (septic) O08.2
endometritis O08.0
genital tract and pelvic infection O08.0
hemorrhage (delayed) (excessive) O08.1
infection
genital tract or pelvic O08.0
kidney 008.83
urinary tract O08.83
intravascular coagulation O08.1
laceration of pelvic organ(s) O08.6
metabolic disorder O08.5
oliguria O08.4
oophoritis O08.0
parametritis O08.0
pelvic peritonitis O08.0
perforation of pelvic organ(s) O08.6

Pregnancy *(continued)*
- ectopic *(continued)*
  - complicated (by) *(continued)*
    - renal failure or shutdown O08.4
    - salpingitis or salpingo-oophoritis O08.0
    - sepsis O08.82
    - shock O08.83
      - septic O08.82
    - specified condition NEC O08.89
    - tubular necrosis (renal) O08.4
    - uremia O08.4
    - urinary infection O08.83
    - venous complication NEC O08.7
      - embolism O08.2
  - cornual O00.80
    - with intrauterine pregnancy O00.81
  - intraligamentous O00.80
    - with intrauterine pregnancy O00.81
  - mural O00.80
    - with intrauterine pregnancy O00.81
  - ovarian O00.20-
    - with intrauterine pregnancy O00.21-
  - specified site NEC O00.80
    - with intrauterine pregnancy O00.81
  - tubal (ruptured) O00.10-
    - with intrauterine pregnancy O00.11-
- examination (normal) Z34.9-
  - high-risk —*see* Pregnancy, supervision of, high-risk
  - first Z34.0-
  - specified Z34.8-
- extrauterine —*see* Pregnancy, ectopic
- fallopian O00.10-
  - with intrauterine pregnancy O00.11-
- false F45.8
- gestational carrier Z33.3
- hidden O09.3-
- high-risk —*see* Pregnancy, supervision of, high-risk
- incidental finding Z33.1
- interstitial O00.80
  - with intrauterine pregnancy O00.81
- intraligamentous O00.80
  - with intrauterine pregnancy O00.81
- intramural O00.80
  - with intrauterine pregnancy O00.81
- intraperitoneal O00.00
  - with intrauterine pregnancy O00.01
- isthmian O00.10-
  - with intrauterine pregnancy O00.11-
- mesometric (mural) O00.80
  - with intrauterine pregnancy O00.81
- molar NEC O02.0
  - complicated (by) O08.9
    - afibrinogenemia O08.1
    - cardiac arrest O08.81
    - chemical damage of pelvic organ(s) O08.6
    - circulatory collapse O08.3
    - defibrination syndrome O08.1
    - electrolyte imbalance O08.5
    - embolism (amniotic fluid) (blood clot) (pulmonary) (septic) O08.2
    - endometritis O08.0

Pregnancy *(continued)*
- molar NEC *(continued)*
  - complicated (by) *(continued)*
    - genital tract and pelvic infection O08.0
    - hemorrhage (delayed) (excessive) O08.1
    - infection
      - genital tract or pelvic O08.0
      - kidney O08.83
      - urinary tract O08.83
    - intravascular coagulation O08.1
    - laceration of pelvic organ(s) O08.6
    - metabolic disorder O08.5
    - oliguria O08.4
    - oophoritis O08.0
    - parametritis O08.0
    - pelvic peritonitis O08.0
    - perforation of pelvic organ(s) O08.6
    - renal failure or shutdown O08.4
    - salpingitis or salpingo-oophoritis O08.0
    - sepsis O08.82
    - shock O08.3
      - septic O08.82
    - specified condition NEC O08.89
    - tubular necrosis (renal) O08.4
    - uremia O08.4
    - urinary infection O08.83
    - venous complication NEC O08.7
      - embolism O08.2
  - hydatidiform (*see also* Mole, hydatidiform) O01.9-
- multiple (gestation) O30.9-
  - greater than quadruplets —*see* Pregnancy, multiple (gestation), specified NEC
  - specified NEC O30.80-
    - with
      - two or more monoamniotic fetuses O30.82-
      - two or more monochorionic fetuses O30.81-
    - two or more monoamniotic fetuses O30.82-
    - two or more monochorionic fetuses O30.81-
    - unable to determine number of placenta and number of amniotic sacs O30.89-
    - unspecified number of placenta and unspecified number of amniotic sacs O30.80-
- mural O00.80
  - with intrauterine pregnancy O00.81
- normal (supervision of) Z34.9-
  - high-risk —*see* Pregnancy, supervision of, high-risk
  - first Z34.0-
  - specified Z34.8-
- ovarian O00.20-
  - with intrauterine pregnancy O00.21-
- postmature (40 to 42 weeks) O48.0
  - more than 42 weeks gestation O48.1
- post-term (40 to 42 weeks) O48.0
- prenatal care only Z34.9-
  - high-risk —*see* Pregnancy, supervision of, high-risk
  - first Z34.0-
  - specified Z34.8-

Pregnancy *(continued)*
- prolonged (more than 42 weeks gestation) O48.1
- quadruplet O30.20-
  - with
    - two or more monoamniotic fetuses O30.22-
    - two or more monochorionic fetuses O30.21-
  - two or more monoamniotic fetuses O30.22-
  - two or more monochorionic fetuses O30.21-
  - unable to determine number of placenta and number of amniotic sacs O30.29-
  - unspecified number of placenta and unspecified number of amniotic sacs O30.20-
- quintuplet —*see* Pregnancy, multiple (gestation), specified NEC
- sextuplet —*see* Pregnancy, multiple (gestation), specified NEC
- supervision of
  - concealed pregnancy O09.3-
  - elderly mother
    - multigravida O09.52-
    - primigravida O09.51-
  - hidden pregnancy O09.3-
  - high-risk O09.9-
    - due to (history of)
      - ectopic pregnancy O09.1-
      - elderly —*see* Pregnancy, supervision, elderly mother
      - grand multiparity O09.4
      - infertility O09.0-
      - insufficient prenatal care O09.3-
      - in utero procedure during previous pregnancy O09.82-
      - in vitro fertilization O09.81-
      - molar pregnancy O09.A-
      - multiple previous pregnancies O09.4-
      - older mother —*see* Pregnancy, supervision of, elderly mother
      - poor reproductive or obstetric history NEC O09.29-
      - pre-term labor O09.21-
      - previous
        - neonatal death O09.29-
      - social problems O09.7-
      - specified NEC O09.89-
      - very young mother —*see* Pregnancy, supervision, young mother
    - resulting from in vitro fertilization O09.81-
  - normal Z34.9-
    - first Z34.0-
    - specified NEC Z34.8-
  - young mother
    - multigravida O09.62-
    - primigravida O09.61-
- triplet O30.10-
  - with
    - two or more monoamniotic fetuses O30.12-
    - two or more monochorionic fetuses O30.11-
  - two or more monoamniotic fetuses O30.12-
  - two or more monochorionic fetuses O30.11-
  - unable to determine number of placenta and number of amniotic sacs O30.19-

Pregnancy *(continued)*
- triplet *(continued)*
  - unspecified number of placenta and unspecified number of amniotic sacs O30.10-
- tubal (with abortion) (with rupture) O00.10-
  - with intrauterine pregnancy O00.11-
- twin O30.00-
  - conjoined O30.02-
  - dichorionic/diamniotic (two placenta, two amniotic sacs) O30.04-
  - monochorionic/diamniotic (one placenta, two amniotic sacs) O30.03-
  - monochorionic/monoamniotic (one placenta, one amniotic sac) O30.01-
  - unable to determine number of placenta and number of amniotic sacs O30.09-
  - unspecified number of placenta and unspecified number of amniotic sacs O30.00-
- unwanted Z64.0
- weeks of gestation
  - 8 weeks Z3A.08
  - 9 weeks Z3A.09
  - 10 weeks Z3A.10
  - 11 weeks Z3A.11
  - 12 weeks Z3A.12
  - 13 weeks Z3A.13
  - 14 weeks Z3A.14
  - 15 weeks Z3A.15
  - 16 weeks Z3A.16
  - 17 weeks Z3A.17
  - 18 weeks Z3A.18
  - 19 weeks Z3A.19
  - 20 weeks Z3A.20
  - 21 weeks Z3A.21
  - 22 weeks Z3A.22
  - 23 weeks Z3A.23
  - 24 weeks Z3A.24
  - 25 weeks Z3A.25
  - 26 weeks Z3A.26
  - 27 weeks Z3A.27
  - 28 weeks Z3A.28
  - 29 weeks Z3A.29
  - 30 weeks Z3A.30
  - 31 weeks Z3A.31
  - 32 weeks Z3A.32
  - 33 weeks Z3A.33
  - 34 weeks Z3A.34
  - 35 weeks Z3A.35
  - 36 weeks Z3A.36
  - 37 weeks Z3A.37
  - 38 weeks Z3A.38
  - 39 weeks Z3A.39
  - 40 weeks Z3A.40
  - 41 weeks Z3A.41
  - 42 weeks Z3A.42
  - greater than 42 weeks Z3A.49
  - less than 8 weeks Z3A.01
  - not specified Z3A.00

Preiser's disease —*see* Osteonecrosis, secondary, due to, trauma, metacarpus

Pre-kwashiorkor —*see* Malnutrition, severe

Preleukemia (syndrome) D46.9

Preluxation, hip, congenital Q65.6

Premature —*see also* condition
- adrenarche E27.0
- aging E34.8
- beats I49.40
  - atrial I49.1

Premature *(continued)*
- beats *(continued)*
  - auricular I49.1
  - supraventricular I49.1
- birth NEC —*see* Preterm, newborn
- closure, foramen ovale Q21.8
- contraction
  - atrial I49.1
  - atrioventricular I49.2
  - auricular I49.1
  - auriculoventricular I49.49
  - heart (extrasystole) I49.49
  - junctional I49.2
  - ventricular I49.3
- delivery (*see also* Pregnancy, complicated by, preterm labor) O60.10
- ejaculation F52.4
- infant NEC —*see* Preterm, newborn
  - light-for-dates —*see* Light for dates
- labor —*see* Pregnancy, complicated by, preterm labor
- lungs P28.0
- menopause E28.319
  - asymptomatic E28.319
  - symptomatic E28.310
- newborn
  - extreme (less than 28 completed weeks) —*see* Immaturity, extreme
  - less than 37 completed weeks —*see* Preterm, newborn
- puberty E30.1
- rupture membranes or amnion —*see* Pregnancy, complicated by, premature rupture of membranes
- senility E34.8
- thelarche E30.8
- ventricular systole I49.3

Prematurity NEC (less than 37 completed weeks) —*see* Preterm, newborn
- extreme (less than 28 completed weeks) —*see* Immaturity, extreme

Premenstrual
- dysphoric disorder (PMDD) F32.81
- tension (syndrome) N94.3

Premolarization, cuspids K00.2

Prenatal
- care, normal pregnancy —*see* Pregnancy, normal
- screening of mother (*see also* Encounter, antenatal screening) Z36.9
- teeth K00.6

Preparatory care for subsequent treatment NEC
- for dialysis Z49.01
  - peritoneal Z49.02

Prepartum —*see* condition

Preponderance, left or right ventricular I51.7

Prepuce —*see* condition

PRES (posterior reversible encephalopathy syndrome) I67.83

Presbycardia R54

Presbycusis, presbyacusia H91.1-

Presbyesophagus K22.8

Presbyophrenia F03

Presbyopia H52.4

Prescription of contraceptives (initial) Z30.019
- barrier Z30.018
- diaphragm Z30.018
- emergency (postcoital) Z30.012
- implantable subdermal Z30.017

Prescription of contraceptives *(continued)*
- injectable Z30.013
- intrauterine contraceptive device Z30.014
- pills Z30.011
- postcoital (emergency) Z30.012
- repeat Z30.40
  - barrier Z30.49
  - diaphragm Z30.49
  - implantable subdermal Z30.46
  - injectable Z30.42
  - pills Z30.41
  - specified type NEC Z30.49
  - transdermal patch hormonal Z30.45
  - vaginal ring hormonal Z30.44
- specified type NEC Z30.018
  - transdermal patch hormonal Z30.016
  - vaginal ring hormonal Z30.015

Presence (of)
- ankle-joint implant (functional) (prosthesis) Z96.66-
- aortocoronary (bypass) graft Z95.1
- arterial-venous shunt (dialysis) Z99.2
- artificial
  - eye (globe) Z97.0
  - heart (fully implantable) (mechanical) Z95.812
    - valve Z95.2
  - larynx Z96.3
  - lens (intraocular) Z96.1
  - limb (complete) (partial) Z97.1-
    - arm Z97.1-
      - bilateral Z97.15
    - leg Z97.1-
      - bilateral Z97.16
- audiological implant (functional) Z96.29
- bladder implant (functional) Z96.0
- bone
  - conduction hearing device Z96.29
  - implant (functional) NEC Z96.7
  - joint (prosthesis) —*see* Presence, joint implant
- cardiac
  - defibrillator (functional) (with synchronous cardiac pacemaker) Z95.810
  - implant or graft Z95.9
    - specified type NEC Z95.818
  - pacemaker Z95.0
  - resynchronization therapy
    - defibrillator Z95.810
    - pacemaker Z95.0
- cardioverter-defibrillator (ICD) Z95.810
- cerebrospinal fluid drainage device Z98.2
- cochlear implant (functional) Z96.21
- contact lens (es) Z97.3
- coronary artery graft or prosthesis Z95.5
- CRT-D (cardiac resynchronization therapy defibrillator) Z95.810
- CRT-P (cardiac resynchronization therapy pacemaker) Z95.0
- CSF shunt Z98.2
- dental prosthesis device Z97.2
- dentures Z97.2
- device (external) NEC Z97.8
  - cardiac NEC Z95.818
  - heart assist Z95.811
  - implanted (functional) Z96.9
    - specified NEC Z96.89
  - prosthetic Z97.8
- ear implant Z96.20
  - cochlear implant Z96.21

Presence *(continued)*
- ear implant *(continued)*
  - myringotomy tube Z96.22
  - specified type NEC Z96.29
- elbow-joint implant (functional) (prosthesis) Z96.62-
- endocrine implant (functional) NEC Z96.49
- eustachian tube stent or device (functional) Z96.29
- external hearing-aid or device Z97.4
- finger-joint implant (functional) (prosthetic) Z96.69-
- functional implant Z96.9
  - specified NEC Z96.89
- graft
  - cardiac NEC Z95.818
  - vascular NEC Z95.828
- hearing-aid or device (external) Z97.4
  - implant (bone) (cochlear) (functional) Z96.21
- heart assist device Z95.811
- heart valve implant (functional) Z95.2
  - prosthetic Z95.2
  - specified type NEC Z95.4
  - xenogenic Z95.3
- hip-joint implant (functional) (prosthesis) Z96.64-
- ICD (cardioverter-defibrillator) Z95.810
- implanted device (artificial) (functional) (prosthetic) Z96.9
  - automatic cardiac defibrillator (with synchronous cardiac pacemaker) Z95.810
  - cardiac pacemaker Z95.0
  - cochlear Z96.21
  - dental Z96.5
  - heart Z95.812
  - heart valve Z95.2
    - prosthetic Z95.2
    - specified NEC Z95.4
    - xenogenic Z95.3
  - insulin pump Z96.41
  - intraocular lens Z96.1
  - joint Z96.60
    - ankle Z96.66-
    - elbow Z96.62-
    - finger Z96.69-
    - hip Z96.64-
    - knee Z96.65-
    - shoulder Z96.61-
    - specified NEC Z96.698
    - wrist Z96.63-
  - larynx Z96.3
  - myringotomy tube Z96.22
  - otological Z96.20
    - cochlear Z96.21
    - eustachian stent Z96.29
    - myringotomy Z96.22
    - specified NEC Z96.29
    - stapes Z96.29
  - skin Z96.81
  - skull plate Z96.7
  - specified NEC Z96.89
  - urogenital Z96.0
- insulin pump (functional) Z96.41
- intestinal bypass or anastomosis Z98.0
- intraocular lens (functional) Z96.1
- intrauterine contraceptive device (IUD) Z97.5
- intravascular implant (functional) (prosthetic) NEC Z95.9
  - coronary artery Z95.5
  - defibrillator (with synchronous cardiac pacemaker) Z95.810

Presence *(continued)*
- intravascular implant *(continued)*
  - peripheral vessel (with angioplasty) Z95.820
- joint implant (prosthetic) (any) Z96.60
  - ankle —*see* Presence, ankle joint implant
  - elbow —*see* Presence, elbow joint implant
  - finger —*see* Presence, finger joint implant
  - hip —*see* Presence, hip joint implant
  - knee —*see* Presence, knee joint implant
  - shoulder —*see* Presence, shoulder joint implant
  - specified joint NEC Z96.698
  - wrist —*see* Presence, wrist joint implant
- knee-joint implant (functional) (prosthesis) Z96.65-
- laryngeal implant (functional) Z96.3
- mandibular implant (dental) Z96.5
- myringotomy tube(s) Z96.22
- orthopedic-joint implant (prosthetic) (any) —*see* Presence, joint implant
- otological implant (functional) Z96.29
- shoulder-joint implant (functional) (prosthesis) Z96.61-
- skull-plate implant Z96.7
- spectacles Z97.3
- stapes implant (functional) Z96.29
- systemic lupus erythematosus [SLE] inhibitor D68.62
- tendon implant (functional) (graft) Z96.7
- tooth root(s) implant Z96.5
- ureteral stent Z96.0
- urethral stent Z96.0
- urogenital implant (functional) Z96.0
- vascular implant or device Z95.9
  - access port device Z95.828
  - specified type NEC Z95.828
- wrist-joint implant (functional) (prosthesis) Z96.63-

Presenile —*see also* condition
- dementia F03
- premature aging E34.8

Presentation, fetal —*see* Delivery, complicated by, malposition

Prespondylolisthesis (congenital) Q76.2

Pressure
- area, skin —*see* Ulcer, pressure, by site
- brachial plexus G54.0
- brain G93.5
  - injury at birth NEC P11.1
- cerebral —*see* Pressure, brain
- chest R07.89
- cone, tentorial G93.5
- hyposystolic —*see also* Hypotension
  - incidental reading, without diagnosis of hypotension R03.1
- increased
  - intracranial (benign) G93.2
    - injury at birth P11.0
  - intraocular H40.05-
- lumbosacral plexus G54.1
- mediastinum J98.59

Pressure *(continued)*
- necrosis (chronic) —*see* Ulcer, pressure, by site
- parental, inappropriate (excessive) Z62.6
- sore (chronic) —*see* Ulcer, pressure, by site
- spinal cord G95.20
- ulcer (chronic) —*see* Ulcer, pressure, by site
- venous, increased I87.8

Pre-syncope R55

Preterm
- delivery (*see also* Pregnancy, complicated by, preterm labor) O60.10
- labor —*see* Pregnancy, complicated by, preterm labor
- newborn (infant) P07.30
  - gestational age
    - 28 completed weeks (28 weeks, 0 days through 28 weeks, 6 days) P07.31
    - 29 completed weeks (29 weeks, 0 days through 29 weeks, 6 days) P07.32
    - 30 completed weeks (30 weeks, 0 days through 30 weeks, 6 days) P07.33
    - 31 completed weeks (31 weeks, 0 days through 31 weeks, 6 days) P07.34
    - 32 completed weeks (32 weeks, 0 days through 32 weeks, 6 days) P07.35
    - 33 completed weeks (33 weeks, 0 days through 33 weeks, 6 days) P07.36
    - 34 completed weeks (34 weeks, 0 days through 34 weeks, 6 days) P07.37
    - 35 completed weeks (35 weeks, 0 days through 35 weeks, 6 days) P07.38
    - 36 completed weeks (36 weeks, 0 days through 36 weeks, 6 days) P07.39

Previa
- placenta (total) (without hemorrhage) O44.0-
  - with hemorrhage O44.1-
  - complete O44.0-
    - with hemorrhage O44.1-
  - low (*see also* Delivery, complicated, by, placenta, low) O44.4-
    - with hemorrhage O44.5-
  - marginal O44.2-
    - with hemorrhage O44.3-
  - partial O44.2-
    - with hemorrhage O44.3-
- vasa O69.4

Priapism N48.30
- due to
  - disease classified elsewhere N48.32
  - drug N48.33
  - specified cause NEC N48.39
  - trauma N48.31

Prickling sensation (skin) R20.2

Prickly heat L74.0

Primary —*see* condition

Primigravida
- elderly, affecting management of pregnancy, labor and delivery (supervision only) —*see* Pregnancy, complicated by, elderly, primigravida
- older, affecting management of pregnancy, labor and delivery (supervision only) —*see* Pregnancy, complicated by, elderly, primigravida
- very young, affecting management of pregnancy, labor and delivery (supervision only) —*see* Pregnancy, complicated by, young mother, primigravida

Primipara
- elderly, affecting management of pregnancy, labor and delivery (supervision only) —*see* Pregnancy, complicated by, elderly, primigravida
- older, affecting management of pregnancy, labor and delivery (supervision only) —*see* Pregnancy, complicated by, elderly, primigravida
- very young, affecting management of pregnancy, labor and delivery (supervision only) —*see* Pregnancy, complicated by, young mother, primigravida

Primus varus (bilateral) Q66.2

PRIND (Prolonged reversible ischemic neurologic deficit) I63.9

Pringle's disease (tuberous sclerosis) Q85.1

Prinzmetal angina I20.1

Prizefighter ear —*see* Cauliflower ear

Problem (with) (related to)
- academic Z55.8
- acculturation Z60.3
- adjustment (to)
  - change of job Z56.1
  - life-cycle transition Z60.0
  - pension Z60.0
  - retirement Z60.0
- adopted child Z62.821
- alcoholism in family Z63.72
- atypical parenting situation Z62.9
- bankruptcy Z59.8
- behavioral (adult) F69
  - drug *see*king Z76.5
- birth of sibling affecting child Z62.898
- care (of)
  - provider dependency Z74.9
    - specified NEC Z74.8
  - sick or handicapped person in family or household Z63.6
- child
  - abuse (affecting the child) —*see* Maltreatment, child
  - custody or support proceedings Z65.3
  - in welfare custody Z62.21
  - in care of non-parental family member Z62.21
  - in foster care Z62.21
  - living in orphanage or group home Z62.22
- child-rearing Z62.9
  - specified NEC Z62.898
- communication (developmental) F80.9
- conflict or discord (with)
  - boss Z56.4
  - classmates Z55.4
  - counselor Z64.4
  - employer Z56.4
  - family Z63.9
    - specified NEC Z63.8
  - probation officer Z64.4
  - social worker Z64.4
  - teachers Z55.4
  - workmates Z56.4
- conviction in legal proceedings Z65.0
  - with imprisonment Z65.1
- counselor Z64.4
- creditors Z59.8
- digestive K92.9
- drug addict in family Z63.72
- ear —*see* Disorder, ear
- economic Z59.9
  - affecting care Z59.9
  - specified NEC Z59.8
- education Z55.9
  - specified NEC Z55.8
- employment Z56.9
  - change of job Z56.1
  - discord Z56.4
  - environment Z56.5
  - sexual harassment Z56.81
  - specified NEC Z56.89
  - stress NEC Z56.6
  - stressful schedule Z56.3
  - threat of job loss Z56.2
  - unemployment Z56.0
- enuresis, child F98.0
- eye H57.9
- failed examinations (school) Z55.2
- falling Z91.81
- family (*see also* Disruption, family) Z63.9-
  - specified NEC Z63.8
- feeding (elderly) (infant) R63.3
  - newborn P92.9
    - breast P92.5
    - overfeeding P92.4
    - slow P92.2
    - specified NEC P92.8
    - underfeeding P92.3
  - nonorganic F50.89
- finance Z59.9
  - specified NEC Z59.8
- foreclosure on loan Z59.8
- foster child Z62.822
- frightening experience(s) in childhood Z62.898
- genital NEC
  - female N94.9
  - male N50.9
- health care Z75.9
  - specified NEC Z75.8
- hearing —*see* Deafness
- homelessness Z59.0
- housing Z59.9
  - inadequate Z59.1
  - isolated Z59.8
  - specified NEC Z59.8
- identity (of childhood) F93.8
- illegitimate pregnancy (unwanted) Z64.0
- illiteracy Z55.0
- impaired mobility Z74.09
- imprisonment or incarceration Z65.1
- inadequate teaching affecting education Z55.8
- inappropriate (excessive) parental pressure Z62.6
- influencing health status NEC Z78.9
- in-law Z63.1
- institutionalization, affecting child Z62.22
- intrafamilial communication Z63.8
- jealousy, child F93.8
- landlord Z59.2
- language (developmental) F80.9
- learning (developmental) F81.9
- legal Z65.3
  - conviction without imprisonment Z65.0
  - imprisonment Z65.1
  - release from prison Z65.2
- life-management Z73.9
  - specified NEC Z73.89
- life-style Z72.9
  - gambling Z72.6
  - high-risk sexual behavior (heterosexual) Z72.51
    - bisexual Z72.53
    - homosexual Z72.52
  - inappropriate eating habits Z72.4
  - self-damaging behavior NEC Z72.89
  - specified NEC Z72.89
  - tobacco use Z72.0
- literacy Z55.9
  - low level Z55.0
  - specified NEC Z55.8
- living alone Z60.2
- lodgers Z59.2
- loss of love relationship in childhood Z62.898
- marital Z63.0
  - involving
    - divorce Z63.5
    - estrangement Z63.5
    - gender identity F66
- mastication K08.89
- medical
  - care, within family Z63.6
  - facilities Z75.9
    - specified NEC Z75.8
- mental F48.9
- multiparity Z64.1
- negative life events in childhood Z62.9
  - altered pattern of family relationships Z62.898
  - frightening experience Z62.898
  - loss of
    - love relationship Z62.898
    - self-esteem Z62.898
  - physical abuse (alleged) —*see* Maltreatment, child
  - removal from home Z62.29
  - specified event NEC Z62.898
- neighbor Z59.2
- neurological NEC R29.818
- new step-parent affecting child Z62.898
- none (feared complaint unfounded) Z71.1
- occupational NEC Z56.89
- parent-child —*see* Conflict, parent-child
- personal hygiene Z91.89
- personality F69
- phase-of-life transition, adjustment Z60.0
- presence of sick or disabled person in family or household Z63.79
  - needing care Z63.6
- primary support group (family) Z63.9
  - specified NEC Z63.8
- probation officer Z64.4
- psychiatric F99
- psychosexual (development) F66
- psychosocial Z65.9
  - religious or spiritual Z65.8
  - specified NEC Z65.8
- relationship Z63.9
  - childhood F93.8
- release from prison Z65.2
- religious or spiritual Z65.8

Problem *(continued)*
removal from home affecting child Z62.29
seeking and accepting known hazardous and harmful
  behavioral or psychological interventions Z65.8
  chemical, nutritional or physical interventions Z65.8
sexual function (nonorganic) F52.9
sight H54.7
sleep disorder, child F51.9
smell *—see* Disturbance, sensation, smell
social
  environment Z60.9
    specified NEC Z60.8
  exclusion and rejection Z60.4
  worker Z64.4
speech R47.9
  developmental F80.9
  specified NEC R47.89
swallowing *—see* Dysphagia
taste *—see* Disturbance, sensation, taste
tic, child F95.0
underachievement in school Z55.3
unemployment Z56.0
  threatened Z56.2
unwanted pregnancy Z64.0
upbringing Z62.9
  specified NEC Z62.898
urinary N39.9
voice production R47.89
work schedule (stressful) Z56.3

Procedure (surgical)
converted
  arthroscopic to open Z53.33
  laparoscopic to open Z53.31
  specified procedure NEC to open Z53.39
  thoracoscopic to open Z53.32
for purpose other than remedying health state Z41.9
  specified NEC Z41.8
not done Z53.9
  because of
    administrative reasons Z53.8
    contraindication Z53.09
      smoking Z53.01
    patient's decision Z53.20
      for reasons of belief or group pressure Z53.1
      left against medical advice (AMA) Z53.21
      specified reason NEC Z53.29
    specified reason NEC Z53.8

Procidentia (uteri) N81.3

Proctalgia K62.89
fugax K59.4
spasmodic K59.4

Proctitis K62.89
amebic (acute) A06.0
chlamydial A56.3
gonococcal A54.6
granulomatous *—see* Enteritis, regional, large intestine
herpetic A60.1
radiation K62.7
tuberculous A18.32
ulcerative (chronic) K51.20
  with
    complication K51.219
      abscess K51.214
      fistula K51.213
      obstruction K51.212
      rectal bleeding K51.211
      specified NEC K51.218

Proctocele
female (without uterine prolapse) N81.6
  with uterine prolapse N81.2
    complete N81.3
male K62.3

Proctocolitis
food-induced eosinophilic K52.82
food protein-induced K52.82
mild protein-induced K52.82
mucosal - *see* Rectosigmoiditis, ulcerative

Proctoptosis K62.3

Proctorrhagia K62.5

Proctosigmoiditis K63.89
ulcerative (chronic) *—see* Rectosigmoiditis, ulcerative

Proctospasm K59.4
psychogenic F45.8

Profichet's disease *—see* Disorder, soft tissue, specified type NEC

Progeria E34.8

Prognathism (mandibular) (maxillary) M26.19

Progonoma (melanotic) *—see* Neoplasm, benign, by site

Progressive *—see* condition

Prolactinoma
specified site *—see* Neoplasm, benign, by site
unspecified site D35.2

Prolapse, prolapsed
anus, anal (canal) (sphincter) K62.2
arm or hand O32.2
  causing obstructed labor O64.4
bladder (mucosa) (sphincter) (acquired)
  congenital Q79.4
  female *—see* Cystocele
  male N32.89
breast implant (prosthetic) T85.49
cecostomy K94.09
cecum K63.4
cervix, cervical (hypertrophied) N81.2
  anterior lip, obstructing labor O65.5
  congenital Q51.828
  postpartal, old N81.2
  stump N81.85
ciliary body (traumatic) *—see* Laceration, eye (ball), with prolapse or loss of interocular tissue
colon (pedunculated) K63.4
colostomy K94.09
disc (intervertebral) *—see* Displacement, intervertebral disc
eye implant (orbital) T85.398
  lens (ocular) *—see* Complications, intraocular lens
fallopian tube N83.4-
gastric (mucosa) K31.89
genital, female N81.9
  specified NEC N81.89
globe, nontraumatic *—see* Luxation, globe
ileostomy bud K94.19
intervertebral disc *—see* Displacement, intervertebral disc
intestine (small) K63.4
iris (traumatic) *—see* Laceration, eye (ball), with prolapse or loss of interocular tissue
  nontraumatic H21.89

Prolapse, prolapsed *(continued)*
kidney N28.83
  congenital Q63.2
laryngeal muscles or ventricle J38.7
liver K76.89
meatus urinarius N36.8
mitral (valve) I34.1
ocular lens implant *—see* Complications, intraocular lens
organ or site, congenital NEC *—see* Malposition, congenital
ovary N83.4-
pelvic floor, female N81.89
perineum, female N81.89
rectum (mucosa) (sphincter) K62.3
  due to trichuris trichuria B79
spleen D73.89
stomach K31.89
umbilical cord
  complicating delivery O69.0
urachus, congenital Q64.4
ureter N28.89
  with obstruction N13.5
    with infection N13.6
ureterovesical orifice N28.89
urethra (acquired) (infected) (mucosa) N36.8
  congenital Q64.71
urinary meatus N36.8
  congenital Q64.72
uterovaginal N81.4
  complete N81.3
  incomplete N81.2
uterus (with prolapse of vagina) N81.4
  complete N81.3
  congenital Q51.818
  first degree N81.2
  in pregnancy or childbirth *—see* Pregnancy, complicated by, abnormal, uterus
  incomplete N81.2
  postpartal (old) N81.4
  second degree N81.2
  third degree N81.3
uveal (traumatic) *—see* Laceration, eye (ball), with prolapse or loss of interocular tissue
vagina (anterior) (wall) *—see* Cystocele
  with prolapse of uterus N81.4
    complete N81.3
    incomplete N81.2
  posterior wall N81.6
  posthysterectomy N99.3
vitreous (humor) H43.0-
  in wound *—see* Laceration, eye (ball), with prolapse or loss of interocular tissue
womb *—see* Prolapse, uterus

Prolapsus, female N81.9
specified NEC N81.89

Proliferation(s)
primary cutaneous CD30-positive large T-cell C86.6
prostate, atypical small acinar N42.32

Proliferative *—see* condition

Prolonged, prolongation (of)
bleeding (time) (idiopathic) R79.1
coagulation (time) R79.1
gestation (over 42 completed weeks)
  mother O48.1
  newborn P08.22
interval I44.0
labor O63.9
  first stage O63.0
  second stage O63.1

Prolonged, prolongation *(continued)*
partial thromboplastin time (PTT) R79.1
pregnancy (more than 42 weeks gestation) O48.1
prothrombin time R79.1
QT interval I45.81
uterine contractions in labor O62.4

Prominence, prominent
auricle (congenital) (ear) Q17.5
ischial spine or sacral promontory
  with disproportion (fetopelvic) O33.0
    causing obstructed labor O65.0
nose (congenital) acquired M95.0

Promiscuity *—see* High, risk, sexual behavior

Pronation
ankle *—see* Deformity, limb, foot, specified NEC
foot *—see also* Deformity, limb, foot, specified NEC
  congenital Q74.2

Prophylactic
administration of
  antibiotics, long-term Z79.2
    short-term use - omit code
  drug (*see also* Long-term (current) drug therapy (use of)) Z79.899-
medication Z79.899
organ removal (for neoplasia management) Z40.00
  breast Z40.01
  fallopian tube(s) Z40.03
    with ovary(s) Z40.02
  ovary(s) Z40.02
  specified site NEC Z40.09
surgery Z40.9
  for risk factors related to malignant neoplasm *—see* Prophylactic, organ removal
  specified NEC Z40.8
vaccination Z23

Propionic acidemia E71.121

Proptosis (ocular) *—see also* Exophthalmos
thyroid *—see* Hyperthyroidism, with goiter

Prosecution, anxiety concerning Z65.3

Prosopagnosia R48.3

Prostadynia N42.81

Prostate, prostatic *—see* condition

Prostatism *—see* Hyperplasia, prostate

Prostatitis (congestive) (suppurative) (with cystitis) N41.9
acute N41.0
cavitary N41.8
chronic N41.1
diverticular N41.8
due to Trichomonas (vaginalis) A59.02
fibrous N41.1
gonococcal (acute) (chronic) A54.22
granulomatous N41.4
hypertrophic N41.1
subacute N41.1
trichomonal A59.02
tuberculous A18.14

Prostatocystitis N41.3

Prostatorrhea N42.89

Prostatosis N42.82

Prostration R53.83
- heat *—see also* Heat, exhaustion
  - anhydrotic T67.3
  - due to
    - salt (and water) depletion T67.4
    - water depletion T67.3
- nervous F48.8
- senile R54

Protanomaly (anomalous trichromat) H53.54

Protanopia (complete) (incomplete) H53.54

Protection (against) (from) *—see* Prophylactic

Protein
- deficiency NEC *—see* Malnutrition
- malnutrition *—see* Malnutrition
- sickness (*see also* Reaction, serum) T80.69

Proteinemia R77.9

Proteinosis
- alveolar (pulmonary) J84.01
- lipid or lipoid (of Urbach) E78.89

Proteinuria R80.9
- Bence Jones R80.3
- complicating pregnancy *—see* Proteinuria, gestational
- gestational
  - complicating
    - childbirth O12.14
    - pregnancy O12.1-
      - with edema O12.2-
    - puerperium O12.15
- idiopathic R80.0
- isolated R80.0
  - with glomerular lesion N06.9
    - dense deposit disease N06.6
    - diffuse
      - crescentic glomerulonephritis N06.7
      - endocapillary proliferative glomerulonephritis N06.4
      - mesangiocapillary glomerulonephritis N06.5
    - focal and segmental hyalinosis or sclerosis N06.1
    - membranous (diffuse) N06.2
    - mesangial proliferative (diffuse) N06.3
    - minimal change N06.0
    - specified pathology NEC N06.8
- orthostatic R80.2
  - with glomerular lesion *—see* Proteinuria, isolated, with glomerular lesion
- persistent R80.1
  - with glomerular lesion *—see* Proteinuria, isolated, with glomerular lesion
- postural R80.2
  - with glomerular lesion *—see* Proteinuria, isolated, with glomerular lesion
- pre-eclamptic *—see* Pre-eclampsia
- puerperal O12.15
- specified type NEC R80.8

Proteolysis, pathologic D65

Proteus (mirabilis) (morganii)**, as cause of disease classified elsewhere** B96.4

Prothrombin gene mutation D68.52

Protoporphyria, erythropoietic E80.0

Protozoal *—see also* condition
- disease B64
  - specified NEC B60.8

Protrusion, protrusio
- acetabuli M24.7
- acetabulum (into pelvis) M24.7
- device, implant or graft (*see also* Complications, by site and type, mechanical) T85.698
  - arterial graft NEC *—see* Complication, cardiovascular device, mechanical, vascular
  - breast (implant) T85.49
  - catheter NEC T85.698
    - cystostomy T83.090
    - dialysis (renal) T82.49
      - intraperitoneal T85.691
    - infusion NEC T82.594
      - spinal (epidural) (subdural) T85.690
    - urinary (*see also* Complications, catheter, urinary), T83.098
  - electronic (electrode) (pulse generator) (stimulator)
    - bone T84.390
    - nervous system *—see* Complication, prosthetic device, mechanical, electronic nervous system stimulator
  - fixation, internal (orthopedic) NEC *—see* Complication, fixation device, mechanical
  - gastrointestinal *—see* Complications, prosthetic device, mechanical, gastrointestinal device
  - genital NEC T83.498
    - intrauterine contraceptive device T83.39
    - penile prosthesis (cylinder) (implanted) (pump) (resevoir) T83.490
    - testicular prosthesis T83.491
  - heart NEC *—see* Complication, cardiovascular device, mechanical
  - joint prosthesis *—see* Complications, joint prosthesis, mechanical, specified NEC, by site
  - ocular NEC *—see* Complications, prosthetic device, mechanical, ocular device
  - orthopedic NEC *—see* Complication, orthopedic, device, mechanical
  - specified NEC T85.628
  - urinary NEC *—see also* Complication, genitourinary, device, urinary, mechanical graft T83.29
  - vascular NEC *—see* Complication, cardiovascular device, mechanical
  - ventricular intracranial shunt T85.09
- intervertebral disc *—see* Displacement, intervertebral disc
- joint prosthesis *—see* Complications, joint prosthesis, mechanical, specified NEC, by site
- nucleus pulposus *—see* Displacement, intervertebral disc

Prune belly (syndrome) Q79.4

Prurigo (ferox) (gravis) (Hebrae) (Hebra's) (mitis) (simplex) L28.2
- Besnier's L20.0
- estivalis L56.4
- nodularis L28.1
- psychogenic F45.8

Pruritus, pruritic (essential) L29.9
- ani, anus L29.0
  - psychogenic F45.8
- anogenital L29.3
  - psychogenic F45.8
- due to onchocerca volvulus B73.1
- gravidarum *—see* Pregnancy, complicated by, specified pregnancy-related condition NEC
- hiemalis L29.8
- neurogenic (any site) F45.8
- perianal L29.0
- psychogenic (any site) F45.8
- scroti, scrotum L29.1
  - psychogenic F45.8
- senile, senilis L29.8
- specified NEC L29.8
  - psychogenic F45.8
- Trichomonas A59.9
- vulva, vulvae L29.2
  - psychogenic F45.8

Pseudarthrosis, pseudoarthrosis (bone) *—see* Nonunion, fracture
- clavicle, congenital Q74.0
- joint, following fusion or arthrodesis M96.0

Pseudoaneurysm *—see* Aneurysm

Pseudoangioma I81

Pseudoangina (pectoris) *—see* Angina

Pseudoarteriosus Q28.8

Pseudoarthrosis *—see* Pseudarthrosis

Pseudobulbar affect (PBA) F48.2

Pseudochromhidrosis L67.8

Pseudocirrhosis, liver, pericardial I31.1

Pseudocowpox B08.03

Pseudocoxalgia M91.3-

Pseudocroup J38.5

Pseudo-Cushing's syndrome, alcohol-induced E24.4

Pseudocyesis F45.8

Pseudocyst
- lung J98.4
- pancreas K86.3
- retina *—see* Cyst, retina

Pseudoelephantiasis neuroarthritica Q82.0

Pseudoexfoliation, capsule (lens) *—see* Cataract, specified NEC

Pseudofolliculitis barbae L73.1

Pseudoglioma H44.89

Pseudohemophilia (Bernuth's) (hereditary) (type B) D68.0
- Type A D69.8
- vascular D69.8

Pseudohermaphroditism Q56.3
- adrenal E25.8
- female Q56.2
  - with adrenocortical disorder E25.8
  - without adrenocortical disorder Q56.2
  - adrenal (congenital) E25.0
  - unspecified E25.9
- male Q56.1
  - with
    - adrenocortical disorder E25.8
    - androgen resistance E34.51
    - cleft scrotum Q56.1
    - feminizing testis E34.51
    - 5-alpha-reductase deficiency E29.1
  - without gonadal disorder Q56.1
  - adrenal E25.8
  - unspecified E25.9

Pseudo-Hurler's polydystrophy E77.0

Pseudohydrocephalus G93.2

Pseudohypertrophic muscular dystrophy (Erb's) G71.0

Pseudohypertrophy, muscle G71.0

Pseudohypoparathyroidism E20.1

Pseudoinsomnia F51.03

Pseudoleukemia, infantile D64.89

Pseudomembranous *—see* condition

Pseudomenses (newborn) P54.6

Pseudomenstruation (newborn) P54.6

Pseudomeningocele (cerebral) (infective) (post-traumatic) G96.19
- postprocedural (spinal) G97.82

Pseudomonas
- aeruginosa, as cause of disease classified elsewhere B96.5
- mallei infection A24.0
  - as cause of disease classified elsewhere B96.5
- pseudomallei, as cause of disease classified elsewhere B96.5

Pseudomyotonia G71.19

Pseudomyxoma peritonei C78.6

Pseudoneuritis, optic (nerve) (disc) (papilla)**, congenital** Q14.2

Pseudo-obstruction intestine (acute) (chronic) (idiopathic) (intermittent secondary) (primary) K59.8

Pseudopapilledema H47.33-
- congenital Q14.2

Pseudoparalysis
- arm or leg R29.818
- atonic, congenital P94.2

Pseudopelade L66.0

Pseudophakia Z96.1

Pseudopolyarthritis, rhizomelic M35.3

Pseudopolycythemia D75.1

Pseudopseudohypoparathyroidism E20.1

Pseudopterygium H11.81-

Pseudoptosis (eyelid) *—see* Blepharochalasis

Pseudopuberty, precocious
- female heterosexual E25.8
- male isosexual E25.8

Pseudorickets (renal) N25.0

Pseudorubella B08.20

Pseudosclerema, newborn P83.88

Pseudosclerosis (brain)
- of Westphal (Strümpell) E83.01
- Jakob's *—see* Creutzfeldt-Jakob disease or syndrome
- spastic *—see* Creutzfeldt-Jakob disease or syndrome

Pseudotetanus *—see* Convulsions

Pseudotetany R29.0
- hysterical F44.5

Pseudotruncus arteriosus Q25.49

Pseudotuberculosis A28.2
- enterocolitis A04.8
- pasteurella (infection) A28.0

Pseudotumor
- cerebri G93.2
- orbital H05.11-

Pseudoxanthoma elasticum Q82.8

- **Psilosis** (sprue) (tropical) K90.1
  - nontropical K90.0
- **Psittacosis** A70
- **Psoitis** M60.88
- **Psoriasis** L40.9
  - arthropathic L40.50
    - arthritis mutilans L40.52
    - distal interphalangeal L40.51
    - juvenile L40.54
    - other specified L40.59
    - spondylitis L40.53
  - buccal K13.29
  - flexural L40.8
  - guttate L40.4
  - mouth K13.29
  - nummular L40.0
  - plaque L40.0
  - psychogenic F54
  - pustular (generalized) L40.1
    - palmaris et plantaris L40.3
  - specified NEC L40.8
  - vulgaris L40.0
- **Psychasthenia** F48.8
- **Psychiatric disorder or problem** F99
- **Psychogenic** *—see also* condition
  - factors associated with physical conditions F54
- **Psychological and behavioral factors affecting medical condition** F59
- **Psychoneurosis, psychoneurotic** *—see also* Neurosis
  - anxiety (state) F41.1
  - depersonalization F48.1
  - hypochondriacal F45.21
  - hysteria F44.9
  - neurasthenic F48.8
  - personality NEC F60.89
- **Psychopathy, psychopathic**
  - affectionless F94.2
  - autistic F84.5
  - constitution, post-traumatic F07.81
  - personality *—see* Disorder, personality
  - sexual *—see* Deviation, sexual
  - state F60.2
- **Psychosexual identity disorder of childhood** F64.2
- **Psychosis, psychotic** F29
  - acute (transient) F23
    - hysterical F44.9
  - affective *—see* Disorder, mood
  - alcoholic F10.959
    - with
      - abuse F10.159
      - anxiety disorder F10.980
        - with
          - abuse F10.180
          - dependence F10.280
      - delirium tremens F10.231
      - delusions F10.950
        - with
          - abuse F10.150
          - dependence F10.250
      - dementia F10.97
        - with dependence F10.27
      - dependence F10.259
      - hallucinosis F10.951
        - with
          - abuse F10.151
          - dependence F10.251
      - mood disorder F10.94
        - with
          - abuse F10.14
          - dependence F10.24
      - paranoia F10.950
        - with
          - abuse F10.150
          - dependence F10.250

Psychosis, psychotic *(continued)*

- alcoholic *(continued)*
  - with *(continued)*
    - persisting amnesia F10.96
      - with dependence F10.26
  - amnestic confabulatory F10.96
    - with dependence F10.26
  - delirium tremens F10.231
  - Korsakoff's, Korsakov's, Korsakow's F10.26
  - paranoid type F10.950
    - with
      - abuse F10.150
      - dependence F10.250
- anergastic *—see* Psychosis, organic
- arteriosclerotic (simple type) (uncomplicated) F01.50
  - with behavioral disturbance F01.51
- childhood F84.0
  - atypical F84.8
- climacteric *—see* Psychosis, involutional
- confusional F29
  - acute or subacute F05
  - reactive F23
- cycloid F23
- depressive *—see* Disorder, depressive
- disintegrative (childhood) F84.3
- drug-induced *—see* F11-F19 with .x59
  - paranoid and hallucinatory states *—see* F11-F19 with .x50 or .x51
- due to or associated with
  - addiction, drug *—see* F11-F19 with .x59
  - dependence
    - alcohol F10.259
    - drug *—see* F11-F19 with .x59
  - epilepsy F06.8
  - Huntington's chorea F06.8
  - ischemia, cerebrovascular (generalized) F06.8
  - multiple sclerosis F06.8
  - physical disease F06.8
  - presenile dementia F03
  - senile dementia F03
  - vascular disease (arteriosclerotic) (cerebral) F01.50
    - with behavioral disturbance F01.51
- epileptic F06.8
- episode F23
  - due to or associated with physical condition F06.8
- exhaustive F43.0
- hallucinatory, chronic F28
- hypomanic F30.8
- hysterical (acute) F44.9
- induced F24
- infantile F84.0
  - atypical F84.8
- infective (acute) (subacute) F05
- involutional F28
  - depressive *—see* Disorder, depressive
  - melancholic *—see* Disorder, depressive
  - paranoid (state) F22
- Korsakoff's, Korsakov's, Korsakow's (nonalcoholic) F04
  - alcoholic F10.96
    - in dependence F10.26
  - induced by other psychoactive substance *—see* categories F11-F19 with .x5x
- mania, manic (single episode) F30.2
  - recurrent type F31.89

Psychosis, psychotic *(continued)*

- manic-depressive *—see* Disorder, bipolar
- menopausal *—see* Psychosis, involutional
- mixed schizophrenic and affective F25.8
- multi-infarct (cerebrovascular) F01.50
  - with behavioral disturbance F01.51
- nonorganic F29
  - specified NEC F28
- organic F09
  - due to or associated with
    - arteriosclerosis (cerebral) *—see* Psychosis, arteriosclerotic
    - cerebrovascular disease, arteriosclerotic *—see* Psychosis, arteriosclerotic
    - childbirth *—see* Psychosis, puerperal
    - Creutzfeldt-Jakob disease or syndrome *—see* Creutzfeldt-Jakob disease or syndrome
    - dependence, alcohol F10.259
    - disease
      - alcoholic liver F10.259
      - brain, arteriosclerotic *—see* Psychosis, arteriosclerotic
      - cerebrovascular F01.50
        - with behavioral disturbance F01.51
      - Creutzfeldt-Jakob *—see* Creutzfeldt-Jakob disease or syndrome
      - endocrine or metabolic F06.8
        - acute or subacute F05
      - liver, alcoholic F10.259
    - epilepsy transient (acute) F05
    - infection
      - brain (intracranial) F06.8
        - acute or subacute F05
    - intoxication
      - alcoholic (acute) F10.259
      - drug F19 with .x59 F11-
    - ischemia, cerebrovascular (generalized) *—see* Psychosis, arteriosclerotic
    - puerperium *—see* Psychosis, puerperal
    - trauma, brain (birth) (from electric current) (surgical) F06.8
      - acute or subacute F05
  - infective F06.8
    - acute or subacute F05
  - post-traumatic F06.8
    - acute or subacute F05
- paranoiac F22
- paranoid (climacteric) (involutional) (menopausal) F22
  - psychogenic (acute) F23
  - schizophrenic F20.0
  - senile F03
- postpartum F53
- presbyophrenic (type) F03
- presenile F03
- psychogenic (paranoid) F23
  - depressive F32.3
- puerperal F53
  - specified type *—see* Psychosis, by type
- reactive (brief) (transient) (emotional stress) (psychological trauma) F23
  - depressive F32.3
    - recurrent F33.3
  - excitative type F30.8
- schizoaffective F25.9
  - depressive type F25.1
  - manic type F25.0

Psychosis, psychotic *(continued)*

- schizophrenia, schizophrenic *—see* Schizophrenia
- schizophrenia-like, in epilepsy F06.2
- schizophreniform F20.81
  - affective type F25.9
  - brief F23
  - confusional type F23
  - mixed type F25.0
- senile NEC F03
  - depressed or paranoid type F03
  - simple deterioration F03
  - specified type - code to condition
- shared F24
- situational (reactive) F23
- symbiotic (childhood) F84.3
- symptomatic F09

- **Psychosomatic** *—see* Disorder, psychosomatic
- **Psychosyndrome, organic** F07.9
- **Psychotic episode due to or associated with physical condition** F06.8
- **Pterygium** (eye) H11.00-
  - amyloid H11.01-
  - central H11.02-
  - colli Q18.3
  - double H11.03-
  - peripheral
    - progressive H11.05-
    - stationary H11.04-
  - recurrent H11.06-
- **Ptilosis** (eyelid) *—see* Madarosis
- **Ptomaine** (poisoning) *—see* Poisoning, food
- **Ptosis** *—see also* Blepharoptosis
  - adiposa (false) *—see* Blepharoptosis
  - breast N64.81
  - cecum K63.4
  - colon K63.4
  - congenital (eyelid) Q10.0
    - specified site NEC *—see* Anomaly, by site
  - eyelid *—see* Blepharoptosis
    - congenital Q10.0
  - gastric K31.89
  - intestine K63.4
  - kidney N28.83
  - liver K76.89
  - renal N28.83
  - splanchnic K63.4
  - spleen D73.89
  - stomach K31.89
  - viscera K63.4
- **PTP** D69.51
- **Ptyalism** (periodic) K11.7
  - hysterical F45.8
  - pregnancy *—see* Pregnancy, complicated by, specified pregnancy-related condition NEC
  - psychogenic F45.8
- **Ptyalolithiasis** K11.5
- **Pubarche, precocious** E30.1
- **Pubertas praecox** E30.1
- **Puberty** (development state) Z00.3
  - bleeding (excessive) N92.2
  - delayed E30.0
  - precocious (constitutional) (cryptogenic) (idiopathic) E30.1
    - central E22.8
    - due to
      - ovarian hyperfunction E28.1
        - estrogen E28.0
      - testicular hyperfunction E29.0

Puberty *(continued)*
- premature E30.1
  - due to
    - adrenal cortical hyperfunction E25.8
    - pineal tumor E34.8
    - pituitary (anterior) hyperfunction E22.8

Puckering, macula *—see* Degeneration, macula, puckering

Pudenda, pudendum *—see* condition

Puente's disease (simple glandular cheilitis) K13.0

Puerperal, puerperium (complicated by, complications)
- abnormal glucose (tolerance test) O99.815
- abscess
  - areola O91.02
    - associated with lactation O91.03
  - Bartholin's gland O86.19
  - breast O91.12
    - associated with lactation O91.13
  - cervix (uteri) O86.11
  - genital organ NEC O86.19
  - kidney O86.21
  - mammary O91.12
    - associated with lactation O91.13
  - nipple O91.02
    - associated with lactation O91.03
  - peritoneum O85
  - subareolar O91.12
    - associated with lactation O91.13
  - urinary tract *—see* Puerperal, infection, urinary
  - uterus O86.12
  - vagina (wall) O86.13
  - vaginorectal O86.13
  - vulvovaginal gland O86.13
- adnexitis O86.19
- afibrinogenemia, or other coagulation defect O72.3
- albuminuria (acute) (subacute) *—see* Proteinuria, gestational
- alcohol use O99.315
- anemia O90.81
  - pre-existing (pre-pregnancy) O99.03
- anesthetic death O89.8
- apoplexy O99.43
- bariatric surgery status O99.845
- blood disorder NEC O99.13
- blood dyscrasia O72.3
- cardiomyopathy O90.3
- cerebrovascular disorder (conditions in I60-I69) O99.43
- cervicitis O86.11
- circulatory system disorder O99.43
- coagulopathy (any) O99.13
  - with hemorrhage O72.3
- complications O90.9
  - specified NEC O90.89
- convulsions *—see* Eclampsia
- cystitis O86.22
- cystopyelitis O86.29
- delirium NEC F05
- diabetes O24.93
  - gestational *—see* Puerperal, gestational diabetes
  - pre-existing O24.33
    - specified NEC O24.83
    - type 1 O24.03
    - type 2 O24.13
- digestive system disorder O99.63

Puerperal, puerperium *(continued)*
- disease O90.9
  - breast NEC O92.29
  - cerebrovascular (acute) O99.43
  - nonobstetric NEC O99.89
  - tubo-ovarian O86.19
  - Valsuani's O99.03
- disorder O90.9
  - biliary tract O26.63
  - lactation O92.70
  - liver O26.63
  - nonobstetric NEC O99.89
- disruption
  - cesarean wound O90.0
  - episiotomy wound O90.1
  - perineal laceration wound O90.1
- drug use O99.325
- eclampsia (with pre-existing hypertension) O15.2
- embolism (pulmonary) (blood clot) *—see* Embolism, obstetric, puerperal
- endocrine, nutritional or metabolic disease NEC O99.285
- endophlebitis *—see* Puerperal, phlebitis
- endotrachelitis O86.11
- failure
  - lactation (complete) O92.3
    - partial O92.4
  - renal, acute O90.4
- fever (of unknown origin) O86.4
  - septic O85
- fissure, nipple O92.12
  - associated with lactation O92.13
- fistula
  - breast (due to mastitis) O91.12
    - associated with lactation O91.13
  - nipple O91.02
    - associated with lactation O91.03
- galactophoritis O91.22
  - associated with lactation O91.23
- galactorrhea O92.6
- gastric banding status O99.845
- gastric bypass status O99.845
- gastrointestinal disease NEC O99.63
- gestational
  - diabetes O24.439
    - diet controlled O24.430
    - insulin (and diet) controlled O24.434
    - oral drug controlled (antidiabetic) (hypoglycemic) O24.435
  - edema O12.05
    - with proteinuria O12.25
  - proteinuria O12.15
- gonorrhea O98.23
- hematoma, subdural O99.43
- hemiplegia, cerebral O99.355
  - due to cerbrovascular disorder O99.43
- hemorrhage O72.1
  - brain O99.43
  - bulbar O99.43
  - cerebellar O99.43
  - cerebral O99.43
  - cortical O99.43
  - delayed or secondary O72.2
  - extradural O99.43
  - internal capsule O99.43
  - intracranial O99.43
  - intrapontine O99.43
  - meningeal O99.43
  - pontine O99.43
  - retained placenta O72.0
  - subarachnoid O99.43
  - subcortical O99.43

Puerperal, puerperium *(continued)*
- hemorrhage *(continued)*
  - subdural O99.43
  - third stage O72.0
  - uterine, delayed O72.2
  - ventricular O99.43
- hemorrhoids O87.2
- hepatorenal syndrome O90.4
- hypertension *—see* Hypertension, complicating, puerperium
- hypertrophy, breast O92.29
- induration breast (fibrous) O92.29
- infection O86.4
  - cervix O86.11
  - generalized O85
  - genital tract NEC O86.19
    - obstetric surgical wound O86.0
  - kidney (bacillus coli) O86.21
  - maternal O98.93
    - carrier state NEC O99.835
    - gonorrhea O98.23
    - human immunodeficiency virus (HIV) O98.73
    - protozoal O98.63
    - sexually transmitted NEC O98.33
    - specified NEC O98.83
    - streptococcus group B (GBS) carrier state O99.825
    - syphilis O98.13
    - tuberculosis O98.03
    - viral hepatitis O98.43
    - viral NEC O98.53
  - nipple O91.02
    - associated with lactation O91.03
  - peritoneum O85
  - renal O86.21
  - specified NEC O86.89
  - urinary (asymptomatic) (tract) NEC O86.20
    - bladder O86.22
    - kidney O86.21
    - specified site NEC O86.29
    - urethra O86.22
  - vagina O86.13
  - vein *—see* Puerperal, phlebitis
- ischemia, cerebral O99.43
- lymphangitis O86.89
  - breast O91.22
    - associated with lactation O91.23
- malignancy O9A.13
- malnutrition O25.3
- mammillitis O91.02
  - associated with lactation O91.03
- mammitis O91.22
  - associated with lactation O91.23
- mania F30.8
- mastitis O91.22
  - associated with lactation O91.23
  - purulent O91.12
    - associated with lactation O91.13
- melancholia *—see* Disorder, depressive
- mental disorder NEC O99.345
- metroperitonitis O85
- metrorrhagia *—see* Hemorrhage, postpartum
- metrosalpingitis O86.19
- metrovaginitis O86.13
- milk leg O87.1
- monoplegia, cerebral O99.43
- mood disturbance O90.6
- necrosis, liver (acute) (subacute) (conditions in subcategory K72.0) O26.63
  - with renal failure O90.4
- nervous system disorder O99.355

Puerperal, puerperium *(continued)*
- neuritis O90.89
- obesity (pre-existing prior to pregnancy) O99.215
- obesity surgery status O99.845
- occlusion, precerebral artery O99.4
- paralysis
  - bladder (sphincter) O90.89
  - cerebral O99.43
- paralytic stroke O99.43
- parametritis O85
- paravaginitis O86.13
- pelviperitonitis O85
- perimetritis O86.12
- perimetrosalpingitis O86.19
- perinephritis O86.21
- periphlebitis *—see* Puerperal phlebitis
- peritoneal infection O85
- peritonitis (pelvic) O85
- perivaginitis O86.13
- phlebitis O87.0
  - deep O87.1
  - pelvic O87.1
  - superficial O87.0
- phlebothrombosis, deep O87.1
- phlegmasia alba dolens O87.1
- placental polyp O90.89
- pneumonia, embolic *—see* Embolism, obstetric, puerperal
- pre-eclampsia *—see* Pre-eclampsia
- psychosis F53
- pyelitis O86.21
- pyelocystitis O86.29
- pyelonephritis O86.21
- pyelonephrosis O86.21
- pyemia O85
- pyocystitis O86.29
- pyohemia O85
- pyometra O86.12
- pyonephritis O86.21
- pyosalpingitis O86.19
- pyrexia (of unknown origin) O86.4
- renal
  - disease NEC O90.89
  - failure O90.4
- respiratory disease NEC O99.53
- retention
  - decidua *—see* Retention, decidua
  - placenta O72.0
  - secundines *—see* Retention, secundines
- retrated nipple O92.02
- salpingo-ovaritis O86.19
- salpingoperitonitis O85
- secondary perineal tear O90.1
- sepsis (pelvic) O85
- sepsis O85
- septic thrombophlebitis O86.81
- skin disorder NEC O99.73
- specified condition NEC O99.89
- stroke O99.43
- subinvolution (uterus) O90.89
- subluxation of symphysis (pubis) O26.73
- suppuration *—see* Puerperal, absces
- tetanus A34
- thelitis O91.02
  - associated with lactation O91.03
- thrombocytopenia O72.3
- thrombophlebitis (superficial) O87.
  - deep O87.1
  - pelvic O87.1
  - septic O86.81
- thrombosis (venous) *—see* Thrombosis, puerperal
- thyroiditis O90.5
- toxemia (eclamptic) (pre-eclamptic) (with convulsions) O15.2
- trauma, non-obstetric O9A.23

Puerperal, puerperium *(continued)*
  trauma, non-obstetric *(continued)*
    caused by abuse (physical) (suspected) O9A.33
      confirmed O9A.33
      psychological (suspected) O9A.53
        confirmed O9A.53
      sexual (suspected) O9A.43
        confirmed O9A.43
  uremia (due to renal failure) O90.4
  urethritis O86.22
  vaginitis O86.13
  varicose veins (legs) O87.4
    vulva or perineum O87.8
  venous O87.9
  vulvitis O86.19
  vulvovaginitis O86.13
  white leg O87.1

Puerperium —*see* Puerperal

Pulmolithiasis J98.4

Pulmonary —*see* condition

Pulpitis (acute) (anachoretic) (chronic) (hyperplastic) (putrescent) (suppurative) (ulcerative) K04.01
  irreversible K04.02
  reversible K04.01

Pulpless tooth K04.99

Pulse
  alternating R00.8
  bigeminal R00.8
  fast R00.0
  feeble, rapid due to shock following injury T79.4
  rapid R00.0
  weak R09.89

Pulsus alternans or trigeminus R00.8

Punch drunk F07.81

Punctum lacrimale occlusion —*see* Obstruction, lacrimal

Puncture
  abdomen, abdominal
    wall S31.139
      with
        foreign body S31.149
        penetration into peritoneal cavity S31.639
          with foreign body S31.649
    wall S31.139
      epigastric region S31.132
        with
          foreign body S31.142
          penetration into peritoneal cavity S31.632
            with foreign body S31.642
      left
        lower quadrant S31.134
          with
            foreign body S31.144
            penetration into peritoneal cavity S31.634
              with foreign body S31.644
        upper quadrant S31.131
          with
            foreign body S31.141
            penetration into peritoneal cavity S31.631
              with foreign body S31.641
      periumbilic region S31.135

Puncture *(continued)*
  abdomen *(continued)*
    wall *(continued)*
      periumbilic region *(continued)*
        with
          foreign body S31.145
          penetration into peritoneal cavity S31.635
            with foreign body S31.645
      right
        lower quadrant S31.133
          with
            foreign body S31.143
            penetration into peritoneal cavity S31.633
              with foreign body S31.643
        upper quadrant S31.130
          with
            foreign body S31.140
            penetration into peritoneal cavity S31.630
              with foreign body S31.640
  accidental, complicating surgery —*see* Complication, accidental puncture or laceration
  alveolar (process) —*see* Puncture, oral cavity
  ankle S91.039
    with
      foreign body S91.049
    left S91.032
      with
        foreign body S91.042
    right S91.031
      with
        foreign body S91.041
  anus S31.833
    with foreign body S31.834
  arm (upper) S41.139
    with foreign body S41.149
    left S41.132
      with foreign body S41.142
    lower —*see* Puncture, forearm
    right S41.131
      with foreign body S41.141
  auditory canal (external) (meatus) —*see* Puncture, ear
  auricle, ear —*see* Puncture, ear
  axilla —*see* Puncture, arm
  back —*see also* Puncture, thorax, back
    lower S31.030
      with
        foreign body S31.040
          with penetration into retroperitoneal space S31.041
        penetration into retroperitoneal space S31.031
  bladder (traumatic) S37.29
    nontraumatic N32.89
  breast S21.039
    with foreign body S21.049
    left S21.032
      with foreign body S21.042
    right S21.031
      with foreign body S21.041
  buttock S31.803
    with foreign body S31.804
    left S31.823
      with foreign body S31.824
    right S31.813
      with foreign body S31.814

Puncture *(continued)*
  by
    device, implant or graft —*see* Complications, by site and type, mechanical
    foreign body left accidentally in operative wound T81.539
    instrument (any) during a procedure, accidental —*see* Puncture, accidental complicating surgery
  calf —*see* Puncture, leg
  canaliculus lacrimalis —*see* Puncture, eyelid
  canthus, eye —*see* Puncture, eyelid
  cervical esophagus S11.23
    with foreign body S11.24
  cheek (external) S01.439
    with foreign body S01.449
    left S01.432
      with foreign body S01.442
    right S01.431
      with foreign body S01.441
    internal —*see* Puncture, oral cavity
  chest wall —*see* Puncture, thorax
  chin —*see* Puncture, head, specified site NEC
  clitoris —*see* Puncture, vulva
  costal region —*see* Puncture, thorax
  digit(s)
    hand —*see* Puncture, finger
    foot —*see* Puncture, toe
  ear (canal) (external) S01.339
    with foreign body S01.349
    left S01.332
      with foreign body S01.342
    right S01.331
      with foreign body S01.341
    drum S09.2-
  elbow S51.039
    with
      foreign body S51.049
    left S51.032
      with
        foreign body S51.042
    right S51.031
      with
        foreign body S51.041
  epididymis —*see* Puncture, testis
  epigastric region —*see* Puncture, abdomen, wall, epigastric
  epiglottis S11.83
    with foreign body S11.84
  esophagus
    cervical S11.23
      with foreign body S11.24
    thoracic S27.818
  eyeball S05.6-
    with foreign body S05.5-
  eyebrow —*see* Puncture, eyelid
  eyelid S01.13-
    with foreign body S01.14-
    left S01.132
      with foreign body S01.142
    right S01.131
      with foreign body S01.141
  face NEC —*see* Puncture, head, specified site NEC
  finger(s) S61.239
    with
      damage to nail S61.339
        with
          foreign body S61.349
      foreign body S61.249
    index S61.238

Puncture *(continued)*
  finger *(continued)*
    index *(continued)*
      with
        damage to nail S61.338
          with
            foreign body S61.348
        foreign body S61.248
      left S61.231
        with
          damage to nail S61.331
            with
              foreign body S61.341
          foreign body S61.241
      right S61.230
        with
          damage to nail S61.330
            with
              foreign body S61.340
          foreign body S61.240
    little S61.238
      with
        damage to nail S61.338
          with
            foreign body S61.348
        foreign body S61.248
      left S61.237
        with
          damage to nail S61.337
            with
              foreign body S61.347
          foreign body S61.247
      right S61.236
        with
          damage to nail S61.336
            with
              foreign body S61.346
          foreign body S61.246
    middle S61.238
      with
        damage to nail S61.338
          with
            foreign body S61.348
        foreign body S61.248
      left S61.233
        with
          damage to nail S61.333
            with
              foreign body S61.343
          foreign body S61.243
      right S61.232
        with
          damage to nail S61.332
            with
              foreign body S61.342
          foreign body S61.242
    ring S61.238
      with
        damage to nail S61.338
          with
            foreign body S61.348
        foreign body S61.248
      left S61.235
        with
          damage to nail S61.335
            with
              foreign body S61.345
          foreign body S61.245
      right S61.234
        with
          damage to nail S61.334
            with
              foreign body S61.344
          foreign body S61.244
  flank S31.139
    with foreign body S31.149
  foot (except toe(s) alone) S91.339
    with foreign body S91.349
    left S91.332

Puncture *(continued)*
foot *(continued)*
left *(continued)*
with foreign body S91.342
right S91.331
with foreign body S91.341
toe —*see* Puncture, toe
forearm S51.839
with
foreign body S51.849
elbow only —*see* Puncture, elbow
left S51.832
with
foreign body S51.842
right S51.831
with
foreign body S51.841
forehead —*see* Puncture, head, specified site NEC
genital organs, external
female S31.532
with foreign body S31.542
vagina —*see* Puncture, vagina
vulva —*see* Puncture, vulva
male S31.531
with foreign body S31.541
penis —*see* Puncture, penis
scrotum —*see* Puncture, scrotum
testis —*see* Puncture, testis
groin —*see* Puncture, abdomen, wall
gum —*see* Puncture, oral cavity
hand S61.439
with
foreign body S61.449
finger —*see* Puncture, finger
left S61.432
with
foreign body S61.442
right S61.431
with
foreign body S61.441
thumb —*see* Puncture, thumb
head S01.93
with foreign body S01.94
cheek —*see* Puncture, cheek
ear —*see* Puncture, ear
eyelid —*see* Puncture, eyelid
lip —*see* Puncture, oral cavity
nose —*see* Puncture, nose
oral cavity —*see* Puncture, oral cavity
scalp S01.03
with foreign body S01.04
specified site NEC S01.83
with foreign body S01.84
temporomandibular area —*see* Puncture, cheek
heart S26.99
with hemopericardium S26.09
without hemopericardium S26.19
heel —*see* Puncture, foot
hip S71.039
with foreign body S71.049
left S71.032
with foreign body S71.042
right S71.031
with foreign body S71.041
hymen —*see* Puncture, vagina
hypochondrium —*see* Puncture, abdomen, wall
hypogastric region —*see* Puncture, abdomen, wall
inguinal region —*see* Puncture, abdomen, wall
instep —*see* Puncture, foot
internal organs —*see* Injury, by site
interscapular region —*see* Puncture, thorax, back

Puncture *(continued)*
intestine
large
colon S36.599
ascending S36.590
descending S36.592
sigmoid S36.593
specified site NEC S36.598
transverse S36.591
rectum S36.69
small S36.499
duodenum S36.490
specified site NEC S36.498
intra-abdominal organ S36.99
gallbladder S36.128
intestine —*see* Puncture, intestine
liver S36.118
pancreas —*see* Puncture, pancreas
peritoneum S36.81
specified site NEC S36.898
spleen S36.09
stomach S36.39
jaw —*see* Puncture, head, specified site NEC
knee S81.039
with foreign body S81.049
left S81.032
with foreign body S81.042
right S81.031
with foreign body S81.041
labium (majus) (minus) —*see* Puncture, vulva
lacrimal duct —*see* Puncture, eyelid
larynx S11.013
with foreign body S11.014
leg (lower) S81.839
with foreign body S81.849
foot —*see* Puncture, foot
knee —*see* Puncture, knee
left S81.832
with foreign body S81.842
right S81.831
with foreign body S81.841
upper —*see* Puncture, thigh
lip S01.531
with foreign body S01.541
loin —*see* Puncture, abdomen, wall
lower back —*see* Puncture, back, lower
lumbar region —*see* Puncture, back, lower
malar region —*see* Puncture, head, specified site NEC
mammary —*see* Puncture, breast
mastoid region —*see* Puncture, head, specified site NEC
mouth —*see* Puncture, oral cavity
nail
finger —*see* Puncture, finger, with damage to nail
toe —*see* Puncture, toe, with damage to nail
nasal (septum) (sinus) —*see* Puncture, nose
nasopharynx —*see* Puncture, head, specified site NEC
neck S11.93
with foreign body S11.94
involving
cervical esophagus —*see* Puncture, cervical esophagus
larynx —*see* Puncture, larynx
pharynx —*see* Puncture, pharynx
thyroid gland —*see* Puncture, thyroid gland
trachea —*see* Puncture, trachea
specified site NEC S11.83
with foreign body S11.84

Puncture *(continued)*
nose (septum) (sinus) S01.23
with foreign body S01.24
ocular —*see* Puncture, eyeball
oral cavity S01.532
with foreign body S01.542
orbit S05.4-
palate —*see* Puncture, oral cavity
palm —*see* Puncture, hand
pancreas S36.299
body S36.291
head S36.290
tail S36.292
pelvis —*see* Puncture, back, lower
penis S31.23
with foreign body S31.24
perineum
female S31.43
with foreign body S31.44
male S31.139
with foreign body S31.149
periocular area (with or without lacrimal passages) —*see* Puncture, eyelid
phalanges
finger —*see* Puncture, finger
toe —*see* Puncture, toe
pharynx S11.23
with foreign body S11.24
pinna —*see* Puncture, ear
popliteal space —*see* Puncture, knee
prepuce —*see* Puncture, penis
pubic region S31.139
with foreign body S31.149
pudendum —*see* Puncture, genital organs, external
rectovaginal septum —*see* Puncture, vagina
sacral region —*see* Puncture, back, lower
sacroiliac region —*see* Puncture, back, lower
salivary gland —*see* Puncture, oral cavity
scalp S01.03
with foreign body S01.04
scapular region —*see* Puncture, shoulder
scrotum S31.33
with foreign body S31.34
shin —*see* Puncture, leg
shoulder S41.039
with foreign body S41.049
left S41.032
with foreign body S41.042
right S41.031
with foreign body S41.041
spermatic cord —*see* Puncture, testis
sternal region —*see* Puncture, thorax, front
submaxillary region —*see* Puncture, head, specified site NEC
submental region —*see* Puncture, head, specified site NEC
subungual
finger(s) —*see* Puncture, finger, with damage to nail
toe —*see* Puncture, toe, with damage to nail
supraclavicular fossa —*see* Puncture, neck, specified site NEC
temple, temporal region —*see* Puncture, head, specified site NEC
temporomandibular area —*see* Puncture, cheek
testis S31.33
with foreign body S31.34
thigh S71.139

Puncture *(continued)*
thigh *(continued)*
with foreign body S71.149
left S71.132
with foreign body S71.142
right S71.131
with foreign body S71.141
thorax, thoracic (wall) S21.93
with foreign body S21.94
back S21.23-
with
foreign body S21.24-
with penetration S21.44
penetration S21.43
breast —*see* Puncture, breast
front S21.13-
with
foreign body S21.14-
with penetration S21.34
penetration S21.33
throat —*see* Puncture, neck
thumb S61.039
with
damage to nail S61.139
with
foreign body S61.149
foreign body S61.049
left S61.032
with
damage to nail S61.132
with
foreign body S61.142
foreign body S61.042
right S61.031
with
damage to nail S61.131
with
foreign body S61.141
foreign body S61.041
thyroid gland S11.13
with foreign body S11.14
toe(s) S91.139
with
damage to nail S91.239
with
foreign body S91.249
foreign body S91.149
great S91.133
with
damage to nail S91.233
with
foreign body S91.243
foreign body S91.143
left S91.132
with
damage to nail S91.232
with
foreign body S91.242
foreign body S91.142
right S91.131
with
damage to nail S91.231
with
foreign body S91.241
foreign body S91.141
lesser S91.136
with
damage to nail S91.236
with
foreign body S91.246
foreign body S91.146
left S91.135
with
damage to nail S91.235
with
foreign body S91.245
foreign body S91.145
right S91.134

uncture *(continued)*
toe(s) *(continued)*
lesser *(continued)*
right *(continued)*
with
damage to nail S91.234
with
foreign body S91.244
foreign body S91.144
tongue —*see* Puncture, oral cavity
trachea S11.023
with foreign body S11.024
tunica vaginalis —*see* Puncture, testis
tympanum, tympanic membrane S09.2-
umbilical region S31.135
with foreign body S31.145
uvula —*see* Puncture, oral cavity
vagina S31.43
with foreign body S31.44
vocal cords S11.033
with foreign body S11.034
vulva S31.43
with foreign body S31.44
wrist S61.539
with
foreign body S61.549
left S61.532
with
foreign body S61.542
right S61.531
with
foreign body S61.541

PUO (pyrexia of unknown origin) R50.9

Pupillary membrane (persistent) Q13.89

Pupillotonia —*see* Anomaly, pupil, function, tonic pupil

Purpura D69.2
abdominal D69.0
allergic D69.0
anaphylactoid D69.0
annularis telangiectodes L81.7
arthritic D69.0
autoerythrocyte sensitization D69.2
autoimmune D69.0
bacterial D69.0
Bateman's (senile) D69.2
capillary fragility (hereditary) (idiopathic) D69.8
cryoglobulinemic D89.1
Devil's pinches D69.2
fibrinolytic —*see* Fibrinolysis
fulminans, fulminous D65
gangrenous D65
hemorrhagic, hemorrhagica D69.3
not due to thrombocytopenia D69.0
Henoch (-Schönlein) (allergic) D69.0
hypergammaglobulinemic (benign) (Waldenström) D89.0
idiopathic (thrombocytopenic) D69.3
nonthrombocytopenic D69.0
immune thrombocytopenic D69.3
infectious D69.0
malignant D69.0
neonatorum P54.5
nervosa D69.0
newborn P54.5
nonthrombocytopenic D69.2
hemorrhagic D69.0
idiopathic D69.0
nonthrombopenic D69.2
peliosis rheumatica D69.0

Purpura *(continued)*
posttransfusion (post-transfusion) (from (fresh) whole blood or blood products) D69.51
primary D69.49
red cell membrane sensitivity D69.2
rheumatica D69.0
Schönlein (-Henoch) (allergic) D69.0
scorbutic E54 *[D77]*
senile D69.2
simplex D69.2
symptomatica D69.0
telangiectasia annularis L81.7
thrombocytopenic D69.49
congenital D69.42
hemorrhagic D69.3
hereditary D69.42
idiopathic D69.3
immune D69.3
neonatal, transitory P61.0
thrombotic M31.1
thrombohemolytic —*see* Fibrinolysis
thrombolytic —*see* Fibrinolysis
thrombopenic D69.49
thrombotic, thrombocytopenic M31.1
toxic D69.0
vascular D69.0
visceral symptoms D69.0

Purpuric spots R23.3

Purulent —*see* condition

Pus
in
stool R19.5
urine N39.0
tube (rupture) —*see* Salpingo-oophoritis

Pustular rash L08.0

Pustule (nonmalignant) L08.9
malignant A22.0

Pustulosis palmaris et plantaris L40.3

Putnam (-Dana) **disease or syndrome** —*see* Degeneration, combined

Putrescent pulp (dental) K04.1

Pyarthritis, pyarthrosis —*see* Arthritis, pyogenic or pyemic
tuberculous —*see* Tuberculosis, joint

Pyelectasis —*see* Hydronephrosis

Pyelitis (congenital) (uremic) —*see also* Pyelonephritis
with
calculus —*see* category N20
with hydronephrosis N13.2
contracted kidney N11.9
acute N10
chronic N11.9
with calculus —*see* category N20
with hydronephrosis N13.2
cystica N28.84
puerperal (postpartum) O86.21
tuberculous A18.11

Pyelocystitis —*see* Pyelonephritis

Pyelonephritis —*see also* Nephritis, tubulo-interstitial
with
calculus —*see* category N20
with hydronephrosis N13.2
contracted kidney N11.9
acute N10
calculous —*see* category N20
with hydronephrosis N13.2

Pyelonephritis *(continued)*
chronic N11.9
with calculus —*see* category N20
with hydronephrosis N13.2
associated with ureteral obstruction or stricture N11.1
nonobstructive N11.8
with reflux (vesicoureteral) N11.0
obstructive N11.1
specified NEC N11.8
in (due to)
brucellosis A23.9 *[N16]*
cryoglobulinemia (mixed) D89.1 *[N16]*
cystinosis E72.04
diphtheria A36.84
glycogen storage disease E74.09 *[N16]*
leukemia NEC C95.9- *[N16]*
lymphoma NEC C85.90 *[N16]*
multiple myeloma C90.0- *[N16]*
obstruction N11.1
Salmonella infection A02.25
sarcoidosis D86.84
sepsis A41.9 *[N16]*
Sjögren's disease M35.04
toxoplasmosis B58.83
transplant rejection T86.91 *[N16]*
Wilson's disease E83.01 *[N16]*
nonobstructive N12
with reflux (vesicoureteral) N11.0
chronic N11.8
syphilitic A52.75

Pyelonephrosis (obstructive) N11.1
chronic N11.9

Pyelophlebitis I80.8

Pyeloureteritis cystica N28.85

Pyemia, pyemic (fever) (infection) (purulent) —*see also* Sepsis
joint —*see* Arthritis, pyogenic or pyemic
liver K75.1
pneumococcal A40.3
portal K75.1
postvaccinal T88.0
puerperal, postpartum, childbirth O85
specified organism NEC A41.89
tuberculous —*see* Tuberculosis, miliary

Pygopagus Q89.4

Pyknoepilepsy (idiopathic) —*see* Pyknolepsy

Pyknolepsy G40.A09
intractable G40.A19
with status epilepticus G40.A11
without status epilepticus G40.A19
not intractable G40.A09
with status epilepticus G40.A01
without status epilepticus G40.A09

Pylephlebitis K75.1

Pyle's syndrome Q78.5

Pylethrombophlebitis K75.1

Pylethrombosis K75.1

Pyloritis K29.90
with bleeding K29.91

Pylorospasm (reflex) **NEC** K31.3
congenital or infantile Q40.0
newborn Q40.0
neurotic F45.8
psychogenic F45.8

Pylorus, pyloric —*see* condition

Pyoarthrosis —*see* Arthritis, pyogenic or pyemic

Pyocele
mastoid —*see* Mastoiditis, acute
sinus (accessory) —*see* Sinusitis
turbinate (bone) J32.9
urethra (*see also* Urethritis) N34.0

Pyocolpos —*see* Vaginitis

Pyocystitis N30.80
with hematuria N30.81

Pyoderma, pyodermia L08.0
gangrenosum L88
newborn P39.4
phagedenic L88
vegetans L08.81

Pyodermatitis L08.0
vegetans L08.81

Pyogenic —*see* condition

Pyohydronephrosis N13.6

Pyometra, pyometrium, pyometritis —*see* Endometritis

Pyomyositis (tropical) —*see* Myositis, infective

Pyonephritis N12

Pyonephrosis N13.6
tuberculous A18.11

Pyo-oophoritis —*see* Salpingo-oophoritis

Pyo-ovarium —*see* Salpingo-oophoritis

Pyopericarditis, pyopericardium I30.1

Pyophlebitis —*see* Phlebitis

Pyopneumopericardium I30.1

Pyopneumothorax (infective) J86.9
with fistula J86.0
tuberculous NEC A15.6

Pyosalpinx, pyosalpingitis —*see also* Salpingo-oophoritis

Pyothorax J86.9
with fistula J86.0
tuberculous NEC A15.6

Pyoureter N28.89
tuberculous A18.11

Pyramidopallidonigral syndrome G20

Pyrexia (of unknown origin) R50.9
atmospheric T67.0
during labor NEC O75.2
heat T67.0
newborn P81.9
environmentally-induced P81.0
persistent R50.9
puerperal O86.4

Pyroglobulinemia NEC E88.09

Pyromania F63.1

Pyrosis R12

Pyuria (bacterial) N39.0

Q

Q fever A78
with pneumonia A78

Quadricuspid aortic valve Q23.8

Quadrilateral fever A78

Quadriparesis —*see* Quadriplegia
meaning muscle weakness M62.81

Quadriplegia G82.50
- complete
  - C1-C4 level G82.51
  - C5-C7 level G82.53
- congenital (cerebral) (spinal) G80.8
  - spastic G80.0
- embolic (current episode) I63.4-
- functional R53.2
- incomplete
  - C1-C4 level G82.52
  - C5-C7 level G82.54
- thrombotic (current episode) I63.3-
- traumatic -- code to injury with seventh character S
  - current episode *—see* Injury, spinal (cord), cervical

Quadruplet, pregnancy *—see* Pregnancy, quadruplet

Quarrelsomeness F60.3

Queensland fever A77.3

Quervain's disease M65.4
- thyroid E06.1

Queyrat's erythroplasia D07.4
- penis D07.4
- specified site *—see* Neoplasm, skin, in situ
- unspecified site D07.4

Quincke's disease or edema T78.3
- hereditary D84.1

Quinsy (gangrenous) J36

Quintan fever A79.0

Quintuplet, pregnancy *—see* Pregnancy, quintuplet

R

Rabbit fever *—see* Tularemia

Rabies A82.9
- contact Z20.3
- exposure to Z20.3
- inoculation reaction *—see* Complications, vaccination
- sylvatic A82.0
- urban A82.1

Rachischisis *—see* Spina bifida

Rachitic *—see also* condition
- deformities of spine (late effect) (sequelae) E64.3
- pelvis (late effect) (sequelae) E64.3
  - with disproportion (fetopelvic) O33.0
    - causing obstructed labor O65.0

Rachitis, rachitism (acute) (tarda) *—see also* Rickets
- renalis N25.0
- sequelae E64.3

Radial nerve *—see* condition

Radiation
- burn *—see* Burn
- effects NOS T66
- sickness NOS T66
- therapy, encounter for Z51.0

Radiculitis (pressure) (vertebrogenic) *—see* Radiculopathy

Radiculomyelitis *—see also* Encephalitis
- toxic, due to
  - Clostridium tetani A35
  - Corynebacterium diphtheriae A36.82

Radiculopathy M54.10
- cervical region M54.12
- cervicothoracic region M54.13

Radiculopathy *(continued)*
- due to
  - disc disorder
    - C3 M50.11
    - C4 M50.11
    - C5 M50.121
    - C6 M50.122
    - C7 M50.123
    - C8 M50.13
  - displacement of intervertebral disc *—see* Disorder, disc, with, radiculopathy
- leg M54.1-
- lumbar region M54.16
- lumbosacral region M54.17
- occipito-atlanto-axial region M54.11
- postherpetic B02.29
- sacrococcygeal region M54.18
- syphilitic A52.11
- thoracic region (with visceral pain) M54.14
- thoracolumbar region M54.15

Radiodermal burns (acute, chronic, or occupational) *—see* Burn

Radiodermatitis L58.9
- acute L58.0
- chronic L58.1

Radiotherapy session Z51.0

RAEB (refractory anemia with excess blasts) D46.2-

Rage, meaning rabies *—see* Rabies

Ragpicker's disease A22.1

Ragsorter's disease A22.1

Raillietiniasis B71.8

Railroad neurosis F48.8

Railway spine F48.8

Raised *—see also* Elevated
- antibody titer R76.0

Rake teeth, tooth M26.39

Rales R09.89

Ramifying renal pelvis Q63.8

Ramsay-Hunt disease or syndrome (*see also* Hunt's disease) B02.21
- meaning dyssynergia cerebellaris myoclonica G11.1

Ranula K11.6
- congenital Q38.4

Rape
- adult
  - confirmed T74.21
  - suspected T76.21
- alleged, observation or examination, ruled out
  - adult Z04.41
  - child Z04.42
- child
  - confirmed T74.22
  - suspected T76.22

Rapid
- feeble pulse, due to shock, following injury T79.4
- heart (beat) R00.0
  - psychogenic F45.8
- second stage (delivery) O62.3
- time-zone change syndrome *—see* Disorder, sleep, circadian rhythm, psychogenic

Rarefaction, bone *—see* Disorder, bone, density and structure, specified NEC

Rash (toxic) R21
- canker A38.9
- diaper L22

Rash *(continued)*
- drug (internal use) L27.0
  - contact (*see also* Dermatitis, due to, drugs, external) L25.1
- following immunization T88.1
- food *—see* Dermatitis, due to, food
- heat L74.0
- napkin (psoriasiform) L22
- nettle *—see* Urticaria
- pustular L08.0
- rose R21
  - epidemic B06.9
- scarlet A38.9
- serum (*see also* Reaction, serum) T80.69
- wandering tongue K14.1

Rasmussen aneurysm *—see* Tuberculosis, pulmonary

Rasmussen encephalitis G04.81

Rat-bite fever A25.9
- due to Streptobacillus moniliformis A25.1
- spirochetal (morsus muris) A25.0

Rathke's pouch tumor D44.3

Raymond (-Céstan) **syndrome** I65.8

Raynaud's disease, phenomenon or syndrome (secondary) I73.00
- with gangrene (symmetric) I73.01

RDS (newborn) (type I) P22.0
- type II P22.1

Reaction *—see also* Disorder
- adaptation *—see* Disorder, adjustment
- adjustment (anxiety) (conduct disorder) (depressiveness) (distress) *—see* Disorder, adjustment
  - with
    - mutism, elective (child) (adolescent) F94.0
- adverse
  - food (any) (ingested) NEC T78.1
    - anaphylactic *—see* Shock, anaphylactic, due to food
- affective *—see* Disorder, mood
- allergic *—see* Allergy
- anaphylactic *—see* Shock, anaphylactic
- anaphylactoid *—see* Shock, anaphylactic
- anesthesia *—see* Anesthesia, complication
- antitoxin (prophylactic) (therapeutic) *—see* Complications, vaccination
- anxiety F41.1
- Arthus *—see* Arthus' phenomenon
- asthenic F48.8
- combat and operational stress F43.0
- compulsive F42.8
- conversion F44.9
- crisis, acute F43.0
- deoxyribonuclease (DNA) (DNase) hypersensitivity D69.2
- depressive (single episode) F32.9
  - affective (single episode) F31.4
    - recurrent episode F33.9
  - neurotic F34.1
  - psychoneurotic F34.1
  - psychotic F32.3
  - recurrent *—see* Disorder, depressive, recurrent
- dissociative F44.9
- drug NEC T88.7
  - addictive *—see* Dependence, drug
    - transmitted via placenta or breast milk *—see* Absorption, drug, addictive, through placenta

Reaction *(continued)*
- drug *(continued)*
  - allergic *—see* Allergy, drug
  - lichenoid L43.2
  - newborn P93.8
    - gray baby syndrome P93.0
  - overdose or poisoning (by accident) *—see* Table of Drug and Chemicals, by drug, poisoning
  - photoallergic L56.1
  - phototoxic L56.0
  - withdrawal *—see* Dependence, b drug, with, withdrawal
    - infant of dependent mother P96.1
    - newborn P96.1
  - wrong substance given or taken (by accident) *—see* Table of Drugs and Chemicals, by drug poisoning
- fear F40.9
  - child (abnormal) F93.8
- febrile nonhemolytic transfusion (FNHTR) R50.84
- fluid loss, cerebrospinal G97.1
- foreign
  - body NEC *—see* Granuloma, foreign body
    - in operative wound (inadvertently left) *—see* Foreign body, accidentally left during a procedure
  - substance accidentally left during a procedure (chemical) (powder) (talc) T81.60
    - aseptic peritonitis T81.61
    - body or object (instrument) (sponge) (swab) *—see* Foreign body, accidentally left during a procedure
    - specified reaction NEC T81.69
- grief *—see* Disorder, adjustment
- Herxheimer's R68.89
- hyperkinetic *—see* Hyperkinesia
- hypochondriacal F45.20
- hypoglycemic, due to insulin E16.0
  - with coma (diabetic) *—see* Diabetes, coma
    - nondiabetic E15
  - therapeutic misadventure *—see* subcategory T38.3
- hypomanic F30.8
- hysterical F44.9
- immunization *—see* Complications, vaccination
- incompatibility
  - ABO blood group (infusion) (transfusion) *—see* Complication(s), transfusion, incompatibility reaction, ABO
    - delayed serologic T80.39
  - minor blood group (Duffy) (E) (K (ell)) (Kidd) (Lewis) (M) (N) (P) (S) T80.89
  - Rh (factor) (infusion) (transfusion *—see* Complication(s), transfusion, incompatibility reaction, Rh (factor)
- inflammatory *—see* Infection
- infusion *—see* Complications, infusion
- inoculation (immune serum) *—see* Complications, vaccination
- insulin T38.3-
- involutional psychotic *—see* Disorder, depressive
- leukemoid D72.823
  - basophilic D72.823
  - lymphocytic D72.823
  - monocytic D72.823

Reaction *(continued)*
- leukemoid *(continued)*
  - myelocytic D72.823
  - neutrophilic D72.823
- LSD (acute)
  - due to drug abuse —*see* Abuse, drug, hallucinogen
  - due to drug dependence —*see* Dependence, drug, hallucinogen
- lumbar puncture G97.1
- manic-depressive —*see* Disorder, bipolar
- neurasthenic F48.8
- neurogenic —*see* Neurosis
- neurotic F48.9
- neurotic-depressive F34.1
- nitritoid —*see* Crisis, nitritoid
- nonspecific
  - to
    - cell mediated immunity measurement of gamma interferon antigen response without active tuberculosis R76.12
    - QuantiFERON-TB test (QFT) without active tuberculosis R76.12
    - tuberculin test (*see also* Reaction, tuberculin skin test) R76.11
- obsessive-compulsive F42.8
- organic, acute or subacute —*see* Delirium
- paranoid (acute) F23
  - chronic F22
  - senile F03
- passive dependency F60.7
- phobic F40.9
- post-traumatic stress, uncomplicated Z73.3
- psychogenic F99
- psychoneurotic —*see also* Neurosis
  - compulsive F42.8
  - depersonalization F48.1
  - depressive F34.1
  - hypochondriacal F45.20
  - neurasthenic F48.8
  - obsessive F42.8
- psychophysiologic —*see* Disorder, somatoform
- psychosomatic —*see* Disorder, somatoform
- psychotic —*see* Psychosis
- scarlet fever toxin —*see* Complications, vaccination
- schizophrenic F23
  - acute (brief) (undifferentiated) F23
  - latent F21
  - undifferentiated (acute) (brief) F23
- serological for syphilis —*see* Serology for syphilis
- serum T80.69
  - anaphylactic (immediate) —*see also* Shock, anaphylactic T80.59
  - specified reaction NEC
    - due to
      - administration of blood and blood products T80.61
      - immunization T80.62
      - serum specified NEC T80.69
      - vaccination T80.62
- situational —*see* Disorder, adjustment
- somatization —*see* Disorder, somatoform
- spinal puncture G97.1
- stress (severe) F43.9

Reaction *(continued)*
- stress (severe) *(continued)*
  - acute (agitation) ("daze") (disorientation) (disturbance of consciousness) (flight reaction) (fugue) F43.0
  - specified NEC F43.8
- surgical procedure —*see* Complications, surgical procedure
- tetanus antitoxin —*see* Complications, vaccination
- toxic, to local anesthesia T88.59
  - in labor and delivery O74.4
  - in pregnancy O29.3X-
  - postpartum, puerperal O89.3
- toxin-antitoxin —*see* Complications, vaccination
- transfusion (blood) (bone marrow) (lymphocytes) (allergic) —*see* Complications, transfusion
- tuberculin skin test, abnormal R76.11
- vaccination (any) —*see* Complications, vaccination
- withdrawing, child or adolescent F93.8

Reactive airway disease —*see* Asthma

Reactive depression —*see* Reaction, depressive

Rearrangement
- chromosomal
  - balanced (in) Q95.9
    - abnormal individual (autosomal) Q95.2
    - non-sex (autosomal) chromosomes Q95.2
    - sex/non-sex chromosomes Q95.3
    - specified NEC Q95.8

Recalcitrant patient —*see* Noncompliance

Recanalization, thrombus —*see* Thrombosis

Recession, receding
- chamber angle (eye) H21.55-
- chin M26.09
- gingival (postinfective) (postoperative)
  - generalized K06.020
    - minimal K06.021
    - moderate K06.022
    - severe K06.023
  - localized K06.010
    - minimal K06.011
    - moderate K06.012
    - severe K06.013

Recklinghausen disease Q85.01
- bones E21.0

Reclus' disease (cystic) —*see* Mastopathy, cystic

Recrudescent typhus (fever) A75.1

Recruitment, auditory H93.21-

Rectalgia K62.89

Rectitis K62.89

Rectocele
- female (without uterine prolapse) N81.6
  - with uterine prolapse N81.4
    - incomplete N81.2
- in pregnancy —*see* Pregnancy, complicated by, abnormal, pelvic organs or tissues NEC
- male K62.3

Rectosigmoid junction —*see* condition

Rectosigmoiditis K63.89
- ulcerative (chronic) K51.30

Rectosigmoiditis *(continued)*
- ulcerative *(continued)*
  - with
    - complication K51.319
      - abscess K51.314
      - fistula K51.313
      - obstruction K51.312
      - rectal bleeding K51.311
      - specified NEC K51.318

Rectourethral —*see* condition

Rectovaginal —*see* condition

Rectovesical —*see* condition

Rectum, rectal —*see* condition

Recurrent —*see* condition
- pregnancy loss —*see* Loss (of), pregnancy, recurrent

Red bugs B88.0

Red-cedar lung or pneumonitis J67.8

Red tide (*see also* Table of Drugs and Chemicals) T65.82-

Reduced
- mobility Z74.09
- ventilatory or vital capacity R94.2

Redundant, redundancy
- anus (congenital) Q43.8
- clitoris N90.89
- colon (congenital) Q43.8
- foreskin (congenital) N47.8
- intestine (congenital) Q43.8
- labia N90.69
- organ or site, congenital NEC —*see* Accessory
- panniculus (abdominal) E65
- prepuce (congenital) N47.8
- pylorus K31.89
- rectum (congenital) Q43.8
- scrotum N50.89
- sigmoid (congenital) Q43.8
- skin L98.7
  - and subcutaneous tissue L98.7
  - of face L57.4
    - eyelids - *see* Blepharochalasis
- stomach K31.89

Reduplication —*see* Duplication

Reflex R29.2
- hyperactive gag J39.2
- pupillary, abnormal —*see* Anomaly, pupil, function
- vasoconstriction I73.9
- vasovagal R55

Reflux K21.9
- acid K21.9
- esophageal K21.9
  - with esophagitis K21.0
  - newborn P78.83
- gastroesophageal K21.9
  - with esophagitis K21.0
- mitral —*see* Insufficiency, mitral
- ureteral —*see* Reflux, vesicoureteral
- vesicoureteral (with scarring) N13.70
  - with
    - nephropathy N13.729
      - with hydroureter N13.739
        - bilateral N13.732
        - unilateral N13.731
      - bilateral N13.722
      - unilateral N13.721
      - without hydroureter N13.729
        - bilateral N13.722
        - unilateral N13.721
    - pyelonephritis (chronic) N11.0
  - congenital Q62.7
  - without nephropathy N13.71

Reforming, artificial openings —*see* Attention to, artificial, opening

Refractive error —*see* Disorder, refraction

Refsum's disease or syndrome G60.1

Refusal of
- food, psychogenic F50.89
- treatment (because of) Z53.20
  - left against medical advice (AMA) Z53.21
  - patient's decision NEC Z53.29
  - reasons of belief or group pressure Z53.1

Regional —*see* condition

Regurgitation R11.10
- aortic (valve) —*see* Insufficiency, aortic
- food —*see also* Vomiting
  - with reswallowing —*see* Rumination
  - newborn P92.1
- gastric contents —*see* Vomiting
- heart —*see* Endocarditis
- mitral (valve) —*see* Insufficiency, mitral
  - congenital Q23.3
- myocardial —*see* Endocarditis
- pulmonary (valve) (heart) I37.1
  - congenital Q22.2
  - syphilitic A52.03
- tricuspid —*see* Insufficiency, tricuspid
- valve, valvular —*see* Endocarditis
  - congenital Q24.8
- vesicoureteral —*see* Reflux, vesicoureteral

Reifenstein syndrome E34.52

Reinsertion
- implantable subdermal contraceptive Z30.46
- intrauterine contraceptive device Z30.433

Reiter's disease, syndrome, or urethritis M02.30
- ankle M02.37-
- elbow M02.32-
- foot joint M02.37-
- hand joint M02.34-
- hip M02.35-
- knee M02.36-
- multiple site M02.39
- shoulder M02.31-
- vertebra M02.38
- wrist M02.33-

Reichmann's disease or syndrome K31.89

Rejection
- food, psychogenic F50.89
- transplant T86.91
  - bone T86.830
    - marrow T86.01
  - cornea T86.840
  - heart T86.21
    - with lung(s) T86.31
  - intestine T86.850
  - kidney T86.11
  - liver T86.41
  - lung(s) T86.810
    - with heart T86.31
  - organ (immune or nonimmune cause) T86.91
  - pancreas T86.890
  - skin (allograft) (autograft) T86.820
  - specified NEC T86.890
  - stem cell (peripheral blood) (umbilical cord) T86.5

Relapsing fever A68.9
- Carter's (Asiatic) A68.1

- **Relapsing fever** *(continued)*
  - Dutton's (West African) A68.1
  - Koch's A68.9
  - louse-borne (epidemic) A68.0
  - Novy's (American) A68.1
  - Obermeyers's (European) A68.0
  - Spirillum A68.9
  - tick-borne (endemic) A68.1
- **Relationship**
  - occlusal
    - open anterior M26.220
    - open posterior M26.221
- **Relaxation**
  - anus (sphincter) K62.89
    - psychogenic F45.8
  - arch (foot) *—see also* Deformity, limb, flat foot
  - back ligaments *—see* Instability, joint, spine
  - bladder (sphincter) N31.2
  - cardioesophageal K21.9
  - cervix *—see* Incompetency, cervix
  - diaphragm J98.6
  - joint (capsule) (ligament) (paralytic) *—see* Flail, joint
    - congenital NEC Q74.8
  - lumbosacral (joint) *—see* subcategory M53.2
  - pelvic floor N81.89
  - perineum N81.89
  - posture R29.3
  - rectum (sphincter) K62.89
  - sacroiliac (joint) *—see* subcategory M53.2
  - scrotum N50.89
  - urethra (sphincter) N36.44
  - vesical N31.2
- **Release from prison, anxiety concerning** Z65.2
- **Remains**
  - canal of Cloquet Q14.0
  - capsule (opaque) Q14.8
- **Remittent fever** (malarial) B54
- **Remnant**
  - canal of Cloquet Q14.0
  - capsule (opaque) Q14.8
  - cervix, cervical stump (acquired) (postoperative) N88.8
  - cystic duct, postcholecystectomy K91.5
  - fingernail L60.8
    - congenital Q84.6
  - meniscus, knee *—see* Derangement, knee, meniscus, specified NEC
  - thyroglossal duct Q89.2
  - tonsil J35.8
    - infected (chronic) J35.01
  - urachus Q64.4
- **Removal** (from) (of)
  - artificial
    - arm Z44.00-
      - complete Z44.01-
      - partial Z44.02-
    - eye Z44.2-
    - leg Z44.10-
      - complete Z44.11-
      - partial Z44.12-
  - breast implant Z45.81
  - cardiac pulse generator (battery) (end-of-life) Z45.010
  - catheter (urinary) (indwelling) Z46.6
    - from artificial opening *—see* Attention to, artificial, opening
    - non-vascular Z46.82
    - vascular NEC Z45.2
  - drains Z48.03
  - device Z46.9
    - contraceptive Z30.432
      - implantable subdermal Z30.46
    - implanted NEC Z45.89
    - specified NEC Z46.89
  - dressing (nonsurgical) Z48.00
    - surgical Z48.01
  - external
    - fixation device - code to fracture with seventh character D
    - prosthesis, prosthetic device Z44.9
      - breast Z44.3-
      - specified NEC Z44.8
  - home in childhood (to foster home or institution) Z62.29
  - ileostomy Z43.2
  - insulin pump Z46.81
  - myringotomy device (stent) (tube) Z45.82
  - nervous system device NEC Z46.2
    - brain neuropacemaker Z46.2
    - visual substitution device Z46.2
      - implanted Z45.31
  - non-vascular catheter Z46.82
  - orthodontic device Z46.4
  - organ, prophylactic (for neoplasia management) *—see* Prophylactic, organ removal
  - staples Z48.02
  - stent
    - ureteral Z46.6
  - suture Z48.02
  - urinary device Z46.6
  - vascular access device or catheter Z45.2
- **Ren**
  - arcuatus Q63.1
  - mobile, mobilis N28.89
    - congenital Q63.8
  - unguliformis Q63.1
- **Renal** *—see* condition
- **Rendu-Osler-Weber disease or syndrome** I78.0
- **Reninoma** D41.0-
- **Renon-Delille syndrome** E23.3
- **Reovirus, as cause of disease classified elsewhere** B97.5
- **Repeated falls NEC** R29.6
- **Replaced chromosome by dicentric ring** Q93.2
- **Replacement by artificial or mechanical device or prosthesis of**
  - bladder Z96.0
  - blood vessel NEC Z95.828
  - bone NEC Z96.7
  - cochlea Z96.21
  - coronary artery Z95.5
  - eustachian tube Z96.29
  - eye globe Z97.0
  - heart Z95.812
    - valve Z95.2
      - prosthetic Z95.2
      - specified NEC Z95.4
      - xenogenic Z95.3
  - intestine Z96.89
  - joint Z96.60
    - hip *—see* Presence, hip joint implant
    - knee *—see* Presence, knee joint implant
    - specified site NEC Z96.698
  - larynx Z96.3
  - lens Z96.1
  - limb(s) *—see* Presence, artificial, limb
  - mandible NEC (for tooth root implant(s)) Z96.5
- **Replacement by artificial or mechanical device or prosthesis of** *(continued)*
  - organ NEC Z96.89
  - peripheral vessel NEC Z95.828
  - stapes Z96.29
  - teeth Z97.2
  - tendon Z96.7
  - tissue NEC Z96.89
  - tooth root(s) Z96.5
  - vessel NEC Z95.828
    - coronary (artery) Z95.5
- **Request for expert evidence** Z04.8
- **Reserve, decreased or low**
  - cardiac *—see* Disease, heart
  - kidney N28.89
- **Residual** *—see also* condition
  - ovary syndrome N99.83
  - state, schizophrenic F20.5
  - urine R39.198
- **Resistance, resistant** (to)
  - activated protein C D68.51
  - complicating pregnancy O26.89
  - insulin E88.81
  - organism(s)
    - to
      - drug Z16.30
        - aminoglycosides Z16.29
        - amoxicillin Z16.11
        - ampicillin Z16.11
        - antibiotic(s) Z16.20
          - multiple Z16.24
          - specified NEC Z16.29
        - antifungal Z16.32
        - antimicrobial (single) Z16.30
          - multiple Z16.35
          - specified NEC Z16.39
        - antimycobacterial (single) Z16.341
          - multiple Z16.342
        - antiparasitic Z16.31
        - antiviral Z16.33
        - beta lactam antibiotics Z16.10
          - specified NEC Z16.19
        - cephalosporins Z16.19
        - extended beta lactamase (ESBL) Z16.12
        - fluoroquinolones Z16.23
        - macrolides Z16.29
        - methicillin *—see* MRSA
        - multiple drugs (MDRO)
          - antibiotics Z16.24
          - antimicrobial Z16.35
          - antimycobacterials Z16.342
        - penicillins Z16.11
        - quinine (and related compounds) Z16.31
        - quinolones Z16.23
        - sulfonamides Z16.29
        - tetracyclines Z16.29
        - tuberculostatics (single) Z16.341
          - multiple Z16.342
        - vancomycin Z16.21
          - related antibiotics Z16.22
  - thyroid hormone E07.89
- **Resorption**
  - dental (roots) K03.3
    - alveoli M26.79
  - teeth (external) (internal) (pathological) (roots) K03.3
- **Respiration**
  - Cheyne-Stokes R06.3
  - decreased due to shock, following injury T79.4
  - disorder of, psychogenic F45.8
  - insufficient, or poor R06.89
    - newborn P28.5
- **Respiration** *(continued)*
  - painful R07.1
  - sighing, psychogenic F45.8
- **Respiratory** *—see also* condition
  - distress syndrome (newborn) (type I) P22.0
    - type II P22.1
  - syncytial virus, as cause of disease classified elsewhere B97.4
- **Respite care** Z75.5
- **Response** (drug)
  - photoallergic L56.1
  - phototoxic L56.0
- **Restenosis**
  - stent
    - vascular
      - end stent
        - adjacent to stent *—see* Arteriosclerosis
        - within the stent
          - coronary T82.855
          - peripheral T82.856
      - in stent
        - coronary vessel T82.855
        - peripheral vessel T82.856
- **Restless legs** (syndrome) G25.81
- **Restlessness** R45.1
- **Restriction of housing space** Z59.1
- **Restoration** (of)
  - dental
    - aesthetically inadequate or displeasing K08.56
    - defective K08.50
      - specified NEC K08.59
    - failure of marginal integrity K08.51
    - failure of periodontal anatomical intergrity K08.54
  - organ continuity from previous sterilization (tuboplasty) (vasoplasty) Z31.0
    - aftercare Z31.42
  - tooth (existing)
    - contours biologically incompatible with oral health K08.54
    - open margins K08.51
    - overhanging K08.52
    - poor aesthetic K08.56
    - poor gingival margins K08.51
  - unsatisfactory, of tooth K08.50
    - specified NEC K08.59
- **Restorative material** (dental)
  - allergy to K08.55
  - fractured K08.539
    - with loss of material K08.531
    - without loss of material K08.530
  - unrepairable overhanging of K08.52
- **Rests, ovarian, in fallopian tube** Q50.6
- **Restzustand** (schizophrenic) F20.5
- **Retained** *—see also* Retention
  - cholelithiasis following cholecystectomy K91.86
  - foreign body fragments (type of) Z18.9
    - acrylics Z18.2
    - animal quill(s) or spines Z18.31
    - cement Z18.83
    - concrete Z18.83
    - crystalline Z18.83
    - depleted isotope Z18.09
    - depleted uranium Z18.01
    - diethylhexylphthalates Z18.2
    - glass Z18.81

Retained *(continued)*
- foreign body fragments *(continued)*
  - isocyanate Z18.2
  - magnetic metal Z18.11
  - metal Z18.10
  - nonmagnectic metal Z18.12
  - nontherapeutic radioactive Z18.09
  - organic NEC Z18.39
  - plastic Z18.2
  - quill(s) (animal) Z18.31
  - radioactive (nontherapeutic) NEC Z18.09
  - specified NEC Z18.89
  - spine(s) (animal) Z18.31
  - stone Z18.83
  - tooth (teeth) Z18.32
  - wood Z18.33
- fragments (type of) Z18.9
  - acrylics Z18.2
  - animal quill(s) or spines Z18.31
  - cement Z18.83
  - concrete Z18.83
  - crystalline Z18.83
  - depleted isotope Z18.09
  - depleted uranium Z18.01
  - diethylhexylphthalates Z18.2
  - glass Z18.81
  - isocyanate Z18.2
  - magnetic metal Z18.11
  - metal Z18.10
  - nonmagnectic metal Z18.12
  - nontherapeutic radioactive Z18.09
  - organic NEC Z18.39
  - plastic Z18.2
  - quill(s) (animal) Z18.31
  - radioactive (nontherapeutic) NEC Z18.09
  - specified NEC Z18.89
  - spine(s) (animal) Z18.31
  - stone Z18.83
  - tooth (teeth) Z18.32
  - wood Z18.33
- gallstones, following cholecystectomy K91.86

Retardation
- development, developmental, specific *—see* Disorder, developmental
- endochondral bone growth *—see* Disorder, bone, development or growth
- growth R62.50
  - due to malnutrition E45
- mental *—see* Disability, intellectual
- motor function, specific F82
- physical (child) R62.52
  - due to malnutrition E45
- reading (specific) F81.0
- spelling (specific) (without reading disorder) F81.81

Retching *—see* Vomiting

Retention *—see also* Retained
- bladder *—see* Retention, urine
- carbon dioxide E87.2
- cholelithiasis following cholecystectomy K91.86
- cyst *—see* Cyst
- dead
  - fetus (at or near term) (mother) O36.4
    - early fetal death O02.1
  - ovum O02.0
- decidua (fragments) (following delivery) (with hemorrhage) O72.2
  - without hemorrhage O73.1
- deciduous tooth K00.6
- dental root K08.3
- fecal *—see* Constipation

Retention *(continued)*
- fetus
  - dead O36.4
    - early O02.1
- fluid R60.9
- foreign body *—see also* Foreign body, retained
  - current trauma - code as Foreign body, by site or type
- gallstones, following cholecystectomy K91.86
- gastric K31.89
- intrauterine contraceptive device, in pregnancy *—see* Pregnancy, complicated by, retention, intrauterine device
- membranes (complicating delivery) (with hemorrhage) O72.2
  - with abortion *—see* Abortion, by type
  - without hemorrhage O73.1
- meniscus *—see* Derangement, meniscus
- menses N94.89
- milk (puerperal, postpartum) O92.79
- nitrogen, extrarenal R39.2
- ovary syndrome N99.83
- placenta (total) (with hemorrhage) O72.0
  - without hemorrhage O73.0
  - portions or fragments (with hemorrhage) O72.2
    - without hemorrhage O73.1
- products of conception
  - early pregnancy (dead fetus) O02.1
  - following
    - delivery (with hemorrhage) O72.2
      - without hemorrhage O73.1
- secundines (following delivery) (with hemorrhage) O72.0
  - without hemorrhage O73.0
  - complicating puerperium (delayed hemorrhage) O72.2
  - partial O72.2
    - without hemorrhage O73.1
- smegma, clitoris N90.89
- urine R33.9
  - due to hyperplasia (hypertrophy) of prostate *—see* Hyperplasia, prostate
  - drug-induced R33.0
  - organic R33.8
    - drug-induced R33.0
  - psychogenic F45.8
  - specified NEC R33.8
- water (in tissues) *—see* Edema

Reticular erythematous mucinosis L98.5

Reticulation, dust *—see* Pneumoconiosis

Reticulocytosis R70.1

Reticuloendotheliosis
- acute infantile C96.0
- leukemic C91.4-
- nonlipid C96.0

Reticulohistiocytoma (giant-cell) D76.3

Reticuloid, actinic L57.1

Reticulosis (skin)
- acute of infancy C96.0
- hemophagocytic, familial D76.1
- histiocytic medullary C96.A
- lipomelanotic I89.8
- malignant (midline) C86.0
- polymorphic C86.0
- Sézary *—see* Sézary disease

Retina, retinal *—see also* condition
- dark area D49.81

Retinitis *—see also* Inflammation, chorioretinal
- albuminurica N18.9 *[H32]*
- diabetic *—see* Diabetes, retinitis
- disciformis *—see* Degeneration, macula
- focal *—see* Inflammation, chorioretinal, focal
- gravidarum *—see* Pregnancy, complicated by, specified pregnancy-related condition NEC
- juxtapapillaris *—see* Inflammation, chorioretinal, focal, juxtapapillary
- luetic *—see* Retinitis, syphilitic
- pigmentosa H35.52
- proliferans *—see* Disorder, globe, degenerative, specified type NEC
- proliferating *—see* Disorder, globe, degenerative, specified type NEC
- renal N18.9 *[H32]*
- syphilitic (early) (secondary) A51.43
  - central, recurrent A52.71
  - congenital (early) A50.01 *[H32]*
  - late A52.71
- tuberculous A18.53

Retinoblastoma C69.2-
- differentiated C69.2-
- undifferentiated C69.2-

Retinochoroiditis *—see also* Inflammation, chorioretinal
- disseminated *—see* Inflammation, chorioretinal, disseminated
  - syphilitic A52.71
- focal *—see* Inflammation, chorioretinal
- juxtapapillaris *—see* Inflammation, chorioretinal, focal, juxtapapillary

Retinopathy (background) H35.00
- arteriosclerotic I70.8 *[H35.0-]*
- atherosclerotic I70.8 *[H35.0-]*
- central serous *—see* Chorioretinopathy, central serous
- Coats H35.02-
- diabetic *—see* Diabetes, retinopathy
- exudative H35.02-
- hypertensive H35.03-
- in (due to)
  - diabetes *—see* Diabetes, retinopathy
  - sickle-cell disorders D57.- H36
- of prematurity H35.10-
  - stage 0 H35.11-
  - stage 1 H35.12-
  - stage 2 H35.13-
  - stage 3 H35.14-
  - stage 4 H35.15-
  - stage 5 H35.16-
- pigmentary, congenital *—see* Dystrophy, retina
- proliferative NEC H35.2-
  - diabetic *—see* Diabetes, retinopathy, proliferative
  - sickle-cell D57.- *[H36]*
- solar H31.02-

Retinoschisis H33.10-
- congenital Q14.1
- specified type NEC H33.19-

Retortamoniasis A07.8

Retractile testis Q55.22

Retraction
- cervix *—see* Retroversion, uterus
- drum (membrane) *—see* Disorder, tympanic membrane, specified NEC
- finger *—see* Deformity, finger

Retraction *(continued)*
- lid H02.539
  - left H02.536
    - lower H02.535
    - upper H02.534
  - right H02.533
    - lower H02.532
    - upper H02.531
- lung J98.4
- mediastinum J98.59
- nipple N64.53
  - associated with
    - lactation O92.03
    - pregnancy O92.01-
    - puerperium O92.02
  - congenital Q83.8
- palmar fascia M72.0
- pleura *—see* Pleurisy
- ring, uterus (Bandl's) (pathological) O62.4
- sternum (congenital) Q76.7
  - acquired M95.4
- uterus *—see* Retroversion, uterus
- valve (heart) *—see* Endocarditis

Retrobulbar *—see* condition

Retrocecal *—see* condition

Retrocession *—see* Retroversion

Retrodisplacement *—see* Retroversion

Retroflection, retroflexion *—see* Retroversion

Retrognathia, retrognathism (mandibular) (maxillary) M26.19

Retrograde menstruation N92.5

Retroperineal *—see* condition

Retroperitoneal *—see* condition

Retroperitonitis K68.9

Retropharyngeal *—see* condition

Retroplacental *—see* condition

Retroposition *—see* Retroversion

Retroprosthetic membrane T85.398

Retrosternal thyroid (congenital) Q89.2

Retroversion, retroverted
- cervix *—see* Retroversion, uterus
- female NEC *—see* Retroversion, uterus
- iris H21.89
- testis (congenital) Q55.29
- uterus (acquired) (acute) (any degree) (asymptomatic) (cervix) (postinfectional) (postpartal, old) N85.4
  - congenital Q51.818
  - in pregnancy O34.53-

Retrovirus, as cause of disease classified elsewhere B97.30
- human
  - immunodeficiency, type 2 (HIV 2) B97.35
  - T-cell lymphotropic
    - type I (HTLV-I) B97.33
    - type II (HTLV-II) B97.34
- lentivirus B97.31
- oncovirus B97.32
- specified NEC B97.39

Retrusion, premaxilla (developmental) M26.09

Rett's disease or syndrome F84.2

Reverse peristalsis R19.2

Reye's syndrome G93.7

Rh (factor)
- hemolytic disease (newborn) P55.0
- incompatibility, immunization or sensitization

Rh *(continued)*
- incompatibility, immunization or *(continued)*
  - affecting management of pregnancy NEC O36.09-
    - anti-D antibody O36.01-
  - newborn P55.0
  - transfusion reaction *—see* Complication(s), transfusion, incompatibility reaction, Rh (factor)
- negative mother affecting newborn P55.0
- titer elevated *—see* Complication(s), transfusion, incompatibility reaction, Rh (factor)
- transfusion reaction *—see* Complication(s), transfusion, incompatibility reaction, Rh (factor)

Rhabdomyolysis (idiopathic) **NEC** M62.82
- traumatic T79.6

Rhabdomyoma *—see also* Neoplasm, connective tissue, benign
- adult *—see* Neoplasm, connective tissue, benign
- fetal *—see* Neoplasm, connective tissue, benign
- glycogenic *—see* Neoplasm, connective tissue, benign

Rhabdomyosarcoma (any type) *—see* Neoplasm, connective tissue, malignant

Rhabdosarcoma *—see* Rhabdomyosarcoma

Rhesus (factor) **incompatibility** *—see* Rh, incompatibility

Rheumatic (acute) (subacute) (chronic)
- adherent pericardium I09.2
- coronary arteritis I01.9
- degeneration, myocardium I09.0
- fever (acute) *—see* Fever, rheumatic
- heart *—see* Disease, heart, rheumatic
- myocardial degeneration *—see* Degeneration, myocardium
- myocarditis (chronic) (inactive) (with chorea) I09.0
  - active or acute I01.2
  - with chorea (acute) (rheumatic) (Sydenham's) I02.0
- pancarditis, acute I01.8
  - with chorea (acute (rheumatic) Sydenham's) I02.0
- pericarditis (active) (acute) (with effusion) (with pneumonia) I01.0
  - with chorea (acute) (rheumatic) (Sydenham's) I02.0
  - chronic or inactive I09.2
- pneumonia I00 *[J17]*
- torticollis M43.6
- typhoid fever A01.09

Rheumatism (articular) (neuralgic) (nonarticular) M79.0
- gout *—see* Arthritis, rheumatoid
- intercostal, meaning Tietze's disease M94.0
- palindromic (any site) M12.30
  - ankle M12.37-
  - elbow M12.32-
  - foot joint M12.37-
  - hand joint M12.34-
  - hip M12.35-
  - knee M12.36-
  - multiple site M12.39

Rheumatism *(continued)*
- palindromic *(continued)*
  - shoulder M12.31-
  - specified joint NEC M12.38
  - vertebrae M12.38
  - wrist M12.33-
- sciatic M54.4-

Rheumatoid *—see also* condition
- arthritis *—see also* Arthritis, rheumatoid
  - with involvement of organs NEC M05.60
    - ankle M05.67-
    - elbow M05.62-
    - foot joint M05.67-
    - hand joint M05.64-
    - hip M05.65-
    - knee M05.66-
    - multiple site M05.69
    - shoulder M05.61-
    - vertebra *—see* Spondylitis, ankylosing
    - wrist M05.63-
  - seronegative *—see* Arthritis, rheumatoid, seronegative
  - seropositive *—see* Arthritis, rheumatoid, seropositive
- carditis M05.30
  - ankle M05.37-
  - elbow M05.32-
  - foot joint M05.37-
  - hand joint M05.34-
  - hip M05.35-
  - knee M05.36-
  - multiple site M05.39
  - shoulder M05.31-
  - vertebra *—see* Spondylitis, ankylosing
  - wrist M05.33-
- endocarditis *—see* Rheumatoid, carditis
- lung (disease) M05.10
  - ankle M05.17-
  - elbow M05.12-
  - foot joint M05.17-
  - hand joint M05.14-
  - hip M05.15-
  - knee M05.16-
  - multiple site M05.19
  - shoulder M05.11-
  - vertebra *—see* Spondylitis, ankylosing
  - wrist M05.13-
- myocarditis *—see* Rheumatoid, carditis
- myopathy M05.40
  - ankle M05.47-
  - elbow M05.42-
  - foot joint M05.47-
  - hand joint M05.44-
  - hip M05.45-
  - knee M05.46-
  - multiple site M05.49
  - shoulder M05.41-
  - vertebra *—see* Spondylitis, ankylosing
  - wrist M05.43-
- pericarditis *—see* Rheumatoid, carditis
- polyarthritis *—see* Arthritis, rheumatoid
- polyneuropathy M05.50
  - ankle M05.57-
  - elbow M05.52-
  - foot joint M05.57-
  - hand joint M05.54-
  - hip M05.55-
  - knee M05.56-
  - multiple site M05.59
  - shoulder M05.51-

Rheumatoid *(continued)*
- polyneuropathy *(continued)*
  - vertebra *—see* Spondylitis, ankylosing
  - wrist M05.53-
- vasculitis M05.20
  - ankle M05.27-
  - elbow M05.22-
  - foot joint M05.27-
  - hand joint M05.24-
  - hip M05.25-
  - knee M05.26-
  - multiple site M05.29
  - shoulder M05.21-
  - vertebra *—see* Spondylitis, ankylosing
  - wrist M05.23-

Rhinitis (atrophic) (catarrhal) (chronic) (croupous) (fibrinous) (granulomatous) (hyperplastic) (hypertrophic) (membranous) (obstructive) (purulent) (suppurative) (ulcerative) J31.0
- with
  - sore throat *—see* Nasopharyngitis
- acute J00
- allergic J30.9
  - with asthma J45.909
    - with
      - exacerbation (acute) J45.901
      - status asthmaticus J45.902
  - due to
    - food J30.5
    - pollen J30.1
  - nonseasonal J30.89
  - perennial J30.89
  - seasonal NEC J30.2
  - specified NEC J30.89
- infective J00
- pneumococcal J00
- syphilitic A52.73
  - congenital A50.05 *[J99]*
- tuberculous A15.8
- vasomotor J30.0

Rhinoantritis (chronic) *—see* Sinusitis, maxillary

Rhinodacryolith *—see* Dacryolith

Rhinolith (nasal sinus) J34.89

Rhinomegaly J34.89

Rhinopharyngitis (acute) (subacute) *—see also* Nasopharyngitis
- chronic J31.1
- destructive ulcerating A66.5
- mutilans A66.5

Rhinophyma L71.1

Rhinorrhea J34.89
- cerebrospinal (fluid) G96.0
- paroxysmal *—see* Rhinitis, allergic
- spasmodic *—see* Rhinitis, allergic

Rhinosalpingitis *—see* Salpingitis, eustachian

Rhinoscleroma A48.8

Rhinosporidiosis B48.1

Rhinovirus infection NEC B34.8

Rhizomelic chondrodysplasia punctata E71.540

Rhythm
- atrioventricular nodal I49.8
- disorder I49.9
  - coronary sinus I49.8
  - ectopic I49.8
  - nodal I49.8
- escape I49.9
- heart, abnormal I49.9
- idioventricular I44.2
- nodal I49.8

Rhythm *(continued)*
- sleep, inversion G47.2-
  - nonorganic origin *—see* Disorder, sleep, circadian rhythm, psychogenic

Rhytidosis facialis L98.8

Rib *—see also* condition
- cervical Q76.5

Riboflavin deficiency E53.0

Rice bodies *—see also* Loose, body, joint
- knee M23.4-

Richter syndrome *—see* Leukemia, chronic lymphocytic, B-cell type

Richter's hernia *—see* Hernia, abdomen, with obstruction

Ricinism *—see* Poisoning, food, noxious, plant

Rickets (active) (acute) (adolescent) (chest wall) (congenital) (current) (infantile) (intestinal) E55.0
- adult *—see* Osteomalacia
- celiac K90.0
- hypophosphatemic with nephrotic-glycosuric dwarfism E72.09
- inactive E64.3
- kidney N25.0
- renal N25.0
- sequelae, any E64.3
- vitamin-D-resistant E83.31 *[M90.80]*

Rickettsial disease A79.9
- specified type NEC A79.89

Rickettsialpox (Rickettsia akari) A79.1

Rickettsiosis A79.9
- due to
  - Ehrlichia sennetsu A79.81
  - Rickettsia akari (rickettsialpox) A79.1
- specified type NEC A79.89
- tick-borne A77.9
- vesicular A79.1

Rider's bone *—see* Ossification, muscle, specified NEC

Ridge, alveolus *—see also* condition
- flabby K06.8

Ridged ear, congenital Q17.3

Riedel's
- lobe, liver Q44.7
- struma, thyroiditis or disease E06.5

Rieger's anomaly or syndrome Q13.81

Riehl's melanosis L81.4

Rietti-Greppi-Micheli anemia D56.9

Rieux's hernia *—see* Hernia, abdomen, specified site NEC

Riga (-Fede) **disease** K14.0

Riggs' disease *—see* Periodontitis

Right aortic arch Q25.47

Right middle lobe syndrome J98.11

Rigid, rigidity *—see also* condition
- abdominal R19.30
  - with severe abdominal pain R10.0
  - epigastric R19.36
  - generalized R19.37
  - left lower quadrant R19.34
  - left upper quadrant R19.32
  - periumbilic R19.35
  - right lower quadrant R19.33
  - right upper quadrant R19.31
- articular, multiple, congenital Q68.8
- cervix (uteri) in pregnancy *—see* Pregnancy, complicated by, abnormal, cervix

Rigid, rigidity *(continued)*
hymen (acquired) (congenital) N89.6
nuchal R29.1
pelvic floor in pregnancy —*see* Pregnancy, complicated by, abnormal, pelvic organs or tissues NEC
perineum or vulva in pregnancy —*see* Pregnancy, complicated by, abnormal, vulva
spine —*see* Dorsopathy, specified NEC
vagina in pregnancy —*see* Pregnancy, complicated by, abnormal, vagina
Rigors R68.89
with fever R50.9
Riley-Day syndrome G90.1
RIND (reversible ischemic neurologic deficit) I63.9
Ring(s)
aorta (vascular) Q25.45
Bandl's O62.4
contraction, complicating delivery O62.4
esophageal, lower (muscular) K22.2
Fleischer's (cornea) H18.04-
hymenal, tight (acquired) (congenital) N89.6
Kayser-Fleischer (cornea) H18.04-
retraction, uterus, pathological O62.4
Schatzki's (esophagus) (lower) K22.2
congenital Q39.3
Soemmerring's —*see* Cataract, secondary
vascular (congenital) Q25.8
aorta Q25.45
Ringed hair (congenital) Q84.1
Ringworm B35.9
beard B35.0
black dot B35.0
body B35.4
Burmese B35.5
corporeal B35.4
foot B35.3
groin B35.6
hand B35.2
honeycomb B35.0
nails B35.1
perianal (area) B35.6
scalp B35.0
specified NEC B35.8
Tokelau B35.5
Rise, venous pressure I87.8
Rising, PSA following treatment for malignant neoplasm of prostate R97.21
Risk
for
dental caries Z91.849
high Z91.843
low Z91.841
moderate Z91.842
suicidal
meaning personal history of attempted suicide Z91.5
meaning suicidal ideation —*see* Ideation, suicidal
Ritter's disease L00
Rivalry, sibling Z62.891
Rivalta's disease A42.2
River blindness B73.01
Robert's pelvis Q74.2
with disproportion (fetopelvic) O33.0
causing obstructed labor O65.0
Robin (-Pierre) **syndrome** Q87.0
Robinow-Silvermann-Smith syndrome Q87.1
Robinson's (hidrotic) **ectodermal dysplasia or syndrome** Q82.4
Robles' disease B73.01
Rocky Mountain (spotted) **fever** A77.0
Roetheln —*see* Rubella
Roger's disease Q21.0
Rokitansky-Aschoff sinuses (gallbladder) K82.8
Rolando's fracture (displaced) S62.22-
nondisplaced S62.22-
Romano-Ward (prolonged QT interval) **syndrome** I45.81
Romberg's disease or syndrome G51.8
Roof, mouth —*see* condition
Rosacea L71.9
acne L71.9
keratitis L71.8
specified NEC L71.8
Rosary, rachitic E55.0
Rose
cold J30.1
fever J30.1
rash R21
epidemic B06.9
Rosenbach's erysipeloid A26.0
Rosenthal's disease or syndrome D68.1
Roseola B09
infantum B08.20
due to human herpesvirus 6 B08.21
due to human herpesvirus 7 B08.22
Rossbach's disease K31.89
psychogenic F45.8
Ross River disease or fever B33.1
Rostan's asthma (cardiac) —*see* Failure, ventricular, left
Rotation
anomalous, incomplete or insufficient, intestine Q43.3
cecum (congenital) Q43.3
colon (congenital) Q43.3
spine, incomplete or insufficient —*see* Dorsopathy, deforming, specified NEC
tooth, teeth, fully erupted M26.35
vertebra, incomplete or insufficient —*see* Dorsopathy, deforming, specified NEC
Rotes Quérol disease or syndrome —*see* Hyperostosis, ankylosing
Roth (-Bernhardt) **disease or syndrome** —*see* Meralgia paraesthetica
Rothmund (-Thomson) **syndrome** Q82.8
Rotor's disease or syndrome E80.6
Round
back (with wedging of vertebrae) —*see* Kyphosis
Round *(continued)*
back *(continued)*
sequelae (late effect) of rickets E64.3
worms (large) (infestation) NEC B82.0
Ascariasis (*see also* Ascariasis) B77.9
Roussy-Lévy syndrome G60.0
Rubella (German measles) B06.9
complication NEC B06.09
neurological B06.00
congenital P35.0
contact Z20.4
exposure to Z20.4
maternal
manifest rubella in infant P35.0
care for (suspected) damage to fetus O35.3
suspected damage to fetus affecting management of pregnancy O35.3
specified complications NEC B06.89
Rubeola (meaning measles) —*see* Measles
meaning rubella —*see* Rubella
Rubeosis, iris —*see* Disorder, iris, vascular
Rubinstein-Taybi syndrome Q87.2
Rudimentary (congenital) —*see also* Agenesis
arm —*see* Defect, reduction, upper limb
bone Q79.9
cervix uteri Q51.828
eye Q11.2
lobule of ear Q17.3
patella Q74.1
respiratory organs in thoracopagus Q89.4
tracheal bronchus Q32.4
uterus Q51.818
in male Q56.1
vagina Q52.0
Ruled out condition —*see* Observation, suspected
Rumination R11.10
with nausea R11.2
disorder of infancy F98.21
neurotic F42.8
newborn P92.1
obsessional F42.8
psychogenic F42.8
Runeberg's disease D51.0
Runny nose R09.89
Rupia (syphilitic) A51.39
congenital A50.06
tertiary A52.79
Rupture, ruptured
abscess (spontaneous) - code by site under Abscess
aneurysm —*see* Aneurysm
anus (sphincter) —*see* Laceration, anus
aorta, aortic I71.8
abdominal I71.3
arch I71.1
ascending I71.1
descending I71.8
abdominal I71.3
thoracic I71.1
syphilitic A52.01
thoracoabdominal I71.5
thorax, thoracic I71.1
transverse I71.1
traumatic —*see* Injury, aorta, laceration, major
Rupture, ruptured *(continued)*
aorta, aortic *(continued)*
valve or cusp (*see also* Endocarditis, aortic) I35.8
appendix (with peritonitis) K35.2
with localized peritonitis K35.3
arteriovenous fistula, brain I60.8
artery I77.2
brain —*see* Hemorrhage, intracranial, intracerebral
coronary —*see* Infarct, myocardium
heart —*see* Infarct, myocardium
pulmonary I28.8
traumatic (complication) —*see* Injury, blood vessel
bile duct (common) (hepatic) K83.2
cystic K82.2
bladder (sphincter) (nontraumatic) (spontaneous) N32.89
following ectopic or molar pregnancy O08.6
obstetrical trauma O71.5
traumatic S37.29
blood vessel —*see also* Hemorrhage
brain —*see* Hemorrhage, intracranial, intracerebral
heart —*see* Infarct, myocardium
traumatic (complication) —*see* Injury, blood vessel, laceration, major, by site
bone —*see* Fracture
bowel (nontraumatic) K63.1
brain
aneurysm (congenital) —*see also* Hemorrhage, intracranial, subarachnoid
syphilitic A52.05
hemorrhagic —*see* Hemorrhage, intracranial, intracerebral
capillaries I78.8
cardiac (auricle) (ventricle) (wall) I23.3
with hemopericardium I23.0
infectional I40.9
traumatic —*see* Injury, heart
cartilage (articular) (current) —*see also* Sprain
knee S83.3-
semilunar —*see* Tear, meniscus
cecum (with peritonitis) K65.0
with peritoneal abscess K35.3
traumatic S36.598
celiac artery, traumatic —*see* Injury, blood vessel, celiac artery, laceration, major
cerebral aneurysm (congenital) (*see* Hemorrhage, intracranial, subarachnoid)
cervix (uteri)
with ectopic or molar pregnancy O08.6
following ectopic or molar pregnancy O08.6
obstetrical trauma O71.3
traumatic S37.69
chordae tendineae NEC I51.1
concurrent with acute myocardial infarction —*see* Infarct, myocardium
following acute myocardial infarction (current complication) I23.4
choroid (direct) (indirect) (traumatic) H31.32-
circle of Willis I60.6
colon (nontraumatic) K63.1
traumatic —*see* Injury, intestine, large
cornea (traumatic) —*see* Injury, eye, laceration

Rupture, ruptured *(continued)*
- coronary (artery) (thrombotic) —*see* Infarct, myocardium
- corpus luteum (infected) (ovary) N83.1-
- cyst —*see* Cyst
- cystic duct K82.2
- Descemet's membrane —*see* Change, corneal membrane, Descemet's, rupture
  - traumatic —*see* Injury, eye, laceration
- diaphragm, traumatic —*see* Injury, intrathoracic, diaphragm
- disc —*see* Rupture, intervertebral disc
- diverticulum (intestine) K57.80
  - with bleeding K57.81
  - bladder N32.3
  - large intestine K57.20
    - with
      - bleeding K57.21
      - small intestine K57.40
        - with bleeding K57.41
  - small intestine K57.00
    - with
      - bleeding K57.01
      - large intestine K57.40
        - with bleeding K57.41
- duodenal stump K31.89
- ear drum (nontraumatic) —*see also* Perforation, tympanum
  - traumatic S09.2-
    - due to blast injury —*see* Injury, blast, ear
- esophagus K22.3
- eye (without prolapse or loss of intraocular tissue) —*see* Injury, eye, laceration
- fallopian tube NEC (nonobstetric) (nontraumatic) N83.8
  - due to pregnancy O00.10-
    - with intrauterine pregnancy O00.11-
- fontanel P13.1
- gallbladder K82.2
  - traumatic S36.128
- gastric —*see also* Rupture, stomach
  - vessel K92.2
- globe (eye) (traumatic) —*see* Injury, eye, laceration
- graafian follicle (hematoma) N83.0-
- heart —*see* Rupture, cardiac
- hymen (nontraumatic) (nonintentional) N89.8
- internal organ, traumatic —*see* Injury, by site
- intervertebral disc —*see* Displacement, intervertebral disc
  - traumatic —*see* Rupture, traumatic, intervertebral disc
- intestine NEC (nontraumatic) K63.1
  - traumatic —*see* Injury, intestine
- iris —*see also* Abnormality, pupillary
  - traumatic —*see* Injury, eye, laceration
- joint capsule, traumatic —*see* Sprain
- kidney (traumatic) S37.06-
  - birth injury P15.8
  - nontraumatic N28.89
- lacrimal duct (traumatic) —*see* Injury, eye, specified site NEC
- lens (cataract) (traumatic) —*see* Cataract, traumatic
- ligament, traumatic —*see* Rupture, traumatic, ligament, by site
- liver S36.116
  - birth injury P15.0
- lymphatic vessel I89.8

Rupture, ruptured *(continued)*
- marginal sinus (placental) (with hemorrhage) —*see* Hemorrhage, antepartum, specified cause NEC
- membrana tympani (nontraumatic) —*see* Perforation, tympanum
- membranes (spontaneous)
  - artificial
    - delayed delivery following O75.5
  - delayed delivery following —*see* Pregnancy, complicated by, premature rupture of membranes
- meningeal artery I60.8
- meniscus (knee) —*see also* Tear, meniscus
  - old —*see* Derangement, meniscus
  - site other than knee - code as Sprain
- mesenteric artery, traumatic —*see* Injury, mesenteric, artery, laceration, major
- mesentery (nontraumatic) K66.8
  - traumatic —*see* Injury, intra-abdominal, specified, site NEC
- mitral (valve) I34.8
- muscle (traumatic) —*see also* Strain
  - diastasis —*see* Diastasis, muscle
  - nontraumatic M62.10
    - ankle M62.17-
    - foot M62.17-
    - forearm M62.13-
    - hand M62.14-
    - lower leg M62.16-
    - pelvic region M62.15-
    - shoulder region M62.11-
    - specified site NEC M62.18
    - thigh M62.15-
    - upper arm M62.12-
  - traumatic —*see* Strain, by site
- musculotendinous junction NEC, nontraumatic —*see* Rupture, tendon, spontaneous
- mycotic aneurysm causing cerebral hemorrhage —*see* Hemorrhage, intracranial, subarachnoid
- myocardium, myocardial —*see* Rupture, cardiac
  - traumatic —*see* Injury, heart
- nontraumatic, meaning hernia —*see* Hernia
- obstructed —*see* Hernia, by site, obstructed
- operation wound —*see* Disruption, wound, operation
- ovary, ovarian N83.8
  - corpus luteum cyst N83.1-
  - follicle (graafian) N83.0-
- oviduct (nonobstetric) (nontraumatic) N83.8
  - due to pregnancy O00.10-
    - with intrauterine pregnancy O00.11-
- pancreas (nontraumatic) K86.89
  - traumatic S36.299
- papillary muscle NEC I51.2
  - following acute myocardial infarction (current complication) I23.5
- pelvic
  - floor, complicating delivery O70.1
  - organ NEC, obstetrical trauma O71.5
- perineum (nonobstetric) (nontraumatic) N90.89
  - complicating delivery —*see* Delivery, complicated, by, laceration, anus (sphincter)
- postoperative wound —*see* Disruption, wound, operation

Rupture, ruptured *(continued)*
- prostate (traumatic) S37.828
- pulmonary
  - artery I28.8
  - valve (heart) I37.8
  - vein I28.8
  - vessel I28.8
- pus tube —*see* Salpingitis
- pyosalpinx —*see* Salpingitis
- rectum (nontraumatic) K63.1
  - traumatic S36.69
- retina, retinal (traumatic) (without detachment) —*see also* Break, retina
  - with detachment —*see* Detachment, retina, with retinal, break
- rotator cuff (nontraumatic) M75.10-
  - complete M75.12-
  - incomplete M75.11-
- sclera —*see* Injury, eye, laceration
- sigmoid (nontraumatic) K63.1
  - traumatic S36.593
- spinal cord —*see also* Injury, spinal cord, by region
  - due to injury at birth P11.5
  - newborn (birth injury) P11.5
- spleen (traumatic) S36.09
  - birth injury P15.1
  - congenital (birth injury) P15.1
  - due to P. vivax malaria B51.0
  - nontraumatic D73.5
  - spontaneous D73.5
- splenic vein R58
  - traumatic —*see* Injury, blood vessel, splenic vein
- stomach (nontraumatic) (spontaneous) K31.89
  - traumatic S36.39
- supraspinatus (complete) (incomplete) (nontraumatic) —*see* Tear, rotator cuff
- symphysis pubis
  - obstetric O71.6
  - traumatic S33.4
- synovium (cyst) M66.10
  - ankle M66.17-
  - elbow M66.12-
  - finger M66.14-
  - foot M66.17-
  - forearm M66.13-
  - hand M66.14-
  - pelvic region M66.15-
  - shoulder region M66.11-
  - specified site NEC M66.18
  - thigh M66.15-
  - toe M66.17-
  - upper arm M66.12-
  - wrist M66.13-
- tendon (traumatic) —*see* Strain
  - nontraumatic (spontaneous) M66.9
    - ankle M66.87-
    - extensor M66.20
      - ankle M66.27-
      - foot M66.27-
      - forearm M66.23-
      - hand M66.24-
      - lower leg M66.26-
      - multiple sites M66.29
      - pelvic region M66.25-
      - shoulder region M66.21-
      - specified site NEC M66.28
      - thigh M66.25-
      - upper arm M66.22-
    - flexor M66.30
      - ankle M66.37-
      - foot M66.37-
      - forearm M66.33-
      - hand M66.34-
      - lower leg M66.36-

Rupture, ruptured *(continued)*
- tendon *(continued)*
  - nontraumatic *(continued)*
    - flexor *(continued)*
      - multiple sites M66.39
      - pelvic region M66.35-
      - shoulder region M66.31-
      - specified site NEC M66.38
      - thigh M66.35-
      - upper arm M66.32-
    - foot M66.87-
    - forearm M66.83-
    - hand M66.84-
    - lower leg M66.86-
    - multiple sites M66.89
    - pelvic region M66.85-
    - shoulder region M66.81-
    - specified
      - site NEC M66.88
      - tendon M66.80
    - thigh M66.85-
    - upper arm M66.82-
- thoracic duct I89.8
- tonsil J35.8
- traumatic
  - aorta —*see* Injury, aorta, laceration, major
  - diaphragm —*see* Injury, intrathoracic, diaphragm
  - external site —*see* Wound, open, by site
  - eye —*see* Injury, eye, laceration
  - internal organ —*see* Injury, by site
  - intervertebral disc
    - cervical S13.0
    - lumbar S33.0
    - thoracic S23.0
  - kidney S37.06-
  - ligament —*see also* Sprain
    - ankle —*see* Sprain, ankle
    - carpus —*see* Rupture, traumatic, ligament, wrist
    - collateral (hand) —*see* Rupture, traumatic, ligament, finger, collateral
    - finger (metacarpophalangeal) (interphalangeal) S63.40-
      - collateral S63.41-
        - index S63.41-
        - little S63.41-
        - middle S63.41-
        - ring S63.41-
      - index S63.40-
      - little S63.40-
      - middle S63.40-
      - palmar S63.42-
        - index S63.42-
        - little S63.42-
        - middle S63.42-
        - ring S63.42-
      - ring S63.40-
      - specified site NEC S63.499
        - index S63.49-
        - little S63.49-
        - middle S63.49-
        - ring S63.49-
      - volar plate S63.43-
        - index S63.43-
        - little S63.43-
        - middle S63.43-
        - ring S63.43-
    - foot —*see* Sprain, foot
    - radial collateral S53.2-
    - radiocarpal —*see* Rupture, traumatic, ligament, wrist, radiocarpal
    - ulnar collateral S53.3-
    - ulnocarpal —*see* Rupture, traumatic, ligament, wrist, ulnocarpal

Rupture, ruptured *(continued)*
traumatic *(continued)*
ligament *(continued)*
wrist S63.30-
collateral S63.31-
radiocarpal S63.32-
specified site NEC S63.39-
ulnocarpal (palmar) S63.33-
liver S36.116
membrana tympani *—see* Rupture, ear drum, traumatic
muscle or tendon *—see* Strain
myocardium *—see* Injury, heart
pancreas S36.299
rectum S36.69
sigmoid S36.593
spleen S36.09
stomach S36.39
symphysis pubis S33.4
tympanum, tympanic (membrane) *—see* Rupture, ear drum, traumatic
ureter S37.19
uterus S37.69
vagina *—see* Injury, vagina
vena cava *—see* Injury, vena cava, laceration, major
tricuspid (heart) (valve) I07.8
tube, tubal (nonobstetric) (nontraumatic) N83.8
abscess *—see* Salpingitis
due to pregnancy O00.10-
with intrauterine pregnancy O00.11-
tympanum, tympanic (membrane) (nontraumatic) (*see also* Perforation, tympanic membrane) H72.9-
traumatic *—see* Rupture, ear drum, traumatic
umbilical cord, complicating delivery O69.89
ureter (traumatic) S37.19
nontraumatic N28.89
urethra (nontraumatic) N36.8
with ectopic or molar pregnancy O08.6
following ectopic or molar pregnancy O08.6
obstetrical trauma O71.5
traumatic S37.39
uterosacral ligament (nonobstetric) (nontraumatic) N83.8
uterus (traumatic) S37.69
before labor O71.0-
during or after labor O71.1
nonpuerperal, nontraumatic N85.8
pregnant (during labor) O71.1
before labor O71.0-
vagina *—see* Injury, vagina
valve, valvular (heart) *—see* Endocarditis
varicose vein *—see* Varix
varix *—see* Varix
vena cava R58
traumatic *—see* Injury, vena cava, laceration, major
vesical (urinary) N32.89
vessel (blood) R58
pulmonary I28.8
traumatic *—see* Injury, blood vessel
viscus R19.8
vulva complicating delivery O70.0

Russell-Silver syndrome Q87.1

Russian spring-summer type encephalitis A84.0

Rust's disease (tuberculous cervical spondylitis) A18.01

Ruvalcaba-Myhre-Smith syndrome E71.440

Rytand-Lipsitch syndrome I44.2

S

Saber, sabre shin or tibia (syphilitic) A50.56 *[M90.8-]*

Sac lacrimal *—see* condition

Saccharomyces infection B37.9

Saccharopinuria E72.3

Saccular *—see* condition

Sacculation
aorta (nonsyphilitic) *—see* Aneurysm, aorta
bladder N32.3
intralaryngeal (congenital) (ventricular) Q31.3
larynx (congenital) (ventricular) Q31.3
organ or site, congenital *—see* Distortion
pregnant uterus *—see* Pregnancy, complicated by, abnormal, uterus
ureter N28.89
urethra N36.1
vesical N32.3

Sachs' amaurotic familial idiocy or disease E75.02

Sachs-Tay disease E75.02

Sacks-Libman disease M32.11

Sacralgia M53.3

Sacralization Q76.49

Sacrodynia M53.3

Sacroiliac joint *—see* condition

Sacroiliitis NEC M46.1

Sacrum *—see* condition

Saddle
back *—see* Lordosis
embolus
abdominal aorta I74.01
pulmonary artery I26.92
with acute cor pulmonale I26.02
injury - code to condition
nose M95.0
due to syphilis A50.57

Sadism (sexual) F65.52

Sadness, postpartal O90.6

Sadomasochism F65.50

Saemisch's ulcer (cornea) *—see* Ulcer, cornea, central

Sagging
skin and subcutaneous tissue (following bariatric surgery weight loss) (following dietary weight loss) L98.7

Sahib disease B55.0

Sailors' skin L57.8

Saint
Anthony's fire *—see* Erysipelas
triad *—see* Hernia, diaphragm
Vitus' dance *—see* Chorea, Sydenham's

Salaam
attack(s) *—see* Epilepsy, spasms
tic R25.8

Salicylism
abuse F55.8
overdose or wrong substance given *—see* Table of Drugs and Chemicals, by drug, poisoning

Salivary duct or gland *—see* condition

Salivation, excessive K11.7

Salmonella *—see* Infection, Salmonella

Salmonellosis A02.0

Salpingitis (catarrhal) (fallopian tube) (nodular) (pseudofollicular) (purulent) (septic) N70.91
with oophoritis N70.93
acute N70.01
with oophoritis N70.03
chlamydial A56.11
chronic N70.11
with oophoritis N70.13
complicating abortion *—see* Abortion, by type, complicated by, salpingitis
ear *—see* Salpingitis, eustachian
eustachian (tube) H68.00-
acute H68.01-
chronic H68.02-
follicularis N70.11
with oophoritis N70.13
gonococcal (acute) (chronic) A54.24
interstitial, chronic N70.11
with oophoritis N70.13
isthmica nodosa N70.11
with oophoritis N70.13
specific (gonococcal) (acute) (chronic) A54.24
tuberculous (acute) (chronic) A18.17
venereal (gonococcal) (acute) (chronic) A54.24

Salpingocele N83.4-

Salpingo-oophoritis (catarrhal) (purulent) (ruptured) (septic) (suppurative) N70.93
acute N70.03
with ectopic or molar pregnancy O08.0
following ectopic or molar pregnancy O08.0
gonococcal A54.24
chronic N70.13
following ectopic or molar pregnancy O08.0
gonococcal (acute) (chronic) A54.24
puerperal O86.19
specific (gonococcal) (acute) (chronic) A54.24
subacute N70.03
tuberculous (acute) (chronic) A18.17
venereal (gonococcal) (acute) (chronic) A54.24

Salpingo-ovaritis *—see* Salpingo-oophoritis

Salpingoperitonitis *—see* Salpingo-oophoritis

Salzmann's nodular dystrophy *—see* Degeneration, cornea, nodular

Sampson's cyst or tumor N80.1

San Joaquin (Valley) **fever** B38.0

Sandblaster's asthma, lung or pneumoconiosis J62.8

Sander's disease (paranoia) F22

Sandfly fever A93.1

Sandhoff's disease E75.01

Sanfilippo (Type B) (Type C) (Type D) **syndrome** E76.22

Sanger-Brown ataxia G11.2

Sao Paulo fever or typhus A77.0

Saponification, mesenteric K65.8

Sarcocele (benign)
syphilitic A52.76
congenital A50.59

Sarcocystosis A07.8

Sarcoepiplocele *—see* Hernia

Sarcoepiplomphalocele Q79.2

Sarcoid *—see also* Sarcoidosis
arthropathy D86.86
Boeck's D86.9
Darier-Roussy D86.3
iridocyclitis D86.83
meningitis D86.81
myocarditis D86.85
myositis D86.87
pyelonephritis D86.84
Spiegler-Fendt L08.89

Sarcoidosis D86.9
with
cranial nerve palsies D86.82
hepatic granuloma D86.89
polyarthritis D86.86
tubulo-interstitial nephropathy D86.84
combined sites NEC D86.89
lung D86.0
and lymph nodes D86.2
lymph nodes D86.1
and lung D86.2
meninges D86.81
skin D86.3
specified type NEC D86.89

Sarcoma (of) *—see also* Neoplasm, connective tissue, malignant
alveolar soft part *—see* Neoplasm, connective tissue, malignant
ameloblastic C41.1
upper jaw (bone) C41.0
botryoid *—see* Neoplasm, connective tissue, malignant
botryoides *—see* Neoplasm, connective tissue, malignant
cerebellar C71.6
circumscribed (arachnoidal) C71.6
circumscribed (arachnoidal) cerebellar C71.6
clear cell *—see also* Neoplasm, connective tissue, malignant
kidney C64.-
dendritic cells (accessory cells) C96.4
embryonal *—see* Neoplasm, connective tissue, malignant
endometrial (stromal) C54.1
isthmus C54.0
epithelioid (cell) *—see* Neoplasm, connective tissue, malignant
Ewing's *—see* Neoplasm, bone, malignant
follicular dendritic cell C96.4
germinoblastic (diffuse) *—see* Lymphoma, diffuse large cell
follicular *—see* Lymphoma, follicular, specified NEC
giant cell (except of bone) *—see also* Neoplasm, connective tissue, malignant
bone *—see* Neoplasm, bone, malignant

Sarcoma *(continued)*
- glomoid —*see* Neoplasm, connective tissue, malignant
- granulocytic C92.3-
- hemangioendothelial —*see* Neoplasm, connective tissue, malignant
- hemorrhagic, multiple —*see* Sarcoma, Kaposi's
- histiocytic C96.A
- Hodgkin —*see* Lymphoma, Hodgkin
- immunoblastic (diffuse) —*see* Lymphoma, diffuse large cell
- interdigitating dendritic cell C96.4
- Kaposi's
  - colon C46.4
  - connective tissue C46.1
  - gastrointestinal organ C46.4
  - lung C46.5-
  - lymph node(s) C46.3
  - palate (hard) (soft) C46.2
  - rectum C46.4
  - skin C46.0
  - specified site NEC C46.7
  - stomach C46.4
  - unspecified site C46.9
- Kupffer cell C22.3
- Langerhans cell C96.4
- leptomeningeal —*see* Neoplasm, meninges, malignant
- liver NEC C22.4
- lymphangioendothelial —*see* Neoplasm, connective tissue, malignant
- lymphoblastic —*see* Lymphoma, lymphoblastic (diffuse)
- lymphocytic —*see* Lymphoma, small cell B-cell
- mast cell C96.22
- melanotic —*see* Melanoma
- meningeal —*see* Neoplasm, meninges, malignant
- meningothelial —*see* Neoplasm, meninges, malignant
- mesenchymal —*see also* Neoplasm, connective tissue, malignant
  - mixed —*see* Neoplasm, connective tissue, malignant
- mesothelial —*see* Mesothelioma
- monstrocellular
  - specified site —*see* Neoplasm, malignant, by site
  - unspecified site C71.9
- myeloid C92.3-
- neurogenic —*see* Neoplasm, nerve, malignant
- odontogenic C41.1
  - upper jaw (bone) C41.0
- osteoblastic —*see* Neoplasm, bone, malignant
- osteogenic —*see also* Neoplasm, bone, malignant
  - juxtacortical —*see* Neoplasm, bone, malignant
  - periosteal —*see* Neoplasm, bone, malignant
- periosteal —*see also* Neoplasm, bone, malignant
  - osteogenic —*see* Neoplasm, bone, malignant
- pleomorphic cell —*see* Neoplasm, connective tissue, malignant
- reticulum cell (diffuse) —*see* Lymphoma, diffuse large cell
  - nodular —*see* Lymphoma, follicular
  - pleomorphic cell type —*see* Lymphoma, diffuse large cell
- rhabdoid —*see* Neoplasm, malignant, by site

Sarcoma *(continued)*
- round cell —*see* Neoplasm, connective tissue, malignant
- small cell —*see* Neoplasm, connective tissue, malignant
- soft tissue —*see* Neoplasm, connective tissue, malignant
- spindle cell —*see* Neoplasm, connective tissue, malignant
- stromal (endometrial) C54.1
  - isthmus C54.0
- synovial —*see also* Neoplasm, connective tissue, malignant
  - biphasic —*see* Neoplasm, connective tissue, malignant
  - epithelioid cell —*see* Neoplasm, connective tissue, malignant
  - spindle cell —*see* Neoplasm, connective tissue, malignant

Sarcomatosis
- meningeal —*see* Neoplasm, meninges, malignant
- specified site NEC —*see* Neoplasm, connective tissue, malignant
- unspecified site C80.1

Sarcopenia (age-related) M62.84

Sarcosinemia E72.59

Sarcosporidiosis (intestinal) A07.8

Satiety, early R68.81

Saturnine —*see* condition

Saturnism
- overdose or wrong substance given or taken —*see* Table of Drugs and Chemicals, by drug, poisoning

Satyriasis F52.8

Sauriasis —*see* Ichthyosis

SBE (subacute bacterial endocarditis) I33.0

Scabs R23.4

Scabies (any site) B86

Scaglietti-Dagnini syndrome E22.0

Scald —*see* Burn

Scalenus anticus (anterior) **syndrome** G54.0

Scales R23.4

Scaling, skin R23.4

Scalp —*see* condition

Scapegoating affecting child Z62.3

Scaphocephaly Q75.0

Scapulalgia M89.8X1

Scapulohumeral myopathy G71.0

Scar, scarring (*see also* Cicatrix) L90.5
- adherent L90.5
- atrophic L90.5
- cervix
  - in pregnancy or childbirth —*see* Pregnancy, complicated by, abnormal cervix
- cheloid L91.0
- chorioretinal H31.00-
  - posterior pole macula H31.01-
  - postsurgical H59.81-
  - solar retinopathy H31.02-
  - specified type NEC H31.09-
- choroid —*see* Scar, chorioretinal
- conjunctiva H11.24-
- cornea H17.9
  - xerophthalmic —*see also* Opacity, cornea
    - vitamin A deficiency E50.6
- duodenum, obstructive K31.5
- hypertrophic L91.0
- keloid L91.0

Scar, scarring *(continued)*
- labia N90.89
- lung (base) J98.4
- macula —*see* Scar, chorioretinal, posterior pole
- muscle M62.89
- myocardium, myocardial I25.2
- painful L90.5
- posterior pole (eye) —*see* Scar, chorioretinal, posterior pole
- retina —*see* Scar, chorioretinal
- trachea J39.8
- transmural uterine, in pregnancy O34.29
- uterus N85.8
  - in pregnancy O34.29
- vagina N89.8
  - postoperative N99.2
- vulva N90.89

Scarabiasis B88.2

Scarlatina (anginosa) (maligna) A38.9
- myocarditis (acute) A38.1
  - old —*see* Myocarditis
- otitis media A38.0
- ulcerosa A38.8

Scarlet fever (albuminuria) (angina) A38.9

Schamberg's disease (progressive pigmentary dermatosis) L81.7

Schatzki's ring (acquired) (esophagus) (lower) K22.2
- congenital Q39.3

Schaufenster krankheit I20.8

Schaumann's
- benign lymphogranulomatosis D86.1
- disease or syndrome —*see* Sarcoidosis

Scheie's syndrome E76.03

Schenck's disease B42.1

Scheuermann's disease or osteochondrosis —*see* Osteochondrosis, juvenile, spine

Schilder (-Flatau) **disease** G37.0

Schilling-type monocytic leukemia C93.0-

Schimmelbusch's disease, cystic mastitis, or hyperplasia —*see* Mastopathy, cystic

Schistosoma infestation —*see* Infestation, Schistosoma

Schistosomiasis B65.9
- with muscle disorder B65.9 *[M63.80]*
  - ankle B65.9 *[M63.87-]*
  - foot B65.9 *[M63.87-]*
  - forearm B65.9 *[M63.83-]*
  - hand B65.9 *[M63.84-]*
  - lower leg B65.9 *[M63.86-]*
  - multiple sites B65.9 *[M63.89]*
  - pelvic region B65.9 *[M63.85-]*
  - shoulder region B65.9 *[M63.81-]*
  - specified site NEC B65.9 *[M63.88]*
  - thigh B65.9 *[M63.85-]*
  - upper arm B65.9 *[M63.82-]*
- Asiatic B65.2
- bladder B65.0
- chestermani B65.8
- colon B65.1
- cutaneous B65.3
- due to
  - S. haematobium B65.0
  - S. japonicum B65.2
  - S. mansoni B65.1
  - S. mattheii B65.8
- Eastern B65.2
- genitourinary tract B65.0

Schistosomiasis *(continued)*
- intestinal B65.1
- lung NEC B65.9 *[J99]*
  - pneumonia B65.9 *[J17]*
- Manson's (intestinal) B65.1
- oriental B65.2
- pulmonary NEC B65.9 *[J99]*
  - pneumonia B65.9
- Schistosoma
  - haematobium B65.0
  - japonicum B65.2
  - mansoni B65.1
- specified type NEC B65.8
- urinary B65.0
- vesical B65.0

Schizencephaly Q04.6

Schizoaffective psychosis F25.9

Schizodontia K00.2

Schizoid personality F60.1

Schizophrenia, schizophrenic F20.9
- acute (brief) (undifferentiated) F23
- atypical (form) F20.3
- borderline F21
- catalepsy F20.2
- catatonic (type) (excited) (withdrawn) F20.2
- cenesthopathic, cenesthesiopathic F20.89
- childhood type F84.5
- chronic undifferentiated F20.5
- cyclic F25.0
- disorganized (type) F20.1
- flexibilitas cerea F20.2
- hebephrenic (type) F20.1
- incipient F21
- latent F21
- negative type F20.5
- paranoid (type) F20.0
- paraphrenic F20.0
- post-psychotic depression F32.89
- prepsychotic F21
- prodromal F21
- pseudoneurotic F21
- pseudopsychopathic F21
- reaction F23
- residual (state) (type) F20.5
- restzustand F20.5
- schizoaffective (type) —*see* Psychosis, schizoaffective
- simple (type) F20.89
- simplex F20.89
- specified type NEC F20.89
- spectrum and other psychotic disorder F29
  - specified NEC F28
- stupor F20.2
- syndrome of childhood F84.5
- undifferentiated (type) F20.3
  - chronic F20.5

Schizothymia (persistent) F60.1

Schlatter-Osgood disease or osteochondrosis —*see* Osteochondrosis, juvenile, tibia

Schlatter's tibia —*see* Osteochondrosis, juvenile, tibia

Schmidt's syndrome (polyglandular, autoimmune) E31.0

Schmincke's carcinoma or tumor —*see* Neoplasm, nasopharynx, malignant

Schmitz (-Stutzer) **dysentery** A03.0

Schmorl's disease or nodes
- lumbar region M51.46
- lumbosacral region M51.47
- sacrococcygeal region M53.3
- thoracic region M51.44
- thoracolumbar region M51.45

nneiderian
papilloma —*see* Neoplasm, nasopharynx, benign
specified site —*see* Neoplasm, benign, by site
unspecified site D14.0
specified site —*see* Neoplasm, malignant, by site
unspecified site C30.0
holte's syndrome (malignant carcinoid) E34.0
holz (-Bielchowsky-Henneberg) **disease or syndrome** E75.25
hönlein (-Henoch) **disease or purpura** (primary) (rheumatic) D69.0
hottmuller's disease A01.4
hroeder's syndrome (endocrine hypertensive) E27.0
hüller-Christian disease or syndrome C96.5
hultze's type acroparesthesia, simple I73.89
hultz's disease or syndrome —*see* Agranulocytosis
hwalbe-Ziehen-Oppenheim disease G24.1
hwannoma —*see also* Neoplasm, nerve, benign
malignant —*see also* Neoplasm, nerve, malignant
with rhabdomyoblastic differentiation —*see* Neoplasm, nerve, malignant
melanocytic —*see* Neoplasm, nerve, benign
pigmented —*see* Neoplasm, nerve, benign
hwannomatosis Q85.03
hwartz (-Jampel) **syndrome** G71.13
hwartz-Bartter syndrome E22.2
hweniger-Buzzi anetoderma L90.1
iatic —*see* condition
iatica (infective)
with lumbago M54.4-
due to intervertebral disc disorder —*see* Disorder, disc, with, radiculopathy
due to displacement of intervertebral disc (with lumbago) —*see* Disorder, disc, with, radiculopathy
wallet M54.3-
imitar syndrome Q26.8
lera —*see* condition
lerectasia H15.84-
leredema
adultorum —*see* Sclerosis, systemic
Buschke's —*see* Sclerosis, systemic
newborn P83.0
lerema (adiposum) (edematosum) (neonatorum) (newborn) P83.0
adultorum —*see* Sclerosis, systemic
leriasis —*see* Scleroderma
leritis H15.00-
with corneal involvement H15.04-
anterior H15.01-
brawny H15.02-
in (due to) zoster B02.34
posterior H15.03-
specified type NEC H15.09-
syphilitic A52.71
tuberculous (nodular) A18.51
lerochoroiditis H31.8

Scleroconjunctivitis —*see* Scleritis
Sclerocystic ovary syndrome E28.2
Sclerodactyly, sclerodactylia L94.3
Scleroderma, sclerodermia (acrosclerotic) (diffuse) (generalized) (progressive) (pulmonary) (*see also* Sclerosis, systemic) M34.9-
circumscribed L94.0
linear L94.1
localized L94.0
newborn P83.88
systemic M34.9
Sclerokeratitis H16.8
tuberculous A18.52
Scleroma nasi A48.8
Scleromalacia (perforans) H15.05-
Scleromyxedema L98.5
Sclérose en plaques G35
Sclerosis, sclerotic
adrenal (gland) E27.8
Alzheimer's —*see* Disease, Alzheimer's
amyotrophic (lateral) G12.21
aorta, aortic I70.0
valve —*see* Endocarditis, aortic
artery, arterial, arteriolar, arteriovascular —*see* Arteriosclerosis
ascending multiple G35
brain (generalized) (lobular) G37.9
artery, arterial I67.2
diffuse G37.0
disseminated G35
insular G35
Krabbe's E75.23
miliary G35
multiple G35
presenile (Alzheimer's) —*see* Disease, Alzheimer's, early onset
senile (arteriosclerotic) I67.2
stem, multiple G35
tuberous Q85.1
bulbar, multiple G35
bundle of His I44.39
cardiac —*see* Disease, heart, ischemic, atherosclerotic
cardiorenal —*see* Hypertension, cardiorenal
cardiovascular —*see also* Disease, cardiovascular
renal —*see* Hypertension, cardiorenal
cerebellar —*see* Sclerosis, brain
cerebral —*see* Sclerosis, brain
cerebrospinal (disseminated) (multiple) G35
cerebrovascular I67.2
choroid —*see* Degeneration, choroid
combined (spinal cord) —*see also* Degeneration, combined
multiple G35
concentric (Balo) G37.5
cornea —*see* Opacity, cornea
coronary (artery) I25.10
with angina pectoris —*see* Arteriosclerosis, coronary (artery),
corpus cavernosum
female N90.89
male N48.6
diffuse (brain) (spinal cord) G37.0
disseminated G35
dorsal G35
dorsolateral (spinal cord) —*see* Degeneration, combined
endometrium N85.5

Sclerosis, sclerotic *(continued)*
extrapyramidal G25.9
eye, nuclear (senile) —*see* Cataract, senile, nuclear
focal and segmental (glomerular) (*see also* N00-N07 with fourth character .1) N05.1
Friedreich's (spinal cord) G11.1
funicular (spermatic cord) N50.89
general (vascular) —*see* Arteriosclerosis
gland (lymphatic) I89.8
hepatic K74.1
alcoholic K70.2
hereditary
cerebellar G11.9
spinal (Friedreich's ataxia) G11.1
hippocampal G93.81
insular G35
kidney —*see* Sclerosis, renal
larynx J38.7
lateral (amyotrophic) (descending) (spinal) G12.21
primary G12.23
lens, senile nuclear —*see* Cataract, senile, nuclear
liver K74.1
with fibrosis K74.2
alcoholic K70.2
alcoholic K70.2
cardiac K76.1
lung —*see* Fibrosis, lung
mastoid —*see* Mastoiditis, chronic
mesial temporal G93.81
mitral I05.8
Mönckeberg's (medial) —*see* Arteriosclerosis, extremities
multiple (brain stem) (cerebral) (generalized) (spinal cord) G35
myocardium, myocardial —*see* Disease, heart, ischemic, atherosclerotic
nuclear (senile), eye —*see* Cataract, senile, nuclear
ovary N83.8
pancreas K86.89
penis N48.6
peripheral arteries —*see* Arteriosclerosis, extremities
plaques G35
pluriglandular E31.8
polyglandular E31.8
posterolateral (spinal cord) —*see* Degeneration, combined
presenile (Alzheimer's) —*see* Disease, Alzheimer's, early onset
primary, lateral G12.23
progressive, systemic M34.0
pulmonary —*see* Fibrosis, lung
artery I27.0
valve (heart) —*see* Endocarditis, pulmonary
renal N26.9
with
cystine storage disease E72.09
hypertensive heart disease (conditions in I11) —*see* Hypertension, cardiorenal
arteriolar (hyaline) (hyperplastic) —*see* Hypertension, kidney
retina (senile) (vascular) H35.00
senile (vascular) —*see* Arteriosclerosis
spinal (cord) (progressive) G95.89
ascending G61.0
combined —*see also* Degeneration, combined
multiple G35
syphilitic A52.11
disseminated G35
dorsolateral —*see* Degeneration, combined

Sclerosis, sclerotic *(continued)*
spinal *(continued)*
hereditary (Friedreich's) (mixed form) G11.1
lateral (amyotrophic) G12.23
multiple G35
posterior (syphilitic) A52.11
stomach K31.89
subendocardial, congenital I42.4
systemic M34.9
with
lung involvement M34.81
myopathy M34.82
polyneuropathy M34.83
drug-induced M34.2
due to chemicals NEC M34.2
progressive M34.0
specified NEC M34.89
temporal (mesial) G93.81
tricuspid (heart) (valve) I07.8
tuberous (brain) Q85.1
tympanic membrane —*see* Disorder, tympanic membrane, specified NEC
valve, valvular (heart) —*see* Endocarditis
vascular —*see* Arteriosclerosis
vein I87.8

Scoliosis (acquired) (postural) M41.9
adolescent (idiopathic) —*see* Scoliosis, idiopathic, adolescent
congenital Q67.5
due to bony malformation Q76.3
failure of segmentation (hemivertebra) Q76.3
hemivertebra fusion Q76.3
postural Q67.5
idiopathic M41.20
adolescent M41.129
cervical region M41.122
cervicothoracic region M41.123
lumbar region M41.126
lumbosacral region M41.127
thoracic region M41.124
thoracolumbar region M41.125
cervical region M41.22
cervicothoracic region M41.23
infantile M41.00
cervical region M41.02
cervicothoracic region M41.03
lumbar region M41.06
lumbosacral region M41.07
sacrococcygeal region M41.08
thoracic region M41.04
thoracolumbar region M41.05
juvenile M41.119
cervical region M41.112
cervicothoracic region M41.113
lumbar region M41.116
lumbosacral region M41.117
thoracic region M41.114
thoracolumbar region M41.115
lumbar region M41.26
lumbosacral region M41.27
thoracic region M41.24
thoracolumbar region M41.25
infantile - *see* Scoliosis, idiopathic, infantile
neuromuscular M41.40
cervical region M41.42
cervicothoracic region M41.43
lumbar region M41.46
lumbosacral region M41.47
occipito-atlanto-axial region M41.41
thoracic region M41.44
thoracolumbar region M41.45
paralytic —*see* Scoliosis, neuromuscular
postradiation therapy M96.5

Scoliosis *(continued)*
- rachitic (late effect or sequelae) E64.3 *[M49.80]*
  - cervical region E64.3 *[M49.82]*
  - cervicothoracic region E64.3 *[M49.83]*
  - lumbar region E64.3 *[M49.86]*
  - lumbosacral region E64.3 *[M49.87]*
  - multiple sites E64.3 *[M49.89]*
  - occipito-atlanto-axial region E64.3 *[M49.81]*
  - sacrococcygeal region E64.3 *[M49.88]*
  - thoracic region E64.3 *[M49.84]*
  - thoracolumbar region E64.3 *[M49.85]*
- sciatic M54.4-
- secondary (to) NEC M41.50
  - cerebral palsy, Friedreich's ataxia, poliomyelitis, neuromuscular disorders *—see* Scoliosis, neuromuscular
  - cervical region M41.52
  - cervicothoracic region M41.53
  - lumbar region M41.56
  - lumbosacral region M41.57
  - thoracic region M41.54
  - thoracolumbar region M41.55
- specified form NEC M41.80
  - cervical region M41.82
  - cervicothoracic region M41.83
  - lumbar region M41.86
  - lumbosacral region M41.87
  - thoracic region M41.84
  - thoracolumbar region M41.85
- thoracogenic M41.30
  - thoracic region M41.34
  - thoracolumbar region M41.35
- tuberculous A18.01

Scoliotic pelvis
- with disproportion (fetopelvic) O33.0
  - causing obstructed labor O65.0

Scorbutus, scorbutic *—see also* Scurvy
- anemia D53.2

Score, NIHSS (National Institutes of Health Stoke Scale) R29.7-

Scotoma (arcuate) (Bjerrum) (central) (ring) *—see also* Defect, visual field, localized, scotoma
- scintillating H53.19

Scratch *—see* Abrasion

Scratchy throat R09.89

Screening (for) Z13.9
- alcoholism Z13.89
- anemia Z13.0
- anomaly, congenital Z13.89
- antenatal, of mother (*see also* Encounter, antenatal screening) Z36.9
- arterial hypertension Z13.6
- arthropod-borne viral disease NEC Z11.59
- bacteriuria, asymptomatic Z13.89
- behavioral disorder Z13.89
- brain injury, traumatic Z13.850
- bronchitis, chronic Z13.83
- brucellosis Z11.2
- cardiovascular disorder Z13.6
- cataract Z13.5
- chlamydial diseases Z11.8
- cholera Z11.0
- chromosomal abnormalities (nonprocreative) NEC Z13.79
- colonoscopy Z12.11
- congenital
  - dislocation of hip Z13.89
  - eye disorder Z13.5
  - malformation or deformation Z13.89
- contamination NEC Z13.88
- cystic fibrosis Z13.228
- dengue fever Z11.59
- dental disorder Z13.84
- depression Z13.89
- developmental handicap Z13.42
  - in early childhood Z13.42
  - infant Z13.41
- diabetes mellitus Z13.1
- diphtheria Z11.2
- disability, intellectual Z13.42
  - infant Z13.41
- disease or disorder Z13.9
  - bacterial NEC Z11.2
    - intestinal infectious Z11.0
    - respiratory tuberculosis Z11.1
  - blood or blood-forming organ Z13.0
  - cardiovascular Z13.6
  - Chagas' Z11.6
  - chlamydial Z11.8
  - dental Z13.89
  - developmental Z13.42
    - in child Z13.42
    - infant Z13.41
  - digestive tract NEC Z13.818
    - lower GI Z13.811
    - upper GI Z13.810
  - ear Z13.5
  - endocrine Z13.29
  - eye Z13.5
  - genitourinary Z13.89
  - heart Z13.6
  - human immunodeficiency virus (HIV) infection Z11.4
  - immunity Z13.0
  - infection
    - intestinal Z11.0
      - specified NEC Z11.6
  - infectious Z11.9
  - mental Z13.89
  - metabolic Z13.228
  - neurological Z13.89
  - nutritional Z13.21
    - metabolic Z13.228
      - lipoid disorders Z13.220
  - protozoal Z11.6
    - intestinal Z11.0
  - respiratory Z13.83
  - rheumatic Z13.828
  - rickettsial Z11.8
  - sexually-transmitted NEC Z11.3
    - human immunodeficiency virus (HIV) Z11.4
  - sickle-cell (trait) Z13.0
  - skin Z13.89
  - specified NEC Z13.89
  - spirochetal Z11.8
  - thyroid Z13.29
  - vascular Z13.6
  - venereal Z11.3
  - viral NEC Z11.59
    - human immunodeficiency virus (HIV) Z11.4
    - intestinal Z11.0
- elevated titer Z13.89
- emphysema Z13.83
- encephalitis, viral (mosquito- or tick-borne) Z11.59
- exposure to contaminants (toxic) Z13.88
- fever
  - dengue Z11.59
  - hemorrhagic Z11.59
  - yellow Z11.59
- filariasis Z11.6
- galactosemia Z13.228
- gastrointestinal condition Z13.818
- genetic (nonprocreative) - for procreative management *—see* Testing, genetic, for procreative management
  - disease carrier status (nonprocreative) Z13.71
  - specified NEC (nonprocreative) Z13.79
- genitourinary condition Z13.89
- glaucoma Z13.5
- gonorrhea Z11.3
- gout Z13.89
- helminthiasis (intestinal) Z11.6
- hematopoietic malignancy Z12.89
- hemoglobinopathies NEC Z13.0
- hemorrhagic fever Z11.59
- Hodgkin disease Z12.89
- human immunodeficiency virus (HIV) Z11.4
- human papillomavirus Z11.51
- hypertension Z13.6
- immunity disorders Z13.0
- infection
  - mycotic Z11.8
  - parasitic Z11.8
- ingestion of radioactive substance Z13.88
- intellectual disability Z13.42
  - infant Z13.41
- intestinal
  - helminthiasis Z11.6
  - infectious disease Z11.0
- leishmaniasis Z11.6
- leprosy Z11.2
- leptospirosis Z11.8
- leukemia Z12.89
- lymphoma Z12.89
- malaria Z11.6
- malnutrition Z13.29
  - metabolic Z13.228
  - nutritional Z13.21
- measles Z11.59
- mental disorder Z13.89
- metabolic errors, inborn Z13.228
- multiphasic Z13.89
- musculoskeletal disorder Z13.828
  - osteoporosis Z13.820
- mycoses Z11.8
- myocardial infarction (acute) Z13.6
- neoplasm (malignant) (of) Z12.9
  - bladder Z12.6
  - blood Z12.89
  - breast Z12.39
    - routine mammogram Z12.31
  - cervix Z12.4
  - colon Z12.11
  - genitourinary organs NEC Z12.79
    - bladder Z12.6
    - cervix Z12.4
    - ovary Z12.73
    - prostate Z12.5
    - testis Z12.71
    - vagina Z12.72
  - hematopoietic system Z12.89
  - intestinal tract Z12.10
    - colon Z12.11
    - rectum Z12.12
    - small intestine Z12.13
  - lung Z12.2
  - lymph (glands) Z12.89
  - nervous system Z12.82
  - oral cavity Z12.81
  - prostate Z12.5
  - rectum Z12.12
  - respiratory organs Z12.2
  - skin Z12.83
  - small intestine Z12.13
  - specified site NEC Z12.89
  - stomach Z12.0
- nephropathy Z13.89
- nervous system disorders NEC Z13.858
- neurological condition Z13.89
- osteoporosis Z13.820
- parasitic infestation Z11.9
  - specified NEC Z11.8
- phenylketonuria Z13.228
- plague Z11.2
- poisoning (chemical) (heavy metal) Z13.88
- poliomyelitis Z11.59
- postnatal, chromosomal abnormalities Z13.89
- prenatal, of mother (*see also* Encounter, antenatal screening) Z36.9
- protozoal disease Z11.6
  - intestinal Z11.0
- pulmonary tuberculosis Z11.1
- radiation exposure Z13.88
- respiratory condition Z13.83
- respiratory tuberculosis Z11.1
- rheumatoid arthritis Z13.828
- rubella Z11.59
- schistosomiasis Z11.6
- sexually-transmitted disease NEC Z11.3
  - human immunodeficiency virus (HIV) Z11.4
- sickle-cell disease or trait Z13.0
- skin condition Z13.89
- sleeping sickness Z11.6
- special Z13.9
  - specified NEC Z13.89
- syphilis Z11.3
- tetanus Z11.2
- trachoma Z11.8
- traumatic brain injury Z13.850
- trypanosomiasis Z11.6
- tuberculosis, respiratory Z11.1
- venereal disease Z11.3
- viral encephalitis (mosquito- or tick-borne) Z11.59
- whooping cough Z11.2
- worms, intestinal Z11.6
- yaws Z11.8
- yellow fever Z11.59

Scrofula, scrofulosis (tuberculosis of cervical lymph glands) A18.2

Scrofulide (primary) (tuberculous) A18.4

Scrofuloderma, scrofulodermia (any site) (primary) A18.4

Scrofulosus lichen (primary) (tuberculous) A18.4

Scrofulous *—see* condition

Scrotal tongue K14.5

Scrotum *—see* condition

Scurvy, scorbutic E54
- anemia D53.2
- gum E54
- infantile E54
- rickets E55.0 *[M90.80]*

Sealpox B08.62

Seasickness T75.3

Seatworm (infection) (infestation) B80

Sebaceous *—see also* condition
- cyst *—see* Cyst, sebaceous

Seborrhea, seborrheic L21.9
- capillitii R23.8
- capitis L21.0
- dermatitis L21.9
  - infantile L21.1
- eczema L21.9
  - infantile L21.1
- sicca L21.0

Seckel's syndrome Q87.1

Seclusion, pupil *—see* Membrane, pupillary

Second hand tobacco smoke
- **exposure** (acute) (chronic) Z77.22
- in the perinatal period P96.81

Secondary
- dentin (in pulp) K04.3
- neoplasm, secondaries *—see* Table of Neoplasms, secondary

Secretion
- antidiuretic hormone, inappropriate E22.2
- catecholamine, by pheochromocytoma E27.5
- hormone
  - antidiuretic, inappropriate (syndrome) E22.2
  - by
    - carcinoid tumor E34.0
    - pheochromocytoma E27.5
  - ectopic NEC E34.2
- urinary
  - excessive R35.8
  - suppression R34

Section
- nerve, traumatic *—see* Injury, nerve

Sedative, hypnotic, or anxiolytic-induced
- anxiety disorder F13.980
- bipolar and related disorder F13.94
- delirium F13.921
- depressive disorder F13.94
- major neurocognitive disorder F13.97
- mild neurocognitive disorder F13.988
- psychotic disorder F13.959
- sexual dysfunction F13.981
- sleep disorder F13.982

Segmentation, incomplete (congenital) *—see also* Fusion
- bone NEC Q78.8
- lumbosacral (joint) (vertebra) Q76.49

Seitelberger's syndrome (infantile neuraxonal dystrophy) G31.89

Seizure(s) (*see also* Convulsions) R56.9
- akinetic *—see* Epilepsy, generalized, specified NEC
- atonic *—see* Epilepsy, generalized, specified NEC
- autonomic (hysterical) F44.5
- convulsive *—see* Convulsions
- cortical (focal) (motor) *—see* Epilepsy, localization-related, symptomatic, with simple partial seizures
- disorder (*see also* Epilepsy) G40.909
- due to stroke *—see* Sequelae (of), disease, cerebrovascular, by type, specified NEC
- epileptic *—see* Epilepsy
- febrile (simple) R56.00
  - with status epilepticus G40.901
  - complex (atypical) (complicated) R56.01
    - with status epilepticus G40.901
- grand mal G40.409
  - intractable G40.419
    - with status epilepticus G40.411
    - without status epilepticus G40.419
  - not intractable G40.409
    - with status epilepticus G40.401
    - without status epilepticus G40.409

Seizure *(continued)*
- heart *—see* Disease, heart
- hysterical F44.5
- intractable G40.919
  - with status epilepticus G40.911
- Jacksonian (focal) (motor type) (sensory type) *—see* Epilepsy, localization-related, symptomatic, with simple partial seizures
- newborn P90
- nonspecific epileptic
  - atonic *—see* Epilepsy, generalized, specified NEC
  - clonic *—see* Epilepsy, generalized, specified NEC
  - myoclonic *—see* Epilepsy, generalized, specified NEC
  - tonic *—see* Epilepsy, generalized, specified NEC
  - tonic-clonic *—see* Epilepsy, generalized, specified NEC
- partial, developing into secondarily generalized seizures
  - complex *—see* Epilepsy, localization-related, symptomatic, with complex partial seizures
  - simple *—see* Epilepsy, localization-related, symptomatic, with simple partial seizures
- petit mal G40.409
  - intractable G40.419
    - with status epilepticus G40.411
    - without status epilepticus G40.419
  - not intractable G40.409
    - with status epilepticus G40.401
    - without status epilepticus G40.409
- post traumatic R56.1
- recurrent G40.909
- specified NEC G40.89
- uncinate *—see* Epilepsy, localization-related, symptomatic, with complex partial seizures

Selenium deficiency, dietary E59

Self-damaging behavior (life-style) Z72.89

Self-harm (attempted)
- history (personal) Z91.5
  - in family Z81.8

Self-mutilation (attempted)
- history (personal) Z91.5
  - in family Z81.8

Self-poisoning
- history (personal) Z91.5
  - in family Z81.8
- observation following (alleged) attempt Z03.6

Semicoma R40.1

Seminal vesiculitis N49.0

Seminoma C62.9-
- specified site *—see* Neoplasm, malignant, by site

Senear-Usher disease or syndrome L10.4

Senectus R54

Senescence (without mention of psychosis) R54

Senile, senility (*see also* condition) R41.81
- with
  - acute confusional state F05
  - mental changes NOS F03
  - psychosis NEC *—see* Psychosis, senile

Senile, senility *(continued)*
- asthenia R54
- cervix (atrophic) N88.8
- debility R54
- endometrium (atrophic) N85.8
- fallopian tube (atrophic) *—see* Atrophy, fallopian tube
- heart (failure) R54
- ovary (atrophic) *—see* Atrophy, ovary
- premature E34.8
- vagina, vaginitis (atrophic) N95.2
- wart L82.1

Sensation
- burning (skin) R20.8
  - tongue K14.6
- loss of R20.8
- prickling (skin) R20.2
- tingling (skin) R20.2

Sense loss
- smell *—see* Disturbance, sensation, smell
- taste *—see* Disturbance, sensation, taste
- touch R20.8

Sensibility disturbance (cortical) (deep) (vibratory) R20.9

Sensitive, sensitivity *—see also* Allergy
- carotid sinus G90.01
- child (excessive) F93.8
- cold, autoimmune D59.1
- dentin K03.89
- gluten (non-celiac) K90.41
- latex Z91.040
- methemoglobin D74.8
- tuberculin, without clinical or radiological symptoms R76.11
- visual
  - glare H53.71
  - impaired contrast H53.72

Sensitiver Beziehungswahn F22

Sensitization, auto-erythrocytic D69.2

Separation
- anxiety, abnormal (of childhood) F93.0
- apophysis, traumatic - code as Fracture, by site
- choroid *—see* Detachment, choroid
- epiphysis, epiphyseal
  - nontraumatic *—see also* Osteochondropathy, specified type NEC
    - upper femoral *—see* Slipped, epiphysis, upper femoral
  - traumatic - code as Fracture, by site
- fracture *—see* Fracture
- infundibulum cardiac from right ventricle by a partition Q24.3
- joint (traumatic) (current) - code by site under Dislocation
- pubic bone, obstetrical trauma O71.6
- retina, retinal *—see* Detachment, retina
- symphysis pubis, obstetrical trauma O71.6
- tracheal ring, incomplete, congenital Q32.1

Sepsis (generalized) (unspecified organism) A41.9
- with
  - organ dysfunction (acute) (multiple) R65.20
    - with septic shock R65.21
- actinomycotic A42.7
- adrenal hemorrhage syndrome (meningococcal) A39.1
- anaerobic A41.4
- Bacillus anthracis A22.7

Sepsis *(continued)*
- Brucella *—see also* Brucellosis A23.9
- candidal B37.7
- cryptogenic A41.9
- due to device, implant or graft T85.79
  - arterial graft NEC T82.7
  - breast (implant) T85.79
  - catheter NEC T85.79
    - dialysis (renal) T82.7
      - intraperitoneal T85.71
    - infusion NEC T82.7
      - spinal (cranial) (epidural) (intrathecal) (spinal) (subarachnoid) (subdural) T85.735
    - urethral (indwelling) T83.511
    - urinary T83.518
  - ectopic or molar pregnancy O08.82
  - electronic (electrode) (pulse generator) (stimulator)
    - bone T84.7
    - cardiac T82.7
    - nervous system T85.738
      - brain T85.731
      - neurostimulator generator T85.734
      - peripheral nerve T85.732
      - spinal cord T85.733
    - urinary T83.590
  - fixation, internal (orthopedic) *—see* Complication, fixation device, infection
  - gastrointestinal (bile duct) (esophagus) T85.79
    - neurostimulator electrode (lead) T85.732
  - genital T83.69
  - heart NEC T82.7
    - valve (prosthesis) T82.6
      - graft T82.7
  - joint prosthesis *—see* Complication, joint prosthesis, infection
  - ocular (corneal graft) (orbital implant) T85.79
  - orthopedic NEC T84.7
    - fixation device, internal *—see* Complication, fixation device, infection
  - specified NEC T85.79
  - vascular T82.7
  - ventricular intracranial (communicating) shunt T85.730
- during labor O75.3
- Enterococcus A41.81
- Erysipelothrix (rhusiopathiae) (erysipeloid) A26.7
- Escherichia coli (E. coli) A41.5
- extraintestinal yersiniosis A28.2
- following
  - abortion (subsequent episode) O08.0
    - current episode *—see* Abortion
  - ectopic or molar pregnancy O08.82
  - immunization T88.0
  - infusion, therapeutic injection or transfusion NEC T80.29
- gangrenous A41.9
- gonococcal A54.86
- Gram-negative (organism) A41.5
  - anaerobic A41.4
- Haemophilus influenzae A41.3
- herpesviral B00.7
- intra-abdominal K65.1
- intraocular *—see* Endophthalmitis, purulent
- Listeria monocytogenes A32.7
- localized - code to specific localized infection
  - in operation wound T81.4

Sepsis *(continued)*
localized - code to specific localized *(continued)*
skin —*see* Abscess
malleus A24.0
melioidosis A24.1
meningeal —*see* Meningitis
meningococcal A39.4
acute A39.2
chronic A39.3
MSSA (Methicillin susceptible Staphylococcus aureus) A41.01
newborn P36.9
due to
anaerobes NEC P36.5
Escherichia coli P36.4
Staphylococcus P36.30
aureus P36.2
specified NEC P36.39
Streptococcus P36.10
group B P36.0
specified NEC P36.19
specified NEC P36.8
Pasteurella multocida A28.0
pelvic, puerperal, postpartum, childbirth O85
postprocedural T81.4
pneumococcal A40.3
puerperal, postpartum, childbirth (pelvic) O85
Salmonella (arizonae) (cholerae-suis) (enteritidis) (typhimurium) A02.1
severe R65.20
with septic shock R65.21
skin, localized —*see* Abscess
Shigella (*see also* Dysentery, bacillary) A03.9
specified organism NEC A41.89
Staphylococcus, staphylococcal A41.2
aureus (methicillin susceptible) (MSSA) A41.01
methicillin resistant (MRSA) A41.02
coagulase-negative A41.1
specified NEC A41.1
Streptococcus, streptococcal A40.9
agalactiae A40.1
group
A A40.0
B A40.1
D A41.81
neonatal P36.10
group B P36.0
specified NEC P36.19
pneumoniae A40.3
pyogenes A40.0
specified NEC A40.8
tracheostomy stoma J95.02
tularemic A21.7
umbilical, umbilical cord (newborn) —*see* Sepsis, newborn
Yersinia pestis A20.7

Septate —*see* Septum

Septic —*see* condition
arm —*see* Cellulitis, upper limb
with lymphangitis —*see* Lymphangitis, acute, upper limb
embolus —*see* Embolism
finger —*see* Cellulitis, digit
with lymphangitis —*see* Lymphangitis, acute, digit
foot —*see* Cellulitis, lower limb
with lymphangitis —*see* Lymphangitis, acute, lower limb
gallbladder (acute) K81.0
hand —*see* Cellulitis, upper limb
with lymphangitis —*see* Lymphangitis, acute, upper limb

Septic *(continued)*
joint —*see* Arthritis, pyogenic or pyemic
leg —*see* Cellulitis, lower limb
with lymphangitis —*see* Lymphangitis, acute, lower limb
nail —*see also* Cellulitis, digit
with lymphangitis —*see* Lymphangitis, acute, digit
sore —*see also* Abscess
throat J02.0
streptococcal J02.0
spleen (acute) D73.89
teeth, tooth (pulpal origin) K04.4
throat —*see* Pharyngitis
thrombus —*see* Thrombosis
toe —*see* Cellulitis, digit
with lymphangitis —*see* Lymphangitis, acute, digit
tonsils, chronic J35.01
with adenoiditis J35.03
uterus —*see* Endometritis

Septicemia A41.9
meaning sepsis —*see* Sepsis

Septum, septate (congenital) —*see also* Anomaly, by site
anal Q42.3
with fistula Q42.2
aqueduct of Sylvius Q03.0
with spina bifida —*see* Spina bifida, by site, with hydrocephalus
uterus (complete) (partial) Q51.2
vagina Q52.10
in pregnancy —*see* Pregnancy, complicated by, abnormal vagina
causing obstructed labor O65.5
longitudinal Q52.129
microperforate
left side Q52.124
right side Q52.123
nonobstruction Q52.120
obstructing Q52.129
left side Q52.122
right side Q52.1221
transverse Q52.11

Sequelae (of) —*see also* condition
abscess, intracranial or intraspinal (conditions in G06) G09
amputation -- code to injury with seventh character S
burn and corrosion -- code to injury with seventh character S
calcium deficiency E64.8
cerebrovascular disease —*see* Sequelae, disease, cerebrovascular
childbirth O94
contusion -- code to injury with seventh character S
corrosion —*see* Sequelae, burn and corrosion
crushing injury -- code to injury with seventh character S
disease
cerebrovascular I69.90
alteration of sensation I69.998
aphasia I69.920
apraxia I69.990
ataxia I69.993
cognitive deficits I69.91
disturbance of vision I69.998
dysarthria I69.922
dysphagia I69.991
dysphasia I69.921
facial droop I69.992
facial weakness I69.992
fluency disorder I69.923
hemiplegia I69.95-
hemorrhage

Sequelae *(continued)*
disease *(continued)*
cerebrovascular *(continued)*
hemorrhage *(continued)*
intracerebral —*see* Sequelae, hemorrhage, intracerebral
intracranial, nontraumatic NEC —*see* Sequelae, hemorrhage, intracranial, nontraumatic
subarachnoid —*see* Sequelae, hemorrhage, subarachnoid
language deficit I69.928
monoplegia
lower limb I69.94-
upper limb I69.93-
paralytic syndrome I69.96-
specified effect NEC I69.998
specified type NEC I69.80
alteration of sensation I69.898
aphasia I69.820
apraxia I69.890
ataxia I69.893
cognitive deficits I69.81
disturbance of vision I69.898
dysarthria I69.822
dysphagia I69.891
dysphasia I69.821
facial droop I69.892
facial weakness I69.892
fluency disorder I69.823
hemiplegia I69.85-
language deficit I69.828
monoplegia
lower limb I69.84-
upper limb I69.83-
paralytic syndrome I69.86-
specified effect NEC I69.898
speech deficit I69.928
speech deficit I69.828
stroke NOS —*see* Sequelae, stroke NOS
dislocation -- code to injury with seventh character S
encephalitis or encephalomyelitis (conditions in G04) G09
in infectious disease NEC B94.8
viral B94.1
external cause -- code to injury with seventh character S
foreign body entering natural orifice -- code to injury with seventh character S
fracture -- code to injury with seventh character S
frostbite -- code to injury with seventh character S
Hansen's disease B92
hemorrhage
intracerebral I69.10
alteration of sensation I69.198
aphasia I69.120
apraxia I69.190
ataxia I69.193
cognitive deficits I69.11
disturbance of vision I69.198
dysarthria I69.122
dysphagia I69.191
dysphasia I69.121
facial droop I69.192
facial weakness I69.192
fluency disorder I69.123
hemiplegia I69.15-
language deficit NEC I69.128
monoplegia
lower limb I69.14-
upper limb I69.13-
paralytic syndrome I69.16-
specified effect NEC I69.198
speech deficit NEC I69.128

Sequelae *(continued)*
hemorrhage *(continued)*
intracranial, nontraumatic NEC I69.20
alteration of sensation I69.298
aphasia I69.220
apraxia I69.290
ataxia I69.293
cognitive deficits I69.21
disturbance of vision I69.298
dysarthria I69.222
dysphagia I69.291
dysphasia I69.221
facial droop I69.292
facial weakness I69.292
fluency disorder I69.223
hemiplegia I69.25-
language deficit NEC I69.228
monoplegia
lower limb I69.24-
upper limb I69.23-
paralytic syndrome I69.26-
specified effect NEC I69.298
speech deficit NEC I69.228
subarachnoid I69.00
alteration of sensation I69.098
aphasia I69.020
apraxia I69.090
ataxia I69.093
cognitive deficits —*see* subcategory I69.01-
disturbance of vision I69.098
dysarthria I69.022
dysphagia I69.091
dysphasia I69.021
facial droop I69.092
facial weakness I69.092
fluency disorder I69.023
hemiplegia I69.05-
language deficit NEC I69.028
monoplegia
lower limb I69.04-
upper limb I69.03-
paralytic syndrome I69.06-
specified effect NEC I69.098
speech deficit NEC I69.028
hepatitis, viral B94.2
hyperalimentation E68
infarction
cerebral I69.30
alteration of sensation I69.398
aphasia I69.320
apraxia I69.390
ataxia I69.393
cognitive deficits I69.31
disturbance of vision I69.398
dysarthria I69.322
dysphagia I69.391
dysphasia I69.321
facial droop I69.392
facial weakness I69.392
fluency disorder I69.323
hemiplegia I69.35-
language deficit NEC I69.328
monoplegia
lower limb I69.34-
upper limb I69.33-
paralytic syndrome I69.36-
specified effect NEC I69.398
speech deficit NEC I69.328
infection, pyogenic, intracranial or intraspinal G09
infectious disease B94.9
specified NEC B94.8
injury -- code to injury with seventh character S
leprosy B92
meningitis
bacterial (conditions in G00) G09
other or unspecified cause (conditions in G03) G09

Sequelae *(continued)*
- muscle (and tendon) injury - code to injury with seventh character S
- myelitis *—see* Sequelae, encephalitis
- niacin deficiency E64.8
- nutritional deficiency E64.9
  - specified NEC E64.8
- obstetrical condition O94
- parasitic disease B94.9
- phlebitis or thrombophlebitis of intracranial or intraspinal venous sinuses and veins (conditions in G08) G09
- poisoning -- code to poisoning with seventh character S
  - nonmedicinal substance *—see* Sequelae, toxic effect, nonmedicinal substance
- poliomyelitis (acute) B91
- pregnancy O94
- protein-energy malnutrition E64.0
- puerperium O94
- rickets E64.3
- selenium deficiency E64.8
- sprain and strain - code to injury with seventh character S
- stroke NOS I69.30
  - alteration in sensation I69.398
  - aphasia I69.320
  - apraxia I69.390
  - ataxia I69.393
  - cognitive deficits I69.31
  - disturbance of vision I69.398
  - dysarthria I69.322
  - dysphagia I69.391
  - dysphasia I69.321
  - facial droop I69.392
  - facial weakness I69.392
  - hemiplegia I69.35-
  - language deficit NEC I69.328
  - monoplegia
    - lower limb I69.34-
    - upper limb I69.33-
  - paralytic syndrome I69.36-
  - specified effect NEC I69.398
  - speech deficit NEC I69.328
- tendon and muscle injury - code to injury with seventh character S
- thiamine deficiency E64.8
- trachoma B94.0
- tuberculosis B90.9
  - bones and joints B90.2
  - central nervous system B90.0
  - genitourinary B90.1
  - pulmonary (respiratory) B90.9
  - specified organs NEC B90.8
- viral
  - encephalitis B94.1
  - hepatitis B94.2
- vitamin deficiency NEC E64.8
  - A E64.1
  - B E64.8
  - C E64.2
- wound, open - code to injury with seventh character S

Sequestration *—see also* Sequestrum
- disk *—see* Displacement, intervertebral disk
- lung, congenital Q33.2

Sequestrum
- bone *—see* Osteomyelitis, chronic
- dental M27.2
- jaw bone M27.2
- orbit *—see* Osteomyelitis, orbit
- sinus (accessory) (nasal) *—see* Sinusitis

Sequoiosis lung or pneumonitis J67.8

Serology for syphilis
- doubtful
  - with signs or symptoms - code by site and stage under Syphilis
  - follow-up of latent syphilis *—see* Syphilis, latent
- negative, with signs or symptoms - code by site and stage under Syphilis
- positive A53.0
  - with signs or symptoms - code by site and stage under Syphilis
- reactivated A53.0

Seroma *—see also* Hematoma
- postprocedural - *see* Complication, postprocedural, seroma
- traumatic, secondary and recurrent T79.2

Seropurulent *—see* condition

Serositis, multiple K65.8
- pericardial I31.1
- peritoneal K65.8

Serous *—see* condition

Sertoli cell
- adenoma
  - specified site *—see* Neoplasm, benign, by site
  - unspecified site
    - female D27.9
    - male D29.20
- carcinoma
  - specified site *—see* Neoplasm, malignant, by site
  - unspecified site (male) C62.9-
    - female C56.9
- tumor
  - with lipid storage
    - specified site *—see* Neoplasm, benign, by site
    - unspecified site
      - female D27.9
      - male D29.20
  - specified site *—see* Neoplasm, benign, by site
  - unspecified site
    - female D27.9
    - male D29.20

Sertoli-Leydig cell tumor *—see* Neoplasm, benign, by site
- specified site *—see* Neoplasm, benign, by site
- unspecified site
  - female D27.9
  - male D29.20

Serum
- allergy, allergic reaction (*see also* Reaction, serum) T80.69
  - shock (*see also* Shock, anaphylactic) T80.59
- arthritis (*see also* Reaction, serum) T80.69
- complication or reaction NEC (*see also* Reaction, serum) T80.69
- disease NEC (*see also* Reaction, serum) T80.69
- hepatitis *—see also* Hepatitis, viral, type B
  - carrier (suspected) of B18.1
- intoxication (*see also* Reaction, serum) T80.69
- neuritis (*see also* Reaction, serum) T80.69
- neuropathy G61.1
- poisoning NEC (*see also* Reaction, serum) T80.69
- rash NEC (*see also* Reaction, serum) T80.69
- reaction NEC (*see also* Reaction, serum) T80.69
- sickness NEC (*see also* Reaction, serum) T80.69
- urticaria (*see also* Reaction, serum) T80.69

Sesamoiditis M25.8-

Sever's disease or osteochondrosis *— see* Osteochondrosis, juvenile, tarsus

Severe sepsis R65.20
- with septic shock R65.21

Sex
- chromosome mosaics Q97.8
  - lines with various numbers of X chromosomes Q97.2
- education Z70.8
- reassignment surgery status Z87.890

Sextuplet pregnancy *—see* Pregnancy, sextuplet

Sexual
- function, disorder of (psychogenic) F52.9
- immaturity (female) (male) E30.0
- impotence (psychogenic) organic origin NEC *—see* Dysfunction, sexual, male
- precocity (constitutional) (cryptogenic) (female) (idiopathic) (male) E30.1

Sexuality, pathologic *—see* Deviation, sexual

Sézary disease C84.1-

Shadow, lung R91.8

Shaking palsy or paralysis *—see* Parkinsonism

Shallowness, acetabulum *—see* Derangement, joint, specified type NEC, hip

Shaver's disease J63.1

Sheath (tendon) *—see* condition

Sheathing, retinal vessels H35.01-

Shedding
- nail L60.8
- premature, primary (deciduous) teeth K00.6

Sheehan's disease or syndrome E23.0

Shelf, rectal K62.89

Shell teeth K00.5

Shellshock (current) F43.0
- lasting state *—see* Disorder, post-traumatic stress

Shield kidney Q63.1

Shift
- auditory threshold (temporary) H93.24-
- mediastinal R93.8

Shifting sleep-work schedule (affecting sleep) G47.26

Shiga (-Kruse) **dysentery** A03.0

Shiga's bacillus A03.0

Shigella (dysentery) *—see* Dysentery, bacillary

Shigellosis A03.9
- Group A A03.0
- Group B A03.1
- Group C A03.2
- Group D A03.3

Shin splints S86.89

Shingles *—see* Herpes, zoster

Shipyard disease or eye B30.0

Shirodkar suture, in pregnancy *—see* Pregnancy, complicated by, incompetent cervix

Shock R57.9
- with ectopic or molar pregnancy O08.3
- adrenal (cortical) (Addisonian) E27.2
- adverse food reaction (anaphylactic) *—see* Shock, anaphylactic, due to food
- allergic *—see* Shock, anaphylactic
- anaphylactic T78.2
  - chemical *—see* Table of Drugs and Chemicals
  - due to drug or medicinal substance
    - correct substance properly administered T88.6
    - overdose or wrong substance given or taken (by accident) *—see* Table of Drugs and Chemicals, by drug, poisoning
  - due to food (nonpoisonous) T78.00
    - additives T78.06
    - dairy products T78.07
    - eggs T78.08
    - fish T78.03
      - shellfish T78.02
    - fruit T78.04
    - milk T78.07
    - nuts T78.05
      - multiple types T78.05
      - peanuts T78.01
    - peanuts T78.01
    - *see*ds T78.05
    - specified type NEC T78.09
    - vegetable T78.04
  - following sting(s) *—see* Venom
  - immunization T80.52
  - serum T80.59
    - blood and blood products T80.51
    - immunization T80.52
    - specified NEC T80.59
    - vaccination T80.52
- anaphylactoid *—see* Shock, anaphylactic
- anesthetic
  - correct substance properly administered T88.2
  - overdose or wrong substance given or taken *—see* Table of Drugs and Chemicals, by drug, poisoning
    - specified anesthetic *—see* Table of Drugs and Chemicals, by drug, poisoning
- cardiogenic R57.0
- chemical substance *—see* Table of Drugs and Chemicals
- complicating ectopic or molar pregnancy O08.3
- culture *—see* Disorder, adjustment
- drug
  - due to correct substance properly administered T88.6
  - overdose or wrong substance given or taken (by accident) *—see* Table of Drugs and Chemicals, by drug, poisoning
- during or after labor and delivery O75.1
- electric T75.4
  - (taser) T75.4
- endotoxic R65.21
  - postprocedural (resulting from a procedure, not elsewhere classified) T81.12

Shock *(continued)*
- following
  - ectopic or molar pregnancy O08.3
  - injury (immediate) (delayed) T79.4
  - labor and delivery O75.1
- food (anaphylactic) —*see* Shock, anaphylactic, due to food
- from electroshock gun (taser) T75.4
- gram-negative R65.21
  - postprocedural (resulting from a procedure, not elsewhere classified) T81.12
- hematologic R57.8
- hemorrhagic R57.8
  - surgery (intraoperative) (postoperative) T81.19
  - trauma T79.4
- hypovolemic R57.1
  - surgical T81.19
  - traumatic T79.4
- insulin E15
  - therapeutic misadventure —*see* subcategory T38.3
- kidney N17.0
  - traumatic (following crushing) T79.5
- lightning T75.01
- liver K72.00
- lung J80
- obstetric O75.1
  - with ectopic or molar pregnancy O08.3
  - following ectopic or molar pregnancy O08.3
- pleural (surgical) T81.19
  - due to trauma T79.4
- postprocedural (postoperative) T81.10
  - with ectopic or molar pregnancy O08.3
  - cardiogenic T81.11
  - endotoxic T81.12
  - following ectopic or molar pregnancy O08.3
  - gram-negative T81.12
  - hypovolemic T81.19
  - septic T81.12
  - specified type NEC T81.19
- psychic F43.0
- septic (due to severe sepsis) R65.21
- specified NEC R57.8
- surgical T81.10
- taser gun (taser) T75.4
- therapeutic misadventure NEC T81.10
- thyroxin
  - overdose or wrong substance given or taken —*see* Table of Drugs and Chemicals, by drug, poisoning
- toxic, syndrome A48.3
- transfusion —*see* Complications, transfusion
- traumatic (immediate) (delayed) T79.4

Shoemaker's chest M95.4

Short, shortening, shortness
- arm (acquired) —*see also* Deformity, limb, unequal length
  - congenital Q71.81-
  - forearm —*see* Deformity, limb, unequal length
- bowel syndrome K91.2
- breath R06.02
- cervical (complicating pregnancy) O26.87-
  - non-gravid uterus N88.3
- common bile duct, congenital Q44.5
- cord (umbilical), complicating delivery O69.3
- cystic duct, congenital Q44.5

Short, shortening, shortness *(continued)*
- esophagus (congenital) Q39.8
- femur (acquired) —*see* Deformity, limb, unequal length, femur
  - congenital —*see* Defect, reduction, lower limb, longitudinal, femur
- frenum, frenulum, linguae (congenital) Q38.1
- hip (acquired) —*see also* Deformity, limb, unequal length
  - congenital Q65.89
- leg (acquired) —*see also* Deformity, limb, unequal length
  - congenital Q72.81-
  - lower leg —*see also* Deformity, limb, unequal length
- limbed stature, with immunodeficiency D82.2
- lower limb (acquired) —*see also* Deformity, limb, unequal length
  - congenital Q72.81-
- organ or site, congenital NEC —*see* Distortion
- palate, congenital Q38.5
- radius (acquired) —*see also* Deformity, limb, unequal length
  - congenital —*see* Defect, reduction, upper limb, longitudinal, radius
- rib syndrome Q77.2
- stature (child) (hereditary) (idiopathic) NEC R62.52
  - constitutional E34.3
  - due to endocrine disorder E34.3
  - Laron-type E34.3
- tendon —*see also* Contraction, tendon
  - with contracture of joint —*see* Contraction, joint
  - Achilles (acquired) M67.0-
    - congenital Q66.89
  - congenital Q79.8
- thigh (acquired) —*see also* Deformity, limb, unequal length, femur
  - congenital —*see* Defect, reduction, lower limb, longitudinal, femur
- tibialis anterior (tendon) —*see* Contraction, tendon
- umbilical cord
  - complicating delivery O69.3
- upper limb, congenital —*see* Defect, reduction, upper limb, specified type NEC
- urethra N36.8
- uvula, congenital Q38.5
- vagina (congenital) Q52.4

Shortsightedness —*see* Myopia

Shoshin (acute fulminating beriberi) E51.11

Shoulder —*see* condition

Shovel-shaped incisors K00.2

Shower, thromboembolic —*see* Embolism

Shunt
- arterial-venous (dialysis) Z99.2
- arteriovenous, pulmonary (acquired) I28.0
  - congenital Q25.72
- cerebral ventricle (communicating) in situ Z98.2
- surgical, prosthetic, with complications —*see* Complications, cardiovascular, device or implant

Shutdown, renal N28.9

Shy-Drager syndrome G90.3

Sialadenitis, sialadenosis (any gland) (chronic) (periodic) (suppurative) —*see* Sialoadenitis

Sialectasia K11.8

Sialidosis E77.1

Sialitis, silitis (any gland) (chronic) (suppurative) —*see* Sialoadenitis

Sialoadenitis (any gland) (periodic) (suppurative) K11.20
- acute K11.21
  - recurrent K11.22
- chronic K11.23

Sialoadenopathy K11.9

Sialoangitis —*see* Sialoadenitis

Sialodochitis (fibrinosa) —*see* Sialoadenitis

Sialodocholithiasis K11.5

Sialolithiasis K11.5

Sialometaplasia, necrotizing K11.8

Sialorrhea —*see also* Ptyalism
- periodic —*see* Sialoadenitis

Sialosis K11.7

Siamese twin Q89.4

Sibling rivalry Z62.891

Sicard's syndrome G52.7

Sicca syndrome M35.00
- with
  - keratoconjunctivitis M35.01
  - lung involvement M35.02
  - myopathy M35.03
  - renal tubulo-interstitial disorders M35.04
- specified organ involvement NEC M35.09

Sick R69
- or handicapped person in family Z63.79
  - needing care at home Z63.6
- sinus (syndrome) I49.5

Sick-euthyroid syndrome E07.81

Sickle-cell
- anemia —*see* Disease, sickle-cell
- trait D57.3

Sicklemia —*see also* Disease, sickle-cell
- trait D57.3

Sickness
- air (travel) T75.3
- airplane T75.3
- alpine T70.29
- altitude T70.20
- Andes T70.29
- aviator's T70.29
- balloon T70.29
- car T75.3
- compressed air T70.3
- decompression T70.3
- green D50.8
- milk —*see* Poisoning, food, noxious
- motion T75.3
- mountain T70.29
  - acute D75.1
- protein (*see also* Reaction, serum) T80.69
- radiation T66
- roundabout (motion) T75.3
- sea T75.3
- serum NEC (*see also* Reaction, serum) T80.69

Sickness *(continued)*
- sleeping (African) B56.9
  - by Trypanosoma B56.9
    - brucei
      - gambiense B56.0
      - rhodesiense B56.1
  - East African B56.1
  - Gambian B56.0
  - Rhodesian B56.1
  - West African B56.0
- swing (motion) T75.3
- train (railway) (travel) T75.3
- travel (any vehicle) T75.3

Sideropenia —*see* Anemia, iron deficiency

Siderosilicosis J62.8

Siderosis (lung) J63.4
- eye (globe) —*see* Disorder, globe, degenerative, siderosis

Siemens' syndrome (ectodermal dysplasia) Q82.8

Sighing R06.89
- psychogenic F45.8

Sigmoid —*see also* condition
- flexure —*see* condition
- kidney Q63.1

Sigmoiditis (*see also* Enteritis) K52.9
- infectious A09
- noninfectious K52.9

Silfversköld's syndrome Q78.9

Silicosiderosis J62.8

Silicosis, silicotic (simple) (complicated) J62.8
- with tuberculosis J65

Silicotuberculosis J65

Silo-fillers' disease J68.8
- bronchitis J68.0
- pneumonitis J68.0
- pulmonary edema J68.1

Silver's syndrome Q87.1

Simian malaria B53.1

Simmonds' cachexia or disease E23.0

Simons' disease or syndrome (progressive lipodystrophy) E88.1

Simple, simplex —*see* condition

Simulation, conscious (of illness) Z76.5

Simultanagnosia (asimultagnosia) R48.3

Sin Nombre virus disease (Hantavirus) (cardio)-**pulmonary syndrome)** B33.4

Sinding-Larsen disease or osteochondrosis —*see* Osteochondrosis, juvenile, patella

Singapore hemorrhagic fever A91

Singer's node or nodule J38.2

Single
- atrium Q21.2
- coronary artery Q24.5
- umbilical artery Q27.0
- ventricle Q20.4

Singultus R06.6
- epidemicus B33.0

Sinus —*see also* Fistula
- abdominal K63.89
- arrest I45.5
- arrhythmia I49.8
- bradycardia R00.1
- branchial cleft (internal) (external) Q18.0
- coccygeal —*see* Sinus, pilonidal
- dental K04.6

Sinus *(continued)*
dermal (congenital) Q06.8
with abscess Q06.8
coccygeal, pilonidal —*see* Sinus, coccygeal
infected, skin NEC L08.89
marginal, ruptured or bleeding —*see* Hemorrhage, antepartum, specified cause NEC
medial, face and neck Q18.8
pause I45.5
pericranii Q01.9
pilonidal (infected) (rectum) L05.92
with abscess L05.02
preauricular Q18.1
rectovaginal N82.3
Rokitansky-Aschoff (gallbladder) K82.8
sacrococcygeal (dermoid) (infected) —*see* Sinus, pilonidal
tachycardia R00.0
paroxysmal I47.1
tarsi syndrome M25.57-
testis N50.89
tract (postinfective) —*see* Fistula
urachus Q64.4

Sinusitis (accessory) (chronic) (hyperplastic) (nasal) (nonpurulent) (purulent) J32.9
acute J01.90
ethmoidal J01.20
recurrent J01.21
frontal J01.10
recurrent J01.11
involving more than one sinus, other than pansinusitis J01.80
recurrent J01.81
maxillary J01.00
recurrent J01.01
pansinusitis J01.40
recurrent J01.41
recurrent J01.91
specified NEC J01.80
recurrent J01.81
sphenoidal J01.30
recurrent J01.31
allergic —*see* Rhinitis, allergic
due to high altitude T70.1
ethmoidal J32.2
acute J01.20
recurrent J01.21
frontal J32.1
acute J01.10
recurrent J01.11
influenzal —*see* Influenza, with, respiratory manifestations NEC
involving more than one sinus but not pansinusitis J32.8
acute J01.80
recurrent J01.81
maxillary J32.0
acute J01.00
recurrent J01.01
sphenoidal J32.3
acute J01.30
recurrent J01.31
tuberculous, any sinus A15.8

Sinusitis-bronchiectasis-situs inversus (syndrome) (triad) Q89.3

Sipple's syndrome E31.22

Sirenomelia (syndrome) Q87.2

Siriasis T67.0

Sirkari's disease B55.0

Siti A65

Situation, psychiatric F99

Situational
disturbance (transient) —*see* Disorder, adjustment
acute F43.0
maladjustment —*see* Disorder, adjustment
reaction —*see* Disorder, adjustment
acute F43.0

Situs inversus or transversus (abdominalis) (thoracis) Q89.3

Sixth disease B08.20
due to human herpesvirus 6 B08.21
due to human herpesvirus 7 B08.22

Sjögren-Larsson syndrome Q87.1

Sjögren's syndrome or disease —*see* Sicca syndrome

Skeletal —*see* condition

Skene's gland —*see* condition

Skenitis —*see* Urethritis

Skerljevo A65

Skevas-Zerfus disease —*see* Toxicity, venom, marine animal, sea anemone

Skin —*see also* condition
clammy R23.1
donor —*see* Donor, skin
hidebound M35.9

Slate-dressers' or slate-miners' lung J62.8

Sleep
apnea —*see* Apnea, sleep
deprivation Z72.820
disorder or disturbance G47.9
child F51.9
nonorganic origin F51.9
specified NEC G47.8
disturbance G47.9
nonorganic origin F51.9
drunkenness F51.9
rhythm inversion G47.2-
terrors F51.4
walking F51.3
hysterical F44.89

Sleep hygiene
abuse Z72.821
inadequate Z72.821
poor Z72.821

Sleeping sickness —*see* Sickness, sleeping

Sleeplessness —*see* Insomnia
menopausal N95.1

Sleep-wake schedule disorder G47.20

Slim disease (in HIV infection) B20

Slipped, slipping
epiphysis (traumatic) —*see also* Osteochondropathy, specified type NEC
capital femoral (traumatic)
acute (on chronic) S79.01-
current traumatic - code as Fracture, by site
upper femoral (nontraumatic) M93.00-
acute M93.01-
on chronic M93.03-
chronic M93.02-
intervertebral disc —*see* Displacement, intervertebral disc
ligature, umbilical P51.8
patella —*see* Disorder, patella, derangement NEC
rib M89.8X8
sacroiliac joint —*see* subcategory M53.2
tendon —*see* Disorder, tendon

Slipped, slipping *(continued)*
ulnar nerve, nontraumatic —*see* Lesion, nerve, ulnar
vertebra NEC —*see* Spondylolisthesis

Slocumb's syndrome E27.0

Sloughing (multiple) (phagedena) (skin) —*see also* Gangrene
abscess —*see* Abscess
appendix K38.8
fascia —*see* Disorder, soft tissue, specified type NEC
scrotum N50.89
tendon —*see* Disorder, tendon
transplanted organ —*see* Rejection, transplant
ulcer —*see* Ulcer, skin

Slow
feeding, newborn P92.2
flow syndrome, coronary I20.8
heart (beat) R00.1

Slowing, urinary stream R39.198

Sluder's neuralgia (syndrome) G44.89

Slurred, slurring speech R47.81

Small (ness)
for gestational age —*see* Small for dates
introitus, vagina N89.6
kidney (unknown cause) N27.9
bilateral N27.1
unilateral N27.0
ovary (congenital) Q50.39
pelvis
with disproportion (fetopelvic) O33.1
causing obstructed labor O65.1
uterus N85.8
white kidney N03.9

Small-and-light-for-dates —*see* Small for dates

Small-for-dates (infant) P05.10
with weight of
499 grams or less P05.11
500-749 grams P05.12
750-999 grams P05.13
1000-1249 grams P05.14
1250-1499 grams P05.15
1500-1749 grams P05.16
1750-1999 grams P05.17
2000-2499 grams P05.18
2500 grams and over P05.19
specified NEC P05.19

Smallpox B03

Smearing, fecal R15.1

Smith-Lemli-Opitz syndrome E78.72

Smith's fracture S52.54-

Smoker —*see* Dependence, drug, nicotine

Smoker's
bronchitis J41.0
cough J41.0
palate K13.24
throat J31.2
tongue K13.24

Smoking
passive Z77.22

Smothering spells R06.81

Snaggle teeth, tooth M26.39

Snapping
finger —*see* Trigger finger
hip —*see* Derangement, joint, specified type NEC, hip
involving the iliotiblial band M76.3-

Snapping *(continued)*
knee —*see* Derangement, knee
involving the iliotiblial band M76.3-

Sneddon-Wilkinson disease or syndrome (sub-corneal pustular dermatosis) L13.1

Sneezing (intractable) R06.7

Sniffing
cocaine
abuse —*see* Abuse, drug, cocaine
dependence —*see* Dependence, drug, cocaine
gasoline
abuse —*see* Abuse, drug, inhalant
dependence —*see* Dependence, drug, inhalant
glue (airplane)
abuse —*see* Abuse, drug, inhalant
drug dependence —*see* Dependence, drug, inhalant

Sniffles
newborn P28.89

Snoring R06.83

Snow blindness —*see* Photokeratitis

Snuffles (non-syphilitic) R06.5
newborn P28.89
syphilitic (infant) A50.05 *[J99]*

Social
exclusion Z60.4
due to discrimination or persecution (perceived) Z60.5
migrant Z59.0
acculturation difficulty Z60.3
rejection Z60.4
due to discrimination or persecution Z60.5
role conflict NEC Z73.5
skills inadequacy NEC Z73.4
transplantation Z60.3

Sodoku A25.0

Soemmerring's ring —*see* Cataract, secondary

Soft —*see also* condition
nails L60.3

Softening
bone —*see* Osteomalacia
brain (necrotic) (progressive) G93.89
congenital Q04.8
embolic I63.4-
hemorrhagic —*see* Hemorrhage, intracranial, intracerebral
occlusive I63.5-
thrombotic I63.3-
cartilage M94.2-
patella M22.4-
cerebellar —*see* Softening, brain
cerebral —*see* Softening, brain
cerebrospinal —*see* Softening, brain
myocardial, heart —*see* Degeneration, myocardial
spinal cord G95.89
stomach K31.89

Soldier's
heart F45.8
patches I31.0

Solitary
cyst, kidney N28.1
kidney, congenital Q60.0

Solvent abuse —*see* Abuse, drug, inhalant
dependence —*see* Dependence, drug, inhalant

Somatization reaction, somatic reaction —*see* Disorder, somatoform
Somnambulism F51.3
hysterical F44.89
Somnolence R40.0
nonorganic origin F51.11
Sonne dysentery A03.3
Soor B37.0
Sore
bed —*see* Ulcer, pressure, by site
chiclero B55.1
Delhi B55.1
desert —*see* Ulcer, skin
eye H57.1-
Lahore B55.1
mouth K13.79
canker K12.0
muscle M79.1
Naga —*see* Ulcer, skin
of skin —*see* Ulcer, skin
oriental B55.1
pressure —*see* Ulcer, pressure, by site
skin L98.9
soft A57
throat (acute) —*see also* Pharyngitis
with influenza, flu, or grippe —*see* Influenza, with, respiratory manifestations NEC
chronic J31.2
coxsackie (virus) B08.5
diphtheritic A36.0
herpesviral B00.2
influenzal —*see* Influenza, with, respiratory manifestations NEC
septic J02.0
streptococcal (ulcerative) J02.0
viral NEC J02.8
coxsackie B08.5
tropical —*see* Ulcer, skin
veldt —*see* Ulcer, skin
Soto's syndrome (cerebral gigantism) Q87.3
South African cardiomyopathy syndrome I42.8
Southeast Asian hemorrhagic fever A91
Spacing
abnormal, tooth, teeth, fully erupted M26.30
excessive, tooth, fully erupted M26.32
Spade-like hand (congenital) Q68.1
Spading nail L60.8
congenital Q84.6
Spanish collar N47.1
Sparganosis B70.1
Spasm(s), **spastic, spasticity** (*see also* condition) R25.2
accommodation —*see* Spasm, of accommodation
ampulla of Vater K83.4
anus, ani (sphincter) (reflex) K59.4
psychogenic F45.8
artery I73.9
cerebral G45.9
Bell's G51.3
bladder (sphincter, external or internal) N32.89
psychogenic F45.8
bronchus, bronchiole J98.01
Spasm(s), spastic, spasticity *(continued)*
cardia K22.0
cardiac I20.1
carpopedal —*see* Tetany
cerebral (arteries) (vascular) G45.9
cervix, complicating delivery O62.4
ciliary body (of accommodation) —*see* Spasm, of accommodation
colon (*see also* Irritable, bowel) K58.9
with diarrhea K58.0
psychogenic F45.8
common duct K83.8
compulsive —*see* Tic
conjugate H51.8
coronary (artery) I20.1
diaphragm (reflex) R06.6
epidemic B33.0
psychogenic F45.8
duodenum K59.8
epidemic diaphragmatic (transient) B33.0
esophagus (diffuse) K22.4
psychogenic F45.8
facial G51.3
fallopian tube N83.8
gastrointestinal (tract) K31.89
psychogenic F45.8
glottis J38.5
hysterical F44.4
psychogenic F45.8
conversion reaction F44.4
reflex through recurrent laryngeal nerve J38.5
habit —*see* Tic
heart I20.1
hemifacial (clonic) G51.3
hourglass —*see* Contraction, hourglass
hysterical F44.4
infantile —*see* Epilepsy, spasms
inferior oblique, eye H51.8
intestinal (*see also* Syndrome, irritable bowel) K58.9
psychogenic F45.8
larynx, laryngeal J38.5
hysterical F44.4
psychogenic F45.8
conversion reaction F44.4
levator palpebrae superioris —*see* Disorder, eyelid function
muscle NEC M62.838
back M62.830
nerve, trigeminal G51.0
nervous F45.8
nodding F98.4
occupational F48.8
oculogyric H51.8
psychogenic F45.8
of accommodation H52.53-
ophthalmic artery —*see* Occlusion, artery, retina
perineal, female N94.89
peroneo-extensor —*see also* Deformity, limb, flat foot
pharynx (reflex) J39.2
hysterical F45.8
psychogenic F45.8
psychogenic F45.8
pylorus NEC K31.3
adult hypertrophic K31.89
congenital or infantile Q40.0
psychogenic F45.8
rectum (sphincter) K59.4
psychogenic F45.8
retinal (artery) —*see* Occlusion, artery, retina
sigmoid (*see also* Syndrome, irritable bowel) K58.9
psychogenic F45.8
Spasm(s), spastic, spasticity *(continued)*
sphincter of Oddi K83.4
stomach K31.89
neurotic F45.8
throat J39.2
hysterical F45.8
psychogenic F45.8
tic F95.9
chronic F95.1
transient of childhood F95.0
tongue K14.8
torsion (progressive) G24.1
trigeminal nerve —*see* Neuralgia, trigeminal
ureter N13.5
urethra (sphincter) N35.9
uterus N85.8
complicating labor O62.4
vagina N94.2
psychogenic F52.5
vascular I73.9
vasomotor I73.9
vein NEC I87.8
viscera —*see* Pain, abdominal
Spasmodic —*see* condition
Spasmophilia —*see* Tetany
Spasmus nutans F98.4
Spastic, spasticity —*see also* Spasm
child (cerebral) (congenital) (paralysis) G80.1
Speaker's throat R49.8
Specific, specified —*see* condition
Speech
defect, disorder, disturbance, impediment R47.9
psychogenic, in childhood and adolescence F98.8
slurring R47.81
specified NEC R47.89
Spencer's disease A08.19
Spens' syndrome (syncope with heart block) I45.9
Sperm counts (fertility testing) Z31.41
postvasectomy Z30.8
reversal Z31.42
Spermatic cord —*see* condition
Spermatocele N43.40
congenital Q55.4
multiple N43.42
single N43.41
Spermatocystitis N49.0
Spermatocytoma C62.9-
specified site —*see* Neoplasm, malignant, by site
Spermatorrhea N50.89
Sphacelus —*see* Gangrene
Sphenoidal —*see* condition
Sphenoiditis (chronic) —*see* Sinusitis, sphenoidal
Sphenopalatine ganglion neuralgia G90.09
Sphericity, increased, lens (congenital) Q12.4
Spherocytosis (congenital) (familial) (hereditary) D58.0
hemoglobin disease D58.0
sickle-cell (disease) D57.8-
Spherophakia Q12.4
Sphincter —*see* condition
Sphincteritis, sphincter of Oddi —*see* Cholangitis
Sphingolipidosis E75.3
specified NEC E75.29
Sphingomyelinosis E75.3
Spicule tooth K00.2
Spider
bite —*see* Toxicity, venom, spider
fingers —*see* Syndrome, Marfan's
nevus I78.1
toes —*see* Syndrome, Marfan's
vascular I78.1
Spiegler-Fendt
benign lymphocytoma L98.8
sarcoid L08.89
Spielmeyer-Vogt disease E75.4
Spina bifida (aperta) Q05.9
with hydrocephalus NEC Q05.4
cervical Q05.5
with hydrocephalus Q05.0
dorsal Q05.6
with hydrocephalus Q05.1
lumbar Q05.7
with hydrocephalus Q05.2
lumbosacral Q05.7
with hydrocephalus Q05.2
occulta Q76.0
sacral Q05.8
with hydrocephalus Q05.3
thoracic Q05.6
with hydrocephalus Q05.1
thoracolumbar Q05.6
with hydrocephalus Q05.1
Spindle, Krukenberg's —*see* Pigmentation, cornea, posterior
Spine, spinal —*see* condition
Spiradenoma (eccrine) —*see* Neoplasm, skin, benign
Spirillosis A25.0
Spirillum
minus A25.0
obermeieri infection A68.0
Spirochetal —*see* condition
Spirochetosis A69.9
arthritic, arthritica A69.9
bronchopulmonary A69.8
icterohemorrhagic A27.0
lung A69.8
Spirometrosis B70.1
Spitting blood —*see* Hemoptysis
Splanchnoptosis K63.4
Spleen, splenic —*see* condition
Splenectasis —*see* Splenomegaly
Splenitis (interstitial) (malignant) (nonspecific) D73.89
malarial (*see also* Malaria) B54 *[D77]*
tuberculous A18.85
Splenocele D73.89
Splenomegaly, splenomegalia (Bengal) (cryptogenic) (idiopathic) (tropical) R16.1
with hepatomegaly R16.2
cirrhotic D73.2
congenital Q89.09
congestive, chronic D73.2
Egyptian B65.1
Gaucher's E75.22
malarial (*see also* Malaria) B54 *[D77]*
neutropenic D73.81
Niemann-Pick —*see* Niemann-Pick disease or syndrome
siderotic D73.2
syphilitic A52.79
congenital (early) A50.08 *[D77]*

Splenopathy D73.9
Splenoptosis D73.89
Splenosis D73.89
Splinter —*see* Foreign body, superficial, by site
Split, splitting
foot Q72.7-
hand Q71.6
heart sounds R01.2
lip, congenital —*see* Cleft, lip
nails L60.3
urinary stream R39.13
Spondylarthrosis —*see* Spondylosis
Spondylitis (chronic) —*see also* Spondylopathy, inflammatory
ankylopoietica —*see* Spondylitis, ankylosing
ankylosing (chronic) M45.9
with lung involvement M45.9 *[J99]*
cervical region M45.2
cervicothoracic region M45.3
juvenile M08.1
lumbar region M45.6
lumbosacral region M45.7
multiple sites M45.0
occipito-atlanto-axial region M45.1
sacrococcygeal region M45.8
thoracic region M45.4
thoracolumbar region M45.5
atrophic (ligamentous) —*see* Spondylitis, ankylosing
deformans (chronic) —*see* Spondylosis
gonococcal A54.41
gouty (*see also* Gout, by type, vertebrae) M10.08
in (due to)
brucellosis A23.9 *[M49.80]*
cervical region A23.9 *[M49.82]*
cervicothoracic region A23.9 *[M49.83]*
lumbar region A23.9 *[M49.86]*
lumbosacral region A23.9 *[M49.87]*
multiple sites A23.9 *[M49.89]*
occipito-atlanto-axial region A23.9 *[M49.81]*
sacrococcygeal region A23.9 *[M49.88]*
thoracic region A23.9 *[M49.84]*
thoracolumbar region A23.9 *[M49.85]*
enterobacteria (*see also* subcategory M49.8) A04.9
tuberculosis A18.01
infectious NEC —*see* Spondylopathy, infective
juvenile ankylosing (chronic) M08.1
Kümmell's —*see* Spondylopathy, traumatic
Marie-Strümpell —*see* Spondylitis, ankylosing
muscularis —*see* Spondylopathy, specified NEC
psoriatic L40.53
rheumatoid —*see* Spondylitis, ankylosing
rhizomelica —*see* Spondylitis, ankylosing
sacroiliac NEC M46.1
senescent, senile —*see* Spondylosis
traumatic (chronic) or post-traumatic —*see* Spondylopathy, traumatic
tuberculous A18.01
typhosa A01.05
Spondylolisthesis (acquired) (degenerative) M43.10
with disproportion (fetopelvic) O33.0
causing obstructed labor O65.0
cervical region M43.12
cervicothoracic region M43.13
congenital Q76.2
lumbar region M43.16
lumbosacral region M43.17
multiple sites M43.19
occipito-atlanto-axial region M43.11
sacrococcygeal region M43.18
thoracic region M43.14
thoracolumbar region M43.15
traumatic (old) M43.10
acute
fifth cervical (displaced) S12.430
nondisplaced S12.431
specified type NEC (displaced) S12.450
nondisplaced S12.451
type III S12.44
fourth cervical (displaced) S12.330
nondisplaced S12.331
specified type NEC (displaced) S12.350
nondisplaced S12.351
type III S12.34
second cervical (displaced) S12.130
nondisplaced S12.131
specified type NEC (displaced) S12.150
nondisplaced S12.151
type III S12.14
seventh cervical (displaced) S12.630
nondisplaced S12.631
specified type NEC (displaced) S12.650
nondisplaced S12.651
type III S12.64
sixth cervical (displaced) S12.530
nondisplaced S12.531
specified type NEC (displaced) S12.550
nondisplaced S12.551
type III S12.54
third cervical (displaced) S12.230
nondisplaced S12.231
specified type NEC (displaced) S12.250
nondisplaced S12.251
type III S12.24
Spondylolysis (acquired) M43.00
cervical region M43.02
cervicothoracic region M43.03
congenital Q76.2
lumbar region M43.06
lumbosacral region M43.07
with disproportion (fetopelvic) O33.0
causing obstructed labor O65.8
multiple sites M43.09
occipito-atlanto-axial region M43.01
sacrococcygeal region M43.08
thoracic region M43.04
thoracolumbar region M43.05
Spondylopathy M48.9
infective NEC M46.50
cervical region M46.52
cervicothoracic region M46.53
lumbar region M46.56
lumbosacral region M46.57
multiple sites M46.59
occipito-atlanto-axial region M46.51
sacrococcygeal region M46.58
thoracic region M46.54
thoracolumbar region M46.55
inflammatory M46.90
cervical region M46.92
cervicothoracic region M46.93
lumbar region M46.96
lumbosacral region M46.97
multiple sites M46.99
occipito-atlanto-axial region M46.91
sacrococcygeal region M46.98
specified type NEC M46.80
cervical region M46.82
cervicothoracic region M46.83
lumbar region M46.86
lumbosacral region M46.87
multiple sites M46.89
occipito-atlanto-axial region M46.81
sacrococcygeal region M46.88
thoracic region M46.84
thoracolumbar region M46.85
thoracic region M46.94
thoracolumbar region M46.95
neuropathic, in
syringomyelia and syringobulbia G95.0
tabes dorsalis A52.11
specified NEC M48.8
traumatic M48.30
cervical region M48.32
cervicothoracic region M48.33
lumbar region M48.36
lumbosacral region M48.37
occipito-atlanto-axial region M48.31
sacrococcygeal region M48.38
thoracic region M48.34
thoracolumbar region M48.35
Spondylosis M47.9
with
disproportion (fetopelvic) O33.0
causing obstructed labor O65.0
myelopathy NEC M47.10
cervical region M47.12
cervicothoracic region M47.13
lumbar region M47.16
occipito-atlanto-axial region M47.11
thoracic region M47.14
thoracolumbar region M47.15
radiculopathy M47.20
cervical region M47.22
cervicothoracic region M47.23
lumbar region M47.26
lumbosacral region M47.27
occipito-atlanto-axial region M47.21
sacrococcygeal region M47.28
thoracic region M47.24
thoracolumbar region M47.25
specified NEC M47.899
cervical region M47.892
cervicothoracic region M47.893
lumbar region M47.896
lumbosacral region M47.897
occipito-atlanto-axial region M47.891
sacrococcygeal region M47.898
thoracic region M47.894
thoracolumbar region M47.895
traumatic —*see* Spondylopathy, traumatic
without myelopathy or radiculopathy M47.819
cervical region M47.812
cervicothoracic region M47.813
lumbar region M47.816
lumbosacral region M47.817
occipito-atlanto-axial region M47.811
sacrococcygeal region M47.818
thoracic region M47.814
thoracolumbar region M47.815
Sponge
inadvertently left in operation wound —*see* Foreign body, accidentally left during a procedure
kidney (medullary) Q61.5
Sponge-diver's disease —*see* Toxicity, venom, marine animal, sea anemone
Spongioblastoma (any type) —*see* Neoplasm, malignant, by site
specified site —*see* Neoplasm, malignant, by site
unspecified site C71.9
Spongioneuroblastoma —*see* Neoplasm, malignant, by site
Spontaneous —*see also* condition
fracture (cause unknown) —*see* Fracture, pathological
Spoon nail L60.3
congenital Q84.6
Sporadic —*see* condition
Sporothrix schenckii infection —*see* Sporotrichosis
Sporotrichosis B42.9
arthritis B42.82
disseminated B42.7
generalized B42.7
lymphocutaneous (fixed) (progressive) B42.1
pulmonary B42.0
specified NEC B42.89
Spots, spotting (in) (of)
Bitot's —*see also* Pigmentation, conjunctiva
in the young child E50.1
vitamin A deficiency E50.1
café, au lait L81.3
Cayenne pepper I78.1
cotton wool, retina —*see* Occlusion, artery, retina
de Morgan's (senile angiomas) I78.1
Fuchs' black (myopic) (*see also* Myopia, degenerative) H44.2-
intermenstrual (regular) N92.0
irregular N92.1
Koplik's B05.9
liver L81.4
pregnancy O26.85-
purpuric R23.3
ruby I78.1
Spotted fever —*see* Fever, spotted
N92.3
Sprain (joint) (ligament)
acromioclavicular joint or ligament S43.5-
ankle S93.40-
calcaneofibular ligament S93.41-
deltoid ligament S93.42-
internal collateral ligament —*see* Sprain, ankle, specified ligament NEC
specified ligament NEC S93.49-
talofibular ligament —*see* Sprain, ankle, specified ligament NEC
tibiofibular ligament S93.43-

Sprain *(continued)*
- anterior longitudinal, cervical S13.4
- atlas, atlanto-axial, atlanto-occipital S13.4
- breast bone —*see* Sprain, sternum
- calcaneofibular —*see* Sprain, ankle
- carpal —*see* Sprain, wrist
- carpometacarpal —*see* Sprain, hand, specified site NEC
- cartilage
  - costal S23.41
  - semilunar (knee) —*see* Sprain, knee, specified site NEC
    - with current tear —*see* Tear, meniscus
  - thyroid region S13.5
  - xiphoid —*see* Sprain, sternum
- cervical, cervicodorsal, cervicothoracic S13.4
- chondrosternal S23.421
- coracoclavicular S43.8-
- coracohumeral S43.41-
- coronary, knee —*see* Sprain, knee, specified site NEC
- costal cartilage S23.41
- cricoarytenoid articulation or ligament S13.5
- cricothyroid articulation S13.5
- cruciate, knee —*see* Sprain, knee, cruciate
- deltoid, ankle —*see* Sprain, ankle
- dorsal (spine) S23.3
- elbow S53.40-
  - radial collateral ligament S53.43-
  - radiohumeral S53.41-
  - rupture
    - radial collateral ligament —*see* Rupture, traumatic, ligament, radial collateral
    - ulnar collateral ligament —*see* Rupture, traumatic, ligament, ulnar collateral
  - specified type NEC S53.49-
  - ulnar collateral ligament S53.44-
  - ulnohumeral S53.42-
- femur, head —*see* Sprain, hip
- fibular collateral, knee —*see* Sprain, knee, collateral
- fibulocalcaneal —*see* Sprain, ankle
- finger(s) S63.61-
  - index S63.61-
  - interphalangeal (joint) S63.63-
    - index S63.63-
    - little S63.63-
    - middle S63.63-
    - ring S63.63-
  - little S63.61-
  - middle S63.61-
  - ring S63.61-
  - metacarpophalangeal (joint) S63.65-
  - specified site NEC S63.69-
    - index S63.69-
    - little S63.69-
    - middle S63.69-
    - ring S63.69-
- foot S93.60-
  - specified ligament NEC S93.69-
  - tarsal ligament S93.61-
  - tarsometatarsal ligament S93.62-
  - toe —*see* Sprain, toe
- hand S63.9-
  - finger —*see* Sprain, finger
  - specified site NEC S63.8
  - thumb —*see* Sprain, thumb
- head S03.9
- hip S73.10-
  - iliofemoral ligament S73.11-
  - ischiocapsular (ligament) S73.12-
  - specified NEC S73.19-

Sprain *(continued)*
- iliofemoral —*see* Sprain, hip
- innominate
  - acetabulum —*see* Sprain, hip
  - sacral junction S33.6
- internal
  - collateral, ankle —*see* Sprain, ankle
  - semilunar cartilage —*see* Sprain, knee, specified site NEC
- interphalangeal
  - finger —*see* Sprain, finger, interphalangeal (joint)
  - toe —*see* Sprain, toe, interphalangeal joint
- ischiocapsular —*see* Sprain, hip
- ischiofemoral —*see* Sprain, hip
- jaw (articular disc) (cartilage) (meniscus) S03.4-
  - old M26.69
- knee S83.9-
  - collateral ligament S83.40-
    - lateral (fibular) S83.42-
    - medial (tibial) S83.41-
  - cruciate ligament S83.50-
    - anterior S83.51-
    - posterior S83.52-
  - lateral (fibular) collateral ligament S83.42-
  - medial (tibial) collateral ligament S83.41-
  - patellar ligament S76.11-
  - specified site NEC S83.8X-
  - superior tibiofibular joint (ligament) S83.6-
- lateral collateral, knee —*see* Sprain, knee, collateral
- lumbar (spine) S33.5
- lumbosacral S33.9
- mandible (articular disc) S03.4-
  - old M26.69
- medial collateral, knee —*see* Sprain, knee, collateral
- meniscus
  - jaw S03.4-
    - old M26.69
  - knee —*see* Sprain, knee, specified site NEC
    - with current tear —*see* Tear, meniscus
      - old —*see* Derangement, knee, meniscus, due to old tear
  - mandible S03.4-
    - old M26.69
- metacarpal (distal) (proximal) —*see* Sprain, hand, specified site NEC
- metacarpophalangeal —*see* Sprain, finger, metacarpophalangeal (joint)
- metatarsophalangeal —*see* Sprain, toe, metatarsophalangeal joint
- midcarpal —*see* Sprain, hand, specified site NEC
- midtarsal —*see* Sprain, foot, specified site NEC
- neck S13.9
  - anterior longitudinal cervical ligament S13.4
  - atlanto-axial joint S13.4
  - atlanto-occipital joint S13.4
  - cervical spine S13.4
  - cricoarytenoid ligament S13.5
  - cricothyroid ligament S13.5
  - specified site NEC S13.8
  - thyroid region (cartilage) S13.5
- nose S03.8
- orbicular, hip —*see* Sprain, hip
- patella —*see* Sprain, knee, specified site NEC
- patellar ligament S76.11-

Sprain *(continued)*
- pelvis NEC S33.8
- phalanx
  - finger —*see* Sprain, finger
  - toe —*see* Sprain, toe
- pubofemoral —*see* Sprain, hip
- radiocarpal —*see* Sprain, wrist
- radiohumeral —*see* Sprain, elbow
- radius, collateral —*see* Rupture, traumatic, ligament, radial collateral
- rib (cage) S23.41
- rotator cuff (capsule) S43.42-
- sacroiliac (region)
  - chronic or old —*see* subcategory M53.2
  - joint S33.6
- scaphoid (hand) —*see* Sprain, hand, specified site NEC
- scapula (r) —*see* Sprain, shoulder girdle, specified site NEC
- semilunar cartilage (knee) —*see* Sprain, knee, specified site NEC
  - with current tear —*see* Tear, meniscus
    - old —*see* Derangement, knee, meniscus, due to old tear
- shoulder joint S43.40-
  - acromioclavicular joint (ligament) —*see* Sprain, acromioclavicular joint
  - blade —*see* Sprain, shoulder, girdle, specified site NEC
  - coracoclavicular joint (ligament) —*see* Sprain, coracoclavicular joint
  - coracohumeral ligament —*see* Sprain, coracohumeral joint
  - girdle S43.9-
    - specified site NEC S43.8-
  - rotator cuff —*see* Sprain, rotator cuff
  - specified site NEC S43.49-
  - sternoclavicular joint (ligament) —*see* Sprain, sternoclavicular joint
- spine
  - cervical S13.4
  - lumbar S33.5
  - thoracic S23.3
- sternoclavicular joint S43.6-
- sternum S23.429
  - chondrosternal joint S23.421
  - specified site NEC S23.428
  - sternoclavicular (joint) (ligament) S23.420
- symphysis
  - jaw S03.4-
    - old M26.69
  - mandibular S03.4-
    - old M26.69
- talofibular —*see* Sprain, ankle
- tarsal —*see* Sprain, foot, specified site NEC
- tarsometatarsal —*see* Sprain, foot, specified site NEC
- temporomandibular S03.4-
  - old M26.69
- thorax S23.9
  - ribs S23.41
  - specified site NEC S23.8
  - spine S23.3
  - sternum —*see* Sprain, sternum
- thumb S63.60-
  - interphalangeal (joint) S63.62-
  - metacarpophalangeal (joint) S63.64-
  - specified site NEC S63.68-
- thyroid cartilage or region S13.5
- tibia (proximal end) —*see* Sprain, knee, specified site NEC

Sprain *(continued)*
- tibial collateral, knee —*see* Sprain, knee, collateral
- tibiofibular
  - distal —*see* Sprain, ankle
  - superior —*see* Sprain, knee, specified site NEC
- toe(s) S93.50-
  - great S93.50-
  - interphalangeal joint S93.51-
    - great S93.51-
    - lesser S93.51-
  - lesser S93.50-
  - metatarsophalangeal joint S93.52-
    - great S93.52-
    - lesser S93.52-
- ulna, collateral —*see* Rupture, traumatic, ligament, ulnar collateral
- ulnohumeral —*see* Sprain, elbow
- wrist S63.50-
  - carpal S63.51-
  - radiocarpal S63.52-
  - specified site NEC S63.59-
- xiphoid cartilage —*see* Sprain, sternum

Sprengel's deformity (congenital) Q74.0

Sprue (tropical) K90.1
- celiac K90.0
- idiopathic K90.49
- meaning thrush B37.0
- nontropical K90.0

Spur, bone —*see also* Enthesopathy
- calcaneal M77.3-
- iliac crest M76.2-
- nose (septum) J34.89

Spurway's syndrome Q78.0

Sputum
- abnormal (amount) (color) (odor) (purulent) R09.3
- blood-stained R04.2
- excessive (cause unknown) R09.3

Squamous —*see also* condition
- epithelium in
  - cervical canal (congenital) Q51.828
  - uterine mucosa (congenital) Q51.818

Squashed nose M95.0
- congenital Q67.4

Squeeze, diver's T70.3

Squint —*see also* Strabismus
- accommodative —*see* Strabismus, convergent concomitant

St. Hubert's disease A82.9

Stab —*see also* Laceration
- internal organs —*see* Injury, by site

Stafne's cyst or cavity M27.0

Staggering gait R26.0
- hysterical F44.4

Staghorn calculus —*see* Calculus, kidney

Stähli's line (cornea) (pigment) —*see* Pigmentation, cornea, anterior

Stain, staining
- meconium (newborn) P96.83
- port wine Q82.5
- tooth, teeth (hard tissues) (extrinsic) K03.6
  - due to
    - accretions K03.6
    - deposits (betel) (black) (green) (materia alba) (orange) (soft) (tobacco) K03.6
    - metals (copper) (silver) K03.7
    - nicotine K03.6

Stain, staining *(continued)*
tooth, teeth *(continued)*
due to *(continued)*
pulpal bleeding K03.7
tobacco K03.6
intrinsic K00.8
Stammering (*see also* Disorder, fluency) F80.81
Standstill
auricular I45.5
cardiac —*see* Arrest, cardiac
sinoatrial I45.5
ventricular —*see* Arrest, cardiac
Stannosis J63.5
Stanton's disease —*see* Melioidosis
Staphylitis (acute) (catarrhal) (chronic) (gangrenous) (membranous) (suppurative) (ulcerative) K12.2
Staphylococcal scalded skin syndrome L00
Staphylococcemia A41.2
Staphylococcus, staphylococcal —*see also* condition
as cause of disease classified elsewhere B95.8
aureus (methicillin susceptible) (MSSA) B95.61
methicillin resistant (MRSA) B95.62
specified NEC, as cause of disease classified elsewhere B95.7
Staphyloma (sclera)
cornea H18.72-
equatorial H15.81-
localized (anterior) H15.82-
posticum H15.83-
ring H15.85-
Stargardt's disease —*see* Dystrophy, retina
Starvation (inanition) (due to lack of food) T73.0
edema —*see* Malnutrition, severe
Stasis
bile (noncalculous) K83.1
bronchus J98.09
with infection —*see* Bronchitis
cardiac —*see* Failure, heart, congestive
cecum K59.8
colon K59.8
dermatitis I87.2
with
varicose ulcer —*see* Varix, leg, with ulcer, with inflammation
varicose veins —*see* Varix, leg, with inflammation
due to postthrombotic syndrome —*see* Syndrome, postthombotic
duodenal K31.5
eczema —*see* Varix, leg, with, inflammation
edema —*see* Hypertension, venous (chronic), idiopathic
foot T69.0-
ileocecal coil K59.8
ileum K59.8
intestinal K59.8
jejunum K59.8
kidney N19
liver (cirrhotic) K76.1
lymphatic I89.8
pneumonia J18.2
pulmonary —*see* Edema, lung
rectal K59.8
renal N19
tubular N17.0

Stasis *(continued)*
ulcer —*see* Varix, leg, with, ulcer
without varicose veins I87.2
urine —*see* Retention, urine
venous I87.8
State (of)
affective and paranoid, mixed, organic psychotic F06.8
agitated R45.1
acute reaction to stress F43.0
anxiety (neurotic) F41.1
apprehension F41.1
burn-out Z73.0
climacteric, female Z78.0
symptomatic N95.1
compulsive F42.8
mixed with obsessional thoughts F42.2
confusional (psychogenic) F44.89
acute —*see also* Delirium
with
arteriosclerotic dementia F01.50
with behavioral disturbance F01.51
senility or dementia F05
alcoholic F10.231
epileptic F05
reactive (from emotional stress, psychological trauma) F44.89
subacute —*see* Delirium
convulsive —*see* Convulsions
crisis F43.0
depressive F32.9
neurotic F34.1
dissociative F44.9
emotional shock (stress) R45.7
hypercoagulation —*see* Hypercoagulable
locked-in G83.5
menopausal Z78.0
symptomatic N95.1
neurotic F48.9
with depersonalization F48.1
obsessional F42.8
oneiroid (schizophrenia-like) F23
organic
hallucinatory (nonalcoholic) F06.0
paranoid (-hallucinatory) F06.2
panic F41.0
paranoid F22
climacteric F22
involutional F22
menopausal F22
organic F06.2
senile F03
simple F22
persistent vegetative R40.3
phobic F40.9
postleukotomy F07.0
pregnant
gestational carrier Z33.3
incidental Z33.1
psychogenic, twilight F44.89
psychopathic (constitutional) F60.2
psychotic, organic —*see also* Psychosis, organic
mixed paranoid and affective F06.8
senile or presenile F03
transient NEC F06.8
with
hallucinations F06.0
depression F06.31
residual schizophrenic F20.5
restlessness R45.1
stress (emotional) R45.7
tension (mental) F48.9
specified NEC F48.8

State *(continued)*
transient organic psychotic NEC F06.8
depressive type F06.31
hallucinatory type F06.0
twilight
epileptic F05
psychogenic F44.89
vegetative, persistent R40.3
vital exhaustion Z73.0
withdrawal, —*see* Withdrawal, state
Status (post) —*see also* Presence (of)
absence, epileptic —*see* Epilepsy, by type, with status epilepticus
administration of tPA (rtPA) in a different facility within the last 24 hours prior to admission to current facility Z92.82
adrenalectomy (unilateral) (bilateral) E89.6
anastomosis Z98.0
angioplasty (peripheral) Z98.62
with implant Z95.820
coronary artery Z98.61
with implant Z95.5
anginosus I20.9
aortocoronary bypass Z95.1
arthrodesis Z98.1
artificial opening (of) Z93.9
gastrointestinal tract Z93.4
specified NEC Z93.8
urinary tract Z93.6
vagina Z93.8
asthmaticus —*see* Asthma, by type, with status asthmaticus
awaiting organ transplant Z76.82
bariatric surgery Z98.84
bed confinement Z74.01
bleb, filtering (vitreous), after glaucoma surgery Z98.83
breast implant Z98.82
removal Z98.86
cataract extraction Z98.4-
cholecystectomy Z90.49
clitorectomy N90.811
with excision of labia minora N90.812
colectomy (complete) (partial) Z90.49
colonization —*see* Carrier (suspected) of
colostomy Z93.3
convulsivus idiopathicus —*see* Epilepsy, by type, with status epilepticus
coronary artery angioplasty —*see* Status, angioplasty, coronary artery
coronary artery bypass graft Z95.1
cystectomy (urinary bladder) Z90.6
cystostomy Z93.50
appendico-vesicostomy Z93.52
cutaneous Z93.51
specified NEC Z93.59
delinquent immunization Z28.3
dental Z98.818
crown Z98.811
fillings Z98.811
restoration Z98.811
sealant Z98.810
specified NEC Z98.818
deployment (current) (military) Z56.82
dialysis (hemodialysis) (peritoneal) Z99.2
do not resuscitate (DNR) Z66
donor —*see* Donor
embedded fragments —*see* Retained, foreign body fragments (type of)

Status *(continued)*
embedded splinter —*see* Retained, foreign body fragments (type of)
enterostomy Z93.4
epileptic, epilepticus (*see also* Epilepsy, by type, with status epilepticus) G40.901
estrogen receptor
negative Z17.1
positive Z17.0
female genital cutting —*see* Female genital mutilation status
female genital mutilation —*see* Female genital mutilation status
filtering (vitreous) bleb after glaucoma surgery Z98.83
gastrectomy (complete) (partial) Z90.3
gastric banding Z98.84
gastric bypass for obesity Z98.84
gastrostomy Z93.1
human immunodeficiency virus (HIV) infection, asymptomatic Z21
hysterectomy (complete) (total) Z90.710
partial (with remaining cervial stump) Z90.711
ileostomy Z93.2
implant
breast Z98.82
infibulation N90.813
intestinal bypass Z98.0
jejunostomy Z93.4
laryngectomy Z90.02
lapsed immunization schedule Z28.3
lymphaticus E32.8
malignancy
castrate resistant prostate Z19.2
hormone resistant Z19.2
hormone sensitive Z19.1
marmoratus G80.3
mastectomy (unilateral) (bilateral) Z90.1-
military deployment status (current) Z56.82
in theater or in support of military war, peacekeeping and humanitarian operations Z56.82
nephrectomy (unilateral) (bilateral) Z90.5
nephrostomy Z93.6
obesity surgery Z98.84
oophorectomy
bilateral Z90.722
unilateral Z90.721
organ replacement
by artificial or mechanical device or prosthesis of
artery Z95.828
bladder Z96.0
blood vessel Z95.828
breast Z97.8
eye globe Z97.0
heart Z95.812
valve Z95.2
intestine Z97.8
joint Z96.60
hip —*see* Presence, hip joint implant
knee —*see* Presence, knee joint implant
specified site NEC Z96.698
kidney Z97.8
larynx Z96.3
lens Z96.1
limbs —*see* Presence, artificial, limb
liver Z97.8
lung Z97.8

Status *(continued)*
- organ replacement *(continued)*
  - by artificial or mechanical device or prosthesis of *(continued)*
    - pancreas Z97.8
  - by organ transplant (heterologous) (homologous) *—see* Transplant
- pacemaker
  - brain Z96.89
  - cardiac Z95.0
  - specified NEC Z96.89
- pancreatectomy Z90.410
  - complete Z90.410
  - partial Z90.411
  - total Z90.410
- physical restraint Z78.1
- pneumonectomy (complete) (partial) Z90.2
- pneumothorax, therapeutic Z98.3
- postcommotio cerebri F07.81
- postoperative (postprocedural) NEC Z98.890
  - breast implant Z98.82
  - dental Z98.818
    - crown Z98.811
    - fillings Z98.811
    - restoration Z98.811
    - sealant Z98.810
    - specified NEC Z98.818
  - pneumothorax, therapeutic Z98.3
  - uterine scar Z98.891
- postpartum (routine follow-up) Z39.2
  - care immediately after delivery Z39.0
- postsurgical (postprocedural) NEC Z98.890
  - pneumothorax, therapeutic Z98.3
- pregnancy, incidental Z33.1
- prosthesis coronary angioplasty Z95.5
- pseudophakia Z96.1
- renal dialysis (hemodialysis) (peritoneal) Z99.2
- retained foreign body *—see* Retained, foreign body fragments (type of)
- reversed jejunal transposition (for bypass) Z98.0
- salpingo-oophorectomy
  - bilateral Z90.722
  - unilateral Z90.721
- sex reassignment surgery status Z87.890
- shunt
  - arteriovenous (for dialysis) Z99.2
  - cerebrospinal fluid Z98.2
  - ventricular (communicating) (for drainage) Z98.2
- splenectomy Z90.81
- thymicolymphaticus E32.8
- thymicus E32.8
- thymolymphaticus E32.8
- thyroidectomy (hypothyroidism) E89.0
- tooth (teeth) extraction (*see also* Absence, teeth, acquired) K08.409
- tPA (rtPA) administration in a different facility within the last 24 hours prior to admission to current facility Z92.82
- tracheostomy Z93.0
- transplant *—see* Transplant
  - organ removed Z98.85
- tubal ligation Z98.51
- underimmunization Z28.3
- ureterostomy Z93.6
- urethrostomy Z93.6
- vagina, artificial Z93.8
- vasectomy Z98.52

Status *(continued)*
- wheelchair confinement Z99.3

Stealing
- child problem F91.8
  - in company with others Z72.810
- pathological (compulsive) F63.2

Steam burn *—see* Burn

Steatocystoma multiplex L72.2

Steatohepatitis (nonalcoholic) (NASH) K75.81

Steatoma L72.3
- eyelid (cystic) *—see* Dermatosis, eyelid
  - infected *—see* Hordeolum

Steatorrhea (chronic) K90.4
- with lacteal obstruction K90.2
- idiopathic (adult) (infantile) K90.9
- pancreatic K90.3
- primary K90.0
- tropical K90.1

Steatosis E88.89
- heart *—see* Degeneration, myocardial
- kidney N28.89
- liver NEC K76.0

Steele-Richardson-Olszewski disease or syndrome G23.1

Steinbrocker's syndrome G90.8

Steinert's disease G71.11

Stein-Leventhal syndrome E28.2

Stein's syndrome E28.2

STEMI (*see also* Infarct, myocardium ST elevation) I21.3

Stenocardia I20.8

Stenocephaly Q75.8

Stenosis, stenotic (cicatricial) *—see also* Stricture
- ampulla of Vater K83.1
- anus, anal (canal) (sphincter) K62.4
  - and rectum K62.4
  - congenital Q42.3
    - with fistula Q42.2
- aorta (ascending) (supraventricular) (congenital) Q25.1
  - arteriosclerotic I70.0
  - calcified I70.0
  - supravalvular Q25.3
- aortic (valve) I35.0
  - with insufficiency I35.2
  - congenital Q23.0
  - rheumatic I06.0
    - with
      - incompetency, insufficiency or regurgitation I06.2
        - with mitral (valve) disease I08.0
          - with tricuspid (valve) disease I08.3
      - mitral (valve) disease I08.0
        - with tricuspid (valve) disease I08.3
      - tricuspid (valve) disease I08.2
        - with mitral (valve) disease I08.3
  - specified cause NEC I35.0
  - syphilitic A52.03
- aqueduct of Sylvius (congenital) Q03.0
  - with spina bifida *—see* Spina bifida, by site, with hydrocephalus
  - acquired G91.1
- artery NEC (*see also* Arteriosclerosis) I77.1
  - celiac I77.4

Stenosis, stenotic *(continued)*
- artery NEC *(continued)*
  - cerebral *—see* Occlusion, artery, cerebral
  - extremities *—see* Arteriosclerosis, extremities
  - precerebral *—see* Occlusion, artery, precerebral
  - pulmonary (congenital) Q25.6
    - acquired I28.8
  - renal I70.1
  - stent
    - coronary T82.855
    - peripheral T82.856
- bile duct (common) (hepatic) K83.1
  - congenital Q44.3
- bladder-neck (acquired) N32.0
  - congenital Q64.31
- brain G93.89
- bronchus J98.09
  - congenital Q32.3
  - syphilitic A52.72
- cardia (stomach) K22.2
  - congenital Q39.3
- cardiovascular *—see* Disease, cardiovascular
- caudal M48.08
- cervix, cervical (canal) N88.2
  - congenital Q51.828
  - in pregnancy or childbirth *—see* Pregnancy, complicated by, abnormal cervix
- colon *—see also* Obstruction, intestine
  - congenital Q42.9
    - specified NEC Q42.8
- colostomy K94.03
- common (bile) duct K83.1
  - congenital Q44.3
- coronary (artery) *—see* Disease, heart, ischemic, atherosclerotic
- cystic duct *—see* Obstruction, gallbladder
- due to presence of device, implant or graft (*see also* Complications, by site and type, specified NEC) T85.858
  - arterial graft NEC T82.858
  - breast (implant) T85.858
  - catheter T85.858
    - dialysis (renal) T82.858
      - intraperitoneal T85.858
    - infusion NEC T82.858
      - spinal (epidural) (subdural) T85.850
    - urinary (indwelling) T83.85
  - fixation, internal (orthopedic) NEC T84.85
  - gastrointestinal (bile duct) (esophagus) T85.858
  - genital NEC T83.85
  - heart NEC T82.857
  - joint prosthesis T84.85
  - ocular (corneal graft) (orbital implant) NEC T85.858
  - orthopedic NEC T84.85
  - specified NEC T85.858
  - urinary NEC T83.85
  - vascular NEC T82.858
  - ventricular intracranial shunt T85.850
- duodenum K31.5
  - congenital Q41.0
- ejaculatory duct NEC N50.89
- endocervical os *—see* Stenosis, cervix
- enterostomy K94.13
- esophagus K22.2
  - congenital Q39.3
  - syphilitic A52.79
    - congenital A50.59 *[K23]*

Stenosis, stenotic *(continued)*
- eustachian tube *—see* Obstruction, eustachian tube
- external ear canal (acquired) H61.30-
  - congenital Q16.1
  - due to
    - inflammation H61.32-
    - trauma H61.31-
  - postprocedural H95.81-
  - specified cause NEC H61.39-
- gallbladder *—see* Obstruction, gallbladder
- glottis J38.6
- heart valve (congenital) Q24.8
  - aortic Q23.0
  - mitral Q23.2
  - pulmonary Q22.1
  - tricuspid Q22.4
- hepatic duct K83.1
- hymen N89.6
- hypertrophic subaortic (idiopathic) I42.1
- ileum (*see also* Obstruction, intestine, specified NEC) K56.699
  - congenital Q41.2
- infundibulum cardia Q24.3
- intervertebral foramina *—see also* Lesion, biomechanical, specified NEC
  - connective tissue M99.79
    - abdomen M99.79
    - cervical region M99.71
    - cervicothoracic M99.71
    - head region M99.70
    - lumbar region M99.73
    - lumbosacral M99.73
    - occipitocervical M99.70
    - sacral region M99.74
    - sacrococcygeal M99.74
    - sacroiliac M99.74
    - specified NEC M99.79
    - thoracic region M99.72
    - thoracolumbar M99.72
  - disc M99.79
    - abdomen M99.79
    - cervical region M99.71
    - cervicothoracic M99.71
    - head region M99.70
    - lower extremity M99.76
    - lumbar region M99.73
    - lumbosacral M99.73
    - occipitocervical M99.70
    - pelvic M99.75
    - rib cage M99.78
    - sacral region M99.74
    - sacrococcygeal M99.74
    - sacroiliac M99.74
    - specified NEC M99.79
    - thoracic region M99.72
    - thoracolumbar M99.72
    - upper extremity M99.77
  - osseous M99.69
    - abdomen M99.69
    - cervical region M99.61
    - cervicothoracic M99.61
    - head region M99.60
    - lower extremity M99.66
    - lumbar region M99.63
    - lumbosacral M99.63
    - occipitocervical M99.60
    - pelvic M99.65
    - rib cage M99.68
    - sacral region M99.64
    - sacrococcygeal M99.64
    - sacroiliac M99.64
    - specified NEC M99.69
    - thoracic region M99.62
    - thoracolumbar M99.62
    - upper extremity M99.67

Stenosis, stenotic *(continued)*
- intervertebral foramina *(continued)*
  - subluxation *—see* Stenosis, intervertebral foramina, Vosseous
- intestine *—see also* Obstruction, intestine
  - congenital (small) Q41.9
    - large Q42.9
      - specified NEC Q42.8
    - specified NEC Q41.8
- jejunum (*see also* Obstruction, intestine, specified NEC) K56.699
  - congenital Q41.1
- lacrimal (passage)
  - canaliculi H04.54-
  - congenital Q10.5
  - duct H04.55-
  - punctum H04.56-
  - sac H04.57-
- lacrimonasal duct *—see* Stenosis, lacrimal, duct
  - congenital Q10.5
- larynx J38.6
  - congenital NEC Q31.8
    - subglottic Q31.1
  - syphilitic A52.73
    - congenital A50.59 *[J99]*
- mitral (chronic) (inactive) (valve) I05.0
  - with
    - aortic valve disease I08.0
    - incompetency, insufficiency or regurgitation I05.2
  - active or acute I01.1
    - with rheumatic or Sydenham's chorea I02.0
  - congenital Q23.2
  - specified cause, except rheumatic I34.2
  - syphilitic A52.03
- myocardium, myocardial *—see also* Degeneration, myocardial
  - hypertrophic subaortic (idiopathic) I42.1
- nares (anterior) (posterior) J34.89
  - congenital Q30.0
- nasal duct *—see also* Stenosis, lacrimal, duct
  - congenital Q10.5
- nasolacrimal duct *—see also* Stenosis, lacrimal, duct
  - congenital Q10.5
- neural canal *—see also* Lesion, biomechanical, specified NEC
  - connective tissue M99.49
    - abdomen M99.49
    - cervical region M99.41
    - cervicothoracic M99.41
    - head region M99.40
    - lower extremity M99.46
    - lumbar region M99.43
    - lumbosacral M99.43
    - occipitocervical M99.40
    - pelvic M99.45
    - rib cage M99.48
    - sacral region M99.44
    - sacrococcygeal M99.44
    - sacroiliac M99.44
    - specified NEC M99.49
    - thoracic region M99.42
    - thoracolumbar M99.42
    - upper extremity M99.47
  - intervertebral disc M99.59
    - abdomen M99.59
    - cervical region M99.51
    - cervicothoracic M99.51
    - head region M99.50
    - lower extremity M99.56
    - lumbar region M99.53
    - lumbosacral M99.53
    - occipitocervical M99.50

Stenosis, stenotic *(continued)*
- neural canal *(continued)*
  - intervertebral disc *(continued)*
    - pelvic M99.55
    - rib cage M99.58
    - sacral region M99.54
    - sacrococcygeal M99.54
    - sacroiliac M99.54
    - specified NEC M99.59
    - thoracic region M99.52
    - thoracolumbar M99.52
    - upper extremity M99.57
  - osseous M99.39
    - abdomen M99.39
    - cervical region M99.31
    - cervicothoracic M99.31
    - head region M99.30
    - lower extremity M99.36
    - lumbar region M99.33
    - lumbosacral M99.33
    - pelvic M99.35
    - rib cage M99.38
    - occipitocervical M99.30
    - sacral region M99.34
    - sacrococcygeal M99.34
    - sacroiliac M99.34
    - specified NEC M99.39
    - thoracic region M99.32
    - thoracolumbar M99.32
    - upper extremity M99.37
  - subluxation M99.29
    - cervical region M99.21
    - cervicothoracic M99.21
    - head region M99.20
    - lower extremity M99.26
    - lumbar region M99.23
    - lumbosacral M99.23
    - occipitocervical M99.20
    - pelvic M99.25
    - rib cage M99.28
    - sacral region M99.24
    - sacrococcygeal M99.24
    - sacroiliac M99.24
    - specified NEC M99.29
    - thoracic region M99.22
    - thoracolumbar M99.22
    - upper extremity M99.27
- organ or site, congenital NEC *—see* Atresia, by site
- papilla of Vater K83.1
- pulmonary (artery) (congenital) Q25.6
  - with ventricular septal defect, transposition of aorta, and hypertrophy of right ventricle Q21.3
  - acquired I28.8
  - in tetralogy of Fallot Q21.3
  - infundibular Q24.3
  - subvalvular Q24.3
  - supravalvular Q25.6
  - valve I37.0
    - with insufficiency I37.2
    - congenital Q22.1
    - rheumatic I09.89
      - with aortic, mitral or tricuspid (valve) disease I08.8
  - vein, acquired I28.8
  - vessel NEC I28.8
- pulmonic (congenital) Q22.1
  - infundibular Q24.3
  - subvalvular Q24.3
- pylorus (hypertrophic) (acquired) K31.1
  - adult K31.1
  - congenital Q40.0
  - infantile Q40.0
- rectum (sphincter) *—see* Stricture, rectum
- renal artery I70.1

Stenosis, stenotic *(continued)*
- renal artery *(continued)*
  - congenital Q27.1
- salivary duct (any) K11.8
- sphincter of Oddi K83.1
- spinal M48.00
  - cervical region M48.02
  - cervicothoracic region M48.03
  - lumbar region (NOS) (without neurogenic claudication) M48.061
    - with neurogenic claudication M48.062
  - lumbosacral region M48.07
  - occipito-atlanto-axial region M48.01
  - sacrococcygeal region M48.08
  - thoracic region M48.04
  - thoracolumbar region M48.05
- stent
  - vascular
    - end stent
      - adjacent to stent - see Arteriosclerosis
    - within the stent
      - coronary T82.855
      - peripheral T82.856
    - in stent
      - coronary vessel T82.855
      - peripheral vessel T82.856
- stomach, hourglass K31.2
- subaortic (congenital) Q24.4
  - hypertrophic (idiopathic) I42.1
- subglottic J38.6
  - congenital Q31.1
  - postprocedural J95.5
- trachea J39.8
  - congenital Q32.1
  - syphilitic A52.73
  - tuberculous NEC A15.5
- tracheostomy J95.03
- tricuspid (valve) I07.0
  - with
    - aortic (valve) disease I08.2
    - incompetency, insufficiency or regurgitation I07.2
      - with aortic (valve) disease I08.2
        - with mitral (valve) disease I08.3
    - mitral (valve) disease I08.1
      - with aortic (valve) disease I08.3
  - congenital Q22.4
  - nonrheumatic I36.0
    - with insufficiency I36.2
- tubal N97.1
- ureter *—see* Atresia, ureter
- ureteropelvic junction, congenital Q62.11
- ureterovesical orifice, congenital Q62.12
- urethra (valve) *—see also* Stricture, urethra
  - congenital Q64.32
- urinary meatus, congenital Q64.33
- vagina N89.5
  - congenital Q52.4
  - in pregnancy *—see* Pregnancy, complicated by, abnormal vagina
    - causing obstructed labor O65.5
- valve (cardiac) (heart) (*see also* Endocarditis) I38
  - congenital Q24.8
    - aortic Q23.0
    - mitral Q23.2
    - pulmonary Q22.1
    - tricuspid Q22.4

Stenosis, stenotic *(continued)*
- vena cava (inferior) (superior) I87.1
  - congenital Q26.0
- vesicourethral orifice Q64.31
- vulva N90.5

Stent jail T82.897

Stercolith (impaction) K56.41
- appendix K38.1

Stercoraceous, stercoral ulcer K63.3
- anus or rectum K62.6

Stereotypies NEC F98.4

Sterility *—see* Infertility

Sterilization *—see* Encounter (for), sterilization

Sternalgia *—see* Angina

Sternopagus Q89.4

Sternum bifidum Q76.7

Steroid
- effects (adverse) (adrenocortical) (iatrogenic)
  - cushingoid E24.2
    - correct substance properly administered *—see* Table of Drugs and Chemicals, by drug, adverse effect
    - overdose or wrong substance given or taken *—see* Table of Drugs and Chemicals, by drug, poisoning
  - diabetes *—see* category E09
    - correct substance properly administered *—see* Table of Drugs and Chemicals, by drug, adverse effect
    - overdose or wrong substance given or taken *—see* Table of Drugs and Chemicals, by drug, poisoning
  - fever R50.2
  - insufficiency E27.3
    - correct substance properly administered *—see* Table of Drugs and Chemicals, by drug, adverse effect
    - overdose or wrong substance given or taken *—see* Table of Drugs and Chemicals, by drug, poisoning
- responder H40.04-

Stevens-Johnson disease or syndrome L51.1
- toxic epidermal necrolysis overlap L51.3

Stewart-Morel syndrome M85.2

Sticker's disease B08.3

Sticky eye *—see* Conjunctivitis, acute, mucopurulent

Stieda's disease *—see* Bursitis, tibial collateral

Stiff neck *—see* Torticollis

Stiff-man syndrome G25.82

Stiffness, joint NEC M25.60-
- ankle M25.67-
- ankylosis *—see* Ankylosis, joint
- contracture *—see* Contraction, joint
- elbow M25.62-
- foot M25.67-
- hand M25.64-
- hip M25.65-
- knee M25.66-
- shoulder M25.61-
- wrist M25.63-

Stigmata congenital syphilis A50.59

Stillbirth P95

Still-Felty syndrome —*see* Felty's syndrome

Still's disease or syndrome (juvenile) M08.20
- adult-onset M06.1
- ankle M08.27-
- elbow M08.22-
- foot joint M08.27-
- hand joint M08.24-
- hip M08.25-
- knee M08.26-
- multiple site M08.29
- shoulder M08.21-
- vertebra M08.28
- wrist M08.23-

Stimulation, ovary E28.1

Sting (venomous) (with allergic or anaphylactic shock) —*see* Table of Drugs and Chemicals, by animal or substance, poisoning

Stippled epiphyses Q78.8

Stitch
- abscess T81.4
- burst (in operation wound) —*see* Disruption, wound, operation

Stokes-Adams disease or syndrome I45.9

Stokes' disease E05.00
- with thyroid storm E05.01

Stokvis (-Talma) **disease** D74.8

Stoma malfunction
- colostomy K94.03
- enterostomy K94.13
- gastrostomy K94.23
- ileostomy K94.13
- tracheostomy J95.03

Stomach —*see* condition

Stomatitis (denture) (ulcerative) K12.1
- angular K13.0
  - due to dietary or vitamin deficiency E53.0
- aphthous K12.0
- bovine B08.61
- candidal B37.0
- catarrhal K12.1
- diphtheritic A36.89
- due to
  - dietary deficiency E53.0
  - thrush B37.0
  - vitamin deficiency
    - B group NEC E53.9
    - B2(riboflavin) E53.0
- epidemic B08.8
- epizootic B08.8
- follicular K12.1
- gangrenous A69.0
- Geotrichum B48.3
- herpesviral, herpetic B00.2
- herpetiformis K12.0
- malignant K12.1
- membranous acute K12.1
- monilial B37.0
- mycotic B37.0
- necrotizing ulcerative A69.0
- parasitic B37.0
- septic K12.1
- spirochetal A69.1
- suppurative (acute) K12.2
- ulceromembranous A69.1
- vesicular K12.1
  - with exanthem (enteroviral) B08.4
  - virus disease A93.8
- Vincent's A69.1

Stomatocytosis D58.8

Stomatomycosis B37.0

Stomatorrhagia K13.79

Stone(s) —*see also* Calculus
- bladder (diverticulum) N21.0
- cystine E72.09
- heart syndrome I50.1
- kidney N20.0
- prostate N42.0
- pulpal (dental) K04.2
- renal N20.0
- salivary gland or duct (any) K11.5
- urethra (impacted) N21.1
- urinary (duct) (impacted) (passage) N20.9
  - bladder (diverticulum) N21.0
  - lower tract N21.9
  - specified NEC N21.8
- xanthine E79.8 *[N22]*

Stonecutter's lung J62.8

Stonemason's asthma, disease, lung or pneumoconiosis J62.8

Stoppage
- heart —*see* Arrest, cardiac
- urine —*see* Retention, urine

Storm, thyroid —*see* Thyrotoxicosis

Strabismus (congenital) (nonparalytic) H50.9
- concomitant H50.40
  - convergent —*see* Strabismus, convergent concomitant
  - divergent —*see* Strabismus, divergent concomitant
- convergent concomitant H50.00
  - accommodative component H50.43
  - alternating H50.05
    - with
      - A pattern H50.06
      - specified nonconcomitances NEC H50.08
      - V pattern H50.07
  - monocular H50.01-
    - with
      - A pattern H50.02-
      - specified nonconcomitances NEC H50.04-
      - V pattern H50.03-
    - intermittent H50.31-
      - alternating H50.32
- cyclotropia H50.41
- divergent concomitant H50.10
  - alternating H50.15
    - with
      - A pattern H50.16
      - specified noncomitances NEC H50.18
      - V pattern H50.17
  - monocular H50.11-
    - with
      - A pattern H50.12-
      - specified noncomitances NEC H50.14-
      - V pattern H50.13-
    - intermittent H50.33
      - alternating H50.34
- Duane's syndrome H50.81-
- due to adhesions, scars H50.69
- heterophoria H50.50
  - alternating H50.55
  - cyclophoria H50.54
  - esophoria H50.51
  - exophoria H50.52
  - vertical H50.53
- heterotropia H50.40
  - intermittent H50.30
- hypertropia H50.2-
- hypotropia —*see* Hypertropia
- latent H50.50
- mechanical H50.60

Strabismus *(continued)*
- mechanical *(continued)*
  - Brown's sheath syndrome H50.61-
  - specified type NEC H50.69
- monofixation syndrome H50.42
- paralytic H49.9
  - abducens nerve H49.2-
  - fourth nerve H49.1-
  - Kearns-Sayre syndrome H49.81-
  - ophthalmoplegia (external)
    - progressive H49.4-
      - with pigmentary retinopathy H49.81-
    - total H49.3-
  - sixth nerve H49.2-
  - specified type NEC H49.88-
  - third nerve H49.0-
  - trochlear nerve H49.1-
- specified type NEC H50.89
- vertical H50.2-

Strain
- back S39.012
- cervical S16.1
- eye NEC —*see* Disturbance, vision, subjective
- heart —*see* Disease, heart
- low back S39.012
- mental NOS Z73.3
  - work-related Z56.6
- muscle (tendon) —*see* Injury, muscle, by site, strain
- neck S16.1
- postural —*see also* Disorder, soft tissue, due to use
- physical NOS Z73.3
  - work-related Z56.6
- psychological NEC Z73.3
- tendon —*see* Injury, muscle, by site, strain

Straining, on urination R39.16

Strand, vitreous —*see* Opacity, vitreous, membranes and strands

Strangulation, strangulated —*see also* Asphyxia, traumatic
- appendix K38.8
- bladder-neck N32.0
- bowel or colon K56.2
- food or foreign body —*see* Foreign body, by site
- hemorrhoids —*see* Hemorrhoids, with complication
- hernia —*see also* Hernia, by site, with obstruction
  - with gangrene —*see* Hernia, by site, with gangrene
- intestine (large) (small) K56.2
  - with hernia —*see also* Hernia, by site, with obstruction
    - with gangrene —*see* Hernia, by site, with gangrene
- mesentery K56.2
- mucus —*see* Asphyxia, mucus
- omentum K56.2
- organ or site, congenital NEC —*see* Atresia, by site
- ovary —*see* Torsion, ovary
- penis N48.89
  - foreign body T19.4
- rupture —*see* Hernia, by site, with obstruction
- stomach due to hernia —*see also* Hernia, by site, with obstruction
  - with gangrene —*see* Hernia, by site, with gangrene
- vesicourethral orifice N32.0

Strangury R30.0

Straw itch B88.0

Strawberry
- gallbladder K82.4
- mark Q82.5
- tongue (red) (white) K14.3

Streak(s)
- macula, angioid H35.33
- ovarian Q50.32

Strephosymbolia F81.0
- secondary to organic lesion R48.8

Streptobacillary fever A25.1

Streptobacillosis A25.1

Streptobacillus moniliformis A25.1

Streptococcus, streptococcal —*see also* condition
- as cause of disease classified elsewhere B95.5
- group
  - A, as cause of disease classified elsewhere B95.0
  - B, as cause of disease classified elsewhere B95.1
  - D, as cause of disease classified elsewhere B95.2
- pneumoniae, as cause of disease classified elsewhere B95.3
- specified NEC, as cause of disease classified elsewhere B95.4

Streptomycosis B47.1

Streptotrichosis A48.8

Stress F43.9
- family —*see* Disruption, family
- fetal P84
  - complicating pregnancy O77.9
    - due to drug administration O77.1
- mental NEC Z73.3
  - work-related Z56.6
- physical NEC Z73.3
  - work-related Z56.6
- polycythemia D75.1
- reaction (*see also* Reaction, stress) F43.9
- work schedule Z56.3

Stretching, nerve —*see* Injury, nerve

Striae albicantes, atrophicae or distensae (cutis) L90.6

Stricture —*see also* Stenosis
- ampulla of Vater K83.1
- anus (sphincter) K62.4
  - congenital Q42.3
    - with fistula Q42.2
  - infantile Q42.3
    - with fistula Q42.2
- aorta (ascending) (congenital) Q25.1
  - arteriosclerotic I70.0
  - calcified I70.0
  - supravalvular, congenital Q25.3
- aortic (valve) —*see* Stenosis, aortic
- aqueduct of Sylvius (congenital) Q03.0
  - with spina bifida —*see* Spina bifida, by site, with hydrocephalus
  - acquired G91.1
- artery I77.1
  - basilar —*see* Occlusion, artery, basilar
  - carotid —*see* Occlusion, artery, carotid
  - celiac I77.4
  - congenital (peripheral) Q27.8
    - cerebral Q28.3
    - coronary Q24.5
    - digestive system Q27.8
    - lower limb Q27.8

Stricture *(continued)*
- artery *(continued)*
  - congenital *(continued)*
    - retinal Q14.1
    - specified site NEC Q27.8
    - umbilical Q27.0
    - upper limb Q27.8
  - coronary *—see* Disease, heart, ischemic, atherosclerotic
    - congenital Q24.5
  - precerebral *—see* Occlusion, artery, precerebral
  - pulmonary (congenital) Q25.6
    - acquired I28.8
  - renal I70.1
  - vertebral *—see* Occlusion, artery, vertebral
- auditory canal (external) (congenital)
  - acquired *—see* Stenosis, external ear canal
- bile duct (common) (hepatic) K83.1
  - congenital Q44.3
  - postoperative K91.89
- bladder N32.89
  - neck N32.0
- bowel *—see* Obstruction, intestine
- brain G93.89
- bronchus J98.09
  - congenital Q32.3
  - syphilitic A52.72
- cardia (stomach) K22.2
  - congenital Q39.3
- cardiac *—see also* Disease, heart
  - orifice (stomach) K22.2
- cecum *—see* Obstruction, intestine
- cervix, cervical (canal) N88.2
  - congenital Q51.828
  - in pregnancy *—see* Pregnancy, complicated by, abnormal cervix
    - causing obstructed labor O65.5
- colon *—see also* Obstruction, intestine
  - congenital Q42.9
    - specified NEC Q42.8
- colostomy K94.03
- common (bile) duct K83.1
- coronary (artery) *—see* Disease, heart, ischemic, atherosclerotic
- cystic duct *—see* Obstruction, gallbladder
- digestive organs NEC, congenital Q45.8
- duodenum K31.5
  - congenital Q41.0
- ear canal (external) (congenital) Q16.1
  - acquired *—see* Stricture, auditory canal, acquired
- ejaculatory duct N50.89
- enterostomy K94.13
- esophagus K22.2
  - congenital Q39.3
  - syphilitic A52.79
    - congenital A50.59 *[K23]*
- eustachian tube *—see also* Obstruction, eustachian tube
  - congenital Q17.8
- fallopian tube N97.1
  - gonococcal A54.24
  - tuberculous A18.17
- gallbladder *—see* Obstruction, gallbladder
- glottis J38.6
- heart *—see also* Disease, heart
  - valve (*see also* Endocarditis) I38
    - aortic Q23.0
    - mitral Q23.2
    - pulmonary Q22.1
    - tricuspid Q22.4
- hepatic duct K83.1
- hourglass, of stomach K31.2

Stricture *(continued)*
- hymen N89.6
- hypopharynx J39.2
- ileum (*see also* Obstruction, intestine, specified NEC) K56.699
  - congenital Q41.2
- intestine *—see also* Obstruction, intestine
  - congenital (small) Q41.9
    - large Q42.9
      - specified NEC Q42.8
    - specified NEC Q41.8
  - ischemic K55.1
- jejunum (*see also* Obstruction, intestine, specified NEC) K56.699
  - congenital Q41.1
- lacrimal passages *—see also* Stenosis, lacrimal
  - congenital Q10.5
- larynx J38.6
  - congenital NEC Q31.8
    - subglottic Q31.1
  - syphilitic A52.73
    - congenital A50.59 *[J99]*
- meatus
  - ear (congenital) Q16.1
    - acquired *—see* Stricture, auditory canal, acquired
  - osseous (ear) (congenital) Q16.1
    - acquired *—see* Stricture, auditory canal, acquired
  - urinarius *—see also* Stricture, urethra
    - congenital Q64.33
- mitral (valve) *—see* Stenosis, mitral
- myocardium, myocardial I51.5
  - hypertrophic subaortic (idiopathic) I42.1
- nares (anterior) (posterior) J34.89
  - congenital Q30.0
- nasal duct *—see also* Stenosis, lacrimal, duct
  - congenital Q10.5
- nasolacrimal duct *—see also* Stenosis, lacrimal, duct
  - congenital Q10.5
- nasopharynx J39.2
  - syphilitic A52.73
- nose J34.89
  - congenital Q30.0
- nostril (anterior) (posterior) J34.89
  - congenital Q30.0
  - syphilitic A52.73
    - congenital A50.59 *[J99]*
- organ or site, congenital NEC *—see* Atresia, by site
- os uteri *—see* Stricture, cervix
- osseous meatus (ear) (congenital) Q16.1
  - acquired *—see* Stricture, auditory canal, acquired
- oviduct *—see* Stricture, fallopian tube
- pelviureteric junction (congenital) Q62.11
  - acquired, with hydronephrosis N13.0
- penis, by foreign body T19.4
- pharynx J39.2
- prostate N42.89
- pulmonary, pulmonic
  - artery (congenital) Q25.6
    - acquired I28.8
    - noncongenital I28.8
  - infundibulum (congenital) Q24.3
  - valve I37.0
    - congenital Q22.1
  - vein, acquired I28.8
  - vessel NEC I28.8

Stricture *(continued)*
- punctum lacrimale *—see also* Stenosis, lacrimal, punctum
  - congenital Q10.5
- pylorus (hypertrophic) K31.1
  - adult K31.1
  - congenital Q40.0
  - infantile Q40.0
- rectosigmoid (*see also* Obstruction, intestine, specified NEC) K56.699
- rectum (sphincter) K62.4
  - congenital Q42.1
    - with fistula Q42.0
  - due to
    - chlamydial lymphogranuloma A55
    - irradiation K91.89
    - lymphogranuloma venereum A55
  - gonococcal A54.6
  - inflammatory (chlamydial) A55
  - syphilitic A52.74
  - tuberculous A18.32
- renal artery I70.1
  - congenital Q27.1
- salivary duct or gland (any) K11.8
- sigmoid (flexure) *—see* Obstruction, intestine
- spermatic cord N50.89
- stoma (following) (of)
  - colostomy K94.03
  - enterostomy K94.13
  - gastrostomy K94.23
  - ileostomy K94.13
  - tracheostomy J95.03
- stomach K31.89
  - congenital Q40.2
  - hourglass K31.2
- subaortic Q24.4
  - hypertrophic (acquired) (idiopathic) I42.1
- subglottic J38.6
- syphilitic NEC A52.79
- trachea J39.8
  - congenital Q32.1
  - syphilitic A52.73
  - tuberculous NEC A15.5
- tracheostomy J95.03
- tricuspid (valve) *—see* Stenosis, tricuspid
- tunica vaginalis N50.89
- ureter (postoperative) N13.5
  - with
    - hydronephrosis N13.1
      - with infection N13.6
    - pyelonephritis (chronic) N11.1
  - congenital *—see* Atresia, ureter
  - tuberculous A18.11
- ureteropelvic junction (congenital) Q62.11
  - acquired, with hydronephrosis N13.0
- ureterovesical orifice N13.5
  - with infection N13.6
- urethra (organic) (spasmodic) N35.9
  - associated with schistosomiasis B65.0 *[N37]*
  - congenital Q64.39
    - valvular (posterior) Q64.2
  - due to
    - infection *—see* Stricture, urethra, postinfective
    - trauma *—see* Stricture, urethra, post-traumatic
  - gonococcal, gonorrheal A54.01

Stricture *(continued)*
- urethra *(continued)*
  - infective NEC *—see* Stricture, urethra, postinfective
  - late effect (sequelae) of injury *—see* Stricture, urethra, post-traumatic
  - postcatheterization *— see* Stricture, urethra, postprocedural
  - postinfective NEC
    - female N35.12
    - male N35.119
      - anterior urethra N35.114
      - bulbous urethra N35.112
      - meatal N35.111
      - membranous urethra N35.113
  - postobstetric N35.021
  - postoperative *—see* Stricture, urethra, postprocedural
  - postprocedural
    - female N99.12
    - male N99.114
      - anterior bulbous urethra N99.113
      - bulbous urethra N99.111
      - fossa navicularis N99.115
      - meatal N99.110
      - membranous urethra N99.112
  - post-traumatic
    - female N35.028
      - due to childbirth N35.021
    - male N35.014
      - anterior urethra N35.013
      - bulbous urethra N35.011
      - meatal N35.010
      - membranous urethra N35.012
  - sequela (late effect) of
    - childbirth N35.021
    - injury *—see* Stricture, urethra, post-traumatic
  - specified cause NEC N35.8
  - syphilitic A52.76
  - traumatic *—see* Stricture, urethra, post-traumatic
  - valvular (posterior), congenital Q64.2
- urinary meatus *—see* Stricture, urethra
- uterus, uterine (synechiae) N85.6
  - os (external) (internal) *—see* Stricture, cervix
- vagina (outlet) *—see* Stenosis, vagina
- valve (cardiac) (heart) *—see also* Endocarditis
  - congenital
    - aortic Q23.0
    - mitral Q23.2
    - pulmonary Q22.1
    - tricuspid Q22.4
- vas deferens N50.89
  - congenital Q55.4
- vein I87.1
- vena cava (inferior) (superior) NEC I87.1
  - congenital Q26.0
- vesicourethral orifice N32.0
  - congenital Q64.31
- vulva (acquired) N90.5

Stridor R06.1
- congenital (larynx) P28.89

Stridulous *—see* condition

Stroke (apoplectic) (brain) (embolic) (ischemic) (paralytic) (thrombotic) I63.9
- cryptogenic (*see also* Infarction, cerebral) I63.9

Stroke *(continued)*
epileptic *—see* Epilepsy
heat T67.0
in evolution I63.9
intraoperative
during cardiac surgery I97.810
during other surgery I97.811
lightning *—see* Lightning
meaning
cerebral hemorrhage - code to Hemorrhage, intracranial
cerebral infarction - code to Infarction, cerebral
postprocedural
following cardiac surgery I97.820
following other surgery I97.821
unspecified (NOS) I63.9

Stromatosis, endometrial D39.0

Strongyloidiasis, strongyloidosis B78.9
cutaneous B78.1
disseminated B78.7
intestinal B78.0

Strophulus pruriginosus L28.2

Struck by lightning *—see* Lightning

Struma *—see also* Goiter
Hashimoto E06.3
lymphomatosa E06.3
nodosa (simplex) E04.9
endemic E01.2
multinodular E01.1
multinodular E04.2
iodine-deficiency related E01.1
toxic or with hyperthyroidism E05.20
with thyroid storm E05.21
multinodular E05.20
with thyroid storm E05.21
uninodular E05.10
with thyroid storm E05.11
toxicosa E05.20
with thyroid storm E05.21
multinodular E05.20
with thyroid storm E05.21
uninodular E05.10
with thyroid storm E05.11
uninodular E04.1
ovarii D27.-
Riedel's E06.5

Strumipriva cachexia E03.4

Strümpell-Marie spine *—see* Spondylitis, ankylosing

Strümpell-Westphal pseudosclerosis E83.01

Stuart deficiency disease (factor X) D68.2

Stuart-Prower factor deficiency (factor X) D68.2

Student's elbow *—see* Bursitis, elbow, olecranon

Stump *—see* Amputation

Stunting, nutritional E45

Stupor (catatonic) R40.1
depressive (single episode) F32.89
recurrent episode F33.8
dissociative F44.2
manic F30.2
manic-depressive F31.89
psychogenic (anergic) F44.2
reaction to exceptional stress (transient) F43.0

Sturge (-Weber) (-Dimitri) (-Kalischer) **disease or syndrome** Q85.8

Stuttering F80.81
adult onset F98.5
childhood onset F80.81
following cerebrovascular disease *—see* Disorder, fluency. following cerebrovascular disease
in conditions classified elsewhere R47.82

Sty, stye (external) (internal) (meibomian) (zeisian) *—see* Hordeolum

Subacidity, gastric K31.89
psychogenic F45.8

Subacute *—see* condition

Subarachnoid *—see* condition

Subcortical *—see* condition

Subcostal syndrome, nerve compression *—see* Mononeuropathy, upper limb, specified site NEC

Subcutaneous, subcuticular *—see* condition

Subdural *—see* condition

Subendocardium *—see* condition

Subependymoma
specified site *—see* Neoplasm, uncertain behavior, by site
unspecified site D43.2

Suberosis J67.3

Subglossitis *—see* Glossitis

Subhemophilia D66

Subinvolution
breast (postlactational) (postpuerperal) N64.89
puerperal O90.89
uterus (chronic) (nonpuerperal) N85.3
puerperal O90.89

Sublingual *—see* condition

Sublinguitis *—see* Sialoadenitis

Subluxatable hip Q65.6

Subluxation *—see also* Dislocation
acromioclavicular S43.11-
ankle S93.0-
atlantoaxial, recurrent M43.4
with myelopathy M43.3
carpometacarpal (joint) NEC S63.05-
thumb S63.04-
complex, vertebral *—see* Complex, subluxation
congenital *—see also* Malposition, congenital
hip *—see* Dislocation, hip, congenital, partial
joint (excluding hip)
lower limb Q68.8
shoulder Q68.8
upper limb Q68.8
elbow (traumatic) S53.10-
anterior S53.11-
lateral S53.14-
medial S53.13-
posterior S53.12-
specified type NEC S53.19-
finger S63.20-
index S63.20-
interphalangeal S63.22-
distal S63.24-
index S63.24-
little S63.24-
middle S63.24-
ring S63.24-
index S63.22-
little S63.22-

Subluxation *(continued)*
finger *(continued)*
interphalangeal *(continued)*
middle S63.22-
proximal S63.23-
index S63.23-
little S63.23-
middle S63.23-
ring S63.23-
ring S63.22-
little S63.20-
metacarpophalangeal S63.21-
index S63.21-
little S63.21-
middle S63.21-
ring S63.21-
middle S63.20-
ring S63.20-
foot S93.30-
specified site NEC S93.33-
tarsal joint S93.31-
tarsometatarsal joint S93.32-
toe *—see* Subluxation, toe
hip S73.00-
anterior S73.03-
obturator S73.02-
central S73.04-
posterior S73.01-
interphalangeal (joint)
finger S63.22-
distal joint S63.24-
index S63.24-
little S63.24-
middle S63.24-
ring S63.24-
index S63.22-
little S63.22-
middle S63.22-
proximal joint S63.23-
index S63.23-
little S63.23-
middle S63.23-
ring S63.23-
ring S63.22-
thumb S63.12-
distal joint S63.14-
proximal joint S63.13-
toe S93.13-
great S93.13-
lesser S93.13-
joint prosthesis *—see* Complications, joint prosthesis, mechanical, displacement, by site
knee S83.10-
cap *—see* Subluxation, patella
patella *—see* Subluxation, patella
proximal tibia
anteriorly S83.11-
laterally S83.14-
medially S83.13-
posteriorly S83.12-
specified type NEC S83.19-
lens *—see* Dislocation, lens, partial
ligament, traumatic *—see* Sprain, by site
metacarpal (bone)
proximal end S63.06-
metacarpophalangeal (joint)
finger S63.21-
index S63.21-
little S63.21-
middle S63.21-
ring S63.21-
thumb S63.11-
metatarsophalangeal joint S93.14-
great toe S93.14-
lesser toe S93.14-

Subluxation *(continued)*
midcarpal (joint) S63.03-
patella S83.00-
lateral S83.01-
recurrent (nontraumatic) *—see* Dislocation, patella, recurrent, incomplete
specified type NEC S83.09-
pathological *—see* Dislocation, pathological
radial head S53.00-
anterior S53.01-
nursemaid's elbow S53.03-
posterior S53.02-
specified type NEC S53.09-
radiocarpal (joint) S63.02-
radioulnar (joint)
distal S63.01-
proximal *—see* Subluxation, elbow
shoulder
congenital Q68.8
girdle S43.30-
scapula S43.31-
specified site NEC S43.39-
traumatic S43.00-
anterior S43.01-
inferior S43.03-
posterior S43.02-
specified type NEC S43.08-
sternoclavicular (joint) S43.20-
anterior S43.21-
posterior S43.22-
symphysis (pubis)
thumb S63.103
interphalangeal joint *—see* Subluxation, interphalangeal (joint), thumb
metacarpophalangeal joint *—see* Subluxation, metacarpophalangeal (joint), thumb
toe(s) S93.10-
great S93.10-
interphalangeal joint S93.13-
metatarsophalangeal joint S93.14-
interphalangeal joint S93.13-
lesser S93.10-
interphalangeal joint S93.13-
metatarsophalangeal joint S93.14-
metatarsophalangeal joint S93.149
ulna
distal end S63.07-
proximal end *—see* Subluxation, elbow
ulnohumeral joint *—see* Subluxation, elbow
vertebral
recurrent NEC *—see* subcategory M43.5
traumatic
cervical S13.100
atlantoaxial joint S13.120
atlantooccipital joint S13.110
atloidooccipital joint S13.110
joint between
C0 and C1 S13.110
C1 and C2 S13.120
C2 and C3 S13.130
C3 and C4 S13.140
C4 and C5 S13.150
C5 and C6 S13.160
C6 and C7 S13.170
C7 and T1 S13.180
occipitoatloid joint S13.110
lumbar S33.100

- **Subluxation** *(continued)*
  - vertebral *(continued)*
    - traumatic *(continued)*
      - lumbar *(continued)*
        - joint between
          - L1 and L2 S33.110
          - L2 and L3 S33.120
          - L3 and L4 S33.130
          - L4 and L5 S33.140
      - thoracic S23.100
        - joint between
          - T1 and T2 S23.110
          - T2 and T3 S23.120
          - T3 and T4 S23.122
          - T4 and T5 S23.130
          - T5 and T6 S23.132
          - T6 and T7 S23.140
          - T7 and T8 S23.142
          - T8 and T9 S23.150
          - T9 and T10 S23.152
          - T10 and T11 S23.160
          - T11 and T12 S23.162
          - T12 and L1 S23.170
  - wrist (carpal bone) S63.00-
    - carpometacarpal joint —*see* Subluxation, carpometacarpal (joint)
    - distal radioulnar joint —*see* Subluxation, radioulnar (joint), distal
    - metacarpal bone, proximal —*see* Subluxation, metacarpal (bone), proximal end
    - midcarpal —*see* Subluxation, midcarpal (joint)
    - radiocarpal joint —*see* Subluxation, radiocarpal (joint)
    - recurrent —*see* Dislocation, recurrent, wrist
    - specified site NEC S63.09-
    - ulna —*see* Subluxation, ulna, distal end
- **Submaxillary** —*see* condition
- **Submersion** (fatal) (nonfatal) T75.1
- **Submucous** —*see* condition
- **Subnormal, subnormality**
  - accommodation (old age) H52.4
  - mental —*see* Disability, intellectual
  - temperature (accidental) T68
- **Subphrenic** —*see* condition
- **Subscapular nerve** —*see* condition
- **Subseptus uterus** Q51.2
- **Subsiding appendicitis** K36
- **Substance (other psychoactive) -induced**
  - anxiety disorder F19.980
  - bipolar and related disorder F19.94
  - delirium F19.921
  - depressive disorder F19.94
  - major neurocognitive disorder F19.97
  - mild neurocognitive disorder F19.988
  - obsessive-compulsive and related disorder F19.988
  - psychotic disorder F19.959
  - sexual dysfunction F19.981
  - sleep disorder F19.982
- **Substernal thyroid** E04.9
  - congenital Q89.2
- **Substitution disorder** F44.9
- **Subtentorial** —*see* condition
- **Subthyroidism** (acquired) —*see also* Hypothyroidism
  - congenital E03.1
- **Succenturiate placenta** O43.19-
- **Sucking thumb, child** (excessive) F98.8
- **Sudamen, sudamina** L74.1
- **Sudanese kala-azar** B55.0
- **Sudden**
  - heart failure —*see* Failure, heart
  - hearing loss —*see* Deafness, sudden
- **Sudeck's atrophy, disease, or syndrome** —*see* Algoneurodystrophy
- **Suffocation** —*see* Asphyxia, traumatic
- **Sugar**
  - blood
    - high (transient) R73.9
    - low (transient) E16.2
  - in urine R81
- **Suicide, suicidal** (attempted) T14.91
  - by poisoning —*see* Table of Drugs and Chemicals
  - history of (personal) Z91.5
    - in family Z81.8
  - ideation —*see* Ideation, suicidal
  - risk
    - meaning personal history of attempted suicide Z91.5
    - meaning suicidal ideation —*see* Ideation, suicidal
  - tendencies
    - meaning personal history of attempted suicide Z91.5
    - meaning suicidal ideation —*see* Ideation, suicidal
  - trauma —*see* nature of injury by site
- **Suipestifer infection** —*see* Infection, salmonella
- **Sulfhemoglobinemia, sulphemoglobinemia** (acquired) (with methemoglobinemia) D74.8
- **Sumatran mite fever** A75.3
- **Summer** —*see* condition
- **Sunburn** L55.9
  - due to
    - tanning bed (acute) L56.8
      - chronic L57.8
    - ultraviolet radiation (acute) L56.8
      - chronic L57.8
  - first degree L55.0
  - second degree L55.1
  - third degree L55.2
- **SUNCT** (short lasting unilateral neuralgiform headache with conjunctival injection and tearing) G44.059
  - intractable G44.051
  - not intractable G44.059
- **Sundowning** F05
- **Sunken acetabulum** —*see* Derangement, joint, specified type NEC, hip
- **Sunstroke** T67.0
- **Superfecundation** —*see* Pregnancy, multiple
- **Superfetation** —*see* Pregnancy, multiple
- **Superinvolution** (uterus) N85.8
- **Supernumerary** (congenital)
  - aortic cusps Q23.8
  - auditory ossicles Q16.3
  - bone Q79.8
  - breast Q83.1
  - carpal bones Q74.0
  - cusps, heart valve NEC Q24.8
    - aortic Q23.8
    - mitral Q23.2
    - pulmonary Q22.3
  - digit(s) Q69.9
  - ear (lobule) Q17.0
  - fallopian tube Q50.6
  - finger Q69.0
  - hymen Q52.4
  - kidney Q63.0
  - lacrimonasal duct Q10.6
  - lobule (ear) Q17.0
  - mitral cusps Q23.2
  - muscle Q79.8
  - nipple(s) Q83.3
  - organ or site not listed —*see* Accessory
  - ossicles, auditory Q16.3
  - ovary Q50.31
  - oviduct Q50.6
  - pulmonary, pulmonic cusps Q22.3
  - rib Q76.6
    - cervical or first (syndrome) Q76.5
  - roots (of teeth) K00.2
  - spleen Q89.09
  - tarsal bones Q74.2
  - teeth K00.1
  - testis Q55.29
  - thumb Q69.1
  - toe Q69.2
  - uterus Q51.2
  - vagina Q52.1
  - vertebra Q76.49
- **Supervision** (of)
  - contraceptive —*see* Prescription, contraceptives
  - dietary (for) Z71.3
    - allergy (food) Z71.3
    - colitis Z71.3
    - diabetes mellitus Z71.3
    - food allergy or intolerance Z71.3
    - gastritis Z71.3
    - hypercholesterolemia Z71.3
    - hypoglycemia Z71.3
    - intolerance (food) Z71.3
    - obesity Z71.3
    - specified NEC Z71.3
  - healthy infant or child Z76.2
    - foundling Z76.1
  - high-risk pregnancy —*see* Pregnancy, complicated by, high, risk
  - lactation Z39.1
  - pregnancy —*see* Pregnancy, supervision of
- **Supplemental teeth** K00.1
- **Suppression**
  - binocular vision H53.34
  - lactation O92.5
  - menstruation N94.89
  - ovarian secretion E28.39
  - renal N28.9
  - urine, urinary secretion R34
- **Suppuration, suppurative** —*see also* condition
  - accessory sinus (chronic) —*see* Sinusitis
  - adrenal gland
  - antrum (chronic) —*see* Sinusitis, maxillary
  - bladder —*see* Cystitis
  - brain G06.0
    - sequelae G09
  - breast N61.1
    - puerperal, postpartum or gestational —*see* Mastitis, obstetric, purulent
  - dental periosteum M27.3
  - ear (middle) —*see also* Otitis, media
    - external NEC —*see* Otitis, externa, infective
    - internal —*see* subcategory H83.0
  - ethmoidal (chronic) (sinus) —*see* Sinusitis, ethmoidal
  - fallopian tube —*see* Salpingo-oophoritis
  - frontal (chronic) (sinus) —*see* Sinusitis, frontal
  - gallbladder (acute) K81.0
  - gum K05.20
    - generalized - *see* Peridontitis, aggressive, generalized
    - localized - *see* Peridontitis, aggressive, localized
  - intracranial G06.0
  - joint —*see* Arthritis, pyogenic or pyemic
  - labyrinthine —*see* subcategory H83.0
  - lung —*see* Abscess, lung
  - mammary gland N61.1
    - puerperal, postpartum O91.12
      - associated with lactation O91.13
  - maxilla, maxillary M27.2
    - sinus (chronic) —*see* Sinusitis, maxillary
  - muscle —*see* Myositis, infective
  - nasal sinus (chronic) —*see* Sinusitis
  - pancreas, acute (*see also* Pancreatitis, acute) K85.80
  - parotid gland —*see* Sialoadenitis
  - pelvis, pelvic
    - female —*see* Disease, pelvis, inflammatory
    - male K65.0
  - pericranial —*see* Osteomyelitis
  - salivary duct or gland (any) —*see* Sialoadenitis
  - sinus (accessory) (chronic) (nasal) —*see* Sinusitis
  - sphenoidal sinus (chronic) —*see* Sinusitis, sphenoidal
  - thymus (gland) E32.1
  - thyroid (gland) E06.0
  - tonsil —*see* Tonsillitis
  - uterus —*see* Endometritis
- **Supraeruption of tooth** (teeth) M26.34
- **Supraglottitis** J04.30
  - with obstruction J04.31
- **Suprarenal** (gland) —*see* condition
- **Suprascapular nerve** —*see* condition
- **Suprasellar** —*see* condition
- **Surfer's knots or nodules** S89.8-
- **Surgical**
  - emphysema T81.82
  - procedures, complication or misadventure —*see* Complications, surgical procedures
  - shock T81.10
- **Surveillance** (of) (for) —*see also* Observation
  - alcohol abuse Z71.41
  - contraceptive —*see* Prescription, contraceptives
  - dietary Z71.3
  - drug abuse Z71.51

Susceptibility to disease, genetic Z15.89
  - malignant neoplasm Z15.09
    - breast Z15.01
    - endometrium Z15.04
    - ovary Z15.02
    - prostate Z15.03
    - specified NEC Z15.09
  - multiple endocrine neoplasia Z15.81

Suspected condition, ruled out *—see also* Observation, suspected
  - amniotic cavity and membrane Z03.71
  - cervical shortening Z03.75
  - fetal anomaly Z03.73
  - fetal growth Z03.74
  - maternal and fetal conditions NEC Z03.79
  - newborn (*see also* Observation, newborn, suspected condition ruled out) Z05.9
  - oligohydramnios Z03.71
  - placental problem Z03.72
  - polyhydramnios Z03.71

Suspended uterus
  - in pregnancy or childbirth *—see* Pregnancy, complicated by, abnormal uterus

Sutton's nevus D22.9

Suture
  - burst (in operation wound) T81.31
    - external operation wound T81.31
    - internal operation wound T81.32
  - inadvertently left in operation wound *—see* Foreign body, accidentally left during a procedure
  - removal Z48.02

Swab inadvertently left in operation wound *—see* Foreign body, accidentally left during a procedure

Swallowed, swallowing
  - difficulty *—see* Dysphagia
  - foreign body *—see* Foreign body, alimentary tract

Swan-neck deformity (finger) *—see* Deformity, finger, swan-neck

Swearing, compulsive F42.8
  - in Gilles de la Tourette's syndrome F95.2

Sweat, sweats
  - fetid L75.0
  - night R61

Sweating, excessive R61

Sweeley-Klionsky disease E75.21

Sweet's disease or dermatosis L98.2

Swelling (of) R60.9
  - abdomen, abdominal (not referable to any particular organ) *—see* Mass, abdominal
  - ankle *—see* Effusion, joint, ankle
  - arm M79.89
    - forearm M79.89
  - breast (*see also* Lump, breast) N63.0
  - Calabar B74.3
  - cervical gland R59.0
  - chest, localized R22.2
  - ear H93.8-
  - extremity (lower) (upper) *—see* Disorder, soft tissue, specified type NEC
  - finger M79.89
  - foot M79.89
  - glands R59.9
    - generalized R59.1
    - localized R59.0
  - hand M79.89
  - head (localized) R22.0

Swelling *(continued)*
  - inflammatory *—see* Inflammation
  - intra-abdominal *—see* Mass, abdominal
  - joint *—see* Effusion, joint
  - leg M79.89
    - lower M79.89
  - limb *—see* Disorder, soft tissue, specified type NEC
  - localized (skin) R22.9
    - chest R22.2
    - head R22.0
    - limb
      - lower *—see* Mass, localized, limb, lower
      - upper *—see* Mass, localized, limb, upper
    - neck R22.1
    - trunk R22.2
  - neck (localized) R22.1
  - pelvic *—see* Mass, abdominal
  - scrotum N50.89
  - splenic *—see* Splenomegaly
  - testis N50.89
  - toe M79.89
  - umbilical R19.09
  - wandering, due to Gnathostoma (spinigerum) B83.1
  - white *—see* Tuberculosis, arthritis

Swift (-Feer) **disease**
  - overdose or wrong substance given or taken *—see* Table of Drugs and Chemicals, by drug, poisoning

Swimmer's
  - cramp T75.1
  - ear H60.33-
  - itch B65.3

Swimming in the head R42

Swollen *—see* Swelling

Swyer syndrome Q99.1

Sycosis L73.8
  - barbae (not parasitic) L73.8
  - contagiosa (mycotic) B35.0
  - lupoides L73.8
  - mycotic B35.0
  - parasitic B35.0
  - vulgaris L73.8

Sydenham's chorea *—see* Chorea, Sydenham's

Sylvatic yellow fever A95.0

Sylvest's disease B33.0

Symblepharon H11.23-
  - congenital Q10.3

Symond's syndrome G93.2

Sympathetic *—see* condition

Sympatheticotonia G90.8

Sympathicoblastoma
  - specified site *—see* Neoplasm, malignant, by site
  - unspecified site C74.90

Sympathogonioma *—see* Sympathicoblastoma

Symphalangy (fingers) (toes) Q70.9

Symptoms NEC R68.89
  - breast NEC N64.59
  - cold J00
  - development NEC R63.8
  - factitious, self-induced *—see* Disorder, factitious
  - genital organs, female R10.2
  - involving
    - abdomen NEC R19.8
    - appearance NEC R46.89
    - awareness R41.9
      - altered mental status R41.82

Symptoms NEC *(continued)*
  - involving *(continued)*
    - awareness *(continued)*
      - amnesia *—see* Amnesia
      - borderline intellectual functioning R41.83
      - coma *—see* Coma
      - disorientation R41.0
      - neurologic neglect syndrome R41.4
      - senile cognitive decline R41.81
      - specified symptom NEC R41.89
    - behavior NEC R46.89
    - cardiovascular system NEC R09.89
    - chest NEC R09.89
    - circulatory system NEC R09.89
    - cognitive functions R41.9
      - altered mental status R41.82
      - amnesia *—see* Amnesia
      - borderline intellectual functioning R41.83
      - coma *—see* Coma
      - disorientation R41.0
      - neurologic neglect syndrome R41.4
      - senile cognitive decline R41.81
      - specified symptom NEC R41.89
    - development NEC R62.50
    - digestive system NEC R19.8
    - emotional state NEC R45.89
      - emotional lability R45.86
    - food and fluid intake R63.8
    - general perceptions and sensations R44.9
      - specified NEC R44.8
    - musculoskeletal system R29.91
      - specified NEC R29.898
    - nervous system R29.90
      - specified NEC R29.818
    - pelvis NEC R19.8
    - respiratory system NEC R09.89
    - skin and integument R23.9
    - urinary system R39.9
  - menopausal N95.1
  - metabolism NEC R63.8
  - neurotic F48.8
  - of infancy R68.19
  - pelvis NEC, female R10.2
  - skin and integument NEC R23.9
  - subcutaneous tissue NEC R23.9
  - viral cold J00

Sympus Q74.2

Syncephalus Q89.4

Synchondrosis
  - abnormal (congenital) Q78.8
  - ischiopubic M91.0

Synchysis (scintillans) (senile) (vitreous body) H43.89

Syncope (near) (pre-) R55
  - anginosa I20.8
  - bradycardia R00.1
  - cardiac R55
  - carotid sinus G90.01
  - due to spinal (lumbar) puncture G97.1
  - heart R55
  - heat T67.1
  - laryngeal R05
  - psychogenic F48.8
  - tussive R05
  - vasoconstriction R55
  - vasodepressor R55
  - vasomotor R55
  - vasovagal R55

Syndactylism, syndactyly Q70.9
  - complex (with synostosis)
    - fingers Q70.0-
    - toes Q70.2-
  - simple (without synostosis)
    - fingers Q70.1-
    - toes Q70.3-

Syndrome *—see also* Disease
  - 5q minus NOS D46.C
  - 48, XXXX Q97.1
  - 49, XXXXX Q97.1
  - abdominal
    - acute R10.0
    - muscle deficiency Q79.4
  - abnormal innervation H02.519
    - left H02.516
      - lower H02.515
      - upper H02.514
    - right H02.513
      - lower H02.512
      - upper H02.511
  - abstinence, neonatal P96.1
  - acid pulmonary aspiration, obstetric O74.0
  - acquired immunodeficiency *—see* Human, immunodeficiency virus (HIV) disease
  - acute abdominal R10.0
  - acute respiratory distress (adult) (child) J80
    - idiopathic J84.114
  - Adair-Dighton Q78.0
  - Adams-Stokes (-Morgagni) I45.9
  - adiposogenital E23.6
  - adrenal
    - hemorrhage (meningococcal) A39.1
    - meningococcic A39.1
  - adrenocortical *—see* Cushing's, syndrome
  - adrenogenital E25.9
    - congenital, associated with enzyme deficiency E25.0
  - afferent loop NEC K91.89
  - Alagille's Q44.7
  - alcohol withdrawal (without convulsions) *—see* Dependence, alcohol, with, withdrawal
  - Alder's D72.0
  - Aldrich (-Wiskott) D82.0
  - alien hand R41.4
  - Alport Q87.81
  - alveolar hypoventilation E66.2
  - alveolocapillary block J84.10
  - amnesic, amnestic (confabulatory) (due to) *—see* Disorder, amnesic
  - amyostatic (Wilson's disease) E83.01
  - androgen insensitivity E34.50
    - complete E34.51
    - partial E34.52
  - androgen resistance (*see also* Syndrome, androgen insensitivity) E34.50
  - Angelman Q93.5
  - anginal *—see* Angina
  - ankyloglossia superior Q38.1
  - anterior
    - chest wall R07.89
    - cord G83.82
    - spinal artery G95.19
      - compression M47.019
        - cervical region M47.012
        - cervicothoracic region M47.013
        - lumbar region M47.016
        - occipito-atlanto-axial region M47.011
        - thoracic region M47.014

- anterior *(continued)*
  - spinal artery *(continued)*
    - compression *(continued)*
      - thoracolumbar region M47.015
  - tibial M76.81-
- antibody deficiency D80.9
  - agammaglobulinemic D80.1
    - hereditary D80.0
  - congenital D80.0
  - hypogammaglobulinemic D80.1
    - hereditary D80.0
- anticardiolipin (-antibody) D68.61
- antidepressant discontinuation T43.205
- antiphospholipid (-antibody) D68.61
- aortic
  - arch M31.4
  - bifurcation I74.09
- aortomesenteric duodenum occlusion K31.5
- apical ballooning (transient left ventricular) I51.81
- arcuate ligament I77.4
- argentaffin, argintaffinoma E34.0
- Arnold-Chiari —*see* Arnold-Chiari disease
- Arrillaga-Ayerza I27.0
- arterial tortuosity Q87.82
- arteriovenous steal T82.898-
- Asherman's N85.6
- aspiration, of newborn —*see* Aspiration, by substance, with pneumonia
  - meconium P24.01
- ataxia-telangiectasia G11.3
- auriculotemporal G50.8
- autoerythrocyte sensitization (Gardner-Diamond) D69.2
- autoimmune polyglandular E31.0
- autoimmune lymphoproliferative [ALPS] D89.82
- autoinflammatory M04.9
  - specified type NEC M04.8
- autosomal —*see* Abnormal, autosomes
- Avellis' G46.8
- Ayerza (-Arrillaga) I27.0
- Babinski-Nageotte G83.89
- Bakwin-Krida Q78.5
- bare lymphocyte D81.6
- Barré-Guillain G61.0
- Barré-Liéou M53.0
- Barrett's —*see* Barrett's, esophagus
- Barsony-Polgar K22.4
- Barsony-Teschendorf K22.4
- Barth E78.71
- Bartter's E26.81
- basal cell nevus Q87.89
- Basedow's E05.00
  - with thyroid storm E05.01
- basilar artery G45.0
- Batten-Steinert G71.11
- battered
  - baby or child —*see* Maltreatment, child, physical abuse
  - spouse —*see* Maltreatment, adult, physical abuse
- Beals Q87.40
- Beau's I51.5
- Beck's I65.8
- Benedikt's G46.3
- Béquez César (-Steinbrinck-Chédiak-Higashi) E70.330
- Bernhardt-Roth —*see* Meralgia paresthetica
- Bernheim's - *see* Failure, heart, right
- big spleen D73.1
- bilateral polycystic ovarian E28.2

- Bing-Horton's —*see* Horton's headache
- Birt-Hogg-Dube syndrome Q87.89
- Björck (-Thorsen) E34.0
- black
  - lung J60
  - widow spider bite —*see* Toxicity, venom, spider, black widow
- Blackfan-Diamond D61.01
- Blau M04.8
- blind loop K90.2
  - congenital Q43.8
  - postsurgical K91.2
- blue sclera Q78.0
- blue toe I75.02-
- Boder-Sedgewick G11.3
- Boerhaave's K22.3
- Borjeson Forssman Lehmann Q89.8
- Bouillaud's I01.9
- Bourneville (-Pringle) Q85.1
- Bouveret (-Hoffman) I47.9
- brachial plexus G54.0
- bradycardia-tachycardia I49.5
- brain (nonpsychotic) F09
  - with psychosis, psychotic reaction F09
  - acute or subacute —*see* Delirium
  - congenital —*see* Disability, intellectual
  - organic F09
    - post-traumatic (nonpsychotic) F07.81
      - psychotic F09
  - personality change F07.0
  - postcontusional F07.81
  - post-traumatic, nonpsychotic F07.81
  - psycho-organic F09
  - psychotic F06.8
- brain stem stroke G46.3
- Brandt's (acrodermatitis enteropathica) E83.2
- broad ligament laceration N83.8
- Brock's J98.11
- bronze baby P83.88
- Brown-Sequard G83.81
- Brugada I49.8
- bubbly lung P27.0
- Buchem's M85.2
- Budd-Chiari I82.0
- bulbar (progressive) G12.22
- Bürger-Grütz E78.3
- Burke's K86.89
- Burnett's (milk-alkali) E83.52
- burning feet E53.9
- Bywaters' T79.5
- Call-Fleming I67.841
- carbohydrate-deficient glycoprotein (CDGS) E77.8
- carcinogenic thrombophlebitis I82.1
- carcinoid E34.0
- cardiac asthma I50.1
- cardiacos negros I27.0
- cardiofaciocutaneous Q87.89
- cardiopulmonary-obesity E66.2
- cardiorenal —*see* Hypertension, cardiorenal
- cardiorespiratory distress (idiopathic), newborn P22.0
- cardiovascular renal —*see* Hypertension, cardiorenal
- carotid
  - artery (hemispheric) (internal) G45.1
  - body G90.01
  - sinus G90.01
- carpal tunnel G56.0-
- Cassidy (-Scholte) E34.0
- cat cry Q93.4
- cat eye Q92.8

- cauda equina G83.4
- causalgia —*see* Causalgia
- celiac K90.0
  - artery compression I77.4
  - axis I77.4
- central pain G89.0
- cerebellar
  - hereditary G11.9
  - stroke G46.4
- cerebellomedullary malformation —*see* Spina bifida
- cerebral
  - artery
    - anterior G46.1
    - middle G46.0
    - posterior G46.2
  - gigantism E22.0
- cervical (root) M53.1
  - disc —*see* Disorder, disc, cervical, with neuritis
  - fusion Q76.1
  - posterior, sympathicus M53.0
  - rib Q76.5
  - sympathetic paralysis G90.2
- cervicobrachial (diffuse) M53.1
- cervicocranial M53.0
- cervicodorsal outlet G54.2
- cervicothoracic outlet G54.0
- Céstan (-Raymond) I65.8
- Charcot's (angina cruris) (intermittent claudication) I73.9
- Charcot-Weiss-Baker G90.09
- CHARGE Q89.8
- Chédiak-Higashi (-Steinbrinck) E70.330
- chest wall R07.1
- Chiari's (hepatic vein thrombosis) I82.0
- Chilaiditi's Q43.3
- child maltreatment —*see* Maltreatment, child
- chondrocostal junction M94.0
- chondroectodermal dysplasia Q77.6
- chromosome 4 short arm deletion Q93.3
- chromosome 5 short arm deletion Q93.4
- chronic
  - infantile neurological, cutaneous and articular (CINCA) M04.2
  - pain G89.4
    - personality F68.8
- Clarke-Hadfield K86.89
- Clerambault's automatism G93.89
- Clouston's (hidrotic ectodermal dysplasia) Q82.4
- clumsiness, clumsy child F82
- cluster headache G44.009
  - intractable G44.001
  - not intractable G44.009
- Coffin-Lowry Q89.8
- cold injury (newborn) P80.0
- combined immunity deficiency D81.9
- compartment (deep) (posterior) (traumatic) T79.A0
  - abdomen T79.A3
  - lower extremity (hip, buttock, thigh, leg, foot, toes) T79.A2
  - nontraumatic
    - abdomen M79.A3
    - lower extremity (hip, buttock, thigh, leg, foot, toes) M79.A2-
    - specified site NEC M79.A9
    - upper extremity (shoulder, arm, forearm, wrist, hand, fingers) M79.A1-

- compartment *(continued)*
  - postprocedural —*see* Syndrome, compartment, nontraumatic
  - specified site NEC T79.A9
  - upper extremity (shoulder, arm, forearm, wrist, hand, fingers) T79.A1
- complex regional pain —*see* Syndrome, pain, complex regional
- compression T79.5
  - anterior spinal —*see* Syndrome, anterior, spinal artery, compression
  - cauda equina G83.4
  - celiac artery I77.4
  - vertebral artery M47.029
    - occipito-atlanto-axial region M47.021
    - cervical region M47.022
- concussion F07.81
- congenital
  - affecting multiple systems NEC Q87.89
  - central alveolar hypoventilation G47.35
  - facial diplegia Q87.0
  - muscular hypertrophy-cerebral Q87.89
  - oculo-auriculovertebral Q87.0
  - oculofacial diplegia (Moebius) Q87.0
  - rubella (manifest) P35.0
- congestion-fibrosis (pelvic), female N94.89
- congestive dysmenorrhea N94.6
- Conn's E26.01
- connective tissue M35.9
  - overlap NEC M35.1
- conus medullaris G95.81
- cord
  - anterior G83.82
  - posterior G83.83
- coronary
  - acute NEC I24.9
  - insufficiency or intermediate I20.0
  - slow flow I20.8
- Costen's (complex) M26.69
- costochondral junction M94.0
- costoclavicular G54.0
- costovertebral E22.0
- Cowden Q85.8
- craniovertebral M53.0
- Creutzfeldt-Jakob —*see* Creutzfeldt-Jakob disease or syndrome
- cri-du-chat Q93.4
- crib death R99
- cricopharyngeal —*see* Dysphagia
- croup J05.0
- CRPS I —*see* Syndrome, pain, complex regional I
- crush T79.5
- cryopyrin-associated periodic M04.2
- cubital tunnel —*see* Lesion, nerve, ulnar
- Curschmann (-Batten) (-Steinert) G71.11
- Cushing's E24.9
  - alcohol-induced E24.4
  - due to
    - alcohol
    - drugs E24.2
    - ectopic ACTH E24.3
    - overproduction of pituitary ACTH E24.0
  - drug-induced E24.2
  - overdose or wrong substance given or taken —*see* Table of Drugs and Chemicals, by drug, poisoning

Syndrome *(continued)*
Cushing's *(continued)*
pituitary-dependent E24.0
specified type NEC E24.8
cryptophthalmos Q87.0
cystic duct stump K91.5
Dana-Putnam D51.0
Danbolt (-Cross) (acrodermatitis enteropathica) E83.2
Dandy-Walker Q03.1
with spina bifida Q07.01
Danlos' Q79.6
defibrination —*see also* Fibrinolysis
with
antepartum hemorrhage —*see* Hemorrhage, antepartum, with coagulation defect
intrapartum hemorrhage —*see* Hemorrhage, complicating, delivery
newborn P60
postpartum O72.3
Degos' I77.89
Déjérine-Roussy G89.0
delayed sleep phase G47.21
demyelinating G37.9
dependence —*see* F10-F19 with fourth character .2
depersonalization (-derealization) F48.1
De Quervain E34.51
de Toni-Fanconi (-Debré) E72.09
with cystinosis E72.04
diabetes mellitus-hypertension-nephrosis —*see* Diabetes, nephrosis
diabetes mellitus in newborn infant P70.2
diabetes-nephrosis —*see* Diabetes, nephrosis
diabetic amyotrophy —*see* Diabetes, amyotrophy
dialysis associated steal T82.898-
Diamond-Blackfan D61.01
Diamond-Gardener D69.2
DIC (diffuse or disseminated intravascular coagulopathy) D65
di George's D82.1
Dighton's Q78.0
disequilibrium E87.8
Döhle body-panmyelopathic D72.0
dorsolateral medullary G46.4
double athetosis G80.3
Down (*see also* Down syndrome) Q90.9
Dresbach's (elliptocytosis) D58.1
Dressler's (postmyocardial infarction) I24.1
postcardiotomy I97.0
drug withdrawal, infant of dependent mother P96.1
dry eye H04.12-
due to abnormality
chromosomal Q99.9
sex
female phenotype Q97.9
male phenotype Q98.9
specified NEC Q99.8
dumping (postgastrectomy) K91.1
nonsurgical K31.89
Dupré's (meningism) R29.1
dysmetabolic X E88.81
dyspraxia, developmental F82
Eagle-Barrett Q79.4
Eaton-Lambert —*see* Syndrome, Lambert-Eaton
Ebstein's Q22.5
ectopic ACTH E24.3
eczema-thrombocytopenia D82.0
Eddowes' Q78.0

Syndrome *(continued)*
effort (psychogenic) F45.8
Eisenmenger's I27.83
Ehlers-Danlos Q79.6
Ekman's Q78.0
electric feet E53.8
Ellis-van Creveld Q77.6
empty nest Z60.0
endocrine-hypertensive E27.0
entrapment —*see* Neuropathy, entrapment
eosinophilia-myalgia M35.8
epileptic —*see also* Epilepsy, by type
absence G40.A09
intractable G40.A19
with status epilepticus G40.A11
without status epilepticus G40.A19
not intractable G40.A09
with status epilepticus G40.A01
without status epilepticus G40.A09
Erdheim-Chester (ECD) E88.89
Erdheim's E22.0
erythrocyte fragmentation D59.4
Evans D69.41
exhaustion F48.8
extrapyramidal G25.9
specified NEC G25.89
eye retraction —*see* Strabismus
eyelid-malar-mandible Q87.0
Faber's D50.9
facial pain, paroxysmal G50.0
Fallot's Q21.3
familial cold autoinflammatory M04.2
familial eczema-thrombocytopenia (Wiskott-Aldrich) D82.0
Fanconi (-de Toni) (-Debré) E72.09
with cystinosis E72.04
Fanconi's (anemia) (congenital pancytopenia) D61.09
fatigue
chronic R53.82
psychogenic F48.8
faulty bowel habit K59.39
Feil-Klippel (brevicollis) Q76.1
Felty's —*see* Felty's syndrome
fertile eunuch E23.0
fetal
alcohol (dysmorphic) Q86.0
hydantoin Q86.1
Fiedler's I40.1
first arch Q87.0
fish odor E72.8
Fisher's G61.0
Fitzhugh-Curtis
due to
Chlamydia trachomatis A74.81
Neisseria gonorrhorea (gonococcal peritonitis) A54.85
Fitz's (*see also* Pancreatitis, acute) K85.80
Flajani (-Basedow) E05.00
with thyroid storm E05.01
flatback —*see* Flatback syndrome
floppy
baby P94.2
iris (intraoeprative) (IFIS) H21.81
mitral valve I34.1
flush E34.0
Foix-Alajouanine G95.19
Fong's Q87.2
food protein-induced enterocolitis K52.21
foramen magnum G93.5

Syndrome *(continued)*
Foster-Kennedy H47.14-
Foville's (peduncular) G46.3
fragile X Q99.2
Franceschetti Q75.4
Frey's
auriculotemporal G50.8
hyperhidrosis L74.52
Friderichsen-Waterhouse A39.1
Froin's G95.89
frontal lobe F07.0
Fukuhara E88.49
functional
bowel K59.9
prepubertal castrate E29.1
Gaisböck's D75.1
ganglion (basal ganglia brain) G25.9
geniculi G51.1
Gardner-Diamond D69.2
gastroesophageal
junction K22.0
laceration-hemorrhage K22.6
gastrojejunal loop obstruction K91.89
Gee-Herter-Heubner K90.0
Gelineau's G47.419
with cataplexy G47.411
genito-anorectal A55
Gerstmann-Sträussler-Scheinker (GSS) A81.82
Gianotti-Crosti L44.4
giant platelet (Bernard-Soulier) D69.1
Gilles de la Tourette's F95.2
goiter-deafness E07.1
Goldberg Q89.8
Goldberg-Maxwell E34.51
Good's D83.8
Gopalan'(burning feet) E53.8
Gorlin's Q87.89
Gougerot-Blum L81.7
Gouley's I31.1
Gower's R55
gray or grey (newborn) P93.0
platelet D69.1
Gubler-Millard G46.3
Guillain-Barré (-Strohl) G61.0
gustatory sweating G50.8
Hadfield-Clarke K86.89
hair tourniquet —*see* Constriction, external, by site
Hamman's J98.19
hand-foot L27.1
hand-shoulder G90.8
hantavirus (cardio)-pulmonary (HPS) (HCPS) B33.4
happy puppet Q93.5
Harada's H30.81-
Hayem-Faber D50.9
headache NEC G44.89
complicated NEC G44.59
Heberden's I20.8
Hedinger's E34.0
Hegglin's D72.0
HELLP (hemolysis, elevated liver enzymes and low platelet count) O14.2-
complicating
childbirth O14.24
puerperium O14.25
hemolytic-uremic D59.3
hemophagocytic, infection-associated D76.2
Henoch-Schönlein D69.0
hepatic flexure K59.8
hepatopulmonary K76.81
hepatorenal K76.7
following delivery O90.4
postoperative or postprocedural K91.83

Syndrome *(continued)*
hepatorenal *(continued)*
postpartum, puerperal O90.4
hepatourologic K76.7
Herter (-Gee) (nontropical sprue) K90.0
Heubner-Herter K90.0
Heyd's K76.7
Hilger's G90.09
histamine-like (fish poisoning) —*see* Poisoning, fish
histiocytic D76.3
histiocytosis NEC D76.3
HIV infection, acute B20
Hoffmann-Werdnig G12.0
Hollander-Simons E88.1
Hoppe-Goldflam G70.00
with exacerbation (acute) G70.01
in crisis G70.01
Horner's G90.2
hungry bone E83.81
hunterian glossitis D51.0
Hutchinson's triad A50.53
hyperabduction G54.0
hyperammonemia-hyperornithinemia-homocitrullinemia E72.4
hypereosinophilic (idiopathic) D72.1
hyperimmunoglobulin D M04.1
hyperimmunoglobulin E (IgE) D82.4
hyperkalemic E87.5
hyperkinetic —*see* Hyperkinesia
hypermobility M35.7
hypernatremia E87.0
hyperosmolarity E87.0
hyperperfusion G97.82
hypersplenic D73.1
hypertransfusion, newborn P61.1
hyperventilation F45.8
hyperviscosity (of serum)
polycythemic D75.1
sclerothymic D58.8
hypoglycemic (familial) (neonatal) E16.2
hypokalemic E87.6
hyponatremic E87.1
hypopituitarism E23.0
hypoplastic left-heart Q23.4
hypopotassemia E87.6
hyposmolality E87.1
hypotension, maternal O26.5-
hypothenar hammer I73.89
hypoventilation, obesity (OHS) E66.2
ICF (intravascular coagulation-fibrinolysis) D65
idiopathic
cardiorespiratory distress, newborn P22.0
nephrotic (infantile) N04.9
iliotibial band M76.3-
immobility, immobilization (paraplegic) M62.3
immune reconstitution D89.3
immune reconstitution inflammatory [IRIS] D89.3
immunity deficiency, combined D81.9
immunodeficiency
acquired —*see* Human, immunodeficiency virus (HIV) disease
combined D81.9
impending coronary I20.0
impingement, shoulder M75.4-
inappropriate secretion of antidiuretic hormone E22.2
infant
of diabetic mother P70.1
gestational diabetes P70.0

Syndrome *(continued)*
- infantilism (pituitary) E23.0
- inferior vena cava I87.1
- inspissated bile (newborn) P59.1
- institutional (childhood) F94.2
- insufficient sleep F51.12
- intermediate coronary (artery) I20.0
- interspinous ligament *—see* Spondylopathy, specified NEC
- intestinal
  - carcinoid E34.0
  - knot K56.2
- intravascular coagulation-fibrinolysis (ICF) D65
- iodine-deficiency, congenital E00.9
  - type
    - mixed E00.2
    - myxedematous E00.1
    - neurological E00.0
- IRDS (idiopathic respiratory distress, newborn) P22.0
- irritable
  - bowel K58.9
    - with
      - constipation K58.1
      - diarrhea K58.0
    - mixed K58.2
    - psychogenic F45.8
    - specified NEC K58.8
  - heart (psychogenic) F45.8
  - weakness F48.8
- ischemic
  - bowel (transient) K55.9
  - chronic K55.1
  - due to mesenteric artery insufficiency K55.1
  - steal T82.898
- IVC (intravascular coagulopathy) D65
- Ivemark's Q89.01
- Jaccoud's *—see* Arthropathy, postrheumatic, chronic
- Jackson's G83.89
- Jakob-Creutzfeldt *—see* Creutzfeldt-Jakob disease or syndrome
- jaw-winking Q07.8
- Jervell-Lange-Nielsen I45.81
- jet lag G47.25
- Job's D71
- Joseph-Diamond-Blackfan D61.01
- jugular foramen G52.7
- Kabuki Q89.8
- Kanner's (autism) F84.0
- Kartagener's Q89.3
- Kelly's D50.1
- Kimmelsteil-Wilson *—see* Diabetes, specified type, with Kimmelsteil-Wilson disease
- Klein (e)-Levine G47.13
- Klippel-Feil (brevicollis) Q76.1
- Köhler-Pellegrini-Steida *—see* Bursitis, tibial collateral
- König's K59.8
- Korsakoff (-Wernicke) (nonalcoholic) F04
  - alcoholic F10.26
- Kostmann's D70.0
- Krabbe's congenital muscle hypoplasia Q79.8
- labyrinthine H83.2
- lacunar NEC G46.7
- Lambert-Eaton G70.80
  - in
    - neoplastic disease G73.1
    - specified disease NEC G70.81
- Landau-Kleffner *—see* Epilepsy, specified NEC
- Larsen's Q74.8
- lateral
  - cutaneous nerve of thigh G57.1-

Syndrome *(continued)*
- lateral *(continued)*
  - medullary G46.4
- Launois' E22.0
- lazy
  - leukocyte D70.8
  - posture M62.3
- Lemiere I80.8
- Lennox-Gastaut G40.812
  - intractable G40.814
    - with status epilepticus G40.813
    - without status epilepticus G40.814
  - not intractable G40.812
    - with status epilepticus G40.811
    - without status epilepticus G40.812
- lenticular, progressive E83.01
- Leopold-Levi's E05.90
- Lev's I44.2
- Li-Fraumeni Z15.01
- Lichtheim's D51.0
- Lightwood's N25.89
- Lignac (de Toni) (-Fanconi) (-Debré) E72.09
  - with cystinosis E72.04
- Likoff's I20.8
- limbic epilepsy personality F07.0
- liver-kidney K76.7
- lobotomy F07.0
- Loffler's J82
- long arm 18 or 21 deletion Q93.89
- long QT I45.81
- Louis-Barré G11.3
- low
  - atmospheric pressure T70.29
  - back M54.5
  - output (cardiac) I50.9
- lower radicular, newborn (birth injury) P14.8
- Luetscher's (dehydration) E86.0
- Lupus anticoagulant D68.62
- Lutembacher's Q21.1
- macrophage activation D76.1
  - due to infection D76.2
- magnesium-deficiency R29.0
- Majeed M04.8
- Mal de Debarquement R42
- malabsorption K90.9
  - postsurgical K91.2
- malformation, congenital, due to
  - alcohol Q86.0
  - exogenous cause NEC Q86.8
  - hydantoin Q86.1
  - warfarin Q86.2
- malignant
  - carcinoid E34.0
  - neuroleptic G21.0
- Mallory-Weiss K22.6
- mandibulofacial dysostosis Q75.4
- manic-depressive *—see* Disorder, bipolar
- maple-syrup-urine E71.0
- Marable's I77.4
- Marfan's Q87.40
  - with
    - cardiovascular manifestations Q87.418
      - aortic dilation Q87.410
    - ocular manifestations Q87.42
    - skeletal manifestations Q87.43
- Marie's (acromegaly) E22.0
- mast cell activation - *see* Activation, mast cell
- maternal hypotension *—see* Syndrome, hypotension, maternal
- May (-Hegglin) D72.0
- McArdle (-Schmidt) (-Pearson) E74.04
- McQuarrie's E16.2

Syndrome *(continued)*
- meconium plug (newborn) P76.0
- median arcuate ligament I77.4
- Meekeren-Ehlers-Danlos Q79.6
- megavitamin-B6 E67.2
- Meige G24.4
- MELAS E88.41
- Mendelson's O74.0
- MERRF (myoclonic epilepsy associated with ragged-red fibers) E88.42
- mesenteric
  - artery (superior) K55.1
  - vascular insufficiency K55.1
- metabolic E88.81
- metastatic carcinoid E34.0
- micrognathia-glossoptosis Q87.0
- midbrain NEC G93.89
- middle lobe (lung) J98.19
- middle radicular G54.0
- migraine (*see also* Migraine) G43.909-
- Mikulicz' K11.8
- milk-alkali E83.52
- Millard-Gubler G46.3
- Miller-Dieker Q93.88
- Miller-Fisher G61.0
- Minkowski-Chauffard D58.0
- Mirizzi's K83.1
- MNGIE (Mitochondrial Neurogastrointestinal Encephalopathy) E88.49
- Möbius, ophthalmoplegic migraine *—see* Migraine, ophthalmoplegic
- monofixation H50.42
- Morel-Moore M85.2
- Morel-Morgagni M85.2
- Morgagni (-Morel) (-Stewart) M85.2
- Morgagni-Adams-Stokes I45.9
- mucocutaneous lymph node (acute febrile) (MCLS) M30.3
- multiple endocrine neoplasia (MEN) *—see* Neoplasia, endocrine, multiple (MEN)
- multiple operations *—see* Disorder, factitious
- Mounier-Kuhn Q32.4
  - with bronchiectasis J47.9
    - with
      - exacerbation (acute) J47.1
      - lower respiratory infection J47.0
  - acquired J98.09
    - with bronchiectasis J47.9
      - with
        - exacerbation (acute) J47.1
        - lower respiratory infection J47.0
- Muckle-Wells M04.2
- myasthenic G70.9
  - in
    - diabetes mellitus *—see* Diabetes, amyotrophy
    - endocrine disease NEC E34.9 *[G73.3]*
    - neoplastic disease (*see also* Neoplasm) D49.9 *[G73.3]*
    - thyrotoxicosis (hyperthyroidism) E05.90 *[G73.3]*
      - with thyroid storm E05.91 *[G73.3]*
- myelodysplastic D46.9
  - with
    - 5q deletion D46.C
    - isolated del (5q) chromosomal abnormality D46.C
  - lesions, low grade D46.20
  - specified NEC D46.Z
- myelopathic pain G89.0

Syndrome *(continued)*
- myeloproliferative (chronic) D47.1
- myofascial pain M79.1
- Naffziger's G54.0
- nail patella Q87.2
- NARP (Neuropathy, Ataxia and Retinitis pigmentosa) E88.49
- neonatal abstinence P96.1
- nephritic *—see also* Nephritis
  - with edema *—see* Nephrosis
  - acute N00.9
  - chronic N03.9
  - rapidly progressive N01.9
- nephrotic (congenital) (*see also* Nephrosis) N04.9
  - with
    - dense deposit disease N04.6
    - diffuse
      - crescentic glomerulonephritis N04.7
      - endocapillary proliferative glomerulonephritis N04.4
      - membranous glomerulonephritis N04.2
      - mesangial proliferative glomerulonephritis N04.3
      - mesangiocapillary glomerulonephritis N04.5
    - focal and segmental glomerular lesions N04.1
    - minor glomerular abnormality N04.0
    - specified morphological changes NEC N04.8
  - diabetic *—see* Diabetes, nephrosis
- neurologic neglect R41.4
- Nezelof's D81.4
- Nonne-Milroy-Meige Q82.0
- Nothnagel's vasomotor acroparesthesia I73.89
- obesity hypoventilation (OHS) E66.2
- oculomotor H51.9
- ophthalmoplegia-cerebellar ataxia *—see* Strabismus, paralytic, third nerve
- oral allergy T78.1
- oral-facial-digital Q87.0
- organic
  - affective F06.30
  - amnesic (not alcohol- or drug-induced) F04
  - brain F09
  - depressive F06.31
  - hallucinosis F06.0
  - personality F07.0
- Ormond's N13.5
- oro-facial-digital Q87.0
- os trigonum Q68.8
- Osler-Weber-Rendu I78.0
- osteoporosis-osteomalacia M83.8
- Osterreicher-Turner Q87.2
- otolith *—see* subcategory H81.8
- oto-palatal-digital Q87.0
- outlet (thoracic) G54.0
- ovary
  - polycystic E28.2
  - resistant E28.39
  - sclerocystic E28.2
- Owren's D68.2
- Paget-Schroetter I82.890
- pain *—see also* Pain
  - complex regional I G90.50
    - lower limb G90.52-
    - specified site NEC G90.59
    - upper limb G90.51-
  - complex regional II *—see* Causalgia
- painful
  - bruising D69.2
  - feet E53.8

- **Syndrome** *(continued)*
  - painful *(continued)*
    - prostate N42.81
  - paralysis agitans *—see* Parkinsonism
  - paralytic G83.9
    - specified NEC G83.89
  - Parinaud's H51.0
  - parkinsonian *—see* Parkinsonism
  - Parkinson's *—see* Parkinsonism
  - paroxysmal facial pain G50.0
  - Parry's E05.00
    - with thyroid storm E05.01
  - Parsonage (-Aldren)-Turner G54.5
  - patella clunk M25.86-
  - Paterson (-Brown) (-Kelly) D50.1
  - pectoral girdle I77.89
  - pectoralis minor I77.89
  - pediatric autoimmune neuropsychiatric disorders associated with streptococcal infections (PANDAS) D89.89
  - Pelger-Huet D72.0
  - pellagra-cerebellar ataxia-renal aminoaciduria E72.02
  - pellagroid E52
  - Pellegrini-Stieda *—see* Bursitis, tibial collateral
  - pelvic congestion-fibrosis, female N94.89
  - penta X Q97.1
  - peptic ulcer *—see* Ulcer, peptic
  - perabduction I77.89
  - periodic fever M04.1
  - periodic fever, aphthous stomatitis, pharyngitis, and adenopathy [PFAPA] M04.8
  - periodic headache, in adults and children *—see* Headache, periodic syndromes in adults and children
  - periurethral fibrosis N13.5
  - phantom limb (without pain) G54.7
    - with pain G54.6
  - pharyngeal pouch D82.1
  - Pick's *see* Disease, Pick's
  - Pickwickian E66.2
  - PIE (pulmonary infiltration with eosinophilia) J82
  - pigmentary pallidal degeneration (progressive) G23.0
  - pineal E34.8
  - pituitary E22.0
  - plantar fascia M72.2
  - placental transfusion *—see* Pregnancy, complicated by, placental transfusion syndromes
  - plateau iris (post-iridectomy) (postprocedural) H21.82
  - Plummer-Vinson D50.1
  - pluricarential of infancy E40
  - plurideficiency E40
  - pluriglandular (compensatory) E31.8
    - autoimmune E31.0
  - pneumatic hammer T75.21
  - polyangiitis overlap M30.8
  - polycarential of infancy E40
  - polyglandular E31.8
    - autoimmune E31.0
  - polysplenia Q89.09
  - pontine NEC G93.89
  - popliteal
    - artery entrapment I77.89
    - web Q87.89
  - postcardiac injury
    - postcardiotomy I97.0
    - postmyocardial infarction I24.1
  - postcardiotomy I97.0
  - post chemoembolization - code to associated conditions
  - postcholecystectomy K91.5
  - postcommissurotomy I97.0

- **Syndrome** *(continued)*
  - postconcussional F07.81
  - postcontusional F07.81
  - postencephalitic F07.89
  - posterior
    - cervical sympathetic M53.0
    - cord G83.83
    - fossa compression G93.5
    - reversible encephalopathy (PRES) I67.83
  - postgastrectomy (dumping) K91.1
  - postgastric surgery K91.1
  - postinfarction I24.1
  - postlaminectomy NEC M96.1
  - postleukotomy F07.0
  - postmastectomy lymphedema I97.2
  - postmyocardial infarction I24.1
  - postoperative NEC T81.9
    - blind loop K90.2
  - postpartum panhypopituitary (Sheehan) E23.0
  - postpolio (myelitic) G14
  - postthrombotic I87.009
    - with
      - inflammation I87.02-
        - with ulcer I87.03-
      - specified complication NEC I87.09-
      - ulcer I87.01-
        - with inflammation I87.03-
    - asymptomatic I87.00-
  - postvagotomy K91.1
  - postvalvulotomy I97.0
  - postviral NEC G93.3
    - fatigue G93.3
  - Potain's K31.0
  - potassium intoxication E87.5
  - precerebral artery (multiple) (bilateral) G45.2
  - preinfarction I20.0
  - preleukemic D46.9
  - premature senility E34.8
  - premenstrual dysphoric F32.89
  - premenstrual tension N94.3
  - Prinzmetal-Massumi R07.1
  - prune belly Q79.4
  - pseudocarpal tunnel (sublimis) *—see* Syndrome, carpal tunnel
  - pseudoparalytica G70.00
    - with exacerbation (acute) G70.01
    - in crisis G70.01
  - pseudo -Turner's Q87.1
  - psycho-organic (nonpsychotic severity) F07.9
    - acute or subacute F05
    - depressive type F06.31
    - hallucinatory type F06.0
    - nonpsychotic severity F07.0
    - specified NEC F07.89
  - pulmonary
    - arteriosclerosis I27.0
    - dysmaturity (Wilson-Mikity) P27.0
    - hypoperfusion (idiopathic) P22.0
    - renal (hemorrhagic) (Goodpasture's) M31.0
  - pure
    - motor lacunar G46.5
    - sensory lacunar G46.6
  - Putnam-Dana D51.0
  - pyogenic arthritis, pyoderma gangrenosum, and acne [PAPA] M04.8
  - pyramidopallidonigral G20
  - pyriformis *—see* Lesion, nerve, sciatic
  - QT interval prolongation I45.81
  - radicular NEC *—see* Radiculopathy
    - upper limbs, newborn (birth injury) P14.3
  - rapid time-zone change G47.25

- **Syndrome** *(continued)*
  - Rasmussen G04.81
  - Raymond (-Céstan) I65.8
  - Raynaud's I73.00
    - with gangrene I73.01
  - RDS (respiratory distress syndrome, newborn) P22.0
  - reactive airways dysfunction J68.3
  - Refsum's G60.1
  - Reifenstein E34.52
  - renal glomerulohyalinosis-diabetic *—see* Diabetes, nephrosis
  - Rendu-Osler-Weber I78.0
  - residual ovary N99.83
  - resistant ovary E28.39
  - respiratory
    - distress
      - acute J80
        - adult J80
        - child J80
        - idiopathic J84.114
      - newborn (idiopathic) (type I) P22.0
        - type II P22.1
  - restless legs G25.81
  - retinoblastoma (familial) C69.2
  - retroperitoneal fibrosis N13.5
  - retroviral seroconversion (acute) Z21
  - Reye's G93.7
  - Richter *—see* Leukemia, chronic lymphocytic, B-cell type
  - Ridley's I50.1
  - right
    - heart, hypoplastic Q22.6
    - ventricular obstruction *—see* Failure, heart, congestive
  - Romano-Ward (prolonged QT interval) I45.81
  - rotator cuff, shoulder (*see also* Tear, rotator cuff) M75.10-
  - Rotes Quérol *—see* Hyperostosis, ankylosing
  - Roth *—see* Meralgia paresthetica
  - rubella (congenital) P35.0
  - Ruvalcaba-Myhre-Smith E71.440
  - Rytand-Lipsitch I44.2
  - salt
    - depletion E87.1
      - due to heat NEC T67.8
        - causing heat exhaustion or prostration T67.4
    - low E87.1
  - salt-losing N28.89
  - Scaglietti-Dagnini E22.0
  - scalenus anticus (anterior) G54.0
  - scapulocostal *—see* Mononeuropathy, upper limb, specified site NEC
  - scapuloperoneal G71.0
  - schizophrenic, of childhood NEC F84.5
  - Schnitzler D47.2
  - Scholte's E34.0
  - Schroeder's E27.0
  - Schüller-Christian C96.5
  - Schwachman's *—see* Syndrome, Shwachman's
  - Schwartz (-Jampel) G71.13
  - Schwartz-Bartter E22.2
  - scimitar Q26.8
  - sclerocystic ovary E28.2
  - Seitelberger's G31.89
  - septicemic adrenal hemorrhage A39.1
  - seroconversion, retroviral (acute) Z21
  - serous meningitis G93.2
  - severe acute respiratory (SARS) J12.81
  - shaken infant T74.4

- **Syndrome** *(continued)*
  - shock (traumatic) T79.4
    - kidney N17.0
      - following crush injury T79.5
    - toxic A48.3
  - shock-lung J80
  - Shone's - code to specific anomalies
  - short
    - bowel K91.2
    - rib Q77.2
  - shoulder-hand *—see* Algoneurodystrophy
  - Shwachman's D70.4
  - sicca *—see* Sicca syndrome
  - sick
    - cell E87.1
    - sinus I49.5
  - sick-euthyroid E07.81
  - sideropenic D50.1
  - Siemens' ectodermal dysplasia Q82.4
  - Silfverskiöld's Q78.9
  - Simons' E88.1
  - sinus tarsi M25.57-
  - sinusitis-bronchiectasis-situs inversus Q89.3
  - Sipple's E31.22
  - sirenomelia Q87.2
  - Slocumb's E27.0
  - slow flow, coronary I20.8
  - Sluder's G44.89
  - Smith-Magenis Q93.88
  - Sneddon-Wilkinson L13.1
  - Sotos' Q87.3
  - South African cardiomyopathy I42.8
  - spasmodic
    - upward movement, eyes H51.8
    - winking F95.8
  - Spen's I45.9
  - splenic
    - agenesis Q89.01
    - flexure K59.8
    - neutropenia D73.81
  - Spurway's Q78.0
  - staphylococcal scalded skin L00
  - steal
    - arteriovenous T82.898-
    - ischemic T82.898-
    - subclavian G45.8
  - Stein-Leventhal E28.2
  - Stein's E28.2
  - Stevens-Johnson syndrome L51.1
    - toxic epidermal necrolysis overlap L51.3
  - Stewart-Morel M85.2
  - Stickler Q89.8
  - stiff baby Q89.8
  - stiff man G25.82
  - Still-Felty *—see* Felty's syndrome
  - Stokes (-Adams) I45.9
  - stone heart I50.1
  - straight back, congenital Q76.49
  - subclavian steal G45.8
  - subcoracoid-pectoralis minor G54.0
  - subcostal nerve compression I77.89
  - subphrenic interposition Q43.3
  - superior
    - cerebellar artery I63.8
    - mesenteric artery K55.1
    - semi-circular canal dehiscence H83.8X-
    - vena cava I87.1
  - supine hypotensive (maternal) *—see* Syndrome, hypotension, maternal
  - suprarenal cortical E27.0
  - supraspinatus (*see also* Tear, rotator cuff) M75.10-
  - Susac G93.49
  - swallowed blood P78.2

Syndrome *(continued)*
- sweat retention L74.0
- Swyer Q99.1
- Symond's G93.2
- sympathetic
  - cervical paralysis G90.2
  - pelvic, female N94.89
- systemic inflammatory response (SIRS), of non-infectious origin (without organ dysfunction) R65.10
  - with acute organ dysfunction R65.11
- tachycardia-bradycardia I49.5
- takotsubo I51.81
- TAR (thrombocytopenia with absent radius) Q87.2
- tarsal tunnel G57.5-
- teething K00.7
- tegmental G93.89
- telangiectasic-pigmentation-cataract Q82.8
- temporal pyramidal apex *—see* Otitis, media, suppurative, acute
- temporomandibular joint-pain-dysfunction M26.62-
- Terry's (*see also* Myopia, degenerative) H44.2-
- testicular feminization (*see also* Syndrome, androgen insensitivity) E34.51
- thalamic pain (hyperesthetic) G89.0
- thoracic outlet (compression) G54.0
- Thorson-Björck E34.0
- thrombocytopenia with absent radius (TAR) Q87.2
- thyroid-adrenocortical insufficiency E31.0
- tibial
  - anterior M76.81-
  - posterior M76.82-
- Tietze's M94.0
- time-zone (rapid) G47.25
- Toni-Fanconi E72.09
  - with cystinosis E72.04
- Touraine's Q79.8
- tourniquet *—see* Constriction, external, by site
- toxic shock A48.3
- transient left ventricular apical ballooning I51.81
- traumatic vasospastic T75.22
- Treacher Collins Q75.4
- triple X, female Q97.0
- trisomy Q92.9
  - 13 Q91.7
    - meiotic nondisjunction Q91.4
    - mitotic nondisjunction Q91.5
    - mosaicism Q91.5
    - translocation Q91.6
  - 18 Q91.3
    - meiotic nondisjunction Q91.0
    - mitotic nondisjunction Q91.1
    - mosaicism Q91.1
    - translocation Q91.2
  - 20 (q)(p) Q92.8
  - 21 Q90.9
    - meiotic nondisjunction Q90.0
    - mitotic nondisjunction Q90.1
    - mosaicism Q90.1
    - translocation Q90.2
  - 22 Q92.8
- tropical wet feet T69.0-
- Trousseau's I82.1
- tumor lysis (following antineoplastic chemotherapy) (spontaneous) NEC E88.3
- tumor necrosis factor receptor associated periodic (TRAPS) M04.1

Syndrome *(continued)*
- Twiddler's (due to)
  - automatic implantable defibrillator T82.198
  - cardiac pacemaker T82.198
- Unverricht (-Lundborg) *—see* Epilepsy, generalized, idiopathic
- upward gaze H51.8
- uremia, chronic (*see also* Disease, kidney, chronic) N18.9
- urethral N34.3
- urethro-oculo-articular *—see* Reiter's disease
- urohepatic K76.7
- vago-hypoglossal G52.7
- vascular NEC in cerebrovascular disease G46.8
- vasoconstriction, reversible cerebrovascular I67.841
- vasomotor I73.9
- vasospastic (traumatic) T75.22
- vasovagal R55
- van Buchem's M85.2
- van der Hoeve's Q78.0
- VATER Q87.2
- velo-cardio-facial Q93.81
- vena cava (inferior) (superior) (obstruction) I87.1
- vertebral
  - artery G45.0
    - compression *—see* Syndrome, anterior, spinal artery, compression
  - steal G45.0
- vertebro-basilar artery G45.0
- vertebrogenic (pain) M54.89
- vertiginous *—see* Disorder, vestibular function
- Vinson-Plummer D50.1
- virus B34.9
- visceral larva migrans B83.0
- visual disorientation H53.8
- vitamin B6 deficiency E53.1
- vitreal corneal H59.01-
- vitreous (touch) H59.01-
- Vogt-Koyanagi H20.82-
- Volkmann's T79.6
- von Schroetter's I82.890
- von Willebrand (-Jürgen) D68.0
- Waldenström-Kjellberg D50.1
- Wallenberg's G46.3
- water retention E87.79
- Waterhouse (-Friderichsen) A39.1
- Weber-Gubler G46.3
- Weber-Leyden G46.3
- Weber's G46.3
- Wegener's M31.30
  - with
    - kidney involvement M31.31
    - lung involvement M31.30
      - with kidney involvement M31.31
- Weingarten's (tropical eosinophilia) J82
- Weiss-Baker G90.09
- Werdnig-Hoffman G12.0
- Wermer's E31.21
- Werner's E34.8
- Wernicke-Korsakoff (nonalcoholic) F04
  - alcoholic F10.26
- West's *—see* Epilepsy, spasms
- Westphal-Strümpell E83.01
- wet
  - feet (maceration) (tropical) T69.0-
  - lung, newborn P22.1
- whiplash S13.4
- whistling face Q87.0
- Wilkie's K55.1
- Wilkinson-Sneddon L13.1

Syndrome *(continued)*
- Willebrand (-Jürgens) D68.0
- Wilson's (hepatolenticular degeneration) E83.01
- Wiskott-Aldrich D82.0
- withdrawal *—see* Withdrawal, state
  - drug
    - infant of dependent mother P96.1
    - therapeutic use, newborn P96.2
- Woakes' (ethmoiditis) J33.1
- Wright's (hyperabduction) G54.0
- X I20.9
- XXXX Q97.1
- XXXXX Q97.1
- XXXXY Q98.1
- XXY Q98.0
- yellow nail L60.5
- Zahorsky's B08.5
- Zellweger syndrome E71.510
- Zellweger-like syndrome E71.541

Synechia (anterior) (iris) (posterior) (pupil) *—see also* Adhesions, iris
- intra-uterine (traumatic) N85.6

Synesthesia R20.8

Syngamiasis, syngamosis B83.3

Synodontia K00.2

Synorchidism, synorchism Q55.1

Synostosis (congenital) Q78.8
- astragalo-scaphoid Q74.2
- radioulnar Q74.0

Synovial sarcoma *—see* Neoplasm, connective tissue, malignant

Synovioma (malignant) *—see also* Neoplasm, connective tissue, malignant
- benign *—see* Neoplasm, connective tissue, benign

Synoviosarcoma *—see* Neoplasm, connective tissue, malignant

Synovitis (*see also* Tenosynovitis) M65.9
- crepitant
  - hand M70.0-
  - wrist M70.03-
- gonococcal A54.49
- gouty *—see* Gout,
- in (due to)
  - crystals M65.8-
  - gonorrhea A54.49
  - syphilis (late) A52.78
  - use, overuse, pressure *—see* Disorder, soft tissue, due to use
- infective NEC *—see* Tenosynovitis, infective NEC
- specified NEC *—see* Tenosynovitis, specified type NEC
- syphilitic A52.78
  - congenital (early) A50.02
- toxic *—see* Synovitis, transient
- transient M67.3-
  - ankle M67.37-
  - elbow M67.32-
  - foot joint M67.37-
  - hand joint M67.34-
  - hip M67.35-
  - knee M67.36-
  - multiple site M67.39
  - pelvic region M67.35-
  - shoulder M67.31-
  - specified joint NEC M67.38
  - wrist M67.33-
- traumatic, current *—see* Sprain
- tuberculous *—see* Tuberculosis, synovitis
- villonodular (pigmented) M12.2-
  - ankle M12.27-

Synovitis *(continued)*
- villonodular *(continued)*
  - elbow M12.22-
  - foot joint M12.27-
  - hand joint M12.24-
  - hip M12.25-
  - knee M12.26-
  - multiple site M12.29
  - pelvic region M12.25-
  - shoulder M12.21-
  - specified joint NEC M12.28
  - vertebrae M12.28
  - wrist M12.23-

Syphilid A51.39
- congenital A50.06
- newborn A50.06
- tubercular (late) A52.79

Syphilis, syphilitic (acquired) A53.9
- abdomen (late) A52.79
- acoustic nerve A52.15
- adenopathy (secondary) A51.49
- adrenal (gland) (with cortical hypofunction) A52.79
- age under 2 years NOS *—see also* Syphilis, congenital, early
  - acquired A51.9
- alopecia (secondary) A51.32
- anemia (late) A52.79 *[D63.8]*
- aneurysm (aorta) (ruptured) A52.01
  - central nervous system A52.05
  - congenital A50.54 *[I79.0]*
- anus (late) A52.74
  - primary A51.1
  - secondary A51.39
- aorta (arch) (abdominal) (thoracic) A52.02
  - aneurysm A52.01
- aortic (insufficiency) (regurgitation) (stenosis) A52.03
  - aneurysm A52.01
- arachnoid (adhesive) (cerebral) (spinal) A52.13
- asymptomatic *—see* Syphilis, latent
- ataxia (locomotor) A52.11
- atrophoderma maculatum A51.39
- auricular fibrillation A52.06
- bladder (late) A52.76
- bone A52.77
  - secondary A51.46
- brain A52.17
- breast (late) A52.79
- bronchus (late) A52.72
- bubo (primary) A51.0
- bulbar palsy A52.19
- bursa (late) A52.78
- cardiac decompensation A52.06
- cardiovascular A52.00
- central nervous system (late) (recurrent) (relapse) (tertiary) A52.3
  - with
    - ataxia A52.11
    - general paralysis A52.17
      - juvenile A50.45
    - paresis (general) A52.17
      - juvenile A50.45
    - tabes (dorsalis) A52.11
      - juvenile A50.45
    - taboparesis A52.17
      - juvenile A50.45
  - aneurysm A52.05
  - congenital A50.40
  - juvenile A50.40
  - remission in (sustained) A52.3
  - serology doubtful, negative, or positive A52.3
  - specified nature or site NEC A52.19

Syphilis, syphilitic *(continued)*
- central nervous system *(continued)*
  - vascular A52.05
- cerebral A52.17
  - meningovascular A52.13
  - nerves (multiple palsies) A52.15
  - sclerosis A52.17
  - thrombosis A52.05
- cerebrospinal (tabetic type) A52.12
- cerebrovascular A52.05
- cervix (late) A52.76
- chancre (multiple) A51.0
  - extragenital A51.2
  - Rollet's A51.0
- Charcot's joint A52.16
- chorioretinitis A51.43
  - congenital A50.01
  - late A52.71
  - prenatal A50.01
- choroiditis *—see* Syphilitic chorioretinitis
- choroidoretinitis *—see* Syphilitic chorioretinitis
- ciliary body (secondary) A51.43
  - late A52.71
- colon (late) A52.74
- combined spinal sclerosis A52.11
- condyloma (latum) A51.31
- congenital A50.9
  - with
    - paresis (general) A50.45
    - tabes (dorsalis) A50.45
    - taboparesis A50.45
  - chorioretinitis, choroiditis A50.01 *[H32]*
  - early, or less than 2 years after birth NEC A50.2
    - with manifestations *—see* Syphilis, congenital, early, symptomatic
    - latent (without manifestations) A50.1
      - negative spinal fluid test A50.1
      - serology positive A50.1
    - symptomatic A50.09
      - cutaneous A50.06
      - mucocutaneous A50.07
      - oculopathy A50.01
      - osteochondropathy A50.02
      - pharyngitis A50.03
      - pneumonia A50.04
      - rhinitis A50.05
      - visceral A50.08
  - interstitial keratitis A50.31
  - juvenile neurosyphilis A50.45
  - late, or 2 years or more after birth NEC A50.7
    - chorioretinitis, choroiditis A50.32
    - interstitial keratitis A50.31
    - juvenile neurosyphilis A50.45
    - latent (without manifestations) A50.6
      - negative spinal fluid test A50.6
      - serology positive A50.6
    - symptomatic or with manifestations NEC A50.59
      - arthropathy A50.55
      - cardiovascular A50.54
      - Clutton's joints A50.51
      - Hutchinson's teeth A50.52
      - Hutchinson's triad A50.53
      - osteochondropathy A50.56
      - saddle nose A50.57
- conjugal A53.9
  - tabes A52.11
- conjunctiva (late) A52.71
- contact Z20.2

Syphilis, syphilitic *(continued)*
- cord bladder A52.19
- cornea, late A52.71
- coronary (artery) (sclerosis) A52.06
- coryza, congenital A50.05
- cranial nerve A52.15
  - multiple palsies A52.15
- cutaneous *—see* Syphilis, skin
- dacryocystitis (late) A52.71
- degeneration, spinal cord A52.12
- dementia paralytica A52.17
  - juvenilis A50.45
- destruction of bone A52.77
- dilatation, aorta A52.01
- due to blood transfusion A53.9
- dura mater A52.13
- ear A52.79
  - inner A52.79
    - nerve (eighth) A52.15
    - neurorecurrence A52.15
- early A51.9
  - cardiovascular A52.00
  - central nervous system A52.3
  - latent (without manifestations) (less than 2 years after infection) A51.5
    - negative spinal fluid test A51.5
    - serological relapse after treatment A51.5
    - serology positive A51.5
  - relapse (treated, untreated) A51.9
  - skin A51.39
  - symptomatic A51.9
    - extragenital chancre A51.2
    - primary, except extragenital chancre A51.0
    - secondary (*see also* Syphilis, secondary) A51.39
      - relapse (treated, untreated) A51.49
  - ulcer A51.39
- eighth nerve (neuritis) A52.15
- endemic A65
- endocarditis A52.03
  - aortic A52.03
  - pulmonary A52.03
- epididymis (late) A52.76
- epiglottis (late) A52.73
- epiphysitis (congenital) (early) A50.02
- episcleritis (late) A52.71
- esophagus A52.79
- eustachian tube A52.73
- exposure to Z20.2
- eye A52.71
- eyelid (late) (with gumma) A52.71
- fallopian tube (late) A52.76
- fracture A52.77
- gallbladder (late) A52.74
- gastric (polyposis) (late) A52.74
- general A53.9
  - paralysis A52.17
    - juvenile A50.45
- genital (primary) A51.0
- glaucoma A52.71
- gumma NEC A52.79
  - cardiovascular system A52.00
  - central nervous system A52.3
  - congenital A50.59
- heart (block) (decompensation) (disease) (failure) A52.06 *[I52]*
  - valve NEC A52.03
- hemianesthesia A52.19
- hemianopsia A52.71
- hemiparesis A52.17
- hemiplegia A52.17
- hepatic artery A52.09
- hepatis A52.74
- hepatomegaly, congenital A50.08

Syphilis, syphilitic *(continued)*
- hereditaria tarda *—see* Syphilis, congenital, late
- hereditary *—see* Syphilis, congenital
- Hutchinson's teeth A50.52
- hyalitis A52.71
- inactive *—see* Syphilis, latent
- infantum *—see* Syphilis, congenital
- inherited *—see* Syphilis, congenital
- internal ear A52.79
- intestine (late) A52.74
- iris, iritis (secondary) A51.43
  - late A52.71
- joint (late) A52.77
- keratitis (congenital) (interstitial) (late) A50.31
- kidney (late) A52.75
- lacrimal passages (late) A52.71
- larynx (late) A52.73
- late A52.9
  - cardiovascular A52.00
  - central nervous system A52.3
  - kidney A52.75
  - latent or 2 years or more after infection (without manifestations) A52.8
    - negative spinal fluid test A52.8
    - serology positive A52.8
  - paresis A52.17
  - specified site NEC A52.79
  - symptomatic or with manifestations A52.79
  - tabes A52.11
- latent A53.0
  - with signs or symptoms - code by site and stage under Syphilis
  - central nervous system A52.2
  - date of infection unspecified A53.0
  - early, or less than 2 years after infection A51.5
  - follow-up of latent syphilis A53.0
    - date of infection unspecified A53.0
    - late, or 2 years or more after infection A52.8
  - late, or 2 years or more after infection A52.8
  - positive serology (only finding) A53.0
    - date of infection unspecified A53.0
    - early, or less than 2 years after infection A51.5
    - late, or 2 years or more after infection A52.8
- lens (late) A52.71
- leukoderma A51.39
  - late A52.79
- lienitis A52.79
- lip A51.39
  - chancre (primary) A51.2
  - late A52.79
- Lissauer's paralysis A52.17
- liver A52.74
- locomotor ataxia A52.11
- lung A52.72
- lymph gland (early) (secondary) A51.49
  - late A52.79
- lymphadenitis (secondary) A51.49
- macular atrophy of skin A51.39
  - striated A52.79
- mediastinum (late) A52.73
- meninges (adhesive) (brain) (spinal cord) A52.13
- meningitis A52.13
  - acute (secondary) A51.41
  - congenital A50.41
- meningoencephalitis A52.14

Syphilis, syphilitic *(continued)*
- meningovascular A52.13
  - congenital A50.41
- mesarteritis A52.09
  - brain A52.04
- middle ear A52.77
- mitral stenosis A52.03
- monoplegia A52.17
- mouth (secondary) A51.39
  - late A52.79
- mucocutaneous (secondary) A51.39
  - late A52.79
- mucous
  - membrane (secondary) A51.39
    - late A52.79
  - patches A51.39
    - congenital A50.07
- mulberry molars A50.52
- muscle A52.78
- myocardium A52.06
- nasal sinus (late) A52.73
- neonatorum *—see* Syphilis, congenital
- nephrotic syndrome (secondary) A51.44
- nerve palsy (any cranial nerve) A52.15
  - multiple A52.15
- nervous system, central A52.3
- neuritis A52.15
  - acoustic A52.15
- neurorecidive of retina A52.19
- neuroretinitis A52.19
- newborn *—see* Syphilis, congenital
- nodular superficial (late) A52.79
- nonvenereal A65
- nose (late) A52.73
  - saddle back deformity A50.57
- occlusive arterial disease A52.09
- oculopathy A52.71
- ophthalmic (late) A52.71
- optic nerve (atrophy) (neuritis) (papilla) A52.15
- orbit (late) A52.71
- organic A53.9
- osseous (late) A52.77
- osteochondritis (congenital) (early) A50.02 *[M90.80]*
- osteoporosis A52.77
- ovary (late) A52.76
- oviduct (late) A52.76
- palate (late) A52.79
- pancreas (late) A52.74
- paralysis A52.17
  - general A52.17
    - juvenile A50.45
- paresis (general) A52.17
  - juvenile A50.45
- paresthesia A52.19
- Parkinson's disease or syndrome A52.19
- paroxysmal tachycardia A52.06
- pemphigus (congenital) A50.06
- penis (chancre) A51.0
  - late A52.76
- pericardium A52.06
- perichondritis, larynx (late) A52.73
- periosteum (late) A52.77
  - congenital (early) A50.02 *[M90.80]*
  - early (secondary) A51.46
- peripheral nerve A52.79
- petrous bone (late) A52.77
- pharynx (late) A52.73
  - secondary A51.39
- pituitary (gland) A52.79
- pleura (late) A52.73
- pneumonia, white A50.04
- pontine lesion A52.17
- portal vein A52.09

Syphilis, syphilitic *(continued)*
- primary A51.0
  - anal A51.1
  - and secondary *—see* Syphilis, secondary
  - central nervous system A52.3
  - extragenital chancre NEC A51.2
  - fingers A51.2
  - genital A51.0
  - lip A51.2
  - specified site NEC A51.2
  - tonsils A51.2
- prostate (late) A52.76
- ptosis (eyelid) A52.71
- pulmonary (late) A52.72
  - artery A52.09
- pyelonephritis (late) A52.75
- recently acquired, symptomatic A51.9
- rectum (late) A52.74
- respiratory tract (late) A52.73
- retina, late A52.71
- retrobulbar neuritis A52.15
- salpingitis A52.76
- sclera (late) A52.71
- sclerosis
  - cerebral A52.17
  - coronary A52.06
  - multiple A52.11
- scotoma (central) A52.71
- scrotum (late) A52.76
- secondary (and primary) A51.49
  - adenopathy A51.49
  - anus A51.39
  - bone A51.46
  - chorioretinitis, choroiditis A51.43
  - hepatitis A51.45
  - liver A51.45
  - lymphadenitis A51.49
  - meningitis (acute) A51.41
  - mouth A51.39
  - mucous membranes A51.39
  - periosteum, periostitis A51.46
  - pharynx A51.39
  - relapse (treated, untreated) A51.49
  - skin A51.39
  - specified form NEC A51.49
  - tonsil A51.39
  - ulcer A51.39
  - viscera NEC A51.49
  - vulva A51.39
- seminal vesicle (late) A52.76
- seronegative with signs or symptoms - code by site and stage under Syphilis
- seropositive
  - with signs or symptoms - code by site and stage under Syphilis
  - follow-up of latent syphilis *—see* Syphilis, latent
  - only finding *—see* Syphilis, latent
- seventh nerve (paralysis) A52.15
- sinus, sinusitis (late) A52.73
- skeletal system A52.77
- skin (with ulceration) (early) (secondary) A51.39
  - late or tertiary A52.79
- small intestine A52.74
- spastic spinal paralysis A52.17
- spermatic cord (late) A52.76
- spinal (cord) A52.12
- spleen A52.79
- splenomegaly A52.79
- spondylitis A52.77
- staphyloma A52.71
- stigmata (congenital) A50.59
- stomach A52.74
- synovium A52.78
- tabes dorsalis (late) A52.11

Syphilis, syphilitic *(continued)*
- tabes dorsalis *(continued)*
  - juvenile A50.45
- tabetic type A52.11
  - juvenile A50.45
- taboparesis A52.17
  - juvenile A50.45
- tachycardia A52.06
- tendon (late) A52.78
- tertiary A52.9
  - with symptoms NEC A52.79
  - cardiovascular A52.00
  - central nervous system A52.3
  - multiple NEC A52.79
  - specified site NEC A52.79
- testis A52.76
- thorax A52.73
- throat A52.73
- thymus (gland) (late) A52.79
- thyroid (late) A52.79
- tongue (late) A52.79
- tonsil (lingual) (late) A52.73
  - primary A51.2
  - secondary A51.39
- trachea (late) A52.73
- tunica vaginalis (late) A52.76
- ulcer (any site) (early) (secondary) A51.39
  - late A52.79
  - perforating A52.79
    - foot A52.11
- urethra (late) A52.76
- urogenital (late) A52.76
- uterus (late) A52.76
- uveal tract (secondary) A51.43
  - late A52.71
- uveitis (secondary) A51.43
  - late A52.71
- uvula (late) (perforated) A52.79
- vagina A51.0
  - late A52.76
- valvulitis NEC A52.03
- vascular A52.00
  - brain (cerebral) A52.05
- ventriculi A52.74
- vesicae urinariae (late) A52.76
- viscera (abdominal) (late) A52.74
  - secondary A51.49
- vitreous (opacities) (late) A52.71
  - hemorrhage A52.71
- vulva A51.0
  - late A52.76
  - secondary A51.39

Syphiloma A52.79
- cardiovascular system A52.00
- central nervous system A52.3
- circulatory system A52.00
- congenital A50.59

Syphilophobia F45.29

Syringadenoma *—see also* Neoplasm, skin, benign
- papillary *—see* Neoplasm, skin, benign

Syringobulbia G95.0

Syringocystadenoma *—see* Neoplasm, skin, benign
- papillary *—see* Neoplasm, skin, benign

Syringoma *—see also* Neoplasm, skin, benign
- chondroid *—see* Neoplasm, skin, benign

Syringomyelia G95.0

Syringomyelitis *—see* Encephalitis

Syringomyelocele *—see* Spina bifida

Syringopontia G95.0

System, systemic *—see also* condition
- disease, combined *—see* Degeneration, combined
- inflammatory response syndrome (SIRS) of non-infectious origin (without organ dysfunction) R65.10
  - with acute organ dysfunction R65.11
- lupus erythematosus M32.9
  - inhibitor present D68.62

T

Tabacism, tabacosis, tabagism *—see also* Poisoning, tobacco
- meaning dependence (without remission) F17.200
  - with
    - disorder F17.299
      - in remission F17.211
      - specified disorder NEC F17.298
      - withdrawal F17.203

Tabardillo A75.9
- flea-borne A75.2
- louse-borne A75.0

Tabes, tabetic A52.10
- with
  - central nervous system syphilis A52.10
  - Charcot's joint A52.16
  - cord bladder A52.19
  - crisis, viscera (any) A52.19
  - paralysis, general A52.17
  - paresis (general) A52.17
  - perforating ulcer (foot) A52.19
- arthropathy (Charcot) A52.16
- bladder A52.19
- bone A52.11
- cerebrospinal A52.12
- congenital A50.45
- conjugal A52.10
- dorsalis A52.11
  - juvenile A50.49
- juvenile A50.49
- latent A52.19
- mesenterica A18.39
- paralysis, insane, general A52.17
- spasmodic A52.17
- syphilis (cerebrospinal) A52.12

Taboparalysis A52.17

Taboparesis (remission) A52.17
- juvenile A50.45

TAC (trigeminal autonomic cephalgia) **NEC** G44.099
- intractable G44.091
- not intractable G44.099

Tache noir S60.22-

Tachyalimentation K91.2

Tachyarrhythmia, tachyrhythmia *—see* Tachycardia

Tachycardia R00.0
- atrial (paroxysmal) I47.1
- auricular I47.1
- AV nodal re-entry (re-entrant) I47.1
- junctional (paroxysmal) I47.1
- newborn P29.11
- nodal (paroxysmal) I47.1
- non-paroxysmal AV nodal I45.89
- paroxysmal (sustained) (nonsustained) I47.9
  - with sinus bradycardia I49.5
  - atrial (PAT) I47.1
  - atrioventricular (AV) (re-entrant) I47.1
    - psychogenic F54
  - junctional I47.1

Tachycardia *(continued)*
- paroxysmal *(continued)*
  - junctional *(continued)*
    - ectopic I47.1
  - nodal I47.1
  - psychogenic (atrial) (supraventricular) (ventricular) F54
  - supraventricular (sustained) I47.1
    - psychogenic F54
  - ventricular I47.2
    - psychogenic F54
- psychogenic F45.8
- sick sinus I49.5
- sinoauricular NOS R00.0
  - paroxysmal I47.1
- sinus [sinusal] NOS R00.0
  - paroxysmal I47.1
- supraventricular I47.1
- ventricular (paroxysmal) (sustained) I47.2
  - psychogenic F54

Tachygastria K31.89

Tachypnea R06.82
- hysterical F45.8
- newborn (idiopathic) (transitory) P22.1
- psychogenic F45.8
- transitory, of newborn P22.1

Taenia (infection) (infestation) B68.9
- diminuta B71.0
- echinococcal infestation B67.90
- mediocanellata B68.1
- nana B71.0
- saginata B68.1
- solium (intestinal form) B68.0
  - larval form *—see* Cysticercosis

Taeniasis (intestine) *—see* Taenia

TACO (transfusion associated circulatory overload) E87.71

Tag (hypertrophied skin) (infected) L91.8
- adenoid J35.8
- anus K64.4
- hemorrhoidal K64.4
- hymen N89.8
- perineal N90.89
- preauricular Q17.0
- sentinel K64.4
- skin L91.8
  - accessory (congenital) Q82.8
  - anus K64.4
  - congenital Q82.8
  - preauricular Q17.0
- tonsil J35.8
- urethra, urethral N36.8
- vulva N90.89

Tahyna fever B33.8

Takahara's disease E80.3

Takayasu's disease or syndrome M31.4

Talcosis (pulmonary) J62.0

Talipes (congenital) Q66.89
- acquired, planus *—see* Deformity, limb, flat foot
- asymmetric Q66.89
- calcaneovalgus Q66.4
- calcaneovarus Q66.1
- calcaneus Q66.89
- cavus Q66.7
- equinovalgus Q66.6
- equinovarus Q66.0
- equinus Q66.89
- percavus Q66.7

Talipes *(continued)*
- planovalgus Q66.6
- planus (acquired) (any degree) —*see also* Deformity, limb, flat foot
  - congenital Q66.5-
  - due to rickets (sequelae) E64.3
- valgus Q66.6
- varus Q66.3

Tall stature, constitutional E34.4

Talma's disease M62.89

Talon noir S90.3-
- hand S60.22-
- heel S90.3-
- toe S90.1-

Tamponade, heart I31.4

Tanapox (virus disease) B08.71

Tangier disease E78.6

Tantrum, child problem F91.8

Tapeworm (infection) (infestation) —*see* Infestation, tapeworm

Tapia's syndrome G52.7

TAR (thrombocytopenia with absent radius) **syndrome** Q87.2

Tarral-Besnier disease L44.0

Tarsal tunnel syndrome —*see* Syndrome, tarsal tunnel

Tarsalgia —*see* Pain, limb, lower

Tarsitis (eyelid) H01.8
- syphilitic A52.71
- tuberculous A18.4

Tartar (teeth) (dental calculus) K03.6

Tattoo (mark) L81.8

Tauri's disease E74.09

Taurodontism K00.2

Taussig-Bing syndrome Q20.1

Taybi's syndrome Q87.2

Tay-Sachs amaurotic familial idiocy or disease E75.02

TBI (traumatic brain injury) S06.9

Teacher's node or nodule J38.2

Tear, torn (traumatic) —*see also* Laceration
- with abortion —*see* Abortion
- annular fibrosis M51.35
- anus, anal (sphincter) S31.831
  - complicating delivery
    - with third degree perineal laceration (*see also* Delivery, complicated, by, laceration, perineum, third degree) O70.20
      - with mucosa O70.3
    - without third degree perineal laceration O70.4
  - nontraumatic (healed) (old) K62.81
- articular cartilage, old —*see* Derangement, joint, articular cartilage, by site
- bladder
  - with ectopic or molar pregnancy O08.6
  - following ectopic or molar pregnancy O08.6
  - obstetrical O71.5
  - traumatic —*see* Injury, bladder
- bowel
  - with ectopic or molar pregnancy O08.6
  - following ectopic or molar pregnancy O08.6
  - obstetrical trauma O71.5

Tear, torn *(continued)*
- broad ligament
  - with ectopic or molar pregnancy O08.6
- broad ligament
  - following ectopic or molar pregnancy O08.6
  - obstetrical trauma O71.6
- bucket handle (knee) (meniscus) —*see* Tear, meniscus
- capsule, joint —*see* Sprain
- cartilage —*see also* Sprain
  - articular, old —*see* Derangement, joint, articular cartilage, by site
- cervix
  - with ectopic or molar pregnancy O08.6
  - following ectopic or molar pregnancy O08.6
  - obstetrical trauma (current) O71.3
  - old N88.1
  - traumatic —*see* Injury, uterus
- dural G97.41
  - nontraumatic G96.11
- internal organ —*see* Injury, by site
- knee cartilage
  - articular (current) S83.3-
  - old —*see* Derangement, knee, meniscus, due to old tear
- ligament —*see* Sprain
- meniscus (knee) (current injury) S83.209
  - bucket-handle S83.20-
  - lateral
    - bucket-handle S83.25-
    - complex S83.27-
    - peripheral S83.26-
    - specified type NEC S83.28-
  - medial
    - bucket-handle S83.21-
    - complex S83.23-
    - peripheral S83.22-
    - specified type NEC S83.24-
  - old —*see* Derangement, knee, meniscus, due to old tear
  - site other than knee - code as Sprain
  - specified type NEC S83.20-
- muscle —*see* Strain
- pelvic
  - floor, complicating delivery O70.1
  - organ NEC, obstetrical trauma O71.5
    - with ectopic or molar pregnancy O08.6
    - following ectopic or molar pregnancy O08.6
- perineal, secondary O90.1
- periurethral tissue, obstetrical trauma O71.82
  - with ectopic or molar pregnancy O08.6
  - following ectopic or molar pregnancy O08.6
- rectovaginal septum —*see* Laceration, vagina
- retina, retinal (without detachment) (horseshoe) —*see also* Break, retina, horseshoe
  - with detachment —*see* Detachment, retina, with retinal, break
- rotator cuff (nontraumatic) M75.10-
  - complete M75.12-
  - incomplete M75.11-
  - traumatic S46.01-
    - capsule S43.42-
- semilunar cartilage, knee —*see* Tear, meniscus

Tear, torn *(continued)*
- supraspinatus (complete) (incomplete) (nontraumatic) (*see also* Tear, rotator cuff) M75.10-
- tendon —*see* Strain
- tentorial, at birth P10.4
- umbilical cord
  - complicating delivery O69.89
- urethra
  - with ectopic or molar pregnancy O08.6
  - following ectopic or molar pregnancy O08.6
  - obstetrical trauma O71.5
- uterus —*see* Injury, uterus
- vagina —*see* Laceration, vagina
- vessel, from catheter —*see* Puncture, accidental complicating surgery
- vulva, complicating delivery O70.0

Tear-stone —*see* Dacryolith

Teeth —*see also* condition
- grinding
  - psychogenic F45.8
  - sleep related G47.63

Teething (syndrome) K00.7

Telangiectasia, telangiectasis (verrucous) I78.1
- ataxic (cerebellar) (Louis-Bar) G11.3
- familial I78.0
- hemorrhagic, hereditary (congenital) (senile) I78.0
- hereditary, hemorrhagic (congenital) (senile) I78.0
- juxtafoveal H35.07-
- macular H35.07-
- macularis eruptiva perstans D47.01
- parafoveal H35.07-
- retinal (idiopathic) (juxtafoveal) (macular) (parafoveal) H35.07-
- spider I78.1

Telephone scatologia F65.89

Telescoped bowel or intestine K56.1
- congenital Q43.8

Temperature
- body, high (of unknown origin) R50.9
- cold, trauma from T69.9
  - newborn P80.0
  - specified effect NEC T69.8

Temple —*see* condition

Temporal —*see* condition

Temporomandibular joint pain-dysfunction syndrome M26.62-

Temporosphenoidal —*see* condition

Tendency
- bleeding —*see* Defect, coagulation
- suicide
  - meaning personal history of attempted suicide Z91.5
  - meaning suicidal ideation —*see* Ideation, suicidal
- to fall R29.6

Tenderness, abdominal R10.819
- epigastric R10.816
- generalized R10.817
- left lower quadrant R10.814
- left upper quadrant R10.812
- periumbilic R10.815
- right lower quadrant R10.813
- right upper quadrant R10.811
- rebound R10.829
  - epigastric R10.826
  - generalized R10.827
  - left lower quadrant R10.824
  - left upper quadrant R10.822
  - periumbilic R10.825

Tenderness, abdominal *(continued)*
- rebound *(continued)*
  - right lower quadrant R10.823
  - right upper quadrant R10.821

Tendinitis, tendonitis —*see also* Enthesopathy
- Achilles M76.6-
- adhesive —*see* Tenosynovitis, specified type NEC
  - shoulder —*see* Capsulitis, adhesive
- bicipital M75.2-
- calcific M65.2-
  - ankle M65.27-
  - foot M65.27-
  - forearm M65.23-
  - hand M65.24-
  - lower leg M65.26-
  - multiple sites M65.29
  - pelvic region M65.25-
  - shoulder M75.3-
  - specified site NEC M65.28
  - thigh M65.25-
  - upper arm M65.22-
- due to use, overuse, pressure —*see also* Disorder, soft tissue, due to use
  - specified NEC —*see* Disorder, soft tissue, due to use, specified NEC
- gluteal M76.0-
- patellar M76.5-
- peroneal M76.7-
- psoas M76.1-
- tibial (posterior) M76.82-
  - anterior M76.81-
- trochanteric —*see* Bursitis, hip, trochanteric

Tendon —*see* condition

Tendosynovitis —*see* Tenosynovitis

Tenesmus (rectal) R19.8
- vesical R30.1

Tennis elbow —*see* Epicondylitis, lateral

Tenonitis —*see also* Tenosynovitis
- eye (capsule) H05.04-

Tenontosynovitis —*see* Tenosynovitis

Tenontothecitis —*see* Tenosynovitis

Tenophyte —*see* Disorder, synovium, specified type NEC

Tenosynovitis (*see also* Synovitis) M65.9
- adhesive —*see* Tenosynovitis, specified type NEC
  - shoulder —*see* Capsulitis, adhesive
- bicipital (calcifying) —*see* Tendinitis, bicipital
- gonococcal A54.49
- in (due to)
  - crystals M65.8-
  - gonorrhea A54.49
  - syphilis (late) A52.78
  - use, overuse, pressure —*see also* Disorder, soft tissue, due to use
    - specified NEC —*see* Disorder, soft tissue, due to use, specified NEC
- infective NEC M65.1-
  - ankle M65.17-
  - foot M65.17-
  - forearm M65.13-
  - hand M65.14-
  - lower leg M65.16-
  - multiple sites M65.19
  - pelvic region M65.15-
  - shoulder region M65.11-

Tenosynovitis *(continued)*
infective *(continued)*
specified site NEC M65.18
thigh M65.15-
upper arm M65.12-
radial styloid M65.4
shoulder region M65.81-
adhesive *—see* Capsulitis, adhesive
specified type NEC M65.88
ankle M65.87-
foot M65.87-
forearm M65.83-
hand M65.84-
lower leg M65.86-
multiple sites M65.89
pelvic region M65.85-
shoulder region M65.81-
specified site NEC M65.88
thigh M65.85-
upper arm M65.82-
tuberculous *—see* Tuberculosis, tenosynovitis

Tenovaginitis *—see* Tenosynovitis

Tension
arterial, high *—see also* Hypertension
without diagnosis of hypertension R03.0
headache G44.209
intractable G44.201
not intractable G44.209
nervous R45.0
pneumothorax J93.0
premenstrual N94.3
state (mental) F48.9

Tentorium *—see* condition

Teratencephalus Q89.8

Teratism Q89.7

Teratoblastoma (malignant) *—see* Neoplasm, malignant, by site

Teratocarcinoma *—see also* Neoplasm, malignant, by site
liver C22.7

Teratoma (solid) *—see also* Neoplasm, uncertain behavior, by site
with embryonal carcinoma, mixed *—see* Neoplasm, malignant, by site
with malignant transformation *—see* Neoplasm, malignant, by site
adult (cystic) *—see* Neoplasm, benign, by site
benign *—see* Neoplasm, benign, by site
combined with choriocarcinoma *—see* Neoplasm, malignant, by site
cystic (adult) *—see* Neoplasm, benign, by site
differentiated *—see* Neoplasm, benign, by site
embryonal *—see also* Neoplasm, malignant, by site
liver C22.7
immature *—see* Neoplasm, malignant, by site
liver C22.7
adult, benign, cystic, differentiated type or mature D13.4
malignant *—see also* Neoplasm, malignant, by site
anaplastic *—see* Neoplasm, malignant, by site
intermediate *—see* Neoplasm, malignant, by site
specified site *—see* Neoplasm, malignant, by site

Teratoma *(continued)*
malignant *(continued)*
intermediate *(continued)*
unspecified site C62.90
undifferentiated *—see* Neoplasm, malignant, by site
mature *—see* Neoplasm, uncertain behavior, by site
malignant *—see* Neoplasm, by site, malignant, by site
ovary D27.-
embryonal, immature or malignant C56-
solid *—see* Neoplasm, uncertain behavior, by site
testis C62.9-
adult, benign, cystic, differentiated type or mature D29.2-
scrotal C62.1-
undescended C62.0-

Termination
anomalous *—see also* Malposition, congenital
right pulmonary vein Q26.3
pregnancy, elective Z33.2

Ternidens diminutus infestation B81.8

Ternidensiasis B81.8

Terror(s) **night** (child) F51.4

Terrorism, victim of Z65.4

Terry's syndrome (*see also* Myopia, degenerative) H44.2-

Tertiary *—see* condition

Test, tests, testing (for)
adequacy (for dialysis)
hemodialysis Z49.31
peritoneal Z49.32
blood pressure Z01.30
abnormal reading *—see* Blood, pressure
blood-alcohol Z04.8
positive *—see* Findings, abnormal, in blood
blood-drug Z04.8
positive *—see* Findings, abnormal, in blood
blood typing Z01.83
Rh typing Z01.83
cardiac pulse generator (battery) Z45.010
fertility Z31.41
genetic
disease carrier status for procreative management
female Z31.430
male Z31.440
male partner of patient with recurrent pregnancy loss Z31.441
procreative management NEC
female Z31.438
male Z31.448
hearing Z01.10
with abnormal findings NEC Z01.118
HIV (human immunodeficiency virus)
nonconclusive (in infants) R75
positive Z21
seropositive Z21
immunity status Z01.84
intelligence NEC Z01.89
laboratory (as part of a general medical examination) Z00.00
with abnormal finding Z00.01
for medicolegal reason NEC Z04.8

Test, tests, testing *(continued)*
male partner of patient with recurrent pregnancy loss Z31.441
Mantoux (for tuberculosis) Z11.1
abnormal result R76.11
pregnancy, positive first pregnancy *—see* Pregnancy, normal, first
procreative Z31.49
fertility Z31.41
skin, diagnostic
allergy Z01.82
special screening examination *—see* Screening, by name of disease
Mantoux Z11.1
tuberculin Z11.1
specified NEC Z01.89
tuberculin Z11.1
abnormal result R76.11
vision Z01.00
with abnormal findings Z01.01
Wassermann Z11.3
positive *—see* Serology for syphilis, positive

Testicle, testicular, testis *—see also* condition
feminization syndrome (*see also* Syndrome, androgen insensitivity) E34.51
migrans Q55.29

Tetanus, tetanic (cephalic) (convulsions) A35
with
abortion A34
ectopic or molar pregnancy O08.0
following ectopic or molar pregnancy O08.0
inoculation reaction (due to serum) *—see* Complications, vaccination
neonatorum A33
obstetrical A34
puerperal, postpartum, childbirth A34

Tetany (due to) R29.0
alkalosis E87.3
associated with rickets E55.0
convulsions R29.0
hysterical F44.5
functional (hysterical) F44.5
hyperkinetic R29.0
hysterical F44.5
hyperpnea R06.4
hysterical F44.5
psychogenic F45.8
hyperventilation (*see also* Hyperventilation) R06.4
hysterical F44.5
neonatal (without calcium or magnesium deficiency) P71.3
parathyroid (gland) E20.9
parathyroprival E89.2
post- (para)thyroidectomy E89.2
postoperative E89.2
pseudotetany R29.0
psychogenic (conversion reaction) F44.5

Tetralogy of Fallot Q21.3

Tetraplegia (chronic) (*see also* Quadriplegia) G82.50

Thailand hemorrhagic fever A91

Thalassanemia *—see* Thalassemia

Thalassemia (anemia) (disease) D56.9
with other hemoglobinopathy D56.8
alpha (major) (severe) (triple gene defect) D56.0
minor D56.3
silent carrier D56.3
trait D56.3

Thalassemia *(continued)*
beta (severe) D56.1
homozygous D56.1
major D56.1
minor D56.3
trait D56.3
delta-beta (homozygous) D56.2
minor D56.3
trait D56.3
dominant D56.8
hemoglobin
C D56.8
E-beta D56.5
intermedia D56.1
major D56.1
minor D56.3
mixed D56.8
sickle-cell *—see* Disease, sickle-cell, thalassemia
specified type NEC D56.8
trait D56.3
variants D56.8

Thanatophoric dwarfism or short stature Q77.1

Thaysen-Gee disease (nontropical sprue) K90.0

Thaysen's disease K90.0

Thecoma D27-
luteinized D27-
malignant C56-

Thelarche, premature E30.8

Thelaziasis B83.8

Thelitis N61.0
puerperal, postpartum or gestational *—see* Infection, nipple

Therapeutic *—see* condition

Therapy
drug, long-term (current) (prophylactic)
agents affecting estrogen receptors and estrogen levels NEC Z79.818
anastrozole (Arimidex) Z79.811
antibiotics Z79.2
short-term use - omit code
anticoagulants Z79.01
anti-inflammatory Z79.1
antiplatelet Z79.02
antithrombotics Z79.02
aromatase inhibitors Z79.811
aspirin Z79.82
birth control pill or patch Z79.3
bisphosphonates Z79.83
contraceptive, oral Z79.3
drug, specified NEC Z79.899
estrogen receptor downregulators Z79.818
Evista Z79.810
exemestane (Aromasin) Z79.811
Fareston Z79.810
fulvestrant (Faslodex) Z79.818
gonadotropin-releasing hormone (GnRH) agonist Z79.818
goserelin acetate (Zoladex) Z79.818
hormone replacement Z79.890
insulin Z79.4
letrozole (Femara) Z79.811
leuprolide acetate (leuprorelin) (Lupron) Z79.818
megestrol acetate (Megace) Z79.818
methadone
for pain management Z79.891
maintenance therapy F11.20
Nolvadex Z79.810
opiate analgesic Z79.891

Therapy *(continued)*
- drug, long-term *(continued)*
  - oral contraceptive Z79.3
  - raloxifene (Evista) Z79.810
  - selective estrogen receptor modulators (SERMs) Z79.810
  - short term - omit code
  - steroids
    - inhaled Z79.51
    - systemic Z79.52
  - tamoxifen (Nolvadex) Z79.810
  - toremifene (Fareston) Z79.810

Thermic *—see* condition

Thermography (abnormal) (*see also* Abnormal, diagnostic imaging) R93.8
- breast R92.8

Thermoplegia T67.0

Thesaurismosis, glycogen *—see* Disease, glycogen storage

Thiamin deficiency E51.9
- specified NEC E51.8

Thiaminic deficiency with beriberi E51.11

Thibierge-Weissenbach syndrome *—see* Sclerosis, systemic

Thickening
- bone *—see* Hypertrophy, bone
- breast N64.59
- endometrium R93.8
- epidermal L85.9
  - specified NEC L85.8
- hymen N89.6
- larynx J38.7
- nail L60.2
  - congenital Q84.5
- periosteal *—see* Hypertrophy, bone
- pleura J92.9
  - with asbestos J92.0
- skin R23.4
- subepiglottic J38.7
- tongue K14.8
- valve, heart *—see* Endocarditis

Thigh *—see* condition

Thinning vertebra *—see* Spondylopathy, specified NEC

Thirst, excessive R63.1
- due to deprivation of water T73.1

Thomsen disease G71.12

Thoracic *—see also* condition
- kidney Q63.2
- outlet syndrome G54.0

Thoracogastroschisis (congenital) Q79.8

Thoracopagus Q89.4

Thorax *—see* condition

Thorn's syndrome N28.89

Thorson-Björck syndrome E34.0

Threadworm (infection) (infestation) B80

Threatened
- abortion O20.0
  - with subsequent abortion O03.9
- job loss, anxiety concerning Z56.2
- labor (without delivery) O47.9
  - at or after 37 completed weeks of gestation O47.1
  - before 37 completed weeks of gestation O47.0-
- loss of job, anxiety concerning Z56.2
- miscarriage O20.0
- unemployment, anxiety concerning Z56.2

Three-day fever A93.1

Threshers' lung J67.0

Thrix annulata (congenital) Q84.1

Throat *—see* condition

Thrombasthenia (Glanzmann) (hemorrhagic) (hereditary) D69.1

Thromboangiitis I73.1
- obliterans (general) I73.1
  - cerebral I67.89
  - vessels
    - brain I67.89
    - spinal cord I67.89

Thromboarteritis *—see* Arteritis

Thromboasthenia (Glanzmann) (hemorrhagic) (hereditary) D69.1

Thrombocytasthenia (Glanzmann) D69.1

Thrombocythemia (essential) (hemorrhagic) (idiopathic) (primary) D47.3

Thrombocytopathy (dystrophic) (granulopenic) D69.1

Thrombocytopenia, thrombocytopenic D69.6
- with absent radius (TAR) Q87.2
- congenital D69.42
- dilutional D69.59
- due to
  - drugs D69.59
  - extracorporeal circulation of blood D69.59
  - (massive) blood transfusion D69.59
  - platelet alloimmunization D69.59
- essential D69.3
- heparin induced (HIT) D75.82
- hereditary D69.42
- idiopathic D69.3
- neonatal, transitory P61.0
  - due to
    - exchange transfusion P61.0
    - idiopathic maternal thrombocytopenia P61.0
    - isoimmunization P61.0
- primary NEC D69.49
  - idiopathic D69.3
- puerperal, postpartum O72.3
- secondary D69.59
- transient neonatal P61.0

Thrombocytosis, essential D47.3
- primary D47.3

Thromboembolism *—see* Embolism

Thrombopathy (Bernard-Soulier) D69.1
- constitutional D68.0
- Willebrand-Jurgens D68.0

Thrombopenia *—see* Thrombocytopenia

Thrombophilia D68.59
- primary NEC D68.59
- secondary NEC D68.69
- specified NEC D68.69

Thrombophlebitis I80.9
- antepartum O22.2-
  - deep O22.3-
  - superficial O22.2-
- cavernous (venous) sinus G08
  - complicating pregnancy O22.5-
  - nonpyogenic I67.6
- cerebral (sinus) (vein) G08
  - nonpyogenic I67.6
  - sequelae G09

Thrombophlebitis *(continued)*
- due to implanted device *—see* Complications, by site and type, specified NEC
- during or resulting from a procedure NEC T81.72
- femoral vein (superficial) I80.1-
- femoropopliteal vein I80.0-
- hepatic (vein) I80.8
- idiopathic, recurrent I82.1
- iliofemoral I80.1-
- intracranial venous sinus (any) G08
  - nonpyogenic I67.6
  - sequelae G09
- intraspinal venous sinuses and veins G08
  - nonpyogenic G95.19
- lateral (venous) sinus G08
  - nonpyogenic I67.6
- leg I80.3
  - superficial I80.0-
- longitudinal (venous) sinus G08
  - nonpyogenic I67.6
- lower extremity I80.299
- migrans, migrating I82.1
- pelvic
  - with ectopic or molar pregnancy O08.0
  - following ectopic or molar pregnancy O08.0
  - puerperal O87.1
- popliteal vein *—see* Phlebitis, leg, deep, popliteal
- portal (vein) K75.1
- postoperative T81.72
- pregnancy *—see* Thrombophlebitis, antepartum
- puerperal, postpartum, childbirth O87.0
  - deep O87.1
  - pelvic O87.1
  - septic O86.81
  - superficial O87.0
- saphenous (greater) (lesser) I80.0-
- sinus (intracranial) G08
  - nonpyogenic I67.6
- specified site NEC I80.8
- tibial vein I80.23-

Thrombosis, thrombotic (bland) (multiple) (progressive) (silent) (vessel) I82.90
- anal K64.5
- antepartum *—see* Thrombophlebitis, antepartum
- aorta, aortic I74.10
  - abdominal I74.09
    - saddle I74.01
  - bifurcation I74.09
  - saddle I74.01
  - specified site NEC I74.19
  - terminal I74.09
  - thoracic I74.11
  - valve *—see* Endocarditis, aortic
- apoplexy I63.3-
- artery, arteries (postinfectional) I74.9
  - auditory, internal *—see* Occlusion, artery, precerebral, specified NEC
  - basilar *—see* Occlusion, artery, basilar
  - carotid (common) (internal) *—see* Occlusion, artery, carotid
  - cerebellar (anterior inferior) (posterior inferior) (superior) *—see* Occlusion, artery, cerebellar
  - cerebral *—see* Occlusion, artery, cerebral
  - choroidal (anterior) *—see* Occlusion, artery, precerebral, specified NEC

Thrombosis, thrombotic *(continued)*
- artery, arteries *(continued)*
  - communicating, posterior *—see* Occlusion, artery, precerebral, specified NEC
  - coronary *—see also* Infarct, myocardium
    - not resulting in infarction I24.0
  - hepatic I74.8
  - hypophyseal *—see* Occlusion, artery, precerebral, specified NEC
  - iliac I74.5
  - limb I74.4
    - lower I74.3
    - upper I74.2
  - meningeal, anterior or posterior *—see* Occlusion, artery, cerebral, specified NEC
  - mesenteric (with gangrene) (*see also* Infarct, intestine) K55.069
  - ophthalmic *—see* Occlusion, artery, retina
  - pontine *—see* Occlusion, artery, precerebral, specified NEC
  - precerebral *—see* Occlusion, artery, precerebral
  - pulmonary (iatrogenic) *—see* Embolism, pulmonary
  - renal N28.0
  - retinal *—see* Occlusion, artery, retina
  - spinal, anterior or posterior G95.11
  - traumatic NEC T14.8
  - vertebral *—see* Occlusion, artery, vertebral
- atrium, auricular *—see also* Infarct, myocardium
  - following acute myocardial infarction (current complication) I23.6
  - not resulting in infarction I51.3
  - old I51.3
- basilar (artery) *—see* Occlusion, artery, basilar
- brain (artery) (stem) *—see also* Occlusion, artery, cerebral
  - due to syphilis A52.05
  - puerperal O99.43
  - sinus *—see* Thrombosis, intracranial venous sinus
- capillary I78.8
- cardiac *—see also* Infarct, myocardium
  - not resulting in infarction I51.3
  - old I51.3
  - valve *—see* Endocarditis
- carotid (artery) (common) (internal) *—see* Occlusion, artery, carotid
- cavernous (venous) sinus *—see* Thrombosis, intracranial venous sinus
- cerebellar artery (anterior inferior) (posterior inferior) (superior) I66.3
- cerebral (artery) *—see* Occlusion, artery, cerebral
- cerebrovenous sinus *—see also* Thrombosis, intracranial venous sinus
  - puerperium O87.3
- chronic I82.91
- coronary (artery) (vein) *—see also* Infarct, myocardium
  - not resulting in infarction I24.0
- corpus cavernosum N48.89
- cortical I66.9

Thrombosis, thrombotic *(continued)*
- deep *—see* Embolism, vein, lower extremity
- due to device, implant or graft (*see also* Complications, by site and type, specified NEC) T85.868
  - arterial graft NEC T82.868
  - breast (implant) T85.868
  - catheter NEC T85.868
    - dialysis (renal) T82.868
      - intraperitoneal T85.868
    - infusion NEC T82.868
      - spinal (epidural) (subdural) T85.860
    - urinary (indwelling) T83.86
  - electronic (electrode) (pulse generator) (stimulator)
    - bone T84.86
    - cardiac T82.867
    - nervous system (brain) (peripheral nerve) (spinal) T85.860
    - urinary T83.86
  - fixation, internal (orthopedic) NEC T84.86
  - gastrointestinal (bile duct) (esophagus) T85.868
  - genital NEC T83.86
  - heart T82.867
  - joint prosthesis T84.86
  - ocular (corneal graft) (orbital implant) NEC T85.868
  - orthopedic NEC T84.86
  - specified NEC T85.868
  - urinary NEC T83.86
  - vascular NEC T82.868
  - ventricular intracranial shunt T85.860
- during the puerperium *—see* Thrombosis, puerperal
- endocardial *—see also* Infarct, myocardium
  - not resulting in infarction I51.3
- eye *—see* Occlusion, retina
- genital organ
  - female NEC N94.89
    - pregnancy *—see* Thrombophlebitis, antepartum
  - male N50.1
- gestational *—see* Phlebopathy, gestational
- heart (chamber) *—see also* Infarct, myocardium
  - not resulting in infarction I51.3
  - old I51.3
- hepatic (vein) I82.0
  - artery I74.8
- history (of) Z86.718
- intestine (with gangrene (*see also* Infarct, intestine)) K55.069
- intracardiac NEC (apical) (atrial) (auricular) (ventricular) (old) I51.3
- intracranial (arterial) I66.9
  - venous sinus (any) G08
    - nonpyogenic origin I67.6
    - puerperium O87.3
- intramural *—see also* Infarct, myocardium
  - not resulting in infarction I51.3
  - old I51.3
- intraspinal venous sinuses and veins G08
  - nonpyogenic G95.19
- kidney (artery) N28.0
- lateral (venous) sinus *—see* Thrombosis, intracranial venous sinus

Thrombosis, thrombotic *(continued)*
- leg *—see* Thrombosis, vein, lower extremity
  - arterial I74.3
- liver (venous) I82.0
  - artery I74.8
  - portal vein I81
- longitudinal (venous) sinus *—see* Thrombosis, intracranial venous sinus
- lower limb *—see* Thrombosis, vein, lower extremity
- lung (iatrogenic) (postoperative) *—see* Embolism, pulmonary
- meninges (brain) (arterial) I66.8
- mesenteric (artery) (with gangrene) (*see also* Infarct, intestine) K55.069
  - vein (inferior) (superior) I81
- mitral I34.8
- mural *—see also* Infarct, myocardium
  - due to syphilis A52.06
  - not resulting in infarction I51.3
  - old I51.3
- omentum (with gangrene) (*see also* Infarct, intestine) K55.069
- ophthalmic *—see* Occlusion, retina
- pampiniform plexus (male) N50.1
- parietal *—see also* Infarct, myocardium
  - not resulting in infarction I24.0
- penis, superficial vein N48.81
- perianal venous K64.5
- peripheral arteries I74.4
  - upper I74.2
- personal history (of) Z86.718
- portal I81
  - due to syphilis A52.09
- precerebral artery *—see* Occlusion, artery, precerebral
- puerperal, postpartum O87.0
  - brain (artery) O99.43
    - venous (sinus) O87.3
  - cardiac O99.43
  - cerebral (artery) O99.43
    - venous (sinus) O87.3
  - superficial O87.0
- pulmonary (artery) (iatrogenic) (postoperative) (vein) *—see* Embolism, pulmonary
- renal (artery) N28.0
  - vein I82.3
- resulting from presence of device, implant or graft *—see* Complications, by site and type, specified NEC
- retina, retinal *—see* Occlusion, retina
- scrotum N50.1
- seminal vesicle N50.1
- sigmoid (venous) sinus *—see* Thrombosis, intracranial venous sinus
- sinus, intracranial (any) *—see* Thrombosis, intracranial venous sinus
- specified site NEC I82.890
  - chronic I82.891
- spermatic cord N50.1
- spinal cord (arterial) G95.11
  - due to syphilis A52.09
  - pyogenic origin G06.1
- spleen, splenic D73.5
  - artery I74.8
- testis N50.1
- tumor *—see* Neoplasm, unspecified behavior, by site
- traumatic NEC T14.8
- tricuspid I07.8
- tunica vaginalis N50.1

Thrombosis, thrombotic *(continued)*
- umbilical cord (vessels), complicating delivery O69.5
- vas deferens N50.1
- vein (acute) I82.90
  - antecubital I82.61-
    - chronic I82.71-
  - axillary I82.A1-
    - chronic I82.A2-
  - basilic I82.61-
    - chronic I82.71-
  - brachial I82.62-
    - chronic I82.72-
  - brachiocephalic (innominate) I82.290
    - chronic I82.291
  - cerebral, nonpyogenic I67.6
  - cephalic I82.61-
    - chronic I82.71-
  - chronic I82.91
  - deep (DVT) I82.40-
    - calf I82.4Z-
      - chronic I82.5Z-
    - lower leg I82.4Z-
      - chronic I82.5Z-
    - thigh I82.4Y-
      - chronic I82.5Y-
    - upper leg I82.4Y
      - chronic I82.5y--
  - femoral I82.41-
    - chronic I82.51-
  - iliac (iliofemoral) I82.42-
    - chronic I82.52-
  - innominate I82.290
    - chronic I82.291
  - internal jugular I82.C1-
    - chronic I82.C2-
  - lower extremity
    - deep I82.40-
      - chronic I82.50-
      - specified NEC I82.49-
        - chronic NEC I82.59-
    - distal
      - deep I82.4Z-
    - proximal
      - deep I82.4Y-
        - chronic I82.5Y-
    - superficial I82.81-
  - perianal K64.5
  - popliteal I82.43-
    - chronic I82.53-
  - radial I82.62-
    - chronic I82.72-
  - renal I82.3
  - saphenous (greater) (lesser) I82.81-
  - specified NEC I82.890
    - chronic NEC I82.891
  - subclavian I82.B1-
    - chronic I82.B2-
  - thoracic NEC I82.290
    - chronic I82.291
  - tibial I82.44-
    - chronic I82.54-
  - ulnar I82.62-
    - chronic I82.72-
  - upper extremity I82.60-
    - chronic I82.70-
    - deep I82.62-
      - chronic I82.72-
    - superficial I82.61-
      - chronic I82.71-
- vena cava
  - inferior I82.220
    - chronic I82.221
  - superior I82.210
    - chronic I82.211
- venous, perianal K64.5
- ventricle *—see also* Infarct, myocardium

Thrombosis, thrombotic *(continued)*
- ventricle *(continued)*
  - following acute myocardial infarction (current complication) I23.6
  - not resulting in infarction I24.0
  - old I51.3

Thrombus *—see* Thrombosis

Thrush *—see also* Candidiasis
- oral B37.0
- newborn P37.5
- vaginal B37.3

Thumb *—see also* condition
- sucking (child problem) F98.8

Thymitis E32.8

Thymoma (benign) D15.0
- malignant C37

Thymus, thymic (gland) *—see* condition

Thyrocele *—see* Goiter

Thyroglossal *—see also* condition
- cyst Q89.2
- duct, persistent Q89.2

Thyroid (gland) (body) *—see also* condition
- hormone resistance E07.89
- lingual Q89.2
- nodule (cystic) (nontoxic) (single) E04.1

Thyroiditis E06.9
- acute (nonsuppurative) (pyogenic) (suppurative) E06.0
- autoimmune E06.3
- chronic (nonspecific) (sclerosing) E06.5
  - with thyrotoxicosis, transient E06.2
  - fibrous E06.5
  - lymphadenoid E06.3
  - lymphocytic E06.3
  - lymphoid E06.3
- de Quervain's E06.1
- drug-induced E06.4
- fibrous (chronic) E06.5
- giant-cell (follicular) E06.1
- granulomatous (de Quervain) (subacute) E06.1
- Hashimoto's (struma lymphomatosa) E06.3
- iatrogenic E06.4
- ligneous E06.5
- lymphocytic (chronic) E06.3
- lymphoid E06.3
- lymphomatous E06.3
- nonsuppurative E06.1
- postpartum, puerperal O90.5
- pseudotuberculous E06.1
- pyogenic E06.0
- radiation E06.4
- Riedel's E06.5
- subacute (granulomatous) E06.1
- suppurative E06.0
- tuberculous A18.81
- viral E06.1
- woody E06.5

Thyrolingual duct, persistent Q89.2

Thyromegaly E01.0

Thyrotoxic
- crisis *—see* Thyrotoxicosis
- heart disease or failure (*see also* Thyrotoxicosis) E05.90 *[I43]*
  - with thyroid storm E05.91 *[I43]*
- storm *—see* Thyrotoxicosis

- **Thyrotoxicosis** (recurrent) E05.90
  - with
    - goiter (diffuse) E05.00
      - with thyroid storm E05.01
      - adenomatous uninodular E05.10
        - with thyroid storm E05.11
      - multinodular E05.20
        - with thyroid storm E05.21
      - nodular E05.20
        - with thyroid storm E05.21
      - uninodular E05.10
        - with thyroid storm E05.11
    - infiltrative
      - dermopathy E05.00
        - with thyroid storm E05.01
      - ophthalmopathy E05.00
        - with thyroid storm E05.01
    - single thyroid nodule E05.10
      - with thyroid storm E05.11
    - thyroid storm E05.91
  - due to
    - ectopic thyroid nodule or tissue E05.30
      - with thyroid storm E05.31
    - ingestion of (excessive) thyroid material E05.40
      - with thyroid storm E05.41
    - overproduction of thyroid-stimulating hormone E05.80
      - with thyroid storm E05.81
    - specified cause NEC E05.80
      - with thyroid storm E05.81
  - factitia E05.40
    - with thyroid storm E05.41
  - heart (*see also* Failure, heart, high-output) E05.90 *[I43]*
    - with thyroid storm (*see* also Failure, heart, high-output) E05.91 *[I43]*
    - failure (*see* also Failure, heart, high-output) E05.90 *[I43]*
  - neonatal (transient) P72.1
  - transient with chronic thyroiditis E06.2
- **Tibia vara** —*see* Osteochondrosis, juvenile, tibia
- **Tic** (disorder) F95.9
  - breathing F95.8
  - child problem F95.0
  - compulsive F95.1
  - de la Tourette F95.2
  - degenerative (generalized) (localized) G25.69
    - facial G25.69
  - disorder
    - chronic
      - motor F95.1
      - vocal F95.1
    - combined vocal and multiple motor F95.2
    - transient F95.0
  - douloureux G50.0
    - atypical G50.1
    - postherpetic, postzoster B02.22
  - drug-induced G25.61
  - eyelid F95.8
  - habit F95.9
    - chronic F95.1
    - transient of childhood F95.0
  - lid, transient of childhood F95.0
  - motor-verbal F95.2
  - occupational F48.8
  - orbicularis F95.8
    - transient of childhood F95.0
  - organic origin G25.69
  - postchoreic G25.69
  - provisional F95.0
  - psychogenic, compulsive F95.1
  - salaam R25.8

- **Tic** *(continued)*
  - spasm (motor or vocal) F95.9
    - chronic F95.1
    - transient of childhood F95.0
  - specified NEC F95.8
- **Tick-borne** —*see* condition
- **Tietze's disease or syndrome** M94.0
- **Tight, tightness**
  - anus K62.89
  - chest R07.89
  - fascia (lata) M62.89
  - foreskin (congenital) N47.1
  - hymen, hymenal ring N89.6
  - introitus (acquired) (congenital) N89.6
  - rectal sphincter K62.89
  - tendon —*see* Short, tendon
  - urethral sphincter N35.9
- **Tilting vertebra** —*see* Dorsopathy, deforming, specified NEC
- **Timidity, child** F93.8
- **Tin-miner's lung** J63.5
- **Tinea** (intersecta) (tarsi) B35.9
  - amiantacea L44.8
  - asbestina B35.0
  - barbae B35.0
  - beard B35.0
  - black dot B35.0
  - blanca B36.2
  - capitis B35.0
  - corporis B35.4
  - cruris B35.6
  - flava B36.0
  - foot B35.3
  - furfuracea B36.0
  - imbricata (Tokelau) B35.5
  - kerion B35.0
  - manuum B35.2
  - microsporic —*see* Dermatophytosis
  - nigra B36.1
  - nodosa —*see* Piedra
  - pedis B35.3
  - scalp B35.0
  - specified NEC B35.8
  - sycosis B35.0
  - tonsurans B35.0
  - trichophytic —*see* Dermatophytosis
  - unguium B35.1
  - versicolor B36.0
- **Tingling sensation** (skin) R20.2
- **Tinnitus NOS** H93.1-
  - audible H93.1-
  - aurium H93.1-
  - pulsatile H93.A-
  - subjective H93.1-
- **Tipped tooth** (teeth) M26.33
- **Tipping**
  - pelvis M95.5
    - with disproportion (fetopelvic) O33.0
      - causing obstructed labor O65.0
  - tooth (teeth), fully erupted M26.33
- **Tiredness** R53.83
- **Tissue** —*see* condition
- **Tobacco** (nicotine)
  - abuse, - *see* Tobacco, use
  - dependence —*see* Dependence, drug, nicotine
  - harmful use Z72.0
  - heart —*see* Tobacco, toxic effect
  - maternal use, affecting newborn P04.2
  - toxic effect —*see* Table of Drugs and Chemicals, by substance, poisoning

- **Tobacco** *(continued)*
  - toxic effect *(continued)*
    - chewing tobacco —*see* Table of Drugs and Chemicals, by substance, poisoning
    - cigarettes —*see* Table of Drugs and Chemicals, by substance, poisoning
  - use Z72.0
    - complicating
      - childbirth O99.334
      - pregnancy O99.33-
      - puerperium O99.335
    - counseling and surveillance Z71.6
    - history Z87.891
  - withdrawal state (*see also* Dependence, drug, nicotine) F17.203
- **Tocopherol deficiency** E56.0
- **Todd's**
  - cirrhosis K74.3
  - paralysis (postepileptic) (transitory) G83.84
- **Toe** —*see* condition
- **Toilet, artificial opening** —*see* Attention to, artificial, opening
- **Tokelau** (ringworm) B35.5
- **Tollwut** —*see* Rabies
- **Tommaselli's disease** R31.9
  - correct substance properly administered —*see* Table of Drugs and Chemicals, by drug, adverse effect
  - overdose or wrong substance given or taken —*see* Table of Drugs and Chemicals, by drug, poisoning
- **Tongue** —*see also* condition
  - tie Q38.1
- **Tonic pupil** —*see* Anomaly, pupil, function, tonic pupil
- **Toni-Fanconi syndrome** (cystinosis) E72.09
  - with cystinosis E72.04
- **Tonsil** —*see* condition
- **Tonsillitis** (acute) (catarrhal) (croupous) (follicular) (gangrenous) (infective) (lacunar) (lingual) (malignant) (membranous) (parenchymatous) (phlegmonous) (pseudomembranous) (purulent) (septic) (subacute) (suppurative) (toxic) (ulcerative) (vesicular) (viral) J03.90
  - chronic J35.01
    - with adenoiditis J35.03
  - diphtheritic A36.0
  - hypertrophic J35.01
    - with adenoiditis J35.03
  - recurrent J03.91
  - specified organism NEC J03.80
    - recurrent J03.81
  - staphylococcal J03.80
    - recurrent J03.81
  - streptococcal J03.00
    - recurrent J03.01
  - tuberculous A15.8
  - Vincent's A69.1
- **Tooth, teeth** —*see* condition
- **Toothache** K08.89
- **Topagnosis** R20.8
- **Tophi** —*see* Gout, chronic
- **TORCH infection** —*see* Infection, congenital
  - without active infection P00.2

- **Torn** —*see* Tear
- **Tornwaldt's cyst or disease** J39.2
- **Torsion**
  - accessory tube —*see* Torsion, fallopian tube
  - adnexa (female) —*see* Torsion, fallopian tube
  - aorta, acquired I77.1
  - appendix epididymis N44.04
  - appendix testis N44.03
  - bile duct (common) (hepatic) K83.8
    - congenital Q44.5
  - bowel, colon or intestine K56.2
  - cervix —*see* Malposition, uterus
  - cystic duct K82.8
  - dystonia —*see* Dystonia, torsion
  - epididymis (appendix) N44.04
  - fallopian tube N83.52-
    - with ovary N83.53
  - gallbladder K82.8
    - congenital Q44.1
  - hydatid of Morgagni
    - female N83.52-
    - male N44.03
  - kidney (pedicle) (leading to infarction) N28.0
  - Meckel's diverticulum (congenital) Q43.0
    - malignant —*see* Table of Neoplasms, small intestine, malignant
  - mesentery K56.2
  - omentum K56.2
  - organ or site, congenital NEC —*see* Anomaly, by site
  - ovary (pedicle) N83.51-
    - with fallopian tube N83.53
    - congenital Q50.2
  - oviduct —*see* Torsion, fallopian tube
  - penis (acquired) N48.82
    - congenital Q55.63
  - spasm —*see* Dystonia, torsion
  - spermatic cord N44.02
    - extravaginal N44.01
    - intravaginal N44.02
  - spleen D73.5
  - testis, testicle N44.00
    - appendix N44.03
  - tibia —*see* Deformity, limb, specified type NEC, lower leg
  - uterus —*see* Malposition, uterus
- **Torticollis** (intermittent) (spastic) M43.6
  - congenital (sternomastoid) Q68.0
  - due to birth injury P15.8
  - hysterical F44.4
  - ocular R29.891
  - psychogenic F45.8
    - conversion reaction F44.4
  - rheumatic M43.6
  - rheumatoid M06.88
  - spasmodic G24.3
  - traumatic, current S13.4
- **Tortipelvis** G24.1
- **Tortuous**
  - aortic arch Q25.46
  - artery I77.1
  - organ or site, congenital NEC —*see* Distortion
  - retinal vessel, congenital Q14.1
  - ureter N13.8
  - urethra N36.8
  - vein —*see* Varix
- **Torture, victim of** Z65.4

Torula, torular (histolytica) (infection) —*see* Cryptococcosis

Torulosis —*see* Cryptococcosis

Torus (mandibularis) (palatinus) M27.0
- fracture —*see* Fracture, by site, torus

Touraine's syndrome Q79.8

Tourette's syndrome F95.2

Tourniquet syndrome —*see* Constriction, external, by site

Tower skull Q75.0
- with exophthalmos Q87.0

Toxemia R68.89
- bacterial —*see* Sepsis
- burn —*see* Burn
- eclamptic (with pre-existing hypertension) —*see* Eclampsia
- erysipelatous —*see* Erysipelas
- fatigue R68.89
- food —*see* Poisoning, food
- gastrointestinal K52.1
- intestinal K52.1
- kidney —*see* Uremia
- malarial —*see* Malaria
- myocardial —*see* Myocarditis, toxic
- of pregnancy —*see* Pre-eclampsia
- pre-eclamptic —*see* Pre-eclampsia
- small intestine K52.1
- staphylococcal, due to food A05.0
- stasis R68.89
- uremic —*see* Uremia
- urinary —*see* Uremia

Toxemica cerebropathia psychica (nonalcoholic) F04
- alcoholic —*see* Alcohol, amnestic disorder

Toxic (poisoning) (*see also* condition) T65.91
- effect —*see* Table of Drugs and Chemicals, by substance, poisoning
- shock syndrome A48.3
- thyroid (gland) —*see* Thyrotoxicosis

Toxicemia —*see* Toxemia

Toxicity —*see* Table of Drugs and Chemicals, by substance, poisoning
- fava bean D55.0
- food, noxious —*see* Poisoning, food
- from drug or nonmedicinal substance —*see* Table of Drugs and Chemicals, by drug

Toxicosis —*see also* Toxemia
- capillary, hemorrhagic D69.0

Toxinfection, gastrointestinal K52.1

Toxocariasis B83.0

Toxoplasma, toxoplasmosis (acquired) B58.9
- with
  - hepatitis B58.1
  - meningoencephalitis B58.2
  - ocular involvement B58.00
  - other organ involvement B58.89
  - pneumonia, pneumonitis B58.3
- congenital (acute) (subacute) (chronic) P37.1
- maternal, manifest toxoplasmosis in infant (acute) (subacute) (chronic) P37.1

tPA (rtPA) **administation in a different facility within the last 24 hours prior to admission to current facility** Z92.82

Trabeculation, bladder N32.89

Trachea —*see* condition

Tracheitis (catarrhal) (infantile) (membranous) (plastic) (septal) (suppurative) (viral) J04.10
- with
  - bronchitis (15 years of age and above) J40
    - acute or subacute —*see* Bronchitis, acute
    - chronic J42
    - tuberculous NEC A15.5
    - under 15 years of age J20.9
  - laryngitis (acute) J04.2
    - chronic J37.1
    - tuberculous NEC A15.5
- acute J04.10
  - with obstruction J04.11
- chronic J42
  - with
    - bronchitis (chronic) J42
    - laryngitis (chronic) J37.1
- diphtheritic (membranous) A36.89
- due to external agent —*see* Inflammation, respiratory, upper, due to
- syphilitic A52.73
- tuberculous A15.5

Trachelitis (nonvenereal) —*see* Cervicitis

Tracheobronchial —*see* condition

Tracheobronchitis (15 years of age and above) —*see also* Bronchitis
- due to
  - Bordetella bronchiseptica A37.80
    - with pneumonia A37.81
  - Francisella tularensis A21.8

Tracheobronchomegaly Q32.4
- with bronchiectasis J47.9
  - with
    - exacerbation (acute) J47.1
    - lower respiratory infection J47.0
- acquired J98.09
  - with bronchiectasis J47.9
    - with
      - exacerbation (acute) J47.1
      - lower respiratory infection J47.0

Tracheobronchopneumonitis —*see* Pneumonia, broncho-

Tracheocele (external) (internal) J39.8
- congenital Q32.1

Tracheomalacia J39.8
- congenital Q32.0

Tracheopharyngitis (acute) J06.9
- chronic J42
- due to external agent —*see* Inflammation, respiratory, upper, due to

Tracheostenosis J39.8

Tracheostomy
- complication —*see* Complication, tracheostomy
- status Z93.0
  - attention to Z43.0
  - malfunctioning J95.03

Trachoma, trachomatous A71.9
- active (stage) A71.1
- contraction of conjunctiva A71.1
- dubium A71.0
- initial (stage) A71.0
- healed or sequelae B94.0
- pannus A71.1
- Türck's J37.0

Traction, vitreomacular H43.82-

Train sickness T75.3

Trait(s)
- Hb-S D57.3
- hemoglobin
  - abnormal NEC D58.2
    - with thalassemia D56.3
  - C —*see* Disease, hemoglobin C
  - S (Hb-S) D57.3
- Lepore D56.3
- personality, accentuated Z73.1
- sickle-cell D57.3
  - with elliptocytosis or spherocytosis D57.3
- type A personality Z73.1

Tramp Z59.0

Trance R41.89
- hysterical F44.89

Transection
- abdomen (partial) S38.3
- aorta (incomplete) —*see also* Injury, aorta
  - complete —*see* Injury, aorta, laceration, major
- carotid artery (incomplete) —*see also* Injury, blood vessel, carotid, laceration
  - complete —*see* Injury, blood vessel, carotid, laceration, major
- celiac artery (incomplete) S35.211
  - branch (incomplete) S35.291
    - complete S35.292
  - complete S35.212
- innominate
  - artery (incomplete) —*see also* Injury, blood vessel, thoracic, innominate, artery, laceration
    - complete —*see* Injury, blood vessel, thoracic, innominate, artery, laceration, major
  - vein (incomplete) —*see also* Injury, blood vessel, thoracic, innominate, vein, laceration
    - complete —*see* Injury, blood vessel, thoracic, innominate, vein, laceration, major
- jugular vein (external) (incomplete) —*see also* Injury, blood vessel, jugular vein, laceration
  - complete —*see* Injury, blood vessel, jugular vein, laceration, major
  - internal (incomplete) —*see also* Injury, blood vessel, jugular vein, internal, laceration
    - complete —*see* Injury, blood vessel, jugular vein, internal, laceration, major
- mesenteric artery (incomplete) —*see also* Injury, mesenteric, artery, laceration
  - complete —*see* Injury, mesenteric artery, laceration, major
- pulmonary vessel (incomplete) —*see also* Injury, blood vessel, thoracic, pulmonary, laceration
  - complete —*see* Injury, blood vessel, thoracic, pulmonary, laceration, major
- subclavian —*see* Transection, innominate
- vena cava (incomplete) —*see also* Injury, vena cava
  - complete —*see* Injury, vena cava, laceration, major
- vertebral artery (incomplete) —*see also* Injury, blood vessel, vertebral, laceration
  - complete —*see* Injury, blood vessel, vertebral, laceration, major

Transaminasemia R74.0

Transfusion
- associated (red blood cell) hemochromatosis E83.111
- blood
  - ABO incompatible —*see* Complication(s), transfusion, incompatibility reaction, ABO
  - minor blood group (Duffy) (E) (K (ell)) (Kidd) (Lewis) (M) (N) (P) (S) T80.89
  - reaction or complication —*see* Complications, transfusion
- fetomaternal (mother) —*see* Pregnancy, complicated by, placenta, transfusion syndrome
- maternofetal (mother) —*see* Pregnancy, complicated by, placenta, transfusion syndrome
- placental (syndrome) (mother) —*see* Pregnancy, complicated by, placenta, transfusion syndrome
- reaction (adverse) —*see* Complications, transfusion
- related acute lung injury (TRALI) J95.84
- twin-to-twin —*see* Pregnancy, complicated by, placenta, transfusion syndrome, fetus to fetus

Transient (meaning homeless) —*see also* condition Z59.0

Translocation
- balanced autosomal Q95.9
  - in normal individual Q95.0
- chromosomes NEC Q99.8
  - balanced and insertion in normal individual Q95.0
- Down syndrome Q90.2
- trisomy
  - 13 Q91.6
  - 18 Q91.2
  - 21 Q90.2

Translucency, iris —*see* Degeneration, iris

Transmission of chemical substances through the placenta —*see* Absorption, chemical, through placenta

Transparency, lung, unilateral J43.0

Transplant (ed) (status) Z94.9
- awaiting organ Z76.82
- bone Z94.6
  - marrow Z94.81
- candidate Z76.82
- complication —*see* Complication, transplant
- cornea Z94.7
- heart Z94.1
  - and lung(s) Z94.3
  - valve Z95.2
    - prosthetic Z95.2
    - specified NEC Z95.4
    - xenogenic Z95.3
- intestine Z94.82
- kidney Z94.0
- liver Z94.4
- lung(s) Z94.2
  - and heart Z94.3
- organ (failure) (infection) (rejection) Z94.9
  - removal status Z98.85
- pancreas Z94.83
- skin Z94.5
- social Z60.3

Transplant *(continued)*
- specified organ or tissue NEC Z94.89
- stem cells Z94.84
- tissue Z94.9

Transplants, ovarian, endometrial N80.1

Transposed *—see* Transposition

Transposition (congenital) *—see also* Malposition, congenital
- abdominal viscera Q89.3
- aorta (dextra) Q20.3
- appendix Q43.8
- colon Q43.8
- corrected Q20.5
- great vessels (complete) (partial) Q20.3
- heart Q24.0
  - with complete transposition of viscera Q89.3
- intestine (large) (small) Q43.8
- reversed jejunal (for bypass) (status) Z98.0
- scrotum Q55.23
- stomach Q40.2
  - with general transposition of viscera Q89.3
- tooth, teeth, fully erupted M26.30
- vessels, great (complete) (partial) Q20.3
- viscera (abdominal) (thoracic) Q89.3

Transsexualism F64.0

Transverse *—see also* condition
- arrest (deep), in labor O64.0
- lie (mother) O32.2
  - causing obstructed labor O64.8

Transvestism, transvestitism (dual-role) F64.1
- fetishistic F65.1

Trapped placenta (with hemorrhage) O72.0
- without hemorrhage O73.0

TRAPS (tumor necrosis factor receptor associated periodic syndrome) M04.1

Trauma, traumatism *—see also* Injury
- acoustic *—see* subcategory H83.3
- birth *—see* Birth, injury
- complicating ectopic or molar pregnancy O08.6
- during delivery O71.9
- following ectopic or molar pregnancy O08.6
- obstetric O71.9
  - specified NEC O71.89
- occlusal
  - primary K08.81
  - secondary K08.82

Traumatic *—see also* condition
- brain injury S06.9

Treacher Collins syndrome Q75.4

Treitz's hernia *—see* Hernia, abdomen, specified site NEC

Trematode infestation *—see* Infestation, fluke

Trematodiasis *—see* Infestation, fluke

Trembling paralysis *—see* Parkinsonism

Tremor(s) R25.1
- drug induced G25.1
- essential (benign) G25.0
- familial G25.0
- hereditary G25.0

Tremor *(continued)*
- hysterical F44.4
- intention G25.2
- medication induced postural G25.1
- mercurial *—see* subcategory T56.1
- Parkinson's *—see* Parkinsonism
- psychogenic (conversion reaction) F44.4
- senilis R54
- specified type NEC G25.2

Trench
- fever A79.0
- foot *—see* Immersion, foot
- mouth A69.1

Treponema pallidum infection *—see* Syphilis

Treponematosis
- due to
  - T. pallidum *—see* Syphilis
  - T. pertenue *—see* Yaws

Triad
- Hutchinson's (congenital syphilis) A50.53
- Kartagener's Q89.3
- Saint's *—see* Hernia, diaphragm

Trichiasis (eyelid) H02.059
- with entropion *—see* Entropion
- left H02.056
  - lower H02.055
  - upper H02.054
- right H02.053
  - lower H02.052
  - upper H02.051

Trichinella spiralis (infection) (infestation) B75

Trichinellosis, trichiniasis, trichinelliasis, trichinosis B75
- with muscle disorder B75 *[M63.80]*
  - ankle B75 *[M63.87-]*
  - foot B75 *[M63.87-]*
  - forearm B75 *[M63.83-]*
  - hand B75 *[M63.84-]*
  - lower leg B75 *[M63.86-]*
  - multiple sites B75 *[M63.89]*
  - pelvic region B75 *[M63.85-]*
  - shoulder region B75 *[M63.81-]*
  - specified site NEC B75 *[M63.88]*
  - thigh B75 *[M63.85-]*
  - upper arm B75 *[M63.82-]*

Trichobezoar T18.9
- intestine T18.3
- stomach T18.2

Trichocephaliasis, trichocephalosis B79

Trichocephalus infestation B79

Trichoclasis L67.8

Trichoepithelioma *—see also* Neoplasm, skin, benign
- malignant *—see* Neoplasm, skin, malignant

Trichofolliculoma *—see* Neoplasm, skin, benign

Tricholemmoma *—see* Neoplasm, skin, benign

Trichomoniasis A59.9
- bladder A59.03
- cervix A59.09
- intestinal A07.8
- prostate A59.02
- seminal vesicles A59.09
- specified site NEC A59.8
- urethra A59.03
- urogenitalis A59.00
- vagina A59.01
- vulva A59.01

Trichomycosis
- axillaris A48.8
- nodosa, nodularis B36.8

Trichonodosis L67.8

Trichophytid, trichophyton infection *—see* Dermatophytosis

Trichophytobezoar T18.9
- intestine T18.3
- stomach T18.2

Trichophytosis *—see* Dermatophytosis

Trichoptilosis L67.8

Trichorrhexis (nodosa) (invaginata) L67.0

Trichosis axillaris A48.8

Trichosporosis nodosa B36.2

Trichostasis spinulosa (congenital) Q84.1

Trichostrongyliasis, trichostrongylosis (small intestine) B81.2

Trichostrongylus infection B81.2

Trichotillomania F63.3

Trichromat, trichromatopsia, anomalous (congenital) H53.55

Trichuriasis B79

Trichuris trichiura (infection) (infestation) (any site) B79

Tricuspid (valve) *—see* condition

Trifid *—see also* Accessory
- kidney (pelvis) Q63.8
- tongue Q38.3

Trigeminal neuralgia *—see* Neuralgia, trigeminal

Trigeminy R00.8

Trigger finger (acquired) M65.30
- congenital Q74.0
- index finger M65.32-
- little finger M65.35-
- middle finger M65.33-
- ring finger M65.34-
- thumb M65.31-

Trigonitis (bladder) (chronic) (pseudomembranous) N30.30
- with hematuria N30.31

Trigonocephaly Q75.0

Trilocular heart *—see* Cor triloculare

Trimethylaminuria E72.52

Tripartite placenta O43.19-

Triphalangeal thumb Q74.0

Triple *—see also* Accessory
- kidneys Q63.0
- uteri Q51.818
- X, female Q97.0

Triplegia G83.89
- congenital G80.8

Triplet (newborn) *—see also* Newborn, triplet
- complicating pregnancy *—see* Pregnancy, triplet

Triplication *—see* Accessory

Triploidy Q92.7

Trismus R25.2
- neonatorum A33
- newborn A33

Trisomy (syndrome) Q92.9
- autosomes Q92.9
- chromosome specified NEC Q92.8
  - partial Q92.2

Trisomy *(continued)*
- chromosome specified NEC *(continued)*
  - partial *(continued)*
    - due to unbalanced translocation Q92.5
  - whole (nonsex chromosome)
    - meiotic nondisjunction Q92.0
    - mitotic nondisjunction Q92.1
    - mosaicism Q92.1
  - specified NEC Q92.8
- due to
  - dicentrics *—see* Extra, marker chromosomes
  - extra rings *—see* Extra, marker chromosomes
  - isochromosomes *—see* Extra, marker chromosomes
- specified NEC Q92.8
- whole chromosome Q92.9
  - meiotic nondisjunction Q92.0
  - mitotic nondisjunction Q92.1
  - mosaicism Q92.1
  - partial Q92.9
  - specified NEC Q92.8
- 13 (partial) Q91.7
  - meiotic nondisjunction Q91.4
  - mitotic nondisjunction Q91.5
  - mosaicism Q91.5
  - translocation Q91.6
- 18 (partial) Q91.3
  - meiotic nondisjunction Q91.0
  - mitotic nondisjunction Q91.1
  - mosaicism Q91.1
  - translocation Q91.2
- 20 Q92.8
- 21 (partial) Q90.9
  - meiotic nondisjunction Q90.0
  - mitotic nondisjunction Q90.1
  - mosaicism Q90.1
  - translocation Q90.2
- 22 Q92.8

Tritanomaly, tritanopia H53.55

Trombiculosis, trombiculiasis, trombidiosis B88.0

Trophedema (congenital) (hereditary) Q82.0

Trophoblastic disease (*see also* Mole, hydatidiform) O01.9

Tropholymphedema Q82.0

Trophoneurosis NEC G96.8
- disseminated M34.9

Tropical *—see* condition

Trouble *—see also* Disease
- heart *—see* Disease, heart
- kidney *—see* Disease, renal
- nervous R45.0
- sinus *—see* Sinusitis

Trousseau's syndrome (thrombophlebitis migrans) I82.1

Truancy, childhood
- from school Z72.810

Truncus
- arteriosus (persistent) Q20.0
- communis Q20.0

Trunk *—see* condition

Trypanosomiasis
- African B56.9
  - by Trypanosoma brucei
    - gambiense B56.0
    - rhodesiense B56.1
- American *—see* Chagas' disease
- Brazilian *—see* Chagas' disease
- by Trypanosoma
  - brucei gambiense B56.0
  - brucei rhodesiense B56.1
  - cruzi *—see* Chagas' disease

Trypanosomiasis *(continued)*
  gambiensis, Gambian B56.0
  rhodesiensis, Rhodesian B56.1
  South American *—see* Chagas' disease
  where
    African trypanosomiasis is prevalent B56.9
    Chagas' disease is prevalent B57.2

T-shaped incisors K00.2

Tsutsugamushi (disease) (fever) A75.3

Tube, tubal, tubular *—see* condition

Tubercle *—see also* Tuberculosis
  brain, solitary A17.81
  Darwin's Q17.8
  Ghon, primary infection A15.7

Tuberculid, tuberculide (indurating, subcutaneous) (lichenoid) (miliary) (papulonecrotic) (primary) (skin) A18.4

Tuberculoma *—see also* Tuberculosis
  brain A17.81
  meninges (cerebral) (spinal) A17.1
  spinal cord A17.81

Tuberculosis, tubercular, tuberculous (calcification) (calcified) (caseous) (chromogenic acid-fast bacilli) (degeneration) (fibrocaseous) (fistula) (interstitial) (isolated circumscribed lesions) (necrosis) (parenchymatous) (ulcerative) A15.9
  with pneumoconiosis (any condition in J60-J64) J65
  abdomen (lymph gland) A18.39
  abscess (respiratory) A15.9
    bone A18.03
      hip A18.02
      knee A18.02
      sacrum A18.01
      specified site NEC A18.03
      spinal A18.01
      vertebra A18.01
    brain A17.81
    breast A18.89
    Cowper's gland A18.15
    dura (mater) (cerebral) (spinal) A17.81
    epidural (cerebral) (spinal) A17.81
    female pelvis A18.17
    frontal sinus A15.8
    genital organs NEC A18.10
    genitourinary A18.10
    gland (lymphatic) *—see* Tuberculosis, lymph gland
    hip A18.02
    intestine A18.32
    ischiorectal A18.32
    joint NEC A18.02
      hip A18.02
      knee A18.02
      specified NEC A18.02
      vertebral A18.01
    kidney A18.11
    knee A18.02
    latent R76.11
    lumbar (spine) A18.01
    lung *—see* Tuberculosis, pulmonary
    meninges (cerebral) (spinal) A17.0
    muscle A18.09
    perianal (fistula) A18.32
    perinephritic A18.11
    perirectal A18.32
    rectum A18.32
    retropharyngeal A15.8
    sacrum A18.01

Tuberculosis, tubercular, tuberculous *(continued)*
  abscess *(continued)*
    scrofulous A18.2
    scrotum A18.15
    skin (primary) A18.4
    spinal cord A17.81
    spine or vertebra (column) A18.01
    subdiaphragmatic A18.31
    testis A18.15
    urinary A18.13
    uterus A18.17
  accessory sinus *—see* Tuberculosis, sinus
  Addison's disease A18.7
  adenitis *—see* Tuberculosis, lymph gland
  adenoids A15.8
  adenopathy *—see* Tuberculosis, lymph gland
  adherent pericardium A18.84
  adnexa (uteri) A18.17
  adrenal (capsule) (gland) A18.7
  alimentary canal A18.32
  anemia A18.89
  ankle (joint) (bone) A18.02
  anus A18.32
  apex, apical *—see* Tuberculosis, pulmonary
  appendicitis, appendix A18.32
  arachnoid A17.0
  artery, arteritis A18.89
    cerebral A18.89
  arthritis (chronic) (synovial) A18.02
    spine or vertebra (column) A18.01
  articular *—see* Tuberculosis, joint
  ascites A18.31
  asthma *—see* Tuberculosis, pulmonary
  axilla, axillary (gland) A18.2
  bladder A18.12
  bone A18.03
    hip A18.02
    knee A18.02
    limb NEC A18.03
    sacrum A18.01
    spine or vertebral column A18.01
  bowel (miliary) A18.32
  brain A17.81
  breast A18.89
  broad ligament A18.17
  bronchi, bronchial, bronchus A15.5
    ectasia, ectasis (bronchiectasis) *—see* Tuberculosis, pulmonary
    fistula A15.5
      primary (progressive) A15.7
    gland or node A15.4
      primary (progressive) A15.7
    lymph gland or node A15.4
      primary (progressive) A15.7
  bronchiectasis *—see* Tuberculosis, pulmonary
  bronchitis A15.5
  bronchopleural A15.6
  bronchopneumonia, bronchopneumonic *—see* Tuberculosis, pulmonary
  bronchorrhagia A15.5
  bronchotracheal A15.5
  bronze disease A18.7
  buccal cavity A18.83
  bulbourethral gland A18.15
  bursa A18.09
  cachexia A15.9
  cardiomyopathy A18.84
  caries *—see* Tuberculosis, bone
  cartilage A18.02
    intervertebral A18.01
  catarrhal *—see* Tuberculosis, respiratory

Tuberculosis, tubercular, tuberculous *(continued)*
  cecum A18.32
  cellulitis (primary) A18.4
  cerebellum A17.81
  cerebral, cerebrum A17.81
  cerebrospinal A17.81
    meninges A17.0
  cervical (lymph gland or node) A18.2
  cervicitis, cervix (uteri) A18.16
  chest *—see* Tuberculosis, respiratory
  chorioretinitis A18.53
  choroid, choroiditis A18.53
  ciliary body A18.54
  colitis A18.32
  collier's J65
  colliquativa (primary) A18.4
  colon A18.32
  complex, primary A15.7
  congenital P37.0
  conjunctiva A18.59
  connective tissue (systemic) A18.89
  contact Z20.1
  cornea (ulcer) A18.52
  Cowper's gland A18.15
  coxae A18.02
  coxalgia A18.02
  cul-de-sac of Douglas A18.17
  curvature, spine A18.01
  cutis (colliquativa) (primary) A18.4
  cyst, ovary A18.18
  cystitis A18.12
  dactylitis A18.03
  diarrhea A18.32
  diffuse *—see* Tuberculosis, miliary
  digestive tract A18.32
  disseminated *—see* Tuberculosis, miliary
  duodenum A18.32
  dura (mater) (cerebral) (spinal) A17.0
    abscess (cerebral) (spinal) A17.81
  dysentery A18.32
  ear (inner) (middle) A18.6
    bone A18.03
    external (primary) A18.4
    skin (primary) A18.4
  elbow A18.02
  emphysema *—see* Tuberculosis, pulmonary
  empyema A15.6
  encephalitis A17.82
  endarteritis A18.89
  endocarditis A18.84
    aortic A18.84
    mitral A18.84
    pulmonary A18.84
    tricuspid A18.84
  endocrine glands NEC A18.82
  endometrium A18.17
  enteric, enterica, enteritis A18.32
  enterocolitis A18.32
  epididymis, epididymitis A18.15
  epidural abscess (cerebral) (spinal) A17.81
  epiglottis A15.5
  episcleritis A18.51
  erythema (induratum) (nodosum) (primary) A18.4
  esophagus A18.83
  eustachian tube A18.6
  exposure (to) Z20.1
  exudative *—see* Tuberculosis, pulmonary
  eye A18.50
  eyelid (primary) (lupus) A18.4
  fallopian tube (acute) (chronic) A18.17
  fascia A18.09

Tuberculosis, tubercular, tuberculous *(continued)*
  fauces A15.8
  female pelvic inflammatory disease A18.17
  finger A18.03
  first infection A15.7
  gallbladder A18.83
  ganglion A18.09
  gastritis A18.83
  gastrocolic fistula A18.32
  gastroenteritis A18.32
  gastrointestinal tract A18.32
  general, generalized *—see* Tuberculosis, miliary
  genital organs A18.10
  genitourinary A18.10
  genu A18.02
  glandula suprarenalis A18.7
  glandular, general A18.2
  glottis A15.5
  grinder's J65
  gum A18.83
  hand A18.03
  heart A18.84
  hematogenous *—see* Tuberculosis, miliary
  hemoptysis *—see* Tuberculosis, pulmonary
  hemorrhage NEC *—see* Tuberculosis, pulmonary
  hemothorax A15.6
  hepatitis A18.83
  hilar lymph nodes A15.4
    primary (progressive) A15.7
  hip (joint) (disease) (bone) A18.02
  hydropneumothorax A15.6
  hydrothorax A15.6
  hypoadrenalism A18.7
  hypopharynx A15.8
  ileocecal (hyperplastic) A18.32
  ileocolitis A18.32
  ileum A18.32
  iliac spine (superior) A18.03
  immunological findings only A15.7
  indurativa (primary) A18.4
  infantile A15.7
  infection A15.9
    without clinical manifestations A15.7
  infraclavicular gland A18.2
  inguinal gland A18.2
  inguinalis A18.2
  intestine (any part) A18.32
  iridocyclitis A18.54
  iris, iritis A18.54
  ischiorectal A18.32
  jaw A18.03
  jejunum A18.32
  joint A18.02
    vertebral A18.01
  keratitis (interstitial) A18.52
  keratoconjunctivitis A18.52
  kidney A18.11
  knee (joint) A18.02
  kyphosis, kyphoscoliosis A18.01
  laryngitis A15.5
  larynx A15.5
  latent R76.11
  leptomeninges, leptomeningitis (cerebral) (spinal) A17.0
  lichenoides (primary) A18.4
  linguae A18.83
  lip A18.83
  liver A18.83
  lordosis A18.01
  lung *—see* Tuberculosis, pulmonary
  lupus vulgaris A18.4
  lymph gland or node (peripheral) A18.2
    abdomen A18.39

Tuberculosis, tubercular, tuberculous *(continued)*
- lymph gland or node *(continued)*
  - bronchial A15.4
    - primary (progressive) A15.7
  - cervical A18.2
  - hilar A15.4
    - primary (progressive) A15.7
  - intrathoracic A15.4
    - primary (progressive) A15.7
  - mediastinal A15.4
    - primary (progressive) A15.7
  - mesenteric A18.39
  - retroperitoneal A18.39
  - tracheobronchial A15.4
    - primary (progressive) A15.7
- lymphadenitis *—see* Tuberculosis, lymph gland
- lymphangitis *—see* Tuberculosis, lymph gland
- lymphatic (gland) (vessel) *—see* Tuberculosis, lymph gland
- mammary gland A18.89
- marasmus A15.9
- mastoiditis A18.03
- mediastinal lymph gland or node A15.4
  - primary (progressive) A15.7
- mediastinitis A15.8
  - primary (progressive) A15.7
- mediastinum A15.8
  - primary (progressive) A15.7
- medulla A17.81
- melanosis, Addisonian A18.7
- meninges, meningitis (basilar) (cerebral) (cerebrospinal) (spinal) A17.0
- meningoencephalitis A17.82
- mesentery, mesenteric (gland or node) A18.39
- miliary A19.9
  - acute A19.2
    - multiple sites A19.1
    - single specified site A19.0
  - chronic A19.8
  - specified NEC A19.8
- millstone makers' J65
- miner's J65
- molder's J65
- mouth A18.83
- multiple A19.9
  - acute A19.1
  - chronic A19.8
- muscle A18.09
- myelitis A17.82
- myocardium, myocarditis A18.84
- nasal (passage) (sinus) A15.8
- nasopharynx A15.8
- neck gland A18.2
- nephritis A18.11
- nerve (mononeuropathy) A17.83
- nervous system A17.9
- nose (septum) A15.8
- ocular A18.50
- omentum A18.31
- oophoritis (acute) (chronic) A18.17
- optic (nerve trunk) (papilla) A18.59
- orbit A18.59
- orchitis A18.15
- organ, specified NEC A18.89
- osseous *—see* Tuberculosis, bone
- osteitis *—see* Tuberculosis, bone
- osteomyelitis *—see* Tuberculosis, bone
- otitis media A18.6
- ovary, ovaritis (acute) (chronic) A18.17
- oviduct (acute) (chronic) A18.17
- pachymeningitis A17.0
- palate (soft) A18.83
- pancreas A18.83
- papulonecrotic (a) (primary) A18.4
- parathyroid glands A18.82
- paronychia (primary) A18.4
- parotid gland or region A18.83
- pelvis (bony) A18.03
- penis A18.15
- peribronchitis A15.5
- pericardium, pericarditis A18.84
- perichondritis, larynx A15.5
- periostitis *—see* Tuberculosis, bone
- perirectal fistula A18.32
- peritoneum NEC A18.31
- peritonitis A18.31
- pharynx, pharyngitis A15.8
- phlyctenulosis (keratoconjunctivitis) A18.52
- phthisis NEC *—see* Tuberculosis, pulmonary
- pituitary gland A18.82
- pleura, pleural, pleurisy, pleuritis (fibrinous) (obliterative) (purulent) (simple plastic) (with effusion) A15.6
  - primary (progressive) A15.7
- pneumonia, pneumonic *—see* Tuberculosis, pulmonary
- pneumothorax (spontaneous) (tense valvular) *—see* Tuberculosis, pulmonary
- polyneuropathy A17.89
- polyserositis A19.9
  - acute A19.1
  - chronic A19.8
- potter's J65
- prepuce A18.15
- primary (complex) A15.7
- proctitis A18.32
- prostate, prostatitis A18.14
- pulmonalis *—see* Tuberculosis, pulmonary
- pulmonary (cavitated) (fibrotic) (infiltrative) (nodular) A15.0
  - childhood type or first infection A15.7
  - primary (complex) A15.7
- pyelitis A18.11
- pyelonephritis A18.11
- pyemia *—see* Tuberculosis, miliary
- pyonephrosis A18.11
- pyopneumothorax A15.6
- pyothorax A15.6
- rectum (fistula) (with abscess) A18.32
- reinfection stage *—see* Tuberculosis, pulmonary
- renal A18.11
- renis A18.11
- respiratory A15.9
  - primary A15.7
  - specified site NEC A15.8
- retina, retinitis A18.53
- retroperitoneal (lymph gland or node) A18.39
- rheumatism NEC A18.09
- rhinitis A15.8
- sacroiliac (joint) A18.01
- sacrum A18.01
- salivary gland A18.83
- salpingitis (acute) (chronic) A18.17
- sandblaster's J65
- sclera A18.51
- scoliosis A18.01
- scrofulous A18.2
- scrotum A18.15
- seminal tract or vesicle A18.15
- senile A15.9
- septic *—see* Tuberculosis, miliary
- shoulder (joint) A18.02
  - blade A18.03
- sigmoid A18.32
- sinus (any nasal) A15.8
  - bone A18.03
  - epididymis A18.15
- skeletal NEC A18.03
- skin (any site) (primary) A18.4
- small intestine A18.32
- soft palate A18.83
- spermatic cord A18.15
- spine, spinal (column) A18.01
  - cord A17.81
  - medulla A17.81
  - membrane A17.0
  - meninges A17.0
- spleen, splenitis A18.85
- spondylitis A18.01
- sternoclavicular joint A18.02
- stomach A18.83
- stonemason's J65
- subcutaneous tissue (cellular) (primary) A18.4
- subcutis (primary) A18.4
- subdeltoid bursa A18.83
- submaxillary (region) A18.83
- supraclavicular gland A18.2
- suprarenal (capsule) (gland) A18.7
- swelling, joint (*see also* category M01) (*see also* Tuberculosis, joint) A18.02
- symphysis pubis A18.02
- synovitis A18.09
  - articular A18.02
  - spine or vertebra A18.01
- systemic *—see* Tuberculosis, miliary
- tarsitis A18.4
- tendon (sheath) *—see* Tuberculosis, tenosynovitis
- tenosynovitis A18.09
  - spine or vertebra A18.01
- testis A18.15
- throat A15.8
- thymus gland A18.82
- thyroid gland A18.81
- tongue A18.83
- tonsil, tonsillitis A15.8
- trachea, tracheal A15.5
  - lymph gland or node A15.4
    - primary (progressive) A15.7
- tracheobronchial A15.5
  - lymph gland or node A15.4
    - primary (progressive) A15.7
- tubal (acute) (chronic) A18.17
- tunica vaginalis A18.15
- ulcer (skin) (primary) A18.4
  - bowel or intestine A18.32
  - specified NEC - code under Tuberculosis, by site
- unspecified site A15.9
- ureter A18.11
- urethra, urethral (gland) A18.13
- urinary organ or tract A18.13
- uterus A18.17
- uveal tract A18.54
- uvula A18.83
- vagina A18.18
- vas deferens A18.15
- verruca, verrucosa (cutis) (primary) A18.4
- vertebra (column) A18.01
- vesiculitis A18.15
- vulva A18.18
- wrist (joint) A18.02

Tuberculum
- Carabelli *—see* Note at K00.2
- occlusal *—see* Note at K00.2
- paramolare K00.2

Tuberosity, enitre maxillary M26.07

Tuberous sclerosis (brain) Q85.1

Tubo-ovarian *—see* condition

Tuboplasty, after previous sterilization Z31.0
- aftercare Z31.42

Tubotympanitis, catarrhal (chronic) *—see* Otitis, media, nonsuppurative, chronic, serous

Tularemia A21.9
- with
  - conjunctivitis A21.1
  - pneumonia A21.2
- abdominal A21.3
- bronchopneumonic A21.2
- conjunctivitis A21.1
- cryptogenic A21.3
- enteric A21.3
- gastrointestinal A21.3
- generalized A21.7
- ingestion A21.3
- intestinal A21.3
- oculoglandular A21.1
- ophthalmic A21.1
- pneumonia (any), pneumonic A21.2
- pulmonary A21.2
- sepsis A21.7
- specified NEC A21.8
- typhoidal A21.7
- ulceroglandular A21.0

Tularensis conjunctivitis A21.1

Tumefaction *—see also* Swelling
- liver *—see* Hypertrophy, liver

Tumor *—see also* Neoplasm, unspecified behavior, by site
- acinar cell *—see* Neoplasm, uncertain behavior, by site
- acinic cell *—see* Neoplasm, uncertain behavior, by site
- adenocarcinoid *—see* Neoplasm, malignant, by site
- adenomatoid *—see also* Neoplasm, benign, by site
  - odontogenic *—see* Cyst, calcifying odontogenic
- adnexal (skin) *—see* Neoplasm, skin, benign, by site
- adrenal
  - cortical (benign) D35.0-
    - malignant C74.0-
  - rest *—see* Neoplasm, benign, by site
- alpha-cell
  - malignant
    - pancreas C25.4
    - specified site NEC *—see* Neoplasm, malignant, by site
    - unspecified site C25.4
  - pancreas D13.7
  - specified site NEC *—see* Neoplasm, benign, by site
  - unspecified site D13.7
- aneurysmal *—see* Aneurysm
- aortic body D44.7
  - malignant C75.5
- Askin's *—see* Neoplasm, connective tissue, malignant
- basal cell (*see also* Neoplasm, skin, uncertain behavior) D48.5
- Bednar *—see* Neoplasm, skin, malignant
- benign (unclassified) *—see* Neoplasm, benign, by site
- beta-cell
  - malignant
    - pancreas C25.4
    - specified site NEC *—see* Neoplasm, malignant, by site

mor *(continued)*
beta-cell *(continued)*
  malignant *(continued)*
    unspecified site C25.4
  pancreas D13.7
  specified site NEC *—see* Neoplasm, benign, by site
  unspecified site D13.7
Brenner D27.9
  borderline malignancy D39.1-
  malignant C56-
  proliferating D39.1-
bronchial alveolar, intravascular D38.1
Brooke's *—see* Neoplasm, skin, benign
brown fat *—see* Lipoma
Burkitt *—see* Lymphoma, Burkitt
calcifying epithelial odontogenic *—see* Cyst, calcifying odontogenic
carcinoid
  benign D3A.00
    appendix D3A.020
    ascending colon D3A.022
    bronchus (lung) D3A.090
    cecum D3A.021
    colon D3A.029
    descending colon D3A.024
    duodenum D3A.010
    foregut NOS D3A.094
    hindgut NOS D3A.096
    ileum D3A.012
    jejunum D3A.011
    kidney D3A.093
    large intestine D3A.029
    lung (bronchus) D3A.090
    midgut NOS D3A.095
    rectum D3A.026
    sigmoid colon D3A.025
    small intestine D3A.019
    specified NEC D3A.098
    stomach D3A.092
    thymus D3A.091
    transverse colon D3A.023
  malignant C7A.00
    appendix C7A.020
    ascending colon C7A.022
    bronchus (lung) C7A.090
    cecum C7A.021
    colon C7A.029
    descending colon C7A.024
    duodenum C7A.010
    foregut NOS C7A.094
    hindgut NOS C7A.096
    ileum C7A.012
    jejunum C7A.011
    kidney C7A.093
    large intestine C7A.029
    lung (bronchus) C7A.090
    midgut NOS C7A.095
    rectum C7A.026
    sigmoid colon C7A.025
    small intestine C7A.019
    specified NEC C7A.098
    stomach C7A.092
    thymus C7A.091
    transverse colon C7A.023
  mesentary metastasis C7B.04
  secondary C7B.00
    bone C7B.03
    distant lymph nodes C7B.01
    liver C7B.02
    peritoneum C7B.04
    specified NEC C7B.09
carotid body D44.6
  malignant C75.4
cells *—see also* Neoplasm, unspecified behavior, by site

Tumor *(continued)*
cells *(continued)*
  benign *—see* Neoplasm, benign, by site
  malignant *—see* Neoplasm, malignant, by site
  uncertain whether benign or malignant *—see* Neoplasm, uncertain behavior, by site
cervix, in pregnancy or childbirth *—see* Pregnancy, complicated by, tumor, cervix
chondromatous giant cell *—see* Neoplasm, bone, benign
chromaffin *—see also* Neoplasm, benign, by site
  malignant *—see* Neoplasm, malignant, by site
Cock's peculiar L72.3
Codman's *—see* Neoplasm, bone, benign
dentigerous, mixed *—see* Cyst, calcifying odontogenic
dermoid *—see* Neoplasm, benign, by site
  with malignant transformation C56-
desmoid (extra-abdominal) *—see also* Neoplasm, connective tissue, uncertain behavior
  abdominal *—see* Neoplasm, connective tissue, uncertain behavior
embolus *—see* Neoplasm, secondary, by site
embryonal (mixed) *—see also* Neoplasm, uncertain behavior, by site
  liver C22.7
endodermal sinus
  specified site *—see* Neoplasm, malignant, by site
  unspecified site
    female C56.-
    male C62.90
epithelial
  benign *—see* Neoplasm, benign, by site
  malignant *—see* Neoplasm, malignant, by site
Ewing's *—see* Neoplasm, bone, malignant, by site
fatty *—see* Lipoma
fibroid *—see* Leiomyoma
G cell
  malignant
    pancreas C25.4
    specified site NEC *—see* Neoplasm, malignant, by site
    unspecified site C25.4
  specified site *—see* Neoplasm, uncertain behavior, by site
  unspecified site D37.8
germ cell *—see also* Neoplasm, malignant, by site
  mixed *—see* Neoplasm, malignant, by site
ghost cell, odontogenic *—see* Cyst, calcifying odontogenic
giant cell *—see also* Neoplasm, uncertain behavior, by site
  bone D48.0
    malignant *—see* Neoplasm, bone, malignant
  chondromatous *—see* Neoplasm, bone, benign
  malignant *—see* Neoplasm, malignant, by site

Tumor *(continued)*
giant cell *(continued)*
  soft parts *—see* Neoplasm, connective tissue, uncertain behavior
    malignant *—see* Neoplasm, connective tissue, malignant
glomus D18.00
  intra-abdominal D18.03
  intracranial D18.02
  jugulare D44.7
    malignant C75.5
  skin D18.01
  specified site NEC D18.09
gonadal stromal *—see* Neoplasm, uncertain behavior, by site
granular cell *—see also* Neoplasm, connective tissue, benign
  malignant *—see* Neoplasm, connective tissue, malignant
granulosa cell D39.1-
  juvenile D39.1-
  malignant C56-
granulosa cell-theca cell D39.1-
  malignant C56-
Grawitz's C64-
hemorrhoidal *—see* Hemorrhoids
hilar cell D27-
hilus cell D27-
Hurthle cell (benign) D34
  malignant C73
hydatid *—see* Echinococcus
hypernephroid *—see also* Neoplasm, uncertain behavior, by site
interstitial cell *—see also* Neoplasm, uncertain behavior, by site
  benign *—see* Neoplasm, benign, by site
  malignant *—see* Neoplasm, malignant, by site
intravascular bronchial alveolar D38.1
islet cell *—see* Neoplasm, benign, by site
  malignant *—see* Neoplasm, malignant, by site
    pancreas C25.4
    specified site NEC *—see* Neoplasm, malignant, by site
    unspecified site C25.4
  pancreas D13.7
  specified site NEC *—see* Neoplasm, benign, by site
  unspecified site D13.7
juxtaglomerular D41.0-
Klatskin's C24.0
Krukenberg's C79.6-
Leydig cell *—see* Neoplasm, uncertain behavior, by site
  benign *—see* Neoplasm, benign, by site
    specified site *—see* Neoplasm, benign, by site
    unspecified site
      female D27.9
      male D29.20
  malignant *—see* Neoplasm, malignant, by site
    specified site *—see* Neoplasm, malignant, by site
    unspecified site
      female C56.9
      male C62.90
  specified site *—see* Neoplasm, uncertain behavior, by site
  unspecified site
    female D39.10
    male D40.10
lipid cell, ovary D27-
lipoid cell, ovary D27-

Tumor *(continued)*
malignant (*see also* Neoplasm, malignant, by site) C80.1
  fusiform cell (type) C80.1
  giant cell (type) C80.1
  localized, plasma cell *—see* Plasmacytoma, solitary
  mixed NEC C80.1
  small cell (type) C80.1
  spindle cell (type) C80.1
  unclassified C80.1
mast cell D47.09
melanotic, neuroectodermal *—see* Neoplasm, benign, by site
Merkel cell *—see* Carcinoma, Merkel cell
mesenchymal
  malignant *—see* Neoplasm, connective tissue, malignant
  mixed *—see* Neoplasm, connective tissue, uncertain behavior
mesodermal, mixed *—see also* Neoplasm, malignant, by site
  liver C22.4
mesonephric *—see also* Neoplasm, uncertain behavior, by site
  malignant *—see* Neoplasm, malignant, by site
metastatic
  from specified site *—see* Neoplasm, malignant, by site
  of specified site *—see* Neoplasm, malignant, by site
  to specified site *—see* Neoplasm, secondary, by site
mixed NEC *—see also* Neoplasm, benign, by site
  malignant *—see* Neoplasm, malignant, by site
mucinous of low malignant potential
  specified site *—see* Neoplasm, malignant, by site
  unspecified site C56.9
mucocarcinoid
  specified site *—see* Neoplasm, malignant, by site
  unspecified site C18.1
mucoepidermoid *—see* Neoplasm, uncertain behavior, by site
Müllerian, mixed
  specified site *—see* Neoplasm, malignant, by site
  unspecified site C54.9
myoepithelial *—see* Neoplasm, benign, by site
neuroectodermal (peripheral) *—see* Neoplasm, malignant, by site
  primitive
    specified site *—see* Neoplasm, malignant, by site
    unspecified site C71.9
neuroendocrine D3A.8
  malignant poorly differentiated C7A.1
  secondary NEC C7B.8
  specified NEC C7A.8
neurogenic olfactory C30.0
nonencapsulated sclerosing C73
odontogenic (adenomatoid) (benign) (calcifying epithelial) (keratocystic) (squamous) *—see* Cyst, calcifying odontogenic
  malignant C41.1
    upper jaw (bone) C41.0
ovarian stromal D39.1-
ovary, in pregnancy *—see* Pregnancy, complicated by

Tumor *(continued)*
- pacinian *—see* Neoplasm, skin, benign
- Pancoast's *—see* Pancoast's syndrome
- papillary *—see also* Papilloma
  - cystic D37.9
  - mucinous of low malignant potential C56-
    - specified site *—see* Neoplasm, malignant, by site
    - unspecified site C56.9
  - serous of low malignant potential
    - specified site *—see* Neoplasm, malignant, by site
    - unspecified site C56.9
- pelvic, in pregnancy or childbirth *—see* Pregnancy, complicated by
- phantom F45.8
- phyllodes D48.6-
  - benign D24-
  - malignant *—see* Neoplasm, breast, malignant
- Pindborg *—see* Cyst, calcifying odontogenic
- placental site trophoblastic D39.2
- plasma cell (malignant) (localized) *—see* Plasmacytoma, solitary
- polyvesicular vitelline
  - specified site *—see* Neoplasm, malignant, by site
  - unspecified site
    - female C56.9
    - male C62.90
- Pott's puffy *—see* Osteomyelitis, specified NEC
- Rathke's pouch D44.3
- retinal anlage *—see* Neoplasm, benign, by site
- salivary gland type, mixed *—see* Neoplasm, salivary gland, benign
  - malignant *—see* Neoplasm, salivary gland, malignant
- Sampson's N80.1
- Schmincke's *—see* Neoplasm, nasopharynx, malignant
- sclerosing stromal D27-
- sebaceous *—see* Cyst, sebaceous
- secondary *—see* Neoplasm, secondary, by site
  - carcinoid C7B.00
    - bone C7B.03
    - distant lymph nodes C7B.01
    - liver C7B.02
    - peritoneum C7B.04
    - specified NEC C7B.09
  - neuroendocrine NEC C7B.8
- serous of low malignant potential
  - specified site *—see* Neoplasm, malignant, by site
  - unspecified site C56.9
- Sertoli cell *—see* Neoplasm, benign, by site
  - with lipid storage
    - specified site *—see* Neoplasm, benign, by site
    - unspecified site
      - female D27.9
      - male D29.20
  - specified site *—see* Neoplasm, benign, by site
  - unspecified site
    - female D27.9
    - male D29.20
- Sertoli-Leydig cell *—see* Neoplasm, benign, by site
  - specified site *—see* Neoplasm, benign, by site
  - unspecified site

Tumor *(continued)*
- Sertoli-Leydig cell *(continued)*
  - unspecified site *(continued)*
    - female D27.9
    - male D29.20
- sex cord (-stromal) *—see* Neoplasm, uncertain behavior, by site
  - with annular tubules D39.1-
- skin appendage *—see* Neoplasm, skin, benign
- smooth muscle *—see* Neoplasm, connective tissue, uncertain behavior
- soft tissue
  - benign *—see* Neoplasm, connective tissue, benign
  - malignant *—see* Neoplasm, connective tissue, malignant
- sternomastoid (congenital) Q68.0
- stromal
  - endometrial D39.0
  - gastric D48.1
    - benign D21.4
    - malignant C16.9
    - uncertain behavior D48.1
  - gastrointestinal C49.A-
    - benign D21.4
    - esophagus C49.A1
    - malignant C49.A0
      - colon C49.A4
      - duodenum C49.A3
      - esophagus C49.A1
      - ileum C49.A3
      - jejunum C49.A3
      - Meckel diverticulum C49.A3
      - large intestine C49.A4
      - omentum C49.A9
      - peritoneum C49.A9
      - rectum C49.A5
      - small intestine C49.A3
      - specified site NEC C49.A9
      - stomach C49.A2
    - rectum C49.A5
    - small intestine C49.A3
    - specified site NEC C49.A9
    - stomach C49.A2
    - uncertain behavior D48.1
  - intestine
    - benign D21.4
    - malignant
      - large C49.A4
      - small C49.A3
    - uncertain behavior D48.1
  - ovarian D39.1-
  - stomach C49.A2
    - benign D21.4
    - malignant C49.A2
    - uncertain behavior D48.1
- testicular D40.10
- sweat gland *—see also* Neoplasm, skin, uncertain behavior
  - benign *—see* Neoplasm, skin, benign
  - malignant *—see* Neoplasm, skin, malignant
- syphilitic, brain A52.17
- testicular stromal D40.1-
- theca cell D27.-
- theca cell-granulosa cell D39.1-
- Triton, malignant *—see* Neoplasm, nerve, malignant
- trophoblastic, placental site D39.2
- turban D23.4
- uterus (body), in pregnancy or childbirth *—see* Pregnancy, complicated by, tumor, uterus
- vagina, in pregnancy or childbirth *—see* Pregnancy, complicated by

Tumor *(continued)*
- varicose *—see* Varix
- von Recklinghausen's *—see* Neurofibromatosis
- vulva or perineum, in pregnancy or childbirth *—see* Pregnancy, complicated by
  - causing obstructed labor O65.5
- Warthin's *—see* Neoplasm, salivary gland, benign
- Wilms' C64-
- yolk sac *—see* Neoplasm, malignant, by site
  - specified site *—see* Neoplasm, malignant, by site
  - unspecified site
    - female C56.9
    - male C62.90

Tumor lysis syndrome (following antineoplastic chemotherapy) (spontaneous) **NEC** E88.3

Tumorlet *—see* Neoplasm, uncertain behavior, by site

Tungiasis B88.1

Tunica vasculosa lentis Q12.2

Turban tumor D23.4

Türck's trachoma J37.0

Turner-Kieser syndrome Q87.2

Turner-like syndrome Q87.1

Turner's
- hypoplasia (tooth) K00.4
- syndrome Q96.9
  - specified NEC Q96.8
- tooth K00.4

Turner-Ullrich syndrome Q96.9

Tussis convulsiva *—see* Whooping cough

Twiddler's syndrome (due to)
- automatic implantable defibrillator T82.198
- cardiac pacemaker T82.198

Twilight state
- epileptic F05
- psychogenic F44.89

Twin (newborn) *—see also* Newborn, twin
- conjoined Q89.4
- pregnancy *—see* Pregnancy, twin

Twinning, teeth K00.2

Twist, twisted
- bowel, colon or intestine K56.2
- hair (congenital) Q84.1
- mesentery K56.2
- omentum K56.2
- organ or site, congenital NEC *—see* Anomaly, by site
- ovarian pedicle *—see* Torsion, ovary

Twitching R25.3

Tylosis (acquired) L84
- buccalis K13.29
- linguae K13.29
- palmaris et plantaris (congenital) (inherited) Q82.8
  - acquired L85.1

Tympanism R14.0

Tympanites (abdominal) (intestinal) R14.0

Tympanitis *—see* Myringitis

Tympanosclerosis *—see* subcategory H74.0

Tympanum *—see* condition

Tympany
- abdomen R14.0
- chest R09.89

Type A behavior pattern Z73.1

Typhlitis *—see* Appendicitis

Typhoenteritis *—see* Typhoid

Typhoid (abortive) (ambulant) (any site) (clinical) (fever) (hemorrhagic) (infection) (intermittent) (malignant) (rheumatic) (Widal negative) A01.00
- with pneumonia A01.03
- abdominal A01.09
- arthritis A01.04
- carrier (suspected) of Z22.0
- cholecystitis (current) A01.09
- endocarditis A01.02
- heart involvement A01.02
- inoculation reaction *—see* Complications, vaccination
- meningitis A01.01
- mesenteric lymph nodes A01.09
- myocarditis A01.02
- osteomyelitis A01.05
- perichondritis, larynx A01.09
- pneumonia A01.03
- spine A01.05
- specified NEC A01.09
- ulcer (perforating) A01.09

Typhomalaria (fever) *—see* Malaria

Typhomania A01.00

Typhoperitonitis A01.09

Typhus (fever) A75.9
- abdominal, abdominalis *—see* Typhoid
- African tick A77.1
- amarillic A95.9
- brain A75.9 *[G94]*
- cerebral A75.9 *[G94]*
- classical A75.0
- due to Rickettsia
  - prowazekii A75.0
    - recrudescent A75.1
  - tsutsugamushi A75.3
  - typhi A75.2
- endemic (flea-borne) A75.2
- epidemic (louse-borne) A75.0
- exanthematic NEC A75.0
- exanthematicus SAI A75.0
  - brillii SAI A75.1
  - mexicanus SAI A75.2
  - typhus murinus A75.2
- flea-borne A75.2
- India tick A77.1
- Kenya (tick) A77.1
- louse-borne A75.0
- Mexican A75.2
- mite-borne A75.3
- murine A75.2
- North Asian tick-borne A77.2
- petechial A75.9
- Queensland tick A77.3
- rat A75.2
- recrudescent A75.1
- recurrens *—see* Fever, relapsing
- Sao Paulo A77.0
- scrub (China) (India) (Malaysia) (New Guinea) A75.3
- shop (of Malaysia) A75.2
- Siberian tick A77.2
- tick-borne A77.9
- tropical (mite-borne) A75.3

Tyrosinemia E70.21
- newborn, transitory P74.5

Tyrosinosis E70.21

Tyrosinuria E70.29

Uhl's anomaly or disease Q24.8

Ulcer, ulcerated, ulcerating, ulceration, ulcerative
- alveolar process M27.3
- amebic (intestine) A06.1
  - skin A06.7
- anastomotic —*see* Ulcer, gastrojejunal
- anorectal K62.6
- antral —*see* Ulcer, stomach
- anus (sphincter) (solitary) K62.6
- aorta —*see* Aneurysm
- aphthous (oral) (recurrent) K12.0
  - genital organ(s)
    - female N76.6
    - male N50.89
- artery I77.2
- atrophic —*see* Ulcer, skin
  - decubitus —*see* Ulcer, pressure, by site
- back L98.429
  - with
    - bone involvement without evidence of necrosis L98.426
    - bone necrosis L98.424
    - exposed fat layer L98.422
    - muscle involvement without evidence of necrosis L98.425
    - muscle necrosis L98.423
    - skin breakdown only L98.421
    - specified severity NEC L98.428
- Barrett's (esophagus) K22.10
  - with bleeding K22.11
- bile duct (common) (hepatic) K83.8
- bladder (solitary) (sphincter) NEC N32.89
  - bilharzial B65.9 *[N33]*
  - in schistosomiasis (bilharzial) B65.9 *[N33]*
  - submucosal —*see* Cystitis, interstitial
  - tuberculous A18.12
- bleeding K27.4
- bone —*see* Osteomyelitis, specified type NEC
- bowel —*see* Ulcer, intestine
- breast N61.1
- bronchus J98.09
- buccal (cavity) (traumatic) K12.1
- Buruli A31.1
- buttock L98.419
  - with
    - bone involvement without evidence of necrosis L98.416
    - bone necrosis L98.414
    - exposed fat layer L98.412
    - muscle involvement without evidence of necrosis L98.415
    - muscle necrosis L98.413
    - skin breakdown only L98.411
    - specified severity NEC L98.418
- cancerous —*see* Neoplasm, malignant, by site
- cardia K22.10
  - with bleeding K22.11
- cardioesophageal (peptic) K22.10
  - with bleeding K22.11
- cecum —*see* Ulcer, intestine
- cervix (uteri) (decubitus) (trophic) N86
  - with cervicitis N72
- chancroidal A57
- chiclero B55.1
- chronic (cause unknown) —*see* Ulcer, skin
- Cochin-China B55.1
- colon —*see* Ulcer, intestine
- conjunctiva H10.89

Ulcer, ulcerated, ulcerating, ulceration, ulcerative *(continued)*
- cornea H16.00-
  - with hypopyon H16.03-
  - central H16.01-
  - dendritic (herpes simplex) B00.52
  - marginal H16.04-
  - Mooren's H16.05-
  - mycotic H16.06-
  - perforated H16.07-
  - ring H16.02-
  - tuberculous (phlyctenular) A18.52
- corpus cavernosum (chronic) N48.5
- crural —*see* Ulcer, lower limb
- Curling's —*see* Ulcer, peptic, acute
- Cushing's —*see* Ulcer, peptic, acute
- cystic duct K82.8
- cystitis (interstitial) —*see* Cystitis, interstitial
- decubitus —*see* Ulcer, pressure, by site
- dendritic, cornea (herpes simplex) B00.52
- diabetes, diabetic —*see* Diabetes, ulcer
- Dieulafoy's K25.0
- due to
  - infection NEC —*see* Ulcer, skin
  - radiation NEC L59.8
  - trophic disturbance (any region) —*see* Ulcer, skin
  - X-ray L58.1
- duodenum, duodenal (eroded) (peptic) K26.9
  - with
    - hemorrhage K26.4
      - and perforation K26.6
    - perforation K26.5
  - acute K26.3
    - with
      - hemorrhage K26.0
        - and perforation K26.2
      - perforation K26.1
  - chronic K26.7
    - with
      - hemorrhage K26.4
        - and perforation K26.6
      - perforation K26.5
- dysenteric A09
- elusive —*see* Cystitis, interstitial
- endocarditis (acute) (chronic) (subacute) I28.8
- epiglottis J38.7
- esophagus (peptic) K22.10
  - with bleeding K22.11
  - due to
    - aspirin K22.10
      - with bleeding K22.11
    - gastrointestinal reflux disease K21.0
    - ingestion of chemical or medicament K22.10
      - with bleeding K22.11
  - fungal K22.10
    - with bleeding K22.11
  - infective K22.10
    - with bleeding K22.11
  - varicose —*see* Varix, esophagus
- eyelid (region) H01.8
- fauces J39.2
- Fenwick (-Hunner) (solitary) —*see* Cystitis, interstitial
- fistulous —*see* Ulcer, skin
- foot (indolent) (trophic) —*see* Ulcer, lower limb
- frambesial, initial A66.0
- frenum (tongue) K14.0
- gallbladder or duct K82.8

Ulcer, ulcerated, ulcerating, ulceration, ulcerative *(continued)*
- gangrenous —*see* Gangrene
- gastric —*see* Ulcer, stomach
- gastrocolic —*see* Ulcer, gastrojejunal
- gastroduodenal —*see* Ulcer, peptic
- gastroesophageal —*see* Ulcer, stomach
- gastrointestinal —*see* Ulcer, gastrojejunal
- gastrojejunal (peptic) K28.9
  - with
    - hemorrhage K28.4
      - and perforation K28.6
    - perforation K28.5
  - acute K28.3
    - with
      - hemorrhage K28.0
        - and perforation K28.2
      - perforation K28.1
  - chronic K28.7
    - with
      - hemorrhage K28.4
        - and perforation K28.6
      - perforation K28.5
- gastrojejunocolic —*see* Ulcer, gastrojejunal
- gingiva K06.8
- gingivitis K05.10
  - nonplaque induced K05.11
  - plaque induced K05.10
- glottis J38.7
- granuloma of pudenda A58
- gum K06.8
- gumma, due to yaws A66.4
- heel —*see* Ulcer, lower limb
- hemorrhoid (*see also* Hemorrhoids, by degree) K64.8
- Hunner's —*see* Cystitis, interstitial
- hypopharynx J39.2
- hypopyon (chronic) (subacute) —*see* Ulcer, cornea, with hypopyon
- hypostaticum —*see* Ulcer, varicose
- ileum —*see* Ulcer, intestine
- intestine, intestinal K63.3
  - with perforation K63.1
  - amebic A06.1
  - duodenal —*see* Ulcer, duodenum
  - granulocytopenic (with hemorrhage) —*see* Neutropenia
  - marginal —*see* Ulcer, gastrojejunal
  - perforating K63.1
    - newborn P78.0
  - primary, small intestine K63.3
  - rectum K62.6
  - stercoraceous, stercoral K63.3
  - tuberculous A18.32
  - typhoid (fever) —*see* Typhoid
  - varicose I86.8
- jejunum, jejunal —*see* Ulcer, gastrojejunal
- keratitis —*see* Ulcer, cornea
- knee —*see* Ulcer, lower limb
- labium (majus) (minus) N76.6
- laryngitis —*see* Laryngitis
- larynx (aphthous) (contact) J38.7
  - diphtheritic A36.2
- leg —*see* Ulcer, lower limb
- lip K13.0
- Lipschütz's N76.6
- lower limb (atrophic) (chronic) (neurogenic) (perforating) (pyogenic) (trophic) (tropical) L97.909
  - with
    - bone involvement without evidence of necrosis L97.906

Ulcer, ulcerated, ulcerating, ulceration, ulcerative *(continued)*
- lower limb *(continued)*
  - with *(continued)*
    - bone necrosis L97.904
    - exposed fat layer L97.902
    - muscle involvement without evidence of necrosis L97.905
    - muscle necrosis L97.903
    - skin breakdown only L97.901
    - specified severity NEC L97.908
  - ankle L97.309
    - with
      - bone involvement without evidence of necrosis L97.306
      - bone necrosis L97.304
      - exposed fat layer L97.302
      - muscle involvement without evidence of necrosis L97.305
      - muscle necrosis L97.303
      - skin breakdown only L97.301
      - specified severity NEC L97.308
    - left L97.329
      - with
        - bone involvement without evidence of necrosis L97.326
        - bone necrosis L97.324
        - exposed fat layer L97.322
        - muscle involvement without evidence of necrosis L97.325
        - muscle necrosis L97.323
        - skin breakdown only L97.321
        - specified severity NEC L97.328
    - right L97.319
      - with
        - bone involvement without evidence of necrosis L97.316
        - bone necrosis L97.314
        - exposed fat layer L97.312
        - muscle involvement without evidence of necrosis L97.315
        - muscle necrosis L97.313
        - skin breakdown only L97.311
        - specified severity NEC L97.318
  - calf L97.209
    - with
      - bone involvement without evidence of necrosis L97.206
      - bone necrosis L97.204
      - exposed fat layer L97.202
      - muscle involvement without evidence of necrosis L97.205
      - muscle necrosis L97.203
      - skin breakdown only L97.201
      - specified severity NEC L97.208
    - left L97.229
      - with
        - bone involvement without evidence of necrosis L97.226
        - bone necrosis L97.224
        - exposed fat layer L97.222
        - muscle involvement without evidence of necrosis L97.225

Ulcer, ulcerated, ulcerating, ulceration, ulcerative *(continued)*
lower limb *(continued)*
calf *(continued)*
left *(continued)*
with *(continued)*
muscle necrosis L97.223
skin breakdown only L97.221
specified severity NEC L97.228
right L97.219
with
bone involvement without evidence of necrosis L97.216
bone necrosis L97.214
exposed fat layer L97.212
muscle involvement without evidence of necrosis L97.215
muscle necrosis L97.213
skin breakdown only L97.211
specified severity NEC L97.218
decubitus *—see* Ulcer, pressure, by site
foot specified NEC L97.509
with
bone involvement without evidence of necrosis L97.506
bone necrosis L97.504
exposed fat layer L97.502
muscle involvement without evidence of necrosis L97.505
muscle necrosis L97.503
skin breakdown only L97.501
specified severity NEC L97.508
left L97.529
with
bone involvement without evidence of necrosis L97.526
bone necrosis L97.524
exposed fat layer L97.522
muscle involvement without evidence of necrosis L97.525
muscle necrosis L97.523
skin breakdown only L97.521
specified severity NEC L97.528
right L97.519
with
bone involvement without evidence of necrosis L97.516
bone necrosis L97.514
exposed fat layer L97.512
muscle involvement without evidence of necrosis L97.515
muscle necrosis L97.513
skin breakdown only L97.511
specified severity NEC L97.518
heel L97.409
with
bone involvement without evidence of necrosis L97.406
bone necrosis L97.404
exposed fat layer L97.402
muscle involvement without evidence of necrosis L97.405
muscle necrosis L97.403

Ulcer, ulcerated, ulcerating, ulceration, ulcerative *(continued)*
lower limb *(continued)*
foot specified NEC L907.509 *(continued)*
with *(continued)*
skin breakdown only L97.401
specified severity NEC L97.408
left L97.429
with
bone involvement without evidence of necrosis L97.426
bone necrosis L97.424
exposed fat layer L97.422
muscle involvement without evidence of necrosis L97.425
muscle necrosis L97.423
skin breakdown only L97.421
specified severity NEC L97.428
right L97.419
with
bone involvement without evidence of necrosis L97.416
bone necrosis L97.414
exposed fat layer L97.412
muscle involvement without evidence of necrosis L97.415
muscle necrosis L97.413
skin breakdown only L97.411
specified severity NEC L97.418
left L97.929
with
bone involvement without evidence of necrosis L97.926
bone necrosis L97.924
exposed fat layer L97.922
muscle involvement without evidence of necrosis L97.925
muscle necrosis L97.923
skin breakdown only L97.921
specified severity NEC L97.928
lower leg NOS L97.909
with
bone involvement without evidence of necrosis L97.906
bone necrosis L97.904
exposed fat layer L97.902
muscle involvement without evidence of necrosis L97.905
muscle necrosis L97.903
skin breakdown only L97.901
specified severity NEC L97.908
left L97.929
with
bone involvement without evidence of necrosis L97.926
bone necrosis L97.924
exposed fat layer L97.922
muscle involvement without evidence of necrosis L97.925
muscle necrosis L97.923
skin breakdown only L97.921

Ulcer, ulcerated, ulcerating, ulceration, ulcerative *(continued)*
lower limb *(continued)*
lower leg NOS *(continued)*
left *(continued)*
with *(continued)*
specified severity NEC L97.928
right L97.919
with
bone involvement without evidence of necrosis L97.916
bone necrosis L97.914
exposed fat layer L97.912
muscle involvement without evidence of necrosis L97.915
muscle necrosis L97.913
skin breakdown only L97.911
specified severity NEC L97.918
specified site NEC L97.809
with
bone involvement without evidence of necrosis L97.806
bone necrosis L97.804
exposed fat layer L97.802
muscle involvement without evidence of necrosis L97.805
muscle necrosis L97.803
skin breakdown only L97.801
specified severity NEC L97.808
left L97.829
with
bone involvement without evidence of necrosis L97.826
bone necrosis L97.824
exposed fat layer L97.822
muscle involvement without evidence of necrosis L97.825
muscle necrosis L97.823
skin breakdown only L97.821
specified severity NEC L97.828
right L97.819
with
bone involvement without evidence of necrosis L97.816
bone necrosis L97.814
exposed fat layer L97.812
muscle involvement without evidence of necrosis L97.815
muscle necrosis L97.813
skin breakdown only L97.811
specified severity NEC L97.818
midfoot L97.409
with
bone involvement without evidence of necrosis L97.406
bone necrosis L97.404
exposed fat layer L97.402
muscle involvement without evidence of necrosis L97.405
muscle necrosis L97.403

Ulcer, ulcerated, ulcerating, ulceration, ulcerative *(continued)*
lower limb *(continued)*
midfoot *(continued)*
with *(continued)*
skin breakdown only L97.401
specified severity NEC L97.408
left L97.429
with
bone involvement without evidence of necrosis L97.426
bone necrosis L97.424
exposed fat layer L97.422
muscle involvement without evidence of necrosis L97.425
muscle necrosis L97.423
skin breakdown only L97.421
specified severity NEC L97.428
right L97.419
with
bone involvement without evidence of necrosis L97.416
bone necrosis L97.414
exposed fat layer L97.412
muscle involvement without evidence of necrosis L97.415
muscle necrosis L97.413
skin breakdown only L97.411
specified severity NEC L97.418
right L97.919
with
bone involvement without evidence of necrosis L97.916
bone necrosis L97.914
exposed fat layer L97.912
muscle involvement without evidence of necrosis L97.915
muscle necrosis L97.913
skin breakdown only L97.911
specified severity NEC L97.918
thigh L97.109
with
bone involvement without evidence of necrosis L97.106
bone necrosis L97.104
exposed fat layer L97.102
muscle involvement without evidence of necrosis L97.105
muscle necrosis L97.103
skin breakdown only L97.101
specified severity NEC L97.108
left L97.129
with
bone involvement without evidence of necrosis L97.126
bone necrosis L97.124
exposed fat layer L97.122
muscle involvement without evidence of necrosis L97.125
muscle necrosis L97.123

Ulcer, ulcerated, ulcerating, ulceration, ulcerative *(continued)*
lower limb *(continued)*
thigh *(continued)*
left *(continued)*
with *(continued)*
muscle necrosis *(continued)*
skin breakdown only L97.121
specified severity NEC L97.128
right L97.119
with
bone involvement without evidence of necrosis L97.116
bone necrosis L97.114
exposed fat layer L97.112
muscle involvement without evidence of necrosis L97.115
muscle necrosis L97.113
skin breakdown only L97.111
specified severity NEC L97.118
toe L97.509
with
bone involvement without evidence of necrosis L97.506
bone necrosis L97.504
exposed fat layer L97.502
muscle involvement without evidence of necrosis L97.505
muscle necrosis L97.503
skin breakdown only L97.501
specified severity NEC L97.508
left L97.529
with
bone involvement without evidence of necrosis L97.526
bone necrosis L97.524
exposed fat layer L97.522
muscle involvement without evidence of necrosis L97.525
muscle necrosis L97.523
skin breakdown only L97.521
specified severity NEC L97.528
right L97.519
with
bone involvement without evidence of necrosis L97.516
bone necrosis L97.514
exposed fat layer L97.512
muscle involvement without evidence of necrosis L97.515
muscle necrosis L97.513
skin breakdown only L97.511
specified severity NEC L97.518
leprous A30.1
syphilitic A52.19
varicose *—see* Varix, leg, with, ulcer
luetic *—see* Ulcer, syphilitic
lung J98.4
tuberculous *—see* Tuberculosis, pulmonary

Ulcer, ulcerated, ulcerating, ulceration, ulcerative *(continued)*
lung *(continued)*
malignant *—see* Neoplasm, malignant, by site
marginal NEC *—see* Ulcer, gastrojejunal
meatus (urinarius) N34.2
Meckel's diverticulum Q43.0
malignant *—see* Table of Neoplasms, small intestine, malignant
Meleney's (chronic undermining) *—see* Ulcer, skin
Mooren's (cornea) *—see* Ulcer, cornea, Mooren's
mycobacterial (skin) A31.1
nasopharynx J39.2
neck, uterus N86
neurogenic NEC *—see* Ulcer, skin
nose, nasal (passage) (infective) (septum) J34.0
skin *—see* Ulcer, skin
spirochetal A69.8
varicose (bleeding) I86.8
oral mucosa (traumatic) K12.1
palate (soft) K12.1
penis (chronic) N48.5
peptic (site unspecified) K27.9
with
hemorrhage K27.4
and perforation K27.6
perforation K27.5
acute K27.3
with
hemorrhage K27.0
and perforation K27.2
perforation K27.1
chronic K27.7
with
hemorrhage K27.4
and perforation K27.6
perforation K27.5
esophagus K22.10
with bleeding K22.11
newborn P78.82
perforating K27.5
skin *—see* Ulcer, skin
peritonsillar J35.8
phagedenic (tropical) *—see* Ulcer, skin
pharynx J39.2
phlebitis *—see* Phlebitis
plaster *—see* Ulcer, pressure, by site
popliteal space *—see* Ulcer, lower limb
postpyloric *—see* Ulcer, duodenum
prepuce N47.7
prepyloric *—see* Ulcer, stomach
pressure (pressure area) L89.9-
ankle L89.5-
back L89.1-
buttock L89.3-
coccyx L89.15-
contiguous site of back, buttock, hip L89.4-
elbow L89.0-
face L89.81-
head L89.81-
heel L89.6-
hip L89.2-
sacral region (tailbone) L89.15-
specified site NEC L89.89-
stage 1 (healing) (pre-ulcer skin changes limited to persistent focal edema)
ankle L89.5-
back L89.1-

Ulcer, ulcerated, ulcerating, ulceration, ulcerative *(continued)*
pressure *(continued)*
stage 1 *(continued)*
buttock L89.3-
coccyx L89.15-
contiguous site of back, buttock, hip L89.4-
elbow L89.0-
face L89.81-
head L89.81-
heel L89.6-
hip L89.2-
sacral region (tailbone) L89.15-
specified site NEC L89.89-
stage 2 (healing) (abrasion, blister, partial thickness skin loss involving epidermis and/ or dermis)
ankle L89.5-
back L89.1-
buttock L89.3-
coccyx L89.15-
contiguous site of back, buttock, hip L89.4-
elbow L89.0-
face L89.81-
head L89.81-
heel L89.6-
hip L89.2-
sacral region (tailbone) L89.15-
specified site NEC L89.89-
stage 3 (healing) (full thickness skin loss involving damage or necrosis of subcutaneous tissue)
ankle L89.5-
back L89.1-
buttock L89.3-
coccyx L89.15-
contiguous site of back, buttock, hip L89.4-
elbow L89.0-
face L89.81-
head L89.81-
heel L89.6-
hip L89.2-
sacral region (tailbone) L89.15-
specified site NEC L89.89-
stage 4 (healing) (necrosis of soft tissues through to underlying muscle, tendon, or bone)
ankle L89.5-
back L89.1-
buttock L89.3-
coccyx L89.15-
contiguous site of back, buttock, hip L89.4-
elbow L89.0-
face L89.81-
head L89.81-
heel L89.6-
hip L89.2-
sacral region (tailbone) L89.15-
specified site NEC L89.89-
unspecified stage
ankle L89.5-
back L89.1-
buttock L89.3-
coccyx L89.15-
contiguous site of back, buttock, hip L89.4-
elbow L89.0-
face L89.81-
head L89.81-
heel L89.6-
hip L89.2-
sacral region (tailbone) L89.15-
specified site NEC L89.89-

Ulcer, ulcerated, ulcerating, ulceration, ulcerative *(continued)*
pressure *(continued)*
unstageable
ankle L89.5-
back L89.1-
buttock L89.3-
coccyx L89.15-
contiguous site of back, buttock, hip L89.4-
elbow L89.0-
face L89.81-
head L89.81-
heel L89.6-
hip L89.2-
sacral region (tailbone) L89.15-
specified site NEC L89.89-
primary of intestine K63.3
with perforation K63.1
prostate N41.9
pyloric *—see* Ulcer, stomach
rectosigmoid K63.3
with perforation K63.1
rectum (sphincter) (solitary) K62.6
stercoraceous, stercoral K62.6
retina *—see* Inflammation, chorioretinal
rodent *—see also* Neoplasm, skin, malignant
sclera *—see* Scleritis
scrofulous (tuberculous) A18.2
scrotum N50.89
tuberculous A18.15
varicose I86.1
seminal vesicle N50.89
sigmoid *—see* Ulcer, intestine
skin (atrophic) (chronic) (neurogenic) (non-healing) (perforating) (pyogenic) (trophic) (tropical) L98.499
with gangrene *—see* Gangrene
amebic A06.7
back *—see* Ulcer, back
buttock *—see* Ulcer, buttock
decubitus *—see* Ulcer, pressure
lower limb *—see* Ulcer, lower limb
mycobacterial A31.1
specified site NEC L98.499
with
bone involvement without evidence of necrosis L98.496
bone necrosis L98.494
exposed fat layer L98.492
muscle involvement without evidence of necrosis L98.495
muscle necrosis L98.493
skin breakdown only L98.491
specified severity NEC L98.498
tuberculous (primary) A18.4
varicose *—see* Ulcer, varicose
sloughing *—see* Ulcer, skin
solitary, anus or rectum (sphincter) K62.6
sore throat J02.9
streptococcal J02.0
spermatic cord N50.89
spine (tuberculous) A18.01
stasis (venous) *—see* Varix, leg, with, ulcer
without varicose veins I87.2
stercoraceous, stercoral K63.3
with perforation K63.1
anus or rectum K62.6
stoma, stomal *—see* Ulcer, gastrojejunal
stomach (eroded) (peptic) (round) K25.9

Ulcer, ulcerated, ulcerating, ulceration, ulcerative *(continued)*
stomach *(continued)*
with
hemorrhage K25.4
and perforation K25.6
perforation K25.5
acute K25.3
with
hemorrhage K25.0
and perforation K25.2
perforation K25.1
chronic K25.7
with
hemorrhage K25.4
and perforation K25.6
perforation K25.5
stomal *—see* Ulcer, gastrojejunal
stomatitis K12.1
stress *—see* Ulcer, peptic
strumous (tuberculous) A18.2
submucosal, bladder *—see* Cystitis, interstitial
syphilitic (any site) (early) (secondary) A51.39
late A52.79
perforating A52.79
foot A52.11
testis N50.89
thigh *—see* Ulcer, lower limb
throat J39.2
diphtheritic A36.0
toe *—see* Ulcer, lower limb
tongue (traumatic) K14.0
tonsil J35.8
diphtheritic A36.0
trachea J39.8
trophic *—see* Ulcer, skin
tropical *—see* Ulcer, skin
tuberculous *—see* Tuberculosis, ulcer
tunica vaginalis N50.89
turbinate J34.89
typhoid (perforating) *—see* Typhoid
unspecified site *—see* Ulcer, skin
urethra (meatus) *—see* Urethritis
uterus N85.8
cervix N86
with cervicitis N72
neck N86
with cervicitis N72
vagina N76.5
in Behçet's disease M35.2 *[N77.0]*
pessary N89.8
valve, heart I33.0
varicose (lower limb, any part) *—see also* Varix, leg, with, ulcer
broad ligament I86.2
esophagus *—see* Varix, esophagus
inflamed or infected *—see* Varix, leg, with ulcer, with inflammation
nasal septum I86.8
perineum I86.3
scrotum I86.1
specified site NEC I86.8
sublingual I86.0
vulva I86.3
vas deferens N50.89
vulva (acute) (infectional) N76.6
in (due to)
Behçet's disease M35.2 *[N77.0]*
herpesviral (herpes simplex) infection A60.04
tuberculosis A18.18
vulvobuccal, recurring N76.6
X-ray L58.1
yaws A66.4

Ulcerosa scarlatina A38.8

Ulcus *—see also* Ulcer
cutis tuberculosum A18.4
duodeni *—see* Ulcer, duodenum

Ulcus *(continued)*
durum (syphilitic) A51.0
extragenital A51.2
gastrojejunale *—see* Ulcer, gastrojejunal
hypostaticum *—see* Ulcer, varicose
molle (cutis) (skin) A57
serpens corneae *—see* Ulcer, cornea, central
ventriculi *—see* Ulcer, stomach

Ulegyria Q04.8

Ulerythema
ophryogenes, congenital Q84.2
sycosiforme L73.8

Ullrich (-Bonnevie) (-Turner) **syndrome** (*see also* Turner's syndrome) Q87.1

Ullrich-Feichtiger syndrome Q87.0

Ulnar *—see* condition

Ulorrhagia, ulorrhea K06.8

Umbilicus, umbilical *—see* condition

Unacceptable
contours of tooth K08.54
morphology of tooth K08.54

Unavailability (of)
bed at medical facility Z75.1
health service-related agencies Z75.4
medical facilities (at) Z75.3
due to
investigation by social service agency Z75.2
lack of services at home Z75.0
remoteness from facility Z75.3
waiting list Z75.1
home Z75.0
outpatient clinic Z75.3
schooling Z55.1
social service agencies Z75.4

Uncinaria americana infestation B76.1

Uncinariasis B76.9

Uncongenial work Z56.5

Unconscious (ness) *—see* Coma

Under observation *—see* Observation

Underachievement in school Z55.3

Underdevelopment *—see also* Undeveloped
nose Q30.1
sexual E30.0

Underdosing (*see also* Tables of Drugs and Chemicals, categories T36-T50, with final character 6) Z91.14
intentional NEC Z91.128
due to financial hardship of patient Z91.120
unintentional NEC Z91.138
due to patient's age related debility Z91.130

Underfeeding, newborn P92.3

Underfill, endodontic M27.53

Underimmunization status Z28.3

Undernourishment *—see* Malnutrition

Undernutrition *—see* Malnutrition

Underweight R63.6
for gestational age *—see* Light for dates

Underwood's disease P83.0

Undescended *—see also* Malposition, congenital
cecum Q43.3
colon Q43.3
testicle *—see* Cryptorchid

Undeveloped, undevelopment *—see also* Hypoplasia
brain (congenital) Q02
cerebral (congenital) Q02
heart Q24.8
lung Q33.6
testis E29.1
uterus E30.0

Undiagnosed (disease) R69

Undulant fever *—see* Brucellosis

Unemployment, anxiety concerning Z56.0
threatened Z56.2

Unequal length (acquired) (limb) *—see also* Deformity, limb, unequal length
leg *—see also* Deformity, limb, unequal length
congenital Q72.9-

Unextracted dental root K08.3

Unguis incarnatus L60.0

Unhappiness R45.2

Unicornate uterus Q51.4
in pregnancy or childbirth O34.00

Unilateral *—see also* condition
development, breast N64.89
organ or site, congenital NEC *—see* Agenesis, by site

Unilocular heart Q20.8

Union, abnormal *—see also* Fusion
larynx and trachea Q34.8

Universal mesentery Q43.3

Unrepairable overhanging of dental restorative materials K08.52

Unsatisfactory
restoration of tooth K08.50
specified NEC K08.59
sample of cytologic smear
anus R85.615
cervix R87.615
vagina R87.625
surroundings Z59.1
work Z56.5

Unsoundness of mind *—see* Psychosis

Unstable
back NEC *—see* Instability, joint, spine
hip (congenital) Q65.6
acquired *—see* Derangement, joint, specified type NEC, hip
joint *—see* Instability, joint
secondary to removal of joint prosthesis M96.89
lie (mother) O32.0
lumbosacral joint (congenital)
acquired *—see* subcategory M53.2
sacroiliac *—see* subcategory M53.2
spine NEC *—see* Instability, joint, spine

Unsteadiness on feet R26.81

Untruthfulness, child problem F91.8

Unverricht (-Lundborg) **disease or epilepsy** *—see* Epilepsy, generalized, idiopathic

Unwanted pregnancy Z64.0

Upbringing, institutional Z62.22
away from parents NEC Z62.29
in care of non-parental family member Z62.21
in foster care Z62.21
in orphanage or group home Z62.22
in welfare custody Z62.21

Upper respiratory *—see* condition

Upset
gastric K30
gastrointestinal K30
psychogenic F45.8
intestinal (large) (small) K59.9
psychogenic F45.8
menstruation N93.9
mental F48.9
stomach K30
psychogenic F45.8

Urachus *—see also* condition
patent or persistent Q64.4

Urbach-Oppenheim disease (necrobiosis lipoidica diabeticorum) *—see* E08-E13 with .620

Urbach's lipoid proteinosis E78.89

Urbach-Wiethe disease E78.89

Urban yellow fever A95.1

Urea
blood, high *—see* Uremia
cycle metabolism disorder *—see* Disorder, urea cycle metabolism

Uremia, uremic N19
with
ectopic or molar pregnancy O08.4
polyneuropathy N18.9 *[G63]*
chronic NOS (*see also* Disease, kidney, chronic) N18.9
due to hypertension *—see* Hypertensive, kidney
complicating
ectopic or molar pregnancy O08.4
congenital P96.0
extrarenal R39.2
following ectopic or molar pregnancy O08.4
newborn P96.0
prerenal R39.2

Ureter, ureteral *—see* condition

Ureteralgia N23

Ureterectasis *—see* Hydroureter

Ureteritis N28.89
cystica N28.86
due to calculus N20.1
with calculus, kidney N20.2
with hydronephrosis N13.2
gonococcal (acute) (chronic) A54.21
nonspecific N28.89

Ureterocele N28.89
congenital (orthotopic) Q62.31
ectopic Q62.32

Ureterolith, ureterolithiasis *—see* Calculus, ureter

Ureterostomy
attention to Z43.6
status Z93.6

Urethra, urethral *—see* condition

Urethralgia R39.89

Urethritis (anterior) (posterior) N34.2
calculous N21.1
candidal B37.41
chlamydial A56.01
diplococcal (gonococcal) A54.01
with abscess (accessory gland) (periurethral) A54.1
gonococcal A54.01
with abscess (accessory gland) (periurethral) A54.1
nongonococcal N34.1
Reiter's *—see* Reiter's disease
nonspecific N34.1
nonvenereal N34.1
postmenopausal N34.2

rethritis *(continued)*
- puerperal O86.22
- Reiter's —*see* Reiter's disease
- specified NEC N34.2
- trichomonal or due to Trichomonas (vaginalis) A59.03

rethrocele N81.0
- with
  - cystocele —*see* Cystocele
  - prolapse of uterus —*see* Prolapse, uterus

rethrolithiasis (with colic or infection) N21.1

rethrorectal —*see* condition

rethrorrhagia N36.8

rethrorrhea R36.9

rethrostomy
- attention to Z43.6
- status Z93.6

rethrotrigonitis —*see* Trigonitis

rethrovaginal —*see* condition

rgency
- fecal R15.2
- hypertensive —*see* Hypertension
- urinary R39.15

rhidrosis, uridrosis L74.8

ric acid in blood (increased) E79.0

ricacidemia (asymptomatic) E79.0

ricemia (asymptomatic) E79.0

ricosuria R82.99

rinary —*see* condition

rination
- frequent R35.0
- painful R30.9

rine
- blood in —*see* Hematuria
- discharge, excessive R35.8
- enuresis, nonorganic origin F98.0
- extravasation R39.0
- frequency R35.0
- incontinence R32
  - nonorganic origin F98.0
- intermittent stream R39.198
- pus in N39.0
- retention or stasis R33.9
  - organic R33.8
    - drug-induced R33.0
  - psychogenic F45.8
- secretion
  - deficient R34
  - excessive R35.8
  - frequency R35.0
- stream
  - intermittent R39.198
  - slowing R39.198
  - splitting R39.13
  - weak R39.12

rinemia —*see* Uremia

rinoma, urethra N36.8

roarthritis, infectious (Reiter's) —*see* Reiter's disease

rodialysis R34

rolithiasis —*see* Calculus, urinary

ronephrosis —*see* Hydronephrosis

ropathy N39.9
- obstructive N13.9
  - specified NEC N13.8
- reflux N13.9
  - specified NEC N13.8
- vesicoureteral reflux-associated —*see* Reflux, vesicoureteral

Urosepsis - code to condition

Urticaria L50.9
- with angioneurotic edema T78.3
  - hereditary D84.1
- allergic L50.0
- cholinergic L50.5
- chronic L50.8
- cold, familial L50.2
- contact L50.6
- dermatographic L50.3
- due to
  - cold or heat L50.2
  - drugs L50.0
  - food L50.0
  - inhalants L50.0
  - plants L50.6
  - serum (*see also* Reaction, serum) T80.69
- factitial L50.3
- familial cold M04.2
- giant T78.3
  - hereditary D84.1
- gigantea T78.3
- idiopathic L50.1
- larynx T78.3
  - hereditary D84.1
- neonatorum P83.88
- nonallergic L50.1
- papulosa (Hebra) L28.2
- pigmentosa D47.01
  - congenital Q82.2
  - of neonatal onset Q82.2
  - of newborn onset Q82.2
- recurrent periodic L50.8
- serum (*see also* Reaction, serum) T80.69
- solar L56.3
- specified type NEC L50.8
- thermal (cold) (heat) L50.2
- vibratory L50.4
- xanthelasmoidea - *see* Urticaria pigmentosa

Use (of)
- alcohol Z72.89
  - with
    - intoxication F10.929
    - sleep disorder F10.982
  - harmful —*see* Abuse, alcohol
- amphetamines —*see* Use, stimulant NEC
- caffeine —*see* Use, stimulant NEC
- cannabis F12.90
  - with
    - anxiety disorder F12.980
    - intoxication F12.929
      - with
        - delirium F12.921
        - perceptual disturbance F12.922
      - uncomplicated F12.920
    - other specified disorder F12.988
    - psychosis F12.959
      - delusions F12.950
      - hallucinations F12.951
    - unspecified disorder F12.99
- cocaine F14.90
  - with
    - anxiety disorder F14.980
    - intoxication F14.929
      - with
        - delirium F14.921
        - perceptual disturbance F14.922
      - uncomplicated F14.920
    - other specified disorder F14.988
    - psychosis F14.959
      - delusions F14.950
      - hallucinations F14.951
    - sexual dysfunction F14.981
    - sleep disorder F14.982

Use *(continued)*
- cocaine *(continued)*
  - with *(continued)*
    - unspecified disorder F14.99
  - harmful —*see* Abuse, drug, cocaine
- drug(s) NEC F19.90
  - with sleep disorder F19.982
  - harmful —*see* Abuse, drug, by type
- hallucinogen NEC F16.90
  - with
    - anxiety disorder F16.980
    - intoxication F16.929
      - with
        - delirium F16.921
      - uncomplicated F16.920
    - mood disorder F16.94
    - other specified disorder F16.988
    - perception disorder (flashbacks) F16.983
    - psychosis F16.959
      - delusions F16.950
      - hallucinations F16.951
    - unspecified disorder F16.99
  - harmful —*see* Abuse, drug, hallucinogen NEC
- inhalants F18.90
  - with
    - anxiety disorder F18.980
    - intoxication F18.929
      - with delirium F18.921
      - uncomplicated F18.920
    - mood disorder F18.94
    - other specified disorder F18.988
    - persisting dementia F18.97
    - psychosis F18.959
      - delusions F18.950
      - hallucinations F18.951
    - unspecified disorder F18.99
  - harmful —*see* Abuse, drug, inhalant
- methadone - *see* Use, opioid
- nonprescribed drugs F19.90
  - harmful —*see* Abuse, non-psychoactive substance
- opioid F11.90
  - with
    - disorder F11.99
      - mood F11.94
      - sleep F11.982
      - specified type NEC F11.988
    - intoxication F11.929
      - with
        - delirium F11.921
        - perceptual disturbance F11.922
      - uncomplicated F11.920
    - withdrawal F11.93
  - harmful —*see* Abuse, drug, opioid
- patent medicines F19.90
  - harmful —*see* Abuse, non-psychoactive substance
- psychoactive drug NEC F19.90
  - with
    - anxiety disorder F19.980
    - intoxication F19.929
      - with
        - delirium F19.921
        - perceptual disturbance F19.922
      - uncomplicated F19.920
    - mood disorder F19.94
    - other specified disorder F19.988
    - persisting
      - amnestic disorder F19.96
      - dementia F19.97
    - psychosis F19.959
      - delusions F19.950

Use *(continued)*
- psychoactive drug NEC *(continued)*
  - with *(continued)*
    - psychosis *(continued)*
      - hallucinations F19.951
    - sexual dysfunction F19.981
    - sleep disorder F19.982
    - unspecified disorder F19.99
    - withdrawal F19.939
      - with
        - delirium F19.931
        - perceptual disturbance F19.932
      - uncomplicated F19.930
  - harmful —*see* Abuse, drug NEC, psychoactive NEC
- sedative, hypnotic, or anxiolytic F13.90
  - with
    - anxiety disorder F13.980
    - intoxication F13.929
      - with
        - delirium F13.921
      - uncomplicated F13.920
    - other specified disorder F13.988
    - persisting
      - amnestic disorder F13.96
      - dementia F13.97
    - psychosis F13.959
      - delusions F13.950
      - hallucinations F13.951
    - sexual dysfunction F13.981
    - sleep disorder F13.982
    - unspecified disorder F13.99
  - harmful —*see* Abuse, drug, sedative, hypnotic, or anxiolytic
- stimulant NEC F15.90
  - with
    - anxiety disorder F15.980
    - intoxication F15.929
      - with
        - delirium F15.921
        - perceptual disturbance F15.922
      - uncomplicated F15.920
    - mood disorder F15.94
    - other specified disorder F15.988
    - psychosis F15.959
      - delusions F15.950
      - hallucinations F15.951
    - sexual dysfunction F15.981
    - sleep disorder F15.982
    - unspecified disorder F15.99
    - withdrawal F15.93
  - harmful —*see* Abuse, drug, stimulant NEC
- volatile solvents (*see also* Use, inhalant) F18.90
  - harmful —*see* Abuse, drug, inhalant
- tobacco Z72.0
  - with dependence —*see* Dependence, drug, nicotine

Usher-Senear disease or syndrome L10.4

Uta B55.1

Uteromegaly N85.2

Uterovaginal —*see* condition

Uterovesical —*see* condition

Uveal —*see* condition

Uveitis (anterior) —*see also* Iridocyclitis
- acute —*see* Iridocyclitis, acute
- chronic —*see* Iridocyclitis, chronic
- due to toxoplasmosis (acquired) B58.09
  - congenital P37.1

Uveitis *(continued)*
- granulomatous *—see* Iridocyclitis, chronic
- heterochromic *—see* Cyclitis, Fuchs' heterochromic
- lens-induced *—see* Iridocyclitis, lens-induced
- posterior *—see* Chorioretinitis
- sympathetic H44.13-
- syphilitic (secondary) A51.43
  - congenital (early) A50.01
    - late A52.71
- tuberculous A18.54

Uveoencephalitis *—see* Inflammation, chorioretinal

Uveokeratitis *—see* Iridocyclitis

Uveoparotitis D86.89

Uvula *—see* condition

Uvulitis (acute) (catarrhal) (chronic) (membranous) (suppurative) (ulcerative) K12.2

V

Vaccination (prophylactic)
- complication or reaction *—see* Complications, vaccination
- delayed Z28.9
- encounter for Z23
- not done *—see* Immunization, not done, because (of)

Vaccinia (generalized) (localized) T88.1
- congenital P35.8
- without vaccination B08.011

Vacuum, in sinus (accessory) (nasal) J34.89

Vagabond, vagabondage Z59.0

Vagabond's disease B85.1

Vagina, vaginal *—see* condition

Vaginalitis (tunica) (testis) N49.1

Vaginismus (reflex) N94.2
- functional F52.5
- nonorganic F52.5
- psychogenic F52.5
- secondary N94.2

Vaginitis (acute) (circumscribed) (diffuse) (emphysematous) (nonvenereal) (ulcerative) N76.0
- with ectopic or molar pregnancy O08.0
- amebic A06.82
- atrophic, postmenopausal N95.2
- bacterial N76.0
- blennorrhagic (gonococcal) A54.02
- candidal B37.3
- chlamydial A56.02
- chronic N76.1
- due to Trichomonas (vaginalis) A59.01
- following ectopic or molar pregnancy O08.0
- gonococcal A54.02
  - with abscess (accessory gland) (periurethral) A54.1
- granuloma A58
- in (due to)
  - candidiasis B37.3
  - herpesviral (herpes simplex) infection A60.04
  - pinworm infection B80 *[N77.1]*
- monilial B37.3
- mycotic (candidal) B37.3

Vaginitis *(continued)*
- postmenopausal atrophic N95.2
- puerperal (postpartum) O86.13
- senile (atrophic) N95.2
- subacute or chronic N76.1
- syphilitic (early) A51.0
  - late A52.76
- trichomonal A59.01
- tuberculous A18.18

Vaginosis *—see* Vaginitis

Vagotonia G52.2

Vagrancy Z59.0

VAIN *—see* Neoplasia, intraepithelial, vagina

Vallecula *—see* condition

Valley fever B38.0

Valsuani's disease *—see* Anemia, obstetric

Valve, valvular (formation) *—see also* condition
- cerebral ventricle (communicating) in situ Z98.2
- cervix, internal os Q51.828
- congenital NEC *—see* Atresia, by site
- ureter (pelvic junction) (vesical orifice) Q62.39
- urethra (congenital) (posterior) Q64.2

Valvulitis (chronic) *—see* Endocarditis

Valvulopathy *—see* Endocarditis

Van Bogaert's leukoencephalopathy (sclerosing) (subacute) A81.1

Van Bogaert-Scherer-Epstein disease or syndrome E75.5

Van Buchem's syndrome M85.2

Van Creveld-von Gierke disease E74.01

Van der Hoeve (-de Kleyn) **syndrome** Q78.0

Van der Woude's syndrome Q38.0

Van Neck's disease or osteochondrosis M91.0

Vanishing lung J44.9

Vapor asphyxia or suffocation T59.9
- specified agent *—see* Table of Drugs and Chemicals

Variance, lethal ball, prosthetic heart valve T82.09

Variants, thalassemic D56.8

Variations in hair color L67.1

Varicella B01.9
- with
  - complications NEC B01.89
  - encephalitis B01.11
  - encephalomyelitis B01.11
  - meningitis B01.0
  - myelitis B01.12
  - pneumonia B01.2
- congenital P35.8

Varices *—see* Varix

Varicocele (scrotum) (thrombosed) I86.1
- ovary I86.2
- perineum I86.3
- spermatic cord (ulcerated) I86.1

Varicose
- aneurysm (ruptured) I77.0
- dermatitis *—see* Varix, leg, with, inflammation
- eczema *—see* Varix, leg, with, inflammation

Varicose *(continued)*
- phlebitis *—see* Varix, with, inflammation
- tumor *—see* Varix
- ulcer (lower limb, any part) *—see also* Varix, leg, with, ulcer
  - anus (*see also* Hemorrhoids) K64.8
  - esophagus *—see* Varix, esophagus
  - inflamed or infected *—see* Varix, leg, with ulcer, with inflammation
  - nasal septum I86.8
  - perineum I86.3
  - scrotum I86.1
  - specified site NEC I86.8
- vein *—see* Varix
- vessel *—see* Varix, leg

Varicosis, varicosities, varicosity *—see* Varix

Variola (major) (minor) B03

Varioloid B03

Varix (lower limb) (ruptured) I83.90
- with
  - edema I83.899
  - inflammation I83.10
    - with ulcer (venous) I83.209
  - pain I83.819
  - specified complication NEC I83.899
  - stasis dermatitis I83.10
    - with ulcer (venous) I83.209
  - swelling I83.899
  - ulcer I83.009
    - with inflammation I83.209
- aneurysmal I77.0
- asymptomatic I83.9-
- bladder I86.2
- broad ligament I86.2
- complicating
  - childbirth (lower extremity) O87.4
    - anus or rectum O87.2
    - genital (vagina, vulva or perineum) O87.8
  - pregnancy (lower extremity) O22.0-
    - anus or rectum O22.4-
    - genital (vagina, vulva or perineum) O22.1-
  - puerperium (lower extremity) O87.4
    - anus or rectum O87.2
    - genital (vagina, vulva, perineum) O87.8
- congenital (any site) Q27.8
- esophagus (idiopathic) (primary) (ulcerated) I85.00
  - bleeding I85.01
  - congenital Q27.8
  - in (due to)
    - alcoholic liver disease I85.10
      - bleeding I85.11
    - cirrhosis of liver I85.10
      - bleeding I85.11
    - portal hypertension I85.10
      - bleeding I85.11
    - schistosomiasis I85.10
      - bleeding I85.11
    - toxic liver disease I85.10
      - bleeding I85.11
  - secondary I85.10
    - bleeding I85.11
- gastric I86.4
- inflamed or infected I83.10
  - ulcerated I83.209
- labia (majora) I86.3
- leg (asymptomatic) I83.90
  - with
    - edema I83.899

Varix *(continued)*
- leg *(continued)*
  - with *(continued)*
    - inflammation I83.10
      - with ulcer *—see* Varix, leg, with, ulcer, with inflammation by site
    - pain I83.819
    - specified complication NEC I83.899
    - swelling I83.899
    - ulcer I83.009
      - with inflammation I83.209
      - ankle I83.003
        - with inflammation I83.203
      - calf I83.002
        - with inflammation I83.202
      - foot NEC I83.005
        - with inflammation I83.205
      - heel I83.004
        - with inflammation I83.204
      - lower leg NEC I83.008
        - with inflammation I83.208
      - midfoot I83.004
        - with inflammation I83.204
      - thigh I83.001
        - with inflammation I83.201
  - bilateral (asymptomatic) I83.93
    - with
      - edema I83.893
      - pain I83.813
      - specified complication NEC I83.893
      - swelling I83.893
      - ulcer I83.0-
        - with inflammation I83.209
  - left (asymptomatic) I83.92
    - with
      - edema I83.892
      - pain I83.812
      - specified complication NEC I83.892
      - swelling I83.892
      - inflammation I83.12
        - with ulcer *—see* Varix, leg, with, ulcer, with inflammation by site
      - ulcer I83.029
        - with inflammation I83.229
        - ankle I83.023
          - with inflammation I83.223
        - calf I83.022
          - with inflammation I83.222
        - foot NEC I83.025
          - with inflammation I83.225
        - heel I83.024
          - with inflammation I83.224
        - lower leg NEC I83.028
          - with inflammation I83.228
        - midfoot I83.024
          - with inflammation I83.224
        - thigh I83.021
          - with inflammation I83.221
  - right (asymptomatic) I83.91
    - with
      - edema I83.891
      - pain I83.811
      - specified complication NEC I83.891
      - swelling I83.891
      - inflammation I83.11

- **Varix** *(continued)*
  - leg *(continued)*
    - right *(continued)*
      - with *(continued)*
        - inflammation *(continued)*
          - with ulcer *—see* Varix, leg, with, ulcer, with inflammation by site
        - ulcer I83.019
          - with inflammation I83.219
          - ankle I83.013
            - with inflammation I83.213
          - calf I83.012
            - with inflammation I83.212
          - foot NEC I83.015
            - with inflammation I83.215
          - heel I83.014
            - with inflammation I83.214
          - lower leg NEC I83.018
            - with inflammation I83.218
          - midfoot I83.014
            - with inflammation I83.214
          - thigh I83.011
            - with inflammation I83.211
  - nasal septum I86.8
  - orbit I86.8
    - congenital Q27.8
  - ovary I86.2
  - papillary I78.1
  - pelvis I86.2
  - perineum I86.3
  - pharynx I86.8
  - placenta O43.89-
  - renal papilla I86.8
  - retina H35.09
  - scrotum (ulcerated) I86.1
  - sigmoid colon I86.8
  - specified site NEC I86.8
  - spinal (cord) (vessels) I86.8
  - spleen, splenic (vein) (with phlebolith) I86.8
  - stomach I86.4
  - sublingual I86.0
  - ulcerated I83.009
    - inflamed or infected I83.209
  - uterine ligament I86.2
  - vagina I86.8
  - vocal cord I86.8
  - vulva I86.3
- **Vas deferens** *—see* condition
- **Vas deferentitis** N49.1
- **Vasa previa** O69.4
  - hemorrhage from, affecting newborn P50.0
- **Vascular** *—see also* condition
  - loop on optic papilla Q14.2
  - spasm I73.9
  - spider I78.1
- **Vascularization, cornea** *—see* Neovascularization, cornea
- **Vasculitis** I77.6
  - allergic D69.0
  - cryoglobulinemic D89.1
  - disseminated I77.6
  - hypocomplementemic M31.8
  - kidney I77.89
  - livedoid L95.0
  - nodular L95.8
  - retina H35.06-
  - rheumatic *—see* Fever, rheumatic
  - rheumatoid *—see* Rheumatoid, vasculitis
- **Vasculitis** *(continued)*
  - rheumatoid *(continued)*
  - skin (limited to) L95.9
    - specified NEC L95.8
  - systemic M31.8
- **Vasculopathy, necrotizing** M31.9
  - cardiac allograft T86.290
  - specified NEC M31.8
- **Vasitis** (nodosa) N49.1
  - tuberculous A18.15
- **Vasodilation** I73.9
- **Vasomotor** *—see* condition
- **Vasoplasty, after previous sterilization** Z31.0
  - aftercare Z31.42
- **Vasospasm** (vasoconstriction) I73.9
  - cerebral (cerebrovascular) (artery) I67.848
    - reversible I67.841
  - coronary I20.1
  - nerve
    - arm *—see* Mononeuropathy, upper limb
    - brachial plexus G54.0
    - cervical plexus G54.2
    - leg *—see* Mononeuropathy, lower limb
  - peripheral NOS I73.9
  - retina (artery) *—see* Occlusion, artery, retina
- **Vasospastic** *—see* condition
- **Vasovagal attack** (paroxysmal) R55
  - psychogenic F45.8
- **VATER syndrome** Q87.2
- **Vater's ampulla** *—see* condition
- **Vegetation, vegetative**
  - adenoid (nasal fossa) J35.8
  - endocarditis (acute) (any valve) (subacute) I33.0
  - heart (mycotic) (valve) I33.0
- **Veil**
  - Jackson's Q43.3
- **Vein, venous** *—see* condition
- **Veldt sore** *—see* Ulcer, skin
- **Velpeau's hernia** *—see* Hernia, femoral
- **Venereal**
  - bubo A55
  - disease A64
  - granuloma inguinale A58
  - lymphogranuloma (Durand-Nicolas-Favre) A55
- **Venofibrosis** I87.8
- **Venom, venomous** *—see* Table of Drugs and Chemicals, by animal or substance, poisoning
- **Venous** *—see* condition
- **Ventilator lung, newborn** P27.8
- **Ventral** *—see* condition
- **Ventricle, ventricular** *—see also* condition
  - escape I49.3
  - inversion Q20.5
- **Ventriculitis** (cerebral) (*see also* Encephalitis) G04.90
- **Ventriculostomy status** Z98.2
- **Vernet's syndrome** G52.7
- **Verneuil's disease** (syphilitic bursitis) A52.78
- **Verruca** (due to HPV) (filiformis) (simplex) (viral) (vulgaris) B07.9
  - acuminata A63.0
  - necrogenica (primary) (tuberculosa) A18.4
  - plana B07.8
  - plantaris B07.0
  - seborrheica L82.1
    - inflamed L82.0
  - senile (seborrheic) L82.1
    - inflamed L82.0
  - tuberculosa (primary) A18.4
  - venereal A63.0
- **Verrucosities** *—see* Verruca
- **Verruga peruana, peruviana** A44.1
- **Version**
  - with extraction
  - cervix *—see* Malposition, uterus
  - uterus (postinfectional) (postpartal, old) *—see* Malposition, uterus
- **Vertebra, vertebral** *—see* condition
- **Vertical talus** (congenital) Q66.80
  - left foot Q66.82
  - right foot Q66.81
- **Vertigo** R42
  - auditory *—see* Vertigo, aural
  - aural H81.31-
  - benign paroxysmal (positional) H81.1-
  - central (origin) H81.4-
  - cerebral H81.4-
  - Dix and Hallpike (epidemic) *—see* Neuronitis, vestibular
  - due to infrasound T75.23
  - epidemic A88.1
    - Dix and Hallpike *—see* Neuronitis, vestibular
    - Pedersen's *—see* Neuronitis, vestibular
    - vestibular neuronitis *—see* Neuronitis, vestibular
  - hysterical F44.89
  - infrasound *—see* subcategory T75.23
  - labyrinthine H81.0
  - laryngeal R05
  - malignant positional H81.4-
  - Ménière's *—see* subcategory H81.0
  - menopausal N95.1
  - otogenic *—see* Vertigo, aural
  - paroxysmal positional, benign *—see* Vertigo, benign paroxysmal
  - Pedersen's (epidemic) *—see* Neuronitis, vestibular
  - peripheral NEC H81.39-
  - positional
    - benign paroxysmal *—see* Vertigo, benign paroxysmal
    - malignant H81.4-
- **Very-low-density-lipoprotein-type (VLDL) hyperlipoproteinemia** E78.1
- **Vesania** *—see* Psychosis
- **Vesical** *—see* condition
- **Vesicle**
  - cutaneous R23.8
  - seminal *—see* condition
  - skin R23.8
- **Vesicocolic** *—see* condition
- **Vesicoperineal** *—see* condition
- **Vesicorectal** *—see* condition
- **Vesicourethrorectal** *—see* condition
- **Vesicovaginal** *—see* condition
- **Vesicular** *—see* condition
- **Vesiculitis** (seminal) N49.0
  - amebic A06.82
  - gonorrheal (acute) (chronic) A54.23
  - trichomonal A59.09
  - tuberculous A18.15
- **Vestibulitis** (ear) *—see also* subcategory H83.0
  - nose (external) J34.89
  - vulvar N94.810
- **Vestibulopathy, acute peripheral** (recurrent) *—see* Neuronitis, vestibular
- **Vestige, vestigial** *—see also* Persistence
  - branchial Q18.0
  - structures in vitreous Q14.0
- **Vibration**
  - adverse effects T75.20
    - pneumatic hammer syndrome T75.21
    - specified effect NEC T75.29
    - vasospastic syndrome T75.22
    - vertigo from infrasound T75.23
  - exposure (occupational) Z57.7
  - vertigo T75.23
- **Vibriosis** A28.9
- **Victim** (of)
  - crime Z65.4
  - disaster Z65.5
  - terrorism Z65.4
  - torture Z65.4
  - war Z65.5
- **Vidal's disease** L28.0
- **Villaret's syndrome** G52.7
- **Villous** *—see* condition
- **VIN** *—see* Neoplasia, intraepithelial, vulva
- **Vincent's infection** (angina) (gingivitis) A69.1
  - stomatitis NEC A69.1
- **Vinson-Plummer syndrome** D50.1
- **Violence, physical** R45.6
- **Viosterol deficiency** *—see* Deficiency, calciferol
- **Vipoma** *—see* Neoplasm, malignant, by site
- **Viremia** B34.9
- **Virilism** (adrenal) E25.9
  - congenital E25.0
- **Virilization** (female) (suprarenal) E25.9
  - congenital E25.0
  - isosexual E28.2
- **Virulent bubo** A57
- **Virus, viral** *—see also* condition
  - as cause of disease classified elsewhere B97.89
  - cytomegalovirus B25.9
  - human immunodeficiency (HIV) *—see* Human, immunodeficiency virus (HIV) disease
  - infection *—see* Infection, virus
  - specified NEC B34.8
  - swine influenza (viruses that normally cause infections in pigs) (*see also* Influenza, due to, identified novel influenza A virus) J09.X2
  - West Nile (fever) A92.30
    - with
      - complications NEC A92.39
      - cranial nerve disorders A92.32
      - encephalitis A92.31
      - encephalomyelitis A92.31

Virus, viral *(continued)*
- West Nile *(continued)*
  - with *(continued)*
    - neurologic manifestation NEC A92.32
    - optic neuritis A92.32
    - polyradiculitis A92.32

Viscera, visceral *—see* condition

Visceroptosis K63.4

Visible peristalsis R19.2

Vision, visual
- binocular, suppression H53.34
- blurred, blurring H53.8
  - hysterical F44.6
- defect, defective NEC H54.7
- disorientation (syndrome) H53.8
- disturbance H53.9
  - hysterical F44.6
- double H53.2
- examination Z01.00
  - with abnormal findings Z01.01
- field, limitation (defect) *—see* Defect, visual field
- hallucinations R44.1
- halos H53.19
- loss *—see* Loss, vision
  - sudden *—see* Disturbance, vision, subjective, loss, sudden
- low (both eyes) *—see* Low, vision
- perception, simultaneous without fusion H53.33

Vitality, lack or want of R53.83
- newborn P96.89

Vitamin deficiency *—see* Deficiency, vitamin

Vitelline duct, persistent Q43.0

Vitiligo L80
- eyelid H02.739
  - left H02.736
    - lower H02.735
    - upper H02.734
  - right H02.733
    - lower H02.732
    - upper H02.731
- pinta A67.2
- vulva N90.89

Vitreal corneal syndrome H59.01-

Vitreoretinopathy, proliferative *—see also* Retinopathy, proliferative
- with retinal detachment *—see* Detachment, retina, traction

Vitreous *—see also* condition
- touch syndrome *—see* Complication, postprocedural, following cataract surgery

Vocal cord *—see* condition

Vogt-Koyanagi syndrome H20.82-

Vogt's disease or syndrome G80.3

Vogt-Spielmeyer amaurotic idiocy or disease E75.4

Voice
- change R49.9
  - specified NEC R49.8
- loss *—see* Aphonia

Volhynian fever A79.0

Volkmann's ischemic contracture or paralysis (complicating trauma) T79.6

Volvulus (bowel) (colon) (intestine) K56.2
- with perforation K56.2
- congenital Q43.8

Volvulus *(continued)*
- duodenum K31.5
- fallopian tube *—see* Torsion, fallopian tube
- oviduct *—see* Torsion, fallopian tube
- stomach (due to absence of gastrocolic ligament) K31.89

Vomiting R11.10
- with nausea R11.2
- asphyxia *—see* Foreign body, by site, causing asphyxia, gastric contents
- bilious (cause unknown) R11.14
  - in newborn P92.01
  - following gastro-intestinal surgery K91.0
- blood *—see* Hematemesis
- causing asphyxia, choking, or suffocation *—see* Foreign body, by site
- cyclical G43.A0
  - with refractory migraine G43.A1
  - intractable G43.A1
  - not intractable G43.A0
  - psychogenic F50.89
  - without refractory migraine G43.A0
- fecal mater R11.13
- following gastrointestinal surgery K91.0
  - psychogenic F50.89
- functional K31.89
- hysterical F50.89
- nervous F50.89
- neurotic F50.89
- newborn NEC P92.09
  - bilious P92.01
- periodic R11.10
  - psychogenic F50.89
- projectile R11.12
- psychogenic F50.89
- uremic *—see* Uremia
- without nausea R11.11

Vomito negro *—see* Fever, yellow

Von Bezold's abscess *—see* Mastoiditis, acute

Von Economo-Cruchet disease A85.8

Von Eulenburg's disease G71.19

Von Gierke's disease E74.01

Von Hippel (-Lindau) **disease or syndrome** Q85.8

Von Jaksch's anemia or disease D64.89

Von Recklinghausen
- disease (neurofibromatosis) Q85.01
  - bones E21.0

Von Schroetter's syndrome I82.890

Von Willebrand (-Jurgens) (-Minot) **disease or syndrome** D68.0

Von Zumbusch's disease L40.1

Voyeurism F65.3

Vrolik's disease Q78.0

Vulva *—see* condition

Vulvismus N94.2

Vulvitis (acute) (allergic) (atrophic) (hypertrophic) (intertriginous) (senile) N76.2
- with ectopic or molar pregnancy O08.0
- adhesive, congenital Q52.79
- blennorrhagic (gonococcal) A54.02

Vulvitis *(continued)*
- blennorrhagic *(continued)*
- candidal B37.3
- chlamydial A56.02
- due to Haemophilus ducreyi A57
- following ectopic or molar pregnancy O08.0
- gonococcal A54.02
  - with abscess (accessory gland) (periurethral) A54.1
- herpesviral A60.04
- leukoplakic N90.4
- monilial B37.3
- puerperal (postpartum) O86.19
- subacute or chronic N76.3
- syphilitic (early) A51.0
  - late A52.76
- trichomonal A59.01
- tuberculous A18.18

Vulvodynia N94.819
- specified NEC N94.818

Vulvorectal *—see* condition

Vulvovaginitis (acute) *—see* Vaginitis

W

Waiting list, person on Z75.1
- for organ transplant Z76.82
- undergoing social agency investigation Z75.2

Waldenström-Kjellberg syndrome D50.1

Waldenström
- hypergammaglobulinemia D89.0
- syndrome or macroglobulinemia C88.0

Walking
- difficulty R26.2
  - psychogenic F44.4
- sleep F51.3
  - hysterical F44.89

Wall, abdominal *—see* condition

Wallenberg's disease or syndrome G46.3

Wallgren's disease I87.8

Wandering
- gallbladder, congenital Q44.1
- in diseases classified elsewhere Z91.83
- kidney, congenital Q63.8
- organ or site, congenital NEC *—see* Malposition, congenital, by site
- pacemaker (heart) I49.8
- spleen D73.89

War neurosis F48.8

Wart (due to HPV) (filiform) (infectious) (viral) B07.9
- anogenital region (venereal) A63.0
- common B07.8
- external genital organs (venereal) A63.0
- flat B07.8
- Hassal-Henle's (of cornea) H18.49
- Peruvian A44.1
- plantar B07.0
- prosector (tuberculous) A18.4
- seborrheic L82.1
  - inflamed L82.0
- senile (seborrheic) L82.1
  - inflamed L82.0
- tuberculous A18.4
- venereal A63.0

Warthin's tumor *—see* Neoplasm, salivary gland, benign

Wassilieff's disease A27.0

Wasting
- disease R64
  - due to malnutrition E41
- extreme (due to malnutrition) E41
- muscle NEC *—see* Atrophy, muscle

Water
- clefts (senile cataract) *—see* Cataract, senile, incipient
- deprivation of T73.1
- intoxication E87.79
- itch B76.9
- lack of T73.1
- loading E87.70
- on
  - brain *—see* Hydrocephalus
  - chest J94.8
- poisoning E87.79

Waterbrash R12

Waterhouse (-Friderichsen) **syndrome or disease** (meningococcal) A39.1

Water-losing nephritis N25.89

Watermelon stomach K31.819
- with hemorrhage K31.811
- without hemorrhage K31.819

Watsoniasis B66.8

Wax in ear *—see* Impaction, cerumen

Weak, weakening, weakness (generalized) R53.1
- arches (acquired) *—see also* Deformity, limb, flat foot
- bladder (sphincter) R32
- facial R29.810
  - following
    - cerebrovascular disease I69.992
      - cerebral infarction I69.392
      - intracerebral hemorrhage I69.192
      - nontraumatic intracranial hemorrhage NEC I69.292
      - specified disease NEC I69.892
      - stroke I69.392
      - subarachnoid hemorrhage I69.092
- foot (double) *—see* Weak, arches
- heart, cardiac *—see* Failure, heart
- mind F70
- muscle M62.81
- myocardium *—see* Failure, heart
- newborn P96.89
- pelvic fundus N81.89
- pubocervical tissue N81.82
- senile R54
- rectovaginal tissue N81.83
- urinary stream R39.12
- valvular *—see* Endocarditis

Wear, worn (with normal or routine use)
- articular bearing surface of internal joint prosthesis *—see* Complications, joint prosthesis, mechanical, wear of articular bearing surfaces, by site
- device, implant or graft *—see* Complications, by site, mechanical complication
- tooth, teeth (approximal) (hard tissues) (interproximal) (occlusal) K03.0

Weather, weathered
- effects of
  - cold T69.9
    - specified effect NEC T69.8
  - hot *—see* Heat
- skin L57.8

Weaver's syndrome Q87.3
Web, webbed (congenital)
  duodenal Q43.8
  esophagus Q39.4
  fingers Q70.1-
  larynx (glottic) (subglottic) Q31.0
  neck (pterygium colli) Q18.3
  Paterson-Kelly D50.1
  popliteal syndrome Q87.89
  toes Q70.3-
Weber-Christian disease M35.6
Weber-Cockayne syndrome (epidermolysis bullosa) Q81.8
Weber-Gubler syndrome G46.3
Weber-Leyden syndrome G46.3
Weber-Osler syndrome I78.0
Weber's paralysis or syndrome G46.3
Wedge-shaped or wedging vertebra —*see* Collapse, vertebra NEC
Wegener's granulomatosis or syndrome M31.30
  with
    kidney involvement M31.31
    lung involvement M31.30
      with kidney involvement M31.31
Wegner's disease A50.02
Weight
  1000-2499 grams at birth (low) —*see* Low, birthweight
  999 grams or less at birth (extremely low) —*see* Low, birthweight, extreme
  and length below 10th percentile for gestational age P05.1-
  below but length above 10th percentile for gestational age P05.0-
  gain (abnormal) (excessive) R63.5
    in pregnancy —*see* Pregnancy, complicated by, excessive weight gain
      low —*see* Pregnancy, complicated by, insufficient, weight gain
  loss (abnormal) (cause unknown) R63.4
Weightlessness (effect of) T75.82
Weil (l)-Marchesani syndrome Q87.1
Weil's disease A27.0
Weingarten's syndrome J82
Weir Mitchell's disease I73.81
Weiss-Baker syndrome G90.09
Wells' disease L98.3
Wen —*see* Cyst, sebaceous
Wenckebach's block or phenomenon I44.1
Werdnig-Hoffmann syndrome (muscular atrophy) G12.0
Werlhof's disease D69.3
Wermer's disease or syndrome E31.21
Werner-His disease A79.0
Werner's disease or syndrome E34.8
Wernicke-Korsakoff's syndrome or psychosis (alcoholic) F10.96
  with dependence F10.26
  drug-induced
    due to drug abuse —*see* Abuse, drug, by type, with amnestic disorder
    due to drug dependence —*see* Dependence, drug, by type, with amnestic disorder
  nonalcoholic F04
Wernicke-Posadas disease B38.9
Wernicke's
  developmental aphasia F80.2
  disease or syndrome E51.2
  encephalopathy E51.2
  polioencephalitis, superior E51.2
West African fever B50.8
Westphal-Strümpell syndrome E83.01
West's syndrome —*see* Epilepsy, spasms
Wet
  feet, tropical (maceration) (syndrome) —*see* Immersion, foot
  lung (syndrome), newborn P22.1
Wharton's duct —*see* condition
Wheal —*see* Urticaria
Wheezing R06.2
Whiplash injury S13.4
Whipple's disease (*see also* subcategory M14.8-) K90.81
Whipworm (disease) (infection) (infestation) B79
Whistling face Q87.0
White —*see also* condition
  kidney, small N03.9
  leg, puerperal, postpartum, childbirth O87.1
  mouth B37.0
  patches of mouth K13.29
  spot lesions, teeth
    chewing surface K02.51
    pit and fissure surface K02.51
    smooth surface K02.61
Whitehead L70.0
Whitlow —*see also* Cellulitis, digit
  with lymphangitis —*see* Lymphangitis, acute, digit
  herpesviral B00.89
Whitmore's disease or fever —*see* Melioidosis
Whooping cough A37.90
  with pneumonia A37.91
    due to Bordetella
      bronchiseptica A37.81
      parapertussis A37.11
      pertussis A37.01
    specified organism NEC A37.81
  due to
    Bordetella
      bronchiseptica A37.80
        with pneumonia A37.81
      parapertussis A37.10
        with pneumonia A37.11
      pertussis A37.00
        with pneumonia A37.01
      specified NEC A37.80
        with pneumonia A37.81
Wichman's asthma J38.5
Wide cranial sutures, newborn P96.3
Widening aorta —*see* Ectasia, aorta
  with aneurysm —*see* Aneurysm, aorta
Wilkie's disease or syndrome K55.1
Wilkinson-Sneddon disease or syndrome L13.1
Willebrand (-Jürgens) **thrombopathy** D68.0
Willige-Hunt disease or syndrome G23.1
Wilms' tumor C64-
Wilson-Mikity syndrome P27.0
Wilson's
  disease or syndrome E83.01
  hepatolenticular degeneration E83.01
  lichen ruber L43.9
Window —*see also* Imperfect, closure
  aorticopulmonary Q21.4
Winter —*see* condition
Wiskott-Aldrich syndrome D82.0
Withdrawal state —*see also* Dependence, drug by type, with withdrawal
  alcohol
    with perceptual disturbances F10.232
    without perceptual disturbances F10.239
  caffeine F15.93
  cannabis F12.288
  newborn
    correct therapeutic substance properly administered P96.2
    infant of dependent mother P96.1
  therapeutic substance, neonatal P96.2
Witts' anemia D50.8
Witzelsucht F07.0
Woakes' ethmoiditis or syndrome J33.1
Wolff-Hirschorn syndrome Q93.3
Wolff-Parkinson-White syndrome I45.6
Wolhynian fever A79.0
Wolman's disease E75.5
Wood lung or pneumonitis J67.8
Woolly, wooly hair (congenital) (nevus) Q84.1
Woolsorter's disease A22.1
Word
  blindness (congenital) (developmental) F81.0
  deafness (congenital) (developmental) H93.25
Worm(s) (infection) (infestation) —*see also* Infestation, helminth
  guinea B72
  in intestine NEC B82.0
Worm-eaten soles A66.3
Worn out —*see* Exhaustion
  cardiac
    defibrillator (with synchronous cardiace pacemaker) Z45.02
    pacemaker
      battery Z45.010
      lead Z45.018
  device, implant or graft —*see* Complications, by site, mechanical
Worried well Z71.1
Worries R45.82
Wound check Z48.0-
  due to injury - code to Injury, by site, using appropriate seventh character for subsequent encounter
Wound, open T14.8-
  abdomen, abdominal
    wall S31.109
      with penetration into peritoneal cavity S31.609
      bite —*see* Bite, abdomen, wall
      epigastric region S31.102
        with penetration into peritoneal cavity S31.602
Wound, open *(continued)*
  abdomen, abdominal *(continued)*
    wall *(continued)*
      epigastric region *(continued)*
        bite —*see* Bite, abdomen, wall, epigastric region
        laceration —*see* Laceration, abdomen, wall, epigastric region
        puncture —*see* Puncture, abdomen, wall, epigastric region
      laceration —*see* Laceration, abdomen, wall
      left
        lower quadrant S31.104
          with penetration into peritoneal cavity S31.604
          bite —*see* Bite, abdomen, wall, left, lower quadrant
          laceration —*see* Laceration, abdomen, wall, left, lower quadrant
          puncture —*see* Puncture, abdomen, wall, left, lower quadrant
        upper quadrant S31.101
          with penetration into peritoneal cavity S31.601
          bite —*see* Bite, abdomen, wall, left, upper quadrant
          laceration —*see* Laceration, abdomen, wall, left, upper quadrant
          puncture —*see* Puncture, abdomen, wall, left, upper quadrant
      periumbilic region S31.105
        with penetration into peritoneal cavity S31.605
        bite —*see* Bite, abdomen, wall, periumbilic region
        laceration —*see* Laceration, abdomen, wall, periumbilic region
        puncture —*see* Puncture, abdomen, wall, periumbilic region
      puncture —*see* Puncture, abdomen, wall
      right
        lower quadrant S31.103
          with penetration into peritoneal cavity S31.603
          bite —*see* Bite, abdomen, wall, right, lower quadrant
          laceration —*see* Laceration, abdomen, wall, right, lower quadrant
          puncture —*see* Puncture, abdomen, wall, right, lower quadrant
        upper quadrant S31.100
          with penetration into peritoneal cavity S31.600
          bite —*see* Bite, abdomen, wall, right, upper quadrant

Wound, open *(continued)*
  abdomen, abdominal *(continued)*
    wall *(continued)*
      right *(continued)*
        upper quadrant *(continued)*
          laceration —*see* Laceration, abdomen, wall, right, upper quadrant
          puncture —*see* Puncture, abdomen, wall, right, upper quadrant
  alveolar (process) —*see* Wound, open, oral cavity
  ankle S91.00-
    bite —*see* Bite, ankle
    laceration —*see* Laceration, ankle
    puncture —*see* Puncture, ankle
  antecubital space —*see* Wound, open, elbow
  anterior chamber, eye —*see* Wound, open, ocular
  anus S31.839
    bite S31.835
    laceration —*see* Laceration, anus
    puncture —*see* Puncture, anus
  arm (upper) S41.10-
    with amputation —*see* Amputation, traumatic, arm
    bite —*see* Bite, arm
    forearm —*see* Wound, open, forearm
    laceration —*see* Laceration, arm
    puncture —*see* Puncture, arm
  auditory canal (external) (meatus) —*see* Wound, open, ear
  auricle, ear —*see* Wound, open, ear
  axilla —*see* Wound, open, arm
  back —*see also* Wound, open, thorax, back
    lower S31.000
      with penetration into retroperitoneal space S31.001
      bite —*see* Bite, back, lower
      laceration —*see* Laceration, back, lower
      puncture —*see* Puncture, back, lower
  bite —*see* Bite
  blood vessel —*see* Injury, blood vessel
  breast S21.00-
    with amputation —*see* Amputation, traumatic, breast
    bite —*see* Bite, breast
    laceration —*see* Laceration, breast
    puncture —*see* Puncture, breast
  buttock S31.809
    bite —*see* Bite, buttock
    laceration —*see* Laceration, buttock
    left S31.829
    puncture —*see* Puncture, buttock
    right S31.819
  calf —*see* Wound, open, leg
  canaliculus lacrimalis —*see* Wound, open, eyelid
  canthus, eye —*see* Wound, open, eyelid
  cervical esophagus S11.20
    bite S11.25
    laceration —*see* Laceration, esophagus, traumatic, cervical
    puncture —*see* Puncture, cervical esophagus
  cheek (external) S01.40-
    bite —*see* Bite, cheek
    laceration —*see* Laceration, cheek

Wound, open *(continued)*
  cheek *(continued)*
    laceration *(continued)*
    puncture —*see* Puncture, cheek
    internal —*see* Wound, open, oral cavity
  chest wall —*see* Wound, open, thorax
  chin —*see* Wound, open, head, specified site NEC
  choroid —*see* Wound, open, ocular
  ciliary body (eye) —*see* Wound, open, ocular
  clitoris S31.40
    with amputation —*see* Amputation, traumatic, clitoris
    bite S31.45
    laceration —*see* Laceration, vulva
    puncture —*see* Puncture, vulva
  conjunctiva —*see* Wound, open, ocular
  cornea —*see* Wound, open, ocular
  costal region —*see* Wound, open, thorax
  Descemet's membrane —*see* Wound, open, ocular
  digit(s)
    foot —*see* Wound, open, toe
    hand —*see* Wound, open, finger
  ear (canal) (external) S01.30-
    with amputation —*see* Amputation, traumatic, ear
    bite —*see* Bite, ear
    laceration —*see* Laceration, ear
    puncture —*see* Puncture, ear
    drum S09.2-
  elbow S51.00-
    bite —*see* Bite, elbow
    laceration —*see* Laceration, elbow
    puncture —*see* Puncture, elbow
  epididymis —*see* Wound, open, testis
  epigastric region S31.102
    with penetration into peritoneal cavity S31.602
    bite —*see* Bite, abdomen, wall, epigastric region
    laceration —*see* Laceration, abdomen, wall, epigastric region
    puncture —*see* Puncture, abdomen, wall, epigastric region
  epiglottis —*see* Wound, open, neck, specified site NEC
  esophagus (thoracic) S27.819
    cervical —*see* Wound, open, cervical esophagus
    laceration S27.813
    specified type NEC S27.818
  eye —*see* Wound, open, ocular
  eyeball —*see* Wound, open, ocular
  eyebrow —*see* Wound, open, eyelid
  eyelid S01.10-
    bite —*see* Bite, eyelid
    laceration —*see* Laceration, eyelid
    puncture —*see* Puncture, eyelid
  face NEC —*see* Wound, open, head, specified site NEC
  finger(s) S61.209
    with
      amputation —*see* Amputation, traumatic, finger
      damage to nail S61.309
    bite —*see* Bite, finger
    index S61.208
      with
        damage to nail S61.308
      left S61.201

Wound, open *(continued)*
  finger *(continued)*
    index *(continued)*
      left *(continued)*
        damage to nail *(continued)*
        with
          damage to nail S61.301
      right S61.200
        with
          damage to nail S61.300
    laceration —*see* Laceration, finger
    little S61.208
      with
        damage to nail S61.308
      left S61.207
        with damage to nail S61.307
      right S61.206
        with damage to nail S61.306
    middle S61.208
      with
        damage to nail S61.308
      left S61.203
        with damage to nail S61.303
      right S61.202
        with damage to nail S61.302
    puncture —*see* Puncture, finger
    ring S61.208
      with
        damage to nail S61.308
      left S61.205
        with damage to nail S61.305
      right S61.204
        with damage to nail S61.304
  flank —*see* Wound, open, abdomen, wall
  foot (except toe(s) alone) S91.30-
    with amputation —*see* Amputation, traumatic, foot
    bite —*see* Bite, foot
    laceration —*see* Laceration, foot
    puncture —*see* Puncture, foot
    toe —*see* Wound, open, toe
  forearm S51.80-
    with
      amputation —*see* Amputation, traumatic, forearm
    bite —*see* Bite, forearm
    elbow only —*see* Wound, open, elbow
    laceration —*see* Laceration, forearm
    puncture —*see* Puncture, forearm
  forehead —*see* Wound, open, head, specified site NEC
  genital organs, external
    with amputation —*see* Amputation, traumatic, genital organs
    bite —*see* Bite, genital organ
    female S31.502
      vagina S31.40
      vulva S31.40
    laceration —*see* Laceration, genital organ
    male S31.501
      penis S31.20
      scrotum S31.30
      testes S31.30
    puncture —*see* Puncture, genital organ
  globe (eye) —*see* Wound, open, ocular
  groin —*see* Wound, open, abdomen, wall
  gum —*see* Wound, open, oral cavity
  hand S61.40-
    with
      amputation —*see* Amputation, traumatic, hand
    bite —*see* Bite, hand

Wound, open *(continued)*
  hand *(continued)*
    finger(s) —*see* Wound, open, finger
    laceration —*see* Laceration, hand
    puncture —*see* Puncture, hand
    thumb —*see* Wound, open, thumb
  head S01.90
    bite —*see* Bite, head
    cheek —*see* Wound, open, cheek
    ear —*see* Wound, open, ear
    eyelid —*see* Wound, open, eyelid
    laceration —*see* Laceration, head
    lip —*see* Wound, open, lip
    nose S01.20
    oral cavity —*see* Wound, open, oral cavity
    puncture —*see* Puncture, head
    scalp —*see* Wound, open, scalp
    specified site NEC S01.80
    temporomandibular area —*see* Wound, open, cheek
  heel —*see* Wound, open, foot
  hip S71.00-
    with amputation —*see* Amputation, traumatic, hip
    bite —*see* Bite, hip
    laceration —*see* Laceration, hip
    puncture —*see* Puncture, hip
  hymen S31.40
    bite —*see* Bite, vulva
    laceration —*see* Laceration, vagina
    puncture —*see* Puncture, vagina
  hypochondrium S31.109
    bite —*see* Bite, hypochondrium
    laceration —*see* Laceration, hypochondrium
    puncture —*see* Puncture, hypochondrium
  hypogastric region S31.109
    bite —*see* Bite, hypogastric region
    laceration —*see* Laceration, hypogastric region
    puncture —*see* Puncture, hypogastric region
  iliac (region) —*see* Wound, open, inguinal region
  inguinal region S31.109
    bite —*see* Bite, abdomen, wall, lower quadrant
    laceration —*see* Laceration, inguinal region
    puncture —*see* Puncture, inguinal region
  instep —*see* Wound, open, foot
  interscapular region —*see* Wound, open, thorax, back
  intraocular —*see* Wound, open, ocular
  iris —*see* Wound, open, ocular
  jaw —*see* Wound, open, head, specified site NEC
  knee S81.00-
    bite —*see* Bite, knee
    laceration —*see* Laceration, knee
    puncture —*see* Puncture, knee
  labium (majus) (minus) —*see* Wound, open, vulva
  laceration —*see* Laceration, by site
  lacrimal duct —*see* Wound, open, eyelid
  larynx S11.019
    bite —*see* Bite, larynx
    laceration —*see* Laceration, larynx
    puncture —*see* Puncture, larynx

, open *(continued)*
wer quadrant S31.104
with penetration into peritoneal cavity S31.604
bite *—see* Bite, abdomen, wall, left, lower quadrant
laceration *—see* Laceration, abdomen, wall, left, lower quadrant
puncture *—see* Puncture, abdomen, wall, left, lower quadrant
per quadrant S31.101
with penetration into peritoneal cavity S31.601
bite *—see* Bite, abdomen, wall, left, upper quadrant
laceration *—see* Laceration, abdomen, wall, left, upper quadrant
puncture *—see* Puncture, abdomen, wall, left, upper quadrant
lower) S81.80-
ith amputation *—see* Amputation, traumatic, leg
kle *—see* Wound, open, ankle
te *—see* Bite, leg
ot *—see* Wound, open, foot
iee *—see* Wound, open, knee
ceration *—see* Laceration, leg
incture *—see* Puncture, leg
e *—see* Wound, open, toe
pper *—see* Wound, open, thigh
01.501
te *—see* Bite, lip
ceration *—see* Laceration, lip
uncture *—see* Puncture, lip
S31.109
te *—see* Bite, abdomen, wall
ceration *—see* Laceration, loin
uncture *—see* Puncture, loin
er back *—see* Wound, open, ack, lower
bar region *—see* Wound, open, ack, lower
ar region *—see* Wound, open, ead, specified site NEC
nmary *—see* Wound, open, reast
toid region *—see* Wound, open, ead, specified site NEC
th *—see* Wound, open, oral avity

nger *—see* Wound, open, finger, with damage to nail
e *—see* Wound, open, toe, with damage to nail
e (neck) *—see* Wound, open, eck
l (septum) (sinus) *—see* Wound, pen, nose
pharynx *—see* Wound, open, ead, specified site NEC
S11.90
te *—see* Bite, neck
nvolving
cervical esophagus S11.20
larynx *—see* Wound, open, larynx
pharynx S11.20
thyroid S11.10
trachea (cervical) S11.029
bite *—see* Bite, trachea
laceration S11.021

Wound, open *(continued)*
neck *(continued)*
involving *(continued)*
trachea *(continued)*
laceration *(continued)*
with foreign body S11.022
puncture S11.023
with foreign body S11.024
laceration *—see* Laceration, neck
puncture *—see* Puncture, neck
specified site NEC S11.80
specified type NEC S11.89
nose (septum) (sinus) S01.20
with amputation *—see* Amputation, traumatic, nose
bite *—see* Bite, nose
laceration *—see* Laceration, nose
puncture *—see* Puncture, nose
ocular S05.90
avulsion (traumatic enucleation) S05.7-
eyeball S05.6-
with foreign body S05.5-
eyelid *—see* Wound, open, eyelid
laceration and rupture S05.3-
with prolapse or loss of intraocular tissue S05.2-
orbit (penetrating) (with or without foreign body) S05.4-
periocular area *—see* Wound, open, eyelid
specified NEC S05.8X-
oral cavity S01.502
bite S01.552
laceration *—see* Laceration, oral cavity
puncture *—see* Puncture, oral cavity
orbit *—see* Wound, open, ocular, orbit
palate *—see* Wound, open, oral cavity
palm *—see* Wound, open, hand
pelvis, pelvic *—see also* Wound, open, back, lower
girdle *—see* Wound, open, hip
penetrating *—see* Puncture, by site
penis S31.20
with amputation *—see* Amputation, traumatic, penis
bite S31.25
laceration *—see* Laceration, penis
puncture *—see* Puncture, penis
perineum
bite *—see* Bite, perineum
female S31.502
laceration *—see* Laceration, perineum
male S31.501
puncture *—see* Puncture, perineum
periocular area (with or without lacrimal passages) *—see* Wound, open, eyelid
periumbilic region S31.105
with penetration into peritoneal cavity S31.605
bite *—see* Bite, abdomen, wall, periumbilic region
laceration *—see* Laceration, abdomen, wall, periumbilic region
puncture *—see* Puncture, abdomen, wall, periumbilic region
phalanges
finger *—see* Wound, open, finger
toe *—see* Wound, open, toe
pharynx S11.20

Wound, open *(continued)*
pinna *—see* Wound, open, ear
popliteal space *—see* Wound, open, knee
prepuce *—see* Wound, open, penis
pubic region *—see* Wound, open, back, lower
pudendum *—see* Wound, open, genital organs, external
puncture wound *—see* Puncture
rectovaginal septum *—see* Wound, open, vagina
right
lower quadrant S31.103
with penetration into peritoneal cavity S31.603
bite *—see* Bite, abdomen, wall, right, lower quadrant
laceration *—see* Laceration, abdomen, wall, right, lower quadrant
puncture *—see* Puncture, abdomen, wall, right, lower quadrant
upper quadrant S31.100
with penetration into peritoneal cavity S31.600
bite *—see* Bite, abdomen, wall, right, upper quadrant
laceration *—see* Laceration, abdomen, wall, right, upper quadrant
puncture *—see* Puncture, abdomen, wall, right, upper quadrant
sacral region *—see* Wound, open, back, lower
sacroiliac region *—see* Wound, open, back, lower
salivary gland *—see* Wound, open, oral cavity
scalp S01.00
bite S01.05
laceration *—see* Laceration, scalp
puncture *—see* Puncture, scalp
scalpel, newborn (birth injury) P15.8
scapular region *—see* Wound, open, shoulder
sclera *—see* Wound, open, ocular
scrotum S31.30
with amputation *—see* Amputation, traumatic, scrotum
bite S31.35
laceration *—see* Laceration, scrotum
puncture *—see* Puncture, scrotum
shin *—see* Wound, open, leg
shoulder S41.00-
with amputation *—see* Amputation, traumatic, arm
bite *—see* Bite, shoulder
laceration *—see* Laceration, shoulder
puncture *—see* Puncture, shoulder
skin NOS T14.8
spermatic cord *—see* Wound, open, testis
sternal region *—see* Wound, open, thorax, front wall
submaxillary region *—see* Wound, open, head, specified site NEC
submental region *—see* Wound, open, head, specified site NEC
subungual
finger(s) *—see* Wound, open, finger
toe(s) *—see* Wound, open, toe
supraclavicular region *—see* Wound, open, neck, specified site NEC

Wound, open *(continued)*
temple, temporal region *—see* Wound, open, head, specified site NEC
temporomandibular area *—see* Wound, open, cheek
testis S31.30
with amputation *—see* Amputation, traumatic, testes
bite S31.35
laceration *—see* Laceration, testis
puncture *—see* Puncture, testis
thigh S71.10-
with amputation *—see* Amputation, traumatic, hip
bite *—see* Bite, thigh
laceration *—see* Laceration, thigh
puncture *—see* Puncture, thigh
thorax, thoracic (wall) S21.90
back S21.20-
with penetration S21.40
bite *—see* Bite, thorax
breast *—see* Wound, open, breast
front S21.10-
with penetration S21.30
laceration *—see* Laceration, thorax
puncture *—see* Puncture, thorax
throat *—see* Wound, open, neck
thumb S61.009
with
amputation *—see* Amputation, traumatic, thumb
damage to nail S61.109
bite *—see* Bite, thumb
laceration *—see* Laceration, thumb
left S61.002
with
damage to nail S61.102
puncture *—see* Puncture, thumb
right S61.001
with
damage to nail S61.101
thyroid (gland) *—see* Wound, open, neck, thyroid
toe(s) S91.109
with
amputation *—see* Amputation, traumatic, toe
damage to nail S91.209
bite *—see* Bite, toe
great S91.103
with
damage to nail S91.203
left S91.102
with
damage to nail S91.202
right S91.101
with
damage to nail S91.201
laceration *—see* Laceration, toe
lesser S91.106
with
damage to nail S91.206
left S91.105
with
damage to nail S91.205
right S91.104
with
damage to nail S91.204
puncture *—see* Puncture, toe
tongue *—see* Wound, open, oral cavity
trachea (cervical region) *—see* Wound, open, neck, trachea
tunica vaginalis *—see* Wound, open, testis

Wound, open *(continued)*
tympanum, tympanic membrane S09.2-
laceration —*see* Laceration, ear, drum
puncture —*see* Puncture, tympanum
umbilical region —*see* Wound, open, abdomen, wall, periumbilic region
uvula —*see* Wound, open, oral cavity
vagina S31.40
bite S31.45
laceration —*see* Laceration, vagina
puncture —*see* Puncture, vagina
vocal cord S11.039
bite —*see* Bite, vocal cord
laceration S11.031
with foreign body S11.032
puncture S11.033
with foreign body S11.034
vitreous (humor) —*see* Wound, open, ocular
vulva S31.40
with amputation —*see* Amputation, traumatic, vulva
bite S31.45
laceration —*see* Laceration, vulva
puncture —*see* Puncture, vulva
wrist S61.50-
bite —*see* Bite, wrist
laceration —*see* Laceration, wrist
puncture —*see* Puncture, wrist

Wound, superficial —*see* Injury —*see also* specified injury type

Wright's syndrome G54.0

Wrist —*see* condition

Wrong drug (by accident) (given in error) —*see* Table of Drugs and Chemicals, by drug, poisoning

Wry neck —*see* Torticollis

Wuchereria (bancrofti) **infestation** B74.0

Wuchereriasis B74.0

Wuchernde Struma Langhans C73

X

Xanthelasma (eyelid) (palpebrarum) H02.60
left H02.66
lower H02.65
upper H02.64
right H02.63
lower H02.62
upper H02.61

Xanthelasmatosis (essential) E78.2

Xanthinuria, hereditary E79.8

Xanthoastrocytoma
specified site —*see* Neoplasm, malignant, by site
unspecified site C71.9

Xanthofibroma —*see* Neoplasm, connective tissue, benign

Xanthogranuloma D76.3

Xanthoma(s), xanthomatosis (primary) (familial) (hereditary) E75.5
with
hyperlipoproteinemia
Type I E78.3
Type III E78.2
Type IV E78.1
Type V E78.3
bone (generalisata) C96.5
cerebrotendinous E75.5
cutaneotendinous E75.5
disseminatum (skin) E78.2
eruptive E78.2
hypercholesterinemic E78.00
hypercholesterolemic E78.00
hyperlipidemic E78.5
joint E75.5
multiple (skin) E78.2
tendon (sheath) E75.5
tubo-eruptive E78.2
tuberosum E78.2
tuberous E78.2
verrucous, oral mucosa K13.4

Xanthosis R23.8

Xenophobia F40.10

Xeroderma —*see also* Ichthyosis
acquired L85.0
eyelid H01.149
left H01.146
lower H01.145
upper H01.144
right H01.143
lower H01.142
upper H01.141
pigmentosum Q82.1
vitamin A deficiency E50.8

Xerophthalmia (vitamin A deficiency) E50.7
unrelated to vitamin A deficiency —*see* Keratoconjunctivitis

Xerosis
conjunctiva H11.14-
with Bitot's spots —*see also* Pigmentation, conjunctiva
vitamin A deficiency E50.1
vitamin A deficiency E50.0
cornea H18.89-
with ulceration —*see* Ulcer, cornea
vitamin A deficiency E50.3
vitamin A deficiency E50.2
cutis L85.3
skin L85.3

Xerostomia K11.7

Xiphopagus Q89.4

XO syndrome Q96.9

X-ray (of)
abnormal findings —*see* Abnormal, diagnostic imaging
breast (mammogram) (routine) Z12.31
chest
routine (as part of a general medical examination) Z00.00
with abnormal findings Z00.01
routine (as part of a general medical examination) Z00.00
with abnormal findings Z00.01

XXXXY syndrome Q98.1

XXY syndrome Q98.0

Y

Yaba pox (virus disease) B08.72

Yatapoxvirus B08.70
specified NEC B08.79

Yawning R06.89
psychogenic F45.8

Yaws A66.9
bone lesions A66.6
butter A66.1
chancre A66.0
cutaneous, less than five years after infection A66.2
early (cutaneous) (macular) (maculopapular) (micropapular) (papular) A66.2
frambeside A66.2
skin lesions NEC A66.2
eyelid A66.2
ganglion A66.6
gangosis, gangosa A66.5
gumma, gummata A66.4
bone A66.6
gummatous
frambeside A66.4
osteitis A66.6
periostitis A66.6
hydrarthrosis (*see also* subcategory M14.8-) A66.6
hyperkeratosis (early) (late) A66.3
initial lesions A66.0
joint lesions (*see also* subcategory M14.8-) A66.6
juxta-articular nodules A66.7
late nodular (ulcerated) A66.4
latent (without clinical manifestations) (with positive serology) A66.8
mother A66.0
mucosal A66.7
multiple papillomata A66.1
nodular, late (ulcerated) A66.4
osteitis A66.6
papilloma, plantar or palmar A66.1
periostitis (hypertrophic) A66.6
specified NEC A66.7
ulcers A66.4
wet crab A66.1

Yeast infection (*see also* Candidiasis) B37.9

Yellow
atrophy (liver) —*see* Failure, hepatic
fever —*see* Fever, yellow
jack —*see* Fever, yellow
jaundice —*see* Jaundice
nail syndrome L60.5

Yersiniosis —*see also* Infection, Yersinia
extraintestinal A28.2
intestinal A04.6

Z

Zahorsky's syndrome (herpangina) B08.5

Zellweger's syndrome Q87.89

Zenker's diverticulum (esophagus) K22.5

Ziehen-Oppenheim disease G24.1

Zieve's syndrome K70.0

Zika NOS A92.5

Zinc
deficiency, dietary E60
metabolism disorder E83.2

Zollinger-Ellison syndrome E16.4

Zona —*see* Herpes, zoster

Zoophobia F40.218

Zoster (herpes) —*see* Herpes, zoster

Zygomycosis B46.9
specified NEC B46.8

Zymotic —*see* condition

Neoplasm Table Guidance

he Neoplasm Table gives the code numbers for neoplasms by anatomical site. For each site there are six possible code numbers according to /hether the neoplasm in question is malignant, benign, in situ, of uncertain behavior, or of unspecified nature. The description of the neoplasm /ill often indicate which of the six columns is appropriate; e.g., malignant melanoma of skin, benign fibroadenoma of breast, carcinoma in situ f cervix uteri.

Where such descriptors are not present, the remainder of the Index should be consulted where guidance is given to the appropriate column or each morphological (histological) variety listed; e.g., Mesonephroma—see Neoplasm, malignant; Embryoma—see also Neoplasm, uncertain ehavior; Disease, Bowen's—see Neoplasm, skin, in situ. However, the guidance in the Index can be overridden if one of the descriptors nentioned above is present; e.g., malignant adenoma of colon is coded to C18.9 and not to D12.6 as the adjective "malignant" overrides the Index ntry "Adenoma—see also Neoplasm, benign."

Codes listed with a dash -, following the code have a required additional character for laterality. The tabular must be reviewed for the omplete code.

Table of Neoplasms

	Malignant Primary	Malignant Secondary	Ca in situ	Benign	Uncertain Behavior	Unspecified Behavior
Neoplasm, neoplastic	C80.1	C79.9	D09.9	D36.9	D48.9	D49.9
A						
abdomen, abdominal	C76.2	C79.8-	D09.8	D36.7	D48.7	D49.89
cavity	C76.2	C79.8-	D09.8	D36.7	D48.7	D49.89
organ	C76.2	C79.8-	D09.8	D36.7	D48.7	D49.89
viscera	C76.2	C79.8-	D09.8	D36.7	D48.7	D49.89
wall—see also Neoplasm, abdomen, wall, skin	C44.509	C79.2	D04.5	D23.5	D48.5	D49.2
connective tissue	C49.4	C79.8-	-	D21.4	D48.1	D49.2
skin	C44.509					
basal cell carcinoma	C44.519	-	-	-	-	-
specified type NEC	C44.599	-	-	-	-	-
squamous cell carcinoma	C44.529	-	-	-	-	-
abdominopelvic	C76.8	C79.8-	-	D36.7	D48.7	D49.89
accessory sinus—see Neoplasm, sinus						
acoustic nerve	C72.4-	C79.49	-	D33.3	D43.3	D49.7
adenoid (pharynx) (tissue)	C11.1	C79.89	D00.08	D10.6	D37.05	D49.0
adipose tissue —see also Neoplasm, connective tissue	C49.4	C79.89	-	D21.9	D48.1	D49.2
adnexa (uterine)	C57.4	C79.89	D07.39	D28.7	D39.8	D49.59
adrenal	C74.9-	C79.7-	D09.3	D35.0-	D44.1-	D49.7
capsule	C74.9-	C79.7-	D09.3	D35.0-	D44.1-	D49.7
cortex	C74.0-	C79.7-	D09.3	D35.0-	D44.1-	D49.7
gland	C74.9-	C79.7-	D09.3	D35.0-	D44.1-	D49.7
medulla	C74.1-	C79.7-	D09.3	D35.0-	D44.1-	D49.7
ala nasi (external)—see also Neoplasm, skin, nose	C44.301	C79.2	D04.39	D23.39	D48.5	D49.2
alimentary canal or tract NEC	C26.9	C78.80	D01.9	D13.9	D37.9	D49.0
alveolar	C03.9	C79.89	D00.03	D10.39	D37.09	D49.0
mucosa	C03.9	C79.89	D00.03	D10.39	D37.09	D49.0
lower	C03.1	C79.89	D00.03	D10.39	D37.09	D49.0
upper	C03.0	C79.89	D00.03	D10.39	D37.09	D49.0
ridge or process	C41.1	C79.51	-	D16.5	D48.0	D49.2
carcinoma	C03.9	C79.8-	-	-	-	-
lower	C03.1	C79.8-	-	-	-	-
upper	C03.0	C79.8-	-	-	-	-
lower	C41.1	C79.51	-	D16.5-	D48.0	D49.2
mucosa	C03.9	C79.89	D00.03	D10.39	D37.09	D49.0
lower	C03.1	C79.89	D00.03	D10.39	D37.09	D49.0
upper	C03.0	C79.89	D00.03	D10.39	D37.09	D49.0
upper	C41.0	C79.51	-	D16.4-	D48.0	D49.2
sulcus	C06.1	C79.89	D00.02	D10.39	D37.09	D49.0
alveolus	C03.9	C79.89	D00.03	D10.39	D37.09	D49.0
lower	C03.1	C79.89	D00.03	D10.39	D37.09	D49.0
upper	C03.0	C79.89	D00.03	D10.39	D37.09	D49.0
ampulla of Vater	C24.1	C78.89	D01.5	D13.5	D37.6	D49.0
ankle NEC	C76.5-	C79.89	D04.7-	D36.7	D48.7	D49.89
anorectum, anorectal (junction)	C21.8	C78.5	D01.3	D12.9	D37.8	D49.0
antecubital fossa or space	C76.4-	C79.89	D04.6-	D36.7	D48.7	D49.89
antrum (Highmore) (maxillary)	C31.0	C78.39	D02.3	D14.0	D38.5	D49.1
pyloric	C16.3	C78.89	D00.2	D13.1	D37.1	D49.0
tympanicum	C30.1	C78.39	D02.3	D14.0	D38.5	D49.1
anus, anal	C21.0	C78.5	D01.3	D12.9	D37.8	D49.0
canal	C21.1	C78.5	D01.3	D12.9	D37.8	D49.0
cloacogenic zone	C21.2	C78.5	D01.3	D12.9	D37.8	D49.0
margin—see also Neoplasm, anus, skin	C44.500	C79.2	D04.5	D23.5	D48.5	D49.2
overlapping lesion with rectosigmoid junction or rectum	C21.8	-	-	-	-	-
skin	C44.500	C79.2	D04.5	D23.5	D48.5	D49.2
basal cell carcinoma	C44.510	-	-	-	-	-
specified type NEC	C44.590	-	-	-	-	-
squamous cell carcinoma	C44.520	-	-	-	-	-
sphincter	C21.1	C78.5	D01.3	D12.9	D37.8	D49.0
aorta (thoracic)	C49.3	C79.89	-	D21.3	D48.1	D49.2
abdominal	C49.4	C79.89	-	D21.4	D48.1	D49.2
aortic body	C75.5	C79.89	-	D35.6	D44.7	D49.7
aponeurosis	C49.9	C79.89	-	D21.9	D48.1	D49.2
palmar	C49.1-	C79.89	-	D21.1-	D48.1	D49.2
plantar	C49.2-	C79.89	-	D21.2-	D48.1	D49.2
appendix	C18.1	C78.5	D01.0	D12.1	D37.3	D49.0
arachnoid	C70.9	C79.49	-	D32.9	D42.9	D49.7
cerebral	C70.0	C79.32	-	D32.0	D42.0	D49.7
spinal	C70.1	C79.49	-	D32.1	D42.1	D49.7
areola	C50.0-	C79.81	D05.-	D24.-	D48.6-	D49.3
arm NEC	C76.4-	C79.89	D04.6-	D36.7	D48.7	D49.89
artery—see Neoplasm, connective tissue						
aryepiglottic fold	C13.1	C79.89	D00.08	D10.7	D37.05	D49.0
hypopharyngeal aspect	C13.1	C79.89	D00.08	D10.7	D37.05	D49.0
laryngeal aspect	C32.1	C78.39	D02.0	D14.1	D38.0	D49.1
marginal zone	C13.1	C79.89	D00.08	D10.7	D37.05	D49.0
arytenoid (cartilage)	C32.3	C78.39	D02.0	D14.1	D38.0	D49.1
fold—see Neoplasm, aryepiglottic						
associated with transplanted organ	C80.2	-	-	-	-	-
atlas	C41.2	C79.51	-	D16.6	D48.0	D49.2
atrium, cardiac	C38.0	C79.89	-	D15.1	D48.7	D49.89
auditory						
canal (external) (skin)	C44.20-	C79.2	D04.2-	D23.2-	D48.5	D49.2
internal	C30.1	C78.39	D02.3	D14.0	D38.5	D49.1
nerve	C72.4-	C79.49	-	D33.3	D43.3	D49.7
tube	C30.1	C78.39	D02.3	D14.0	D38.5	D49.1
opening	C11.2	C79.89	D00.08	D10.6	D37.05	D49.0

	Malignant Primary	Malignant Secondary	Ca in situ	Benign	Uncertain Behavior	Unspecified Behavior
auricle, ear—see also Neoplasm, skin, ear	C44.20-	C79.2	D04.2-	D23.2-	D48.5	D49.2
auricular canal (external)—see also Neoplasm, skin, ear	C44.20-	C79.2	D04.2-	D23.2-	D48.5	D49.2
internal	C30.1	C78.39	D02.3	D14.0	D38.5	D49.2
autonomic nerve or nervous system NEC (see Neoplasm, nerve, peripheral)						
axilla, axillary	C76.1	C79.89	D09.8	D36.7	D48.7	D49.89
fold—see also Neoplasm, skin, trunk	C44.509	C79.2	D04.5	D23.5	D48.5	D49.2
B						
back NEC	C76.8	C79.89	D04.5	D36.7	D48.7	D49.89
Bartholin's gland	C51.0	C79.82	D07.1	D28.0	D39.8	D49.59
basal ganglia	C71.0	C79.31	-	D33.0	D43.0	D49.6
basis pedunculi	C71.7	C79.31	-	D33.1	D43.1	D49.6
bile or biliary (tract)	C24.9	C78.89	D01.5	D13.5	D37.6	D49.0
canaliculi (biliferi) (intrahepatic)	C22.1	C78.7	D01.5	D13.4	D37.6	D49.0
canals, interlobular	C22.1	C78.89	D01.5	D13.4	D37.6	D49.0
duct or passage (common) (cystic) (extrahepatic)	C24.0	C78.89	D01.5	D13.5	D37.6	D49.0
interlobular	C22.1	C78.89	D01.5	D13.4	D37.6	D49.0
intrahepatic	C22.1	C78.7	D01.5	D13.4	D37.6	D49.0
and extrahepatic	C24.8	C78.89	D01.5	D13.5	D37.6	D49.0
bladder (urinary)	C67.9	C79.11	D09.0	D30.3	D41.4	D49.4
dome	C67.1	C79.11	D09.0	D30.3	D41.4	D49.4
neck	C67.5	C79.11	D09.0	D30.3	D41.4	D49.4
orifice	C67.9	C79.11	D09.0	D30.3	D41.4	D49.4
ureteric	C67.6	C79.11	D09.0	D30.3	D41.4	D49.4
urethral	C67.5	C79.11	D09.0	D30.3	D41.4	D49.4
overlapping lesion	C67.8	-	-	-	-	-
sphincter	C67.8	C79.11	D09.0	D30.3	D41.4	D49.4
trigone	C67.0	C79.11	D09.0	D30.3	D41.4	D49.4
urachus	C67.7	C79.11	D09.0	D30.3	D41.4	D49.4
wall	C67.9	C79.11	D09.0	D30.3	D41.4	D49.4
anterior	C67.3	C79.11	D09.0	D30.3	D41.4	D49.4
lateral	C67.2	C79.11	D09.0	D30.3	D41.4	D49.4
posterior	C67.4	C79.11	D09.0	D30.3	D41.4	D49.4
blood vessel—see Neoplasm, connective tissue						
bone (periosteum)	C41.9	C79.51	-	D16.9	D48.0	D49.2
acetabulum	C41.4	C79.51	-	D16.8	D48.0	D49.2
ankle	C40.3-	C79.51	-	D16.3-	-	-
arm NEC	C40.0-	C79.51	-	D16.0-	-	-
astragalus	C40.3-	C79.51	-	D16.3-	-	-
atlas	C41.2	C79.51	-	D16.6	D48.0	D49.2
axis	C41.2	C79.51	-	D16.6	D48.0	D49.2
back NEC	C41.2	C79.51	-	D16.6	D48.0	D49.2
calcaneus	C40.3-	C79.51	-	D16.3-	-	-
calvarium	C41.0	C79.51	-	D16.4	D48.0	D49.2
carpus (any)	C40.1-	C79.51	-	D16.1-	-	-
cartilage NEC	C41.9	C79.51	-	D16.9	D48.0	D49.2
bone — *continued*						
clavicle	C41.3	C79.51	-	D16.7	D48.0	D49.2
clivus	C41.0	C79.51	-	D16.4	D48.0	D49.2
coccygeal vertebra	C41.4	C79.51	-	D16.8	D48.0	D49.2
coccyx	C41.4	C79.51	-	D16.8	D48.0	D49.2
costal cartilage	C41.3	C79.51	-	D16.7	D48.0	D49.2
costovertebral joint	C41.3	C79.51	-	D16.7	D48.0	D49.2
cranial	C41.0	C79.51	-	D16.4	D48.0	D49.2
cuboid	C40.3-	C79.51	-	D16.3-	-	-
cuneiform	C41.9	C79.51	-	D16.9	D48.0	D49.2
elbow	C40.0-	C79.51	-	D16.0-	-	-
ethmoid (labyrinth)	C41.0	C79.51	-	D16.4	D48.0	D49.2
face	C41.0	C79.51	-	D16.4	D48.0	D49.2
femur (any part)	C40.2-	C79.51	-	D16.2-	-	-
fibula (any part)	C40.2-	C79.51	-	D16.2-	-	-
finger (any)	C40.1-	C79.51	-	D16.1-	-	-
foot	C40.3-	C79.51	-	D16.3-	-	-
forearm	C40.0-	C79.51	-	D16.0-	-	-
frontal	C41.0	C79.51	-	D16.4	D48.0	D49.2
hand	C40.1-	C79.51	-	D16.1-	-	-
heel	C40.3-	C79.51	-	D16.3-	-	-
hip	C41.4	C79.51	-	D16.8	D48.0	D49.2
humerus (any part)	C40.0-	C79.51	-	D16.0-	-	-
hyoid	C41.0	C79.51	-	D16.4	D48.0	D49.2
ilium	C41.4	C79.51	-	D16.8	D48.0	D49.2
innominate	C41.4	C79.51	-	D16.8	D48.0	D49.2
intervertebral cartilage or disc	C41.2	C79.51	-	D16.6	D48.0	D49.2
ischium	C41.4	C79.51	-	D16.8	D48.0	D49.2
jaw (lower)	C41.1	C79.51	-	D16.5	D48.0	D49.2
knee	C40.2-	C79.51	-	D16.2-	-	-
leg NEC	C40.2-	C79.51	-	D16.2-	-	-
limb NEC	C40.9-	C79.51	-	D16.9	-	-
lower (long bones)	C40.2-	C79.51	-	D16.2-	-	-
short bones	C40.3-	C79.51	-	D16.3-	-	-
upper (long bones)	C40.0-	C79.51	-	D16.0-	-	-
short bones	C40.1-	C79.51	-	D16.1-	-	-
malar	C41.0	C79.51	-	D16.4	D48.0	D49.2
mandible	C41.1	C79.51	-	D16.5	D48.0	D49.2
marrow NEC (any bone)	C96.9	C79.52	-	-	D47.9	D49.89
mastoid	C41.0	C79.51	-	D16.4	D48.0	D49.2
maxilla, maxillary (superior)	C41.0	C79.51	-	D16.4	D48.0	D49.2
inferior	C41.1	C79.51	-	D16.4	D48.0	D49.2
metacarpus (any)	C40.1-	C79.51	-	D16.1-	-	-
metatarsus (any)	C40.3-	C79.51	-	D16.3-	-	-
navicular						
ankle	C40.3-	C79.51	-	-	-	-
hand	C40.1-	C79.51	-	-	-	-
nose, nasal	C41.0	C79.51	-	D16.4	D48.0	D49.2
occipital	C41.0	C79.51	-	D16.4	D48.0	D49.2
orbit	C41.0	C79.51	-	D16.4	D48.0	D49.2

	Malignant Primary	Malignant Secondary	Ca in situ	Benign	Uncertain Behavior	Unspecified Behavior
bone — *continued*						
overlapping sites	C40.8-	-	-	-	-	-
parietal	C41.0	C79.51	-	D16.4	D48.0	D49.2
patella	C40.2-	C79.51	-	-	-	-
pelvic	C41.4	C79.51	-	D16.8	D48.0	D49.2
phalanges						
foot	C40.3-	C79.51	-	-	-	-
hand	C40.1-	C79.51	-	-	-	-
pubic	C41.4	C79.51	-	D16.8	D48.0	D49.2
radius (any part)	C40.0-	C79.51	-	D16.0-	-	-
rib	C41.3	C79.51	-	D16.7	D48.0	D49.2
sacral vertebra	C41.4	C79.51	-	D16.8	D48.0	D49.2
sacrum	C41.4	C79.51	-	D16.8	D48.0	D49.2
scaphoid					-	-
of ankle	C40.3-	C79.51	-	-	-	-
of hand	C40.1-	C79.51	-	-	-	-
scapula (any part)	C40.0-	C79.51	-	D16.0-	-	-
sella turcica	C41.0	C79.51	-	D16.4	D48.0	D49.2
shoulder	C40.0-	C79.51	-	D16.0-	-	-
skull	C41.0	C79.51	-	D16.4	D48.0	D49.2
sphenoid	C41.0	C79.51	-	D16.4	D48.0	D49.2
spine, spinal (column)	C41.2	C79.51	-	D16.6	D48.0	D49.2
coccyx	C41.4	C79.51	-	D16.8	D48.0	D49.2
sacrum	C41.4	C79.51	-	D16.8	D48.0	D49.2
sternum	C41.3	C79.51	-	D16.7	D48.0	D49.2
tarsus (any)	C40.3-	C79.51	-	-	-	-
temporal	C41.0	C79.51	-	D16.4	D48.0	D49.2
thumb	C40.1-	C79.51	-	-	-	-
tibia (any part)	C40.2-	C79.51	-	-	-	-
toe (any)	C40.3-	C79.51	-	-	-	-
trapezium	C40.1-	C79.51	-	-	-	-
trapezoid	C40.1-	C79.51	-	-	-	-
turbinate	C41.0	C79.51	-	D16.4	D48.0	D49.2
ulna (any part)	C40.0-	C79.51	-	D16.0-	-	-
unciform	C40.1-	C79.51	-	-	-	-
vertebra (column)	C41.2	C79.51	-	D16.6	D48.0	D49.2
coccyx	C41.4	C79.51	-	D16.8	D48.0	D49.2
sacrum	C41.4	C79.51	-	D16.8	D48.0	D49.2
vomer	C41.0	C79.51	-	D16.4	D48.0	D49.2
wrist	C40.1-	C79.51	-	-	-	-
xiphoid process	C41.3	C79.51	-	D16.7	D48.0	D49.2
zygomatic	C41.0	C79.51	-	D16.4	D48.0	D49.2
book-leaf (mouth)	C06.89	C79.89	D00.00	D10.39	D37.09	D49.0
bowel—see Neoplasm, intestine						
brachial plexus	C47.1-	C79.89	-	D36.12	D48.2	D49.2
brain NEC	C71.9	C79.31	-	D33.2	D43.2	D49.6
basal ganglia	C71.0	C79.31	-	D33.0	D43.0	D49.6
cerebellopontine angle	C71.6	C79.31	-	D33.1	D43.1	D49.6
cerebellum NOS	C71.6	C79.31	-	D33.1	D43.1	D49.6
cerebrum	C71.0	C79.31	-	D33.0	D43.0	D49.6
choroid plexus	C71.7	C79.31	-	D33.1	D43.1	D49.6
corpus callosum	C71.8	C79.31	-	D33.2	D43.2	D49.6

	Malignant Primary	Malignant Secondary	Ca in situ	Benign	Uncertain Behavior	Unspecified Behavior
brain NEC — *continued*						
corpus striatum	C71.0	C79.31	-	D33.0	D43.0	D49.6
cortex (cerebral)	C71.0	C79.31	-	D33.0	D43.0	D49.6
frontal lobe	C71.1	C79.31	-	D33.0	D43.0	D49.6
globus pallidus	C71.0	C79.31	-	D33.0	D43.0	D49.6
hippocampus	C71.2	C79.31	-	D33.0	D43.0	D49.6
hypothalamus	C71.0	C79.31	-	D33.0	D43.0	D49.6
internal capsule	C71.0	C79.31	-	D33.0	D43.0	D49.6
medulla oblongata	C71.7	C79.31	-	D33.1	D43.1	D49.6
meninges	C70.0	C79.32	-	D32.0	D42.0	D49.7
midbrain	C71.7	C79.31	-	D33.1	D43.1	D49.6
occipital lobe	C71.4	C79.31	-	D33.0	D43.0	D49.6
overlapping lesion	C71.8	C79.31	-	-	-	-
parietal lobe	C71.3	C79.31	-	D33.0	D43.0	D49.6
peduncle	C71.7	C79.31	-	D33.1	D43.1	D49.6
pons	C71.7	C79.31	-	D33.1	D43.1	D49.6
stem	C71.7	C79.31	-	D33.1	D43.1	D49.6
tapetum	C71.8	C79.31	-	D33.2	D43.2	D49.6
temporal lobe	C71.2	C79.31	-	D33.0	D43.0	D49.6
thalamus	C71.0	C79.31	-	D33.0	D43.0	D49.6
uncus	C71.2	C79.31	-	D33.0	D43.0	D49.6
ventricle (floor)	C71.5	C79.31	-	D33.0	D43.0	D49.6
fourth	C71.7	C79.31	-	D33.1	D43.1	D49.6
branchial (cleft) (cyst) (vestiges)	C10.4	C79.89	D00.08	D10.5	D37.05	D49.0
breast (connective tissue) (glandular tissue) (soft parts)	C50.9-	C79.81	D05.-	D24.-	D48.6-	D49.3
areola	C50.0-	C79.81	D05.-	D24.-	D48.6-	D49.3
axillary tail	C50.6-	C79.81	D05.-	D24.-	D48.6-	D49.3
central portion	C50.1-	C79.81	D05.-	D24.-	D48.6-	D49.3
inner	C50.8-	C79.81	D05.-	D24.-	D48.6-	D49.3
lower	C50.8-	C79.81	D05.-	D24.-	D48.6-	D49.3
lower-inner quadrant	C50.3-	C79.81	D05.-	D24.-	D48.6-	D49.3
lower-outer quadrant	C50.5-	C79.81	D05.-	D24.-	D48.6-	D49.3
mastectomy site (skin)—see also Neoplasm, breast, skin	C44.501	C79.2	-	-	-	-
specified as breast tissue	C50.8-	C79.81	-	-	-	-
midline	C50.8-	C79.81	D05.-	D24.-	D48.6-	D49.3
nipple	C50.0-	C79.81	D05.-	D24.-	D48.6-	D49.3
outer	C50.8-	C79.81	D05.-	D24.-	D48.6-	D49.3
overlapping lesion	C50.8-	-	-	-	-	-
skin	C44.501	C79.2	D04.5	D23.5	D48.5	D49.2
basal cell carcinoma	C44.511	-	-	-	-	-
specified type NEC	C44.591	-	-	-	-	-
squamous cell carcinoma	C44.521	-	-	-	-	-
tail (axillary)	C50.6-	C79.81	D05.-	D24.-	D48.6-	D49.3
upper	C50.8-	C79.81	D05.-	D24.-	D48.6-	D49.3
upper-inner quadrant	C50.2-	C79.81	D05.-	D24.-	D48.6-	D49.3
upper-outer quadrant	C50.4-	C79.81	D05.-	D24.-	D48.6-	D49.3
broad ligament	C57.1-	C79.82	D07.39	D28.2	D39.8	D49.59

	Malignant Primary	Malignant Secondary	Ca in situ	Benign	Uncertain Behavior	Unspecified Behavior
bronchiogenic, bronchogenic (lung)	C34.9-	C78.0-	D02.2-	D14.3-	D38.1	D49.1
bronchiole	C34.9-	C78.0-	D02.2-	D14.3-	D38.1	D49.1
bronchus	C34.9-	C78.0-	D02.2-	D14.3-	D38.1	D49.1
carina	C34.0-	C78.0-	D02.2-	D14.3-	D38.1	D49.1
lower lobe of lung	C34.3-	C78.0-	D02.2-	D14.3-	D38.1	D49.1
main	C34.0-	C78.0-	D02.2-	D14.3-	D38.1	D49.1
middle lobe of lung	C34.2	C78.0-	D02.21	D14.31	D38.1	D49.1
overlapping lesion	C34.8-	-	-	-	-	-
upper lobe of lung	C34.1-	C78.0-	D02.2-	D14.3-	D38.1	D49.1
brow	C44.309	C79.2	D04.39	D23.39	D48.5	D49.2
basal cell carcinoma	C44.319	-	-	-	-	-
specified type NEC	C44.399	-	-	-	-	-
squamous cell carcinoma	C44.329	-	-	-	-	-
buccal (cavity)	C06.9	C79.89	D00.00	D10.39	D37.09	D49.0
commissure	C06.0	C79.89	D00.02	D10.39	D37.09	D49.0
groove (lower) (upper)	C06.1	C79.89	D00.02	D10.39	D37.09	D49.0
mucosa	C06.0	C79.89	D00.02	D10.39	D37.09	D49.0
sulcus (lower) (upper)	C06.1	C79.89	D00.02	D10.39	D37.09	D49.0
bulbourethral gland	C68.0	C79.19	D09.19	D30.4	D41.3	D49.59
bursa—see Neoplasm, connective tissue						
buttock NEC	C76.3	C79.89	D04.5	D36.7	D48.7	D49.89
C						
calf	C76.5-	C79.89	D04.7-	D36.7	D48.7	D49.89
calvarium	C41.0	C79.51	-	D16.4	D48.0	D49.2
calyx, renal	C65.-	C79.0-	D09.19	D30.1-	D41.1-	D49.51-
canal						
anal	C21.1	C78.5	D01.3	D12.9	D37.8	D49.0
auditory (external)—see also Neoplasm, skin, ear	C44.20-	C79.2	D04.2-	D23.2-	D48.5	D49.2
auricular (external)—see also Neoplasm, skin, ear	C44.20-	C79.2	D04.2-	D23.2-	D48.5	D49.2
canaliculi, biliary (biliferi) (intrahepatic)	C22.1	C78.7	D01.5	D13.4	D37.6	D49.0
canthus (eye) (inner) (outer)	C44.10-	C79.2	D04.1-	D23.1-	D48.5	D49.2
basal cell carcinoma	C44.11-	-	-	-	-	-
specified type NEC	C44.19-	-	-	-	-	-
squamous cell carcinoma	C44.12-	-	-	-	-	-
capillary—see Neoplasm, connective tissue						
caput coli	C18.0	C78.5	D01.0	D12.0	D37.4	D49.0
carcinoid—see Tumor, carcinoid						
cardia (gastric)	C16.0	C78.89	D00.2	D13.1	D37.1	D49.0
cardiac orifice (stomach)	C16.0	C78.89	D00.2	D13.1	D37.1	D49.0
cardio-esophageal junction	C16.0	C78.89	D00.2	D13.1	D37.1	D49.0
cardio-esophagus	C16.0	C78.89	D00.2	D13.1	D37.1	D49.0
carina (bronchus)	C34.0-	C78.0-	D02.2-	D14.3-	D38.1	D49.1
carotid (artery)	C49.0	C79.89	-	D21.0	D48.1	D49.2
body	C75.4	C79.89	-	D35.5	D44.6	D49.7
carpus (any bone)	C40.1-	C79.51	-	D16.1-	-	-
cartilage (articular) (joint) NEC—see also Neoplasm, bone	C41.9	C79.51	-	D16.9	D48.0	D49.2
arytenoid	C32.3	C78.39	D02.0	D14.1	D38.0	D49.1

	Malignant Primary	Malignant Secondary	Ca in situ	Benign	Uncertain Behavior	Unspecified Behavior
cartilage NEC — *continued*						
auricular	C49.0	C79.89	-	D21.0	D48.1	D49.2
bronchi	C34.0-	C78.39	-	D14.3-	D38.1	D49.1
costal	C41.3	C79.51	-	D16.7	D48.0	D49.2
cricoid	C32.3	C78.39	D02.0	D14.1	D38.0	D49.1
cuneiform	C32.3	C78.39	D02.0	D14.1	D38.0	D49.1
ear (external)	C49.0	C79.89	-	D21.0	D48.1	D49.2
ensiform	C41.3	C79.51	-	D16.7	D48.0	D49.2
epiglottis	C32.1	C78.39	D02.0	D14.1	D38.0	D49.1
anterior surface	C10.1	C79.89	D00.08	D10.5	D37.05	D49.0
eyelid	C49.0	C79.89	-	D21.0	D48.1	D49.2
intervertebral	C41.2	C79.51	-	D16.6	D48.0	D49.2
larynx, laryngeal	C32.3	C78.39	D02.0	D14.1	D38.0	D49.1
nose, nasal	C30.0	C78.39	D02.3	D14.0	D38.5	D49.1
pinna	C49.0	C79.89	-	D21.0	D48.1	D49.2
rib	C41.3	C79.51	-	D16.7	D48.0	D49.2
semilunar (knee)	C40.2-	C79.51	-	D16.2-	D48.0	D49.2
thyroid	C32.3	C78.39	D02.0	D14.1	D38.0	D49.1
trachea	C33	C78.39	D02.1	D14.2	D38.1	D49.1
cauda equina	C72.1	C79.49	-	D33.4	D43.4	D49.7
cavity						
buccal	C06.9	C79.89	D00.00	D10.30	D37.09	D49.0
nasal	C30.0	C78.39	D02.3	D14.0	D38.5	D49.1
oral	C06.9	C79.89	D00.00	D10.30	D37.09	D49.0
peritoneal	C48.2	C78.6	-	D20.1	D48.4	D49.0
tympanic	C30.1	C78.39	D02.3	D14.0	D38.5	D49.1
cecum	C18.0	C78.5	D01.0	D12.0	D37.4	D49.0
central nervous system	C72.9	C79.40	-	-	-	-
cerebellopontine (angle)	C71.6	C79.31	-	D33.1	D43.1	D49.6
cerebellum, cerebellar	C71.6	C79.31	-	D33.1	D43.1	D49.6
cerebrum, cerebral (cortex) (hemisphere) (white matter)	C71.0	C79.31	-	D33.0	D43.0	D49.6
meninges	C70.0	C79.32	-	D32.0	D42.0	D49.7
peduncle	C71.7	C79.31	-	D33.1	D43.1	D49.6
ventricle	C71.5	C79.31	-	D33.0	D43.0	D49.6
fourth	C71.7	C79.31	-	D33.1	D43.1	D49.6
cervical region	C76.0	C79.89	D09.8	D36.7	D48.7	D49.89
cervix (cervical) (uteri) (uterus)	C53.9	C79.82	D06.9	D26.0	D39.0	D49.59
canal	C53.0	C79.82	D06.0	D26.0	D39.0	D49.59
endocervix (canal) (gland)	C53.0	C79.82	D06.0	D26.0	D39.0	D49.59
exocervix	C53.1	C79.82	D06.1	D26.0	D39.0	D49.59
external os	C53.1	C79.82	D06.1	D26.0	D39.0	D49.59
internal os	C53.0	C79.82	D06.0	D26.0	D39.0	D49.59
nabothian gland	C53.0	C79.82	D06.0	D26.0	D39.0	D49.59
overlapping lesion	C53.8	-	-	-	-	-
squamocolumnar junction	C53.8	C79.82	D06.7	D26.0	D39.0	D49.59
stump	C53.8	C79.82	D06.7	D26.0	D39.0	D49.59
cheek	C76.0	C79.89	D09.8	D36.7	D48.7	D49.89
external	C44.309	C79.2	D04.39	D23.39	D48.5	D49.2
basal cell carcinoma	C44.319	-	-	-	-	-
specified type NEC	C44.399	-	-	-	-	-

	Malignant Primary	Malignant Secondary	Ca in situ	Benign	Uncertain Behavior	Unspecified Behavior
cheek, external — *continued*						
squamous cell carcinoma	C44.329	-	-	-	-	-
inner aspect	C06.0	C79.89	D00.02	D10.39	D37.09	D49.0
internal	C06.0	C79.89	D00.02	D10.39	D37.09	D49.0
mucosa	C06.0	C79.89	D00.02	D10.39	D37.09	D49.0
chest (wall) NEC	C76.1	C79.89	D09.8	D36.7	D48.7	D49.89
chiasma opticum	C72.3-	C79.49	-	D33.3	D43.3	D49.7
chin	C44.309	C79.2	D04.39	D23.39	D48.5	D49.2
basal cell carcinoma	C44.319	-	-	-	-	-
specified type NEC	C44.399	-	-	-	-	-
squamous cell carcinoma	C44.329	-	-	-	-	-
choana	C11.3	C79.89	D00.08	D10.6	D37.05	D49.0
cholangiole	C22.1	C78.89	D01.5	D13.4	D37.6	D49.0
choledochal duct	C24.0	C78.89	D01.5	D13.5	D37.6	D49.0
choroid	C69.3-	C79.49	D09.2-	D31.3-	D48.7	D49.81
plexus	C71.5	C79.31	-	D33.0	D43.0	D49.6
ciliary body	C69.4-	C79.49	D09.2-	D31.4-	D48.7	D49.89
clavicle	C41.3	C79.51	-	D16.7	D48.0	D49.2
clitoris	C51.2	C79.82	D07.1	D28.0	D39.8	D49.59
clivus	C41.0	C79.51	-	D16.4-	D48.0	D49.2
cloacogenic zone	C21.2	C78.5	D01.3	D12.9	D37.8	D49.0
coccygeal						
body or glomus	C49.5	C79.89	-	D21.5	D48.1	D49.2
vertebra	C41.4	C79.51	-	D16.8	D48.0	D49.2
coccyx	C41.4	C79.51	-	D16.8	D48.0	D49.2
colon—see also Neoplasm, intestine, large	C18.9	C78.5	-	-	-	-
with rectum	C19	C78.5	D01.1	D12.7	D37.5	D49.0
column, spinal—see Neoplasm, spine						
columnella—see also Neoplasm, skin, face	C44.390	C79.2	D04.39	D23.39	D48.5	D49.2
commissure						
labial, lip	C00.6	C79.89	D00.01	D10.39	D37.01	D49.0
laryngeal	C32.0	C78.39	D02.0	D14.1	D38.0	D49.1
common (bile) duct	C24.0	C78.89	D01.5	D13.5	D37.6	D49.0
concha—see also Neoplasm, skin, ear	C44.20-	C79.2	D04.2-	D23.2-	D48.5	D49.2
nose	C30.0	C78.39	D02.3	D14.0	D38.5	D49.1
conjunctiva	C69.0-	C79.49	D09.2-	D31.0-	D48.7	D49.89
connective tissue NEC	C49.9	C79.89	-	D21.9	D48.1	D49.2
Note: For neoplasms of connective tissue (blood vessel, bursa, fascia, ligament, muscle, peripheral nerves, sympathetic and parasympathetic nerves and ganglia, synovia, tendon, etc.) or of morphological types that indicate connective tissue, code according to the list under "Neoplasm, connective tissue". For sites that do not appear in this list, code to neoplasm of that site; e.g., fibrosarcoma, pancreas (C25.9)						

	Malignant Primary	Malignant Secondary	Ca in situ	Benign	Uncertain Behavior	Unspecified Behavior
connective tissue NEC — *continued*						
Note: Morphological types that indicate connective tissue appear in their proper place in the alphabetic index with the instruction "see Neoplasm, connective tissue …."						
abdomen	C49.4	C79.89	-	D21.4	D48.1	D49.2
abdominal wall	C49.4	C79.89	-	D21.4	D48.1	D49.2
ankle	C49.2-	C79.89	-	D21.2-	D48.1	D49.2
antecubital fossa or space	C49.1-	C79.89	-	D21.1-	D48.1	D49.2
arm	C49.1-	C79.89	-	D21.1-	D48.1	D49.2
auricle (ear)	C49.0	C79.89	-	D21.0	D48.1	D49.2
axilla	C49.3	C79.89	-	D21.3	D48.1	D49.2
back	C49.6	C79.89	-	D21.6	D48.1	D49.2
breast—see Neoplasm, breast						
buttock	C49.5	C79.89	-	D21.5	D48.1	D49.2
calf	C49.2-	C79.89	-	D21.2-	D48.1	D49.2
cervical region	C49.0	C79.89	-	D21.0	D48.1	D49.2
cheek	C49.0	C79.89	-	D21.0	D48.1	D49.2
chest (wall)	C49.3	C79.89	-	D21.3	D48.1	D49.2
chin	C49.0	C79.89	-	D21.0	D48.1	D49.2
diaphragm	C49.3	C79.89	-	D21.3	D48.1	D49.2
ear (external)	C49.0	C79.89	-	D21.0	D48.1	D49.2
elbow	C49.1-	C79.89	-	D21.1-	D48.1	D49.2
extrarectal	C49.5	C79.89	-	D21.5	D48.1	D49.2
extremity	C49.9	C79.89	-	D21.9	D48.1	D49.2
lower	C49.2-	C79.89	-	D21.2-	D48.1	D49.2
upper	C49.1-	C79.89	-	D21.1-	D48.1	D49.2
eyelid	C49.0	C79.89	-	D21.0	D48.1	D49.2
face	C49.0	C79.89	-	D21.0	D48.1	D49.2
finger	C49.1-	C79.89	-	D21.1-	D48.1	D49.2
flank	C49.6	C79.89	-	D21.6	D48.1	D49.2
foot	C49.2-	C79.89	-	D21.2-	D48.1	D49.2
forearm	C49.1-	C79.89	-	D21.1-	D48.1	D49.2
forehead	C49.0	C79.89	-	D21.0	D48.1	D49.2
gastric	C49.4	C79.89	-	D21.4	D48.1	D49.2
gastrointestinal	C49.4	C79.89	-	D21.4	D48.1	D49.2
gluteal region	C49.5	C79.89	-	D21.5	D48.1	D49.2
great vessels NEC	C49.3	C79.89	-	D21.3	D48.1	D49.2
groin	C49.5	C79.89	-	D21.5	D48.1	D49.2
hand	C49.1-	C79.89	-	D21.1-	D48.1	D49.2
head	C49.0	C79.89	-	D21.0	D48.1	D49.2
heel	C49.2-	C79.89	-	D21.2-	D48.1	D49.2
hip	C49.2-	C79.89	-	D21.2-	D48.1	D49.2
hypochondrium	C49.4	C79.89	-	D21.4	D48.1	D49.2
iliopsoas muscle	C49.5	C79.89	-	D21.5	D48.1	D49.2
infraclavicular region	C49.3	C79.89	-	D21.3	D48.1	D49.2
inguinal (canal) (region)	C49.5	C79.89	-	D21.5	D48.1	D49.2
intestinal	C49.4	C79.89	-	D21.4	D48.1	D49.2
intrathoracic	C49.3	C79.89	-	D21.3	D48.1	D49.2
ischiorectal fossa	C49.5	C79.89	-	D21.5	D48.1	D49.2

	Malignant Primary	Malignant Secondary	Ca in situ	Benign	Uncertain Behavior	Unspecified Behavior
connective tissue NEC — *continued*						
jaw	C03.9	C79.89	D00.03	D10.39	D48.1	D49.0
knee	C49.2-	C79.89	-	D21.2-	D48.1	D49.2
leg	C49.2-	C79.89	-	D21.2-	D48.1	D49.2
limb NEC	C49.9	C79.89	-	D21.9	D48.1	D49.2
lower	C49.2-	C79.89	-	D21.2-	D48.1	D49.2
upper	C49.1-	C79.89	-	D21.1-	D48.1	D49.2
nates	C49.5	C79.89	-	D21.5	D48.1	D49.2
neck	C49.0	C79.89	-	D21.0	D48.1	D49.2
orbit	C69.6-	C79.49	D09.2-	D31.6-	D48.1	D49.89
overlapping lesion	C49.8	-	-	-	-	-
pararectal	C49.5	C79.89	-	D21.5	D48.1	D49.2
para-urethral	C49.5	C79.89	-	D21.5	D48.1	D49.2
paravaginal	C49.5	C79.89	-	D21.5	D48.1	D49.2
pelvis (floor)	C49.5	C79.89	-	D21.5	D48.1	D49.2
pelvo-abdominal	C49.8	C79.89	-	D21.6	D48.1	D49.2
perineum	C49.5	C79.89	-	D21.5	D48.1	D49.2
perirectal (tissue)	C49.5	C79.89	-	D21.5	D48.1	D49.2
periurethral (tissue)	C49.5	C79.89	-	D21.5	D48.1	D49.2
popliteal fossa or space	C49.2-	C79.89	-	D21.2-	D48.1	D49.2
presacral	C49.5	C79.89	-	D21.5	D48.1	D49.2
psoas muscle	C49.4	C79.89	-	D21.4	D48.1	D49.2
pterygoid fossa	C49.0	C79.89	-	D21.0	D48.1	D49.2
rectovaginal septum or wall	C49.5	C79.89	-	D21.5	D48.1	D49.2
rectovesical	C49.5	C79.89	-	D21.5	D48.1	D49.2
retroperitoneum	C48.0	C78.6	-	D20.0	D48.3	D49.0
sacrococcygeal region	C49.5	C79.89	-	D21.5	D48.1	D49.2
scalp	C49.0	C79.89	-	D21.0	D48.1	D49.2
scapular region	C49.3	C79.89	-	D21.3	D48.1	D49.2
shoulder	C49.1-	C79.89	-	D21.1-	D48.1	D49.2
skin (dermis) NEC—see also Neoplasm, skin, by site	C44.90	C79.2	D04.9	D23.9	D48.5	D49.2
stomach	C49.4	C79.89	-	D21.4	D48.1	D49.2
submental	C49.0	C79.89	-	D21.0	D48.1	D49.2
supraclavicular region	C49.0	C79.89	-	D21.0	D48.1	D49.2
temple	C49.0	C79.89	-	D21.0	D48.1	D49.2
temporal region	C49.0	C79.89	-	D21.0	D48.1	D49.2
thigh	C49.2-	C79.89	-	D21.2-	D48.1	D49.2
thoracic (duct) (wall)	C49.3	C79.89	-	D21.3	D48.1	D49.2
thorax	C49.3	C79.89	-	D21.3	D48.1	D49.2
thumb	C49.1-	C79.89	-	D21.1-	D48.1	D49.2
toe	C49.2-	C79.89	-	D21.2-	D48.1	D49.2
trunk	C49.6	C79.89	-	D21.6	D48.1	D49.2
umbilicus	C49.4	C79.89	-	D21.4	D48.1	D49.2
vesicorectal	C49.5	C79.89	-	D21.5	D48.1	D49.2
wrist	C49.1-	C79.89	-	D21.1-	D48.1	D49.2
conus medullaris	C72.0	C79.49	-	D33.4	D43.4	D49.7
cord (true) (vocal)	C32.0	C78.39	D02.0	D14.1	D38.0	D49.1
false	C32.1	C78.39	D02.0	D14.1	D38.0	D49.1
spermatic	C63.1-	C79.82	D07.69	D29.8	D40.8	D49.59

	Malignant Primary	Malignant Secondary	Ca in situ	Benign	Uncertain Behavior	Unspecified Behavior
cord (true) (vocal) — *continued*						
spinal (cervical) (lumbar) (thoracic)	C72.0	C79.49	-	D33.4	D43.4	D49.7
cornea (limbus)	C69.1-	C79.49	D09.2-	D31.1-	D48.7	D49.89
corpus						
albicans	C56.-	C79.6-	D07.39	D27.-	D39.1-	D49.59
callosum, brain	C71.0	C79.31	-	D33.2	D43.2	D49.6
cavernosum	C60.2	C79.82	D07.4	D29.0	D40.8	D49.59
gastric	C16.2	C78.89	D00.2	D13.1	D37.1	D49.0
overlapping sites	C54.8	-	-	-	-	-
penis	C60.2	C79.82	D07.4	D29.0	D40.8	D49.59
striatum, cerebrum	C71.0	C79.31	-	D33.0	D43.0	D49.6
uteri	C54.9	C79.82	D07.0	D26.1	D39.0	D49.59
isthmus	C54.0	C79.82	D07.0	D26.1	D39.0	D49.59
cortex						
adrenal	C74.0-	C79.7-	D09.3	D35.0-	D44.1-	D49.7
cerebral	C71.0	C79.31	-	D33.0	D43.0	D49.6
costal cartilage	C41.3	C79.51	-	D16.7	D48.0	D49.2
costovertebral joint	C41.3	C79.51	-	D16.7	D48.0	D49.2
Cowper's gland	C68.0	C79.19	D09.19	D30.4	D41.3	D49.59
cranial (fossa, any)	C71.9	C79.31	-	D33.2	D43.2	D49.6
meninges	C70.0	C79.32	-	D32.0	D42.0	D49.7
nerve	C72.50	C79.49	-	D33.3	D43.3	D49.7
specified NEC	C72.59	C79.49	-	D33.3	D43.3	D49.7
craniobuccal pouch	C75.2	C79.89	D09.3	D35.2	D44.3	D49.7
craniopharyngeal (duct) (pouch)	C75.2	C79.89	D09.3	D35.3	D44.4	D49.7
cricoid	C13.0	C79.89	D00.08	D10.7	D37.05	D49.0
cartilage	C32.3	C78.39	D02.0	D14.1	D38.0	D49.1
cricopharynx	C13.0	C79.89	D00.08	D10.7	D37.05	D49.0
crypt of Morgagni	C21.8	C78.5	D01.3	D12.9	D37.8	D49.0
crystalline lens	C69.4-	C79.49	D09.2-	D31.4-	D48.7	D49.89
cul-de-sac (Douglas')	C48.1	C78.6	-	D20.1	D48.4	D49.0
cuneiform cartilage	C32.3	C78.39	D02.0	D14.1	D38.0	D49.1
cutaneous—see Neoplasm, skin						
cutis—see Neoplasm, skin						
cystic (bile) duct (common)	C24.0	C78.89	D01.5	D13.5	D37.6	D49.0
D						
dermis—see Neoplasm, skin						
diaphragm	C49.3	C79.89	-	D21.3	D48.1	D49.2
digestive organs, system, tube, or tract NEC	C26.9	C78.89	D01.9	D13.9	D37.9	D49.0
disc, intervertebral	C41.2	C79.51	-	D16.6	D48.0	D49.2
disease, generalized	C80.0	-	-	-	-	-
disseminated	C80.0	-	-	-	-	-
Douglas' cul-de-sac or pouch	C48.1	C78.6	-	D20.1	D48.4	D49.0
duodenojejunal junction	C17.8	C78.4	D01.49	D13.39	D37.2	D49.0
duodenum	C17.0	C78.4	D01.49	D13.2	D37.2	D49.0
dura (cranial) (mater)	C70.9	C79.49	-	D32.9	D42.9	D49.7
cerebral	C70.0	C79.32	-	D32.0	D42.0	D49.7
spinal	C70.1	C79.49	-	D32.1	D42.1	D49.7

	Malignant Primary	Malignant Secondary	Ca in situ	Benign	Uncertain Behavior	Unspecified Behavior
E						
ear (external)—see also Neoplasm, skin, ear	C44.20-	C79.2	D04.2-	D23.2-	D48.5	D49.2
auricle or auris—see also Neoplasm, skin, ear	C44.20-	C79.2	D04.2-	D23.2-	D48.5	D49.2
canal, external—see also Neoplasm, skin, ear	C44.20-	C79.2	D04.2-	D23.2-	D48.5	D49.2
cartilage	C49.0	C79.89	-	D21.0	D48.1	D49.2
external meatus—see also Neoplasm, skin, ear	C44.20-	C79.2	D04.2-	D23.2-	D48.5	D49.2
inner	C30.1	C78.39	D02.3	D14.0	D38.5	D49.1
lobule—see also Neoplasm, skin, ear	C44.20-	C79.2	D04.2-	D23.2-	D48.5	D49.2
middle	C30.1	C78.39	D02.3	D14.0	D38.5	D49.1
overlapping lesion with accessory sinuses	C31.8	-	-	-	-	-
skin	C44.20-	C79.2	D04.2-	D23.2-	D48.5	D49.2
basal cell carcinoma	C44.21-	-	-	-	-	-
specified type NEC	C44.29-	-	-	-	-	-
squamous cell carcinoma	C44.22-	-	-	-	-	-
earlobe	C44.20-	C79.2	D04.2-	D23.2-	D48.5	D49.2
basal cell carcinoma	C44.21-	-	-	-	-	-
specified type NEC	C44.29-	-	-	-	-	-
squamous cell carcinoma	C44.22-	-	-	-	-	-
ejaculatory duct	C63.7	C79.82	D07.69	D29.8	D40.8	D49.59
elbow NEC	C76.4-	C79.89	D04.6-	D36.7	D48.7	D49.89
endocardium	C38.0	C79.89	-	D15.1	D48.7	D49.89
endocervix (canal) (gland)	C53.0	C79.82	D06.0	D26.0	D39.0	D49.59
endocrine gland NEC	C75.9	C79.89	D09.3	D35.9	D44.9	D49.7
pluriglandular	C75.8	C79.89	D09.3	D35.7	D44.9	D49.7
endometrium (gland) (stroma)	C54.1	C79.82	D07.0	D26.1	D39.0	D49.59
ensiform cartilage	C41.3	C79.51	-	D16.7	D48.0	D49.2
enteric—see Neoplasm, intestine						
ependyma (brain)	C71.5	C79.31	-	D33.0	D43.0	D49.6
fourth ventricle	C71.7	C79.31	-	D33.1	D43.1	D49.6
epicardium	C38.0	C79.89	-	D15.1	D48.7	D49.89
epididymis	C63.0-	C79.82	D07.69	D29.3-	D40.8	D49.59
epidural	C72.9	C79.49	-	D33.9	D43.9	D49.7
epiglottis	C32.1	C78.39	D02.0	D14.1	D38.0	D49.1
anterior aspect or surface	C10.1	C79.89	D00.08	D10.5	D37.05	D49.0
cartilage	C32.3	C78.39	D02.0	D14.1	D38.0	D49.1
free border (margin)	C10.1	C79.89	D00.08	D10.5	D37.05	D49.0
junctional region	C10.8	C79.89	D00.08	D10.5	D37.05	D49.0
posterior (laryngeal) surface	C32.1	C78.39	D02.0	D14.1	D38.0	D49.1
suprahyoid portion	C32.1	C78.39	D02.0	D14.1	D38.0	D49.1
esophagogastric junction	C16.0	C78.89	D00.2	D13.1	D37.1	D49.0
esophagus	C15.9	C78.89	D00.1	D13.0	D37.8	D49.0
abdominal	C15.5	C78.89	D00.1	D13.0	D37.8	D49.0
cervical	C15.3	C78.89	D00.1	D13.0	D37.8	D49.0
distal (third)	C15.5	C78.89	D00.1	D13.0	D37.8	D49.0
lower (third)	C15.5	C78.89	D00.1	D13.0	D37.8	D49.0
esophagus — *continued*						
middle (third)	C15.4	C78.89	D00.1	D13.0	D37.8	D49.0
overlapping lesion	C15.8	-	-	-	-	-
proximal (third)	C15.3	C78.89	D00.1	D13.0	D37.8	D49.0
thoracic	C15.4	C78.89	D00.1	D13.0	D37.8	D49.0
upper (third)	C15.3	C78.89	D00.1	D13.0	D37.8	D49.0
ethmoid (sinus)	C31.1	C78.39	D02.3	D14.0	D38.5	D49.1
bone or labyrinth	C41.0	C79.51	-	D16.4-	D48.0	D49.2
eustachian tube	C30.1	C78.39	D02.3	D14.0	D38.5	D49.1
exocervix	C53.1	C79.82	D06.1	D26.0	D39.0	D49.59
external						
meatus (ear)—see also Neoplasm, skin, ear	C44.20-	C79.2	D04.2-	D23.2-	D48.5	D49.2
os, cervix uteri	C53.1	C79.82	D06.1	D26.0	D39.0	D49.59
extradural	C72.9	C79.49	-	D33.9	D43.9	D49.7
extrahepatic (bile) duct	C24.0	C78.89	D01.5	D13.5	D37.6	D49.0
overlapping lesion with gallbladder	C24.8	-	-	-	-	-
extraocular muscle	C69.6-	C79.49	D09.2-	D31.6-	D48.7	D49.89
extrarectal	C76.3	C79.89	D09.8	D36.7	D48.7	D49.89
extremity	C76.8	C79.89	D04.8	D36.7	D48.7	D49.89
lower	C76.5-	C79.89	D04.7-	D36.7	D48.7	D49.89
upper	C76.4-	C79.89	D04.6-	D36.7	D48.7	D49.89
eye NEC	C69.9-	C79.49	D09.2-	D31.9	D48.7	D49.89
overlapping sites	C69.8-	-	-	-	-	-
eyeball	C69.9-	C79.49	D09.2-	D31.9-	D48.7	D49.89
eyebrow	C44.309	C79.2	D04.39	D23.39	D48.5	D49.2
basal cell carcinoma	C44.319	-	-	-	-	-
specified type NEC	C44.399	-	-	-	-	-
squamous cell carcinoma	C44.329	-	-	-	-	-
eyelid (lower) (skin) (upper)	C44.10-	-	-	-	-	-
basal cell carcinoma	C44.11-	-	-	-	-	-
specified type NEC	C44.19-	-	-	-	-	-
squamous cell carcinoma	C44.12-	-	-	-	-	-
cartilage	C49.0	C79.89	-	D21.0	D48.1	D49.2
F						
face NEC	C76.0	C79.89	D04.39	D36.7	D48.7	D49.89
fallopian tube (accessory)	C57.0-	C79.82	D07.39	D28.2	D39.8	D49.59
falx (cerebella) (cerebri)	C70.0	C79.32	-	D32.0	D42.0	D49.7
fascia—see also Neoplasm, connective tissue						
palmar	C49.1-	C79.89	-	D21.1-	D48.1	D49.2
plantar	C49.2-	C79.89	-	D21.2-	D48.1	D49.2
fatty tissue—see Neoplasm, connective tissue						
fauces, faucial NEC	C10.9	C79.89	D00.08	D10.5	D37.05	D49.0
pillars	C09.1	C79.89	D00.08	D10.5	D37.05	D49.0
tonsil	C09.9	C79.89	D00.08	D10.4	D37.05	D49.0
femur (any part)	C40.2-	-	-	D16.2-	-	-
fetal membrane	C58	C79.82	D07.0	D26.7	D39.2	D49.59
fibrous tissue—see Neoplasm, connective tissue						
fibula (any part)	C40.2-	C79.51	-	D16.2-	-	-

	Malignant Primary	Malignant Secondary	Ca in situ	Benign	Uncertain Behavior	Unspecified Behavior
filum terminale	C72.0	C79.49	-	D33.4	D43.4	D49.7
finger NEC	C76.4-	C79.89	D04.6-	D36.7	D48.7	D49.89
flank NEC	C76.8	C79.89	D04.5	D36.7	D48.7	D49.89
follicle, nabothian	C53.0	C79.82	D06.0	D26.0	D39.0	D49.59
foot NEC	C76.5-	C79.89	D04.7-	D36.7	D48.7	D49.89
forearm NEC	C76.4-	C79.89	D04.6-	D36.7	D48.7	D49.89
forehead (skin)	C44.309	C79.2	D04.39	D23.39	D48.5	D49.2
basal cell carcinoma	C44.319	-	-	-	-	-
specified type NEC	C44.399	-	-	-	-	-
squamous cell carcinoma	C44.329	-	-	-	-	-
foreskin	C60.0	C79.82	D07.4	D29.0	D40.8	D49.59
fornix						
pharyngeal	C11.3	C79.89	D00.08	D10.6	D37.05	D49.0
vagina	C52	C79.82	D07.2	D28.1	D39.8	D49.59
fossa (of)						
anterior (cranial)	C71.9	C79.31	-	D33.2	D43.2	D49.6
cranial	C71.9	C79.31	-	D33.2	D43.2	D49.6
ischiorectal	C76.3	C79.89	D09.8	D36.7	D48.7	D49.89
middle (cranial)	C71.9	C79.31	-	D33.2	D43.2	D49.6
piriform	C12	C79.89	D00.08	D10.7	D37.05	D49.0
pituitary	C75.1	C79.89	D09.3	D35.2	D44.3	D49.7
posterior (cranial)	C71.9	C79.31	-	D33.2	D43.2	D49.6
pterygoid	C49.0	C79.89	-	D21.0	D48.1	D49.2
pyriform	C12	C79.89	D00.08	D10.7	D37.05	D49.0
Rosenmuller	C11.2	C79.89	D00.08	D10.6	D37.05	D49.0
tonsillar	C09.0	C79.89	D00.08	D10.5	D37.05	D49.0
fourchette	C51.9	C79.82	D07.1	D28.0	D39.8	D49.59
frenulum						
labii—see Neoplasm, lip, internal						
linguae	C02.2	C79.89	D00.07	D10.1	D37.02	D49.0
frontal						
bone	C41.0	C79.51	-	D16.4	D48.0	D49.2
lobe, brain	C71.1	C79.31	-	D33.0	D43.0	D49.6
pole	C71.1	C79.31	-	D33.0	D43.0	D49.6
sinus	C31.2	C78.39	D02.3	D14.0	D38.5	D49.1
fundus						
stomach	C16.1	C78.89	D00.2	D13.1	D37.1	D49.0
uterus	C54.3	C79.82	D07.0	D26.1	D39.0	D49.59
G						
gall duct (extrahepatic)	C24.0	C78.89	D01.5	D13.5	D37.6	D49.0
intrahepatic	C22.1	C78.7	D01.5	D13.4	D37.6	D49.0
gallbladder	C23	C78.89	D01.5	D13.5	D37.6	D49.0
overlapping lesion with extrahepatic bile ducts	C24.8	-	-	-	-	-
ganglia—see also Neoplasm, nerve, peripheral	C47.9	C79.89	-	D36.10	D48.2	D49.2
basal	C71.0	C79.31	-	D33.0	D43.0	D49.6
cranial nerve	C72.50	C79.49	-	D33.3	D43.3	D49.7
Gartner's duct	C52	C79.82	D07.2	D28.1	D39.8	D49.59
gastric—see Neoplasm, stomach						
gastrocolic	C26.9	C78.89	D01.9	D13.9	D37.9	D49.0
gastroesophageal junction	C16.0	C78.89	D00.2	D13.1	D37.1	D49.0
gastrointestinal (tract) NEC	C26.9	C78.89	D01.9	D13.9	D37.9	D49.0
generalized	C80.0	-	-	-	-	-
genital organ or tract						
female NEC	C57.9	C79.82	D07.30	D28.9	D39.9	D49.59
overlapping lesion	C57.8	-	-	-	-	-
specified site NEC	C57.7	C79.82	D07.39	D28.7	D39.8	D49.59
male NEC	C63.9	C79.82	D07.60	D29.9	D40.9	D49.59
overlapping lesion	C63.8	-	-	-	-	-
specified site NEC	C63.7	C79.82	D07.69	D29.8	D40.8	D49.59
genitourinary tract						
female	C57.9	C79.82	D07.30	D28.9	D39.9	D49.59
male	C63.9	C79.82	D07.60	D29.9	D40.9	D49.59
gingiva (alveolar) (marginal)	C03.9	C79.89	D00.03	D10.39	D37.09	D49.0
lower	C03.1	C79.89	D00.03	D10.39	D37.09	D49.0
mandibular	C03.1	C79.89	D00.03	D10.39	D37.09	D49.0
maxillary	C03.0	C79.89	D00.03	D10.39	D37.09	D49.0
upper	C03.0	C79.89	D00.03	D10.39	D37.09	D49.0
gland, glandular (lymphatic) (system)—see also Neoplasm, lymph gland						
endocrine NEC	C75.9	C79.89	D09.3	D35.9	D44.9	D49.7
salivary—see Neoplasm, salivary gland						
glans penis	C60.1	C79.82	D07.4	D29.0	D40.8	D49.59
globus pallidus	C71.0	C79.31	-	D33.0	D43.0	D49.6
glomus						
coccygeal	C49.5	C79.89	-	D21.5	D48.1	D49.2
jugularis	C75.5	C79.89	-	D35.6	D44.7	D49.7
glosso-epiglottic fold(s)	C10.1	C79.89	D00.08	D10.5	D37.05	D49.0
glossopalatine fold	C09.1	C79.89	D00.08	D10.5	D37.05	D49.0
glossopharyngeal sulcus	C09.0	C79.89	D00.08	D10.5	D37.05	D49.0
glottis	C32.0	C78.39	D02.0	D14.1	D38.0	D49.1
gluteal region	C76.3	C79.89	D04.5	D36.7	D48.7	D49.89
great vessels NEC	C49.3	C79.89	-	D21.3	D48.1	D49.2
groin NEC	C76.3	C79.89	D04.5	D36.7	D48.7	D49.89
gum	C03.9	C79.89	D00.03	D10.39	D37.09	D49.0
lower	C03.1	C79.89	D00.03	D10.39	D37.09	D49.0
upper	C03.0	C79.89	D00.03	D10.39	D37.09	D49.0
H						
hand NEC	C76.4-	C79.89	D04.6-	D36.7	D48.7	D49.89
head NEC	C76.0	C79.89	D04.4	D36.7	D48.7	D49.89
heart	C38.0	C79.89	-	D15.1	D48.7	D49.89
heel NEC	C76.5-	C79.89	D04.7-	D36.7	D48.7	D49.89
helix—see also Neoplasm, skin, ear	C44.20-	C79.2	D04.2-	D23.2-	D48.5	D49.2
hematopoietic, hemopoietic tissue NEC	C96.9	-	-	-	-	-
specified NEC	C96.Z	-	-	-	-	-
hemisphere, cerebral	C71.0	C79.31	-	D33.0	D43.0	D49.6
hemorrhoidal zone	C21.1	C78.5	D01.3	D12.9	D37.8	D49.0
hepatic—see also Index to disease, by histology	C22.9	C78.7	D01.5	D13.4	D37.6	D49.0
duct (bile)	C24.0	C78.89	D01.5	D13.5	D37.6	D49.0

	Malignant Primary	Malignant Secondary	Ca in situ	Benign	Uncertain Behavior	Unspecified Behavior
hepatic — *continued*						
flexure (colon)	C18.3	C78.5	D01.0	D12.3	D37.4	D49.0
primary	C22.8	C78.7	D01.5	D13.4	D37.6	D49.0
hepatobiliary	C24.9	C78.89	D01.5	D13.5	D37.6	D49.0
hepatoblastoma	C22.2	C78.7	D01.5	D13.4	D37.6	D49.0
hepatoma	C22.0	C78.7	D01.5	D13.4	D37.6	D49.0
hilus of lung	C34.0-	C78.0-	D02.2-	D14.3-	D38.1	D49.1
hip NEC	C76.5-	C79.89	D04.7-	D36.7	D48.7	D49.89
hippocampus, brain	C71.2	C79.31	-	D33.0	D43.0	D49.6
humerus (any part)	C40.0-	C79.51	-	D16.0-	-	-
hymen	C52	C79.82	D07.2	D28.1	D39.8	D49.59
hypopharynx, hypopharyngeal NEC	C13.9	C79.89	D00.08	D10.7	D37.05	D49.0
overlapping lesion	C13.8	-	-	-	-	-
postcricoid region	C13.0	C79.89	D00.08	D10.7	D37.05	D49.0
posterior wall	C13.2	C79.89	D00.08	D10.7	D37.05	D49.0
pyriform fossa (sinus)	C12	C79.89	D00.08	D10.7	D37.05	D49.0
hypophysis	C75.1	C79.89	D09.3	D35.2	D44.3	D49.7
hypothalamus	C71.0	C79.31	-	D33.0	D43.0	D49.6
I						
ileocecum, ileocecal (coil) (junction) (valve)	C18.0	C78.5	D01.0	D12.0	D37.4	D49.0
ileum	C17.2	C78.4	D01.49	D13.39	D37.2	D49.0
ilium	C41.4	C79.51	-	D16.8	D48.0	D49.2
immunoproliferative NEC	C88.9	-	-	-	-	-
infraclavicular (region)	C76.1	C79.89	D04.5	D36.7	D48.7	D49.89
inguinal (region)	C76.3	C79.89	D04.5	D36.7	D48.7	D49.89
insula	C71.0	C79.31	-	D33.0	D43.0	D49.6
insular tissue (pancreas)	C25.4	C78.89	D01.7	D13.7	D37.8	D49.0
brain	C71.0	C79.31	-	D33.0	D43.0	D49.6
interarytenoid fold	C13.1	C79.89	D00.08	D10.7	D37.05	D49.0
hypopharyngeal aspect	C13.1	C79.89	D00.08	D10.7	D37.05	D49.0
laryngeal aspect	C32.1	C78.39	D02.0	D14.1	D38.0	D49.1
marginal zone	C13.1	C79.89	D00.08	D10.7	D37.05	D49.0
interdental papillae	C03.9	C79.89	D00.03	D10.39	D37.09	D49.0
lower	C03.1	C79.89	D00.03	D10.39	D37.09	D49.0
upper	C03.0	C79.89	D00.03	D10.39	D37.09	D49.0
internal						
capsule	C71.0	C79.31	-	D33.0	D43.0	D49.6
os (cervix)	C53.0	C79.82	D06.0	D26.0	D39.0	D49.59
intervertebral cartilage or disc	C41.2	C79.51	-	D16.6	D48.0	D49.2
intestine, intestinal	C26.0	C78.80	D01.40	D13.9	D37.8	D49.0
large	C18.9	C78.5	D01.0	D12.6	D37.4	D49.0
appendix	C18.1	C78.5	D01.0	D12.1	D37.3	D49.0
caput coli	C18.0	C78.5	D01.0	D12.0	D37.4	D49.0
cecum	C18.0	C78.5	D01.0	D12.0	D37.4	D49.0
colon	C18.9	C78.5	D01.0	D12.6	D37.4	D49.0
and rectum	C19	C78.5	D01.1	D12.7	D37.5	D49.0
ascending	C18.2	C78.5	D01.0	D12.2	D37.4	D49.0
caput	C18.0	C78.5	D01.0	D12.0	D37.4	D49.0
descending	C18.6	C78.5	D01.0	D12.4	D37.4	D49.0

	Malignant Primary	Malignant Secondary	Ca in situ	Benign	Uncertain Behavior	Unspecified Behavior
intestine, intestinal, large — *continued*						
distal	C18.6	C78.5	D01.0	D12.4	D37.4	D49.0
left	C18.6	C78.5	D01.0	D12.4	D37.4	D49.0
overlapping lesion	C18.8	-	-	-	-	-
pelvic	C18.7	C78.5	D01.0	D12.5	D37.4	D49.0
right	C18.2	C78.5	D01.0	D12.2	D37.4	D49.0
sigmoid (flexure)	C18.7	C78.5	D01.0	D12.5	D37.4	D49.0
transverse	C18.4	C78.5	D01.0	D12.3	D37.4	D49.0
hepatic flexure	C18.3	C78.5	D01.0	D12.3	D37.4	D49.0
ileocecum, ileocecal (coil) (valve)	C18.0	C78.5	D01.0	D12.0	D37.4	D49.0
overlapping lesion	C18.8	-	-	-	-	-
sigmoid flexure (lower) (upper)	C18.7	C78.5	D01.0	D12.5	D37.4	D49.0
splenic flexure	C18.5	C78.5	D01.0	D12.3	D37.4	D49.0
small	C17.9	C78.4	D01.40	D13.30	D37.2	D49.0
duodenum	C17.0	C78.4	D01.49	D13.2	D37.2	D49.0
ileum	C17.2	C78.4	D01.49	D13.39	D37.2	D49.0
jejunum	C17.1	C78.4	D01.49	D13.39	D37.2	D49.0
overlapping lesion	C17.8	-	-	-	-	-
tract NEC	C26.0	C78.89	D01.40	D13.9	D37.8	D49.0
intra-abdominal	C76.2	C79.89	D09.8	D36.7	D48.7	D49.89
intracranial NEC	C71.9	C79.31	-	D33.2	D43.2	D49.6
intrahepatic (bile) duct	C22.1	C78.7	D01.5	D13.4	D37.6	D49.0
intraocular	C69.9-	C79.49	D09.2-	D31.9-	D48.7	D49.89
intraorbital	C69.6-	C79.49	D09.2-	D31.6-	D48.7	D49.89
intrasellar	C75.1	C79.89	D09.3	D35.2	D44.3	D49.7
intrathoracic (cavity) (organs)	C76.1	C79.89	D09.8	D15.9	D48.7	D49.89
specified NEC	C76.1	C79.89	D09.8	D15.7	-	-
iris	C69.4-	C79.49	D09.2-	D31.4-	D48.7	D49.89
ischiorectal (fossa)	C76.3	C79.89	D09.8	D36.7	D48.7	D49.89
ischium	C41.4	C79.51	-	D16.8	D48.0	D49.2
island of Reil	C71.0	C79.31	-	D33.0	D43.0	D49.6
islands or islets of Langerhans	C25.4	C78.89	D01.7	D13.7	D37.8	D49.0
isthmus uteri	C54.0	C79.82	D07.0	D26.1	D39.0	D49.59
J						
jaw	C76.0	C79.89	D09.8	D36.7	D48.7	D49.89
bone	C41.1	C79.51	-	D16.5	D48.0	D49.2
lower	C41.1	C79.51	-	D16.5	-	-
upper	C41.0	C79.51	-	D16.4	-	-
carcinoma (any type) (lower) (upper)	C76.0	C79.89	-	-	-	-
skin—see also Neoplasm, skin, face	C44.309	C79.2	D04.39	D23.39	D48.5	D49.2
soft tissues	C03.9	C79.89	D00.03	D10.39	D37.09	D49.0
lower	C03.1	C79.89	D00.03	D10.39	D37.09	D49.0
upper	C03.0	C79.89	D00.03	D10.39	D37.09	D49.0
jejunum	C17.1	C78.4	D01.49	D13.39	D37.2	D49.0
joint NEC—see also Neoplasm, bone	C41.9	C79.51	-	D16.9	D48.0	D49.2
acromioclavicular	C40.0-	C79.51	-	D16.0-	-	-

	Malignant Primary	Malignant Secondary	Ca in situ	Benign	Uncertain Behavior	Unspecified Behavior
joint NEC — *continued*						
bursa or synovial membrane—see Neoplasm, connective tissue						
costovertebral	C41.3	C79.51	-	D16.7	D48.0	D49.2
sternocostal	C41.3	C79.51	-	D16.7	D48.0	D49.2
temporomandibular	C41.1	C79.51	-	D16.5	D48.0	D49.2
junction						
anorectal	C21.8	C78.5	D01.3	D12.9	D37.8	D49.0
cardioesophageal	C16.0	C78.89	D00.2	D13.1	D37.1	D49.0
esophagogastric	C16.0	C78.89	D00.2	D13.1	D37.1	D49.0
gastroesophageal	C16.0	C78.89	D00.2	D13.1	D37.1	D49.0
hard and soft palate	C05.9	C79.89	D00.00	D10.39	D37.09	D49.0
ileocecal	C18.0	C78.5	D01.0	D12.0	D37.4	D49.0
pelvirectal	C19	C78.5	D01.1	D12.7	D37.5	D49.0
pelviureteric	C65.-	C79.0-	D09.19	D30.1-	D41.1-	D49.59
rectosigmoid	C19	C78.5	D01.1	D12.7	D37.5	D49.0
squamocolumnar, of cervix	C53.8	C79.82	D06.7	D26.0	D39.0	D49.59
K						
Kaposi's sarcoma—see Kaposi's, sarcoma						
kidney (parenchymal)	C64.-	C79.0-	D09.19	D30.0-	D41.0-	D49.51-
calyx	C65.-	C79.0-	D09.19	D30.1-	D41.1-	D49.51-
hilus	C65.-	C79.0-	D09.19	D30.1-	D41.1-	D49.51-
pelvis	C65.-	C79.0-	D09.19	D30.1-	D41.1-	D49.51-
knee NEC	C76.5-	C79.89	D04.7-	D36.7	D48.7	D49.89
L						
labia (skin)	C51.9	C79.82	D07.1	D28.0	D39.8	D49.59
majora	C51.0	C79.82	D07.1	D28.0	D39.8	D49.59
minora	C51.1	C79.82	D07.1	D28.0	D39.8	D49.59
labial—see also Neoplasm, lip	C00.9	C79.89	D00.01	D10.0	D37.01	D49.0
sulcus (lower) (upper)	C06.1	C79.89	D00.02	D10.39	D37.09	D49.0
labium (skin)	C51.9	C79.82	D07.1	D28.0	D39.8	D49.59
majus	C51.0	C79.82	D07.1	D28.0	D39.8	D49.59
minus	C51.1	C79.82	D07.1	D28.0	D39.8	D49.59
lacrimal						
canaliculi	C69.5-	C79.49	D09.2-	D31.5-	D48.7	D49.89
duct (nasal)	C69.5-	C79.49	D09.2-	D31.5-	D48.7	D49.89
gland	C69.5-	C79.49	D09.2-	D31.5-	D48.7	D49.89
punctum	C69.5-	C79.49	D09.2-	D31.5-	D48.7	D49.89
sac	C69.5-	C79.49	D09.2-	D31.5-	D48.7	D49.89
Langerhans, islands or islets	C25.4	C78.89	D01.7	D13.7	D37.8	D49.0
laryngopharynx	C13.9	C79.89	D00.08	D10.7	D37.05	D49.0
larynx, laryngeal NEC	C32.9	C78.39	D02.0	D14.1	D38.0	D49.1
aryepiglottic fold	C32.1	C78.39	D02.0	D14.1	D38.0	D49.1
cartilage (arytenoid) (cricoid) (cuneiform) (thyroid)	C32.3	C78.39	D02.0	D14.1	D38.0	D49.1
commissure (anterior) (posterior)	C32.0	C78.39	D02.0	D14.1	D38.0	D49.1

	Malignant Primary	Malignant Secondary	Ca in situ	Benign	Uncertain Behavior	Unspecified Behavior
larynx, laryngeal NEC — *continued*						
extrinsic NEC	C32.1	C78.39	D02.0	D14.1	D38.0	D49.1
meaning hypopharynx	C13.9	C79.89	D00.08	D10.7	D37.05	D49.0
interarytenoid fold	C32.1	C78.39	D02.0	D14.1	D38.0	D49.1
intrinsic	C32.0	C78.39	D02.0	D14.1	D38.0	D49.1
overlapping lesion	C32.8	-	-	-	-	-
ventricular band	C32.1	C78.39	D02.0	D14.1	D38.0	D49.1
leg NEC	C76.5-	C79.89	D04.7-	D36.7	D48.7	D49.89
lens, crystalline	C69.4-	C79.49	D09.2-	D31.4-	D48.7	D49.89
lid (lower) (upper)	C44.10-	C79.2	D04.1-	D23.1-	D48.5	D49.2
basal cell carcinoma	C44.11-	-	-	-	-	-
specified type NEC	C44.19-	-	-	-	-	-
squamous cell carcinoma	C44.12-	-	-	-	-	-
ligament—see also Neoplasm, connective tissue						
broad	C57.1-	C79.82	D07.39	D28.2	D39.8	D49.59
Mackenrodt's	C57.7	C79.82	D07.39	D28.7	D39.8	D49.59
non-uterine—see Neoplasm, connective tissue						
round	C57.2-	C79.82	-	D28.2	D39.8	D49.59
sacro-uterine	C57.3	C79.82	-	D28.2	D39.8	D49.59
uterine	C57.3	C79.82	-	D28.2	D39.8	D49.59
utero-ovarian	C57.7	C79.82	D07.39	D28.2	D39.8	D49.59
uterosacral	C57.3	C79.82	-	D28.2	D39.8	D49.59
limb	C76.8	C79.89	D04.8	D36.7	D48.7	D49.89
lower	C76.5-	C79.89	D04.7-	D36.7	D48.7	D49.89
upper	C76.4-	C79.89	D04.6-	D36.7	D48.7	D49.89
limbus of cornea	C69.1-	C79.49	D09.2-	D31.1-	D48.7	D49.89
lingual NEC—see also Neoplasm, tongue	C02.9	C79.89	D00.07	D10.1	D37.02	D49.0
lingula, lung	C34.1-	C78.0-	D02.2-	D14.3-	D38.1	D49.1
lip	C00.9	C79.89	D00.01	D10.0	D37.01	D49.0
buccal aspect—see Neoplasm, lip, internal						
commissure	C00.6	C79.89	D00.01	D10.0	D37.01	D49.0
external	C00.2	C79.89	D00.01	D10.0	D37.01	D49.0
lower	C00.1	C79.89	D00.01	D10.0	D37.01	D49.0
upper	C00.0	C79.89	D00.01	D10.0	D37.01	D49.0
frenulum—see Neoplasm, lip, internal						
inner aspect—see Neoplasm, lip, internal						
internal	C00.5	C79.89	D00.01	D10.0	D37.01	D49.0
lower	C00.4	C79.89	D00.01	D10.0	D37.01	D49.0
upper	C00.3	C79.89	D00.01	D10.0	D37.01	D49.0
lipstick area	C00.2	C79.89	D00.01	D10.0	D37.01	D49.0
lower	C00.1	C79.89	D00.01	D10.0	D37.01	D49.0
upper	C00.0	C79.89	D00.01	D10.0	D37.01	D49.0
lower	C00.1	C79.89	D00.01	D10.0	D37.01	D49.0
internal	C00.4	C79.89	D00.01	D10.0	D37.01	D49.0
mucosa—see Neoplasm, lip, intervnal						

	Malignant Primary	Malignant Secondary	Ca in situ	Benign	Uncertain Behavior	Unspecified Behavior
lip — *continued*						
oral aspect—see Neoplasm, lip, internal						
overlapping lesion	C00.8	-	-	-	-	-
with oral cavity or pharynx	C14.8	-	-	-	-	-
skin (commissure) (lower) (upper)	C44.00	C79.2	D04.0	D23.0	D48.5	D49.2
basal cell carcinoma	C44.01	-	-	-	-	-
specified type NEC	C44.09	-	-	-	-	-
squamous cell carcinoma	C44.02	-	-	-	-	-
upper	C00.0	C79.89	D00.01	D10.0	D37.01	D49.0
internal	C00.3	C79.89	D00.01	D10.0	D37.01	D49.0
vermilion border	C00.2	C79.89	D00.01	D10.0	D37.01	D49.0
lower	C00.1	C79.89	D00.01	D10.0	D37.01	D49.0
upper	C00.0	C79.89	D00.01	D10.0	D37.01	D49.0
lipomatous—see Lipoma, by site						
liver—see also Index to disease, by histology	C22.9	C78.7	D01.5	D13.4	D37.6	D49.0
primary	C22.8	C78.7	D01.5	D13.4	D37.6	D49.0
lumbosacral plexus	C47.5	C79.89	-	D36.16	D48.2	D49.2
lung	C34.9-	C78.0-	D02.2-	D14.3-	D38.1	D49.1
azygos lobe	C34.1-	C78.0-	D02.2-	D14.3-	D38.1	D49.1
carina	C34.0-	C78.0-	D02.2-	D14.3-	D38.1	D49.1
hilus	C34.0-	C78.0-	D02.2-	D14.3-	D38.1	D49.1
linqula	C34.1-	C78.0-	D02.2-	D14.3-	D38.1	D49.1
lobe NEC	C34.9-	C78.0-	D02.2-	D14.3-	D38.1	D49.1
lower lobe	C34.3-	C78.0-	D02.2-	D14.3-	D38.1	D49.1
main bronchus	C34.0-	C78.0-	D02.2-	D14.3-	D38.1	D49.1
mesothelioma—see Mesothelioma						
middle lobe	C34.2	C78.0-	D02.21	D14.31	D38.1	D49.1
overlapping lesion	C34.8-	-	-	-	-	-
upper lobe	C34.1-	C78.0-	D02.2-	D14.3-	D38.1	D49.1
lymph, lymphatic channel NEC	C49.9	C79.89	-	D21.9	D48.1	D49.2
gland (secondary)	-	C77.9	-	D36.0	D48.7	D49.89
abdominal	-	C77.2	-	D36.0	D48.7	D49.89
aortic	-	C77.2	-	D36.0	D48.7	D49.89
arm	-	C77.3	-	D36.0	D48.7	D49.89
auricular (anterior) (posterior)	-	C77.0	-	D36.0	D48.7	D49.89
axilla, axillary	-	C77.3	-	D36.0	D48.7	D49.89
brachial	-	C77.3	-	D36.0	D48.7	D49.89
bronchial	-	C77.1	-	D36.0	D48.7	D49.89
bronchopulmonary	-	C77.1	-	D36.0	D48.7	D49.89
celiac	-	C77.2	-	D36.0	D48.7	D49.89
cervical	-	C77.0	-	D36.0	D48.7	D49.89
cervicofacial	-	C77.0	-	D36.0	D48.7	D49.89
Cloquet	-	C77.4	-	D36.0	D48.7	D49.89
colic	-	C77.2	-	D36.0	D48.7	D49.89
common duct	-	C77.2	-	D36.0	D48.7	D49.89
cubital	-	C77.3	-	D36.0	D48.7	D49.89

	Malignant Primary	Malignant Secondary	Ca in situ	Benign	Uncertain Behavior	Unspecified Behavior
lymph, lymphatic channel NEC, gland — *continued*						
diaphragmatic	-	C77.1	-	D36.0	D48.7	D49.89
epigastric, inferior	-	C77.1	-	D36.0	D48.7	D49.89
epitrochlear	-	C77.3	-	D36.0	D48.7	D49.89
esophageal	-	C77.1	-	D36.0	D48.7	D49.89
face	-	C77.0	-	D36.0	D48.7	D49.89
femoral	-	C77.4	-	D36.0	D48.7	D49.89
gastric	-	C77.2	-	D36.0	D48.7	D49.89
groin	-	C77.4	-	D36.0	D48.7	D49.89
head	-	C77.0	-	D36.0	D48.7	D49.89
hepatic	-	C77.2	-	D36.0	D48.7	D49.89
hilar (pulmonary)	-	C77.1	-	D36.0	D48.7	D49.89
splenic	-	C77.2	-	D36.0	D48.7	D49.89
hypogastric	-	C77.5	-	D36.0	D48.7	D49.89
ileocolic	-	C77.2	-	D36.0	D48.7	D49.89
iliac	-	C77.5	-	D36.0	D48.7	D49.89
infraclavicular	-	C77.3	-	D36.0	D48.7	D49.89
inguina, inguinal	-	C77.4	-	D36.0	D48.7	D49.89
innominate	-	C77.1	-	D36.0	D48.7	D49.89
intercostal	-	C77.1	-	D36.0	D48.7	D49.89
intestinal	-	C77.2	-	D36.0	D48.7	D49.89
intrabdominal	-	C77.2	-	D36.0	D48.7	D49.89
intrapelvic	-	C77.5	-	D36.0	D48.7	D49.89
intrathoracic	-	C77.1	-	D36.0	D48.7	D49.89
jugular	-	C77.0	-	D36.0	D48.7	D49.89
leg	-	C77.4	-	D36.0	D48.7	D49.89
limb						
lower	-	C77.4	-	D36.0	D48.7	D49.89
upper	-	C77.3	-	D36.0	D48.7	D49.89
lower limb	-	C77.4	-	D36.0	D48.7	D49.89
lumbar	-	C77.2	-	D36.0	D48.7	D49.89
mandibular	-	C77.0	-	D36.0	D48.7	D49.89
mediastinal	-	C77.1	-	D36.0	D48.7	D49.89
mesenteric (inferior) (superior)	-	C77.2	-	D36.0	D48.7	D49.89
midcolic	-	C77.2	-	D36.0	D48.7	D49.89
multiple sites in categories C77.0 - C77.5	-	C77.8	-	D36.0	D48.7	D49.89
neck	-	C77.0	-	D36.0	D48.7	D49.89
obturator	-	C77.5	-	D36.0	D48.7	D49.89
occipital	-	C77.0	-	D36.0	D48.7	D49.89
pancreatic	-	C77.2	-	D36.0	D48.7	D49.89
para-aortic	-	C77.2	-	D36.0	D48.7	D49.89
paracervical	-	C77.5	-	D36.0	D48.7	D49.89
parametrial	-	C77.5	-	D36.0	D48.7	D49.89
parasternal	-	C77.1	-	D36.0	D48.7	D49.89
parotid	-	C77.0	-	D36.0	D48.7	D49.89
pectoral	-	C77.3	-	D36.0	D48.7	D49.89
pelvic	-	C77.5	-	D36.0	D48.7	D49.89
peri-aortic	-	C77.2	-	D36.0	D48.7	D49.89
peripancreatic	-	C77.2	-	D36.0	D48.7	D49.89

	Malignant Primary	Malignant Secondary	Ca in situ	Benign	Uncertain Behavior	Unspecified Behavior
lymph, lymphatic channel NEC, gland — *continued*						
popliteal	-	C77.4	-	D36.0	D48.7	D49.89
porta hepatis	-	C77.2	-	D36.0	D48.7	D49.89
portal	-	C77.2	-	D36.0	D48.7	D49.89
preauricular	-	C77.0	-	D36.0	D48.7	D49.89
prelaryngeal	-	C77.0	-	D36.0	D48.7	D49.89
presymphysial	-	C77.5	-	D36.0	D48.7	D49.89
pretracheal	-	C77.0	-	D36.0	D48.7	D49.89
primary (any site) NEC	C96.9	-	-	-	-	-
pulmonary (hiler)	-	C77.1	-	D36.0	D48.7	D49.89
pyloric	-	C77.2	-	D36.0	D48.7	D49.89
retroperitoneal	-	C77.2	-	D36.0	D48.7	D49.89
retropharyngeal	-	C77.0	-	D36.0	D48.7	D49.89
Rosenmuller's	-	C77.4	-	D36.0	D48.7	D49.89
sacral	-	C77.5	-	D36.0	D48.7	D49.89
scalene	-	C77.0	-	D36.0	D48.7	D49.89
site NEC	-	C77.9	-	D36.0	D48.7	D49.89
splenic (hilar)	-	C77.2	-	D36.0	D48.7	D49.89
subclavicular	-	C77.3	-	D36.0	D48.7	D49.89
subinguinal	-	C77.4	-	D36.0	D48.7	D49.89
sublingual	-	C77.0	-	D36.0	D48.7	D49.89
submandibular	-	C77.0	-	D36.0	D48.7	D49.89
submaxillary	-	C77.0	-	D36.0	D48.7	D49.89
submental	-	C77.0	-	D36.0	D48.7	D49.89
subscapular	-	C77.3	-	D36.0	D48.7	D49.89
supraclavicular	-	C77.0	-	D36.0	D48.7	D49.89
thoracic	-	C77.1	-	D36.0	D48.7	D49.89
tibial	-	C77.4	-	D36.0	D48.7	D49.89
tracheal	-	C77.1	-	D36.0	D48.7	D49.89
tracheobronchial	-	C77.1	-	D36.0	D48.7	D49.89
upper limb	-	C77.3	-	D36.0	D48.7	D49.89
Virchow's	-	C77.0	-	D36.0	D48.7	D49.89
node—see also Neoplasm, lymph gland						
primary NEC	C96.9	-	-	-	-	-
vessel—see also Neoplasm, connective tissue	C49.9	C79.89	-	D21.9	D48.1	D49.2
M						
Mackenrodt's ligament	C57.7	C79.82	D07.39	D28.7	D39.8	D49.59
malar	C41.0	C79.51	-	D16.4	D48.0	D49.2
region—see Neoplasm, cheek						
mammary gland—see Neoplasm, breast						
mandible	C41.1	C79.51	-	D16.5	D48.0	D49.2
alveolar						
mucosa (carcinoma)	C03.1	C79.89	D00.03	D10.39	D37.09	D49.0
ridge or process	C41.1	C79.51	-	D16.5	D48.0	D49.2
marrow (bone) NEC	C96.9	C79.52	-	-	D47.9	D49.89
mastectomy site (skin)—see also Neoplasm, breast, skin	C44.501	C79.2	-	-	-	-
specified as breast tissue	C50.8-	C79.81	-	-	-	-
mastoid (air cells) (antrum) (cavity)	C30.1	C78.39	D02.3	D14.0	D38.5	D49.1
bone or process	C41.0	C79.51	-	D16.4	D48.0	D49.2
maxilla, maxillary (superior)	C41.0	C79.51	-	D16.4	D48.0	D49.2
alveolar						
mucosa	C03.0	C79.89	D00.03	D10.39	D37.09	D49.0
ridge or process (carcinoma)	C41.0	C79.51	-	D16.4	D48.0	D49.2
antrum	C31.0	C78.39	D02.3	D14.0	D38.5	D49.1
carcinoma	C03.0	C79.51	-	-	-	-
inferior—see Neoplasm, mandible						
sinus	C31.0	C78.39	D02.3	D14.0	D38.5	D49.1
meatus external (ear)—see also Neoplasm, skin, ear	C44.20-	C79.2	D04.2-	D23.2-	D48.5	D49.2
Meckel diverticulum, malignant	C17.3	C78.4	D01.49	D13.39	D37.2	D49.0
mediastinum, mediastinal	C38.3	C78.1	-	D15.2	D38.3	D49.89
anterior	C38.1	C78.1	-	D15.2	D38.3	D49.89
posterior	C38.2	C78.1	-	D15.2	D38.3	D49.89
medulla						
adrenal	C74.1-	C79.7-	D09.3	D35.0-	D44.1-	D49.7
oblongata	C71.7	C79.31	-	D33.1	D43.1	D49.6
meibomian gland	C44.10-	C79.2	D04.1-	D23.1-	D48.5	D49.2
basal cell carcinoma	C44.11-	-	-	-	-	-
specified type NEC	C44.19-	-	-	-	-	-
squamous cell carcinoma	C44.12-	-	-	-	-	-
melanoma—see Melanoma						
meninges	C70.9	C79.49	-	D32.9	D42.9	D49.7
brain	C70.0	C79.32	-	D32.0	D42.0	D49.7
cerebral	C70.0	C79.32	-	D32.0	D42.0	D49.7
crainial	C70.0	C79.32	-	D32.0	D42.0	D49.7
intracranial	C70.0	C79.32	-	D32.0	D42.0	D49.7
spinal (cord)	C70.1	C79.49	-	D32.1	D42.1	D49.7
meniscus, knee joint (lateral) (medial)	C40.2-	C79.51	-	D16.2-	D48.0	D49.2
Merkel cell—see Carcinoma, Merkel cell						
mesentery, mesenteric	C48.1	C78.6	-	D20.1	D48.4	D49.0
mesoappendix	C48.1	C78.6	-	D20.1	D48.4	D49.0
mesocolon	C48.1	C78.6	-	D20.1	D48.4	D49.0
mesopharynx—see Neoplasm, oropharynx						
mesosalpinx	C57.1-	C79.82	D07.39	D28.2	D39.8	D49.59
mesothelial tissue—see Mesothelioma						
mesothelioma—see Mesothelioma						
mesovarium	C57.1-	C79.82	D07.39	D28.2	D39.8	D49.59
metacarpus (any bone)	C40.1-	C79.51	-	D16.1-	-	-
metastatic NEC—see also Neoplasm, by site, secondary	-	C79.9	-	-	-	-
metatarsus (any bone)	C40.3-	C79.51	-	D16.3-	-	-
midbrain	C71.7	C79.31	-	D33.1	D43.1	D49.6
milk duct—see Neoplasm, breast						

	Malignant Primary	Malignant Secondary	Ca in situ	Benign	Uncertain Behavior	Unspecified Behavior
mons						
pubis	C51.9	C79.82	D07.1	D28.0	D39.8	D49.59
veneris	C51.9	C79.82	D07.1	D28.0	D39.8	D49.59
motor tract	C72.9	C79.49	-	D33.9	D43.9	D49.7
brain	C71.9	C79.31	-	D33.2	D43.2	D49.6
cauda equina	C72.1	C79.49	-	D33.4	D43.4	D49.7
spinal	C72.0	C79.49	-	D33.4	D43.4	D49.7
mouth	C06.9	C79.89	D00.00	D10.30	D37.09	D49.0
book-leaf	C06.89	C79.89	-	-	-	-
floor	C04.9	C79.89	D00.06	D10.2	D37.09	D49.0
anterior portion	C04.0	C79.89	D00.06	D10.2	D37.09	D49.0
lateral portion	C04.1	C79.89	D00.06	D10.2	D37.09	D49.0
overlapping lesion	C04.8	-	-	-	-	-
overlapping NEC	C06.80	-	-	-	-	-
roof	C05.9	C79.89	D00.00	D10.39	D37.09	D49.0
specified part NEC	C06.89	C79.89	D00.00	D10.39	D37.09	D49.0
vestibule	C06.1	C79.89	D00.00	D10.39	D37.09	D49.0
mucosa						
alveolar (ridge or process)	C03.9	C79.89	D00.03	D10.39	D37.09	D49.0
lower	C03.1	C79.89	D00.03	D10.39	D37.09	D49.0
upper	C03.0	C79.89	D00.03	D10.39	D37.09	D49.0
buccal	C06.0	C79.89	D00.02	D10.39	D37.09	D49.0
cheek	C06.0	C79.89	D00.02	D10.39	D37.09	D49.0
lip—see Neoplasm, lip, internal						
nasal	C30.0	C78.39	D02.3	D14.0	D38.5	D49.1
oral	C06.0	C79.89	D00.02	D10.39	D37.09	D49.0
Mullerian duct						
female	C57.7	C79.82	D07.39	D28.7	D39.8	D49.59
male	C63.7	C79.82	D07.69	D29.8	D40.8	D49.59
muscle—see also Neoplasm, connective tissue						
extraocular	C69.6-	C79.49	D09.2-	D31.6-	D48.7	D49.89
myocardium	C38.0	C79.89	-	D15.1	D48.7	D49.89
myometrium	C54.2	C79.82	D07.0	D26.1	D39.0	D49.59
myopericardium	C38.0	C79.89	-	D15.1	D48.7	D49.89
N						
nabothian gland (follicle)	C53.0	C79.82	D06.0	D26.0	D39.0	D49.59
nail—see also Neoplasm, skin, limb	C44.90	C79.2	D04.9	D23.9	D48.5	D49.2
finger—see also Neoplasm, skin, limb, upper	C44.60-	C79.2	D04.6-	D23.6-	D48.5	D49.2
toe—see also Neoplasm, skin, limb, lower	C44.70-	C79.2	D04.7-	D23.7-	D48.5	D49.2
nares, naris (anterior) (posterior)	C30.0	C78.39	D02.3	D14.0	D38.5	D49.1
nasal—see Neoplasm, nose						
nasolabial groove—see also Neoplasm, skin, face	C44.309	C79.2	D04.39	D23.39	D48.5	D49.2
nasolacrimal duct	C69.5-	C79.49	D09.2-	D31.5-	D48.7	D49.89
nasopharynx, nasopharyngeal	C11.9	C79.89	D00.08	D10.6	D37.05	D49.0
floor	C11.3	C79.89	D00.08	D10.6	D37.05	D49.0
overlapping lesion	C11.8	-	-	-	-	-
nasopharynx, nasopharyngeal — *continued*						
roof	C11.0	C79.89	D00.08	D10.6	D37.05	D49.0
wall	C11.9	C79.89	D00.08	D10.6	D37.05	D49.0
anterior	C11.3	C79.89	D00.08	D10.6	D37.05	D49.0
lateral	C11.2	C79.89	D00.08	D10.6	D37.05	D49.0
posterior	C11.1	C79.89	D00.08	D10.6	D37.05	D49.0
superior	C11.0	C79.89	D00.08	D10.6	D37.05	D49.0
nates—see also Neoplasm, skin, trunk	C44.509	C79.2	D04.5	D23.5	D48.5	D49.2
neck NEC	C76.0	C79.89	D09.8	D36.7	D48.7	D49.89
skin	C44.40	-	-	-	-	-
basal cell carcinoma	C44.41	-	-	-	-	-
specified type NEC	C44.49	-	-	-	-	-
squamous cell carcinoma	C44.42	-	-	-	-	-
nerve (ganglion)	C47.9	C79.89	-	D36.10	D48.2	D49.2
abducens	C72.59	C79.49	-	D33.3	D43.3	D49.7
accessory (spinal)	C72.59	C79.49	-	D33.3	D43.3	D49.7
acoustic	C72.4-	C79.49	-	D33.3	D43.3	D49.7
auditory	C72.4-	C79.49	-	D33.3	D43.3	D49.7
autonomic NEC—see also Neoplasm, nerve, peripheral	C47.9	C79.89	-	D36.10	D48.2	D49.2
brachial	C47.1-	C79.89	-	D36.12	D48.2	D49.2
cranial	C72.50	C79.49	-	D33.3	D43.3	D49.7
specified NEC	C72.59	C79.49	-	D33.3	D43.3	D49.7
facial	C72.59	C79.49	-	D33.3	D43.3	D49.7
femoral	C47.2-	C79.89	-	D36.13	D48.2	D49.2
ganglion NEC—see also Neoplasm, nerve, peripheral	C47.9	C79.89	-	D36.10	D48.2	D49.2
glossopharyngeal	C72.59	C79.49	-	D33.3	D43.3	D49.7
hypoglossal	C72.59	C79.49	-	D33.3	D43.3	D49.7
intercostal	C47.3	C79.89	-	D36.14	D48.2	D49.2
lumbar	C47.6	C79.89	-	D36.17	D48.2	D49.2
median	C47.1-	C79.89	-	D36.12	D48.2	D49.2
obturator	C47.2-	C79.89	-	D36.13	D48.2	D49.2
oculomotor	C72.59	C79.49	-	D33.3	D43.3	D49.7
olfactory	C47.2-	C79.49	-	D33.3	D43.3	D49.7
optic	C72.3-	C79.49	-	D33.3	D43.3	D49.7
parasympathetic NEC	C47.9	C79.89	-	D36.10	D48.2	D49.2
peripheral NEC	C47.9	C79.89	-	D36.10	D48.2	D49.2
abdomen	C47.4	C79.89	-	D36.15	D48.2	D49.2
abdominal wall	C47.4	C79.89	-	D36.15	D48.2	D49.2
ankle	C47.2-	C79.89	-	D36.13	D48.2	D49.2
antecubital fossa or space	C47.1-	C79.89	-	D36.12	D48.2	D49.2
arm	C47.1-	C79.89	-	D36.12	D48.2	D49.2
auricle (ear)	C47.0	C79.89	-	D36.11	D48.2	D49.2
axilla	C47.3	C79.89	-	D36.12	D48.2	D49.2
back	C47.6	C79.89	-	D36.17	D48.2	D49.2
buttock	C47.5	C79.89	-	D36.16	D48.2	D49.2
calf	C47.2-	C79.89	-	D36.13	D48.2	D49.2

	Malignant Primary	Malignant Secondary	Ca in situ	Benign	Uncertain Behavior	Unspecified Behavior
nerve (ganglion), peripheral NEC — *continued*						
cervical region	C47.0	C79.89	-	D36.11	D48.2	D49.2
cheek	C47.0	C79.89	-	D36.11	D48.2	D49.2
chest (wall)	C47.3	C79.89	-	D36.14	D48.2	D49.2
chin	C47.0	C79.89	-	D36.11	D48.2	D49.2
ear (external)	C47.0	C79.89	-	D36.11	D48.2	D49.2
elbow	C47.1-	C79.89	-	D36.12	D48.2	D49.2
extrarectal	C47.5	C79.89	-	D36.16	D48.2	D49.2
extremity	C47.9	C79.89	-	D36.10	D48.2	D49.2
lower	C47.2-	C79.89	-	D36.13	D48.2	D49.2
upper	C47.1-	C79.89	-	D36.12	D48.2	D49.2
eyelid	C47.0	C79.89	-	D36.11	D48.2	D49.2
face	C47.0	C79.89	-	D36.11	D48.2	D49.2
finger	C47.1-	C79.89	-	D36.12	D48.2	D49.2
flank	C47.6	C79.89	-	D36.17	D48.2	D49.2
foot	C47.2-	C79.89	-	D36.13	D48.2	D49.2
forearm	C47.1-	C79.89	-	D36.12	D48.2	D49.2
forehead	C47.0	C79.89	-	D36.11	D48.2	D49.2
gluteal region	C47.5	C79.89	-	D36.16	D48.2	D49.2
groin	C47.5	C79.89	-	D36.16	D48.2	D49.2
hand	C47.1-	C79.89	-	D36.12	D48.2	D49.2
head	C47.0	C79.89	-	D36.11	D48.2	D49.2
heel	C47.2-	C79.89	-	D36.13	D48.2	D49.2
hip	C47.2-	C79.89	-	D36.13	D48.2	D49.2
infraclavicular region	C47.3	C79.89	-	D36.14	D48.2	D49.2
inguinal (canal) (region)	C47.5	C79.89	-	D36.16	D48.2	D49.2
intrathoracic	C47.3	C79.89	-	D36.14	D48.2	D49.2
ischiorectal fossa	C47.5	C79.89	-	D36.16	D48.2	D49.2
knee	C47.2-	C79.89	-	D36.13	D48.2	D49.2
leg	C47.2-	C79.89	-	D36.13	D48.2	D49.2
limb NEC	C47.9	C79.89	-	D36.10	D48.2	D49.2
lower	C47.2-	C79.89	-	D36.13	D48.2	D49.2
upper	C47.1-	C79.89	-	D36.12	D48.2	D49.2
nates	C47.5	C79.89	-	D36.16	D48.2	D49.2
neck	C47.0	C79.89	-	D36.11	D48.2	D49.2
orbit	C69.6-	C79.49	-	D31.6-	D48.7	D49.2
pararectal	C47.5	C79.89	-	D36.16	D48.2	D49.2
paraurethral	C47.5	C79.89	-	D36.16	D48.2	D49.2
paravaginal	C47.5	C79.89	-	D36.16	D48.2	D49.2
pelvis (floor)	C47.5	C79.89	-	D36.16	D48.2	D49.2
pelvoabdominal	C47.8	C79.89	-	D36.17	D48.2	D49.2
perineum	C47.5	C79.89	-	D36.16	D48.2	D49.2
perirectal (tissue)	C47.5	C79.89	-	D36.16	D48.2	D49.2
periurethral (tissue)	C47.5	C79.89	-	D36.16	D48.2	D49.2
popliteal fossa or space	C47.2-	C79.89	-	D36.13	D48.2	D49.2
presacral	C47.5	C79.89	-	D36.16	D48.2	D49.2
pterygoid fossa	C47.0	C79.89	-	D36.11	D48.2	D49.2
rectovaginal septum or wall	C47.5	C79.89	-	D36.16	D48.2	D49.2
rectovesical	C47.5	C79.89	-	D36.16	D48.2	D49.2
sacrococcygeal region	C47.5	C79.89	-	D36.16	D48.2	D49.2
scalp	C47.0	C79.89	-	D36.11	D48.2	D49.2

	Malignant Primary	Malignant Secondary	Ca in situ	Benign	Uncertain Behavior	Unspecified Behavior
nerve (ganglion), peripheral NEC — *continued*						
scapular region	C47.3	C79.89	-	D36.14	D48.2	D49.2
shoulder	C47.1-	C79.89	-	D36.12	D48.2	D49.2
submental	C47.0	C79.89	-	D36.11	D48.2	D49.2
supraclavicular region	C47.0	C79.89	-	D36.11	D48.2	D49.2
temple	C47.0	C79.89	-	D36.11	D48.2	D49.2
temporal region	C47.0	C79.89	-	D36.11	D48.2	D49.2
thigh	C47.2-	C79.89	-	D36.13	D48.2	D49.2
thoracic (duct) (wall)	C47.3	C79.89	-	D36.14	D48.2	D49.2
thorax	C47.3	C79.89	-	D36.14	D48.2	D49.2
thumb	C47.1-	C79.89	-	D36.12	D48.2	D49.2
toe	C47.2-	C79.89	-	D36.13	D48.2	D49.2
trunk	C47.6	C79.89	-	D36.17	D48.2	D49.2
umbilicus	C47.4	C79.89	-	D36.15	D48.2	D49.2
vesicorectal	C47.5	C79.89	-	D36.16	D48.2	D49.2
wrist	C47.1-	C79.89	-	D36.12	D48.2	D49.2
radial	C47.1-	C79.89	-	D36.12	D48.2	D49.2
sacral	C47.5	C79.89	-	D36.16	D48.2	D49.2
sciatic	C47.2-	C79.89	-	D36.13	D48.2	D49.2
spinal NEC	C47.9	C79.89	-	D36.10	D48.2	D49.2
accessory	C72.59	C79.49	-	D33.3	D43.3	D49.7
sympathetic NEC—see also Neoplasm, nerve, peripheral	C47.9	C79.89	-	D36.10	D48.2	D49.2
trigeminal	C72.59	C79.49	-	D33.3	D43.3	D49.7
trochlear	C72.59	C79.49	-	D33.3	D43.3	D49.7
ulnar	C47.1-	C79.89	-	D36.12	D48.2	D49.2
vagus	C72.59	C79.49	-	D33.3	D43.3	D49.7
nervous system (central)	C72.9	C79.40	-	D33.9	D43.9	D49.7
autonomic—see Neoplasm, nerve, peripheral						
parasympathetic—see Neoplasm, nerve, peripheral						
specified site NEC	-	C79.49	-	D33.7	D43.8	-
sympathetic—see Neoplasm, nerve, peripheral						
nevus—see Nevus						
nipple	C50.0-	C79.81	D05.-	D24.-	-	-
nose, nasal	C76.0	C79.89	D09.8	D36.7	D48.7	D49.89
ala (external) (nasi)—see also Neoplasm, nose, skin	C44.301	C79.2	D04.39	D23.39	D48.5	D49.2
bone	C41.0	C79.51	-	D16.4	D48.0	D49.2
cartilage	C30.0	C78.39	D02.3	D14.0	D38.5	D49.1
cavity	C30.0	C78.39	D02.3	D14.0	D38.5	D49.1
choana	C11.3	C79.89	D00.08	D10.6	D37.05	D49.0
external (skin)—see also Neoplasm, nose, skin	C44.301	C79.2	D04.39	D23.39	D48.5	D49.2
fossa	C30.0	C78.39	D02.3	D14.0	D38.5	D49.1
internal	C30.0	C78.39	D02.3	D14.0	D38.5	D49.1
mucosa	C30.0	C78.39	D02.3	D14.0	D38.5	D49.1
septum	C30.0	C78.39	D02.3	D14.0	D38.5	D49.1
posterior margin	C11.3	C79.89	D00.08	D10.6	D37.05	D49.0

	Malignant Primary	Malignant Secondary	Ca in situ	Benign	Uncertain Behavior	Unspecified Behavior
nose, nasal — *continued*						
sinus—see Neoplasm, sinus						
skin	C44.301	C79.2	D04.39	D23.39	D48.5	D49.2
basal cell carcinoma	C44.311	-	-	-	-	-
specified type NEC	C44.391	-	-	-	-	-
squamous cell carcinoma	C44.321	-	-	-	-	-
turbinate (mucosa)	C30.0	C78.39	D02.3	D14.0	D38.5	D49.1
bone	C41.0	C79.51	-	D16.4	D48.0	D49.2
vestibule	C30.0	C78.39	D02.3	D14.0	D38.5	D49.1
nostril	C30.0	C78.39	D02.3	D14.0	D38.5	D49.1
nucleus pulposus	C41.2	C79.51	-	D16.6	D48.0	D49.2
O						
occipital						
bone	C41.0	C79.51	-	D16.4	D48.0	D49.2
lobe or pole, brain	C71.4	C79.31	-	D33.0	D43.0	D49.6
odontogenic—see Neoplasm, jaw bone						
olfactory nerve or bulb	C72.2-	C79.49	-	D33.3	D43.3	D49.7
olive (brain)	C71.7	C79.31	-	D33.1	D43.1	D49.6
omentum	C48.1	C78.6	-	D20.1	D48.4	D49.0
operculum (brain)	C71.0	C79.31	-	D33.0	D43.0	D49.6
optic nerve, chiasm, or tract	C72.3-	C79.49	-	D33.3	D43.3	D49.7
oral (cavity)	C06.9	C79.89	D00.00	D10.30	D37.09	D49.0
ill-defined	C14.8	C79.89	D00.00	D10.30	D37.09	D49.0
mucosa	C06.0	C79.89	D00.02	D10.39	D37.09	D49.0
orbit	C69.6-	C79.49	D09.2-	D31.6-	D48.7	D49.89
autonomic nerve	C69.6-	C79.49	-	D31.6-	D48.7	D49.2
bone	C41.0	C79.51	-	D16.4	D48.0	D49.2
eye	C69.6-	C79.49	D09.2-	D31.6-	D48.7	D49.89
peripheral nerves	C69.6-	C79.49	-	D31.6-	D48.7	D49.2
soft parts	C69.6-	C79.49	D09.2-	D31.6-	D48.7	D49.89
organ of Zuckerkandl	C75.5	C79.89	-	D35.6	D44.7	D49.7
oropharynx	C10.9	C79.89	D00.08	D10.5	D37.05	D49.0
branchial cleft (vestige)	C10.4	C79.89	D00.08	D10.5	D37.05	D49.0
junctional region	C10.8	C79.89	D00.08	D10.5	D37.05	D49.0
lateral wall	C10.2	C79.89	D00.08	D10.5	D37.05	D49.0
overlapping lesion	C10.8	-	-	-	-	-
pillars or fauces	C09.1	C79.89	D00.08	D10.5	D37.05	D49.0
posterior wall	C10.3	C79.89	D00.08	D10.5	D37.05	D49.0
vallecula	C10.0	C79.89	D00.08	D10.5	D37.05	D49.0
os						
external	C53.1	C79.82	D06.1	D26.0	D39.0	D49.59
internal	C53.0	C79.82	D06.0	D26.0	D39.0	D49.59
ovary	C56.-	C79.6-	D07.39	D27.-	D39.1-	D49.59
oviduct	C57.0-	C79.82	D07.39	D28.2	D39.8	D49.59
P						
palate	C05.9	C79.89	D00.00	D10.39	D37.09	D49.0
hard	C05.0	C79.89	D00.05	D10.39	D37.09	D49.0
junction of hard and soft palate	C05.9	C79.89	D00.00	D10.39	D37.09	D49.0
overlapping lesions	C05.8	-	-	-	-	-
soft	C05.1	C79.89	D00.04	D10.39	D37.09	D49.0

	Malignant Primary	Malignant Secondary	Ca in situ	Benign	Uncertain Behavior	Unspecified Behavior
palate — *continued*						
nasopharyngeal surface	C11.3	C79.89	D00.08	D10.6	D37.05	D49.0
posterior surface	C11.3	C79.89	D00.08	D10.6	D37.05	D49.0
superior surface	C11.3	C79.89	D00.08	D10.6	D37.05	D49.0
palatoglossal arch	C09.1	C79.89	D00.00	D10.5	D37.09	D49.0
palatopharyngeal arch	C09.1	C79.89	D00.00	D10.5	D37.09	D49.0
pallium	C71.0	C79.31	-	D33.0	D43.0	D49.6
palpebra	C44.10-	C79.2	D04.1-	D23.1-	D48.5	D49.2
basal cell carcinoma	C44.11-	-	-	-	-	-
specified type NEC	C44.19-	-	-	-	-	-
squamous cell carcinoma	C44.12-	-	-	-	-	-
pancreas	C25.9	C78.89	D01.7	D13.6	D37.8	D49.0
body	C25.1	C78.89	D01.7	D13.6	D37.8	D49.0
duct (of Santorini) (of Wirsung)	C25.3	C78.89	D01.7	D13.6	D37.8	D49.0
ectopic tissue	C25.7	C78.89	-	D13.6	D37.8	D49.0
head	C25.0	C78.89	D01.7	D13.6	D37.8	D49.0
islet cells	C25.4	C78.89	D01.7	D13.7	D37.8	D49.0
neck	C25.7	C78.89	D01.7	D13.6	D37.8	D49.0
overlapping lesion	C25.8	-	-	-	-	-
tail	C25.2	C78.89	D01.7	D13.6	D37.8	D49.0
para-aortic body	C75.5	C79.89	-	D35.6	D44.7	D49.7
paraganglion NEC	C75.5	C79.89	-	D35.6	D44.7	D49.7
parametrium	C57.3	C79.82	-	D28.2	D39.8	D49.59
paranephric	C48.0	C78.6	-	D20.0	D48.3	D49.0
pararectal	C76.3	C79.89	-	D36.7	D48.7	D49.89
parasagittal (region)	C76.0	C79.89	D09.8	D36.7	D48.7	D49.89
parasellar	C72.9	C79.49	-	D33.9	D43.8	D49.7
parathyroid (gland)	C75.0	C79.89	D09.3	D35.1	D44.2	D49.7
paraurethral	C76.3	C79.89	-	D36.7	D48.7	D49.89
gland	C68.1	C79.19	D09.19	D30.8	D41.8	D49.59
paravaginal	C76.3	C79.89	-	D36.7	D48.7	D49.89
parenchyma, kidney	C64.-	C79.0-	D09.19	D30.0-	D41.0-	D49.51-
parietal						
bone	C41.0	C79.51	-	D16.4	D48.0	D49.2
lobe, brain	C71.3	C79.31	-	D33.0	D43.0	D49.6
paroophoron	C57.1-	C79.82	D07.39	D28.2	D39.8	D49.59
parotid (duct) (gland)	C07	C79.89	D00.00	D11.0	D37.030	D49.0
parovarium	C57.1-	C79.82	D07.39	D28.2	D39.8	D49.59
patella	C40.20	C79.51	-	-	-	-
peduncle, cerebral	C71.7	C79.31	-	D33.1	D43.1	D49.6
pelvirectal junction	C19	C78.5	D01.1	D12.7	D37.5	D49.0
pelvis, pelvic	C76.3	C79.89	D09.8	D36.7	D48.7	D49.89
bone	C41.4	C79.51	-	D16.8	D48.0	D49.2
floor	C76.3	C79.89	D09.8	D36.7	D48.7	D49.89
renal	C65.-	C79.0-	D09.19	D30.1-	D41.1-	D49.51-
viscera	C76.3	C79.89	D09.8	D36.7	D48.7	D49.89
wall	C76.3	C79.89	D09.8	D36.7	D48.7	D49.89
pelvo-abdominal	C76.8	C79.89	D09.8	D36.7	D48.7	D49.89
penis	C60.9	C79.82	D07.4	D29.0	D40.8	D49.59
body	C60.2	C79.82	D07.4	D29.0	D40.8	D49.59
corpus (cavernosum)	C60.2	C79.82	D07.4	D29.0	D40.8	D49.59

	Malignant Primary	Malignant Secondary	Ca in situ	Benign	Uncertain Behavior	Unspecified Behavior
penis — *continued*						
glans	C60.1	C79.82	D07.4	D29.0	D40.8	D49.59
overlapping sites	C60.8	-	-	-	-	-
skin NEC	C60.9	C79.82	D07.4	D29.0	D40.8	D49.59
periadrenal (tissue)	C48.0	C78.6	-	D20.0	D48.3	D49.0
perianal (skin)—see also Neoplasm, anus, skin	C44.500	C79.2	D04.5	D23.5	D48.5	D49.2
pericardium	C38.0	C79.89	-	D15.1	D48.7	D49.89
perinephric	C48.0	C78.6	-	D20.0	D48.3	D49.0
perineum	C76.3	C79.89	D09.8	D36.7	D48.7	D49.89
periodontal tissue NEC	C03.9	C79.89	D00.03	D10.39	D37.09	D49.0
periosteum—see Neoplasm, bone						
peripancreatic	C48.0	C78.6	-	D20.0	D48.3	D49.0
peripheral nerve NEC	C47.9	C79.89	-	D36.10	D48.2	D49.2
perirectal (tissue)	C76.3	C79.89	-	D36.7	D48.7	D49.89
perirenal (tissue)	C48.0	C78.6	-	D20.0	D48.3	D49.0
peritoneum, peritoneal (cavity)	C48.2	C78.6	-	D20.1	D48.4	D49.0
benign mesothelial tissue—see Mesothelioma, benign						
overlapping lesion	C48.8	-	-	-	-	-
with digestive organs	C26.9	-	-	-	-	-
parietal	C48.1	C78.6	-	D20.1	D48.4	D49.0
pelvic	C48.1	C78.6	-	D20.1	D48.4	D49.0
specified part NEC	C48.1	C78.6	-	D20.1	D48.4	D49.0
peritonsillar (tissue)	C76.0	C79.89	D09.8	D36.7	D48.7	D49.89
periurethral tissue	C76.3	C79.89	-	D36.7	D48.7	D49.89
phalanges						
foot	C40.3-	C79.51	-	D16.3-	-	-
hand	C40.1-	C79.51	-	D16.1-	-	-
pharynx, pharyngeal	C14.0	C79.89	D00.08	D10.9	D37.05	D49.0
bursa	C11.1	C79.89	D00.08	D10.6	D37.05	D49.0
fornix	C11.3	C79.89	D00.08	D10.6	D37.05	D49.0
recess	C11.2	C79.89	D00.08	D10.6	D37.05	D49.0
region	C14.0	C79.89	D00.08	D10.9	D37.05	D49.0
tonsil	C11.1	C79.89	D00.08	D10.6	D37.05	D49.0
wall (lateral) (posterior)	C14.0	C79.89	D00.08	D10.9	D37.05	D49.0
pia mater	C70.9	C79.40	-	D32.9	D42.9	D49.7
cerebral	C70.0	C79.32	-	D32.0	D42.0	D49.7
cranial	C70.0	C79.32	-	D32.0	D42.0	D49.7
spinal	C70.1	C79.49	-	D32.1	D42.1	D49.7
pillars of fauces	C09.1	C79.89	D00.08	D10.5	D37.05	D49.0
pineal (body) (gland)	C75.3	C79.89	D09.3	D35.4	D44.5	D49.7
pinna (ear) NEC—see also Neoplasm, skin, ear	C44.20-	C79.2	D04.2-	D23.2-	D48.5	D49.2
piriform fossa or sinus	C12	C79.89	D00.08	D10.7	D37.05	D49.0
pituitary (body) (fossa) (gland) (lobe)	C75.1	C79.89	D09.3	D35.2	D44.3	D49.7
placenta	C58	C79.82	D07.0	D26.7	D39.2	D49.59
pleura, pleural (cavity)	C38.4	C78.2	-	D19.0	D38.2	D49.1
overlapping lesion with heart or mediastinum	C38.8	-	-	-	-	-
parietal	C38.4	C78.2	-	D19.0	D38.2	D49.1

	Malignant Primary	Malignant Secondary	Ca in situ	Benign	Uncertain Behavior	Unspecified Behavior
pleura, pleural — *continued*						
visceral	C38.4	C78.2	-	D19.0	D38.2	D49.1
plexus						
brachial	C47.1-	C79.89	-	D36.12	D48.2	D49.2
cervical	C47.0	C79.89	-	D36.11	D48.2	D49.2
choroid	C71.5	C79.31	-	D33.0	D43.0	D49.6
lumbosacral	C47.5	C79.89	-	D36.16	D48.2	D49.2
sacral	C47.5	C79.89	-	D36.16	D48.2	D49.2
pluriendocrine	C75.8	C79.89	D09.3	D35.7	D44.9	D49.7
pole						
frontal	C71.1	C79.31	-	D33.0	D43.0	D49.6
occipital	C71.4	C79.31	-	D33.0	D43.0	D49.6
pons (varolii)	C71.7	C79.31	-	D33.1	D43.1	D49.6
popliteal fossa or space	C76.5-	C79.89	D04.7-	D36.7	D48.7	D49.89
postcricoid (region)	C13.0	C79.89	D00.08	D10.7	D37.05	D49.0
posterior fossa (cranial)	C71.9	C79.31	-	D33.2	D43.2	D49.6
postnasal space	C11.9	C79.89	D00.08	D10.6	D37.05	D49.0
prepuce	C60.0	C79.82	D07.4	D29.0	D40.8	D49.59
prepylorus	C16.4	C78.89	D00.2	D13.1	D37.1	D49.0
presacral (region)	C76.3	C79.89	-	D36.7	D48.7	D49.89
prostate (gland)	C61	C79.82	D07.5	D29.1	D40.0	D49.59
utricle	C68.0	C79.19	D09.19	D30.4	D41.3	D49.59
pterygoid fossa	C49.0	C79.89	-	D21.0	D48.1	D49.2
pubic bone	C41.4	C79.51	-	D16.8	D48.0	D49.2
pudenda, pudendum (femaie)	C51.9	C79.82	D07.1	D28.0	D39.8	D49.59
pulmonary—see also Neoplasm, lung	C34.9-	C78.0-	D02.2-	D14.3-	D38.1	D49.1
putamen	C71.0	C79.31	-	D33.0	D43.0	D49.6
pyloric						
antrum	C16.3	C78.89	D00.2	D13.1	D37.1	D49.0
canal	C16.4	C78.89	D00.2	D13.1	D37.1	D49.0
pylorus	C16.4	C78.89	D00.2	D13.1	D37.1	D49.0
pyramid (brain)	C71.7	C79.31	-	D33.1	D43.1	D49.6
pyriform fossa or sinus	C12	C79.89	D00.08	D10.7	D37.05	D49.0
R						
radius (any part)	C40.0-	C79.51	-	D16.0-	-	-
Rathke's pouch	C75.1	C79.89	D09.3	D35.2	D44.3	D49.7
rectosigmoid (junction)	C19	C78.5	D01.1	D12.7	D37.5	D49.0
overlapping lesion with anus or rectum	C21.8	-	-	-	-	-
rectouterine pouch	C48.1	C78.6	-	D20.1	D48.4	D49.0
rectovaginal septum or wall	C76.3	C79.89	D09.8	D36.7	D48.7	D49.89
rectovesical septum	C76.3	C79.89	D09.8	D36.7	D48.7	D49.89
rectum (ampulla)	C20	C78.5	D01.2	D12.8	D37.5	D49.0
and colon	C19	C78.5	D01.1	D12.7	D37.5	D49.0
overlapping lesion with anus or rectosigmoid junction	C21.8	-	-	-	-	-
renal	C64.-	C79.0-	D09.19	D30.0-	D41.0-	D49.51-
calyx	C65.-	C79.0-	D09.19	D30.1-	D41.1-	D49.51-
hilus	C65.-	C79.0-	D09.19	D30.1-	D41.1-	D49.51-

	Malignant Primary	Malignant Secondary	Ca in situ	Benign	Uncertain Behavior	Unspecified Behavior
renal — *continued*						
parenchyma	C64.-	C79.0-	D09.19	D30.0-	D41.0-	D49.51-
pelvis	C65.-	C79.0-	D09.19	D30.1-	D41.1-	D49.51-
respiratory						
organs or system NEC	C39.9	C78.30	D02.4	D14.4	D38.6	D49.1
tract NEC	C39.9	C78.30	D02.4	D14.4	D38.5	D49.1
upper	C39.0	C78.30	D02.4	D14.4	D38.5	D49.1
retina	C69.2-	C79.49	D09.2-	D31.2-	D48.7	D49.81
retrobulbar	C69.6-	C79.49	-	D31.6-	D48.7	D49.89
retrocecal	C48.0	C78.6	-	D20.0	D48.3	D49.0
retromolar (area) (triangle) (trigone)	C06.2	C79.89	D00.00	D10.39	D37.09	D49.0
retro-orbital	C76.0	C79.89	D09.8	D36.7	D48.7	D49.89
retroperitoneal (space) (tissue)	C48.0	C78.6	-	D20.0	D48.3	D49.0
retroperitoneum	C48.0	C78.6	-	D20.0	D48.3	D49.0
retropharyngeal	C14.0	C79.89	D00.08	D10.9	D37.05	D49.0
retrovesical (septum)	C76.3	C79.89	D09.8	D36.7	D48.7	D49.89
rhinencephalon	C71.0	C79.31	-	D33.0	D43.0	D49.6
rib	C41.3	C79.51	-	D16.7	D48.0	D49.2
Rosenmuller's fossa	C11.2	C79.89	D00.08	D10.6	D37.05	D49.0
round ligament	C57.2-	C79.82	-	D28.2	D39.8	D49.59
S						
sacrococcyx, sacrococcygeal	C41.4	C79.51		D16.8	D48.0	D49.2
region	C76.3	C79.89	D09.8	D36.7	D48.7	D49.89
sacrouterine ligament	C57.3	C79.82	-	D28.2	D39.8	D49.59
sacrum, sacral (vertebra)	C41.4	C79.51	-	D16.8	D48.0	D49.2
salivary gland or duct (major)	C08.9	C79.89	D00.00	D11.9	D37.039	D49.0
minor NEC	C06.9	C79.89	D00.00	D10.39	D37.04	D49.0
overlapping lesion	C08.9	-	-	-	-	-
parotid	C07	C79.89	D00.00	D11.0	D37.030	D49.0
pluriglandular	C08.9	C79.89	D00.00	D11.9	D37.039	D49.0
sublingual	C08.1	C79.89	D00.00	D11.7	D37.031	D49.0
submandibular	C08.0	C79.89	D00.00	D11.7	D37.032	D49.0
submaxillary	C08.0	C79.89	D00.00	D11.7	D37.032	D49.0
salpinx (uterine)	C57.0-	C79.82	D07.39	D28.2	D39.8	D49.59
Santorini's duct	C25.3	C78.89	D01.7	D13.6	D37.8	D49.0
scalp	C44.40	C79.2	D04.4	D23.4	D48.5	D49.2
basal cell carcinoma	C44.41	-	-	-	-	-
specified type NEC	C44.49	-	-	-	-	-
squamous cell carcinoma	C44.42	-	-	-	-	-
scapula (any part)	C40.0-	C79.51	-	D16.0-	-	-
scapular region	C76.1	C79.89	D09.8	D36.7	D48.7	D49.89
scar NEC—see *also* Neoplasm, skin, by site	C44.90	C79.2	D04.9	D23.9	D48.5	D49.2
sciatic nerve	C47.2-	C79.89	-	D36.13	D48.2	D49.2
sclera	C69.4-	C79.49	D09.2-	D31.4-	D48.7	D49.89
scrotum (skin)	C63.2	C79.82	D07.61	D29.4	D40.8	D49.59
sebaceous gland—see Neoplasm, skin						
sella turcica	C75.1	C79.89	D09.3	D35.2	D44.3	D49.7
bone	C41.0	C79.51	-	D16.4	D48.0	D49.2
semilunar cartilage (knee)	C40.2-	C79.51	-	D16.2-	D48.0	D49.2

	Malignant Primary	Malignant Secondary	Ca in situ	Benign	Uncertain Behavior	Unspecified Behavior
seminal vesicle	C63.7	C79.82	D07.69	D29.8	D40.8	D49.59
septum						
nasal	C30.0	C78.39	D02.3	D14.0	D38.5	D49.1
posterior margin	C11.3	C79.89	D00.08	D10.6	D37.05	D49.0
rectovaginal	C76.3	C79.89	D09.8	D36.7	D48.7	D49.89
rectovesical	C76.3	C79.89	D09.8	D36.7	D48.7	D49.89
urethrovaginal	C57.9	C79.82	D07.30	D28.9	D39.9	D49.59
vesicovaginal	C57.9	C79.82	D07.30	D28.9	D39.9	D49.59
shoulder NEC	C76.4-	C79.89	D04.6-	D36.7	D48.7	D49.89
sigmoid flexure (lower) (upper)	C18.7	C78.5	D01.0	D12.5	D37.4	D49.0
sinus (accessory)	C31.9	C78.39	D02.3	D14.0	D38.5	D49.1
bone (any)	C41.0	C79.51	-	D16.4	D48.0	D49.2
ethmoidal	C31.1	C78.39	D02.3	D14.0	D38.5	D49.1
frontal	C31.2	C78.39	D02.3	D14.0	D38.5	D49.1
maxillary	C31.0	C78.39	D02.3	D14.0	D38.5	D49.1
nasal, paranasal NEC	C31.9	C78.39	D02.3	D14.0	D38.5	D49.1
overlapping lesion	C31.8	-	-	-	-	-
pyriform	C12	C79.89	D00.08	D10.7	D37.05	D49.0
sphenoid	C31.3	C78.39	D02.3	D14.0	D38.5	D49.1
skeleton, skeletal NEC	C41.9	C79.51	-	D16.9	D48.0	D49.2
Skene's gland	C68.1	C79.19	D09.19	D30.8	D41.8	D49.59
skin NOS	C44.90	C79.2	D04.9	D23.9	D48.5	D49.2
abdominal wall	C44.509	C79.2	D04.5	D23.5	D48.5	D49.2
basal cell carcinoma	C44.519	-	-	-	-	-
specified type NEC	C44.599	-	-	-	-	-
squamous cell carcinoma	C44.529	-	-	-	-	-
ala nasi—see also Neoplasm, nose, skin	C44.301	C79.2	D04.39	D23.39	D48.5	D49.2
ankle—see also Neoplasm, skin, limb, lower	C44.70-	C79.2	D04.7-	D23.7-	D48.5	D49.2
antecubital space—see also Neoplasm, skin, limb, upper	C44.60-	C79.2	D04.6-	D23.6-	D48.5	D49.2
anus	C44.500	C79.2	D04.5	D23.5	D48.5	D49.2
basal cell carcinoma	C44.510	-	-	-	-	-
specified type NEC	C44.590	-	-	-	-	-
squamous cell carcinoma	C44.520	-	-	-	-	-
arm—see also Neoplasm, skin, limb, upper	C44.60-	C79.2	D04.6-	D23.6-	D48.5	D49.2
auditory canal (external)—see also Neoplasm, skin, ear	C44.20-	C79.2	D04.2-	D23.2-	D48.5	D49.2
auricle (ear)—see also Neoplasm, skin, ear	C44.20-	C79.2	D04.2-	D23.2-	D48.5	D49.2
auricular canal (external)—see also Neoplasm, skin, ear	C44.20-	C79.2	D04.2-	D23.2-	D48.5	D49.2
axilla, axillary fold—see also Neoplasm, skin, trunk	C44.509	C79.2	D04.5	D23.5	D48.5	D49.2
back—see also Neoplasm, skin, trunk	C44.509	C79.2	D04.5	D23.5	D48.5	D49.2
basal cell carcinoma	C44.91					
breast	C44.501	C79.2	D04.5	D23.5	D48.5	D49.2

	Malignant Primary	Malignant Secondary	Ca in situ	Benign	Uncertain Behavior	Unspecified Behavior
skin NOS, breast — *continued*						
basal cell carcinoma	C44.511	-	-	-	-	-
specified type NEC	C44.591	-	-	-	-	-
squamous cell carcinoma	C44.521	-	-	-	-	-
brow—see also Neoplasm, skin, face	C44.309	C79.2	D04.39	D23.39	D48.5	D49.2
buttock—see also Neoplasm, skin, trunk	C44.509	C79.2	D04.5	D23.5	D48.5	D49.2
calf—see also Neoplasm, skin, limb, lower	C44.70-	C79.2	D04.7-	D23.7-	D48.5	D49.2
canthus (eye) (inner) (outer)	C44.10-	C79.2	D04.1-	D23.1-	D48.5	D49.2
basal cell carcinoma	C44.11-	-	-	-	-	-
specified type NEC	C44.19-	-	-	-	-	-
squamous cell carcinoma	C44.12-	-	-	-	-	-
cervical region—see also Neoplasm, skin, neck	C44.40	C79.2	D04.4	D23.4	D48.5	D49.2
cheek (external) —see also Neoplasm, skin, face	C44.309	C79.2	D04.39	D23.39	D48.5	D49.2
chest (wall)—see also Neoplasm, skin, trunk	C44.509	C79.2	D04.5	D23.5	D48.5	D49.2
chin—see also Neoplasm, skin, face	C44.309	C79.2	D04.39	D23.39	D48.5	D49.2
clavicular area—see also Neoplasm, skin, trunk	C44.509	C79.2	D04.5	D23.5	D48.5	D49.2
clitoris	C51.2	C79.82	D07.1	D28.0	D39.8	D49.59
columnella—see also Neoplasm, skin, face	C44.309	C79.2	D04.39	D23.39	D48.5	D49.2
concha—see also Neoplasm, skin, ear	C44.20-	C79.2	D04.2-	D23.2-	D48.5	D49.2
ear (external)	C44.20-	C79.2	D04.2-	D23.2-	D48.5	D49.2
basal cell carcinoma	C44.21-	-	-	-	-	-
specified type NEC	C44.29-	-	-	-	-	-
squamous cell carcinoma	C44.22-	-	-	-	-	-
elbow—see also Neoplasm, skin, limb, upper	C44.60-	C79.2	D04.6-	D23.6-	D48.5	D49.2
eyebrow—see also Neoplasm, skin, face	C44.309	C79.2	D04.39	D23.39	D48.5	D49.2
eyelid	C44.10-	C79.2	D04.1-	D23.1-	D48.5	D49.2
basal cell carcinoma	C44.11-	-	-	-	-	-
specified type NEC	C44.19-	-	-	-	-	-
squamous cell carcinoma	C44.12-	-	-	-	-	-
face NOS	C44.300	C79.2	D04.30	D23.30	D48.5	D49.2
basal cell carcinoma	C44.310	-	-	-	-	-
specified type NEC	C44.390	-	-	-	-	-
squamous cell carcinoma	C44.320	-	-	-	-	-
female genital organs (external)	C51.9	C79.82	D07.1	D28.0	D39.8	D49.59
clitoris	C51.2	C79.82	D07.1	D28.0	D39.8	D49.59
labium NEC	C51.9	C79.82	D07.1	D28.0	D39.8	D49.59
skin NOS, female genital organs — *continued*						
majus	C51.0	C79.82	D07.1	D28.0	D39.8	D49.59
minus	C51.1	C79.82	D07.1	D28.0	D39.8	D49.59
pudendum	C51.9	C79.82	D07.1	D28.0	D39.8	D49.59
vulva	C51.9	C79.82	D07.1	D28.0	D39.8	D49.59
finger—see also Neoplasm, skin, limb, upper	C44.60-	C79.2	D04.6-	D23.6-	D48.5	D49.2
flank—see also Neoplasm, skin, trunk	C44.509	C79.2	D04.5	D23.5	D48.5	D49.2
foot—see also Neoplasm, skin, limb, lower	C44.70-	C79.2	D04.7-	D23.7-	D48.5	D49.2
forearm—see also Neoplasm, skin, limb, upper	C44.60-	C79.2	D04.6-	D23.6-	D48.5	D49.2
forehead—see also *Neoplasm, skin, face*	C44.309	C79.2	D04.39	D23.39	D48.5	D49.2
glabella—see also Neoplasm, skin, face	C44.309	C79.2	D04.39	D23.39	D48.5	D49.2
gluteal region—see also Neoplasm, skin, trunk	C44.509	C79.2	D04.5	D23.5	D48.5	D49.2
groin—see also Neoplasm, skin, trunk	C44.509	C79.2	D04.5	D23.5	D48.5	D49.2
hand—see also Neoplasm, skin, limb, upper	C44.60-	C79.2	D04.6-	D23.6-	D48.5	D49.2
head NEC—see also Neoplasm, skin, scalp	C44.40	C79.2	D04.4	D23.4	D48.5	D49.2
heel—see also Neoplasm, skin, limb, lower	C44.70-	C79.2	D04.7-	D23.7-	D48.5	D49.2
helix—see also Neoplasm, skin, ear	C44.20-	C79.2	D04.2-	D23.2-	D48.5	D49.2
hip—see also Neoplasm, skin, limb, lower	C44.70-	C79.2	D04.7-	D23.7-	D48.5	D49.2
infraclavicular region—see also Neoplasm, skin, trunk	C44.509	C79.2	D04.5	D23.5	D48.5	D49.2
inguinal region—see also Neoplasm, skin, trunk	C44.509	C79.2	D04.5	D23.5	D48.5	D49.2
jaw—see also Neoplasm, skin, face	C44.309	C79.2	D04.39	D23.39	D48.5	D49.2
Kaposi's sarcoma —see Kaposi's, sarcoma, skin						
knee—see also Neoplasm, skin, limb, lower	C44.70-	C79.2	D04.7-	D23.7-	D48.5	D49.2
labia						
majora	C51.0	C79.82	D07.1	D28.0	D39.8	D49.59
minora	C51.1	C79.82	D07.1	D28.0	D39.8	D49.59
leg—see also Neoplasm, skin, limb, lower	C44.70-	C79.2	D04.7-	D23.7-	D48.5	D49.2
lid (lower) (upper)	C44.10-	C79.2	D04.1-	D23.1-	D48.5	D49.2
basal cell carcinoma	C44.11-	-	-	-	-	-
specified type NEC	C44.19-	-	-	-	-	-
squamous cell carcinoma	C44.12-	-	-	-	-	-
limb NEC	C44.90	C79.2	D04.9	D23.9	D48.5	D49.2
basal cell carcinoma	C44.91					

	Malignant Primary	Malignant Secondary	Ca in situ	Benign	Uncertain Behavior	Unspecified Behavior
skin NOS, limb NEC — *continued*						
lower	C44.70-	C79.2	D04.7-	D23.7-	D48.5	D49.2
basal cell carcinoma	C44.71-	-	-	-	-	-
specified type NEC	C44.79-	-	-	-	-	-
squamous cell carcinoma	C44.72-	-	-	-	-	-
upper	C44.60-	C79.2	D04.6-	D23.6-	D48.5	D49.2
basal cell carcinoma	C44.61-	-	-	-	-	-
specified type NEC	C44.69-	-	-	-	-	-
squamous cell carcinoma	C44.62-	-	-	-	-	-
lip (lower) (upper)	C44.00	C79.2	D04.0	D23.0	D48.5	D49.2
basal cell carcinoma	C44.01	-	-	-	-	-
specified type NEC	C44.09	-	-	-	-	-
squamous cell carcinoma	C44.02	-	-	-	-	-
male genital organs	C63.9	C79.82	D07.60	D29.9	D40.8	D49.59
penis	C60.9	C79.82	D07.4	D29.0	D40.8	D49.59
prepuce	C60.0	C79.82	D07.4	D29.0	D40.8	D49.59
scrotum	C63.2	C79.82	D07.61	D29.4	D40.8	D49.59
mastectomy site (skin)—see also Neoplasm, skin, breast	C44.501	C79.2	-	-	-	-
specified as breast tissue	C50.8-	C79.81	-	-	-	-
meatus, acoustic (external)—see also Neoplasm, skin, ear	C44.20-	C79.2	D04.2-	D23.2-	D48.5	D49.2
melanotic—see Melanoma						
Merkel cell—see Carcinoma, Merkel cell						
nates—see also Neoplasm, skin, trunk	C44.509	C79.2	D04.5	D23.5	D48.5	D49.2
neck	C44.40	C79.2	D04.4	D23.4	D48.5	D49.2
basal cell carcinoma	C44.41	-	-	-	-	-
specified type NEC	C44.49	-	-	-	-	-
squamous cell carcinoma	C44.42	-	-	-	-	-
nevus—see Nevus, skin						
nose (external)—see also Neoplasm, nose, skin	C44.301	C79.2	D04.39	D23.39	D48.5	D49.2
overlapping lesion	C44.80	-	-	-	-	-
basal cell carcinoma	C44.81	-	-	-	-	-
specified type NEC	C44.89	-	-	-	-	-
squamous cell carcinoma	C44.82	-	-	-	-	-
palm—see also Neoplasm, skin, limb, upper	C44.60-	C79.2	D04.6-	D23.6-	D48.5	D49.2
palpebra	C44.10-	C79.2	D04.1-	D23.1-	D48.5	D49.2
basal cell carcinoma	C44.11-	-	-	-	-	-
specified type NEC	C44.19-	-	-	-	-	-
squamous cell carcinoma	C44.12-	-	-	-	-	-
penis NEC	C60.9	C79.82	D07.4	D29.0	D40.8	D49.59
perianal—see also Neoplasm, skin, anus	C44.500	C79.2	D04.5	D23.5	D48.5	D49.2

	Malignant Primary	Malignant Secondary	Ca in situ	Benign	Uncertain Behavior	Unspecified Behavior
skin NOS — *continued*						
perineum—see also Neoplasm, skin, anus	C44.500	C79.2	D04.5	D23.5	D48.5	D49.2
pinna—see also Neoplasm, skin, ear	C44.20-	C79.2	D04.2-	D23.2-	D48.5	D49.2
plantar—see also Neoplasm, skin, limb, lower	C44.70-	C79.2	D04.7-	D23.7-	D48.5	D49.2
popliteal fossa or space—see also Neoplasm, skin, limb, lower	C44.70-	C79.2	D04.7-	D23.7-	D48.5	D49.2
prepuce	C60.0	C79.82	D07.4	D29.0	D40.8	D49.59
pubes—see also Neoplasm, skin, trunk	C44.509	C79.2	D04.5	D23.5	D48.5	D49.2
sacrococcygeal region—see also Neoplasm, skin, trunk	C44.509	C79.2	D04.5	D23.5	D48.5	D49.2
scalp	C44.40	C79.2	D04.4	D23.4	D48.5	D49.2
basal cell carcinoma	C44.41	-	-	-	-	-
specified type NEC	C44.49	-	-	-	-	-
squamous cell carcinoma	C44.42	-	-	-	-	-
scapular region—see also Neoplasm, skin, trunk	C44.509	C79.2	D04.5	D23.5	D48.5	D49.2
scrotum	C63.2	C79.82	D07.61	D29.4	D40.8	D49.59
shoulder—see also Neoplasm, skin, limb, upper	C44.60-	C79.2	D04.6-	D23.6-	D48.5	D49.2
sole (foot)—see also Neoplasm, skin, limb, lower	C44.70-	C79.2	D04.7-	D23.7-	D48.5	D49.2
specified sites NEC	C44.80	C79.2	D04.8	D23.9	D48.5	D49.2
basal cell carcinoma	C44.81	-	-	-	-	-
specified type NEC	C44.89	-	-	-	-	-
squamous cell carcinoma	C44.82	-	-	-	-	-
specified type NEC	C44.99	-	-	-	-	-
squamous cell carcinoma	C44.92	-	-	-	-	-
submammary fold—see also Neoplasm, skin, trunk	C44.509	C79.2	D04.5	D23.5	D48.5	D49.2
supraclavicular region—see also Neoplasm, skin, neck	C44.40	C79.2	D04.4	D23.4	D48.5	D49.2
temple—see also Neoplasm, skin, face	C44.309	C79.2	D04.39	D23.39	D48.5	D49.2
thigh—see also Neoplasm, skin, limb, lower	C44.70-	C79.2	D04.7-	D23.7-	D48.5	D49.2
thoracic wall—see also Neoplasm, skin, trunk	C44.509	C79.2	D04.5	D23.5	D48.5	D49.2
thumb—see also Neoplasm, skin, limb, upper	C44.60-	C79.2	D04.6-	D23.6-	D48.5	D49.2
toe—see also Neoplasm, skin, limb, lower	C44.70-	C79.2	D04.7-	D23.7-	D48.5	D49.2
tragus—see also Neoplasm, skin, ear	C44.20-	C79.2	D04.2-	D23.2-	D48.5	D49.2
trunk	C44.509	C79.2	D04.5	D23.5	D48.5	D49.2
basal cell carcinoma	C44.519	-	-	-	-	-
specified type NEC	C44.599	-	-	-	-	-

	Malignant Primary	Malignant Secondary	Ca in situ	Benign	Uncertain Behavior	Unspecified Behavior
skin NOS, trunk — *continued*						
squamous cell carcinoma	C44.529	-	-	-	-	-
umbilicus—see also Neoplasm, skin, trunk	C44.509	C79.2	D04.5	D23.5	D48.5	D49.2
vulva	C51.9	C79.82	D07.1	D28.0	D39.8	D49.59
overlapping lesion	C51.8	-	-	-	-	-
wrist—see also Neoplasm, skin, limb, upper	C44.60-	C79.2	D04.6-	D23.6-	D48.5	D49.2
skull	C41.0	C79.51	-	D16.4	D48.0	D49.2
soft parts or tissues—see Neoplasm, connective tissue						
specified site NEC	C76.8	C79.89	D09.8	D36.7	D48.7	D49.89
spermatic cord	C63.1-	C79.82	D07.69	D29.8	D40.8	D49.59
sphenoid	C31.3	C78.39	D02.3	D14.0	D38.5	D49.1
bone	C41.0	C79.51	-	D16.4	D48.0	D49.2
sinus	C31.3	C78.39	D02.3	D14.0	D38.5	D49.1
sphincter						
anal	C21.1	C78.5	D01.3	D12.9	D37.8	D49.0
of Oddi	C24.0	C78.89	D01.5	D13.5	D37.6	D49.0
spine, spinal (column)	C41.2	C79.51	-	D16.6	D48.0	D49.2
bulb	C71.7	C79.31	-	D33.1	D43.1	D49.6
coccyx	C41.4	C79.51	-	D16.8	D48.0	D49.2
cord (cervical) (lumbar) (sacral) (thoracic)	C72.0	C79.49	-	D33.4	D43.4	D49.7
dura mater	C70.1	C79.49	-	D32.1	D42.1	D49.7
lumbosacral	C41.2	C79.51	-	D16.6	D48.0	D49.2
marrow NEC	C96.9	C79.52	-	-	D47.9	D49.89
membrane	C70.1	C79.49	-	D32.1	D42.1	D49.7
meninges	C70.1	C79.49	-	D32.1	D42.1	D49.7
nerve (root)	C47.9	C79.89	-	D36.10	D48.2	D49.2
pia mater	C70.1	C79.49	-	D32.1	D42.1	D49.7
root	C47.9	C79.89	-	D36.10	D48.2	D49.2
sacrum	C41.4	C79.51	-	D16.8	D48.0	D49.2
spleen, splenic NEC	C26.1	C78.89	D01.7	D13.9	D37.8	D49.0
flexure (colon)	C18.5	C78.5	D01.0	D12.3	D37.4	D49.0
stem, brain	C71.7	C79.31	-	D33.1	D43.1	D49.6
Stensen's duct	C07	C79.89	D00.00	D11.0	D37.030	D49.0
sternum	C41.3	C79.51	-	D16.7	D48.0	D49.2
stomach	C16.9	C78.89	D00.2	D13.1	D37.1	D49.0
antrum (pyloric)	C16.3	C78.89	D00.2	D13.1	D37.1	D49.0
body	C16.2	C78.89	D00.2	D13.1	D37.1	D49.0
cardia	C16.0	C78.89	D00.2	D13.1	D37.1	D49.0
cardiac orifice	C16.0	C78.89	D00.2	D13.1	D37.1	D49.0
corpus	C16.2	C78.89	D00.2	D13.1	D37.1	D49.0
fundus	C16.1	C78.89	D00.2	D13.1	D37.1	D49.0
greater curvature NEC	C16.6	C78.89	D00.2	D13.1	D37.1	D49.0
lesser curvature NEC	C16.5	C78.89	D00.2	D13.1	D37.1	D49.0
overlapping lesion	C16.8	-	-	-	-	-
prepylorus	C16.4	C78.89	D00.2	D13.1	D37.1	D49.0
pylorus	C16.4	C78.89	D00.2	D13.1	D37.1	D49.0
wall NEC	C16.9	C78.89	D00.2	D13.1	D37.1	D49.0
anterior NEC	C16.8	C78.89	D00.2	D13.1	D37.1	D49.0
stomach, wall NEC — *continued*						
posterior NEC	C16.8	C78.89	D00.2	D13.1	D37.1	D49.0
stroma, endometrial	C54.1	C79.82	D07.0	D26.1	D39.0	D49.59
stump, cervical	C53.8	C79.82	D06.7	D26.0	D39.0	D49.59
subcutaneous (nodule) (tissue) NEC—see Neoplasm, connective tissue						
subdural	C70.9	C79.32	-	D32.9	D42.9	D49.7
subglottis, subglottic	C32.2	C78.39	D02.0	D14.1	D38.0	D49.1
sublingual	C04.9	C79.89	D00.06	D10.2	D37.09	D49.0
gland or duct	C08.1	C79.89	D00.00	D11.7	D37.031	D49.0
submandibular gland	C08.0	C79.89	D00.00	D11.7	D37.032	D49.0
submaxillary gland or duct	C08.0	C79.89	D00.00	D11.7	D37.032	D49.0
submental	C76.0	C79.89	D09.8	D36.7	D48.7	D49.89
subpleural	C34.9-	C78.0-	D02.2-	D14.3-	D38.1	D49.1
substernal	C38.1	C78.1	-	D15.2	D38.3	D49.89
sudoriferous, sudoriparous gland, site unspecified	C44.90	C79.2	D04.9	D23.9	D48.5	D49.2
specified site—see Neoplasm, skin						
supraclavicular region	C76.0	C79.89	D09.8	D36.7	D48.7	D49.89
supraglottis	C32.1	C78.39	D02.0	D14.1	D38.0	D49.1
suprarenal	C74.9-	C79.7-	D09.3	D35.0-	D44.1-	D49.7
capsule	C74.9-	C79.7-	D09.3	D35.0-	D44.1-	D49.7
cortex	C74.0-	C79.7-	D09.3	D35.0-	D44.1-	D49.7
gland	C74.9-	C79.7-	D09.3	D35.0-	D44.1-	D49.7
medulla	C74.1-	C79.7-	D09.3	D35.0-	D44.1-	D49.7
suprasellar (region)	C71.9	C79.31	-	D33.2	D43.2	D49.6
supratentorial (brain) NEC	C71.0	C79.31	-	D33.0	D43.0	D49.6
sweat gland (apocrine) (eccrine), site unspecified	C44.90	C79.2	D04.9	D23.9	D48.5	D49.2
specified site—see Neoplasm, skin						
sympathetic nerve or nervous system NEC	C47.9	C79.89	-	D36.10	D48.2	D49.2
symphysis pubis	C41.4	C79.51	-	D16.8	D48.0	D49.2
synovial membrane—see Neoplasm, connective tissue						
T						
tapetum, brain	C71.8	C79.31	-	D33.2	D43.2	D49.6
tarsus (any bone)	C40.3-	C79.51	-	D16.3-	-	-
temple (skin)—see also Neoplasm, skin, face	C44.309	C79.2	D04.39	D23.39	D48.5	D49.2
temporal						
bone	C41.0	C79.51	-	D16.4	D48.0	D49.2
lobe or pole	C71.2	C79.31	-	D33.0	D43.0	D49.6
region	C76.0	C79.89	D09.8	D36.7	D48.7	D49.89
skin—see also Neoplasm, skin, face	C44.309	C79.2	D04.39	D23.39	D48.5	D49.2
tendon (sheath)—see Neoplasm, connective tissue						
tentorium (cerebelli)	C70.0	C79.32	-	D32.0	D42.0	D49.7
testis, testes	C62.9-	C79.82	D07.69	D29.2-	D40.1-	D49.59
descended	C62.1-	C79.82	D07.69	D29.2-	D40.1-	D49.59
ectopic	C62.0-	C79.82	D07.69	D29.2-	D40.1-	D49.59

	Malignant Primary	Malignant Secondary	Ca in situ	Benign	Uncertain Behavior	Unspecified Behavior
testis, testes — *continued*						
retained	C62.0-	C79.82	D07.69	D29.2-	D40.1-	D49.59
scrotal	C62.1-	C79.82	D07.69	D29.2-	D40.1-	D49.59
undescended	C62.0-	C79.82	D07.69	D29.2-	D40.1-	D49.59
unspecified whether descended or undescended	C62.9-	C79.82	D07.69	D29.2-	D40.1-	D49.59
thalamus	C71.0	C79.31	-	D33.0	D43.0	D49.6
thigh NEC	C76.5-	C79.89	D04.7-	D36.7	D48.7	D49.89
thorax, thoracic (cavity) (organs NEC)	C76.1	C79.89	D09.8	D36.7	D48.7	D49.89
duct	C49.3	C79.89	-	D21.3	D48.1	D49.2
wall NEC	C76.1	C79.89	D09.8	D36.7	D48.7	D49.89
throat	C14.0	C79.89	D00.08	D10.9	D37.05	D49.0
thumb NEC	C76.4-	C79.89	D04.6-	D36.7	D48.7	D49.89
thymus (gland)	C37	C79.89	D09.3	D15.0	D38.4	D49.89
thyroglossal duct	C73	C79.89	D09.3	D34	D44.0	D49.7
thyroid (gland)	C73	C79.89	D09.3	D34	D44.0	D49.7
cartilage	C32.3	C78.39	D02.0	D14.1	D38.0	D49.1
tibia (any part)	C40.2-	C79.51	-	D16.2-	-	-
toe NEC	C76.5-	C79.89	D04.7-	D36.7	D48.7	D49.89
tongue	C02.9	C79.89	D00.07	D10.1	D37.02	D49.0
anterior (two-thirds) NEC	C02.3	C79.89	D00.07	D10.1	D37.02	D49.0
dorsal surface	C02.0	C79.89	D00.07	D10.1	D37.02	D49.0
ventral surface	C02.2	C79.89	D00.07	D10.1	D37.02	D49.0
base (dorsal surface)	C01	C79.89	D00.07	D10.1	D37.02	D49.0
border (lateral)	C02.1	C79.89	D00.07	D10.1	D37.02	D49.0
dorsal surface NEC	C02.0	C79.89	D00.07	D10.1	D37.02	D49.0
fixed part NEC	C01	C79.89	D00.07	D10.1	D37.02	D49.0
foreamen cecum	C02.0	C79.89	D00.07	D10.1	D37.02	D49.0
frenulum linguae	C02.2	C79.89	D00.07	D10.1	D37.02	D49.0
junctional zone	C02.8	C79.89	D00.07	D10.1	D37.02	D49.0
margin (lateral)	C02.1	C79.89	D00.07	D10.1	D37.02	D49.0
midline NEC	C02.0	C79.89	D00.07	D10.1	D37.02	D49.0
mobile part NEC	C02.3	C79.89	D00.07	D10.1	D37.02	D49.0
overlapping lesion	C02.8	-	-	-	-	-
posterior (third)	C01	C79.89	D00.07	D10.1	D37.02	D49.0
root	C01	C79.89	D00.07	D10.1	D37.02	D49.0
surface (dorsal)	C02.0	C79.89	D00.07	D10.1	D37.02	D49.0
base	C01	C79.89	D00.07	D10.1	D37.02	D49.0
ventral	C02.2	C79.89	D00.07	D10.1	D37.02	D49.0
tip	C02.1	C79.89	D00.07	D10.1	D37.02	D49.0
tonsil	C02.4	C79.89	D00.07	D10.1	D37.02	D49.0
tonsil	C09.9	C79.89	D00.08	D10.4	D37.05	D49.0
fauces, faucial	C09.9	C79.89	D00.08	D10.4	D37.05	D49.0
lingual	C02.4	C79.89	D00.07	D10.1	D37.02	D49.0
overlapping sites	C09.8	-	-	-	-	-
palatine	C09.9	C79.89	D00.08	D10.4	D37.05	D49.0
pharyngeal	C11.1	C79.89	D00.08	D10.6	D37.05	D49.0
pillar (anterior) (posterior)	C09.1	C79.89	D00.08	D10.5	D37.05	D49.0
tonsillar fossa	C09.0	C79.89	D00.08	D10.5	D37.05	D49.0
tooth socket NEC	C03.9	C79.89	D00.03	D10.39	D37.09	D49.0
trachea (cartilage) (mucosa)	C33	C78.39	D02.1	D14.2	D38.1	D49.1
overlapping lesion with bronchus or lung	C34.8-	-	-	-	-	-

	Malignant Primary	Malignant Secondary	Ca in situ	Benign	Uncertain Behavior	Unspecified Behavior
tracheobronchial	C34.8-	C78.39	D02.1	D14.2	D38.1	D49.1
overlapping lesion with lung	C34.8-	-	-	-	-	-
tragus—see also Neoplasm, skin, ear	C44.20-	C79.2	D04.2-	D23.2-	D48.5	D49.2
trunk NEC	C76.8	C79.89	D04.5	D36.7	D48.7	D49.89
tubo-ovarian	C57.8	C79.82	D07.39	D28.7	D39.8	D49.59
tunica vaginalis	C63.7	C79.82	D07.69	D29.8	D40.8	D49.59
turbinate (bone)	C41.0	C79.51	-	D16.4	D48.0	D49.2
nasal	C30.0	C78.39	D02.3	D14.0	D38.5	D49.1
tympanic cavity	C30.1	C78.39	D02.3	D14.0	D38.5	D49.1
U						
ulna (any part)	C40.0-	C79.51	-	D16.0-	-	-
umbilicus, umbilical—see also Neoplasm, skin, trunk	C44.509	C79.2	D04.5	D23.5	D48.5	D49.2
uncus, brain	C71.2	C79.31	-	D33.0	D43.0	D49.6
unknown site or unspecified	C80.1	C79.9	D09.9	D36.9	D48.9	D49.9
urachus	C67.7	C79.11	D09.0	D30.3	D41.4	D49.4
ureter, ureteral	C66.-	C79.19	D09.19	D30.2-	D41.2-	D49.59
orifice (bladder)	C67.6	C79.11	D09.0	D30.3	D41.4	D49.4
ureter-bladder (junction)	C67.6	C79.11	D09.0	D30.3	D41.4	D49.4
urethra, urethral (gland)	C68.0	C79.19	D09.19	D30.4	D41.3	D49.59
orifice, internal	C67.5	C79.11	D09.0	D30.3	D41.4	D49.4
urethrovaginal (septum)	C57.9	C79.82	D07.30	D28.9	D39.8	D49.59
urinary organ or system	C68.9	C79.10	D09.10	D30.9	D41.9	D49.59
bladder—see Neoplasm, bladder						
overlapping lesion	C68.8	-	-	-	-	-
specified sites NEC	C68.8	C79.19	D09.19	D30.8	D41.8	D49.59
utero-ovarian	C57.8	C79.82	D07.39	D28.7	D39.8	D49.59
ligament	C57.1	C79.82	D07.39	D28.2	D39.8	D49.59
uterosacral ligament	C57.3	C79.82	-	D28.2	D39.8	D49.59
uterus, uteri, uterine	C55	C79.82	D07.0	D26.9	D39.0	D49.59
adnexa NEC	C57.4	C79.82	D07.39	D28.7	D39.8	D49.59
body	C54.9	C79.82	D07.0	D26.1	D39.0	D49.59
cervix	C53.9	C79.82	D06.9	D26.0	D39.0	D49.59
cornu	C54.9	C79.82	D07.0	D26.1	D39.0	D49.59
corpus	C54.9	C79.82	D07.0	D26.1	D39.0	D49.59
endocervix (canal) (gland)	C53.0	C79.82	D06.0	D26.0	D39.0	D49.59
endometrium	C54.1	C79.82	D07.0	D26.1	D39.0	D49.59
exocervix	C53.1	C79.82	D06.1	D26.0	D39.0	D49.59
external os	C53.1	C79.82	D06.1	D26.0	D39.0	D49.59
fundus	C54.3	C79.82	D07.0	D26.1	D39.0	D49.59
internal os	C53.0	C79.82	D06.0	D26.0	D39.0	D49.59
isthmus	C54.0	C79.82	D07.0	D26.1	D39.0	D49.59
ligament	C57.3	C79.82	-	D28.2	D39.8	D49.59
broad	C57.1	C79.82	D07.39	D28.2	D39.8	D49.59
round	C57.2	C79.82	-	D28.2	D39.8	D49.59
lower segment	C54.0	C79.82	D07.0	D26.1	D39.0	D49.59
myometrium	C54.2	C79.82	D07.0	D26.1	D39.0	D49.59
overlapping sites	C54.8	-	-	-	-	-
squamocolumnar junction	C53.8	C79.82	D06.7	D26.0	D39.0	D49.59
tube	C57.0-	C79.82	D07.39	D28.2	D39.8	D49.59

	Malignant Primary	Malignant Secondary	Ca in situ	Benign	Uncertain Behavior	Unspecified Behavior
utricle, prostatic	C68.0	C79.19	D09.19	D30.4	D41.3	D49.59
uveal tract	C69.4-	C79.49	D09.2-	D31.4-	D48.7	D49.89
uvula	C05.2	C79.89	D00.04	D10.39	D37.09	D49.0
V						
vagina, vaginal (fornix) (vault) (wall)	C52	C79.82	D07.2	D28.1	D39.8	D49.59
vaginovesical	C57.9	C79.82	D07.30	D28.9	D39.9	D49.59
septum	C57.9	C79.82	D07.30	D28.9	D39.9	D49.59
vallecula (epigiottis)	C10.0	C79.89	D00.08	D10.5	D37.05	D49.0
vas deferens	C63.1-	C79.82	D07.69	D29.8	D40.8	D49.59
vascular—see Neoplasm, connective tissue						
Vater's ampulla	C24.1	C78.89	D01.5	D13.5	D37.6	D49.0
vein, venous—see Neoplasm, connective tissue						
vena cava (abdominal) (inferior)	C49.4	C79.89	-	D21.4	D48.1	D49.2
superior	C49.3	C79.89	-	D21.3	D48.1	D49.2
ventricle (cerebral) (floor) (lateral) (third)	C71.5	C79.31	-	D33.0	D43.0	D49.6
cardiac (left) (right)	C38.0	C79.89	-	D15.1	D48.7	D49.89
fourth	C71.7	C79.31	-	D33.1	D43.1	D49.6
ventricular band of larynx	C32.1	C78.39	D02.0	D14.1	D38.0	D49.1
ventriculus—see Neoplasm, stomach						
vermillion border—see Neoplasm, lip						
vermis, cerebellum	C71.6	C79.31	-	D33.1	D43.1	D49.6
vertebra (column)	C41.2	C79.51	-	D16.6	D48.0	D49.2
coccyx	C41.4	C79.51	-	D16.8	D48.0	D49.2
marrow NEC	C96.9	C79.52	-	-	D47.9	D49.89
sacrum	C41.4	C79.51	-	D16.8	D48.0	D49.2
vesical—see Neoplasm, bladder						
vesicle, seminal	C63.7	C79.82	D07.69	D29.8	D40.8	D49.59
vesicocervical tissue	C57.9	C79.82	D07.30	D28.9	D39.9	D49.59
vesicorectal	C76.3	C79.82	D09.8	D36.7	D48.7	D49.89
vesicovaginal	C57.9	C79.82	D07.30	D28.9	D39.9	D49.59
septum	C57.9	C79.82	D07.30	D28.9	D39.8	D49.59
vessel (blood)—see Neoplasm, connective tissue						
vestibular gland, greater	C51.0	C79.82	D07.1	D28.0	D39.8	D49.59
vestibule						
mouth	C06.1	C79.89	D00.00	D10.39	D37.09	D49.0
nose	C30.0	C78.39	D02.3	D14.0	D38.5	D49.1
Virchow's gland	C77.0	C77.0	-	D36.0	D48.7	D49.89
viscera NEC	C76.8	C79.89	D09.8	D36.7	D48.7	D49.89
vocal cords (true)	C32.0	C78.39	D02.0	D14.1	D38.0	D49.1
false	C32.1	C78.39	D02.0	D14.1	D38.0	D49.1
vomer	C41.0	C79.51	-	D16.4	D48.0	D49.2
vulva	C51.9	C79.82	D07.1	D28.0	D39.8	D49.59
vulvovaginal gland	C51.0	C79.82	D07.1	D28.0	D39.8	D49.59
W						
Waldeyer's ring	C14.2	C79.89	D00.08	D10.9	D37.05	D49.0
Wharton's duct	C08.0	C79.89	D00.00	D11.7	D37.032	D49.0
white matter (central) (cerebral)	C71.0	C79.31	-	D33.0	D43.0	D49.6
windpipe	C33	C78.39	D02.1	D14.2	D38.1	D49.1
Wirsung's duct	C25.3	C78.89	D01.7	D13.6	D37.8	D49.0
wolffian (body) (duct)						
female	C57.7	C79.82	D07.39	D28.7	D39.8	D49.59
male	C63.7	C79.82	D07.69	D29.8	D40.8	D49.59
womb—see Neoplasm, uterus						
wrist NEC	C76.4-	C79.89	D04.6-	D36.7	D48.7	D49.89
X						
xiphoid process	C41.3	C79.51	-	D16.7	D48.0	D49.2
Z						
Zuckerkandl organ	C75.5	C79.89	-	D35.6	D44.7	D49.7

Table of Drugs and Chemicals

Substance	Poisoning, Accidental (unintentional)	Poisoning, Intentional self-harm	Poisoning, Assault	Poisoning, Undetermined	Adverse effect	Underdosing
1-propanol	T51.3X1	T51.3X2	T51.3X3	T51.3X4	—	—
2-propanol	T51.2X1	T51.2X2	T51.2X3	T51.2X4	—	—
2,4-D (dichlorophen-oxyacetic acid)	T60.3X1	T60.3X2	T60.3X3	T60.3X4	—	—
2,4-toluene diisocyanate	T65.0X1	T65.0X2	T65.0X3	T65.0X4	—	—
2,4,5-T (trichloro-phenoxyacetic acid)	T60.1X1	T60.1X2	T60.1X3	T60.1X4	—	—
14-hydroxydihydro-morphinone	T40.2X1	T40.2X2	T40.2X3	T40.2X4	T40.2X5	T40.2X6
A						
ABOB	T37.5X1	T37.5X2	T37.5X3	T37.5X4	T37.5X5	T37.5X6
Abrine	T62.2X1	T62.2X2	T62.2X3	T62.2X4	—	—
Abrus (seed)	T62.2X1	T62.2X2	T62.2X3	T62.2X4	—	—
Absinthe	T51.0X1	T51.0X2	T51.0X3	T51.0X4	—	—
beverage	T51.0X1	T51.0X2	T51.0X3	T51.0X4	—	—
Acaricide	T60.8X1	T60.8X2	T60.8X3	T60.8X4	—	—
Acebutolol	T44.7X1	T44.7X2	T44.7X3	T44.7X4	T44.7X5	T44.7X6
Acecarbromal	T42.6X1	T42.6X2	T42.6X3	T42.6X4	T42.6X5	T42.6X6
Aceclidine	T44.1X1	T44.1X2	T44.1X3	T44.1X4	T44.1X5	T44.1X6
Acedapsone	T37.0X1	T37.0X2	T37.0X3	T37.0X4	T37.0X5	T37.0X6
Acefylline piperazine	T48.6X1	T48.6X2	T48.6X3	T48.6X4	T48.6X5	T48.6X6
Acemorphan	T40.2X1	T40.2X2	T40.2X3	T40.2X4	T40.2X5	T40.2X6
Acenocoumarin	T45.511	T45.512	T45.513	T45.514	T45.515	T45.516
Acenocoumarol	T45.511	T45.512	T45.513	T45.514	T45.515	T45.516
Acepifylline	T48.6X1	T48.6X2	T48.6X3	T48.6X4	T48.6X5	T48.6X6
Acepromazine	T43.3X1	T43.3X2	T43.3X3	T43.3X4	T43.3X5	T43.3X6
Acesulfamethoxy-pyridazine	T37.0X1	T37.0X2	T37.0X3	T37.0X4	T37.0X5	T37.0X6
Acetal	T52.8X1	T52.8X2	T52.8X3	T52.8X4	—	—
Acetaldehyde (vapor)	T52.8X1	T52.8X2	T52.8X3	T52.8X4	—	—
liquid	T65.891	T65.892	T65.893	T65.894	—	—
P-Acetamidophenol	T39.1X1	T39.1X2	T39.1X3	T39.1X4	T39.1X5	T39.1X6
Acetaminophen	T39.1X1	T39.1X2	T39.1X3	T39.1X4	T39.1X5	T39.1X6
Acetaminosalol	T39.1X1	T39.1X2	T39.1X3	T39.1X4	T39.1X5	T39.1X6
Acetanilide	T39.1X1	T39.1X2	T39.1X3	T39.1X4	T39.1X5	T39.1X6
Acetarsol	T37.3X1	T37.3X2	T37.3X3	T37.3X4	T37.3X5	T37.3X6
Acetazolamide	T50.2X1	T50.2X2	T50.2X3	T50.2X4	T50.2X5	T50.2X6
Acetiamine	T45.2X1	T45.2X2	T45.2X3	T45.2X4	T45.2X5	T45.2X6
Acetic						
acid	T54.2X1	T54.2X2	T54.2X3	T54.2X4	—	—
with sodium acetate (ointment)	T49.3X1	T49.3X2	T49.3X3	T49.3X4	T49.3X5	T49.3X6
ester (solvent) (vapor)	T52.8X1	T52.8X2	T52.8X3	T52.8X4	—	—
irrigating solution	T50.3X1	T50.3X2	T50.3X3	T50.3X4	T50.3X5	T50.3X6
medicinal (lotion)	T49.2X1	T49.2X2	T49.2X3	T49.2X4	T49.2X5	T49.2X6
anhydride	T65.891	T65.892	T65.893	T65.894	—	—
ether (vapor)	T52.8X1	T52.8X2	T52.8X3	T52.8X4	—	—
Acetohexamide	T38.3X1	T38.3X2	T38.3X3	T38.3X4	T38.3X5	T38.3X6
Acetohydroxamic acid	T50.991	T50.992	T50.993	T50.994	T50.995	T50.996
Acetomenaphthone	T45.7X1	T45.7X2	T45.7X3	T45.7X4	T45.7X5	T45.7X6
Acetomorphine	T40.1X1	T40.1X2	T40.1X3	T40.1X4	—	—
Acetone (oils)	T52.4X1	T52.4X2	T52.4X3	T52.4X4	—	—
chlorinated	T52.4X1	T52.4X2	T52.4X3	T52.4X4	—	—
vapor	T52.4X1	T52.4X2	T52.4X3	T52.4X4	—	—
Acetonitrile	T52.8X1	T52.8X2	T52.8X3	T52.8X4	—	—
Acetophenazine	T43.3X1	T43.3X2	T43.3X3	T43.3X4	T43.3X5	T43.3X6
Acetophenetedin	T39.1X1	T39.1X2	T39.1X3	T39.1X4	T39.1X5	T39.1X6
Acetophenone	T52.4X1	T52.4X2	T52.4X3	T52.4X4	—	—
Acetorphine	T40.2X1	T40.2X2	T40.2X3	T40.2X4	—	—
Acetosulfone (sodium)	T37.1X1	T37.1X2	T37.1X3	T37.1X4	T37.1X5	T37.1X6
Acetrizoate (sodium)	T50.8X1	T50.8X2	T50.8X3	T50.8X4	T50.8X5	T50.8X6
Acetrizoic acid	T50.8X1	T50.8X2	T50.8X3	T50.8X4	T50.8X5	T50.8X6
Acetyl						
bromide	T53.6X1	T53.6X2	T53.6X3	T53.6X4	—	—
chloride	T53.6X1	T53.6X2	T53.6X3	T53.6X4	—	—
Acetylcarbromal	T42.6X1	T42.6X2	T42.6X3	T42.6X4	T42.6X5	T42.6X6
Acetylcholine						
chloride	T44.1X1	T44.1X2	T44.1X3	T44.1X4	T44.1X5	T44.1X6
derivative	T44.1X1	T44.1X2	T44.1X3	T44.1X4	T44.1X5	T44.1X6
Acetylcysteine	T48.4X1	T48.4X2	T48.4X3	T48.4X4	T48.4X5	T48.4X6
Acetyldigitoxin	T46.0X1	T46.0X2	T46.0X3	T46.0X4	T46.0X5	T46.0X6
Acetyldigoxin	T46.0X1	T46.0X2	T46.0X3	T46.0X4	T46.0X5	T46.0X6
Acetyldihydrocodeine	T40.2X1	T40.2X2	T40.2X3	T40.2X4	—	—
Acetyldihydroco-deinone	T40.2X1	T40.2X2	T40.2X3	T40.2X4	—	—
Acetylene (gas)	T59.891	T59.892	T59.893	T59.894	—	—
dichloride	T53.6X1	T53.6X2	T53.6X3	T53.6X4	—	—
incomplete combustion of	T58.11	T58.12	T58.13	T58.14	—	—
industrial	T59.891	T59.892	T59.893	T59.894	—	—
tetrachloride	T53.6X1	T53.6X2	T53.6X3	T53.6X4	—	—
vapor	T53.6X1	T53.6X2	T53.6X3	T53.6X4	—	—
Acetylpheneturide	T42.6X1	T42.6X2	T42.6X3	T42.6X4	T42.6X5	T42.6X6
Acetylphenylhydra-zine	T39.8X1	T39.8X2	T39.8X3	T39.8X4	T39.8X5	T39.8X6
Acetylsalicylic acid (salts)	T39.011	T39.012	T39.013	T39.014	T39.015	T39.016
enteric coated	T39.011	T39.012	T39.013	T39.014	T39.015	T39.016
Acetylsulfamethoxy-pyridazine	T37.0X1	T37.0X2	T37.0X3	T37.0X4	T37.0X5	T37.0X6
Achromycin	T36.4X1	T36.4X2	T36.4X3	T36.4X4	T36.4X5	T36.4X6
ophthalmic preparation	T49.5X1	T49.5X2	T49.5X3	T49.5X4	T49.5X5	T49.5X6
topical NEC	T49.0X1	T49.0X2	T49.0X3	T49.0X4	T49.0X5	T49.0X6
Aciclovir	T37.5X1	T37.5X2	T37.5X3	T37.5X4	T37.5X5	T37.5X6
Acid (corrosive) NEC	T54.2X1	T54.2X2	T54.2X3	T54.2X4	—	—
Acidifying agent NEC	T50.901	T50.902	T50.903	T50.904	T50.905	T50.906
Acipimox	T46.6X1	T46.6X2	T46.6X3	T46.6X4	T46.6X5	T46.6X6
Acitretin	T50.991	T50.992	T50.993	T50.994	T50.995	T50.996
Aclarubicin	T45.1X1	T45.1X2	T45.1X3	T45.1X4	T45.1X5	T45.1X6

Substance	Poisoning, Accidental (unintentional)	Poisoning, Intentional self-harm	Poisoning, Assault	Poisoning, Undetermined	Adverse effect	Underdosing
Aclatonium napadisilate	T48.1X1	T48.1X2	T48.1X3	T48.1X4	T48.1X5	T48.1X6
Aconite (wild)	T46.991	T46.992	T46.993	T46.994	T46.995	T46.996
Aconitine	T46.991	T46.992	T46.993	T46.994	T46.995	T46.996
Aconitum ferox	T46.991	T46.992	T46.993	T46.994	T46.995	T46.996
Acridine	T65.6X1	T65.6X2	T65.6X3	T65.6X4	—	—
vapor	T59.891	T59.892	T59.893	T59.894	—	—
Acriflavine	T37.91	T37.92	T37.93	T37.94	T37.95	T37.96
Acriflavinium chloride	T49.0X1	T49.0X2	T49.0X3	T49.0X4	T49.0X5	T49.0X6
Acrinol	T49.0X1	T49.0X2	T49.0X3	T49.0X4	T49.0X5	T49.0X6
Acrisorcin	T49.0X1	T49.0X2	T49.0X3	T49.0X4	T49.0X5	T49.0X6
Acrivastine	T45.0X1	T45.0X2	T45.0X3	T45.0X4	T45.0X5	T45.0X6
Acrolein (gas)	T59.891	T59.892	T59.893	T59.894	—	—
liquid	T54.1X1	T54.1X2	T54.1X3	T54.1X4	—	—
Acrylamide	T65.891	T65.892	T65.893	T65.894	—	—
Acrylic resin	T49.3X1	T49.3X2	T49.3X3	T49.3X4	T49.3X5	T49.3X6
Acrylonitrile	T65.891	T65.892	T65.893	T65.894	—	—
Actaea spicata	T62.2X1	T62.2X2	T62.2X3	T62.2X4	—	—
berry	T62.1X1	T62.1X2	T62.1X3	T62.1X4	—	—
Acterol	T37.3X1	T37.3X2	T37.3X3	T37.3X4	T37.3X5	T37.3X6
ACTH	T38.811	T38.812	T38.813	T38.814	T38.815	T38.816
Actinomycin C	T45.1X1	T45.1X2	T45.1X3	T45.1X4	T45.1X5	T45.1X6
Actinomycin D	T45.1X1	T45.1X2	T45.1X3	T45.1X4	T45.1X5	T45.1X6
Activated charcoal—see also Charcoal, medicinal	T47.6X1	T47.6X2	T47.6X3	T47.6X4	T47.6X5	T47.6X6
Acyclovir	T37.5X1	T37.5X2	T37.5X3	T37.5X4	T37.5X5	T37.5X6
Adenine	T45.2X1	T45.2X2	T45.2X3	T45.2X4	T45.2X5	T45.2X6
arabinoside	T37.5X1	T37.5X2	T37.5X3	T37.5X4	T37.5X5	T37.5X6
Adenosine (phosphate)	T46.2X1	T46.2X2	T46.2X3	T46.2X4	T46.2X5	T46.2X6
ADH	T38.891	T38.892	T38.893	T38.894	T38.895	T38.896
Adhesive NEC	T65.891	T65.892	T65.893	T65.894	—	—
Adicillin	T36.0X1	T36.0X2	T36.0X3	T36.0X4	T36.0X5	T36.0X6
Adiphenine	T44.3X1	T44.3X2	T44.3X3	T44.3X4	T44.3X5	T44.3X6
Adipiodone	T50.8X1	T50.8X2	T50.8X3	T50.8X4	T50.8X5	T50.8X6
Adjunct, pharmaceutical	T50.901	T50.902	T50.903	T50.904	T50.905	T50.906
Adrenal (extract, cortex or medulla) (glucocorticoids) (hormones) (mineralocorticoids)	T38.0X1	T38.0X2	T38.0X3	T38.0X4	T38.0X5	T38.0X6
ENT agent	T49.6X1	T49.6X2	T49.6X3	T49.6X4	T49.6X5	T49.6X6
ophthalmic preparation	T49.5X1	T49.5X2	T49.5X3	T49.5X4	T49.5X5	T49.5X6
topical NEC	T49.0X1	T49.0X2	T49.0X3	T49.0X4	T49.0X5	T49.0X6
Adrenaline	T44.5X1	T44.5X2	T44.5X3	T44.5X4	T44.5X5	T44.5X6
Adrenalin—see Adrenaline						
Adrenergic NEC	T44.901	T44.902	T44.903	T44.904	T44.905	T44.906
blocking agent NEC	T44.8X1	T44.8X2	T44.8X3	T44.8X4	T44.8X5	T44.8X6
beta, heart	T44.7X1	T44.7X2	T44.7X3	T44.7X4	T44.7X5	T44.7X6
specified NEC	T44.991	T44.992	T44.993	T44.994	T44.995	T44.996
Adrenochrome						
(mono) semicarbazone	T46.991	T46.992	T46.993	T46.994	T46.995	T46.996
derivative	T46.991	T46.992	T46.993	T46.994	T46.995	T46.996
Adrenocorticotrophic hormone	T38.811	T38.812	T38.813	T38.814	T38.815	T38.816
Adrenocorticotro-phin	T38.811	T38.812	T38.813	T38.814	T38.815	T38.816
Adriamycin	T45.1X1	T45.1X2	T45.1X3	T45.1X4	T45.1X5	T45.1X6
Aerosol spray NEC	T65.91	T65.92	T65.93	T65.94	—	—
Aerosporin	T36.8X1	T36.8X2	T36.8X3	T36.8X4	T36.8X5	T36.8X6
ENT agent	T49.6X1	T49.6X2	T49.6X3	T49.6X4	T49.6X5	T49.6X6
ophthalmic preparation	T49.5X1	T49.5X2	T49.5X3	T49.5X4	T49.5X5	T49.5X6
topical NEC	T49.0X1	T49.0X2	T49.0X3	T49.0X4	T49.0X5	T49.0X6
Aethusa cynapium	T62.2X1	T62.2X2	T62.2X3	T62.2X4	—	—
Afghanistan black	T40.7X1	T40.7X2	T40.7X3	T40.7X4	T40.7X5	T40.7X6
Aflatoxin	T64.01	T64.02	T64.03	T64.04	—	—
Afloqualone	T42.8X1	T42.8X2	T42.8X3	T42.8X4	T42.8X5	T42.8X6
African boxwood	T62.2X1	T62.2X2	T62.2X3	T62.2X4	—	—
Agar	T47.4X1	T47.4X2	T47.4X3	T47.4X4	T47.4X5	T47.4X6
Agonist						
predominantly						
alpha-adrenoreceptor	T44.4X1	T44.4X2	T44.4X3	T44.4X4	T44.4X5	T44.4X6
beta-adrenoreceptor	T44.5X1	T44.5X2	T44.5X3	T44.5X4	T44.5X5	T44.5X6
Agricultural agent NEC	T65.91	T65.92	T65.93	T65.94	—	—
Agrypnal	T42.3X1	T42.3X2	T42.3X3	T42.3X4	T42.3X5	T42.3X6
AHLG	T50.Z11	T50.Z12	T50.Z13	T50.Z14	T50.Z15	T50.Z16
Air contaminant (s), source/type NOS	T65.91	T65.92	T65.93	T65.94	—	—
Ajmaline	T46.2X1	T46.2X2	T46.2X3	T46.2X4	T46.2X5	T46.2X6
Akee	T62.1X1	T62.1X2	T62.1X3	T62.1X4	—	—
Akrinol	T49.0X1	T49.0X2	T49.0X3	T49.0X4	T49.0X5	T49.0X6
Akritoin	T37.8X1	T37.8X2	T37.8X3	T37.8X4	T37.8X5	T37.8X6
Alacepril	T46.4X1	T46.4X2	T46.4X3	T46.4X4	T46.4X5	T46.4X6
Alantolactone	T37.4X1	T37.4X2	T37.4X3	T37.4X4	T37.4X5	T37.4X6
Albamycin	T36.8X1	T36.8X2	T36.8X3	T36.8X4	T36.8X5	T36.8X6
Albendazole	T37.4X1	T37.4X2	T37.4X3	T37.4X4	T37.4X5	T37.4X6
Albumin						
bovine	T45.8X1	T45.8X2	T45.8X3	T45.8X4	T45.8X5	T45.8X6
human serum	T45.8X1	T45.8X2	T45.8X3	T45.8X4	T45.8X5	T45.8X6
salt-poor	T45.8X1	T45.8X2	T45.8X3	T45.8X4	T45.8X5	T45.8X6
normal human serum	T45.8X1	T45.8X2	T45.8X3	T45.8X4	T45.8X5	T45.8X6
Albuterol	T48.6X1	T48.6X2	T48.6X3	T48.6X4	T48.6X5	T48.6X6
Albutoin	T42.0X1	T42.0X2	T42.0X3	T42.0X4	T42.0X5	T42.0X6
Alclometasone	T49.0X1	T49.0X2	T49.0X3	T49.0X4	T49.0X5	T49.0X6
Alcohol	T51.91	T51.92	T51.93	T51.94	—	—
absolute	T51.0X1	T51.0X2	T51.0X3	T51.0X4	—	—
beverage	T51.0X1	T51.0X2	T51.0X3	T51.0X4	—	—
allyl	T51.8X1	T51.8X2	T51.8X3	T51.8X4	—	—
amyl	T51.3X1	T51.3X2	T51.3X3	T51.3X4	—	—
antifreeze	T51.1X1	T51.1X2	T51.1X3	T51.1X4	—	—
beverage	T51.0X1	T51.0X2	T51.0X3	T51.0X4	—	—
butyl	T51.3X1	T51.3X2	T51.3X3	T51.3X4	—	—
dehydrated	T51.0X1	T51.0X2	T51.0X3	T51.0X4	—	—
beverage	T51.0X1	T51.0X2	T51.0X3	T51.0X4	—	—
denatured	T51.0X1	T51.0X2	T51.0X3	T51.0X4	—	—
deterrent NEC	T50.6X1	T50.6X2	T50.6X3	T50.6X4	T50.6X5	T50.6X6

Substance	Poisoning, Accidental (unintentional)	Poisoning, Intentional self-harm	Poisoning, Assault	Poisoning, Undetermined	Adverse effect	Underdosing
Alcohol — *Continued*						
diagnostic (gastric function)	T50.8X1	T50.8X2	T50.8X3	T50.8X4	T50.8X5	T50.8X6
ethyl	T51.0X1	T51.0X2	T51.0X3	T51.0X4	—	—
beverage	T51.0X1	T51.0X2	T51.0X3	T51.0X4	—	—
grain	T51.0X1	T51.0X2	T51.0X3	T51.0X4	—	—
beverage	T51.0X1	T51.0X2	T51.0X3	T51.0X4	—	—
industrial	T51.0X1	T51.0X2	T51.0X3	T51.0X4	—	—
isopropyl	T51.2X1	T51.2X2	T51.2X3	T51.2X4	—	—
methyl	T51.1X1	T51.1X2	T51.1X3	T51.1X4	—	—
preparation for consumption	T51.0X1	T51.0X2	T51.0X3	T51.0X4	—	—
propyl	T51.3X1	T51.3X2	T51.3X3	T51.3X4	—	—
secondary	T51.2X1	T51.2X2	T51.2X3	T51.2X4	—	—
radiator	T51.1X1	T51.1X2	T51.1X3	T51.1X4	—	—
rubbing	T51.2X1	T51.2X2	T51.2X3	T51.2X4	—	—
specified type NEC	T51.8X1	T51.8X2	T51.8X3	T51.8X4	—	—
surgical	T51.0X1	T51.0X2	T51.0X3	T51.0X4	—	—
vapor (from any type of Alcohol)	T59.891	T59.892	T59.893	T59.894	—	—
wood	T51.1X1	T51.1X2	T51.1X3	T51.1X4	—	—
Alcuronium (chloride)	T48.1X1	T48.1X2	T48.1X3	T48.1X4	T48.1X5	T48.1X6
Aldactone	T50.0X1	T50.0X2	T50.0X3	T50.0X4	T50.0X5	T50.0X6
Aldesulfone sodium	T37.1X1	T37.1X2	T37.1X3	T37.1X4	T37.1X5	T37.1X6
Aldicarb	T60.0X1	T60.0X2	T60.0X3	T60.0X4	—	—
Aldomet	T46.5X1	T46.5X2	T46.5X3	T46.5X4	T46.5X5	T46.5X6
Aldosterone	T50.0X1	T50.0X2	T50.0X3	T50.0X4	T50.0X5	T50.0X6
Aldrin (dust)	T60.1X1	T60.1X2	T60.1X3	T60.1X4	—	—
Aleve—see Naproxen						
Alexitol sodium	T47.1X1	T47.1X2	T47.1X3	T47.1X4	T47.1X5	T47.1X6
Alfacalcidol	T45.2X1	T45.2X2	T45.2X3	T45.2X4	T45.2X5	T45.2X6
Alfadolone	T41.1X1	T41.1X2	T41.1X3	T41.1X4	T41.1X5	T41.1X6
Alfaxalone	T41.1X1	T41.1X2	T41.1X3	T41.1X4	T41.1X5	T41.1X6
Alfentanil	T40.4X1	T40.4X2	T40.4X3	T40.4X4	T40.4X5	T40.4X6
Alfuzosin (hydrochloride)	T44.8X1	T44.8X2	T44.8X3	T44.8X4	T44.8X5	T44.8X6
Algae (harmful) (toxin)	T65.821	T65.822	T65.823	T65.824	—	—
Algeldrate	T47.1X1	T47.1X2	T47.1X3	T47.1X4	T47.1X5	T47.1X6
Algin	T47.8X1	T47.8X2	T47.8X3	T47.8X4	T47.8X5	T47.8X6
Alglucerase	T45.3X1	T45.3X2	T45.3X3	T45.3X4	T45.3X5	T45.3X6
Alidase	T45.3X1	T45.3X2	T45.3X3	T45.3X4	T45.3X5	T45.3X6
Alimemazine	T43.3X1	T43.3X2	T43.3X3	T43.3X4	T43.3X5	T43.3X6
Aliphatic thiocyanates	T65.0X1	T65.0X2	T65.0X3	T65.0X4	—	—
Alizapride	T45.0X1	T45.0X2	T45.0X3	T45.0X4	T45.0X5	T45.0X6
Alkali (caustic)	T54.3X1	T54.3X2	T54.3X3	T54.3X4	—	—
Alkaline antiseptic solution (aromatic)	T49.6X1	T49.6X2	T49.6X3	T49.6X4	T49.6X5	T49.6X6
Alkalinizing agents (medicinal)	T50.901	T50.902	T50.903	T50.904	T50.905	T50.906
Alkalizing agent NEC	T50.901	T50.902	T50.903	T50.904	T50.905	T50.906
Alka-seltzer	T39.011	T39.012	T39.013	T39.014	T39.015	T39.016
Alkavervir	T46.5X1	T46.5X2	T46.5X3	T46.5X4	T46.5X5	T46.5X6
Alkonium (bromide)	T49.0X1	T49.0X2	T49.0X3	T49.0X4	T49.0X5	T49.0X6

Substance	Poisoning, Accidental (unintentional)	Poisoning, Intentional self-harm	Poisoning, Assault	Poisoning, Undetermined	Adverse effect	Underdosing
Alkylating drug NEC	T45.1X1	T45.1X2	T45.1X3	T45.1X4	T45.1X5	T45.1X6
antimyeloprolifera-tive	T45.1X1	T45.1X2	T45.1X3	T45.1X4	T45.1X5	T45.1X6
lymphatic	T45.1X1	T45.1X2	T45.1X3	T45.1X4	T45.1X5	T45.1X6
Alkylisocyanate	T65.0X1	T65.0X2	T65.0X3	T65.0X4	—	—
Allantoin	T49.4X1	T49.4X2	T49.4X3	T49.4X4	T49.4X5	T49.4X6
Allegron	T43.011	T43.012	T43.013	T43.014	T43.015	T43.016
Allethrin	T49.0X1	T49.0X2	T49.0X3	T49.0X4	T49.0X5	T49.0X6
Allobarbital	T42.3X1	T42.3X2	T42.3X3	T42.3X4	T42.3X5	T42.3X6
Allopurinol	T50.4X1	T50.4X2	T50.4X3	T50.4X4	T50.4X5	T50.4X6
Allyl						
Alcohol	T51.8X1	T51.8X2	T51.8X3	T51.8X4	—	—
disulfide	T46.6X1	T46.6X2	T46.6X3	T46.6X4	T46.6X5	T46.6X6
Allylestrenol	T38.5X1	T38.5X2	T38.5X3	T38.5X4	T38.5X5	T38.5X6
Allylisopropyl-acetylurea	T42.6X1	T42.6X2	T42.6X3	T42.6X4	T42.6X5	T42.6X6
Allylisopropyl-malonylurea	T42.3X1	T42.3X2	T42.3X3	T42.3X4	T42.3X5	T42.3X6
Allylthiourea	T49.3X1	T49.3X2	T49.3X3	T49.3X4	T49.3X5	T49.3X6
Allyltribromide	T42.6X1	T42.6X2	T42.6X3	T42.6X4	T42.6X5	T42.6X6
Allypropymal	T42.3X1	T42.3X2	T42.3X3	T42.3X4	T42.3X5	T42.3X6
Almagate	T47.1X1	T47.1X2	T47.1X3	T47.1X4	T47.1X5	T47.1X6
Almasilate	T47.1X1	T47.1X2	T47.1X3	T47.1X4	T47.1X5	T47.1X6
Almitrine	T50.7X1	T50.7X2	T50.7X3	T50.7X4	T50.7X5	T50.7X6
Aloes	T47.2X1	T47.2X2	T47.2X3	T47.2X4	T47.2X5	T47.2X6
Aloglutamol	T47.1X1	T47.1X2	T47.1X3	T47.1X4	T47.1X5	T47.1X6
Aloin	T47.2X1	T47.2X2	T47.2X3	T47.2X4	T47.2X5	T47.2X6
Aloxidone	T42.2X1	T42.2X2	T42.2X3	T42.2X4	T42.2X5	T42.2X6
Alpha						
acetyldigoxin	T46.0X1	T46.0X2	T46.0X3	T46.0X4	T46.0X5	T46.0X6
adrenergic blocking drug	T44.6X1	T44.6X2	T44.6X3	T44.6X4	T44.6X5	T44.6X6
amylase	T45.3X1	T45.3X2	T45.3X3	T45.3X4	T45.3X5	T45.3X6
tocoferol (acetate)	T45.2X1	T45.2X2	T45.2X3	T45.2X4	T45.2X5	T45.2X6
tocopherol	T45.2X1	T45.2X2	T45.2X3	T45.2X4	T45.2X5	T45.2X6
Alphadolone	T41.1X1	T41.1X2	T41.1X3	T41.1X4	T41.1X5	T41.1X6
Alphaprodine	T40.4X1	T40.4X2	T40.4X3	T40.4X4	T40.4X5	T40.4X6
Alphaxalone	T41.1X1	T41.1X2	T41.1X3	T41.1X4	T41.1X5	T41.1X6
Alprazolam	T42.4X1	T42.4X2	T42.4X3	T42.4X4	T42.4X5	T42.4X6
Alprenolol	T44.7X1	T44.7X2	T44.7X3	T44.7X4	T44.7X5	T44.7X6
Alprostadil	T46.7X1	T46.7X2	T46.7X3	T46.7X4	T46.7X5	T46.7X6
Alsactide	T38.811	T38.812	T38.813	T38.814	T38.815	T38.816
Alseroxylon	T46.5X1	T46.5X2	T46.5X3	T46.5X4	T46.5X5	T46.5X6
Alteplase	T45.611	T45.612	T45.613	T45.614	T45.615	T45.616
Altizide	T50.2X1	T50.2X2	T50.2X3	T50.2X4	T50.2X5	T50.2X6
Altretamine	T45.1X1	T45.1X2	T45.1X3	T45.1X4	T45.1X5	T45.1X6
Alum (medicinal)	T49.4X1	T49.4X2	T49.4X3	T49.4X4	T49.4X5	T49.4X6
nonmedicinal (ammonium) (potassium)	T56.891	T56.892	T56.893	T56.894	—	—
Aluminium, aluminum						
acetate	T49.2X1	T49.2X2	T49.2X3	T49.2X4	T49.2X5	T49.2X6
solution	T49.0X1	T49.0X2	T49.0X3	T49.0X4	T49.0X5	T49.0X6

Substance	Poisoning, Accidental (unintentional)	Poisoning, Intentional self-harm	Poisoning, Assault	Poisoning, Undetermined	Adverse effect	Underdosing
Aluminium, aluminum — *Continued*						
aspirin	T39.011	T39.012	T39.013	T39.014	T39.015	T39.016
bis (acetylsalicylate)	T39.011	T39.012	T39.013	T39.014	T39.015	T39.016
carbonate (gel, basic)	T47.1X1	T47.1X2	T47.1X3	T47.1X4	T47.1X5	T47.1X6
chlorhydroxide-complex	T47.1X1	T47.1X2	T47.1X3	T47.1X4	T47.1X5	T47.1X6
chloride	T49.2X1	T49.2X2	T49.2X3	T49.2X4	T49.2X5	T49.2X6
clofibrate	T46.6X1	T46.6X2	T46.6X3	T46.6X4	T46.6X5	T46.6X6
diacetate	T49.2X1	T49.2X2	T49.2X3	T49.2X4	T49.2X5	T49.2X6
glycinate	T47.1X1	T47.1X2	T47.1X3	T47.1X4	T47.1X5	T47.1X6
hydroxide (gel)	T47.1X1	T47.1X2	T47.1X3	T47.1X4	T47.1X5	T47.1X6
hydroxide-magnesium carb. gel	T47.1X1	T47.1X2	T47.1X3	T47.1X4	T47.1X5	T47.1X6
magnesium silicate	T47.1X1	T47.1X2	T47.1X3	T47.1X4	T47.1X5	T47.1X6
nicotinate	T46.7X1	T46.7X2	T46.7X3	T46.7X4	T46.7X5	T46.7X6
ointment (surgical) (topical)	T49.3X1	T49.3X2	T49.3X3	T49.3X4	T49.3X5	T49.3X6
phosphate	T47.1X1	T47.1X2	T47.1X3	T47.1X4	T47.1X5	T47.1X6
salicylate	T39.091	T39.092	T39.093	T39.094	T39.095	T39.096
silicate	T47.1X1	T47.1X2	T47.1X3	T47.1X4	T47.1X5	T47.1X6
sodium silicate	T47.1X1	T47.1X2	T47.1X3	T47.1X4	T47.1X5	T47.1X6
subacetate	T49.2X1	T49.2X2	T49.2X3	T49.2X4	T49.2X5	T49.2X6
sulfate	T49.0X1	T49.0X2	T49.0X3	T49.0X4	T49.0X5	T49.0X6
tannate	T47.6X1	T47.6X2	T47.6X3	T47.6X4	T47.6X5	T47.6X6
topical NEC	T49.3X1	T49.3X2	T49.3X3	T49.3X4	T49.3X5	T49.3X6
Alurate	T42.3X1	T42.3X2	T42.3X3	T42.3X4	T42.3X5	T42.3X6
Alverine	T44.3X1	T44.3X2	T44.3X3	T44.3X4	T44.3X5	T44.3X6
Alvodine	T40.2X1	T40.2X2	T40.2X3	T40.2X4	T40.2X5	T40.2X6
Amanita phalloides	T62.0X1	T62.0X2	T62.0X3	T62.0X4	—	—
Amanitine	T62.0X1	T62.0X2	T62.0X3	T62.0X4	—	—
Amantadine	T42.8X1	T42.8X2	T42.8X3	T42.8X4	T42.8X5	T42.8X6
Ambazone	T49.6X1	T49.6X2	T49.6X3	T49.6X4	T49.6X5	T49.6X6
Ambenonium (chloride)	T44.0X1	T44.0X2	T44.0X3	T44.0X4	T44.0X5	T44.0X6
Ambroxol	T48.4X1	T48.4X2	T48.4X3	T48.4X4	T48.4X5	T48.4X6
Ambuphylline	T48.6X1	T48.6X2	T48.6X3	T48.6X4	T48.6X5	T48.6X6
Ambutonium bromide	T44.3X1	T44.3X2	T44.3X3	T44.3X4	T44.3X5	T44.3X6
Amcinonide	T49.0X1	T49.0X2	T49.0X3	T49.0X4	T49.0X5	T49.0X6
Amdinocilline	T36.0X1	T36.0X2	T36.0X3	T36.0X4	T36.0X5	T36.0X6
Ametazole	T50.8X1	T50.8X2	T50.8X3	T50.8X4	T50.8X5	T50.8X6
Amethocaine	T41.3X1	T41.3X2	T41.3X3	T41.3X4	T41.3X5	T41.3X6
regional	T41.3X1	T41.3X2	T41.3X3	T41.3X4	T41.3X5	T41.3X6
spinal	T41.3X1	T41.3X2	T41.3X3	T41.3X4	T41.3X5	T41.3X6
Amethopterin	T45.1X1	T45.1X2	T45.1X3	T45.1X4	T45.1X5	T45.1X6
Amezinium metilsulfate	T44.991	T44.992	T44.993	T44.994	T44.995	T44.996
Amfebutamone	T43.291	T43.292	T43.293	T43.294	T43.295	T43.296
Amfepramone	T50.5X1	T50.5X2	T50.5X3	T50.5X4	T50.5X5	T50.5X6
Amfetamine	T43.621	T43.622	T43.623	T43.624	T43.625	T43.626
Amfetaminil	T43.621	T43.622	T43.623	T43.624	T43.625	T43.626
Amfomycin	T36.8X1	T36.8X2	T36.8X3	T36.8X4	T36.8X5	T36.8X6
Amidefrine mesilate	T48.5X1	T48.5X2	T48.5X3	T48.5X4	T48.5X5	T48.5X6
Amidone	T40.3X1	T40.3X2	T40.3X3	T40.3X4	T40.3X5	T40.3X6
Amidopyrine	T39.2X1	T39.2X2	T39.2X3	T39.2X4	T39.2X5	T39.2X6
Amidotrizoate	T50.8X1	T50.8X2	T50.8X3	T50.8X4	T50.8X5	T50.8X6
Amiflamine	T43.1X1	T43.1X2	T43.1X3	T43.1X4	T43.1X5	T43.1X6
Amikacin	T36.5X1	T36.5X2	T36.5X3	T36.5X4	T36.5X5	T36.5X6
Amikhelline	T46.3X1	T46.3X2	T46.3X3	T46.3X4	T46.3X5	T46.3X6
Amiloride	T50.2X1	T50.2X2	T50.2X3	T50.2X4	T50.2X5	T50.2X6
Aminacrine	T49.0X1	T49.0X2	T49.0X3	T49.0X4	T49.0X5	T49.0X6
Amineptine	T43.011	T43.012	T43.013	T43.014	T43.015	T43.016
Aminitrozole	T37.3X1	T37.3X2	T37.3X3	T37.3X4	T37.3X5	T37.3X6
Amino acids	T50.3X1	T50.3X2	T50.3X3	T50.3X4	T50.3X5	T50.3X6
Aminoacetic acid (derivatives)	T50.3X1	T50.3X2	T50.3X3	T50.3X4	T50.3X5	T50.3X6
Aminoacridine	T49.0X1	T49.0X2	T49.0X3	T49.0X4	T49.0X5	T49.0X6
Aminobenzoic acid(-p)	T49.3X1	T49.3X2	T49.3X3	T49.3X4	T49.3X5	T49.3X6
4-Aminobutyric acid	T43.8X1	T43.8X2	T43.8X3	T43.8X4	T43.8X5	T43.8X6
Aminocaproic acid	T45.621	T45.622	T45.623	T45.624	T45.625	T45.626
Aminoethyl-isothiourium	T45.8X1	T45.8X2	T45.8X3	T45.8X4	T45.8X5	T45.8X6
Aminofenazone	T39.2X1	T39.2X2	T39.2X3	T39.2X4	T39.2X5	T39.2X6
Aminoglutethimide	T45.1X1	T45.1X2	T45.1X3	T45.1X4	T45.1X5	T45.1X6
Aminohippuric acid	T50.8X1	T50.8X2	T50.8X3	T50.8X4	T50.8X5	T50.8X6
Aminomethylbenzoic acid	T45.691	T45.692	T45.693	T45.694	T45.695	T45.696
Aminometradine	T50.2X1	T50.2X2	T50.2X3	T50.2X4	T50.2X5	T50.2X6
Aminopentamide	T44.3X1	T44.3X2	T44.3X3	T44.3X4	T44.3X5	T44.3X6
Aminophenazone	T39.2X1	T39.2X2	T39.2X3	T39.2X4	T39.2X5	T39.2X6
Aminophenol	T54.0X1	T54.0X2	T54.0X3	T54.0X4	—	—
4-Aminophenol derivatives	T39.1X1	T39.1X2	T39.1X3	T39.1X4	T39.1X5	T39.1X6
Aminophenylpyri-done	T43.591	T43.592	T43.593	T43.594	T43.595	T43.596
Aminophylline	T48.6X1	T48.6X2	T48.6X3	T48.6X4	T48.6X5	T48.6X6
Aminopterin sodium	T45.1X1	T45.1X2	T45.1X3	T45.1X4	T45.1X5	T45.1X6
Aminopyrine	T39.2X1	T39.2X2	T39.2X3	T39.2X4	T39.2X5	T39.2X6
8-Aminoquinoline drugs	T37.2X1	T37.2X2	T37.2X3	T37.2X4	T37.2X5	T37.2X6
Aminorex	T50.5X1	T50.5X2	T50.5X3	T50.5X4	T50.5X5	T50.5X6
Aminosalicylic acid	T37.1X1	T37.1X2	T37.1X3	T37.1X4	T37.1X5	T37.1X6
Aminosalylum	T37.1X1	T37.1X2	T37.1X3	T37.1X4	T37.1X5	T37.1X6
Amiodarone	T46.2X1	T46.2X2	T46.2X3	T46.2X4	T46.2X5	T46.2X6
Amiphenazole	T50.7X1	T50.7X2	T50.7X3	T50.7X4	T50.7X5	T50.7X6
Amiquinsin	T46.5X1	T46.5X2	T46.5X3	T46.5X4	T46.5X5	T46.5X6
Amisometradine	T50.2X1	T50.2X2	T50.2X3	T50.2X4	T50.2X5	T50.2X6
Amisulpride	T43.591	T43.592	T43.593	T43.594	T43.595	T43.596
Amitriptyline	T43.011	T43.012	T43.013	T43.014	T43.015	T43.016
Amitriptylinoxide	T43.011	T43.012	T43.013	T43.014	T43.015	T43.016
Amlexanox	T48.6X1	T48.6X2	T48.6X3	T48.6X4	T48.6X5	T48.6X6
Ammonia (fumes) (gas) (vapor)	T59.891	T59.892	T59.893	T59.894	—	—
aromatic spirit	T48.991	T48.992	T48.993	T48.994	T48.995	T48.996
liquid (household)	T54.3X1	T54.3X2	T54.3X3	T54.3X4	—	—
Ammoniated mercury	T49.0X1	T49.0X2	T49.0X3	T49.0X4	T49.0X5	T49.0X6

Substance	Poisoning, Accidental (unintentional)	Poisoning, Intentional self-harm	Poisoning, Assault	Poisoning, Undetermined	Adverse effect	Underdosing
Ammonium						
acid tartrate	T49.5X1	T49.5X2	T49.5X3	T49.5X4	T49.5X5	T49.5X6
bromide	T42.6X1	T42.6X2	T42.6X3	T42.6X4	T42.6X5	T42.6X6
carbonate	T54.3X1	T54.3X2	T54.3X3	T54.3X4	—	—
chloride	T50.991	T50.992	T50.993	T50.994	T50.995	T50.996
expectorant	T48.4X1	T48.4X2	T48.4X3	T48.4X4	T48.4X5	T48.4X6
compounds (household) NEC	T54.3X1	T54.3X2	T54.3X3	T54.3X4	—	—
fumes (any usage)	T59.891	T59.892	T59.893	T59.894	—	—
industrial	T54.3X1	T54.3X2	T54.3X3	T54.3X4	—	—
ichthyosulronate	T49.4X1	T49.4X2	T49.4X3	T49.4X4	T49.4X5	T49.4X6
mandelate	T37.91	T37.92	T37.93	T37.94	T37.95	T37.96
sulfamate	T60.3X1	T60.3X2	T60.3X3	T60.3X4	—	—
sulfonate resin	T47.8X1	T47.8X2	T47.8X3	T47.8X4	T47.8X5	T47.8X6
Amobarbital (sodium)	T42.3X1	T42.3X2	T42.3X3	T42.3X4	T42.3X5	T42.3X6
Amodiaquine	T37.2X1	T37.2X2	T37.2X3	T37.2X4	T37.2X5	T37.2X6
Amopyroquin(e)	T37.2X1	T37.2X2	T37.2X3	T37.2X4	T37.2X5	T37.2X6
Amoxapine	T43.011	T43.012	T43.013	T43.014	T43.015	T43.016
Amoxicillin	T36.0X1	T36.0X2	T36.0X3	T36.0X4	T36.0X5	T36.0X6
Amperozide	T43.591	T43.592	T43.593	T43.594	T43.595	T43.596
Amphenidone	T43.591	T43.592	T43.593	T43.594	T43.595	T43.596
Amphetamine NEC	T43.621	T43.622	T43.623	T43.624	T43.625	T43.626
Amphomycin	T36.8X1	T36.8X2	T36.8X3	T36.8X4	T36.8X5	T36.8X6
Amphotalide	T37.4X1	T37.4X2	T37.4X3	T37.4X4	T37.4X5	T37.4X6
Amphotericin B	T36.7X1	T36.7X2	T36.7X3	T36.7X4	T36.7X5	T36.7X6
topical	T49.0X1	T49.0X2	T49.0X3	T49.0X4	T49.0X5	T49.0X6
Ampicillin	T36.0X1	T36.0X2	T36.0X3	T36.0X4	T36.0X5	T36.0X6
Amprotropine	T44.3X1	T44.3X2	T44.3X3	T44.3X4	T44.3X5	T44.3X6
Amsacrine	T45.1X1	T45.1X2	T45.1X3	T45.1X4	T45.1X5	T45.1X6
Amygdaline	T62.2X1	T62.2X2	T62.2X3	T62.2X4	—	—
Amyl						
acetate	T52.8X1	T52.8X2	T52.8X3	T52.8X4	—	—
vapor	T59.891	T59.892	T59.893	T59.894	—	—
alcohol	T51.3X1	T51.3X2	T51.3X3	T51.3X4	—	—
chloride	T53.6X1	T53.6X2	T53.6X3	T53.6X4	—	—
formate	T52.8X1	T52.8X2	T52.8X3	T52.8X4	—	—
nitrite	T46.3X1	T46.3X2	T46.3X3	T46.3X4	T46.3X5	T46.3X6
propionate	T65.891	T65.892	T65.893	T65.894	—	—
Amylase	T47.5X1	T47.5X2	T47.5X3	T47.5X4	T47.5X5	T47.5X6
Amyleine, regional	T41.3X1	T41.3X2	T41.3X3	T41.3X4	T41.3X5	T41.3X6
Amylene						
dichloride	T53.6X1	T53.6X2	T53.6X3	T53.6X4	—	—
hydrate	T51.3X1	T51.3X2	T51.3X3	T51.3X4	—	—
Amylmetacresol	T49.6X1	T49.6X2	T49.6X3	T49.6X4	T49.6X5	T49.6X6
Amylobarbitone	T42.3X1	T42.3X2	T42.3X3	T42.3X4	T42.3X5	T42.3X6
Amylocaine, regional	T41.3X1	T41.3X2	T41.3X3	T41.3X4	T41.3X5	T41.3X6
infiltration (subcutaneous)	T41.3X1	T41.3X2	T41.3X3	T41.3X4	T41.3X5	T41.3X6
nerve block (peripheral) (plexus)	T41.3X1	T41.3X2	T41.3X3	T41.3X4	T41.3X5	T41.3X6
spinal	T41.3X1	T41.3X2	T41.3X3	T41.3X4	T41.3X5	T41.3X6
topical (surface)	T41.3X1	T41.3X2	T41.3X3	T41.3X4	T41.3X5	T41.3X6
Amylopectin	T47.6X1	T47.6X2	T47.6X3	T47.6X4	T47.6X5	T47.6X6
Amytal (sodium)	T42.3X1	T42.3X2	T42.3X3	T42.3X4	T42.3X5	T42.3X6
Anabolic steroid	T38.7X1	T38.7X2	T38.7X3	T38.7X4	T38.7X5	T38.7X6
Analeptic NEC	T50.7X1	T50.7X2	T50.7X3	T50.7X4	T50.7X5	T50.7X6
Analgesic	T39.91	T39.92	T39.93	T39.94	T39.95	T39.96
anti-inflammatory NEC	T39.91	T39.92	T39.93	T39.94	T39.95	T39.96
propionic acid derivative	T39.311	T39.312	T39.313	T39.314	T39.315	T39.316
antirheumatic NEC	T39.4X1	T39.4X2	T39.4X3	T39.4X4	T39.4X5	T39.4X6
aromatic NEC	T39.1X1	T39.1X2	T39.1X3	T39.1X4	T39.1X5	T39.1X6
narcotic NEC	T40.601	T40.602	T40.603	T40.604	T40.605	T40.606
combination	T40.601	T40.602	T40.603	T40.604	T40.605	T40.606
obstetric	T40.601	T40.602	T40.603	T40.604	T40.605	T40.606
non-narcotic NEC	T39.91	T39.92	T39.93	T39.94	T39.95	T39.96
combination	T39.91	T39.92	T39.93	T39.94	T39.95	T39.96
pyrazole	T39.2X1	T39.2X2	T39.2X3	T39.2X4	T39.2X5	T39.2X6
specified NEC	T39.8X1	T39.8X2	T39.8X3	T39.8X4	T39.8X5	T39.8X6
Analgin	T39.2X1	T39.2X2	T39.2X3	T39.2X4	T39.2X5	T39.2X6
Anamirta cocculus	T62.1X1	T62.1X2	T62.1X3	T62.1X4	—	—
Ancillin	T36.0X1	T36.0X2	T36.0X3	T36.0X4	T36.0X5	T36.0X6
Ancrod	T45.691	T45.692	T45.693	T45.694	T45.695	T45.696
Androgen	T38.7X1	T38.7X2	T38.7X3	T38.7X4	T38.7X5	T38.7X6
Androgen-estrogen mixture	T38.7X1	T38.7X2	T38.7X3	T38.7X4	T38.7X5	T38.7X6
Androstalone	T38.7X1	T38.7X2	T38.7X3	T38.7X4	T38.7X5	T38.7X6
Androstanolone	T38.7X1	T38.7X2	T38.7X3	T38.7X4	T38.7X5	T38.7X6
Androsterone	T38.7X1	T38.7X2	T38.7X3	T38.7X4	T38.7X5	T38.7X6
Anemone pulsatilla	T62.2X1	T62.2X2	T62.2X3	T62.2X4	—	—
Anesthesia						
caudal	T41.3X1	T41.3X2	T41.3X3	T41.3X4	T41.3X5	T41.3X6
endotracheal	T41.0X1	T41.0X2	T41.0X3	T41.0X4	T41.0X5	T41.0X6
epidural	T41.3X1	T41.3X2	T41.3X3	T41.3X4	T41.3X5	T41.3X6
inhalation	T41.0X1	T41.0X2	T41.0X3	T41.0X4	T41.0X5	T41.0X6
local	T41.3X1	T41.3X2	T41.3X3	T41.3X4	T41.3X5	T41.3X6
mucosal	T41.3X1	T41.3X2	T41.3X3	T41.3X4	T41.3X5	T41.3X6
muscle relaxation	T48.1X1	T48.1X2	T48.1X3	T48.1X4	T48.1X5	T48.1X6
nerve blocking	T41.3X1	T41.3X2	T41.3X3	T41.3X4	T41.3X5	T41.3X6
plexus blocking	T41.3X1	T41.3X2	T41.3X3	T41.3X4	T41.3X5	T41.3X6
potentiated	T41.201	T41.202	T41.203	T41.204	T41.205	T41.206
rectal	T41.201	T41.202	T41.203	T41.204	T41.205	T41.206
general	T41.201	T41.202	T41.203	T41.204	T41.205	T41.206
local	T41.3X1	T41.3X2	T41.3X3	T41.3X4	T41.3X5	T41.3X6
regional	T41.3X1	T41.3X2	T41.3X3	T41.3X4	T41.3X5	T41.3X6
surface	T41.3X1	T41.3X2	T41.3X3	T41.3X4	T41.3X5	T41.3X6
Anesthetic NEC —see also Anesthesia	T41.41	T41.42	T41.43	T41.44	T41.45	T41.46
with muscle relaxant	T41.201	T41.202	T41.203	T41.204	T41.205	T41.206
general	T41.201	T41.202	T41.203	T41.204	T41.205	T41.206
local	T41.3X1	T41.3X2	T41.3X3	T41.3X4	T41.3X5	T41.3X6
gaseous NEC	T41.0X1	T41.0X2	T41.0X3	T41.0X4	T41.0X5	T41.0X6
general NEC	T41.201	T41.202	T41.203	T41.204	T41.205	T41.206

Substance	Poisoning, Accidental (unintentional)	Poisoning, Intentional self-harm	Poisoning, Assault	Poisoning, Undetermined	Adverse effect	Underdosing
Anesthetic NEC — *Continued*						
halogenated hydrocarbon derivatives NEC	T41.0X1	T41.0X2	T41.0X3	T41.0X4	T41.0X5	T41.0X6
infiltration NEC	T41.3X1	T41.3X2	T41.3X3	T41.3X4	T41.3X5	T41.3X6
intravenous NEC	T41.1X1	T41.1X2	T41.1X3	T41.1X4	T41.1X5	T41.1X6
local NEC	T41.3X1	T41.3X2	T41.3X3	T41.3X4	T41.3X5	T41.3X6
rectal	T41.201	T41.202	T41.203	T41.204	T41.205	T41.206
general	T41.201	T41.202	T41.203	T41.204	T41.205	T41.206
local	T41.3X1	T41.3X2	T41.3X3	T41.3X4	T41.3X5	T41.3X6
regional NEC	T41.3X1	T41.3X2	T41.3X3	T41.3X4	T41.3X5	T41.3X6
spinal NEC	T41.3X1	T41.3X2	T41.3X3	T41.3X4	T41.3X5	T41.3X6
thiobarbiturate	T41.1X1	T41.1X2	T41.1X3	T41.1X4	T41.1X5	T41.1X6
topical	T41.3X1	T41.3X2	T41.3X3	T41.3X4	T41.3X5	T41.3X6
Aneurine	T45.2X1	T45.2X2	T45.2X3	T45.2X4	T45.2X5	T45.2X6
Angio-Conray	T50.8X1	T50.8X2	T50.8X3	T50.8X4	T50.8X5	T50.8X6
Angiotensin	T44.5X1	T44.5X2	T44.5X3	T44.5X4	T44.5X5	T44.5X6
Angiotensinamide	T44.991	T44.992	T44.993	T44.994	T44.995	T44.996
Anhydrohydroxy-progesterone	T38.5X1	T38.5X2	T38.5X3	T38.5X4	T38.5X5	T38.5X6
Anhydron	T50.2X1	T50.2X2	T50.2X3	T50.2X4	T50.2X5	T50.2X6
Anileridine	T40.4X1	T40.4X2	T40.4X3	T40.4X4	T40.4X5	T40.4X6
Aniline (dye) (liquid)	T65.3X1	T65.3X2	T65.3X3	T65.3X4	—	—
analgesic	T39.1X1	T39.1X2	T39.1X3	T39.1X4	T39.1X5	T39.1X6
derivatives, therapeutic NEC	T39.1X1	T39.1X2	T39.1X3	T39.1X4	T39.1X5	T39.1X6
vapor	T65.3X1	T65.3X2	T65.3X3	T65.3X4	—	—
Aniscoropine	T44.3X1	T44.3X2	T44.3X3	T44.3X4	T44.3X5	T44.3X6
Anise oil	T47.5X1	T47.5X2	T47.5X3	T47.5X4	T47.5X5	T47.5X6
Anisidine	T65.3X1	T65.3X2	T65.3X3	T65.3X4	—	—
Anisindione	T45.511	T45.512	T45.513	T45.514	T45.515	T45.516
Anisotropine methyl-bromide	T44.3X1	T44.3X2	T44.3X3	T44.3X4	T44.3X5	T44.3X6
Anistreplase	T45.611	T45.612	T45.613	T45.614	T45.615	T45.616
Anorexiant (central)	T50.5X1	T50.5X2	T50.5X3	T50.5X4	T50.5X5	T50.5X6
Anorexic agents	T50.5X1	T50.5X2	T50.5X3	T50.5X4	T50.5X5	T50.5X6
Ansamycin	T36.6X1	T36.6X2	T36.6X3	T36.6X4	T36.6X5	T36.6X6
Ant (bite) (sting)	T63.421	T63.422	T63.423	T63.424	—	—
Ant poison—see Insecticide						
Antabuse	T50.6X1	T50.6X2	T50.6X3	T50.6X4	T50.6X5	T50.6X6
Antacid NEC	T47.1X1	T47.1X2	T47.1X3	T47.1X4	T47.1X5	T47.1X6
Antagonist						
Aldosterone	T50.0X1	T50.0X2	T50.0X3	T50.0X4	T50.0X5	T50.0X6
alpha-adrenoreceptor	T44.6X1	T44.6X2	T44.6X3	T44.6X4	T44.6X5	T44.6X6
anticoagulant	T45.7X1	T45.7X2	T45.7X3	T45.7X4	T45.7X5	T45.7X6
beta-adrenoreceptor	T44.7X1	T44.7X2	T44.7X3	T44.7X4	T44.7X5	T44.7X6
extrapyramidal NEC	T44.3X1	T44.3X2	T44.3X3	T44.3X4	T44.3X5	T44.3X6
folic acid	T45.1X1	T45.1X2	T45.1X3	T45.1X4	T45.1X5	T45.1X6
H2 receptor	T47.0X1	T47.0X2	T47.0X3	T47.0X4	T47.0X5	T47.0X6
heavy metal	T45.8X1	T45.8X2	T45.8X3	T45.8X4	T45.8X5	T45.8X6
narcotic analgesic	T50.7X1	T50.7X2	T50.7X3	T50.7X4	T50.7X5	T50.7X6
opiate	T50.7X1	T50.7X2	T50.7X3	T50.7X4	T50.7X5	T50.7X6
pyrimidine	T45.1X1	T45.1X2	T45.1X3	T45.1X4	T45.1X5	T45.1X6
serotonin	T46.5X1	T46.5X2	T46.5X3	T46.5X4	T46.5X5	T46.5X6
Antazolin(e)	T45.0X1	T45.0X2	T45.0X3	T45.0X4	T45.0X5	T45.0X6
Anterior pituitary hormone NEC	T38.811	T38.812	T38.813	T38.814	T38.815	T38.816
Anthelmintic NEC	T37.4X1	T37.4X2	T37.4X3	T37.4X4	T37.4X5	T37.4X6
Anthiolimine	T37.4X1	T37.4X2	T37.4X3	T37.4X4	T37.4X5	T37.4X6
Anthralin	T49.4X1	T49.4X2	T49.4X3	T49.4X4	T49.4X5	T49.4X6
Anthramycin	T45.1X1	T45.1X2	T45.1X3	T45.1X4	T45.1X5	T45.1X6
Antiadrenergic NEC	T44.8X1	T44.8X2	T44.8X3	T44.8X4	T44.8X5	T44.8X6
Antiallergic NEC	T45.0X1	T45.0X2	T45.0X3	T45.0X4	T45.0X5	T45.0X6
Anti-anemic (drug) (preparation)	T45.8X1	T45.8X2	T45.8X3	T45.8X4	T45.8X5	T45.8X6
Antiandrogen NEC	T38.6X1	T38.6X2	T38.6X3	T38.6X4	T38.6X5	T38.6X6
Antianxiety drug NEC	T43.501	T43.502	T43.503	T43.504	T43.505	T43.506
Antiaris toxicaria	T65.891	T65.892	T65.893	T65.894	—	—
Antiarteriosclerotic drug	T46.6X1	T46.6X2	T46.6X3	T46.6X4	T46.6X5	T46.6X6
Antiasthmatic drug NEC	T48.6X1	T48.6X2	T48.6X3	T48.6X4	T48.6X5	T48.6X6
Antibiotic NEC	T36.91	T36.92	T36.93	T36.94	T36.95	T36.96
aminoglycoside	T36.5X1	T36.5X2	T36.5X3	T36.5X4	T36.5X5	T36.5X6
anticancer	T45.1X1	T45.1X2	T45.1X3	T45.1X4	T45.1X5	T45.1X6
antifungal	T36.7X1	T36.7X2	T36.7X3	T36.7X4	T36.7X5	T36.7X6
antimycobacterial	T36.5X1	T36.5X2	T36.5X3	T36.5X4	T36.5X5	T36.5X6
antineoplastic	T45.1X1	T45.1X2	T45.1X3	T45.1X4	T45.1X5	T45.1X6
cephalosporin (group)	T36.1X1	T36.1X2	T36.1X3	T36.1X4	T36.1X5	T36.1X6
chloramphenicol (group)	T36.2X1	T36.2X2	T36.2X3	T36.2X4	T36.2X5	T36.2X6
ENT	T49.6X1	T49.6X2	T49.6X3	T49.6X4	T49.6X5	T49.6X6
eye	T49.5X1	T49.5X2	T49.5X3	T49.5X4	T49.5X5	T49.5X6
fungicidal (local)	T49.0X1	T49.0X2	T49.0X3	T49.0X4	T49.0X5	T49.0X6
intestinal	T36.8X1	T36.8X2	T36.8X3	T36.8X4	T36.8X5	T36.8X6
b-lactam NEC	T36.1X1	T36.1X2	T36.1X3	T36.1X4	T36.1X5	T36.1X6
local	T49.0X1	T49.0X2	T49.0X3	T49.0X4	T49.0X5	T49.0X6
macrolides	T36.3X1	T36.3X2	T36.3X3	T36.3X4	T36.3X5	T36.3X6
polypeptide	T36.8X1	T36.8X2	T36.8X3	T36.8X4	T36.8X5	T36.8X6
specified NEC	T36.8X1	T36.8X2	T36.8X3	T36.8X4	T36.8X5	T36.8X6
tetracycline (group)	T36.4X1	T36.4X2	T36.4X3	T36.4X4	T36.4X5	T36.4X6
throat	T49.6X1	T49.6X2	T49.6X3	T49.6X4	T49.6X5	T49.6X6
Anticancer agents NEC	T45.1X1	T45.1X2	T45.1X3	T45.1X4	T45.1X5	T45.1X6
Anticholesterolemic drug NEC	T46.6X1	T46.6X2	T46.6X3	T46.6X4	T46.6X5	T46.6X6
Anticholinergic NEC	T44.3X1	T44.3X2	T44.3X3	T44.3X4	T44.3X5	T44.3X6
Anticholinesterase	T44.0X1	T44.0X2	T44.0X3	T44.0X4	T44.0X5	T44.0X6
organophosphorus	T44.0X1	T44.0X2	T44.0X3	T44.0X4	T44.0X5	T44.0X6
insecticide	T60.0X1	T60.0X2	T60.0X3	T60.0X4	—	—
nerve gas	T59.891	T59.892	T59.893	T59.894	—	—
reversible	T44.0X1	T44.0X2	T44.0X3	T44.0X4	T44.0X5	T44.0X6
ophthalmological	T49.5X1	T49.5X2	T49.5X3	T49.5X4	T49.5X5	T49.5X6
Anticoagulant NEC	T45.511	T45.512	T45.513	T45.514	T45.515	T45.516
Antagonist	T45.7X1	T45.7X2	T45.7X3	T45.7X4	T45.7X5	T45.7X6

Substance	Poisoning, Accidental (unintentional)	Poisoning, Intentional self-harm	Poisoning, Assault	Poisoning, Undetermined	Adverse effect	Underdosing
Anti-common-cold drug NEC	T48.5X1	T48.5X2	T48.5X3	T48.5X4	T48.5X5	T48.5X6
Anticonvulsant	T42.71	T42.72	T42.73	T42.74	T42.75	T42.76
barbiturate	T42.3X1	T42.3X2	T42.3X3	T42.3X4	T42.3X5	T42.3X6
combination (with barbiturate)	T42.3X1	T42.3X2	T42.3X3	T42.3X4	T42.3X5	T42.3X6
hydantoin	T42.0X1	T42.0X2	T42.0X3	T42.0X4	T42.0X5	T42.0X6
hypnotic NEC	T42.6X1	T42.6X2	T42.6X3	T42.6X4	T42.6X5	T42.6X6
oxazolidinedione	T42.2X1	T42.2X2	T42.2X3	T42.2X4	T42.2X5	T42.2X6
pyrimidinedione	T42.6X1	T42.6X2	T42.6X3	T42.6X4	T42.6X5	T42.6X6
specified NEC	T42.6X1	T42.6X2	T42.6X3	T42.6X4	T42.6X5	T42.6X6
succinimide	T42.2X1	T42.2X2	T42.2X3	T42.2X4	T42.2X5	T42.2X6
Anti-D immunoglobulin (human)	T50.Z11	T50.Z12	T50.Z13	T50.Z14	T50.Z15	T50.Z16
Antidepressant	T43.201	T43.202	T43.203	T43.204	T43.205	T43.206
monoamine oxidase inhibitor	T43.1X1	T43.1X2	T43.1X3	T43.1X4	T43.1X5	T43.1X6
selective serotonin norepinephrine reuptake inhibitor	T43.211	T43.212	T43.213	T43.214	T43.215	T43.216
selective serotonin reuptake inhibitor	T43.221	T43.222	T43.223	T43.224	T43.225	T43.226
specified NEC	T43.291	T43.292	T43.293	T43.294	T43.295	T43.296
tetracyclic	T43.021	T43.022	T43.023	T43.024	T43.025	T43.026
triazolopyridine	T43.211	T43.212	T43.213	T43.214	T43.215	T43.216
tricyclic	T43.011	T43.012	T43.013	T43.014	T43.015	T43.016
Antidiabetic NEC	T38.3X1	T38.3X2	T38.3X3	T38.3X4	T38.3X5	T38.3X6
biguanide	T38.3X1	T38.3X2	T38.3X3	T38.3X4	T38.3X5	T38.3X6
and sulfonyl combined	T38.3X1	T38.3X2	T38.3X3	T38.3X4	T38.3X5	T38.3X6
combined	T38.3X1	T38.3X2	T38.3X3	T38.3X4	T38.3X5	T38.3X6
sulfonylurea	T38.3X1	T38.3X2	T38.3X3	T38.3X4	T38.3X5	T38.3X6
Antidiarrheal drug NEC	T47.6X1	T47.6X2	T47.6X3	T47.6X4	T47.6X5	T47.6X6
absorbent	T47.6X1	T47.6X2	T47.6X3	T47.6X4	T47.6X5	T47.6X6
Antidiphtheria serum	T50.Z11	T50.Z12	T50.Z13	T50.Z14	T50.Z15	T50.Z16
Antidiuretic hormone	T38.891	T38.892	T38.893	T38.894	T38.895	T38.896
Antidote NEC	T50.6X1	T50.6X2	T50.6X3	T50.6X4	T50.6X5	T50.6X6
heavy metal	T45.8X1	T45.8X2	T45.8X3	T45.8X4	T45.8X5	T45.8X6
Antidysrhythmic NEC	T46.2X1	T46.2X2	T46.2X3	T46.2X4	T46.2X5	T46.2X6
Antiemetic drug	T45.0X1	T45.0X2	T45.0X3	T45.0X4	T45.0X5	T45.0X6
Antiepilepsy agent	T42.71	T42.72	T42.73	T42.74	T42.75	T42.76
combination	T42.5X1	T42.5X2	T42.5X3	T42.5X4	T42.5X5	T42.5X6
mixed	T42.5X1	T42.5X2	T42.5X3	T42.5X4	T42.5X5	T42.5X6
specified, NEC	T42.6X1	T42.6X2	T42.6X3	T42.6X4	T42.6X5	T42.6X6
Antiestrogen NEC	T38.6X1	T38.6X2	T38.6X3	T38.6X4	T38.6X5	T38.6X6
Antifertility pill	T38.4X1	T38.4X2	T38.4X3	T38.4X4	T38.4X5	T38.4X6
Antifibrinolytic drug	T45.621	T45.622	T45.623	T45.624	T45.625	T45.626
Antifilarial drug	T37.4X1	T37.4X2	T37.4X3	T37.4X4	T37.4X5	T37.4X6
Antiflatulent	T47.5X1	T47.5X2	T47.5X3	T47.5X4	T47.5X5	T47.5X6
Antifreeze	T65.91	T65.92	T65.93	T65.94	—	—
alcohol	T51.1X1	T51.1X2	T51.1X3	T51.1X4	—	—
ethylene glycol	T51.8X1	T51.8X2	T51.8X3	T51.8X4	—	—
Antifungal						
antibiotic (systemic)	T36.7X1	T36.7X2	T36.7X3	T36.7X4	T36.7X5	T36.7X6
anti-infective NEC	T37.91	T37.92	T37.93	T37.94	T37.95	T37.96
disinfectant, local	T49.0X1	T49.0X2	T49.0X3	T49.0X4	T49.0X5	T49.0X6
nonmedicinal (spray)	T60.3X1	T60.3X2	T60.3X3	T60.3X4	—	—
topical	T49.0X1	T49.0X2	T49.0X3	T49.0X4	T49.0X5	T49.0X6
Anti-gastric-secretion drug NEC	T47.1X1	T47.1X2	T47.1X3	T47.1X4	T47.1X5	T47.1X6
Antigonadotrophin NEC	T38.6X1	T38.6X2	T38.6X3	T38.6X4	T38.6X5	T38.6X6
Antihallucinogen	T43.501	T43.502	T43.503	T43.504	T43.505	T43.506
Antihelmintics	T37.4X1	T37.4X2	T37.4X3	T37.4X4	T37.4X5	T37.4X6
Antihemophilic						
factor	T45.8X1	T45.8X2	T45.8X3	T45.8X4	T45.8X5	T45.8X6
fraction	T45.8X1	T45.8X2	T45.8X3	T45.8X4	T45.8X5	T45.8X6
globulin concentrate	T45.7X1	T45.7X2	T45.7X3	T45.7X4	T45.7X5	T45.7X6
human plasma	T45.8X1	T45.8X2	T45.8X3	T45.8X4	T45.8X5	T45.8X6
plasma, dried	T45.7X1	T45.7X2	T45.7X3	T45.7X4	T45.7X5	T45.7X6
Antihemorrhoidal preparation	T49.2X1	T49.2X2	T49.2X3	T49.2X4	T49.2X5	T49.2X6
Antiheparin drug	T45.7X1	T45.7X2	T45.7X3	T45.7X4	T45.7X5	T45.7X6
Antihistamine	T45.0X1	T45.0X2	T45.0X3	T45.0X4	T45.0X5	T45.0X6
Antihookworm drug	T37.4X1	T37.4X2	T37.4X3	T37.4X4	T37.4X5	T37.4X6
Anti-human lymphocytic globulin	T50.Z11	T50.Z12	T50.Z13	T50.Z14	T50.Z15	T50.Z16
Antihyperlipidemic drug	T46.6X1	T46.6X2	T46.6X3	T46.6X4	T46.6X5	T46.6X6
Antihypertensive drug NEC	T46.5X1	T46.5X2	T46.5X3	T46.5X4	T46.5X5	T46.5X6
Anti-infective NEC	T37.91	T37.92	T37.93	T37.94	T37.95	T37.96
anthelmintic	T37.4X1	T37.4X2	T37.4X3	T37.4X4	T37.4X5	T37.4X6
antibiotics	T36.91	T36.92	T36.93	T36.94	T36.95	T36.96
specified NEC	T36.8X1	T36.8X2	T36.8X3	T36.8X4	T36.8X5	T36.8X6
antimalarial	T37.2X1	T37.2X2	T37.2X3	T37.2X4	T37.2X5	T37.2X6
antimycobacterial NEC	T37.1X1	T37.1X2	T37.1X3	T37.1X4	T37.1X5	T37.1X6
antibiotics	T36.5X1	T36.5X2	T36.5X3	T36.5X4	T36.5X5	T36.5X6
antiprotozoal NEC	T37.3X1	T37.3X2	T37.3X3	T37.3X4	T37.3X5	T37.3X6
blood	T37.2X1	T37.2X2	T37.2X3	T37.2X4	T37.2X5	T37.2X6
antiviral	T37.5X1	T37.5X2	T37.5X3	T37.5X4	T37.5X5	T37.5X6
arsenical	T37.8X1	T37.8X2	T37.8X3	T37.8X4	T37.8X5	T37.8X6
bismuth, local	T49.0X1	T49.0X2	T49.0X3	T49.0X4	T49.0X5	T49.0X6
ENT	T49.6X1	T49.6X2	T49.6X3	T49.6X4	T49.6X5	T49.6X6
eye NEC	T49.5X1	T49.5X2	T49.5X3	T49.5X4	T49.5X5	T49.5X6
heavy metals NEC	T37.8X1	T37.8X2	T37.8X3	T37.8X4	T37.8X5	T37.8X6
local NEC	T49.0X1	T49.0X2	T49.0X3	T49.0X4	T49.0X5	T49.0X6
specified NEC	T49.0X1	T49.0X2	T49.0X3	T49.0X4	T49.0X5	T49.0X6
mixed	T37.91	T37.92	T37.93	T37.94	T37.95	T37.96
ophthalmic preparation	T49.5X1	T49.5X2	T49.5X3	T49.5X4	T49.5X5	T49.5X6
topical NEC	T49.0X1	T49.0X2	T49.0X3	T49.0X4	T49.0X5	T49.0X6
Anti-inflammatory drug NEC	T39.391	T39.392	T39.393	T39.394	T39.395	T39.396
local	T49.0X1	T49.0X2	T49.0X3	T49.0X4	T49.0X5	T49.0X6

Substance	Poisoning, Accidental (unintentional)	Poisoning, Intentional self-harm	Poisoning, Assault	Poisoning, Undetermined	Adverse effect	Underdosing
Anti-inflammatory drug NEC — *Continued*						
nonsteroidal NEC	T39.391	T39.392	T39.393	T39.394	T39.395	T39.396
propionic acid derivative	T39.311	T39.312	T39.313	T39.314	T39.315	T39.316
specified NEC	T39.391	T39.392	T39.393	T39.394	T39.395	T39.396
Antikaluretic	T50.3X1	T50.3X2	T50.3X3	T50.3X4	T50.3X5	T50.3X6
Antiknock (tetraethyl lead)	T56.0X1	T56.0X2	T56.0X3	T56.0X4	—	—
Antilipemic drug NEC	T46.6X1	T46.6X2	T46.6X3	T46.6X4	T46.6X5	T46.6X6
Antimalarial	T37.2X1	T37.2X2	T37.2X3	T37.2X4	T37.2X5	T37.2X6
prophylactic NEC	T37.2X1	T37.2X2	T37.2X3	T37.2X4	T37.2X5	T37.2X6
pyrimidine derivative	T37.2X1	T37.2X2	T37.2X3	T37.2X4	T37.2X5	T37.2X6
Antimetabolite	T45.1X1	T45.1X2	T45.1X3	T45.1X4	T45.1X5	T45.1X6
Antimitotic agent	T45.1X1	T45.1X2	T45.1X3	T45.1X4	T45.1X5	T45.1X6
Antimony (compounds) (vapor)NEC	T56.891	T56.892	T56.893	T56.894	—	—
anti-infectives	T37.8X1	T37.8X2	T37.8X3	T37.8X4	T37.8X5	T37.8X6
dimercaptosuccinate	T37.3X1	T37.3X2	T37.3X3	T37.3X4	T37.3X5	T37.3X6
hydride	T56.891	T56.892	T56.893	T56.894	—	—
pesticide (vapor)	T60.8X1	T60.8X2	T60.8X3	T60.8X4	—	—
potassium (sodium) tartrate	T37.8X1	T37.8X2	T37.8X3	T37.8X4	T37.8X5	T37.8X6
sodium dimercaptosuccinate	T37.3X1	T37.3X2	T37.3X3	T37.3X4	T37.3X5	T37.3X6
tartrated	T37.8X1	T37.8X2	T37.8X3	T37.8X4	T37.8X5	T37.8X6
Antimuscarinic NEC	T44.3X1	T44.3X2	T44.3X3	T44.3X4	T44.3X5	T44.3X6
Antimycobacterial drug NEC	T37.1X1	T37.1X2	T37.1X3	T37.1X4	T37.1X5	T37.1X6
antibiotics	T36.5X1	T36.5X2	T36.5X3	T36.5X4	T36.5X5	T36.5X6
combination	T37.1X1	T37.1X2	T37.1X3	T37.1X4	T37.1X5	T37.1X6
Antinausea drug	T45.0X1	T45.0X2	T45.0X3	T45.0X4	T45.0X5	T45.0X6
Antinematode drug	T37.4X1	T37.4X2	T37.4X3	T37.4X4	T37.4X5	T37.4X6
Antineoplastic NEC	T45.1X1	T45.1X2	T45.1X3	T45.1X4	T45.1X5	T45.1X6
alkaloidal	T45.1X1	T45.1X2	T45.1X3	T45.1X4	T45.1X5	T45.1X6
antibiotics	T45.1X1	T45.1X2	T45.1X3	T45.1X4	T45.1X5	T45.1X6
combination	T45.1X1	T45.1X2	T45.1X3	T45.1X4	T45.1X5	T45.1X6
estrogen	T38.5X1	T38.5X2	T38.5X3	T38.5X4	T38.5X5	T38.5X6
steroid	T38.7X1	T38.7X2	T38.7X3	T38.7X4	T38.7X5	T38.7X6
Antiparasitic drug (systemic)	T37.91	T37.92	T37.93	T37.94	T37.95	T37.96
local	T49.0X1	T49.0X2	T49.0X3	T49.0X4	T49.0X5	T49.0X6
specified NEC	T37.8X1	T37.8X2	T37.8X3	T37.8X4	T37.8X5	T37.8X6
Antiparkinsonism drug NEC	T42.8X1	T42.8X2	T42.8X3	T42.8X4	T42.8X5	T42.8X6
Antiperspirant NEC	T49.2X1	T49.2X2	T49.2X3	T49.2X4	T49.2X5	T49.2X6
Antiphlogistic NEC	T39.4X1	T39.4X2	T39.4X3	T39.4X4	T39.4X5	T39.4X6
Antiplatyhelmintic drug	T37.4X1	T37.4X2	T37.4X3	T37.4X4	T37.4X5	T37.4X6
Antiprotozoal drug NEC	T37.3X1	T37.3X2	T37.3X3	T37.3X4	T37.3X5	T37.3X6
blood	T37.2X1	T37.2X2	T37.2X3	T37.2X4	T37.2X5	T37.2X6
local	T49.0X1	T49.0X2	T49.0X3	T49.0X4	T49.0X5	T49.0X6
Antipruritic drug NEC	T49.1X1	T49.1X2	T49.1X3	T49.1X4	T49.1X5	T49.1X6
Antipsychotic drug	T43.501	T43.502	T43.503	T43.504	T43.505	T43.506
specified NEC	T43.591	T43.592	T43.593	T43.594	T43.595	T43.596

Substance	Poisoning, Accidental (unintentional)	Poisoning, Intentional self-harm	Poisoning, Assault	Poisoning, Undetermined	Adverse effect	Underdosing
Antipyretic	T39.91	T39.92	T39.93	T39.94	T39.95	T39.96
specified NEC	T39.8X1	T39.8X2	T39.8X3	T39.8X4	T39.8X5	T39.8X6
Antipyrine	T39.2X1	T39.2X2	T39.2X3	T39.2X4	T39.2X5	T39.2X6
Antirabies hyperimmune serum	T50.Z11	T50.Z12	T50.Z13	T50.Z14	T50.Z15	T50.Z16
Antirheumatic NEC	T39.4X1	T39.4X2	T39.4X3	T39.4X4	T39.4X5	T39.4X6
Antirigidity drug NEC	T42.8X1	T42.8X2	T42.8X3	T42.8X4	T42.8X5	T42.8X6
Antischistosomal drug	T37.4X1	T37.4X2	T37.4X3	T37.4X4	T37.4X5	T37.4X6
Antiscorpion sera	T50.Z11	T50.Z12	T50.Z13	T50.Z14	T50.Z15	T50.Z16
Antiseborrheics	T49.4X1	T49.4X2	T49.4X3	T49.4X4	T49.4X5	T49.4X6
Antiseptics (external) (medicinal)	T49.0X1	T49.0X2	T49.0X3	T49.0X4	T49.0X5	T49.0X6
Antistine	T45.0X1	T45.0X2	T45.0X3	T45.0X4	T45.0X5	T45.0X6
Antitapeworm drug	T37.4X1	T37.4X2	T37.4X3	T37.4X4	T37.4X5	T37.4X6
Antitetanus immunoglobulin	T50.Z11	T50.Z12	T50.Z13	T50.Z14	T50.Z15	T50.Z16
Antithrombotic	T45.521	T45.522	T45.523	T45.524	T45.525	T45.526
Antithyroid drug NEC	T38.2X1	T38.2X2	T38.2X3	T38.2X4	T38.2X5	T38.2X6
Antitoxin	T50.Z11	T50.Z12	T50.Z13	T50.Z14	T50.Z15	T50.Z16
diphtheria	T50.Z11	T50.Z12	T50.Z13	T50.Z14	T50.Z15	T50.Z16
gas gangrene	T50.Z11	T50.Z12	T50.Z13	T50.Z14	T50.Z15	T50.Z16
tetanus	T50.Z11	T50.Z12	T50.Z13	T50.Z14	T50.Z15	T50.Z16
Antitrichomonal drug	T37.3X1	T37.3X2	T37.3X3	T37.3X4	T37.3X5	T37.3X6
Antituberculars	T37.1X1	T37.1X2	T37.1X3	T37.1X4	T37.1X5	T37.1X6
antibiotics	T36.5X1	T36.5X2	T36.5X3	T36.5X4	T36.5X5	T36.5X6
Antitussive NEC	T48.3X1	T48.3X2	T48.3X3	T48.3X4	T48.3X5	T48.3X6
codeine mixture	T40.2X1	T40.2X2	T40.2X3	T40.2X4	T40.2X5	T40.2X6
opiate	T40.2X1	T40.2X2	T40.2X3	T40.2X4	T40.2X5	T40.2X6
Antivaricose drug	T46.8X1	T46.8X2	T46.8X3	T46.8X4	T46.8X5	T46.8X6
Antivenin, antivenom (sera)	T50.Z11	T50.Z12	T50.Z13	T50.Z14	T50.Z15	T50.Z16
crotaline	T50.Z11	T50.Z12	T50.Z13	T50.Z14	T50.Z15	T50.Z16
spider bite	T50.Z11	T50.Z12	T50.Z13	T50.Z14	T50.Z15	T50.Z16
Antivertigo drug	T45.0X1	T45.0X2	T45.0X3	T45.0X4	T45.0X5	T45.0X6
Antiviral drug NEC	T37.5X1	T37.5X2	T37.5X3	T37.5X4	T37.5X5	T37.5X6
eye	T49.5X1	T49.5X2	T49.5X3	T49.5X4	T49.5X5	T49.5X6
Antiwhipworm drug	T37.4X1	T37.4X2	T37.4X3	T37.4X4	T37.4X5	T37.4X6
Antrol—see also by specific chemical substance	T60.91	T60.92	T60.93	T60.94	—	—
fungicide	T60.91	T60.92	T60.93	T60.94	—	—
ANTU (alpha naphthylthiourea)	T60.4X1	T60.4X2	T60.4X3	T60.4X4	—	—
Apalcillin	T36.0X1	T36.0X2	T36.0X3	T36.0X4	T36.0X5	T36.0X6
APC	T48.5X1	T48.5X2	T48.5X3	T48.5X4	T48.5X5	T48.5X6
Aplonidine	T44.4X1	T44.4X2	T44.4X3	T44.4X4	T44.4X5	T44.4X6
Apomorphine	T47.7X1	T47.7X2	T47.7X3	T47.7X4	T47.7X5	T47.7X6
Appetite depressants, central	T50.5X1	T50.5X2	T50.5X3	T50.5X4	T50.5X5	T50.5X6
Apraclonidine (hydrochloride)	T44.4X1	T44.4X2	T44.4X3	T44.4X4	T44.4X5	T44.4X6
Apresoline	T46.5X1	T46.5X2	T46.5X3	T46.5X4	T46.5X5	T46.5X6
Aprindine	T46.2X1	T46.2X2	T46.2X3	T46.2X4	T46.2X5	T46.2X6
Aprobarbital	T42.3X1	T42.3X2	T42.3X3	T42.3X4	T42.3X5	T42.3X6
Apronalide	T42.6X1	T42.6X2	T42.6X3	T42.6X4	T42.6X5	T42.6X6

Substance	Poisoning, Accidental (unintentional)	Poisoning, Intentional self-harm	Poisoning, Assault	Poisoning, Undetermined	Adverse effect	Underdosing
Aprotinin	T45.621	T45.622	T45.623	T45.624	T45.625	T45.626
Aptocaine	T41.3X1	T41.3X2	T41.3X3	T41.3X4	T41.3X5	T41.3X6
Aqua fortis	T54.2X1	T54.2X2	T54.2X3	T54.2X4	—	—
Ara-A	T37.5X1	T37.5X2	T37.5X3	T37.5X4	T37.5X5	T37.5X6
Ara-C	T45.1X1	T45.1X2	T45.1X3	T45.1X4	T45.1X5	T45.1X6
Arachis oil	T49.3X1	T49.3X2	T49.3X3	T49.3X4	T49.3X5	T49.3X6
cathartic	T47.4X1	T47.4X2	T47.4X3	T47.4X4	T47.4X5	T47.4X6
Aralen	T37.2X1	T37.2X2	T37.2X3	T37.2X4	T37.2X5	T37.2X6
Arecoline	T44.1X1	T44.1X2	T44.1X3	T44.1X4	T44.1X5	T44.1X6
Arginine	T50.991	T50.992	T50.993	T50.994	T50.995	T50.996
glutamate	T50.991	T50.992	T50.993	T50.994	T50.995	T50.996
Argyrol	T49.0X1	T49.0X2	T49.0X3	T49.0X4	T49.0X5	T49.0X6
ENT agent	T49.6X1	T49.6X2	T49.6X3	T49.6X4	T49.6X5	T49.6X6
ophthalmic preparation	T49.5X1	T49.5X2	T49.5X3	T49.5X4	T49.5X5	T49.5X6
Aristocort	T38.0X1	T38.0X2	T38.0X3	T38.0X4	T38.0X5	T38.0X6
ENT agent	T49.6X1	T49.6X2	T49.6X3	T49.6X4	T49.6X5	T49.6X6
ophthalmic preparation	T49.5X1	T49.5X2	T49.5X3	T49.5X4	T49.5X5	T49.5X6
topical NEC	T49.0X1	T49.0X2	T49.0X3	T49.0X4	T49.0X5	T49.0X6
Aromatics, corrosive	T54.1X1	T54.1X2	T54.1X3	T54.1X4	—	—
disinfectants	T54.1X1	T54.1X2	T54.1X3	T54.1X4	—	—
Arsenate of lead	T57.0X1	T57.0X2	T57.0X3	T57.0X4	—	—
herbicide	T57.0X1	T57.0X2	T57.0X3	T57.0X4	—	—
Arsenic, arsenicals (compounds) (dust) (vapor) NEC	T57.0X1	T57.0X2	T57.0X3	T57.0X4	—	—
anti-infectives	T37.8X1	T37.8X2	T37.8X3	T37.8X4	T37.8X5	T37.8X6
pesticide (dust) (fumes)	T57.0X1	T57.0X2	T57.0X3	T57.0X4	—	—
Arsine (gas)	T57.0X1	T57.0X2	T57.0X3	T57.0X4	—	—
Arsphenamine (silver)	T37.8X1	T37.8X2	T37.8X3	T37.8X4	T37.8X5	T37.8X6
Arsthinol	T37.3X1	T37.3X2	T37.3X3	T37.3X4	T37.3X5	T37.3X6
Artane	T44.3X1	T44.3X2	T44.3X3	T44.3X4	T44.3X5	T44.3X6
Arthropod (venomous) NEC	T63.481	T63.482	T63.483	T63.484	—	—
Articaine	T41.3X1	T41.3X2	T41.3X3	T41.3X4	T41.3X5	T41.3X6
Asbestos	T57.8X1	T57.8X2	T57.8X3	T57.8X4	—	—
Ascaridole	T37.4X1	T37.4X2	T37.4X3	T37.4X4	T37.4X5	T37.4X6
Ascorbic acid	T45.2X1	T45.2X2	T45.2X3	T45.2X4	T45.2X5	T45.2X6
Asiaticoside	T49.0X1	T49.0X2	T49.0X3	T49.0X4	T49.0X5	T49.0X6
Asparaginase	T45.1X1	T45.1X2	T45.1X3	T45.1X4	T45.1X5	T45.1X6
Aspidium (oleoresin)	T37.4X1	T37.4X2	T37.4X3	T37.4X4	T37.4X5	T37.4X6
Aspirin (aluminum) (soluble)	T39.011	T39.012	T39.013	T39.014	T39.015	T39.016
Aspoxicillin	T36.0X1	T36.0X2	T36.0X3	T36.0X4	T36.0X5	T36.0X6
Astemizole	T45.0X1	T45.0X2	T45.0X3	T45.0X4	T45.0X5	T45.0X6
Astringent (local)	T49.2X1	T49.2X2	T49.2X3	T49.2X4	T49.2X5	T49.2X6
specified NEC	T49.2X1	T49.2X2	T49.2X3	T49.2X4	T49.2X5	T49.2X6
Astromicin	T36.5X1	T36.5X2	T36.5X3	T36.5X4	T36.5X5	T36.5X6
Ataractic drug NEC	T43.501	T43.502	T43.503	T43.504	T43.505	T43.506
Atenolol	T44.7X1	T44.7X2	T44.7X3	T44.7X4	T44.7X5	T44.7X6
Atonia drug, intestinal	T47.4X1	T47.4X2	T47.4X3	T47.4X4	T47.4X5	T47.4X6
Atophan	T50.4X1	T50.4X2	T50.4X3	T50.4X4	T50.4X5	T50.4X6

Substance	Poisoning, Accidental (unintentional)	Poisoning, Intentional self-harm	Poisoning, Assault	Poisoning, Undetermined	Adverse effect	Underdosing
Atracurium besilate	T48.1X1	T48.1X2	T48.1X3	T48.1X4	T48.1X5	T48.1X6
Atropine	T44.3X1	T44.3X2	T44.3X3	T44.3X4	T44.3X5	T44.3X6
derivative	T44.3X1	T44.3X2	T44.3X3	T44.3X4	T44.3X5	T44.3X6
methonitrate	T44.3X1	T44.3X2	T44.3X3	T44.3X4	T44.3X5	T44.3X6
Attapulgite	T47.6X1	T47.6X2	T47.6X3	T47.6X4	T47.6X5	T47.6X6
Auramine	T65.891	T65.892	T65.893	T65.894	—	—
dye	T65.6X1	T65.6X2	T65.6X3	T65.6X4	—	—
fungicide	T60.3X1	T60.3X2	T60.3X3	T60.3X4	—	—
Auranofin	T39.4X1	T39.4X2	T39.4X3	T39.4X4	T39.4X5	T39.4X6
Aurantiin	T46.991	T46.992	T46.993	T46.994	T46.995	T46.996
Aureomycin	T36.4X1	T36.4X2	T36.4X3	T36.4X4	T36.4X5	T36.4X6
ophthalmic preparation	T49.5X1	T49.5X2	T49.5X3	T49.5X4	T49.5X5	T49.5X6
topical NEC	T49.0X1	T49.0X2	T49.0X3	T49.0X4	T49.0X5	T49.0X6
Aurothioglucose	T39.4X1	T39.4X2	T39.4X3	T39.4X4	T39.4X5	T39.4X6
Aurothioglycanide	T39.4X1	T39.4X2	T39.4X3	T39.4X4	T39.4X5	T39.4X6
Aurothiomalate sodium	T39.4X1	T39.4X2	T39.4X3	T39.4X4	T39.4X5	T39.4X6
Aurotioprol	T39.4X1	T39.4X2	T39.4X3	T39.4X4	T39.4X5	T39.4X6
Automobile fuel	T52.0X1	T52.0X2	T52.0X3	T52.0X4	—	—
Autonomic nervous system agent NEC	T44.901	T44.902	T44.903	T44.904	T44.905	T44.906
Avlosulfon	T37.1X1	T37.1X2	T37.1X3	T37.1X4	T37.1X5	T37.1X6
Avomine	T42.6X1	T42.6X2	T42.6X3	T42.6X4	T42.6X5	T42.6X6
Axerophthol	T45.2X1	T45.2X2	T45.2X3	T45.2X4	T45.2X5	T45.2X6
Azacitidine	T45.1X1	T45.1X2	T45.1X3	T45.1X4	T45.1X5	T45.1X6
Azacyclonol	T43.591	T43.592	T43.593	T43.594	T43.595	T43.596
Azadirachta	T60.2X1	T60.2X2	T60.2X3	T60.2X4	—	—
Azanidazole	T37.3X1	T37.3X2	T37.3X3	T37.3X4	T37.3X5	T37.3X6
Azapetine	T46.7X1	T46.7X2	T46.7X3	T46.7X4	T46.7X5	T46.7X6
Azapropazone	T39.2X1	T39.2X2	T39.2X3	T39.2X4	T39.2X5	T39.2X6
Azaribine	T45.1X1	T45.1X2	T45.1X3	T45.1X4	T45.1X5	T45.1X6
Azaserine	T45.1X1	T45.1X2	T45.1X3	T45.1X4	T45.1X5	T45.1X6
Azatadine	T45.0X1	T45.0X2	T45.0X3	T45.0X4	T45.0X5	T45.0X6
Azatepa	T45.1X1	T45.1X2	T45.1X3	T45.1X4	T45.1X5	T45.1X6
Azathioprine	T45.1X1	T45.1X2	T45.1X3	T45.1X4	T45.1X5	T45.1X6
Azelaic acid	T49.0X1	T49.0X2	T49.0X3	T49.0X4	T49.0X5	T49.0X6
Azelastine	T45.0X1	T45.0X2	T45.0X3	T45.0X4	T45.0X5	T45.0X6
Azidocillin	T36.0X1	T36.0X2	T36.0X3	T36.0X4	T36.0X5	T36.0X6
Azidothymidine	T37.5X1	T37.5X2	T37.5X3	T37.5X4	T37.5X5	T37.5X6
Azinphos (ethyl) (methyl)	T60.0X1	T60.0X2	T60.0X3	T60.0X4	—	—
Aziridine (chelating)	T54.1X1	T54.1X2	T54.1X3	T54.1X4	—	—
Azithromycin	T36.3X1	T36.3X2	T36.3X3	T36.3X4	T36.3X5	T36.3X6
Azlocillin	T36.0X1	T36.0X2	T36.0X3	T36.0X4	T36.0X5	T36.0X6
Azobenzene smoke	T65.3X1	T65.3X2	T65.3X3	T65.3X4	—	—
acaricide	T60.8X1	T60.8X2	T60.8X3	T60.8X4	—	—
Azosulfamide	T37.0X1	T37.0X2	T37.0X3	T37.0X4	T37.0X5	T37.0X6
AZT	T37.5X1	T37.5X2	T37.5X3	T37.5X4	T37.5X5	T37.5X6
Aztreonam	T36.1X1	T36.1X2	T36.1X3	T36.1X4	T36.1X5	T36.1X6
Azulfidine	T37.0X1	T37.0X2	T37.0X3	T37.0X4	T37.0X5	T37.0X6
Azuresin	T50.8X1	T50.8X2	T50.8X3	T50.8X4	T50.8X5	T50.8X6

Substance	Poisoning, Accidental (unintentional)	Poisoning, Intentional self-harm	Poisoning, Assault	Poisoning, Undetermined	Adverse effect	Underdosing
B						
Bacampicillin	T36.0X1	T36.0X2	T36.0X3	T36.0X4	T36.0X5	T36.0X6
Bacillus						
lactobacillus	T47.8X1	T47.8X2	T47.8X3	T47.8X4	T47.8X5	T47.8X6
subtilis	T47.6X1	T47.6X2	T47.6X3	T47.6X4	T47.6X5	T47.6X6
Bacimycin	T49.0X1	T49.0X2	T49.0X3	T49.0X4	T49.0X5	T49.0X6
ophthalmic preparation	T49.5X1	T49.5X2	T49.5X3	T49.5X4	T49.5X5	T49.5X6
Bacitracin zinc	T49.0X1	T49.0X2	T49.0X3	T49.0X4	T49.0X5	T49.0X6
with neomycin	T49.0X1	T49.0X2	T49.0X3	T49.0X4	T49.0X5	T49.0X6
ENT agent	T49.6X1	T49.6X2	T49.6X3	T49.6X4	T49.6X5	T49.6X6
ophthalmic preparation	T49.5X1	T49.5X2	T49.5X3	T49.5X4	T49.5X5	T49.5X6
topical NEC	T49.0X1	T49.0X2	T49.0X3	T49.0X4	T49.0X5	T49.0X6
Baclofen	T42.8X1	T42.8X2	T42.8X3	T42.8X4	T42.8X5	T42.8X6
Baking soda	T50.991	T50.992	T50.993	T50.994	T50.995	T50.996
BAL	T45.8X1	T45.8X2	T45.8X3	T45.8X4	T45.8X5	T45.8X6
Bambuterol	T48.6X1	T48.6X2	T48.6X3	T48.6X4	T48.6X5	T48.6X6
Bamethan (sulfate)	T46.7X1	T46.7X2	T46.7X3	T46.7X4	T46.7X5	T46.7X6
Bamifylline	T48.6X1	T48.6X2	T48.6X3	T48.6X4	T48.6X5	T48.6X6
Bamipine	T45.0X1	T45.0X2	T45.0X3	T45.0X4	T45.0X5	T45.0X6
Baneberry—see Actauseea spicata						
Banewort—see Belladonna						
Barbenyl	T42.3X1	T42.3X2	T42.3X3	T42.3X4	T42.3X5	T42.3X6
Barbexaclone	T42.6X1	T42.6X2	T42.6X3	T42.6X4	T42.6X5	T42.6X6
Barbital	T42.3X1	T42.3X2	T42.3X3	T42.3X4	T42.3X5	T42.3X6
sodium	T42.3X1	T42.3X2	T42.3X3	T42.3X4	T42.3X5	T42.3X6
Barbitone	T42.3X1	T42.3X2	T42.3X3	T42.3X4	T42.3X5	T42.3X6
Barbiturate NEC	T42.3X1	T42.3X2	T42.3X3	T42.3X4	T42.3X5	T42.3X6
with tranquilizer	T42.3X1	T42.3X2	T42.3X3	T42.3X4	T42.3X5	T42.3X6
anesthetic (intravenous)	T41.1X1	T41.1X2	T41.1X3	T41.1X4	T41.1X5	T41.1X6
Barium (carbonate) (chloride) (sulfite)	T57.8X1	T57.8X2	T57.8X3	T57.8X4	—	—
diagnostic agent	T50.8X1	T50.8X2	T50.8X3	T50.8X4	T50.8X5	T50.8X6
pesticide	T60.4X1	T60.4X2	T60.4X3	T60.4X4	—	—
rodenticide	T60.4X1	T60.4X2	T60.4X3	T60.4X4	—	—
sulfate (medicinal)	T50.8X1	T50.8X2	T50.8X3	T50.8X4	T50.8X5	T50.8X6
Barrier cream	T49.3X1	T49.3X2	T49.3X3	T49.3X4	T49.3X5	T49.3X6
Basic fuchsin	T49.0X1	T49.0X2	T49.0X3	T49.0X4	T49.0X5	T49.0X6
Battery acid or fluid	T54.2X1	T54.2X2	T54.2X3	T54.2X4	—	—
Bay rum	T51.8X1	T51.8X2	T51.8X3	T51.8X4	—	—
BCG (vaccine)	T50.A91	T50.A92	T50.A93	T50.A94	T50.A95	T50.A96
BCNU	T45.1X1	T45.1X2	T45.1X3	T45.1X4	T45.1X5	T45.1X6
Bearsfoot	T62.2X1	T62.2X2	T62.2X3	T62.2X4	—	—
Beclamide	T42.6X1	T42.6X2	T42.6X3	T42.6X4	T42.6X5	T42.6X6
Beclomethasone	T44.5X1	T44.5X2	T44.5X3	T44.5X4	T44.5X5	T44.5X6
Bee (sting) (venom)	T63.441	T63.442	T63.443	T63.444	—	—
Befunolol	T49.5X1	T49.5X2	T49.5X3	T49.5X4	T49.5X5	T49.5X6
Bekanamycin	T36.5X1	T36.5X2	T36.5X3	T36.5X4	T36.5X5	T36.5X6
Belladonna—see also Nightshade						
alkaloids	T44.3X1	T44.3X2	T44.3X3	T44.3X4	T44.3X5	T44.3X6
extract	T44.3X1	T44.3X2	T44.3X3	T44.3X4	T44.3X5	T44.3X6
herb	T44.3X1	T44.3X2	T44.3X3	T44.3X4	T44.3X5	T44.3X6
Bemegride	T50.7X1	T50.7X2	T50.7X3	T50.7X4	T50.7X5	T50.7X6
Benactyzine	T44.3X1	T44.3X2	T44.3X3	T44.3X4	T44.3X5	T44.3X6
Benadryl	T45.0X1	T45.0X2	T45.0X3	T45.0X4	T45.0X5	T45.0X6
Benaprizine	T44.3X1	T44.3X2	T44.3X3	T44.3X4	T44.3X5	T44.3X6
Benazepril	T46.4X1	T46.4X2	T46.4X3	T46.4X4	T46.4X5	T46.4X6
Bencyclane	T46.7X1	T46.7X2	T46.7X3	T46.7X4	T46.7X5	T46.7X6
Bendazol	T46.3X1	T46.3X2	T46.3X3	T46.3X4	T46.3X5	T46.3X6
Bendrofluazide	T50.2X1	T50.2X2	T50.2X3	T50.2X4	T50.2X5	T50.2X6
Bendroflumethiazide	T50.2X1	T50.2X2	T50.2X3	T50.2X4	T50.2X5	T50.2X6
Benemid	T50.4X1	T50.4X2	T50.4X3	T50.4X4	T50.4X5	T50.4X6
Benethamine penicillin	T36.0X1	T36.0X2	T36.0X3	T36.0X4	T36.0X5	T36.0X6
Benexate	T47.1X1	T47.1X2	T47.1X3	T47.1X4	T47.1X5	T47.1X6
Benfluorex	T46.6X1	T46.6X2	T46.6X3	T46.6X4	T46.6X5	T46.6X6
Benfotiamine	T45.2X1	T45.2X2	T45.2X3	T45.2X4	T45.2X5	T45.2X6
Benisone	T49.0X1	T49.0X2	T49.0X3	T49.0X4	T49.0X5	T49.0X6
Benomyl	T60.0X1	T60.0X2	T60.0X3	T60.0X4	—	—
Benoquin	T49.8X1	T49.8X2	T49.8X3	T49.8X4	T49.8X5	T49.8X6
Benoxinate	T41.3X1	T41.3X2	T41.3X3	T41.3X4	T41.3X5	T41.3X6
Benperidol	T43.4X1	T43.4X2	T43.4X3	T43.4X4	T43.4X5	T43.4X6
Benproperine	T48.3X1	T48.3X2	T48.3X3	T48.3X4	T48.3X5	T48.3X6
Benserazide	T42.8X1	T42.8X2	T42.8X3	T42.8X4	T42.8X5	T42.8X6
Bentazepam	T42.4X1	T42.4X2	T42.4X3	T42.4X4	T42.4X5	T42.4X6
Bentiromide	T50.8X1	T50.8X2	T50.8X3	T50.8X4	T50.8X5	T50.8X6
Bentonite	T49.3X1	T49.3X2	T49.3X3	T49.3X4	T49.3X5	T49.3X6
Benzalbutyramide	T46.6X1	T46.6X2	T46.6X3	T46.6X4	T46.6X5	T46.6X6
Benzalkonium (chloride)	T49.0X1	T49.0X2	T49.0X3	T49.0X4	T49.0X5	T49.0X6
ophthalmic preparation	T49.5X1	T49.5X2	T49.5X3	T49.5X4	T49.5X5	T49.5X6
Benzamidosali cylate (calcium)	T37.1X1	T37.1X2	T37.1X3	T37.1X4	T37.1X5	T37.1X6
Benzamine	T41.3X1	T41.3X2	T41.3X3	T41.3X4	T41.3X5	T41.3X6
lactate	T49.1X1	T49.1X2	T49.1X3	T49.1X4	T49.1X5	T49.1X6
Benzamphetamine	T50.5X1	T50.5X2	T50.5X3	T50.5X4	T50.5X5	T50.5X6
Benzapril hydrochloride	T46.5X1	T46.5X2	T46.5X3	T46.5X4	T46.5X5	T46.5X6
Benzathine benzylpenicillin	T36.0X1	T36.0X2	T36.0X3	T36.0X4	T36.0X5	T36.0X6
Benzathine penicillin	T36.0X1	T36.0X2	T36.0X3	T36.0X4	T36.0X5	T36.0X6
Benzatropine	T42.8X1	T42.8X2	T42.8X3	T42.8X4	T42.8X5	T42.8X6
Benzbromarone	T50.4X1	T50.4X2	T50.4X3	T50.4X4	T50.4X5	T50.4X6
Benzcarbimine	T45.1X1	T45.1X2	T45.1X3	T45.1X4	T45.1X5	T45.1X6
Benzedrex	T44.991	T44.992	T44.993	T44.994	T44.995	T44.996
Benzedrine (amphetamine)	T43.621	T43.622	T43.623	T43.624	T43.625	T43.626
Benzenamine	T65.3X1	T65.3X2	T65.3X3	T65.3X4	—	—
Benzene	T52.1X1	T52.1X2	T52.1X3	T52.1X4	—	—
homologues (acetyl) (dimethyl) (methyl) (solvent)	T52.2X1	T52.2X2	T52.2X3	T52.2X4	—	—

Substance	Poisoning, Accidental (unintentional)	Poisoning, Intentional self-harm	Poisoning, Assault	Poisoning, Undetermined	Adverse effect	Underdosing
Benzethonium (chloride)	T49.0X1	T49.0X2	T49.0X3	T49.0X4	T49.0X5	T49.0X6
Benzfetamine	T50.5X1	T50.5X2	T50.5X3	T50.5X4	T50.5X5	T50.5X6
Benzhexol	T44.3X1	T44.3X2	T44.3X3	T44.3X4	T44.3X5	T44.3X6
Benzhydramine (chloride)	T45.0X1	T45.0X2	T45.0X3	T45.0X4	T45.0X5	T45.0X6
Benzidine	T65.891	T65.892	T65.893	T65.894	—	—
Benzilonium bromide	T44.3X1	T44.3X2	T44.3X3	T44.3X4	T44.3X5	T44.3X6
Benzimidazole	T60.3X1	T60.3X2	T60.3X3	T60.3X4	—	—
Benzin(e)—see Ligroin						
Benziodarone	T46.3X1	T46.3X2	T46.3X3	T46.3X4	T46.3X5	T46.3X6
Benznidazole	T37.3X1	T37.3X2	T37.3X3	T37.3X4	T37.3X5	T37.3X6
Benzocaine	T41.3X1	T41.3X2	T41.3X3	T41.3X4	T41.3X5	T41.3X6
Benzodiapin	T42.4X1	T42.4X2	T42.4X3	T42.4X4	T42.4X5	T42.4X6
Benzodiazepine NEC	T42.4X1	T42.4X2	T42.4X3	T42.4X4	T42.4X5	T42.4X6
Benzoic acid	T49.0X1	T49.0X2	T49.0X3	T49.0X4	T49.0X5	T49.0X6
with salicylic acid	T49.0X1	T49.0X2	T49.0X3	T49.0X4	T49.0X5	T49.0X6
Benzoin (tincture)	T48.5X1	T48.5X2	T48.5X3	T48.5X4	T48.5X5	T48.5X6
Benzol (benzene)	T52.1X1	T52.1X2	T52.1X3	T52.1X4	—	—
vapor	T52.0X1	T52.0X2	T52.0X3	T52.0X4	—	—
Benzomorphan	T40.2X1	T40.2X2	T40.2X3	T40.2X4	T40.2X5	T40.2X6
Benzonatate	T48.3X1	T48.3X2	T48.3X3	T48.3X4	T48.3X5	T48.3X6
Benzophenones	T49.3X1	T49.3X2	T49.3X3	T49.3X4	T49.3X5	T49.3X6
Benzopyrone	T46.991	T46.992	T46.993	T46.994	T46.995	T46.996
Benzothiadiazides	T50.2X1	T50.2X2	T50.2X3	T50.2X4	T50.2X5	T50.2X6
Benzoxonium chloride	T49.0X1	T49.0X2	T49.0X3	T49.0X4	T49.0X5	T49.0X6
Benzoyl peroxide	T49.0X1	T49.0X2	T49.0X3	T49.0X4	T49.0X5	T49.0X6
Benzoylpas calcium	T37.1X1	T37.1X2	T37.1X3	T37.1X4	T37.1X5	T37.1X6
Benzperidin	T43.591	T43.592	T43.593	T43.594	T43.595	T43.596
Benzperidol	T43.591	T43.592	T43.593	T43.594	T43.595	T43.596
Benzphetamine	T50.5X1	T50.5X2	T50.5X3	T50.5X4	T50.5X5	T50.5X6
Benzpyrinium bromide	T44.1X1	T44.1X2	T44.1X3	T44.1X4	T44.1X5	T44.1X6
Benzquinamide	T45.0X1	T45.0X2	T45.0X3	T45.0X4	T45.0X5	T45.0X6
Benzthiazide	T50.2X1	T50.2X2	T50.2X3	T50.2X4	T50.2X5	T50.2X6
Benztropine						
anticholinergic	T44.3X1	T44.3X2	T44.3X3	T44.3X4	T44.3X5	T44.3X6
antiparkinson	T42.8X1	T42.8X2	T42.8X3	T42.8X4	T42.8X5	T42.8X6
Benzydamine	T49.0X1	T49.0X2	T49.0X3	T49.0X4	T49.0X5	T49.0X6
Benzyl						
acetate	T52.8X1	T52.8X2	T52.8X3	T52.8X4	—	—
alcohol	T49.0X1	T49.0X2	T49.0X3	T49.0X4	T49.0X5	T49.0X6
benzoate	T49.0X1	T49.0X2	T49.0X3	T49.0X4	T49.0X5	T49.0X6
Benzoic acid	T49.0X1	T49.0X2	T49.0X3	T49.0X4	T49.0X5	T49.0X6
morphine	T40.2X1	T40.2X2	T40.2X3	T40.2X4	—	—
nicotinate	T46.6X1	T46.6X2	T46.6X3	T46.6X4	T46.6X5	T46.6X6
penicillin	T36.0X1	T36.0X2	T36.0X3	T36.0X4	T36.0X5	T36.0X6
Benzylhydrochl-orthia-zide	T50.2X1	T50.2X2	T50.2X3	T50.2X4	T50.2X5	T50.2X6
Benzylpenicillin	T36.0X1	T36.0X2	T36.0X3	T36.0X4	T36.0X5	T36.0X6
Benzylthiouracil	T38.2X1	T38.2X2	T38.2X3	T38.2X4	T38.2X5	T38.2X6
Bephenium hydroxy-naphthoate	T37.4X1	T37.4X2	T37.4X3	T37.4X4	T37.4X5	T37.4X6

Substance	Poisoning, Accidental (unintentional)	Poisoning, Intentional self-harm	Poisoning, Assault	Poisoning, Undetermined	Adverse effect	Underdosing
Bepridil	T46.1X1	T46.1X2	T46.1X3	T46.1X4	T46.1X5	T46.1X6
Bergamot oil	T65.891	T65.892	T65.893	T65.894	—	—
Bergapten	T50.991	T50.992	T50.993	T50.994	T50.995	T50.996
Berries, poisonous	T62.1X1	T62.1X2	T62.1X3	T62.1X4	—	—
Beryllium (compounds)	T56.7X1	T56.7X2	T56.7X3	T56.7X4	—	—
b-acetyldigoxin	T46.0X1	T46.0X2	T46.0X3	T46.0X4	T46.0X5	T46.0X6
beta adrenergic blocking agent, heart	T44.7X1	T44.7X2	T44.7X3	T44.7X4	T44.7X5	T44.7X6
b-benzalbutyramide	T46.6X1	T46.6X2	T46.6X3	T46.6X4	T46.6X5	T46.6X6
Betacarotene	T45.2X1	T45.2X2	T45.2X3	T45.2X4	T45.2X5	T45.2X6
b-eucaine	T49.1X1	T49.1X2	T49.1X3	T49.1X4	T49.1X5	T49.1X6
Beta-Chlor	T42.6X1	T42.6X2	T42.6X3	T42.6X4	T42.6X5	T42.6X6
b-galactosidase	T47.5X1	T47.5X2	T47.5X3	T47.5X4	T47.5X5	T47.5X6
Betahistine	T46.7X1	T46.7X2	T46.7X3	T46.7X4	T46.7X5	T46.7X6
Betaine	T47.5X1	T47.5X2	T47.5X3	T47.5X4	T47.5X5	T47.5X6
Betamethasone	T49.0X1	T49.0X2	T49.0X3	T49.0X4	T49.0X5	T49.0X6
topical	T49.0X1	T49.0X2	T49.0X3	T49.0X4	T49.0X5	T49.0X6
Betamicin	T36.8X1	T36.8X2	T36.8X3	T36.8X4	T36.8X5	T36.8X6
Betanidine	T46.5X1	T46.5X2	T46.5X3	T46.5X4	T46.5X5	T46.5X6
b-sitosterol(s)	T46.6X1	T46.6X2	T46.6X3	T46.6X4	T46.6X5	T46.6X6
Betaxolol	T44.7X1	T44.7X2	T44.7X3	T44.7X4	T44.7X5	T44.7X6
Betazole	T50.8X1	T50.8X2	T50.8X3	T50.8X4	T50.8X5	T50.8X6
Bethanechol	T44.1X1	T44.1X2	T44.1X3	T44.1X4	T44.1X5	T44.1X6
chloride	T44.1X1	T44.1X2	T44.1X3	T44.1X4	T44.1X5	T44.1X6
Bethanidine	T46.5X1	T46.5X2	T46.5X3	T46.5X4	T46.5X5	T46.5X6
Betoxycaine	T41.3X1	T41.3X2	T41.3X3	T41.3X4	T41.3X5	T41.3X6
Betula oil	T49.3X1	T49.3X2	T49.3X3	T49.3X4	T49.3X5	T49.3X6
Bevantolol	T44.7X1	T44.7X2	T44.7X3	T44.7X4	T44.7X5	T44.7X6
Bevonium metilsulfate	T44.3X1	T44.3X2	T44.3X3	T44.3X4	T44.3X5	T44.3X6
Bezafibrate	T46.6X1	T46.6X2	T46.6X3	T46.6X4	T46.6X5	T46.6X6
Bezitramide	T40.4X1	T40.4X2	T40.4X3	T40.4X4	T40.4X5	T40.4X6
BHA	T50.991	T50.992	T50.993	T50.994	T50.995	T50.996
Bhang	T40.7X1	T40.7X2	T40.7X3	T40.7X4	T40.7X5	T40.7X6
BHC (medicinal)	T49.0X1	T49.0X2	T49.0X3	T49.0X4	T49.0X5	T49.0X6
nonmedicinal (vapor)	T53.6X1	T53.6X2	T53.6X3	T53.6X4	—	—
Bialamicol	T37.3X1	T37.3X2	T37.3X3	T37.3X4	T37.3X5	T37.3X6
Bibenzonium bromide	T48.3X1	T48.3X2	T48.3X3	T48.3X4	T48.3X5	T48.3X6
Bibrocathol	T49.5X1	T49.5X2	T49.5X3	T49.5X4	T49.5X5	T49.5X6
Bichloride of mercury—see Mercury, chloride						
Bichromates (calcium) (potassium) (sodium) (crystals)	T57.8X1	T57.8X2	T57.8X3	T57.8X4	—	—
fumes	T56.2X1	T56.2X2	T56.2X3	T56.2X4	—	—
Biclotymol	T49.6X1	T49.6X2	T49.6X3	T49.6X4	T49.6X5	T49.6X6
Bicucculine	T50.7X1	T50.7X2	T50.7X3	T50.7X4	T50.7X5	T50.7X6
Bifemelane	T43.291	T43.292	T43.293	T43.294	T43.295	T43.296
Biguanide derivatives, oral	T38.3X1	T38.3X2	T38.3X3	T38.3X4	T38.3X5	T38.3X6
Bile salts	T47.5X1	T47.5X2	T47.5X3	T47.5X4	T47.5X5	T47.5X6
Biligrafin	T50.8X1	T50.8X2	T50.8X3	T50.8X4	T50.8X5	T50.8X6
Bilopaque	T50.8X1	T50.8X2	T50.8X3	T50.8X4	T50.8X5	T50.8X6

Substance	Poisoning, Accidental (unintentional)	Poisoning, Intentional self-harm	Poisoning, Assault	Poisoning, Undetermined	Adverse effect	Underdosing
Binifibrate	T46.6X1	T46.6X2	T46.6X3	T46.6X4	T46.6X5	T46.6X6
Binitrobenzol	T65.3X1	T65.3X2	T65.3X3	T65.3X4	—	—
Bioflavonoid(s)	T46.991	T46.992	T46.993	T46.994	T46.995	T46.996
Biological substance NEC	T50.901	T50.902	T50.903	T50.904	T50.905	T50.906
Biotin	T45.2X1	T45.2X2	T45.2X3	T45.2X4	T45.2X5	T45.2X6
Biperiden	T44.3X1	T44.3X2	T44.3X3	T44.3X4	T44.3X5	T44.3X6
Bisacodyl	T47.2X1	T47.2X2	T47.2X3	T47.2X4	T47.2X5	T47.2X6
Bisbentiamine	T45.2X1	T45.2X2	T45.2X3	T45.2X4	T45.2X5	T45.2X6
Bisbutiamine	T45.2X1	T45.2X2	T45.2X3	T45.2X4	T45.2X5	T45.2X6
Bisdequalinium (salts) (diacetate)	T49.6X1	T49.6X2	T49.6X3	T49.6X4	T49.6X5	T49.6X6
Bishydroxycoumarin	T45.511	T45.512	T45.513	T45.514	T45.515	T45.516
Bismarsen	T37.8X1	T37.8X2	T37.8X3	T37.8X4	T37.8X5	T37.8X6
Bismuth salts	T47.6X1	T47.6X2	T47.6X3	T47.6X4	T47.6X5	T47.6X6
aluminate	T47.1X1	T47.1X2	T47.1X3	T47.1X4	T47.1X5	T47.1X6
anti-infectives	T37.8X1	T37.8X2	T37.8X3	T37.8X4	T37.8X5	T37.8X6
formic iodide	T49.0X1	T49.0X2	T49.0X3	T49.0X4	T49.0X5	T49.0X6
glycolylarsenate	T49.0X1	T49.0X2	T49.0X3	T49.0X4	T49.0X5	T49.0X6
nonmedicinal (compounds) NEC	T65.91	T65.92	T65.93	T65.94	—	—
subcarbonate	T47.6X1	T47.6X2	T47.6X3	T47.6X4	T47.6X5	T47.6X6
subsalicylate	T37.8X1	T37.8X2	T37.8X3	T37.8X4	T37.8X5	T37.8X6
sulfarsphenamine	T37.8X1	T37.8X2	T37.8X3	T37.8X4	T37.8X5	T37.8X6
Bisoprolol	T44.7X1	T44.7X2	T44.7X3	T44.7X4	T44.7X5	T44.7X6
Bisoxatin	T47.2X1	T47.2X2	T47.2X3	T47.2X4	T47.2X5	T47.2X6
Bisulepin (hydro-chloride)	T45.0X1	T45.0X2	T45.0X3	T45.0X4	T45.0X5	T45.0X6
Bithionol	T37.8X1	T37.8X2	T37.8X3	T37.8X4	T37.8X5	T37.8X6
anthelminthic	T37.4X1	T37.4X2	T37.4X3	T37.4X4	T37.4X5	T37.4X6
Bitolterol	T48.6X1	T48.6X2	T48.6X3	T48.6X4	T48.6X5	T48.6X6
Bitoscanate	T37.4X1	T37.4X2	T37.4X3	T37.4X4	T37.4X5	T37.4X6
Bitter almond oil	T62.8X1	T62.8X2	T62.8X3	T62.8X4	—	—
Bittersweet	T62.2X1	T62.2X2	T62.2X3	T62.2X4	—	—
Black						
flag	T60.91	T60.92	T60.93	T60.94	—	—
henbane	T62.2X1	T62.2X2	T62.2X3	T62.2X4	—	—
leaf (40)	T60.91	T60.92	T60.93	T60.94	—	—
widow spider (bite)	T63.311	T63.312	T63.313	T63.314	—	—
antivenin	T50.Z11	T50.Z12	T50.Z13	T50.Z14	T50.Z15	T50.Z16
Blast furnace gas (carbon monoxide from)	T58.8X1	T58.8X2	T58.8X3	T58.8X4	—	—
Bleach	T54.91	T54.92	T54.93	T54.94	—	—
Bleaching agent (medicinal)	T49.4X1	T49.4X2	T49.4X3	T49.4X4	T49.4X5	T49.4X6
Bleomycin	T45.1X1	T45.1X2	T45.1X3	T45.1X4	T45.1X5	T45.1X6
Blockain	T41.3X1	T41.3X2	T41.3X3	T41.3X4	T41.3X5	T41.3X6
infiltration (subcutaneous)	T41.3X1	T41.3X2	T41.3X3	T41.3X4	T41.3X5	T41.3X6
nerve block (peripheral) (plexus)	T41.3X1	T41.3X2	T41.3X3	T41.3X4	T41.3X5	T41.3X6
topical (surface)	T41.3X1	T41.3X2	T41.3X3	T41.3X4	T41.3X5	T41.3X6
Blockers, calcium channel	T46.1X1	T46.1X2	T46.1X3	T46.1X4	T46.1X5	T46.1X6

Substance	Poisoning, Accidental (unintentional)	Poisoning, Intentional self-harm	Poisoning, Assault	Poisoning, Undetermined	Adverse effect	Underdosing
Blood (derivatives) (natural) (plasma) (whole)	T45.8X1	T45.8X2	T45.8X3	T45.8X4	T45.8X5	T45.8X6
dried	T45.8X1	T45.8X2	T45.8X3	T45.8X4	T45.8X5	T45.8X6
drug affecting NEC	T45.91	T45.92	T45.93	T45.94	T45.95	T45.96
expander NEC	T45.8X1	T45.8X2	T45.8X3	T45.8X4	T45.8X5	T45.8X6
fraction NEC	T45.8X1	T45.8X2	T45.8X3	T45.8X4	T45.8X5	T45.8X6
substitute (macromolecular)	T45.8X1	T45.8X2	T45.8X3	T45.8X4	T45.8X5	T45.8X6
Blue velvet	T40.2X1	T40.2X2	T40.2X3	T40.2X4	—	—
Bone meal	T62.8X1	T62.8X2	T62.8X3	T62.8X4	—	—
Bonine	T45.0X1	T45.0X2	T45.0X3	T45.0X4	T45.0X5	T45.0X6
Bopindolol	T44.7X1	T44.7X2	T44.7X3	T44.7X4	T44.7X5	T44.7X6
Boracic acid	T49.0X1	T49.0X2	T49.0X3	T49.0X4	T49.0X5	T49.0X6
ENT agent	T49.6X1	T49.6X2	T49.6X3	T49.6X4	T49.6X5	T49.6X6
ophthalmic preparation	T49.5X1	T49.5X2	T49.5X3	T49.5X4	T49.5X5	T49.5X6
Borane complex	T57.8X1	T57.8X2	T57.8X3	T57.8X4	—	—
Borate (s)	T57.8X1	T57.8X2	T57.8X3	T57.8X4	—	—
buffer	T50.991	T50.992	T50.993	T50.994	T50.995	T50.996
cleanser	T54.91	T54.92	T54.93	T54.94	—	—
sodium	T57.8X1	T57.8X2	T57.8X3	T57.8X4	—	—
Borax (cleanser)	T54.91	T54.92	T54.93	T54.94	—	—
Bordeaux mixture	T60.3X1	T60.3X2	T60.3X3	T60.3X4	—	—
Boric acid	T49.0X1	T49.0X2	T49.0X3	T49.0X4	T49.0X5	T49.0X6
ENT agent	T49.6X1	T49.6X2	T49.6X3	T49.6X4	T49.6X5	T49.6X6
ophthalmic preparation	T49.5X1	T49.5X2	T49.5X3	T49.5X4	T49.5X5	T49.5X6
Bornaprine	T44.3X1	T44.3X2	T44.3X3	T44.3X4	T44.3X5	T44.3X6
Boron	T57.8X1	T57.8X2	T57.8X3	T57.8X4	—	—
hydride NEC	T57.8X1	T57.8X2	T57.8X3	T57.8X4	—	—
fumes or gas	T57.8X1	T57.8X2	T57.8X3	T57.8X4	—	—
trifluoride	T59.891	T59.892	T59.893	T59.894	—	—
Botox	T48.291	T48.292	T48.293	T48.294	T48.295	T48.296
Botulinus anti-toxin (type A, B)	T50.Z11	T50.Z12	T50.Z13	T50.Z14	T50.Z15	T50.Z16
Brake fluid vapor	T59.891	T59.892	T59.893	T59.894	—	—
Brallobarbital	T42.3X1	T42.3X2	T42.3X3	T42.3X4	T42.3X5	T42.3X6
Bran (wheat)	T47.4X1	T47.4X2	T47.4X3	T47.4X4	T47.4X5	T47.4X6
Brass (fumes)	T56.891	T56.892	T56.893	T56.894	—	—
Brasso	T52.0X1	T52.0X2	T52.0X3	T52.0X4	—	—
Bretylium tosilate	T46.2X1	T46.2X2	T46.2X3	T46.2X4	T46.2X5	T46.2X6
Brevital (sodium)	T41.1X1	T41.1X2	T41.1X3	T41.1X4	T41.1X5	T41.1X6
Brinase	T45.3X1	T45.3X2	T45.3X3	T45.3X4	T45.3X5	T45.3X6
British antilewisite	T45.8X1	T45.8X2	T45.8X3	T45.8X4	T45.8X5	T45.8X6
Brodifacoum	T60.4X1	T60.4X2	T60.4X3	T60.4X4	—	—
Bromal (hydrate)	T42.6X1	T42.6X2	T42.6X3	T42.6X4	T42.6X5	T42.6X6
Bromazepam	T42.4X1	T42.4X2	T42.4X3	T42.4X4	T42.4X5	T42.4X6
Bromazine	T45.0X1	T45.0X2	T45.0X3	T45.0X4	T45.0X5	T45.0X6
Brombenzylcyanide	T59.3X1	T59.3X2	T59.3X3	T59.3X4	—	—
Bromelains	T45.3X1	T45.3X2	T45.3X3	T45.3X4	T45.3X5	T45.3X6
Bromethalin	T60.4X1	T60.4X2	T60.4X3	T60.4X4	—	—
Bromhexine	T48.4X1	T48.4X2	T48.4X3	T48.4X4	T48.4X5	T48.4X6
Bromide salts	T42.6X1	T42.6X2	T42.6X3	T42.6X4	T42.6X5	T42.6X6

Substance	Poisoning, Accidental (unintentional)	Poisoning, Intentional self-harm	Poisoning, Assault	Poisoning, Undetermined	Adverse effect	Underdosing
Bromindione	T45.511	T45.512	T45.513	T45.514	T45.515	T45.516
Bromine						
compounds (medicinal)	T42.6X1	T42.6X2	T42.6X3	T42.6X4	T42.6X5	T42.6X6
sedative	T42.6X1	T42.6X2	T42.6X3	T42.6X4	T42.6X5	T42.6X6
vapor	T59.891	T59.892	T59.893	T59.894	—	—
Bromisoval	T42.6X1	T42.6X2	T42.6X3	T42.6X4	T42.6X5	T42.6X6
Bromisovalum	T42.6X1	T42.6X2	T42.6X3	T42.6X4	T42.6X5	T42.6X6
Bromobenzylcyanide	T59.3X1	T59.3X2	T59.3X3	T59.3X4	—	—
Bromochloro-salicylani-lide	T49.0X1	T49.0X2	T49.0X3	T49.0X4	T49.0X5	T49.0X6
Bromocriptine	T42.8X1	T42.8X2	T42.8X3	T42.8X4	T42.8X5	T42.8X6
Bromodiphenhy-dramine	T45.0X1	T45.0X2	T45.0X3	T45.0X4	T45.0X5	T45.0X6
Bromoform	T42.6X1	T42.6X2	T42.6X3	T42.6X4	T42.6X5	T42.6X6
Bromophenol blue reagent	T50.991	T50.992	T50.993	T50.994	T50.995	T50.996
Bromopride	T47.8X1	T47.8X2	T47.8X3	T47.8X4	T47.8X5	T47.8X6
Bromosalicyl chloranitide	T49.0X1	T49.0X2	T49.0X3	T49.0X4	T49.0X5	T49.0X6
Bromosalicyl hydroxamic acid	T37.1X1	T37.1X2	T37.1X3	T37.1X4	T37.1X5	T37.1X6
Bromo-seltzer	T39.1X1	T39.1X2	T39.1X3	T39.1X4	T39.1X5	T39.1X6
Bromoxynil	T60.3X1	T60.3X2	T60.3X3	T60.3X4	—	—
Bromperidol	T43.4X1	T43.4X2	T43.4X3	T43.4X4	T43.4X5	T43.4X6
Brompheniramine	T45.0X1	T45.0X2	T45.0X3	T45.0X4	T45.0X5	T45.0X6
Bromsulfophthalein	T50.8X1	T50.8X2	T50.8X3	T50.8X4	T50.8X5	T50.8X6
Bromural	T42.6X1	T42.6X2	T42.6X3	T42.6X4	T42.6X5	T42.6X6
Bromvaletone	T42.6X1	T42.6X2	T42.6X3	T42.6X4	T42.6X5	T42.6X6
Bronchodilator NEC	T48.6X1	T48.6X2	T48.6X3	T48.6X4	T48.6X5	T48.6X6
Brotizolam	T42.4X1	T42.4X2	T42.4X3	T42.4X4	T42.4X5	T42.4X6
Brovincamine	T46.7X1	T46.7X2	T46.7X3	T46.7X4	T46.7X5	T46.7X6
Brown recluse spider (bite) (venom)	T63.331	T63.332	T63.333	T63.334	—	—
Brown spider (bite) (venom)	T63.391	T63.392	T63.393	T63.394	—	—
Broxaterol	T48.6X1	T48.6X2	T48.6X3	T48.6X4	T48.6X5	T48.6X6
Broxuridine	T45.1X1	T45.1X2	T45.1X3	T45.1X4	T45.1X5	T45.1X6
Broxyquinoline	T37.8X1	T37.8X2	T37.8X3	T37.8X4	T37.8X5	T37.8X6
Bruceine	T48.291	T48.292	T48.293	T48.294	T48.295	T48.296
Brucia	T62.2X1	T62.2X2	T62.2X3	T62.2X4	—	—
Brucine	T65.1X1	T65.1X2	T65.1X3	T65.1X4	—	—
Brunswick green—see Copper						
Bruten—see Ibuprofen						
Bryonia	T47.2X1	T47.2X2	T47.2X3	T47.2X4	T47.2X5	T47.2X6
Buclizine	T45.0X1	T45.0X2	T45.0X3	T45.0X4	T45.0X5	T45.0X6
Buclosamide	T49.0X1	T49.0X2	T49.0X3	T49.0X4	T49.0X5	T49.0X6
Budesonide	T44.5X1	T44.5X2	T44.5X3	T44.5X4	T44.5X5	T44.5X6
Budralazine	T46.5X1	T46.5X2	T46.5X3	T46.5X4	T46.5X5	T46.5X6
Bufferin	T39.011	T39.012	T39.013	T39.014	T39.015	T39.016
Buflomedil	T46.7X1	T46.7X2	T46.7X3	T46.7X4	T46.7X5	T46.7X6
Buformin	T38.3X1	T38.3X2	T38.3X3	T38.3X4	T38.3X5	T38.3X6
Bufotenine	T40.991	T40.992	T40.993	T40.994	—	—
Bufrolin	T48.6X1	T48.6X2	T48.6X3	T48.6X4	T48.6X5	T48.6X6
Bufylline	T48.6X1	T48.6X2	T48.6X3	T48.6X4	T48.6X5	T48.6X6

Substance	Poisoning, Accidental (unintentional)	Poisoning, Intentional self-harm	Poisoning, Assault	Poisoning, Undetermined	Adverse effect	Underdosing
Bulk filler	T50.5X1	T50.5X2	T50.5X3	T50.5X4	T50.5X5	T50.5X6
cathartic	T47.4X1	T47.4X2	T47.4X3	T47.4X4	T47.4X5	T47.4X6
Bumetanide	T50.1X1	T50.1X2	T50.1X3	T50.1X4	T50.1X5	T50.1X6
Bunaftine	T46.2X1	T46.2X2	T46.2X3	T46.2X4	T46.2X5	T46.2X6
Bunamiodyl	T50.8X1	T50.8X2	T50.8X3	T50.8X4	T50.8X5	T50.8X6
Bunazosin	T44.6X1	T44.6X2	T44.6X3	T44.6X4	T44.6X5	T44.6X6
Bunitrolol	T44.7X1	T44.7X2	T44.7X3	T44.7X4	T44.7X5	T44.7X6
Buphenine	T46.7X1	T46.7X2	T46.7X3	T46.7X4	T46.7X5	T46.7X6
Bupivacaine	T41.3X1	T41.3X2	T41.3X3	T41.3X4	T41.3X5	T41.3X6
infiltration (subcutaneous)	T41.3X1	T41.3X2	T41.3X3	T41.3X4	T41.3X5	T41.3X6
nerve block (peripheral) (plexus)	T41.3X1	T41.3X2	T41.3X3	T41.3X4	T41.3X5	T41.3X6
spinal	T41.3X1	T41.3X2	T41.3X3	T41.3X4	T41.3X5	T41.3X6
Bupranolol	T44.7X1	T44.7X2	T44.7X3	T44.7X4	T44.7X5	T44.7X6
Buprenorphine	T40.4X1	T40.4X2	T40.4X3	T40.4X4	T40.4X5	T40.4X6
Bupropion	T43.291	T43.292	T43.293	T43.294	T43.295	T43.296
Burimamide	T47.1X1	T47.1X2	T47.1X3	T47.1X4	T47.1X5	T47.1X6
Buserelin	T38.891	T38.892	T38.893	T38.894	T38.895	T38.896
Buspirone	T43.591	T43.592	T43.593	T43.594	T43.595	T43.596
Busulfan, busulphan	T45.1X1	T45.1X2	T45.1X3	T45.1X4	T45.1X5	T45.1X6
Butabarbital (sodium)	T42.3X1	T42.3X2	T42.3X3	T42.3X4	T42.3X5	T42.3X6
Butabarbitone	T42.3X1	T42.3X2	T42.3X3	T42.3X4	T42.3X5	T42.3X6
Butabarpal	T42.3X1	T42.3X2	T42.3X3	T42.3X4	T42.3X5	T42.3X6
Butacaine	T41.3X1	T41.3X2	T41.3X3	T41.3X4	T41.3X5	T41.3X6
Butalamine	T46.7X1	T46.7X2	T46.7X3	T46.7X4	T46.7X5	T46.7X6
Butalbital	T42.3X1	T42.3X2	T42.3X3	T42.3X4	T42.3X5	T42.3X6
Butallylonal	T42.3X1	T42.3X2	T42.3X3	T42.3X4	T42.3X5	T42.3X6
Butamben	T41.3X1	T41.3X2	T41.3X3	T41.3X4	T41.3X5	T41.3X6
Butamirate	T48.3X1	T48.3X2	T48.3X3	T48.3X4	T48.3X5	T48.3X6
Butane (distributed in mobile container)	T59.891	T59.892	T59.893	T59.894	—	—
distributed through pipes	T59.891	T59.892	T59.893	T59.894	—	—
incomplete combustion	T58.11	T58.12	T58.13	T58.14	—	—
Butanilicaine	T41.3X1	T41.3X2	T41.3X3	T41.3X4	T41.3X5	T41.3X6
Butanol	T51.3X1	T51.3X2	T51.3X3	T51.3X4	—	—
Butanone, 2-butanone	T52.4X1	T52.4X2	T52.4X3	T52.4X4	—	—
Butantrone	T49.4X1	T49.4X2	T49.4X3	T49.4X4	T49.4X5	T49.4X6
Butaperazine	T43.3X1	T43.3X2	T43.3X3	T43.3X4	T43.3X5	T43.3X6
Butazolidin	T39.2X1	T39.2X2	T39.2X3	T39.2X4	T39.2X5	T39.2X6
Butetamate	T48.6X1	T48.6X2	T48.6X3	T48.6X4	T48.6X5	T48.6X6
Butethal	T42.3X1	T42.3X2	T42.3X3	T42.3X4	T42.3X5	T42.3X6
Butethamate	T44.3X1	T44.3X2	T44.3X3	T44.3X4	T44.3X5	T44.3X6
Buthalitone (sodium)	T41.1X1	T41.1X2	T41.1X3	T41.1X4	T41.1X5	T41.1X6
Butisol (sodium)	T42.3X1	T42.3X2	T42.3X3	T42.3X4	T42.3X5	T42.3X6
Butizide	T50.2X1	T50.2X2	T50.2X3	T50.2X4	T50.2X5	T50.2X6
Butobarbital	T42.3X1	T42.3X2	T42.3X3	T42.3X4	T42.3X5	T42.3X6
sodium	T42.3X1	T42.3X2	T42.3X3	T42.3X4	T42.3X5	T42.3X6
Butobarbitone	T42.3X1	T42.3X2	T42.3X3	T42.3X4	T42.3X5	T42.3X6
Butoconazole (nitrate)	T49.0X1	T49.0X2	T49.0X3	T49.0X4	T49.0X5	T49.0X6
Butorphanol	T40.4X1	T40.4X2	T40.4X3	T40.4X4	T40.4X5	T40.4X6

Substance	Poisoning, Accidental (unintentional)	Poisoning, Intentional self-harm	Poisoning, Assault	Poisoning, Undetermined	Adverse effect	Underdosing
Butriptyline	T43.011	T43.012	T43.013	T43.014	T43.015	T43.016
Butropium bromide	T44.3X1	T44.3X2	T44.3X3	T44.3X4	T44.3X5	T44.3X6
Butter of antimony—see Antimony						
Buttercups	T62.2X1	T62.2X2	T62.2X3	T62.2X4	—	—
Butyl						
acetate (secondary)	T52.8X1	T52.8X2	T52.8X3	T52.8X4	—	—
alcohol	T51.3X1	T51.3X2	T51.3X3	T51.3X4	—	—
aminobenzoate	T41.3X1	T41.3X2	T41.3X3	T41.3X4	T41.3X5	T41.3X6
butyrate	T52.8X1	T52.8X2	T52.8X3	T52.8X4	—	—
carbinol	T51.3X1	T51.3X2	T51.3X3	T51.3X4	—	—
carbitol	T52.3X1	T52.3X2	T52.3X3	T52.3X4	—	—
cellosolve	T52.3X1	T52.3X2	T52.3X3	T52.3X4	—	—
chloral (hydrate)	T42.6X1	T42.6X2	T42.6X3	T42.6X4	T42.6X5	T42.6X6
formate	T52.8X1	T52.8X2	T52.8X3	T52.8X4	—	—
lactate	T52.8X1	T52.8X2	T52.8X3	T52.8X4	—	—
propionate	T52.8X1	T52.8X2	T52.8X3	T52.8X4	—	—
scopolamine bromide	T44.3X1	T44.3X2	T44.3X3	T44.3X4	T44.3X5	T44.3X6
thiobarbital sodium	T41.1X1	T41.1X2	T41.1X3	T41.1X4	T41.1X5	T41.1X6
Butylated hydroxy-anisole	T50.991	T50.992	T50.993	T50.994	T50.995	T50.996
Butylchloral hydrate	T42.6X1	T42.6X2	T42.6X3	T42.6X4	T42.6X5	T42.6X6
Butyltoluene	T52.2X1	T52.2X2	T52.2X3	T52.2X4	—	—
Butyn	T41.3X1	T41.3X2	T41.3X3	T41.3X4	T41.3X5	T41.3X6
Butyrophenone(-based tranquilizers)	T43.4X1	T43.4X2	T43.4X3	T43.4X4	T43.4X5	T43.4X6
C						
Cabergoline	T42.8X1	T42.8X2	T42.8X3	T42.8X4	T42.8X5	T42.8X6
Cacodyl, cacodylic acid	T57.0X1	T57.0X2	T57.0X3	T57.0X4	—	—
Cactinomycin	T45.1X1	T45.1X2	T45.1X3	T45.1X4	T45.1X5	T45.1X6
Cade oil	T49.4X1	T49.4X2	T49.4X3	T49.4X4	T49.4X5	T49.4X6
Cadexomer iodine	T49.0X1	T49.0X2	T49.0X3	T49.0X4	T49.0X5	T49.0X6
Cadmium (chloride) (fumes) (oxide)	T56.3X1	T56.3X2	T56.3X3	T56.3X4	—	—
sulfide (medicinal) NEC	T49.4X1	T49.4X2	T49.4X3	T49.4X4	T49.4X5	T49.4X6
Cadralazine	T46.5X1	T46.5X2	T46.5X3	T46.5X4	T46.5X5	T46.5X6
Caffeine	T43.611	T43.612	T43.613	T43.614	T43.615	T43.616
Calabar bean	T62.2X1	T62.2X2	T62.2X3	T62.2X4	—	—
Caladium seguinum	T62.2X1	T62.2X2	T62.2X3	T62.2X4	—	—
Calamine (lotion)	T49.3X1	T49.3X2	T49.3X3	T49.3X4	T49.3X5	T49.3X6
Calcifediol	T45.2X1	T45.2X2	T45.2X3	T45.2X4	T45.2X5	T45.2X6
Calciferol	T45.2X1	T45.2X2	T45.2X3	T45.2X4	T45.2X5	T45.2X6
Calcitonin	T50.991	T50.992	T50.993	T50.994	T50.995	T50.996
Calcitriol	T45.2X1	T45.2X2	T45.2X3	T45.2X4	T45.2X5	T45.2X6
Calcium	T50.3X1	T50.3X2	T50.3X3	T50.3X4	T50.3X5	T50.3X6
actylsalicylate	T39.011	T39.012	T39.013	T39.014	T39.015	T39.016
benzamidosalicylate	T37.1X1	T37.1X2	T37.1X3	T37.1X4	T37.1X5	T37.1X6
bromide	T42.6X1	T42.6X2	T42.6X3	T42.6X4	T42.6X5	T42.6X6
bromolactobionate	T42.6X1	T42.6X2	T42.6X3	T42.6X4	T42.6X5	T42.6X6
carbaspirin	T39.011	T39.012	T39.013	T39.014	T39.015	T39.016
carbimide	T50.6X1	T50.6X2	T50.6X3	T50.6X4	T50.6X5	T50.6X6
Calcium — *Continued*						
carbonate	T47.1X1	T47.1X2	T47.1X3	T47.1X4	T47.1X5	T47.1X6
chloride	T50.991	T50.992	T50.993	T50.994	T50.995	T50.996
anhydrous	T50.991	T50.992	T50.993	T50.994	T50.995	T50.996
cyanide	T57.8X1	T57.8X2	T57.8X3	T57.8X4	—	—
dioctyl sulfosuccinate	T47.4X1	T47.4X2	T47.4X3	T47.4X4	T47.4X5	T47.4X6
disodium edathamil	T45.8X1	T45.8X2	T45.8X3	T45.8X4	T45.8X5	T45.8X6
disodium edetate	T45.8X1	T45.8X2	T45.8X3	T45.8X4	T45.8X5	T45.8X6
dobesilate	T46.991	T46.992	T46.993	T46.994	T46.995	T46.996
EDTA	T45.8X1	T45.8X2	T45.8X3	T45.8X4	T45.8X5	T45.8X6
ferrous citrate	T45.4X1	T45.4X2	T45.4X3	T45.4X4	T45.4X5	T45.4X6
folinate	T45.8X1	T45.8X2	T45.8X3	T45.8X4	T45.8X5	T45.8X6
glubionate	T50.3X1	T50.3X2	T50.3X3	T50.3X4	T50.3X5	T50.3X6
gluconate	T50.3X1	T50.3X2	T50.3X3	T50.3X4	T50.3X5	T50.3X6
gluconoga-lactogluconate	T50.3X1	T50.3X2	T50.3X3	T50.3X4	T50.3X5	T50.3X6
hydrate, hydroxide	T54.3X1	T54.3X2	T54.3X3	T54.3X4	—	—
hypochlorite	T54.3X1	T54.3X2	T54.3X3	T54.3X4	—	—
iodide	T48.4X1	T48.4X2	T48.4X3	T48.4X4	T48.4X5	T48.4X6
ipodate	T50.8X1	T50.8X2	T50.8X3	T50.8X4	T50.8X5	T50.8X6
lactate	T50.3X1	T50.3X2	T50.3X3	T50.3X4	T50.3X5	T50.3X6
leucovorin	T45.8X1	T45.8X2	T45.8X3	T45.8X4	T45.8X5	T45.8X6
mandelate	T37.91	T37.92	T37.93	T37.94	T37.95	T37.96
oxide	T54.3X1	T54.3X2	T54.3X3	T54.3X4	—	—
pantothenate	T45.2X1	T45.2X2	T45.2X3	T45.2X4	T45.2X5	T45.2X6
phosphate	T50.3X1	T50.3X2	T50.3X3	T50.3X4	T50.3X5	T50.3X6
salicylate	T39.091	T39.092	T39.093	T39.094	T39.095	T39.096
salts	T50.3X1	T50.3X2	T50.3X3	T50.3X4	T50.3X5	T50.3X6
Calculus-dissolving drug	T50.991	T50.992	T50.993	T50.994	T50.995	T50.996
Calomel	T49.0X1	T49.0X2	T49.0X3	T49.0X4	T49.0X5	T49.0X6
Caloric agent	T50.3X1	T50.3X2	T50.3X3	T50.3X4	T50.3X5	T50.3X6
Calusterone	T38.7X1	T38.7X2	T38.7X3	T38.7X4	T38.7X5	T38.7X6
Camazepam	T42.4X1	T42.4X2	T42.4X3	T42.4X4	T42.4X5	T42.4X6
Camomile	T49.0X1	T49.0X2	T49.0X3	T49.0X4	T49.0X5	T49.0X6
Camoquin	T37.2X1	T37.2X2	T37.2X3	T37.2X4	T37.2X5	T37.2X6
Camphor						
insecticide	T60.2X1	T60.2X2	T60.2X3	T60.2X4	—	—
medicinal	T49.8X1	T49.8X2	T49.8X3	T49.8X4	T49.8X5	T49.8X6
Camylofin	T44.3X1	T44.3X2	T44.3X3	T44.3X4	T44.3X5	T44.3X6
Cancer chemotherapy drug regimen	T45.1X1	T45.1X2	T45.1X3	T45.1X4	T45.1X5	T45.1X6
Candeptin	T49.0X1	T49.0X2	T49.0X3	T49.0X4	T49.0X5	T49.0X6
Candicidin	T49.0X1	T49.0X2	T49.0X3	T49.0X4	T49.0X5	T49.0X6
Cannabinol	T40.7X1	T40.7X2	T40.7X3	T40.7X4	T40.7X5	T40.7X6
Cannabis (derivatives)	T40.7X1	T40.7X2	T40.7X3	T40.7X4	T40.7X5	T40.7X6
Canned heat	T51.1X1	T51.1X2	T51.1X3	T51.1X4	—	—
Canrenoic acid	T50.0X1	T50.0X2	T50.0X3	T50.0X4	T50.0X5	T50.0X6
Canrenone	T50.0X1	T50.0X2	T50.0X3	T50.0X4	T50.0X5	T50.0X6
Cantharides, cantharidin, cantharis	T49.8X1	T49.8X2	T49.8X3	T49.8X4	T49.8X5	T49.8X6
Canthaxanthin	T50.991	T50.992	T50.993	T50.994	T50.995	T50.996
Capillary-active drug NEC	T46.901	T46.902	T46.903	T46.904	T46.905	T46.906

Substance	Poisoning, Accidental (unintentional)	Poisoning, Intentional self-harm	Poisoning, Assault	Poisoning, Undetermined	Adverse effect	Underdosing
Capreomycin	T36.8X1	T36.8X2	T36.8X3	T36.8X4	T36.8X5	T36.8X6
Capsicum	T49.4X1	T49.4X2	T49.4X3	T49.4X4	T49.4X5	T49.4X6
Captafol	T60.3X1	T60.3X2	T60.3X3	T60.3X4	—	—
Captan	T60.3X1	T60.3X2	T60.3X3	T60.3X4	—	—
Captodiame, captodiamine	T43.591	T43.592	T43.593	T43.594	T43.595	T43.596
Captopril	T46.4X1	T46.4X2	T46.4X3	T46.4X4	T46.4X5	T46.4X6
Caramiphen	T44.3X1	T44.3X2	T44.3X3	T44.3X4	T44.3X5	T44.3X6
Carazolol	T44.7X1	T44.7X2	T44.7X3	T44.7X4	T44.7X5	T44.7X6
Carbachol	T44.1X1	T44.1X2	T44.1X3	T44.1X4	T44.1X5	T44.1X6
Carbacrylamine (resin)	T50.3X1	T50.3X2	T50.3X3	T50.3X4	T50.3X5	T50.3X6
Carbamate (insecticide)	T60.0X1	T60.0X2	T60.0X3	T60.0X4	—	—
Carbamate (sedative)	T42.6X1	T42.6X2	T42.6X3	T42.6X4	T42.6X5	T42.6X6
herbicide	T60.0X1	T60.0X2	T60.0X3	T60.0X4	—	—
insecticide	T60.0X1	T60.0X2	T60.0X3	T60.0X4	—	—
Carbamazepine	T42.1X1	T42.1X2	T42.1X3	T42.1X4	T42.1X5	T42.1X6
Carbamide	T47.3X1	T47.3X2	T47.3X3	T47.3X4	T47.3X5	T47.3X6
peroxide	T49.0X1	T49.0X2	T49.0X3	T49.0X4	T49.0X5	T49.0X6
topical	T49.8X1	T49.8X2	T49.8X3	T49.8X4	T49.8X5	T49.8X6
Carbamylcholine chloride	T44.1X1	T44.1X2	T44.1X3	T44.1X4	T44.1X5	T44.1X6
Carbaril	T60.0X1	T60.0X2	T60.0X3	T60.0X4	—	—
Carbarsone	T37.3X1	T37.3X2	T37.3X3	T37.3X4	T37.3X5	T37.3X6
Carbaryl	T60.0X1	T60.0X2	T60.0X3	T60.0X4	—	—
Carbaspirin	T39.011	T39.012	T39.013	T39.014	T39.015	T39.016
Carbazochrome (salicylate) (sodium sulfonate)	T49.4X1	T49.4X2	T49.4X3	T49.4X4	T49.4X5	T49.4X6
Carbenicillin	T36.0X1	T36.0X2	T36.0X3	T36.0X4	T36.0X5	T36.0X6
Carbenoxolone	T47.1X1	T47.1X2	T47.1X3	T47.1X4	T47.1X5	T47.1X6
Carbetapentane	T48.3X1	T48.3X2	T48.3X3	T48.3X4	T48.3X5	T48.3X6
Carbethyl salicylate	T39.091	T39.092	T39.093	T39.094	T39.095	T39.096
Carbidopa (with levodopa)	T42.8X1	T42.8X2	T42.8X3	T42.8X4	T42.8X5	T42.8X6
Carbimazole	T38.2X1	T38.2X2	T38.2X3	T38.2X4	T38.2X5	T38.2X6
Carbinol	T51.1X1	T51.1X2	T51.1X3	T51.1X4	—	—
Carbinoxamine	T45.0X1	T45.0X2	T45.0X3	T45.0X4	T45.0X5	T45.0X6
Carbiphene	T39.8X1	T39.8X2	T39.8X3	T39.8X4	T39.8X5	T39.8X6
Carbitol	T52.3X1	T52.3X2	T52.3X3	T52.3X4	—	—
Carbo medicinalis	T47.6X1	T47.6X2	T47.6X3	T47.6X4	T47.6X5	T47.6X6
Carbocaine	T41.3X1	T41.3X2	T41.3X3	T41.3X4	T41.3X5	T41.3X6
infiltration (subcutaneous)	T41.3X1	T41.3X2	T41.3X3	T41.3X4	T41.3X5	T41.3X6
nerve block (peripheral) (plexus)	T41.3X1	T41.3X2	T41.3X3	T41.3X4	T41.3X5	T41.3X6
topical (surface)	T41.3X1	T41.3X2	T41.3X3	T41.3X4	T41.3X5	T41.3X6
Carbocisteine	T48.4X1	T48.4X2	T48.4X3	T48.4X4	T48.4X5	T48.4X6
Carbocromen	T46.3X1	T46.3X2	T46.3X3	T46.3X4	T46.3X5	T46.3X6
Carbol fuchsin	T49.0X1	T49.0X2	T49.0X3	T49.0X4	T49.0X5	T49.0X6
Carbolic acid—see also Phenol	T54.0X1	T54.0X2	T54.0X3	T54.0X4	—	—
Carbolonium (bromide)	T48.1X1	T48.1X2	T48.1X3	T48.1X4	T48.1X5	T48.1X6
Carbomycin	T36.8X1	T36.8X2	T36.8X3	T36.8X4	T36.8X5	T36.8X6

Substance	Poisoning, Accidental (unintentional)	Poisoning, Intentional self-harm	Poisoning, Assault	Poisoning, Undetermined	Adverse effect	Underdosing
Carbon						
bisulfide (liquid)	T65.4X1	T65.4X2	T65.4X3	T65.4X4	—	—
vapor	T65.4X1	T65.4X2	T65.4X3	T65.4X4	—	—
dioxide (gas)	T59.7X1	T59.7X2	T59.7X3	T59.7X4	—	—
medicinal	T41.5X1	T41.5X2	T41.5X3	T41.5X4	T41.5X5	T41.5X6
nonmedicinal	T59.7X1	T59.7X2	T59.7X3	T59.7X4	—	—
snow	T49.4X1	T49.4X2	T49.4X3	T49.4X4	T49.4X5	T49.4X6
disulfide (liquid)	T65.4X1	T65.4X2	T65.4X3	T65.4X4	—	—
vapor	T65.4X1	T65.4X2	T65.4X3	T65.4X4	—	—
monoxide (from incomplete combustion)	T58.91	T58.92	T58.93	T58.94	—	—
blast furnace gas	T58.8X1	T58.8X2	T58.8X3	T58.8X4	—	—
butane (distributed in mobile container)	T58.11	T58.12	T58.13	T58.14	—	—
distributed through pipes	T58.11	T58.12	T58.13	T58.14	—	—
charcoal fumes	T58.2X1	T58.2X2	T58.2X3	T58.2X4	—	—
coal	T58.2X1	T58.2X2	T58.2X3	T58.2X4	—	—
coke (in domestic stoves, fireplaces)	T58.2X1	T58.2X2	T58.2X3	T58.2X4	—	—
gas (piped)	T58.11	T58.12	T58.13	T58.14	—	—
solid (in domestic stoves, fireplaces)	T58.2X1	T58.2X2	T58.2X3	T58.2X4	—	—
exhaust gas (motor) not in transit	T58.01	T58.02	T58.03	T58.04	—	—
combustion engine, any not in watercraft	T58.01	T58.02	T58.03	T58.04	—	—
farm tractor, not in transit	T58.01	T58.02	T58.03	T58.04	—	—
gas engine	T58.01	T58.02	T58.03	T58.04	—	—
motor pump	T58.01	T58.02	T58.03	T58.04	—	—
motor vehicle, not in transit	T58.01	T58.02	T58.03	T58.04	—	—
fuel (in domestic use)	T58.2X1	T58.2X2	T58.2X3	T58.2X4	—	—
gas (piped)	T58.11	T58.12	T58.13	T58.14	—	—
in mobile container	T58.11	T58.12	T58.13	T58.14	—	—
piped (natural)	T58.11	T58.12	T58.13	T58.14	—	—
utility	T58.11	T58.12	T58.13	T58.14	—	—
in mobile container	T58.11	T58.12	T58.13	T58.14	—	—
illuminating gas	T58.11	T58.12	T58.13	T58.14	—	—
industrial fuels or gases, any	T58.8X1	T58.8X2	T58.8X3	T58.8X4	—	—
kerosene (in domestic stoves, fireplaces)	T58.2X1	T58.2X2	T58.2X3	T58.2X4	—	—
kiln gas or vapor	T58.8X1	T58.8X2	T58.8X3	T58.8X4	—	—
motor exhaust gas, not in transit	T58.01	T58.02	T58.03	T58.04	—	—
piped gas (manufactured) (natural)	T58.11	T58.12	T58.13	T58.14	—	—
producer gas	T58.8X1	T58.8X2	T58.8X3	T58.8X4	—	—
propane (distributed in mobile container)	T58.11	T58.12	T58.13	T58.14	—	—
distributed through pipes	T58.11	T58.12	T58.13	T58.14	—	—

Substance	Poisoning, Accidental (unintentional)	Poisoning, Intentional self-harm	Poisoning, Assault	Poisoning, Undetermined	Adverse effect	Underdosing
Carbon — *Continued*						
specified source NEC	T58.8X1	T58.8X2	T58.8X3	T58.8X4	—	—
stove gas	T58.11	T58.12	T58.13	T58.14	—	—
piped	T58.11	T58.12	T58.13	T58.14	—	—
utility gas	T58.11	T58.12	T58.13	T58.14	—	—
piped	T58.11	T58.12	T58.13	T58.14	—	—
water gas	T58.11	T58.12	T58.13	T58.14	—	—
wood (in domestic stoves, fireplaces)	T58.2X1	T58.2X2	T58.2X3	T58.2X4	—	—
tetrachloride (vapor) NEC	T53.0X1	T53.0X2	T53.0X3	T53.0X4	—	—
liquid (cleansing agent) NEC	T53.0X1	T53.0X2	T53.0X3	T53.0X4	—	—
solvent	T53.0X1	T53.0X2	T53.0X3	T53.0X4	—	—
Carbonic acid gas	T59.7X1	T59.7X2	T59.7X3	T59.7X4	—	—
anhydrase inhibitor NEC	T50.2X1	T50.2X2	T50.2X3	T50.2X4	T50.2X5	T50.2X6
Carbophenothion	T60.0X1	T60.0X2	T60.0X3	T60.0X4	—	—
Carboplatin	T45.1X1	T45.1X2	T45.1X3	T45.1X4	T45.1X5	T45.1X6
Carboprost	T48.0X1	T48.0X2	T48.0X3	T48.0X4	T48.0X5	T48.0X6
Carboquone	T45.1X1	T45.1X2	T45.1X3	T45.1X4	T45.1X5	T45.1X6
Carbowax	T49.3X1	T49.3X2	T49.3X3	T49.3X4	T49.3X5	T49.3X6
Carboxymethyl-cellulose	T47.4X1	T47.4X2	T47.4X3	T47.4X4	T47.4X5	T47.4X6
S-Carboxymethyl-cysteine	T48.4X1	T48.4X2	T48.4X3	T48.4X4	T48.4X5	T48.4X6
Carbrital	T42.3X1	T42.3X2	T42.3X3	T42.3X4	T42.3X5	T42.3X6
Carbromal	T42.6X1	T42.6X2	T42.6X3	T42.6X4	T42.6X5	T42.6X6
Carbutamide	T38.3X1	T38.3X2	T38.3X3	T38.3X4	T38.3X5	T38.3X6
Carbuterol	T48.6X1	T48.6X2	T48.6X3	T48.6X4	T48.6X5	T48.6X6
Cardiac						
depressants	T46.2X1	T46.2X2	T46.2X3	T46.2X4	T46.2X5	T46.2X6
rhythm regulator	T46.2X1	T46.2X2	T46.2X3	T46.2X4	T46.2X5	T46.2X6
specified NEC	T46.2X1	T46.2X2	T46.2X3	T46.2X4	T46.2X5	T46.2X6
Cardiografin	T50.8X1	T50.8X2	T50.8X3	T50.8X4	T50.8X5	T50.8X6
Cardio-green	T50.8X1	T50.8X2	T50.8X3	T50.8X4	T50.8X5	T50.8X6
Cardiotonic (glycoside)NEC	T46.0X1	T46.0X2	T46.0X3	T46.0X4	T46.0X5	T46.0X6
Cardiovascular drug NEC	T46.901	T46.902	T46.903	T46.904	T46.905	T46.906
Cardrase	T50.2X1	T50.2X2	T50.2X3	T50.2X4	T50.2X5	T50.2X6
Carfecillin	T36.0X1	T36.0X2	T36.0X3	T36.0X4	T36.0X5	T36.0X6
Carfenazine	T43.3X1	T43.3X2	T43.3X3	T43.3X4	T43.3X5	T43.3X6
Carfusin	T49.0X1	T49.0X2	T49.0X3	T49.0X4	T49.0X5	T49.0X6
Carindacillin	T36.0X1	T36.0X2	T36.0X3	T36.0X4	T36.0X5	T36.0X6
Carisoprodol	T42.8X1	T42.8X2	T42.8X3	T42.8X4	T42.8X5	T42.8X6
Carmellose	T47.4X1	T47.4X2	T47.4X3	T47.4X4	T47.4X5	T47.4X6
Carminative	T47.5X1	T47.5X2	T47.5X3	T47.5X4	T47.5X5	T47.5X6
Carmofur	T45.1X1	T45.1X2	T45.1X3	T45.1X4	T45.1X5	T45.1X6
Carmustine	T45.1X1	T45.1X2	T45.1X3	T45.1X4	T45.1X5	T45.1X6
Carotene	T45.2X1	T45.2X2	T45.2X3	T45.2X4	T45.2X5	T45.2X6
Carphenazine	T43.3X1	T43.3X2	T43.3X3	T43.3X4	T43.3X5	T43.3X6
Carpipramine	T42.4X1	T42.4X2	T42.4X3	T42.4X4	T42.4X5	T42.4X6
Carprofen	T39.311	T39.312	T39.313	T39.314	T39.315	T39.316
Carpronium chloride	T44.3X1	T44.3X2	T44.3X3	T44.3X4	T44.3X5	T44.3X6

Substance	Poisoning, Accidental (unintentional)	Poisoning, Intentional self-harm	Poisoning, Assault	Poisoning, Undetermined	Adverse effect	Underdosing
Carrageenan	T47.8X1	T47.8X2	T47.8X3	T47.8X4	T47.8X5	T47.8X6
Carteolol	T44.7X1	T44.7X2	T44.7X3	T44.7X4	T44.7X5	T44.7X6
Carter's Little Pills	T47.2X1	T47.2X2	T47.2X3	T47.2X4	T47.2X5	T47.2X6
Cascara (sagrada)	T47.2X1	T47.2X2	T47.2X3	T47.2X4	T47.2X5	T47.2X6
Cassava	T62.2X1	T62.2X2	T62.2X3	T62.2X4	—	—
Castellani's paint	T49.0X1	T49.0X2	T49.0X3	T49.0X4	T49.0X5	T49.0X6
Castor						
bean	T62.2X1	T62.2X2	T62.2X3	T62.2X4	—	—
oil	T47.2X1	T47.2X2	T47.2X3	T47.2X4	T47.2X5	T47.2X6
Catalase	T45.3X1	T45.3X2	T45.3X3	T45.3X4	T45.3X5	T45.3X6
Caterpillar (sting)	T63.431	T63.432	T63.433	T63.434	—	—
Catha (edulis) (tea)	T43.691	T43.692	T43.693	T43.694	—	—
Cathartic NEC	T47.4X1	T47.4X2	T47.4X3	T47.4X4	T47.4X5	T47.4X6
anthacene derivative	T47.2X1	T47.2X2	T47.2X3	T47.2X4	T47.2X5	T47.2X6
bulk	T47.4X1	T47.4X2	T47.4X3	T47.4X4	T47.4X5	T47.4X6
contact	T47.2X1	T47.2X2	T47.2X3	T47.2X4	T47.2X5	T47.2X6
emollient NEC	T47.4X1	T47.4X2	T47.4X3	T47.4X4	T47.4X5	T47.4X6
irritant NEC	T47.2X1	T47.2X2	T47.2X3	T47.2X4	T47.2X5	T47.2X6
mucilage	T47.4X1	T47.4X2	T47.4X3	T47.4X4	T47.4X5	T47.4X6
saline	T47.3X1	T47.3X2	T47.3X3	T47.3X4	T47.3X5	T47.3X6
vegetable	T47.2X1	T47.2X2	T47.2X3	T47.2X4	T47.2X5	T47.2X6
Cathine	T50.5X1	T50.5X2	T50.5X3	T50.5X4	T50.5X5	T50.5X6
Cathomycin	T36.8X1	T36.8X2	T36.8X3	T36.8X4	T36.8X5	T36.8X6
Cation exchange resin	T50.3X1	T50.3X2	T50.3X3	T50.3X4	T50.3X5	T50.3X6
Caustic(s) NEC	T54.91	T54.92	T54.93	T54.94	—	—
alkali	T54.3X1	T54.3X2	T54.3X3	T54.3X4	—	—
hydroxide	T54.3X1	T54.3X2	T54.3X3	T54.3X4	—	—
potash	T54.3X1	T54.3X2	T54.3X3	T54.3X4	—	—
soda	T54.3X1	T54.3X2	T54.3X3	T54.3X4	—	—
specified NEC	T54.91	T54.92	T54.93	T54.94	—	—
Ceepryn	T49.0X1	T49.0X2	T49.0X3	T49.0X4	T49.0X5	T49.0X6
ENT agent	T49.6X1	T49.6X2	T49.6X3	T49.6X4	T49.6X5	T49.6X6
lozenges	T49.6X1	T49.6X2	T49.6X3	T49.6X4	T49.6X5	T49.6X6
Cefacetrile	T36.1X1	T36.1X2	T36.1X3	T36.1X4	T36.1X5	T36.1X6
Cefaclor	T36.1X1	T36.1X2	T36.1X3	T36.1X4	T36.1X5	T36.1X6
Cefadroxil	T36.1X1	T36.1X2	T36.1X3	T36.1X4	T36.1X5	T36.1X6
Cefalexin	T36.1X1	T36.1X2	T36.1X3	T36.1X4	T36.1X5	T36.1X6
Cefaloglycin	T36.1X1	T36.1X2	T36.1X3	T36.1X4	T36.1X5	T36.1X6
Cefaloridine	T36.1X1	T36.1X2	T36.1X3	T36.1X4	T36.1X5	T36.1X6
Cefalosporins	T36.1X1	T36.1X2	T36.1X3	T36.1X4	T36.1X5	T36.1X6
Cefalotin	T36.1X1	T36.1X2	T36.1X3	T36.1X4	T36.1X5	T36.1X6
Cefamandole	T36.1X1	T36.1X2	T36.1X3	T36.1X4	T36.1X5	T36.1X6
Cefamycin antibiotic	T36.1X1	T36.1X2	T36.1X3	T36.1X4	T36.1X5	T36.1X6
Cefapirin	T36.1X1	T36.1X2	T36.1X3	T36.1X4	T36.1X5	T36.1X6
Cefatrizine	T36.1X1	T36.1X2	T36.1X3	T36.1X4	T36.1X5	T36.1X6
Cefazedone	T36.1X1	T36.1X2	T36.1X3	T36.1X4	T36.1X5	T36.1X6
Cefazolin	T36.1X1	T36.1X2	T36.1X3	T36.1X4	T36.1X5	T36.1X6
Cefbuperazone	T36.1X1	T36.1X2	T36.1X3	T36.1X4	T36.1X5	T36.1X6
Cefetamet	T36.1X1	T36.1X2	T36.1X3	T36.1X4	T36.1X5	T36.1X6
Cefixime	T36.1X1	T36.1X2	T36.1X3	T36.1X4	T36.1X5	T36.1X6

Substance	Poisoning, Accidental (unintentional)	Poisoning, Intentional self-harm	Poisoning, Assault	Poisoning, Undetermined	Adverse effect	Underdosing
Cefmenoxime	T36.1X1	T36.1X2	T36.1X3	T36.1X4	T36.1X5	T36.1X6
Cefmetazole	T36.1X1	T36.1X2	T36.1X3	T36.1X4	T36.1X5	T36.1X6
Cefminox	T36.1X1	T36.1X2	T36.1X3	T36.1X4	T36.1X5	T36.1X6
Cefonicid	T36.1X1	T36.1X2	T36.1X3	T36.1X4	T36.1X5	T36.1X6
Cefoperazone	T36.1X1	T36.1X2	T36.1X3	T36.1X4	T36.1X5	T36.1X6
Ceforanide	T36.1X1	T36.1X2	T36.1X3	T36.1X4	T36.1X5	T36.1X6
Cefotaxime	T36.1X1	T36.1X2	T36.1X3	T36.1X4	T36.1X5	T36.1X6
Cefotetan	T36.1X1	T36.1X2	T36.1X3	T36.1X4	T36.1X5	T36.1X6
Cefotiam	T36.1X1	T36.1X2	T36.1X3	T36.1X4	T36.1X5	T36.1X6
Cefoxitin	T36.1X1	T36.1X2	T36.1X3	T36.1X4	T36.1X5	T36.1X6
Cefpimizole	T36.1X1	T36.1X2	T36.1X3	T36.1X4	T36.1X5	T36.1X6
Cefpiramide	T36.1X1	T36.1X2	T36.1X3	T36.1X4	T36.1X5	T36.1X6
Cefradine	T36.1X1	T36.1X2	T36.1X3	T36.1X4	T36.1X5	T36.1X6
Cefroxadine	T36.1X1	T36.1X2	T36.1X3	T36.1X4	T36.1X5	T36.1X6
Cefsulodin	T36.1X1	T36.1X2	T36.1X3	T36.1X4	T36.1X5	T36.1X6
Ceftazidime	T36.1X1	T36.1X2	T36.1X3	T36.1X4	T36.1X5	T36.1X6
Cefteram	T36.1X1	T36.1X2	T36.1X3	T36.1X4	T36.1X5	T36.1X6
Ceftezole	T36.1X1	T36.1X2	T36.1X3	T36.1X4	T36.1X5	T36.1X6
Ceftizoxime	T36.1X1	T36.1X2	T36.1X3	T36.1X4	T36.1X5	T36.1X6
Ceftriaxone	T36.1X1	T36.1X2	T36.1X3	T36.1X4	T36.1X5	T36.1X6
Cefuroxime	T36.1X1	T36.1X2	T36.1X3	T36.1X4	T36.1X5	T36.1X6
Cefuzonam	T36.1X1	T36.1X2	T36.1X3	T36.1X4	T36.1X5	T36.1X6
Celestone	T38.0X1	T38.0X2	T38.0X3	T38.0X4	T38.0X5	T38.0X6
topical	T49.0X1	T49.0X2	T49.0X3	T49.0X4	T49.0X5	T49.0X6
Celiprolol	T44.7X1	T44.7X2	T44.7X3	T44.7X4	T44.7X5	T44.7X6
Cell stimulants and proliferants	T49.8X1	T49.8X2	T49.8X3	T49.8X4	T49.8X5	T49.8X6
Cellosolve	T52.91	T52.92	T52.93	T52.94	—	—
Cellulose						
cathartic	T47.4X1	T47.4X2	T47.4X3	T47.4X4	T47.4X5	T47.4X6
hydroxyethyl	T47.4X1	T47.4X2	T47.4X3	T47.4X4	T47.4X5	T47.4X6
nitrates (topical)	T49.3X1	T49.3X2	T49.3X3	T49.3X4	T49.3X5	T49.3X6
oxidized	T49.4X1	T49.4X2	T49.4X3	T49.4X4	T49.4X5	T49.4X6
Centipede (bite)	T63.411	T63.412	T63.413	T63.414	—	—
Central nervous system						
depressants	T42.71	T42.72	T42.73	T42.74	T42.75	T42.76
anesthetic (general) NEC	T41.201	T41.202	T41.203	T41.204	T41.205	T41.206
gases NEC	T41.0X1	T41.0X2	T41.0X3	T41.0X4	T41.0X5	T41.0X6
intravenous	T41.1X1	T41.1X2	T41.1X3	T41.1X4	T41.1X5	T41.1X6
barbiturates	T42.3X1	T42.3X2	T42.3X3	T42.3X4	T42.3X5	T42.3X6
benzodiazepines	T42.4X1	T42.4X2	T42.4X3	T42.4X4	T42.4X5	T42.4X6
bromides	T42.6X1	T42.6X2	T42.6X3	T42.6X4	T42.6X5	T42.6X6
cannabis sativa	T40.7X1	T40.7X2	T40.7X3	T40.7X4	T40.7X5	T40.7X6
chloral hydrate	T42.6X1	T42.6X2	T42.6X3	T42.6X4	T42.6X5	T42.6X6
ethanol	T51.0X1	T51.0X2	T51.0X3	T51.0X4	—	—
hallucinogenics	T40.901	T40.902	T40.903	T40.904	T40.905	T40.906
hypnotics	T42.71	T42.72	T42.73	T42.74	T42.75	T42.76
specified NEC	T42.6X1	T42.6X2	T42.6X3	T42.6X4	T42.6X5	T42.6X6
muscle relaxants	T42.8X1	T42.8X2	T42.8X3	T42.8X4	T42.8X5	T42.8X6
Central nervous system — *Continued*						
paraldehyde	T42.6X1	T42.6X2	T42.6X3	T42.6X4	T42.6X5	T42.6X6
sedatives; sedative-hypnotics	T42.71	T42.72	T42.73	T42.74	T42.75	T42.76
mixed NEC	T42.6X1	T42.6X2	T42.6X3	T42.6X4	T42.6X5	T42.6X6
specified NEC	T42.6X1	T42.6X2	T42.6X3	T42.6X4	T42.6X5	T42.6X6
muscle-tone depressants	T42.8X1	T42.8X2	T42.8X3	T42.8X4	T42.8X5	T42.8X6
stimulants	T43.601	T43.602	T43.603	T43.604	T43.605	T43.606
amphetamines	T43.621	T43.622	T43.623	T43.624	T43.625	T43.626
analeptics	T50.7X1	T50.7X2	T50.7X3	T50.7X4	T50.7X5	T50.7X6
antidepressants	T43.201	T43.202	T43.203	T43.204	T43.205	T43.206
opiate antagonists	T50.7X1	T50.7X2	T50.7X3	T50.7X4	T50.7X5	T50.7X6
specified NEC	T43.691	T43.692	T43.693	T43.694	T43.695	T43.696
Cephalexin	T36.1X1	T36.1X2	T36.1X3	T36.1X4	T36.1X5	T36.1X6
Cephaloglycin	T36.1X1	T36.1X2	T36.1X3	T36.1X4	T36.1X5	T36.1X6
Cephaloridine	T36.1X1	T36.1X2	T36.1X3	T36.1X4	T36.1X5	T36.1X6
Cephalosporins	T36.1X1	T36.1X2	T36.1X3	T36.1X4	T36.1X5	T36.1X6
N(adicillin)	T36.0X1	T36.0X2	T36.0X3	T36.0X4	T36.0X5	T36.0X6
Cephalothin	T36.1X1	T36.1X2	T36.1X3	T36.1X4	T36.1X5	T36.1X6
Cephalotin	T36.1X1	T36.1X2	T36.1X3	T36.1X4	T36.1X5	T36.1X6
Cephradine	T36.1X1	T36.1X2	T36.1X3	T36.1X4	T36.1X5	T36.1X6
Cerbera (odallam)	T62.2X1	T62.2X2	T62.2X3	T62.2X4	—	—
Cerberin	T46.0X1	T46.0X2	T46.0X3	T46.0X4	T46.0X5	T46.0X6
Cerebral stimulants	T43.601	T43.602	T43.603	T43.604	T43.605	T43.606
psychotherapeutic	T43.601	T43.602	T43.603	T43.604	T43.605	T43.606
specified NEC	T43.691	T43.692	T43.693	T43.694	T43.695	T43.696
Cerium oxalate	T45.0X1	T45.0X2	T45.0X3	T45.0X4	T45.0X5	T45.0X6
Cerous oxalate	T45.0X1	T45.0X2	T45.0X3	T45.0X4	T45.0X5	T45.0X6
Ceruletide	T50.8X1	T50.8X2	T50.8X3	T50.8X4	T50.8X5	T50.8X6
Cetalkonium (chloride)	T49.0X1	T49.0X2	T49.0X3	T49.0X4	T49.0X5	T49.0X6
Cethexonium chloride	T49.0X1	T49.0X2	T49.0X3	T49.0X4	T49.0X5	T49.0X6
Cetiedil	T46.7X1	T46.7X2	T46.7X3	T46.7X4	T46.7X5	T46.7X6
Cetirizine	T45.0X1	T45.0X2	T45.0X3	T45.0X4	T45.0X5	T45.0X6
Cetomacrogol	T50.991	T50.992	T50.993	T50.994	T50.995	T50.996
Cetotiamine	T45.2X1	T45.2X2	T45.2X3	T45.2X4	T45.2X5	T45.2X6
Cetoxime	T45.0X1	T45.0X2	T45.0X3	T45.0X4	T45.0X5	T45.0X6
Cetraxate	T47.1X1	T47.1X2	T47.1X3	T47.1X4	T47.1X5	T47.1X6
Cetrimide	T49.0X1	T49.0X2	T49.0X3	T49.0X4	T49.0X5	T49.0X6
Cetrimonium (bromide)	T49.0X1	T49.0X2	T49.0X3	T49.0X4	T49.0X5	T49.0X6
Cetylpyridinium chloride	T49.0X1	T49.0X2	T49.0X3	T49.0X4	T49.0X5	T49.0X6
ENT agent	T49.6X1	T49.6X2	T49.6X3	T49.6X4	T49.6X5	T49.6X6
lozenges	T49.6X1	T49.6X2	T49.6X3	T49.6X4	T49.6X5	T49.6X6
Cevadilla—see Sabadilla						
Cevitamic acid	T45.2X1	T45.2X2	T45.2X3	T45.2X4	T45.2X5	T45.2X6
Chalk, precipitated	T47.1X1	T47.1X2	T47.1X3	T47.1X4	T47.1X5	T47.1X6
Chamomile	T49.0X1	T49.0X2	T49.0X3	T49.0X4	T49.0X5	T49.0X6
Ch'an su	T46.0X1	T46.0X2	T46.0X3	T46.0X4	T46.0X5	T46.0X6

Substance	Poisoning, Accidental (unintentional)	Poisoning, Intentional self-harm	Poisoning, Assault	Poisoning, Undetermined	Adverse effect	Underdosing
Charcoal	T47.6X1	T47.6X2	T47.6X3	T47.6X4	T47.6X5	T47.6X6
activated—see also Charcoal, medicinal	T47.6X1	T47.6X2	T47.6X3	T47.6X4	T47.6X5	T47.6X6
fumes (Carbon monoxide)	T58.2X1	T58.2X2	T58.2X3	T58.2X4	—	—
industrial	T58.8X1	T58.8X2	T58.8X3	T58.8X4	—	—
medicinal (activated)	T47.6X1	T47.6X2	T47.6X3	T47.6X4	T47.6X5	T47.6X6
antidiarrheal	T47.6X1	T47.6X2	T47.6X3	T47.6X4	T47.6X5	T47.6X6
poison control	T47.8X1	T47.8X2	T47.8X3	T47.8X4	T47.8X5	T47.8X6
specified use other than for diarrhea	T47.8X1	T47.8X2	T47.8X3	T47.8X4	T47.8X5	T47.8X6
topical	T49.8X1	T49.8X2	T49.8X3	T49.8X4	T49.8X5	T49.8X6
Chaulmosulfone	T37.1X1	T37.1X2	T37.1X3	T37.1X4	T37.1X5	T37.1X6
Chelating agent NEC	T50.6X1	T50.6X2	T50.6X3	T50.6X4	T50.6X5	T50.6X6
Chelidonium majus	T62.2X1	T62.2X2	T62.2X3	T62.2X4	—	—
Chemical substance NEC	T65.91	T65.92	T65.93	T65.94	—	—
Chenodeoxycholic acid	T47.5X1	T47.5X2	T47.5X3	T47.5X4	T47.5X5	T47.5X6
Chenodiol	T47.5X1	T47.5X2	T47.5X3	T47.5X4	T47.5X5	T47.5X6
Chenopodium	T37.4X1	T37.4X2	T37.4X3	T37.4X4	T37.4X5	T37.4X6
Cherry laurel	T62.2X1	T62.2X2	T62.2X3	T62.2X4	—	—
Chinidin(e)	T46.2X1	T46.2X2	T46.2X3	T46.2X4	T46.2X5	T46.2X6
Chiniofon	T37.8X1	T37.8X2	T37.8X3	T37.8X4	T37.8X5	T37.8X6
Chlophedianol	T48.3X1	T48.3X2	T48.3X3	T48.3X4	T48.3X5	T48.3X6
Chloral	T42.6X1	T42.6X2	T42.6X3	T42.6X4	T42.6X5	T42.6X6
derivative	T42.6X1	T42.6X2	T42.6X3	T42.6X4	T42.6X5	T42.6X6
hydrate	T42.6X1	T42.6X2	T42.6X3	T42.6X4	T42.6X5	T42.6X6
Chloralamide	T42.6X1	T42.6X2	T42.6X3	T42.6X4	T42.6X5	T42.6X6
Chloralodol	T42.6X1	T42.6X2	T42.6X3	T42.6X4	T42.6X5	T42.6X6
Chloralose	T60.4X1	T60.4X2	T60.4X3	T60.4X4	—	—
Chlorambucil	T45.1X1	T45.1X2	T45.1X3	T45.1X4	T45.1X5	T45.1X6
Chloramine	T57.8X1	T57.8X2	T57.8X3	T57.8X4	—	—
T	T49.0X1	T49.0X2	T49.0X3	T49.0X4	T49.0X5	T49.0X6
topical	T49.0X1	T49.0X2	T49.0X3	T49.0X4	T49.0X5	T49.0X6
Chloramphenicol	T36.2X1	T36.2X2	T36.2X3	T36.2X4	T36.2X5	T36.2X6
ENT agent	T49.6X1	T49.6X2	T49.6X3	T49.6X4	T49.6X5	T49.6X6
ophthalmic preparation	T49.5X1	T49.5X2	T49.5X3	T49.5X4	T49.5X5	T49.5X6
topical NEC	T49.0X1	T49.0X2	T49.0X3	T49.0X4	T49.0X5	T49.0X6
Chlorate (potassium) (sodium) NEC	T60.3X1	T60.3X2	T60.3X3	T60.3X4	—	—
herbicide	T60.3X1	T60.3X2	T60.3X3	T60.3X4	—	—
Chlorazanil	T50.2X1	T50.2X2	T50.2X3	T50.2X4	T50.2X5	T50.2X6
Chlorbenzene, chlorbenzol	T53.7X1	T53.7X2	T53.7X3	T53.7X4	—	—
Chlorbenzoxamine	T44.3X1	T44.3X2	T44.3X3	T44.3X4	T44.3X5	T44.3X6
Chlorbutol	T42.6X1	T42.6X2	T42.6X3	T42.6X4	T42.6X5	T42.6X6
Chlorcyclizine	T45.0X1	T45.0X2	T45.0X3	T45.0X4	T45.0X5	T45.0X6
Chlordan(e) (dust)	T60.1X1	T60.1X2	T60.1X3	T60.1X4	—	—
Chlordantoin	T49.0X1	T49.0X2	T49.0X3	T49.0X4	T49.0X5	T49.0X6
Chlordiazepoxide	T42.4X1	T42.4X2	T42.4X3	T42.4X4	T42.4X5	T42.4X6
Chlordiethyl benzamide	T49.3X1	T49.3X2	T49.3X3	T49.3X4	T49.3X5	T49.3X6
Chloresium	T49.8X1	T49.8X2	T49.8X3	T49.8X4	T49.8X5	T49.8X6
Chlorethiazol	T42.6X1	T42.6X2	T42.6X3	T42.6X4	T42.6X5	T42.6X6
Chlorethyl—see Ethyl chloride						
Chloretone	T42.6X1	T42.6X2	T42.6X3	T42.6X4	T42.6X5	T42.6X6
Chlorex	T53.6X1	T53.6X2	T53.6X3	T53.6X4	—	—
insecticide	T60.1X1	T60.1X2	T60.1X3	T60.1X4	—	—
Chlorfenvinphos	T60.0X1	T60.0X2	T60.0X3	T60.0X4	—	—
Chlorhexadol	T42.6X1	T42.6X2	T42.6X3	T42.6X4	T42.6X5	T42.6X6
Chlorhexamide	T45.1X1	T45.1X2	T45.1X3	T45.1X4	T45.1X5	T45.1X6
Chlorhexidine	T49.0X1	T49.0X2	T49.0X3	T49.0X4	T49.0X5	T49.0X6
Chlorhydro-xyquinolin	T49.0X1	T49.0X2	T49.0X3	T49.0X4	T49.0X5	T49.0X6
Chloride of lime (bleach)	T54.3X1	T54.3X2	T54.3X3	T54.3X4	—	—
Chlorimipramine	T43.011	T43.012	T43.013	T43.014	T43.015	T43.016
Chlorinated						
camphene	T53.6X1	T53.6X2	T53.6X3	T53.6X4	—	—
diphenyl	T53.7X1	T53.7X2	T53.7X3	T53.7X4	—	—
hydrocarbons NEC	T53.91	T53.92	T53.93	T53.94	—	—
solvents	T53.91	T53.92	T53.93	T53.94	—	—
lime (bleach)	T54.3X1	T54.3X2	T54.3X3	T54.3X4	—	—
and boric acid solution	T49.0X1	T49.0X2	T49.0X3	T49.0X4	T49.0X5	T49.0X6
naphthalene (insecticide)	T60.1X1	T60.1X2	T60.1X3	T60.1X4	—	—
industrial (non-pesticide)	T53.7X1	T53.7X2	T53.7X3	T53.7X4	—	—
pesticide NEC	T60.8X1	T60.8X2	T60.8X3	T60.8X4	—	—
soda—see also sodium hypochlorite						
solution	T49.0X1	T49.0X2	T49.0X3	T49.0X4	T49.0X5	T49.0X6
Chlorine (fumes) (gas)	T59.4X1	T59.4X2	T59.4X3	T59.4X4	—	—
bleach	T54.3X1	T54.3X2	T54.3X3	T54.3X4	—	—
compound gas NEC	T59.4X1	T59.4X2	T59.4X3	T59.4X4	—	—
disinfectant	T59.4X1	T59.4X2	T59.4X3	T59.4X4	—	—
releasing agents NEC	T59.4X1	T59.4X2	T59.4X3	T59.4X4	—	—
Chlorisondamine chloride	T46.991	T46.992	T46.993	T46.994	T46.995	T46.996
Chlormadinone	T38.5X1	T38.5X2	T38.5X3	T38.5X4	T38.5X5	T38.5X6
Chlormephos	T60.0X1	T60.0X2	T60.0X3	T60.0X4	—	—
Chlormerodrin	T50.2X1	T50.2X2	T50.2X3	T50.2X4	T50.2X5	T50.2X6
Chlormethiazole	T42.6X1	T42.6X2	T42.6X3	T42.6X4	T42.6X5	T42.6X6
Chlormethine	T45.1X1	T45.1X2	T45.1X3	T45.1X4	T45.1X5	T45.1X6
Chlormethyle-necycline	T36.4X1	T36.4X2	T36.4X3	T36.4X4	T36.4X5	T36.4X6
Chlormezanone	T42.6X1	T42.6X2	T42.6X3	T42.6X4	T42.6X5	T42.6X6
Chloroacetic acid	T60.3X1	T60.3X2	T60.3X3	T60.3X4	—	—
Chloroacetone	T59.3X1	T59.3X2	T59.3X3	T59.3X4	—	—
Chloroacetophenone	T59.3X1	T59.3X2	T59.3X3	T59.3X4	—	—
Chloroaniline	T53.7X1	T53.7X2	T53.7X3	T53.7X4	—	—
Chlorobenzene, chlorobenzol	T53.7X1	T53.7X2	T53.7X3	T53.7X4	—	—
Chlorobromo methane (fire extinguisher)	T53.6X1	T53.6X2	T53.6X3	T53.6X4	—	—
Chlorobutanol	T49.0X1	T49.0X2	T49.0X3	T49.0X4	T49.0X5	T49.0X6
Chlorocresol	T49.0X1	T49.0X2	T49.0X3	T49.0X4	T49.0X5	T49.0X6
Chlorodehydro-methyltestosterone	T38.7X1	T38.7X2	T38.7X3	T38.7X4	T38.7X5	T38.7X6

Substance	Poisoning, Accidental (unintentional)	Poisoning, Intentional self-harm	Poisoning, Assault	Poisoning, Undetermined	Adverse effect	Underdosing
Chlorodinitro-benzene	T53.7X1	T53.7X2	T53.7X3	T53.7X4	—	—
dust or vapor	T53.7X1	T53.7X2	T53.7X3	T53.7X4	—	—
Chlorodiphenyl	T53.7X1	T53.7X2	T53.7X3	T53.7X4	—	—
Chloroethane—see Ethyl chloride						
Chloroethylene	T53.6X1	T53.6X2	T53.6X3	T53.6X4	—	—
Chlorofluorocarbons	T53.5X1	T53.5X2	T53.5X3	T53.5X4	—	—
Chloroform (fumes) (vapor)	T53.1X1	T53.1X2	T53.1X3	T53.1X4	—	—
anesthetic	T41.0X1	T41.0X2	T41.0X3	T41.0X4	T41.0X5	T41.0X6
solvent	T53.1X1	T53.1X2	T53.1X3	T53.1X4	—	—
water, concentrated	T41.0X1	T41.0X2	T41.0X3	T41.0X4	T41.0X5	T41.0X6
Chloroguanide	T37.2X1	T37.2X2	T37.2X3	T37.2X4	T37.2X5	T37.2X6
Chloromycetin	T36.2X1	T36.2X2	T36.2X3	T36.2X4	T36.2X5	T36.2X6
ENT agent	T49.6X1	T49.6X2	T49.6X3	T49.6X4	T49.6X5	T49.6X6
ophthalmic preparation	T49.5X1	T49.5X2	T49.5X3	T49.5X4	T49.5X5	T49.5X6
otic solution	T49.6X1	T49.6X2	T49.6X3	T49.6X4	T49.6X5	T49.6X6
topical NEC	T49.0X1	T49.0X2	T49.0X3	T49.0X4	T49.0X5	T49.0X6
Chloronitrobenzene	T53.7X1	T53.7X2	T53.7X3	T53.7X4	—	—
dust or vapor	T53.7X1	T53.7X2	T53.7X3	T53.7X4	—	—
Chlorophacinone	T60.4X1	T60.4X2	T60.4X3	T60.4X4	—	—
Chlorophenol	T53.7X1	T53.7X2	T53.7X3	T53.7X4	—	—
Chlorophenothane	T60.1X1	T60.1X2	T60.1X3	T60.1X4	—	—
Chlorophyll	T50.991	T50.992	T50.993	T50.994	T50.995	T50.996
Chloropicrin (fumes)	T53.6X1	T53.6X2	T53.6X3	T53.6X4	—	—
fumigant	T60.8X1	T60.8X2	T60.8X3	T60.8X4	—	—
fungicide	T60.3X1	T60.3X2	T60.3X3	T60.3X4	—	—
pesticide	T60.8X1	T60.8X2	T60.8X3	T60.8X4	—	—
Chloroprocaine	T41.3X1	T41.3X2	T41.3X3	T41.3X4	T41.3X5	T41.3X6
infiltration (subcutaneous)	T41.3X1	T41.3X2	T41.3X3	T41.3X4	T41.3X5	T41.3X6
nerve block (peripheral) (plexus)	T41.3X1	T41.3X2	T41.3X3	T41.3X4	T41.3X5	T41.3X6
spinal	T41.3X1	T41.3X2	T41.3X3	T41.3X4	T41.3X5	T41.3X6
Chloroptic	T49.5X1	T49.5X2	T49.5X3	T49.5X4	T49.5X5	T49.5X6
Chloropurine	T45.1X1	T45.1X2	T45.1X3	T45.1X4	T45.1X5	T45.1X6
Chloropyramine	T45.0X1	T45.0X2	T45.0X3	T45.0X4	T45.0X5	T45.0X6
Chloropyrifos	T60.0X1	T60.0X2	T60.0X3	T60.0X4	—	—
Chloropyrilene	T45.0X1	T45.0X2	T45.0X3	T45.0X4	T45.0X5	T45.0X6
Chloroquine	T37.2X1	T37.2X2	T37.2X3	T37.2X4	T37.2X5	T37.2X6
Chlorothalonil	T60.3X1	T60.3X2	T60.3X3	T60.3X4	—	—
Chlorothen	T45.0X1	T45.0X2	T45.0X3	T45.0X4	T45.0X5	T45.0X6
Chlorothiazide	T50.2X1	T50.2X2	T50.2X3	T50.2X4	T50.2X5	T50.2X6
Chlorothymol	T49.4X1	T49.4X2	T49.4X3	T49.4X4	T49.4X5	T49.4X6
Chlorotrianisene	T38.5X1	T38.5X2	T38.5X3	T38.5X4	T38.5X5	T38.5X6
Chlorovinyldichloro-arsine, not in war	T57.0X1	T57.0X2	T57.0X3	T57.0X4	—	—
Chloroxine	T49.4X1	T49.4X2	T49.4X3	T49.4X4	T49.4X5	T49.4X6
Chloroxylenol	T49.0X1	T49.0X2	T49.0X3	T49.0X4	T49.0X5	T49.0X6
Chlorphenamine	T45.0X1	T45.0X2	T45.0X3	T45.0X4	T45.0X5	T45.0X6
Chlorphenesin	T42.8X1	T42.8X2	T42.8X3	T42.8X4	T42.8X5	T42.8X6
topical (antifungal)	T49.0X1	T49.0X2	T49.0X3	T49.0X4	T49.0X5	T49.0X6
Chlorpheniramine	T45.0X1	T45.0X2	T45.0X3	T45.0X4	T45.0X5	T45.0X6

Substance	Poisoning, Accidental (unintentional)	Poisoning, Intentional self-harm	Poisoning, Assault	Poisoning, Undetermined	Adverse effect	Underdosing
Chlorphenoxamine	T45.0X1	T45.0X2	T45.0X3	T45.0X4	T45.0X5	T45.0X6
Chlorphentermine	T50.5X1	T50.5X2	T50.5X3	T50.5X4	T50.5X5	T50.5X6
Chlorprocaine—see Chloroprocaine						
Chlorproguanil	T37.2X1	T37.2X2	T37.2X3	T37.2X4	T37.2X5	T37.2X6
Chlorpromazine	T43.3X1	T43.3X2	T43.3X3	T43.3X4	T43.3X5	T43.3X6
Chlorpropamide	T38.3X1	T38.3X2	T38.3X3	T38.3X4	T38.3X5	T38.3X6
Chlorprothixene	T43.4X1	T43.4X2	T43.4X3	T43.4X4	T43.4X5	T43.4X6
Chlorquinaldol	T49.0X1	T49.0X2	T49.0X3	T49.0X4	T49.0X5	T49.0X6
Chlorquinol	T49.0X1	T49.0X2	T49.0X3	T49.0X4	T49.0X5	T49.0X6
Chlortalidone	T50.2X1	T50.2X2	T50.2X3	T50.2X4	T50.2X5	T50.2X6
Chlortetracycline	T36.4X1	T36.4X2	T36.4X3	T36.4X4	T36.4X5	T36.4X6
Chlorthalidone	T50.2X1	T50.2X2	T50.2X3	T50.2X4	T50.2X5	T50.2X6
Chlorthiophos	T60.0X1	T60.0X2	T60.0X3	T60.0X4	—	—
Chlortrianisene	T38.5X1	T38.5X2	T38.5X3	T38.5X4	T38.5X5	T38.5X6
Chlor-Trimeton	T45.0X1	T45.0X2	T45.0X3	T45.0X4	T45.0X5	T45.0X6
Chlorthion	T60.0X1	T60.0X2	T60.0X3	T60.0X4	—	—
Chlorzoxazone	T42.8X1	T42.8X2	T42.8X3	T42.8X4	T42.8X5	T42.8X6
Choke damp	T59.7X1	T59.7X2	T59.7X3	T59.7X4	—	—
Cholagogues	T47.5X1	T47.5X2	T47.5X3	T47.5X4	T47.5X5	T47.5X6
Cholebrine	T50.8X1	T50.8X2	T50.8X3	T50.8X4	T50.8X5	T50.8X6
Cholecalciferol	T45.2X1	T45.2X2	T45.2X3	T45.2X4	T45.2X5	T45.2X6
Cholecystokinin	T50.8X1	T50.8X2	T50.8X3	T50.8X4	T50.8X5	T50.8X6
Cholera vaccine	T50.A91	T50.A92	T50.A93	T50.A94	T50.A95	T50.A96
Choleretic	T47.5X1	T47.5X2	T47.5X3	T47.5X4	T47.5X5	T47.5X6
Cholesterol-lowering agents	T46.6X1	T46.6X2	T46.6X3	T46.6X4	T46.6X5	T46.6X6
Cholestyramine (resin)	T46.6X1	T46.6X2	T46.6X3	T46.6X4	T46.6X5	T46.6X6
Cholic acid	T47.5X1	T47.5X2	T47.5X3	T47.5X4	T47.5X5	T47.5X6
Choline	T48.6X1	T48.6X2	T48.6X3	T48.6X4	T48.6X5	T48.6X6
chloride	T50.991	T50.992	T50.993	T50.994	T50.995	T50.996
dihydrogen citrate	T50.991	T50.992	T50.993	T50.994	T50.995	T50.996
salicylate	T39.091	T39.092	T39.093	T39.094	T39.095	T39.096
theophyllinate	T48.6X1	T48.6X2	T48.6X3	T48.6X4	T48.6X5	T48.6X6
Cholinergic (drug) NEC	T44.1X1	T44.1X2	T44.1X3	T44.1X4	T44.1X5	T44.1X6
muscle tone enhancer	T44.1X1	T44.1X2	T44.1X3	T44.1X4	T44.1X5	T44.1X6
organophosphorus	T44.0X1	T44.0X2	T44.0X3	T44.0X4	T44.0X5	T44.0X6
insecticide	T60.0X1	T60.0X2	T60.0X3	T60.0X4	—	—
nerve gas	T59.891	T59.892	T59.893	T59.894	—	—
trimethyl ammonium propanediol	T44.1X1	T44.1X2	T44.1X3	T44.1X4	T44.1X5	T44.1X6
Cholinesterase reactivator	T50.6X1	T50.6X2	T50.6X3	T50.6X4	T50.6X5	T50.6X6
Cholografin	T50.8X1	T50.8X2	T50.8X3	T50.8X4	T50.8X5	T50.8X6
Chorionic gonadotropin	T38.891	T38.892	T38.893	T38.894	T38.895	T38.896
Chromate	T56.2X1	T56.2X2	T56.2X3	T56.2X4	—	—
dust or mist	T56.2X1	T56.2X2	T56.2X3	T56.2X4	—	—
lead—see also lead	T56.0X1	T56.0X2	T56.0X3	T56.0X4	—	—
paint	T56.0X1	T56.0X2	T56.0X3	T56.0X4	—	—
Chromic						
acid	T56.2X1	T56.2X2	T56.2X3	T56.2X4	—	—
dust or mist	T56.2X1	T56.2X2	T56.2X3	T56.2X4	—	—

Substance	Poisoning, Accidental (unintentional)	Poisoning, Intentional self-harm	Poisoning, Assault	Poisoning, Undetermined	Adverse effect	Underdosing
hromic — *Continued*						
phosphate 32P	T45.1X1	T45.1X2	T45.1X3	T45.1X4	T45.1X5	T45.1X6
hromium	T56.2X1	T56.2X2	T56.2X3	T56.2X4	—	—
mpounds—see Chromate						
sesquioxide	T50.8X1	T50.8X2	T50.8X3	T50.8X4	T50.8X5	T50.8X6
hromomycin A3	T45.1X1	T45.1X2	T45.1X3	T45.1X4	T45.1X5	T45.1X6
hromonar	T46.3X1	T46.3X2	T46.3X3	T46.3X4	T46.3X5	T46.3X6
hromyl chloride	T56.2X1	T56.2X2	T56.2X3	T56.2X4	—	—
hrysarobin	T49.4X1	T49.4X2	T49.4X3	T49.4X4	T49.4X5	T49.4X6
hrysazin	T47.2X1	T47.2X2	T47.2X3	T47.2X4	T47.2X5	T47.2X6
hymar	T45.3X1	T45.3X2	T45.3X3	T45.3X4	T45.3X5	T45.3X6
ophthalmic preparation	T49.5X1	T49.5X2	T49.5X3	T49.5X4	T49.5X5	T49.5X6
hymopapain	T45.3X1	T45.3X2	T45.3X3	T45.3X4	T45.3X5	T45.3X6
hymotrypsin	T45.3X1	T45.3X2	T45.3X3	T45.3X4	T45.3X5	T45.3X6
ophthalmic preparation	T49.5X1	T49.5X2	T49.5X3	T49.5X4	T49.5X5	T49.5X6
ianidanol	T50.991	T50.992	T50.993	T50.994	T50.995	T50.996
ianopramine	T43.011	T43.012	T43.013	T43.014	T43.015	T43.016
ibenzoline	T46.2X1	T46.2X2	T46.2X3	T46.2X4	T46.2X5	T46.2X6
iclacillin	T36.0X1	T36.0X2	T36.0X3	T36.0X4	T36.0X5	T36.0X6
iclobarbital—see exobarbital						
iclonicate	T46.7X1	T46.7X2	T46.7X3	T46.7X4	T46.7X5	T46.7X6
iclopirox (olamine)	T49.0X1	T49.0X2	T49.0X3	T49.0X4	T49.0X5	T49.0X6
iclosporin	T45.1X1	T45.1X2	T45.1X3	T45.1X4	T45.1X5	T45.1X6
icuta maculata or virosa	T62.2X1	T62.2X2	T62.2X3	T62.2X4	—	—
icutoxin	T62.2X1	T62.2X2	T62.2X3	T62.2X4	—	—
igarette lighter fluid	T52.0X1	T52.0X2	T52.0X3	T52.0X4	—	—
igarettes (tobacco)	T65.221	T65.222	T65.223	T65.224	—	—
iguatoxin	T61.01	T61.02	T61.03	T61.04	—	—
ilazapril	T46.4X1	T46.4X2	T46.4X3	T46.4X4	T46.4X5	T46.4X6
imetidine	T47.0X1	T47.0X2	T47.0X3	T47.0X4	T47.0X5	T47.0X6
imetropium bromide	T44.3X1	T44.3X2	T44.3X3	T44.3X4	T44.3X5	T44.3X6
inchocaine	T41.3X1	T41.3X2	T41.3X3	T41.3X4	T41.3X5	T41.3X6
topical (surface)	T41.3X1	T41.3X2	T41.3X3	T41.3X4	T41.3X5	T41.3X6
inchona	T37.2X1	T37.2X2	T37.2X3	T37.2X4	T37.2X5	T37.2X6
inchonine alkaloids	T37.2X1	T37.2X2	T37.2X3	T37.2X4	T37.2X5	T37.2X6
inchophen	T50.4X1	T50.4X2	T50.4X3	T50.4X4	T50.4X5	T50.4X6
inepazide	T46.7X1	T46.7X2	T46.7X3	T46.7X4	T46.7X5	T46.7X6
innamedrine	T48.5X1	T48.5X2	T48.5X3	T48.5X4	T48.5X5	T48.5X6
innarizine	T45.0X1	T45.0X2	T45.0X3	T45.0X4	T45.0X5	T45.0X6
inoxacin	T37.8X1	T37.8X2	T37.8X3	T37.8X4	T37.8X5	T37.8X6
iprofibrate	T46.6X1	T46.6X2	T46.6X3	T46.6X4	T46.6X5	T46.6X6
iprofloxacin	T36.8X1	T36.8X2	T36.8X3	T36.8X4	T36.8X5	T36.8X6
isapride	T47.8X1	T47.8X2	T47.8X3	T47.8X4	T47.8X5	T47.8X6
isplatin	T45.1X1	T45.1X2	T45.1X3	T45.1X4	T45.1X5	T45.1X6
Citalopram	T43.221	T43.222	T43.223	T43.224	T43.225	T43.226
Citanest	T41.3X1	T41.3X2	T41.3X3	T41.3X4	T41.3X5	T41.3X6
infiltration (subcutaneous)	T41.3X1	T41.3X2	T41.3X3	T41.3X4	T41.3X5	T41.3X6
nerve block (peripheral) (plexus)	T41.3X1	T41.3X2	T41.3X3	T41.3X4	T41.3X5	T41.3X6

Substance	Poisoning, Accidental (unintentional)	Poisoning, Intentional self-harm	Poisoning, Assault	Poisoning, Undetermined	Adverse effect	Underdosing
Citric acid	T47.5X1	T47.5X2	T47.5X3	T47.5X4	T47.5X5	T47.5X6
Citrovorum (factor)	T45.8X1	T45.8X2	T45.8X3	T45.8X4	T45.8X5	T45.8X6
Claviceps purpurea	T62.2X1	T62.2X2	T62.2X3	T62.2X4	—	—
Clavulanic acid	T36.1X1	T36.1X2	T36.1X3	T36.1X4	T36.1X5	T36.1X6
Cleaner, cleansing agent, type not specified	T65.891	T65.892	T65.893	T65.894	—	—
of paint or varnish	T52.91	T52.92	T52.93	T52.94	—	—
specified type NEC	T65.891	T65.892	T65.893	T65.894	—	—
Clebopride	T47.8X1	T47.8X2	T47.8X3	T47.8X4	T47.8X5	T47.8X6
Clefamide	T37.3X1	T37.3X2	T37.3X3	T37.3X4	T37.3X5	T37.3X6
Clemastine	T45.0X1	T45.0X2	T45.0X3	T45.0X4	T45.0X5	T45.0X6
Clematis vitalba	T62.2X1	T62.2X2	T62.2X3	T62.2X4	—	—
Clemizole	T45.0X1	T45.0X2	T45.0X3	T45.0X4	T45.0X5	T45.0X6
penicillin	T36.0X1	T36.0X2	T36.0X3	T36.0X4	T36.0X5	T36.0X6
Clenbuterol	T48.6X1	T48.6X2	T48.6X3	T48.6X4	T48.6X5	T48.6X6
Clidinium bromide	T44.3X1	T44.3X2	T44.3X3	T44.3X4	T44.3X5	T44.3X6
Clindamycin	T36.8X1	T36.8X2	T36.8X3	T36.8X4	T36.8X5	T36.8X6
Clinofibrate	T46.6X1	T46.6X2	T46.6X3	T46.6X4	T46.6X5	T46.6X6
Clioquinol	T37.8X1	T37.8X2	T37.8X3	T37.8X4	T37.8X5	T37.8X6
Cliradon	T40.2X1	T40.2X2	T40.2X3	T40.2X4	—	—
Clobazam	T42.4X1	T42.4X2	T42.4X3	T42.4X4	T42.4X5	T42.4X6
Clobenzorex	T50.5X1	T50.5X2	T50.5X3	T50.5X4	T50.5X5	T50.5X6
Clobetasol	T49.0X1	T49.0X2	T49.0X3	T49.0X4	T49.0X5	T49.0X6
Clobetasone	T49.0X1	T49.0X2	T49.0X3	T49.0X4	T49.0X5	T49.0X6
Clobutinol	T48.3X1	T48.3X2	T48.3X3	T48.3X4	T48.3X5	T48.3X6
Clocortolone	T38.0X1	T38.0X2	T38.0X3	T38.0X4	T38.0X5	T38.0X6
Clodantoin	T49.0X1	T49.0X2	T49.0X3	T49.0X4	T49.0X5	T49.0X6
Clodronic acid	T50.991	T50.992	T50.993	T50.994	T50.995	T50.996
Clofazimine	T37.1X1	T37.1X2	T37.1X3	T37.1X4	T37.1X5	T37.1X6
Clofedanol	T48.3X1	T48.3X2	T48.3X3	T48.3X4	T48.3X5	T48.3X6
Clofenamide	T50.2X1	T50.2X2	T50.2X3	T50.2X4	T50.2X5	T50.2X6
Clofenotane	T49.0X1	T49.0X2	T49.0X3	T49.0X4	T49.0X5	T49.0X6
Clofezone	T39.2X1	T39.2X2	T39.2X3	T39.2X4	T39.2X5	T39.2X6
Clofibrate	T46.6X1	T46.6X2	T46.6X3	T46.6X4	T46.6X5	T46.6X6
Clofibride	T46.6X1	T46.6X2	T46.6X3	T46.6X4	T46.6X5	T46.6X6
Cloforex	T50.5X1	T50.5X2	T50.5X3	T50.5X4	T50.5X5	T50.5X6
Clomethiazole	T42.6X1	T42.6X2	T42.6X3	T42.6X4	T42.6X5	T42.6X6
Clometocillin	T36.0X1	T36.0X2	T36.0X3	T36.0X4	T36.0X5	T36.0X6
Clomifene	T38.5X1	T38.5X2	T38.5X3	T38.5X4	T38.5X5	T38.5X6
Clomiphene	T38.5X1	T38.5X2	T38.5X3	T38.5X4	T38.5X5	T38.5X6
Clomipramine	T43.011	T43.012	T43.013	T43.014	T43.015	T43.016
Clomocycline	T36.4X1	T36.4X2	T36.4X3	T36.4X4	T36.4X5	T36.4X6
Clonazepam	T42.4X1	T42.4X2	T42.4X3	T42.4X4	T42.4X5	T42.4X6
Clonidine	T46.5X1	T46.5X2	T46.5X3	T46.5X4	T46.5X5	T46.5X6
Clonixin	T39.8X1	T39.8X2	T39.8X3	T39.8X4	T39.8X5	T39.8X6
Clopamide	T50.2X1	T50.2X2	T50.2X3	T50.2X4	T50.2X5	T50.2X6
Clopenthixol	T43.4X1	T43.4X2	T43.4X3	T43.4X4	T43.4X5	T43.4X6
Cloperastine	T48.3X1	T48.3X2	T48.3X3	T48.3X4	T48.3X5	T48.3X6
Clophedianol	T48.3X1	T48.3X2	T48.3X3	T48.3X4	T48.3X5	T48.3X6
Cloponone	T36.2X1	T36.2X2	T36.2X3	T36.2X4	T36.2X5	T36.2X6

Substance	Poisoning, Accidental (unintentional)	Poisoning, Intentional self-harm	Poisoning, Assault	Poisoning, Undetermined	Adverse effect	Underdosing
Clopednol	T38.0X1	T38.0X2	T38.0X3	T38.0X4	T38.0X5	T38.0X6
Cloral betaine	T42.6X1	T42.6X2	T42.6X3	T42.6X4	T42.6X5	T42.6X6
Cloramfenicol	T36.2X1	T36.2X2	T36.2X3	T36.2X4	T36.2X5	T36.2X6
Clorazepate (dipotassium)	T42.4X1	T42.4X2	T42.4X3	T42.4X4	T42.4X5	T42.4X6
Clorexolone	T50.2X1	T50.2X2	T50.2X3	T50.2X4	T50.2X5	T50.2X6
Clorfenamine	T45.0X1	T45.0X2	T45.0X3	T45.0X4	T45.0X5	T45.0X6
Clorgiline	T43.1X1	T43.1X2	T43.1X3	T43.1X4	T43.1X5	T43.1X6
Clorotepine	T44.3X1	T44.3X2	T44.3X3	T44.3X4	T44.3X5	T44.3X6
Clorox (bleach)	T54.91	T54.92	T54.93	T54.94	—	—
Clorprenaline	T48.6X1	T48.6X2	T48.6X3	T48.6X4	T48.6X5	T48.6X6
Clortermine	T50.5X1	T50.5X2	T50.5X3	T50.5X4	T50.5X5	T50.5X6
Clotiapine	T43.591	T43.592	T43.593	T43.594	T43.595	T43.596
Clotiazepam	T42.4X1	T42.4X2	T42.4X3	T42.4X4	T42.4X5	T42.4X6
Clotibric acid	T46.6X1	T46.6X2	T46.6X3	T46.6X4	T46.6X5	T46.6X6
Clotrimazole	T49.0X1	T49.0X2	T49.0X3	T49.0X4	T49.0X5	T49.0X6
Cloxacillin	T36.0X1	T36.0X2	T36.0X3	T36.0X4	T36.0X5	T36.0X6
Cloxazolam	T42.4X1	T42.4X2	T42.4X3	T42.4X4	T42.4X5	T42.4X6
Cloxiquine	T49.0X1	T49.0X2	T49.0X3	T49.0X4	T49.0X5	T49.0X6
Clozapine	T42.4X1	T42.4X2	T42.4X3	T42.4X4	T42.4X5	T42.4X6
Coagulant NEC	T45.7X1	T45.7X2	T45.7X3	T45.7X4	T45.7X5	T45.7X6
Coal (carbon monoxide from)—see also Carbon, monoxide, coal	T58.2X1	T58.2X2	T58.2X3	T58.2X4	—	—
oil—see Kerosene						
tar	T49.1X1	T49.1X2	T49.1X3	T49.1X4	T49.1X5	T49.1X6
fumes	T59.891	T59.892	T59.893	T59.894	—	—
medicinal (ointment)	T49.4X1	T49.4X2	T49.4X3	T49.4X4	T49.4X5	T49.4X6
analgesics NEC	T39.2X1	T39.2X2	T39.2X3	T39.2X4	T39.2X5	T39.2X6
naphtha (solvent)	T52.0X1	T52.0X2	T52.0X3	T52.0X4	—	—
Cobalamine	T45.2X1	T45.2X2	T45.2X3	T45.2X4	T45.2X5	T45.2X6
Cobalt (nonmedicinal) (fumes) (industrial)	T56.891	T56.892	T56.893	T56.894	—	—
medicinal (trace) (chloride)	T45.8X1	T45.8X2	T45.8X3	T45.8X4	T45.8X5	T45.8X6
Cobra (venom)	T63.041	T63.042	T63.043	T63.044	—	—
Coca (leaf)	T40.5X1	T40.5X2	T40.5X3	T40.5X4	T40.5X5	T40.5X6
Cocaine	T40.5X1	T40.5X2	T40.5X3	T40.5X4	T40.5X5	T40.5X6
topical anesthetic	T41.3X1	T41.3X2	T41.3X3	T41.3X4	T41.3X5	T41.3X6
Cocarboxylase	T45.3X1	T45.3X2	T45.3X3	T45.3X4	T45.3X5	T45.3X6
Coccidioidin	T50.8X1	T50.8X2	T50.8X3	T50.8X4	T50.8X5	T50.8X6
Cocculus indicus	T62.1X1	T62.1X2	T62.1X3	T62.1X4	—	—
Cochineal	T65.6X1	T65.6X2	T65.6X3	T65.6X4	—	—
medicinal products	T50.991	T50.992	T50.993	T50.994	T50.995	T50.996
Codeine	T40.2X1	T40.2X2	T40.2X3	T40.2X4	T40.2X5	T40.2X6
Cod-liver oil	T45.2X1	T45.2X2	T45.2X3	T45.2X4	T45.2X5	T45.2X6
Coenzyme A	T50.991	T50.992	T50.993	T50.994	T50.995	T50.996
Coffee	T62.8X1	T62.8X2	T62.8X3	T62.8X4	—	—
Cogalactoiso-merase	T50.991	T50.992	T50.993	T50.994	T50.995	T50.996
Cogentin	T44.3X1	T44.3X2	T44.3X3	T44.3X4	T44.3X5	T44.3X6
Coke fumes or gas (carbon monoxide)	T58.2X1	T58.2X2	T58.2X3	T58.2X4	—	—
industrial use	T58.8X1	T58.8X2	T58.8X3	T58.8X4	—	—
Colace	T47.4X1	T47.4X2	T47.4X3	T47.4X4	T47.4X5	T47.4X6

Substance	Poisoning, Accidental (unintentional)	Poisoning, Intentional self-harm	Poisoning, Assault	Poisoning, Undetermined	Adverse effect	Underdosing
Colaspase	T45.1X1	T45.1X2	T45.1X3	T45.1X4	T45.1X5	T45.1X
Colchicine	T50.4X1	T50.4X2	T50.4X3	T50.4X4	T50.4X5	T50.4X
Colchicum	T62.2X1	T62.2X2	T62.2X3	T62.2X4	—	—
Cold cream	T49.3X1	T49.3X2	T49.3X3	T49.3X4	T49.3X5	T49.3X
Colecalciferol	T45.2X1	T45.2X2	T45.2X3	T45.2X4	T45.2X5	T45.2X
Colestipol	T46.6X1	T46.6X2	T46.6X3	T46.6X4	T46.6X5	T46.6X
Colestyramine	T46.6X1	T46.6X2	T46.6X3	T46.6X4	T46.6X5	T46.6X
Colimycin	T36.8X1	T36.8X2	T36.8X3	T36.8X4	T36.8X5	T36.8X
Colistimethate	T36.8X1	T36.8X2	T36.8X3	T36.8X4	T36.8X5	T36.8X
Colistin	T36.8X1	T36.8X2	T36.8X3	T36.8X4	T36.8X5	T36.8X
sulfate (eye preparation)	T49.5X1	T49.5X2	T49.5X3	T49.5X4	T49.5X5	T49.5X
Collagen	T50.991	T50.992	T50.993	T50.994	T50.995	T50.99
Collagenase	T49.4X1	T49.4X2	T49.4X3	T49.4X4	T49.4X5	T49.4X
Collodion	T49.3X1	T49.3X2	T49.3X3	T49.3X4	T49.3X5	T49.3X
Colocynth	T47.2X1	T47.2X2	T47.2X3	T47.2X4	T47.2X5	T47.2X
Colophony adhesive	T49.3X1	T49.3X2	T49.3X3	T49.3X4	T49.3X5	T49.3X
Colorant—see also Dye	T50.991	T50.992	T50.993	T50.994	T50.995	T50.99
Coloring matter—see Dye(s)						
Combustion gas (after combustion)—see Carbon, monoxide						
prior to combustion	T59.891	T59.892	T59.893	T59.894	—	—
Compazine	T43.3X1	T43.3X2	T43.3X3	T43.3X4	T43.3X5	T43.3X
Compound						
42 (warfarin)	T60.4X1	T60.4X2	T60.4X3	T60.4X4	—	—
269 (endrin)	T60.1X1	T60.1X2	T60.1X3	T60.1X4	—	—
497 (dieldrin)	T60.1X1	T60.1X2	T60.1X3	T60.1X4	—	—
1080 (sodium fluoroacetate)	T60.4X1	T60.4X2	T60.4X3	T60.4X4	—	—
3422 (parathion)	T60.0X1	T60.0X2	T60.0X3	T60.0X4	—	—
3911 (phorate)	T60.0X1	T60.0X2	T60.0X3	T60.0X4	—	—
3956 (toxaphene)	T60.1X1	T60.1X2	T60.1X3	T60.1X4	—	—
4049 (malathion)	T60.0X1	T60.0X2	T60.0X3	T60.0X4	—	—
4069 (malathion)	T60.0X1	T60.0X2	T60.0X3	T60.0X4	—	—
4124 (dicapthon)	T60.0X1	T60.0X2	T60.0X3	T60.0X4	—	—
E (cortisone)	T38.0X1	T38.0X2	T38.0X3	T38.0X4	T38.0X5	T38.0X
F (hydrocortisone)	T38.0X1	T38.0X2	T38.0X3	T38.0X4	T38.0X5	T38.0X
Congener, avwnabolic	T38.7X1	T38.7X2	T38.7X3	T38.7X4	T38.7X5	T38.7X
Congo red	T50.8X1	T50.8X2	T50.8X3	T50.8X4	T50.8X5	T50.8X
Coniine, conine	T62.2X1	T62.2X2	T62.2X3	T62.2X4	—	—
Conium (maculatum)	T62.2X1	T62.2X2	T62.2X3	T62.2X4	—	—
Conjugated estrogenic substances	T38.5X1	T38.5X2	T38.5X3	T38.5X4	T38.5X5	T38.5X
Contac	T48.5X1	T48.5X2	T48.5X3	T48.5X4	T48.5X5	T48.5X
Contact lens solution	T49.5X1	T49.5X2	T49.5X3	T49.5X4	T49.5X5	T49.5X
Contraceptive (oral)	T38.4X1	T38.4X2	T38.4X3	T38.4X4	T38.4X5	T38.4X
vaginal	T49.8X1	T49.8X2	T49.8X3	T49.8X4	T49.8X5	T49.8X
Contrast medium, radiography	T50.8X1	T50.8X2	T50.8X3	T50.8X4	T50.8X5	T50.8X
Convallaria glycosides	T46.0X1	T46.0X2	T46.0X3	T46.0X4	T46.0X5	T46.0X

Substance	Poisoning, Accidental (unintentional)	Poisoning, Intentional self-harm	Poisoning, Assault	Poisoning, Undetermined	Adverse effect	Underdosing
Convallaria majalis	T62.2X1	T62.2X2	T62.2X3	T62.2X4	—	—
berry	T62.1X1	T62.1X2	T62.1X3	T62.1X4	—	—
Copper (dust) (fumes) (nonmedicinal) NEC	T56.4X1	T56.4X2	T56.4X3	T56.4X4	—	—
arsenate, arsenite	T57.0X1	T57.0X2	T57.0X3	T57.0X4	—	—
insecticide	T60.2X1	T60.2X2	T60.2X3	T60.2X4	—	—
emetic	T47.7X1	T47.7X2	T47.7X3	T47.7X4	T47.7X5	T47.7X6
fungicide	T60.3X1	T60.3X2	T60.3X3	T60.3X4	—	—
gluconate	T49.0X1	T49.0X2	T49.0X3	T49.0X4	T49.0X5	T49.0X6
insecticide	T60.2X1	T60.2X2	T60.2X3	T60.2X4	—	—
medicinal (trace)	T45.8X1	T45.8X2	T45.8X3	T45.8X4	T45.8X5	T45.8X6
oleate	T49.0X1	T49.0X2	T49.0X3	T49.0X4	T49.0X5	T49.0X6
sulfate	T56.4X1	T56.4X2	T56.4X3	T56.4X4	—	—
cupric	T56.4X1	T56.4X2	T56.4X3	T56.4X4	—	—
fungicide	T60.3X1	T60.3X2	T60.3X3	T60.3X4	—	—
medicinal						
ear	T49.6X1	T49.6X2	T49.6X3	T49.6X4	T49.6X5	T49.6X6
emetic	T47.7X1	T47.7X2	T47.7X3	T47.7X4	T47.7X5	T47.7X6
eye	T49.5X1	T49.5X2	T49.5X3	T49.5X4	T49.5X5	T49.5X6
cuprous	T56.4X1	T56.4X2	T56.4X3	T56.4X4	—	—
fungicide	T60.3X1	T60.3X2	T60.3X3	T60.3X4	—	—
medicinal						
ear	T49.6X1	T49.6X2	T49.6X3	T49.6X4	T49.6X5	T49.6X6
emetic	T47.7X1	T47.7X2	T47.7X3	T47.7X4	T47.7X5	T47.7X6
eye	T49.5X1	T49.5X2	T49.5X3	T49.5X4	T49.5X5	T49.5X6
Copperhead snake (bite) (venom)	T63.061	T63.062	T63.063	T63.064	—	—
Coral (sting)	T63.691	T63.692	T63.693	T63.694	—	—
snake (bite) (venom)	T63.021	T63.022	T63.023	T63.024	—	—
Corbadrine	T49.6X1	T49.6X2	T49.6X3	T49.6X4	T49.6X5	T49.6X6
Cordite	T65.891	T65.892	T65.893	T65.894	—	—
vapor	T59.891	T59.892	T59.893	T59.894	—	—
Cordran	T49.0X1	T49.0X2	T49.0X3	T49.0X4	T49.0X5	T49.0X6
Corn cures	T49.4X1	T49.4X2	T49.4X3	T49.4X4	T49.4X5	T49.4X6
Corn starch	T49.3X1	T49.3X2	T49.3X3	T49.3X4	T49.3X5	T49.3X6
Cornhusker's lotion	T49.3X1	T49.3X2	T49.3X3	T49.3X4	T49.3X5	T49.3X6
Coronary vasodilator NEC	T46.3X1	T46.3X2	T46.3X3	T46.3X4	T46.3X5	T46.3X6
Corrosive NEC	T54.91	T54.92	T54.93	T54.94	—	—
acid NEC	T54.2X1	T54.2X2	T54.2X3	T54.2X4	—	—
aromatics	T54.1X1	T54.1X2	T54.1X3	T54.1X4	—	—
disinfectant	T54.1X1	T54.1X2	T54.1X3	T54.1X4	—	—
fumes NEC	T54.91	T54.92	T54.93	T54.94	—	—
specified NEC	T54.91	T54.92	T54.93	T54.94	—	—
sublimate	T56.1X1	T56.1X2	T56.1X3	T56.1X4	—	—
Cortate	T38.0X1	T38.0X2	T38.0X3	T38.0X4	T38.0X5	T38.0X6
Cort-Dome	T38.0X1	T38.0X2	T38.0X3	T38.0X4	T38.0X5	T38.0X6
ENT agent	T49.6X1	T49.6X2	T49.6X3	T49.6X4	T49.6X5	T49.6X6
ophthalmic preparation	T49.5X1	T49.5X2	T49.5X3	T49.5X4	T49.5X5	T49.5X6
topical NEC	T49.0X1	T49.0X2	T49.0X3	T49.0X4	T49.0X5	T49.0X6

Substance	Poisoning, Accidental (unintentional)	Poisoning, Intentional self-harm	Poisoning, Assault	Poisoning, Undetermined	Adverse effect	Underdosing
Cortef	T38.0X1	T38.0X2	T38.0X3	T38.0X4	T38.0X5	T38.0X6
ENT agent	T49.6X1	T49.6X2	T49.6X3	T49.6X4	T49.6X5	T49.6X6
ophthalmic preparation	T49.5X1	T49.5X2	T49.5X3	T49.5X4	T49.5X5	T49.5X6
topical NEC	T49.0X1	T49.0X2	T49.0X3	T49.0X4	T49.0X5	T49.0X6
Corticosteroid	T38.0X1	T38.0X2	T38.0X3	T38.0X4	T38.0X5	T38.0X6
ENT agent	T49.6X1	T49.6X2	T49.6X3	T49.6X4	T49.6X5	T49.6X6
mineral	T50.0X1	T50.0X2	T50.0X3	T50.0X4	T50.0X5	T50.0X6
ophthalmic	T49.5X1	T49.5X2	T49.5X3	T49.5X4	T49.5X5	T49.5X6
topical NEC	T49.0X1	T49.0X2	T49.0X3	T49.0X4	T49.0X5	T49.0X6
Corticotropin	T38.811	T38.812	T38.813	T38.814	T38.815	T38.816
Cortisol	T49.0X1	T49.0X2	T49.0X3	T49.0X4	T49.0X5	T49.0X6
ENT agent	T49.6X1	T49.6X2	T49.6X3	T49.6X4	T49.6X5	T49.6X6
ophthalmic preparation	T49.5X1	T49.5X2	T49.5X3	T49.5X4	T49.5X5	T49.5X6
topical NEC	T49.0X1	T49.0X2	T49.0X3	T49.0X4	T49.0X5	T49.0X6
Cortisone (acetate)	T38.0X1	T38.0X2	T38.0X3	T38.0X4	T38.0X5	T38.0X6
ENT agent	T49.6X1	T49.6X2	T49.6X3	T49.6X4	T49.6X5	T49.6X6
ophthalmic preparation	T49.5X1	T49.5X2	T49.5X3	T49.5X4	T49.5X5	T49.5X6
topical NEC	T49.0X1	T49.0X2	T49.0X3	T49.0X4	T49.0X5	T49.0X6
Cortivazol	T38.0X1	T38.0X2	T38.0X3	T38.0X4	T38.0X5	T38.0X6
Cortogen	T38.0X1	T38.0X2	T38.0X3	T38.0X4	T38.0X5	T38.0X6
ENT agent	T49.6X1	T49.6X2	T49.6X3	T49.6X4	T49.6X5	T49.6X6
ophthalmic preparation	T49.5X1	T49.5X2	T49.5X3	T49.5X4	T49.5X5	T49.5X6
Cortone	T38.0X1	T38.0X2	T38.0X3	T38.0X4	T38.0X5	T38.0X6
ENT agent	T49.6X1	T49.6X2	T49.6X3	T49.6X4	T49.6X5	T49.6X6
ophthalmic preparation	T49.5X1	T49.5X2	T49.5X3	T49.5X4	T49.5X5	T49.5X6
Cortril	T38.0X1	T38.0X2	T38.0X3	T38.0X4	T38.0X5	T38.0X6
ENT agent	T49.6X1	T49.6X2	T49.6X3	T49.6X4	T49.6X5	T49.6X6
ophthalmic preparation	T49.5X1	T49.5X2	T49.5X3	T49.5X4	T49.5X5	T49.5X6
topical NEC	T49.0X1	T49.0X2	T49.0X3	T49.0X4	T49.0X5	T49.0X6
Corynebacterium parvum	T45.1X1	T45.1X2	T45.1X3	T45.1X4	T45.1X5	T45.1X6
Cosmetic preparation	T49.8X1	T49.8X2	T49.8X3	T49.8X4	T49.8X5	T49.8X6
Cosmetics	T49.8X1	T49.8X2	T49.8X3	T49.8X4	T49.8X5	T49.8X6
Cosyntropin	T38.811	T38.812	T38.813	T38.814	T38.815	T38.816
Cotarnine	T45.7X1	T45.7X2	T45.7X3	T45.7X4	T45.7X5	T45.7X6
Co-trimoxazole	T36.8X1	T36.8X2	T36.8X3	T36.8X4	T36.8X5	T36.8X6
Cottonseed oil	T49.3X1	T49.3X2	T49.3X3	T49.3X4	T49.3X5	T49.3X6
Cough mixture (syrup)	T48.4X1	T48.4X2	T48.4X3	T48.4X4	T48.4X5	T48.4X6
containing opiates	T40.2X1	T40.2X2	T40.2X3	T40.2X4	T40.2X5	T40.2X6
expectorants	T48.4X1	T48.4X2	T48.4X3	T48.4X4	T48.4X5	T48.4X6
Coumadin	T45.511	T45.512	T45.513	T45.514	T45.515	T45.516
rodenticide	T60.4X1	T60.4X2	T60.4X3	T60.4X4	—	—
Coumaphos	T60.0X1	T60.0X2	T60.0X3	T60.0X4	—	—
Coumarin	T45.511	T45.512	T45.513	T45.514	T45.515	T45.516
Coumetarol	T45.511	T45.512	T45.513	T45.514	T45.515	T45.516
Cowbane	T62.2X1	T62.2X2	T62.2X3	T62.2X4	—	—
Cozyme	T45.2X1	T45.2X2	T45.2X3	T45.2X4	T45.2X5	T45.2X6
Crack	T40.5X1	T40.5X2	T40.5X3	T40.5X4	—	—
Crataegus extract	T46.0X1	T46.0X2	T46.0X3	T46.0X4	T46.0X5	T46.0X6
Creolin	T54.1X1	T54.1X2	T54.1X3	T54.1X4	—	—
disinfectant	T54.1X1	T54.1X2	T54.1X3	T54.1X4	—	—

Substance	Poisoning, Accidental (unintentional)	Poisoning, Intentional self-harm	Poisoning, Assault	Poisoning, Undetermined	Adverse effect	Underdosing
Creosol (compound)	T49.0X1	T49.0X2	T49.0X3	T49.0X4	T49.0X5	T49.0X6
Creosote (coal tar) (beechwood)	T49.0X1	T49.0X2	T49.0X3	T49.0X4	T49.0X5	T49.0X6
medicinal (expectorant)	T48.4X1	T48.4X2	T48.4X3	T48.4X4	T48.4X5	T48.4X6
syrup	T48.4X1	T48.4X2	T48.4X3	T48.4X4	T48.4X5	T48.4X6
Cresol(s)	T49.0X1	T49.0X2	T49.0X3	T49.0X4	T49.0X5	T49.0X6
and soap solution	T49.0X1	T49.0X2	T49.0X3	T49.0X4	T49.0X5	T49.0X6
Cresyl acetate	T49.0X1	T49.0X2	T49.0X3	T49.0X4	T49.0X5	T49.0X6
Cresylic acid	T49.0X1	T49.0X2	T49.0X3	T49.0X4	T49.0X5	T49.0X6
Crimidine	T60.4X1	T60.4X2	T60.4X3	T60.4X4	—	—
Croconazole	T37.8X1	T37.8X2	T37.8X3	T37.8X4	T37.8X5	T37.8X6
Cromoglicic acid	T48.6X1	T48.6X2	T48.6X3	T48.6X4	T48.6X5	T48.6X6
Cromolyn	T48.6X1	T48.6X2	T48.6X3	T48.6X4	T48.6X5	T48.6X6
Cromonar	T46.3X1	T46.3X2	T46.3X3	T46.3X4	T46.3X5	T46.3X6
Cropropamide	T39.8X1	T39.8X2	T39.8X3	T39.8X4	T39.8X5	T39.8X6
with crotethamide	T50.7X1	T50.7X2	T50.7X3	T50.7X4	T50.7X5	T50.7X6
Crotamiton	T49.0X1	T49.0X2	T49.0X3	T49.0X4	T49.0X5	T49.0X6
Crotethamide	T39.8X1	T39.8X2	T39.8X3	T39.8X4	T39.8X5	T39.8X6
with cropropamide	T50.7X1	T50.7X2	T50.7X3	T50.7X4	T50.7X5	T50.7X6
Croton (oil)	T47.2X1	T47.2X2	T47.2X3	T47.2X4	T47.2X5	T47.2X6
chloral	T42.6X1	T42.6X2	T42.6X3	T42.6X4	T42.6X5	T42.6X6
Crude oil	T52.0X1	T52.0X2	T52.0X3	T52.0X4	—	—
Cryogenine	T39.8X1	T39.8X2	T39.8X3	T39.8X4	T39.8X5	T39.8X6
Cryolite (vapor)	T60.1X1	T60.1X2	T60.1X3	T60.1X4	—	—
insecticide	T60.1X1	T60.1X2	T60.1X3	T60.1X4	—	—
Cryptenamine (tannates)	T46.5X1	T46.5X2	T46.5X3	T46.5X4	T46.5X5	T46.5X6
Crystal violet	T49.0X1	T49.0X2	T49.0X3	T49.0X4	T49.0X5	T49.0X6
Cuckoopint	T62.2X1	T62.2X2	T62.2X3	T62.2X4	—	—
Cumetharol	T45.511	T45.512	T45.513	T45.514	T45.515	T45.516
Cupric						
acetate	T60.3X1	T60.3X2	T60.3X3	T60.3X4	—	—
acetoarsenite	T57.0X1	T57.0X2	T57.0X3	T57.0X4	—	—
arsenate	T57.0X1	T57.0X2	T57.0X3	T57.0X4	—	—
gluconate	T49.0X1	T49.0X2	T49.0X3	T49.0X4	T49.0X5	T49.0X6
oleate	T49.0X1	T49.0X2	T49.0X3	T49.0X4	T49.0X5	T49.0X6
sulfate	T56.4X1	T56.4X2	T56.4X3	T56.4X4	—	—
Cuprous sulfate—see also Copper sulfate	T56.4X1	T56.4X2	T56.4X3	T56.4X4	—	—
Curare, curarine	T48.1X1	T48.1X2	T48.1X3	T48.1X4	T48.1X5	T48.1X6
Cyamemazine	T43.3X1	T43.3X2	T43.3X3	T43.3X4	T43.3X5	T43.3X6
Cyamopsis tetragono-loba	T46.6X1	T46.6X2	T46.6X3	T46.6X4	T46.6X5	T46.6X6
Cyanacetyl hydrazide	T37.1X1	T37.1X2	T37.1X3	T37.1X4	T37.1X5	T37.1X6
Cyanic acid (gas)	T59.891	T59.892	T59.893	T59.894	—	—
Cyanide(s) (compounds) (potassium) (sodium) NEC	T65.0X1	T65.0X2	T65.0X3	T65.0X4	—	—
dust or gas (inhalation) NEC	T57.3X1	T57.3X2	T57.3X3	T57.3X4	—	—
fumigant	T65.0X1	T65.0X2	T65.0X3	T65.0X4	—	—
hydrogen	T57.3X1	T57.3X2	T57.3X3	T57.3X4	—	—
mercuric—see *Mercury*						
pesticide (dust) (fumes)	T65.0X1	T65.0X2	T65.0X3	T65.0X4	—	—

Substance	Poisoning, Accidental (unintentional)	Poisoning, Intentional self-harm	Poisoning, Assault	Poisoning, Undetermined	Adverse effect	Underdosing
Cyanoacrylate adhesive	T49.3X1	T49.3X2	T49.3X3	T49.3X4	T49.3X5	T49.3X
Cyanocobalamin	T45.8X1	T45.8X2	T45.8X3	T45.8X4	T45.8X5	T45.8X
Cyanogen (chloride) (gas) NEC	T59.891	T59.892	T59.893	T59.894	—	—
Cyclacillin	T36.0X1	T36.0X2	T36.0X3	T36.0X4	T36.0X5	T36.0X
Cyclaine	T41.3X1	T41.3X2	T41.3X3	T41.3X4	T41.3X5	T41.3X
Cyclamate	T50.991	T50.992	T50.993	T50.994	T50.995	T50.99
Cyclamen europaeum	T62.2X1	T62.2X2	T62.2X3	T62.2X4	—	—
Cyclandelate	T46.7X1	T46.7X2	T46.7X3	T46.7X4	T46.7X5	T46.7X
Cyclazocine	T50.7X1	T50.7X2	T50.7X3	T50.7X4	T50.7X5	T50.7X
Cyclizine	T45.0X1	T45.0X2	T45.0X3	T45.0X4	T45.0X5	T45.0X
Cyclobarbital	T42.3X1	T42.3X2	T42.3X3	T42.3X4	T42.3X5	T42.3X
Cyclobarbitone	T42.3X1	T42.3X2	T42.3X3	T42.3X4	T42.3X5	T42.3X
Cyclobenzaprine	T48.1X1	T48.1X2	T48.1X3	T48.1X4	T48.1X5	T48.1X
Cyclodrine	T44.3X1	T44.3X2	T44.3X3	T44.3X4	T44.3X5	T44.3X
Cycloguanil embonate	T37.2X1	T37.2X2	T37.2X3	T37.2X4	T37.2X5	T37.2X
Cyclohexane	T52.8X1	T52.8X2	T52.8X3	T52.8X4	—	—
Cyclohexanol	T51.8X1	T51.8X2	T51.8X3	T51.8X4	—	—
Cyclohexanone	T52.4X1	T52.4X2	T52.4X3	T52.4X4	—	—
Cycloheximide	T60.3X1	T60.3X2	T60.3X3	T60.3X4	—	—
Cyclohexyl acetate	T52.8X1	T52.8X2	T52.8X3	T52.8X4	—	—
Cycloleucin	T45.1X1	T45.1X2	T45.1X3	T45.1X4	T45.1X5	T45.1X
Cyclomethycaine	T41.3X1	T41.3X2	T41.3X3	T41.3X4	T41.3X5	T41.3X
Cyclopentamine	T44.4X1	T44.4X2	T44.4X3	T44.4X4	T44.4X5	T44.4X
Cyclopenthiazide	T50.2X1	T50.2X2	T50.2X3	T50.2X4	T50.2X5	T50.2X
Cyclopentolate	T44.3X1	T44.3X2	T44.3X3	T44.3X4	T44.3X5	T44.3X
Cyclophosphamide	T45.1X1	T45.1X2	T45.1X3	T45.1X4	T45.1X5	T45.1X
Cycloplegic drug	T49.5X1	T49.5X2	T49.5X3	T49.5X4	T49.5X5	T49.5X
Cyclopropane	T41.291	T41.292	T41.293	T41.294	T41.295	T41.29
Cyclopyrabital	T39.8X1	T39.8X2	T39.8X3	T39.8X4	T39.8X5	T39.8X
Cycloserine	T37.1X1	T37.1X2	T37.1X3	T37.1X4	T37.1X5	T37.1X
Cyclosporin	T45.1X1	T45.1X2	T45.1X3	T45.1X4	T45.1X5	T45.1X
Cyclothiazide	T50.2X1	T50.2X2	T50.2X3	T50.2X4	T50.2X5	T50.2X
Cycrimine	T44.3X1	T44.3X2	T44.3X3	T44.3X4	T44.3X5	T44.3X
Cyhalothrin	T60.1X1	T60.1X2	T60.1X3	T60.1X4	—	—
Cymarin	T46.0X1	T46.0X2	T46.0X3	T46.0X4	T46.0X5	T46.0X
Cypermethrin	T60.1X1	T60.1X2	T60.1X3	T60.1X4	—	—
Cyphenothrin	T60.2X1	T60.2X2	T60.2X3	T60.2X4	—	—
Cyproheptadine	T45.0X1	T45.0X2	T45.0X3	T45.0X4	T45.0X5	T45.0X
Cyproterone	T38.6X1	T38.6X2	T38.6X3	T38.6X4	T38.6X5	T38.6X
Cysteamine	T50.6X1	T50.6X2	T50.6X3	T50.6X4	T50.6X5	T50.6X
Cytarabine	T45.1X1	T45.1X2	T45.1X3	T45.1X4	T45.1X5	T45.1X
Cytisus						
laburnum	T62.2X1	T62.2X2	T62.2X3	T62.2X4	—	—
scoparius	T62.2X1	T62.2X2	T62.2X3	T62.2X4	—	—
Cytochrome C	T47.5X1	T47.5X2	T47.5X3	T47.5X4	T47.5X5	T47.5X
Cytomel	T38.1X1	T38.1X2	T38.1X3	T38.1X4	T38.1X5	T38.1X
Cytosine arabinoside	T45.1X1	T45.1X2	T45.1X3	T45.1X4	T45.1X5	T45.1X
Cytoxan	T45.1X1	T45.1X2	T45.1X3	T45.1X4	T45.1X5	T45.1X

Substance	Poisoning, Accidental (unintentional)	Poisoning, Intentional self-harm	Poisoning, Assault	Poisoning, Undetermined	Adverse effect	Underdosing
Cytozyme	T45.7X1	T45.7X2	T45.7X3	T45.7X4	T45.7X5	T45.7X6
2,4-D	T60.3X1	T60.3X2	T60.3X3	T60.3X4	—	—
D						
Dacarbazine	T45.1X1	T45.1X2	T45.1X3	T45.1X4	T45.1X5	T45.1X6
Dactinomycin	T45.1X1	T45.1X2	T45.1X3	T45.1X4	T45.1X5	T45.1X6
DADPS	T37.1X1	T37.1X2	T37.1X3	T37.1X4	T37.1X5	T37.1X6
Dakin's solution	T49.0X1	T49.0X2	T49.0X3	T49.0X4	T49.0X5	T49.0X6
Dalapon (sodium)	T60.3X1	T60.3X2	T60.3X3	T60.3X4	—	—
Dalmane	T42.4X1	T42.4X2	T42.4X3	T42.4X4	T42.4X5	T42.4X6
Danazol	T38.6X1	T38.6X2	T38.6X3	T38.6X4	T38.6X5	T38.6X6
Danilone	T45.511	T45.512	T45.513	T45.514	T45.515	T45.516
Danthron	T47.2X1	T47.2X2	T47.2X3	T47.2X4	T47.2X5	T47.2X6
Dantrolene	T42.8X1	T42.8X2	T42.8X3	T42.8X4	T42.8X5	T42.8X6
Dantron	T47.2X1	T47.2X2	T47.2X3	T47.2X4	T47.2X5	T47.2X6
Daphne (gnidium) (mezereum)	T62.2X1	T62.2X2	T62.2X3	T62.2X4	—	—
berry	T62.1X1	T62.1X2	T62.1X3	T62.1X4	—	—
Dapsone	T37.1X1	T37.1X2	T37.1X3	T37.1X4	T37.1X5	T37.1X6
Daraprim	T37.2X1	T37.2X2	T37.2X3	T37.2X4	T37.2X5	T37.2X6
Darnel	T62.2X1	T62.2X2	T62.2X3	T62.2X4	—	—
Darvon	T39.8X1	T39.8X2	T39.8X3	T39.8X4	T39.8X5	T39.8X6
Daunomycin	T45.1X1	T45.1X2	T45.1X3	T45.1X4	T45.1X5	T45.1X6
Daunorubicin	T45.1X1	T45.1X2	T45.1X3	T45.1X4	T45.1X5	T45.1X6
DBI	T38.3X1	T38.3X2	T38.3X3	T38.3X4	T38.3X5	T38.3X6
D-Con	T60.91	T60.92	T60.93	T60.94	—	—
insecticide	T60.2X1	T60.2X2	T60.2X3	T60.2X4	—	—
rodenticide	T60.4X1	T60.4X2	T60.4X3	T60.4X4	—	—
DDAVP	T38.891	T38.892	T38.893	T38.894	T38.895	T38.896
DDE (bis (chlorophenyl)-dichloroethylene)	T60.2X1	T60.2X2	T60.2X3	T60.2X4	—	—
DDS	T37.1X1	T37.1X2	T37.1X3	T37.1X4	T37.1X5	T37.1X6
DDT (dust)	T60.1X1	T60.1X2	T60.1X3	T60.1X4	—	—
Deadly nightshade—see also Belladonna	T62.2X1	T62.2X2	T62.2X3	T62.2X4	—	—
berry	T62.1X1	T62.1X2	T62.1X3	T62.1X4	—	—
Deamino-D-arginine vasopressin	T38.891	T38.892	T38.893	T38.894	T38.895	T38.896
Deanol (aceglumate)	T50.991	T50.992	T50.993	T50.994	T50.995	T50.996
Debrisoquine	T46.5X1	T46.5X2	T46.5X3	T46.5X4	T46.5X5	T46.5X6
Decaborane	T57.8X1	T57.8X2	T57.8X3	T57.8X4	—	—
fumes	T59.891	T59.892	T59.893	T59.894	—	—
Decadron	T38.0X1	T38.0X2	T38.0X3	T38.0X4	T38.0X5	T38.0X6
ENT agent	T49.6X1	T49.6X2	T49.6X3	T49.6X4	T49.6X5	T49.6X6
ophthalmic preparation	T49.5X1	T49.5X2	T49.5X3	T49.5X4	T49.5X5	T49.5X6
topical NEC	T49.0X1	T49.0X2	T49.0X3	T49.0X4	T49.0X5	T49.0X6
Decahydro-naphthalene	T52.8X1	T52.8X2	T52.8X3	T52.8X4	—	—
Decalin	T52.8X1	T52.8X2	T52.8X3	T52.8X4	—	—
Decametho-nium (bromide)	T48.1X1	T48.1X2	T48.1X3	T48.1X4	T48.1X5	T48.1X6
Decholin	T47.5X1	T47.5X2	T47.5X3	T47.5X4	T47.5X5	T47.5X6
Declomycin	T36.4X1	T36.4X2	T36.4X3	T36.4X4	T36.4X5	T36.4X6
Decongestant, nasal (mucosa)	T48.5X1	T48.5X2	T48.5X3	T48.5X4	T48.5X5	T48.5X6
combination	T48.5X1	T48.5X2	T48.5X3	T48.5X4	T48.5X5	T48.5X6
Deet	T60.8X1	T60.8X2	T60.8X3	T60.8X4	—	—
Deferoxamine	T45.8X1	T45.8X2	T45.8X3	T45.8X4	T45.8X5	T45.8X6
Deflazacort	T38.0X1	T38.0X2	T38.0X3	T38.0X4	T38.0X5	T38.0X6
Deglycyrrhizinized extract of licorice	T48.4X1	T48.4X2	T48.4X3	T48.4X4	T48.4X5	T48.4X6
Dehydrocholic acid	T47.5X1	T47.5X2	T47.5X3	T47.5X4	T47.5X5	T47.5X6
Dehydroemetine	T37.3X1	T37.3X2	T37.3X3	T37.3X4	T37.3X5	T37.3X6
Dekalin	T52.8X1	T52.8X2	T52.8X3	T52.8X4	—	—
Delalutin	T38.5X1	T38.5X2	T38.5X3	T38.5X4	T38.5X5	T38.5X6
Delorazepam	T42.4X1	T42.4X2	T42.4X3	T42.4X4	T42.4X5	T42.4X6
Delphinium	T62.2X1	T62.2X2	T62.2X3	T62.2X4	—	—
Deltamethrin	T60.1X1	T60.1X2	T60.1X3	T60.1X4	—	—
Deltasone	T38.0X1	T38.0X2	T38.0X3	T38.0X4	T38.0X5	T38.0X6
Deltra	T38.0X1	T38.0X2	T38.0X3	T38.0X4	T38.0X5	T38.0X6
Delvinal	T42.3X1	T42.3X2	T42.3X3	T42.3X4	T42.3X5	T42.3X6
Demecarium (bromide)	T49.5X1	T49.5X2	T49.5X3	T49.5X4	T49.5X5	T49.5X6
Demeclocycline	T36.4X1	T36.4X2	T36.4X3	T36.4X4	T36.4X5	T36.4X6
Demecolcine	T45.1X1	T45.1X2	T45.1X3	T45.1X4	T45.1X5	T45.1X6
Demegestone	T38.5X1	T38.5X2	T38.5X3	T38.5X4	T38.5X5	T38.5X6
Demelanizing agents	T49.8X1	T49.8X2	T49.8X3	T49.8X4	T49.8X5	T49.8X6
Demephion -O and -S	T60.0X1	T60.0X2	T60.0X3	T60.0X4	—	—
Demerol	T40.2X1	T40.2X2	T40.2X3	T40.2X4	T40.2X5	T40.2X6
Demethylchlor-tetracycline	T36.4X1	T36.4X2	T36.4X3	T36.4X4	T36.4X5	T36.4X6
Demethyltetracycline	T36.4X1	T36.4X2	T36.4X3	T36.4X4	T36.4X5	T36.4X6
Demeton -O and -S	T60.0X1	T60.0X2	T60.0X3	T60.0X4	—	—
Demulcent (external)	T49.3X1	T49.3X2	T49.3X3	T49.3X4	T49.3X5	T49.3X6
specified NEC	T49.3X1	T49.3X2	T49.3X3	T49.3X4	T49.3X5	T49.3X6
Demulen	T38.4X1	T38.4X2	T38.4X3	T38.4X4	T38.4X5	T38.4X6
Denatured alcohol	T51.0X1	T51.0X2	T51.0X3	T51.0X4	—	—
Dendrid	T49.5X1	T49.5X2	T49.5X3	T49.5X4	T49.5X5	T49.5X6
Dental drug, topical application NEC	T49.7X1	T49.7X2	T49.7X3	T49.7X4	T49.7X5	T49.7X6
Dentifrice	T49.7X1	T49.7X2	T49.7X3	T49.7X4	T49.7X5	T49.7X6
Deodorant spray (feminine hygiene)	T49.8X1	T49.8X2	T49.8X3	T49.8X4	T49.8X5	T49.8X6
Deoxycortone	T50.0X1	T50.0X2	T50.0X3	T50.0X4	T50.0X5	T50.0X6
2-Deoxy-5-fluorouridine	T45.1X1	T45.1X2	T45.1X3	T45.1X4	T45.1X5	T45.1X6
5-Deoxy-5-fluorouridine	T45.1X1	T45.1X2	T45.1X3	T45.1X4	T45.1X5	T45.1X6
Deoxyribonuclease (pancreatic)	T45.3X1	T45.3X2	T45.3X3	T45.3X4	T45.3X5	T45.3X6
Depilatory	T49.4X1	T49.4X2	T49.4X3	T49.4X4	T49.4X5	T49.4X6
Deprenalin	T42.8X1	T42.8X2	T42.8X3	T42.8X4	T42.8X5	T42.8X6
Deprenyl	T42.8X1	T42.8X2	T42.8X3	T42.8X4	T42.8X5	T42.8X6
Depressant, appetite	T50.5X1	T50.5X2	T50.5X3	T50.5X4	T50.5X5	T50.5X6
Depressant						
appetite (central)	T50.5X1	T50.5X2	T50.5X3	T50.5X4	T50.5X5	T50.5X6
cardiac	T46.2X1	T46.2X2	T46.2X3	T46.2X4	T46.2X5	T46.2X6

Substance	Poisoning, Accidental (unintentional)	Poisoning, Intentional self-harm	Poisoning, Assault	Poisoning, Undetermined	Adverse effect	Underdosing
Depressant — *Continued*						
central nervous system (anesthetic)—see also Central nervous system, depressants	T42.71	T42.72	T42.73	T42.74	T42.75	T42.76
general anesthetic	T41.201	T41.202	T41.203	T41.204	T41.205	T41.206
muscle tone	T42.8X1	T42.8X2	T42.8X3	T42.8X4	T42.8X5	T42.8X6
muscle tone, central	T42.8X1	T42.8X2	T42.8X3	T42.8X4	T42.8X5	T42.8X6
psychotherapeutic	T43.501	T43.502	T43.503	T43.504	T43.505	T43.506
Deptropine	T45.0X1	T45.0X2	T45.0X3	T45.0X4	T45.0X5	T45.0X6
Dequalinium (chloride)	T49.0X1	T49.0X2	T49.0X3	T49.0X4	T49.0X5	T49.0X6
Derris root	T60.2X1	T60.2X2	T60.2X3	T60.2X4	—	—
Deserpidine	T46.5X1	T46.5X2	T46.5X3	T46.5X4	T46.5X5	T46.5X6
Desferrioxamine	T45.8X1	T45.8X2	T45.8X3	T45.8X4	T45.8X5	T45.8X6
Desipramine	T43.011	T43.012	T43.013	T43.014	T43.015	T43.016
Deslanoside	T46.0X1	T46.0X2	T46.0X3	T46.0X4	T46.0X5	T46.0X6
Desloughing agent	T49.4X1	T49.4X2	T49.4X3	T49.4X4	T49.4X5	T49.4X6
Desmethy-limipramine	T43.011	T43.012	T43.013	T43.014	T43.015	T43.016
Desmopressin	T38.891	T38.892	T38.893	T38.894	T38.895	T38.896
Desocodeine	T40.2X1	T40.2X2	T40.2X3	T40.2X4	T40.2X5	T40.2X6
Desogestrel	T38.5X1	T38.5X2	T38.5X3	T38.5X4	T38.5X5	T38.5X6
Desomorphine	T40.2X1	T40.2X2	T40.2X3	T40.2X4	—	—
Desonide	T49.0X1	T49.0X2	T49.0X3	T49.0X4	T49.0X5	T49.0X6
Desoximetasone	T49.0X1	T49.0X2	T49.0X3	T49.0X4	T49.0X5	T49.0X6
Desoxycorticosteroid	T50.0X1	T50.0X2	T50.0X3	T50.0X4	T50.0X5	T50.0X6
Desoxycortone	T50.0X1	T50.0X2	T50.0X3	T50.0X4	T50.0X5	T50.0X6
Desoxyephedrine	T43.621	T43.622	T43.623	T43.624	T43.625	T43.626
Detaxtran	T46.6X1	T46.6X2	T46.6X3	T46.6X4	T46.6X5	T46.6X6
Detergent	T49.2X1	T49.2X2	T49.2X3	T49.2X4	T49.2X5	T49.2X6
external medication	T49.2X1	T49.2X2	T49.2X3	T49.2X4	T49.2X5	T49.2X6
local	T49.2X1	T49.2X2	T49.2X3	T49.2X4	T49.2X5	T49.2X6
medicinal	T49.2X1	T49.2X2	T49.2X3	T49.2X4	T49.2X5	T49.2X6
nonmedicinal	T55.1X1	T55.1X2	T55.1X3	T55.1X4	—	—
specified NEC	T55.1X1	T55.1X2	T55.1X3	T55.1X4	—	—
Deterrent, alcohol	T50.6X1	T50.6X2	T50.6X3	T50.6X4	T50.6X5	T50.6X6
Detoxifying agent	T50.6X1	T50.6X2	T50.6X3	T50.6X4	T50.6X5	T50.6X6
Detrothyronine	T38.1X1	T38.1X2	T38.1X3	T38.1X4	T38.1X5	T38.1X6
Dettol (external medication)	T49.0X1	T49.0X2	T49.0X3	T49.0X4	T49.0X5	T49.0X6
Dexamethasone	T38.0X1	T38.0X2	T38.0X3	T38.0X4	T38.0X5	T38.0X6
ENT agent	T49.6X1	T49.6X2	T49.6X3	T49.6X4	T49.6X5	T49.6X6
ophthalmic preparation	T49.5X1	T49.5X2	T49.5X3	T49.5X4	T49.5X5	T49.5X6
topical NEC	T49.0X1	T49.0X2	T49.0X3	T49.0X4	T49.0X5	T49.0X6
Dexamfetamine	T43.621	T43.622	T43.623	T43.624	T43.625	T43.626
Dexamphetamine	T43.621	T43.622	T43.623	T43.624	T43.625	T43.626
Dexbrom-pheniramine	T45.0X1	T45.0X2	T45.0X3	T45.0X4	T45.0X5	T45.0X6
Dexchlorpheniramine	T45.0X1	T45.0X2	T45.0X3	T45.0X4	T45.0X5	T45.0X6
Dexedrine	T43.621	T43.622	T43.623	T43.624	T43.625	T43.626
Dexetimide	T44.3X1	T44.3X2	T44.3X3	T44.3X4	T44.3X5	T44.3X6
Dexfenfluramine	T50.5X1	T50.5X2	T50.5X3	T50.5X4	T50.5X5	T50.5X6
Dexpanthenol	T45.2X1	T45.2X2	T45.2X3	T45.2X4	T45.2X5	T45.2X6
Dextran (40) (70) (150)	T45.8X1	T45.8X2	T45.8X3	T45.8X4	T45.8X5	T45.8X6

Substance	Poisoning, Accidental (unintentional)	Poisoning, Intentional self-harm	Poisoning, Assault	Poisoning, Undetermined	Adverse effect	Underdosing
Dextriferron	T45.4X1	T45.4X2	T45.4X3	T45.4X4	T45.4X5	T45.4X
Dextro calcium pantothenate	T45.2X1	T45.2X2	T45.2X3	T45.2X4	T45.2X5	T45.2X
Dextro pantothenyl alcohol	T45.2X1	T45.2X2	T45.2X3	T45.2X4	T45.2X5	T45.2X
Dextroamphetamine	T43.621	T43.622	T43.623	T43.624	T43.625	T43.62
Dextromethorphan	T48.3X1	T48.3X2	T48.3X3	T48.3X4	T48.3X5	T48.3X
Dextromoramide	T40.4X1	T40.4X2	T40.4X3	T40.4X4	—	—
topical	T49.8X1	T49.8X2	T49.8X3	T49.8X4	T49.8X5	T49.8X
Dextropropoxyphene	T40.4X1	T40.4X2	T40.4X3	T40.4X4	T40.4X5	T40.4X
Dextrorphan	T40.2X1	T40.2X2	T40.2X3	T40.2X4	T40.2X5	T40.2X
Dextrose	T50.3X1	T50.3X2	T50.3X3	T50.3X4	T50.3X5	T50.3X
concentrated solution, intravenous	T46.8X1	T46.8X2	T46.8X3	T46.8X4	T46.8X5	T46.8X
Dextrothyroxin	T38.1X1	T38.1X2	T38.1X3	T38.1X4	T38.1X5	T38.1X
Dextrothyroxine sodium	T38.1X1	T38.1X2	T38.1X3	T38.1X4	T38.1X5	T38.1X
DFP	T44.0X1	T44.0X2	T44.0X3	T44.0X4	T44.0X5	T44.0X
DHE	T37.3X1	T37.3X2	T37.3X3	T37.3X4	T37.3X5	T37.3X
45	T46.5X1	T46.5X2	T46.5X3	T46.5X4	T46.5X5	T46.5X
Diabinese	T38.3X1	T38.3X2	T38.3X3	T38.3X4	T38.3X5	T38.3X
Diacetone alcohol	T52.4X1	T52.4X2	T52.4X3	T52.4X4	—	—
Diacetyl monoxime	T50.991	T50.992	T50.993	T50.994	—	—
Diacetylmorphine	T40.1X1	T40.1X2	T40.1X3	T40.1X4	—	—
Diachylon plaster	T49.4X1	T49.4X2	T49.4X3	T49.4X4	T49.4X5	T49.4X
Diaethylst-ilboestrolum	T38.5X1	T38.5X2	T38.5X3	T38.5X4	T38.5X5	T38.5X
Diagnostic agent NEC	T50.8X1	T50.8X2	T50.8X3	T50.8X4	T50.8X5	T50.8X
Dial (soap)	T49.2X1	T49.2X2	T49.2X3	T49.2X4	T49.2X5	T49.2X
sedative	T42.3X1	T42.3X2	T42.3X3	T42.3X4	T42.3X5	T42.3X
Dialkyl carbonate	T52.91	T52.92	T52.93	T52.94	—	—
Diallylbarbituric acid	T42.3X1	T42.3X2	T42.3X3	T42.3X4	T42.3X5	T42.3X
Diallymal	T42.3X1	T42.3X2	T42.3X3	T42.3X4	T42.3X5	T42.3X
Dialysis solution (intraperitoneal)	T50.3X1	T50.3X2	T50.3X3	T50.3X4	T50.3X5	T50.3X
Diaminodi-phenylsulfone	T37.1X1	T37.1X2	T37.1X3	T37.1X4	T37.1X5	T37.1X
Diamorphine	T40.1X1	T40.1X2	T40.1X3	T40.1X4	—	—
Diamox	T50.2X1	T50.2X2	T50.2X3	T50.2X4	T50.2X5	T50.2X6
Diamthazole	T49.0X1	T49.0X2	T49.0X3	T49.0X4	T49.0X5	T49.0X6
Dianthone	T47.2X1	T47.2X2	T47.2X3	T47.2X4	T47.2X5	T47.2X6
Diaphenylsulfone	T37.0X1	T37.0X2	T37.0X3	T37.0X4	T37.0X5	T37.0X6
Diasone (sodium)	T37.1X1	T37.1X2	T37.1X3	T37.1X4	T37.1X5	T37.1X6
Diastase	T47.5X1	T47.5X2	T47.5X3	T47.5X4	T47.5X5	T47.5X6
Diatrizoate	T50.8X1	T50.8X2	T50.8X3	T50.8X4	T50.8X5	T50.8X6
Diazepam	T42.4X1	T42.4X2	T42.4X3	T42.4X4	T42.4X5	T42.4X6
Diazinon	T60.0X1	T60.0X2	T60.0X3	T60.0X4	—	—
Diazomethane (gas)	T59.891	T59.892	T59.893	T59.894	—	—
Diazoxide	T46.5X1	T46.5X2	T46.5X3	T46.5X4	T46.5X5	T46.5X6
Dibekacin	T36.5X1	T36.5X2	T36.5X3	T36.5X4	T36.5X5	T36.5X6
Dibenamine	T44.6X1	T44.6X2	T44.6X3	T44.6X4	T44.6X5	T44.6X6
Dibenzepin	T43.011	T43.012	T43.013	T43.014	T43.015	T43.016
Dibenzheptropine	T45.0X1	T45.0X2	T45.0X3	T45.0X4	T45.0X5	T45.0X6
Dibenzyline	T44.6X1	T44.6X2	T44.6X3	T44.6X4	T44.6X5	T44.6X6
Diborane (gas)	T59.891	T59.892	T59.893	T59.894	—	—

Substance	Poisoning, Accidental (unintentional)	Poisoning, Intentional self-harm	Poisoning, Assault	Poisoning, Undetermined	Adverse effect	Underdosing
Dibromoch-loropropane	T60.8X1	T60.8X2	T60.8X3	T60.8X4	—	—
Dibromodulcitol	T45.1X1	T45.1X2	T45.1X3	T45.1X4	T45.1X5	T45.1X6
Dibromoethane	T53.6X1	T53.6X2	T53.6X3	T53.6X4	—	—
Dibromomannitol	T45.1X1	T45.1X2	T45.1X3	T45.1X4	T45.1X5	T45.1X6
Dibromopropamidine isethionate	T49.0X1	T49.0X2	T49.0X3	T49.0X4	T49.0X5	T49.0X6
Dibrompropamidine	T49.0X1	T49.0X2	T49.0X3	T49.0X4	T49.0X5	T49.0X6
Dibucaine	T41.3X1	T41.3X2	T41.3X3	T41.3X4	T41.3X5	T41.3X6
topical (surface)	T41.3X1	T41.3X2	T41.3X3	T41.3X4	T41.3X5	T41.3X6
Dibunate sodium	T48.3X1	T48.3X2	T48.3X3	T48.3X4	T48.3X5	T48.3X6
Dibutoline sulfate	T44.3X1	T44.3X2	T44.3X3	T44.3X4	T44.3X5	T44.3X6
Dicamba	T60.3X1	T60.3X2	T60.3X3	T60.3X4	—	—
Dicapthon	T60.0X1	T60.0X2	T60.0X3	T60.0X4	—	—
Dichlobenil	T60.3X1	T60.3X2	T60.3X3	T60.3X4	—	—
Dichlone	T60.3X1	T60.3X2	T60.3X3	T60.3X4	—	—
Dichloralphenozone	T42.6X1	T42.6X2	T42.6X3	T42.6X4	T42.6X5	T42.6X6
Dichlorbenzidine	T65.3X1	T65.3X2	T65.3X3	T65.3X4	—	—
Dichlorhydrin	T52.8X1	T52.8X2	T52.8X3	T52.8X4	—	—
Dichlorhydroxy-quinoline	T37.8X1	T37.8X2	T37.8X3	T37.8X4	T37.8X5	T37.8X6
Dichlorobenzene	T53.7X1	T53.7X2	T53.7X3	T53.7X4	—	—
Dichlorobenzyl alcohol	T49.6X1	T49.6X2	T49.6X3	T49.6X4	T49.6X5	T49.6X6
Dichlorodifluoro-methane	T53.5X1	T53.5X2	T53.5X3	T53.5X4	—	—
Dichloroethane	T52.8X1	T52.8X2	T52.8X3	T52.8X4	—	—
sym-Dichloroethyl ether	T53.6X1	T53.6X2	T53.6X3	T53.6X4	—	—
Dichloroethyl sulfide, not in war	T59.891	T59.892	T59.893	T59.894	—	—
Dichloroethylene	T53.6X1	T53.6X2	T53.6X3	T53.6X4	—	—
Dichloroformoxine, not in war	T59.891	T59.892	T59.893	T59.894	—	—
Dichlorohydrin, alpha-dichlorohydrin	T52.8X1	T52.8X2	T52.8X3	T52.8X4	—	—
Dichloromethane (solvent)	T53.4X1	T53.4X2	T53.4X3	T53.4X4	—	—
vapor	T53.4X1	T53.4X2	T53.4X3	T53.4X4	—	—
Dichloronaphtho-quinone	T60.3X1	T60.3X2	T60.3X3	T60.3X4	—	—
Dichlorophen	T37.4X1	T37.4X2	T37.4X3	T37.4X4	T37.4X5	T37.4X6
2,4-Dichlorophenoxy-acetic acid	T60.3X1	T60.3X2	T60.3X3	T60.3X4	—	—
Dichloropropene	T60.3X1	T60.3X2	T60.3X3	T60.3X4	—	—
Dichloropropionic acid	T60.3X1	T60.3X2	T60.3X3	T60.3X4	—	—
Dichlorphenamide	T50.2X1	T50.2X2	T50.2X3	T50.2X4	T50.2X5	T50.2X6
Dichlorvos	T60.0X1	T60.0X2	T60.0X3	T60.0X4	—	—
Diclofenac	T39.391	T39.392	T39.393	T39.394	T39.395	T39.396
Diclofenamide	T50.2X1	T50.2X2	T50.2X3	T50.2X4	T50.2X5	T50.2X6
Diclofensine	T43.291	T43.292	T43.293	T43.294	T43.295	T43.296
Diclonixine	T39.8X1	T39.8X2	T39.8X3	T39.8X4	T39.8X5	T39.8X6
Dicloxacillin	T36.0X1	T36.0X2	T36.0X3	T36.0X4	T36.0X5	T36.0X6
Dicophane	T49.0X1	T49.0X2	T49.0X3	T49.0X4	T49.0X5	T49.0X6
Dicoumarol, dicoumarin, dicumarol	T45.511	T45.512	T45.513	T45.514	T45.515	T45.516
Dicrotophos	T60.0X1	T60.0X2	T60.0X3	T60.0X4	—	—
Dicyanogen (gas)	T65.0X1	T65.0X2	T65.0X3	T65.0X4	—	—
Dicyclomine	T44.3X1	T44.3X2	T44.3X3	T44.3X4	T44.3X5	T44.3X6
Dicycloverine	T44.3X1	T44.3X2	T44.3X3	T44.3X4	T44.3X5	T44.3X6
Dideoxycytidine	T37.5X1	T37.5X2	T37.5X3	T37.5X4	T37.5X5	T37.5X6
Dideoxyinosine	T37.5X1	T37.5X2	T37.5X3	T37.5X4	T37.5X5	T37.5X6
Dieldrin (vapor)	T60.1X1	T60.1X2	T60.1X3	T60.1X4	—	—
Diemal	T42.3X1	T42.3X2	T42.3X3	T42.3X4	T42.3X5	T42.3X6
Dienestrol	T38.5X1	T38.5X2	T38.5X3	T38.5X4	T38.5X5	T38.5X6
Dienoestrol	T38.5X1	T38.5X2	T38.5X3	T38.5X4	T38.5X5	T38.5X6
Dietetic drug NEC	T50.901	T50.902	T50.903	T50.904	T50.905	T50.906
Diethazine	T42.8X1	T42.8X2	T42.8X3	T42.8X4	T42.8X5	T42.8X6
Diethyl						
barbituric acid	T42.3X1	T42.3X2	T42.3X3	T42.3X4	T42.3X5	T42.3X6
carbamazine	T37.4X1	T37.4X2	T37.4X3	T37.4X4	T37.4X5	T37.4X6
carbinol	T51.3X1	T51.3X2	T51.3X3	T51.3X4	—	—
carbonate	T52.8X1	T52.8X2	T52.8X3	T52.8X4	—	—
ether (vapor)—see also ether	T41.0X1	T41.0X2	T41.0X3	T41.0X4	T41.0X5	T41.0X6
oxide	T52.8X1	T52.8X2	T52.8X3	T52.8X4	—	—
propion	T50.5X1	T50.5X2	T50.5X3	T50.5X4	T50.5X5	T50.5X6
stilbestrol	T38.5X1	T38.5X2	T38.5X3	T38.5X4	T38.5X5	T38.5X6
toluamide (nonmedicinal)	T60.8X1	T60.8X2	T60.8X3	T60.8X4	—	—
medicinal	T49.3X1	T49.3X2	T49.3X3	T49.3X4	T49.3X5	T49.3X6
Diethylcarbamazine	T37.4X1	T37.4X2	T37.4X3	T37.4X4	T37.4X5	T37.4X6
Diethylene						
dioxide	T52.8X1	T52.8X2	T52.8X3	T52.8X4	—	—
glycol (monoacetate) (monobutyl ether) (monoethyl ether)	T52.3X1	T52.3X2	T52.3X3	T52.3X4	—	—
Diethylhexy-lphthalate	T65.891	T65.892	T65.893	T65.894	—	—
Diethylpropion	T50.5X1	T50.5X2	T50.5X3	T50.5X4	T50.5X5	T50.5X6
Diethylstilbestrol	T38.5X1	T38.5X2	T38.5X3	T38.5X4	T38.5X5	T38.5X6
Diethylstilboestrol	T38.5X1	T38.5X2	T38.5X3	T38.5X4	T38.5X5	T38.5X6
Diethylsulfone-diethylmethane	T42.6X1	T42.6X2	T42.6X3	T42.6X4	T42.6X5	T42.6X6
Diethyltoluamide	T49.0X1	T49.0X2	T49.0X3	T49.0X4	T49.0X5	T49.0X6
Diethyltryptamine (DET)	T40.991	T40.992	T40.993	T40.994	—	—
Difebarbamate	T42.3X1	T42.3X2	T42.3X3	T42.3X4	T42.3X5	T42.3X6
Difencloxazine	T40.2X1	T40.2X2	T40.2X3	T40.2X4	T40.2X5	T40.2X6
Difenidol	T45.0X1	T45.0X2	T45.0X3	T45.0X4	T45.0X5	T45.0X6
Difenoxin	T47.6X1	T47.6X2	T47.6X3	T47.6X4	T47.6X5	T47.6X6
Difetarsone	T37.3X1	T37.3X2	T37.3X3	T37.3X4	T37.3X5	T37.3X6
Diffusin	T45.3X1	T45.3X2	T45.3X3	T45.3X4	T45.3X5	T45.3X6
Diflorasone	T49.0X1	T49.0X2	T49.0X3	T49.0X4	T49.0X5	T49.0X6
Diflos	T44.0X1	T44.0X2	T44.0X3	T44.0X4	T44.0X5	T44.0X6
Diflubenzuron	T60.1X1	T60.1X2	T60.1X3	T60.1X4	—	—
Diflucortolone	T49.0X1	T49.0X2	T49.0X3	T49.0X4	T49.0X5	T49.0X6
Diflunisal	T39.091	T39.092	T39.093	T39.094	T39.095	T39.096
Difluoromethyldopa	T42.8X1	T42.8X2	T42.8X3	T42.8X4	T42.8X5	T42.8X6
Difluorophate	T44.0X1	T44.0X2	T44.0X3	T44.0X4	T44.0X5	T44.0X6
Digestant NEC	T47.5X1	T47.5X2	T47.5X3	T47.5X4	T47.5X5	T47.5X6
Digitalin(e)	T46.0X1	T46.0X2	T46.0X3	T46.0X4	T46.0X5	T46.0X6

Substance	Poisoning, Accidental (unintentional)	Poisoning, Intentional self-harm	Poisoning, Assault	Poisoning, Undetermined	Adverse effect	Underdosing
Digitalis (leaf) (glycoside)	T46.0X1	T46.0X2	T46.0X3	T46.0X4	T46.0X5	T46.0X6
lanata	T46.0X1	T46.0X2	T46.0X3	T46.0X4	T46.0X5	T46.0X6
purpurea	T46.0X1	T46.0X2	T46.0X3	T46.0X4	T46.0X5	T46.0X6
Digitoxin	T46.0X1	T46.0X2	T46.0X3	T46.0X4	T46.0X5	T46.0X6
Digitoxose	T46.0X1	T46.0X2	T46.0X3	T46.0X4	T46.0X5	T46.0X6
Digoxin	T46.0X1	T46.0X2	T46.0X3	T46.0X4	T46.0X5	T46.0X6
Digoxine	T46.0X1	T46.0X2	T46.0X3	T46.0X4	T46.0X5	T46.0X6
Dihydralazine	T46.5X1	T46.5X2	T46.5X3	T46.5X4	T46.5X5	T46.5X6
Dihydrazine	T46.5X1	T46.5X2	T46.5X3	T46.5X4	T46.5X5	T46.5X6
Dihydrocodeine	T40.2X1	T40.2X2	T40.2X3	T40.2X4	T40.2X5	T40.2X6
Dihydrocodeinone	T40.2X1	T40.2X2	T40.2X3	T40.2X4	T40.2X5	T40.2X6
Dihydroergocornine	T46.7X1	T46.7X2	T46.7X3	T46.7X4	T46.7X5	T46.7X6
Dihydroergocristine (mesilate)	T46.7X1	T46.7X2	T46.7X3	T46.7X4	T46.7X5	T46.7X6
Dihydroergokryptine	T46.7X1	T46.7X2	T46.7X3	T46.7X4	T46.7X5	T46.7X6
Dihydroergotamine	T46.5X1	T46.5X2	T46.5X3	T46.5X4	T46.5X5	T46.5X6
Dihydroergotoxine	T46.7X1	T46.7X2	T46.7X3	T46.7X4	T46.7X5	T46.7X6
mesilate	T46.7X1	T46.7X2	T46.7X3	T46.7X4	T46.7X5	T46.7X6
Dihydrohydroxy-codeinone	T40.2X1	T40.2X2	T40.2X3	T40.2X4	T40.2X5	T40.2X6
Dihydrohydroxy-morphinone	T40.2X1	T40.2X2	T40.2X3	T40.2X4	T40.2X5	T40.2X6
Dihydroisocodeine	T40.2X1	T40.2X2	T40.2X3	T40.2X4	T40.2X5	T40.2X6
Dihydromorphine	T40.2X1	T40.2X2	T40.2X3	T40.2X4	—	—
Dihydromorphinone	T40.2X1	T40.2X2	T40.2X3	T40.2X4	T40.2X5	T40.2X6
Dihydrostreptomycin	T36.5X1	T36.5X2	T36.5X3	T36.5X4	T36.5X5	T36.5X6
Dihydrotachysterol	T45.2X1	T45.2X2	T45.2X3	T45.2X4	T45.2X5	T45.2X6
Dihydroxyaluminum aminoacetate	T47.1X1	T47.1X2	T47.1X3	T47.1X4	T47.1X5	T47.1X6
Dihydroxyaluminum sodium carbonate	T47.1X1	T47.1X2	T47.1X3	T47.1X4	T47.1X5	T47.1X6
Dihydroxyanthra-quinone	T47.2X1	T47.2X2	T47.2X3	T47.2X4	T47.2X5	T47.2X6
Dihydroxycodeinone	T40.2X1	T40.2X2	T40.2X3	T40.2X4	T40.2X5	T40.2X6
Dihydroxypropyl theophylline	T50.2X1	T50.2X2	T50.2X3	T50.2X4	T50.2X5	T50.2X6
Diiodohydroxyquin	T37.8X1	T37.8X2	T37.8X3	T37.8X4	T37.8X5	T37.8X6
topical	T49.0X1	T49.0X2	T49.0X3	T49.0X4	T49.0X5	T49.0X6
Diiodo-hydroxyquinoline	T37.8X1	T37.8X2	T37.8X3	T37.8X4	T37.8X5	T37.8X6
Diiodotyrosine	T38.2X1	T38.2X2	T38.2X3	T38.2X4	T38.2X5	T38.2X6
Diisopromine	T44.3X1	T44.3X2	T44.3X3	T44.3X4	T44.3X5	T44.3X6
Diisopropylamine	T46.3X1	T46.3X2	T46.3X3	T46.3X4	T46.3X5	T46.3X6
Diisopropyl-fluorophos-phonate	T44.0X1	T44.0X2	T44.0X3	T44.0X4	T44.0X5	T44.0X6
Dilantin	T42.0X1	T42.0X2	T42.0X3	T42.0X4	T42.0X5	T42.0X6
Dilaudid	T40.2X1	T40.2X2	T40.2X3	T40.2X4	T40.2X5	T40.2X6
Dilazep	T46.3X1	T46.3X2	T46.3X3	T46.3X4	T46.3X5	T46.3X6
Dill	T47.5X1	T47.5X2	T47.5X3	T47.5X4	T47.5X5	T47.5X6
Diloxanide	T37.3X1	T37.3X2	T37.3X3	T37.3X4	T37.3X5	T37.3X6
Diltiazem	T46.1X1	T46.1X2	T46.1X3	T46.1X4	T46.1X5	T46.1X6
Dimazole	T49.0X1	T49.0X2	T49.0X3	T49.0X4	T49.0X5	T49.0X6
Dimefline	T50.7X1	T50.7X2	T50.7X3	T50.7X4	T50.7X5	T50.7X6
Dimefox	T60.0X1	T60.0X2	T60.0X3	T60.0X4	—	—
Dimemorfan	T48.3X1	T48.3X2	T48.3X3	T48.3X4	T48.3X5	T48.3X6

Substance	Poisoning, Accidental (unintentional)	Poisoning, Intentional self-harm	Poisoning, Assault	Poisoning, Undetermined	Adverse effect	Underdosing
Dimenhydrinate	T45.0X1	T45.0X2	T45.0X3	T45.0X4	T45.0X5	T45.0X
Dimercaprol (British anti-lewisite)	T45.8X1	T45.8X2	T45.8X3	T45.8X4	T45.8X5	T45.8X
Dimercaptopropanol	T45.8X1	T45.8X2	T45.8X3	T45.8X4	T45.8X5	T45.8X
Dimestrol	T38.5X1	T38.5X2	T38.5X3	T38.5X4	T38.5X5	T38.5X
Dimetane	T45.0X1	T45.0X2	T45.0X3	T45.0X4	T45.0X5	T45.0X
Dimethicone	T47.1X1	T47.1X2	T47.1X3	T47.1X4	T47.1X5	T47.1X
Dimethindene	T45.0X1	T45.0X2	T45.0X3	T45.0X4	T45.0X5	T45.0X
Dimethisoquin	T49.1X1	T49.1X2	T49.1X3	T49.1X4	T49.1X5	T49.1X
Dimethisterone	T38.5X1	T38.5X2	T38.5X3	T38.5X4	T38.5X5	T38.5X
Dimethoate	T60.0X1	T60.0X2	T60.0X3	T60.0X4	—	—
Dimethocaine	T41.3X1	T41.3X2	T41.3X3	T41.3X4	T41.3X5	T41.3X
Dimethoxanate	T48.3X1	T48.3X2	T48.3X3	T48.3X4	T48.3X5	T48.3X
Dimethyl						
arsine, arsinic acid	T57.0X1	T57.0X2	T57.0X3	T57.0X4	—	—
carbinol	T51.2X1	T51.2X2	T51.2X3	T51.2X4	—	—
carbonate	T52.8X1	T52.8X2	T52.8X3	T52.8X4	—	—
diguanide	T38.3X1	T38.3X2	T38.3X3	T38.3X4	T38.3X5	T38.3X
ketone	T52.4X1	T52.4X2	T52.4X3	T52.4X4	—	—
vapor	T52.4X1	T52.4X2	T52.4X3	T52.4X4	—	—
meperidine	T40.2X1	T40.2X2	T40.2X3	T40.2X4	T40.2X5	T40.2X
parathion	T60.0X1	T60.0X2	T60.0X3	T60.0X4	—	—
phthlate	T49.3X1	T49.3X2	T49.3X3	T49.3X4	T49.3X5	T49.3X
polysiloxane	T47.8X1	T47.8X2	T47.8X3	T47.8X4	T47.8X5	T47.8X
sulfate (fumes)	T59.891	T59.892	T59.893	T59.894	—	—
liquid	T65.891	T65.892	T65.893	T65.894	—	—
sulfoxide (nonmedicinal)	T52.8X1	T52.8X2	T52.8X3	T52.8X4	—	—
medicinal	T49.4X1	T49.4X2	T49.4X3	T49.4X4	T49.4X5	T49.4X
tryptamine	T40.991	T40.992	T40.993	T40.994	—	—
tubocurarine	T48.1X1	T48.1X2	T48.1X3	T48.1X4	T48.1X5	T48.1X
Dimethylamine sulfate	T49.4X1	T49.4X2	T49.4X3	T49.4X4	T49.4X5	T49.4X
Dimethylformamide	T52.8X1	T52.8X2	T52.8X3	T52.8X4	—	—
Dimethyltubocurari-nium chloride	T48.1X1	T48.1X2	T48.1X3	T48.1X4	T48.1X5	T48.1X
Dimeticone	T47.1X1	T47.1X2	T47.1X3	T47.1X4	T47.1X5	T47.1X
Dimetilan	T60.0X1	T60.0X2	T60.0X3	T60.0X4	—	—
Dimetindene	T45.0X1	T45.0X2	T45.0X3	T45.0X4	T45.0X5	T45.0X
Dimetotiazine	T43.3X1	T43.3X2	T43.3X3	T43.3X4	T43.3X5	T43.3X
Dimorpholamine	T50.7X1	T50.7X2	T50.7X3	T50.7X4	T50.7X5	T50.7X
Dimoxyline	T46.3X1	T46.3X2	T46.3X3	T46.3X4	T46.3X5	T46.3X
Dinitrobenzene	T65.3X1	T65.3X2	T65.3X3	T65.3X4	—	—
vapor	T59.891	T59.892	T59.893	T59.894	—	—
Dinitrobenzol	T65.3X1	T65.3X2	T65.3X3	T65.3X4	—	—
vapor	T59.891	T59.892	T59.893	T59.894	—	—
Dinitrobutylphenol	T65.3X1	T65.3X2	T65.3X3	T65.3X4	—	—
Dinitro (-ortho-)cresol (pesticide) (spray)	T65.3X1	T65.3X2	T65.3X3	T65.3X4	—	—
Dinitro-cyclohexylphenol	T65.3X1	T65.3X2	T65.3X3	T65.3X4	—	—
Dinitrophenol	T65.3X1	T65.3X2	T65.3X3	T65.3X4	—	—
Dinoprost	T48.0X1	T48.0X2	T48.0X3	T48.0X4	T48.0X5	T48.0X

Substance	Poisoning, Accidental (unintentional)	Poisoning, Intentional self-harm	Poisoning, Assault	Poisoning, Undetermined	Adverse effect	Underdosing
inoprostone	T48.0X1	T48.0X2	T48.0X3	T48.0X4	T48.0X5	T48.0X6
inoseb	T60.3X1	T60.3X2	T60.3X3	T60.3X4	—	—
ioctyl sulfosuccinate alcium) (sodium)	T47.4X1	T47.4X2	T47.4X3	T47.4X4	T47.4X5	T47.4X6
iodone	T50.8X1	T50.8X2	T50.8X3	T50.8X4	T50.8X5	T50.8X6
iodoquin	T37.8X1	T37.8X2	T37.8X3	T37.8X4	T37.8X5	T37.8X6
ionin	T40.2X1	T40.2X2	T40.2X3	T40.2X4	T40.2X5	T40.2X6
iosmin	T46.991	T46.992	T46.993	T46.994	T46.995	T46.996
ioxane	T52.8X1	T52.8X2	T52.8X3	T52.8X4	—	—
ioxathion	T60.0X1	T60.0X2	T60.0X3	T60.0X4	—	—
ioxin	T53.7X1	T53.7X2	T53.7X3	T53.7X4	—	—
ioxopromethazine	T43.3X1	T43.3X2	T43.3X3	T43.3X4	T43.3X5	T43.3X6
ioxyline	T46.3X1	T46.3X2	T46.3X3	T46.3X4	T46.3X5	T46.3X6
ipentene	T52.8X1	T52.8X2	T52.8X3	T52.8X4	—	—
iperodon	T41.3X1	T41.3X2	T41.3X3	T41.3X4	T41.3X5	T41.3X6
iphacinone	T60.4X1	T60.4X2	T60.4X3	T60.4X4	—	—
iphemanil	T44.3X1	T44.3X2	T44.3X3	T44.3X4	T44.3X5	T44.3X6
metilsulfate	T44.3X1	T44.3X2	T44.3X3	T44.3X4	T44.3X5	T44.3X6
iphenadione	T45.511	T45.512	T45.513	T45.514	T45.515	T45.516
rodenticide	T60.4X1	T60.4X2	T60.4X3	T60.4X4	—	—
iphenhydramine	T45.0X1	T45.0X2	T45.0X3	T45.0X4	T45.0X5	T45.0X6
iphenidol	T45.0X1	T45.0X2	T45.0X3	T45.0X4	T45.0X5	T45.0X6
iphenoxylate	T47.6X1	T47.6X2	T47.6X3	T47.6X4	T47.6X5	T47.6X6
iphenylamine	T65.3X1	T65.3X2	T65.3X3	T65.3X4	—	—
iphenylbutazone	T39.2X1	T39.2X2	T39.2X3	T39.2X4	T39.2X5	T39.2X6
iphenyl-chloroarsine, not war	T57.0X1	T57.0X2	T57.0X3	T57.0X4	—	—
iphenylhydantoin	T42.0X1	T42.0X2	T42.0X3	T42.0X4	T42.0X5	T42.0X6
iphenylmethane dye	T52.1X1	T52.1X2	T52.1X3	T52.1X4	—	—
iphenylpyraline	T45.0X1	T45.0X2	T45.0X3	T45.0X4	T45.0X5	T45.0X6
iphtheria						
antitoxin	T50.Z11	T50.Z12	T50.Z13	T50.Z14	T50.Z15	T50.Z16
toxoid	T50.A91	T50.A92	T50.A93	T50.A94	T50.A95	T50.A96
with tetanus toxoid	T50.A21	T50.A22	T50.A23	T50.A24	T50.A25	T50.A26
with pertussis component	T50.A11	T50.A12	T50.A13	T50.A14	T50.A15	T50.A16
vaccine	T50.A91	T50.A92	T50.A93	T50.A94	T50.A95	T50.A96
combination						
including pertussis	T50.A11	T50.A12	T50.A13	T50.A14	T50.A15	T50.A16
without pertussis	T50.A21	T50.A22	T50.A23	T50.A24	T50.A25	T50.A26
iphylline	T50.2X1	T50.2X2	T50.2X3	T50.2X4	T50.2X5	T50.2X6
ipipanone	T40.4X1	T40.4X2	T40.4X3	T40.4X4	—	—
ipivefrine	T49.5X1	T49.5X2	T49.5X3	T49.5X4	T49.5X5	T49.5X6
iplovax	T50.B91	T50.B92	T50.B93	T50.B94	T50.B95	T50.B96
iprophylline	T50.2X1	T50.2X2	T50.2X3	T50.2X4	T50.2X5	T50.2X6
ipropyline	T48.291	T48.292	T48.293	T48.294	T48.295	T48.296
ipyridamole	T46.3X1	T46.3X2	T46.3X3	T46.3X4	T46.3X5	T46.3X6
ipyrone	T39.2X1	T39.2X2	T39.2X3	T39.2X4	T39.2X5	T39.2X6
iquat (dibromide)	T60.3X1	T60.3X2	T60.3X3	T60.3X4	—	—
isinfectant	T65.891	T65.892	T65.893	T65.894	—	—
alkaline	T54.3X1	T54.3X2	T54.3X3	T54.3X4	—	—

Substance	Poisoning, Accidental (unintentional)	Poisoning, Intentional self-harm	Poisoning, Assault	Poisoning, Undetermined	Adverse effect	Underdosing
Disinfectant — *Continued*						
aromatic	T54.1X1	T54.1X2	T54.1X3	T54.1X4	—	—
intestinal	T37.8X1	T37.8X2	T37.8X3	T37.8X4	T37.8X5	T37.8X6
Disipal	T42.8X1	T42.8X2	T42.8X3	T42.8X4	T42.8X5	T42.8X6
Disodium edetate	T50.6X1	T50.6X2	T50.6X3	T50.6X4	T50.6X5	T50.6X6
Disoprofol	T41.291	T41.292	T41.293	T41.294	T41.295	T41.296
Disopyramide	T46.2X1	T46.2X2	T46.2X3	T46.2X4	T46.2X5	T46.2X6
Distigmine (bromide)	T44.0X1	T44.0X2	T44.0X3	T44.0X4	T44.0X5	T44.0X6
Disulfamide	T50.2X1	T50.2X2	T50.2X3	T50.2X4	T50.2X5	T50.2X6
Disulfanilamide	T37.0X1	T37.0X2	T37.0X3	T37.0X4	T37.0X5	T37.0X6
Disulfiram	T50.6X1	T50.6X2	T50.6X3	T50.6X4	T50.6X5	T50.6X6
Disulfoton	T60.0X1	T60.0X2	T60.0X3	T60.0X4	—	—
Dithiazanine iodide	T37.4X1	T37.4X2	T37.4X3	T37.4X4	T37.4X5	T37.4X6
Dithiocarbamate	T60.0X1	T60.0X2	T60.0X3	T60.0X4	—	—
Dithranol	T49.4X1	T49.4X2	T49.4X3	T49.4X4	T49.4X5	T49.4X6
Diucardin	T50.2X1	T50.2X2	T50.2X3	T50.2X4	T50.2X5	T50.2X6
Diupres	T50.2X1	T50.2X2	T50.2X3	T50.2X4	T50.2X5	T50.2X6
Diuretic NEC	T50.2X1	T50.2X2	T50.2X3	T50.2X4	T50.2X5	T50.2X6
benzothiadiazine	T50.2X1	T50.2X2	T50.2X3	T50.2X4	T50.2X5	T50.2X6
carbonic acid anhydrase inhibitors	T50.2X1	T50.2X2	T50.2X3	T50.2X4	T50.2X5	T50.2X6
furfuryl NEC	T50.2X1	T50.2X2	T50.2X3	T50.2X4	T50.2X5	T50.2X6
loop (high-ceiling)	T50.1X1	T50.1X2	T50.1X3	T50.1X4	T50.1X5	T50.1X6
mercurial NEC	T50.2X1	T50.2X2	T50.2X3	T50.2X4	T50.2X5	T50.2X6
osmotic	T50.2X1	T50.2X2	T50.2X3	T50.2X4	T50.2X5	T50.2X6
purine NEC	T50.2X1	T50.2X2	T50.2X3	T50.2X4	T50.2X5	T50.2X6
saluretic NEC	T50.2X1	T50.2X2	T50.2X3	T50.2X4	T50.2X5	T50.2X6
sulfonamide	T50.2X1	T50.2X2	T50.2X3	T50.2X4	T50.2X5	T50.2X6
thiazide NEC	T50.2X1	T50.2X2	T50.2X3	T50.2X4	T50.2X5	T50.2X6
xanthine	T50.2X1	T50.2X2	T50.2X3	T50.2X4	T50.2X5	T50.2X6
Diurgin	T50.2X1	T50.2X2	T50.2X3	T50.2X4	T50.2X5	T50.2X6
Diuril	T50.2X1	T50.2X2	T50.2X3	T50.2X4	T50.2X5	T50.2X6
Diuron	T60.3X1	T60.3X2	T60.3X3	T60.3X4	—	—
Divalproex	T42.6X1	T42.6X2	T42.6X3	T42.6X4	T42.6X5	T42.6X6
Divinyl ether	T41.0X1	T41.0X2	T41.0X3	T41.0X4	T41.0X5	T41.0X6
Dixanthogen	T49.0X1	T49.0X2	T49.0X3	T49.0X4	T49.0X5	T49.0X6
Dixyrazine	T43.3X1	T43.3X2	T43.3X3	T43.3X4	T43.3X5	T43.3X6
D-lysergic acid diethylamide	T40.8X1	T40.8X2	T40.8X3	T40.8X4	—	—
DMCT	T36.4X1	T36.4X2	T36.4X3	T36.4X4	T36.4X5	T36.4X6
DMSO—see Dimethyl sulfoxide						
DNBP	T60.3X1	T60.3X2	T60.3X3	T60.3X4	—	—
DNOC	T65.3X1	T65.3X2	T65.3X3	T65.3X4	—	—
Dobutamine	T44.5X1	T44.5X2	T44.5X3	T44.5X4	T44.5X5	T44.5X6
DOCA	T38.0X1	T38.0X2	T38.0X3	T38.0X4	T38.0X5	T38.0X6
Docusate sodium	T47.4X1	T47.4X2	T47.4X3	T47.4X4	T47.4X5	T47.4X6
Dodicin	T49.0X1	T49.0X2	T49.0X3	T49.0X4	T49.0X5	T49.0X6
Dofamium chloride	T49.0X1	T49.0X2	T49.0X3	T49.0X4	T49.0X5	T49.0X6
Dolophine	T40.3X1	T40.3X2	T40.3X3	T40.3X4	T40.3X5	T40.3X6
Doloxene	T39.8X1	T39.8X2	T39.8X3	T39.8X4	T39.8X5	T39.8X6

Substance	Poisoning, Accidental (unintentional)	Poisoning, Intentional self-harm	Poisoning, Assault	Poisoning, Undetermined	Adverse effect	Underdosing
Domestic gas (after combustion)—see Gas, utility						
prior to combustion	T59.891	T59.892	T59.893	T59.894	—	—
Domiodol	T48.4X1	T48.4X2	T48.4X3	T48.4X4	T48.4X5	T48.4X6
Domiphen (bromide)	T49.0X1	T49.0X2	T49.0X3	T49.0X4	T49.0X5	T49.0X6
Domperidone	T45.0X1	T45.0X2	T45.0X3	T45.0X4	T45.0X5	T45.0X6
Dopa	T42.8X1	T42.8X2	T42.8X3	T42.8X4	T42.8X5	T42.8X6
Dopamine	T44.991	T44.992	T44.993	T44.994	T44.995	T44.996
Doriden	T42.6X1	T42.6X2	T42.6X3	T42.6X4	T42.6X5	T42.6X6
Dormiral	T42.3X1	T42.3X2	T42.3X3	T42.3X4	T42.3X5	T42.3X6
Dormison	T42.6X1	T42.6X2	T42.6X3	T42.6X4	T42.6X5	T42.6X6
Dornase	T48.4X1	T48.4X2	T48.4X3	T48.4X4	T48.4X5	T48.4X6
Dorsacaine	T41.3X1	T41.3X2	T41.3X3	T41.3X4	T41.3X5	T41.3X6
Dosulepin	T43.011	T43.012	T43.013	T43.014	T43.015	T43.016
Dothiepin	T43.011	T43.012	T43.013	T43.014	T43.015	T43.016
Doxantrazole	T48.6X1	T48.6X2	T48.6X3	T48.6X4	T48.6X5	T48.6X6
Doxapram	T50.7X1	T50.7X2	T50.7X3	T50.7X4	T50.7X5	T50.7X6
Doxazosin	T44.6X1	T44.6X2	T44.6X3	T44.6X4	T44.6X5	T44.6X6
Doxepin	T43.011	T43.012	T43.013	T43.014	T43.015	T43.016
Doxifluridine	T45.1X1	T45.1X2	T45.1X3	T45.1X4	T45.1X5	T45.1X6
Doxorubicin	T45.1X1	T45.1X2	T45.1X3	T45.1X4	T45.1X5	T45.1X6
Doxycycline	T36.4X1	T36.4X2	T36.4X3	T36.4X4	T36.4X5	T36.4X6
Doxylamine	T45.0X1	T45.0X2	T45.0X3	T45.0X4	T45.0X5	T45.0X6
Dramamine	T45.0X1	T45.0X2	T45.0X3	T45.0X4	T45.0X5	T45.0X6
Drano (drain cleaner)	T54.3X1	T54.3X2	T54.3X3	T54.3X4	—	—
Dressing, live pulp	T49.7X1	T49.7X2	T49.7X3	T49.7X4	T49.7X5	T49.7X6
Drocode	T40.2X1	T40.2X2	T40.2X3	T40.2X4	T40.2X5	T40.2X6
Dromoran	T40.2X1	T40.2X2	T40.2X3	T40.2X4	T40.2X5	T40.2X6
Dromostanolone	T38.7X1	T38.7X2	T38.7X3	T38.7X4	T38.7X5	T38.7X6
Dronabinol	T40.7X1	T40.7X2	T40.7X3	T40.7X4	T40.7X5	T40.7X6
Droperidol	T43.591	T43.592	T43.593	T43.594	T43.595	T43.596
Dropropizine	T48.3X1	T48.3X2	T48.3X3	T48.3X4	T48.3X5	T48.3X6
Drostanolone	T38.7X1	T38.7X2	T38.7X3	T38.7X4	T38.7X5	T38.7X6
Drotaverine	T44.3X1	T44.3X2	T44.3X3	T44.3X4	T44.3X5	T44.3X6
Drotrecogin alfa	T45.511	T45.512	T45.513	T45.514	T45.515	T45.516
Drug NEC	T50.901	T50.902	T50.903	T50.904	T50.905	T50.906
specified NEC	T50.991	T50.992	T50.993	T50.994	T50.995	T50.996
DTIC	T45.1X1	T45.1X2	T45.1X3	T45.1X4	T45.1X5	T45.1X6
Duboisine	T44.3X1	T44.3X2	T44.3X3	T44.3X4	T44.3X5	T44.3X6
Dulcolax	T47.2X1	T47.2X2	T47.2X3	T47.2X4	T47.2X5	T47.2X6
Duponol (C) (EP)	T49.2X1	T49.2X2	T49.2X3	T49.2X4	T49.2X5	T49.2X6
Durabolin	T38.7X1	T38.7X2	T38.7X3	T38.7X4	T38.7X5	T38.7X6
Dyclone	T41.3X1	T41.3X2	T41.3X3	T41.3X4	T41.3X5	T41.3X6
Dyclonine	T41.3X1	T41.3X2	T41.3X3	T41.3X4	T41.3X5	T41.3X6
Dydrogesterone	T38.5X1	T38.5X2	T38.5X3	T38.5X4	T38.5X5	T38.5X6
Dye NEC	T65.6X1	T65.6X2	T65.6X3	T65.6X4	—	—
antiseptic	T49.0X1	T49.0X2	T49.0X3	T49.0X4	T49.0X5	T49.0X6
diagnostic agents	T50.8X1	T50.8X2	T50.8X3	T50.8X4	T50.8X5	T50.8X6
pharmaceutical NEC	T50.901	T50.902	T50.903	T50.904	T50.905	T50.906
Dyflos	T44.0X1	T44.0X2	T44.0X3	T44.0X4	T44.0X5	T44.0X6

Substance	Poisoning, Accidental (unintentional)	Poisoning, Intentional self-harm	Poisoning, Assault	Poisoning, Undetermined	Adverse effect	Underdosing
Dymelor	T38.3X1	T38.3X2	T38.3X3	T38.3X4	T38.3X5	T38.3X
Dynamite	T65.3X1	T65.3X2	T65.3X3	T65.3X4	—	—
fumes	T59.891	T59.892	T59.893	T59.894	—	—
Dyphylline	T44.3X1	T44.3X2	T44.3X3	T44.3X4	T44.3X5	T44.3X
E						
Ear drug NEC	T49.6X1	T49.6X2	T49.6X3	T49.6X4	T49.6X5	T49.6X
Ear preparations	T49.6X1	T49.6X2	T49.6X3	T49.6X4	T49.6X5	T49.6X
Echothiophate, echothiopate, ecothiopate	T49.5X1	T49.5X2	T49.5X3	T49.5X4	T49.5X5	T49.5X
Econazole	T49.0X1	T49.0X2	T49.0X3	T49.0X4	T49.0X5	T49.0X
Ecothiopate iodide	T49.5X1	T49.5X2	T49.5X3	T49.5X4	T49.5X5	T49.5X
Ecstasy	T43.621	T43.622	T43.623	T43.624	T43.625	T43.62
Ectylurea	T42.6X1	T42.6X2	T42.6X3	T42.6X4	T42.6X5	T42.6X
Edathamil disodium	T45.8X1	T45.8X2	T45.8X3	T45.8X4	T45.8X5	T45.8X
Edecrin	T50.1X1	T50.1X2	T50.1X3	T50.1X4	T50.1X5	T50.1X
Edetate, disodium (calcium)	T45.8X1	T45.8X2	T45.8X3	T45.8X4	T45.8X5	T45.8X
Edoxudine	T49.5X1	T49.5X2	T49.5X3	T49.5X4	T49.5X5	T49.5X
Edrophonium	T44.0X1	T44.0X2	T44.0X3	T44.0X4	T44.0X5	T44.0X
chloride	T44.0X1	T44.0X2	T44.0X3	T44.0X4	T44.0X5	T44.0X
EDTA	T50.6X1	T50.6X2	T50.6X3	T50.6X4	T50.6X5	T50.6X
Eflornithine	T37.2X1	T37.2X2	T37.2X3	T37.2X4	T37.2X5	T37.2X
Efloxate	T46.3X1	T46.3X2	T46.3X3	T46.3X4	T46.3X5	T46.3X
Elase	T49.8X1	T49.8X2	T49.8X3	T49.8X4	T49.8X5	T49.8X
Elastase	T47.5X1	T47.5X2	T47.5X3	T47.5X4	T47.5X5	T47.5X
Elaterium	T47.2X1	T47.2X2	T47.2X3	T47.2X4	T47.2X5	T47.2X
Elcatonin	T50.991	T50.992	T50.993	T50.994	T50.995	T50.99
Elder	T62.2X1	T62.2X2	T62.2X3	T62.2X4	—	—
berry,(unripe)	T62.1X1	T62.1X2	T62.1X3	T62.1X4	—	—
Electrolyte balance drug	T50.3X1	T50.3X2	T50.3X3	T50.3X4	T50.3X5	T50.3X
Electrolytes NEC	T50.3X1	T50.3X2	T50.3X3	T50.3X4	T50.3X5	T50.3X
Electrolytic agent NEC	T50.3X1	T50.3X2	T50.3X3	T50.3X4	T50.3X5	T50.3X
Elemental diet	T50.901	T50.902	T50.903	T50.904	T50.905	T50.90
Elliptinium acetate	T45.1X1	T45.1X2	T45.1X3	T45.1X4	T45.1X5	T45.1X
Embramine	T45.0X1	T45.0X2	T45.0X3	T45.0X4	T45.0X5	T45.0X
Emepronium (salts)	T44.3X1	T44.3X2	T44.3X3	T44.3X4	T44.3X5	T44.3X
bromide	T44.3X1	T44.3X2	T44.3X3	T44.3X4	T44.3X5	T44.3X
Emetic NEC	T47.7X1	T47.7X2	T47.7X3	T47.7X4	T47.7X5	T47.7X
Emetine	T37.3X1	T37.3X2	T37.3X3	T37.3X4	T37.3X5	T37.3X
Emollient NEC	T49.3X1	T49.3X2	T49.3X3	T49.3X4	T49.3X5	T49.3X
Emorfazone	T39.8X1	T39.8X2	T39.8X3	T39.8X4	T39.8X5	T39.8X
Emylcamate	T43.591	T43.592	T43.593	T43.594	T43.595	T43.59
Enalapril	T46.4X1	T46.4X2	T46.4X3	T46.4X4	T46.4X5	T46.4X
Enalaprilat	T46.4X1	T46.4X2	T46.4X3	T46.4X4	T46.4X5	T46.4X
Encainide	T46.2X1	T46.2X2	T46.2X3	T46.2X4	T46.2X5	T46.2X
Endocaine	T41.3X1	T41.3X2	T41.3X3	T41.3X4	T41.3X5	T41.3X
Endosulfan	T60.2X1	T60.2X2	T60.2X3	T60.2X4	—	—
Endothall	T60.3X1	T60.3X2	T60.3X3	T60.3X4	—	—
Endralazine	T46.5X1	T46.5X2	T46.5X3	T46.5X4	T46.5X5	T46.5X
Endrin	T60.1X1	T60.1X2	T60.1X3	T60.1X4	—	—

Substance	Poisoning, Accidental (unintentional)	Poisoning, Intentional self-harm	Poisoning, Assault	Poisoning, Undetermined	Adverse effect	Underdosing
nflurane	T41.0X1	T41.0X2	T41.0X3	T41.0X4	T41.0X5	T41.0X6
nhexymal	T42.3X1	T42.3X2	T42.3X3	T42.3X4	T42.3X5	T42.3X6
nocitabine	T45.1X1	T45.1X2	T45.1X3	T45.1X4	T45.1X5	T45.1X6
novid	T38.4X1	T38.4X2	T38.4X3	T38.4X4	T38.4X5	T38.4X6
noxacin	T36.8X1	T36.8X2	T36.8X3	T36.8X4	T36.8X5	T36.8X6
noxaparin (sodium)	T45.511	T45.512	T45.513	T45.514	T45.515	T45.516
npiprazole	T43.591	T43.592	T43.593	T43.594	T43.595	T43.596
nprofylline	T48.6X1	T48.6X2	T48.6X3	T48.6X4	T48.6X5	T48.6X6
nprostil	T47.1X1	T47.1X2	T47.1X3	T47.1X4	T47.1X5	T47.1X6
NT preparations nti-infectives)	T49.6X1	T49.6X2	T49.6X3	T49.6X4	T49.6X5	T49.6X6
nterogastrone	T38.891	T38.892	T38.893	T38.894	T38.895	T38.896
nviomycin	T36.8X1	T36.8X2	T36.8X3	T36.8X4	T36.8X5	T36.8X6
nzodase	T45.3X1	T45.3X2	T45.3X3	T45.3X4	T45.3X5	T45.3X6
nzyme NEC	T45.3X1	T45.3X2	T45.3X3	T45.3X4	T45.3X5	T45.3X6
depolymerizing	T49.8X1	T49.8X2	T49.8X3	T49.8X4	T49.8X5	T49.8X6
fibrolytic	T45.3X1	T45.3X2	T45.3X3	T45.3X4	T45.3X5	T45.3X6
gastric	T47.5X1	T47.5X2	T47.5X3	T47.5X4	T47.5X5	T47.5X6
intestinal	T47.5X1	T47.5X2	T47.5X3	T47.5X4	T47.5X5	T47.5X6
local action	T49.4X1	T49.4X2	T49.4X3	T49.4X4	T49.4X5	T49.4X6
proteolytic	T49.4X1	T49.4X2	T49.4X3	T49.4X4	T49.4X5	T49.4X6
thrombolytic	T45.3X1	T45.3X2	T45.3X3	T45.3X4	T45.3X5	T45.3X6
PAB	T41.3X1	T41.3X2	T41.3X3	T41.3X4	T41.3X5	T41.3X6
panutin	T42.0X1	T42.0X2	T42.0X3	T42.0X4	T42.0X5	T42.0X6
phedra	T44.991	T44.992	T44.993	T44.994	T44.995	T44.996
phedrine	T44.991	T44.992	T44.993	T44.994	T44.995	T44.996
pichlorhydrin, pichlorohydrin	T52.8X1	T52.8X2	T52.8X3	T52.8X4	—	—
picillin	T36.0X1	T36.0X2	T36.0X3	T36.0X4	T36.0X5	T36.0X6
piestriol	T38.5X1	T38.5X2	T38.5X3	T38.5X4	T38.5X5	T38.5X6
pilim—see Sodium alproate						
pimestrol	T38.5X1	T38.5X2	T38.5X3	T38.5X4	T38.5X5	T38.5X6
pinephrine	T44.5X1	T44.5X2	T44.5X3	T44.5X4	T44.5X5	T44.5X6
pirubicin	T45.1X1	T45.1X2	T45.1X3	T45.1X4	T45.1X5	T45.1X6
pitiostanol	T38.7X1	T38.7X2	T38.7X3	T38.7X4	T38.7X5	T38.7X6
pitizide	T50.2X1	T50.2X2	T50.2X3	T50.2X4	T50.2X5	T50.2X6
PN	T60.0X1	T60.0X2	T60.0X3	T60.0X4	—	—
PO	T45.8X1	T45.8X2	T45.8X3	T45.8X4	T45.8X5	T45.8X6
poetin alpha	T45.8X1	T45.8X2	T45.8X3	T45.8X4	T45.8X5	T45.8X6
pomediol	T50.991	T50.992	T50.993	T50.994	T50.995	T50.996
poprostenol	T45.521	T45.522	T45.523	T45.524	T45.525	T45.526
poxy resin	T65.891	T65.892	T65.893	T65.894	—	—
prazinone	T48.4X1	T48.4X2	T48.4X3	T48.4X4	T48.4X5	T48.4X6
psilon amino-caproic acid	T45.621	T45.622	T45.623	T45.624	T45.625	T45.626
psom salt	T47.3X1	T47.3X2	T47.3X3	T47.3X4	T47.3X5	T47.3X6
ptazocine	T40.4X1	T40.4X2	T40.4X3	T40.4X4	T40.4X5	T40.4X6
quanil	T43.591	T43.592	T43.593	T43.594	T43.595	T43.596
quisetum	T62.2X1	T62.2X2	T62.2X3	T62.2X4	—	—
diuretic	T50.2X1	T50.2X2	T50.2X3	T50.2X4	T50.2X5	T50.2X6
rgobasine	T48.0X1	T48.0X2	T48.0X3	T48.0X4	T48.0X5	T48.0X6
Ergocalciferol	T45.2X1	T45.2X2	T45.2X3	T45.2X4	T45.2X5	T45.2X6
Ergoloid mesylates	T46.7X1	T46.7X2	T46.7X3	T46.7X4	T46.7X5	T46.7X6
Ergometrine	T48.0X1	T48.0X2	T48.0X3	T48.0X4	T48.0X5	T48.0X6
Ergonovine	T48.0X1	T48.0X2	T48.0X3	T48.0X4	T48.0X5	T48.0X6
Ergot NEC	T64.81	T64.82	T64.83	T64.84	—	—
derivative	T48.0X1	T48.0X2	T48.0X3	T48.0X4	T48.0X5	T48.0X6
medicinal (alkaloids)	T48.0X1	T48.0X2	T48.0X3	T48.0X4	T48.0X5	T48.0X6
prepared	T48.0X1	T48.0X2	T48.0X3	T48.0X4	T48.0X5	T48.0X6
Ergotamine	T46.5X1	T46.5X2	T46.5X3	T46.5X4	T46.5X5	T46.5X6
Ergotocine	T48.0X1	T48.0X2	T48.0X3	T48.0X4	T48.0X5	T48.0X6
Ergotrate	T48.0X1	T48.0X2	T48.0X3	T48.0X4	T48.0X5	T48.0X6
Eritrityl tetranitrate	T46.3X1	T46.3X2	T46.3X3	T46.3X4	T46.3X5	T46.3X6
Erythrityl tetranitrate	T46.3X1	T46.3X2	T46.3X3	T46.3X4	T46.3X5	T46.3X6
Erythrol tetranitrate	T46.3X1	T46.3X2	T46.3X3	T46.3X4	T46.3X5	T46.3X6
Erythromycin (salts)	T36.3X1	T36.3X2	T36.3X3	T36.3X4	T36.3X5	T36.3X6
ophthalmic preparation	T49.5X1	T49.5X2	T49.5X3	T49.5X4	T49.5X5	T49.5X6
topical NEC	T49.0X1	T49.0X2	T49.0X3	T49.0X4	T49.0X5	T49.0X6
Erythropoietin	T45.8X1	T45.8X2	T45.8X3	T45.8X4	T45.8X5	T45.8X6
human	T45.8X1	T45.8X2	T45.8X3	T45.8X4	T45.8X5	T45.8X6
Escin	T46.991	T46.992	T46.993	T46.994	T46.995	T46.996
Esculin	T45.2X1	T45.2X2	T45.2X3	T45.2X4	T45.2X5	T45.2X6
Esculoside	T45.2X1	T45.2X2	T45.2X3	T45.2X4	T45.2X5	T45.2X6
ESDT (ether-soluble tar distillate)	T49.1X1	T49.1X2	T49.1X3	T49.1X4	T49.1X5	T49.1X6
Eserine	T49.5X1	T49.5X2	T49.5X3	T49.5X4	T49.5X5	T49.5X6
Esflurbiprofen	T39.311	T39.312	T39.313	T39.314	T39.315	T39.316
Eskabarb	T42.3X1	T42.3X2	T42.3X3	T42.3X4	T42.3X5	T42.3X6
Eskalith	T43.8X1	T43.8X2	T43.8X3	T43.8X4	T43.8X5	T43.8X6
Esmolol	T44.7X1	T44.7X2	T44.7X3	T44.7X4	T44.7X5	T44.7X6
Estanozolol	T38.7X1	T38.7X2	T38.7X3	T38.7X4	T38.7X5	T38.7X6
Estazolam	T42.4X1	T42.4X2	T42.4X3	T42.4X4	T42.4X5	T42.4X6
Estradiol	T38.5X1	T38.5X2	T38.5X3	T38.5X4	T38.5X5	T38.5X6
with testosterone	T38.7X1	T38.7X2	T38.7X3	T38.7X4	T38.7X5	T38.7X6
benzoate	T38.5X1	T38.5X2	T38.5X3	T38.5X4	T38.5X5	T38.5X6
Estramustine	T45.1X1	T45.1X2	T45.1X3	T45.1X4	T45.1X5	T45.1X6
Estriol	T38.5X1	T38.5X2	T38.5X3	T38.5X4	T38.5X5	T38.5X6
Estrogen	T38.5X1	T38.5X2	T38.5X3	T38.5X4	T38.5X5	T38.5X6
with progesterone	T38.5X1	T38.5X2	T38.5X3	T38.5X4	T38.5X5	T38.5X6
conjugated	T38.5X1	T38.5X2	T38.5X3	T38.5X4	T38.5X5	T38.5X6
Estrone	T38.5X1	T38.5X2	T38.5X3	T38.5X4	T38.5X5	T38.5X6
Estropipate	T38.5X1	T38.5X2	T38.5X3	T38.5X4	T38.5X5	T38.5X6
Etacrynate sodium	T50.1X1	T50.1X2	T50.1X3	T50.1X4	T50.1X5	T50.1X6
Etacrynic acid	T50.1X1	T50.1X2	T50.1X3	T50.1X4	T50.1X5	T50.1X6
Etafedrine	T48.6X1	T48.6X2	T48.6X3	T48.6X4	T48.6X5	T48.6X6
Etafenone	T46.3X1	T46.3X2	T46.3X3	T46.3X4	T46.3X5	T46.3X6
Etambutol	T37.1X1	T37.1X2	T37.1X3	T37.1X4	T37.1X5	T37.1X6
Etamiphyllin	T48.6X1	T48.6X2	T48.6X3	T48.6X4	T48.6X5	T48.6X6
Etamivan	T50.7X1	T50.7X2	T50.7X3	T50.7X4	T50.7X5	T50.7X6
Etamsylate	T45.7X1	T45.7X2	T45.7X3	T45.7X4	T45.7X5	T45.7X6
Etebenecid	T50.4X1	T50.4X2	T50.4X3	T50.4X4	T50.4X5	T50.4X6

Substance	Poisoning, Accidental (unintentional)	Poisoning, Intentional self-harm	Poisoning, Assault	Poisoning, Undetermined	Adverse effect	Underdosing
Ethacridine	T49.0X1	T49.0X2	T49.0X3	T49.0X4	T49.0X5	T49.0X6
Ethacrynic acid	T50.1X1	T50.1X2	T50.1X3	T50.1X4	T50.1X5	T50.1X6
Ethadione	T42.2X1	T42.2X2	T42.2X3	T42.2X4	T42.2X5	T42.2X6
Ethambutol	T37.1X1	T37.1X2	T37.1X3	T37.1X4	T37.1X5	T37.1X6
Ethamide	T50.2X1	T50.2X2	T50.2X3	T50.2X4	T50.2X5	T50.2X6
Ethamivan	T50.7X1	T50.7X2	T50.7X3	T50.7X4	T50.7X5	T50.7X6
Ethamsylate	T45.7X1	T45.7X2	T45.7X3	T45.7X4	T45.7X5	T45.7X6
Ethanol	T51.0X1	T51.0X2	T51.0X3	T51.0X4	—	—
beverage	T51.0X1	T51.0X2	T51.0X3	T51.0X4	—	—
Ethanolamine oleate	T46.8X1	T46.8X2	T46.8X3	T46.8X4	T46.8X5	T46.8X6
Ethaverine	T44.3X1	T44.3X2	T44.3X3	T44.3X4	T44.3X5	T44.3X6
Ethchlorvynol	T42.6X1	T42.6X2	T42.6X3	T42.6X4	T42.6X5	T42.6X6
Ethebenecid	T50.4X1	T50.4X2	T50.4X3	T50.4X4	T50.4X5	T50.4X6
Ether (vapor)	T41.0X1	T41.0X2	T41.0X3	T41.0X4	T41.0X5	T41.0X6
anesthetic	T41.0X1	T41.0X2	T41.0X3	T41.0X4	T41.0X5	T41.0X6
divinyl	T41.0X1	T41.0X2	T41.0X3	T41.0X4	T41.0X5	T41.0X6
ethyl (medicinal)	T41.0X1	T41.0X2	T41.0X3	T41.0X4	T41.0X5	T41.0X6
nonmedicinal	T52.8X1	T52.8X2	T52.8X3	T52.8X4	—	—
petroleum—see Ligroin						
solvent	T52.8X1	T52.8X2	T52.8X3	T52.8X4	—	—
Ethiazide	T50.2X1	T50.2X2	T50.2X3	T50.2X4	T50.2X5	T50.2X6
Ethidium chloride (vapor)	T59.891	T59.892	T59.893	T59.894	—	—
Ethinamate	T42.6X1	T42.6X2	T42.6X3	T42.6X4	T42.6X5	T42.6X6
Ethinylestradiol, ethinyloestradiol	T38.5X1	T38.5X2	T38.5X3	T38.5X4	T38.5X5	T38.5X6
with						
levonorgestrel	T38.4X1	T38.4X2	T38.4X3	T38.4X4	T38.4X5	T38.4X6
norethisterone	T38.4X1	T38.4X2	T38.4X3	T38.4X4	T38.4X5	T38.4X6
Ethiodized oil (131 I)	T50.8X1	T50.8X2	T50.8X3	T50.8X4	T50.8X5	T50.8X6
Ethion	T60.0X1	T60.0X2	T60.0X3	T60.0X4	—	—
Ethionamide	T37.1X1	T37.1X2	T37.1X3	T37.1X4	T37.1X5	T37.1X6
Ethioniamide	T37.1X1	T37.1X2	T37.1X3	T37.1X4	T37.1X5	T37.1X6
Ethisterone	T38.5X1	T38.5X2	T38.5X3	T38.5X4	T38.5X5	T38.5X6
Ethobral	T42.3X1	T42.3X2	T42.3X3	T42.3X4	T42.3X5	T42.3X6
Ethocaine (infiltration) (topical)	T41.3X1	T41.3X2	T41.3X3	T41.3X4	T41.3X5	T41.3X6
nerve block (peripheral) (plexus)	T41.3X1	T41.3X2	T41.3X3	T41.3X4	T41.3X5	T41.3X6
spinal	T41.3X1	T41.3X2	T41.3X3	T41.3X4	T41.3X5	T41.3X6
Ethoheptazine	T40.4X1	T40.4X2	T40.4X3	T40.4X4	T40.4X5	T40.4X6
Ethopropazine	T44.3X1	T44.3X2	T44.3X3	T44.3X4	T44.3X5	T44.3X6
Ethosuximide	T42.2X1	T42.2X2	T42.2X3	T42.2X4	T42.2X5	T42.2X6
Ethotoin	T42.0X1	T42.0X2	T42.0X3	T42.0X4	T42.0X5	T42.0X6
Ethoxazene	T37.91	T37.92	T37.93	T37.94	T37.95	T37.96
Ethoxazorutoside	T46.991	T46.992	T46.993	T46.994	T46.995	T46.996
2-Ethoxyethanol	T52.3X1	T52.3X2	T52.3X3	T52.3X4	—	—
Ethoxzolamide	T50.2X1	T50.2X2	T50.2X3	T50.2X4	T50.2X5	T50.2X6
Ethyl						
acetate	T52.8X1	T52.8X2	T52.8X3	T52.8X4	—	—
alcohol	T51.0X1	T51.0X2	T51.0X3	T51.0X4	—	—
beverage	T51.0X1	T51.0X2	T51.0X3	T51.0X4	—	—

Substance	Poisoning, Accidental (unintentional)	Poisoning, Intentional self-harm	Poisoning, Assault	Poisoning, Undetermined	Adverse effect	Underdosing
Ethyl — *Continued*						
aldehyde (vapor)	T59.891	T59.892	T59.893	T59.894	—	—
liquid	T52.8X1	T52.8X2	T52.8X3	T52.8X4	—	—
aminobenzoate	T41.3X1	T41.3X2	T41.3X3	T41.3X4	T41.3X5	T41.3X
aminophenothiazine	T43.3X1	T43.3X2	T43.3X3	T43.3X4	T43.3X5	T43.3X
benzoate	T52.8X1	T52.8X2	T52.8X3	T52.8X4	—	—
biscoumacetate	T45.511	T45.512	T45.513	T45.514	T45.515	T45.51
bromide (anesthetic)	T41.0X1	T41.0X2	T41.0X3	T41.0X4	T41.0X5	T41.0X
carbamate	T45.1X1	T45.1X2	T45.1X3	T45.1X4	T45.1X5	T45.1X
carbinol	T51.3X1	T51.3X2	T51.3X3	T51.3X4	—	—
carbonate	T52.8X1	T52.8X2	T52.8X3	T52.8X4	—	—
chaulmoograte	T37.1X1	T37.1X2	T37.1X3	T37.1X4	T37.1X5	T37.1X
chloride (anesthetic)	T41.0X1	T41.0X2	T41.0X3	T41.0X4	T41.0X5	T41.0X
anesthetic (local)	T41.3X1	T41.3X2	T41.3X3	T41.3X4	T41.3X5	T41.3X
inhaled	T41.0X1	T41.0X2	T41.0X3	T41.0X4	T41.0X5	T41.0X
local	T49.4X1	T49.4X2	T49.4X3	T49.4X4	T49.4X5	T49.4X
solvent	T53.6X1	T53.6X2	T53.6X3	T53.6X4	—	—
dibunate	T48.3X1	T48.3X2	T48.3X3	T48.3X4	T48.3X5	T48.3X
dichloroarsine (vapor)	T57.0X1	T57.0X2	T57.0X3	T57.0X4	—	—
estranol	T38.7X1	T38.7X2	T38.7X3	T38.7X4	T38.7X5	T38.7X
ether—see also ether	T52.8X1	T52.8X2	T52.8X3	T52.8X4	—	—
formate NEC (solvent)	T52.0X1	T52.0X2	T52.0X3	T52.0X4	—	—
fumarate	T49.4X1	T49.4X2	T49.4X3	T49.4X4	T49.4X5	T49.4X
hydroxyisobutyrate NEC (solvent)	T52.8X1	T52.8X2	T52.8X3	T52.8X4	—	—
iodoacetate	T59.3X1	T59.3X2	T59.3X3	T59.3X4	—	—
lactate NEC (solvent)	T52.8X1	T52.8X2	T52.8X3	T52.8X4	—	—
loflazepate	T42.4X1	T42.4X2	T42.4X3	T42.4X4	T42.4X5	T42.4X
mercuric chloride	T56.1X1	T56.1X2	T56.1X3	T56.1X4	—	—
methylcarbinol	T51.8X1	T51.8X2	T51.8X3	T51.8X4	—	—
morphine	T40.2X1	T40.2X2	T40.2X3	T40.2X4	T40.2X5	T40.2X
noradrenaline	T48.6X1	T48.6X2	T48.6X3	T48.6X4	T48.6X5	T48.6X
oxybutyrate NEC (solvent)	T52.8X1	T52.8X2	T52.8X3	T52.8X4	—	—
Ethylene (gas)	T59.891	T59.892	T59.893	T59.894	—	—
anesthetic (general)	T41.0X1	T41.0X2	T41.0X3	T41.0X4	T41.0X5	T41.0X
chlorohydrin	T52.8X1	T52.8X2	T52.8X3	T52.8X4	—	—
vapor	T53.6X1	T53.6X2	T53.6X3	T53.6X4	—	—
dichloride	T52.8X1	T52.8X2	T52.8X3	T52.8X4	—	—
vapor	T53.6X1	T53.6X2	T53.6X3	T53.6X4	—	—
dinitrate	T52.3X1	T52.3X2	T52.3X3	T52.3X4	—	—
glycol(s)	T52.8X1	T52.8X2	T52.8X3	T52.8X4	—	—
dinitrate	T52.3X1	T52.3X2	T52.3X3	T52.3X4	—	—
monobutyl ether	T52.3X1	T52.3X2	T52.3X3	T52.3X4	—	—
imine	T54.1X1	T54.1X2	T54.1X3	T54.1X4	—	—
oxide (fumigant) (nonmedicinal)	T59.891	T59.892	T59.893	T59.894	—	—
medicinal	T49.0X1	T49.0X2	T49.0X3	T49.0X4	T49.0X5	T49.0X
Ethylenediamine theophylline	T48.6X1	T48.6X2	T48.6X3	T48.6X4	T48.6X5	T48.6X
Ethylenediaminetetra-acetic acid	T50.6X1	T50.6X2	T50.6X3	T50.6X4	T50.6X5	T50.6X

Substance	Poisoning, Accidental (unintentional)	Poisoning, Intentional self-harm	Poisoning, Assault	Poisoning, Undetermined	Adverse effect	Underdosing
hylen-edinitrilotetra-etate	T50.6X1	T50.6X2	T50.6X3	T50.6X4	T50.6X5	T50.6X6
hylestrenol	T38.7X1	T38.7X2	T38.7X3	T38.7X4	T38.7X5	T38.7X6
hylhydro-xycellulose	T47.4X1	T47.4X2	T47.4X3	T47.4X4	T47.4X5	T47.4X6
hylidene						
chloride NEC	T53.6X1	T53.6X2	T53.6X3	T53.6X4	—	—
diacetate	T60.3X1	T60.3X2	T60.3X3	T60.3X4	—	—
licoumarin	T45.511	T45.512	T45.513	T45.514	T45.515	T45.516
dicoumarol	T45.511	T45.512	T45.513	T45.514	T45.515	T45.516
diethyl ether	T52.0X1	T52.0X2	T52.0X3	T52.0X4	—	—
hylmorphine	T40.2X1	T40.2X2	T40.2X3	T40.2X4	T40.2X5	T40.2X6
hylnorepinephrine	T48.6X1	T48.6X2	T48.6X3	T48.6X4	T48.6X5	T48.6X6
hylparachloro-enoxyisobutyrate	T46.6X1	T46.6X2	T46.6X3	T46.6X4	T46.6X5	T46.6X6
hynodiol	T38.4X1	T38.4X2	T38.4X3	T38.4X4	T38.4X5	T38.4X6
with mestranol diacetate	T38.4X1	T38.4X2	T38.4X3	T38.4X4	T38.4X5	T38.4X6
idocaine	T41.3X1	T41.3X2	T41.3X3	T41.3X4	T41.3X5	T41.3X6
infiltration (subcutaneous)	T41.3X1	T41.3X2	T41.3X3	T41.3X4	T41.3X5	T41.3X6
nerve (peripheral) (plexus)	T41.3X1	T41.3X2	T41.3X3	T41.3X4	T41.3X5	T41.3X6
idronate	T50.991	T50.992	T50.993	T50.994	T50.995	T50.996
idronic acid (disodium t)	T50.991	T50.992	T50.993	T50.994	T50.995	T50.996
ifoxine	T42.6X1	T42.6X2	T42.6X3	T42.6X4	T42.6X5	T42.6X6
ilefrine	T44.4X1	T44.4X2	T44.4X3	T44.4X4	T44.4X5	T44.4X6
ilfen	T42.3X1	T42.3X2	T42.3X3	T42.3X4	T42.3X5	T42.3X6
inodiol	T38.4X1	T38.4X2	T38.4X3	T38.4X4	T38.4X5	T38.4X6
iroxate	T46.6X1	T46.6X2	T46.6X3	T46.6X4	T46.6X5	T46.6X6
izolam	T42.4X1	T42.4X2	T42.4X3	T42.4X4	T42.4X5	T42.4X6
odolac	T39.391	T39.392	T39.393	T39.394	T39.395	T39.396
ofamide	T37.3X1	T37.3X2	T37.3X3	T37.3X4	T37.3X5	T37.3X6
ofibrate	T46.6X1	T46.6X2	T46.6X3	T46.6X4	T46.6X5	T46.6X6
ofylline	T46.7X1	T46.7X2	T46.7X3	T46.7X4	T46.7X5	T46.7X6
clofibrate	T46.6X1	T46.6X2	T46.6X3	T46.6X4	T46.6X5	T46.6X6
oglucid	T45.1X1	T45.1X2	T45.1X3	T45.1X4	T45.1X5	T45.1X6
omidate	T41.1X1	T41.1X2	T41.1X3	T41.1X4	T41.1X5	T41.1X6
omide	T39.8X1	T39.8X2	T39.8X3	T39.8X4	T39.8X5	T39.8X6
omidoline	T44.3X1	T44.3X2	T44.3X3	T44.3X4	T44.3X5	T44.3X6
oposide	T45.1X1	T45.1X2	T45.1X3	T45.1X4	T45.1X5	T45.1X6
orphine	T40.2X1	T40.2X2	T40.2X3	T40.2X4	T40.2X5	T40.2X6
oval	T42.3X1	T42.3X2	T42.3X3	T42.3X4	T42.3X5	T42.3X6
ozolin	T50.1X1	T50.1X2	T50.1X3	T50.1X4	T50.1X5	T50.1X6
retinate	T50.991	T50.992	T50.993	T50.994	T50.995	T50.996
ryptamine	T43.691	T43.692	T43.693	T43.694	T43.695	T43.696
ybenzatropine	T44.3X1	T44.3X2	T44.3X3	T44.3X4	T44.3X5	T44.3X6
ynodiol	T38.4X1	T38.4X2	T38.4X3	T38.4X4	T38.4X5	T38.4X6
ucaine	T41.3X1	T41.3X2	T41.3X3	T41.3X4	T41.3X5	T41.3X6
ucalyptus oil	T49.7X1	T49.7X2	T49.7X3	T49.7X4	T49.7X5	T49.7X6
ucatropine	T49.5X1	T49.5X2	T49.5X3	T49.5X4	T49.5X5	T49.5X6
ucodal	T40.2X1	T40.2X2	T40.2X3	T40.2X4	T40.2X5	T40.2X6

Substance	Poisoning, Accidental (unintentional)	Poisoning, Intentional self-harm	Poisoning, Assault	Poisoning, Undetermined	Adverse effect	Underdosing
Euneryl	T42.3X1	T42.3X2	T42.3X3	T42.3X4	T42.3X5	T42.3X6
Euphthalmine	T44.3X1	T44.3X2	T44.3X3	T44.3X4	T44.3X5	T44.3X6
Eurax	T49.0X1	T49.0X2	T49.0X3	T49.0X4	T49.0X5	T49.0X6
Euresol	T49.4X1	T49.4X2	T49.4X3	T49.4X4	T49.4X5	T49.4X6
Euthroid	T38.1X1	T38.1X2	T38.1X3	T38.1X4	T38.1X5	T38.1X6
Evans blue	T50.8X1	T50.8X2	T50.8X3	T50.8X4	T50.8X5	T50.8X6
Evipal	T42.3X1	T42.3X2	T42.3X3	T42.3X4	T42.3X5	T42.3X6
sodium	T41.1X1	T41.1X2	T41.1X3	T41.1X4	T41.1X5	T41.1X6
Evipan	T42.3X1	T42.3X2	T42.3X3	T42.3X4	T42.3X5	T42.3X6
sodium	T41.1X1	T41.1X2	T41.1X3	T41.1X4	T41.1X5	T41.1X6
Exalamide	T49.0X1	T49.0X2	T49.0X3	T49.0X4	T49.0X5	T49.0X6
Exalgin	T39.1X1	T39.1X2	T39.1X3	T39.1X4	T39.1X5	T39.1X6
Excipients, pharmaceutical	T50.901	T50.902	T50.903	T50.904	T50.905	T50.906
Exhaust gas (engine) (motor vehicle)	T58.01	T58.02	T58.03	T58.04	—	—
Ex-Lax (phenolphthalein)	T47.2X1	T47.2X2	T47.2X3	T47.2X4	T47.2X5	T47.2X6
Expectorant NEC	T48.4X1	T48.4X2	T48.4X3	T48.4X4	T48.4X5	T48.4X6
Extended insulin zinc suspension	T38.3X1	T38.3X2	T38.3X3	T38.3X4	T38.3X5	T38.3X6
External medications (skin) (mucous membrane)	T49.91	T49.92	T49.93	T49.94	T49.95	T49.96
dental agent	T49.7X1	T49.7X2	T49.7X3	T49.7X4	T49.7X5	T49.7X6
ENT agent	T49.6X1	T49.6X2	T49.6X3	T49.6X4	T49.6X5	T49.6X6
ophthalmic preparation	T49.5X1	T49.5X2	T49.5X3	T49.5X4	T49.5X5	T49.5X6
specified NEC	T49.8X1	T49.8X2	T49.8X3	T49.8X4	T49.8X5	T49.8X6
Extrapyramidal antagonist NEC	T44.3X1	T44.3X2	T44.3X3	T44.3X4	T44.3X5	T44.3X6
Eye agents (anti-infective)	T49.5X1	T49.5X2	T49.5X3	T49.5X4	T49.5X5	T49.5X6
Eye drug NEC	T49.5X1	T49.5X2	T49.5X3	T49.5X4	T49.5X5	T49.5X6
F						
FAC (fluorouracil + doxorubicin + cyclophosphamide)	T45.1X1	T45.1X2	T45.1X3	T45.1X4	T45.1X5	T45.1X6
Factor						
I (fibrinogen)	T45.8X1	T45.8X2	T45.8X3	T45.8X4	T45.8X5	T45.8X6
III (thromboplastin)	T45.8X1	T45.8X2	T45.8X3	T45.8X4	T45.8X5	T45.8X6
VIII (antihemophilic Factor) (concentrate)	T45.8X1	T45.8X2	T45.8X3	T45.8X4	T45.8X5	T45.8X6
IX complex	T45.7X1	T45.7X2	T45.7X3	T45.7X4	T45.7X5	T45.7X6
human	T45.8X1	T45.8X2	T45.8X3	T45.8X4	T45.8X5	T45.8X6
Famotidine	T47.0X1	T47.0X2	T47.0X3	T47.0X4	T47.0X5	T47.0X6
Fat suspension, intravenous	T50.991	T50.992	T50.993	T50.994	T50.995	T50.996
Fazadinium bromide	T48.1X1	T48.1X2	T48.1X3	T48.1X4	T48.1X5	T48.1X6
Febarbamate	T42.3X1	T42.3X2	T42.3X3	T42.3X4	T42.3X5	T42.3X6
Fecal softener	T47.4X1	T47.4X2	T47.4X3	T47.4X4	T47.4X5	T47.4X6
Fedrilate	T48.3X1	T48.3X2	T48.3X3	T48.3X4	T48.3X5	T48.3X6
Felodipine	T46.1X1	T46.1X2	T46.1X3	T46.1X4	T46.1X5	T46.1X6
Felypressin	T38.891	T38.892	T38.893	T38.894	T38.895	T38.896
Femoxetine	T43.221	T43.222	T43.223	T43.224	T43.225	T43.226
Fenalcomine	T46.3X1	T46.3X2	T46.3X3	T46.3X4	T46.3X5	T46.3X6
Fenamisal	T37.1X1	T37.1X2	T37.1X3	T37.1X4	T37.1X5	T37.1X6

Substance	Poisoning, Accidental (unintentional)	Poisoning, Intentional self-harm	Poisoning, Assault	Poisoning, Undetermined	Adverse effect	Underdosing
Fenazone	T39.2X1	T39.2X2	T39.2X3	T39.2X4	T39.2X5	T39.2X6
Fenbendazole	T37.4X1	T37.4X2	T37.4X3	T37.4X4	T37.4X5	T37.4X6
Fenbutrazate	T50.5X1	T50.5X2	T50.5X3	T50.5X4	T50.5X5	T50.5X6
Fencamfamine	T43.691	T43.692	T43.693	T43.694	T43.695	T43.696
Fendiline	T46.1X1	T46.1X2	T46.1X3	T46.1X4	T46.1X5	T46.1X6
Fenetylline	T43.691	T43.692	T43.693	T43.694	T43.695	T43.696
Fenflumizole	T39.391	T39.392	T39.393	T39.394	T39.395	T39.396
Fenfluramine	T50.5X1	T50.5X2	T50.5X3	T50.5X4	T50.5X5	T50.5X6
Fenobarbital	T42.3X1	T42.3X2	T42.3X3	T42.3X4	T42.3X5	T42.3X6
Fenofibrate	T46.6X1	T46.6X2	T46.6X3	T46.6X4	T46.6X5	T46.6X6
Fenoprofen	T39.311	T39.312	T39.313	T39.314	T39.315	T39.316
Fenoterol	T48.6X1	T48.6X2	T48.6X3	T48.6X4	T48.6X5	T48.6X6
Fenoverine	T44.3X1	T44.3X2	T44.3X3	T44.3X4	T44.3X5	T44.3X6
Fenoxazoline	T48.5X1	T48.5X2	T48.5X3	T48.5X4	T48.5X5	T48.5X6
Fenproporex	T50.5X1	T50.5X2	T50.5X3	T50.5X4	T50.5X5	T50.5X6
Fenquizone	T50.2X1	T50.2X2	T50.2X3	T50.2X4	T50.2X5	T50.2X6
Fentanyl	T40.4X1	T40.4X2	T40.4X3	T40.4X4	T40.4X5	T40.4X6
Fentazin	T43.3X1	T43.3X2	T43.3X3	T43.3X4	T43.3X5	T43.3X6
Fenthion	T60.0X1	T60.0X2	T60.0X3	T60.0X4	—	—
Fenticlor	T49.0X1	T49.0X2	T49.0X3	T49.0X4	T49.0X5	T49.0X6
Fenylbutazone	T39.2X1	T39.2X2	T39.2X3	T39.2X4	T39.2X5	T39.2X6
Feprazone	T39.2X1	T39.2X2	T39.2X3	T39.2X4	T39.2X5	T39.2X6
Fer de lance (bite) (venom)	T63.061	T63.062	T63.063	T63.064	—	—
Ferric—see also Iron						
chloride	T45.4X1	T45.4X2	T45.4X3	T45.4X4	T45.4X5	T45.4X6
citrate	T45.4X1	T45.4X2	T45.4X3	T45.4X4	T45.4X5	T45.4X6
hydroxide						
colloidal	T45.4X1	T45.4X2	T45.4X3	T45.4X4	T45.4X5	T45.4X6
polymaltose	T45.4X1	T45.4X2	T45.4X3	T45.4X4	T45.4X5	T45.4X6
pyrophosphate	T45.4X1	T45.4X2	T45.4X3	T45.4X4	T45.4X5	T45.4X6
Ferritin	T45.4X1	T45.4X2	T45.4X3	T45.4X4	T45.4X5	T45.4X6
Ferrocholinate	T45.4X1	T45.4X2	T45.4X3	T45.4X4	T45.4X5	T45.4X6
Ferrodextrane	T45.4X1	T45.4X2	T45.4X3	T45.4X4	T45.4X5	T45.4X6
Ferropolimaler	T45.4X1	T45.4X2	T45.4X3	T45.4X4	T45.4X5	T45.4X6
Ferrous—see also Iron						
phosphate	T45.4X1	T45.4X2	T45.4X3	T45.4X4	T45.4X5	T45.4X6
salt	T45.4X1	T45.4X2	T45.4X3	T45.4X4	T45.4X5	T45.4X6
with folic acid	T45.4X1	T45.4X2	T45.4X3	T45.4X4	T45.4X5	T45.4X6
Ferrous fumerate, gluconate, lactate, salt NEC, sulfate (medicinal)	T45.4X1	T45.4X2	T45.4X3	T45.4X4	T45.4X5	T45.4X6
Ferrovanadium (fumes)	T59.891	T59.892	T59.893	T59.894	—	—
Ferrum—see Iron						
Fertilizers NEC	T65.891	T65.892	T65.893	T65.894	—	—
with herbicide mixture	T60.3X1	T60.3X2	T60.3X3	T60.3X4	—	—
Fetoxilate	T47.6X1	T47.6X2	T47.6X3	T47.6X4	T47.6X5	T47.6X6
Fiber, dietary	T47.4X1	T47.4X2	T47.4X3	T47.4X4	T47.4X5	T47.4X6
Fiberglass	T65.831	T65.832	T65.833	T65.834	—	—
Fibrinogen (human)	T45.8X1	T45.8X2	T45.8X3	T45.8X4	T45.8X5	T45.8X6
Fibrinolysin (human)	T45.691	T45.692	T45.693	T45.694	T45.695	T45.696

Substance	Poisoning, Accidental (unintentional)	Poisoning, Intentional self-harm	Poisoning, Assault	Poisoning, Undetermined	Adverse effect	Underdosing
Fibrinolysis						
affecting drug	T45.601	T45.602	T45.603	T45.604	T45.605	T45.60
inhibitor NEC	T45.621	T45.622	T45.623	T45.624	T45.625	T45.62
Fibrinolytic drug	T45.611	T45.612	T45.613	T45.614	T45.615	T45.61
Filix mas	T37.4X1	T37.4X2	T37.4X3	T37.4X4	T37.4X5	T37.4X
Filtering cream	T49.3X1	T49.3X2	T49.3X3	T49.3X4	T49.3X5	T49.3X
Fiorinal	T39.011	T39.012	T39.013	T39.014	T39.015	T39.01
Firedamp	T59.891	T59.892	T59.893	T59.894	—	—
Fish, noxious, nonbacterial	T61.91	T61.92	T61.93	T61.94	—	—
ciguatera	T61.01	T61.02	T61.03	T61.04	—	—
scombroid	T61.11	T61.12	T61.13	T61.14	—	—
shell	T61.781	T61.782	T61.783	T61.784	—	—
specified NEC	T61.771	T61.772	T61.773	T61.774	—	—
Flagyl	T37.3X1	T37.3X2	T37.3X3	T37.3X4	T37.3X5	T37.3X
Flavine adenine dinucleotide	T45.2X1	T45.2X2	T45.2X3	T45.2X4	T45.2X5	T45.2X
Flavodic acid	T46.991	T46.992	T46.993	T46.994	T46.995	T46.99
Flavoxate	T44.3X1	T44.3X2	T44.3X3	T44.3X4	T44.3X5	T44.3X
Flaxedil	T48.1X1	T48.1X2	T48.1X3	T48.1X4	T48.1X5	T48.1X
Flaxseed (medicinal)	T49.3X1	T49.3X2	T49.3X3	T49.3X4	T49.3X5	T49.3X
Flecainide	T46.2X1	T46.2X2	T46.2X3	T46.2X4	T46.2X5	T46.2X
Fleroxacin	T36.8X1	T36.8X2	T36.8X3	T36.8X4	T36.8X5	T36.8X
Floctafenine	T39.8X1	T39.8X2	T39.8X3	T39.8X4	T39.8X5	T39.8X
Flomax	T44.6X1	T44.6X2	T44.6X3	T44.6X4	T44.6X5	T44.6X
Flomoxef	T36.1X1	T36.1X2	T36.1X3	T36.1X4	T36.1X5	T36.1X
Flopropione	T44.3X1	T44.3X2	T44.3X3	T44.3X4	T44.3X5	T44.3X
Florantyrone	T47.5X1	T47.5X2	T47.5X3	T47.5X4	T47.5X5	T47.5X
Floraquin	T37.8X1	T37.8X2	T37.8X3	T37.8X4	T37.8X5	T37.8X
Florinef	T38.0X1	T38.0X2	T38.0X3	T38.0X4	T38.0X5	T38.0X
ENT agent	T49.6X1	T49.6X2	T49.6X3	T49.6X4	T49.6X5	T49.6X
ophthalmic preparation	T49.5X1	T49.5X2	T49.5X3	T49.5X4	T49.5X5	T49.5X
topical NEC	T49.0X1	T49.0X2	T49.0X3	T49.0X4	T49.0X5	T49.0X
Flowers of sulfur	T49.4X1	T49.4X2	T49.4X3	T49.4X4	T49.4X5	T49.4X
Floxuridine	T45.1X1	T45.1X2	T45.1X3	T45.1X4	T45.1X5	T45.1X
Fluanisone	T43.4X1	T43.4X2	T43.4X3	T43.4X4	T43.4X5	T43.4X
Flubendazole	T37.4X1	T37.4X2	T37.4X3	T37.4X4	T37.4X5	T37.4X
Fluclorolone acetonide	T49.0X1	T49.0X2	T49.0X3	T49.0X4	T49.0X5	T49.0X
Flucloxacillin	T36.0X1	T36.0X2	T36.0X3	T36.0X4	T36.0X5	T36.0X
Fluconazole	T37.8X1	T37.8X2	T37.8X3	T37.8X4	T37.8X5	T37.8X
Flucytosine	T37.8X1	T37.8X2	T37.8X3	T37.8X4	T37.8X5	T37.8X
Fludeoxyglucose (18F)	T50.8X1	T50.8X2	T50.8X3	T50.8X4	T50.8X5	T50.8X
Fludiazepam	T42.4X1	T42.4X2	T42.4X3	T42.4X4	T42.4X5	T42.4X
Fludrocortisone	T50.0X1	T50.0X2	T50.0X3	T50.0X4	T50.0X5	T50.0X
ENT agent	T49.6X1	T49.6X2	T49.6X3	T49.6X4	T49.6X5	T49.6X
ophthalmic preparation	T49.5X1	T49.5X2	T49.5X3	T49.5X4	T49.5X5	T49.5X
topical NEC	T49.0X1	T49.0X2	T49.0X3	T49.0X4	T49.0X5	T49.0X
Fludroxycortide	T49.0X1	T49.0X2	T49.0X3	T49.0X4	T49.0X5	T49.0X
Flufenamic acid	T39.391	T39.392	T39.393	T39.394	T39.395	T39.39
Fluindione	T45.511	T45.512	T45.513	T45.514	T45.515	T45.51
Flumequine	T37.8X1	T37.8X2	T37.8X3	T37.8X4	T37.8X5	T37.8X

Substance	Poisoning, Accidental (unintentional)	Poisoning, Intentional self-harm	Poisoning, Assault	Poisoning, Undetermined	Adverse effect	Underdosing
methasone	T49.0X1	T49.0X2	T49.0X3	T49.0X4	T49.0X5	T49.0X6
methiazide	T50.2X1	T50.2X2	T50.2X3	T50.2X4	T50.2X5	T50.2X6
midin	T37.5X1	T37.5X2	T37.5X3	T37.5X4	T37.5X5	T37.5X6
narizine	T46.7X1	T46.7X2	T46.7X3	T46.7X4	T46.7X5	T46.7X6
nidazole	T37.8X1	T37.8X2	T37.8X3	T37.8X4	T37.8X5	T37.8X6
nisolide	T48.6X1	T48.6X2	T48.6X3	T48.6X4	T48.6X5	T48.6X6
nitrazepam	T42.4X1	T42.4X2	T42.4X3	T42.4X4	T42.4X5	T42.4X6
ocinolone etonide)	T49.0X1	T49.0X2	T49.0X3	T49.0X4	T49.0X5	T49.0X6
ocinonide	T49.0X1	T49.0X2	T49.0X3	T49.0X4	T49.0X5	T49.0X6
ocortin (butyl)	T49.0X1	T49.0X2	T49.0X3	T49.0X4	T49.0X5	T49.0X6
ocortolone	T49.0X1	T49.0X2	T49.0X3	T49.0X4	T49.0X5	T49.0X6
ohydrocortisone	T38.0X1	T38.0X2	T38.0X3	T38.0X4	T38.0X5	T38.0X6
NT agent	T49.6X1	T49.6X2	T49.6X3	T49.6X4	T49.6X5	T49.6X6
phthalmic preparation	T49.5X1	T49.5X2	T49.5X3	T49.5X4	T49.5X5	T49.5X6
opical NEC	T49.0X1	T49.0X2	T49.0X3	T49.0X4	T49.0X5	T49.0X6
onid	T49.0X1	T49.0X2	T49.0X3	T49.0X4	T49.0X5	T49.0X6
opromazine	T43.3X1	T43.3X2	T43.3X3	T43.3X4	T43.3X5	T43.3X6
oracetate	T60.8X1	T60.8X2	T60.8X3	T60.8X4	—	—
orescein	T50.8X1	T50.8X2	T50.8X3	T50.8X4	T50.8X5	T50.8X6
orhydrocortisone	T50.0X1	T50.0X2	T50.0X3	T50.0X4	T50.0X5	T50.0X6
oride (nonmedicin al) sticide) (sodium) NEC	T60.8X1	T60.8X2	T60.8X3	T60.8X4	—	—
ydrogen—see Hydrofluoric acid						
nedicinal NEC	T50.991	T50.992	T50.993	T50.994	T50.995	T50.996
dental use	T49.7X1	T49.7X2	T49.7X3	T49.7X4	T49.7X5	T49.7X6
ot pesticide NEC	T54.91	T54.92	T54.93	T54.94	—	—
tannous	T49.7X1	T49.7X2	T49.7X3	T49.7X4	T49.7X5	T49.7X6
orinated corticosteroids	T38.0X1	T38.0X2	T38.0X3	T38.0X4	T38.0X5	T38.0X6
orine (gas)	T59.5X1	T59.5X2	T59.5X3	T59.5X4	—	—
alt—see Fluoride(s)						
oristan	T49.7X1	T49.7X2	T49.7X3	T49.7X4	T49.7X5	T49.7X6
ormetholone	T49.0X1	T49.0X2	T49.0X3	T49.0X4	T49.0X5	T49.0X6
oroacetate	T60.8X1	T60.8X2	T60.8X3	T60.8X4	—	—
orocarbon monomer	T53.6X1	T53.6X2	T53.6X3	T53.6X4	—	—
orocytosine	T37.8X1	T37.8X2	T37.8X3	T37.8X4	T37.8X5	T37.8X6
orodeoxyuridine	T45.1X1	T45.1X2	T45.1X3	T45.1X4	T45.1X5	T45.1X6
orometholone	T49.0X1	T49.0X2	T49.0X3	T49.0X4	T49.0X5	T49.0X6
phthalmic preparation	T49.5X1	T49.5X2	T49.5X3	T49.5X4	T49.5X5	T49.5X6
orophosphate secticide	T60.0X1	T60.0X2	T60.0X3	T60.0X4	—	—
orosol	T46.3X1	T46.3X2	T46.3X3	T46.3X4	T46.3X5	T46.3X6
orouracil	T45.1X1	T45.1X2	T45.1X3	T45.1X4	T45.1X5	T45.1X6
orphenylalanine	T49.5X1	T49.5X2	T49.5X3	T49.5X4	T49.5X5	T49.5X6
othane	T41.0X1	T41.0X2	T41.0X3	T41.0X4	T41.0X5	T41.0X6
oxetine	T43.221	T43.222	T43.223	T43.224	T43.225	T43.226
oxymesterone	T38.7X1	T38.7X2	T38.7X3	T38.7X4	T38.7X5	T38.7X6
penthixol	T43.4X1	T43.4X2	T43.4X3	T43.4X4	T43.4X5	T43.4X6
pentixol	T43.4X1	T43.4X2	T43.4X3	T43.4X4	T43.4X5	T43.4X6
phenazine	T43.3X1	T43.3X2	T43.3X3	T43.3X4	T43.3X5	T43.3X6

Substance	Poisoning, Accidental (unintentional)	Poisoning, Intentional self-harm	Poisoning, Assault	Poisoning, Undetermined	Adverse effect	Underdosing
Fluprednidene	T49.0X1	T49.0X2	T49.0X3	T49.0X4	T49.0X5	T49.0X6
Fluprednisolone	T38.0X1	T38.0X2	T38.0X3	T38.0X4	T38.0X5	T38.0X6
Fluradoline	T39.8X1	T39.8X2	T39.8X3	T39.8X4	T39.8X5	T39.8X6
Flurandrenolide	T49.0X1	T49.0X2	T49.0X3	T49.0X4	T49.0X5	T49.0X6
Flurandrenolone	T49.0X1	T49.0X2	T49.0X3	T49.0X4	T49.0X5	T49.0X6
Flurazepam	T42.4X1	T42.4X2	T42.4X3	T42.4X4	T42.4X5	T42.4X6
Flurbiprofen	T39.311	T39.312	T39.313	T39.314	T39.315	T39.316
Flurobate	T49.0X1	T49.0X2	T49.0X3	T49.0X4	T49.0X5	T49.0X6
Fluroxene	T41.0X1	T41.0X2	T41.0X3	T41.0X4	T41.0X5	T41.0X6
Fluspirilene	T43.591	T43.592	T43.593	T43.594	T43.595	T43.596
Flutamide	T38.6X1	T38.6X2	T38.6X3	T38.6X4	T38.6X5	T38.6X6
Flutazolam	T42.4X1	T42.4X2	T42.4X3	T42.4X4	T42.4X5	T42.4X6
Fluticasone propionate	T38.0X1	T38.0X2	T38.0X3	T38.0X4	T38.0X5	T38.0X6
Flutoprazepam	T42.4X1	T42.4X2	T42.4X3	T42.4X4	T42.4X5	T42.4X6
Flutropium bromide	T48.6X1	T48.6X2	T48.6X3	T48.6X4	T48.6X5	T48.6X6
Fluvoxamine	T43.221	T43.222	T43.223	T43.224	T43.225	T43.226
Folacin	T45.8X1	T45.8X2	T45.8X3	T45.8X4	T45.8X5	T45.8X6
Folic acid	T45.8X1	T45.8X2	T45.8X3	T45.8X4	T45.8X5	T45.8X6
with ferrous salt	T45.2X1	T45.2X2	T45.2X3	T45.2X4	T45.2X5	T45.2X6
antagonist	T45.1X1	T45.1X2	T45.1X3	T45.1X4	T45.1X5	T45.1X6
Folinic acid	T45.8X1	T45.8X2	T45.8X3	T45.8X4	T45.8X5	T45.8X6
Folium stramoniae	T48.6X1	T48.6X2	T48.6X3	T48.6X4	T48.6X5	T48.6X6
Follicle-stimulating hormone, human	T38.811	T38.812	T38.813	T38.814	T38.815	T38.816
Folpet	T60.3X1	T60.3X2	T60.3X3	T60.3X4	—	—
Fominoben	T48.3X1	T48.3X2	T48.3X3	T48.3X4	T48.3X5	T48.3X6
Food, foodstuffs, noxious, nonbacterial, NEC	T62.91	T62.92	T62.93	T62.94	—	—
berries	T62.1X1	T62.1X2	T62.1X3	T62.1X4	—	—
fish—see also Fish	T61.91	T61.92	T61.93	T61.94	—	—
mushrooms	T62.0X1	T62.0X2	T62.0X3	T62.0X4	—	—
plants	T62.2X1	T62.2X2	T62.2X3	T62.2X4	—	—
seafood	T61.91	T61.92	T61.93	T61.94	—	—
specified NEC	T61.8X1	T61.8X2	T61.8X3	T61.8X4	—	—
seeds	T62.2X1	T62.2X2	T62.2X3	T62.2X4	—	—
shellfish	T61.781	T61.782	T61.783	T61.784	—	—
specified NEC	T62.8X1	T62.8X2	T62.8X3	T62.8X4	—	—
Fool's parsley	T62.2X1	T62.2X2	T62.2X3	T62.2X4	—	—
Formaldehyde (solution), gas or vapor	T59.2X1	T59.2X2	T59.2X3	T59.2X4	—	—
fungicide	T60.3X1	T60.3X2	T60.3X3	T60.3X4	—	—
Formalin	T59.2X1	T59.2X2	T59.2X3	T59.2X4	—	—
fungicide	T60.3X1	T60.3X2	T60.3X3	T60.3X4	—	—
vapor	T59.2X1	T59.2X2	T59.2X3	T59.2X4	—	—
Formic acid	T54.2X1	T54.2X2	T54.2X3	T54.2X4	—	—
vapor	T59.891	T59.892	T59.893	T59.894	—	—
Foscarnet sodium	T37.5X1	T37.5X2	T37.5X3	T37.5X4	T37.5X5	T37.5X6
Fosfestrol	T38.5X1	T38.5X2	T38.5X3	T38.5X4	T38.5X5	T38.5X6
Fosfomycin	T36.8X1	T36.8X2	T36.8X3	T36.8X4	T36.8X5	T36.8X6
Fosfonet sodium	T37.5X1	T37.5X2	T37.5X3	T37.5X4	T37.5X5	T37.5X6

Substance	Poisoning, Accidental (unintentional)	Poisoning, Intentional self-harm	Poisoning, Assault	Poisoning, Undetermined	Adverse effect	Underdosing
Fosinopril	T46.4X1	T46.4X2	T46.4X3	T46.4X4	T46.4X5	T46.4X6
sodium	T46.4X1	T46.4X2	T46.4X3	T46.4X4	T46.4X5	T46.4X6
Fowler's solution	T57.0X1	T57.0X2	T57.0X3	T57.0X4	—	—
Foxglove	T62.2X1	T62.2X2	T62.2X3	T62.2X4	—	—
Framycetin	T36.5X1	T36.5X2	T36.5X3	T36.5X4	T36.5X5	T36.5X6
Frangula	T47.2X1	T47.2X2	T47.2X3	T47.2X4	T47.2X5	T47.2X6
extract	T47.2X1	T47.2X2	T47.2X3	T47.2X4	T47.2X5	T47.2X6
Frei antigen	T50.8X1	T50.8X2	T50.8X3	T50.8X4	T50.8X5	T50.8X6
Freon	T53.5X1	T53.5X2	T53.5X3	T53.5X4	—	—
Fructose	T50.3X1	T50.3X2	T50.3X3	T50.3X4	T50.3X5	T50.3X6
Frusemide	T50.1X1	T50.1X2	T50.1X3	T50.1X4	T50.1X5	T50.1X6
FSH	T38.811	T38.812	T38.813	T38.814	T38.815	T38.816
Ftorafur	T45.1X1	T45.1X2	T45.1X3	T45.1X4	T45.1X5	T45.1X6
Fuel						
automobile	T52.0X1	T52.0X2	T52.0X3	T52.0X4	—	—
exhaust gas, not in transit	T58.01	T58.02	T58.03	T58.04	—	—
vapor NEC	T52.0X1	T52.0X2	T52.0X3	T52.0X4	—	—
gas (domestic use)—see also Carbon, monoxide, fuel, utility	T59.891	T59.892	T59.893	T59.894	—	—
utility	T59.891	T59.892	T59.893	T59.894	—	—
in mobile container	T59.891	T59.892	T59.893	T59.894	—	—
incomplete combustion of—see Carbon, monoxide, fuel, utility						
piped (natural)	T59.891	T59.892	T59.893	T59.894	—	—
industrial, incomplete combustion	T58.8X1	T58.8X2	T58.8X3	T58.8X4	—	—
Fugillin	T36.8X1	T36.8X2	T36.8X3	T36.8X4	T36.8X5	T36.8X6
Fulminate of mercury	T56.1X1	T56.1X2	T56.1X3	T56.1X4	—	—
Fulvicin	T36.7X1	T36.7X2	T36.7X3	T36.7X4	T36.7X5	T36.7X6
Fumadil	T36.8X1	T36.8X2	T36.8X3	T36.8X4	T36.8X5	T36.8X6
Fumagillin	T36.8X1	T36.8X2	T36.8X3	T36.8X4	T36.8X5	T36.8X6
Fumaric acid	T49.4X1	T49.4X2	T49.4X3	T49.4X4	T49.4X5	T49.4X6
Fumes (from)	T59.91	T59.92	T59.93	T59.94	—	—
carbon monoxide—see Carbon, monoxide						
charcoal (domestic use)—see Charcoal, fumes						
chloroform—see Chloroform						
coke (in domestic stoves, fireplaces)—see Coke fumes						
corrosive NEC	T54.91	T54.92	T54.93	T54.94	—	—
ether—see ether						
freons	T53.5X1	T53.5X2	T53.5X3	T53.5X4	—	—
hydrocarbons	T59.891	T59.892	T59.893	T59.894	—	—
petroleum (liquefied)	T59.891	T59.892	T59.893	T59.894	—	—
distributed through pipes (pure or mixed with air)	T59.891	T59.892	T59.893	T59.894	—	—
lead—see lead						

Substance	Poisoning, Accidental (unintentional)	Poisoning, Intentional self-harm	Poisoning, Assault	Poisoning, Undetermined	Adverse effect	Underdosing
Fumes — *Continued*						
metal—see Metals, or the specified metal						
nitrogen dioxide	T59.0X1	T59.0X2	T59.0X3	T59.0X4	—	—
pesticides—see Pesticides						
petroleum (liquefied)	T59.891	T59.892	T59.893	T59.894	—	—
distributed through pipes (pure or mixed with air)	T59.891	T59.892	T59.893	T59.894	—	—
polyester	T59.891	T59.892	T59.893	T59.894	—	—
specified source NEC—see also substance specified	T59.891	T59.892	T59.893	T59.894	—	—
sulfur dioxide	T59.1X1	T59.1X2	T59.1X3	T59.1X4	—	—
Fumigant NEC	T60.91	T60.92	T60.93	T60.94	—	—
Fungi, noxious, used as food	T62.0X1	T62.0X2	T62.0X3	T62.0X4	—	—
Fungicide NEC (nonmedicinal)	T60.3X1	T60.3X2	T60.3X3	T60.3X4	—	—
Fungizone	T36.7X1	T36.7X2	T36.7X3	T36.7X4	T36.7X5	T36.7X
topical	T49.0X1	T49.0X2	T49.0X3	T49.0X4	T49.0X5	T49.0X
Furacin	T49.0X1	T49.0X2	T49.0X3	T49.0X4	T49.0X5	T49.0X
Furadantin	T37.91	T37.92	T37.93	T37.94	T37.95	T37.9
Furazolidone	T37.8X1	T37.8X2	T37.8X3	T37.8X4	T37.8X5	T37.8X
Furazolium chloride	T49.0X1	T49.0X2	T49.0X3	T49.0X4	T49.0X5	T49.0X
Furfural	T52.8X1	T52.8X2	T52.8X3	T52.8X4	—	—
Furnace (coal burning) (domestic), gas from	T58.2X1	T58.2X2	T58.2X3	T58.2X4	—	—
industrial	T58.8X1	T58.8X2	T58.8X3	T58.8X4	—	—
Furniture polish	T65.891	T65.892	T65.893	T65.894	—	—
Furosemide	T50.1X1	T50.1X2	T50.1X3	T50.1X4	T50.1X5	T50.1X
Furoxone	T37.91	T37.92	T37.93	T37.94	T37.95	T37.9
Fursultiamine	T45.2X1	T45.2X2	T45.2X3	T45.2X4	T45.2X5	T45.2X
Fusafungine	T36.8X1	T36.8X2	T36.8X3	T36.8X4	T36.8X5	T36.8X
Fusel oil (any) (amyl) (butyl) (propyl), vapor	T51.3X1	T51.3X2	T51.3X3	T51.3X4	—	—
Fusidate (ethanolamine) (sodium)	T36.8X1	T36.8X2	T36.8X3	T36.8X4	T36.8X5	T36.8X
Fusidic acid	T36.8X1	T36.8X2	T36.8X3	T36.8X4	T36.8X5	T36.8X
Fytic acid, nonasodium	T50.6X1	T50.6X2	T50.6X3	T50.6X4	T50.6X5	T50.6X
G						
GABA	T43.8X1	T43.8X2	T43.8X3	T43.8X4	T43.8X5	T43.8X
Gadopentetic acid	T50.8X1	T50.8X2	T50.8X3	T50.8X4	T50.8X5	T50.8X
Galactose	T50.3X1	T50.3X2	T50.3X3	T50.3X4	T50.3X5	T50.3X
b-Galactosidase	T47.5X1	T47.5X2	T47.5X3	T47.5X4	T47.5X5	T47.5X
Galantamine	T44.0X1	T44.0X2	T44.0X3	T44.0X4	T44.0X5	T44.0X
Gallamine (triethiodide)	T48.1X1	T48.1X2	T48.1X3	T48.1X4	T48.1X5	T48.1X
Gallium citrate	T50.991	T50.992	T50.993	T50.994	T50.995	T50.99
Gallopamil	T46.1X1	T46.1X2	T46.1X3	T46.1X4	T46.1X5	T46.1X
Gamboge	T47.2X1	T47.2X2	T47.2X3	T47.2X4	T47.2X5	T47.2X
Gamimune	T50.Z11	T50.Z12	T50.Z13	T50.Z14	T50.Z15	T50.Z1
Gamma globulin	T50.Z11	T50.Z12	T50.Z13	T50.Z14	T50.Z15	T50.Z1
Gamma-aminobutyric acid	T43.8X1	T43.8X2	T43.8X3	T43.8X4	T43.8X5	T43.8X

Substance	Poisoning, Accidental (unintentional)	Poisoning, Intentional self-harm	Poisoning, Assault	Poisoning, Undetermined	Adverse effect	Underdosing
amma-benzene exachloride (medicinal)	T49.0X1	T49.0X2	T49.0X3	T49.0X4	T49.0X5	T49.0X6
nonmedicinal, vapor	T53.6X1	T53.6X2	T53.6X3	T53.6X4	—	—
amma-BHC (medicinal)—e also Gamma-benzene exachloride	T49.0X1	T49.0X2	T49.0X3	T49.0X4	T49.0X5	T49.0X6
amulin	T50.Z11	T50.Z12	T50.Z13	T50.Z14	T50.Z15	T50.Z16
anciclovir (sodium)	T37.5X1	T37.5X2	T37.5X3	T37.5X4	T37.5X5	T37.5X6
anglionic blocking rug NEC	T44.2X1	T44.2X2	T44.2X3	T44.2X4	T44.2X5	T44.2X6
specified NEC	T44.2X1	T44.2X2	T44.2X3	T44.2X4	T44.2X5	T44.2X6
anja	T40.7X1	T40.7X2	T40.7X3	T40.7X4	T40.7X5	T40.7X6
aramycin	T36.5X1	T36.5X2	T36.5X3	T36.5X4	T36.5X5	T36.5X6
ophthalmic preparation	T49.5X1	T49.5X2	T49.5X3	T49.5X4	T49.5X5	T49.5X6
topical NEC	T49.0X1	T49.0X2	T49.0X3	T49.0X4	T49.0X5	T49.0X6
ardenal	T42.3X1	T42.3X2	T42.3X3	T42.3X4	T42.3X5	T42.3X6
ardepanyl	T42.3X1	T42.3X2	T42.3X3	T42.3X4	T42.3X5	T42.3X6
as NEC	T59.91	T59.92	T59.93	T59.94	—	—
acetylene	T59.891	T59.892	T59.893	T59.894	—	—
incomplete combustion of	T58.11	T58.12	T58.13	T58.14	—	—
air contaminants, source or type not specified	T59.91	T59.92	T59.93	T59.94	—	—
anesthetic	T41.0X1	T41.0X2	T41.0X3	T41.0X4	T41.0X5	T41.0X6
blast furnace	T58.8X1	T58.8X2	T58.8X3	T58.8X4	—	—
butane—see butane						
carbon monoxide—see Carbon, monoxide						
chlorine	T59.4X1	T59.4X2	T59.4X3	T59.4X4	—	—
coal	T58.2X1	T58.2X2	T58.2X3	T58.2X4	—	—
cyanide	T57.3X1	T57.3X2	T57.3X3	T57.3X4	—	—
dicyanogen	T65.0X1	T65.0X2	T65.0X3	T65.0X4	—	—
domestic—see Domestic gas						
exhaust	T58.01	T58.02	T58.03	T58.04	—	—
from utility (for cooking, heating, or lighting) (after combustion)—see Carbon, monoxide, fuel, utility						
prior to combustion	T59.891	T59.892	T59.893	T59.894	—	—
from wood- or coal-burning stove or fireplace	T58.2X1	T58.2X2	T58.2X3	T58.2X4	—	—
fuel (domestic use) (after combustion)—see also Carbon, monoxide, fuel						
industrial use	T58.8X1	T58.8X2	T58.8X3	T58.8X4	—	—
prior to combustion	T59.891	T59.892	T59.893	T59.894	—	—
utility	T59.891	T59.892	T59.893	T59.894	—	—
in mobile container	T59.891	T59.892	T59.893	T59.894	—	—
incomplete combustion of—see Carbon, monoxide, fuel, utility						
piped (natural)	T59.891	T59.892	T59.893	T59.894	—	—

Substance	Poisoning, Accidental (unintentional)	Poisoning, Intentional self-harm	Poisoning, Assault	Poisoning, Undetermined	Adverse effect	Underdosing
Gas — *Continued*						
garage	T58.01	T58.02	T58.03	T58.04	—	—
hydrocarbon NEC	T59.891	T59.892	T59.893	T59.894	—	—
incomplete combustion of—see Carbon, monoxide, fuel, utility						
liquefied—see butane						
piped	T59.891	T59.892	T59.893	T59.894	—	—
hydrocyanic acid	T65.0X1	T65.0X2	T65.0X3	T65.0X4	—	—
illuminating (after combustion)	T58.11	T58.12	T58.13	T58.14	—	—
prior to combustion	T59.891	T59.892	T59.893	T59.894	—	—
incomplete combustion, any—see Carbon, monoxide						
kiln	T58.8X1	T58.8X2	T58.8X3	T58.8X4	—	—
lacrimogenic	T59.3X1	T59.3X2	T59.3X3	T59.3X4	—	—
liquefied petroleum—see butane						
marsh	T59.891	T59.892	T59.893	T59.894	—	—
motor exhaust, not in transit	T58.01	T58.02	T58.03	T58.04	—	—
mustard, not in war	T59.891	T59.892	T59.893	T59.894	—	—
natural	T59.891	T59.892	T59.893	T59.894	—	—
nerve, not in war	T59.91	T59.92	T59.93	T59.94	—	—
oil	T52.0X1	T52.0X2	T52.0X3	T52.0X4	—	—
petroleum (liquefied) (distributed in mobile containers)	T59.891	T59.892	T59.893	T59.894	—	—
piped (pure or mixed with air)	T59.891	T59.892	T59.893	T59.894	—	—
piped (manufactured) (natural) NEC	T59.891	T59.892	T59.893	T59.894	—	—
producer	T58.8X1	T58.8X2	T58.8X3	T58.8X4	—	—
propane—see propane						
refrigerant (chlorofluoro-carbon)	T53.5X1	T53.5X2	T53.5X3	T53.5X4	—	—
not chlorofluoro-carbon	T59.891	T59.892	T59.893	T59.894	—	—
sewer	T59.91	T59.92	T59.93	T59.94	—	—
specified source NEC	T59.91	T59.92	T59.93	T59.94	—	—
stove (after combustion)	T58.11	T58.12	T58.13	T58.14	—	—
prior to combustion	T59.891	T59.892	T59.893	T59.894	—	—
tear	T59.3X1	T59.3X2	T59.3X3	T59.3X4	—	—
therapeutic	T41.5X1	T41.5X2	T41.5X3	T41.5X4	T41.5X5	T41.5X6
utility (for cooking, heating, or lighting) (piped) NEC	T59.891	T59.892	T59.893	T59.894	—	—
in mobile container	T59.891	T59.892	T59.893	T59.894	—	—
incomplete combustion of—see Carbon, monoxide, fuel, utilty						
piped (natural)	T59.891	T59.892	T59.893	T59.894	—	—
water	T58.11	T58.12	T58.13	T58.14	—	—
incomplete combustion of—see Carbon, monoxide, fuel, utility						

Substance	Poisoning, Accidental (unintentional)	Poisoning, Intentional self-harm	Poisoning, Assault	Poisoning, Undetermined	Adverse effect	Underdosing
Gaseous substance—see Gas						
Gasoline	T52.0X1	T52.0X2	T52.0X3	T52.0X4	—	—
vapor	T52.0X1	T52.0X2	T52.0X3	T52.0X4	—	—
Gastric enzymes	T47.5X1	T47.5X2	T47.5X3	T47.5X4	T47.5X5	T47.5X6
Gastrografin	T50.8X1	T50.8X2	T50.8X3	T50.8X4	T50.8X5	T50.8X6
Gastrointestinal drug	T47.91	T47.92	T47.93	T47.94	T47.95	T47.96
biological	T47.8X1	T47.8X2	T47.8X3	T47.8X4	T47.8X5	T47.8X6
specified NEC	T47.8X1	T47.8X2	T47.8X3	T47.8X4	T47.8X5	T47.8X6
Gaultheria procumbens	T62.2X1	T62.2X2	T62.2X3	T62.2X4	—	—
Gefarnate	T44.3X1	T44.3X2	T44.3X3	T44.3X4	T44.3X5	T44.3X6
Gelatin (intravenous)	T45.8X1	T45.8X2	T45.8X3	T45.8X4	T45.8X5	T45.8X6
absorbable (sponge)	T45.7X1	T45.7X2	T45.7X3	T45.7X4	T45.7X5	T45.7X6
Gelfilm	T49.8X1	T49.8X2	T49.8X3	T49.8X4	T49.8X5	T49.8X6
Gelfoam	T45.7X1	T45.7X2	T45.7X3	T45.7X4	T45.7X5	T45.7X6
Gelsemine	T50.991	T50.992	T50.993	T50.994	T50.995	T50.996
Gelsemium (sempervirens)	T62.2X1	T62.2X2	T62.2X3	T62.2X4	—	—
Gemeprost	T48.0X1	T48.0X2	T48.0X3	T48.0X4	T48.0X5	T48.0X6
Gemfibrozil	T46.6X1	T46.6X2	T46.6X3	T46.6X4	T46.6X5	T46.6X6
Gemonil	T42.3X1	T42.3X2	T42.3X3	T42.3X4	T42.3X5	T42.3X6
Gentamicin	T36.5X1	T36.5X2	T36.5X3	T36.5X4	T36.5X5	T36.5X6
ophthalmic preparation	T49.5X1	T49.5X2	T49.5X3	T49.5X4	T49.5X5	T49.5X6
topical NEC	T49.0X1	T49.0X2	T49.0X3	T49.0X4	T49.0X5	T49.0X6
Gentian	T47.5X1	T47.5X2	T47.5X3	T47.5X4	T47.5X5	T47.5X6
violet	T49.0X1	T49.0X2	T49.0X3	T49.0X4	T49.0X5	T49.0X6
Gepefrine	T44.4X1	T44.4X2	T44.4X3	T44.4X4	T44.4X5	T44.4X6
Gestonorone caproate	T38.5X1	T38.5X2	T38.5X3	T38.5X4	T38.5X5	T38.5X6
Gexane	T49.0X1	T49.0X2	T49.0X3	T49.0X4	T49.0X5	T49.0X6
Gila monster (venom)	T63.111	T63.112	T63.113	T63.114	—	—
Ginger	T47.5X1	T47.5X2	T47.5X3	T47.5X4	T47.5X5	T47.5X6
Jamaica—see Jamaica, ginger						
Gitalin	T46.0X1	T46.0X2	T46.0X3	T46.0X4	T46.0X5	T46.0X6
amorphous	T46.0X1	T46.0X2	T46.0X3	T46.0X4	T46.0X5	T46.0X6
Gitaloxin	T46.0X1	T46.0X2	T46.0X3	T46.0X4	T46.0X5	T46.0X6
Gitoxin	T46.0X1	T46.0X2	T46.0X3	T46.0X4	T46.0X5	T46.0X6
Glafenine	T39.8X1	T39.8X2	T39.8X3	T39.8X4	T39.8X5	T39.8X6
Glandular extract (medicinal) NEC	T50.Z91	T50.Z92	T50.Z93	T50.Z94	T50.Z95	T50.Z96
Glaucarubin	T37.3X1	T37.3X2	T37.3X3	T37.3X4	T37.3X5	T37.3X6
Glibenclamide	T38.3X1	T38.3X2	T38.3X3	T38.3X4	T38.3X5	T38.3X6
Glibornuride	T38.3X1	T38.3X2	T38.3X3	T38.3X4	T38.3X5	T38.3X6
Gliclazide	T38.3X1	T38.3X2	T38.3X3	T38.3X4	T38.3X5	T38.3X6
Glimidine	T38.3X1	T38.3X2	T38.3X3	T38.3X4	T38.3X5	T38.3X6
Glipizide	T38.3X1	T38.3X2	T38.3X3	T38.3X4	T38.3X5	T38.3X6
Gliquidone	T38.3X1	T38.3X2	T38.3X3	T38.3X4	T38.3X5	T38.3X6
Glisolamide	T38.3X1	T38.3X2	T38.3X3	T38.3X4	T38.3X5	T38.3X6
Glisoxepide	T38.3X1	T38.3X2	T38.3X3	T38.3X4	T38.3X5	T38.3X6
Globin zinc insulin	T38.3X1	T38.3X2	T38.3X3	T38.3X4	T38.3X5	T38.3X6

Substance	Poisoning, Accidental (unintentional)	Poisoning, Intentional self-harm	Poisoning, Assault	Poisoning, Undetermined	Adverse effect	Underdosing
Globulin						
antilymphocytic	T50.Z11	T50.Z12	T50.Z13	T50.Z14	T50.Z15	T50.Z1
antirhesus	T50.Z11	T50.Z12	T50.Z13	T50.Z14	T50.Z15	T50.Z1
antivenin	T50.Z11	T50.Z12	T50.Z13	T50.Z14	T50.Z15	T50.Z1
antiviral	T50.Z11	T50.Z12	T50.Z13	T50.Z14	T50.Z15	T50.Z1
Glucagon	T38.3X1	T38.3X2	T38.3X3	T38.3X4	T38.3X5	T38.3X
Glucocorticoids	T38.0X1	T38.0X2	T38.0X3	T38.0X4	T38.0X5	T38.0X
Glucocorticosteroid	T38.0X1	T38.0X2	T38.0X3	T38.0X4	T38.0X5	T38.0X
Gluconic acid	T50.991	T50.992	T50.993	T50.994	T50.995	T50.99
Glucosamine sulfate	T39.4X1	T39.4X2	T39.4X3	T39.4X4	T39.4X5	T39.4X
Glucose	T50.3X1	T50.3X2	T50.3X3	T50.3X4	T50.3X5	T50.3X
with sodium chloride	T50.3X1	T50.3X2	T50.3X3	T50.3X4	T50.3X5	T50.3X
Glucosulfone sodium	T37.1X1	T37.1X2	T37.1X3	T37.1X4	T37.1X5	T37.1X
Glucurolactone	T47.8X1	T47.8X2	T47.8X3	T47.8X4	T47.8X5	T47.8X
Glue NEC	T52.8X1	T52.8X2	T52.8X3	T52.8X4	—	—
Glutamic acid	T47.5X1	T47.5X2	T47.5X3	T47.5X4	T47.5X5	T47.5X
Glutaral (medicinal)	T49.0X1	T49.0X2	T49.0X3	T49.0X4	T49.0X5	T49.0X
nonmedicinal	T65.891	T65.892	T65.893	T65.894	—	—
Glutaraldehyde (nonmedicinal)	T65.891	T65.892	T65.893	T65.894	—	—
medicinal	T49.0X1	T49.0X2	T49.0X3	T49.0X4	T49.0X5	T49.0X
Glutathione	T50.6X1	T50.6X2	T50.6X3	T50.6X4	T50.6X5	T50.6X
Glutethimide	T42.6X1	T42.6X2	T42.6X3	T42.6X4	T42.6X5	T42.6X
Glyburide	T38.3X1	T38.3X2	T38.3X3	T38.3X4	T38.3X5	T38.3X
Glycerin	T47.4X1	T47.4X2	T47.4X3	T47.4X4	T47.4X5	T47.4X
Glycerol	T47.4X1	T47.4X2	T47.4X3	T47.4X4	T47.4X5	T47.4X
borax	T49.6X1	T49.6X2	T49.6X3	T49.6X4	T49.6X5	T49.6X
intravenous	T50.3X1	T50.3X2	T50.3X3	T50.3X4	T50.3X5	T50.3X
iodinated	T48.4X1	T48.4X2	T48.4X3	T48.4X4	T48.4X5	T48.4X
Glycerophosphate	T50.991	T50.992	T50.993	T50.994	T50.995	T50.99
Glyceryl						
guaiacolate	T48.4X1	T48.4X2	T48.4X3	T48.4X4	T48.4X5	T48.4X
nitrate	T46.3X1	T46.3X2	T46.3X3	T46.3X4	T46.3X5	T46.3X
triacetate (topical)	T49.0X1	T49.0X2	T49.0X3	T49.0X4	T49.0X5	T49.0X
trinitrate	T46.3X1	T46.3X2	T46.3X3	T46.3X4	T46.3X5	T46.3X
Glycine	T50.3X1	T50.3X2	T50.3X3	T50.3X4	T50.3X5	T50.3X
Glyclopyramide	T38.3X1	T38.3X2	T38.3X3	T38.3X4	T38.3X5	T38.3X
Glycobiarsol	T37.3X1	T37.3X2	T37.3X3	T37.3X4	T37.3X5	T37.3X
Glycols (ether)	T52.3X1	T52.3X2	T52.3X3	T52.3X4	—	—
Glyconiazide	T37.1X1	T37.1X2	T37.1X3	T37.1X4	T37.1X5	T37.1X
Glycopyrrolate	T44.3X1	T44.3X2	T44.3X3	T44.3X4	T44.3X5	T44.3X
Glycopyrronium	T44.3X1	T44.3X2	T44.3X3	T44.3X4	T44.3X5	T44.3X
bromide	T44.3X1	T44.3X2	T44.3X3	T44.3X4	T44.3X5	T44.3X
Glycoside, cardiac (stimulant)	T46.0X1	T46.0X2	T46.0X3	T46.0X4	T46.0X5	T46.0X
Glycyclamide	T38.3X1	T38.3X2	T38.3X3	T38.3X4	T38.3X5	T38.3X
Glycyrrhiza extract	T48.4X1	T48.4X2	T48.4X3	T48.4X4	T48.4X5	T48.4X
Glycyrrhizic acid	T48.4X1	T48.4X2	T48.4X3	T48.4X4	T48.4X5	T48.4X
Glycyrrhizinate potassium	T48.4X1	T48.4X2	T48.4X3	T48.4X4	T48.4X5	T48.4X
Glymidine sodium	T38.3X1	T38.3X2	T38.3X3	T38.3X4	T38.3X5	T38.3X

Substance	Poisoning, Accidental (unintentional)	Poisoning, Intentional self-harm	Poisoning, Assault	Poisoning, Undetermined	Adverse effect	Underdosing
lyphosate	T60.3X1	T60.3X2	T60.3X3	T60.3X4	—	—
lyphylline	T48.6X1	T48.6X2	T48.6X3	T48.6X4	T48.6X5	T48.6X6
old						
colloidal (198Au)	T45.1X1	T45.1X2	T45.1X3	T45.1X4	T45.1X5	T45.1X6
salts	T39.4X1	T39.4X2	T39.4X3	T39.4X4	T39.4X5	T39.4X6
olden sulfide of antimony	T56.891	T56.892	T56.893	T56.894	—	—
oldylocks	T62.2X1	T62.2X2	T62.2X3	T62.2X4	—	—
onadal tissue extract	T38.901	T38.902	T38.903	T38.904	T38.905	T38.906
female	T38.5X1	T38.5X2	T38.5X3	T38.5X4	T38.5X5	T38.5X6
male	T38.7X1	T38.7X2	T38.7X3	T38.7X4	T38.7X5	T38.7X6
onadorelin	T38.891	T38.892	T38.893	T38.894	T38.895	T38.896
onadotropin	T38.891	T38.892	T38.893	T38.894	T38.895	T38.896
chorionic	T38.891	T38.892	T38.893	T38.894	T38.895	T38.896
pituitary	T38.811	T38.812	T38.813	T38.814	T38.815	T38.816
oserelin	T45.1X1	T45.1X2	T45.1X3	T45.1X4	T45.1X5	T45.1X6
rain alcohol	T51.0X1	T51.0X2	T51.0X3	T51.0X4	—	—
ramicidin	T49.0X1	T49.0X2	T49.0X3	T49.0X4	T49.0X5	T49.0X6
ranisetron	T45.0X1	T45.0X2	T45.0X3	T45.0X4	T45.0X5	T45.0X6
ratiola officinalis	T62.2X1	T62.2X2	T62.2X3	T62.2X4	—	—
rease	T65.891	T65.892	T65.893	T65.894	—	—
reen hellebore	T62.2X1	T62.2X2	T62.2X3	T62.2X4	—	—
reen soap	T49.2X1	T49.2X2	T49.2X3	T49.2X4	T49.2X5	T49.2X6
rifulvin	T36.7X1	T36.7X2	T36.7X3	T36.7X4	T36.7X5	T36.7X6
riseofulvin	T36.7X1	T36.7X2	T36.7X3	T36.7X4	T36.7X5	T36.7X6
owth hormone	T38.811	T38.812	T38.813	T38.814	T38.815	T38.816
aiac reagent	T50.991	T50.992	T50.993	T50.994	T50.995	T50.996
aiacol derivatives	T48.4X1	T48.4X2	T48.4X3	T48.4X4	T48.4X5	T48.4X6
aifenesin	T48.4X1	T48.4X2	T48.4X3	T48.4X4	T48.4X5	T48.4X6
aimesal	T48.4X1	T48.4X2	T48.4X3	T48.4X4	T48.4X5	T48.4X6
aiphenesin	T48.4X1	T48.4X2	T48.4X3	T48.4X4	T48.4X5	T48.4X6
amecycline	T36.4X1	T36.4X2	T36.4X3	T36.4X4	T36.4X5	T36.4X6
anabenz	T46.5X1	T46.5X2	T46.5X3	T46.5X4	T46.5X5	T46.5X6
anacline	T46.5X1	T46.5X2	T46.5X3	T46.5X4	T46.5X5	T46.5X6
anadrel	T46.5X1	T46.5X2	T46.5X3	T46.5X4	T46.5X5	T46.5X6
anatol	T37.2X1	T37.2X2	T37.2X3	T37.2X4	T37.2X5	T37.2X6
anethidine	T46.5X1	T46.5X2	T46.5X3	T46.5X4	T46.5X5	T46.5X6
anfacine	T46.5X1	T46.5X2	T46.5X3	T46.5X4	T46.5X5	T46.5X6
ano	T65.891	T65.892	T65.893	T65.894	—	—
anochlor	T46.5X1	T46.5X2	T46.5X3	T46.5X4	T46.5X5	T46.5X6
anoclor	T46.5X1	T46.5X2	T46.5X3	T46.5X4	T46.5X5	T46.5X6
anoctine	T46.5X1	T46.5X2	T46.5X3	T46.5X4	T46.5X5	T46.5X6
anoxabenz	T46.5X1	T46.5X2	T46.5X3	T46.5X4	T46.5X5	T46.5X6
anoxan	T46.5X1	T46.5X2	T46.5X3	T46.5X4	T46.5X5	T46.5X6
ar gum (medicinal)	T46.6X1	T46.6X2	T46.6X3	T46.6X4	T46.6X5	T46.6X6
H						
chimycin	T36.7X1	T36.7X2	T36.7X3	T36.7X4	T36.7X5	T36.7X6
ir						
lye	T49.4X1	T49.4X2	T49.4X3	T49.4X4	T49.4X5	T49.4X6
reparation NEC	T49.4X1	T49.4X2	T49.4X3	T49.4X4	T49.4X5	T49.4X6
lazepam	T42.4X1	T42.4X2	T42.4X3	T42.4X4	T42.4X5	T42.4X6

Substance	Poisoning, Accidental (unintentional)	Poisoning, Intentional self-harm	Poisoning, Assault	Poisoning, Undetermined	Adverse effect	Underdosing
Halcinolone	T49.0X1	T49.0X2	T49.0X3	T49.0X4	T49.0X5	T49.0X6
Halcinonide	T49.0X1	T49.0X2	T49.0X3	T49.0X4	T49.0X5	T49.0X6
Halethazole	T49.0X1	T49.0X2	T49.0X3	T49.0X4	T49.0X5	T49.0X6
Hallucinogen NEC	T40.901	T40.902	T40.903	T40.904	T40.905	T40.906
Halofantrine	T37.2X1	T37.2X2	T37.2X3	T37.2X4	T37.2X5	T37.2X6
Halofenate	T46.6X1	T46.6X2	T46.6X3	T46.6X4	T46.6X5	T46.6X6
Halometasone	T49.0X1	T49.0X2	T49.0X3	T49.0X4	T49.0X5	T49.0X6
Haloperidol	T43.4X1	T43.4X2	T43.4X3	T43.4X4	T43.4X5	T43.4X6
Haloprogin	T49.0X1	T49.0X2	T49.0X3	T49.0X4	T49.0X5	T49.0X6
Halotex	T49.0X1	T49.0X2	T49.0X3	T49.0X4	T49.0X5	T49.0X6
Halothane	T41.0X1	T41.0X2	T41.0X3	T41.0X4	T41.0X5	T41.0X6
Haloxazolam	T42.4X1	T42.4X2	T42.4X3	T42.4X4	T42.4X5	T42.4X6
Halquinols	T49.0X1	T49.0X2	T49.0X3	T49.0X4	T49.0X5	T49.0X6
Hamamelis	T49.2X1	T49.2X2	T49.2X3	T49.2X4	T49.2X5	T49.2X6
Haptendextran	T45.8X1	T45.8X2	T45.8X3	T45.8X4	T45.8X5	T45.8X6
Harmonyl	T46.5X1	T46.5X2	T46.5X3	T46.5X4	T46.5X5	T46.5X6
Hartmann's solution	T50.3X1	T50.3X2	T50.3X3	T50.3X4	T50.3X5	T50.3X6
Hashish	T40.7X1	T40.7X2	T40.7X3	T40.7X4	T40.7X5	T40.7X6
Hawaiian Woodrose seeds	T40.991	T40.992	T40.993	T40.994	—	—
HCB	T60.3X1	T60.3X2	T60.3X3	T60.3X4	—	—
HCH	T53.6X1	T53.6X2	T53.6X3	T53.6X4	—	—
medicinal	T49.0X1	T49.0X2	T49.0X3	T49.0X4	T49.0X5	T49.0X6
HCN	T57.3X1	T57.3X2	T57.3X3	T57.3X4	—	—
Headache cures, drugs, powders NEC	T50.901	T50.902	T50.903	T50.904	T50.905	T50.906
Heavenly Blue (morning glory)	T40.991	T40.992	T40.993	T40.994	—	—
Heavy metal antidote	T45.8X1	T45.8X2	T45.8X3	T45.8X4	T45.8X5	T45.8X6
Hedaquinium	T49.0X1	T49.0X2	T49.0X3	T49.0X4	T49.0X5	T49.0X6
Hedge hyssop	T62.2X1	T62.2X2	T62.2X3	T62.2X4	—	—
Heet	T49.8X1	T49.8X2	T49.8X3	T49.8X4	T49.8X5	T49.8X6
Helenin	T37.4X1	T37.4X2	T37.4X3	T37.4X4	T37.4X5	T37.4X6
Helium (nonmedicinal) NEC	T59.891	T59.892	T59.893	T59.894	—	—
medicinal	T48.991	T48.992	T48.993	T48.994	T48.995	T48.996
Hellebore (black) (green) (white)	T62.2X1	T62.2X2	T62.2X3	T62.2X4	—	—
Hematin	T45.8X1	T45.8X2	T45.8X3	T45.8X4	T45.8X5	T45.8X6
Hematinic preparation	T45.8X1	T45.8X2	T45.8X3	T45.8X4	T45.8X5	T45.8X6
Hematological agent	T45.91	T45.92	T45.93	T45.94	T45.95	T45.96
specified NEC	T45.8X1	T45.8X2	T45.8X3	T45.8X4	T45.8X5	T45.8X6
Hemlock	T62.2X1	T62.2X2	T62.2X3	T62.2X4	—	—
Hemostatic	T45.621	T45.622	T45.623	T45.624	T45.625	T45.626
drug, systemic	T45.621	T45.622	T45.623	T45.624	T45.625	T45.626
Hemostyptic	T49.4X1	T49.4X2	T49.4X3	T49.4X4	T49.4X5	T49.4X6
Henbane	T62.2X1	T62.2X2	T62.2X3	T62.2X4	—	—
Heparin (sodium)	T45.511	T45.512	T45.513	T45.514	T45.515	T45.516
action reverser	T45.7X1	T45.7X2	T45.7X3	T45.7X4	T45.7X5	T45.7X6
Heparin-fraction	T45.511	T45.512	T45.513	T45.514	T45.515	T45.516
Heparinoid (systemic)	T45.511	T45.512	T45.513	T45.514	T45.515	T45.516
Hepatic secretion stimulant	T47.8X1	T47.8X2	T47.8X3	T47.8X4	T47.8X5	T47.8X6

Substance	Poisoning, Accidental (unintentional)	Poisoning, Intentional self-harm	Poisoning, Assault	Poisoning, Undetermined	Adverse effect	Underdosing
Hepatitis B						
immune globulin	T50.Z11	T50.Z12	T50.Z13	T50.Z14	T50.Z15	T50.Z16
vaccine	T50.B91	T50.B92	T50.B93	T50.B94	T50.B95	T50.B96
Hepronicate	T46.7X1	T46.7X2	T46.7X3	T46.7X4	T46.7X5	T46.7X6
Heptabarb	T42.3X1	T42.3X2	T42.3X3	T42.3X4	T42.3X5	T42.3X6
Heptabarbital	T42.3X1	T42.3X2	T42.3X3	T42.3X4	T42.3X5	T42.3X6
Heptabarbitone	T42.3X1	T42.3X2	T42.3X3	T42.3X4	T42.3X5	T42.3X6
Heptachlor	T60.1X1	T60.1X2	T60.1X3	T60.1X4	—	—
Heptalgin	T40.2X1	T40.2X2	T40.2X3	T40.2X4	T40.2X5	T40.2X6
Heptaminol	T46.3X1	T46.3X2	T46.3X3	T46.3X4	T46.3X5	T46.3X6
Herbicide NEC	T60.3X1	T60.3X2	T60.3X3	T60.3X4	—	—
Heroin	T40.1X1	T40.1X2	T40.1X3	T40.1X4	—	—
Herplex	T49.5X1	T49.5X2	T49.5X3	T49.5X4	T49.5X5	T49.5X6
HES	T45.8X1	T45.8X2	T45.8X3	T45.8X4	T45.8X5	T45.8X6
Hesperidin	T46.991	T46.992	T46.993	T46.994	T46.995	T46.996
Hetacillin	T36.0X1	T36.0X2	T36.0X3	T36.0X4	T36.0X5	T36.0X6
Hetastarch	T45.8X1	T45.8X2	T45.8X3	T45.8X4	T45.8X5	T45.8X6
HETP	T60.0X1	T60.0X2	T60.0X3	T60.0X4	—	—
Hexachlorobenzene (vapor)	T60.3X1	T60.3X2	T60.3X3	T60.3X4	—	—
Hexachlorocyclohexane	T53.6X1	T53.6X2	T53.6X3	T53.6X4	—	—
Hexachlorophene	T49.0X1	T49.0X2	T49.0X3	T49.0X4	T49.0X5	T49.0X6
Hexadiline	T46.3X1	T46.3X2	T46.3X3	T46.3X4	T46.3X5	T46.3X6
Hexadimethrine (bromide)	T45.7X1	T45.7X2	T45.7X3	T45.7X4	T45.7X5	T45.7X6
Hexadylamine	T46.3X1	T46.3X2	T46.3X3	T46.3X4	T46.3X5	T46.3X6
Hexaethyl tetraphosphate	T60.0X1	T60.0X2	T60.0X3	T60.0X4	—	—
Hexafluorenium bromide	T48.1X1	T48.1X2	T48.1X3	T48.1X4	T48.1X5	T48.1X6
Hexafluronium (bromide)	T48.1X1	T48.1X2	T48.1X3	T48.1X4	T48.1X5	T48.1X6
Hexa-germ	T49.2X1	T49.2X2	T49.2X3	T49.2X4	T49.2X5	T49.2X6
Hexahydrobenzol	T52.8X1	T52.8X2	T52.8X3	T52.8X4	—	—
Hexahydrocresol(s)	T51.8X1	T51.8X2	T51.8X3	T51.8X4	—	—
arsenide	T57.0X1	T57.0X2	T57.0X3	T57.0X4	—	—
arseniurated	T57.0X1	T57.0X2	T57.0X3	T57.0X4	—	—
cyanide	T57.3X1	T57.3X2	T57.3X3	T57.3X4	—	—
gas	T59.891	T59.892	T59.893	T59.894	—	—
Fluoride (liquid)	T57.8X1	T57.8X2	T57.8X3	T57.8X4	—	—
vapor	T59.891	T59.892	T59.893	T59.894	—	—
phophorated	T60.0X1	T60.0X2	T60.0X3	T60.0X4	—	—
sulfate	T57.8X1	T57.8X2	T57.8X3	T57.8X4	—	—
sulfide (gas)	T59.6X1	T59.6X2	T59.6X3	T59.6X4	—	—
arseniurated	T57.0X1	T57.0X2	T57.0X3	T57.0X4	—	—
sulfurated	T57.8X1	T57.8X2	T57.8X3	T57.8X4	—	—
Hexahydrophenol	T51.8X1	T51.8X2	T51.8X3	T51.8X4	—	—
Hexalen	T51.8X1	T51.8X2	T51.8X3	T51.8X4	—	—
Hexamethonium bromide	T44.2X1	T44.2X2	T44.2X3	T44.2X4	T44.2X5	T44.2X6
Hexamethylene	T52.8X1	T52.8X2	T52.8X3	T52.8X4	—	—
Hexamethylmelamine	T45.1X1	T45.1X2	T45.1X3	T45.1X4	T45.1X5	T45.1X6
Hexamidine	T49.0X1	T49.0X2	T49.0X3	T49.0X4	T49.0X5	T49.0X6
Hexamine (mandelate)	T37.8X1	T37.8X2	T37.8X3	T37.8X4	T37.8X5	T37.8X6
Hexanone, 2-hexanone	T52.4X1	T52.4X2	T52.4X3	T52.4X4	—	—
Hexanuorenium	T48.1X1	T48.1X2	T48.1X3	T48.1X4	T48.1X5	T48.1X
Hexapropymate	T42.6X1	T42.6X2	T42.6X3	T42.6X4	T42.6X5	T42.6X
Hexasonium iodide	T44.3X1	T44.3X2	T44.3X3	T44.3X4	T44.3X5	T44.3X
Hexcarbacholine bromide	T48.1X1	T48.1X2	T48.1X3	T48.1X4	T48.1X5	T48.1X
Hexemal	T42.3X1	T42.3X2	T42.3X3	T42.3X4	T42.3X5	T42.3X
Hexestrol	T38.5X1	T38.5X2	T38.5X3	T38.5X4	T38.5X5	T38.5X
Hexethal (sodium)	T42.3X1	T42.3X2	T42.3X3	T42.3X4	T42.3X5	T42.3X
Hexetidine	T37.8X1	T37.8X2	T37.8X3	T37.8X4	T37.8X5	T37.8X
Hexobarbital	T42.3X1	T42.3X2	T42.3X3	T42.3X4	T42.3X5	T42.3X
rectal	T41.291	T41.292	T41.293	T41.294	T41.295	T41.29
sodium	T41.1X1	T41.1X2	T41.1X3	T41.1X4	T41.1X5	T41.1X
Hexobendine	T46.3X1	T46.3X2	T46.3X3	T46.3X4	T46.3X5	T46.3X
Hexocyclium	T44.3X1	T44.3X2	T44.3X3	T44.3X4	T44.3X5	T44.3X
metilsulfate	T44.3X1	T44.3X2	T44.3X3	T44.3X4	T44.3X5	T44.3X
Hexoestrol	T38.5X1	T38.5X2	T38.5X3	T38.5X4	T38.5X5	T38.5X
Hexone	T52.4X1	T52.4X2	T52.4X3	T52.4X4	—	—
Hexoprenaline	T48.6X1	T48.6X2	T48.6X3	T48.6X4	T48.6X5	T48.6X
Hexylcaine	T41.3X1	T41.3X2	T41.3X3	T41.3X4	T41.3X5	T41.3X
Hexylresorcinol	T52.2X1	T52.2X2	T52.2X3	T52.2X4	—	—
HGH (human growth hormone)	T38.811	T38.812	T38.813	T38.814	T38.815	T38.81
Hinkle's pills	T47.2X1	T47.2X2	T47.2X3	T47.2X4	T47.2X5	T47.2X
Histalog	T50.8X1	T50.8X2	T50.8X3	T50.8X4	T50.8X5	T50.8X
Histamine (phosphate)	T50.8X1	T50.8X2	T50.8X3	T50.8X4	T50.8X5	T50.8X
Histoplasmin	T50.8X1	T50.8X2	T50.8X3	T50.8X4	T50.8X5	T50.8X
Holly berries	T62.2X1	T62.2X2	T62.2X3	T62.2X4	—	—
Homatropine	T44.3X1	T44.3X2	T44.3X3	T44.3X4	T44.3X5	T44.3X
methylbromide	T44.3X1	T44.3X2	T44.3X3	T44.3X4	T44.3X5	T44.3X
Homochlorcyclizine	T45.0X1	T45.0X2	T45.0X3	T45.0X4	T45.0X5	T45.0X
Homosalate	T49.3X1	T49.3X2	T49.3X3	T49.3X4	T49.3X5	T49.3X
Homo-tet	T50.Z11	T50.Z12	T50.Z13	T50.Z14	T50.Z15	T50.Z1
Hormone	T38.801	T38.802	T38.803	T38.804	T38.805	T38.80
adrenal cortical steroids	T38.0X1	T38.0X2	T38.0X3	T38.0X4	T38.0X5	T38.0X
androgenic	T38.7X1	T38.7X2	T38.7X3	T38.7X4	T38.7X5	T38.7X
anterior pituitary NEC	T38.811	T38.812	T38.813	T38.814	T38.815	T38.81
antidiabetic agents	T38.3X1	T38.3X2	T38.3X3	T38.3X4	T38.3X5	T38.3X
antidiuretic	T38.891	T38.892	T38.893	T38.894	T38.895	T38.89
cancer therapy	T45.1X1	T45.1X2	T45.1X3	T45.1X4	T45.1X5	T45.1X
follicle stimulating	T38.811	T38.812	T38.813	T38.814	T38.815	T38.81
gonadotropic	T38.891	T38.892	T38.893	T38.894	T38.895	T38.89
pituitary	T38.811	T38.812	T38.813	T38.814	T38.815	T38.81
growth	T38.811	T38.812	T38.813	T38.814	T38.815	T38.81
luteinizing	T38.811	T38.812	T38.813	T38.814	T38.815	T38.81
ovarian	T38.5X1	T38.5X2	T38.5X3	T38.5X4	T38.5X5	T38.5X
oxytocic	T48.0X1	T48.0X2	T48.0X3	T48.0X4	T48.0X5	T48.0X
parathyroid (derivatives)	T50.991	T50.992	T50.993	T50.994	T50.995	T50.99
pituitary (posterior) NEC	T38.891	T38.892	T38.893	T38.894	T38.895	T38.89
anterior	T38.811	T38.812	T38.813	T38.814	T38.815	T38.81
specified, NEC	T38.891	T38.892	T38.893	T38.894	T38.895	T38.89
thyroid	T38.1X1	T38.1X2	T38.1X3	T38.1X4	T38.1X5	T38.1X

Substance	Poisoning, Accidental (unintentional)	Poisoning, Intentional self-harm	Poisoning, Assault	Poisoning, Undetermined	Adverse effect	Underdosing
Hornet (sting)	T63.451	T63.452	T63.453	T63.454	—	—
Horse anti-human lymphocytic serum	T50.Z11	T50.Z12	T50.Z13	T50.Z14	T50.Z15	T50.Z16
Horticulture agent NEC	T65.91	T65.92	T65.93	T65.94	—	—
with pesticide	T60.91	T60.92	T60.93	T60.94	—	—
Human						
albumin	T45.8X1	T45.8X2	T45.8X3	T45.8X4	T45.8X5	T45.8X6
growth hormone (HGH)	T38.811	T38.812	T38.813	T38.814	T38.815	T38.816
immune serum	T50.Z11	T50.Z12	T50.Z13	T50.Z14	T50.Z15	T50.Z16
Hyaluronidase	T45.3X1	T45.3X2	T45.3X3	T45.3X4	T45.3X5	T45.3X6
Hyazyme	T45.3X1	T45.3X2	T45.3X3	T45.3X4	T45.3X5	T45.3X6
Hycodan	T40.2X1	T40.2X2	T40.2X3	T40.2X4	T40.2X5	T40.2X6
Hydantoin derivative NEC	T42.0X1	T42.0X2	T42.0X3	T42.0X4	T42.0X5	T42.0X6
Hydeltra	T38.0X1	T38.0X2	T38.0X3	T38.0X4	T38.0X5	T38.0X6
Hydergine	T44.6X1	T44.6X2	T44.6X3	T44.6X4	T44.6X5	T44.6X6
Hydrabamine penicillin	T36.0X1	T36.0X2	T36.0X3	T36.0X4	T36.0X5	T36.0X6
Hydralazine	T46.5X1	T46.5X2	T46.5X3	T46.5X4	T46.5X5	T46.5X6
Hydrargaphen	T49.0X1	T49.0X2	T49.0X3	T49.0X4	T49.0X5	T49.0X6
Hydrargyri amino-chloridum	T49.0X1	T49.0X2	T49.0X3	T49.0X4	T49.0X5	T49.0X6
Hydrastine	T48.291	T48.292	T48.293	T48.294	T48.295	T48.296
Hydrazine	T54.1X1	T54.1X2	T54.1X3	T54.1X4	—	—
monoamine oxidase inhibitors	T43.1X1	T43.1X2	T43.1X3	T43.1X4	T43.1X5	T43.1X6
Hydrazoic acid, azides	T54.2X1	T54.2X2	T54.2X3	T54.2X4	—	—
Hydriodic acid	T48.4X1	T48.4X2	T48.4X3	T48.4X4	T48.4X5	T48.4X6
Hydrocarbon gas	T59.891	T59.892	T59.893	T59.894	—	—
incomplete combustion of—see Carbon, monoxide, fuel, utility						
liquefied (mobile container)	T59.891	T59.892	T59.893	T59.894	—	—
piped (natural)	T59.891	T59.892	T59.893	T59.894	—	—
Hydrochloric acid (liquid)	T54.2X1	T54.2X2	T54.2X3	T54.2X4	—	—
medicinal (digestant)	T47.5X1	T47.5X2	T47.5X3	T47.5X4	T47.5X5	T47.5X6
vapor	T59.891	T59.892	T59.893	T59.894	—	—
Hydrochlorothiazide	T50.2X1	T50.2X2	T50.2X3	T50.2X4	T50.2X5	T50.2X6
Hydrocodone	T40.2X1	T40.2X2	T40.2X3	T40.2X4	T40.2X5	T40.2X6
Hydrocortisone (derivatives)	T38.0X1	T38.0X2	T38.0X3	T38.0X4	T38.0X5	T38.0X6
aceponate	T49.0X1	T49.0X2	T49.0X3	T49.0X4	T49.0X5	T49.0X6
ENT agent	T49.6X1	T49.6X2	T49.6X3	T49.6X4	T49.6X5	T49.6X6
ophthalmic preparation	T49.5X1	T49.5X2	T49.5X3	T49.5X4	T49.5X5	T49.5X6
topical NEC	T49.0X1	T49.0X2	T49.0X3	T49.0X4	T49.0X5	T49.0X6
Hydrocortone	T38.0X1	T38.0X2	T38.0X3	T38.0X4	T38.0X5	T38.0X6
ENT agent	T49.6X1	T49.6X2	T49.6X3	T49.6X4	T49.6X5	T49.6X6
ophthalmic preparation	T49.5X1	T49.5X2	T49.5X3	T49.5X4	T49.5X5	T49.5X6
topical NEC	T49.0X1	T49.0X2	T49.0X3	T49.0X4	T49.0X5	T49.0X6
Hydrocyanic acid (liquid)	T57.3X1	T57.3X2	T57.3X3	T57.3X4	—	—
gas	T65.0X1	T65.0X2	T65.0X3	T65.0X4	—	—
Hydroflumethiazide	T50.2X1	T50.2X2	T50.2X3	T50.2X4	T50.2X5	T50.2X6

Substance	Poisoning, Accidental (unintentional)	Poisoning, Intentional self-harm	Poisoning, Assault	Poisoning, Undetermined	Adverse effect	Underdosing
Hydrofluoric acid (liquid)	T54.2X1	T54.2X2	T54.2X3	T54.2X4	—	—
vapor	T59.891	T59.892	T59.893	T59.894	—	—
Hydrogen	T59.891	T59.892	T59.893	T59.894	—	—
arsenide	T57.0X1	T57.0X2	T57.0X3	T57.0X4	—	—
arseniureted	T57.0X1	T57.0X2	T57.0X3	T57.0X4	—	—
chloride	T57.8X1	T57.8X2	T57.8X3	T57.8X4	—	—
cyanide (salts)	T57.3X1	T57.3X2	T57.3X3	T57.3X4	—	—
gas	T57.3X1	T57.3X2	T57.3X3	T57.3X4	—	—
Fluoride	T59.5X1	T59.5X2	T59.5X3	T59.5X4	—	—
vapor	T59.5X1	T59.5X2	T59.5X3	T59.5X4	—	—
peroxide	T49.0X1	T49.0X2	T49.0X3	T49.0X4	T49.0X5	T49.0X6
phosphureted	T57.1X1	T57.1X2	T57.1X3	T57.1X4	—	—
sulfide	T59.6X1	T59.6X2	T59.6X3	T59.6X4	—	—
arseniureted	T57.0X1	T57.0X2	T57.0X3	T57.0X4	—	—
sulfureted	T59.6X1	T59.6X2	T59.6X3	T59.6X4	—	—
Hydromethylpyridine	T46.7X1	T46.7X2	T46.7X3	T46.7X4	T46.7X5	T46.7X6
Hydromorphinol	T40.2X1	T40.2X2	T40.2X3	T40.2X4	—	—
Hydromorphinone	T40.2X1	T40.2X2	T40.2X3	T40.2X4	T40.2X5	T40.2X6
Hydromorphone	T40.2X1	T40.2X2	T40.2X3	T40.2X4	T40.2X5	T40.2X6
Hydromox	T50.2X1	T50.2X2	T50.2X3	T50.2X4	T50.2X5	T50.2X6
Hydrophilic lotion	T49.3X1	T49.3X2	T49.3X3	T49.3X4	T49.3X5	T49.3X6
Hydroquinidine	T46.2X1	T46.2X2	T46.2X3	T46.2X4	T46.2X5	T46.2X6
Hydroquinone	T52.2X1	T52.2X2	T52.2X3	T52.2X4	—	—
vapor	T59.891	T59.892	T59.893	T59.894	—	—
Hydrosulfuric acid (gas)	T59.6X1	T59.6X2	T59.6X3	T59.6X4	—	—
Hydrotalcite	T47.1X1	T47.1X2	T47.1X3	T47.1X4	T47.1X5	T47.1X6
Hydrous wool fat	T49.3X1	T49.3X2	T49.3X3	T49.3X4	T49.3X5	T49.3X6
Hydroxide, caustic	T54.3X1	T54.3X2	T54.3X3	T54.3X4	—	—
Hydroxocobalamin	T45.8X1	T45.8X2	T45.8X3	T45.8X4	T45.8X5	T45.8X6
Hydroxyamp-hetamine	T49.5X1	T49.5X2	T49.5X3	T49.5X4	T49.5X5	T49.5X6
Hydroxycarbamide	T45.1X1	T45.1X2	T45.1X3	T45.1X4	T45.1X5	T45.1X6
Hydroxychloroquine	T37.8X1	T37.8X2	T37.8X3	T37.8X4	T37.8X5	T37.8X6
Hydroxydihydro-codeinone	T40.2X1	T40.2X2	T40.2X3	T40.2X4	T40.2X5	T40.2X6
Hydroxyestrone	T38.5X1	T38.5X2	T38.5X3	T38.5X4	T38.5X5	T38.5X6
Hydroxyethyl starch	T45.8X1	T45.8X2	T45.8X3	T45.8X4	T45.8X5	T45.8X6
Hydroxyme-thylpentanone	T52.4X1	T52.4X2	T52.4X3	T52.4X4	—	—
Hydroxyphenamate	T43.591	T43.592	T43.593	T43.594	T43.595	T43.596
Hydroxypheny-lbutazone	T39.2X1	T39.2X2	T39.2X3	T39.2X4	T39.2X5	T39.2X6
Hydroxyprogesterone	T38.5X1	T38.5X2	T38.5X3	T38.5X4	T38.5X5	T38.5X6
caproate	T38.5X1	T38.5X2	T38.5X3	T38.5X4	T38.5X5	T38.5X6
Hydroxyquinoline (derivatives) NEC	T37.8X1	T37.8X2	T37.8X3	T37.8X4	T37.8X5	T37.8X6
Hydroxystilbamidine	T37.3X1	T37.3X2	T37.3X3	T37.3X4	T37.3X5	T37.3X6
Hydroxytoluene (nonmedicinal)	T54.0X1	T54.0X2	T54.0X3	T54.0X4	—	—
medicinal	T49.0X1	T49.0X2	T49.0X3	T49.0X4	T49.0X5	T49.0X6
Hydroxyurea	T45.1X1	T45.1X2	T45.1X3	T45.1X4	T45.1X5	T45.1X6
Hydroxyzine	T43.591	T43.592	T43.593	T43.594	T43.595	T43.596
Hyoscine	T44.3X1	T44.3X2	T44.3X3	T44.3X4	T44.3X5	T44.3X6
Hyoscyamine	T44.3X1	T44.3X2	T44.3X3	T44.3X4	T44.3X5	T44.3X6

Substance	Poisoning, Accidental (unintentional)	Poisoning, Intentional self-harm	Poisoning, Assault	Poisoning, Undetermined	Adverse effect	Underdosing
Hyoscyamus	T44.3X1	T44.3X2	T44.3X3	T44.3X4	T44.3X5	T44.3X6
dry extract	T44.3X1	T44.3X2	T44.3X3	T44.3X4	T44.3X5	T44.3X6
Hypaque	T50.8X1	T50.8X2	T50.8X3	T50.8X4	T50.8X5	T50.8X6
Hypertussis	T50.Z11	T50.Z12	T50.Z13	T50.Z14	T50.Z15	T50.Z16
Hypnotic	T42.71	T42.72	T42.73	T42.74	T42.75	T42.76
anticonvulsant	T42.71	T42.72	T42.73	T42.74	T42.75	T42.76
specified NEC	T42.6X1	T42.6X2	T42.6X3	T42.6X4	T42.6X5	T42.6X6
Hypochlorite	T49.0X1	T49.0X2	T49.0X3	T49.0X4	T49.0X5	T49.0X6
Hypophysis, posterior	T38.891	T38.892	T38.893	T38.894	T38.895	T38.896
Hypotensive NEC	T46.5X1	T46.5X2	T46.5X3	T46.5X4	T46.5X5	T46.5X6
Hypromellose	T49.5X1	T49.5X2	T49.5X3	T49.5X4	T49.5X5	T49.5X6
I						
Ibacitabine	T37.5X1	T37.5X2	T37.5X3	T37.5X4	T37.5X5	T37.5X6
Ibopamine	T44.991	T44.992	T44.993	T44.994	T44.995	T44.996
Ibufenac	T39.311	T39.312	T39.313	T39.314	T39.315	T39.316
Ibuprofen	T39.311	T39.312	T39.313	T39.314	T39.315	T39.316
Ibuproxam	T39.311	T39.312	T39.313	T39.314	T39.315	T39.316
Ibuterol	T48.6X1	T48.6X2	T48.6X3	T48.6X4	T48.6X5	T48.6X6
Ichthammol	T49.0X1	T49.0X2	T49.0X3	T49.0X4	T49.0X5	T49.0X6
Ichthyol	T49.4X1	T49.4X2	T49.4X3	T49.4X4	T49.4X5	T49.4X6
Idarubicin	T45.1X1	T45.1X2	T45.1X3	T45.1X4	T45.1X5	T45.1X6
Idrocilamide	T42.8X1	T42.8X2	T42.8X3	T42.8X4	T42.8X5	T42.8X6
Ifenprodil	T46.7X1	T46.7X2	T46.7X3	T46.7X4	T46.7X5	T46.7X6
Ifosfamide	T45.1X1	T45.1X2	T45.1X3	T45.1X4	T45.1X5	T45.1X6
Iletin	T38.3X1	T38.3X2	T38.3X3	T38.3X4	T38.3X5	T38.3X6
Ilex	T62.2X1	T62.2X2	T62.2X3	T62.2X4	—	—
Illuminating gas (after combustion)	T58.11	T58.12	T58.13	T58.14	—	—
prior to combustion	T59.891	T59.892	T59.893	T59.894	—	—
Ilopan	T45.2X1	T45.2X2	T45.2X3	T45.2X4	T45.2X5	T45.2X6
Iloprost	T46.7X1	T46.7X2	T46.7X3	T46.7X4	T46.7X5	T46.7X6
Ilotycin	T36.3X1	T36.3X2	T36.3X3	T36.3X4	T36.3X5	T36.3X6
ophthalmic preparation	T49.5X1	T49.5X2	T49.5X3	T49.5X4	T49.5X5	T49.5X6
topical NEC	T49.0X1	T49.0X2	T49.0X3	T49.0X4	T49.0X5	T49.0X6
Imidazole-4-carboxamide	T45.1X1	T45.1X2	T45.1X3	T45.1X4	T45.1X5	T45.1X6
Imipenem	T36.0X1	T36.0X2	T36.0X3	T36.0X4	T36.0X5	T36.0X6
Imipramine	T43.011	T43.012	T43.013	T43.014	T43.015	T43.016
Iminostilbene	T42.1X1	T42.1X2	T42.1X3	T42.1X4	T42.1X5	T42.1X6
Immu-G	T50.Z11	T50.Z12	T50.Z13	T50.Z14	T50.Z15	T50.Z16
Immuglobin	T50.Z11	T50.Z12	T50.Z13	T50.Z14	T50.Z15	T50.Z16
Immune						
globulin	T50.Z11	T50.Z12	T50.Z13	T50.Z14	T50.Z15	T50.Z16
serum globulin	T50.Z11	T50.Z12	T50.Z13	T50.Z14	T50.Z15	T50.Z16
Immunoglobin human (intravenous) (normal)	T50.Z11	T50.Z12	T50.Z13	T50.Z14	T50.Z15	T50.Z16
unmodified	T50.Z11	T50.Z12	T50.Z13	T50.Z14	T50.Z15	T50.Z16
Immunosuppressive drug	T45.1X1	T45.1X2	T45.1X3	T45.1X4	T45.1X5	T45.1X6
Immu-tetanus	T50.Z11	T50.Z12	T50.Z13	T50.Z14	T50.Z15	T50.Z16
Indalpine	T43.221	T43.222	T43.223	T43.224	T43.225	T43.226
Indanazoline	T48.5X1	T48.5X2	T48.5X3	T48.5X4	T48.5X5	T48.5X6

Substance	Poisoning, Accidental (unintentional)	Poisoning, Intentional self-harm	Poisoning, Assault	Poisoning, Undetermined	Adverse effect	Underdosing
Indandione (derivatives)	T45.511	T45.512	T45.513	T45.514	T45.515	T45.516
Indapamide	T46.5X1	T46.5X2	T46.5X3	T46.5X4	T46.5X5	T46.5X6
Indendione (derivatives)	T45.511	T45.512	T45.513	T45.514	T45.515	T45.516
Indenolol	T44.7X1	T44.7X2	T44.7X3	T44.7X4	T44.7X5	T44.7X6
Inderal	T44.7X1	T44.7X2	T44.7X3	T44.7X4	T44.7X5	T44.7X6
Indian						
hemp	T40.7X1	T40.7X2	T40.7X3	T40.7X4	T40.7X5	T40.7X6
tobacco	T62.2X1	T62.2X2	T62.2X3	T62.2X4	—	—
Indigo carmine	T50.8X1	T50.8X2	T50.8X3	T50.8X4	T50.8X5	T50.8X6
Indobufen	T45.521	T45.522	T45.523	T45.524	T45.525	T45.526
Indocin	T39.2X1	T39.2X2	T39.2X3	T39.2X4	T39.2X5	T39.2X6
Indocyanine green	T50.8X1	T50.8X2	T50.8X3	T50.8X4	T50.8X5	T50.8X6
Indometacin	T39.391	T39.392	T39.393	T39.394	T39.395	T39.396
Indomethacin	T39.391	T39.392	T39.393	T39.394	T39.395	T39.396
farnesil	T39.4X1	T39.4X2	T39.4X3	T39.4X4	T39.4X5	T39.4X6
Indoramin	T44.6X1	T44.6X2	T44.6X3	T44.6X4	T44.6X5	T44.6X6
Industrial						
alcohol	T51.0X1	T51.0X2	T51.0X3	T51.0X4	—	—
fumes	T59.891	T59.892	T59.893	T59.894	—	—
solvents (fumes) (vapors)	T52.91	T52.92	T52.93	T52.94	—	—
Influenza vaccine	T50.B91	T50.B92	T50.B93	T50.B94	T50.B95	T50.B96
Ingested substance NEC	T65.91	T65.92	T65.93	T65.94	—	—
INH	T37.1X1	T37.1X2	T37.1X3	T37.1X4	T37.1X5	T37.1X6
Inhalation, gas (noxious)—see Gas						
Inhibitor						
angiotensin-converting enzyme	T46.4X1	T46.4X2	T46.4X3	T46.4X4	T46.4X5	T46.4X6
carbonic anhydrase	T50.2X1	T50.2X2	T50.2X3	T50.2X4	T50.2X5	T50.2X6
fibrinolysis	T45.621	T45.622	T45.623	T45.624	T45.625	T45.626
monoamine oxidase NEC	T43.1X1	T43.1X2	T43.1X3	T43.1X4	T43.1X5	T43.1X6
hydrazine	T43.1X1	T43.1X2	T43.1X3	T43.1X4	T43.1X5	T43.1X6
postsynaptic	T43.8X1	T43.8X2	T43.8X3	T43.8X4	T43.8X5	T43.8X6
prothrombin synthesis	T45.511	T45.512	T45.513	T45.514	T45.515	T45.516
Ink	T65.891	T65.892	T65.893	T65.894	—	—
Inorganic substance NEC	T57.91	T57.92	T57.93	T57.94	—	—
Inosine pranobex	T37.5X1	T37.5X2	T37.5X3	T37.5X4	T37.5X5	T37.5X6
Inositol	T50.991	T50.992	T50.993	T50.994	T50.995	T50.996
nicotinate	T46.7X1	T46.7X2	T46.7X3	T46.7X4	T46.7X5	T46.7X6
Inproquone	T45.1X1	T45.1X2	T45.1X3	T45.1X4	T45.1X5	T45.1X6
Insect (sting), venomous	T63.481	T63.482	T63.483	T63.484	—	—
ant	T63.421	T63.422	T63.423	T63.424	—	—
bee	T63.441	T63.442	T63.443	T63.444	—	—
caterpillar	T63.431	T63.432	T63.433	T63.434	—	—
hornet	T63.451	T63.452	T63.453	T63.454	—	—
wasp	T63.461	T63.462	T63.463	T63.464	—	—
Insecticide NEC	T60.91	T60.92	T60.93	T60.94	—	—
carbamate	T60.0X1	T60.0X2	T60.0X3	T60.0X4	—	—
chlorinated	T60.1X1	T60.1X2	T60.1X3	T60.1X4	—	—
mixed	T60.91	T60.92	T60.93	T60.94	—	—

Substance	Poisoning, Accidental (unintentional)	Poisoning, Intentional self-harm	Poisoning, Assault	Poisoning, Undetermined	Adverse effect	Underdosing
secticide NEC — *ontinued*						
organochlorine	T60.1X1	T60.1X2	T60.1X3	T60.1X4	—	—
organophosphorus	T60.0X1	T60.0X2	T60.0X3	T60.0X4	—	—
sular tissue extract	T38.3X1	T38.3X2	T38.3X3	T38.3X4	T38.3X5	T38.3X6
sulin (amorphous) lobin) (isophane) ente) (NPH) (Semilente) Jltralente)	T38.3X1	T38.3X2	T38.3X3	T38.3X4	T38.3X5	T38.3X6
defalan	T38.3X1	T38.3X2	T38.3X3	T38.3X4	T38.3X5	T38.3X6
human	T38.3X1	T38.3X2	T38.3X3	T38.3X4	T38.3X5	T38.3X6
injection, soluble	T38.3X1	T38.3X2	T38.3X3	T38.3X4	T38.3X5	T38.3X6
biphasic	T38.3X1	T38.3X2	T38.3X3	T38.3X4	T38.3X5	T38.3X6
intermediate acting	T38.3X1	T38.3X2	T38.3X3	T38.3X4	T38.3X5	T38.3X6
protamine zinc	T38.3X1	T38.3X2	T38.3X3	T38.3X4	T38.3X5	T38.3X6
slow acting	T38.3X1	T38.3X2	T38.3X3	T38.3X4	T38.3X5	T38.3X6
zinc						
protamine injection	T38.3X1	T38.3X2	T38.3X3	T38.3X4	T38.3X5	T38.3X6
suspension (amorphous) (crystalline)	T38.3X1	T38.3X2	T38.3X3	T38.3X4	T38.3X5	T38.3X6
terferon (alpha) (beta) amma)	T37.5X1	T37.5X2	T37.5X3	T37.5X4	T37.5X5	T37.5X6
testinal motility control rug	T47.6X1	T47.6X2	T47.6X3	T47.6X4	T47.6X5	T47.6X6
biological	T47.8X1	T47.8X2	T47.8X3	T47.8X4	T47.8X5	T47.8X6
tranarcon	T41.1X1	T41.1X2	T41.1X3	T41.1X4	T41.1X5	T41.1X6
travenous						
amino acids	T50.991	T50.992	T50.993	T50.994	T50.995	T50.996
fat suspension	T50.991	T50.992	T50.993	T50.994	T50.995	T50.996
ulin	T50.8X1	T50.8X2	T50.8X3	T50.8X4	T50.8X5	T50.8X6
vert sugar	T50.3X1	T50.3X2	T50.3X3	T50.3X4	T50.3X5	T50.3X6
za—see Naproxen						
benzamic acid	T50.8X1	T50.8X2	T50.8X3	T50.8X4	T50.8X5	T50.8X6
carmic acid	T50.8X1	T50.8X2	T50.8X3	T50.8X4	T50.8X5	T50.8X6
cetamic acid	T50.8X1	T50.8X2	T50.8X3	T50.8X4	T50.8X5	T50.8X6
damide	T50.8X1	T50.8X2	T50.8X3	T50.8X4	T50.8X5	T50.8X6
dide NEC—see also dine	T49.0X1	T49.0X2	T49.0X3	T49.0X4	T49.0X5	T49.0X6
mercury (ointment)	T49.0X1	T49.0X2	T49.0X3	T49.0X4	T49.0X5	T49.0X6
methylate	T49.0X1	T49.0X2	T49.0X3	T49.0X4	T49.0X5	T49.0X6
potassium (expectorant) NEC	T48.4X1	T48.4X2	T48.4X3	T48.4X4	T48.4X5	T48.4X6
dinated						
contrast medium	T50.8X1	T50.8X2	T50.8X3	T50.8X4	T50.8X5	T50.8X6
glycerol	T48.4X1	T48.4X2	T48.4X3	T48.4X4	T48.4X5	T48.4X6
human serum albumin (131I)	T50.8X1	T50.8X2	T50.8X3	T50.8X4	T50.8X5	T50.8X6
dine (antiseptic, external) incture) NEC	T49.0X1	T49.0X2	T49.0X3	T49.0X4	T49.0X5	T49.0X6
125—see also Radiation sickness, and Exposure to radioactivce isotopes	T50.8X1	T50.8X2	T50.8X3	T50.8X4	T50.8X5	T50.8X6
therapeutic	T50.991	T50.992	T50.993	T50.994	T50.995	T50.996

Substance	Poisoning, Accidental (unintentional)	Poisoning, Intentional self-harm	Poisoning, Assault	Poisoning, Undetermined	Adverse effect	Underdosing
Iodine — *Continued*						
131—see also Radiation sickness, and Exposure to radioactivce isotopes	T50.8X1	T50.8X2	T50.8X3	T50.8X4	T50.8X5	T50.8X6
therapeutic	T38.2X1	T38.2X2	T38.2X3	T38.2X4	T38.2X5	T38.2X6
diagnostic	T50.8X1	T50.8X2	T50.8X3	T50.8X4	T50.8X5	T50.8X6
for thyroid conditions (antithyroid)	T38.2X1	T38.2X2	T38.2X3	T38.2X4	T38.2X5	T38.2X6
solution	T49.0X1	T49.0X2	T49.0X3	T49.0X4	T49.0X5	T49.0X6
vapor	T59.891	T59.892	T59.893	T59.894	—	—
Iodipamide	T50.8X1	T50.8X2	T50.8X3	T50.8X4	T50.8X5	T50.8X6
Iodized (poppy seed) oil	T50.8X1	T50.8X2	T50.8X3	T50.8X4	T50.8X5	T50.8X6
Iodobismitol	T37.8X1	T37.8X2	T37.8X3	T37.8X4	T37.8X5	T37.8X6
Iodochlorhyd-roxyquin	T37.8X1	T37.8X2	T37.8X3	T37.8X4	T37.8X5	T37.8X6
topical	T49.0X1	T49.0X2	T49.0X3	T49.0X4	T49.0X5	T49.0X6
Iodochlorhydroxy-quinoline	T37.8X1	T37.8X2	T37.8X3	T37.8X4	T37.8X5	T37.8X6
Iodocholesterol (131I)	T50.8X1	T50.8X2	T50.8X3	T50.8X4	T50.8X5	T50.8X6
Iodoform	T49.0X1	T49.0X2	T49.0X3	T49.0X4	T49.0X5	T49.0X6
Iodohippuric acid	T50.8X1	T50.8X2	T50.8X3	T50.8X4	T50.8X5	T50.8X6
Iodopanoic acid	T50.8X1	T50.8X2	T50.8X3	T50.8X4	T50.8X5	T50.8X6
Iodophthalein (sodium)	T50.8X1	T50.8X2	T50.8X3	T50.8X4	T50.8X5	T50.8X6
Iodopyracet	T50.8X1	T50.8X2	T50.8X3	T50.8X4	T50.8X5	T50.8X6
Iodoquinol	T37.8X1	T37.8X2	T37.8X3	T37.8X4	T37.8X5	T37.8X6
Iodoxamic acid	T50.8X1	T50.8X2	T50.8X3	T50.8X4	T50.8X5	T50.8X6
Iofendylate	T50.8X1	T50.8X2	T50.8X3	T50.8X4	T50.8X5	T50.8X6
Ioglycamic acid	T50.8X1	T50.8X2	T50.8X3	T50.8X4	T50.8X5	T50.8X6
Iohexol	T50.8X1	T50.8X2	T50.8X3	T50.8X4	T50.8X5	T50.8X6
Ion exchange resin						
anion	T47.8X1	T47.8X2	T47.8X3	T47.8X4	T47.8X5	T47.8X6
cation	T50.3X1	T50.3X2	T50.3X3	T50.3X4	T50.3X5	T50.3X6
cholestyramine	T46.6X1	T46.6X2	T46.6X3	T46.6X4	T46.6X5	T46.6X6
intestinal	T47.8X1	T47.8X2	T47.8X3	T47.8X4	T47.8X5	T47.8X6
Iopamidol	T50.8X1	T50.8X2	T50.8X3	T50.8X4	T50.8X5	T50.8X6
Iopanoic acid	T50.8X1	T50.8X2	T50.8X3	T50.8X4	T50.8X5	T50.8X6
Iophenoic acid	T50.8X1	T50.8X2	T50.8X3	T50.8X4	T50.8X5	T50.8X6
Iopodate, sodium	T50.8X1	T50.8X2	T50.8X3	T50.8X4	T50.8X5	T50.8X6
Iopodic acid	T50.8X1	T50.8X2	T50.8X3	T50.8X4	T50.8X5	T50.8X6
Iopromide	T50.8X1	T50.8X2	T50.8X3	T50.8X4	T50.8X5	T50.8X6
Iopydol	T50.8X1	T50.8X2	T50.8X3	T50.8X4	T50.8X5	T50.8X6
Iotalamic acid	T50.8X1	T50.8X2	T50.8X3	T50.8X4	T50.8X5	T50.8X6
Iothalamate	T50.8X1	T50.8X2	T50.8X3	T50.8X4	T50.8X5	T50.8X6
Iothiouracil	T38.2X1	T38.2X2	T38.2X3	T38.2X4	T38.2X5	T38.2X6
Iotrol	T50.8X1	T50.8X2	T50.8X3	T50.8X4	T50.8X5	T50.8X6
Iotrolan	T50.8X1	T50.8X2	T50.8X3	T50.8X4	T50.8X5	T50.8X6
Iotroxate	T50.8X1	T50.8X2	T50.8X3	T50.8X4	T50.8X5	T50.8X6
Iotroxic acid	T50.8X1	T50.8X2	T50.8X3	T50.8X4	T50.8X5	T50.8X6
Ioversol	T50.8X1	T50.8X2	T50.8X3	T50.8X4	T50.8X5	T50.8X6
Ioxaglate	T50.8X1	T50.8X2	T50.8X3	T50.8X4	T50.8X5	T50.8X6
Ioxaglic acid	T50.8X1	T50.8X2	T50.8X3	T50.8X4	T50.8X5	T50.8X6
Ioxitalamic acid	T50.8X1	T50.8X2	T50.8X3	T50.8X4	T50.8X5	T50.8X6
Ipecac	T47.7X1	T47.7X2	T47.7X3	T47.7X4	T47.7X5	T47.7X6

Substance	Poisoning, Accidental (unintentional)	Poisoning, Intentional self-harm	Poisoning, Assault	Poisoning, Undetermined	Adverse effect	Underdosing
Ipecacuanha	T48.4X1	T48.4X2	T48.4X3	T48.4X4	T48.4X5	T48.4X6
Ipodate, calcium	T50.8X1	T50.8X2	T50.8X3	T50.8X4	T50.8X5	T50.8X6
Ipral	T42.3X1	T42.3X2	T42.3X3	T42.3X4	T42.3X5	T42.3X6
Ipratropium (bromide)	T48.6X1	T48.6X2	T48.6X3	T48.6X4	T48.6X5	T48.6X6
Ipriflavone	T46.3X1	T46.3X2	T46.3X3	T46.3X4	T46.3X5	T46.3X6
Iprindole	T43.011	T43.012	T43.013	T43.014	T43.015	T43.016
Iproclozide	T43.1X1	T43.1X2	T43.1X3	T43.1X4	T43.1X5	T43.1X6
Iprofenin	T50.8X1	T50.8X2	T50.8X3	T50.8X4	T50.8X5	T50.8X6
Iproheptine	T49.2X1	T49.2X2	T49.2X3	T49.2X4	T49.2X5	T49.2X6
Iproniazid	T43.1X1	T43.1X2	T43.1X3	T43.1X4	T43.1X5	T43.1X6
Iproplatin	T45.1X1	T45.1X2	T45.1X3	T45.1X4	T45.1X5	T45.1X6
Iproveratril	T46.1X1	T46.1X2	T46.1X3	T46.1X4	T46.1X5	T46.1X6
Iron (compounds) (medicinal) NEC	T45.4X1	T45.4X2	T45.4X3	T45.4X4	T45.4X5	T45.4X6
ammonium	T45.4X1	T45.4X2	T45.4X3	T45.4X4	T45.4X5	T45.4X6
dextran injection	T45.4X1	T45.4X2	T45.4X3	T45.4X4	T45.4X5	T45.4X6
nonmedicinal	T56.891	T56.892	T56.893	T56.894	—	—
salts	T45.4X1	T45.4X2	T45.4X3	T45.4X4	T45.4X5	T45.4X6
sorbitex	T45.4X1	T45.4X2	T45.4X3	T45.4X4	T45.4X5	T45.4X6
sorbitol citric acid complex	T45.4X1	T45.4X2	T45.4X3	T45.4X4	T45.4X5	T45.4X6
Irrigating fluid (vaginal)	T49.8X1	T49.8X2	T49.8X3	T49.8X4	T49.8X5	T49.8X6
eye	T49.5X1	T49.5X2	T49.5X3	T49.5X4	T49.5X5	T49.5X6
Isepamicin	T36.5X1	T36.5X2	T36.5X3	T36.5X4	T36.5X5	T36.5X6
Isoaminile (citrate)	T48.3X1	T48.3X2	T48.3X3	T48.3X4	T48.3X5	T48.3X6
Isoamyl nitrite	T46.3X1	T46.3X2	T46.3X3	T46.3X4	T46.3X5	T46.3X6
Isobenzan	T60.1X1	T60.1X2	T60.1X3	T60.1X4	—	—
Isobutyl acetate	T52.8X1	T52.8X2	T52.8X3	T52.8X4	—	—
Isocarboxazid	T43.1X1	T43.1X2	T43.1X3	T43.1X4	T43.1X5	T43.1X6
Isoconazole	T49.0X1	T49.0X2	T49.0X3	T49.0X4	T49.0X5	T49.0X6
Isocyanate	T65.0X1	T65.0X2	T65.0X3	T65.0X4	—	—
Isoephedrine	T44.991	T44.992	T44.993	T44.994	T44.995	T44.996
Isoetarine	T48.6X1	T48.6X2	T48.6X3	T48.6X4	T48.6X5	T48.6X6
Isoethadione	T42.2X1	T42.2X2	T42.2X3	T42.2X4	T42.2X5	T42.2X6
Isoetharine	T44.5X1	T44.5X2	T44.5X3	T44.5X4	T44.5X5	T44.5X6
Isoflurane	T41.0X1	T41.0X2	T41.0X3	T41.0X4	T41.0X5	T41.0X6
Isoflurophate	T44.0X1	T44.0X2	T44.0X3	T44.0X4	T44.0X5	T44.0X6
Isomaltose, ferric complex	T45.4X1	T45.4X2	T45.4X3	T45.4X4	T45.4X5	T45.4X6
Isometheptene	T44.3X1	T44.3X2	T44.3X3	T44.3X4	T44.3X5	T44.3X6
Isoniazid	T37.1X1	T37.1X2	T37.1X3	T37.1X4	T37.1X5	T37.1X6
with						
rifampicin	T36.6X1	T36.6X2	T36.6X3	T36.6X4	T36.6X5	T36.6X6
thioacetazone	T37.1X1	T37.1X2	T37.1X3	T37.1X4	T37.1X5	T37.1X6
Isonicotinic acid hydrazide	T37.1X1	T37.1X2	T37.1X3	T37.1X4	T37.1X5	T37.1X6
Isonipecaine	T40.4X1	T40.4X2	T40.4X3	T40.4X4	T40.4X5	T40.4X6
Isopentaquine	T37.2X1	T37.2X2	T37.2X3	T37.2X4	T37.2X5	T37.2X6
Isophane insulin	T38.3X1	T38.3X2	T38.3X3	T38.3X4	T38.3X5	T38.3X6
Isophorone	T65.891	T65.892	T65.893	T65.894	—	—
Isophosphamide	T45.1X1	T45.1X2	T45.1X3	T45.1X4	T45.1X5	T45.1X6
Isopregnenone	T38.5X1	T38.5X2	T38.5X3	T38.5X4	T38.5X5	T38.5X6
Isoprenaline	T48.6X1	T48.6X2	T48.6X3	T48.6X4	T48.6X5	T48.6X6
Isopromethazine	T43.3X1	T43.3X2	T43.3X3	T43.3X4	T43.3X5	T43.3X6

Substance	Poisoning, Accidental (unintentional)	Poisoning, Intentional self-harm	Poisoning, Assault	Poisoning, Undetermined	Adverse effect	Underdosing
Isopropamide	T44.3X1	T44.3X2	T44.3X3	T44.3X4	T44.3X5	T44.3X
iodide	T44.3X1	T44.3X2	T44.3X3	T44.3X4	T44.3X5	T44.3X
Isopropanol	T51.2X1	T51.2X2	T51.2X3	T51.2X4	—	—
Isopropyl						
acetate	T52.8X1	T52.8X2	T52.8X3	T52.8X4	—	—
alcohol	T51.2X1	T51.2X2	T51.2X3	T51.2X4	—	—
medicinal	T49.4X1	T49.4X2	T49.4X3	T49.4X4	T49.4X5	T49.4X
ether	T52.8X1	T52.8X2	T52.8X3	T52.8X4	—	—
Isopropylamino-phenazone	T39.2X1	T39.2X2	T39.2X3	T39.2X4	T39.2X5	T39.2X
Isoproterenol	T48.6X1	T48.6X2	T48.6X3	T48.6X4	T48.6X5	T48.6X
Isosorbide dinitrate	T46.3X1	T46.3X2	T46.3X3	T46.3X4	T46.3X5	T46.3X
Isothipendyl	T45.0X1	T45.0X2	T45.0X3	T45.0X4	T45.0X5	T45.0X
Isotretinoin	T50.991	T50.992	T50.993	T50.994	T50.995	T50.99
Isoxazolyl penicillin	T36.0X1	T36.0X2	T36.0X3	T36.0X4	T36.0X5	T36.0X
Isoxicam	T39.391	T39.392	T39.393	T39.394	T39.395	T39.39
Isoxsuprine	T46.7X1	T46.7X2	T46.7X3	T46.7X4	T46.7X5	T46.7X
Ispagula	T47.4X1	T47.4X2	T47.4X3	T47.4X4	T47.4X5	T47.4X
husk	T47.4X1	T47.4X2	T47.4X3	T47.4X4	T47.4X5	T47.4X
Isradipine	T46.1X1	T46.1X2	T46.1X3	T46.1X4	T46.1X5	T46.1X
I-thyroxine sodium	T38.1X1	T38.1X2	T38.1X3	T38.1X4	T38.1X5	T38.1X
Itraconazole	T37.8X1	T37.8X2	T37.8X3	T37.8X4	T37.8X5	T37.8X
Itramin tosilate	T46.3X1	T46.3X2	T46.3X3	T46.3X4	T46.3X5	T46.3X
Ivermectin	T37.4X1	T37.4X2	T37.4X3	T37.4X4	T37.4X5	T37.4X
Izoniazid	T37.1X1	T37.1X2	T37.1X3	T37.1X4	T37.1X5	T37.1X
with thioacetazone	T37.1X1	T37.1X2	T37.1X3	T37.1X4	T37.1X5	T37.1X
J						
Jalap	T47.2X1	T47.2X2	T47.2X3	T47.2X4	T47.2X5	T47.2X
Jamaica						
dogwood (bark)	T39.8X1	T39.8X2	T39.8X3	T39.8X4	T39.8X5	T39.8X
ginger	T65.891	T65.892	T65.893	T65.894	—	—
root	T62.2X1	T62.2X2	T62.2X3	T62.2X4	—	—
Jatropha	T62.2X1	T62.2X2	T62.2X3	T62.2X4	—	—
curcas	T62.2X1	T62.2X2	T62.2X3	T62.2X4	—	—
Jectofer	T45.4X1	T45.4X2	T45.4X3	T45.4X4	T45.4X5	T45.4X
Jellyfish (sting)	T63.621	T63.622	T63.623	T63.624	—	—
Jequirity (bean)	T62.2X1	T62.2X2	T62.2X3	T62.2X4	—	—
Jimson weed (stramonium)	T62.2X1	T62.2X2	T62.2X3	T62.2X4	—	—
seeds	T62.2X1	T62.2X2	T62.2X3	T62.2X4	—	—
Josamycin	T36.3X1	T36.3X2	T36.3X3	T36.3X4	T36.3X5	T36.3X
Juniper tar	T49.1X1	T49.1X2	T49.1X3	T49.1X4	T49.1X5	T49.1X
K						
Kallidinogenase	T46.7X1	T46.7X2	T46.7X3	T46.7X4	T46.7X5	T46.7X
Kallikrein	T46.7X1	T46.7X2	T46.7X3	T46.7X4	T46.7X5	T46.7X
Kanamycin	T36.5X1	T36.5X2	T36.5X3	T36.5X4	T36.5X5	T36.5X
Kantrex	T36.5X1	T36.5X2	T36.5X3	T36.5X4	T36.5X5	T36.5X
Kaolin	T47.6X1	T47.6X2	T47.6X3	T47.6X4	T47.6X5	T47.6X
light	T47.6X1	T47.6X2	T47.6X3	T47.6X4	T47.6X5	T47.6X
Karaya (gum)	T47.4X1	T47.4X2	T47.4X3	T47.4X4	T47.4X5	T47.4X
Kebuzone	T39.2X1	T39.2X2	T39.2X3	T39.2X4	T39.2X5	T39.2X
Kelevan	T60.1X1	T60.1X2	T60.1X3	T60.1X4	—	—

Substance	Poisoning, Accidental (unintentional)	Poisoning, Intentional self-harm	Poisoning, Assault	Poisoning, Undetermined	Adverse effect	Underdosing
Kemithal	T41.1X1	T41.1X2	T41.1X3	T41.1X4	T41.1X5	T41.1X6
Kenacort	T38.0X1	T38.0X2	T38.0X3	T38.0X4	T38.0X5	T38.0X6
Keratolytic drug NEC	T49.4X1	T49.4X2	T49.4X3	T49.4X4	T49.4X5	T49.4X6
anthracene	T49.4X1	T49.4X2	T49.4X3	T49.4X4	T49.4X5	T49.4X6
Keratoplastic NEC	T49.4X1	T49.4X2	T49.4X3	T49.4X4	T49.4X5	T49.4X6
Kerosene, kerosine (fuel) (solvent) NEC	T52.0X1	T52.0X2	T52.0X3	T52.0X4	—	—
insecticide	T52.0X1	T52.0X2	T52.0X3	T52.0X4	—	—
vapor	T52.0X1	T52.0X2	T52.0X3	T52.0X4	—	—
Ketamine	T41.291	T41.292	T41.293	T41.294	T41.295	T41.296
Ketazolam	T42.4X1	T42.4X2	T42.4X3	T42.4X4	T42.4X5	T42.4X6
Ketazon	T39.2X1	T39.2X2	T39.2X3	T39.2X4	T39.2X5	T39.2X6
Ketobemidone	T40.4X1	T40.4X2	T40.4X3	T40.4X4	—	—
Ketoconazole	T49.0X1	T49.0X2	T49.0X3	T49.0X4	T49.0X5	T49.0X6
Ketols	T52.4X1	T52.4X2	T52.4X3	T52.4X4	—	—
Ketone oils	T52.4X1	T52.4X2	T52.4X3	T52.4X4	—	—
Ketoprofen	T39.311	T39.312	T39.313	T39.314	T39.315	T39.316
Ketorolac	T39.8X1	T39.8X2	T39.8X3	T39.8X4	T39.8X5	T39.8X6
Ketotifen	T45.0X1	T45.0X2	T45.0X3	T45.0X4	T45.0X5	T45.0X6
Khat	T43.691	T43.692	T43.693	T43.694	—	—
Khellin	T46.3X1	T46.3X2	T46.3X3	T46.3X4	T46.3X5	T46.3X6
Khelloside	T46.3X1	T46.3X2	T46.3X3	T46.3X4	T46.3X5	T46.3X6
Kiln gas or vapor (carbon monoxide)	T58.8X1	T58.8X2	T58.8X3	T58.8X4	—	—
Kitasamycin	T36.3X1	T36.3X2	T36.3X3	T36.3X4	T36.3X5	T36.3X6
Konsyl	T47.4X1	T47.4X2	T47.4X3	T47.4X4	T47.4X5	T47.4X6
Kosam seed	T62.2X1	T62.2X2	T62.2X3	T62.2X4	—	—
Krait (venom)	T63.091	T63.092	T63.093	T63.094	—	—
Kwell (insecticide)	T60.1X1	T60.1X2	T60.1X3	T60.1X4	—	—
anti-infective (topical)	T49.0X1	T49.0X2	T49.0X3	T49.0X4	T49.0X5	T49.0X6
L						
Labetalol	T44.8X1	T44.8X2	T44.8X3	T44.8X4	T44.8X5	T44.8X6
Laburnum (seeds)	T62.2X1	T62.2X2	T62.2X3	T62.2X4	—	—
leaves	T62.2X1	T62.2X2	T62.2X3	T62.2X4	—	—
Lachesine	T49.5X1	T49.5X2	T49.5X3	T49.5X4	T49.5X5	T49.5X6
Lacidipine	T46.5X1	T46.5X2	T46.5X3	T46.5X4	T46.5X5	T46.5X6
Lacquer	T65.6X1	T65.6X2	T65.6X3	T65.6X4	—	—
Lacrimogenic gas	T59.3X1	T59.3X2	T59.3X3	T59.3X4	—	—
Lactated potassic saline	T50.3X1	T50.3X2	T50.3X3	T50.3X4	T50.3X5	T50.3X6
Lactic acid	T49.8X1	T49.8X2	T49.8X3	T49.8X4	T49.8X5	T49.8X6
Lactobacillus						
acidophilus	T47.6X1	T47.6X2	T47.6X3	T47.6X4	T47.6X5	T47.6X6
compound	T47.6X1	T47.6X2	T47.6X3	T47.6X4	T47.6X5	T47.6X6
bifidus, lyophilized	T47.6X1	T47.6X2	T47.6X3	T47.6X4	T47.6X5	T47.6X6
bulgaricus	T47.6X1	T47.6X2	T47.6X3	T47.6X4	T47.6X5	T47.6X6
sporogenes	T47.6X1	T47.6X2	T47.6X3	T47.6X4	T47.6X5	T47.6X6
Lactoflavin	T45.2X1	T45.2X2	T45.2X3	T45.2X4	T45.2X5	T45.2X6
Lactose (as excipient)	T50.901	T50.902	T50.903	T50.904	T50.905	T50.906
Lactuca (virosa) (extract)	T42.6X1	T42.6X2	T42.6X3	T42.6X4	T42.6X5	T42.6X6
Lactucarium	T42.6X1	T42.6X2	T42.6X3	T42.6X4	T42.6X5	T42.6X6
Lactulose	T47.3X1	T47.3X2	T47.3X3	T47.3X4	T47.3X5	T47.3X6
Laevo—see Levo-						
Lanatosides	T46.0X1	T46.0X2	T46.0X3	T46.0X4	T46.0X5	T46.0X6
Lanolin	T49.3X1	T49.3X2	T49.3X3	T49.3X4	T49.3X5	T49.3X6
Largactil	T43.3X1	T43.3X2	T43.3X3	T43.3X4	T43.3X5	T43.3X6
Larkspur	T62.2X1	T62.2X2	T62.2X3	T62.2X4	—	—
Laroxyl	T43.011	T43.012	T43.013	T43.014	T43.015	T43.016
Lasix	T50.1X1	T50.1X2	T50.1X3	T50.1X4	T50.1X5	T50.1X6
Lassar's paste	T49.4X1	T49.4X2	T49.4X3	T49.4X4	T49.4X5	T49.4X6
Latamoxef	T36.1X1	T36.1X2	T36.1X3	T36.1X4	T36.1X5	T36.1X6
Latex	T65.811	T65.812	T65.813	T65.814	—	—
Lathyrus (seed)	T62.2X1	T62.2X2	T62.2X3	T62.2X4	—	—
Laudanum	T40.0X1	T40.0X2	T40.0X3	T40.0X4	T40.0X5	T40.0X6
Laudexium	T48.1X1	T48.1X2	T48.1X3	T48.1X4	T48.1X5	T48.1X6
Laughing gas	T41.0X1	T41.0X2	T41.0X3	T41.0X4	T41.0X5	T41.0X6
Laurel, black or cherry	T62.2X1	T62.2X2	T62.2X3	T62.2X4	—	—
Laurolinium	T49.0X1	T49.0X2	T49.0X3	T49.0X4	T49.0X5	T49.0X6
Lauryl sulfoacetate	T49.2X1	T49.2X2	T49.2X3	T49.2X4	T49.2X5	T49.2X6
Laxative NEC	T47.4X1	T47.4X2	T47.4X3	T47.4X4	T47.4X5	T47.4X6
osmotic	T47.3X1	T47.3X2	T47.3X3	T47.3X4	T47.3X5	T47.3X6
saline	T47.3X1	T47.3X2	T47.3X3	T47.3X4	T47.3X5	T47.3X6
stimulant	T47.2X1	T47.2X2	T47.2X3	T47.2X4	T47.2X5	T47.2X6
L-dopa	T42.8X1	T42.8X2	T42.8X3	T42.8X4	T42.8X5	T42.8X6
Lead (dust) (fumes) (vapor) NEC	T56.0X1	T56.0X2	T56.0X3	T56.0X4	—	—
acetate	T49.2X1	T49.2X2	T49.2X3	T49.2X4	T49.2X5	T49.2X6
alkyl (fuel additive)	T56.0X1	T56.0X2	T56.0X3	T56.0X4	—	—
anti-infectives	T37.8X1	T37.8X2	T37.8X3	T37.8X4	T37.8X5	T37.8X6
antiknock compound (tetraethyl)	T56.0X1	T56.0X2	T56.0X3	T56.0X4	—	—
arsenate, arsenite (dust) (herbicide) (insecticide) (vapor)	T57.0X1	T57.0X2	T57.0X3	T57.0X4	—	—
carbonate	T56.0X1	T56.0X2	T56.0X3	T56.0X4	—	—
paint	T56.0X1	T56.0X2	T56.0X3	T56.0X4	—	—
chromate	T56.0X1	T56.0X2	T56.0X3	T56.0X4	—	—
paint	T56.0X1	T56.0X2	T56.0X3	T56.0X4	—	—
dioxide	T56.0X1	T56.0X2	T56.0X3	T56.0X4	—	—
inorganic	T56.0X1	T56.0X2	T56.0X3	T56.0X4	—	—
iodide	T56.0X1	T56.0X2	T56.0X3	T56.0X4	—	—
pigment (paint)	T56.0X1	T56.0X2	T56.0X3	T56.0X4	—	—
monoxide (dust)	T56.0X1	T56.0X2	T56.0X3	T56.0X4	—	—
paint	T56.0X1	T56.0X2	T56.0X3	T56.0X4	—	—
organic	T56.0X1	T56.0X2	T56.0X3	T56.0X4	—	—
oxide	T56.0X1	T56.0X2	T56.0X3	T56.0X4	—	—
paint	T56.0X1	T56.0X2	T56.0X3	T56.0X4	—	—
paint	T56.0X1	T56.0X2	T56.0X3	T56.0X4	—	—
salts	T56.0X1	T56.0X2	T56.0X3	T56.0X4	—	—
specified compound NEC	T56.0X1	T56.0X2	T56.0X3	T56.0X4	—	—
tetra-ethyl	T56.0X1	T56.0X2	T56.0X3	T56.0X4	—	—
Lebanese red	T40.7X1	T40.7X2	T40.7X3	T40.7X4	T40.7X5	T40.7X6
Lefetamine	T39.8X1	T39.8X2	T39.8X3	T39.8X4	T39.8X5	T39.8X6

Substance	Poisoning, Accidental (unintentional)	Poisoning, Intentional self-harm	Poisoning, Assault	Poisoning, Undetermined	Adverse effect	Underdosing
Lenperone	T43.4X1	T43.4X2	T43.4X3	T43.4X4	T43.4X5	T43.4X6
Lente lietin (insulin)	T38.3X1	T38.3X2	T38.3X3	T38.3X4	T38.3X5	T38.3X6
Leptazol	T50.7X1	T50.7X2	T50.7X3	T50.7X4	T50.7X5	T50.7X6
Leptophos	T60.0X1	T60.0X2	T60.0X3	T60.0X4	—	—
Leritine	T40.2X1	T40.2X2	T40.2X3	T40.2X4	T40.2X5	T40.2X6
Letosteine	T48.4X1	T48.4X2	T48.4X3	T48.4X4	T48.4X5	T48.4X6
Letter	T38.1X1	T38.1X2	T38.1X3	T38.1X4	T38.1X5	T38.1X6
Lettuce opium	T42.6X1	T42.6X2	T42.6X3	T42.6X4	T42.6X5	T42.6X6
Leucinocaine	T41.3X1	T41.3X2	T41.3X3	T41.3X4	T41.3X5	T41.3X6
Leucocianidol	T46.991	T46.992	T46.993	T46.994	T46.995	T46.996
Leucovorin (factor)	T45.8X1	T45.8X2	T45.8X3	T45.8X4	T45.8X5	T45.8X6
Leukeran	T45.1X1	T45.1X2	T45.1X3	T45.1X4	T45.1X5	T45.1X6
Leuprolide	T38.891	T38.892	T38.893	T38.894	T38.895	T38.896
Levalbuterol	T48.6X1	T48.6X2	T48.6X3	T48.6X4	T48.6X5	T48.6X6
Levallorphan	T50.7X1	T50.7X2	T50.7X3	T50.7X4	T50.7X5	T50.7X6
Levamisole	T37.4X1	T37.4X2	T37.4X3	T37.4X4	T37.4X5	T37.4X6
Levanil	T42.6X1	T42.6X2	T42.6X3	T42.6X4	T42.6X5	T42.6X6
Levarterenol	T44.4X1	T44.4X2	T44.4X3	T44.4X4	T44.4X5	T44.4X6
Levdropropizine	T48.3X1	T48.3X2	T48.3X3	T48.3X4	T48.3X5	T48.3X6
Levobunolol	T49.5X1	T49.5X2	T49.5X3	T49.5X4	T49.5X5	T49.5X6
Levocabastine (hydrochloride)	T45.0X1	T45.0X2	T45.0X3	T45.0X4	T45.0X5	T45.0X6
Levocarnitine	T50.991	T50.992	T50.993	T50.994	T50.995	T50.996
Levodopa	T42.8X1	T42.8X2	T42.8X3	T42.8X4	T42.8X5	T42.8X6
with carbidopa	T42.8X1	T42.8X2	T42.8X3	T42.8X4	T42.8X5	T42.8X6
Levo-dromoran	T40.2X1	T40.2X2	T40.2X3	T40.2X4	T40.2X5	T40.2X6
Levoglutamide	T50.991	T50.992	T50.993	T50.994	T50.995	T50.996
Levoid	T38.1X1	T38.1X2	T38.1X3	T38.1X4	T38.1X5	T38.1X6
Levo-iso-methadone	T40.3X1	T40.3X2	T40.3X3	T40.3X4	T40.3X5	T40.3X6
Levomepromazine	T43.3X1	T43.3X2	T43.3X3	T43.3X4	T43.3X5	T43.3X6
Levonordefrin	T49.6X1	T49.6X2	T49.6X3	T49.6X4	T49.6X5	T49.6X6
Levonorgestrel	T38.4X1	T38.4X2	T38.4X3	T38.4X4	T38.4X5	T38.4X6
with ethinylestradiol	T38.5X1	T38.5X2	T38.5X3	T38.5X4	T38.5X5	T38.5X6
Levopromazine	T43.3X1	T43.3X2	T43.3X3	T43.3X4	T43.3X5	T43.3X6
Levoprome	T42.6X1	T42.6X2	T42.6X3	T42.6X4	T42.6X5	T42.6X6
Levopropoxyphene	T40.4X1	T40.4X2	T40.4X3	T40.4X4	T40.4X5	T40.4X6
Levopropylhexedrine	T50.5X1	T50.5X2	T50.5X3	T50.5X4	T50.5X5	T50.5X6
Levoproxyphylline	T48.6X1	T48.6X2	T48.6X3	T48.6X4	T48.6X5	T48.6X6
Levorphanol	T40.4X1	T40.4X2	T40.4X3	T40.4X4	T40.4X5	T40.4X6
Levothyroxine	T38.1X1	T38.1X2	T38.1X3	T38.1X4	T38.1X5	T38.1X6
sodium	T38.1X1	T38.1X2	T38.1X3	T38.1X4	T38.1X5	T38.1X6
Levsin	T44.3X1	T44.3X2	T44.3X3	T44.3X4	T44.3X5	T44.3X6
Levulose	T50.3X1	T50.3X2	T50.3X3	T50.3X4	T50.3X5	T50.3X6
Lewisite (gas), not in war	T57.0X1	T57.0X2	T57.0X3	T57.0X4	—	—
Librium	T42.4X1	T42.4X2	T42.4X3	T42.4X4	T42.4X5	T42.4X6
Lidex	T49.0X1	T49.0X2	T49.0X3	T49.0X4	T49.0X5	T49.0X6
Lidocaine	T41.3X1	T41.3X2	T41.3X3	T41.3X4	T41.3X5	T41.3X6
regional	T41.3X1	T41.3X2	T41.3X3	T41.3X4	T41.3X5	T41.3X6
spinal	T41.3X1	T41.3X2	T41.3X3	T41.3X4	T41.3X5	T41.3X6
Lidofenin	T50.8X1	T50.8X2	T50.8X3	T50.8X4	T50.8X5	T50.8X6

Substance	Poisoning, Accidental (unintentional)	Poisoning, Intentional self-harm	Poisoning, Assault	Poisoning, Undetermined	Adverse effect	Underdosing
Lidoflazine	T46.1X1	T46.1X2	T46.1X3	T46.1X4	T46.1X5	T46.1X
Lighter fluid	T52.0X1	T52.0X2	T52.0X3	T52.0X4	—	—
Lignin hemicellulose	T47.6X1	T47.6X2	T47.6X3	T47.6X4	T47.6X5	T47.6X
Lignocaine	T41.3X1	T41.3X2	T41.3X3	T41.3X4	T41.3X5	T41.3X
regional	T41.3X1	T41.3X2	T41.3X3	T41.3X4	T41.3X5	T41.3X
spinal	T41.3X1	T41.3X2	T41.3X3	T41.3X4	T41.3X5	T41.3X
Ligroin(e) (solvent)	T52.0X1	T52.0X2	T52.0X3	T52.0X4	—	—
vapor	T59.891	T59.892	T59.893	T59.894	—	—
Ligustrum vulgare	T62.2X1	T62.2X2	T62.2X3	T62.2X4	—	—
Lily of the valley	T62.2X1	T62.2X2	T62.2X3	T62.2X4	—	—
Lime (chloride)	T54.3X1	T54.3X2	T54.3X3	T54.3X4	—	—
Limonene	T52.8X1	T52.8X2	T52.8X3	T52.8X4	—	—
Lincomycin	T36.8X1	T36.8X2	T36.8X3	T36.8X4	T36.8X5	T36.8X
Lindane (insecticide) (nonmedicinal) (vapor)	T53.6X1	T53.6X2	T53.6X3	T53.6X4	—	—
medicinal	T49.0X1	T49.0X2	T49.0X3	T49.0X4	T49.0X5	T49.0X
Liniments NEC	T49.91	T49.92	T49.93	T49.94	T49.95	T49.96
Linoleic acid	T46.6X1	T46.6X2	T46.6X3	T46.6X4	T46.6X5	T46.6X
Linolenic acid	T46.6X1	T46.6X2	T46.6X3	T46.6X4	T46.6X5	T46.6X
Linseed	T47.4X1	T47.4X2	T47.4X3	T47.4X4	T47.4X5	T47.4X
Liothyronine	T38.1X1	T38.1X2	T38.1X3	T38.1X4	T38.1X5	T38.1X
Liotrix	T38.1X1	T38.1X2	T38.1X3	T38.1X4	T38.1X5	T38.1X
Lipancreatin	T47.5X1	T47.5X2	T47.5X3	T47.5X4	T47.5X5	T47.5X
Lipo-alprostadil	T46.7X1	T46.7X2	T46.7X3	T46.7X4	T46.7X5	T46.7X
Lipo-Lutin	T38.5X1	T38.5X2	T38.5X3	T38.5X4	T38.5X5	T38.5X
Lipotropic drug NEC	T50.901	T50.902	T50.903	T50.904	T50.905	T50.90
Liquefied petroleum gases	T59.891	T59.892	T59.893	T59.894	—	—
piped (pure or mixed with air)	T59.891	T59.892	T59.893	T59.894	—	—
Liquid						
paraffin	T47.4X1	T47.4X2	T47.4X3	T47.4X4	T47.4X5	T47.4X
petrolatum	T47.4X1	T47.4X2	T47.4X3	T47.4X4	T47.4X5	T47.4X
topical	T49.3X1	T49.3X2	T49.3X3	T49.3X4	T49.3X5	T49.3X
specified NEC	T65.891	T65.892	T65.893	T65.894	—	—
substance	T65.91	T65.92	T65.93	T65.94	—	—
Liquor creosolis compositus	T65.891	T65.892	T65.893	T65.894	—	—
Liquorice	T48.4X1	T48.4X2	T48.4X3	T48.4X4	T48.4X5	T48.4X
extract	T47.8X1	T47.8X2	T47.8X3	T47.8X4	T47.8X5	T47.8X
Lisinopril	T46.4X1	T46.4X2	T46.4X3	T46.4X4	T46.4X5	T46.4X
Lisuride	T42.8X1	T42.8X2	T42.8X3	T42.8X4	T42.8X5	T42.8X
Lithane	T43.8X1	T43.8X2	T43.8X3	T43.8X4	T43.8X5	T43.8X
Lithium	T56.891	T56.892	T56.893	T56.894	—	—
gluconate	T43.591	T43.592	T43.593	T43.594	T43.595	T43.59
salts (carbonate)	T43.591	T43.592	T43.593	T43.594	T43.595	T43.59
Lithonate	T43.8X1	T43.8X2	T43.8X3	T43.8X4	T43.8X5	T43.8X
Liver						
extract	T45.8X1	T45.8X2	T45.8X3	T45.8X4	T45.8X5	T45.8X
for parenteral use	T45.8X1	T45.8X2	T45.8X3	T45.8X4	T45.8X5	T45.8X
fraction 1	T45.8X1	T45.8X2	T45.8X3	T45.8X4	T45.8X5	T45.8X
hydrolysate	T45.8X1	T45.8X2	T45.8X3	T45.8X4	T45.8X5	T45.8X

Substance	Poisoning, Accidental (unintentional)	Poisoning, Intentional self-harm	Poisoning, Assault	Poisoning, Undetermined	Adverse effect	Underdosing
Lizard (bite) (venom)	T63.121	T63.122	T63.123	T63.124	—	—
LMD	T45.8X1	T45.8X2	T45.8X3	T45.8X4	T45.8X5	T45.8X6
Lobelia	T62.2X1	T62.2X2	T62.2X3	T62.2X4	—	—
Lobeline	T50.7X1	T50.7X2	T50.7X3	T50.7X4	T50.7X5	T50.7X6
Local action drug NEC	T49.8X1	T49.8X2	T49.8X3	T49.8X4	T49.8X5	T49.8X6
Locorten	T49.0X1	T49.0X2	T49.0X3	T49.0X4	T49.0X5	T49.0X6
Lofepramine	T43.011	T43.012	T43.013	T43.014	T43.015	T43.016
Lolium temulentum	T62.2X1	T62.2X2	T62.2X3	T62.2X4	—	—
Lomotil	T47.6X1	T47.6X2	T47.6X3	T47.6X4	T47.6X5	T47.6X6
Lomustine	T45.1X1	T45.1X2	T45.1X3	T45.1X4	T45.1X5	T45.1X6
Lonidamine	T45.1X1	T45.1X2	T45.1X3	T45.1X4	T45.1X5	T45.1X6
Loperamide	T47.6X1	T47.6X2	T47.6X3	T47.6X4	T47.6X5	T47.6X6
Loprazolam	T42.4X1	T42.4X2	T42.4X3	T42.4X4	T42.4X5	T42.4X6
Lorajmine	T46.2X1	T46.2X2	T46.2X3	T46.2X4	T46.2X5	T46.2X6
Loratidine	T45.0X1	T45.0X2	T45.0X3	T45.0X4	T45.0X5	T45.0X6
Lorazepam	T42.4X1	T42.4X2	T42.4X3	T42.4X4	T42.4X5	T42.4X6
Lorcainide	T46.2X1	T46.2X2	T46.2X3	T46.2X4	T46.2X5	T46.2X6
Lormetazepam	T42.4X1	T42.4X2	T42.4X3	T42.4X4	T42.4X5	T42.4X6
Lotions NEC	T49.91	T49.92	T49.93	T49.94	T49.95	T49.96
Lotusate	T42.3X1	T42.3X2	T42.3X3	T42.3X4	T42.3X5	T42.3X6
Lovastatin	T46.6X1	T46.6X2	T46.6X3	T46.6X4	T46.6X5	T46.6X6
Lowila	T49.2X1	T49.2X2	T49.2X3	T49.2X4	T49.2X5	T49.2X6
Loxapine	T43.591	T43.592	T43.593	T43.594	T43.595	T43.596
Lozenges (throat)	T49.6X1	T49.6X2	T49.6X3	T49.6X4	T49.6X5	T49.6X6
LSD	T40.8X1	T40.8X2	T40.8X3	T40.8X4	—	—
L-Tryptophan—see amino acid						
Lubricant, eye	T49.5X1	T49.5X2	T49.5X3	T49.5X4	T49.5X5	T49.5X6
Lubricating oil NEC	T52.0X1	T52.0X2	T52.0X3	T52.0X4	—	—
Lucanthone	T37.4X1	T37.4X2	T37.4X3	T37.4X4	T37.4X5	T37.4X6
Luminal	T42.3X1	T42.3X2	T42.3X3	T42.3X4	T42.3X5	T42.3X6
Lung irritant (gas) NEC	T59.91	T59.92	T59.93	T59.94	—	—
Luteinizing hormone	T38.811	T38.812	T38.813	T38.814	T38.815	T38.816
Lutocylol	T38.5X1	T38.5X2	T38.5X3	T38.5X4	T38.5X5	T38.5X6
Lutromone	T38.5X1	T38.5X2	T38.5X3	T38.5X4	T38.5X5	T38.5X6
Lututrin	T48.291	T48.292	T48.293	T48.294	T48.295	T48.296
Lye (concentrated)	T54.3X1	T54.3X2	T54.3X3	T54.3X4	—	—
Lygranum (skin test)	T50.8X1	T50.8X2	T50.8X3	T50.8X4	T50.8X5	T50.8X6
Lymecycline	T36.4X1	T36.4X2	T36.4X3	T36.4X4	T36.4X5	T36.4X6
Lymphogranuloma venereum antigen	T50.8X1	T50.8X2	T50.8X3	T50.8X4	T50.8X5	T50.8X6
Lynestrenol	T38.4X1	T38.4X2	T38.4X3	T38.4X4	T38.4X5	T38.4X6
Lyovac Sodium Edecrin	T50.1X1	T50.1X2	T50.1X3	T50.1X4	T50.1X5	T50.1X6
Lypressin	T38.891	T38.892	T38.893	T38.894	T38.895	T38.896
Lysergic acid diethylamide	T40.8X1	T40.8X2	T40.8X3	T40.8X4	—	—
Lysergide	T40.8X1	T40.8X2	T40.8X3	T40.8X4	—	—
Lysine vasopressin	T38.891	T38.892	T38.893	T38.894	T38.895	T38.896
Lysol	T54.1X1	T54.1X2	T54.1X3	T54.1X4	—	—
Lysozyme	T49.0X1	T49.0X2	T49.0X3	T49.0X4	T49.0X5	T49.0X6
Lytta (vitatta)	T49.8X1	T49.8X2	T49.8X3	T49.8X4	T49.8X5	T49.8X6

Substance	Poisoning, Accidental (unintentional)	Poisoning, Intentional self-harm	Poisoning, Assault	Poisoning, Undetermined	Adverse effect	Underdosing
M						
Mace	T59.3X1	T59.3X2	T59.3X3	T59.3X4	—	—
Macrogol	T50.991	T50.992	T50.993	T50.994	T50.995	T50.996
Macrolide						
anabolic drug	T38.7X1	T38.7X2	T38.7X3	T38.7X4	T38.7X5	T38.7X6
antibiotic	T36.3X1	T36.3X2	T36.3X3	T36.3X4	T36.3X5	T36.3X6
Mafenide	T49.0X1	T49.0X2	T49.0X3	T49.0X4	T49.0X5	T49.0X6
Magaldrate	T47.1X1	T47.1X2	T47.1X3	T47.1X4	T47.1X5	T47.1X6
Magic mushroom	T40.991	T40.992	T40.993	T40.994	—	—
Magnamycin	T36.8X1	T36.8X2	T36.8X3	T36.8X4	T36.8X5	T36.8X6
Magnesia magma	T47.1X1	T47.1X2	T47.1X3	T47.1X4	T47.1X5	T47.1X6
Magnesium NEC	T56.891	T56.892	T56.893	T56.894	—	—
carbonate	T47.1X1	T47.1X2	T47.1X3	T47.1X4	T47.1X5	T47.1X6
citrate	T47.4X1	T47.4X2	T47.4X3	T47.4X4	T47.4X5	T47.4X6
hydroxide	T47.1X1	T47.1X2	T47.1X3	T47.1X4	T47.1X5	T47.1X6
oxide	T47.1X1	T47.1X2	T47.1X3	T47.1X4	T47.1X5	T47.1X6
peroxide	T49.0X1	T49.0X2	T49.0X3	T49.0X4	T49.0X5	T49.0X6
salicylate	T39.091	T39.092	T39.093	T39.094	T39.095	T39.096
silicofluoride	T50.3X1	T50.3X2	T50.3X3	T50.3X4	T50.3X5	T50.3X6
sulfate	T47.4X1	T47.4X2	T47.4X3	T47.4X4	T47.4X5	T47.4X6
thiosulfate	T45.0X1	T45.0X2	T45.0X3	T45.0X4	T45.0X5	T45.0X6
trisilicate	T47.1X1	T47.1X2	T47.1X3	T47.1X4	T47.1X5	T47.1X6
Malathion (medicinal)	T49.0X1	T49.0X2	T49.0X3	T49.0X4	T49.0X5	T49.0X6
insecticide	T60.0X1	T60.0X2	T60.0X3	T60.0X4	—	—
Male fern extract	T37.4X1	T37.4X2	T37.4X3	T37.4X4	T37.4X5	T37.4X6
M-AMSA	T45.1X1	T45.1X2	T45.1X3	T45.1X4	T45.1X5	T45.1X6
Mandelic acid	T37.8X1	T37.8X2	T37.8X3	T37.8X4	T37.8X5	T37.8X6
Manganese (dioxide) (salts)	T57.2X1	T57.2X2	T57.2X3	T57.2X4	—	—
medicinal	T50.991	T50.992	T50.993	T50.994	T50.995	T50.996
Mannitol	T47.3X1	T47.3X2	T47.3X3	T47.3X4	T47.3X5	T47.3X6
hexanitrate	T46.3X1	T46.3X2	T46.3X3	T46.3X4	T46.3X5	T46.3X6
Mannomustine	T45.1X1	T45.1X2	T45.1X3	T45.1X4	T45.1X5	T45.1X6
MAO inhibitors	T43.1X1	T43.1X2	T43.1X3	T43.1X4	T43.1X5	T43.1X6
Mapharsen	T37.8X1	T37.8X2	T37.8X3	T37.8X4	T37.8X5	T37.8X6
Maphenide	T49.0X1	T49.0X2	T49.0X3	T49.0X4	T49.0X5	T49.0X6
Maprotiline	T43.021	T43.022	T43.023	T43.024	T43.025	T43.026
Marcaine	T41.3X1	T41.3X2	T41.3X3	T41.3X4	T41.3X5	T41.3X6
infiltration (subcutaneous)	T41.3X1	T41.3X2	T41.3X3	T41.3X4	T41.3X5	T41.3X6
nerve block (peripheral) (plexus)	T41.3X1	T41.3X2	T41.3X3	T41.3X4	T41.3X5	T41.3X6
Marezine	T45.0X1	T45.0X2	T45.0X3	T45.0X4	T45.0X5	T45.0X6
Marihuana	T40.7X1	T40.7X2	T40.7X3	T40.7X4	T40.7X5	T40.7X6
Marijuana	T40.7X1	T40.7X2	T40.7X3	T40.7X4	T40.7X5	T40.7X6
Marine (sting)	T63.691	T63.692	T63.693	T63.694	—	—
animals (sting)	T63.691	T63.692	T63.693	T63.694	—	—
plants (sting)	T63.711	T63.712	T63.713	T63.714	—	—
Marplan	T43.1X1	T43.1X2	T43.1X3	T43.1X4	T43.1X5	T43.1X6
Marsh gas	T59.891	T59.892	T59.893	T59.894	—	—
Marsilid	T43.1X1	T43.1X2	T43.1X3	T43.1X4	T43.1X5	T43.1X6

Substance	Poisoning, Accidental (unintentional)	Poisoning, Intentional self-harm	Poisoning, Assault	Poisoning, Undetermined	Adverse effect	Underdosing
Matulane	T45.1X1	T45.1X2	T45.1X3	T45.1X4	T45.1X5	T45.1X6
Mazindol	T50.5X1	T50.5X2	T50.5X3	T50.5X4	T50.5X5	T50.5X6
MCPA	T60.3X1	T60.3X2	T60.3X3	T60.3X4	—	—
MDMA	T43.621	T43.622	T43.623	T43.624	T43.625	T43.626
Meadow saffron	T62.2X1	T62.2X2	T62.2X3	T62.2X4	—	—
Measles virus vaccine (attenuated)	T50.B91	T50.B92	T50.B93	T50.B94	T50.B95	T50.B96
Meat, noxious	T62.8X1	T62.8X2	T62.8X3	T62.8X4	—	—
Meballymal	T42.3X1	T42.3X2	T42.3X3	T42.3X4	T42.3X5	T42.3X6
Mebanazine	T43.1X1	T43.1X2	T43.1X3	T43.1X4	T43.1X5	T43.1X6
Mebaral	T42.3X1	T42.3X2	T42.3X3	T42.3X4	T42.3X5	T42.3X6
Mebendazole	T37.4X1	T37.4X2	T37.4X3	T37.4X4	T37.4X5	T37.4X6
Mebeverine	T44.3X1	T44.3X2	T44.3X3	T44.3X4	T44.3X5	T44.3X6
Mebhydrolin	T45.0X1	T45.0X2	T45.0X3	T45.0X4	T45.0X5	T45.0X6
Mebumal	T42.3X1	T42.3X2	T42.3X3	T42.3X4	T42.3X5	T42.3X6
Mebutamate	T43.591	T43.592	T43.593	T43.594	T43.595	T43.596
Mecamylamine	T44.2X1	T44.2X2	T44.2X3	T44.2X4	T44.2X5	T44.2X6
Mechlorethamine	T45.1X1	T45.1X2	T45.1X3	T45.1X4	T45.1X5	T45.1X6
Mecillinam	T36.0X1	T36.0X2	T36.0X3	T36.0X4	T36.0X5	T36.0X6
Meclizine (hydrochloride)	T45.0X1	T45.0X2	T45.0X3	T45.0X4	T45.0X5	T45.0X6
Meclocycline	T36.4X1	T36.4X2	T36.4X3	T36.4X4	T36.4X5	T36.4X6
Meclofenamate	T39.391	T39.392	T39.393	T39.394	T39.395	T39.396
Meclofenamic acid	T39.391	T39.392	T39.393	T39.394	T39.395	T39.396
Meclofenoxate	T43.691	T43.692	T43.693	T43.694	T43.695	T43.696
Meclozine	T45.0X1	T45.0X2	T45.0X3	T45.0X4	T45.0X5	T45.0X6
Mecobalamin	T45.8X1	T45.8X2	T45.8X3	T45.8X4	T45.8X5	T45.8X6
Mecoprop	T60.3X1	T60.3X2	T60.3X3	T60.3X4	—	—
Mecrilate	T49.3X1	T49.3X2	T49.3X3	T49.3X4	T49.3X5	T49.3X6
Mecysteine	T48.4X1	T48.4X2	T48.4X3	T48.4X4	T48.4X5	T48.4X6
Medazepam	T42.4X1	T42.4X2	T42.4X3	T42.4X4	T42.4X5	T42.4X6
Medicament NEC	T50.901	T50.902	T50.903	T50.904	T50.905	T50.906
Medinal	T42.3X1	T42.3X2	T42.3X3	T42.3X4	T42.3X5	T42.3X6
Medomin	T42.3X1	T42.3X2	T42.3X3	T42.3X4	T42.3X5	T42.3X6
Medrogestone	T38.5X1	T38.5X2	T38.5X3	T38.5X4	T38.5X5	T38.5X6
Medroxalol	T44.8X1	T44.8X2	T44.8X3	T44.8X4	T44.8X5	T44.8X6
Medroxyprogesteron eacetate (depot)	T38.5X1	T38.5X2	T38.5X3	T38.5X4	T38.5X5	T38.5X6
Medrysone	T49.0X1	T49.0X2	T49.0X3	T49.0X4	T49.0X5	T49.0X6
Mefenamic acid	T39.391	T39.392	T39.393	T39.394	T39.395	T39.396
Mefenorex	T50.5X1	T50.5X2	T50.5X3	T50.5X4	T50.5X5	T50.5X6
Mefloquine	T37.2X1	T37.2X2	T37.2X3	T37.2X4	T37.2X5	T37.2X6
Mefruside	T50.2X1	T50.2X2	T50.2X3	T50.2X4	T50.2X5	T50.2X6
Megahallucinogen	T40.901	T40.902	T40.903	T40.904	T40.905	T40.906
Megestrol	T38.5X1	T38.5X2	T38.5X3	T38.5X4	T38.5X5	T38.5X6
Meglumine						
antimoniate	T37.8X1	T37.8X2	T37.8X3	T37.8X4	T37.8X5	T37.8X6
diatrizoate	T50.8X1	T50.8X2	T50.8X3	T50.8X4	T50.8X5	T50.8X6
iodipamide	T50.8X1	T50.8X2	T50.8X3	T50.8X4	T50.8X5	T50.8X6
iotroxate	T50.8X1	T50.8X2	T50.8X3	T50.8X4	T50.8X5	T50.8X6

Substance	Poisoning, Accidental (unintentional)	Poisoning, Intentional self-harm	Poisoning, Assault	Poisoning, Undetermined	Adverse effect	Underdosing
MEK (methyl ethyl ketone)	T52.4X1	T52.4X2	T52.4X3	T52.4X4	—	—
Meladinin	T49.3X1	T49.3X2	T49.3X3	T49.3X4	T49.3X5	T49.3X
Meladrazine	T44.3X1	T44.3X2	T44.3X3	T44.3X4	T44.3X5	T44.3X
Melaleuca alternifolia oil	T49.0X1	T49.0X2	T49.0X3	T49.0X4	T49.0X5	T49.0X
Melanizing agents	T49.3X1	T49.3X2	T49.3X3	T49.3X4	T49.3X5	T49.3X
Melanocyte-stimulating hormone	T38.891	T38.892	T38.893	T38.894	T38.895	T38.89
Melarsonyl potassium	T37.3X1	T37.3X2	T37.3X3	T37.3X4	T37.3X5	T37.3X
Melarsoprol	T37.3X1	T37.3X2	T37.3X3	T37.3X4	T37.3X5	T37.3X
Melia azedarach	T62.2X1	T62.2X2	T62.2X3	T62.2X4	—	—
Melitracen	T43.011	T43.012	T43.013	T43.014	T43.015	T43.01
Mellaril	T43.3X1	T43.3X2	T43.3X3	T43.3X4	T43.3X5	T43.3X
Meloxine	T49.3X1	T49.3X2	T49.3X3	T49.3X4	T49.3X5	T49.3X
Melperone	T43.4X1	T43.4X2	T43.4X3	T43.4X4	T43.4X5	T43.4X
Melphalan	T45.1X1	T45.1X2	T45.1X3	T45.1X4	T45.1X5	T45.1X
Memantine	T43.8X1	T43.8X2	T43.8X3	T43.8X4	T43.8X5	T43.8X
Menadiol	T45.7X1	T45.7X2	T45.7X3	T45.7X4	T45.7X5	T45.7X
sodium sulfate	T45.7X1	T45.7X2	T45.7X3	T45.7X4	T45.7X5	T45.7X
Menadione	T45.7X1	T45.7X2	T45.7X3	T45.7X4	T45.7X5	T45.7X
sodium bisulfite	T45.7X1	T45.7X2	T45.7X3	T45.7X4	T45.7X5	T45.7X
Menaphthone	T45.7X1	T45.7X2	T45.7X3	T45.7X4	T45.7X5	T45.7X
Menaquinone	T45.7X1	T45.7X2	T45.7X3	T45.7X4	T45.7X5	T45.7X
Menatetrenone	T45.7X1	T45.7X2	T45.7X3	T45.7X4	T45.7X5	T45.7X
Meningococcal vaccine	T50.A91	T50.A92	T50.A93	T50.A94	T50.A95	T50.A9
Menningovax (-AC) (-C)	T50.A91	T50.A92	T50.A93	T50.A94	T50.A95	T50.A9
Menotropins	T38.811	T38.812	T38.813	T38.814	T38.815	T38.81
Menthol	T48.5X1	T48.5X2	T48.5X3	T48.5X4	T48.5X5	T48.5X
Mepacrine	T37.2X1	T37.2X2	T37.2X3	T37.2X4	T37.2X5	T37.2X
Meparfynol	T42.6X1	T42.6X2	T42.6X3	T42.6X4	T42.6X5	T42.6X
Mepartricin	T36.7X1	T36.7X2	T36.7X3	T36.7X4	T36.7X5	T36.7X
Mepazine	T43.3X1	T43.3X2	T43.3X3	T43.3X4	T43.3X5	T43.3X
Mepenzolate	T44.3X1	T44.3X2	T44.3X3	T44.3X4	T44.3X5	T44.3X
bromide	T44.3X1	T44.3X2	T44.3X3	T44.3X4	T44.3X5	T44.3X
Meperidine	T40.4X1	T40.4X2	T40.4X3	T40.4X4	T40.4X5	T40.4X
Mephebarbital	T42.3X1	T42.3X2	T42.3X3	T42.3X4	T42.3X5	T42.3X
Mephenamin (e)	T42.8X1	T42.8X2	T42.8X3	T42.8X4	T42.8X5	T42.8X
Mephenesin	T42.8X1	T42.8X2	T42.8X3	T42.8X4	T42.8X5	T42.8X
Mephenhydramine	T45.0X1	T45.0X2	T45.0X3	T45.0X4	T45.0X5	T45.0X
Mephenoxalone	T42.8X1	T42.8X2	T42.8X3	T42.8X4	T42.8X5	T42.8X
Mephentermine	T44.991	T44.992	T44.993	T44.994	T44.995	T44.99
Mephenytoin	T42.0X1	T42.0X2	T42.0X3	T42.0X4	T42.0X5	T42.0X
with phenobarbital	T42.3X1	T42.3X2	T42.3X3	T42.3X4	T42.3X5	T42.3X
Mephobarbital	T42.3X1	T42.3X2	T42.3X3	T42.3X4	T42.3X5	T42.3X
Mephosfolan	T60.0X1	T60.0X2	T60.0X3	T60.0X4	—	—
Mepindolol	T44.7X1	T44.7X2	T44.7X3	T44.7X4	T44.7X5	T44.7X
Mepiperphenidol	T44.3X1	T44.3X2	T44.3X3	T44.3X4	T44.3X5	T44.3X
Mepitiostane	T38.7X1	T38.7X2	T38.7X3	T38.7X4	T38.7X5	T38.7X
Mepivacaine	T41.3X1	T41.3X2	T41.3X3	T41.3X4	T41.3X5	T41.3X
epidural	T41.3X1	T41.3X2	T41.3X3	T41.3X4	T41.3X5	T41.3X

Substance	Poisoning, Accidental (unintentional)	Poisoning, Intentional self-harm	Poisoning, Assault	Poisoning, Undetermined	Adverse effect	Underdosing
Meprednisone	T38.0X1	T38.0X2	T38.0X3	T38.0X4	T38.0X5	T38.0X6
Meprobam	T43.591	T43.592	T43.593	T43.594	T43.595	T43.596
Meprobamate	T43.591	T43.592	T43.593	T43.594	T43.595	T43.596
Meproscillarin	T46.0X1	T46.0X2	T46.0X3	T46.0X4	T46.0X5	T46.0X6
Meprylcaine	T41.3X1	T41.3X2	T41.3X3	T41.3X4	T41.3X5	T41.3X6
Meptazinol	T39.8X1	T39.8X2	T39.8X3	T39.8X4	T39.8X5	T39.8X6
Mepyramine	T45.0X1	T45.0X2	T45.0X3	T45.0X4	T45.0X5	T45.0X6
Mequitazine	T43.3X1	T43.3X2	T43.3X3	T43.3X4	T43.3X5	T43.3X6
Meralluride	T50.2X1	T50.2X2	T50.2X3	T50.2X4	T50.2X5	T50.2X6
Merbaphen	T50.2X1	T50.2X2	T50.2X3	T50.2X4	T50.2X5	T50.2X6
Merbromin	T49.0X1	T49.0X2	T49.0X3	T49.0X4	T49.0X5	T49.0X6
Mercaptoben-zothiazole salts	T49.0X1	T49.0X2	T49.0X3	T49.0X4	T49.0X5	T49.0X6
Mercaptomerin	T50.2X1	T50.2X2	T50.2X3	T50.2X4	T50.2X5	T50.2X6
Mercaptopurine	T45.1X1	T45.1X2	T45.1X3	T45.1X4	T45.1X5	T45.1X6
Mercumatilin	T50.2X1	T50.2X2	T50.2X3	T50.2X4	T50.2X5	T50.2X6
Mercuramide	T50.2X1	T50.2X2	T50.2X3	T50.2X4	T50.2X5	T50.2X6
Mercurochrome	T49.0X1	T49.0X2	T49.0X3	T49.0X4	T49.0X5	T49.0X6
Mercurophylline	T50.2X1	T50.2X2	T50.2X3	T50.2X4	T50.2X5	T50.2X6
Mercury, mercurial, mercuric, mercurous (compounds) (cyanide) (fumes) (nonmedicinal) (vapor) NEC	T56.1X1	T56.1X2	T56.1X3	T56.1X4	—	—
ammoniated	T49.0X1	T49.0X2	T49.0X3	T49.0X4	T49.0X5	T49.0X6
anti-infective						
local	T49.0X1	T49.0X2	T49.0X3	T49.0X4	T49.0X5	T49.0X6
systemic	T37.8X1	T37.8X2	T37.8X3	T37.8X4	T37.8X5	T37.8X6
topical	T49.0X1	T49.0X2	T49.0X3	T49.0X4	T49.0X5	T49.0X6
chloride (ammoniated)	T49.0X1	T49.0X2	T49.0X3	T49.0X4	T49.0X5	T49.0X6
fungicide	T56.1X1	T56.1X2	T56.1X3	T56.1X4	—	—
diuretic NEC	T50.2X1	T50.2X2	T50.2X3	T50.2X4	T50.2X5	T50.2X6
fungicide	T56.1X1	T56.1X2	T56.1X3	T56.1X4	—	—
organic (fungicide)	T56.1X1	T56.1X2	T56.1X3	T56.1X4	—	—
oxide, yellow	T49.0X1	T49.0X2	T49.0X3	T49.0X4	T49.0X5	T49.0X6
Mersalyl	T50.2X1	T50.2X2	T50.2X3	T50.2X4	T50.2X5	T50.2X6
Merthiolate	T49.0X1	T49.0X2	T49.0X3	T49.0X4	T49.0X5	T49.0X6
ophthalmic preparation	T49.5X1	T49.5X2	T49.5X3	T49.5X4	T49.5X5	T49.5X6
Meruvax	T50.B91	T50.B92	T50.B93	T50.B94	T50.B95	T50.B96
Mesalazine	T47.8X1	T47.8X2	T47.8X3	T47.8X4	T47.8X5	T47.8X6
Mescal buttons	T40.991	T40.992	T40.993	T40.994	—	—
Mescaline	T40.991	T40.992	T40.993	T40.994	—	—
Mesna	T48.4X1	T48.4X2	T48.4X3	T48.4X4	T48.4X5	T48.4X6
Mesoglycan	T46.6X1	T46.6X2	T46.6X3	T46.6X4	T46.6X5	T46.6X6
Mesoridazine	T43.3X1	T43.3X2	T43.3X3	T43.3X4	T43.3X5	T43.3X6
Mestanolone	T38.7X1	T38.7X2	T38.7X3	T38.7X4	T38.7X5	T38.7X6
Mesterolone	T38.7X1	T38.7X2	T38.7X3	T38.7X4	T38.7X5	T38.7X6
Mestranol	T38.5X1	T38.5X2	T38.5X3	T38.5X4	T38.5X5	T38.5X6
Mesulergine	T42.8X1	T42.8X2	T42.8X3	T42.8X4	T42.8X5	T42.8X6
Mesulfen	T49.0X1	T49.0X2	T49.0X3	T49.0X4	T49.0X5	T49.0X6
Mesuximide	T42.2X1	T42.2X2	T42.2X3	T42.2X4	T42.2X5	T42.2X6

Substance	Poisoning, Accidental (unintentional)	Poisoning, Intentional self-harm	Poisoning, Assault	Poisoning, Undetermined	Adverse effect	Underdosing
Metabutethamine	T41.3X1	T41.3X2	T41.3X3	T41.3X4	T41.3X5	T41.3X6
Metactesylacetate	T49.0X1	T49.0X2	T49.0X3	T49.0X4	T49.0X5	T49.0X6
Metacycline	T36.4X1	T36.4X2	T36.4X3	T36.4X4	T36.4X5	T36.4X6
Metaldehyde (snail killer) NEC	T60.8X1	T60.8X2	T60.8X3	T60.8X4	—	—
Metals (heavy) (nonmedicinal)	T56.91	T56.92	T56.93	T56.94	—	—
dust, fumes, or vapor NEC	T56.91	T56.92	T56.93	T56.94	—	—
light NEC	T56.91	T56.92	T56.93	T56.94	—	—
dust, fumes, or vapor NEC	T56.91	T56.92	T56.93	T56.94	—	—
specified NEC	T56.891	T56.892	T56.893	T56.894	—	—
thallium	T56.811	T56.812	T56.813	T56.814	—	—
Metamfetamine	T43.621	T43.622	T43.623	T43.624	T43.625	T43.626
Metamizole sodium	T39.2X1	T39.2X2	T39.2X3	T39.2X4	T39.2X5	T39.2X6
Metampicillin	T36.0X1	T36.0X2	T36.0X3	T36.0X4	T36.0X5	T36.0X6
Metamucil	T47.4X1	T47.4X2	T47.4X3	T47.4X4	T47.4X5	T47.4X6
Metandienone	T38.7X1	T38.7X2	T38.7X3	T38.7X4	T38.7X5	T38.7X6
Metandrostenolone	T38.7X1	T38.7X2	T38.7X3	T38.7X4	T38.7X5	T38.7X6
Metaphen	T49.0X1	T49.0X2	T49.0X3	T49.0X4	T49.0X5	T49.0X6
Metaphos	T60.0X1	T60.0X2	T60.0X3	T60.0X4	—	—
Metapramine	T43.011	T43.012	T43.013	T43.014	T43.015	T43.016
Metaproterenol	T48.291	T48.292	T48.293	T48.294	T48.295	T48.296
Metaraminol	T44.4X1	T44.4X2	T44.4X3	T44.4X4	T44.4X5	T44.4X6
Metaxalone	T42.8X1	T42.8X2	T42.8X3	T42.8X4	T42.8X5	T42.8X6
Metenolone	T38.7X1	T38.7X2	T38.7X3	T38.7X4	T38.7X5	T38.7X6
Metergoline	T42.8X1	T42.8X2	T42.8X3	T42.8X4	T42.8X5	T42.8X6
Metescufylline	T46.991	T46.992	T46.993	T46.994	T46.995	T46.996
Metetoin	T42.0X1	T42.0X2	T42.0X3	T42.0X4	T42.0X5	T42.0X6
Metformin	T38.3X1	T38.3X2	T38.3X3	T38.3X4	T38.3X5	T38.3X6
Methacholine	T44.1X1	T44.1X2	T44.1X3	T44.1X4	T44.1X5	T44.1X6
Methacycline	T36.4X1	T36.4X2	T36.4X3	T36.4X4	T36.4X5	T36.4X6
Methadone	T40.3X1	T40.3X2	T40.3X3	T40.3X4	T40.3X5	T40.3X6
Methallenestril	T38.5X1	T38.5X2	T38.5X3	T38.5X4	T38.5X5	T38.5X6
Methallenoestril	T38.5X1	T38.5X2	T38.5X3	T38.5X4	T38.5X5	T38.5X6
Methamphetamine	T43.621	T43.622	T43.623	T43.624	T43.625	T43.626
Methampyrone	T39.2X1	T39.2X2	T39.2X3	T39.2X4	T39.2X5	T39.2X6
Methandienone	T38.7X1	T38.7X2	T38.7X3	T38.7X4	T38.7X5	T38.7X6
Methandriol	T38.7X1	T38.7X2	T38.7X3	T38.7X4	T38.7X5	T38.7X6
Methandrostenolone	T38.7X1	T38.7X2	T38.7X3	T38.7X4	T38.7X5	T38.7X6
Methane	T59.891	T59.892	T59.893	T59.894	—	—
Methanethiol	T59.891	T59.892	T59.893	T59.894	—	—
Methaniazide	T37.1X1	T37.1X2	T37.1X3	T37.1X4	T37.1X5	T37.1X6
Methanol (vapor)	T51.1X1	T51.1X2	T51.1X3	T51.1X4	—	—
Methantheline	T44.3X1	T44.3X2	T44.3X3	T44.3X4	T44.3X5	T44.3X6
Methanthelinium bromide	T44.3X1	T44.3X2	T44.3X3	T44.3X4	T44.3X5	T44.3X6
Methaphenilene	T45.0X1	T45.0X2	T45.0X3	T45.0X4	T45.0X5	T45.0X6
Methapyrilene	T45.0X1	T45.0X2	T45.0X3	T45.0X4	T45.0X5	T45.0X6
Methaqualone (compound)	T42.6X1	T42.6X2	T42.6X3	T42.6X4	T42.6X5	T42.6X6
Metharbital	T42.3X1	T42.3X2	T42.3X3	T42.3X4	T42.3X5	T42.3X6
Methazolamide	T50.2X1	T50.2X2	T50.2X3	T50.2X4	T50.2X5	T50.2X6

Substance	Poisoning, Accidental (unintentional)	Poisoning, Intentional self-harm	Poisoning, Assault	Poisoning, Undetermined	Adverse effect	Underdosing
Methdilazine	T43.3X1	T43.3X2	T43.3X3	T43.3X4	T43.3X5	T43.3X6
Methedrine	T43.621	T43.622	T43.623	T43.624	T43.625	T43.626
Methenamine (mandelate)	T37.8X1	T37.8X2	T37.8X3	T37.8X4	T37.8X5	T37.8X6
Methenolone	T38.7X1	T38.7X2	T38.7X3	T38.7X4	T38.7X5	T38.7X6
Methergine	T48.0X1	T48.0X2	T48.0X3	T48.0X4	T48.0X5	T48.0X6
Methetoin	T42.0X1	T42.0X2	T42.0X3	T42.0X4	T42.0X5	T42.0X6
Methiacil	T38.2X1	T38.2X2	T38.2X3	T38.2X4	T38.2X5	T38.2X6
Methicillin	T36.0X1	T36.0X2	T36.0X3	T36.0X4	T36.0X5	T36.0X6
Methimazole	T38.2X1	T38.2X2	T38.2X3	T38.2X4	T38.2X5	T38.2X6
Methiodal sodium	T50.8X1	T50.8X2	T50.8X3	T50.8X4	T50.8X5	T50.8X6
Methionine	T50.991	T50.992	T50.993	T50.994	T50.995	T50.996
Methisazone	T37.5X1	T37.5X2	T37.5X3	T37.5X4	T37.5X5	T37.5X6
Methisoprinol	T37.5X1	T37.5X2	T37.5X3	T37.5X4	T37.5X5	T37.5X6
Methitural	T42.3X1	T42.3X2	T42.3X3	T42.3X4	T42.3X5	T42.3X6
Methixene	T44.3X1	T44.3X2	T44.3X3	T44.3X4	T44.3X5	T44.3X6
Methobarbital, methobarbitone	T42.3X1	T42.3X2	T42.3X3	T42.3X4	T42.3X5	T42.3X6
Methocarbamol	T42.8X1	T42.8X2	T42.8X3	T42.8X4	T42.8X5	T42.8X6
skeletal muscle relaxant	T48.1X1	T48.1X2	T48.1X3	T48.1X4	T48.1X5	T48.1X6
Methohexital	T41.1X1	T41.1X2	T41.1X3	T41.1X4	T41.1X5	T41.1X6
Methohexitone	T41.1X1	T41.1X2	T41.1X3	T41.1X4	T41.1X5	T41.1X6
Methoin	T42.0X1	T42.0X2	T42.0X3	T42.0X4	T42.0X5	T42.0X6
Methopholine	T39.8X1	T39.8X2	T39.8X3	T39.8X4	T39.8X5	T39.8X6
Methopromazine	T43.3X1	T43.3X2	T43.3X3	T43.3X4	T43.3X5	T43.3X6
Methorate	T48.3X1	T48.3X2	T48.3X3	T48.3X4	T48.3X5	T48.3X6
Methoserpidine	T46.5X1	T46.5X2	T46.5X3	T46.5X4	T46.5X5	T46.5X6
Methotrexate	T45.1X1	T45.1X2	T45.1X3	T45.1X4	T45.1X5	T45.1X6
Methotrimeprazine	T43.3X1	T43.3X2	T43.3X3	T43.3X4	T43.3X5	T43.3X6
Methoxa-Dome	T49.3X1	T49.3X2	T49.3X3	T49.3X4	T49.3X5	T49.3X6
Methoxamine	T44.4X1	T44.4X2	T44.4X3	T44.4X4	T44.4X5	T44.4X6
Methoxsalen	T50.991	T50.992	T50.993	T50.994	T50.995	T50.996
Methoxyaniline	T65.3X1	T65.3X2	T65.3X3	T65.3X4	—	—
Methoxybenzyl penicillin	T36.0X1	T36.0X2	T36.0X3	T36.0X4	T36.0X5	T36.0X6
Methoxychlor	T53.7X1	T53.7X2	T53.7X3	T53.7X4	—	—
Methoxy-DDT	T53.7X1	T53.7X2	T53.7X3	T53.7X4	—	—
2-Methoxyethanol	T52.3X1	T52.3X2	T52.3X3	T52.3X4	—	—
Methoxyflurane	T41.0X1	T41.0X2	T41.0X3	T41.0X4	T41.0X5	T41.0X6
Methoxyphenamine	T48.6X1	T48.6X2	T48.6X3	T48.6X4	T48.6X5	T48.6X6
Methoxypromazine	T43.3X1	T43.3X2	T43.3X3	T43.3X4	T43.3X5	T43.3X6
5-Methoxypsoralen (5-MOP)	T50.991	T50.992	T50.993	T50.994	T50.995	T50.996
8-Methoxypsoralen (8-MOP)	T50.991	T50.992	T50.993	T50.994	T50.995	T50.996
Methscopolamine bromide	T44.3X1	T44.3X2	T44.3X3	T44.3X4	T44.3X5	T44.3X6
Methsuximide	T42.2X1	T42.2X2	T42.2X3	T42.2X4	T42.2X5	T42.2X6
Methyclothiazide	T50.2X1	T50.2X2	T50.2X3	T50.2X4	T50.2X5	T50.2X6
Methyl						
acetate	T52.4X1	T52.4X2	T52.4X3	T52.4X4	—	—
acetone	T52.4X1	T52.4X2	T52.4X3	T52.4X4	—	—
acrylate	T65.891	T65.892	T65.893	T65.894	—	—
alcohol	T51.1X1	T51.1X2	T51.1X3	T51.1X4	—	—

Substance	Poisoning, Accidental (unintentional)	Poisoning, Intentional self-harm	Poisoning, Assault	Poisoning, Undetermined	Adverse effect	Underdosing
Methyl — *Continued*						
aminophenol	T65.3X1	T65.3X2	T65.3X3	T65.3X4	—	—
amphetamine	T43.621	T43.622	T43.623	T43.624	T43.625	T43.62
androstanolone	T38.7X1	T38.7X2	T38.7X3	T38.7X4	T38.7X5	T38.7X
atropine	T44.3X1	T44.3X2	T44.3X3	T44.3X4	T44.3X5	T44.3X
benzene	T52.2X1	T52.2X2	T52.2X3	T52.2X4	—	—
benzoate	T52.8X1	T52.8X2	T52.8X3	T52.8X4	—	—
benzol	T52.2X1	T52.2X2	T52.2X3	T52.2X4	—	—
bromide (gas)	T59.891	T59.892	T59.893	T59.894	—	—
fumigant	T60.8X1	T60.8X2	T60.8X3	T60.8X4	—	—
butanol	T51.3X1	T51.3X2	T51.3X3	T51.3X4	—	—
carbinol	T51.1X1	T51.1X2	T51.1X3	T51.1X4	—	—
carbonate	T52.8X1	T52.8X2	T52.8X3	T52.8X4	—	—
CCNU	T45.1X1	T45.1X2	T45.1X3	T45.1X4	T45.1X5	T45.1X
cellosolve	T52.91	T52.92	T52.93	T52.94	—	—
cellulose	T47.4X1	T47.4X2	T47.4X3	T47.4X4	T47.4X5	T47.4X
chloride (gas)	T59.891	T59.892	T59.893	T59.894	—	—
chloroformate	T59.3X1	T59.3X2	T59.3X3	T59.3X4	—	—
cyclohexane	T52.8X1	T52.8X2	T52.8X3	T52.8X4	—	—
cyclohexanol	T51.8X1	T51.8X2	T51.8X3	T51.8X4	—	—
cyclohexanone	T52.8X1	T52.8X2	T52.8X3	T52.8X4	—	—
cyclohexyl acetate	T52.8X1	T52.8X2	T52.8X3	T52.8X4	—	—
demeton	T60.0X1	T60.0X2	T60.0X3	T60.0X4	—	—
dihydromorphinone	T40.2X1	T40.2X2	T40.2X3	T40.2X4	T40.2X5	T40.2X
ergometrine	T48.0X1	T48.0X2	T48.0X3	T48.0X4	T48.0X5	T48.0X
ergonovine	T48.0X1	T48.0X2	T48.0X3	T48.0X4	T48.0X5	T48.0X
ethyl ketone	T52.4X1	T52.4X2	T52.4X3	T52.4X4	—	—
glucamine antimonate	T37.8X1	T37.8X2	T37.8X3	T37.8X4	T37.8X5	T37.8X
hydrazine	T65.891	T65.892	T65.893	T65.894	—	—
iodide	T65.891	T65.892	T65.893	T65.894	—	—
isobutyl ketone	T52.4X1	T52.4X2	T52.4X3	T52.4X4	—	—
isothiocyanate	T60.3X1	T60.3X2	T60.3X3	T60.3X4	—	—
mercaptan	T59.891	T59.892	T59.893	T59.894	—	—
morphine NEC	T40.2X1	T40.2X2	T40.2X3	T40.2X4	T40.2X5	T40.2X
nicotinate	T49.4X1	T49.4X2	T49.4X3	T49.4X4	T49.4X5	T49.4X
paraben	T49.0X1	T49.0X2	T49.0X3	T49.0X4	T49.0X5	T49.0X
parafynol	T42.6X1	T42.6X2	T42.6X3	T42.6X4	T42.6X5	T42.6X
parathion	T60.0X1	T60.0X2	T60.0X3	T60.0X4	—	—
peridol	T43.4X1	T43.4X2	T43.4X3	T43.4X4	T43.4X5	T43.4X
phenidate	T43.631	T43.632	T43.633	T43.634	T43.635	T43.63
prednisolone	T38.0X1	T38.0X2	T38.0X3	T38.0X4	T38.0X5	T38.0X
ENT agent	T49.6X1	T49.6X2	T49.6X3	T49.6X4	T49.6X5	T49.6X
ophthalmic preparation	T49.5X1	T49.5X2	T49.5X3	T49.5X4	T49.5X5	T49.5X
topical NEC	T49.0X1	T49.0X2	T49.0X3	T49.0X4	T49.0X5	T49.0X
propylcarbinol	T51.3X1	T51.3X2	T51.3X3	T51.3X4	—	—
rosaniline NEC	T49.0X1	T49.0X2	T49.0X3	T49.0X4	T49.0X5	T49.0X
salicylate	T49.2X1	T49.2X2	T49.2X3	T49.2X4	T49.2X5	T49.2X
sulfate (fumes)	T59.891	T59.892	T59.893	T59.894	—	—
liquid	T52.8X1	T52.8X2	T52.8X3	T52.8X4	—	—
sulfonal	T42.6X1	T42.6X2	T42.6X3	T42.6X4	T42.6X5	T42.6X

Substance	Poisoning, Accidental (unintentional)	Poisoning, Intentional self-harm	Poisoning, Assault	Poisoning, Undetermined	Adverse effect	Underdosing
Methyl — *Continued*						
testosterone	T38.7X1	T38.7X2	T38.7X3	T38.7X4	T38.7X5	T38.7X6
thiouracil	T38.2X1	T38.2X2	T38.2X3	T38.2X4	T38.2X5	T38.2X6
Methylamphetamine	T43.621	T43.622	T43.623	T43.624	T43.625	T43.626
Methylated spirit	T51.1X1	T51.1X2	T51.1X3	T51.1X4	—	—
Methylatropine nitrate	T44.3X1	T44.3X2	T44.3X3	T44.3X4	T44.3X5	T44.3X6
Methylbenactyzium bromide	T44.3X1	T44.3X2	T44.3X3	T44.3X4	T44.3X5	T44.3X6
Methylbenzethonium chloride	T49.0X1	T49.0X2	T49.0X3	T49.0X4	T49.0X5	T49.0X6
Methylcellulose	T47.4X1	T47.4X2	T47.4X3	T47.4X4	T47.4X5	T47.4X6
laxative	T47.4X1	T47.4X2	T47.4X3	T47.4X4	T47.4X5	T47.4X6
Methylchlorophenoxy-acetic acid	T60.3X1	T60.3X2	T60.3X3	T60.3X4	—	—
Methyldopa	T46.5X1	T46.5X2	T46.5X3	T46.5X4	T46.5X5	T46.5X6
Methyldopate	T46.5X1	T46.5X2	T46.5X3	T46.5X4	T46.5X5	T46.5X6
Methylene						
blue	T50.6X1	T50.6X2	T50.6X3	T50.6X4	T50.6X5	T50.6X6
chloride or dichloride (solvent) NEC	T53.4X1	T53.4X2	T53.4X3	T53.4X4	—	—
Methylenedioxy-amphetamine	T43.621	T43.622	T43.623	T43.624	T43.625	T43.626
Methylenedioxy-methamphetamine	T43.621	T43.622	T43.623	T43.624	T43.625	T43.626
Methylergometrine	T48.0X1	T48.0X2	T48.0X3	T48.0X4	T48.0X5	T48.0X6
Methylergonovine	T48.0X1	T48.0X2	T48.0X3	T48.0X4	T48.0X5	T48.0X6
Methylestrenolone	T38.5X1	T38.5X2	T38.5X3	T38.5X4	T38.5X5	T38.5X6
Methylethyl cellulose	T50.991	T50.992	T50.993	T50.994	T50.995	T50.996
Methylhexabital	T42.3X1	T42.3X2	T42.3X3	T42.3X4	T42.3X5	T42.3X6
Methylmorphine	T40.2X1	T40.2X2	T40.2X3	T40.2X4	T40.2X5	T40.2X6
Methylparaben (ophthalmic)	T49.5X1	T49.5X2	T49.5X3	T49.5X4	T49.5X5	T49.5X6
Methylparafynol	T42.6X1	T42.6X2	T42.6X3	T42.6X4	T42.6X5	T42.6X6
Methylpentynol, methylpenthynol	T42.6X1	T42.6X2	T42.6X3	T42.6X4	T42.6X5	T42.6X6
Methylphenidate	T43.631	T43.632	T43.633	T43.634	T43.635	T43.636
Methylphenobarbital	T42.3X1	T42.3X2	T42.3X3	T42.3X4	T42.3X5	T42.3X6
Methylpolysiloxane	T47.1X1	T47.1X2	T47.1X3	T47.1X4	T47.1X5	T47.1X6
Methylprednisolone— see Methyl, prednisolone						
Methylrosaniline	T49.0X1	T49.0X2	T49.0X3	T49.0X4	T49.0X5	T49.0X6
Methylrosanilinium chloride	T49.0X1	T49.0X2	T49.0X3	T49.0X4	T49.0X5	T49.0X6
Methyltestosterone	T38.7X1	T38.7X2	T38.7X3	T38.7X4	T38.7X5	T38.7X6
Methylthionine chloride	T50.6X1	T50.6X2	T50.6X3	T50.6X4	T50.6X5	T50.6X6
Methylthioninium chloride	T50.6X1	T50.6X2	T50.6X3	T50.6X4	T50.6X5	T50.6X6
Methylthiouracil	T38.2X1	T38.2X2	T38.2X3	T38.2X4	T38.2X5	T38.2X6
Methyprylon	T42.6X1	T42.6X2	T42.6X3	T42.6X4	T42.6X5	T42.6X6
Methysergide	T46.5X1	T46.5X2	T46.5X3	T46.5X4	T46.5X5	T46.5X6
Metiamide	T47.1X1	T47.1X2	T47.1X3	T47.1X4	T47.1X5	T47.1X6
Meticillin	T36.0X1	T36.0X2	T36.0X3	T36.0X4	T36.0X5	T36.0X6
Meticrane	T50.2X1	T50.2X2	T50.2X3	T50.2X4	T50.2X5	T50.2X6
Metildigoxin	T46.0X1	T46.0X2	T46.0X3	T46.0X4	T46.0X5	T46.0X6

Substance	Poisoning, Accidental (unintentional)	Poisoning, Intentional self-harm	Poisoning, Assault	Poisoning, Undetermined	Adverse effect	Underdosing
Metipranolol	T49.5X1	T49.5X2	T49.5X3	T49.5X4	T49.5X5	T49.5X6
Metirosine	T46.5X1	T46.5X2	T46.5X3	T46.5X4	T46.5X5	T46.5X6
Metisazone	T37.5X1	T37.5X2	T37.5X3	T37.5X4	T37.5X5	T37.5X6
Metixene	T44.3X1	T44.3X2	T44.3X3	T44.3X4	T44.3X5	T44.3X6
Metizoline	T48.5X1	T48.5X2	T48.5X3	T48.5X4	T48.5X5	T48.5X6
Metoclopramide	T45.0X1	T45.0X2	T45.0X3	T45.0X4	T45.0X5	T45.0X6
Metofenazate	T43.3X1	T43.3X2	T43.3X3	T43.3X4	T43.3X5	T43.3X6
Metofoline	T39.8X1	T39.8X2	T39.8X3	T39.8X4	T39.8X5	T39.8X6
Metolazone	T50.2X1	T50.2X2	T50.2X3	T50.2X4	T50.2X5	T50.2X6
Metopon	T40.2X1	T40.2X2	T40.2X3	T40.2X4	T40.2X5	T40.2X6
Metoprine	T45.1X1	T45.1X2	T45.1X3	T45.1X4	T45.1X5	T45.1X6
Metoprolol	T44.7X1	T44.7X2	T44.7X3	T44.7X4	T44.7X5	T44.7X6
Metrifonate	T60.0X1	T60.0X2	T60.0X3	T60.0X4	—	—
Metrizamide	T50.8X1	T50.8X2	T50.8X3	T50.8X4	T50.8X5	T50.8X6
Metrizoic acid	T50.8X1	T50.8X2	T50.8X3	T50.8X4	T50.8X5	T50.8X6
Metronidazole	T37.8X1	T37.8X2	T37.8X3	T37.8X4	T37.8X5	T37.8X6
Metycaine	T41.3X1	T41.3X2	T41.3X3	T41.3X4	T41.3X5	T41.3X6
infiltration (subcutaneous)	T41.3X1	T41.3X2	T41.3X3	T41.3X4	T41.3X5	T41.3X6
nerve block (peripheral) (plexus)	T41.3X1	T41.3X2	T41.3X3	T41.3X4	T41.3X5	T41.3X6
topical (surface)	T41.3X1	T41.3X2	T41.3X3	T41.3X4	T41.3X5	T41.3X6
Metyrapone	T50.8X1	T50.8X2	T50.8X3	T50.8X4	T50.8X5	T50.8X6
Mevinphos	T60.0X1	T60.0X2	T60.0X3	T60.0X4	—	—
Mexazolam	T42.4X1	T42.4X2	T42.4X3	T42.4X4	T42.4X5	T42.4X6
Mexenone	T49.3X1	T49.3X2	T49.3X3	T49.3X4	T49.3X5	T49.3X6
Mexiletine	T46.2X1	T46.2X2	T46.2X3	T46.2X4	T46.2X5	T46.2X6
Mezereon	T62.2X1	T62.2X2	T62.2X3	T62.2X4	—	—
berries	T62.1X1	T62.1X2	T62.1X3	T62.1X4	—	—
Mezlocillin	T36.0X1	T36.0X2	T36.0X3	T36.0X4	T36.0X5	T36.0X6
Mianserin	T43.021	T43.022	T43.023	T43.024	T43.025	T43.026
Micatin	T49.0X1	T49.0X2	T49.0X3	T49.0X4	T49.0X5	T49.0X6
Miconazole	T49.0X1	T49.0X2	T49.0X3	T49.0X4	T49.0X5	T49.0X6
Micronomicin	T36.5X1	T36.5X2	T36.5X3	T36.5X4	T36.5X5	T36.5X6
Midazolam	T42.4X1	T42.4X2	T42.4X3	T42.4X4	T42.4X5	T42.4X6
Midecamycin	T36.3X1	T36.3X2	T36.3X3	T36.3X4	T36.3X5	T36.3X6
Mifepristone	T38.6X1	T38.6X2	T38.6X3	T38.6X4	T38.6X5	T38.6X6
Milk of magnesia	T47.1X1	T47.1X2	T47.1X3	T47.1X4	T47.1X5	T47.1X6
Millipede (tropical) (venomous)	T63.411	T63.412	T63.413	T63.414	—	—
Miltown	T43.591	T43.592	T43.593	T43.594	T43.595	T43.596
Milverine	T44.3X1	T44.3X2	T44.3X3	T44.3X4	T44.3X5	T44.3X6
Minaprine	T43.291	T43.292	T43.293	T43.294	T43.295	T43.296
Minaxolone	T41.291	T41.292	T41.293	T41.294	T41.295	T41.296
Mineral						
acids	T54.2X1	T54.2X2	T54.2X3	T54.2X4	—	—
oil (laxative) (medicinal)	T47.4X1	T47.4X2	T47.4X3	T47.4X4	T47.4X5	T47.4X6
emulsion	T47.2X1	T47.2X2	T47.2X3	T47.2X4	T47.2X5	T47.2X6
nonmedicinal	T52.0X1	T52.0X2	T52.0X3	T52.0X4	—	—
topical	T49.3X1	T49.3X2	T49.3X3	T49.3X4	T49.3X5	T49.3X6
salt NEC	T50.3X1	T50.3X2	T50.3X3	T50.3X4	T50.3X5	T50.3X6
spirits	T52.0X1	T52.0X2	T52.0X3	T52.0X4	—	—

Substance	Poisoning, Accidental (unintentional)	Poisoning, Intentional self-harm	Poisoning, Assault	Poisoning, Undetermined	Adverse effect	Underdosing
Mineralocorticosteroid	T50.0X1	T50.0X2	T50.0X3	T50.0X4	T50.0X5	T50.0X6
Minocycline	T36.4X1	T36.4X2	T36.4X3	T36.4X4	T36.4X5	T36.4X6
Minoxidil	T46.7X1	T46.7X2	T46.7X3	T46.7X4	T46.7X5	T46.7X6
Miokamycin	T36.3X1	T36.3X2	T36.3X3	T36.3X4	T36.3X5	T36.3X6
Miotic drug	T49.5X1	T49.5X2	T49.5X3	T49.5X4	T49.5X5	T49.5X6
Mipafox	T60.0X1	T60.0X2	T60.0X3	T60.0X4	—	—
Mirex	T60.1X1	T60.1X2	T60.1X3	T60.1X4	—	—
Mirtazapine	T43.021	T43.022	T43.023	T43.024	T43.025	T43.026
Misonidazole	T37.3X1	T37.3X2	T37.3X3	T37.3X4	T37.3X5	T37.3X6
Misoprostol	T47.1X1	T47.1X2	T47.1X3	T47.1X4	T47.1X5	T47.1X6
Mithramycin	T45.1X1	T45.1X2	T45.1X3	T45.1X4	T45.1X5	T45.1X6
Mitobronitol	T45.1X1	T45.1X2	T45.1X3	T45.1X4	T45.1X5	T45.1X6
Mitoguazone	T45.1X1	T45.1X2	T45.1X3	T45.1X4	T45.1X5	T45.1X6
Mitolactol	T45.1X1	T45.1X2	T45.1X3	T45.1X4	T45.1X5	T45.1X6
Mitomycin	T45.1X1	T45.1X2	T45.1X3	T45.1X4	T45.1X5	T45.1X6
Mitopodozide	T45.1X1	T45.1X2	T45.1X3	T45.1X4	T45.1X5	T45.1X6
Mitotane	T45.1X1	T45.1X2	T45.1X3	T45.1X4	T45.1X5	T45.1X6
Mitoxantrone	T45.1X1	T45.1X2	T45.1X3	T45.1X4	T45.1X5	T45.1X6
Mivacurium chloride	T48.1X1	T48.1X2	T48.1X3	T48.1X4	T48.1X5	T48.1X6
Miyari bacteria	T47.6X1	T47.6X2	T47.6X3	T47.6X4	T47.6X5	T47.6X6
Moclobemide	T43.1X1	T43.1X2	T43.1X3	T43.1X4	T43.1X5	T43.1X6
Moderil	T46.5X1	T46.5X2	T46.5X3	T46.5X4	T46.5X5	T46.5X6
Mofebutazone	T39.2X1	T39.2X2	T39.2X3	T39.2X4	T39.2X5	T39.2X6
Mogadon—see Nitrazepam						
Molindone	T43.591	T43.592	T43.593	T43.594	T43.595	T43.596
Molsidomine	T46.3X1	T46.3X2	T46.3X3	T46.3X4	T46.3X5	T46.3X6
Mometasone	T49.0X1	T49.0X2	T49.0X3	T49.0X4	T49.0X5	T49.0X6
Monistat	T49.0X1	T49.0X2	T49.0X3	T49.0X4	T49.0X5	T49.0X6
Monkshood	T62.2X1	T62.2X2	T62.2X3	T62.2X4	—	—
Monoamine oxidase inhibitor NEC	T43.1X1	T43.1X2	T43.1X3	T43.1X4	T43.1X5	T43.1X6
hydrazine	T43.1X1	T43.1X2	T43.1X3	T43.1X4	T43.1X5	T43.1X6
Monobenzone	T49.4X1	T49.4X2	T49.4X3	T49.4X4	T49.4X5	T49.4X6
Monochloroacetic acid	T60.3X1	T60.3X2	T60.3X3	T60.3X4	—	—
Monochlorobenzene	T53.7X1	T53.7X2	T53.7X3	T53.7X4	—	—
Monoethanolamine	T46.8X1	T46.8X2	T46.8X3	T46.8X4	T46.8X5	T46.8X6
oleate	T46.8X1	T46.8X2	T46.8X3	T46.8X4	T46.8X5	T46.8X6
Monooctanoin	T50.991	T50.992	T50.993	T50.994	T50.995	T50.996
Monophenylbutazone	T39.2X1	T39.2X2	T39.2X3	T39.2X4	T39.2X5	T39.2X6
Monosodium glutamate	T65.891	T65.892	T65.893	T65.894	—	—
Monosulfiram	T49.0X1	T49.0X2	T49.0X3	T49.0X4	T49.0X5	T49.0X6
Monoxide, carbon—see Carbon, monoxide						
Monoxidine hydrochloride	T46.1X1	T46.1X2	T46.1X3	T46.1X4	T46.1X5	T46.1X6
Monuron	T60.3X1	T60.3X2	T60.3X3	T60.3X4	—	—
Moperone	T43.4X1	T43.4X2	T43.4X3	T43.4X4	T43.4X5	T43.4X6
Mopidamol	T45.1X1	T45.1X2	T45.1X3	T45.1X4	T45.1X5	T45.1X6
MOPP (mechloreth-amine + vincristine + prednisone + procarba-zine)	T45.1X1	T45.1X2	T45.1X3	T45.1X4	T45.1X5	T45.1X6
Morfin	T40.2X1	T40.2X2	T40.2X3	T40.2X4	T40.2X5	T40.2X
Morinamide	T37.1X1	T37.1X2	T37.1X3	T37.1X4	T37.1X5	T37.1X
Morning glory seeds	T40.991	T40.992	T40.993	T40.994	—	—
Moroxydine	T37.5X1	T37.5X2	T37.5X3	T37.5X4	T37.5X5	T37.5X
Morphazinamide	T37.1X1	T37.1X2	T37.1X3	T37.1X4	T37.1X5	T37.1X
Morphine	T40.2X1	T40.2X2	T40.2X3	T40.2X4	T40.2X5	T40.2X
antagonist	T50.7X1	T50.7X2	T50.7X3	T50.7X4	T50.7X5	T50.7X
Morpholinylethyl-morphine	T40.2X1	T40.2X2	T40.2X3	T40.2X4	—	—
Morsuximide	T42.2X1	T42.2X2	T42.2X3	T42.2X4	T42.2X5	T42.2X
Mosapramine	T43.591	T43.592	T43.593	T43.594	T43.595	T43.59
Moth balls—see also Pesticides	T60.2X1	T60.2X2	T60.2X3	T60.2X4	—	—
naphthalene	T60.2X1	T60.2X2	T60.2X3	T60.2X4	—	—
paradichlorobenzene	T60.1X1	T60.1X2	T60.1X3	T60.1X4	—	—
Motor exhaust gas	T58.01	T58.02	T58.03	T58.04	—	—
Mouthwash (antiseptic) (zincchloride)	T49.6X1	T49.6X2	T49.6X3	T49.6X4	T49.6X5	T49.6X
Moxastine	T45.0X1	T45.0X2	T45.0X3	T45.0X4	T45.0X5	T45.0X
Moxaverine	T44.3X1	T44.3X2	T44.3X3	T44.3X4	T44.3X5	T44.3X
Moxisylyte	T46.7X1	T46.7X2	T46.7X3	T46.7X4	T46.7X5	T46.7X
Mucilage, plant	T47.4X1	T47.4X2	T47.4X3	T47.4X4	T47.4X5	T47.4X
Mucolytic drug	T48.4X1	T48.4X2	T48.4X3	T48.4X4	T48.4X5	T48.4X
Mucomyst	T48.4X1	T48.4X2	T48.4X3	T48.4X4	T48.4X5	T48.4X
Mucous membrane agents (external)	T49.91	T49.92	T49.93	T49.94	T49.95	T49.96
specified NEC	T49.8X1	T49.8X2	T49.8X3	T49.8X4	T49.8X5	T49.8X
Mumps						
immune globulin (human)	T50.Z11	T50.Z12	T50.Z13	T50.Z14	T50.Z15	T50.Z1
skin test antigen	T50.8X1	T50.8X2	T50.8X3	T50.8X4	T50.8X5	T50.8X
vaccine	T50.B91	T50.B92	T50.B93	T50.B94	T50.B95	T50.B9
Mumpsvax	T50.B91	T50.B92	T50.B93	T50.B94	T50.B95	T50.B9
Mupirocin	T49.0X1	T49.0X2	T49.0X3	T49.0X4	T49.0X5	T49.0X
Muriatic acid—see Hydrochloric acid						
Muromonab-CD3	T45.1X1	T45.1X2	T45.1X3	T45.1X4	T45.1X5	T45.1X
Muscle-action drug NEC	T48.201	T48.202	T48.203	T48.204	T48.205	T48.20
Muscle affecting agents NEC	T48.201	T48.202	T48.203	T48.204	T48.205	T48.20
oxytocic	T48.0X1	T48.0X2	T48.0X3	T48.0X4	T48.0X5	T48.0X
relaxants	T48.201	T48.202	T48.203	T48.204	T48.205	T48.20
central nervous system	T42.8X1	T42.8X2	T42.8X3	T42.8X4	T42.8X5	T42.8X
skeletal	T48.1X1	T48.1X2	T48.1X3	T48.1X4	T48.1X5	T48.1X
smooth	T44.3X1	T44.3X2	T44.3X3	T44.3X4	T44.3X5	T44.3X
Muscle relaxant—see Relaxant, muscle						
Muscle-tone depressant, central NEC	T42.8X1	T42.8X2	T42.8X3	T42.8X4	T42.8X5	T42.8X
specified NEC	T42.8X1	T42.8X2	T42.8X3	T42.8X4	T42.8X5	T42.8X
Mushroom, noxious	T62.0X1	T62.0X2	T62.0X3	T62.0X4	—	—
Mussel, noxious	T61.781	T61.782	T61.783	T61.784	—	—

Substance	Poisoning, Accidental (unintentional)	Poisoning, Intentional self-harm	Poisoning, Assault	Poisoning, Undetermined	Adverse effect	Underdosing
Mustard (emetic)	T47.7X1	T47.7X2	T47.7X3	T47.7X4	T47.7X5	T47.7X6
black	T47.7X1	T47.7X2	T47.7X3	T47.7X4	T47.7X5	T47.7X6
gas, not in war	T59.91	T59.92	T59.93	T59.94	—	—
nitrogen	T45.1X1	T45.1X2	T45.1X3	T45.1X4	T45.1X5	T45.1X6
Mustine	T45.1X1	T45.1X2	T45.1X3	T45.1X4	T45.1X5	T45.1X6
M-vac	T45.1X1	T45.1X2	T45.1X3	T45.1X4	T45.1X5	T45.1X6
Mycifradin	T36.5X1	T36.5X2	T36.5X3	T36.5X4	T36.5X5	T36.5X6
topical	T49.0X1	T49.0X2	T49.0X3	T49.0X4	T49.0X5	T49.0X6
Mycitracin	T36.8X1	T36.8X2	T36.8X3	T36.8X4	T36.8X5	T36.8X6
ophthalmic preparation	T49.5X1	T49.5X2	T49.5X3	T49.5X4	T49.5X5	T49.5X6
Mycostatin	T36.7X1	T36.7X2	T36.7X3	T36.7X4	T36.7X5	T36.7X6
topical	T49.0X1	T49.0X2	T49.0X3	T49.0X4	T49.0X5	T49.0X6
Mycotoxins	T64.81	T64.82	T64.83	T64.84	—	—
aflatoxin	T64.01	T64.02	T64.03	T64.04	—	—
specified NEC	T64.81	T64.82	T64.83	T64.84	—	—
Mydriacyl	T44.3X1	T44.3X2	T44.3X3	T44.3X4	T44.3X5	T44.3X6
Mydriatic drug	T49.5X1	T49.5X2	T49.5X3	T49.5X4	T49.5X5	T49.5X6
Myelobromal	T45.1X1	T45.1X2	T45.1X3	T45.1X4	T45.1X5	T45.1X6
Myleran	T45.1X1	T45.1X2	T45.1X3	T45.1X4	T45.1X5	T45.1X6
Myochrysin(e)	T39.2X1	T39.2X2	T39.2X3	T39.2X4	T39.2X5	T39.2X6
Myoneural blocking agents	T48.1X1	T48.1X2	T48.1X3	T48.1X4	T48.1X5	T48.1X6
Myralact	T49.0X1	T49.0X2	T49.0X3	T49.0X4	T49.0X5	T49.0X6
Myristica fragrans	T62.2X1	T62.2X2	T62.2X3	T62.2X4	—	—
Myristicin	T65.891	T65.892	T65.893	T65.894	—	—
Mysoline	T42.3X1	T42.3X2	T42.3X3	T42.3X4	T42.3X5	T42.3X6
N						
Nabilone	T40.7X1	T40.7X2	T40.7X3	T40.7X4	T40.7X5	T40.7X6
Nabumetone	T39.391	T39.392	T39.393	T39.394	T39.395	T39.396
Nadolol	T44.7X1	T44.7X2	T44.7X3	T44.7X4	T44.7X5	T44.7X6
Nafcillin	T36.0X1	T36.0X2	T36.0X3	T36.0X4	T36.0X5	T36.0X6
Nafoxidine	T38.6X1	T38.6X2	T38.6X3	T38.6X4	T38.6X5	T38.6X6
Naftazone	T46.991	T46.992	T46.993	T46.994	T46.995	T46.996
Naftidrofuryl (oxalate)	T46.7X1	T46.7X2	T46.7X3	T46.7X4	T46.7X5	T46.7X6
Naftifine	T49.0X1	T49.0X2	T49.0X3	T49.0X4	T49.0X5	T49.0X6
Nail polish remover	T52.91	T52.92	T52.93	T52.94	—	—
Nalbuphine	T40.4X1	T40.4X2	T40.4X3	T40.4X4	T40.4X5	T40.4X6
Naled	T60.0X1	T60.0X2	T60.0X3	T60.0X4	—	—
Nalidixic acid	T37.8X1	T37.8X2	T37.8X3	T37.8X4	T37.8X5	T37.8X6
Nalorphine	T50.7X1	T50.7X2	T50.7X3	T50.7X4	T50.7X5	T50.7X6
Naloxone	T50.7X1	T50.7X2	T50.7X3	T50.7X4	T50.7X5	T50.7X6
Naltrexone	T50.7X1	T50.7X2	T50.7X3	T50.7X4	T50.7X5	T50.7X6
Namenda	T43.8X1	T43.8X2	T43.8X3	T43.8X4	T43.8X5	T43.8X6
Nandrolone	T38.7X1	T38.7X2	T38.7X3	T38.7X4	T38.7X5	T38.7X6
Naphazoline	T48.5X1	T48.5X2	T48.5X3	T48.5X4	T48.5X5	T48.5X6
Naphtha (painters') (petroleum)	T52.0X1	T52.0X2	T52.0X3	T52.0X4	—	—
solvent	T52.0X1	T52.0X2	T52.0X3	T52.0X4	—	—
vapor	T52.0X1	T52.0X2	T52.0X3	T52.0X4	—	—
Naphthalene (non-chlorinated)	T60.2X1	T60.2X2	T60.2X3	T60.2X4	—	—

Substance	Poisoning, Accidental (unintentional)	Poisoning, Intentional self-harm	Poisoning, Assault	Poisoning, Undetermined	Adverse effect	Underdosing
Naphthalene — *Continued*						
chlorinated	T60.1X1	T60.1X2	T60.1X3	T60.1X4	—	—
vapor	T60.1X1	T60.1X2	T60.1X3	T60.1X4	—	—
insecticide or moth repellent	T60.2X1	T60.2X2	T60.2X3	T60.2X4	—	—
chlorinated	T60.1X1	T60.1X2	T60.1X3	T60.1X4	—	—
vapor	T60.2X1	T60.2X2	T60.2X3	T60.2X4	—	—
chlorinated	T60.1X1	T60.1X2	T60.1X3	T60.1X4	—	—
Naphthol	T65.891	T65.892	T65.893	T65.894	—	—
Naphthylamine	T65.891	T65.892	T65.893	T65.894	—	—
Naphthylthiourea (ANTU)	T60.4X1	T60.4X2	T60.4X3	T60.4X4	—	—
Naprosyn—see Naproxen						
Naproxen	T39.311	T39.312	T39.313	T39.314	T39.315	T39.316
Narcotic (drug)	T40.601	T40.602	T40.603	T40.604	T40.605	T40.606
analgesic NEC	T40.601	T40.602	T40.603	T40.604	T40.605	T40.606
antagonist	T50.7X1	T50.7X2	T50.7X3	T50.7X4	T50.7X5	T50.7X6
specified NEC	T40.691	T40.692	T40.693	T40.694	T40.695	T40.696
synthetic	T40.4X1	T40.4X2	T40.4X3	T40.4X4	T40.4X5	T40.4X6
Narcotine	T48.3X1	T48.3X2	T48.3X3	T48.3X4	T48.3X5	T48.3X6
Nardil	T43.1X1	T43.1X2	T43.1X3	T43.1X4	T43.1X5	T43.1X6
Nasal drug NEC	T49.6X1	T49.6X2	T49.6X3	T49.6X4	T49.6X5	T49.6X6
Natamycin	T49.0X1	T49.0X2	T49.0X3	T49.0X4	T49.0X5	T49.0X6
Natrium cyanide—see Cyanide (s)						
Natural						
blood (product)	T45.8X1	T45.8X2	T45.8X3	T45.8X4	T45.8X5	T45.8X6
gas (piped)	T59.891	T59.892	T59.893	T59.894	—	—
incomplete combustion	T58.11	T58.12	T58.13	T58.14	—	—
Nealbarbital	T42.3X1	T42.3X2	T42.3X3	T42.3X4	T42.3X5	T42.3X6
Nectadon	T48.3X1	T48.3X2	T48.3X3	T48.3X4	T48.3X5	T48.3X6
Nedocromil	T48.6X1	T48.6X2	T48.6X3	T48.6X4	T48.6X5	T48.6X6
Nefopam	T39.8X1	T39.8X2	T39.8X3	T39.8X4	T39.8X5	T39.8X6
Nematocyst (sting)	T63.691	T63.692	T63.693	T63.694	—	—
Nembutal	T42.3X1	T42.3X2	T42.3X3	T42.3X4	T42.3X5	T42.3X6
Nemonapride	T43.591	T43.592	T43.593	T43.594	T43.595	T43.596
Neoarsphenamine	T37.8X1	T37.8X2	T37.8X3	T37.8X4	T37.8X5	T37.8X6
Neocinchophen	T50.4X1	T50.4X2	T50.4X3	T50.4X4	T50.4X5	T50.4X6
Neomycin (derivatives)	T36.5X1	T36.5X2	T36.5X3	T36.5X4	T36.5X5	T36.5X6
with						
bacitracin	T49.0X1	T49.0X2	T49.0X3	T49.0X4	T49.0X5	T49.0X6
neostigmine	T44.0X1	T44.0X2	T44.0X3	T44.0X4	T44.0X5	T44.0X6
ENT agent	T49.6X1	T49.6X2	T49.6X3	T49.6X4	T49.6X5	T49.6X6
ophthalmic preparation	T49.5X1	T49.5X2	T49.5X3	T49.5X4	T49.5X5	T49.5X6
topical NEC	T49.0X1	T49.0X2	T49.0X3	T49.0X4	T49.0X5	T49.0X6
Neonal	T42.3X1	T42.3X2	T42.3X3	T42.3X4	T42.3X5	T42.3X6
Neoprontosil	T37.0X1	T37.0X2	T37.0X3	T37.0X4	T37.0X5	T37.0X6
Neosalvarsan	T37.8X1	T37.8X2	T37.8X3	T37.8X4	T37.8X5	T37.8X6
Neosilversalvarsan	T37.8X1	T37.8X2	T37.8X3	T37.8X4	T37.8X5	T37.8X6
Neosporin	T36.8X1	T36.8X2	T36.8X3	T36.8X4	T36.8X5	T36.8X6
ENT agent	T49.6X1	T49.6X2	T49.6X3	T49.6X4	T49.6X5	T49.6X6

Substance	Poisoning, Accidental (unintentional)	Poisoning, Intentional self-harm	Poisoning, Assault	Poisoning, Undetermined	Adverse effect	Underdosing
Neosporin — *Continued*						
opthalmic preparation	T49.5X1	T49.5X2	T49.5X3	T49.5X4	T49.5X5	T49.5X6
topical NEC	T49.0X1	T49.0X2	T49.0X3	T49.0X4	T49.0X5	T49.0X6
Neostigmine bromide	T44.0X1	T44.0X2	T44.0X3	T44.0X4	T44.0X5	T44.0X6
Neraval	T42.3X1	T42.3X2	T42.3X3	T42.3X4	T42.3X5	T42.3X6
Neravan	T42.3X1	T42.3X2	T42.3X3	T42.3X4	T42.3X5	T42.3X6
Nerium oleander	T62.2X1	T62.2X2	T62.2X3	T62.2X4	—	—
Nerve gas, not in war	T59.91	T59.92	T59.93	T59.94	—	—
Nesacaine	T41.3X1	T41.3X2	T41.3X3	T41.3X4	T41.3X5	T41.3X6
infiltration (subcutaneous)	T41.3X1	T41.3X2	T41.3X3	T41.3X4	T41.3X5	T41.3X6
nerve block (peripheral) (plexus)	T41.3X1	T41.3X2	T41.3X3	T41.3X4	T41.3X5	T41.3X6
Netilmicin	T36.5X1	T36.5X2	T36.5X3	T36.5X4	T36.5X5	T36.5X6
Neurobarb	T42.3X1	T42.3X2	T42.3X3	T42.3X4	T42.3X5	T42.3X6
Neuroleptic drug NEC	T43.501	T43.502	T43.503	T43.504	T43.505	T43.506
Neuromuscular blocking drug	T48.1X1	T48.1X2	T48.1X3	T48.1X4	T48.1X5	T48.1X6
Neutral insulin injection	T38.3X1	T38.3X2	T38.3X3	T38.3X4	T38.3X5	T38.3X6
Neutral spirits	T51.0X1	T51.0X2	T51.0X3	T51.0X4	—	—
beverage	T51.0X1	T51.0X2	T51.0X3	T51.0X4	—	—
Niacin	T46.7X1	T46.7X2	T46.7X3	T46.7X4	T46.7X5	T46.7X6
Niacinamide	T45.2X1	T45.2X2	T45.2X3	T45.2X4	T45.2X5	T45.2X6
Nialamide	T43.1X1	T43.1X2	T43.1X3	T43.1X4	T43.1X5	T43.1X6
Niaprazine	T42.6X1	T42.6X2	T42.6X3	T42.6X4	T42.6X5	T42.6X6
Nicametate	T46.7X1	T46.7X2	T46.7X3	T46.7X4	T46.7X5	T46.7X6
Nicardipine	T46.1X1	T46.1X2	T46.1X3	T46.1X4	T46.1X5	T46.1X6
Nicergoline	T46.7X1	T46.7X2	T46.7X3	T46.7X4	T46.7X5	T46.7X6
Nickel (carbonyl) (tetra-carbonyl) (fumes) (vapor)	T56.891	T56.892	T56.893	T56.894	—	—
Nickelocene	T56.891	T56.892	T56.893	T56.894	—	—
Niclosamide	T37.4X1	T37.4X2	T37.4X3	T37.4X4	T37.4X5	T37.4X6
Nicofuranose	T46.7X1	T46.7X2	T46.7X3	T46.7X4	T46.7X5	T46.7X6
Nicomorphine	T40.2X1	T40.2X2	T40.2X3	T40.2X4	—	—
Nicorandil	T46.3X1	T46.3X2	T46.3X3	T46.3X4	T46.3X5	T46.3X6
Nicotiana (plant)	T62.2X1	T62.2X2	T62.2X3	T62.2X4	—	—
Nicotinamide	T45.2X1	T45.2X2	T45.2X3	T45.2X4	T45.2X5	T45.2X6
Nicotine (insecticide) (spray) (sulfate) NEC	T60.2X1	T60.2X2	T60.2X3	T60.2X4	—	—
from tobacco	T65.291	T65.292	T65.293	T65.294	—	—
cigarettes	T65.221	T65.222	T65.223	T65.224	—	—
not insecticide	T65.291	T65.292	T65.293	T65.294	—	—
Nicotinic acid	T46.7X1	T46.7X2	T46.7X3	T46.7X4	T46.7X5	T46.7X6
Nicotinyl alcohol	T46.7X1	T46.7X2	T46.7X3	T46.7X4	T46.7X5	T46.7X6
Nicoumalone	T45.511	T45.512	T45.513	T45.514	T45.515	T45.516
Nifedipine	T46.1X1	T46.1X2	T46.1X3	T46.1X4	T46.1X5	T46.1X6
Nifenazone	T39.2X1	T39.2X2	T39.2X3	T39.2X4	T39.2X5	T39.2X6
Nifuraldezone	T37.91	T37.92	T37.93	T37.94	T37.95	T37.96
Nifuratel	T37.8X1	T37.8X2	T37.8X3	T37.8X4	T37.8X5	T37.8X6
Nifurtimox	T37.3X1	T37.3X2	T37.3X3	T37.3X4	T37.3X5	T37.3X6
Nifurtoinol	T37.8X1	T37.8X2	T37.8X3	T37.8X4	T37.8X5	T37.8X6
Nightshade, deadly (solanum)—see also Belladonna	T62.2X1	T62.2X2	T62.2X3	T62.2X4	—	—
berry	T62.1X1	T62.1X2	T62.1X3	T62.1X4	—	—
Nikethamide	T50.7X1	T50.7X2	T50.7X3	T50.7X4	T50.7X5	T50.7X6
Nilstat	T36.7X1	T36.7X2	T36.7X3	T36.7X4	T36.7X5	T36.7X6
topical	T49.0X1	T49.0X2	T49.0X3	T49.0X4	T49.0X5	T49.0X6
Nilutamide	T38.6X1	T38.6X2	T38.6X3	T38.6X4	T38.6X5	T38.6X6
Nimesulide	T39.391	T39.392	T39.393	T39.394	T39.395	T39.396
Nimetazepam	T42.4X1	T42.4X2	T42.4X3	T42.4X4	T42.4X5	T42.4X6
Nimodipine	T46.1X1	T46.1X2	T46.1X3	T46.1X4	T46.1X5	T46.1X6
Nimorazole	T37.3X1	T37.3X2	T37.3X3	T37.3X4	T37.3X5	T37.3X6
Nimustine	T45.1X1	T45.1X2	T45.1X3	T45.1X4	T45.1X5	T45.1X6
Niridazole	T37.4X1	T37.4X2	T37.4X3	T37.4X4	T37.4X5	T37.4X6
Nisentil	T40.2X1	T40.2X2	T40.2X3	T40.2X4	T40.2X5	T40.2X6
Nisoldipine	T46.1X1	T46.1X2	T46.1X3	T46.1X4	T46.1X5	T46.1X6
Nitramine	T65.3X1	T65.3X2	T65.3X3	T65.3X4	—	—
Nitrate, organic	T46.3X1	T46.3X2	T46.3X3	T46.3X4	T46.3X5	T46.3X6
Nitrazepam	T42.4X1	T42.4X2	T42.4X3	T42.4X4	T42.4X5	T42.4X6
Nitrefazole	T50.6X1	T50.6X2	T50.6X3	T50.6X4	T50.6X5	T50.6X6
Nitrendipine	T46.1X1	T46.1X2	T46.1X3	T46.1X4	T46.1X5	T46.1X6
Nitric						
acid (liquid)	T54.2X1	T54.2X2	T54.2X3	T54.2X4	—	—
vapor	T59.891	T59.892	T59.893	T59.894	—	—
oxide (gas)	T59.0X1	T59.0X2	T59.0X3	T59.0X4	—	—
Nitrimidazine	T37.3X1	T37.3X2	T37.3X3	T37.3X4	T37.3X5	T37.3X6
Nitrite, amyl (medicinal) (vapor)	T46.3X1	T46.3X2	T46.3X3	T46.3X4	T46.3X5	T46.3X6
Nitroaniline	T65.3X1	T65.3X2	T65.3X3	T65.3X4	—	—
vapor	T59.891	T59.892	T59.893	T59.894	—	—
Nitrobenzene, nitrobenzol	T65.3X1	T65.3X2	T65.3X3	T65.3X4	—	—
vapor	T65.3X1	T65.3X2	T65.3X3	T65.3X4	—	—
Nitrocellulose	T65.891	T65.892	T65.893	T65.894	—	—
lacquer	T65.891	T65.892	T65.893	T65.894	—	—
Nitrodiphenyl	T65.3X1	T65.3X2	T65.3X3	T65.3X4	—	—
Nitrofural	T49.0X1	T49.0X2	T49.0X3	T49.0X4	T49.0X5	T49.0X6
Nitrofurantoin	T37.8X1	T37.8X2	T37.8X3	T37.8X4	T37.8X5	T37.8X6
Nitrofurazone	T49.0X1	T49.0X2	T49.0X3	T49.0X4	T49.0X5	T49.0X6
Nitrogen	T59.0X1	T59.0X2	T59.0X3	T59.0X4	—	—
mustard	T45.1X1	T45.1X2	T45.1X3	T45.1X4	T45.1X5	T45.1X6
Nitroglycerin, nitro-glycerol (medicinal)	T46.3X1	T46.3X2	T46.3X3	T46.3X4	T46.3X5	T46.3X6
nonmedicinal	T65.5X1	T65.5X2	T65.5X3	T65.5X4	—	—
fumes	T65.5X1	T65.5X2	T65.5X3	T65.5X4	—	—
Nitroglycol	T52.3X1	T52.3X2	T52.3X3	T52.3X4	—	—
Nitrohydrochloric acid	T54.2X1	T54.2X2	T54.2X3	T54.2X4	—	—
Nitromersol	T49.0X1	T49.0X2	T49.0X3	T49.0X4	T49.0X5	T49.0X6
Nitronaphthalene	T65.891	T65.892	T65.893	T65.894	—	—
Nitrophenol	T54.0X1	T54.0X2	T54.0X3	T54.0X4	—	—
Nitropropane	T52.8X1	T52.8X2	T52.8X3	T52.8X4	—	—
Nitroprusside	T46.5X1	T46.5X2	T46.5X3	T46.5X4	T46.5X5	T46.5X6

Substance	Poisoning, Accidental (unintentional)	Poisoning, Intentional self-harm	Poisoning, Assault	Poisoning, Undetermined	Adverse effect	Underdosing
Nitrosodimethylamine	T65.3X1	T65.3X2	T65.3X3	T65.3X4	—	—
Nitrothiazol	T37.4X1	T37.4X2	T37.4X3	T37.4X4	T37.4X5	T37.4X6
Nitrotoluene, nitrotoluol	T65.3X1	T65.3X2	T65.3X3	T65.3X4	—	—
vapor	T65.3X1	T65.3X2	T65.3X3	T65.3X4	—	—
Nitrous						
acid (liquid)	T54.2X1	T54.2X2	T54.2X3	T54.2X4	—	—
fumes	T59.891	T59.892	T59.893	T59.894	—	—
ether spirit	T46.3X1	T46.3X2	T46.3X3	T46.3X4	T46.3X5	T46.3X6
oxide	T41.0X1	T41.0X2	T41.0X3	T41.0X4	T41.0X5	T41.0X6
Nitroxoline	T37.8X1	T37.8X2	T37.8X3	T37.8X4	T37.8X5	T37.8X6
Nitrozone	T49.0X1	T49.0X2	T49.0X3	T49.0X4	T49.0X5	T49.0X6
Nizatidine	T47.0X1	T47.0X2	T47.0X3	T47.0X4	T47.0X5	T47.0X6
Nizofenone	T43.8X1	T43.8X2	T43.8X3	T43.8X4	T43.8X5	T43.8X6
Noctec	T42.6X1	T42.6X2	T42.6X3	T42.6X4	T42.6X5	T42.6X6
Noludar	T42.6X1	T42.6X2	T42.6X3	T42.6X4	T42.6X5	T42.6X6
Nomegestrol	T38.5X1	T38.5X2	T38.5X3	T38.5X4	T38.5X5	T38.5X6
Nomifensine	T43.291	T43.292	T43.293	T43.294	T43.295	T43.296
Nonoxinol	T49.8X1	T49.8X2	T49.8X3	T49.8X4	T49.8X5	T49.8X6
Nonylphenoxy (polyethoxy-ethanol)	T49.8X1	T49.8X2	T49.8X3	T49.8X4	T49.8X5	T49.8X6
Noptil	T42.3X1	T42.3X2	T42.3X3	T42.3X4	T42.3X5	T42.3X6
Noradrenaline	T44.4X1	T44.4X2	T44.4X3	T44.4X4	T44.4X5	T44.4X6
Noramidopyrine	T39.2X1	T39.2X2	T39.2X3	T39.2X4	T39.2X5	T39.2X6
methanesulfonate sodium	T39.2X1	T39.2X2	T39.2X3	T39.2X4	T39.2X5	T39.2X6
Norbormide	T60.4X1	T60.4X2	T60.4X3	T60.4X4	—	—
Nordazepam	T42.4X1	T42.4X2	T42.4X3	T42.4X4	T42.4X5	T42.4X6
Norepinephrine	T44.4X1	T44.4X2	T44.4X3	T44.4X4	T44.4X5	T44.4X6
Norethandrolone	T38.7X1	T38.7X2	T38.7X3	T38.7X4	T38.7X5	T38.7X6
Norethindrone	T38.4X1	T38.4X2	T38.4X3	T38.4X4	T38.4X5	T38.4X6
Norethisterone (acetate) (enantate)	T38.4X1	T38.4X2	T38.4X3	T38.4X4	T38.4X5	T38.4X6
with ethinylestradiol	T38.5X1	T38.5X2	T38.5X3	T38.5X4	T38.5X5	T38.5X6
Noretynodrel	T38.5X1	T38.5X2	T38.5X3	T38.5X4	T38.5X5	T38.5X6
Norfenefrine	T44.4X1	T44.4X2	T44.4X3	T44.4X4	T44.4X5	T44.4X6
Norfloxacin	T36.8X1	T36.8X2	T36.8X3	T36.8X4	T36.8X5	T36.8X6
Norgestrel	T38.4X1	T38.4X2	T38.4X3	T38.4X4	T38.4X5	T38.4X6
Norgestrienone	T38.4X1	T38.4X2	T38.4X3	T38.4X4	T38.4X5	T38.4X6
Norlestrin	T38.4X1	T38.4X2	T38.4X3	T38.4X4	T38.4X5	T38.4X6
Norlutin	T38.4X1	T38.4X2	T38.4X3	T38.4X4	T38.4X5	T38.4X6
Normal serum albumin (human), salt-poor	T45.8X1	T45.8X2	T45.8X3	T45.8X4	T45.8X5	T45.8X6
Normethandrone	T38.5X1	T38.5X2	T38.5X3	T38.5X4	T38.5X5	T38.5X6
Normison—see Benzodiazepines						
Normorphine	T40.2X1	T40.2X2	T40.2X3	T40.2X4	—	—
Norpseudoephedrine	T50.5X1	T50.5X2	T50.5X3	T50.5X4	T50.5X5	T50.5X6
Nortestosterone (furanpro pionate)	T38.7X1	T38.7X2	T38.7X3	T38.7X4	T38.7X5	T38.7X6
Nortriptyline	T43.011	T43.012	T43.013	T43.014	T43.015	T43.016
Noscapine	T48.3X1	T48.3X2	T48.3X3	T48.3X4	T48.3X5	T48.3X6
Nose preparations	T49.6X1	T49.6X2	T49.6X3	T49.6X4	T49.6X5	T49.6X6
Novobiocin	T36.5X1	T36.5X2	T36.5X3	T36.5X4	T36.5X5	T36.5X6
Novocain (infiltration) (topical)	T41.3X1	T41.3X2	T41.3X3	T41.3X4	T41.3X5	T41.3X6
nerve block (peripheral) (plexus)	T41.3X1	T41.3X2	T41.3X3	T41.3X4	T41.3X5	T41.3X6
spinal	T41.3X1	T41.3X2	T41.3X3	T41.3X4	T41.3X5	T41.3X6
Noxious foodstuff	T62.91	T62.92	T62.93	T62.94	—	—
specified NEC	T62.8X1	T62.8X2	T62.8X3	T62.8X4	—	—
Noxiptiline	T43.011	T43.012	T43.013	T43.014	T43.015	T43.016
Noxytiolin	T49.0X1	T49.0X2	T49.0X3	T49.0X4	T49.0X5	T49.0X6
NPH Iletin (insulin)	T38.3X1	T38.3X2	T38.3X3	T38.3X4	T38.3X5	T38.3X6
Numorphan	T40.2X1	T40.2X2	T40.2X3	T40.2X4	T40.2X5	T40.2X6
Nunol	T42.3X1	T42.3X2	T42.3X3	T42.3X4	T42.3X5	T42.3X6
Nupercaine (spinal anesthetic)	T41.3X1	T41.3X2	T41.3X3	T41.3X4	T41.3X5	T41.3X6
topical (surface)	T41.3X1	T41.3X2	T41.3X3	T41.3X4	T41.3X5	T41.3X6
Nutmeg oil (liniment)	T49.3X1	T49.3X2	T49.3X3	T49.3X4	T49.3X5	T49.3X6
Nutritional supplement	T50.901	T50.902	T50.903	T50.904	T50.905	T50.906
Nux vomica	T65.1X1	T65.1X2	T65.1X3	T65.1X4	—	—
Nydrazid	T37.1X1	T37.1X2	T37.1X3	T37.1X4	T37.1X5	T37.1X6
Nylidrin	T46.7X1	T46.7X2	T46.7X3	T46.7X4	T46.7X5	T46.7X6
Nystatin	T36.7X1	T36.7X2	T36.7X3	T36.7X4	T36.7X5	T36.7X6
topical	T49.0X1	T49.0X2	T49.0X3	T49.0X4	T49.0X5	T49.0X6
Nytol	T45.0X1	T45.0X2	T45.0X3	T45.0X4	T45.0X5	T45.0X6
O						
Obidoxime chloride	T50.6X1	T50.6X2	T50.6X3	T50.6X4	T50.6X5	T50.6X6
Octafonium (chloride)	T49.3X1	T49.3X2	T49.3X3	T49.3X4	T49.3X5	T49.3X6
Octamethyl pyrophos-phoramide	T60.0X1	T60.0X2	T60.0X3	T60.0X4	—	—
Octanoin	T50.991	T50.992	T50.993	T50.994	T50.995	T50.996
Octatropine methyl-bromide	T44.3X1	T44.3X2	T44.3X3	T44.3X4	T44.3X5	T44.3X6
Octotiamine	T45.2X1	T45.2X2	T45.2X3	T45.2X4	T45.2X5	T45.2X6
Octoxinol (9)	T49.8X1	T49.8X2	T49.8X3	T49.8X4	T49.8X5	T49.8X6
Octreotide	T38.991	T38.992	T38.993	T38.994	T38.995	T38.996
Octyl nitrite	T46.3X1	T46.3X2	T46.3X3	T46.3X4	T46.3X5	T46.3X6
Oestradiol	T38.5X1	T38.5X2	T38.5X3	T38.5X4	T38.5X5	T38.5X6
Oestriol	T38.5X1	T38.5X2	T38.5X3	T38.5X4	T38.5X5	T38.5X6
Oestrogen	T38.5X1	T38.5X2	T38.5X3	T38.5X4	T38.5X5	T38.5X6
Oestrone	T38.5X1	T38.5X2	T38.5X3	T38.5X4	T38.5X5	T38.5X6
Ofloxacin	T36.8X1	T36.8X2	T36.8X3	T36.8X4	T36.8X5	T36.8X6
Oil (of)	T65.891	T65.892	T65.893	T65.894	—	—
bitter almond	T62.8X1	T62.8X2	T62.8X3	T62.8X4	—	—
cloves	T49.7X1	T49.7X2	T49.7X3	T49.7X4	T49.7X5	T49.7X6
colors	T65.6X1	T65.6X2	T65.6X3	T65.6X4	—	—
fumes	T59.891	T59.892	T59.893	T59.894	—	—
lubricating	T52.0X1	T52.0X2	T52.0X3	T52.0X4	—	—
Niobe	T52.8X1	T52.8X2	T52.8X3	T52.8X4	—	—
vitriol (liquid)	T54.2X1	T54.2X2	T54.2X3	T54.2X4	—	—
fumes	T54.2X1	T54.2X2	T54.2X3	T54.2X4	—	—
wintergreen (bitter) NEC	T49.3X1	T49.3X2	T49.3X3	T49.3X4	T49.3X5	T49.3X6

Substance	Poisoning, Accidental (unintentional)	Poisoning, Intentional self-harm	Poisoning, Assault	Poisoning, Undetermined	Adverse effect	Underdosing
Oily preparation (for skin)	T49.3X1	T49.3X2	T49.3X3	T49.3X4	T49.3X5	T49.3X6
Ointment NEC	T49.3X1	T49.3X2	T49.3X3	T49.3X4	T49.3X5	T49.3X6
Olanzapine	T43.591	T43.592	T43.593	T43.594	T43.595	T43.596
Oleander	T62.2X1	T62.2X2	T62.2X3	T62.2X4	—	—
Oleandomycin	T36.3X1	T36.3X2	T36.3X3	T36.3X4	T36.3X5	T36.3X6
Oleandrin	T46.0X1	T46.0X2	T46.0X3	T46.0X4	T46.0X5	T46.0X6
Oleic acid	T46.6X1	T46.6X2	T46.6X3	T46.6X4	T46.6X5	T46.6X6
Oleovitamin A	T45.2X1	T45.2X2	T45.2X3	T45.2X4	T45.2X5	T45.2X6
Oleum ricini	T47.2X1	T47.2X2	T47.2X3	T47.2X4	T47.2X5	T47.2X6
Olive oil (medicinal) NEC	T47.4X1	T47.4X2	T47.4X3	T47.4X4	T47.4X5	T47.4X6
Olivomycin	T45.1X1	T45.1X2	T45.1X3	T45.1X4	T45.1X5	T45.1X6
Olsalazine	T47.8X1	T47.8X2	T47.8X3	T47.8X4	T47.8X5	T47.8X6
Omeprazole	T47.1X1	T47.1X2	T47.1X3	T47.1X4	T47.1X5	T47.1X6
OMPA	T60.0X1	T60.0X2	T60.0X3	T60.0X4	—	—
Oncovin	T45.1X1	T45.1X2	T45.1X3	T45.1X4	T45.1X5	T45.1X6
Ondansetron	T45.0X1	T45.0X2	T45.0X3	T45.0X4	T45.0X5	T45.0X6
Ophthaine	T41.3X1	T41.3X2	T41.3X3	T41.3X4	T41.3X5	T41.3X6
Ophthetic	T41.3X1	T41.3X2	T41.3X3	T41.3X4	T41.3X5	T41.3X6
Opiate NEC	T40.601	T40.602	T40.603	T40.604	T40.605	T40.606
antagonists	T50.7X1	T50.7X2	T50.7X3	T50.7X4	T50.7X5	T50.7X6
Opioid NEC	T40.2X1	T40.2X2	T40.2X3	T40.2X4	T40.2X5	T40.2X6
Opipramol	T43.011	T43.012	T43.013	T43.014	T43.015	T43.016
Opium alkaloids (total)	T40.0X1	T40.0X2	T40.0X3	T40.0X4	T40.0X5	T40.0X6
standardized powdered	T40.0X1	T40.0X2	T40.0X3	T40.0X4	T40.0X5	T40.0X6
tincture (camphorated)	T40.0X1	T40.0X2	T40.0X3	T40.0X4	T40.0X5	T40.0X6
Oracon	T38.4X1	T38.4X2	T38.4X3	T38.4X4	T38.4X5	T38.4X6
Oragrafin	T50.8X1	T50.8X2	T50.8X3	T50.8X4	T50.8X5	T50.8X6
Oral contraceptives	T38.4X1	T38.4X2	T38.4X3	T38.4X4	T38.4X5	T38.4X6
Oral rehydration salts	T50.3X1	T50.3X2	T50.3X3	T50.3X4	T50.3X5	T50.3X6
Orazamide	T50.991	T50.992	T50.993	T50.994	T50.995	T50.996
Orciprenaline	T48.291	T48.292	T48.293	T48.294	T48.295	T48.296
Organidin	T48.4X1	T48.4X2	T48.4X3	T48.4X4	T48.4X5	T48.4X6
Organonitrate NEC	T46.3X1	T46.3X2	T46.3X3	T46.3X4	T46.3X5	T46.3X6
Organophosphates	T60.0X1	T60.0X2	T60.0X3	T60.0X4	—	—
Orimune	T50.B91	T50.B92	T50.B93	T50.B94	T50.B95	T50.B96
Orinase	T38.3X1	T38.3X2	T38.3X3	T38.3X4	T38.3X5	T38.3X6
Ormeloxifene	T38.6X1	T38.6X2	T38.6X3	T38.6X4	T38.6X5	T38.6X6
Ornidazole	T37.3X1	T37.3X2	T37.3X3	T37.3X4	T37.3X5	T37.3X6
Ornithine aspartate	T50.991	T50.992	T50.993	T50.994	T50.995	T50.996
Ornoprostil	T47.1X1	T47.1X2	T47.1X3	T47.1X4	T47.1X5	T47.1X6
Orphenadrine (hydrochloride)	T42.8X1	T42.8X2	T42.8X3	T42.8X4	T42.8X5	T42.8X6
Ortal (sodium)	T42.3X1	T42.3X2	T42.3X3	T42.3X4	T42.3X5	T42.3X6
Orthoboric acid	T49.0X1	T49.0X2	T49.0X3	T49.0X4	T49.0X5	T49.0X6
ENT agent	T49.6X1	T49.6X2	T49.6X3	T49.6X4	T49.6X5	T49.6X6
ophthalmic preparation	T49.5X1	T49.5X2	T49.5X3	T49.5X4	T49.5X5	T49.5X6
Orthocaine	T41.3X1	T41.3X2	T41.3X3	T41.3X4	T41.3X5	T41.3X6
Orthodichlorobenzene	T53.7X1	T53.7X2	T53.7X3	T53.7X4	—	—
Ortho-Novum	T38.4X1	T38.4X2	T38.4X3	T38.4X4	T38.4X5	T38.4X6
Orthotolidine (reagent)	T54.2X1	T54.2X2	T54.2X3	T54.2X4	—	—

Substance	Poisoning, Accidental (unintentional)	Poisoning, Intentional self-harm	Poisoning, Assault	Poisoning, Undetermined	Adverse effect	Underdosing
Osmic acid (liquid)	T54.2X1	T54.2X2	T54.2X3	T54.2X4	—	—
fumes	T54.2X1	T54.2X2	T54.2X3	T54.2X4	—	—
Osmotic diuretics	T50.2X1	T50.2X2	T50.2X3	T50.2X4	T50.2X5	T50.2X6
Otilonium bromide	T44.3X1	T44.3X2	T44.3X3	T44.3X4	T44.3X5	T44.3X6
Otorhinolaryngological drug NEC	T49.6X1	T49.6X2	T49.6X3	T49.6X4	T49.6X5	T49.6X6
Ouabain(e)	T46.0X1	T46.0X2	T46.0X3	T46.0X4	T46.0X5	T46.0X6
Ovarian						
hormone	T38.5X1	T38.5X2	T38.5X3	T38.5X4	T38.5X5	T38.5X6
stimulant	T38.5X1	T38.5X2	T38.5X3	T38.5X4	T38.5X5	T38.5X6
Ovral	T38.4X1	T38.4X2	T38.4X3	T38.4X4	T38.4X5	T38.4X6
Ovulen	T38.4X1	T38.4X2	T38.4X3	T38.4X4	T38.4X5	T38.4X6
Oxacillin	T36.0X1	T36.0X2	T36.0X3	T36.0X4	T36.0X5	T36.0X6
Oxalic acid	T54.2X1	T54.2X2	T54.2X3	T54.2X4	—	—
ammonium salt	T50.991	T50.992	T50.993	T50.994	T50.995	T50.996
Oxamniquine	T37.4X1	T37.4X2	T37.4X3	T37.4X4	T37.4X5	T37.4X6
Oxanamide	T43.591	T43.592	T43.593	T43.594	T43.595	T43.596
Oxandrolone	T38.7X1	T38.7X2	T38.7X3	T38.7X4	T38.7X5	T38.7X6
Oxantel	T37.4X1	T37.4X2	T37.4X3	T37.4X4	T37.4X5	T37.4X6
Oxapium iodide	T44.3X1	T44.3X2	T44.3X3	T44.3X4	T44.3X5	T44.3X6
Oxaprotiline	T43.021	T43.022	T43.023	T43.024	T43.025	T43.026
Oxaprozin	T39.311	T39.312	T39.313	T39.314	T39.315	T39.316
Oxatomide	T45.0X1	T45.0X2	T45.0X3	T45.0X4	T45.0X5	T45.0X6
Oxazepam	T42.4X1	T42.4X2	T42.4X3	T42.4X4	T42.4X5	T42.4X6
Oxazimedrine	T50.5X1	T50.5X2	T50.5X3	T50.5X4	T50.5X5	T50.5X6
Oxazolam	T42.4X1	T42.4X2	T42.4X3	T42.4X4	T42.4X5	T42.4X6
Oxazolidine derivatives	T42.2X1	T42.2X2	T42.2X3	T42.2X4	T42.2X5	T42.2X6
Oxazolidinedione (derivative)	T42.2X1	T42.2X2	T42.2X3	T42.2X4	T42.2X5	T42.2X6
Ox bile extract	T47.5X1	T47.5X2	T47.5X3	T47.5X4	T47.5X5	T47.5X6
Oxcarbazepine	T42.1X1	T42.1X2	T42.1X3	T42.1X4	T42.1X5	T42.1X6
Oxedrine	T44.4X1	T44.4X2	T44.4X3	T44.4X4	T44.4X5	T44.4X6
Oxeladin (citrate)	T48.3X1	T48.3X2	T48.3X3	T48.3X4	T48.3X5	T48.3X6
Oxendolone	T38.5X1	T38.5X2	T38.5X3	T38.5X4	T38.5X5	T38.5X6
Oxetacaine	T41.3X1	T41.3X2	T41.3X3	T41.3X4	T41.3X5	T41.3X6
Oxethazine	T41.3X1	T41.3X2	T41.3X3	T41.3X4	T41.3X5	T41.3X6
Oxetorone	T39.8X1	T39.8X2	T39.8X3	T39.8X4	T39.8X5	T39.8X6
Oxiconazole	T49.0X1	T49.0X2	T49.0X3	T49.0X4	T49.0X5	T49.0X6
Oxidizing agent NEC	T54.91	T54.92	T54.93	T54.94	—	—
Oxipurinol	T50.4X1	T50.4X2	T50.4X3	T50.4X4	T50.4X5	T50.4X6
Oxitriptan	T43.291	T43.292	T43.293	T43.294	T43.295	T43.296
Oxitropium bromide	T48.6X1	T48.6X2	T48.6X3	T48.6X4	T48.6X5	T48.6X6
Oxodipine	T46.1X1	T46.1X2	T46.1X3	T46.1X4	T46.1X5	T46.1X6
Oxolamine	T48.3X1	T48.3X2	T48.3X3	T48.3X4	T48.3X5	T48.3X6
Oxolinic acid	T37.8X1	T37.8X2	T37.8X3	T37.8X4	T37.8X5	T37.8X6
Oxomemazine	T43.3X1	T43.3X2	T43.3X3	T43.3X4	T43.3X5	T43.3X6
Oxophenarsine	T37.3X1	T37.3X2	T37.3X3	T37.3X4	T37.3X5	T37.3X6
Oxprenolol	T44.7X1	T44.7X2	T44.7X3	T44.7X4	T44.7X5	T44.7X6
Oxsoralen	T49.3X1	T49.3X2	T49.3X3	T49.3X4	T49.3X5	T49.3X6
Oxtriphylline	T48.6X1	T48.6X2	T48.6X3	T48.6X4	T48.6X5	T48.6X6

Substance	Poisoning, Accidental (unintentional)	Poisoning, Intentional self-harm	Poisoning, Assault	Poisoning, Undetermined	Adverse effect	Underdosing
Oxybate sodium	T41.291	T41.292	T41.293	T41.294	T41.295	T41.296
Oxybuprocaine	T41.3X1	T41.3X2	T41.3X3	T41.3X4	T41.3X5	T41.3X6
Oxybutynin	T44.3X1	T44.3X2	T44.3X3	T44.3X4	T44.3X5	T44.3X6
Oxychlorosene	T49.0X1	T49.0X2	T49.0X3	T49.0X4	T49.0X5	T49.0X6
Oxycodone	T40.2X1	T40.2X2	T40.2X3	T40.2X4	T40.2X5	T40.2X6
Oxyfedrine	T46.3X1	T46.3X2	T46.3X3	T46.3X4	T46.3X5	T46.3X6
Oxygen	T41.5X1	T41.5X2	T41.5X3	T41.5X4	T41.5X5	T41.5X6
Oxylone	T49.0X1	T49.0X2	T49.0X3	T49.0X4	T49.0X5	T49.0X6
ophthalmic preparation	T49.5X1	T49.5X2	T49.5X3	T49.5X4	T49.5X5	T49.5X6
Oxymesterone	T38.7X1	T38.7X2	T38.7X3	T38.7X4	T38.7X5	T38.7X6
Oxymetazoline	T48.5X1	T48.5X2	T48.5X3	T48.5X4	T48.5X5	T48.5X6
Oxymetholone	T38.7X1	T38.7X2	T38.7X3	T38.7X4	T38.7X5	T38.7X6
Oxymorphone	T40.2X1	T40.2X2	T40.2X3	T40.2X4	T40.2X5	T40.2X6
Oxypertine	T43.591	T43.592	T43.593	T43.594	T43.595	T43.596
Oxyphenbutazone	T39.2X1	T39.2X2	T39.2X3	T39.2X4	T39.2X5	T39.2X6
Oxyphencyclimine	T44.3X1	T44.3X2	T44.3X3	T44.3X4	T44.3X5	T44.3X6
Oxyphenisatine	T47.2X1	T47.2X2	T47.2X3	T47.2X4	T47.2X5	T47.2X6
Oxyphenonium bromide	T44.3X1	T44.3X2	T44.3X3	T44.3X4	T44.3X5	T44.3X6
Oxypolygelatin	T45.8X1	T45.8X2	T45.8X3	T45.8X4	T45.8X5	T45.8X6
Oxyquinoline (derivatives)	T37.8X1	T37.8X2	T37.8X3	T37.8X4	T37.8X5	T37.8X6
Oxytetracycline	T36.4X1	T36.4X2	T36.4X3	T36.4X4	T36.4X5	T36.4X6
Oxytocic drug NEC	T48.0X1	T48.0X2	T48.0X3	T48.0X4	T48.0X5	T48.0X6
Oxytocin (synthetic)	T48.0X1	T48.0X2	T48.0X3	T48.0X4	T48.0X5	T48.0X6
Ozone	T59.891	T59.892	T59.893	T59.894	—	—
P						
PABA	T49.3X1	T49.3X2	T49.3X3	T49.3X4	T49.3X5	T49.3X6
Packed red cells	T45.8X1	T45.8X2	T45.8X3	T45.8X4	T45.8X5	T45.8X6
Padimate	T49.3X1	T49.3X2	T49.3X3	T49.3X4	T49.3X5	T49.3X6
Paint NEC	T65.6X1	T65.6X2	T65.6X3	T65.6X4	—	—
cleaner	T52.91	T52.92	T52.93	T52.94	—	—
fumes NEC	T59.891	T59.892	T59.893	T59.894	—	—
lead (fumes)	T56.0X1	T56.0X2	T56.0X3	T56.0X4	—	—
solvent NEC	T52.8X1	T52.8X2	T52.8X3	T52.8X4	—	—
stripper	T52.8X1	T52.8X2	T52.8X3	T52.8X4	—	—
Palfium	T40.2X1	T40.2X2	T40.2X3	T40.2X4	—	—
Palm kernel oil	T50.991	T50.992	T50.993	T50.994	T50.995	T50.996
Paludrine	T37.2X1	T37.2X2	T37.2X3	T37.2X4	T37.2X5	T37.2X6
PAM (pralidoxime)	T50.6X1	T50.6X2	T50.6X3	T50.6X4	T50.6X5	T50.6X6
Pamaquine (naphthoute)	T37.2X1	T37.2X2	T37.2X3	T37.2X4	T37.2X5	T37.2X6
Panadol	T39.1X1	T39.1X2	T39.1X3	T39.1X4	T39.1X5	T39.1X6
Pancreatic						
digestive secretion stimulant	T47.8X1	T47.8X2	T47.8X3	T47.8X4	T47.8X5	T47.8X6
dornase	T45.3X1	T45.3X2	T45.3X3	T45.3X4	T45.3X5	T45.3X6
Pancreatin	T47.5X1	T47.5X2	T47.5X3	T47.5X4	T47.5X5	T47.5X6
Pancrelipase	T47.5X1	T47.5X2	T47.5X3	T47.5X4	T47.5X5	T47.5X6
Pancuronium (bromide)	T48.1X1	T48.1X2	T48.1X3	T48.1X4	T48.1X5	T48.1X6
Pangamic acid	T45.2X1	T45.2X2	T45.2X3	T45.2X4	T45.2X5	T45.2X6
Panthenol	T45.2X1	T45.2X2	T45.2X3	T45.2X4	T45.2X5	T45.2X6
topical	T49.8X1	T49.8X2	T49.8X3	T49.8X4	T49.8X5	T49.8X6

Substance	Poisoning, Accidental (unintentional)	Poisoning, Intentional self-harm	Poisoning, Assault	Poisoning, Undetermined	Adverse effect	Underdosing
Pantopon	T40.0X1	T40.0X2	T40.0X3	T40.0X4	T40.0X5	T40.0X6
Pantothenic acid	T45.2X1	T45.2X2	T45.2X3	T45.2X4	T45.2X5	T45.2X6
Panwarfin	T45.511	T45.512	T45.513	T45.514	T45.515	T45.516
Papain	T47.5X1	T47.5X2	T47.5X3	T47.5X4	T47.5X5	T47.5X6
digestant	T47.5X1	T47.5X2	T47.5X3	T47.5X4	T47.5X5	T47.5X6
Papaveretum	T40.0X1	T40.0X2	T40.0X3	T40.0X4	T40.0X5	T40.0X6
Papaverine	T44.3X1	T44.3X2	T44.3X3	T44.3X4	T44.3X5	T44.3X6
Para-acetamidophenol	T39.1X1	T39.1X2	T39.1X3	T39.1X4	T39.1X5	T39.1X6
Para-aminobenzoic acid	T49.3X1	T49.3X2	T49.3X3	T49.3X4	T49.3X5	T49.3X6
Para-aminophenol derivatives	T39.1X1	T39.1X2	T39.1X3	T39.1X4	T39.1X5	T39.1X6
Para-aminosalicylic acid	T37.1X1	T37.1X2	T37.1X3	T37.1X4	T37.1X5	T37.1X6
Paracetaldehyde	T42.6X1	T42.6X2	T42.6X3	T42.6X4	T42.6X5	T42.6X6
Paracetamol	T39.1X1	T39.1X2	T39.1X3	T39.1X4	T39.1X5	T39.1X6
Parachlorophenol (camphorated)	T49.0X1	T49.0X2	T49.0X3	T49.0X4	T49.0X5	T49.0X6
Paracodin	T40.2X1	T40.2X2	T40.2X3	T40.2X4	T40.2X5	T40.2X6
Paradione	T42.2X1	T42.2X2	T42.2X3	T42.2X4	T42.2X5	T42.2X6
Paraffin(s) (wax)	T52.0X1	T52.0X2	T52.0X3	T52.0X4	—	—
liquid (medicinal)	T47.4X1	T47.4X2	T47.4X3	T47.4X4	T47.4X5	T47.4X6
nonmedicinal	T52.0X1	T52.0X2	T52.0X3	T52.0X4	—	—
Paraformaldehyde	T60.3X1	T60.3X2	T60.3X3	T60.3X4	—	—
Paraldehyde	T42.6X1	T42.6X2	T42.6X3	T42.6X4	T42.6X5	T42.6X6
Paramethadione	T42.2X1	T42.2X2	T42.2X3	T42.2X4	T42.2X5	T42.2X6
Paramethasone	T38.0X1	T38.0X2	T38.0X3	T38.0X4	T38.0X5	T38.0X6
acetate	T49.0X1	T49.0X2	T49.0X3	T49.0X4	T49.0X5	T49.0X6
Paraoxon	T60.0X1	T60.0X2	T60.0X3	T60.0X4	—	—
Paraquat	T60.3X1	T60.3X2	T60.3X3	T60.3X4	—	—
Parasympatholytic NEC	T44.3X1	T44.3X2	T44.3X3	T44.3X4	T44.3X5	T44.3X6
Parasympathomimetic drug NEC	T44.1X1	T44.1X2	T44.1X3	T44.1X4	T44.1X5	T44.1X6
Parathion	T60.0X1	T60.0X2	T60.0X3	T60.0X4	—	—
Parathormone	T50.991	T50.992	T50.993	T50.994	T50.995	T50.996
Parathyroid extract	T50.991	T50.992	T50.993	T50.994	T50.995	T50.996
Paratyphoid vaccine	T50.A91	T50.A92	T50.A93	T50.A94	T50.A95	T50.A96
Paredrine	T44.4X1	T44.4X2	T44.4X3	T44.4X4	T44.4X5	T44.4X6
Paregoric	T40.0X1	T40.0X2	T40.0X3	T40.0X4	T40.0X5	T40.0X6
Pargyline	T46.5X1	T46.5X2	T46.5X3	T46.5X4	T46.5X5	T46.5X6
Paris green	T57.0X1	T57.0X2	T57.0X3	T57.0X4	—	—
insecticide	T57.0X1	T57.0X2	T57.0X3	T57.0X4	—	—
Parnate	T43.1X1	T43.1X2	T43.1X3	T43.1X4	T43.1X5	T43.1X6
Paromomycin	T36.5X1	T36.5X2	T36.5X3	T36.5X4	T36.5X5	T36.5X6
Paroxypropione	T45.1X1	T45.1X2	T45.1X3	T45.1X4	T45.1X5	T45.1X6
Parzone	T40.2X1	T40.2X2	T40.2X3	T40.2X4	T40.2X5	T40.2X6
PAS	T37.1X1	T37.1X2	T37.1X3	T37.1X4	T37.1X5	T37.1X6
Pasiniazid	T37.1X1	T37.1X2	T37.1X3	T37.1X4	T37.1X5	T37.1X6
PBB (polybrominated biphenyls)	T65.891	T65.892	T65.893	T65.894	—	—
PCB	T65.891	T65.892	T65.893	T65.894	—	—
PCP						
meaning pentachlorophenol	T60.1X1	T60.1X2	T60.1X3	T60.1X4	—	—

Substance	Poisoning, Accidental (unintentional)	Poisoning, Intentional self-harm	Poisoning, Assault	Poisoning, Undetermined	Adverse effect	Underdosing
PCP — *Continued*						
fungicide	T60.3X1	T60.3X2	T60.3X3	T60.3X4	—	—
herbicide	T60.3X1	T60.3X2	T60.3X3	T60.3X4	—	—
insecticide	T60.1X1	T60.1X2	T60.1X3	T60.1X4	—	—
meaning phencyclidine	T40.991	T40.992	T40.993	T40.994	—	—
Peach kernel oil (emulsion)	T47.4X1	T47.4X2	T47.4X3	T47.4X4	T47.4X5	T47.4X6
Peanut oil (emulsion) NEC	T47.4X1	T47.4X2	T47.4X3	T47.4X4	T47.4X5	T47.4X6
topical	T49.3X1	T49.3X2	T49.3X3	T49.3X4	T49.3X5	T49.3X6
Pearly Gates (morning glory seeds)	T40.991	T40.992	T40.993	T40.994	—	—
Pecazine	T43.3X1	T43.3X2	T43.3X3	T43.3X4	T43.3X5	T43.3X6
Pectin	T47.6X1	T47.6X2	T47.6X3	T47.6X4	T47.6X5	T47.6X6
Pefloxacin	T37.8X1	T37.8X2	T37.8X3	T37.8X4	T37.8X5	T37.8X6
Pegademase, bovine	T50.Z91	T50.Z92	T50.Z93	T50.Z94	T50.Z95	T50.Z96
Pelletierine tannate	T37.4X1	T37.4X2	T37.4X3	T37.4X4	T37.4X5	T37.4X6
Pemirolast (potassium)	T48.6X1	T48.6X2	T48.6X3	T48.6X4	T48.6X5	T48.6X6
Pemoline	T50.7X1	T50.7X2	T50.7X3	T50.7X4	T50.7X5	T50.7X6
Pempidine	T44.2X1	T44.2X2	T44.2X3	T44.2X4	T44.2X5	T44.2X6
Penamecillin	T36.0X1	T36.0X2	T36.0X3	T36.0X4	T36.0X5	T36.0X6
Penbutolol	T44.7X1	T44.7X2	T44.7X3	T44.7X4	T44.7X5	T44.7X6
Penethamate	T36.0X1	T36.0X2	T36.0X3	T36.0X4	T36.0X5	T36.0X6
Penfluridol	T43.591	T43.592	T43.593	T43.594	T43.595	T43.596
Penflutizide	T50.2X1	T50.2X2	T50.2X3	T50.2X4	T50.2X5	T50.2X6
Pengitoxin	T46.0X1	T46.0X2	T46.0X3	T46.0X4	T46.0X5	T46.0X6
Penicillamine	T50.6X1	T50.6X2	T50.6X3	T50.6X4	T50.6X5	T50.6X6
Penicillin (any)	T36.0X1	T36.0X2	T36.0X3	T36.0X4	T36.0X5	T36.0X6
Penicillinase	T45.3X1	T45.3X2	T45.3X3	T45.3X4	T45.3X5	T45.3X6
Penicilloyl polylysine	T50.8X1	T50.8X2	T50.8X3	T50.8X4	T50.8X5	T50.8X6
Penimepicycline	T36.4X1	T36.4X2	T36.4X3	T36.4X4	T36.4X5	T36.4X6
Pentachloroethane	T53.6X1	T53.6X2	T53.6X3	T53.6X4	—	—
Pentachloronaphthalene	T53.7X1	T53.7X2	T53.7X3	T53.7X4	—	—
Pentachlorophenol (pesticide)	T60.1X1	T60.1X2	T60.1X3	T60.1X4	—	—
fungicide	T60.3X1	T60.3X2	T60.3X3	T60.3X4	—	—
herbicide	T60.3X1	T60.3X2	T60.3X3	T60.3X4	—	—
insecticide	T60.1X1	T60.1X2	T60.1X3	T60.1X4	—	—
Pentaerythritol	T46.3X1	T46.3X2	T46.3X3	T46.3X4	T46.3X5	T46.3X6
chloral	T42.6X1	T42.6X2	T42.6X3	T42.6X4	T42.6X5	T42.6X6
tetranitrate NEC	T46.3X1	T46.3X2	T46.3X3	T46.3X4	T46.3X5	T46.3X6
Pentaerythrityl tetranitrate	T46.3X1	T46.3X2	T46.3X3	T46.3X4	T46.3X5	T46.3X6
Pentagastrin	T50.8X1	T50.8X2	T50.8X3	T50.8X4	T50.8X5	T50.8X6
Pentalin	T53.6X1	T53.6X2	T53.6X3	T53.6X4	—	—
Pentamethonium bromide	T44.2X1	T44.2X2	T44.2X3	T44.2X4	T44.2X5	T44.2X6
Pentamidine	T37.3X1	T37.3X2	T37.3X3	T37.3X4	T37.3X5	T37.3X6
Pentanol	T51.3X1	T51.3X2	T51.3X3	T51.3X4	—	—
Pentapyrrolinium (bitartrate)	T44.2X1	T44.2X2	T44.2X3	T44.2X4	T44.2X5	T44.2X6
Pentaquine	T37.2X1	T37.2X2	T37.2X3	T37.2X4	T37.2X5	T37.2X6
Pentazocine	T40.4X1	T40.4X2	T40.4X3	T40.4X4	T40.4X5	T40.4X6
Pentetrazole	T50.7X1	T50.7X2	T50.7X3	T50.7X4	T50.7X5	T50.7X6
Penthienate bromide	T44.3X1	T44.3X2	T44.3X3	T44.3X4	T44.3X5	T44.3X6

Substance	Poisoning, Accidental (unintentional)	Poisoning, Intentional self-harm	Poisoning, Assault	Poisoning, Undetermined	Adverse effect	Underdosing
Pentifylline	T46.7X1	T46.7X2	T46.7X3	T46.7X4	T46.7X5	T46.7X6
Pentobarbital	T42.3X1	T42.3X2	T42.3X3	T42.3X4	T42.3X5	T42.3X6
sodium	T42.3X1	T42.3X2	T42.3X3	T42.3X4	T42.3X5	T42.3X6
Pentobarbitone	T42.3X1	T42.3X2	T42.3X3	T42.3X4	T42.3X5	T42.3X6
Pentolonium tartrate	T44.2X1	T44.2X2	T44.2X3	T44.2X4	T44.2X5	T44.2X6
Pentosan polysulfate (sodium)	T39.8X1	T39.8X2	T39.8X3	T39.8X4	T39.8X5	T39.8X6
Pentostatin	T45.1X1	T45.1X2	T45.1X3	T45.1X4	T45.1X5	T45.1X6
Pentothal	T41.1X1	T41.1X2	T41.1X3	T41.1X4	T41.1X5	T41.1X6
Pentoxifylline	T46.7X1	T46.7X2	T46.7X3	T46.7X4	T46.7X5	T46.7X6
Pentoxyverine	T48.3X1	T48.3X2	T48.3X3	T48.3X4	T48.3X5	T48.3X6
Pentrinat	T46.3X1	T46.3X2	T46.3X3	T46.3X4	T46.3X5	T46.3X6
Pentylenetetrazole	T50.7X1	T50.7X2	T50.7X3	T50.7X4	T50.7X5	T50.7X6
Pentylsalicylamide	T37.1X1	T37.1X2	T37.1X3	T37.1X4	T37.1X5	T37.1X6
Pentymal	T42.3X1	T42.3X2	T42.3X3	T42.3X4	T42.3X5	T42.3X6
Peplomycin	T45.1X1	T45.1X2	T45.1X3	T45.1X4	T45.1X5	T45.1X6
Peppermint (oil)	T47.5X1	T47.5X2	T47.5X3	T47.5X4	T47.5X5	T47.5X6
Pepsin	T47.5X1	T47.5X2	T47.5X3	T47.5X4	T47.5X5	T47.5X6
digestant	T47.5X1	T47.5X2	T47.5X3	T47.5X4	T47.5X5	T47.5X6
Pepstatin	T47.1X1	T47.1X2	T47.1X3	T47.1X4	T47.1X5	T47.1X6
Peptavlon	T50.8X1	T50.8X2	T50.8X3	T50.8X4	T50.8X5	T50.8X6
Perazine	T43.3X1	T43.3X2	T43.3X3	T43.3X4	T43.3X5	T43.3X6
Percaine (spinal)	T41.3X1	T41.3X2	T41.3X3	T41.3X4	T41.3X5	T41.3X6
topical (surface)	T41.3X1	T41.3X2	T41.3X3	T41.3X4	T41.3X5	T41.3X6
Perchloroethylene	T53.3X1	T53.3X2	T53.3X3	T53.3X4	—	—
medicinal	T37.4X1	T37.4X2	T37.4X3	T37.4X4	T37.4X5	T37.4X6
vapor	T53.3X1	T53.3X2	T53.3X3	T53.3X4	—	—
Percodan	T40.2X1	T40.2X2	T40.2X3	T40.2X4	T40.2X5	T40.2X6
Percogesic—see also acetaminophen	T45.0X1	T45.0X2	T45.0X3	T45.0X4	T45.0X5	T45.0X6
Percorten	T38.0X1	T38.0X2	T38.0X3	T38.0X4	T38.0X5	T38.0X6
Pergolide	T42.8X1	T42.8X2	T42.8X3	T42.8X4	T42.8X5	T42.8X6
Pergonal	T38.811	T38.812	T38.813	T38.814	T38.815	T38.816
Perhexilene	T46.3X1	T46.3X2	T46.3X3	T46.3X4	T46.3X5	T46.3X6
Perhexiline (maleate)	T46.3X1	T46.3X2	T46.3X3	T46.3X4	T46.3X5	T46.3X6
Periactin	T45.0X1	T45.0X2	T45.0X3	T45.0X4	T45.0X5	T45.0X6
Periciazine	T43.3X1	T43.3X2	T43.3X3	T43.3X4	T43.3X5	T43.3X6
Periclor	T42.6X1	T42.6X2	T42.6X3	T42.6X4	T42.6X5	T42.6X6
Perindopril	T46.4X1	T46.4X2	T46.4X3	T46.4X4	T46.4X5	T46.4X6
Perisoxal	T39.8X1	T39.8X2	T39.8X3	T39.8X4	T39.8X5	T39.8X6
Peritoneal dialysis solution	T50.3X1	T50.3X2	T50.3X3	T50.3X4	T50.3X5	T50.3X6
Peritrate	T46.3X1	T46.3X2	T46.3X3	T46.3X4	T46.3X5	T46.3X6
Perlapine	T42.4X1	T42.4X2	T42.4X3	T42.4X4	T42.4X5	T42.4X6
Permanganate	T65.891	T65.892	T65.893	T65.894	—	—
Permethrin	T60.1X1	T60.1X2	T60.1X3	T60.1X4	—	—
Pernocton	T42.3X1	T42.3X2	T42.3X3	T42.3X4	T42.3X5	T42.3X6
Pernoston	T42.3X1	T42.3X2	T42.3X3	T42.3X4	T42.3X5	T42.3X6
Peronine	T40.2X1	T40.2X2	T40.2X3	T40.2X4	—	—
Perphenazine	T43.3X1	T43.3X2	T43.3X3	T43.3X4	T43.3X5	T43.3X6
Pertofrane	T43.011	T43.012	T43.013	T43.014	T43.015	T43.016

Substance	Poisoning, Accidental (unintentional)	Poisoning, Intentional self-harm	Poisoning, Assault	Poisoning, Undetermined	Adverse effect	Underdosing
Pertussis						
immune serum (human)	T50.Z11	T50.Z12	T50.Z13	T50.Z14	T50.Z15	T50.Z16
vaccine (with diphtheria toxoid) (with tetanus toxoid)	T50.A11	T50.A12	T50.A13	T50.A14	T50.A15	T50.A16
Peruvian balsam	T49.0X1	T49.0X2	T49.0X3	T49.0X4	T49.0X5	T49.0X6
Peruvoside	T46.0X1	T46.0X2	T46.0X3	T46.0X4	T46.0X5	T46.0X6
Pesticide (dust) (fumes) (vapor) NEC	T60.91	T60.92	T60.93	T60.94	—	—
arsenic	T57.0X1	T57.0X2	T57.0X3	T57.0X4	—	—
chlorinated	T60.1X1	T60.1X2	T60.1X3	T60.1X4	—	—
cyanide	T65.0X1	T65.0X2	T65.0X3	T65.0X4	—	—
kerosene	T52.0X1	T52.0X2	T52.0X3	T52.0X4	—	—
mixture (of compounds)	T60.91	T60.92	T60.93	T60.94	—	—
naphthalene	T60.2X1	T60.2X2	T60.2X3	T60.2X4	—	—
organochlorine (compounds)	T60.1X1	T60.1X2	T60.1X3	T60.1X4	—	—
petroleum (distillate) (products) NEC	T60.8X1	T60.8X2	T60.8X3	T60.8X4	—	—
specified ingredient NEC	T60.8X1	T60.8X2	T60.8X3	T60.8X4	—	—
strychnine	T65.1X1	T65.1X2	T65.1X3	T65.1X4	—	—
thallium	T60.4X1	T60.4X2	T60.4X3	T60.4X4	—	—
Pethidine	T40.4X1	T40.4X2	T40.4X3	T40.4X4	T40.4X5	T40.4X6
Petrichloral	T42.6X1	T42.6X2	T42.6X3	T42.6X4	T42.6X5	T42.6X6
Petrol	T52.0X1	T52.0X2	T52.0X3	T52.0X4	—	—
vapor	T52.0X1	T52.0X2	T52.0X3	T52.0X4	—	—
Petrolatum	T49.3X1	T49.3X2	T49.3X3	T49.3X4	T49.3X5	T49.3X6
hydrophilic	T49.3X1	T49.3X2	T49.3X3	T49.3X4	T49.3X5	T49.3X6
liquid	T47.4X1	T47.4X2	T47.4X3	T47.4X4	T47.4X5	T47.4X6
topical	T49.3X1	T49.3X2	T49.3X3	T49.3X4	T49.3X5	T49.3X6
nonmedicinal	T52.0X1	T52.0X2	T52.0X3	T52.0X4	—	—
red veterinary	T49.3X1	T49.3X2	T49.3X3	T49.3X4	T49.3X5	T49.3X6
white	T49.3X1	T49.3X2	T49.3X3	T49.3X4	T49.3X5	T49.3X6
Petroleum (products) NEC	T52.0X1	T52.0X2	T52.0X3	T52.0X4	—	—
benzine(s)—see Ligroin						
ether—see Ligroin						
jelly—see Petrolatum						
naphtha—see Ligroin						
pesticide	T60.8X1	T60.8X2	T60.8X3	T60.8X4	—	—
solids	T52.0X1	T52.0X2	T52.0X3	T52.0X4	—	—
solvents	T52.0X1	T52.0X2	T52.0X3	T52.0X4	—	—
vapor	T52.0X1	T52.0X2	T52.0X3	T52.0X4	—	—
Peyote	T40.991	T40.992	T40.993	T40.994	—	—
Phanodorm, phanodorn	T42.3X1	T42.3X2	T42.3X3	T42.3X4	T42.3X5	T42.3X6
Phanquinone	T37.3X1	T37.3X2	T37.3X3	T37.3X4	T37.3X5	T37.3X6
Phanquone	T37.3X1	T37.3X2	T37.3X3	T37.3X4	T37.3X5	T37.3X6
Pharmaceutical						
adjunct NEC	T50.901	T50.902	T50.903	T50.904	T50.905	T50.906
excipient NEC	T50.901	T50.902	T50.903	T50.904	T50.905	T50.906
sweetener	T50.901	T50.902	T50.903	T50.904	T50.905	T50.906
viscous agent	T50.901	T50.902	T50.903	T50.904	T50.905	T50.906

Substance	Poisoning, Accidental (unintentional)	Poisoning, Intentional self-harm	Poisoning, Assault	Poisoning, Undetermined	Adverse effect	Underdosing
Phemitone	T42.3X1	T42.3X2	T42.3X3	T42.3X4	T42.3X5	T42.3X6
Phenacaine	T41.3X1	T41.3X2	T41.3X3	T41.3X4	T41.3X5	T41.3X6
Phenacemide	T42.6X1	T42.6X2	T42.6X3	T42.6X4	T42.6X5	T42.6X6
Phenacetin	T39.1X1	T39.1X2	T39.1X3	T39.1X4	T39.1X5	T39.1X6
Phenadoxone	T40.2X1	T40.2X2	T40.2X3	T40.2X4	—	—
Phenaglycodol	T43.591	T43.592	T43.593	T43.594	T43.595	T43.596
Phenantoin	T42.0X1	T42.0X2	T42.0X3	T42.0X4	T42.0X5	T42.0X6
Phenaphthazine reagent	T50.991	T50.992	T50.993	T50.994	T50.995	T50.996
Phenazocine	T40.4X1	T40.4X2	T40.4X3	T40.4X4	T40.4X5	T40.4X6
Phenazone	T39.2X1	T39.2X2	T39.2X3	T39.2X4	T39.2X5	T39.2X6
Phenazopyridine	T39.8X1	T39.8X2	T39.8X3	T39.8X4	T39.8X5	T39.8X6
Phenbenicillin	T36.0X1	T36.0X2	T36.0X3	T36.0X4	T36.0X5	T36.0X6
Phenbutrazate	T50.5X1	T50.5X2	T50.5X3	T50.5X4	T50.5X5	T50.5X6
Phencyclidine	T40.991	T40.992	T40.993	T40.994	T40.995	T40.996
Phendimetrazine	T50.5X1	T50.5X2	T50.5X3	T50.5X4	T50.5X5	T50.5X6
Phenelzine	T43.1X1	T43.1X2	T43.1X3	T43.1X4	T43.1X5	T43.1X6
Phenemal	T42.3X1	T42.3X2	T42.3X3	T42.3X4	T42.3X5	T42.3X6
Phenergan	T42.6X1	T42.6X2	T42.6X3	T42.6X4	T42.6X5	T42.6X6
Pheneticillin	T36.0X1	T36.0X2	T36.0X3	T36.0X4	T36.0X5	T36.0X6
Pheneturide	T42.6X1	T42.6X2	T42.6X3	T42.6X4	T42.6X5	T42.6X6
Phenformin	T38.3X1	T38.3X2	T38.3X3	T38.3X4	T38.3X5	T38.3X6
Phenglutarimide	T44.3X1	T44.3X2	T44.3X3	T44.3X4	T44.3X5	T44.3X6
Phenicarbazide	T39.8X1	T39.8X2	T39.8X3	T39.8X4	T39.8X5	T39.8X6
Phenindamine	T45.0X1	T45.0X2	T45.0X3	T45.0X4	T45.0X5	T45.0X6
Phenindione	T45.511	T45.512	T45.513	T45.514	T45.515	T45.516
Pheniprazine	T43.1X1	T43.1X2	T43.1X3	T43.1X4	T43.1X5	T43.1X6
Pheniramine	T45.0X1	T45.0X2	T45.0X3	T45.0X4	T45.0X5	T45.0X6
Phenisatin	T47.2X1	T47.2X2	T47.2X3	T47.2X4	T47.2X5	T47.2X6
Phenmetrazine	T50.5X1	T50.5X2	T50.5X3	T50.5X4	T50.5X5	T50.5X6
Phenobal	T42.3X1	T42.3X2	T42.3X3	T42.3X4	T42.3X5	T42.3X6
Phenobarbital	T42.3X1	T42.3X2	T42.3X3	T42.3X4	T42.3X5	T42.3X6
with						
mephenytoin	T42.3X1	T42.3X2	T42.3X3	T42.3X4	T42.3X5	T42.3X6
phenytoin	T42.3X1	T42.3X2	T42.3X3	T42.3X4	T42.3X5	T42.3X6
sodium	T42.3X1	T42.3X2	T42.3X3	T42.3X4	T42.3X5	T42.3X6
Phenobarbitone	T42.3X1	T42.3X2	T42.3X3	T42.3X4	T42.3X5	T42.3X6
Phenobutiodil	T50.8X1	T50.8X2	T50.8X3	T50.8X4	T50.8X5	T50.8X6
Phenoctide	T49.0X1	T49.0X2	T49.0X3	T49.0X4	T49.0X5	T49.0X6
Phenol	T49.0X1	T49.0X2	T49.0X3	T49.0X4	T49.0X5	T49.0X6
disinfectant	T54.0X1	T54.0X2	T54.0X3	T54.0X4	—	—
in oil injection	T46.8X1	T46.8X2	T46.8X3	T46.8X4	T46.8X5	T46.8X6
medicinal	T49.1X1	T49.1X2	T49.1X3	T49.1X4	T49.1X5	T49.1X6
nonmedicinal NEC	T54.0X1	T54.0X2	T54.0X3	T54.0X4	—	—
pesticide	T60.8X1	T60.8X2	T60.8X3	T60.8X4	—	—
red	T50.8X1	T50.8X2	T50.8X3	T50.8X4	T50.8X5	T50.8X6
Phenolic preparation	T49.1X1	T49.1X2	T49.1X3	T49.1X4	T49.1X5	T49.1X6
Phenolphthalein	T47.2X1	T47.2X2	T47.2X3	T47.2X4	T47.2X5	T47.2X6
Phenolsulfonphthalein	T50.8X1	T50.8X2	T50.8X3	T50.8X4	T50.8X5	T50.8X6
Phenomorphan	T40.2X1	T40.2X2	T40.2X3	T40.2X4	—	—
Phenonyl	T42.3X1	T42.3X2	T42.3X3	T42.3X4	T42.3X5	T42.3X6

Substance	Poisoning, Accidental (unintentional)	Poisoning, Intentional self-harm	Poisoning, Assault	Poisoning, Undetermined	Adverse effect	Underdosing
Phenoperidine	T40.4X1	T40.4X2	T40.4X3	T40.4X4	—	—
Phenopyrazone	T46.991	T46.992	T46.993	T46.994	T46.995	T46.996
Phenoquin	T50.4X1	T50.4X2	T50.4X3	T50.4X4	T50.4X5	T50.4X6
Phenothiazine (psychotropic) NEC	T43.3X1	T43.3X2	T43.3X3	T43.3X4	T43.3X5	T43.3X6
insecticide	T60.2X1	T60.2X2	T60.2X3	T60.2X4	—	—
Phenothrin	T49.0X1	T49.0X2	T49.0X3	T49.0X4	T49.0X5	T49.0X6
Phenoxybenzamine	T46.7X1	T46.7X2	T46.7X3	T46.7X4	T46.7X5	T46.7X6
Phenoxyethanol	T49.0X1	T49.0X2	T49.0X3	T49.0X4	T49.0X5	T49.0X6
Phenoxymethyl penicillin	T36.0X1	T36.0X2	T36.0X3	T36.0X4	T36.0X5	T36.0X6
Phenprobamate	T42.8X1	T42.8X2	T42.8X3	T42.8X4	T42.8X5	T42.8X6
Phenprocoumon	T45.511	T45.512	T45.513	T45.514	T45.515	T45.516
Phensuximide	T42.2X1	T42.2X2	T42.2X3	T42.2X4	T42.2X5	T42.2X6
Phentermine	T50.5X1	T50.5X2	T50.5X3	T50.5X4	T50.5X5	T50.5X6
Phenthicillin	T36.0X1	T36.0X2	T36.0X3	T36.0X4	T36.0X5	T36.0X6
Phentolamine	T46.7X1	T46.7X2	T46.7X3	T46.7X4	T46.7X5	T46.7X6
Phenyl						
butazone	T39.2X1	T39.2X2	T39.2X3	T39.2X4	T39.2X5	T39.2X6
enediamine	T65.3X1	T65.3X2	T65.3X3	T65.3X4	—	—
hydrazine	T65.3X1	T65.3X2	T65.3X3	T65.3X4	—	—
antineoplastic	T45.1X1	T45.1X2	T45.1X3	T45.1X4	T45.1X5	T45.1X6
mercuric compounds—see Mercury						
salicylate	T49.3X1	T49.3X2	T49.3X3	T49.3X4	T49.3X5	T49.3X6
Phenylalanine mustard	T45.1X1	T45.1X2	T45.1X3	T45.1X4	T45.1X5	T45.1X6
Phenylbutazone	T39.2X1	T39.2X2	T39.2X3	T39.2X4	T39.2X5	T39.2X6
Phenylenediamine	T65.3X1	T65.3X2	T65.3X3	T65.3X4	—	—
Phenylephrine	T44.4X1	T44.4X2	T44.4X3	T44.4X4	T44.4X5	T44.4X6
Phenylethylbiguanide	T38.3X1	T38.3X2	T38.3X3	T38.3X4	T38.3X5	T38.3X6
Phenylmercuric						
acetate	T49.0X1	T49.0X2	T49.0X3	T49.0X4	T49.0X5	T49.0X6
borate	T49.0X1	T49.0X2	T49.0X3	T49.0X4	T49.0X5	T49.0X6
nitrate	T49.0X1	T49.0X2	T49.0X3	T49.0X4	T49.0X5	T49.0X6
Phenylmethylbarbitone	T42.3X1	T42.3X2	T42.3X3	T42.3X4	T42.3X5	T42.3X6
Phenylpropanol	T47.5X1	T47.5X2	T47.5X3	T47.5X4	T47.5X5	T47.5X6
Phenylpropanolamine	T44.991	T44.992	T44.993	T44.994	T44.995	T44.996
Phenylsulfthion	T60.0X1	T60.0X2	T60.0X3	T60.0X4	—	—
Phenyltoloxamine	T45.0X1	T45.0X2	T45.0X3	T45.0X4	T45.0X5	T45.0X6
Phenyramidol, phenyramidon	T39.8X1	T39.8X2	T39.8X3	T39.8X4	T39.8X5	T39.8X6
Phenytoin	T42.0X1	T42.0X2	T42.0X3	T42.0X4	T42.0X5	T42.0X6
with Phenobarbital	T42.3X1	T42.3X2	T42.3X3	T42.3X4	T42.3X5	T42.3X6
pHisoHex	T49.2X1	T49.2X2	T49.2X3	T49.2X4	T49.2X5	T49.2X6
Pholcodine	T48.3X1	T48.3X2	T48.3X3	T48.3X4	T48.3X5	T48.3X6
Pholedrine	T46.991	T46.992	T46.993	T46.994	T46.995	T46.996
Phorate	T60.0X1	T60.0X2	T60.0X3	T60.0X4	—	—
Phosdrin	T60.0X1	T60.0X2	T60.0X3	T60.0X4	—	—
Phosfolan	T60.0X1	T60.0X2	T60.0X3	T60.0X4	—	—
Phosgene (gas)	T59.891	T59.892	T59.893	T59.894	—	—
Phosphamidon	T60.0X1	T60.0X2	T60.0X3	T60.0X4	—	—

Substance	Poisoning, Accidental (unintentional)	Poisoning, Intentional self-harm	Poisoning, Assault	Poisoning, Undetermined	Adverse effect	Underdosing
Phosphate	T65.891	T65.892	T65.893	T65.894	—	—
laxative	T47.4X1	T47.4X2	T47.4X3	T47.4X4	T47.4X5	T47.4X6
organic	T60.0X1	T60.0X2	T60.0X3	T60.0X4	—	—
solvent	T52.91	T52.92	T52.93	T52.94	—	—
tricresyl	T65.891	T65.892	T65.893	T65.894	—	—
Phosphine	T57.1X1	T57.1X2	T57.1X3	T57.1X4	—	—
fumigant	T57.1X1	T57.1X2	T57.1X3	T57.1X4	—	—
Phospholine	T49.5X1	T49.5X2	T49.5X3	T49.5X4	T49.5X5	T49.5X6
Phosphoric acid	T54.2X1	T54.2X2	T54.2X3	T54.2X4	—	—
Phosphorus (compound) NEC	T57.1X1	T57.1X2	T57.1X3	T57.1X4	—	—
pesticide	T60.0X1	T60.0X2	T60.0X3	T60.0X4	—	—
Phthalates	T65.891	T65.892	T65.893	T65.894	—	—
Phthalic anhydride	T65.891	T65.892	T65.893	T65.894	—	—
Phthalimidoglutarimide	T42.6X1	T42.6X2	T42.6X3	T42.6X4	T42.6X5	T42.6X6
Phthalylsulfathiazole	T37.0X1	T37.0X2	T37.0X3	T37.0X4	T37.0X5	T37.0X6
Phylloquinone	T45.7X1	T45.7X2	T45.7X3	T45.7X4	T45.7X5	T45.7X6
Physeptone	T40.3X1	T40.3X2	T40.3X3	T40.3X4	T40.3X5	T40.3X6
Physostigma venenosum	T62.2X1	T62.2X2	T62.2X3	T62.2X4	—	—
Physostigmine	T49.5X1	T49.5X2	T49.5X3	T49.5X4	T49.5X5	T49.5X6
Phytolacca decandra	T62.2X1	T62.2X2	T62.2X3	T62.2X4	—	—
berries	T62.1X1	T62.1X2	T62.1X3	T62.1X4	—	—
Phytomenadione	T45.7X1	T45.7X2	T45.7X3	T45.7X4	T45.7X5	T45.7X6
Phytonadione	T45.7X1	T45.7X2	T45.7X3	T45.7X4	T45.7X5	T45.7X6
Picoperine	T48.3X1	T48.3X2	T48.3X3	T48.3X4	T48.3X5	T48.3X6
Picosulfate (sodium)	T47.2X1	T47.2X2	T47.2X3	T47.2X4	T47.2X5	T47.2X6
Picric (acid)	T54.2X1	T54.2X2	T54.2X3	T54.2X4	—	—
Picrotoxin	T50.7X1	T50.7X2	T50.7X3	T50.7X4	T50.7X5	T50.7X6
Piketoprofen	T49.0X1	T49.0X2	T49.0X3	T49.0X4	T49.0X5	T49.0X6
Pilocarpine	T44.1X1	T44.1X2	T44.1X3	T44.1X4	T44.1X5	T44.1X6
Pilocarpus (jaborandi) extract	T44.1X1	T44.1X2	T44.1X3	T44.1X4	T44.1X5	T44.1X6
Pilsicainide (hydrochloride)	T46.2X1	T46.2X2	T46.2X3	T46.2X4	T46.2X5	T46.2X6
Pimaricin	T36.7X1	T36.7X2	T36.7X3	T36.7X4	T36.7X5	T36.7X6
Pimeclone	T50.7X1	T50.7X2	T50.7X3	T50.7X4	T50.7X5	T50.7X6
Pimelic ketone	T52.8X1	T52.8X2	T52.8X3	T52.8X4	—	—
Pimethixene	T45.0X1	T45.0X2	T45.0X3	T45.0X4	T45.0X5	T45.0X6
Piminodine	T40.2X1	T40.2X2	T40.2X3	T40.2X4	T40.2X5	T40.2X6
Pimozide	T43.591	T43.592	T43.593	T43.594	T43.595	T43.596
Pinacidil	T46.5X1	T46.5X2	T46.5X3	T46.5X4	T46.5X5	T46.5X6
Pinaverium bromide	T44.3X1	T44.3X2	T44.3X3	T44.3X4	T44.3X5	T44.3X6
Pinazepam	T42.4X1	T42.4X2	T42.4X3	T42.4X4	T42.4X5	T42.4X6
Pindolol	T44.7X1	T44.7X2	T44.7X3	T44.7X4	T44.7X5	T44.7X6
Pindone	T60.4X1	T60.4X2	T60.4X3	T60.4X4	—	—
Pine oil (disinfectant)	T65.891	T65.892	T65.893	T65.894	—	—
Pinkroot	T37.4X1	T37.4X2	T37.4X3	T37.4X4	T37.4X5	T37.4X6
Pipadone	T40.2X1	T40.2X2	T40.2X3	T40.2X4	—	—
Pipamazine	T45.0X1	T45.0X2	T45.0X3	T45.0X4	T45.0X5	T45.0X6
Pipamperone	T43.4X1	T43.4X2	T43.4X3	T43.4X4	T43.4X5	T43.4X6
Pipazetate	T48.3X1	T48.3X2	T48.3X3	T48.3X4	T48.3X5	T48.3X6

Substance	Poisoning, Accidental (unintentional)	Poisoning, Intentional self-harm	Poisoning, Assault	Poisoning, Undetermined	Adverse effect	Underdosing
Pipemidic acid	T37.8X1	T37.8X2	T37.8X3	T37.8X4	T37.8X5	T37.8X6
Pipenzolate bromide	T44.3X1	T44.3X2	T44.3X3	T44.3X4	T44.3X5	T44.3X6
Piperacetazine	T43.3X1	T43.3X2	T43.3X3	T43.3X4	T43.3X5	T43.3X6
Piperacillin	T36.0X1	T36.0X2	T36.0X3	T36.0X4	T36.0X5	T36.0X6
Piperazine	T37.4X1	T37.4X2	T37.4X3	T37.4X4	T37.4X5	T37.4X6
estrone sulfate	T38.5X1	T38.5X2	T38.5X3	T38.5X4	T38.5X5	T38.5X6
Piper cubeba	T62.2X1	T62.2X2	T62.2X3	T62.2X4	—	—
Piperidione	T48.3X1	T48.3X2	T48.3X3	T48.3X4	T48.3X5	T48.3X6
Piperidolate	T44.3X1	T44.3X2	T44.3X3	T44.3X4	T44.3X5	T44.3X6
Piperocaine	T41.3X1	T41.3X2	T41.3X3	T41.3X4	T41.3X5	T41.3X6
infiltration (subcutaneous)	T41.3X1	T41.3X2	T41.3X3	T41.3X4	T41.3X5	T41.3X6
nerve block (peripheral) (plexus)	T41.3X1	T41.3X2	T41.3X3	T41.3X4	T41.3X5	T41.3X6
topical (surface)	T41.3X1	T41.3X2	T41.3X3	T41.3X4	T41.3X5	T41.3X6
Piperonyl butoxide	T60.8X1	T60.8X2	T60.8X3	T60.8X4	—	—
Pipethanate	T44.3X1	T44.3X2	T44.3X3	T44.3X4	T44.3X5	T44.3X6
Pipobroman	T45.1X1	T45.1X2	T45.1X3	T45.1X4	T45.1X5	T45.1X6
Pipotiazine	T43.3X1	T43.3X2	T43.3X3	T43.3X4	T43.3X5	T43.3X6
Pipoxizine	T45.0X1	T45.0X2	T45.0X3	T45.0X4	T45.0X5	T45.0X6
Pipradrol	T43.691	T43.692	T43.693	T43.694	T43.695	T43.696
Piprinhydrinate	T45.0X1	T45.0X2	T45.0X3	T45.0X4	T45.0X5	T45.0X6
Pirarubicin	T45.1X1	T45.1X2	T45.1X3	T45.1X4	T45.1X5	T45.1X6
Pirazinamide	T37.1X1	T37.1X2	T37.1X3	T37.1X4	T37.1X5	T37.1X6
Pirbuterol	T48.6X1	T48.6X2	T48.6X3	T48.6X4	T48.6X5	T48.6X6
Pirenzepine	T47.1X1	T47.1X2	T47.1X3	T47.1X4	T47.1X5	T47.1X6
Piretanide	T50.1X1	T50.1X2	T50.1X3	T50.1X4	T50.1X5	T50.1X6
Piribedil	T42.8X1	T42.8X2	T42.8X3	T42.8X4	T42.8X5	T42.8X6
Piridoxilate	T46.3X1	T46.3X2	T46.3X3	T46.3X4	T46.3X5	T46.3X6
Piritramide	T40.4X1	T40.4X2	T40.4X3	T40.4X4	—	—
Piromidic acid	T37.8X1	T37.8X2	T37.8X3	T37.8X4	T37.8X5	T37.8X6
Piroxicam	T39.391	T39.392	T39.393	T39.394	T39.395	T39.396
beta-cyclodextrin complex	T39.8X1	T39.8X2	T39.8X3	T39.8X4	T39.8X5	T39.8X6
Pirozadil	T46.6X1	T46.6X2	T46.6X3	T46.6X4	T46.6X5	T46.6X6
Piscidia (bark) (erythrina)	T39.8X1	T39.8X2	T39.8X3	T39.8X4	T39.8X5	T39.8X6
Pitch	T65.891	T65.892	T65.893	T65.894	—	—
Pitkin's solution	T41.3X1	T41.3X2	T41.3X3	T41.3X4	T41.3X5	T41.3X6
Pitocin	T48.0X1	T48.0X2	T48.0X3	T48.0X4	T48.0X5	T48.0X6
Pitressin (tannate)	T38.891	T38.892	T38.893	T38.894	T38.895	T38.896
Pituitary extracts (posterior)	T38.891	T38.892	T38.893	T38.894	T38.895	T38.896
anterior	T38.811	T38.812	T38.813	T38.814	T38.815	T38.816
Pituitrin	T38.891	T38.892	T38.893	T38.894	T38.895	T38.896
Pivampicillin	T36.0X1	T36.0X2	T36.0X3	T36.0X4	T36.0X5	T36.0X6
Pivmecillinam	T36.0X1	T36.0X2	T36.0X3	T36.0X4	T36.0X5	T36.0X6
Placental hormone	T38.891	T38.892	T38.893	T38.894	T38.895	T38.896
Placidyl	T42.6X1	T42.6X2	T42.6X3	T42.6X4	T42.6X5	T42.6X6
Plague vaccine	T50.A91	T50.A92	T50.A93	T50.A94	T50.A95	T50.A96
Plant						
food or fertilizer NEC	T65.891	T65.892	T65.893	T65.894	—	—
containing herbicide	T60.3X1	T60.3X2	T60.3X3	T60.3X4	—	—

Substance	Poisoning, Accidental (unintentional)	Poisoning, Intentional self-harm	Poisoning, Assault	Poisoning, Undetermined	Adverse effect	Underdosing
Plant — *Continued*						
noxious, used as food	T62.2X1	T62.2X2	T62.2X3	T62.2X4	—	—
berries	T62.1X1	T62.1X2	T62.1X3	T62.1X4	—	—
seeds	T62.2X1	T62.2X2	T62.2X3	T62.2X4	—	—
specified type NEC	T62.2X1	T62.2X2	T62.2X3	T62.2X4	—	—
Plasma	T45.8X1	T45.8X2	T45.8X3	T45.8X4	T45.8X5	T45.8X6
expander NEC	T45.8X1	T45.8X2	T45.8X3	T45.8X4	T45.8X5	T45.8X6
protein fraction (human)	T45.8X1	T45.8X2	T45.8X3	T45.8X4	T45.8X5	T45.8X6
Plasmanate	T45.8X1	T45.8X2	T45.8X3	T45.8X4	T45.8X5	T45.8X6
Plasminogen (tissue) activator	T45.611	T45.612	T45.613	T45.614	T45.615	T45.616
Plaster dressing	T49.3X1	T49.3X2	T49.3X3	T49.3X4	T49.3X5	T49.3X6
Plastic dressing	T49.3X1	T49.3X2	T49.3X3	T49.3X4	T49.3X5	T49.3X6
Plegicil	T43.3X1	T43.3X2	T43.3X3	T43.3X4	T43.3X5	T43.3X6
Plicamycin	T45.1X1	T45.1X2	T45.1X3	T45.1X4	T45.1X5	T45.1X6
Podophyllotoxin	T49.8X1	T49.8X2	T49.8X3	T49.8X4	T49.8X5	T49.8X6
Podophyllum (resin)	T49.4X1	T49.4X2	T49.4X3	T49.4X4	T49.4X5	T49.4X6
Poison NEC	T65.91	T65.92	T65.93	T65.94	—	—
Poisonous berries	T62.1X1	T62.1X2	T62.1X3	T62.1X4	—	—
Pokeweed (any part)	T62.2X1	T62.2X2	T62.2X3	T62.2X4	—	—
Poldine metilsulfate	T44.3X1	T44.3X2	T44.3X3	T44.3X4	T44.3X5	T44.3X6
Polidexide (sulfate)	T46.6X1	T46.6X2	T46.6X3	T46.6X4	T46.6X5	T46.6X6
Polidocanol	T46.8X1	T46.8X2	T46.8X3	T46.8X4	T46.8X5	T46.8X6
Poliomyelitis vaccine	T50.B91	T50.B92	T50.B93	T50.B94	T50.B95	T50.B96
Polish (car) (floor) (furniture) (metal) (porcelain) (silver)	T65.891	T65.892	T65.893	T65.894	—	
abrasive	T65.891	T65.892	T65.893	T65.894	—	—
porcelain	T65.891	T65.892	T65.893	T65.894	—	—
Poloxalkol	T47.4X1	T47.4X2	T47.4X3	T47.4X4	T47.4X5	T47.4X6
Poloxamer	T47.4X1	T47.4X2	T47.4X3	T47.4X4	T47.4X5	T47.4X6
Polyaminostyrene resins	T50.3X1	T50.3X2	T50.3X3	T50.3X4	T50.3X5	T50.3X6
Polycarbophil	T47.4X1	T47.4X2	T47.4X3	T47.4X4	T47.4X5	T47.4X6
Polychlorinated biphenyl	T65.891	T65.892	T65.893	T65.894	—	—
Polycycline	T36.4X1	T36.4X2	T36.4X3	T36.4X4	T36.4X5	T36.4X6
Polyester fumes	T59.891	T59.892	T59.893	T59.894	—	—
Polyester resin hardener	T52.91	T52.92	T52.93	T52.94	—	—
fumes	T59.891	T59.892	T59.893	T59.894	—	—
Polyestradiol phosphate	T38.5X1	T38.5X2	T38.5X3	T38.5X4	T38.5X5	T38.5X6
Polyethanolamine alkyl sulfate	T49.2X1	T49.2X2	T49.2X3	T49.2X4	T49.2X5	T49.2X6
Polyethylene adhesive	T49.3X1	T49.3X2	T49.3X3	T49.3X4	T49.3X5	T49.3X6
Polyferose	T45.4X1	T45.4X2	T45.4X3	T45.4X4	T45.4X5	T45.4X6
Polygeline	T45.8X1	T45.8X2	T45.8X3	T45.8X4	T45.8X5	T45.8X6
Polymyxin	T36.8X1	T36.8X2	T36.8X3	T36.8X4	T36.8X5	T36.8X6
B	T36.8X1	T36.8X2	T36.8X3	T36.8X4	T36.8X5	T36.8X6
ENT agent	T49.6X1	T49.6X2	T49.6X3	T49.6X4	T49.6X5	T49.6X6
ophthalmic preparation	T49.5X1	T49.5X2	T49.5X3	T49.5X4	T49.5X5	T49.5X6
topical NEC	T49.0X1	T49.0X2	T49.0X3	T49.0X4	T49.0X5	T49.0X6
E sulfate (eye preparation)	T49.5X1	T49.5X2	T49.5X3	T49.5X4	T49.5X5	T49.5X6

Substance	Poisoning, Accidental (unintentional)	Poisoning, Intentional self-harm	Poisoning, Assault	Poisoning, Undetermined	Adverse effect	Underdosing
Polynoxylin	T49.0X1	T49.0X2	T49.0X3	T49.0X4	T49.0X5	T49.0X6
Polyoestradiol phosphate	T38.5X1	T38.5X2	T38.5X3	T38.5X4	T38.5X5	T38.5X6
Polyoxymethyleneurea	T49.0X1	T49.0X2	T49.0X3	T49.0X4	T49.0X5	T49.0X6
Polysilane	T47.8X1	T47.8X2	T47.8X3	T47.8X4	T47.8X5	T47.8X6
Polytetrafluoroethylene (inhaled)	T59.891	T59.892	T59.893	T59.894	—	—
Polythiazide	T50.2X1	T50.2X2	T50.2X3	T50.2X4	T50.2X5	T50.2X6
Polyvidone	T45.8X1	T45.8X2	T45.8X3	T45.8X4	T45.8X5	T45.8X6
Polyvinylpyrrolidone	T45.8X1	T45.8X2	T45.8X3	T45.8X4	T45.8X5	T45.8X6
Pontocaine (hydrochloride) (infiltration) (topical)	T41.3X1	T41.3X2	T41.3X3	T41.3X4	T41.3X5	T41.3X6
nerve block (peripheral) (plexus)	T41.3X1	T41.3X2	T41.3X3	T41.3X4	T41.3X5	T41.3X6
spinal	T41.3X1	T41.3X2	T41.3X3	T41.3X4	T41.3X5	T41.3X6
Porfiromycin	T45.1X1	T45.1X2	T45.1X3	T45.1X4	T45.1X5	T45.1X6
Posterior pituitary hormone NEC	T38.891	T38.892	T38.893	T38.894	T38.895	T38.896
Pot	T40.7X1	T40.7X2	T40.7X3	T40.7X4	T40.7X5	T40.7X6
Potash (caustic)	T54.3X1	T54.3X2	T54.3X3	T54.3X4	—	—
Potassic saline injection (lactated)	T50.3X1	T50.3X2	T50.3X3	T50.3X4	T50.3X5	T50.3X6
Potassium (salts) NEC	T50.3X1	T50.3X2	T50.3X3	T50.3X4	T50.3X5	T50.3X6
aminobenzoate	T45.8X1	T45.8X2	T45.8X3	T45.8X4	T45.8X5	T45.8X6
aminosalicylate	T37.1X1	T37.1X2	T37.1X3	T37.1X4	T37.1X5	T37.1X6
antimony 'tartrate'	T37.8X1	T37.8X2	T37.8X3	T37.8X4	T37.8X5	T37.8X6
arsenite (solution)	T57.0X1	T57.0X2	T57.0X3	T57.0X4	—	—
bichromate	T56.2X1	T56.2X2	T56.2X3	T56.2X4	—	—
bisulfate	T47.3X1	T47.3X2	T47.3X3	T47.3X4	T47.3X5	T47.3X6
bromide	T42.6X1	T42.6X2	T42.6X3	T42.6X4	T42.6X5	T42.6X6
canrenoate	T50.0X1	T50.0X2	T50.0X3	T50.0X4	T50.0X5	T50.0X6
carbonate	T54.3X1	T54.3X2	T54.3X3	T54.3X4	—	—
chlorate NEC	T65.891	T65.892	T65.893	T65.894	—	—
chloride	T50.3X1	T50.3X2	T50.3X3	T50.3X4	T50.3X5	T50.3X6
citrate	T50.991	T50.992	T50.993	T50.994	T50.995	T50.996
cyanide	T65.0X1	T65.0X2	T65.0X3	T65.0X4	—	—
ferric hexacyano-ferrate (medicinal)	T50.6X1	T50.6X2	T50.6X3	T50.6X4	T50.6X5	T50.6X6
nonmedicinal	T65.891	T65.892	T65.893	T65.894	—	—
Fluoride	T57.8X1	T57.8X2	T57.8X3	T57.8X4	—	—
glucaldrate	T47.1X1	T47.1X2	T47.1X3	T47.1X4	T47.1X5	T47.1X6
hydroxide	T54.3X1	T54.3X2	T54.3X3	T54.3X4	—	—
iodate	T49.0X1	T49.0X2	T49.0X3	T49.0X4	T49.0X5	T49.0X6
iodide	T48.4X1	T48.4X2	T48.4X3	T48.4X4	T48.4X5	T48.4X6
nitrate	T57.8X1	T57.8X2	T57.8X3	T57.8X4	—	—
oxalate	T65.891	T65.892	T65.893	T65.894	—	—
perchlorate (nonmedicinal) NEC	T65.891	T65.892	T65.893	T65.894	—	—
antithyroid	T38.2X1	T38.2X2	T38.2X3	T38.2X4	T38.2X5	T38.2X6
medicinal	T38.2X1	T38.2X2	T38.2X3	T38.2X4	T38.2X5	T38.2X6
Permanganate (nonmedicinal)	T65.891	T65.892	T65.893	T65.894	—	—
medicinal	T49.0X1	T49.0X2	T49.0X3	T49.0X4	T49.0X5	T49.0X6

Substance	Poisoning, Accidental (unintentional)	Poisoning, Intentional self-harm	Poisoning, Assault	Poisoning, Undetermined	Adverse effect	Underdosing
Potassium — *Continued*						
sulfate	T47.2X1	T47.2X2	T47.2X3	T47.2X4	T47.2X5	T47.2X
Potassium-removing resin	T50.3X1	T50.3X2	T50.3X3	T50.3X4	T50.3X5	T50.3X
Potassium-retaining drug	T50.3X1	T50.3X2	T50.3X3	T50.3X4	T50.3X5	T50.3X
Povidone	T45.8X1	T45.8X2	T45.8X3	T45.8X4	T45.8X5	T45.8X
iodine	T49.0X1	T49.0X2	T49.0X3	T49.0X4	T49.0X5	T49.0X
Practolol	T44.7X1	T44.7X2	T44.7X3	T44.7X4	T44.7X5	T44.7X
Prajmalium bitartrate	T46.2X1	T46.2X2	T46.2X3	T46.2X4	T46.2X5	T46.2X
Pralidoxime (iodide)	T50.6X1	T50.6X2	T50.6X3	T50.6X4	T50.6X5	T50.6X
chloride	T50.6X1	T50.6X2	T50.6X3	T50.6X4	T50.6X5	T50.6X
Pramiverine	T44.3X1	T44.3X2	T44.3X3	T44.3X4	T44.3X5	T44.3X6
Pramocaine	T49.1X1	T49.1X2	T49.1X3	T49.1X4	T49.1X5	T49.1X6
Pramoxine	T49.1X1	T49.1X2	T49.1X3	T49.1X4	T49.1X5	T49.1X
Prasterone	T38.7X1	T38.7X2	T38.7X3	T38.7X4	T38.7X5	T38.7X
Pravastatin	T46.6X1	T46.6X2	T46.6X3	T46.6X4	T46.6X5	T46.6X
Prazepam	T42.4X1	T42.4X2	T42.4X3	T42.4X4	T42.4X5	T42.4X
Praziquantel	T37.4X1	T37.4X2	T37.4X3	T37.4X4	T37.4X5	T37.4X
Prazitone	T43.291	T43.292	T43.293	T43.294	T43.295	T43.296
Prazosin	T44.6X1	T44.6X2	T44.6X3	T44.6X4	T44.6X5	T44.6X6
Prednicarbate	T49.0X1	T49.0X2	T49.0X3	T49.0X4	T49.0X5	T49.0X
Prednimustine	T45.1X1	T45.1X2	T45.1X3	T45.1X4	T45.1X5	T45.1X6
Prednisolone	T38.0X1	T38.0X2	T38.0X3	T38.0X4	T38.0X5	T38.0X6
ENT agent	T49.6X1	T49.6X2	T49.6X3	T49.6X4	T49.6X5	T49.6X
ophthalmic preparation	T49.5X1	T49.5X2	T49.5X3	T49.5X4	T49.5X5	T49.5X
steaglate	T49.0X1	T49.0X2	T49.0X3	T49.0X4	T49.0X5	T49.0X6
topical NEC	T49.0X1	T49.0X2	T49.0X3	T49.0X4	T49.0X5	T49.0X6
Prednisone	T38.0X1	T38.0X2	T38.0X3	T38.0X4	T38.0X5	T38.0X6
Prednylidene	T38.0X1	T38.0X2	T38.0X3	T38.0X4	T38.0X5	T38.0X6
Pregnandiol	T38.5X1	T38.5X2	T38.5X3	T38.5X4	T38.5X5	T38.5X6
Pregneninolone	T38.5X1	T38.5X2	T38.5X3	T38.5X4	T38.5X5	T38.5X6
Preludin	T43.691	T43.692	T43.693	T43.694	T43.695	T43.696
Premarin	T38.5X1	T38.5X2	T38.5X3	T38.5X4	T38.5X5	T38.5X6
Premedication anesthetic	T41.201	T41.202	T41.203	T41.204	T41.205	T41.206
Prenalterol	T44.5X1	T44.5X2	T44.5X3	T44.5X4	T44.5X5	T44.5X6
Prenoxdiazine	T48.3X1	T48.3X2	T48.3X3	T48.3X4	T48.3X5	T48.3X6
Prenylamine	T46.3X1	T46.3X2	T46.3X3	T46.3X4	T46.3X5	T46.3X6
Preparation H	T49.8X1	T49.8X2	T49.8X3	T49.8X4	T49.8X5	T49.8X6
Preparation, local	T49.4X1	T49.4X2	T49.4X3	T49.4X4	T49.4X5	T49.4X6
Preservative (nonmedicinal)	T65.891	T65.892	T65.893	T65.894	—	—
medicinal	T50.901	T50.902	T50.903	T50.904	T50.905	T50.906
wood	T60.91	T60.92	T60.93	T60.94	—	—
Prethcamide	T50.7X1	T50.7X2	T50.7X3	T50.7X4	T50.7X5	T50.7X6
Pride of China	T62.2X1	T62.2X2	T62.2X3	T62.2X4	—	—
Pridinol	T44.3X1	T44.3X2	T44.3X3	T44.3X4	T44.3X5	T44.3X6
Prifinium bromide	T44.3X1	T44.3X2	T44.3X3	T44.3X4	T44.3X5	T44.3X6
Prilocaine	T41.3X1	T41.3X2	T41.3X3	T41.3X4	T41.3X5	T41.3X6
infiltration (subcutaneous)	T41.3X1	T41.3X2	T41.3X3	T41.3X4	T41.3X5	T41.3X6
nerve block (peripheral) (plexus)	T41.3X1	T41.3X2	T41.3X3	T41.3X4	T41.3X5	T41.3X6
regional	T41.3X1	T41.3X2	T41.3X3	T41.3X4	T41.3X5	T41.3X6

Substance	Poisoning, Accidental (unintentional)	Poisoning, Intentional self-harm	Poisoning, Assault	Poisoning, Undetermined	Adverse effect	Underdosing
Primaquine	T37.2X1	T37.2X2	T37.2X3	T37.2X4	T37.2X5	T37.2X6
Primidone	T42.6X1	T42.6X2	T42.6X3	T42.6X4	T42.6X5	T42.6X6
Primula (veris)	T62.2X1	T62.2X2	T62.2X3	T62.2X4	—	—
Prinadol	T40.2X1	T40.2X2	T40.2X3	T40.2X4	T40.2X5	T40.2X6
Priscol, Priscoline	T44.6X1	T44.6X2	T44.6X3	T44.6X4	T44.6X5	T44.6X6
Pristinamycin	T36.3X1	T36.3X2	T36.3X3	T36.3X4	T36.3X5	T36.3X6
Privet	T62.2X1	T62.2X2	T62.2X3	T62.2X4	—	—
berries	T62.1X1	T62.1X2	T62.1X3	T62.1X4	—	—
Privine	T44.4X1	T44.4X2	T44.4X3	T44.4X4	T44.4X5	T44.4X6
Pro-Banthine	T44.3X1	T44.3X2	T44.3X3	T44.3X4	T44.3X5	T44.3X6
Probarbital	T42.3X1	T42.3X2	T42.3X3	T42.3X4	T42.3X5	T42.3X6
Probenecid	T50.4X1	T50.4X2	T50.4X3	T50.4X4	T50.4X5	T50.4X6
Probucol	T46.6X1	T46.6X2	T46.6X3	T46.6X4	T46.6X5	T46.6X6
Procainamide	T46.2X1	T46.2X2	T46.2X3	T46.2X4	T46.2X5	T46.2X6
Procaine	T41.3X1	T41.3X2	T41.3X3	T41.3X4	T41.3X5	T41.3X6
benzylpenicillin	T36.0X1	T36.0X2	T36.0X3	T36.0X4	T36.0X5	T36.0X6
nerve block (periphreal) (plexus)	T41.3X1	T41.3X2	T41.3X3	T41.3X4	T41.3X5	T41.3X6
penicillin G	T36.0X1	T36.0X2	T36.0X3	T36.0X4	T36.0X5	T36.0X6
regional	T41.3X1	T41.3X2	T41.3X3	T41.3X4	T41.3X5	T41.3X6
spinal	T41.3X1	T41.3X2	T41.3X3	T41.3X4	T41.3X5	T41.3X6
Procalmidol	T43.591	T43.592	T43.593	T43.594	T43.595	T43.596
Procarbazine	T45.1X1	T45.1X2	T45.1X3	T45.1X4	T45.1X5	T45.1X6
Procaterol	T44.5X1	T44.5X2	T44.5X3	T44.5X4	T44.5X5	T44.5X6
Prochlorperazine	T43.3X1	T43.3X2	T43.3X3	T43.3X4	T43.3X5	T43.3X6
Procyclidine	T44.3X1	T44.3X2	T44.3X3	T44.3X4	T44.3X5	T44.3X6
Producer gas	T58.8X1	T58.8X2	T58.8X3	T58.8X4	—	—
Profadol	T40.4X1	T40.4X2	T40.4X3	T40.4X4	T40.4X5	T40.4X6
Profenamine	T44.3X1	T44.3X2	T44.3X3	T44.3X4	T44.3X5	T44.3X6
Profenil	T44.3X1	T44.3X2	T44.3X3	T44.3X4	T44.3X5	T44.3X6
Proflavine	T49.0X1	T49.0X2	T49.0X3	T49.0X4	T49.0X5	T49.0X6
Progabide	T42.6X1	T42.6X2	T42.6X3	T42.6X4	T42.6X5	T42.6X6
Progesterone	T38.5X1	T38.5X2	T38.5X3	T38.5X4	T38.5X5	T38.5X6
Progestin	T38.5X1	T38.5X2	T38.5X3	T38.5X4	T38.5X5	T38.5X6
oral contraceptive	T38.4X1	T38.4X2	T38.4X3	T38.4X4	T38.4X5	T38.4X6
Progestogen NEC	T38.5X1	T38.5X2	T38.5X3	T38.5X4	T38.5X5	T38.5X6
Progestone	T38.5X1	T38.5X2	T38.5X3	T38.5X4	T38.5X5	T38.5X6
Proglumide	T47.1X1	T47.1X2	T47.1X3	T47.1X4	T47.1X5	T47.1X6
Proguanil	T37.2X1	T37.2X2	T37.2X3	T37.2X4	T37.2X5	T37.2X6
Prolactin	T38.811	T38.812	T38.813	T38.814	T38.815	T38.816
Prolintane	T43.691	T43.692	T43.693	T43.694	T43.695	T43.696
Proloid	T38.1X1	T38.1X2	T38.1X3	T38.1X4	T38.1X5	T38.1X6
Proluton	T38.5X1	T38.5X2	T38.5X3	T38.5X4	T38.5X5	T38.5X6
Promacetin	T37.1X1	T37.1X2	T37.1X3	T37.1X4	T37.1X5	T37.1X6
Promazine	T43.3X1	T43.3X2	T43.3X3	T43.3X4	T43.3X5	T43.3X6
Promedol	T40.2X1	T40.2X2	T40.2X3	T40.2X4	—	—
Promegestone	T38.5X1	T38.5X2	T38.5X3	T38.5X4	T38.5X5	T38.5X6
Promethazine (teoclate)	T43.3X1	T43.3X2	T43.3X3	T43.3X4	T43.3X5	T43.3X6
Promin	T37.1X1	T37.1X2	T37.1X3	T37.1X4	T37.1X5	T37.1X6

Substance	Poisoning, Accidental (unintentional)	Poisoning, Intentional self-harm	Poisoning, Assault	Poisoning, Undetermined	Adverse effect	Underdosing
Pronase	T45.3X1	T45.3X2	T45.3X3	T45.3X4	T45.3X5	T45.3X6
Pronestyl (hydrochloride)	T46.2X1	T46.2X2	T46.2X3	T46.2X4	T46.2X5	T46.2X6
Pronetalol	T44.7X1	T44.7X2	T44.7X3	T44.7X4	T44.7X5	T44.7X6
Prontosil	T37.0X1	T37.0X2	T37.0X3	T37.0X4	T37.0X5	T37.0X6
Propachlor	T60.3X1	T60.3X2	T60.3X3	T60.3X4	—	—
Propafenone	T46.2X1	T46.2X2	T46.2X3	T46.2X4	T46.2X5	T46.2X6
Propallylonal	T42.3X1	T42.3X2	T42.3X3	T42.3X4	T42.3X5	T42.3X6
Propamidine	T49.0X1	T49.0X2	T49.0X3	T49.0X4	T49.0X5	T49.0X6
Propane (distributed in mobile container)	T59.891	T59.892	T59.893	T59.894	—	—
distributed through pipes	T59.891	T59.892	T59.893	T59.894	—	—
incomplete combustion	T58.11	T58.12	T58.13	T58.14	—	—
Propanidid	T41.291	T41.292	T41.293	T41.294	T41.295	T41.296
Propanil	T60.3X1	T60.3X2	T60.3X3	T60.3X4	—	—
1-Propanol	T51.3X1	T51.3X2	T51.3X3	T51.3X4	—	—
2-Propanol	T51.2X1	T51.2X2	T51.2X3	T51.2X4	—	—
Propantheline	T44.3X1	T44.3X2	T44.3X3	T44.3X4	T44.3X5	T44.3X6
bromide	T44.3X1	T44.3X2	T44.3X3	T44.3X4	T44.3X5	T44.3X6
Proparacaine	T41.3X1	T41.3X2	T41.3X3	T41.3X4	T41.3X5	T41.3X6
Propatylnitrate	T46.3X1	T46.3X2	T46.3X3	T46.3X4	T46.3X5	T46.3X6
Propicillin	T36.0X1	T36.0X2	T36.0X3	T36.0X4	T36.0X5	T36.0X6
Propiolactone	T49.0X1	T49.0X2	T49.0X3	T49.0X4	T49.0X5	T49.0X6
Propiomazine	T45.0X1	T45.0X2	T45.0X3	T45.0X4	T45.0X5	T45.0X6
Propionaldehyde (medicinal)	T42.6X1	T42.6X2	T42.6X3	T42.6X4	T42.6X5	T42.6X6
Propionate (calcium) (sodium)	T49.0X1	T49.0X2	T49.0X3	T49.0X4	T49.0X5	T49.0X6
Propion gel	T49.0X1	T49.0X2	T49.0X3	T49.0X4	T49.0X5	T49.0X6
Propitocaine	T41.3X1	T41.3X2	T41.3X3	T41.3X4	T41.3X5	T41.3X6
infiltration (subcutaneous)	T41.3X1	T41.3X2	T41.3X3	T41.3X4	T41.3X5	T41.3X6
nerve block (peripheral) (plexus)	T41.3X1	T41.3X2	T41.3X3	T41.3X4	T41.3X5	T41.3X6
Propofol	T41.291	T41.292	T41.293	T41.294	T41.295	T41.296
Propoxur	T60.0X1	T60.0X2	T60.0X3	T60.0X4	—	—
Propoxycaine	T41.3X1	T41.3X2	T41.3X3	T41.3X4	T41.3X5	T41.3X6
infiltration (subcutaneous)	T41.3X1	T41.3X2	T41.3X3	T41.3X4	T41.3X5	T41.3X6
nerve block (peripheral) (plexus)	T41.3X1	T41.3X2	T41.3X3	T41.3X4	T41.3X5	T41.3X6
topical (surface)	T41.3X1	T41.3X2	T41.3X3	T41.3X4	T41.3X5	T41.3X6
Propoxyphene	T40.4X1	T40.4X2	T40.4X3	T40.4X4	T40.4X5	T40.4X6
Propranolol	T44.7X1	T44.7X2	T44.7X3	T44.7X4	T44.7X5	T44.7X6
Propyl						
alcohol	T51.3X1	T51.3X2	T51.3X3	T51.3X4	—	—
carbinol	T51.3X1	T51.3X2	T51.3X3	T51.3X4	—	—
hexadrine	T44.4X1	T44.4X2	T44.4X3	T44.4X4	T44.4X5	T44.4X6
iodone	T50.8X1	T50.8X2	T50.8X3	T50.8X4	T50.8X5	T50.8X6
thiouracil	T38.2X1	T38.2X2	T38.2X3	T38.2X4	T38.2X5	T38.2X6
Propylaminopheno-thiazine	T43.3X1	T43.3X2	T43.3X3	T43.3X4	T43.3X5	T43.3X6
Propylene	T59.891	T59.892	T59.893	T59.894	—	—
Propylhexedrine	T48.5X1	T48.5X2	T48.5X3	T48.5X4	T48.5X5	T48.5X6
Propyliodone	T50.8X1	T50.8X2	T50.8X3	T50.8X4	T50.8X5	T50.8X6

Substance	Poisoning, Accidental (unintentional)	Poisoning, Intentional self-harm	Poisoning, Assault	Poisoning, Undetermined	Adverse effect	Underdosing
Propylparaben (ophthalmic)	T49.5X1	T49.5X2	T49.5X3	T49.5X4	T49.5X5	T49.5X6
Propylthiouracil	T38.2X1	T38.2X2	T38.2X3	T38.2X4	T38.2X5	T38.2X6
Propyphenazone	T39.2X1	T39.2X2	T39.2X3	T39.2X4	T39.2X5	T39.2X6
Proquazone	T39.391	T39.392	T39.393	T39.394	T39.395	T39.396
Proscillaridin	T46.0X1	T46.0X2	T46.0X3	T46.0X4	T46.0X5	T46.0X6
Prostacyclin	T45.521	T45.522	T45.523	T45.524	T45.525	T45.526
Prostaglandin (I2)	T45.521	T45.522	T45.523	T45.524	T45.525	T45.526
E1	T46.7X1	T46.7X2	T46.7X3	T46.7X4	T46.7X5	T46.7X6
E2	T48.0X1	T48.0X2	T48.0X3	T48.0X4	T48.0X5	T48.0X6
F2 alpha	T48.0X1	T48.0X2	T48.0X3	T48.0X4	T48.0X5	T48.0X6
Prostigmin	T44.0X1	T44.0X2	T44.0X3	T44.0X4	T44.0X5	T44.0X6
Prosultiamine	T45.2X1	T45.2X2	T45.2X3	T45.2X4	T45.2X5	T45.2X6
Protamine sulfate	T45.7X1	T45.7X2	T45.7X3	T45.7X4	T45.7X5	T45.7X6
zinc insulin	T38.3X1	T38.3X2	T38.3X3	T38.3X4	T38.3X5	T38.3X6
Protease	T47.5X1	T47.5X2	T47.5X3	T47.5X4	T47.5X5	T47.5X6
Protectant, skin NEC	T49.3X1	T49.3X2	T49.3X3	T49.3X4	T49.3X5	T49.3X6
Protein hydrolysate	T50.991	T50.992	T50.993	T50.994	T50.995	T50.996
Prothiaden—see Dothiepin hydrochloride						
Prothionamide	T37.1X1	T37.1X2	T37.1X3	T37.1X4	T37.1X5	T37.1X6
Prothipendyl	T43.591	T43.592	T43.593	T43.594	T43.595	T43.596
Prothoate	T60.0X1	T60.0X2	T60.0X3	T60.0X4	—	—
Prothrombin						
activator	T45.7X1	T45.7X2	T45.7X3	T45.7X4	T45.7X5	T45.7X6
synthesis inhibitor	T45.511	T45.512	T45.513	T45.514	T45.515	T45.516
Protionamide	T37.1X1	T37.1X2	T37.1X3	T37.1X4	T37.1X5	T37.1X6
Protirelin	T38.891	T38.892	T38.893	T38.894	T38.895	T38.896
Protokylol	T48.6X1	T48.6X2	T48.6X3	T48.6X4	T48.6X5	T48.6X6
Protopam	T50.6X1	T50.6X2	T50.6X3	T50.6X4	T50.6X5	T50.6X6
Protoveratrine (s) (A) (B)	T46.5X1	T46.5X2	T46.5X3	T46.5X4	T46.5X5	T46.5X6
Protriptyline	T43.011	T43.012	T43.013	T43.014	T43.015	T43.016
Provera	T38.5X1	T38.5X2	T38.5X3	T38.5X4	T38.5X5	T38.5X6
Provitamin A	T45.2X1	T45.2X2	T45.2X3	T45.2X4	T45.2X5	T45.2X6
Proxibarbal	T42.3X1	T42.3X2	T42.3X3	T42.3X4	T42.3X5	T42.3X6
Proxymetacaine	T41.3X1	T41.3X2	T41.3X3	T41.3X4	T41.3X5	T41.3X6
Proxyphylline	T48.6X1	T48.6X2	T48.6X3	T48.6X4	T48.6X5	T48.6X6
Prozac—see Fluoxetine hydrochloride						
Prunus						
laurocerasus	T62.2X1	T62.2X2	T62.2X3	T62.2X4	—	—
virginiana	T62.2X1	T62.2X2	T62.2X3	T62.2X4	—	—
Prussian blue						
commercial	T65.891	T65.892	T65.893	T65.894	—	—
therapeutic	T50.6X1	T50.6X2	T50.6X3	T50.6X4	T50.6X5	T50.6X6
Prussic acid	T65.0X1	T65.0X2	T65.0X3	T65.0X4	—	—
vapor	T57.3X1	T57.3X2	T57.3X3	T57.3X4	—	—
Pseudoephedrine	T44.991	T44.992	T44.993	T44.994	T44.995	T44.996
Psilocin	T40.991	T40.992	T40.993	T40.994	—	—
Psilocybin	T40.991	T40.992	T40.993	T40.994	—	—
Psilocybine	T40.991	T40.992	T40.993	T40.994	—	—

Substance	Poisoning, Accidental (unintentional)	Poisoning, Intentional self-harm	Poisoning, Assault	Poisoning, Undetermined	Adverse effect	Underdosing
Psoralene (nonmedicinal)	T65.891	T65.892	T65.893	T65.894	—	—
Psoralens (medicinal)	T50.991	T50.992	T50.993	T50.994	T50.995	T50.996
PSP (phenolsulfon-phthalein)	T50.8X1	T50.8X2	T50.8X3	T50.8X4	T50.8X5	T50.8X6
Psychodysleptic drug NEC	T40.901	T40.902	T40.903	T40.904	T40.905	T40.906
Psychostimulant	T43.601	T43.602	T43.603	T43.604	T43.605	T43.606
amphetamine	T43.621	T43.622	T43.623	T43.624	T43.625	T43.626
caffeine	T43.611	T43.612	T43.613	T43.614	T43.615	T43.616
methylphenidate	T43.631	T43.632	T43.633	T43.634	T43.635	T43.636
specified NEC	T43.691	T43.692	T43.693	T43.694	T43.695	T43.696
Psychotherapeutic drug NEC	T43.91	T43.92	T43.93	T43.94	T43.95	T43.96
antidepressants—see also Antidepressant	T43.201	T43.202	T43.203	T43.204	T43.205	T43.206
specified NEC	T43.8X1	T43.8X2	T43.8X3	T43.8X4	T43.8X5	T43.8X6
tranquilizers NEC	T43.501	T43.502	T43.503	T43.504	T43.505	T43.506
Psychotomimetic agents	T40.901	T40.902	T40.903	T40.904	T40.905	T40.906
Psychotropic drug NEC	T43.91	T43.92	T43.93	T43.94	T43.95	T43.96
specified NEC	T43.8X1	T43.8X2	T43.8X3	T43.8X4	T43.8X5	T43.8X6
Psyllium hydrophilic mucilloid	T47.4X1	T47.4X2	T47.4X3	T47.4X4	T47.4X5	T47.4X6
Pteroylglutamic acid	T45.8X1	T45.8X2	T45.8X3	T45.8X4	T45.8X5	T45.8X6
Pteroyltriglutamate	T45.1X1	T45.1X2	T45.1X3	T45.1X4	T45.1X5	T45.1X6
PTFE—see Polytetra-fluoroethylene						
Pulp						
devitalizing paste	T49.7X1	T49.7X2	T49.7X3	T49.7X4	T49.7X5	T49.7X6
dressing	T49.7X1	T49.7X2	T49.7X3	T49.7X4	T49.7X5	T49.7X6
Pulsatilla	T62.2X1	T62.2X2	T62.2X3	T62.2X4	—	—
Pumpkin seed extract	T37.4X1	T37.4X2	T37.4X3	T37.4X4	T37.4X5	T37.4X6
Purex (bleach)	T54.91	T54.92	T54.93	T54.94	—	—
Purgative NEC—see also Cathartic	T47.4X1	T47.4X2	T47.4X3	T47.4X4	T47.4X5	T47.4X6
Purine analogue (antineoplastic)	T45.1X1	T45.1X2	T45.1X3	T45.1X4	T45.1X5	T45.1X6
Purine diuretics	T50.2X1	T50.2X2	T50.2X3	T50.2X4	T50.2X5	T50.2X6
Purinethol	T45.1X1	T45.1X2	T45.1X3	T45.1X4	T45.1X5	T45.1X6
PVP	T45.8X1	T45.8X2	T45.8X3	T45.8X4	T45.8X5	T45.8X6
Pyrabital	T39.8X1	T39.8X2	T39.8X3	T39.8X4	T39.8X5	T39.8X6
Pyramidon	T39.2X1	T39.2X2	T39.2X3	T39.2X4	T39.2X5	T39.2X6
Pyrantel	T37.4X1	T37.4X2	T37.4X3	T37.4X4	T37.4X5	T37.4X6
Pyrathiazine	T45.0X1	T45.0X2	T45.0X3	T45.0X4	T45.0X5	T45.0X6
Pyrazinamide	T37.1X1	T37.1X2	T37.1X3	T37.1X4	T37.1X5	T37.1X6
Pyrazinoic acid (amide)	T37.1X1	T37.1X2	T37.1X3	T37.1X4	T37.1X5	T37.1X6
Pyrazole (derivatives)	T39.2X1	T39.2X2	T39.2X3	T39.2X4	T39.2X5	T39.2X6
Pyrazolone analgesic NEC	T39.2X1	T39.2X2	T39.2X3	T39.2X4	T39.2X5	T39.2X6
Pyrethrin, pyrethrum (nonmedicinal)	T60.2X1	T60.2X2	T60.2X3	T60.2X4	—	—
Pyrethrum extract	T49.0X1	T49.0X2	T49.0X3	T49.0X4	T49.0X5	T49.0X6
Pyribenzamine	T45.0X1	T45.0X2	T45.0X3	T45.0X4	T45.0X5	T45.0X6

Substance	Poisoning, Accidental (unintentional)	Poisoning, Intentional self-harm	Poisoning, Assault	Poisoning, Undetermined	Adverse effect	Underdosing
Pyridine	T52.8X1	T52.8X2	T52.8X3	T52.8X4	—	—
aldoxime methiodide	T50.6X1	T50.6X2	T50.6X3	T50.6X4	T50.6X5	T50.6X6
aldoxime methyl chloride	T50.6X1	T50.6X2	T50.6X3	T50.6X4	T50.6X5	T50.6X6
vapor	T59.891	T59.892	T59.893	T59.894	—	—
Pyridium	T39.8X1	T39.8X2	T39.8X3	T39.8X4	T39.8X5	T39.8X6
Pyridostigmine bromide	T44.0X1	T44.0X2	T44.0X3	T44.0X4	T44.0X5	T44.0X6
Pyridoxal phosphate	T45.2X1	T45.2X2	T45.2X3	T45.2X4	T45.2X5	T45.2X6
Pyridoxine	T45.2X1	T45.2X2	T45.2X3	T45.2X4	T45.2X5	T45.2X6
Pyrilamine	T45.0X1	T45.0X2	T45.0X3	T45.0X4	T45.0X5	T45.0X6
Pyrimethamine	T37.2X1	T37.2X2	T37.2X3	T37.2X4	T37.2X5	T37.2X6
with sulfadoxine	T37.2X1	T37.2X2	T37.2X3	T37.2X4	T37.2X5	T37.2X6
Pyrimidine antagonist	T45.1X1	T45.1X2	T45.1X3	T45.1X4	T45.1X5	T45.1X6
Pyriminil	T60.4X1	T60.4X2	T60.4X3	T60.4X4	—	—
Pyrithione zinc	T49.4X1	T49.4X2	T49.4X3	T49.4X4	T49.4X5	T49.4X6
Pyrithyldione	T42.6X1	T42.6X2	T42.6X3	T42.6X4	T42.6X5	T42.6X6
Pyrogallic acid	T49.0X1	T49.0X2	T49.0X3	T49.0X4	T49.0X5	T49.0X6
Pyrogallol	T49.0X1	T49.0X2	T49.0X3	T49.0X4	T49.0X5	T49.0X6
Pyroxylin	T49.3X1	T49.3X2	T49.3X3	T49.3X4	T49.3X5	T49.3X6
Pyrrobutamine	T45.0X1	T45.0X2	T45.0X3	T45.0X4	T45.0X5	T45.0X6
Pyrrolizidine alkaloids	T62.8X1	T62.8X2	T62.8X3	T62.8X4	—	—
Pyrvinium chloride	T37.4X1	T37.4X2	T37.4X3	T37.4X4	T37.4X5	T37.4X6
PZI	T38.3X1	T38.3X2	T38.3X3	T38.3X4	T38.3X5	T38.3X6
Q						
Quaalude	T42.6X1	T42.6X2	T42.6X3	T42.6X4	T42.6X5	T42.6X6
Quarternary ammonium						
anti-infective	T49.0X1	T49.0X2	T49.0X3	T49.0X4	T49.0X5	T49.0X6
ganglion blocking	T44.2X1	T44.2X2	T44.2X3	T44.2X4	T44.2X5	T44.2X6
parasympatholytic	T44.3X1	T44.3X2	T44.3X3	T44.3X4	T44.3X5	T44.3X6
Quazepam	T42.4X1	T42.4X2	T42.4X3	T42.4X4	T42.4X5	T42.4X6
Quicklime	T54.3X1	T54.3X2	T54.3X3	T54.3X4	—	—
Quillaja extract	T48.4X1	T48.4X2	T48.4X3	T48.4X4	T48.4X5	T48.4X6
Quinacrine	T37.2X1	T37.2X2	T37.2X3	T37.2X4	T37.2X5	T37.2X6
Quinaglute	T46.2X1	T46.2X2	T46.2X3	T46.2X4	T46.2X5	T46.2X6
Quinalbarbital	T42.3X1	T42.3X2	T42.3X3	T42.3X4	T42.3X5	T42.3X6
Quinalbarbitone sodium	T42.3X1	T42.3X2	T42.3X3	T42.3X4	T42.3X5	T42.3X6
Quinalphos	T60.0X1	T60.0X2	T60.0X3	T60.0X4	—	—
Quinapril	T46.4X1	T46.4X2	T46.4X3	T46.4X4	T46.4X5	T46.4X6
Quinestradiol	T38.5X1	T38.5X2	T38.5X3	T38.5X4	T38.5X5	T38.5X6
Quinestradol	T38.5X1	T38.5X2	T38.5X3	T38.5X4	T38.5X5	T38.5X6
Quinestrol	T38.5X1	T38.5X2	T38.5X3	T38.5X4	T38.5X5	T38.5X6
Quinethazone	T50.2X1	T50.2X2	T50.2X3	T50.2X4	T50.2X5	T50.2X6
Quingestanol	T38.4X1	T38.4X2	T38.4X3	T38.4X4	T38.4X5	T38.4X6
Quinidine	T46.2X1	T46.2X2	T46.2X3	T46.2X4	T46.2X5	T46.2X6
Quinine	T37.2X1	T37.2X2	T37.2X3	T37.2X4	T37.2X5	T37.2X6
Quiniobine	T37.8X1	T37.8X2	T37.8X3	T37.8X4	T37.8X5	T37.8X6
Quinisocaine	T49.1X1	T49.1X2	T49.1X3	T49.1X4	T49.1X5	T49.1X6
Quinocide	T37.2X1	T37.2X2	T37.2X3	T37.2X4	T37.2X5	T37.2X6
Quinoline (derivatives) NEC	T37.8X1	T37.8X2	T37.8X3	T37.8X4	T37.8X5	T37.8X6
Quinupramine	T43.011	T43.012	T43.013	T43.014	T43.015	T43.016
Quotane	T41.3X1	T41.3X2	T41.3X3	T41.3X4	T41.3X5	T41.3X6

Substance	Poisoning, Accidental (unintentional)	Poisoning, Intentional self-harm	Poisoning, Assault	Poisoning, Undetermined	Adverse effect	Underdosing
R						
Rabies						
immune globulin (human)	T50.Z11	T50.Z12	T50.Z13	T50.Z14	T50.Z15	T50.Z16
vaccine	T50.B91	T50.B92	T50.B93	T50.B94	T50.B95	T50.B96
Racemoramide	T40.2X1	T40.2X2	T40.2X3	T40.2X4	—	—
Racemorphan	T40.2X1	T40.2X2	T40.2X3	T40.2X4	T40.2X5	T40.2X6
Racepinefrin	T44.5X1	T44.5X2	T44.5X3	T44.5X4	T44.5X5	T44.5X6
Raclopride	T43.591	T43.592	T43.593	T43.594	T43.595	T43.596
Radiator alcohol	T51.1X1	T51.1X2	T51.1X3	T51.1X4	—	—
Radioactive drug NEC	T50.8X1	T50.8X2	T50.8X3	T50.8X4	T50.8X5	T50.8X6
Radio-opaque (drugs) (materials)	T50.8X1	T50.8X2	T50.8X3	T50.8X4	T50.8X5	T50.8X6
Ramifenazone	T39.2X1	T39.2X2	T39.2X3	T39.2X4	T39.2X5	T39.2X6
Ramipril	T46.4X1	T46.4X2	T46.4X3	T46.4X4	T46.4X5	T46.4X6
Ranitidine	T47.0X1	T47.0X2	T47.0X3	T47.0X4	T47.0X5	T47.0X6
Ranunculus	T62.2X1	T62.2X2	T62.2X3	T62.2X4	—	—
Rat poison NEC	T60.4X1	T60.4X2	T60.4X3	T60.4X4	—	—
Rattlesnake (venom)	T63.011	T63.012	T63.013	T63.014	—	—
Raubasine	T46.7X1	T46.7X2	T46.7X3	T46.7X4	T46.7X5	T46.7X6
Raudixin	T46.5X1	T46.5X2	T46.5X3	T46.5X4	T46.5X5	T46.5X6
Rautensin	T46.5X1	T46.5X2	T46.5X3	T46.5X4	T46.5X5	T46.5X6
Rautina	T46.5X1	T46.5X2	T46.5X3	T46.5X4	T46.5X5	T46.5X6
Rautotal	T46.5X1	T46.5X2	T46.5X3	T46.5X4	T46.5X5	T46.5X6
Rauwiloid	T46.5X1	T46.5X2	T46.5X3	T46.5X4	T46.5X5	T46.5X6
Rauwoldin	T46.5X1	T46.5X2	T46.5X3	T46.5X4	T46.5X5	T46.5X6
Rauwolfia (alkaloids)	T46.5X1	T46.5X2	T46.5X3	T46.5X4	T46.5X5	T46.5X6
Razoxane	T45.1X1	T45.1X2	T45.1X3	T45.1X4	T45.1X5	T45.1X6
Realgar	T57.0X1	T57.0X2	T57.0X3	T57.0X4	—	—
Recombinant(R)—see specific protein						
Red blood cells, packed	T45.8X1	T45.8X2	T45.8X3	T45.8X4	T45.8X5	T45.8X6
Red squill (scilliroside)	T60.4X1	T60.4X2	T60.4X3	T60.4X4	—	—
Reducing agent, industrial NEC	T65.891	T65.892	T65.893	T65.894	—	—
Refrigerant gas (chlorofluoro-carbon)	T53.5X1	T53.5X2	T53.5X3	T53.5X4	—	—
not chlorofluoro-carbon	T59.891	T59.892	T59.893	T59.894	—	—
Regroton	T50.2X1	T50.2X2	T50.2X3	T50.2X4	T50.2X5	T50.2X6
Rehydration salts (oral)	T50.3X1	T50.3X2	T50.3X3	T50.3X4	T50.3X5	T50.3X6
Rela	T42.8X1	T42.8X2	T42.8X3	T42.8X4	T42.8X5	T42.8X6
Relaxant, muscle						
anesthetic	T48.1X1	T48.1X2	T48.1X3	T48.1X4	T48.1X5	T48.1X6
central nervous system	T42.8X1	T42.8X2	T42.8X3	T42.8X4	T42.8X5	T42.8X6
skeletal NEC	T48.1X1	T48.1X2	T48.1X3	T48.1X4	T48.1X5	T48.1X6
smooth NEC	T44.3X1	T44.3X2	T44.3X3	T44.3X4	T44.3X5	T44.3X6
Remoxipride	T43.591	T43.592	T43.593	T43.594	T43.595	T43.596
Renese	T50.2X1	T50.2X2	T50.2X3	T50.2X4	T50.2X5	T50.2X6
Renografin	T50.8X1	T50.8X2	T50.8X3	T50.8X4	T50.8X5	T50.8X6
Replacement solution	T50.3X1	T50.3X2	T50.3X3	T50.3X4	T50.3X5	T50.3X6
Reproterol	T48.6X1	T48.6X2	T48.6X3	T48.6X4	T48.6X5	T48.6X6
Rescinnamine	T46.5X1	T46.5X2	T46.5X3	T46.5X4	T46.5X5	T46.5X6

Substance	Poisoning, Accidental (unintentional)	Poisoning, Intentional self-harm	Poisoning, Assault	Poisoning, Undetermined	Adverse effect	Underdosing
Reserpin(e)	T46.5X1	T46.5X2	T46.5X3	T46.5X4	T46.5X5	T46.5X6
Resorcin, resorcinol (nonmedicinal)	T65.891	T65.892	T65.893	T65.894	—	—
medicinal	T49.4X1	T49.4X2	T49.4X3	T49.4X4	T49.4X5	T49.4X6
Respaire	T48.4X1	T48.4X2	T48.4X3	T48.4X4	T48.4X5	T48.4X6
Respiratory drug NEC	T48.901	T48.902	T48.903	T48.904	T48.905	T48.906
antiasthmatic NEC	T48.6X1	T48.6X2	T48.6X3	T48.6X4	T48.6X5	T48.6X6
anti-common-cold NEC	T48.5X1	T48.5X2	T48.5X3	T48.5X4	T48.5X5	T48.5X6
expectorant NEC	T48.4X1	T48.4X2	T48.4X3	T48.4X4	T48.4X5	T48.4X6
stimulant	T48.901	T48.902	T48.903	T48.904	T48.905	T48.906
Retinoic acid	T49.0X1	T49.0X2	T49.0X3	T49.0X4	T49.0X5	T49.0X6
Retinol	T45.2X1	T45.2X2	T45.2X3	T45.2X4	T45.2X5	T45.2X6
Rh(D) immune globulin (human)	T50.Z11	T50.Z12	T50.Z13	T50.Z14	T50.Z15	T50.Z16
Rhodine	T39.011	T39.012	T39.013	T39.014	T39.015	T39.016
RhoGAM	T50.Z11	T50.Z12	T50.Z13	T50.Z14	T50.Z15	T50.Z16
Rhubarb						
dry extract	T47.2X1	T47.2X2	T47.2X3	T47.2X4	T47.2X5	T47.2X6
tincture, compound	T47.2X1	T47.2X2	T47.2X3	T47.2X4	T47.2X5	T47.2X6
Ribavirin	T37.5X1	T37.5X2	T37.5X3	T37.5X4	T37.5X5	T37.5X6
Riboflavin	T45.2X1	T45.2X2	T45.2X3	T45.2X4	T45.2X5	T45.2X6
Ribostamycin	T36.5X1	T36.5X2	T36.5X3	T36.5X4	T36.5X5	T36.5X6
Ricin	T62.2X1	T62.2X2	T62.2X3	T62.2X4	—	—
Ricinus communis	T62.2X1	T62.2X2	T62.2X3	T62.2X4	—	—
Rickettsial vaccine NEC	T50.A91	T50.A92	T50.A93	T50.A94	T50.A95	T50.A96
Rifabutin	T36.6X1	T36.6X2	T36.6X3	T36.6X4	T36.6X5	T36.6X6
Rifamide	T36.6X1	T36.6X2	T36.6X3	T36.6X4	T36.6X5	T36.6X6
Rifampicin	T36.6X1	T36.6X2	T36.6X3	T36.6X4	T36.6X5	T36.6X6
with isoniazid	T37.1X1	T37.1X2	T37.1X3	T37.1X4	T37.1X5	T37.1X6
Rifampin	T36.6X1	T36.6X2	T36.6X3	T36.6X4	T36.6X5	T36.6X6
Rifamycin	T36.6X1	T36.6X2	T36.6X3	T36.6X4	T36.6X5	T36.6X6
Rifaximin	T36.6X1	T36.6X2	T36.6X3	T36.6X4	T36.6X5	T36.6X6
Rimantadine	T37.5X1	T37.5X2	T37.5X3	T37.5X4	T37.5X5	T37.5X6
Rimazolium metilsulfate	T39.8X1	T39.8X2	T39.8X3	T39.8X4	T39.8X5	T39.8X6
Rimifon	T37.1X1	T37.1X2	T37.1X3	T37.1X4	T37.1X5	T37.1X6
Rimiterol	T48.6X1	T48.6X2	T48.6X3	T48.6X4	T48.6X5	T48.6X6
Ringer (lactate) solution	T50.3X1	T50.3X2	T50.3X3	T50.3X4	T50.3X5	T50.3X6
Ristocetin	T36.8X1	T36.8X2	T36.8X3	T36.8X4	T36.8X5	T36.8X6
Ritalin	T43.631	T43.632	T43.633	T43.634	T43.635	T43.636
Ritodrine	T44.5X1	T44.5X2	T44.5X3	T44.5X4	T44.5X5	T44.5X6
Roach killer—see Insecticide						
Rociverine	T44.3X1	T44.3X2	T44.3X3	T44.3X4	T44.3X5	T44.3X6
Rocky Mountain spotted fever vaccine	T50.A91	T50.A92	T50.A93	T50.A94	T50.A95	T50.A96
Rodenticide NEC	T60.4X1	T60.4X2	T60.4X3	T60.4X4	—	—
Rohypnol	T42.4X1	T42.4X2	T42.4X3	T42.4X4	T42.4X5	T42.4X6
Rokitamycin	T36.3X1	T36.3X2	T36.3X3	T36.3X4	T36.3X5	T36.3X6
Rolaids	T47.1X1	T47.1X2	T47.1X3	T47.1X4	T47.1X5	T47.1X6
Rolitetracycline	T36.4X1	T36.4X2	T36.4X3	T36.4X4	T36.4X5	T36.4X6
Romilar	T48.3X1	T48.3X2	T48.3X3	T48.3X4	T48.3X5	T48.3X6
Ronifibrate	T46.6X1	T46.6X2	T46.6X3	T46.6X4	T46.6X5	T46.6X6
Rosaprostol	T47.1X1	T47.1X2	T47.1X3	T47.1X4	T47.1X5	T47.1X6
Rose bengal sodium (131I)	T50.8X1	T50.8X2	T50.8X3	T50.8X4	T50.8X5	T50.8X6
Rose water ointment	T49.3X1	T49.3X2	T49.3X3	T49.3X4	T49.3X5	T49.3X6
Rosoxacin	T37.8X1	T37.8X2	T37.8X3	T37.8X4	T37.8X5	T37.8X6
Rotenone	T60.2X1	T60.2X2	T60.2X3	T60.2X4	—	—
Rotoxamine	T45.0X1	T45.0X2	T45.0X3	T45.0X4	T45.0X5	T45.0X6
Rough-on-rats	T60.4X1	T60.4X2	T60.4X3	T60.4X4	—	—
Roxatidine	T47.0X1	T47.0X2	T47.0X3	T47.0X4	T47.0X5	T47.0X6
Roxithromycin	T36.3X1	T36.3X2	T36.3X3	T36.3X4	T36.3X5	T36.3X6
Rt-PA	T45.611	T45.612	T45.613	T45.614	T45.615	T45.616
Rubbing alcohol	T51.2X1	T51.2X2	T51.2X3	T51.2X4	—	—
Rubefacient	T49.4X1	T49.4X2	T49.4X3	T49.4X4	T49.4X5	T49.4X6
Rubella vaccine	T50.B91	T50.B92	T50.B93	T50.B94	T50.B95	T50.B96
Rubeola vaccine	T50.B91	T50.B92	T50.B93	T50.B94	T50.B95	T50.B96
Rubidium chloride Rb82	T50.8X1	T50.8X2	T50.8X3	T50.8X4	T50.8X5	T50.8X6
Rubidomycin	T45.1X1	T45.1X2	T45.1X3	T45.1X4	T45.1X5	T45.1X6
Rue	T62.2X1	T62.2X2	T62.2X3	T62.2X4	—	—
Rufocromomycin	T45.1X1	T45.1X2	T45.1X3	T45.1X4	T45.1X5	T45.1X6
Russel's viper venin	T45.7X1	T45.7X2	T45.7X3	T45.7X4	T45.7X5	T45.7X6
Ruta (graveolens)	T62.2X1	T62.2X2	T62.2X3	T62.2X4	—	—
Rutinum	T46.991	T46.992	T46.993	T46.994	T46.995	T46.996
Rutoside	T46.991	T46.992	T46.993	T46.994	T46.995	T46.996
S						
Sabadilla (plant)	T62.2X1	T62.2X2	T62.2X3	T62.2X4	—	—
pesticide	T60.2X1	T60.2X2	T60.2X3	T60.2X4	—	—
Saccharated iron oxide	T45.8X1	T45.8X2	T45.8X3	T45.8X4	T45.8X5	T45.8X6
Saccharin	T50.901	T50.902	T50.903	T50.904	T50.905	T50.906
Saccharomyces boulardii	T47.6X1	T47.6X2	T47.6X3	T47.6X4	T47.6X5	T47.6X6
Safflower oil	T46.6X1	T46.6X2	T46.6X3	T46.6X4	T46.6X5	T46.6X6
Safrazine	T43.1X1	T43.1X2	T43.1X3	T43.1X4	T43.1X5	T43.1X6
Salazosulfapyridine	T37.0X1	T37.0X2	T37.0X3	T37.0X4	T37.0X5	T37.0X6
Salbutamol	T48.6X1	T48.6X2	T48.6X3	T48.6X4	T48.6X5	T48.6X6
Salicylamide	T39.091	T39.092	T39.093	T39.094	T39.095	T39.096
Salicylate NEC	T39.091	T39.092	T39.093	T39.094	T39.095	T39.096
methyl	T49.3X1	T49.3X2	T49.3X3	T49.3X4	T49.3X5	T49.3X6
theobromine calcium	T50.2X1	T50.2X2	T50.2X3	T50.2X4	T50.2X5	T50.2X6
Salicylazosulfapyridine	T37.0X1	T37.0X2	T37.0X3	T37.0X4	T37.0X5	T37.0X6
Salicylhydroxamic acid	T49.0X1	T49.0X2	T49.0X3	T49.0X4	T49.0X5	T49.0X6
Salicylic acid	T49.4X1	T49.4X2	T49.4X3	T49.4X4	T49.4X5	T49.4X6
with benzoic acid	T49.4X1	T49.4X2	T49.4X3	T49.4X4	T49.4X5	T49.4X6
congeners	T39.091	T39.092	T39.093	T39.094	T39.095	T39.096
derivative	T39.091	T39.092	T39.093	T39.094	T39.095	T39.096
salts	T39.091	T39.092	T39.093	T39.094	T39.095	T39.096
Salinazid	T37.1X1	T37.1X2	T37.1X3	T37.1X4	T37.1X5	T37.1X6
Salmeterol	T48.6X1	T48.6X2	T48.6X3	T48.6X4	T48.6X5	T48.6X6
Salol	T49.3X1	T49.3X2	T49.3X3	T49.3X4	T49.3X5	T49.3X6
Salsalate	T39.091	T39.092	T39.093	T39.094	T39.095	T39.096
Salt substitute	T50.901	T50.902	T50.903	T50.904	T50.905	T50.906

Substance	Poisoning, Accidental (unintentional)	Poisoning, Intentional self-harm	Poisoning, Assault	Poisoning, Undetermined	Adverse effect	Underdosing
Salt-replacing drug	T50.901	T50.902	T50.903	T50.904	T50.905	T50.906
Salt-retaining mineralocorticoid	T50.0X1	T50.0X2	T50.0X3	T50.0X4	T50.0X5	T50.0X6
Saluretic NEC	T50.2X1	T50.2X2	T50.2X3	T50.2X4	T50.2X5	T50.2X6
Saluron	T50.2X1	T50.2X2	T50.2X3	T50.2X4	T50.2X5	T50.2X6
Salvarsan 606 (neosilver) (silver)	T37.8X1	T37.8X2	T37.8X3	T37.8X4	T37.8X5	T37.8X6
Sambucus canadensis	T62.2X1	T62.2X2	T62.2X3	T62.2X4	—	—
berry	T62.1X1	T62.1X2	T62.1X3	T62.1X4	—	—
Sandril	T46.5X1	T46.5X2	T46.5X3	T46.5X4	T46.5X5	T46.5X6
Sanguinaria canadensis	T62.2X1	T62.2X2	T62.2X3	T62.2X4	—	—
Saniflush (cleaner)	T54.2X1	T54.2X2	T54.2X3	T54.2X4	—	—
Santonin	T37.4X1	T37.4X2	T37.4X3	T37.4X4	T37.4X5	T37.4X6
Santyl	T49.8X1	T49.8X2	T49.8X3	T49.8X4	T49.8X5	T49.8X6
Saralasin	T46.5X1	T46.5X2	T46.5X3	T46.5X4	T46.5X5	T46.5X6
Sarcolysin	T45.1X1	T45.1X2	T45.1X3	T45.1X4	T45.1X5	T45.1X6
Sarkomycin	T45.1X1	T45.1X2	T45.1X3	T45.1X4	T45.1X5	T45.1X6
Saroten	T43.011	T43.012	T43.013	T43.014	T43.015	T43.016
Saturnine—see Lead						
Savin (oil)	T49.4X1	T49.4X2	T49.4X3	T49.4X4	T49.4X5	T49.4X6
Scammony	T47.2X1	T47.2X2	T47.2X3	T47.2X4	T47.2X5	T47.2X6
Scarlet red	T49.8X1	T49.8X2	T49.8X3	T49.8X4	T49.8X5	T49.8X6
Scheele's green	T57.0X1	T57.0X2	T57.0X3	T57.0X4	—	—
insecticide	T57.0X1	T57.0X2	T57.0X3	T57.0X4	—	—
Schizontozide (blood) (tissue)	T37.2X1	T37.2X2	T37.2X3	T37.2X4	T37.2X5	T37.2X6
Schradan	T60.0X1	T60.0X2	T60.0X3	T60.0X4	—	—
Schweinfurth green	T57.0X1	T57.0X2	T57.0X3	T57.0X4	—	—
insecticide	T57.0X1	T57.0X2	T57.0X3	T57.0X4	—	—
Scilla, rat poison	T60.4X1	T60.4X2	T60.4X3	T60.4X4	—	—
Scillaren	T60.4X1	T60.4X2	T60.4X3	T60.4X4	—	—
Sclerosing agent	T46.8X1	T46.8X2	T46.8X3	T46.8X4	T46.8X5	T46.8X6
Scombrotoxin	T61.11	T61.12	T61.13	T61.14	—	—
Scopolamine	T44.3X1	T44.3X2	T44.3X3	T44.3X4	T44.3X5	T44.3X6
Scopolia extract	T44.3X1	T44.3X2	T44.3X3	T44.3X4	T44.3X5	T44.3X6
Scouring powder	T65.891	T65.892	T65.893	T65.894	—	—
Sea						
anemone (sting)	T63.631	T63.632	T63.633	T63.634	—	—
cucumber (sting)	T63.691	T63.692	T63.693	T63.694	—	—
snake (bite) (venom)	T63.091	T63.092	T63.093	T63.094	—	—
urchin spine (puncture)	T63.691	T63.692	T63.693	T63.694	—	—
Seafood	T61.91	T61.92	T61.93	T61.94	—	—
specified NEC	T61.8X1	T61.8X2	T61.8X3	T61.8X4	—	—
Secbutabarbital	T42.3X1	T42.3X2	T42.3X3	T42.3X4	T42.3X5	T42.3X6
Secbutabarbitone	T42.3X1	T42.3X2	T42.3X3	T42.3X4	T42.3X5	T42.3X6
Secnidazole	T37.3X1	T37.3X2	T37.3X3	T37.3X4	T37.3X5	T37.3X6
Secobarbital	T42.3X1	T42.3X2	T42.3X3	T42.3X4	T42.3X5	T42.3X6
Seconal	T42.3X1	T42.3X2	T42.3X3	T42.3X4	T42.3X5	T42.3X6
Secretin	T50.8X1	T50.8X2	T50.8X3	T50.8X4	T50.8X5	T50.8X6
Sedative NEC	T42.71	T42.72	T42.73	T42.74	T42.75	T42.76
mixed NEC	T42.6X1	T42.6X2	T42.6X3	T42.6X4	T42.6X5	T42.6X6

Substance	Poisoning, Accidental (unintentional)	Poisoning, Intentional self-harm	Poisoning, Assault	Poisoning, Undetermined	Adverse effect	Underdosing
Sedormid	T42.6X1	T42.6X2	T42.6X3	T42.6X4	T42.6X5	T42.6X6
Seed disinfectant or dressing	T60.8X1	T60.8X2	T60.8X3	T60.8X4	—	—
Seeds (poisonous)	T62.2X1	T62.2X2	T62.2X3	T62.2X4	—	—
Selegiline	T42.8X1	T42.8X2	T42.8X3	T42.8X4	T42.8X5	T42.8X6
Selenium NEC	T56.891	T56.892	T56.893	T56.894	—	—
disulfide or sulfide	T49.4X1	T49.4X2	T49.4X3	T49.4X4	T49.4X5	T49.4X6
fumes	T59.891	T59.892	T59.893	T59.894	—	—
sulfide	T49.4X1	T49.4X2	T49.4X3	T49.4X4	T49.4X5	T49.4X6
Selenomethionine (75Se)	T50.8X1	T50.8X2	T50.8X3	T50.8X4	T50.8X5	T50.8X6
Selsun	T49.4X1	T49.4X2	T49.4X3	T49.4X4	T49.4X5	T49.4X6
Semustine	T45.1X1	T45.1X2	T45.1X3	T45.1X4	T45.1X5	T45.1X6
Senega syrup	T48.4X1	T48.4X2	T48.4X3	T48.4X4	T48.4X5	T48.4X6
Senna	T47.2X1	T47.2X2	T47.2X3	T47.2X4	T47.2X5	T47.2X6
Sennoside A+B	T47.2X1	T47.2X2	T47.2X3	T47.2X4	T47.2X5	T47.2X6
Septisol	T49.2X1	T49.2X2	T49.2X3	T49.2X4	T49.2X5	T49.2X6
Seractide	T38.811	T38.812	T38.813	T38.814	T38.815	T38.816
Serax	T42.4X1	T42.4X2	T42.4X3	T42.4X4	T42.4X5	T42.4X6
Serenesil	T42.6X1	T42.6X2	T42.6X3	T42.6X4	T42.6X5	T42.6X6
Serenium (hydrochloride)	T37.91	T37.92	T37.93	T37.94	T37.95	T37.96
Serepax—see Oxazepam						
Sermorelin	T38.891	T38.892	T38.893	T38.894	T38.895	T38.896
Sernyl	T41.1X1	T41.1X2	T41.1X3	T41.1X4	T41.1X5	T41.1X6
Serotonin	T50.991	T50.992	T50.993	T50.994	T50.995	T50.996
Serpasil	T46.5X1	T46.5X2	T46.5X3	T46.5X4	T46.5X5	T46.5X6
Serrapeptase	T45.3X1	T45.3X2	T45.3X3	T45.3X4	T45.3X5	T45.3X6
Serum						
antibotulinus	T50.Z11	T50.Z12	T50.Z13	T50.Z14	T50.Z15	T50.Z16
anticytotoxic	T50.Z11	T50.Z12	T50.Z13	T50.Z14	T50.Z15	T50.Z16
antidiphtheria	T50.Z11	T50.Z12	T50.Z13	T50.Z14	T50.Z15	T50.Z16
antimeningococcus	T50.Z11	T50.Z12	T50.Z13	T50.Z14	T50.Z15	T50.Z16
anti-Rh	T50.Z11	T50.Z12	T50.Z13	T50.Z14	T50.Z15	T50.Z16
anti-snake-bite	T50.Z11	T50.Z12	T50.Z13	T50.Z14	T50.Z15	T50.Z16
antitetanic	T50.Z11	T50.Z12	T50.Z13	T50.Z14	T50.Z15	T50.Z16
antitoxic	T50.Z11	T50.Z12	T50.Z13	T50.Z14	T50.Z15	T50.Z16
complement (inhibitor)	T45.8X1	T45.8X2	T45.8X3	T45.8X4	T45.8X5	T45.8X6
convalescent	T50.Z11	T50.Z12	T50.Z13	T50.Z14	T50.Z15	T50.Z16
hemolytic complement	T45.8X1	T45.8X2	T45.8X3	T45.8X4	T45.8X5	T45.8X6
immune (human)	T50.Z11	T50.Z12	T50.Z13	T50.Z14	T50.Z15	T50.Z16
protective NEC	T50.Z11	T50.Z12	T50.Z13	T50.Z14	T50.Z15	T50.Z16
Setastine	T45.0X1	T45.0X2	T45.0X3	T45.0X4	T45.0X5	T45.0X6
Setoperone	T43.591	T43.592	T43.593	T43.594	T43.595	T43.596
Sewer gas	T59.91	T59.92	T59.93	T59.94	—	—
Shampoo	T55.0X1	T55.0X2	T55.0X3	T55.0X4	—	—
Shellfish, noxious, nonbacterial	T61.781	T61.782	T61.783	T61.784	—	—
Sildenafil	T46.7X1	T46.7X2	T46.7X3	T46.7X4	T46.7X5	T46.7X6
Silibinin	T50.991	T50.992	T50.993	T50.994	T50.995	T50.996
Silicone NEC	T65.891	T65.892	T65.893	T65.894	—	—
medicinal	T49.3X1	T49.3X2	T49.3X3	T49.3X4	T49.3X5	T49.3X6

Substance	Poisoning, Accidental (unintentional)	Poisoning, Intentional self-harm	Poisoning, Assault	Poisoning, Undetermined	Adverse effect	Underdosing
Silvadene	T49.0X1	T49.0X2	T49.0X3	T49.0X4	T49.0X5	T49.0X6
Silver	T49.0X1	T49.0X2	T49.0X3	T49.0X4	T49.0X5	T49.0X6
anti-infectives	T49.0X1	T49.0X2	T49.0X3	T49.0X4	T49.0X5	T49.0X6
arsphenamine	T37.8X1	T37.8X2	T37.8X3	T37.8X4	T37.8X5	T37.8X6
colloidal	T49.0X1	T49.0X2	T49.0X3	T49.0X4	T49.0X5	T49.0X6
nitrate	T49.0X1	T49.0X2	T49.0X3	T49.0X4	T49.0X5	T49.0X6
ophthalmic preparation	T49.5X1	T49.5X2	T49.5X3	T49.5X4	T49.5X5	T49.5X6
toughened (keratolytic)	T49.4X1	T49.4X2	T49.4X3	T49.4X4	T49.4X5	T49.4X6
nonmedicinal (dust)	T56.891	T56.892	T56.893	T56.894	—	—
protein	T49.5X1	T49.5X2	T49.5X3	T49.5X4	T49.5X5	T49.5X6
salvarsan	T37.8X1	T37.8X2	T37.8X3	T37.8X4	T37.8X5	T37.8X6
sulfadiazine	T49.4X1	T49.4X2	T49.4X3	T49.4X4	T49.4X5	T49.4X6
Silymarin	T50.991	T50.992	T50.993	T50.994	T50.995	T50.996
Simaldrate	T47.1X1	T47.1X2	T47.1X3	T47.1X4	T47.1X5	T47.1X6
Simazine	T60.3X1	T60.3X2	T60.3X3	T60.3X4	—	—
Simethicone	T47.1X1	T47.1X2	T47.1X3	T47.1X4	T47.1X5	T47.1X6
Simfibrate	T46.6X1	T46.6X2	T46.6X3	T46.6X4	T46.6X5	T46.6X6
Simvastatin	T46.6X1	T46.6X2	T46.6X3	T46.6X4	T46.6X5	T46.6X6
Sincalide	T50.8X1	T50.8X2	T50.8X3	T50.8X4	T50.8X5	T50.8X6
Sinequan	T43.011	T43.012	T43.013	T43.014	T43.015	T43.016
Singoserp	T46.5X1	T46.5X2	T46.5X3	T46.5X4	T46.5X5	T46.5X6
Sintrom	T45.511	T45.512	T45.513	T45.514	T45.515	T45.516
Sisomicin	T36.5X1	T36.5X2	T36.5X3	T36.5X4	T36.5X5	T36.5X6
Sitosterols	T46.6X1	T46.6X2	T46.6X3	T46.6X4	T46.6X5	T46.6X6
Skeletal muscle relaxants	T48.1X1	T48.1X2	T48.1X3	T48.1X4	T48.1X5	T48.1X6
Skin						
agents (external)	T49.91	T49.92	T49.93	T49.94	T49.95	T49.96
specified NEC	T49.8X1	T49.8X2	T49.8X3	T49.8X4	T49.8X5	T49.8X6
test antigen	T50.8X1	T50.8X2	T50.8X3	T50.8X4	T50.8X5	T50.8X6
Sleep-eze	T45.0X1	T45.0X2	T45.0X3	T45.0X4	T45.0X5	T45.0X6
Sleeping draught, pill	T42.71	T42.72	T42.73	T42.74	T42.75	T42.76
Smallpox vaccine	T50.B11	T50.B12	T50.B13	T50.B14	T50.B15	T50.B16
Smelter fumes NEC	T56.91	T56.92	T56.93	T56.94	—	—
Smog	T59.1X1	T59.1X2	T59.1X3	T59.1X4	—	—
Smoke NEC	T59.811	T59.812	T59.813	T59.814	—	—
Smooth muscle relaxant	T44.3X1	T44.3X2	T44.3X3	T44.3X4	T44.3X5	T44.3X6
Snail killer NEC	T60.8X1	T60.8X2	T60.8X3	T60.8X4	—	—
Snake venom or bite	T63.001	T63.002	T63.003	T63.004	—	—
hemocoagulase	T45.7X1	T45.7X2	T45.7X3	T45.7X4	T45.7X5	T45.7X6
Snuff	T65.211	T65.212	T65.213	T65.214	—	—
Soap (powder) (product)	T55.0X1	T55.0X2	T55.0X3	T55.0X4	—	—
enema	T47.4X1	T47.4X2	T47.4X3	T47.4X4	T47.4X5	T47.4X6
medicinal, soft	T49.2X1	T49.2X2	T49.2X3	T49.2X4	T49.2X5	T49.2X6
superfatted	T49.2X1	T49.2X2	T49.2X3	T49.2X4	T49.2X5	T49.2X6
Sobrerol	T48.4X1	T48.4X2	T48.4X3	T48.4X4	T48.4X5	T48.4X6
Soda (caustic)	T54.3X1	T54.3X2	T54.3X3	T54.3X4	—	—
bicarb	T47.1X1	T47.1X2	T47.1X3	T47.1X4	T47.1X5	T47.1X6
chlorinated—see Sodium, hypochlorite						

Substance	Poisoning, Accidental (unintentional)	Poisoning, Intentional self-harm	Poisoning, Assault	Poisoning, Undetermined	Adverse effect	Underdosing
Sodium						
acetosulfone	T37.1X1	T37.1X2	T37.1X3	T37.1X4	T37.1X5	T37.1X6
acetrizoate	T50.8X1	T50.8X2	T50.8X3	T50.8X4	T50.8X5	T50.8X6
acid phosphate	T50.3X1	T50.3X2	T50.3X3	T50.3X4	T50.3X5	T50.3X6
alginate	T47.8X1	T47.8X2	T47.8X3	T47.8X4	T47.8X5	T47.8X6
amidotrizoate	T50.8X1	T50.8X2	T50.8X3	T50.8X4	T50.8X5	T50.8X6
aminopterin	T45.1X1	T45.1X2	T45.1X3	T45.1X4	T45.1X5	T45.1X6
amylosulfate	T47.8X1	T47.8X2	T47.8X3	T47.8X4	T47.8X5	T47.8X6
amytal	T42.3X1	T42.3X2	T42.3X3	T42.3X4	T42.3X5	T42.3X6
antimony gluconate	T37.3X1	T37.3X2	T37.3X3	T37.3X4	T37.3X5	T37.3X6
arsenate	T57.0X1	T57.0X2	T57.0X3	T57.0X4	—	—
aurothiomalate	T39.4X1	T39.4X2	T39.4X3	T39.4X4	T39.4X5	T39.4X6
aurothiosulfate	T39.4X1	T39.4X2	T39.4X3	T39.4X4	T39.4X5	T39.4X6
barbiturate	T42.3X1	T42.3X2	T42.3X3	T42.3X4	T42.3X5	T42.3X6
basic phosphate	T47.4X1	T47.4X2	T47.4X3	T47.4X4	T47.4X5	T47.4X6
bicarbonate	T47.1X1	T47.1X2	T47.1X3	T47.1X4	T47.1X5	T47.1X6
bichromate	T57.8X1	T57.8X2	T57.8X3	T57.8X4	—	—
biphosphate	T50.3X1	T50.3X2	T50.3X3	T50.3X4	T50.3X5	T50.3X6
bisulfate	T65.891	T65.892	T65.893	T65.894	—	—
borate						
cleanser	T57.8X1	T57.8X2	T57.8X3	T57.8X4	—	—
eye	T49.5X1	T49.5X2	T49.5X3	T49.5X4	T49.5X5	T49.5X6
therapeutic	T49.8X1	T49.8X2	T49.8X3	T49.8X4	T49.8X5	T49.8X6
bromide	T42.6X1	T42.6X2	T42.6X3	T42.6X4	T42.6X5	T42.6X6
cacodylate (nonmedicinal) NEC	T50.8X1	T50.8X2	T50.8X3	T50.8X4	T50.8X5	T50.8X6
anti-infective	T37.8X1	T37.8X2	T37.8X3	T37.8X4	T37.8X5	T37.8X6
herbicide	T60.3X1	T60.3X2	T60.3X3	T60.3X4	—	—
calcium edetate	T45.8X1	T45.8X2	T45.8X3	T45.8X4	T45.8X5	T45.8X6
carbonate NEC	T54.3X1	T54.3X2	T54.3X3	T54.3X4	—	—
chlorate NEC	T65.891	T65.892	T65.893	T65.894	—	—
herbicide	T54.91	T54.92	T54.93	T54.94	—	—
chloride	T50.3X1	T50.3X2	T50.3X3	T50.3X4	T50.3X5	T50.3X6
with glucose	T50.3X1	T50.3X2	T50.3X3	T50.3X4	T50.3X5	T50.3X6
chromate	T65.891	T65.892	T65.893	T65.894	—	—
citrate	T50.991	T50.992	T50.993	T50.994	T50.995	T50.996
cromoglicate	T48.6X1	T48.6X2	T48.6X3	T48.6X4	T48.6X5	T48.6X6
cyanide	T65.0X1	T65.0X2	T65.0X3	T65.0X4	—	—
cyclamate	T50.3X1	T50.3X2	T50.3X3	T50.3X4	T50.3X5	T50.3X6
dehydrocholate	T45.8X1	T45.8X2	T45.8X3	T45.8X4	T45.8X5	T45.8X6
diatrizoate	T50.8X1	T50.8X2	T50.8X3	T50.8X4	T50.8X5	T50.8X6
dibunate	T48.4X1	T48.4X2	T48.4X3	T48.4X4	T48.4X5	T48.4X6
dioctyl sulfosuccinate	T47.4X1	T47.4X2	T47.4X3	T47.4X4	T47.4X5	T47.4X6
dipantoyl ferrate	T45.8X1	T45.8X2	T45.8X3	T45.8X4	T45.8X5	T45.8X6
edetate	T45.8X1	T45.8X2	T45.8X3	T45.8X4	T45.8X5	T45.8X6
ethacrynate	T50.1X1	T50.1X2	T50.1X3	T50.1X4	T50.1X5	T50.1X6
feredetate	T45.8X1	T45.8X2	T45.8X3	T45.8X4	T45.8X5	T45.8X6
Fluoride—see Fluoride						
fluoroacetate (dust) (pesticide)	T60.4X1	T60.4X2	T60.4X3	T60.4X4	—	—
free salt	T50.3X1	T50.3X2	T50.3X3	T50.3X4	T50.3X5	T50.3X6

Substance	Poisoning, Accidental (unintentional)	Poisoning, Intentional self-harm	Poisoning, Assault	Poisoning, Undetermined	Adverse effect	Underdosing
Sodium — *Continued*						
fusidate	T36.8X1	T36.8X2	T36.8X3	T36.8X4	T36.8X5	T36.8X6
glucaldrate	T47.1X1	T47.1X2	T47.1X3	T47.1X4	T47.1X5	T47.1X6
glucosulfone	T37.1X1	T37.1X2	T37.1X3	T37.1X4	T37.1X5	T37.1X6
glutamate	T45.8X1	T45.8X2	T45.8X3	T45.8X4	T45.8X5	T45.8X6
hydrogen carbonate	T50.3X1	T50.3X2	T50.3X3	T50.3X4	T50.3X5	T50.3X6
hydroxide	T54.3X1	T54.3X2	T54.3X3	T54.3X4	—	—
hypochlorite (bleach) NEC	T54.3X1	T54.3X2	T54.3X3	T54.3X4	—	—
disinfectant	T54.3X1	T54.3X2	T54.3X3	T54.3X4	—	—
medicinal (anti-infective) (external)	T49.0X1	T49.0X2	T49.0X3	T49.0X4	T49.0X5	T49.0X6
vapor	T54.3X1	T54.3X2	T54.3X3	T54.3X4	—	—
hyposulfite	T49.0X1	T49.0X2	T49.0X3	T49.0X4	T49.0X5	T49.0X6
indigotin disulfonate	T50.8X1	T50.8X2	T50.8X3	T50.8X4	T50.8X5	T50.8X6
iodide	T50.991	T50.992	T50.993	T50.994	T50.995	T50.996
I-131	T50.8X1	T50.8X2	T50.8X3	T50.8X4	T50.8X5	T50.8X6
therapeutic	T38.2X1	T38.2X2	T38.2X3	T38.2X4	T38.2X5	T38.2X6
iodohippurate (131I)	T50.8X1	T50.8X2	T50.8X3	T50.8X4	T50.8X5	T50.8X6
iopodate	T50.8X1	T50.8X2	T50.8X3	T50.8X4	T50.8X5	T50.8X6
iothalamate	T50.8X1	T50.8X2	T50.8X3	T50.8X4	T50.8X5	T50.8X6
iron edetate	T45.4X1	T45.4X2	T45.4X3	T45.4X4	T45.4X5	T45.4X6
lactate (compound solution)	T45.8X1	T45.8X2	T45.8X3	T45.8X4	T45.8X5	T45.8X6
lauryl (sulfate)	T49.2X1	T49.2X2	T49.2X3	T49.2X4	T49.2X5	T49.2X6
L-triiodothyronine	T38.1X1	T38.1X2	T38.1X3	T38.1X4	T38.1X5	T38.1X6
magnesium citrate	T50.991	T50.992	T50.993	T50.994	T50.995	T50.996
mersalate	T50.2X1	T50.2X2	T50.2X3	T50.2X4	T50.2X5	T50.2X6
metasilicate	T65.891	T65.892	T65.893	T65.894	—	—
metrizoate	T50.8X1	T50.8X2	T50.8X3	T50.8X4	T50.8X5	T50.8X6
monofluoroacetate (pesticide)	T60.1X1	T60.1X2	T60.1X3	T60.1X4	—	—
morrhuate	T46.8X1	T46.8X2	T46.8X3	T46.8X4	T46.8X5	T46.8X6
nafcillin	T36.0X1	T36.0X2	T36.0X3	T36.0X4	T36.0X5	T36.0X6
nitrate (oxidizing agent)	T65.891	T65.892	T65.893	T65.894	—	—
nitrite	T50.6X1	T50.6X2	T50.6X3	T50.6X4	T50.6X5	T50.6X6
nitroferricyanide	T46.5X1	T46.5X2	T46.5X3	T46.5X4	T46.5X5	T46.5X6
nitroprusside	T46.5X1	T46.5X2	T46.5X3	T46.5X4	T46.5X5	T46.5X6
oxalate	T65.891	T65.892	T65.893	T65.894	—	—
oxide/peroxide	T65.891	T65.892	T65.893	T65.894	—	—
oxybate	T41.291	T41.292	T41.293	T41.294	T41.295	T41.296
para-aminohippurate	T50.8X1	T50.8X2	T50.8X3	T50.8X4	T50.8X5	T50.8X6
perborate (nonmedicinal) NEC	T65.891	T65.892	T65.893	T65.894	—	—
medicinal	T49.0X1	T49.0X2	T49.0X3	T49.0X4	T49.0X5	T49.0X6
soap	T55.0X1	T55.0X2	T55.0X3	T55.0X4	—	—
percarbonate—see Sodium, perborate						
pertechnetate Tc99m	T50.8X1	T50.8X2	T50.8X3	T50.8X4	T50.8X5	T50.8X6
phosphate						
cellulose	T45.8X1	T45.8X2	T45.8X3	T45.8X4	T45.8X5	T45.8X6
dibasic	T47.2X1	T47.2X2	T47.2X3	T47.2X4	T47.2X5	T47.2X6
monobasic	T47.2X1	T47.2X2	T47.2X3	T47.2X4	T47.2X5	T47.2X6
Sodium — *Continued*						
phytate	T50.6X1	T50.6X2	T50.6X3	T50.6X4	T50.6X5	T50.6X6
picosulfate	T47.2X1	T47.2X2	T47.2X3	T47.2X4	T47.2X5	T47.2X6
polyhydroxyaluminium monocarbonate	T47.1X1	T47.1X2	T47.1X3	T47.1X4	T47.1X5	T47.1X6
polystyrene sulfonate	T50.3X1	T50.3X2	T50.3X3	T50.3X4	T50.3X5	T50.3X6
propionate	T49.0X1	T49.0X2	T49.0X3	T49.0X4	T49.0X5	T49.0X6
propyl hydroxybenzoate	T50.991	T50.992	T50.993	T50.994	T50.995	T50.996
psylliate	T46.8X1	T46.8X2	T46.8X3	T46.8X4	T46.8X5	T46.8X6
removing resins	T50.3X1	T50.3X2	T50.3X3	T50.3X4	T50.3X5	T50.3X6
salicylate	T39.091	T39.092	T39.093	T39.094	T39.095	T39.096
salt NEC	T50.3X1	T50.3X2	T50.3X3	T50.3X4	T50.3X5	T50.3X6
selenate	T60.2X1	T60.2X2	T60.2X3	T60.2X4	—	—
stibogluconate	T37.3X1	T37.3X2	T37.3X3	T37.3X4	T37.3X5	T37.3X6
sulfate	T47.4X1	T47.4X2	T47.4X3	T47.4X4	T47.4X5	T47.4X6
sulfoxone	T37.1X1	T37.1X2	T37.1X3	T37.1X4	T37.1X5	T37.1X6
tetradecyl sulfate	T46.8X1	T46.8X2	T46.8X3	T46.8X4	T46.8X5	T46.8X6
thiopental	T41.1X1	T41.1X2	T41.1X3	T41.1X4	T41.1X5	T41.1X6
thiosalicylate	T39.091	T39.092	T39.093	T39.094	T39.095	T39.096
thiosulfate	T50.6X1	T50.6X2	T50.6X3	T50.6X4	T50.6X5	T50.6X6
tolbutamide	T38.3X1	T38.3X2	T38.3X3	T38.3X4	T38.3X5	T38.3X6
(L)-triiodothyronine	T38.1X1	T38.1X2	T38.1X3	T38.1X4	T38.1X5	T38.1X6
tyropanoate	T50.8X1	T50.8X2	T50.8X3	T50.8X4	T50.8X5	T50.8X6
valproate	T42.6X1	T42.6X2	T42.6X3	T42.6X4	T42.6X5	T42.6X6
versenate	T50.6X1	T50.6X2	T50.6X3	T50.6X4	T50.6X5	T50.6X6
Sodium-free salt	T50.901	T50.902	T50.903	T50.904	T50.905	T50.906
Sodium-removing resin	T50.3X1	T50.3X2	T50.3X3	T50.3X4	T50.3X5	T50.3X6
Soft soap	T55.0X1	T55.0X2	T55.0X3	T55.0X4	—	—
Solanine	T62.2X1	T62.2X2	T62.2X3	T62.2X4	—	—
berries	T62.1X1	T62.1X2	T62.1X3	T62.1X4	—	—
Solanum dulcamara	T62.2X1	T62.2X2	T62.2X3	T62.2X4	—	—
berries	T62.1X1	T62.1X2	T62.1X3	T62.1X4	—	—
Solapsone	T37.1X1	T37.1X2	T37.1X3	T37.1X4	T37.1X5	T37.1X6
Solar lotion	T49.3X1	T49.3X2	T49.3X3	T49.3X4	T49.3X5	T49.3X6
Solasulfone	T37.1X1	T37.1X2	T37.1X3	T37.1X4	T37.1X5	T37.1X6
Soldering fluid	T65.891	T65.892	T65.893	T65.894	—	—
Solid substance	T65.91	T65.92	T65.93	T65.94	—	—
specified NEC	T65.891	T65.892	T65.893	T65.894	—	—
Solvent, industrial NEC	T52.91	T52.92	T52.93	T52.94	—	—
naphtha	T52.0X1	T52.0X2	T52.0X3	T52.0X4	—	—
petroleum	T52.0X1	T52.0X2	T52.0X3	T52.0X4	—	—
specified NEC	T52.8X1	T52.8X2	T52.8X3	T52.8X4	—	—
Soma	T42.8X1	T42.8X2	T42.8X3	T42.8X4	T42.8X5	T42.8X6
Somatorelin	T38.891	T38.892	T38.893	T38.894	T38.895	T38.896
Somatostatin	T38.991	T38.992	T38.993	T38.994	T38.995	T38.996
Somatotropin	T38.811	T38.812	T38.813	T38.814	T38.815	T38.816
Somatrem	T38.811	T38.812	T38.813	T38.814	T38.815	T38.816
Somatropin	T38.811	T38.812	T38.813	T38.814	T38.815	T38.816
Sominex	T45.0X1	T45.0X2	T45.0X3	T45.0X4	T45.0X5	T45.0X6
Somnos	T42.6X1	T42.6X2	T42.6X3	T42.6X4	T42.6X5	T42.6X6

Substance	Poisoning, Accidental (unintentional)	Poisoning, Intentional self-harm	Poisoning, Assault	Poisoning, Undetermined	Adverse effect	Underdosing
Somonal	T42.3X1	T42.3X2	T42.3X3	T42.3X4	T42.3X5	T42.3X6
Soneryl	T42.3X1	T42.3X2	T42.3X3	T42.3X4	T42.3X5	T42.3X6
Soothing syrup	T50.901	T50.902	T50.903	T50.904	T50.905	T50.906
Sopor	T42.6X1	T42.6X2	T42.6X3	T42.6X4	T42.6X5	T42.6X6
Soporific	T42.71	T42.72	T42.73	T42.74	T42.75	T42.76
Soporific drug	T42.71	T42.72	T42.73	T42.74	T42.75	T42.76
specified type NEC	T42.6X1	T42.6X2	T42.6X3	T42.6X4	T42.6X5	T42.6X6
Sorbide nitrate	T46.3X1	T46.3X2	T46.3X3	T46.3X4	T46.3X5	T46.3X6
Sorbitol	T47.4X1	T47.4X2	T47.4X3	T47.4X4	T47.4X5	T47.4X6
Sotalol	T44.7X1	T44.7X2	T44.7X3	T44.7X4	T44.7X5	T44.7X6
Sotradecol	T46.8X1	T46.8X2	T46.8X3	T46.8X4	T46.8X5	T46.8X6
Soysterol	T46.6X1	T46.6X2	T46.6X3	T46.6X4	T46.6X5	T46.6X6
Spacoline	T44.3X1	T44.3X2	T44.3X3	T44.3X4	T44.3X5	T44.3X6
Spanish fly	T49.8X1	T49.8X2	T49.8X3	T49.8X4	T49.8X5	T49.8X6
Sparine	T43.3X1	T43.3X2	T43.3X3	T43.3X4	T43.3X5	T43.3X6
Sparteine	T48.0X1	T48.0X2	T48.0X3	T48.0X4	T48.0X5	T48.0X6
Spasmolytic						
anticholinergics	T44.3X1	T44.3X2	T44.3X3	T44.3X4	T44.3X5	T44.3X6
autonomic	T44.3X1	T44.3X2	T44.3X3	T44.3X4	T44.3X5	T44.3X6
bronchial NEC	T48.6X1	T48.6X2	T48.6X3	T48.6X4	T48.6X5	T48.6X6
quaternary ammonium	T44.3X1	T44.3X2	T44.3X3	T44.3X4	T44.3X5	T44.3X6
skeletal muscle NEC	T48.1X1	T48.1X2	T48.1X3	T48.1X4	T48.1X5	T48.1X6
Spectinomycin	T36.5X1	T36.5X2	T36.5X3	T36.5X4	T36.5X5	T36.5X6
Speed	T43.621	T43.622	T43.623	T43.624	T43.625	T43.626
Spermicide	T49.8X1	T49.8X2	T49.8X3	T49.8X4	T49.8X5	T49.8X6
Spider (bite) (venom)	T63.391	T63.392	T63.393	T63.394	—	—
antivenin	T50.Z11	T50.Z12	T50.Z13	T50.Z14	T50.Z15	T50.Z16
Spigelia (root)	T37.4X1	T37.4X2	T37.4X3	T37.4X4	T37.4X5	T37.4X6
Spindle inactivator	T50.4X1	T50.4X2	T50.4X3	T50.4X4	T50.4X5	T50.4X6
Spiperone	T43.4X1	T43.4X2	T43.4X3	T43.4X4	T43.4X5	T43.4X6
Spiramycin	T36.3X1	T36.3X2	T36.3X3	T36.3X4	T36.3X5	T36.3X6
Spirapril	T46.4X1	T46.4X2	T46.4X3	T46.4X4	T46.4X5	T46.4X6
Spirilene	T43.591	T43.592	T43.593	T43.594	T43.595	T43.596
Spirit(s) (neutral) NEC	T51.0X1	T51.0X2	T51.0X3	T51.0X4	—	—
beverage	T51.0X1	T51.0X2	T51.0X3	T51.0X4	—	—
industrial	T51.0X1	T51.0X2	T51.0X3	T51.0X4	—	—
mineral	T52.0X1	T52.0X2	T52.0X3	T52.0X4	—	—
of salt—see Hydrochloric acid						
surgical	T51.0X1	T51.0X2	T51.0X3	T51.0X4	—	—
Spironolactone	T50.0X1	T50.0X2	T50.0X3	T50.0X4	T50.0X5	T50.0X6
Spiroperidol	T43.4X1	T43.4X2	T43.4X3	T43.4X4	T43.4X5	T43.4X6
Sponge, absorbable (gelatin)	T45.7X1	T45.7X2	T45.7X3	T45.7X4	T45.7X5	T45.7X6
Sporostacin	T49.0X1	T49.0X2	T49.0X3	T49.0X4	T49.0X5	T49.0X6
Spray (aerosol)	T65.91	T65.92	T65.93	T65.94	—	—
cosmetic	T65.891	T65.892	T65.893	T65.894	—	—
medicinal NEC	T50.901	T50.902	T50.903	T50.904	T50.905	T50.906
pesticides—see Pesticides						
specified content—see specific substance						

Substance	Poisoning, Accidental (unintentional)	Poisoning, Intentional self-harm	Poisoning, Assault	Poisoning, Undetermined	Adverse effect	Underdosing
Spurge flax	T62.2X1	T62.2X2	T62.2X3	T62.2X4	—	—
Spurges	T62.2X1	T62.2X2	T62.2X3	T62.2X4	—	—
Sputum viscosity-lowering drug	T48.4X1	T48.4X2	T48.4X3	T48.4X4	T48.4X5	T48.4X6
Squill	T46.0X1	T46.0X2	T46.0X3	T46.0X4	T46.0X5	T46.0X6
rat poison	T60.4X1	T60.4X2	T60.4X3	T60.4X4	—	—
Squirting cucumber (cathartic)	T47.2X1	T47.2X2	T47.2X3	T47.2X4	T47.2X5	T47.2X6
Stains	T65.6X1	T65.6X2	T65.6X3	T65.6X4	—	—
Stannous fluoride	T49.7X1	T49.7X2	T49.7X3	T49.7X4	T49.7X5	T49.7X6
Stanolone	T38.7X1	T38.7X2	T38.7X3	T38.7X4	T38.7X5	T38.7X6
Stanozolol	T38.7X1	T38.7X2	T38.7X3	T38.7X4	T38.7X5	T38.7X6
Staphisagria or stavesacre (pediculicide)	T49.0X1	T49.0X2	T49.0X3	T49.0X4	T49.0X5	T49.0X6
Starch	T50.901	T50.902	T50.903	T50.904	T50.905	T50.906
Stelazine	T43.3X1	T43.3X2	T43.3X3	T43.3X4	T43.3X5	T43.3X6
Stemetil	T43.3X1	T43.3X2	T43.3X3	T43.3X4	T43.3X5	T43.3X6
Stepronin	T48.4X1	T48.4X2	T48.4X3	T48.4X4	T48.4X5	T48.4X6
Sterculia	T47.4X1	T47.4X2	T47.4X3	T47.4X4	T47.4X5	T47.4X6
Sternutator gas	T59.891	T59.892	T59.893	T59.894	—	—
Steroid	T38.0X1	T38.0X2	T38.0X3	T38.0X4	T38.0X5	T38.0X6
anabolic	T38.7X1	T38.7X2	T38.7X3	T38.7X4	T38.7X5	T38.7X6
androgenic	T38.7X1	T38.7X2	T38.7X3	T38.7X4	T38.7X5	T38.7X6
antineoplastic, hormone	T38.7X1	T38.7X2	T38.7X3	T38.7X4	T38.7X5	T38.7X6
estrogen	T38.5X1	T38.5X2	T38.5X3	T38.5X4	T38.5X5	T38.5X6
ENT agent	T49.6X1	T49.6X2	T49.6X3	T49.6X4	T49.6X5	T49.6X6
ophthalmic preparation	T49.5X1	T49.5X2	T49.5X3	T49.5X4	T49.5X5	T49.5X6
topical NEC	T49.0X1	T49.0X2	T49.0X3	T49.0X4	T49.0X5	T49.0X6
Stibine	T56.891	T56.892	T56.893	T56.894	—	—
Stibogluconate	T37.3X1	T37.3X2	T37.3X3	T37.3X4	T37.3X5	T37.3X6
Stibophen	T37.4X1	T37.4X2	T37.4X3	T37.4X4	T37.4X5	T37.4X6
Stilbamidine (isetionate)	T37.3X1	T37.3X2	T37.3X3	T37.3X4	T37.3X5	T37.3X6
Stilbestrol	T38.5X1	T38.5X2	T38.5X3	T38.5X4	T38.5X5	T38.5X6
Stilboestrol	T38.5X1	T38.5X2	T38.5X3	T38.5X4	T38.5X5	T38.5X6
Stimulant						
central nervous system—see also Psychostimulant	T43.601	T43.602	T43.603	T43.604	T43.605	T43.606
analeptics	T50.7X1	T50.7X2	T50.7X3	T50.7X4	T50.7X5	T50.7X6
opiate antagonist	T50.7X1	T50.7X2	T50.7X3	T50.7X4	T50.7X5	T50.7X6
psychotherapeutic NEC—see also Psychotherapeutic drug	T43.601	T43.602	T43.603	T43.604	T43.605	T43.606
specified NEC	T43.691	T43.692	T43.693	T43.694	T43.695	T43.696
respiratory	T48.901	T48.902	T48.903	T48.904	T48.905	T48.906
Stone-dissolving drug	T50.901	T50.902	T50.903	T50.904	T50.905	T50.906
Storage battery (cells) (acid)	T54.2X1	T54.2X2	T54.2X3	T54.2X4	—	—
Stovaine	T41.3X1	T41.3X2	T41.3X3	T41.3X4	T41.3X5	T41.3X6
infiltration (subcutaneous)	T41.3X1	T41.3X2	T41.3X3	T41.3X4	T41.3X5	T41.3X6
nerve block (peripheral) (plexus)	T41.3X1	T41.3X2	T41.3X3	T41.3X4	T41.3X5	T41.3X6
spinal	T41.3X1	T41.3X2	T41.3X3	T41.3X4	T41.3X5	T41.3X6
topical (surface)	T41.3X1	T41.3X2	T41.3X3	T41.3X4	T41.3X5	T41.3X6

Substance	Poisoning, Accidental (unintentional)	Poisoning, Intentional self-harm	Poisoning, Assault	Poisoning, Undetermined	Adverse effect	Underdosing
Stovarsal	T37.8X1	T37.8X2	T37.8X3	T37.8X4	T37.8X5	T37.8X6
Stove gas—see Gas, stove						
Stoxil	T49.5X1	T49.5X2	T49.5X3	T49.5X4	T49.5X5	T49.5X6
Stramonium	T48.6X1	T48.6X2	T48.6X3	T48.6X4	T48.6X5	T48.6X6
natural state	T62.2X1	T62.2X2	T62.2X3	T62.2X4	—	—
Streptodornase	T45.3X1	T45.3X2	T45.3X3	T45.3X4	T45.3X5	T45.3X6
Streptoduocin	T36.5X1	T36.5X2	T36.5X3	T36.5X4	T36.5X5	T36.5X6
Streptokinase	T45.611	T45.612	T45.613	T45.614	T45.615	T45.616
Streptomycin (derivative)	T36.5X1	T36.5X2	T36.5X3	T36.5X4	T36.5X5	T36.5X6
Streptonivicin	T36.5X1	T36.5X2	T36.5X3	T36.5X4	T36.5X5	T36.5X6
Streptovarycin	T36.5X1	T36.5X2	T36.5X3	T36.5X4	T36.5X5	T36.5X6
Streptozocin	T45.1X1	T45.1X2	T45.1X3	T45.1X4	T45.1X5	T45.1X6
Streptozotocin	T45.1X1	T45.1X2	T45.1X3	T45.1X4	T45.1X5	T45.1X6
Stripper (paint) (solvent)	T52.8X1	T52.8X2	T52.8X3	T52.8X4	—	—
Strobane	T60.1X1	T60.1X2	T60.1X3	T60.1X4	—	—
Strofantina	T46.0X1	T46.0X2	T46.0X3	T46.0X4	T46.0X5	T46.0X6
Strophanthin (g) (k)	T46.0X1	T46.0X2	T46.0X3	T46.0X4	T46.0X5	T46.0X6
Strophanthus	T46.0X1	T46.0X2	T46.0X3	T46.0X4	T46.0X5	T46.0X6
Strophantin	T46.0X1	T46.0X2	T46.0X3	T46.0X4	T46.0X5	T46.0X6
Strophantin-g	T46.0X1	T46.0X2	T46.0X3	T46.0X4	T46.0X5	T46.0X6
Strychnine (nonmedicinal) (pesticide) (salts)	T65.1X1	T65.1X2	T65.1X3	T65.1X4	—	—
medicinal	T48.291	T48.292	T48.293	T48.294	T48.295	T48.296
Strychnos (ignatii)—see Strychnine						
Styramate	T42.8X1	T42.8X2	T42.8X3	T42.8X4	T42.8X5	T42.8X6
Styrene	T65.891	T65.892	T65.893	T65.894	—	—
Succinimide, antiepileptic or anticonvulsant	T42.2X1	T42.2X2	T42.2X3	T42.2X4	T42.2X5	T42.2X6
mercuric—see Mercury						
Succinylcholine	T48.1X1	T48.1X2	T48.1X3	T48.1X4	T48.1X5	T48.1X6
Succinylsulfathiazole	T37.0X1	T37.0X2	T37.0X3	T37.0X4	T37.0X5	T37.0X6
Sucralfate	T47.1X1	T47.1X2	T47.1X3	T47.1X4	T47.1X5	T47.1X6
Sucrose	T50.3X1	T50.3X2	T50.3X3	T50.3X4	T50.3X5	T50.3X6
Sufentanil	T40.4X1	T40.4X2	T40.4X3	T40.4X4	T40.4X5	T40.4X6
Sulbactam	T36.0X1	T36.0X2	T36.0X3	T36.0X4	T36.0X5	T36.0X6
Sulbenicillin	T36.0X1	T36.0X2	T36.0X3	T36.0X4	T36.0X5	T36.0X6
Sulbentine	T49.0X1	T49.0X2	T49.0X3	T49.0X4	T49.0X5	T49.0X6
Sulfacetamide	T49.0X1	T49.0X2	T49.0X3	T49.0X4	T49.0X5	T49.0X6
ophthalmic preparation	T49.5X1	T49.5X2	T49.5X3	T49.5X4	T49.5X5	T49.5X6
Sulfachlorpyridazine	T37.0X1	T37.0X2	T37.0X3	T37.0X4	T37.0X5	T37.0X6
Sulfacitine	T37.0X1	T37.0X2	T37.0X3	T37.0X4	T37.0X5	T37.0X6
Sulfadiasulfone sodium	T37.0X1	T37.0X2	T37.0X3	T37.0X4	T37.0X5	T37.0X6
Sulfadiazine	T37.0X1	T37.0X2	T37.0X3	T37.0X4	T37.0X5	T37.0X6
silver (topical)	T49.0X1	T49.0X2	T49.0X3	T49.0X4	T49.0X5	T49.0X6
Sulfadimethoxine	T37.0X1	T37.0X2	T37.0X3	T37.0X4	T37.0X5	T37.0X6
Sulfadimidine	T37.0X1	T37.0X2	T37.0X3	T37.0X4	T37.0X5	T37.0X6
Sulfadoxine	T37.0X1	T37.0X2	T37.0X3	T37.0X4	T37.0X5	T37.0X6
with pyrimethamine	T37.2X1	T37.2X2	T37.2X3	T37.2X4	T37.2X5	T37.2X6
Sulfaethidole	T37.0X1	T37.0X2	T37.0X3	T37.0X4	T37.0X5	T37.0X6
Sulfafurazole	T37.0X1	T37.0X2	T37.0X3	T37.0X4	T37.0X5	T37.0X6
Sulfaguanidine	T37.0X1	T37.0X2	T37.0X3	T37.0X4	T37.0X5	T37.0X6
Sulfalene	T37.0X1	T37.0X2	T37.0X3	T37.0X4	T37.0X5	T37.0X6
Sulfaloxate	T37.0X1	T37.0X2	T37.0X3	T37.0X4	T37.0X5	T37.0X6
Sulfaloxic acid	T37.0X1	T37.0X2	T37.0X3	T37.0X4	T37.0X5	T37.0X6
Sulfamazone	T39.2X1	T39.2X2	T39.2X3	T39.2X4	T39.2X5	T39.2X6
Sulfamerazine	T37.0X1	T37.0X2	T37.0X3	T37.0X4	T37.0X5	T37.0X6
Sulfameter	T37.0X1	T37.0X2	T37.0X3	T37.0X4	T37.0X5	T37.0X6
Sulfamethazine	T37.0X1	T37.0X2	T37.0X3	T37.0X4	T37.0X5	T37.0X6
Sulfamethizole	T37.0X1	T37.0X2	T37.0X3	T37.0X4	T37.0X5	T37.0X6
Sulfamethoxazole	T37.0X1	T37.0X2	T37.0X3	T37.0X4	T37.0X5	T37.0X6
with trimethoprim	T36.8X1	T36.8X2	T36.8X3	T36.8X4	T36.8X5	T36.8X6
Sulfamethoxydiazine	T37.0X1	T37.0X2	T37.0X3	T37.0X4	T37.0X5	T37.0X6
Sulfamethoxypyridazine	T37.0X1	T37.0X2	T37.0X3	T37.0X4	T37.0X5	T37.0X6
Sulfamethylthiazole	T37.0X1	T37.0X2	T37.0X3	T37.0X4	T37.0X5	T37.0X6
Sulfametoxydiazine	T37.0X1	T37.0X2	T37.0X3	T37.0X4	T37.0X5	T37.0X6
Sulfamidopyrine	T39.2X1	T39.2X2	T39.2X3	T39.2X4	T39.2X5	T39.2X6
Sulfamonomethoxine	T37.0X1	T37.0X2	T37.0X3	T37.0X4	T37.0X5	T37.0X6
Sulfamoxole	T37.0X1	T37.0X2	T37.0X3	T37.0X4	T37.0X5	T37.0X6
Sulfamylon	T49.0X1	T49.0X2	T49.0X3	T49.0X4	T49.0X5	T49.0X6
Sulfan blue (diagnostic dye)	T50.8X1	T50.8X2	T50.8X3	T50.8X4	T50.8X5	T50.8X6
Sulfanilamide	T37.0X1	T37.0X2	T37.0X3	T37.0X4	T37.0X5	T37.0X6
Sulfanilylguanidine	T37.0X1	T37.0X2	T37.0X3	T37.0X4	T37.0X5	T37.0X6
Sulfaperin	T37.0X1	T37.0X2	T37.0X3	T37.0X4	T37.0X5	T37.0X6
Sulfaphenazole	T37.0X1	T37.0X2	T37.0X3	T37.0X4	T37.0X5	T37.0X6
Sulfaphenylthiazole	T37.0X1	T37.0X2	T37.0X3	T37.0X4	T37.0X5	T37.0X6
Sulfaproxyline	T37.0X1	T37.0X2	T37.0X3	T37.0X4	T37.0X5	T37.0X6
Sulfapyridine	T37.0X1	T37.0X2	T37.0X3	T37.0X4	T37.0X5	T37.0X6
Sulfapyrimidine	T37.0X1	T37.0X2	T37.0X3	T37.0X4	T37.0X5	T37.0X6
Sulfarsphenamine	T37.8X1	T37.8X2	T37.8X3	T37.8X4	T37.8X5	T37.8X6
Sulfasalazine	T37.0X1	T37.0X2	T37.0X3	T37.0X4	T37.0X5	T37.0X6
Sulfasuxidine	T37.0X1	T37.0X2	T37.0X3	T37.0X4	T37.0X5	T37.0X6
Sulfasymazine	T37.0X1	T37.0X2	T37.0X3	T37.0X4	T37.0X5	T37.0X6
Sulfated amylopectin	T47.8X1	T47.8X2	T47.8X3	T47.8X4	T47.8X5	T47.8X6
Sulfathiazole	T37.0X1	T37.0X2	T37.0X3	T37.0X4	T37.0X5	T37.0X6
Sulfatostearate	T49.2X1	T49.2X2	T49.2X3	T49.2X4	T49.2X5	T49.2X6
Sulfinpyrazone	T50.4X1	T50.4X2	T50.4X3	T50.4X4	T50.4X5	T50.4X6
Sulfiram	T49.0X1	T49.0X2	T49.0X3	T49.0X4	T49.0X5	T49.0X6
Sulfisomidine	T37.0X1	T37.0X2	T37.0X3	T37.0X4	T37.0X5	T37.0X6
Sulfisoxazole	T37.0X1	T37.0X2	T37.0X3	T37.0X4	T37.0X5	T37.0X6
ophthalmic preparation	T49.5X1	T49.5X2	T49.5X3	T49.5X4	T49.5X5	T49.5X6
Sulfobromophthalein (sodium)	T50.8X1	T50.8X2	T50.8X3	T50.8X4	T50.8X5	T50.8X6
Sulfobromphthalein	T50.8X1	T50.8X2	T50.8X3	T50.8X4	T50.8X5	T50.8X6
Sulfogaiacol	T48.4X1	T48.4X2	T48.4X3	T48.4X4	T48.4X5	T48.4X6
Sulfomyxin	T36.8X1	T36.8X2	T36.8X3	T36.8X4	T36.8X5	T36.8X6
Sulfonal	T42.6X1	T42.6X2	T42.6X3	T42.6X4	T42.6X5	T42.6X6
Sulfonamide NEC	T37.0X1	T37.0X2	T37.0X3	T37.0X4	T37.0X5	T37.0X6
eye	T49.5X1	T49.5X2	T49.5X3	T49.5X4	T49.5X5	T49.5X6
Sulfonazide	T37.1X1	T37.1X2	T37.1X3	T37.1X4	T37.1X5	T37.1X6
Sulfones	T37.1X1	T37.1X2	T37.1X3	T37.1X4	T37.1X5	T37.1X6

Substance	Poisoning, Accidental (unintentional)	Poisoning, Intentional self-harm	Poisoning, Assault	Poisoning, Undetermined	Adverse effect	Underdosing
Sulfonethylmethane	T42.6X1	T42.6X2	T42.6X3	T42.6X4	T42.6X5	T42.6X6
Sulfonmethane	T42.6X1	T42.6X2	T42.6X3	T42.6X4	T42.6X5	T42.6X6
Sulfonphthal, sulfonphthol	T50.8X1	T50.8X2	T50.8X3	T50.8X4	T50.8X5	T50.8X6
Sulfonylurea derivatives, oral	T38.3X1	T38.3X2	T38.3X3	T38.3X4	T38.3X5	T38.3X6
Sulforidazine	T43.3X1	T43.3X2	T43.3X3	T43.3X4	T43.3X5	T43.3X6
Sulfoxone	T37.1X1	T37.1X2	T37.1X3	T37.1X4	T37.1X5	T37.1X6
Sulfur, sulfurated, sulfuric, sulfurous, sulfuryl (compounds NEC) (medicinal)	T49.4X1	T49.4X2	T49.4X3	T49.4X4	T49.4X5	T49.4X6
acid	T54.2X1	T54.2X2	T54.2X3	T54.2X4	—	—
dioxide (gas)	T59.1X1	T59.1X2	T59.1X3	T59.1X4	—	—
ether—see Ether(s)						
hydrogen	T59.6X1	T59.6X2	T59.6X3	T59.6X4	—	—
medicinal (keratolytic) (ointment) NEC	T49.4X1	T49.4X2	T49.4X3	T49.4X4	T49.4X5	T49.4X6
ointment	T49.0X1	T49.0X2	T49.0X3	T49.0X4	T49.0X5	T49.0X6
pesticide (vapor)	T60.91	T60.92	T60.93	T60.94	—	—
vapor NEC	T59.891	T59.892	T59.893	T59.894	—	—
Sulfuric acid	T54.2X1	T54.2X2	T54.2X3	T54.2X4	—	—
Sulglicotide	T47.1X1	T47.1X2	T47.1X3	T47.1X4	T47.1X5	T47.1X6
Sulindac	T39.391	T39.392	T39.393	T39.394	T39.395	T39.396
Sulisatin	T47.2X1	T47.2X2	T47.2X3	T47.2X4	T47.2X5	T47.2X6
Sulisobenzone	T49.3X1	T49.3X2	T49.3X3	T49.3X4	T49.3X5	T49.3X6
Sulkowitch's reagent	T50.8X1	T50.8X2	T50.8X3	T50.8X4	T50.8X5	T50.8X6
Sulmetozine	T44.3X1	T44.3X2	T44.3X3	T44.3X4	T44.3X5	T44.3X6
Suloctidil	T46.7X1	T46.7X2	T46.7X3	T46.7X4	T46.7X5	T46.7X6
Sulph-—see also Sulf-						
Sulphadiazine	T37.0X1	T37.0X2	T37.0X3	T37.0X4	T37.0X5	T37.0X6
Sulphadimethoxine	T37.0X1	T37.0X2	T37.0X3	T37.0X4	T37.0X5	T37.0X6
Sulphadimidine	T37.0X1	T37.0X2	T37.0X3	T37.0X4	T37.0X5	T37.0X6
Sulphadione	T37.1X1	T37.1X2	T37.1X3	T37.1X4	T37.1X5	T37.1X6
Sulphafurazole	T37.0X1	T37.0X2	T37.0X3	T37.0X4	T37.0X5	T37.0X6
Sulphamethizole	T37.0X1	T37.0X2	T37.0X3	T37.0X4	T37.0X5	T37.0X6
Sulphamethoxazole	T37.0X1	T37.0X2	T37.0X3	T37.0X4	T37.0X5	T37.0X6
Sulphan blue	T50.8X1	T50.8X2	T50.8X3	T50.8X4	T50.8X5	T50.8X6
Sulphaphenazole	T37.0X1	T37.0X2	T37.0X3	T37.0X4	T37.0X5	T37.0X6
Sulphapyridine	T37.0X1	T37.0X2	T37.0X3	T37.0X4	T37.0X5	T37.0X6
Sulphasalazine	T37.0X1	T37.0X2	T37.0X3	T37.0X4	T37.0X5	T37.0X6
Sulphinpyrazone	T50.4X1	T50.4X2	T50.4X3	T50.4X4	T50.4X5	T50.4X6
Sulpiride	T43.591	T43.592	T43.593	T43.594	T43.595	T43.596
Sulprostone	T48.0X1	T48.0X2	T48.0X3	T48.0X4	T48.0X5	T48.0X6
Sulpyrine	T39.2X1	T39.2X2	T39.2X3	T39.2X4	T39.2X5	T39.2X6
Sultamicillin	T36.0X1	T36.0X2	T36.0X3	T36.0X4	T36.0X5	T36.0X6
Sulthiame	T42.6X1	T42.6X2	T42.6X3	T42.6X4	T42.6X5	T42.6X6
Sultiame	T42.6X1	T42.6X2	T42.6X3	T42.6X4	T42.6X5	T42.6X6
Sultopride	T43.591	T43.592	T43.593	T43.594	T43.595	T43.596
Sumatriptan	T39.8X1	T39.8X2	T39.8X3	T39.8X4	T39.8X5	T39.8X6
Sunflower seed oil	T46.6X1	T46.6X2	T46.6X3	T46.6X4	T46.6X5	T46.6X6
Superinone	T48.4X1	T48.4X2	T48.4X3	T48.4X4	T48.4X5	T48.4X6

Substance	Poisoning, Accidental (unintentional)	Poisoning, Intentional self-harm	Poisoning, Assault	Poisoning, Undetermined	Adverse effect	Underdosing
Suprofen	T39.311	T39.312	T39.313	T39.314	T39.315	T39.316
Suramin (sodium)	T37.4X1	T37.4X2	T37.4X3	T37.4X4	T37.4X5	T37.4X6
Surfacaine	T41.3X1	T41.3X2	T41.3X3	T41.3X4	T41.3X5	T41.3X6
Surital	T41.1X1	T41.1X2	T41.1X3	T41.1X4	T41.1X5	T41.1X6
Sutilains	T45.3X1	T45.3X2	T45.3X3	T45.3X4	T45.3X5	T45.3X6
Suxamethonium (chloride)	T48.1X1	T48.1X2	T48.1X3	T48.1X4	T48.1X5	T48.1X6
Suxethonium (chloride)	T48.1X1	T48.1X2	T48.1X3	T48.1X4	T48.1X5	T48.1X6
Suxibuzone	T39.2X1	T39.2X2	T39.2X3	T39.2X4	T39.2X5	T39.2X6
Sweet niter spirit	T46.3X1	T46.3X2	T46.3X3	T46.3X4	T46.3X5	T46.3X6
Sweet oil (birch)	T49.3X1	T49.3X2	T49.3X3	T49.3X4	T49.3X5	T49.3X6
Sweetener	T50.901	T50.902	T50.903	T50.904	T50.905	T50.906
Sym-dichloroethyl ether	T53.6X1	T53.6X2	T53.6X3	T53.6X4	—	—
Sympatholytic NEC	T44.8X1	T44.8X2	T44.8X3	T44.8X4	T44.8X5	T44.8X6
haloalkylamine	T44.8X1	T44.8X2	T44.8X3	T44.8X4	T44.8X5	T44.8X6
Sympathomimetic NEC	T44.901	T44.902	T44.903	T44.904	T44.905	T44.906
anti-common-cold	T48.5X1	T48.5X2	T48.5X3	T48.5X4	T48.5X5	T48.5X6
bronchodilator	T48.6X1	T48.6X2	T48.6X3	T48.6X4	T48.6X5	T48.6X6
specified NEC	T44.991	T44.992	T44.993	T44.994	T44.995	T44.996
Synagis	T50.B91	T50.B92	T50.B93	T50.B94	T50.B95	T50.B96
Synalar	T49.0X1	T49.0X2	T49.0X3	T49.0X4	T49.0X5	T49.0X6
Synthroid	T38.1X1	T38.1X2	T38.1X3	T38.1X4	T38.1X5	T38.1X6
Syntocinon	T48.0X1	T48.0X2	T48.0X3	T48.0X4	T48.0X5	T48.0X6
Syrosingopine	T46.5X1	T46.5X2	T46.5X3	T46.5X4	T46.5X5	T46.5X6
Systemic drug	T45.91	T45.92	T45.93	T45.94	T45.95	T45.96
specified NEC	T45.8X1	T45.8X2	T45.8X3	T45.8X4	T45.8X5	T45.8X6
2,4,5-T	T60.3X1	T60.3X2	T60.3X3	T60.3X4	—	—
T						
Tablets—see also specified substance	T50.901	T50.902	T50.903	T50.904	T50.905	T50.906
Tace	T38.5X1	T38.5X2	T38.5X3	T38.5X4	T38.5X5	T38.5X6
Tacrine	T44.0X1	T44.0X2	T44.0X3	T44.0X4	T44.0X5	T44.0X6
Tadalafil	T46.7X1	T46.7X2	T46.7X3	T46.7X4	T46.7X5	T46.7X6
Talampicillin	T36.0X1	T36.0X2	T36.0X3	T36.0X4	T36.0X5	T36.0X6
Talbutal	T42.3X1	T42.3X2	T42.3X3	T42.3X4	T42.3X5	T42.3X6
Talc powder	T49.3X1	T49.3X2	T49.3X3	T49.3X4	T49.3X5	T49.3X6
Talcum	T49.3X1	T49.3X2	T49.3X3	T49.3X4	T49.3X5	T49.3X6
Taleranol	T38.6X1	T38.6X2	T38.6X3	T38.6X4	T38.6X5	T38.6X6
Tamoxifen	T38.6X1	T38.6X2	T38.6X3	T38.6X4	T38.6X5	T38.6X6
Tamsulosin	T44.6X1	T44.6X2	T44.6X3	T44.6X4	T44.6X5	T44.6X6
Tandearil, tanderil	T39.2X1	T39.2X2	T39.2X3	T39.2X4	T39.2X5	T39.2X6
Tannic acid	T49.2X1	T49.2X2	T49.2X3	T49.2X4	T49.2X5	T49.2X6
medicinal (astringent)	T49.2X1	T49.2X2	T49.2X3	T49.2X4	T49.2X5	T49.2X6
Tannin—see Tannic acid						
Tansy	T62.2X1	T62.2X2	T62.2X3	T62.2X4	—	—
TAO	T36.3X1	T36.3X2	T36.3X3	T36.3X4	T36.3X5	T36.3X6
Tapazole	T38.2X1	T38.2X2	T38.2X3	T38.2X4	T38.2X5	T38.2X6
Tar NEC	T52.0X1	T52.0X2	T52.0X3	T52.0X4	—	—
camphor	T60.1X1	T60.1X2	T60.1X3	T60.1X4	—	—
distillate	T49.1X1	T49.1X2	T49.1X3	T49.1X4	T49.1X5	T49.1X6
fumes	T59.891	T59.892	T59.893	T59.894	—	—

Substance	Poisoning, Accidental (unintentional)	Poisoning, Intentional self-harm	Poisoning, Assault	Poisoning, Undetermined	Adverse effect	Underdosing
Tar NEC — *Continued*						
medicinal	T49.1X1	T49.1X2	T49.1X3	T49.1X4	T49.1X5	T49.1X6
ointment	T49.1X1	T49.1X2	T49.1X3	T49.1X4	T49.1X5	T49.1X6
Taractan	T43.591	T43.592	T43.593	T43.594	T43.595	T43.596
Tarantula (venomous)	T63.321	T63.322	T63.323	T63.324	—	—
Tartar emetic	T37.8X1	T37.8X2	T37.8X3	T37.8X4	T37.8X5	T37.8X6
Tartaric acid	T65.891	T65.892	T65.893	T65.894	—	—
Tartrate, laxative	T47.4X1	T47.4X2	T47.4X3	T47.4X4	T47.4X5	T47.4X6
Tartrated antimony (anti-infective)	T37.8X1	T37.8X2	T37.8X3	T37.8X4	T37.8X5	T37.8X6
Tauromustine	T45.1X1	T45.1X2	T45.1X3	T45.1X4	T45.1X5	T45.1X6
TCA—see Trichloroacetic acid						
TCDD	T53.7X1	T53.7X2	T53.7X3	T53.7X4	—	—
TDI (vapor)	T65.0X1	T65.0X2	T65.0X3	T65.0X4	—	—
Tear						
gas	T59.3X1	T59.3X2	T59.3X3	T59.3X4	—	—
solution	T49.5X1	T49.5X2	T49.5X3	T49.5X4	T49.5X5	T49.5X6
Teclothiazide	T50.2X1	T50.2X2	T50.2X3	T50.2X4	T50.2X5	T50.2X6
Teclozan	T37.3X1	T37.3X2	T37.3X3	T37.3X4	T37.3X5	T37.3X6
Tegafur	T45.1X1	T45.1X2	T45.1X3	T45.1X4	T45.1X5	T45.1X6
Tegretol	T42.1X1	T42.1X2	T42.1X3	T42.1X4	T42.1X5	T42.1X6
Teicoplanin	T36.8X1	T36.8X2	T36.8X3	T36.8X4	T36.8X5	T36.8X6
Telepaque	T50.8X1	T50.8X2	T50.8X3	T50.8X4	T50.8X5	T50.8X6
Tellurium	T56.891	T56.892	T56.893	T56.894	—	—
fumes	T56.891	T56.892	T56.893	T56.894	—	—
TEM	T45.1X1	T45.1X2	T45.1X3	T45.1X4	T45.1X5	T45.1X6
Temazepam	T42.4X1	T42.4X2	T42.4X3	T42.4X4	T42.4X5	T42.4X6
Temocillin	T36.0X1	T36.0X2	T36.0X3	T36.0X4	T36.0X5	T36.0X6
Tenamfetamine	T43.621	T43.622	T43.623	T43.624	T43.625	T43.626
Teniposide	T45.1X1	T45.1X2	T45.1X3	T45.1X4	T45.1X5	T45.1X6
Tenitramine	T46.3X1	T46.3X2	T46.3X3	T46.3X4	T46.3X5	T46.3X6
Tenoglicin	T48.4X1	T48.4X2	T48.4X3	T48.4X4	T48.4X5	T48.4X6
Tenonitrozole	T37.3X1	T37.3X2	T37.3X3	T37.3X4	T37.3X5	T37.3X6
Tenoxicam	T39.391	T39.392	T39.393	T39.394	T39.395	T39.396
TEPA	T45.1X1	T45.1X2	T45.1X3	T45.1X4	T45.1X5	T45.1X6
TEPP	T60.0X1	T60.0X2	T60.0X3	T60.0X4	—	—
Teprotide	T46.5X1	T46.5X2	T46.5X3	T46.5X4	T46.5X5	T46.5X6
Terazosin	T44.6X1	T44.6X2	T44.6X3	T44.6X4	T44.6X5	T44.6X6
Terbufos	T60.0X1	T60.0X2	T60.0X3	T60.0X4	—	—
Terbutaline	T48.6X1	T48.6X2	T48.6X3	T48.6X4	T48.6X5	T48.6X6
Terconazole	T49.0X1	T49.0X2	T49.0X3	T49.0X4	T49.0X5	T49.0X6
Terfenadine	T45.0X1	T45.0X2	T45.0X3	T45.0X4	T45.0X5	T45.0X6
Teriparatide (acetate)	T50.991	T50.992	T50.993	T50.994	T50.995	T50.996
Terizidone	T37.1X1	T37.1X2	T37.1X3	T37.1X4	T37.1X5	T37.1X6
Terlipressin	T38.891	T38.892	T38.893	T38.894	T38.895	T38.896
Terodiline	T46.3X1	T46.3X2	T46.3X3	T46.3X4	T46.3X5	T46.3X6
Teroxalene	T37.4X1	T37.4X2	T37.4X3	T37.4X4	T37.4X5	T37.4X6
Terpin(cis) hydrate	T48.4X1	T48.4X2	T48.4X3	T48.4X4	T48.4X5	T48.4X6
Terramycin	T36.4X1	T36.4X2	T36.4X3	T36.4X4	T36.4X5	T36.4X6
Tertatolol	T44.7X1	T44.7X2	T44.7X3	T44.7X4	T44.7X5	T44.7X6
Tessalon	T48.3X1	T48.3X2	T48.3X3	T48.3X4	T48.3X5	T48.3X6
Testolactone	T38.7X1	T38.7X2	T38.7X3	T38.7X4	T38.7X5	T38.7X6
Testosterone	T38.7X1	T38.7X2	T38.7X3	T38.7X4	T38.7X5	T38.7X6
Tetanus toxoid or vaccine	T50.A91	T50.A92	T50.A93	T50.A94	T50.A95	T50.A96
antitoxin	T50.Z11	T50.Z12	T50.Z13	T50.Z14	T50.Z15	T50.Z16
immune globulin (human)	T50.Z11	T50.Z12	T50.Z13	T50.Z14	T50.Z15	T50.Z16
toxoid	T50.A91	T50.A92	T50.A93	T50.A94	T50.A95	T50.A96
with diphtheria toxoid	T50.A21	T50.A22	T50.A23	T50.A24	T50.A25	T50.A26
with pertussis	T50.A11	T50.A12	T50.A13	T50.A14	T50.A15	T50.A16
Tetrabenazine	T43.591	T43.592	T43.593	T43.594	T43.595	T43.596
Tetracaine	T41.3X1	T41.3X2	T41.3X3	T41.3X4	T41.3X5	T41.3X6
nerve block (peripheral) (plexus)	T41.3X1	T41.3X2	T41.3X3	T41.3X4	T41.3X5	T41.3X6
regional	T41.3X1	T41.3X2	T41.3X3	T41.3X4	T41.3X5	T41.3X6
spinal	T41.3X1	T41.3X2	T41.3X3	T41.3X4	T41.3X5	T41.3X6
Tetrachlorethylene—see Tetrachloroethylene						
Tetrachlormethiazide	T50.2X1	T50.2X2	T50.2X3	T50.2X4	T50.2X5	T50.2X6
2,3,7,8-Tetrachlorodi-benzo-p-dioxin	T53.7X1	T53.7X2	T53.7X3	T53.7X4	—	—
Tetrachloroethane	T53.6X1	T53.6X2	T53.6X3	T53.6X4	—	—
vapor	T53.6X1	T53.6X2	T53.6X3	T53.6X4	—	—
paint or varnish	T53.6X1	T53.6X2	T53.6X3	T53.6X4	—	—
Tetrachloroethylene (liquid)	T53.3X1	T53.3X2	T53.3X3	T53.3X4	—	—
medicinal	T37.4X1	T37.4X2	T37.4X3	T37.4X4	T37.4X5	T37.4X6
vapor	T53.3X1	T53.3X2	T53.3X3	T53.3X4	—	—
Tetrachloromethane—see Carbon tetrachloride						
Tetracosactide	T38.811	T38.812	T38.813	T38.814	T38.815	T38.816
Tetracosactrin	T38.811	T38.812	T38.813	T38.814	T38.815	T38.816
Tetracycline	T36.4X1	T36.4X2	T36.4X3	T36.4X4	T36.4X5	T36.4X6
ophthalmic preparation	T49.5X1	T49.5X2	T49.5X3	T49.5X4	T49.5X5	T49.5X6
topical NEC	T49.0X1	T49.0X2	T49.0X3	T49.0X4	T49.0X5	T49.0X6
Tetradifon	T60.8X1	T60.8X2	T60.8X3	T60.8X4	—	—
Tetradotoxin	T61.771	T61.772	T61.773	T61.774	—	—
Tetraethyl						
lead	T56.0X1	T56.0X2	T56.0X3	T56.0X4	—	—
pyrophosphate	T60.0X1	T60.0X2	T60.0X3	T60.0X4	—	—
Tetraethylammonium chloride	T44.2X1	T44.2X2	T44.2X3	T44.2X4	T44.2X5	T44.2X6
Tetraethylthiuram disulfide	T50.6X1	T50.6X2	T50.6X3	T50.6X4	T50.6X5	T50.6X6
Tetrahydroamino-acridine	T44.0X1	T44.0X2	T44.0X3	T44.0X4	T44.0X5	T44.0X6
Tetrahydrocannabinol	T40.7X1	T40.7X2	T40.7X3	T40.7X4	T40.7X5	T40.7X6
Tetrahydrofuran	T52.8X1	T52.8X2	T52.8X3	T52.8X4	—	—
Tetrahydronaphthalene	T52.8X1	T52.8X2	T52.8X3	T52.8X4	—	—
Tetrahydrozoline	T49.5X1	T49.5X2	T49.5X3	T49.5X4	T49.5X5	T49.5X6
Tetralin	T52.8X1	T52.8X2	T52.8X3	T52.8X4	—	—
Tetramethrin	T60.2X1	T60.2X2	T60.2X3	T60.2X4	—	—

Substance	Poisoning, Accidental (unintentional)	Poisoning, Intentional self-harm	Poisoning, Assault	Poisoning, Undetermined	Adverse effect	Underdosing
Tetramethylthiuram (disulfide) NEC	T60.3X1	T60.3X2	T60.3X3	T60.3X4	—	—
medicinal	T49.0X1	T49.0X2	T49.0X3	T49.0X4	T49.0X5	T49.0X6
Tetramisole	T37.4X1	T37.4X2	T37.4X3	T37.4X4	T37.4X5	T37.4X6
Tetranicotinoyl fructose	T46.7X1	T46.7X2	T46.7X3	T46.7X4	T46.7X5	T46.7X6
Tetrazepam	T42.4X1	T42.4X2	T42.4X3	T42.4X4	T42.4X5	T42.4X6
Tetronal	T42.6X1	T42.6X2	T42.6X3	T42.6X4	T42.6X5	T42.6X6
Tetryl	T65.3X1	T65.3X2	T65.3X3	T65.3X4	—	—
Tetrylammonium chloride	T44.2X1	T44.2X2	T44.2X3	T44.2X4	T44.2X5	T44.2X6
Tetryzoline	T49.5X1	T49.5X2	T49.5X3	T49.5X4	T49.5X5	T49.5X6
Thalidomide	T45.1X1	T45.1X2	T45.1X3	T45.1X4	T45.1X5	T45.1X6
Thallium (compounds) (dust) NEC	T56.811	T56.812	T56.813	T56.814	—	—
pesticide	T60.4X1	T60.4X2	T60.4X3	T60.4X4	—	—
THC	T40.7X1	T40.7X2	T40.7X3	T40.7X4	T40.7X5	T40.7X6
Thebacon	T48.3X1	T48.3X2	T48.3X3	T48.3X4	T48.3X5	T48.3X6
Thebaine	T40.2X1	T40.2X2	T40.2X3	T40.2X4	T40.2X5	T40.2X6
Thenoic acid	T49.6X1	T49.6X2	T49.6X3	T49.6X4	T49.6X5	T49.6X6
Thenyldiamine	T45.0X1	T45.0X2	T45.0X3	T45.0X4	T45.0X5	T45.0X6
Theobromine (calcium salicylate)	T48.6X1	T48.6X2	T48.6X3	T48.6X4	T48.6X5	T48.6X6
sodium salicylate	T48.6X1	T48.6X2	T48.6X3	T48.6X4	T48.6X5	T48.6X6
Theophyllamine	T48.6X1	T48.6X2	T48.6X3	T48.6X4	T48.6X5	T48.6X6
Theophylline	T48.6X1	T48.6X2	T48.6X3	T48.6X4	T48.6X5	T48.6X6
aminobenzoic acid	T48.6X1	T48.6X2	T48.6X3	T48.6X4	T48.6X5	T48.6X6
ethylenediamine	T48.6X1	T48.6X2	T48.6X3	T48.6X4	T48.6X5	T48.6X6
piperazine p-amino-benzoate	T48.6X1	T48.6X2	T48.6X3	T48.6X4	T48.6X5	T48.6X6
Thiabendazole	T37.4X1	T37.4X2	T37.4X3	T37.4X4	T37.4X5	T37.4X6
Thialbarbital	T41.1X1	T41.1X2	T41.1X3	T41.1X4	T41.1X5	T41.1X6
Thiamazole	T38.2X1	T38.2X2	T38.2X3	T38.2X4	T38.2X5	T38.2X6
Thiambutosine	T37.1X1	T37.1X2	T37.1X3	T37.1X4	T37.1X5	T37.1X6
Thiamine	T45.2X1	T45.2X2	T45.2X3	T45.2X4	T45.2X5	T45.2X6
Thiamphenicol	T36.2X1	T36.2X2	T36.2X3	T36.2X4	T36.2X5	T36.2X6
Thiamylal	T41.1X1	T41.1X2	T41.1X3	T41.1X4	T41.1X5	T41.1X6
sodium	T41.1X1	T41.1X2	T41.1X3	T41.1X4	T41.1X5	T41.1X6
Thiazesim	T43.291	T43.292	T43.293	T43.294	T43.295	T43.296
Thiazides (diuretics)	T50.2X1	T50.2X2	T50.2X3	T50.2X4	T50.2X5	T50.2X6
Thiazinamium metilsulfate	T43.3X1	T43.3X2	T43.3X3	T43.3X4	T43.3X5	T43.3X6
Thiethylperazine	T43.3X1	T43.3X2	T43.3X3	T43.3X4	T43.3X5	T43.3X6
Thimerosal	T49.0X1	T49.0X2	T49.0X3	T49.0X4	T49.0X5	T49.0X6
ophthalmic preparation	T49.5X1	T49.5X2	T49.5X3	T49.5X4	T49.5X5	T49.5X6
Thioacetazone	T37.1X1	T37.1X2	T37.1X3	T37.1X4	T37.1X5	T37.1X6
with isoniazid	T37.1X1	T37.1X2	T37.1X3	T37.1X4	T37.1X5	T37.1X6
Thiobarbital sodium	T41.1X1	T41.1X2	T41.1X3	T41.1X4	T41.1X5	T41.1X6
Thiobarbiturate anesthetic	T41.1X1	T41.1X2	T41.1X3	T41.1X4	T41.1X5	T41.1X6
Thiobismol	T37.8X1	T37.8X2	T37.8X3	T37.8X4	T37.8X5	T37.8X6
Thiobutabarbital sodium	T41.1X1	T41.1X2	T41.1X3	T41.1X4	T41.1X5	T41.1X6
Thiocarbamate (insecticide)	T60.0X1	T60.0X2	T60.0X3	T60.0X4	—	—
Thiocarbamide	T38.2X1	T38.2X2	T38.2X3	T38.2X4	T38.2X5	T38.2X6

Substance	Poisoning, Accidental (unintentional)	Poisoning, Intentional self-harm	Poisoning, Assault	Poisoning, Undetermined	Adverse effect	Underdosing
Thiocarbarsone	T37.8X1	T37.8X2	T37.8X3	T37.8X4	T37.8X5	T37.8X6
Thiocarlide	T37.1X1	T37.1X2	T37.1X3	T37.1X4	T37.1X5	T37.1X6
Thioctamide	T50.991	T50.992	T50.993	T50.994	T50.995	T50.996
Thioctic acid	T50.991	T50.992	T50.993	T50.994	T50.995	T50.996
Thiofos	T60.0X1	T60.0X2	T60.0X3	T60.0X4	—	—
Thioglycolate	T49.4X1	T49.4X2	T49.4X3	T49.4X4	T49.4X5	T49.4X6
Thioglycolic acid	T65.891	T65.892	T65.893	T65.894	—	—
Thioguanine	T45.1X1	T45.1X2	T45.1X3	T45.1X4	T45.1X5	T45.1X6
Thiomercaptomerin	T50.2X1	T50.2X2	T50.2X3	T50.2X4	T50.2X5	T50.2X6
Thiomerin	T50.2X1	T50.2X2	T50.2X3	T50.2X4	T50.2X5	T50.2X6
Thiomersal	T49.0X1	T49.0X2	T49.0X3	T49.0X4	T49.0X5	T49.0X6
Thionazin	T60.0X1	T60.0X2	T60.0X3	T60.0X4	—	—
Thiopental (sodium)	T41.1X1	T41.1X2	T41.1X3	T41.1X4	T41.1X5	T41.1X6
Thiopentone (sodium)	T41.1X1	T41.1X2	T41.1X3	T41.1X4	T41.1X5	T41.1X6
Thiopropazate	T43.3X1	T43.3X2	T43.3X3	T43.3X4	T43.3X5	T43.3X6
Thioproperazine	T43.3X1	T43.3X2	T43.3X3	T43.3X4	T43.3X5	T43.3X6
Thioridazine	T43.3X1	T43.3X2	T43.3X3	T43.3X4	T43.3X5	T43.3X6
Thiosinamine	T49.3X1	T49.3X2	T49.3X3	T49.3X4	T49.3X5	T49.3X6
Thiotepa	T45.1X1	T45.1X2	T45.1X3	T45.1X4	T45.1X5	T45.1X6
Thiothixene	T43.4X1	T43.4X2	T43.4X3	T43.4X4	T43.4X5	T43.4X6
Thiouracil (benzyl) (methyl) (propyl)	T38.2X1	T38.2X2	T38.2X3	T38.2X4	T38.2X5	T38.2X6
Thiourea	T38.2X1	T38.2X2	T38.2X3	T38.2X4	T38.2X5	T38.2X6
Thiphenamil	T44.3X1	T44.3X2	T44.3X3	T44.3X4	T44.3X5	T44.3X6
Thiram	T60.3X1	T60.3X2	T60.3X3	T60.3X4	—	—
medicinal	T49.2X1	T49.2X2	T49.2X3	T49.2X4	T49.2X5	T49.2X6
Thonzylamine (systemic)	T45.0X1	T45.0X2	T45.0X3	T45.0X4	T45.0X5	T45.0X6
mucosal decongestant	T48.5X1	T48.5X2	T48.5X3	T48.5X4	T48.5X5	T48.5X6
Thorazine	T43.3X1	T43.3X2	T43.3X3	T43.3X4	T43.3X5	T43.3X6
Thorium dioxide suspension	T50.8X1	T50.8X2	T50.8X3	T50.8X4	T50.8X5	T50.8X6
Thornapple	T62.2X1	T62.2X2	T62.2X3	T62.2X4	—	—
Throat drug NEC	T49.6X1	T49.6X2	T49.6X3	T49.6X4	T49.6X5	T49.6X6
Thrombin	T45.7X1	T45.7X2	T45.7X3	T45.7X4	T45.7X5	T45.7X6
Thrombolysin	T45.611	T45.612	T45.613	T45.614	T45.615	T45.616
Thromboplastin	T45.7X1	T45.7X2	T45.7X3	T45.7X4	T45.7X5	T45.7X6
Thurfyl nicotinate	T46.7X1	T46.7X2	T46.7X3	T46.7X4	T46.7X5	T46.7X6
Thymol	T49.0X1	T49.0X2	T49.0X3	T49.0X4	T49.0X5	T49.0X6
Thymopentin	T37.5X1	T37.5X2	T37.5X3	T37.5X4	T37.5X5	T37.5X6
Thymoxamine	T46.7X1	T46.7X2	T46.7X3	T46.7X4	T46.7X5	T46.7X6
Thymus extract	T38.891	T38.892	T38.893	T38.894	T38.895	T38.896
Thyreotrophic hormone	T38.811	T38.812	T38.813	T38.814	T38.815	T38.816
Thyroglobulin	T38.1X1	T38.1X2	T38.1X3	T38.1X4	T38.1X5	T38.1X6
Thyroid (hormone)	T38.1X1	T38.1X2	T38.1X3	T38.1X4	T38.1X5	T38.1X6
Thyrolar	T38.1X1	T38.1X2	T38.1X3	T38.1X4	T38.1X5	T38.1X6
Thyrotrophin	T38.811	T38.812	T38.813	T38.814	T38.815	T38.816
Thyrotropic hormone	T38.811	T38.812	T38.813	T38.814	T38.815	T38.816
Thyroxine	T38.1X1	T38.1X2	T38.1X3	T38.1X4	T38.1X5	T38.1X6
Tiabendazole	T37.4X1	T37.4X2	T37.4X3	T37.4X4	T37.4X5	T37.4X6
Tiamizide	T50.2X1	T50.2X2	T50.2X3	T50.2X4	T50.2X5	T50.2X6

Substance	Poisoning, Accidental (unintentional)	Poisoning, Intentional self-harm	Poisoning, Assault	Poisoning, Undetermined	Adverse effect	Underdosing
Tianeptine	T43.291	T43.292	T43.293	T43.294	T43.295	T43.296
Tiapamil	T46.1X1	T46.1X2	T46.1X3	T46.1X4	T46.1X5	T46.1X6
Tiapride	T43.591	T43.592	T43.593	T43.594	T43.595	T43.596
Tiaprofenic acid	T39.311	T39.312	T39.313	T39.314	T39.315	T39.316
Tiaramide	T39.8X1	T39.8X2	T39.8X3	T39.8X4	T39.8X5	T39.8X6
Ticarcillin	T36.0X1	T36.0X2	T36.0X3	T36.0X4	T36.0X5	T36.0X6
Ticlatone	T49.0X1	T49.0X2	T49.0X3	T49.0X4	T49.0X5	T49.0X6
Ticlopidine	T45.521	T45.522	T45.523	T45.524	T45.525	T45.526
Ticrynafen	T50.1X1	T50.1X2	T50.1X3	T50.1X4	T50.1X5	T50.1X6
Tidiacic	T50.991	T50.992	T50.993	T50.994	T50.995	T50.996
Tiemonium	T44.3X1	T44.3X2	T44.3X3	T44.3X4	T44.3X5	T44.3X6
iodide	T44.3X1	T44.3X2	T44.3X3	T44.3X4	T44.3X5	T44.3X6
Tienilic acid	T50.1X1	T50.1X2	T50.1X3	T50.1X4	T50.1X5	T50.1X6
Tifenamil	T44.3X1	T44.3X2	T44.3X3	T44.3X4	T44.3X5	T44.3X6
Tigan	T45.0X1	T45.0X2	T45.0X3	T45.0X4	T45.0X5	T45.0X6
Tigloidine	T44.3X1	T44.3X2	T44.3X3	T44.3X4	T44.3X5	T44.3X6
Tilactase	T47.5X1	T47.5X2	T47.5X3	T47.5X4	T47.5X5	T47.5X6
Tiletamine	T41.291	T41.292	T41.293	T41.294	T41.295	T41.296
Tilidine	T40.4X1	T40.4X2	T40.4X3	T40.4X4	—	—
Timepidium bromide	T44.3X1	T44.3X2	T44.3X3	T44.3X4	T44.3X5	T44.3X6
Timiperone	T43.4X1	T43.4X2	T43.4X3	T43.4X4	T43.4X5	T43.4X6
Timolol	T44.7X1	T44.7X2	T44.7X3	T44.7X4	T44.7X5	T44.7X6
Tin (chloride) (dust) (oxide) NEC	T56.6X1	T56.6X2	T56.6X3	T56.6X4	—	—
anti-infectives	T37.8X1	T37.8X2	T37.8X3	T37.8X4	T37.8X5	T37.8X6
Tincture, iodine—see Iodine						
Tindal	T43.3X1	T43.3X2	T43.3X3	T43.3X4	T43.3X5	T43.3X6
Tinidazole	T37.3X1	T37.3X2	T37.3X3	T37.3X4	T37.3X5	T37.3X6
Tinoridine	T39.8X1	T39.8X2	T39.8X3	T39.8X4	T39.8X5	T39.8X6
Tiocarlide	T37.1X1	T37.1X2	T37.1X3	T37.1X4	T37.1X5	T37.1X6
Tioclomarol	T45.511	T45.512	T45.513	T45.514	T45.515	T45.516
Tioconazole	T49.0X1	T49.0X2	T49.0X3	T49.0X4	T49.0X5	T49.0X6
Tioguanine	T45.1X1	T45.1X2	T45.1X3	T45.1X4	T45.1X5	T45.1X6
Tiopronin	T50.991	T50.992	T50.993	T50.994	T50.995	T50.996
Tiotixene	T43.4X1	T43.4X2	T43.4X3	T43.4X4	T43.4X5	T43.4X6
Tioxolone	T49.4X1	T49.4X2	T49.4X3	T49.4X4	T49.4X5	T49.4X6
Tipepidine	T48.3X1	T48.3X2	T48.3X3	T48.3X4	T48.3X5	T48.3X6
Tiquizium bromide	T44.3X1	T44.3X2	T44.3X3	T44.3X4	T44.3X5	T44.3X6
Tiratricol	T38.1X1	T38.1X2	T38.1X3	T38.1X4	T38.1X5	T38.1X6
Tisopurine	T50.4X1	T50.4X2	T50.4X3	T50.4X4	T50.4X5	T50.4X6
Titanium (compounds) (vapor)	T56.891	T56.892	T56.893	T56.894	—	—
dioxide	T49.3X1	T49.3X2	T49.3X3	T49.3X4	T49.3X5	T49.3X6
ointment	T49.3X1	T49.3X2	T49.3X3	T49.3X4	T49.3X5	T49.3X6
oxide	T49.3X1	T49.3X2	T49.3X3	T49.3X4	T49.3X5	T49.3X6
tetrachloride	T56.891	T56.892	T56.893	T56.894	—	—
Titanocene	T56.891	T56.892	T56.893	T56.894	—	—
Titroid	T38.1X1	T38.1X2	T38.1X3	T38.1X4	T38.1X5	T38.1X6
Tizanidine	T42.8X1	T42.8X2	T42.8X3	T42.8X4	T42.8X5	T42.8X6
TMTD	T60.3X1	T60.3X2	T60.3X3	T60.3X4	—	—
TNT (fumes)	T65.3X1	T65.3X2	T65.3X3	T65.3X4	—	—
Toadstool	T62.0X1	T62.0X2	T62.0X3	T62.0X4	—	—
Tobacco NEC	T65.291	T65.292	T65.293	T65.294	—	—
cigarettes	T65.221	T65.222	T65.223	T65.224	—	—
Indian	T62.2X1	T62.2X2	T62.2X3	T62.2X4	—	—
smoke, second-hand	T65.221	T65.222	T65.223	T65.224	—	—
Tobramycin	T36.5X1	T36.5X2	T36.5X3	T36.5X4	T36.5X5	T36.5X6
Tocainide	T46.2X1	T46.2X2	T46.2X3	T46.2X4	T46.2X5	T46.2X6
Tocoferol	T45.2X1	T45.2X2	T45.2X3	T45.2X4	T45.2X5	T45.2X6
Tocopherol	T45.2X1	T45.2X2	T45.2X3	T45.2X4	T45.2X5	T45.2X6
acetate	T45.2X1	T45.2X2	T45.2X3	T45.2X4	T45.2X5	T45.2X6
Tocosamine	T48.0X1	T48.0X2	T48.0X3	T48.0X4	T48.0X5	T48.0X6
Todralazine	T46.5X1	T46.5X2	T46.5X3	T46.5X4	T46.5X5	T46.5X6
Tofisopam	T42.4X1	T42.4X2	T42.4X3	T42.4X4	T42.4X5	T42.4X6
Tofranil	T43.011	T43.012	T43.013	T43.014	T43.015	T43.016
Toilet deodorizer	T65.891	T65.892	T65.893	T65.894	—	—
Tolamolol	T44.7X1	T44.7X2	T44.7X3	T44.7X4	T44.7X5	T44.7X6
Tolazamide	T38.3X1	T38.3X2	T38.3X3	T38.3X4	T38.3X5	T38.3X6
Tolazoline	T46.7X1	T46.7X2	T46.7X3	T46.7X4	T46.7X5	T46.7X6
Tolbutamide (sodium)	T38.3X1	T38.3X2	T38.3X3	T38.3X4	T38.3X5	T38.3X6
Tolciclate	T49.0X1	T49.0X2	T49.0X3	T49.0X4	T49.0X5	T49.0X6
Tolmetin	T39.391	T39.392	T39.393	T39.394	T39.395	T39.396
Tolnaftate	T49.0X1	T49.0X2	T49.0X3	T49.0X4	T49.0X5	T49.0X6
Tolonidine	T46.5X1	T46.5X2	T46.5X3	T46.5X4	T46.5X5	T46.5X6
Toloxatone	T42.6X1	T42.6X2	T42.6X3	T42.6X4	T42.6X5	T42.6X6
Tolperisone	T44.3X1	T44.3X2	T44.3X3	T44.3X4	T44.3X5	T44.3X6
Tolserol	T42.8X1	T42.8X2	T42.8X3	T42.8X4	T42.8X5	T42.8X6
Toluene (liquid)	T52.2X1	T52.2X2	T52.2X3	T52.2X4	—	—
diisocyanate	T65.0X1	T65.0X2	T65.0X3	T65.0X4	—	—
Toluidine	T65.891	T65.892	T65.893	T65.894	—	—
vapor	T59.891	T59.892	T59.893	T59.894	—	—
Toluol (liquid)	T52.2X1	T52.2X2	T52.2X3	T52.2X4	—	—
vapor	T52.2X1	T52.2X2	T52.2X3	T52.2X4	—	—
Toluylenediamine	T65.3X1	T65.3X2	T65.3X3	T65.3X4	—	—
Tolylene-2,4-diisocyanate	T65.0X1	T65.0X2	T65.0X3	T65.0X4	—	—
Tonic NEC	T50.901	T50.902	T50.903	T50.904	T50.905	T50.906
Topical action drug NEC	T49.91	T49.92	T49.93	T49.94	T49.95	T49.96
ear, nose or throat	T49.6X1	T49.6X2	T49.6X3	T49.6X4	T49.6X5	T49.6X6
eye	T49.5X1	T49.5X2	T49.5X3	T49.5X4	T49.5X5	T49.5X6
skin	T49.91	T49.92	T49.93	T49.94	T49.95	T49.96
specified NEC	T49.8X1	T49.8X2	T49.8X3	T49.8X4	T49.8X5	T49.8X6
Toquizine	T44.3X1	T44.3X2	T44.3X3	T44.3X4	T44.3X5	T44.3X6
Toremifene	T38.6X1	T38.6X2	T38.6X3	T38.6X4	T38.6X5	T38.6X6
Tosylchloramide sodium	T49.8X1	T49.8X2	T49.8X3	T49.8X4	T49.8X5	T49.8X6
Toxaphene (dust) (spray)	T60.1X1	T60.1X2	T60.1X3	T60.1X4	—	—
Toxin, diphtheria (Schick Test)	T50.8X1	T50.8X2	T50.8X3	T50.8X4	T50.8X5	T50.8X6
Toxoid						
combined	T50.A21	T50.A22	T50.A23	T50.A24	T50.A25	T50.A26
diphtheria	T50.A91	T50.A92	T50.A93	T50.A94	T50.A95	T50.A96
tetanus	T50.A91	T50.A92	T50.A93	T50.A94	T50.A95	T50.A96

Substance	Poisoning, Accidental (unintentional)	Poisoning, Intentional self-harm	Poisoning, Assault	Poisoning, Undetermined	Adverse effect	Underdosing
Trace element NEC	T45.8X1	T45.8X2	T45.8X3	T45.8X4	T45.8X5	T45.8X6
Tractor fuel NEC	T52.0X1	T52.0X2	T52.0X3	T52.0X4	—	—
Tragacanth	T50.991	T50.992	T50.993	T50.994	T50.995	T50.996
Tramadol	T40.4X1	T40.4X2	T40.4X3	T40.4X4	T40.4X5	T40.4X6
Tramazoline	T48.5X1	T48.5X2	T48.5X3	T48.5X4	T48.5X5	T48.5X6
Tranexamic acid	T45.621	T45.622	T45.623	T45.624	T45.625	T45.626
Tranilast	T45.0X1	T45.0X2	T45.0X3	T45.0X4	T45.0X5	T45.0X6
Tranquilizer NEC	T43.501	T43.502	T43.503	T43.504	T43.505	T43.506
with hypnotic or sedative	T42.6X1	T42.6X2	T42.6X3	T42.6X4	T42.6X5	T42.6X6
benzodiazepine NEC	T42.4X1	T42.4X2	T42.4X3	T42.4X4	T42.4X5	T42.4X6
butyrophenone NEC	T43.4X1	T43.4X2	T43.4X3	T43.4X4	T43.4X5	T43.4X6
carbamate	T43.591	T43.592	T43.593	T43.594	T43.595	T43.596
dimethylamine	T43.3X1	T43.3X2	T43.3X3	T43.3X4	T43.3X5	T43.3X6
ethylamine	T43.3X1	T43.3X2	T43.3X3	T43.3X4	T43.3X5	T43.3X6
hydroxyzine	T43.591	T43.592	T43.593	T43.594	T43.595	T43.596
major NEC	T43.501	T43.502	T43.503	T43.504	T43.505	T43.506
penothiazine NEC	T43.3X1	T43.3X2	T43.3X3	T43.3X4	T43.3X5	T43.3X6
phenothiazine-based	T43.3X1	T43.3X2	T43.3X3	T43.3X4	T43.3X5	T43.3X6
piperazine NEC	T43.3X1	T43.3X2	T43.3X3	T43.3X4	T43.3X5	T43.3X6
piperidine	T43.3X1	T43.3X2	T43.3X3	T43.3X4	T43.3X5	T43.3X6
propylamine	T43.3X1	T43.3X2	T43.3X3	T43.3X4	T43.3X5	T43.3X6
specified NEC	T43.591	T43.592	T43.593	T43.594	T43.595	T43.596
thioxanthene NEC	T43.591	T43.592	T43.593	T43.594	T43.595	T43.596
Tranxene	T42.4X1	T42.4X2	T42.4X3	T42.4X4	T42.4X5	T42.4X6
Tranylcypromine	T43.1X1	T43.1X2	T43.1X3	T43.1X4	T43.1X5	T43.1X6
Trapidil	T46.3X1	T46.3X2	T46.3X3	T46.3X4	T46.3X5	T46.3X6
Trasentine	T44.3X1	T44.3X2	T44.3X3	T44.3X4	T44.3X5	T44.3X6
Travert	T50.3X1	T50.3X2	T50.3X3	T50.3X4	T50.3X5	T50.3X6
Trazodone	T43.211	T43.212	T43.213	T43.214	T43.215	T43.216
Trecator	T37.1X1	T37.1X2	T37.1X3	T37.1X4	T37.1X5	T37.1X6
Treosulfan	T45.1X1	T45.1X2	T45.1X3	T45.1X4	T45.1X5	T45.1X6
Tretamine	T45.1X1	T45.1X2	T45.1X3	T45.1X4	T45.1X5	T45.1X6
Tretinoin	T49.0X1	T49.0X2	T49.0X3	T49.0X4	T49.0X5	T49.0X6
Tretoquinol	T48.6X1	T48.6X2	T48.6X3	T48.6X4	T48.6X5	T48.6X6
Triacetin	T49.0X1	T49.0X2	T49.0X3	T49.0X4	T49.0X5	T49.0X6
Triacetoxyanthracene	T49.4X1	T49.4X2	T49.4X3	T49.4X4	T49.4X5	T49.4X6
Triacetyloleandomycin	T36.3X1	T36.3X2	T36.3X3	T36.3X4	T36.3X5	T36.3X6
Triamcinolone	T38.0X1	T38.0X2	T38.0X3	T38.0X4	T38.0X5	T38.0X6
ENT agent	T49.6X1	T49.6X2	T49.6X3	T49.6X4	T49.6X5	T49.6X6
hexacetonide	T49.0X1	T49.0X2	T49.0X3	T49.0X4	T49.0X5	T49.0X6
ophthalmic preparation	T49.5X1	T49.5X2	T49.5X3	T49.5X4	T49.5X5	T49.5X6
topical NEC	T49.0X1	T49.0X2	T49.0X3	T49.0X4	T49.0X5	T49.0X6
Triampyzine	T44.3X1	T44.3X2	T44.3X3	T44.3X4	T44.3X5	T44.3X6
Triamterene	T50.2X1	T50.2X2	T50.2X3	T50.2X4	T50.2X5	T50.2X6
Triazine (herbicide)	T60.3X1	T60.3X2	T60.3X3	T60.3X4	—	—
Triaziquone	T45.1X1	T45.1X2	T45.1X3	T45.1X4	T45.1X5	T45.1X6
Triazolam	T42.4X1	T42.4X2	T42.4X3	T42.4X4	T42.4X5	T42.4X6
Triazole (herbicide)	T60.3X1	T60.3X2	T60.3X3	T60.3X4	—	—
Tribenoside	T46.991	T46.992	T46.993	T46.994	T46.995	T46.996

Substance	Poisoning, Accidental (unintentional)	Poisoning, Intentional self-harm	Poisoning, Assault	Poisoning, Undetermined	Adverse effect	Underdosing
Tribromacetaldehyde	T42.6X1	T42.6X2	T42.6X3	T42.6X4	T42.6X5	T42.6X6
Tribromoethanol, rectal	T41.291	T41.292	T41.293	T41.294	T41.295	T41.296
Tribromomethane	T42.6X1	T42.6X2	T42.6X3	T42.6X4	T42.6X5	T42.6X6
Trichlorethane	T53.2X1	T53.2X2	T53.2X3	T53.2X4	—	—
Trichlorethylene	T53.2X1	T53.2X2	T53.2X3	T53.2X4	—	—
Trichlorfon	T60.0X1	T60.0X2	T60.0X3	T60.0X4	—	—
Trichlormethiazide	T50.2X1	T50.2X2	T50.2X3	T50.2X4	T50.2X5	T50.2X6
Trichlormethine	T45.1X1	T45.1X2	T45.1X3	T45.1X4	T45.1X5	T45.1X6
Trichloroacetic acid, Trichloracetic acid	T54.2X1	T54.2X2	T54.2X3	T54.2X4	—	—
medicinal	T49.4X1	T49.4X2	T49.4X3	T49.4X4	T49.4X5	T49.4X6
Trichloroethane	T53.2X1	T53.2X2	T53.2X3	T53.2X4	—	—
Trichloroethanol	T42.6X1	T42.6X2	T42.6X3	T42.6X4	T42.6X5	T42.6X6
Trichloroethyl phosphate	T42.6X1	T42.6X2	T42.6X3	T42.6X4	T42.6X5	T42.6X6
Trichloroethylene (liquid) (vapor)	T53.2X1	T53.2X2	T53.2X3	T53.2X4	—	—
anesthetic (gas)	T41.0X1	T41.0X2	T41.0X3	T41.0X4	T41.0X5	T41.0X6
vapor NEC	T53.2X1	T53.2X2	T53.2X3	T53.2X4	—	—
Trichlorofluoromethane NEC	T53.5X1	T53.5X2	T53.5X3	T53.5X4	—	—
Trichloronate	T60.0X1	T60.0X2	T60.0X3	T60.0X4	—	—
2,4,5-Trichlorophenoxyacetic acid	T60.3X1	T60.3X2	T60.3X3	T60.3X4	—	—
Trichloropropane	T53.6X1	T53.6X2	T53.6X3	T53.6X4	—	—
Trichlorotriethylamine	T45.1X1	T45.1X2	T45.1X3	T45.1X4	T45.1X5	T45.1X6
Trichomonacides NEC	T37.3X1	T37.3X2	T37.3X3	T37.3X4	T37.3X5	T37.3X6
Trichomycin	T36.7X1	T36.7X2	T36.7X3	T36.7X4	T36.7X5	T36.7X6
Triclobisonium chloride	T49.0X1	T49.0X2	T49.0X3	T49.0X4	T49.0X5	T49.0X6
Triclocarban	T49.0X1	T49.0X2	T49.0X3	T49.0X4	T49.0X5	T49.0X6
Triclofos	T42.6X1	T42.6X2	T42.6X3	T42.6X4	T42.6X5	T42.6X6
Triclosan	T49.0X1	T49.0X2	T49.0X3	T49.0X4	T49.0X5	T49.0X6
Tricresyl phosphate	T65.891	T65.892	T65.893	T65.894	—	—
solvent	T52.91	T52.92	T52.93	T52.94	—	—
Tricyclamol chloride	T44.3X1	T44.3X2	T44.3X3	T44.3X4	T44.3X5	T44.3X6
Tridesilon	T49.0X1	T49.0X2	T49.0X3	T49.0X4	T49.0X5	T49.0X6
Tridihexethyl iodide	T44.3X1	T44.3X2	T44.3X3	T44.3X4	T44.3X5	T44.3X6
Tridione	T42.2X1	T42.2X2	T42.2X3	T42.2X4	T42.2X5	T42.2X6
Trientine	T45.8X1	T45.8X2	T45.8X3	T45.8X4	T45.8X5	T45.8X6
Triethanolamine NEC	T54.3X1	T54.3X2	T54.3X3	T54.3X4	—	—
detergent	T54.3X1	T54.3X2	T54.3X3	T54.3X4	—	—
trinitrate (biphosphate)	T46.3X1	T46.3X2	T46.3X3	T46.3X4	T46.3X5	T46.3X6
Triethanomelamine	T45.1X1	T45.1X2	T45.1X3	T45.1X4	T45.1X5	T45.1X6
Triethylenemelamine	T45.1X1	T45.1X2	T45.1X3	T45.1X4	T45.1X5	T45.1X6
Triethylenephosphoramide	T45.1X1	T45.1X2	T45.1X3	T45.1X4	T45.1X5	T45.1X6
Triethylenethiophosphoramide	T45.1X1	T45.1X2	T45.1X3	T45.1X4	T45.1X5	T45.1X6
Trifluoperazine	T43.3X1	T43.3X2	T43.3X3	T43.3X4	T43.3X5	T43.3X6
Trifluoroethyl vinyl ether	T41.0X1	T41.0X2	T41.0X3	T41.0X4	T41.0X5	T41.0X6
Trifluperidol	T43.4X1	T43.4X2	T43.4X3	T43.4X4	T43.4X5	T43.4X6
Triflupromazine	T43.3X1	T43.3X2	T43.3X3	T43.3X4	T43.3X5	T43.3X6

Substance	Poisoning, Accidental (unintentional)	Poisoning, Intentional self-harm	Poisoning, Assault	Poisoning, Undetermined	Adverse effect	Underdosing
Trifluridine	T37.5X1	T37.5X2	T37.5X3	T37.5X4	T37.5X5	T37.5X6
Triflusal	T45.521	T45.522	T45.523	T45.524	T45.525	T45.526
Trihexyphenidyl	T44.3X1	T44.3X2	T44.3X3	T44.3X4	T44.3X5	T44.3X6
Triiodothyronine	T38.1X1	T38.1X2	T38.1X3	T38.1X4	T38.1X5	T38.1X6
Trilene	T41.0X1	T41.0X2	T41.0X3	T41.0X4	T41.0X5	T41.0X6
Trilostane	T38.991	T38.992	T38.993	T38.994	T38.995	T38.996
Trimebutine	T44.3X1	T44.3X2	T44.3X3	T44.3X4	T44.3X5	T44.3X6
Trimecaine	T41.3X1	T41.3X2	T41.3X3	T41.3X4	T41.3X5	T41.3X6
Trimeprazine (tartrate)	T44.3X1	T44.3X2	T44.3X3	T44.3X4	T44.3X5	T44.3X6
Trimetaphan camsilate	T44.2X1	T44.2X2	T44.2X3	T44.2X4	T44.2X5	T44.2X6
Trimetazidine	T46.7X1	T46.7X2	T46.7X3	T46.7X4	T46.7X5	T46.7X6
Trimethadione	T42.2X1	T42.2X2	T42.2X3	T42.2X4	T42.2X5	T42.2X6
Trimethaphan	T44.2X1	T44.2X2	T44.2X3	T44.2X4	T44.2X5	T44.2X6
Trimethidinium	T44.2X1	T44.2X2	T44.2X3	T44.2X4	T44.2X5	T44.2X6
Trimethobenzamide	T45.0X1	T45.0X2	T45.0X3	T45.0X4	T45.0X5	T45.0X6
Trimethoprim	T37.8X1	T37.8X2	T37.8X3	T37.8X4	T37.8X5	T37.8X6
with sulfamethoxazole	T36.8X1	T36.8X2	T36.8X3	T36.8X4	T36.8X5	T36.8X6
Trimethylcarbinol	T51.3X1	T51.3X2	T51.3X3	T51.3X4	—	—
Trimethylpsoralen	T49.3X1	T49.3X2	T49.3X3	T49.3X4	T49.3X5	T49.3X6
Trimeton	T45.0X1	T45.0X2	T45.0X3	T45.0X4	T45.0X5	T45.0X6
Trimetrexate	T45.1X1	T45.1X2	T45.1X3	T45.1X4	T45.1X5	T45.1X6
Trimipramine	T43.011	T43.012	T43.013	T43.014	T43.015	T43.016
Trimustine	T45.1X1	T45.1X2	T45.1X3	T45.1X4	T45.1X5	T45.1X6
Trinitrine	T46.3X1	T46.3X2	T46.3X3	T46.3X4	T46.3X5	T46.3X6
Trinitrobenzol	T65.3X1	T65.3X2	T65.3X3	T65.3X4	—	—
Trinitrophenol	T65.3X1	T65.3X2	T65.3X3	T65.3X4	—	—
Trinitrotoluene (fumes)	T65.3X1	T65.3X2	T65.3X3	T65.3X4	—	—
Trional	T42.6X1	T42.6X2	T42.6X3	T42.6X4	T42.6X5	T42.6X6
Triorthocresyl phosphate	T65.891	T65.892	T65.893	T65.894	—	—
Trioxide of arsenic	T57.0X1	T57.0X2	T57.0X3	T57.0X4	—	—
Trioxysalen	T49.4X1	T49.4X2	T49.4X3	T49.4X4	T49.4X5	T49.4X6
Tripamide	T50.2X1	T50.2X2	T50.2X3	T50.2X4	T50.2X5	T50.2X6
Triparanol	T46.6X1	T46.6X2	T46.6X3	T46.6X4	T46.6X5	T46.6X6
Tripelennamine	T45.0X1	T45.0X2	T45.0X3	T45.0X4	T45.0X5	T45.0X6
Triperiden	T44.3X1	T44.3X2	T44.3X3	T44.3X4	T44.3X5	T44.3X6
Triperidol	T43.4X1	T43.4X2	T43.4X3	T43.4X4	T43.4X5	T43.4X6
Triphenylphosphate	T65.891	T65.892	T65.893	T65.894	—	—
Triple						
bromides	T42.6X1	T42.6X2	T42.6X3	T42.6X4	T42.6X5	T42.6X6
carbonate	T47.1X1	T47.1X2	T47.1X3	T47.1X4	T47.1X5	T47.1X6
vaccine						
DPT	T50.A11	T50.A12	T50.A13	T50.A14	T50.A15	T50.A16
including pertussis	T50.A11	T50.A12	T50.A13	T50.A14	T50.A15	T50.A16
MMR	T50.B91	T50.B92	T50.B93	T50.B94	T50.B95	T50.B96
Triprolidine	T45.0X1	T45.0X2	T45.0X3	T45.0X4	T45.0X5	T45.0X6
Trisodium hydrogen edetate	T50.6X1	T50.6X2	T50.6X3	T50.6X4	T50.6X5	T50.6X6
Trisoralen	T49.3X1	T49.3X2	T49.3X3	T49.3X4	T49.3X5	T49.3X6
Trisulfapyrimidines	T37.0X1	T37.0X2	T37.0X3	T37.0X4	T37.0X5	T37.0X6

Substance	Poisoning, Accidental (unintentional)	Poisoning, Intentional self-harm	Poisoning, Assault	Poisoning, Undetermined	Adverse effect	Underdosing
Trithiozine	T44.3X1	T44.3X2	T44.3X3	T44.3X4	T44.3X5	T44.3X6
Tritiozine	T44.3X1	T44.3X2	T44.3X3	T44.3X4	T44.3X5	T44.3X6
Tritoqualine	T45.0X1	T45.0X2	T45.0X3	T45.0X4	T45.0X5	T45.0X6
Trofosfamide	T45.1X1	T45.1X2	T45.1X3	T45.1X4	T45.1X5	T45.1X6
Troleandomycin	T36.3X1	T36.3X2	T36.3X3	T36.3X4	T36.3X5	T36.3X6
Trolnitrate (phosphate)	T46.3X1	T46.3X2	T46.3X3	T46.3X4	T46.3X5	T46.3X6
Tromantadine	T37.5X1	T37.5X2	T37.5X3	T37.5X4	T37.5X5	T37.5X6
Trometamol	T50.2X1	T50.2X2	T50.2X3	T50.2X4	T50.2X5	T50.2X6
Tromethamine	T50.2X1	T50.2X2	T50.2X3	T50.2X4	T50.2X5	T50.2X6
Tronothane	T41.3X1	T41.3X2	T41.3X3	T41.3X4	T41.3X5	T41.3X6
Tropacine	T44.3X1	T44.3X2	T44.3X3	T44.3X4	T44.3X5	T44.3X6
Tropatepine	T44.3X1	T44.3X2	T44.3X3	T44.3X4	T44.3X5	T44.3X6
Tropicamide	T44.3X1	T44.3X2	T44.3X3	T44.3X4	T44.3X5	T44.3X6
Trospium chloride	T44.3X1	T44.3X2	T44.3X3	T44.3X4	T44.3X5	T44.3X6
Troxerutin	T46.991	T46.992	T46.993	T46.994	T46.995	T46.996
Troxidone	T42.2X1	T42.2X2	T42.2X3	T42.2X4	T42.2X5	T42.2X6
Tryparsamide	T37.3X1	T37.3X2	T37.3X3	T37.3X4	T37.3X5	T37.3X6
Trypsin	T45.3X1	T45.3X2	T45.3X3	T45.3X4	T45.3X5	T45.3X6
Tryptizol	T43.011	T43.012	T43.013	T43.014	T43.015	T43.016
TSH	T38.811	T38.812	T38.813	T38.814	T38.815	T38.816
Tuaminoheptane	T48.5X1	T48.5X2	T48.5X3	T48.5X4	T48.5X5	T48.5X6
Tuberculin, purified protein derivative (PPD)	T50.8X1	T50.8X2	T50.8X3	T50.8X4	T50.8X5	T50.8X6
Tubocurare	T48.1X1	T48.1X2	T48.1X3	T48.1X4	T48.1X5	T48.1X6
Tubocurarine (chloride)	T48.1X1	T48.1X2	T48.1X3	T48.1X4	T48.1X5	T48.1X6
Tulobuterol	T48.6X1	T48.6X2	T48.6X3	T48.6X4	T48.6X5	T48.6X6
Turpentine (spirits of)	T52.8X1	T52.8X2	T52.8X3	T52.8X4	—	—
vapor	T52.8X1	T52.8X2	T52.8X3	T52.8X4	—	—
Tybamate	T43.591	T43.592	T43.593	T43.594	T43.595	T43.596
Tyloxapol	T48.4X1	T48.4X2	T48.4X3	T48.4X4	T48.4X5	T48.4X6
Tymazoline	T48.5X1	T48.5X2	T48.5X3	T48.5X4	T48.5X5	T48.5X6
Typhoid-paratyphoid vaccine	T50.A91	T50.A92	T50.A93	T50.A94	T50.A95	T50.A96
Typhus vaccine	T50.A91	T50.A92	T50.A93	T50.A94	T50.A95	T50.A96
Tyropanoate	T50.8X1	T50.8X2	T50.8X3	T50.8X4	T50.8X5	T50.8X6
Tyrothricin	T49.6X1	T49.6X2	T49.6X3	T49.6X4	T49.6X5	T49.6X6
ENT agent	T49.6X1	T49.6X2	T49.6X3	T49.6X4	T49.6X5	T49.6X6
ophthalmic preparation	T49.5X1	T49.5X2	T49.5X3	T49.5X4	T49.5X5	T49.5X6
U						
Ufenamate	T39.391	T39.392	T39.393	T39.394	T39.395	T39.396
Ultraviolet light protectant	T49.3X1	T49.3X2	T49.3X3	T49.3X4	T49.3X5	T49.3X6
Undecenoic acid	T49.0X1	T49.0X2	T49.0X3	T49.0X4	T49.0X5	T49.0X6
Undecoylium	T49.0X1	T49.0X2	T49.0X3	T49.0X4	T49.0X5	T49.0X6
Undecylenic acid (derivatives)	T49.0X1	T49.0X2	T49.0X3	T49.0X4	T49.0X5	T49.0X6
Unna's boot	T49.3X1	T49.3X2	T49.3X3	T49.3X4	T49.3X5	T49.3X6
Unsaturated fatty acid	T46.6X1	T46.6X2	T46.6X3	T46.6X4	T46.6X5	T46.6X6
Uracil mustard	T45.1X1	T45.1X2	T45.1X3	T45.1X4	T45.1X5	T45.1X6
Uramustine	T45.1X1	T45.1X2	T45.1X3	T45.1X4	T45.1X5	T45.1X6
Urapidil	T46.5X1	T46.5X2	T46.5X3	T46.5X4	T46.5X5	T46.5X6

Substance	Poisoning, Accidental (unintentional)	Poisoning, Intentional self-harm	Poisoning, Assault	Poisoning, Undetermined	Adverse effect	Underdosing
Urari	T48.1X1	T48.1X2	T48.1X3	T48.1X4	T48.1X5	T48.1X6
Urate oxidase	T50.4X1	T50.4X2	T50.4X3	T50.4X4	T50.4X5	T50.4X6
Urea	T47.3X1	T47.3X2	T47.3X3	T47.3X4	T47.3X5	T47.3X6
peroxide	T49.0X1	T49.0X2	T49.0X3	T49.0X4	T49.0X5	T49.0X6
stibamine	T37.4X1	T37.4X2	T37.4X3	T37.4X4	T37.4X5	T37.4X6
topical	T49.8X1	T49.8X2	T49.8X3	T49.8X4	T49.8X5	T49.8X6
Urethane	T45.1X1	T45.1X2	T45.1X3	T45.1X4	T45.1X5	T45.1X6
Urginea (maritima) (scilla)—see Squill						
Uric acid metabolism drug NEC	T50.4X1	T50.4X2	T50.4X3	T50.4X4	T50.4X5	T50.4X6
Uricosuric agent	T50.4X1	T50.4X2	T50.4X3	T50.4X4	T50.4X5	T50.4X6
Urinary anti-infective	T37.8X1	T37.8X2	T37.8X3	T37.8X4	T37.8X5	T37.8X6
Urofollitropin	T38.811	T38.812	T38.813	T38.814	T38.815	T38.816
Urokinase	T45.611	T45.612	T45.613	T45.614	T45.615	T45.616
Urokon	T50.8X1	T50.8X2	T50.8X3	T50.8X4	T50.8X5	T50.8X6
Ursodeoxycholic acid	T50.991	T50.992	T50.993	T50.994	T50.995	T50.996
Ursodiol	T50.991	T50.992	T50.993	T50.994	T50.995	T50.996
Urtica	T62.2X1	T62.2X2	T62.2X3	T62.2X4	—	—
Utility gas—see Gas, utility						
V						
Vaccine NEC	T50.Z91	T50.Z92	T50.Z93	T50.Z94	T50.Z95	T50.Z96
antineoplastic	T50.Z91	T50.Z92	T50.Z93	T50.Z94	T50.Z95	T50.Z96
bacterial NEC	T50.A91	T50.A92	T50.A93	T50.A94	T50.A95	T50.A96
with						
other bacterial component	T50.A21	T50.A22	T50.A23	T50.A24	T50.A25	T50.A26
pertussis component	T50.A11	T50.A12	T50.A13	T50.A14	T50.A15	T50.A16
viral-rickettsial component	T50.A21	T50.A22	T50.A23	T50.A24	T50.A25	T50.A26
mixed NEC	T50.A21	T50.A22	T50.A23	T50.A24	T50.A25	T50.A26
BCG	T50.A91	T50.A92	T50.A93	T50.A94	T50.A95	T50.A96
cholera	T50.A91	T50.A92	T50.A93	T50.A94	T50.A95	T50.A96
diphtheria	T50.A91	T50.A92	T50.A93	T50.A94	T50.A95	T50.A96
with tetanus	T50.A21	T50.A22	T50.A23	T50.A24	T50.A25	T50.A26
and pertussis	T50.A11	T50.A12	T50.A13	T50.A14	T50.A15	T50.A16
influenza	T50.B91	T50.B92	T50.B93	T50.B94	T50.B95	T50.B96
measles	T50.B91	T50.B92	T50.B93	T50.B94	T50.B95	T50.B96
with mumps and rubella	T50.B91	T50.B92	T50.B93	T50.B94	T50.B95	T50.B96
meningococcal	T50.A91	T50.A92	T50.A93	T50.A94	T50.A95	T50.A96
mumps	T50.B91	T50.B92	T50.B93	T50.B94	T50.B95	T50.B96
paratyphoid	T50.A91	T50.A92	T50.A93	T50.A94	T50.A95	T50.A96
pertussis	T50.A11	T50.A12	T50.A13	T50.A14	T50.A15	T50.A16
with diphtheria	T50.A11	T50.A12	T50.A13	T50.A14	T50.A15	T50.A16
and tetanus	T50.A11	T50.A12	T50.A13	T50.A14	T50.A15	T50.A16
with other component	T50.A11	T50.A12	T50.A13	T50.A14	T50.A15	T50.A16
plague	T50.A91	T50.A92	T50.A93	T50.A94	T50.A95	T50.A96
poliomyelitis	T50.B91	T50.B92	T50.B93	T50.B94	T50.B95	T50.B96
poliovirus	T50.B91	T50.B92	T50.B93	T50.B94	T50.B95	T50.B96
rabies	T50.B91	T50.B92	T50.B93	T50.B94	T50.B95	T50.B96
respiratory syncytial virus	T50.B91	T50.B92	T50.B93	T50.B94	T50.B95	T50.B96

Substance	Poisoning, Accidental (unintentional)	Poisoning, Intentional self-harm	Poisoning, Assault	Poisoning, Undetermined	Adverse effect	Underdosing
Vaccine NEC — *Continued*						
rickettsial NEC	T50.A91	T50.A92	T50.A93	T50.A94	T50.A95	T50.A96
with						
bacterial component	T50.A21	T50.A22	T50.A23	T50.A24	T50.A25	T50.A26
Rocky Mountain spotted fever	T50.A91	T50.A92	T50.A93	T50.A94	T50.A95	T50.A96
rubella	T50.B91	T50.B92	T50.B93	T50.B94	T50.B95	T50.B96
sabin oral	T50.B91	T50.B92	T50.B93	T50.B94	T50.B95	T50.B96
smallpox	T50.B11	T50.B12	T50.B13	T50.B14	T50.B15	T50.B16
TAB	T50.A91	T50.A92	T50.A93	T50.A94	T50.A95	T50.A96
tetanus	T50.A91	T50.A92	T50.A93	T50.A94	T50.A95	T50.A96
typhoid	T50.A91	T50.A92	T50.A93	T50.A94	T50.A95	T50.A96
typhus	T50.A91	T50.A92	T50.A93	T50.A94	T50.A95	T50.A96
viral NEC	T50.B91	T50.B92	T50.B93	T50.B94	T50.B95	T50.B96
yellow fever	T50.B91	T50.B92	T50.B93	T50.B94	T50.B95	T50.B96
Vaccinia immune globulin	T50.Z11	T50.Z12	T50.Z13	T50.Z14	T50.Z15	T50.Z16
Vaginal contraceptives	T49.8X1	T49.8X2	T49.8X3	T49.8X4	T49.8X5	T49.8X6
Valerian						
root	T42.6X1	T42.6X2	T42.6X3	T42.6X4	T42.6X5	T42.6X6
tincture	T42.6X1	T42.6X2	T42.6X3	T42.6X4	T42.6X5	T42.6X6
Valethamate bromide	T44.3X1	T44.3X2	T44.3X3	T44.3X4	T44.3X5	T44.3X6
Valisone	T49.0X1	T49.0X2	T49.0X3	T49.0X4	T49.0X5	T49.0X6
Valium	T42.4X1	T42.4X2	T42.4X3	T42.4X4	T42.4X5	T42.4X6
Valmid	T42.6X1	T42.6X2	T42.6X3	T42.6X4	T42.6X5	T42.6X6
Valnoctamide	T42.6X1	T42.6X2	T42.6X3	T42.6X4	T42.6X5	T42.6X6
Valproate (sodium)	T42.6X1	T42.6X2	T42.6X3	T42.6X4	T42.6X5	T42.6X6
Valproic acid	T42.6X1	T42.6X2	T42.6X3	T42.6X4	T42.6X5	T42.6X6
Valpromide	T42.6X1	T42.6X2	T42.6X3	T42.6X4	T42.6X5	T42.6X6
Vanadium	T56.891	T56.892	T56.893	T56.894	—	—
Vancomycin	T36.8X1	T36.8X2	T36.8X3	T36.8X4	T36.8X5	T36.8X6
Vapor—see also Gas	T59.91	T59.92	T59.93	T59.94	—	—
kiln (carbon monoxide)	T58.8X1	T58.8X2	T58.8X3	T58.8X4	—	—
lead—see lead						
specified source NEC	T59.891	T59.892	T59.893	T59.894	—	—
Vardenafil	T46.7X1	T46.7X2	T46.7X3	T46.7X4	T46.7X5	T46.7X6
Varicose reduction drug	T46.8X1	T46.8X2	T46.8X3	T46.8X4	T46.8X5	T46.8X6
Varnish	T65.4X1	T65.4X2	T65.4X3	T65.4X4	—	—
cleaner	T52.91	T52.92	T52.93	T52.94	—	—
Vaseline	T49.3X1	T49.3X2	T49.3X3	T49.3X4	T49.3X5	T49.3X6
Vasodilan	T46.7X1	T46.7X2	T46.7X3	T46.7X4	T46.7X5	T46.7X6
Vasodilator						
coronary NEC	T46.3X1	T46.3X2	T46.3X3	T46.3X4	T46.3X5	T46.3X6
peripheral NEC	T46.7X1	T46.7X2	T46.7X3	T46.7X4	T46.7X5	T46.7X6
Vasopressin	T38.891	T38.892	T38.893	T38.894	T38.895	T38.896
Vasopressor drugs	T38.891	T38.892	T38.893	T38.894	T38.895	T38.896
Vecuronium bromide	T48.1X1	T48.1X2	T48.1X3	T48.1X4	T48.1X5	T48.1X6
Vegetable extract, astringent	T49.2X1	T49.2X2	T49.2X3	T49.2X4	T49.2X5	T49.2X6
Venlafaxine	T43.211	T43.212	T43.213	T43.214	T43.215	T43.216

Substance	Poisoning, Accidental (unintentional)	Poisoning, Intentional self-harm	Poisoning, Assault	Poisoning, Undetermined	Adverse effect	Underdosing
Venom, venomous (bite) (sting)	T63.91	T63.92	T63.93	T63.94	—	—
amphibian NEC	T63.831	T63.832	T63.833	T63.834	—	—
animal NEC	T63.891	T63.892	T63.893	T63.894	—	—
ant	T63.421	T63.422	T63.423	T63.424	—	—
arthropod NEC	T63.481	T63.482	T63.483	T63.484	—	—
bee	T63.441	T63.442	T63.443	T63.444	—	—
centipede	T63.411	T63.412	T63.413	T63.414	—	—
fish	T63.591	T63.592	T63.593	T63.594	—	—
frog	T63.811	T63.812	T63.813	T63.814	—	—
hornet	T63.451	T63.452	T63.453	T63.454	—	—
insect NEC	T63.481	T63.482	T63.483	T63.484	—	—
lizard	T63.121	T63.122	T63.123	T63.124	—	—
marine						
animals	T63.691	T63.692	T63.693	T63.694	—	—
bluebottle	T63.611	T63.612	T63.613	T63.614	—	—
jellyfish NEC	T63.621	T63.622	T63.623	T63.624	—	—
Portugese Man-o-war	T63.611	T63.612	T63.613	T63.614	—	—
sea anemone	T63.631	T63.632	T63.633	T63.634	—	—
specified NEC	T63.691	T63.692	T63.693	T63.694	—	—
fish	T63.591	T63.592	T63.593	T63.594	—	—
plants	T63.711	T63.712	T63.713	T63.714	—	—
sting ray	T63.511	T63.512	T63.513	T63.514	—	—
millipede (tropical)	T63.411	T63.412	T63.413	T63.414	—	—
plant NEC	T63.791	T63.792	T63.793	T63.794	—	—
marine	T63.711	T63.712	T63.713	T63.714	—	—
reptile	T63.191	T63.192	T63.193	T63.194	—	—
gila monster	T63.111	T63.112	T63.113	T63.114	—	—
lizard NEC	T63.121	T63.122	T63.123	T63.124	—	—
scorpion	T63.2X1	T63.2X2	T63.2X3	T63.2X4	—	—
snake	T63.001	T63.002	T63.003	T63.004	—	—
African NEC	T63.081	T63.082	T63.083	T63.084	—	—
American (North) (South) NEC	T63.061	T63.062	T63.063	T63.064	—	—
Asian	T63.081	T63.082	T63.083	T63.084	—	—
Australian	T63.071	T63.072	T63.073	T63.074	—	—
cobra	T63.041	T63.042	T63.043	T63.044	—	—
coral snake	T63.021	T63.022	T63.023	T63.024	—	—
rattlesnake	T63.011	T63.012	T63.013	T63.014	—	—
specified NEC	T63.091	T63.092	T63.093	T63.094	—	—
taipan	T63.031	T63.032	T63.033	T63.034	—	—
specified NEC	T63.891	T63.892	T63.893	T63.894	—	—
spider	T63.301	T63.302	T63.303	T63.304	—	—
black widow	T63.311	T63.312	T63.313	T63.314	—	—
brown recluse	T63.331	T63.332	T63.333	T63.334	—	—
specified NEC	T63.391	T63.392	T63.393	T63.394	—	—
tarantula	T63.321	T63.322	T63.323	T63.324	—	—
sting ray	T63.511	T63.512	T63.513	T63.514	—	—
toad	T63.821	T63.822	T63.823	T63.824	—	—
wasp	T63.461	T63.462	T63.463	T63.464	—	—
Venous sclerosing drug NEC	T46.8X1	T46.8X2	T46.8X3	T46.8X4	T46.8X5	T46.8X6

Substance	Poisoning, Accidental (unintentional)	Poisoning, Intentional self-harm	Poisoning, Assault	Poisoning, Undetermined	Adverse effect	Underdosing
Ventolin—see Albuterol						
Veramon	T42.3X1	T42.3X2	T42.3X3	T42.3X4	T42.3X5	T42.3X6
Verapamil	T46.1X1	T46.1X2	T46.1X3	T46.1X4	T46.1X5	T46.1X6
Veratrine	T46.5X1	T46.5X2	T46.5X3	T46.5X4	T46.5X5	T46.5X6
Veratrum						
album	T62.2X1	T62.2X2	T62.2X3	T62.2X4	—	—
alkaloids	T46.5X1	T46.5X2	T46.5X3	T46.5X4	T46.5X5	T46.5X6
viride	T62.2X1	T62.2X2	T62.2X3	T62.2X4	—	—
Verdigris	T60.3X1	T60.3X2	T60.3X3	T60.3X4	—	—
Veronal	T42.3X1	T42.3X2	T42.3X3	T42.3X4	T42.3X5	T42.3X6
Veroxil	T37.4X1	T37.4X2	T37.4X3	T37.4X4	T37.4X5	T37.4X6
Versenate	T50.6X1	T50.6X2	T50.6X3	T50.6X4	T50.6X5	T50.6X6
Versidyne	T39.8X1	T39.8X2	T39.8X3	T39.8X4	T39.8X5	T39.8X6
Vetrabutine	T48.0X1	T48.0X2	T48.0X3	T48.0X4	T48.0X5	T48.0X6
Vidarabine	T37.5X1	T37.5X2	T37.5X3	T37.5X4	T37.5X5	T37.5X6
Vienna						
green	T57.0X1	T57.0X2	T57.0X3	T57.0X4	—	—
insecticide	T60.2X1	T60.2X2	T60.2X3	T60.2X4	—	—
red	T57.0X1	T57.0X2	T57.0X3	T57.0X4	—	—
pharmaceutical dye	T50.991	T50.992	T50.993	T50.994	T50.995	T50.996
Vigabatrin	T42.6X1	T42.6X2	T42.6X3	T42.6X4	T42.6X5	T42.6X6
Viloxazine	T43.291	T43.292	T43.293	T43.294	T43.295	T43.296
Viminol	T39.8X1	T39.8X2	T39.8X3	T39.8X4	T39.8X5	T39.8X6
Vinbarbital, vinbarbitone	T42.3X1	T42.3X2	T42.3X3	T42.3X4	T42.3X5	T42.3X6
Vinblastine	T45.1X1	T45.1X2	T45.1X3	T45.1X4	T45.1X5	T45.1X6
Vinburnine	T46.7X1	T46.7X2	T46.7X3	T46.7X4	T46.7X5	T46.7X6
Vincamine	T45.1X1	T45.1X2	T45.1X3	T45.1X4	T45.1X5	T45.1X6
Vincristine	T45.1X1	T45.1X2	T45.1X3	T45.1X4	T45.1X5	T45.1X6
Vindesine	T45.1X1	T45.1X2	T45.1X3	T45.1X4	T45.1X5	T45.1X6
Vinesthene, vinethene	T41.0X1	T41.0X2	T41.0X3	T41.0X4	T41.0X5	T41.0X6
Vinorelbine tartrate	T45.1X1	T45.1X2	T45.1X3	T45.1X4	T45.1X5	T45.1X6
Vinpocetine	T46.7X1	T46.7X2	T46.7X3	T46.7X4	T46.7X5	T46.7X6
Vinyl						
acetate	T65.891	T65.892	T65.893	T65.894	—	—
bital	T42.3X1	T42.3X2	T42.3X3	T42.3X4	T42.3X5	T42.3X6
bromide	T65.891	T65.892	T65.893	T65.894	—	—
chloride	T59.891	T59.892	T59.893	T59.894	—	—
ether	T41.0X1	T41.0X2	T41.0X3	T41.0X4	T41.0X5	T41.0X6
Vinylbital	T42.3X1	T42.3X2	T42.3X3	T42.3X4	T42.3X5	T42.3X6
Vinylidene chloride	T65.891	T65.892	T65.893	T65.894	—	—
Vioform	T37.8X1	T37.8X2	T37.8X3	T37.8X4	T37.8X5	T37.8X6
topical	T49.0X1	T49.0X2	T49.0X3	T49.0X4	T49.0X5	T49.0X6
Viomycin	T36.8X1	T36.8X2	T36.8X3	T36.8X4	T36.8X5	T36.8X6
Viosterol	T45.2X1	T45.2X2	T45.2X3	T45.2X4	T45.2X5	T45.2X6
Viper (venom)	T63.091	T63.092	T63.093	T63.094	—	—
Viprynium	T37.4X1	T37.4X2	T37.4X3	T37.4X4	T37.4X5	T37.4X6
Viquidil	T46.7X1	T46.7X2	T46.7X3	T46.7X4	T46.7X5	T46.7X6
Viral vaccine NEC	T50.B91	T50.B92	T50.B93	T50.B94	T50.B95	T50.B96
Virginiamycin	T36.8X1	T36.8X2	T36.8X3	T36.8X4	T36.8X5	T36.8X6
Virugon	T37.5X1	T37.5X2	T37.5X3	T37.5X4	T37.5X5	T37.5X6
Viscous agent	T50.901	T50.902	T50.903	T50.904	T50.905	T50.906

Substance	Poisoning, Accidental (unintentional)	Poisoning, Intentional self-harm	Poisoning, Assault	Poisoning, Undetermined	Adverse effect	Underdosing
Visine	T49.5X1	T49.5X2	T49.5X3	T49.5X4	T49.5X5	T49.5X6
Visnadine	T46.3X1	T46.3X2	T46.3X3	T46.3X4	T46.3X5	T46.3X6
Vitamin NEC	T45.2X1	T45.2X2	T45.2X3	T45.2X4	T45.2X5	T45.2X6
A	T45.2X1	T45.2X2	T45.2X3	T45.2X4	T45.2X5	T45.2X6
B NEC	T45.2X1	T45.2X2	T45.2X3	T45.2X4	T45.2X5	T45.2X6
nicotinic acid	T46.7X1	T46.7X2	T46.7X3	T46.7X4	T46.7X5	T46.7X6
B1	T45.2X1	T45.2X2	T45.2X3	T45.2X4	T45.2X5	T45.2X6
B2	T45.2X1	T45.2X2	T45.2X3	T45.2X4	T45.2X5	T45.2X6
B6	T45.2X1	T45.2X2	T45.2X3	T45.2X4	T45.2X5	T45.2X6
B12	T45.2X1	T45.2X2	T45.2X3	T45.2X4	T45.2X5	T45.2X6
B15	T45.2X1	T45.2X2	T45.2X3	T45.2X4	T45.2X5	T45.2X6
C	T45.2X1	T45.2X2	T45.2X3	T45.2X4	T45.2X5	T45.2X6
D	T45.2X1	T45.2X2	T45.2X3	T45.2X4	T45.2X5	T45.2X6
D2	T45.2X1	T45.2X2	T45.2X3	T45.2X4	T45.2X5	T45.2X6
D3	T45.2X1	T45.2X2	T45.2X3	T45.2X4	T45.2X5	T45.2X6
E	T45.2X1	T45.2X2	T45.2X3	T45.2X4	T45.2X5	T45.2X6
E acetate	T45.2X1	T45.2X2	T45.2X3	T45.2X4	T45.2X5	T45.2X6
hematopoietic	T45.8X1	T45.8X2	T45.8X3	T45.8X4	T45.8X5	T45.8X6
K NEC	T45.7X1	T45.7X2	T45.7X3	T45.7X4	T45.7X5	T45.7X6
K1	T45.7X1	T45.7X2	T45.7X3	T45.7X4	T45.7X5	T45.7X6
K2	T45.7X1	T45.7X2	T45.7X3	T45.7X4	T45.7X5	T45.7X6
PP	T45.2X1	T45.2X2	T45.2X3	T45.2X4	T45.2X5	T45.2X6
ulceroprotectant	T47.1X1	T47.1X2	T47.1X3	T47.1X4	T47.1X5	T47.1X6
Vleminckx's solution	T49.4X1	T49.4X2	T49.4X3	T49.4X4	T49.4X5	T49.4X6
Voltaren—see Diclofenac sodium						
W						
Warfarin	T45.511	T45.512	T45.513	T45.514	T45.515	T45.516
rodenticide	T60.4X1	T60.4X2	T60.4X3	T60.4X4	—	—
sodium	T45.511	T45.512	T45.513	T45.514	T45.515	T45.516
Wasp (sting)	T63.461	T63.462	T63.463	T63.464	—	—
Water						
balance drug	T50.3X1	T50.3X2	T50.3X3	T50.3X4	T50.3X5	T50.3X6
distilled	T50.3X1	T50.3X2	T50.3X3	T50.3X4	T50.3X5	T50.3X6
gas—see Gas, water						
incomplete combustion of—see Carbon, monoxide, fuel, utility						
hemlock	T62.2X1	T62.2X2	T62.2X3	T62.2X4	—	—
moccasin (venom)	T63.061	T63.062	T63.063	T63.064	—	—
purified	T50.3X1	T50.3X2	T50.3X3	T50.3X4	T50.3X5	T50.3X6
Wax (paraffin) (petroleum)	T52.0X1	T52.0X2	T52.0X3	T52.0X4	—	—
automobile	T65.891	T65.892	T65.893	T65.894	—	—
floor	T52.0X1	T52.0X2	T52.0X3	T52.0X4	—	—
Weed killers NEC	T60.3X1	T60.3X2	T60.3X3	T60.3X4	—	—
Welldorm	T42.6X1	T42.6X2	T42.6X3	T42.6X4	T42.6X5	T42.6X6
White						
arsenic	T57.0X1	T57.0X2	T57.0X3	T57.0X4	—	—
hellebore	T62.2X1	T62.2X2	T62.2X3	T62.2X4	—	—
lotion (keratolytic)	T49.4X1	T49.4X2	T49.4X3	T49.4X4	T49.4X5	T49.4X6
spirit	T52.0X1	T52.0X2	T52.0X3	T52.0X4	—	—
Whitewash	T65.891	T65.892	T65.893	T65.894	—	—
Whole blood (human)	T45.8X1	T45.8X2	T45.8X3	T45.8X4	T45.8X5	T45.8X6
Wild						
black cherry	T62.2X1	T62.2X2	T62.2X3	T62.2X4	—	—
poisonous plants NEC	T62.2X1	T62.2X2	T62.2X3	T62.2X4	—	—
Window cleaning fluid	T65.891	T65.892	T65.893	T65.894	—	—
Wintergreen (oil)	T49.3X1	T49.3X2	T49.3X3	T49.3X4	T49.3X5	T49.3X6
Wisterine	T62.2X1	T62.2X2	T62.2X3	T62.2X4	—	—
Witch hazel	T49.2X1	T49.2X2	T49.2X3	T49.2X4	T49.2X5	T49.2X6
Wood alcohol or spirit	T51.1X1	T51.1X2	T51.1X3	T51.1X4	—	—
Wool fat (hydrous)	T49.3X1	T49.3X2	T49.3X3	T49.3X4	T49.3X5	T49.3X6
Woorali	T48.1X1	T48.1X2	T48.1X3	T48.1X4	T48.1X5	T48.1X6
Wormseed, American	T37.4X1	T37.4X2	T37.4X3	T37.4X4	T37.4X5	T37.4X6
X						
Xamoterol	T44.5X1	T44.5X2	T44.5X3	T44.5X4	T44.5X5	T44.5X6
Xanthine diuretics	T50.2X1	T50.2X2	T50.2X3	T50.2X4	T50.2X5	T50.2X6
Xanthinol nicotinate	T46.7X1	T46.7X2	T46.7X3	T46.7X4	T46.7X5	T46.7X6
Xanthotoxin	T49.3X1	T49.3X2	T49.3X3	T49.3X4	T49.3X5	T49.3X6
Xantinol nicotinate	T46.7X1	T46.7X2	T46.7X3	T46.7X4	T46.7X5	T46.7X6
Xantocillin	T36.0X1	T36.0X2	T36.0X3	T36.0X4	T36.0X5	T36.0X6
Xenon (127Xe) (133Xe)	T50.8X1	T50.8X2	T50.8X3	T50.8X4	T50.8X5	T50.8X6
Xenysalate	T49.4X1	T49.4X2	T49.4X3	T49.4X4	T49.4X5	T49.4X6
Xibornol	T37.8X1	T37.8X2	T37.8X3	T37.8X4	T37.8X5	T37.8X6
Xigris	T45.511	T45.512	T45.513	T45.514	T45.515	T45.516
Xipamide	T50.2X1	T50.2X2	T50.2X3	T50.2X4	T50.2X5	T50.2X6
Xylene (vapor)	T52.2X1	T52.2X2	T52.2X3	T52.2X4	—	—
Xylocaine (infiltration) (topical)	T41.3X1	T41.3X2	T41.3X3	T41.3X4	T41.3X5	T41.3X6
nerve block (peripheral) (plexus)	T41.3X1	T41.3X2	T41.3X3	T41.3X4	T41.3X5	T41.3X6
spinal	T41.3X1	T41.3X2	T41.3X3	T41.3X4	T41.3X5	T41.3X6
Xylol (vapor)	T52.2X1	T52.2X2	T52.2X3	T52.2X4	—	—
Xylometazoline	T48.5X1	T48.5X2	T48.5X3	T48.5X4	T48.5X5	T48.5X6
Y						
Yeast	T45.2X1	T45.2X2	T45.2X3	T45.2X4	T45.2X5	T45.2X6
dried	T45.2X1	T45.2X2	T45.2X3	T45.2X4	T45.2X5	T45.2X6
Yellow						
fever vaccine	T50.B91	T50.B92	T50.B93	T50.B94	T50.B95	T50.B96
jasmine	T62.2X1	T62.2X2	T62.2X3	T62.2X4	—	—
phenolphthalein	T47.2X1	T47.2X2	T47.2X3	T47.2X4	T47.2X5	T47.2X6
Yew	T62.2X1	T62.2X2	T62.2X3	T62.2X4	—	—
Yohimbic acid	T40.991	T40.992	T40.993	T40.994	T40.995	T40.996
Z						
Zactane	T39.8X1	T39.8X2	T39.8X3	T39.8X4	T39.8X5	T39.8X6
Zalcitabine	T37.5X1	T37.5X2	T37.5X3	T37.5X4	T37.5X5	T37.5X6
Zaroxolyn	T50.2X1	T50.2X2	T50.2X3	T50.2X4	T50.2X5	T50.2X6
Zephiran (topical)	T49.0X1	T49.0X2	T49.0X3	T49.0X4	T49.0X5	T49.0X6
ophthalmic preparation	T49.5X1	T49.5X2	T49.5X3	T49.5X4	T49.5X5	T49.5X6
Zeranol	T38.7X1	T38.7X2	T38.7X3	T38.7X4	T38.7X5	T38.7X6
Zerone	T51.1X1	T51.1X2	T51.1X3	T51.1X4	—	—
Zidovudine	T37.5X1	T37.5X2	T37.5X3	T37.5X4	T37.5X5	T37.5X6
Zimeldine	T43.221	T43.222	T43.223	T43.224	T43.225	T43.226

Substance	Poisoning, Accidental (unintentional)	Poisoning, Intentional self-harm	Poisoning, Assault	Poisoning, Undetermined	Adverse effect	Underdosing
Zinc (compounds) (fumes) (vapor) NEC	T56.5X1	T56.5X2	T56.5X3	T56.5X4	—	—
anti-infectives	T49.0X1	T49.0X2	T49.0X3	T49.0X4	T49.0X5	T49.0X6
antivaricose	T46.8X1	T46.8X2	T46.8X3	T46.8X4	T46.8X5	T46.8X6
bacitracin	T49.0X1	T49.0X2	T49.0X3	T49.0X4	T49.0X5	T49.0X6
chloride (mouthwash)	T49.6X1	T49.6X2	T49.6X3	T49.6X4	T49.6X5	T49.6X6
chromate	T56.5X1	T56.5X2	T56.5X3	T56.5X4	—	—
gelatin	T49.3X1	T49.3X2	T49.3X3	T49.3X4	T49.3X5	T49.3X6
oxide	T49.3X1	T49.3X2	T49.3X3	T49.3X4	T49.3X5	T49.3X6
plaster	T49.3X1	T49.3X2	T49.3X3	T49.3X4	T49.3X5	T49.3X6
peroxide	T49.0X1	T49.0X2	T49.0X3	T49.0X4	T49.0X5	T49.0X6
pesticides	T56.5X1	T56.5X2	T56.5X3	T56.5X4	—	—
phosphide	T60.4X1	T60.4X2	T60.4X3	T60.4X4	—	—
pyrithionate	T49.4X1	T49.4X2	T49.4X3	T49.4X4	T49.4X5	T49.4X6
stearate	T49.3X1	T49.3X2	T49.3X3	T49.3X4	T49.3X5	T49.3X6
sulfate	T49.5X1	T49.5X2	T49.5X3	T49.5X4	T49.5X5	T49.5X6
ENT agent	T49.6X1	T49.6X2	T49.6X3	T49.6X4	T49.6X5	T49.6X6
ophthalmic solution	T49.5X1	T49.5X2	T49.5X3	T49.5X4	T49.5X5	T49.5X6
Zinc (compounds) (fumes) (vapor) NEC — *Continued*						
topical NEC	T49.0X1	T49.0X2	T49.0X3	T49.0X4	T49.0X5	T49.0X6
undecylenate	T49.0X1	T49.0X2	T49.0X3	T49.0X4	T49.0X5	T49.0X6
Zineb	T60.0X1	T60.0X2	T60.0X3	T60.0X4	—	—
Zinostatin	T45.1X1	T45.1X2	T45.1X3	T45.1X4	T45.1X5	T45.1X6
Zipeprol	T48.3X1	T48.3X2	T48.3X3	T48.3X4	T48.3X5	T48.3X6
Zofenopril	T46.4X1	T46.4X2	T46.4X3	T46.4X4	T46.4X5	T46.4X6
Zolpidem	T42.6X1	T42.6X2	T42.6X3	T42.6X4	T42.6X5	T42.6X6
Zomepirac	T39.391	T39.392	T39.393	T39.394	T39.395	T39.396
Zopiclone	T42.6X1	T42.6X2	T42.6X3	T42.6X4	T42.6X5	T42.6X6
Zorubicin	T45.1X1	T45.1X2	T45.1X3	T45.1X4	T45.1X5	T45.1X6
Zotepine	T43.591	T43.592	T43.593	T43.594	T43.595	T43.596
Zovant	T45.511	T45.512	T45.513	T45.514	T45.515	T45.516
Zoxazolamine	T42.8X1	T42.8X2	T42.8X3	T42.8X4	T42.8X5	T42.8X6
Zuclopenthixol	T43.4X1	T43.4X2	T43.4X3	T43.4X4	T43.4X5	T43.4X6
Zygadenus (venenosus)	T62.2X1	T62.2X2	T62.2X3	T62.2X4	—	—
Zyprexa	T43.591	T43.592	T43.593	T43.594	T43.595	T43.596

External Cause of Injuries Index

A

Abandonment (causing exposure to weather conditions) (with intent to injure or kill) NEC X58

Abuse (adult) (child) (mental) (physical) (sexual) X58

Accident (to) X58
- aircraft (in transit) (powered) *—see also* Accident, transport, aircraft
  - due to, caused by cataclysm *—see* Forces of nature, by type
- animal-rider *—see* Accident, transport, animal-rider
- animal-drawn vehicle *—see* Accident, transport, animal-drawn vehicle occupant
- automobile *—see* Accident, transport, car occupant
- bare foot water skiier V94.4
- boat, boating *—see also* Accident, watercraft
  - striking swimmer
    - powered V94.11
    - unpowered V94.12
- bus *—see* Accident, transport, bus occupant
- cable car, not on rails V98.0
  - on rails *—see* Accident, transport, streetcar occupant
- car *—see* Accident, transport, car occupant
- caused by, due to
  - animal NEC W64
  - chain hoist W24.0
  - cold (excessive) *—see* Exposure, cold
  - corrosive liquid, substance *—see* Table of Drugs and Chemicals
  - cutting or piercing instrument *—see* Contact, with, by type of instrument
  - drive belt W24.0
  - electric
    - current *—see* Exposure, electric current
    - motor *—see also* Contact, with, by type of machine W31.3
      - current (of) W86.8
  - environmental factor NEC X58
  - explosive material *—see* Explosion
  - fire, flames *—see* Exposure, fire
  - firearm missile *—see* Discharge, firearm by type
  - heat (excessive) *—see* Heat
  - hot *—see* Contact, with, hot
  - ignition *—see* Ignition
  - lifting device W24.0
  - lightning *—see subcategory* T75.0
    - causing fire *—see* Exposure, fire
  - machine, machinery *—see* Contact, with, by type of machine
  - natural factor NEC X58
  - pulley (block) W24.0
  - radiation *—see* Radiation
  - steam X13.1
    - inhalation X13.0
    - pipe X16
  - thunderbolt *—see subcategory* T75.0
    - causing fire *—see* Exposure, fire
  - transmission device W24.1
- coach *—see* Accident, transport, bus occupant

Accident *(continued)*
- coal car *—see* Accident, transport, industrial vehicle occupant
- diving *—see also* Fall, into, water
  - with
    - drowning or submersion *—see* Drowning
- forklift *—see* Accident, transport, industrial vehicle occupant
- heavy transport vehicle NOS *—see* Accident, transport, truck occupant
- ice yacht V98.2
- in
  - medical, surgical procedure
    - as, or due to misadventure *—see* Misadventure
    - causing an abnormal reaction or later complication without mention of misadventure *—see also* Complication of or following, by type of procedure Y84.9
- land yacht V98.1
- late effect of *—see* W00-X58 with 7th character S
- logging car *—see* Accident, transport, industrial vehicle occupant
- machine, machinery *—see also* Contact, with, by type of machine
  - on board watercraft V93.69
    - explosion *—see* Explosion, in, watercraft
    - fire *—see* Burn, on board watercraft
    - powered craft V93.63
      - ferry boat V93.61
      - fishing boat V93.62
      - jetskis V93.63
      - liner V93.61
      - merchant ship V93.60
      - passenger ship V93.61
      - sailboat V93.64
- mine tram *—see* Accident, transport, industrial vehicle occupant
- mobility scooter (motorized) *—see* Accident, transport, pedestrian, conveyance, specified type NEC
- motor scooter *—see* Accident, transport, motorcyclist
- motor vehicle NOS (traffic) *—see also* Accident, transport V89.2
  - nontraffic V89.0
  - three-wheeled NOS *—see* Accident, transport, three-wheeled motor vehicle occupant
- motorcycle NOS *—see* Accident, transport, motorcyclist
- nonmotor vehicle NOS (nontraffic) *—see also* Accident, transport V89.1
  - traffic NOS V89.3
- nontraffic (victim's mode of transport NOS) V88.9
  - collision (between) V88.7
    - bus and truck V88.5
    - car and:
      - bus V88.3
      - pickup V88.2
      - three-wheeled motor vehicle V88.0
      - train V88.6
      - truck V88.4
      - two-wheeled motor vehicle V88.0
      - van V88.2

Accident *(continued)*
- nontraffic *(continued)*
  - collision *(continued)*
    - specified vehicle NEC and:
      - three-wheeled motor vehicle V88.1
      - two-wheeled motor vehicle V88.1
  - known mode of transport *—see* Accident, transport, by type of vehicle
  - noncollision V88.8
- on board watercraft V93.89
  - powered craft V93.83
    - ferry boat V93.81
    - fishing boat V93.82
    - jetskis V93.83
    - liner V93.81
    - merchant ship V93.80
    - passenger ship V93.81
  - unpowered craft V93.88
    - canoe V93.85
    - inflatable V93.86
      - in tow
        - recreational V94.31
        - specified NEC V94.32
    - kayak V93.85
    - sailboat V93.84
    - surf-board V93.88
    - water skis V93.87
    - windsurfer V93.88
- parachutist V97.29
  - entangled in object V97.21
  - injured on landing V97.22
- pedal cycle *—see* Accident, transport, pedal cyclist
- pedestrian (on foot)
  - with
    - another pedestrian W51
      - with fall W03
        - due to ice or snow W00.0
      - on pedestrian conveyance NEC V00.09
    - roller skater (in-line) V00.01
    - skate boarder V00.02
    - transport vehicle *—see* Accident, transport
  - on pedestrian conveyance *—see* Accident, transport, pedestrian, conveyance
- pick-up truck or van *—see* Accident, transport, pickup truck occupant
- quarry truck *—see* Accident, transport, industrial vehicle occupant
- railway vehicle (any) (in motion) *—see* Accident, transport, railway vehicle occupant
  - due to cataclysm *—see* Forces of nature, by type
- scooter (non-motorized) *—see* Accident, transport, pedestrian, conveyance, scooter
- sequelae of *—see* W00-X58 with 7th character S
- skateboard *—see* Accident, transport, pedestrian, conveyance, skateboard
- ski (ing) *—see* Accident, transport, pedestrian, conveyance
  - lift V98.3
- specified cause NEC X58
- streetcar *—see* Accident, transport, streetcar occupant
- traffic (victim's mode of transport NOS) V87.9

Accident *(continued)*
- traffic *(continued)*
  - collision (between) V87.7
    - bus and truck V87.5
    - car and:
      - bus V87.3
      - pickup V87.2
      - three-wheeled motor vehicle V87.0
      - train V87.6
      - truck V87.4
      - two-wheeled motor vehicle V87.0
      - van V87.2
    - specified vehicle NEC and:
      - three-wheeled motor vehicle V87.1
      - two-wheeled motor vehicle V87.1
  - known mode of transport *—see* Accident, transport, by type of vehicle
  - noncollision V87.8
- transport (involving injury to) V99
  - 18 wheeler *—see* Accident, transport, truck occupant
  - agricultural vehicle occupant (nontraffic) V84.9
    - driver V84.5
    - hanger-on V84.7
    - passenger V84.6
    - traffic V84.3
      - driver V84.0
      - hanger-on V84.2
      - passenger V84.1
    - while boarding or alighting V84.4
  - aircraft NEC V97.89
    - military NEC V97.818
      - with civlian aircraft V97.810
      - civilian injured by V97.811
    - occupant injured (in)
      - nonpowered craft accident V96.9
        - balloon V96.00
          - collision V96.03
          - crash V96.01
          - explosion V96.05
          - fire V96.04
          - forced landing V96.02
          - specified type NEC V96.09
        - glider V96.20
          - collision V96.23
          - crash V96.21
          - explosion V96.25
          - fire V96.24
          - forced landing V96.22
          - specified type NEC V96.29
        - hang glider V96.10
          - collision V96.13
          - crash V96.11
          - explosion V96.15
          - fire V96.14
          - forced landing V96.12
          - specified type NEC V96.19
        - specified craft NEC V96.8
      - powered craft accident V95.9
        - fixed wing NEC
          - commercial V95.30
            - collision V95.33
            - crash V95.31
            - explosion V95.35

Accident *(continued)*
transport *(continued)*
aircraft NEC *(continued)*
occupant injured *(continued)*
powered craft accident *(continued)*
fixed wing NEC *(continued)*
commercial *(continued)*
fire V95.34
forced landing V95.32
specified type NEC V95.39
private V95.20
collision V95.23
crash V95.21
explosion V95.25
fire V95.24
forced landing V95.22
specified type NEC V95.29
glider V95.10
collision V95.13
crash V95.11
explosion V95.15
fire V95.14
forced landing V95.12
specified type NEC V95.19
helicopter V95.00
collision V95.03
crash V95.01
explosion V95.05
fire V95.04
forced landing V95.02
specified type NEC V95.09
spacecraft V95.40
collision V95.43
crash V95.41
explosion V95.45
fire V95.44
forced landing V95.42
specified type NEC V95.49
specified craft NEC V95.8
ultralight V95.10
collision V95.13
crash V95.11
explosion V95.15
fire V95.14
forced landing V95.12
specified type NEC V95.19
specified accident NEC V97.0
while boarding or alighting V97.1
person (injured by)
falling from, in or on aircraft V97.0
machinery on aircraft V97.89
on ground with aircraft involvement V97.39
rotating propeller V97.32
struck by object falling from aircraft V97.31
sucked into aircraft jet V97.33
while boarding or alighting aircraft V97.1
airport (battery-powered) passenger vehicle —*see* Accident, transport, industrial vehicle occupant
all-terrain vehicle occupant (nontraffic) V86.95
driver V86.55
dune buggy —*see* Accident, transport, dune buggy occupant
hanger-on V86.75
passenger V86.65

Accident *(continued)*
transport *(continued)*
all-terrain vehicle occupant *(continued)*
snowmobile —*see* Accident, transport, snowmobile occupant
specified type NEC V86.99
traffic V86.35
driver V86.05
hanger-on V86.25
passenger V86.15
while boarding or alighting V86.45
ambulance occupant (traffic) V86.31
driver V86.01
hanger-on V86.21
nontraffic V86.91
driver V86.51
hanger-on V86.71
passenger V86.61
passenger V86.11
while boarding or alighting V86.41
animal-drawn vehicle occupant (in) V80.929
collision (with)
animal V80.12
being ridden V80.711
animal-drawn vehicle V80.721
bus V80.42
car V80.42
fixed or stationary object V80.82
military vehicle V80.920
nonmotor vehicle V80.791
pedal cycle V80.22
pedestrian V80.12
pickup V80.42
railway train or vehicle V80.62
specified motor vehicle NEC V80.52
streetcar V80.731
truck V80.42
two- or three-wheeled motor vehicle V80.32
van V80.42
noncollision V80.02
specified circumstance NEC V80.928
animal-rider V80.919
collision (with)
animal V80.11
being ridden V80.710
animal-drawn vehicle V80.720
bus V80.41
car V80.41
fixed or stationary object V80.81
military vehicle V80.910
nonmotor vehicle V80.790
pedal cycle V80.21
pedestrian V80.11
pickup V80.41
railway train or vehicle V80.61
specified motor vehicle NEC V80.51
streetcar V80.730
truck V80.41
two- or three-wheeled motor vehicle V80.31
van V80.41
noncollision V80.018
specified as horse rider V80.010
specified circumstance NEC V80.918

Accident *(continued)*
transport *(continued)*
armored car —*see* Accident, transport, truck occupant
battery-powered truck (baggage) (mail) —*see* Accident, transport, industrial vehicle occupant
bus occupant V79.9
collision (with)
animal (traffic) V70.9
being ridden (traffic) V76.9
nontraffic V76.3
while boarding or alighting V76.4
nontraffic V70.3
while boarding or alighting V70.4
animal-drawn vehicle (traffic) V76.9
nontraffic V76.3
while boarding or alighting V76.4
bus (traffic) V74.9
nontraffic V74.3
while boarding or alighting V74.4
car (traffic) V73.9
nontraffic V73.3
while boarding or alighting V73.4
motor vehicle NOS (traffic) V79.60
nontraffic V79.20
specified type NEC (traffic) V79.69
nontraffic V79.29
pedal cycle (traffic) V71.9
nontraffic V71.3
while boarding or alighting V71.4
pickup truck (traffic) V73.9
nontraffic V73.3
while boarding or alighting V73.4
railway vehicle (traffic) V75.9
nontraffic V75.3
while boarding or alighting V75.4
specified vehicle NEC (traffic) V76.9
nontraffic V76.3
while boarding or alighting V76.4
stationary object (traffic) V77.9
nontraffic V77.3
while boarding or alighting V77.4
streetcar (traffic) V76.9
nontraffic V76.3
while boarding or alighting V76.4
three wheeled motor vehicle (traffic) V72.9
nontraffic V72.3
while boarding or alighting V72.4
truck (traffic) V74.9
nontraffic V74.3
while boarding or alighting V74.4
two wheeled motor vehicle (traffic) V72.9
nontraffic V72.3
while boarding or alighting V72.4
van (traffic) V73.9
nontraffic V73.3
while boarding or alighting V73.4

Accident *(continued)*
transport *(continued)*
bus occupant *(continued)*
driver
collision (with)
animal (traffic) V70.5
being ridden (traffic) V76.5
nontraffic V76.0
nontraffic V70.0
animal-drawn vehicle (traffic) V76.5
nontraffic V76.0
bus (traffic) V74.5
nontraffic V74.0
car (traffic) V73.5
nontraffic V73.0
motor vehicle NOS (traffic) V79.40
nontraffic V79.00
specified type NEC (traffic) V79.49
nontraffic V79.09
pedal cycle (traffic) V71.5
nontraffic V71.0
pickup truck (traffic) V73.5
nontraffic V73.0
railway vehicle (traffic) V75.5
nontraffic V75.0
specified vehicle NEC (traffic) V76.5
nontraffic V76.0
stationary object (traffic) V77.5
nontraffic V77.0
streetcar (traffic) V76.5
nontraffic V76.0
three wheeled motor vehicle (traffic) V72.5
nontraffic V72.0
truck (traffic) V74.5
nontraffic V74.0
two wheeled motor vehicle (traffic) V72.5
nontraffic V72.0
van (traffic) V73.5
nontraffic V73.0
noncollision accident (traffic) V78.5
nontraffic V78.0
noncollision accident (traffic) V78.9
nontraffic V78.3
while boarding or alighting V78.4
nontraffic V79.3
hanger-on
collision (with)
animal (traffic) V70.7
being ridden (traffic) V76.7
nontraffic V76.2
nontraffic V70.2
animal-drawn vehicle (traffic) V76.7
nontraffic V76.2
bus (traffic) V74.7
nontraffic V74.2
car (traffic) V73.7
nontraffic V73.2
pedal cycle (traffic) V71.7
nontraffic V71.2
pickup truck (traffic) V73.7
nontraffic V73.2
railway vehicle (traffic) V75.7
nontraffic V75.2
specified vehicle NEC (traffic) V76.7
nontraffic V76.2

Accident *(continued)*
transport *(continued)*
bus occupant *(continued)*
hanger-on *(continued)*
collision *(continued)*
stationary object (traffic) V77.7
nontraffic V77.2
streetcar (traffic) V76.7
nontraffic V76.2
three wheeled motor vehicle (traffic) V72.7
nontraffic V72.2
truck (traffic) V74.7
nontraffic V74.2
two wheeled motor vehicle (traffic) V72.7
nontraffic V72.2
van (traffic) V73.7
nontraffic V73.2
noncollision accident (traffic) V78.7
nontraffic V78.2
passenger
collision (with)
animal (traffic) V70.6
being ridden (traffic) V76.6
nontraffic V76.1
nontraffic V70.1
animal-drawn vehicle (traffic) V76.6
nontraffic V76.1
bus (traffic) V74.6
nontraffic V74.1
car (traffic) V73.6
nontraffic V73.1
motor vehicle NOS (traffic) V79.50
nontraffic V79.10
specified type NEC (traffic) V79.59
nontraffic V79.19
pedal cycle (traffic) V71.6
nontraffic V71.1
pickup truck (traffic) V73.6
nontraffic V73.1
railway vehicle (traffic) V75.6
nontraffic V75.1
specified vehicle NEC (traffic) V76.6
nontraffic V76.1
stationary object (traffic) V77.6
nontraffic V77.1
streetcar (traffic) V76.6
nontraffic V76.1
three wheeled motor vehicle (traffic) V72.6
nontraffic V72.1
truck (traffic) V74.6
nontraffic V74.1
two wheeled motor vehicle (traffic) V72.6
nontraffic V72.1
van (traffic) V73.6
nontraffic V73.1
noncollision accident (traffic) V78.6
nontraffic V78.1
specified type NEC V79.88
military vehicle V79.81
cable car, not on rails V98.0
on rails *—see* Accident, transport, streetcar occupant
car occupant V49.9
ambulance occupant *—see* Accident, transport, ambulance occupant
collision (with)

Accident *(continued)*
transport *(continued)*
car occupant *(continued)*
collision *(continued)*
animal (traffic) V40.9
being ridden (traffic) V46.9
nontraffic V46.3
while boarding or alighting V46.4
nontraffic V40.3
while boarding or alighting V40.4
animal-drawn vehicle (traffic) V46.9
nontraffic V46.3
while boarding or alighting V46.4
bus (traffic) V44.9
nontraffic V44.3
while boarding or alighting V44.4
car (traffic) V43.92
nontraffic V43.32
while boarding or alighting V43.42
motor vehicle NOS (traffic) V49.60
nontraffic V49.20
specified type NEC (traffic) V49.69
nontraffic V49.29
pedal cycle (traffic) V41.9
nontraffic V41.3
while boarding or alighting V41.4
pickup truck (traffic) V43.93
nontraffic V43.33
while boarding or alighting V43.43
railway vehicle (traffic) V45.9
nontraffic V45.3
while boarding or alighting V45.4
specified vehicle NEC (traffic) V46.9
nontraffic V46.3
while boarding or alighting V46.4
sport utility vehicle (traffic) V43.91
nontraffic V43.31
while boarding or alighting V43.41
stationary object (traffic) V47.9
nontraffic V47.3
while boarding or alighting V47.4
streetcar (traffic) V46.9
nontraffic V46.3
while boarding or alighting V46.4
three wheeled motor vehicle (traffic) V42.9
nontraffic V42.3
while boarding or alighting V42.4
truck (traffic) V44.9
nontraffic V44.3
while boarding or alighting V44.4
two wheeled motor vehicle (traffic) V42.9
nontraffic V42.3
while boarding or alighting V42.4
van (traffic) V43.94
nontraffic V43.34
while boarding or alighting V43.44

Accident *(continued)*
transport *(continued)*
car occupant *(continued)*
driver
collision (with)
animal (traffic) V40.5
being ridden (traffic) V46.5
nontraffic V46.0
nontraffic V40.0
animal-drawn vehicle (traffic) V46.5
nontraffic V46.0
bus (traffic) V44.5
nontraffic V44.0
car (traffic) V43.52
nontraffic V43.02
motor vehicle NOS (traffic) V49.40
nontraffic V49.00
specified type NEC (traffic) V49.49
nontraffic V49.09
pedal cycle (traffic) V41.5
nontraffic V41.0
pickup truck (traffic) V43.53
nontraffic V43.03
railway vehicle (traffic) V45.5
nontraffic V45.0
specified vehicle NEC (traffic) V46.5
nontraffic V46.0
sport utility vehicle (traffic) V43.51
nontraffic V43.01
stationary object (traffic) V47.5
nontraffic V47.0
streetcar (traffic) V46.5
nontraffic V46.0
three wheeled motor vehicle (traffic) V42.5
nontraffic V42.0
truck (traffic) V44.5
nontraffic V44.0
two wheeled motor vehicle (traffic) V42.5
nontraffic V42.0
van (traffic) V43.54
nontraffic V43.04
noncollision accident (traffic) V48.5
nontraffic V48.0
noncollision accident (traffic) V48.9
nontraffic V48.3
while boarding or alighting V48.4
nontraffic V49.3
hanger-on
collision (with)
animal (traffic) V40.7
being ridden (traffic) V46.7
nontraffic V46.2
nontraffic V40.2
animal-drawn vehicle (traffic) V46.7
nontraffic V46.2
bus (traffic) V44.7
nontraffic V44.2
car (traffic) V43.72
nontraffic V43.22
pedal cycle (traffic) V41.7
nontraffic V41.2
pickup truck (traffic) V43.73
nontraffic V43.23

Accident *(continued)*
transport *(continued)*
car occupant *(continued)*
hanger-on *(continued)*
collision *(continued)*
railway vehicle (traffic) V45.7
nontraffic V45.2
specified vehicle NEC (traffic) V46.7
nontraffic V46.2
sport utility vehicle (traffic) V43.71
nontraffic V43.21
stationary object (traffic) V47.7
nontraffic V47.2
streetcar (traffic) V46.7
nontraffic V46.2
three wheeled motor vehicle (traffic) V42.7
nontraffic V42.2
truck (traffic) V44.7
nontraffic V44.2
two wheeled motor vehicle (traffic) V42.7
nontraffic V42.2
van (traffic) V43.74
nontraffic V43.24
noncollision accident (traffic) V48.7
nontraffic V48.2
passenger
collision (with)
animal (traffic) V40.6
being ridden (traffic) V46.6
nontraffic V46.1
nontraffic V40.1
animal-drawn vehicle (traffic) V46.6
nontraffic V46.1
bus (traffic) V44.6
nontraffic V44.1
car (traffic) V43.62
nontraffic V43.12
motor vehicle NOS (traffic) V49.50
nontraffic V49.10
specified type NEC (traffic) V49.59
nontraffic V49.19
pedal cycle (traffic) V41.6
nontraffic V41.1
pickup truck (traffic) V43.63
nontraffic V43.13
railway vehicle (traffic) V45.6
nontraffic V45.1
specified vehicle NEC (traffic) V46.6
nontraffic V46.1
sport utility vehicle (traffic) V43.61
nontraffic V43.11
stationary object (traffic) V47.6
nontraffic V47.1
streetcar (traffic) V46.6
nontraffic V46.1
three wheeled motor vehicle (traffic) V42.6
nontraffic V42.1
truck (traffic) V44.6
nontraffic V44.1
two wheeled motor vehicle (traffic) V42.6
nontraffic V42.1
van (traffic) V43.64
nontraffic V43.14

Accident *(continued)*
transport *(continued)*
car occupant *(continued)*
passenger *(continued)*
noncollision accident (traffic) V48.6
nontraffic V48.1
specified type NEC V49.88
military vehicle V49.81
coal car *—see* Accident, transport, industrial vehicle occupant
construction vehicle occupant (nontraffic) V85.9
driver V85.5
hanger-on V85.7
passenger V85.6
traffic V85.3
driver V85.0
hanger-on V85.2
passenger V85.1
while boarding or alighting V85.4
dirt bike rider (nontraffic) V86.96
driver V86.56
hanger-on V86.76
passenger V86.66
traffic V86.36
driver V86.06
hanger-on V86.26
passenger V86.16
while boarding or alighting V86.46
motor/cross bike rider (*see also* Accident, transport, dirt bike rider) V86.96
due to cataclysm *—see* Forces of nature, by type
dune buggy occupant (nontraffic) V86.93
driver V86.53
hanger-on V86.73
passenger V86.63
traffic V86.33
driver V86.03
hanger-on V86.23
passenger V86.13
while boarding or alighting V86.43
forklift *—see* Accident, transport, industrial vehicle occupant
go cart *—see* Accident, transport, all-terrain vehicle occupant
golf cart *—see* Accident, transport, all-terrain vehicle occupant
heavy transport vehicle occupant *—see* Accident, transport, truck occupant
ice yacht V98.2
industrial vehicle occupant (nontraffic) V83.9
driver V83.5
hanger-on V83.7
passenger V83.6
traffic V83.3
driver V83.0
hanger-on V83.2
passenger V83.1
while boarding or alighting V83.4
interurban electric car *—see* Accident, transport, streetcar
land yacht V98.1
logging car *—see* Accident, transport, industrial vehicle occupant
military vehicle occupant (traffic) V86.34
driver V86.04
hanger-on V86.24

Accident *(continued)*
transport *(continued)*
military vehicle occupant *(continued)*
nontraffic V86.94
driver V86.54
hanger-on V86.74
passenger V86.64
passenger V86.14
while boarding or alighting V86.44
mine tram *—see* Accident, transport, industrial vehicle occupant
motorcoach *—see* Accident, transport, bus occupant
motorcyclist V29.9
collision (with)
animal (traffic) V20.9
being ridden (traffic) V26.9
nontraffic V26.2
while boarding or alighting V26.3
nontraffic V20.2
while boarding or alighting V20.3
animal-drawn vehicle (traffic) V26.9
nontraffic V26.2
while boarding or alighting V26.3
bus (traffic) V24.9
nontraffic V24.2
while boarding or alighting V24.3
car (traffic) V23.9
nontraffic V23.2
while boarding or alighting V23.3
motor vehicle NOS (traffic) V29.60
nontraffic V29.20
specified type NEC (traffic) V29.69
nontraffic V29.29
pedal cycle (traffic) V21.9
nontraffic V21.2
while boarding or alighting V21.3
pickup truck (traffic) V23.9
nontraffic V23.2
while boarding or alighting V23.3
railway vehicle (traffic) V25.9
nontraffic V25.2
while boarding or alighting V25.3
specified vehicle NEC (traffic) V26.9
nontraffic V26.2
while boarding or alighting V26.3
stationary object (traffic) V27.9
nontraffic V27.2
while boarding or alighting V27.3
streetcar (traffic) V26.9
nontraffic V26.2
while boarding or alighting V26.3
three wheeled motor vehicle (traffic) V22.9
nontraffic V22.2
while boarding or alighting V22.3
truck (traffic) V24.9
nontraffic V24.2
while boarding or alighting V24.3

Accident *(continued)*
transport *(continued)*
motorcyclist *(continued)*
collision *(continued)*
two wheeled motor vehicle (traffic) V22.9
nontraffic V22.2
while boarding or alighting V22.3
van (traffic) V23.9
nontraffic V23.2
while boarding or alighting V23.3
driver
collision (with)
animal (traffic) V20.4
being ridden (traffic) V26.4
nontraffic V26.0
nontraffic V20.0
animal-drawn vehicle (traffic) V26.4
nontraffic V26.0
bus (traffic) V24.4
nontraffic V24.0
car (traffic) V23.4
nontraffic V23.0
motor vehicle NOS (traffic) V29.40
nontraffic V29.00
specified type NEC (traffic) V29.49
nontraffic V29.09
pedal cycle (traffic) V21.4
nontraffic V21.0
pickup truck (traffic) V23.4
nontraffic V23.0
railway vehicle (traffic) V25.4
nontraffic V25.0
specified vehicle NEC (traffic) V26.4
nontraffic V26.0
stationary object (traffic) V27.4
nontraffic V27.0
streetcar (traffic) V26.4
nontraffic V26.0
three wheeled motor vehicle (traffic) V22.4
nontraffic V22.0
truck (traffic) V24.4
nontraffic V24.0
two wheeled motor vehicle (traffic) V22.4
nontraffic V22.0
van (traffic) V23.4
nontraffic V23.0
noncollision accident (traffic) V28.4
nontraffic V28.0
noncollision accident (traffic) V28.9
nontraffic V28.2
while boarding or alighting V28.3
nontraffic V29.3
passenger
collision (with)
animal (traffic) V20.5
being ridden (traffic) V26.5
nontraffic V26.1
nontraffic V20.1
animal-drawn vehicle (traffic) V26.5
nontraffic V26.1
bus (traffic) V24.5
nontraffic V24.1

Accident *(continued)*
transport *(continued)*
motorcyclist *(continued)*
passenger *(continued)*
collision *(continued)*
car (traffic) V23.5
nontraffic V23.1
motor vehicle NOS (traffic) V29.50
nontraffic V29.10
specified type NEC (traffic) V29.59
nontraffic V29.19
pedal cycle (traffic) V21.5
nontraffic V21.1
pickup truck (traffic) V23.5
nontraffic V23.1
railway vehicle (traffic) V25.5
nontraffic V25.1
specified vehicle NEC (traffic) V26.5
nontraffic V26.1
stationary object (traffic) V27.5
nontraffic V27.1
streetcar (traffic) V26.5
nontraffic V26.1
three wheeled motor vehicle (traffic) V22.5
nontraffic V22.1
truck (traffic) V24.5
nontraffic V24.1
two wheeled motor vehicle (traffic) V22.5
nontraffic V22.1
van (traffic) V23.5
nontraffic V23.1
noncollision accident (traffic) V28.5
nontraffic V28.1
specified type NEC V29.88
military vehicle V29.81
motor vehicle NEC occupant (traffic) V89.2
occupant (of)
aircraft (powered) V95.9
fixed wing
commercial *—see* Accident, transport, aircraft, occupant, powered, fixed wing, commercial
private *—see* Accident, transport, aircraft, occupant, powered, fixed wing, private
nonpowered V96.9
specified NEC V95.8
airport battery-powered vehicle *—see* Accident, transport, industrial vehicle occupant
all-terrain vehicle (ATV) *—see* Accident, transport, all-terrain vehicle occupant
animal-drawn vehicle *—see* Accident, transport, animal-drawn vehicle occupant
automobile *—see* Accident, transport, car occupant
balloon V96.00
battery-powered vehicle *—see* Accident, transport, industrial vehicle occupant
bicycle *—see* Accident, transport, pedal cyclist
motorized *—see* Accident, transport, motorcycle rider
boat NEC *—see* Accident, watercraft

Accident *(continued)*
transport *(continued)*
occupant *(continued)*
bulldozer —*see* Accident, transport, construction vehicle occupant
bus —*see* Accident, transport, bus occupant
cable car (on rails) —*see also* Accident, transport, streetcar occupant
not on rails V98.0
car —*see also* Accident, transport, car occupant
cable (on rails) —*see also* Accident, transport, streetcar occupant
not on rails V98.0
coach —*see* Accident, transport, bus occupant
coal-car —*see* Accident, transport, industrial vehicle occupant
digger —*see* Accident, transport, construction vehicle occupant
dump truck —*see* Accident, transport, construction vehicle occupant
earth-leveler —*see* Accident, transport, construction vehicle occupant
farm machinery (self-propelled) —*see* Accident, transport, agricultural vehicle occupant
forklift —*see* Accident, transport, industrial vehicle occupant
glider (unpowered) V96.20
hang V96.10
powered (microlight) (ultralight) —*see* Accident, transport, aircraft, occupant, powered, glider
glider (unpowered) NEC V96.20
hang-glider V96.10
harvester —*see* Accident, transport, agricultural vehicle occupant
heavy (transport) vehicle —*see* Accident, transport, truck occupant
helicopter —*see* Accident, transport, aircraft, occupant, helicopter
ice-yacht V98.2
kite (carrying person) V96.8
land-yacht V98.1
logging car —*see* Accident, transport, industrial vehicle occupant
mechanical shovel —*see* Accident, transport, construction vehicle occupant
microlight —*see* Accident, transport, aircraft, occupant, powered, glider
minibus —*see* Accident, transport, pickup truck occupant
minivan —*see* Accident, transport, pickup truck occupant
moped —*see* Accident, transport, motorcycle
motor scooter —*see* Accident, transport, motorcycle
motorcycle (with sidecar) —*see* Accident, transport, motorcycle
off-road motor-vehicle (*see also* Accident, transport, all-terrain vehicle occupant) V86.99

Accident *(continued)*
transport *(continued)*
occupant *(continued)*
pedal cycle —*see also* Accident, transport, pedal cyclist
pick-up (truck) —*see* Accident, transport, pickup truck occupant
railway (train) (vehicle) (subterranean) (elevated) —*see* Accident, transport, railway vehicle occupant
rickshaw —*see* Accident, transport, pedal cycle
motorized —*see* Accident, transport, three-wheeled motor vehicle
pedal driven —*see* Accident, transport, pedal cyclist
road-roller —*see* Accident, transport, construction vehicle occupant
ship NOS V94.9
ski-lift (chair) (gondola) V98.3
snowmobile —*see* Accident, transport, snowmobile occupant
spacecraft, spaceship —*see* Accident, transport, aircraft, occupant, spacecraft
sport utility vehicle —*see* Accident, transport, pickup truck occupant
streetcar (interurban) (operating on public street or highway) —*see* Accident, transport, streetcar occupant
SUV —*see* Accident, transport, pickup truck occupant
téléférique V98.0
three-wheeled vehicle (motorized) —*see also* Accident, transport, three-wheeled motor vehicle occupant
nonmotorized —*see* Accident, transport, pedal cycle
tractor (farm) (and trailer) —*see* Accident, transport, agricultural vehicle occupant
train —*see* Accident, transport, railway vehicle occupant
tram —*see* Accident, transport, streetcar occupant
in mine or quarry —*see* Accident, transport, industrial vehicle occupant
tricycle —*see* Accident, transport, pedal cycle
motorized —*see* Accident, transport, three-wheeled motor vehicle
trolley —*see* Accident, transport, streetcar occupant
in mine or quarry —*see* Accident, transport, industrial vehicle occupant
tub, in mine or quarry —*see* Accident, transport, industrial vehicle occupant
ultralight —*see* Accident, transport, aircraft, occupant, powered, glider
van —*see* Accident, transport, van occupant
vehicle NEC V89.9
heavy transport —*see* Accident, transport, truck occupant
motor (traffic) NEC V89.2
nontraffic NEC V89.0

Accident *(continued)*
transport *(continued)*
occupant *(continued)*
watercraft NOS V94.9
causing drowning —*see* Drowning, resulting from accident to boat
off-road motor-vehicle (*see also* Accident, transport, all-terrain occupant) V86.99
parachutist V97.29
after accident to aircraft —*see* Accident, transport, aircraft
entangled in object V97.21
injured on landing V97.22
pedal cyclist V19.9
collision (with)
animal (traffic) V10.9
being ridden (traffic) V16.9
nontraffic V16.2
while boarding or alighting V16.3
nontraffic V10.2
while boarding or alighting V10.3
animal-drawn vehicle (traffic) V16.9
nontraffic V16.2
while boarding or alighting V16.3
bus (traffic) V14.9
nontraffic V14.2
while boarding or alighting V14.3
car (traffic) V13.9
nontraffic V13.2
while boarding or alighting V13.3
motor vehicle NOS (traffic) V19.60
nontraffic V19.20
specified type NEC (traffic) V19.69
nontraffic V19.29
pedal cycle (traffic) V11.9
nontraffic V11.2
while boarding or alighting V11.3
pickup truck (traffic) V13.9
nontraffic V13.2
while boarding or alighting V13.3
railway vehicle (traffic) V15.9
nontraffic V15.2
while boarding or alighting V15.3
specified vehicle NEC (traffic) V16.9
nontraffic V16.2
while boarding or alighting V16.3
stationary object (traffic) V17.9
nontraffic V17.2
while boarding or alighting V17.3
streetcar (traffic) V16.9
nontraffic V16.2
while boarding or alighting V16.3
three wheeled motor vehicle (traffic) V12.9
nontraffic V12.2
while boarding or alighting V12.3
truck (traffic) V14.9
nontraffic V14.2
while boarding or alighting V14.3
two wheeled motor vehicle (traffic) V12.9
nontraffic V12.2
while boarding or alighting V12.3

Accident *(continued)*
transport *(continued)*
pedal cyclist *(continued)*
collision *(continued)*
van (traffic) V13.9
nontraffic V13.2
while boarding or alighti V13.3
driver
collision (with)
animal (traffic) V10.4
being ridden (traffic) V16.4
nontraffic V16.0
nontraffic V10.0
animal-drawn vehicle (traffic) V16.4
nontraffic V16.0
bus (traffic) V14.4
nontraffic V14.0
car (traffic) V13.4
nontraffic V13.0
motor vehicle NOS (traffi V19.40
nontraffic V19.00
specified type NEC (traffic) V19.49
nontraffic V19.09
pedal cycle (traffic) V11.
nontraffic V11.0
pickup truck (traffic) tV13
nontraffic V13.0
railway vehicle (traffic) V15.4
nontraffic V15.0
specified vehicle NEC (traffic) V16.4
nontraffic V16.0
stationary object (traffic) V17.4
nontraffic V17.0
streetcar (traffic) V16.4
nontraffic V16.0
three wheeled motor vehicle (traffic) V12.4
nontraffic V12.0
truck (traffic) V14.4
nontraffic V14.0
two wheeled motor vehic (traffic) V12.4
nontraffic V12.0
van (traffic) V13.4
nontraffic V13.0
noncollision accident (traffic V18.4
nontraffic V18.0
noncollision accident (traffic) V18.9
nontraffic V18.2
while boarding or alighting V18.3
nontraffic V19.3
passenger
collision (with)
animal (traffic) V10.5
being ridden (traffic) V16.5
nontraffic V16.1
nontraffic V10.1
animal-drawn vehicle (traffic) V16.5
nontraffic V16.1
bus (traffic) V14.5
nontraffic V14.1
car (traffic) V13.5
nontraffic V13.1
motor vehicle NOS (traffic) V19.50
nontraffic V19.10
specified type NEC (traffic) V19.59

Accident *(continued)*
transport *(continued)*
pedal cyclist *(continued)*
passenger *(continued)*
collision *(continued)*
motor vehicle NOS *(continued)*
specified type NEC *(continued)*
nontraffic V19.19
pedal cycle (traffic) V11.5
nontraffic V11.1
pickup truck (traffic) V13.5
nontraffic V13.1
railway vehicle (traffic) V15.5
nontraffic V15.1
specified vehicle NEC (traffic) V16.5
nontraffic V16.1
stationary object (traffic) V17.5
nontraffic V17.1
streetcar (traffic) V16.5
nontraffic V16.1
three wheeled motor vehicle (traffic) V12.5
nontraffic V12.1
truck (traffic) V14.5
nontraffic V14.1
two wheeled motor vehicle (traffic) V12.5
nontraffic V12.1
van (traffic) V13.5
nontraffic V13.1
noncollision accident (traffic) V18.5
nontraffic V18.1
specified type NEC V19.88
military vehicle V19.81
pedestrian
conveyance (occupant) V09.9
babystroller V00.828
collision (with) V09.9
animal being ridden or animal drawn vehicle V06.99
nontraffic V06.09
traffic V06.19
bus or heavy transport V04.99
nontraffic V04.09
traffic V04.19
car V03.99
nontraffic V03.09
traffic V03.19
pedal cycle V01.99
nontraffic V01.09
traffic V01.19
pick-up truck or van V03.99
nontraffic V03.09
traffic V03.19
railway (train) (vehicle) V05.99
nontraffic V05.09
traffic V05.19
streetcar V06.99
nontraffic V06.09
traffic V06.19
stationary object V00.822
two- or three-wheeled motor vehicle V02.99
nontraffic V02.09
traffic V02.19
vehicle V09.9
animal-drawn V06.99
nontraffic V06.09

Accident *(continued)*
transport *(continued)*
pedestrian *(continued)*
conveyance *(continued)*
babystroller *(continued)*
collision *(continued)*
vehicle *(continued)*
animal-drawn *(continued)*
traffic V06.19
motor
nontraffic V09.00
traffic V09.20
fall V00.821
nontraffic V09.1
involving motor vehicle NEC V09.00
traffic V09.3
involving motor vehicle NEC V09.20
flat-bottomed NEC V00.388
collision (with) V09.9
animal being ridden or animal drawn vehicle V06.99
nontraffic V06.09
traffic V06.19
bus or heavy transport V04.99
nontraffic V04.09
traffic V04.19
car V03.99
nontraffic V03.09
traffic V03.19
pedal cycle V01.99
nontraffic V01.09
traffic V01.19
pick-up truck or van V03.99
nontraffic V03.09
traffic V03.19
railway (train) (vehicle) V05.99
nontraffic V05.09
traffic V05.19
stationary object V00.382
streetcar V06.99
nontraffic V06.09
traffic V06.19
two- or three-wheeled motor vehicle V02.99
nontraffic V02.09
traffic V02.19
vehicle V09.9
animal-drawn V06.99
nontraffic V06.09
traffic V06.19
motor
nontraffic V09.00
traffic V09.20
fall V00.381
nontraffic V09.1
involving motor vehicle NEC V09.00
snow
board *—see* Accident, transport, pedestrian, conveyance, snow board
ski *—see* Accident, transport, pedestrian, conveyance, skis (snow)
traffic V09.3
involving motor vehicle NEC V09.20
gliding type NEC V00.288
collision (with) V09.9

Accident *(continued)*
transport *(continued)*
pedestrian *(continued)*
conveyance *(continued)*
gliding type NEC *(continued)*
collision *(continued)*
animal being ridden or animal drawn vehicle V06.99
nontraffic V06.09
traffic V06.19
bus or heavy transport V04.99
nontraffic V04.09
traffic V04.19
car V03.99
nontraffic V03.09
traffic V03.19
pedal cycle V01.99
nontraffic V01.09
traffic V01.19
pick-up truck or van V03.99
nontraffic V03.09
traffic V03.19
railway (train) (vehicle) V05.99
nontraffic V05.09
traffic V05.19
stationary object V00.282
streetcar V06.99
nontraffic V06.09
traffic V06.19
two- or three-wheeled motor vehicle V02.99
nontraffic V02.09
traffic V02.19
vehicle V09.9
animal-drawn V06.99
nontraffic V06.09
traffic V06.19
motor
nontraffic V09.00
traffic V09.20
fall V00.281
heelies *—see* Accident, transport, pedestrian, conveyance, heelies
ice skate *—see* Accident, transport, pedestrian, conveyance, ice skate
nontraffic V09.1
involving motor vehicle NEC V09.00
sled *—see* Accident, transport, pedestrian, conveyance, sled
traffic V09.3
involving motor vehicle NEC V09.20
wheelies *—see* Accident, transport, pedestrian, conveyance, heelies
heelies V00.158
colliding with stationary object V00.152
fall V00.151
ice skates V00.218
collision (with) V09.9
animal being ridden or animal drawn vehicle V06.99
nontraffic V06.09
traffic V06.19
bus or heavy transport V04.99
nontraffic V04.09
traffic V04.19
car V03.99
nontraffic V03.09

Accident *(continued)*
transport *(continued)*
pedestrian *(continued)*
conveyance *(continued)*
ice skates *(continued)*
collision *(continued)*
car *(continued)*
traffic V03.19
pedal cycle V01.99
nontraffic V01.09
traffic V01.19
pick-up truck or van V03.99
nontraffic V03.09
traffic V03.19
railway (train) (vehicle) V05.99
nontraffic V05.09
traffic V05.19
streetcar V06.99
nontraffic V06.09
traffic V06.19
stationary object V00.212
two- or three-wheeled motor vehicle V02.99
nontraffic V02.09
traffic V02.19
vehicle V09.9
animal-drawn V06.99
nontraffic V06.09
traffic V06.19
motor
nontraffic V09.00
traffic V09.20
fall V00.211
nontraffic V09.1
involving motor vehicle NEC V09.00
traffic V09.3
involving motor vehicle NEC V09.20
motorized mobility scooter V00.838
collision with stationary object V00.832
fall from V00.831
nontraffic V09.1
involving motor vehicle V09.00
military V09.01
specified type NEC V09.09
roller skates (non in-line) V00.128
collision (with) V09.9
animal being ridden or animal drawn vehicle V06.91
nontraffic V06.01
traffic V06.11
bus or heavy transport V04.91
nontraffic V04.01
traffic V04.11
car V03.91
nontraffic V03.01
traffic V03.11
pedal cycle V01.91
nontraffic V01.01
traffic V01.11
pick-up truck or van V03.91
nontraffic V03.01
traffic V03.11
railway (train) (vehicle) V05.91
nontraffic V05.01
traffic V05.11
streetcar V06.91

- **Accident** *(continued)*
  - transport *(continued)*
    - pedestrian *(continued)*
      - conveyance *(continued)*
        - roller skates *(continued)*
          - collision *(continued)*
            - streetcar *(continued)*
              - nontraffic V06.01
              - traffic V06.11
            - stationary object V00.122
            - two- or three-wheeled motor vehicle V02.91
              - nontraffic V02.01
              - traffic V02.11
            - vehicle V09.9
              - animal-drawn V06.91
                - nontraffic V06.01
                - traffic V06.11
              - motor
                - nontraffic V09.00
                - traffic V09.20
          - fall V00.121
          - in-line V00.118
            - collision —*see also* Accident, transport, pedestrian, conveyance occupant, roller skates, collision with stationary object V00.112
            - fall V00.111
          - nontraffic V09.1
            - involving motor vehicle NEC V09.00
          - traffic V09.3
            - involving motor vehicle NEC V09.20
        - rolling shoes V00.158
          - colliding with stationary object V00.152
          - fall V00.151
        - rolling type NEC V00.188
          - collision (with) V09.9
            - animal being ridden or animal drawn vehicle V06.99
              - nontraffic V06.09
              - traffic V06.19
            - bus or heavy transport V04.99
              - nontraffic V04.09
              - traffic V04.19
            - car V03.99
              - nontraffic V03.09
              - traffic V03.19
            - pedal cycle V01.99
              - nontraffic V01.09
              - traffic V01.19
            - pick-up truck or van V03.99
              - nontraffic V03.09
              - traffic V03.19
            - railway (train) (vehicle) V05.99
              - nontraffic V05.09
              - traffic V05.19
            - stationary object V00.182
            - streetcar V06.99
              - nontraffic V06.09
              - traffic V06.19
            - two- or three-wheeled motor vehicle V02.99
              - nontraffic V02.09
              - traffic V02.19
            - vehicle V09.9
              - animal-drawn V06.99
                - nontraffic V06.09
                - traffic V06.19

Accident *(continued)*
- transport *(continued)*
  - pedestrian *(continued)*
    - conveyance *(continued)*
      - rolling type NEC *(continued)*
        - collision *(continued)*
          - vehicle *(continued)*
            - motor
              - nontraffic V09.00
              - traffic V09.20
        - fall V00.181
        - in-line roller skate —*see* Accident, transport, pedestrian, conveyance, roller skate, in-line
        - nontraffic V09.1
          - involving motor vehicle NEC V09.00
        - roller skate —*see* Accident, transport, pedestrian, conveyance, roller skate
        - scooter (non-motorized) —*see* Accident, transport, pedestrian, conveyance, scooter
        - skateboard —*see* Accident, transport, pedestrian, conveyance, skateboard
        - traffic V09.3
          - involving motor vehicle NEC V09.20
      - scooter (non-motorized) V00.148
        - collision (with) V09.9
          - animal being ridden or animal drawn vehicle V06.99
            - nontraffic V06.09
            - traffic V06.19
          - bus or heavy transport V04.99
            - nontraffic V04.09
            - traffic V04.19
          - car V03.99
            - nontraffic V03.09
            - traffic V03.19
          - pedal cycle V01.99
            - nontraffic V01.09
            - traffic V01.19
          - pick-up truck or van V03.99
            - nontraffic V03.09
            - traffic V03.19
          - railway (train) (vehicle) V05.99
            - nontraffic V05.09
            - traffic V05.19
          - streetcar V06.99
            - nontraffic V06.09
            - traffic V06.19
          - stationary object V00.142
          - two- or three-wheeled motor vehicle V02.99
            - nontraffic V02.09
            - traffic V02.19
          - vehicle V09.9
            - animal-drawn V06.99
              - nontraffic V06.09
              - traffic V06.19
            - motor
              - nontraffic V09.00
              - traffic V09.20
        - fall V00.141
        - nontraffic V09.1
          - involving motor vehicle NEC V09.00
        - traffic V09.3
          - involving motor vehicle NEC V09.20

Accident *(continued)*
- transport *(continued)*
  - pedestrian *(continued)*
    - conveyance *(continued)*
      - skate board V00.138
        - collision (with) V09.9
          - animal being ridden or animal drawn vehicle V06.92
            - nontraffic V06.02
            - traffic V06.12
          - bus or heavy transport V04.92
            - nontraffic V04.02
            - traffic V04.12
          - car V03.92
            - nontraffic V03.02
            - traffic V03.12
          - pedal cycle V01.92
            - nontraffic V01.02
            - traffic V01.12
          - pick-up truck or van V03.92
            - nontraffic V03.02
            - traffic V03.12
          - railway (train) (vehicle) V05.92
            - nontraffic V05.02
            - traffic V05.12
          - streetcar V06.92
            - nontraffic V06.02
            - traffic V06.12
          - stationary object V00.132
          - two- or three-wheeled motor vehicle V02.92
            - nontraffic V02.02
            - traffic V02.12
          - vehicle V09.9
            - animal-drawn V06.92
              - nontraffic V06.02
              - traffic V06.12
            - motor
              - nontraffic V09.00
              - traffic V09.20
        - fall V00.131
        - nontraffic V09.1
          - involving motor vehicle NEC V09.00
        - traffic V09.3
          - involving motor vehicle NEC V09.20
      - sled V00.228
        - collision (with) V09.9
          - animal being ridden or animal drawn vehicle V06.99
            - nontraffic V06.09
            - traffic V06.19
          - bus or heavy transport V04.99
            - nontraffic V04.09
            - traffic V04.19
          - car V03.99
            - nontraffic V03.09
            - traffic V03.19
          - pedal cycle V01.99
            - nontraffic V01.09
            - traffic V01.19
          - pick-up truck or van V03.99
            - nontraffic V03.09
            - traffic V03.19
          - railway (train) (vehicle) V05.99
            - nontraffic V05.09
            - traffic V05.19
          - streetcar V06.99
            - nontraffic V06.09
            - traffic V06.19
          - stationary object V00.222

Accident *(continued)*
- transport *(continued)*
  - pedestrian *(continued)*
    - conveyance *(continued)*
      - sled *(continued)*
        - collision *(continued)*
          - two- or three-wheeled motor vehicle V02.9
            - nontraffic V02.09
            - traffic V02.19
          - vehicle V09.9
            - animal-drawn V06.9
              - nontraffic V06.09
              - traffic V06.19
            - motor
              - nontraffic V09.00
              - traffic V09.20
        - fall V00.221
        - nontraffic V09.1
          - involving motor vehicle NEC V09.00
        - traffic V09.3
          - involving motor vehicle NEC V09.20
      - skis (snow) V00.328
        - collision (with) V09.9
          - animal being ridden or animal drawn vehicle V06.99
            - nontraffic V06.09
            - traffic V06.19
          - bus or heavy transport V04.99
            - nontraffic V04.09
            - traffic V04.19
          - car V03.99
            - nontraffic V03.09
            - traffic V03.19
          - pedal cycle V01.99
            - nontraffic V01.09
            - traffic V01.19
          - pick-up truck or van V03.99
            - nontraffic V03.09
            - traffic V03.19
          - railway (train) (vehicle) V05.99
            - nontraffic V05.09
            - traffic V05.19
          - streetcar V06.99
            - nontraffic V06.09
            - traffic V06.19
          - stationary object V00.322
          - two- or three-wheeled motor vehicle V02.99
            - nontraffic V02.09
            - traffic V02.19
          - vehicle V09.9
            - animal-drawn V06.99
              - nontraffic V06.09
              - traffic V06.19
            - motor
              - nontraffic V09.00
              - traffic V09.20
        - fall V00.321
        - nontraffic V09.1
          - involving motor vehicle NEC V09.00
        - traffic V09.3
          - involving motor vehicle NEC V09.20
      - snow board V00.318
        - collision (with) V09.9
          - animal being ridden or animal drawn vehicle V06.99
            - nontraffic V06.09
            - traffic V06.19

Accident *(continued)*
transport *(continued)*
pedestrian *(continued)*
conveyance *(continued)*
snow board *(continued)*
collision *(continued)*
bus or heavy transport V04.99
nontraffic V04.09
traffic V04.19
car V03.99
nontraffic V03.09
traffic V03.19
pedal cycle V01.99
nontraffic V01.09
traffic V01.19
pick-up truck or van V03.99
nontraffic V03.09
traffic V03.19
railway (train) (vehicle) V05.99
nontraffic V05.09
traffic V05.19
streetcar V06.99
nontraffic V06.09
traffic V06.19
stationary object V00.312
two- or three-wheeled motor vehicle V02.99
nontraffic V02.09
traffic V02.19
vehicle V09.9
animal-drawn V06.99
nontraffic V06.09
traffic V06.19
motor
nontraffic V09.00
traffic V09.20
fall V00.311
nontraffic V09.1
involving motor vehicle NEC V09.00
traffic V09.3
involving motor vehicle NEC V09.20
specified type NEC V00.898
collision (with) V09.9
animal being ridden or animal drawn vehicle V06.99
nontraffic V06.09
traffic V06.19
bus or heavy transport V04.99
nontraffic V04.09
traffic V04.19
car V03.99
nontraffic V03.09
traffic V03.19
pedal cycle V01.99
nontraffic V01.09
traffic V01.19
pick-up truck or van V03.99
nontraffic V03.09
traffic V03.19
railway (train) (vehicle) V05.99
nontraffic V05.09
traffic V05.19
streetcar V06.99
nontraffic V06.09
traffic V06.19
stationary object V00.892
two- or three-wheeled motor vehicle V02.99
nontraffic V02.09
traffic V02.19

Accident *(continued)*
transport *(continued)*
pedestrian *(continued)*
conveyance *(continued)*
specified type NEC *(continued)*
collision *(continued)*
vehicle V09.9
animal-drawn V06.99
nontraffic V06.09
traffic V06.19
motor
nontraffic V09.00
traffic V09.20
fall V00.891
nontraffic V09.1
involving motor vehicle NEC V09.00
traffic V09.3
involving motor vehicle NEC V09.20
traffic V09.3
involving motor vehicle V09.20
military V09.21
specified type NEC V09.29
wheelchair (powered) V00.818
collision (with) V09.9
animal being ridden or animal drawn vehicle V06.99
nontraffic V06.09
traffic V06.19
bus or heavy transport V04.99
nontraffic V04.09
traffic V04.19
car V03.99
nontraffic V03.09
traffic V03.19
pedal cycle V01.99
nontraffic V01.09
traffic V01.19
pick-up truck or van V03.99
nontraffic V03.09
traffic V03.19
railway (train) (vehicle) V05.99
nontraffic V05.09
traffic V05.19
streetcar V06.99
nontraffic V06.09
traffic V06.19
stationary object V00.812
two- or three-wheeled motor vehicle V02.99
nontraffic V02.09
traffic V02.19
vehicle V09.9
animal-drawn V06.99
nontraffic V06.09
traffic V06.19
motor
nontraffic V09.00
traffic V09.20
fall V00.811
nontraffic V09.1
involving motor vehicle NEC V09.00
traffic V09.3
involving motor vehicle NEC V09.20
wheeled shoe V00.158
colliding with stationary object V00.152
fall V00.151

Accident *(continued)*
transport *(continued)*
pedestrian *(continued)*
on foot —*see also* Accident, pedestrian
collision (with)
animal being ridden or animal drawn vehicle V06.90
nontraffic V06.00
traffic V06.10
bus or heavy transport V04.90
nontraffic V04.00
traffic V04.10
car V03.90
nontraffic V03.00
traffic V03.10
pedal cycle V01.90
nontraffic V01.00
traffic V01.10
pick-up truck or van V03.90
nontraffic V03.00
traffic V03.10
railway (train) (vehicle) V05.90
nontraffic V05.00
traffic V05.10
streetcar V06.90
nontraffic V06.00
traffic V06.10
two- or three-wheeled motor vehicle V02.90
nontraffic V02.00
traffic V02.10
vehicle V09.9
animal-drawn V06.90
nontraffic V06.00
traffic V06.10
motor
nontraffic V09.00
traffic V09.20
nontraffic V09.1
involving motor vehicle V09.00
military V09.01
specified type NEC V09.09
traffic V09.3
involving motor vehicle V09.20
military V09.21
specified type NEC V09.29
person NEC (unknown way or transportation) V99
collision (between)
bus (with)
heavy transport vehicle (traffic) V87.5
nontraffic V88.5
car (with)
nontraffic V88.5
bus (traffic) V87.3
nontraffic V88.3
heavy transport vehicle (traffic) V87.4
nontraffic V88.4
pick-up truck or van (traffic) V87.2
nontraffic V88.2
train or railway vehicle (traffic) V87.6
nontraffic V88.6
two- or three-wheeled motor vehicle (traffic) V87.0
nontraffic V88.0
motor vehicle (traffic) NEC V87.7
nontraffic V88.7

Accident *(continued)*
transport *(continued)*
person NEC *(continued)*
collision *(continued)*
two-or three-wheeled vehicle (with) (traffic)
motor vehicle NEC V87.1
nontraffic V88.1
nonmotor vehicle (collision) (noncollision) (traffic) V87.9
nontraffic V88.9
pickup truck occupant V59.9
collision (with)
animal (traffic) V50.9
being ridden (traffic) V56.9
nontraffic V56.3
while boarding or alighting V56.4
nontraffic V50.3
while boarding or alighting V50.4
animal-drawn vehicle (traffic) V56.9
nontraffic V56.3
while boarding or alighting V56.4
bus (traffic) V54.9
nontraffic V54.3
while boarding or alighting V54.4
car (traffic) V53.9
nontraffic V53.3
while boarding or alighting V53.4
motor vehicle NOS (traffic) V59.60
nontraffic V59.20
specified type NEC (traffic) V59.69
nontraffic V59.29
pedal cycle (traffic) V51.9
nontraffic V51.3
while boarding or alighting V51.4
pickup truck (traffic) V53.9
nontraffic V53.3
while boarding or alighting V53.4
railway vehicle (traffic) V55.9
nontraffic V55.3
while boarding or alighting V55.4
specified vehicle NEC (traffic) V56.9
nontraffic V56.3
while boarding or alighting V56.4
stationary object (traffic) V57.9
nontraffic V57.3
while boarding or alighting V57.4
streetcar (traffic) V56.9
nontraffic V56.3
while boarding or alighting V56.4
three wheeled motor vehicle (traffic) V52.9
nontraffic V52.3
while boarding or alighting V52.4
truck (traffic) V54.9
nontraffic V54.3
while boarding or alighting V54.4
two wheeled motor vehicle (traffic) V52.9
nontraffic V52.3
while boarding or alighting V52.4

Accident *(continued)*
- transport *(continued)*
  - pickup truck occupant *(continued)*
    - collision *(continued)*
      - van (traffic) V53.9
        - nontraffic V53.3
        - while boarding or alighting V53.4
    - driver
      - collision (with)
        - animal (traffic) V50.5
          - being ridden (traffic) V56.5
            - nontraffic V56.0
          - nontraffic V50.0
        - animal-drawn vehicle (traffic) V56.5
          - nontraffic V56.0
        - bus (traffic) V54.5
          - nontraffic V54.0
        - car (traffic) V53.5
          - nontraffic V53.0
        - motor vehicle NOS (traffic) V59.40
          - nontraffic V59.00
          - specified type NEC (traffic) V59.49
            - nontraffic V59.09
        - pedal cycle (traffic) V51.5
          - nontraffic V51.0
        - pickup truck (traffic) V53.5
          - nontraffic V53.0
        - railway vehicle (traffic) V55.5
          - nontraffic V55.0
        - specified vehicle NEC (traffic) V56.5
          - nontraffic V56.0
        - stationary object (traffic) V57.5
          - nontraffic V57.0
        - streetcar (traffic) V56.5
          - nontraffic V56.0
        - three wheeled motor vehicle (traffic) V52.5
          - nontraffic V52.0
        - truck (traffic) V54.5
          - nontraffic V54.0
        - two wheeled motor vehicle (traffic) V52.5
          - nontraffic V52.0
        - van (traffic) V53.5
          - nontraffic V53.0
      - noncollision accident (traffic) V58.5
        - nontraffic V58.0
    - noncollision accident (traffic) V58.9
      - nontraffic V58.3
      - while boarding or alighting V58.4
    - nontraffic V59.3
    - hanger-on
      - collision (with)
        - animal (traffic) V50.7
          - being ridden (traffic) V56.7
            - nontraffic V56.2
          - nontraffic V50.2
        - animal-drawn vehicle (traffic) V56.7
          - nontraffic V56.2
        - bus (traffic) V54.7
          - nontraffic V54.2
        - car (traffic) V53.7
          - nontraffic V53.2
        - pedal cycle (traffic) V51.7
          - nontraffic V51.2
        - pickup truck (traffic) V53.7
          - nontraffic V53.2

Accident *(continued)*
- transport *(continued)*
  - pickup truck occupant *(continued)*
    - hanger-on *(continued)*
      - collision *(continued)*
        - railway vehicle (traffic) V55.7
          - nontraffic V55.2
        - specified vehicle NEC (traffic) V56.7
          - nontraffic V56.2
        - stationary object (traffic) V57.7
          - nontraffic V57.2
        - streetcar (traffic) V56.7
          - nontraffic V56.2
        - three wheeled motor vehicle (traffic) V52.7
          - nontraffic V52.2
        - truck (traffic) V54.7
          - nontraffic V54.2
        - two wheeled motor vehicle (traffic) V52.7
          - nontraffic V52.2
        - van (traffic) V53.7
          - nontraffic V53.2
      - noncollision accident (traffic) V58.7
        - nontraffic V58.2
    - passenger
      - collision (with)
        - animal (traffic) V50.6
          - being ridden (traffic) V56.6
            - nontraffic V56.1
          - nontraffic V50.1
        - animal-drawn vehicle (traffic) V56.6
          - nontraffic V56.1
        - bus (traffic) V54.6
          - nontraffic V54.1
        - car (traffic) V53.6
          - nontraffic V53.1
        - motor vehicle NOS (traffic) V59.50
          - nontraffic V59.10
          - specified type NEC (traffic) V59.59
            - nontraffic V59.19
        - pedal cycle (traffic) V51.6
          - nontraffic V51.1
        - pickup truck (traffic) V53.6
          - nontraffic V53.1
        - railway vehicle (traffic) V55.6
          - nontraffic V55.1
        - specified vehicle NEC (traffic) V56.6
          - nontraffic V56.1
        - stationary object (traffic) V57.6
          - nontraffic V57.1
        - streetcar (traffic) V56.6
          - nontraffic V56.1
        - three wheeled motor vehicle (traffic) V52.6
          - nontraffic V52.1
        - truck (traffic) V54.6
          - nontraffic V54.1
        - two wheeled motor vehicle (traffic) V52.6
          - nontraffic V52.1
        - van (traffic) V53.6
          - nontraffic V53.1
      - noncollision accident (traffic) V58.6
        - nontraffic V58.1
    - specified type NEC V59.88
      - military vehicle V59.81

Accident *(continued)*
- transport *(continued)*
  - quarry truck —*see* Accident, transport, industrial vehicle occupant
  - race car —*see* Accident, transport, motor vehicle NEC occupant
  - railway vehicle occupant V81.9
    - collision (with) V81.3
      - motor vehicle (non-military) (traffic) V81.1
        - military V81.83
        - nontraffic V81.0
      - rolling stock V81.2
      - specified object NEC V81.3
    - during derailment V81.7
      - with antecedent collision —*see* Accident, transport, railway vehicle occupant, collision
    - explosion V81.81
    - fall (in railway vehicle) V81.5
      - during derailment V81.7
        - with antecedent collision —*see* Accident, transport, railway vehicle occupant, collision
      - from railway vehicle V81.6
        - during derailment V81.7
          - with antecedent collision —*see* Accident, transport, railway vehicle occupant, collision
      - while boarding or alighting V81.4
    - fire V81.81
    - object falling onto train V81.82
    - specified type NEC V81.89
    - while boarding or alighting V81.4
  - ski lift V98.3
  - snowmobile occupant (nontraffic) V86.92
    - driver V86.52
    - hanger-on V86.72
    - passenger V86.62
    - traffic V86.32
      - driver V86.02
      - hanger-on V86.22
      - passenger V86.12
    - while boarding or alighting V86.42
  - specified NEC V98.8
  - sport utility vehicle occupant —*see also* Accident, transport, pickup truck occupant
  - streetcar occupant V82.9
    - collision (with) V82.3
      - motor vehicle (traffic) V82.1
        - nontraffic V82.0
      - rolling stock V82.2
    - during derailment V82.7
      - with antecedent collision —*see* Accident, transport, streetcar occupant, collision
    - fall (in streetcar) V82.5
      - during derailment V82.7
        - with antecedent collision —*see* Accident, transport, streetcar occupant, collision
      - from streetcar V82.6
        - during derailment V82.7
          - with antecedent collision —*see* Accident, transport, streetcar occupant, collision
        - while boarding or alighting V82.4

Accident *(continued)*
- transport *(continued)*
  - streetcar occupant *(continued)*
    - fall *(continued)*
      - while boarding or alighting V82.4
    - specified type NEC V82.8
    - while boarding or alighting V82
  - three-wheeled motor vehicle occupant V39.9
    - collision (with)
      - animal (traffic) V30.9
        - being ridden (traffic) V36.9
          - nontraffic V36.3
          - while boarding or alighting V36.4
        - nontraffic V30.3
        - while boarding or alighti V30.4
      - animal-drawn vehicle (traffic) V36.9
        - nontraffic V36.3
        - while boarding or alighti V36.4
      - bus (traffic) V34.9
        - nontraffic V34.3
        - while boarding or alighti V34.4
      - car (traffic) V33.9
        - nontraffic V33.3
        - while boarding or alightir V33.4
      - motor vehicle NOS (traffic) V39.60
        - nontraffic V39.20
        - specified type NEC (traffic) V39.69
          - nontraffic V39.29
      - pedal cycle (traffic) V31.9
        - nontraffic V31.3
        - while boarding or alightin V31.4
      - pickup truck (traffic) V33.9
        - nontraffic V33.3
        - while boarding or alightir V33.4
      - railway vehicle (traffic) V35.9
        - nontraffic V35.3
        - while boarding or alightin V35.4
      - specified vehicle NEC (traffic) V36.9
        - nontraffic V36.3
        - while boarding or alightin V36.4
      - stationary object (traffic) V37.9
        - nontraffic V37.3
        - while boarding or alightin V37.4
      - streetcar (traffic) V36.9
        - nontraffic V36.3
        - while boarding or alightin V36.4
      - three wheeled motor vehicle (traffic) V32.9
        - nontraffic V32.3
        - while boarding or alightin V32.4
      - truck (traffic) V34.9
        - nontraffic V34.3
        - while boarding or alightin V34.4
      - two wheeled motor vehicle (traffic) V32.9
        - nontraffic V32.3
        - while boarding or alightin V32.4

Accident *(continued)*
transport *(continued)*
three-wheeled motor vehicle
occupant *(continued)*
collision *(continued)*
van (traffic) V33.9
nontraffic V33.3
while boarding or alighting V33.4
driver
collision (with)
animal (traffic) V30.5
being ridden (traffic) V36.5
nontraffic V36.0
nontraffic V30.0
animal-drawn vehicle (traffic) V36.5
nontraffic V36.0
bus (traffic) V34.5
nontraffic V34.0
car (traffic) V33.5
nontraffic V33.0
motor vehicle NOS (traffic) V39.40
nontraffic V39.00
specified type NEC (traffic) V39.49
nontraffic V39.09
pedal cycle (traffic) V31.5
nontraffic V31.0
pickup truck (traffic) V33.5
nontraffic V33.0
railway vehicle (traffic) V35.5
nontraffic V35.0
specified vehicle NEC (traffic) V36.5
nontraffic V36.0
stationary object (traffic) V37.5
nontraffic V37.0
streetcar (traffic) V36.5
nontraffic V36.0
three wheeled motor vehicle (traffic) V32.5
nontraffic V32.0
truck (traffic) V34.5
nontraffic V34.0
two wheeled motor vehicle (traffic) V32.5
nontraffic V32.0
van (traffic) V33.5
nontraffic V33.0
noncollision accident (traffic) V38.5
nontraffic V38.0
noncollision accident (traffic) V38.9
nontraffic V38.3
while boarding or alighting V38.4
nontraffic V39.3
hanger-on
collision (with)
animal (traffic) V30.7
being ridden (traffic) V36.7
nontraffic V36.2
nontraffic V30.2
animal-drawn vehicle (traffic) V36.7
nontraffic V36.2
bus (traffic) V34.7
nontraffic V34.2
car (traffic) V33.7
nontraffic V33.2
pedal cycle (traffic) V31.7
nontraffic V31.2

Accident *(continued)*
transport *(continued)*
three-wheeled motor vehicle
occupant *(continued)*
hanger-on *(continued)*
collision *(continued)*
pickup truck (traffic) V33.7
nontraffic V33.2
railway vehicle (traffic) V35.7
nontraffic V35.2
specified vehicle NEC (traffic) V36.7
nontraffic V36.2
stationary object (traffic) V37.7
nontraffic V37.2
streetcar (traffic) V36.7
nontraffic V36.2
three wheeled motor vehicle (traffic) V32.7
nontraffic V32.2
truck (traffic) V34.7
nontraffic V34.2
two wheeled motor vehicle (traffic) V32.7
nontraffic V32.2
van (traffic) V33.7
nontraffic V33.2
noncollision accident (traffic) V38.7
nontraffic V38.2
passenger
collision (with)
animal (traffic) V30.6
being ridden (traffic) V36.6
nontraffic V36.1
nontraffic V30.1
animal-drawn vehicle (traffic) V36.6
nontraffic V36.1
bus (traffic) V34.6
nontraffic V34.1
car (traffic) V33.6
nontraffic V33.1
motor vehicle NOS (traffic) V39.50
nontraffic V39.10
specified type NEC (traffic) V39.59
nontraffic V39.19
pedal cycle (traffic) V31.6
nontraffic V31.1
pickup truck (traffic) V33.6
nontraffic V33.1
railway vehicle (traffic) V35.6
nontraffic V35.1
specified vehicle NEC (traffic) V36.6
nontraffic V36.1
stationary object (traffic) V37.6
nontraffic V37.1
streetcar (traffic) V36.6
nontraffic V36.1
three wheeled motor vehicle (traffic) V32.6
nontraffic V32.1
truck (traffic) V34.6
nontraffic V34.1
two wheeled motor vehicle (traffic) V32.6
nontraffic V32.1
van (traffic) V33.6
nontraffic V33.1
noncollision accident (traffic) V38.6
nontraffic V38.1

Accident *(continued)*
transport *(continued)*
three-wheeled motor vehicle
occupant *(continued)*
specified type NEC V39.89
military vehicle V39.81
tractor (farm) (and trailer) *—see* Accident, transport, agricultural vehicle occupant
tram *—see* Accident, transport, streetcar
in mine or quarry *—see* Accident, transport, industrial vehicle occupant
trolley *—see* Accident, transport, streetcar
in mine or quarry *—see* Accident, transport, industrial vehicle occupant
truck (heavy) occupant V69.9
collision (with)
animal (traffic) V60.9
being ridden (traffic) V66.9
nontraffic V66.3
while boarding or alighting V66.4
nontraffic V60.3
while boarding or alighting V60.4
animal-drawn vehicle (traffic) V66.9
nontraffic V66.3
while boarding or alighting V66.4
bus (traffic) V64.9
nontraffic V64.3
while boarding or alighting V64.4
car (traffic) V63.9
nontraffic V63.3
while boarding or alighting V63.4
motor vehicle NOS (traffic) V69.60
nontraffic V69.20
specified type NEC (traffic) V69.69
nontraffic V69.29
pedal cycle (traffic) V61.9
nontraffic V61.3
while boarding or alighting V61.4
pickup truck (traffic) V63.9
nontraffic V63.3
while boarding or alighting V63.4
railway vehicle (traffic) V65.9
nontraffic V65.3
while boarding or alighting V65.4
specified vehicle NEC (traffic) V66.9
nontraffic V66.3
while boarding or alighting V66.4
stationary object (traffic) V67.9
nontraffic V67.3
while boarding or alighting V67.4
streetcar (traffic) V66.9
nontraffic V66.3
while boarding or alighting V66.4
three wheeled motor vehicle (traffic) V62.9
nontraffic V62.3
while boarding or alighting V62.4

Accident *(continued)*
transport *(continued)*
truck occupant *(continued)*
collision *(continued)*
truck (traffic) V64.9
nontraffic V64.3
while boarding or alighting V64.4
two wheeled motor vehicle (traffic) V62.9
nontraffic V62.3
while boarding or alighting V62.4
van (traffic) V63.9
nontraffic V63.3
while boarding or alighting V63.4
driver
collision (with)
animal (traffic) V60.5
being ridden (traffic) V66.5
nontraffic V66.0
nontraffic V60.0
animal-drawn vehicle (traffic) V66.5
nontraffic V66.0
bus (traffic) V64.5
nontraffic V64.0
car (traffic) V63.5
nontraffic V63.0
motor vehicle NOS (traffic) V69.40
nontraffic V69.00
specified type NEC (traffic) V69.49
nontraffic V69.09
pedal cycle (traffic) V61.5
nontraffic V61.0
pickup truck (traffic) V63.5
nontraffic V63.0
railway vehicle (traffic) V65.5
nontraffic V65.0
specified vehicle NEC (traffic) V66.5
nontraffic V66.0
stationary object (traffic) V67.5
nontraffic V67.0
streetcar (traffic) V66.5
nontraffic V66.0
three wheeled motor vehicle (traffic) V62.5
nontraffic V62.0
truck (traffic) V64.5
nontraffic V64.0
two wheeled motor vehicle (traffic) V62.5
nontraffic V62.0
van (traffic) V63.5
nontraffic V63.0
noncollision accident (traffic) V68.5
nontraffic V68.0
dump *—see* Accident, transport, construction vehicle occupant
hanger-on
collision (with)
animal (traffic) V60.7
being ridden (traffic) V66.7
nontraffic V66.2
nontraffic V60.2
animal-drawn vehicle (traffic) V66.7
nontraffic V66.2
bus (traffic) V64.7
nontraffic V64.2

Accident *(continued)*
transport *(continued)*
truck occupant *(continued)*
hanger-on *(continued)*
collision *(continued)*
car (traffic) V63.7
nontraffic V63.2
pedal cycle (traffic) V61.7
nontraffic V61.2
pickup truck (traffic) V63.7
nontraffic V63.2
railway vehicle (traffic) V65.7
nontraffic V65.2
specified vehicle NEC (traffic) V66.7
nontraffic V66.2
stationary object (traffic) V67.7
nontraffic V67.2
streetcar (traffic) V66.7
nontraffic V66.2
three wheeled motor vehicle (traffic) V62.7
nontraffic V62.2
truck (traffic) V64.7
nontraffic V64.2
two wheeled motor vehicle (traffic) V62.7
nontraffic V62.2
van (traffic) V63.7
nontraffic V63.2
noncollision accident (traffic) V68.7
nontraffic V68.2
noncollision accident (traffic) V68.9
nontraffic V68.3
while boarding or alighting V68.4
nontraffic V69.3
passenger
collision (with)
animal (traffic) V60.6
being ridden (traffic) V66.6
nontraffic V66.1
nontraffic V60.1
animal-drawn vehicle (traffic) V66.6
nontraffic V66.1
bus (traffic) V64.6
nontraffic V64.1
car (traffic) V63.6
nontraffic V63.1
motor vehicle NOS (traffic) V69.50
nontraffic V69.10
specified type NEC (traffic) V69.59
nontraffic V69.19
pedal cycle (traffic) V61.6
nontraffic V61.1
pickup truck (traffic) V63.6
nontraffic V63.1
railway vehicle (traffic) V65.6
nontraffic V65.1
specified vehicle NEC (traffic) V66.6
nontraffic V66.1
stationary object (traffic) V67.6
nontraffic V67.1
streetcar (traffic) V66.6
nontraffic V66.1
three wheeled motor vehicle (traffic) V62.6
nontraffic V62.1
truck (traffic) V64.6
nontraffic V64.1

Accident *(continued)*
transport *(continued)*
truck occupant *(continued)*
passenger *(continued)*
collision *(continued)*
two wheeled motor vehicle (traffic) V62.6
nontraffic V62.1
van (traffic) V63.6
nontraffic V63.1
noncollision accident (traffic) V68.6
nontraffic V68.1
pickup —*see* Accident, transport, pickup truck occupant
specified type NEC V69.88
military vehicle V69.81
van occupant V59.9
collision (with)
animal (traffic) V50.9
being ridden (traffic) V56.9
nontraffic V56.3
while boarding or alighting V56.4
nontraffic V50.3
while boarding or alighting V50.4
animal-drawn vehicle (traffic) V56.9
nontraffic V56.3
while boarding or alighting V56.4
bus (traffic) V54.9
nontraffic V54.3
while boarding or alighting V54.4
car (traffic) V53.9
nontraffic V53.3
while boarding or alighting V53.4
motor vehicle NOS (traffic) V59.60
nontraffic V59.20
specified type NEC (traffic) V59.69
nontraffic V59.29
pedal cycle (traffic) V51.9
nontraffic V51.3
while boarding or alighting V51.4
pickup truck (traffic) V53.9
nontraffic V53.3
while boarding or alighting V53.4
railway vehicle (traffic) V55.9
nontraffic V55.3
while boarding or alighting V55.4
specified vehicle NEC (traffic) V56.9
nontraffic V56.3
while boarding or alighting V56.4
stationary object (traffic) V57.9
nontraffic V57.3
while boarding or alighting V57.4
streetcar (traffic) V56.9
nontraffic V56.3
while boarding or alighting V56.4
three wheeled motor vehicle (traffic) V52.9
nontraffic V52.3
while boarding or alighting V52.4
truck (traffic) V54.9
nontraffic V54.3

Accident *(continued)*
transport *(continued)*
van occupant *(continued)*
collision *(continued)*
truck *(continued)*
while boarding or alighting V54.4
two wheeled motor vehicle (traffic) V52.9
nontraffic V52.3
while boarding or alighting V52.4
van (traffic) V53.9
nontraffic V53.3
while boarding or alighting V53.4
driver
collision (with)
animal (traffic) V50.5
being ridden (traffic) V56.5
nontraffic V56.0
nontraffic V50.0
animal-drawn vehicle (traffic) V56.5
nontraffic V56.0
bus (traffic) V54.5
nontraffic V54.0
car (traffic) V53.5
nontraffic V53.0
motor vehicle NOS (traffic) V59.40
nontraffic V59.00
specified type NEC (traffic) V59.49
nontraffic V59.09
pedal cycle (traffic) V51.5
nontraffic V51.0
pickup truck (traffic) V53.5
nontraffic V53.0
railway vehicle (traffic) V55.5
nontraffic V55.0
specified vehicle NEC (traffic) V56.5
nontraffic V56.0
stationary object (traffic) V57.5
nontraffic V57.0
streetcar (traffic) V56.5
nontraffic V56.0
three wheeled motor vehicle (traffic) V52.5
nontraffic V52.0
truck (traffic) V54.5
nontraffic V54.0
two wheeled motor vehicle (traffic) V52.5
driver
nontraffic V52.0
van (traffic) V53.5
nontraffic V53.0
noncollision accident (traffic) V58.5
nontraffic V58.0
noncollision accident (traffic) V58.9
nontraffic V58.3
while boarding or alighting V58.4
nontraffic V59.3
hanger-on
collision (with)
animal (traffic) V50.7
being ridden (traffic) V56.7
nontraffic V56.2
nontraffic V50.2
animal-drawn vehicle (traffic) V56.7
nontraffic V56.2

Accident *(continued)*
transport *(continued)*
van occupant *(continued)*
hanger-on *(continued)*
collision *(continued)*
bus (traffic) V54.7
nontraffic V54.2
car (traffic) V53.7
nontraffic V53.2
pedal cycle (traffic) V51.
nontraffic V51.2
pickup truck (traffic) V53.7
nontraffic V53.2
railway vehicle (traffic) V55.7
nontraffic V55.2
specified vehicle NEC (traffic) V56.7
nontraffic V56.2
stationary object (traffic) V57.7
nontraffic V57.2
streetcar (traffic) V56.7
nontraffic V56.2
three wheeled motor vehicle (traffic) V52.7
nontraffic V52.2
truck (traffic) V54.7
nontraffic V54.2
two wheeled motor vehic
(traffic) V52.7
nontraffic V52.2
van (traffic) V53.7
nontraffic V53.2
noncollision accident (traffi
V58.7
nontraffic V58.2
passenger
collision (with)
animal (traffic) V50.6
being ridden (traffic) V56.6
nontraffic V56.1
nontraffic V50.1
animal-drawn vehicle (traffic) V56.6
nontraffic V56.1
bus (traffic) V54.6
nontraffic V54.1
car (traffic) V53.6
nontraffic V53.1
motor vehicle NOS (traffic) V59.50
nontraffic V59.10
specified type NEC (traffic) V59.59
nontraffic V59.19
pedal cycle (traffic) V51.6
nontraffic V51.1
pickup truck (traffic) V53.6
nontraffic V53.1
railway vehicle (traffic) V55.6
nontraffic V55.1
specified vehicle NEC (traffic) V56.6
nontraffic V56.1
stationary object (traffic) V57.6
nontraffic V57.1
streetcar (traffic) V56.6
nontraffic V56.1
three wheeled motor vehicle (traffic) V52.6
nontraffic V52.1
truck (traffic) V54.6
nontraffic V54.1

ccident *(continued)*
transport *(continued)*
  van occupant *(continued)*
    passenger *(continued)*
      collision *(continued)*
        two wheeled motor vehicle (traffic) V52.6
          nontraffic V52.1
        van (traffic) V53.6
          nontraffic V53.1
      noncollision accident (traffic) V58.6
        nontraffic V58.1
    specified type NEC V59.88
      military vehicle V59.81
  watercraft occupant —*see* Accident, watercraft
vehicle NEC V89.9
  animal-drawn NEC —*see* Accident, transport, animal-drawn vehicle occupant
  special
    agricultural —*see* Accident, transport, agricultural vehicle occupant
    construction —*see* Accident, transport, construction vehicle occupant
    industrial —*see* Accident, transport, industrial vehicle occupant
  three-wheeled NEC (motorized) —*see* Accident, transport, three-wheeled motor vehicle occupant
watercraft V94.9
  causing
    drowning —*see* Drowning, due to, accident to, watercraft
    injury NEC V91.89
      crushed between craft and object V91.19
        powered craft V91.13
          ferry boat V91.11
          fishing boat V91.12
          jetskis V91.13
          liner V91.11
          merchant ship V91.10
          passenger ship V91.11
        unpowered craft V91.18
          canoe V91.15
          inflatable V91.16
          kayak V91.15
          sailboat V91.14
          surf-board V91.18
          windsurfer V91.18
      fall on board V91.29
        powered craft V91.23
          ferry boat V91.21
          fishing boat V91.22
          jetskis V91.23
          liner V91.21
          merchant ship V91.20
          passenger ship V91.21
        unpowered craft
          canoe V91.25
          inflatable V91.26
          kayak V91.25
          sailboat V91.24
      fire on board causing burn V91.09
        powered craft V91.03
          ferry boat V91.01
          fishing boat V91.02
          jetskis V91.03
          liner V91.01
          merchant ship V91.00
          passenger ship V91.01

Accident *(continued)*
  watercraft *(continued)*
    causing *(continued)*
      drowning *(continued)*
        fire on board *(continued)*
          unpowered craft V91.08
            canoe V91.05
            inflatable V91.06
            kayak V91.05
            sailboat V91.04
            surf-board V91.08
            water skis V91.07
            windsurfer V91.08
        hit by falling object V91.39
          powered craft V91.33
            ferry boat V91.31
            fishing boat V91.32
            jetskis V91.33
            liner V91.31
            merchant ship V91.30
            passenger ship V91.31
          unpowered craft V91.38
            canoe V91.35
            inflatable V91.36
            kayak V91.35
            sailboat V91.34
            surf-board V91.38
            water skis V91.37
            windsurfer V91.38
        specified type NEC V91.89
          powered craft V91.83
            ferry boat V91.81
            fishing boat V91.82
            jetskis V91.83
            liner V91.81
            merchant ship V91.80
            passenger ship V91.81
          unpowered craft V91.88
            canoe V91.85
            inflatable V91.86
            kayak V91.85
            sailboat V91.84
            surf-board V91.88
            water skis V91.87
            windsurfer V91.88
    due to, caused by cataclysm —*see* Forces of nature, by type
    military NEC V94.818
      with civilian watercraft V94.810
      civilian in water injured by V94.811
    nonpowered, struck by
      nonpowered vessel V94.22
      powered vessel V94.21
    specified type NEC V94.89
    striking swimmer
      powered V94.11
      unpowered V94.12

Acid throwing (assault) Y08.89

Activity (involving) (of victim at time of event) Y93.9
  aerobic and step exercise (class) Y93.A3
  alpine skiing Y93.23
  animal care NEC Y93.K9
  arts and handcrafts NEC Y93.D9
  athletics NEC Y93.79
  athletics played as a team or group NEC Y93.69
  athletics played individually NEC Y93.59
  baking Y93.G3
  ballet Y93.41
  barbells Y93.B3
  BASE (Building, Antenna, Span, Earth) jumping Y93.33
  baseball Y93.64
  basketball Y93.67
  bathing (personal) Y93.E1
  beach volleyball Y93.68

Activity *(continued)*
  bike riding Y93.55
  blackout game Y93.85
  boogie boarding Y93.18
  bowling Y93.54
  boxing Y93.71
  brass instrument playing Y93.J4
  building construction Y93.H3
  bungee jumping Y93.34
  calisthenics Y93.A2
  canoeing (in calm and turbulent water) Y93.16
  capture the flag Y93.6A
  cardiorespiratory exercise NEC Y93.A9
  caregiving (providing) NEC Y93 F9
    bathing Y93.F1
    lifting Y93.F2
  cellular
    communication device Y93.C2
    telephone Y93.C2
  challenge course Y93.A5
  cheerleading Y93.45
  choking game Y93.85
  circuit training Y93.A4
  cleaning
    floor Y93.E5
  climbing NEC Y93.39
    mountain Y93.31
    rock Y93.31
    wall Y93.31
  clothing care and maintenance NEC Y93.E9
  combatives Y93.75
  computer
    keyboarding Y93.C1
    technology NEC Y93.C9
  confidence course Y93.A5
  construction (building) Y93.H3
  cooking and baking Y93.G3
  cool down exercises Y93.A2
  cricket Y93.69
  crocheting Y93.D1
  cross country skiing Y93.24
  dancing (all types) Y93.41
  digging
    dirt Y93.H1
  dirt digging Y93.H1
  dishwashing Y93.G1
  diving (platform) (springboard) Y93.12
    underwater Y93.15
  dodge ball Y93.6A
  downhill skiing Y93.23
  drum playing Y93.J2
  dumbbells Y93.B3
  electronic
    devices NEC Y93.C9
      hand held interactive Y93.C2
    game playing (using) (with)
      interactive device Y93.C2
      keyboard or other stationary device Y93.C1
  elliptical machine Y93.A1
  exercise(s)
    machines ((primarily) for)
      cardiorespiratory conditioning Y93.A1
      muscle strengthening Y93.B1
    muscle strengthening (non-machine) NEC Y93.B9
  external motion NEC Y93.I9
    rollercoaster Y93.I1
  fainting game Y93.85
  field hockey Y93.65
  figure skating (pairs) (singles) Y93.21
  flag football Y93.62
  floor mopping and cleaning Y93.E5
  food preparation and clean up Y93.G1
  football (American) NOS Y93.61
    flag Y93.62

Activity *(continued)*
  football NOS *(continued)*
    tackle Y93.61
    touch Y93.62
  four square Y93.6A
  free weights Y93.B3
  frisbee (ultimate) Y93.74
  furniture
    building Y93.D3
    finishing Y93.D3
    repair Y93.D3
  game playing (electronic)
    using keyboard or other stationary device Y93.C1
    using interactive device Y93.C2
  gardening Y93.H2
  golf Y93.53
  grass drills Y93.A6
  grilling and smoking food Y93.G2
  grooming and shearing an animal Y93.K3
  guerilla drills Y93.A6
  gymnastics (rhythmic) Y93.43
  handball Y93.73
  handcrafts NEC Y93.D9
  hand held interactive electronic device Y93.C2
  hang gliding Y93.35
  hiking (on level or elevated terrain) Y93.01
  hockey (ice) Y93.22
    field Y93.65
  horseback riding Y93.52
  household (interior) maintenance NEC Y93.E9
  ice NEC Y93.29
    dancing Y93.21
    hockey Y93.22
    skating Y93.21
  inline roller skating Y93.51
  ironing Y93.E4
  judo Y93.75
  jumping (off) NEC Y93.39
    BASE (Building, Antenna, Span, Earth) Y93.33
    bungee Y93.34
    jacks Y93.A2
    rope Y93.56
  jumping jacks Y93.A2
  jumping rope Y93.56
  karate Y93.75
  kayaking (in calm and turbulent water) Y93.16
  keyboarding (computer) Y93.C1
  kickball Y93.6A
  knitting Y93.D1
  lacrosse Y93.65
  land maintenance NEC Y93.H9
  landscaping Y93.H2
  laundry Y93.E2
  machines (exercise)
    primarily for cardiorespiratory conditioning Y93.A1
    primarily for muscle strengthening Y93.B1
  maintenance
    exterior building NEC Y93.H9
    household (interior) NEC Y93.E9
    land Y93.H9
    property Y93.H9
  marching (on level or elevated terrain) Y93.01
  martial arts Y93.75
  microwave oven Y93.G3
  milking an animal Y93.K2
  mopping (floor) Y93.E5
  mountain climbing Y93.31
  muscle strengthening
    exercises (non-machine) NEC Y93.B9
    machines Y93.B1

Activity *(continued)*
  musical keyboard (electronic)
    playing Y93.J1
  nordic skiing Y93.24
  obstacle course Y93.A5
  oven (microwave) Y93.G3
  packing up and unpacking in moving to a new residence Y93.E6
  parasailing Y93.19
  pass out game Y93.85
  percussion instrument playing NEC Y93.J2
  personal
    bathing and showering Y93.E1
    hygiene NEC Y93.E8
    showering Y93.E1
  physical games generally associated with school recess, summer camp and children Y93.6A
  physical training NEC Y93.A9
  piano playing Y93.J1
  pilates Y93.B4
  platform diving Y93.12
  playing musical instrument
    brass instrument Y93.J4
    drum Y93.J2
    musical keyboard (electronic) Y93.J1
    percussion instrument NEC Y93.J2
    piano Y93.J1
    string instrument Y93.J3
    winds instrument Y93.J4
  property maintenance
    exterior NEC Y93.H9
    interior NEC Y93.E9
  pruning (garden and lawn) Y93.H2
  pull-ups Y93.B2
  push-ups Y93.B2
  racquetball Y93.73
  rafting (in calm and turbulent water) Y93.16
  raking (leaves) Y93.H1
  rappelling Y93.32
  refereeing a sports activity Y93.81
  residential relocation Y93.E6
  rhythmic gymnastics Y93.43
  rhythmic movement NEC Y93.49
  riding
    horseback Y93.52
    rollercoaster Y93.I1
  rock climbing Y93.31
  rollercoaster riding Y93.I1
  roller skating (inline) Y93.51
  rough housing and horseplay Y93.83
  rowing (in calm and turbulent water) Y93.16
  rugby Y93.63
  running Y93.02
  SCUBA diving Y93.15
  sewing Y93.D2
  shoveling Y93.H1
    dirt Y93.H1
    snow Y93.H1
  showering (personal) Y93.E1
  sit-ups Y93.B2
  skateboarding Y93.51
  skating (ice) Y93.21
    roller Y93.51
  skiing (alpine) (downhill) Y93.23
    cross country Y93.24
    nordic Y93.24
    water Y93.17
  sledding (snow) Y93.23
  sleeping (sleep) Y93.84
  smoking and grilling food Y93.G2
  snorkeling Y93.15
  snow NEC Y93.29
    boarding Y93.23
    shoveling Y93.H1
    sledding Y93.23
    tubing Y93.23
  soccer Y93.66
  softball Y93.64

Activity *(continued)*
  specified NEC Y93.89
  spectator at an event Y93.82
  sports NEC Y93.79
    sports played as a team or group NEC Y93.69
    sports played individually NEC Y93.59
  springboard diving Y93.12
  squash Y93.73
  stationary bike Y93.A1
  step (stepping) exercise (class) Y93.A3
  stepper machine Y93.A1
  stove Y93.G3
  string instrument playing Y93.J3
  surfing Y93.18
    wind Y93.18
  swimming Y93.11
  tackle football Y93.61
  tap dancing Y93.41
  tennis Y93.73
  tobogganing Y93.23
  touch football Y93.62
  track and field events (non-running) Y93.57
    running Y93.02
  trampoline Y93.44
  treadmill Y93.A1
  trimming shrubs Y93.H2
  tubing (in calm and turbulent water) Y93.16
    snow Y93.23
  ultimate frisbee Y93.74
  underwater diving Y93.15
  unpacking in moving to a new residence Y93.E6
  use of stove, oven and microwave oven Y93.G3
  vacuuming Y93.E3
  volleyball (beach) (court) Y93.68
  wake boarding Y93.17
  walking an animal Y93.K1
  walking (on level or elevated terrain) Y93.01
    an animal Y93.K1
  wall climbing Y93.31
  warm up and cool down exercises Y93.A2
  water NEC Y93.19
    aerobics Y93.14
    craft NEC Y93.19
    exercise Y93.14
    polo Y93.13
    skiing Y93.17
    sliding Y93.18
    survival training and testing Y93.19
  weeding (garden and lawn) Y93.H2
  wind instrument playing Y93.J4
  windsurfing Y93.18
  wrestling Y93.72
  yoga Y93.42

Adverse effect of drugs *—see* Table of Drugs and Chemicals

Aerosinusitis *—see* Air, pressure

After-effect, late *—see* Sequelae

Air
  blast in war operations *—see* War operations, air blast
  pressure
    change, rapid
      during
        ascent W94.29
          while (in) (surfacing from)
            aircraft W94.23
            deep water diving W94.21
            underground W94.22

Air *(continued)*
  pressure *(continued)*
    change, rapid *(continued)*
      during *(continued)*
        descent W94.39
          in
            aircraft W94.31
            water W94.32
    high, prolonged W94.0
    low, prolonged W94.12
      due to residence or long visit at high altitude W94.11

Alpine sickness W94.11

Altitude sickness W94.11

Anaphylactic shock, anaphylaxis *—see* Table of Drugs and Chemicals

Andes disease W94.11

Arachnidism, arachnoidism X58

Arson (with intent to injure or kill) X97

Asphyxia, asphyxiation
  by
    food (bone) (seed) *—see* categories T17 and T18
    gas *—see also* Table of Drugs and Chemicals
      legal

Asphyxia, asphyxiation *(continued)*
        execution *—see* Legal, intervention, gas
        intervention *—see* Legal, intervention, gas
  from
    fire *—see also* Exposure, fire
      in war operations *—see* War operations, fire
    ignition *—see* Ignition
    vomitus T17.81
  in war operations *—see* War operations, restriction of airway

Aspiration
  food (any type) (into respiratory tract) (with asphyxia, obstruction respiratory tract, suffocation) *—see* categories T17 and T18
  foreign body *—see* Foreign body, aspiration
  vomitus (with asphyxia, obstruction respiratory tract, suffocation) T17.81

Assassination (attempt) *—see* Assault

Assault (homicidal) (by) (in) Y09
  arson X97
  bite (of human being) Y04.1
  bodily force Y04.8
    bite Y04.1
    bumping into Y04.2
    sexual *—see* subcategories T74.0, T76.0
    unarmed fight Y04.0
  bomb X96.9
    antipersonnel X96.0
    fertilizer X96.3
    gasoline X96.1
    letter X96.2
    petrol X96.1
    pipe X96.3
    specified NEC X96.8
  brawl (hand) (fists) (foot) (unarmed) Y04.0
  burning, burns (by fire) NEC X97
    acid Y08.89
    caustic, corrosive substance Y08.89
    chemical from swallowing caustic, corrosive substance *—see* Table of Drugs and Chemicals
    cigarette(s) X97
    hot object X98.9

Assault *(continued)*
  burning, burns NEC *(continued)*
    hot object *(continued)*
      fluid NEC X98.2
      household appliance X98.3
      specified NEC X98.8
      steam X98.0
      tap water X98.1
      vapors X98.0
    scalding *—see* Assault, burning
    steam X98.0
    vitriol Y08.89
  caustic, corrosive substance (gas) Y08.89
  crashing of
    aircraft Y08.81
    motor vehicle Y03.8
      pushed in front of Y02.0
      run over Y03.0
      specified NEC Y03.8
  cutting or piercing instrument X99.9
    dagger X99.2
    glass X99.0
    knife X99.1
    specified NEC X99.8
    sword X99.2
  dagger X99.2
  drowning (in) X92.9
    bathtub X92.0
    natural water X92.3
    specified NEC X92.8
    swimming pool X92.1
      following fall X92.2
  dynamite X96.8
  explosive(s) (material) X96.9
  fight (hand) (fists) (foot) (unarmed) Y04.0
    with weapon *—see* Assault, by type of weapon
  fire X97
  firearm X95.9
    airgun X95.01
    handgun X93
    hunting rifle X94.1
    larger X94.9
      specified NEC X94.8
    machine gun X94.2
    shotgun X94.0
    specified NEC X95.8
  gunshot (wound) NEC *—see* Assault, firearm, by type
  incendiary device X97
  injury Y09
    to child due to criminal abortion attempt NEC Y08.89
  knife X99.1
  late effect of *—see* X92-Y08 with 7th character S
  placing before moving object NEC Y02.8
    motor vehicle Y02.0
  poisoning *—see* categories T36-T65 with 7th character S
  puncture, any part of body *—see* Assault, cutting or piercing instrument
  pushing
    before moving object NEC Y02.8
      motor vehicle Y02.0
      subway train Y02.1
      train Y02.1
    from high place Y01
  rape T74.2-
  scalding *—see* Assault, burning
  sequelae of *—see* X92-Y08 with 7th character S
  sexual (by bodily force) T74.2-
  shooting *—see* Assault, firearm
  specified means NEC Y08.89

sault *(continued)*
- stab, any part of body —*see* Assault, cutting or piercing instrument
- steam X98.0
- striking against
  - other person Y04.2
  - sports equipment Y08.09
    - baseball bat Y08.02
    - hockey stick Y08.01
- struck by
  - sports equipment Y08.09
    - baseball bat Y08.02
    - hockey stick Y08.01
- submersion —*see* Assault, drowning
- violence Y09
- weapon Y09
  - blunt Y00
  - cutting or piercing —*see* Assault, cutting or piercing instrument
  - firearm —*see* Assault, firearm
- wound Y09
  - cutting —*see* Assault, cutting or piercing instrument
  - gunshot —*see* Assault, firearm
  - knife X99.1
  - piercing —*see* Assault, cutting or piercing instrument
  - puncture —*see* Assault, cutting or piercing instrument
  - stab —*see* Assault, cutting or piercing instrument

ttack by mammals NEC W55.89

valanche —*see* Landslide

viator's disease —*see* Air, pressure

rotitis, barodontalgia, barosinusitis, barotrauma (otitic) (sinus) —*see* Air, pressure

ttered (baby) (child) (person) (syndrome) X58

yonet wound W26.1
- in
  - legal intervention —*see* Legal, intervention, sharp object, bayonet
  - war operations —*see* War operations, combat
- stated as undetermined whether accidental or intentional Y28.8
- suicide (attempt) X78.2

ean in nose —*see* categories T17 and T18

d set on fire NEC —*see* Exposure, fire, uncontrolled, building, bed

heading (by guillotine)
- homicide X99.9
- legal execution —*see* Legal, intervention

ending, injury in (prolonged) (static) X50.1

ends —*see* Air, pressure, change

te, bitten by
- alligator W58.01
- arthropod (nonvenomous) NEC W57
- bull W55.21
- cat W55.01
- cow W55.21
- crocodile W58.11
- dog W54.0
- goat W55.31
- hoof stock NEC W55.31
- horse W55.11
- human being (accidentally) W50.3
  - with intent to injure or kill Y04.1
  - as, or caused by, a crowd or human stampede (with fall) W52
  - assault Y04.1

Bite, bitten by *(continued)*
- human being *(continued)*
  - homicide (attempt) Y04.1
  - in
    - fight Y04.1
- insect (nonvenomous) W57
- lizard (nonvenomous) W59.01
- mammal NEC W55.81
  - marine W56.31
- marine animal (nonvenomous) W56.81
- millipede W57
- moray eel W56.51
- mouse W53.01
- person(s) (accidentally) W50.3
  - with intent to injure or kill Y04.1
  - as, or caused by, a crowd or human stampede (with fall) W52
  - assault Y04.1
  - homicide (attempt) Y04.1
  - in
    - fight Y04.1
- pig W55.41
- raccoon W55.51
- rat W53.11
- reptile W59.81
  - lizard W59.01
  - snake W59.11
  - turtle W59.21
    - terrestrial W59.81
- rodent W53.81
  - mouse W53.01
  - rat W53.11
  - specified NEC W53.81
  - squirrel W53.21
- shark W56.41
- sheep W55.31
- snake (nonvenomous) W59.11
- spider (nonvenomous) W57
- squirrel W53.21

Blast (air) **in war operations** —*see* War operations, blast

Blizzard X37.2

Blood alcohol level Y90.9
- less than 20mg/100ml Y90.0
- presence in blood, level not specified Y90.9
- 20-39mg/100ml Y90.1
- 40-59mg/100ml Y90.2
- 60-79mg/100ml Y90.3
- 80-99mg/100ml Y90.4
- 100-119mg/100ml Y90.5
- 120-199mg/100ml Y90.6
- 200-239mg/100ml Y90.7

Blow X58
- by law-enforcing agent, police (on duty) —*see* Legal, intervention, manhandling
  - blunt object —*see* Legal, intervention, blunt object

Blowing up —*see* Explosion

Brawl (hand) (fists) (foot) Y04.0

Breakage (accidental) (part of)
- ladder (causing fall) W11
- scaffolding (causing fall) W12

Broken
- glass, contact with —*see* Contact, with, glass
- power line (causing electric shock) W85

Bumping against, into (accidentally)
- object NEC W22.8
  - with fall —*see* Fall, due to, bumping against, object
  - caused by crowd or human stampede (with fall) W52
  - sports equipment W21.9
- person(s) W51
  - with fall W03
    - due to ice or snow W00.0
  - assault Y04.2

Bumping against, into *(continued)*
- person(s) *(continued)*
  - caused by, a crowd or human stampede (with fall) W52
  - homicide (attempt) Y04.2
- sports equipment W21.9

Burn, burned, burning (accidental) (by) (from) (on)
- acid NEC —*see* Table of Drugs and Chemicals
- bed linen —*see* Exposure, fire, uncontrolled, in building, bed
- blowtorch X08.8
  - with ignition of clothing NEC X06.2
    - nightwear X05
- bonfire, campfire (controlled) —*see also* Exposure, fire, controlled, not in building
  - uncontrolled —*see* Exposure, fire, uncontrolled, not in building
- candle X08.8
  - with ignition of clothing NEC X06.2
    - nightwear X05
- caustic liquid, substance (external) (internal) NEC —*see* Table of Drugs and Chemicals
- chemical (external) (internal) —*see also* Table of Drugs and Chemicals
  - in war operations —*see* War operations. fire
- cigar(s) or cigarette(s) X08.8
  - with ignition of clothing NEC X06.2
    - nightwear X05
- clothes, clothing NEC (from controlled fire) X06.2
  - with conflagration —*see* Exposure, fire, uncontrolled, building
    - not in building or structure —*see* Exposure, fire, uncontrolled, not in building
- cooker (hot) X15.8
  - stated as undetermined whether accidental or intentional Y27.3
  - suicide (attempt) X77.3
- electric blanket X16
- engine (hot) X17
- fire, flames —*see* Exposure, fire
- flare, Very pistol —*see* Discharge, firearm NEC
- heat
  - from appliance (electrical) (household) X15.8
    - cooker X15.8
    - hotplate X15.2
    - kettle X15.8
    - light bulb X15.8
    - saucepan X15.3
    - skillet X15.3
    - stove X15.0
    - stated as undetermined whether accidental or intentional Y27.3
    - suicide (attempt) X77.3
    - toaster X15.1
  - in local application or packing during medical or surgical procedure Y63.5
- heating
  - appliance, radiator or pipe X16
- homicide (attempt) —*see* Assault, burning
- hot
  - air X14.1
  - cooker X15.8
  - drink X10.0
  - engine X17
  - fat X10.2
  - fluid NEC X12
  - food X10.1
  - gases X14.1
  - heating appliance X16

Burn, burned, burning *(continued)*
- hot *(continued)*
  - household appliance NEC X15.8
  - kettle X15.8
  - liquid NEC X12
  - machinery X17
  - metal (molten) (liquid) NEC X18
  - object (not producing fire or flames) NEC X19
  - oil (cooking) X10.2
  - pipe(s) X16
  - radiator X16
  - saucepan (glass) (metal) X15.3
  - stove (kitchen) X15.0
  - substance NEC X19
    - caustic or corrosive NEC —*see* Table of Drugs and Chemicals
  - toaster X15.1
  - tool X17
  - vapor X13.1
  - water (tap) —*see* Contact, with, hot, tap water
- hotplate X15.2
  - suicide (attempt) X77.3
- ignition —*see* Ignition
- in war operations —*see* War operations, fire
- inflicted by other person X97
  - by hot objects, hot vapor, and steam —*see* Assault, burning, hot object
- internal, from swallowed caustic, corrosive liquid, substance —*see* Table of Drugs and Chemicals
- iron (hot) X15.8
  - stated as undetermined whether accidental or intentional Y27.3
  - suicide (attempt) X77.3
- kettle (hot) X15.8
  - stated as undetermined whether accidental or intentional Y27.3
  - suicide (attempt) X77.3
- lamp (flame) X08.8
  - with ignition of clothing NEC X06.2
    - nightwear X05
- lighter (cigar) (cigarette) X08.8
  - with ignition of clothing NEC X06.2
    - nightwear X05
- lightning —*see* subcategory T75.0
  - causing fire —*see* Exposure, fire
- liquid (boiling) (hot) NEC X12
  - stated as undetermined whether accidental or intentional Y27.2
  - suicide (attempt) X77.2
- local application of externally applied substance in medical or surgical care Y63.5
- machinery (hot) X17
- matches X08.8
  - with ignition of clothing NEC X06.2
    - nightwear X05
- mattress —*see* Exposure, fire, uncontrolled, building, bed
- medicament, externally applied Y63.5
- metal (hot) (liquid) (molten) NEC X18
- nightwear (nightclothes, nightdress, gown, pajamas, robe) X05
- object (hot) NEC X19
- on board watercraft
  - due to
    - accident to watercraft V91.09
      - powered craft V91.03
        - ferry boat V91.01
        - fishing boat V91.02

Burn, burned, burning *(continued)*
- on board watercraft *(continued)*
  - due to *(continued)*
    - accident to watercraft *(continued)*
      - powered craft *(continued)*
        - jetskis V91.03
        - liner V91.01
        - merchant ship V91.00
        - passenger ship V91.01
      - unpowered craft V91.08
        - canoe V91.05
        - inflatable V91.06
        - kayak V91.05
        - sailboat V91.04
        - surf-board V91.08
        - water skis V91.07
        - windsurfer V91.08
    - fire on board V93.09
      - ferry boat V93.01
      - fishing boat V93.02
      - jetskis V93.03
      - liner V93.01
      - merchant ship V93.00
      - passenger ship V93.01
      - powered craft NEC V93.03
      - sailboat V93.04
    - specified heat source NEC on board V93.19
      - ferry boat V93.11
      - fishing boat V93.12
      - jetskis V93.13
      - liner V93.11
      - merchant ship V93.10
      - passenger ship V93.11
      - powered craft NEC V93.13
      - sailboat V93.14
- pipe (hot) X16
  - smoking X08.8
    - with ignition of clothing NEC X06.2
      - nightwear X05
- powder —*see* Powder burn
- radiator (hot) X16
- saucepan (hot) (glass) (metal) X15.3
  - stated as undetermined whether accidental or intentional Y27.3
  - suicide (attempt) X77.3
- self-inflicted X76
  - stated as undetermined whether accidental or intentional Y26
- steam X13.1
  - pipe X16
    - stated as undetermined whether accidental or intentional Y27.8
  - stated as undetermined whether accidental or intentional Y27.0
  - suicide (attempt) X77.0
- stove (hot) (kitchen) X15.0
  - stated as undetermined whether accidental or intentional Y27.3
  - suicide (attempt) X77.3
- substance (hot) NEC X19
  - boiling X12
    - stated as undetermined whether accidental or intentional Y27.2
    - suicide (attempt) X77.2
  - molten (metal) X18
- suicide (attempt) NEC X76
  - hot
    - household appliance X77.3
    - object X77.9
- therapeutic misadventure
  - heat in local application or packing during medical or surgical procedure Y63.5
  - overdose of radiation Y63.2
- toaster (hot) X15.1
  - stated as undetermined whether accidental or intentional Y27.3

Burn, burned, burning *(continued)*
- toaster *(continued)*
  - suicide (attempt) X77.3
- tool (hot) X17
- torch, welding X08.8
  - with ignition of clothing NEC X06.2
    - nightwear X05
- trash fire (controlled) —*see* Exposure, fire, controlled, not in building
  - uncontrolled —*see* Exposure, fire, uncontrolled, not in building
- vapor (hot) X13.1
  - stated as undetermined whether accidental or intentional Y27.0
  - suicide (attempt) X77.0
- Very pistol —*see* Discharge, firearm NEC

Butted by animal W55.82
- bull W55.22
- cow W55.22
- goat W55.32
- horse W55.12
- pig W55.42
- sheep W55.32

C

Caisson disease —*see* Air, pressure, change

Campfire (exposure to) (controlled) —*see also* Exposure, fire, controlled, not in building
- uncontrolled —*see* Exposure, fire, uncontrolled, not in building

Capital punishment (any means) —*see* Legal, intervention

Car sickness T75.3

Casualty (not due to war) NEC X58
- war —*see* War operations

Cat
- bite W55.01
- scratch W55.03

Cataclysm, cataclysmic (any injury) NEC —*see* Forces of nature

Catching fire —*see* Exposure, fire

Caught
- between
  - folding object W23.0
  - objects (moving) (stationary and moving) W23.0
    - and machinery —*see* Contact, with, by type of machine
    - stationary W23.1
  - sliding door and door frame W23.0
- by, in
  - machinery (moving parts of) —*see* Contact, with, by type of machine
  - washing-machine wringer W23.0
- under packing crate (due to losing grip) W23.1

Cave-in caused by cataclysmic earth surface movement or eruption —*see* Landslide

Change(s) in air pressure —*see* Air, pressure, change

Choked, choking (on) (any object except food or vomitus)
- food (bone) (seed) —*see* categories T17 and T18
- vomitus T17.81-

Civil insurrection —*see* War operations

Cloudburst (any injury) X37.8

Cold, exposure to (accidental) (excessive) (extreme) (natural) (place) NEC —*see* Exposure, cold

Collapse
- building W20.1
  - burning (uncontrolled fire) X00.2
- dam or man-made structure (causing earth movement) X36.0
- machinery —*see* Contact, with, by type of machine
- structure W20.1
  - burning (uncontrolled fire) X00.2

Collision (accidental) NEC —*see also* Accident, transport V89.9
- pedestrian W51
  - with fall W03
  - due to ice or snow W00.0
    - involving pedestrian conveyance —*see* Accident, transport, pedestrian, conveyance
  - and
    - crowd or human stampede (with fall) W52
    - object W22.8
      - with fall —*see* Fall, due to, bumping against, object
- person(s) —*see* Collision, pedestrian
- transport vehicle NEC V89.9
  - and
    - avalanche, fallen or not moving —*see* Accident, transport
      - falling or moving —*see* Landslide
    - landslide, fallen or not moving —*see* Accident, transport
      - falling or moving —*see* Landslide
  - due to cataclysm —*see* Forces of nature, by type
  - intentional, purposeful suicide (attempt) —*see* Suicide, collision

Combustion, spontaneous —*see* Ignition

Complication (delayed) of or following (medical or surgical procedure) Y84.9
- with misadventure —*see* Misadventure
- amputation of limb(s) Y83.5
- anastomosis (arteriovenous) (blood vessel) (gastrojejunal) (tendon) (natural or artificial material) Y83.2
- aspiration (of fluid) Y84.4
  - tissue Y84.8
- biopsy Y84.8
- blood
  - sampling Y84.7
  - transfusion
    - procedure Y84.8
- bypass Y83.2
- catheterization (urinary) Y84.6
  - cardiac Y84.0
- colostomy Y83.3
- cystostomy Y83.3
- dialysis (kidney) Y84.1
- drug —*see* Table of Drugs and Chemicals
- due to misadventure —*see* Misadventure
- duodenostomy Y83.3
- electroshock therapy Y84.3
- external stoma, creation of Y83.3
- formation of external stoma Y83.3
- gastrostomy Y83.3
- graft Y83.2
- hypothermia (medically-induced) Y84.8
- implant, implantation (of)
  - artificial
    - internal device (cardiac pacemaker) (electrodes in brain) (heart valve prosthesis) (orthopedic) Y83.1
    - material or tissue (for anastomosis or bypass) Y83.2

Complication *(continued)*
- implant, implantation *(continued)*
  - artificial *(continued)*
    - material or tissue *(continued)*
      - with creation of external stoma Y83.3
  - natural tissues (for anastomosis or bypass) Y83.2
    - with creation of external stoma Y83.3
- infusion
  - procedure Y84.8
- injection —*see* Table of Drugs and Chemicals
  - procedure Y84.8
- insertion of gastric or duodenal sound Y84.5
- insulin-shock therapy Y84.3
- paracentesis (abdominal) (thoracic) (aspirative) Y84.4
- procedures other than surgical operation —*see* Complication of or following, by type of procedure
- radiological procedure or therapy Y84.2
- removal of organ (partial) (total) NEC Y83.6
- sampling
  - blood Y84.7
  - fluid NEC Y84.4
  - tissue Y84.8
- shock therapy Y84.3
- surgical operation NEC —*see also* Complication of or following, by type of operation Y83.9
  - reconstructive NEC Y83.4
    - with
      - anastomosis, bypass or graft Y83.2
      - formation of external stoma Y83.3
  - specified NEC Y83.8
- transfusion —*see also* Table of Drugs and Chemicals
  - procedure Y84.8
- transplant, transplantation (heart) (kidney) (liver) (whole organ, any) Y83.0
  - partial organ Y83.4
- ureterostomy Y83.3
- vaccination —*see also* Table of Drugs and Chemicals
  - procedure Y84.8

Compression
- divers' squeeze —*see* Air, pressure, change
- trachea by
  - food (lodged in esophagus) —*see* categories T17 and T18
  - vomitus (lodged in esophagus) T17.81-

Conflagration —*see* Exposure, fire, uncontrolled

Constriction (external)
- hair W49.01
- jewelry W49.04
- ring W49.04
- rubber band W49.03
- specified item NEC W49.09
- string W49.02
- thread W49.02

Contact (accidental)
- with
  - abrasive wheel (metalworking) W31.1
  - alligator W58.09
    - bite W58.01
    - crushing W58.03
    - strike W58.02

Contact *(continued)*
  with *(continued)*
    amphibian W62.9
      frog W62.0
      toad W62.1
    animal (nonvenomous) NEC W64
      marine W56.89
        bite W56.81
        dolphin *—see* Contact, with, dolphin
        fish NEC *—see* Contact, with, fish
        mammal *—see* Contact, with, mammal, marine
        orca *—see* Contact, with, orca
        sea lion *—see* Contact, with, sea lion
        shark *—see* Contact, with, shark
        strike W56.82
    animate mechanical force NEC W64
    arrow W21.89
      not thrown, projected or falling W45.8
    arthropods (nonvenomous) W57
    axe W27.0
    band-saw (industrial) W31.2
    bayonet *—see* Bayonet wound
    bee(s) X58
    bench-saw (industrial) W31.2
    bird W61.99
      bite W61.91
      chicken *—see* Contact, with, chicken
      duck *—see* Contact, with, duck
      goose *—see* Contact, with, goose
      macaw *—see* Contact, with, macaw
      parrot *—see* Contact, with, parrot
      psittacine *—see* Contact, with, psittacine
      strike W61.92
      turkey *—see* Contact, with, turkey
    blender W29.0
    boiling water X12
      stated as undetermined whether accidental or intentional Y27.2
      suicide (attempt) X77.2
    bore, earth-drilling or mining (land) (seabed) W31.0
    buffalo *—see* Contact, with, hoof stock NEC
    bull W55.29
      bite W55.21
      gored W55.22
      strike W55.22
    bumper cars W31.81
    camel *—see* Contact, with, hoof stock NEC
    can
      lid W26.8
      opener W27.4
        powered W29.0
    cat W55.09
      bite W55.01
      scratch W55.03
    caterpillar (venomous) X58
    centipede (venomous) X58
    chain
      hoist W24.0
        agricultural operations W30.89
      saw W29.3
    chicken W61.39
      peck W61.33
      strike W61.32
    chisel W27.0
    circular saw W31.2
    cobra X58

Contact *(continued)*
  with *(continued)*
    combine (harvester) W30.0
    conveyer belt W24.1
    cooker (hot) X15.8
      stated as undetermined whether accidental or intentional Y27.3
      suicide (attempt) X77.3
    coral X58
    cotton gin W31.82
    cow W55.29
      bite W55.21
      strike W55.22
    crane W24.0
      agricultural operations W30.89
    crocodile W58.19
      bite W58.11
      crushing W58.13
      strike W58.12
    dagger W26.1
      stated as undetermined whether accidental or intentional Y28.2
      suicide (attempt) X78.2
    dairy equipment W31.82
    dart W21.89
      not thrown, projected or falling W45.8
    deer *—see* Contact, with, hoof stock NEC
    derrick W24.0
      agricultural operations W30.89
        hay W30.2
    dog W54.8
      bite W54.0
      strike W54.1
    dolphin W56.09
      bite W56.01
      strike W56.02
    donkey *—see* Contact, with, hoof stock NEC
    drill (powered) W29.8
      earth (land) (seabed) W31.0
      nonpowered W27.8
    drive belt W24.0
      agricultural operations W30.89
    dry ice *—see* Exposure, cold, man-made
    dryer (clothes) (powered) (spin) W29.2
    duck W61.69
      bite W61.61
      strike W61.62
    earth (-)
      drilling machine (industrial) W31.0
      scraping machine in stationary use W31.83
    edge of stiff paper W26.2
    electric
      beater W29.0
      blanket X16
      fan W29.2
        commercial W31.82
      knife W29.1
      mixer W29.0
    elevator (building) W24.0
      agricultural operations W30.89
        grain W30.3
    engine(s), hot NEC X17
    excavating machine W31.0
    farm machine W30.9
    feces *—see* Contact, with, by type of animal
    fer de lance X58
    fish W56.59
      bite W56.51
      shark *—see* Contact, with, shark
      strike W56.52
    flying horses W31.81
    forging (metalworking) machine W31.1
    fork W27.4

Contact *(continued)*
  with *(continued)*
    forklift (truck) W24.0
      agricultural operations W30.89
    frog W62.0
    garden
      cultivator (powered) W29.3
        riding W30.89
      fork W27.1
    gas turbine W31.3
    Gila monster X58
    giraffe *—see* Contact, with, hoof stock NEC
    glass (sharp) (broken) W25
      with subsequent fall W18.02
      assault X99.0
      due to fall *—see* Fall, by type
      stated as undetermined whether accidental or intentional Y28.0
      suicide (attempt) X78.0
    goat W55.39
      bite W55.31
      strike W55.32
    goose W61.59
      bite W61.51
      strike W61.52
    hand
      saw W27.0
      tool (not powered) NEC W27.8
        powered W29.8
    harvester W30.0
    hay-derrick W30.2
    heat NEC X19
      from appliance (electrical) (household) *—see* Contact, with, hot, household appliance
        heating appliance X16
    heating
      appliance (hot) X16
      pad (electric) X16
    hedge-trimmer (powered) W29.3
    hoe W27.1
    hoist (chain) (shaft) NEC W24.0
      agricultural W30.89
    hoof stock NEC W55.39
      bite W55.31
      strike W55.32
    hornet(s) X58
    horse W55.19
      bite W55.11
      strike W55.12
    hot
      air X14.1
        inhalation X14.0
      cooker X15.8
      drinks X10.0
      engine X17
      fats X10.2
      fluids NEC X12
        assault X98.2
        suicide (attempt) X77.2
        undetermined whether accidental or intentional Y27.2
      food X10.1
      gases X14.1
        inhalation X14.0
      heating appliance X16
      household appliance X15.8
        assault X98.3
        cooker X15.8
        hotplate X15.2
        kettle X15.8
        light bulb X15.8
        object NEC X19
          assault X98.8
          stated as undetermined whether accidental or intentional Y27.9
          suicide (attempt) X77.8
        saucepan X15.3

Contact *(continued)*
  with *(continued)*
    hot *(continued)*
      household appliance *(continued)*
        skillet X15.3
        stove X15.0
        stated as undetermined whether accidental or intentional Y27.3
        suicide (attempt) X77.3
        toaster X15.1
      kettle X15.8
      light bulb X15.8
      liquid NEC (*see also* Burn) X12
        drinks X10.0
        stated as undetermined whether accidental or intentional Y27.2
        suicide (attempt) X77.2
        tap water X11.8
          stated as undetermined whether accidental or intentional Y27.1
          suicide (attempt) X77.1
      machinery X17
      metal (molten) (liquid) NEC X18
      object (not producing fire or flames) NEC X19
      oil (cooking) X10.2
      pipe X16
      plate X15.2
      radiator X16
      saucepan (glass) (metal) X15.3
      skillet X15.3
      stove (kitchen) X15.0
      substance NEC X19
      tap-water X11.8
        assault X98.1
        heated on stove X12
          stated as undetermined whether accidental or intentional Y27.2
          suicide (attempt) X77.2
        in bathtub X11.0
        running X11.1
        stated as undetermined whether accidental or intentional Y27.1
        suicide (attempt) X77.1
      toaster X15.1
      tool X17
      vapors X13.1
        inhalation X13.0
      water (tap) X11.8
        boiling X12
          stated as undetermined whether accidental or intentional Y27.2
          suicide (attempt) X77.2
        heated on stove X12
          stated as undetermined whether accidental or intentional Y27.2
          suicide (attempt) X77.2
        in bathtub X11.0
        running X11.1
        stated as undetermined whether accidental or intentional Y27.1
        suicide (attempt) X77.1
    hotplate X15.2
    ice-pick W27.4
    insect (nonvenomous) NEC W57
    kettle (hot) X15.8
    knife W26.0
      assault X99.1
      electric W29.1
      stated as undetermined whether accidental or intentional Y28.1
      suicide (attempt) X78.1

Contact *(continued)*
  with *(continued)*
    lathe (metalworking) W31.1
      turnings W45.8
      woodworking W31.2
    lawnmower (powered) (ridden) W28
      causing electrocution W86.8
        suicide (attempt) X83.1
      unpowered W27.1
    lift, lifting (devices) W24.0
      agricultural operations W30.89
      shaft W24.0
    liquefied gas —*see* Exposure, cold, man-made
    liquid air, hydrogen, nitrogen —*see* Exposure, cold, man-made
    lizard (nonvenomous) W59.09
      bite W59.01
      strike W59.02
    llama —*see* Contact, with, hoof stock NEC
    macaw W61.19
      bite W61.11
      strike W61.12
    machine, machinery W31.9
      abrasive wheel W31.1
      agricultural including animal-powered W30.9
        combine harvester W30.0
        grain storage elevator W30.3
        hay derrick W30.2
        power take-off device W30.1
        reaper W30.0
        specified NEC W30.89
        thresher W30.0
        transport vehicle, stationary W30.81
      band saw W31.2
      bench saw W31.2
      circular saw W31.2
      commercial NEC W31.82
      drilling, metal (industrial) W31.1
      earth-drilling W31.0
      earthmoving or scraping W31.89
      excavating W31.89
      forging machine W31.1
      gas turbine W31.3
      hot X17
      internal combustion engine W31.3
      land drill W31.0
      lathe W31.1
      lifting (devices) W24.0
      metal drill W31.1
      metalworking (industrial) W31.1
      milling, metal W31.1
      mining W31.0
      molding W31.2
      overhead plane W31.2
      power press, metal W31.1
      prime mover W31.3
      printing W31.89
      radial saw W31.2
      recreational W31.81
      roller-coaster W31.81
      rolling mill, metal W31.1
      sander W31.2
      seabed drill W31.0
      shaft
        hoist W31.0
        lift W31.0
      specified NEC W31.89
      spinning W31.89
      steam engine W31.3
      transmission W24.1
      undercutter W31.0
      water driven turbine W31.3
      weaving W31.89
      woodworking or forming (industrial) W31.2

Contact *(continued)*
  with *(continued)*
    mammal (feces) (urine) W55.89
      bull —*see* Contact, with, bull
      cat —*see* Contact, with, cat
      cow —*see* Contact, with, cow
      goat —*see* Contact, with, goat
      hoof stock —*see* Contact, with, hoof stock
      horse —*see* Contact, with, horse
      marine W56.39
        dolphin —*see* Contact, with, dolphin
        orca —*see* Contact, with, orca
        sea lion —*see* Contact, with, sea lion
        specified NEC W56.39
          bite W56.31
          strike W56.32
      pig —*see* Contact, with, pig
      raccoon —*see* Contact, with, raccoon
      rodent —*see* Contact, with, rodent
      sheep —*see* Contact, with, sheep
      specified NEC W55.89
        bite W55.81
        strike W55.82
    marine
      animal W56.89
        bite W56.81
        dolphin —*see* Contact, with, dolphin
        fish NEC —*see* Contact, with, fish
        mammal —*see* Contact, with, mammal, marine
        orca —*see* Contact, with, orca
        sea lion —*see* Contact, with, sea lion
        shark —*see* Contact, with, shark
        strike W56.82
    meat
      grinder (domestic) W29.0
        industrial W31.82
        nonpowered W27.4
      slicer (domestic) W29.0
        industrial W31.82
    merry go round W31.81
    metal, hot (liquid) (molten) NEC X18
    millipede W57
    nail W45.0
      gun W29.4
    needle (sewing) W27.3
      hypodermic W46.0
        contaminated W46.1
    object (blunt) NEC
      hot NEC X19
      legal intervention —*see* Legal, intervention, blunt object
      sharp NEC W45.8
        inflicted by other person NEC W45.8
          stated as
            intentional homicide (attempt) —*see* Assault, cutting or piercing instrument
        legal intervention —*see* Legal, intervention, sharp object
        self-inflicted X78.9
    orca W56.29
      bite W56.21
      strike W56.22
    overhead plane W31.2
    paper (as sharp object) W26.2
    paper-cutter W27.5
    parrot W61.09
      bite W61.01
      strike W61.02

Contact *(continued)*
  with *(continued)*
    pig W55.49
      bite W55.41
      strike W55.42
    pipe, hot X16
    pitchfork W27.1
    plane (metal) (wood) W27.0
      overhead W31.2
    plant thorns, spines, sharp leaves or other mechanisms W60
    powered
      garden cultivator W29.3
      household appliance, implement, or machine W29.8
      saw (industrial) W31.2
        hand W29.8
    printing machine W31.89
    psittacine bird W61.29
      bite W61.21
      macaw —*see* Contact, with, macaw
      parrot —*see* Contact, with, parrot
      strike W61.22
    pulley (block) (transmission) W24.0
      agricultural operations W30.89
    raccoon W55.59
      bite W55.51
      strike W55.52
    radial-saw (industrial) W31.2
    radiator (hot) X16
    rake W27.1
    rattlesnake X58
    reaper W30.0
    reptile W59.89
      lizard —*see* Contact, with, lizard
      snake —*see* Contact, with, snake
      specified NEC W59.89
        bite W59.81
        crushing W59.83
        strike W59.82
      turtle —*see* Contact, with, turtle
    rivet gun (powered) W29.4
    road scraper —*see* Accident, transport, construction vehicle
    rodent (feces) (urine) W53.89
      bite W53.81
      mouse W53.09
        bite W53.01
      rat W53.19
        bite W53.11
      specified NEC W53.89
        bite W53.81
      squirrel W53.29
        bite W53.21
    roller coaster W31.81
    rope NEC W24.0
      agricultural operations W30.89
    saliva —*see* Contact, with, by type of animal
    sander W29.8
      industrial W31.2
    saucepan (hot) (glass) (metal) X15.3
    saw W27.0
      band (industrial) W31.2
      bench (industrial) W31.2
      chain W29.3
      hand W27.0
    sawing machine, metal W31.1
    scissors W27.2
    scorpion X58
    screwdriver W27.0
      powered W29.8
    sea
      anemone, cucumber or urchin (spine) X58
      lion W56.19
        bite W56.11
        strike W56.12
    serpent —*see* Contact, with, snake, by type

Contact *(continued)*
  with *(continued)*
    sewing-machine (electric) (powered) W29.2
      not powered W27.8
    shaft (hoist) (lift) (transmission) NEC W24.0
      agricultural W30.89
    shark W56.49
      bite W56.41
      strike W56.42
    sharp object(s) W26.9
      specified NEC W26.8
    shears (hand) W27.2
      powered (industrial) W31.1
        domestic W29.2
    sheep W55.39
      bite W55.31
      strike W55.32
    shovel W27.8
      steam —*see* Accident, transport, construction vehicl
    snake (nonvenomous) W59.19
      bite W59.11
      crushing W59.13
      strike W59.12
    spade W27.1
    spider (venomous) X58
    spin-drier W29.2
    spinning machine W31.89
    splinter W45.8
    sports equipment W21.9
    staple gun (powered) W29.8
    steam X13.1
      engine W31.3
      inhalation X13.0
      pipe X16
      shovel W31.89
    stove (hot) (kitchen) X15.0
    substance, hot NEC X19
      molten (metal) X18
    sword W26.1
      assault X99.2
      stated as undetermined whether accidental or intentional Y28.2
      suicide (attempt) X78.2
    tarantula X58
    thresher W30.0
    tin can lid W26.8
    toad W62.1
    toaster (hot) X15.1
    tool W27.8
      hand (not powered) W27.8
        auger W27.0
        axe W27.0
        can opener W27.4
        chisel W27.0
        fork W27.4
        garden W27.1
        handsaw W27.0
        hoe W27.1
        ice-pick W27.4
        kitchen utensil W27.4
        manual
          lawn mower W27.1
          sewing machine W27.8
        meat grinder W27.4
        needle (sewing) W27.3
          hypodermic W46.0
            contaminated W46.1
        paper cutter W27.5
        pitchfork W27.1
        rake W27.1
        scissors W27.2
        screwdriver W27.0
        specified NEC W27.8
        workbench W27.0
      hot X17
      powered W29.8

- **Contact** *(continued)*
  - with *(continued)*
    - tool *(continued)*
      - powered *(continued)*
        - blender W29.0
          - commercial W31.82
        - can opener W29.0
          - commercial W31.82
        - chainsaw W29.3
        - clothes dryer W29.2
          - commercial W31.82
        - dishwasher W29.2
          - commercial W31.82
        - edger W29.3
        - electric fan W29.2
          - commercial W31.82
        - electric knife W29.1
        - food processor W29.0
          - commercial W31.82
        - garbage disposal W29.0
          - commercial W31.82
        - garden tool W29.3
        - hedge trimmer W29.3
        - ice maker W29.0
          - commercial W31.82
        - kitchen appliance W29.0
          - commercial W31.82
        - lawn mower W28
        - meat grinder W29.0
          - commercial W31.82
        - mixer W29.0
          - commercial W31.82
        - rototiller W29.3
        - sewing machine W29.2
          - commercial W31.82
        - washing machine W29.2
          - commercial W31.82
    - transmission device (belt, cable, chain, gear, pinion, shaft) W24.1
      - agricultural operations W30.89
    - turbine (gas) (water-driven) W31.3
    - turkey W61.49
      - peck W61.43
      - strike W61.42
    - turtle (nonvenomous) W59.29
      - bite W59.21
      - strike W59.22
      - terrestrial W59.89
        - bite W59.81
        - crushing W59.83
        - strike W59.82
    - under-cutter W31.0
    - urine —*see* Contact, with, by type of animal
    - vehicle
      - agricultural use (transport) —*see* Accident, transport, agricultural vehicle
        - not on public highway W30.81
      - industrial use (transport) —*see* Accident, transport, industrial vehicle
        - not on public highway W31.83
      - off-road use (transport) —*see* Accident, transport, all-terrain or off-road vehicle
        - not on public highway W31.83
      - special construction use (transport) —*see* Accident, transport, construction vehicle
        - not on public highway W31.83
    - venomous
      - animal X58
      - arthropods X58
      - lizard X58
      - marine animal NEC X58
      - marine plant NEC X58
      - millipedes (tropical) X58

- **Contact** *(continued)*
  - with *(continued)*
    - venomous *(continued)*
      - plant(s) X58
      - snake X58
      - spider X58
    - viper X58
    - washing-machine (powered) W29.2
    - wasp X58
    - weaving-machine W31.89
    - winch W24.0
      - agricultural operations W30.89
    - wire NEC W24.0
      - agricultural operations W30.89
    - wood slivers W45.8
    - yellow jacket X58
    - zebra —*see* Contact, with, hoof stock NEC
  - pressure X50.9
  - stress X50.9

- **Coup de soleil** X32

- **Crash**
  - aircraft (in transit) (powered) V95.9
    - balloon V96.01
    - fixed wing NEC (private) V95.21
      - commercial V95.31
    - glider V96.21
      - hang V96.11
      - powered V95.11
    - helicopter V95.01
    - in war operations —*see* War operations, destruction of aircraft
    - microlight V95.11
    - nonpowered V96.9
      - specified NEC V96.8
    - powered NEC V95.8
    - stated as
      - homicide (attempt) Y08.81
      - suicide (attempt) X83.0
    - ultralight V95.11
  - spacecraft V95.41
  - transport vehicle NEC —*see also* Accident, transport V89.9
    - homicide (attempt) Y03.8
    - motor NEC (traffic) V89.2
      - homicide (attempt) Y03.8
      - suicide (attempt) —*see* Suicide, collision

- **Cruelty** (mental) (physical) (sexual) X58

- **Crushed** (accidentally) X58
  - between objects (moving) (stationary and moving) W23.0
    - stationary W23.1
  - by
    - alligator W58.03
    - avalanche NEC —*see* Landslide
    - cave-in W20.0
      - caused by cataclysmic earth surface movement —*see* Landslide
    - crocodile W58.13
    - crowd or human stampede W52
    - falling
      - aircraft V97.39
        - in war operations —*see* War operations, destruction of aircraft
      - earth, material W20.0
        - caused by cataclysmic earth surface movement —*see* Landslide
      - object NEC W20.8
    - landslide NEC —*see* Landslide
    - lizard (nonvenomous) W59.09
    - machinery —*see* Contact, with, by type of machine
    - reptile NEC W59.89
    - snake (nonvenomous) W59.13

- **Crushed** *(continued)*
  - in
    - machinery —*see* Contact, with, by type of machine

- **Cut, cutting** (any part of body) (accidental) —*see also* Contact, with, by object or machine
  - during medical or surgical treatment
    - as misadventure —*see* Index to Diseases and Injuries, Complications
  - homicide (attempt) —*see* Assault, cutting or piercing instrument
  - inflicted by other person —*see* Assault, cutting or piercing instrument
  - legal
    - execution —*see* Legal, intervention
    - intervention —*see* Legal, intervention, sharp object
  - machine NEC —*see also* Contact, with, by type of machine W31.9
  - self-inflicted —*see* Suicide, cutting or piercing instrument
  - suicide (attempt) —*see* Suicide, cutting or piercing instrument

- **Cyclone** (any injury) X37.1

D

- **Decapitation** (accidental circumstances) NEC X58
  - homicide X99.9
  - legal execution —*see* Legal, intervention

- **Dehydration from lack of water** X58

- **Deprivation** X58

- **Derailment** (accidental)
  - railway (rolling stock) (train) (vehicle) (without antecedent collision) V81.7
    - with antecedent collision —*see* Accident, transport, railway vehicle occupant
  - streetcar (without antecedent collision) V82.7
    - with antecedent collision —*see* Accident, transport, streetcar occupant

- **Descent**
  - parachute (voluntary) (without accident to aircraft) V97.29
    - due to accident to aircraft —*see* Accident, transport, aircraft

- **Desertion** X58

- **Destitution** X58

- **Disability, late effect or sequela of injury** —*see* Sequelae

- **Discharge** (accidental)
  - airgun W34.010
    - assault X95.01
    - homicide (attempt) X95.01
    - stated as undetermined whether accidental or intentional Y24.0
    - suicide (attempt) X74.01
  - BB gun —*see* Discharge, airgun
  - firearm (accidental) W34.00
    - assault X95.9
    - handgun (pistol) (revolver) W32.0
      - assault X93
      - homicide (attempt) X93
      - legal intervention —*see* Legal, intervention, firearm, handgun
      - stated as undetermined whether accidental or intentional Y22
      - suicide (attempt) X72

- **Discharge** *(continued)*
  - firearm *(continued)*
    - homicide (attempt) X95.9
    - hunting rifle W33.02
      - assault X94.1
      - homicide (attempt) X94.1
      - legal intervention
        - injuring
          - bystander Y35.032
          - law enforcement personnel Y35.031
          - suspect Y35.033
      - stated as undetermined whether accidental or intentional Y23.1
      - suicide (attempt) X73.1
    - larger W33.00
      - assault X94.9
      - homicide (attempt) X94.9
      - hunting rifle —*see* Discharge, firearm, hunting rifle
    - legal intervention —*see* Legal, intervention, firearm by type of firearm
      - machine gun —*see* Discharge, firearm, machine gun
      - shotgun —*see* Discharge, firearm, shotgun
        - assault X94.8
        - homicide (attempt) X94.8
        - legal intervention
          - injuring
            - bystander Y35.092
            - law enforcement personnel Y35.091
            - suspect Y35.093
        - stated as undetermined whether accidental or intentional Y23.8
      - specified NEC W33.09
        - suicide (attempt) X73.8
      - stated as undetermined whether accidental or intentional Y23.9
      - suicide (attempt) X73.9
    - legal intervention
      - injuring
        - bystander Y35.002
        - law enforcement personnel Y35.001
        - suspect Y35.03
      - using rubber bullet
        - injuring
          - bystander Y35.042
          - law enforcement personnel Y35.041
          - suspect Y35.043
    - machine gun W33.03
      - assault X94.2
      - homicide (attempt) X94.2
      - legal intervention —*see* Legal, intervention, firearm, machine gun
      - stated as undetermined whether accidental or intentional Y23.3
      - suicide (attempt) X73.2
    - pellet gun —*see* Discharge, airgun
    - shotgun W33.01
      - assault X94.0
      - homicide (attempt) X94.0
      - legal intervention —*see* Legal, intervention, firearm, specified NEC
      - stated as undetermined whether accidental or intentional Y23.0
      - suicide (attempt) X73.0
    - specified NEC W34.09
      - assault X95.8
      - homicide (attempt) X95.8
      - legal intervention —*see* Legal, intervention, firearm, specified NEC

- **Discharge** *(continued)*
  - firearm *(continued)*
    - specified NEC *(continued)*
      - stated as undetermined whether accidental or intentional Y24.8
      - suicide (attempt) X74.8
    - stated as undetermined whether accidental or intentional Y24.9
    - suicide (attempt) X74.9
    - Very pistol W34.09
      - assault X95.8
      - homicide (attempt) X95.8
      - stated as undetermined whether accidental or intentional Y24.8
      - suicide (attempt) X74.8
  - firework(s) W39
    - stated as undetermined whether accidental or intentional Y25
  - gas-operated gun NEC W34.018
    - airgun *—see* Discharge, airgun
    - assault X95.09
    - homicide (attempt) X95.09
    - paintball gun *—see* Discharge, paintball gun
    - stated as undetermined whether accidental or intentional Y24.8
    - suicide (attempt) X74.09
  - gun NEC *—see also* Discharge, firearm NEC
    - air *—see* Discharge, airgun
    - BB *—see* Discharge, airgun
    - for single hand use *—see* Discharge, firearm, handgun
    - hand *—see* Discharge, firearm, handgun
    - machine *—see* Discharge, firearm, machine gun
    - other specified *—see* Discharge, firearm NEC
    - paintball *—see* Discharge, paintball gun
    - pellet *—see* Discharge, airgun
  - handgun *—see* Discharge, firearm, handgun
  - machine gun *—see* Discharge, firearm, machine gun
  - paintball gun W34.011
    - assault X95.02
    - homicide (attempt) X95.02
    - stated as undetermined whether accidental or intentional Y24.8
    - suicide (attempt) X74.02
  - pistol *—see* Discharge, firearm, handgun
    - flare *—see* Discharge, firearm, Very pistol
    - pellet *—see* Discharge, airgun
    - Very *—see* Discharge, firearm, Very pistol
  - revolver *—see* Discharge, firearm, handgun
  - rifle (hunting) *—see* Discharge, firearm, hunting rifle
  - shotgun *—see* Discharge, firearm, shotgun
  - spring-operated gun NEC W34.018
    - assault X95.09
    - homicide (attempt) X95.09
    - stated as undetermined whether accidental or intentional Y24.8
    - suicide (attempt) X74.09
- **Disease**
  - Andes W94.11
  - aviator's *—see* Air, pressure
  - range W94.11
- **Diver's disease, palsy, paralysis, squeeze** *—see* Air, pressure
- **Diving** (into water) *—see* Accident, diving
- **Dog bite** W54.0
- **Dragged by transport vehicle NEC** *—see also* Accident, transport V09.9
- **Drinking poison** (accidental) *—see* Table of Drugs and Chemicals
- **Dropped** (accidentally) while being carriedor supported by other person W04
- **Drowning** (accidental) W74
  - assault X92.9
  - due to
    - accident (to)
      - machinery *—see* Contact, with, by type of machine
      - watercraft V90.89
        - burning V90.29
          - powered V90.23
            - fishing boat V90.22
            - jetskis V90.23
            - merchant ship V90.20
            - passenger ship V90.21
          - unpowered V90.28
            - canoe V90.25
            - inflatable V90.26
            - kayak V90.25
            - sailboat V90.24
            - water skis V90.27
        - crushed V90.39
          - powered V90.33
            - fishing boat V90.32
            - jetskis V90.33
            - merchant ship V90.30
            - passenger ship V90.31
          - unpowered V90.38
            - canoe V90.35
            - inflatable V90.36
            - kayak V90.35
            - sailboat V90.34
            - water skis V90.37
        - overturning V90.09
          - powered V90.03
            - fishing boat V90.02
            - jetskis V90.03
            - merchant ship V90.00
            - passenger ship V90.01
          - unpowered V90.08
            - canoe V90.05
            - inflatable V90.06
            - kayak V90.05
            - sailboat V90.04
        - sinking V90.19
          - powered V90.13
            - fishing boat V90.12
            - jetskis V90.13
            - merchant ship V90.10
            - passenger ship V90.11
          - unpowered V90.18
            - canoe V90.15
            - inflatable V90.16
            - kayak V90.15
            - sailboat V90.14
        - specified type NEC V90.89
          - powered V90.83
            - fishing boat V90.82
            - jetskis V90.83
            - merchant ship V90.80
            - passenger ship V90.81
          - unpowered V90.88
            - canoe V90.85
            - inflatable V90.86
            - kayak V90.85
            - sailboat V90.84
            - water skis V90.87
    - avalanche *—see* Landslide
    - cataclysmic
      - earth surface movement NEC *—see* Forces of nature, earth movement
- **Drowning** *(continued)*
  - due to *(continued)*
    - cataclysmic *(continued)*
      - storm *—see* Forces of nature, cataclysmic storm
    - cloudburst X37.8
    - cyclone X37.1
    - fall overboard (from) V92.09
      - powered craft V92.03
        - ferry boat V92.01
        - fishing boat V92.02
        - jetskis V92.03
        - liner V92.01
        - merchant ship V92.00
        - passenger ship V92.01
      - unpowered craft V92.08
        - canoe V92.05
        - inflatable V92.06
        - kayak V92.05
        - sailboat V92.04
        - surf-board V92.08
        - water skis V92.07
        - windsurfer V92.08
      - resulting from
        - accident to watercraft *—see* Drowning, due to, accident to, watercraft
        - being washed overboard (from) V92.29
          - powered craft V92.23
            - ferry boat V92.21
            - fishing boat V92.22
            - jetskis V92.23
            - liner V92.21
            - merchant ship V92.20
            - passenger ship V92.21
          - unpowered craft V92.28
            - canoe V92.25
            - inflatable V92.26
            - kayak V92.25
            - sailboat V92.24
            - surf-board V92.28
            - water skis V92.27
            - windsurfer V92.28
        - motion of watercraft V92.19
          - powered craft V92.13
            - ferry boat V92.11
            - fishing boat V92.12
            - jetskis V92.13
            - liner V92.11
            - merchant ship V92.10
            - passenger ship V92.11
          - unpowered craft
            - canoe V92.15
            - inflatable V92.16
            - kayak V92.15
            - sailboat V92.14
    - hurricane X37.0
    - jumping into water from watercraft (involved in accident) *—see also* Drowning, due to, accident to, watercraft
      - without accident to or on watercraft W16.711
    - tidal wave NEC *—see* Forces of nature, tidal wave
    - torrential rain X37.8
  - following
    - fall
      - into
        - bathtub W16.211
        - bucket W16.221
        - fountain *—see* Drowning, following, fall, into, water, specified NEC
        - quarry *—see* Drowning, following, fall, into, water, specified NEC
        - reservoir *—see* Drowning, following, fall, into, water, specified NEC
- **Drowning** *(continued)*
  - following *(continued)*
    - fall *(continued)*
      - into *(continued)*
        - swimming-pool W16.011
          - striking
            - bottom W16.021
            - wall W16.031
          - stated as undetermined whether accidental or intentional Y21.3
          - suicide (attempt) X71.2
        - water NOS W16.41
          - natural (lake) (open sea) (river) (stream) (pond) W16.111
            - striking
              - bottom W16.121
              - side W16.131
          - specified NEC W16.311
            - striking
              - bottom W16.321
              - wall W16.331
      - overboard NEC *—see* Drowning, due to, fall overboard
    - jump or dive
      - from boat W16.711
        - striking bottom W16.721
      - into
        - fountain *—see* Drowning, following, jump or dive, into, water, specified NEC
        - quarry *—see* Drowning, following, jump or dive, into, water, specified NEC
        - reservoir *—see* Drowning, following, jump or dive, into, water, specified NEC
        - swimming-pool W16.511
          - striking
            - bottom W16.521
            - wall W16.531
          - suicide (attempt) X71.2
        - water NOS W16.91
          - natural (lake) (open sea) (river) (stream) (pond) W16.611
          - specified NEC W16.811
            - striking
              - bottom W16.821
              - wall W16.831
          - striking bottom W16.621
  - homicide (attempt) X92.9
  - in
    - bathtub (accidental) W65
      - assault X92.0
      - following fall W16.211
        - stated as undetermined whether accidental or intentional Y21.1
      - stated as undetermined whether accidental or intentional Y21.0
      - suicide (attempt) X71.0
    - lake *—see* Drowning, in, natural water
    - natural water (lake) (open sea) (river) (stream) (pond) W69
      - assault X92.3
      - following
        - dive or jump W16.611
          - striking bottom W16.621
        - fall W16.111
          - striking
            - bottom W16.121
            - side W16.131
      - stated as undetermined whether accidental or intentional Y21.4
      - suicide (attempt) X71.3

rowning *(continued)*
in *(continued)*
quarry —*see* Drowning, in, specified place NEC
quenching tank —*see* Drowning, in, specified place NEC
reservoir —*see* Drowning, in, specified place NEC
river —*see* Drowning, in, natural water
sea —*see* Drowning, in, natural water
specified place NEC W73
assault X92.8
following
dive or jump W16.811
striking
bottom W16.821
wall W16.831
fall W16.311
striking
bottom W16.321
wall W16.331
stated as undetermined whether accidental or intentional Y21.8
suicide (attempt) X71.8
stream —*see* Drowning, in, natural water
swimming-pool W67
assault X92.1
following fall X92.2
following
dive or jump W16.511
striking
bottom W16.521
wall W16.531
fall W16.011
striking
bottom W16.021
wall W16.031
stated as undetermined whether accidental or intentional Y21.2
following fall Y21.3
suicide (attempt) X71.1
following fall X71.2
war operations —*see* War operations, restriction of airway
resulting from accident to watercraft *see* Drowning, due to, accident, watercraft
self-inflicted X71.9
stated as undetermined whether accidental or intentional Y21.9
suicide (attempt) X71.9

E

arth (surface) movement NEC —*see* Forces of nature, earth movement
arth falling (on) W20.0
caused by cataclysmic earth surface movement or eruption —*see* Landslide
arthquake (any injury) X34
ffect(s) (adverse) of
air pressure (any)- —*see* Air, pressure
cold, excessive (exposure to) —*see* Exposure, cold
heat (excessive) —*see* Heat
hot place (weather) —*see* Heat
insolation X30
late —*see* Sequelae
motion —*see* Motion
nuclear explosion or weapon in war operations —*see* War operations, nuclear weapon
radiation —*see* Radiation
travel —*see* Travel

Electric shock (accidental) (by) (in) —*see* Exposure, electric current
Electrocution (accidental) —*see* Exposure, electric current
Endotracheal tube wrongly placed during anesthetic procedure
Entanglement
in
bed linen, causing suffocation —*see* categories T71
wheel of pedal cycle V19.88
Entry of foreign body or material —*see* Foreign body
Environmental pollution related condition —*see* Z57
Execution, legal (any method) —*see* Legal, intervention
Exhaustion
cold —*see* Exposure, cold
due to excessive exertion (*see also* Overexertion) X50.9
heat —*see* Heat
Explosion (accidental) (of) (with secondary fire) W40.9
acetylene W40.1
aerosol can W36.1
air tank (compressed) (in machinery) W36.2
aircraft (in transit) (powered) NEC V95.9
balloon V96.05
fixed wing NEC (private) V95.25
commercial V95.35
glider V96.25
hang V96.15
powered V95.15
helicopter V95.05
in war operations —*see* War operations, destruction of aircraft
microlight V95.15
nonpowered V96.9
specified NEC V96.8
powered NEC V95.8
stated as
homicide (attempt) Y03.8
suicide (attempt) X83.0
ultralight V95.15
anesthetic gas in operating room W40.1
antipersonnel bomb W40.8
assault X96.0
homicide (attempt) X96.0
suicide (attempt) X75
assault X96.9
bicycle tire W37.0
blasting (cap) (materials) W40.0
boiler (machinery), not on transport vehicle W35
on watercraft —*see* Explosion, in, watercraft
butane W40.1
caused by other person X96.9
coal gas W40.1
detonator W40.0
dump (munitions) W40.8
dynamite W40.0
in
assault X96.8
homicide (attempt) X96.8
legal intervention
injuring
bystander Y35.112
law enforcement personnel Y35.111
suspect Y35.113
suicide (attempt) X75
explosive (material) W40.9
gas W40.1

Explosion *(continued)*
explosive *(continued)*
in blasting operation W40.0
specified NEC W40.8
in
assault X96.8
homicide (attempt) X96.8
legal intervention
injuring
bystander Y35.192
law enforcement personnel Y35.191
suspect Y35.193
suicide (attempt) X75
factory (munitions) W40.8
fertilizer bomb W40.8
assault X96.3
homicide (attempt) X96.3
suicide (attempt) X75
firearm (parts) NEC W34.19
airgun W34.110
BB gun W34.110
gas, air or spring-operated gun NEC W34.118
hangun W32.1
hunting rifle W33.12
larger firearm W33.10
specified NEC W33.19
machine gun W33.13
paintball gun W34.111
pellet gun W34.110
shotgun W33.11
Very pistol [flare] W34.19
fire-damp W40.1
fireworks W39
gas (coal) (explosive) W40.1
cylinder W36.9
aerosol can W36.1
air tank W36.2
pressurized W36.3
specified NEC W36.8
gasoline (fumes) (tank) not in moving motor vehicle W40.1
bomb W40.8
assault X96.1
homicide (attempt) X96.1
suicide (attempt) X75
in motor vehicle —*see* Accident, transport, by type of vehicle
grain store W40.8
grenade W40.8
in
assault X96.8
homicide (attempt) X96.8
legal intervention
injuring
bystander Y35.192
law enforcement personnel Y35.191
suspect Y35.193
suicide (attempt) X75
handgun (parts) —*see* Explosion, firearm, hangun (parts)
homicide (attempt) X96.9
antipersonnel bomb —*see* Explosion, antipersonnel bomb
fertilizer bomb —*see* Explosion, fertilizer bomb
gasoline bomb —*see* Explosion, gasoline bomb
letter bomb —*see* Explosion, letter bomb
pipe bomb —*see* Explosion, pipe bomb
specified NEC X96.8
hose, pressurized W37.8
hot water heater, tank (in machinery) W35
on watercraft —*see* Explosion, in, watercraft

Explosion *(continued)*
in, on
dump W40.8
factory W40.8
mine (of explosive gases) NEC W40.1
watercraft V93.59
powered craft V93.53
ferry boat V93.51
fishing boat V93.52
jetskis V93.53
liner V93.51
merchant ship V93.50
passenger ship V93.51
sailboat V93.54
letter bomb W40.8
assault X96.2
homicide (attempt) X96.2
suicide (attempt) X75
machinery —*see also* Contact, with, by type of machine
on board watercraft —*see* Explosion, in, watercraft
pressure vessel —*see* Explosion, by type of vessel
methane W40.1
mine W40.1
missile NEC W40.8
mortar bomb W40.8
in
assault X96.8
homicide (attempt) X96.8
legal intervention
injuring
bystander Y35.192
law enforcement personnel Y35.191
suspect Y35.193
suicide (attempt) X75
munitions (dump) (factory) W40.8
pipe, pressurized W37.8
bomb W40.8
assault X96.4
homicide (attempt) X96.4
suicide (attempt) X75
pressure, pressurized
cooker W38
gas tank (in machinery) W36.3
hose W37.8
pipe W37.8
specified device NEC W38
tire W37.8
bicycle W37.0
vessel (in machinery) W38
propane W40.1
self-inflicted X75
shell (artillery) NEC W40.8
during war operations —*see* War operations, explosion
in
legal intervention
injuring
bystander Y35.122
law enforcement personnel Y35.121
suspect Y35.123
war —*see* War operations, explosion
spacecraft V95.45
stated as undetermined whether accidental or intentional Y25
steam or water lines (in machinery) W37.8
stove W40.9
suicide (attempt) X75
tire, pressurized W37.8
bicycle W37.0
undetermined whether accidental or intentional Y25
vehicle tire NEC W37.8
bicycle W37.0

Explosion *(continued)*
- war operations —*see* War operations, explosion

Exposure (to) X58
- air pressure change —*see* Air, pressure
- cold (accidental) (excessive) (extreme) (natural) (place) X31
  - assault Y08.89
  - due to
    - man-made conditions W93.8
      - dry ice (contact) W93.01
        - inhalation W93.02
      - liquid air (contact) (hydrogen) (nitrogen) W93.11
        - inhalation W93.12
      - refrigeration unit (deep freeze) W93.2
      - suicide (attempt) X83.2
    - weather (conditions) X31
  - homicide (attempt) Y08.89
  - self-inflicted X83.2
- due to abandonment or neglect X58
- electric current W86.8
  - appliance (faulty) W86.8
    - domestic W86.0
  - caused by other person Y08.89
  - conductor (faulty) W86.1
  - control apparatus (faulty) W86.1
  - electric power generating plant, distribution station W86.1
  - electroshock gun —*see* Exposure, electric current, taser
  - high-voltage cable W85
  - homicide (attempt) Y08.89
  - legal execution —*see* Legal, intervention, specified means NEC
  - lightning —*see* subcategory T75.0
  - live rail W86.8
  - misadventure in medical or surgical procedure in electroshock therapy Y63.4
  - motor (electric) (faulty) W86.8
    - domestic W86.0
  - self-inflicted X83.1
  - specified NEC W86.8
    - domestic W86.0
  - stun gun —*see* Exposure, electric current, taser
  - suicide (attempt) X83.1
  - taser W86.8
    - assault Y08.89
    - legal intervention —*see* categories Y35
    - self-harm (intentional) X83.8
    - undetermined intent Y33
  - third rail W86.8
  - transformer (faulty) W86.1
  - transmission lines W85
- environmental tobacco smoke X58
- excessive
  - cold —*see* Exposure, cold
  - heat (natural) NEC X30
    - man-made W92
- factor(s) NOS X58
  - environmental NEC X58
    - man-made NEC W99
    - natural NEC —*see* Forces of nature
  - specified NEC X58
- fire, flames (accidental) X08.8
  - assault X97
  - campfire —*see* Exposure, fire, controlled, not in building
  - controlled (in)
    - with ignition (of) clothing —*see also* Ignition, clothes X06.2
      - nightwear X05
    - bonfire —*see* Exposure, fire, controlled, not in building

Exposure *(continued)*
- fire, flames *(continued)*
  - controlled *(continued)*
    - brazier (in building or structure) —*see also* Exposure, fire, controlled, building
      - not in building or structure —*see* Exposure, fire, controlled, not in building
    - building or structure X02.0
      - with
        - fall from building X02.3
        - injury due to building collapse X02.2
        - from building X02.5
        - smoke inhalation X02.1
      - hit by object from building X02.4
      - specified mode of injury NEC X02.8
    - fireplace, furnace or stove —*see* Exposure, fire, controlled, building
    - not in building or structure X03.0
      - with
        - fall X03.3
        - smoke inhalation X03.1
      - hit by object X03.4
      - specified mode of injury NEC X03.8
    - trash —*see* Exposure, fire, controlled, not in building
  - fireplace —*see* Exposure, fire, controlled, building
  - fittings or furniture (in building or structure) (uncontrolled) —*see* Exposure, fire, uncontrolled, building
  - forest (uncontrolled) —*see* Exposure, fire, uncontrolled, not in building
  - grass (uncontrolled) —*see* Exposure, fire, uncontrolled, not in building
  - hay (uncontrolled) —*see* Exposure, fire, uncontrolled, not in building
  - homicide (attempt) X97
  - ignition of highly flammable material X04
  - in, of, on, starting in
    - machinery —*see* Contact, with, by type of machine
    - motor vehicle (in motion) —*see also* Accident, transport, occupant by type of vehicle V87.8
      - with collision —*see* Collision
    - railway rolling stock, train, vehicle V81.81
      - with collision —*see* Accident, transport, railway vehicle occupant
    - street car (in motion) V82.8
      - with collision —*see* Accident, transport, streetcar occupant
    - transport vehicle NEC —*see also* Accident, transport
      - with collision —*see* Collision
    - war operations —*see also* War operations, fire
      - from nuclear explosion —*see* War operations, nuclear weapons
    - watercraft (in transit) (not in transit) V91.09
      - localized —*see* Burn, on board watercraft, due to, fire on board

Exposure *(continued)*
- fire, flames *(continued)*
  - in, of, on, starting in *(continued)*
    - watercraft *(continued)*
      - powered craft V91.03
        - ferry boat V91.01
        - fishing boat V91.02
        - jet skis V91.03
        - liner V91.01
        - merchant ship V91.00
        - passenger ship V91.01
      - unpowered craft V91.08
        - canoe V91.05
        - inflatable V91.06
        - kayak V91.05
        - sailboat V91.04
        - surf-board V91.08
        - waterskis V91.07
        - windsurfer V91.08
  - lumber (uncontrolled) —*see* Exposure, fire, uncontrolled, not in building
  - mine (uncontrolled) —*see* Exposure, fire, uncontrolled, not in building
  - prairie (uncontrolled) —*see* Exposure, fire, uncontrolled, not in building
  - resulting from
    - explosion —*see* Explosion
    - lightning X08.8
  - self-inflicted X76
  - specified NEC X08.8
  - started by other person X97
  - stated as undetermined whether accidental or intentional Y26
  - stove —*see* Exposure, fire, controlled, building
  - suicide (attempt) X76
  - tunnel (uncontrolled) —*see* Exposure, fire, uncontrolled, not in building
  - uncontrolled
    - in building or structure X00.0
      - with
        - fall from building X00.3
        - injury due to building collapse X00.2
      - jump from building X00.5
        - smoke inhalation X00.1
      - bed X08.00
        - due to
          - cigarette X08.01
          - specified material NEC X08.09
      - furniture NEC X08.20
        - due to
          - cigarette X08.21
          - specified material NEC X08.29
      - hit by object from building X00.4
      - sofa X08.10
        - due to
          - cigarette X08.11
          - specified material NEC X08.19
      - specified mode of injury NEC X00.8
    - not in building or structure (any) X01.0
      - with
        - fall X01.3
        - smoke inhalation X01.1
      - hit by object X01.4
      - specified mode of injury NEC X01.8
    - undetermined whether accidental or intentional Y26
- forces of nature NEC —*see* Forces of nature

Exposure *(continued)*
- G-forces (abnormal) W49.9
- gravitational forces (abnormal) W49.9
- heat (natural) NEC —*see* Heat
- high-pressure jet (hydraulic) (pneumatic) W49.9
- hydraulic jet W49.9
- inanimate mechanical force W49.9
- jet, high-pressure (hydraulic) (pneumatic) W49.9
- lightning —*see* subcategory T75.0
  - causing fire —*see* Exposure, fire
- mechanical forces NEC W49.9
  - animate NEC W64
  - inanimate NEC W49.9
- noise W42.9
  - supersonic W42.0
- noxious substance —*see* Table of Drugs and Chemical
- pneumatic jet W49.9
- prolonged in deep-freeze unit or refrigerator W93.2
- radiation —*see* Radiation
- smoke —*see also* Exposure, fire
  - tobacco, second hand Z77.22
- specified factors NEC X58
- sunlight X32
  - man-made (sun lamp) W89.8
    - tanning bed W89.1
- supersonic waves W42.0
- transmission line(s), electric W85
- vibration W49.9
- waves
  - infrasound W49.9
  - sound W42.9
  - supersonic W42.0
- weather NEC —*see* Forces of nature

External cause status Y99.9
- child assisting in compensated work for family Y99.8
- civilian activity done for financial or other compensation Y99.0
- civilian activity done for income or pay Y99.0
- family member assisting in compensated work for other family member Y99.8
- hobby not done for income Y99.8
- leisure activity Y99.8
- military activity Y99.1
- off-duty activity of military personnel Y99.8
- recreation or sport not for income or while a student Y99.8
- specified NEC Y99.8
- student activity Y99.8
- volunteer activity Y99.2

F

Factors, supplemental
- alcohol
  - blood level
    - less than 20mg/100ml Y90.0
    - presence in blood, level not specified Y90.9
    - 20-39mg/100ml Y90.1
    - 40-59mg/100ml Y90.2
    - 60-79mg/100ml Y90.3
    - 80-99mg/100ml Y90.4
    - 100-119mg/100ml Y90.5
    - 120-199mg/100ml Y90.6
    - 200-239mg/100ml Y90.7
    - 240mg/100ml or more Y90.8
  - presence in blood, but level not specified Y90.9
- environmental-pollution-related condition- *see* Z57
- nosocomial condition Y95
- work-related condition Y99.0

ilure
in suture or ligature during surgical procedure Y65.2
mechanical, of instrument or apparatus (any) (during any medical or surgical procedure) Y65.8
sterile precautions (during medical and surgical care) *—see* Misadventure, failure, sterile precautions, by type of procedure
to
introduce tube or instrument Y65.4
endotracheal tube during anesthesia Y65.3
make curve (transport vehicle) NEC *—see* Accident, transport
remove tube or instrument Y65.4
ll, falling (accidental) W19
building W20.1
burning (uncontrolled fire) X00.3
down
embankment W17.81
escalator W10.0
hill W17.81
ladder W11
ramp W10.2
stairs, steps W10.9
due to
bumping against
object W18.00
sharp glass W18.02
specified NEC W18.09
sports equipment W18.01
person W03
due to ice or snow W00.0
on pedestrian conveyance *—see* Accident, transport, pedestrian, conveyance
collision with another person W03
due to ice or snow W00.0
involving pedestrian conveyance *—see* Accident, transport, pedestrian, conveyance
grocery cart tipping over W17.82
ice or snow W00.9
from one level to another W00.2
on stairs or steps W00.1
involving pedestrian conveyance *—see* Accident, transport, pedestrian, conveyance
on same level W00.0
slipping (on moving sidewalk) W01.0
with subsequent striking against object W01.10
furniture W01.190
sharp object W01.119
glass W01.110
power tool or machine W01.111
specified NEC W01.118
specified NEC W01.198
striking against
object W18.00
sharp glass W18.02
specified NEC W18.09
sports equipment W18.01
person W03
due to ice or snow W00.0
on pedestrian conveyance *—see* Accident, transport, pedestrian, conveyance
earth (with asphyxia or suffocation (by pressure)) *—see* Earth, falling
from, off, out of
aircraft NEC (with accident to aircraft NEC) V97.0
while boarding or alighting V97.1

Fall, falling *(continued)*
from, off, out of *(continued)*
balcony W13.0
bed W06
boat, ship, watercraft NEC (with drowning or submersion) *—see* Drowning, due to, fall overboard
with hitting bottom or object V94.0
bridge W13.1
building W13.9
burning (uncontrolled fire) X00.3
cavity W17.2
chair W07
cherry picker W17.89
cliff W15
dock W17.4
embankment W17.81
escalator W10.0
flagpole W13.8
furniture NEC W08
grocery cart W17.82
haystack W17.89
high place NEC W17.89
stated as undetermined whether accidental or intentional Y30
hole W17.2
incline W10.2
ladder W11
lifting device W17.89
machine, machinery *—see also* Contact, with, by type of machine
not in operation W17.89
manhole W17.1
mobile elevated work platform [MEWP] W17.89
motorized mobility scooter W05.2
one level to another NEC W17.89
intentional, purposeful, suicide (attempt) X80
stated as undetermined whether accidental or intentional Y30
pit W17.2
playground equipment W09.8
jungle gym W09.2
slide W09.0
swing W09.1
quarry W17.89
railing W13.9
ramp W10.2
roof W13.2
scaffolding W12
scooter (nonmotorized) W05.1
motorized mobility W05.2
sky lift W17.89
stairs, steps W10.9
curb W10.1
due to ice or snow W00.1
escalator W10.0
incline W10.2
ramp W10.2
sidewalk curb W10.1
specified NEC W10.8
stepladder W11
storm drain W17.1
streetcar NEC V82.6
with antecedent collision *—see* Accident, transport, streetcar occupant
while boarding or alighting V82.4
structure NEC W13.8
burning (uncontrolled fire) X00.3
table W08
toilet W18.11
with subsequent striking against object W18.12
train NEC V81.6

Fall, falling *(continued)*
from, off, out of *(continued)*
train NEC *(continued)*
during derailment (without antecedent collision) V81.7
with antecedent collision *—see* Accident, transport, railway vehicle occupant
while boarding or alighting V81.4
transport vehicle after collision *—see* Accident, transport, by type of vehicle, collision
tree W14
vehicle (in motion) NEC *—see also* Accident, transport V89.9
motor NEC *—see also* Accident, transport, occupant, by type of vehicle V87.8
stationary W17.89
while boarding or alighting *—see* Accident, transport, by type of vehicle, while boarding or alighting
viaduct W13.8
wall W13.8
watercraft *—see also* Drowning, due to, fall overboard
with hitting bottom or object V94.0
well W17.0
wheelchair, non-moving W05.0
powered *—see* Accident, transport, pedestrian, conveyance occupant, specified type NEC
window W13.4
in, on
aircraft NEC V97.0
with accident to aircraft V97.0
while boarding or alighting V97.1
bathtub (empty) W18.2
filled W16.212
causing drowning W16.211
escalator W10.0
incline W10.2
ladder W11
machine, machinery *—see* Contact, with, by type of machine
object, edged, pointed or sharp (with cut) *—see* Fall, by type
playground equipment W09.8
jungle gym W09.2
slide W09.0
swing W09.1
ramp W10.2
scaffolding W12
shower W18.2
causing drowning W16.211
staircase, stairs, steps W10.9
curb W10.1
due to ice or snow W00.1
escalator W10.0
incline W10.2
specified NEC W10.8
streetcar (without antecedent collision) V82.5
with antecedent collision *—see* Accident, transport, streetcar occupant
while boarding or alighting V82.4
train (without antecedent collision) V81.5
with antecedent collision *—see* Accident, transport, railway vehicle occupant
during derailment (without antecedent collision) V81.7

Fall, falling *(continued)*
in, on *(continued)*
train *(continued)*
during derailment *(continued)*
with antecedent collision *—see* Accident, transport, railway vehicle occupant
while boarding or alighting V81.4
transport vehicle after collision *—see* Accident, transport, by type of vehicle, collision
watercraft V93.39
due to
accident to craft V91.29
powered craft V91.23
ferry boat V91.21
fishing boat V91.22
jetskis V91.23
liner V91.21
merchant ship V91.20
passenger ship V91.21
unpowered craft
canoe V91.25
inflatable V91.26
kayak V91.25
sailboat V91.24
powered craft V93.33
ferry boat V93.31
fishing boat V93.32
jetskis V93.33
liner V93.31
merchant ship V93.30
passenger ship V93.31
unpowered craft V93.38
canoe V93.35
inflatable V93.36
kayak V93.35
sailboat V93.34
surf-board V93.38
windsurfer V93.38
into
cavity W17.2
dock W17.4
fire *—see* Exposure, fire, by type
haystack W17.89
hole W17.2
manhole W17.1
moving part of machinery *—see* Contact, with, by type of machine
ocean *—see* Fall, into, water
opening in surface NEC W17.89
pit W17.2
pond *—see* Fall, into, water
quarry W17.89
river *—see* Fall, into, water
shaft W17.89
storm drain W17.1
stream *—see* Fall, into, water
swimming pool *—see also* Fall, into, water, in, swimming pool
empty W17.3
tank W17.89
water W16.42
causing drowning W16.41
from watercraft *—see* Drowning, due to, fall overboard
hitting diving board W21.4
in
bathtub W16.212
causing drowning W16.211
bucket W16.222
causing drowning W16.221
natural body of water W16.112
causing drowning W16.111
striking
bottom W16.122

Fall, falling *(continued)*
into *(continued)*
water *(continued)*
in *(continued)*
natural body of water *(continued)*
striking *(continued)*
bottom *(continued)*
causing drowning W16.121
side W16.132
causing drowning W16.131
specified water NEC W16.312
causing drowning W16.311
striking
bottom W16.322
causing drowning W16.321
wall W16.332
causing drowning W16.331
swimming pool W16.012
causing drowning W16.011
striking
bottom W16.022
causing drowning W16.021
wall W16.032
causing drowning W16.031
utility bucket W16.222
causing drowning W16.221
well W17.0
involving
bed W06
chair W07
furniture NEC W08
glass —*see* Fall, by type
playground equipment W09.8
jungle gym W09.2
slide W09.0
swing W09.1
roller blades —*see* Accident, transport, pedestrian, conveyance
skateboard(s) —*see* Accident, transport, pedestrian, conveyance
skates (ice) (in line) (roller) —*see* Accident, transport, pedestrian, conveyance
skis —*see* Accident, transport, pedestrian, conveyance
table W08
wheelchair, non-moving W05.0
powered —*see* Accident, transport, pedestrian, conveyance, specified type NEC
object —*see* Struck by, object, falling
off
toilet W18.11
with subsequent striking against object W18.12
on same level W18.30
due to
specified NEC W18.39
stepping on an object W18.31
out of
bed W06
building NEC W13.8
chair W07
furniture NEC W08
wheelchair, non-moving W05.0
powered —*see* Accident, transport, pedestrian, conveyance, specified type NEC
window W13.4
over
animal W01.0
cliff W15

Fall, falling *(continued)*
over *(continued)*
embankment W17.81
small object W01.0
rock W20.8
same level W18.30
from
being crushed, pushed, or stepped on by a crowd or human stampede W52
collision, pushing, shoving, by or with other person W03
slipping, stumbling, tripping W01.0
involving ice or snow W00.0
involving skates (ice) (roller), skateboard, skis —*see* Accident, transport, pedestrian, conveyance
snowslide (avalanche) —*see* Landslide
stone W20.8
structure W20.1
burning (uncontrolled fire) X00.3
through
bridge W13.1
floor W13.3
roof W13.2
wall W13.8
window W13.4
timber W20.8
tree (caused by lightning) W20.8
while being carried or supported by other person(s) W04

Fallen on by
animal (not being ridden) NEC W55.89

Felo-de-se —*see* Suicide

Fight (hand) (fists) (foot) —*see* Assault, fight

Fire (accidental) —*see* Exposure, fire

Firearm discharge —*see* Discharge, firearm

Fireball effects from nuclear explosion in war operations —*see* War operations, nuclear weapons

Fireworks (explosion) W39

Flash burns from explosion —*see* Explosion

Flood (any injury) (caused by) X38
collapse of man-made structure causing earth movement X36.0
tidal wave —*see* Forces of nature, tidal wave

Food (any type) in
air passages (with asphyxia, obstruction, or suffocation) —*see* categories T17 and T18
alimentary tract causing asphyxia (due to compression of trachea) —*see* categories T17 and T18

Forces of nature X39.8
avalanche X36.1
causing transport accident —*see* Accident, transport, by type of vehicle
blizzard X37.2
cataclysmic storm X37.9
with flood X38
blizzard X37.2
cloudburst X37.8
cyclone X37.1
dust storm X37.3
hurricane X37.0
specified storm NEC X37.8
storm surge X37.0
tornado X37.1

Forces of nature *(continued)*
cataclysmic storm *(continued)*
twister X37.1
typhoon X37.0
cloudburst X37.8
cold (natural) X31
cyclone X37.1
dam collapse causing earth movementX36.0
dust storm X37.3
earth movement X36.1
earthquake X34
caused by dam or structure collapse X36.0
earthquake X34
flood (caused by) X38
dam collapse X36.0
tidal wave —*see* Forces of nature, tidal wave
heat (natural) X30
hurricane X37.0
landslide X36.1
causing transport accident —*see* Accident, transport, by type of vehicle
lightning —*see subcategory* T75.0
causing fire —*see* Exposure, fire
mudslide X36.1
causing transport accident —*see* Accident, transport, by type of vehicle
radiation (natural) X39.08
radon X39.01
radon X39.01
specified force NEC X39.8
storm surge X37.0
structure collapse causing earth movement X36.0
sunlight X32
tidal wave X37.41
due to
earthquake X37.41
landslide X37.43
storm X37.42
volcanic eruption X37.41
tornado X37.1
tsunami X37.41
twister X37.1
typhoon X37.0
volcanic eruption X35

Foreign body
aspiration —*see* Index to Diseases and Injuries, Foreign body, respiratory tract
embedded in skin W45.-
entering through skin W45.8
can lid W26.8
nail W45.0
paper W26.2
specified NEC W45.8
splinter W45.8

Forest fire (exposure to) —*see* Exposure, fire, uncontrolled, not in building

Found injured X58
from exposure (to) —*see* Exposure
on
highway, road (way), street V89.9
railway right of way V81.9

Fracture (circumstances unknown or unspecified) X58
due to specified cause NEC X58

Freezing —*see* Exposure, cold

Frostbite X31
due to man-made conditions —*see* Exposure, cold, man-made

Frozen —*see* Exposure, cold

G

Gored by bull W55.22

Gunshot wound W34.00

H

Hailstones, injured by X39.8

Hanged herself or himself —*see* Hanging, self-inflicted

Hanging (accidental) —*see also* category T71
legal execution —*see* Legal, intervention, specified means NE

Heat (effects of) (excessive) X30
due to
man-made conditions W92
on board watercraft V93.29
fishing boat V93.22
merchant ship V93.20
passenger ship V93.21
sailboat V93.24
specified powered craft NEC V93.23
weather (conditions) X30
from
electric heating apparatus causing burning X16
nuclear explosion in war operations —*see* War operations, nuclear weapons
inappropriate in local application or packing in medical or surgical procedure Y63.5

Hemorrhage
delayed following medical or surgical treatment without mention of misadventure —*see* Index to Diseases and Injuries, Complication(s)
during medical or surgical treatment as misadventure —*see* Index to Diseases and Injuries, Complication(s)

High
altitude (effects) —*see* Air, pressure, low
level of radioactivity, effects —*see* Radiation
pressure (effects) —*see* Air, pressure, high
temperature, effects —*see* Heat

Hit, hitting (accidental) by —*see* Struck by

Hitting against —*see* Striking against

Homicide (attempt) (justifiable) —*see* Assault

Hot
place, effects —*see also* Heat
weather, effects X30

House fire (uncontrolled) —*see* Exposure, fire, uncontrolled, building

Humidity, causing problem X39.8

Hunger X58

Hurricane (any injury) X37.0

Hypobarism, hypobaropathy —*see* Air, pressure, low

I

Ictus
caloris —*see also* Heat
solaris X30

Ignition (accidental)
- *—see also* Exposure, fire X08.8
- anesthetic gas in operating room W40.1
- apparel X06.2
  - from highly flammable material X04
  - nightwear X05
- bed linen (sheets) (spreads) (pillows) (mattress) *—see* Exposure, fire, uncontrolled, building, bed
- benzine X04
- clothes, clothing NEC (from controlled fire) X06.2
  - from
    - highly flammable material X04
- ether X04
  - in operating room W40.1
- explosive material *—see* Explosion
- gasoline X04
- jewelry (plastic) (any) X06.0
- kerosene X04
- material
  - explosive *—see* Explosion
  - highly flammable with secondary explosion X04
- nightwear X05
- paraffin X04
- petrol X04

Immersion (accidental)
- *—see also* Drowning
- hand or foot due to cold (excessive) X31

Implantation of quills of porcupine W55.89

Inanition (from) (hunger) X58
- thirst X58

Inappropriate operation performed
- correct operation on wrong side or body part (wrong side) (wrong site) Y65.53
- operation intended for another patient done on wrong patient Y65.52
- wrong operation performed on correct patient Y65.51

Inattention after, at birth (homicidal intent) (infanticidal intent) X58

Incident, adverse
- device
  - anesthesiology Y70.8
    - accessory Y70.2
    - diagnostic Y70.0
    - miscellaneous Y70.8
    - monitoring Y70.0
    - prosthetic Y70.2
    - rehabilitative Y70.1
    - surgical Y70.3
    - therapeutic Y70.1
  - cardiovascular Y71.8
    - accessory Y71.2
    - diagnostic Y71.0
    - miscellaneous Y71.8
    - monitoring Y71.0
    - prosthetic Y71.2
    - rehabilitative Y71.1
    - surgical Y71.3
    - therapeutic Y71.1
  - gastroenterology Y73.8
    - accessory Y73.2
    - diagnostic Y73.0
    - miscellaneous Y73.8
    - monitoring Y73.0
    - prosthetic Y73.2
    - rehabilitative Y73.1
    - surgical Y73.3
    - therapeutic Y73.1
  - general
    - hospital Y74.8
      - accessory Y74.2

Incident, adverse *(continued)*
- device *(continued)*
  - general *(continued)*
    - hospital *(continued)*
      - diagnostic Y74.0
      - miscellaneous Y74.8
      - monitoring Y74.0
      - prosthetic Y74.2
      - rehabilitative Y74.1
      - surgical Y74.3
      - therapeutic Y74.1
    - surgical Y81.8
      - accessory Y81.2
      - diagnostic Y81.0
      - miscellaneous Y81.8
      - monitoring Y81.0
      - prosthetic Y81.2
      - rehabilitative Y81.1
      - surgical Y81.3
      - therapeutic Y81.1
  - gynecological Y76.8
    - accessory Y76.2
    - diagnostic Y76.0
    - miscellaneous Y76.8
    - monitoring Y76.0
    - prosthetic Y76.2
    - rehabilitative Y76.1
    - surgical Y76.3
    - therapeutic Y76.1
  - medical Y82.9
    - specified type NEC Y82.8
  - neurological Y75.8
    - accessory Y75.2
    - diagnostic Y75.0
    - miscellaneous Y75.8
    - monitoring Y75.0
    - prosthetic Y75.2
    - rehabilitative Y75.1
    - surgical Y75.3
    - therapeutic Y75.1
  - obstetrical Y76.8
    - accessory Y76.2
    - diagnostic Y76.0
    - miscellaneous Y76.8
    - monitoring Y76.0
    - prosthetic Y76.2
    - rehabilitative Y76.1
    - surgical Y76.3
    - therapeutic Y76.1
  - ophthalmic Y77.8
    - accessory Y77.2
    - diagnostic Y77.0
    - miscellaneous Y77.8
    - monitoring Y77.0
    - prosthetic Y77.2
    - rehabilitative Y77.1
    - surgical Y77.3
    - therapeutic Y77.1
  - orthopedic Y79.8
    - accessory Y79.2
    - diagnostic Y79.0
    - miscellaneous Y79.8
    - monitoring Y79.0
    - prosthetic Y79.2
    - rehabilitative Y79.1
    - surgical Y79.3
    - therapeutic Y79.1
  - otorhinolaryngological Y72.8
    - accessory Y72.2
    - diagnostic Y72.0
    - miscellaneous Y72.8
    - monitoring Y72.0
    - prosthetic Y72.2
    - rehabilitative Y72.1
    - surgical Y72.3
    - therapeutic Y72.1
  - personal use Y74.8
    - accessory Y74.2
    - diagnostic Y74.0
    - miscellaneous Y74.8
    - monitoring Y74.0

Incident, adverse *(continued)*
- device *(continued)*
  - personal use *(continued)*
    - prosthetic Y74.2
    - rehabilitative Y74.1
    - surgical Y74.3
    - therapeutic Y74.1
  - physical medicine Y80.8
    - accessory Y80.2
    - diagnostic Y80.0
    - miscellaneous Y80.8
    - monitoring Y80.0
    - prosthetic Y80.2
    - rehabilitative Y80.1
    - surgical Y80.3
    - therapeutic Y80.1
  - plastic surgical Y81.8
    - accessory Y81.2
    - diagnostic Y81.0
    - miscellaneous Y81.8
    - monitoring Y81.0
    - prosthetic Y81.2
    - rehabilitative Y81.1
    - surgical Y81.3
    - therapeutic Y81.1
  - radiological Y78.8
    - accessory Y78.2
    - diagnostic Y78.0
    - miscellaneous Y78.8
    - monitoring Y78.0
    - prosthetic Y78.2
    - rehabilitative Y78.1
    - surgical Y78.3
    - therapeutic Y78.1
  - urology Y73.8
    - accessory Y73.2
    - diagnostic Y73.0
    - miscellaneous Y73.8
    - monitoring Y73.0
    - prosthetic Y73.2
    - rehabilitative Y73.1
    - surgical Y73.3
    - therapeutic Y73.1

Incineration (accidental)
- *—see* Exposure, fire

Infanticide *—see* Assault

Infrasound waves (causing injury) W49.9

Ingestion
- foreign body (causing injury) (with obstruction) *—see* Foreign body, alimentary canal
- poisonous
  - plant(s) X58
  - substance NEC *—see* Table of Drugs and Chemicals

Inhalation
- excessively cold substance, man-made *—see* Exposure, cold, man-made
- food (any type) (into respiratory tract) (with asphyxia, obstruction respiratory tract, suffocation) *—see* categories T17 and T18
- foreign body *—see* Foreign body, aspiration
- gastric contents (with asphyxia, obstruction respiratory passage, suffocation) T17.81-
- hot air or gases X14.0
- liquid air, hydrogen, nitrogen W93.12
  - suicide (attempt) X83.2
- steam X13.0
  - assault X98.0
  - stated as undetermined whether accidental or intentional Y27.0
  - suicide (attempt) X77.0
- toxic gas *—see* Table of Drugs and Chemicals

Inhalation *(continued)*
- vomitus (with asphyxia, obstruction respiratory passage, suffocation) T17.81-

Injury, injured (accidental(ly))
- NOS X58
- by, caused by, from
  - assault *—see* Assault
  - law-enforcing agent, police, in course of legal intervention *—see* Legal intervention
  - suicide (attempt) X83.8
- due to, in
  - civil insurrection *—see* War operations
  - fight *—see also* Assault, fight Y04.0
  - war operations *—see* War operations
- homicide *—see also* Assault Y09
- inflicted (by)
  - in course of arrest (attempted), suppression of disturbance, maintenance of order, by law-enforcing agents *—see* Legal intervention
  - other person
    - stated as
      - accidental X58
      - intentional, homicide (attempt) *—see* Assault
      - undetermined whether accidental or intentional Y33
- purposely (inflicted) by other person(s) *—see* Assault
- self-inflicted X83.8
  - stated as accidental X58
- specified cause NEC X58
- undetermined whether accidental or intentional Y33

Insolation, effects X30

Insufficient nourishment X58

Interruption of respiration (by)
- food (lodged in esophagus) *—see* categories T17 and T18
- vomitus (lodged in esophagus) T17.81-

Intervention, legal *—see* Legal intervention

Intoxication
- drug *—see* Table of Drugs and Chemicals
- poison *—see* Table of Drugs and Chemicals

J

Jammed (accidentally)
- between objects (moving) (stationary and moving) W23.0
  - stationary W23.1

Jumped, jumping
- before moving object NEC X81.8
  - motor vehicle X81.0
  - subway train X81.1
  - train X81.1
  - undetermined whether accidental or intentional Y31
- from
  - boat (into water) voluntarily, without accident (to or on boat) W16.712
    - with
      - accident to or on boat *—see* Accident, watercraft
      - drowning or submersion W16.711
        - suicide (attempt) X71.3
    - striking bottom W16.722

Jumped, jumping *(continued)*
- from *(continued)*
  - boat (into water) voluntarily, without accident *(continued)*
    - striking bottom *(continued)*
      - causing drowning W16.721
  - building *—see also* Jumped, from, high place W13.9
    - burning (uncontrolled fire) X00.5
  - high place NEC W17.89
    - suicide (attempt) X80
    - undetermined whether accidental or intentional Y30
  - structure *—see also* Jumped, from, high place W13.9
    - burning (uncontrolled fire) X00.5
- into water W16.92
  - causing drowning W16.91
  - from, off watercraft *—see* Jumped, from, boat
  - in
    - natural body W16.612
      - causing drowning W16.611
      - striking bottom W16.622
        - causing drowning W16.621
    - specified place NEC W16.812
      - causing drowning W16.811
      - striking
        - bottom W16.822
          - causing drowning W16.821
        - wall W16.832
          - causing drowning W16.831
    - swimming pool W16.512
      - causing drowning W16.511
      - striking
        - bottom W16.522
          - causing drowning W16.521
        - wall W16.532
          - causing drowning W16.531
  - suicide (attempt) X71.3

K

Kicked by
- animal NEC W55.82
- person(s) (accidentally) W50.1
  - with intent to injure or kill Y04.0
  - as, or caused by, a crowd or human stampede (with fall) W52
  - assault Y04.0
  - homicide (attempt) Y04.0
  - in
    - fight Y04.0
    - legal intervention
      - injuring
        - bystander Y35.812
        - law enforcement personnel Y35.811
        - suspect Y35.813

Kicking
- against
  - object W22.8
    - sports equipment W21.9
    - stationary W22.09
      - sports equipment W21.89
  - person *—see* Striking against, person
  - sports equipment W21.9
- carpet stretcher with knee X50.3

Killed, killing (accidentally)
- NOS *—see also* Injury X58
- in action *—see* War operations
  - brawl, fight (hand) (fists) (foot) Y04.0
    - by weapon *—see also* Assault
      - cutting, piercing *—see* Assault, cutting or piercing instrument

Killed, killing *(continued)*
- in action *(continued)*
  - brawl, fight *(continued)*
    - by weapon *(continued)*
      - firearm *—see* Discharge, firearm, by type, homicide
- self
  - stated as
    - accident NOS X58
    - suicide *—see* Suicide
    - undetermined whether accidental or intentional Y33

Kneeling (prolonged) (static) X50.1

Knocked down (accidentally) (by)
- NOS X58
- animal (not being ridden) NEC *—see also* Struck by, by type of animal
- crowd or human stampede W52
- person W51
  - in brawl, fight Y04.0
- transport vehicle NEC *—see also* Accident, transport V09.9

L

Laceration NEC *—see* Injury

Lack of
- care (helpless person) (infant) (newborn) X58
- food except as result of abandonment or neglect X58
  - due to abandonment or neglect X58
- water except as result of transport accident X58
  - due to transport accident *—see* Accident, transport, by type
  - helpless person, infant, newborn X58

Landslide (falling on transport vehicle) X36.1
- caused by collapse of man-made structure X36.0

Late effect *—see* Sequelae

Legal
- execution (any method) *—see* Legal, intervention
- intervention (by)
  - baton *—see* Legal, intervention, blunt object, baton
  - bayonet *—see* Legal, intervention, sharp object, bayonet
  - blow *—see* Legal, intervention, manhandling
  - blunt object
    - baton
      - injuring
        - bystander Y35.312
        - law enforcement personnel Y35.311
        - suspect Y35.313
    - injuring
      - bystander Y35.302
      - law enforcement personnel Y35.301
      - suspect Y35.303
    - specified NEC
      - injuring
        - bystander Y35.392
        - law enforcement personnel Y35.391
        - suspect Y35.393
    - stave
      - injuring
        - bystander Y35.392
        - law enforcement personnel Y35.391
        - suspect Y35.393
  - bomb *—see* Legal, intervention, explosive

Legal *(continued)*
- intervention *(continued)*
  - cutting or piercing instrument *—see* Legal, intervention, sharp object
  - dynamite *—see* Legal, intervention, explosive, dynamite
  - explosive(s)
    - dynamite
      - injuring
        - bystander Y35.112
        - law enforcement personnel Y35.111
        - suspect Y35.113
    - grenade
      - injuring
        - bystander Y35.192
        - law enforcement personnel Y35.191
        - suspect Y35.193
    - injuring
      - bystander Y35.102
      - law enforcement personnel Y35.101
      - suspect Y35.103
    - mortar bomb
      - injuring
        - bystander Y35.192
        - law enforcement personnel Y35.191
        - suspect Y35.193
    - shell
      - injuring
        - bystander Y35.122
        - law enforcement personnel Y35.121
        - suspect Y35.123
    - specified NEC
      - injuring
        - bystander Y35.192
        - law enforcement personnel Y35.191
        - suspect Y35.193
  - firearm(s) (discharge)
    - handgun
      - injuring
        - bystander Y35.022
        - law enforcement personnel Y35.021
        - suspect Y35.023
    - injuring
      - bystander Y35.002
      - law enforcement personnel Y35.001
      - suspect Y35.003
    - machine gun
      - injuring
        - bystander Y35.012
        - law enforcement personnel Y35.011
        - suspect Y35.013
    - rifle pellet
      - injuring
        - bystander Y35.032
        - law enforcement personnel Y35.031
        - suspect Y35.033
    - rubber bullet
      - injuring
        - bystander Y35.042
        - law enforcement personnel Y35.041
        - suspect Y35.043
    - shotgun *—see* Legal, intervention, firearm, specified NEC
    - specified NEC
      - injuring
        - bystander Y35.092
        - law enforcement personnel Y35.091
        - suspect Y35.093

Legal *(continued)*
- intervention *(continued)*
  - gas (asphyxiation) (poisoning)
    - injuring
      - bystander Y35.202
      - law enforcement personnel Y35.201
      - suspect Y35.203
    - specified NEC
      - injuring
        - bystander Y35.292
        - law enforcement personnel Y35.291
        - suspect Y35.293
    - tear gas
      - injuring
        - bystander Y35.212
        - law enforcement personnel Y35.211
        - suspect Y35.213
  - grenade *—see* Legal, intervention explosive, grenade
  - injuring
    - bystander Y35.92
    - law enforcement personnel Y35.91
    - suspect Y35.93
  - late effect (of) *—see* with 7th character S Y35
  - manhandling
    - injuring
      - bystander Y35.812
      - law enforcement personnel Y35.811
      - suspect Y35.813
  - sequelae (of) *—see* with 7th character S Y35
  - sharp objects
    - bayonet
      - injuring
        - bystander Y35.412
        - law enforcement personnel Y35.411
        - suspect Y35.413
    - injuring
      - bystander Y35.402
      - law enforcement personnel Y35.401
      - suspect Y35.403
    - specified NEC
      - injuring
        - bystander Y35.492
        - law enforcement personnel Y35.491
        - suspect Y35.493
  - specified means NEC
    - injuring
      - bystander Y35.892
      - law enforcement personnel Y35.891
      - suspect Y35.893
  - stabbing *—see* Legal, intervention sharp object
  - stave *—see* Legal, intervention, blunt object, stave
  - tear gas *—see* Legal, intervention, gas, tear gas
  - truncheon *—see* Legal, intervention, blunt object, stave

Lifting - *see also* Overexertion
- heavy objects X50.0
- weights X50.0

Lightning (shock) (stroke) (struck by) *—see* subcategory T75.0
- causing fire *—see* Exposure, fire

Loss of control (transport vehicle) NEC *—see* Accident, transport

Lost at sea NOS *—see* Drowning, due to, fall overboard

Low
pressure (effects) *—see* Air, pressure, low
temperature (effects) *—see* Exposure, cold
Lying before train, vehicle or other moving object X81.8
subway train X81.1
train X81.1
undetermined whether accidental or intentional Y31
Lynching *—see* Assault

M

Malfunction (mechanism or component) (of)
firearm W34.10
airgun W34.110
BB gun W34.110
gas, air or spring-operated gun NEC W34.118
handgun W32.1
hunting rifle W33.12
larger firearm W33.10
specified NEC W33.19
machine gun W33.13
paintball gun W34.111
pellet gun W34.110
shotgun W33.11
specified NEC W34.19
Very pistol [flare] W34.19
handgun *—see* Malfunction, firearm, handgun
Maltreatment *—see* Perpetrator
Mangled (accidentally) NOS X58
Manhandling (in brawl, fight) Y04.0
legal intervention *—see* Legal, intervention, manhandling
Manslaughter (nonaccidental) *—see* Assault
Mauled by animal NEC W55.89
Medical procedure, complication
of (delayed or as an abnormal reaction without mention of misadventure) *—see* Complication of or following, by specified type of procedure
due to or as a result of misadventure *—see* Misadventure
Melting (due to fire) *—see also* Exposure, fire
apparel NEC X06.3
clothes, clothing NEC X06.3
nightwear X05
fittings or furniture (burning building) (uncontrolled fire) X00.8
nightwear X05
plastic jewelry X06.1
Mental cruelty X58
Military operations (injuries to military and civilians occuring during peacetime on military property and during routine military exercises and operations) (by) (from) (involving) Y37.90-
air blast Y37.20-
aircraft
destruction *—see* Military operations, destruction of aircraft
airway restriction *—see* Military operations, restriction of airways
asphyxiation *—see* Military operations, restriction of airways
biological weapons Y37.6X-
blast Y37.20-
blast fragments Y37.20-
blast wave Y37.20-
Military operations *(continued)*
blast wind Y37.20-
bomb Y37.20-
dirty Y37.50-
gasoline Y37.31-
incendiary Y37.31-
petrol Y37.31-
bullet Y37.43-
incendiary Y37.32-
rubber Y37.41-
chemical weapons Y37.7X-
combat
hand to hand (unarmed) combat Y37.44-
using blunt or piercing object Y37.45-
conflagration *—see* Military operations, fire
conventional warfare NEC Y37.49-
depth-charge Y37.01-
destruction of aircraft Y37.10-
due to
air to air missile Y37.11-
collision with other aircraft Y37.12-
detonation (accidental) of onboard munitions and explosives Y37.14-
enemy fire or explosives Y37.11-
explosive placed on aircraft Y37.11-
onboard fire Y37.13-
rocket propelled grenade [RPG] Y37.11-
small arms fire Y37.11-
surface to air missile Y37.11-
specified NEC Y37.19-
detonation (accidental) of
onboard marine weapons Y37.05-
own munitions or munitions launch device Y37.24-
dirty bomb Y37.50-
explosion (of) Y37.20-
aerial bomb Y37.21-
bomb NOS *—see also* Military operations, bomb(s) Y37.20-
fragments Y37.20-
grenade Y37.29-
guided missile Y37.22-
improvised explosive device [IED] (person-borne) (roadside) (vehicle-borne) Y37.23-
land mine Y37.29-
marine mine (at sea) (in harbor) Y37.02-
marine weapon Y37.00-
specified NEC Y37.09-
own munitions or munitions launch device (accidental) Y37.24-
sea-based artillery shell Y37.03-
specified NEC Y37.29-
torpedo Y37.04-
fire Y37.30-
specified NEC Y37.39-
firearms
discharge Y37.43-
pellets Y37.42-
flamethrower Y37.33-
fragments (from) (of)
improvised explosive device [IED] (person-borne) (roadside) (vehicle-borne) Y37.26-
munitions Y37.25-
specified NEC Y37.29-
weapons Y37.27-
friendly fire Y37.92-
hand to hand (unarmed) combat Y37.44-
hot substances *—see* Military operations, fire
Military operations *(continued)*
incendiary bullet Y37.32-
nuclear weapon (effects of) Y37.50-
acute radiation exposure Y37.54-
blast pressure Y37.51-
direct blast Y37.51-
direct heat Y37.53-
fallout exposure Y37.54-
fireball Y37.53-
indirect blast (struck or crushed by blast debris) (being thrown by blast) Y37.52-
ionizing radiation (immediate exposure) Y37.54-
nuclear radiation Y37.54-
radiation
ionizing (immediate exposure) Y37.54-
nuclear Y37.54-
thermal Y37.53-
specified NEC Y37.59-
secondary effects Y37.54-
thermal radiation Y37.53-
restriction of air (airway)
intentional Y37.46-
unintentional Y37.47-
rubber bullets Y37.41-
shrapnel NOS Y37.29-
suffocation *—see* Military operations, restriction of airways
unconventional warfare NEC Y37.7X-
underwater blast NOS Y37.00-
warfare
conventional NEC Y37.49-
unconventional NEC Y37.7X-
weapons
biological weapons Y37.6X-
chemical Y37.7X-
nuclear (effects of) Y37.50-
acute radiation exposure Y37.54-
blast pressure Y37.51-
direct blast Y37.51-
direct heat Y37.53-
fallout exposure Y37.54-
fireball Y37.53-
radiation
ionizing (immediate exposure) Y37.54-
nuclear Y37.54-
thermal Y37.53-
secondary effects Y37.54-
specified NEC Y37.59-
of mass destruction [WMD] Y37.91-
weapon of mass destruction [WMD] Y37.91-
Misadventure(s) to patient(s) during surgical or medical care Y69
contaminated medical or biological substance (blood, drug, fluid) Y64.9
administered (by) NEC Y64.9
immunization Y64.1
infusion Y64.0
injection Y64.1
specified means NEC Y64.8
transfusion Y64.0
vaccination Y64.1
excessive amount of blood or other fluid during transfusion or infusion Y63.0
failure
in dosage Y63.9
electroshock therapy Y63.4
inappropriate temperature (too hot or too cold) in local application and packing Y63.5
Misadventure(s) to patient(s) during surgical or medical care *(continued)*
failure *(continued)*
in dosage *(continued)*
infusion
excessive amount of fluid Y63.0
incorrect dilution of fluid Y63.1
insulin-shock therapy Y63.4
nonadministration of necessary drug or biological substance Y63.6
overdose *—see* Table of Drugs and Chemicals
radiation, in therapy Y63.2
radiation
overdose Y63.2
specified procedure NEC Y63.8
transfusion
excessive amount of blood Y63.0
mechanical, of instrument or apparatus (any) (during any procedure) Y65.8
sterile precautions (during procedure) Y62.9
aspiration of fluid or tissue (by puncture or catheterization, except heart) Y62.6
biopsy (except needle aspiration) Y62.8
needle (aspirating) Y62.6
blood sampling Y62.6
catheterization Y62.6
heart Y62.5
dialysis (kidney) Y62.2
endoscopic examination Y62.4
enema Y62.8
immunization Y62.3
infusion Y62.1
injection Y62.3
needle biopsy Y62.6
paracentesis (abdominal) (thoracic) Y62.6
perfusion Y62.2
puncture (lumbar) Y62.6
removal of catheter or packing Y62.8
specified procedure NEC Y62.8
surgical operation Y62.0
transfusion Y62.1
vaccination Y62.3
suture or ligature during surgical procedure Y65.2
to introduce or to remove tube or instrument *—see* Failure, to
hemorrhage *—see* Index to Diseases and Injuries, Complication(s)
inadvertent exposure of patient to radiation Y63.3
inappropriate
operation performed *—see* Inappropriate operation performed
temperature (too hot or too cold) in local application or packing Y63.5
infusion *—see also* Misadventure, by type, infusion Y69
excessive amount of fluid Y63.0
incorrect dilution of fluid Y63.1
wrong fluid Y65.1
mismatched blood in transfusion Y65.0
nonadministration of necessary drug or biological substance Y63.6
overdose *—see* Table of Drugs and Chemicals
radiation (in therapy) Y63.2
perforation *—see* Index to Diseases and Injuries, Complication(s)

Misadventure(s) to patient(s) during surgical or medical care *(continued)*
- performance of inappropriate operation —*see* Inappropriate operation performed
- puncture —*see* Index to Diseases and Injuries, Complication(s)
- specified type NEC Y65.8
  - failure
    - suture or ligature during surgical operation Y65.2
    - to introduce or to remove tube or instrument —*see* Failure, to
  - infusion of wrong fluid Y65.1
  - performance of inappropriate operation —*see* Inappropriate operation performed
  - transfusion of mismatched blood Y65.0
  - wrong
    - drug given in error —*see* Table of Drugs and Chemicals
    - fluid in infusion Y65.1
    - placement of endotracheal tube during anesthetic procedure Y65.3
- transfusion —*see* Misadventure, by type, transfusion
  - excessive amount of blood Y63.0
  - mismatched blood Y65.0
- wrong
  - drug given in error —*see* Table of Drugs and Chemicals
  - fluid in infusion Y65.1
  - placement of endotracheal tube during anesthetic procedure Y65.3

Mismatched blood in transfusion Y65.0

Motion sickness T75.3

Mountain sickness W94.11

Mudslide (of cataclysmic nature) —*see* Landslide

Murder (attempt) —*see* Assault

N

Nail
- contact with W45.0
  - gun W29.4
- embedded in skin W45.0

Neglect (criminal) (homicidal intent) X58

Noise (causing injury) (pollution) W42.9
- supersonic W42.0

Nonadministration (of)
- drug or biological substance (necessary) Y63.6
- surgical and medical care Y66

Nosocomial condition Y95

O

Object
- falling
  - from, in, on, hitting
    - machinery —*see* Contact, with, by type of machine
- set in motion by
  - accidental explosion or rupture of pressure vessel W38
  - firearm —*see* Discharge, firearm, by type
  - machine (ry) —*see* Contact, with, by type of machine

Overdose (drug) —*see* Table of Drugs and Chemicals
- radiation Y63.2

Overexertion X50.9
- from
  - prolonged static or awkward postures X50.1
  - repetitive movements X50.3
  - specified strenuous movements or postures NEC X50.9
  - strenuous movement or load X50.0

Overexposure (accidental) (to)
- cold —*see also* Exposure, cold X31
  - due to man-made conditions —*see* Exposure, cold, man-made
- heat —*see also* Heat X30
- radiation —*see* Radiation
- radioactivity W88.0
- sun (sunburn) X32
- weather NEC —*see* Forces of nature
- wind NEC —*see* Forces of nature

Overheated —*see* Heat

Overturning (accidental)
- machinery —*see* Contact, with, by type of machine
- transport vehicle NEC —*see also* Accident, transport V89.9
- watercraft (causing drowning, submersion) —*see also* Drowning, due to, accident to, watercraft, overturning
  - causing injury except drowning or submersion —*see* Accident, watercraft, causing, injury NEC

P

Parachute descent (voluntary) (without accident to aircraft) V97.29
- due to accident to aircraft —*see* Accident, transport, aircraft

Pecked by bird W61.99

Perforation during medical or surgical treatment as misadventure —*see* Index to Diseases and Injuries, Complication(s)

Perpetrator, perpetration, of assault, maltreatment and neglect (by) Y07.9
- boyfriend Y07.03
- brother Y07.410
  - stepbrother Y07.435
- coach Y07.53
- cousin
  - female Y07.491
  - male Y07.490
- daycare provider Y07.519
  - at-home
    - adult care Y07.512
    - childcare Y07.510
  - care center
    - adult care Y07.513
    - childcare Y07.511
- family member NEC Y07.499
- father Y07.11
  - adoptive Y07.13
  - foster Y07.420
  - stepfather Y07.430
- foster father Y07.420
- foster mother Y07.421
- girl friend Y07.04
- healthcare provider Y07.529
  - mental health Y07.521
  - specified NEC Y07.528
- husband Y07.01
- instructor Y07.53
- mother Y07.12
  - adoptive Y07.14
  - foster Y07.421
  - stepmother Y07.433

Perpetrator, perpetration, of assault, maltreatment and neglect *(continued)*
- nonfamily member Y07.50
  - specified NEC Y07.59
- nurse Y07.528
- occupational therapist Y07.528
- partner of parent
  - female Y07.434
  - male Y07.432
- physical therapist Y07.528
- sister Y07.411
- speech therapist Y07.528
- stepbrother Y07.435
- stepfather Y07.430
- stepmother Y07.433
- stepsister Y07.436
- teacher Y07.53
- wife Y07.02

Piercing —*see* Contact, with, by type of object or machine

Pinched
- between objects (moving) (stationary and moving) W23.0
  - stationary W23.1

Pinned under machine (ry) —*see* Contact, with, by type of machine

Place of occurrence Y92.9
- abandoned house Y92.89
- airplane Y92.813
- airport Y92.520
- ambulatory health services establishment NEC Y92.538
- ambulatory surgery center Y92.530
- amusement park Y92.831
- apartment (co-op) —*see* Place of occurrence, residence, apartment
- assembly hall Y92.29
- bank Y92.510
- barn Y92.71
- baseball field Y92.320
- basketball court Y92.310
- beach Y92.832
- boarding house —*see* Place of occurrence, residence, boarding house
- boat Y92.814
- bowling alley Y92.39
- bridge Y92.89
- building under construction Y92.61
- bus Y92.811
  - station Y92.521
- cafe Y92.511
- campsite Y92.833
- campus —*see* Place of occurrence, school
- canal Y92.89
- car Y92.810
- casino Y92.59
- children's home —*see* Place of occurrence, residence, institutional, orphanage
- church Y92.22
- cinema Y92.26
- clubhouse Y92.29
- coal pit Y92.64
- college (community) Y92.214
- condominium —*see* Place of occurrence, residence, apartment
- construction area —*see* Place of occurrence, industrial and construction area
- convalescent home —*see* Place of occurrence, residence, institutional, nursing home
- court-house Y92.240
- cricket ground Y92.328
- cultural building Y92.258
  - art gallery Y92.250

Place of occurrence *(continued)*
- cultural building *(continued)*
  - museum Y92.251
  - music hall Y92.252
  - opera house Y92.253
  - specified NEC Y92.258
  - theater Y92.254
- dancehall Y92.252
- day nursery Y92.210
- dentist office Y92.531
- derelict house Y92.89
- desert Y92.820
- dock NOS Y92.89
- dockyard Y92.62
- doctor's office Y92.531
- dormitory —*see* Place of occurrence residence, institutional, school dormitory
- dry dock Y92.62
- factory (building) (premises) Y92.63
- farm (land under cultivation) (outbuildings) Y92.79
  - barn Y92.71
  - chicken coop Y92.72
  - field Y92.73
  - hen house Y92.72
  - house —*see* Place of occurrence, residence, house
  - orchard Y92.74
  - specified NEC Y92.79
- football field Y92.321
- forest Y92.821
- freeway Y92.411
- gallery Y92.250
- garage (commercial) Y92.59
  - boarding house Y92.044
  - military base Y92.135
  - mobile home Y92.025
  - nursing home Y92.124
  - orphanage Y92.114
  - private house Y92.015
  - reform school Y92.155
- gas station Y92.524
- gasworks Y92.69
- golf course Y92.39
- gravel pit Y92.64
- grocery Y92.512
- gymnasium Y92.39
- handball court Y92.318
- harbor Y92.89
- harness racing course Y92.39
- healthcare provider office Y92.531
- highway (interstate) Y92.411
- hill Y92.828
- hockey rink Y92.330
- home —*see* Place of occurrence, residence
- hospice —*see* Place of occurrence, residence, institutional, nursing home
- hospital Y92.239
  - cafeteria Y92.233
  - corridor Y92.232
  - operating room Y92.234
  - patient
    - bathroom Y92.231
    - room Y92.230
  - specified NEC Y92.238
- hotel Y92.59
- house —*see also* Place of occurrence, residence
  - abandoned Y92.89
  - under construction Y92.61
- industrial and construction area (yard) Y92.69
  - building under construction Y92.61
  - dock Y92.62
  - dry dock Y92.62
  - factory Y92.63
  - gasworks Y92.69
  - mine Y92.64

Place of occurrence *(continued)*
- industrial and construction area *(continued)*
  - oil rig Y92.65
  - pit Y92.64
  - power station Y92.69
  - shipyard Y92.62
  - specified NEC Y92.69
  - tunnel under construction Y92.69
  - workshop Y92.69
- kindergarten Y92.211
- lacrosse field Y92.328
- lake Y92.828
- library Y92.241
- mall Y92.59
- market Y92.512
- marsh Y92.828
- military
  - base —*see* Place of occurrence, residence, institutional, military base
  - training ground Y92.84
- mine Y92.64
- mosque Y92.22
- motel Y92.59
- motorway (interstate) Y92.411
- mountain Y92.828
- movie-house Y92.26
- museum Y92.251
- music-hall Y92.252
- not applicable Y92.9
- nuclear power station Y92.69
- nursing home —*see* Place of occurrence, residence, institutional, nursing home
- office building Y92.59
- offshore installation Y92.65
- oil rig Y92.65
- old people's home —*see* Place of occurrence, residence, institutional, specified NEC
- opera-house Y92.253
- orphanage —*see* Place of occurrence, residence, institutional, orphanage
- outpatient surgery center Y92.530
- park (public) Y92.830
  - amusement Y92.831
- parking garage Y92.89
  - lot Y92.481
- pavement Y92.480
- physician office Y92.531
- polo field Y92.328
- pond Y92.828
- post office Y92.242
- power station Y92.69
- prairie Y92.828
- prison —*see* Place of occurrence, residence, institutional, prison
- public
  - administration building Y92.248
    - city hall Y92.243
    - courthouse Y92.240
    - library Y92.241
    - post office Y92.242
    - specified NEC Y92.248
  - building NEC Y92.29
  - hall Y92.29
  - place NOS Y92.89
- race course Y92.39
- radio station Y92.59
- railway line (bridge) Y92.85
- ranch (outbuildings) —*see* Place of occurrence, farm
- recreation area Y92.838
  - amusement park Y92.831
  - beach Y92.832
  - campsite Y92.833
  - park (public) Y92.830
  - seashore Y92.832
  - specified NEC Y92.838

Place of occurrence *(continued)*
- religious institution Y92.22
- reform school —*see* Place of occurrence, residence, institutional, reform school
- residence (non-institutional) (private) Y92.009
  - apartment Y92.039
    - bathroom Y92.031
    - bedroom Y92.032
    - kitchen Y92.030
    - specified NEC Y92.038
  - bathroom Y92.002
  - bedroom Y92.003
  - boarding house Y92.049
    - bathroom Y92.041
    - bedroom Y92.042
    - driveway Y92.043
    - garage Y92.044
    - garden Y92.046
    - kitchen Y92.040
    - specified NEC Y92.048
    - swimming pool Y92.045
    - yard Y92.046
  - dining room Y92.001
  - garden Y92.007
  - home Y92.009
  - house, single family Y92.019
    - bathroom Y92.012
    - bedroom Y92.013
    - dining room Y92.011
    - driveway Y92.014
    - garage Y92.015
    - garden Y92.017
    - kitchen Y92.010
    - specified NEC Y92.018
    - swimming pool Y92.016
    - yard Y92.017
  - institutional Y92.10
    - children's home —*see* Place of occurrence, residence, institutional, orphanage
    - hospice —*see* Place of occurrence, residence, institutional, nursing home
    - military base Y92.139
      - barracks Y92.133
      - garage Y92.135
      - garden Y92.137
      - kitchen Y92.130
      - mess hall Y92.131
      - specified NEC Y92.138
      - swimming pool Y92.136
      - yard Y92.137
    - nursing home Y92.129
      - bathroom Y92.121
      - bedroom Y92.122
      - driveway Y92.123
      - garage Y92.124
      - garden Y92.126
      - kitchen Y92.120
      - specified NEC Y92.128
      - swimming pool Y92.125
      - yard Y92.126
    - orphanage Y92.119
      - bathroom Y92.111
      - bedroom Y92.112
      - driveway Y92.113
      - garage Y92.114
      - garden Y92.116
      - kitchen Y92.110
      - specified NEC Y92.118
      - swimming pool Y92.115
      - yard Y92.116
    - prison Y92.149
      - bathroom Y92.142
      - cell Y92.143
      - courtyard Y92.147
      - dining room Y92.141
      - kitchen Y92.140

Place of occurrence *(continued)*
- residence *(continued)*
  - institutional *(continued)*
    - prison *(continued)*
      - specified NEC Y92.148
      - swimming pool Y92.146
    - reform school Y92.159
      - bathroom Y92.152
      - bedroom Y92.153
      - dining room Y92.151
      - driveway Y92.154
      - garage Y92.155
      - garden Y92.157
      - kitchen Y92.150
      - specified NEC Y92.158
      - swimming pool Y92.156
      - yard Y92.157
    - school dormitory Y92.169
      - bathroom Y92.162
      - bedroom Y92.163
      - dining room Y92.161
      - kitchen Y92.160
      - specified NEC Y92.168
    - specified NEC Y92.199
      - bathroom Y92.192
      - bedroom Y92.193
      - dining room Y92.191
      - driveway Y92.194
      - garage Y92.195
      - garden Y92.197
      - kitchen Y92.190
      - specified NEC Y92.198
      - swimming pool Y92.196
      - yard Y92.197
  - kitchen Y92.000
  - mobile home Y92.029
    - bathroom Y92.022
    - bedroom Y92.023
    - dining room Y92.021
    - driveway Y92.024
    - garage Y92.025
    - garden Y92.027
    - kitchen Y92.020
    - specified NEC Y92.028
    - swimming pool Y92.026
    - yard Y92.027
  - specified place in residence NEC Y92.008
  - specified residence type NEC Y92.099
    - bathroom Y92.091
    - bedroom Y92.092
    - driveway Y92.093
    - garage Y92.094
    - garden Y92.096
    - kitchen Y92.090
    - specified NEC Y92.098
    - swimming pool Y92.095
    - yard Y92.096
- restaurant Y92.511
- riding school Y92.39
- river Y92.828
- road Y92.488
- rodeo ring Y92.39
- rugby field Y92.328
- same day surgery center Y92.530
- sand pit Y92.64
- school (private) (public) (state) Y92.219
  - college Y92.214
  - daycare center Y92.210
  - elementary school Y92.211
  - high school Y92.213
  - kindergarten Y92.211
  - middle school Y92.212
  - specified NEC Y92.218
  - trace school Y92.215
  - university Y92.214
  - vocational school Y92.215
- sea (shore) Y92.832
- senior citizen center Y92.29

Place of occurrence *(continued)*
- service area
  - airport Y92.520
  - bus station Y92.521
  - gas station Y92.524
  - highway rest stop Y92.523
  - railway station Y92.522
- shipyard Y92.62
- shop (commercial) Y92.513
- sidewalk Y92.480
- silo Y92.79
- skating rink (roller) Y92.331
  - ice Y92.330
- slaughter house Y92.86
- soccer field Y92.322
- specified place NEC Y92.89
- sports area Y92.39
  - athletic
    - court Y92.318
      - basketball Y92.310
      - specified NEC Y92.318
      - squash Y92.311
      - tennis Y92.312
    - field Y92.328
      - baseball Y92.320
      - cricket ground Y92.328
      - football Y92.321
      - hockey Y92.328
      - soccer Y92.322
      - specified NEC Y92.328
  - golf course Y92.39
  - gymnasium Y92.39
  - riding school Y92.39
  - skating rink (roller) Y92.331
    - ice Y92.330
  - stadium Y92.39
  - swimming pool Y92.34
- squash court Y92.311
- stadium Y92.39
- steeplechasing course Y92.39
- store Y92.512
- stream Y92.828
- street and highway Y92.410
  - bike path Y92.482
  - freeway Y92.411
  - highway ramp Y92.415
  - interstate highway Y92.411
  - local residential or business street Y92.414
  - motorway Y92.411
  - parkway Y92.412
  - parking lot Y92.481
  - sidewalk Y92.480
  - specified NEC Y92.488
  - state road Y92.413
- subway car Y92.816
- supermarket Y92.512
- swamp Y92.828
- swimming pool (public) Y92.34
  - private (at) Y92.095
    - boarding house Y92.045
    - military base Y92.136
    - mobile home Y92.026
    - nursing home Y92.125
    - orphanage Y92.115
    - prison Y92.146
    - reform school Y92.156
    - single family residence Y92.016
- synagogue Y92.22
- television station Y92.59
- tennis court Y92.312
- theater Y92.254
- trade area Y92.59
  - bank Y92.510
  - cafe Y92.511
  - casino Y92.59
  - garage Y92.59
  - hotel Y92.59
  - market Y92.512
  - office building Y92.59
  - radio station Y92.59

Place of occurrence *(continued)*
trade area *(continued)*
restaurant Y92.511
shop Y92.513
shopping mall Y92.59
store Y92.512
supermarket Y92.512
television station Y92.59
warehouse Y92.59
trailer park, residential *—see* Place of occurrence, residence, mobile home
trailer site NOS Y92.89
train Y92.815
station Y92.522
truck Y92.812
tunnel under construction Y92.69
urgent (health) care center Y92.532
university Y92.214
vehicle (transport) Y92.818
airplane Y92.813
boat Y92.814
bus Y92.811
car Y92.810
specified NEC Y92.818
subway car Y92.816
train Y92.815
truck Y92.812
warehouse Y92.59
water reservoir Y92.89
wilderness area Y92.828
desert Y92.820
forest Y92.821
marsh Y92.828
mountain Y92.828
prairie Y92.828
specified NEC Y92.828
swamp Y92.828
workshop Y92.69
yard, private Y92.096
boarding house Y92.046
single family house Y92.017
mobile home Y92.027
youth center Y92.29
zoo (zoological garden) Y92.834

Plumbism *—see* Table of Drugs and Chemicals, lead

Poisoning (accidental) (by) *—see also* Table of Drugs and Chemicals
by plant, thorns, spines, sharp leaves or other mechanisms NEC X58
carbon monoxide
generated by
motor vehicle *—see* Accident, transport
watercraft (in transit) (not in transit) V93.89
ferry boat V93.81
fishing boat V93.82
jet skis V93.83
liner V93.81
merchant ship V93.80
passenger ship V93.81
powered craft NEC V93.83
caused by injection of poisons into skin by plant thorns, spines, sharp leaves X58
marine or sea plants (venomous) X58
exhaust gas
generated by
motor vehicle *—see* Accident, transport
watercraft (in transit) (not in transit) V93.89
ferry boat V93.81
fishing boat V93.82
jet skis V93.83
liner V93.81

Poisoning *(continued)*
exhaust gas *(continued)*
generated by *(continued)*
watercraft *(continued)*
merchant ship V93.80
passenger ship V93.81
powered craft NEC V93.83
fumes or smoke due to
explosion *—see also* Explosion W40.9
fire *—see* Exposure, fire
ignition *—see* Ignition
gas
in legal intervention *—see* Legal, intervention, gas
legal execution *—see* Legal, intervention, gas
in war operations *—see* War operations

Powder burn (by) (from)
airgun W34.110
BB gun W34.110
firearn NEC W34.19
gas, air or spring-operated gun NEC W34.118
handgun W32.1
hunting rifle W33.12
larger firearm W33.10
specified NEC W33.19
machine gun W33.13
paintball gun W34.111
pellet gun W34.110
shotgun W33.11
Very pistol [flare] W34.19

Premature cessation (of) surgical and medical care Y66

Privation (food) (water) X58

Procedure (operation)
correct, on wrong side or body part (wrong side) (wrong site) Y65.53
intended for another patient
done on wrong patient Y65.52
performed on patient not scheduled for surgery Y65.52
performed on wrong patient Y65.52
wrong, performed on correct patient Y65.51

Prolonged
sitting in transport vehicle *—see* Travel, by type of vehicle
stay in
high altitude as cause of anoxia, barodontalgia, barotitis or hypoxia W94.11
weightless environment X52

Pulling, excessive *(see also* Overexertion) X50.9

Puncture, puncturing *—see also* Contact, with, by type of object or machine
by
plant thorns, spines, sharp leaves or other mechanisms NEC W60
during medical or surgical treatment as misadventure *—see* Index to Diseases and Injuries, Complication(s)

Pushed, pushing (accidental) (injury in)
by other person(s) (accidental) W51
with fall W03
due to ice or snow W00.0
as, or caused by, a crowd or human stampede (with fall) W52
before moving object NEC Y02.8
motor vehicle Y02.0
subway train Y02.1
train Y02.1
from

Pushed, pushing *(continued)*
by other person *(continued)*
from *(continued)*
high place NEC
in accidental circumstances W17.89
stated as
intentional, homicide (attempt) Y01
undetermined whether accidental or intentional Y30
transport vehicle NEC *—see also* Accident, transport V89.9
stated as
intentional, homicide (attempt) Y08.89
overexertion X50.9

R

Radiation (exposure to)
arc lamps W89.0
atomic power plant (malfunction) NEC W88.1
complication of or abnormal reaction to medical radiotherapy Y84.2
electromagnetic, ionizing W88.0
gamma rays W88.1
in
war operations (from or following nuclear explosion) *—see* War operations
inadvertent exposure of patient (receiving test or therapy) Y63.3
infrared (heaters and lamps) W90.1
excessive heat from W92
ionized, ionizing (particles, artificially accelerated)
radioisotopes W88.1
specified NEC W88.8
x-rays W88.0
isotopes, radioactive *—see* Radiation, radioactive isotopes
laser(s) W90.2
in war operations *—see* War operations
misadventure in medical care Y63.2
light sources (man-made visible and ultraviolet) W89.9
natural X32
specified NEC W89.8
tanning bed W89.1
welding light W89.0
man-made visible light W89.9
specified NEC W89.8
tanning bed W89.1
welding light W89.0
microwave W90.8
misadventure in medical or surgical procedure Y63.2
natural NEC X39.08
radon X39.01
overdose (in medical or surgical procedure) Y63.2
radar W90.0
radioactive isotopes (any) W88.1
atomic power plant malfunction W88.1
misadventure in medical or surgical treatment Y63.2
radiofrequency W90.0
radium NEC W88.1
sun X32
ultraviolet (light) (man-made) W89.9
natural X32
specified NEC W89.8
tanning bed W89.1
welding light W89.0

Radiation *(continued)*
welding arc, torch, or light W89.0
excessive heat from W92
x-rays (hard) (soft) W88.0

Range disease W94.11

Rape (attempted) T74.2-

Rat bite W53.11

Reaching (prolonged) (static) X50.1

Reaction, abnormal to medical procedure *—see also* Complication of or following, by type of procedure Y84.9
with misadventure *—see* Misadventure
biologicals *—see* Table of Drugs and Chemicals
drugs *—see* Table of Drugs and Chemicals
vaccine *—see* Table of Drugs and Chemicals

Recoil
airgun W34.110
BB gun W34.110
firearn NEC W34.19
gas, air or spring-operated gun NEC W34.118
handgun W32.1
hunting rifle W33.12
larger firearm W33.10
specified NEC W33.19
machine gun W33.13
paintball gun W34.111
pellet W34.110
shotgun W33.11
Very pistol [flare] W34.19

Reduction in
atmospheric pressure *—see* Air, pressure, change

Rock falling on or hitting (accidentally) (person) W20.8
in cave-in W20.0

Run over (accidentally) (by)
animal (not being ridden) NEC W55.89
machinery *—see* Contact, with, by specified type of machine
transport vehicle NEC *—see also* Accident, transport V09.9
intentional homicide (attempt) Y03.0
motor NEC V09.20
intentional homicide (attempt) Y03.0

Running
before moving object X81.8
motor vehicle X81.0

Running off, away
animal (being ridden) *—see also* Accident, transport V80.918
not being ridden W55.89
animal-drawn vehicle NEC *—see also* Accident, transport V80.928
highway, road (way), street
transport vehicle NEC *—see also* Accident, transport V89.9

Rupture pressurized devices —*see* Explosion, by type of device

S

Saturnism *—see* Table of Drugs and Chemicals, lead

Scald, scalding (accidental) (by) (from) (in) X19
air (hot) X14.1
gases (hot) X14.1
homicide (attempt) *—see* Assault, burning, hot object

Scald, scalding *(continued)*
inflicted by other person
stated as intentional, homicide (attempt) —*see* Assault, burning, hot object
liquid (boiling) (hot) NEC X12
stated as undetermined whether accidental or intentional Y27.2
suicide (attempt) X77.2
local application of externally applied substance in medical or surgical care Y63.5
metal (molten) (liquid) (hot) NEC X18
self-inflicted X77.9
stated as undetermined whether accidental or intentional Y27.8
steam X13.1
assault X98.0
stated as undetermined whether accidental or intentional Y27.0
suicide (attempt) X77.0
suicide (attempt) X77.9
vapor (hot) X13.1
assault X98.0
stated as undetermined whether accidental or intentional Y27.0
suicide (attempt) X77.0

Scratched by
cat W55.03
person(s) (accidentally) W50.4
with intent to injure or kill Y04.0
as, or caused by, a crowd or human stampede (with fall) W52
assault Y04.0
homicide (attempt) Y04.0
in
fight Y04.0
legal intervention
injuring
bystander Y35.892
law enforcement personnel Y35.891
suspect Y35.893

Seasickness T75.3

Self-harm NEC —*see also* External cause by type, undetermined whether accidental or intentional
intentional —*see* Suicide
poisoning NEC —*see* Table of drugs and biologicals, accident

Self-inflicted (injury) NEC —*see also* External cause by type, undetermined whether accidental or intentional
intentional —*see* Suicide
poisoning NEC —*see* Table of drugs and biologicals, accident

Sequelae (of)
accident NEC —*see* W00-X58 with 7th character S
assault (homicidal) (any means) —*see* X92-Y08 with 7th character S
homicide, attempt (any means) —*see* X92-Y08 with 7th character S
injury undetermined whether accidentally or purposely inflicted —*see* Y21-Y33 with 7th character S
intentional self-harm (classifiable to X71-X83) —*see* X71-X83 with 7th character S
legal intervention —*see* with 7th character S Y35
motor vehicle accident —*see* V00-V99 with 7th character S

Sequelae *(continued)*
suicide, attempt (any means) —*see* X71-X83 with 7th character S
transport accident —*see* V00-V99 with 7th character S
war operations —*see* War operations

Shock
electric —*see* Exposure, electric current
from electric appliance (any) (faulty) W86.8
domestic W86.0
suicide (attempt) X83.1

Shooting, shot (accidental(ly)) —*see also* Discharge, firearm, by type
herself or himself —*see* Discharge, firearm by type, self-inflicted
homicide (attempt) —*see* Discharge, firearm by type, homicide
in war operations —*see* War operations
inflicted by other person —*see* Discharge, firearm by type, homicide
accidental —*see* Discharge, firearm, by type of firearm
legal
execution —*see* Legal, intervention, firearm
intervention —*see* Legal, intervention, firearm
self-inflicted —*see* Discharge, firearm by type, suicide
accidental —*see* Discharge, firearm, by type of firearm
suicide (attempt) —*see* Discharge, firearm by type, suicide

Shoving (accidentally) by other person —*see* Pushed, by other person

Sickness
alpine W94.11
motion —*see* Motion
mountain W94.11

Sinking (accidental)
watercraft (causing drowning, submersion) —*see also* Drowning, due to, accident to, watercraft, sinking
causing injury except drowning or submersion —*see* Accident, watercraft, causing, injury NEC

Siriasis X32

Sitting (prolonged) (static) X50.1

Slashed wrists —*see* Cut, self-inflicted

Slipping (accidental) (on same level) (with fall) W01.0
on
ice W00.0
with skates —*see* Accident, transport, pedestrian, conveyance
mud W01.0
oil W01.0
snow W00.0
with skis —*see* Accident, transport, pedestrian, conveyance
surface (slippery) (wet) NEC W01.0
without fall W18.40
due to
specified NEC W18.49
stepping from one level to another W18.43
stepping into hole or opening W18.42
stepping on object W18.41

Sliver, wood, contact with W45.8

Smoldering (due to fire) —*see* Exposure, fire

Sodomy (attempted) by force T74.2-

Sound waves (causing injury) W42.9
supersonic W42.0

Splinter, contact with W45.8

Stab, stabbing —*see* Cut

Standing (prolonged) (static) X50.1

Starvation X58

Status of external cause Y99.9
child assisting in compensated work for family Y99.8
civilian activity done for financial or other compensation Y99.0
civilian activity done for income or pay Y99.0
family member assisting in compensated work for other family member Y99.8
hobby not done for income Y99.8
leisure activity Y99.8
military activity Y99.1
off-duty activity of military personnel Y99.8
recreation or sport not for income or while a student Y99.8
specified NEC Y99.8
student activity Y99.8
volunteer activity Y99.2

Stepped on
by
animal (not being ridden) NEC W55.89
crowd or human stampede W52
person W50.0

Stepping on
object W22.8
with fall W18.31
sports equipment W21.9
stationary W22.09
sports equipment W21.89
person W51
by crowd or human stampede W52
sports equipment W21.9

Sting
arthropod, nonvenomous W57
insect, nonvenomous W57

Storm (cataclysmic) —see Forces of nature, cataclysmic storm

Straining, excessive —(*see also* Overexertion) X50.9

Strangling —*see* Strangulation

Strangulation (accidental) —*see* categories T71

Strenuous movements (*see also* Overexertion) X50.9

Striking against
airbag (automobile) W22.10
driver side W22.11
front passenger side W22.12
specified NEC W22.19
bottom when
diving or jumping into water (in) W16.822
causing drowning W16.821
from boat W16.722
causing drowning W16.721
natural body W16.622
causing drowning W16.821
swimming pool W16.522
causing drowning W16.521
falling into water (in) W16.322
causing drowning W16.321

Striking against *(continued)*
bottom when *(continued)*
falling into water *(continued)*
fountain —*see* Striking against, bottom when, falling into water, specified NEC
natural body W16.122
causing drowning W16.121
reservoir —*see* Striking against, bottom when, falling into water, specified NEC
specified NEC W16.322
causing drowning W16.321
swimming pool W16.022
causing drowning W16.021
diving board (swimming-pool) W21.4
object W22.8
with
drowning or submersion —*see* Drowning
fall —*see* Fall, due to, bumping against, object
caused by crowd or human stampede (with fall) W52
furniture W22.03
lamppost W22.02
sports equipment W21.9
stationary W22.09
sports equipment W21.89
wall W22.01
person(s) W51
with fall W03
due to ice or snow W00.0
as, or caused by, a crowd or human stampede (with fall) W52
assault Y04.2
homicide (attempt) Y04.2
sports equipment W21.9
wall (when) W22.01
diving or jumping into water (in) W16.832
causing drowning W16.831
swimming pool W16.532
causing drowning W16.531
falling into water (in) W16.332
causing drowning W16.331
fountain —*see* Striking against, wall when, falling into water, specified NEC
natural body W16.132
causing drowning W16.131
reservoir —*see* Striking against, wall when, falling into water, specified NEC
specified NEC W16.332
causing drowning W16.331
swimming pool W16.032
causing drowning W16.031
swimming pool (when) W22.042
causing drowning W22.041
diving or jumping into water W16.532
causing drowning W16.531
falling into water W16.032
causing drowning W16.031

Struck (accidentally) by
airbag (automobile) W22.10
driver side W22.11
front passenger side W22.12
specified NEC W22.19
alligator W58.02
animal (not being ridden) NEC W55.89
avalanche —*see* Landslide
ball (hit) (thrown) W21.00
assault Y08.09
baseball W21.03
basketball W21.05
golf ball W21.04
football W21.01
soccer W21.02

- **Struck** *(continued)*
  - ball *(continued)*
    - softball W21.07
    - specified NEC W21.09
    - volleyball W21.06
  - bat or racquet
    - baseball bat W21.11
      - assault Y08.02
    - golf club W21.13
      - assault Y08.09
    - specified NEC W21.19
      - assault Y08.09
    - tennis racquet W21.12
      - assault Y08.09
  - bullet *—see also* Discharge, firearm by type
    - in war operations *—see* War operations
  - crocodile W58.12
  - dog W54.1
  - flare, Very pistol *—see* Discharge, firearm NEC
  - hailstones X39.8
  - hockey (ice)
    - field
      - puck W21.221
      - stick W21.211
    - puck W21.220
    - stick W21.210
      - assault Y08.01
  - landslide *—see* Landslide
  - law-enforcement agent (on duty) *—see* Legal, intervention, manhandling
    - with blunt object *—see* Legal, intervention, blunt object
  - lightning *—see subcategory* T75.0
    - causing fire *—see* Exposure, fire
  - machine *—see* Contact, with, by type of machine
  - mammal NEC W55.89
    - marine W56.32
  - marine animal W56.82
  - missile
    - firearm *—see* Discharge, firearm by type
    - in war operations *—see* War operations, missile
  - object W22.8
    - blunt W22.8
      - assault Y00
      - suicide (attempt) X79
      - undetermined whether accidental or intentional Y29
    - falling W20.8
      - from, in, on
        - building W20.1
          - burning (uncontrolled fire) X00.4
        - cataclysmic
          - earth surface movement NEC *—see* Landslide
          - storm *—see* Forces of nature, cataclysmic storm
        - cave-in W20.0
        - earthquake X34
        - machine (in operation) *—see* Contact, with, by type of machine
        - structure W20.1
          - burning X00.4
        - transport vehicle (in motion) *—see* Accident, transport, by type of vehicle
        - watercraft V93.49
          - due to
            - accident to craft V91.39
              - powered craft V91.33
                - ferry boat V91.31
                - fishing boat V91.32
                - jetskis V91.33
                - liner V91.31

- **Struck** *(continued)*
  - object *(continued)*
    - falling *(continued)*
      - from, in, on *(continued)*
        - watercraft *(continued)*
          - due to *(continued)*
            - accident to craft *(continued)*
              - powered craft *(continued)*
                - merchant ship V91.30
                - passenger ship V91.31
              - unpowered craft V91.38
                - canoe V91.35
                - inflatable V91.36
                - kayak V91.35
                - sailboat V91.34
                - surf-board V91.38
                - windsurfer V91.38
            - powered craft V93.43
              - ferry boat V93.41
              - fishing boat V93.42
              - jetskis V93.43
              - liner V93.41
              - merchant ship V93.40
              - passenger ship V93.41
            - unpowered craft V93.48
              - sailboat V93.44
              - surf-board V93.48
              - windsurfer V93.48
    - moving NEC W20.8
    - projected W20.8
      - assault Y00
      - in sports W21.9
        - assault Y08.09
        - ball W21.00
          - baseball W21.03
          - basketball W21.05
          - football W21.01
          - golf ball W21.04
          - soccer W21.02
          - softball W21.07
          - specified NEC W21.09
          - volleyball W21.06
        - bat or racquet
          - baseball bat W21.11
            - assault Y08.02
          - golf club W21.13
            - assault Y08.09
          - specified NEC W21.19
            - assault Y08.09
          - tennis racquet W21.12
            - assault Y08.09
        - hockey (ice)
          - field
            - puck W21.221
            - stick W21.211
          - puck W21.220
          - stick W21.210
            - assault Y08.01
        - specified NEC W21.89
    - set in motion by explosion *—see* Explosion
    - thrown W20.8
      - assault Y00
      - in sports W21.9
        - assault Y08.09
        - ball W21.00
          - baseball W21.03
          - basketball W21.05
          - football W21.01
          - golf ball W21.04
          - soccer W21.02
          - soft ball W21.07
          - specified NEC W21.09
          - volleyball W21.06

- **Struck** *(continued)*
  - object *(continued)*
    - thrown *(continued)*
      - in sports *(continued)*
        - bat or racquet
          - baseball bat W21.11
            - assault Y08.02
          - golf club W21.13
            - assault Y08.09
          - specified NEC W21.19
            - assault Y08.09
          - tennis racquet W21.12
            - assault Y08.09
        - hockey (ice)
          - field
            - puck W21.221
            - stick W21.211
          - puck W21.220
          - stick W21.210
            - assault Y08.01
        - specified NEC W21.89
  - other person(s) W50.0
    - with
      - blunt object W22.8
        - intentional, homicide (attempt) Y00
        - sports equipment W21.9
        - undetermined whether accidental or intentional Y29
      - fall W03
        - due to ice or snow W00.0
    - as, or caused by, a crowd or human stampede (with fall) W52
    - assault Y04.2
    - homicide (attempt) Y04.2
    - in legal intervention
      - injuring
        - bystander Y35.812
        - law enforcement personnel Y35.811
        - suspect Y35.813
    - sports equipment W21.9
  - police (on duty) *—see* Legal, intervention, manhandling
    - with blunt object *—see* Legal, intervention, blunt object
  - sports equipment W21.9
    - assault Y08.09
    - ball W21.00
      - baseball W21.03
      - basketball W21.05
      - football W21.01
      - golf ball W21.04
      - soccer W21.02
      - soft ball W21.07
      - specified NEC W21.09
      - volleyball W21.06
    - bat or racquet
      - baseball bat W21.11
        - assault Y08.02
      - golf club W21.13
        - assault Y08.09
      - specified NEC W21.19
      - tennis racquet W21.12
        - assault Y08.09
    - cleats (shoe) W21.31
    - foot wear NEC W21.39
    - football helmet W21.81
    - hockey (ice)
      - field
        - puck W21.221
        - stick W21.211
      - puck W21.220
      - stick W21.210
        - assault Y08.01
    - skate blades W21.32
    - specified NEC W21.89
      - assault Y08.09
  - thunderbolt *—see subcategory* T75.0
    - causing fire *—see* Exposure, fire

- **Struck** *(continued)*
  - transport vehicle NEC *—see also* Accident, transport V09.9
    - intentional, homicide (attempt) Y03.0
    - motor NEC *—see also* Accident, transport V09.20
      - homicide Y03.0
  - vehicle (transport) NEC *—see* Accident, transport, by type of vehicle
    - stationary (falling from jack, hydraulic lift, ramp) W20.8

- **Stumbling**
  - over
    - animal NEC W01.0
      - with fall W18.09
    - carpet, rug or (small) object W22.
      - with fall W18.09
    - person W51
      - with fall W03
        - due to ice or snow W00.0
  - without fall W18.40
    - due to
      - specified NEC W18.49
      - stepping from one level to another W18.43
      - stepping into hole or opening W18.42
      - stepping on object W18.41

- **Submersion** (accidental) *—see* Drowning

- **Suffocation** (accidental) (by external means) (by pressure) (mechanical) *—see also* category T71
  - due to, by
    - avalanche *—see* Landslide
    - explosion *—see* Explosion
    - fire *—see* Exposure, fire
    - food, any type (aspiration) (ingestion) (inhalation) *—see* categories T17 and T18
    - ignition *—see* Ignition
    - landslide *—see* Landslide
    - machine (ry) *—see* Contact, with, by type of machine
    - vomitus (aspiration) (inhalation) T17.81-
  - in
    - burning building X00.8

- **Suicide, suicidal** (attempted) (by) X83.8
  - blunt object X79
  - burning, burns X76
    - hot object X77.9
      - fluid NEC X77.2
      - household appliance X77.3
      - specified NEC X77.8
      - steam X77.0
      - tap water X77.1
      - vapors X77.0
  - caustic substance *—see* Table of Drugs and Chemicals
  - cold, extreme X83.2
  - collision of motor vehicle with
    - motor vehicle X82.0
    - specified NEC X82.8
    - train X82.1
    - tree X82.2
  - crashing of aircraft X83.0
  - cut (any part of body) X78.9
  - cutting or piercing instrument X78.9
    - dagger X78.2
    - glass X78.0
    - knife X78.1
    - specified NEC X78.8
    - sword X78.2
  - drowning (in) X71.9

Suicide, suicidal *(continued)*
drowning *(continued)*
bathtub X71.0
natural water X71.3
specified NEC X71.8
swimming pool X71.1
following fall X71.2
electrocution X83.1
explosive(s) (material) X75
fire, flames X76
firearm X74.9
airgun X74.01
handgun X72
hunting rifle X73.1
larger X73.9
specified NEC X73.8
machine gun X73.2
shotgun X73.0
specified NEC X74.8
hanging X83.8
hot object —*see* Suicide, burning, hot object
jumping
before moving object X81.8
motor vehicle X81.0
subway train X81.1
train X81.1
from high place X80
late effect of attempt —*see* X71-X83 with 7th character S
lying before moving object, train, vehicle X81.8
poisoning —*see* Table of Drugs and Chemicals
puncture (any part of body) —*see* Suicide, cutting or piercing instrument
scald —*see* Suicide, burning, hot object
sequelae of attempt —*see* X71-X83 with 7th character S
sharp object (any) —*see* Suicide, cutting or piercing instrument
shooting —*see* Suicide, firearm
specified means NEC X83.8
stab (any part of body) —*see* Suicide, cutting or piercing instrument
steam, hot vapors X77.0
strangulation X83.8
submersion —*see* Suicide, drowning
suffocation X83.8
wound NEC X83.8

Sunstroke X32

Supersonic waves (causing injury) W42.0

Surgical procedure, complication of (delayed or as an abnormal reaction without mention of misadventure) —*see also* Complication of
or following, by type of procedure
due to or as a result of misadventure —*see* Misadventure

Swallowed, swallowing
foreign body —*see* Foreign body, alimentary canal
poison —*see* Table of Drugs and Chemicals
substance
caustic or corrosive —*see* Table of Drugs and Chemicals
poisonous —*see* Table of Drugs and Chemicals

T

Tackle in sport W03

Terrorism (involving) Y38.80
biological weapons Y38.6X-
chemical weapons Y38.7X-

Terrorism *(continued)*
conflagration Y38.3X-
drowning and submersion Y38.89-
explosion Y38.2X-
destruction of aircraft Y38.1X-
marine weapons Y38.0X-
fire Y38.3X-
firearms Y38.4X-
hot substances Y38.3X-
lasers Y38.89-
nuclear weapons Y38.3X-
piercing or stabbing instruments Y38.89-
secondary effects Y38.9X-
specified method NEC Y38.89-
suicide bomber Y38.81-

Thirst X58

Threat to breathing
aspiration —*see* Aspiration
due to cave-in, falling earth or substance NEC —*see categories* T71

Thrown (accidentally)
against part (any) of or object in transport vehicle (in motion) NEC —*see also* Accident, transport
from
high place, homicide (attempt) Y01
machinery —*see* Contact, with, by type of machine
transport vehicle NEC —*see also* Accident, transport V89.9
off —*see* Thrown, from

Thunderbolt —*see* subcategory T75.0
causing fire —*see* Exposure, fire

Tidal wave (any injury) NEC —*see* Forces of nature, tidal wave

Took
overdose (drug) —*see* Table of Drugs and Chemicals
poison —*see* Table of Drugs and Chemicals

Tornado (any injury) X37.1

Torrential rain (any injury) X37.8

Torture X58

Trampled by animal NEC W55.89

Trapped (accidentally)
between objects (moving) (stationary and moving) —*see* Caught
by part (any) of
motorcycle V29.88
pedal cycle V19.88
transport vehicle NEC —*see also* Accident, transport V89.9

Travel (effects) (sickness) T75.3

Tree falling on or hitting (accidentally) (person) W20.8

Tripping
over
animal W01.0
with fall W01.0
carpet, rug or (small) object W22.8
with fall W18.09
person W51
with fall W03
due to ice or snow W00.0
without fall W18.40
due to
specified NEC W18.49
stepping from one level to another W18.43
stepping into hole or opening W18.42
stepping on object W18.41

Twisted by person(s) (accidentally) W50.2

Twisted by person *(continued)*
with intent to injure or kill Y04.0
as, or caused by, a crowd or human stampede (with fall) W52
assault Y04.0
homicide (attempt) Y04.0
in
fight Y04.0
legal intervention —*see* Legal, intervention, manhandling

Twisting (prolonged) (static) X50.1

U

Underdosing of necessary drugs, medicaments or biological substances Y63.6

Undetermined intent (contact) (exposure)
automobile collision Y32
blunt object Y29
drowning (submersion) (in) Y21.9
bathtub Y21.0
after fall Y21.1
natural water (lake) (ocean) (pond) (river) (stream) Y21.4
specified place NEC Y21.8
swimming pool Y21.2
after fall Y21.3
explosive material Y25
fall, jump or push from high place Y30
falling, lying or running before moving object Y31
fire Y26
firearm discharge Y24.9
airgun (BB) (pellet) Y24.0
handgun (pistol) (revolver) Y22
hunting rifle Y23.1
larger Y23.9
hunting rifle Y23.1
machine gun Y23.3
military Y23.2
shotgun Y23.0
specified type NEC Y23.8
machine gun Y23.3
military Y23.2
shotgun Y23.0
specified type NEC Y24.8
Very pistol Y24.8
hot object Y27.9
fluid NEC Y27.2
household appliance Y27.3
specified object NEC Y27.8
steam Y27.0
tap water Y27.1
vapor Y27.0
jump, fall or push from high place Y30
lying, falling or running before moving object Y31
motor vehicle crash Y32
push, fall or jump from high place Y30
running, falling or lying before moving object Y31
sharp object Y28.9
dagger Y28.2
glass Y28.0
knife Y28.1
specified object NEC Y28.8
sword Y28.2
smoke Y26
specified event NEC Y33

Use of hand as hammer X50.3

V

Vibration (causing injury) W49.9

Victim (of)
avalanche —*see* Landslide

Victim *(continued)*
earth movements NEC —*see* Forces of nature, earth movement
earthquake X34
flood —*see* Flood
landslide —*see* Landslide
lightning —*see subcategory* T75.0
causing fire —*see* Exposure, fire
storm (cataclysmic) NEC —*see* Forces of nature, cataclysmic storm
volcanic eruption X35

Volcanic eruption (any injury) X35

Vomitus, gastric contents in air passages (with asphyxia, obstruction or suffocation) T17.81-

W

Walked into stationary object (any) W22.09
furniture W22.03
lamppost W22.02
wall W22.01

War operations (injuries to military personnel and civilians during war, civil insurrection and peacekeeping missions) (by) (from) (involving) Y36.90
after cessation of hostilities Y36.89-
explosion (of)
bomb placed during war operations Y36.82-
mine placed during war operations Y36.81-
specified NEC Y36.88-
air blast Y36.20-
aircraft
destruction —*see* War operations, destruction of aircraft
airway restriction —*see* War operations, restriction of airways
asphyxiation —*see* War operations, restriction of airways
biological weapons Y36.6X-
blast Y36.20-
blast fragments Y36.20-
blast wave Y36.20-
blast wind Y36.20-
bomb Y36.20-
dirty Y36.50-
gasoline Y36.31-
incendiary Y36.31-
petrol Y36.31-
bullet Y36.43-
incendiary Y36.32-
rubber Y36.41-
chemical weapons Y36.7X-
combat
hand to hand (unarmed) combat Y36.44-
using blunt or piercing object Y36.45-
conflagration —*see* War operations, fire
conventional warfare NEC Y36.49-
depth-charge Y36.01-
destruction of aircraft Y36.10-
due to
air to air missile Y36.11-
collision with other aircraft Y36.12-
detonation (accidental) of onboard munitions and explosives Y36.14-
enemy fire or explosives Y36.11-
explosive placed on aircraft Y36.11-
onboard fire Y36.13-

War operations *(continued)*
destruction of aircraft *(continued)*
due to *(continued)*
rocket propelled grenade [RPG] Y36.11-
small arms fire Y36.11-
surface to air missile Y36.11-
specified NEC Y36.19-
detonation (accidental) of
onboard marine weapons Y36.05-
own munitions or munitions launch device Y36.24-
dirty bomb Y36.50-
explosion (of) Y36.20-
after cessation of hostilities
bomb placed during war operations Y36.82-
mine placed during war operations Y36.81-
aerial bomb Y36.21-
bomb NOS *—see also* War operations, bomb(s) Y36.20-
own munitions or munitions launch device (accidental) Y36.24-
fragments Y36.20-
grenade Y36.29-
guided missile Y36.22-
improvised explosive device [IED] (person-borne) (roadside) (vehicle-borne) Y36.23-
land mine Y36.29-
marine mine (at sea) (in harbor) Y36.02-
marine weapon Y36.00-
specified NEC Y36.09-
sea-based artillery shell Y36.03-

War operations *(continued)*
explosion *(continued)*
specified NEC Y36.29-
torpedo Y36.04-
fire Y36.30-
specified NEC Y36.39-
firearms
discharge Y36.43-
pellets Y36.42-
flamethrower Y36.33-
fragments (from) (of)
improvised explosive device [IED] (person-borne) (roadside) (vehicle-borne) Y36.26-
munitions Y36.25-
specified NEC Y36.29-
weapons Y36.27-
friendly fire Y36.92
hand to hand (unarmed) combat Y36.44-
hot substances *—see* War operations, fire
incendiary bullet Y36.32-
nuclear weapon (effects of) Y36.50-
acute radiation exposure Y36.54-
blast pressure Y36.51-
direct blast Y36.51-
direct heat Y36.53-
fallout exposure Y36.54-
fireball Y36.53-
indirect blast (struck or crushed by blast debris) (being thrown by blast) Y36.52-
ionizing radiation (immediate exposure) Y36.54-
nuclear radiation Y36.54-

War operations *(continued)*
nuclear weapon *(continued)*
radiation
ionizing (immediate exposure) Y36.54-
nuclear Y36.54-
thermal Y36.53-
specified NEC Y36.59-
secondary effects Y36.54-
thermal radiation Y36.53-
restriction of air (airway)
intentional Y36.46-
unintentional Y36.47-
rubber bullets Y36.41-
shrapnel NOS Y36.29-
suffocation *—see* War operations, restriction of airways
unconventional warfare NEC Y36.7X-
underwater blast NOS Y36.00-
warfare
conventional NEC Y36.49-
unconventional NEC Y36.7X-
weapons
biological weapons Y36.6X-
chemical Y36.7X-
nuclear (effects of) Y36.50-
acute radiation exposure Y36.54-
blast pressure Y36.51-
direct blast Y36.51-
direct heat Y36.53-
fallout exposure Y36.54-
fireball Y36.53-
radiation
ionizing (immediate exposure) Y36.54-
nuclear Y36.54-
thermal Y36.53-

War operations *(continued)*
weapons *(continued)*
nuclear *(continued)*
secondary effects Y36.54-
specified NEC Y36.59-
of mass destruction [WMD] Y36.
weapon of mass destruction [WMD
Y36.91

Washed
away by flood *—see* Flood
off road by storm (transport vehicle) *—see* Forces of nature, cataclysmic storm

Weather exposure NEC
—see Forces of nature

Weightlessness (causing injury) (effects of) (in spacecraft, real or simulated) X52

Work related condition Y99.0

Wound (accidental) NEC
—see also Injury X58
battle *—see also* War operations Y36.90
gunshot *—see* Discharge, firearm by type

Wreck transport vehicle NEC
—see also Accident, transport V89.

Wrong
device implanted into correct surgical site Y65.51
fluid in infusion Y65.1
procedure (operation) on correct patient Y65.51
patient, procedure performed on Y65.52

ʼable of Contents

1. Certain infectious and parasitic diseases (A00-B99)
2. Neoplasms (C00-D49)
3. Diseases of the blood and blood-forming organs and certain disorders involving the immune mechanism (D50-D89)
4. Endocrine, nutritional and metabolic diseases (E00-E89)
5. Mental, Behavioral and Neurodevelopmental disorders (F01-F99)
6. Diseases of the nervous system (G00-G99)
7. Diseases of the eye and adnexa (H00-H59)
8. Diseases of the ear and mastoid process (H60-H95)
9. Diseases of the circulatory system (I00-I99)
10. Diseases of the respiratory system (J00-J99)
11. Diseases of the digestive system (K00-K95)
12. Diseases of the skin and subcutaneous tissue (L00-L99)
13. Diseases of the musculoskeletal system and connective tissue (M00-M99)
14. Diseases of the genitourinary system (N00-N99)
15. Pregnancy, childbirth and the puerperium (O00-O9A)
16. Certain conditions originating in the perinatal period (P00-P96)
17. Congenital malformations, deformations and chromosomal abnormalities (Q00-Q99)
18. Symptoms, signs and abnormal clinical and laboratory findings, not elsewhere classified (R00-R99)
19. Injury, poisoning and certain other consequences of external causes (S00-T88)
20. External causes of morbidity (V00-Y99)
21. Factors influencing health status and contact with health services (Z00-Z99)

nstructional Notations

ncludes:

he word 'Includes' appears immediately under certain categories to further define, or give examples of, the content of the category.

ːxcludes Notes

ne ICD-10-CM has two types of excludes notes. Each note has a different definition for use but they are both similar in that they indicate that codes excluded from each her are independent of each other.

ːxcludes1

type 1 Excludes note is a pure excludes. It means 'NOT CODED HERE!' An Excludes1 note indicates that the code excluded should never be used at the same time as the ɔde above the Excludes1 note. An Excludes1 is used when two conditions cannot occur together, such as a congenital form versus an acquired form of the same condition.

ːxcludes2

type 2 excludes note represents 'Not included here'. An Excludes2 note indicates that the condition excluded is not part of the condition it is excluded from but a patient ay have both conditions at the same time. When an Excludes2 note appears under a code it is acceptable to use both the code and the excluded code together.

ːode First/Use Additional Code notes (etiology/manifestation paired codes)

ertain conditions have both an underlying etiology and multiple body system manifestations due to the underlying etiology. For such conditions the ICD-10-CM has a ɔding convention that requires the underlying condition be sequenced first followed by the manifestation. Wherever such a combination exists there is a 'use additional ɔde' note at the etiology code, and a 'code first' note at the manifestation code. These instructional notes indicate the proper sequencing order of the codes, etiology ɔllowed by manifestation.

 most cases the manifestation codes will have in the code title, 'in diseases classified elsewhere.' Codes with this title are a component of the etiology/ manifestation ɔnvention. The code title indicates that it is a manifestation code. 'In diseases classified elsewhere' codes are never permitted to be used as first listed or principal diagnosis ɔdes. They must be used in conjunction with an underlying condition code and they must be listed following the underlying condition.

ːode Also

"code also" note instructs that two codes may be required to fully describe a condition, but this note does not provide sequencing direction. **The sequencing depends on e circumstances of the encounter**.

th characters and placeholder X

ertain ICD-10-CM categories have applicable 7th characters. The applicable 7th character is required for all codes within the category, or as the notes in the Tabular List struct. The 7th character must always be the 7th character in the data field. If a code that requires a 7th character is not 6 characters, a placeholder X must be used to fill the empty characters.

Chapter 1: Certain Infectious and Parasitic Diseases (A00-B99)

Includes: diseases generally recognized as communicable or transmissible

Use additional code to identify resistance to antimicrobial drugs (Z16-)

Excludes1: *certain localized infections - see body system-related chapters*

Excludes2: *carrier or suspected carrier of infectious disease (Z22.-)*
infectious and parasitic diseases specific to the perinatal period (P35-P39)
infectious and parasitic diseases complicating pregnancy, childbirth and the puerperium (O98.-)
influenza and other acute respiratory infections (J00-J22)

This chapter contains the following category blocks:

A00-A09	Intestinal infectious diseases
A15-A19	Tuberculosis
A20-A28	Certain zoonotic bacterial diseases
A30-A49	Other bacterial diseases
A50-A64	Infections with a predominantly sexual mode of transmission
A65-A69	Other spirochetal diseases
A70-A74	Other diseases caused by chlamydiae
A75-A79	Rickettsioses
A80-A89	Viral and prion infections of the central nervous system
A90-A99	Arthropod-borne viral fevers and viral hemorrhagic fevers
B00-B09	Viral infections characterized by skin and mucous membrane lesions
B10	Other human herpesviruses
B15-B19	Viral hepatitis
B20	Human immunodeficiency virus [HIV] disease
B25-B34	Other viral diseases
B35-B49	Mycoses
B50-B64	Protozoal diseases
B65-B83	Helminthiases
B85-B89	Pediculosis, acariasis and other infestations
B90-B94	Sequelae of infectious and parasitic diseases
B95-B97	Bacterial and viral infectious agents
B99	Other infectious diseases

C. Chapter-Specific Coding Guidelines

In addition to general coding guidelines, there are guidelines for specific diagnoses and/or conditions in the classification. Unless otherwise indicated, these guidelines apply to all health care settings. Please refer to Section II for guidelines on the selection of principal diagnosis.

1. Chapter 1: Certain Infectious and Parasitic Diseases (A00-B99)

a. Human Immunodeficiency Virus (HIV) Infections

1) Code only confirmed cases

Code only confirmed cases of HIV infection/illness. This is an exception to the hospital inpatient guideline Section II, H.

In this context, "confirmation" does not require documentation of positive serology or culture for HIV; the provider's diagnostic statement that the patient is HIV positive, or has an HIV-related illness is sufficient.

2) Selection and sequencing of HIV codes

(a) Patient admitted for HIV-related condition

If a patient is admitted for an HIV-related condition, the principal diagnosis should be B20, Human immunodeficiency virus [HIV] disease followed by additional diagnosis codes for all reported HIV-related conditions.

(b) Patient with HIV disease admitted for unrelated condition

If a patient with HIV disease is admitted for an unrelated condition (such as a traumatic injury), the code for the unrelated condition (e.g., the nature of injury code) should be the principal diagnosis. Other diagnoses would be B20 followed by additional diagnosis codes for all reported HIV-related conditions.

(c) Whether the patient is newly diagnosed

Whether the patient is newly diagnosed or has had previous admissions/encounters for HIV conditions is irrelevant to the sequencing decision.

(d) Asymptomatic human immunodeficiency virus

Z21, Asymptomatic human immunodeficiency virus [HIV] infection status, is to be applied when the patient without any documentation of symptoms is listed as being "HIV positive," "known HIV," "HIV test positive," or similar terminology. Do not use this code if the term "AIDS" is used or if the patient is treated for any HIV-related illness or is described as having any condition(s) resulting from his/her HIV positive status; use B20 in these cases.

(e) Patients with inconclusive HIV serology

Patients with inconclusive HIV serology, but no definitive diagnosis c manifestations of the illness, may be assigned code R75, Inconclusiv laboratory evidence of human immunodeficiency virus [HIV].

(f) Previously diagnosed HIV-related illness

Patients with any known prior diagnosis of an HIV-related illness shoul be coded to B20. Once a patient has developed an HIV-related illnes the patient should always be assigned code B20 on every subseque admission/encounter. Patients previously diagnosed with any HI illness (B20) should never be assigned to R75 or Z21, Asymptomati human immunodeficiency virus [HIV] infection status.

(g) HIV Infection in Pregnancy, Childbirth and the Puerperium

During pregnancy, childbirth or the puerperium, a patient admitte (or presenting for a health care encounter) because of an HIV-relate illness should receive a principal diagnosis code of O98.7-, Huma immunodeficiency [HIV] disease complicating pregnancy, childbirth an the puerperium, followed by B20 and the code(s) for the HIV-relate illness(es).

Codes from Chapter 15 always take sequencing priority.

Patients with asymptomatic HIV infection status admitted (or presentin for a health care encounter) during pregnancy, childbirth, or th puerperium should receive codes of O98.7- and Z21.

(h) Encounters for testing for HIV

If a patient is being seen to determine his/her HIV status, use code Z11.4 Encounter for screening for human immunodeficiency virus [HIV]. Us additional codes for any associated high risk behavior.

If a patient with signs or symptoms is being seen for HIV testing, cod the signs and symptoms. An additional counseling code Z71.7, Huma immunodeficiency virus [HIV] counseling, may be used if counseling i provided during the encounter for the test.

When a patient returns to be informed of his/her HIV test results and th test result is negative, use code Z71.7, Human immunodeficiency viru [HIV] counseling.

If the results are positive, see previous guidelines and assign codes a appropriate.

b. Infectious agents as the cause of diseases classified to other chapters

Certain infections are classified in chapters other than Chapter 1 and n organism is identified as part of the infection code. In these instances, it i necessary to use an additional code from Chapter 1 to identify the organism A code from category B95, Streptococcus, Staphylococcus, and Enterococcu as the cause of diseases classified to other chapters, B96, Other bacterial agent as the cause of diseases classified to other chapters, or B97, Viral agents as th cause of diseases classified to other chapters, is to be used as an additional cod to identify the organism. An instructional note will be found at the infectio code advising that an additional organism code is required.

c. Infections resistant to antibiotics

Many bacterial infections are resistant to current antibiotics. It is necessary t identify all infections documented as antibiotic resistant. Assign a code fro category Z16, Resistance to antimicrobial drugs, following the infection cod only if the infection code does not identify drug resistance.

d. Sepsis, Severe Sepsis, and Septic Shock

1) Coding of Sepsis and Severe Sepsis

(a) Sepsis

For a diagnosis of sepsis, assign the appropriate code for the underlyin systemic infection. If the type of infection or causal organism is nc further specified, assign code A41.9, Sepsis, unspecified organism.

A code from subcategory R65.2, Severe sepsis, should not be assigne unless severe sepsis or an associated acute organ dysfunction i documented.

(i) Negative or inconclusive blood cultures and sepsis

Negative or inconclusive blood cultures do not preclude a diagnosi of sepsis in patients with clinical evidence of the condition, howeve the provider should be queried.

(ii) Urosepsis

The term urosepsis is a nonspecific term. It is not to be considere synonymous with sepsis. It has no default code in the Alphabeti Index. Should a provider use this term, he/she must be queried fo clarification.

(iii) Sepsis with organ dysfunction

If a patient has sepsis and associated acute organ dysfunction c multiple organ dysfunction (MOD), follow the instructions fc coding severe sepsis.

(iv) Acute organ dysfunction that is not clearly associated with the sepsis

If a patient has sepsis and an acute organ dysfunction, but the medical record documentation indicates that the acute organ dysfunction is related to a medical condition other than the sepsis, do not assign a code from subcategory R65.2, Severe sepsis. An acute organ dysfunction must be associated with the sepsis in order to assign the severe sepsis code. If the documentation is not clear as to whether an acute organ dysfunction is related to the sepsis or another medical condition, query the provider.

(b) Severe sepsis

The coding of severe sepsis requires a minimum of 2 codes: first a code for the underlying systemic infection, followed by a code from subcategory R65.2, Severe sepsis. If the causal organism is not documented, assign code A41.9, Sepsis, unspecified organism, for the infection. Additional code(s) for the associated acute organ dysfunction are also required.

Due to the complex nature of severe sepsis, some cases may require querying the provider prior to assignment of the codes.

2) Septic shock

(a) Septic shock generally refers to circulatory failure associated with severe sepsis, and therefore, it represents a type of acute organ dysfunction.

For cases of septic shock, the code for the systemic infection should be sequenced first, followed by code R65.21, Severe sepsis with septic shock or code T81.12, Postprocedural septic shock. Any additional codes for the other acute organ dysfunctions should also be assigned. As noted in the sequencing instructions in the Tabular List, the code for septic shock cannot be assigned as a principal diagnosis.

3) Sequencing of severe sepsis

If severe sepsis is present on admission, and meets the definition of principal diagnosis, the underlying systemic infection should be assigned as principal diagnosis followed by the appropriate code from subcategory R65.2 as required by the sequencing rules in the Tabular List. A code from subcategory R65.2 can never be assigned as a principal diagnosis.

When severe sepsis develops during an encounter (it was not present on admission) the underlying systemic infection and the appropriate code from subcategory R65.2 should be assigned as secondary diagnoses.

Severe sepsis may be present on admission but the diagnosis may not be confirmed until sometime after admission. If the documentation is not clear whether severe sepsis was present on admission, the provider should be queried.

4) Sepsis and severe sepsis with a localized infection

If the reason for admission is both sepsis or severe sepsis and a localized infection, such as pneumonia or cellulitis, a code(s) for the underlying systemic infection should be assigned first and the code for the localized infection should be assigned as a secondary diagnosis. If the patient has severe sepsis, a code from subcategory R65.2 should also be assigned as a secondary diagnosis. If the patient is admitted with a localized infection, such as pneumonia, and sepsis/severe sepsis doesn't develop until after admission, the localized infection should be assigned first, followed by the appropriate sepsis/severe sepsis codes.

5) Sepsis due to a postprocedural infection

(a) Documentation of causal relationship

As with all postprocedural complications, code assignment is based on the provider's documentation of the relationship between the infection and the procedure.

(b) Sepsis due to a postprocedural infection

For such cases, the postprocedural infection code, such as, T80.2, Infections following infusion, transfusion, and therapeutic injection, T81.4, Infection following a procedure, T88.0, Infection following immunization, or O86.0, Infection of obstetric surgical wound, should be coded first, followed by the code for the specific infection. If the patient has severe sepsis the appropriate code from subcategory R65.2 should also be assigned with the additional code(s) for any acute organ dysfunction.

(c) Postprocedural infection and postprocedural septic shock

In cases where a postprocedural infection has occurred and has resulted in severe sepsis and postprocedural septic shock, the code for the precipitating complication such as code T81.4, Infection following a procedure, or O86.0, Infection of obstetrical surgical wound should be coded first followed by code R65.20, Severe sepsis without septic shock. A code for the systemic infection should also be assigned.

If a postprocedural infection has resulted in postprocedural septic shock, the code for the precipitating complication such as code T81.4, Infection following a procedure, or O96.0, Infection of obstetrical surgical wound should be coded first followed by code T81.12-, Postprocedural septic shock. A code for the systemic infection should also be assigned.

6) Sepsis and severe sepsis associated with a noninfectious process (condition)

In some cases a noninfectious process (condition), such as trauma, may lead to an infection which can result in sepsis or severe sepsis. If sepsis or severe sepsis is documented as associated with a noninfectious condition, such as a burn or serious injury, and this condition meets the definition for principal diagnosis, the code for the noninfectious condition should be sequenced first, followed by the code for the resulting infection. If severe sepsis, is present a code from subcategory R65.2 should also be assigned with any associated organ dysfunction(s) codes. It is not necessary to assign a code from subcategory R65.1, Systemic inflammatory response syndrome (SIRS) of non-infectious origin, for these cases.

If the infection meets the definition of principal diagnosis it should be sequenced before the non-infectious condition. When both the associated non-infectious condition and the infection meet the definition of principal diagnosis either may be assigned as principal diagnosis.

Only one code from category R65, Symptoms and signs specifically associated with systemic inflammation and infection, should be assigned. Therefore, when a non-infectious condition leads to an infection resulting in severe sepsis, assign the appropriate code from subcategory R65.2, Severe sepsis. Do not additionally assign a code from subcategory R65.1, Systemic inflammatory response syndrome (SIRS) of non-infectious origin.

See Section I.C.18. SIRS due to non-infectious process

7) Sepsis and septic shock complicating abortion, pregnancy, childbirth, and the puerperium

See Section I.C.15. Sepsis and septic shock complicating abortion, pregnancy, childbirth and the puerperium

8) Newborn sepsis

See Section I.C.16. f. Bacterial sepsis of Newborn

e. Methicillin Resistant *Staphylococcus aureus* (MRSA) Conditions

1) Selection and sequencing of MRSA codes

(a) Combination codes for MRSA infection

When a patient is diagnosed with an infection that is due to methicillin resistant Staphylococcus aureus (MRSA), and that infection has a combination code that includes the causal organism (e.g., sepsis, pneumonia) assign the appropriate combination code for the condition (e.g., code A41.02, Sepsis due to Methicillin resistant Staphylococcus aureus or code J15.212, Pneumonia due to Methicillin resistant Staphylococcus aureus). Do not assign code B95.62, Methicillin resistant Staphylococcus aureus infection as the cause of diseases classified elsewhere, as an additional code because the combination code includes the type of infection and the MRSA organism. Do not assign a code from subcategory Z16.11, Resistance to penicillins, as an additional diagnosis.

See Section C.1. for instructions on coding and sequencing of sepsis and severe sepsis.

(b) Other codes for MRSA infection

When there is documentation of a current infection (e.g., wound infection, stitch abscess, urinary tract infection) due to MRSA, and that infection does not have a combination code that includes the causal organism, assign the appropriate code to identify the condition along with code B95.62, Methicillin resistant Staphylococcus aureus infection as the cause of diseases classified elsewhere for the MRSA infection. Do not assign a code from subcategory Z16.11, Resistance to penicillins.

(c) Methicillin susceptible Staphylococcus aureus (MSSA) and MRSA colonization

The condition or state of being colonized or carrying MSSA or MRSA is called colonization or carriage, while an individual person is described as being colonized or being a carrier. Colonization means that MSSA or MSRA is present on or in the body without necessarily causing illness. A positive MRSA colonization test might be documented by the provider as "MRSA screen positive" or "MRSA nasal swab positive".

Assign code Z22.322, Carrier or suspected carrier of Methicillin resistant Staphylococcus aureus, for patients documented as having MRSA colonization. Assign code Z22.321, Carrier or suspected carrier of Methicillin susceptible Staphylococcus aureus, for patient documented as having MSSA colonization. Colonization is not necessarily indicative of a disease process or as the cause of a specific condition the patient may have unless documented as such by the provider.

(d) MRSA colonization and infection

If a patient is documented as having both MRSA colonization and infection during a hospital admission, code Z22.322, Carrier or suspected carrier of Methicillin resistant Staphylococcus aureus, and a code for the MRSA infection may both be assigned.

f. Zika virus infections

1) Code only confirmed cases

Code only a confirmed diagnosis of Zika virus (A92.5, Zika virus disease) as documented by the provider. This is an exception to the hospital inpatient guideline Section II, H.

In this context, "confirmation" does not require documentation of the type of test performed; the physician's diagnostic statement that the condition is confirmed is sufficient. This code should be assigned regardless of the stated mode of transmission.

If the provider documents "suspected", "possible" or "provable" Zika, do not assign code A92.5. Assign a code(s) explaining the reason for encounter (such as fever, rash, or joint pain) or Z20.828, Contact with and (suspected) exposure to other viral communicable diseases.

Intestinal infectious diseases (A00-A09)

A00 Cholera

CC **A00.0 Cholera due to Vibrio cholerae 01, biovar cholerae**
Classical cholera
CC Exclusion see Appendix A PDX collection 0002

CC **A00.1 Cholera due to Vibrio cholerae 01, biovar eltor**
Cholera eltor
CC Exclusion see Appendix A PDX collection 0002

CC **A00.9 Cholera, unspecified**
CC Exclusion see Appendix A PDX collection 0002

A01 Typhoid and paratyphoid fevers

\+ **A01.0 Typhoid fever**
Infection due to Salmonella typhi

CC **A01.00 Typhoid fever, unspecified**
CC Exclusion see Appendix A PDX collection 0003

CC **A01.01 Typhoid meningitis**
CC Exclusion see Appendix A PDX collection 0003

CC **A01.02 Typhoid fever with heart involvement**
Typhoid endocarditis
Typhoid myocarditis
CC Exclusion see Appendix A PDX collection 0003

CC **A01.03 Typhoid pneumonia**
CC Exclusion see Appendix A PDX collection 0003

CC **A01.04 Typhoid arthritis**
CC Exclusion see Appendix A PDX collection 0003

CC **A01.05 Typhoid osteomyelitis**
CC Exclusion see Appendix A PDX collection 0003

CC **A01.09 Typhoid fever with other complications**
CC Exclusion see Appendix A PDX collection 0003

CC **A01.1 Paratyphoid fever A**
CC Exclusion see Appendix A PDX collection 0003

CC **A01.2 Paratyphoid fever B**
CC Exclusion see Appendix A PDX collection 0003

CC **A01.3 Paratyphoid fever C**
CC Exclusion see Appendix A PDX collection 0003

CC **A01.4 Paratyphoid fever, unspecified**
Infection due to Salmonella paratyphi NOS
CC Exclusion see Appendix A PDX collection 0003

A02 Other salmonella infections

Includes: infection or foodborne intoxication due to any Salmonella species other than S. typhi and S. paratyphi

CC **A02.0 Salmonella enteritis**
Salmonellosis
CC Exclusion see Appendix A PDX collection 0004

MCC **A02.1 Salmonella sepsis**
MCC Exclusion see Appendix A PDX collection 0005
Review coding guideline C.1.d

\+ **A02.2 Localized salmonella infections**

A02.20 Localized salmonella infection, unspecified

MCC **A02.21 Salmonella meningitis**
MCC Exclusion see Appendix A PDX collection 0006

MCC **A02.22 Salmonella pneumonia**
MCC Exclusion see Appendix A PDX collection 0007

CC **A02.23 Salmonella arthritis**
CC Exclusion see Appendix A PDX collection 0008

CC **A02.24 Salmonella osteomyelitis**
CC Exclusion see Appendix A PDX collection 0009

CC **A02.25 Salmonella pyelonephritis**
Salmonella tubulo-interstitial nephropathy
CC Exclusion see Appendix A PDX collection 0010

CC **A02.29 Salmonella with other localized infection**
CC Exclusion see Appendix A PDX collection 0010

CC **A02.8 Other specified salmonella infections**
CC Exclusion see Appendix A PDX collection 0011

CC **A02.9 Salmonella infection, unspecified**
CC Exclusion see Appendix A PDX collection 0012

A03 Shigellosis

CC **A03.0 Shigellosis due to Shigella dysenteriae**
Group A shigellosis [Shiga-Kruse dysentery]
CC Exclusion see Appendix A PDX collection 0013

A03.1 Shigellosis due to Shigella flexneri
Group B shigellosis

A03.2 Shigellosis due to Shigella boydii
Group C shigellosis

A03.3 Shigellosis due to Shigella sonnei
Group D shigellosis

A03.8 Other shigellosis

A03.9 Shigellosis, unspecified
Bacillary dysentery NOS

A04 Other bacterial intestinal infections

Excludes1: *bacterial foodborne intoxications, NEC (A05.-)*
tuberculous enteritis (A18.32)

CC **A04.0 Enteropathogenic Escherichia coli infection**
CC Exclusion see Appendix A PDX collection 0014

CC **A04.1 Enterotoxigenic Escherichia coli infection**
CC Exclusion see Appendix A PDX collection 0014

CC **A04.2 Enteroinvasive Escherichia coli infection**
CC Exclusion see Appendix A PDX collection 0014

CC **A04.3 Enterohemorrhagic Escherichia coli infection**
CC Exclusion see Appendix A PDX collection 0014

CC **A04.4 Other intestinal Escherichia coli infections**
Escherichia coli enteritis NOS
CC Exclusion see Appendix A PDX collection 0014

CC **A04.5 Campylobacter enteritis**
CC Exclusion see Appendix A PDX collection 0015

CC **A04.6 Enteritis due to Yersinia enterocolitica**
Excludes1: *extraintestinal yersiniosis (A28.2)*
CC Exclusion see Appendix A PDX collection 0015

\+ **A04.7 Enterocolitis due to Clostridium difficile**
Foodborne intoxication by Clostridium difficile
Pseudomembraneous colitis

CC **A04.71 Enterocolitis due to clostridium difficile, recurrent**
CC Exclusion see Appendix A PDX collection 0015

CC **A04.72 Enterocolitis due to clostridium difficile, not specified as recurrent**
CC Exclusion see Appendix A PDX collection 0015

CC **A04.8 Other specified bacterial intestinal infections**
CC Exclusion see Appendix A PDX collection 0015

CC **A04.9 Bacterial intestinal infection, unspecified**
Bacterial enteritis NOS
CC Exclusion see Appendix A PDX collection 0016

A05 Other bacterial foodborne intoxications, not elsewhere classified

Excludes1: *Clostridium difficile foodborne intoxication and infection (A04.7-)*
Escherichia coli infection (A04.0-A04.4)
listeriosis (A32.-)
salmonella foodborne intoxication and infection (A02.-)
toxic effect of noxious foodstuffs (T61-T62)

CC **A05.0 Foodborne staphylococcal intoxication**
CC Exclusion see Appendix A PDX collection 0017

CC **A05.1 Botulism food poisoning**
Botulism NOS
Classical foodborne intoxication due to Clostridium botulinum
Excludes1: *infant botulism (A48.51)*
wound botulism (A48.52)
CC Exclusion see Appendix A PDX collection 0018

CC **A05.2 Foodborne Clostridium perfringens [Clostridium welchii] intoxication**
Enteritis necroticans
Pig-bel
CC Exclusion see Appendix A PDX collection 0019

CC **A05.3 Foodborne Vibrio parahaemolyticus intoxication**
CC Exclusion see Appendix A PDX collection 0017

CC **A05.4 Foodborne Bacillus cereus intoxication**
CC Exclusion see Appendix A PDX collection 0017

CC **A05.5 Foodborne Vibrio vulnificus intoxication**
CC Exclusion see Appendix A PDX collection 0017

CC **A05.8 Other specified bacterial foodborne intoxications**
CC Exclusion see Appendix A PDX collection 0017

A05.9 Bacterial foodborne intoxication, unspecified

A06 Amebiasis

Includes: infection due to Entamoeba histolytica
Excludes1: *other protozoal intestinal diseases (A07.-)*
Excludes2: *acanthamebiasis (B60.1-)*
Naegleriasis (B60.2)

CC **A06.0 Acute amebic dysentery**
Acute amebiasis
Intestinal amebiasis NOS
CC Exclusion see Appendix A PDX collection 0020

CC **A06.1 Chronic intestinal amebiasis**
CC Exclusion see Appendix A PDX collection 0020

CC **A06.2 Amebic nondysenteric colitis**
CC Exclusion see Appendix A PDX collection 0021

CC **A06.3 Ameboma of intestine**
Ameboma NOS
CC Exclusion see Appendix A PDX collection 0022

MCC **A06.4 Amebic liver abscess**
Hepatic amebiasis
MCC Exclusion see Appendix A PDX collection 0023

MCC **A06.5 Amebic lung abscess**
Amebic abscess of lung (and liver)
MCC Exclusion see Appendix A PDX collection 0024

MCC **A06.6 Amebic brain abscess**
Amebic abscess of brain (and liver) (and lung)
MCC Exclusion see Appendix A PDX collection 0025

A06.7 Cutaneous amebiasis

\+ **A06.8 Amebic infection of other sites**

CC **A06.81 Amebic cystitis**
CC Exclusion see Appendix A PDX collection 0022

CC **A06.82 Other amebic genitourinary infections**
Amebic balanitis
Amebic vesiculitis
Amebic vulvovaginitis
CC Exclusion see Appendix A PDX collection 0022

CC **A06.89 Other amebic infections**
Amebic appendicitis
Amebic splenic abscess
CC Exclusion see Appendix A PDX collection 0022

A06.9 Amebiasis, unspecified

A07 Other protozoal intestinal diseases

A07.0 Balantidiasis
Balantidial dysentery

CC **A07.1 Giardiasis [lambliasis]**
CC Exclusion see Appendix A PDX collection 0026

CC **A07.2 Cryptosporidiosis**
CC Exclusion see Appendix A PDX collection 0026

CC **A07.3 Isosporiasis**
Infection due to Isospora belli and Isospora hominis
Intestinal coccidiosis
Isosporosis
CC Exclusion see Appendix A PDX collection 0026

CC **A07.4 Cyclosporiasis**
CC Exclusion see Appendix A PDX collection 0027

CC **A07.8 Other specified protozoal intestinal diseases**
Intestinal microsporidiosis
Intestinal trichomoniasis
Sarcocystosis
Sarcosporidiosis
CC Exclusion see Appendix A PDX collection 0026

CC **A07.9 Protozoal intestinal disease, unspecified**
Flagellate diarrhea
Protozoal colitis
Protozoal diarrhea
Protozoal dysentery
CC Exclusion see Appendix A PDX collection 0026

A08 Viral and other specified intestinal infections

Excludes1: *influenza with involvement of gastrointestinal tract (J09.X3, J10.2, J11.2)*

CC **A08.0 Rotaviral enteritis**
CC Exclusion see Appendix A PDX collection 0028

\+ **A08.1 Acute gastroenteropathy due to Norwalk agent and other small round viruses**

CC **A08.11 Acute gastroenteropathy due to Norwalk agent**
Acute gastroenteropathy due to Norovirus
Acute gastroenteropathy due to Norwalk-like agent
CC Exclusion see Appendix A PDX collection 0028

CC **A08.19 Acute gastroenteropathy due to other small round viruses**
Acute gastroenteropathy due to small round virus [SRV] NOS
CC Exclusion see Appendix A PDX collection 0028

CC **A08.2 Adenoviral enteritis**
CC Exclusion see Appendix A PDX collection 0028

\+ **A08.3 Other viral enteritis**

CC **A08.31 Calicivirus enteritis**
CC Exclusion see Appendix A PDX collection 0028

CC **A08.32 Astrovirus enteritis**
CC Exclusion see Appendix A PDX collection 0028

CC **A08.39 Other viral enteritis**
Coxsackie virus enteritis
Echovirus enteritis
Enterovirus enteritis NEC
Torovirus enteritis
CC Exclusion see Appendix A PDX collection 0028

A08.4 Viral intestinal infection, unspecified
Viral enteritis NOS
Viral gastroenteritis NOS
Viral gastroenteropathy NOS
AHA CC: 3Q, 2016, 12

A08.8 Other specified intestinal infections

CC **A09 Infectious gastroenteritis and colitis, unspecified**

Infectious colitis NOS
Infectious enteritis NOS
Infectious gastroenteritis NOS
Excludes1: *colitis NOS (K52.9)*
diarrhea NOS (R19.7)
enteritis NOS (K52.9)
gastroenteritis NOS (K52.9)
noninfective gastroenteritis and colitis, unspecified (K52.9)
CC Exclusion see Appendix A PDX collection 0017
Valid 3-character code, no further characters required

Tuberculosis (A15-A19)

Includes: infections due to Mycobacterium tuberculosis and Mycobacterium bovis

Excludes1: *congenital tuberculosis (P37.0)*
nonspecific reaction to test for tuberculosis without active tuberculosis (R76.1-)
pneumoconiosis associated with tuberculosis, any type in A15 (J65)
positive PPD (R76.11)
positive tuberculin skin test without active tuberculosis (R76.11)
sequelae of tuberculosis (B90.-)
silicotuberculosis (J65)

A15 Respiratory tuberculosis

CC **A15.0 Tuberculosis of lung**
Tuberculous bronchiectasis
Tuberculous fibrosis of lung
Tuberculous pneumonia
Tuberculous pneumothorax
CC Exclusion see Appendix A PDX collection 0029

CC **A15.4 Tuberculosis of intrathoracic lymph nodes**
Tuberculosis of hilar lymph nodes
Tuberculosis of mediastinal lymph nodes
Tuberculosis of tracheobronchial lymph nodes
Excludes1: *tuberculosis specified as primary (A15.7)*
CC Exclusion see Appendix A PDX collection 0029

CC **A15.5 Tuberculosis of larynx, trachea and bronchus**
Tuberculosis of bronchus
Tuberculosis of glottis
Tuberculosis of larynx
Tuberculosis of trachea
CC Exclusion see Appendix A PDX collection 0029

CC **A15.6 Tuberculous pleurisy**
Tuberculosis of pleura Tuberculous empyema
Excludes1: *primary respiratory tuberculosis (A15.7)*
CC Exclusion see Appendix A PDX collection 0029

CC **A15.7 Primary respiratory tuberculosis**
CC Exclusion see Appendix A PDX collection 0030

CC **A15.8 Other respiratory tuberculosis**
Mediastinal tuberculosis
Nasopharyngeal tuberculosis
Tuberculosis of nose
Tuberculosis of sinus [any nasal]
CC Exclusion see Appendix A PDX collection 0031

CC **A15.9 Respiratory tuberculosis unspecified**
CC Exclusion see Appendix A PDX collection 0031

A17 Tuberculosis of nervous system

MCC **A17.0 Tuberculous meningitis**
Tuberculosis of meninges (cerebral)(spinal)
Tuberculous leptomeningitis
Excludes1: *tuberculous meningoencephalitis (A17.82)*
MCC Exclusion see Appendix A PDX collection 0032

MCC **A17.1 Meningeal tuberculoma**
Tuberculoma of meninges (cerebral) (spinal)
Excludes2: *tuberculoma of brain and spinal cord (A17.81)*
MCC Exclusion see Appendix A PDX collection 0032

\+ **A17.8 Other tuberculosis of nervous system**

MCC **A17.81 Tuberculoma of brain and spinal cord**
Tuberculous abscess of brain and spinal cord
MCC Exclusion see Appendix A PDX collection 0033

MCC **A17.82 Tuberculous meningoencephalitis**
Tuberculous myelitis
MCC Exclusion see Appendix A PDX collection 0033

MCC **A17.83 Tuberculous neuritis**
Tuberculous mononeuropathy
No MCC Exclusions

MCC **A17.89 Other tuberculosis of nervous system**
Tuberculous polyneuropathy
MCC Exclusion see Appendix A PDX collection 0034

CC **A17.9 Tuberculosis of nervous system, unspecified**
CC Exclusion see Appendix A PDX collection 0035

A18 Tuberculosis of other organs

\+ **A18.0 Tuberculosis of bones and joints**

CC **A18.01 Tuberculosis of spine**
Pott's disease or curvature of spine
Tuberculous arthritis
Tuberculous osteomyelitis of spine
Tuberculous spondylitis
CC Exclusion see Appendix A PDX collection 0036

CC **A18.02 Tuberculous arthritis of other joints**
Tuberculosis of hip (joint)
Tuberculosis of knee (joint)
CC Exclusion see Appendix A PDX collection 0037

CC **A18.03 Tuberculosis of other bones**
Tuberculous mastoiditis
Tuberculous osteomyelitis
CC Exclusion see Appendix A PDX collection 0038

CC **A18.09 Other musculoskeletal tuberculosis**
Tuberculous myositis
Tuberculous synovitis
Tuberculous tenosynovitis
CC Exclusion see Appendix A PDX collection 0039

\+ **A18.1 Tuberculosis of genitourinary system**

CC **A18.10 Tuberculosis of genitourinary system, unspecified**
CC Exclusion see Appendix A PDX collection 0040

CC **A18.11 Tuberculosis of kidney and ureter**
CC Exclusion see Appendix A PDX collection 0041

CC **A18.12 Tuberculosis of bladder**
CC Exclusion see Appendix A PDX collection 0041

CC **A18.13 Tuberculosis of other urinary organs**
Tuberculous urethritis
CC Exclusion see Appendix A PDX collection 0041

● ♂ CC **A18.14 Tuberculosis of prostate**
CC Exclusion see Appendix A PDX collection 0042

♂ CC **A18.15 Tuberculosis of other male genital organs**
CC Exclusion see Appendix A PDX collection 0042

♀ CC **A18.16 Tuberculosis of cervix**
CC Exclusion see Appendix A PDX collection 0043

♀ CC **A18.17 Tuberculous female pelvic inflammatory disease**
Tuberculous endometritis
Tuberculous oophoritis and salpingitis
CC Exclusion see Appendix A PDX collection 0043

♀ CC **A18.18 Tuberculosis of other female genital organs**
Tuberculous ulceration of vulva
CC Exclusion see Appendix A PDX collection 0043

CC **A18.2 Tuberculous peripheral lymphadenopathy**
Tuberculous adenitis
Excludes2: *tuberculosis of bronchial and mediastinal lymph nodes (A15.4)*
tuberculosis of mesenteric and retroperitoneal lymph nodes (A18.39)
tuberculous tracheobronchial adenopathy (A15.4)
CC Exclusion see Appendix A PDX collection 0044

\+ **A18.3 Tuberculosis of intestines, peritoneum and mesenteric glands**

MCC **A18.31 Tuberculous peritonitis**
Tuberculous ascites
MCC Exclusion see Appendix A PDX collection 0045

CC **A18.32 Tuberculous enteritis**
Tuberculosis of anus and rectum
Tuberculosis of intestine (large) (small)
CC Exclusion see Appendix A PDX collection 0045

CC **A18.39 Retroperitoneal tuberculosis**
Tuberculosis of mesenteric glands
Tuberculosis of retroperitoneal (lymph glands)
CC Exclusion see Appendix A PDX collection 0045

CC **A18.4 Tuberculosis of skin and subcutaneous tissue**
Erythema induratum, tuberculous
Lupus excedens
Lupus vulgaris NOS
Lupus vulgaris of eyelid
Scrofuloderma
Tuberculosis of external ear
Excludes2: *lupus erythematosus (L93.-)*
lupus NOS (M32.9)
systemic (M32.-)
CC Exclusion see Appendix A PDX collection 0030

\+ **A18.5 Tuberculosis of eye**
Excludes2: *lupus vulgaris of eyelid (A18.4)*

CC **A18.50 Tuberculosis of eye, unspecified**
CC Exclusion see Appendix A PDX collection 0046

CC **A18.51 Tuberculous episcleritis**
CC Exclusion see Appendix A PDX collection 0046

CC **A18.52 Tuberculous keratitis**
Tuberculous interstitial keratitis
Tuberculous keratoconjunctivitis (interstitial) (phlyctenular)
CC Exclusion see Appendix A PDX collection 0046

CC **A18.53 Tuberculous chorioretinitis**
CC Exclusion see Appendix A PDX collection 0046

CC **A18.54 Tuberculous iridocyclitis**
CC Exclusion see Appendix A PDX collection 0046

CC **A18.59 Other tuberculosis of eye**
Tuberculous conjunctivitis
CC Exclusion see Appendix A PDX collection 0046

CC **A18.6 Tuberculosis of (inner) (middle) ear**
Tuberculous otitis media
Excludes2: *tuberculosis of external ear (A18.4)*
tuberculous mastoiditis (A18.03)
CC Exclusion see Appendix A PDX collection 0047

CC **A18.7 Tuberculosis of adrenal glands**
Tuberculous Addison's disease
CC Exclusion see Appendix A PDX collection 0048

\+ **A18.8 Tuberculosis of other specified organs**

CC **A18.81 Tuberculosis of thyroid gland**
CC Exclusion see Appendix A PDX collection 0049

CC **A18.82 Tuberculosis of other endocrine glands**
Tuberculosis of pituitary gland
Tuberculosis of thymus gland
CC Exclusion see Appendix A PDX collection 0035

CC **A18.83 Tuberculosis of digestive tract organs, not elsewhere classified**
Excludes1: *tuberculosis of intestine (A18.32)*
CC Exclusion see Appendix A PDX collection 0045

CC **A18.84 Tuberculosis of heart**
Tuberculous cardiomyopathy
Tuberculous endocarditis
Tuberculous myocarditis
Tuberculous pericarditis
CC Exclusion see Appendix A PDX collection 0035

CC **A18.85 Tuberculosis of spleen**
CC Exclusion see Appendix A PDX collection 0050

CC **A18.89 Tuberculosis of other sites**
Tuberculosis of muscle
Tuberculous cerebral arteritis
CC Exclusion see Appendix A PDX collection 0035

A19 Miliary tuberculosis

Includes: disseminated tuberculosis
generalized tuberculosis
tuberculous polyserositis

MCC **A19.0 Acute miliary tuberculosis of a single specified site**
MCC Exclusion see Appendix A PDX collection 0051

MCC **A19.1 Acute miliary tuberculosis of multiple sites**
MCC Exclusion see Appendix A PDX collection 0051

MCC **A19.2 Acute miliary tuberculosis, unspecified**
MCC Exclusion see Appendix A PDX collection 0051

MCC **A19.8 Other miliary tuberculosis**
MCC Exclusion see Appendix A PDX collection 0051

MCC **A19.9 Miliary tuberculosis, unspecified**
MCC Exclusion see Appendix A PDX collection 0051

Certain zoonotic bacterial diseases (A20-A28)

A20 Plague

Includes: infection due to Yersinia pestis

MCC **A20.0 Bubonic plague**
MCC Exclusion see Appendix A PDX collection 0052

MCC **A20.1 Cellulocutaneous plague**
MCC Exclusion see Appendix A PDX collection 0052

MCC **A20.2 Pneumonic plague**
MCC Exclusion see Appendix A PDX collection 0053

MCC **A20.3 Plague meningitis**
MCC Exclusion see Appendix A PDX collection 0054

MCC **A20.7 Septicemic plague**
MCC Exclusion see Appendix A PDX collection 0055
Review coding guideline C.1.d

MCC **A20.8 Other forms of plague**
Abortive plague
Asymptomatic plague
Pestis minor
MCC Exclusion see Appendix A PDX collection 0054

MCC **A20.9 Plague, unspecified**
MCC Exclusion see Appendix A PDX collection 0056

A21 Tularemia

Includes: deer-fly fever
infection due to Francisella tularensis
rabbit fever

CC **A21.0 Ulceroglandular tularemia**
CC Exclusion see Appendix A PDX collection 0057

CC **A21.1 Oculoglandular tularemia**
Ophthalmic tularemia
CC Exclusion see Appendix A PDX collection 0058

CC **A21.2 Pulmonary tularemia**
CC Exclusion see Appendix A PDX collection 0059

CC **A21.3 Gastrointestinal tularemia**
Abdominal tularemia
CC Exclusion see Appendix A PDX collection 0060

CC **A21.7 Generalized tularemia**
CC Exclusion see Appendix A PDX collection 0061
Review coding guideline C.1.d

CC **A21.8 Other forms of tularemia**
CC Exclusion see Appendix A PDX collection 0061

CC **A21.9 Tularemia, unspecified**
CC Exclusion see Appendix A PDX collection 0061

A22 Anthrax

Includes: infection due to Bacillus anthracis

CC **A22.0 Cutaneous anthrax**
Malignant carbuncle
Malignant pustule
CC Exclusion see Appendix A PDX collection 0062

MCC **A22.1 Pulmonary anthrax**
Inhalation anthrax
Ragpicker's disease
Woolsorter's disease
MCC Exclusion see Appendix A PDX collection 0063

CC **A22.2 Gastrointestinal anthrax**
CC Exclusion see Appendix A PDX collection 0064

MCC **A22.7 Anthrax sepsis**
MCC Exclusion see Appendix A PDX collection 0005
Review coding guideline C.1.d

CC **A22.8 Other forms of anthrax**
Anthrax meningitis
CC Exclusion see Appendix A PDX collection 0065

CC **A22.9 Anthrax, unspecified**
CC Exclusion see Appendix A PDX collection 0066

A23 Brucellosis

Includes: Malta fever
Mediterranean fever
undulant fever

A23.0 Brucellosis due to Brucella melitensis

A23.1 Brucellosis due to Brucella abortus

A23.2 Brucellosis due to Brucella suis

A23.3 Brucellosis due to Brucella canis

CC **A23.8 Other brucellosis**
CC Exclusion see Appendix A PDX collection 0067

CC **A23.9 Brucellosis, unspecified**
CC Exclusion see Appendix A PDX collection 0067
Review coding guideline C.1.d

A24 Glanders and melioidosis

CC **A24.0 Glanders**
Infection due to Pseudomonas mallei
Malleus
CC Exclusion see Appendix A PDX collection 0068
Review coding guideline C.1.d

CC **A24.1 Acute and fulminating melioidosis**
Melioidosis pneumonia
Melioidosis sepsis
CC Exclusion see Appendix A PDX collection 0069
Review coding guideline C.1.d

CC **A24.2 Subacute and chronic melioidosis**
CC Exclusion see Appendix A PDX collection 0069

CC **A24.3 Other melioidosis**
CC Exclusion see Appendix A PDX collection 0069

CC **A24.9 Melioidosis, unspecified**
Infection due to Pseudomonas pseudomallei NOS
Whitmore's disease
CC Exclusion see Appendix A PDX collection 0069

A25 Rat-bite fevers

CC **A25.0 Spirillosis**
Sodoku
CC Exclusion see Appendix A PDX collection 0070

CC **A25.1 Streptobacillosis**
Epidemic arthritic erythema
Haverhill fever
Streptobacillary rat-bite fever
CC Exclusion see Appendix A PDX collection 0070

CC **A25.9 Rat-bite fever, unspecified**
CC Exclusion see Appendix A PDX collection 0070

A26 Erysipeloid

A26.0 Cutaneous erysipeloid
Erythema migrans

MCC **A26.7 Erysipelothrix sepsis**
MCC Exclusion see Appendix A PDX collection 0071
Review coding guideline C.1.d

A26.8 Other forms of erysipeloid

A26.9 Erysipeloid, unspecified

A27 Leptospirosis

CC **A27.0 Leptospirosis icterohemorrhagica**
Leptospiral or spirochetal jaundice (hemorrhagic)
Weil's disease
CC Exclusion see Appendix A PDX collection 0072

\+ **A27.8 Other forms of leptospirosis**

MCC **A27.81 Aseptic meningitis in leptospirosis**
MCC Exclusion see Appendix A PDX collection 0073

CC **A27.89 Other forms of leptospirosis**
CC Exclusion see Appendix A PDX collection 0072

CC **A27.9 Leptospirosis, unspecified**
CC Exclusion see Appendix A PDX collection 0072

A28 Other zoonotic bacterial diseases, not elsewhere classified

CC **A28.0 Pasteurellosis**
CC Exclusion see Appendix A PDX collection 0074
Review coding guideline C.1.d

CC **A28.1 Cat-scratch disease**
Cat-scratch fever
CC Exclusion see Appendix A PDX collection 0075

CC **A28.2 Extraintestinal yersiniosis**
Excludes1: *enteritis due to Yersinia enterocolitica (A04.6)*
plague (A20.-)
CC Exclusion see Appendix A PDX collection 0074
Review coding guideline C.1.d

CC **A28.8 Other specified zoonotic bacterial diseases, not elsewhere classified**
CC Exclusion see Appendix A PDX collection 0074

CC **A28.9 Zoonotic bacterial disease, unspecified**
CC Exclusion see Appendix A PDX collection 0074

Other bacterial diseases (A30-A49)

A30 Leprosy [Hansen's disease]

Includes: infection due to Mycobacterium leprae
Excludes1: *sequelae of leprosy (B92)*

CC **A30.0 Indeterminate leprosy**
I leprosy
CC Exclusion see Appendix A PDX collection 0076

CC **A30.1 Tuberculoid leprosy**
TT leprosy
CC Exclusion see Appendix A PDX collection 0077

CC A30.2 **Borderline tuberculoid leprosy**
BT leprosy
CC Exclusion see Appendix A PDX collection 0078

CC A30.3 **Borderline leprosy**
BB leprosy
CC Exclusion see Appendix A PDX collection 0078

CC A30.4 **Borderline lepromatous leprosy**
BL leprosy
CC Exclusion see Appendix A PDX collection 0078

CC A30.5 **Lepromatous leprosy**
LL leprosy
CC Exclusion see Appendix A PDX collection 0079

CC A30.8 **Other forms of leprosy**
CC Exclusion see Appendix A PDX collection 0080

CC A30.9 **Leprosy, unspecified**
CC Exclusion see Appendix A PDX collection 0081

A31 Infection due to other mycobacteria

Excludes2: *leprosy (A30.-)*
tuberculosis (A15-A19)

CC A31.0 **Pulmonary mycobacterial infection**
Infection due to Mycobacterium avium
Infection due to Mycobacterium intracellulare [Battey bacillus]
Infection due to Mycobacterium kansasii
CC Exclusion see Appendix A PDX collection 0082

CC A31.1 **Cutaneous mycobacterial infection**
Buruli ulcer
Infection due to Mycobacterium marinum
Infection due to Mycobacterium ulcerans
CC Exclusion see Appendix A PDX collection 0083

CC A31.2 **Disseminated mycobacterium avium-intracellulare complex (DMAC)**
MAC sepsis
CC Exclusion see Appendix A PDX collection 0083

CC A31.8 **Other mycobacterial infections**
CC Exclusion see Appendix A PDX collection 0083

CC A31.9 **Mycobacterial infection, unspecified**
Atypical mycobacterial infection NOS
Mycobacteriosis NOS
CC Exclusion see Appendix A PDX collection 0083

A32 Listeriosis

Includes: listerial foodborne infection
Excludes1: *neonatal (disseminated) listeriosis (P37.2)*

CC A32.0 **Cutaneous listeriosis**
CC Exclusion see Appendix A PDX collection 0074

\+ A32.1 **Listerial meningitis and meningoencephalitis**

CC A32.11 **Listerial meningitis**
CC Exclusion see Appendix A PDX collection 0074

CC A32.12 **Listerial meningoencephalitis**
CC Exclusion see Appendix A PDX collection 0074

MCC A32.7 **Listerial sepsis**
MCC Exclusion see Appendix A PDX collection 0071
Review coding guideline C.1.d

\+ A32.8 **Other forms of listeriosis**

CC A32.81 **Oculoglandular listeriosis**
CC Exclusion see Appendix A PDX collection 0074

CC A32.82 **Listerial endocarditis**
CC Exclusion see Appendix A PDX collection 0074

CC A32.89 **Other forms of listeriosis**
Listerial cerebral arteritis
CC Exclusion see Appendix A PDX collection 0074

CC A32.9 **Listeriosis, unspecified**
CC Exclusion see Appendix A PDX collection 0074

A33 Tetanus neonatorum
MCC ●
MCC Exclusion see Appendix A PDX collection 0084
Valid 3-character code, no further characters required

A34 Obstetrical tetanus
♀ CC ●
CC Exclusion see Appendix A PDX collection 0085
Valid 3-character code, no further characters required

A35 Other tetanus
MCC
Tetanus NOS
Excludes1: *obstetrical tetanus (A34)*
tetanus neonatorum (A33)
MCC Exclusion see Appendix A PDX collection 0086
Valid 3-character code, no further characters required

A36 Diphtheria

CC A36.0 **Pharyngeal diphtheria**
Diphtheritic membranous angina
Tonsillar diphtheria
CC Exclusion see Appendix A PDX collection 0087

CC A36.1 **Nasopharyngeal diphtheria**
CC Exclusion see Appendix A PDX collection 0087

CC A36.2 **Laryngeal diphtheria**
Diphtheritic laryngotracheitis
CC Exclusion see Appendix A PDX collection 0087

CC A36.3 **Cutaneous diphtheria**
Excludes2: *erythrasma (L08.1)*
CC Exclusion see Appendix A PDX collection 0087

\+ A36.8 **Other diphtheria**

CC A36.81 **Diphtheritic cardiomyopathy**
Diphtheritic myocarditis
CC Exclusion see Appendix A PDX collection 0088

CC A36.82 **Diphtheritic radiculomyelitis**
CC Exclusion see Appendix A PDX collection 0087

CC A36.83 **Diphtheritic polyneuritis**
CC Exclusion see Appendix A PDX collection 0087

CC A36.84 **Diphtheritic tubulo-interstitial nephropathy**
CC Exclusion see Appendix A PDX collection 0087

CC A36.85 **Diphtheritic cystitis**
CC Exclusion see Appendix A PDX collection 0087

CC A36.86 **Diphtheritic conjunctivitis**
CC Exclusion see Appendix A PDX collection 0087

CC A36.89 **Other diphtheritic complications**
Diphtheritic peritonitis
CC Exclusion see Appendix A PDX collection 0087

CC A36.9 **Diphtheria, unspecified**
CC Exclusion see Appendix A PDX collection 0087

A37 Whooping cough

\+ A37.0 **Whooping cough due to Bordetella pertussis**

CC A37.00 **Whooping cough due to Bordetella pertussis without pneumonia**
CC Exclusion see Appendix A PDX collection 0089

MCC A37.01 **Whooping cough due to Bordetella pertussis with pneumonia**
MCC Exclusion see Appendix A PDX collection 0090

\+ A37.1 **Whooping cough due to Bordetella parapertussis**

CC A37.10 **Whooping cough due to Bordetella parapertussis without pneumonia**
CC Exclusion see Appendix A PDX collection 0089

MCC A37.11 **Whooping cough due to Bordetella parapertussis with pneumonia**
MCC Exclusion see Appendix A PDX collection 0090

\+ A37.8 **Whooping cough due to other Bordetella species**

CC A37.80 **Whooping cough due to other Bordetella species without pneumonia**
CC Exclusion see Appendix A PDX collection 0089

MCC A37.81 **Whooping cough due to other Bordetella species with pneumonia**
MCC Exclusion see Appendix A PDX collection 0090

\+ A37.9 **Whooping cough, unspecified species**

CC A37.90 **Whooping cough, unspecified species without pneumonia**
CC Exclusion see Appendix A PDX collection 0089

MCC A37.91 **Whooping cough, unspecified species with pneumonia**
MCC Exclusion see Appendix A PDX collection 0090

A38 Scarlet fever

Includes: scarlatina
Excludes2: *streptococcal sore throat (J02.0)*

CC A38.0 **Scarlet fever with otitis media**
CC Exclusion see Appendix A PDX collection 0091

CC A38.1 **Scarlet fever with myocarditis**
CC Exclusion see Appendix A PDX collection 0091

CC A38.8 **Scarlet fever with other complications**
CC Exclusion see Appendix A PDX collection 0091

CC A38.9 **Scarlet fever, uncomplicated**
Scarlet fever, NOS
CC Exclusion see Appendix A PDX collection 0091

A39 Meningococcal infection

MCC A39.0 **Meningococcal meningitis**
MCC Exclusion see Appendix A PDX collection 0092

MCC A39.1 **Waterhouse-Friderichsen syndrome**
Meningococcal hemorrhagic adrenalitis
Meningococcic adrenal syndrome
MCC Exclusion see Appendix A PDX collection 0093
Review coding guideline C.1.d

MCC A39.2 **Acute meningococcemia**
MCC Exclusion see Appendix A PDX collection 0094
Review coding guideline C.1.d

MCC A39.3 **Chronic meningococcemia**
MCC Exclusion see Appendix A PDX collection 0094
Review coding guideline C.1.d

MCC **A39.4 Meningococcemia, unspecified**
MCC Exclusion see Appendix A PDX collection 0094
Review coding guideline C.1.d
+ **A39.5 Meningococcal heart disease**
MCC **A39.50 Meningococcal carditis, unspecified**
MCC Exclusion see Appendix A PDX collection 0095
MCC **A39.51 Meningococcal endocarditis**
MCC Exclusion see Appendix A PDX collection 0096
MCC **A39.52 Meningococcal myocarditis**
MCC Exclusion see Appendix A PDX collection 0097
MCC **A39.53 Meningococcal pericarditis**
MCC Exclusion see Appendix A PDX collection 0098
+ **A39.8 Other meningococcal infections**
MCC **A39.81 Meningococcal encephalitis**
MCC Exclusion see Appendix A PDX collection 0099
CC **A39.82 Meningococcal retrobulbar neuritis**
CC Exclusion see Appendix A PDX collection 0100
CC **A39.83 Meningococcal arthritis**
CC Exclusion see Appendix A PDX collection 0101
CC **A39.84 Postmeningococcal arthritis**
CC Exclusion see Appendix A PDX collection 0101
CC **A39.89 Other meningococcal infections**
Meningococcal conjunctivitis
CC Exclusion see Appendix A PDX collection 0102
CC **A39.9 Meningococcal infection, unspecified**
Meningococcal disease NOS
CC Exclusion see Appendix A PDX collection 0102

A40 Streptococcal sepsis

Code first:
postprocedural streptococcal sepsis (T81.4-)
streptococcal sepsis during labor (O75.3)
streptococcal sepsis following abortion or ectopic or molar pregnancy (O03-O07, O08.0)
streptococcal sepsis following immunization (T88.0)
streptococcal sepsis following infusion, transfusion or therapeutic injection (T80.2-)

Excludes1: *neonatal (P36.0-P36.1)*
puerperal sepsis (O85)
sepsis due to Streptococcus, group D (A41.81)
Review coding guideline C.1.d

MCC **A40.0 Sepsis due to streptococcus, group A**
MCC Exclusion see Appendix A PDX collection 0071
MCC **A40.1 Sepsis due to streptococcus, group B**
MCC Exclusion see Appendix A PDX collection 0071
MCC **A40.3 Sepsis due to Streptococcus pneumoniae**
Pneumococcal sepsis
No MCC Exclusions
MCC **A40.8 Other streptococcal sepsis**
MCC Exclusion see Appendix A PDX collection 0071
MCC **A40.9 Streptococcal sepsis, unspecified**
MCC Exclusion see Appendix A PDX collection 0071

A41 Other sepsis

Code first:
postprocedural sepsis (T81.4-)
sepsis during labor (O75.3)
sepsis following abortion, ectopic or molar pregnancy (O03-O07, O08.0)
sepsis following immunization (T88.0)
sepsis following infusion, transfusion or therapeutic injection (T80.2-)

Excludes1: *bacteremia NOS (R78.81)*
neonatal (P36.-)
puerperal sepsis (O85)
streptococcal sepsis (A40.-)

Excludes2: *sepsis (due to) (in) actinomycotic (A42.7)*
sepsis (due to) (in) anthrax (A22.7)
sepsis (due to) (in) candidal (B37.7)
sepsis (due to) (in) Erysipelothrix (A26.7)
sepsis (due to) (in) extraintestinal yersiniosis (A28.2)
sepsis (due to) (in) gonococcal (A54.86)
sepsis (due to) (in) herpesviral (B00.7)
sepsis (due to) (in) listerial (A32.7)
sepsis (due to) (in) melioidosis (A24.1)
sepsis (due to) (in) meningococcal (A39.2-A39.4)
sepsis (due to) (in) plague (A20.7)
sepsis (due to) (in) tularemia (A21.7)
toxic shock syndrome (A48.3)
Review coding guideline C.1.d

+ **A41.0 Sepsis due to Staphylococcus aureus**
MCC **A41.01 Sepsis due to Methicillin susceptible Staphylococcus aureus**
MSSA sepsis
Staphylococcus aureus sepsis NOS
MCC Exclusion see Appendix A PDX collection 0071
MCC **A41.02 Sepsis due to Methicillin resistant Staphylococcus aureus**
MCC Exclusion see Appendix A PDX collection 0071
Review coding guideline C.1.e.1.a
MCC **A41.1 Sepsis due to other specified staphylococcus**
Coagulase negative staphylococcus sepsis
MCC Exclusion see Appendix A PDX collection 0071
MCC **A41.2 Sepsis due to unspecified staphylococcus**
MCC Exclusion see Appendix A PDX collection 0071
MCC **A41.3 Sepsis due to Hemophilus influenzae**
MCC Exclusion see Appendix A PDX collection 0071
MCC **A41.4 Sepsis due to anaerobes**
Excludes1: *gas gangrene (A48.0)*
MCC Exclusion see Appendix A PDX collection 0071
+ **A41.5 Sepsis due to other Gram-negative organisms**
MCC **A41.50 Gram-negative sepsis, unspecified**
Gram-negative sepsis NOS
MCC Exclusion see Appendix A PDX collection 0071
MCC **A41.51 Sepsis due to Escherichia coli [E. coli]**
MCC Exclusion see Appendix A PDX collection 0071
MCC **A41.52 Sepsis due to Pseudomonas**
Pseudomonas aeroginosa
MCC Exclusion see Appendix A PDX collection 0071
MCC **A41.53 Sepsis due to Serratia**
MCC Exclusion see Appendix A PDX collection 0071
MCC **A41.59 Other Gram-negative sepsis**
MCC Exclusion see Appendix A PDX collection 0071
+ **A41.8 Other specified sepsis**
MCC **A41.81 Sepsis due to Enterococcus**
MCC Exclusion see Appendix A PDX collection 0071
MCC **A41.89 Other specified sepsis**
MCC Exclusion see Appendix A PDX collection 0071
AHA CC: 3Q, 2016, 9-14
MCC **A41.9 Sepsis, unspecified organism**
Septicemia NOS
MCC Exclusion see Appendix A PDX collection 0071

A42 Actinomycosis

Excludes1: *actinomycetoma (B47.1)*
CC **A42.0 Pulmonary actinomycosis**
CC Exclusion see Appendix A PDX collection 0103
CC **A42.1 Abdominal actinomycosis**
CC Exclusion see Appendix A PDX collection 0104
CC **A42.2 Cervicofacial actinomycosis**
CC Exclusion see Appendix A PDX collection 0105
MCC **A42.7 Actinomycotic sepsis**
MCC Exclusion see Appendix A PDX collection 0071
Review coding guideline C.1.d
+ **A42.8 Other forms of actinomycosis**
CC **A42.81 Actinomycotic meningitis**
CC Exclusion see Appendix A PDX collection 0106
CC **A42.82 Actinomycotic encephalitis**
CC Exclusion see Appendix A PDX collection 0106
CC **A42.89 Other forms of actinomycosis**
CC Exclusion see Appendix A PDX collection 0106
CC **A42.9 Actinomycosis, unspecified**
CC Exclusion see Appendix A PDX collection 0106

A43 Nocardiosis

CC **A43.0 Pulmonary nocardiosis**
CC Exclusion see Appendix A PDX collection 0103
CC **A43.1 Cutaneous nocardiosis**
CC Exclusion see Appendix A PDX collection 0107
CC **A43.8 Other forms of nocardiosis**
CC Exclusion see Appendix A PDX collection 0106
CC **A43.9 Nocardiosis, unspecified**
CC Exclusion see Appendix A PDX collection 0106

A44 Bartonellosis

CC **A44.0 Systemic bartonellosis**
Oroya fever
CC Exclusion see Appendix A PDX collection 0108
CC **A44.1 Cutaneous and mucocutaneous bartonellosis**
Verruga peruana
CC Exclusion see Appendix A PDX collection 0108
CC **A44.8 Other forms of bartonellosis**
CC Exclusion see Appendix A PDX collection 0108
CC **A44.9 Bartonellosis, unspecified**
CC Exclusion see Appendix A PDX collection 0108

A46 Erysipelas

Excludes1: postpartum or puerperal erysipelas (O86.89)
Valid 3-character code, no further characters required

A48 Other bacterial diseases, not elsewhere classified

Excludes1: actinomycetoma (B47.1)

MCC **A48.0 Gas gangrene**
Clostridial cellulitis
Clostridial myonecrosis
MCC Exclusion see Appendix A PDX collection 0109

MCC **A48.1 Legionnaires' disease**
MCC Exclusion see Appendix A PDX collection 0110

A48.2 Nonpneumonic Legionnaires' disease [Pontiac fever]

MCC **A48.3 Toxic shock syndrome**
Use additional code to identify the organism (B95, B96)
Excludes1: endotoxic shock NOS (R57.8)
sepsis NOS (A41.9)
MCC Exclusion see Appendix A PDX collection 0111

A48.4 Brazilian purpuric fever
Systemic Hemophilus aegyptius infection

\+ **A48.5 Other specified botulism**
Non-foodborne intoxication due to toxins of Clostridium botulinum [C. botulinum]
Excludes1: food poisoning due to toxins of Clostridium botulinum (A05.1)

• CC **A48.51 Infant botulism**
CC Exclusion see Appendix A PDX collection 0018

CC **A48.52 Wound botulism**
Non-foodborne botulism NOS
Use additional code for associated wound
CC Exclusion see Appendix A PDX collection 0018

A48.8 Other specified bacterial diseases

A49 Bacterial infection of unspecified site

Excludes1: bacterial agents as the cause of diseases classified elsewhere (B95-B96)
chlamydial infection NOS (A74.9)
meningococcal infection NOS (A39.9)
rickettsial infection NOS (A79.9)
spirochetal infection NOS (A69.9)

\+ **A49.0 Staphylococcal infection, unspecified site**

A49.01 Methicillin susceptible Staphylococcus aureus infection, unspecified site
Methicillin susceptible Staphylococcus aureus (MSSA) infection
Staphylococcus aureus infection NOS

A49.02 Methicillin resistant Staphylococcus aureus infection, unspecified site
Methicillin resistant Staphylococcus aureus (MRSA) infection

A49.1 Streptococcal infection, unspecified site
A49.2 Hemophilus influenzae infection, unspecified site
A49.3 Mycoplasma infection, unspecified site
A49.8 Other bacterial infections of unspecified site
A49.9 Bacterial infection, unspecified
Excludes1: bacteremia NOS (R78.81)

Infections with a predominantly sexual mode of transmission (A50-A64)

Excludes1: human immunodeficiency virus [HIV] disease (B20)
nonspecific and nongonococcal urethritis (N34.1)
Reiter's disease (M02.3-)

A50 Congenital syphilis

\+ **A50.0 Early congenital syphilis, symptomatic**
Any congenital syphilitic condition specified as early or manifest less than two years after birth.

CC **A50.01 Early congenital syphilitic oculopathy**
CC Exclusion see Appendix A PDX collection 0112

CC **A50.02 Early congenital syphilitic osteochondropathy**
CC Exclusion see Appendix A PDX collection 0112

CC **A50.03 Early congenital syphilitic pharyngitis**
Early congenital syphilitic laryngitis
CC Exclusion see Appendix A PDX collection 0112

CC **A50.04 Early congenital syphilitic pneumonia**
CC Exclusion see Appendix A PDX collection 0112

CC **A50.05 Early congenital syphilitic rhinitis**
CC Exclusion see Appendix A PDX collection 0112

CC **A50.06 Early cutaneous congenital syphilis**
CC Exclusion see Appendix A PDX collection 0112

CC **A50.07 Early mucocutaneous congenital syphilis**
CC Exclusion see Appendix A PDX collection 0112

CC **A50.08 Early visceral congenital syphilis**
CC Exclusion see Appendix A PDX collection 0112

CC **A50.09 Other early congenital syphilis, symptomatic**
CC Exclusion see Appendix A PDX collection 0112

A50.1 Early congenital syphilis, latent
Congenital syphilis without clinical manifestations, with positive serological reaction and negative spinal fluid test, less than two years after birth.

CC **A50.2 Early congenital syphilis, unspecified**
Congenital syphilis NOS less than two years after birth.
CC Exclusion see Appendix A PDX collection 0113

\+ **A50.3 Late congenital syphilitic oculopathy**
Excludes1: Hutchinson's triad (A50.53)

CC **A50.30 Late congenital syphilitic oculopathy, unspecified**
CC Exclusion see Appendix A PDX collection 0112

CC **A50.31 Late congenital syphilitic interstitial keratitis**
CC Exclusion see Appendix A PDX collection 0112

CC **A50.32 Late congenital syphilitic chorioretinitis**
CC Exclusion see Appendix A PDX collection 0112

CC **A50.39 Other late congenital syphilitic oculopathy**
CC Exclusion see Appendix A PDX collection 0112

\+ **A50.4 Late congenital neurosyphilis [juvenile neurosyphilis]**
Use additional code to identify any associated mental disorder
Excludes1: Hutchinson's triad (A50.53)

CC **A50.40 Late congenital neurosyphilis, unspecified**
Juvenile neurosyphilis NOS
CC Exclusion see Appendix A PDX collection 0114

MCC **A50.41 Late congenital syphilitic meningitis**
MCC Exclusion see Appendix A PDX collection 0115

MCC **A50.42 Late congenital syphilitic encephalitis**
MCC Exclusion see Appendix A PDX collection 0114

CC **A50.43 Late congenital syphilitic polyneuropathy**
CC Exclusion see Appendix A PDX collection 0114

CC **A50.44 Late congenital syphilitic optic nerve atrophy**
CC Exclusion see Appendix A PDX collection 0112

CC **A50.45 Juvenile general paresis**
Dementia paralytica juvenilis
Juvenile tabetoparetic neurosyphilis
CC Exclusion see Appendix A PDX collection 0114

CC **A50.49 Other late congenital neurosyphilis**
Juvenile tabes dorsalis
CC Exclusion see Appendix A PDX collection 0114

\+ **A50.5 Other late congenital syphilis, symptomatic**
Any congenital syphilitic condition specified as late or manifest two years or more after birth.

CC **A50.51 Clutton's joints**
CC Exclusion see Appendix A PDX collection 0112

CC **A50.52 Hutchinson's teeth**
CC Exclusion see Appendix A PDX collection 0112

CC **A50.53 Hutchinson's triad**
CC Exclusion see Appendix A PDX collection 0112

CC **A50.54 Late congenital cardiovascular syphilis**
CC Exclusion see Appendix A PDX collection 0112

CC **A50.55 Late congenital syphilitic arthropathy**
CC Exclusion see Appendix A PDX collection 0112

CC **A50.56 Late congenital syphilitic osteochondropathy**
CC Exclusion see Appendix A PDX collection 0112

CC **A50.57 Syphilitic saddle nose**
CC Exclusion see Appendix A PDX collection 0112

CC **A50.59 Other late congenital syphilis, symptomatic**
CC Exclusion see Appendix A PDX collection 0112

A50.6 Late congenital syphilis, latent
Congenital syphilis without clinical manifestations, with positive serological reaction and negative spinal fluid test, two years or more after birth.

A50.7 Late congenital syphilis, unspecified
Congenital syphilis NOS two years or more after birth.

A50.9 Congenital syphilis, unspecified

A51 Early syphilis

A51.0 Primary genital syphilis
Syphilitic chancre NOS

A51.1 Primary anal syphilis
A51.2 Primary syphilis of other sites

\+ **A51.3 Secondary syphilis of skin and mucous membranes**

CC **A51.31 Condyloma latum**
CC Exclusion see Appendix A PDX collection 0112

CC **A51.32 Syphilitic alopecia**
CC Exclusion see Appendix A PDX collection 0116

CC **A51.39 Other secondary syphilis of skin**
Syphilitic leukoderma
Syphilitic mucous patch
Excludes1: late syphilitic leukoderma (A52.79)
CC Exclusion see Appendix A PDX collection 0112

+ A51.4 Other secondary syphilis

MCC A51.41 **Secondary syphilitic meningitis**
MCC Exclusion see Appendix A PDX collection 0117

♀ CC A51.42 **Secondary syphilitic female pelvic disease**
CC Exclusion see Appendix A PDX collection 0113

CC A51.43 **Secondary syphilitic oculopathy**
Secondary syphilitic chorioretinitis
Secondary syphilitic iridocyclitis, iritis
Secondary syphilitic uveitis
CC Exclusion see Appendix A PDX collection 0112

CC A51.44 **Secondary syphilitic nephritis**
CC Exclusion see Appendix A PDX collection 0113

CC A51.45 **Secondary syphilitic hepatitis**
CC Exclusion see Appendix A PDX collection 0118

CC A51.46 **Secondary syphilitic osteopathy**
CC Exclusion see Appendix A PDX collection 0119

CC A51.49 **Other secondary syphilitic conditions**
Secondary syphilitic lymphadenopathy
Secondary syphilitic myositis
No CC Exclusions

A51.5 **Early syphilis, latent**
Syphilis (acquired) without clinical manifestations, with positive serological reaction and negative spinal fluid test, less than two years after infection.

A51.9 **Early syphilis, unspecified**

A52 Late syphilis

+ A52.0 **Cardiovascular and cerebrovascular syphilis**

CC A52.00 **Cardiovascular syphilis, unspecified**
CC Exclusion see Appendix A PDX collection 0114

CC A52.01 **Syphilitic aneurysm of aorta**
CC Exclusion see Appendix A PDX collection 0114

CC A52.02 **Syphilitic aortitis**
CC Exclusion see Appendix A PDX collection 0114

CC A52.03 **Syphilitic endocarditis**
Syphilitic aortic valve incompetence or stenosis
Syphilitic mitral valve stenosis
Syphilitic pulmonary valve regurgitation
CC Exclusion see Appendix A PDX collection 0114

CC A52.04 **Syphilitic cerebral arteritis**
CC Exclusion see Appendix A PDX collection 0114

CC A52.05 **Other cerebrovascular syphilis**
Syphilitic cerebral aneurysm (ruptured) (non-ruptured)
Syphilitic cerebral thrombosis
CC Exclusion see Appendix A PDX collection 0114

CC A52.06 **Other syphilitic heart involvement**
Syphilitic coronary artery disease
Syphilitic myocarditis
Syphilitic pericarditis
CC Exclusion see Appendix A PDX collection 0114

CC A52.09 **Other cardiovascular syphilis**
CC Exclusion see Appendix A PDX collection 0114

+ A52.1 **Symptomatic neurosyphilis**

CC A52.10 **Symptomatic neurosyphilis, unspecified**
CC Exclusion see Appendix A PDX collection 0114

CC A52.11 **Tabes dorsalis**
Locomotor ataxia (progressive)
Tabetic neurosyphilis
CC Exclusion see Appendix A PDX collection 0114

CC A52.12 **Other cerebrospinal syphilis**
CC Exclusion see Appendix A PDX collection 0114

MCC A52.13 **Late syphilitic meningitis**
MCC Exclusion see Appendix A PDX collection 0115

MCC A52.14 **Late syphilitic encephalitis**
MCC Exclusion see Appendix A PDX collection 0114

CC A52.15 **Late syphilitic neuropathy**
Late syphilitic acoustic neuritis
Late syphilitic optic (nerve) atrophy
Late syphilitic polyneuropathy
Late syphilitic retrobulbar neuritis
CC Exclusion see Appendix A PDX collection 0114

CC A52.16 **Charcôt's arthropathy (tabetic)**
CC Exclusion see Appendix A PDX collection 0114

CC A52.17 **General paresis**
Dementia paralytica
CC Exclusion see Appendix A PDX collection 0114

CC A52.19 **Other symptomatic neurosyphilis**
Syphilitic parkinsonism
CC Exclusion see Appendix A PDX collection 0114

CC A52.2 **Asymptomatic neurosyphilis**
CC Exclusion see Appendix A PDX collection 0114

CC A52.3 **Neurosyphilis, unspecified**
Gumma (syphilitic)
Syphilis (late)
Syphiloma
CC Exclusion see Appendix A PDX collection 0114

+ A52.7 **Other symptomatic late syphilis**

CC A52.71 **Late syphilitic oculopathy**
Late syphilitic chorioretinitis
Late syphilitic episcleritis
CC Exclusion see Appendix A PDX collection 0120

CC A52.72 **Syphilis of lung and bronchus**
CC Exclusion see Appendix A PDX collection 0116

CC A52.73 **Symptomatic late syphilis of other respiratory organs**
CC Exclusion see Appendix A PDX collection 0116

CC A52.74 **Syphilis of liver and other viscera**
Late syphilitic peritonitis
CC Exclusion see Appendix A PDX collection 0116

CC A52.75 **Syphilis of kidney and ureter**
Syphilitic glomerular disease
CC Exclusion see Appendix A PDX collection 0116

CC A52.76 **Other genitourinary symptomatic late syphilis**
Late syphilitic female pelvic inflammatory disease
CC Exclusion see Appendix A PDX collection 0116

CC A52.77 **Syphilis of bone and joint**
CC Exclusion see Appendix A PDX collection 0116

CC A52.78 **Syphilis of other musculoskeletal tissue**
Late syphilitic bursitis
Syphilis [stage unspecified] of bursa
Syphilis [stage unspecified] of muscle
Syphilis [stage unspecified] of synovium
Syphilis [stage unspecified] of tendon
CC Exclusion see Appendix A PDX collection 0116

CC A52.79 **Other symptomatic late syphilis**
Late syphilitic leukoderma
Syphilis of adrenal gland
Syphilis of pituitary gland
Syphilis of thyroid gland
Syphilitic splenomegaly
Excludes1: *syphilitic leukoderma (secondary) (A51.39)*
CC Exclusion see Appendix A PDX collection 0116

A52.8 **Late syphilis, latent**
Syphilis (acquired) without clinical manifestations, with positive serological reaction and negative spinal fluid test, two years or more after infection

A52.9 **Late syphilis, unspecified**

A53 Other and unspecified syphilis

A53.0 **Latent syphilis, unspecified as early or late**
Latent syphilis NOS
Positive serological reaction for syphilis

A53.9 **Syphilis, unspecified**
Infection due to Treponema pallidum NOS
Syphilis (acquired) NOS
Excludes1: *syphilis NOS under two years of age (A50.2)*

A54 Gonococcal infection

+ A54.0 **Gonococcal infection of lower genitourinary tract without periurethral or accessory gland abscess**
Excludes1: *gonococcal infection with genitourinary gland abscess (A54.1)*
gonococcal infection with periurethral abscess (A54.1)

CC A54.00 **Gonococcal infection of lower genitourinary tract, unspecified**
CC Exclusion see Appendix A PDX collection 0121

CC A54.01 **Gonococcal cystitis and urethritis, unspecified**
CC Exclusion see Appendix A PDX collection 0121

♀ CC A54.02 **Gonococcal vulvovaginitis, unspecified**
CC Exclusion see Appendix A PDX collection 0121

♀ CC A54.03 **Gonococcal cervicitis, unspecified**
CC Exclusion see Appendix A PDX collection 0121

CC A54.09 **Other gonococcal infection of lower genitourinary tract**
CC Exclusion see Appendix A PDX collection 0121

CC A54.1 **Gonococcal infection of lower genitourinary tract with periurethral and accessory gland abscess**
Gonococcal Bartholin's gland abscess
CC Exclusion see Appendix A PDX collection 0121

+ A54.2 **Gonococcal pelviperitonitis and other gonococcal genitourinary infection**

CC A54.21 **Gonococcal infection of kidney and ureter**
CC Exclusion see Appendix A PDX collection 0121

♂ CC **A54.22 Gonococcal prostatitis**
CC Exclusion see Appendix A PDX collection 0121

♂ CC **A54.23 Gonococcal infection of other male genital organs**
Gonococcal epididymitis
Gonococcal orchitis
CC Exclusion see Appendix A PDX collection 0121

♀ CC **A54.24 Gonococcal female pelvic inflammatory disease**
Gonococcal pelviperitonitis
Excludes1: *gonococcal peritonitis (A54.85)*
CC Exclusion see Appendix A PDX collection 0121

CC **A54.29 Other gonococcal genitourinary infections**
CC Exclusion see Appendix A PDX collection 0121

\+ **A54.3 Gonococcal infection of eye**

CC **A54.30 Gonococcal infection of eye, unspecified**
CC Exclusion see Appendix A PDX collection 0116

CC **A54.31 Gonococcal conjunctivitis**
Ophthalmia neonatorum due to gonococcus
CC Exclusion see Appendix A PDX collection 0116

CC **A54.32 Gonococcal iridocyclitis**
CC Exclusion see Appendix A PDX collection 0116

CC **A54.33 Gonococcal keratitis**
CC Exclusion see Appendix A PDX collection 0116

CC **A54.39 Other gonococcal eye infection**
Gonococcal endophthalmia
CC Exclusion see Appendix A PDX collection 0116

\+ **A54.4 Gonococcal infection of musculoskeletal system**

CC **A54.40 Gonococcal infection of musculoskeletal system, unspecified**
CC Exclusion see Appendix A PDX collection 0122

CC **A54.41 Gonococcal spondylopathy**
CC Exclusion see Appendix A PDX collection 0122

CC **A54.42 Gonococcal arthritis**
Excludes2: *gonococcal infection of spine (A54.41)*
CC Exclusion see Appendix A PDX collection 0122

CC **A54.43 Gonococcal osteomyelitis**
Excludes2: *gonococcal infection of spine (A54.41)*
CC Exclusion see Appendix A PDX collection 0122

CC **A54.49 Gonococcal infection of other musculoskeletal tissue**
Gonococcal bursitis
Gonococcal myositis
Gonococcal synovitis
Gonococcal tenosynovitis
CC Exclusion see Appendix A PDX collection 0122

A54.5 Gonococcal pharyngitis

A54.6 Gonococcal infection of anus and rectum

\+ **A54.8 Other gonococcal infections**

MCC **A54.81 Gonococcal meningitis**
MCC Exclusion see Appendix A PDX collection 0117

CC **A54.82 Gonococcal brain abscess**
CC Exclusion see Appendix A PDX collection 0123

CC **A54.83 Gonococcal heart infection**
Gonococcal endocarditis
Gonococcal myocarditis
Gonococcal pericarditis
CC Exclusion see Appendix A PDX collection 0124

CC **A54.84 Gonococcal pneumonia**
CC Exclusion see Appendix A PDX collection 0123

CC **A54.85 Gonococcal peritonitis**
Excludes1: *gonococcal pelviperitonitis (A54.24)*
CC Exclusion see Appendix A PDX collection 0125

MCC **A54.86 Gonococcal sepsis**
MCC Exclusion see Appendix A PDX collection 0071
Review coding guideline C.1.d

CC **A54.89 Other gonococcal infections**
Gonococcal keratoderma
Gonococcal lymphadenitis
CC Exclusion see Appendix A PDX collection 0123

CC **A54.9 Gonococcal infection, unspecified**
CC Exclusion see Appendix A PDX collection 0123

A55 Chlamydial lymphogranuloma (venereum)

Climatic or tropical bubo
Durand-Nicolas-Favre disease
Esthiomene
Lymphogranuloma inguinale
Valid 3-character code, no further characters required

A56 Other sexually transmitted chlamydial diseases

Includes: sexually transmitted diseases due to Chlamydia trachomatis
Excludes1: *neonatal chlamydial conjunctivitis (P39.1)*
neonatal chlamydial pneumonia (P23.1)
Excludes2: *chlamydial lymphogranuloma (A55)*
conditions classified to A74.-

\+ **A56.0 Chlamydial infection of lower genitourinary tract**

A56.00 Chlamydial infection of lower genitourinary tract, unspecified

A56.01 Chlamydial cystitis and urethritis

♀ **A56.02 Chlamydial vulvovaginitis**

A56.09 Other chlamydial infection of lower genitourinary tract
Chlamydial cervicitis

\+ **A56.1 Chlamydial infection of pelviperitoneum and other genitourinary organs**

♀ **A56.11 Chlamydial female pelvic inflammatory disease**

A56.19 Other chlamydial genitourinary infection
Chlamydial epididymitis
Chlamydial orchitis

A56.2 Chlamydial infection of genitourinary tract, unspecified

A56.3 Chlamydial infection of anus and rectum

A56.4 Chlamydial infection of pharynx

A56.8 Sexually transmitted chlamydial infection of other sites

A57 Chancroid

Ulcus molle
Valid 3-character code, no further characters required

A58 Granuloma inguinale

Donovanosis
Valid 3-character code, no further characters required

A59 Trichomoniasis

Excludes2: *intestinal trichomoniasis (A07.8)*

\+ **A59.0 Urogenital trichomoniasis**

A59.00 Urogenital trichomoniasis, unspecified
Fluor (vaginalis) due to Trichomonas
Leukorrhea (vaginalis) due to Trichomonas

♀ **A59.01 Trichomonal vulvovaginitis**

♂ **A59.02 Trichomonal prostatitis**

A59.03 Trichomonal cystitis and urethritis

A59.09 Other urogenital trichomoniasis
Trichomonas cervicitis

A59.8 Trichomoniasis of other sites

A59.9 Trichomoniasis, unspecified

A60 Anogenital herpesviral [herpes simplex] infections

\+ **A60.0 Herpesviral infection of genitalia and urogenital tract**

A60.00 Herpesviral infection of urogenital system, unspecified

♂ **A60.01 Herpesviral infection of penis**

♂ **A60.02 Herpesviral infection of other male genital organs**

♀ **A60.03 Herpesviral cervicitis**

♀ **A60.04 Herpesviral vulvovaginitis**
Herpesviral [herpes simplex] ulceration
Herpesviral [herpes simplex] vaginitis
Herpesviral [herpes simplex] vulvitis

A60.09 Herpesviral infection of other urogenital tract

A60.1 Herpesviral infection of perianal skin and rectum

A60.9 Anogenital herpesviral infection, unspecified

A63 Other predominantly sexually transmitted diseases, not elsewhere classified

Excludes2: *molluscum contagiosum (B08.1)*
papilloma of cervix (D26.0)

A63.0 Anogenital (venereal) warts
Anogenital warts due to (human) papillomavirus [HPV]
Condyloma acuminatum

A63.8 Other specified predominantly sexually transmitted diseases

A64 Unspecified sexually transmitted disease

Valid 3-character code, no further characters required

Other spirochetal diseases (A65-A69)

Excludes2: *leptospirosis (A27.-)*
syphilis (A50-A53)

A65 Nonvenereal syphilis

Bejel
Endemic syphilis
Njovera
Valid 3-character code, no further characters required

A66 Yaws

Includes: bouba
frambesia (tropica)
pian

A66.0 Initial lesions of yaws
Chancre of yaws
Frambesia, initial or primary
Initial frambesial ulcer
Mother yaw

A66.1 Multiple papillomata and wet crab yaws
Frambesioma
Pianoma
Plantar or palmar papilloma of yaws

A66.2 Other early skin lesions of yaws
Cutaneous yaws, less than five years after infection
Early yaws (cutaneous)(macular)(maculopapular)(micropapular)(papular)
Frambeside of early yaws

A66.3 Hyperkeratosis of yaws
Ghoul hand
Hyperkeratosis, palmar or plantar (early) (late) due to yaws
Worm-eaten soles

A66.4 Gummata and ulcers of yaws
Gummatous frambeside
Nodular late yaws (ulcerated)

A66.5 Gangosa
Rhinopharyngitis mutilans

A66.6 Bone and joint lesions of yaws
Yaws ganglion
Yaws goundou
Yaws gumma, bone
Yaws gummatous osteitis or periostitis
Yaws hydrarthrosis
Yaws osteitis
Yaws periostitis (hypertrophic)

A66.7 Other manifestations of yaws
Juxta-articular nodules of yaws
Mucosal yaws

A66.8 Latent yaws
Yaws without clinical manifestations, with positive serology

A66.9 Yaws, unspecified

A67 Pinta [carate]

A67.0 Primary lesions of pinta
Chancre (primary) of pinta
Papule (primary) of pinta

A67.1 Intermediate lesions of pinta
Erythematous plaques of pinta
Hyperchromic lesions of pinta
Hyperkeratosis of pinta
Pintids

A67.2 Late lesions of pinta
Achromic skin lesions of pinta
Cicatricial skin lesions of pinta
Dyschromic skin lesions of pinta

A67.3 Mixed lesions of pinta
Achromic with hyperchromic skin lesions of pinta [carate]

A67.9 Pinta, unspecified

A68 Relapsing fevers

Includes: recurrent fever
Excludes2: *Lyme disease (A69.2-)*

CC **A68.0 Louse-borne relapsing fever**
Relapsing fever due to Borrelia recurrentis
CC Exclusion see Appendix A PDX collection 0108

CC **A68.1 Tick-borne relapsing fever**
Relapsing fever due to any Borrelia species other than Borrelia recurrentis
CC Exclusion see Appendix A PDX collection 0108

CC **A68.9 Relapsing fever, unspecified**
CC Exclusion see Appendix A PDX collection 0108

A69 Other spirochetal infections

A69.0 Necrotizing ulcerative stomatitis
Cancrum oris
Fusospirochetal gangrene
Noma
Stomatitis gangrenosa

CC **A69.1 Other Vincent's infections**
Fusospirochetal pharyngitis
Necrotizing ulcerative (acute) gingivitis
Necrotizing ulcerative (acute) gingivostomatitis
Spirochetal stomatitis
Trench mouth
Vincent's angina
Vincent's gingivitis
CC Exclusion see Appendix A PDX collection 0126

\+ **A69.2 Lyme disease**
Erythema chronicum migrans due to Borrelia burgdorferi

CC **A69.20 Lyme disease, unspecified**
CC Exclusion see Appendix A PDX collection 0108

CC **A69.21 Meningitis due to Lyme disease**
CC Exclusion see Appendix A PDX collection 0108

CC **A69.22 Other neurologic disorders in Lyme disease**
Cranial neuritis
Meningoencephalitis
Polyneuropathy
CC Exclusion see Appendix A PDX collection 0108

CC **A69.23 Arthritis due to Lyme disease**
CC Exclusion see Appendix A PDX collection 0108

CC **A69.29 Other conditions associated with Lyme disease**
Myopericarditis due to Lyme disease
CC Exclusion see Appendix A PDX collection 0108
AHA CC: 3Q, 2016, 12

A69.8 Other specified spirochetal infections

A69.9 Spirochetal infection, unspecified

Other diseases caused by chlamydiae (A70-A74)

Excludes1: *sexually transmitted chlamydial diseases (A55-A56)*

CC **A70 Chlamydia psittaci infections**

Ornithosis
Parrot fever
Psittacosis
CC Exclusion see Appendix A PDX collection 0127
Valid 3-character code, no further characters required

A71 Trachoma

Excludes1: *sequelae of trachoma (B94.0)*

A71.0 Initial stage of trachoma
Trachoma dubium

A71.1 Active stage of trachoma
Granular conjunctivitis (trachomatous)
Trachomatous follicular conjunctivitis
Trachomatous pannus

A71.9 Trachoma, unspecified

A74 Other diseases caused by chlamydiae

Excludes1: *neonatal chlamydial conjunctivitis (P39.1)*
neonatal chlamydial pneumonia (P23.1)
Reiter's disease (M02.3-)
sexually transmitted chlamydial diseases (A55-A56)
Excludes2: *chlamydial pneumonia (J16.0)*

A74.0 Chlamydial conjunctivitis
Paratrachoma

\+ **A74.8 Other chlamydial diseases**

A74.81 Chlamydial peritonitis

A74.89 Other chlamydial diseases

A74.9 Chlamydial infection, unspecified
Chlamydiosis NOS

Rickettsioses (A75-A79)

A75 Typhus fever

Excludes1: *rickettsiosis due to Ehrlichia sennetsu (A79.81)*

CC **A75.0 Epidemic louse-borne typhus fever due to Rickettsia prowazekii**
Classical typhus (fever)
Epidemic (louse-borne) typhus
CC Exclusion see Appendix A PDX collection 0108

CC **A75.1 Recrudescent typhus [Brill's disease]**
Brill-Zinsser disease
CC Exclusion see Appendix A PDX collection 0108

CC **A75.2 Typhus fever due to Rickettsia typhi**
Murine (flea-borne) typhus
CC Exclusion see Appendix A PDX collection 0108
CC **A75.3 Typhus fever due to Rickettsia tsutsugamushi**
Scrub (mite-borne) typhus
Tsutsugamushi fever
CC Exclusion see Appendix A PDX collection 0108
CC **A75.9 Typhus fever, unspecified**
Typhus (fever) NOS
CC Exclusion see Appendix A PDX collection 0128

A77 **Spotted fever [tick-borne rickettsioses]**

CC **A77.0 Spotted fever due to Rickettsia rickettsii**
Rocky Mountain spotted fever
Sao Paulo fever
CC Exclusion see Appendix A PDX collection 0108
CC **A77.1 Spotted fever due to Rickettsia conorii**
African tick typhus
Boutonneuse fever
India tick typhus
Kenya tick typhus
Marseilles fever
Mediterranean tick fever
CC Exclusion see Appendix A PDX collection 0108
CC **A77.2 Spotted fever due to Rickettsia siberica**
North Asian tick fever
Siberian tick typhus
CC Exclusion see Appendix A PDX collection 0108
CC **A77.3 Spotted fever due to Rickettsia australis**
Queensland tick typhus
CC Exclusion see Appendix A PDX collection 0108
+ **A77.4 Ehrlichiosis**
Excludes1: *Rickettsiosis due to Ehrlichia sennetsu (A79.81)*
CC **A77.40 Ehrlichiosis, unspecified**
CC Exclusion see Appendix A PDX collection 0108
CC **A77.41 Ehrlichiosis chafeensis [E. chafeensis]**
CC Exclusion see Appendix A PDX collection 0108
CC **A77.49 Other ehrlichiosis**
CC Exclusion see Appendix A PDX collection 0108
CC **A77.8 Other spotted fevers**
CC Exclusion see Appendix A PDX collection 0108
CC **A77.9 Spotted fever, unspecified**
Tick-borne typhus NOS
CC Exclusion see Appendix A PDX collection 0108

CC A78 **Q fever**
Infection due to Coxiella burnetii
Nine Mile fever
Quadrilateral fever
CC Exclusion see Appendix A PDX collection 0108
Valid 3-character code, no further characters required

A79 **Other rickettsioses**

CC **A79.0 Trench fever**
Quintan fever
Wolhynian fever
CC Exclusion see Appendix A PDX collection 0108
CC **A79.1 Rickettsialpox due to Rickettsia akari**
Kew Garden fever
Vesicular rickettsiosis
CC Exclusion see Appendix A PDX collection 0129
A79.8 Other specified rickettsioses
CC **A79.81 Rickettsiosis due to Ehrlichia sennetsu**
Excludes1: *rickettsiosis due to Ehrlichia sennetsu (A79.81)*
CC Exclusion see Appendix A PDX collection 0129
CC **A79.89 Other specified rickettsioses**
CC Exclusion see Appendix A PDX collection 0129
CC **A79.9 Rickettsiosis, unspecified**
Rickettsial infection NOS
CC Exclusion see Appendix A PDX collection 0129

Viral and prion infections of the central nervous system (A80-A89)

Excludes1: *postpolio syndrome (G14)*
sequelae of poliomyelitis (B91)
sequelae of viral encephalitis (B94.1)

A80 **Acute poliomyelitis**

MCC **A80.0 Acute paralytic poliomyelitis, vaccine-associated**
MCC Exclusion see Appendix A PDX collection 0130
MCC **A80.1 Acute paralytic poliomyelitis, wild virus, imported**
MCC Exclusion see Appendix A PDX collection 0130
MCC **A80.2 Acute paralytic poliomyelitis, wild virus, indigenous**
MCC Exclusion see Appendix A PDX collection 0130
+ **A80.3 Acute paralytic poliomyelitis, other and unspecified**
MCC **A80.30 Acute paralytic poliomyelitis, unspecified**
MCC Exclusion see Appendix A PDX collection 0130
MCC **A80.39 Other acute paralytic poliomyelitis**
MCC Exclusion see Appendix A PDX collection 0130
A80.4 Acute nonparalytic poliomyelitis
A80.9 Acute poliomyelitis, unspecified

A81 **Atypical virus infections of central nervous system**

Includes: diseases of the central nervous system caused by prions
Use additional code to identify:
dementia with behavioral disturbance (F02.81)
dementia without behavioral disturbance (F02.80)

+ **A81.0 Creutzfeldt-Jakob disease**
CC **A81.00 Creutzfeldt-Jakob disease, unspecified**
Jakob-Creutzfeldt disease, unspecified
CC Exclusion see Appendix A PDX collection 0131
CC **A81.01 Variant Creutzfeldt-Jakob disease**
CJD
CC Exclusion see Appendix A PDX collection 0131
CC **A81.09 Other Creutzfeldt-Jakob disease**
CJD
Familial Creutzfeldt-Jakob disease
Iatrogenic Creutzfeldt-Jakob disease
Sporadic Creutzfeldt-Jakob disease
Subacute spongiform encephalopathy (with dementia)
CC Exclusion see Appendix A PDX collection 0131
CC **A81.1 Subacute sclerosing panencephalitis**
Dawson's inclusion body encephalitis
Van Bogaert's sclerosing leukoencephalopathy
CC Exclusion see Appendix A PDX collection 0132
CC **A81.2 Progressive multifocal leukoencephalopathy**
Multifocal leukoencephalopathy NOS
CC Exclusion see Appendix A PDX collection 0133
+ **A81.8 Other atypical virus infections of central nervous system**
CC **A81.81 Kuru**
CC Exclusion see Appendix A PDX collection 0134
CC **A81.82 Gerstmann-Sträussler-Scheinker syndrome**
GSS syndrome
CC Exclusion see Appendix A PDX collection 0135
CC **A81.83 Fatal familial insomnia**
FFI
CC Exclusion see Appendix A PDX collection 0135
CC **A81.89 Other atypical virus infections of central nervous system**
CC Exclusion see Appendix A PDX collection 0135
CC **A81.9 Atypical virus infection of central nervous system, unspecified**
Prion diseases of the central nervous system NOS
CC Exclusion see Appendix A PDX collection 0134

A82 **Rabies**

CC **A82.0 Sylvatic rabies**
CC Exclusion see Appendix A PDX collection 0136
CC **A82.1 Urban rabies**
CC Exclusion see Appendix A PDX collection 0136
CC **A82.9 Rabies, unspecified**
CC Exclusion see Appendix A PDX collection 0136

A83 **Mosquito-borne viral encephalitis**

Includes: mosquito-borne viral meningoencephalitis
Excludes2: *Venezuelan equine encephalitis (A92.2)*
West Nile fever (A92.3-)
West Nile virus (A92.3-)

MCC **A83.0 Japanese encephalitis**
MCC Exclusion see Appendix A PDX collection 0137
MCC **A83.1 Western equine encephalitis**
MCC Exclusion see Appendix A PDX collection 0137
MCC **A83.2 Eastern equine encephalitis**
MCC Exclusion see Appendix A PDX collection 0137
MCC **A83.3 St Louis encephalitis**
MCC Exclusion see Appendix A PDX collection 0137
MCC **A83.4 Australian encephalitis**
Kunjin virus disease
MCC Exclusion see Appendix A PDX collection 0137
MCC **A83.5 California encephalitis**
California meningoencephalitis
La Crosse encephalitis
MCC Exclusion see Appendix A PDX collection 0137
MCC **A83.6 Rocio virus disease**
MCC Exclusion see Appendix A PDX collection 0137

MCC **A83.8 Other mosquito-borne viral encephalitis**
MCC Exclusion see Appendix A PDX collection 0137

MCC **A83.9 Mosquito-borne viral encephalitis, unspecified**
MCC Exclusion see Appendix A PDX collection 0137

A84 Tick-borne viral encephalitis

Includes: tick-borne viral meningoencephalitis

MCC **A84.0 Far Eastern tick-borne encephalitis [Russian spring-summer encephalitis]**
MCC Exclusion see Appendix A PDX collection 0137

MCC **A84.1 Central European tick-borne encephalitis**
MCC Exclusion see Appendix A PDX collection 0137

MCC **A84.8 Other tick-borne viral encephalitis**
Louping ill
Powassan virus disease
MCC Exclusion see Appendix A PDX collection 0137

MCC **A84.9 Tick-borne viral encephalitis, unspecified**
MCC Exclusion see Appendix A PDX collection 0137

A85 Other viral encephalitis, not elsewhere classified

Includes: specified viral encephalomyelitis NEC
specified viral meningoencephalitis NEC

Excludes1: *benign myalgic encephalomyelitis (G93.3)*
encephalitis due to cytomegalovirus (B25.8)
encephalitis due to herpesvirus NEC (B10.0-)
encephalitis due to herpesvirus [herpes simplex] (B00.4)
encephalitis due to measles virus (B05.0)
encephalitis due to mumps virus (B26.2)
encephalitis due to poliomyelitis virus (A80.-)
encephalitis due to zoster (B02.0)
lymphocytic choriomeningitis (A87.2)

CC **A85.0 Enteroviral encephalitis**
Enteroviral encephalomyelitis
CC Exclusion see Appendix A PDX collection 0138

CC **A85.1 Adenoviral encephalitis**
Adenoviral meningoencephalitis
CC Exclusion see Appendix A PDX collection 0138

MCC **A85.2 Arthropod-borne viral encephalitis, unspecified**
Excludes1: *West nile virus with encephalitis (A92.31)*
MCC Exclusion see Appendix A PDX collection 0137

CC **A85.8 Other specified viral encephalitis**
Encephalitis lethargica
Von Economo-Cruchet disease
CC Exclusion see Appendix A PDX collection 0138

CC **A86 Unspecified viral encephalitis**

Viral encephalomyelitis NOS
Viral meningoencephalitis NOS
CC Exclusion see Appendix A PDX collection 0139
Valid 3-character code, no further characters required

A87 Viral meningitis

Excludes1: *meningitis due to herpesvirus [herpes simplex] (B00.3)*
meningitis due to herpesvirus [herpes simplex] (B00.3)
meningitis due to measles virus (B05.1)
meningitis due to mumps virus (B26.1)
meningitis due to poliomyelitis virus (A80.-)
meningitis due to zoster (B02.1)

CC **A87.0 Enteroviral meningitis**
Coxsackievirus meningitis
Echovirus meningitis
CC Exclusion see Appendix A PDX collection 0140

CC **A87.1 Adenoviral meningitis**
CC Exclusion see Appendix A PDX collection 0140

CC **A87.2 Lymphocytic choriomeningitis**
Lymphocytic meningoencephalitis
CC Exclusion see Appendix A PDX collection 0141

CC **A87.8 Other viral meningitis**
CC Exclusion see Appendix A PDX collection 0140

CC **A87.9 Viral meningitis, unspecified**
CC Exclusion see Appendix A PDX collection 0140

A88 Other viral infections of central nervous system, not elsewhere classified

Excludes1: *viral encephalitis NOS (A86)*
viral meningitis NOS (A87.9)

CC **A88.0 Enteroviral exanthematous fever [Boston exanthem]**
CC Exclusion see Appendix A PDX collection 0137

A88.1 Epidemic vertigo

CC **A88.8 Other specified viral infections of central nervous system**
CC Exclusion see Appendix A PDX collection 0138

CC **A89 Unspecified viral infection of central nervous system**

CC Exclusion see Appendix A PDX collection 0139
Valid 3-character code, no further characters required

Arthropod-borne viral fevers and viral hemorrhagic fevers (A90-A99)

CC **A90 Dengue fever [classical dengue]**

Excludes1: *dengue hemorrhagic fever (A91)*
CC Exclusion see Appendix A PDX collection 0142
AHA CC: 3Q, 2016, 13
Valid 3-character code, no further characters required

CC **A91 Dengue hemorrhagic fever**

CC Exclusion see Appendix A PDX collection 0143
Valid 3-character code, no further characters required

A92 Other mosquito-borne viral fevers

Excludes1: *Ross River disease (B33.1)*

CC **A92.0 Chikungunya virus disease**
Chikungunya (hemorrhagic) fever
CC Exclusion see Appendix A PDX collection 0143

CC **A92.1 O'nyong-nyong fever**
CC Exclusion see Appendix A PDX collection 0144

CC **A92.2 Venezuelan equine fever**
Venezuelan equine encephalitis
Venezuelan equine encephalomyelitis virus disease
CC Exclusion see Appendix A PDX collection 0144

\+ **A92.3 West Nile virus infection**
West Nile fever

MCC **A92.30 West Nile virus infection, unspecified**
West Nile fever NOS
West Nile fever without complications
West Nile virus NOS
MCC Exclusion see Appendix A PDX collection 0145

MCC **A92.31 West Nile virus infection with encephalitis**
West Nile encephalitis
West Nile encephalomyelitis
MCC Exclusion see Appendix A PDX collection 0145
AHA CC: 3Q, 2016, 12-13

MCC **A92.32 West Nile virus infection with other neurologic manifestation**
Use additional code to specify the neurologic manifestation
MCC Exclusion see Appendix A PDX collection 0145

MCC **A92.39 West Nile virus infection with other complications**
Use additional code to specify the other conditions
MCC Exclusion see Appendix A PDX collection 0145

CC **A92.4 Rift Valley fever**
CC Exclusion see Appendix A PDX collection 0144

CC **A92.5 Zika virus disease**
Zika virus fever
Zika virus infection
Zika NOS
CC Exclusion see Appendix A PDX collection 0144
Review coding guideline C.1.f
AHA CC: 4Q, 2016, 4-7

CC **A92.8 Other specified mosquito-borne viral fevers**
CC Exclusion see Appendix A PDX collection 0144

CC **A92.9 Mosquito-borne viral fever, unspecified**
CC Exclusion see Appendix A PDX collection 0143

A93 Other arthropod-borne viral fevers, not elsewhere classified

CC **A93.0 Oropouche virus disease**
Oropouche fever
CC Exclusion see Appendix A PDX collection 0144

CC **A93.1 Sandfly fever**
Pappataci fever
Phlebotomus fever
CC Exclusion see Appendix A PDX collection 0143

CC **A93.2 Colorado tick fever**
CC Exclusion see Appendix A PDX collection 0143

CC **A93.8 Other specified arthropod-borne viral fevers**
Piry virus disease
Vesicular stomatitis virus disease [Indiana fever]
CC Exclusion see Appendix A PDX collection 0143

CC **A94 Unspecified arthropod-borne viral fever**

Arboviral fever NOS
Arbovirus infection NOS
CC Exclusion see Appendix A PDX collection 0143
Valid 3-character code, no further characters required

A95 Yellow fever

CC **A95.0 Sylvatic yellow fever**
Jungle yellow fever
CC Exclusion see Appendix A PDX collection 0146

CC **A95.1 Urban yellow fever**
CC Exclusion see Appendix A PDX collection 0146

CC **A95.9 Yellow fever, unspecified**
CC Exclusion see Appendix A PDX collection 0146

A96 Arenaviral hemorrhagic fever

CC **A96.0 Junin hemorrhagic fever**
Argentinian hemorrhagic fever
CC Exclusion see Appendix A PDX collection 0147

CC **A96.1 Machupo hemorrhagic fever**
Bolivian hemorrhagic fever
CC Exclusion see Appendix A PDX collection 0147

A96.2 Lassa fever

CC **A96.8 Other arenaviral hemorrhagic fevers**
CC Exclusion see Appendix A PDX collection 0147

CC **A96.9 Arenaviral hemorrhagic fever, unspecified**
CC Exclusion see Appendix A PDX collection 0147

A98 Other viral hemorrhagic fevers, not elsewhere classified

Excludes1: *chikungunya hemorrhagic fever (A92.0)*
dengue hemorrhagic fever (A91)

CC **A98.0 Crimean-Congo hemorrhagic fever**
Central Asian hemorrhagic fever
CC Exclusion see Appendix A PDX collection 0143

CC **A98.1 Omsk hemorrhagic fever**
CC Exclusion see Appendix A PDX collection 0143

CC **A98.2 Kyasanur Forest disease**
CC Exclusion see Appendix A PDX collection 0143

A98.3 Marburg virus disease

A98.4 Ebola virus disease

CC **A98.5 Hemorrhagic fever with renal syndrome**
Epidemic hemorrhagic fever
Korean hemorrhagic fever
Russian hemorrhagic fever
Hantaan virus disease
Hantavirus disease with renal manifestations
Nephropathia epidemica
Songo fever
Excludes1: *hantavirus (cardio)-pulmonary syndrome (B33.4)*
CC Exclusion see Appendix A PDX collection 0148

CC **A98.8 Other specified viral hemorrhagic fevers**
CC Exclusion see Appendix A PDX collection 0143

CC **A99 Unspecified viral hemorrhagic fever**
CC Exclusion see Appendix A PDX collection 0143
Valid 3-character code, no further characters

Viral infections characterized by skin and mucous membrane lesions (B00-B09)

B00 Herpesviral [herpes simplex] infections

Excludes1: *congenital herpesviral infections (P35.2)*
Excludes2: *anogenital herpesviral infection (A60.-)*
gammaherpesviral mononucleosis (B27.0-)
herpangina (B08.5)

B00.0 Eczema herpeticum
Kaposi's varicelliform eruption

B00.1 Herpesviral vesicular dermatitis
Herpes simplex facialis
Herpes simplex labialis
Herpes simplex otitis externa
Vesicular dermatitis of ear
Vesicular dermatitis of lip

CC **B00.2 Herpesviral gingivostomatitis and pharyngotonsillitis**
Herpesviral pharyngitis
CC Exclusion see Appendix A PDX collection 0149

MCC **B00.3 Herpesviral meningitis**
MCC Exclusion see Appendix A PDX collection 0150

MCC **B00.4 Herpesviral encephalitis**
Herpesviral meningoencephalitis
Simian B disease
Excludes1: *herpesviral encephalitis due to herpesvirus 6 and 7 (B10.01, B10.09)*
non-simplex herpesviral encephalitis (B10.0-)
MCC Exclusion see Appendix A PDX collection 0151

\+ **B00.5 Herpesviral ocular disease**

CC **B00.50 Herpesviral ocular disease, unspecified**
CC Exclusion see Appendix A PDX collection 0152

CC **B00.51 Herpesviral iridocyclitis**
Herpesviral iritis
Herpesviral uveitis, anterior
CC Exclusion see Appendix A PDX collection 0152

CC **B00.52 Herpesviral keratitis**
Herpesviral keratoconjunctivitis
CC Exclusion see Appendix A PDX collection 0152

CC **B00.53 Herpesviral conjunctivitis**
CC Exclusion see Appendix A PDX collection 0152

CC **B00.59 Other herpesviral disease of eye**
Herpesviral dermatitis of eyelid
CC Exclusion see Appendix A PDX collection 0152

MCC **B00.7 Disseminated herpesviral disease**
Herpesviral sepsis
MCC Exclusion see Appendix A PDX collection 0153
Review coding guideline C.1.d

\+ **B00.8 Other forms of herpesviral infections**

CC **B00.81 Herpesviral hepatitis**
CC Exclusion see Appendix A PDX collection 0154

MCC **B00.82 Herpes simplex myelitis**
MCC Exclusion see Appendix A PDX collection 0155

CC **B00.89 Other herpesviral infection**
Herpesviral whitlow
CC Exclusion see Appendix A PDX collection 0156

B00.9 Herpesviral infection, unspecified
Herpes simplex infection NOS

B01 Varicella [chickenpox]

CC **B01.0 Varicella meningitis**
CC Exclusion see Appendix A PDX collection 0157

\+ **B01.1 Varicella encephalitis, myelitis and encephalomyelitis**
Postchickenpox encephalitis, myelitis and encephalomyelitis

MCC **B01.11 Varicella encephalitis and encephalomyelitis**
Postchickenpox encephalitis and encephalomyelitis
MCC Exclusion see Appendix A PDX collection 0158

MCC **B01.12 Varicella myelitis**
Postchickenpox myelitis
MCC Exclusion see Appendix A PDX collection 0159

MCC **B01.2 Varicella pneumonia**
MCC Exclusion see Appendix A PDX collection 0160

\+ **B01.8 Varicella with other complications**

CC **B01.81 Varicella keratitis**
CC Exclusion see Appendix A PDX collection 0157

CC **B01.89 Other varicella complications**
CC Exclusion see Appendix A PDX collection 0157

CC **B01.9 Varicella without complication**
Varicella NOS
CC Exclusion see Appendix A PDX collection 0157

B02 Zoster [herpes zoster]

Includes: shingles
zona

CC **B02.0 Zoster encephalitis**
Zoster meningoencephalitis
CC Exclusion see Appendix A PDX collection 0161

MCC **B02.1 Zoster meningitis**
MCC Exclusion see Appendix A PDX collection 0162

\+ **B02.2 Zoster with other nervous system involvement**

CC **B02.21 Postherpetic geniculate ganglionitis**
CC Exclusion see Appendix A PDX collection 0161

CC **B02.22 Postherpetic trigeminal neuralgia**
CC Exclusion see Appendix A PDX collection 0161

CC **B02.23 Postherpetic polyneuropathy**
CC Exclusion see Appendix A PDX collection 0161

MCC **B02.24 Postherpetic myelitis**
Herpes zoster myelitis
MCC Exclusion see Appendix A PDX collection 0163

CC **B02.29 Other postherpetic nervous system involvement**
Postherpetic radiculopathy
CC Exclusion see Appendix A PDX collection 0161

\+ **B02.3 Zoster ocular disease**

CC **B02.30 Zoster ocular disease, unspecified**
CC Exclusion see Appendix A PDX collection 0164

CC **B02.31 Zoster conjunctivitis**
CC Exclusion see Appendix A PDX collection 0164

CC **B02.32 Zoster iridocyclitis**
CC Exclusion see Appendix A PDX collection 0164

CC **B02.33 Zoster keratitis**
Herpes zoster keratoconjunctivitis
CC Exclusion see Appendix A PDX collection 0164

CC **B02.34 Zoster scleritis**
CC Exclusion see Appendix A PDX collection 0164

CC **B02.39 Other herpes zoster eye disease**
Zoster blepharitis
CC Exclusion see Appendix A PDX collection 0164

CC **B02.7 Disseminated zoster**
CC Exclusion see Appendix A PDX collection 0165

CC **B02.8 Zoster with other complications**
Herpes zoster otitis externa
CC Exclusion see Appendix A PDX collection 0165

B02.9 Zoster without complications
Zoster NOS

CC **B03 Smallpox**

NOTE In 1980 the 33rd World Health Assembly declared that smallpox had been eradicated.
The classification is maintained for surveillance purposes.
CC Exclusion see Appendix A PDX collection 0166
Valid 3-character code, no further characters required

CC **B04 Monkeypox**

CC Exclusion see Appendix A PDX collection 0167
Valid 3-character code, no further characters required

B05 Measles

Includes: morbilli
Excludes1: *subacute sclerosing panencephalitis (A81.1)*

MCC **B05.0 Measles complicated by encephalitis**
Postmeasles encephalitis
MCC Exclusion see Appendix A PDX collection 0168

CC **B05.1 Measles complicated by meningitis**
Postmeasles meningitis
CC Exclusion see Appendix A PDX collection 0169

MCC **B05.2 Measles complicated by pneumonia**
Postmeasles pneumonia
MCC Exclusion see Appendix A PDX collection 0170

B05.3 Measles complicated by otitis media
Postmeasles otitis media

CC **B05.4 Measles with intestinal complications**
CC Exclusion see Appendix A PDX collection 0169

\+ **B05.8 Measles with other complications**

CC **B05.81 Measles keratitis and keratoconjunctivitis**
CC Exclusion see Appendix A PDX collection 0171

CC **B05.89 Other measles complications**
CC Exclusion see Appendix A PDX collection 0169

B05.9 Measles without complication
Measles NOS

B06 Rubella [German measles]

Excludes1: *congenital rubella (P35.0)*

\+ **B06.0 Rubella with neurological complications**

CC **B06.00 Rubella with neurological complication, unspecified**
CC Exclusion see Appendix A PDX collection 0172

MCC **B06.01 Rubella encephalitis**
Rubella meningoencephalitis
MCC Exclusion see Appendix A PDX collection 0172

CC **B06.02 Rubella meningitis**
CC Exclusion see Appendix A PDX collection 0172

CC **B06.09 Other neurological complications of rubella**
CC Exclusion see Appendix A PDX collection 0172

\+ **B06.8 Rubella with other complications**

CC **B06.81 Rubella pneumonia**
CC Exclusion see Appendix A PDX collection 0172

CC **B06.82 Rubella arthritis**
CC Exclusion see Appendix A PDX collection 0173

CC **B06.89 Other rubella complications**
CC Exclusion see Appendix A PDX collection 0172

B06.9 Rubella without complication
Rubella NOS

B07 Viral warts

Includes: verruca simplex
verruca vulgaris
viral warts due to human papillomavirus
Excludes2: *anogenital (venereal) warts (A63.0)*
papilloma of bladder (D41.4)
papilloma of cervix (D26.0)
papilloma larynx (D14.1)

B07.0 Plantar wart
Verruca plantaris

B07.8 Other viral warts
Common wart
Flat wart
Verruca plana

B07.9 Viral wart, unspecified

B08 Other viral infections characterized by skin and mucous membrane lesions, not elsewhere classified

Excludes1: *vesicular stomatitis virus disease (A93.8)*

B08.0 Other orthopoxvirus infections
Excludes2: *monkeypox (B04)*

\+ **B08.01 Cowpox and vaccinia not from vaccine**

B08.010 Cowpox

B08.011 Vaccinia not from vaccine
Excludes1: *vaccinia (from vaccination) (generalized) (T88.1)*

B08.02 Orf virus disease
Contagious pustular dermatitis
Ecthyma contagiosum

B08.03 Pseudocowpox [milker's node]

B08.04 Paravaccinia, unspecified

B08.09 Other orthopoxvirus infections
Orthopoxvirus infection NOS

B08.1 Molluscum contagiosum

\+ **B08.2 Exanthema subitum [sixth disease]**
Roseola infantum

• **B08.20 Exanthema subitum [sixth disease], unspecified**
Roseola infantum, unspecified

• **B08.21 Exanthema subitum [sixth disease] due to human herpesvirus 6**
Roseola infantum due to human herpesvirus 6

• **B08.22 Exanthema subitum [sixth disease] due to human herpesvirus 7**
Roseola infantum due to human herpesvirus 7

CC **B08.3 Erythema infectiosum [fifth disease]**
CC Exclusion see Appendix A PDX collection 0174

B08.4 Enteroviral vesicular stomatitis with exanthem
Hand, foot and mouth disease

B08.5 Enteroviral vesicular pharyngitis
Herpangina

\+ **B08.6 Parapoxvirus infections**

B08.60 Parapoxvirus infection, unspecified

B08.61 Bovine stomatitis

B08.62 Sealpox

B08.69 Other parapoxvirus infections

\+ **B08.7 Yatapoxvirus infections**

B08.70 Yatapoxvirus infection, unspecified

CC **B08.71 Tanapox virus disease**
CC Exclusion see Appendix A PDX collection 0167

B08.72 Yaba pox virus disease
Yaba monkey tumor disease

B08.79 Other yatapoxvirus infections

B08.8 Other specified viral infections characterized by skin and mucous membrane lesions
Enteroviral lymphonodular pharyngitis
Foot-and-mouth disease
Poxvirus NEC

B09 Unspecified viral infection characterized by skin and mucous membrane lesions

Viral enanthema NOS
Viral exanthema NOS
Valid 3-character code, no further characters required

Other human herpesviruses (B10)

B10 Other human herpesviruses

Excludes2: *cytomegalovirus (B25.9)*
Epstein-Barr virus (B27.0-)
herpes NOS (B00.9)
herpes simplex (B00.-)
herpes zoster (B02.-)
human herpesvirus NOS (B00.-)
human herpesvirus 1 and 2 (B00.-)
human herpesvirus 3 (B01.-, B02.-)
human herpesvirus 4 (B27.0-)
human herpesvirus 5 (B25.-)
varicella (B01.-)
zoster (B02.-)

\+ **B10.0 Other human herpesvirus encephalitis**
Excludes2: *herpes encephalitis NOS (B00.4)*
herpes simplex encephalitis (B00.4)
human herpesvirus encephalitis (B00.4)
simian B herpes virus encephalitis (B00.4)

MCC **B10.01 Human herpesvirus 6 encephalitis**
MCC Exclusion see Appendix A PDX collection 0151

MCC **B10.09 Other human herpesvirus encephalitis**
Human herpesvirus 7 encephalitis
MCC Exclusion see Appendix A PDX collection 0151

\+ **B10.8 Other human herpesvirus infection**
B10.81 Human herpesvirus 6 infection
B10.82 Human herpesvirus 7 infection
B10.89 Other human herpesvirus infection
Human herpesvirus 8 infection
Kaposi's sarcoma-associated herpesvirus infection

Viral hepatitis (B15-B19)

Excludes1: *sequelae of viral hepatitis (B94.2)*

Excludes2: *cytomegaloviral hepatitis (B25.1)*
herpesviral [herpes simplex] hepatitis (B00.81)

B15 Acute hepatitis A

MCC **B15.0 Hepatitis A with hepatic coma**
MCC Exclusion see Appendix A PDX collection 0175

CC **B15.9 Hepatitis A without hepatic coma**
Hepatitis A (acute)(viral) NOS
CC Exclusion see Appendix A PDX collection 0175

B16 Acute hepatitis B

MCC **B16.0 Acute hepatitis B with delta-agent with hepatic coma**
MCC Exclusion see Appendix A PDX collection 0175

CC **B16.1 Acute hepatitis B with delta-agent without hepatic coma**
CC Exclusion see Appendix A PDX collection 0175

MCC **B16.2 Acute hepatitis B without delta-agent with hepatic coma**
MCC Exclusion see Appendix A PDX collection 0175

CC **B16.9 Acute hepatitis B without delta-agent and without hepatic coma**
Hepatitis B (acute) (viral) NOS
CC Exclusion see Appendix A PDX collection 0175
AHA CC: 3Q, 2016, 13

B17 Other acute viral hepatitis

CC **B17.0 Acute delta-(super) infection of hepatitis B carrier**
CC Exclusion see Appendix A PDX collection 0175

\+ **B17.1 Acute hepatitis C**

CC **B17.10 Acute hepatitis C without hepatic coma**
Acute hepatitis C NOS
CC Exclusion see Appendix A PDX collection 0175

MCC **B17.11 Acute hepatitis C with hepatic coma**
MCC Exclusion see Appendix A PDX collection 0175

CC **B17.2 Acute hepatitis E**
CC Exclusion see Appendix A PDX collection 0175

CC **B17.8 Other specified acute viral hepatitis**
Hepatitis non-A non-B (acute) (viral) NEC
CC Exclusion see Appendix A PDX collection 0175

CC **B17.9 Acute viral hepatitis, unspecified**
Acute hepatitis NOS
Acute infectious hepatitis NOS
CC Exclusion see Appendix A PDX collection 0175

B18 Chronic viral hepatitis

Includes: Carrier of viral hepatitis

CC **B18.0 Chronic viral hepatitis B with delta-agent**
CC Exclusion see Appendix A PDX collection 0175

CC **B18.1 Chronic viral hepatitis B without delta-agent**
Carrier of viral hepatitis B
Chronic (viral) hepatitis B
CC Exclusion see Appendix A PDX collection 0175

B18.2 Chronic viral hepatitis C
Carrier of viral hepatitis C
AHA CC: 1Q, 2017, 41

CC **B18.8 Other chronic viral hepatitis**
Carrier of other viral hepatitis
CC Exclusion see Appendix A PDX collection 0175

CC **B18.9 Chronic viral hepatitis, unspecified**
Carrier of unspecified viral hepatitis
CC Exclusion see Appendix A PDX collection 0175

B19 Unspecified viral hepatitis

MCC **B19.0 Unspecified viral hepatitis with hepatic coma**
MCC Exclusion see Appendix A PDX collection 0175

\+ **B19.1 Unspecified viral hepatitis B**

CC **B19.10 Unspecified viral hepatitis B without hepatic coma**
Unspecified viral hepatitis B NOS
CC Exclusion see Appendix A PDX collection 0175

MCC **B19.11 Unspecified viral hepatitis B with hepatic coma**
MCC Exclusion see Appendix A PDX collection 0175

\+ **B19.2 Unspecified viral hepatitis C**
B19.20 Unspecified viral hepatitis C without hepatic coma
Viral hepatitis C NOS

MCC **B19.21 Unspecified viral hepatitis C with hepatic coma**
MCC Exclusion see Appendix A PDX collection 0175

CC **B19.9 Unspecified viral hepatitis without hepatic coma**
Viral hepatitis NOS
CC Exclusion see Appendix A PDX collection 0175

Human immunodeficiency virus [HIV] disease (B20)

B20 Human immunodeficiency virus [HIV] disease
MCC

Includes: acquired immune deficiency syndrome [AIDS]
AIDS-related complex [ARC]
HIV infection, symptomatic

Code first Human immunodeficiency virus [HIV] disease complicating pregnancy, childbirth and the puerperium, if applicable (O98.7-)

Use additional code(s) to identify all manifestations of HIV infection

Excludes1: *asymptomatic human immunodeficiency virus [HIV] infection status (Z21)*
exposure to HIV virus (Z20.6)
inconclusive serologic evidence of HIV (R75)

MCC Exclusion see Appendix A PDX collection 0176
Review coding guideline C.1.a
Valid 3-character code, no further characters required

Other viral diseases (B25-B34)

B25 Cytomegaloviral disease

Excludes1: *congenital cytomegalovirus infection (P35.1)*
cytomegaloviral mononucleosis (B27.1-)

MCC **B25.0 Cytomegaloviral pneumonitis**
MCC Exclusion see Appendix A PDX collection 0110

CC **B25.1 Cytomegaloviral hepatitis**
No CC Exclusions

MCC **B25.2 Cytomegaloviral pancreatitis**
MCC Exclusion see Appendix A PDX collection 0177

CC **B25.8 Other cytomegaloviral diseases**
Cytomegaloviral encephalitis
CC Exclusion see Appendix A PDX collection 0178

CC **B25.9 Cytomegaloviral disease, unspecified**
CC Exclusion see Appendix A PDX collection 0178

B26 Mumps

Includes: epidemic parotitis
infectious parotitis

♂ CC **B26.0 Mumps orchitis**
CC Exclusion see Appendix A PDX collection 0179

MCC **B26.1 Mumps meningitis**
MCC Exclusion see Appendix A PDX collection 0180

MCC **B26.2 Mumps encephalitis**
MCC Exclusion see Appendix A PDX collection 0181

CC **B26.3 Mumps pancreatitis**
CC Exclusion see Appendix A PDX collection 0182

\+ **B26.8 Mumps with other complications**

CC **B26.81 Mumps hepatitis**
CC Exclusion see Appendix A PDX collection 0183

CC **B26.82 Mumps myocarditis**
CC Exclusion see Appendix A PDX collection 0184

CC **B26.83 Mumps nephritis**
CC Exclusion see Appendix A PDX collection 0184

CC **B26.84 Mumps polyneuropathy**
CC Exclusion see Appendix A PDX collection 0185

CC **B26.85 Mumps arthritis**
CC Exclusion see Appendix A PDX collection 0184

CC **B26.89 Other mumps complications**
CC Exclusion see Appendix A PDX collection 0184

B26.9 Mumps without complication
Mumps NOS
Mumps parotitis NOS

B27 Infectious mononucleosis

Includes: glandular fever
monocytic angina
Pfeiffer's disease

\+ **B27.0 Gammaherpesviral mononucleosis**
Mononucleosis due to Epstein-Barr virus
B27.00 Gammaherpesviral mononucleosis without complication
B27.01 Gammaherpesviral mononucleosis with polyneuropathy

B27.02 Gammaherpesviral mononucleosis with meningitis
B27.09 Gammaherpesviral mononucleosis with other complications
Hepatomegaly in gammaherpesviral mononucleosis

+ B27.1 Cytomegaloviral mononucleosis
B27.10 Cytomegaloviral mononucleosis without complications
B27.11 Cytomegaloviral mononucleosis with polyneuropathy
B27.12 Cytomegaloviral mononucleosis with meningitis
B27.19 Cytomegaloviral mononucleosis with other complication
Hepatomegaly in cytomegaloviral mononucleosis

+ B27.8 Other infectious mononucleosis
B27.80 Other infectious mononucleosis without complication
B27.81 Other infectious mononucleosis with polyneuropathy
B27.82 Other infectious mononucleosis with meningitis
B27.89 Other infectious mononucleosis with other complication
Hepatomegaly in other infectious mononucleosis

+ B27.9 Infectious mononucleosis, unspecified
B27.90 Infectious mononucleosis, unspecified without complication
B27.91 Infectious mononucleosis, unspecified with polyneuropathy
B27.92 Infectious mononucleosis, unspecified with meningitis
B27.99 Infectious mononucleosis, unspecified with other complication
Hepatomegaly in unspecified infectious mononucleosis

B30 Viral conjunctivitis

Excludes1: *herpesviral [herpes simplex] ocular disease (B00.5)*
ocular zoster (B02.3)

B30.0 Keratoconjunctivitis due to adenovirus
Epidemic keratoconjunctivitis
Shipyard eye

B30.1 Conjunctivitis due to adenovirus
Acute adenoviral follicular conjunctivitis
Swimming-pool conjunctivitis

B30.2 Viral pharyngoconjunctivitis

B30.3 Acute epidemic hemorrhagic conjunctivitis (enteroviral)
Conjunctivitis due to coxsackievirus 24
Conjunctivitis due to enterovirus 70
Hemorrhagic conjunctivitis (acute)(epidemic)

B30.8 Other viral conjunctivitis
Newcastle conjunctivitis

B30.9 Viral conjunctivitis, unspecified

B33 Other viral diseases, not elsewhere classified

B33.0 Epidemic myalgia
Bornholm disease

CC **B33.1 Ross River disease**
Epidemic polyarthritis and exanthema
Ross River fever
CC Exclusion see Appendix A PDX collection 0144

+ **B33.2 Viral carditis**
Coxsackie (virus) carditis

CC **B33.20 Viral carditis, unspecified**
CC Exclusion see Appendix A PDX collection 0186

CC **B33.21 Viral endocarditis**
CC Exclusion see Appendix A PDX collection 0187

CC **B33.22 Viral myocarditis**
CC Exclusion see Appendix A PDX collection 0186

CC **B33.23 Viral pericarditis**
CC Exclusion see Appendix A PDX collection 0188

B33.24 Viral cardiomyopathy

B33.3 Retrovirus infections, not elsewhere classified
Retrovirus infection NOS

CC **B33.4 Hantavirus (cardio)-pulmonary syndrome [HPS] [HCPS]**
Hantavirus disease with pulmonary manifestations
Sin nombre virus disease
Use additional code to identify any associated acute kidney failure (N17.9)
Excludes1: *hantavirus disease with renal manifestations (A98.5)*
hemorrhagic fever with renal manifestations (A98.5)
CC Exclusion see Appendix A PDX collection 0189

B33.8 Other specified viral diseases
Excludes1: *anogenital human papillomavirus infection (A63.0)*
viral warts due to human papillomavirus infection (B07)

B34 Viral infection of unspecified site

Excludes1: *anogenital human papillomavirus infection (A63.0)*
cytomegaloviral disease NOS (B25.9)
herpesvirus [herpes simplex] infection NOS (B00.9)
retrovirus infection NOS (B33.3)
viral agents as the cause of diseases classified elsewhere (B97.-)
viral warts due to human papillomavirus infection (B07)

B34.0 Adenovirus infection, unspecified

B34.1 Enterovirus infection, unspecified
Coxsackievirus infection NOS
Echovirus infection NOS

B34.2 Coronavirus infection, unspecified
Excludes1: *pneumonia due to SARS-associated coronavirus (J12.81)*

CC **B34.3 Parvovirus infection, unspecified**
CC Exclusion see Appendix A PDX collection 0174

B34.4 Papovavirus infection, unspecified

B34.8 Other viral infections of unspecified site

B34.9 Viral infection, unspecified
Viremia NOS
AHA CC: 3Q, 2016, 10

Mycoses (B35-B49)

Excludes2: *hypersensitivity pneumonitis due to organic dust (J67.-)*
mycosis fungoides (C84.0-)

B35 Dermatophytosis

Includes: favus
infections due to species of Epidermophyton, Micro-sporum and Trichophyton
tinea, any type except those in B36.-

B35.0 Tinea barbae and tinea capitis
Beard ringworm
Kerion
Scalp ringworm
Sycosis, mycotic

B35.1 Tinea unguium
Dermatophytic onychia
Dermatophytosis of nail
Onychomycosis
Ringworm of nails

B35.2 Tinea manuum
Dermatophytosis of hand
Hand ringworm

B35.3 Tinea pedis
Athlete's foot
Dermatophytosis of foot
Foot ringworm

B35.4 Tinea corporis
Ringworm of the body

B35.5 Tinea imbricata
Tokelau

B35.6 Tinea cruris
Dhobi itch
Groin ringworm
Jock itch

B35.8 Other dermatophytoses
Disseminated dermatophytosis
Granulomatous dermatophytosis

B35.9 Dermatophytosis, unspecified
Ringworm NOS

B36 Other superficial mycoses

B36.0 Pityriasis versicolor
Tinea flava
Tinea versicolor

B36.1 Tinea nigra
Keratomycosis nigricans palmaris
Microsporosis nigra
Pityriasis nigra

B36.2 White piedra
Tinea blanca

B36.3 Black piedra

B36.8 Other specified superficial mycoses

B36.9 Superficial mycosis, unspecified

B37 Candidiasis
Includes: candidosis
moniliasis
Excludes1: neonatal candidiasis (P37.5)
CC **B37.0 Candidal stomatitis**
Oral thrush
CC Exclusion see Appendix A PDX collection 0190
MCC **B37.1 Pulmonary candidiasis**
Candidal bronchitis
Candidal pneumonia
MCC Exclusion see Appendix A PDX collection 0190
B37.2 Candidiasis of skin and nail
Candidal onychia
Candidal paronychia
Excludes2: diaper dermatitis (L22)
♀ **B37.3 Candidiasis of vulva and vagina**
Candidal vulvovaginitis
Monilial vulvovaginitis
Vaginal thrush
\+ **B37.4 Candidiasis of other urogenital sites**
CC **B37.41 Candidal cystitis and urethritis**
CC Exclusion see Appendix A PDX collection 0191
HAC see Appendix B for HAC conditional logic
♂ **B37.42 Candidal balanitis**
CC **B37.49 Other urogenital candidiasis**
Candidal pyelonephritis
CC Exclusion see Appendix A PDX collection 0191
HAC see Appendix B for HAC conditional logic
MCC **B37.5 Candidal meningitis**
MCC Exclusion see Appendix A PDX collection 0192
MCC **B37.6 Candidal endocarditis**
MCC Exclusion see Appendix A PDX collection 0190
MCC **B37.7 Candidal sepsis**
Disseminated candidiasis
Systemic candidiasis
MCC Exclusion see Appendix A PDX collection 0193
Review coding guideline C.1.d
AHA CC: 4Q, 2014, 46
\+ **B37.8 Candidiasis of other sites**
CC **B37.81 Candidal esophagitis**
CC Exclusion see Appendix A PDX collection 0190
CC **B37.82 Candidal enteritis**
Candidal proctitis
CC Exclusion see Appendix A PDX collection 0190
CC **B37.83 Candidal cheilitis**
CC Exclusion see Appendix A PDX collection 0190
CC **B37.84 Candidal otitis externa**
CC Exclusion see Appendix A PDX collection 0190
CC **B37.89 Other sites of candidiasis**
Candidal osteomyelitis
CC Exclusion see Appendix A PDX collection 0194
B37.9 Candidiasis, unspecified
Thrush NOS

B38 Coccidioidomycosis
CC **B38.0 Acute pulmonary coccidioidomycosis**
CC Exclusion see Appendix A PDX collection 0195
CC **B38.1 Chronic pulmonary coccidioidomycosis**
CC Exclusion see Appendix A PDX collection 0196
CC **B38.2 Pulmonary coccidioidomycosis, unspecified**
CC Exclusion see Appendix A PDX collection 0196
CC **B38.3 Cutaneous coccidioidomycosis**
CC Exclusion see Appendix A PDX collection 0197
MCC **B38.4 Coccidioidomycosis meningitis**
MCC Exclusion see Appendix A PDX collection 0198
CC **B38.7 Disseminated coccidioidomycosis**
Generalized coccidioidomycosis
CC Exclusion see Appendix A PDX collection 0199
\+ **B38.8 Other forms of coccidioidomycosis**
♂ CC **B38.81 Prostatic coccidioidomycosis**
CC Exclusion see Appendix A PDX collection 0197
CC **B38.89 Other forms of coccidioidomycosis**
CC Exclusion see Appendix A PDX collection 0199
CC **B38.9 Coccidioidomycosis, unspecified**
CC Exclusion see Appendix A PDX collection 0199

B39 Histoplasmosis
Code first associated AIDS (B20)
Use additional code for any associated manifestations, such as:
endocarditis (I39)
meningitis (G02)
pericarditis (I32)
retinitis (H32)
MCC **B39.0 Acute pulmonary histoplasmosis capsulati**
MCC Exclusion see Appendix A PDX collection 0200
MCC **B39.1 Chronic pulmonary histoplasmosis capsulati**
MCC Exclusion see Appendix A PDX collection 0200
MCC **B39.2 Pulmonary histoplasmosis capsulati, unspecified**
MCC Exclusion see Appendix A PDX collection 0200
CC **B39.3 Disseminated histoplasmosis capsulati**
Generalized histoplasmosis capsulati
CC Exclusion see Appendix A PDX collection 0201
B39.4 Histoplasmosis capsulati, unspecified
American histoplasmosis
B39.5 Histoplasmosis duboisii
African histoplasmosis
B39.9 Histoplasmosis, unspecified

B40 Blastomycosis
Excludes1: Brazilian blastomycosis (B41.-)
keloidal blastomycosis (B48.0)
CC **B40.0 Acute pulmonary blastomycosis**
CC Exclusion see Appendix A PDX collection 0202
CC **B40.1 Chronic pulmonary blastomycosis**
CC Exclusion see Appendix A PDX collection 0202
CC **B40.2 Pulmonary blastomycosis, unspecified**
CC Exclusion see Appendix A PDX collection 0202
CC **B40.3 Cutaneous blastomycosis**
CC Exclusion see Appendix A PDX collection 0202
CC **B40.7 Disseminated blastomycosis**
Generalized blastomycosis
CC Exclusion see Appendix A PDX collection 0202
\+ **B40.8 Other forms of blastomycosis**
CC **B40.81 Blastomycotic meningoencephalitis**
Meningomyelitis due to blastomycosis
CC Exclusion see Appendix A PDX collection 0202
CC **B40.89 Other forms of blastomycosis**
CC Exclusion see Appendix A PDX collection 0202
CC **B40.9 Blastomycosis, unspecified**
CC Exclusion see Appendix A PDX collection 0202

B41 Paracoccidioidomycosis
Includes: Brazilian blastomycosis
Lutz' disease
CC **B41.0 Pulmonary paracoccidioidomycosis**
CC Exclusion see Appendix A PDX collection 0203
CC **B41.7 Disseminated paracoccidioidomycosis**
Generalized paracoccidioidomycosis
CC Exclusion see Appendix A PDX collection 0203
CC **B41.8 Other forms of paracoccidioidomycosis**
CC Exclusion see Appendix A PDX collection 0203
CC **B41.9 Paracoccidioidomycosis, unspecified**
CC Exclusion see Appendix A PDX collection 0203

B42 Sporotrichosis
B42.0 Pulmonary sporotrichosis
B42.1 Lymphocutaneous sporotrichosis
B42.7 Disseminated sporotrichosis
Generalized sporotrichosis
\+ **B42.8 Other forms of sporotrichosis**
B42.81 Cerebral sporotrichosis
Meningitis due to sporotrichosis
B42.82 Sporotrichosis arthritis
B42.89 Other forms of sporotrichosis
B42.9 Sporotrichosis, unspecified

B43 Chromomycosis and pheomycotic abscess
B43.0 Cutaneous chromomycosis
Dermatitis verrucosa
B43.1 Pheomycotic brain abscess
Cerebral chromomycosis
B43.2 Subcutaneous pheomycotic abscess and cyst
B43.8 Other forms of chromomycosis
B43.9 Chromomycosis, unspecified

B44 Aspergillosis
Includes: aspergilloma
MCC **B44.0 Invasive pulmonary aspergillosis**
MCC Exclusion see Appendix A PDX collection 0110

CC **B44.1 Other pulmonary aspergillosis**
CC Exclusion see Appendix A PDX collection 0204
CC **B44.2 Tonsillar aspergillosis**
CC Exclusion see Appendix A PDX collection 0204
CC **B44.7 Disseminated aspergillosis**
Generalized aspergillosis
CC Exclusion see Appendix A PDX collection 0204
+ **B44.8 Other forms of aspergillosis**
CC **B44.81 Allergic bronchopulmonary aspergillosis**
CC Exclusion see Appendix A PDX collection 0205
CC **B44.89 Other forms of aspergillosis**
CC Exclusion see Appendix A PDX collection 0204
CC **B44.9 Aspergillosis, unspecified**
CC Exclusion see Appendix A PDX collection 0204

B45 Cryptococcosis

CC **B45.0 Pulmonary cryptococcosis**
CC Exclusion see Appendix A PDX collection 0206
MCC **B45.1 Cerebral cryptococcosis**
Cryptococcal meningitis
Cryptococcosis meningocerebralis
MCC Exclusion see Appendix A PDX collection 0207
CC **B45.2 Cutaneous cryptococcosis**
CC Exclusion see Appendix A PDX collection 0206
CC **B45.3 Osseous cryptococcosis**
CC Exclusion see Appendix A PDX collection 0206
CC **B45.7 Disseminated cryptococcosis**
Generalized cryptococcosis
CC Exclusion see Appendix A PDX collection 0206
CC **B45.8 Other forms of cryptococcosis**
CC Exclusion see Appendix A PDX collection 0206
CC **B45.9 Cryptococcosis, unspecified**
CC Exclusion see Appendix A PDX collection 0206

B46 Zygomycosis

MCC **B46.0 Pulmonary mucormycosis**
MCC Exclusion see Appendix A PDX collection 0208
MCC **B46.1 Rhinocerebral mucormycosis**
MCC Exclusion see Appendix A PDX collection 0208
MCC **B46.2 Gastrointestinal mucormycosis**
MCC Exclusion see Appendix A PDX collection 0208
MCC **B46.3 Cutaneous mucormycosis**
Subcutaneous mucormycosis
MCC Exclusion see Appendix A PDX collection 0208
MCC **B46.4 Disseminated mucormycosis**
Generalized mucormycosis
MCC Exclusion see Appendix A PDX collection 0208
MCC **B46.5 Mucormycosis, unspecified**
MCC Exclusion see Appendix A PDX collection 0208
MCC **B46.8 Other zygomycoses**
Entomophthoromycosis
MCC Exclusion see Appendix A PDX collection 0208
MCC **B46.9 Zygomycosis, unspecified**
Phycomycosis NOS
MCC Exclusion see Appendix A PDX collection 0208

B47 Mycetoma

CC **B47.0 Eumycetoma**
Madura foot, mycotic
Maduromycosis
CC Exclusion see Appendix A PDX collection 0209
CC **B47.1 Actinomycetoma**
CC Exclusion see Appendix A PDX collection 0106
CC **B47.9 Mycetoma, unspecified**
Madura foot NOS
CC Exclusion see Appendix A PDX collection 0210

B48 Other mycoses, not elsewhere classified

B48.0 Lobomycosis
Keloidal blastomycosis
Lobo's disease
B48.1 Rhinosporidiosis
CC **B48.2 Allescheriasis**
Infection due to Pseudallescheria boydii
Excludes1: *eumycetoma (B47.0)*
CC Exclusion see Appendix A PDX collection 0211
CC **B48.3 Geotrichosis**
Geotrichum stomatitis
CC Exclusion see Appendix A PDX collection 0212
CC **B48.4 Penicillosis**
CC Exclusion see Appendix A PDX collection 0204
CC **B48.8 Other specified mycoses**
Adiaspiromycosis
Infection of tissue and organs by Alternaria
Infection of tissue and organs by Drechslera
Infection of tissue and organs by Fusarium
Infection of tissue and organs by saprophytic fungi NEC
CC Exclusion see Appendix A PDX collection 0213
AHA CC: 2Q, 2014, 13; 4Q, 2014, 46

CC B49 Unspecified mycosis

Fungemia NOS
CC Exclusion see Appendix A PDX collection 0212
Valid 3-character code, no further characters required

Protozoal diseases (B50-B64)

Excludes1: *amebiasis (A06.-)*
other protozoal intestinal diseases (A07.-)

B50 Plasmodium falciparum malaria

Includes: mixed infections of Plasmodium falciparum with any other Plasmodium species
CC **B50.0 Plasmodium falciparum malaria with cerebral complications**
Cerebral malaria NOS
CC Exclusion see Appendix A PDX collection 0214
CC **B50.8 Other severe and complicated Plasmodium falciparum malaria**
Severe or complicated Plasmodium falciparum malaria NOS
CC Exclusion see Appendix A PDX collection 0214
MCC **B50.9 Plasmodium falciparum malaria, unspecified**
MCC Exclusion see Appendix A PDX collection 0214

B51 Plasmodium vivax malaria

Includes: mixed infections of Plasmodium vivax with other Plasmodium species, except Plasmodium falciparum
Excludes1: *plasmodium vivav with Plasmodium falciparum (B50.-)*
CC **B51.0 Plasmodium vivax malaria with rupture of spleen**
CC Exclusion see Appendix A PDX collection 0214
CC **B51.8 Plasmodium vivax malaria with other complications**
CC Exclusion see Appendix A PDX collection 0214
CC **B51.9 Plasmodium vivax malaria without complication**
Plasmodium vivax malaria NOS
CC Exclusion see Appendix A PDX collection 0215

B52 Plasmodium malariae malaria

Includes: mixed infections of Plasmodium malariae with other Plasmodium species, except Plasmodium falciparum and Plasmodium vivax
Excludes1: *Plasmodium falciparum (B50.-)*
Plasmodium vivax (B51.-)
CC **B52.0 Plasmodium malariae malaria with nephropathy**
CC Exclusion see Appendix A PDX collection 0216
CC **B52.8 Plasmodium malariae malaria with other complications**
CC Exclusion see Appendix A PDX collection 0214
CC **B52.9 Plasmodium malariae malaria without complication**
Plasmodium malariae malaria NOS
CC Exclusion see Appendix A PDX collection 0214

B53 Other specified malaria

CC **B53.0 Plasmodium ovale malaria**
Excludes1: *Plasmodium ovale with Plasmodium falciparum (B50.-)*
Plasmodium ovale with Plasmodium malariae (B52.-)
Plasmodium ovale with Plasmodium vivax (B51.-)
CC Exclusion see Appendix A PDX collection 0214
CC **B53.1 Malaria due to simian plasmodia**
Excludes1: *Malaria due to simian plasmodia with Plasmodium falciparum (B50.-)*
Malaria due to simian plasmodia with Plasmodium malariae (B52.-)
Malaria due to simian plasmodia with Plasmodium ovale (B53.0)
Malaria due to simian plasmodia with Plasmodium vivax (B51.-)
CC Exclusion see Appendix A PDX collection 0214
CC **B53.8 Other malaria, not elsewhere classified**
CC Exclusion see Appendix A PDX collection 0214

CC B54 Unspecified malaria

CC Exclusion see Appendix A PDX collection 0217
Valid 3-character code, no further characters required

B55 Leishmaniasis

CC **B55.0 Visceral leishmaniasis**
Kala-azar
Post-kala-azar dermal leishmaniasis
CC Exclusion see Appendix A PDX collection 0218
CC **B55.1 Cutaneous leishmaniasis**
CC Exclusion see Appendix A PDX collection 0218

CC **B55.2 Mucocutaneous leishmaniasis**
CC Exclusion see Appendix A PDX collection 0218
CC **B55.9 Leishmaniasis, unspecified**
CC Exclusion see Appendix A PDX collection 0218

B56 African trypanosomiasis

CC **B56.0 Gambiense trypanosomiasis**
Infection due to Trypanosoma brucei gambiense
West African sleeping sickness
CC Exclusion see Appendix A PDX collection 0218
CC **B56.1 Rhodesiense trypanosomiasis**
East African sleeping sickness
Infection due to Trypanosoma brucei rhodesiense
CC Exclusion see Appendix A PDX collection 0218
CC **B56.9 African trypanosomiasis, unspecified**
Sleeping sickness NOS
CC Exclusion see Appendix A PDX collection 0218

B57 Chagas' disease

Includes: American trypanosomiasis
infection due to Trypanosoma cruzi
CC **B57.0 Acute Chagas' disease with heart involvement**
Acute Chagas' disease with myocarditis
CC Exclusion see Appendix A PDX collection 0219
CC **B57.1 Acute Chagas' disease without heart involvement**
Acute Chagas' disease NOS
CC Exclusion see Appendix A PDX collection 0218
CC **B57.2 Chagas' disease (chronic) with heart involvement**
American trypanosomiasis NOS
Chagas' disease (chronic) NOS
Chagas' disease (chronic) with myocarditis
Trypanosomiasis NOS
CC Exclusion see Appendix A PDX collection 0219
\+ **B57.3 Chagas' disease (chronic) with digestive system involvement**
CC **B57.30 Chagas' disease with digestive system involvement, unspecified**
CC Exclusion see Appendix A PDX collection 0218
CC **B57.31 Megaesophagus in Chagas' disease**
CC Exclusion see Appendix A PDX collection 0218
CC **B57.32 Megacolon in Chagas' disease**
CC Exclusion see Appendix A PDX collection 0218
CC **B57.39 Other digestive system involvement in Chagas' disease**
CC Exclusion see Appendix A PDX collection 0218
\+ **B57.4 Chagas' disease (chronic) with nervous system involvement**
CC **B57.40 Chagas' disease with nervous system involvement, unspecified**
CC Exclusion see Appendix A PDX collection 0218
CC **B57.41 Meningitis in Chagas' disease**
CC Exclusion see Appendix A PDX collection 0218
CC **B57.42 Meningoencephalitis in Chagas' disease**
CC Exclusion see Appendix A PDX collection 0218
CC **B57.49 Other nervous system involvement in Chagas' disease**
CC Exclusion see Appendix A PDX collection 0218
CC **B57.5 Chagas' disease (chronic) with other organ involvement**
CC Exclusion see Appendix A PDX collection 0218

B58 Toxoplasmosis

Includes: infection due to Toxoplasma gondii
Excludes1: *congenital toxoplasmosis (P37.1)*
\+ **B58.0 Toxoplasma oculopathy**
CC **B58.00 Toxoplasma oculopathy, unspecified**
CC Exclusion see Appendix A PDX collection 0220
CC **B58.01 Toxoplasma chorioretinitis**
CC Exclusion see Appendix A PDX collection 0221
CC **B58.09 Other toxoplasma oculopathy**
Toxoplasma uveitis
CC Exclusion see Appendix A PDX collection 0222
CC **B58.1 Toxoplasma hepatitis**
CC Exclusion see Appendix A PDX collection 0223
MCC **B58.2 Toxoplasma meningoencephalitis**
MCC Exclusion see Appendix A PDX collection 0224
MCC **B58.3 Pulmonary toxoplasmosis**
MCC Exclusion see Appendix A PDX collection 0225
\+ **B58.8 Toxoplasmosis with other organ involvement**
MCC **B58.81 Toxoplasma myocarditis**
MCC Exclusion see Appendix A PDX collection 0226
CC **B58.82 Toxoplasma myositis**
CC Exclusion see Appendix A PDX collection 0220
CC **B58.83 Toxoplasma tubulo-interstitial nephropathy**
Toxoplasma pyelonephritis
CC Exclusion see Appendix A PDX collection 0220
CC **B58.89 Toxoplasmosis with other organ involvement**
CC Exclusion see Appendix A PDX collection 0220
CC **B58.9 Toxoplasmosis, unspecified**
CC Exclusion see Appendix A PDX collection 0227

B59 Pneumocystosis
MCC
Pneumonia due to Pneumocystis carinii
Pneumonia due to Pneumocystis jiroveci
MCC Exclusion see Appendix A PDX collection 0228
Valid 3-character code, no further characters required

B60 Other protozoal diseases, not elsewhere classified

Excludes1: *cryptosporidiosis (A07.2)*
intestinal microsporidiosis (A07.8)
isosporiasis (A07.3)
CC **B60.0 Babesiosis**
Piroplasmosis
CC Exclusion see Appendix A PDX collection 0218
\+ **B60.1 Acanthamebiasis**
CC **B60.10 Acanthamebiasis, unspecified**
CC Exclusion see Appendix A PDX collection 0229
B60.11 Meningoencephalitis due to Acanthamoeba (culbertsoni)
B60.12 Conjunctivitis due to Acanthamoeba
B60.13 Keratoconjunctivitis due to Acanthamoeba
CC **B60.19 Other acanthamebic disease**
CC Exclusion see Appendix A PDX collection 0229
CC **B60.2 Naegleriasis**
Primary amebic meningoencephalitis
CC Exclusion see Appendix A PDX collection 0229
B60.8 Other specified protozoal diseases
Microsporidiosis

B64 Unspecified protozoal disease

Valid 3-character code, no further characters required

Helminthiases (B65-B83)

B65 Schistosomiasis [bilharziasis]

Includes: snail fever
CC **B65.0 Schistosomiasis due to Schistosoma haematobium [urinary schistosomiasis]**
CC Exclusion see Appendix A PDX collection 0230
CC **B65.1 Schistosomiasis due to Schistosoma mansoni [intestinal schistosomiasis]**
CC Exclusion see Appendix A PDX collection 0230
CC **B65.2 Schistosomiasis due to Schistosoma japonicum**
Asiatic schistosomiasis
CC Exclusion see Appendix A PDX collection 0230
CC **B65.3 Cercarial dermatitis**
Swimmer's itch
CC Exclusion see Appendix A PDX collection 0230
CC **B65.8 Other schistosomiasis**
Infection due to Schistosoma intercalatum
Infection due to Schistosoma mattheei
Infection due to Schistosoma mekongi
CC Exclusion see Appendix A PDX collection 0230
CC **B65.9 Schistosomiasis, unspecified**
CC Exclusion see Appendix A PDX collection 0230

B66 Other fluke infections

CC **B66.0 Opisthorchiasis**
Infection due to cat liver fluke
Infection due to Opisthorchis (felineus)(viverrini)
CC Exclusion see Appendix A PDX collection 0231
CC **B66.1 Clonorchiasis**
Chinese liver fluke disease
Infection due to Clonorchis sinensis
Oriental liver fluke disease
CC Exclusion see Appendix A PDX collection 0231
CC **B66.2 Dicroceliasis**
Infection due to Dicrocoelium dendriticum
Lancet fluke infection
CC Exclusion see Appendix A PDX collection 0231
CC **B66.3 Fascioliasis**
Infection due to Fasciola gigantica
Infection due to Fasciola hepatica
Infection due to Fasciola indica
Sheep liver fluke disease
CC Exclusion see Appendix A PDX collection 0231
CC **B66.4 Paragonimiasis**
Infection due to Paragonimus species
Lung fluke disease
Pulmonary distomiasis
CC Exclusion see Appendix A PDX collection 0231

CC **B66.5 Fasciolopsiasis**
Infection due to Fasciolopsis buski
Intestinal distomiasis
CC Exclusion see Appendix A PDX collection 0231

CC **B66.8 Other specified fluke infections**
Echinostomiasis
Heterophyiasis
Metagonimiasis
Nanophyetiasis
Watsoniasis
CC Exclusion see Appendix A PDX collection 0231

B66.9 Fluke infection, unspecified

B67 Echinococcosis

Includes: hydatidosis

CC **B67.0 Echinococcus granulosus infection of liver**
CC Exclusion see Appendix A PDX collection 0232

CC **B67.1 Echinococcus granulosus infection of lung**
CC Exclusion see Appendix A PDX collection 0233

CC **B67.2 Echinococcus granulosus infection of bone**
CC Exclusion see Appendix A PDX collection 0234

\+ **B67.3 Echinococcus granulosus infection, other and multiple sites**

CC **B67.31 Echinococcus granulosus infection, thyroid gland**
CC Exclusion see Appendix A PDX collection 0235

CC **B67.32 Echinococcus granulosus infection, multiple sites**
CC Exclusion see Appendix A PDX collection 0234

CC **B67.39 Echinococcus granulosus infection, other sites**
CC Exclusion see Appendix A PDX collection 0234

CC **B67.4 Echinococcus granulosus infection, unspecified**
Dog tapeworm (infection)
CC Exclusion see Appendix A PDX collection 0236

CC **B67.5 Echinococcus multilocularis infection of liver**
CC Exclusion see Appendix A PDX collection 0237

\+ **B67.6 Echinococcus multilocularis infection, other and multiple sites**

CC **B67.61 Echinococcus multilocularis infection, multiple sites**
CC Exclusion see Appendix A PDX collection 0238

CC **B67.69 Echinococcus multilocularis infection, other sites**
CC Exclusion see Appendix A PDX collection 0238

CC **B67.7 Echinococcus multilocularis infection, unspecified**
CC Exclusion see Appendix A PDX collection 0239

CC **B67.8 Echinococcosis, unspecified, of liver**
CC Exclusion see Appendix A PDX collection 0240

\+ **B67.9 Echinococcosis, other and unspecified**

CC **B67.90 Echinococcosis, unspecified**
Echinococcosis NOS
CC Exclusion see Appendix A PDX collection 0240

CC **B67.99 Other echinococcosis**
CC Exclusion see Appendix A PDX collection 0240

B68 Taeniasis

Excludes1: *cysticercosis (B69.-)*

CC **B68.0 Taenia solium taeniasis**
Pork tapeworm (infection)
CC Exclusion see Appendix A PDX collection 0241

CC **B68.1 Taenia saginata taeniasis**
Beef tapeworm (infection)
Infection due to adult tapeworm Taenia saginata
CC Exclusion see Appendix A PDX collection 0242

CC **B68.9 Taeniasis, unspecified**
CC Exclusion see Appendix A PDX collection 0242

B69 Cysticercosis

Includes: cysticerciasis infection due to larval form of Taenia solium

CC **B69.0 Cysticercosis of central nervous system**
CC Exclusion see Appendix A PDX collection 0242

CC **B69.1 Cysticercosis of eye**
CC Exclusion see Appendix A PDX collection 0242

\+ **B69.8 Cysticercosis of other sites**

CC **B69.81 Myositis in cysticercosis**
CC Exclusion see Appendix A PDX collection 0242

CC **B69.89 Cysticercosis of other sites**
CC Exclusion see Appendix A PDX collection 0242

CC **B69.9 Cysticercosis, unspecified**
CC Exclusion see Appendix A PDX collection 0242

B70 Diphyllobothriasis and sparganosis

CC **B70.0 Diphyllobothriasis**
Diphyllobothrium (adult) (latum) (pacificum) infection
Fish tapeworm (infection)
Excludes2: *larval diphyllobothriasis (B70.1)*
CC Exclusion see Appendix A PDX collection 0242

CC **B70.1 Sparganosis**
Infection due to Sparganum (mansoni) (proliferum)
Infection due to Spirometra larva
Larval diphyllobothriasis
Spirometrosis
CC Exclusion see Appendix A PDX collection 0242

B71 Other cestode infections

CC **B71.0 Hymenolepiasis**
Dwarf tapeworm infection
Rat tapeworm (infection)
CC Exclusion see Appendix A PDX collection 0242

CC **B71.1 Dipylidiasis**
CC Exclusion see Appendix A PDX collection 0242

CC **B71.8 Other specified cestode infections**
Coenurosis
CC Exclusion see Appendix A PDX collection 0242

B71.9 Cestode infection, unspecified
Tapeworm (infection) NOS

CC B72 Dracunculiasis

Includes: guinea worm infection
infection due to Dracunculus medinensis
CC Exclusion see Appendix A PDX collection 0243
Valid 3-character code, no further characters required

B73 Onchocerciasis

Includes: onchocerca volvulus infection
onchocercosis
river blindness

\+ **B73.0 Onchocerciasis with eye disease**

CC **B73.00 Onchocerciasis with eye involvement, unspecified**
CC Exclusion see Appendix A PDX collection 0243

CC **B73.01 Onchocerciasis with endophthalmitis**
CC Exclusion see Appendix A PDX collection 0243

CC **B73.02 Onchocerciasis with glaucoma**
CC Exclusion see Appendix A PDX collection 0243

CC **B73.09 Onchocerciasis with other eye involvement**
Infestation of eyelid due to onchocerciasis
CC Exclusion see Appendix A PDX collection 0243

CC **B73.1 Onchocerciasis without eye disease**
CC Exclusion see Appendix A PDX collection 0243

B74 Filariasis

Excludes2: *onchocerciasis (B73)*
tropical (pulmonary) eosinophilia NOS (J82)

CC **B74.0 Filariasis due to Wuchereria bancrofti**
Bancroftian elephantiasis
Bancroftian filariasis
CC Exclusion see Appendix A PDX collection 0243

CC **B74.1 Filariasis due to Brugia malayi**
CC Exclusion see Appendix A PDX collection 0243

CC **B74.2 Filariasis due to Brugia timori**
CC Exclusion see Appendix A PDX collection 0243

CC **B74.3 Loiasis**
Calabar swelling
Eyeworm disease of Africa
Loa loa infection
CC Exclusion see Appendix A PDX collection 0243

CC **B74.4 Mansonelliasis**
Infection due to Mansonella ozzardi
Infection due to Mansonella perstans
Infection due to Mansonella streptocerca
CC Exclusion see Appendix A PDX collection 0243

CC **B74.8 Other filariases**
Dirofilariasis
CC Exclusion see Appendix A PDX collection 0243

CC **B74.9 Filariasis, unspecified**
CC Exclusion see Appendix A PDX collection 0243

CC B75 Trichinellosis

Includes: infection due to Trichinella species
trichiniasis
CC Exclusion see Appendix A PDX collection 0244
Valid 3-character code, no further characters required

B76 Hookworm diseases

Includes: uncinariasis

CC **B76.0 Ancylostomiasis**
Infection due to Ancylostoma species
CC Exclusion see Appendix A PDX collection 0245

CC **B76.1 Necatoriasis**
Infection due to Necator americanus
CC Exclusion see Appendix A PDX collection 0245

CC **B76.8 Other hookworm diseases**
CC Exclusion see Appendix A PDX collection 0245

CC **B76.9 Hookworm disease, unspecified**
Cutaneous larva migrans NOS
CC Exclusion see Appendix A PDX collection 0245

B77 Ascariasis

Includes: ascaridiasis
roundworm infection

CC **B77.0 Ascariasis with intestinal complications**
CC Exclusion see Appendix A PDX collection 0246

\+ **B77.8 Ascariasis with other complications**

MCC **B77.81 Ascariasis pneumonia**
MCC Exclusion see Appendix A PDX collection 0247

CC **B77.89 Ascariasis with other complications**
CC Exclusion see Appendix A PDX collection 0246

CC **B77.9 Ascariasis, unspecified**
CC Exclusion see Appendix A PDX collection 0246

B78 Strongyloidiasis

Excludes1: *trichostrongyliasis (B81.2)*

CC **B78.0 Intestinal strongyloidiasis**
CC Exclusion see Appendix A PDX collection 0246

B78.1 Cutaneous strongyloidiasis

CC **B78.7 Disseminated strongyloidiasis**
CC Exclusion see Appendix A PDX collection 0246

CC **B78.9 Strongyloidiasis, unspecified**
CC Exclusion see Appendix A PDX collection 0246

CC **B79 Trichuriasis**

Includes: trichocephaliasis
whipworm (disease)(infection)

CC Exclusion see Appendix A PDX collection 0246
Valid 3-character code, no further characters required

CC **B80 Enterobiasis**

Includes: oxyuriasis
pinworm infection
threadworm infection

CC Exclusion see Appendix A PDX collection 0246
Valid 3-character code, no further characters required

B81 Other intestinal helminthiases, not elsewhere classified

Excludes1: *angiostrongyliasis due to:*
Angiostrongylus cantonensis (B83.2)
Parastrongylus cantonensis (B83.2)

CC **B81.0 Anisakiasis**
Infection due to Anisakis larva
CC Exclusion see Appendix A PDX collection 0246

CC **B81.1 Intestinal capillariasis**
Capillariasis NOS
Infection due to Capillaria philippinensis
Excludes2: *hepatic capillariasis (B83.8)*
CC Exclusion see Appendix A PDX collection 0246

CC **B81.2 Trichostrongyliasis**
CC Exclusion see Appendix A PDX collection 0246

CC **B81.3 Intestinal angiostrongyliasis**
Angiostrongyliasis due to:
Angiostrongylus costaricensis
Parastrongylus cantonensis
CC Exclusion see Appendix A PDX collection 0248

CC **B81.4 Mixed intestinal helminthiases**
Infection due to intestinal helminths classified to more than one of the categories B65.0-B81.3 and B81.8
Mixed helminthiasis NOS
CC Exclusion see Appendix A PDX collection 0248

CC **B81.8 Other specified intestinal helminthiases**
Infection due to Oesophagostomum species [esophagostomiasis]
Infection due to Ternidens diminutus [ternidensiasis]
CC Exclusion see Appendix A PDX collection 0248

B82 Unspecified intestinal parasitism

CC **B82.0 Intestinal helminthiasis, unspecified**
CC Exclusion see Appendix A PDX collection 0248

B82.9 Intestinal parasitism, unspecified

B83 Other helminthiases

Excludes1: *capillariasis NOS (B81.1)*
Excludes2: *intestinal capillariasis (B81.1)*

B83.0 Visceral larva migrans
Toxocariasis

B83.1 Gnathostomiasis
Wandering swelling

B83.2 Angiostrongyliasis due to Parastrongylus cantonensis
Eosinophilic meningoencephalitis due to Parastrongylus cantonensis
Excludes2: *intestinal angiostrongyliasis (B81.3)*

B83.3 Syngamiasis
Syngamosis

B83.4 Internal hirudiniasis
Excludes2: *external hirudiniasis (B88.3)*

B83.8 Other specified helminthiases
Acanthocephaliasis
Gongylonemiasis
Hepatic capillariasis
Metastrongyliasis
Thelaziasis

B83.9 Helminthiasis, unspecified
Worms NOS
Excludes1: *intestinal helminthiasis NOS (B82.0)*

Pediculosis, acariasis and other infestations (B85-B89)

B85 Pediculosis and phthiriasis

B85.0 Pediculosis due to Pediculus humanus capitis
Head-louse infestation

B85.1 Pediculosis due to Pediculus humanus corporis
Body-louse infestation

B85.2 Pediculosis, unspecified

B85.3 Phthiriasis
Infestation by crab-louse
Infestation by Phthirus pubis

B85.4 Mixed pediculosis and phthiriasis
Infestation classifiable to more than one of the categories B85.0-B85.3

B86 Scabies

Sarcoptic itch
Valid 3-character code, no further characters required

B87 Myiasis

Includes: infestation by larva of flies

B87.0 Cutaneous myiasis
Creeping myiasis

B87.1 Wound myiasis
Traumatic myiasis

B87.2 Ocular myiasis

B87.3 Nasopharyngeal myiasis
Laryngeal myiasis

B87.4 Aural myiasis

\+ **B87.8 Myiasis of other sites**

B87.81 Genitourinary myiasis

B87.82 Intestinal myiasis

B87.89 Myiasis of other sites

B87.9 Myiasis, unspecified

B88 Other infestations

B88.0 Other acariasis
Acarine dermatitis
Dermatitis due to Demodex species
Dermatitis due to Dermanyssus gallinae
Dermatitis due to Liponyssoides sanguineus
Trombiculosis
Excludes2: *scabies (B86)*

B88.1 Tungiasis [sandflea infestation]

B88.2 Other arthropod infestations
Scarabiasis

B88.3 External hirudiniasis
Leech infestation NOS
Excludes2: *internal hirudiniasis (B83.4)*

B88.8 Other specified infestations
Ichthyoparasitism due to Vandellia cirrhosa
Linguatulosis
Porocephaliasis

B88.9 Infestation, unspecified
Infestation (skin) NOS
Infestation by mites NOS
Skin parasites NOS

B89 Unspecified parasitic disease

Valid 3-character code, no further characters required

Sequelae of infectious and parasitic diseases (B90-B94)

NOTE Categories B90-B94 are to be used to indicate conditions in categories A00-B89 as the cause of sequelae, which are themselves classified elsewhere. The 'sequelae' include conditions specified as such; they also include residuals of diseases classifiable to the above categories if there is evidence that the disease itself is no longer present. Codes from these categories are not to be used for chronic infections. Code chronic current infections to active infectious disease as appropriate.

ode first condition resulting from (sequela) the infectious or parasitic disease

B90 Sequelae of tuberculosis

B90.0 Sequelae of central nervous system tuberculosis
B90.1 Sequelae of genitourinary tuberculosis
B90.2 Sequelae of tuberculosis of bones and joints
B90.8 Sequelae of tuberculosis of other organs
Excludes2: *sequelae of respiratory tuberculosis (B90.9)*
B90.9 Sequelae of respiratory and unspecified tuberculosis
Sequelae of tuberculosis NOS

B91 Sequelae of poliomyelitis

Excludes1: *postpolio syndrome (G14)*
Valid 3-character code, no further characters required

B92 Sequelae of leprosy

Valid 3-character code, no further characters required

B94 Sequelae of other and unspecified infectious and parasitic diseases

B94.0 Sequelae of trachoma
B94.1 Sequelae of viral encephalitis
B94.2 Sequelae of viral hepatitis
B94.8 Sequelae of other specified infectious and parasitic diseases
B94.9 Sequelae of unspecified infectious and parasitic disease

acterial and viral infectious agents (B95-B97)

OTE These categories are provided for use as supplementary or additional codes to identify the infectious agent(s) in diseases classified elsewhere.

B95 Streptococcus, Staphylococcus, and Enterococcus as the cause of diseases classified elsewhere

Review coding guideline C.1.b
B95.0 Streptococcus, group A, as the cause of diseases classified elsewhere
B95.1 Streptococcus, group B, as the cause of diseases classified elsewhere
B95.2 Enterococcus as the cause of diseases classified elsewhere
B95.3 Streptococcus pneumoniae as the cause of diseases classified elsewhere
B95.4 Other streptococcus as the cause of diseases classified elsewhere
B95.5 Unspecified streptococcus as the cause of diseases classified elsewhere
\+ **B95.6 Staphylococcus aureus as the cause of diseases classified elsewhere**
B95.61 Methicillin susceptible Staphylococcus aureus infection as the cause of diseases classified elsewhere
Methicillin susceptible Staphylococcus aureus (MSSA) infection as the cause of diseases classified elsewhere
Staphylococcus aureus infection NOS as the cause of diseases classified elsewhere
B95.62 Methicillin resistant Staphylococcus aureus infection as the cause of diseases classified elsewhere
Methicillin resistant staphylococcus aureus (MRSA) infection as the cause of diseases classified elsewhere
Review coding guidelines C.1.e.1.a and C.1.e.1.b
AHA CC: 1Q, 2016, 12-13
B95.7 Other staphylococcus as the cause of diseases classified elsewhere
B95.8 Unspecified staphylococcus as the cause of diseases classified elsewhere

B96 Other bacterial agents as the cause of diseases classified elsewhere

Review coding guideline C.1.b
B96.0 Mycoplasma pneumoniae [M. pneumoniae] as the cause of diseases classified elsewhere
Pleuro-pneumonia-like-organism [PPLO]
B96.1 Klebsiella pneumoniae [K. pneumoniae] as the cause of diseases classified elsewhere
\+ **B96.2 Escherichia coli [E. coli] as the cause of diseases classified elsewhere**
B96.20 Unspecified Escherichia coli [E. coli] as the cause of diseases classified elsewhere
Escherichia coli [E. coli] NOS
B96.21 Shiga toxin-producing Escherichia coli [E. coli] (STEC) O157 as the cause of diseases classified elsewhere
E. coli O157:H- (nonmotile) with confirmation of Shiga toxin
E. coli O157 with confirmation of Shiga toxin when H antigen is unknown, or is not H7
O157:H7 Escherichia coli [E.coli] with or without confirmation of Shiga toxin-production
Shiga toxin-producing Escherichia coli [E.coli] O157:H7 with or without confirmation of Shiga toxin-production
STEC O157:H7 with or without confirmation of Shiga toxin-production
B96.22 Other specified Shiga toxin-producing Escherichia coli [E. coli] (STEC) as the cause of diseases classified elsewhere
Non-O157 Shiga toxin-producing Escherichia coli [E.coli]
Non-O157 Shiga toxin-producing Escherichia coli [E.coli] with known O group
B96.23 Unspecified Shiga toxin-producing Escherichia coli [E. coli] (STEC) as the cause of diseases classified elsewhere
Shiga toxin-producing Escherichia coli [E. coli] with unspecified O group
STEC NOS
B96.29 Other Escherichia coli [E. coli] as the cause of diseases classified elsewhere
Non-Shiga toxin-producing E. coli
B96.3 Hemophilus influenzae [H. influenzae] as the cause of diseases classified elsewhere
B96.4 Proteus (mirabilis) (morganii) as the cause of diseases classified elsewhere
B96.5 Pseudomonas (aeruginosa) (mallei) (pseudomallei) as the cause of diseases classified elsewhere
AHA CC: 1Q, 2015, 18-19
B96.6 Bacteroides fragilis [B. fragilis] as the cause of diseases classified elsewhere
B96.7 Clostridium perfringens [C. perfringens] as the cause of diseases classified elsewhere
\+ **B96.8 Other specified bacterial agents as the cause of diseases classified elsewhere**
B96.81 Helicobacter pylori [H. pylori] as the cause of diseases classified elsewhere
B96.82 Vibrio vulnificus as the cause of diseases classified elsewhere
B96.89 Other specified bacterial agents as the cause of diseases classified elsewhere

B97 Viral agents as the cause of diseases classified elsewhere

Review coding guideline C.1.b
B97.0 Adenovirus as the cause of diseases classified elsewhere
\+ **B97.1 Enterovirus as the cause of diseases classified elsewhere**
B97.10 Unspecified enterovirus as the cause of diseases classified elsewhere
B97.11 Coxsackievirus as the cause of diseases classified elsewhere
B97.12 Echovirus as the cause of diseases classified elsewhere
B97.19 Other enterovirus as the cause of diseases classified elsewhere
\+ **B97.2 Coronavirus as the cause of diseases classified elsewhere**
CC **B97.21 SARS-associated coronavirus as the cause of diseases classified elsewhere**
Excludes1: *pneumonia due to SARS-associated coronavirus (J12.81)*
CC Exclusion see Appendix A PDX collection 0249
B97.29 Other coronavirus as the cause of diseases classified elsewhere
\+ **B97.3 Retrovirus as the cause of diseases classified elsewhere**
Excludes1: *Human immunodeficiency virus [HIV] disease (B20)*
B97.30 Unspecified retrovirus as the cause of diseases classified elsewhere
B97.31 Lentivirus as the cause of diseases classified elsewhere
B97.32 Oncovirus as the cause of diseases classified elsewhere

CC **B97.33** **Human T-cell lymphotrophic virus, type I [HTLV-I] as the cause of diseases classified elsewhere**
CC Exclusion see Appendix A PDX collection 0250

CC **B97.34** **Human T-cell lymphotrophic virus, type II [HTLV-II] as the cause of diseases classified elsewhere**
CC Exclusion see Appendix A PDX collection 0251

CC **B97.35** **Human immunodeficiency virus, type 2 [HIV 2] as the cause of diseases classified elsewhere**
CC Exclusion see Appendix A PDX collection 0252

B97.39 **Other retrovirus as the cause of diseases classified elsewhere**

B97.4 **Respiratory syncytial virus as the cause of diseases classified elsewhere**

B97.5 **Reovirus as the cause of diseases classified elsewhere**

B97.6 **Parvovirus as the cause of diseases classified elsewhere**

B97.7 **Papillomavirus as the cause of diseases classified elsewhere**

+ **B97.8** **Other viral agents as the cause of diseases classified elsewhere**

B97.81 **Human metapneumovirus as the cause of diseases classified elsewhere**

B97.89 **Other viral agents as the cause of diseases classified elsewhere**
AHA CC: 3Q, 2016, 9-14

Other infectious diseases (B99)

B99 Other and unspecified infectious diseases

B99.8 **Other infectious disease**

B99.9 **Unspecified infectious disease**

'hapter 2: Neoplasms (C00-D49)

OTE **Functional activity**

All neoplasms are classified in this chapter, whether they are functionally active or not. An additional code from Chapter 4 may be used, to identify functional activity associated with any neoplasm.

Morphology [Histology]

Chapter 2 classifies neoplasms primarily by site (topography), with broad groupings for behavior, malignant, in situ, benign, etc. The Table of Neoplasms should be used to identify the correct topography code. In a few cases, such as for malignant melanoma and certain neuroendocrine tumors, the morphology (histologic type) is included in the category and codes.

Primary malignant neoplasms overlapping site boundaries

A primary malignant neoplasm that overlaps two or more contiguous (next to each other) sites should be classified to the subcategory/ code .8 ('overlapping lesion'), unless the combination is specifically indexed elsewhere. For multiple neoplasms of the same site that are not contiguous, such as tumors in different quadrants of the same breast, codes for each site should be assigned.

Malignant neoplasm of ectopic tissue

Malignant neoplasms of ectopic tissue are to be coded to the site mentioned, e.g., ectopic pancreatic malignant neoplasms are coded to pancreas, unspecified (C25.9).

nis chapter contains the following category blocks:

C00-C14	Malignant neoplasms of lip, oral cavity and pharynx
C15-C26	Malignant neoplasms of digestive organs
C30-C39	Malignant neoplasms of respiratory and intrathoracic organs
C40-C41	Malignant neoplasms of bone and articular cartilage
C43-C44	Melanoma and other malignant neoplasms of skin
C45-C49	Malignant neoplasms of mesothelial and soft tissue
C50	Malignant neoplasms of breast
C51-C58	Malignant neoplasms of female genital organs
C60-C63	Malignant neoplasms of male genital organs
C64-C68	Malignant neoplasms of urinary tract
C69-C72	Malignant neoplasms of eye, brain and other parts of central nervous system
C73-C75	Malignant neoplasms of thyroid and other endocrine glands
C7A	Malignant neuroendocrine tumors
C7B	Secondary neuroendocrine tumors
C76-C80	Malignant neoplasms of ill-defined, other secondary and unspecified sites
C81-C96	Malignant neoplasms of lymphoid, hematopoietic and related tissue
D00-D09	In situ neoplasms
D10-D36	Benign neoplasms, except benign neuroendocrine tumors
D3A	Benign neuroendocrine tumors
D37-D48	Neoplasms of uncertain behavior, polycythemia vera and myelodysplastic syndromes
D49	Neoplasms of unspecified behavior

'. Chapter-Specific Coding Guidelines

ı addition to general coding guidelines, there are guidelines for specific diagnoses nd/or conditions in the classification. Unless otherwise indicated, these guidelines pply to all health care settings. Please refer to Section II for guidelines on the election of principal diagnosis.

. Chapter 2: Neoplasms (C00-D49)

General guidelines

Chapter 2 of the ICD-10-CM contains the codes for most benign and all malignant neoplasms. Certain benign neoplasms, such as prostatic adenomas, may be found in the specific body system chapters. To properly code a neoplasm it is necessary to determine from the record if the neoplasm is benign, in-situ, malignant, or of uncertain histologic behavior. If malignant, any secondary (metastatic) sites should also be determined.

Primary malignant neoplasms overlapping site boundaries

A primary malignant neoplasm that overlaps two or more contiguous (next to each other) sites should be classified to the subcategory/code .8 ('overlapping lesion'), unless the combination is specifically indexed elsewhere. For multiple neoplasms of the same site that are not contiguous such as tumors in different quadrants of the same breast, codes for each site should be assigned.

Malignant neoplasm of ectopic tissue

Malignant neoplasms of ectopic tissue are to be coded to the site of origin mentioned, e.g., ectopic pancreatic malignant neoplasms involving the stomach are coded to **malignant neoplasm of** pancreas, unspecified (C25.9).

The neoplasm table in the Alphabetic Index should be referenced first. However, if the histological term is documented, that term should be referenced first, rather than going immediately to the Neoplasm Table, in order to determine which column in the Neoplasm Table is appropriate. For example, if the documentation indicates "adenoma," refer to the term in the Alphabetic Index to review the entries under this term and the instructional note to "see also neoplasm, by site, benign." The table provides the proper code based on the type of neoplasm and the site. It is important to select the proper column in the table that corresponds to the type of neoplasm. The Tabular List should then be referenced to verify that the correct code has been selected from the table and that a more specific site code does not exist.

See Section I.C.21. Factors influencing health status and contact with health services, Status, for information regarding Z15.0, codes for genetic susceptibility to cancer.

a. Treatment directed at the malignancy

If the treatment is directed at the malignancy, designate the malignancy as the principal diagnosis.

The only exception to this guideline is if a patient admission/encounter is solely for the administration of chemotherapy, immunotherapy or **external beam** radiation therapy, assign the appropriate Z51.-- code as the first-listed or principal diagnosis, and the diagnosis or problem for which the service is being performed as a secondary diagnosis.

b. Treatment of secondary site

When a patient is admitted because of a primary neoplasm with metastasis and treatment is directed toward the secondary site only, the secondary neoplasm is designated as the principal diagnosis even though the primary malignancy is still present.

c. Coding and sequencing of complications

Coding and sequencing of complications associated with the malignancies or with the therapy thereof are subject to the following guidelines:

1) Anemia associated with malignancy

When admission/encounter is for management of an anemia associated with the malignancy, and the treatment is only for anemia, the appropriate code for the malignancy is sequenced as the principal or first-listed diagnosis followed by the appropriate code for the anemia (such as code D63.0, Anemia in neoplastic disease).

2) Anemia associated with chemotherapy, immunotherapy and radiation therapy

When the admission/encounter is for management of an anemia associated with an adverse effect of the administration of chemotherapy or immunotherapy and the only treatment is for the anemia, the anemia code is sequenced first followed by the appropriate codes for the neoplasm and the adverse effect (T45.1X5-, Adverse effect of antineoplastic and immunosuppressive drugs).

When the admission/encounter is for management of an anemia associated with an adverse effect of radiotherapy, the anemia code should be sequenced first, followed by the appropriate neoplasm code and code Y84.2, Radiological procedure and radiotherapy as the cause of abnormal reaction of the patient, or of later complication, without mention of misadventure at the time of the procedure.

3) Management of dehydration due to the malignancy

When the admission/encounter is for management of dehydration due to the malignancy and only the dehydration is being treated (intravenous rehydration), the dehydration is sequenced first, followed by the code(s) for the malignancy.

4) Treatment of a complication resulting from a surgical procedure

When the admission/encounter is for treatment of a complication resulting from a surgical procedure, designate the complication as the principal or first-listed diagnosis if treatment is directed at resolving the complication.

d. Primary malignancy previously excised

When a primary malignancy has been previously excised or eradicated from its site and there is no further treatment directed to that site and there is no evidence of any existing primary malignancy, a code from category Z85, Personal history of malignant neoplasm, should be used to indicate the former site of the malignancy. Any mention of extension, invasion, or metastasis to another site is coded as a secondary malignant neoplasm to that site. The secondary site may be the principal or first-listed with the Z85 code used as a secondary code.

e. Admissions/Encounters involving chemotherapy, immunotherapy and radiation therapy

1) Episode of care involves surgical removal of neoplasm

When an episode of care involves the surgical removal of a neoplasm, primary or secondary site, followed by adjunct chemotherapy or radiation treatment during the same episode of care, the code for the neoplasm should be assigned as principal or first-listed diagnosis.

2) **Patient admission/encounter solely for administration of chemotherapy, immunotherapy and radiation therapy**

If a patient admission/encounter is solely for the administration of chemotherapy, immunotherapy or **external beam** radiation therapy assign code Z51.0, Encounter for antineoplastic radiation therapy, or Z51.11, Encounter for antineoplastic chemotherapy, or Z51.12, Encounter for antineoplastic immunotherapy as the first-listed or principal diagnosis. If a patient receives more than one of these therapies during the same admission more than one of these codes may be assigned, in any sequence.

The malignancy for which the therapy is being administered should be assigned as a secondary diagnosis.

If a patient admission/encounter is for the insertion or implantation of radioactive elements (e.g., brachytherapy) the appropriate code for the malignancy is sequenced as the principal or first-listed diagnosis. Code Z51.0 should not be assigned.

3) **Patient admitted for radiation therapy, chemotherapy or immunotherapy and develops complications**

When a patient is admitted for the purpose of **external beam** radiotherapy, immunotherapy or chemotherapy and develops complications such as uncontrolled nausea and vomiting or dehydration, the principal or first-listed diagnosis is Z51.0, Encounter for antineoplastic radiation therapy, or Z51.11, Encounter for antineoplastic chemotherapy, or Z51.12, Encounter for antineoplastic immunotherapy followed by any codes for the complications.

When a patient is admitted for the purpose of insertion or implantation of radioactive elements (e.g., brachytherapy) and develops complications such as uncontrolled nausea and vomiting or dehydration, the principal or first-listed diagnosis is the appropriate code for the malignancy followed by any codes for the complications.

f. Admission/encounter to determine extent of malignancy

When the reason for admission/encounter is to determine the extent of the malignancy, or for a procedure such as paracentesis or thoracentesis, the primary malignancy or appropriate metastatic site is designated as the principal or first-listed diagnosis, even though chemotherapy or radiotherapy is administered.

g. Symptoms, signs, and abnormal findings listed in Chapter 18 associated with neoplasms

Symptoms, signs, and ill-defined conditions listed in Chapter 18 characteristic of, or associated with, an existing primary or secondary site malignancy cannot be used to replace the malignancy as principal or first-listed diagnosis, regardless of the number of admissions or encounters for treatment and care of the neoplasm.

See section I.C.21. Factors influencing health status and contact with health services, Encounter for prophylactic organ removal.

h. Admission/encounter for pain control/management

See Section I.C.6. for information on coding admission/encounter for pain control/management.

i. Malignancy in two or more noncontiguous sites

A patient may have more than one malignant tumor in the same organ. These tumors may represent different primaries or metastatic disease, depending on the site. Should the documentation be unclear, the provider should be queried as to the status of each tumor so that the correct codes can be assigned.

j. Disseminated malignant neoplasm, unspecified

Code C80.0, Disseminated malignant neoplasm, unspecified, is for use only in those cases where the patient has advanced metastatic disease and no known primary or secondary sites are specified. It should not be used in place of assigning codes for the primary site and all known secondary sites.

k. Malignant neoplasm without specification of site

Code C80.1, Malignant (primary) neoplasm, unspecified, equates to Cancer, unspecified. This code should only be used when no determination can be made as to the primary site of a malignancy. This code should rarely be used in the inpatient setting.

l. Sequencing of neoplasm codes

1) **Encounter for treatment of primary malignancy**

If the reason for the encounter is for treatment of a primary malignancy, assign the malignancy as the principal/first-listed diagnosis. The primary site is to be sequenced first, followed by any metastatic sites.

2) **Encounter for treatment of secondary malignancy**

When an encounter is for a primary malignancy with metastasis and treatment is directed toward the metastatic (secondary) site(s) only, the metastatic site(s) is designated as the principal/first-listed diagnosis. The primary malignancy is coded as an additional code.

3) **Malignant neoplasm in a pregnant patient**

When a pregnant woman has a malignant neoplasm, a code fro subcategory O9A.1-, Malignant neoplasm complicating pregnanc childbirth, and the puerperium, should be sequenced first, followed by th appropriate code from Chapter 2 to indicate the type of neoplasm.

4) **Encounter for complication associated with a neoplasm**

When an encounter is for management of a complication associate with a neoplasm, such as dehydration, and the treatment is only for th complication, the complication is coded first, followed by the appropria code(s) for the neoplasm.

The exception to this guideline is anemia. When the admission/encount is for management of an anemia associated with the malignancy, and th treatment is only for anemia, the appropriate code for the malignanc is sequenced as the principal or first-listed diagnosis followed by co D63.0, Anemia in neoplastic disease.

5) **Complication from surgical procedure for treatment of a neoplasm**

When an encounter is for treatment of a complication resulting from surgical procedure performed for the treatment of the neoplasm, designa the complication as the principal/first- listed diagnosis. See guidelir regarding the coding of a current malignancy versus personal history determine if the code for the neoplasm should also be assigned.

6) **Pathologic fracture due to a neoplasm**

When an encounter is for a pathological fracture due to a neoplasm, an the focus of treatment is the fracture, a code from subcategory M84.5 Pathological fracture in neoplastic disease, should be sequenced firs followed by the code for the neoplasm.

If the focus of treatment is the neoplasm with an associated pathologic fracture, the neoplasm code should be sequenced first, followed by a cod from M84.5 for the pathological fracture.

m. Current malignancy versus personal history of malignancy

When a primary malignancy has been excised but further treatment, such a an additional surgery for the malignancy, radiation therapy or chemotherap is directed to that site, the primary malignancy code should be used unt treatment is completed.

When a primary malignancy has been previously excised or eradicated fror its site, there is no further treatment (of the malignancy) directed to that site and there is no evidence of any existing primary malignancy, a code fror category Z85, Personal history of malignant neoplasm, should be used t indicate the former site of the malignancy.

See Section I.C.21. Factors influencing health status and contact with healt services, History (of)

n. Leukemia, Multiple Myeloma, and Malignant Plasma Cell Neoplasm in remission versus personal history

The categories for leukemia, and category C90, Multiple myeloma an malignant plasma cell neoplasms, have codes indicating whether or not th leukemia has achieved remission. There are also codes Z85.6, Personal histor of leukemia, and Z85.79, Personal history of other malignant neoplasms o lymphoid, hematopoietic and related tissues. If the documentation is unclea as to whether the leukemia has achieved remission, the provider should b queried.

See Section I.C.21. Factors influencing health status and contact with healt services, History (of)

o. Aftercare following surgery for neoplasm

See Section I.C.21. Factors influencing health status and contact with healt services, Aftercare

p. Follow-up care for completed treatment of a malignancy

See Section I.C.21. Factors influencing health status and contact with healt services, Follow-up

q. Prophylactic organ removal for prevention of malignancy

See Section I.C. 21, Factors influencing health status and contact with healt services, Prophylactic organ removal

r. Malignant neoplasm associated with transplanted organ

A malignant neoplasm of a transplanted organ should be coded as a transplant complication. Assign first the appropriate code from category T86.-, Complications of transplanted organs and tissue, followed by code C80.2, Malignant neoplasm associated with transplanted organ. Use ar additional code for the specific malignancy.

Malignant neoplasms (C00-C96)

Malignant neoplasms, stated or presumed to be primary (of specified sites), and certain specified histologies, except neuroendocrine, and of lymphoid, hematopoietic and related tissue (C00-C75)

Malignant neoplasms of lip, oral cavity and pharynx (C00-C14)

C00 Malignant neoplasm of lip

Use additional code to identify:
alcohol abuse and dependence (F10.-)
history of tobacco dependence (Z87.891)
tobacco dependence (F17.-)
tobacco use (Z72.0)

Excludes1: *malignant melanoma of lip (C43.0)*
Merkel cell carcinoma of lip (C4A.0)
other and unspecified malignant neoplasm of skin of lip (C44.0-)

C00.0 Malignant neoplasm of external upper lip
Malignant neoplasm of lipstick area of upper lip
Malignant neoplasm of upper lip NOS
Malignant neoplasm of vermilion border of upper lip

C00.1 Malignant neoplasm of external lower lip
Malignant neoplasm of lower lip NOS
Malignant neoplasm of lipstick area of lower lip
Malignant neoplasm of vermilion border of lower lip

C00.2 Malignant neoplasm of external lip, unspecified
Malignant neoplasm of vermilion border of lip NOS

C00.3 Malignant neoplasm of upper lip, inner aspect
Malignant neoplasm of buccal aspect of upper lip
Malignant neoplasm of frenulum of upper lip
Malignant neoplasm of mucosa of upper lip
Malignant neoplasm of oral aspect of upper lip

C00.4 Malignant neoplasm of lower lip, inner aspect
Malignant neoplasm of buccal aspect of lower lip
Malignant neoplasm of frenulum of lower lip
Malignant neoplasm of mucosa of lower lip
Malignant neoplasm of oral aspect of lower lip

C00.5 Malignant neoplasm of lip, unspecified, inner aspect
Malignant neoplasm of buccal aspect of lip, unspecified
Malignant neoplasm of frenulum of lip, unspecified
Malignant neoplasm of mucosa of lip, unspecified
Malignant neoplasm of oral aspect of lip, unspecified

C00.6 Malignant neoplasm of commissure of lip, unspecified

C00.8 Malignant neoplasm of overlapping sites of lip

C00.9 Malignant neoplasm of lip, unspecified

C01 Malignant neoplasm of base of tongue

Malignant neoplasm of dorsal surface of base of tongue
Malignant neoplasm of fixed part of tongue NOS
Malignant neoplasm of posterior third of tongue

Use additional code to identify:
alcohol abuse and dependence (F10.-)
history of tobacco dependence (Z87.891)
tobacco dependence (F17.-)
tobacco use (Z72.0)

Valid 3-character code, no further characters required

C02 Malignant neoplasm of other and unspecified parts of tongue

Use additional code to identify:
alcohol abuse and dependence (F10.-)
history of tobacco dependence (Z87.891)
tobacco dependence (F17.-)
tobacco use (Z72.0)

C02.0 Malignant neoplasm of dorsal surface of tongue
Malignant neoplasm of anterior two-thirds of tongue, dorsal surface
Excludes2: *malignant neoplasm of dorsal surface of base of tongue (C01)*

C02.1 Malignant neoplasm of border of tongue
Malignant neoplasm of tip of tongue

C02.2 Malignant neoplasm of ventral surface of tongue
Malignant neoplasm of anterior two-thirds of tongue, ventral surface
Malignant neoplasm of frenulum linguae

C02.3 Malignant neoplasm of anterior two-thirds of tongue, part unspecified
Malignant neoplasm of middle third of tongue NOS
Malignant neoplasm of mobile part of tongue NOS

C02.4 Malignant neoplasm of lingual tonsil
Excludes2: *malignant neoplasm of tonsil NOS (C09.9)*

C02.8 Malignant neoplasm of overlapping sites of tongue
Malignant neoplasm of two or more contiguous sites of tongue

C02.9 Malignant neoplasm of tongue, unspecified

C03 Malignant neoplasm of gum

Includes: malignant neoplasm of alveolar (ridge) mucosa
malignant neoplasm of gingiva

Use additional code to identify:
alcohol abuse and dependence (F10.-)
history of tobacco dependence (Z87.891)
tobacco dependence (F17.-)
tobacco use (Z72.0)

Excludes2: *malignant odontogenic neoplasms (C41.0-C41.1)*

C03.0 Malignant neoplasm of upper gum

C03.1 Malignant neoplasm of lower gum

C03.9 Malignant neoplasm of gum, unspecified

C04 Malignant neoplasm of floor of mouth

Use additional code to identify:
alcohol abuse and dependence (F10.-)
history of tobacco dependence (Z87.891)
tobacco dependence (F17.-)
tobacco use (Z72.0)

C04.0 Malignant neoplasm of anterior floor of mouth
Malignant neoplasm of anterior to the premolar-canine junction

C04.1 Malignant neoplasm of lateral floor of mouth

C04.8 Malignant neoplasm of overlapping sites of floor of mouth

C04.9 Malignant neoplasm of floor of mouth, unspecified

C05 Malignant neoplasm of palate

Use additional code to identify:
alcohol abuse and dependence (F10.-)
history of tobacco dependence (Z87.891)
tobacco dependence (F17.-)
tobacco use (Z72.0)

Excludes1: *Kaposi's sarcoma of palate (C46.2)*

C05.0 Malignant neoplasm of hard palate

C05.1 Malignant neoplasm of soft palate
Excludes2: *malignant neoplasm of nasopharyngeal surface of soft palate (C11.3)*

C05.2 Malignant neoplasm of uvula

C05.8 Malignant neoplasm of overlapping sites of palate

C05.9 Malignant neoplasm of palate, unspecified
Malignant neoplasm of roof of mouth

C06 Malignant neoplasm of other and unspecified parts of mouth

Use additional code to identify:
alcohol abuse and dependence (F10.-)
history of tobacco dependence (Z87.891)
tobacco dependence (F17.-)
tobacco use (Z72.0)

C06.0 Malignant neoplasm of cheek mucosa
Malignant neoplasm of buccal mucosa NOS
Malignant neoplasm of internal cheek

C06.1 Malignant neoplasm of vestibule of mouth
Malignant neoplasm of buccal sulcus (upper) (lower)
Malignant neoplasm of labial sulcus (upper) (lower)

C06.2 Malignant neoplasm of retromolar area

\+ **C06.8 Malignant neoplasm of overlapping sites of other and unspecified parts of mouth**

C06.80 Malignant neoplasm of overlapping sites of unspecified parts of mouth

C06.89 Malignant neoplasm of overlapping sites of other parts of mouth
'book leaf' neoplasm [ventral surface of tongue and floor of mouth]

C06.9 Malignant neoplasm of mouth, unspecified
Malignant neoplasm of minor salivary gland, unspecified site
Malignant neoplasm of oral cavity NOS

C07 Malignant neoplasm of parotid gland

Use additional code to identify:
alcohol abuse and dependence (F10.-)
exposure to environmental tobacco smoke (Z77.22)
exposure to tobacco smoke in the perinatal period (P96.81)
history of tobacco dependence (Z87.891)
occupational exposure to environmental tobacco smoke (Z57.31)
tobacco dependence (F17.-)
tobacco use (Z72.0)

Valid 3-character code, no further characters required

C08 Malignant neoplasm of other and unspecified major salivary glands

Includes: malignant neoplasm of salivary ducts
Use additional code to identify:
alcohol abuse and dependence (F10.-)
exposure to environmental tobacco smoke (Z77.22)
exposure to tobacco smoke in the perinatal period (P96.81)
history of tobacco dependence (Z87.891)
occupational exposure to environmental tobacco smoke (Z57.31)
tobacco dependence (F17.-)
tobacco use (Z72.0)

Excludes1: *malignant neoplasms of specified minor salivary glands which are classified according to their anatomical location*

Excludes2: *malignant neoplasms of minor salivary glands NOS (C06.9)*
malignant neoplasm of parotid gland (C07)

C08.0 Malignant neoplasm of submandibular gland
Malignant neoplasm of submaxillary gland

C08.1 Malignant neoplasm of sublingual gland

C08.9 Malignant neoplasm of major salivary gland, unspecified
Malignant neoplasm of salivary gland (major) NOS

C09 Malignant neoplasm of tonsil

Use additional code to identify:
alcohol abuse and dependence (F10.-)
exposure to environmental tobacco smoke (Z77.22)
exposure to tobacco smoke in the perinatal period (P96.81)
history of tobacco dependence (Z87.891)
occupational exposure to environmental tobacco smoke (Z57.31)
tobacco dependence (F17.-)
tobacco use (Z72.0)

Excludes2: *malignant neoplasm of lingual tonsil (C02.4)*
malignant neoplasm of pharyngeal tonsil (C11.1)

C09.0 Malignant neoplasm of tonsillar fossa

C09.1 Malignant neoplasm of tonsillar pillar (anterior) (posterior)

C09.8 Malignant neoplasm of overlapping sites of tonsil

C09.9 Malignant neoplasm of tonsil, unspecified
Malignant neoplasm of tonsil NOS
Malignant neoplasm of faucial tonsils
Malignant neoplasm of palatine tonsils

C10 Malignant neoplasm of oropharynx

Use additional code to identify:
alcohol abuse and dependence (F10.-)
exposure to environmental tobacco smoke (Z77.22)
exposure to tobacco smoke in the perinatal period (P96.81)
history of tobacco dependence (Z87.891)
occupational exposure to environmental tobacco smoke (Z57.31)
tobacco dependence (F17.-)
tobacco use (Z72.0)

Excludes2: *malignant neoplasm of tonsil (C09.-)*

C10.0 Malignant neoplasm of vallecula

C10.1 Malignant neoplasm of anterior surface of epiglottis
Malignant neoplasm of epiglottis, free border [margin]
Malignant neoplasm of glossoepiglottic fold(s)
Excludes2: *malignant neoplasm of epiglottis (suprahyoid portion) NOS (C32.1)*

C10.2 Malignant neoplasm of lateral wall of oropharynx

C10.3 Malignant neoplasm of posterior wall of oropharynx

C10.4 Malignant neoplasm of branchial cleft
Malignant neoplasm of branchial cyst [site of neoplasm]

C10.8 Malignant neoplasm of overlapping sites of oropharynx
Malignant neoplasm of junctional region of oropharynx

C10.9 Malignant neoplasm of oropharynx, unspecified

C11 Malignant neoplasm of nasopharynx

Use additional code to identify:
exposure to environmental tobacco smoke (Z77.22)
exposure to tobacco smoke in the perinatal period (P96.81)
history of tobacco dependence (Z87.891)
occupational exposure to environmental tobacco smoke (Z57.31)
tobacco dependence (F17.-)
tobacco use (Z72.0)

C11.0 Malignant neoplasm of superior wall of nasopharynx
Malignant neoplasm of roof of nasopharynx

C11.1 Malignant neoplasm of posterior wall of nasopharynx
Malignant neoplasm of adenoid
Malignant neoplasm of pharyngeal tonsil

C11.2 Malignant neoplasm of lateral wall of nasopharynx
Malignant neoplasm of fossa of Rosenmüller
Malignant neoplasm of opening of auditory tube
Malignant neoplasm of pharyngeal recess

C11.3 Malignant neoplasm of anterior wall of nasopharynx
Malignant neoplasm of floor of nasopharynx
Malignant neoplasm of nasopharyngeal (anterior) (posterior) surface of soft palate
Malignant neoplasm of posterior margin of nasal choana
Malignant neoplasm of posterior margin of nasal septum

C11.8 Malignant neoplasm of overlapping sites of nasopharynx

C11.9 Malignant neoplasm of nasopharynx, unspecified
Malignant neoplasm of nasopharyngeal wall NOS

C12 Malignant neoplasm of pyriform sinus

Malignant neoplasm of pyriform fossa
Use additional code to identify:
exposure to environmental tobacco smoke (Z77.22)
exposure to tobacco smoke in the perinatal period (P96.81)
history of tobacco dependence (Z87.891)
occupational exposure to environmental tobacco smoke (Z57.31)
tobacco dependence (F17.-)
tobacco use (Z72.0)
Valid 3-character code, no further characters required

C13 Malignant neoplasm of hypopharynx

Use additional code to identify:
exposure to environmental tobacco smoke (Z77.22)
exposure to tobacco smoke in the perinatal period (P96.81)
history of tobacco dependence (Z87.891)
occupational exposure to environmental tobacco smoke (Z57.31)
tobacco dependence (F17.-)
tobacco use (Z72.0)

Excludes2: *malignant neoplasm of pyriform sinus (C12)*

C13.0 Malignant neoplasm of postcricoid region

C13.1 Malignant neoplasm of aryepiglottic fold, hypopharyngeal aspect
Malignant neoplasm of aryepiglottic fold NOS
Malignant neoplasm of interarytenoid fold NOS
Malignant neoplasm of aryepiglottic fold, marginal zone
Malignant neoplasm of interarytenoid fold, marginal zone
Excludes2: *malignant neoplasm of aryepiglottic fold or interarytenoid fold, laryngeal aspect (C32.1)*

C13.2 Malignant neoplasm of posterior wall of hypopharynx

C13.8 Malignant neoplasm of overlapping sites of hypopharynx

C13.9 Malignant neoplasm of hypopharynx, unspecified
Malignant neoplasm of hypopharyngeal wall NOS

C14 Malignant neoplasm of other and ill-defined sites in the lip, oral cavity and pharynx

Use additional code to identify:
alcohol abuse and dependence (F10.-)
exposure to environmental tobacco smoke (Z77.22)
exposure to tobacco smoke in the perinatal period (P96.81)
history of tobacco dependence (Z87.891)
occupational exposure to environmental tobacco smoke (Z57.31)
tobacco dependence (F17.-)
tobacco use (Z72.0)

Excludes1: *malignant neoplasm of oral cavity NOS (C06.9)*

C14.0 Malignant neoplasm of pharynx, unspecified

C14.2 Malignant neoplasm of Waldeyer's ring

C14.8 Malignant neoplasm of overlapping sites of lip, oral cavity and pharynx
Primary malignant neoplasm of two or more contiguous sites of lip, oral cavity and pharynx
Excludes1: *'book leaf' neoplasm [ventral surface of tongue and floor of mouth] (C06.89)*

Malignant neoplasms of digestive organs (C15-C26)

Excludes1: *Kaposi's sarcoma of gastrointestinal sites (C46.4)*

Excludes2: *gastrointestinal stromal tumors (C49.A-)*

C15 Malignant neoplasm of esophagus

Use additional code to identify:
alcohol abuse and dependence (F10.-)

CC **C15.3 Malignant neoplasm of upper third of esophagus**
CC Exclusion see Appendix A PDX collection 0253

CC **C15.4 Malignant neoplasm of middle third of esophagus**
CC Exclusion see Appendix A PDX collection 0253

CC **C15.5 Malignant neoplasm of lower third of esophagus**
Excludes1: *malignant neoplasm of cardio-esophageal junction (C16.0)*
CC Exclusion see Appendix A PDX collection 0253

CC **C15.8 Malignant neoplasm of overlapping sites of esophagus**
CC Exclusion see Appendix A PDX collection 0253

CC **C15.9 Malignant neoplasm of esophagus, unspecified**
CC Exclusion see Appendix A PDX collection 0253

C16 Malignant neoplasm of stomach

Use additional code to identify:
alcohol abuse and dependence (F10.-)
Excludes2: *malignant carcinoid tumor of the stomach (C7A.092)*

CC **C16.0 Malignant neoplasm of cardia**
Malignant neoplasm of cardiac orifice
Malignant neoplasm of cardio-esophageal junction
Malignant neoplasm of esophagus and stomach
Malignant neoplasm of gastro-esophageal junction
CC Exclusion see Appendix A PDX collection 0254

CC **C16.1 Malignant neoplasm of fundus of stomach**
CC Exclusion see Appendix A PDX collection 0254

CC **C16.2 Malignant neoplasm of body of stomach**
CC Exclusion see Appendix A PDX collection 0254

CC **C16.3 Malignant neoplasm of pyloric antrum**
Malignant neoplasm of gastric antrum
CC Exclusion see Appendix A PDX collection 0254

CC **C16.4 Malignant neoplasm of pylorus**
Malignant neoplasm of prepylorus
Malignant neoplasm of pyloric canal
CC Exclusion see Appendix A PDX collection 0254

CC **C16.5 Malignant neoplasm of lesser curvature of stomach, unspecified**
Malignant neoplasm of lesser curvature of stomach, not classifiable to C16.1-C16.4
CC Exclusion see Appendix A PDX collection 0254

CC **C16.6 Malignant neoplasm of greater curvature of stomach, unspecified**
Malignant neoplasm of greater curvature of stomach, not classifiable to C16.0-C16.4
CC Exclusion see Appendix A PDX collection 0254

CC **C16.8 Malignant neoplasm of overlapping sites of stomach**
CC Exclusion see Appendix A PDX collection 0254

CC **C16.9 Malignant neoplasm of stomach, unspecified**
Gastric cancer NOS
CC Exclusion see Appendix A PDX collection 0254

C17 Malignant neoplasm of small intestine

Excludes1: *malignant carcinoid tumors of the small intestine (C7A.01)*

CC **C17.0 Malignant neoplasm of duodenum**
CC Exclusion see Appendix A PDX collection 0255

CC **C17.1 Malignant neoplasm of jejunum**
CC Exclusion see Appendix A PDX collection 0256

CC **C17.2 Malignant neoplasm of ileum**
Excludes1: *malignant neoplasm of ileocecal valve (C18.0)*
CC Exclusion see Appendix A PDX collection 0257

CC **C17.3 Meckel's diverticulum, malignant**
Excludes1: *Meckel's diverticulum, congenital (Q43.0)*
CC Exclusion see Appendix A PDX collection 0258

CC **C17.8 Malignant neoplasm of overlapping sites of small intestine**
CC Exclusion see Appendix A PDX collection 0259

CC **C17.9 Malignant neoplasm of small intestine, unspecified**
CC Exclusion see Appendix A PDX collection 0259

C18 Malignant neoplasm of colon

Excludes1: *malignant carcinoid tumors of the colon (C7A.02-)*

CC **C18.0 Malignant neoplasm of cecum**
Malignant neoplasm of ileocecal valve
CC Exclusion see Appendix A PDX collection 0260

CC **C18.1 Malignant neoplasm of appendix**
CC Exclusion see Appendix A PDX collection 0261

CC **C18.2 Malignant neoplasm of ascending colon**
CC Exclusion see Appendix A PDX collection 0262

CC **C18.3 Malignant neoplasm of hepatic flexure**
CC Exclusion see Appendix A PDX collection 0263

CC **C18.4 Malignant neoplasm of transverse colon**
CC Exclusion see Appendix A PDX collection 0264

CC **C18.5 Malignant neoplasm of splenic flexure**
CC Exclusion see Appendix A PDX collection 0265

CC **C18.6 Malignant neoplasm of descending colon**
CC Exclusion see Appendix A PDX collection 0266

CC **C18.7 Malignant neoplasm of sigmoid colon**
Malignant neoplasm of sigmoid (flexure)
Excludes1: *malignant neoplasm of rectosigmoid junction (C19)*
CC Exclusion see Appendix A PDX collection 0267

CC **C18.8 Malignant neoplasm of overlapping sites of colon**
CC Exclusion see Appendix A PDX collection 0268

CC **C18.9 Malignant neoplasm of colon, unspecified**
Malignant neoplasm of large intestine NOS
CC Exclusion see Appendix A PDX collection 0268

CC C19 Malignant neoplasm of rectosigmoid junction

Malignant neoplasm of colon with rectum
Malignant neoplasm of rectosigmoid (colon)
Excludes1: *malignant carcinoid tumors of the colon (C7A.02-)*
CC Exclusion see Appendix A PDX collection 0269
Valid 3-character code, no further characters required

CC C20 Malignant neoplasm of rectum

Malignant neoplasm of rectal ampulla
Excludes1: *malignant carcinoid tumor of the rectum (C7A.026)*
CC Exclusion see Appendix A PDX collection 0270
Valid 3-character code, no further characters required

C21 Malignant neoplasm of anus and anal canal

Excludes2: *malignant carcinoid tumors of the colon (C7A.02-)*
malignant melanoma of anal margin (C43.51)
malignant melanoma of anal skin (C43.51)
malignant melanoma of perianal skin (C43.51)
other and unspecified malignant neoplasm of anal margin (C44.500, C44.510, C44.520, C44.590)
other and unspecified malignant neoplasm of anal skin (C44.500, C44.510, C44.520, C44.590)
other and unspecified malignant neoplasm of perianal skin (C44.500, C44.510, C44.520, C44.590)

CC **C21.0 Malignant neoplasm of anus, unspecified**
CC Exclusion see Appendix A PDX collection 0271

CC **C21.1 Malignant neoplasm of anal canal**
Malignant neoplasm of anal sphincter
CC Exclusion see Appendix A PDX collection 0271

CC **C21.2 Malignant neoplasm of cloacogenic zone**
CC Exclusion see Appendix A PDX collection 0272

CC **C21.8 Malignant neoplasm of overlapping sites of rectum, anus and anal canal**
Malignant neoplasm of anorectal junction
Malignant neoplasm of anorectum
Primary malignant neoplasm of two or more contiguous sites of rectum, anus and anal canal
CC Exclusion see Appendix A PDX collection 0272

C22 Malignant neoplasm of liver and intrahepatic bile ducts

Excludes1: *malignant neoplasm of biliary tract NOS (C24.9)*
secondary malignant neoplasm of liver and intrahepatic bile duct (C78.7)
Use additional code to identify:
alcohol abuse and dependence (F10.-)
hepatitis B (B16.-, B18.0-B18.1)
hepatitis C (B17.1-, B18.2)

CC **C22.0 Liver cell carcinoma**
Hepatocellular carcinoma
Hepatoma
CC Exclusion see Appendix A PDX collection 0273
AHA CC: 1Q, 2016, 18-19

CC **C22.1 Intrahepatic bile duct carcinoma**
Cholangiocarcinoma
Excludes1: *malignant neoplasm of hepatic duct (C24.0)*
CC Exclusion see Appendix A PDX collection 0273

CC **C22.2 Hepatoblastoma**
CC Exclusion see Appendix A PDX collection 0273

CC **C22.3 Angiosarcoma of liver**
Kupffer cell sarcoma
CC Exclusion see Appendix A PDX collection 0273

CC **C22.4 Other sarcomas of liver**
CC Exclusion see Appendix A PDX collection 0273

CC **C22.7 Other specified carcinomas of liver**
CC Exclusion see Appendix A PDX collection 0273

CC **C22.8 Malignant neoplasm of liver, primary, unspecified as to type**
CC Exclusion see Appendix A PDX collection 0273

CC **C22.9 Malignant neoplasm of liver, not specified as primary or secondary**
CC Exclusion see Appendix A PDX collection 0273

CC C23 Malignant neoplasm of gallbladder

CC Exclusion see Appendix A PDX collection 0274
Valid 3-character code, no further characters required

C24 Malignant neoplasm of other and unspecified parts of biliary tract

Excludes1: *malignant neoplasm of intrahepatic bile duct (C22.1)*

CC **C24.0 Malignant neoplasm of extrahepatic bile duct**
Malignant neoplasm of biliary duct or passage NOS
Malignant neoplasm of common bile duct
Malignant neoplasm of cystic duct
Malignant neoplasm of hepatic duct
CC Exclusion see Appendix A PDX collection 0275

CC **C24.1 Malignant neoplasm of ampulla of Vater**
CC Exclusion see Appendix A PDX collection 0276

CC **C24.8 Malignant neoplasm of overlapping sites of biliary tract**
Malignant neoplasm involving both intrahepatic and extrahepatic bile ducts
Primary malignant neoplasm of two or more contiguous sites of biliary tract
CC Exclusion see Appendix A PDX collection 0277

CC **C24.9 Malignant neoplasm of biliary tract, unspecified**
CC Exclusion see Appendix A PDX collection 0277

C25 Malignant neoplasm of pancreas

Code also exocrine pancreatic insufficiency (K86.81)

Use additional code to identify:
alcohol abuse and dependence (F10.-)

CC **C25.0 Malignant neoplasm of head of pancreas**
CC Exclusion see Appendix A PDX collection 0278

CC **C25.1 Malignant neoplasm of body of pancreas**
CC Exclusion see Appendix A PDX collection 0278

CC **C25.2 Malignant neoplasm of tail of pancreas**
CC Exclusion see Appendix A PDX collection 0278

CC **C25.3 Malignant neoplasm of pancreatic duct**
CC Exclusion see Appendix A PDX collection 0278

CC **C25.4 Malignant neoplasm of endocrine pancreas**
Malignant neoplasm of islets of Langerhans
Use additional code to identify any functional activity.
CC Exclusion see Appendix A PDX collection 0278

CC **C25.7 Malignant neoplasm of other parts of pancreas**
Malignant neoplasm of neck of pancreas
CC Exclusion see Appendix A PDX collection 0278

CC **C25.8 Malignant neoplasm of overlapping sites of pancreas**
CC Exclusion see Appendix A PDX collection 0278

CC **C25.9 Malignant neoplasm of pancreas, unspecified**
CC Exclusion see Appendix A PDX collection 0278

C26 Malignant neoplasm of other and ill-defined digestive organs

Excludes1: *malignant neoplasm of peritoneum and retroperitoneum (C48.-)*

C26.0 Malignant neoplasm of intestinal tract, part unspecified
Malignant neoplasm of intestine NOS

C26.1 Malignant neoplasm of spleen
Excludes1: *Hodgkin lymphoma (C81.-)*
non-Hodgkin lymphoma (C82-C85)

C26.9 Malignant neoplasm of ill-defined sites within the digestive system
Malignant neoplasm of alimentary canal or tract NOS
Malignant neoplasm of gastrointestinal tract NOS
Excludes1: *malignant neoplasm of abdominal NOS (C76.2)*
malignant neoplasm of intra-abdominal NOS (C76.2)

Malignant neoplasms of respiratory and intrathoracic organs (C30-C39)

Includes: malignant neoplasm of middle ear

Excludes1: *mesothelioma (C45.-)*

C30 Malignant neoplasm of nasal cavity and middle ear

C30.0 Malignant neoplasm of nasal cavity
Malignant neoplasm of cartilage of nose
Malignant neoplasm of nasal concha
Malignant neoplasm of internal nose
Malignant neoplasm of septum of nose
Malignant neoplasm of vestibule of nose
Excludes1: *malignant neoplasm of nasal bone (C41.0)*
malignant neoplasm of nose NOS (C76.0)
malignant neoplasm of olfactory bulb (C72.2-)
malignant neoplasm of posterior margin of nasal septum and choana (C11.3)
malignant melanoma of skin of nose (C43.31)
malignant neoplasm of turbinates (C41.0)
other and unspecified malignant neoplasm of skin of nose C44.301, C44.311, C44.321, C44.391)

C30.1 Malignant neoplasm of middle ear
Malignant neoplasm of antrum tympanicum
Malignant neoplasm of auditory tube
Malignant neoplasm of eustachian tube
Malignant neoplasm of inner ear
Malignant neoplasm of mastoid air cells
Malignant neoplasm of tympanic cavity
Excludes1: *malignant neoplasm of auricular canal (external) (C43.2-,C44.2-)*
malignant neoplasm of bone of ear (meatus) (C41.0)
malignant neoplasm of cartilage of ear (C49.0)
malignant melanoma of skin of (external) ear (C43.2-)
other and unspecified malignant neoplasm of skin of (external) ear (C44.2-)

C31 Malignant neoplasm of accessory sinuses

C31.0 Malignant neoplasm of maxillary sinus
Malignant neoplasm of antrum (Highmore) (maxillary)

C31.1 Malignant neoplasm of ethmoidal sinus

C31.2 Malignant neoplasm of frontal sinus

C31.3 Malignant neoplasm of sphenoid sinus

C31.8 Malignant neoplasm of overlapping sites of accessory sinuses

C31.9 Malignant neoplasm of accessory sinus, unspecified

C32 Malignant neoplasm of larynx

Use additional code to identify:
alcohol abuse and dependence (F10.-)
exposure to environmental tobacco smoke (Z77.22)
exposure to tobacco smoke in the perinatal period (P96.81)
history of tobacco dependence (Z87.891)
occupational exposure to environmental tobacco smoke (Z57.31)
tobacco dependence (F17.-)
tobacco use (Z72.0)

C32.0 Malignant neoplasm of glottis
Malignant neoplasm of intrinsic larynx
Malignant neoplasm of laryngeal commissure (anterior) (posterior)
Malignant neoplasm of vocal cord (true) NOS

C32.1 Malignant neoplasm of supraglottis
Malignant neoplasm of aryepiglottic fold or interarytenoid fold laryngeal aspect
Malignant neoplasm of epiglottis (suprahyoid portion) NOS
Malignant neoplasm of extrinsic larynx
Malignant neoplasm of false vocal cord
Malignant neoplasm of posterior (laryngeal) surface of epiglottis
Malignant neoplasm of ventricular bands
Excludes2: *malignant neoplasm of anterior surface of epiglottis (C10.1)*
malignant neoplasm of aryepiglottic fold or interarytenoid fold, hypopharyngeal aspect (C13.1)
malignant neoplasm of aryepiglottic fold or interarytenoid fold, marginal zone (C13.1)
malignant neoplasm of aryepiglottic fold or interarytenoid fold NOS (C13.1)

C32.2 Malignant neoplasm of subglottis

C32.3 Malignant neoplasm of laryngeal cartilage

C32.8 Malignant neoplasm of overlapping sites of larynx

C32.9 Malignant neoplasm of larynx, unspecified

CC **C33 Malignant neoplasm of trachea**

Use additional code to identify:
exposure to environmental tobacco smoke (Z77.22)
exposure to tobacco smoke in the perinatal period (P96.81)
history of tobacco dependence (Z87.891)
occupational exposure to environmental tobacco smoke (Z57.31)
tobacco dependence (F17.-)
tobacco use (Z72.0)
CC Exclusion see Appendix A PDX collection 0279
Valid 3-character code, no further characters required

Lungs

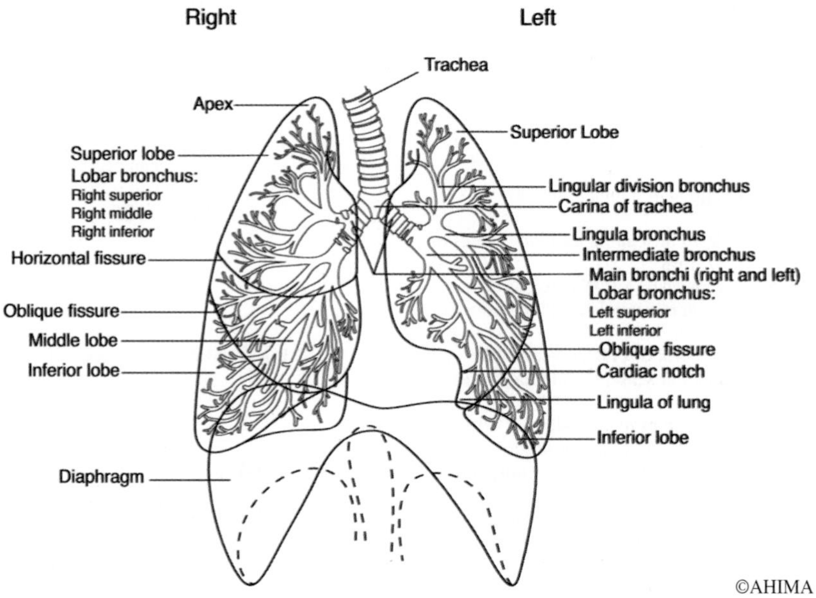

©AHIMA

C34 Malignant neoplasm of bronchus and lung

Use additional code to identify:
exposure to environmental tobacco smoke (Z77.22)
exposure to tobacco smoke in the perinatal period (P96.81)
history of tobacco dependence (Z87.891)
occupational exposure to environmental tobacco smoke (Z57.31)
tobacco dependence (F17.-)
tobacco use (Z72.0)

Excludes1: *Kaposi's sarcoma of lung (C46.5-)*
malignant carcinoid tumor of the bronchus and lung (C7A.090)

\+ **C34.0 Malignant neoplasm of main bronchus**
Malignant neoplasm of carina
Malignant neoplasm of hilus (of lung)

CC **C34.00 Malignant neoplasm of unspecified main bronchus**
CC Exclusion see Appendix A PDX collection 0280

CC **C34.01 Malignant neoplasm of right main bronchus**
CC Exclusion see Appendix A PDX collection 0280

CC **C34.02 Malignant neoplasm of left main bronchus**
CC Exclusion see Appendix A PDX collection 0280

\+ **C34.1 Malignant neoplasm of upper lobe, bronchus or lung**

CC **C34.10 Malignant neoplasm of upper lobe, unspecified bronchus or lung**
CC Exclusion see Appendix A PDX collection 0281

CC **C34.11 Malignant neoplasm of upper lobe, right bronchus or lung**
CC Exclusion see Appendix A PDX collection 0281

CC **C34.12 Malignant neoplasm of upper lobe, left bronchus or lung**
CC Exclusion see Appendix A PDX collection 0281

CC **C34.2 Malignant neoplasm of middle lobe, bronchus or lung**
CC Exclusion see Appendix A PDX collection 0282

\+ **C34.3 Malignant neoplasm of lower lobe, bronchus or lung**

CC **C34.30 Malignant neoplasm of lower lobe, unspecified bronchus or lung**
CC Exclusion see Appendix A PDX collection 0283

CC **C34.31 Malignant neoplasm of lower lobe, right bronchus or lung**
CC Exclusion see Appendix A PDX collection 0283

CC **C34.32 Malignant neoplasm of lower lobe, left bronchus or lung**
CC Exclusion see Appendix A PDX collection 0283

\+ **C34.8 Malignant neoplasm of overlapping sites of bronchus and lung**

CC **C34.80 Malignant neoplasm of overlapping sites of unspecified bronchus and lung**
CC Exclusion see Appendix A PDX collection 0284

CC **C34.81 Malignant neoplasm of overlapping sites of right bronchus and lung**
CC Exclusion see Appendix A PDX collection 0284

CC **C34.82 Malignant neoplasm of overlapping sites of left bronchus and lung**
CC Exclusion see Appendix A PDX collection 0284

\+ **C34.9 Malignant neoplasm of unspecified part of bronchus or lung**

CC **C34.90 Malignant neoplasm of unspecified part of unspecified bronchus or lung**
Lung cancer NOS
CC Exclusion see Appendix A PDX collection 0284
AHA CC: 2Q, 2014, 10

CC **C34.91 Malignant neoplasm of unspecified part of right bronchus or lung**
CC Exclusion see Appendix A PDX collection 0284

CC **C34.92 Malignant neoplasm of unspecified part of left bronchus or lung**
CC Exclusion see Appendix A PDX collection 0284

CC **C37 Malignant neoplasm of thymus**

Excludes1: *malignant carcinoid tumor of the thymus (C7A.091)*
CC Exclusion see Appendix A PDX collection 0285
Valid 3-character code, no further characters required

C38 Malignant neoplasm of heart, mediastinum and pleura

Excludes1: *mesothelioma (C45.-)*

CC **C38.0 Malignant neoplasm of heart**
Malignant neoplasm of pericardium
Excludes1: *malignant neoplasm of great vessels (C49.3)*
CC Exclusion see Appendix A PDX collection 0286

CC **C38.1 Malignant neoplasm of anterior mediastinum**
CC Exclusion see Appendix A PDX collection 0287

CC **C38.2 Malignant neoplasm of posterior mediastinum**
CC Exclusion see Appendix A PDX collection 0287

CC **C38.3 Malignant neoplasm of mediastinum, part unspecified**
CC Exclusion see Appendix A PDX collection 0287

CC **C38.4 Malignant neoplasm of pleura**
CC Exclusion see Appendix A PDX collection 0288

CC **C38.8 Malignant neoplasm of overlapping sites of heart, mediastinum and pleura**
CC Exclusion see Appendix A PDX collection 0287

C39 Malignant neoplasm of other and ill-defined sites in the respiratory system and intrathoracic organs

Use additional code to identify:
exposure to environmental tobacco smoke (Z77.22)
exposure to tobacco smoke in the perinatal period (P96.81)
history of tobacco dependence (Z87.891)
occupational exposure to environmental tobacco smoke (Z57.31)
tobacco dependence (F17.-)
tobacco use (Z72.0)

Excludes1: *intrathoracic malignant neoplasm NOS (C76.1)*
thoracic malignant neoplasm NOS (C76.1)

C39.0 Malignant neoplasm of upper respiratory tract, part unspecified

C39.9 Malignant neoplasm of lower respiratory tract, part unspecified
Malignant neoplasm of respiratory tract NOS

Malignant neoplasms of bone and articular cartilage (C40-C41)

Includes: malignant neoplasm of cartilage (articular) (joint)
malignant neoplasm of periosteum

Excludes1: *malignant neoplasm of bone marrow NOS (C96.9)*
malignant neoplasm of synovia (C49.-)

C40 Malignant neoplasm of bone and articular cartilage of limbs

Use additional code to identify major osseous defect, if applicable (M89.7-)

\+ **C40.0 Malignant neoplasm of scapula and long bones of upper limb**

CC **C40.00 Malignant neoplasm of scapula and long bones of unspecified upper limb**
CC Exclusion see Appendix A PDX collection 0289

CC **C40.01 Malignant neoplasm of scapula and long bones of right upper limb**
CC Exclusion see Appendix A PDX collection 0289

CC **C40.02 Malignant neoplasm of scapula and long bones of left upper limb**
CC Exclusion see Appendix A PDX collection 0289

\+ **C40.1 Malignant neoplasm of short bones of upper limb**

CC **C40.10 Malignant neoplasm of short bones of unspecified upper limb**
CC Exclusion see Appendix A PDX collection 0290

CC **C40.11 Malignant neoplasm of short bones of right upper limb**
CC Exclusion see Appendix A PDX collection 0290

CC **C40.12 Malignant neoplasm of short bones of left upper limb**
CC Exclusion see Appendix A PDX collection 0290

\+ **C40.2 Malignant neoplasm of long bones of lower limb**

CC **C40.20 Malignant neoplasm of long bones of unspecified lower limb**
CC Exclusion see Appendix A PDX collection 0291

CC **C40.21 Malignant neoplasm of long bones of right lower limb**
CC Exclusion see Appendix A PDX collection 0291

CC **C40.22 Malignant neoplasm of long bones of left lower limb**
CC Exclusion see Appendix A PDX collection 0291

\+ **C40.3 Malignant neoplasm of short bones of lower limb**

CC **C40.30 Malignant neoplasm of short bones of unspecified lower limb**
CC Exclusion see Appendix A PDX collection 0292

CC **C40.31 Malignant neoplasm of short bones of right lower limb**
CC Exclusion see Appendix A PDX collection 0292

CC **C40.32 Malignant neoplasm of short bones of left lower limb**
CC Exclusion see Appendix A PDX collection 0292

\+ **C40.8 Malignant neoplasm of overlapping sites of bone and articular cartilage of limb**

CC **C40.80 Malignant neoplasm of overlapping sites of bone and articular cartilage of unspecified limb**
CC Exclusion see Appendix A PDX collection 0293

CC **C40.81 Malignant neoplasm of overlapping sites of bone and articular cartilage of right limb**
CC Exclusion see Appendix A PDX collection 0293

CC **C40.82 Malignant neoplasm of overlapping sites of bone and articular cartilage of left limb**
CC Exclusion see Appendix A PDX collection 0293

\+ **C40.9 Malignant neoplasm of unspecified bones and articular cartilage of limb**

CC **C40.90 Malignant neoplasm of unspecified bones and articular cartilage of unspecified limb**
CC Exclusion see Appendix A PDX collection 0293

CC **C40.91 Malignant neoplasm of unspecified bones and articular cartilage of right limb**
CC Exclusion see Appendix A PDX collection 0293

CC **C40.92 Malignant neoplasm of unspecified bones and articular cartilage of left limb**
CC Exclusion see Appendix A PDX collection 0293

C41 Malignant neoplasm of bone and articular cartilage of other and unspecified sites

Excludes1: *malignant neoplasm of bones of limbs (C40.-)*
malignant neoplasm of cartilage of ear (C49.0)
malignant neoplasm of cartilage of eyelid (C49.0)
malignant neoplasm of cartilage of larynx (C32.3)
malignant neoplasm of cartilage of limbs (C40.-)
malignant neoplasm of cartilage of nose (C30.0)

CC **C41.0 Malignant neoplasm of bones of skull and face**
Malignant neoplasm of maxilla (superior)
Malignant neoplasm of orbital bone
Excludes2: *carcinoma, any type except intraosseous or odontogenic of:*
maxillary sinus (C31.0)
upper jaw (C03.0)
malignant neoplasm of jaw bone (lower) (C41.
CC Exclusion see Appendix A PDX collection 0294

CC **C41.1 Malignant neoplasm of mandible**
Malignant neoplasm of inferior maxilla
Malignant neoplasm of lower jaw bone
Excludes2: *carcinoma, any type except intraosseous or odontogenic of:*
jaw NOS (C03.9)
lower (C03.1)
malignant neoplasm of upper jaw bone (C41.0
CC Exclusion see Appendix A PDX collection 0295

CC **C41.2 Malignant neoplasm of vertebral column**
Excludes1: *malignant neoplasm of sacrum and coccyx (C41.*
CC Exclusion see Appendix A PDX collection 0296

CC **C41.3 Malignant neoplasm of ribs, sternum and clavicle**
CC Exclusion see Appendix A PDX collection 0297

CC **C41.4 Malignant neoplasm of pelvic bones, sacrum and coccyx**
CC Exclusion see Appendix A PDX collection 0298

CC **C41.9 Malignant neoplasm of bone and articular cartilage, unspecified**
CC Exclusion see Appendix A PDX collection 0293

Melanoma and other malignant neoplasms of skin (C43-C44)

C43 Malignant melanoma of skin

Excludes1: *melanoma in situ (D03.-)*
Excludes2: *malignant melanoma of skin of genital organs (C51-C52, C60.-, C63.-)*
Merkel cell carcinoma (C4A.-)
sites other than skin-code to malignant neoplasm of the si

C43.0 Malignant melanoma of lip
Excludes1: *malignant neoplasm of vermilion border of lip (C00.0-C00.2)*

\+ **C43.1 Malignant melanoma of eyelid, including canthus**
C43.10 Malignant melanoma of unspecified eyelid, includin canthus
C43.11 Malignant melanoma of right eyelid, including canthus
C43.12 Malignant melanoma of left eyelid, including canthus

\+ **C43.2 Malignant melanoma of ear and external auricular canal**
C43.20 Malignant melanoma of unspecified ear and externa auricular canal
C43.21 Malignant melanoma of right ear and external auricular canal
C43.22 Malignant melanoma of left ear and external auricular canal

\+ **C43.3 Malignant melanoma of other and unspecified parts of face**
C43.30 Malignant melanoma of unspecified part of face
C43.31 Malignant melanoma of nose
C43.39 Malignant melanoma of other parts of face

C43.4 Malignant melanoma of scalp and neck

\+ **C43.5 Malignant melanoma of trunk**
Excludes2: *malignant neoplasm of anus NOS (C21.0)*
malignant neoplasm of scrotum (C63.2)
C43.51 Malignant melanoma of anal skin
Malignant melanoma of anal margin
Malignant melanoma of perianal skin
C43.52 Malignant melanoma of skin of breast
C43.59 Malignant melanoma of other part of trunk

\+ **C43.6 Malignant melanoma of upper limb, including shoulder**
C43.60 Malignant melanoma of unspecified upper limb, including shoulder
C43.61 Malignant melanoma of right upper limb, including shoulder
C43.62 Malignant melanoma of left upper limb, including shoulder

\+ **C43.7 Malignant melanoma of lower limb, including hip**
C43.70 Malignant melanoma of unspecified lower limb, including hip
C43.71 Malignant melanoma of right lower limb, including hip
C43.72 Malignant melanoma of left lower limb, including hip

C43.8 Malignant melanoma of overlapping sites of skin
C43.9 Malignant melanoma of skin, unspecified
Malignant melanoma of unspecified site of skin
Melanoma (malignant) NOS

C4A Merkel cell carcinoma

C4A.0 Merkel cell carcinoma of lip
Excludes1: malignant neoplasm of vermilion border of lip (C00.0-C00.2)
+ **C4A.1** Merkel cell carcinoma of eyelid, including canthus
C4A.10 Merkel cell carcinoma of unspecified eyelid, including canthus
C4A.11 Merkel cell carcinoma of right eyelid, including canthus
C4A.12 Merkel cell carcinoma of left eyelid, including canthus
+ **C4A.2** Merkel cell carcinoma of ear and external auricular canal
C4A.20 Merkel cell carcinoma of unspecified ear and external auricular canal
C4A.21 Merkel cell carcinoma of right ear and external auricular canal
C4A.22 Merkel cell carcinoma of left ear and external auricular canal
+ **C4A.3** Merkel cell carcinoma of other and unspecified parts of face
C4A.30 Merkel cell carcinoma of unspecified part of face
C4A.31 Merkel cell carcinoma of nose
C4A.39 Merkel cell carcinoma of other parts of face
C4A.4 Merkel cell carcinoma of scalp and neck
+ **C4A.5** Merkel cell carcinoma of trunk
Excludes2: malignant neoplasm of anus NOS (C21.0)
malignant neoplasm of scrotum (C63.2)
C4A.51 Merkel cell carcinoma of anal skin
Merkel cell carcinoma of anal margin
Merkel cell carcinoma of perianal skin
C4A.52 Merkel cell carcinoma of skin of breast
C4A.59 Merkel cell carcinoma of other part of trunk
+ **C4A.6** Merkel cell carcinoma of upper limb, including shoulder
C4A.60 Merkel cell carcinoma of unspecified upper limb, including shoulder
C4A.61 Merkel cell carcinoma of right upper limb, including shoulder
C4A.62 Merkel cell carcinoma of left upper limb, including shoulder
+ **C4A.7** Merkel cell carcinoma of lower limb, including hip
C4A.70 Merkel cell carcinoma of unspecified lower limb, including hip
C4A.71 Merkel cell carcinoma of right lower limb, including hip
C4A.72 Merkel cell carcinoma of left lower limb, including hip
C4A.8 Merkel cell carcinoma of overlapping sites
C4A.9 Merkel cell carcinoma, unspecified
Merkel cell carcinoma of unspecified site
Merkel cell carcinoma NOS

C44 Other and unspecified malignant neoplasm of skin

Includes: malignant neoplasm of sebaceous glands
malignant neoplasm of sweat glands
Excludes1: Kaposi's sarcoma of skin (C46.0)
malignant melanoma of skin (C43.-)
malignant neoplasm of skin of genital organs (C51-C52, C60.-, C63.2)
Merkel cell carcinoma (C4A.-)
+ **C44.0** Other and unspecified malignant neoplasm of skin of lip
Excludes1: malignant neoplasm of lip (C00.-)
C44.00 Unspecified malignant neoplasm of skin of lip
C44.01 Basal cell carcinoma of skin of lip
C44.02 Squamous cell carcinoma of skin of lip
C44.09 Other specified malignant neoplasm of skin of lip
+ **C44.1** Other and unspecified malignant neoplasm of skin of eyelid, including canthus
Excludes1: connective tissue of eyelid (C49.0)
+ **C44.10** Unspecified malignant neoplasm of skin of eyelid, including canthus
C44.101 Unspecified malignant neoplasm of skin of unspecified eyelid, including canthus
C44.102 Unspecified malignant neoplasm of skin of right eyelid, including canthus
C44.109 Unspecified malignant neoplasm of skin of left eyelid, including canthus
+ **C44.11** Basal cell carcinoma of skin of eyelid, including canthus
C44.111 Basal cell carcinoma of skin of unspecified eyelid, including canthus
C44.112 Basal cell carcinoma of skin of right eyelid, including canthus
C44.119 Basal cell carcinoma of skin of left eyelid, including canthus
+ **C44.12** Squamous cell carcinoma of skin of eyelid, including canthus
C44.121 Squamous cell carcinoma of skin of unspecified eyelid, including canthus
C44.122 Squamous cell carcinoma of skin of right eyelid, including canthus
C44.129 Squamous cell carcinoma of skin of left eyelid, including canthus
+ **C44.19** Other specified malignant neoplasm of skin of eyelid, including canthus
C44.191 Other specified malignant neoplasm of skin of unspecified eyelid, including canthus
C44.192 Other specified malignant neoplasm of skin of right eyelid, including canthus
C44.199 Other specified malignant neoplasm of skin of left eyelid, including canthus
+ **C44.2** Other and unspecified malignant neoplasm of skin of ear and external auricular canal
Excludes1: connective tissue of ear (C49.0)
+ **C44.20** Unspecified malignant neoplasm of skin of ear and external auricular canal
C44.201 Unspecified malignant neoplasm of skin of unspecified ear and external auricular canal
C44.202 Unspecified malignant neoplasm of skin of right ear and external auricular canal
C44.209 Unspecified malignant neoplasm of skin of left ear and external auricular canal
+ **C44.21** Basal cell carcinoma of skin of ear and external auricular canal
C44.211 Basal cell carcinoma of skin of unspecified ear and external auricular canal
C44.212 Basal cell carcinoma of skin of right ear and external auricular canal
C44.219 Basal cell carcinoma of skin of left ear and external auricular canal
+ **C44.22** Squamous cell carcinoma of skin of ear and external auricular canal
C44.221 Squamous cell carcinoma of skin of unspecified ear and external auricular canal
C44.222 Squamous cell carcinoma of skin of right ear and external auricular canal
C44.229 Squamous cell carcinoma of skin of left ear and external auricular canal
+ **C44.29** Other specified malignant neoplasm of skin of ear and external auricular canal
C44.291 Other specified malignant neoplasm of skin of unspecified ear and external auricular canal
C44.292 Other specified malignant neoplasm of skin of right ear and external auricular canal
C44.299 Other specified malignant neoplasm of skin of left ear and external auricular canal
+ **C44.3** Other and unspecified malignant neoplasm of skin of other and unspecified parts of face
+ **C44.30** Unspecified malignant neoplasm of skin of other and unspecified parts of face
C44.300 Unspecified malignant neoplasm of skin of unspecified part of face
C44.301 Unspecified malignant neoplasm of skin of nose
C44.309 Unspecified malignant neoplasm of skin of other parts of face
+ **C44.31** Basal cell carcinoma of skin of other and unspecified parts of face
C44.310 Basal cell carcinoma of skin of unspecified parts of face
C44.311 Basal cell carcinoma of skin of nose
C44.319 Basal cell carcinoma of skin of other parts of face
AHA CC: 1Q, 2017, 4

+ **C44.32 Squamous cell carcinoma of skin of other and unspecified parts of face**
  - **C44.320 Squamous cell carcinoma of skin of unspecified parts of face**
  - **C44.321 Squamous cell carcinoma of skin of nose**
  - **C44.329 Squamous cell carcinoma of skin of other parts of face**
+ **C44.39 Other specified malignant neoplasm of skin of other and unspecified parts of face**
  - **C44.390 Other specified malignant neoplasm of skin of unspecified parts of face**
  - **C44.391 Other specified malignant neoplasm of skin of nose**
  - **C44.399 Other specified malignant neoplasm of skin of other parts of face**

+ **C44.4 Other and unspecified malignant neoplasm of skin of scalp and neck**
  - **C44.40 Unspecified malignant neoplasm of skin of scalp and neck**
  - **C44.41 Basal cell carcinoma of skin of scalp and neck**
  - **C44.42 Squamous cell carcinoma of skin of scalp and neck**
  - **C44.49 Other specified malignant neoplasm of skin of scalp and neck**

+ **C44.5 Other and unspecified malignant neoplasm of skin of trunk**
  Excludes1: *anus NOS (C21.0)*
  scrotum (C63.2)
+ **C44.50 Unspecified malignant neoplasm of skin of trunk**
  - **C44.500 Unspecified malignant neoplasm of anal skin**
    Unspecified malignant neoplasm of anal margin
    Unspecified malignant neoplasm of perianal skin
  - **C44.501 Unspecified malignant neoplasm of skin of breast**
  - **C44.509 Unspecified malignant neoplasm of skin of other part of trunk**
+ **C44.51 Basal cell carcinoma of skin of trunk**
  - **C44.510 Basal cell carcinoma of anal skin**
    Basal cell carcinoma of anal margin
    Basal cell carcinoma of perianal skin
  - **C44.511 Basal cell carcinoma of skin of breast**
  - **C44.519 Basal cell carcinoma of skin of other part of trunk**
+ **C44.52 Squamous cell carcinoma of skin of trunk**
  - **C44.520 Squamous cell carcinoma of anal skin**
    Squamous cell carcinoma of anal margin
    Squamous cell carcinoma of perianal skin
  - **C44.521 Squamous cell carcinoma of skin of breast**
  - **C44.529 Squamous cell carcinoma of skin of other part of trunk**
+ **C44.59 Other specified malignant neoplasm of skin of trunk**
  - **C44.590 Other specified malignant neoplasm of anal skin**
    Other specified malignant neoplasm of anal margin
    Other specified malignant neoplasm of perianal skin
  - **C44.591 Other specified malignant neoplasm of skin of breast**
  - **C44.599 Other specified malignant neoplasm of skin of other part of trunk**

+ **C44.6 Other and unspecified malignant neoplasm of skin of upper limb, including shoulder**
+ **C44.60 Unspecified malignant neoplasm of skin of upper limb, including shoulder**
  - **C44.601 Unspecified malignant neoplasm of skin of unspecified upper limb, including shoulder**
  - **C44.602 Unspecified malignant neoplasm of skin of right upper limb, including shoulder**
  - **C44.609 Unspecified malignant neoplasm of skin of left upper limb, including shoulder**
+ **C44.61 Basal cell carcinoma of skin of upper limb, including shoulder**
  - **C44.611 Basal cell carcinoma of skin of unspecified upper limb, including shoulder**
  - **C44.612 Basal cell carcinoma of skin of right upper limb, including shoulder**
  - **C44.619 Basal cell carcinoma of skin of left upper limb, including shoulder**
+ **C44.62 Squamous cell carcinoma of skin of upper limb, including shoulder**
  - **C44.621 Squamous cell carcinoma of skin of unspecified upper limb, including shoulde**
  - **C44.622 Squamous cell carcinoma of skin of right upper limb, including shoulder**
  - **C44.629 Squamous cell carcinoma of skin of left upper limb, including shoulder**
+ **C44.69 Other specified malignant neoplasm of skin of uppe limb, including shoulder**
  - **C44.691 Other specified malignant neoplasm of skin of unspecified upper limb, including shoulde**
  - **C44.692 Other specified malignant neoplasm of ski of right upper limb, including shoulder**
  - **C44.699 Other specified malignant neoplasm of ski of left upper limb, including shoulder**

+ **C44.7 Other and unspecified malignant neoplasm of skin of lower limb, including hip**
+ **C44.70 Unspecified malignant neoplasm of skin of lower limb, including hip**
  - **C44.701 Unspecified malignant neoplasm of skin of unspecified lower limb, including hip**
  - **C44.702 Unspecified malignant neoplasm of skin of right lower limb, including hip**
  - **C44.709 Unspecified malignant neoplasm of skin of left lower limb, including hip**
+ **C44.71 Basal cell carcinoma of skin of lower limb, including hip**
  - **C44.711 Basal cell carcinoma of skin of unspecified lower limb, including hip**
  - **C44.712 Basal cell carcinoma of skin of right lower limb, including hip**
  - **C44.719 Basal cell carcinoma of skin of left lower limb, including hip**
+ **C44.72 Squamous cell carcinoma of skin of lower limb, including hip**
  - **C44.721 Squamous cell carcinoma of skin of unspecified lower limb, including hip**
  - **C44.722 Squamous cell carcinoma of skin of right lower limb, including hip**
  - **C44.729 Squamous cell carcinoma of skin of left lower limb, including hip**
+ **C44.79 Other specified malignant neoplasm of skin of lower limb, including hip**
  - **C44.791 Other specified malignant neoplasm of ski of unspecified lower limb, including hip**
  - **C44.792 Other specified malignant neoplasm of ski of right lower limb, including hip**
  - **C44.799 Other specified malignant neoplasm of ski of left lower limb, including hip**

+ **C44.8 Other and unspecified malignant neoplasm of overlapping site of skin**
  - **C44.80 Unspecified malignant neoplasm of overlapping sites of skin**
  - **C44.81 Basal cell carcinoma of overlapping sites of skin**
  - **C44.82 Squamous cell carcinoma of overlapping sites of skin**
  - **C44.89 Other specified malignant neoplasm of overlapping sites of skin**

+ **C44.9 Other and unspecified malignant neoplasm of skin, unspecified**
  - **C44.90 Unspecified malignant neoplasm of skin, unspecified**
    Malignant neoplasm of unspecified site of skin
  - **C44.91 Basal cell carcinoma of skin, unspecified**
  - **C44.92 Squamous cell carcinoma of skin, unspecified**
  - **C44.99 Other specified malignant neoplasm of skin, unspecified**

Malignant neoplasms of mesothelial and soft tissue (C45-C49)

C45 Mesothelioma

CC **C45.0 Mesothelioma of pleura**
Excludes1: *other malignant neoplasm of pleura (C38.4)*
CC Exclusion see Appendix A PDX collection 0288
AHA CC: 2Q, 2017, 11

CC **C45.1 Mesothelioma of peritoneum**
Mesothelioma of cul-de-sac
Mesothelioma of mesentery
Mesothelioma of mesocolon
Mesothelioma of omentum
Mesothelioma of peritoneum (parietal) (pelvic)
Excludes1: *other malignant neoplasm of soft tissue of peritoneum (C48.-)*
CC Exclusion see Appendix A PDX collection 0299

CC **C45.2** **Mesothelioma of pericardium**
Excludes1: *other malignant neoplasm of pericardium (C38.0)*
CC Exclusion see Appendix A PDX collection 0286
C45.7 **Mesothelioma of other sites**
C45.9 **Mesothelioma, unspecified**

C46 Kaposi's sarcoma

Code first any human immunodeficiency virus [HIV] disease (B20)

CC **C46.0** **Kaposi's sarcoma of skin**
CC Exclusion see Appendix A PDX collection 0300

CC **C46.1** **Kaposi's sarcoma of soft tissue**
Kaposi's sarcoma of blood vessel
Kaposi's sarcoma of connective tissue
Kaposi's sarcoma of fascia
Kaposi's sarcoma of ligament
Kaposi's sarcoma of lymphatic(s) NEC
Kaposi's sarcoma of muscle
Excludes2: *Kaposi's sarcoma of lymph glands and nodes (C46.3)*
CC Exclusion see Appendix A PDX collection 0301

CC **C46.2** **Kaposi's sarcoma of palate**
CC Exclusion see Appendix A PDX collection 0302

CC **C46.3** **Kaposi's sarcoma of lymph nodes**
CC Exclusion see Appendix A PDX collection 0303

CC **C46.4** **Kaposi's sarcoma of gastrointestinal sites**
CC Exclusion see Appendix A PDX collection 0304

\+ **C46.5** **Kaposi's sarcoma of lung**

CC **C46.50** **Kaposi's sarcoma of unspecified lung**
CC Exclusion see Appendix A PDX collection 0284

CC **C46.51** **Kaposi's sarcoma of right lung**
CC Exclusion see Appendix A PDX collection 0284

CC **C46.52** **Kaposi's sarcoma of left lung**
CC Exclusion see Appendix A PDX collection 0284

CC **C46.7** **Kaposi's sarcoma of other sites**
CC Exclusion see Appendix A PDX collection 0305

CC **C46.9** **Kaposi's sarcoma, unspecified**
Kaposi's sarcoma of unspecified site
CC Exclusion see Appendix A PDX collection 0306

C47 Malignant neoplasm of peripheral nerves and autonomic nervous system

Includes: malignant neoplasm of sympathetic and parasympathetic nerves and ganglia
Excludes1: *Kaposi's sarcoma of soft tissue (C46.1)*

CC **C47.0** **Malignant neoplasm of peripheral nerves of head, face and neck**
Excludes1: *malignant neoplasm of peripheral nerves of orbit (C69.6-)*
CC Exclusion see Appendix A PDX collection 0307

\+ **C47.1** **Malignant neoplasm of peripheral nerves of upper limb, including shoulder**

CC **C47.10** **Malignant neoplasm of peripheral nerves of unspecified upper limb, including shoulder**
CC Exclusion see Appendix A PDX collection 0307

CC **C47.11** **Malignant neoplasm of peripheral nerves of right upper limb, including shoulder**
CC Exclusion see Appendix A PDX collection 0307

CC **C47.12** **Malignant neoplasm of peripheral nerves of left upper limb, including shoulder**
CC Exclusion see Appendix A PDX collection 0307

\+ **C47.2** **Malignant neoplasm of peripheral nerves of lower limb, including hip**

CC **C47.20** **Malignant neoplasm of peripheral nerves of unspecified lower limb, including hip**
CC Exclusion see Appendix A PDX collection 0307

CC **C47.21** **Malignant neoplasm of peripheral nerves of right lower limb, including hip**
CC Exclusion see Appendix A PDX collection 0307

CC **C47.22** **Malignant neoplasm of peripheral nerves of left lower limb, including hip**
CC Exclusion see Appendix A PDX collection 0307

CC **C47.3** **Malignant neoplasm of peripheral nerves of thorax**
CC Exclusion see Appendix A PDX collection 0307

CC **C47.4** **Malignant neoplasm of peripheral nerves of abdomen**
CC Exclusion see Appendix A PDX collection 0307

CC **C47.5** **Malignant neoplasm of peripheral nerves of pelvis**
CC Exclusion see Appendix A PDX collection 0307

CC **C47.6** **Malignant neoplasm of peripheral nerves of trunk, unspecified**
Malignant neoplasm of peripheral nerves of unspecified part of trunk
CC Exclusion see Appendix A PDX collection 0307

CC **C47.8** **Malignant neoplasm of overlapping sites of peripheral nerves and autonomic nervous system**
CC Exclusion see Appendix A PDX collection 0307

CC **C47.9** **Malignant neoplasm of peripheral nerves and autonomic nervous system, unspecified**
Malignant neoplasm of unspecified site of peripheral nerves and autonomic nervous system
CC Exclusion see Appendix A PDX collection 0307

C48 Malignant neoplasm of retroperitoneum and peritoneum

Excludes1: *Kaposi's sarcoma of connective tissue (C46.1)*
mesothelioma (C45.-)

CC **C48.0** **Malignant neoplasm of retroperitoneum**
CC Exclusion see Appendix A PDX collection 0308

CC **C48.1** **Malignant neoplasm of specified parts of peritoneum**
Malignant neoplasm of cul-de-sac
Malignant neoplasm of mesentery
Malignant neoplasm of mesocolon
Malignant neoplasm of omentum
Malignant neoplasm of parietal peritoneum
Malignant neoplasm of pelvic peritoneum
CC Exclusion see Appendix A PDX collection 0299

CC **C48.2** **Malignant neoplasm of peritoneum, unspecified**
CC Exclusion see Appendix A PDX collection 0299

CC **C48.8** **Malignant neoplasm of overlapping sites of retroperitoneum and peritoneum**
CC Exclusion see Appendix A PDX collection 0299

C49 Malignant neoplasm of other connective and soft tissue

Includes: malignant neoplasm of blood vessel
malignant neoplasm of bursa
malignant neoplasm of cartilage
malignant neoplasm of fascia
malignant neoplasm of fat
malignant neoplasm of ligament, except uterine
malignant neoplasm of lymphatic vessel
malignant neoplasm of muscle
malignant neoplasm of synovia
malignant neoplasm of tendon (sheath)
Excludes1: *malignant neoplasm of cartilage (of):*
articular (C40-C41)
larynx (C32.3)
nose (C30.0)
malignant neoplasm of connective tissue of breast (C50.-)
Excludes2: *Kaposi's sarcoma of soft tissue (C46.1)*
malignant neoplasm of heart (C38.0)
malignant neoplasm of peripheral nerves and autonomic nervous system (C47.-)
malignant neoplasm of peritoneum (C48.2)
malignant neoplasm of retroperitoneum (C48.0)
malignant neoplasm of uterine ligament (C57.3)
mesothelioma (C45.-)

CC **C49.0** **Malignant neoplasm of connective and soft tissue of head, face and neck**
Malignant neoplasm of connective tissue of ear
Malignant neoplasm of connective tissue of eyelid
Excludes1: *connective tissue of orbit (C69.6-)*
CC Exclusion see Appendix A PDX collection 0307

\+ **C49.1** **Malignant neoplasm of connective and soft tissue of upper limb, including shoulder**

CC **C49.10** **Malignant neoplasm of connective and soft tissue of unspecified upper limb, including shoulder**
CC Exclusion see Appendix A PDX collection 0307

CC **C49.11** **Malignant neoplasm of connective and soft tissue of right upper limb, including shoulder**
CC Exclusion see Appendix A PDX collection 0307

CC **C49.12** **Malignant neoplasm of connective and soft tissue of left upper limb, including shoulder**
CC Exclusion see Appendix A PDX collection 0307

\+ **C49.2** **Malignant neoplasm of connective and soft tissue of lower limb, including hip**

CC **C49.20** **Malignant neoplasm of connective and soft tissue of unspecified lower limb, including hip**
CC Exclusion see Appendix A PDX collection 0307

CC **C49.21** **Malignant neoplasm of connective and soft tissue of right lower limb, including hip**
CC Exclusion see Appendix A PDX collection 0307

CC **C49.22** **Malignant neoplasm of connective and soft tissue of left lower limb, including hip**
CC Exclusion see Appendix A PDX collection 0307

CC **C49.3 Malignant neoplasm of connective and soft tissue of thorax**
Malignant neoplasm of axilla
Malignant neoplasm of diaphragm
Malignant neoplasm of great vessels
Excludes1: *malignant neoplasm of breast (C50.-)*
malignant neoplasm of heart (C38.0)
malignant neoplasm of mediastinum (C38.1-C38.3)
malignant neoplasm of thymus (C37)
CC Exclusion see Appendix A PDX collection 0307
AHA CC: 3Q, 2015, 19-20

CC **C49.4 Malignant neoplasm of connective and soft tissue of abdomen**
Malignant neoplasm of abdominal wall
Malignant neoplasm of hypochondrium
CC Exclusion see Appendix A PDX collection 0307

CC **C49.5 Malignant neoplasm of connective and soft tissue of pelvis**
Malignant neoplasm of buttock
Malignant neoplasm of groin
Malignant neoplasm of perineum
CC Exclusion see Appendix A PDX collection 0307

CC **C49.6 Malignant neoplasm of connective and soft tissue of trunk, unspecified**
Malignant neoplasm of back NOS
CC Exclusion see Appendix A PDX collection 0307

CC **C49.8 Malignant neoplasm of overlapping sites of connective and soft tissue**
Primary malignant neoplasm of two or more contiguous sites of connective and soft tissue
CC Exclusion see Appendix A PDX collection 0307

CC **C49.9 Malignant neoplasm of connective and soft tissue, unspecified**
CC Exclusion see Appendix A PDX collection 0307

+ **C49.A Gastrointestinal stromal tumor**
AHA CC: 4Q, 2016, 8

CC **C49.A0 Gastrointestinal stromal tumor, unspecified site**
CC Exclusion see Appendix A PDX collection 0307

CC **C49.A1 Gastrointestinal stromal tumor of esophagus**
CC Exclusion see Appendix A PDX collection 0307

CC **C49.A2 Gastrointestinal stromal tumor of stomach**
CC Exclusion see Appendix A PDX collection 0307

CC **C49.A3 Gastrointestinal stromal tumor of small intestine**
CC Exclusion see Appendix A PDX collection 0307

CC **C49.A4 Gastrointestinal stromal tumor of large intestine**
CC Exclusion see Appendix A PDX collection 0307

CC **C49.A5 Gastrointestinal stromal tumor of rectum**
CC Exclusion see Appendix A PDX collection 0307

CC **C49.A9 Gastrointestinal stromal tumor of other sites**
CC Exclusion see Appendix A PDX collection 0307

Malignant neoplasms of breast (C50)

C50 Malignant neoplasm of breast

Includes: connective tissue of breast
Paget's disease of breast
Paget's disease of nipple

Use additional code to identify estrogen receptor status (Z17.0, Z17.1)

Excludes1: *skin of breast (C44.501, C44.511, C44.521, C44.591)*

+ **C50.0 Malignant neoplasm of nipple and areola**
+ **C50.01 Malignant neoplasm of nipple and areola, female**
♀ **C50.011 Malignant neoplasm of nipple and areola, right female breast**
♀ **C50.012 Malignant neoplasm of nipple and areola, left female breast**
♀ **C50.019 Malignant neoplasm of nipple and areola, unspecified female breast**
+ **C50.02 Malignant neoplasm of nipple and areola, male**
♂ **C50.021 Malignant neoplasm of nipple and areola, right male breast**
♂ **C50.022 Malignant neoplasm of nipple and areola, left male breast**
♂ **C50.029 Malignant neoplasm of nipple and areola, unspecified male breast**

+ **C50.1 Malignant neoplasm of central portion of breast**
+ **C50.11 Malignant neoplasm of central portion of breast, female**
♀ **C50.111 Malignant neoplasm of central portion of right female breast**
♀ **C50.112 Malignant neoplasm of central portion of left female breast**
♀ **C50.119 Malignant neoplasm of central portion of unspecified female breast**
+ **C50.12 Malignant neoplasm of central portion of breast, male**
♂ **C50.121 Malignant neoplasm of central portion of right male breast**
♂ **C50.122 Malignant neoplasm of central portion of left male breast**
♂ **C50.129 Malignant neoplasm of central portion of unspecified male breast**

+ **C50.2 Malignant neoplasm of upper-inner quadrant of breast**
+ **C50.21 Malignant neoplasm of upper-inner quadrant of breast, female**
♀ **C50.211 Malignant neoplasm of upper-inner quadrant of right female breast**
♀ **C50.212 Malignant neoplasm of upper-inner quadrant of left female breast**
♀ **C50.219 Malignant neoplasm of upper-inner quadrant of unspecified female breast**
+ **C50.22 Malignant neoplasm of upper-inner quadrant of breast, male**
♂ **C50.221 Malignant neoplasm of upper-inner quadrant of right male breast**
♂ **C50.222 Malignant neoplasm of upper-inner quadrant of left male breast**
♂ **C50.229 Malignant neoplasm of upper-inner quadrant of unspecified male breast**

+ **C50.3 Malignant neoplasm of lower-inner quadrant of breast**
+ **C50.31 Malignant neoplasm of lower-inner quadrant of breast, female**
♀ **C50.311 Malignant neoplasm of lower-inner quadrant of right female breast**
♀ **C50.312 Malignant neoplasm of lower-inner quadrant of left female breast**
♀ **C50.319 Malignant neoplasm of lower-inner quadrant of unspecified female breast**
+ **C50.32 Malignant neoplasm of lower-inner quadrant of breast, male**
♂ **C50.321 Malignant neoplasm of lower-inner quadrant of right male breast**
♂ **C50.322 Malignant neoplasm of lower-inner quadrant of left male breast**
♂ **C50.329 Malignant neoplasm of lower-inner quadrant of unspecified male breast**

+ **C50.4 Malignant neoplasm of upper-outer quadrant of breast**
+ **C50.41 Malignant neoplasm of upper-outer quadrant of breast, female**
♀ **C50.411 Malignant neoplasm of upper-outer quadrant of right female breast**
♀ **C50.412 Malignant neoplasm of upper-outer quadrant of left female breast**
♀ **C50.419 Malignant neoplasm of upper-outer quadrant of unspecified female breast**
+ **C50.42 Malignant neoplasm of upper-outer quadrant of breast, male**
♂ **C50.421 Malignant neoplasm of upper-outer quadrant of right male breast**
♂ **C50.422 Malignant neoplasm of upper-outer quadrant of left male breast**
♂ **C50.429 Malignant neoplasm of upper-outer quadrant of unspecified male breast**

+ **C50.5 Malignant neoplasm of lower-outer quadrant of breast**
+ **C50.51 Malignant neoplasm of lower-outer quadrant of breast, female**
♀ **C50.511 Malignant neoplasm of lower-outer quadrant of right female breast**
♀ **C50.512 Malignant neoplasm of lower-outer quadrant of left female breast**
♀ **C50.519 Malignant neoplasm of lower-outer quadrant of unspecified female breast**
+ **C50.52 Malignant neoplasm of lower-outer quadrant of breast, male**
♂ **C50.521 Malignant neoplasm of lower-outer quadrant of right male breast**
♂ **C50.522 Malignant neoplasm of lower-outer quadrant of left male breast**
♂ **C50.529 Malignant neoplasm of lower-outer quadrant of unspecified male breast**

+ **C50.6 Malignant neoplasm of axillary tail of breast**
+ **C50.61 Malignant neoplasm of axillary tail of breast, female**
♀ **C50.611 Malignant neoplasm of axillary tail of right female breast**
♀ **C50.612 Malignant neoplasm of axillary tail of left female breast**
♀ **C50.619 Malignant neoplasm of axillary tail of unspecified female breast**

+ C50.62 **Malignant neoplasm of axillary tail of breast, male**
- ♂ C50.621 **Malignant neoplasm of axillary tail of right male breast**
- ♂ C50.622 **Malignant neoplasm of axillary tail of left male breast**
- ♂ C50.629 **Malignant neoplasm of axillary tail of unspecified male breast**

+ C50.8 **Malignant neoplasm of overlapping sites of breast**

+ C50.81 **Malignant neoplasm of overlapping sites of breast, female**
- ♀ C50.811 **Malignant neoplasm of overlapping sites of right female breast**
- ♀ C50.812 **Malignant neoplasm of overlapping sites of left female breast**
- ♀ C50.819 **Malignant neoplasm of overlapping sites of unspecified female breast**

+ C50.82 **Malignant neoplasm of overlapping sites of breast, male**
- ♂ C50.821 **Malignant neoplasm of overlapping sites of right male breast**
- ♂ C50.822 **Malignant neoplasm of overlapping sites of left male breast**
- ♂ C50.829 **Malignant neoplasm of overlapping sites of unspecified male breast**

+ C50.9 **Malignant neoplasm of breast of unspecified site**

+ C50.91 **Malignant neoplasm of breast of unspecified site, female**
- ♀ C50.911 **Malignant neoplasm of unspecified site of right female breast**
- ♀ C50.912 **Malignant neoplasm of unspecified site of left female breast**
- ♀ C50.919 **Malignant neoplasm of unspecified site of unspecified female breast**

+ C50.92 **Malignant neoplasm of breast of unspecified site, male**
- ♂ C50.921 **Malignant neoplasm of unspecified site of right male breast**
- ♂ C50.922 **Malignant neoplasm of unspecified site of left male breast**
- ♂ C50.929 **Malignant neoplasm of unspecified site of unspecified male breast**

Ialignant neoplasms of female genital organs (C51-C58)

ncludes: malignant neoplasm of skin of female genital organs

C51 Malignant neoplasm of vulva

Excludes1: *carcinoma in situ of vulva (D07.1)*

- ♀ C51.0 **Malignant neoplasm of labium majus**
  Malignant neoplasm of Bartholin's [greater vestibular] gland
- ♀ C51.1 **Malignant neoplasm of labium minus**
- ♀ C51.2 **Malignant neoplasm of clitoris**
- ♀ C51.8 **Malignant neoplasm of overlapping sites of vulva**
- ♀ C51.9 **Malignant neoplasm of vulva, unspecified**
  Malignant neoplasm of external female genitalia NOS
  Malignant neoplasm of pudendum

♀ C52 Malignant neoplasm of vagina

Excludes1: *carcinoma in situ of vagina (D07.2)*
Valid 3-character code, no further characters required

C53 Malignant neoplasm of cervix uteri

Excludes1: *carcinoma in situ of cervix uteri (D06.-)*

- ♀ C53.0 **Malignant neoplasm of endocervix**
- ♀ C53.1 **Malignant neoplasm of exocervix**
- ♀ C53.8 **Malignant neoplasm of overlapping sites of cervix uteri**
- ♀ C53.9 **Malignant neoplasm of cervix uteri, unspecified**

C54 Malignant neoplasm of corpus uteri

- ♀ C54.0 **Malignant neoplasm of isthmus uteri**
  Malignant neoplasm of lower uterine segment
- ♀ C54.1 **Malignant neoplasm of endometrium**
- ♀ C54.2 **Malignant neoplasm of myometrium**
- ♀ C54.3 **Malignant neoplasm of fundus uteri**
- ♀ C54.8 **Malignant neoplasm of overlapping sites of corpus uteri**
- ♀ C54.9 **Malignant neoplasm of corpus uteri, unspecified**

♀ C55 Malignant neoplasm of uterus, part unspecified

Valid 3-character code, no further characters required

C56 Malignant neoplasm of ovary

Use additional code to identify any functional activity

- CC ♀ C56.1 **Malignant neoplasm of right ovary**
  CC Exclusion see Appendix A PDX collection 0309
- CC ♀ C56.2 **Malignant neoplasm of left ovary**
  CC Exclusion see Appendix A PDX collection 0309
- CC ♀ C56.9 **Malignant neoplasm of unspecified ovary**
  CC Exclusion see Appendix A PDX collection 0309

C57 Malignant neoplasm of other and unspecified female genital organs

+ C57.0 **Malignant neoplasm of fallopian tube**
  Malignant neoplasm of oviduct
  Malignant neoplasm of uterine tube
  - ♀ C57.00 **Malignant neoplasm of unspecified fallopian tube**
  - ♀ C57.01 **Malignant neoplasm of right fallopian tube**
  - ♀ C57.02 **Malignant neoplasm of left fallopian tube**

+ C57.1 **Malignant neoplasm of broad ligament**
  - ♀ C57.10 **Malignant neoplasm of unspecified broad ligament**
  - ♀ C57.11 **Malignant neoplasm of right broad ligament**
  - ♀ C57.12 **Malignant neoplasm of left broad ligament**

+ C57.2 **Malignant neoplasm of round ligament**
  - ♀ C57.20 **Malignant neoplasm of unspecified round ligament**
  - ♀ C57.21 **Malignant neoplasm of right round ligament**
  - ♀ C57.22 **Malignant neoplasm of left round ligament**

- ♀ C57.3 **Malignant neoplasm of parametrium**
  Malignant neoplasm of uterine ligament NOS
- ♀ C57.4 **Malignant neoplasm of uterine adnexa, unspecified**
- ♀ C57.7 **Malignant neoplasm of other specified female genital organs**
  Malignant neoplasm of wolffian body or duct
- ♀ C57.8 **Malignant neoplasm of overlapping sites of female genital organs**
  Primary malignant neoplasm of two or more contiguous sites of the female genital organs whose point of origin cannot be determined
  Primary tubo-ovarian malignant neoplasm whose point of origin cannot be determined
  Primary utero-ovarian malignant neoplasm whose point of origin cannot be determined
- ♀ C57.9 **Malignant neoplasm of female genital organ, unspecified**
  Malignant neoplasm of female genitourinary tract NOS

• ♀ C58 Malignant neoplasm of placenta

Includes: choriocarcinoma NOS
chorionepithelioma NOS

Excludes1: *chorioadenoma (destruens) (D39.2)*
hydatidiform mole NOS (O01.9)
invasive hydatidiform mole (D39.2)
male choriocarcinoma NOS (C62.9-)
malignant hydatidiform mole (D39.2)

Valid 3-character code, no further characters required

Malignant neoplasms of male genital organs (C60-C63)

Includes: malignant neoplasm of skin of male genital organs

C60 Malignant neoplasm of penis

- ♂ C60.0 **Malignant neoplasm of prepuce**
  Malignant neoplasm of foreskin
- ♂ C60.1 **Malignant neoplasm of glans penis**
- ♂ C60.2 **Malignant neoplasm of body of penis**
  Malignant neoplasm of corpus cavernosum
- ♂ C60.8 **Malignant neoplasm of overlapping sites of penis**
- ♂ C60.9 **Malignant neoplasm of penis, unspecified**
  Malignant neoplasm of skin of penis NOS

♂ C61 Malignant neoplasm of prostate

Use additional code to identify:
hormone sensitivity status (Z19.1-Z19.2)
rising PSA following treatment for malignant neoplasm of prostate (R97.21)

Excludes1: *malignant neoplasm of seminal vesicle (C63.7)*

AHA CC: 1Q, 2017, 17-18

Valid 3-character code, no further characters required

C62 Malignant neoplasm of testis

Use additional code to identify any functional activity

+ C62.0 **Malignant neoplasm of undescended testis**
  Malignant neoplasm of ectopic testis
  Malignant neoplasm of retained testis
  - ♂ C62.00 **Malignant neoplasm of unspecified undescended testis**
  - ♂ C62.01 **Malignant neoplasm of undescended right testis**
  - ♂ C62.02 **Malignant neoplasm of undescended left testis**

+ C62.1 **Malignant neoplasm of descended testis**
  Malignant neoplasm of scrotal testis
  - ♂ C62.10 **Malignant neoplasm of unspecified descended testis**
  - ♂ C62.11 **Malignant neoplasm of descended right testis**
  - ♂ C62.12 **Malignant neoplasm of descended left testis**

+ C62.9 **Malignant neoplasm of testis, unspecified whether descended or undescended**
  - ♂ C62.90 **Malignant neoplasm of unspecified testis, unspecified whether descended or undescended**
    Malignant neoplasm of testis NOS
  - ♂ C62.91 **Malignant neoplasm of right testis, unspecified whether descended or undescended**
  - ♂ C62.92 **Malignant neoplasm of left testis, unspecified whether descended or undescended**

C63 Malignant neoplasm of other and unspecified male genital organs

+ C63.0 **Malignant neoplasm of epididymis**
  - ♂ C63.00 **Malignant neoplasm of unspecified epididymis**
  - ♂ C63.01 **Malignant neoplasm of right epididymis**
  - ♂ C63.02 **Malignant neoplasm of left epididymis**
+ C63.1 **Malignant neoplasm of spermatic cord**
  - ♂ C63.10 **Malignant neoplasm of unspecified spermatic cord**
  - ♂ C63.11 **Malignant neoplasm of right spermatic cord**
  - ♂ C63.12 **Malignant neoplasm of left spermatic cord**

♂ C63.2 **Malignant neoplasm of scrotum**
Malignant neoplasm of skin of scrotum

♂ C63.7 **Malignant neoplasm of other specified male genital organs**
Malignant neoplasm of seminal vesicle
Malignant neoplasm of tunica vaginalis

♂ C63.8 **Malignant neoplasm of overlapping sites of male genital organs**
Primary malignant neoplasm of two or more contiguous sites of male genital organs whose point of origin cannot be determined

♂ C63.9 **Malignant neoplasm of male genital organ, unspecified**
Malignant neoplasm of male genitourinary tract NOS

Malignant neoplasms of urinary tract (C64-C68)

C64 Malignant neoplasm of kidney, except renal pelvis

Excludes1: *malignant carcinoid tumor of the kidney (C7A.093)*
malignant neoplasm of renal calyces (C65.-)
malignant neoplasm of renal pelvis (C65.-)

CC C64.1 **Malignant neoplasm of right kidney, except renal pelvis**
CC Exclusion see Appendix A PDX collection 0310

CC C64.2 **Malignant neoplasm of left kidney, except renal pelvis**
CC Exclusion see Appendix A PDX collection 0310

CC C64.9 **Malignant neoplasm of unspecified kidney, except renal pelvis**
CC Exclusion see Appendix A PDX collection 0310

C65 Malignant neoplasm of renal pelvis

Includes: malignant neoplasm of pelviureteric junction
malignant neoplasm of renal calyces

CC C65.1 **Malignant neoplasm of right renal pelvis**
CC Exclusion see Appendix A PDX collection 0310

CC C65.2 **Malignant neoplasm of left renal pelvis**
CC Exclusion see Appendix A PDX collection 0310

CC C65.9 **Malignant neoplasm of unspecified renal pelvis**
CC Exclusion see Appendix A PDX collection 0310

C66 Malignant neoplasm of ureter

Excludes1: *malignant neoplasm of ureteric orifice of bladder (C67.6)*

CC C66.1 **Malignant neoplasm of right ureter**
CC Exclusion see Appendix A PDX collection 0311

CC C66.2 **Malignant neoplasm of left ureter**
CC Exclusion see Appendix A PDX collection 0311

CC C66.9 **Malignant neoplasm of unspecified ureter**
CC Exclusion see Appendix A PDX collection 0311

C67 Malignant neoplasm of bladder

C67.0 **Malignant neoplasm of trigone of bladder**
C67.1 **Malignant neoplasm of dome of bladder**
C67.2 **Malignant neoplasm of lateral wall of bladder**
C67.3 **Malignant neoplasm of anterior wall of bladder**
C67.4 **Malignant neoplasm of posterior wall of bladder**
C67.5 **Malignant neoplasm of bladder neck**
Malignant neoplasm of internal urethral orifice
C67.6 **Malignant neoplasm of ureteric orifice**
C67.7 **Malignant neoplasm of urachus**
C67.8 **Malignant neoplasm of overlapping sites of bladder**
C67.9 **Malignant neoplasm of bladder, unspecified**
AHA CC: 1Q, 2016, 19; 1Q, 2017, 6

C68 Malignant neoplasm of other and unspecified urinary organs

Excludes1: *malignant neoplasm of female genitourinary tract NOS (C57.9)*
malignant neoplasm of male genitourinary tract NOS (C63.9)

CC C68.0 **Malignant neoplasm of urethra**
Excludes1: *malignant neoplasm of urethral orifice of bladder (C67.5)*
CC Exclusion see Appendix A PDX collection 0312

CC C68.1 **Malignant neoplasm of paraurethral glands**
CC Exclusion see Appendix A PDX collection 0312

CC C68.8 **Malignant neoplasm of overlapping sites of urinary organs**
Primary malignant neoplasm of two or more contiguous sites urinary organs whose point of origin cannot be determined
CC Exclusion see Appendix A PDX collection 0313

CC C68.9 **Malignant neoplasm of urinary organ, unspecified**
Malignant neoplasm of urinary system NOS
CC Exclusion see Appendix A PDX collection 0313

Malignant neoplasms of eye, brain and other parts of central nervous system (C69-C72)

C69 Malignant neoplasm of eye and adnexa

Excludes1: *malignant neoplasm of connective tissue of eyelid (C49.0)*
malignant neoplasm of eyelid (skin) (C43.1-, C44.1-)
malignant neoplasm of optic nerve (C72.3-)

+ C69.0 **Malignant neoplasm of conjunctiva**
  - C69.00 **Malignant neoplasm of unspecified conjunctiva**
  - C69.01 **Malignant neoplasm of right conjunctiva**
  - C69.02 **Malignant neoplasm of left conjunctiva**
+ C69.1 **Malignant neoplasm of cornea**
  - C69.10 **Malignant neoplasm of unspecified cornea**
  - C69.11 **Malignant neoplasm of right cornea**
  - C69.12 **Malignant neoplasm of left cornea**
+ C69.2 **Malignant neoplasm of retina**
  Excludes1: *dark area on retina (D49.81)*
  neoplasm of unspecified behavior of retina and choroid (D49.81)
  retinal freckle (D49.81)
  - C69.20 **Malignant neoplasm of unspecified retina**
  - C69.21 **Malignant neoplasm of right retina**
  - C69.22 **Malignant neoplasm of left retina**
+ C69.3 **Malignant neoplasm of choroid**
  - C69.30 **Malignant neoplasm of unspecified choroid**
  - C69.31 **Malignant neoplasm of right choroid**
  - C69.32 **Malignant neoplasm of left choroid**
+ C69.4 **Malignant neoplasm of ciliary body**
  - C69.40 **Malignant neoplasm of unspecified ciliary body**
  - C69.41 **Malignant neoplasm of right ciliary body**
  - C69.42 **Malignant neoplasm of left ciliary body**
+ C69.5 **Malignant neoplasm of lacrimal gland and duct**
  Malignant neoplasm of lacrimal sac
  Malignant neoplasm of nasolacrimal duct
  - C69.50 **Malignant neoplasm of unspecified lacrimal gland and duct**
  - C69.51 **Malignant neoplasm of right lacrimal gland and du**
  - C69.52 **Malignant neoplasm of left lacrimal gland and duct**
+ C69.6 **Malignant neoplasm of orbit**
  Malignant neoplasm of connective tissue of orbit
  Malignant neoplasm of extraocular muscle
  Malignant neoplasm of peripheral nerves of orbit
  Malignant neoplasm of retrobulbar tissue
  Malignant neoplasm of retro-ocular tissue
  Excludes1: *malignant neoplasm of orbital bone (C41.0)*
  - C69.60 **Malignant neoplasm of unspecified orbit**
  - C69.61 **Malignant neoplasm of right orbit**
  - C69.62 **Malignant neoplasm of left orbit**
+ C69.8 **Malignant neoplasm of overlapping sites of eye and adnexa**
  - C69.80 **Malignant neoplasm of overlapping sites of unspecified eye and adnexa**
  - C69.81 **Malignant neoplasm of overlapping sites of right ey and adnexa**
  - C69.82 **Malignant neoplasm of overlapping sites of left eye and adnexa**
+ C69.9 **Malignant neoplasm of unspecified site of eye**
  Malignant neoplasm of eyeball
  - C69.90 **Malignant neoplasm of unspecified site of unspecified eye**
  - C69.91 **Malignant neoplasm of unspecified site of right eye**
  - C69.92 **Malignant neoplasm of unspecified site of left eye**

C70 Malignant neoplasm of meninges

CC C70.0 **Malignant neoplasm of cerebral meninges**
CC Exclusion see Appendix A PDX collection 0314

CC C70.1 **Malignant neoplasm of spinal meninges**
CC Exclusion see Appendix A PDX collection 0315

CC C70.9 **Malignant neoplasm of meninges, unspecified**
CC Exclusion see Appendix A PDX collection 0314

C71 Malignant neoplasm of brain

Excludes1: *malignant neoplasm of cranial nerves (C72.2-C72.5)*
retrobulbar malignant neoplasm (C69.6-)

CC **C71.0 Malignant neoplasm of cerebrum, except lobes and ventricles**
Malignant neoplasm of supratentorial NOS
CC Exclusion see Appendix A PDX collection 0316

CC **C71.1 Malignant neoplasm of frontal lobe**
CC Exclusion see Appendix A PDX collection 0316

CC **C71.2 Malignant neoplasm of temporal lobe**
CC Exclusion see Appendix A PDX collection 0316

CC **C71.3 Malignant neoplasm of parietal lobe**
CC Exclusion see Appendix A PDX collection 0316

CC **C71.4 Malignant neoplasm of occipital lobe**
CC Exclusion see Appendix A PDX collection 0316

CC **C71.5 Malignant neoplasm of cerebral ventricle**
Excludes1: *malignant neoplasm of fourth cerebral ventricle (C71.7)*
CC Exclusion see Appendix A PDX collection 0316

CC **C71.6 Malignant neoplasm of cerebellum**
CC Exclusion see Appendix A PDX collection 0316

CC **C71.7 Malignant neoplasm of brain stem**
Malignant neoplasm of fourth cerebral ventricle
Infratentorial malignant neoplasm NOS
CC Exclusion see Appendix A PDX collection 0316

CC **C71.8 Malignant neoplasm of overlapping sites of brain**
CC Exclusion see Appendix A PDX collection 0316

CC **C71.9 Malignant neoplasm of brain, unspecified**
CC Exclusion see Appendix A PDX collection 0316
AHA CC: 3Q, 2014, 3-4

C72 Malignant neoplasm of spinal cord, cranial nerves and other parts of central nervous system

Excludes1: *malignant neoplasm of meninges (C70.-)*
malignant neoplasm of peripheral nerves and autonomic nervous system (C47.-)

CC **C72.0 Malignant neoplasm of spinal cord**
CC Exclusion see Appendix A PDX collection 0317

CC **C72.1 Malignant neoplasm of cauda equina**
CC Exclusion see Appendix A PDX collection 0317

\+ **C72.2 Malignant neoplasm of olfactory nerve**
Malignant neoplasm of olfactory bulb

CC **C72.20 Malignant neoplasm of unspecified olfactory nerve**
CC Exclusion see Appendix A PDX collection 0318

CC **C72.21 Malignant neoplasm of right olfactory nerve**
CC Exclusion see Appendix A PDX collection 0318

CC **C72.22 Malignant neoplasm of left olfactory nerve**
CC Exclusion see Appendix A PDX collection 0318

\+ **C72.3 Malignant neoplasm of optic nerve**

CC **C72.30 Malignant neoplasm of unspecified optic nerve**
CC Exclusion see Appendix A PDX collection 0318

CC **C72.31 Malignant neoplasm of right optic nerve**
CC Exclusion see Appendix A PDX collection 0318

CC **C72.32 Malignant neoplasm of left optic nerve**
CC Exclusion see Appendix A PDX collection 0318

\+ **C72.4 Malignant neoplasm of acoustic nerve**

CC **C72.40 Malignant neoplasm of unspecified acoustic nerve**
CC Exclusion see Appendix A PDX collection 0318

CC **C72.41 Malignant neoplasm of right acoustic nerve**
CC Exclusion see Appendix A PDX collection 0318

CC **C72.42 Malignant neoplasm of left acoustic nerve**
CC Exclusion see Appendix A PDX collection 0318

\+ **C72.5 Malignant neoplasm of other and unspecified cranial nerves**

CC **C72.50 Malignant neoplasm of unspecified cranial nerve**
Malignant neoplasm of cranial nerve NOS
CC Exclusion see Appendix A PDX collection 0318

CC **C72.59 Malignant neoplasm of other cranial nerves**
CC Exclusion see Appendix A PDX collection 0318

CC **C72.9 Malignant neoplasm of central nervous system, unspecified**
Malignant neoplasm of unspecified site of central nervous system
Malignant neoplasm of nervous system NOS
CC Exclusion see Appendix A PDX collection 0319

alignant neoplasms of thyroid and other endocrine glands :73-C75)

C73 Malignant neoplasm of thyroid gland

Use additional code to identify any functional activity
Valid 3-character code, no further characters required

C74 Malignant neoplasm of adrenal gland

\+ **C74.0 Malignant neoplasm of cortex of adrenal gland**

CC **C74.00 Malignant neoplasm of cortex of unspecified adrenal gland**
CC Exclusion see Appendix A PDX collection 0320

CC **C74.01 Malignant neoplasm of cortex of right adrenal gland**
CC Exclusion see Appendix A PDX collection 0320

CC **C74.02 Malignant neoplasm of cortex of left adrenal gland**
CC Exclusion see Appendix A PDX collection 0320

\+ **C74.1 Malignant neoplasm of medulla of adrenal gland**

CC **C74.10 Malignant neoplasm of medulla of unspecified adrenal gland**
CC Exclusion see Appendix A PDX collection 0320

CC **C74.11 Malignant neoplasm of medulla of right adrenal gland**
CC Exclusion see Appendix A PDX collection 0320

CC **C74.12 Malignant neoplasm of medulla of left adrenal gland**
CC Exclusion see Appendix A PDX collection 0320

\+ **C74.9 Malignant neoplasm of unspecified part of adrenal gland**

CC **C74.90 Malignant neoplasm of unspecified part of unspecified adrenal gland**
CC Exclusion see Appendix A PDX collection 0320

CC **C74.91 Malignant neoplasm of unspecified part of right adrenal gland**
CC Exclusion see Appendix A PDX collection 0320

CC **C74.92 Malignant neoplasm of unspecified part of left adrenal gland**
CC Exclusion see Appendix A PDX collection 0320

C75 Malignant neoplasm of other endocrine glands and related structures

Excludes1: *malignant carcinoid tumors (C7A.0-)*
malignant neoplasm of adrenal gland (C74.-)
malignant neoplasm of endocrine pancreas (C25.4)
malignant neoplasm of islets of Langerhans (C25.4)
malignant neoplasm of ovary (C56.-)
malignant neoplasm of testis (C62.-)
malignant neoplasm of thymus (C37)
malignant neoplasm of thyroid gland (C73)
malignant neuroendocrine tumors (C7A.-)

CC **C75.0 Malignant neoplasm of parathyroid gland**
CC Exclusion see Appendix A PDX collection 0321

CC **C75.1 Malignant neoplasm of pituitary gland**
CC Exclusion see Appendix A PDX collection 0322

CC **C75.2 Malignant neoplasm of craniopharyngeal duct**
CC Exclusion see Appendix A PDX collection 0322

CC **C75.3 Malignant neoplasm of pineal gland**
CC Exclusion see Appendix A PDX collection 0323

CC **C75.4 Malignant neoplasm of carotid body**
CC Exclusion see Appendix A PDX collection 0324

CC **C75.5 Malignant neoplasm of aortic body and other paraganglia**
CC Exclusion see Appendix A PDX collection 0325

CC **C75.8 Malignant neoplasm with pluriglandular involvement, unspecified**
CC Exclusion see Appendix A PDX collection 0326

CC **C75.9 Malignant neoplasm of endocrine gland, unspecified**
CC Exclusion see Appendix A PDX collection 0326

Malignant neuroendocrine tumors (C7A)

C7A Malignant neuroendocrine tumors

Code also any associated multiple endocrine neoplasia [MEN] syndromes (E31.2-)

Use additional code to identify any associated endocrine syndrome, such as:
carcinoid syndrome (E34.0)

Excludes2: *malignant pancreatic islet cell tumors (C25.4)*
Merkel cell carcinoma (C4A.-)

\+ **C7A.0 Malignant carcinoid tumors**

CC **C7A.00 Malignant carcinoid tumor of unspecified site**
CC Exclusion see Appendix A PDX collection 0346

\+ **C7A.01 Malignant carcinoid tumors of the small intestine**

CC **C7A.010 Malignant carcinoid tumor of the duodenum**
CC Exclusion see Appendix A PDX collection 0347

CC **C7A.011 Malignant carcinoid tumor ofthe jejunum**
CC Exclusion see Appendix A PDX collection 0348

CC **C7A.012 Malignant carcinoid tumor of the ileum**
CC Exclusion see Appendix A PDX collection 0349

CC **C7A.019 Malignant carcinoid tumor of the small intestine, unspecified portion**
CC Exclusion see Appendix A PDX collection 0350

\+ **C7A.02 Malignant carcinoid tumors of the appendix, large intestine, and rectum**

CC **C7A.020 Malignant carcinoid tumor of the appendix**
CC Exclusion see Appendix A PDX collection 0351

CC **C7A.021 Malignant carcinoid tumor of the cecum**
CC Exclusion see Appendix A PDX collection 0352

<u>**Lymphatic System**</u>

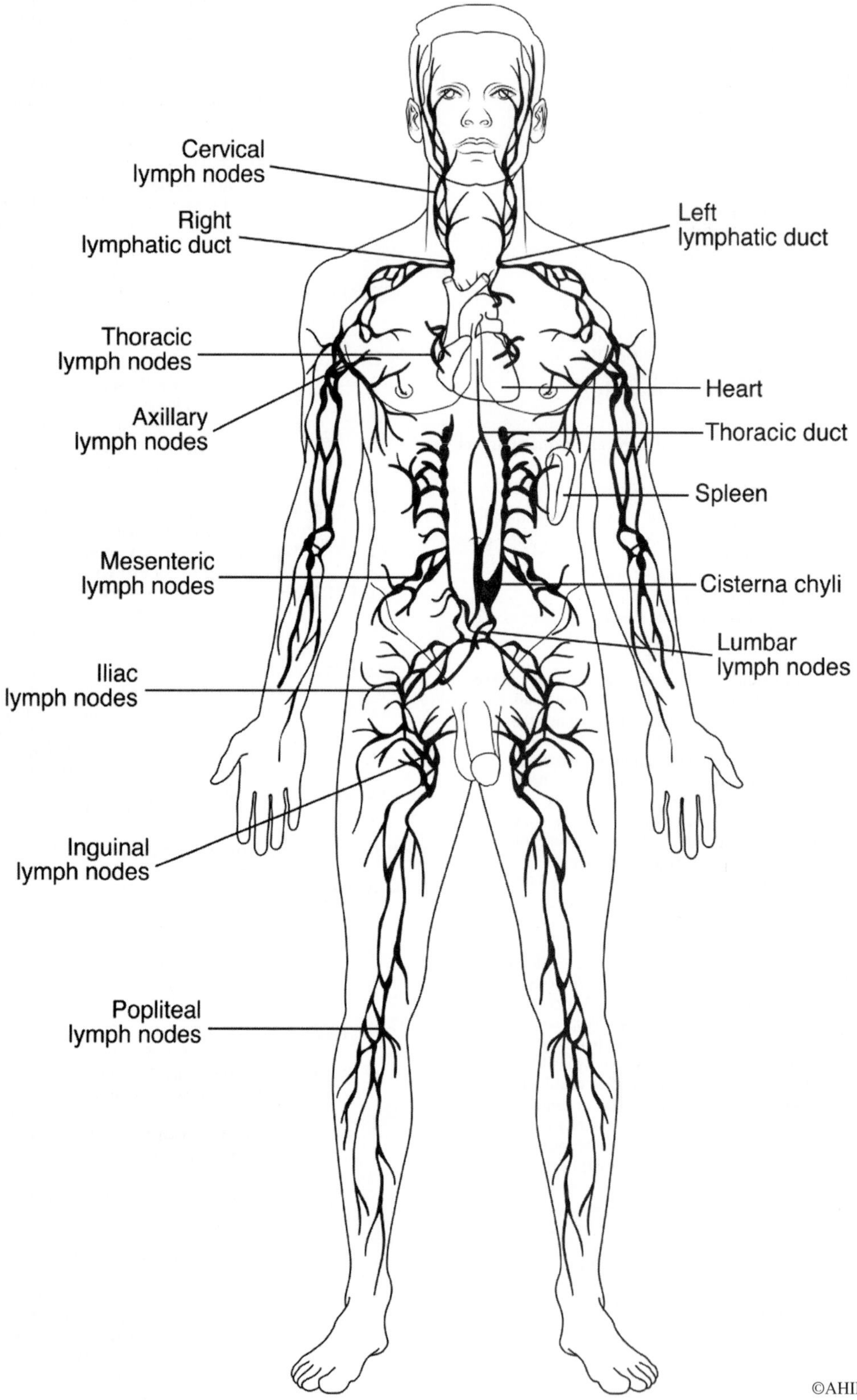
Cervical lymph nodes
Right lymphatic duct
Left lymphatic duct
Thoracic lymph nodes
Axillary lymph nodes
Heart
Thoracic duct
Spleen
Mesenteric lymph nodes
Cisterna chyli
Lumbar lymph nodes
Iliac lymph nodes
Inguinal lymph nodes
Popliteal lymph nodes

CC **C7A.022** **Malignant carcinoid tumor of the ascending colon**
CC Exclusion see Appendix A PDX collection 0353
CC **C7A.023** **Malignant carcinoid tumor of the transverse colon**
CC Exclusion see Appendix A PDX collection 0354
CC **C7A.024** **Malignant carcinoid tumor of the descending colon**
CC Exclusion see Appendix A PDX collection 0355
CC **C7A.025** **Malignant carcinoid tumor of the sigmoid colon**
CC Exclusion see Appendix A PDX collection 0356
CC **C7A.026** **Malignant carcinoid tumor of the rectum**
CC Exclusion see Appendix A PDX collection 0357
CC **C7A.029** **Malignant carcinoid tumor of the large intestine, unspecified portion**
Malignant carcinoid tumor of the colon NOS
CC Exclusion see Appendix A PDX collection 0358
+ **C7A.09** **Malignant carcinoid tumors of other sites**
CC **C7A.090** **Malignant carcinoid tumor of the bronchus and lung**
CC Exclusion see Appendix A PDX collection 0359
CC **C7A.091** **Malignant carcinoid tumor of the thymus**
CC Exclusion see Appendix A PDX collection 0360
CC **C7A.092** **Malignant carcinoid tumor of the stomach**
CC Exclusion see Appendix A PDX collection 0361
CC **C7A.093** **Malignant carcinoid tumor of the kidney**
CC Exclusion see Appendix A PDX collection 0362
CC **C7A.094** **Malignant carcinoid tumor of the foregut, unspecified**
CC Exclusion see Appendix A PDX collection 0361
CC **C7A.095** **Malignant carcinoid tumor of the midgut, unspecified**
CC Exclusion see Appendix A PDX collection 0361
CC **C7A.096** **Malignant carcinoid tumor of the hindgut, unspecified**
CC Exclusion see Appendix A PDX collection 0361
CC **C7A.098** **Malignant carcinoid tumors of other sites**
CC Exclusion see Appendix A PDX collection 0346

CC **C7A.1** **Malignant poorly differentiated neuroendocrine tumors**
Malignant poorly differentiated neuroendocrine tumor NOS
Malignant poorly differentiated neuroendocrine carcinoma, any site
High grade neuroendocrine carcinoma, any site
CC Exclusion see Appendix A PDX collection 0346
CC **C7A.8** **Other malignant neuroendocrine tumors**
CC Exclusion see Appendix A PDX collection 0346

condary neuroendocrine tumors (C7B)

C7B Secondary neuroendocrine tumors
Use additional code to identify any functional activity
+ **C7B.0** **Secondary carcinoid tumors**
C7B.00 **Secondary carcinoid tumors, unspecified site**
CC **C7B.01** **Secondary carcinoid tumors of distant lymph nodes**
CC Exclusion see Appendix A PDX collection 0363
CC **C7B.02** **Secondary carcinoid tumors of liver**
CC Exclusion see Appendix A PDX collection 0364
CC **C7B.03** **Secondary carcinoid tumors of bone**
CC Exclusion see Appendix A PDX collection 0365
CC **C7B.04** **Secondary carcinoid tumors of peritoneum**
Mesentary metastasis of carcinoid tumor
CC Exclusion see Appendix A PDX collection 0366
CC **C7B.09** **Secondary carcinoid tumors of other sites**
CC Exclusion see Appendix A PDX collection 0367
C7B.1 **Secondary Merkel cell carcinoma**
Merkel cell carcinoma nodal presentation
Merkel cell carcinoma visceral metastatic presentation
CC **C7B.8** **Other secondary neuroendocrine tumors**
CC Exclusion see Appendix A PDX collection 0367

Malignant neoplasms of ill-defined, other secondary and unspecified sites (C76-C80)

Review coding guidelines C.2.b and C.2.l.2

C76 Malignant neoplasm of other and ill-defined sites
Excludes1: *malignant neoplasm of female genitourinary tract NOS (C57.9)*
malignant neoplasm of male genitourinary tract NOS (C63.9)
malignant neoplasm of lymphoid, hematopoietic and related tissue (C81-C96)
malignant neoplasm of skin (C44.-)
malignant neoplasm of unspecified site NOS (C80.1)
C76.0 **Malignant neoplasm of head, face and neck**
Malignant neoplasm of cheek NOS
Malignant neoplasm of nose NOS
C76.1 **Malignant neoplasm of thorax**
Intrathoracic malignant neoplasm NOS
Malignant neoplasm of axilla NOS
Thoracic malignant neoplasm NOS
C76.2 **Malignant neoplasm of abdomen**
C76.3 **Malignant neoplasm of pelvis**
Malignant neoplasm of groin NOS
Malignant neoplasm of sites overlapping systems within the pelvis
Rectovaginal (septum) malignant neoplasm
Rectovesical (septum) malignant neoplasm
+ **C76.4** **Malignant neoplasm of upper limb**
C76.40 **Malignant neoplasm of unspecified upper limb**
C76.41 **Malignant neoplasm of right upper limb**
C76.42 **Malignant neoplasm of left upper limb**
+ **C76.5** **Malignant neoplasm of lower limb**
C76.50 **Malignant neoplasm of unspecified lower limb**
C76.51 **Malignant neoplasm of right lower limb**
C76.52 **Malignant neoplasm of left lower limb**
C76.8 **Malignant neoplasm of other specified ill-defined sites**
Malignant neoplasm of overlapping ill-defined sites

+ **C77 Secondary and unspecified malignant neoplasm of lymph nodes**
Excludes1: *malignant neoplasm of lymph nodes, specified as primary (C81-C86, C88, C96.-)*
mesentary metastasis of carcinoid tumor (C7B.04)
secondary carcinoid tumors of distant lymph nodes (C7B.01)
CC **C77.0** **Secondary and unspecified malignant neoplasm of lymph nodes of head, face and neck**
Secondary and unspecified malignant neoplasm of supraclavicular lymph nodes
CC Exclusion see Appendix A PDX collection 0303
CC **C77.1** **Secondary and unspecified malignant neoplasm of intrathoracic lymph nodes**
CC Exclusion see Appendix A PDX collection 0303
CC **C77.2** **Secondary and unspecified malignant neoplasm of intra-abdominal lymph nodes**
CC Exclusion see Appendix A PDX collection 0303
CC **C77.3** **Secondary and unspecified malignant neoplasm of axilla and upper limb lymph nodes**
Secondary and unspecified malignant neoplasm of pectoral lymph nodes
CC Exclusion see Appendix A PDX collection 0303
CC **C77.4** **Secondary and unspecified malignant neoplasm of inguinal and lower limb lymph nodes**
CC Exclusion see Appendix A PDX collection 0303
CC **C77.5** **Secondary and unspecified malignant neoplasm of intrapelvic lymph nodes**
CC Exclusion see Appendix A PDX collection 0303
CC **C77.8** **Secondary and unspecified malignant neoplasm of lymph nodes of multiple regions**
CC Exclusion see Appendix A PDX collection 0303
CC **C77.9** **Secondary and unspecified malignant neoplasm of lymph node, unspecified**
CC Exclusion see Appendix A PDX collection 0303

C78 Secondary malignant neoplasm of respiratory and digestive organs
Excludes1: *secondary carcinoid tumors of liver (C7B.02)*
secondary carcinoid tumors of peritoneum (C7B.04)
Excludes2: *lymph node metastases (C77.0)*
+ **C78.0** **Secondary malignant neoplasm of lung**
CC **C78.00** **Secondary malignant neoplasm of unspecified lung**
CC Exclusion see Appendix A PDX collection 0327
CC **C78.01** **Secondary malignant neoplasm of right lung**
CC Exclusion see Appendix A PDX collection 0327

CC **C78.02** **Secondary malignant neoplasm of left lung**
CC Exclusion see Appendix A PDX collection 0327

CC **C78.1** **Secondary malignant neoplasm of mediastinum**
CC Exclusion see Appendix A PDX collection 0328

CC **C78.2** **Secondary malignant neoplasm of pleura**
CC Exclusion see Appendix A PDX collection 0329

+ **C78.3** **Secondary malignant neoplasm of other and unspecified respiratory organs**

CC **C78.30** **Secondary malignant neoplasm of unspecified respiratory organ**
CC Exclusion see Appendix A PDX collection 0330

CC **C78.39** **Secondary malignant neoplasm of other respiratory organs**
CC Exclusion see Appendix A PDX collection 0330

CC **C78.4** **Secondary malignant neoplasm of small intestine**
CC Exclusion see Appendix A PDX collection 0331

CC **C78.5** **Secondary malignant neoplasm of large intestine and rectum**
CC Exclusion see Appendix A PDX collection 0332

CC **C78.6** **Secondary malignant neoplasm of retroperitoneum and peritoneum**
CC Exclusion see Appendix A PDX collection 0333
AHA CC: 2Q, 2017, 12

CC **C78.7** **Secondary malignant neoplasm of liver and intrahepatic bile duct**
CC Exclusion see Appendix A PDX collection 0334

+ **C78.8** **Secondary malignant neoplasm of other and unspecified digestive organs**

CC **C78.80** **Secondary malignant neoplasm of unspecified digestive organ**
CC Exclusion see Appendix A PDX collection 0335

CC **C78.89** **Secondary malignant neoplasm of other digestive organs**
Code also exocrine pancreatic insufficiency (K86.81)
CC Exclusion see Appendix A PDX collection 0335

C79 Secondary malignant neoplasm of other and unspecified sites

Excludes1: *secondary carcinoid tumors (C7B.-)*
secondary neuroendocrine tumors (C7B.-)

+ **C79.0** **Secondary malignant neoplasm of kidney and renal pelvis**

CC **C79.00** **Secondary malignant neoplasm of unspecified kidney and renal pelvis**
CC Exclusion see Appendix A PDX collection 0336

CC **C79.01** **Secondary malignant neoplasm of right kidney and renal pelvis**
CC Exclusion see Appendix A PDX collection 0336

CC **C79.02** **Secondary malignant neoplasm of left kidney and renal pelvis**
CC Exclusion see Appendix A PDX collection 0336

+ **C79.1** **Secondary malignant neoplasm of bladder and other and unspecified urinary organs**

CC **C79.10** **Secondary malignant neoplasm of unspecified urinary organs**
CC Exclusion see Appendix A PDX collection 0336

CC **C79.11** **Secondary malignant neoplasm of bladder**
Excludes2: *lymph node metastases (C77.0)*
CC Exclusion see Appendix A PDX collection 0336

CC **C79.19** **Secondary malignant neoplasm of other urinary organs**
CC Exclusion see Appendix A PDX collection 0336

CC **C79.2** **Secondary malignant neoplasm of skin**
Excludes1: *secondary Merkel cell carcinoma (C7B.1)*
CC Exclusion see Appendix A PDX collection 0337

+ **C79.3** **Secondary malignant neoplasm of brain and cerebral meninges**

CC **C79.31** **Secondary malignant neoplasm of brain**
CC Exclusion see Appendix A PDX collection 0338

CC **C79.32** **Secondary malignant neoplasm of cerebral meninges**
CC Exclusion see Appendix A PDX collection 0339

+ **C79.4** **Secondary malignant neoplasm of other and unspecified parts of nervous system**

CC **C79.40** **Secondary malignant neoplasm of unspecified part of nervous system**
CC Exclusion see Appendix A PDX collection 0339

CC **C79.49** **Secondary malignant neoplasm of other parts of nervous system**
CC Exclusion see Appendix A PDX collection 0339

+ **C79.5** **Secondary malignant neoplasm of bone and bone marrow**
Excludes1: *secondary carcinoid tumors of bone (C7B.03)*

CC **C79.51** **Secondary malignant neoplasm of bone**
CC Exclusion see Appendix A PDX collection 0340

CC **C79.52** **Secondary malignant neoplasm of bone marrow**
CC Exclusion see Appendix A PDX collection 0340

+ **C79.6** **Secondary malignant neoplasm of ovary**

CC ♀ **C79.60** **Secondary malignant neoplasm of unspecified ovary**
CC Exclusion see Appendix A PDX collection 0341

CC ♀ **C79.61** **Secondary malignant neoplasm of right ovary**
CC Exclusion see Appendix A PDX collection 0341

CC ♀ **C79.62** **Secondary malignant neoplasm of left ovary**
CC Exclusion see Appendix A PDX collection 0341

+ **C79.7** **Secondary malignant neoplasm of adrenal gland**

CC **C79.70** **Secondary malignant neoplasm of unspecified adrenal gland**
CC Exclusion see Appendix A PDX collection 0342

CC **C79.71** **Secondary malignant neoplasm of right adrenal gla**
CC Exclusion see Appendix A PDX collection 0342

CC **C79.72** **Secondary malignant neoplasm of left adrenal gla**
CC Exclusion see Appendix A PDX collection 0342

+ **C79.8** **Secondary malignant neoplasm of other specified sites**

CC **C79.81** **Secondary malignant neoplasm of breast**
CC Exclusion see Appendix A PDX collection 0343

CC **C79.82** **Secondary malignant neoplasm of genital organs**
CC Exclusion see Appendix A PDX collection 0344

CC **C79.89** **Secondary malignant neoplasm of other specified si**
CC Exclusion see Appendix A PDX collection 0345
AHA CC: 2Q, 2017, 11

CC **C79.9** **Secondary malignant neoplasm of unspecified site**
Metastatic cancer NOS
Metastatic disease NOS
Excludes1: *carcinomatosis NOS (C80.0)*
generalized cancer NOS (C80.0)
malignant (primary) neoplasm of unspecified sit (C80.1)
CC Exclusion see Appendix A PDX collection 0345

C80 Malignant neoplasm without specification of site

Excludes1: *malignant carcinoid tumor of unspecified site (C7A.00)*
malignant neoplasm of specified multiple sites- code to each site

CC **C80.0** **Disseminated malignant neoplasm, unspecified**
Carcinomatosis NOS
Generalized cancer, unspecified site (primary) (secondary)
Generalized malignancy, unspecified site (primary) (secondar
CC Exclusion see Appendix A PDX collection 0345
Review coding guideline C.2.j

C80.1 **Malignant (primary) neoplasm, unspecified**
Cancer NOS
Cancer unspecified site (primary)
Carcinoma unspecified site (primary)
Malignancy unspecified site (primary)
Excludes1: *secondary malignant neoplasm of unspecified si (C79.9)*
Review coding guideline C.2.k

CC **C80.2** **Malignant neoplasm associated with transplanted organ**
Code first complication of transplanted organ (T86.-)
Use additional code to identify the specific malignancy
CC Exclusion see Appendix A PDX collection 0345
Review coding guideline C.2.r

Malignant neoplasms of lymphoid, hematopoietic and relate tissue (C81-C96)

Excludes2: *Kaposi's sarcoma of lymph nodes (C46.3)*
secondary and unspecified neoplasm of lymph nodes (C77.-)
secondary neoplasm of bone marrow (C79.52)
secondary neoplasm of spleen (C78.89)

C81 Hodgkin lymphoma

Excludes1: *personal history of Hodgkin lymphoma (Z85.71)*

+ **C81.0** **Nodular lymphocyte predominant Hodgkin lymphoma**

CC **C81.00** **Nodular lymphocyte predominant Hodgkin lymphoma, unspecified site**
CC Exclusion see Appendix A PDX collection 0368

CC **C81.01** **Nodular lymphocyte predominant Hodgkin lymphoma, lymph nodes of head, face, and neck**
CC Exclusion see Appendix A PDX collection 0369

CC **C81.02** **Nodular lymphocyte predominant Hodgkin lymphoma, intrathoracic lymph nodes**
CC Exclusion see Appendix A PDX collection 0370

CC **C81.03** **Nodular lymphocyte predominant Hodgkin lymphoma, intra-abdominal lymph nodes**
CC Exclusion see Appendix A PDX collection 0371

CC **C81.04** **Nodular lymphocyte predominant Hodgkin lymphoma, lymph nodes of axilla and upper limb**
CC Exclusion see Appendix A PDX collection 0372

CC **C81.05** **Nodular lymphocyte predominant Hodgkin lymphoma, lymph nodes of inguinal region and lower limb**
CC Exclusion see Appendix A PDX collection 0373

CC **C81.06** **Nodular lymphocyte predominant Hodgkin lymphoma, intrapelvic lymph nodes**
CC Exclusion see Appendix A PDX collection 0374

CC **C81.07** **Nodular lymphocyte predominant Hodgkin lymphoma, spleen**
CC Exclusion see Appendix A PDX collection 0375

CC **C81.08** **Nodular lymphocyte predominant Hodgkin lymphoma, lymph nodes of multiple sites**
CC Exclusion see Appendix A PDX collection 0368

CC **C81.09** **Nodular lymphocyte predominant Hodgkin lymphoma, extranodal and solid organ sites**
CC Exclusion see Appendix A PDX collection 0368

\+ **C81.1 Nodular sclerosis Hodgkin lymphoma**
Nodular sclerosis classical Hodgkin lymphoma

CC **C81.10** **Nodular sclerosis Hodgkin lymphoma, unspecified site**
CC Exclusion see Appendix A PDX collection 0376

CC **C81.11** **Nodular sclerosis Hodgkin lymphoma, lymph nodes of head, face, and neck**
CC Exclusion see Appendix A PDX collection 0377

CC **C81.12** **Nodular sclerosis Hodgkin lymphoma, intrathoracic lymph nodes**
CC Exclusion see Appendix A PDX collection 0378

CC **C81.13** **Nodular sclerosis Hodgkin lymphoma, intra-abdominal lymph nodes**
CC Exclusion see Appendix A PDX collection 0379

CC **C81.14** **Nodular sclerosis Hodgkin lymphoma, lymph nodes of axilla and upper limb**
CC Exclusion see Appendix A PDX collection 0380

CC **C81.15** **Nodular sclerosis Hodgkin lymphoma, lymph nodes of inguinal region and lower limb**
CC Exclusion see Appendix A PDX collection 0381

CC **C81.16** **Nodular sclerosis Hodgkin lymphoma, intrapelvic lymph nodes**
CC Exclusion see Appendix A PDX collection 0382

CC **C81.17** **Nodular sclerosis Hodgkin lymphoma, spleen**
CC Exclusion see Appendix A PDX collection 0383

CC **C81.18** **Nodular sclerosis Hodgkin lymphoma, lymph nodes of multiple sites**
CC Exclusion see Appendix A PDX collection 0376

CC **C81.19** **Nodular sclerosis Hodgkin lymphoma, extranodal and solid organ sites**
CC Exclusion see Appendix A PDX collection 0376

\+ **C81.2 Mixed cellularity Hodgkin lymphoma**
Mixed cellularity classical Hodgkin lymphoma

CC **C81.20** **Mixed cellularity Hodgkin lymphoma, unspecified site**
CC Exclusion see Appendix A PDX collection 0384

CC **C81.21** **Mixed cellularity Hodgkin lymphoma, lymph nodes of head, face, and neck**
CC Exclusion see Appendix A PDX collection 0385

CC **C81.22** **Mixed cellularity Hodgkin lymphoma, intrathoracic lymph nodes**
CC Exclusion see Appendix A PDX collection 0386

CC **C81.23** **Mixed cellularity Hodgkin lymphoma, intra-abdominal lymph nodes**
CC Exclusion see Appendix A PDX collection 0387

CC **C81.24** **Mixed cellularity Hodgkin lymphoma, lymph nodes of axilla and upper limb**
CC Exclusion see Appendix A PDX collection 0388

CC **C81.25** **Mixed cellularity Hodgkin lymphoma, lymph nodes of inguinal region and lower limb**
CC Exclusion see Appendix A PDX collection 0389

CC **C81.26** **Mixed cellularity Hodgkin lymphoma, intrapelvic lymph nodes**
CC Exclusion see Appendix A PDX collection 0390

CC **C81.27** **Mixed cellularity Hodgkin lymphoma, spleen**
CC Exclusion see Appendix A PDX collection 0391

CC **C81.28** **Mixed cellularity Hodgkin lymphoma, lymph nodes of multiple sites**
CC Exclusion see Appendix A PDX collection 0384

CC **C81.29** **Mixed cellularity Hodgkin lymphoma, extranodal and solid organ sites**
CC Exclusion see Appendix A PDX collection 0384

\+ **C81.3 Lymphocyte depleted Hodgkin lymphoma**
Lymphocyte depleted classical Hodgkin lymphoma

CC **C81.30** **Lymphocyte depleted Hodgkin lymphoma, unspecified site**
CC Exclusion see Appendix A PDX collection 0392

CC **C81.31** **Lymphocyte depleted Hodgkin lymphoma, lymph nodes of head, face, and neck**
CC Exclusion see Appendix A PDX collection 0393

CC **C81.32** **Lymphocyte depleted Hodgkin lymphoma, intrathoracic lymph nodes**
CC Exclusion see Appendix A PDX collection 0394

CC **C81.33** **Lymphocyte depleted Hodgkin lymphoma, intra-abdominal lymph nodes**
CC Exclusion see Appendix A PDX collection 0395

CC **C81.34** **Lymphocyte depleted Hodgkin lymphoma, lymph nodes of axilla and upper limb**
CC Exclusion see Appendix A PDX collection 0396

CC **C81.35** **Lymphocyte depleted Hodgkin lymphoma, lymph nodes of inguinal region and lower limb**
CC Exclusion see Appendix A PDX collection 0397

CC **C81.36** **Lymphocyte depleted Hodgkin lymphoma, intrapelvic lymph nodes**
CC Exclusion see Appendix A PDX collection 0398

CC **C81.37** **Lymphocyte depleted Hodgkin lymphoma, spleen**
CC Exclusion see Appendix A PDX collection 0399

CC **C81.38** **Lymphocyte depleted Hodgkin lymphoma, lymph nodes of multiple sites**
CC Exclusion see Appendix A PDX collection 0400

CC **C81.39** **Lymphocyte depleted Hodgkin lymphoma, extranodal and solid organ sites**
CC Exclusion see Appendix A PDX collection 0392

\+ **C81.4 Lymphocyte-rich Hodgkin lymphoma**
Lymphocyte-rich classical Hodgkin lymphoma
Excludes1: *nodular lymphocyte predominant Hodgkin lymphoma (C81.0-)*

CC **C81.40** **Lymphocyte-rich Hodgkin lymphoma, unspecified site**
CC Exclusion see Appendix A PDX collection 0368

CC **C81.41** **Lymphocyte-rich Hodgkin lymphoma, lymph nodes of head, face, and neck**
CC Exclusion see Appendix A PDX collection 0369

CC **C81.42** **Lymphocyte-rich Hodgkin lymphoma, intrathoracic lymph nodes**
CC Exclusion see Appendix A PDX collection 0370

CC **C81.43** **Lymphocyte-rich Hodgkin lymphoma, intra-abdominal lymph nodes**
CC Exclusion see Appendix A PDX collection 0371

CC **C81.44** **Lymphocyte-rich Hodgkin lymphoma, lymph nodes of axilla and upper limb**
CC Exclusion see Appendix A PDX collection 0372

CC **C81.45** **Lymphocyte-rich Hodgkin lymphoma, lymph nodes of inguinal region and lower limb**
CC Exclusion see Appendix A PDX collection 0373

CC **C81.46** **Lymphocyte-rich Hodgkin lymphoma, intrapelvic lymph nodes**
CC Exclusion see Appendix A PDX collection 0374

CC **C81.47** **Lymphocyte-rich Hodgkin lymphoma, spleen**
CC Exclusion see Appendix A PDX collection 0375

CC **C81.48** **Lymphocyte-rich Hodgkin lymphoma, lymph nodes of multiple sites**
CC Exclusion see Appendix A PDX collection 0368

CC **C81.49** **Lymphocyte-rich Hodgkin lymphoma, extranodal and solid organ sites**
CC Exclusion see Appendix A PDX collection 0368

\+ **C81.7 Other Hodgkin lymphoma**
Classical Hodgkin lymphoma NOS
Other classical Hodgkin lymphoma

CC **C81.70** **Other Hodgkin lymphoma, unspecified site**
CC Exclusion see Appendix A PDX collection 0401

CC **C81.71** **Other Hodgkin lymphoma, lymph nodes of head, face, and neck**
CC Exclusion see Appendix A PDX collection 0402

CC **C81.72** **Other Hodgkin lymphoma, intrathoracic lymph nodes**
CC Exclusion see Appendix A PDX collection 0403

CC **C81.73** **Other Hodgkin lymphoma, intra-abdominal lymph nodes**
CC Exclusion see Appendix A PDX collection 0404

CC **C81.74** **Other Hodgkin lymphoma, lymph nodes of axilla and upper limb**
CC Exclusion see Appendix A PDX collection 0405

CC **C81.75** **Other Hodgkin lymphoma, lymph nodes of inguinal region and lower limb**
CC Exclusion see Appendix A PDX collection 0406

CC **C81.76** **Other Hodgkin lymphoma, intrapelvic lymph nodes**
CC Exclusion see Appendix A PDX collection 0407

CC **C81.77** **Other Hodgkin lymphoma, spleen**
CC Exclusion see Appendix A PDX collection 0408

CC **C81.78** **Other Hodgkin lymphoma, lymph nodes of multiple sites**
CC Exclusion see Appendix A PDX collection 0401

CC **C81.79** **Other Hodgkin lymphoma, extranodal and solid organ sites**
CC Exclusion see Appendix A PDX collection 0401

+ C81.9 Hodgkin lymphoma, unspecified
- CC **C81.90** Hodgkin lymphoma, unspecified, unspecified site
  CC Exclusion see Appendix A PDX collection 0409
- CC **C81.91** Hodgkin lymphoma, unspecified, lymph nodes of head, face, and neck
  CC Exclusion see Appendix A PDX collection 0410
- CC **C81.92** Hodgkin lymphoma, unspecified, intrathoracic lymph nodes
  CC Exclusion see Appendix A PDX collection 0411
- CC **C81.93** Hodgkin lymphoma, unspecified, intra-abdominal lymph nodes
  CC Exclusion see Appendix A PDX collection 0412
- CC **C81.94** Hodgkin lymphoma, unspecified, lymph nodes of axilla and upper limb
  CC Exclusion see Appendix A PDX collection 0413
- CC **C81.95** Hodgkin lymphoma, unspecified, lymph nodes of inguinal region and lower limb
  CC Exclusion see Appendix A PDX collection 0414
- CC **C81.96** Hodgkin lymphoma, unspecified, intrapelvic lymph nodes
  CC Exclusion see Appendix A PDX collection 0415
- CC **C81.97** Hodgkin lymphoma, unspecified, spleen
  CC Exclusion see Appendix A PDX collection 0416
- CC **C81.98** Hodgkin lymphoma, unspecified, lymph nodes of multiple sites
  CC Exclusion see Appendix A PDX collection 0409
- CC **C81.99** Hodgkin lymphoma, unspecified, extranodal and solid organ sites
  No CC Exclusions

C82 Follicular lymphoma

Includes: follicular lymphoma with or without diffuse areas
Excludes1: *mature T/NK-cell lymphomas (C84.-)*
personal history of non-Hodgkin lymphoma (Z85.72)

+ C82.0 Follicular lymphoma grade I
- CC **C82.00** Follicular lymphoma grade I, unspecified site
  CC Exclusion see Appendix A PDX collection 0417
- CC **C82.01** Follicular lymphoma grade I, lymph nodes of head, face, and neck
  CC Exclusion see Appendix A PDX collection 0418
- CC **C82.02** Follicular lymphoma grade I, intrathoracic lymph nodes
  CC Exclusion see Appendix A PDX collection 0419
- CC **C82.03** Follicular lymphoma grade I, intra-abdominal lymph nodes
  CC Exclusion see Appendix A PDX collection 0420
- CC **C82.04** Follicular lymphoma grade I, lymph nodes of axilla and upper limb
  CC Exclusion see Appendix A PDX collection 0421
- CC **C82.05** Follicular lymphoma grade I, lymph nodes of inguinal region and lower limb
  CC Exclusion see Appendix A PDX collection 0422
- CC **C82.06** Follicular lymphoma grade I, intrapelvic lymph nodes
  CC Exclusion see Appendix A PDX collection 0423
- CC **C82.07** Follicular lymphoma grade I, spleen
  CC Exclusion see Appendix A PDX collection 0424
- CC **C82.08** Follicular lymphoma grade I, lymph nodes of multiple sites
  CC Exclusion see Appendix A PDX collection 0425
- CC **C82.09** Follicular lymphoma grade I, extranodal and solid organ sites
  CC Exclusion see Appendix A PDX collection 0417

+ C82.1 Follicular lymphoma grade II
- CC **C82.10** Follicular lymphoma grade II, unspecified site
  CC Exclusion see Appendix A PDX collection 0417
- CC **C82.11** Follicular lymphoma grade II, lymph nodes of head, face, and neck
  CC Exclusion see Appendix A PDX collection 0418
- CC **C82.12** Follicular lymphoma grade II, intrathoracic lymph nodes
  CC Exclusion see Appendix A PDX collection 0419
- CC **C82.13** Follicular lymphoma grade II, intra-abdominal lymph nodes
  CC Exclusion see Appendix A PDX collection 0420
- CC **C82.14** Follicular lymphoma grade II, lymph nodes of axilla and upper limb
  CC Exclusion see Appendix A PDX collection 0421
- CC **C82.15** Follicular lymphoma grade II, lymph nodes of inguinal region and lower limb
  CC Exclusion see Appendix A PDX collection 0422
- CC **C82.16** Follicular lymphoma grade II, intrapelvic lymph nodes
  CC Exclusion see Appendix A PDX collection 0423
- CC **C82.17** Follicular lymphoma grade II, spleen
  CC Exclusion see Appendix A PDX collection 0424
- CC **C82.18** Follicular lymphoma grade II, lymph nodes of multiple sites
  CC Exclusion see Appendix A PDX collection 0425
- CC **C82.19** Follicular lymphoma grade II, extranodal and solid organ sites
  CC Exclusion see Appendix A PDX collection 0417

+ C82.2 Follicular lymphoma grade III, unspecified
- CC **C82.20** Follicular lymphoma grade III, unspecified, unspecified site
  CC Exclusion see Appendix A PDX collection 0417
- CC **C82.21** Follicular lymphoma grade III, unspecified, lymph nodes of head, face, and neck
  CC Exclusion see Appendix A PDX collection 0418
- CC **C82.22** Follicular lymphoma grade III, unspecified, intrathoracic lymph nodes
  CC Exclusion see Appendix A PDX collection 0419
- CC **C82.23** Follicular lymphoma grade III, unspecified, intra-abdominal lymph nodes
  CC Exclusion see Appendix A PDX collection 0420
- CC **C82.24** Follicular lymphoma grade III, unspecified, lymph nodes of axilla and upper limb
  CC Exclusion see Appendix A PDX collection 0421
- CC **C82.25** Follicular lymphoma grade III, unspecified, lymph nodes of inguinal region and lower limb
  CC Exclusion see Appendix A PDX collection 0422
- CC **C82.26** Follicular lymphoma grade III, unspecified, intrapelvic lymph nodes
  CC Exclusion see Appendix A PDX collection 0423
- CC **C82.27** Follicular lymphoma grade III, unspecified, spleen
  CC Exclusion see Appendix A PDX collection 0424
- CC **C82.28** Follicular lymphoma grade III, unspecified, lymph nodes of multiple sites
  CC Exclusion see Appendix A PDX collection 0425
- CC **C82.29** Follicular lymphoma grade III, unspecified, extranodal and solid organ sites
  CC Exclusion see Appendix A PDX collection 0417

+ C82.3 Follicular lymphoma grade IIIa
- CC **C82.30** Follicular lymphoma grade IIIa, unspecified site
  CC Exclusion see Appendix A PDX collection 0417
- CC **C82.31** Follicular lymphoma grade IIIa, lymph nodes of head, face, and neck
  CC Exclusion see Appendix A PDX collection 0418
- CC **C82.32** Follicular lymphoma grade IIIa, intrathoracic lymph nodes
  CC Exclusion see Appendix A PDX collection 0419
- CC **C82.33** Follicular lymphoma grade IIIa, intra-abdominal lymph nodes
  CC Exclusion see Appendix A PDX collection 0420
- CC **C82.34** Follicular lymphoma grade IIIa, lymph nodes of axilla and upper limb
  CC Exclusion see Appendix A PDX collection 0421
- CC **C82.35** Follicular lymphoma grade IIIa, lymph nodes of inguinal region and lower limb
  CC Exclusion see Appendix A PDX collection 0422
- CC **C82.36** Follicular lymphoma grade IIIa, intrapelvic lymph nodes
  CC Exclusion see Appendix A PDX collection 0423
- CC **C82.37** Follicular lymphoma grade IIIa, spleen
  CC Exclusion see Appendix A PDX collection 0424
- CC **C82.38** Follicular lymphoma grade IIIa, lymph nodes of multiple sites
  CC Exclusion see Appendix A PDX collection 0425
- CC **C82.39** Follicular lymphoma grade IIIa, extranodal and solid organ sites
  CC Exclusion see Appendix A PDX collection 0417

+ C82.4 Follicular lymphoma grade IIIb
- CC **C82.40** Follicular lymphoma grade IIIb, unspecified site
  CC Exclusion see Appendix A PDX collection 0417
- CC **C82.41** Follicular lymphoma grade IIIb, lymph nodes of head, face, and neck
  CC Exclusion see Appendix A PDX collection 0418
- CC **C82.42** Follicular lymphoma grade IIIb, intrathoracic lymph nodes
  CC Exclusion see Appendix A PDX collection 0419
- CC **C82.43** Follicular lymphoma grade IIIb, intra-abdominal lymph nodes
  CC Exclusion see Appendix A PDX collection 0420

CC **C82.44** **Follicular lymphoma grade IIIb, lymph nodes of axilla and upper limb**
CC Exclusion see Appendix A PDX collection 0421
CC **C82.45** **Follicular lymphoma grade IIIb, lymph nodes of inguinal region and lower limb**
CC Exclusion see Appendix A PDX collection 0422
CC **C82.46** **Follicular lymphoma grade IIIb, intrapelvic lymph nodes**
CC Exclusion see Appendix A PDX collection 0423
CC **C82.47** **Follicular lymphoma grade IIIb, spleen**
CC Exclusion see Appendix A PDX collection 0424
CC **C82.48** **Follicular lymphoma grade IIIb, lymph nodes of multiple sites**
CC Exclusion see Appendix A PDX collection 0425
CC **C82.49** **Follicular lymphoma grade IIIb, extranodal and solid organ sites**
CC Exclusion see Appendix A PDX collection 0417
+ **C82.5** **Diffuse follicle center lymphoma**
CC **C82.50** **Diffuse follicle center lymphoma, unspecified site**
CC Exclusion see Appendix A PDX collection 0426
CC **C82.51** **Diffuse follicle center lymphoma, lymph nodes of head, face, and neck**
CC Exclusion see Appendix A PDX collection 0427
CC **C82.52** **Diffuse follicle center lymphoma, intrathoracic lymph nodes**
CC Exclusion see Appendix A PDX collection 0428
CC **C82.53** **Diffuse follicle center lymphoma, intra-abdominal lymph nodes**
CC Exclusion see Appendix A PDX collection 0429
CC **C82.54** **Diffuse follicle center lymphoma, lymph nodes of axilla and upper limb**
CC Exclusion see Appendix A PDX collection 0430
CC **C82.55** **Diffuse follicle center lymphoma, lymph nodes of inguinal region and lower limb**
CC Exclusion see Appendix A PDX collection 0431
CC **C82.56** **Diffuse follicle center lymphoma, intrapelvic lymph nodes**
CC Exclusion see Appendix A PDX collection 0432
CC **C82.57** **Diffuse follicle center lymphoma, spleen**
CC Exclusion see Appendix A PDX collection 0433
CC **C82.58** **Diffuse follicle center lymphoma, lymph nodes of multiple sites**
CC Exclusion see Appendix A PDX collection 0434
CC **C82.59** **Diffuse follicle center lymphoma, extranodal and solid organ sites**
CC Exclusion see Appendix A PDX collection 0426
+ **C82.6** **Cutaneous follicle center lymphoma**
CC **C82.60** **Cutaneous follicle center lymphoma, unspecified site**
CC Exclusion see Appendix A PDX collection 0417
CC **C82.61** **Cutaneous follicle center lymphoma, lymph nodes of head, face, and neck**
CC Exclusion see Appendix A PDX collection 0418
CC **C82.62** **Cutaneous follicle center lymphoma, intrathoracic lymph nodes**
CC Exclusion see Appendix A PDX collection 0419
CC **C82.63** **Cutaneous follicle center lymphoma, intra-abdominal lymph nodes**
CC Exclusion see Appendix A PDX collection 0420
CC **C82.64** **Cutaneous follicle center lymphoma, lymph nodes of axilla and upper limb**
CC Exclusion see Appendix A PDX collection 0421
CC **C82.65** **Cutaneous follicle center lymphoma, lymph nodes of inguinal region and lower limb**
CC Exclusion see Appendix A PDX collection 0422
CC **C82.66** **Cutaneous follicle center lymphoma, intrapelvic lymph nodes**
CC Exclusion see Appendix A PDX collection 0423
CC **C82.67** **Cutaneous follicle center lymphoma, spleen**
CC Exclusion see Appendix A PDX collection 0424
CC **C82.68** **Cutaneous follicle center lymphoma, lymph nodes of multiple sites**
CC Exclusion see Appendix A PDX collection 0425
CC **C82.69** **Cutaneous follicle center lymphoma, extranodal and solid organ sites**
CC Exclusion see Appendix A PDX collection 0417
+ **C82.8** **Other types of follicular lymphoma**
CC **C82.80** **Other types of follicular lymphoma, unspecified site**
CC Exclusion see Appendix A PDX collection 0417
CC **C82.81** **Other types of follicular lymphoma, lymph nodes of head, face, and neck**
CC Exclusion see Appendix A PDX collection 0418
CC **C82.82** **Other types of follicular lymphoma, intrathoracic lymph nodes**
CC Exclusion see Appendix A PDX collection 0419
CC **C82.83** **Other types of follicular lymphoma, intra-abdominal lymph nodes**
CC Exclusion see Appendix A PDX collection 0420
CC **C82.84** **Other types of follicular lymphoma, lymph nodes of axilla and upper limb**
CC Exclusion see Appendix A PDX collection 0421
CC **C82.85** **Other types of follicular lymphoma, lymph nodes of inguinal region and lower limb**
CC Exclusion see Appendix A PDX collection 0422
CC **C82.86** **Other types of follicular lymphoma, intrapelvic lymph nodes**
CC Exclusion see Appendix A PDX collection 0423
CC **C82.87** **Other types of follicular lymphoma, spleen**
CC Exclusion see Appendix A PDX collection 0424
CC **C82.88** **Other types of follicular lymphoma, lymph nodes of multiple sites**
CC Exclusion see Appendix A PDX collection 0425
CC **C82.89** **Other types of follicular lymphoma, extranodal and solid organ sites**
CC Exclusion see Appendix A PDX collection 0417
+ **C82.9** **Follicular lymphoma, unspecified**
CC **C82.90** **Follicular lymphoma, unspecified, unspecified site**
CC Exclusion see Appendix A PDX collection 0417
CC **C82.91** **Follicular lymphoma, unspecified, lymph nodes of head, face, and neck**
CC Exclusion see Appendix A PDX collection 0418
CC **C82.92** **Follicular lymphoma, unspecified, intrathoracic lymph nodes**
CC Exclusion see Appendix A PDX collection 0419
CC **C82.93** **Follicular lymphoma, unspecified, intra-abdominal lymph nodes**
CC Exclusion see Appendix A PDX collection 0420
CC **C82.94** **Follicular lymphoma, unspecified, lymph nodes of axilla and upper limb**
CC Exclusion see Appendix A PDX collection 0421
CC **C82.95** **Follicular lymphoma, unspecified, lymph nodes of inguinal region and lower limb**
CC Exclusion see Appendix A PDX collection 0422
CC **C82.96** **Follicular lymphoma, unspecified, intrapelvic lymph nodes**
CC Exclusion see Appendix A PDX collection 0423
CC **C82.97** **Follicular lymphoma, unspecified, spleen**
CC Exclusion see Appendix A PDX collection 0424
CC **C82.98** **Follicular lymphoma, unspecified, lymph nodes of multiple sites**
CC Exclusion see Appendix A PDX collection 0425
CC **C82.99** **Follicular lymphoma, unspecified, extranodal and solid organ sites**
CC Exclusion see Appendix A PDX collection 0417

C83 Non-follicular lymphoma

Excludes1: *personal history of non-Hodgkin lymphoma (Z85.72)*

+ **C83.0** **Small cell B-cell lymphoma**
Lymphoplasmacytic lymphoma
Nodal marginal zone lymphoma
Non-leukemic variant of B-CLL
Splenic marginal zone lymphoma
Excludes1: *chronic lymphocytic leukemia (C91.1)*
mature T/NK-cell lymphomas (C84.-)
Waldenström macroglobulinemia (C88.0)
CC **C83.00** **Small cell B-cell lymphoma, unspecified site**
CC Exclusion see Appendix A PDX collection 0435
CC **C83.01** **Small cell B-cell lymphoma, lymph nodes of head, face, and neck**
CC Exclusion see Appendix A PDX collection 0436
CC **C83.02** **Small cell B-cell lymphoma, intrathoracic lymph nodes**
CC Exclusion see Appendix A PDX collection 0437
CC **C83.03** **Small cell B-cell lymphoma, intra-abdominal lymph nodes**
CC Exclusion see Appendix A PDX collection 0438
CC **C83.04** **Small cell B-cell lymphoma, lymph nodes of axilla and upper limb**
CC Exclusion see Appendix A PDX collection 0439
CC **C83.05** **Small cell B-cell lymphoma, lymph nodes of inguinal region and lower limb**
CC Exclusion see Appendix A PDX collection 0440
CC **C83.06** **Small cell B-cell lymphoma, intrapelvic lymph nodes**
CC Exclusion see Appendix A PDX collection 0441
CC **C83.07** **Small cell B-cell lymphoma, spleen**
CC Exclusion see Appendix A PDX collection 0442
CC **C83.08** **Small cell B-cell lymphoma, lymph nodes of multiple sites**
CC Exclusion see Appendix A PDX collection 0435

CC **C83.09 Small cell B-cell lymphoma, extranodal and solid organ sites**
CC Exclusion see Appendix A PDX collection 0435

+ **C83.1 Mantle cell lymphoma**
Centrocytic lymphoma
Malignant lymphomatous polyposis

CC **C83.10 Mantle cell lymphoma, unspecified site**
CC Exclusion see Appendix A PDX collection 0426

CC **C83.11 Mantle cell lymphoma, lymph nodes of head, face, and neck**
CC Exclusion see Appendix A PDX collection 0427

CC **C83.12 Mantle cell lymphoma, intrathoracic lymph nodes**
CC Exclusion see Appendix A PDX collection 0428

CC **C83.13 Mantle cell lymphoma, intra-abdominal lymph nodes**
CC Exclusion see Appendix A PDX collection 0429

CC **C83.14 Mantle cell lymphoma, lymph nodes of axilla and upper limb**
CC Exclusion see Appendix A PDX collection 0430

CC **C83.15 Mantle cell lymphoma, lymph nodes of inguinal region and lower limb**
CC Exclusion see Appendix A PDX collection 0431

CC **C83.16 Mantle cell lymphoma, intrapelvic lymph nodes**
CC Exclusion see Appendix A PDX collection 0432

CC **C83.17 Mantle cell lymphoma, spleen**
CC Exclusion see Appendix A PDX collection 0433

CC **C83.18 Mantle cell lymphoma, lymph nodes of multiple sites**
CC Exclusion see Appendix A PDX collection 0434

CC **C83.19 Mantle cell lymphoma, extranodal and solid organ sites**
CC Exclusion see Appendix A PDX collection 0426

+ **C83.3 Diffuse large B-cell lymphoma**
Anaplastic diffuse large B-cell lymphoma
CD30-positive diffuse large B-cell lymphoma
Centroblastic diffuse large B-cell lymphoma
Diffuse large B-cell lymphoma, subtype not specified
Immunoblastic diffuse large B-cell lymphoma
Plasmablastic diffuse large B-cell lymphoma
Diffuse large B-cell lymphoma, subtype not specified
T-cell rich diffuse large B-cell lymphoma
Excludes1: *mediastinal (thymic) large B-cell lymphoma (C85.2-)*
mature T/NK-cell lymphomas (C84.-)

CC **C83.30 Diffuse large B-cell lymphoma, unspecified site**
CC Exclusion see Appendix A PDX collection 0443

CC **C83.31 Diffuse large B-cell lymphoma, lymph nodes of head, face, and neck**
CC Exclusion see Appendix A PDX collection 0444

CC **C83.32 Diffuse large B-cell lymphoma, intrathoracic lymph nodes**
CC Exclusion see Appendix A PDX collection 0445

CC **C83.33 Diffuse large B-cell lymphoma, intra-abdominal lymph nodes**
CC Exclusion see Appendix A PDX collection 0446

CC **C83.34 Diffuse large B-cell lymphoma, lymph nodes of axilla and upper limb**
CC Exclusion see Appendix A PDX collection 0447

CC **C83.35 Diffuse large B-cell lymphoma, lymph nodes of inguinal region and lower limb**
CC Exclusion see Appendix A PDX collection 0448

CC **C83.36 Diffuse large B-cell lymphoma, intrapelvic lymph nodes**
CC Exclusion see Appendix A PDX collection 0449

CC **C83.37 Diffuse large B-cell lymphoma, spleen**
CC Exclusion see Appendix A PDX collection 0450

CC **C83.38 Diffuse large B-cell lymphoma, lymph nodes of multiple sites**
CC Exclusion see Appendix A PDX collection 0443

CC **C83.39 Diffuse large B-cell lymphoma, extranodal and solid organ sites**
CC Exclusion see Appendix A PDX collection 0443

+ **C83.5 Lymphoblastic (diffuse) lymphoma**
B-precursor lymphoma
Lymphoblastic B-cell lymphoma
Lymphoblastic lymphoma NOS
Lymphoblastic T-cell lymphoma
T-precursor lymphoma

CC **C83.50 Lymphoblastic (diffuse) lymphoma, unspecified site**
CC Exclusion see Appendix A PDX collection 0451

CC **C83.51 Lymphoblastic (diffuse) lymphoma, lymph nodes of head, face, and neck**
CC Exclusion see Appendix A PDX collection 0452

CC **C83.52 Lymphoblastic (diffuse) lymphoma, intrathoracic lymph nodes**
CC Exclusion see Appendix A PDX collection 0453

CC **C83.53 Lymphoblastic (diffuse) lymphoma, intra-abdominal lymph nodes**
CC Exclusion see Appendix A PDX collection 0454

CC **C83.54 Lymphoblastic (diffuse) lymphoma, lymph nodes of axilla and upper limb**
CC Exclusion see Appendix A PDX collection 0455

CC **C83.55 Lymphoblastic (diffuse) lymphoma, lymph nodes of inguinal region and lower limb**
CC Exclusion see Appendix A PDX collection 0456

CC **C83.56 Lymphoblastic (diffuse) lymphoma, intrapelvic lymph nodes**
CC Exclusion see Appendix A PDX collection 0457

CC **C83.57 Lymphoblastic (diffuse) lymphoma, spleen**
CC Exclusion see Appendix A PDX collection 0458

CC **C83.58 Lymphoblastic (diffuse) lymphoma, lymph nodes of multiple sites**
CC Exclusion see Appendix A PDX collection 0451

CC **C83.59 Lymphoblastic (diffuse) lymphoma, extranodal and solid organ sites**
CC Exclusion see Appendix A PDX collection 0451

+ **C83.7 Burkitt lymphoma**
Atypical Burkitt lymphoma
Burkitt-like lymphoma
Excludes1: *mature B-cell leukemia Burkitt type (C91.A-)*

CC **C83.70 Burkitt lymphoma, unspecified site**
CC Exclusion see Appendix A PDX collection 0459

CC **C83.71 Burkitt lymphoma, lymph nodes of head, face, and neck**
CC Exclusion see Appendix A PDX collection 0460

CC **C83.72 Burkitt lymphoma, intrathoracic lymph nodes**
CC Exclusion see Appendix A PDX collection 0461

CC **C83.73 Burkitt lymphoma, intra-abdominal lymph nodes**
CC Exclusion see Appendix A PDX collection 0462

CC **C83.74 Burkitt lymphoma, lymph nodes of axilla and upper limb**
CC Exclusion see Appendix A PDX collection 0463

CC **C83.75 Burkitt lymphoma, lymph nodes of inguinal region and lower limb**
CC Exclusion see Appendix A PDX collection 0464

CC **C83.76 Burkitt lymphoma, intrapelvic lymph nodes**
CC Exclusion see Appendix A PDX collection 0465

CC **C83.77 Burkitt lymphoma, spleen**
CC Exclusion see Appendix A PDX collection 0466

CC **C83.78 Burkitt lymphoma, lymph nodes of multiple sites**
CC Exclusion see Appendix A PDX collection 0459

CC **C83.79 Burkitt lymphoma, extranodal and solid organ sites**
CC Exclusion see Appendix A PDX collection 0459

+ **C83.8 Other non-follicular lymphoma**
Intravascular large B-cell lymphoma
Lymphoid granulomatosis
Primary effusion B-cell lymphoma
Excludes1: *mediastinal (thymic) large B-cell lymphoma (C85.2-)*
T-cell rich B-cell lymphoma (C83.3-)

CC **C83.80 Other non-follicular lymphoma, unspecified site**
CC Exclusion see Appendix A PDX collection 0435

CC **C83.81 Other non-follicular lymphoma, lymph nodes of head, face, and neck**
CC Exclusion see Appendix A PDX collection 0436

CC **C83.82 Other non-follicular lymphoma, intrathoracic lymph nodes**
CC Exclusion see Appendix A PDX collection 0437

CC **C83.83 Other non-follicular lymphoma, intra-abdominal lymph nodes**
CC Exclusion see Appendix A PDX collection 0438

CC **C83.84 Other non-follicular lymphoma, lymph nodes of axilla and upper limb**
CC Exclusion see Appendix A PDX collection 0439

CC **C83.85 Other non-follicular lymphoma, lymph nodes of inguinal region and lower limb**
CC Exclusion see Appendix A PDX collection 0440

CC **C83.86 Other non-follicular lymphoma, intrapelvic lymph nodes**
CC Exclusion see Appendix A PDX collection 0441

CC **C83.87 Other non-follicular lymphoma, spleen**
CC Exclusion see Appendix A PDX collection 0442

CC **C83.88 Other non-follicular lymphoma, lymph nodes of multiple sites**
CC Exclusion see Appendix A PDX collection 0435

CC **C83.89** **Other non-follicular lymphoma, extranodal and solid organ sites**
CC Exclusion see Appendix A PDX collection 0435

\+ **C83.9 Non-follicular (diffuse) lymphoma, unspecified**

CC **C83.90** **Non-follicular (diffuse) lymphoma, unspecified, unspecified site**
CC Exclusion see Appendix A PDX collection 0435

CC **C83.91** **Non-follicular (diffuse) lymphoma, unspecified, lymph nodes of head, face, and neck**
CC Exclusion see Appendix A PDX collection 0436

CC **C83.92** **Non-follicular (diffuse) lymphoma, unspecified, intrathoracic lymph nodes**
CC Exclusion see Appendix A PDX collection 0437

CC **C83.93** **Non-follicular (diffuse) lymphoma, unspecified, intra-abdominal lymph nodes**
CC Exclusion see Appendix A PDX collection 0438

CC **C83.94** **Non-follicular (diffuse) lymphoma, unspecified, lymph nodes of axilla and upper limb**
CC Exclusion see Appendix A PDX collection 0439

CC **C83.95** **Non-follicular (diffuse) lymphoma, unspecified, lymph nodes of inguinal region and lower limb**
CC Exclusion see Appendix A PDX collection 0440

CC **C83.96** **Non-follicular (diffuse) lymphoma, unspecified, intrapelvic lymph nodes**
CC Exclusion see Appendix A PDX collection 0441

CC **C83.97** **Non-follicular (diffuse) lymphoma, unspecified, spleen**
CC Exclusion see Appendix A PDX collection 0442

CC **C83.98** **Non-follicular (diffuse) lymphoma, unspecified, lymph nodes of multiple sites**
CC Exclusion see Appendix A PDX collection 0435

CC **C83.99** **Non-follicular (diffuse) lymphoma, unspecified, extranodal and solid organ sites**
CC Exclusion see Appendix A PDX collection 0435

C84 Mature T/NK-cell lymphomas

Excludes1: *personal history of non-Hodgkin lymphoma (Z85.72)*

\+ **C84.0 Mycosis fungoides**

Excludes1: *peripheral T-cell lymphoma, not classified (C84.4-)*

CC **C84.00** **Mycosis fungoides, unspecified site**
CC Exclusion see Appendix A PDX collection 0467

CC **C84.01** **Mycosis fungoides, lymph nodes of head, face, and neck**
CC Exclusion see Appendix A PDX collection 0468

CC **C84.02** **Mycosis fungoides, intrathoracic lymph nodes**
CC Exclusion see Appendix A PDX collection 0469

CC **C84.03** **Mycosis fungoides, intra-abdominal lymph nodes**
CC Exclusion see Appendix A PDX collection 0470

CC **C84.04** **Mycosis fungoides, lymph nodes of axilla and upper limb**
CC Exclusion see Appendix A PDX collection 0471

CC **C84.05** **Mycosis fungoides, lymph nodes of inguinal region and lower limb**
CC Exclusion see Appendix A PDX collection 0472

CC **C84.06** **Mycosis fungoides, intrapelvic lymph nodes**
CC Exclusion see Appendix A PDX collection 0473

CC **C84.07** **Mycosis fungoides, spleen**
CC Exclusion see Appendix A PDX collection 0474

CC **C84.08** **Mycosis fungoides, lymph nodes of multiple sites**
CC Exclusion see Appendix A PDX collection 0475

CC **C84.09** **Mycosis fungoides, extranodal and solid organ sites**
CC Exclusion see Appendix A PDX collection 0467

\+ **C84.1 Sézary disease**

CC **C84.10** **Sézary disease, unspecified site**
CC Exclusion see Appendix A PDX collection 0476

CC **C84.11** **Sézary disease, lymph nodes of head, face, and neck**
CC Exclusion see Appendix A PDX collection 0477

CC **C84.12** **Sézary disease, intrathoracic lymph nodes**
CC Exclusion see Appendix A PDX collection 0478

CC **C84.13** **Sézary disease, intra-abdominal lymph nodes**
CC Exclusion see Appendix A PDX collection 0479

CC **C84.14** **Sézary disease, lymph nodes of axilla and upper limb**
CC Exclusion see Appendix A PDX collection 0480

CC **C84.15** **Sézary disease, lymph nodes of inguinal region and lower limb**
CC Exclusion see Appendix A PDX collection 0481

CC **C84.16** **Sézary disease, intrapelvic lymph nodes**
CC Exclusion see Appendix A PDX collection 0482

CC **C84.17** **Sézary disease, spleen**
CC Exclusion see Appendix A PDX collection 0483

CC **C84.18** **Sézary disease, lymph nodes of multiple sites**
CC Exclusion see Appendix A PDX collection 0484

CC **C84.19** **Sézary disease, extranodal and solid organ sites**
CC Exclusion see Appendix A PDX collection 0476

\+ **C84.4 Peripheral T-cell lymphoma, not classified**

Lennert's lymphoma
Lymphoepithelioid lymphoma
Mature T-cell lymphoma, not elsewhere classified

CC **C84.40** **Peripheral T-cell lymphoma, not classified, unspecified site**
CC Exclusion see Appendix A PDX collection 0426

CC **C84.41** **Peripheral T-cell lymphoma, not classified, lymph nodes of head, face, and neck**
CC Exclusion see Appendix A PDX collection 0427

CC **C84.42** **Peripheral T-cell lymphoma, not classified, intrathoracic lymph nodes**
CC Exclusion see Appendix A PDX collection 0428

CC **C84.43** **Peripheral T-cell lymphoma, not classified, intra-abdominal lymph nodes**
CC Exclusion see Appendix A PDX collection 0429

CC **C84.44** **Peripheral T-cell lymphoma, not classified, lymph nodes of axilla and upper limb**
CC Exclusion see Appendix A PDX collection 0430

CC **C84.45** **Peripheral T-cell lymphoma, not classified, lymph nodes of inguinal region and lower limb**
CC Exclusion see Appendix A PDX collection 0431

CC **C84.46** **Peripheral T-cell lymphoma, not classified, intrapelvic lymph nodes**
CC Exclusion see Appendix A PDX collection 0432

CC **C84.47** **Peripheral T-cell lymphoma, not classified, spleen**
CC Exclusion see Appendix A PDX collection 0433

CC **C84.48** **Peripheral T-cell lymphoma, not classified, lymph nodes of multiple sites**
CC Exclusion see Appendix A PDX collection 0434

CC **C84.49** **Peripheral T-cell lymphoma, not classified, extranodal and solid organ sites**
CC Exclusion see Appendix A PDX collection 0426

\+ **C84.6 Anaplastic large cell lymphoma, ALK-positive**

Anaplastic large cell lymphoma, CD30-positive

CC **C84.60** **Anaplastic large cell lymphoma, ALK-positive, unspecified site**
CC Exclusion see Appendix A PDX collection 0426

CC **C84.61** **Anaplastic large cell lymphoma, ALK-positive, lymph nodes of head, face, and neck**
CC Exclusion see Appendix A PDX collection 0427

CC **C84.62** **Anaplastic large cell lymphoma, ALK-positive, intrathoracic lymph nodes**
CC Exclusion see Appendix A PDX collection 0428

CC **C84.63** **Anaplastic large cell lymphoma, ALK-positive, intra-abdominal lymph nodes**
CC Exclusion see Appendix A PDX collection 0429

CC **C84.64** **Anaplastic large cell lymphoma, ALK-positive, lymph nodes of axilla and upper limb**
CC Exclusion see Appendix A PDX collection 0430

CC **C84.65** **Anaplastic large cell lymphoma, ALK-positive, lymph nodes of inguinal region and lower limb**
CC Exclusion see Appendix A PDX collection 0431

CC **C84.66** **Anaplastic large cell lymphoma, ALK-positive, intrapelvic lymph nodes**
CC Exclusion see Appendix A PDX collection 0432

CC **C84.67** **Anaplastic large cell lymphoma, ALK-positive, spleen**
CC Exclusion see Appendix A PDX collection 0433

CC **C84.68** **Anaplastic large cell lymphoma, ALK-positive, lymph nodes of multiple sites**
CC Exclusion see Appendix A PDX collection 0434

CC **C84.69** **Anaplastic large cell lymphoma, ALK-positive, extranodal and solid organ sites**
CC Exclusion see Appendix A PDX collection 0426

\+ **C84.7 Anaplastic large cell lymphoma, ALK-negative**

Excludes1: *primary cutaneous CD30-positive T-cell proliferations (C86.6-)*

CC **C84.70** **Anaplastic large cell lymphoma, ALK-negative, unspecified site**
CC Exclusion see Appendix A PDX collection 0426

CC **C84.71** **Anaplastic large cell lymphoma, ALK-negative, lymph nodes of head, face, and neck**
CC Exclusion see Appendix A PDX collection 0427

CC **C84.72** **Anaplastic large cell lymphoma, ALK-negative, intrathoracic lymph nodes**
CC Exclusion see Appendix A PDX collection 0428

CC **C84.73** **Anaplastic large cell lymphoma, ALK-negative, intra-abdominal lymph nodes**
CC Exclusion see Appendix A PDX collection 0429

CC **C84.74** **Anaplastic large cell lymphoma, ALK-negative, lymph nodes of axilla and upper limb**
CC Exclusion see Appendix A PDX collection 0430

CC **C84.75** **Anaplastic large cell lymphoma, ALK-negative, lymph nodes of inguinal region and lower limb**
CC Exclusion see Appendix A PDX collection 0431

CC **C84.76** **Anaplastic large cell lymphoma, ALK-negative, intrapelvic lymph nodes**
CC Exclusion see Appendix A PDX collection 0432

CC **C84.77** **Anaplastic large cell lymphoma, ALK-negative, spleen**
CC Exclusion see Appendix A PDX collection 0433

CC **C84.78** **Anaplastic large cell lymphoma, ALK-negative, lymph nodes of multiple sites**
CC Exclusion see Appendix A PDX collection 0434

CC **C84.79** **Anaplastic large cell lymphoma, ALK-negative, extranodal and solid organ sites**
CC Exclusion see Appendix A PDX collection 0426

+ **C84.A Cutaneous T-cell lymphoma, unspecified**

CC **C84.A0** **Cutaneous T-cell lymphoma, unspecified, unspecified site**
CC Exclusion see Appendix A PDX collection 0426

CC **C84.A1** **Cutaneous T-cell lymphoma, unspecified lymph nodes of head, face, and neck**
CC Exclusion see Appendix A PDX collection 0427

CC **C84.A2** **Cutaneous T-cell lymphoma, unspecified, intrathoracic lymph nodes**
CC Exclusion see Appendix A PDX collection 0428

CC **C84.A3** **Cutaneous T-cell lymphoma, unspecified, intra-abdominal lymph nodes**
CC Exclusion see Appendix A PDX collection 0429

CC **C84.A4** **Cutaneous T-cell lymphoma, unspecified, lymph nodes of axilla and upper limb**
CC Exclusion see Appendix A PDX collection 0430

CC **C84.A5** **Cutaneous T-cell lymphoma, unspecified, lymph nodes of inguinal region and lower limb**
CC Exclusion see Appendix A PDX collection 0431

CC **C84.A6** **Cutaneous T-cell lymphoma, unspecified, intrapelvic lymph nodes**
CC Exclusion see Appendix A PDX collection 0432

CC **C84.A7** **Cutaneous T-cell lymphoma, unspecified, spleen**
CC Exclusion see Appendix A PDX collection 0433

CC **C84.A8** **Cutaneous T-cell lymphoma, unspecified, lymph nodes of multiple sites**
CC Exclusion see Appendix A PDX collection 0434

CC **C84.A9** **Cutaneous T-cell lymphoma, unspecified, extranodal and solid organ sites**
CC Exclusion see Appendix A PDX collection 0426

+ **C84.Z Other mature T/NK-cell lymphomas**

NOTE If T-cell lineage or involvement is mentioned in conjunction with a specific lymphoma, code to the more specific description.

Excludes1: *angioimmunoblastic T-cell lymphoma (C86.5)*
blastic NK-cell lymphoma (C86.4)
enteropathy-type T-cell lymphoma (C86.2)
extranodal NK-cell lymphoma, nasal type (C86.0)
hepatosplenic T-cell lymphoma (C86.1)
primary cutaneous CD30-positive T-cell proliferations (C86.6)
subcutaneous panniculitis-like T-cell lymphoma (C86.3)
T-cell leukemia (C91.1-)

CC **C84.Z0** **Other mature T/NK-cell lymphomas, unspecified site**
CC Exclusion see Appendix A PDX collection 0426

CC **C84.Z1** **Other mature T/NK-cell lymphomas, lymph nodes of head, face, and neck**
CC Exclusion see Appendix A PDX collection 0427

CC **C84.Z2** **Other mature T/NK-cell lymphomas, intrathoracic lymph nodes**
CC Exclusion see Appendix A PDX collection 0428

CC **C84.Z3** **Other mature T/NK-cell lymphomas, intra-abdominal lymph nodes**
CC Exclusion see Appendix A PDX collection 0429

CC **C84.Z4** **Other mature T/NK-cell lymphomas, lymph nodes of axilla and upper limb**
CC Exclusion see Appendix A PDX collection 0430

CC **C84.Z5** **Other mature T/NK-cell lymphomas, lymph nodes of inguinal region and lower limb**
CC Exclusion see Appendix A PDX collection 0431

CC **C84.Z6** **Other mature T/NK-cell lymphomas, intrapelvic lymph nodes**
CC Exclusion see Appendix A PDX collection 0432

CC **C84.Z7** **Other mature T/NK-cell lymphomas, spleen**
CC Exclusion see Appendix A PDX collection 0433

CC **C84.Z8** **Other mature T/NK-cell lymphomas, lymph nodes of multiple sites**
CC Exclusion see Appendix A PDX collection 0434

CC **C84.Z9** **Other mature T/NK-cell lymphomas, extranodal and solid organ sites**
CC Exclusion see Appendix A PDX collection 0426

+ **C84.9 Mature T/NK-cell lymphomas, unspecified**

NK/T cell lymphoma NOS

Excludes1: *mature T-cell lymphoma, not elsewhere classified (C84.4-)*

CC **C84.90** **Mature T/NK-cell lymphomas, unspecified, unspecified site**
CC Exclusion see Appendix A PDX collection 0426

CC **C84.91** **Mature T/NK-cell lymphomas, unspecified, lymph nodes of head, face, and neck**
CC Exclusion see Appendix A PDX collection 0427

CC **C84.92** **Mature T/NK-cell lymphomas, unspecified, intrathoracic lymph nodes**
CC Exclusion see Appendix A PDX collection 0428

CC **C84.93** **Mature T/NK-cell lymphomas, unspecified, intra-abdominal lymph nodes**
CC Exclusion see Appendix A PDX collection 0429

CC **C84.94** **Mature T/NK-cell lymphomas, unspecified, lymph nodes of axilla and upper limb**
CC Exclusion see Appendix A PDX collection 0430

CC **C84.95** **Mature T/NK-cell lymphomas, unspecified, lymph nodes of inguinal region and lower limb**
CC Exclusion see Appendix A PDX collection 0431

CC **C84.96** **Mature T/NK-cell lymphomas, unspecified, intrapelvic lymph nodes**
CC Exclusion see Appendix A PDX collection 0432

CC **C84.97** **Mature T/NK-cell lymphomas, unspecified, spleen**
CC Exclusion see Appendix A PDX collection 0433

CC **C84.98** **Mature T/NK-cell lymphomas, unspecified, lymph nodes of multiple sites**
CC Exclusion see Appendix A PDX collection 0434

CC **C84.99** **Mature T/NK-cell lymphomas, unspecified, extranodal and solid organ sites**
CC Exclusion see Appendix A PDX collection 0426

C85 Other specified and unspecified types of non-Hodgkin lymphoma

Excludes1: *other specified types of T/NK-cell lymphoma (C86.-)*
personal history of non-Hodgkin lymphoma (Z85.72)

+ **C85.1 Unspecified B-cell lymphoma**

NOTE If B-cell lineage or involvement is mentioned in conjunction with a specific lymphoma, code to the more specific description.

CC **C85.10** **Unspecified B-cell lymphoma, unspecified site**
CC Exclusion see Appendix A PDX collection 0426

CC **C85.11** **Unspecified B-cell lymphoma, lymph nodes of head, face, and neck**
CC Exclusion see Appendix A PDX collection 0427

CC **C85.12** **Unspecified B-cell lymphoma, intrathoracic lymph nodes**
CC Exclusion see Appendix A PDX collection 0428

CC **C85.13** **Unspecified B-cell lymphoma, intra-abdominal lymph nodes**
CC Exclusion see Appendix A PDX collection 0429

CC **C85.14** **Unspecified B-cell lymphoma, lymph nodes of axilla and upper limb**
CC Exclusion see Appendix A PDX collection 0430

CC **C85.15** **Unspecified B-cell lymphoma, lymph nodes of inguinal region and lower limb**
CC Exclusion see Appendix A PDX collection 0431

CC **C85.16** **Unspecified B-cell lymphoma, intrapelvic lymph nodes**
CC Exclusion see Appendix A PDX collection 0432

CC **C85.17** **Unspecified B-cell lymphoma, spleen**
CC Exclusion see Appendix A PDX collection 0433

CC **C85.18** **Unspecified B-cell lymphoma, lymph nodes of multiple sites**
CC Exclusion see Appendix A PDX collection 0434

CC **C85.19** **Unspecified B-cell lymphoma, extranodal and solid organ sites**
CC Exclusion see Appendix A PDX collection 0426

+ **C85.2 Mediastinal (thymic) large B-cell lymphoma**

CC **C85.20** **Mediastinal (thymic) large B-cell lymphoma, unspecified site**
CC Exclusion see Appendix A PDX collection 0426

CC **C85.21** **Mediastinal (thymic) large B-cell lymphoma, lymph nodes of head, face, and neck**
CC Exclusion see Appendix A PDX collection 0427

CC **C85.22** **Mediastinal (thymic) large B-cell lymphoma, intrathoracic lymph nodes**
CC Exclusion see Appendix A PDX collection 0428

CC **C85.23** **Mediastinal (thymic) large B-cell lymphoma, intra-abdominal lymph nodes**
CC Exclusion see Appendix A PDX collection 0429

CC **C85.24** **Mediastinal (thymic) large B-cell lymphoma, lymph nodes of axilla and upper limb**
CC Exclusion see Appendix A PDX collection 0430

CC **C85.25** **Mediastinal (thymic) large B-cell lymphoma, lymph nodes of inguinal region and lower limb**
CC Exclusion see Appendix A PDX collection 0431

CC **C85.26** **Mediastinal (thymic) large B-cell lymphoma, intrapelvic lymph nodes**
CC Exclusion see Appendix A PDX collection 0432

CC **C85.27** **Mediastinal (thymic) large B-cell lymphoma, spleen**
CC Exclusion see Appendix A PDX collection 0433

CC **C85.28** **Mediastinal (thymic) large B-cell lymphoma, lymph nodes of multiple sites**
CC Exclusion see Appendix A PDX collection 0434

CC **C85.29** **Mediastinal (thymic) large B-cell lymphoma, extranodal and solid organ sites**
CC Exclusion see Appendix A PDX collection 0426

+ **C85.8** **Other specified types of non-Hodgkin lymphoma**

CC **C85.80** **Other specified types of non-Hodgkin lymphoma, unspecified site**
CC Exclusion see Appendix A PDX collection 0426

CC **C85.81** **Other specified types of non-Hodgkin lymphoma, lymph nodes of head, face, and neck**
CC Exclusion see Appendix A PDX collection 0427

CC **C85.82** **Other specified types of non-Hodgkin lymphoma, intrathoracic lymph nodes**
CC Exclusion see Appendix A PDX collection 0428

CC **C85.83** **Other specified types of non-Hodgkin lymphoma, intra-abdominal lymph nodes**
CC Exclusion see Appendix A PDX collection 0429

CC **C85.84** **Other specified types of non-Hodgkin lymphoma, lymph nodes of axilla and upper limb**
CC Exclusion see Appendix A PDX collection 0430

CC **C85.85** **Other specified types of non-Hodgkin lymphoma, lymph nodes of inguinal region and lower limb**
CC Exclusion see Appendix A PDX collection 0431

CC **C85.86** **Other specified types of non-Hodgkin lymphoma, intrapelvic lymph nodes**
CC Exclusion see Appendix A PDX collection 0432

CC **C85.87** **Other specified types of non-Hodgkin lymphoma, spleen**
CC Exclusion see Appendix A PDX collection 0433

CC **C85.88** **Other specified types of non-Hodgkin lymphoma, lymph nodes of multiple sites**
CC Exclusion see Appendix A PDX collection 0434

CC **C85.89** **Other specified types of non-Hodgkin lymphoma, extranodal and solid organ sites**
CC Exclusion see Appendix A PDX collection 0426

+ **C85.9** **Non-Hodgkin lymphoma, unspecified**
Lymphoma NOS
Malignant lymphoma NOS
Non-Hodgkin lymphoma NOS

CC **C85.90** **Non-Hodgkin lymphoma, unspecified, unspecified site**
CC Exclusion see Appendix A PDX collection 0426

CC **C85.91** **Non-Hodgkin lymphoma, unspecified, lymph nodes of head, face, and neck**
CC Exclusion see Appendix A PDX collection 0427

CC **C85.92** **Non-Hodgkin lymphoma, unspecified, intrathoracic lymph nodes**
CC Exclusion see Appendix A PDX collection 0428

CC **C85.93** **Non-Hodgkin lymphoma, unspecified, intra-abdominal lymph nodes**
CC Exclusion see Appendix A PDX collection 0429

CC **C85.94** **Non-Hodgkin lymphoma, unspecified, lymph nodes of axilla and upper limb**
CC Exclusion see Appendix A PDX collection 0430

CC **C85.95** **Non-Hodgkin lymphoma, unspecified, lymph nodes of inguinal region and lower limb**
CC Exclusion see Appendix A PDX collection 0431

CC **C85.96** **Non-Hodgkin lymphoma, unspecified, intrapelvic lymph nodes**
CC Exclusion see Appendix A PDX collection 0432

CC **C85.97** **Non-Hodgkin lymphoma, unspecified, spleen**
CC Exclusion see Appendix A PDX collection 0433

CC **C85.98** **Non-Hodgkin lymphoma, unspecified, lymph nodes of multiple sites**
CC Exclusion see Appendix A PDX collection 0434

CC **C85.99** **Non-Hodgkin lymphoma, unspecified, extranodal and solid organ sites**
CC Exclusion see Appendix A PDX collection 0426

C86 Other specified types of T/NK-cell lymphoma

Excludes1: *anaplastic large cell lymphoma, ALK negative (C84.7-)*
anaplastic large cell lymphoma, ALK positive (C84.6-)
mature T/NK-cell lymphomas (C84.-)
other specified types of non-Hodgkin lymphoma (C85.8-)

CC **C86.0** **Extranodal NK/T-cell lymphoma, nasal type**
CC Exclusion see Appendix A PDX collection 0427

CC **C86.1** **Hepatosplenic T-cell lymphoma**
Alpha-beta and gamma delta types
CC Exclusion see Appendix A PDX collection 0433

CC **C86.2** **Enteropathy-type (intestinal) T-cell lymphoma**
Enteropathy associated T-cell lymphoma
CC Exclusion see Appendix A PDX collection 0429

CC **C86.3** **Subcutaneous panniculitis-like T-cell lymphoma**
CC Exclusion see Appendix A PDX collection 0429

CC **C86.4** **Blastic NK-cell lymphoma**
Blastic plasmacytoid dendritic cell neoplasm (BPDCN)
CC Exclusion see Appendix A PDX collection 0426

CC **C86.5** **Angioimmunoblastic T-cell lymphoma**
Angioimmunoblastic lymphadenopathy with dysproteinemia (AILD)
CC Exclusion see Appendix A PDX collection 0435

CC **C86.6** **Primary cutaneous CD30-positive T-cell proliferations**
Lymphomatoid papulosis
Primary cutaneous anaplastic large cell lymphoma
Primary cutaneous CD30-positive large T-cell lymphoma
CC Exclusion see Appendix A PDX collection 0435

C88 Malignant immunoproliferative diseases and certain other B-cell lymphomas

Excludes1: *B-cell lymphoma, unspecified (C85.1-)*
personal history of other malignant neoplasms of lymphoid, hematopoietic and related tissues (Z85.79)

C88.0 **Waldenström macroglobulinemia**
Lymphoplasmacytic lymphoma with IgM-production
Macroglobulinemia (idiopathic) (primary)
Excludes1: *small cell B-cell lymphoma (C83.0)*

CC **C88.2** **Heavy chain disease**
Franklin disease
Gamma heavy chain disease
Mu heavy chain disease
CC Exclusion see Appendix A PDX collection 0485

CC **C88.3** **Immunoproliferative small intestinal disease**
Alpha heavy chain disease
Mediterranean lymphoma
CC Exclusion see Appendix A PDX collection 0485

CC **C88.4** **Extranodal marginal zone B-cell lymphoma of mucosa-associated lymphoid tissue [MALT-lymphoma]**
Lymphoma of skin-associated lymphoid tissue [SALT-lymphoma]
Lymphoma of bronchial-associated lymphoid tissue [BALT-lymphoma]
Excludes1: *high malignant (diffuse large B-cell) lymphoma (C83.3-)*
CC Exclusion see Appendix A PDX collection 0426

CC **C88.8** **Other malignant immunoproliferative diseases**
CC Exclusion see Appendix A PDX collection 0486

CC **C88.9** **Malignant immunoproliferative disease, unspecified**
Immunoproliferative disease NOS
CC Exclusion see Appendix A PDX collection 0485

C90 Multiple myeloma and malignant plasma cell neoplasms

Excludes1: *personal history of other malignant neoplasms of lymphoid, hematopoietic and related tissues (Z85.79)*

+ **C90.0** **Multiple myeloma**
Kahler's disease
Medullary plasmacytoma
Myelomatosis
Plasma cell myeloma
Excludes1: *solitary myeloma (C90.3-)*
solitary plasmactyoma (C90.3-)

CC **C90.00** **Multiple myeloma not having achieved remission**
Multiple myeloma with failed remission
Multiple myeloma NOS
CC Exclusion see Appendix A PDX collection 0485

CC **C90.01** **Multiple myeloma in remission**
CC Exclusion see Appendix A PDX collection 0485

CC **C90.02** **Multiple myeloma in relapse**
CC Exclusion see Appendix A PDX collection 0485

+ **C90.1** **Plasma cell leukemia**
Plasmacytic leukemia

CC **C90.10** **Plasma cell leukemia not having achieved remission**
Plasma cell leukemia with failed remission
Plasma cell leukemia NOS
CC Exclusion see Appendix A PDX collection 0485

CC **C90.11 Plasma cell leukemia in remission**
CC Exclusion see Appendix A PDX collection 0485

CC **C90.12 Plasma cell leukemia in relapse**
CC Exclusion see Appendix A PDX collection 0485

+ **C90.2 Extramedullary plasmacytoma**

CC **C90.20 Extramedullary plasmacytoma not having achieved remission**
Extramedullary plasmacytoma with failed remission
Extramedullary plasmacytoma NOS
CC Exclusion see Appendix A PDX collection 0485

CC **C90.21 Extramedullary plasmacytoma in remission**
CC Exclusion see Appendix A PDX collection 0485

CC **C90.22 Extramedullary plasmacytoma in relapse**
CC Exclusion see Appendix A PDX collection 0485

+ **C90.3 Solitary plasmacytoma**
Localized malignant plasma cell tumor NOS
Plasmacytoma NOS
Solitary myeloma

CC **C90.30 Solitary plasmacytoma not having achieved remission**
Solitary plasmacytoma with failed remission
Solitary plasmacytoma NOS
CC Exclusion see Appendix A PDX collection 0485

CC **C90.31 Solitary plasmacytoma in remission**
CC Exclusion see Appendix A PDX collection 0485

CC **C90.32 Solitary plasmacytoma in relapse**
CC Exclusion see Appendix A PDX collection 0485

C91 Lymphoid leukemia

Excludes1: *personal history of leukemia (Z85.6)*

+ **C91.0 Acute lymphoblastic leukemia [ALL]**
NOTE Code C91.0 should only be used for T-cell and B-cell precursor leukemia

CC **C91.00 Acute lymphoblastic leukemia not having achieved remission**
Acute lymphoblastic leukemia with failed remission
Acute lymphoblastic leukemia NOS
CC Exclusion see Appendix A PDX collection 0485

CC **C91.01 Acute lymphoblastic leukemia, in remission**
CC Exclusion see Appendix A PDX collection 0485

CC **C91.02 Acute lymphoblastic leukemia, in relapse**
CC Exclusion see Appendix A PDX collection 0485

+ **C91.1 Chronic lymphocytic leukemia of B-cell type**
Lymphoplasmacytic leukemia
Richter syndrome
Excludes1: *lymphoplasmacytic lymphoma (C83.0-)*

CC **C91.10 Chronic lymphocytic leukemia of B-cell type not having achieved remission**
Chronic lymphocytic leukemia of B-cell type with failed remission
Chronic lymphocytic leukemia of B-cell type NOS
CC Exclusion see Appendix A PDX collection 0485

CC **C91.11 Chronic lymphocytic leukemia of B-cell type in remission**
CC Exclusion see Appendix A PDX collection 0485

CC **C91.12 Chronic lymphocytic leukemia of B-cell type in relapse**
CC Exclusion see Appendix A PDX collection 0485

+ **C91.3 Prolymphocytic leukemia of B-cell type**

CC **C91.30 Prolymphocytic leukemia of B-cell type not having achieved remission**
Prolymphocytic leukemia of B-cell type with failed remission
Prolymphocytic leukemia of B-cell type NOS
CC Exclusion see Appendix A PDX collection 0485

CC **C91.31 Prolymphocytic leukemia of B-cell type, in remission**
CC Exclusion see Appendix A PDX collection 0485

CC **C91.32 Prolymphocytic leukemia of B-cell type, in relapse**
CC Exclusion see Appendix A PDX collection 0485

+ **C91.4 Hairy cell leukemia**
Leukemic reticuloendotheliosis

CC **C91.40 Hairy cell leukemia not having achieved remission**
Hairy cell leukemia with failed remission
Hairy cell leukemia NOS
CC Exclusion see Appendix A PDX collection 0487

CC **C91.41 Hairy cell leukemia, in remission**
CC Exclusion see Appendix A PDX collection 0487

CC **C91.42 Hairy cell leukemia, in relapse**
CC Exclusion see Appendix A PDX collection 0487

+ **C91.5 Adult T-cell lymphoma/leukemia (HTLV-1-associated)**
Acute variant of adult T-cell lymphoma/leukemia (HTLV-1-associated)
Chronic variant of adult T-cell lymphoma/leukemia (HTLV-1-associated)
Lymphomatoid variant of adult T-cell lymphoma/leukemia (HTLV-1-associated)
Smouldering variant of adult T-cell lymphoma/leukemia (HTLV-1-associated)

• CC **C91.50 Adult T-cell lymphoma/leukemia (HTLV-1-associated) not having achieved remission**
Adult T-cell lymphoma/leukemia (HTLV-1-associated) with failed remission
Adult T-cell lymphoma/leukemia (HTLV-1-associated) NOS
CC Exclusion see Appendix A PDX collection 0485

• CC **C91.51 Adult T-cell lymphoma/leukemia (HTLV-1-associated), in remission**
CC Exclusion see Appendix A PDX collection 0485

• CC **C91.52 Adult T-cell lymphoma/leukemia (HTLV-1-associated), in relapse**
CC Exclusion see Appendix A PDX collection 0485

+ **C91.6 Prolymphocytic leukemia of T-cell type**

CC **C91.60 Prolymphocytic leukemia of T-cell type not having achieved remission**
Prolymphocytic leukemia of T-cell type with failed remission
Prolymphocytic leukemia of T-cell type NOS
CC Exclusion see Appendix A PDX collection 0485

CC **C91.61 Prolymphocytic leukemia of T-cell type, in remission**
CC Exclusion see Appendix A PDX collection 0485

CC **C91.62 Prolymphocytic leukemia of T-cell type, in relapse**
CC Exclusion see Appendix A PDX collection 0485

+ **C91.A Mature B-cell leukemia Burkitt-type**
Excludes1: *Burkitt lymphoma (C83.7-)*

CC **C91.A0 Mature B-cell leukemia Burkitt-type not having achieved remission**
Mature B-cell leukemia Burkitt-type with failed remission
Mature B-cell leukemia Burkitt-type NOS
CC Exclusion see Appendix A PDX collection 0485

CC **C91.A1 Mature B-cell leukemia Burkitt-type, in remission**
CC Exclusion see Appendix A PDX collection 0485

CC **C91.A2 Mature B-cell leukemia Burkitt-type, in relapse**
CC Exclusion see Appendix A PDX collection 0485

+ **C91.Z Other lymphoid leukemia**
T-cell large granular lymphocytic leukemia (associated with rheumatoid arthritis)

CC **C91.Z0 Other lymphoid leukemia not having achieved remission**
Other lymphoid leukemia with failed remission
Other lymphoid leukemia NOS
CC Exclusion see Appendix A PDX collection 0485

CC **C91.Z1 Other lymphoid leukemia, in remission**
CC Exclusion see Appendix A PDX collection 0485

CC **C91.Z2 Other lymphoid leukemia, in relapse**
CC Exclusion see Appendix A PDX collection 0485

+ **C91.9 Lymphoid leukemia, unspecified**

CC **C91.90 Lymphoid leukemia, unspecified not having achieved remission**
Lymphoid leukemia with failed remission
Lymphoid leukemia NOS
CC Exclusion see Appendix A PDX collection 0485

CC **C91.91 Lymphoid leukemia, unspecified, in remission**
CC Exclusion see Appendix A PDX collection 0485

CC **C91.92 Lymphoid leukemia, unspecified, in relapse**
CC Exclusion see Appendix A PDX collection 0485

C92 Myeloid leukemia

Includes: granulocytic leukemia
myelogenous leukemia
Excludes1: *personal history of leukemia (Z85.6)*

+ **C92.0 Acute myeloblastic leukemia**
Acute myeloblastic leukemia, minimal differentiation
Acute myeloblastic leukemia (with maturation)
Acute myeloblastic leukemia 1/ETO
Acute myeloblastic leukemia M0
Acute myeloblastic leukemia M1
Acute myeloblastic leukemia M2
Acute myeloblastic leukemia with t(8;21)
Acute myeloblastic leukemia (without a FAB classification) NOS
Refractory anemia with excess blasts in transformation [RAEB T]
Excludes1: *acute exacerbation of chronic myeloid leukemia (C92.10)*
refractory anemia with excess of blasts not in transformation (D46.2-)

CC **C92.00 Acute myeloblastic leukemia, not having achieved remission**
Acute myeloblastic leukemia with failed remission
Acute myeloblastic leukemia NOS
CC Exclusion see Appendix A PDX collection 0485

CC **C92.01 Acute myeloblastic leukemia, in remission**
CC Exclusion see Appendix A PDX collection 0485

CC **C92.02 Acute myeloblastic leukemia, in relapse**
CC Exclusion see Appendix A PDX collection 0485

+ **C92.1 Chronic myeloid leukemia, BCR/ABL-positive**
Chronic myelogenous leukemia, Philadelphia chromosome (Ph1) positive
Chronic myelogenous leukemia, t(9;22) (q34;q11)
Chronic myelogenous leukemia with crisis of blast cells
Excludes1: *atypical chronic myeloid leukemia BCR/ABL-negative (C92.2-)*
chronic myelomonocytic leukemia (C93.1-)
chronic myeloproliferative disease (D47.1)

CC **C92.10 Chronic myeloid leukemia, BCR/ABL-positive, not having achieved remission**
Chronic myeloid leukemia, BCR/ABL-positive with failed remission
Chronic myeloid leukemia, BCR/ABL-positive NOS
CC Exclusion see Appendix A PDX collection 0485
AHA CC: 1Q, 2017, 7

CC **C92.11 Chronic myeloid leukemia, BCR/ABL-positive, in remission**
CC Exclusion see Appendix A PDX collection 0485

CC **C92.12 Chronic myeloid leukemia, BCR/ABL-positive, in relapse**
CC Exclusion see Appendix A PDX collection 0485

+ **C92.2 Atypical chronic myeloid leukemia, BCR/ABL-negative**

CC **C92.20 Atypical chronic myeloid leukemia, BCR/ABL-negative, not having achieved remission**
Atypical chronic myeloid leukemia, BCR/ABL-negative with failed remission
Atypical chronic myeloid leukemia, BCR/ABL-negative NOS
CC Exclusion see Appendix A PDX collection 0485

CC **C92.21 Atypical chronic myeloid leukemia, BCR/ABL-negative, in remission**
CC Exclusion see Appendix A PDX collection 0485

CC **C92.22 Atypical chronic myeloid leukemia, BCR/ABL-negative, in relapse**
CC Exclusion see Appendix A PDX collection 0485

+ **C92.3 Myeloid sarcoma**
A malignant tumor of immature myeloid cells
Chloroma
Granulocytic sarcoma

CC **C92.30 Myeloid sarcoma, not having achieved remission**
Myeloid sarcoma with failed remission
Myeloid sarcoma NOS
CC Exclusion see Appendix A PDX collection 0485

CC **C92.31 Myeloid sarcoma, in remission**
CC Exclusion see Appendix A PDX collection 0485

CC **C92.32 Myeloid sarcoma, in relapse**
CC Exclusion see Appendix A PDX collection 0485

+ **C92.4 Acute promyelocytic leukemia**
AML M3
AML Me with t(15;17) and variants

CC **C92.40 Acute promyelocytic leukemia, not having achieved remission**
Acute promyelocytic leukemia with failed remission
Acute promyelocytic leukemia NOS
CC Exclusion see Appendix A PDX collection 0485

CC **C92.41 Acute promyelocytic leukemia, in remission**
CC Exclusion see Appendix A PDX collection 0485

CC **C92.42 Acute promyelocytic leukemia, in relapse**
CC Exclusion see Appendix A PDX collection 0485

+ **C92.5 Acute myelomonocytic leukemia**
AML M4
AML M4 Eo with inv(16) or t(16;16)

CC **C92.50 Acute myelomonocytic leukemia, not having achieved remission**
Acute myelomonocytic leukemia with failed remission
Acute myelomonocytic leukemia NOS
CC Exclusion see Appendix A PDX collection 0485

CC **C92.51 Acute myelomonocytic leukemia, in remission**
CC Exclusion see Appendix A PDX collection 0485

CC **C92.52 Acute myelomonocytic leukemia, in relapse**
CC Exclusion see Appendix A PDX collection 0485

+ **C92.6 Acute myeloid leukemia with 11q23-abnormality**
Acute myeloid leukemia with variation of MLL-gene

CC **C92.60 Acute myeloid leukemia with 11q23-abnormality not having achieved remission**
Acute myeloid leukemia with 11q23-abnormality with failed remission
Acute myeloid leukemia with 11q23-abnormality NOS
CC Exclusion see Appendix A PDX collection 0485

CC **C92.61 Acute myeloid leukemia with 11q23-abnormality in remission**
CC Exclusion see Appendix A PDX collection 0485

CC **C92.62 Acute myeloid leukemia with 11q23-abnormality in relapse**
CC Exclusion see Appendix A PDX collection 0485

+ **C92.A Acute myeloid leukemia with multilineage dysplasia**
Acute myeloid leukemia with dysplasia of remaining hematopoesis and/or myelodysplastic disease in its history

CC **C92.A0 Acute myeloid leukemia with multilineage dysplasia, not having achieved remission**
Acute myeloid leukemia with multilineage dysplasia with failed remission
Acute myeloid leukemia with multilineage dysplasia NOS
CC Exclusion see Appendix A PDX collection 0485

CC **C92.A1 Acute myeloid leukemia with multilineage dysplasia, in remission**
CC Exclusion see Appendix A PDX collection 0485

CC **C92.A2 Acute myeloid leukemia with multilineage dysplasia, in relapse**
CC Exclusion see Appendix A PDX collection 0485

+ **C92.Z Other myeloid leukemia**

CC **C92.Z0 Other myeloid leukemia not having achieved remission**
Myeloid leukemia NEC with failed remission
Myeloid leukemia NEC
CC Exclusion see Appendix A PDX collection 0485

CC **C92.Z1 Other myeloid leukemia, in remission**
CC Exclusion see Appendix A PDX collection 0485

CC **C92.Z2 Other myeloid leukemia, in relapse**
CC Exclusion see Appendix A PDX collection 0485

+ **C92.9 Myeloid leukemia, unspecified**

CC **C92.90 Myeloid leukemia, unspecified, not having achieved remission**
Myeloid leukemia, unspecified with failed remission
Myeloid leukemia, unspecified NOS
CC Exclusion see Appendix A PDX collection 0485

CC **C92.91 Myeloid leukemia, unspecified in remission**
CC Exclusion see Appendix A PDX collection 0485

CC **C92.92 Myeloid leukemia, unspecified in relapse**
CC Exclusion see Appendix A PDX collection 0485

C93 Monocytic leukemia

Includes: monocytoid leukemia
Excludes1: *personal history of leukemia (Z85.6)*

+ **C93.0 Acute monoblastic/monocytic leukemia**
AML M5
AML M5a
AML M5b

CC **C93.00 Acute monoblastic/monocytic leukemia, not having achieved remission**
Acute monoblastic/monocytic leukemia with failed remission
Acute monoblastic/monocytic leukemia NOS
CC Exclusion see Appendix A PDX collection 0485

CC **C93.01 Acute monoblastic/monocytic leukemia, in remission**
CC Exclusion see Appendix A PDX collection 0485

CC **C93.02** **Acute monoblastic/monocytic leukemia, in relapse**
CC Exclusion see Appendix A PDX collection 0485

\+ **C93.1 Chronic myelomonocytic leukemia**
Chronic monocytic leukemia
CMML-1
CMML-2
CMML with eosinophilia

CC **C93.10** **Chronic myelomonocytic leukemia not having achieved remission**
Chronic myelomonocytic leukemia with failed remission
Chronic myelomonocytic leukemia NOS
CC Exclusion see Appendix A PDX collection 0485

CC **C93.11** **Chronic myelomonocytic leukemia, in remission**
CC Exclusion see Appendix A PDX collection 0485

CC **C93.12** **Chronic myelomonocytic leukemia, in relapse**
CC Exclusion see Appendix A PDX collection 0485

\+ **C93.3 Juvenile myelomonocytic leukemia**

• CC **C93.30** **Juvenile myelomonocytic leukemia, not having achieved remission**
Juvenile myelomonocytic leukemia with failed remission
Juvenile myelomonocytic leukemia NOS
CC Exclusion see Appendix A PDX collection 0485

• CC **C93.31** **Juvenile myelomonocytic leukemia, in remission**
CC Exclusion see Appendix A PDX collection 0485

• CC **C93.32** **Juvenile myelomonocytic leukemia, in relapse**
CC Exclusion see Appendix A PDX collection 0485

\+ **C93.Z Other monocytic leukemia**

CC **C93.Z0** **Other monocytic leukemia, not having achieved remission**
Other monocytic leukemia NOS
CC Exclusion see Appendix A PDX collection 0485

CC **C93.Z1** **Other monocytic leukemia, in remission**
CC Exclusion see Appendix A PDX collection 0485

CC **C93.Z2** **Other monocytic leukemia, in relapse**
CC Exclusion see Appendix A PDX collection 0485

\+ **C93.9 Monocytic leukemia, unspecified**

CC **C93.90** **Monocytic leukemia, unspecified, not having achieved remission**
Monocytic leukemia, unspecified with failed remission
Monocytic leukemia, unspecified NOS
CC Exclusion see Appendix A PDX collection 0485

CC **C93.91** **Monocytic leukemia, unspecified in remission**
CC Exclusion see Appendix A PDX collection 0485

CC **C93.92** **Monocytic leukemia, unspecified in relapse**
CC Exclusion see Appendix A PDX collection 0485

C94 Other leukemias of specified cell type

Excludes1: *leukemic reticuloendotheliosis (C91.4-)*
myelodysplastic syndromes (D46.-)
personal history of leukemia (Z85.6)
plasma cell leukemia (C90.1-)

\+ **C94.0 Acute erythroid leukemia**
Acute myeloid leukemia M6(a)(b)
Erythroleukemia

CC **C94.00** **Acute erythroid leukemia, not having achieved remission**
Acute erythroid leukemia with failed remission
Acute erythroid leukemia NOS
CC Exclusion see Appendix A PDX collection 0485

CC **C94.01** **Acute erythroid leukemia, in remission**
CC Exclusion see Appendix A PDX collection 0485

CC **C94.02** **Acute erythroid leukemia, in relapse**
CC Exclusion see Appendix A PDX collection 0485

\+ **C94.2 Acute megakaryoblastic leukemia**
Acute myeloid leukemia M7
Acute megakaryocytic leukemia

CC **C94.20** **Acute megakaryoblastic leukemia not having achieved remission**
Acute megakaryoblastic leukemia with failed remission
Acute megakaryoblastic leukemia NOS
CC Exclusion see Appendix A PDX collection 0485

CC **C94.21** **Acute megakaryoblastic leukemia, in remission**
CC Exclusion see Appendix A PDX collection 0485

CC **C94.22** **Acute megakaryoblastic leukemia, in relapse**
CC Exclusion see Appendix A PDX collection 0485

\+ **C94.3 Mast cell leukemia**

CC **C94.30** **Mast cell leukemia not having achieved remission**
Mast cell leukemia with failed remission
Mast cell leukemia NOS
CC Exclusion see Appendix A PDX collection 0485

CC **C94.31** **Mast cell leukemia, in remission**
CC Exclusion see Appendix A PDX collection 0485

CC **C94.32** **Mast cell leukemia, in relapse**
CC Exclusion see Appendix A PDX collection 0485

\+ **C94.4 Acute panmyelosis with myelofibrosis**
Acute myelofibrosis
Excludes1: *myelofibrosis NOS (D75.81)*
secondary myelofibrosis NOS (D75.81)

CC **C94.40** **Acute panmyelosis with myelofibrosis not having achieved remission**
Acute myelofibrosis NOS
Acute panmyelosis with myelofibrosis with failed remission
Acute panmyelosis NOS
CC Exclusion see Appendix A PDX collection 0488

CC **C94.41** **Acute panmyelosis with myelofibrosis, in remission**
CC Exclusion see Appendix A PDX collection 0488

CC **C94.42** **Acute panmyelosis with myelofibrosis, in relapse**
CC Exclusion see Appendix A PDX collection 0488

CC **C94.6** **Myelodysplastic disease, not classified**
Myeloproliferative disease, not classified
CC Exclusion see Appendix A PDX collection 0488

\+ **C94.8 Other specified leukemias**
Aggressive NK-cell leukemia
Acute basophilic leukemia

CC **C94.80** **Other specified leukemias not having achieved remission**
Other specified leukemia with failed remission
Other specified leukemias NOS
CC Exclusion see Appendix A PDX collection 0485

CC **C94.81** **Other specified leukemias, in remission**
CC Exclusion see Appendix A PDX collection 0485

CC **C94.82** **Other specified leukemias, in relapse**
CC Exclusion see Appendix A PDX collection 0485

C95 Leukemia of unspecified cell type

Excludes1: *personal history of leukemia (Z85.6)*

\+ **C95.0 Acute leukemia of unspecified cell type**
Acute bilineal leukemia
Acute mixed lineage leukemia
Biphenotypic acute leukemia
Stem cell leukemia of unclear lineage
Excludes1: *acute exacerbation of unspecified chronic leukem (C95.10)*

CC **C95.00** **Acute leukemia of unspecified cell type not having achieved remission**
Acute leukemia of unspecified cell type with failed remission
Acute leukemia NOS
CC Exclusion see Appendix A PDX collection 0485

CC **C95.01** **Acute leukemia of unspecified cell type, in remission**
CC Exclusion see Appendix A PDX collection 0485

CC **C95.02** **Acute leukemia of unspecified cell type, in relapse**
CC Exclusion see Appendix A PDX collection 0485

\+ **C95.1 Chronic leukemia of unspecified cell type**

CC **C95.10** **Chronic leukemia of unspecified cell type not havin achieved remission**
Chronic leukemia of unspecified cell type with failed remission
Chronic leukemia NOS
CC Exclusion see Appendix A PDX collection 0485

CC **C95.11** **Chronic leukemia of unspecified cell type, in remission**
CC Exclusion see Appendix A PDX collection 0485

CC **C95.12** **Chronic leukemia of unspecified cell type, in relaps**
CC Exclusion see Appendix A PDX collection 0485

\+ **C95.9 Leukemia, unspecified**

CC **C95.90** **Leukemia, unspecified not having achieved remissi**
Leukemia, unspecified with failed remission
Leukemia NOS
CC Exclusion see Appendix A PDX collection 0485

CC **C95.91** **Leukemia, unspecified, in remission**
CC Exclusion see Appendix A PDX collection 0485

CC **C95.92** **Leukemia, unspecified, in relapse**
CC Exclusion see Appendix A PDX collection 0485

C96 Other and unspecified malignant neoplasms of lymphoid, hematopoietic and related tissue

Excludes1: *personal history of other malignant neoplasms of lymphoid, hematopoietic and related tissues (Z85.79)*

CC **C96.0 Multifocal and multisystemic (disseminated) Langerhans-cell histiocytosis**

Histiocytosis X, multisystemic
Letterer-Siwe disease

Excludes1: *adult pulmonary Langerhans cell histiocytosis (J84.82)*
multifocal and unisystemic Langerhans-cell histiocytosis (C96.5)
unifocal Langerhans-cell histiocytosis (C96.6)

CC Exclusion see Appendix A PDX collection 0489

\+ **C96.2 Malignant mast cell neoplasm**

Excludes1: *indolent mastocytosis (D47.02)*
mast cell leukemia (C94.30)
mastocytosis (congenital) (cutaneous) (Q82.2)

CC **C96.20 Malignant mast cell neoplasm, unspecified**
CC Exclusion see Appendix A PDX collection 0490

CC **C96.21 Aggressive systemic mastocytosis**
CC Exclusion see Appendix A PDX collection 0490

CC **C96.22 Mast cell sarcoma**
CC Exclusion see Appendix A PDX collection 0490

CC **C96.29 Other malignant mast cell neoplasm**
CC Exclusion see Appendix A PDX collection 0490

CC **C96.4 Sarcoma of dendritic cells (accessory cells)**

Follicular dendritic cell sarcoma
Interdigitating dendritic cell sarcoma
Langerhans cell sarcoma

CC Exclusion see Appendix A PDX collection 0491

CC **C96.5 Multifocal and unisystemic Langerhans-cell histiocytosis**

Hand-Schüller-Christian disease
Histiocytosis X, multifocal

Excludes1: *multifocal and multisystemic (disseminated) Langerhans-cell histiocytosis (C96.0)*
unifocal Langerhans-cell histiocytosis (C96.6)

CC Exclusion see Appendix A PDX collection 0492

CC **C96.6 Unifocal Langerhans-cell histiocytosis**

Eosinophilic granuloma
Histiocytosis X, unifocal
Histiocytosis X NOS
Langerhans-cell histiocytosis NOS

Excludes1: *multifocal and multisysemic (disseminated) Langerhans-cell histiocytosis (C96.0)*
multifocal and unisystemic Langerhans-cell histiocytosis (C96.5)

CC Exclusion see Appendix A PDX collection 0492

CC **C96.A Histiocytic sarcoma**

Malignant histiocytosis

CC Exclusion see Appendix A PDX collection 0493

CC **C96.Z Other specified malignant neoplasms of lymphoid, hematopoietic and related tissue**
CC Exclusion see Appendix A PDX collection 0491

CC **C96.9 Malignant neoplasm of lymphoid, hematopoietic and related tissue, unspecified**
CC Exclusion see Appendix A PDX collection 0491

situ neoplasms (D00-D09)

cludes: Bowen's disease
erythroplasia
grade III intraepithelial neoplasia
Queyrat's erythroplasia

D00 Carcinoma in situ of oral cavity, esophagus and stomach

Excludes1: *melanoma in situ (D03.-)*

\+ **D00.0 Carcinoma in situ of lip, oral cavity and pharynx**

Use additional code to identify:
exposure to environmental tobacco smoke (Z77.22)
exposure to tobacco smoke in the perinatal period (P96.81)
history of tobacco dependence (Z87.891)
occupational exposure to environmental tobacco smoke (Z57.31)
tobacco dependence (F17.-)
tobacco use (Z72.0)

Excludes1: *carcinoma in situ of aryepiglottic fold or interarytenoid fold, laryngeal aspect (D02.0)*
carcinoma in situ of epiglottis NOS (D02.0)
carcinoma in situ of epiglottis suprahyoid portion (D02.0)
carcinoma in situ of skin of lip (D03.0, D04.0)

D00.00 Carcinoma in situ of oral cavity, unspecified site

D00.01 Carcinoma in situ of labial mucosa and vermilion border

D00.02 Carcinoma in situ of buccal mucosa

D00.03 Carcinoma in situ of gingiva and edentulous alveolar ridge

D00.04 Carcinoma in situ of soft palate

D00.05 Carcinoma in situ of hard palate

D00.06 Carcinoma in situ of floor of mouth

D00.07 Carcinoma in situ of tongue

D00.08 Carcinoma in situ of pharynx

Carcinoma in situ of aryepiglottic fold NOS
Carcinoma in situ of hypopharyngeal aspect of aryepiglottic fold
Carcinoma in situ of marginal zone of aryepiglottic fold

D00.1 Carcinoma in situ of esophagus

D00.2 Carcinoma in situ of stomach

D01 Carcinoma in situ of other and unspecified digestive organs

Excludes1: *melanoma in situ (D03.-)*

D01.0 Carcinoma in situ of colon

Excludes1: *carcinoma in situ of rectosigmoid junction (D01.1)*

D01.1 Carcinoma in situ of rectosigmoid junction

D01.2 Carcinoma in situ of rectum

D01.3 Carcinoma in situ of anus and anal canal

Anal intraepithelial neoplasia III [AIN III]
Severe dysplasia of anus

Excludes1: *anal intraepithelial neoplasia I and II [AIN I and AIN II] (K62.82)*
carcinoma in situ of anal margin (D04.5)
carcinoma in situ of anal skin (D04.5)
carcinoma in situ of perianal skin (D04.5)

\+ **D01.4 Carcinoma in situ of other and unspecified parts of intestine**

Excludes1: carcinoma in situ of ampulla of Vater (D01.5)

D01.40 Carcinoma in situ of unspecified part of intestine

D01.49 Carcinoma in situ of other parts of intestine

D01.5 Carcinoma in situ of liver, gallbladder and bile ducts

Carcinoma in situ of ampulla of Vater

D01.7 Carcinoma in situ of other specified digestive organs

Carcinoma in situ of pancreas

D01.9 Carcinoma in situ of digestive organ, unspecified

D02 Carcinoma in situ of middle ear and respiratory system

Use additional code to identify:
exposure to environmental tobacco smoke (Z77.22)
exposure to tobacco smoke in the perinatal period (P96.81)
history of tobacco dependence (Z87.891)
occupational exposure to environmental tobacco smoke (Z57.31)
tobacco dependence (F17.-)
tobacco use (Z72.0)

Excludes1: *melanoma in situ (D03.-)*

D02.0 Carcinoma in situ of larynx

Carcinoma in situ of aryepiglottic fold or interarytenoid fold, laryngeal aspect
Carcinoma in situ of epiglottis (suprahyoid portion)

Excludes1: *carcinoma in situ of aryepiglottic fold or interarytenoid fold NOS (D00.08)*
carcinoma in situ of hypopharyngeal aspect (D00.08)
carcinoma in situ of marginal zone (D00.08)

D02.1 Carcinoma in situ of trachea

\+ **D02.2 Carcinoma in situ of bronchus and lung**

D02.20 Carcinoma in situ of unspecified bronchus and lung

D02.21 Carcinoma in situ of right bronchus and lung

D02.22 Carcinoma in situ of left bronchus and lung

D02.3 Carcinoma in situ of other parts of respiratory system

Carcinoma in situ of accessory sinuses
Carcinoma in situ of middle ear
Carcinoma in situ of nasal cavities

Excludes1: *carcinoma in situ of ear (external) (skin) (D04.2-)*
carcinoma in situ of nose NOS D09.8
carcinoma in situ of skin of nose (D04.3)

D02.4 Carcinoma in situ of respiratory system, unspecified

D03 Melanoma in situ

D03.0 Melanoma in situ of lip

\+ **D03.1 Melanoma in situ of eyelid, including canthus**

D03.10 Melanoma in situ of unspecified eyelid, including canthus

D03.11 Melanoma in situ of right eyelid, including canthus

D03.12 Melanoma in situ of left eyelid, including canthus

\+ **D03.2 Melanoma in situ of ear and external auricular canal**

D03.20 Melanoma in situ of unspecified ear and external auricular canal

D03.21 Melanoma in situ of right ear and external auricular canal
D03.22 Melanoma in situ of left ear and external auricular canal
+ D03.3 Melanoma in situ of other and unspecified parts of face
D03.30 Melanoma in situ of unspecified part of face
D03.39 Melanoma in situ of other parts of face
D03.4 Melanoma in situ of scalp and neck
+ D03.5 Melanoma in situ of trunk
D03.51 Melanoma in situ of anal skin
Melanoma in situ of anal margin
Melanoma in situ of perianal skin
D03.52 Melanoma in situ of breast (skin) (soft tissue)
D03.59 Melanoma in situ of other part of trunk
+ D03.6 Melanoma in situ of upper limb, including shoulder
D03.60 Melanoma in situ of unspecified upper limb, including shoulder
D03.61 Melanoma in situ of right upper limb, including shoulder
D03.62 Melanoma in situ of left upper limb, including shoulder
+ D03.7 Melanoma in situ of lower limb, including hip
D03.70 Melanoma in situ of unspecified lower limb, including hip
D03.71 Melanoma in situ of right lower limb, including hip
D03.72 Melanoma in situ of left lower limb, including hip
D03.8 Melanoma in situ of other sites
Melanoma in situ of scrotum
Excludes1: *carcinoma in situ of scrotum (D07.61)*
D03.9 Melanoma in situ, unspecified

D04 Carcinoma in situ of skin

Excludes1: *erythroplasia of Queyrat (penis) NOS (D07.4)*
melanoma in situ (D03.-)

D04.0 Carcinoma in situ of skin of lip
Excludes1: *carcinoma in situ of vermilion border of lip (D00.01)*
+ D04.1 Carcinoma in situ of skin of eyelid, including canthus
D04.10 Carcinoma in situ of skin of unspecified eyelid, including canthus
D04.11 Carcinoma in situ of skin of right eyelid, including canthus
D04.12 Carcinoma in situ of skin of left eyelid, including canthus
+ D04.2 Carcinoma in situ of skin of ear and external auricular canal
D04.20 Carcinoma in situ of skin of unspecified ear and external auricular canal
D04.21 Carcinoma in situ of skin of right ear and external auricular canal
D04.22 Carcinoma in situ of skin of left ear and external auricular canal
+ D04.3 Carcinoma in situ of skin of other and unspecified parts of face
D04.30 Carcinoma in situ of skin of unspecified part of face
D04.39 Carcinoma in situ of skin of other parts of face
D04.4 Carcinoma in situ of skin of scalp and neck
D04.5 Carcinoma in situ of skin of trunk
Carcinoma in situ of anal margin
Carcinoma in situ of anal skin
Carcinoma in situ of perianal skin
Carcinoma in situ of skin of breast
Excludes1: *carcinoma in situ of anus NOS (D01.3)*
carcinoma in situ of scrotum (D07.61)
carcinoma in situ of skin of genital organs (D07.-)
+ D04.6 Carcinoma in situ of skin of upper limb, including shoulder
D04.60 Carcinoma in situ of skin of unspecified upper limb, including shoulder
D04.61 Carcinoma in situ of skin of right upper limb, including shoulder
D04.62 Carcinoma in situ of skin of left upper limb, including shoulder
+ D04.7 Carcinoma in situ of skin of lower limb, including hip
D04.70 Carcinoma in situ of skin of unspecified lower limb, including hip
D04.71 Carcinoma in situ of skin of right lower limb, including hip
D04.72 Carcinoma in situ of skin of left lower limb, including hip
D04.8 Carcinoma in situ of skin of other sites
D04.9 Carcinoma in situ of skin, unspecified

D05 Carcinoma in situ of breast

Excludes1: *carcinoma in situ of skin of breast (D04.5)*
melanoma in situ of breast (skin) (D03.5)
Paget's disease of breast or nipple (C50.-)

+ D05.0 Lobular carcinoma in situ of breast
D05.00 Lobular carcinoma in situ of unspecified breast
D05.01 Lobular carcinoma in situ of right breast
D05.02 Lobular carcinoma in situ of left breast
+ D05.1 Intraductal carcinoma in situ of breast
D05.10 Intraductal carcinoma in situ of unspecified breast
D05.11 Intraductal carcinoma in situ of right breast
D05.12 Intraductal carcinoma in situ of left breast
+ D05.8 Other specified type of carcinoma in situ of breast
D05.80 Other specified type of carcinoma in situ of unspecified breast
D05.81 Other specified type of carcinoma in situ of right breast
D05.82 Other specified type of carcinoma in situ of left brea
+ D05.9 Unspecified type of carcinoma in situ of breast
D05.90 Unspecified type of carcinoma in situ of unspecified breast
D05.91 Unspecified type of carcinoma in situ of right breas
D05.92 Unspecified type of carcinoma in situ of left breast

D06 Carcinoma in situ of cervix uteri

Includes: cervical adenocarcinoma in situ
cervical intraepithelial glandular neoplasia
cervical intraepithelial neoplasia III [CIN III]
severe dysplasia of cervix uteri
Excludes1: *cervical intraepithelial neoplasia II [CIN II] (N87.1)*
cytologic evidence of malignancy of cervix without histologic confirmation (R87.614)
high grade squamous intraepithelial lesion (HGSIL) of cervix (R87.613)
melanoma in situ of cervix (D03.5)
moderate cervical dysplasia (N87.1)

♀ D06.0 Carcinoma in situ of endocervix
♀ D06.1 Carcinoma in situ of exocervix
♀ D06.7 Carcinoma in situ of other parts of cervix
♀ D06.9 Carcinoma in situ of cervix, unspecified

D07 Carcinoma in situ of other and unspecified genital organs

Excludes1: *melanoma in situ of trunk (D03.5)*

♀ D07.0 Carcinoma in situ of endometrium
♀ D07.1 Carcinoma in situ of vulva
Severe dysplasia of vulva
Vulvar intraepithelial neoplasia III [VIN III]
Excludes1: *moderate dysplasia of vulva (N90.1)*
vulvar intraepithelial neoplasia II [VIN II] (N90.
♀ D07.2 Carcinoma in situ of vagina
Severe dysplasia of vagina
Vaginal intraepithelial neoplasia III [VAIN III]
Excludes1: *moderate dysplasia of vagina (N89.1)*
vaginal intraepithelial neoplasia II [VIN II] (N89.
+ D07.3 Carcinoma in situ of other and unspecified female genital organs
♀ D07.30 Carcinoma in situ of unspecified female genital orga
♀ D07.39 Carcinoma in situ of other female genital organs
♂ D07.4 Carcinoma in situ of penis
Erythroplasia of Queyrat NOS
♂ D07.5 Carcinoma in situ of prostate
Prostatic intraepithelial neoplasia III (PIN III)
Severe dysplasia of prostate
Excludes1: *dysplasia (mild) (moderate) of prostate (N42.3-)*
prostatic intraepithelial neoplasia II [PIN II] (N42.3
+ D07.6 Carcinoma in situ of other and unspecified male genital orga
♂ D07.60 Carcinoma in situ of unspecified male genital organ
♂ D07.61 Carcinoma in situ of scrotum
♂ D07.69 Carcinoma in situ of other male genital organs

D09 Carcinoma in situ of other and unspecified sites

Excludes1: *melanoma in situ (D03.-)*

D09.0 Carcinoma in situ of bladder
+ D09.1 Carcinoma in situ of other and unspecified urinary organs
D09.10 Carcinoma in situ of unspecified urinary organ
D09.19 Carcinoma in situ of other urinary organs
+ D09.2 Carcinoma in situ of eye
Excludes1: *carcinoma in situ of skin of eyelid (D04.1-)*
D09.20 Carcinoma in situ of unspecified eye
D09.21 Carcinoma in situ of right eye
D09.22 Carcinoma in situ of left eye

D09.3 Carcinoma in situ of thyroid and other endocrine glands
Excludes1: *carcinoma in situ of endocrine pancreas (D01.7)*
carcinoma in situ of ovary (D07.39)
carcinoma in situ of testis (D07.69)
D09.8 Carcinoma in situ of other specified sites
D09.9 Carcinoma in situ, unspecified

enign neoplasms, except benign neuroendocrine tumors 10-D36)

D10 Benign neoplasm of mouth and pharynx

D10.0 Benign neoplasm of lip
Benign neoplasm of lip (frenulum) (inner aspect) (mucosa) (vermilion border)
Excludes1: *benign neoplasm of skin of lip (D22.0, D23.0)*
D10.1 Benign neoplasm of tongue
Benign neoplasm of lingual tonsil
D10.2 Benign neoplasm of floor of mouth
\+ **D10.3 Benign neoplasm of other and unspecified parts of mouth**
D10.30 Benign neoplasm of unspecified part of mouth
D10.39 Benign neoplasm of other parts of mouth
Benign neoplasm of minor salivary gland NOS
Excludes1: *benign odontogenic neoplasms (D16.4-D16.5)*
benign neoplasm of mucosa of lip (D10.0)
benign neoplasm of nasopharyngeal surface of soft palate (D10.6)
D10.4 Benign neoplasm of tonsil
Benign neoplasm of tonsil (faucial) (palatine)
Excludes1: *benign neoplasm of lingual tonsil (D10.1)*
benign neoplasm of pharyngeal tonsil (D10.6)
benign neoplasm of tonsillar fossa (D10.5)
benign neoplasm of tonsillar pillars (D10.5)
D10.5 Benign neoplasm of other parts of oropharynx
Benign neoplasm of epiglottis, anterior aspect
Benign neoplasm of tonsillar fossa
Benign neoplasm of tonsillar pillars
Benign neoplasm of vallecula
Excludes1: *benign neoplasm of epiglottis NOS (D14.1)*
benign neoplasm of epiglottis, suprahyoid portion (D14.1)
D10.6 Benign neoplasm of nasopharynx
Benign neoplasm of pharyngeal tonsil
Benign neoplasm of posterior margin of septum and choanae
D10.7 Benign neoplasm of hypopharynx
D10.9 Benign neoplasm of pharynx, unspecified

D11 Benign neoplasm of major salivary glands

Excludes1: *benign neoplasms of specified minor salivary glands which are classified according to their anatomical location*
benign neoplasms of minor salivary glands NOS (D10.39)
D11.0 Benign neoplasm of parotid gland
D11.7 Benign neoplasm of other major salivary glands
Benign neoplasm of sublingual salivary gland
Benign neoplasm of submandibular salivary gland
D11.9 Benign neoplasm of major salivary gland, unspecified

D12 Benign neoplasm of colon, rectum, anus and anal canal

Excludes1: *benign carcinoid tumors of the large intestine, and rectum (D3A.02-)*
D12.0 Benign neoplasm of cecum
Benign neoplasm of ileocecal valve
D12.1 Benign neoplasm of appendix
Excludes1: *benign carcinoid tumor of the appendix (D3A.020)*
D12.2 Benign neoplasm of ascending colon
D12.3 Benign neoplasm of transverse colon
Benign neoplasm of hepatic flexure
Benign neoplasm of splenic flexure
D12.4 Benign neoplasm of descending colon
D12.5 Benign neoplasm of sigmoid colon
D12.6 Benign neoplasm of colon, unspecified
Adenomatosis of colon
Benign neoplasm of large intestine NOS
Polyposis (hereditary) of colon
Excludes1: *inflammatory polyp of colon (K51.4-)*
polyp of colon NOS (K63.5)
AHA CC: 1Q, 2017, 8-9
D12.7 Benign neoplasm of rectosigmoid junction
D12.8 Benign neoplasm of rectum
Excludes1: *benign carcinoid tumor of the rectum (D3A.026)*
D12.9 Benign neoplasm of anus and anal canal
Benign neoplasm of anus NOS
Excludes1: *benign neoplasm of anal margin (D22.5, D23.5)*
benign neoplasm of anal skin (D22.5, D23.5)
benign neoplasm of perianal skin (D22.5, D23.5)

D13 Benign neoplasm of other and ill-defined parts of digestive system

Excludes1: *benign stromal tumors of digestive system (D21.4)*
D13.0 Benign neoplasm of esophagus
D13.1 Benign neoplasm of stomach
Excludes1: *benign carcinoid tumor of the stomach (D3A.092)*
D13.2 Benign neoplasm of duodenum
Excludes1: *benign carcinoid tumor of the duodenum (D3A.010)*
\+ **D13.3 Benign neoplasm of other and unspecified parts of small intestine**
Excludes1: *benign carcinoid tumors of the small intestine(D3A.01-)*
benign neoplasm of ileocecal valve (D12.0)
D13.30 Benign neoplasm of unspecified part of small intestine
D13.39 Benign neoplasm of other parts of small intestine
D13.4 Benign neoplasm of liver
Benign neoplasm of intrahepatic bile ducts
D13.5 Benign neoplasm of extrahepatic bile ducts
D13.6 Benign neoplasm of pancreas
Excludes1: *benign neoplasm of endocrine pancreas (D13.7)*
D13.7 Benign neoplasm of endocrine pancreas
Islet cell tumor
Benign neoplasm of islets of Langerhans
Use additional code to identify any functional activity.
D13.9 Benign neoplasm of ill-defined sites within the digestive system
Benign neoplasm of digestive system NOS
Benign neoplasm of intestine NOS
Benign neoplasm of spleen

D14 Benign neoplasm of middle ear and respiratory system

D14.0 Benign neoplasm of middle ear, nasal cavity and accessory sinuses
Benign neoplasm of cartilage of nose
Excludes1: *benign neoplasm of auricular canal (external) (D22.2-, D23.2-)*
benign neoplasm of bone of ear (D16.4)
benign neoplasm of bone of nose (D16.4)
benign neoplasm of cartilage of ear (D21.0)
benign neoplasm of ear (external)(skin) (D22.2-, D23.2-)
benign neoplasm of nose NOS (D36.7)
benign neoplasm of skin of nose (D22.39, D23.39)
benign neoplasm of olfactory bulb (D33.3)
benign neoplasm of posterior margin of septum and choanae (D10.6)
polyp of accessory sinus (J33.8)
polyp of ear (middle) (H74.4)
polyp of nasal (cavity) (J33.-)
D14.1 Benign neoplasm of larynx
Adenomatous polyp of larynx
Benign neoplasm of epiglottis (suprahyoid portion)
Excludes1: *benign neoplasm of epiglottis, anterior aspect (D10.5)*
polyp (nonadenomatous) of vocal cord or larynx (J38.1)
D14.2 Benign neoplasm of trachea
\+ **D14.3 Benign neoplasm of bronchus and lung**
Excludes1: *benign carcinoid tumor of the bronchus and lung (D3A.090)*
D14.30 Benign neoplasm of unspecified bronchus and lung
D14.31 Benign neoplasm of right bronchus and lung
D14.32 Benign neoplasm of left bronchus and lung
D14.4 Benign neoplasm of respiratory system, unspecified

D15 Benign neoplasm of other and unspecified intrathoracic organs

Excludes1: *benign neoplasm of mesothelial tissue (D19.-)*
D15.0 Benign neoplasm of thymus
Excludes1: *benign carcinoid tumor of the thymus (D3A.091)*
D15.1 Benign neoplasm of heart
Excludes1: *benign neoplasm of great vessels (D21.3)*
D15.2 Benign neoplasm of mediastinum
D15.7 Benign neoplasm of other specified intrathoracic organs
D15.9 Benign neoplasm of intrathoracic organ, unspecified

D16 Benign neoplasm of bone and articular cartilage

Excludes1: *benign neoplasm of connective tissue of ear (D21.0)*
benign neoplasm of connective tissue of eyelid (D21.0)
benign neoplasm of connective tissue of larynx (D14.1)
benign neoplasm of connective tissue of nose (D14.0)
benign neoplasm of synovia (D21.-)

+ **D16.0 Benign neoplasm of scapula and long bones of upper limb**
  - **D16.00 Benign neoplasm of scapula and long bones of unspecified upper limb**
  - **D16.01 Benign neoplasm of scapula and long bones of right upper limb**
  - **D16.02 Benign neoplasm of scapula and long bones of left upper limb**

+ **D16.1 Benign neoplasm of short bones of upper limb**
  - **D16.10 Benign neoplasm of short bones of unspecified upper limb**
  - **D16.11 Benign neoplasm of short bones of right upper limb**
  - **D16.12 Benign neoplasm of short bones of left upper limb**

+ **D16.2 Benign neoplasm of long bones of lower limb**
  - **D16.20 Benign neoplasm of long bones of unspecified lower limb**
  - **D16.21 Benign neoplasm of long bones of right lower limb**
  - **D16.22 Benign neoplasm of long bones of left lower limb**

+ **D16.3 Benign neoplasm of short bones of lower limb**
  - **D16.30 Benign neoplasm of short bones of unspecified lower limb**
  - **D16.31 Benign neoplasm of short bones of right lower limb**
  - **D16.32 Benign neoplasm of short bones of left lower limb**

D16.4 Benign neoplasm of bones of skull and face
Benign neoplasm of maxilla (superior)
Benign neoplasm of orbital bone
Keratocyst of maxilla
Keratocystic odontogenic tumor of maxilla
Excludes2: *benign neoplasm of lower jaw bone (D16.5)*

D16.5 Benign neoplasm of lower jaw bone
Keratocyst of mandible
Keratocystic odontogenic tumor of mandible

D16.6 Benign neoplasm of vertebral column
Excludes1: *benign neoplasm of sacrum and coccyx (D16.8)*

D16.7 Benign neoplasm of ribs, sternum and clavicle

D16.8 Benign neoplasm of pelvic bones, sacrum and coccyx

D16.9 Benign neoplasm of bone and articular cartilage, unspecified

D17 Benign lipomatous neoplasm

D17.0 Benign lipomatous neoplasm of skin and subcutaneous tissue of head, face and neck

D17.1 Benign lipomatous neoplasm of skin and subcutaneous tissue of trunk

+ **D17.2 Benign lipomatous neoplasm of skin and subcutaneous tissue of limb**
  - **D17.20 Benign lipomatous neoplasm of skin and subcutaneous tissue of unspecified limb**
  - **D17.21 Benign lipomatous neoplasm of skin and subcutaneous tissue of right arm**
  - **D17.22 Benign lipomatous neoplasm of skin and subcutaneous tissue of left arm**
  - **D17.23 Benign lipomatous neoplasm of skin and subcutaneous tissue of right leg**
  - **D17.24 Benign lipomatous neoplasm of skin and subcutaneous tissue of left leg**

+ **D17.3 Benign lipomatous neoplasm of skin and subcutaneous tissue of other and unspecified sites**
  - **D17.30 Benign lipomatous neoplasm of skin and subcutaneous tissue of unspecified sites**
  - **D17.39 Benign lipomatous neoplasm of skin and subcutaneous tissue of other sites**

D17.4 Benign lipomatous neoplasm of intrathoracic organs

D17.5 Benign lipomatous neoplasm of intra-abdominal organs
Excludes1: *benign lipomatous neoplasm of peritoneum and retroperitoneum (D17.79)*

♂ **D17.6 Benign lipomatous neoplasm of spermatic cord**

+ **D17.7 Benign lipomatous neoplasm of other sites**
  - **D17.71 Benign lipomatous neoplasm of kidney**
  - **D17.72 Benign lipomatous neoplasm of other genitourinary organ**
  - **D17.79 Benign lipomatous neoplasm of other sites**
    Benign lipomatous neoplasm of peritoneum
    Benign lipomatous neoplasm of retroperitoneum

D17.9 Benign lipomatous neoplasm, unspecified
Lipoma NOS

D18 Hemangioma and lymphangioma, any site

Excludes1: *benign neoplasm of glomus jugulare (D35.6)*
blue or pigmented nevus (D22.-)
nevus NOS (D22.-)
vascular nevus (Q82.5)

+ **D18.0 Hemangioma**
Angioma NOS
Cavernous nevus
  - **D18.00 Hemangioma unspecified site**
  - **D18.01 Hemangioma of skin and subcutaneous tissue**
  - **D18.02 Hemangioma of intracranial structures**
  - **D18.03 Hemangioma of intra-abdominal structures**
  - **D18.09 Hemangioma of other sites**

D18.1 Lymphangioma, any site

D19 Benign neoplasm of mesothelial tissue

D19.0 Benign neoplasm of mesothelial tissue of pleura

D19.1 Benign neoplasm of mesothelial tissue of peritoneum

D19.7 Benign neoplasm of mesothelial tissue of other sites

D19.9 Benign neoplasm of mesothelial tissue, unspecified
Benign mesothelioma NOS

D20 Benign neoplasm of soft tissue of retroperitoneum and peritoneum

Excludes1: *benign lipomatous neoplasm of peritoneum and retroperitoneum (D17.79)*
benign neoplasm of mesothelial tissue (D19.-)

D20.0 Benign neoplasm of soft tissue of retroperitoneum

D20.1 Benign neoplasm of soft tissue of peritoneum

D21 Other benign neoplasms of connective and other soft tissue

Includes: benign neoplasm of blood vessel
benign neoplasm of bursa
benign neoplasm of cartilage
benign neoplasm of fascia
benign neoplasm of fat
benign neoplasm of ligament, except uterine
benign neoplasm of lymphatic channel
benign neoplasm of muscle
benign neoplasm of synovia
benign neoplasm of tendon (sheath)
benign stromal tumors

Excludes1: *benign neoplasm of articular cartilage (D16.-)*
benign neoplasm of cartilage of larynx (D14.1)
benign neoplasm of cartilage of nose (D14.0)
benign neoplasm of connective tissue of breast (D24.-)
benign neoplasm of peripheral nerves and autonomic nervous system (D36.1-)
benign neoplasm of peritoneum (D20.1)
benign neoplasm of retroperitoneum (D20.0)
benign neoplasm of uterine ligament, any (D28.2)
benign neoplasm of vascular tissue (D18.-)
hemangioma (D18.0-)
lipomatous neoplasm (D17.-)
lymphangioma (D18.1)
uterine leiomyoma (D25.-)

D21.0 Benign neoplasm of connective and other soft tissue of head, face and neck
Benign neoplasm of connective tissue of ear
Benign neoplasm of connective tissue of eyelid
Excludes1: *benign neoplasm of connective tissue of orbit (D31.6-)*

+ **D21.1 Benign neoplasm of connective and other soft tissue of upper limb, including shoulder**
  - **D21.10 Benign neoplasm of connective and other soft tissue of unspecified upper limb, including shoulder**
  - **D21.11 Benign neoplasm of connective and other soft tissue of right upper limb, including shoulder**
  - **D21.12 Benign neoplasm of connective and other soft tissue of left upper limb, including shoulder**

+ **D21.2 Benign neoplasm of connective and other soft tissue of lower limb, including hip**
  - **D21.20 Benign neoplasm of connective and other soft tissue of unspecified lower limb, including hip**
  - **D21.21 Benign neoplasm of connective and other soft tissue of right lower limb, including hip**
  - **D21.22 Benign neoplasm of connective and other soft tissue of left lower limb, including hip**

D21.3 Benign neoplasm of connective and other soft tissue of thorax
Benign neoplasm of axilla
Benign neoplasm of diaphragm
Benign neoplasm of great vessels
Excludes1: *benign neoplasm of heart (D15.1)*
benign neoplasm of mediastinum (D15.2)
benign neoplasm of thymus (D15.0)

D21.4 Benign neoplasm of connective and other soft tissue of abdomen
Benign stromal tumors of abdomen

D21.5 Benign neoplasm of connective and other soft tissue of pelvis
Excludes1: *benign neoplasm of any uterine ligament (D28.2)*
uterine leiomyoma (D25.-)

D21.6 Benign neoplasm of connective and other soft tissue of trunk, unspecified
Benign neoplasm of back NOS

D21.9 Benign neoplasm of connective and other soft tissue, unspecified

D22 Melanocytic nevi

Includes: atypical nevus
blue hairy pigmented nevus
nevus NOS

D22.0 Melanocytic nevi of lip
+ **D22.1 Melanocytic nevi of eyelid, including canthus**
D22.10 Melanocytic nevi of unspecified eyelid, including canthus
D22.11 Melanocytic nevi of right eyelid, including canthus
D22.12 Melanocytic nevi of left eyelid, including canthus
+ **D22.2 Melanocytic nevi of ear and external auricular canal**
D22.20 Melanocytic nevi of unspecified ear and external auricular canal
D22.21 Melanocytic nevi of right ear and external auricular canal
D22.22 Melanocytic nevi of left ear and external auricular canal
+ **D22.3 Melanocytic nevi of other and unspecified parts of face**
D22.30 Melanocytic nevi of unspecified part of face
D22.39 Melanocytic nevi of other parts of face
D22.4 Melanocytic nevi of scalp and neck
D22.5 Melanocytic nevi of trunk
Melanocytic nevi of anal margin
Melanocytic nevi of anal skin
Melanocytic nevi of perianal skin
Melanocytic nevi of skin of breast
+ **D22.6 Melanocytic nevi of upper limb, including shoulder**
D22.60 Melanocytic nevi of unspecified upper limb, including shoulder
D22.61 Melanocytic nevi of right upper limb, including shoulder
D22.62 Melanocytic nevi of left upper limb, including shoulder
+ **D22.7 Melanocytic nevi of lower limb, including hip**
D22.70 Melanocytic nevi of unspecified lower limb, including hip
D22.71 Melanocytic nevi of right lower limb, including hip
D22.72 Melanocytic nevi of left lower limb, including hip
D22.9 Melanocytic nevi, unspecified

D23 Other benign neoplasms of skin

Includes: benign neoplasm of hair follicles
benign neoplasm of sebaceous glands
benign neoplasm of sweat glands
Excludes1: *benign lipomatous neoplasms of skin (D17.0-D17.3)*
melanocytic nevi (D22.-)

D23.0 Other benign neoplasm of skin of lip
Excludes1: *benign neoplasm of vermilion border of lip (D10.0)*
+ **D23.1 Other benign neoplasm of skin of eyelid, including canthus**
D23.10 Other benign neoplasm of skin of unspecified eyelid, including canthus
D23.11 Other benign neoplasm of skin of right eyelid, including canthus
D23.12 Other benign neoplasm of skin of left eyelid, including canthus
+ **D23.2 Other benign neoplasm of skin of ear and external auricular canal**
D23.20 Other benign neoplasm of skin of unspecified ear and external auricular canal
D23.21 Other benign neoplasm of skin of right ear and external auricular canal
D23.22 Other benign neoplasm of skin of left ear and external auricular canal
+ **D23.3 Other benign neoplasm of skin of other and unspecified parts of face**
D23.30 Other benign neoplasm of skin of unspecified part of face
D23.39 Other benign neoplasm of skin of other parts of face
D23.4 Other benign neoplasm of skin of scalp and neck
D23.5 Other benign neoplasm of skin of trunk
Other benign neoplasm of anal margin
Other benign neoplasm of anal skin
Other benign neoplasm of perianal skin
Other benign neoplasm of skin of breast
Excludes1: *benign neoplasm of anus NOS (D12.9)*
+ **D23.6 Other benign neoplasm of skin of upper limb, including shoulder**
D23.60 Other benign neoplasm of skin of unspecified upper limb, including shoulder
D23.61 Other benign neoplasm of skin of right upper limb, including shoulder
D23.62 Other benign neoplasm of skin of left upper limb, including shoulder
+ **D23.7 Other benign neoplasm of skin of lower limb, including hip**
D23.70 Other benign neoplasm of skin of unspecified lower limb, including hip
D23.71 Other benign neoplasm of skin of right lower limb, including hip
D23.72 Other benign neoplasm of skin of left lower limb, including hip
D23.9 Other benign neoplasm of skin, unspecified

D24 Benign neoplasm of breast

Includes: benign neoplasm of connective tissue of breast
benign neoplasm of soft parts of breast
fibroadenoma of breast
Excludes2: *adenofibrosis of breast (N60.2)*
benign cyst of breast (N60.-)
benign mammary dysplasia (N60.-)
benign neoplasm of skin of breast (D22.5, D23.5)
fibrocystic disease of breast (N60.-)

D24.1 Benign neoplasm of right breast
AHA CC: 1Q, 2017, 5-6
D24.2 Benign neoplasm of left breast
D24.9 Benign neoplasm of unspecified breast

D25 Leiomyoma of uterus

Includes: uterine fibroid
uterine fibromyoma
uterine myoma

♀ **D25.0 Submucous leiomyoma of uterus**
♀ **D25.1 Intramural leiomyoma of uterus**
Interstitial leiomyoma of uterus
♀ **D25.2 Subserosal leiomyoma of uterus**
Subperitoneal leiomyoma of uterus
♀ **D25.9 Leiomyoma of uterus, unspecified**

D26 Other benign neoplasms of uterus

♀ **D26.0 Other benign neoplasm of cervix uteri**
♀ **D26.1 Other benign neoplasm of corpus uteri**
♀ **D26.7 Other benign neoplasm of other parts of uterus**
♀ **D26.9 Other benign neoplasm of uterus, unspecified**

D27 Benign neoplasm of ovary

Use additional code to identify any functional activity.
Excludes2: *corpus albicans cyst (N83.2-)*
corpus luteum cyst (N83.1-)
endometrial cyst (N80.1)
follicular (atretic) cyst (N83.0-)
graafian follicle cyst (N83.0-)
ovarian cyst NEC (N83.2-)
ovarian retention cyst (N83.2-)

♀ **D27.0 Benign neoplasm of right ovary**
♀ **D27.1 Benign neoplasm of left ovary**
♀ **D27.9 Benign neoplasm of unspecified ovary**

D28 Benign neoplasm of other and unspecified female genital organs

Includes: adenomatous polyp
benign neoplasm of skin of female genital organs
benign teratoma
Excludes1: *epoophoron cyst (Q50.5)*
fimbrial cyst (Q50.4)
Gartner's duct cyst (Q52.4)
parovarian cyst (Q50.5)

♀ **D28.0 Benign neoplasm of vulva**
♀ **D28.1 Benign neoplasm of vagina**
♀ **D28.2 Benign neoplasm of uterine tubes and ligaments**
Benign neoplasm of fallopian tube
Benign neoplasm of uterine ligament (broad) (round)
♀ **D28.7 Benign neoplasm of other specified female genital organs**
♀ **D28.9 Benign neoplasm of female genital organ, unspecified**

D29 Benign neoplasm of male genital organs

Includes: benign neoplasm of skin of male genital organs
♂ **D29.0 Benign neoplasm of penis**
♂ **D29.1 Benign neoplasm of prostate**
Excludes1: *enlarged prostate (N40.-)*
\+ **D29.2 Benign neoplasm of testis**
Use additional code to identify any functional activity.
♂ **D29.20 Benign neoplasm of unspecified testis**
♂ **D29.21 Benign neoplasm of right testis**
♂ **D29.22 Benign neoplasm of left testis**
\+ **D29.3 Benign neoplasm of epididymis**
♂ **D29.30 Benign neoplasm of unspecified epididymis**
♂ **D29.31 Benign neoplasm of right epididymis**
♂ **D29.32 Benign neoplasm of left epididymis**
♂ **D29.4 Benign neoplasm of scrotum**
Benign neoplasm of skin of scrotum
♂ **D29.8 Benign neoplasm of other specified male genital organs**
Benign neoplasm of seminal vesicle
Benign neoplasm of spermatic cord
Benign neoplasm of tunica vaginalis
♂ **D29.9 Benign neoplasm of male genital organ, unspecified**

D30 Benign neoplasm of urinary organs

\+ **D30.0 Benign neoplasm of kidney**
Excludes1: *benign carcinoid tumor of the kidney (D3A.093)*
benign neoplasm of renal calyces (D30.1-)
benign neoplasm of renal pelvis (D30.1-)
D30.00 Benign neoplasm of unspecified kidney
D30.01 Benign neoplasm of right kidney
D30.02 Benign neoplasm of left kidney
\+ **D30.1 Benign neoplasm of renal pelvis**
D30.10 Benign neoplasm of unspecified renal pelvis
D30.11 Benign neoplasm of right renal pelvis
D30.12 Benign neoplasm of left renal pelvis
\+ **D30.2 Benign neoplasm of ureter**
Excludes1: *benign neoplasm of ureteric orifice of bladder (D30.3)*
D30.20 Benign neoplasm of unspecified ureter
D30.21 Benign neoplasm of right ureter
D30.22 Benign neoplasm of left ureter
D30.3 Benign neoplasm of bladder
Benign neoplasm of ureteric orifice of bladder
Benign neoplasm of urethral orifice of bladder
D30.4 Benign neoplasm of urethra
Excludes1: *benign neoplasm of urethral orifice of bladder (D30.3)*
D30.8 Benign neoplasm of other specified urinary organs
Benign neoplasm of paraurethral glands
D30.9 Benign neoplasm of urinary organ, unspecified
Benign neoplasm of urinary system NOS

D31 Benign neoplasm of eye and adnexa

Excludes1: *benign neoplasm of connective tissue of eyelid (D21.0)*
benign neoplasm of optic nerve (D33.3)
benign neoplasm of skin of eyelid (D22.1-, D23.1-)
\+ **D31.0 Benign neoplasm of conjunctiva**
D31.00 Benign neoplasm of unspecified conjunctiva
D31.01 Benign neoplasm of right conjunctiva
D31.02 Benign neoplasm of left conjunctiva
\+ **D31.1 Benign neoplasm of cornea**
D31.10 Benign neoplasm of unspecified cornea
D31.11 Benign neoplasm of right cornea
D31.12 Benign neoplasm of left cornea
\+ **D31.2 Benign neoplasm of retina**
Excludes1: *dark area on retina (D49.81)*
hemangioma of retina (D49.81)
neoplasm of unspecified behavior of retina and choroid (D49.81)
retinal freckle (D49.81)
D31.20 Benign neoplasm of unspecified retina
D31.21 Benign neoplasm of right retina
D31.22 Benign neoplasm of left retina
\+ **D31.3 Benign neoplasm of choroid**
D31.30 Benign neoplasm of unspecified choroid
D31.31 Benign neoplasm of right choroid
D31.32 Benign neoplasm of left choroid
\+ **D31.4 Benign neoplasm of ciliary body**
D31.40 Benign neoplasm of unspecified ciliary body
D31.41 Benign neoplasm of right ciliary body
D31.42 Benign neoplasm of left ciliary body
\+ **D31.5 Benign neoplasm of lacrimal gland and duct**
Benign neoplasm of lacrimal sac
Benign neoplasm of nasolacrimal duct
D31.50 Benign neoplasm of unspecified lacrimal gland and duct
D31.51 Benign neoplasm of right lacrimal gland and duct
D31.52 Benign neoplasm of left lacrimal gland and duct
\+ **D31.6 Benign neoplasm of unspecified site of orbit**
Benign neoplasm of connective tissue of orbit
Benign neoplasm of extraocular muscle
Benign neoplasm of peripheral nerves of orbit
Benign neoplasm of retrobulbar tissue
Benign neoplasm of retro-ocular tissue
Excludes1: *benign neoplasm of orbital bone (D16.4)*
D31.60 Benign neoplasm of unspecified site of unspecified orbit
D31.61 Benign neoplasm of unspecified site of right orbit
D31.62 Benign neoplasm of unspecified site of left orbit
\+ **D31.9 Benign neoplasm of unspecified part of eye**
Benign neoplasm of eyeball
D31.90 Benign neoplasm of unspecified part of unspecified eye
D31.91 Benign neoplasm of unspecified part of right eye
D31.92 Benign neoplasm of unspecified part of left eye

D32 Benign neoplasm of meninges

D32.0 Benign neoplasm of cerebral meninges
D32.1 Benign neoplasm of spinal meninges
D32.9 Benign neoplasm of meninges, unspecified
Meningioma NOS

D33 Benign neoplasm of brain and other parts of central nervous system

Excludes1: *angioma (D18.0-)*
benign neoplasm of meninges (D32.-)
benign neoplasm of peripheral nerves and autonomic nervous system (D36.1-)
hemangioma (D18.0-)
neurofibromatosis (Q85.0-)
retro-ocular benign neoplasm (D31.6-)
D33.0 Benign neoplasm of brain, supratentorial
Benign neoplasm of cerebral ventricle
Benign neoplasm of cerebrum
Benign neoplasm of frontal lobe
Benign neoplasm of occipital lobe
Benign neoplasm of parietal lobe
Benign neoplasm of temporal lobe
Excludes1: *benign neoplasm of fourth ventricle (D33.1)*
D33.1 Benign neoplasm of brain, infratentorial
Benign neoplasm of brain stem
Benign neoplasm of cerebellum
Benign neoplasm of fourth ventricle
D33.2 Benign neoplasm of brain, unspecified
D33.3 Benign neoplasm of cranial nerves
Benign neoplasm of olfactory bulb
D33.4 Benign neoplasm of spinal cord
D33.7 Benign neoplasm of other specified parts of central nervous system
D33.9 Benign neoplasm of central nervous system, unspecified
Benign neoplasm of nervous system (central) NOS

D34 Benign neoplasm of thyroid gland

Use additional code to identify any functional activity
Valid 3-character code, no further characters required

D35 Benign neoplasm of other and unspecified endocrine glands

Use additional code to identify any functional activity
Excludes1: *benign neoplasm of endocrine pancreas (D13.7)*
benign neoplasm of ovary (D27.-)
benign neoplasm of testis (D29.2.-)
benign neoplasm of thymus (D15.0)

+ **D35.0 Benign neoplasm of adrenal gland**
  - **D35.00 Benign neoplasm of unspecified adrenal gland**
  - **D35.01 Benign neoplasm of right adrenal gland**
  - **D35.02 Benign neoplasm of left adrenal gland**

D35.1 Benign neoplasm of parathyroid gland

D35.2 Benign neoplasm of pituitary gland
AHA CC: 3Q, 2014, 22-23

D35.3 Benign neoplasm of craniopharyngeal duct

D35.4 Benign neoplasm of pineal gland

D35.5 Benign neoplasm of carotid body

D35.6 Benign neoplasm of aortic body and other paraganglia
Benign tumor of glomus jugulare

D35.7 Benign neoplasm of other specified endocrine glands

D35.9 Benign neoplasm of endocrine gland, unspecified
Benign neoplasm of unspecified endocrine gland

D36 Benign neoplasm of other and unspecified sites

D36.0 Benign neoplasm of lymph nodes
Excludes1: *lymphangioma (D18.1)*

+ **D36.1 Benign neoplasm of peripheral nerves and autonomic nervous system**
Excludes1: *benign neoplasm of peripheral nerves of orbit (D31.6-)*
neurofibromatosis (Q85.0-)
  - **D36.10 Benign neoplasm of peripheral nerves and autonomic nervous system, unspecified**
  - **D36.11 Benign neoplasm of peripheral nerves and autonomic nervous system of face, head, and neck**
  - **D36.12 Benign neoplasm of peripheral nerves and autonomic nervous system, upper limb, including shoulder**
  - **D36.13 Benign neoplasm of peripheral nerves and autonomic nervous system of lower limb, including hip**
  - **D36.14 Benign neoplasm of peripheral nerves and autonomic nervous system of thorax**
  - **D36.15 Benign neoplasm of peripheral nerves and autonomic nervous system of abdomen**
  - **D36.16 Benign neoplasm of peripheral nerves and autonomic nervous system of pelvis**
  - **D36.17 Benign neoplasm of peripheral nerves and autonomic nervous system of trunk, unspecified**

D36.7 Benign neoplasm of other specified sites
Benign neoplasm of nose NOS

D36.9 Benign neoplasm, unspecified site

enign neuroendocrine tumors (D3A)

D3A Benign neuroendocrine tumors

Code also any associated multiple endocrine neoplasia [MEN] syndromes (E31.2-)

Use additional code to identify any associated endocrine syndrome, such as:
carcinoid syndrome (E34.0)

Excludes2: *benign pancreatic islet cell tumors (D13.7)*

+ **D3A.0 Benign carcinoid tumors**
  - **D3A.00 Benign carcinoid tumor of unspecified site**
    Carcinoid tumor NOS
  - + **D3A.01 Benign carcinoid tumors of the small intestine**
    - **D3A.010 Benign carcinoid tumor of the duodenum**
    - **D3A.011 Benign carcinoid tumor of the jejunum**
    - **D3A.012 Benign carcinoid tumor of the ileum**
    - **D3A.019 Benign carcinoid tumor of the small intestine, unspecified portion**
  - + **D3A.02 Benign carcinoid tumors of the appendix, large intestine, and rectum**
    - **D3A.020 Benign carcinoid tumor of the appendix**
    - **D3A.021 Benign carcinoid tumor of the cecum**
    - **D3A.022 Benign carcinoid tumor of the ascending colon**
    - **D3A.023 Benign carcinoid tumor of the transverse colon**
    - **D3A.024 Benign carcinoid tumor of the descending colon**
    - **D3A.025 Benign carcinoid tumor of the sigmoid colon**
    - **D3A.026 Benign carcinoid tumor of the rectum**
    - **D3A.029 Benign carcinoid tumor of the large intestine, unspecified portion**
      Benign carcinoid tumor of the colon NOS
  - + **D3A.09 Benign carcinoid tumors of other sites**
    - **D3A.090 Benign carcinoid tumor of the bronchus and lung**
    - **D3A.091 Benign carcinoid tumor of the thymus**
    - **D3A.092 Benign carcinoid tumor of the stomach**
    - **D3A.093 Benign carcinoid tumor of the kidney**
    - **D3A.094 Benign carcinoid tumor of the foregut, unspecified**
    - **D3A.095 Benign carcinoid tumor of the midgut, unspecified**
    - **D3A.096 Benign carcinoid tumor of the hindgut, unspecified**
    - **D3A.098 Benign carcinoid tumors of other sites**

D3A.8 Other benign neuroendocrine tumors
Neuroendocrine tumor NOS

Neoplasms of uncertain behavior, polycythemia vera and myelodysplastic syndromes (D37-D48)

NOTE Categories D37-D44, and D48 classify by site neoplasms of uncertain behavior, i.e., histologic confirmation whether the neoplasm is malignant or benign cannot be made.

Excludes1: *neoplasms of unspecified behavior (D49.-)*

D37 Neoplasm of uncertain behavior of oral cavity and digestive organs

Excludes1: *stromal tumors of uncertain behavior of digestive system (D48.1)*

+ **D37.0 Neoplasm of uncertain behavior of lip, oral cavity and pharynx**
Excludes1: *neoplasm of uncertain behavior of aryepiglottic fold or interarytenoid fold, laryngeal aspect (D38.0)*
neoplasm of uncertain behavior of epiglottis NOS (D38.0)
neoplasm of uncertain behavior of skin of lip (D48.5)
neoplasm of uncertain behavior of suprahyoid portion of epiglottis (D38.0)
  - **D37.01 Neoplasm of uncertain behavior of lip**
    Neoplasm of uncertain behavior of vermilion border of lip
  - **D37.02 Neoplasm of uncertain behavior of tongue**
  - + **D37.03 Neoplasm of uncertain behavior of the major salivary glands**
    - **D37.030 Neoplasm of uncertain behavior of the parotid salivary glands**
    - **D37.031 Neoplasm of uncertain behavior of the sublingual salivary glands**
    - **D37.032 Neoplasm of uncertain behavior of the submandibular salivary glands**
    - **D37.039 Neoplasm of uncertain behavior of the major salivary glands, unspecified**
  - **D37.04 Neoplasm of uncertain behavior of the minor salivary glands**
    Neoplasm of uncertain behavior of submucosal salivary glands of lip
    Neoplasm of uncertain behavior of submucosal salivary glands of cheek
    Neoplasm of uncertain behavior of submucosal salivary glands of hard palate
    Neoplasm of uncertain behavior of submucosal salivary glands of soft palate
  - **D37.05 Neoplasm of uncertain behavior of pharynx**
    Neoplasm of uncertain behavior of aryepiglottic fold of pharynx NOS
    Neoplasm of uncertain behavior of hypopharyngeal aspect of aryepiglottic fold of pharynx
    Neoplasm of uncertain behavior of marginal zone of aryepiglottic fold of pharynx
  - **D37.09 Neoplasm of uncertain behavior of other specified sites of the oral cavity**

D37.1 Neoplasm of uncertain behavior of stomach

D37.2 Neoplasm of uncertain behavior of small intestine

D37.3 Neoplasm of uncertain behavior of appendix

D37.4 Neoplasm of uncertain behavior of colon

D37.5 Neoplasm of uncertain behavior of rectum
Neoplasm of uncertain behavior of rectosigmoid junction

D37.6 Neoplasm of uncertain behavior of liver, gallbladder and bile ducts
Neoplasm of uncertain behavior of ampulla of Vater

D37.8 Neoplasm of uncertain behavior of other specified digestive organs
Neoplasm of uncertain behavior of anal canal
Neoplasm of uncertain behavior of anal sphincter
Neoplasm of uncertain behavior of anus NOS
Neoplasm of uncertain behavior of esophagus
Neoplasm of uncertain behavior of intestine NOS
Neoplasm of uncertain behavior of pancreas
Excludes1: *neoplasm of uncertain behavior of anal margin (D48.5)*
neoplasm of uncertain behavior of anal skin (D48.5)
neoplasm of uncertain behavior of perianal skin (D48.5)

D37.9 Neoplasm of uncertain behavior of digestive organ, unspecified

D38 Neoplasm of uncertain behavior of middle ear and respiratory and intrathoracic organs

Excludes1: *neoplasm of uncertain behavior of heart (D48.7)*

D38.0 Neoplasm of uncertain behavior of larynx
Neoplasm of uncertain behavior of aryepiglottic fold or interarytenoid fold, laryngeal aspect
Neoplasm of uncertain behavior of epiglottis (suprahyoid portion)
Excludes1: *neoplasm of uncertain behavior of aryepiglottic fold or interarytenoid fold NOS (D37.05)*
neoplasm of uncertain behavior of hypopharyngeal aspect of aryepiglottic fold (D37.05)
neoplasm of uncertain behavior of marginal zone of aryepiglottic fold (D37.05)

D38.1 Neoplasm of uncertain behavior of trachea, bronchus and lung
D38.2 Neoplasm of uncertain behavior of pleura
D38.3 Neoplasm of uncertain behavior of mediastinum
D38.4 Neoplasm of uncertain behavior of thymus
D38.5 Neoplasm of uncertain behavior of other respiratory organs
Neoplasm of uncertain behavior of accessory sinuses
Neoplasm of uncertain behavior of cartilage of nose
Neoplasm of uncertain behavior of middle ear
Neoplasm of uncertain behavior of nasal cavities
Excludes1: *neoplasm of uncertain behavior of ear (external) (skin) (D48.5)*
neoplasm of uncertain behavior of nose NOS (D48.7)
neoplasm of uncertain behavior of skin of nose (D48.5)

D38.6 Neoplasm of uncertain behavior of respiratory organ, unspecified

D39 Neoplasm of uncertain behavior of female genital organs

♀ **D39.0 Neoplasm of uncertain behavior of uterus**
\+ **D39.1 Neoplasm of uncertain behavior of ovary**
Use additional code to identify any functional activity.
♀ **D39.10 Neoplasm of uncertain behavior of unspecified ovary**
♀ **D39.11 Neoplasm of uncertain behavior of right ovary**
♀ **D39.12 Neoplasm of uncertain behavior of left ovary**
• ♀ **D39.2 Neoplasm of uncertain behavior of placenta**
Chorioadenoma destruens
Invasive hydatidiform mole
Malignant hydatidiform mole
Excludes1: *hydatidiform mole NOS (O01.9)*
♀ **D39.8 Neoplasm of uncertain behavior of other specified female genital organs**
Neoplasm of uncertain behavior of skin of female genital organs
♀ **D39.9 Neoplasm of uncertain behavior of female genital organ, unspecified**

D40 Neoplasm of uncertain behavior of male genital organs

♂ **D40.0 Neoplasm of uncertain behavior of prostate**
\+ **D40.1 Neoplasm of uncertain behavior of testis**
♂ **D40.10 Neoplasm of uncertain behavior of unspecified testis**
♂ **D40.11 Neoplasm of uncertain behavior of right testis**
♂ **D40.12 Neoplasm of uncertain behavior of left testis**
♂ **D40.8 Neoplasm of uncertain behavior of other specified male genital organs**
Neoplasm of uncertain behavior of skin of male genital organs
♂ **D40.9 Neoplasm of uncertain behavior of male genital organ, unspecified**

D41 Neoplasm of uncertain behavior of urinary organs

\+ **D41.0 Neoplasm of uncertain behavior of kidney**
Excludes1: *neoplasm of uncertain behavior of renal pelvis (D41.1-)*
D41.00 Neoplasm of uncertain behavior of unspecified kidney
D41.01 Neoplasm of uncertain behavior of right kidney
D41.02 Neoplasm of uncertain behavior of left kidney
\+ **D41.1 Neoplasm of uncertain behavior of renal pelvis**
D41.10 Neoplasm of uncertain behavior of unspecified renal pelvis
D41.11 Neoplasm of uncertain behavior of right renal pelvis
D41.12 Neoplasm of uncertain behavior of left renal pelvis
\+ **D41.2 Neoplasm of uncertain behavior of ureter**
D41.20 Neoplasm of uncertain behavior of unspecified ureter
D41.21 Neoplasm of uncertain behavior of right ureter
D41.22 Neoplasm of uncertain behavior of left ureter
D41.3 Neoplasm of uncertain behavior of urethra
D41.4 Neoplasm of uncertain behavior of bladder
D41.8 Neoplasm of uncertain behavior of other specified urinary organs
D41.9 Neoplasm of uncertain behavior of unspecified urinary organ

D42 Neoplasm of uncertain behavior of meninges

D42.0 Neoplasm of uncertain behavior of cerebral meninges
D42.1 Neoplasm of uncertain behavior of spinal meninges
D42.9 Neoplasm of uncertain behavior of meninges, unspecified

D43 Neoplasm of uncertain behavior of brain and central nervous system

Excludes1: *neoplasm of uncertain behavior of peripheral nerves and autonomic nervous system (D48.2)*

D43.0 Neoplasm of uncertain behavior of brain, supratentorial
Neoplasm of uncertain behavior of cerebral ventricle
Neoplasm of uncertain behavior of cerebrum
Neoplasm of uncertain behavior of frontal lobe
Neoplasm of uncertain behavior of occipital lobe
Neoplasm of uncertain behavior of parietal lobe
Neoplasm of uncertain behavior of temporal lobe
Excludes1: *neoplasm of uncertain behavior of fourth ventricle (D43.1)*
D43.1 Neoplasm of uncertain behavior of brain, infratentorial
Neoplasm of uncertain behavior of brain stem
Neoplasm of uncertain behavior of cerebellum
Neoplasm of uncertain behavior of fourth ventricle
D43.2 Neoplasm of uncertain behavior of brain, unspecified
D43.3 Neoplasm of uncertain behavior of cranial nerves
D43.4 Neoplasm of uncertain behavior of spinal cord
D43.8 Neoplasm of uncertain behavior of other specified parts of central nervous system
D43.9 Neoplasm of uncertain behavior of central nervous system, unspecified
Neoplasm of uncertain behavior of nervous system (central) NOS

D44 Neoplasm of uncertain behavior of endocrine glands

Excludes1: *multiple endocrine adenomatosis (E31.2-)*
multiple endocrine neoplasia (E31.2-)
neoplasm of uncertain behavior of endocrine pancreas (D37.8)
neoplasm of uncertain behavior of ovary (D39.1-)
neoplasm of uncertain behavior of testis (D40.1-)
neoplasm of uncertain behavior of thymus (D38.4)

D44.0 Neoplasm of uncertain behavior of thyroid gland
\+ **D44.1 Neoplasm of uncertain behavior of adrenal gland**
Use additional code to identify any functional activity.
D44.10 Neoplasm of uncertain behavior of unspecified adrenal gland
D44.11 Neoplasm of uncertain behavior of right adrenal gland
D44.12 Neoplasm of uncertain behavior of left adrenal gland
D44.2 Neoplasm of uncertain behavior of parathyroid gland
D44.3 Neoplasm of uncertain behavior of pituitary gland
Use additional code to identify any functional activity.
D44.4 Neoplasm of uncertain behavior of craniopharyngeal duct
D44.5 Neoplasm of uncertain behavior of pineal gland
D44.6 Neoplasm of uncertain behavior of carotid body
D44.7 Neoplasm of uncertain behavior of aortic body and other paraganglia
AHA CC: 4Q, 2016, 26
D44.9 Neoplasm of uncertain behavior of unspecified endocrine gland

D45 Polycythemia vera

Excludes1: *familial polycythemia (D75.0)*
secondary polycythemia (D75.1)
Valid 3-character code, no further characters required

D46 Myelodysplastic syndromes

Use additional code for adverse effect, if applicable, to identify drug (T36-T50 with fifth or sixth character 5)
Excludes2: *drug-induced aplastic anemia (D61.1)*

D46.0 Refractory anemia without ring sideroblasts, so stated
Refractory anemia without sideroblasts, without excess of blasts

D46.1 Refractory anemia with ring sideroblasts
RARS

+ **D46.2 Refractory anemia with excess of blasts [RAEB]**

D46.20 Refractory anemia with excess of blasts, unspecified
RAEB NOS

D46.21 Refractory anemia with excess of blasts 1
RAEB 1

CC **D46.22 Refractory anemia with excess of blasts 2**
RAEB 2
CC Exclusion see Appendix A PDX collection 0488

D46.A Refractory cytopenia with multilineage dysplasia

D46.B Refractory cytopenia with multilineage dysplasia and ring sideroblasts
RCMD RS

CC **D46.C Myelodysplastic syndrome with isolated del(5q) chromosomal abnormality**
Myelodysplastic syndrome with 5q deletion
5q minus syndrome NOS
CC Exclusion see Appendix A PDX collection 0488

D46.4 Refractory anemia, unspecified

D46.Z Other myelodysplastic syndromes
Excludes1: *chronic myelomonocytic leukemia (C93.1-)*

D46.9 Myelodysplastic syndrome, unspecified
Myelodysplasia NOS

D47 Other neoplasms of uncertain behavior of lymphoid, hematopoietic and related tissue

D47.0 Mast cell neoplasms of uncertain behavior
Excludes1: *congenital cutaneous mastocytosis (Q82.2-)*
histiocytic neoplasms of uncertain behavior (D47.Z9)
malignant mast cell neoplasm (C96.2-)

CC **D47.01 Cutaneous mastocytosis**
Diffuse cutaneous mastocytosis
Maculopapular cutaneous mastocytosis
Solitary mastocytoma
Telangiectasia macularis eruptiva perstans
Urticaria pigmentosa
Excludes1: *congenital (diffuse) (maculopapular) cutaneous mastocytosis (Q82.2)*
congenital urticaria pigmentosa (Q82.2)
extracutaneous mastocytoma (D47.09)
CC Exclusion see Appendix A PDX collection 0494

CC **D47.02 Systemic mastocytosis**
Indolent systemic mastocytosis
Isolated bone marrow mastocytosis
Smoldering systemic mastocytosis
Systemic mastocytosis, with an associated hematological non-mast cell lineage disease (SM-AHNMD)
Code also, if applicable, any associated hematological non-mast cell lineage disease, such as:
acute myeloid leukemia (C92.6-, C92.A-)
chronic myelomonocytic leukemia (C93.1-)
essential thrombocytosis (D47.3)
hypereosinophilic syndrome (D72.1)
myelodysplastic syndrome (D46.9)
myeloproliferative syndrome (D47.1)
non-Hodgkin lymphoma (C82-C85)
plasma cell myeloma (C90.0-)
polycythemia vera (D45)
Excludes1: *aggressive systemic mastocytosis (C96.21)*
mast cell leukemia (C94.3-)
CC Exclusion see Appendix A PDX collection 0494

CC **D47.09 Other mast cell neoplasms of uncertain behavior**
Extracutaneous mastocytoma
Mast cell tumor NOS
Mastocytoma NOS
Mastocytosis NOS
CC Exclusion see Appendix A PDX collection 0494
Excludes1: *malignant mast cell tumor (C96.2)*
mastocytosis (congenital) (cutaneous) (Q82.2)

CC **D47.1 Chronic myeloproliferative disease**
Chronic neutrophilic leukemia
Myeloproliferative disease, unspecified
Excludes1: *atypical chronic myeloid leukemia BCR/ABL-negative (C92.2-)*
chronic myeloid leukemia BCR/ABL-positive (C92.1-)
myelofibrosis NOS (D75.81)
myelophthisic anemia (D61.82)
myelophthisis (D61.82)
secondary myelofibrosis NOS (D75.81)
CC Exclusion see Appendix A PDX collection 0488

D47.2 Monoclonal gammopathy
Monoclonal gammopathy of undetermined significance [MGUS]

D47.3 Essential (hemorrhagic) thrombocythemia
Essential thrombocytosis
Idiopathic hemorrhagic thrombocythemia

D47.4 Osteomyelofibrosis
Chronic idiopathic myelofibrosis
Myelofibrosis (idiopathic) (with myeloid metaplasia)
Myelosclerosis (megakaryocytic) with myeloid metaplasia
Secondary myelofibrosis in myeloproliferative disease
Excludes1: *acute myelofibrosis (C94.4-)*

+ **D47.Z Other specified neoplasms of uncertain behavior of lymphoid, hematopoietic and related tissue**

CC **D47.Z1 Post-transplant lymphoproliferative disorder (PTLD)**
Code first complications of transplanted organs and tissue (T86.-)
CC Exclusion see Appendix A PDX collection 0495

CC **D47.Z2 Castleman disease**
Code also if applicable human herpesvirus 8 infection (B10.89)
Excludes2: *Kaposi's sarcoma (C46-)*
CC Exclusion see Appendix A PDX collection 0488
AHA CC: 4Q, 2016, 8

CC **D47.Z9 Other specified neoplasms of uncertain behavior of lymphoid, hematopoietic and related tissue**
Histiocytic tumors of uncertain behavior
CC Exclusion see Appendix A PDX collection 0488

CC **D47.9 Neoplasm of uncertain behavior of lymphoid, hematopoietic and related tissue, unspecified**
Lymphoproliferative disease NOS
CC Exclusion see Appendix A PDX collection 0488

D48 Neoplasm of uncertain behavior of other and unspecified sites

Excludes1: *neurofibromatosis (nonmalignant) (Q85.0-)*

D48.0 Neoplasm of uncertain behavior of bone and articular cartilage
Excludes1: *neoplasm of uncertain behavior of cartilage of ear (D48.1)*
neoplasm of uncertain behavior of cartilage of larynx (D38.0)
neoplasm of uncertain behavior of cartilage of nose (D38.5)
neoplasm of uncertain behavior of connective tissue of eyelid (D48.1)
neoplasm of uncertain behavior of synovia (D48.1)

D48.1 Neoplasm of uncertain behavior of connective and other soft tissue
Neoplasm of uncertain behavior of connective tissue of ear
Neoplasm of uncertain behavior of connective tissue of eyelid
Stromal tumors of uncertain behavior of digestive system
Excludes1: *neoplasm of uncertain behavior of articular cartilage (D48.0)*
neoplasm of uncertain behavior of cartilage of larynx (D38.0)
neoplasm of uncertain behavior of cartilage of nose (D38.5)
neoplasm of uncertain behavior of connective tissue of breast (D48.6-)

D48.2 Neoplasm of uncertain behavior of peripheral nerves and autonomic nervous system

Excludes1: *neoplasm of uncertain behavior of peripheral nerves of orbit (D48.7)*

D48.3 Neoplasm of uncertain behavior of retroperitoneum

D48.4 Neoplasm of uncertain behavior of peritoneum

D48.5 Neoplasm of uncertain behavior of skin

Neoplasm of uncertain behavior of anal margin
Neoplasm of uncertain behavior of anal skin
Neoplasm of uncertain behavior of perianal skin
Neoplasm of uncertain behavior of skin of breast

Excludes1: *neoplasm of uncertain behavior of anus NOS (D37.8)*
neoplasm of uncertain behavior of skin of genital organs (D39.8, D40.8)
neoplasm of uncertain behavior of vermilion border of lip (D37.0)

\+ **D48.6 Neoplasm of uncertain behavior of breast**

Neoplasm of uncertain behavior of connective tissue of breast
Cystosarcoma phyllodes

Excludes1: *neoplasm of uncertain behavior of skin of breast (D48.5)*

D48.60 Neoplasm of uncertain behavior of unspecified breast

D48.61 Neoplasm of uncertain behavior of right breast

D48.62 Neoplasm of uncertain behavior of left breast

D48.7 Neoplasm of uncertain behavior of other specified sites

Neoplasm of uncertain behavior of eye
Neoplasm of uncertain behavior of heart
Neoplasm of uncertain behavior of peripheral nerves of orbit

Excludes1: *neoplasm of uncertain behavior of connective tissue (D48.1)*
neoplasm of uncertain behavior of skin of eyelid (D48.5)

D48.9 Neoplasm of uncertain behavior, unspecified

Neoplasms of unspecified behavior (D49)

D49 Neoplasms of unspecified behavior

NOTE Category D49 classifies by site neoplasms ofunspecified morphology and behavior. The term'mass', unless otherwise stated, is not to be regarded as a neoplastic growth.

Includes: 'growth' NOS
neoplasm NOS
new growth NOS
tumor NOS

Excludes1: *neoplasms of uncertain behavior (D37-D44, D48)*

D49.0 Neoplasm of unspecified behavior of digestive system

Excludes1: *neoplasm of unspecified behavior of margin of anus (D49.2)*
neoplasm of unspecified behavior of perianal skin (D49.2)
neoplasm of unspecified behavior of skin of anus (D49.2)

D49.1 Neoplasm of unspecified behavior of respiratory system

D49.2 Neoplasm of unspecified behavior of bone, soft tissue, and skin

Excludes1: *neoplasm of unspecified behavior of anal canal (D49.0)*
neoplasm of unspecified behavior of anus NOS (D49.0)
neoplasm of unspecified behavior of bone marrow (D49.89)
neoplasm of unspecified behavior of cartilage of larynx (D49.1)
neoplasm of unspecified behavior of cartilage of nose (D49.1)
neoplasm of unspecified behavior of connective tissue of breast (D49.3)
neoplasm of unspecified behavior of skin of genital organs (D49.59)
neoplasm of unspecified behavior of vermilion border of lip (D49.0)

D49.3 Neoplasm of unspecified behavior of breast

Excludes1: *neoplasm of unspecified behavior of skin of breast (D49.2)*

D49.4 Neoplasm of unspecified behavior of bladder

\+ **D49.5 Neoplasm of unspecified behavior of other genitourinary organs**

AHA CC: 4Q, 2016, 9

\+ **D49.51 Neoplasm of unspecified behavior of kidney**

D49.511 Neoplasm of unspecified behavior of right kidney

D49.512 Neoplasm of unspecified behavior of left kidney

D49.519 Neoplasm of unspecified behavior of unspecified kidney

D49.59 Neoplasm unspecified behavior of other genitourinary organ

D49.6 Neoplasm of unspecified behavior of brain

Excludes1: *neoplasm of unspecified behavior of cerebral meninges (D49.7)*
neoplasm of unspecified behavior of cranial nerve (D49.7)

D49.7 Neoplasm of unspecified behavior of endocrine glands and other parts of nervous system

Excludes1: *neoplasm of unspecified behavior of peripheral, sympathetic, and parasympathetic nerves and ganglia (D49.2)*

\+ **D49.8 Neoplasm of unspecified behavior of other specified sites**

Excludes1: *neoplasm of unspecified behavior of eyelid (skin) (D49.2)*
neoplasm of unspecified behavior of eyelid cartilage (D49.2)
neoplasm of unspecified behavior of great vessels (D49.2)
neoplasm of unspecified behavior of optic nerve (D49.7)

D49.81 Neoplasm of unspecified behavior of retina and choroid

Dark area on retina
Retinal freckle

D49.89 Neoplasm of unspecified behavior of other specified sites

D49.9 Neoplasm of unspecified behavior of unspecified site

Chapter 3: Diseases of the Blood and Blood-Forming Organs and Certain Disorders Involving the Immune Mechanism (D50-D89)

Excludes2: *autoimmune disease (systemic) NOS (M35.9)*
certain conditions originating in the perinatal period (P00-P96)
complications of pregnancy, childbirth and the puerperium (O00-O9A)
congenital malformations, deformations and chromosomal abnormalities (Q00-Q99)
endocrine, nutritional and metabolic diseases (E00-E88)
human immunodeficiency virus [HIV] disease (B20)
injury, poisoning and certain other consequences of external causes (S00-T88)
neoplasms (C00-D49)
symptoms, signs and abnormal clinical and laboratory findings, not elsewhere classified (R00-R94)

This chapter contains the following category blocks:

D50-D53 Nutritional anemias
D55-D59 Hemolytic anemias
D60-D64 Aplastic and other anemias and other bone marrow failure syndromes
D65-D69 Coagulation defects, purpura and other hemorrhagic conditions
D70-D77 Other disorders of blood and blood-forming organs
D78 Intraoperative and postprocedural complications of the spleen
D80-D89 Certain disorders involving the immune mechanism

. Chapter-Specific Coding Guidelines

In addition to general coding guidelines, there are guidelines for specific diagnoses and/or conditions in the classification. Unless otherwise indicated, these guidelines apply to all health care settings. Please refer to Section II for guidelines on the selection of principal diagnosis.

Chapter 3: Diseases of the Blood and Blood-Forming Organs and Certain Disorders Involving the Immune Mechanism (D50-D89)

Reserved for future guideline expansion

Nutritional anemias (D50-D53)

D50 Iron deficiency anemia

Includes: asiderotic anemia
hypochromic anemia

D50.0 Iron deficiency anemia secondary to blood loss (chronic)
Posthemorrhagic anemia (chronic)
Excludes1: *acute posthemorrhagic anemia (D62)*
congenital anemia from fetal blood loss (P61.3)

D50.1 Sideropenic dysphagia
Kelly-Paterson syndrome
Plummer-Vinson syndrome

D50.8 Other iron deficiency anemias
Iron deficiency anemia due to inadequate dietary iron intake

D50.9 Iron deficiency anemia, unspecified

D51 Vitamin B12 deficiency anemia

Excludes1: *vitamin B12 deficiency (E53.8)*

D51.0 Vitamin B12 deficiency anemia due to intrinsic factor deficiency
Addison anemia
Biermer anemia
Pernicious (congenital) anemia
Congenital intrinsic factor deficiency

D51.1 Vitamin B12 deficiency anemia due to selective vitamin B12 malabsorption with proteinuria
Imerslund (Gräsbeck) syndrome
Megaloblastic hereditary anemia

D51.2 Transcobalamin II deficiency

D51.3 Other dietary vitamin B12 deficiency anemia
Vegan anemia

D51.8 Other vitamin B12 deficiency anemias

D51.9 Vitamin B12 deficiency anemia, unspecified

D52 Folate deficiency anemia

Excludes1: *folate deficiency without anemia (E53.8)*

D52.0 Dietary folate deficiency anemia
Nutritional megaloblastic anemia

D52.1 Drug-induced folate deficiency anemia
Use additional code for adverse effect, if applicable, to identify drug (T36-T50 with fifth or sixth character 5)

D52.8 Other folate deficiency anemias

D52.9 Folate deficiency anemia, unspecified
Folic acid deficiency anemia NOS

D53 Other nutritional anemias

Includes: megaloblastic anemia unresponsive to vitamin B12 or folate therapy

D53.0 Protein deficiency anemia
Amino-acid deficiency anemia
Orotaciduric anemia
Excludes1: *Lesch-Nyhan syndrome (E79.1)*

D53.1 Other megaloblastic anemias, not elsewhere classified
Megaloblastic anemia NOS
Excludes1: *Di Guglielmo's disease (C94.0)*

D53.2 Scorbutic anemia
Excludes1: *scurvy (E54)*

D53.8 Other specified nutritional anemias
Anemia associated with deficiency of copper
Anemia associated with deficiency of molybdenum
Anemia associated with deficiency of zinc
Excludes1: *nutritional deficiencies without anemia, such as:*
copper deficiency NOS (E61.0)
molybdenum deficiency NOS (E61.5)
zinc deficiency NOS (E60)

D53.9 Nutritional anemia, unspecified
Simple chronic anemia
Excludes1: *anemia NOS (D64.9)*

Hemolytic anemias (D55-D59)

D55 Anemia due to enzyme disorders

Excludes1: *drug-induced enzyme deficiency anemia (D59.2)*

D55.0 Anemia due to glucose-6-phosphate dehydrogenase [G6PD] deficiency
Favism
G6PD deficiency anemia

D55.1 Anemia due to other disorders of glutathione metabolism
Anemia (due to) enzyme deficiencies, except G6PD, related to the hexose monophosphate [HMP] shunt pathway
Anemia (due to) hemolytic nonspherocytic (hereditary), type I

D55.2 Anemia due to disorders of glycolytic enzymes
Hemolytic nonspherocytic (hereditary) anemia, type II
Hexokinase deficiency anemia
Pyruvate kinase [PK] deficiency anemia
Triose-phosphate isomerase deficiency anemia
Excludes1: *disorders of glycolysis not associated with anemia (E74.8)*

D55.3 Anemia due to disorders of nucleotide metabolism

D55.8 Other anemias due to enzyme disorders

D55.9 Anemia due to enzyme disorder, unspecified

D56 Thalassemia

Excludes1: *sickle-cell thalassemia (D57.4-)*

D56.0 Alpha thalassemia
Alpha thalassemia major
Hemoglobin H Constant Spring
Hemoglobin H disease
Hydrops fetalis due to alpha thalassemia
Severe alpha thalassemia
Triple gene defect alpha thalassemia
Use additional code, if applicable, for hydrops fetalis due to alpha thalassemia (P56.99)
Excludes1: *alpha thalassemia trait or minor (D56.3)*
asymptomatic alpha thalassemia (D56.3)
hydrops fetalis due to isoimmunization (P56.0)
hydrops fetalis not due to immune hemolysis (P83.2)

D56.1 Beta thalassemia
Beta thalassemia major
Cooley's anemia
Homozygous beta thalassemia
Severe beta thalassemia
Thalassemia intermedia
Thalassemia major
Excludes1: *beta thalassemia minor (D56.3)*
beta thalassemia trait (D56.3)
delta-beta thalassemia (D56.2)
hemoglobin E-beta thalassemia (D56.5)
sickle-cell beta thalassemia (D57.4-)

D56.2 Delta-beta thalassemia
Homozygous delta-beta thalassemia
Excludes1: *delta-beta thalassemia minor (D56.3)*
delta-beta thalassemia trait (D56.3)

D56.3 Thalassemia minor
Alpha thalassemia minor
Alpha thalassemia silent carrier
Alpha thalassemia trait
Beta thalassemia minor
Beta thalassemia trait
Delta-beta thalassemia minor
Delta-beta thalassemia trait
Thalassemia trait NOS
Excludes1: *alpha thalassemia (D56.0)*
beta thalassemia (D56.1)
delta-beta thalassemia (D56.2)
hemoglobin E-beta thalassemia (D56.5)
sickle-cell trait (D57.3)

D56.4 Hereditary persistence of fetal hemoglobin [HPFH]

D56.5 Hemoglobin E-beta thalassemia
Excludes1: *beta thalassemia (D56.1)*
beta thalassemia minor (D56.3)
beta thalassemia trait (D56.3)
delta-beta thalassemia (D56.2)
delta-beta thalassemia trait (D56.3)
hemoglobin E disease (D58.2)
other hemoglobinopathies (D58.2)
sickle-cell beta thalassemia (D57.4-)

D56.8 Other thalassemias
Dominant thalassemia
Hemoglobin C thalassemia
Mixed thalassemia
Thalassemia with other hemoglobinopathy
Excludes1: *hemoglobin C disease (D58.2)*
hemoglobin E disease (D58.2)
other hemoglobinopathies (D58.2)
sickle-cell anemia (D57.-)
sickle-cell thalassemia (D57.4)

D56.9 Thalassemia, unspecified
Mediterranean anemia (with other hemoglobinopathy)

D57 Sickle-cell disorders

Use additional code for any associated fever (R50.81)
Excludes1: *other hemoglobinopathies (D58.-)*

+ **D57.0 Hb-SS disease with crisis**
Sickle-cell disease NOS with crisis
Hb-SS disease with vasoocclusive pain

MCC **D57.00 Hb-SS disease with crisis, unspecified**
MCC Exclusion see Appendix A PDX collection 0496

MCC **D57.01 Hb-SS disease with acute chest syndrome**
MCC Exclusion see Appendix A PDX collection 0496

MCC **D57.02 Hb-SS disease with splenic sequestration**
MCC Exclusion see Appendix A PDX collection 0496

D57.1 Sickle-cell disease without crisis
Hb-SS disease without crisis
Sickle-cell anemia NOS
Sickle-cell disease NOS
Sickle-cell disorder NOS

+ **D57.2 Sickle-cell/Hb-C disease**
Hb-SC disease
Hb-S/Hb-C disease

D57.20 Sickle-cell/Hb-C disease without crisis

D57.21 Sickle-cell/Hb-C disease with crisis

MCC **D57.211 Sickle-cell/Hb-C disease with acute chest syndrome**
MCC Exclusion see Appendix A PDX collection 0496

MCC **D57.212 Sickle-cell/Hb-C disease with splenic sequestration**
MCC Exclusion see Appendix A PDX collection 0496

MCC **D57.219 Sickle-cell/Hb-C disease with crisis, unspecified**
Sickle-cell/Hb-C disease with crisis NOS
MCC Exclusion see Appendix A PDX collection 0496

D57.3 Sickle-cell trait
Hb-S trait
Heterozygous hemoglobin S

+ **D57.4 Sickle-cell thalassemia**
Sickle-cell beta thalassemia
Thalassemia Hb-S disease

D57.40 Sickle-cell thalassemia without crisis
Microdrepanocytosis
Sickle-cell thalassemia NOS

+ **D57.41 Sickle-cell thalassemia with crisis**
Sickle-cell thalassemia with vasoocclusive pain

MCC **D57.411 Sickle-cell thalassemia with acute chest syndrome**
MCC Exclusion see Appendix A PDX collection 0496

MCC **D57.412 Sickle-cell thalassemia with splenic sequestration**
MCC Exclusion see Appendix A PDX collection 0496

MCC **D57.419 Sickle-cell thalassemia with crisis, unspecified**
Sickle-cell thalassemia with crisis NOS
MCC Exclusion see Appendix A PDX collection 0496

+ **D57.8 Other sickle-cell disorders**
Hb-SD disease
Hb-SE disease

D57.80 Other sickle-cell disorders without crisis

+ **D57.81 Other sickle-cell disorders with crisis**

MCC **D57.811 Other sickle-cell disorders with acute chest syndrome**
MCC Exclusion see Appendix A PDX collection 0496

MCC **D57.812 Other sickle-cell disorders with splenic sequestration**
MCC Exclusion see Appendix A PDX collection 0496

MCC **D57.819 Other sickle-cell disorders with crisis, unspecified**
Other sickle-cell disorders with crisis NOS
MCC Exclusion see Appendix A PDX collection 0496

D58 Other hereditary hemolytic anemias

Excludes1: *hemolytic anemia of the newborn (P55.-)*

D58.0 Hereditary spherocytosis
Acholuric (familial) jaundice
Congenital (spherocytic) hemolytic icterus
Minkowski-Chauffard syndrome

D58.1 Hereditary elliptocytosis
Elliptocytosis (congenital)
Ovalocytosis (congenital) (hereditary)

D58.2 Other hemoglobinopathies
Abnormal hemoglobin NOS
Congenital Heinz body anemia
Hb-C disease
Hb-D disease
Hb-E disease
Hemoglobinopathy NOS
Unstable hemoglobin hemolytic disease
Excludes1: *familial polycythemia (D75.0)*
Hb-M disease (D74.0)
hemoglobin E-beta thalassemia (D56.5)
hereditary persistence of fetal hemoglobin [HPFH] (D56.4)
high-altitude polycythemia (D75.1)
methemoglobinemia (D74.-)
other hemoglobinopathies with thalassemia (D56.8)

CC **D58.8 Other specified hereditary hemolytic anemias**
Stomatocytosis
CC Exclusion see Appendix A PDX collection 0497

CC **D58.9 Hereditary hemolytic anemia, unspecified**
CC Exclusion see Appendix A PDX collection 0497

D59 Acquired hemolytic anemia

CC **D59.0 Drug-induced autoimmune hemolytic anemia**
Use additional code for adverse effect, if applicable, to identify drug (T36-T50 with fifth or sixth character 5)
CC Exclusion see Appendix A PDX collection 0496

CC **D59.1 Other autoimmune hemolytic anemias**
Autoimmune hemolytic disease (cold type) (warm type)
Chronic cold hemagglutinin disease
Cold agglutinin disease
Cold agglutinin hemoglobinuria
Cold type (secondary) (symptomatic) hemolytic anemia
Warm type (secondary) (symptomatic) hemolytic anemia
Excludes1: *Evans syndrome (D69.41)*
hemolytic disease of newborn (P55.-)
paroxysmal cold hemoglobinuria (D59.6)
CC Exclusion see Appendix A PDX collection 0496

CC **D59.2 Drug-induced nonautoimmune hemolytic anemia**
Drug-induced enzyme deficiency anemia
Use additional code for adverse effect, if applicable, to identify drug (T36-T50 with fifth or sixth character 5)
CC Exclusion see Appendix A PDX collection 0496

MCC **D59.3 Hemolytic-uremic syndrome**
Use additional code to identify associated:
E. coli infection (B96.2-)
Pneumococcal pneumonia (J13)
Shigella dysenteriae (A03.9)
MCC Exclusion see Appendix A PDX collection 0496

CC **D59.4 Other nonautoimmune hemolytic anemias**
Mechanical hemolytic anemia
Microangiopathic hemolytic anemia
Toxic hemolytic anemia
CC Exclusion see Appendix A PDX collection 0496

D59.5 Paroxysmal nocturnal hemoglobinuria [Marchiafava-Micheli]
Excludes1: *hemoglobinuria NOS (R82.3)*

D59.6 Hemoglobinuria due to hemolysis from other external causes
Hemoglobinuria from exertion
March hemoglobinuria
Paroxysmal cold hemoglobinuria
Use additional code (Chapter 20) to identify external cause
Excludes1: *hemoglobinuria NOS (R82.3)*

D59.8 Other acquired hemolytic anemias

CC **D59.9 Acquired hemolytic anemia, unspecified**
Idiopathic hemolytic anemia, chronic
CC Exclusion see Appendix A PDX collection 0496

Aplastic and other anemias and other bone marrow failure syndromes (D60-D64)

D60 Acquired pure red cell aplasia [erythroblastopenia]

Includes: red cell aplasia (acquired) (adult) (with thymoma)
Excludes1: *congenital red cell aplasia (D61.01)*

MCC **D60.0 Chronic acquired pure red cell aplasia**
MCC Exclusion see Appendix A PDX collection 0496

MCC **D60.1 Transient acquired pure red cell aplasia**
MCC Exclusion see Appendix A PDX collection 0496

MCC **D60.8 Other acquired pure red cell aplasias**
MCC Exclusion see Appendix A PDX collection 0496

MCC **D60.9 Acquired pure red cell aplasia, unspecified**
MCC Exclusion see Appendix A PDX collection 0496

D61 Other aplastic anemias and other bone marrow failure syndromes

Excludes1: *neutropenia (D70.-)*

\+ **D61.0 Constitutional aplastic anemia**

CC **D61.01 Constitutional (pure) red blood cell aplasia**
Blackfan-Diamond syndrome
Congenital (pure) red cell aplasia
Familial hypoplastic anemia
Primary (pure) red cell aplasia
Red cell (pure) aplasia of infants
Excludes1: *acquired red cell aplasia (D60.9)*
CC Exclusion see Appendix A PDX collection 0498

CC **D61.09 Other constitutional aplastic anemia**
Fanconi's anemia
Pancytopenia with malformations
CC Exclusion see Appendix A PDX collection 0499

MCC **D61.1 Drug-induced aplastic anemia**
Use additional code for adverse effect, if applicable, to identify drug (T36-T50 with fifth or sixth character 5)
MCC Exclusion see Appendix A PDX collection 0496

MCC **D61.2 Aplastic anemia due to other external agents**
Code first, if applicable, toxic effects of substances chiefly nonmedicinal as to source (T51-T65)
MCC Exclusion see Appendix A PDX collection 0496

MCC **D61.3 Idiopathic aplastic anemia**
MCC Exclusion see Appendix A PDX collection 0496

\+ **D61.8 Other specified aplastic anemias and other bone marrow failure syndromes**

\+ **D61.81 Pancytopenia**
Excludes1: *pancytopenia (due to) (with) aplastic anemia (D61.9)*
pancytopenia (due to) (with) bone marrow infiltration (D61.82)
pancytopenia (due to) (with) congenital (pure) red cell aplasia (D61.01)
pancytopenia (due to) (with) hairy cell leukemia (C91.4-)
pancytopenia (due to) (with) human immunodeficiency virus disease (B20.-)
pancytopenia (due to) (with) leukoerythroblastic anemia (D61.82)
pancytopenia (due to) (with) myeloproliferative disease (D47.1)
Excludes2: *pancytopenia (due to) (with) myelodysplastic syndromes (D46.-)*

MCC **D61.810 Antineoplastic chemotherapy induced pancytopenia**
Excludes2: *aplastic anemia due to antineoplasticchemotherapy (D61.1)*
MCC Exclusion see Appendix A PDX collection 0500

MCC **D61.811 Other drug-induced pancytopenia**
Excludes2: *aplastic anemia due to drugs (D61.1)*
MCC Exclusion see Appendix A PDX collection 0500

CC **D61.818 Other pancytopenia**
CC Exclusion see Appendix A PDX collection 0500

CC **D61.82 Myelophthisis**
Leukoerythroblastic anemia
Myelophthisic anemia
Panmyelophthisis
Code also the underlying disorder, such as:
malignant neoplasm of breast (C50.-)
tuberculosis (A15.-)
Excludes1: *idiopathic myelofibrosis (D47.1)*
myelofibrosis NOS (D75.81)
myelofibrosis with myeloid metaplasia (D47.4)
primary myelofibrosis (D47.1)
secondary myelofibrosis (D75.81)
CC Exclusion see Appendix A PDX collection 0500

MCC **D61.89 Other specified aplastic anemias and other bone marrow failure syndromes**
MCC Exclusion see Appendix A PDX collection 0496

CC **D61.9 Aplastic anemia, unspecified**
Hypoplastic anemia NOS
Medullary hypoplasia
CC Exclusion see Appendix A PDX collection 0496

CC **D62 Acute posthemorrhagic anemia**

Excludes1: *anemia due to chronic blood loss (D50.0)*
blood loss anemia NOS (D50.0)
congenital anemia from fetal blood loss (P61.3)
CC Exclusion see Appendix A PDX collection 0501
Valid 3-character code, no further characters required

D63 Anemia in chronic diseases classified elsewhere

D63.0 Anemia in neoplastic disease
Code first neoplasm (C00-D49)
Excludes1: *aplastic anemia due to antineoplastic chemotherapy (D61.1)*
Excludes2: *anemia due to antineoplastic chemotherapy (D64.81)*
Review coding guidelines C.2.c.1, C.2.c.2 and C.2.l.4

D63.1 Anemia in chronic kidney disease
Erythropoietin resistant anemia (EPO resistant anemia)
Code first underlying chronic kidney disease (CKD) (N18.-)

D63.8 Anemia in other chronic diseases classified elsewhere
Code first underlying disease, such as:
diphyllobothriasis (B70.0)
hookworm disease (B76.0-B76.9)
hypothyroidism (E00.0-E03.9)
malaria (B50.0-B54)
symptomatic late syphilis (A52.79)
tuberculosis (A18.89)

D64 Other anemias

Excludes1: *refractory anemia (D46.-)*
refractory anemia with excess blasts in transformation [RAEB T] (C92.0-)

D64.0 Hereditary sideroblastic anemia
Sex-linked hypochromic sideroblastic anemia

D64.1 Secondary sideroblastic anemia due to disease
Code first underlying disease

D64.2 Secondary sideroblastic anemia due to drugs and toxins
Code first poisoning due to drug or toxin, if applicable (T36-T65 with fifth or sixth character 1-4 or 6)

Use additional code for adverse effect, if applicable, to identify drug (T36-T50 with fifth or sixth character 5)

D64.3 Other sideroblastic anemias
Sideroblastic anemia NOS
Pyridoxine-responsive sideroblastic anemia NEC

D64.4 Congenital dyserythropoietic anemia
Dyshematopoietic anemia (congenital)
Excludes1: *Blackfan-Diamond syndrome (D61.01)*
Di Guglielmo's disease (C94.0)

+ D64.8 Other specified anemias

D64.81 Anemia due to antineoplastic chemotherapy
Antineoplastic chemotherapy induced anemia
Excludes1: *aplastic anemia due to antineoplastic chemotherapy (D61.1)*
Excludes2: *anemia in neoplastic disease (D63.0)*
AHA CC: 4Q, 2014, 22-23

D64.89 Other specified anemias
Infantile pseudoleukemia

D64.9 Anemia, unspecified

Coagulation defects, purpura and other hemorrhagic conditions (D65-D69)

MCC **D65 Disseminated intravascular coagulation [defibrination syndrome]**
Afibrinogenemia, acquired
Consumption coagulopathy
Diffuse or disseminated intravascular coagulation [DIC]
Fibrinolytic hemorrhage, acquired
Fibrinolytic purpura
Purpura fulminans
Excludes1: *disseminated intravascular coagulation (complicating):*
abortion or ectopic or molar pregnancy (O00-O07, O08.1)
in newborn (P60)
pregnancy, childbirth and the puerperium (O45.0, O46.0, O67.0, O72.3)
MCC Exclusion see Appendix A PDX collection 0502
Valid 3-character code, no further characters required

MCC **D66 Hereditary factor VIII deficiency**
Classical hemophilia
Deficiency factor VIII (with functional defect)
Hemophilia NOS
Hemophilia A
Excludes1: *factor VIII deficiency with vascular defect (D68.0)*
MCC Exclusion see Appendix A PDX collection 0502
Valid 3-character code, no further characters required

MCC **D67 Hereditary factor IX deficiency**
Christmas disease
Factor IX deficiency (with functional defect)
Hemophilia B
Plasma thromboplastin component [PTC] deficiency
MCC Exclusion see Appendix A PDX collection 0502
Valid 3-character code, no further characters required

D68 Other coagulation defects

Excludes1: *abnormal coagulation profile (R79.1)*
coagulation defects complicating abortion or ectopic or molar pregnancy (O00-O07, O08.1)
coagulation defects complicating pregnancy, childbirth and the puerperium (O45.0, O46.0, O67.0, O72.3)

CC **D68.0 Von Willebrand's disease**
Angiohemophilia
Factor VIII deficiency with vascular defect
Vascular hemophilia
Excludes1: *capillary fragility (hereditary) (D69.8)*
factor VIII deficiency NOS (D66)
factor VIII deficiency with functional defect (D66)
CC Exclusion see Appendix A PDX collection 0502

CC **D68.1 Hereditary factor XI deficiency**
Hemophilia C
Plasma thromboplastin antecedent [PTA] deficiency
Rosenthal's disease
CC Exclusion see Appendix A PDX collection 0502

CC **D68.2 Hereditary deficiency of other clotting factors**
AC globulin deficiency
Congenital afibrinogenemia
Deficiency of factor I [fibrinogen]
Deficiency of factor II [prothrombin]
Deficiency of factor V [labile]
Deficiency of factor VII [stable]
Deficiency of factor X [Stuart-Prower]
Deficiency of factor XII [Hageman]
Deficiency of factor XIII [fibrin stabilizing]
Dysfibrinogenemia (congenital)
Hypoproconvertinemia
Owren's disease
Proaccelerin deficiency
CC Exclusion see Appendix A PDX collection 0502

+ D68.3 Hemorrhagic disorder due to circulating anticoagulants

+ D68.31 Hemorrhagic disorder due to intrinsic circulating anticoagulants, antibodies, or inhibitors

CC **D68.311 Acquired hemophilia**
Autoimmune hemophilia
Autoimmune inhibitors to clotting factors
Secondary hemophilia
CC Exclusion see Appendix A PDX collection 0503

CC **D68.312 Antiphospholipid antibody with hemorrhagic disorder**
Lupus anticoagulant (LAC) with hemorrhagic disorder
Systemic lupus erythematosus [SLE] inhibitor with hemorrhagic disorder
Excludes1: *antiphospholipid antibody, finding without diagnosis (R76.0)*
antiphospholipid antibody syndrome (D68.61)
antiphospholipid antibody with hypercoagulable state (D68.61)
lupus anticoagulant (LAC) finding without diagnosis (R76.0)
lupus anticoagulant (LAC) with hypercoagulable state (D68.62)
systemic lupus erythematosus [SLE] inhibitor finding without diagnosis (R76.0)
systemic lupus erythematosus [SLE] inhibitor with hypercoagulable state (D68.62)
CC Exclusion see Appendix A PDX collection 0504

CC **D68.318 Other hemorrhagic disorder due to intrinsic circulating anticoagulants, antibodies, or inhibitors**
Antithromboplastinemia
Antithromboplastinogenemia
Hemorrhagic disorder due to intrinsic increase in antithrombin
Hemorrhagic disorder due to intrinsic increase in anti-VIIIa
Hemorrhagic disorder due to intrinsic increase in anti-IXa
Hemorrhagic disorder due to intrinsic increase in anti-XIa
CC Exclusion see Appendix A PDX collection 050

CC **D68.32 Hemorrhagic disorder due to extrinsic circulating anticoagulants**
Drug-induced hemorrhagic disorder
Hemorrhagic disorder due to increase in anti-IIa
Hemorrhagic disorder due to increase in anti-Xa
Hyperheparinemia
Use additional code for adverse effect, if applicable, to identify drug (T45.515, T45.525)
CC Exclusion see Appendix A PDX collection 0502
AHA CC: 1Q, 2016, 14-15

CC **D68.4 Acquired coagulation factor deficiency**
Deficiency of coagulation factor due to liver disease
Deficiency of coagulation factor due to vitamin K deficiency
Excludes1: *vitamin K deficiency of newborn (P53)*
CC Exclusion see Appendix A PDX collection 0502

\+ **D68.5 Primary thrombophilia**
Primary hypercoagulable states
Excludes1: *antiphospholipid syndrome (D68.61)*
lupus anticoagulant (D68.62)
secondary activated protein C resistance (D68.69)
secondary antiphospholipid antibody syndrome (D68.69)
secondary lupus anticoagulant with hypercoagulable state (D68.69)
secondary systemic lupus erythematosus [SLE] inhibitor with hypercoagulable state (D68.69)
systemic lupus erythematosus [SLE] inhibitor finding without diagnosis (R76.0)
systemic lupus erythematosus [SLE] inhibitor with hemorrhagic disorder (D68.312)
thrombotic thrombocytopenic purpura (M31.1)

CC **D68.51 Activated protein C resistance**
Factor V Leiden mutation
CC Exclusion see Appendix A PDX collection 0505

CC **D68.52 Prothrombin gene mutation**
CC Exclusion see Appendix A PDX collection 0505

CC **D68.59 Other primary thrombophilia**
Antithrombin III deficiency
Hypercoagulable state NOS
Primary hypercoagulable state NEC
Primary thrombophilia NEC
Protein C deficiency
Protein S deficiency
Thrombophilia NOS
CC Exclusion see Appendix A PDX collection 0505

\+ **D68.6 Other thrombophilia**
Other hypercoagulable states
Excludes1: *diffuse or disseminated intravascular coagulation [DIC] (D65)*
heparin induced thrombocytopenia (HIT) (D75.82)
hyperhomocysteinemia (E72.11)

CC **D68.61 Antiphospholipid syndrome**
Anticardiolipin syndrome
Antiphospholipid antibody syndrome
Excludes1: *anti-phospholipid antibody, finding without diagnosis (R76.0)*
anti-phospholipid antibody with hemorrhagic disorder (D68.312)
lupus anticoagulant syndrome (D68.62)
CC Exclusion see Appendix A PDX collection 0505

CC **D68.62 Lupus anticoagulant syndrome**
Lupus anticoagulant
Presence of systemic lupus erythematosus [SLE] inhibitor
Excludes1: *anticardiolipin syndrome (D68.61)*
antiphospholipid syndrome (D68.61)
lupus anticoagulant (LAC) finding without diagnosis (R76.0)
lupus anticoagulant (LAC) with hemorrhagic disorder (D68.312)
CC Exclusion see Appendix A PDX collection 0505

CC **D68.69 Other thrombophilia**
Hypercoagulable states NEC
Secondary hypercoagulable state NOS
CC Exclusion see Appendix A PDX collection 0505

CC **D68.8 Other specified coagulation defects**
Excludes1: *hemorrhagic disease of newborn (P53)*
CC Exclusion see Appendix A PDX collection 0502

CC **D68.9 Coagulation defect, unspecified**
CC Exclusion see Appendix A PDX collection 0502

D69 Purpura and other hemorrhagic conditions

Excludes1: *benign hypergammaglobulinemic purpura (D89.0)*
cryoglobulinemic purpura (D89.1)
essential (hemorrhagic) thrombocythemia (D47.3)
hemorrhagic thrombocythemia (D47.3)
purpura fulminans (D65)
thrombotic thrombocytopenic purpura (M31.1)
Waldenström hypergammaglobulinemic purpura (D89.0)

CC **D69.0 Allergic purpura**
Allergic vasculitis
Nonthrombocytopenic hemorrhagic purpura
Nonthrombocytopenic idiopathic purpura
Purpura anaphylactoid
Purpura Henoch(-Schönlein)
Purpura rheumatica
Vascular purpura
Excludes1: *thrombocytopenic hemorrhagic purpura (D69.3)*
CC Exclusion see Appendix A PDX collection 0502

D69.1 Qualitative platelet defects
Bernard-Soulier [giant platelet] syndrome
Glanzmann's disease
Grey platelet syndrome
Thromboasthenia (hemorrhagic) (hereditary)
Thrombocytopathy
Excludes1: *von Willebrand's disease (D68.0)*

D69.2 Other nonthrombocytopenic purpura
Purpura NOS
Purpura simplex
Senile purpura

CC **D69.3 Immune thrombocytopenic purpura**
Hemorrhagic (thrombocytopenic) purpura
Idiopathic thrombocytopenic purpura
Tidal platelet dysgenesis
CC Exclusion see Appendix A PDX collection 0502

\+ **D69.4 Other primary thrombocytopenia**
Excludes1: *transient neonatal thrombocytopenia (P61.0)*
Wiskott-Aldrich syndrome (D82.0)

CC **D69.41 Evans syndrome**
CC Exclusion see Appendix A PDX collection 0502

CC **D69.42 Congenital and hereditary thrombocytopenia purpura**
Congenital thrombocytopenia
Hereditary thrombocytopenia
Code first congential or hereditary disorder, such as:
thrombocytopenia with absent radius (TAR syndrome) (Q87.2)
CC Exclusion see Appendix A PDX collection 0502

D69.49 Other primary thrombocytopenia
Megakaryocytic hypoplasia
Primary thrombocytopenia NOS

\+ **D69.5 Secondary thrombocytopenia**
Excludes1: *heparin induced thrombocytopenia (HIT) (D75.82)*
transient thrombocytopenia of newborn (P61.0)

D69.51 Posttransfusion purpura
Posttransfusion purpura from whole blood (fresh) or blood products PTP

D69.59 Other secondary thrombocytopenia
AHA CC: 4Q, 2014, 22-23

D69.6 Thrombocytopenia, unspecified

D69.8 Other specified hemorrhagic conditions
Capillary fragility (hereditary)
Vascular pseudohemophilia

D69.9 Hemorrhagic condition, unspecified

Other disorders of blood and blood-forming organs (D70-D77)

D70 Neutropenia

Includes: agranulocytosis
decreased absolute neurophile count (ANC)
Use additional code for any associated:
fever (R50.81)
mucositis (J34.81, K12.3-, K92.81, N76.81)
Excludes1: *neutropenic splenomegaly (D73.81)*
transient neonatal neutropenia (P61.5)

D70.0 Congenital agranulocytosis
Congenital neutropenia
Infantile genetic agranulocytosis
Kostmann's disease

D70.1 Agranulocytosis secondary to cancer chemotherapy
Use additional code for adverse effect, if applicable, to identify drug (T45.1X5)

Code also underlying neoplasm
AHA CC: 4Q, 2014, 22-23

D70.2 Other drug-induced agranulocytosis
Use additional code for adverse effect, if applicable, to identify drug (T36-T50 with fifth or sixth character 5)

D70.3 Neutropenia due to infection

D70.4 Cyclic neutropenia
Cyclic hematopoiesis
Periodic neutropenia
D70.8 Other neutropenia
D70.9 Neutropenia, unspecified

D71 Functional disorders of polymorphonuclear neutrophils
Cell membrane receptor complex [CR3] defect
Chronic (childhood) granulomatous disease
Congenital dysphagocytosis
Progressive septic granulomatosis
Valid 3-character code, no further characters required

D72 Other disorders of white blood cells
Excludes1: *basophilia (D72.824)*
immunity disorders (D80-D89)
neutropenia (D70)
preleukemia (syndrome) (D46.9)
D72.0 Genetic anomalies of leukocytes
Alder (granulation) (granulocyte) anomaly
Alder syndrome
Hereditary leukocytic hypersegmentation
Hereditary leukocytic hyposegmentation
Hereditary leukomelanopathy
May-Hegglin (granulation) (granulocyte) anomaly
May-Hegglin syndrome
Pelger-Huët (granulation) (granulocyte) anomaly
Pelger-Huët syndrome
Excludes1: *Chédiak (-Steinbrinck)-Higashi syndrome (E70.330)*
D72.1 Eosinophilia
Allergic eosinophilia
Hereditary eosinophilia
Excludes1: *Löffler's syndrome (J82)*
pulmonary eosinophilia (J82)
\+ **D72.8 Other specified disorders of white blood cells**
Excludes1: *leukemia (C91-C95)*
\+ **D72.81 Decreased white blood cell count**
Excludes1: *neutropenia (D70.-)*
D72.810 Lymphocytopenia
Decreased lymphocytes
D72.818 Other decreased white blood cell count
Basophilic leukopenia
Eosinophilic leukopenia
Monocytopenia
Other decreased leukocytes
Plasmacytopenia
D72.819 Decreased white blood cell count, unspecified
Decreased leukocytes, unspecified
Leukocytopenia, unspecified
Leukopenia
Excludes1: *malignant leukopenia (D70.9)*
\+ **D72.82 Elevated white blood cell count**
Excludes1: *eosinophilia (D72.1)*
D72.820 Lymphocytosis (symptomatic)
Elevated lymphocytes
D72.821 Monocytosis (symptomatic)
Excludes1: *infectious mononucleosis (B27.-)*
D72.822 Plasmacytosis
D72.823 Leukemoid reaction
Basophilic leukemoid reaction
Leukemoid reaction NOS
Lymphocytic leukemoid reaction
Monocytic leukemoid reaction
Myelocytic leukemoid reaction
Neutrophilic leukemoid reaction
D72.824 Basophilia
D72.825 Bandemia
Bandemia without diagnosis of specific infection
Excludes1: *confirmed infection - code to infection*
leukemia (C91.-, C92.-, C93.-, C94.-, C95.-)
D72.828 Other elevated white blood cell count
D72.829 Elevated white blood cell count, unspecified
Elevated leukocytes, unspecified
Leukocytosis, unspecified
D72.89 Other specified disorders of white blood cells
Abnormality of white blood cells NEC
D72.9 Disorder of white blood cells, unspecified
Abnormal leukocyte differential NOS

D73 Diseases of spleen
D73.0 Hyposplenism
Atrophy of spleen
Excludes1: *asplenia (congenital) (Q89.01)*
postsurgical absence of spleen (Z90.81)
D73.1 Hypersplenism
Excludes1: *neutropenic splenomegaly (D73.81)*
primary splenic neutropenia (D73.81)
splenitis, splenomegaly in late syphilis (A52.79)
splenitis, splenomegaly in tuberculosis (A18.85)
splenomegaly NOS (R16.1)
splenomegaly congenital (Q89.0)
D73.2 Chronic congestive splenomegaly
D73.3 Abscess of spleen
D73.4 Cyst of spleen
D73.5 Infarction of spleen
Splenic rupture, nontraumatic
Torsion of spleen
Excludes1: *rupture of spleen due to Plasmodium vivax malari[a] (B51.0)*
traumatic rupture of spleen (S36.03-)
\+ **D73.8 Other diseases of spleen**
D73.81 Neutropenic splenomegaly
Werner-Schultz disease
D73.89 Other diseases of spleen
Fibrosis of spleen NOS
Perisplenitis
Splenitis NOS
D73.9 Disease of spleen, unspecified

D74 Methemoglobinemia
CC **D74.0 Congenital methemoglobinemia**
Congenital NADH-methemoglobin reductase deficiency
Hemoglobin-M [Hb-M] disease
Methemoglobinemia, hereditary
CC Exclusion see Appendix A PDX collection 0506
CC **D74.8 Other methemoglobinemias**
Acquired methemoglobinemia (with sulfhemoglobinemia)
Toxic methemoglobinemia
CC Exclusion see Appendix A PDX collection 0506
CC **D74.9 Methemoglobinemia, unspecified**
CC Exclusion see Appendix A PDX collection 0506

D75 Other and unspecified diseases of blood and blood-forming organs
Excludes2: *acute lymphadenitis (L04.-)*
chronic lymphadenitis (I88.1)
enlarged lymph nodes (R59.-)
hypergammaglobulinemia NOS (D89.2)
lymphadenitis NOS (I88.9)
mesenteric lymphadenitis (acute) (chronic) (I88.0)
D75.0 Familial erythrocytosis
Benign polycythemia
Familial polycythemia
Excludes1: *hereditary ovalocytosis (D58.1)*
D75.1 Secondary polycythemia
Acquired polycythemia
Emotional polycythemia
Erythrocytosis NOS
Hypoxemic polycythemia
Nephrogenous polycythemia
Polycythemia due to erythropoietin
Polycythemia due to fall in plasma volume
Polycythemia due to high altitude
Polycythemia due to stress
Polycythemia NOS
Relative polycythemia
Excludes1: *polycythemia neonatorum (P61.1)*
polycythemia vera (D45)
\+ **D75.8 Other specified diseases of blood and blood-forming organs**
CC **D75.81 Myelofibrosis**
Myelofibrosis NOS
Secondary myelofibrosis NOS
Code first the underlying disorder, such as:
malignant neoplasm of breast (C50.-)
Use additional code, if applicable, for associated therapy-related myelodysplastic syndrome (D46.-)

Use additional code for adverse effect, if applicable, to identify drug (T45.1X5)

Excludes1: *acute myelofibrosis (C94.4-)*
idiopathic myelofibrosis (D47.1)
leukoerythroblastic anemia (D61.82)
myelofibrosis with myeloid metaplasia (D47.4)
myelophthisic anemia (D61.82)
myelophthisis (D61.82)
primary myelofibrosis (D47.1)

CC Exclusion see Appendix A PDX collection 0488

D75.82 Heparin induced thrombocytopenia (HIT)

D75.89 Other specified diseases of blood and blood-forming organs

D75.9 Disease of blood and blood-forming organs, unspecified

D76 Other specified diseases with participation of lymphoreticular and reticulohistiocytic tissue

Excludes1: *(Abt-) Letterer-Siwe disease (C96.0)*
eosinophilic granuloma (C96.6)
Hand-Schüller-Christian disease (C96.5)
histiocytic medullary reticulosis (C96.9)
histiocytic sarcoma (C96.A)
histiocytosis X, multifocal (C96.5)
histiocytosis X, unifocal (C96.6)
Langerhans-cell histiocytosis, multifocal (C96.5)
Langerhans-cell histiocytosis NOS (C96.6)
Langerhans-cell histiocytosis, unifocal (C96.6)
leukemic reticuloendotheliosis (C91.4-)
lipomelanotic reticulosis (I89.8)
malignant histiocytosis (C96.A)
malignant reticulosis (C86.0)
nonlipid reticuloendotheliosis (C96.0)

CC **D76.1 Hemophagocytic lymphohistiocytosis**
Familial hemophagocytic reticulosis
Histiocytoses of mononuclear phagocytes
CC Exclusion see Appendix A PDX collection 0507

CC **D76.2 Hemophagocytic syndrome, infection-associated**
Use additional code to identify infectious agent or disease.
CC Exclusion see Appendix A PDX collection 0507

CC **D76.3 Other histiocytosis syndromes**
Reticulohistiocytoma (giant-cell)
Sinus histiocytosis with massive lymphadenopathy
Xanthogranuloma
CC Exclusion see Appendix A PDX collection 0507

D77 Other disorders of blood and blood-forming organs in diseases classified elsewhere

Code first underlying disease, such as:
amyloidosis (E85.-)
congenital early syphilis (A50.0)
echinococcosis (B67.0-B67.9)
malaria (B50.0-B54)
schistosomiasis [bilharziasis] (B65.0-B65.9)
vitamin C deficiency (E54)

Excludes1: *rupture of spleen due to Plasmodium vivax malaria (B51.0)*
splenitis, splenomegaly in late syphilis (A52.79)
splenitis, splenomegaly in tuberculosis (A18.85)

Valid 3-character code, no further characters required

ntraoperative and postprocedural complications of the pleen (D78)

D78 Intraoperative and postprocedural complications of the spleen

AHA CC: 4Q, 2016, 9-10

\+ **D78.0 Intraoperative hemorrhage and hematoma of the spleen complicating a procedure**

Excludes1: *intraoperative hemorrhage and hematoma of the spleen due to accidental puncture or laceration during a procedure (D78.1-)*

CC **D78.01 Intraoperative hemorrhage and hematoma of the spleen complicating a procedure on the spleen**
CC Exclusion see Appendix A PDX collection 0508

CC **D78.02 Intraoperative hemorrhage and hematoma of the spleen complicating other procedure**
CC Exclusion see Appendix A PDX collection 0508

\+ **D78.1 Accidental puncture and laceration of the spleen during a procedure**

CC **D78.11 Accidental puncture and laceration of the spleen during a procedure on the spleen**
CC Exclusion see Appendix A PDX collection 0509

CC **D78.12 Accidental puncture and laceration of the spleen during other procedure**
CC Exclusion see Appendix A PDX collection 0509

\+ **D78.2 Postprocedural hemorrhage of the spleen following a procedure**

CC **D78.21 Postprocedural hemorrhage of the spleen following a procedure on the spleen**
CC Exclusion see Appendix A PDX collection 0508

CC **D78.22 Postprocedural hemorrhage of the spleen following other procedure**
CC Exclusion see Appendix A PDX collection 0508

\+ **D78.3 Postprocedural hematoma and seroma of the spleen following a procedure**

CC **D78.31 Postprocedural hematoma of the spleen following a procedure on the spleen**
CC Exclusion see Appendix A PDX collection 0508

CC **D78.32 Postprocedural hematoma of the spleen following other procedure**
CC Exclusion see Appendix A PDX collection 0508

CC **D78.33 Postprocedural seroma of the spleen following a procedure on the spleen**
CC Exclusion see Appendix A PDX collection 0508

CC **D78.34 Postprocedural seroma of the spleen following other procedure**
CC Exclusion see Appendix A PDX collection 0508

\+ **D78.8 Other intraoperative and postprocedural complications of the spleen**
Use additional code, if applicable, to further specify disorder

CC **D78.81 Other intraoperative complications of the spleen**
CC Exclusion see Appendix A PDX collection 0510

CC **D78.89 Other postprocedural complications of the spleen**
CC Exclusion see Appendix A PDX collection 0510

Certain disorders involving the immune mechanism (D80-D89)

Includes: defects in the complement system
immunodeficiency disorders, except human immunodeficiency virus [HIV] disease sarcoidosis

Excludes1: *autoimmune disease (systemic) NOS (M35.9)*
functional disorders of polymorphonuclear neutrophils (D71)
human immunodeficiency virus [HIV] disease (B20)

D80 Immunodeficiency with predominantly antibody defects

CC **D80.0 Hereditary hypogammaglobulinemia**
Autosomal recessive agammaglobulinemia (Swiss type)
X-linked agammaglobulinemia [Bruton] (with growth hormone deficiency)
CC Exclusion see Appendix A PDX collection 0511

CC **D80.1 Nonfamilial hypogammaglobulinemia**
Agammaglobulinemia with immunoglobulin-bearing B-lymphocytes
Common variable agammaglobulinemia [CVAgamma]
Hypogammaglobulinemia NOS
CC Exclusion see Appendix A PDX collection 0512

CC **D80.2 Selective deficiency of immunoglobulin A [IgA]**
CC Exclusion see Appendix A PDX collection 0512

CC **D80.3 Selective deficiency of immunoglobulin G [IgG] subclasses**
CC Exclusion see Appendix A PDX collection 0511

CC **D80.4 Selective deficiency of immunoglobulin M [IgM]**
CC Exclusion see Appendix A PDX collection 0511

CC **D80.5 Immunodeficiency with increased immunoglobulin M [IgM]**
CC Exclusion see Appendix A PDX collection 0511

CC **D80.6 Antibody deficiency with near-normal immunoglobulins or with hyperimmunoglobulinemia**
CC Exclusion see Appendix A PDX collection 0511

CC **D80.7 Transient hypogammaglobulinemia of infancy**
CC Exclusion see Appendix A PDX collection 0511

CC **D80.8 Other immunodeficiencies with predominantly antibody defects**
Kappa light chain deficiency
CC Exclusion see Appendix A PDX collection 0511

CC **D80.9 Immunodeficiency with predominantly antibody defects, unspecified**
CC Exclusion see Appendix A PDX collection 0511

D81 Combined immunodeficiencies

Excludes1: *autosomal recessive agammaglobulinemia (Swiss type) (D80.0)*

CC **D81.0 Severe combined immunodeficiency [SCID] with reticular dysgenesis**
CC Exclusion see Appendix A PDX collection 0511

CC **D81.1 Severe combined immunodeficiency [SCID] with low T- and B-cell numbers**
CC Exclusion see Appendix A PDX collection 0511

CC **D81.2 Severe combined immunodeficiency [SCID] with low or normal B-cell numbers**
CC Exclusion see Appendix A PDX collection 0511

CC **D81.3 Adenosine deaminase [ADA] deficiency**
CC Exclusion see Appendix A PDX collection 0513

CC **D81.4 Nezelof's syndrome**
CC Exclusion see Appendix A PDX collection 0511
CC **D81.5 Purine nucleoside phosphorylase [PNP] deficiency**
CC Exclusion see Appendix A PDX collection 0513
CC **D81.6 Major histocompatibility complex class I deficiency**
Bare lymphocyte syndrome
CC Exclusion see Appendix A PDX collection 0511
CC **D81.7 Major histocompatibility complex class II deficiency**
CC Exclusion see Appendix A PDX collection 0511
+ **D81.8 Other combined immunodeficiencies**
+ **D81.81 Biotin-dependent carboxylase deficiency**
Multiple carboxylase deficiency
Excludes1: *biotin-dependent carboxylase deficiency due to dietary deficiency of biotin (E53.8)*
D81.810 Biotinidase deficiency
D81.818 Other biotin-dependent carboxylase deficiency
Holocarboxylase synthetase deficiency
Other multiple carboxylase deficiency
D81.819 Biotin-dependent carboxylase deficiency, unspecified
Multiple carboxylase deficiency, unspecified
CC **D81.89 Other combined immunodeficiencies**
CC Exclusion see Appendix A PDX collection 0511
CC **D81.9 Combined immunodeficiency, unspecified**
Severe combined immunodeficiency disorder [SCID] NOS
CC Exclusion see Appendix A PDX collection 0511

D82 Immunodeficiency associated with other major defects
Excludes1: *ataxia telangiectasia [Louis-Bar] (G11.3)*
CC **D82.0 Wiskott-Aldrich syndrome**
Immunodeficiency with thrombocytopenia and eczema
CC Exclusion see Appendix A PDX collection 0511
CC **D82.1 Di George's syndrome**
Pharyngeal pouch syndrome
Thymic alymphoplasia
Thymic aplasia or hypoplasia with immunodeficiency
CC Exclusion see Appendix A PDX collection 0511
D82.2 Immunodeficiency with short-limbed stature
D82.3 Immunodeficiency following hereditary defective response to Epstein-Barr virus
X-linked lymphoproliferative disease
D82.4 Hyperimmunoglobulin E [IgE] syndrome
D82.8 Immunodeficiency associated with other specified major defects
D82.9 Immunodeficiency associated with major defect, unspecified

D83 Common variable immunodeficiency
CC **D83.0 Common variable immunodeficiency with predominant abnormalities of B-cell numbers and function**
CC Exclusion see Appendix A PDX collection 0511
CC **D83.1 Common variable immunodeficiency with predominant immunoregulatory T-cell disorders**
CC Exclusion see Appendix A PDX collection 0511
CC **D83.2 Common variable immunodeficiency with autoantibodies to B- or T-cells**
CC Exclusion see Appendix A PDX collection 0511
CC **D83.8 Other common variable immunodeficiencies**
CC Exclusion see Appendix A PDX collection 0511
CC **D83.9 Common variable immunodeficiency, unspecified**
CC Exclusion see Appendix A PDX collection 0511

D84 Other immunodeficiencies
D84.0 Lymphocyte function antigen-1 [LFA-1] defect
D84.1 Defects in the complement system
C1 esterase inhibitor [C1-INH] deficiency
CC **D84.8 Other specified immunodeficiencies**
CC Exclusion see Appendix A PDX collection 0511
CC **D84.9 Immunodeficiency, unspecified**
CC Exclusion see Appendix A PDX collection 0511

D86 Sarcoidosis
D86.0 Sarcoidosis of lung
D86.1 Sarcoidosis of lymph nodes
D86.2 Sarcoidosis of lung with sarcoidosis of lymph nodes
D86.3 Sarcoidosis of skin
+ **D86.8 Sarcoidosis of other sites**
D86.81 Sarcoid meningitis
D86.82 Multiple cranial nerve palsies in sarcoidosis
D86.83 Sarcoid iridocyclitis
D86.84 Sarcoid pyelonephritis
Tubulo-interstitial nephropathy in sarcoidosis
D86.85 Sarcoid myocarditis
D86.86 Sarcoid arthropathy
Polyarthritis in sarcoidosis
D86.87 Sarcoid myositis
D86.89 Sarcoidosis of other sites
Hepatic granuloma
Uveoparotid fever [Heerfordt]
D86.9 Sarcoidosis, unspecified

D89 Other disorders involving the immune mechanism, not elsewhere classified
Excludes1: *hyperglobulinemia NOS (R77.1)*
monoclonal gammopathy (of undetermined significance) (D47.2
Excludes2: *transplant failure and rejection (T86.-)*
D89.0 Polyclonal hypergammaglobulinemia
Benign hypergammaglobulinemic purpura
Polyclonal gammopathy NOS
D89.1 Cryoglobulinemia
Cryoglobulinemic purpura
Cryoglobulinemic vasculitis
Essential cryoglobulinemia
Idiopathic cryoglobulinemia
Mixed cryoglobulinemia
Primary cryoglobulinemia
Secondary cryoglobulinemia
D89.2 Hypergammaglobulinemia, unspecified
D89.3 Immune reconstitution syndrome
Immune reconstitution inflammatory syndrome [IRIS]
Use additional code for adverse effect, if applicable, to identify drug (T36-T50 with fifth or sixth character 5)
Add the following new codes after D89.3.
+ **D89.4 Mast cell activation syndrome and related disorders**
Excludes1: *aggressive systemic mastocytosis (C96.21)*
congenital cutaneous mastocytosis (Q82.2)
(indolent) systemic mastocytosis (D47.02)
malignant mast cell neoplasm (C96.2-)
malignant mastocytoma (C96.29)
mast cell sarcoma (C96.22)
mastocytoma NOS *(D47.09)*
(non-congenital) cutaneous mastocytosis (D47.01)
other mast cell neoplasms of uncertain behavior (D47.09)
systemic mastocytosis associated with a clonal hematologic non-mast cell lineage disease (SM-AHNMD) (D47.02)
AHA CC: 4Q, 2016, 11
D89.40 Mast cell activation, unspecified
Mast cell activation disorder, unspecified
Mast cell activation syndrome, NOS
D89.41 Monoclonal mast cell activation syndrome
D89.42 Idiopathic mast cell activation syndrome
D89.43 Secondary mast cell activation
Secondary mast cell activation syndrome
Code also underlying etiology, if known
D89.49 Other mast cell activation disorder
Other mast cell activation syndrome
+ **D89.8 Other specified disorders involving the immune mechanism, not elsewhere classified**
+ **D89.81 Graft-versus-host disease**
Code first underlying cause, such as:
complications of transplanted organs and tissues (T86.-
complications of blood transfusion (T80.89)

Use additional code to identify associated manifestations, such as:
desquamative dermatitis (L30.8)
diarrhea (R19.7)
elevated bilirubin (R17)
hair loss (L65.9)
CC **D89.810 Acute graft-versus-host disease**
CC Exclusion see Appendix A PDX collection 051
CC **D89.811 Chronic graft-versus-host disease**
CC Exclusion see Appendix A PDX collection 051
CC **D89.812 Acute on chronic graft-versus-host disease**
CC Exclusion see Appendix A PDX collection 051
CC **D89.813 Graft-versus-host disease, unspecified**
CC Exclusion see Appendix A PDX collection 051
D89.82 Autoimmune lymphoproliferative syndrome [ALPS]
D89.89 Other specified disorders involving the immune mechanism, not elsewhere classified
Excludes1: *human immunodeficiency virus disease (B20*
D89.9 Disorder involving the immune mechanism, unspecified
Immune disease NOS
AHA CC: 3Q, 2015, 22

Chapter 4: Endocrine, Nutritional and Metabolic Disease (E00-E89)

NOTE All neoplasms, whether functionally active or not, are classified in Chapter 2. Appropriate codes in this chapter (i.e. E05.8, E07.0, E16-E31, E34.-) may be used as additional codes to indicate either functional activity by neoplasms and ectopic endocrine tissue or hyperfunction and hypofunction of endocrine glands associated with neoplasms and other conditions classified elsewhere.

Excludes1: *transitory endocrine and metabolic disorders specific to newborn (P70-P74)*

This chapter contains the following category blocks:

- E00-E07 Disorders of thyroid gland
- E08-E13 Diabetes mellitus
- E15-E16 Other disorders of glucose regulation and pancreatic internal secretion
- E20-E35 Disorders of other endocrine glands
- E36 Intraoperative complications of endocrine system
- E40-E46 Malnutrition
- E50-E64 Other nutritional deficiencies
- E65-E68 Overweight, obesity and other hyperalimentation
- E70-E88 Metabolic disorders
- E89 Postprocedural endocrine and metabolic complications and disorders, not elsewhere classified

C. Chapter-Specific Coding Guidelines

In addition to general coding guidelines, there are guidelines for specific diagnoses and/or conditions in the classification. Unless otherwise indicated, these guidelines apply to all health care settings. Please refer to Section II for guidelines on the selection of principal diagnosis.

4. Chapter 4: Endocrine, Nutritional and Metabolic Diseases (E00-E89)

a. Diabetes mellitus

The diabetes mellitus codes are combination codes that include the type of diabetes mellitus, the body system affected, and the complications affecting that body system. As many codes within a particular category as are necessary to describe all of the complications of the disease may be used. They should be sequenced based on the reason for a particular encounter. Assign as many codes from categories E08 – E13 as needed to identify all of the associated conditions that the patient has.

1) Type of diabetes

The age of a patient is not the sole determining factor, though most type 1 diabetics develop the condition before reaching puberty. For this reason type 1 diabetes mellitus is also referred to as juvenile diabetes.

2) Type of diabetes mellitus not documented

If the type of diabetes mellitus is not documented in the medical record the default is E11.-, Type 2 diabetes mellitus.

3) Diabetes mellitus and the use of insulin and oral hypoglycemics

If the documentation in a medical record does not indicate the type of diabetes but does indicate that the patient uses insulin, code E11-, Type 2 diabetes mellitus, should be assigned. **An additional code should be assigned from category Z79 to identify the long-term (current) use of insulin or oral hypoglycemic drugs. If the patient is treated with both oral medications and insulin, only the code for long-term (current) use of insulin should be assigned. Code Z79.4 should not be assigned if insulin is given temporarily to bring a type 2 patient's blood sugar under control during an encounter.**

4) Diabetes mellitus in pregnancy and gestational diabetes

See Section I.C.15. Diabetes mellitus in pregnancy.

See Section I.C.15. Gestational (pregnancy induced) diabetes

5) Complications due to insulin pump malfunction

(a) Underdose of insulin due to insulin pump failure

An underdose of insulin due to an insulin pump failure should be assigned to a code from subcategory T85.6, Mechanical complication of other specified internal and external prosthetic devices, implants and grafts, that specifies the type of pump malfunction, as the principal or first-listed code, followed by code T38.3x6-, Underdosing of insulin and oral hypoglycemic [antidiabetic] drugs. Additional codes for the type of diabetes mellitus and any associated complications due to the underdosing should also be assigned.

(b) Overdose of insulin due to insulin pump failure

The principal or first-listed code for an encounter due to an insulin pump malfunction resulting in an overdose of insulin, should also be T85.6-, Mechanical complication of other specified internal and external prosthetic devices, implants and grafts, followed by code T38.3x1-, Poisoning by insulin and oral hypoglycemic [antidiabetic] drugs, accidental (unintentional).

6) Secondary diabetes mellitus

Codes under categories E08, Diabetes mellitus due to underlying condition, E09, Drug or chemical induced diabetes mellitus, and E13, Other specified diabetes mellitus, identify complications/manifestations associated with secondary diabetes mellitus. Secondary diabetes is always caused by another condition or event (e.g., cystic fibrosis, malignant neoplasm of pancreas, pancreatectomy, adverse effect of drug, or poisoning).

(a) Secondary diabetes mellitus and the use of insulin or *oral* hypoglycemic drugs

For patients with secondary diabetes mellitus who routinely use insulin or oral hypoglycemic drugs, an additional code from category Z79 should be assigned to identify the long-term (current) use of insulin or oral hypoglycemic drugs. If the patient is treated with both oral medications and insulin, only the code for long-term (current) use of insulin should be assigned. Code Z79.4 should not be assigned if insulin is given temporarily to bring a secondary diabetic patient's blood sugar under control during an encounter.

(b) Assigning and sequencing secondary diabetes codes and its causes

The sequencing of the secondary diabetes codes in relationship to codes for the cause of the diabetes is based on the Tabular List instructions for categories E08, E09 and E13.

(i) Secondary diabetes mellitus due to pancreatectomy

For postpancreatectomy diabetes mellitus (lack of insulin due to the surgical removal of all or part of the pancreas), assign code E89.1, Postprocedural hypoinsulinemia. Assign a code from category E13 and a code from subcategory Z90.41-, Acquired absence of pancreas, as additional codes.

(ii) Secondary diabetes due to drugs

Secondary diabetes may be caused by an adverse effect of correctly administered medications, poisoning or sequela of poisoning.

See section I.C.19.e for coding of adverse effects and poisoning, and section I.C.20 for external cause code reporting.

Disorders of thyroid gland (E00-E07)

E00 Congenital iodine-deficiency syndrome

Use additional code (F70-F79) to identify associated intellectual disabilities.

Excludes1: *subclinical iodine-deficiency hypothyroidism (E02)*

E00.0 Congenital iodine-deficiency syndrome, neurological type
Endemic cretinism, neurological type

E00.1 Congenital iodine-deficiency syndrome, myxedematous type
Endemic hypothyroid cretinism
Endemic cretinism, myxedematous type

E00.2 Congenital iodine-deficiency syndrome, mixed type
Endemic cretinism, mixed type

E00.9 Congenital iodine-deficiency syndrome, unspecified
Congenital iodine-deficiency hypothyroidism NOS
Endemic cretinism NOS

E01 Iodine-deficiency related thyroid disorders and allied conditions

Excludes1: *congenital iodine-deficiency syndrome (E00.-)*
subclinical iodine-deficiency hypothyroidism (E02)

E01.0 Iodine-deficiency related diffuse (endemic) goiter

E01.1 Iodine-deficiency related multinodular (endemic) goiter
Iodine-deficiency related nodular goiter

E01.2 Iodine-deficiency related (endemic) goiter, unspecified
Endemic goiter NOS

E01.8 Other iodine-deficiency related thyroid disorders and allied conditions
Acquired iodine-deficiency hypothyroidism NOS

E02 Subclinical iodine-deficiency hypothyroidism

Valid 3-character code, no further characters required

E03 Other hypothyroidism

Excludes1: *iodine-deficiency related hypothyroidism (E00-E02)*
postprocedural hypothyroidism (E89.0)

E03.0 Congenital hypothyroidism with diffuse goiter
Congenital parenchymatous goiter (nontoxic)
Congenital goiter (nontoxic) NOS
Excludes1: *transitory congenital goiter with normal function (P72.0)*

E03.1 Congenital hypothyroidism without goiter
Aplasia of thyroid (with myxedema)
Congenital atrophy of thyroid
Congenital hypothyroidism NOS

Endocrine System

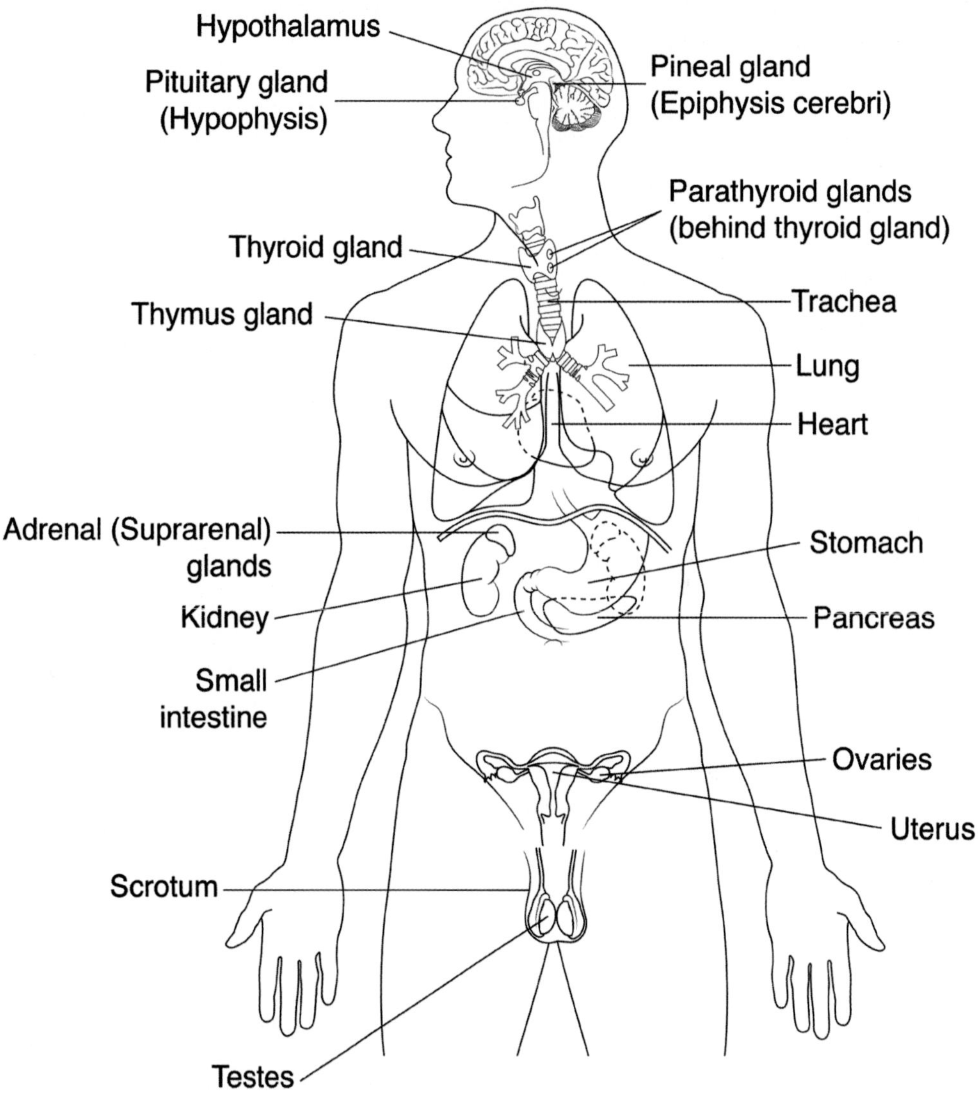

©AHIMA

E03.2 **Hypothyroidism due to medicaments and other exogenous substances**
Code first poisoning due to drug or toxin, if applicable (T36-T65 with fifth or sixth character 1-4 or 6)

Use additional code for adverse effect, if applicable, to identify drug (T36-T50 with fifth or sixth character 5)

E03.3 **Postinfectious hypothyroidism**

E03.4 **Atrophy of thyroid (acquired)**
Excludes1: *congenital atrophy of thyroid (E03.1)*

MCC **E03.5** **Myxedema coma**
MCC Exclusion see Appendix A PDX collection 0515

E03.8 **Other specified hypothyroidism**

E03.9 **Hypothyroidism, unspecified**
Myxedema NOS

E04 **Other nontoxic goiter**
Excludes1: *congenital goiter (NOS) (diffuse) (parenchymatous) (E03.0)*
iodine-deficiency related goiter (E00-E02)

E04.0 **Nontoxic diffuse goiter**
Diffuse (colloid) nontoxic goiter
Simple nontoxic goiter

E04.1 **Nontoxic single thyroid nodule**
Colloid nodule (cystic) (thyroid)
Nontoxic uninodular goiter
Thyroid (cystic) nodule NOS

E04.2 **Nontoxic multinodular goiter**
Cystic goiter NOS
Multinodular (cystic) goiter NOS

E04.8 **Other specified nontoxic goiter**

E04.9 **Nontoxic goiter, unspecified**
Goiter NOS
Nodular goiter (nontoxic) NOS

E05 **Thyrotoxicosis [hyperthyroidism]**
Excludes1: *chronic thyroiditis with transient thyrotoxicosis (E06.2)*
neonatal thyrotoxicosis (P72.1)

\+ E05.0 **Thyrotoxicosis with diffuse goiter**
Exophthalmic or toxic goiter NOS
Graves' disease
Toxic diffuse goiter

E05.00 **Thyrotoxicosis with diffuse goiter without thyrotoxic crisis or storm**

MCC **E05.01** **Thyrotoxicosis with diffuse goiter with thyrotoxic crisis or storm**
MCC Exclusion see Appendix A PDX collection 0516

\+ E05.1 **Thyrotoxicosis with toxic single thyroid nodule**
Thyrotoxicosis with toxic uninodular goiter

E05.10 **Thyrotoxicosis with toxic single thyroid nodule without thyrotoxic crisis or storm**

MCC **E05.11** **Thyrotoxicosis with toxic single thyroid nodule with thyrotoxic crisis or storm**
MCC Exclusion see Appendix A PDX collection 0516

+ E05.2 **Thyrotoxicosis with toxic multinodular goiter**
Toxic nodular goiter NOS
E05.20 **Thyrotoxicosis with toxic multinodular goiter without thyrotoxic crisis or storm**
MCC **E05.21** **Thyrotoxicosis with toxic multinodular goiter with thyrotoxic crisis or storm**
MCC Exclusion see Appendix A PDX collection 0516
+ E05.3 **Thyrotoxicosis from ectopic thyroid tissue**
E05.30 **Thyrotoxicosis from ectopic thyroid tissue without thyrotoxic crisis or storm**
MCC **E05.31** **Thyrotoxicosis from ectopic thyroid tissue with thyrotoxic crisis or storm**
MCC Exclusion see Appendix A PDX collection 0516
+ E05.4 **Thyrotoxicosis factitia**
E05.40 **Thyrotoxicosis factitia without thyrotoxic crisis or storm**
MCC **E05.41** **Thyrotoxicosis factitia with thyrotoxic crisis or storm**
MCC Exclusion see Appendix A PDX collection 0516
+ E05.8 **Other thyrotoxicosis**
Overproduction of thyroid-stimulating hormone
E05.80 **Other thyrotoxicosis without thyrotoxic crisis or storm**
MCC **E05.81** **Other thyrotoxicosis with thyrotoxic crisis or storm**
MCC Exclusion see Appendix A PDX collection 0516
+ E05.9 **Thyrotoxicosis, unspecified**
Hyperthyroidism NOS
E05.90 **Thyrotoxicosis, unspecified without thyrotoxic crisis or storm**
MCC **E05.91** **Thyrotoxicosis, unspecified with thyrotoxic crisis or storm**
MCC Exclusion see Appendix A PDX collection 0516

E06 Thyroiditis

Excludes1: *postpartum thyroiditis (O90.5)*

CC **E06.0** **Acute thyroiditis**
Abscess of thyroid
Pyogenic thyroiditis
Suppurative thyroiditis
Use additional code (B95-B97) to identify infectious agent.
CC Exclusion see Appendix A PDX collection 0517

E06.1 **Subacute thyroiditis**
de Quervain thyroiditis
Giant-cell thyroiditis
Granulomatous thyroiditis
Nonsuppurative thyroiditis
Viral thyroiditis
Excludes1: *autoimmune thyroiditis (E06.3)*

E06.2 **Chronic thyroiditis with transient thyrotoxicosis**
Excludes1: *autoimmune thyroiditis (E06.3)*

E06.3 **Autoimmune thyroiditis**
Hashimoto's thyroiditis
Hashitoxicosis (transient)
Lymphadenoid goiter
Lymphocytic thyroiditis
Struma lymphomatosa

E06.4 **Drug-induced thyroiditis**
Use additional code for adverse effect, if applicable, to identify drug (T36-T50 with fifth or sixth character 5)

E06.5 **Other chronic thyroiditis**
Chronic fibrous thyroiditis
Chronic thyroiditis NOS
Ligneous thyroiditis
Riedel thyroiditis

E06.9 **Thyroiditis, unspecified**

E07 Other disorders of thyroid

E07.0 **Hypersecretion of calcitonin**
C-cell hyperplasia of thyroid
Hypersecretion of thyrocalcitonin

E07.1 **Dyshormogenetic goiter**
Familial dyshormogenetic goiter
Pendred's syndrome
Excludes1: *transitory congenital goiter with normal function (P72.0)*

+ **E07.8** **Other specified disorders of thyroid**
E07.81 **Sick-euthyroid syndrome**
Euthyroid sick-syndrome
E07.89 **Other specified disorders of thyroid**
Abnormality of thyroid-binding globulin
Hemorrhage of thyroid
Infarction of thyroid

E07.9 **Disorder of thyroid, unspecified**

Diabetes mellitus (E08-E13)

Review coding guideline C.4.a

E08 Diabetes mellitus due to underlying condition

Code first the underlying condition, such as:
congenital rubella (P35.0)
Cushing's syndrome (E24.-)
cystic fibrosis (E84.-)
malignant neoplasm (C00-C96)
malnutrition (E40-E46)
pancreatitis and other diseases of the pancreas (K85-K86.-)

Use additional code to identify control using:
insulin (Z79.4)
oral antidiabetic drugs (Z79.84)
oral hypoglycemic drugs (Z79.84)

Excludes1: *drug or chemical induced diabetes mellitus (E09.-)*
gestational diabetes (O24.4-)
neonatal diabetes mellitus (P70.2)
postpancreatectomy diabetes mellitus (E13.-)
postprocedural diabetes mellitus (E13.-)
secondary diabetes mellitus NEC (E13.-)
type 1 diabetes mellitus (E10.-)
type 2 diabetes mellitus (E11.-)

Review coding guideline C.4.a.6.a

+ **E08.0** **Diabetes mellitus due to underlying condition with hyperosmolarity**
MCC **E08.00** **Diabetes mellitus due to underlying condition with hyperosmolarity without nonketotic hyperglycemic-hyperosmolar coma (NKHHC)**
MCC Exclusion see Appendix A PDX collection 0518
HAC see Appendix B for HAC conditional logic
MCC **E08.01** **Diabetes mellitus due to underlying condition with hyperosmolarity with coma**
MCC Exclusion see Appendix A PDX collection 0518
HAC see Appendix B for HAC conditional logic

+ **E08.1** **Diabetes mellitus due to underlying condition with ketoacidosis**
MCC **E08.10** **Diabetes mellitus due to underlying condition with ketoacidosis without coma**
MCC Exclusion see Appendix A PDX collection 0518
HAC see Appendix B for HAC conditional logic
MCC **E08.11** **Diabetes mellitus due to underlying condition with ketoacidosis with coma**
MCC Exclusion see Appendix A PDX collection 0518

+ **E08.2** **Diabetes mellitus due to underlying condition with kidney complications**
E08.21 **Diabetes mellitus due to underlying condition with diabetic nephropathy**
Diabetes mellitus due to underlying condition with intercapillary glomerulosclerosis
Diabetes mellitus due to underlying condition with intracapillary glomerulonephrosis
Diabetes mellitus due to underlying condition with Kimmelstiel-Wilson disease
E08.22 **Diabetes mellitus due to underlying condition with diabetic chronic kidney disease**
Use additional code to identify stage of chronic kidney disease (N18.1-N18.6)
E08.29 **Diabetes mellitus due to underlying condition with other diabetic kidney complication**
Renal tubular degeneration in diabetes mellitus due to underlying condition

+ **E08.3** **Diabetes mellitus due to underlying condition with ophthalmic complications**
AHA CC: 4Q, 2016, 11-13
+ **E08.31** **Diabetes mellitus due to underlying condition with unspecified diabetic retinopathy**
E08.311 **Diabetes mellitus due to underlying condition with unspecified diabetic retinopathy with macular edema**
E08.319 **Diabetes mellitus due to underlying condition with unspecified diabetic retinopathy without macular edema**

+ **E08.32 Diabetes mellitus due to underlying condition with mild nonproliferative diabetic retinopathy**
Diabetes mellitus due to underlying condition with nonproliferative diabetic retinopathy NOS

One of the following 7th characters is to be assigned to codes in subcategory **E08.32** to designate laterality of the disease:
1 right eye
2 left eye
3 bilateral
9 unspecified eye

+7th **E08.321 Diabetes mellitus due to underlying condition with mild nonproliferative diabetic retinopathy with macular edema**
+7th **E08.329 Diabetes mellitus due to underlying condition with mild nonproliferative diabetic retinopathy without macular edema**
+ **E08.33 Diabetes mellitus due to underlying condition with moderate nonproliferative diabetic retinopathy**

One of the following 7th characters is to be assigned to codes in subcategory **E08.33** to designate laterality of the disease:
1 right eye
2 left eye
3 bilateral
9 unspecified eye

+7th **E08.331 Diabetes mellitus due to underlying condition with moderate nonproliferative diabetic retinopathy with macular edema**
+7th **E08.339 Diabetes mellitus due to underlying condition with moderate nonproliferative diabetic retinopathy without macular edema**
+ **E08.34 Diabetes mellitus due to underlying condition with severe nonproliferative diabetic retinopathy**

One of the following 7th characters is to be assigned to codes in subcategory **E08.34** to designate laterality of the disease:
1 right eye
2 left eye
3 bilateral
9 unspecified eye

+7th **E08.341 Diabetes mellitus due to underlying condition with severe nonproliferative diabetic retinopathy with macular edema**
+7th **E08.349 Diabetes mellitus due to underlying condition with severe nonproliferative diabetic retinopathy without macular edema**
+ **E08.35 Diabetes mellitus due to underlying condition with proliferative diabetic retinopathy**

One of the following 7th characters is to be assigned to codes in subcategory **E08.35** to designate laterality of the disease:
1 right eye
2 left eye
3 bilateral
9 unspecified eye

+7th **E08.351 Diabetes mellitus due to underlying condition with proliferative diabetic retinopathy with macular edema**
+7th **E08.352 Diabetes mellitus due to underlying condition with proliferative diabetic retinopathy with traction retinal detachment involving the macula**
+7th **E08.353 Diabetes mellitus due to underlying condition with proliferative diabetic retinopathy with traction retinal detachment not involving the macula**
+7th **E08.354 Diabetes mellitus due to underlying condition with proliferative diabetic retinopathy with combined traction retinal detachment and rhegmatogenous retinal detachment**
+7th **E08.355 Diabetes mellitus due to underlying condition with stable proliferative diabetic retinopathy**
+7th **E08.359 Diabetes mellitus due to underlying condition with proliferative diabetic retinopathy without macular edema**
E08.36 Diabetes mellitus due to underlying condition with diabetic cataract
X+7th **E08.37 Diabetes mellitus due to underlying condition with diabetic macular edema, resolved following treatment**

One of the following 7th characters is to be assigned to codes in subcategory **E08.37** to designate laterality of the disease:
1 right eye
2 left eye
3 bilateral
9 unspecified eye

E08.39 Diabetes mellitus due to underlying condition with other diabetic ophthalmic complication
Use additional code to identify manifestation, such as:
diabetic glaucoma (H40-H42)
+ **E08.4 Diabetes mellitus due to underlying condition with neurological complications**
E08.40 Diabetes mellitus due to underlying condition with diabetic neuropathy, unspecified
E08.41 Diabetes mellitus due to underlying condition with diabetic mononeuropathy
E08.42 Diabetes mellitus due to underlying condition with diabetic polyneuropathy
Diabetes mellitus due to underlying condition with diabetic neuralgia
E08.43 Diabetes mellitus due to underlying condition with diabetic autonomic (poly)neuropathy
Diabetes mellitus due to underlying condition with diabetic gastroparesis
AHA CC: 3Q, 2013, 114-115
E08.44 Diabetes mellitus due to underlying condition with diabetic amyotrophy
E08.49 Diabetes mellitus due to underlying condition with other diabetic neurological complication
+ **E08.5 Diabetes mellitus due to underlying condition with circulatory complications**
E08.51 Diabetes mellitus due to underlying condition with diabetic peripheral angiopathy without gangrene
CC **E08.52 Diabetes mellitus due to underlying condition with diabetic peripheral angiopathy with gangrene**
Diabetes mellitus due to underlying condition with diabetic gangrene
CC Exclusion see Appendix A PDX collection 0519
E08.59 Diabetes mellitus due to underlying condition with other circulatory complications
+ **E08.6 Diabetes mellitus due to underlying condition with other specified complications**
+ **E08.61 Diabetes mellitus due to underlying condition with diabetic arthropathy**
E08.610 Diabetes mellitus due to underlying condition with diabetic neuropathic arthropathy
Diabetes mellitus due to underlying condition with Charcôt's joints
E08.618 Diabetes mellitus due to underlying condition with other diabetic arthropathy
+ **E08.62 Diabetes mellitus due to underlying condition with skin complications**
E08.620 Diabetes mellitus due to underlying condition with diabetic dermatitis
Diabetes mellitus due to underlying condition with diabetic necrobiosis lipoidica
E08.621 Diabetes mellitus due to underlying condition with foot ulcer
Use additional code to identify site of ulcer (L97.4-, L97.5-)
E08.622 Diabetes mellitus due to underlying condition with other skin ulcer
Use additional code to identify site of ulcer (L97.1-L97.9, L98.41-L98.49)
E08.628 Diabetes mellitus due to underlying condition with other skin complications

+ E08.63 **Diabetes mellitus due to underlying condition with oral complications**

E08.630 **Diabetes mellitus due to underlying condition with periodontal disease**

E08.638 **Diabetes mellitus due to underlying condition with other oral complications**

+ E08.64 **Diabetes mellitus due to underlying condition with hypoglycemia**

MCC E08.641 **Diabetes mellitus due to underlying condition with hypoglycemia with coma**

MCC Exclusion see Appendix A PDX collection 0518

E08.649 **Diabetes mellitus due to underlying condition with hypoglycemia without coma**

E08.65 **Diabetes mellitus due to underlying condition with hyperglycemia**

E08.69 **Diabetes mellitus due to underlying condition with other specified complication**

Use additional code to identify complication

E08.8 **Diabetes mellitus due to underlying condition with unspecified complications**

E08.9 **Diabetes mellitus due to underlying condition without complications**

E09 Drug or chemical induced diabetes mellitus

Code first poisoning due to drug or toxin, if applicable (T36-T65 with fifth or sixth character 1-4 or 6)

Use additional code for adverse effect, if applicable, to identify drug (T36-T50 with fifth or sixth character 5)

Use additional code to identify control using:
insulin (Z79.4)
oral antidiabetic drugs (Z79.84)
oral hypoglycemic drugs (Z79.84)

Excludes1: *diabetes mellitus due to underlying condition (E08.-)*
gestational diabetes (O24.4-)
neonatal diabetes mellitus (P70.2)
postpancreatectomy diabetes mellitus (E13.-)
postprocedural diabetes mellitus (E13.-)
secondary diabetes mellitus NEC (E13.-)
type 1 diabetes mellitus (E10.-)
type 2 diabetes mellitus (E11.-)

Review coding guideline C.4.a.6.a

+ E09.0 **Drug or chemical induced diabetes mellitus with hyperosmolarity**

MCC E09.00 **Drug or chemical induced diabetes mellitus with hyperosmolarity without nonketotic hyperglycemic-hyperosmolar coma (NKHHC)**

MCC Exclusion see Appendix A PDX collection 0518

HAC see Appendix B for HAC conditional logic

MCC E09.01 **Drug or chemical induced diabetes mellitus with hyperosmolarity with coma**

MCC Exclusion see Appendix A PDX collection 0518

HAC see Appendix B for HAC conditional logic

+ E09.1 **Drug or chemical induced diabetes mellitus with ketoacidosis**

MCC E09.10 **Drug or chemical induced diabetes mellitus with ketoacidosis without coma**

MCC Exclusion see Appendix A PDX collection 0518

HAC see Appendix B for HAC conditional logic

MCC E09.11 **Drug or chemical induced diabetes mellitus with ketoacidosis with coma**

MCC Exclusion see Appendix A PDX collection 0518

+ E09.2 **Drug or chemical induced diabetes mellitus with kidney complications**

E09.21 **Drug or chemical induced diabetes mellitus with diabetic nephropathy**

Drug or chemical induced diabetes mellitus with intercapillary glomerulosclerosis

Drug or chemical induced diabetes mellitus with intracapillary glomerulonephrosis

Drug or chemical induced diabetes mellitus with Kimmelstiel-Wilson disease

E09.22 **Drug or chemical induced diabetes mellitus with diabetic chronic kidney disease**

Use additional code to identify stage of chronic kidney disease (N18.1-N18.6)

E09.29 **Drug or chemical induced diabetes mellitus with other diabetic kidney complication**

Drug or chemical induced diabetes mellitus with renal tubular degeneration

+ E09.3 **Drug or chemical induced diabetes mellitus with ophthalmic complications**

AHA CC: 4Q, 2016, 11-13

+ E09.31 **Drug or chemical induced diabetes mellitus with unspecified diabetic retinopathy**

E09.311 **Drug or chemical induced diabetes mellitus with unspecified diabetic retinopathy with macular edema**

E09.319 **Drug or chemical induced diabetes mellitus with unspecified diabetic retinopathy without macular edema**

+ E09.32 **Drug or chemical induced diabetes mellitus with mild nonproliferative diabetic retinopathy**

Drug or chemical induced diabetes mellitus with nonproliferative diabetic retinopathy NOS

One of the following 7th characters is to be assigned to codes in subcategory **E09.32** to designate laterality of the disease:
1 right eye
2 left eye
3 bilateral
9 unspecified eye

+7th E09.321 **Drug or chemical induced diabetes mellitus with mild nonproliferative diabetic retinopathy with macular edema**

+7th E09.329 **Drug or chemical induced diabetes mellitus with mild nonproliferative diabetic retinopathy without macular edema**

+7th E09.33 **Drug or chemical induced diabetes mellitus with moderate nonproliferative diabetic retinopathy**

One of the following 7th characters is to be assigned to codes in subcategory **E09.33** to designate laterality of the disease:
1 right eye
2 left eye
3 bilateral
9 unspecified eye

+7th E09.331 **Drug or chemical induced diabetes mellitus with moderate nonproliferative diabetic retinopathy with macular edema**

+7th E09.339 **Drug or chemical induced diabetes mellitus with moderate nonproliferative diabetic retinopathy without macular edema**

+ E09.34 **Drug or chemical induced diabetes mellitus with severe nonproliferative diabetic retinopathy**

One of the following 7th characters is to be assigned to codes in subcategory **E09.34** to designate laterality of the disease:
1 right eye
2 left eye
3 bilateral
9 unspecified eye

+7th E09.341 **Drug or chemical induced diabetes mellitus with severe nonproliferative diabetic retinopathy with macular edema**

+7th E09.349 **Drug or chemical induced diabetes mellitus with severe nonproliferative diabetic retinopathy without macular edema**

+ E09.35 **Drug or chemical induced diabetes mellitus with proliferative diabetic retinopathy**

One of the following 7th characters is to be assigned to codes in subcategory **E09.35** to designate laterality of the disease:
1 right eye
2 left eye
3 bilateral
9 unspecified eye

+7th E09.351 **Drug or chemical induced diabetes mellitus with proliferative diabetic retinopathy with macular edema**

+7th **E09.352 Drug or chemical induced diabetes mellitus with proliferative diabetic retinopathy with traction retinal detachment involving the macula**

+7th **E09.353 Drug or chemical induced diabetes mellitus with proliferative diabetic retinopathy with traction retinal detachment not involving the macula**

+7th **E09.354 Drug or chemical induced diabetes mellitus with proliferative diabetic retinopathy with combined traction retinal detachment and rhegmatogenous retinal detachment**

+7th **E09.355 Drug or chemical induced diabetes mellitus with stable proliferative diabetic retinopathy**

+7th **E09.359 Drug or chemical induced diabetes mellitus with proliferative diabetic retinopathy without macular edema**

E09.36 Drug or chemical induced diabetes mellitus with diabetic cataract

X+7th **E09.37 Drug or chemical induced diabetes mellitus with diabetic macular edema, resolved following treatment**

One of the following 7th characters is to be assigned to codes in subcategory **E09.37** to designate laterality of the disease:
1 right eye
2 left eye
3 bilateral
9 unspecified eye

E09.39 Drug or chemical induced diabetes mellitus with other diabetic ophthalmic complication
Use additional code to identify manifestation, such as:
diabetic glaucoma (H40-H42)

+ **E09.4 Drug or chemical induced diabetes mellitus with neurological complications**

E09.40 Drug or chemical induced diabetes mellitus with neurological complications with diabetic neuropathy, unspecified

E09.41 Drug or chemical induced diabetes mellitus with neurological complications with diabetic mononeuropathy

E09.42 Drug or chemical induced diabetes mellitus with neurological complications with diabetic polyneuropathy
Drug or chemical induced diabetes mellitus with diabetic neuralgia

E09.43 Drug or chemical induced diabetes mellitus with neurological complications with diabetic autonomic (poly)neuropathy
Drug or chemical induced diabetes mellitus with diabetic gastroparesis
AHA CC: 3Q, 2013, 114-115

E09.44 Drug or chemical induced diabetes mellitus with neurological complications with diabetic amyotrophy

E09.49 Drug or chemical induced diabetes mellitus with neurological complications with other diabetic neurological complication

+ **E09.5 Drug or chemical induced diabetes mellitus with circulatory complications**

E09.51 Drug or chemical induced diabetes mellitus with diabetic peripheral angiopathy without gangrene

CC **E09.52 Drug or chemical induced diabetes mellitus with diabetic peripheral angiopathy with gangrene**
Drug or chemical induced diabetes mellitus with diabetic gangrene
CC Exclusion see Appendix A PDX collection 0519

E09.59 Drug or chemical induced diabetes mellitus with other circulatory complications

+ **E09.6 Drug or chemical induced diabetes mellitus with other specified complications**

+ **E09.61 Drug or chemical induced diabetes mellitus with diabetic arthropathy**

E09.610 Drug or chemical induced diabetes mellitus with diabetic neuropathic arthropathy
Drug or chemical induced diabetes mellitus with Charcôt's joints

E09.618 Drug or chemical induced diabetes mellitus with other diabetic arthropathy

+ **E09.62 Drug or chemical induced diabetes mellitus with skin complications**

E09.620 Drug or chemical induced diabetes mellitus with diabetic dermatitis
Drug or chemical induced diabetes mellitus with diabetic necrobiosis lipoidica

E09.621 Drug or chemical induced diabetes mellitus with foot ulcer
Use additional code to identify site of ulcer (L97.4-, L97.5-)

E09.622 Drug or chemical induced diabetes mellitus with other skin ulcer
Use additional code to identify site of ulcer (L97.1-L97.9, L98.41-L98.49)

E09.628 Drug or chemical induced diabetes mellitus with other skin complications

+ **E09.63 Drug or chemical induced diabetes mellitus with oral complications**

E09.630 Drug or chemical induced diabetes mellitus with periodontal disease

E09.638 Drug or chemical induced diabetes mellitus with other oral complications

+ **E09.64 Drug or chemical induced diabetes mellitus with hypoglycemia**

MCC **E09.641 Drug or chemical induced diabetes mellitus with hypoglycemia with coma**
MCC Exclusion see Appendix A PDX collection 0518

E09.649 Drug or chemical induced diabetes mellitus with hypoglycemia without coma

E09.65 Drug or chemical induced diabetes mellitus with hyperglycemia

E09.69 Drug or chemical induced diabetes mellitus with other specified complication
Use additional code to identify complication

E09.8 Drug or chemical induced diabetes mellitus with unspecified complications

E09.9 Drug or chemical induced diabetes mellitus without complications

E10 Type 1 diabetes mellitus

Includes: brittle diabetes (mellitus)
diabetes (mellitus) due to autoimmune process
diabetes (mellitus) due to immune mediated pancreatic islet beta-cell destruction
idiopathic diabetes (mellitus)
juvenile onset diabetes (mellitus)
ketosis-prone diabetes (mellitus)

Excludes1: *diabetes mellitus due to underlying condition (E08.-)*
drug or chemical induced diabetes mellitus (E09.-)
gestational diabetes (O24.4-)
hyperglycemia NOS (R73.9)
neonatal diabetes mellitus (P70.2)
postpancreatectomy diabetes mellitus (E13.-)
postprocedural diabetes mellitus (E13.-)
secondary diabetes mellitus NEC (E13.-)
type 2 diabetes mellitus (E11.-)

+ **E10.1 Type 1 diabetes mellitus with ketoacidosis**

MCC **E10.10 Type 1 diabetes mellitus with ketoacidosis without coma**
MCC Exclusion see Appendix A PDX collection 0520
HAC see Appendix B for HAC conditional logic
AHA CC: 3Q, 2013, 20

MCC **E10.11 Type 1 diabetes mellitus with ketoacidosis with coma**
MCC Exclusion see Appendix A PDX collection 0520

+ **E10.2 Type 1 diabetes mellitus with kidney complications**

E10.21 Type 1 diabetes mellitus with diabetic nephropathy
Type 1 diabetes mellitus with intercapillary glomerulosclerosis
Type 1 diabetes mellitus with intracapillary glomerulonephrosis
Type 1 diabetes mellitus with Kimmelstiel-Wilson disease

E10.22 Type 1 diabetes mellitus with diabetic chronic kidney disease
Use additional code to identify stage of chronic kidney disease (N18.1-N18.6)

E10.29 Type 1 diabetes mellitus with other diabetic kidney complication
Type 1 diabetes mellitus with renal tubular degeneration

+ **E10.3 Type 1 diabetes mellitus with ophthalmic complications**
AHA CC: 4Q, 2016, 11-13

+ **E10.31 Type 1 diabetes mellitus with unspecified diabetic retinopathy**

E10.311 Type 1 diabetes mellitus with unspecified diabetic retinopathy with macular edema

E10.319 Type 1 diabetes mellitus with unspecified diabetic retinopathy without macular edema

+ **E10.32 Type 1 diabetes mellitus with mild nonproliferative diabetic retinopathy**
Type 1 diabetes mellitus with nonproliferative diabetic retinopathy NOS

One of the following 7th characters is to be assigned to codes in subcategory **E10.32** to designate laterality of the disease:
1 right eye
2 left eye
3 bilateral
9 unspecified eye

+7th **E10.321 Type 1 diabetes mellitus with mild nonproliferative diabetic retinopathy with macular edema**

+7th **E10.329 Type 1 diabetes mellitus with mild nonproliferative diabetic retinopathy without macular edema**

+ **E10.33 Type 1 diabetes mellitus with moderate nonproliferative diabetic retinopathy**

One of the following 7th characters is to be assigned to codes in subcategory **E10.33** to designate laterality of the disease:
1 right eye
2 left eye
3 bilateral
9 unspecified eye

+7th **E10.331 Type 1 diabetes mellitus with moderate nonproliferative diabetic retinopathy with macular edema**

+7th **E10.339 Type 1 diabetes mellitus with moderate nonproliferative diabetic retinopathy without macular edema**

+ **E10.34 Type 1 diabetes mellitus with severe nonproliferative diabetic retinopathy**

One of the following 7th characters is to be assigned to codes in subcategory **E10.34** to designate laterality of the disease:
1 right eye
2 left eye
3 bilateral
9 unspecified eye

+7th **E10.341 Type 1 diabetes mellitus with severe nonproliferative diabetic retinopathy with macular edema**

+7th **E10.349 Type 1 diabetes mellitus with severe nonproliferative diabetic retinopathy without macular edema**

+ **E10.35 Type 1 diabetes mellitus with proliferative diabetic retinopathy**

One of the following 7th characters is to be assigned to codes in subcategory **E10.35** to designate laterality of the disease:
1 right eye
2 left eye
3 bilateral
9 unspecified eye

+7th **E10.351 Type 1 diabetes mellitus with proliferative diabetic retinopathy with macular edema**

+7th **E10.352 Type 1 diabetes mellitus with proliferative diabetic retinopathy with traction retinal detachment involving the macula**

+7th **E10.353 Type 1 diabetes mellitus with proliferative diabetic retinopathy with traction retinal detachment not involving the macula**

+7th **E10.354 Type 1 diabetes mellitus with proliferative diabetic retinopathy with combined traction retinal detachment and rhegmatogenous retinal detachment**

+7th **E10.355 Type 1 diabetes mellitus with stable proliferative diabetic retinopathy**

+7th **E10.359 Type 1 diabetes mellitus with proliferative diabetic retinopathy without macular edema**

E10.36 Type 1 diabetes mellitus with diabetic cataract

X+7th **E10.37 Type 1 diabetes mellitus with diabetic macular edema, resolved following treatment**

One of the following 7th characters is to be assigned to codes in subcategory **E10.37** to designate laterality of the disease:
1 right eye
2 left eye
3 bilateral
9 unspecified eye

E10.39 Type 1 diabetes mellitus with other diabetic ophthalmic complication
Use additional code to identify manifestation, such as:
diabetic glaucoma (H40-H42)

+ **E10.4 Type 1 diabetes mellitus with neurological complications**

E10.40 Type 1 diabetes mellitus with diabetic neuropathy, unspecified

E10.41 Type 1 diabetes mellitus with diabetic mononeuropathy

E10.42 Type 1 diabetes mellitus with diabetic polyneuropathy
Type 1 diabetes mellitus with diabetic neuralgia

E10.43 Type 1 diabetes mellitus with diabetic autonomic (poly)neuropathy
Type 1 diabetes mellitus with diabetic gastroparesis
AHA CC: 3Q, 2013, 114-115

E10.44 Type 1 diabetes mellitus with diabetic amyotrophy

E10.49 Type 1 diabetes mellitus with other diabetic neurological complication

+ **E10.5 Type 1 diabetes mellitus with circulatory complications**

E10.51 Type 1 diabetes mellitus with diabetic peripheral angiopathy without gangrene

CC **E10.52 Type 1 diabetes mellitus with diabetic peripheral angiopathy with gangrene**
Type 1 diabetes mellitus with diabetic gangrene
CC Exclusion see Appendix A PDX collection 0519

E10.59 Type 1 diabetes mellitus with other circulatory complications

+ **E10.6 Type 1 diabetes mellitus with other specified complications**

+ **E10.61 Type 1 diabetes mellitus with diabetic arthropathy**

E10.610 Type 1 diabetes mellitus with diabetic neuropathic arthropathy
Type 1 diabetes mellitus with Charcôt's joints

E10.618 Type 1 diabetes mellitus with other diabetic arthropathy

+ **E10.62 Type 1 diabetes mellitus with skin complications**

E10.620 Type 1 diabetes mellitus with diabetic dermatitis
Type 1 diabetes mellitus with diabetic necrobiosis lipoidica

E10.621 Type 1 diabetes mellitus with foot ulcer
Use additional code to identify site of ulcer (L97.4-, L97.5-)

E10.622 Type 1 diabetes mellitus with other skin ulcer
Use additional code to identify site of ulcer (L97.1-L97.9, L98.41-L98.49)

E10.628 Type 1 diabetes mellitus with other skin complications

+ **E10.63 Type 1 diabetes mellitus with oral complications**

E10.630 Type 1 diabetes mellitus with periodontal disease

E10.638 Type 1 diabetes mellitus with other oral complications

+ **E10.64 Type 1 diabetes mellitus with hypoglycemia**

MCC **E10.641 Type 1 diabetes mellitus with hypoglycemia with coma**
MCC Exclusion see Appendix A PDX collection 0520

E10.649 Type 1 diabetes mellitus with hypoglycemia without coma
AHA CC: 1Q, 2016, 13

E10.65 Type 1 diabetes mellitus with hyperglycemia

E10.69 Type 1 diabetes mellitus with other specified complication
Use additional code to identify complication

E10.8 Type 1 diabetes mellitus with unspecified complications

E10.9 Type 1 diabetes mellitus without complications

E11 Type 2 diabetes mellitus

Includes: diabetes (mellitus) due to insulin secretory defect
diabetes NOS
insulin resistant diabetes (mellitus)

Use additional code to identify control using:
insulin (Z79.4)
oral antidiabetic drugs (Z79.84)
oral hypoglycemic drugs (Z79.84)

Excludes1: *diabetes mellitus due to underlying condition (E08.-)*
drug or chemical induced diabetes mellitus (E09.-)
gestational diabetes (O24.4-)
neonatal diabetes mellitus (P70.2)
postpancreatectomy diabetes mellitus (E13.-)
postprocedural diabetes mellitus (E13.-)
secondary diabetes mellitus NEC (E13.-)
type 1 diabetes mellitus (E10.-)

Review coding guidelines C.4.a.2 and C.4.a.3

\+ **E11.0 Type 2 diabetes mellitus with hyperosmolarity**

MCC **E11.00 Type 2 diabetes mellitus with hyperosmolarity without nonketotic hyperglycemic-hyperosmolar coma (NKHHC)**
MCC Exclusion see Appendix A PDX collection 0518
HAC see Appendix B for HAC conditional logic

MCC **E11.01 Type 2 diabetes mellitus with hyperosmolarity with coma**
MCC Exclusion see Appendix A PDX collection 0518
HAC see Appendix B for HAC conditional logic

\+ **E11.1 Type 2 diabetes mellitus with ketoacidosis**

MCC **E11.10 Type 2 diabetes mellitus with ketoacidosis without coma**
MCC Exclusion see Appendix A PDX collection 0518

MCC **E11.11 Type 2 diabetes mellitus with ketoacidosis with coma**
MCC Exclusion see Appendix A PDX collection 0518

\+ **E11.2 Type 2 diabetes mellitus with kidney complications**

E11.21 Type 2 diabetes mellitus with diabetic nephropathy
Type 2 diabetes mellitus with intercapillary glomerulosclerosis
Type 2 diabetes mellitus with intracapillary glomerulonephrosis
Type 2 diabetes mellitus with Kimmelstiel-Wilson disease

E11.22 Type 2 diabetes mellitus with diabetic chronic kidney disease
Use additional code to identify stage of chronic kidney disease (N18.1-N18.6)

E11.29 Type 2 diabetes mellitus with other diabetic kidney complication
Type 2 diabetes mellitus with renal tubular degeneration

\+ **E11.3 Type 2 diabetes mellitus with ophthalmic complications**
AHA CC: 4Q, 2016, 11-13

\+ **E11.31 Type 2 diabetes mellitus with unspecified diabetic retinopathy**

E11.311 Type 2 diabetes mellitus with unspecified diabetic retinopathy with macular edema

E11.319 Type 2 diabetes mellitus with unspecified diabetic retinopathy without macular edema
AHA CC: 3Q, 2013, 20

\+ **E11.32 Type 2 diabetes mellitus with mild nonproliferative diabetic retinopathy**
Type 2 diabetes mellitus with nonproliferative diabetic retinopathy NOS

One of the following 7th characters is to be assigned to codes in subcategory **E11.32** to designate laterality of the disease:
1 right eye
2 left eye
3 bilateral
9 unspecified eye

+7th **E11.321 Type 2 diabetes mellitus with mild nonproliferative diabetic retinopathy with macular edema**

+7th **E11.329 Type 2 diabetes mellitus with mild nonproliferative diabetic retinopathy without macular edema**

\+ **E11.33 Type 2 diabetes mellitus with moderate nonproliferative diabetic retinopathy**

One of the following 7th characters is to be assigned to codes in subcategory **E11.33** to designate laterality of the disease:
1 right eye
2 left eye
3 bilateral
9 unspecified eye

+7th **E11.331 Type 2 diabetes mellitus with moderate nonproliferative diabetic retinopathy with macular edema**

+7th **E11.339 Type 2 diabetes mellitus with moderate nonproliferative diabetic retinopathy without macular edema**

\+ **E11.34 Type 2 diabetes mellitus with severe nonproliferative diabetic retinopathy**

One of the following 7th characters is to be assigned to codes in subcategory **E11.34** to designate laterality of the disease:
1 right eye
2 left eye
3 bilateral
9 unspecified eye

+7th **E11.341 Type 2 diabetes mellitus with severe nonproliferative diabetic retinopathy with macular edema**

+7th **E11.349 Type 2 diabetes mellitus with severe nonproliferative diabetic retinopathy without macular edema**

\+ **E11.35 Type 2 diabetes mellitus with proliferative diabetic retinopathy**

One of the following 7th characters is to be assigned to codes in subcategory **E11.35** to designate laterality of the disease:
1 right eye
2 left eye
3 bilateral
9 unspecified eye

+7th **E11.351 Type 2 diabetes mellitus with proliferative diabetic retinopathy with macular edema**

+7th **E11.352 Type 2 diabetes mellitus with proliferative diabetic retinopathy with traction retinal detachment involving the macula**

+7th **E11.353 Type 2 diabetes mellitus with proliferative diabetic retinopathy with traction retinal detachment not involving the macula**

+7th **E11.354 Type 2 diabetes mellitus with proliferative diabetic retinopathy with combined traction retinal detachment and rhegmatogenous retinal detachment**

+7th **E11.355 Type 2 diabetes mellitus with stable proliferative diabetic retinopathy**

+7th **E11.359 Type 2 diabetes mellitus with proliferative diabetic retinopathy without macular edema**

E11.36 Type 2 diabetes mellitus with diabetic cataract

X+7th **E11.37 Type 2 diabetes mellitus with diabetic macular edema, resolved following treatment**

One of the following 7th characters is to be assigned to codes in subcategory **E11.37** to designate laterality of the disease:
1 right eye
2 left eye
3 bilateral
9 unspecified eye

E11.39 Type 2 diabetes mellitus with other diabetic ophthalmic complication
Use additional code to identify manifestation, such as:
diabetic glaucoma (H40-H42)

+ E11.4 **Type 2 diabetes mellitus with neurological complications**

E11.40 **Type 2 diabetes mellitus with diabetic neuropathy, unspecified**

AHA CC: 4Q, 2013, 129

E11.41 **Type 2 diabetes mellitus with diabetic mononeuropathy**

E11.42 **Type 2 diabetes mellitus with diabetic polyneuropathy**

Type 2 diabetes mellitus with diabetic neuralgia

E11.43 **Type 2 diabetes mellitus with diabetic autonomic (poly)neuropathy**

AHA CC: 4Q, 2013, 114-115

Type 2 diabetes mellitus with diabetic gastroparesis

E11.44 **Type 2 diabetes mellitus with diabetic amyotrophy**

E11.49 **Type 2 diabetes mellitus with other diabetic neurological complication**

+ E11.5 **Type 2 diabetes mellitus with circulatory complications**

E11.51 **Type 2 diabetes mellitus with diabetic peripheral angiopathy without gangrene**

CC **E11.52** **Type 2 diabetes mellitus with diabetic peripheral angiopathy with gangrene**

Type 2 diabetes mellitus with diabetic gangrene

CC Exclusion see Appendix A PDX collection 0519

E11.59 **Type 2 diabetes mellitus with other circulatory complications**

+ E11.6 **Type 2 diabetes mellitus with other specified complications**

+ E11.61 **Type 2 diabetes mellitus with diabetic arthropathy**

E11.610 **Type 2 diabetes mellitus with diabetic neuropathic arthropathy**

Type 2 diabetes mellitus with Charcôt's joints

E11.618 **Type 2 diabetes mellitus with other diabetic arthropathy**

+ E11.62 **Type 2 diabetes mellitus with skin complications**

E11.620 **Type 2 diabetes mellitus with diabetic dermatitis**

Type 2 diabetes mellitus with diabetic necrobiosis lipoidica

E11.621 **Type 2 diabetes mellitus with foot ulcer**

Use additional code to identify site of ulcer (L97.4-, L97.5-)

AHA CC: 1Q, 2016, 12-13

E11.622 **Type 2 diabetes mellitus with other skin ulcer**

Use additional code to identify site of ulcer (L97.1-L97.9, L98.41-L98.49)

E11.628 **Type 2 diabetes mellitus with other skin complications**

+ E11.63 **Type 2 diabetes mellitus with oral complications**

E11.630 **Type 2 diabetes mellitus with periodontal disease**

E11.638 **Type 2 diabetes mellitus with other oral complications**

+ E11.64 **Type 2 diabetes mellitus with hypoglycemia**

MCC **E11.641** **Type 2 diabetes mellitus with hypoglycemia with coma**

MCC Exclusion see Appendix A PDX collection 0518

E11.649 **Type 2 diabetes mellitus with hypoglycemia without coma**

AHA CC: 3Q, 2015, 21; 3Q, 2016, 42

E11.65 **Type 2 diabetes mellitus with hyperglycemia**

AHA CC: 3Q, 2013, 20

E11.69 **Type 2 diabetes mellitus with other specified complication**

Use additional code to identify complication

AHA CC: 4Q, 2016, 141-142

E11.8 **Type 2 diabetes mellitus with unspecified complications**

E11.9 **Type 2 diabetes mellitus without complications**

AHA CC: 4Q, 2013, 128

E13 Other specified diabetes mellitus

Includes: diabetes mellitus due to genetic defects of beta-cell function
diabetes mellitus due to genetic defects in insulin action
postpancreatectomy diabetes mellitus postprocedural
diabetes mellitus secondary diabetes mellitus NEC

Use additional code to identify control using:
insulin (Z79.4)
oral antidiabetic drugs (Z79.84)
oral hypoglycemic drugs (Z79.84)

Excludes1: *diabetes (mellitus) due to autoimmune process (E10.-)*
diabetes (mellitus) due to immune mediated pancreatic islet beta-cell destruction (E10.-)
diabetes mellitus due to underlying condition (E08.-)
drug or chemical induced diabetes mellitus (E09.-)
gestational diabetes (O24.4-)
neonatal diabetes mellitus (P70.2)
type 1 diabetes mellitus (E10.-)

Review coding guidelines C.4.a.6.a and C.4.a.6.b.i

+ E13.0 **Other specified diabetes mellitus with hyperosmolarity**

MCC **E13.00** **Other specified diabetes mellitus with hyperosmolarity without nonketotic hyperglycemic-hyperosmolar coma (NKHHC)**

Excludes2: *type 2 diabetes mellitus (E11.-)*

MCC Exclusion see Appendix A PDX collection 0518

HAC see Appendix B for HAC conditional logic

MCC **E13.01** **Other specified diabetes mellitus with hyperosmolarity with coma**

MCC Exclusion see Appendix A PDX collection 0518

HAC see Appendix B for HAC conditional logic

+ E13.1 **Other specified diabetes mellitus with ketoacidosis**

MCC **E13.10** **Other specified diabetes mellitus with ketoacidosis without coma**

MCC Exclusion see Appendix A PDX collection 0518

HAC see Appendix B for HAC conditional logic

AHA CC: 1Q, 2013, 26-27; 2Q, 2016,10

MCC **E13.11** **Other specified diabetes mellitus with ketoacidosis with coma**

MCC Exclusion see Appendix A PDX collection 0518

+ E13.2 **Other specified diabetes mellitus with kidney complications**

E13.21 **Other specified diabetes mellitus with diabetic nephropathy**

Other specified diabetes mellitus with intercapillary glomerulosclerosis

Other specified diabetes mellitus with intracapillary glomerulonephrosis

Other specified diabetes mellitus with Kimmelstiel-Wilson disease

E13.22 **Other specified diabetes mellitus with diabetic chronic kidney disease**

Use additional code to identify stage of chronic kidney disease (N18.1-N18.6)

E13.29 **Other specified diabetes mellitus with other diabetic kidney complication**

Other specified diabetes mellitus with renal tubular degeneration

+ E13.3 **Other specified diabetes mellitus with ophthalmic complications**

AHA CC: 4Q, 2016, 11-13

+ E13.31 **Other specified diabetes mellitus with unspecified diabetic retinopathy**

E13.311 **Other specified diabetes mellitus with unspecified diabetic retinopathy with macular edema**

E13.319 **Other specified diabetes mellitus with unspecified diabetic retinopathy without macular edema**

+ E13.32 **Other specified diabetes mellitus with mild nonproliferative diabetic retinopathy**

Other specified diabetes mellitus with nonproliferative diabetic retinopathy NOS

> One of the following 7th characters is to be assigned to codes in subcategory **E13.32** to designate laterality of the disease:
> 1 right eye
> 2 left eye
> 3 bilateral
> 9 unspecified eye

+7th **E13.321** **Other specified diabetes mellitus with mild nonproliferative diabetic retinopathy with macular edema**

+7th **E13.329** **Other specified diabetes mellitus with mild nonproliferative diabetic retinopathy without macular edema**

\+ **E13.33** **Other specified diabetes mellitus with moderate nonproliferative diabetic retinopathy**

One of the following 7th characters is to be assigned to codes in subcategory **E13.33** to designate laterality of the disease:
1 right eye
2 left eye
3 bilateral
9 unspecified eye

+7th **E13.331** **Other specified diabetes mellitus with moderate nonproliferative diabetic retinopathy with macular edema**

+7th **E13.339** **Other specified diabetes mellitus with moderate nonproliferative diabetic retinopathy without macular edema**

\+ **E13.34** **Other specified diabetes mellitus with severe nonproliferative diabetic retinopathy**

One of the following 7th characters is to be assigned to codes in subcategory **E13.34** to designate laterality of the disease:
1 right eye
2 left eye
3 bilateral
9 unspecified eye

+7th **E13.341** **Other specified diabetes mellitus with severe nonproliferative diabetic retinopathy with macular edema**

+7th **E13.349** **Other specified diabetes mellitus with severe nonproliferative diabetic retinopathy without macular edema**

\+ **E13.35** **Other specified diabetes mellitus with proliferative diabetic retinopathy**

One of the following 7th characters is to be assigned to codes in subcategory **E13.35** to designate laterality of the disease:
1 right eye
2 left eye
3 bilateral
9 unspecified eye

+7th **E13.351** **Other specified diabetes mellitus with proliferative diabetic retinopathy with macular edema**

+7th **E13.352** **Other specified diabetes mellitus with proliferative diabetic retinopathy with traction retinal detachment involving the macula**

+7th **E13.353** **Other specified diabetes mellitus with proliferative diabetic retinopathy with traction retinal detachment not involving the macula**

+7th **E13.354** **Other specified diabetes mellitus with proliferative diabetic retinopathy with combined traction retinal detachment and rhegmatogenous retinal detachment**

+7th **E13.355** **Other specified diabetes mellitus with stable proliferative diabetic retinopathy**

+7th **E13.359** **Other specified diabetes mellitus with proliferative diabetic retinopathy without macular edema**

E13.36 **Other specified diabetes mellitus with diabetic cataract**

X+7th **E13.37** **Other specified diabetes mellitus with diabetic macular edema, resolved following treatment**

One of the following 7th characters is to be assigned to codes in subcategory **E13.37** to designate laterality of the disease:
1 right eye
2 left eye
3 bilateral
9 unspecified eye

E13.39 **Other specified diabetes mellitus with other diabetic ophthalmic complication**
Use additional code to identify manifestation, such as:
diabetic glaucoma (H40-H42)

\+ **E13.4** **Other specified diabetes mellitus with neurological complications**

E13.40 **Other specified diabetes mellitus with diabetic neuropathy, unspecified**
AHA CC: 4Q, 2013, 129

E13.41 **Other specified diabetes mellitus with diabetic mononeuropathy**

E13.42 **Other specified diabetes mellitus with diabetic polyneuropathy**
Other specified diabetes mellitus with diabetic neuralgia

E13.43 **Other specified diabetes mellitus with diabetic autonomic (poly)neuropathy**
Other specified diabetes mellitus with diabetic gastroparesis
AHA CC: 4Q, 2013, 114-115

E13.44 **Other specified diabetes mellitus with diabetic amyotrophy**

E13.49 **Other specified diabetes mellitus with other diabetic neurological complication**

\+ **E13.5** **Other specified diabetes mellitus with circulatory complications**

E13.51 **Other specified diabetes mellitus with diabetic peripheral angiopathy without gangrene**

CC **E13.52** **Other specified diabetes mellitus with diabetic peripheral angiopathy with gangrene**
Other specified diabetes mellitus with diabetic gangrene
CC Exclusion see Appendix A PDX collection 0519

E13.59 **Other specified diabetes mellitus with other circulatory complications**

\+ **E13.6** **Other specified diabetes mellitus with other specified complications**

\+ **E13.61** **Other specified diabetes mellitus with diabetic arthropathy**

E13.610 **Other specified diabetes mellitus with diabetic neuropathic arthropathy**
Other specified diabetes mellitus with Charcôt's joints

E13.618 **Other specified diabetes mellitus with other diabetic arthropathy**

\+ **E13.62** **Other specified diabetes mellitus with skin complications**

E13.620 **Other specified diabetes mellitus with diabetic dermatitis**
Other specified diabetes mellitus with diabetic necrobiosis lipoidica

E13.621 **Other specified diabetes mellitus with foot ulcer**
Use additional code to identify site of ulcer (L97.4-, L97.5-)

E13.622 **Other specified diabetes mellitus with other skin ulcer**
Use additional code to identify site of ulcer (L97.1-L97.9, L98.41-L98.49)

E13.628 **Other specified diabetes mellitus with other skin complications**

\+ **E13.63** **Other specified diabetes mellitus with oral complications**

E13.630 **Other specified diabetes mellitus with periodontal disease**

E13.638 **Other specified diabetes mellitus with other oral complications**

\+ **E13.64** **Other specified diabetes mellitus with hypoglycemia**

MCC **E13.641** **Other specified diabetes mellitus with hypoglycemia with coma**
MCC Exclusion see Appendix A PDX collection 0518

E13.649 **Other specified diabetes mellitus with hypoglycemia without coma**

E13.65 **Other specified diabetes mellitus with hyperglycemia**

E13.69 **Other specified diabetes mellitus with other specified complication**
Use additional code to identify complication

E13.8 **Other specified diabetes mellitus with unspecified complications**

E13.9 **Other specified diabetes mellitus without complications**

...her disorders of glucose regulation and pancreatic internal ...cretion (E15-E16)

E15 Nondiabetic hypoglycemic coma

Includes: drug-induced insulin coma in nondiabetic
hyperinsulinism with hypoglycemic coma
hypoglycemic coma NOS

CC Exclusion see Appendix A PDX collection 0520

HAC see Appendix B for HAC conditional logic

Valid 3-character code, no further characters required

E16 Other disorders of pancreatic internal secretion

E16.0 Drug-induced hypoglycemia without coma
Use additional code for adverse effect, if applicable, to identify drug (T36-T50 with fifth or sixth character 5)
Excludes1: *diabetes with hypoglycemia without coma (E09.649)*

E16.1 Other hypoglycemia
Functional hyperinsulinism
Functional nonhyperinsulinemic hypoglycemia
Hyperinsulinism NOS
Hyperplasia of pancreatic islet beta cells NOS
Excludes1: *diabetes with hypoglycemia (E08.649, E10.649, E11.649, E13.649)*
hypoglycemia in infant of diabetic mother (P70.1)
neonatal hypoglycemia (P70.4)

E16.2 Hypoglycemia, unspecified
Excludes1: *diabetes with hypoglycemia (E08.649, E10.649, E11.649, E13.649)*

E16.3 Increased secretion of glucagon
Hyperplasia of pancreatic endocrine cells with glucagon excess

E16.4 Increased secretion of gastrin
Hypergastrinemia
Hyperplasia of pancreatic endocrine cells with gastrin excess
Zollinger-Ellison syndrome

E16.8 Other specified disorders of pancreatic internal secretion
Increased secretion from endocrine pancreas of growth hormone-releasing hormone
Increased secretion from endocrine pancreas of pancreatic polypeptide
Increased secretion from endocrine pancreas of somatostatin
Increased secretion from endocrine pancreas of vasoactive-intestinal polypeptide

E16.9 Disorder of pancreatic internal secretion, unspecified
Islet-cell hyperplasia NOS
Pancreatic endocrine cell hyperplasia NOS

...isorders of other endocrine glands (E20-E35)

Excludes1: *galactorrhea (N64.3)*
gynecomastia (N62)

E20 Hypoparathyroidism

Excludes1: *Di George's syndrome (D82.1)*
postprocedural hypoparathyroidism (E89.2)
tetany NOS (R29.0)
transitory neonatal hypoparathyroidism (P71.4)

E20.0 Idiopathic hypoparathyroidism
E20.1 Pseudohypoparathyroidism
E20.8 Other hypoparathyroidism
E20.9 Hypoparathyroidism, unspecified
Parathyroid tetany

E21 Hyperparathyroidism and other disorders of parathyroid gland

Excludes1: *adult osteomalacia (M83.-)*
ectopic hyperparathyroidism (E34.2)
familial hypocalciuric hypercalcemia (E83.52)
hungry bone syndrome (E83.81)
infantile and juvenile osteomalacia (E55.0)

E21.0 Primary hyperparathyroidism
Hyperplasia of parathyroid
Osteitis fibrosa cystica generalisata [von Recklinghausen's disease of bone]

E21.1 Secondary hyperparathyroidism, not elsewhere classified
Excludes1: *secondary hyperparathyroidism of renal origin (N25.81)*

E21.2 Other hyperparathyroidism
Tertiary hyperparathyroidism
Excludes1: *familial hypocalciuric hypercalcemia (E83.52)*

E21.3 Hyperparathyroidism, unspecified
E21.4 Other specified disorders of parathyroid gland
E21.5 Disorder of parathyroid gland, unspecified

E22 Hyperfunction of pituitary gland

Excludes1: *Cushing's syndrome (E24.-)*
Nelson's syndrome (E24.1)
overproduction of ACTH not associated with Cushing's disease (E27.0)
overproduction of pituitary ACTH (E24.0)
overproduction of thyroid-stimulating hormone (E05.8-)

E22.0 Acromegaly and pituitary gigantism
Overproduction of growth hormone
Excludes1: *constitutional gigantism (E34.4)*
constitutional tall stature (E34.4)
increased secretion from endocrine pancreas of growth hormone-releasing hormone (E16.8)

CC **E22.1 Hyperprolactinemia**
Use additional code for adverse effect, if applicable, to identify drug (T36-T50 with fifth or sixth character 5)
CC Exclusion see Appendix A PDX collection 0521

CC **E22.2 Syndrome of inappropriate secretion of antidiuretic hormone**
CC Exclusion see Appendix A PDX collection 0522

CC **E22.8 Other hyperfunction of pituitary gland**
Central precocious puberty
CC Exclusion see Appendix A PDX collection 0521

CC **E22.9 Hyperfunction of pituitary gland, unspecified**
CC Exclusion see Appendix A PDX collection 0521

E23 Hypofunction and other disorders of the pituitary gland

Includes: the listed conditions whether the disorder is in the pituitary or the hypothalamus
Excludes1: *postprocedural hypopituitarism (E89.3)*

CC **E23.0 Hypopituitarism**
Fertile eunuch syndrome
Hypogonadotropic hypogonadism
Idiopathic growth hormone deficiency
Isolated deficiency of gonadotropin
Isolated deficiency of growth hormone
Isolated deficiency of pituitary hormone
Kallmann's syndrome
Lorain-Levi short stature
Necrosis of pituitary gland (postpartum)
Panhypopituitarism
Pituitary cachexia
Pituitary insufficiency NOS
Pituitary short stature
Sheehan's syndrome
Simmonds' disease
CC Exclusion see Appendix A PDX collection 0523

E23.1 Drug-induced hypopituitarism
Use additional code for adverse effect, if applicable, to identify drug (T36-T50 with fifth or sixth character 5)

CC **E23.2 Diabetes insipidus**
Excludes1: *nephrogenic diabetes insipidus (N25.1)*
CC Exclusion see Appendix A PDX collection 0524

E23.3 Hypothalamic dysfunction, not elsewhere classified
Excludes1: *Prader-Willi syndrome (Q87.1)*
Russell-Silver syndrome (Q87.1)

E23.6 Other disorders of pituitary gland
Abscess of pituitary
Adiposogenital dystrophy

E23.7 Disorder of pituitary gland, unspecified

E24 Cushing's syndrome

Excludes1: *congenital adrenal hyperplasia (E25.0)*

CC **E24.0 Pituitary-dependent Cushing's disease**
Overproduction of pituitary ACTH
Pituitary-dependent hypercorticalism
CC Exclusion see Appendix A PDX collection 0525

E24.1 Nelson's syndrome

CC **E24.2 Drug-induced Cushing's syndrome**
Use additional code for adverse effect, if applicable, to identify drug (T36-T50 with fifth or sixth character 5)
CC Exclusion see Appendix A PDX collection 0525

CC **E24.3 Ectopic ACTH syndrome**
CC Exclusion see Appendix A PDX collection 0525

CC **E24.4 Alcohol-induced pseudo-Cushing's syndrome**
CC Exclusion see Appendix A PDX collection 0525

CC **E24.8 Other Cushing's syndrome**
CC Exclusion see Appendix A PDX collection 0525

CC **E24.9 Cushing's syndrome, unspecified**
CC Exclusion see Appendix A PDX collection 0525

E25 Adrenogenital disorders

Includes: adrenogenital syndromes, virilizing or feminizing, whether acquired or due to adrenal hyperplasia consequent on inborn enzyme defects in hormone synthesis
Female adrenal pseudohermaphroditism
Female heterosexual precocious pseudopuberty
Male isosexual precocious pseudopuberty
Male macrogenitosomia praecox
Male sexual precocity with adrenal hyperplasia
Male virilization (female)

Excludes1: *indeterminate sex and pseudohermaphroditism (Q56)*
chromosomal abnormalities (Q90-Q99)

E25.0 Congenital adrenogenital disorders associated with enzyme deficiency
Congenital adrenal hyperplasia
21-Hydroxylase deficiency
Salt-losing congenital adrenal hyperplasia

E25.8 Other adrenogenital disorders
Idiopathic adrenogenital disorder
Use additional code for adverse effect, if applicable, to identify drug (T36-T50 with fifth or sixth character 5)

E25.9 Adrenogenital disorder, unspecified
Adrenogenital syndrome NOS

E26 Hyperaldosteronism

+ **E26.0 Primary hyperaldosteronism**
E26.01 Conn's syndrome
Code also adrenal adenoma (D35.0-)
E26.02 Glucocorticoid-remediable aldosteronism
Familial aldosteronism type I
E26.09 Other primary hyperaldosteronism
Primary aldosteronism due to adrenal hyperplasia (bilateral)

E26.1 Secondary hyperaldosteronism

+ **E26.8 Other hyperaldosteronism**
E26.81 Bartter's syndrome
E26.89 Other hyperaldosteronism

E26.9 Hyperaldosteronism, unspecified
Aldosteronism NOS
Hyperaldosteronism NOS

E27 Other disorders of adrenal gland

CC **E27.0 Other adrenocortical overactivity**
Overproduction of ACTH, not associated with Cushing's disease
Premature adrenarche
Excludes1: *Cushing's syndrome (E24.-)*
CC Exclusion see Appendix A PDX collection 0526

CC **E27.1 Primary adrenocortical insufficiency**
Addison's disease
Autoimmune adrenalitis
Excludes1: *Addison only phenotype adrenoleukodystrophy (E71.528)*
amyloidosis (E85.-)
tuberculous Addison's disease (A18.7)
Waterhouse-Friderichsen syndrome (A39.1)
CC Exclusion see Appendix A PDX collection 0526

CC **E27.2 Addisonian crisis**
Adrenal crisis
Adrenocortical crisis
CC Exclusion see Appendix A PDX collection 0526

CC **E27.3 Drug-induced adrenocortical insufficiency**
Use additional code for adverse effect, if applicable, to identify drug (T36-T50 with fifth or sixth character 5)
CC Exclusion see Appendix A PDX collection 0526

+ **E27.4 Other and unspecified adrenocortical insufficiency**
Excludes1: *adrenoleukodystrophy [Addison-Schilder] (E71.528)*
Waterhouse-Friderichsen syndrome (A39.1)

CC **E27.40 Unspecified adrenocortical insufficiency**
Adrenocortical insufficiency NOS
Hypoaldosteronism
CC Exclusion see Appendix A PDX collection 0526

CC **E27.49 Other adrenocortical insufficiency**
Adrenal hemorrhage
Adrenal infarction
CC Exclusion see Appendix A PDX collection 0526

CC **E27.5 Adrenomedullary hyperfunction**
Adrenomedullary hyperplasia
Catecholamine hypersecretion
CC Exclusion see Appendix A PDX collection 0526

E27.8 Other specified disorders of adrenal gland
Abnormality of cortisol-binding globulin

E27.9 Disorder of adrenal gland, unspecified

E28 Ovarian dysfunction

Excludes1: *isolated gonadotropin deficiency (E23.0)*
postprocedural ovarian failure (E89.4-)

♀ **E28.0 Estrogen excess**
Use additional code for adverse effect, if applicable, to identif drug (T36-T50 with fifth or sixth character 5)

♀ **E28.1 Androgen excess**
Hypersecretion of ovarian androgens
Use additional code for adverse effect, if applicable, to identif drug (T36-T50 with fifth or sixth character 5)

♀ **E28.2 Polycystic ovarian syndrome**
Sclerocystic ovary syndrome
Stein-Leventhal syndrome

+ **E28.3 Primary ovarian failure**
Excludes1: *pure gonadal dysgenesis (Q99.1)*
Turner's syndrome (Q96.-)

+ **E28.31 Premature menopause**
• ♀ **E28.310 Symptomatic premature menopause**
Symptoms such as flushing, sleeplessness, headache, lack of concentration, associated with premature menopause
• ♀ **E28.319 Asymptomatic premature menopause**
Premature menopause NOS

♀ **E28.39 Other primary ovarian failure**
Decreased estrogen
Resistant ovary syndrome

♀ **E28.8 Other ovarian dysfunction**
Ovarian hyperfunction NOS
Excludes1: *postprocedural ovarian failure (E89.4-)*

♀ **E28.9 Ovarian dysfunction, unspecified**

E29 Testicular dysfunction

Excludes1: *androgen insensitivity syndrome (E34.5-)*
azoospermia or oligospermia NOS (N46.0-N46.1)
isolated gonadotropin deficiency (E23.0)
Klinefelter's syndrome (Q98.0-Q98.1, Q98.4)

♂ **E29.0 Testicular hyperfunction**
Hypersecretion of testicular hormones

♂ **E29.1 Testicular hypofunction**
Defective biosynthesis of testicular androgen NOS
5-delta-Reductase deficiency (with male pseudohermaphroditism)
Testicular hypogonadism NOS
Use additional code for adverse effect, if applicable, to identify drug (T36-T50 with fifth or sixth character 5)
Excludes1: *postprocedural testicular hypofunction (E89.5)*

♂ **E29.8 Other testicular dysfunction**

♂ **E29.9 Testicular dysfunction, unspecified**

E30 Disorders of puberty, not elsewhere classified

E30.0 Delayed puberty
Constitutional delay of puberty
Delayed sexual development

• **E30.1 Precocious puberty**
Precocious menstruation
Excludes1: *Albright (-McCune) (-Sternberg) syndrome (Q78.*
central precocious puberty (E22.8)
congenital adrenal hyperplasia (E25.0)
female heterosexual precocious pseudopuberty (E25.-)
male isosexual precocious pseudopuberty (E25.-)

• **E30.8 Other disorders of puberty**
Premature thelarche

E30.9 Disorder of puberty, unspecified

E31 Polyglandular dysfunction

Excludes1: *ataxia telangiectasia [Louis-Bar] (G11.3)*
dystrophia myotonica [Steinert] (G71.11)
pseudohypoparathyroidism (E20.1)

E31.0 Autoimmune polyglandular failure
Schmidt's syndrome

E31.1 Polyglandular hyperfunction
Excludes1: *multiple endocrine adenomatosis (E31.2-)*
multiple endocrine neoplasia (E31.2-)

+ **E31.2 Multiple endocrine neoplasia [MEN] syndromes**
Multiple endocrine adenomatosis
Code also any associated malignancies and other conditions associated with the syndromes

E31.20 Multiple endocrine neoplasia [MEN] syndrome, unspecified
Multiple endocrine adenomatosis NOS
Multiple endocrine neoplasia [MEN] syndrome NOS
E31.21 Multiple endocrine neoplasia [MEN] type I
Wermer's syndrome
E31.22 Multiple endocrine neoplasia [MEN] type IIA
Sipple's syndrome
E31.23 Multiple endocrine neoplasia [MEN] type IIB
E31.8 Other polyglandular dysfunction
E31.9 Polyglandular dysfunction, unspecified

E32 Diseases of thymus
Excludes1: *aplasia or hypoplasia of thymus with immunodeficiency (D82.1)*
myasthenia gravis (G70.0)
E32.0 Persistent hyperplasia of thymus
Hypertrophy of thymus
CC **E32.1 Abscess of thymus**
CC Exclusion see Appendix A PDX collection 0527
E32.8 Other diseases of thymus
Excludes1: *aplasia or hypoplasia with immunodeficiency (D82.1)*
thymoma (D15.0)
E32.9 Disease of thymus, unspecified

E34 Other endocrine disorders
Excludes1: *pseudohypoparathyroidism (E20.1)*
CC **E34.0 Carcinoid syndrome**
NOTE May be used as an additional code to identify functional activity associated with a carcinoid tumor.
CC Exclusion see Appendix A PDX collection 0528
E34.1 Other hypersecretion of intestinal hormones
E34.2 Ectopic hormone secretion, not elsewhere classified
Excludes1: *ectopic ACTH syndrome (E24.3)*
E34.3 Short stature due to endocrine disorder
Constitutional short stature
Laron-type short stature
Excludes1: *achondroplastic short stature (Q77.4)*
hypochondroplastic short stature (Q77.4)
nutritional short stature (E45)
pituitary short stature (E23.0)
progeria (E34.8)
renal short stature (N25.0)
Russell-Silver syndrome (Q87.1)
short-limbed stature with immunodeficiency (D82.2)
short stature in specific dysmorphic syndromes - code to syndrome - see Alphabetical Index
short stature NOS (R62.52)
E34.4 Constitutional tall stature
Constitutional gigantism
\+ **E34.5 Androgen insensitivity syndrome**
E34.50 Androgen insensitivity syndrome, unspecified
Androgen insensitivity NOS
E34.51 Complete androgen insensitivity syndrome
Complete androgen insensitivity
de Quervain syndrome
Goldberg-Maxwell syndrome
E34.52 Partial androgen insensitivity syndrome
Partial androgen insensitivity
Reifenstein syndrome
E34.8 Other specified endocrine disorders
Pineal gland dysfunction
Progeria
Excludes2: *pseudohypoparathyroidism (E20.1)*
E34.9 Endocrine disorder, unspecified
Endocrine disturbance NOS
Hormone disturbance NOS

E35 Disorders of endocrine glands in diseases classified elsewhere
Code first underlying disease, such as:
late congenital syphilis of thymus gland [Dubois disease] (A50.5)

Use additional code, if applicable, to identify:
sequelae of tuberculosis of other organs (B90.8)
Excludes1: *Echinococcus granulosus infection of thyroid gland (B67.3)*
meningococcal hemorrhagic adrenalitis (A39.1)
syphilis of endocrine gland (A52.79)
tuberculosis of adrenal gland, except calcification (A18.7)
tuberculosis of endocrine gland NEC (A18.82)
tuberculosis of thyroid gland (A18.81)
Waterhouse-Friderichsen syndrome (A39.1)
Valid 3-character code, no further characters required

Intraoperative complications of endocrine system (E36)

E36 Intraoperative complications of endocrine system
Excludes2: *postprocedural endocrine and metabolic complications and disorders, not elsewhere classified (E89.-)*
\+ **E36.0 Intraoperative hemorrhage and hematoma of an endocrine system organ or structure complicating a procedure**
Excludes1: *intraoperative hemorrhage and hematoma of an endocrine system organ or structure due to accidental puncture or laceration during a procedure (E36.1-)*
CC **E36.01 Intraoperative hemorrhage and hematoma of an endocrine system organ or structure complicating an endocrine system procedure**
CC Exclusion see Appendix A PDX collection 0529
CC **E36.02 Intraoperative hemorrhage and hematoma of an endocrine system organ or structure complicating other procedure**
CC Exclusion see Appendix A PDX collection 0529
\+ **E36.1 Accidental puncture and laceration of an endocrine system organ or structure during a procedure**
CC **E36.11 Accidental puncture and laceration of an endocrine system organ or structure during an endocrine system procedure**
CC Exclusion see Appendix A PDX collection 0509
CC **E36.12 Accidental puncture and laceration of an endocrine system organ or structure during other procedure**
CC Exclusion see Appendix A PDX collection 0509
E36.8 Other intraoperative complications of endocrine system
Use additional code, if applicable, to further specify disorder

Malnutrition (E40-E46)

Excludes1: *intestinal malabsorption (K90.-)*
sequelae of protein-calorie malnutrition (E64.0)
Excludes2: *nutritional anemias (D50-D53)*
starvation (T73.0)

MCC **E40 Kwashiorkor**
Severe malnutrition with nutritional edema with dyspigmentation of skin and hair
Excludes1: *marasmic kwashiorkor (E42)*
MCC Exclusion see Appendix A PDX collection 0530
Valid 3-character code, no further characters required

MCC **E41 Nutritional marasmus**
Severe malnutrition with marasmus
Excludes1: *marasmic kwashiorkor (E42)*
MCC Exclusion see Appendix A PDX collection 0530
Valid 3-character code, no further characters required

MCC **E42 Marasmic kwashiorkor**
Intermediate form severe protein-calorie malnutrition
Severe protein-calorie malnutrition with signs of both kwashiorkor and marasmus
MCC Exclusion see Appendix A PDX collection 0530
Valid 3-character code, no further characters required

MCC **E43 Unspecified severe protein-calorie malnutrition**
Starvation edema
MCC Exclusion see Appendix A PDX collection 0530
Valid 3-character code, no further characters required

E44 Protein-calorie malnutrition of moderate and mild degree
CC **E44.0 Moderate protein-calorie malnutrition**
CC Exclusion see Appendix A PDX collection 0530
CC **E44.1 Mild protein-calorie malnutrition**
CC Exclusion see Appendix A PDX collection 0530

CC **E45** **Retarded development following protein-calorie malnutrition**

Nutritional short stature
Nutritional stunting
Physical retardation due to malnutrition
CC Exclusion see Appendix A PDX collection 0530
Valid 3-character code, no further characters required

CC **E46** **Unspecified protein-calorie malnutrition**

Malnutrition NOS
Protein-calorie imbalance NOS
Excludes1: *nutritional deficiency NOS (E63.9)*
CC Exclusion see Appendix A PDX collection 0530
Valid 3-character code, no further characters required

Other nutritional deficiencies (E50-E64)

Excludes2: *nutritional anemias (D50-D53)*

E50 Vitamin A deficiency

Excludes1: *sequelae of vitamin A deficiency (E64.1)*
E50.0 Vitamin A deficiency with conjunctival xerosis
E50.1 Vitamin A deficiency with Bitot's spot and conjunctival xerosis
Bitot's spot in the young child
E50.2 Vitamin A deficiency with corneal xerosis
E50.3 Vitamin A deficiency with corneal ulceration and xerosis
E50.4 Vitamin A deficiency with keratomalacia
E50.5 Vitamin A deficiency with night blindness
E50.6 Vitamin A deficiency with xerophthalmic scars of cornea
E50.7 Other ocular manifestations of vitamin A deficiency
Xerophthalmia NOS
E50.8 Other manifestations of vitamin A deficiency
Follicular keratosis
Xeroderma
E50.9 Vitamin A deficiency, unspecified
Hypovitaminosis A NOS

E51 Thiamine deficiency

Excludes1: *sequelae of thiamine deficiency (E64.8)*
\+ **E51.1 Beriberi**
CC **E51.11 Dry beriberi**
Beriberi NOS
Beriberi with polyneuropathy
CC Exclusion see Appendix A PDX collection 0531
CC **E51.12 Wet beriberi**
Beriberi with cardiovascular manifestations
Cardiovascular beriberi
Shoshin disease
CC Exclusion see Appendix A PDX collection 0531
CC **E51.2 Wernicke's encephalopathy**
CC Exclusion see Appendix A PDX collection 0531
CC **E51.8 Other manifestations of thiamine deficiency**
CC Exclusion see Appendix A PDX collection 0531
CC **E51.9 Thiamine deficiency, unspecified**
CC Exclusion see Appendix A PDX collection 0531

E52 Niacin deficiency [pellagra]

Niacin (-tryptophan) deficiency
Nicotinamide deficiency
Pellagra (alcoholic)
Excludes1: *sequelae of niacin deficiency (E64.8)*
Valid 3-character code, no further characters required

E53 Deficiency of other B group vitamins

Excludes1: *sequelae of vitamin B deficiency (E64.8)*
CC **E53.0 Riboflavin deficiency**
Ariboflavinosis
Vitamin B2 deficiency
CC Exclusion see Appendix A PDX collection 0531
E53.1 Pyridoxine deficiency
Vitamin B6 deficiency
Excludes1: *pyridoxine-responsive sideroblastic anemia (D64.3)*
E53.8 Deficiency of other specified B group vitamins
Biotin deficiency
Cyanocobalamin deficiency
Folate deficiency
Folic acid deficiency
Pantothenic acid deficiency
Vitamin B12 deficiency
Excludes1: *folate deficiency anemia (D52.-)*
vitamin B12 deficiency anemia (D51.-)
E53.9 Vitamin B deficiency, unspecified

E54 Ascorbic acid deficiency

Deficiency of vitamin C
Scurvy
Excludes1: *scorbutic anemia (D53.2)*
sequelae of vitamin C deficiency (E64.2)
Valid 3-character code, no further characters required

E55 Vitamin D deficiency

Excludes1: *adult osteomalacia (M83.-)*
osteoporosis (M80.-)
sequelae of rickets (E64.3)
CC **E55.0 Rickets, active**
Infantile osteomalacia
Juvenile osteomalacia
Excludes1: *celiac rickets (K90.0)*
Crohn's rickets (K50.-)
hereditary vitamin D-dependent rickets (E83.32)
inactive rickets (E64.3)
renal rickets (N25.0)
sequelae of rickets (E64.3)
vitamin D-resistant rickets (E83.31)
CC Exclusion see Appendix A PDX collection 0532
E55.9 Vitamin D deficiency, unspecified
Avitaminosis D

E56 Other vitamin deficiencies

Excludes1: *sequelae of other vitamin deficiencies (E64.8)*
E56.0 Deficiency of vitamin E
E56.1 Deficiency of vitamin K
Excludes1: *deficiency of coagulation factor due to vitamin K deficiency (D68.4)*
vitamin K deficiency of newborn (P53)
E56.8 Deficiency of other vitamins
E56.9 Vitamin deficiency, unspecified

E58 Dietary calcium deficiency

Excludes1: *disorders of calcium metabolism (E83.5-)*
sequelae of calcium deficiency (E64.8)
Valid 3-character code, no further characters required

E59 Dietary selenium deficiency

Keshan disease
Excludes1: *sequelae of selenium deficiency (E64.8)*
Valid 3-character code, no further characters required

E60 Dietary zinc deficiency

Valid 3-character code, no further characters required

E61 Deficiency of other nutrient elements

Use additional code for adverse effect, if applicable, to identify drug (T36-T50 with fifth or sixth character 5)
Excludes1: *disorders of mineral metabolism (E83.-)*
iodine deficiency related thyroid disorders (E00-E02)
sequelae of malnutrition and other nutritional deficiencies (E64.-)
E61.0 Copper deficiency
E61.1 Iron deficiency
Excludes1: *iron deficiency anemia (D50.-)*
E61.2 Magnesium deficiency
E61.3 Manganese deficiency
E61.4 Chromium deficiency
E61.5 Molybdenum deficiency
E61.6 Vanadium deficiency
E61.7 Deficiency of multiple nutrient elements
E61.8 Deficiency of other specified nutrient elements
E61.9 Deficiency of nutrient element, unspecified

E63 Other nutritional deficiencies

Excludes1: *dehydration (E86.0)*
failure to thrive, adult (R62.7)
failure to thrive, child (R62.51)
feeding problems in newborn (P92.-)
sequelae of malnutrition and other nutritional deficiencies (E64.-)
E63.0 Essential fatty acid [EFA] deficiency
E63.1 Imbalance of constituents of food intake
E63.8 Other specified nutritional deficiencies
E63.9 Nutritional deficiency, unspecified

E64 Sequelae of malnutrition and other nutritional deficiencies

NOTE This category is to be used to indicate conditions in categories E43, E44, E46, E50-E63 as the cause of sequelae, which are themselves classified elsewhere. The 'sequelae' include conditions specified as such; they also include the late effects of diseases classifiable to the above categories if the disease itself is no longer present

Code first condition resulting from (sequela) of malnutrition and other nutritional deficiencies

CC **E64.0 Sequelae of protein-calorie malnutrition**

Excludes2: *retarded development following protein-calorie malnutrition (E45)*

CC Exclusion see Appendix A PDX collection 0530

E64.1 Sequelae of vitamin A deficiency

E64.2 Sequelae of vitamin C deficiency

E64.3 Sequelae of rickets

E64.8 Sequelae of other nutritional deficiencies

E64.9 Sequelae of unspecified nutritional deficiency

Overweight, obesity and other hyperalimentation (E65-E68)

E65 Localized adiposity

Fat pad

Valid 3-character code, no further characters required

E66 Overweight and obesity

Code first obesity complicating pregnancy, childbirth and the puerperium, if applicable (O99.21-)

Use additional code to identify body mass index (BMI), if known (Z68.-)

Excludes1: *adiposogenital dystrophy (E23.6)*
lipomatosis NOS (E88.2)
lipomatosis dolorosa [Dercum] (E88.2)
Prader-Willi syndrome (Q87.1)

+ **E66.0 Obesity due to excess calories**

E66.01 Morbid (severe) obesity due to excess calories

Excludes1: *morbid (severe) obesity with alveolar hypoventilation (E66.2)*

HAC see Appendix B for HAC conditional logic

E66.09 Other obesity due to excess calories

E66.1 Drug-induced obesity

Use additional code for adverse effect, if applicable, to identify drug (T36-T50 with fifth or sixth character 5)

CC **E66.2 Morbid (severe) obesity with alveolar hypoventilation**

Obesity hypoventilation syndrome (OHS)

Pickwickian syndrome

CC Exclusion see Appendix A PDX collection 0533

E66.3 Overweight

E66.8 Other obesity

E66.9 Obesity, unspecified

Obesity NOS

AHA CC: 4Q, 2013, 129

E67 Other hyperalimentation

Excludes1: *hyperalimentation NOS (R63.2)*
sequelae of hyperalimentation (E68)

E67.0 Hypervitaminosis A

E67.1 Hypercarotinemia

E67.2 Megavitamin-B6 syndrome

E67.3 Hypervitaminosis D

E67.8 Other specified hyperalimentation

E68 Sequelae of hyperalimentation

Code first condition resulting from (sequela) of hyperalimentation

Valid 3-character code, no further characters required

Metabolic disorders (E70-E88)

Excludes1: *androgen insensitivity syndrome (E34.5-)*
congenital adrenal hyperplasia (E25.0)
Ehlers-Danlos syndrome (Q79.6)
hemolytic anemias attributable to enzyme disorders (D55.-)
Marfan's syndrome (Q87.4)
5-alpha-reductase deficiency (E29.1)

E70 Disorders of aromatic amino-acid metabolism

CC **E70.0 Classical phenylketonuria**

CC Exclusion see Appendix A PDX collection 0534

CC **E70.1 Other hyperphenylalaninemias**

CC Exclusion see Appendix A PDX collection 0534

+ **E70.2 Disorders of tyrosine metabolism**

Excludes1: *transitory tyrosinemia of newborn (P74.5)*

CC **E70.20 Disorder of tyrosine metabolism, unspecified**

CC Exclusion see Appendix A PDX collection 0534

CC **E70.21 Tyrosinemia**

Hypertyrosinemia

CC Exclusion see Appendix A PDX collection 0534

CC **E70.29 Other disorders of tyrosine metabolism**

Alkaptonuria

Ochronosis

CC Exclusion see Appendix A PDX collection 0534

+ **E70.3 Albinism**

CC **E70.30 Albinism, unspecified**

CC Exclusion see Appendix A PDX collection 0534

+ **E70.31 Ocular albinism**

CC **E70.310 X-linked ocular albinism**

CC Exclusion see Appendix A PDX collection 0534

CC **E70.311 Autosomal recessive ocular albinism**

CC Exclusion see Appendix A PDX collection 0534

CC **E70.318 Other ocular albinism**

CC Exclusion see Appendix A PDX collection 0534

CC **E70.319 Ocular albinism, unspecified**

CC Exclusion see Appendix A PDX collection 0534

+ **E70.32 Oculocutaneous albinism**

Excludes1: *Chediak-Higashi syndrome (E70.330)*
Hermansky-Pudlak syndrome (E70.331)

CC **E70.320 Tyrosinase negative oculocutaneous albinism**

Albinism I

Oculocutaneous albinism ty-neg

CC Exclusion see Appendix A PDX collection 0534

CC **E70.321 Tyrosinase positive oculocutaneous albinism**

Albinism II

Oculocutaneous albinism ty-pos

CC Exclusion see Appendix A PDX collection 0534

CC **E70.328 Other oculocutaneous albinism**

Cross syndrome

CC Exclusion see Appendix A PDX collection 0534

CC **E70.329 Oculocutaneous albinism, unspecified**

CC Exclusion see Appendix A PDX collection 0534

+ **E70.33 Albinism with hematologic abnormality**

CC **E70.330 Chediak-Higashi syndrome**

CC Exclusion see Appendix A PDX collection 0534

CC **E70.331 Hermansky-Pudlak syndrome**

CC Exclusion see Appendix A PDX collection 0534

CC **E70.338 Other albinism with hematologic abnormality**

CC Exclusion see Appendix A PDX collection 0534

CC **E70.339 Albinism with hematologic abnormality, unspecified**

CC Exclusion see Appendix A PDX collection 0534

CC **E70.39 Other specified albinism**

Piebaldism

CC Exclusion see Appendix A PDX collection 0534

+ **E70.4 Disorders of histidine metabolism**

CC **E70.40 Disorders of histidine metabolism, unspecified**

CC Exclusion see Appendix A PDX collection 0534

CC **E70.41 Histidinemia**

CC Exclusion see Appendix A PDX collection 0534

CC **E70.49 Other disorders of histidine metabolism**

CC Exclusion see Appendix A PDX collection 0534

CC **E70.5** **Disorders of tryptophan metabolism**
CC Exclusion see Appendix A PDX collection 0534

CC **E70.8** **Other disorders of aromatic amino-acid metabolism**
CC Exclusion see Appendix A PDX collection 0534

CC **E70.9** **Disorder of aromatic amino-acid metabolism, unspecified**
CC Exclusion see Appendix A PDX collection 0534

E71 Disorders of branched-chain amino-acid metabolism and fatty-acid metabolism

CC **E71.0** **Maple-syrup-urine disease**
CC Exclusion see Appendix A PDX collection 0534

\+ E71.1 **Other disorders of branched-chain amino-acid metabolism**

\+ E71.11 **Branched-chain organic acidurias**

CC **E71.110** **Isovaleric acidemia**
CC Exclusion see Appendix A PDX collection 0534

CC **E71.111** **3-methylglutaconic aciduria**
CC Exclusion see Appendix A PDX collection 0534

CC **E71.118** **Other branched-chain organic acidurias**
CC Exclusion see Appendix A PDX collection 0534

\+ E71.12 **Disorders of propionate metabolism**

CC **E71.120** **Methylmalonic acidemia**
CC Exclusion see Appendix A PDX collection 0534

CC **E71.121** **Propionic acidemia**
CC Exclusion see Appendix A PDX collection 0534

CC **E71.128** **Other disorders of propionate metabolism**
CC Exclusion see Appendix A PDX collection 0534

CC **E71.19** **Other disorders of branched-chain amino-acid metabolism**
Hyperleucine-isoleucinemia
Hypervalinemia
CC Exclusion see Appendix A PDX collection 0534

CC **E71.2** **Disorder of branched-chain amino-acid metabolism, unspecified**
CC Exclusion see Appendix A PDX collection 0534

\+ E71.3 **Disorders of fatty-acid metabolism**
Excludes1: *peroxisomal disorders (E71.5)*
Refsum's disease (G60.1)
Schilder's disease (G37.0)
Excludes2: *carnitine deficiency due to inborn error of metabolism (E71.42)*

E71.30 **Disorder of fatty-acid metabolism, unspecified**

\+ E71.31 **Disorders of fatty-acid oxidation**

CC **E71.310** **Long chain/very long chain acyl CoA dehydrogenase deficiency**
LCAD
VLCAD
CC Exclusion see Appendix A PDX collection 0535

CC **E71.311** **Medium chain acyl CoA dehydrogenase deficiency**
MCAD
CC Exclusion see Appendix A PDX collection 0535

CC **E71.312** **Short chain acyl CoA dehydrogenase deficiency**
SCAD
CC Exclusion see Appendix A PDX collection 0535

CC **E71.313** **Glutaric aciduria type II**
Glutaric aciduria type II A
Glutaric aciduria type II B
Glutaric aciduria type II C
Excludes1: *glutaric aciduria (type 1) NOS (E72.3)*
CC Exclusion see Appendix A PDX collection 0535

CC **E71.314** **Muscle carnitine palmitoyltransferase deficiency**
CC Exclusion see Appendix A PDX collection 0535

CC **E71.318** **Other disorders of fatty-acid oxidation**
CC Exclusion see Appendix A PDX collection 0535

CC **E71.32** **Disorders of ketone metabolism**
CC Exclusion see Appendix A PDX collection 0535

CC **E71.39** **Other disorders of fatty-acid metabolism**
CC Exclusion see Appendix A PDX collection 0492

\+ E71.4 **Disorders of carnitine metabolism**
Excludes1: *Muscle carnitine palmitoyltransferase deficiency (E71.314)*

E71.40 **Disorder of carnitine metabolism, unspecified**

E71.41 **Primary carnitine deficiency**

E71.42 **Carnitine deficiency due to inborn errors of metabolism**
Code also associated inborn error or metabolism

E71.43 **Iatrogenic carnitine deficiency**
Carnitine deficiency due to hemodialysis
Carnitine deficiency due to Valproic acid therapy

\+ E71.44 **Other secondary carnitine deficiency**

E71.440 **Ruvalcaba-Myhre-Smith syndrome**

E71.448 **Other secondary carnitine deficiency**

\+ E71.5 **Peroxisomal disorders**
Excludes1: *Schilder's disease (G37.0)*

CC **E71.50** **Peroxisomal disorder, unspecified**
CC Exclusion see Appendix A PDX collection 0536

\+ E71.51 **Disorders of peroxisome biogenesis**
Group 1 peroxisomal disorders
Excludes1: *Refsum's disease (G60.1)*

CC **E71.510** **Zellweger syndrome**
CC Exclusion see Appendix A PDX collection 0536

CC **E71.511** **Neonatal adrenoleukodystrophy**
Excludes1: *X-linked adrenoleukodystrophy (E71.42-)*
CC Exclusion see Appendix A PDX collection 0536

CC **E71.518** **Other disorders of peroxisome biogenesis**
CC Exclusion see Appendix A PDX collection 0536

\+ E71.52 **X-linked adrenoleukodystrophy**

CC **E71.520** **Childhood cerebral X-linked adrenoleukodystrophy**
CC Exclusion see Appendix A PDX collection 0536

CC **E71.521** **Adolescent X-linked adrenoleukodystrophy**
CC Exclusion see Appendix A PDX collection 0536

CC **E71.522** **Adrenomyeloneuropathy**
CC Exclusion see Appendix A PDX collection 0536

CC **E71.528** **Other X-linked adrenoleukodystrophy**
Addison only phenotype adrenoleukodystrophy
Addison-Schilder adrenoleukodystrophy
CC Exclusion see Appendix A PDX collection 0536

CC **E71.529** **X-linked adrenoleukodystrophy, unspecified type**
CC Exclusion see Appendix A PDX collection 0536

CC **E71.53** **Other group 2 peroxisomal disorders**
CC Exclusion see Appendix A PDX collection 0536

\+ E71.54 **Other peroxisomal disorders**

CC **E71.540** **Rhizomelic chondrodysplasia punctata**
Excludes1: *chondrodysplasia punctata NOS (Q77.3)*
CC Exclusion see Appendix A PDX collection 0536

CC **E71.541** **Zellweger-like syndrome**
CC Exclusion see Appendix A PDX collection 0536

CC **E71.542** **Other group 3 peroxisomal disorders**
CC Exclusion see Appendix A PDX collection 0536

CC **E71.548** **Other peroxisomal disorders**
CC Exclusion see Appendix A PDX collection 0536

E72 Other disorders of amino-acid metabolism

Excludes1: *disorders of:*
aromatic amino-acid metabolism (E70.-)
branched-chain amino-acid metabolism (E71.0-E71.2)
fatty-acid metabolism (E71.3)
purine and pyrimidine metabolism (E79.-)
gout (M1A.-, M10.-)

\+ E72.0 **Disorders of amino-acid transport**
Excludes1: *disorders of tryptophan metabolism (E70.5)*

CC **E72.00** **Disorders of amino-acid transport, unspecified**
CC Exclusion see Appendix A PDX collection 0534

CC **E72.01** **Cystinuria**
CC Exclusion see Appendix A PDX collection 0534

CC **E72.02** **Hartnup's disease**
CC Exclusion see Appendix A PDX collection 0534

CC **E72.03** **Lowe's syndrome**
Use additional code for associated glaucoma (H42)
No CC Exclusions

CC **E72.04** **Cystinosis**
Fanconi (-de Toni) (-Debré) syndrome with cystinosis
Excludes1: *Fanconi (-de Toni) (-Debré) syndrome without cystinosis (E72.09)*
CC Exclusion see Appendix A PDX collection 0534

CC **E72.09** **Other disorders of amino-acid transport**
Fanconi (-de Toni) (-Debré) syndrome, unspecified
CC Exclusion see Appendix A PDX collection 0534

\+ **E72.1** **Disorders of sulfur-bearing amino-acid metabolism**
Excludes1: *cystinosis (E72.04)*
cystinuria (E72.01)
transcobalamin II deficiency (D51.2)

CC **E72.10** **Disorders of sulfur-bearing amino-acid metabolism, unspecified**
CC Exclusion see Appendix A PDX collection 0534

CC **E72.11** **Homocystinuria**
Cystathionine synthase deficiency
CC Exclusion see Appendix A PDX collection 0534

CC **E72.12** **Methylenetetrahydrofolate reductase deficiency**
CC Exclusion see Appendix A PDX collection 0534

CC **E72.19** **Other disorders of sulfur-bearing amino-acid metabolism**
Cystathioninuria
Methioninemia
Sulfite oxidase deficiency
CC Exclusion see Appendix A PDX collection 0534

\+ **E72.2** **Disorders of urea cycle metabolism**
Excludes1: *disorders of ornithine metabolism (E72.4)*

CC **E72.20** **Disorder of urea cycle metabolism, unspecified**
Hyperammonemia
Excludes1: *hyperammonemia-hyperornithinemia-homocitrullinemia syndrome E72.4*
transient hyperammonemia of newborn (P74.6)
CC Exclusion see Appendix A PDX collection 0534

CC **E72.21** **Argininemia**
CC Exclusion see Appendix A PDX collection 0534

CC **E72.22** **Arginosuccinic aciduria**
CC Exclusion see Appendix A PDX collection 0534

CC **E72.23** **Citrullinemia**
CC Exclusion see Appendix A PDX collection 0534

CC **E72.29** **Other disorders of urea cycle metabolism**
CC Exclusion see Appendix A PDX collection 0534

CC **E72.3** **Disorders of lysine and hydroxylysine metabolism**
Glutaric aciduria NOS
Glutaric aciduria (type I)
Hydroxylysinemia
Hyperlysinemia
Excludes1: *glutaric aciduria type II (E71.313)*
Refsum's disease (G60.1)
Zellweger syndrome (E71.510)
CC Exclusion see Appendix A PDX collection 0534

CC **E72.4** **Disorders of ornithine metabolism**
Hyperammonemia-Hyperornithinemia-Homocitrullinemia syndrome
Ornithinemia (types I, II)
Ornithine transcarbamylase deficiency
Excludes1: *hereditary choroidal dystrophy (H31.2-)*
CC Exclusion see Appendix A PDX collection 0534

\+ **E72.5** **Disorders of glycine metabolism**

CC **E72.50** **Disorder of glycine metabolism, unspecified**
CC Exclusion see Appendix A PDX collection 0534

CC **E72.51** **Non-ketotic hyperglycinemia**
CC Exclusion see Appendix A PDX collection 0534

CC **E72.52** **Trimethylaminuria**
CC Exclusion see Appendix A PDX collection 0534

CC **E72.53** **Hyperoxaluria**
Oxalosis
Oxaluria
CC Exclusion see Appendix A PDX collection 0534

CC **E72.59** **Other disorders of glycine metabolism**
D-glycericacidemia
Hyperhydroxyprolinemia
Hyperprolinemia (types I, II)
Sarcosinemia
CC Exclusion see Appendix A PDX collection 0534

CC **E72.8** **Other specified disorders of amino-acid metabolism**
Disorders of beta-amino-acid metabolism
Disorders of gamma-glutamyl cycle
CC Exclusion see Appendix A PDX collection 0534

CC **E72.9** **Disorder of amino-acid metabolism, unspecified**
CC Exclusion see Appendix A PDX collection 0534

E73 Lactose intolerance

E73.0 **Congenital lactase deficiency**
E73.1 **Secondary lactase deficiency**
E73.8 **Other lactose intolerance**
E73.9 **Lactose intolerance, unspecified**

E74 Other disorders of carbohydrate metabolism

Excludes1: *diabetes mellitus (E08-E13)*
NOS (E16.2)
increased secretion of glucagon (E16.3)
mucopolysaccharidosis (E76.0-E76.3)

\+ **E74.0** **Glycogen storage disease**

CC **E74.00** **Glycogen storage disease, unspecified**
CC Exclusion see Appendix A PDX collection 0534

CC **E74.01** **von Gierke disease**
Type I glycogen storage disease
CC Exclusion see Appendix A PDX collection 0534

CC **E74.02** **Pompe disease**
Cardiac glycogenosis
Type II glycogen storage disease
CC Exclusion see Appendix A PDX collection 0534

CC **E74.03** **Cori disease**
Forbes disease
Type III glycogen storage disease
CC Exclusion see Appendix A PDX collection 0534

CC **E74.04** **McArdle disease**
Type V glycogen storage disease
CC Exclusion see Appendix A PDX collection 0534

CC **E74.09** **Other glycogen storage disease**
Andersen disease
Hers disease
Tauri disease
Glycogen storage disease, types 0, IV, VI-XI
Liver phosphorylase deficiency
Muscle phosphofructokinase deficiency
CC Exclusion see Appendix A PDX collection 0534

\+ **E74.1** **Disorders of fructose metabolism**
Excludes1: *muscle phosphofructokinase deficiency (E74.09)*

E74.10 **Disorder of fructose metabolism, unspecified**
E74.11 **Essential fructosuria**
Fructokinase deficiency
E74.12 **Hereditary fructose intolerance**
Fructosemia
E74.19 **Other disorders of fructose metabolism**
Fructose-1, 6-diphosphatase deficiency

\+ **E74.2** **Disorders of galactose metabolism**

CC **E74.20** **Disorders of galactose metabolism, unspecified**
CC Exclusion see Appendix A PDX collection 0534

CC **E74.21** **Galactosemia**
CC Exclusion see Appendix A PDX collection 0534

CC **E74.29** **Other disorders of galactose metabolism**
Galactokinase deficiency
CC Exclusion see Appendix A PDX collection 0534

\+ **E74.3** **Other disorders of intestinal carbohydrate absorption**
Excludes2: *lactose intolerance (E73.-)*

E74.31 **Sucrase-isomaltase deficiency**
E74.39 **Other disorders of intestinal carbohydrate absorption**
Disorder of intestinal carbohydrate absorption NOS
Glucose-galactose malabsorption
Sucrase deficiency

CC **E74.4** **Disorders of pyruvate metabolism and gluconeogenesis**
Deficiency of phosphoenolpyruvate carboxykinase
Deficiency of pyruvate carboxylase
Deficiency of pyruvate dehydrogenase
Excludes1: *disorders of pyruvate metabolism and gluconeogenesis with anemia (D55.-)*
Leigh's syndrome (G31.82)
CC Exclusion see Appendix A PDX collection 0534

CC **E74.8** **Other specified disorders of carbohydrate metabolism**
Essential pentosuria
Renal glycosuria
CC Exclusion see Appendix A PDX collection 0534

E74.9 **Disorder of carbohydrate metabolism, unspecified**

E75 **Disorders of sphingolipid metabolism and other lipid storage disorders**

Excludes1: *mucolipidosis, types I-III (E77.0-E77.1)*
Refsum's disease (G60.1)

\+ E75.0 **GM2 gangliosidosis**
CC **E75.00 GM2 gangliosidosis, unspecified**
CC Exclusion see Appendix A PDX collection 0537
CC **E75.01 Sandhoff disease**
CC Exclusion see Appendix A PDX collection 0537
CC **E75.02 Tay-Sachs disease**
CC Exclusion see Appendix A PDX collection 0537
CC **E75.09 Other GM2 gangliosidosis**
Adult GM2 gangliosidosis
Juvenile GM2 gangliosidosis
CC Exclusion see Appendix A PDX collection 0537

\+ E75.1 **Other and unspecified gangliosidosis**
CC **E75.10 Unspecified gangliosidosis**
Gangliosidosis NOS
CC Exclusion see Appendix A PDX collection 0537
CC **E75.11 Mucolipidosis IV**
CC Exclusion see Appendix A PDX collection 0537
CC **E75.19 Other gangliosidosis**
GM1 gangliosidosis
GM3 gangliosidosis
CC Exclusion see Appendix A PDX collection 0537

\+ E75.2 **Other sphingolipidosis**
Excludes1: *adrenoleukodystrophy [Addison-Schilder] (E71.528)*
E75.21 Fabry (-Anderson) disease
E75.22 Gaucher disease
CC **E75.23 Krabbe disease**
CC Exclusion see Appendix A PDX collection 0538
\+ E75.24 **Niemann-Pick disease**
E75.240 Niemann-Pick disease type A
E75.241 Niemann-Pick disease type B
E75.242 Niemann-Pick disease type C
E75.243 Niemann-Pick disease type D
E75.248 Other Niemann-Pick disease
E75.249 Niemann-Pick disease, unspecified
CC **E75.25 Metachromatic leukodystrophy**
CC Exclusion see Appendix A PDX collection 0538
CC **E75.29 Other sphingolipidosis**
Farber's syndrome
Sulfatase deficiency
Sulfatide lipidosis
CC Exclusion see Appendix A PDX collection 0538

E75.3 Sphingolipidosis, unspecified

CC **E75.4 Neuronal ceroid lipofuscinosis**
Batten disease
Bielschowsky-Jansky disease
Kufs disease
Spielmeyer-Vogt disease
CC Exclusion see Appendix A PDX collection 0537

E75.5 Other lipid storage disorders
Cerebrotendinous cholesterosis [van Bogaert-Scherer-Epstein]
Wolman's disease

E75.6 Lipid storage disorder, unspecified

E76 **Disorders of glycosaminoglycan metabolism**

\+ E76.0 **Mucopolysaccharidosis, type I**
CC **E76.01 Hurler's syndrome**
CC Exclusion see Appendix A PDX collection 0539
CC **E76.02 Hurler-Scheie syndrome**
CC Exclusion see Appendix A PDX collection 0539
CC **E76.03 Scheie's syndrome**
CC Exclusion see Appendix A PDX collection 0539

CC **E76.1 Mucopolysaccharidosis, type II**
Hunter's syndrome
CC Exclusion see Appendix A PDX collection 0539

\+ E76.2 **Other mucopolysaccharidoses**
\+ E76.21 **Morquio mucopolysaccharidoses**
CC **E76.210 Morquio A mucopolysaccharidoses**
Classic Morquio syndrome
Morquio syndrome A
Mucopolysaccharidosis, type IVA
CC Exclusion see Appendix A PDX collection 0539
CC **E76.211 Morquio B mucopolysaccharidoses**
Morquio-like mucopolysaccharidoses
Morquio-like syndrome
Morquio syndrome B
Mucopolysaccharidosis, type IVB
CC Exclusion see Appendix A PDX collection 0539
CC **E76.219 Morquio mucopolysaccharidoses, unspecified**
Morquio syndrome
Mucopolysaccharidosis, type IV
CC Exclusion see Appendix A PDX collection 0539
CC **E76.22 Sanfilippo mucopolysaccharidoses**
Mucopolysaccharidosis, type III (A) (B) (C) (D)
Sanfilippo A syndrome
Sanfilippo B syndrome
Sanfilippo C syndrome
Sanfilippo D syndrome
CC Exclusion see Appendix A PDX collection 0539
CC **E76.29 Other mucopolysaccharidoses**
beta-Glucuronidase deficiency
Maroteaux-Lamy (mild) (severe) syndrome
Mucopolysaccharidosis, types VI, VII
CC Exclusion see Appendix A PDX collection 0539

CC **E76.3 Mucopolysaccharidosis, unspecified**
CC Exclusion see Appendix A PDX collection 0539

CC **E76.8 Other disorders of glucosaminoglycan metabolism**
CC Exclusion see Appendix A PDX collection 0539

CC **E76.9 Glucosaminoglycan metabolism disorder, unspecified**
CC Exclusion see Appendix A PDX collection 0539

E77 **Disorders of glycoprotein metabolism**

E77.0 Defects in post-translational modification of lysosomal enzymes
Mucolipidosis II [I-cell disease]
Mucolipidosis III [pseudo-Hurler polydystrophy]

E77.1 Defects in glycoprotein degradation
Aspartylglucosaminuria
Fucosidosis
Mannosidosis
Sialidosis [mucolipidosis I]

E77.8 Other disorders of glycoprotein metabolism

E77.9 Disorder of glycoprotein metabolism, unspecified

E78 **Disorders of lipoprotein metabolism and other lipidemias**

Excludes1: *sphingolipidosis (E75.0-E75.3)*

\+ E78.0 **Pure hypercholesterolemia**
E78.00 Pure hypercholesterolemia, unspecified
Fedrickson's hyperlipoproteinemia, type IIa
Hyperbetalipoproteinemia
Low-density-lipoprotein-type [LDL] hyperlipoproteinemia
(Pure) hypercholesterolemia, NOS
AHA CC: 4Q, 2016, 13-14
E78.01 Familial hypercholesterolemia

E78.1 Pure hyperglyceridemia
Elevated fasting triglycerides
Endogenous hyperglyceridemia
Fredrickson's hyperlipoproteinemia, type IV
Hyperlipidemia, group B
Hyperprebetalipoproteinemia
Very-low-density-lipoprotein-type [VLDL] hyperlipoproteinemia

E78.2 Mixed hyperlipidemia
Broad- or floating-betalipoproteinemia
Combined hyperlipidemia NOS
Elevated cholesterol with elevated triglycerides NEC
Fredrickson's hyperlipoproteinemia, type IIb or III
Hyperbetalipoproteinemia with prebetalipoproteinemia
Hypercholesteremia with endogenous hyperglyceridemia
Hyperlipidemia, group C
Tubo-eruptive xanthoma
Xanthoma tuberosum
Excludes1: *cerebrotendinous cholesterosis [van Bogaert-Scherer-Epstein] (E75.5)*
familial combined hyperlipidemia (E78.4)

E78.3 Hyperchylomicronemia
Chylomicron retention disease
Fredrickson's hyperlipoproteinemia, type I or V
Hyperlipidemia, group D
Mixed hyperglyceridemia

E78.4 Other hyperlipidemia
Familial combined hyperlipidemia

E78.5 Hyperlipidemia, unspecified

E78.6 **Lipoprotein deficiency**
Abetalipoproteinemia
Depressed HDL cholesterol
High-density lipoprotein deficiency
Hypoalphalipoproteinemia
Hypobetalipoproteinemia (familial)
Lecithin cholesterol acyltransferase deficiency
Tangier disease

\+ E78.7 **Disorders of bile acid and cholesterol metabolism**
Excludes1: *Niemann-Pick disease type C (E75.242)*
E78.70 **Disorder of bile acid and cholesterol metabolism, unspecified**
CC E78.71 **Barth syndrome**
CC Exclusion see Appendix A PDX collection 0540
CC E78.72 **Smith-Lemli-Opitz syndrome**
CC Exclusion see Appendix A PDX collection 0540
E78.79 **Other disorders of bile acid and cholesterol metabolism**

\+ E78.8 **Other disorders of lipoprotein metabolism**
E78.81 **Lipoid dermatoarthritis**
E78.89 **Other lipoprotein metabolism disorders**
E78.9 **Disorder of lipoprotein metabolism, unspecified**

E79 **Disorders of purine and pyrimidine metabolism**
Excludes1: *Ataxia-telangiectasia (Q87.1)*
Bloom's syndrome (Q82.8)
Cockayne's syndrome (Q87.1)
calculus of kidney (N20.0)
combined immunodeficiency disorders (D81.-)
Fanconi's anemia (D61.09)
gout (M1A.-, M10.-)
orotaciduric anemia (D53.0)
progeria (E34.8)
Werner's syndrome (E34.8)
xeroderma pigmentosum (Q82.1)

E79.0 **Hyperuricemia without signs of inflammatory arthritis and tophaceous disease**
Asymptomatic hyperuricemia
CC E79.1 **Lesch-Nyhan syndrome**
HGPRT deficiency
CC Exclusion see Appendix A PDX collection 0513
CC E79.2 **Myoadenylate deaminase deficiency**
CC Exclusion see Appendix A PDX collection 0513
CC E79.8 **Other disorders of purine and pyrimidine metabolism**
Hereditary xanthinuria
CC Exclusion see Appendix A PDX collection 0513
CC E79.9 **Disorder of purine and pyrimidine metabolism, unspecified**
CC Exclusion see Appendix A PDX collection 0513

E80 **Disorders of porphyrin and bilirubin metabolism**
Includes: defects of catalase and peroxidase
CC E80.0 **Hereditary erythropoietic porphyria**
Congenital erythropoietic porphyria
Erythropoietic protoporphyria
CC Exclusion see Appendix A PDX collection 0513
CC E80.1 **Porphyria cutanea tarda**
CC Exclusion see Appendix A PDX collection 0513
\+ E80.2 **Other and unspecified porphyria**
CC E80.20 **Unspecified porphyria**
Porphyria NOS
CC Exclusion see Appendix A PDX collection 0513
CC E80.21 **Acute intermittent (hepatic) porphyria**
CC Exclusion see Appendix A PDX collection 0513
CC E80.29 **Other porphyria**
Hereditary coproporphyria
CC Exclusion see Appendix A PDX collection 0513
CC E80.3 **Defects of catalase and peroxidase**
Acatalasia [Takahara]
CC Exclusion see Appendix A PDX collection 0492
E80.4 **Gilbert syndrome**
E80.5 **Crigler-Najjar syndrome**
E80.6 **Other disorders of bilirubin metabolism**
Dubin-Johnson syndrome
Rotor's syndrome
E80.7 **Disorder of bilirubin metabolism, unspecified**

E83 **Disorders of mineral metabolism**
Excludes1: *dietary mineral deficiency (E58-E61)*
parathyroid disorders (E20-E21)
vitamin D deficiency (E55.-)

\+ E83.0 **Disorders of copper metabolism**
E83.00 **Disorder of copper metabolism, unspecified**
E83.01 **Wilson's disease**
Code also associated Kayser Fleischer ring (H18.04-)
E83.09 **Other disorders of copper metabolism**
Menkes' (kinky hair) (steely hair) disease

\+ E83.1 **Disorders of iron metabolism**
Excludes1: *iron deficiency anemia (D50.-)*
sideroblastic anemia (D64.0-D64.3)
E83.10 **Disorder of iron metabolism, unspecified**
\+ E83.11 **Hemochromatosis**
Excludes1: *GALD (P78.84)*
Gestational alloimmune liver disease (P78.84)
Neonatal hemochromatosis (P78.84)
E83.110 **Hereditary hemochromatosis**
Bronzed diabetes
Pigmentary cirrhosis (of liver)
Primary (hereditary) hemochromatosis
E83.111 **Hemochromatosis due to repeated red blood cell transfusions**
Iron overload due to repeated red blood cell transfusions
Transfusion (red blood cell) associated hemochromatosis
E83.118 **Other hemochromatosis**
E83.119 **Hemochromatosis, unspecified**
E83.19 **Other disorders of iron metabolism**
Use additional code, if applicable, for idiopathic pulmonary hemosiderosis (J84.03)

E83.2 **Disorders of zinc metabolism**
Acrodermatitis enteropathica

\+ E83.3 **Disorders of phosphorus metabolism and phosphatases**
Excludes1: *adult osteomalacia (M83.-)*
osteoporosis (M80.-)
E83.30 **Disorder of phosphorus metabolism, unspecified**
E83.31 **Familial hypophosphatemia**
Vitamin D-resistant osteomalacia
Vitamin D-resistant rickets
Excludes1: *vitamin D-deficiency rickets (E55.0)*
E83.32 **Hereditary vitamin D-dependent rickets (type 1) (type 2)**
25-hydroxyvitamin D 1-alpha-hydroxylase deficiency
Pseudovitamin D deficiency
Vitamin D receptor defect
E83.39 **Other disorders of phosphorus metabolism**
Acid phosphatase deficiency
Hypophosphatasia

\+ E83.4 **Disorders of magnesium metabolism**
E83.40 **Disorders of magnesium metabolism, unspecified**
E83.41 **Hypermagnesemia**
AHA CC: 4Q, 2016, 54-55
E83.42 **Hypomagnesemia**
E83.49 **Other disorders of magnesium metabolism**

\+ E83.5 **Disorders of calcium metabolism**
Excludes1: *chondrocalcinosis (M11.1-M11.2)*
hungry bone syndrome (E83.81)
hyperparathyroidism (E21.0-E21.3)
E83.50 **Unspecified disorder of calcium metabolism**
E83.51 **Hypocalcemia**
E83.52 **Hypercalcemia**
Familial hypocalciuric hypercalcemia
E83.59 **Other disorders of calcium metabolism**
Idiopathic hypercalciuria

\+ E83.8 **Other disorders of mineral metabolism**
E83.81 **Hungry bone syndrome**
E83.89 **Other disorders of mineral metabolism**
E83.9 **Disorder of mineral metabolism, unspecified**

E84 **Cystic fibrosis**
Code also exocrine pancreatic insufficiency (K86.81)
Includes: mucoviscidosis
MCC E84.0 **Cystic fibrosis with pulmonary manifestations**
Use additional code to identify any infectious organism present, such as:
Pseudomonas (B96.5)
MCC Exclusion see Appendix A PDX collection 0541
\+ E84.1 **Cystic fibrosis with intestinal manifestations**
• MCC E84.11 **Meconium ileus in cystic fibrosis**
Excludes1: *meconium ileus not due to cystic fibrosis (P76.0)*
MCC Exclusion see Appendix A PDX collection 0541
CC E84.19 **Cystic fibrosis with other intestinal manifestations**
Distal intestinal obstruction syndrome
CC Exclusion see Appendix A PDX collection 0541

CC **E84.8 Cystic fibrosis with other manifestations**
CC Exclusion see Appendix A PDX collection 0541

CC **E84.9 Cystic fibrosis, unspecified**
CC Exclusion see Appendix A PDX collection 0541

E85 Amyloidosis

Excludes2: *Alzheimer's disease (G30.0-)*

CC **E85.0 Non-neuropathic heredofamilial amyloidosis**
Hereditary amyloid nephropathy
Code also associated disorders, such as:
autoinflammatory syndromes (M04.-)
Excludes2: *Transthyretin-related (ATTR) familial amyloid cardiomyopathy (E85.4)*
CC Exclusion see Appendix A PDX collection 0542

CC **E85.1 Neuropathic heredofamilial amyloidosis**
Amyloid polyneuropathy (Portuguese)
Transthyretin-related (ATTR) familial amyloid polyneuropathy
CC Exclusion see Appendix A PDX collection 0542
AHA CC: 4Q, 2012, 99-101

CC **E85.2 Heredofamilial amyloidosis, unspecified**
CC Exclusion see Appendix A PDX collection 0542

CC **E85.3 Secondary systemic amyloidosis**
Hemodialysis-associated amyloidosis
CC Exclusion see Appendix A PDX collection 0542

CC **E85.4 Organ-limited amyloidosis**
Localized amyloidosis
Transthyretin-related (ATTR) familial amyloid cardiomyopathy
CC Exclusion see Appendix A PDX collection 0542

\+ **E85.8 Other amyloidosis**

CC **E85.81 Light chain (AL) amyloidosis**
CC Exclusion see Appendix A PDX collection 0542

CC **E85.82 Wild-type transthyretin-related (ATTR) amyloidosis**
Senile systemic amyloidosis (SSA)
CC Exclusion see Appendix A PDX collection 0542

CC **E85.89 Other amyloidosis**
CC Exclusion see Appendix A PDX collection 0542

CC **E85.9 Amyloidosis, unspecified**
CC Exclusion see Appendix A PDX collection 0542

E86 Volume depletion

Use Additional code(s) for any associated disorders of electrolyte and acid-base balance (E87.-)

Excludes1: *dehydration of newborn (P74.1)*
hypovolemic shock NOS (R57.1)
postprocedural hypovolemic shock (T81.19)
traumatic hypovolemic shock (T79.4)

E86.0 Dehydration
Review coding guidelines C.2.c.3
AHA CC: 1Q, 2014, 7

E86.1 Hypovolemia
Depletion of volume of plasma

E86.9 Volume depletion, unspecified

E87 Other disorders of fluid, electrolyte and acid-base balance

Excludes1: *diabetes insipidus (E23.2)*
electrolyte imbalance associated with hyperemesis gravidarum (O21.1)
electrolyte imbalance following ectopic or molar pregnancy (O08.5)
familial periodic paralysis (G72.3)

CC **E87.0 Hyperosmolality and hypernatremia**
Sodium [Na] excess
Sodium [Na] overload
CC Exclusion see Appendix A PDX collection 0543
AHA CC: 1Q, 2014, 7

CC **E87.1 Hypo-osmolality and hyponatremia**
Sodium [Na] deficiency
Excludes1: *syndrome of inappropriate secretion of antidiuretic hormone (E22.2)*
CC Exclusion see Appendix A PDX collection 0543
AHA CC: 1Q, 2014, 7

CC **E87.2 Acidosis**
Acidosis NOS
Lactic acidosis
Metabolic acidosis
Respiratory acidosis
Excludes1: *diabetic acidosis - see categories E08-E10, E13 with ketoacidosis*
CC Exclusion see Appendix A PDX collection 0543

CC **E87.3 Alkalosis**
Alkalosis NOS
Metabolic alkalosis
Respiratory alkalosis
CC Exclusion see Appendix A PDX collection 0543

CC **E87.4 Mixed disorder of acid-base balance**
CC Exclusion see Appendix A PDX collection 0543

E87.5 Hyperkalemia
Potassium [K] excess
Potassium [K] overload

E87.6 Hypokalemia
Potassium [K] deficiency

\+ **E87.7 Fluid overload**
Excludes1: *edema NOS (R60.9)*
fluid retention (R60.9)

E87.70 Fluid overload, unspecified

E87.71 Transfusion associated circulatory overload
Fluid overload due to transfusion (blood) (blood components)
TACO

E87.79 Other fluid overload

E87.8 Other disorders of electrolyte and fluid balance, not elsewhere classified
Electrolyte imbalance NOS
Hyperchloremia
Hypochloremia

E88 Other and unspecified metabolic disorders

Use additional codes for associated conditions
Excludes1: *histiocytosis X (chronic) (C96.6)*

\+ **E88.0 Disorders of plasma-protein metabolism, not elsewhere classified**
Excludes1: *disorder of lipoprotein metabolism (E78.-)*
monoclonal gammopathy (of undetermined significance) (D47.2)
polyclonal hypergammaglobulinemia (D89.0)
Waldenström macroglobulinemia (C88.0)

E88.01 Alpha-1-antitrypsin deficiency
AAT deficiency

E88.09 Other disorders of plasma-protein metabolism, not elsewhere classified
Bisalbuminemia

E88.1 Lipodystrophy, not elsewhere classified
Lipodystrophy NOS
Excludes1: *Whipple's disease (K90.81)*

E88.2 Lipomatosis, not elsewhere classified
Lipomatosis NOS
Lipomatosis (Check) dolorosa [Dercum]

MCC **E88.3 Tumor lysis syndrome**
Tumor lysis syndrome (spontaneous)
Tumor lysis syndrome following antineoplastic drug chemotherapy
Use additional code for adverse effect, if applicable, to identify drug (T45.1X5)
MCC Exclusion see Appendix A PDX collection 0544

\+ **E88.4 Mitochondrial metabolism disorders**
Excludes1: disorders of pyruvate metabolism (E74.4)
Kearns-Sayre syndrome (H49.81)
Leber's disease (H47.22)
Leigh's encephalopathy (G31.82)
Mitochondrial myopathy, NEC (G71.3)
Reye's syndrome (G93.7)

CC **E88.40 Mitochondrial metabolism disorder, unspecified**
CC Exclusion see Appendix A PDX collection 0545

CC **E88.41 MELAS syndrome**
Mitochondrial myopathy, encephalopathy, lactic acidosis and stroke-like episodes
CC Exclusion see Appendix A PDX collection 0545

CC **E88.42 MERRF syndrome**
Myoclonic epilepsy associated with ragged-red fibers
Code also progressive myoclonic epilepsy (G40.3-)
CC Exclusion see Appendix A PDX collection 0545

CC **E88.49 Other mitochondrial metabolism disorders**
CC Exclusion see Appendix A PDX collection 0545

\+ **E88.8 Other specified metabolic disorders**

E88.81 Metabolic syndrome
Dysmetabolic syndrome X
Use additional codes for associated manifestations, such as:
obesity (E66.-)

E88.89 Other specified metabolic disorders
Launois-Bensaude adenolipomatosis
Excludes1: *adult pulmonary Langerhans cell histiocytosis (J84.82)*

E88.9 Metabolic disorder, unspecified

ostprocedural endocrine and metabolic complications and isorders, not elsewhere classified (E89)

E89 Postprocedural endocrine and metabolic complications and disorders, not elsewhere classified

Excludes2: *intraoperative complications of endocrine system organ or structure (E36.0-, E36.1-, E36.8)*

E89.0 Postprocedural hypothyroidism
Postirradiation hypothyroidism
Postsurgical hypothyroidism

CC **E89.1 Postprocedural hypoinsulinemia**
Postpancreatectomy hyperglycemia
Postsurgical hypoinsulinemia
Use additional code, if applicable, to identify:
acquired absence of pancreas (Z90.41-)
diabetes mellitus (postpancreatectomy) (postprocedural) (E13.-)
insulin use (Z79.4)
Excludes1: *transient postprocedural hyperglycemia (R73.9)*
transient postprocedural hypoglycemia (E16.2)
CC Exclusion see Appendix A PDX collection 0520
Review coding guideline C.4.a.6.b.i

E89.2 Postprocedural hypoparathyroidism
Parathyroprival tetany

E89.3 Postprocedural hypopituitarism
Postirradiation hypopituitarism

+ **E89.4 Postprocedural ovarian failure**

♀ **E89.40 Asymptomatic postprocedural ovarian failure**
Postprocedural ovarian failure NOS

♀ **E89.41 Symptomatic postprocedural ovarian failure**
Symptoms such as flushing, sleeplessness, headache, lack of concentration, associated with postprocedural menopause

♂ **E89.5 Postprocedural testicular hypofunction**

CC **E89.6 Postprocedural adrenocortical (-medullary) hypofunction**
CC Exclusion see Appendix A PDX collection 0526

+ **E89.8 Other postprocedural endocrine and metabolic complications and disorders**
AHA CC: 4Q, 2016, 9-10

+ **E89.81 Postprocedural hemorrhage of an endocrine system organ or structure following a procedure**

CC **E89.810 Postprocedural hemorrhage of an endocrine system organ or structure following an endocrine system procedure**
CC Exclusion see Appendix A PDX collection 0546

CC **E89.811 Postprocedural hemorrhage of an endocrine system organ or structure following other procedure**
CC Exclusion see Appendix A PDX collection 0546

+ **E89.82 Postprocedural hematoma and seroma of an endocrine system organ or structre**

CC **E89.820 Postprocedural hematoma of an endocrine system organ or structure following an endocrine system procedure**
CC Exclusion see Appendix A PDX collection 0546

CC **E89.821 Postprocedural hematoma of an endocrine system organ or structure following other procedure**
CC Exclusion see Appendix A PDX collection 0546

CC **E89.822 Postprocedural seroma of an endocrine system organ or structure following an endocrine system procedure**
CC Exclusion see Appendix A PDX collection 0546

CC **E89.823 Postprocedural seroma of an endocrine system organ or structure following other procedure**
CC Exclusion see Appendix A PDX collection 0546

CC **E89.89 Other postprocedural endocrine and metabolic complications and disorders**
Use additional code, if applicable, to further specify disorder
CC Exclusion see Appendix A PDX collection 0546

Chapter 5: Mental, Behavioral and Neurodevelopmental Disorders (F01-F99)

Includes: disorders of psychological development

Excludes2: *symptoms, signs and abnormal clinical laboratory findings, not elsewhere classified (R00-R99)*

This chapter contains the following category blocks:

F01-F09	Mental disorders due to known physiological conditions
F10-F19	Mental and behavioral disorders due to psychoactive substance use
F20-F29	Schizophrenia, schizotypal, delusional, and other non-mood psychotic disorders
F30-F39	Mood [affective] disorders
F40-F48	Anxiety, dissociative, stress-related, somatoform and other nonpsychotic mental disorders
F50-F59	Behavioral syndromes associated with physiological disturbances and physical factors
F60-F69	Disorders of adult personality and behavior
F70-F79	Intellectual disabilities
F80-F89	Pervasive and specific developmental disorders
F90-F98	Behavioral and emotional disorders with onset usually occurring in childhood and adolescence
F99	Unspecified mental disorder

C. Chapter-Specific Coding Guidelines

In addition to general coding guidelines, there are guidelines for specific diagnoses and/or conditions in the classification. Unless otherwise indicated, these guidelines apply to all health care settings. Please refer to Section II for guidelines on the selection of principal diagnosis.

5. Chapter 5: Mental, Behavioral and Neurodevelopmental Disorders (F01-F99)

a. Pain disorders related to psychological factors

Assign code F45.41, for pain that is exclusively related to psychological disorders. As indicated by the Excludes 1 note under category G89, a code from category G89 should not be assigned with code F45.41

Code F45.42, Pain disorders with related psychological factors, should be used with a code from category G89, Pain, not elsewhere classified, if there is documentation of a psychological component for a patient with acute or chronic pain.

See Section I.C.6. Pain

b. Mental and behavioral disorders due to psychoactive substance use

1) In Remission

Selection of codes for “in remission” for categories F10-F19, Mental and behavioral disorders due to psychoactive substance use (categories F10-F19 with **-.11,** -.21) requires the provider’s clinical judgment. The appropriate codes for “in remission” are assigned only on the basis of provider documentation (as defined in the Official Guidelines for Coding and Reporting), **unless otherwise instructed by the classification.**

Mild substance use disorders in early or sustained remission are classified to the appropriate codes for substance abuse in remission, and moderate or severe substance use disorders in early or sustained remission are classified to the appropriate codes for substance dependence in remission.

2) Psychoactive Substance Use, Abuse And Dependence

When the provider documentation refers to use, abuse and dependence of the same substance (e.g. alcohol, opioid, cannabis, etc.), only one code should be assigned to identify the pattern of use based on the following hierarchy:

- If both use and abuse are documented, assign only the code for abuse
- If both abuse and dependence are documented, assign only the code for dependence
- If use, abuse and dependence are all documented, assign only the code for dependence
- If both use and dependence are documented, assign only the code for dependence.

3) Psychoactive Substance Use *Disorders*

As with all other diagnoses, the codes for psychoactive substance use **disorders** (F10.9-, F11.9-, F12.9-, F13.9-, F14.9-, F15.9-, F16.9-) should only be assigned based on provider documentation and when they meet the definition of a reportable diagnosis (see Section III, Reporting Additional Diagnoses). The codes are to be used only when the psychoactive substance use is associated with a **physical,** mental or behavioral disorder, and such a relationship is documented by the provider.

Mental disorders due to known physiological conditions (F01-F09)

NOTE This block comprises a range of mental disorders grouped together on the basis of their having in common a demonstrable etiology in cerebral disease, brain injury, or other insult leading to cerebral dysfunction. The dysfunction may be primary, as in diseases, injuries, and insults that affe the brain directly and selectively; or secondary, as in systemic diseases and disorders that attack the brain only as one of the multiple organs or systems of the body that are involved.

F01 Vascular dementia

Vascular dementia as a result of infarction of the brain due to vascular disease, including hypertensive cerebrovascular disease.

Includes: arteriosclerotic dementia

Code first the underlying physiological condition or sequelae of cerebrovascular disease.

\+ **F01.5 Vascular dementia**

• **F01.50 Vascular dementia without behavioral disturbance**

Major neurocognitive disorder without behavioral disturbance

• CC **F01.51 Vascular dementia with behavioral disturbance**

Major neurocognitive disorder due to vascular disease with behavioral disturbance
Major neurocognitive disorder with aggressive behavi
Major neurocognitive disorder with combative behavic
Major neurocognitive disorder with violent behavior
Vascular dementia with aggressive behavior
Vascular dementia with combative behavior
Vascular dementia with violent behavior

Use additional code, if applicable, to identify wandering in vascular dementia (Z91.83)

CC Exclusion see Appendix A PDX collection 0547

F02 Dementia in other diseases classified elsewhere

Includes: Major neurocognitive disorder in other diseases classified elsewhere

Code first the underlying physiological condition, such as:
Alzheimer’s (G30.-)
cerebral lipidosis (E75.4)
Creutzfeldt-Jakob disease (A81.0-)
dementia with Lewy bodies (G31.83)
dementia with Parkinsonism (G31.83)
epilepsy and recurrent seizures (G40.-)
frontotemporal dementia (G31.09)
hepatolenticular degeneration (E83.0)
human immunodeficiency virus [HIV] disease (B20)
Huntington’s disease (G10)
hypercalcemia (E83.52)
hypothyroidism, acquired (E00-E03.-)
intoxications (T36-T65)
Jakob-Creutzfeldt disease (A81.0-)
multiple sclerosis (G35)
neurosyphilis (A52.17)
niacin deficiency [pellagra] (E52)
Parkinson’s disease (G20)
Pick’s disease (G31.01)
polyarteritis nodosa (M30.0)
prion disease (A81.9)
systemic lupus erythematosus (M32.-)
traumatic brain injury (S06.-)
trypanosomiasis (B56.-, B57.-)
vitamin B deficiency (E53.8)

Excludes2: *dementia in alcohol and psychoactive substance disorders (F10-F19, with .17, .27, .97)*
vascular dementia (F01.5-)

\+ **F02.8 Dementia in other diseases classified elsewhere**

F02.80 Dementia in other diseases classified elsewhere without behavioral disturbance

Dementia in other diseases classified elsewhere NOS
Major neurocognitive disorder in other diseases classified elsewhere

AHA CC: 2Q, 2016, 6; 4Q, 2016, 141; 1Q, 2017, 43-44

CC **F02.81 Dementia in other diseases classified elsewhere with behavioral disturbance**
Dementia in other diseases classified elsewhere with aggressive behavior
Dementia in other diseases classified elsewhere with combative behavior
Dementia in other diseases classified elsewhere with violent behavior
Major neurocognitive disorder in other diseases classified elsewhere with aggressive behavior
Major neurocognitive disorder in other diseases classified elsewhere with combative behavior
Major neurocognitive disorder in other diseases classified elsewhere with violent behavior
Use additional code, if applicable, to identify wandering in dementia in conditions classified elsewhere (Z91.83)
CC Exclusion see Appendix A PDX collection 0548
AHA CC: 2Q, 2017, 7-8

F03 Unspecified dementia
Presenile dementia NOS
Presenile psychosis NOS
Primary degenerative dementia NOS
Senile dementia NOS
Senile dementia depressed or paranoid type
Senile psychosis NOS
Excludes1: *senility NOS (R41.81)*
Excludes2: *mild memory disturbance due to known physiological condition (F06.8)*
senile dementia with delirium or acute confusional state (F05)

\+ **F03.9 Unspecified dementia**

• **F03.90 Unspecified dementia without behavioral disturbance**
Dementia NOS
AHA CC: 4Q, 2012, 92-93

• CC **F03.91 Unspecified dementia with behavioral disturbance**
Unspecified dementia with aggressive behavior
Unspecified dementia with combative behavior
Unspecified dementia with violent behavior
Use additional code, if applicable, to identify wandering in unspecified dementia (Z91.83)
CC Exclusion see Appendix A PDX collection 0548

F04 Amnestic disorder due to known physiological condition
Korsakov's psychosis or syndrome, nonalcoholic
Code first the underlying physiological condition
Excludes1: *amnesia NOS (R41.3)*
anterograde amnesia (R41.1)
dissociative amnesia (F44.0)
retrograde amnesia (R41.2)
Excludes2: *alcohol-induced or unspecified Korsakov's syndrome (F10.26, F10.96)*
Korsakov's syndrome induced by other psychoactive substances (F13.26, F13.96, F19.16, F19.26, F19.96)
Valid 3-character code, no further characters required

CC **F05 Delirium due to known physiological condition**
Acute or subacute brain syndrome
Acute or subacute confusional state (nonalcoholic)
Acute or subacute infective psychosis
Acute or subacute organic reaction
Acute or subacute psycho-organic syndrome
Delirium of mixed etiology
Delirium superimposed on dementia
Sundowning
Code first the underlying physiological condition
Excludes1: *delirium NOS (R41.0)*
Excludes2: *delirium tremens alcohol-induced or unspecified (F10.231, F10.921)*
CC Exclusion see Appendix A PDX collection 0549
Valid 3-character code, no further characters required

F06 Other mental disorders due to known physiological condition
Includes: mental disorders due to endocrine disorder
mental disorders due to exogenous hormone
mental disorders due to exogenous toxic substance
mental disorders due to primary cerebral disease
mental disorders due to somatic illness
mental disorders due to systemic disease affecting the brain
Code first the underlying physiological condition
Excludes1: *unspecified dementia (F03)*
Excludes2: *delirium due to known physiological condition (F05)*
dementia as classified in F01-F02
other mental disorders associated with alcohol and other psychoactive substances (F10-F19)

CC **F06.0 Psychotic disorder with hallucinations due to known physiological condition**
Organic hallucinatory state (nonalcoholic)
Excludes2: *hallucinations and perceptual disturbance induced by alcohol and other psychoactive substances (F10-F19 with .151, .251, .951)*
schizophrenia (F20.-)
CC Exclusion see Appendix A PDX collection 0550

F06.1 Catatonic disorder due to known physiological condition
Catatonia associated with another mental disorder
Catatonia NOS
Excludes1: *catatonic stupor (R40.1)*
stupor NOS (R40.1)
Excludes2: *catatonic schizophrenia (F20.2)*
dissociative stupor (F44.2)

CC **F06.2 Psychotic disorder with delusions due to known physiological condition**
Paranoid and paranoid-hallucinatory organic states
Schizophrenia-like psychosis in epilepsy
Excludes2: *alcohol and drug-induced psychotic disorder (F10-F19 with .150, .250, .950)*
brief psychotic disorder (F23)
delusional disorder (F22)
schizophrenia (F20.-)
CC Exclusion see Appendix A PDX collection 0550

\+ **F06.3 Mood disorder due to known physiological condition**
Excludes2: *mood disorders due to alcohol and other psychoactive substances (F10-F19 with .14, .24, .94)*
mood disorders, not due to known physiological condition or unspecified (F30-F39)

F06.30 Mood disorder due to known physiological condition, unspecified

F06.31 Mood disorder due to known physiological condition with depressive features
Depressive disorder due to known physiological condition, with depressive features

F06.32 Mood disorder due to known physiological condition with major depressive-like episode
Depressive disorder due to known physiological condition, with major depressive-like episode

F06.33 Mood disorder due to known physiological condition with manic features
Bipolar and related disorder due to a known physiological condition, with manic features
Bipolar and related disorder due to known physiological condition, with manic- or hypomanic-like episodes

F06.34 Mood disorder due to known physiological condition with mixed features
Bipolar and related disorder due to known physiological condition, with mixed features
Depressive disorder due to known physiological condition, with mixed features

F06.4 Anxiety disorder due to known physiological condition
Excludes2: *anxiety disorders due to alcohol and other psychoactive substances (F10-F19 with .180, .280, .980)*
anxiety disorders, not due to known physiological condition or unspecified (F40.-, F41.-)

F06.8 Other specified mental disorders due to known physiological condition
Epileptic psychosis NOS
Obsessive-compulsive and related disorder due to a known physiological condition
Organic dissociative disorder
Organic emotionally labile [asthenic] disorder

F07 Personality and behavioral disorders due to known physiological condition

Code first the underlying physiological condition

F07.0 Personality change due to known physiological condition

Frontal lobe syndrome
Limbic epilepsy personality syndrome
Lobotomy syndrome
Organic personality disorder
Organic pseudopsychopathic personality
Organic pseudoretarded personality
Postleucotomy syndrome
Code first underlying physiological condition

Excludes1: *mild cognitive impairment (G31.84)*
postconcussional syndrome (F07.81)
postencephalitic syndrome (F07.89)
signs and symptoms involving emotional state (R45.-)

Excludes2: *specific personality disorder (F60.-)*

+ **F07.8 Other personality and behavioral disorders due to known physiological condition**

F07.81 Postconcussional syndrome

Postcontusional syndrome (encephalopathy)
Post-traumatic brain syndrome, nonpsychotic
Use additional code to identify associated post-traumatic headache, if applicable (G44.3-)

Excludes1: *current concussion (brain) (S06.0-)*
postencephalitic syndrome (F07.89)

F07.89 Other personality and behavioral disorders due to known physiological condition

Postencephalitic syndrome
Right hemispheric organic affective disorder

F07.9 Unspecified personality and behavioral disorder due to known physiological condition

Organic psychosyndrome

F09 Unspecified mental disorder due to known physiological condition

Mental disorder NOS due to known physiological condition
Organic brain syndrome NOS
Organic mental disorder NOS
Organic psychosis NOS
Symptomatic psychosis NOS
Code first the underlying physiological condition

Excludes1: *psychosis NOS (F29)*

Valid 3-character code, no further characters required

Mental and behavioral disorders due to psychoactive substance use (F10-F19)

Review coding guideline C.5.b

F10 Alcohol related disorders

Use additional code for blood alcohol level, if applicable (Y90.-)

+ **F10.1 Alcohol abuse**

Excludes1: *alcohol dependence (F10.2-)*
alcohol use, unspecified (F10.9-)

F10.10 Alcohol abuse, uncomplicated

Alcohol use disorder, mild

F10.11 Alcohol abuse, in remission

Alcohol use disorder, mild, in early remission
Alcohol use disorder, mild, in sustained remission

+ **F10.12 Alcohol abuse with intoxication**

F10.120 Alcohol abuse with intoxication, uncomplicated

CC **F10.121 Alcohol abuse with intoxication delirium**

CC Exclusion see Appendix A PDX collection 0550

F10.129 Alcohol abuse with intoxication, unspecified

CC **F10.14 Alcohol abuse with alcohol-induced mood disorder**

Alcohol use disorder, mild, with alcohol-induced bipolar or related disorder
Alcohol use disorder, mild, with alcohol-induced depressive disorder

CC Exclusion see Appendix A PDX collection 0550

+ **F10.15 Alcohol abuse with alcohol-induced psychotic disorder**

F10.150 Alcohol abuse with alcohol-induced psychotic disorder with delusions

CC **F10.151 Alcohol abuse with alcohol-induced psychotic disorder with hallucinations**

CC Exclusion see Appendix A PDX collection 0550

CC **F10.159 Alcohol abuse with alcohol-induced psychotic disorder, unspecified**

CC Exclusion see Appendix A PDX collection 0550

+ **F10.18 Alcohol abuse with other alcohol-induced disorders**

CC **F10.180 Alcohol abuse with alcohol-induced anxiety disorder**

CC Exclusion see Appendix A PDX collection 0550

CC **F10.181 Alcohol abuse with alcohol-induced sexual dysfunction**

CC Exclusion see Appendix A PDX collection 0550

F10.182 Alcohol abuse with alcohol-induced sleep disorder

CC **F10.188 Alcohol abuse with other alcohol-induced disorder**

CC Exclusion see Appendix A PDX collection 0550

CC **F10.19 Alcohol abuse with unspecified alcohol-induced disorder**

CC Exclusion see Appendix A PDX collection 0550

+ **F10.2 Alcohol dependence**

Excludes1: *alcohol abuse (F10.1-)*
alcohol use, unspecified (F10.9-)

Excludes2: *toxic effect of alcohol (T51.0-)*

F10.20 Alcohol dependence, uncomplicated

Alcohol use disorder, moderate
Alcohol use disorder, severe

F10.21 Alcohol dependence, in remission

Alcohol use disorder, moderate, in early remission
Alcohol use disorder, moderate, in sustained remission
Alcohol use disorder, severe, in early remission
Alcohol use disorder, severe, in sustained remission

+ **F10.22 Alcohol dependence with intoxication**

Acute drunkenness (in alcoholism)

Excludes2: *alcohol dependence with withdrawal (F10.23-)*

F10.220 Alcohol dependence with intoxication, uncomplicated

CC **F10.221 Alcohol dependence with intoxication delirium**

CC Exclusion see Appendix A PDX collection 0550

F10.229 Alcohol dependence with intoxication, unspecified

+ **F10.23 Alcohol dependence with withdrawal**

Excludes2: *Alcohol dependence with intoxication (F10.22-)*

CC **F10.230 Alcohol dependence with withdrawal, uncomplicated**

CC Exclusion see Appendix A PDX collection 0550

CC **F10.231 Alcohol dependence with withdrawal delirium**

CC Exclusion see Appendix A PDX collection 0550

CC **F10.232 Alcohol dependence with withdrawal with perceptual disturbance**

CC Exclusion see Appendix A PDX collection 0550

CC **F10.239 Alcohol dependence with withdrawal, unspecified**

CC Exclusion see Appendix A PDX collection 0550

CC **F10.24 Alcohol dependence with alcohol-induced mood disorder**

Alcohol use disorder, moderate, with alcohol-induced bipolar or related disorder
Alcohol use disorder, moderate, with alcohol-induced depressive disorder
Alcohol use disorder, severe, with alcohol-induced bipolar or related disorder
Alcohol use disorder, severe, with alcohol-induced depressive disorder

CC Exclusion see Appendix A PDX collection 0550

+ **F10.25 Alcohol dependence with alcohol-induced psychotic disorder**
F10.250 Alcohol dependence with alcohol-induced psychotic disorder with delusions
CC **F10.251 Alcohol dependence with alcohol-induced psychotic disorder with hallucinations**
CC Exclusion see Appendix A PDX collection 0550
CC **F10.259 Alcohol dependence with alcohol-induced psychotic disorder, unspecified**
CC Exclusion see Appendix A PDX collection 0550
F10.26 Alcohol dependence with alcohol-induced persisting amnestic disorder
Alcohol use disorder, moderate, with alcohol-induced major neurocognitive disorder, amnestic-confabulatory type
Alcohol use disorder, severe, with alcohol-induced major neurocognitive disorder, amnestic-confabulatory type
CC **F10.27 Alcohol dependence with alcohol-induced persisting dementia**
Alcohol use disorder, moderate, with alcohol-induced major neurocognitive disorder, nonamnestic-confabulatory type
Alcohol use disorder, severe, with alcohol-induced major neurocognitive disorder, nonamnestic-confabulatory type
CC Exclusion see Appendix A PDX collection 0550
+ **F10.28 Alcohol dependence with other alcohol-induced disorders**
CC **F10.280 Alcohol dependence with alcohol-induced anxiety disorder**
CC Exclusion see Appendix A PDX collection 0550
CC **F10.281 Alcohol dependence with alcohol-induced sexual dysfunction**
CC Exclusion see Appendix A PDX collection 0550
F10.282 Alcohol dependence with alcohol-induced sleep disorder
CC **F10.288 Alcohol dependence with other alcohol-induced disorder**
Alcohol use disorder, moderate, with alcohol-induced mild neurocognitive disorder
Alcohol use disorder, severe, with alcohol-induced mild neurocognitive disorder
CC Exclusion see Appendix A PDX collection 0550
CC **F10.29 Alcohol dependence with unspecified alcohol-induced disorder**
CC Exclusion see Appendix A PDX collection 0550
+ **F10.9 Alcohol use, unspecified**
Excludes1: *alcohol abuse (F10.1-)*
alcohol dependence (F10.2-)
+ **F10.92 Alcohol use, unspecified with intoxication**
F10.920 Alcohol use, unspecified with intoxication, uncomplicated
CC **F10.921 Alcohol use, unspecified with intoxication delirium**
CC Exclusion see Appendix A PDX collection 0550
F10.929 Alcohol use, unspecified with intoxication, unspecified
CC **F10.94 Alcohol use, unspecified with alcohol-induced mood disorder**
Alcohol-induced bipolar or related disorder, without use disorder
Alcohol-induced depressive disorder, without use disorder
CC Exclusion see Appendix A PDX collection 0550
+ **F10.95 Alcohol use, unspecified with alcohol-induced psychotic disorder**
F10.950 Alcohol use, unspecified with alcohol-induced psychotic disorder with delusions
CC **F10.951 Alcohol use, unspecified with alcohol-induced psychotic disorder with hallucinations**
CC Exclusion see Appendix A PDX collection 0550
CC **F10.959 Alcohol use, unspecified with alcohol-induced psychotic disorder, unspecified**
Alcohol-induced psychotic disorder without use disorder
CC Exclusion see Appendix A PDX collection 0550
F10.96 Alcohol use, unspecified with alcohol-induced persisting amnestic disorder
Alcohol-induced major neurocognitive disorder, amnestic-confabulatory type, without use disorder
F10.97 Alcohol use, unspecified with alcohol-induced persisting dementia
Alcohol-induced major neurocognitive disorder, nonamnestic-confabulatory type, without use disorder
+ **F10.98 Alcohol use, unspecified with other alcohol-induced disorders**
CC **F10.980 Alcohol use, unspecified with alcohol-induced anxiety disorder**
Alcohol-induced anxiety disorder, without use disorder
CC Exclusion see Appendix A PDX collection 0550
CC **F10.981 Alcohol use, unspecified with alcohol-induced sexual dysfunction**
Alcohol-induced sexual dysfunction, without use disorder
CC Exclusion see Appendix A PDX collection 0550
F10.982 Alcohol use, unspecified with alcohol-induced sleep disorder
Alcohol-induced sleep disorder, without use disorder
CC **F10.988 Alcohol use, unspecified with other alcohol-induced disorder**
Alcohol-induced mild neurocognitive disorder, without use disorder
CC Exclusion see Appendix A PDX collection 0550
CC **F10.99 Alcohol use, unspecified with unspecified alcohol-induced disorder**
CC Exclusion see Appendix A PDX collection 0550

F11 Opioid related disorders

+ **F11.1 Opioid abuse**
Excludes1: *opioid dependence (F11.2-)*
opioid use, unspecified (F11.9-)
F11.10 Opioid abuse, uncomplicated
Opioid use disorder, mild
F11.11 Opioid abuse, in remission
Opioid use disorder, mild, in early remission
Opioid use disorder, mild, in sustained remission
+ **F11.12 Opioid abuse with intoxication**
F11.120 Opioid abuse with intoxication, uncomplicated
CC **F11.121 Opioid abuse with intoxication delirium**
CC Exclusion see Appendix A PDX collection 0550
F11.122 Opioid abuse with intoxication with perceptual disturbance
F11.129 Opioid abuse with intoxication, unspecified
F11.14 Opioid abuse with opioid-induced mood disorder
Opioid use disorder, mild, with opioid-induced depressive disorder
+ **F11.15 Opioid abuse with opioid-induced psychotic disorder**
CC **F11.150 Opioid abuse with opioid-induced psychotic disorder with delusions**
CC Exclusion see Appendix A PDX collection 0550
CC **F11.151 Opioid abuse with opioid-induced psychotic disorder with hallucinations**
CC Exclusion see Appendix A PDX collection 0550
F11.159 Opioid abuse with opioid-induced psychotic disorder, unspecified

+ **F11.18 Opioid abuse with other opioid-induced disorder**
  - **F11.181 Opioid abuse with opioid-induced sexual dysfunction**
  - **F11.182 Opioid abuse with opioid-induced sleep disorder**
  - **F11.188 Opioid abuse with other opioid-induced disorder**
- **F11.19 Opioid abuse with unspecified opioid-induced disorder**

+ **F11.2 Opioid dependence**
  Excludes1: *opioid abuse (F11.1-)*
  opioid use, unspecified (F11.9-)
  Excludes2: *opioid poisoning (T40.0-T40.2-)*
- CC **F11.20 Opioid dependence, uncomplicated**
  Opioid use disorder, moderate
  Opioid use disorder, severe
  No CC Exclusions
- **F11.21 Opioid dependence, in remission**
  Opioid use disorder, moderate, in early remission
  Opioid use disorder, moderate, in sustained remission
  Opioid use disorder, severe, in early remission
  Opioid use disorder, severe, in sustained remission
+ **F11.22 Opioid dependence with intoxication**
  Excludes1: *opioid dependence with withdrawal (F11.23)*
  - **F11.220 Opioid dependence with intoxication, uncomplicated**
  - CC **F11.221 Opioid dependence with intoxication delirium**
    CC Exclusion see Appendix A PDX collection 0550
  - CC **F11.222 Opioid dependence with intoxication with perceptual disturbance**
    No CC Exclusions
  - **F11.229 Opioid dependence with intoxication, unspecified**
- CC **F11.23 Opioid dependence with withdrawal**
  Excludes1: *opioid dependence with intoxication (F11.22-)*
  CC Exclusion see Appendix A PDX collection 0550
- **F11.24 Opioid dependence with opioid-induced mood disorder**
  Opioid use disorder, moderate, with opioid-induced depressive disorder
+ **F11.25 Opioid dependence with opioid-induced psychotic disorder**
  - CC **F11.250 Opioid dependence with opioid-induced psychotic disorder with delusions**
    CC Exclusion see Appendix A PDX collection 0550
  - CC **F11.251 Opioid dependence with opioid-induced psychotic disorder with hallucinations**
    CC Exclusion see Appendix A PDX collection 0550
  - CC **F11.259 Opioid dependence with opioid-induced psychotic disorder, unspecified**
    No CC Exclusions
+ **F11.28 Opioid dependence with other opioid-induced disorder**
  - CC **F11.281 Opioid dependence with opioid-induced sexual dysfunction**
    No CC Exclusions
  - CC **F11.282 Opioid dependence with opioid-induced sleep disorder**
    No CC Exclusions
  - CC **F11.288 Opioid dependence with other opioid-induced disorder**
    No CC Exclusions
- **F11.29 Opioid dependence with unspecified opioid-induced disorder**

+ **F11.9 Opioid use, unspecified**
  Excludes1: *opioid abuse (F11.1-)*
  opioid dependence (F11.2-)
- **F11.90 Opioid use, unspecified, uncomplicated**
+ **F11.92 Opioid use, unspecified with intoxication**
  Excludes1: *opioid use, unspecified with withdrawal (F11.93)*
  - **F11.920 Opioid use, unspecified with intoxication, uncomplicated**
  - CC **F11.921 Opioid use, unspecified with intoxication delirium**
    Opioid use delirium
    CC Exclusion see Appendix A PDX collection 0550
  - **F11.922 Opioid use, unspecified with intoxication with perceptual disturbance**
  - **F11.929 Opioid use, unspecified with intoxication unspecified**
- CC **F11.93 Opioid use, unspecified with withdrawal**
  Excludes1: *opioid use, unspecified with intoxication (F11.92-)*
  CC Exclusion see Appendix A PDX collection 0550
- **F11.94 Opioid use, unspecified with opioid-induced mood disorder**
  Opioid-induced depressive disorder, without use disorder
+ **F11.95 Opioid use, unspecified with opioid-induced psychotic disorder**
  - CC **F11.950 Opioid use, unspecified with opioid-induced psychotic disorder with delusions**
    CC Exclusion see Appendix A PDX collection 0550
  - CC **F11.951 Opioid use, unspecified with opioid-induced psychotic disorder with hallucinations**
    CC Exclusion see Appendix A PDX collection 0550
  - **F11.959 Opioid use, unspecified with opioid-induced psychotic disorder, unspecified**
+ **F11.98 Opioid use, unspecified with other specified opioid-induced disorder**
  - **F11.981 Opioid use, unspecified with opioid-induced sexual dysfunction**
    Opioid-induced sexual dysfunction, without use disorder
  - **F11.982 Opioid use, unspecified with opioid-induced sleep disorder**
    Opioid-induced sleep disorder, without use disorder
  - **F11.988 Opioid use, unspecified with other opioid-induced disorder**
    Opioid-induced anxiety disorder, without use disorder
- **F11.99 Opioid use, unspecified with unspecified opioid-induced disorder**

F12 Cannabis related disorders

Includes: marijuana

+ **F12.1 Cannabis abuse**
  Excludes1: *cannabis dependence (F12.2-)*
  cannabis use, unspecified (F12.9-)
- **F12.10 Cannabis abuse, uncomplicated**
  Cannabis use disorder, mild
- **F12.11 Cannabis abuse, in remission**
  Cannabis use disorder, mild, in early remission
  Cannabis use disorder, mild, in sustained remission
+ **F12.12 Cannabis abuse with intoxication**
  - **F12.120 Cannabis abuse with intoxication, uncomplicated**
  - CC **F12.121 Cannabis abuse with intoxication delirium**
    CC Exclusion see Appendix A PDX collection 0550
  - **F12.122 Cannabis abuse with intoxication with perceptual disturbance**
  - **F12.129 Cannabis abuse with intoxication, unspecified**
+ **F12.15 Cannabis abuse with psychotic disorder**
  - CC **F12.150 Cannabis abuse with psychotic disorder with delusions**
    CC Exclusion see Appendix A PDX collection 0550
  - CC **F12.151 Cannabis abuse with psychotic disorder with hallucinations**
    CC Exclusion see Appendix A PDX collection 0550
  - **F12.159 Cannabis abuse with psychotic disorder, unspecified**

+ F12.18 **Cannabis abuse with other cannabis-induced disorder**
F12.180 **Cannabis abuse with cannabis-induced anxiety disorder**
F12.188 **Cannabis abuse with other cannabis-induced disorder**
Cannabis use disorder, mild, with cannabis-induced sleep disorder
F12.19 **Cannabis abuse with unspecified cannabis-induced disorder**
+ F12.2 **Cannabis dependence**
Excludes1: *cannabis abuse (F12.1-)*
cannabis use, unspecified (F12.9-)
Excludes2: *cannabis poisoning (T40.7-)*
F12.20 **Cannabis dependence, uncomplicated**
Cannabis use disorder, moderate
Cannabis use disorder, severe
F12.21 **Cannabis dependence, in remission**
Cannabis use disorder, moderate, in early remission
Cannabis use disorder, moderate, in sustained remission
Cannabis use disorder, severe, in early remission
Cannabis use disorder, severe, in sustained remission
+ F12.22 **Cannabis dependence with intoxication**
F12.220 **Cannabis dependence with intoxication, uncomplicated**
CC F12.221 **Cannabis dependence with intoxication delirium**
CC Exclusion see Appendix A PDX collection 0550
F12.222 **Cannabis dependence with intoxication with perceptual disturbance**
F12.229 **Cannabis dependence with intoxication, unspecified**
+ F12.25 **Cannabis dependence with psychotic disorder**
CC F12.250 **Cannabis dependence with psychotic disorder with delusions**
CC Exclusion see Appendix A PDX collection 0550
CC F12.251 **Cannabis dependence with psychotic disorder with hallucinations**
CC Exclusion see Appendix A PDX collection 0550
F12.259 **Cannabis dependence with psychotic disorder, unspecified**
+ F12.28 **Cannabis dependence with other cannabis-induced disorder**
F12.280 **Cannabis dependence with cannabis-induced anxiety disorder**
F12.288 **Cannabis dependence with other cannabis-induced disorder**
Cannabis use disorder, moderate, with cannabis-induced sleep disorder
Cannabis use disorder, severe, with cannabis-induced sleep disorder
Cannabis withdrawal
F12.29 **Cannabis dependence with unspecified cannabis-induced disorder**
+ F12.9 **Cannabis use, unspecified**
Excludes1: *cannabis abuse (F12.1-)*
cannabis dependence (F12.2-)
F12.90 **Cannabis use, unspecified, uncomplicated**
+ F12.92 **Cannabis use, unspecified with intoxication**
F12.920 **Cannabis use, unspecified with intoxication, uncomplicated**
CC F12.921 **Cannabis use, unspecified with intoxication delirium**
CC Exclusion see Appendix A PDX collection 0550
F12.922 **Cannabis use, unspecified with intoxication with perceptual disturbance**
F12.929 **Cannabis use, unspecified with intoxication, unspecified**
+ F12.95 **Cannabis use, unspecified with psychotic disorder**
CC F12.950 **Cannabis use, unspecified with psychotic disorder with delusions**
CC Exclusion see Appendix A PDX collection 0550
CC F12.951 **Cannabis use, unspecified with psychotic disorder with hallucinations**
CC Exclusion see Appendix A PDX collection 0550
F12.959 **Cannabis use, unspecified with psychotic disorder, unspecified**
Cannabis-induced psychotic disorder, without use disorder
+ F12.98 **Cannabis use, unspecified with other cannabis-induced disorder**
F12.980 **Cannabis use, unspecified with anxiety disorder**
Cannabis-induced anxiety disorder, without use disorder
F12.988 **Cannabis use, unspecified with other cannabis-induced disorder**
Cannabis-induced sleep disorder, without use disorder
F12.99 **Cannabis use, unspecified with unspecified cannabis-induced disorder**

F13 Sedative, hypnotic, or anxiolytic related disorders

+ F13.1 **Sedative, hypnotic or anxiolytic-related abuse**
Excludes1: *sedative, hypnotic or anxiolytic-related dependence (F13.2-)*
sedative, hypnotic, or anxiolytic use, unspecified (F13.9-)
F13.10 **Sedative, hypnotic or anxiolytic abuse, uncomplicated**
Sedative, hypnotic, or anxiolytic use disorder, mild
F13.11 **Sedative, hypnotic or anxiolytic abuse, in remission**
Sedative, hypnotic or anxiolytic use disorder, mild, in early remission
Sedative, hypnotic or anxiolytic use disorder, mild, in sustained remission
+ F13.12 **Sedative, hypnotic or anxiolytic abuse with intoxication**
F13.120 **Sedative, hypnotic or anxiolytic abuse with intoxication, uncomplicated**
CC F13.121 **Sedative, hypnotic or anxiolytic abuse with intoxication delirium**
CC Exclusion see Appendix A PDX collection 0550
F13.129 **Sedative, hypnotic or anxiolytic abuse with intoxication, unspecified**
F13.14 **Sedative, hypnotic or anxiolytic abuse with sedative, hypnotic or anxiolytic-induced mood disorder**
Sedative, hypnotic, or anxiolytic use disorder, mild, with sedative, hypnotic, or anxiolytic-induced bipolar or related disorder
Sedative, hypnotic, or anxiolytic use disorder, mild, with sedative, hypnotic, or anxiolytic-induced depressive disorder
+ F13.15 **Sedative, hypnotic or anxiolytic abuse with sedative, hypnotic or anxiolytic-induced psychotic disorder**
CC F13.150 **Sedative, hypnotic or anxiolytic abuse with sedative, hypnotic or anxiolytic-induced psychotic disorder with delusions**
CC Exclusion see Appendix A PDX collection 0550
CC F13.151 **Sedative, hypnotic or anxiolytic abuse with sedative, hypnotic or anxiolytic-induced psychotic disorder with hallucinations**
CC Exclusion see Appendix A PDX collection 0550
F13.159 **Sedative, hypnotic or anxiolytic abuse with sedative, hypnotic or anxiolytic-induced psychotic disorder, unspecified**
+ F13.18 **Sedative, hypnotic or anxiolytic abuse with other sedative, hypnotic or anxiolytic-induced disorders**
F13.180 **Sedative, hypnotic or anxiolytic abuse with sedative, hypnotic or anxiolytic-induced anxiety disorder**
F13.181 **Sedative, hypnotic or anxiolytic abuse with sedative, hypnotic or anxiolytic-induced sexual dysfunction**
F13.182 **Sedative, hypnotic or anxiolytic abuse with sedative, hypnotic or anxiolytic-induced sleep disorder**
F13.188 **Sedative, hypnotic or anxiolytic abuse with other sedative, hypnotic or anxiolytic-induced disorder**
F13.19 **Sedative, hypnotic or anxiolytic abuse with unspecified sedative, hypnotic or anxiolytic-induced disorder**

+ F13.2 Sedative, hypnotic or anxiolytic-related dependence
Excludes1: *sedative, hypnotic or anxiolytic-related abuse (F13.1-)*
sedative, hypnotic, or anxiolytic use, unspecified (F13.9-)
Excludes2: *sedative, hypnotic, or anxiolytic poisoning (T42.-)*

CC **F13.20 Sedative, hypnotic or anxiolytic dependence, uncomplicated**
No CC Exclusions

F13.21 Sedative, hypnotic or anxiolytic dependence, in remission
Sedative, hypnotic or anxiolytic use disorder, moderate, in early remission
Sedative, hypnotic or anxiolytic use disorder, moderate, in sustained remission
Sedative, hypnotic or anxiolytic use disorder, severe, in early remission
Sedative, hypnotic or anxiolytic use disorder, severe, in sustained remission

+ F13.22 Sedative, hypnotic or anxiolytic dependence with intoxication
Excludes1: *sedative, hypnotic or anxiolytic dependencewithwithdrawal(F13.23-)*

F13.220 Sedative, hypnotic or anxiolytic dependence with intoxication, uncomplicated

CC **F13.221 Sedative, hypnotic or anxiolytic dependence with intoxication delirium**
CC Exclusion see Appendix A PDX collection 0550

F13.229 Sedative, hypnotic or anxiolytic dependence with intoxication, unspecified

+ F13.23 Sedative, hypnotic or anxiolytic dependence with withdrawal
Sedative, hypnotic, or anxiolytic use disorder, moderate
Sedative, hypnotic, or anxiolytic use disorder, severe
Excludes1: *sedative, hypnotic or anxiolytic dependencewithintoxication(F13.22-)*

CC **F13.230 Sedative, hypnotic or anxiolytic dependence with withdrawal, uncomplicated**
CC Exclusion see Appendix A PDX collection 0550

CC **F13.231 Sedative, hypnotic or anxiolytic dependence with withdrawal delirium**
CC Exclusion see Appendix A PDX collection 0550

CC **F13.232 Sedative, hypnotic or anxiolytic dependence with withdrawal with perceptual disturbance**
Sedative, hypnotic, or anxiolytic withdrawal with perceptual disturbances
CC Exclusion see Appendix A PDX collection 0550

CC **F13.239 Sedative, hypnotic or anxiolytic dependence with withdrawal, unspecified**
Sedative, hypnotic, or anxiolytic withdrawal without perceptual disturbances
CC Exclusion see Appendix A PDX collection 0550

F13.24 Sedative, hypnotic or anxiolytic dependence with sedative, hypnotic or anxiolytic-induced mood disorder
Sedative, hypnotic, or anxiolytic use disorder, moderate, with sedative, hypnotic, or anxiolytic-induced bipolar or related disorder
Sedative, hypnotic, or anxiolytic use disorder, moderate, with sedative, hypnotic, or anxiolytic-induced depressive disorder
Sedative, hypnotic, or anxiolytic use disorder, severe, with sedative, hypnotic, or anxiolytic-induced bipolar or related disorder
Sedative, hypnotic, or anxiolytic use disorder, severe, with sedative, hypnotic, or anxiolytic-induced depressive disorder

+ F13.25 Sedative, hypnotic or anxiolytic dependence with sedative, hypnotic or anxiolytic-induced psychotic disorder

CC **F13.250 Sedative, hypnotic or anxiolytic dependence with sedative, hypnotic or anxiolytic-induced psychotic disorder with delusions**
CC Exclusion see Appendix A PDX collection 0550

CC **F13.251 Sedative, hypnotic or anxiolytic dependence with sedative, hypnotic or anxiolytic-induced psychotic disorder with hallucinations**
CC Exclusion see Appendix A PDX collection 0550

CC **F13.259 Sedative, hypnotic or anxiolytic dependence with sedative, hypnotic or anxiolytic-induced psychotic disorder, unspecified**
No CC Exclusions

CC **F13.26 Sedative, hypnotic or anxiolytic dependence with sedative, hypnotic or anxiolytic-induced persisting amnestic disorder**
No CC Exclusions

CC **F13.27 Sedative, hypnotic or anxiolytic dependence with sedative, hypnotic or anxiolytic-induced persisting dementia**
Sedative, hypnotic, or anxiolytic use disorder, moderate, with sedative, hypnotic, or anxiolytic-induced major neurocognitive disorder
Sedative, hypnotic, or anxiolytic use disorder, severe, with sedative, hypnotic, or anxiolytic-induced major neurocognitive disorder
CC Exclusion see Appendix A PDX collection 0550

+ F13.28 Sedative, hypnotic or anxiolytic dependence with other sedative, hypnotic or anxiolytic-induced disorders

CC **F13.280 Sedative, hypnotic or anxiolytic dependence with sedative, hypnotic or anxiolytic-induced anxiety disorder**
No CC Exclusions

CC **F13.281 Sedative, hypnotic or anxiolytic dependence with sedative, hypnotic or anxiolytic-induced sexual dysfunction**
No CC Exclusions

CC **F13.282 Sedative, hypnotic or anxiolytic dependence with sedative, hypnotic or anxiolytic-induced sleep disorder**
No CC Exclusions

CC **F13.288 Sedative, hypnotic or anxiolytic dependence with other sedative, hypnotic or anxiolytic-induced disorder**
Sedative, hypnotic, or anxiolytic use disorder, moderate, with sedative, hypnotic, or anxiolytic-induced mild neurocognitive disorder
Sedative, hypnotic, or anxiolytic use disorder, severe, with sedative, hypnotic, or anxiolytic-induced mild neurocognitive disorder
No CC Exclusions

F13.29 Sedative, hypnotic or anxiolytic dependence with unspecified sedative, hypnotic or anxiolytic-induced disorder

+ F13.9 Sedative, hypnotic or anxiolytic-related use, unspecified
Excludes1: *sedative, hypnotic or anxiolytic-related abuse (F13.1-)*
sedative, hypnotic or anxiolytic-related dependence (F13.2-)

F13.90 Sedative, hypnotic, or anxiolytic use, unspecified, uncomplicated

+ F13.92 Sedative, hypnotic or anxiolytic use, unspecified with intoxication
Excludes1: *sedative, hypnotic or anxiolytic use, unspecified with withdrawal (F13.93-)*

F13.920 Sedative, hypnotic or anxiolytic use, unspecified with intoxication, uncomplicated

CC **F13.921 Sedative, hypnotic or anxiolytic use, unspecified with intoxication delirium**
Sedative, hypnotic, or anxiolytic-induced delirium
CC Exclusion see Appendix A PDX collection 0550

F13.929 Sedative, hypnotic or anxiolytic use, unspecified with intoxication, unspecified

+ **F13.93 Sedative, hypnotic or anxiolytic use, unspecified with withdrawal**
Excludes1: *sedative, hypnotic or anxiolytic use, unspecifiedwithintoxication(F13.92-)*

CC **F13.930 Sedative, hypnotic or anxiolytic use, unspecified with withdrawal, uncomplicated**
CC Exclusion see Appendix A PDX collection 0550

CC **F13.931 Sedative, hypnotic or anxiolytic use, unspecified with withdrawal delirium**
CC Exclusion see Appendix A PDX collection 0550

CC **F13.932 Sedative, hypnotic or anxiolytic use, unspecified with withdrawal with perceptual disturbances**
CC Exclusion see Appendix A PDX collection 0550

CC **F13.939 Sedative, hypnotic or anxiolytic use, unspecified with withdrawal, unspecified**
CC Exclusion see Appendix A PDX collection 0550

F13.94 Sedative, hypnotic or anxiolytic use, unspecified with sedative, hypnotic or anxiolytic-induced mood disorder
Sedative, hypnotic, or anxiolytic-induced bipolar or related disorder, without use disorder
Sedative, hypnotic, or anxiolytic-induced depressive disorder, without use disorder

+ **F13.95 Sedative, hypnotic or anxiolytic use, unspecified with sedative, hypnotic or anxiolytic-induced psychotic disorder**

CC **F13.950 Sedative, hypnotic or anxiolytic use, unspecified with sedative, hypnotic or anxiolytic-induced psychotic disorder with delusions**
CC Exclusion see Appendix A PDX collection 0550

CC **F13.951 Sedative, hypnotic or anxiolytic use, unspecified with sedative, hypnotic or anxiolytic-induced psychotic disorder with hallucinations**
CC Exclusion see Appendix A PDX collection 0550

F13.959 Sedative, hypnotic or anxiolytic use, unspecified with sedative, hypnotic or anxiolytic-induced psychotic disorder, unspecified
Sedative, hypnotic, or anxiolytic-induced psychotic disorder, without use disorder

F13.96 Sedative, hypnotic or anxiolytic use, unspecified with sedative, hypnotic or anxiolytic-induced persisting amnestic disorder

CC **F13.97 Sedative, hypnotic or anxiolytic use, unspecified with sedative, hypnotic or anxiolytic-induced persisting dementia**
Sedative, hypnotic, or anxiolytic-induced major neurocognitive disorder, without use disorder
CC Exclusion see Appendix A PDX collection 0550

+ **F13.98 Sedative, hypnotic or anxiolytic use, unspecified with other sedative, hypnotic or anxiolytic-induced disorders**

F13.980 Sedative, hypnotic or anxiolytic use, unspecified with sedative, hypnotic or anxiolytic-induced anxiety disorder
Sedative, hypnotic, or anxiolytic-induced anxiety disorder, without use disorder

F13.981 Sedative, hypnotic or anxiolytic use, unspecified with sedative, hypnotic or anxiolytic-induced sexual dysfunction
Sedative, hypnotic, or anxiolytic-induced sexual dysfunction, without use disorder

F13.982 Sedative, hypnotic or anxiolytic use, unspecified with sedative, hypnotic or anxiolytic-induced sleep disorder
Sedative, hypnotic, or anxiolytic-induced sleep, without use disorder

F13.988 Sedative, hypnotic or anxiolytic use, unspecified with other sedative, hypnotic or anxiolytic-induced disorder
Sedative, hypnotic, or anxiolytic-induced mild neurocognitive disorder

F13.99 Sedative, hypnotic or anxiolytic use, unspecified with unspecified sedative, hypnotic or anxiolytic-induced disorder

F14 Cocaine related disorders

Excludes2: *other stimulant-related disorders (F15.-)*

+ **F14.1 Cocaine abuse**
Excludes1: *cocaine dependence (F14.2-)*
cocaine use, unspecified (F14.9-)

F14.10 Cocaine abuse, uncomplicated
Cocaine use disorder, mild

F14.11 Cocaine abuse, in remission
Cocaine use disorder, mild, in early remission
Cocaine use disorder, mild, in sustained remission

+ **F14.12 Cocaine abuse with intoxication**

F14.120 Cocaine abuse with intoxication, uncomplicated

CC **F14.121 Cocaine abuse with intoxication with delirium**
CC Exclusion see Appendix A PDX collection 0550

F14.122 Cocaine abuse with intoxication with perceptual disturbance

F14.129 Cocaine abuse with intoxication, unspecified

F14.14 Cocaine abuse with cocaine-induced mood disorder
Cocaine use disorder, mild, with cocaine-induced bipolar or related disorder
Cocaine use disorder, mild, with cocaine-induced depressive disorder

+ **F14.15 Cocaine abuse with cocaine-induced psychotic disorder**

CC **F14.150 Cocaine abuse with cocaine-induced psychotic disorder with delusions**
CC Exclusion see Appendix A PDX collection 0550

CC **F14.151 Cocaine abuse with cocaine-induced psychotic disorder with hallucinations**
CC Exclusion see Appendix A PDX collection 0550

F14.159 Cocaine abuse with cocaine-induced psychotic disorder, unspecified

+ **F14.18 Cocaine abuse with other cocaine-induced disorder**

F14.180 Cocaine abuse with cocaine-induced anxiety disorder

F14.181 Cocaine abuse with cocaine-induced sexual dysfunction

F14.182 Cocaine abuse with cocaine-induced sleep disorder

F14.188 Cocaine abuse with other cocaine-induced disorder
Cocaine use disorder, mild, with cocaine-induced obsessive compulsive or related disorder

F14.19 Cocaine abuse with unspecified cocaine-induced disorder

+ **F14.2 Cocaine dependence**
Excludes1: *cocaine abuse (F14.1-)*
cocaine use, unspecified (F14.9-)
Excludes2: *cocaine poisoning (T40.5-)*

CC **F14.20 Cocaine dependence, uncomplicated**
Cocaine use disorder, moderate
Cocaine use disorder, severe
No CC Exclusions

F14.21 Cocaine dependence, in remission
Cocaine use disorder, moderate, in early remission
Cocaine use disorder, moderate, in sustained remission
Cocaine use disorder, severe, in early remission
Cocaine use disorder, severe, in sustained remission
AHA CC: 2Q, 2017, 26-28

+ **F14.22 Cocaine dependence with intoxication**
  Excludes1: cocaine dependence with withdrawal (F14.23)
  F14.220 Cocaine dependence with intoxication, uncomplicated
  CC **F14.221 Cocaine dependence with intoxication delirium**
  CC Exclusion see Appendix A PDX collection 0550
  CC **F14.222 Cocaine dependence with intoxication with perceptual disturbance**
  No CC Exclusions
  CC **F14.229 Cocaine dependence with intoxication, unspecified**
  No CC Exclusions

CC **F14.23 Cocaine dependence with withdrawal**
  Excludes1: cocaine dependence with intoxication (F14.22-)
  CC Exclusion see Appendix A PDX collection 0550

F14.24 Cocaine dependence with cocaine-induced mood disorder
  Cocaine use disorder, moderate, with cocaine-induced bipolar or related disorder
  Cocaine use disorder, moderate, with cocaine-induced depressive disorder
  Cocaine use disorder, severe, with cocaine-induced bipolar or related disorder
  Cocaine use disorder, severe, with cocaine-induced depressive disorder

+ **F14.25 Cocaine dependence with cocaine-induced psychotic disorder**
  CC **F14.250 Cocaine dependence with cocaine-induced psychotic disorder with delusions**
  CC Exclusion see Appendix A PDX collection 0550
  CC **F14.251 Cocaine dependence with cocaine-induced psychotic disorder with hallucinations**
  CC Exclusion see Appendix A PDX collection 0550
  CC **F14.259 Cocaine dependence with cocaine-induced psychotic disorder, unspecified**
  No CC Exclusions

+ **F14.28 Cocaine dependence with other cocaine-induced disorder**
  CC **F14.280 Cocaine dependence with cocaine-induced anxiety disorder**
  No CC Exclusions
  CC **F14.281 Cocaine dependence with cocaine-induced sexual dysfunction**
  No CC Exclusions
  CC **F14.282 Cocaine dependence with cocaine-induced sleep disorder**
  No CC Exclusions
  CC **F14.288 Cocaine dependence with other cocaine-induced disorder**
  Cocaine use disorder, moderate, with cocaine-induced obsessive compulsive or related disorder
  Cocaine use disorder, severe, with cocaine-induced obsessive compulsive or related disorder
  No CC Exclusions

F14.29 Cocaine dependence with unspecified cocaine-induced disorder

+ **F14.9 Cocaine use, unspecified**
  Excludes1: cocaine abuse (F14.1-)
  cocaine dependence (F14.2-)

F14.90 Cocaine use, unspecified, uncomplicated

+ **F14.92 Cocaine use, unspecified with intoxication**
  F14.920 Cocaine use, unspecified with intoxication, uncomplicated
  CC **F14.921 Cocaine use, unspecified with intoxication delirium**
  CC Exclusion see Appendix A PDX collection 0550
  F14.922 Cocaine use, unspecified with intoxication with perceptual disturbance
  F14.929 Cocaine use, unspecified with intoxication, unspecified

F14.94 Cocaine use, unspecified with cocaine-induced mood disorder
  Cocaine-induced bipolar or related disorder, without use disorder
  Cocaine-induced depressive disorder, without use disorder

+ **F14.95 Cocaine use, unspecified with cocaine-induced psychotic disorder**
  CC **F14.950 Cocaine use, unspecified with cocaine-induced psychotic disorder with delusions**
  CC Exclusion see Appendix A PDX collection 0550
  CC **F14.951 Cocaine use, unspecified with cocaine-induced psychotic disorder with hallucinations**
  CC Exclusion see Appendix A PDX collection 0550
  F14.959 Cocaine use, unspecified with cocaine-induced psychotic disorder, unspecified
  Cocaine-induced psychotic disorder, without use disorder

+ **F14.98 Cocaine use, unspecified with other specified cocaine-induced disorder**
  F14.980 Cocaine use, unspecified with cocaine-induced anxiety disorder
  Cocaine-induced anxiety disorder, without use disorder
  F14.981 Cocaine use, unspecified with cocaine-induced sexual dysfunction
  Cocaine-induced sexual dysfunction, without use disorder
  F14.982 Cocaine use, unspecified with cocaine-induced sleep disorder
  Cocaine-induced sleep disorder, without use disorder
  F14.988 Cocaine use, unspecified with other cocaine-induced disorder
  Cocaine-induced obsessive compulsive or related disorder

F14.99 Cocaine use, unspecified with unspecified cocaine-induced disorder

F15 Other stimulant related disorders

Includes: amphetamine-related disorders
caffeine
Excludes2: *cocaine-related disorders (F14.-)*

+ **F15.1 Other stimulant abuse**
  Excludes1: other stimulant dependence (F15.2-)
  other stimulant use, unspecified (F15.9-)

F15.10 Other stimulant abuse, uncomplicated
  Amphetamine type substance use disorder, mild
  Other or unspecified stimulant use disorder, mild

F15.11 Other stimulant abuse, in remission
  Amphetamine type substance use disorder, mild, in early remission
  Amphetamine type substance use disorder, mild, in sustained remission
  Other or unspecified stimulant use disorder, mild, in early remission
  Other or unspecified stimulant use disorder, mild, in sustained remission

+ **F15.12 Other stimulant abuse with intoxication**
  F15.120 Other stimulant abuse with intoxication, uncomplicated
  CC **F15.121 Other stimulant abuse with intoxication delirium**
  CC Exclusion see Appendix A PDX collection 0550
  F15.122 Other stimulant abuse with intoxication with perceptual disturbance
  Amphetamine or other stimulant use disorder, mild, with amphetamine or other stimulant intoxication, with perceptual disturbances
  F15.129 Other stimulant abuse with intoxication, unspecified
  Amphetamine or other stimulant use disorder, mild, with amphetamine or other stimulant intoxication, without perceptual disturbances

F15.14 Other stimulant abuse with stimulant-induced mood disorder
Amphetamine or other stimulant use disorder, mild, with amphetamine or other stimulant-induced bipolar or related disorder
Amphetamine or other stimulant use disorder, mild, with amphetamine or other stimulant-induced depressive disorder

+ **F15.15 Other stimulant abuse with stimulant-induced psychotic disorder**

CC **F15.150 Other stimulant abuse with stimulant-induced psychotic disorder with delusions**
CC Exclusion see Appendix A PDX collection 0550

CC **F15.151 Other stimulant abuse with stimulant-induced psychotic disorder with hallucinations**
CC Exclusion see Appendix A PDX collection 0550

F15.159 Other stimulant abuse with stimulant-induced psychotic disorder, unspecified

+ **F15.18 Other stimulant abuse with other stimulant-induced disorder**

F15.180 Other stimulant abuse with stimulant-induced anxiety disorder

F15.181 Other stimulant abuse with stimulant-induced sexual dysfunction

F15.182 Other stimulant abuse with stimulant-induced sleep disorder

F15.188 Other stimulant abuse with other stimulant-induced disorder
Amphetamine or other stimulant use disorder, mild, with amphetamine or other stimulant-induced obsessive-compulsive or related disorder

F15.19 Other stimulant abuse with unspecified stimulant-induced disorder

+ **F15.2 Other stimulant dependence**
Excludes1: *other stimulant abuse (F15.1-)*
other stimulant use, unspecified (F15.9-)

CC **F15.20 Other stimulant dependence, uncomplicated**
Amphetamine type substance use disorder, moderate
Amphetamine type substance use disorder, severe
Other or unspecified stimulant use disorder, moderate
Other or unspecified stimulant use disorder, severe
No CC Exclusions

F15.21 Other stimulant dependence, in remission
Amphetamine type substance use disorder, moderate, in early remission
Amphetamine type substance use disorder, moderate, in sustained remission
Amphetamine type substance use disorder, severe, in early remission
Amphetamine type substance use disorder, severe, in sustained remission
Other or unspecified stimulant use disorder, moderate, in early remission
Other or unspecified stimulant use disorder, moderate, in sustained remission
Other or unspecified stimulant use disorder, severe, in early remission
Other or unspecified stimulant use disorder, severe, in sustained remission

+ **F15.22 Other stimulant dependence with intoxication**
Excludes1: *other stimulant dependence with withdrawal (F15.23)*

F15.220 Other stimulant dependence with intoxication, uncomplicated

CC **F15.221 Other stimulant dependence with intoxication delirium**
CC Exclusion see Appendix A PDX collection 0550

CC **F15.222 Other stimulant dependence with intoxication with perceptual disturbance**
Amphetamine or other stimulant use disorder, moderate, with amphetamine or other stimulant intoxication, with perceptual disturbances
Amphetamine or other stimulant use disorder, severe, with amphetamine or other stimulant intoxication, with perceptual disturbances
No CC Exclusions

F15.229 Other stimulant dependence with intoxication, unspecified
Amphetamine or other stimulant use disorder, moderate, with amphetamine or other stimulant intoxication, without perceptual disturbances
Amphetamine or other stimulant use disorder, severe, with amphetamine or other stimulant intoxication, without perceptual disturbances

CC **F15.23 Other stimulant dependence with withdrawal**
Amphetamine or other stimulant withdrawal
Excludes1: *other stimulant dependence with intoxication (F15.22-)*
CC Exclusion see Appendix A PDX collection 0550

F15.24 Other stimulant dependence with stimulant-induced mood disorder
Amphetamine or other stimulant use disorder, moderate, with amphetamine or other stimulant-induced bipolar or related disorder
Amphetamine or other stimulant use disorder, moderate, with amphetamine or other stimulant-induced depressive disorder
Amphetamine or other stimulant use disorder, severe, with amphetamine or other stimulant-induced bipolar or related disorder
Amphetamine or other stimulant use disorder, severe, with amphetamine or other stimulant-induced depressive disorder

+ **F15.25 Other stimulant dependence with stimulant-induced psychotic disorder**

CC **F15.250 Other stimulant dependence with stimulant-induced psychotic disorder with delusions**
CC Exclusion see Appendix A PDX collection 0550

CC **F15.251 Other stimulant dependence with stimulant-induced psychotic disorder with hallucinations**
CC Exclusion see Appendix A PDX collection 0550

CC **F15.259 Other stimulant dependence with stimulant-induced psychotic disorder, unspecified**
No CC Exclusions

+ **F15.28 Other stimulant dependence with other stimulant-induced disorder**

CC **F15.280 Other stimulant dependence with stimulant-induced anxiety disorder**
No CC Exclusions

CC **F15.281 Other stimulant dependence with stimulant-induced sexual dysfunction**
No CC Exclusions

CC **F15.282 Other stimulant dependence with stimulant-induced sleep disorder**
No CC Exclusions

CC **F15.288 Other stimulant dependence with other stimulant-induced disorder**
Amphetamine or other stimulant use disorder, moderate, with amphetamine or other stimulant-induced obsessive-compulsive or related disorder
Amphetamine or other stimulant use disorder, severe, with amphetamine or other stimulant-induced obsessive-compulsive or related disorder
No CC Exclusions

F15.29 Other stimulant dependence with unspecified stimulant-induced disorder

+ F15.9 **Other stimulant use, unspecified**
Excludes1: *other stimulant abuse (F15.1-)*
other stimulant dependence (F15.2-)
F15.90 **Other stimulant use, unspecified, uncomplicated**
+ F15.92 **Other stimulant use, unspecified with intoxication**
Excludes1: *other stimulant use, unspecified with withdrawal (F15.93)*
F15.920 **Other stimulant use, unspecified with intoxication, uncomplicated**
CC F15.921 **Other stimulant use, unspecified with intoxication delirium**
Amphetamine or other stimulant-induced delirium
CC Exclusion see Appendix A PDX collection 0550
F15.922 **Other stimulant use, unspecified with intoxication with perceptual disturbance**
F15.929 **Other stimulant use, unspecified with intoxication, unspecified**
Caffeine intoxication
CC F15.93 **Other stimulant use, unspecified with withdrawal**
Caffeine withdrawal
Excludes1: *other stimulant use, unspecified with intoxication (F15.92-)*
CC Exclusion see Appendix A PDX collection 0550
F15.94 **Other stimulant use, unspecified with stimulant-induced mood disorder**
Amphetamine or other stimulant-induced bipolar or related disorder, without use disorder
Amphetamine or other stimulant-induced depressive disorder, without use disorder
+ F15.95 **Other stimulant use, unspecified with stimulant-induced psychotic disorder**
CC F15.950 **Other stimulant use, unspecified with stimulant-induced psychotic disorder with delusions**
CC Exclusion see Appendix A PDX collection 0550
CC F15.951 **Other stimulant use, unspecified with stimulant-induced psychotic disorder with hallucinations**
CC Exclusion see Appendix A PDX collection 0550
F15.959 **Other stimulant use, unspecified with stimulant-induced psychotic disorder, unspecified**
Amphetamine or other stimulant-induced psychotic disorder, without use disorder
+ F15.98 **Other stimulant use, unspecified with other stimulant-induced disorder**
F15.980 **Other stimulant use, unspecified with stimulant-induced anxiety disorder**
Amphetamine or other stimulant-induced anxiety disorder, without use disorder
Caffeine induced anxiety disorder, without use disorder
F15.981 **Other stimulant use, unspecified with stimulant-induced sexual dysfunction**
Amphetamine or other stimulant-induced sexual dysfunction, without use disorder
F15.982 **Other stimulant use, unspecified with stimulant-induced sleep disorder**
Amphetamine or other stimulant-induced sleep disorder, without use disorder
Caffeine induced sleep disorder, without use disorder
F15.988 **Other stimulant use, unspecified with other stimulant-induced disorder**
Amphetamine or other stimulant-induced obsessive-comppulsive or related disorder, without use disorder
F15.99 **Other stimulant use, unspecified with unspecified stimulant-induced disorder**

F16 Hallucinogen related disorders

Includes: ecstasy
PCP
phencyclidine
+ F16.1 **Hallucinogen abuse**
Excludes1: *hallucinogen dependence (F16.2-)*
hallucinogen use, unspecified (F16.9-)
F16.10 **Hallucinogen abuse, uncomplicated**
Other hallucinogen use disorder, mild
Phencyclidine use disorder, mild
F16.11 **Hallucinogen abuse, in remission**
Other hallucinogen use disorder, mild, in early remission
Other hallucinogen use disorder, mild, in sustained remission
Phencyclidine use disorder, mild, in early remission
Phencyclidine use disorder, mild, in sustained remission
+ F16.12 **Hallucinogen abuse with intoxication**
F16.120 **Hallucinogen abuse with intoxication, uncomplicated**
CC F16.121 **Hallucinogen abuse with intoxication with delirium**
CC Exclusion see Appendix A PDX collection 0550
F16.122 **Hallucinogen abuse with intoxication with perceptual disturbance**
F16.129 **Hallucinogen abuse with intoxication, unspecified**
F16.14 **Hallucinogen abuse with hallucinogen-induced mood disorder**
Other hallucinogen use disorder, mild, with other hallucinogen-induced bipolar or related disorder
Other hallucinogen use disorder, mild, with other hallucinogen-induced depressive disorder
Phencyclidine use disorder, mild, with other hallucinogen-induced bipolar or related disorder
Phencyclidine use disorder, mild, with other hallucinogen-induced depressive disorder
+ F16.15 **Hallucinogen abuse with hallucinogen-induced psychotic disorder**
CC F16.150 **Hallucinogen abuse with hallucinogen-induced psychotic disorder with delusions**
CC Exclusion see Appendix A PDX collection 0550
CC F16.151 **Hallucinogen abuse with hallucinogen-induced psychotic disorder with hallucinations**
CC Exclusion see Appendix A PDX collection 0550
F16.159 **Hallucinogen abuse with hallucinogen-induced psychotic disorder, unspecified**
+ F16.18 **Hallucinogen abuse with other hallucinogen-induced disorder**
F16.180 **Hallucinogen abuse with hallucinogen-induced anxiety disorder**
F16.183 **Hallucinogen abuse with hallucinogen persisting perception disorder (flashbacks)**
F16.188 **Hallucinogen abuse with other hallucinogen-induced disorder**
F16.19 **Hallucinogen abuse with unspecified hallucinogen-induced disorder**
+ F16.2 **Hallucinogen dependence**
Excludes1: *hallucinogen abuse (F16.1-)*
hallucinogen use, unspecified (F16.9-)
CC F16.20 **Hallucinogen dependence, uncomplicated**
Other hallucinogen use disorder, moderate
Other hallucinogen use disorder, severe
Phencyclidine use disorder, moderate
Phencyclidine use disorder, severe
No CC Exclusions
F16.21 **Hallucinogen dependence, in remission**
Other hallucinogen use disorder, moderate, in early remission
Other hallucinogen use disorder, moderate, in sustained remission
Other hallucinogen use disorder, severe, in early remission
Other hallucinogen use disorder, severe, in sustained remission

Phencyclidine use disorder, moderate, in early remission
Phencyclidine use disorder, moderate, in sustained remission
Phencyclidine use disorder, severe, in early remission
Phencyclidine use disorder, severe, in sustained remission

+ **F16.22 Hallucinogen dependence with intoxication**

F16.220 Hallucinogen dependence with intoxication, uncomplicated

CC **F16.221 Hallucinogen dependence with intoxication with delirium**
CC Exclusion see Appendix A PDX collection 0550

F16.229 Hallucinogen dependence with intoxication, unspecified

F16.24 Hallucinogen dependence with hallucinogen-induced mood disorder
Other hallucinogen use disorder, moderate, with other hallucinogen-induced bipolar or related disorder
Other hallucinogen use disorder, moderate, with other hallucinogen-induced depressive disorder
Other hallucinogen use disorder, severe, with other hallucinogen-induced bipolar or related disorder
Other hallucinogen use disorder, severe, with other hallucinogen-induced depressive disorder
Phencyclidine use disorder, moderate, with other phencyclidine-induced bipolar or related disorder
Phencyclidine use disorder, moderate, with other phencyclidine-induced depressive disorder
Phencyclidine use disorder, severe, with other phencyclidine-induced bipolar or related disorder
Phencyclidine use disorder, severe, with other phencyclidine-induced depressive disorder

+ **F16.25 Hallucinogen dependence with hallucinogen-induced psychotic disorder**

CC **F16.250 Hallucinogen dependence with hallucinogen-induced psychotic disorder with delusions**
CC Exclusion see Appendix A PDX collection 0550

CC **F16.251 Hallucinogen dependence with hallucinogen-induced psychotic disorder with hallucinations**
CC Exclusion see Appendix A PDX collection 0550

CC **F16.259 Hallucinogen dependence with hallucinogen-induced psychotic disorder, unspecified**
No CC Exclusions

+ **F16.28 Hallucinogen dependence with other hallucinogen-induced disorder**

CC **F16.280 Hallucinogen dependence with hallucinogen-induced anxiety disorder**
No CC Exclusions

CC **F16.283 Hallucinogen dependence with hallucinogen persisting perception disorder (flashbacks)**
No CC Exclusions

CC **F16.288 Hallucinogen dependence with other hallucinogen-induced disorder**
No CC Exclusions

F16.29 Hallucinogen dependence with unspecified hallucinogen-induced disorder

+ **F16.9 Hallucinogen use, unspecified**

Excludes1: *hallucinogen abuse (F16.1-)*
hallucinogen dependence (F16.2-)

F16.90 Hallucinogen use, unspecified, uncomplicated

+ **F16.92 Hallucinogen use, unspecified with intoxication**

F16.920 Hallucinogen use, unspecified with intoxication, uncomplicated

CC **F16.921 Hallucinogen use, unspecified with intoxication with delirium**
Other hallucinogen intoxication delirium
CC Exclusion see Appendix A PDX collection 0550

F16.929 Hallucinogen use, unspecified with intoxication, unspecified

F16.94 Hallucinogen use, unspecified with hallucinogen-induced mood disorder
Other hallucinogen-induced bipolar or related disorder, without use disorder
Other hallucinogen-induced depressive disorder, without use disorder
Phencyclidine-induced bipolar or related disorder, without use disorder
Phencyclidine-induced depressive disorder, without use disorder

+ **F16.95 Hallucinogen use, unspecified with hallucinogen-induced psychotic disorder**

CC **F16.950 Hallucinogen use, unspecified with hallucinogen-induced psychotic disorder with delusions**
CC Exclusion see Appendix A PDX collection 0550

CC **F16.951 Hallucinogen use, unspecified with hallucinogen-induced psychotic disorder with hallucinations**
CC Exclusion see Appendix A PDX collection 0550

F16.959 Hallucinogen use, unspecified with hallucinogen-induced psychotic disorder, unspecified
Other hallucinogen-induced psychotic disorder, without use disorder
Phencyclidine-induced psychotic disorder, without use disorder

+ **F16.98 Hallucinogen use, unspecified with other specified hallucinogen-induced disorder**

F16.980 Hallucinogen use, unspecified with hallucinogen-induced anxiety disorder
Other hallucinogen-induced anxiety disorder, without use disorder
Phencyclidine-induced anxiety disorder, without use disorder

F16.983 Hallucinogen use, unspecified with hallucinogen persisting perception disorder (flashbacks)

F16.988 Hallucinogen use, unspecified with other hallucinogen-induced disorder

F16.99 Hallucinogen use, unspecified with unspecified hallucinogen-induced disorder

F17 Nicotine dependence

Excludes1: *history of tobacco dependence (Z87.891)*
tobacco use NOS (Z72.0)

Excludes2: *tobacco use (smoking) during pregnancy, childbirth and the puerperium (O99.33-)*
toxic effect of nicotine (T65.2-)

Review coding guideline C.15.1.2

+ **F17.2 Nicotine dependence**

+ **F17.20 Nicotine dependence, unspecified**

F17.200 Nicotine dependence, unspecified, uncomplicated
Tobacco use disorder, mild
Tobacco use disorder, moderate
Tobacco use disorder, severe
AHA CC: 4Q, 2013, 108; 1Q, 2016, 36-37

F17.201 Nicotine dependence, unspecified, in remission
Tobacco use disorder, mild, in early remission
Tobacco use disorder, mild, in sustained remission
Tobacco use disorder, moderate, in early remission
Tobacco use disorder, moderate, in sustained remission
Tobacco use disorder, severe, in early remission
Tobacco use disorder, severe, in sustained remission

CC **F17.203 Nicotine dependence unspecified, with withdrawal**
Tobacco withdrawal
CC Exclusion see Appendix A PDX collection 0550

F17.208 **Nicotine dependence, unspecified, with other nicotine-induced disorders**

F17.209 **Nicotine dependence, unspecified, with unspecified nicotine-induced disorders**

+ **F17.21** **Nicotine dependence, cigarettes**

F17.210 **Nicotine dependence, cigarettes, uncomplicated**

AHA CC: 4Q, 2013, 109; 2Q, 2017, 28-29

F17.211 **Nicotine dependence, cigarettes, in remission**

Tobacco use disorder, cigarettes, mild, in early remission

Tobacco use disorder, cigarettes, mild, in sustained remission

Tobacco use disorder, cigarettes, moderate, in early remission

Tobacco use disorder, cigarettes, moderate, in sustained remission

Tobacco use disorder, cigarettes, severe, in early remission

Tobacco use disorder, cigarettes, severe, in sustained remission

CC **F17.213** **Nicotine dependence, cigarettes, with withdrawal**

CC Exclusion see Appendix A PDX collection 0550

F17.218 **Nicotine dependence, cigarettes, with other nicotine-induced disorders**

F17.219 **Nicotine dependence, cigarettes, with unspecified nicotine-induced disorders**

+ **F17.22** **Nicotine dependence, chewing tobacco**

F17.220 **Nicotine dependence, chewing tobacco, uncomplicated**

F17.221 **Nicotine dependence, chewing tobacco, in remission**

Tobacco use disorder, chewing tobacco, mild, in early remission

Tobacco use disorder, chewing tobacco, mild, in sustained remission

Tobacco use disorder, chewing tobacco, moderate, in early remission

Tobacco use disorder, chewing tobacco, moderate, in sustained remission

Tobacco use disorder, chewing tobacco, severe, in early remission

Tobacco use disorder, chewing tobacco, severe, in sustained remission

CC **F17.223** **Nicotine dependence, chewing tobacco, with withdrawal**

CC Exclusion see Appendix A PDX collection 0550

F17.228 **Nicotine dependence, chewing tobacco, with other nicotine-induced disorders**

F17.229 **Nicotine dependence, chewing tobacco, with unspecified nicotine-induced disorders**

+ **F17.29** **Nicotine dependence, other tobacco product**

F17.290 **Nicotine dependence, other tobacco product, uncomplicated**

AHA CC: 2Q, 2017, 28-29

F17.291 **Nicotine dependence, other tobacco product, in remission**

Tobacco use disorder, other tobacco product, mild, in early remission

Tobacco use disorder, other tobacco product, mild, in sustained remission

Tobacco use disorder, other tobacco product, moderate, in early remission

Tobacco use disorder, other tobacco product, moderate, in sustained remission

Tobacco use disorder, other tobacco product, severe, in early remission

Tobacco use disorder, other tobacco product, severe, in sustained remission

CC **F17.293** **Nicotine dependence, other tobacco product, with withdrawal**

CC Exclusion see Appendix A PDX collection 0550

F17.298 **Nicotine dependence, other tobacco product, with other nicotine-induced disorders**

F17.299 **Nicotine dependence, other tobacco product, with unspecified nicotine-induced disorders**

F18 Inhalant related disorders

Includes: volatile solvents

+ **F18.1** **Inhalant abuse**

Excludes1: *inhalant dependence (F18.2-)*
inhalant use, unspecified (F18.9-)

F18.10 **Inhalant abuse, uncomplicated**

Inhalant use disorder, mild

F18.11 **Inhalant abuse, in remission**

Inhalant use disorder, mild, in early remission

Inhalant use disorder, mild, in sustained remission

+ **F18.12** **Inhalant abuse with intoxication**

F18.120 **Inhalant abuse with intoxication, uncomplicated**

CC **F18.121** **Inhalant abuse with intoxication delirium**

CC Exclusion see Appendix A PDX collection 0550

F18.129 **Inhalant abuse with intoxication, unspecified**

F18.14 **Inhalant abuse with inhalant-induced mood disorder**

Inhalant use disorder, mild, with inhalant-induced depressive disorder

+ **F18.15** **Inhalant abuse with inhalant-induced psychotic disorder**

CC **F18.150** **Inhalant abuse with inhalant-induced psychotic disorder with delusions**

CC Exclusion see Appendix A PDX collection 0550

CC **F18.151** **Inhalant abuse with inhalant-induced psychotic disorder with hallucinations**

CC Exclusion see Appendix A PDX collection 0550

F18.159 **Inhalant abuse with inhalant-induced psychotic disorder, unspecified**

CC **F18.17** **Inhalant abuse with inhalant-induced dementia**

Inhalant use disorder, mild, with inhalant-induced major neurocognitive disorder

CC Exclusion see Appendix A PDX collection 0550

+ **F18.18** **Inhalant abuse with other inhalant-induced disorders**

F18.180 **Inhalant abuse with inhalant-induced anxiety disorder**

F18.188 **Inhalant abuse with other inhalant-induced disorder**

Inhalant use disorder, mild, with inhalant-induced mild neurocognitive disorder

F18.19 **Inhalant abuse with unspecified inhalant-induced disorder**

+ **F18.2** **Inhalant dependence**

Excludes1: *inhalant abuse (F18.1-)*
inhalant use, unspecified (F18.9-)

CC **F18.20** **Inhalant dependence, uncomplicated**

Inhalant use disorder, moderate

Inhalant use disorder, severe

No CC Exclusions

F18.21 **Inhalant dependence, in remission**

Inhalant use disorder, moderate, in early remission

Inhalant use disorder, moderate, in sustained remission

Inhalant use disorder, severe, in early remission

Inhalant use disorder, severe, in sustained remission

+ **F18.22** **Inhalant dependence with intoxication**

F18.220 **Inhalant dependence with intoxication, uncomplicated**

CC **F18.221** **Inhalant dependence with intoxication delirium**

CC Exclusion see Appendix A PDX collection 0550

F18.229 **Inhalant dependence with intoxication, unspecified**

F18.24 **Inhalant dependence with inhalant-induced mood disorder**

Inhalant use disorder, moderate, with inhalant-induced depressive disorder

Inhalant use disorder, severe, with inhalant-induced depressive disorder

+ F18.25 **Inhalant dependence with inhalant-induced psychotic disorder**
  - CC **F18.250** **Inhalant dependence with inhalant-induced psychotic disorder with delusions**
    - CC Exclusion see Appendix A PDX collection 0550
  - CC **F18.251** **Inhalant dependence with inhalant-induced psychotic disorder with hallucinations**
    - CC Exclusion see Appendix A PDX collection 0550
  - CC **F18.259** **Inhalant dependence with inhalant-induced psychotic disorder, unspecified**
    - No CC Exclusions

CC **F18.27** **Inhalant dependence with inhalant-induced dementia**
- Inhalant use disorder, moderate, with inhalant-induced major neurocognitive disorder
- Inhalant use disorder, severe, with inhalant-induced major neurocognitive disorder
- CC Exclusion see Appendix A PDX collection 0550

+ F18.28 **Inhalant dependence with other inhalant-induced disorders**
  - CC **F18.280** **Inhalant dependence with inhalant-induced anxiety disorder**
    - No CC Exclusions
  - CC **F18.288** **Inhalant dependence with other inhalant-induced disorder**
    - Inhalant use disorder, moderate, with inhalant-induced mild neurocognitive disorder
    - Inhalant use disorder, severe, with inhalant-induced mild neurocognitive disorder
    - No CC Exclusions

F18.29 **Inhalant dependence with unspecified inhalant-induced disorder**

+ F18.9 **Inhalant use, unspecified**
  - ***Excludes1:*** *inhalant abuse (F18.1-)*
    inhalant dependence (F18.2-)

F18.90 **Inhalant use, unspecified, uncomplicated**

+ F18.92 **Inhalant use, unspecified with intoxication**
  - **F18.920** **Inhalant use, unspecified with intoxication, uncomplicated**
  - CC **F18.921** **Inhalant use, unspecified with intoxication with delirium**
    - CC Exclusion see Appendix A PDX collection 0550
  - **F18.929** **Inhalant use, unspecified with intoxication, unspecified**

F18.94 **Inhalant use, unspecified with inhalant-induced mood disorder**
- Inhalant-induced depressive disorder

+ F18.95 **Inhalant use, unspecified with inhalant-induced psychotic disorder**
  - CC **F18.950** **Inhalant use, unspecified with inhalant-induced psychotic disorder with delusions**
    - CC Exclusion see Appendix A PDX collection 0550
  - CC **F18.951** **Inhalant use, unspecified with inhalant-induced psychoticdisorder with hallucinations**
    - CC Exclusion see Appendix A PDX collection 0550
  - **F18.959** **Inhalant use, unspecified with inhalant-induced psychotic disorder, unspecified**

CC **F18.97** **Inhalant use, unspecified with inhalant-induced persisting dementia**
- Inhalant-induced major neurocognitive disorder
- CC Exclusion see Appendix A PDX collection 0550

+ F18.98 **Inhalant use, unspecified with other inhalant-induced disorders**
  - **F18.980** **Inhalant use, unspecified with inhalant-induced anxiety disorder**
  - **F18.988** **Inhalant use, unspecified with other inhalant-induced disorder**
    - Inhalant-induced mild neurocognitive disorder

F18.99 **Inhalant use, unspecified with unspecified inhalant-induced disorder**

F19 Other psychoactive substance related disorders

Includes: polysubstance drug use (indiscriminate drug use)

+ F19.1 **Other psychoactive substance abuse**
  - ***Excludes1:*** *other psychoactive substance dependence (F19.2-)*
    other psychoactive substance use, unspecified (F19.9-)

F19.10 **Other psychoactive substance abuse, uncomplicated**
- Other (or unknown) substance use disorder, mild

F19.11 **Other psychoactive substance abuse, in remission**
- Other (or unknown) substance use disorder, mild, in early remission
- Other (or unknown) substance use disorder, mild, in sustained remission

+ F19.12 **Other psychoactive substance abuse with intoxication**
  - **F19.120** **Other psychoactive substance abuse with intoxication, uncomplicated**
  - CC **F19.121** **Other psychoactive substance abuse with intoxication delirium**
    - CC Exclusion see Appendix A PDX collection 0550
  - **F19.122** **Other psychoactive substance abuse with intoxication with perceptual disturbances**
  - **F19.129** **Other psychoactive substance abuse with intoxication, unspecified**

F19.14 **Other psychoactive substance abuse with psychoactive substance-induced mood disorder**
- Other (or unknown) substance use disorder, mild, with other (or known) substance-induced bipolar or related disorder
- Other (or unknown) substance use disorder, mild, with other (or known) substance-induced depressive disorder

+ F19.15 **Other psychoactive substance abuse with psychoactive substance-induced psychotic disorder**
  - CC **F19.150** **Other psychoactive substance abuse with psychoactive substance-induced psychotic disorder with delusions**
    - CC Exclusion see Appendix A PDX collection 0550
  - CC **F19.151** **Other psychoactive substance abuse with psychoactive substance-induced psychotic disorder with hallucinations**
    - CC Exclusion see Appendix A PDX collection 0550
  - **F19.159** **Other psychoactive substance abuse with psychoactive substance-induced psychotic disorder, unspecified**

F19.16 **Other psychoactive substance abuse with psychoactive substance-induced persisting amnestic disorder**

CC **F19.17** **Other psychoactive substance abuse with psychoactive substance-induced persisting dementia**
- Other (or unknown) substance use disorder, mild, with other (or known) substance-induced major neurocognitive disorder
- CC Exclusion see Appendix A PDX collection 0550

+ F19.18 **Other psychoactive substance abuse with other psychoactive substance-induced disorders**
  - **F19.180** **Other psychoactive substance abuse with psychoactive substance-induced anxiety disorder**
  - **F19.181** **Other psychoactive substance abuse with psychoactive substance-induced sexual dysfunction**
  - **F19.182** **Other psychoactive substance abuse with psychoactive substance-induced sleep disorder**
  - **F19.188** **Other psychoactive substance abuse with other psychoactive substance-induced disorder**
    - Other (or unknown) substance use disorder, mild, with other (or known) substance-induced mild neurocognitive disorder
    - Other (or unknown) substance use disorder, mild, with other (or known) substance-induced obsessive-compulsive disorder

F19.19 **Other psychoactive substance abuse with unspecified psychoactive substance-induced disorder**

+ F19.2 **Other psychoactive substance dependence**
  Excludes1: *other psychoactive substance abuse (F19.1-)*
  other psychoactive substance use, unspecified (F19.9-)

CC **F19.20** **Other psychoactive substance dependence, uncomplicated**
  Other (or unknown) substance use disorder, moderate
  Other (or unknown) substance use disorder, severe
  No CC Exclusions

F19.21 **Other psychoactive substance dependence, in remission**
  Other (or unknown) substance use disorder, moderate, in early remission
  Other (or unknown) substance use disorder, moderate, in sustained remission
  Other (or unknown) substance use disorder, severe, in early remission
  Other (or unknown) substance use disorder, severe, in sustained remission

+ F19.22 **Other psychoactive substance dependence with intoxication**
  Excludes1: *other psychoactive substance dependence with withdrawal (F19.23-)*

F19.220 **Other psychoactive substance dependence with intoxication, uncomplicated**

CC **F19.221** **Other psychoactive substance dependence with intoxication delirium**
  CC Exclusion see Appendix A PDX collection 0550

CC **F19.222** **Other psychoactive substance dependence with intoxication with perceptual disturbance**
  No CC Exclusions

F19.229 **Other psychoactive substance dependence with intoxication, unspecified**

+ F19.23 **Other psychoactive substance dependence with withdrawal**
  Excludes1: *other psychoactive substance dependence with intoxication (F19.22-)*

CC **F19.230** **Other psychoactive substance dependence with withdrawal, uncomplicated**
  CC Exclusion see Appendix A PDX collection 0550

CC **F19.231** **Other psychoactive substance dependence with withdrawal delirium**
  CC Exclusion see Appendix A PDX collection 0550

CC **F19.232** **Other psychoactive substance dependence with withdrawal with perceptual disturbance**
  CC Exclusion see Appendix A PDX collection 0550

CC **F19.239** **Other psychoactive substance dependence with withdrawal, unspecified**
  CC Exclusion see Appendix A PDX collection 0550

F19.24 **Other psychoactive substance dependence with psychoactive substance-induced mood disorder**
  Other (or known) substance use disorder, moderate, with other (or unknown) substance-induced bipolar or related disorder
  Other (or known) substance use disorder, moderate, with other (or unknown) substance-induced depressive disorder
  Other (or known) substance use disorder, severe, with other (or unknown) substance-induced bipolar or related disorder
  Other (or known) substance use disorder, severe, with other (or unknown) substance-induced depressive disorder

+ F19.25 **Other psychoactive substance dependence with psychoactive substance-induced psychotic disorder**

CC **F19.250** **Other psychoactive substance dependence with psychoactive substance-induced psychotic disorder with delusions**
  CC Exclusion see Appendix A PDX collection 0550

CC **F19.251** **Other psychoactive substance dependence with psychoactive substance-induced psychotic disorder with hallucinations**
  CC Exclusion see Appendix A PDX collection 0550

CC **F19.259** **Other psychoactive substance dependence with psychoactive substance-induced psychotic disorder, unspecified**
  No CC Exclusions

CC **F19.26** **Other psychoactive substance dependence with psychoactive substance-induced persisting amnestic disorder**
  No CC Exclusions

CC **F19.27** **Other psychoactive substance dependence with psychoactive substance-induced persisting dementia**
  Other (or unknown) substance use disorder, moderate, with other (or known) substance-induced major neurocognitive disorder
  Other (or unknown) substance use disorder, severe, with other (or known) substance-induced major neurocognitive disorder
  CC Exclusion see Appendix A PDX collection 0550

+ F19.28 **Other psychoactive substance dependence with other psychoactive substance-induced disorders**

CC **F19.280** **Other psychoactive substance dependence with psychoactive substance-induced anxiety disorder**
  No CC Exclusions

CC **F19.281** **Other psychoactive substance dependence with psychoactive substance-induced sexual dysfunction**
  No CC Exclusions

CC **F19.282** **Other psychoactive substance dependence with psychoactive substance-induced sleep disorder**
  No CC Exclusions

CC **F19.288** **Other psychoactive substance dependence with other psychoactive substance-induced disorder**
  Other (or unknown) substance use disorder, moderate, with other (or known) substance-induced mild neurocognitive disorder
  Other (or unknown) substance use disorder, moderate, with other (or known) substance-induced obsessive-compulsive disorder
  Other (or unknown) substance use disorder, severe, with other (or known) substance-induced mild neurocognitive disorder
  Other (or unknown) substance use disorder, severe, with other (or known) substance-induced obsessive-compulsive disorder
  No CC Exclusions

F19.29 **Other psychoactive substance dependence with unspecified psychoactive substance-induced disorder**

+ F19.9 **Other psychoactive substance use, unspecified**
  Excludes1: *other psychoactive substance abuse (F19.1-)*
  other psychoactive substance dependence (F19.2-)

F19.90 **Other psychoactive substance use, unspecified, uncomplicated**

+ F19.92 **Other psychoactive substance use, unspecified with intoxication**
  Excludes1: *other psychoactive substance use, unspecified with withdrawal (F19.93)*

F19.920 **Other psychoactive substance use, unspecified with intoxication, uncomplicated**

CC **F19.921** **Other psychoactive substance use, unspecified with intoxication with delirium**
  Other (or unknown) substance-induced delirium
  CC Exclusion see Appendix A PDX collection 0550

F19.922 **Other psychoactive substance use, unspecified with intoxication with perceptual disturbance**

F19.929 **Other psychoactive substance use, unspecified with intoxication, unspecified**

+ F19.93 **Other psychoactive substance use, unspecified with withdrawal**

Excludes1: *other psychoactive substance use, unspecifiedwithintoxication(F19.92-)*

CC **F19.930** **Other psychoactive substance use, unspecified with withdrawal, uncomplicated**
CC Exclusion see Appendix A PDX collection 0550

CC **F19.931** **Other psychoactive substance use, unspecified with withdrawal delirium**
CC Exclusion see Appendix A PDX collection 0550

CC **F19.932** **Other psychoactive substance use, unspecified with withdrawal with perceptual disturbance**
CC Exclusion see Appendix A PDX collection 0550

CC **F19.939** **Other psychoactive substance use, unspecified with withdrawal, unspecified**
CC Exclusion see Appendix A PDX collection 0550

F19.94 **Other psychoactive substance use, unspecified with psychoactive substance-induced mood disorder**
Other (or unknown) substance-induced bipolar or related disorder, without use disorder
Other (or unknown) substance-induced depressive disorder, without use disorder

+ F19.95 **Other psychoactive substance use, unspecified with psychoactive substance-induced psychotic disorder**

CC **F19.950** **Other psychoactive substance use, unspecified with psychoactive substance-induced psychotic disorder with delusions**
CC Exclusion see Appendix A PDX collection 0550

CC **F19.951** **Other psychoactive substance use, unspecified with psychoactive substance-induced psychotic disorder with hallucinations**
CC Exclusion see Appendix A PDX collection 0550

F19.959 **Other psychoactive substance use, unspecified with psychoactive substance-induced psychotic disorder, unspecified**
Other (or unknown) substance-induced psychotic disorder, without use disorder

F19.96 **Other psychoactive substance use, unspecified with psychoactive substance-induced persisting amnestic disorder**

CC **F19.97** **Other psychoactive substance use, unspecified with psychoactive substance-induced persisting dementia**
Other (or unknown) substance-induced major neurocognitive disorder, without use disorder
CC Exclusion see Appendix A PDX collection 0550

+ F19.98 **Other psychoactive substance use, unspecified with other psychoactive substance-induced disorders**

F19.980 **Other psychoactive substance use, unspecified with psychoactive substance-induced anxiety disorder**
Other (or unknown) substance-induced anxiety disorder, without use disorder

F19.981 **Other psychoactive substance use, unspecified with psychoactive substance-induced sexual dysfunction**
Other (or unknown) substance-induced sexual dysfunction, without use disorder

F19.982 **Other psychoactive substance use, unspecified with psychoactive substance-induced sleep disorder**
Other (or unknown) substance-induced sleep disorder, without use disorder

F19.988 **Other psychoactive substance use, unspecified with other psychoactive substance-induced disorder**
Other (or unknown) substance-induced mild neurocognitive disorder, without use disorder
Other (or unknown) substance-induced obsessive-compulsive or related disorder, without use disorder

F19.99 **Other psychoactive substance use, unspecified with unspecified psychoactive substance-induced disorder**

Schizophrenia, schizotypal, delusional, and other non-mood psychotic disorders (F20-F29)

F20 Schizophrenia

Excludes1: *brief psychotic disorder (F23)*
cyclic schizophrenia (F25.0)
mood [affective] disorders with psychotic symptoms (F30.2, F31.2, F31.5, F31.64, F32.3, F33.3)
schizoaffective disorder (F25.-)
schizophrenic reaction NOS (F23)

Excludes2: *schizophrenic reaction in:*
alcoholism (F10.15-, F10.25-, F10.95-)
brain disease (F06.2)
epilepsy (F06.2)
psychoactive drug use (F11-F19 with .15. .25, .95)
schizotypal disorder (F21)

CC **F20.0** **Paranoid schizophrenia**
Paraphrenic schizophrenia
Excludes1: *involutional paranoid state (F22)*
paranoia (F22)
CC Exclusion see Appendix A PDX collection 0551

CC **F20.1** **Disorganized schizophrenia**
Hebephrenic schizophrenia
Hebephrenia
CC Exclusion see Appendix A PDX collection 0551

CC **F20.2** **Catatonic schizophrenia**
Schizophrenic catalepsy
Schizophrenic catatonia
Schizophrenic flexibilitas cerea
Excludes1: *catatonic stupor (R40.1)*
CC Exclusion see Appendix A PDX collection 0551

F20.3 **Undifferentiated schizophrenia**
Atypical schizophrenia
Excludes1: *acute schizophrenia-like psychotic disorder (F23)*
Excludes2: *post-schizophrenic depression (F32.89)*

CC **F20.5** **Residual schizophrenia**
Restzustand (schizophrenic)
Schizophrenic residual state
CC Exclusion see Appendix A PDX collection 0551

+ F20.8 **Other schizophrenia**

CC **F20.81** **Schizophreniform disorder**
Schizophreniform psychosis NOS
CC Exclusion see Appendix A PDX collection 0551

CC **F20.89** **Other schizophrenia**
Cenesthopathic schizophrenia
Simple schizophrenia
CC Exclusion see Appendix A PDX collection 0551

F20.9 **Schizophrenia, unspecified**

F21 Schizotypal disorder

Borderline schizophrenia
Latent schizophrenia
Latent schizophrenic reaction
Prepsychotic schizophrenia
Prodromal schizophrenia
Pseudoneurotic schizophrenia
Pseudopsychopathic schizophrenia
Schizotypal personality disorder
Excludes2: *Asperger's syndrome (F84.5)*
schizoid personality disorder (F60.1)
Valid 3-character code, no further characters required

F22 Delusional disorders

Delusional dysmorphophobia
Involutional paranoid state
Paranoia
Paranoia querulans
Paranoid psychosis
Paranoid state
Paraphrenia (late)
Sensitiver Beziehungswahn
Excludes1: *mood [affective] disorders with psychotic symptoms (F30.2, F31.2, F31.5, F31.64, F32.3, F33.3)*
paranoid schizophrenia (F20.0)
Excludes2: *paranoid personality disorder (F60.0)*
paranoid psychosis, psychogenic (F23)
paranoid reaction (F23)
Valid 3-character code, no further characters required

CC **F23 Brief psychotic disorder**

Paranoid reaction
Psychogenic paranoid psychosis
Excludes2: *mood [affective] disorders with psychotic symptoms (F30.2, F31.2, F31.5, F31.64, F32.3, F33.3)*
No CC Exclusions
Valid 3-character code, no further characters required

F24 Shared psychotic disorder

Folie à deux
Induced paranoid disorder
Induced psychotic disorder
Valid 3-character code, no further characters required

F25 Schizoaffective disorders

Excludes1: *mood [affective] disorders with psychotic symptoms (F30.2, F31.2, F31.5, F31.64, F32.3, F33.3)*
schizophrenia (F20.-)

F25.0 Schizoaffective disorder, bipolar type
Cyclic schizophrenia
Schizoaffective disorder, manic type
Schizoaffective disorder, mixed type
Schizoaffective psychosis, bipolar type

F25.1 Schizoaffective disorder, depressive type
Schizoaffective psychosis, depressive type

F25.8 Other schizoaffective disorders

F25.9 Schizoaffective disorder, unspecified
Schizoaffective psychosis NOS

F28 Other psychotic disorder not due to a substance or known physiological condition

Chronic hallucinatory psychosis
Other specified schizophrenia spectrum and other psychotic disorder
Valid 3-character code, no further characters required

F29 Unspecified psychosis not due to a substance or known physiological condition

Psychosis NOS
Unspecified schizophrenia spectrum and other psychotic disorder
Excludes1: *mental disorder NOS (F99)*
unspecified mental disorder due to known physiological condition (F09)
Valid 3-character code, no further characters required

Mood [affective] disorders (F30-F39)

F30 Manic episode

Includes: bipolar disorder, single manic episode
mixed affective episode
Excludes1: *bipolar disorder (F31.-)*
major depressive disorder, single episode (F32.-)
major depressive disorder, recurrent (F33.-)

\+ **F30.1 Manic episode without psychotic symptoms**

CC **F30.10 Manic episode without psychotic symptoms, unspecified**
CC Exclusion see Appendix A PDX collection 0551

CC **F30.11 Manic episode without psychotic symptoms, mild**
CC Exclusion see Appendix A PDX collection 0551

CC **F30.12 Manic episode without psychotic symptoms, moderate**
CC Exclusion see Appendix A PDX collection 0551

CC **F30.13 Manic episode, severe, without psychotic symptoms**
CC Exclusion see Appendix A PDX collection 0552

CC **F30.2 Manic episode, severe with psychotic symptoms**
Manic stupor
Mania with mood-congruent psychotic symptoms
Mania with mood-incongruent psychotic symptoms
CC Exclusion see Appendix A PDX collection 0551

F30.3 Manic episode in partial remission

F30.4 Manic episode in full remission

F30.8 Other manic episodes
Hypomania

CC **F30.9 Manic episode, unspecified**
Mania NOS
CC Exclusion see Appendix A PDX collection 0551

F31 Bipolar disorder

Includes: bipolar I disorder
bipolar type I disorder
manic-depressive illness
manic-depressive psychosis
manic-depressive reaction
Excludes1: *bipolar disorder, single manic episode (F30.-)*
major depressive disorder, single episode (F32.-)
major depressive disorder, recurrent (F33.-)
Excludes2: *cyclothymia (F34.0)*

CC **F31.0 Bipolar disorder, current episode hypomanic**
CC Exclusion see Appendix A PDX collection 0551

\+ **F31.1 Bipolar disorder, current episode manic without psychotic features**

CC **F31.10 Bipolar disorder, current episode manic without psychotic features, unspecified**
CC Exclusion see Appendix A PDX collection 0551

CC **F31.11 Bipolar disorder, current episode manic without psychotic features, mild**
CC Exclusion see Appendix A PDX collection 0551

CC **F31.12 Bipolar disorder, current episode manic without psychotic features, moderate**
CC Exclusion see Appendix A PDX collection 0551

CC **F31.13 Bipolar disorder, current episode manic without psychotic features, severe**
CC Exclusion see Appendix A PDX collection 0553

CC **F31.2 Bipolar disorder, current episode manic severe with psychoti[c] features**
Bipolar disorder, current episode manic with mood-congruent psychotic symptoms
Bipolar disorder, current episode manic with mood-incongrue[nt] psychotic symptoms
Bipolar I disorder, current or most recent episode manic, with psychotic features
CC Exclusion see Appendix A PDX collection 0551

\+ **F31.3 Bipolar disorder, current episode depressed, mild or modera[te] severity**

CC **F31.30 Bipolar disorder, current episode depressed, mild o[r] moderate severity, unspecified**
CC Exclusion see Appendix A PDX collection 0551

CC **F31.31 Bipolar disorder, current episode depressed, mild**
CC Exclusion see Appendix A PDX collection 0551

CC **F31.32 Bipolar disorder, current episode depressed, modera[te]**
CC Exclusion see Appendix A PDX collection 0551

CC **F31.4 Bipolar disorder, current episode depressed, severe, without psychotic features**
CC Exclusion see Appendix A PDX collection 0554

CC **F31.5 Bipolar disorder, current episode depressed, severe, with psychotic features**
Bipolar disorder, current episode depressed with mood-incongruent psychotic symptoms
Bipolar disorder, current episode depressed with mood-congruent psychotic symptoms
Bipolar I disorder, current or most recent episode depressed, with psychotic features
CC Exclusion see Appendix A PDX collection 0551

\+ **F31.6 Bipolar disorder, current episode mixed**

CC **F31.60 Bipolar disorder, current episode mixed, unspecifie[d]**
CC Exclusion see Appendix A PDX collection 0551

CC **F31.61 Bipolar disorder, current episode mixed, mild**
CC Exclusion see Appendix A PDX collection 0551

CC **F31.62 Bipolar disorder, current episode mixed, moderate**
CC Exclusion see Appendix A PDX collection 0551

CC **F31.63 Bipolar disorder, current episode mixed, severe, without psychotic features**
CC Exclusion see Appendix A PDX collection 0554

CC **F31.64 Bipolar disorder, current episode mixed, severe, wi[th] psychotic features**
Bipolar disorder, current episode mixed with mood-congruent psychotic symptoms
Bipolar disorder, current episode mixed with mood-incongruent psychotic symptoms
CC Exclusion see Appendix A PDX collection 0551

\+ **F31.7 Bipolar disorder, currently in remission**

F31.70 Bipolar disorder, currently in remission, most rece[nt] episode unspecified

F31.71 Bipolar disorder, in partial remission, most recent episode hypomanic

F31.72 Bipolar disorder, in full remission, most recent episode hypomanic

F31.73 Bipolar disorder, in partial remission, most recent episode manic

F31.74 Bipolar disorder, in full remission, most recent episode manic

F31.75 Bipolar disorder, in partial remission, most recent episode depressed

F31.76 Bipolar disorder, in full remission, most recent episode depressed

F31.77 Bipolar disorder, in partial remission, most recent episode mixed

F31.78 Bipolar disorder, in full remission, most recent episode mixed

+ **F31.8 Other bipolar disorders**

CC **F31.81 Bipolar II disorder**
Bipolar disorder, type 2
CC Exclusion see Appendix A PDX collection 0551

CC **F31.89 Other bipolar disorder**
Recurrent manic episodes NOS
CC Exclusion see Appendix A PDX collection 0551

F31.9 Bipolar disorder, unspecified
Manic depression

F32 Major depressive disorder, single episode

Includes: single episode of agitated depression
single episode of depressive reaction
single episode of major depression
single episode of psychogenic depression
single episode of reactive depression
single episode of vital depression

Excludes1: *bipolar disorder (F31.-)*
manic episode (F30.-)
recurrent depressive disorder (F33.-)

Excludes2: *adjustment disorder (F43.2)*

CC **F32.0 Major depressive disorder, single episode, mild**
CC Exclusion see Appendix A PDX collection 0555

CC **F32.1 Major depressive disorder, single episode, moderate**
CC Exclusion see Appendix A PDX collection 0555

CC **F32.2 Major depressive disorder, single episode, severe without psychotic features**
CC Exclusion see Appendix A PDX collection 0555

CC **F32.3 Major depressive disorder, single episode, severe with psychotic features**
Single episode of major depression with mood-congruent psychotic symptoms
Single episode of major depression with mood-incongruent psychotic symptoms
Single episode of major depression with psychotic symptoms
Single episode of psychogenic depressive psychosis
Single episode of psychotic depression
Single episode of reactive depressive psychosis
CC Exclusion see Appendix A PDX collection 0555

F32.4 Major depressive disorder, single episode, in partial remission

F32.5 Major depressive disorder, single episode, in full remission

+ **F32.8 Other depressive episodes**
AHA CC: 4Q, 2016, 14

♀ **F32.81 Premenstrual dysphoric disorder**
Excludes1: *premenstrual tension syndrome (N94.3)*

F32.89 Other specified depressive episodes
Atypical depression
Post-schizophrenic depression
Single episode of 'masked' depression NOS

F32.9 Major depressive disorder, single episode, unspecified
Depression NOS
Depressive disorder NOS
Major depression NOS
AHA CC: 4Q, 2013, 107-108

F33 Major depressive disorder, recurrent

Includes: recurrent episodes of depressive reaction
recurrent episodes of endogenous depression
recurrent episodes of major depression
recurrent episodes of psychogenic depression
recurrent episodes of reactive depression
recurrent episodes of seasonal depressive disorder
recurrent episodes of vital depression

Excludes1: *bipolar disorder (F31.-)*
manic episode (F30.-)

CC **F33.0 Major depressive disorder, recurrent, mild**
CC Exclusion see Appendix A PDX collection 0555

CC **F33.1 Major depressive disorder, recurrent, moderate**
CC Exclusion see Appendix A PDX collection 0555

CC **F33.2 Major depressive disorder, recurrent severe without psychotic features**
CC Exclusion see Appendix A PDX collection 0555

CC **F33.3 Major depressive disorder, recurrent, severe with psychotic symptoms**
Endogenous depression with psychotic symptoms
Major depressive disorder, recurrent, with psychotic features
Recurrent severe episodes of major depression with mood-congruent psychotic symptoms
Recurrent severe episodes of major depression with mood-incongruent psychotic symptoms
Recurrent severe episodes of major depression with psychotic symptoms
Recurrent severe episodes of psychogenic depressive psychosis
Recurrent severe episodes of psychotic depression
Recurrent severe episodes of reactive depressive psychosis
CC Exclusion see Appendix A PDX collection 0551

+ **F33.4 Major depressive disorder, recurrent, in remission**

CC **F33.40 Major depressive disorder, recurrent, in remission, unspecified**
CC Exclusion see Appendix A PDX collection 0555

F33.41 Major depressive disorder, recurrent, in partial remission

F33.42 Major depressive disorder, recurrent, in full remission

CC **F33.8 Other recurrent depressive disorders**
Recurrent brief depressive episodes
CC Exclusion see Appendix A PDX collection 0551

CC **F33.9 Major depressive disorder, recurrent, unspecified**
Monopolar depression NOS
CC Exclusion see Appendix A PDX collection 0555

F34 Persistent mood [affective] disorders

F34.0 Cyclothymic disorder
Affective personality disorder
Cycloid personality
Cyclothymia
Cyclothymic personality

F34.1 Dysthymic disorder
Depressive neurosis
Depressive personality disorder
Dysthymia
Neurotic depression
Persistent depressive disorder
Persistent anxiety depression
Excludes2: *anxiety depression (mild or not persistent) (F41.8)*

+ **F34.8 Other persistent mood [affective] disorders**
AHA CC: 4Q, 2016, 14

CC **F34.81 Disruptive mood dysregulation disorder**
CC Exclusion see Appendix A PDX collection 0551

CC **F34.89 Other specified persistent mood disorders**
CC Exclusion see Appendix A PDX collection 0551

CC **F34.9 Persistent mood [affective] disorder, unspecified**
CC Exclusion see Appendix A PDX collection 0551

F39 Unspecified mood [affective] disorder

Affective psychosis NOS
Valid 3-character code, no further characters required

Anxiety, dissociative, stress-related, somatoform and other nonpsychotic mental disorders (F40-F48)

F40 Phobic anxiety disorders

+ **F40.0 Agoraphobia**

F40.00 Agoraphobia, unspecified

F40.01 Agoraphobia with panic disorder
Panic disorder with agoraphobia
Excludes1: *panic disorder without agoraphobia (F41.0)*

F40.02 Agoraphobia without panic disorder

+ **F40.1 Social phobias**
Anthropophobia
Social anxiety disorder
Social anxiety disorder of childhood
Social neurosis

F40.10 Social phobia, unspecified

F40.11 Social phobia, generalized

+ **F40.2 Specific (isolated) phobias**
Excludes2: *dysmorphophobia (nondelusional) (F45.22)*
nosophobia (F45.22)

+ **F40.21 Animal type phobia**

F40.210 Arachnophobia
Fear of spiders

F40.218 Other animal type phobia

+ **F40.22 Natural environment type phobia**

F40.220 Fear of thunderstorms

F40.228 Other natural environment type phobia

+ **F40.23 Blood, injection, injury type phobia**
  - **F40.230 Fear of blood**
  - **F40.231 Fear of injections and transfusions**
  - **F40.232 Fear of other medical care**
  - **F40.233 Fear of injury**

+ **F40.24 Situational type phobia**
  - **F40.240 Claustrophobia**
  - **F40.241 Acrophobia**
  - **F40.242 Fear of bridges**
  - **F40.243 Fear of flying**
  - **F40.248 Other situational type phobia**

+ **F40.29 Other specified phobia**
  - **F40.290 Androphobia**
    Fear of men
  - **F40.291 Gynephobia**
    Fear of women
  - **F40.298 Other specified phobia**

F40.8 Other phobic anxiety disorders
Phobic anxiety disorder of childhood

F40.9 Phobic anxiety disorder, unspecified
Phobia NOS
Phobic state NOS

F41 Other anxiety disorders

Excludes2: *anxiety in:*
acute stress reaction (F43.0)
transient adjustment reaction (F43.2)
neurasthenia (F48.8)
psychophysiologic disorders (F45.-)
separation anxiety (F93.0)

F41.0 Panic disorder [episodic paroxysmal anxiety]
Panic attack
Panic state
Excludes1: *panic disorder with agoraphobia (F40.01)*

F41.1 Generalized anxiety disorder
Anxiety neurosis
Anxiety reaction
Anxiety state
Overanxious disorder
Excludes2: *neurasthenia (F48.8)*

F41.3 Other mixed anxiety disorders

F41.8 Other specified anxiety disorders
Anxiety depression (mild or not persistent)
Anxiety hysteria
Mixed anxiety and depressive disorder

F41.9 Anxiety disorder, unspecified
Anxiety NOS

F42 Obsessive-compulsive disorder

Excludes2: *obsessive-compulsive personality (disorder) (F60.5)*
obsessive-compulsive symptoms occurring in depression (F32-F33)
obsessive-compulsive symptoms occurring in schizophrenia (F20.-)

AHA CC: 4Q, 2016, 14-15

F42.2 Mixed obsessional thoughts and acts

F42.3 Hoarding disorder

F42.4 Excoriation (skin-picking) disorder
Excludes1: *factitial dermatitis (L98.1)*
other specified behavioral and emotional disorders with onset usually occurring in early childhood and adolescence (F98.8)

F42.8 Other obsessive compulsive disorder
Anancastic neurosis
Obsessive-compulsive neurosis

F42.9 Obsessive-compulsive disorder, unspecified

F43 Reaction to severe stress, and adjustment disorders

F43.0 Acute stress reaction
Acute crisis reaction
Acute reaction to stress
Combat and operational stress reaction
Combat fatigue
Crisis state
Psychic shock

+ **F43.1 Post-traumatic stress disorder (PTSD)**
  Traumatic neurosis
  - **F43.10 Post-traumatic stress disorder, unspecified**
  - **F43.11 Post-traumatic stress disorder, acute**
  - **F43.12 Post-traumatic stress disorder, chronic**

+ **F43.2 Adjustment disorders**
  Culture shock
  Grief reaction
  Hospitalism in children
  Excludes2: *separation anxiety disorder of childhood (F93.0)*
  - **F43.20 Adjustment disorder, unspecified**
  - **F43.21 Adjustment disorder with depressed mood**
    AHA CC: 1Q, 2014, 25
  - **F43.22 Adjustment disorder with anxiety**
  - **F43.23 Adjustment disorder with mixed anxiety and depressed mood**
  - **F43.24 Adjustment disorder with disturbance of conduct**
  - **F43.25 Adjustment disorder with mixed disturbance of emotions and conduct**
  - **F43.29 Adjustment disorder with other symptoms**

F43.8 Other reactions to severe stress
Other specified trauma and stressor-related disorder

F43.9 Reaction to severe stress, unspecified
Trauma and stressor-related disorder, NOS

F44 Dissociative and conversion disorders

Includes: conversion hysteria
conversion reaction
hysteria
hysterical psychosis

Excludes2: *malingering [conscious simulation] (Z76.5)*

F44.0 Dissociative amnesia
Excludes1: *amnesia NOS (R41.3)*
anterograde amnesia (R41.1)
dissociative amnesia with dissociative fugue (F44.1)
retrograde amnesia (R41.2)
Excludes2: *alcohol-or other psychoactive substance-induced amnestic disorder (F10, F13, F19 with .26, .96)*
amnestic disorder due to known physiological condition (F04)
postictal amnesia in epilepsy (G40.-)

F44.1 Dissociative fugue
Dissociative amnesia with dissociative fugue
Excludes2: *postictal fugue in epilepsy (G40.-)*

F44.2 Dissociative stupor
Excludes1: *catatonic stupor (R40.1)*
stupor NOS (R40.1)
Excludes2: *catatonic disorder due to known physiological condition (F06.1)*
depressive stupor (F32, F33)
manic stupor (F30, F31)

F44.4 Conversion disorder with motor symptom or deficit
Conversion disorder with abnormal movement
Conversion disorder with speech symptoms
Conversion disorder with swallowing symptoms
Conversion disorder with weakness/paralysis
Dissociative motor disorders
Psychogenic aphonia
Psychogenic dysphonia

F44.5 Conversion disorder with seizures or convulsions
Conversion disorder with attacks or seizures
Dissociative convulsions

F44.6 Conversion disorder with sensory symptom or deficit
Conversion disorder with anesthesia or sensory loss
Conversion disorder with special sensory symptoms
Dissociative anesthesia and sensory loss
Psychogenic deafness

F44.7 Conversion disorder with mixed symptom presentation

+ **F44.8 Other dissociative and conversion disorders**
  - **F44.81 Dissociative identity disorder**
    Multiple personality disorder
  - **F44.89 Other dissociative and conversion disorders**
    Ganser's syndrome
    Psychogenic confusion
    Psychogenic twilight state
    Trance and possession disorders

F44.9 Dissociative and conversion disorder, unspecified
Dissociative disorder NOS

F45 Somatoform disorders

Excludes2: *dissociative and conversion disorders (F44.-)*
factitious disorders (F68.1-)
hair-plucking (F63.3)
lalling (F80.0)
lisping (F80.0)
malingering [conscious simulation] (Z76.5)
nail-biting (F98.8)
psychological or behavioral factors associated with disorders or diseases classified elsewhere (F54)
sexual dysfunction, not due to a substance or known physiological condition (F52.-)
thumb-sucking (F98.8)
tic disorders (in childhood and adolescence) (F95.-)
Tourette's syndrome (F95.2)
trichotillomania (F63.3)

F45.0 Somatization disorder
Briquet's disorder
Multiple psychosomatic disorder

F45.1 Undifferentiated somatoform disorder
Somatic symptom disorder
Undifferentiated psychosomatic disorder

+ **F45.2 Hypochondriacal disorders**
Excludes2: *delusional dysmorphophobia (F22)*
fixed delusions about bodily functions or shape (F22)

F45.20 Hypochondriacal disorder, unspecified

F45.21 Hypochondriasis
Hypochondriacal neurosis
Illness anxiety disorder

F45.22 Body dysmorphic disorder
Dysmorphophobia (nondelusional)
Nosophobia

F45.29 Other hypochondriacal disorders

+ **F45.4 Pain disorders related to psychological factors**
Excludes1: *pain NOS (R52)*

F45.41 Pain disorder exclusively related to psychological factors
Somatoform pain disorder (persistent)
Review coding guideline C.5.a

F45.42 Pain disorder with related psychological factors
Code also associated acute or chronic pain (G89.-)
Review coding guideline C.5.a

F45.8 Other somatoform disorders
Psychogenic dysmenorrhea
Psychogenic dysphagia, including 'globus hystericus'
Psychogenic pruritus
Psychogenic torticollis
Somatoform autonomic dysfunction
Teeth grinding
Excludes1: *sleep related teeth grinding (G47.63)*

F45.9 Somatoform disorder, unspecified
Psychosomatic disorder NOS

F48 Other nonpsychotic mental disorders

F48.1 Depersonalization-derealization syndrome

F48.2 Pseudobulbar affect
Involuntary emotional expression disorder
Code first underlying cause, if known, such as:
amyotrophic lateral sclerosis (G12.21)
multiple sclerosis (G35)
sequelae of cerebrovascular disease (I69.-)
sequelae of traumatic intracranial injury (S06.-)

F48.8 Other specified nonpsychotic mental disorders
Dhat syndrome
Neurasthenia
Occupational neurosis, including writer's cramp
Psychasthenia
Psychasthenic neurosis
Psychogenic syncope

F48.9 Nonpsychotic mental disorder, unspecified
Neurosis NOS

Behavioral syndromes associated with physiological disturbances and physical factors (F50-F59)

F50 Eating disorders

Excludes1: *anorexia NOS (R63.0)*
feeding difficulties (R63.3)
feeding problems of newborn (P92.-)
polyphagia (R63.2)
Excludes2: *feeding disorder in infancy or childhood (F98.2-)*

+ **F50.0 Anorexia nervosa**
Excludes1: *loss of appetite (R63.0)*
psychogenic loss of appetite (F50.89)

CC **F50.00 Anorexia nervosa, unspecified**
CC Exclusion see Appendix A PDX collection 0556

CC **F50.01 Anorexia nervosa, restricting type**
CC Exclusion see Appendix A PDX collection 0556

CC **F50.02 Anorexia nervosa, binge eating/purging type**
Excludes1: *bulimia nervosa (F50.2)*
CC Exclusion see Appendix A PDX collection 0556

CC **F50.2 Bulimia nervosa**
Bulimia NOS
Hyperorexia nervosa
Excludes1: *anorexia nervosa, binge eating/purging type (F50.02)*
CC Exclusion see Appendix A PDX collection 0557

+ **F50.8 Other eating disorders**
Excludes2: *pica of infancy and childhood (F98.3)*
AHA CC: 4Q, 2016, 15-16

F50.81 Binge eating disorder

F50.82 Avoidant/restrictive food intake disorder

F50.89 Other specified eating disorder
Pica in adults
Psychogenic loss of appetite

F50.9 Eating disorder, unspecified
Atypical anorexia nervosa
Atypical bulimia nervosa
Feeding or eating disorder, unspecified
Other specified feeding disorder

F51 Sleep disorders not due to a substance or known physiological condition

Excludes2: *organic sleep disorders (G47.-)*

+ **F51.0 Insomnia not due to a substance or known physiological condition**
Excludes2: *alcohol related insomnia (F10.182, F10.282, F10.982)*
drug-related insomnia (F11.182, F11.282, F11.982, F13.182, F13.282, F13.982, F14.182, F14.282, F14.982, F15.182, F15.282, F15.982, F19.182, F19.282, F19.982)
insomnia NOS (G47.0-)
insomnia due to known physiological condition (G47.0-)
organic insomnia (G47.0-)
sleep deprivation (Z72.820)

F51.01 Primary insomnia
Idiopathic insomnia

F51.02 Adjustment insomnia

F51.03 Paradoxical insomnia

F51.04 Psychophysiologic insomnia

F51.05 Insomnia due to other mental disorder
Code also associated mental disorder

F51.09 Other insomnia not due to a substance or known physiological condition

+ **F51.1 Hypersomnia not due to a substance or known physiological condition**
Excludes2: *alcohol related hypersomnia (F10.182, F10.282, F10.982)*
drug-related hypersomnia (F11.182, F11.282, F11.982, F13.182, F13.282, F13.982, F14.182, F14.282, F14.982, F15.182, F15.282, F15.982, F19.182, F19.282, F19.982)
hypersomnia NOS (G47.10)
hypersomnia due to known physiological condition (G47.10)
idiopathic hypersomnia (G47.11, G47.12)
narcolepsy (G47.4-)

F51.11 Primary hypersomnia

F51.12 Insufficient sleep syndrome
Excludes1: *sleep deprivation (Z72.820)*

F51.13 Hypersomnia due to other mental disorder
Code also associated mental disorder
F51.19 Other hypersomnia not due to a substance or known physiological condition
F51.3 Sleepwalking [somnambulism]
Non-rapid eye movement sleep arousal disorders, sleepwalking type
F51.4 Sleep terrors [night terrors]
Non-rapid eye movement sleep arousal disorders, sleep terror type
F51.5 Nightmare disorder
Dream anxiety disorder
F51.8 Other sleep disorders not due to a substance or known physiological condition
F51.9 Sleep disorder not due to a substance or known physiological condition, unspecified
Emotional sleep disorder NOS

F52 Sexual dysfunction not due to a substance or known physiological condition
Excludes2: *Dhat syndrome (F48.8)*
F52.0 Hypoactive sexual desire disorder
Lack or loss of sexual desire
Male hypoactive sexual desire disorder
Sexual anhedonia
Excludes1: *decreased libido (R68.82)*
F52.1 Sexual aversion disorder
Sexual aversion and lack of sexual enjoyment
\+ **F52.2 Sexual arousal disorders**
Failure of genital response
♂ **F52.21 Male erectile disorder**
Erectile disorder
Psychogenic impotence
Excludes1: *impotence of organic origin (N52.-)*
impotence NOS (N52.-)
♀ **F52.22 Female sexual arousal disorder**
Female sexual interest/arousal disorder
\+ **F52.3 Orgasmic disorder**
Inhibited orgasm
Psychogenic anorgasmy
♀ **F52.31 Female orgasmic disorder**
♂ **F52.32 Male orgasmic disorder**
Delayed ejaculation
♂ **F52.4 Premature ejaculation**
♀ **F52.5 Vaginismus not due to a substance or known physiological condition**
Psychogenic vaginismus
Excludes2: *vaginismus (due to a known physiological condition) (N94.2)*
F52.6 Dyspareunia not due to a substance or known physiological condition
Genito-pelvic pain penetration disorder
Psychogenic dyspareunia
Excludes2: *dyspareunia (due to a known physiological condition) (N94.1-)*
F52.8 Other sexual dysfunction not due to a substance or known physiological condition
Excessive sexual drive
Nymphomania
Satyriasis
F52.9 Unspecified sexual dysfunction not due to a substance or known physiological condition
Sexual dysfunction NOS

• ♀ **F53 Puerperal psychosis**
Postpartum depression
Excludes1: *mood disorders with psychotic features (F30.2, F31.2, F31.5, F31.64, F32.3, F33.3)*
postpartum dysphoria (O90.6)
psychosis in schizophrenia, schizotypal, delusional, and other psychotic disorders (F20-F29)
Valid 3-character code, no further characters required

F54 Psychological and behavioral factors associated with disorders or diseases classified elsewhere
Psychological factors affecting physical conditions
Code first the associated physical disorder, such as:
asthma (J45.-)
dermatitis (L23-L25)
gastric ulcer (K25.-)
mucous colitis (K58.-)
ulcerative colitis (K51.-)
urticaria (L50.-)
Excludes2: *tension-type headache (G44.2)*
Valid 3-character code, no further characters required

F55 Abuse of non-psychoactive substances
Excludes2: *abuse of psychoactive substances (F10-F19)*
F55.0 Abuse of antacids
F55.1 Abuse of herbal or folk remedies
F55.2 Abuse of laxatives
F55.3 Abuse of steroids or hormones
F55.4 Abuse of vitamins
F55.8 Abuse of other non-psychoactive substances

F59 Unspecified behavioral syndromes associated with physiological disturbances and physical factors
Psychogenic physiological dysfunction NOS
Valid 3-character code, no further characters required

Disorders of adult personality and behavior (F60-F69)

F60 Specific personality disorders
F60.0 Paranoid personality disorder
Expansive paranoid personality (disorder)
Fanatic personality (disorder)
Querulant personality (disorder)
Paranoid personality (disorder)
Sensitive paranoid personality (disorder)
Excludes2: *paranoia (F22)*
paranoia querulans (F22)
paranoid psychosis (F22)
paranoid schizophrenia (F20.0)
paranoid state (F22)
F60.1 Schizoid personality disorder
Excludes2: *Asperger's syndrome (F84.5)*
delusional disorder (F22)
schizoid disorder of childhood (F84.5)
schizophrenia (F20.-)
schizotypal disorder (F21)
F60.2 Antisocial personality disorder
Amoral personality (disorder)
Asocial personality (disorder)
Dissocial personality disorder
Psychopathic personality (disorder)
Sociopathic personality (disorder)
Excludes1: *conduct disorders (F91.-)*
Excludes2: *borderline personality disorder (F60.3)*
F60.3 Borderline personality disorder
Aggressive personality (disorder)
Emotionally unstable personality disorder
Explosive personality (disorder)
Excludes2: *antisocial personality disorder (F60.2)*
F60.4 Histrionic personality disorder
Hysterical personality (disorder)
Psychoinfantile personality (disorder)
F60.5 Obsessive-compulsive personality disorder
Anankastic personality (disorder)
Compulsive personality (disorder)
Obsessional personality (disorder)
Excludes2: *obsessive-compulsive disorder (F42.-)*
F60.6 Avoidant personality disorder
Anxious personality disorder
F60.7 Dependent personality disorder
Asthenic personality (disorder)
Inadequate personality (disorder)
Passive personality (disorder)

+ **F60.8 Other specific personality disorders**
  - **F60.81 Narcissistic personality disorder**
  - **F60.89 Other specific personality disorders**
    - Eccentric personality disorder
    - 'Haltlose' type personality disorder
    - Immature personality disorder
    - Passive-aggressive personality disorder
    - Psychoneurotic personality disorder
    - Self-defeating personality disorder

F60.9 Personality disorder, unspecified
- Character disorder NOS
- Character neurosis NOS
- Pathological personality NOS

F63 Impulse disorders

Excludes2: *habitual excessive use of alcohol or psychoactive substances (F10-F19)*
impulse disorders involving sexual behavior (F65.-)

F63.0 Pathological gambling
- Compulsive gambling
- Gambling disorder
- **Excludes1:** *gambling and betting NOS (Z72.6)*
- **Excludes2:** *excessive gambling by manic patients (F30, F31)*
  gambling in antisocial personality disorder (F60.2)

F63.1 Pyromania
- Pathological fire-setting
- **Excludes2:** *fire-setting (by) (in):*
  adult with antisocial personality disorder (F60.2)
  alcohol or psychoactive substance intoxication (F10-F19)
  conduct disorders (F91.-)
  mental disorders due to known physiological condition (F01-F09)
  schizophrenia (F20.-)

F63.2 Kleptomania
- Pathological stealing
- **Excludes1:** *shoplifting as the reason for observation for suspected mental disorder (Z03.8)*
- **Excludes2:** *depressive disorder with stealing (F31-F33)*
  stealing due to underlying mental condition-code to mental condition
  stealing in mental disorders due to known physiological condition (F01-F09)

F63.3 Trichotillomania
- Hair plucking
- **Excludes2:** *other stereotyped movement disorder (F98.4)*

+ **F63.8 Other impulse disorders**
  - **F63.81 Intermittent explosive disorder**
  - **F63.89 Other impulse disorders**

F63.9 Impulse disorder, unspecified
- Impulse control disorder NOS

F64 Gender identity disorders

AHA CC: 4Q, 2016, 16

F64.0 Transsexualism
- Gender identify disorder in adolescence and adulthood
- Gender dysphoria in adolescents and adults

F64.1 Dual role transvestism
- Use additional code to identify sex reassignment status (Z87.890)
- **Excludes1:** *gender identity disorder in childhood (F64.2)*
- **Excludes2:** *fetishistic transvestism (F65.1)*

• **F64.2 Gender identity disorder of childhood**
- Gender dysphoria in children
- **Excludes1:** *gender identity disorder in adolescence and adulthood (F64.0)*
- **Excludes2:** *sexual maturation disorder (F66)*

F64.8 Other gender identity disorders
- Other specified gender dysphoria

F64.9 Gender identity disorder, unspecified
- Gender dysphoria, unspecified
- Gender-role disorder NOS

F65 Paraphilias

F65.0 Fetishism
- Fetishistic disorder

F65.1 Transvestic fetishism
- Fetishistic transvestism
- Transvestic disorder

F65.2 Exhibitionism
- Exhibitionistic disorder

F65.3 Voyeurism
- Voyeuristic disorder

F65.4 Pedophilia
- Pedophilic disorder

+ **F65.5 Sadomasochism**
  - **F65.50 Sadomasochism, unspecified**
  - **F65.51 Sexual masochism**
    - Sexual masochism disorder
  - **F65.52 Sexual sadism**
    - Sexual sadism disorder

+ **F65.8 Other paraphilias**
  - **F65.81 Frotteurism**
    - Frotteuristic disorder
  - **F65.89 Other paraphilias**
    - Necrophilia
    - Other specified paraphilic disorder

F65.9 Paraphilia, unspecified
- Paraphillic disorder, unspecified
- Sexual deviation NOS

F66 Other sexual disorders

- Sexual maturation disorder
- Sexual relationship disorder

Valid 3-character code, no further characters required

F68 Other disorders of adult personality and behavior

+ **F68.1 Factitious disorder**
  - Compensation neurosis
  - Elaboration of physical symptoms for psychological reasons
  - Hospital hopper syndrome
  - Münchausen's syndrome
  - Peregrinating patient
  - **Excludes2:** *factitial dermatitis (L98.1)*
    person feigning illness (with obvious motivation) (Z76.5)
  - CC **F68.10 Factitious disorder, unspecified**
  - **F68.11 Factitious disorder with predominantly psychological signs and symptoms**
    CC Exclusion see Appendix A PDX collection 0550
  - CC **F68.12 Factitious disorder with predominantly physical signs and symptoms**
    CC Exclusion see Appendix A PDX collection 0551
  - **F68.13 Factitious disorder with combined psychological and physical signs and symptoms**

F68.8 Other specified disorders of adult personality and behavior

• F69 Unspecified disorder of adult personality and behavior

Valid 3-character code, no further characters required

Intellectual Disabilities (F70-F79)

Code first any associated physical or developmental disorders

Excludes1: *borderline intellectual functioning, IQ above 70 to 84 (R41.83)*

F70 Mild intellectual disabilities

- IQ level 50-55 to approximately 70
- Mild mental subnormality

Valid 3-character code, no further characters required

F71 Moderate intellectual disabilities

- IQ level 35-40 to 50-55
- Moderate mental subnormality

Valid 3-character code, no further characters required

CC F72 Severe intellectual disabilities

- IQ 20-25 to 35-40
- Severe mental subnormality

CC Exclusion see Appendix A PDX collection 0558
Valid 3-character code, no further characters required

CC F73 Profound intellectual disabilities

- IQ level below 20-25
- Profound mental subnormality

CC Exclusion see Appendix A PDX collection 0558
Valid 3-character code, no further characters required

F78 Other intellectual disabilities

Valid 3-character code, no further characters required

F79 Unspecified intellectual disabilities

- Mental deficiency NOS
- Mental subnormality NOS

Valid 3-character code, no further characters required

Pervasive and specific developmental disorders (F80-F89)

F80 Specific developmental disorders of speech and language

F80.0 Phonological disorder
Dyslalia
Functional speech articulation disorder
Lalling
Lisping
Phonological developmental disorder
Speech articulation developmental disorder
Speech-sound disorder
Excludes1: *speech articulation impairment due to aphasia NOS (R47.01)*
speech articulation impairment due to apraxia (R48.2)
Excludes2: *speech articulation impairment due to hearing loss (F80.4)*
speech articulation impairment due to intellectual disabilities (F70-F79)
speech articulation impairment with expressive language developmental disorder (F80.1)
speech articulation impairment with mixed receptive expressive language developmental disorder (F80.2)

F80.1 Expressive language disorder
Developmental dysphasia or aphasia, expressive type
Excludes1: *mixed receptive-expressive language disorder (F80.2)*
dysphasia and aphasia NOS (R47.-)
Excludes2: *acquired aphasia with epilepsy [Landau-Kleffner] (G40.80-)*
selective mutism (F94.0)
intellectual disabilities (F70-F79)
pervasive developmental disorders (F84.-)

F80.2 Mixed receptive-expressive language disorder
Developmental dysphasia or aphasia, receptive type
Developmental Wernicke's aphasia
Excludes1: *central auditory processing disorder (H93.25)*
dysphasia or aphasia NOS (R47.-)
expressive language disorder (F80.1)
expressive type dysphasia or aphasia (F80.1)
word deafness (H93.25)
Excludes2: *acquired aphasia with epilepsy [Landau-Kleffner] (G40.80-)*
pervasive developmental disorders (F84.-)
selective mutism (F94.0)
intellectual disabilities (F70-F79)

F80.4 Speech and language development delay due to hearing loss
Code also type of hearing loss (H90.-, H91.-)

\+ **F80.8 Other developmental disorders of speech and language**

F80.81 Childhood onset fluency disorder
Cluttering NOS
Stuttering NOS
Excludes1: *adult onset fluency disorder (F98.5)*
fluency disorder in conditions classified elsewhere (R47.82)
fluency disorder (stuttering) following cerebrovascular disease (I69. with final characters -23)

F80.82 Social pragmatic communication disorder
Excludes1: *Asperger's syndrome (F84.5)*
autistic disorder (F84.0)
AHA CC: 4Q, 2016, 16

F80.89 Other developmental disorders of speech and language
AHA CC: 1Q, 2017, 27-28

F80.9 Developmental disorder of speech and language, unspecified
Communication disorder NOS
Language disorder NOS

F81 Specific developmental disorders of scholastic skills

F81.0 Specific reading disorder
'Backward reading'
Developmental dyslexia
Specific learning disorder, with impairment in reading
Specific reading retardation
Excludes1: *alexia NOS (R48.0)*
dyslexia NOS (R48.0)

F81.2 Mathematics disorder
Developmental acalculia
Developmental arithmetical disorder
Developmental Gerstmann's syndrome
Specific learning disorder, with impairment in mathematics
Excludes1: *acalculia NOS (R48.8)*
Excludes2: *arithmetical difficulties associated with a reading disorder (F81.0)*
arithmetical difficulties associated with a spelling disorder (F81.81)
arithmetical difficulties due to inadequate teachin[g] (Z55.8)

\+ **F81.8 Other developmental disorders of scholastic skills**

F81.81 Disorder of written expression
Specific learning disorder, with impairment in written expression
Specific spelling disorder

F81.89 Other developmental disorders of scholastic skills

F81.9 Developmental disorder of scholastic skills, unspecified
Knowledge acquisition disability NOS
Learning disability NOS
Learning disorder NOS

F82 Specific developmental disorder of motor function

Clumsy child syndrome
Developmental coordination disorder
Developmental dyspraxia
Excludes1: *abnormalities of gait and mobility (R26.-)*
lack of coordination (R27.-)
Excludes2: *lack of coordination secondary to intellectual disabilities (F70-F79)*
Valid 3-character code, no further characters required

F84 Pervasive developmental disorders

Use additional code to identify any associated medical condition and intellectual disabilities.

CC **F84.0 Autistic disorder**
Autism spectrum disorder
Infantile autism
Infantile psychosis
Kanner's syndrome
Excludes1: *Asperger's syndrome (F84.5)*
CC Exclusion see Appendix A PDX collection 0551
AHA CC: 1Q, 2017, 27-28

CC **F84.2 Rett's syndrome**
Excludes1: *Asperger's syndrome (F84.5)*
Autistic disorder (F84.0)
Other childhood disintegrative disorder (F84.3)
CC Exclusion see Appendix A PDX collection 0537

• CC **F84.3 Other childhood disintegrative disorder**
Dementia infantilis
Disintegrative psychosis
Heller's syndrome
Symbiotic psychosis
Use additional code to identify any associated neurological condition.
Excludes1: *Asperger's syndrome (F84.5)*
Autistic disorder (F84.0)
Rett's syndrome (F84.2)
CC Exclusion see Appendix A PDX collection 0551

CC **F84.5 Asperger's syndrome**
Asperger's disorder
Autistic psychopathy
Schizoid disorder of childhood
CC Exclusion see Appendix A PDX collection 0551

CC **F84.8 Other pervasive developmental disorders**
Overactive disorder associated with intellectual disabilities an[d] stereotyped movements
CC Exclusion see Appendix A PDX collection 0551

CC **F84.9 Pervasive developmental disorder, unspecified**
Atypical autism
CC Exclusion see Appendix A PDX collection 0551

F88 Other disorders of psychological development

Developmental agnosia
Global developmental delay
Other specified neurodevelopmental disorder
Valid 3-character code, no further characters required

F89 Unspecified disorder of psychological development

Developmental disorder NOS
Neurodevelopmental disorder NOS
Valid 3-character code, no further characters required

Behavioral and emotional disorders with onset usually occurring in childhood and adolescence (F90-F98)

NOTE Codes within categories F90-F98 may be used regardless of the age of a patient. These disorders generally have onset within the childhood or adolescent years, but may continue throughout life or not be diagnosed until adulthood

F90 Attention-deficit hyperactivity disorders

Includes: attention deficit disorder with hyperactivity
attention deficit syndrome with hyperactivity
Excludes2: *anxiety disorders (F40.-, F41.-)*
mood [affective] disorders (F30-F39)
pervasive developmental disorders (F84.-)
schizophrenia (F20.-)

F90.0 Attention-deficit hyperactivity disorder, predominantly inattentive type
Attention-deficit/hyperactivity disorder, predominantly inattentive presentation

F90.1 Attention-deficit hyperactivity disorder, predominantly hyperactive type
Attention-deficit/hyperactivity disorder, predominantly hyperactive impulsive presentation

F90.2 Attention-deficit hyperactivity disorder, combined type
Attention-deficit/hyperactivity disorder, combined presentation

F90.8 Attention-deficit hyperactivity disorder, other type

F90.9 Attention-deficit hyperactivity disorder, unspecified type
Attention-deficit hyperactivity disorder of childhood or adolescence NOS
Attention-deficit hyperactivity disorder NOS

F91 Conduct disorders

Excludes1: *antisocial behavior (Z72.81-)*
antisocial personality disorder (F60.2)
Excludes2: *conduct problems associated with attention-deficit hyperactivity disorder (F90.-)*
mood [affective] disorders (F30-F39)
pervasive developmental disorders (F84.-)
schizophrenia (F20.-)

F91.0 Conduct disorder confined to family context

F91.1 Conduct disorder, childhood-onset type
Unsocialized conduct disorder
Conduct disorder, solitary aggressive type
Unsocialized aggressive disorder

F91.2 Conduct disorder, adolescent-onset type
Socialized conduct disorder
Conduct disorder, group type

F91.3 Oppositional defiant disorder

F91.8 Other conduct disorders
Other specified conduct disorder
Other specified disruptive disorder

F91.9 Conduct disorder, unspecified
Behavioral disorder NOS
Conduct disorder NOS
Disruptive behavior disorder NOS
Disruptive disorder NOS

F93 Emotional disorders with onset specific to childhood

F93.0 Separation anxiety disorder of childhood
Excludes2: *mood [affective] disorders (F30-F39)*
nonpsychotic mental disorders (F40-F48)
phobic anxiety disorder of childhood (F40.8)
social phobia (F40.1)

F93.8 Other childhood emotional disorders
Identity disorder
Excludes2: *gender identity disorder of childhood (F64.2)*

F93.9 Childhood emotional disorder, unspecified

F94 Disorders of social functioning with onset specific to childhood and adolescence

F94.0 Selective mutism
Elective mutism
Excludes2: *pervasive developmental disorders (F84.-)*
schizophrenia (F20.-)
specific developmental disorders of speech and language (F80.-)
transient mutism as part of separation anxiety in young children (F93.0)

F94.1 Reactive attachment disorder of childhood
Use additional code to identify any associated failure to thrive or growth retardation
Excludes1: *disinhibited attachment disorder of childhood (F94.2)*
normal variation in pattern of selective attachment
Excludes2: *Asperger's syndrome (F84.5)*
maltreatment syndromes (T74.-)
sexual or physical abuse in childhood, resulting in psychosocial problems (Z62.81-)

F94.2 Disinhibited attachment disorder of childhood
Affectionless psychopathy
Institutional syndrome
Excludes1: *reactive attachment disorder of childhood (F94.1)*
Excludes2: *Asperger's syndrome (F84.5)*
attention-deficit hyperactivity disorders (F90.-)
hospitalism in children (F43.2-)

F94.8 Other childhood disorders of social functioning

F94.9 Childhood disorder of social functioning, unspecified

F95 Tic disorder

F95.0 Transient tic disorder
Provisional tic disorder

F95.1 Chronic motor or vocal tic disorder

F95.2 Tourette's disorder
Combined vocal and multiple motor tic disorder [de la Tourette]
Tourette's syndrome

F95.8 Other tic disorders

F95.9 Tic disorder, unspecified
Tic NOS

F98 Other behavioral and emotional disorders with onset usually occurring in childhood and adolescence

Excludes2: *breath-holding spells (R06.89)*
gender identity disorder of childhood (F64.2)
Kleine-Levin syndrome (G47.13)
obsessive-compulsive disorder (F42.-)
sleep disorders not due to a substance or known physiological condition (F51.-)

F98.0 Enuresis not due to a substance or known physiological condition
Enuresis (primary) (secondary) of nonorganic origin
Functional enuresis
Psychogenic enuresis
Urinary incontinence of nonorganic origin
Excludes1: *enuresis NOS (R32)*

F98.1 Encopresis not due to a substance or known physiological condition
Functional encopresis
Incontinence of feces of nonorganic origin
Psychogenic encopresis
Use additional code to identify the cause of any coexisting constipation.
Excludes1: *encopresis NOS (R15.-)*

\+ **F98.2 Other feeding disorders of infancy and childhood**
Excludes1: *feeding difficulties (R63.3)*
Excludes2: *anorexia nervosa and other eating disorders (F50.-)*
feeding problems of newborn (P92.-)
pica of infancy or childhood (F98.3)

F98.21 Rumination disorder of infancy

F98.29 Other feeding disorders of infancy and early childhood

F98.3 Pica of infancy and childhood

F98.4 Stereotyped movement disorders
Stereotype/habit disorder
Excludes1: *abnormal involuntary movements (R25.-)*
Excludes2: *compulsions in obsessive-compulsive disorder (F42.-)*
hair plucking (F63.3)
movement disorders of organic origin (G20-G25)
nail-biting (F98.8)
nose-picking (F98.8)
stereotypies that are part of a broader psychiatric condition (F01-F95)
thumb-sucking (F98.8)
tic disorders (F95.-)
trichotillomania (F63.3)

F98.5 Adult onset fluency disorder

Excludes1: *childhood onset fluency disorder (F80.81)*
dysphasia (R47.02)
fluency disorder in conditions classified elsewhere (R47.82)
fluency disorder (stuttering) following cerebrovascular disease (I69. with final characters -23)
tic disorders (F95.-)

F98.8 Other specified behavioral and emotional disorders with onset usually occurring in childhood and adolescence

Excessive masturbation
Nail-biting
Nose-picking
Thumb-sucking

F98.9 Unspecified behavioral and emotional disorders with onset usually occurring in childhood and adolescence

Unspecified mental disorder (F99)

F99 Mental disorder, not otherwise specified

Mental illness NOS

Excludes1: *unspecified mental disorder due to known physiological condition (F09)*

Valid 3-character code, no further characters required

Chapter 6: Diseases of the Nervous System (G00-G99)

Excludes2: *certain conditions originating in the perinatal period (P04-P96)*
certain infectious and parasitic diseases (A00-B99)
complications of pregnancy, childbirth and the puerperium (O00-O9A)
congenital malformations, deformations, and chromosomal abnormalities (Q00-Q99)
endocrine, nutritional and metabolic diseases (E00-E88)
injury, poisoning and certain other consequences of external causes (S00-T88)
neoplasms (C00-D49)
symptoms, signs and abnormal clinical and laboratory findings, not elsewhere classified (R00-R94)

This chapter contains the following category blocks:

G00-G09	Inflammatory diseases of the central nervous system
G10-G14	Systemic atrophies primarily affecting the central nervous system
G20-G26	Extrapyramidal and movement disorders
G30-G32	Other degenerative diseases of the nervous system
G35-G37	Demyelinating diseases of the central nervous system
G40-G47	Episodic and paroxysmal disorders
G50-G59	Nerve, nerve root and plexus disorders
G60-G65	Polyneuropathies and other disorders of the peripheral nervous system
G70-G73	Diseases of myoneural junction and muscle
G80-G83	Cerebral palsy and other paralytic syndromes
G89-G99	Other disorders of the nervous system

Chapter-Specific Coding Guidelines

In addition to general coding guidelines, there are guidelines for specific diagnoses and/or conditions in the classification. Unless otherwise indicated, these guidelines apply to all health care settings. Please refer to Section II for guidelines on the selection of principal diagnosis.

Chapter 6: Diseases of the Nervous System (G00-G99)

a. Dominant/nondominant side

Codes from category G81, Hemiplegia and hemiparesis, and subcategories, G83.1, Monoplegia of lower limb, G83.2, Monoplegia of upper limb, and G83.3, Monoplegia, unspecified, identify whether the dominant or nondominant side is affected. Should the affected side be documented, but not specified as dominant or nondominant, and the classification system does not indicate a default, code selection is as follows:

- For ambidextrous patients, the default should be dominant.
- If the left side is affected, the default is non-dominant.
- If the right side is affected, the default is dominant.

b. Pain-Category G89

1) General coding information

Codes in category G89, Pain, not elsewhere classified, may be used in conjunction with codes from other categories and chapters to provide more detail about acute or chronic pain and neoplasm-related pain, unless otherwise indicated below.

If the pain is not specified as acute or chronic, post- thoracotomy, post procedural, or neoplasm-related, do not assign codes from category G89.

A code from category G89 should not be assigned if the underlying (definitive) diagnosis is known, unless the reason for the encounter is pain control/management and not management of the underlying condition.

When an admission or encounter is for a procedure aimed at treating the underlying condition (e.g., spinal fusion, kyphoplasty), a code for the underlying condition (e.g., vertebral fracture, spinal stenosis) should be assigned as the principal diagnosis. No code from category G89 should be assigned.

(a) Category G89 Codes as Principal or First-Listed Diagnosis

Category G89 codes are acceptable as principal diagnosis or the first-listed code:

- When pain control or pain management is the reason for the admission/encounter (e.g., a patient with displaced intervertebral disc, nerve impingement and severe back pain presents for injection of steroid into the spinal canal). The underlying cause of the pain should be reported as an additional diagnosis, if known.
- When a patient is admitted for the insertion of a neurostimulator for pain control, assign the appropriate pain code as the principal or first-listed diagnosis. When an admission or encounter is for a procedure aimed at treating the underlying condition and a neurostimulator is inserted for pain control during the same admission/encounter, a code for the underlying condition should be assigned as the principal diagnosis and the appropriate pain code should be assigned as a secondary diagnosis.

(b) Use of Category G89 Codes in Conjunction with Site Specific Pain Codes

(i) Assigning Category G89 and Site-Specific Pain Codes

Codes from category G89 may be used in conjunction with codes that identify the site of pain (including codes from chapter 18) if the category G89 code provides additional information. For example, if the code describes the site of the pain, but does not fully describe whether the pain is acute or chronic, then both codes should be assigned.

(ii) Sequencing of Category G89 Codes with Site- Specific Pain Codes

The sequencing of category G89 codes with site-specific pain codes (including chapter 18 codes), is dependent on the circumstances of the encounter/admission as follows:

- If the encounter is for pain control or pain management, assign the code from category G89 followed by the code identifying the specific site of pain (e.g., encounter for pain management for acute neck pain from trauma is assigned code G89.11, Acute pain due to trauma, followed by code M54.2, Cervicalgia, to identify the site of pain).
- If the encounter is for any other reason except pain control or pain management, and a related definitive diagnosis has not been established (confirmed) by the provider, assign the code for the specific site of pain first, followed by the appropriate code from category G89.

2) Pain due to devices, implants and grafts

See Section I.C.19. Pain due to medical devices

3) Postoperative Pain

The provider's documentation should be used to guide the coding of postoperative pain, as well *as Section III. Reporting Additional Diagnoses and Section IV. Diagnostic Coding* and *Reporting in the Outpatient Setting.*

The default for post-thoracotomy and other postoperative pain not specified as acute or chronic is the code for the acute form.

Routine or expected postoperative pain immediately after surgery should not be coded.

(a) Postoperative pain not associated with specific postoperative complication

Postoperative pain not associated with a specific postoperative complication is assigned to the appropriate postoperative pain code in category G89.

(b) Postoperative pain associated with specific postoperative complication

Postoperative pain associated with a specific postoperative complication (such as painful wire sutures) is assigned to the appropriate code(s) found in Chapter 19, Injury, poisoning, and certain other consequences of external causes. If appropriate, use additional code(s) from category G89 to identify acute or chronic pain (G89.18 or G89.28).

4) Chronic pain

Chronic pain is classified to subcategory G89.2. There is no time frame defining when pain becomes chronic pain. The provider's documentation should be used to guide use of these codes.

5) Neoplasm Related Pain

Code G89.3 is assigned to pain documented as being related, associated or due to cancer, primary or secondary malignancy, or tumor. This code is assigned regardless of whether the pain is acute or chronic.

This code may be assigned as the principal or first- listed code when the stated reason for the admission/encounter is documented as pain control/pain management. The underlying neoplasm should be reported as an additional diagnosis.

When the reason for the admission/encounter is management of the neoplasm and the pain associated with the neoplasm is also documented, code G89.3 may be assigned as an additional diagnosis. It is not necessary to assign an additional code for the site of the pain.

See Section I.C.2 for instructions on the sequencing of neoplasms for all other stated reasons for the admission/encounter (except for pain control/pain management).

6) Chronic pain syndrome

Central pain syndrome (G89.0) and chronic pain syndrome (G89.4) are different than the term "chronic pain," and therefore codes should only be used when the provider has specifically documented this condition.

See Section I.C.5. Pain disorders related to psychological factors

Inflammatory diseases of the central nervous system (G00-G09)

G00 Bacterial meningitis, not elsewhere classified

Includes: bacterial arachnoiditis
bacterial leptomeningitis
bacterial meningitis
bacterial pachymeningitis

Excludes1: *bacterial meningoencephalitis (G04.2)*
bacterial meningomyelitis (G04.2)

MCC **G00.0 Hemophilus meningitis**
Meningitis due to Hemophilus influenzae
MCC Exclusion see Appendix A PDX collection 0207

MCC **G00.1 Pneumococcal meningitis**
Meningtitis due to Streptococcal pneumoniae
MCC Exclusion see Appendix A PDX collection 0207

MCC **G00.2 Streptococcal meningitis**
Use additional code to further identify organism (B95.0-B95.5)
MCC Exclusion see Appendix A PDX collection 0207

MCC **G00.3 Staphylococcal meningitis**
Use additional code to further identify organism (B95.61-B95.8)
MCC Exclusion see Appendix A PDX collection 0207

MCC **G00.8 Other bacterial meningitis**
Meningitis due to Escherichia coli
Meningitis due to Friedländer's bacillus
Meningitis due to Klebsiella
Use additional code to further identify organism (B96.-)
MCC Exclusion see Appendix A PDX collection 0207

MCC **G00.9 Bacterial meningitis, unspecified**
Meningitis due to gram-negative bacteria, unspecified
Purulent meningitis NOS
Pyogenic meningitis NOS
Suppurative meningitis NOS
MCC Exclusion see Appendix A PDX collection 0207

MCC **G01 Meningitis in bacterial diseases classified elsewhere**

Code first underlying disease

Excludes1: *meningitis (in):*
gonococcal (A54.81)
leptospirosis (A27.81)
listeriosis (A32.11)
Lyme disease (A69.21)
meningococcal (A39.0)
neurosyphilis (A52.13)
tuberculosis (A17.0)
meningoencephalitis and meningomyelitis in bacterial diseases classified elsewhere (G05)

MCC Exclusion see Appendix A PDX collection 0207
Valid 3-character code, no further characters required

MCC **G02 Meningitis in other infectious and parasitic diseases classified elsewhere**

Code first underlying disease, such as:
African trypanosomiasis (B56.-)
poliovirus infection (A80.-)

Excludes1: *candidal meningitis (B37.5)*
coccidioidomycosis meningitis (B38.4)
cryptococcal meningitis (B45.1)
herpesviral [herpes simplex] meningitis (B00.3)
infectious mononucleosis complicated by meningitis (B27.- with fourth character 2)
measles complicated by meningitis (B05.1)
meningoencephalitis and meningomyelitis in other infectious and parasitic diseases classified elsewhere (G05)
mumps meningitis (B26.1)
rubella meningitis (B06.02)
varicella [chickenpox] meningitis (B01.0)
zoster meningitis (B02.1)

MCC Exclusion see Appendix A PDX collection 0559
Valid 3-character code, no further characters required

G03 Meningitis due to other and unspecified causes

Includes: arachnoiditis NOS
leptomeningitis NOS
meningitis NOS
pachymeningitis NOS

Excludes1: *meningoencephalitis (G04.-)*
meningomyelitis (G04.-)

MCC **G03.0 Nonpyogenic meningitis**
Aseptic meningitis
Nonbacterial meningitis
MCC Exclusion see Appendix A PDX collection 0207

CC **G03.1 Chronic meningitis**
CC Exclusion see Appendix A PDX collection 0207

CC **G03.2 Benign recurrent meningitis [Mollaret]**
CC Exclusion see Appendix A PDX collection 0140

MCC **G03.8 Meningitis due to other specified causes**
MCC Exclusion see Appendix A PDX collection 0207

MCC **G03.9 Meningitis, unspecified**
Arachnoiditis (spinal) NOS
MCC Exclusion see Appendix A PDX collection 0207

G04 Encephalitis, myelitis and encephalomyelitis

Includes: acute ascending myelitis
meningoencephalitis
meningomyelitis

Excludes1: *encephalopathy NOS (G93.40)*

Excludes2: *acute transverse myelitis (G37.3-)*
alcoholic encephalopathy (G31.2)
benign myalgic encephalomyelitis (G93.3)
multiple sclerosis (G35)
subacute necrotizing myelitis (G37.4)
toxic encephalitis (G92)
toxic encephalopathy (G92)

\+ **G04.0 Acute disseminated encephalitis and encephalomyelitis (ADEM)**

Excludes1: *acute necrotizing hemorrhagic encephalopathy (G04.3-)*
other noninfectious acute disseminated encephalomyelitis (noninfectious ADEM) (G04.81)

MCC **G04.00 Acute disseminated encephalitis and encephalomyelitis, unspecified**
MCC Exclusion see Appendix A PDX collection 0560

MCC **G04.01 Postinfectious acute disseminated encephalitis and encephalomyelitis (postinfectious ADEM)**
Excludes1: *post chickenpox encephalitis (B01.1)*
post measles encephalitis (B05.0)
post measles myelitis (B05.1)
MCC Exclusion see Appendix A PDX collection 0560

MCC **G04.02 Postimmunization acute disseminated encephalitis myelitis and encephalomyelitis**
Encephalitis, post immunization
Encephalomyelitis, post immunization
Use additional code to identify the vaccine (T50.A-, T50.B-, T50.Z-)
No MCC Exclusions

CC **G04.1 Tropical spastic paraplegia**
CC Exclusion see Appendix A PDX collection 0561

MCC **G04.2 Bacterial meningoencephalitis and meningomyelitis, not elsewhere classified**
MCC Exclusion see Appendix A PDX collection 0207

\+ **G04.3 Acute necrotizing hemorrhagic encephalopathy**
Excludes1: *acute disseminated encephalitis and encephalomyelitis (G04.0-)*

MCC **G04.30 Acute necrotizing hemorrhagic encephalopathy, unspecified**
No MCC Exclusions

MCC **G04.31 Postinfectious acute necrotizing hemorrhagic encephalopathy**
MCC Exclusion see Appendix A PDX collection 0560

MCC **G04.32 Postimmunization acute necrotizing hemorrhagic encephalopathy**
Use additional code to identify the vaccine (T50.A-, T50.B-, T50.Z-)
No MCC Exclusions

MCC **G04.39 Other acute necrotizing hemorrhagic encephalopathy**
Code also underlying etiology, if applicable
No MCC Exclusions

\+ **G04.8 Other encephalitis, myelitis and encephalomyelitis**
Code also any associated seizure (G40.-, R56.9)

MCC **G04.81 Other encephalitis and encephalomyelitis**
Noninfectious acute disseminated encephalomyelitis (noninfectious ADEM)
MCC Exclusion see Appendix A PDX collection 0560

MCC **G04.89 Other myelitis**
MCC Exclusion see Appendix A PDX collection 0560

\+ **G04.9 Encephalitis, myelitis and encephalomyelitis, unspecified**

MCC **G04.90 Encephalitis and encephalomyelitis, unspecified**
Ventriculitis (cerebral) NOS
MCC Exclusion see Appendix A PDX collection 0562

MCC **G04.91 Myelitis, unspecified**
MCC Exclusion see Appendix A PDX collection 0562

G05 Encephalitis, myelitis and encephalomyelitis in diseases classified elsewhere

Code first underlying disease, such as:
human immunodeficiency virus [HIV] disease (B20)
poliovirus (A80.-)
suppurative otitis media (H66.01-H66.4)
trichinellosis (B75)

Excludes1: *adenoviral encephalitis, myelitis and encephalomyelitis (A85.1)*
congenital toxoplasmosis encephalitis, myelitis and encephalomyelitis (P37.1)
cytomegaloviral encephalitis, myelitis and encephalomyelitis (B25.8)
encephalitis, myelitis and encephalomyelitis (in) measles (B05.0)
encephalitis, myelitis and encephalomyelitis (in) systemic lupus erythematosus (M32.19)
enteroviral encephalitis, myelitis and encephalomyelitis (A85.0)
eosinophilic meningoencephalitis (B83.2)
herpesviral [herpes simplex] encephalitis, myelitis and encephalomyelitis (B00.4)
listerial encephalitis, myelitis and encephalomyelitis (A32.12)
meningococcal encephalitis, myelitis and encephalomyelitis (A39.81)
mumps encephalitis, myelitis and encephalomyelitis (B26.2)
postchickenpox encephalitis, myelitis and encephalomyelitis (B01.1-)
rubella encephalitis, myelitis and encephalomyelitis (B06.01)
toxoplasmosis encephalitis, myelitis and encephalomyelitis (B58.2)
zoster encephalitis, myelitis and encephalomyelitis (B02.0)

MCC **G05.3 Encephalitis and encephalomyelitis in diseases classified elsewhere**
Meningoencephalitis in diseases classified elsewhere
MCC Exclusion see Appendix A PDX collection 0560

MCC **G05.4 Myelitis in diseases classified elsewhere**
Meningomyelitis in diseases classified elsewhere
MCC Exclusion see Appendix A PDX collection 0560

G06 Intracranial and intraspinal abscess and granuloma

Use additional code (B95-B97) to identify infectious agent.

MCC **G06.0 Intracranial abscess and granuloma**
Brain [any part] abscess (embolic)
Cerebellar abscess (embolic)
Cerebral abscess (embolic)
Intracranial epidural abscess or granuloma
Intracranial extradural abscess or granuloma
Intracranial subdural abscess or granuloma
Otogenic abscess (embolic)
Excludes1: *tuberculous intracranial abscess and granuloma (A17.81)*
MCC Exclusion see Appendix A PDX collection 0563

MCC **G06.1 Intraspinal abscess and granuloma**
Abscess (embolic) of spinal cord [any part]
Intraspinal epidural abscess or granuloma
Intraspinal extradural abscess or granuloma
Intraspinal subdural abscess or granuloma
Excludes1: *tuberculous intraspinal abscess and granuloma (A17.81)*
MCC Exclusion see Appendix A PDX collection 0564

MCC **G06.2 Extradural and subdural abscess, unspecified**
MCC Exclusion see Appendix A PDX collection 0565

G07 MCC **Intracranial and intraspinal abscess and granuloma in diseases classified elsewhere**

Code first underlying disease such as:
schistosomiasis granuloma of brain (B65.-)

Excludes1: *abscess of brain:*
amebic (A06.6)
chromomycotic (B43.1)
gonococcal (A54.82)
tuberculous (A17.81)
tuberculoma of meninges (A17.1)
MCC Exclusion see Appendix A PDX collection 0565
Valid 3-character code, no further characters required

MCC **G08 Intracranial and intraspinal phlebitis and thrombophlebitis**

Septic embolism of intracranial or intraspinal venous sinuses and veins
Septic endophlebitis of intracranial or intraspinal venous sinuses and veins
Septic phlebitis of intracranial or intraspinal venous sinuses and veins
Septic thrombophlebitis of intracranial or intraspinal venous sinuses and veins
Septic thrombosis of intracranial or intraspinal venous sinuses and veins
Excludes1: *intracranial phlebitis and thrombophlebitis complicating:*
abortion, ectopic or molar pregnancy (O00-O07, O08.7)
pregnancy, childbirth and the puerperium (O22.5, O87.3)
nonpyogenic intracranial phlebitis and thrombophlebitis (I67.6)
Excludes2: *intracranial phlebitis and thrombophlebitis complicating nonpyogenic intraspinal phlebitis and thrombophlebitis (G95.1)*
MCC Exclusion see Appendix A PDX collection 0565
Valid 3-character code, no further characters required

G09 Sequelae of inflammatory diseases of central nervous system

NOTE Category G09 is to be used to indicate conditions whose primary classification is to G00-G08 as the cause of sequelae, themselves classifiable elsewhere. The 'sequelae' include conditions specified as residuals.

Code first condition resulting from (sequela) of inflammatory diseases of central nervous system
Valid 3-character code, no further characters required

Systemic atrophies primarily affecting the central nervous system (G10-G14)

CC **G10 Huntington's disease**
Huntington's chorea
Huntington's dementia
Code also dementia in other diseases classified elsewhere without behavioral disturbance (F02.80)
CC Exclusion see Appendix A PDX collection 0566
Valid 3-character code, no further characters required

G11 Hereditary ataxia

Excludes2: *cerebral palsy (G80.-)*
hereditary and idiopathic neuropathy (G60.-)
metabolic disorders (E70-E88)

CC **G11.0 Congenital nonprogressive ataxia**
CC Exclusion see Appendix A PDX collection 0567

CC **G11.1 Early-onset cerebellar ataxia**
Early-onset cerebellar ataxia with essential tremor
Early-onset cerebellar ataxia with myoclonus [Hunt's ataxia]
Early-onset cerebellar ataxia with retained tendon reflexes
Friedreich's ataxia (autosomal recessive)
X-linked recessive spinocerebellar ataxia
CC Exclusion see Appendix A PDX collection 0567

• CC **G11.2 Late-onset cerebellar ataxia**
CC Exclusion see Appendix A PDX collection 0567

CC **G11.3 Cerebellar ataxia with defective DNA repair**
Ataxia telangiectasia [Louis-Bar]
Excludes2: *Cockayne's syndrome (Q87.1)*
other disorders of purine and pyrimidine metabolism (E79.-)
xeroderma pigmentosum (Q82.1)
CC Exclusion see Appendix A PDX collection 0567

CC **G11.4 Hereditary spastic paraplegia**
CC Exclusion see Appendix A PDX collection 0568

CC **G11.8 Other hereditary ataxias**
CC Exclusion see Appendix A PDX collection 0567

CC **G11.9 Hereditary ataxia, unspecified**
Hereditary cerebellar ataxia NOS
Hereditary cerebellar degeneration
Hereditary cerebellar disease
Hereditary cerebellar syndrome
CC Exclusion see Appendix A PDX collection 0569

G12 Spinal muscular atrophy and related syndromes

CC **G12.0 Infantile spinal muscular atrophy, type I [Werdnig-Hoffman]**
CC Exclusion see Appendix A PDX collection 0570

CC **G12.1 Other inherited spinal muscular atrophy**
Adult form spinal muscular atrophy
Childhood form, type II spinal muscular atrophy
Distal spinal muscular atrophy
Juvenile form, type III spinal muscular atrophy [Kugelberg-Welander]
Progressive bulbar palsy of childhood [Fazio-Londe]
Scapuloperoneal form spinal muscular atrophy
CC Exclusion see Appendix A PDX collection 0570

+ **G12.2 Motor neuron disease**

CC **G12.20 Motor neuron disease, unspecified**
CC Exclusion see Appendix A PDX collection 0570

• CC **G12.21 Amyotrophic lateral sclerosis**
CC Exclusion see Appendix A PDX collection 0570

CC **G12.22 Progressive bulbar palsy**
CC Exclusion see Appendix A PDX collection 0570

CC **G12.23 Primary lateral sclerosis**
CC Exclusion see Appendix A PDX collection 0570

CC **G12.24 Familial motor neuron disease**
CC Exclusion see Appendix A PDX collection 0570

CC **G12.25 Progressive spinal muscle atrophy**
CC Exclusion see Appendix A PDX collection 0570

CC **G12.29 Other motor neuron disease**
CC Exclusion see Appendix A PDX collection 0570

CC **G12.8 Other spinal muscular atrophies and related syndromes**
CC Exclusion see Appendix A PDX collection 0570

CC **G12.9 Spinal muscular atrophy, unspecified**
CC Exclusion see Appendix A PDX collection 0570

G13 Systemic atrophies primarily affecting central nervous system in diseases classified elsewhere

G13.0 Paraneoplastic neuromyopathy and neuropathy
Carcinomatous neuromyopathy
Sensorial paraneoplastic neuropathy [Denny Brown]
Code first underlying neoplasm (C00-D49)

G13.1 Other systemic atrophy primarily affecting central nervous system in neoplastic disease
Paraneoplastic limbic encephalopathy
Code first underlying neoplasm (C00-D49)

G13.2 Systemic atrophy primarily affecting the central nervous system in myxedema
Code first underlying disease, such as:
hypothyroidism (E03.-)
myxedematous congenital iodine deficiency (E00.1)

G13.8 Systemic atrophy primarily affecting central nervous system in other diseases classified elsewhere
Code first underlying disease

G14 Postpolio syndrome

Includes: postpolio myelitic syndrome
Excludes1: *sequelae of poliomyelitis (B91)*
Valid 3-character code, no further characters required

Extrapyramidal and movement disorders (G20-G26)

G20 Parkinson's disease

Hemiparkinsonism
Idiopathic Parkinsonism or Parkinson's disease
Paralysis agitans
Parkinsonism or Parkinson's disease NOS
Primary Parkinsonism or Parkinson's disease
Excludes1: *dementia with Parkinsonism (G31.83)*
AHA CC: 2Q, 2016, 6-7; 2Q, 2017, 7-8
Valid 3-character code, no further characters required

G21 Secondary parkinsonism

Excludes1: *dementia with Parkinsonism (G31.83)*
Huntington's disease (G10)
Shy-Drager syndrome (G90.3)
syphilitic Parkinsonism (A52.19)

MCC **G21.0 Malignant neuroleptic syndrome**
Use additional code for adverse effect, if applicable, to identify drug (T43.3X5, T43.4X5, T43.505, T43.595)
Excludes1: *neuroleptic induced parkinsonism (G21.11)*
MCC Exclusion see Appendix A PDX collection 0571

+ **G21.1 Other drug-induced secondary parkinsonism**

CC **G21.11 Neuroleptic induced parkinsonism**
Use additional code for adverse effect, if applicable, to identify drug (T43.3X5, T43.4X5, T43.505, T43.59
Excludes1: *malignant neuroleptic syndrome (G21.0)*
CC Exclusion see Appendix A PDX collection 0572

CC **G21.19 Other drug induced secondary parkinsonism**
Other medication-induced parkinsonism
Use additional code for adverse effect, if applicable, to identify drug (T36-T50 with fifth or sixth character
CC Exclusion see Appendix A PDX collection 0572

CC **G21.2 Secondary parkinsonism due to other external agents**
Code first (T51-T65) to identify external agent
CC Exclusion see Appendix A PDX collection 0572

CC **G21.3 Postencephalitic parkinsonism**
CC Exclusion see Appendix A PDX collection 0572

G21.4 Vascular parkinsonism

CC **G21.8 Other secondary parkinsonism**
CC Exclusion see Appendix A PDX collection 0572

CC **G21.9 Secondary parkinsonism, unspecified**
CC Exclusion see Appendix A PDX collection 0572

G23 Other degenerative diseases of basal ganglia

Excludes2: *multi-system degeneration of the autonomic nervous syste (G90.3)*

CC **G23.0 Hallervorden-Spatz disease**
Pigmentary pallidal degeneration
CC Exclusion see Appendix A PDX collection 0573

CC **G23.1 Progressive supranuclear ophthalmoplegia [Steele-Richardson-Olszewski]**
Progressive supranuclear palsy
CC Exclusion see Appendix A PDX collection 0573

CC **G23.2 Striatonigral degeneration**
CC Exclusion see Appendix A PDX collection 0573

CC **G23.8 Other specified degenerative diseases of basal ganglia**
Calcification of basal ganglia
CC Exclusion see Appendix A PDX collection 0573

CC **G23.9 Degenerative disease of basal ganglia, unspecified**
CC Exclusion see Appendix A PDX collection 0573

G24 Dystonia

Includes: dyskinesia
Excludes2: *athetoid cerebral palsy (G80.3)*

+ **G24.0 Drug induced dystonia**
Use additional code code for adverse effect, if applicable, to identify drug (T36-T50 with fifth or sixth character 5)

G24.01 Drug induced subacute dyskinesia
Drug induced blepharospasm
Drug induced orofacial dyskinesia
Neuroleptic induced tardive dyskinesia
Tardive dyskinesia

CC **G24.02 Drug induced acute dystonia**
Acute dystonic reaction to drugs
Neuroleptic induced acute dystonia
CC Exclusion see Appendix A PDX collection 0574

CC **G24.09 Other drug induced dystonia**
CC Exclusion see Appendix A PDX collection 0574

G24.1 Genetic torsion dystonia
Dystonia deformans progressiva
Dystonia musculorum deformans
Familial torsion dystonia
Idiopathic familial dystonia
Idiopathic (torsion) dystonia NOS
(Schwalbe-) Ziehen-Oppenheim disease

CC **G24.2 Idiopathic nonfamilial dystonia**
CC Exclusion see Appendix A PDX collection 0574

G24.3 Spasmodic torticollis
Excludes1: *congenital torticollis (Q68.0)*
hysterical torticollis (F44.4)
ocular torticollis (R29.891)
psychogenic torticollis (F45.8)
torticollis NOS (M43.6)
traumatic recurrent torticollis (S13.4)

G24.4 Idiopathic orofacial dystonia
Orofacial dyskinesia
Excludes1: *drug induced orofacial dyskinesia (G24.01)*

G24.5 Blepharospasm
Excludes1: *drug induced blepharospasm (G24.01)*

CC **G24.8 Other dystonia**
Acquired torsion dystonia NOS
CC Exclusion see Appendix A PDX collection 0574

G24.9 Dystonia, unspecified
Dyskinesia NOS

G25 Other extrapyramidal and movement disorders

Excludes2: *sleep related movement disorders (G47.6-)*

G25.0 Essential tremor
Familial tremor
Excludes1: *tremor NOS (R25.1)*

G25.1 Drug-induced tremor
Use additional code for adverse effect, if applicable, to identify drug (T36-T50 with fifth or sixth character 5)

G25.2 Other specified forms of tremor
Intention tremor

G25.3 Myoclonus
Drug-induced myoclonus
Palatal myoclonus
Use additional code for adverse effect, if applicable, to identify drug (T36-T50 with fifth or sixth character 5)
Excludes1: *facial myokymia (G51.4)*
myoclonic epilepsy (G40.-)

G25.4 Drug-induced chorea
Use additional code for adverse effect, if applicable, to identify drug (T36-T50 with fifth or sixth character 5)

G25.5 Other chorea
Chorea NOS
Excludes1: *chorea NOS with heart involvement (I02.0)*
Huntington's chorea (G10)
rheumatic chorea (I02.-)
Sydenham's chorea (I02.-)

+ **G25.6 Drug induced tics and other tics of organic origin**

G25.61 Drug induced tics
Use additional code for adverse effect, if applicable, to identify drug (T36-T50 with fifth or sixth character 5)

G25.69 Other tics of organic origin
Excludes1: *habit spasm (F95.9)*
tic NOS (F95.9)
Tourette's syndrome (F95.2)

+ **G25.7 Other and unspecified drug induced movement disorders**
Use additional code for adverse effect, if applicable, to identify drug (T36-T50 with fifth or sixth character 5)

G25.70 Drug induced movement disorder, unspecified

G25.71 Drug induced akathisia
Drug induced acathisia
Neuroleptic induced acute akathisia
Tardive akathisia

G25.79 Other drug induced movement disorders

+ **G25.8 Other specified extrapyramidal and movement disorders**

G25.81 Restless legs syndrome

CC **G25.82 Stiff-man syndrome**
CC Exclusion see Appendix A PDX collection 0575

G25.83 Benign shuddering attacks

G25.89 Other specified extrapyramidal and movement disorders

CC **G25.9 Extrapyramidal and movement disorder, unspecified**
CC Exclusion see Appendix A PDX collection 0575

G26 Extrapyramidal and movement disorders in diseases classified elsewhere

Code first underlying disease
Valid 3-character code, no further characters required

Other degenerative diseases of the nervous system (G30-G32)

G30 Alzheimer's disease

Includes: Alzheimer's dementia senile and presenile forms
Use additional code to identify:
delirium, if applicable (F05)
dementia with behavioral disturbance (F02.81)
dementia without behavioral disturbance (F02.80)
Excludes1: *senile degeneration of brain NEC (G31.1)*
senile dementia NOS (F03)
senility NOS (R41.81)

G30.0 Alzheimer's disease with early onset

• **G30.1 Alzheimer's disease with late onset**

G30.8 Other Alzheimer's disease

G30.9 Alzheimer's disease, unspecified
AHA CC: 4Q, 2012, 95-96; 2Q, 2016, 6; 1Q, 2017, 43-44

G31 Other degenerative diseases of nervous system, not elsewhere classified

Use additional code to identify:
dementia with behavioral disturbance (F02.81)
dementia without behavioral disturbance (F02.80)
Excludes2: *Reye's syndrome (G93.7)*

+ **G31.0 Frontotemporal dementia**

G31.01 Pick's disease
Primary progressive aphasia
Progressive isolated aphasia

G31.09 Other frontotemporal dementia
Frontal dementia

G31.1 Senile degeneration of brain, not elsewhere classified
Excludes1: *Alzheimer's disease (G30.-)*
senility NOS (R41.81)

G31.2 Degeneration of nervous system due to alcohol
Alcoholic cerebellar ataxia
Alcoholic cerebellar degeneration
Alcoholic cerebral degeneration
Alcoholic encephalopathy
Dysfunction of the autonomic nervous system due to alcohol
Code also associated alcoholism (F10.-)

+ **G31.8 Other specified degenerative diseases of nervous system**

CC **G31.81 Alpers disease**
Grey-matter degeneration
CC Exclusion see Appendix A PDX collection 0537

CC **G31.82 Leigh's disease**
Subacute necrotizing encephalopathy
CC Exclusion see Appendix A PDX collection 0537

G31.83 Dementia with Lewy bodies
Dementia with Parkinsonism
Lewy body dementia
Lewy body disease
AHA CC: 4Q, 2016, 141

G31.84 Mild cognitive impairment, so stated
Mild neurocognitive disorder
Excludes1: *age related cognitive decline (R41.81)*
altered mental status (R41.82)
cerebral degeneration (G31.9)
change in mental status (R41.82)
cognitive deficits following (sequelae of) cerebral hemorrhage or infarction (I69.01-, I69.11-, I69.21-, I69.31-, I69.81-, I69.91-)
cognitive impairment due to intracranial or head injury (S06.-)
dementia (F01.-, F02.-, F03)
mild memory disturbance (F06.8)
neurologic neglect syndrome (R41.4)
personality change, nonpsychotic (F68.8)

G31.85 Corticobasal degeneration

G31.89 Other specified degenerative diseases of nervous system

G31.9 Degenerative disease of nervous system, unspecified

G32 Other degenerative disorders of nervous system in diseases classified elsewhere

CC **G32.0 Subacute combined degeneration of spinal cord in diseases classified elsewhere**
Dana-Putnam syndrome
Sclerosis of spinal cord (combined) (dorsolateral) (posterolateral)
Code first underlying disease, such as:
anemia (D51.9)
dietary (D51.3)
pernicious (D51.0)
vitamin B12 deficiency (E53.8)
Excludes1: *syphilitic combined degeneration of spinal cord (A52.11)*
CC Exclusion see Appendix A PDX collection 0576

+ **G32.8 Other specified degenerative disorders of nervous system in diseases classified elsewhere**
  Code first underlying disease, such as:
  amyloidosis cerebral degeneration (E85.-)
  cerebral degeneration (due to) hypothyroidism (E00.0-E03.9)
  cerebral degeneration (due to) neoplasm (C00-D49)
  cerebral degeneration (due to) vitamin B deficiency, except thiamine (E52-E53.-)
  non-celiac gluten ataxia (M35.9)
  Excludes1: *superior hemorrhagic polioencephalitis [Wernicke's encephalopathy] (E51.2)*

CC **G32.81 Cerebellar ataxia in diseases classified elsewhere**
  Code first underlying disease, such as:
  celiac disease (with gluten ataxia) (K90.0)
  cerebellar ataxia (in) neoplastic disease (paraneoplastic cerebellar degeneration) (C00-D49)
  non-celiac gluten ataxia (M35.9)
  Excludes1: *systemic atrophy primarily affecting the central nervous system in alcoholic cerebellar ataxia (G31.2)*
  systemic atrophy primarily affecting the central nervous system in myxedema (G13.2)
  CC Exclusion see Appendix A PDX collection 0567

G32.89 Other specified degenerative disorders of nervous system in diseases classified elsewhere
  Degenerative encephalopathy in diseases classified elsewhere

Demyelinating diseases of the central nervous system (G35-G37)

G35 Multiple sclerosis
  Disseminated multiple sclerosis
  Generalized multiple sclerosis
  Multiple sclerosis NOS
  Multiple sclerosis of brain stem
  Multiple sclerosis of cord
  Valid 3-character code, no further characters required

G36 Other acute disseminated demyelination
  Excludes1: *postinfectious encephalitis and encephalomyelitis NOS (G04.01)*

CC **G36.0 Neuromyelitis optica [Devic]**
  Demyelination in optic neuritis
  Excludes1: *optic neuritis NOS (H46)*
  CC Exclusion see Appendix A PDX collection 0577

CC **G36.1 Acute and subacute hemorrhagic leukoencephalitis [Hurst]**
  CC Exclusion see Appendix A PDX collection 0578

CC **G36.8 Other specified acute disseminated demyelination**
  CC Exclusion see Appendix A PDX collection 0578

CC **G36.9 Acute disseminated demyelination, unspecified**
  CC Exclusion see Appendix A PDX collection 0578

G37 Other demyelinating diseases of central nervous system

CC **G37.0 Diffuse sclerosis of central nervous system**
  Periaxial encephalitis
  Schilder's disease
  Excludes1: *X linked adrenoleukodystrophy (E71.52-)*
  CC Exclusion see Appendix A PDX collection 0579

CC **G37.1 Central demyelination of corpus callosum**
  CC Exclusion see Appendix A PDX collection 0578

CC **G37.2 Central pontine myelinolysis**
  CC Exclusion see Appendix A PDX collection 0578

CC **G37.3 Acute transverse myelitis in demyelinating disease of central nervous system**
  Acute transverse myelitis NOS
  Acute transverse myelopathy
  Excludes1: *multiple sclerosis (G35)*
  neuromyelitis optica [Devic] (G36.0)
  CC Exclusion see Appendix A PDX collection 0580

MCC **G37.4 Subacute necrotizing myelitis of central nervous system**
  MCC Exclusion see Appendix A PDX collection 0562

CC **G37.5 Concentric sclerosis [Balo] of central nervous system**
  CC Exclusion see Appendix A PDX collection 0579

CC **G37.8 Other specified demyelinating diseases of central nervous system**
  CC Exclusion see Appendix A PDX collection 0578

CC **G37.9 Demyelinating disease of central nervous system, unspecified**
  CC Exclusion see Appendix A PDX collection 0578

Episodic and paroxysmal disorders (G40-G47)

G40 Epilepsy and recurrent seizures
  NOTE the following terms are to be considered equivalent to intractable: pharmacoresistant (pharmacologically resistant), treatment resistant, refractory (medically) and poorly controlled
  Excludes1: *conversion disorder with seizures (F44.5)*
  convulsions NOS (R56.9)
  post traumatic seizures (R56.1)
  seizure (convulsive) NOS (R56.9)
  seizure of newborn (P90)
  Excludes2: *hippocampal sclerosis (G93.81)*
  mesial temporal sclerosis (G93.81)
  temporal sclerosis (G93.81)
  Todd's paralysis (G83.84)

+ **G40.0 Localization-related (focal) (partial) idiopathic epilepsy and epileptic syndromes with seizures of localized onset**
  Benign childhood epilepsy with centrotemporal EEG spikes
  Childhood epilepsy with occipital EEG paroxysms
  Excludes1: *adult onset localization-related epilepsy (G40.1-, G40.2-)*

+ **G40.00 Localization-related (focal) (partial) idiopathic epilepsy and epileptic syndromes with seizures of localized onset, not intractable**
  Localization-related (focal) (partial) idiopathic epilepsy and epileptic syndromes with seizures of localized onset without intractability

CC **G40.001 Localization-related (focal) (partial) idiopathic epilepsy and epileptic syndromes with seizures of localized onset not intractable, with status epilepticus**
  CC Exclusion see Appendix A PDX collection 0581

CC **G40.009 Localization-related (focal) (partial) idiopathic epilepsy and epileptic syndromes with seizures of localized onset, not intractable, without status epilepticus**
  Localization-related (focal) (partial) idiopathic epilepsy and epileptic syndromes with seizures of localized onset NOS
  CC Exclusion see Appendix A PDX collection 0581

+ **G40.01 Localization-related (focal) (partial) idiopathic epilepsy and epileptic syndromes with seizures of localized onset, intractable**

CC **G40.011 Localization-related (focal) (partial) idiopathic epilepsy and epileptic syndromes with seizures of localized onset intractable, with status epilepticus**
  CC Exclusion see Appendix A PDX collection 0582

CC **G40.019 Localization-related (focal) (partial) idiopathic epilepsy and epileptic syndromes with seizures of localized onset, intractable, without status epilepticus**
  CC Exclusion see Appendix A PDX collection 0582

+ **G40.1 Localization-related (focal) (partial) symptomatic epilepsy and epileptic syndromes with simple partial seizures**
  Attacks without alteration of consciousness
  Epilepsia partialis continua [Kozhevnikof]
  Simple partial seizures developing into secondarily generalized seizures

+ **G40.10 Localization-related (focal) (partial) symptomatic epilepsy and epileptic syndromes with simple partial seizures, not intractable**
  Localization-related (focal) (partial) symptomatic epilepsy and epileptic syndromes with simple partial seizures without intractability

CC **G40.101 Localization-related (focal) (partial) symptomatic epilepsy and epileptic syndromes with simple partial seizures, not intractable, with status epilepticus**
  CC Exclusion see Appendix A PDX collection 0581

CC G40.109 **Localization-related (focal) (partial) symptomatic epilepsy and epileptic syndromes with simple partial seizures, not intractable, without status epilepticus**
Localization-related (focal) (partial) symptomatic epilepsy and epileptic syndromes with simple partial seizures NOS
CC Exclusion see Appendix A PDX collection 0581

+ G40.11 **Localization-related (focal) (partial) symptomatic epilepsy and epileptic syndromes with simple partial seizures, intractable**

CC G40.111 **Localization-related (focal) (partial) symptomatic epilepsy and epileptic syndromes with simple partial seizures, intractable, with status epilepticus**
CC Exclusion see Appendix A PDX collection 0582

CC G40.119 **Localization-related (focal) (partial) symptomatic epilepsy and epileptic syndromes with simple partial seizures, intractable, without status epilepticus**
CC Exclusion see Appendix A PDX collection 0582

+ G40.2 **Localization-related (focal) (partial) symptomatic epilepsy and epileptic syndromes with complex partial seizures**
Attacks with alteration of consciousness, often with automatisms
Complex partial seizures developing into secondarily generalized seizures

+ G40.20 **Localization-related (focal) (partial) symptomatic epilepsy and epileptic syndromes with complex partial seizures, not intractable**
Localization-related (focal) (partial) symptomatic epilepsy and epileptic syndromes with complex partial seizures without intractability

CC G40.201 **Localization-related (focal) (partial) symptomatic epilepsy and epileptic syndromes with complex partial seizures, not intractable, with status epilepticus**
CC Exclusion see Appendix A PDX collection 0581

CC G40.209 **Localization-related (focal) (partial) symptomatic epilepsy and epileptic syndromes with complex partial seizures, not intractable, without status epilepticus**
Localization-related (focal) (partial) symptomatic epilepsy and epileptic syndromes with complex partial seizures NOS
CC Exclusion see Appendix A PDX collection 0581

+ G40.21 **Localization-related (focal) (partial) symptomatic epilepsy and epileptic syndromes with complex partial seizures, intractable**

CC G40.211 **Localization-related (focal) (partial) symptomatic epilepsy and epileptic syndromes with complex partial seizures, intractable, with status epilepticus**
CC Exclusion see Appendix A PDX collection 0582

CC G40.219 **Localization-related (focal) (partial) symptomatic epilepsy and epileptic syndromes with complex partial seizures, intractable, without status epilepticus**
CC Exclusion see Appendix A PDX collection 0582

+ G40.3 **Generalized idiopathic epilepsy and epileptic syndromes**
Code also MERRF syndrome, if applicable (E88.42)

+ G40.30 **Generalized idiopathic epilepsy and epileptic syndromes, not intractable**
Generalized idiopathic epilepsy and epileptic syndromes without intractability

MCC G40.301 **Generalized idiopathic epilepsy and epileptic syndromes, not intractable, with status epilepticus**
MCC Exclusion see Appendix A PDX collection 0583

G40.309 **Generalized idiopathic epilepsy and epileptic syndromes, not intractable, without status epilepticus**
Generalized idiopathic epilepsy and epileptic syndromes NOS

+ G40.31 **Generalized idiopathic epilepsy and epileptic syndromes, intractable**

MCC G40.311 **Generalized idiopathic epilepsy and epileptic syndromes, intractable, with status epilepticus**
MCC Exclusion see Appendix A PDX collection 0583

MCC G40.319 **Generalized idiopathic epilepsy and epileptic syndromes, intractable, without status epilepticus**
MCC Exclusion see Appendix A PDX collection 0583

+ G40.A **Absence epileptic syndrome**
Childhood absence epilepsy [pyknolepsy]
Juvenile absence epilepsy
Absence epileptic syndrome, NOS

+ G40.A0 **Absence epileptic syndrome, not intractable**

G40.A01 **Absence epileptic syndrome, not intractable, with status epilepticus**

G40.A09 **Absence epileptic syndrome, not intractable, without status epilepticus**

+ G40.A1 **Absence epileptic syndrome, intractable**

CC G40.A11 **Absence epileptic syndrome, intractable, with status epilepticus**
CC Exclusion see Appendix A PDX collection 0582

CC G40.A19 **Absence epileptic syndrome, intractable, without status epilepticus**
CC Exclusion see Appendix A PDX collection 0582

+ G40.B **Juvenile myoclonic epilepsy [impulsive petit mal]**

+ G40.B0 **Juvenile myoclonic epilepsy, not intractable**

CC G40.B01 **Juvenile myoclonic epilepsy, not intractable, with status epilepticus**
CC Exclusion see Appendix A PDX collection 0582

CC G40.B09 **Juvenile myoclonic epilepsy, not intractable, without status epilepticus**
CC Exclusion see Appendix A PDX collection 0582

+ G40.B1 **Juvenile myoclonic epilepsy, intractable**

CC G40.B11 **Juvenile myoclonic epilepsy, intractable, with status epilepticus**
CC Exclusion see Appendix A PDX collection 0582

CC G40.B19 **Juvenile myoclonic epilepsy, intractable, without status epilepticus**
CC Exclusion see Appendix A PDX collection 0582

+ G40.4 **Other generalized epilepsy and epileptic syndromes**
Epilepsy with grand mal seizures on awakening
Epilepsy with myoclonic absences
Epilepsy with myoclonic-astatic seizures
Grand mal seizure NOS
Nonspecific atonic epileptic seizures
Nonspecific clonic epileptic seizures
Nonspecific myoclonic epileptic seizures
Nonspecific tonic epileptic seizures
Nonspecific tonic-clonic epileptic seizures
Symptomatic early myoclonic encephalopathy

+ G40.40 **Other generalized epilepsy and epileptic syndromes, not intractable**
Other generalized epilepsy and epileptic syndromes without intractability
Other generalized epilepsy and epileptic syndromes NOS

G40.401 **Other generalized epilepsy and epileptic syndromes, not intractable, with status epilepticus**

G40.409 **Other generalized epilepsy and epileptic syndromes, not intractable, without status epilepticus**

+ **G40.41 Other generalized epilepsy and epileptic syndromes, intractable**
  - CC **G40.411 Other generalized epilepsy and epileptic syndromes, intractable, with status epilepticus**
    - **CC Exclusion see Appendix A PDX collection 0582**
  - CC **G40.419 Other generalized epilepsy and epileptic syndromes, intractable, without status epilepticus**
    - **CC Exclusion see Appendix A PDX collection 0582**

+ **G40.5 Epileptic seizures related to external causes**

Epileptic seizures related to alcohol
Epileptic seizures related to drugs
Epileptic seizures related to hormonal changes
Epileptic seizures related to sleep deprivation
Epileptic seizures related to stress

Use additional code for adverse effect, if applicable, to identify drug (T36-T50 with fifth or sixth character 5)

Code also if applicable, associated epilepsy and recurrent seizures (G40.-)

+ **G40.50 Epileptic seizures related to external causes, not intractable**
  - CC **G40.501 Epileptic seizures related to external causes, not intractable, with status epilepticus**
    - **CC Exclusion see Appendix A PDX collection 0582**
  - CC **G40.509 Epileptic seizures related to external causes, not intractable, without status epilepticus**
    - Epileptic seizures related to external causes, NOS
    - **CC Exclusion see Appendix A PDX collection 0582**

+ **G40.8 Other epilepsy and recurrent seizures**

Epilepsies and epileptic syndromes undetermined as to whether they are focal or generalized
Landau-Kleffner syndrome

+ **G40.80 Other epilepsy**
  - CC **G40.801 Other epilepsy, not intractable, with status epilepticus**
    - Other epilepsy without intractability with status epilepticus
    - **CC Exclusion see Appendix A PDX collection 0582**
  - CC **G40.802 Other epilepsy, not intractable, without status epilepticus**
    - Other epilepsy NOS
    - Other epilepsy without intractability without status epilepticus
    - **CC Exclusion see Appendix A PDX collection 0582**
  - CC **G40.803 Other epilepsy, intractable, with status epilepticus**
    - **CC Exclusion see Appendix A PDX collection 0582**
  - CC **G40.804 Other epilepsy, intractable, without status epilepticus**
    - **CC Exclusion see Appendix A PDX collection 0582**

+ **G40.81 Lennox-Gastaut syndrome**
  - CC **G40.811 Lennox-Gastaut syndrome, not intractable, with status epilepticus**
    - **CC Exclusion see Appendix A PDX collection 0582**
  - CC **G40.812 Lennox-Gastaut syndrome, not intractable, without status epilepticus**
    - **CC Exclusion see Appendix A PDX collection 0582**
  - CC **G40.813 Lennox-Gastaut syndrome, intractable, with status epilepticus**
    - **CC Exclusion see Appendix A PDX collection 0582**
  - CC **G40.814 Lennox-Gastaut syndrome, intractable, without status epilepticus**
    - **CC Exclusion see Appendix A PDX collection 0582**

+ **G40.82 Epileptic spasms**

Infantile spasms
Salaam attacks
West's syndrome

  - CC **G40.821 Epileptic spasms, not intractable, with status epilepticus**
    - **CC Exclusion see Appendix A PDX collection 0582**
  - CC **G40.822 Epileptic spasms, not intractable, without status epilepticus**
    - **CC Exclusion see Appendix A PDX collection 0582**
  - CC **G40.823 Epileptic spasms, intractable, with status epilepticus**
    - **CC Exclusion see Appendix A PDX collection 0582**
  - CC **G40.824 Epileptic spasms, intractable, without status epilepticus**
    - **CC Exclusion see Appendix A PDX collection 0582**

CC **G40.89 Other seizures**

Excludes1: *post traumatic seizures (R56.1)*
recurrent seizures NOS (G40.909)
seizure NOS (R56.9)

CC Exclusion see Appendix A PDX collection 0582

+ **G40.9 Epilepsy, unspecified**

+ **G40.90 Epilepsy, unspecified, not intractable**

Epilepsy, unspecified, without intractability

  - **G40.901 Epilepsy, unspecified, not intractable, with status epilepticus**
  - **G40.909 Epilepsy, unspecified, not intractable, without status epilepticus**
    - Epilepsy NOS
    - Epileptic convulsions NOS
    - Epileptic fits NOS
    - Epileptic seizures NOS
    - Recurrent seizures NOS
    - Seizure disorder NOS

+ **G40.91 Epilepsy, unspecified, intractable**

Intractable seizure disorder NOS

  - CC **G40.911 Epilepsy, unspecified, intractable, with status epilepticus**
    - **CC Exclusion see Appendix A PDX collection 0582**
  - CC **G40.919 Epilepsy, unspecified, intractable, without status epilepticus**
    - **CC Exclusion see Appendix A PDX collection 0582**

G43 Migraine

NOTE The following terms are to be considered equivalent to intractable: pharmacoresistant (pharmacologically resistant), treatment resistant, refractory (medically) and poorly controlled

Use additional code for adverse effect, if applicable, to identify drug (T36-T50 with fifth or sixth character 5)

Excludes1: *headache NOS (R51)*
lower half migraine (G44.00)

Excludes2: *headache syndromes (G44.-)*

+ **G43.0 Migraine without aura**

Common migraine

Excludes1: *chronic migraine without aura (G43.7-)*

+ **G43.00 Migraine without aura, not intractable**

Migraine without aura without mention of refractory migraine

  - **G43.001 Migraine without aura, not intractable, with status migrainosus**
  - **G43.009 Migraine without aura, not intractable, without status migrainosus**
    - Migraine without aura NOS

+ **G43.01 Migraine without aura, intractable**

Migraine without aura with refractory migraine

  - **G43.011 Migraine without aura, intractable, with status migrainosus**
  - **G43.019 Migraine without aura, intractable, without status migrainosus**

+ G43.1 **Migraine with aura**
Basilar migraine
Classical migraine
Migraine equivalents
Migraine preceded or accompanied by transient focal neurological phenomena
Migraine triggered seizures
Migraine with acute-onset aura
Migraine with aura without headache (migraine equivalents)
Migraine with prolonged aura
Migraine with typical aura
Retinal migraine
Code also any associated seizure (G40.-, R56.9)
Excludes1: *persistent migraine aura (G43.5-, G43.6-)*

+ G43.10 **Migraine with aura, not intractable**
Migraine with aura without mention of refractory migraine
G43.101 **Migraine with aura, not intractable, with status migrainosus**
G43.109 **Migraine with aura, not intractable, without status migrainosus**
Migraine with aura NOS

+ G43.11 **Migraine with aura, intractable**
Migraine with aura with refractory migraine
G43.111 **Migraine with aura, intractable, with status migrainosus**
G43.119 **Migraine with aura, intractable, without status migrainosus**

+ G43.4 **Hemiplegic migraine**
Familial migraine
Sporadic migraine

+ G43.40 **Hemiplegic migraine, not intractable**
Hemiplegic migraine without refractory migraine
G43.401 **Hemiplegic migraine, not intractable, with status migrainosus**
G43.409 **Hemiplegic migraine, not intractable, without status migrainosus**
Hemiplegic migraine NOS

+ G43.41 **Hemiplegic migraine, intractable**
Hemiplegic migraine with refractory migraine
G43.411 **Hemiplegic migraine, intractable, with status migrainosus**
G43.419 **Hemiplegic migraine, intractable, without status migrainosus**

+ G43.5 **Persistent migraine aura without cerebral infarction**

+ G43.50 **Persistent migraine aura without cerebral infarction, not intractable**
Persistent migraine aura without cerebral infarction, without refractory migraine
G43.501 **Persistent migraine aura without cerebral infarction, not intractable, with status migrainosus**
G43.509 **Persistent migraine aura without cerebral infarction, not intractable, without status migrainosus**
Persistent migraine aura NOS

+ G43.51 **Persistent migraine aura without cerebral infarction, intractable**
Persistent migraine aura without cerebral infarction, with refractory migraine
G43.511 **Persistent migraine aura without cerebral infarction, intractable, with status migrainosus**
G43.519 **Persistent migraine aura without cerebral infarction, intractable, without status migrainosus**

+ G43.6 **Persistent migraine aura with cerebral infarction**
Code also the type of cerebral infarction (I63.-)

+ G43.60 **Persistent migraine aura with cerebral infarction, not intractable**
Persistent migraine aura with cerebral infarction, without refractory migraine
CC G43.601 **Persistent migraine aura with cerebral infarction, not intractable, with status migrainosus**
CC Exclusion see Appendix A PDX collection 0584
CC G43.609 **Persistent migraine aura with cerebral infarction, not intractable, without status migrainosus**
CC Exclusion see Appendix A PDX collection 0585

+ G43.61 **Persistent migraine aura with cerebral infarction, intractable**
Persistent migraine aura with cerebral infarction, with refractory migraine
CC G43.611 **Persistent migraine aura with cerebral infarction, intractable, with status migrainosus**
CC Exclusion see Appendix A PDX collection 0584
CC G43.619 **Persistent migraine aura with cerebral infarction, intractable, without status migrainosus**
CC Exclusion see Appendix A PDX collection 0584

+ G43.7 **Chronic migraine without aura**
Transformed migraine
Excludes1: *migraine without aura (G43.0-)*

+ G43.70 **Chronic migraine without aura, not intractable**
Chronic migraine without aura, without refractory migraine
G43.701 **Chronic migraine without aura, not intractable, with status migrainosus**
G43.709 **Chronic migraine without aura, not intractable, without status migrainosus**
Chronic migraine without aura NOS

+ G43.71 **Chronic migraine without aura, intractable**
Chronic migraine without aura, with refractory migraine
G43.711 **Chronic migraine without aura, intractable, with status migrainosus**
G43.719 **Chronic migraine without aura, intractable, without status migrainosus**

+ G43.A **Cyclical vomiting**
G43.A0 **Cyclical vomiting, not intractable**
Cyclical vomiting, without refractory migraine
G43.A1 **Cyclical vomiting, intractable**
Cyclical vomiting, with refractory migraine

+ G43.B **Ophthalmoplegic migraine**
G43.B0 **Ophthalmoplegic migraine, not intractable**
Ophthalmoplegic migraine, without refractory migraine
G43.B1 **Ophthalmoplegic migraine, intractable**
Ophthalmoplegic migraine, with refractory migraine

+ G43.C **Periodic headache syndromes in child or adult**
G43.C0 **Periodic headache syndromes in child or adult, not intractable**
Periodic headache syndromes in child or adult, without refractory migraine
G43.C1 **Periodic headache syndromes in child or adult, intractable**
Periodic headache syndromes in child or adult, with refractory migraine

+ G43.D **Abdominal migraine**
G43.D0 **Abdominal migraine, not intractable**
Abdominal migraine, without refractory migraine
G43.D1 **Abdominal migraine, intractable**
Abdominal migraine, with refractory migraine

+ G43.8 **Other migraine**

+ G43.80 **Other migraine, not intractable**
Other migraine, without refractory migraine
G43.801 **Other migraine, not intractable, with status migrainosus**
G43.809 **Other migraine, not intractable, without status migrainosus**

+ G43.81 **Other migraine, intractable**
Other migraine, with refractory migraine
G43.811 **Other migraine, intractable, with status migrainosus**
G43.819 **Other migraine, intractable, without status migrainosus**

+ **G43.82 Menstrual migraine, not intractable**
  Menstrual headache, not intractable
  Menstrual migraine, without refractory migraine
  Menstrually related migraine, not intractable
  Pre-menstrual headache, not intractable
  Pre-menstrual migraine, not intractable
  Pure menstrual migraine, not intractable
  Code also associated premenstrual tension syndrome (N94.3)
  ♀ **G43.821 Menstrual migraine, not intractable, with status migrainosus**
  ♀ **G43.829 Menstrual migraine, not intractable, without status migrainosus**
  Menstrual migraine NOS
+ **G43.83 Menstrual migraine, intractable**
  Menstrual headache, intractable
  Menstrual migraine, with refractory migraine
  Menstrually related migraine, intractable
  Pre-menstrual headache, intractable
  Pre-menstrual migraine, intractable
  Pure menstrual migraine, intractable
  Code also associated premenstrual tension syndrome (N94.3)
  ♀ **G43.831 Menstrual migraine, intractable, with status migrainosus**
  ♀ **G43.839 Menstrual migraine, intractable, without status migrainosus**
+ **G43.9 Migraine, unspecified**
+ **G43.90 Migraine, unspecified, not intractable**
  Migraine, unspecified, without refractory migraine
  G43.901 Migraine, unspecified, not intractable, with status migrainosus
  Status migrainosus NOS
  G43.909 Migraine, unspecified, not intractable, without status migrainosus
  Migraine NOS
+ **G43.91 Migraine, unspecified, intractable**
  Migraine, unspecified, with refractory migraine
  G43.911 Migraine, unspecified, intractable, with status migrainosus
  G43.919 Migraine, unspecified, intractable, without status migrainosus

G44 Other headache syndromes

Excludes1: *headache NOS (R51)*
Excludes2: *atypical facial pain (G50.1)*
headache due to lumbar puncture (G97.1)
migraines (G43.-)
trigeminal neuralgia (G50.0)

+ **G44.0 Cluster headaches and other trigeminal autonomic cephalgias (TAC)**
+ **G44.00 Cluster headache syndrome, unspecified**
  Ciliary neuralgia
  Cluster headache NOS
  Histamine cephalgia
  Lower half migraine
  Migrainous neuralgia
  G44.001 Cluster headache syndrome, unspecified, intractable
  G44.009 Cluster headache syndrome, unspecified, not intractable
  Cluster headache syndrome NOS
+ **G44.01 Episodic cluster headache**
  G44.011 Episodic cluster headache, intractable
  G44.019 Episodic cluster headache, not intractable
  Episodic cluster headache NOS
+ **G44.02 Chronic cluster headache**
  G44.021 Chronic cluster headache, intractable
  G44.029 Chronic cluster headache, not intractable
  Chronic cluster headache NOS
+ **G44.03 Episodic paroxysmal hemicrania**
  Paroxysmal hemicrania NOS
  G44.031 Episodic paroxysmal hemicrania, intractable
  G44.039 Episodic paroxysmal hemicrania, not intractable
  Episodic paroxysmal hemicrania NOS
+ **G44.04 Chronic paroxysmal hemicrania**
  G44.041 Chronic paroxysmal hemicrania, intractable
  G44.049 Chronic paroxysmal hemicrania, not intractable
  Chronic paroxysmal hemicrania NOS
+ **G44.05 Short lasting unilateral neuralgiform headache with conjunctival injection and tearing (SUNCT)**
  G44.051 Short lasting unilateral neuralgiform headache with conjunctival injection and tearing (SUNCT), intractable
  G44.059 Short lasting unilateral neuralgiform headache with conjunctival injection and tearing (SUNCT), not intractable
  Short lasting unilateral neuralgiform headache with conjunctival injection and tearing (SUNCT) NOS
+ **G44.09 Other trigeminal autonomic cephalgias (TAC)**
  G44.091 Other trigeminal autonomic cephalgias (TAC), intractable
  G44.099 Other trigeminal autonomic cephalgias (TAC), not intractable

G44.1 Vascular headache, not elsewhere classified
Excludes2: *cluster headache (G44.0)*
complicated headache syndromes (G44.5-)
drug-induced headache (G44.4-)
migraine (G43.-)
other specified headache syndromes (G44.8-)
post-traumatic headache (G44.3-)
tension-type headache (G44.2-)

+ **G44.2 Tension-type headache**
+ **G44.20 Tension-type headache, unspecified**
  G44.201 Tension-type headache, unspecified, intractable
  G44.209 Tension-type headache, unspecified, not intractable
  Tension headache NOS
+ **G44.21 Episodic tension-type headache**
  G44.211 Episodic tension-type headache, intractable
  G44.219 Episodic tension-type headache, not intractable
  Episodic tension-type headache NOS
+ **G44.22 Chronic tension-type headache**
  G44.221 Chronic tension-type headache, intractabl
  G44.229 Chronic tension-type headache, not intractable
  Chronic tension-type headache NOS
+ **G44.3 Post-traumatic headache**
+ **G44.30 Post-traumatic headache, unspecified**
  G44.301 Post-traumatic headache, unspecified, intractable
  G44.309 Post-traumatic headache, unspecified, not intractable
  Post-traumatic headache NOS
+ **G44.31 Acute post-traumatic headache**
  G44.311 Acute post-traumatic headache, intractab
  G44.319 Acute post-traumatic headache, not intractable
  Acute post-traumatic headache NOS
+ **G44.32 Chronic post-traumatic headache**
  G44.321 Chronic post-traumatic headache, intractable
  G44.329 Chronic post-traumatic headache, not intractable
  Chronic post-traumatic headache NOS
+ **G44.4 Drug-induced headache, not elsewhere classified**
  Medication overuse headache
  Use additional code for adverse effect, if applicable, to identify drug (T36-T50 with fifth or sixth character 5)
  G44.40 Drug-induced headache, not elsewhere classified, no intractable
  G44.41 Drug-induced headache, not elsewhere classified, intractable
+ **G44.5 Complicated headache syndromes**
  G44.51 Hemicrania continua
  G44.52 New daily persistent headache (NDPH)
  G44.53 Primary thunderclap headache
  G44.59 Other complicated headache syndrome

+ G44.8 **Other specified headache syndromes**
G44.81 **Hypnic headache**
G44.82 **Headache associated with sexual activity**
Orgasmic headache
Preorgasmic headache
G44.83 **Primary cough headache**
G44.84 **Primary exertional headache**
G44.85 **Primary stabbing headache**
G44.89 **Other headache syndrome**

G45 Transient cerebral ischemic attacks and related syndromes

Excludes1: *neonatal cerebral ischemia (P91.0)*
transient retinal artery occlusion (H34.0-)

CC G45.0 **Vertebro-basilar artery syndrome**
CC Exclusion see Appendix A PDX collection 0586
CC G45.1 **Carotid artery syndrome (hemispheric)**
CC Exclusion see Appendix A PDX collection 0586
CC G45.2 **Multiple and bilateral precerebral artery syndromes**
CC Exclusion see Appendix A PDX collection 0586
CC G45.3 **Amaurosis fugax**
CC Exclusion see Appendix A PDX collection 0587
G45.4 **Transient global amnesia**
Excludes1: *amnesia NOS (R41.3)*
CC G45.8 **Other transient cerebral ischemic attacks and related syndromes**
CC Exclusion see Appendix A PDX collection 0586
CC G45.9 **Transient cerebral ischemic attack, unspecified**
Spasm of cerebral artery
TIA
Transient cerebral ischemia NOS
CC Exclusion see Appendix A PDX collection 0586

G46 Vascular syndromes of brain in cerebrovascular diseases

Code first underlying cerebrovascular disease (I60-I69)

CC G46.0 **Middle cerebral artery syndrome**
CC Exclusion see Appendix A PDX collection 0586
CC G46.1 **Anterior cerebral artery syndrome**
CC Exclusion see Appendix A PDX collection 0586
CC G46.2 **Posterior cerebral artery syndrome**
CC Exclusion see Appendix A PDX collection 0586
G46.3 **Brain stem stroke syndrome**
Benedikt syndrome
Claude syndrome
Foville syndrome
Millard-Gubler syndrome
Wallenberg syndrome
Weber syndrome
G46.4 **Cerebellar stroke syndrome**
G46.5 **Pure motor lacunar syndrome**
G46.6 **Pure sensory lacunar syndrome**
G46.7 **Other lacunar syndromes**
G46.8 **Other vascular syndromes of brain in cerebrovascular diseases**

G47 Sleep disorders

Excludes2: *nightmares (F51.5)*
nonorganic sleep disorders (F51.-)
sleep terrors (F51.4)
sleepwalking (F51.3)

+ G47.0 **Insomnia**
Excludes2: *alcohol related insomnia (F10.182, F10.282, F10.982)*
drug-related insomnia (F11.182, F11.282, F11.982, F13.182, F13.282, F13.982, F14.182, F14.282, F14.982, F15.182, F15.282, F15.982, F19.182, F19.282, F19.982)
idiopathic insomnia (F51.01)
insomnia due to a mental disorder (F51.05)
insomnia not due to a substance or known physiological condition (F51.0-)
nonorganic insomnia (F51.0-)
primary insomnia (F51.01)
sleep apnea (G47.3-)
G47.00 **Insomnia, unspecified**
Insomnia NOS
G47.01 **Insomnia due to medical condition**
Code also associated medical condition
G47.09 **Other insomnia**

+ G47.1 **Hypersomnia**
Excludes2: *alcohol-related hypersomnia (F10.182, F10.282, F10.982)*
drug-related hypersomnia (F11.182, F11.282, F11.982, F13.182, F13.282, F13.982, F14.182, F14.282, F14.982, F15.182, F15.282, F15.982, F19.182, F19.282, F19.982)
hypersomnia due to a mental disorder (F51.13)
hypersomnia not due to a substance or known physiological condition (F51.1-)
primary hypersomnia (F51.11)
sleep apnea (G47.3-)
G47.10 **Hypersomnia, unspecified**
Hypersomnia NOS
G47.11 **Idiopathic hypersomnia with long sleep time**
Idiopathic hypersomnia NOS
G47.12 **Idiopathic hypersomnia without long sleep time**
G47.13 **Recurrent hypersomnia**
Kleine-Levin syndrome
Menstrual related hypersomnia
G47.14 **Hypersomnia due to medical condition**
Code also associated medical condition
G47.19 **Other hypersomnia**

+ G47.2 **Circadian rhythm sleep disorders**
Disorders of the sleep wake schedule
Inversion of nyctohemeral rhythm
Inversion of sleep rhythm
G47.20 **Circadian rhythm sleep disorder, unspecified type**
Sleep wake schedule disorder NOS
G47.21 **Circadian rhythm sleep disorder, delayed sleep phase type**
Delayed sleep phase syndrome
G47.22 **Circadian rhythm sleep disorder, advanced sleep phase type**
G47.23 **Circadian rhythm sleep disorder, irregular sleep wake type**
Irregular sleep-wake pattern
G47.24 **Circadian rhythm sleep disorder, free running type**
Circadian rhythm sleep disorder, non-24-hour sleep-wake type
G47.25 **Circadian rhythm sleep disorder, jet lag type**
G47.26 **Circadian rhythm sleep disorder, shift work type**
G47.27 **Circadian rhythm sleep disorder in conditions classified elsewhere**
Code first underlying condition
G47.29 **Other circadian rhythm sleep disorder**

+ G47.3 **Sleep apnea**
Code also any associated underlying condition
Excludes1: *apnea NOS (R06.81)*
Cheyne-Stokes breathing (R06.3)
pickwickian syndrome (E66.2)
sleep apnea of newborn (P28.3)
G47.30 **Sleep apnea, unspecified**
Sleep apnea NOS
G47.31 **Primary central sleep apnea**
Idiopathic central sleep apnea
G47.32 **High altitude periodic breathing**
G47.33 **Obstructive sleep apnea (adult) (pediatric)**
Obstructive sleep apnea hypopnea
Excludes1: *obstructive sleep apnea of newborn (P28.3)*
G47.34 **Idiopathic sleep related nonobstructive alveolar hypoventilation**
Sleep related hypoxia
G47.35 **Congenital central alveolar hypoventilation syndrome**
G47.36 **Sleep related hypoventilation in conditions classified elsewhere**
Sleep related hypoxemia in conditions classified elsewhere
Code first underlying condition
G47.37 **Central sleep apnea in conditions classified elsewhere**
Code first underlying condition
G47.39 **Other sleep apnea**

Brain

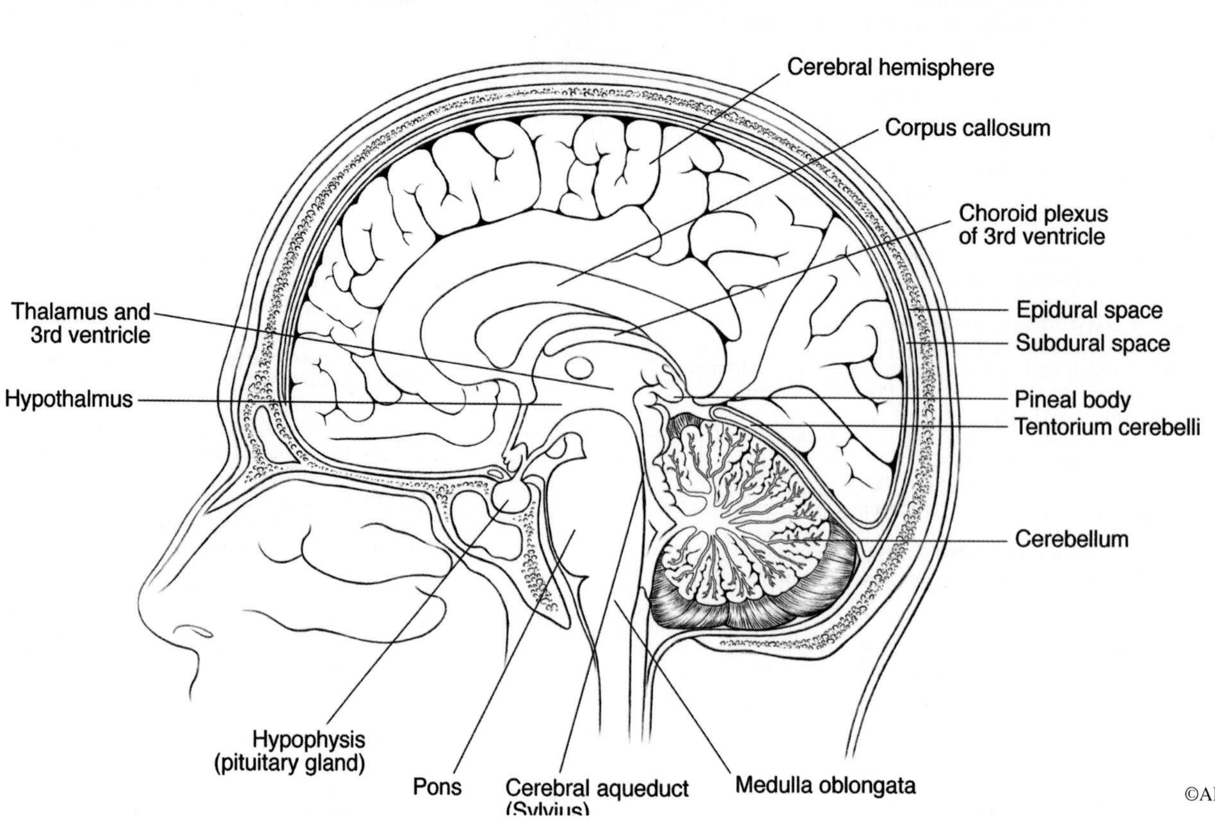
Cerebral hemisphere
Corpus callosum
Choroid plexus
of 3rd ventricle
Thalamus and
3rd ventricle
Epidural space
Subdural space
Hypothalmus
Pineal body
Tentorium cerebelli
Cerebellum
Hypophysis
(pituitary gland)
Pons
Cerebral aqueduct
(Sylvius)
Medulla oblongata

©AHIMA

Cranial Nerves

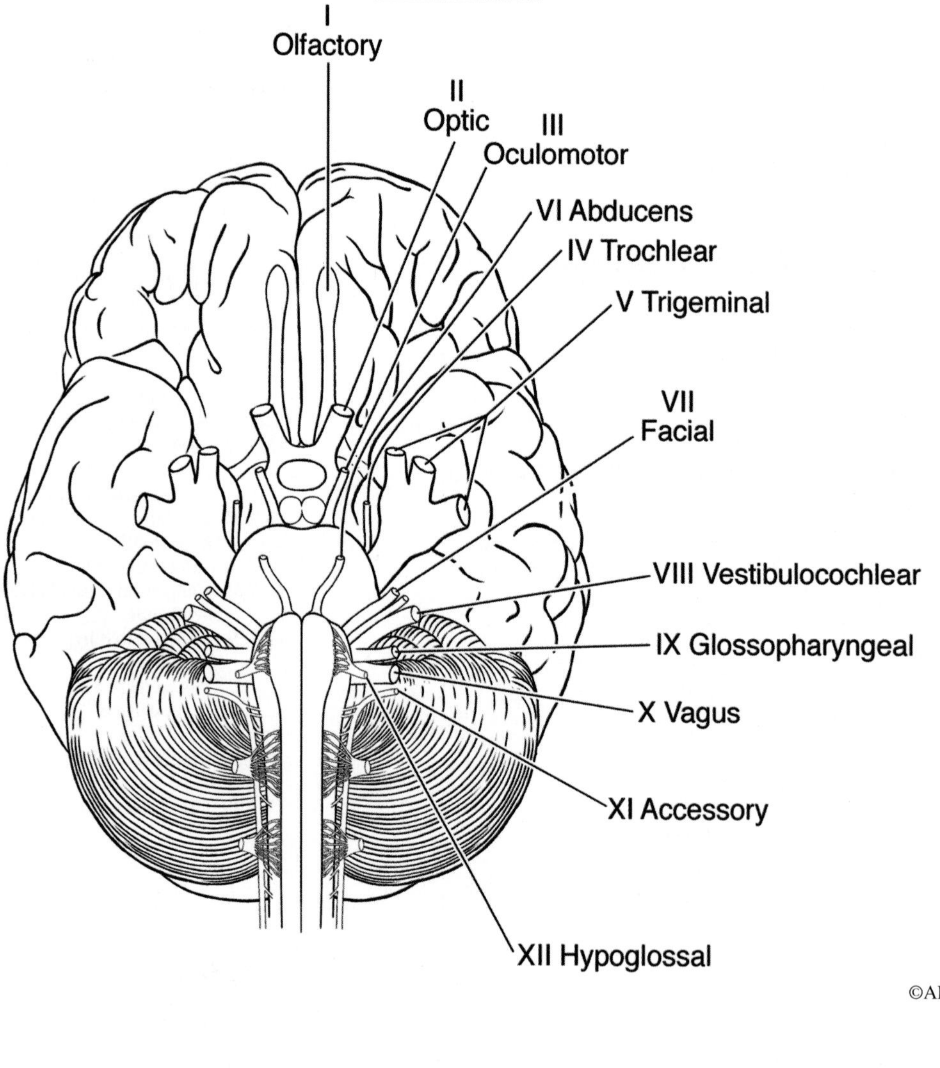
I
Olfactory
II
Optic
III
Oculomotor
VI Abducens
IV Trochlear
V Trigeminal
VII
Facial
VIII Vestibulocochlear
IX Glossopharyngeal
X Vagus
XI Accessory
XII Hypoglossal

©AHIMA

Peripheral Nervous System

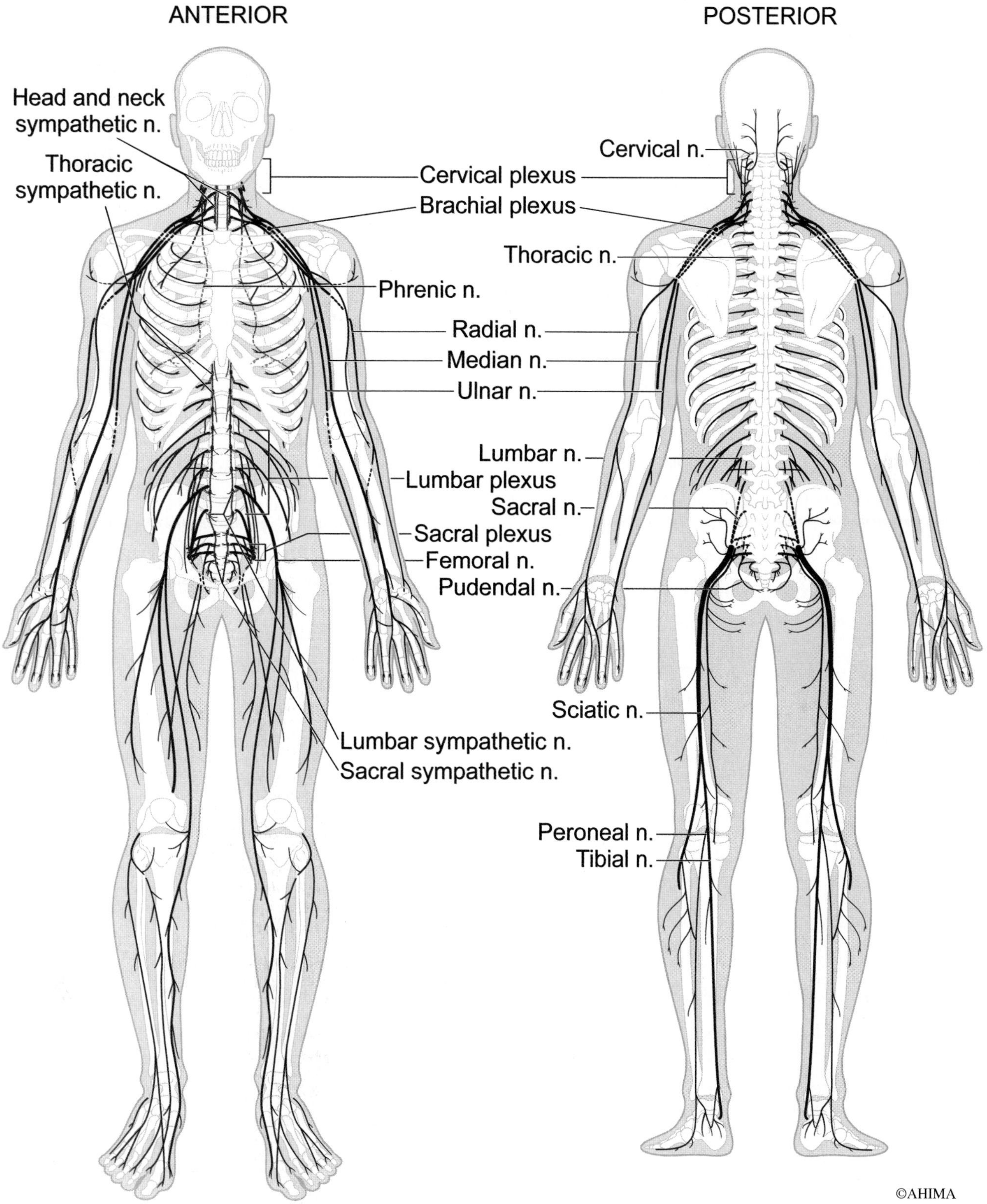

ANTERIOR
POSTERIOR
Head and neck sympathetic n.
Thoracic sympathetic n.
Cervical plexus
Brachial plexus
Phrenic n.
Radial n.
Median n.
Ulnar n.
Lumbar plexus
Sacral plexus
Femoral n.
Lumbar sympathetic n.
Sacral sympathetic n.
Cervical n.
Thoracic n.
Lumbar n.
Sacral n.
Pudendal n.
Sciatic n.
Peroneal n.
Tibial n.

+ G47.4 **Narcolepsy and cataplexy**
  + G47.41 **Narcolepsy**
    - **G47.411 Narcolepsy with cataplexy**
    - **G47.419 Narcolepsy without cataplexy**
      Narcolepsy NOS
  + G47.42 **Narcolepsy in conditions classified elsewhere**
    Code first underlying condition
    - **G47.421 Narcolepsy in conditions classified elsewhere with cataplexy**
    - **G47.429 Narcolepsy in conditions classified elsewhere without cataplexy**
+ G47.5 **Parasomnia**
  Excludes1: *alcohol induced parasomnia (F10.182, F10.282, F10.982)*
  drug induced parasomnia (F11.182, F11.282, F11.982, F13.182, F13.282, F13.982, F14.182, F14.282, F14.982, F15.182, F15.282, F15.982, F19.182, F19.282, F19.982)
  parasomnia not due to a substance or known physiological condition (F51.8)
  - **G47.50 Parasomnia, unspecified**
    Parasomnia NOS
  - **G47.51 Confusional arousals**
  - **G47.52 REM sleep behavior disorder**
  - **G47.53 Recurrent isolated sleep paralysis**
  - **G47.54 Parasomnia in conditions classified elsewhere**
    Code first underlying condition
  - **G47.59 Other parasomnia**
+ G47.6 **Sleep related movement disorders**
  Excludes2: *restless legs syndrome (G25.81)*
  - **G47.61 Periodic limb movement disorder**
  - **G47.62 Sleep related leg cramps**
  - **G47.63 Sleep related bruxism**
    Excludes1: *psychogenic bruxism (F45.8)*
  - **G47.69 Other sleep related movement disorders**
- **G47.8 Other sleep disorders**
  Other specified sleep-wake disorder
- **G47.9 Sleep disorder, unspecified**
  Sleep disorder NOS
  Unspecified sleep-wake disorder

Nerve, nerve root and plexus disorders (G50-G59)

Excludes1: *current traumatic nerve, nerve root and plexus disorders - see Injury, nerve by body region*
neuralgia NOS (M79.2)
neuritis NOS (M79.2)
peripheral neuritis in pregnancy (O26.82-)
radiculitis NOS (M54.1-)

G50 Disorders of trigeminal nerve

Includes: disorders of 5th cranial nerve
- **G50.0 Trigeminal neuralgia**
  Syndrome of paroxysmal facial pain
  Tic douloureux
- **G50.1 Atypical facial pain**
- **G50.8 Other disorders of trigeminal nerve**
- **G50.9 Disorder of trigeminal nerve, unspecified**

G51 Facial nerve disorders

Includes: disorders of 7th cranial nerve
- **G51.0 Bell's palsy**
  Facial palsy
- **G51.1 Geniculate ganglionitis**
  Excludes1: *postherpetic geniculate ganglionitis (B02.21)*
- **G51.2 Melkersson's syndrome**
  Melkersson-Rosenthal syndrome
- **G51.3 Clonic hemifacial spasm**
- **G51.4 Facial myokymia**
- **G51.8 Other disorders of facial nerve**
- **G51.9 Disorder of facial nerve, unspecified**

G52 Disorders of other cranial nerves

Excludes2: *disorders of acoustic [8th] nerve (H93.3)*
disorders of optic [2nd] nerve (H46, H47.0)
paralytic strabismus due to nerve palsy (H49.0-H49.2)
- **G52.0 Disorders of olfactory nerve**
  Disorders of 1st cranial nerve
- **G52.1 Disorders of glossopharyngeal nerve**
  Disorder of 9th cranial nerve
  Glossopharyngeal neuralgia
- **G52.2 Disorders of vagus nerve**
  Disorders of pneumogastric [10th] nerve
- **G52.3 Disorders of hypoglossal nerve**
  Disorders of 12th cranial nerve
- **G52.7 Disorders of multiple cranial nerves**
  Polyneuritis cranialis
- **G52.8 Disorders of other specified cranial nerves**
- **G52.9 Cranial nerve disorder, unspecified**

G53 Cranial nerve disorders in diseases classified elsewhere

Code first underlying disease, such as:
neoplasm (C00-D49)
Excludes1: *multiple cranial nerve palsy in sarcoidosis (D86.82)*
multiple cranial nerve palsy in syphilis (A52.15)
postherpetic geniculate ganglionitis (B02.21)
postherpetic trigeminal neuralgia (B02.22)
Valid 3-character code, no further characters required

G54 Nerve root and plexus disorders

Excludes1: *current traumatic nerve root and plexus disorders - see nerve injury by body region*
intervertebral disc disorders (M50-M51)
neuralgia or neuritis NOS (M79.2)
neuritis or radiculitis brachial NOS (M54.13)
neuritis or radiculitis lumbar NOS (M54.16)
neuritis or radiculitis lumbosacral NOS (M54.17)
neuritis or radiculitis thoracic NOS (M54.14)
radiculitis NOS (M54.10)
radiculopathy NOS (M54.10)
spondylosis (M47.-)
- **G54.0 Brachial plexus disorders**
  Thoracic outlet syndrome
- **G54.1 Lumbosacral plexus disorders**
- **G54.2 Cervical root disorders, not elsewhere classified**
- **G54.3 Thoracic root disorders, not elsewhere classified**
- **G54.4 Lumbosacral root disorders, not elsewhere classified**
- **G54.5 Neuralgic amyotrophy**
  Parsonage-Aldren-Turner syndrome
  Shoulder-girdle neuritis
  Excludes1: *neuralgic amyotrophy in diabetes mellitus (E08-E13 with .44)*
- **G54.6 Phantom limb syndrome with pain**
- **G54.7 Phantom limb syndrome without pain**
  Phantom limb syndrome NOS
- **G54.8 Other nerve root and plexus disorders**
- **G54.9 Nerve root and plexus disorder, unspecified**

G55 Nerve root and plexus compressions in diseases classified elsewhere

Code first underlying disease, such as:
neoplasm (C00-D49)
Excludes1: *nerve root compression (due to) (in) ankylosing spondylitis (M45.-)*
nerve root compression (due to) (in) ankylosing spondylitis (M45.-)
nerve root compression (due to) (in) dorsopathies (M53.-, M54.-)
nerve root compression (due to) (in) intervertebral disc disorders (M50.1.-, M51.1.-)
nerve root compression (due to) (in) spondylopathies (M46.-, M48.-)
Valid 3-character code, no further characters required

G56 Mononeuropathies of upper limb

Excludes1: *current traumatic nerve disorder - see nerve injury by body region*
AHA CC: 4Q, 2016, 17-18
+ G56.0 **Carpal tunnel syndrome**
  - **G56.00 Carpal tunnel syndrome, unspecified upper limb**
  - **G56.01 Carpal tunnel syndrome, right upper limb**
  - **G56.02 Carpal tunnel syndrome, left upper limb**
  - **G56.03 Carpal tunnel syndrome, bilateral upper limbs**
+ G56.1 **Other lesions of median nerve**
  - **G56.10 Other lesions of median nerve, unspecified upper limb**
  - **G56.11 Other lesions of median nerve, right upper limb**
  - **G56.12 Other lesions of median nerve, left upper limb**
  - **G56.13 Other lesions of median nerve, bilateral upper limbs**
+ G56.2 **Lesion of ulnar nerve**
  Tardy ulnar nerve palsy
  - **G56.20 Lesion of ulnar nerve, unspecified upper limb**
  - **G56.21 Lesion of ulnar nerve, right upper limb**
  - **G56.22 Lesion of ulnar nerve, left upper limb**
  - **G56.23 Lesion of ulnar nerve, bilateral upper limbs**

+ G56.3 **Lesion of radial nerve**
- G56.30 **Lesion of radial nerve, unspecified upper limb**
- G56.31 **Lesion of radial nerve, right upper limb**
- G56.32 **Lesion of radial nerve, left upper limb**
- G56.33 **Lesion of radial nerve, bilateral upper limbs**

+ G56.4 **Causalgia of upper limb**

Complex regional pain syndrome II of upper limb

Excludes1: *complex regional pain syndrome I of lower limb (G90.52-)*
complex regional pain syndrome I of upper limb (G90.51-)
complex regional pain syndrome II of lower limb (G57.7-)
reflex sympathetic dystrophy of lower limb (G90.52-)
reflex sympathetic dystrophy of upper limb (G90.51-)

- G56.40 **Causalgia of unspecified upper limb**
- G56.41 **Causalgia of right upper limb**
- G56.42 **Causalgia of left upper limb**
- G56.43 **Causalgia of bilateral upper limbs**

+ G56.8 **Other specified mononeuropathies of upper limb**

Interdigital neuroma of upper limb

- G56.80 **Other specified mononeuropathies of unspecified upper limb**
- G56.81 **Other specified mononeuropathies of right upper limb**
- G56.82 **Other specified mononeuropathies of left upper limb**
- G56.83 **Other specified mononeuropathies of bilateral upper limbs**

+ G56.9 **Unspecified mononeuropathy of upper limb**
- G56.90 **Unspecified mononeuropathy of unspecified upper limb**
- G56.91 **Unspecified mononeuropathy of right upper limb**
- G56.92 **Unspecified mononeuropathy of left upper limb**
- G56.93 **Unspecified mononeuropathy of bilateral upper limbs**

G57 Mononeuropathies of lower limb

Excludes1: *current traumatic nerve disorder - see nerve injury by body region*

AHA CC: 4Q, 2016, 17-18

+ G57.0 **Lesion of sciatic nerve**

Excludes1: *sciatica NOS (M54.3-)*

Excludes2: *sciatica attributed to intervertebral disc disorder (M51.1.-)*

- G57.00 **Lesion of sciatic nerve, unspecified lower limb**
- G57.01 **Lesion of sciatic nerve, right lower limb**
- G57.02 **Lesion of sciatic nerve, left lower limb**
- G57.03 **Lesion of sciatic nerve, bilateral lower limbs**

+ G57.1 **Meralgia paresthetica**

Lateral cutaneous nerve of thigh syndrome

- G57.10 **Meralgia paresthetica, unspecified lower limb**
- G57.11 **Meralgia paresthetica, right lower limb**
- G57.12 **Meralgia paresthetica, left lower limb**
- G57.13 **Meralgia paresthetica, bilateral lower limbs**

+ G57.2 **Lesion of femoral nerve**
- G57.20 **Lesion of femoral nerve, unspecified lower limb**
- G57.21 **Lesion of femoral nerve, right lower limb**
- G57.22 **Lesion of femoral nerve, left lower limb**
- G57.23 **Lesion of femoral nerve, bilateral lower limbs**

+ G57.3 **Lesion of lateral popliteal nerve**

Peroneal nerve palsy

- G57.30 **Lesion of lateral popliteal nerve, unspecified lower limb**
- G57.31 **Lesion of lateral popliteal nerve, right lower limb**
- G57.32 **Lesion of lateral popliteal nerve, left lower limb**
- G57.33 **Lesion of lateral popliteal nerve, bilateral lower limbs**

+ G57.4 **Lesion of medial popliteal nerve**
- G57.40 **Lesion of medial popliteal nerve, unspecified lower limb**
- G57.41 **Lesion of medial popliteal nerve, right lower limb**
- G57.42 **Lesion of medial popliteal nerve, left lower limb**
- G57.43 **Lesion of medial popliteal nerve, bilateral lower limbs**

+ G57.5 **Tarsal tunnel syndrome**
- G57.50 **Tarsal tunnel syndrome, unspecified lower limb**
- G57.51 **Tarsal tunnel syndrome, right lower limb**
- G57.52 **Tarsal tunnel syndrome, left lower limb**
- G57.53 **Tarsal tunnel syndrome, bilateral lower limbs**

+ G57.6 **Lesion of plantar nerve**

Morton's metatarsalgia

- G57.60 **Lesion of plantar nerve, unspecified lower limb**
- G57.61 **Lesion of plantar nerve, right lower limb**
- G57.62 **Lesion of plantar nerve, left lower limb**
- G57.63 **Lesion of plantar nerve, bilateral lower limbs**

+ G57.7 **Causalgia of lower limb**

Complex regional pain syndrome II of lower limb

Excludes1: *complex regional pain syndrome I of lower limb (G90.52-)*
complex regional pain syndrome I of upper limb (G90.51-)
complex regional pain syndrome II of upper limb (G56.4-)
reflex sympathetic dystrophy of lower limb (G90.52-)
reflex sympathetic dystrophy of upper limb (G90.51-)

- G57.70 **Causalgia of unspecified lower limb**
- G57.71 **Causalgia of right lower limb**
- G57.72 **Causalgia of left lower limb**
- G57.73 **Causalgia of bilateral lower limbs**

+ G57.8 **Other specified mononeuropathies of lower limb**

Interdigital neuroma of lower limb

- G57.80 **Other specified mononeuropathies of unspecified lower limb**
- G57.81 **Other specified mononeuropathies of right lower limb**
- G57.82 **Other specified mononeuropathies of left lower limb**
- G57.83 **Other specified mononeuropathies of bilateral lower limbs**

+ G57.9 **Unspecified mononeuropathy of lower limb**
- G57.90 **Unspecified mononeuropathy of unspecified lower limb**
- G57.91 **Unspecified mononeuropathy of right lower limb**
- G57.92 **Unspecified mononeuropathy of left lower limb**
- G57.93 **Unspecified mononeuropathy of bilateral lower limbs**

G58 Other mononeuropathies

- G58.0 **Intercostal neuropathy**
- G58.7 **Mononeuritis multiplex**
- G58.8 **Other specified mononeuropathies**
- G58.9 **Mononeuropathy, unspecified**

G59 Mononeuropathy in diseases classified elsewhere

Code first underlying disease

Excludes1: *diabetic mononeuropathy (E08-E13 with .41)*
syphilitic nerve paralysis (A52.19)
syphilitic neuritis (A52.15)
tuberculous mononeuropathy (A17.83)

Valid 3-character code, no further characters required

Polyneuropathies and other disorders of the peripheral nervous system (G60-G65)

Excludes1: *neuralgia NOS (M79.2)*
neuritis NOS (M79.2)
peripheral neuritis in pregnancy (O26.82-)
radiculitis NOS (M54.10)

G60 Hereditary and idiopathic neuropathy

G60.0 **Hereditary motor and sensory neuropathy**

Charcot-Marie-Tooth disease
Déjérine-Sottas disease
Hereditary motor and sensory neuropathy, types I-IV
Hypertrophic neuropathy of infancy
Peroneal muscular atrophy (axonal type) (hypertrophic type)
Roussy-Levy syndrome

CC G60.1 **Refsum's disease**

Infantile Refsum disease

CC Exclusion see Appendix A PDX collection 0588

G60.2 **Neuropathy in association with hereditary ataxia**

G60.3 **Idiopathic progressive neuropathy**

G60.8 **Other hereditary and idiopathic neuropathies**

Dominantly inherited sensory neuropathy
Morvan's disease
Nelaton's syndrome
Recessively inherited sensory neuropathy

G60.9 **Hereditary and idiopathic neuropathy, unspecified**

G61 Inflammatory polyneuropathy

CC **G61.0 Guillain-Barre syndrome**
Acute (post-)infective polyneuritis
Miller Fisher Syndrome
CC Exclusion see Appendix A PDX collection 0092
AHA CC: 2Q, 2014, 4

G61.1 Serum neuropathy
Use additional code for adverse effect, if applicable, to identify serum (T50.-)

G61.8 Other inflammatory polyneuropathies

CC **G61.81 Chronic inflammatory demyelinating polyneuritis**
CC Exclusion see Appendix A PDX collection 0589

G61.82 Multifocal motor neuropathy
MMN
AHA CC: 4Q, 2016, 18

G61.89 Other inflammatory polyneuropathies

G61.9 Inflammatory polyneuropathy, unspecified

G62 Other and unspecified polyneuropathies

G62.0 Drug-induced polyneuropathy
Use additional code for adverse effect, if applicable, to identify drug (T36-T50 with fifth or sixth character 5)

G62.1 Alcoholic polyneuropathy

G62.2 Polyneuropathy due to other toxic agents
Code first (T51-T65) to identify toxic agent

+ **G62.8 Other specified polyneuropathies**

CC **G62.81 Critical illness polyneuropathy**
Acute motor neuropathy
CC Exclusion see Appendix A PDX collection 0590

G62.82 Radiation-induced polyneuropathy
Use additional external cause code (W88-W90, X39.0-) to identify cause

G62.89 Other specified polyneuropathies
AHA CC: 2Q, 2016, 11

G62.9 Polyneuropathy, unspecified
Neuropathy NOS

G63 Polyneuropathy in diseases classified elsewhere

Code first underlying disease, such as:
amyloidosis (E85.-)
endocrine disease, except diabetes (E00-E07, E15-E16, E20-E34)
metabolic diseases (E70-E88)
neoplasm (C00-D49)
nutritional deficiency (E40-E64)

Excludes1: *polyneuropathy (in):*
diabetes mellitus (E08-E13 with .42)
diphtheria (A36.83)
infectious mononucleosis (B27.0-B27.9 with 1)
Lyme disease (A69.22)
mumps (B26.84)
postherpetic (B02.23)
rheumatoid arthritis (M05.33)
scleroderma (M34.83)
systemic lupus erythematosus (M32.19)

AHA CC: 4Q, 2012, 99-101
Valid 3-character code, no further characters required

G64 Other disorders of peripheral nervous system

Disorder of peripheral nervous system NOS
Valid 3-character code, no further characters required

G65 Sequelae of inflammatory and toxic polyneuropathies

Code first condition resulting from (sequela) of inflammatory and toxic polyneuropathies

G65.0 Sequelae of Guillain-Barré syndrome

G65.1 Sequelae of other inflammatory polyneuropathy

G65.2 Sequelae of toxic polyneuropathy

Diseases of myoneural junction and muscle (G70-G73)

G70 Myasthenia gravis and other myoneural disorders

Excludes1: *botulism (A05.1, A48.51-A48.52)*
transient neonatal myasthenia gravis (P94.0)

+ **G70.0 Myasthenia gravis**

G70.00 Myasthenia gravis without (acute) exacerbation
Myasthenia gravis NOS

MCC **G70.01 Myasthenia gravis with (acute) exacerbation**
Myasthenia gravis in crisis
MCC Exclusion see Appendix A PDX collection 0591

G70.1 Toxic myoneural disorders
Code first (T51-T65) to identify toxic agent

G70.2 Congenital and developmental myasthenia

+ **G70.8 Other specified myoneural disorders**

CC **G70.80 Lambert-Eaton syndrome, unspecified**
Lambert-Eaton syndrome NOS
CC Exclusion see Appendix A PDX collection 0591

CC **G70.81 Lambert-Eaton syndrome in disease classified elsewhere**
Code first underlying disease
Excludes1: *Lambert-Eaton syndrome in neoplastic disease (G73.1)*
CC Exclusion see Appendix A PDX collection 0591

G70.89 Other specified myoneural disorders

G70.9 Myoneural disorder, unspecified

G71 Primary disorders of muscles

Excludes2: *arthrogryposis multiplex congenita (Q74.3)*
metabolic disorders (E70-E88)
myositis (M60.-)

CC **G71.0 Muscular dystrophy**
Autosomal recessive, childhood type, muscular dystrophy resembling Duchenne or Becker muscular dystrophy
Benign [Becker] muscular dystrophy
Benign scapuloperoneal muscular dystrophy with early contractures [Emery-Dreifuss]
Congenital muscular dystrophy NOS
Congenital muscular dystrophy with specific morphological abnormalities of the muscle fiber
Distal muscular dystrophy
Facioscapulohumeral muscular dystrophy
Limb-girdle muscular dystrophy
Ocular muscular dystrophy
Oculopharyngeal muscular dystrophy
Scapuloperoneal muscular dystrophy
Severe [Duchenne] muscular dystrophy
CC Exclusion see Appendix A PDX collection 0592

+ **G71.1 Myotonic disorders**

G71.11 Myotonic muscular dystrophy
Dystrophia myotonica [Steinert]
Myotonia atrophica
Myotonic dystrophy
Proximal myotonic myopathy (PROMM)
Steinert disease

G71.12 Myotonia congenita
Acetazolamide responsive myotonia congenita
Dominant myotonia congenita [Thomsen disease]
Myotonia levior
Recessive myotonia congenita [Becker disease]

G71.13 Myotonic chondrodystrophy
Chondrodystrophic myotonia
Congenital myotonic chondrodystrophy
Schwartz-Jampel disease

G71.14 Drug induced myotonia
Use additional code for adverse effect, if applicable, to identify drug (T36-T50 with fifth or sixth character 5)

G71.19 Other specified myotonic disorders
Myotonia fluctuans
Myotonia permanens
Neuromyotonia [Isaacs]
Paramyotonia congenita (of von Eulenburg)
Pseudomyotonia
Symptomatic myotonia

CC **G71.2 Congenital myopathies**
Central core disease
Fiber-type disproportion
Minicore disease
Multicore disease
Myotubular (centronuclear) myopathy
Nemaline myopathy
Excludes1: *arthrogryposis multiplex congenita (Q74.3)*
CC Exclusion see Appendix A PDX collection 0592

G71.3 Mitochondrial myopathy, not elsewhere classified
Excludes1: *Kearns-Sayre syndrome (H49.81)*
Leber's disease (H47.21)
Leigh's encephalopathy (G31.82)
mitochondrial metabolism disorders (E88.4.-)
Reye's syndrome (G93.7)

G71.8 Other primary disorders of muscles

G71.9 Primary disorder of muscle, unspecified
Hereditary myopathy NOS

G72 **Other and unspecified myopathies**

Excludes1: *arthrogryposis multiplex congenita (Q74.3)*
dermatopolymyositis (M33.-)
ischemic infarction of muscle (M62.2-)
myositis (M60.-)
polymyositis (M33.2.-)

CC **G72.0 Drug-induced myopathy**
Use additional code for adverse effect, if applicable, to identify drug (T36-T50 with fifth or sixth character 5)
CC Exclusion see Appendix A PDX collection 0593

CC **G72.1 Alcoholic myopathy**
Use additional code to identify alcoholism (F10.-)
CC Exclusion see Appendix A PDX collection 0593

CC **G72.2 Myopathy due to other toxic agents**
Code first (T51-T65) to identify toxic agent
CC Exclusion see Appendix A PDX collection 0593

G72.3 Periodic paralysis
Familial periodic paralysis
Hyperkalemic periodic paralysis (familial)
Hypokalemic periodic paralysis (familial)
Myotonic periodic paralysis (familial)
Normokalemic paralysis (familial)
Potassium sensitive periodic paralysis
Excludes1: *paramyotonia congenita (of von Eulenburg) (G71.19)*

\+ **G72.4 Inflammatory and immune myopathies, not elsewhere classified**
G72.41 Inclusion body myositis [IBM]
G72.49 Other inflammatory and immune myopathies, not elsewhere classified
Inflammatory myopathy NOS

\+ **G72.8 Other specified myopathies**
CC **G72.81 Critical illness myopathy**
Acute necrotizing myopathy
Acute quadriplegic myopathy
Intensive care (ICU) myopathy
Myopathy of critical illness
CC Exclusion see Appendix A PDX collection 0594
G72.89 Other specified myopathies

G72.9 Myopathy, unspecified

G73 **Disorders of myoneural junction and muscle in diseases classified elsewhere**

CC **G73.1 Lambert-Eaton syndrome in neoplastic disease**
Code first underlying neoplasm (C00-D49)
Excludes1: *Lambert-Eaton syndrome not associated with neoplasm (G70.80-G70.81)*
CC Exclusion see Appendix A PDX collection 0591

CC **G73.3 Myasthenic syndromes in other diseases classified elsewhere**
Code first underlying disease, such as:
neoplasm (C00-D49)
thyrotoxicosis (E05.-)
CC Exclusion see Appendix A PDX collection 0591

G73.7 Myopathy in diseases classified elsewhere
Code first underlying disease, such as:
hyperparathyroidism (E21.0, E21.3)
hypoparathyroidism (E20.-)
glycogen storage disease (E74.0)
lipid storage disorders (E75.-)
Excludes1: *myopathy in:*
rheumatoid arthritis (M05.32)
sarcoidosis (D86.87)
scleroderma (M34.82)
sicca syndrome [Sjögren] (M35.03)
systemic lupus erythematosus (M32.19)

Cerebral palsy and other paralytic syndromes (G80-G83)

G80 **Cerebral palsy**

Excludes1: *hereditary spastic paraplegia (G11.4)*

MCC **G80.0 Spastic quadriplegic cerebral palsy**
Congenital spastic paralysis (cerebral)
MCC Exclusion see Appendix A PDX collection 0595

CC **G80.1 Spastic diplegic cerebral palsy**
Spastic cerebral palsy NOS
CC Exclusion see Appendix A PDX collection 0596

CC **G80.2 Spastic hemiplegic cerebral palsy**
CC Exclusion see Appendix A PDX collection 0597

CC **G80.3 Athetoid cerebral palsy**
Double athetosis (syndrome)
Dyskinetic cerebral palsy
Dystonic cerebral palsy
Vogt disease
CC Exclusion see Appendix A PDX collection 0598

G80.4 Ataxic cerebral palsy

G80.8 Other cerebral palsy
Mixed cerebral palsy syndromes

G80.9 Cerebral palsy, unspecified
Cerebral palsy NOS

G81 **Hemiplegia and hemiparesis**

NOTE This category is to be used only when hemiplegia (complete) (incomplete) is reported without further specification, or is stated to be old or longstanding but of unspecified cause. The category is also for use in multiple coding to identify these types of hemiplegia resulting from any cause.

Excludes1: *congenital cerebral palsy (G80.-)*
hemiplegia and hemiparesis due to sequela of cerebrovascular disease (I69.05-, I69.15-, I69.25-, I69.35-, I69.85-, I69.95-)

Review coding guideline C.6.a

\+ **G81.0 Flaccid hemiplegia**
CC **G81.00 Flaccid hemiplegia affecting unspecified side**
CC Exclusion see Appendix A PDX collection 0561
CC **G81.01 Flaccid hemiplegia affecting right dominant side**
CC Exclusion see Appendix A PDX collection 0561
CC **G81.02 Flaccid hemiplegia affecting left dominant side**
CC Exclusion see Appendix A PDX collection 0561
CC **G81.03 Flaccid hemiplegia affecting right nondominant side**
CC Exclusion see Appendix A PDX collection 0561
CC **G81.04 Flaccid hemiplegia affecting left nondominant side**
CC Exclusion see Appendix A PDX collection 0561

\+ **G81.1 Spastic hemiplegia**
CC **G81.10 Spastic hemiplegia affecting unspecified side**
CC Exclusion see Appendix A PDX collection 0561
CC **G81.11 Spastic hemiplegia affecting right dominant side**
CC Exclusion see Appendix A PDX collection 0561
CC **G81.12 Spastic hemiplegia affecting left dominant side**
CC Exclusion see Appendix A PDX collection 0561
CC **G81.13 Spastic hemiplegia affecting right nondominant side**
CC Exclusion see Appendix A PDX collection 0561
CC **G81.14 Spastic hemiplegia affecting left nondominant side**
CC Exclusion see Appendix A PDX collection 0561

\+ **G81.9 Hemiplegia, unspecified**
CC **G81.90 Hemiplegia, unspecified affecting unspecified side**
CC Exclusion see Appendix A PDX collection 0561
CC **G81.91 Hemiplegia, unspecified affecting right dominant side**
CC Exclusion see Appendix A PDX collection 0561
CC **G81.92 Hemiplegia, unspecified affecting left dominant side**
CC Exclusion see Appendix A PDX collection 0561
CC **G81.93 Hemiplegia, unspecified affecting right nondominant side**
CC Exclusion see Appendix A PDX collection 0561
CC **G81.94 Hemiplegia, unspecified affecting left nondominant side**
CC Exclusion see Appendix A PDX collection 0561
AHA CC: 1Q, 2015, 26

G82 **Paraplegia (paraparesis) and quadriplegia (quadriparesis)**

NOTE This category is to be used only when the listed conditions are reported without further specification, or are stated to be old or longstanding but of unspecified cause. The category is also for use in multiple coding to identify these conditions resulting from any cause

Excludes1: *congenital cerebral palsy (G80.-)*
functional quadriplegia (R53.2)
hysterical paralysis (F44.4)

\+ **G82.2 Paraplegia**
Paralysis of both lower limbs NOS
Paraparesis (lower) NOS
Paraplegia (lower) NOS
CC **G82.20 Paraplegia, unspecified**
CC Exclusion see Appendix A PDX collection 0561
CC **G82.21 Paraplegia, complete**
CC Exclusion see Appendix A PDX collection 0561
CC **G82.22 Paraplegia, incomplete**
CC Exclusion see Appendix A PDX collection 0561

\+ **G82.5 Quadriplegia**

MCC **G82.50 Quadriplegia, unspecified**
MCC Exclusion see Appendix A PDX collection 0595

MCC **G82.51 Quadriplegia, C1-C4 complete**
MCC Exclusion see Appendix A PDX collection 0595

MCC **G82.52 Quadriplegia, C1-C4 incomplete**
MCC Exclusion see Appendix A PDX collection 0595

MCC **G82.53 Quadriplegia, C5-C7 complete**
MCC Exclusion see Appendix A PDX collection 0595

MCC **G82.54 Quadriplegia, C5-C7 incomplete**
MCC Exclusion see Appendix A PDX collection 0595

G83 Other paralytic syndromes

NOTE This category is to be used only when the listed conditions are reported without further specification, or are stated to be old or longstanding but of unspecified cause. The category is also for use in multiple coding to identify these conditions resulting from any cause.

Includes: paralysis (complete) (incomplete), except as in G80-G82

CC **G83.0 Diplegia of upper limbs**
Diplegia (upper)
Paralysis of both upper limbs
CC Exclusion see Appendix A PDX collection 0599

\+ **G83.1 Monoplegia of lower limb**
Paralysis of lower limb
Excludes1: *monoplegia of lower limbs due to sequela of cerebrovascular disease (I69.04-, I69.14-, I69.24-, I69.34-, I69.84-, I69.94-)*
Review coding guideline C.6.a

G83.10 Monoplegia of lower limb affecting unspecified side
G83.11 Monoplegia of lower limb affecting right dominant side
G83.12 Monoplegia of lower limb affecting left dominant side
G83.13 Monoplegia of lower limb affecting right nondominant side
G83.14 Monoplegia of lower limb affecting left nondominant side

\+ **G83.2 Monoplegia of upper limb**
Paralysis of upper limb
Excludes1: *monoplegia of upper limbs due to sequela of cerebrovascular disease (I69.03-, I69.13-, I69.23-, I69.33-, I69.83-, I69.93-)*
Review coding guideline C.6.a

G83.20 Monoplegia of upper limb affecting unspecified side
G83.21 Monoplegia of upper limb affecting right dominant side
G83.22 Monoplegia of upper limb affecting left dominant side
G83.23 Monoplegia of upper limb affecting right nondominant side
G83.24 Monoplegia of upper limb affecting left nondominant side

\+ **G83.3 Monoplegia, unspecified**
Review coding guideline C.6.a

G83.30 Monoplegia, unspecified affecting unspecified side
G83.31 Monoplegia, unspecified affecting right dominant side
G83.32 Monoplegia, unspecified affecting left dominant side
G83.33 Monoplegia, unspecified affecting right nondominant side
G83.34 Monoplegia, unspecified affecting left nondominant side

CC **G83.4 Cauda equina syndrome**
Neurogenic bladder due to cauda equina syndrome
Excludes1: *cord bladder NOS (G95.89)*
neurogenic bladder NOS (N31.9)
CC Exclusion see Appendix A PDX collection 0600

MCC **G83.5 Locked-in state**
MCC Exclusion see Appendix A PDX collection 0601

\+ **G83.8 Other specified paralytic syndromes**
Excludes1: *paralytic syndromes due to current spinal cord injury-code to spinal cord injury (S14, S24, S34)*

G83.81 Brown-Séquard syndrome
G83.82 Anterior cord syndrome
G83.83 Posterior cord syndrome
G83.84 Todd's paralysis (postepileptic)
G83.89 Other specified paralytic syndromes

G83.9 Paralytic syndrome, unspecified

Other disorders of the nervous system (G89-G99)

G89 **Pain, not elsewhere classified**

Code also related psychological factors associated with pain (F45.42)

Excludes1: *generalized pain NOS (R52)*
pain disorders exclusively related to psychological factors (F45.41)
pain NOS (R52)

Excludes2: *atypical face pain (G50.1)*
headache syndromes (G44.-)
localized pain, unspecified type - code to pain by site, such as:
abdomen pain (R10.-)
back pain (M54.9)
breast pain (N64.4)
chest pain (R07.1-R07.9)
ear pain (H92.0-)
eye pain (H57.1)
headache (R51)
joint pain (M25.5-)
limb pain (M79.6-)
lumbar region pain (M54.5)
painful urination (R30.9)
pelvic and perineal pain (R10.2)
shoulder pain (M25.51-)
spine pain (M54.-)
throat pain (R07.0)
tongue pain (K14.6)
tooth pain (K08.8)
renal colic (N23)
migraines (G43.-)
myalgia (M79.1)
pain from prosthetic devices, implants, and grafts (T82.84, T83.84, T84.84, T85.84-)
phantom limb syndrome with pain (G54.6)
vulvar vestibulitis (N94.810)
vulvodynia (N94.81-)

Review coding guideline C.5.a
Review coding guidelines C.6.b.1 and C.6.b.3
Review coding guideline C.19.g.2

G89.0 Central pain syndrome
Déjérine-Roussy syndrome
Myelopathic pain syndrome
Thalamic pain syndrome (hyperesthetic)
Review coding guideline C.6.b.6

\+ **G89.1 Acute pain, not elsewhere classified**

G89.11 Acute pain due to trauma
G89.12 Acute post-thoracotomy pain
Post-thoracotomy pain NOS
G89.18 Other acute postprocedural pain
Postoperative pain NOS
Postprocedural pain NOS

\+ **G89.2 Chronic pain, not elsewhere classified**
Excludes1: *causalgia, lower limb (G57.7-)*
causalgia, upper limb (G56.4-)
central pain syndrome (G89.0)
chronic pain syndrome (G89.4)
complex regional pain syndrome II, lower limb (G57.7-)
complex regional pain syndrome II, upper limb (G56.4-)
neoplasm related chronic pain (G89.3)
reflex sympathetic dystrophy (G90.5-)
Review coding guideline C.6.b.4

G89.21 Chronic pain due to trauma
G89.22 Chronic post-thoracotomy pain
G89.28 Other chronic postprocedural pain
Other chronic postoperative pain
G89.29 Other chronic pain

G89.3 Neoplasm related pain (acute) (chronic)
Cancer associated pain
Pain due to malignancy (primary) (secondary)
Tumor associated pain
Review coding guideline C.6.b.5

G89.4 Chronic pain syndrome
Chronic pain associated with significant psychosocial dysfunction
Review coding guideline C.6.b.6

G90 Disorders of autonomic nervous system

Excludes1: *dysfunction of the autonomic nervous system due to alcohol (G31.2)*

\+ **G90.0 Idiopathic peripheral autonomic neuropathy**

G90.01 Carotid sinus syncope
Carotid sinus syndrome

G90.09 Other idiopathic peripheral autonomic neuropathy
Idiopathic peripheral autonomic neuropathy NOS

G90.1 Familial dysautonomia [Riley-Day]

G90.2 Horner's syndrome
Bernard(-Horner) syndrome
Cervical sympathetic dystrophy or paralysis

CC **G90.3 Multi-system degeneration of the autonomic nervous system**
Neurogenic orthostatic hypotension [Shy-Drager]
Excludes1: *orthostatic hypotension NOS (I95.1)*
CC Exclusion see Appendix A PDX collection 0573

G90.4 Autonomic dysreflexia
Use additional code to identify the cause, such as:
fecal impaction (K56.41)
pressure ulcer (pressure area) (L89.-)
urinary tract infection (N39.0)

\+ **G90.5 Complex regional pain syndrome I (CRPS I)**
Reflex sympathetic dystrophy
Excludes1: *causalgia of lower limb (G57.7-)*
causalgia of upper limb (G56.4-)
complex regional pain syndrome II of lower limb (G57.7-)
complex regional pain syndrome II of upper limb (G56.4-)

CC **G90.50 Complex regional pain syndrome I, unspecified**
CC Exclusion see Appendix A PDX collection 0602

\+ **G90.51 Complex regional pain syndrome I of upper limb**

CC **G90.511 Complex regional pain syndrome I of right upper limb**
CC Exclusion see Appendix A PDX collection 0603

CC **G90.512 Complex regional pain syndrome I of left upper limb**
CC Exclusion see Appendix A PDX collection 0603

CC **G90.513 Complex regional pain syndrome I of upper limb, bilateral**
CC Exclusion see Appendix A PDX collection 0603

CC **G90.519 Complex regional pain syndrome I of unspecified upper limb**
CC Exclusion see Appendix A PDX collection 0603

\+ **G90.52 Complex regional pain syndrome I of lower limb**

CC **G90.521 Complex regional pain syndrome I of right lower limb**
CC Exclusion see Appendix A PDX collection 0603

CC **G90.522 Complex regional pain syndrome I of left lower limb**
CC Exclusion see Appendix A PDX collection 0603

CC **G90.523 Complex regional pain syndrome I of lower limb, bilateral**
CC Exclusion see Appendix A PDX collection 0603

CC **G90.529 Complex regional pain syndrome I of unspecified lower limb**
CC Exclusion see Appendix A PDX collection 0603

CC **G90.59 Complex regional pain syndrome I of other specified site**
CC Exclusion see Appendix A PDX collection 0603

G90.8 Other disorders of autonomic nervous system

G90.9 Disorder of the autonomic nervous system, unspecified

G91 Hydrocephalus

Includes: acquired hydrocephalus
Excludes1: *Arnold-Chiari syndrome with hydrocephalus (Q07.-)*
congenital hydrocephalus (Q03.-)
spina bifida with hydrocephalus (Q05.-)

CC **G91.0 Communicating hydrocephalus**
Secondary normal pressure hydrocephalus
CC Exclusion see Appendix A PDX collection 0604

CC **G91.1 Obstructive hydrocephalus**
CC Exclusion see Appendix A PDX collection 0605

CC **G91.2 (Idiopathic) normal pressure hydrocephalus**
Normal pressure hydrocephalus NOS
CC Exclusion see Appendix A PDX collection 0604

CC **G91.3 Post-traumatic hydrocephalus, unspecified**
CC Exclusion see Appendix A PDX collection 0605

G91.4 Hydrocephalus in diseases classified elsewhere
Code first underlying condition, such as:
congenital syphilis (A50.4-)
neoplasm (C00-D49)
Excludes1: *hydrocephalus due to congenital toxoplasmosis (P37.1)*
AHA CC: 3Q, 2014, 3-4

CC **G91.8 Other hydrocephalus**
CC Exclusion see Appendix A PDX collection 0605

CC **G91.9 Hydrocephalus, unspecified**
CC Exclusion see Appendix A PDX collection 0605

MCC **G92 Toxic encephalopathy**

Toxic encephalitis
Toxic metabolic encephalopathy
Code first, if applicable, drug induced (T36-T50) (T51-T65) to identify toxic agent
MCC Exclusion see Appendix A PDX collection 0606
AHA CC: 1Q, 2017, 39-40
Valid 3-character code, no further characters required

G93 Other disorders of brain

G93.0 Cerebral cysts
Arachnoid cyst
Porencephalic cyst, acquired
Excludes1: *acquired periventricular cysts of newborn (P91.1)*
congenital cerebral cysts (Q04.6)

CC **G93.1 Anoxic brain damage, not elsewhere classified**
Excludes1: *cerebral anoxia due to anesthesia during labor and delivery (O74.3)*
cerebral anoxia due to anesthesia during the puerperium (O89.2)
neonatal anoxia (P84)
CC Exclusion see Appendix A PDX collection 0607

G93.2 Benign intracranial hypertension
Excludes1: *hypertensive encephalopathy (I67.4)*

G93.3 Postviral fatigue syndrome
Benign myalgic encephalomyelitis
Excludes1: *chronic fatigue syndrome NOS (R53.82)*

\+ **G93.4 Other and unspecified encephalopathy**
Excludes1: alcoholic encephalopathy (G31.2)
encephalopathy in diseases classified elsewhere (G94)
hypertensive encephalopathy (I67.4)
toxic (metabolic) encephalopathy (G92)
AHA CC: 2Q, 2017, 8-9

MCC **G93.40 Encephalopathy, unspecified**
MCC Exclusion see Appendix A PDX collection 0608

MCC **G93.41 Metabolic encephalopathy**
Septic encephalopathy
MCC Exclusion see Appendix A PDX collection 0609
AHA CC: 3Q, 2015, 21; 3Q, 2016, 42

MCC **G93.49 Other encephalopathy**
Encephalopathy NEC
MCC Exclusion see Appendix A PDX collection 0610
AHA CC: 2Q, 2017, 9

MCC **G93.5 Compression of brain**
Arnold-Chiari type 1 compression of brain
Compression of brain (stem)
Herniation of brain (stem)
Excludes1: *diffuse traumatic compression of brain (S06.2-)*
focal traumatic compression of brain (S06.3-)
MCC Exclusion see Appendix A PDX collection 0611

MCC **G93.6 Cerebral edema**
Excludes1: *cerebral edema due to birth injury (P11.0)*
traumatic cerebral edema (S06.1-)
MCC Exclusion see Appendix A PDX collection 0612

• MCC **G93.7 Reye's syndrome**
Code first poisoning due to salicylates, if applicable (T39.0-, with sixth character 1-4)
Use additional code for adverse effect due to salicylates, if applicable (T39.0-, with sixth character 5)
MCC Exclusion see Appendix A PDX collection 0613

+ G93.8 **Other specified disorders of brain**
G93.81 **Temporal sclerosis**
Hippocampal sclerosis
Mesial temporal sclerosis
MCC G93.82 **Brain death**
MCC Exclusion see Appendix A PDX collection 0515
G93.89 **Other specified disorders of brain**
Postradiation encephalopathy
AHA CC: 4Q, 2016, 4-7
G93.9 **Disorder of brain, unspecified**

G94 Other disorders of brain in diseases classified elsewhere

Code first underlying disease
Excludes1: *encephalopathy in congenital syphilis (A50.49)*
encephalopathy in influenza (J09.X9, J10.81, J11.81)
encephalopathy in syphilis (A52.19)
hydrocephalus in diseases classified elsewhere (G91.4)
AHA CC: 2Q, 2017, 8-9
Valid 3-character code, no further characters required

G95 Other and unspecified diseases of spinal cord

Excludes2: *myelitis (G04.-)*
CC G95.0 **Syringomyelia and syringobulbia**
CC Exclusion see Appendix A PDX collection 0614
+ G95.1 **Vascular myelopathies**
Excludes2: *intraspinal phlebitis and thrombophlebitis, except non-pyogenic (G08)*
MCC G95.11 **Acute infarction of spinal cord (embolic) (nonembolic)**
Anoxia of spinal cord
Arterial thrombosis of spinal cord
MCC Exclusion see Appendix A PDX collection 0603
MCC G95.19 **Other vascular myelopathies**
Edema of spinal cord
Hematomyelia
Nonpyogenic intraspinal phlebitis and thrombophlebitis
Subacute necrotic myelopathy
MCC Exclusion see Appendix A PDX collection 0603
+ G95.2 **Other and unspecified cord compression**
CC G95.20 **Unspecified cord compression**
CC Exclusion see Appendix A PDX collection 0615
CC G95.29 **Other cord compression**
CC Exclusion see Appendix A PDX collection 0615
+ G95.8 **Other specified diseases of spinal cord**
Excludes1: *neurogenic bladder NOS (N31.9)*
neurogenic bladder due to cauda equina syndrome (G83.4)
neuromuscular dysfunction of bladder without spinal cord lesion (N31.-)
CC G95.81 **Conus medullaris syndrome**
CC Exclusion see Appendix A PDX collection 0603
CC G95.89 **Other specified diseases of spinal cord**
Cord bladder NOS
Drug-induced myelopathy
Radiation-induced myelopathy
Excludes1: *myelopathy NOS (G95.9)*
CC Exclusion see Appendix A PDX collection 0603
CC G95.9 **Disease of spinal cord, unspecified**
Myelopathy NOS
CC Exclusion see Appendix A PDX collection 0615

G96 Other disorders of central nervous system

CC G96.0 **Cerebrospinal fluid leak**
Excludes1: *cerebrospinal fluid leak from spinal puncture (G97.0)*
CC Exclusion see Appendix A PDX collection 0616
+ G96.1 **Disorders of meninges, not elsewhere classified**
CC G96.11 **Dural tear**
Excludes1: *accidental puncture or laceration of dura during a procedure (G97.41)*
CC Exclusion see Appendix A PDX collection 0509
AHA CC: 4Q, 2014, 24
G96.12 **Meningeal adhesions (cerebral) (spinal)**
G96.19 **Other disorders of meninges, not elsewhere classified**
G96.8 **Other specified disorders of central nervous system**
G96.9 **Disorder of central nervous system, unspecified**

G97 Intraoperative and postprocedural complications and disorders of nervous system, not elsewhere classified

Excludes2: *intraoperative and postprocedural cerebrovascular infarction (I97.81-, I97.82-)*
AHA CC: 4Q, 2016, 9-10
CC G97.0 **Cerebrospinal fluid leak from spinal puncture**
CC Exclusion see Appendix A PDX collection 0617
G97.1 **Other reaction to spinal and lumbar puncture**
Headache due to lumbar puncture
CC G97.2 **Intracranial hypotension following ventricular shunting**
CC Exclusion see Appendix A PDX collection 0617
+ G97.3 **Intraoperative hemorrhage and hematoma of a nervous system organ or structure complicating a procedure**
Excludes1: *intraoperative hemorrhage and hematoma of a nervous system organ or structure due to accidental puncture and laceration during a procedure (G97.4-)*
CC G97.31 **Intraoperative hemorrhage and hematoma of a nervous system organ or structure complicating a nervous system procedure**
CC Exclusion see Appendix A PDX collection 0618
CC G97.32 **Intraoperative hemorrhage and hematoma of a nervous system organ or structure complicating other procedure**
CC Exclusion see Appendix A PDX collection 0618
+ G97.4 **Accidental puncture and laceration of a nervous system organ or structure during a procedure**
CC G97.41 **Accidental puncture or laceration of dura during a procedure**
Incidental (inadvertent) durotomy
CC Exclusion see Appendix A PDX collection 0509
CC G97.48 **Accidental puncture and laceration of other nervous system organ or structure during a nervous system procedure**
CC Exclusion see Appendix A PDX collection 0509
CC G97.49 **Accidental puncture and laceration of other nervous system organ or structure during other procedure**
CC Exclusion see Appendix A PDX collection 0509
+ G97.5 **Postprocedural hemorrhage of a nervous system organ or structure following a procedure**
CC G97.51 **Postprocedural hemorrhage of a nervous system organ or structure following a nervous system procedure**
CC Exclusion see Appendix A PDX collection 0619
CC G97.52 **Postprocedural hemorrhage of a nervous system organ or structure following other procedure**
CC Exclusion see Appendix A PDX collection 0619
+ G97.6 **Postprocedural hematoma and seroma of a nervous system organ or structure following a procedure**
CC G97.61 **Postprocedural hematoma of a nervous system organ or structure following a nervous system procedure**
CC Exclusion see Appendix A PDX collection 0619
CC G97.62 **Postprocedural hematoma of a nervous system organ or structure following other procedure**
CC Exclusion see Appendix A PDX collection 0619
CC G97.63 **Postprocedural seroma of a nervous system organ or structure following a nervous system procedure**
CC Exclusion see Appendix A PDX collection 0619
CC G97.64 **Postprocedural seroma of a nervous system organ or structure following other procedure**
CC Exclusion see Appendix A PDX collection 0619
+ G97.8 **Other intraoperative and postprocedural complications and disorders of nervous system**
Use additional code to further specify disorder
CC G97.81 **Other intraoperative complications of nervous system**
CC Exclusion see Appendix A PDX collection 0617
CC G97.82 **Other postprocedural complications and disorders of nervous system**
CC Exclusion see Appendix A PDX collection 0617

G98 Other disorders of nervous system not elsewhere classified

Includes: nervous system disorder NOS
G98.0 **Neurogenic arthritis, not elsewhere classified**
Nonsyphilitic neurogenic arthropathy NEC
Nonsyphilitic neurogenic spondylopathy NEC
Excludes1: *spondylopathy (in):*
syringomyelia and syringobulbia (G95.0)
tabes dorsalis (A52.11)
G98.8 **Other disorders of nervous system**
Nervous system disorder NOS

G99 **Other disorders of nervous system in diseases classified elsewhere**

CC **G99.0 Autonomic neuropathy in diseases classified elsewhere**

Code first underlying disease, such as:
amyloidosis (E85.-)
gout (M1A.-, M10.-)
hyperthyroidism (E05.-)

Excludes1: *diabetic autonomic neuropathy (E08-E13 with .43)*

CC Exclusion see Appendix A PDX collection 0620

CC **G99.2 Myelopathy in diseases classified elsewhere**

Code first underlying disease, such as:
neoplasm (C00-D49)

Excludes1: *myelopathy in:*
intervertebral disease (M50.0-, M51.0-)
spondylosis (M47.0-, M47.1-)

CC Exclusion see Appendix A PDX collection 0603

G99.8 Other specified disorders of nervous system in diseases classified elsewhere

Code first underlying disorder, such as:
amyloidosis (E85.-)
avitaminosis (E56.9)

Excludes1: *nervous system involvement in:*
cysticercosis (B69.0)
rubella (B06.0-)
syphilis (A52.1-)

Chapter 7: Diseases of the Eye and Adnexa (H00-H59)

NOTE Use an external cause code following the code for the eye condition, if applicable, to identify the cause of the eye condition

Excludes2: *certain conditions originating in the perinatal period (P04-P96)*
certain infectious and parasitic diseases (A00-B99)
complications of pregnancy, childbirth and the puerperium (O00-O9A)
congenital malformations, deformations, and chromosomal abnormalities (Q00-Q99)
diabetes mellitus related eye conditions (E09.3-, E10.3-, E11.3-, E13.3-)
endocrine, nutritional and metabolic diseases (E00-E88)
injury (trauma) of eye and orbit (S05.-)
injury, poisoning and certain other consequences of external causes (S00-T88)
neoplasms (C00-D49)
symptoms, signs and abnormal clinical and laboratory findings, not elsewhere classified (R00-R94)
syphilis related eye disorders (A50.01, A50.3-, A51.43, A52.71)

This chapter contains the following category blocks:

H00-H05	Disorders of eyelid, lacrimal system and orbit
H10-H11	Disorders of conjunctiva
H15-H22	Disorders of sclera, cornea, iris and ciliary body
H25-H28	Disorders of lens
H30-H36	Disorders of choroid and retina
H40-H42	Glaucoma
H43-H44	Disorders of vitreous body and globe
H46-H47	Disorders of optic nerve and visual pathways
H49-H52	Disorders of ocular muscles, binocular movement, accommodation and refraction
H53-H54	Visual disturbances and blindness
H55-H57	Other disorders of eye and adnexa
H59	Intraoperative and postprocedural complications and disorders of eye and adnexa, not elsewhere classified

C. Chapter-Specific Coding Guidelines

In addition to general coding guidelines, there are guidelines for specific diagnoses and/or conditions in the classification. Unless otherwise indicated, these guidelines apply to all health care settings. Please refer to Section II for guidelines on the selection of principal diagnosis.

7. Chapter 7: Diseases of the Eye and Adnexa (H00-H59)

a. Glaucoma

1) Assigning Glaucoma Codes

Assign as many codes from category H40, Glaucoma, as needed to identify the type of glaucoma, the affected eye, and the glaucoma stage.

2) Bilateral glaucoma with same type and stage

When a patient has bilateral glaucoma and both eyes are documented as being the same type and stage, and there is a code for bilateral glaucoma, report only the code for the type of glaucoma, bilateral, with the seventh character for the stage.

When a patient has bilateral glaucoma and both eyes are documented as being the same type and stage, and the classification does not provide a code for bilateral glaucoma (i.e. subcategories H40.10, H40.11 and H40.20) report only one code for the type of glaucoma with the appropriate seventh character for the stage.

3) Bilateral glaucoma stage with different types or stages

When a patient has bilateral glaucoma and each eye is documented as having a different type or stage, and the classification distinguishes laterality, assign the appropriate code for each eye rather than the code for bilateral glaucoma.

When a patient has bilateral glaucoma and each eye is documented as having a different type, and the classification does not distinguish laterality (i.e. subcategories H40.10, H40.11 and H40.20), assign one code for each type of glaucoma with the appropriate seventh character for the stage.

When a patient has bilateral glaucoma and each eye is documented as having the same type, but different stage, and the classification does not distinguish laterality (i.e. subcategories H40.10, H40.11 and H40.20), assign a code for the type of glaucoma for each eye with the seventh character for the specific glaucoma stage documented for each eye.

4) Patient admitted with glaucoma and stage evolves during the admission

If a patient is admitted with glaucoma and the stage progresses during the admission, assign the code for highest stage documented.

5) Indeterminate stage glaucoma

Assignment of the seventh character "4" for "indeterminate stage" should be based on the clinical documentation. The seventh character "4" is used for glaucomas whose stage cannot be clinically determined. This seventh character should not be confused with the seventh character "0", unspecified, which should be assigned when there is no documentation regarding the stage of the glaucoma.

b. Blindness

If "blindness" or "low vision" of both eyes is documented but the visual impairment category is not documented, assign code H54.3, Unqualified visual loss, both eyes. If "blindness" or "low vision" in one eye is documented but the visual impairment category is not documented, assign a code from H54.6-, Unqualified visual loss, one eye. If "blindness" or "visual loss" is documented without any information about whether one or both eyes are affected, assign code H54.7, Unspecified visual loss.

Disorders of eyelid, lacrimal system and orbit (H00-H05)

Excludes2: *open wound of eyelid (S01.1-)*
superficial injury of eyelid (S00.1-, S00.2-)

H00 Hordeolum and chalazion

+ **H00.0 Hordeolum (externum) (internum) of eyelid**
  + **H00.01 Hordeolum externum**
    Hordeolum NOS
    Stye
    H00.011 Hordeolum externum right upper eyelid
    H00.012 Hordeolum externum right lower eyelid
    H00.013 Hordeolum externum right eye, unspecified eyelid
    H00.014 Hordeolum externum left upper eyelid
    H00.015 Hordeolum externum left lower eyelid
    H00.016 Hordeolum externum left eye, unspecified eyelid
    H00.019 Hordeolum externum unspecified eye, unspecified eyelid
  + **H00.02 Hordeolum internum**
    Infection of meibomian gland
    H00.021 Hordeolum internum right upper eyelid
    H00.022 Hordeolum internum right lower eyelid
    H00.023 Hordeolum internum right eye, unspecified eyelid
    H00.024 Hordeolum internum left upper eyelid
    H00.025 Hordeolum internum left lower eyelid
    H00.026 Hordeolum internum left eye, unspecified eyelid
    H00.029 Hordeolum internum unspecified eye, unspecified eyelid
  + **H00.03 Abscess of eyelid**
    Furuncle of eyelid
    H00.031 Abscess of right upper eyelid
    H00.032 Abscess of right lower eyelid
    H00.033 Abscess of eyelid right eye, unspecified eyelid
    H00.034 Abscess of left upper eyelid
    H00.035 Abscess of left lower eyelid
    H00.036 Abscess of eyelid left eye, unspecified eyelid
    H00.039 Abscess of eyelid unspecified eye, unspecified eyelid
+ **H00.1 Chalazion**
  Meibomian (gland) cyst
  Excludes2: *infected meibomian gland (H00.02-)*
  H00.11 Chalazion right upper eyelid
  H00.12 Chalazion right lower eyelid
  H00.13 Chalazion right eye, unspecified eyelid
  H00.14 Chalazion left upper eyelid
  H00.15 Chalazion left lower eyelid
  H00.16 Chalazion left eye, unspecified eyelid
  H00.19 Chalazion unspecified eye, unspecified eyelid

H01 Other inflammation of eyelid

+ **H01.0 Blepharitis**
  Excludes1: *blepharoconjunctivitis (H10.5-)*
  + **H01.00 Unspecified blepharitis**
    H01.001 Unspecified blepharitis right upper eyelid
    H01.002 Unspecified blepharitis right lower eyelid
    H01.003 Unspecified blepharitis right eye, unspecified eyelid
    H01.004 Unspecified blepharitis left upper eyelid
    H01.005 Unspecified blepharitis left lower eyelid
    H01.006 Unspecified blepharitis left eye, unspecified eyelid
    H01.009 Unspecified blepharitis unspecified eye, unspecified eyelid
  + **H01.01 Ulcerative blepharitis**
    H01.011 Ulcerative blepharitis right upper eyelid
    H01.012 Ulcerative blepharitis right lower eyelid
    H01.013 Ulcerative blepharitis right eye, unspecified eyelid

Eye

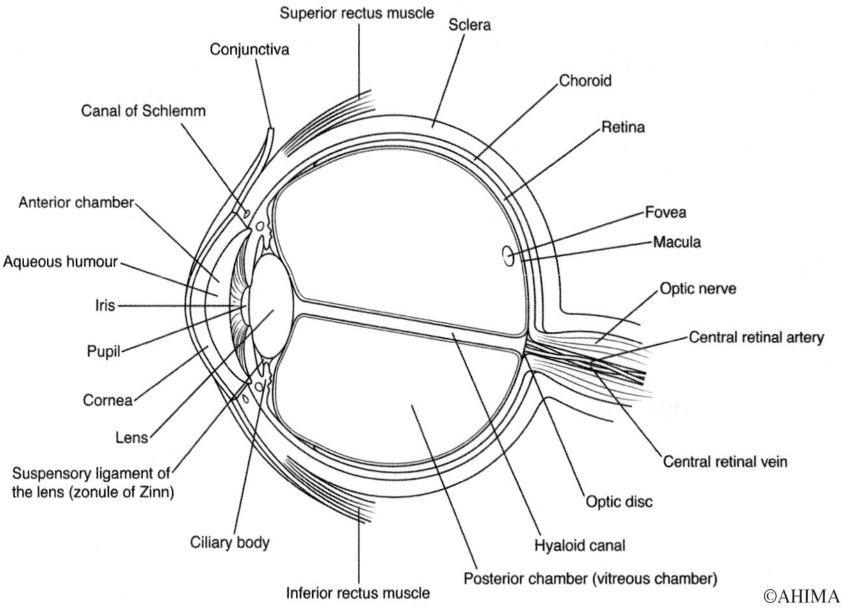

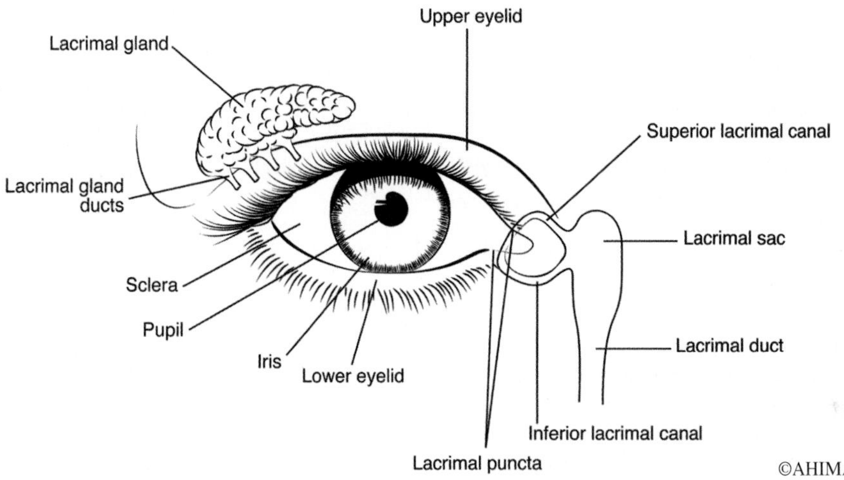

Muscles of the Eye

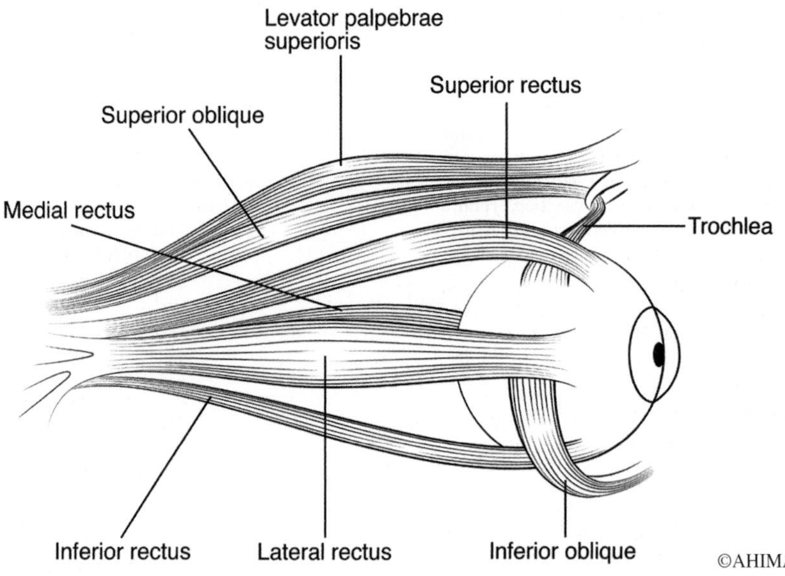

H01.014 Ulcerative blepharitis left upper eyelid
H01.015 Ulcerative blepharitis left lower eyelid
H01.016 Ulcerative blepharitis left eye, unspecified eyelid
H01.019 Ulcerative blepharitis unspecified eye, unspecified eyelid

+ H01.02 Squamous blepharitis
H01.021 Squamous blepharitis right upper eyelid
H01.022 Squamous blepharitis right lower eyelid
H01.023 Squamous blepharitis right eye, unspecified eyelid
H01.024 Squamous blepharitis left upper eyelid
H01.025 Squamous blepharitis left lower eyelid
H01.026 Squamous blepharitis left eye, unspecified eyelid
H01.029 Squamous blepharitis unspecified eye, unspecified eyelid

+ H01.1 Noninfectious dermatoses of eyelid

+ H01.11 Allergic dermatitis of eyelid
Contact dermatitis of eyelid
H01.111 Allergic dermatitis of right upper eyelid
H01.112 Allergic dermatitis of right lower eyelid
H01.113 Allergic dermatitis of right eye, unspecified eyelid
H01.114 Allergic dermatitis of left upper eyelid
H01.115 Allergic dermatitis of left lower eyelid
H01.116 Allergic dermatitis of left eye, unspecified eyelid
H01.119 Allergic dermatitis of unspecified eye, unspecified eyelid

+ H01.12 Discoid lupus erythematosus of eyelid
H01.121 Discoid lupus erythematosus of right upper eyelid
H01.122 Discoid lupus erythematosus of right lower eyelid
H01.123 Discoid lupus erythematosus of right eye, unspecified eyelid
H01.124 Discoid lupus erythematosus of left upper eyelid
H01.125 Discoid lupus erythematosus of left lower eyelid
H01.126 Discoid lupus erythematosus of left eye, unspecified eyelid
H01.129 Discoid lupus erythematosus of unspecified eye, unspecified eyelid

+ H01.13 Eczematous dermatitis of eyelid
H01.131 Eczematous dermatitis of right upper eyelid
H01.132 Eczematous dermatitis of right lower eyelid
H01.133 Eczematous dermatitis of right eye, unspecified eyelid
H01.134 Eczematous dermatitis of left upper eyelid
H01.135 Eczematous dermatitis of left lower eyelid
H01.136 Eczematous dermatitis of left eye, unspecified eyelid
H01.139 Eczematous dermatitis of unspecified eye, unspecified eyelid

+ H01.14 Xeroderma of eyelid
H01.141 Xeroderma of right upper eyelid
H01.142 Xeroderma of right lower eyelid
H01.143 Xeroderma of right eye, unspecified eyelid
H01.144 Xeroderma of left upper eyelid
H01.145 Xeroderma of left lower eyelid
H01.146 Xeroderma of left eye, unspecified eyelid
H01.149 Xeroderma of unspecified eye, unspecified eyelid

H01.8 Other specified inflammations of eyelid

H01.9 Unspecified inflammation of eyelid
Inflammation of eyelid NOS

H02 Other disorders of eyelid

Excludes1: *congenital malformations of eyelid (Q10.0-Q10.3)*

+ H02.0 Entropion and trichiasis of eyelid

+ H02.00 Unspecified entropion of eyelid
H02.001 Unspecified entropion of right upper eyelid
H02.002 Unspecified entropion of right lower eyelid
H02.003 Unspecified entropion of right eye, unspecified eyelid
H02.004 Unspecified entropion of left upper eyelid
H02.005 Unspecified entropion of left lower eyelid
H02.006 Unspecified entropion of left eye, unspecified eyelid
H02.009 Unspecified entropion of unspecified eye, unspecified eyelid

+ H02.01 Cicatricial entropion of eyelid
H02.011 Cicatricial entropion of right upper eyelid
H02.012 Cicatricial entropion of right lower eyelid
H02.013 Cicatricial entropion of right eye, unspecified eyelid
H02.014 Cicatricial entropion of left upper eyelid
H02.015 Cicatricial entropion of left lower eyelid
H02.016 Cicatricial entropion of left eye, unspecified eyelid
H02.019 Cicatricial entropion of unspecified eye, unspecified eyelid

+ H02.02 Mechanical entropion of eyelid
H02.021 Mechanical entropion of right upper eyelid
H02.022 Mechanical entropion of right lower eyelid
H02.023 Mechanical entropion of right eye, unspecified eyelid
H02.024 Mechanical entropion of left upper eyelid
H02.025 Mechanical entropion of left lower eyelid
H02.026 Mechanical entropion of left eye, unspecified eyelid
H02.029 Mechanical entropion of unspecified eye, unspecified eyelid

+ H02.03 Senile entropion of eyelid
• H02.031 Senile entropion of right upper eyelid
• H02.032 Senile entropion of right lower eyelid
• H02.033 Senile entropion of right eye, unspecified eyelid
• H02.034 Senile entropion of left upper eyelid
• H02.035 Senile entropion of left lower eyelid
• H02.036 Senile entropion of left eye, unspecified eyelid
• H02.039 Senile entropion of unspecified eye, unspecified eyelid

+ H02.04 Spastic entropion of eyelid
H02.041 Spastic entropion of right upper eyelid
H02.042 Spastic entropion of right lower eyelid
H02.043 Spastic entropion of right eye, unspecified eyelid
H02.044 Spastic entropion of left upper eyelid
H02.045 Spastic entropion of left lower eyelid
H02.046 Spastic entropion of left eye, unspecified eyelid
H02.049 Spastic entropion of unspecified eye, unspecified eyelid

+ H02.05 Trichiasis without entropion
H02.051 Trichiasis without entropion right upper eyelid
H02.052 Trichiasis without entropion right lower eyelid
H02.053 Trichiasis without entropion right eye, unspecified eyelid
H02.054 Trichiasis without entropion left upper eyelid
H02.055 Trichiasis without entropion left lower eyelid
H02.056 Trichiasis without entropion left eye, unspecified eyelid
H02.059 Trichiasis without entropion unspecified eye, unspecified eyelid

+ H02.1 Ectropion of eyelid

+ H02.10 Unspecified ectropion of eyelid
H02.101 Unspecified ectropion of right upper eyelid
H02.102 Unspecified ectropion of right lower eyelid
H02.103 Unspecified ectropion of right eye, unspecified eyelid
H02.104 Unspecified ectropion of left upper eyelid
H02.105 Unspecified ectropion of left lower eyelid
H02.106 Unspecified ectropion of left eye, unspecified eyelid
H02.109 Unspecified ectropion of unspecified eye, unspecified eyelid

+ H02.11 Cicatricial ectropion of eyelid
H02.111 Cicatricial ectropion of right upper eyelid
H02.112 Cicatricial ectropion of right lower eyelid
H02.113 Cicatricial ectropion of right eye, unspecified eyelid

H02.114 Cicatricial ectropion of left upper eyelid
H02.115 Cicatricial ectropion of left lower eyelid
H02.116 Cicatricial ectropion of left eye, unspecified eyelid
H02.119 Cicatricial ectropion of unspecified eye, unspecified eyelid
+ H02.12 Mechanical ectropion of eyelid
H02.121 Mechanical ectropion of right upper eyelid
H02.122 Mechanical ectropion of right lower eyelid
H02.123 Mechanical ectropion of right eye, unspecified eyelid
H02.124 Mechanical ectropion of left upper eyelid
H02.125 Mechanical ectropion of left lower eyelid
H02.126 Mechanical ectropion of left eye, unspecified eyelid
H02.129 Mechanical ectropion of unspecified eye, unspecified eyelid
+ H02.13 Senile ectropion of eyelid
• H02.131 Senile ectropion of right upper eyelid
• H02.132 Senile ectropion of right lower eyelid
• H02.133 Senile ectropion of right eye, unspecified eyelid
• H02.134 Senile ectropion of left upper eyelid
• H02.135 Senile ectropion of left lower eyelid
• H02.136 Senile ectropion of left eye, unspecified eyelid
• H02.139 Senile ectropion of unspecified eye, unspecified eyelid
+ H02.14 Spastic ectropion of eyelid
H02.141 Spastic ectropion of right upper eyelid
H02.142 Spastic ectropion of right lower eyelid
H02.143 Spastic ectropion of right eye, unspecified eyelid
H02.144 Spastic ectropion of left upper eyelid
H02.145 Spastic ectropion of left lower eyelid
H02.146 Spastic ectropion of left eye, unspecified eyelid
H02.149 Spastic ectropion of unspecified eye, unspecified eyelid
+ H02.2 Lagophthalmos
+ H02.20 Unspecified lagophthalmos
H02.201 Unspecified lagophthalmos right upper eyelid
H02.202 Unspecified lagophthalmos right lower eyelid
H02.203 Unspecified lagophthalmos right eye, unspecified eyelid
H02.204 Unspecified lagophthalmos left upper eyelid
H02.205 Unspecified lagophthalmos left lower eyelid
H02.206 Unspecified lagophthalmos left eye, unspecified eyelid
H02.209 Unspecified lagophthalmos unspecified eye, unspecified eyelid
+ H02.21 Cicatricial lagophthalmos
H02.211 Cicatricial lagophthalmos right upper eyelid
H02.212 Cicatricial lagophthalmos right lower eyelid
H02.213 Cicatricial lagophthalmos right eye, unspecified eyelid
H02.214 Cicatricial lagophthalmos left upper eyelid
H02.215 Cicatricial lagophthalmos left lower eyelid
H02.216 Cicatricial lagophthalmos left eye, unspecified eyelid
H02.219 Cicatricial lagophthalmos unspecified eye, unspecified eyelid
+ H02.22 Mechanical lagophthalmos
H02.221 Mechanical lagophthalmos right upper eyelid
H02.222 Mechanical lagophthalmos right lower eyelid
H02.223 Mechanical lagophthalmos right eye, unspecified eyelid
H02.224 Mechanical lagophthalmos left upper eyelid
H02.225 Mechanical lagophthalmos left lower eyelid
H02.226 Mechanical lagophthalmos left eye, unspecified eyelid
H02.229 Mechanical lagophthalmos unspecified eye, unspecified eyelid
+ H02.23 Paralytic lagophthalmos
H02.231 Paralytic lagophthalmos right upper eyelid
H02.232 Paralytic lagophthalmos right lower eyelid
H02.233 Paralytic lagophthalmos right eye, unspecified eyelid
H02.234 Paralytic lagophthalmos left upper eyelid
H02.235 Paralytic lagophthalmos left lower eyelid
H02.236 Paralytic lagophthalmos left eye, unspecified eyelid
H02.239 Paralytic lagophthalmos unspecified eye, unspecified eyelid
+ H02.3 Blepharochalasis
Pseudoptosis
H02.30 Blepharochalasis unspecified eye, unspecified eyelid
H02.31 Blepharochalasis right upper eyelid
H02.32 Blepharochalasis right lower eyelid
H02.33 Blepharochalasis right eye, unspecified eyelid
H02.34 Blepharochalasis left upper eyelid
H02.35 Blepharochalasis left lower eyelid
H02.36 Blepharochalasis left eye, unspecified eyelid
+ H02.4 Ptosis of eyelid
+ H02.40 Unspecified ptosis of eyelid
H02.401 Unspecified ptosis of right eyelid
H02.402 Unspecified ptosis of left eyelid
H02.403 Unspecified ptosis of bilateral eyelids
H02.409 Unspecified ptosis of unspecified eyelid
+ H02.41 Mechanical ptosis of eyelid
H02.411 Mechanical ptosis of right eyelid
H02.412 Mechanical ptosis of left eyelid
H02.413 Mechanical ptosis of bilateral eyelids
H02.419 Mechanical ptosis of unspecified eyelid
+ H02.42 Myogenic ptosis of eyelid
H02.421 Myogenic ptosis of right eyelid
H02.422 Myogenic ptosis of left eyelid
H02.423 Myogenic ptosis of bilateral eyelids
H02.429 Myogenic ptosis of unspecified eyelid
+ H02.43 Paralytic ptosis of eyelid
Neurogenic ptosis of eyelid
H02.431 Paralytic ptosis of right eyelid
H02.432 Paralytic ptosis of left eyelid
H02.433 Paralytic ptosis of bilateral eyelids
H02.439 Paralytic ptosis unspecified eyelid
+ H02.5 Other disorders affecting eyelid function
Excludes2: *blepharospasm (G24.5)*
organic tic (G25.69)
psychogenic tic (F95.-)
+ H02.51 Abnormal innervation syndrome
H02.511 Abnormal innervation syndrome right upper eyelid
H02.512 Abnormal innervation syndrome right lower eyelid
H02.513 Abnormal innervation syndrome right eye, unspecified eyelid
H02.514 Abnormal innervation syndrome left upper eyelid
H02.515 Abnormal innervation syndrome left lower eyelid
H02.516 Abnormal innervation syndrome left eye, unspecified eyelid
H02.519 Abnormal innervation syndrome unspecified eye, unspecified eyelid
+ H02.52 Blepharophimosis
Ankyloblepharon
H02.521 Blepharophimosis right upper eyelid
H02.522 Blepharophimosis right lower eyelid
H02.523 Blepharophimosis right eye, unspecified eyelid
H02.524 Blepharophimosis left upper eyelid
H02.525 Blepharophimosis left lower eyelid
H02.526 Blepharophimosis left eye, unspecified eyelid
H02.529 Blepharophimosis unspecified eye, unspecified lid
+ H02.53 Eyelid retraction
Eyelid lag
H02.531 Eyelid retraction right upper eyelid
H02.532 Eyelid retraction right lower eyelid
H02.533 Eyelid retraction right eye, unspecified eyelid
H02.534 Eyelid retraction left upper eyelid
H02.535 Eyelid retraction left lower eyelid

H02.536 Eyelid retraction left eye, unspecified eyelid
H02.539 Eyelid retraction unspecified eye, unspecified lid
H02.59 Other disorders affecting eyelid function
Deficient blink reflex
Sensory disorders
+ H02.6 Xanthelasma of eyelid
H02.60 Xanthelasma of unspecified eye, unspecified eyelid
H02.61 Xanthelasma of right upper eyelid
H02.62 Xanthelasma of right lower eyelid
H02.63 Xanthelasma of right eye, unspecified eyelid
H02.64 Xanthelasma of left upper eyelid
H02.65 Xanthelasma of left lower eyelid
H02.66 Xanthelasma of left eye, unspecified eyelid
+ H02.7 Other and unspecified degenerative disorders of eyelid and periocular area
H02.70 Unspecified degenerative disorders of eyelid and periocular area
+ H02.71 Chloasma of eyelid and periocular area
Dyspigmentation of eyelid
Hyperpigmentation of eyelid
H02.711 Chloasma of right upper eyelid and periocular area
H02.712 Chloasma of right lower eyelid and periocular area
H02.713 Chloasma of right eye, unspecified eyelid and periocular area
H02.714 Chloasma of left upper eyelid and periocular area
H02.715 Chloasma of left lower eyelid and periocular area
H02.716 Chloasma of left eye, unspecified eyelid and periocular area
H02.719 Chloasma of unspecified eye, unspecified eyelid and periocular area
+ H02.72 Madarosis of eyelid and periocular area
Hypotrichosis of eyelid
H02.721 Madarosis of right upper eyelid and periocular area
H02.722 Madarosis of right lower eyelid and periocular area
H02.723 Madarosis of right eye, unspecified eyelid and periocular area
H02.724 Madarosis of left upper eyelid and periocular area
H02.725 Madarosis of left lower eyelid and periocular area
H02.726 Madarosis of left eye, unspecified eyelid and periocular area
H02.729 Madarosis of unspecified eye, unspecified eyelid and periocular area
+ H02.73 Vitiligo of eyelid and periocular area
Hypopigmentation of eyelid
H02.731 Vitiligo of right upper eyelid and periocular area
H02.732 Vitiligo of right lower eyelid and periocular area
H02.733 Vitiligo of right eye, unspecified eyelid and periocular area
H02.734 Vitiligo of left upper eyelid and periocular area
H02.735 Vitiligo of left lower eyelid and periocular area
H02.736 Vitiligo of left eye, unspecified eyelid and periocular area
H02.739 Vitiligo of unspecified eye, unspecified eyelid and periocular area
H02.79 Other degenerative disorders of eyelid and periocular area
+ H02.8 Other specified disorders of eyelid
+ H02.81 Retained foreign body in eyelid
Use additional code to identify the type of retained foreign body (Z18.-)
Excludes1: *laceration of eyelid with foreign body (S01.12-)*
retained intraocular foreign body (H44.6-, H44.7-)
superficial foreign body of eyelid and periocular area (S00.25-)
H02.811 Retained foreign body in right upper eyelid
H02.812 Retained foreign body in right lower eyelid
H02.813 Retained foreign body in right eye, unspecified eyelid
H02.814 Retained foreign body in left upper eyelid
H02.815 Retained foreign body in left lower eyelid
H02.816 Retained foreign body in left eye, unspecified eyelid
H02.819 Retained foreign body in unspecified eye, unspecified eyelid
+ H02.82 Cysts of eyelid
Sebaceous cyst of eyelid
H02.821 Cysts of right upper eyelid
H02.822 Cysts of right lower eyelid
H02.823 Cysts of right eye, unspecified eyelid
H02.824 Cysts of left upper eyelid
H02.825 Cysts of left lower eyelid
H02.826 Cysts of left eye, unspecified eyelid
H02.829 Cysts of unspecified eye, unspecified eyelid
+ H02.83 Dermatochalasis of eyelid
H02.831 Dermatochalasis of right upper eyelid
H02.832 Dermatochalasis of right lower eyelid
H02.833 Dermatochalasis of right eye, unspecified eyelid
H02.834 Dermatochalasis of left upper eyelid
H02.835 Dermatochalasis of left lower eyelid
H02.836 Dermatochalasis of left eye, unspecified eyelid
H02.839 Dermatochalasis of unspecified eye, unspecified eyelid
+ H02.84 Edema of eyelid
Hyperemia of eyelid
H02.841 Edema of right upper eyelid
H02.842 Edema of right lower eyelid
H02.843 Edema of right eye, unspecified eyelid
H02.844 Edema of left upper eyelid
H02.845 Edema of left lower eyelid
H02.846 Edema of left eye, unspecified eyelid
H02.849 Edema of unspecified eye, unspecified eyelid
+ H02.85 Elephantiasis of eyelid
H02.851 Elephantiasis of right upper eyelid
H02.852 Elephantiasis of right lower eyelid
H02.853 Elephantiasis of right eye, unspecified eyelid
H02.854 Elephantiasis of left upper eyelid
H02.855 Elephantiasis of left lower eyelid
H02.856 Elephantiasis of left eye, unspecified eyelid
H02.859 Elephantiasis of unspecified eye, unspecified eyelid
+ H02.86 Hypertrichosis of eyelid
H02.861 Hypertrichosis of right upper eyelid
H02.862 Hypertrichosis of right lower eyelid
H02.863 Hypertrichosis of right eye, unspecified eyelid
H02.864 Hypertrichosis of left upper eyelid
H02.865 Hypertrichosis of left lower eyelid
H02.866 Hypertrichosis of left eye, unspecified eyelid
H02.869 Hypertrichosis of unspecified eye, unspecified eyelid
+ H02.87 Vascular anomalies of eyelid
H02.871 Vascular anomalies of right upper eyelid
H02.872 Vascular anomalies of right lower eyelid
H02.873 Vascular anomalies of right eye, unspecified eyelid
H02.874 Vascular anomalies of left upper eyelid
H02.875 Vascular anomalies of left lower eyelid
H02.876 Vascular anomalies of left eye, unspecified eyelid
H02.879 Vascular anomalies of unspecified eye, unspecified eyelid
H02.89 Other specified disorders of eyelid
Hemorrhage of eyelid
H02.9 Unspecified disorder of eyelid
Disorder of eyelid NOS

H04 Disorders of lacrimal system

Excludes1: *congenital malformations of lacrimal system (Q10.4-Q10.6)*

+ **H04.0 Dacryoadenitis**
  + **H04.00 Unspecified dacryoadenitis**
    - **H04.001 Unspecified dacryoadenitis, right lacrimal gland**
    - **H04.002 Unspecified dacryoadenitis, left lacrimal gland**
    - **H04.003 Unspecified dacryoadenitis, bilateral lacrimal glands**
    - **H04.009 Unspecified dacryoadenitis, unspecified lacrimal gland**
  + **H04.01 Acute dacryoadenitis**
    - **H04.011 Acute dacryoadenitis, right lacrimal gland**
    - **H04.012 Acute dacryoadenitis, left lacrimal gland**
    - **H04.013 Acute dacryoadenitis, bilateral lacrimal glands**
    - **H04.019 Acute dacryoadenitis, unspecified lacrimal gland**
  + **H04.02 Chronic dacryoadenitis**
    - **H04.021 Chronic dacryoadenitis, right lacrimal gland**
    - **H04.022 Chronic dacryoadenitis, left lacrimal gland**
    - **H04.023 Chronic dacryoadenitis, bilateral lacrimal gland**
    - **H04.029 Chronic dacryoadenitis, unspecified lacrimal gland**
  + **H04.03 Chronic enlargement of lacrimal gland**
    - **H04.031 Chronic enlargement of right lacrimal gland**
    - **H04.032 Chronic enlargement of left lacrimal gland**
    - **H04.033 Chronic enlargement of bilateral lacrimal glands**
    - **H04.039 Chronic enlargement of unspecified lacrimal gland**
+ **H04.1 Other disorders of lacrimal gland**
  + **H04.11 Dacryops**
    - **H04.111 Dacryops of right lacrimal gland**
    - **H04.112 Dacryops of left lacrimal gland**
    - **H04.113 Dacryops of bilateral lacrimal glands**
    - **H04.119 Dacryops of unspecified lacrimal gland**
  + **H04.12 Dry eye syndrome**

    Tear film insufficiency, NOS
    - **H04.121 Dry eye syndrome of right lacrimal gland**
    - **H04.122 Dry eye syndrome of left lacrimal gland**
    - **H04.123 Dry eye syndrome of bilateral lacrimal glands**
    - **H04.129 Dry eye syndrome of unspecified lacrimal gland**
  + **H04.13 Lacrimal cyst**

    Lacrimal cystic degeneration
    - **H04.131 Lacrimal cyst, right lacrimal gland**
    - **H04.132 Lacrimal cyst, left lacrimal gland**
    - **H04.133 Lacrimal cyst, bilateral lacrimal glands**
    - **H04.139 Lacrimal cyst, unspecified lacrimal gland**
  + **H04.14 Primary lacrimal gland atrophy**
    - **H04.141 Primary lacrimal gland atrophy, right lacrimal gland**
    - **H04.142 Primary lacrimal gland atrophy, left lacrimal gland**
    - **H04.143 Primary lacrimal gland atrophy, bilateral lacrimal glands**
    - **H04.149 Primary lacrimal gland atrophy, unspecified lacrimal gland**
  + **H04.15 Secondary lacrimal gland atrophy**
    - **H04.151 Secondary lacrimal gland atrophy, right lacrimal gland**
    - **H04.152 Secondary lacrimal gland atrophy, left lacrimal gland**
    - **H04.153 Secondary lacrimal gland atrophy, bilateral lacrimal glands**
    - **H04.159 Secondary lacrimal gland atrophy, unspecified lacrimal gland**
  + **H04.16 Lacrimal gland dislocation**
    - **H04.161 Lacrimal gland dislocation, right lacrimal gland**
    - **H04.162 Lacrimal gland dislocation, left lacrimal gland**
    - **H04.163 Lacrimal gland dislocation, bilateral lacrimal glands**
    - **H04.169 Lacrimal gland dislocation, unspecified lacrimal gland**
  - **H04.19 Other specified disorders of lacrimal gland**
+ **H04.2 Epiphora**
  + **H04.20 Unspecified epiphora**
    - **H04.201 Unspecified epiphora, right lacrimal gland**
    - **H04.202 Unspecified epiphora, left lacrimal gland**
    - **H04.203 Unspecified epiphora, bilateral lacrimal glands**
    - **H04.209 Unspecified epiphora, unspecified lacrimal gland**
  + **H04.21 Epiphora due to excess lacrimation**
    - **H04.211 Epiphora due to excess lacrimation, right lacrimal gland**
    - **H04.212 Epiphora due to excess lacrimation, left lacrimal gland**
    - **H04.213 Epiphora due to excess lacrimation, bilateral lacrimal glands**
    - **H04.219 Epiphora due to excess lacrimation, unspecified lacrimal gland**
  + **H04.22 Epiphora due to insufficient drainage**
    - **H04.221 Epiphora due to insufficient drainage, right lacrimal gland**
    - **H04.222 Epiphora due to insufficient drainage, left lacrimal gland**
    - **H04.223 Epiphora due to insufficient drainage, bilateral lacrimal glands**
    - **H04.229 Epiphora due to insufficient drainage, unspecified lacrimal gland**
+ **H04.3 Acute and unspecified inflammation of lacrimal passages**

  Excludes1: *neonatal dacryocystitis (P39.1)*
  + **H04.30 Unspecified dacryocystitis**
    - **H04.301 Unspecified dacryocystitis of right lacrimal passage**
    - **H04.302 Unspecified dacryocystitis of left lacrimal passage**
    - **H04.303 Unspecified dacryocystitis of bilateral lacrimal passages**
    - **H04.309 Unspecified dacryocystitis of unspecified lacrimal passage**
  + **H04.31 Phlegmonous dacryocystitis**
    - **H04.311 Phlegmonous dacryocystitis of right lacrimal passage**
    - **H04.312 Phlegmonous dacryocystitis of left lacrimal passage**
    - **H04.313 Phlegmonous dacryocystitis of bilateral lacrimal passages**
    - **H04.319 Phlegmonous dacryocystitis of unspecified lacrimal passage**
  + **H04.32 Acute dacryocystitis**

    Acute dacryopericystitis
    - **H04.321 Acute dacryocystitis of right lacrimal passage**
    - **H04.322 Acute dacryocystitis of left lacrimal passage**
    - **H04.323 Acute dacryocystitis of bilateral lacrimal passages**
    - **H04.329 Acute dacryocystitis of unspecified lacrimal passage**
  + **H04.33 Acute lacrimal canaliculitis**
    - **H04.331 Acute lacrimal canaliculitis of right lacrimal passage**
    - **H04.332 Acute lacrimal canaliculitis of left lacrimal passage**
    - **H04.333 Acute lacrimal canaliculitis of bilateral lacrimal passages**
    - **H04.339 Acute lacrimal canaliculitis of unspecified lacrimal passage**
+ **H04.4 Chronic inflammation of lacrimal passages**
  + **H04.41 Chronic dacryocystitis**
    - **H04.411 Chronic dacryocystitis of right lacrimal passage**
    - **H04.412 Chronic dacryocystitis of left lacrimal passage**
    - **H04.413 Chronic dacryocystitis of bilateral lacrimal passages**
    - **H04.419 Chronic dacryocystitis of unspecified lacrimal passage**

+ H04.42 Chronic lacrimal canaliculitis
- **H04.421 Chronic lacrimal canaliculitis of right lacrimal passage**
- **H04.422 Chronic lacrimal canaliculitis of left lacrimal passage**
- **H04.423 Chronic lacrimal canaliculitis of bilateral lacrimal passages**
- **H04.429 Chronic lacrimal canaliculitis of unspecified lacrimal passage**

+ H04.43 Chronic lacrimal mucocele
- **H04.431 Chronic lacrimal mucocele of right lacrimal passage**
- **H04.432 Chronic lacrimal mucocele of left lacrimal passage**
- **H04.433 Chronic lacrimal mucocele of bilateral lacrimal passages**
- **H04.439 Chronic lacrimal mucocele of unspecified lacrimal passage**

+ H04.5 Stenosis and insufficiency of lacrimal passages

+ H04.51 Dacryolith
- **H04.511 Dacryolith of right lacrimal passage**
- **H04.512 Dacryolith of left lacrimal passage**
- **H04.513 Dacryolith of bilateral lacrimal passages**
- **H04.519 Dacryolith of unspecified lacrimal passage**

+ H04.52 Eversion of lacrimal punctum
- **H04.521 Eversion of right lacrimal punctum**
- **H04.522 Eversion of left lacrimal punctum**
- **H04.523 Eversion of bilateral lacrimal punctum**
- **H04.529 Eversion of unspecified lacrimal punctum**

+ H04.53 Neonatal obstruction of nasolacrimal duct

Excludes1: *congenital stenosis and stricture of lacrimal duct (Q10.5)*

- • **H04.531 Neonatal obstruction of right nasolacrimal duct**
- • **H04.532 Neonatal obstruction of left nasolacrimal duct**
- • **H04.533 Neonatal obstruction of bilateral nasolacrimal duct**
- • **H04.539 Neonatal obstruction of unspecified nasolacrimal duct**

+ H04.54 Stenosis of lacrimal canaliculi
- **H04.541 Stenosis of right lacrimal canaliculi**
- **H04.542 Stenosis of left lacrimal canaliculi**
- **H04.543 Stenosis of bilateral lacrimal canaliculi**
- **H04.549 Stenosis of unspecified lacrimal canaliculi**

+ H04.55 Acquired stenosis of nasolacrimal duct
- **H04.551 Acquired stenosis of right nasolacrimal duct**
- **H04.552 Acquired stenosis of left nasolacrimal duct**
- **H04.553 Acquired stenosis of bilateral nasolacrimal duct**
- **H04.559 Acquired stenosis of unspecified nasolacrimal duct**

+ H04.56 Stenosis of lacrimal punctum
- **H04.561 Stenosis of right lacrimal punctum**
- **H04.562 Stenosis of left lacrimal punctum**
- **H04.563 Stenosis of bilateral lacrimal punctum**
- **H04.569 Stenosis of unspecified lacrimal punctum**

+ H04.57 Stenosis of lacrimal sac
- **H04.571 Stenosis of right lacrimal sac**
- **H04.572 Stenosis of left lacrimal sac**
- **H04.573 Stenosis of bilateral lacrimal sac**
- **H04.579 Stenosis of unspecified lacrimal sac**

+ H04.6 Other changes of lacrimal passages

+ H04.61 Lacrimal fistula
- **H04.611 Lacrimal fistula right lacrimal passage**
- **H04.612 Lacrimal fistula left lacrimal passage**
- **H04.613 Lacrimal fistula bilateral lacrimal passages**
- **H04.619 Lacrimal fistula unspecified lacrimal passage**

H04.69 Other changes of lacrimal passages

+ H04.8 Other disorders of lacrimal system

+ H04.81 Granuloma of lacrimal passages
- **H04.811 Granuloma of right lacrimal passage**
- **H04.812 Granuloma of left lacrimal passage**
- **H04.813 Granuloma of bilateral lacrimal passages**
- **H04.819 Granuloma of unspecified lacrimal passage**

H04.89 Other disorders of lacrimal system

H04.9 Disorder of lacrimal system, unspecified

H05 Disorders of orbit

Excludes1: *congenital malformation of orbit (Q10.7)*

+ H05.0 Acute inflammation of orbit

H05.00 Unspecified acute inflammation of orbit

+ H05.01 Cellulitis of orbit

Abscess of orbit

- CC **H05.011 Cellulitis of right orbit**
  CC Exclusion see Appendix A PDX collection 0621
- CC **H05.012 Cellulitis of left orbit**
  CC Exclusion see Appendix A PDX collection 0621
- CC **H05.013 Cellulitis of bilateral orbits**
  CC Exclusion see Appendix A PDX collection 0621
- CC **H05.019 Cellulitis of unspecified orbit**
  CC Exclusion see Appendix A PDX collection 0621

+ H05.02 Osteomyelitis of orbit
- CC **H05.021 Osteomyelitis of right orbit**
  CC Exclusion see Appendix A PDX collection 0622
- CC **H05.022 Osteomyelitis of left orbit**
  CC Exclusion see Appendix A PDX collection 0622
- CC **H05.023 Osteomyelitis of bilateral orbits**
  CC Exclusion see Appendix A PDX collection 0622
- CC **H05.029 Osteomyelitis of unspecified orbit**
  CC Exclusion see Appendix A PDX collection 0622

+ H05.03 Periostitis of orbit
- CC **H05.031 Periostitis of right orbit**
  CC Exclusion see Appendix A PDX collection 0623
- CC **H05.032 Periostitis of left orbit**
  CC Exclusion see Appendix A PDX collection 0623
- CC **H05.033 Periostitis of bilateral orbits**
  CC Exclusion see Appendix A PDX collection 0623
- CC **H05.039 Periostitis of unspecified orbit**
  CC Exclusion see Appendix A PDX collection 0623

+ H05.04 Tenonitis of orbit
- **H05.041 Tenonitis of right orbit**
- **H05.042 Tenonitis of left orbit**
- **H05.043 Tenonitis of bilateral orbits**
- **H05.049 Tenonitis of unspecified orbit**

+ H05.1 Chronic inflammatory disorders of orbit

H05.10 Unspecified chronic inflammatory disorders of orbit

+ H05.11 Granuloma of orbit

Pseudotumor (inflammatory) of orbit

- **H05.111 Granuloma of right orbit**
- **H05.112 Granuloma of left orbit**
- **H05.113 Granuloma of bilateral orbits**
- **H05.119 Granuloma of unspecified orbit**

+ H05.12 Orbital myositis
- **H05.121 Orbital myositis, right orbit**
- **H05.122 Orbital myositis, left orbit**
- **H05.123 Orbital myositis, bilateral**
- **H05.129 Orbital myositis, unspecified orbit**

+ H05.2 Exophthalmic conditions

H05.20 Unspecified exophthalmos

+ H05.21 Displacement (lateral) of globe
- **H05.211 Displacement (lateral) of globe, right eye**
- **H05.212 Displacement (lateral) of globe, left eye**
- **H05.213 Displacement (lateral) of globe, bilateral**
- **H05.219 Displacement (lateral) of globe, unspecified eye**

+ H05.22 Edema of orbit

Orbital congestion

- **H05.221 Edema of right orbit**
- **H05.222 Edema of left orbit**
- **H05.223 Edema of bilateral orbit**
- **H05.229 Edema of unspecified orbit**

+ H05.23 Hemorrhage of orbit
- **H05.231 Hemorrhage of right orbit**
- **H05.232 Hemorrhage of left orbit**
- **H05.233 Hemorrhage of bilateral orbit**
- **H05.239 Hemorrhage of unspecified orbit**

+ **H05.24 Constant exophthalmos**
H05.241 Constant exophthalmos, right eye
H05.242 Constant exophthalmos, left eye
H05.243 Constant exophthalmos, bilateral
H05.249 Constant exophthalmos, unspecified eye
+ **H05.25 Intermittent exophthalmos**
H05.251 Intermittent exophthalmos, right eye
H05.252 Intermittent exophthalmos, left eye
H05.253 Intermittent exophthalmos, bilateral
H05.259 Intermittent exophthalmos, unspecified eye
+ **H05.26 Pulsating exophthalmos**
H05.261 Pulsating exophthalmos, right eye
H05.262 Pulsating exophthalmos, left eye
H05.263 Pulsating exophthalmos, bilateral
H05.269 Pulsating exophthalmos, unspecified eye
+ **H05.3 Deformity of orbit**
Excludes1: *congenital deformity of orbit (Q10.7)*
hypertelorism (Q75.2)
H05.30 Unspecified deformity of orbit
+ **H05.31 Atrophy of orbit**
H05.311 Atrophy of right orbit
H05.312 Atrophy of left orbit
H05.313 Atrophy of bilateral orbit
H05.319 Atrophy of unspecified orbit
+ **H05.32 Deformity of orbit due to bone disease**
Code also associated bone disease
H05.321 Deformity of right orbit due to bone disease
H05.322 Deformity of left orbit due to bone disease
H05.323 Deformity of bilateral orbits due to bone disease
H05.329 Deformity of unspecified orbit due to bone disease
+ **H05.33 Deformity of orbit due to trauma or surgery**
H05.331 Deformity of right orbit due to trauma or surgery
H05.332 Deformity of left orbit due to trauma or surgery
H05.333 Deformity of bilateral orbits due to trauma or surgery
H05.339 Deformity of unspecified orbit due to trauma or surgery
+ **H05.34 Enlargement of orbit**
H05.341 Enlargement of right orbit
H05.342 Enlargement of left orbit
H05.343 Enlargement of bilateral orbits
H05.349 Enlargement of unspecified orbit
+ **H05.35 Exostosis of orbit**
H05.351 Exostosis of right orbit
H05.352 Exostosis of left orbit
H05.353 Exostosis of bilateral orbits
H05.359 Exostosis of unspecified orbit
+ **H05.4 Enophthalmos**
+ **H05.40 Unspecified enophthalmos**
H05.401 Unspecified enophthalmos, right eye
H05.402 Unspecified enophthalmos, left eye
H05.403 Unspecified enophthalmos, bilateral
H05.409 Unspecified enophthalmos, unspecified eye
+ **H05.41 Enophthalmos due to atrophy of orbital tissue**
H05.411 Enophthalmos due to atrophy of orbital tissue, right eye
H05.412 Enophthalmos due to atrophy of orbital tissue, left eye
H05.413 Enophthalmos due to atrophy of orbital tissue, bilateral
H05.419 Enophthalmos due to atrophy of orbital tissue, unspecified eye
+ **H05.42 Enophthalmos due to trauma or surgery**
H05.421 Enophthalmos due to trauma or surgery, right eye
H05.422 Enophthalmos due to trauma or surgery, left eye
H05.423 Enophthalmos due to trauma or surgery, bilateral
H05.429 Enophthalmos due to trauma or surgery, unspecified eye
+ **H05.5 Retained (old) foreign body following penetrating wound of orbit**
Retrobulbar foreign body
Use additional code to identify the type of retained foreign body (Z18.-)
Excludes1: *current penetrating wound of orbit (S05.4-)*
Excludes2: *retained foreign body of eyelid (H02.81-)*
retained intraocular foreign body (H44.6-, H44.7-)
H05.50 Retained (old) foreign body following penetrating wound of unspecified orbit
H05.51 Retained (old) foreign body following penetrating wound of right orbit
H05.52 Retained (old) foreign body following penetrating wound of left orbit
H05.53 Retained (old) foreign body following penetrating wound of bilateral orbits
+ **H05.8 Other disorders of orbit**
+ **H05.81 Cyst of orbit**
Encephalocele of orbit
H05.811 Cyst of right orbit
H05.812 Cyst of left orbit
H05.813 Cyst of bilateral orbits
H05.819 Cyst of unspecified orbit
+ **H05.82 Myopathy of extraocular muscles**
H05.821 Myopathy of extraocular muscles, right orbit
H05.822 Myopathy of extraocular muscles, left orbit
H05.823 Myopathy of extraocular muscles, bilateral
H05.829 Myopathy of extraocular muscles, unspecified orbit
H05.89 Other disorders of orbit
H05.9 Unspecified disorder of orbit

Disorders of conjunctiva (H10-H11)

H10 Conjunctivitis

Excludes1: *keratoconjunctivitis (H16.2-)*
+ **H10.0 Mucopurulent conjunctivitis**
+ **H10.01 Acute follicular conjunctivitis**
H10.011 Acute follicular conjunctivitis, right eye
H10.012 Acute follicular conjunctivitis, left eye
H10.013 Acute follicular conjunctivitis, bilateral
H10.019 Acute follicular conjunctivitis, unspecified eye
+ **H10.02 Other mucopurulent conjunctivitis**
H10.021 Other mucopurulent conjunctivitis, right eye
H10.022 Other mucopurulent conjunctivitis, left eye
H10.023 Other mucopurulent conjunctivitis, bilateral
H10.029 Other mucopurulent conjunctivitis, unspecified eye
+ **H10.1 Acute atopic conjunctivitis**
Acute papillary conjunctivitis
H10.10 Acute atopic conjunctivitis, unspecified eye
H10.11 Acute atopic conjunctivitis, right eye
H10.12 Acute atopic conjunctivitis, left eye
H10.13 Acute atopic conjunctivitis, bilateral
+ **H10.2 Other acute conjunctivitis**
+ **H10.21 Acute toxic conjunctivitis**
Acute chemical conjunctivitis
Code first (T51-T65) to identify chemical and intent
Excludes1: *burn and corrosion of eye and adnexa (T26.-)*
H10.211 Acute toxic conjunctivitis, right eye
H10.212 Acute toxic conjunctivitis, left eye
H10.213 Acute toxic conjunctivitis, bilateral
H10.219 Acute toxic conjunctivitis, unspecified eye
+ **H10.22 Pseudomembranous conjunctivitis**
H10.221 Pseudomembranous conjunctivitis, right eye
H10.222 Pseudomembranous conjunctivitis, left eye
H10.223 Pseudomembranous conjunctivitis, bilateral
H10.229 Pseudomembranous conjunctivitis, unspecified eye
+ **H10.23 Serous conjunctivitis, except viral**
Excludes1: *viral conjunctivitis (B30.-)*
H10.231 Serous conjunctivitis, except viral, right eye

H10.232 Serous conjunctivitis, except viral, left eye
H10.233 Serous conjunctivitis, except viral, bilateral
H10.239 Serous conjunctivitis, except viral, unspecified eye

+ H10.3 Unspecified acute conjunctivitis
Excludes1: *ophthalmia neonatorum NOS (P39.1)*
H10.30 Unspecified acute conjunctivitis, unspecified eye
H10.31 Unspecified acute conjunctivitis, right eye
H10.32 Unspecified acute conjunctivitis, left eye
H10.33 Unspecified acute conjunctivitis, bilateral

+ H10.4 Chronic conjunctivitis
+ H10.40 Unspecified chronic conjunctivitis
H10.401 Unspecified chronic conjunctivitis, right eye
H10.402 Unspecified chronic conjunctivitis, left eye
H10.403 Unspecified chronic conjunctivitis, bilateral
H10.409 Unspecified chronic conjunctivitis, unspecified eye
+ H10.41 Chronic giant papillary conjunctivitis
H10.411 Chronic giant papillary conjunctivitis, right eye
H10.412 Chronic giant papillary conjunctivitis, left eye
H10.413 Chronic giant papillary conjunctivitis, bilateral
H10.419 Chronic giant papillary conjunctivitis, unspecified eye
+ H10.42 Simple chronic conjunctivitis
H10.421 Simple chronic conjunctivitis, right eye
H10.422 Simple chronic conjunctivitis, left eye
H10.423 Simple chronic conjunctivitis, bilateral
H10.429 Simple chronic conjunctivitis, unspecified eye
+ H10.43 Chronic follicular conjunctivitis
H10.431 Chronic follicular conjunctivitis, right eye
H10.432 Chronic follicular conjunctivitis, left eye
H10.433 Chronic follicular conjunctivitis, bilateral
H10.439 Chronic follicular conjunctivitis, unspecified eye
H10.44 Vernal conjunctivitis
Excludes1: *vernal keratoconjunctivitis with limbar and corneal involvement (H16.26-)*
H10.45 Other chronic allergic conjunctivitis

+ H10.5 Blepharoconjunctivitis
+ H10.50 Unspecified blepharoconjunctivitis
H10.501 Unspecified blepharoconjunctivitis, right eye
H10.502 Unspecified blepharoconjunctivitis, left eye
H10.503 Unspecified blepharoconjunctivitis, bilateral
H10.509 Unspecified blepharoconjunctivitis, unspecified eye
+ H10.51 Ligneous conjunctivitis
H10.511 Ligneous conjunctivitis, right eye
H10.512 Ligneous conjunctivitis, left eye
H10.513 Ligneous conjunctivitis, bilateral
H10.519 Ligneous conjunctivitis, unspecified eye
+ H10.52 Angular blepharoconjunctivitis
H10.521 Angular blepharoconjunctivitis, right eye
H10.522 Angular blepharoconjunctivitis, left eye
H10.523 Angular blepharoconjunctivitis, bilateral
H10.529 Angular blepharoconjunctivitis, unspecified eye
+ H10.53 Contact blepharoconjunctivitis
H10.531 Contact blepharoconjunctivitis, right eye
H10.532 Contact blepharoconjunctivitis, left eye
H10.533 Contact blepharoconjunctivitis, bilateral
H10.539 Contact blepharoconjunctivitis, unspecified eye

+ H10.8 Other conjunctivitis
+ H10.81 Pingueculitis
Excludes1: *pinguecula (H11.15-)*
H10.811 Pingueculitis, right eye
H10.812 Pingueculitis, left eye
H10.813 Pingueculitis, bilateral
H10.819 Pingueculitis, unspecified eye
H10.89 Other conjunctivitis

H10.9 Unspecified conjunctivitis

H11 Other disorders of conjunctiva

Excludes1: *keratoconjunctivitis (H16.2-)*

+ H11.0 Pterygium of eye
Excludes1: *pseudopterygium (H11.81-)*
+ H11.00 Unspecified pterygium of eye
H11.001 Unspecified pterygium of right eye
H11.002 Unspecified pterygium of left eye
H11.003 Unspecified pterygium of eye, bilateral
H11.009 Unspecified pterygium of unspecified eye
+ H11.01 Amyloid pterygium
H11.011 Amyloid pterygium of right eye
H11.012 Amyloid pterygium of left eye
H11.013 Amyloid pterygium of eye, bilateral
H11.019 Amyloid pterygium of unspecified eye
+ H11.02 Central pterygium of eye
H11.021 Central pterygium of right eye
H11.022 Central pterygium of left eye
H11.023 Central pterygium of eye, bilateral
H11.029 Central pterygium of unspecified eye
+ H11.03 Double pterygium of eye
H11.031 Double pterygium of right eye
H11.032 Double pterygium of left eye
H11.033 Double pterygium of eye, bilateral
H11.039 Double pterygium of unspecified eye
+ H11.04 Peripheral pterygium of eye, stationary
H11.041 Peripheral pterygium, stationary, right eye
H11.042 Peripheral pterygium, stationary, left eye
H11.043 Peripheral pterygium, stationary, bilateral
H11.049 Peripheral pterygium, stationary, unspecified eye
+ H11.05 Peripheral pterygium of eye, progressive
H11.051 Peripheral pterygium, progressive, right eye
H11.052 Peripheral pterygium, progressive, left eye
H11.053 Peripheral pterygium, progressive, bilateral
H11.059 Peripheral pterygium, progressive, unspecified eye
+ H11.06 Recurrent pterygium of eye
H11.061 Recurrent pterygium of right eye
H11.062 Recurrent pterygium of left eye
H11.063 Recurrent pterygium of eye, bilateral
H11.069 Recurrent pterygium of unspecified eye

+ H11.1 Conjunctival degenerations and deposits
Excludes2: *pseudopterygium (H11.81)*
H11.10 Unspecified conjunctival degenerations
+ H11.11 Conjunctival deposits
H11.111 Conjunctival deposits, right eye
H11.112 Conjunctival deposits, left eye
H11.113 Conjunctival deposits, bilateral
H11.119 Conjunctival deposits, unspecified eye
+ H11.12 Conjunctival concretions
H11.121 Conjunctival concretions, right eye
H11.122 Conjunctival concretions, left eye
H11.123 Conjunctival concretions, bilateral
H11.129 Conjunctival concretions, unspecified eye
+ H11.13 Conjunctival pigmentations
Conjunctival argyrosis [argyria]
H11.131 Conjunctival pigmentations, right eye
H11.132 Conjunctival pigmentations, left eye
H11.133 Conjunctival pigmentations, bilateral
H11.139 Conjunctival pigmentations, unspecified eye
+ H11.14 Conjunctival xerosis, unspecified
Excludes1: *xerosis of conjunctiva due to vitamin A deficiency (E50.0, E50.1)*
H11.141 Conjunctival xerosis, unspecified, right eye
H11.142 Conjunctival xerosis, unspecified, left eye
H11.143 Conjunctival xerosis, unspecified, bilateral
H11.149 Conjunctival xerosis, unspecified, unspecified eye
+ H11.15 Pinguecula
Excludes1: pingueculitis (H10.81-)
H11.151 Pinguecula, right eye
H11.152 Pinguecula, left eye
H11.153 Pinguecula, bilateral
H11.159 Pinguecula, unspecified eye

+ **H11.2 Conjunctival scars**
+ **H11.21 Conjunctival adhesions and strands (localized)**
H11.211 Conjunctival adhesions and strands (localized), right eye
H11.212 Conjunctival adhesions and strands (localized), left eye
H11.213 Conjunctival adhesions and strands (localized), bilateral
H11.219 Conjunctival adhesions and strands (localized), unspecified eye
+ **H11.22 Conjunctival granuloma**
H11.221 Conjunctival granuloma, right eye
H11.222 Conjunctival granuloma, left eye
H11.223 Conjunctival granuloma, bilateral
H11.229 Conjunctival granuloma, unspecified
+ **H11.23 Symblepharon**
H11.231 Symblepharon, right eye
H11.232 Symblepharon, left eye
H11.233 Symblepharon, bilateral
H11.239 Symblepharon, unspecified eye
+ **H11.24 Scarring of conjunctiva**
H11.241 Scarring of conjunctiva, right eye
H11.242 Scarring of conjunctiva, left eye
H11.243 Scarring of conjunctiva, bilateral
H11.249 Scarring of conjunctiva, unspecified eye
+ **H11.3 Conjunctival hemorrhage**
Subconjunctival hemorrhage
H11.30 Conjunctival hemorrhage, unspecified eye
H11.31 Conjunctival hemorrhage, right eye
H11.32 Conjunctival hemorrhage, left eye
H11.33 Conjunctival hemorrhage, bilateral
+ **H11.4 Other conjunctival vascular disorders and cysts**
+ **H11.41 Vascular abnormalities of conjunctiva**
Conjunctival aneurysm
H11.411 Vascular abnormalities of conjunctiva, right eye
H11.412 Vascular abnormalities of conjunctiva, left eye
H11.413 Vascular abnormalities of conjunctiva, bilateral
H11.419 Vascular abnormalities of conjunctiva, unspecified eye
+ **H11.42 Conjunctival edema**
H11.421 Conjunctival edema, right eye
H11.422 Conjunctival edema, left eye
H11.423 Conjunctival edema, bilateral
H11.429 Conjunctival edema, unspecified eye
+ **H11.43 Conjunctival hyperemia**
H11.431 Conjunctival hyperemia, right eye
H11.432 Conjunctival hyperemia, left eye
H11.433 Conjunctival hyperemia, bilateral
H11.439 Conjunctival hyperemia, unspecified eye
+ **H11.44 Conjunctival cysts**
H11.441 Conjunctival cysts, right eye
H11.442 Conjunctival cysts, left eye
H11.443 Conjunctival cysts, bilateral
H11.449 Conjunctival cysts, unspecified eye
+ **H11.8 Other specified disorders of conjunctiva**
+ **H11.81 Pseudopterygium of conjunctiva**
H11.811 Pseudopterygium of conjunctiva, right eye
H11.812 Pseudopterygium of conjunctiva, left eye
H11.813 Pseudopterygium of conjunctiva, bilateral
H11.819 Pseudopterygium of conjunctiva, unspecified eye
+ **H11.82 Conjunctivochalasis**
H11.821 Conjunctivochalasis, right eye
H11.822 Conjunctivochalasis, left eye
H11.823 Conjunctivochalasis, bilateral
H11.829 Conjunctivochalasis, unspecified eye
H11.89 Other specified disorders of conjunctiva
H11.9 Unspecified disorder of conjunctiva

isorders of sclera, cornea, iris and ciliary body (H15-H22)

+ **H15 Disorders of sclera**
+ **H15.0 Scleritis**
+ **H15.00 Unspecified scleritis**
H15.001 Unspecified scleritis, right eye
H15.002 Unspecified scleritis, left eye
H15.003 Unspecified scleritis, bilateral
H15.009 Unspecified scleritis, unspecified eye
+ **H15.01 Anterior scleritis**
H15.011 Anterior scleritis, right eye
H15.012 Anterior scleritis, left eye
H15.013 Anterior scleritis, bilateral
H15.019 Anterior scleritis, unspecified eye
+ **H15.02 Brawny scleritis**
H15.021 Brawny scleritis, right eye
H15.022 Brawny scleritis, left eye
H15.023 Brawny scleritis, bilateral
H15.029 Brawny scleritis, unspecified eye
+ **H15.03 Posterior scleritis**
Sclerotenonitis
H15.031 Posterior scleritis, right eye
H15.032 Posterior scleritis, left eye
H15.033 Posterior scleritis, bilateral
H15.039 Posterior scleritis, unspecified eye
+ **H15.04 Scleritis with corneal involvement**
H15.041 Scleritis with corneal involvement, right eye
H15.042 Scleritis with corneal involvement, left eye
H15.043 Scleritis with corneal involvement, bilateral
H15.049 Scleritis with corneal involvement, unspecified eye
+ **H15.05 Scleromalacia perforans**
H15.051 Scleromalacia perforans, right eye
H15.052 Scleromalacia perforans, left eye
H15.053 Scleromalacia perforans, bilateral
H15.059 Scleromalacia perforans, unspecified eye
+ **H15.09 Other scleritis**
Scleral abscess
H15.091 Other scleritis, right eye
H15.092 Other scleritis, left eye
H15.093 Other scleritis, bilateral
H15.099 Other scleritis, unspecified eye
+ **H15.1 Episcleritis**
+ **H15.10 Unspecified episcleritis**
H15.101 Unspecified episcleritis, right eye
H15.102 Unspecified episcleritis, left eye
H15.103 Unspecified episcleritis, bilateral
H15.109 Unspecified episcleritis, unspecified eye
+ **H15.11 Episcleritis periodica fugax**
H15.111 Episcleritis periodica fugax, right eye
H15.112 Episcleritis periodica fugax, left eye
H15.113 Episcleritis periodica fugax, bilateral
H15.119 Episcleritis periodica fugax, unspecified eye
+ **H15.12 Nodular episcleritis**
H15.121 Nodular episcleritis, right eye
H15.122 Nodular episcleritis, left eye
H15.123 Nodular episcleritis, bilateral
H15.129 Nodular episcleritis, unspecified eye
+ **H15.8 Other disorders of sclera**
Excludes2: *blue sclera (Q13.5)*
degenerative myopia (H44.2-)
+ **H15.81 Equatorial staphyloma**
H15.811 Equatorial staphyloma, right eye
H15.812 Equatorial staphyloma, left eye
H15.813 Equatorial staphyloma, bilateral
H15.819 Equatorial staphyloma, unspecified eye
+ **H15.82 Localized anterior staphyloma**
H15.821 Localized anterior staphyloma, right eye
H15.822 Localized anterior staphyloma, left eye
H15.823 Localized anterior staphyloma, bilateral
H15.829 Localized anterior staphyloma, unspecified eye
+ **H15.83 Staphyloma posticum**
H15.831 Staphyloma posticum, right eye
H15.832 Staphyloma posticum, left eye
H15.833 Staphyloma posticum, bilateral
H15.839 Staphyloma posticum, unspecified eye
+ **H15.84 Scleral ectasia**
H15.841 Scleral ectasia, right eye
H15.842 Scleral ectasia, left eye
H15.843 Scleral ectasia, bilateral
H15.849 Scleral ectasia, unspecified eye
+ **H15.85 Ring staphyloma**
H15.851 Ring staphyloma, right eye
H15.852 Ring staphyloma, left eye
H15.853 Ring staphyloma, bilateral
H15.859 Ring staphyloma, unspecified eye
H15.89 Other disorders of sclera
H15.9 Unspecified disorder of sclera

H16 Keratitis

+ **H16.0 Corneal ulcer**
  + **H16.00 Unspecified corneal ulcer**
    - **H16.001 Unspecified corneal ulcer, right eye**
    - **H16.002 Unspecified corneal ulcer, left eye**
    - **H16.003 Unspecified corneal ulcer, bilateral**
    - **H16.009 Unspecified corneal ulcer, unspecified eye**
  + **H16.01 Central corneal ulcer**
    - **H16.011 Central corneal ulcer, right eye**
    - **H16.012 Central corneal ulcer, left eye**
    - **H16.013 Central corneal ulcer, bilateral**
    - **H16.019 Central corneal ulcer, unspecified eye**
  + **H16.02 Ring corneal ulcer**
    - **H16.021 Ring corneal ulcer, right eye**
    - **H16.022 Ring corneal ulcer, left eye**
    - **H16.023 Ring corneal ulcer, bilateral**
    - **H16.029 Ring corneal ulcer, unspecified eye**
  + **H16.03 Corneal ulcer with hypopyon**
    - **H16.031 Corneal ulcer with hypopyon, right eye**
    - **H16.032 Corneal ulcer with hypopyon, left eye**
    - **H16.033 Corneal ulcer with hypopyon, bilateral**
    - **H16.039 Corneal ulcer with hypopyon, unspecified eye**
  + **H16.04 Marginal corneal ulcer**
    - **H16.041 Marginal corneal ulcer, right eye**
    - **H16.042 Marginal corneal ulcer, left eye**
    - **H16.043 Marginal corneal ulcer, bilateral**
    - **H16.049 Marginal corneal ulcer, unspecified eye**
  + **H16.05 Mooren's corneal ulcer**
    - **H16.051 Mooren's corneal ulcer, right eye**
    - **H16.052 Mooren's corneal ulcer, left eye**
    - **H16.053 Mooren's corneal ulcer, bilateral**
    - **H16.059 Mooren's corneal ulcer, unspecified eye**
  + **H16.06 Mycotic corneal ulcer**
    - **H16.061 Mycotic corneal ulcer, right eye**
    - **H16.062 Mycotic corneal ulcer, left eye**
    - **H16.063 Mycotic corneal ulcer, bilateral**
    - **H16.069 Mycotic corneal ulcer, unspecified eye**
  + **H16.07 Perforated corneal ulcer**
    - **H16.071 Perforated corneal ulcer, right eye**
    - **H16.072 Perforated corneal ulcer, left eye**
    - **H16.073 Perforated corneal ulcer, bilateral**
    - **H16.079 Perforated corneal ulcer, unspecified eye**
+ **H16.1 Other and unspecified superficial keratitis without conjunctivitis**
  + **H16.10 Unspecified superficial keratitis**
    - **H16.101 Unspecified superficial keratitis, right eye**
    - **H16.102 Unspecified superficial keratitis, left eye**
    - **H16.103 Unspecified superficial keratitis, bilateral**
    - **H16.109 Unspecified superficial keratitis, unspecified eye**
  + **H16.11 Macular keratitis**
    Areolar keratitis
    Nummular keratitis
    Stellate keratitis
    Striate keratitis
    - **H16.111 Macular keratitis, right eye**
    - **H16.112 Macular keratitis, left eye**
    - **H16.113 Macular keratitis, bilateral**
    - **H16.119 Macular keratitis, unspecified eye**
  + **H16.12 Filamentary keratitis**
    - **H16.121 Filamentary keratitis, right eye**
    - **H16.122 Filamentary keratitis, left eye**
    - **H16.123 Filamentary keratitis, bilateral**
    - **H16.129 Filamentary keratitis, unspecified eye**
  + **H16.13 Photokeratitis**
    Snow blindness
    Welders keratitis
    - **H16.131 Photokeratitis, right eye**
    - **H16.132 Photokeratitis, left eye**
    - **H16.133 Photokeratitis, bilateral**
    - **H16.139 Photokeratitis, unspecified eye**
  + **H16.14 Punctate keratitis**
    - **H16.141 Punctate keratitis, right eye**
    - **H16.142 Punctate keratitis, left eye**
    - **H16.143 Punctate keratitis, bilateral**
    - **H16.149 Punctate keratitis, unspecified eye**
+ **H16.2 Keratoconjunctivitis**
  + **H16.20 Unspecified keratoconjunctivitis**
    Superficial keratitis with conjunctivitis NOS
    - **H16.201 Unspecified keratoconjunctivitis, right eye**
    - **H16.202 Unspecified keratoconjunctivitis, left eye**
    - **H16.203 Unspecified keratoconjunctivitis, bilateral**
    - **H16.209 Unspecified keratoconjunctivitis, unspecified eye**
  + **H16.21 Exposure keratoconjunctivitis**
    - **H16.211 Exposure keratoconjunctivitis, right eye**
    - **H16.212 Exposure keratoconjunctivitis, left eye**
    - **H16.213 Exposure keratoconjunctivitis, bilateral**
    - **H16.219 Exposure keratoconjunctivitis, unspecified eye**
  + **H16.22 Keratoconjunctivitis sicca, not specified as Sjögren's**
    Excludes1: *Sjögren's syndrome (M35.01)*
    - **H16.221 Keratoconjunctivitis sicca, not specified as Sjögren's, right eye**
    - **H16.222 Keratoconjunctivitis sicca, not specified as Sjögren's, left eye**
    - **H16.223 Keratoconjunctivitis sicca, not specified as Sjögren's, bilateral**
    - **H16.229 Keratoconjunctivitis sicca, not specified as Sjögren's, unspecified eye**
  + **H16.23 Neurotrophic keratoconjunctivitis**
    - **H16.231 Neurotrophic keratoconjunctivitis, right eye**
    - **H16.232 Neurotrophic keratoconjunctivitis, left eye**
    - **H16.233 Neurotrophic keratoconjunctivitis, bilateral**
    - **H16.239 Neurotrophic keratoconjunctivitis, unspecified eye**
  + **H16.24 Ophthalmia nodosa**
    - **H16.241 Ophthalmia nodosa, right eye**
    - **H16.242 Ophthalmia nodosa, left eye**
    - **H16.243 Ophthalmia nodosa, bilateral**
    - **H16.249 Ophthalmia nodosa, unspecified eye**
  + **H16.25 Phlyctenular keratoconjunctivitis**
    - **H16.251 Phlyctenular keratoconjunctivitis, right eye**
    - **H16.252 Phlyctenular keratoconjunctivitis, left eye**
    - **H16.253 Phlyctenular keratoconjunctivitis, bilateral**
    - **H16.259 Phlyctenular keratoconjunctivitis, unspecified eye**
  + **H16.26 Vernal keratoconjunctivitis, with limbar and corneal involvement**
    Excludes1: *vernal conjunctivitis without limbar and corneal involvement (H10.44)*
    - **H16.261 Vernal keratoconjunctivitis, with limbar and corneal involvement, right eye**
    - **H16.262 Vernal keratoconjunctivitis, with limbar and corneal involvement, left eye**
    - **H16.263 Vernal keratoconjunctivitis, with limbar and corneal involvement, bilateral**
    - **H16.269 Vernal keratoconjunctivitis, with limbar and corneal involvement, unspecified eye**
  + **H16.29 Other keratoconjunctivitis**
    - **H16.291 Other keratoconjunctivitis, right eye**
    - **H16.292 Other keratoconjunctivitis, left eye**
    - **H16.293 Other keratoconjunctivitis, bilateral**
    - **H16.299 Other keratoconjunctivitis, unspecified eye**
+ **H16.3 Interstitial and deep keratitis**
  + **H16.30 Unspecified interstitial keratitis**
    - **H16.301 Unspecified interstitial keratitis, right eye**
    - **H16.302 Unspecified interstitial keratitis, left eye**
    - **H16.303 Unspecified interstitial keratitis, bilateral**
    - **H16.309 Unspecified interstitial keratitis, unspecified eye**
  + **H16.31 Corneal abscess**
    - **H16.311 Corneal abscess, right eye**
    - **H16.312 Corneal abscess, left eye**
    - **H16.313 Corneal abscess, bilateral**
    - **H16.319 Corneal abscess, unspecified eye**
  + **H16.32 Diffuse interstitial keratitis**
    Cogan's syndrome
    - **H16.321 Diffuse interstitial keratitis, right eye**
    - **H16.322 Diffuse interstitial keratitis, left eye**
    - **H16.323 Diffuse interstitial keratitis, bilateral**
    - **H16.329 Diffuse interstitial keratitis, unspecified eye**
  + **H16.33 Sclerosing keratitis**
    - **H16.331 Sclerosing keratitis, right eye**
    - **H16.332 Sclerosing keratitis, left eye**
    - **H16.333 Sclerosing keratitis, bilateral**
    - **H16.339 Sclerosing keratitis, unspecified eye**

+ **H16.39 Other interstitial and deep keratitis**
H16.391 Other interstitial and deep keratitis, right eye
H16.392 Other interstitial and deep keratitis, left eye
H16.393 Other interstitial and deep keratitis, bilateral
H16.399 Other interstitial and deep keratitis, unspecified eye

+ **H16.4 Corneal neovascularization**
+ **H16.40 Unspecified corneal neovascularization**
H16.401 Unspecified corneal neovascularization, right eye
H16.402 Unspecified corneal neovascularization, left eye
H16.403 Unspecified corneal neovascularization, bilateral
H16.409 Unspecified corneal neovascularization, unspecified eye
+ **H16.41 Ghost vessels (corneal)**
H16.411 Ghost vessels (corneal), right eye
H16.412 Ghost vessels (corneal), left eye
H16.413 Ghost vessels (corneal), bilateral
H16.419 Ghost vessels (corneal), unspecified eye
+ **H16.42 Pannus (corneal)**
H16.421 Pannus (corneal), right eye
H16.422 Pannus (corneal), left eye
H16.423 Pannus (corneal), bilateral
H16.429 Pannus (corneal), unspecified eye
+ **H16.43 Localized vascularization of cornea**
H16.431 Localized vascularization of cornea, right eye
H16.432 Localized vascularization of cornea, left eye
H16.433 Localized vascularization of cornea, bilateral
H16.439 Localized vascularization of cornea, unspecified eye
+ **H16.44 Deep vascularization of cornea**
H16.441 Deep vascularization of cornea, right eye
H16.442 Deep vascularization of cornea, left eye
H16.443 Deep vascularization of cornea, bilateral
H16.449 Deep vascularization of cornea, unspecified eye

H16.8 Other keratitis
H16.9 Unspecified keratitis

H17 Corneal scars and opacities

+ **H17.0 Adherent leukoma**
H17.00 Adherent leukoma, unspecified eye
H17.01 Adherent leukoma, right eye
H17.02 Adherent leukoma, left eye
H17.03 Adherent leukoma, bilateral
+ **H17.1 Central corneal opacity**
H17.10 Central corneal opacity, unspecified eye
H17.11 Central corneal opacity, right eye
H17.12 Central corneal opacity, left eye
H17.13 Central corneal opacity, bilateral
+ **H17.8 Other corneal scars and opacities**
+ **H17.81 Minor opacity of cornea**
Corneal nebula
H17.811 Minor opacity of cornea, right eye
H17.812 Minor opacity of cornea, left eye
H17.813 Minor opacity of cornea, bilateral
H17.819 Minor opacity of cornea, unspecified eye
+ **H17.82 Peripheral opacity of cornea**
H17.821 Peripheral opacity of cornea, right eye
H17.822 Peripheral opacity of cornea, left eye
H17.823 Peripheral opacity of cornea, bilateral
H17.829 Peripheral opacity of cornea, unspecified eye
H17.89 Other corneal scars and opacities
H17.9 Unspecified corneal scar and opacity

H18 Other disorders of cornea

+ **H18.0 Corneal pigmentations and deposits**
+ **H18.00 Unspecified corneal deposit**
H18.001 Unspecified corneal deposit, right eye
H18.002 Unspecified corneal deposit, left eye
H18.003 Unspecified corneal deposit, bilateral
H18.009 Unspecified corneal deposit, unspecified eye
+ **H18.01 Anterior corneal pigmentations**
Staehli's line
H18.011 Anterior corneal pigmentations, right eye
H18.012 Anterior corneal pigmentations, left eye
H18.013 Anterior corneal pigmentations, bilateral
H18.019 Anterior corneal pigmentations, unspecified eye
+ **H18.02 Argentous corneal deposits**
H18.021 Argentous corneal deposits, right eye
H18.022 Argentous corneal deposits, left eye
H18.023 Argentous corneal deposits, bilateral
H18.029 Argentous corneal deposits, unspecified eye
+ **H18.03 Corneal deposits in metabolic disorders**
Code also associated metabolic disorder
H18.031 Corneal deposits in metabolic disorders, right eye
H18.032 Corneal deposits in metabolic disorders, left eye
H18.033 Corneal deposits in metabolic disorders, bilateral
H18.039 Corneal deposits in metabolic disorders, unspecified eye
+ **H18.04 Kayser-Fleischer ring**
Code also associated Wilson's disease (E83.01)
H18.041 Kayser-Fleischer ring, right eye
H18.042 Kayser-Fleischer ring, left eye
H18.043 Kayser-Fleischer ring, bilateral
H18.049 Kayser-Fleischer ring, unspecified eye
+ **H18.05 Posterior corneal pigmentations**
Krukenberg's spindle
H18.051 Posterior corneal pigmentations, right eye
H18.052 Posterior corneal pigmentations, left eye
H18.053 Posterior corneal pigmentations, bilateral
H18.059 Posterior corneal pigmentations, unspecified eye
+ **H18.06 Stromal corneal pigmentations**
Hematocornea
H18.061 Stromal corneal pigmentations, right eye
H18.062 Stromal corneal pigmentations, left eye
H18.063 Stromal corneal pigmentations, bilateral
H18.069 Stromal corneal pigmentations, unspecified eye
+ **H18.1 Bullous keratopathy**
H18.10 Bullous keratopathy, unspecified eye
H18.11 Bullous keratopathy, right eye
H18.12 Bullous keratopathy, left eye
H18.13 Bullous keratopathy, bilateral
+ **H18.2 Other and unspecified corneal edema**
H18.20 Unspecified corneal edema
+ **H18.21 Corneal edema secondary to contact lens**
Excludes2: *other corneal disorders due to contact lens (H18.82-)*
H18.211 Corneal edema secondary to contact lens, right eye
H18.212 Corneal edema secondary to contact lens, left eye
H18.213 Corneal edema secondary to contact lens, bilateral
H18.219 Corneal edema secondary to contact lens, unspecified eye
+ **H18.22 Idiopathic corneal edema**
H18.221 Idiopathic corneal edema, right eye
H18.222 Idiopathic corneal edema, left eye
H18.223 Idiopathic corneal edema, bilateral
H18.229 Idiopathic corneal edema, unspecified eye
+ **H18.23 Secondary corneal edema**
H18.231 Secondary corneal edema, right eye
H18.232 Secondary corneal edema, left eye
H18.233 Secondary corneal edema, bilateral
H18.239 Secondary corneal edema, unspecified eye

+ **H18.3 Changes of corneal membranes**
  - **H18.30 Unspecified corneal membrane change**
  - + **H18.31 Folds and rupture in Bowman's membrane**
    - **H18.311 Folds and rupture in Bowman's membrane, right eye**
    - **H18.312 Folds and rupture in Bowman's membrane, left eye**
    - **H18.313 Folds and rupture in Bowman's membrane, bilateral**
    - **H18.319 Folds and rupture in Bowman's membrane, unspecified eye**
  - + **H18.32 Folds in Descemet's membrane**
    - **H18.321 Folds in Descemet's membrane, right eye**
    - **H18.322 Folds in Descemet's membrane, left eye**
    - **H18.323 Folds in Descemet's membrane, bilateral**
    - **H18.329 Folds in Descemet's membrane, unspecified eye**
  - + **H18.33 Rupture in Descemet's membrane**
    - **H18.331 Rupture in Descemet's membrane, right eye**
    - **H18.332 Rupture in Descemet's membrane, left eye**
    - **H18.333 Rupture in Descemet's membrane, bilateral**
    - **H18.339 Rupture in Descemet's membrane, unspecified eye**

+ **H18.4 Corneal degeneration**
  - **Excludes1:** *Mooren's ulcer (H16.0-)*
    recurrent erosion of cornea (H18.83-)
  - **H18.40 Unspecified corneal degeneration**
  - + **H18.41 Arcus senilis**
    - Senile corneal changes
    - **H18.411 Arcus senilis, right eye**
    - **H18.412 Arcus senilis, left eye**
    - **H18.413 Arcus senilis, bilateral**
    - **H18.419 Arcus senilis, unspecified eye**
  - + **H18.42 Band keratopathy**
    - **H18.421 Band keratopathy, right eye**
    - **H18.422 Band keratopathy, left eye**
    - **H18.423 Band keratopathy, bilateral**
    - **H18.429 Band keratopathy, unspecified eye**
  - **H18.43 Other calcerous corneal degeneration**
  - + **H18.44 Keratomalacia**
    - **Excludes1:** *keratomalacia due to vitamin A deficiency (E50.4)*
    - **H18.441 Keratomalacia, right eye**
    - **H18.442 Keratomalacia, left eye**
    - **H18.443 Keratomalacia, bilateral**
    - **H18.449 Keratomalacia, unspecified eye**
  - + **H18.45 Nodular corneal degeneration**
    - **H18.451 Nodular corneal degeneration, right eye**
    - **H18.452 Nodular corneal degeneration, left eye**
    - **H18.453 Nodular corneal degeneration, bilateral**
    - **H18.459 Nodular corneal degeneration, unspecified eye**
  - + **H18.46 Peripheral corneal degeneration**
    - **H18.461 Peripheral corneal degeneration, right eye**
    - **H18.462 Peripheral corneal degeneration, left eye**
    - **H18.463 Peripheral corneal degeneration, bilateral**
    - **H18.469 Peripheral corneal degeneration, unspecified eye**
  - **H18.49 Other corneal degeneration**

+ **H18.5 Hereditary corneal dystrophies**
  - **H18.50 Unspecified hereditary corneal dystrophies**
  - **H18.51 Endothelial corneal dystrophy**
    - Fuchs' dystrophy
  - **H18.52 Epithelial (juvenile) corneal dystrophy**
  - **H18.53 Granular corneal dystrophy**
  - **H18.54 Lattice corneal dystrophy**
  - **H18.55 Macular corneal dystrophy**
  - **H18.59 Other hereditary corneal dystrophies**

+ **H18.6 Keratoconus**
  - + **H18.60 Keratoconus, unspecified**
    - **H18.601 Keratoconus, unspecified, right eye**
    - **H18.602 Keratoconus, unspecified, left eye**
    - **H18.603 Keratoconus, unspecified, bilateral**
    - **H18.609 Keratoconus, unspecified, unspecified eye**
  - + **H18.61 Keratoconus, stable**
    - **H18.611 Keratoconus, stable, right eye**
    - **H18.612 Keratoconus, stable, left eye**
    - **H18.613 Keratoconus, stable, bilateral**
    - **H18.619 Keratoconus, stable, unspecified eye**
  - + **H18.62 Keratoconus, unstable**
    - Acute hydrops
    - **H18.621 Keratoconus, unstable, right eye**
    - **H18.622 Keratoconus, unstable, left eye**
    - **H18.623 Keratoconus, unstable, bilateral**
    - **H18.629 Keratoconus, unstable, unspecified eye**

+ **H18.7 Other and unspecified corneal deformities**
  - **Excludes1:** *congenital malformations of cornea (Q13.3-Q13.4*
  - **H18.70 Unspecified corneal deformity**
  - + **H18.71 Corneal ectasia**
    - **H18.711 Corneal ectasia, right eye**
    - **H18.712 Corneal ectasia, left eye**
    - **H18.713 Corneal ectasia, bilateral**
    - **H18.719 Corneal ectasia, unspecified eye**
  - + **H18.72 Corneal staphyloma**
    - **H18.721 Corneal staphyloma, right eye**
    - **H18.722 Corneal staphyloma, left eye**
    - **H18.723 Corneal staphyloma, bilateral**
    - **H18.729 Corneal staphyloma, unspecified eye**
  - + **H18.73 Descemetocele**
    - **H18.731 Descemetocele, right eye**
    - **H18.732 Descemetocele, left eye**
    - **H18.733 Descemetocele, bilateral**
    - **H18.739 Descemetocele, unspecified eye**
  - + **H18.79 Other corneal deformities**
    - **H18.791 Other corneal deformities, right eye**
    - **H18.792 Other corneal deformities, left eye**
    - **H18.793 Other corneal deformities, bilateral**
    - **H18.799 Other corneal deformities, unspecified eye**

+ **H18.8 Other specified disorders of cornea**
  - + **H18.81 Anesthesia and hypoesthesia of cornea**
    - **H18.811 Anesthesia and hypoesthesia of cornea, right eye**
    - **H18.812 Anesthesia and hypoesthesia of cornea, left eye**
    - **H18.813 Anesthesia and hypoesthesia of cornea, bilateral**
    - **H18.819 Anesthesia and hypoesthesia of cornea, unspecified eye**
  - + **H18.82 Corneal disorder due to contact lens**
    - **Excludes2:** *corneal edema due to contact lens (H18.21-)*
    - **H18.821 Corneal disorder due to contact lens, right eye**
    - **H18.822 Corneal disorder due to contact lens, left eye**
    - **H18.823 Corneal disorder due to contact lens, bilateral**
    - **H18.829 Corneal disorder due to contact lens, unspecified eye**
  - + **H18.83 Recurrent erosion of cornea**
    - **H18.831 Recurrent erosion of cornea, right eye**
    - **H18.832 Recurrent erosion of cornea, left eye**
    - **H18.833 Recurrent erosion of cornea, bilateral**
    - **H18.839 Recurrent erosion of cornea, unspecified eye**
  - + **H18.89 Other specified disorders of cornea**
    - **H18.891 Other specified disorders of cornea, right eye**
    - **H18.892 Other specified disorders of cornea, left eye**
    - **H18.893 Other specified disorders of cornea, bilateral**
    - **H18.899 Other specified disorders of cornea, unspecified eye**

H18.9 Unspecified disorder of cornea

H20 Iridocyclitis

+ **H20.0 Acute and subacute iridocyclitis**
  Acute anterior uveitis
  Acute cyclitis
  Acute iritis
  Subacute anterior uveitis
  Subacute cyclitis
  Subacute iritis
  Excludes1: *iridocyclitis, iritis, uveitis (due to) (in) diabetes mellitus (E08-E13 with .39)*
  iridocyclitis, iritis, uveitis (due to) (in) diphtheria (A36.89)
  iridocyclitis, iritis, uveitis (due to) (in) gonococcal (A54.32)
  iridocyclitis, iritis, uveitis (due to) (in) herpes (simplex) (B00.51)
  iridocyclitis, iritis, uveitis (due to) (in) herpes zoster (B02.32)
  iridocyclitis, iritis, uveitis (due to) (in) late congenital syphilis (A50.39)
  iridocyclitis, iritis, uveitis (due to) (in) late syphilis (A52.71)
  iridocyclitis, iritis, uveitis (due to) (in) sarcoidosis (D86.83)
  iridocyclitis, iritis, uveitis (due to) (in) syphilis (A51.43)
  iridocyclitis, iritis, uveitis (due to) (in) toxoplasmosis (B58.09)
  iridocyclitis, iritis, uveitis (due to) (in) tuberculosis (A18.54)

CC **H20.00 Unspecified acute and subacute iridocyclitis**
  CC Exclusion see Appendix A PDX collection 0624

+ **H20.01 Primary iridocyclitis**
  CC **H20.011 Primary iridocyclitis, right eye**
    CC Exclusion see Appendix A PDX collection 0624
  CC **H20.012 Primary iridocyclitis, left eye**
    CC Exclusion see Appendix A PDX collection 0624
  CC **H20.013 Primary iridocyclitis, bilateral**
    CC Exclusion see Appendix A PDX collection 0624
  CC **H20.019 Primary iridocyclitis, unspecified eye**
    CC Exclusion see Appendix A PDX collection 0624

+ **H20.02 Recurrent acute iridocyclitis**
  CC **H20.021 Recurrent acute iridocyclitis, right eye**
    CC Exclusion see Appendix A PDX collection 0624
  CC **H20.022 Recurrent acute iridocyclitis, left eye**
    CC Exclusion see Appendix A PDX collection 0624
  CC **H20.023 Recurrent acute iridocyclitis, bilateral**
    CC Exclusion see Appendix A PDX collection 0624
  CC **H20.029 Recurrent acute iridocyclitis, unspecified eye**
    CC Exclusion see Appendix A PDX collection 0624

+ **H20.03 Secondary infectious iridocyclitis**
  CC **H20.031 Secondary infectious iridocyclitis, right eye**
    CC Exclusion see Appendix A PDX collection 0624
  CC **H20.032 Secondary infectious iridocyclitis, left eye**
    CC Exclusion see Appendix A PDX collection 0624
  CC **H20.033 Secondary infectious iridocyclitis, bilateral**
    CC Exclusion see Appendix A PDX collection 0624
  CC **H20.039 Secondary infectious iridocyclitis, unspecified eye**
    CC Exclusion see Appendix A PDX collection 0624

+ **H20.04 Secondary noninfectious iridocyclitis**
  H20.041 Secondary noninfectious iridocyclitis, right eye
  H20.042 Secondary noninfectious iridocyclitis, left eye
  H20.043 Secondary noninfectious iridocyclitis, bilateral
  H20.049 Secondary noninfectious iridocyclitis, unspecified eye

+ **H20.05 Hypopyon**
  H20.051 Hypopyon, right eye
  H20.052 Hypopyon, left eye
  H20.053 Hypopyon, bilateral
  H20.059 Hypopyon, unspecified eye

+ **H20.1 Chronic iridocyclitis**
  Use additional code for any associated cataract (H26.21-)
  Excludes2: *posterior cyclitis (H30.2-)*
  H20.10 Chronic iridocyclitis, unspecified eye
  H20.11 Chronic iridocyclitis, right eye
  H20.12 Chronic iridocyclitis, left eye
  H20.13 Chronic iridocyclitis, bilateral

+ **H20.2 Lens-induced iridocyclitis**
  H20.20 Lens-induced iridocyclitis, unspecified eye
  H20.21 Lens-induced iridocyclitis, right eye
  H20.22 Lens-induced iridocyclitis, left eye
  H20.23 Lens-induced iridocyclitis, bilateral

+ **H20.8 Other iridocyclitis**
  Excludes2: *glaucomatocyclitis crises (H40.4-)*
  posterior cyclitis (H30.2-)
  sympathetic uveitis (H44.13-)

+ **H20.81 Fuchs' heterochromic cyclitis**
  H20.811 Fuchs' heterochromic cyclitis, right eye
  H20.812 Fuchs' heterochromic cyclitis, left eye
  H20.813 Fuchs' heterochromic cyclitis, bilateral
  H20.819 Fuchs' heterochromic cyclitis, unspecified eye

+ **H20.82 Vogt-Koyanagi syndrome**
  H20.821 Vogt-Koyanagi syndrome, right eye
  H20.822 Vogt-Koyanagi syndrome, left eye
  H20.823 Vogt-Koyanagi syndrome, bilateral
  H20.829 Vogt-Koyanagi syndrome, unspecified eye

CC **H20.9 Unspecified iridocyclitis**
  Uveitis NOS
  CC Exclusion see Appendix A PDX collection 0624

H21 Other disorders of iris and ciliary body

Excludes2: *sympathetic uveitis (H44.1-)*

+ **H21.0 Hyphema**
  Excludes1: *traumatic hyphema (S05.1-)*
  H21.00 Hyphema, unspecified eye
  H21.01 Hyphema, right eye
  H21.02 Hyphema, left eye
  H21.03 Hyphema, bilateral

+ **H21.1 Other vascular disorders of iris and ciliary body**
  Neovascularization of iris or ciliary body
  Rubeosis iridis
  Rubeosis of iris

+ **H21.1X Other vascular disorders of iris and ciliary body**
  H21.1X1 Other vascular disorders of iris and ciliary body, right eye
  H21.1X2 Other vascular disorders of iris and ciliary body, left eye
  H21.1X3 Other vascular disorders of iris and ciliary body, bilateral
  H21.1X9 Other vascular disorders of iris and ciliary body, unspecified eye

+ **H21.2 Degeneration of iris and ciliary body**

+ **H21.21 Degeneration of chamber angle**
  H21.211 Degeneration of chamber angle, right eye
  H21.212 Degeneration of chamber angle, left eye
  H21.213 Degeneration of chamber angle, bilateral
  H21.219 Degeneration of chamber angle, unspecified eye

+ **H21.22 Degeneration of ciliary body**
  H21.221 Degeneration of ciliary body, right eye
  H21.222 Degeneration of ciliary body, left eye
  H21.223 Degeneration of ciliary body, bilateral
  H21.229 Degeneration of ciliary body, unspecified eye

+ **H21.23 Degeneration of iris (pigmentary)**
  Translucency of iris
  H21.231 Degeneration of iris (pigmentary), right eye
  H21.232 Degeneration of iris (pigmentary), left eye
  H21.233 Degeneration of iris (pigmentary), bilateral
  H21.239 Degeneration of iris (pigmentary), unspecified eye

+ **H21.24 Degeneration of pupillary margin**
  H21.241 Degeneration of pupillary margin, right eye
  H21.242 Degeneration of pupillary margin, left eye
  H21.243 Degeneration of pupillary margin, bilateral
  H21.249 Degeneration of pupillary margin, unspecified eye

+ **H21.25 Iridoschisis**
  - **H21.251 Iridoschisis, right eye**
  - **H21.252 Iridoschisis, left eye**
  - **H21.253 Iridoschisis, bilateral**
  - **H21.259 Iridoschisis, unspecified eye**

+ **H21.26 Iris atrophy (essential) (progressive)**
  - **H21.261 Iris atrophy (essential) (progressive), right eye**
  - **H21.262 Iris atrophy (essential) (progressive), left eye**
  - **H21.263 Iris atrophy (essential) (progressive), bilateral**
  - **H21.269 Iris atrophy (essential) (progressive), unspecified eye**

+ **H21.27 Miotic pupillary cyst**
  - **H21.271 Miotic pupillary cyst, right eye**
  - **H21.272 Miotic pupillary cyst, left eye**
  - **H21.273 Miotic pupillary cyst, bilateral**
  - **H21.279 Miotic pupillary cyst, unspecified eye**

H21.29 Other iris atrophy

+ **H21.3 Cyst of iris, ciliary body and anterior chamber**

Excludes2: *miotic pupillary cyst (H21.27-)*

+ **H21.30 Idiopathic cysts of iris, ciliary body or anterior chamber**

  Cyst of iris, ciliary body or anterior chamber NOS
  - **H21.301 Idiopathic cysts of iris, ciliary body or anterior chamber, right eye**
  - **H21.302 Idiopathic cysts of iris, ciliary body or anterior chamber, left eye**
  - **H21.303 Idiopathic cysts of iris, ciliary body or anterior chamber, bilateral**
  - **H21.309 Idiopathic cysts of iris, ciliary body or anterior chamber, unspecified eye**

+ **H21.31 Exudative cysts of iris or anterior chamber**
  - **H21.311 Exudative cysts of iris or anterior chamber, right eye**
  - **H21.312 Exudative cysts of iris or anterior chamber, left eye**
  - **H21.313 Exudative cysts of iris or anterior chamber, bilateral**
  - **H21.319 Exudative cysts of iris or anterior chamber, unspecified eye**

+ **H21.32 Implantation cysts of iris, ciliary body or anterior chamber**
  - **H21.321 Implantation cysts of iris, ciliary body or anterior chamber, right eye**
  - **H21.322 Implantation cysts of iris, ciliary body or anterior chamber, left eye**
  - **H21.323 Implantation cysts of iris, ciliary body or anterior chamber, bilateral**
  - **H21.329 Implantation cysts of iris, ciliary body or anterior chamber, unspecified eye**

+ **H21.33 Parasitic cyst of iris, ciliary body or anterior chamber**
  - CC **H21.331 Parasitic cyst of iris, ciliary body or anterior chamber, right eye**
    CC Exclusion see Appendix A PDX collection 0625
  - CC **H21.332 Parasitic cyst of iris, ciliary body or anterior chamber, left eye**
    CC Exclusion see Appendix A PDX collection 0625
  - CC **H21.333 Parasitic cyst of iris, ciliary body or anterior chamber, bilateral**
    CC Exclusion see Appendix A PDX collection 0625
  - CC **H21.339 Parasitic cyst of iris, ciliary body or anterior chamber, unspecified eye**
    CC Exclusion see Appendix A PDX collection 0625

+ **H21.34 Primary cyst of pars plana**
  - **H21.341 Primary cyst of pars plana, right eye**
  - **H21.342 Primary cyst of pars plana, left eye**
  - **H21.343 Primary cyst of pars plana, bilateral**
  - **H21.349 Primary cyst of pars plana, unspecified eye**

+ **H21.35 Exudative cyst of pars plana**
  - **H21.351 Exudative cyst of pars plana, right eye**
  - **H21.352 Exudative cyst of pars plana, left eye**
  - **H21.353 Exudative cyst of pars plana, bilateral**
  - **H21.359 Exudative cyst of pars plana, unspecified eye**

+ **H21.4 Pupillary membranes**

  Iris bombé
  Pupillary occlusion
  Pupillary seclusion

  Excludes1: *congenital pupillary membranes (Q13.8)*
  - **H21.40 Pupillary membranes, unspecified eye**
  - **H21.41 Pupillary membranes, right eye**
  - **H21.42 Pupillary membranes, left eye**
  - **H21.43 Pupillary membranes, bilateral**

+ **H21.5 Other and unspecified adhesions and disruptions of iris and ciliary body**

  Excludes1: *corectopia (Q13.2)*

+ **H21.50 Unspecified adhesions of iris**

  Synechia (iris) NOS
  - **H21.501 Unspecified adhesions of iris, right eye**
  - **H21.502 Unspecified adhesions of iris, left eye**
  - **H21.503 Unspecified adhesions of iris, bilateral**
  - **H21.509 Unspecified adhesions of iris and ciliary body, unspecified eye**

+ **H21.51 Anterior synechiae (iris)**
  - **H21.511 Anterior synechiae (iris), right eye**
  - **H21.512 Anterior synechiae (iris), left eye**
  - **H21.513 Anterior synechiae (iris), bilateral**
  - **H21.519 Anterior synechiae (iris), unspecified eye**

+ **H21.52 Goniosynechiae**
  - **H21.521 Goniosynechiae, right eye**
  - **H21.522 Goniosynechiae, left eye**
  - **H21.523 Goniosynechiae, bilateral**
  - **H21.529 Goniosynechiae, unspecified eye**

+ **H21.53 Iridodialysis**
  - **H21.531 Iridodialysis, right eye**
  - **H21.532 Iridodialysis, left eye**
  - **H21.533 Iridodialysis, bilateral**
  - **H21.539 Iridodialysis, unspecified eye**

+ **H21.54 Posterior synechiae (iris)**
  - **H21.541 Posterior synechiae (iris), right eye**
  - **H21.542 Posterior synechiae (iris), left eye**
  - **H21.543 Posterior synechiae (iris), bilateral**
  - **H21.549 Posterior synechiae (iris), unspecified eye**

+ **H21.55 Recession of chamber angle**
  - **H21.551 Recession of chamber angle, right eye**
  - **H21.552 Recession of chamber angle, left eye**
  - **H21.553 Recession of chamber angle, bilateral**
  - **H21.559 Recession of chamber angle, unspecified eye**

+ **H21.56 Pupillary abnormalities**

  Deformed pupil
  Ectopic pupil
  Rupture of sphincter, pupil

  Excludes1: *congenital deformity of pupil (Q13.2-)*
  - **H21.561 Pupillary abnormality, right eye**
  - **H21.562 Pupillary abnormality, left eye**
  - **H21.563 Pupillary abnormality, bilateral**
  - **H21.569 Pupillary abnormality, unspecified eye**

+ **H21.8 Other specified disorders of iris and ciliary body**
  - **H21.81 Floppy iris syndrome**

    Intraoperative floppy iris syndrome (IFIS)
    Use additional code for adverse effect, if applicable, to identify drug (T36-T50 with fifth or sixth character 5)
  - **H21.82 Plateau iris syndrome (post-iridectomy) (postprocedural)**
  - **H21.89 Other specified disorders of iris and ciliary body**

H21.9 Unspecified disorder of iris and ciliary body

H22 Disorders of iris and ciliary body in diseases classified elsewhere

Code first underlying disease, such as:
- gout (M1A.-, M10.-)
- leprosy (A30.-)
- parasitic disease (B89)

Valid 3-character code, no further characters required

Disorders of lens (H25-H28)

H25 Age-related cataract

Senile cataract

Excludes2: capsular glaucoma with pseudoexfoliation of lens (H40.1-)

+ **H25.0 Age-related incipient cataract**

+ **H25.01 Cortical age-related cataract**
  - • **H25.011 Cortical age-related cataract, right eye**
  - • **H25.012 Cortical age-related cataract, left eye**

• H25.013 Cortical age-related cataract, bilateral
• H25.019 Cortical age-related cataract, unspecified eye
+ H25.03 Anterior subcapsular polar age-related cataract
• H25.031 Anterior subcapsular polar age-related cataract, right eye
• H25.032 Anterior subcapsular polar age-related cataract, left eye
• H25.033 Anterior subcapsular polar age-related cataract, bilateral
• H25.039 Anterior subcapsular polar age-related cataract, unspecified eye
+ H25.04 Posterior subcapsular polar age-related cataract
• H25.041 Posterior subcapsular polar age-related cataract, right eye
• H25.042 Posterior subcapsular polar age-related cataract, left eye
• H25.043 Posterior subcapsular polar age-related cataract, bilateral
• H25.049 Posterior subcapsular polar age-related cataract, unspecified eye
+ H25.09 Other age-related incipient cataract
Coronary age-related cataract
Punctate age-related cataract
Water clefts
• H25.091 Other age-related incipient cataract, right eye
• H25.092 Other age-related incipient cataract, left eye
• H25.093 Other age-related incipient cataract, bilateral
• H25.099 Other age-related incipient cataract, unspecified eye
+ H25.1 Age-related nuclear cataract
Cataracta brunescens
Nuclear sclerosis cataract
• H25.10 Age-related nuclear cataract, unspecified eye
• H25.11 Age-related nuclear cataract, right eye
• H25.12 Age-related nuclear cataract, left eye
AHA CC: 1Q, 2016, 32-33
• H25.13 Age-related nuclear cataract, bilateral
AHA CC: 1Q, 2016, 32-33
+ H25.2 Age-related cataract, morgagnian type
Age-related hypermature cataract
• H25.20 Age-related cataract, morgagnian type, unspecified eye
• H25.21 Age-related cataract, morgagnian type, right eye
• H25.22 Age-related cataract, morgagnian type, left eye
• H25.23 Age-related cataract, morgagnian type, bilateral
+ H25.8 Other age-related cataract
+ H25.81 Combined forms of age-related cataract
• H25.811 Combined forms of age-related cataract, right eye
• H25.812 Combined forms of age-related cataract, left eye
• H25.813 Combined forms of age-related cataract, bilateral
• H25.819 Combined forms of age-related cataract, unspecified eye
• H25.89 Other age-related cataract
• H25.9 Unspecified age-related cataract

H26 Other cataract

Excludes1: *congenital cataract (Q12.0)*
+ H26.0 Infantile and juvenile cataract
+ H26.00 Unspecified infantile and juvenile cataract
• H26.001 Unspecified infantile and juvenile cataract, right eye
• H26.002 Unspecified infantile and juvenile cataract, left eye
• H26.003 Unspecified infantile and juvenile cataract, bilateral
• H26.009 Unspecified infantile and juvenile cataract, unspecified eye
+ H26.01 Infantile and juvenile cortical, lamellar, or zonular cataract
• H26.011 Infantile and juvenile cortical, lamellar, or zonular cataract, right eye
• H26.012 Infantile and juvenile cortical, lamellar, or zonular cataract, left eye
• H26.013 Infantile and juvenile cortical, lamellar, or zonular cataract, bilateral
• H26.019 Infantile and juvenile cortical, lamellar, or zonular cataract, unspecified eye
+ H26.03 Infantile and juvenile nuclear cataract
• H26.031 Infantile and juvenile nuclear cataract, right eye
• H26.032 Infantile and juvenile nuclear cataract, left eye
• H26.033 Infantile and juvenile nuclear cataract, bilateral
• H26.039 Infantile and juvenile nuclear cataract, unspecified eye
+ H26.04 Anterior subcapsular polar infantile and juvenile cataract
• H26.041 Anterior subcapsular polar infantile and juvenile cataract, right eye
• H26.042 Anterior subcapsular polar infantile and juvenile cataract, left eye
• H26.043 Anterior subcapsular polar infantile and juvenile cataract, bilateral
• H26.049 Anterior subcapsular polar infantile and juvenile cataract, unspecified eye
+ H26.05 Posterior subcapsular polar infantile and juvenile cataract
• H26.051 Posterior subcapsular polar infantile and juvenile cataract, right eye
• H26.052 Posterior subcapsular polar infantile and juvenile cataract, left eye
• H26.053 Posterior subcapsular polar infantile and juvenile cataract, bilateral
• H26.059 Posterior subcapsular polar infantile and juvenile cataract, unspecified eye
+ H26.06 Combined forms of infantile and juvenile cataract
• H26.061 Combined forms of infantile and juvenile cataract, right eye
• H26.062 Combined forms of infantile and juvenile cataract, left eye
• H26.063 Combined forms of infantile and juvenile cataract, bilateral
• H26.069 Combined forms of infantile and juvenile cataract, unspecified eye
• H26.09 Other infantile and juvenile cataract
+ H26.1 Traumatic cataract
Use additional code (Chapter 20) to identify external cause
+ H26.10 Unspecified traumatic cataract
H26.101 Unspecified traumatic cataract, right eye
H26.102 Unspecified traumatic cataract, left eye
H26.103 Unspecified traumatic cataract, bilateral
H26.109 Unspecified traumatic cataract, unspecified eye
+ H26.11 Localized traumatic opacities
H26.111 Localized traumatic opacities, right eye
H26.112 Localized traumatic opacities, left eye
H26.113 Localized traumatic opacities, bilateral
H26.119 Localized traumatic opacities, unspecified eye
+ H26.12 Partially resolved traumatic cataract
H26.121 Partially resolved traumatic cataract, right eye
H26.122 Partially resolved traumatic cataract, left eye
H26.123 Partially resolved traumatic cataract, bilateral
H26.129 Partially resolved traumatic cataract, unspecified eye
+ H26.13 Total traumatic cataract
H26.131 Total traumatic cataract, right eye
H26.132 Total traumatic cataract, left eye
H26.133 Total traumatic cataract, bilateral
H26.139 Total traumatic cataract, unspecified eye
+ H26.2 Complicated cataract
H26.20 Unspecified complicated cataract
Cataracta complicata NOS
+ H26.21 Cataract with neovascularization
Code also associated condition, such as:
chronic iridocyclitis (H20.1-)
H26.211 Cataract with neovascularization, right eye
H26.212 Cataract with neovascularization, left eye
H26.213 Cataract with neovascularization, bilateral

H26.219 **Cataract with neovascularization, unspecified eye**

+ **H26.22 Cataract secondary to ocular disorders (degenerative) (inflammatory)**

Code also associated ocular disorder

H26.221 **Cataract secondary to ocular disorders (degenerative) (inflammatory), right eye**

H26.222 **Cataract secondary to ocular disorders (degenerative) (inflammatory), left eye**

H26.223 **Cataract secondary to ocular disorders (degenerative) (inflammatory), bilateral**

H26.229 **Cataract secondary to ocular disorders (degenerative) (inflammatory), unspecified eye**

+ **H26.23 Glaucomatous flecks (subcapsular)**

Code first underlying glaucoma (H40-H42)

H26.231 **Glaucomatous flecks (subcapsular), right eye**

H26.232 **Glaucomatous flecks (subcapsular), left eye**

H26.233 **Glaucomatous flecks (subcapsular), bilateral**

H26.239 **Glaucomatous flecks (subcapsular), unspecified eye**

+ **H26.3 Drug-induced cataract**

Toxic cataract

Use additional code for adverse effect, if applicable, to identify drug (T36-T50 with fifth or sixth character 5)

H26.30 **Drug-induced cataract, unspecified eye**

H26.31 **Drug-induced cataract, right eye**

H26.32 **Drug-induced cataract, left eye**

H26.33 **Drug-induced cataract, bilateral**

+ **H26.4 Secondary cataract**

H26.40 **Unspecified secondary cataract**

+ **H26.41 Soemmering's ring**

H26.411 **Soemmering's ring, right eye**

H26.412 **Soemmering's ring, left eye**

H26.413 **Soemmering's ring, bilateral**

H26.419 **Soemmering's ring, unspecified eye**

+ **H26.49 Other secondary cataract**

H26.491 **Other secondary cataract, right eye**

H26.492 **Other secondary cataract, left eye**

H26.493 **Other secondary cataract, bilateral**

H26.499 **Other secondary cataract, unspecified eye**

H26.8 **Other specified cataract**

H26.9 **Unspecified cataract**

H27 Other disorders of lens

Excludes1: *congenital lens malformations (Q12.-)*
mechanical complications of intraocular lens implant (T85.2)
pseudophakia (Z96.1)

+ **H27.0 Aphakia**

Acquired absence of lens

Acquired aphakia

Aphakia due to trauma

Excludes1: *cataract extraction status (Z98.4-)*
congenital absence of lens (Q12.3)
congenital aphakia (Q12.3)

H27.00 **Aphakia, unspecified eye**

H27.01 **Aphakia, right eye**

H27.02 **Aphakia, left eye**

H27.03 **Aphakia, bilateral**

+ **H27.1 Dislocation of lens**

H27.10 **Unspecified dislocation of lens**

+ **H27.11 Subluxation of lens**

H27.111 **Subluxation of lens, right eye**

H27.112 **Subluxation of lens, left eye**

H27.113 **Subluxation of lens, bilateral**

H27.119 **Subluxation of lens, unspecified eye**

+ **H27.12 Anterior dislocation of lens**

H27.121 **Anterior dislocation of lens, right eye**

H27.122 **Anterior dislocation of lens, left eye**

H27.123 **Anterior dislocation of lens, bilateral**

H27.129 **Anterior dislocation of lens, unspecified eye**

+ **H27.13 Posterior dislocation of lens**

H27.131 **Posterior dislocation of lens, right eye**

H27.132 **Posterior dislocation of lens, left eye**

H27.133 **Posterior dislocation of lens, bilateral**

H27.139 **Posterior dislocation of lens, unspecified eye**

H27.8 **Other specified disorders of lens**

H27.9 **Unspecified disorder of lens**

H28 Cataract in diseases classified elsewhere

Code first underlying disease, such as:
hypoparathyroidism (E20.-)
myotonia (G71.1-)
myxedema (E03.-)
protein-calorie malnutrition (E40-E46)

Excludes1: *cataract in diabetes mellitus (E08.36, E09.36, E10.36, E11.36, E13.36)*

Valid 3-character code, no further characters required

Disorders of choroid and retina (H30-H36)

H30 Chorioretinal inflammation

+ **H30.0 Focal chorioretinal inflammation**

Focal chorioretinitis

Focal choroiditis

Focal retinitis

Focal retinochoroiditis

+ **H30.00 Unspecified focal chorioretinal inflammation**

Focal chorioretinitis NOS

Focal choroiditis NOS

Focal retinitis NOS

Focal retinochoroiditis NOS

H30.001 **Unspecified focal chorioretinal inflammation, right eye**

H30.002 **Unspecified focal chorioretinal inflammation, left eye**

H30.003 **Unspecified focal chorioretinal inflammation, bilateral**

H30.009 **Unspecified focal chorioretinal inflammation, unspecified eye**

+ **H30.01 Focal chorioretinal inflammation, juxtapapillary**

H30.011 **Focal chorioretinal inflammation, juxtapapillary, right eye**

H30.012 **Focal chorioretinal inflammation, juxtapapillary, left eye**

H30.013 **Focal chorioretinal inflammation, juxtapapillary, bilateral**

H30.019 **Focal chorioretinal inflammation, juxtapapillary, unspecified eye**

+ **H30.02 Focal chorioretinal inflammation of posterior pole**

H30.021 **Focal chorioretinal inflammation of posterior pole, right eye**

H30.022 **Focal chorioretinal inflammation of posterior pole, left eye**

H30.023 **Focal chorioretinal inflammation of posterior pole, bilateral**

H30.029 **Focal chorioretinal inflammation of posterior pole, unspecified eye**

+ **H30.03 Focal chorioretinal inflammation, peripheral**

H30.031 **Focal chorioretinal inflammation, peripheral, right eye**

H30.032 **Focal chorioretinal inflammation, peripheral, left eye**

H30.033 **Focal chorioretinal inflammation, peripheral, bilateral**

H30.039 **Focal chorioretinal inflammation, peripheral, unspecified eye**

+ **H30.04 Focal chorioretinal inflammation, macular or paramacular**

H30.041 **Focal chorioretinal inflammation, macular or paramacular, right eye**

H30.042 **Focal chorioretinal inflammation, macular or paramacular, left eye**

H30.043 **Focal chorioretinal inflammation, macular or paramacular, bilateral**

H30.049 **Focal chorioretinal inflammation, macular or paramacular, unspecified eye**

+ **H30.1 Disseminated chorioretinal inflammation**

Disseminated chorioretinitis

Disseminated choroiditis

Disseminated retinitis

Disseminated retinochoroiditis

Excludes2: *exudative retinopathy (H35.02-)*

+ **H30.10 Unspecified disseminated chorioretinal inflammation**

Disseminated chorioretinitis NOS

Disseminated choroiditis NOS

Disseminated retinitis NOS

Disseminated retinochoroiditis NOS

CC **H30.101 Unspecified disseminated chorioretinal inflammation, right eye**
CC Exclusion see Appendix A PDX collection 0626

CC **H30.102 Unspecified disseminated chorioretinal inflammation, left eye**
CC Exclusion see Appendix A PDX collection 0626

CC **H30.103 Unspecified disseminated chorioretinal inflammation, bilateral**
CC Exclusion see Appendix A PDX collection 0626

CC **H30.109 Unspecified disseminated chorioretinal inflammation, unspecified eye**
CC Exclusion see Appendix A PDX collection 0626

+ **H30.11 Disseminated chorioretinal inflammation of posterior pole**

CC **H30.111 Disseminated chorioretinal inflammation of posterior pole, right eye**
CC Exclusion see Appendix A PDX collection 0626

CC **H30.112 Disseminated chorioretinal inflammation of posterior pole, left eye**
CC Exclusion see Appendix A PDX collection 0626

CC **H30.113 Disseminated chorioretinal inflammation of posterior pole, bilateral**
CC Exclusion see Appendix A PDX collection 0626

CC **H30.119 Disseminated chorioretinal inflammation of posterior pole, unspecified eye**
CC Exclusion see Appendix A PDX collection 0626

+ **H30.12 Disseminated chorioretinal inflammation, peripheral**

CC **H30.121 Disseminated chorioretinal inflammation, peripheral right eye**
CC Exclusion see Appendix A PDX collection 0626

CC **H30.122 Disseminated chorioretinal inflammation, peripheral, left eye**
CC Exclusion see Appendix A PDX collection 0626

CC **H30.123 Disseminated chorioretinal inflammation, peripheral, bilateral**
CC Exclusion see Appendix A PDX collection 0626

CC **H30.129 Disseminated chorioretinal inflammation, peripheral, unspecified eye**
CC Exclusion see Appendix A PDX collection 0626

+ **H30.13 Disseminated chorioretinal inflammation, generalized**

CC **H30.131 Disseminated chorioretinal inflammation, generalized, right eye**
CC Exclusion see Appendix A PDX collection 0626

CC **H30.132 Disseminated chorioretinal inflammation, generalized, left eye**
CC Exclusion see Appendix A PDX collection 0626

CC **H30.133 Disseminated chorioretinal inflammation, generalized, bilateral**
CC Exclusion see Appendix A PDX collection 0626

CC **H30.139 Disseminated chorioretinal inflammation, generalized, unspecified eye**
CC Exclusion see Appendix A PDX collection 0626

+ **H30.14 Acute posterior multifocal placoid pigment epitheliopathy**

CC **H30.141 Acute posterior multifocal placoid pigment epitheliopathy, right eye**
CC Exclusion see Appendix A PDX collection 0626

CC **H30.142 Acute posterior multifocal placoid pigment epitheliopathy, left eye**
CC Exclusion see Appendix A PDX collection 0626

CC **H30.143 Acute posterior multifocal placoid pigment epitheliopathy, bilateral**
CC Exclusion see Appendix A PDX collection 0626

CC **H30.149 Acute posterior multifocal placoid pigment epitheliopathy, unspecified eye**
CC Exclusion see Appendix A PDX collection 0626

+ **H30.2 Posterior cyclitis**
Pars planitis

H30.20 Posterior cyclitis, unspecified eye
H30.21 Posterior cyclitis, right eye
H30.22 Posterior cyclitis, left eye
H30.23 Posterior cyclitis, bilateral

+ **H30.8 Other chorioretinal inflammations**

+ **H30.81 Harada's disease**

H30.811 Harada's disease, right eye
H30.812 Harada's disease, left eye
H30.813 Harada's disease, bilateral
H30.819 Harada's disease, unspecified eye

+ **H30.89 Other chorioretinal inflammations**

CC **H30.891 Other chorioretinal inflammations, right eye**
CC Exclusion see Appendix A PDX collection 0626

CC **H30.892 Other chorioretinal inflammations, left eye**
CC Exclusion see Appendix A PDX collection 0626

CC **H30.893 Other chorioretinal inflammations, bilateral**
CC Exclusion see Appendix A PDX collection 0626

CC **H30.899 Other chorioretinal inflammations, unspecified eye**
CC Exclusion see Appendix A PDX collection 0626

+ **H30.9 Unspecified chorioretinal inflammation**
Chorioretinitis NOS
Choroiditis NOS
Neuroretinitis NOS
Retinitis NOS
Retinochoroiditis NOS

CC **H30.90 Unspecified chorioretinal inflammation, unspecified eye**
CC Exclusion see Appendix A PDX collection 0626

CC **H30.91 Unspecified chorioretinal inflammation, right eye**
CC Exclusion see Appendix A PDX collection 0626

CC **H30.92 Unspecified chorioretinal inflammation, left eye**
CC Exclusion see Appendix A PDX collection 0626

CC **H30.93 Unspecified chorioretinal inflammation, bilateral**
CC Exclusion see Appendix A PDX collection 0626

H31 Other disorders of choroid

+ **H31.0 Chorioretinal scars**
Excludes2: *postsurgical chorioretinal scars (H59.81-)*

+ **H31.00 Unspecified chorioretinal scars**

H31.001 Unspecified chorioretinal scars, righ eye
H31.002 Unspecified chorioretinal scars, left eye
H31.003 Unspecified chorioretinal scars, bilateral
H31.009 Unspecified chorioretinal scars, unspecified eye

+ **H31.01 Macula scars of posterior pole (postinflammatory) (post-traumatic)**
Excludes1: *postprocedural chorioretinal scar (H59.81-)*

H31.011 Macula scars of posterior pole (postinflammatory) (post-traumatic), right eye
H31.012 Macula scars of posterior pole (postinflammatory) (post-traumatic), left eye
H31.013 Macula scars of posterior pole (postinflammatory) (post-traumatic), bilateral
H31.019 Macula scars of posterior pole (postinflammatory) (post-traumatic), unspecified eye

+ **H31.02 Solar retinopathy**

H31.021 Solar retinopathy, right eye
H31.022 Solar retinopathy, left eye
H31.023 Solar retinopathy, bilateral
H31.029 Solar retinopathy, unspecified eye

+ **H31.09 Other chorioretinal scars**

H31.091 Other chorioretinal scars, right eye
H31.092 Other chorioretinal scars, left eye
H31.093 Other chorioretinal scars, bilateral
H31.099 Other chorioretinal scars, unspecified eye

+ **H31.1 Choroidal degeneration**
  Excludes2: angioid streaks of macula (H35.33)
  + **H31.10 Unspecified choroidal degeneration**
    Choroidal sclerosis NOS
    H31.101 Choroidal degeneration, unspecified, right eye
    H31.102 Choroidal degeneration, unspecified, left eye
    H31.103 Choroidal degeneration, unspecified, bilateral
    H31.109 Choroidal degeneration, unspecified, unspecified eye
  + **H31.11 Age-related choroidal atrophy**
    • **H31.111 Age-related choroidal atrophy, right eye**
    • **H31.112 Age-related choroidal atrophy, left eye**
    • **H31.113 Age-related choroidal atrophy, bilateral**
    • **H31.119 Age-related choroidal atrophy, unspecified eye**
  + **H31.12 Diffuse secondary atrophy of choroid**
    H31.121 Diffuse secondary atrophy of choroid, right eye
    H31.122 Diffuse secondary atrophy of choroid, left eye
    H31.123 Diffuse secondary atrophy of choroid, bilateral
    H31.129 Diffuse secondary atrophy of choroid, unspecified eye

+ **H31.2 Hereditary choroidal dystrophy**
  Excludes2: hyperornithinemia (E72.4)
  ornithinemia (E72.4)
  H31.20 Hereditary choroidal dystrophy, unspecified
  H31.21 Choroideremia
  H31.22 Choroidal dystrophy (central areolar) (generalized) (peripapillary)
  H31.23 Gyrate atrophy, choroid
  H31.29 Other hereditary choroidal dystrophy

+ **H31.3 Choroidal hemorrhage and rupture**
  + **H31.30 Unspecified choroidal hemorrhage**
    H31.301 Unspecified choroidal hemorrhage, right eye
    H31.302 Unspecified choroidal hemorrhage, left eye
    H31.303 Unspecified choroidal hemorrhage, bilateral
    H31.309 Unspecified choroidal hemorrhage, unspecified eye
  + **H31.31 Expulsive choroidal hemorrhage**
    H31.311 Expulsive choroidal hemorrhage, right eye
    H31.312 Expulsive choroidal hemorrhage, left eye
    H31.313 Expulsive choroidal hemorrhage, bilateral
    H31.319 Expulsive choroidal hemorrhage, unspecified eye
  + **H31.32 Choroidal rupture**
    CC **H31.321 Choroidal rupture, right eye**
      CC Exclusion see Appendix A PDX collection 0627
    CC **H31.322 Choroidal rupture, left eye**
      CC Exclusion see Appendix A PDX collection 0627
    CC **H31.323 Choroidal rupture, bilateral**
      CC Exclusion see Appendix A PDX collection 0627
    CC **H31.329 Choroidal rupture, unspecified eye**
      CC Exclusion see Appendix A PDX collection 0627

+ **H31.4 Choroidal detachment**
  + **H31.40 Unspecified choroidal detachment**
    CC **H31.401 Unspecified choroidal detachment, right eye**
      CC Exclusion see Appendix A PDX collection 0627
    CC **H31.402 Unspecified choroidal detachment, left eye**
      CC Exclusion see Appendix A PDX collection 0627
    CC **H31.403 Unspecified choroidal detachment, bilateral**
      CC Exclusion see Appendix A PDX collection 0627
    CC **H31.409 Unspecified choroidal detachment, unspecified eye**
      CC Exclusion see Appendix A PDX collection 0627
  + **H31.41 Hemorrhagic choroidal detachment**
    CC **H31.411 Hemorrhagic choroidal detachment, right eye**
      CC Exclusion see Appendix A PDX collection 0627
    CC **H31.412 Hemorrhagic choroidal detachment, left eye**
      CC Exclusion see Appendix A PDX collection 0627
    CC **H31.413 Hemorrhagic choroidal detachment, bilateral**
      CC Exclusion see Appendix A PDX collection 0627
    CC **H31.419 Hemorrhagic choroidal detachment, unspecified eye**
      CC Exclusion see Appendix A PDX collection 0627
  + **H31.42 Serous choroidal detachment**
    CC **H31.421 Serous choroidal detachment, right eye**
      CC Exclusion see Appendix A PDX collection 0627
    CC **H31.422 Serous choroidal detachment, left eye**
      CC Exclusion see Appendix A PDX collection 0627
    CC **H31.423 Serous choroidal detachment, bilateral**
      CC Exclusion see Appendix A PDX collection 0627
    CC **H31.429 Serous choroidal detachment, unspecified eye**
      CC Exclusion see Appendix A PDX collection 0627

H31.8 Other specified disorders of choroid
H31.9 Unspecified disorder of choroid

H32 Chorioretinal disorders in diseases classified elsewhere

Code first underlying disease, such as:
congenital toxoplasmosis (P37.1)
histoplasmosis (B39.-)
leprosy (A30.-)
Excludes1: chorioretinitis (in):
toxoplasmosis (acquired) (B58.01)
tuberculosis (A18.53)
Valid 3-character code, no further characters required

H33 Retinal detachments and breaks

Excludes1: detachment of retinal pigment epithelium (H35.72-, H35.73-)

+ **H33.0 Retinal detachment with retinal break**
  Rhegmatogenous retinal detachment
  Excludes1: serous retinal detachment (without retinal break) (H33.2-)
  + **H33.00 Unspecified retinal detachment with retinal break**
    H33.001 Unspecified retinal detachment with retinal break, right eye
    H33.002 Unspecified retinal detachment with retinal break, left eye
    H33.003 Unspecified retinal detachment with retinal break, bilateral
    H33.009 Unspecified retinal detachment with retinal break, unspecified eye
  + **H33.01 Retinal detachment with single break**
    H33.011 Retinal detachment with single break, right eye
    H33.012 Retinal detachment with single break, left eye
    H33.013 Retinal detachment with single break, bilateral
    H33.019 Retinal detachment with single break, unspecified eye
  + **H33.02 Retinal detachment with multiple breaks**
    H33.021 Retinal detachment with multiple breaks, right eye
    H33.022 Retinal detachment with multiple breaks, left eye
    H33.023 Retinal detachment with multiple breaks, bilateral
    H33.029 Retinal detachment with multiple breaks, unspecified eye
  + **H33.03 Retinal detachment with giant retinal tear**
    H33.031 Retinal detachment with giant retinal tear, right eye
    H33.032 Retinal detachment with giant retinal tear, left eye

H33.033 Retinal detachment with giant retinal tear, bilateral
H33.039 Retinal detachment with giant retinal tear, unspecified eye
+ H33.04 Retinal detachment with retinal dialysis
H33.041 Retinal detachment with retinal dialysis, right eye
H33.042 Retinal detachment with retinal dialysis, left eye
H33.043 Retinal detachment with retinal dialysis, bilateral
H33.049 Retinal detachment with retinal dialysis, unspecified eye
+ H33.05 Total retinal detachment
H33.051 Total retinal detachment, right eye
H33.052 Total retinal detachment, left eye
H33.053 Total retinal detachment, bilateral
H33.059 Total retinal detachment, unspecified eye
+ H33.1 Retinoschisis and retinal cysts
Excludes1: *congenital retinoschisis (Q14.1)*
microcystoid degeneration of retina (H35.42-)
+ H33.10 Unspecified retinoschisis
H33.101 Unspecified retinoschisis, right eye
H33.102 Unspecified retinoschisis, left eye
H33.103 Unspecified retinoschisis, bilateral
H33.109 Unspecified retinoschisis, unspecified eye
+ H33.11 Cyst of ora serrata
H33.111 Cyst of ora serrata, right eye
H33.112 Cyst of ora serrata, left eye
H33.113 Cyst of ora serrata, bilateral
H33.119 Cyst of ora serrata, unspecified eye
+ H33.12 Parasitic cyst of retina
CC H33.121 Parasitic cyst of retina, right eye
CC Exclusion see Appendix A PDX collection 0625
CC H33.122 Parasitic cyst of retina, left eye
CC Exclusion see Appendix A PDX collection 0625
CC H33.123 Parasitic cyst of retina, bilateral
CC Exclusion see Appendix A PDX collection 0625
CC H33.129 Parasitic cyst of retina, unspecified eye
CC Exclusion see Appendix A PDX collection 0625
+ H33.19 Other retinoschisis and retinal cysts
Pseudocyst of retina
H33.191 Other retinoschisis and retinal cysts, right eye
H33.192 Other retinoschisis and retinal cysts, left eye
H33.193 Other retinoschisis and retinal cysts, bilateral
H33.199 Other retinoschisis and retinal cysts, unspecified eye
+ H33.2 Serous retinal detachment
Retinal detachment NOS
Retinal detachment without retinal break
Excludes1: *central serous chorioretinopathy (H35.71-)*
CC H33.20 Serous retinal detachment, unspecified eye
CC Exclusion see Appendix A PDX collection 0628
CC H33.21 Serous retinal detachment, right eye
CC Exclusion see Appendix A PDX collection 0628
CC H33.22 Serous retinal detachment, left eye
CC Exclusion see Appendix A PDX collection 0628
CC H33.23 Serous retinal detachment, bilateral
CC Exclusion see Appendix A PDX collection 0628
+ H33.3 Retinal breaks without detachment
Excludes1: *chorioretinal scars after surgery for detachment (H59.81-)*
peripheral retinal degeneration without break (H35.4-)
+ H33.30 Unspecified retinal break
H33.301 Unspecified retinal break, right eye
H33.302 Unspecified retinal break, left eye
H33.303 Unspecified retinal break, bilateral
H33.309 Unspecified retinal break, unspecified eye
+ H33.31 Horseshoe tear of retina without detachment
Operculum of retina without detachment
H33.311 Horseshoe tear of retina without detachment, right eye
H33.312 Horseshoe tear of retina without detachment, left eye
H33.313 Horseshoe tear of retina without detachment, bilateral
H33.319 Horseshoe tear of retina without detachment, unspecified eye
+ H33.32 Round hole of retina without detachment
H33.321 Round hole, right eye
H33.322 Round hole, left eye
H33.323 Round hole, bilateral
H33.329 Round hole, unspecified eye
+ H33.33 Multiple defects of retina without detachment
H33.331 Multiple defects of retina without detachment, right eye
H33.332 Multiple defects of retina without detachment, left eye
H33.333 Multiple defects of retina without detachment, bilateral
H33.339 Multiple defects of retina without detachment, unspecified eye
+ H33.4 Traction detachment of retina
Proliferative vitreo-retinopathy with retinal detachment
CC H33.40 Traction detachment of retina, unspecified eye
CC Exclusion see Appendix A PDX collection 0628
CC H33.41 Traction detachment of retina, right eye
CC Exclusion see Appendix A PDX collection 0628
CC H33.42 Traction detachment of retina, left eye
CC Exclusion see Appendix A PDX collection 0628
CC H33.43 Traction detachment of retina, bilateral
CC Exclusion see Appendix A PDX collection 0628
CC H33.8 Other retinal detachments
CC Exclusion see Appendix A PDX collection 0628

H34 Retinal vascular occlusions

Excludes1: *amaurosis fugax (G45.3)*
+ H34.0 Transient retinal artery occlusion
CC H34.00 Transient retinal artery occlusion, unspecified eye
CC Exclusion see Appendix A PDX collection 0587
CC H34.01 Transient retinal artery occlusion, right eye
CC Exclusion see Appendix A PDX collection 0587
CC H34.02 Transient retinal artery occlusion, left eye
CC Exclusion see Appendix A PDX collection 0587
CC H34.03 Transient retinal artery occlusion, bilateral
CC Exclusion see Appendix A PDX collection 0587
+ H34.1 Central retinal artery occlusion
CC H34.10 Central retinal artery occlusion, unspecified eye
CC Exclusion see Appendix A PDX collection 0587
CC H34.11 Central retinal artery occlusion, right eye
CC Exclusion see Appendix A PDX collection 0587
CC H34.12 Central retinal artery occlusion, left eye
CC Exclusion see Appendix A PDX collection 0587
CC H34.13 Central retinal artery occlusion, bilateral
CC Exclusion see Appendix A PDX collection 0587
+ H34.2 Other retinal artery occlusions
+ H34.21 Partial retinal artery occlusion
Hollenhorst's plaque
Retinal microembolism
CC H34.211 Partial retinal artery occlusion, right eye
CC Exclusion see Appendix A PDX collection 0587
CC H34.212 Partial retinal artery occlusion, left eye
CC Exclusion see Appendix A PDX collection 0587
CC H34.213 Partial retinal artery occlusion, bilateral
CC Exclusion see Appendix A PDX collection 0587
CC H34.219 Partial retinal artery occlusion, unspecified eye
CC Exclusion see Appendix A PDX collection 0587
+ H34.23 Retinal artery branch occlusion
CC H34.231 Retinal artery branch occlusion, right eye
CC Exclusion see Appendix A PDX collection 0587
CC H34.232 Retinal artery branch occlusion, left eye
CC Exclusion see Appendix A PDX collection 0587
CC H34.233 Retinal artery branch occlusion, bilateral
CC Exclusion see Appendix A PDX collection 0587
CC H34.239 Retinal artery branch occlusion, unspecified eye
CC Exclusion see Appendix A PDX collection 0587

+ **H34.8 Other retinal vascular occlusions**
AHA CC: 4Q, 2016, 19

+ **H34.81 Central retinal vein occlusion**

One of the following 7th characters is to be assigned to codes in subcategory **H34.81** to designate the severity of the occlusion:
0 with macular edema
1 with retinal neovascularization
2 stable
Old central retinal vein occlusion

+7th CC **H34.811 Central retinal vein occlusion, right eye**
CC Exclusion see Appendix A PDX collection 0587

+7th CC **H34.812 Central retinal vein occlusion, left eye**
CC Exclusion see Appendix A PDX collection 0587

+7th CC **H34.813 Central retinal vein occlusion, bilateral**
CC Exclusion see Appendix A PDX collection 0587

+7th CC **H34.819 Central retinal vein occlusion, unspecified eye**
CC Exclusion see Appendix A PDX collection 0587

+ **H34.82 Venous engorgement**
Incipient retinal vein occlusion
Partial retinal vein occlusion
H34.821 Venous engorgement, right eye
H34.822 Venous engorgement, left eye
H34.823 Venous engorgement, bilateral
H34.829 Venous engorgement, unspecified eye

+ **H34.83 Tributary (branch) retinal vein occlusion**

One of the following 7th characters is to be assigned to codes in subcategory **H34.83** to designate the severity of the occlusion:
0 with macular edema
1 with retinal neovascularization
2 stable
Old central retinal vein occlusion

+7th **H34.831 Tributary (branch) retinal vein occlusion, right eye**
+7th **H34.832 Tributary (branch) retinal vein occlusion, left eye**
+7th **H34.833 Tributary (branch) retinal vein occlusion, bilateral**
+7th **H34.839 Tributary (branch) retinal vein occlusion, unspecified eye**

CC **H34.9 Unspecified retinal vascular occlusion**
CC Exclusion see Appendix A PDX collection 0587

H35 Other retinal disorders

Excludes2: *diabetic retinal disorders (E08.311-E08.359, E09.311-E09.359, E10.311-E10.359, E11.311-E11.359, E13.311-E13.359)*

+ **H35.0 Background retinopathy and retinal vascular changes**
Review coding guideline C.9.a.5
Code also any associated hypertension (I10)
H35.00 Unspecified background retinopathy

+ **H35.01 Changes in retinal vascular appearance**
Retinal vascular sheathing
H35.011 Changes in retinal vascular appearance, right eye
H35.012 Changes in retinal vascular appearance, left eye
H35.013 Changes in retinal vascular appearance, bilateral
H35.019 Changes in retinal vascular appearance, unspecified eye

+ **H35.02 Exudative retinopathy**
Coats retinopathy
H35.021 Exudative retinopathy, right eye
H35.022 Exudative retinopathy, left eye
H35.023 Exudative retinopathy, bilateral
H35.029 Exudative retinopathy, unspecified eye

+ **H35.03 Hypertensive retinopathy**
H35.031 Hypertensive retinopathy, right eye
H35.032 Hypertensive retinopathy, left eye
H35.033 Hypertensive retinopathy, bilateral
H35.039 Hypertensive retinopathy, unspecified eye

+ **H35.04 Retinal micro-aneurysms, unspecified**
H35.041 Retinal micro-aneurysms, unspecified, right eye
H35.042 Retinal micro-aneurysms, unspecified, left eye
H35.043 Retinal micro-aneurysms, unspecified, bilateral
H35.049 Retinal micro-aneurysms, unspecified, unspecified eye

+ **H35.05 Retinal neovascularization, unspecified**
H35.051 Retinal neovascularization, unspecified, right eye
H35.052 Retinal neovascularization, unspecified, left eye
H35.053 Retinal neovascularization, unspecified, bilateral
H35.059 Retinal neovascularization, unspecified, unspecified eye

+ **H35.06 Retinal vasculitis**
Eales disease
Retinal perivasculitis
H35.061 Retinal vasculitis, right eye
H35.062 Retinal vasculitis, left eye
H35.063 Retinal vasculitis, bilateral
H35.069 Retinal vasculitis, unspecified eye

+ **H35.07 Retinal telangiectasis**
H35.071 Retinal telangiectasis, right eye
H35.072 Retinal telangiectasis, left eye
H35.073 Retinal telangiectasis, bilateral
H35.079 Retinal telangiectasis, unspecified eye

H35.09 Other intraretinal microvascular abnormalities
Retinal varices

+ **H35.1 Retinopathy of prematurity**

+ **H35.10 Retinopathy of prematurity, unspecified**
Retinopathy of prematurity NOS
H35.101 Retinopathy of prematurity, unspecified, right eye
H35.102 Retinopathy of prematurity, unspecified, left eye
H35.103 Retinopathy of prematurity, unspecified, bilateral
H35.109 Retinopathy of prematurity, unspecified, unspecified eye

+ **H35.11 Retinopathy of prematurity, stage 0**
H35.111 Retinopathy of prematurity, stage 0, right eye
H35.112 Retinopathy of prematurity, stage 0, left eye
H35.113 Retinopathy of prematurity, stage 0, bilateral
H35.119 Retinopathy of prematurity, stage 0, unspecified eye

+ **H35.12 Retinopathy of prematurity, stage 1**
H35.121 Retinopathy of prematurity, stage 1, right eye
H35.122 Retinopathy of prematurity, stage 1, left eye
H35.123 Retinopathy of prematurity, stage 1, bilateral
H35.129 Retinopathy of prematurity, stage 1, unspecified eye

+ **H35.13 Retinopathy of prematurity, stage 2**
H35.131 Retinopathy of prematurity, stage 2, right eye
H35.132 Retinopathy of prematurity, stage 2, left eye
H35.133 Retinopathy of prematurity, stage 2, bilateral
H35.139 Retinopathy of prematurity, stage 2, unspecified eye

+ **H35.14 Retinopathy of prematurity, stage 3**
H35.141 Retinopathy of prematurity, stage 3, right eye
H35.142 Retinopathy of prematurity, stage 3, left eye
H35.143 Retinopathy of prematurity, stage 3, bilateral
H35.149 Retinopathy of prematurity, stage 3, unspecified eye

+ **H35.15 Retinopathy of prematurity, stage 4**
H35.151 Retinopathy of prematurity, stage 4, right eye
H35.152 Retinopathy of prematurity, stage 4, left eye
H35.153 Retinopathy of prematurity, stage 4, bilateral

H35.159 Retinopathy of prematurity, stage 4, unspecified eye

+ H35.16 Retinopathy of prematurity, stage 5

H35.161 Retinopathy of prematurity, stage 5, right eye

H35.162 Retinopathy of prematurity, stage 5, left eye

H35.163 Retinopathy of prematurity, stage 5, bilateral

H35.169 Retinopathy of prematurity, stage 5, unspecified eye

+ H35.17 Retrolental fibroplasia

H35.171 Retrolental fibroplasia, right eye

H35.172 Retrolental fibroplasia, left eye

H35.173 Retrolental fibroplasia, bilateral

H35.179 Retrolental fibroplasia, unspecified eye

+ H35.2 Other non-diabetic proliferative retinopathy

Proliferative vitreo-retinopathy

Excludes1: *proliferative vitreo-retinopathy with retinal detachment (H33.4-)*

H35.20 Other non-diabetic proliferative retinopathy, unspecified eye

H35.21 Other non-diabetic proliferative retinopathy, right eye

H35.22 Other non-diabetic proliferative retinopathy, left eye

H35.23 Other non-diabetic proliferative retinopathy, bilateral

+ H35.3 Degeneration of macula and posterior pole

AHA CC: 4Q, 2016, 20-21

• H35.30 Unspecified macular degeneration

Age-related macular degeneration

+ H35.31 Nonexudative age-related macular degeneration

Atrophic age-related macular degeneration

Dry age-related macular degeneration

One of the following 7th characters is to be assigned to codes in subcategory **H35.31** to designate the stage of the disease:

0 stage unspecified
1 early dry stage
2 intermediate dry stage
3 advanced atrophic without subfoveal involvement advanced dry stage
4 advanced atrophic with sobfoveal involvement

• +7th H35.311 Nonexudative age-related macular degeneration, right eye

AHA CC: 4Q, 2016, 21

• +7th H35.312 Nonexudative age-related macular degeneration, left eye

AHA CC: 4Q, 2016, 21

• +7th H35.313 Nonexudative age-related macular degeneration, bilateral

• +7th H35.319 Nonexudative age-related macular degeneration, unspecified eye

+ H35.32 Exudative age-related macular degeneration

Wet age-related macular degeneration

One of the following 7th characters is to be assigned to codes in subcategory **H35.32** to designate the stage of the disease:

0 stage unspecified
1 with active choroidal neovascularization
2 with inactive choroidal neovascularization with involuted or regressed neovascularization
3 with inactive scar

• +7th H35.321 Exudative age-related macular degeneration, right eye

• +7th H35.322 Exudative age-related macular degeneration, left eye

• +7th H35.323 Exudative age-related macular degeneration, bilateral

• +7th H35.329 Exudative age-related macular degeneration, unspecified eye

H35.33 Angioid streaks of macula

+ H35.34 Macular cyst, hole, or pseudohole

H35.341 Macular cyst, hole, or pseudohole, right eye

H35.342 Macular cyst, hole, or pseudohole, left eye

H35.343 Macular cyst, hole, or pseudohole, bilateral

H35.349 Macular cyst, hole, or pseudohole, unspecified eye

+ H35.35 Cystoid macular degeneration

Excludes1: cystoid macular edema following cataract surgery (H59.03-)

H35.351 Cystoid macular degeneration, right eye

H35.352 Cystoid macular degeneration, left eye

H35.353 Cystoid macular degeneration, bilateral

H35.359 Cystoid macular degeneration, unspecified eye

+ H35.36 Drusen (degenerative) of macula

H35.361 Drusen (degenerative) of macula, right eye

H35.362 Drusen (degenerative) of macula, left eye

AHA CC: 4Q, 2016, 21

H35.363 Drusen (degenerative) of macula, bilateral

AHA CC: 4Q, 2016, 21; 1Q, 2017, 51

H35.369 Drusen (degenerative) of macula, unspecified eye

+ H35.37 Puckering of macula

H35.371 Puckering of macula, right eye

H35.372 Puckering of macula, left eye

H35.373 Puckering of macula, bilateral

H35.379 Puckering of macula, unspecified eye

+ H35.38 Toxic maculopathy

Code first poisoning due to drug or toxin, if applicable (T36-T65 with fifth or sixth character 1-4 or 6)

Use additional code for adverse effect, if applicable, to identify drug (T36-T50 with fifth or sixth character 5)

H35.381 Toxic maculopathy, right eye

H35.382 Toxic maculopathy, left eye

H35.383 Toxic maculopathy, bilateral

H35.389 Toxic maculopathy, unspecified eye

+ H35.4 Peripheral retinal degeneration

Excludes1: *hereditary retinal degeneration (dystrophy) (H35.5-)*
peripheral retinal degeneration with retinal break (H33.3-)

H35.40 Unspecified peripheral retinal degeneration

+ H35.41 Lattice degeneration of retina

Palisade degeneration of retina

H35.411 Lattice degeneration of retina, right eye

H35.412 Lattice degeneration of retina, left eye

H35.413 Lattice degeneration of retina, bilateral

H35.419 Lattice degeneration of retina, unspecified eye

+ H35.42 Microcystoid degeneration of retina

H35.421 Microcystoid degeneration of retina, right eye

H35.422 Microcystoid degeneration of retina, left eye

H35.423 Microcystoid degeneration of retina, bilateral

H35.429 Microcystoid degeneration of retina, unspecified eye

+ H35.43 Paving stone degeneration of retina

H35.431 Paving stone degeneration of retina, right eye

H35.432 Paving stone degeneration of retina, left eye

H35.433 Paving stone degeneration of retina, bilateral

H35.439 Paving stone degeneration of retina, unspecified eye

+ H35.44 Age-related reticular degeneration of retina

• H35.441 Age-related reticular degeneration of retina, right eye

• H35.442 Age-related reticular degeneration of retina, left eye

• H35.443 Age-related reticular degeneration of retina, bilateral

• H35.449 Age-related reticular degeneration of retina, unspecified eye

+ H35.45 Secondary pigmentary degeneration

H35.451 Secondary pigmentary degeneration, right eye

H35.452 Secondary pigmentary degeneration, left eye

H35.453 Secondary pigmentary degeneration, bilateral

H35.459 Secondary pigmentary degeneration, unspecified eye

+ H35.46 Secondary vitreoretinal degeneration

H35.461 Secondary vitreoretinal degeneration, right eye

H35.462 Secondary vitreoretinal degeneration, left eye

H35.463 Secondary vitreoretinal degeneration, bilateral
H35.469 Secondary vitreoretinal degeneration, unspecified eye
+ H35.5 Hereditary retinal dystrophy
Excludes1: *dystrophies primarily involving Bruch's membrane (H31.1-)*
H35.50 Unspecified hereditary retinal dystrophy
H35.51 Vitreoretinal dystrophy
H35.52 Pigmentary retinal dystrophy
Albipunctate retinal dystrophy
Retinitis pigmentosa
Tapetoretinal dystrophy
H35.53 Other dystrophies primarily involving the sensory retina
Stargardt's disease
H35.54 Dystrophies primarily involving the retinal pigment epithelium
Vitelliform retinal dystrophy
+ H35.6 Retinal hemorrhage
H35.60 Retinal hemorrhage, unspecified eye
H35.61 Retinal hemorrhage, right eye
H35.62 Retinal hemorrhage, left eye
H35.63 Retinal hemorrhage, bilateral
+ H35.7 Separation of retinal layers
Excludes1: *retinal detachment (serous) (H33.2-)*
rhegmatogenous retinal detachment (H33.0-)
CC H35.70 Unspecified separation of retinal layers
CC Exclusion see Appendix A PDX collection 0628
+ H35.71 Central serous chorioretinopathy
H35.711 Central serous chorioretinopathy, right eye
H35.712 Central serous chorioretinopathy, left eye
H35.713 Central serous chorioretinopathy, bilateral
H35.719 Central serous chorioretinopathy, unspecified eye
+ H35.72 Serous detachment of retinal pigment epithelium
CC H35.721 Serous detachment of retinal pigment epithelium, right eye
CC Exclusion see Appendix A PDX collection 0628
CC H35.722 Serous detachment of retinal pigment epithelium, left eye
CC Exclusion see Appendix A PDX collection 0628
CC H35.723 Serous detachment of retinal pigment epithelium, bilateral
CC Exclusion see Appendix A PDX collection 0628
CC H35.729 Serous detachment of retinal pigment epithelium, unspecified eye
CC Exclusion see Appendix A PDX collection 0628
+ H35.73 Hemorrhagic detachment of retinal pigment epithelium
CC H35.731 Hemorrhagic detachment of retinal pigment epithelium, right eye
CC Exclusion see Appendix A PDX collection 0628
CC H35.732 Hemorrhagic detachment of retinal pigment epithelium, left eye
CC Exclusion see Appendix A PDX collection 0628
CC H35.733 Hemorrhagic detachment of retinal pigment epithelium, bilateral
CC Exclusion see Appendix A PDX collection 0628
CC H35.739 Hemorrhagic detachment of retinal pigment epithelium, unspecified eye
CC Exclusion see Appendix A PDX collection 0628
+ H35.8 Other specified retinal disorders
Excludes2: *retinal hemorrhage (H35.6-)*
H35.81 Retinal edema
Retinal cotton wool spots
CC H35.82 Retinal ischemia
CC Exclusion see Appendix A PDX collection 0629
H35.89 Other specified retinal disorders
H35.9 Unspecified retinal disorder

H36 Retinal disorders in diseases classified elsewhere
Code first underlying disease, such as:
lipid storage disorders (E75.-)
sickle-cell disorders (D57.-)
Excludes1: *arteriosclerotic retinopathy (H35.0-)*
diabetic retinopathy (E08.3-, E09.3-, E10.3-, E11.3-, E13.
Valid 3-character code, no further characters required

Glaucoma (H40-H42)

H40 Glaucoma

Excludes1: *absolute glaucoma (H44.51-)*
congenital glaucoma (Q15.0)
traumatic glaucoma due to birth injury (P15.3)
Review coding guideline C.7.a
+ H40.0 Glaucoma suspect
+ H40.00 Preglaucoma, unspecified
H40.001 Preglaucoma, unspecified, right eye
H40.002 Preglaucoma, unspecified, left eye
H40.003 Preglaucoma, unspecified, bilateral
H40.009 Preglaucoma, unspecified, unspecified eye
+ H40.01 Open angle with borderline findings, low risk
Open angle, low risk
H40.011 Open angle with borderline findings, low risk, right eye
H40.012 Open angle with borderline findings, low risk, left eye
H40.013 Open angle with borderline findings, low risk, bilateral
H40.019 Open angle with borderline findings, low risk, unspecified eye
+ H40.02 Open angle with borderline findings, high risk
Open angle, high risk
H40.021 Open angle with borderline findings, high risk, right eye
H40.022 Open angle with borderline findings, high risk, left eye
H40.023 Open angle with borderline findings, high risk, bilateral
H40.029 Open angle with borderline findings, high risk, unspecified eye
+ H40.03 Anatomical narrow angle
Primary angle closure suspect
H40.031 Anatomical narrow angle, right eye
H40.032 Anatomical narrow angle, left eye
H40.033 Anatomical narrow angle, bilateral
H40.039 Anatomical narrow angle, unspecified eye
+ H40.04 Steroid responder
H40.041 Steroid responder, right eye
H40.042 Steroid responder, left eye
H40.043 Steroid responder, bilateral
H40.049 Steroid responder, unspecified eye
+ H40.05 Ocular hypertension
H40.051 Ocular hypertension, right eye
H40.052 Ocular hypertension, left eye
H40.053 Ocular hypertension, bilateral
H40.059 Ocular hypertension, unspecified eye
+ H40.06 Primary angle closure without glaucoma damage
H40.061 Primary angle closure without glaucoma damage, right eye
H40.062 Primary angle closure without glaucoma damage, left eye
H40.063 Primary angle closure without glaucoma damage, bilateral
H40.069 Primary angle closure without glaucoma damage, unspecified eye
+ H40.1 Open-angle glaucoma
AHA CC: 4Q, 2016, 22
X+7th H40.10 Unspecified open-angle glaucoma

One of the following 7th characters is to be assigned to code **H40.10** to designate the stage of glaucoma
0 stage unspecified
1 mild stage
2 moderate stage
3 severe stage
4 indeterminate stage

+ **H40.11 Primary open-angle glaucoma**
  Chronic simple glaucoma

  One of the following 7th characters is to be assigned to each code in subcategory **H40.11** to designate the stage of glaucoma
  0 stage unspecified
  1 mild stage
  2 moderate stage
  3 severe stage
  4 indeterminate stage

  +7th **H40.111 Primary open-angle glaucoma, right eye**
  +7th **H40.112 Primary open-angle glaucoma, left eye**
  +7th **H40.113 Primary open-angle glaucoma, bilateral**
  +7th **H40.119 Primary open-angle glaucoma, unspecified eye**

+ **H40.12 Low-tension glaucoma**

  One of the following 7th characters is to be assigned to each code in subcategory **H40.12** to designate the stage of glaucoma
  0 stage unspecified
  1 mild stage
  2 moderate stage
  3 severe stage
  4 indeterminate stage

  +7th **H40.121 Low-tension glaucoma, right eye**
  +7th **H40.122 Low-tension glaucoma, left eye**
  +7th **H40.123 Low-tension glaucoma, bilateral**
  +7th **H40.129 Low-tension glaucoma, unspecified eye**

+ **H40.13 Pigmentary glaucoma**

  One of the following 7th characters is to be assigned to each code in subcategory **H40.13** to designate the stage of glaucoma
  0 stage unspecified
  1 mild stage
  2 moderate stage
  3 severe stage
  4 indeterminate stage

  +7th **H40.131 Pigmentary glaucoma, right eye**
  +7th **H40.132 Pigmentary glaucoma, left eye**
  +7th **H40.133 Pigmentary glaucoma, bilateral**
  +7th **H40.139 Pigmentary glaucoma, unspecified eye**

+ **H40.14 Capsular glaucoma with pseudoexfoliation of lens**

  One of the following 7th characters is to be assigned to each code in subcategory **H40.14** to designate the stage of glaucoma
  0 stage unspecified
  1 mild stage
  2 moderate stage
  3 severe stage
  4 indeterminate stage

  +7th **H40.141 Capsular glaucoma with pseudoexfoliation of lens, right eye**
  +7th **H40.142 Capsular glaucoma with pseudoexfoliation of lens, left eye**
  +7th **H40.143 Capsular glaucoma with pseudoexfoliation of lens, bilateral**
  +7th **H40.149 Capsular glaucoma with pseudoexfoliation of lens, unspecified eye**

+ **H40.15 Residual stage of open-angle glaucoma**
  H40.151 Residual stage of open-angle glaucoma, right eye
  H40.152 Residual stage of open-angle glaucoma, left eye
  H40.153 Residual stage of open-angle glaucoma, bilateral
  H40.159 Residual stage of open-angle glaucoma, unspecified eye

+ **H40.2 Primary angle-closure glaucoma**
  Excludes1: *aqueous misdirection (H40.83-)*
  malignant glaucoma (H40.83-)

  X+7th **H40.20 Unspecified primary angle-closure glaucoma**

  One of the following 7th characters is to be assigned to code **H40.20** to designate the stage of glaucoma
  0 stage unspecified
  1 mild stage
  2 moderate stage
  3 severe stage
  4 indeterminate stage

+ **H40.21 Acute angle-closure glaucoma**
  Acute angle-closure glaucoma attack
  Acute angle-closure glaucoma crisis
  CC **H40.211 Acute angle-closure glaucoma, right eye**
  CC Exclusion see Appendix A PDX collection 0630
  CC **H40.212 Acute angle-closure glaucoma, left eye**
  CC Exclusion see Appendix A PDX collection 0630
  CC **H40.213 Acute angle-closure glaucoma, bilateral**
  CC Exclusion see Appendix A PDX collection 0630
  CC **H40.219 Acute angle-closure glaucoma, unspecified eye**
  CC Exclusion see Appendix A PDX collection 0630

+ **H40.22 Chronic angle-closure glaucoma**
  Chronic primary angle closure glaucoma

  One of the following 7th characters is to be assigned to each code in subcategory **H40.22** to designate the stage of glaucoma
  0 stage unspecified
  1 mild stage
  2 moderate stage
  3 severe stage
  4 indeterminate stage

  +7th **H40.221 Chronic angle-closure glaucoma, right eye**
  +7th **H40.222 Chronic angle-closure glaucoma, left eye**
  +7th **H40.223 Chronic angle-closure glaucoma, bilateral**
  +7th **H40.229 Chronic angle-closure glaucoma, unspecified eye**

+ **H40.23 Intermittent angle-closure glaucoma**
  H40.231 Intermittent angle-closure glaucoma, right eye
  H40.232 Intermittent angle-closure glaucoma, left eye
  H40.233 Intermittent angle-closure glaucoma, bilateral
  H40.239 Intermittent angle-closure glaucoma, unspecified eye

+ **H40.24 Residual stage of angle-closure glaucoma**
  H40.241 Residual stage of angle-closure glaucoma, right eye
  H40.242 Residual stage of angle-closure glaucoma, left eye
  H40.243 Residual stage of angle-closure glaucoma, bilateral
  H40.249 Residual stage of angle-closure glaucoma, unspecified eye

+ **H40.3 Glaucoma secondary to eye trauma**
  Code also underlying condition

  One of the following 7th characters is to be assigned to each code in subcategory **H40.3** to designate the stage of glaucoma
  0 stage unspecified
  1 mild stage
  2 moderate stage
  3 severe stage
  4 indeterminate stage

  X+7th **H40.30 Glaucoma secondary to eye trauma, unspecified eye**
  X+7th **H40.31 Glaucoma secondary to eye trauma, right eye**
  X+7th **H40.32 Glaucoma secondary to eye trauma, left eye**
  X+7th **H40.33 Glaucoma secondary to eye trauma, bilateral**

+ **H40.4 Glaucoma secondary to eye inflammation**
  Code also underlying condition

  One of the following 7th characters is to be assigned to each code in subcategory **H40.4** to designate the stage of glaucoma
  0 stage unspecified
  1 mild stage
  2 moderate stage
  3 severe stage
  4 indeterminate stage

  X+7th **H40.40 Glaucoma secondary to eye inflammation, unspecified eye**
  X+7th **H40.41 Glaucoma secondary to eye inflammation, right eye**
  X+7th **H40.42 Glaucoma secondary to eye inflammation, left eye**
  X+7th **H40.43 Glaucoma secondary to eye inflammation, bilateral**

+ **H40.5 Glaucoma secondary to other eye disorders**
Code also underlying eye disorder

One of the following 7th characters is to be assigned to each code in subcategory **H40.5** to designate the stage of glaucoma
0 stage unspecified
1 mild stage
2 moderate stage
3 severe stage
4 indeterminate stage

X+7th **H40.50 Glaucoma secondary to other eye disorders, unspecified eye**
X+7th **H40.51 Glaucoma secondary to other eye disorders, right eye**
X+7th **H40.52 Glaucoma secondary to other eye disorders, left eye**
X+7th **H40.53 Glaucoma secondary to other eye disorders, bilateral**

+ **H40.6 Glaucoma secondary to drugs**
Use additional code for adverse effect, if applicable, to identify drug (T36-T50 with fifth or sixth character 5)

One of the following 7th characters is to be assigned to each code in subcategory **H40.6** to designate the stage of glaucoma
0 stage unspecified
1 mild stage
2 moderate stage
3 severe stage
4 indeterminate stage

X+7th **H40.60 Glaucoma secondary to drugs, unspecified eye**
X+7th **H40.61 Glaucoma secondary to drugs, right eye**
X+7th **H40.62 Glaucoma secondary to drugs, left eye**
X+7th **H40.63 Glaucoma secondary to drugs, bilateral**

+ **H40.8 Other glaucoma**
+ **H40.81 Glaucoma with increased episcleral venous pressure**
H40.811 Glaucoma with increased episcleral venous pressure, right eye
H40.812 Glaucoma with increased episcleral venous pressure, left eye
H40.813 Glaucoma with increased episcleral venous pressure, bilateral
H40.819 Glaucoma with increased episcleral venous pressure, unspecified eye
+ **H40.82 Hypersecretion glaucoma**
H40.821 Hypersecretion glaucoma, right eye
H40.822 Hypersecretion glaucoma, left eye
H40.823 Hypersecretion glaucoma, bilateral
H40.829 Hypersecretion glaucoma, unspecified eye
+ **H40.83 Aqueous misdirection**
Malignant glaucoma
H40.831 Aqueous misdirection, right eye
H40.832 Aqueous misdirection, left eye
H40.833 Aqueous misdirection, bilateral
H40.839 Aqueous misdirection, unspecified eye
H40.89 Other specified glaucoma
H40.9 Unspecified glaucoma

H42 Glaucoma in diseases classified elsewhere

Code first underlying condition, such as:
amyloidosis (E85.-)
aniridia (Q13.1)
glaucoma (in) diabetes mellitus (E08.39, E09.39, E10.39, E11.39, E13.39)
Lowe's syndrome (E72.03)
Reiger's anomaly (Q13.81)
specified metabolic disorder (E70-E88)

Excludes1: *glaucoma (in) onchocerciasis (B73.02)*
glaucoma (in) syphilis (A52.71)
glaucoma (in) tuberculous (A18.59)

Valid 3-character code, no further characters required

Disorders of vitreous body and globe (H43-H44)

H43 Disorders of vitreous body

+ **H43.0 Vitreous prolapse**
Excludes1: *vitreous syndrome following cataract surgery (H59.0-)*
traumatic vitreous prolapse (S05.2-)
H43.00 Vitreous prolapse, unspecified eye
H43.01 Vitreous prolapse, right eye
H43.02 Vitreous prolapse, left eye
H43.03 Vitreous prolapse, bilateral
+ **H43.1 Vitreous hemorrhage**
H43.10 Vitreous hemorrhage, unspecified eye
H43.11 Vitreous hemorrhage, right eye
H43.12 Vitreous hemorrhage, left eye
H43.13 Vitreous hemorrhage, bilateral
+ **H43.2 Crystalline deposits in vitreous body**
H43.20 Crystalline deposits in vitreous body, unspecified e
H43.21 Crystalline deposits in vitreous body, right eye
H43.22 Crystalline deposits in vitreous body, left eye
H43.23 Crystalline deposits in vitreous body, bilateral
+ **H43.3 Other vitreous opacities**
+ **H43.31 Vitreous membranes and strands**
H43.311 Vitreous membranes and strands, right e
H43.312 Vitreous membranes and strands, left eye
H43.313 Vitreous membranes and strands, bilater
H43.319 Vitreous membranes and strands, unspecified eye
+ **H43.39 Other vitreous opacities**
Vitreous floaters
H43.391 Other vitreous opacities, right eye
H43.392 Other vitreous opacities, left eye
H43.393 Other vitreous opacities, bilateral
H43.399 Other vitreous opacities, unspecified eye
+ **H43.8 Other disorders of vitreous body**
Excludes1: *proliferative vitreo-retinopathy with retinal detachment (H33.4-)*
Excludes2: *vitreous abscess (H44.02-)*
+ **H43.81 Vitreous degeneration**
Vitreous detachment
H43.811 Vitreous degeneration, right eye
H43.812 Vitreous degeneration, left eye
H43.813 Vitreous degeneration, bilateral
H43.819 Vitreous degeneration, unspecified eye
+ **H43.82 Vitreomacular adhesion**
Vitreomacular traction
• **H43.821 Vitreomacular adhesion, right eye**
• **H43.822 Vitreomacular adhesion, left eye**
• **H43.823 Vitreomacular adhesion, bilateral**
• **H43.829 Vitreomacular adhesion, unspecified eye**
H43.89 Other disorders of vitreous body
H43.9 Unspecified disorder of vitreous body

H44 Disorders of globe

Includes: disorders affecting multiple structures of eye

+ **H44.0 Purulent endophthalmitis**
Use additional code to identify organism
Excludes1: *bleb associated endophthalmitis (H59.4-)*
+ **H44.00 Unspecified purulent endophthalmitis**
CC **H44.001 Unspecified purulent endophthalmitis, right eye**
CC Exclusion see Appendix A PDX collection 06
CC **H44.002 Unspecified purulent endophthalmitis, lef eye**
CC Exclusion see Appendix A PDX collection 0625
CC **H44.003 Unspecified purulent endophthalmitis, bilateral**
CC Exclusion see Appendix A PDX collection 0625
CC **H44.009 Unspecified purulent endophthalmitis, unspecified eye**
CC Exclusion see Appendix A PDX collection 06
+ **H44.01 Panophthalmitis (acute)**
CC **H44.011 Panophthalmitis (acute), right eye**
CC Exclusion see Appendix A PDX collection 0625
CC **H44.012 Panophthalmitis (acute), left eye**
CC Exclusion see Appendix A PDX collection 0625
CC **H44.013 Panophthalmitis (acute), bilateral**
CC Exclusion see Appendix A PDX collection 0625
CC **H44.019 Panophthalmitis (acute), unspecified eye**
CC Exclusion see Appendix A PDX collection 06
+ **H44.02 Vitreous abscess (chronic)**
CC **H44.021 Vitreous abscess (chronic), right eye**
CC Exclusion see Appendix A PDX collection 06
CC **H44.022 Vitreous abscess (chronic), left eye**
CC Exclusion see Appendix A PDX collection 0631
CC **H44.023 Vitreous abscess (chronic), bilateral**
CC Exclusion see Appendix A PDX collection 06
CC **H44.029 Vitreous abscess (chronic), unspecified ey**
CC Exclusion see Appendix A PDX collection 06

+ **H44.1 Other endophthalmitis**

Excludes1: *bleb associated endophthalmitis (H59.4-)*

Excludes2: *ophthalmia nodosa (H16.2-)*

+ **H44.11 Panuveitis**
  - CC **H44.111 Panuveitis, right eye**
    CC Exclusion see Appendix A PDX collection 0632
  - CC **H44.112 Panuveitis, left eye**
    CC Exclusion see Appendix A PDX collection 0632
  - CC **H44.113 Panuveitis, bilateral**
    CC Exclusion see Appendix A PDX collection 0632
  - CC **H44.119 Panuveitis, unspecified eye**
    CC Exclusion see Appendix A PDX collection 0632
+ **H44.12 Parasitic endophthalmitis, unspecified**
  - CC **H44.121 Parasitic endophthalmitis, unspecified, right eye**
    CC Exclusion see Appendix A PDX collection 0625
  - CC **H44.122 Parasitic endophthalmitis, unspecified, left eye**
    CC Exclusion see Appendix A PDX collection 0625
  - CC **H44.123 Parasitic endophthalmitis, unspecified, bilateral**
    CC Exclusion see Appendix A PDX collection 0625
  - CC **H44.129 Parasitic endophthalmitis, unspecified, unspecified eye**
    CC Exclusion see Appendix A PDX collection 0625
+ **H44.13 Sympathetic uveitis**
  - CC **H44.131 Sympathetic uveitis, right eye**
    CC Exclusion see Appendix A PDX collection 0632
  - CC **H44.132 Sympathetic uveitis, left eye**
    CC Exclusion see Appendix A PDX collection 0632
  - CC **H44.133 Sympathetic uveitis, bilateral**
    CC Exclusion see Appendix A PDX collection 0632
  - CC **H44.139 Sympathetic uveitis, unspecified eye**
    CC Exclusion see Appendix A PDX collection 0632

CC **H44.19 Other endophthalmitis**
CC Exclusion see Appendix A PDX collection 0625

+ **H44.2 Degenerative myopia**

Malignant myopia

H44.20 Degenerative myopia, unspecified eye
H44.21 Degenerative myopia, right eye
H44.22 Degenerative myopia, left eye
H44.23 Degenerative myopia, bilateral

+ **H44.2A Degenerative myopia with choroidal neovascularization**
  Use additional code for any associated choroid disorders (H31.-)
  - **H44.2A1 Degenerative myopia with choroidal neovascularization, right eye**
  - **H44.2A2 Degenerative myopia with choroidal neovascularization, left eye**
  - **H44.2A3 Degenerative myopia with choroidal neovascularization, bilateral eye**
  - **H44.2A9 Degenerative myopia with choroidal neovascularization, unspecified eye**
+ **H44.2B Degenerative myopia with macular hole**
  - **H44.2B1 Degenerative myopia with macular hole, right eye**
  - **H44.2B2 Degenerative myopia with macular hole, left eye**
  - **H44.2B3 Degenerative myopia with macular hole, bilateral eye**
  - **H44.2B9 Degenerative myopia with macular hole, unspecified eye**
+ **H44.2C Degenerative myopia with retinal detachment**
  Use additional code to identify the retinal detachment (H33.-)
  - **H44.2C1 Degenerative myopia with retinal detachment, right eye**
  - **H44.2C2 Degenerative myopia with retinal detachment, left eye**
  - **H44.2C3 Degenerative myopia with retinal detachment, bilateral eye**
  - **H44.2C9 Degenerative myopia with retinal detachment, unspecified eye**
+ **H44.2D Degenerative myopia with foveoschisis**
  - **H44.2D1 Degenerative myopia with foveoschisis, right eye**
  - **H44.2D2 Degenerative myopia with foveoschisis, left eye**
  - **H44.2D3 Degenerative myopia with foveoschisis, bilateral eye**
  - **H44.2D9 Degenerative myopia with foveoschisis, unspecified eye**
+ **H44.2E Degenerative myopia with other maculopathy**
  - **H44.2E1 Degenerative myopia with other maculopathy, right eye**
  - **H44.2E2 Degenerative myopia with other maculopathy, left eye**
  - **H44.2E3 Degenerative myopia with other maculopathy, bilateral eye**
  - **H44.2E9 Degenerative myopia with other maculopathy, unspecified eye**

+ **H44.3 Other and unspecified degenerative disorders of globe**

H44.30 Unspecified degenerative disorder of globe

+ **H44.31 Chalcosis**
  - **H44.311 Chalcosis, right eye**
  - **H44.312 Chalcosis, left eye**
  - **H44.313 Chalcosis, bilateral**
  - **H44.319 Chalcosis, unspecified eye**
+ **H44.32 Siderosis of eye**
  - **H44.321 Siderosis of eye, right eye**
  - **H44.322 Siderosis of eye, left eye**
  - **H44.323 Siderosis of eye, bilateral**
  - **H44.329 Siderosis of eye, unspecified eye**
+ **H44.39 Other degenerative disorders of globe**
  - **H44.391 Other degenerative disorders of globe, right eye**
  - **H44.392 Other degenerative disorders of globe, left eye**
  - **H44.393 Other degenerative disorders of globe, bilateral**
  - **H44.399 Other degenerative disorders of globe, unspecified eye**

+ **H44.4 Hypotony of eye**

H44.40 Unspecified hypotony of eye

+ **H44.41 Flat anterior chamber hypotony of eye**
  - **H44.411 Flat anterior chamber hypotony of right eye**
  - **H44.412 Flat anterior chamber hypotony of left eye**
  - **H44.413 Flat anterior chamber hypotony of eye, bilateral**
  - **H44.419 Flat anterior chamber hypotony of unspecified eye**
+ **H44.42 Hypotony of eye due to ocular fistula**
  - **H44.421 Hypotony of right eye due to ocular fistula**
  - **H44.422 Hypotony of left eye due to ocular fistula**
  - **H44.423 Hypotony of eye due to ocular fistula, bilateral**
  - **H44.429 Hypotony of unspecified eye due to ocular fistula**
+ **H44.43 Hypotony of eye due to other ocular disorders**
  - **H44.431 Hypotony of eye due to other ocular disorders, right eye**
  - **H44.432 Hypotony of eye due to other ocular disorders, left eye**
  - **H44.433 Hypotony of eye due to other ocular disorders, bilateral**
  - **H44.439 Hypotony of eye due to other ocular disorders, unspecified eye**
+ **H44.44 Primary hypotony of eye**
  - **H44.441 Primary hypotony of right eye**
  - **H44.442 Primary hypotony of left eye**
  - **H44.443 Primary hypotony of eye, bilateral**
  - **H44.449 Primary hypotony of unspecified eye**

+ **H44.5 Degenerated conditions of globe**

H44.50 Unspecified degenerated conditions of globe

+ **H44.51 Absolute glaucoma**
  - **H44.511 Absolute glaucoma, right eye**
  - **H44.512 Absolute glaucoma, left eye**
  - **H44.513 Absolute glaucoma, bilateral**
  - **H44.519 Absolute glaucoma, unspecified eye**

+ **H44.52 Atrophy of globe**
  Phthisis bulbi
  - **H44.521 Atrophy of globe, right eye**
  - **H44.522 Atrophy of globe, left eye**
  - **H44.523 Atrophy of globe, bilateral**
  - **H44.529 Atrophy of globe, unspecified eye**

+ **H44.53 Leucocoria**
  - **H44.531 Leucocoria, right eye**
  - **H44.532 Leucocoria, left eye**
  - **H44.533 Leucocoria, bilateral**
  - **H44.539 Leucocoria, unspecified eye**

+ **H44.6 Retained (old) intraocular foreign body, magnetic**
  Use additional code to identify magnetic foreign body (Z18.11)
  Excludes1: *current intraocular foreign body (S05.-)*
  Excludes2: *retained foreign body in eyelid (H02.81-)*
  retained (old) foreign body following penetrating wound of orbit (H05.5-)
  retained (old) intraocular foreign body, nonmagnetic (H44.7-)

+ **H44.60 Unspecified retained (old) intraocular foreign body, magnetic**
  - **H44.601 Unspecified retained (old) intraocular foreign body, magnetic, right eye**
  - **H44.602 Unspecified retained (old) intraocular foreign body, magnetic, left eye**
  - **H44.603 Unspecified retained (old) intraocular foreign body, magnetic, bilateral**
  - **H44.609 Unspecified retained (old) intraocular foreign body, magnetic, unspecified eye**

+ **H44.61 Retained (old) magnetic foreign body in anterior chamber**
  - **H44.611 Retained (old) magnetic foreign body in anterior chamber, right eye**
  - **H44.612 Retained (old) magnetic foreign body in anterior chamber, left eye**
  - **H44.613 Retained (old) magnetic foreign body in anterior chamber, bilateral**
  - **H44.619 Retained (old) magnetic foreign body in anterior chamber, unspecified eye**

+ **H44.62 Retained (old) magnetic foreign body in iris or ciliary body**
  - **H44.621 Retained (old) magnetic foreign body in iris or ciliary body, right eye**
  - **H44.622 Retained (old) magnetic foreign body in iris or ciliary body, left eye**
  - **H44.623 Retained (old) magnetic foreign body in iris or ciliary body, bilateral**
  - **H44.629 Retained (old) magnetic foreign body in iris or ciliary body, unspecified eye**

+ **H44.63 Retained (old) magnetic foreign body in lens**
  - **H44.631 Retained (old) magnetic foreign body in lens, right eye**
  - **H44.632 Retained (old) magnetic foreign body in lens, left eye**
  - **H44.633 Retained (old) magnetic foreign body in lens, bilateral**
  - **H44.639 Retained (old) magnetic foreign body in lens, unspecified eye**

+ **H44.64 Retained (old) magnetic foreign body in posterior wall of globe**
  - **H44.641 Retained (old) magnetic foreign body in posterior wall of globe, right eye**
  - **H44.642 Retained (old) magnetic foreign body in posterior wall of globe, left eye**
  - **H44.643 Retained (old) magnetic foreign body in posterior wall of globe, bilateral**
  - **H44.649 Retained (old) magnetic foreign body in posterior wall of globe, unspecified eye**

+ **H44.65 Retained (old) magnetic foreign body in vitreous body**
  - **H44.651 Retained (old) magnetic foreign body in vitreous body, right eye**
  - **H44.652 Retained (old) magnetic foreign body in vitreous body, left eye**
  - **H44.653 Retained (old) magnetic foreign body in vitreous body, bilateral**
  - **H44.659 Retained (old) magnetic foreign body in vitreous body, unspecified eye**

+ **H44.69 Retained (old) intraocular foreign body, magnetic, in other or multiple sites**
  - **H44.691 Retained (old) intraocular foreign body, magnetic, in other or multiple sites, right eye**
  - **H44.692 Retained (old) intraocular foreign body, magnetic, in other or multiple sites, left ey**
  - **H44.693 Retained (old) intraocular foreign body, magnetic, in other or multiple sites, bilateral**
  - **H44.699 Retained (old) intraocular foreign body, magnetic, in other or multiple sites, unspecified eye**

+ **H44.7 Retained (old) intraocular foreign body, nonmagnetic**
  Use additional code to identify nonmagnetic foreign body (Z18.01-Z18.10, Z18.12, Z18.2-Z18.9)
  Excludes1: *current intraocular foreign body (S05.-)*
  Excludes2: *retained foreign body in eyelid (H02.81-)*
  retained (old) foreign body following penetrating wound of orbit (H05.5-)
  retained (old) intraocular foreign body, magnetic (H44.6-)

+ **H44.70 Unspecified retained (old) intraocular foreign body, nonmagnetic**
  - **H44.701 Unspecified retained (old) intraocular foreign body, nonmagnetic, right eye**
  - **H44.702 Unspecified retained (old) intraocular foreign body, nonmagnetic, left eye**
  - **H44.703 Unspecified retained (old) intraocular foreign body, nonmagnetic, bilateral**
  - **H44.709 Unspecified retained (old) intraocular foreign body, nonmagnetic, unspecified ey**
    Retained (old) intraocular foreign body NO

+ **H44.71 Retained (nonmagnetic) (old) foreign body in anterior chamber**
  - **H44.711 Retained (nonmagnetic) (old) foreign body in anterior chamber, right eye**
  - **H44.712 Retained (nonmagnetic) (old) foreign body in anterior chamber, left eye**
  - **H44.713 Retained (nonmagnetic) (old) foreign body in anterior chamber, bilateral**
  - **H44.719 Retained (nonmagnetic) (old) foreign body in anterior chamber, unspecified eye**

+ **H44.72 Retained (nonmagnetic) (old) foreign body in iris or ciliary body**
  - **H44.721 Retained (nonmagnetic) (old) foreign body in iris or ciliary body, right eye**
  - **H44.722 Retained (nonmagnetic) (old) foreign body in iris or ciliary body, left eye**
  - **H44.723 Retained (nonmagnetic) (old) foreign body in iris or ciliary body, bilateral**
  - **H44.729 Retained (nonmagnetic) (old) foreign body in iris or ciliary body, unspecified eye**

+ **H44.73 Retained (nonmagnetic) (old) foreign body in lens**
  - **H44.731 Retained (nonmagnetic) (old) foreign body in lens, right eye**
  - **H44.732 Retained (nonmagnetic) (old) foreign body in lens, left eye**
  - **H44.733 Retained (nonmagnetic) (old) foreign body in lens, bilateral**
  - **H44.739 Retained (nonmagnetic) (old) foreign body in lens, unspecified eye**

+ **H44.74 Retained (nonmagnetic) (old) foreign body in posterior wall of globe**
  - **H44.741 Retained (nonmagnetic) (old) foreign body in posterior wall of globe, right eye**
  - **H44.742 Retained (nonmagnetic) (old) foreign body in posterior wall of globe, left eye**
  - **H44.743 Retained (nonmagnetic) (old) foreign body in posterior wall of globe, bilateral**
  - **H44.749 Retained (nonmagnetic) (old) foreign body in posterior wall of globe, unspecified eye**

+ **H44.75 Retained (nonmagnetic) (old) foreign body in vitreous body**
  - **H44.751 Retained (nonmagnetic) (old) foreign body in vitreous body, right eye**
  - **H44.752 Retained (nonmagnetic) (old) foreign body in vitreous body, left eye**
  - **H44.753 Retained (nonmagnetic) (old) foreign body in vitreous body, bilateral**
  - **H44.759 Retained (nonmagnetic) (old) foreign body in vitreous body, unspecified eye**

+ H44.79 Retained (old) intraocular foreign body, nonmagnetic, in other or multiple sites
H44.791 Retained (old) intraocular foreign body, nonmagnetic, in other or multiple sites, right eye
H44.792 Retained (old) intraocular foreign body, nonmagnetic, in other or multiple sites, left eye
H44.793 Retained (old) intraocular foreign body, nonmagnetic, in other or multiple sites, bilateral
H44.799 Retained (old) intraocular foreign body, nonmagnetic, in other or multiple sites, unspecified eye
+ H44.8 Other disorders of globe
+ H44.81 Hemophthalmos
H44.811 Hemophthalmos, right eye
H44.812 Hemophthalmos, left eye
H44.813 Hemophthalmos, bilateral
H44.819 Hemophthalmos, unspecified eye
+ H44.82 Luxation of globe
H44.821 Luxation of globe, right eye
H44.822 Luxation of globe, left eye
H44.823 Luxation of globe, bilateral
H44.829 Luxation of globe, unspecified eye
H44.89 Other disorders of globe
H44.9 Unspecified disorder of globe

isorders of optic nerve and visual pathways (H46-H47)

H46 Optic neuritis

Excludes2: *ischemic optic neuropathy (H47.01-)*
neuromyelitis optica [Devic] (G36.0)

+ H46.0 Optic papillitis
CC H46.00 Optic papillitis, unspecified eye
CC Exclusion see Appendix A PDX collection 0633
CC H46.01 Optic papillitis, right eye
CC Exclusion see Appendix A PDX collection 0633
CC H46.02 Optic papillitis, left eye
CC Exclusion see Appendix A PDX collection 0633
CC H46.03 Optic papillitis, bilateral
CC Exclusion see Appendix A PDX collection 0633
+ H46.1 Retrobulbar neuritis
Retrobulbar neuritis NOS
Excludes1: *syphilitic retrobulbar neuritis (A52.15)*
CC H46.10 Retrobulbar neuritis, unspecified eye
CC Exclusion see Appendix A PDX collection 0633
CC H46.11 Retrobulbar neuritis, right eye
CC Exclusion see Appendix A PDX collection 0633
CC H46.12 Retrobulbar neuritis, left eye
CC Exclusion see Appendix A PDX collection 0633
CC H46.13 Retrobulbar neuritis, bilateral
CC Exclusion see Appendix A PDX collection 0633
H46.2 Nutritional optic neuropathy
H46.3 Toxic optic neuropathy
Code first (T51-T65) to identify cause
CC H46.8 Other optic neuritis
CC Exclusion see Appendix A PDX collection 0633
CC H46.9 Unspecified optic neuritis
CC Exclusion see Appendix A PDX collection 0633

H47 Other disorders of optic [2nd] nerve and visual pathways

+ H47.0 Disorders of optic nerve, not elsewhere classified
+ H47.01 Ischemic optic neuropathy
H47.011 Ischemic optic neuropathy, right eye
H47.012 Ischemic optic neuropathy, left eye
H47.013 Ischemic optic neuropathy, bilateral
H47.019 Ischemic optic neuropathy, unspecified eye
+ H47.02 Hemorrhage in optic nerve sheath
H47.021 Hemorrhage in optic nerve sheath, right eye
H47.022 Hemorrhage in optic nerve sheath, left eye
H47.023 Hemorrhage in optic nerve sheath, bilateral
H47.029 Hemorrhage in optic nerve sheath, unspecified eye
+ H47.03 Optic nerve hypoplasia
H47.031 Optic nerve hypoplasia, right eye
H47.032 Optic nerve hypoplasia, left eye
H47.033 Optic nerve hypoplasia, bilateral
H47.039 Optic nerve hypoplasia, unspecified eye
+ H47.09 Other disorders of optic nerve, not elsewhere classified
Compression of optic nerve
H47.091 Other disorders of optic nerve, not elsewhere classified, right eye
H47.092 Other disorders of optic nerve, not elsewhere classified, left eye
H47.093 Other disorders of optic nerve, not elsewhere classified, bilateral
H47.099 Other disorders of optic nerve, not elsewhere classified, unspecified eye
+ H47.1 Papilledema
CC H47.10 Unspecified papilledema
CC Exclusion see Appendix A PDX collection 0634
CC H47.11 Papilledema associated with increased intracranial pressure
CC Exclusion see Appendix A PDX collection 0634
H47.12 Papilledema associated with decreased ocular pressure
H47.13 Papilledema associated with retinal disorder
+ H47.14 Foster-Kennedy syndrome
H47.141 Foster-Kennedy syndrome, right eye
H47.142 Foster-Kennedy syndrome, left eye
H47.143 Foster-Kennedy syndrome, bilateral
H47.149 Foster-Kennedy syndrome, unspecified eye
+ H47.2 Optic atrophy
H47.20 Unspecified optic atrophy
+ H47.21 Primary optic atrophy
H47.211 Primary optic atrophy, right eye
H47.212 Primary optic atrophy, left eye
H47.213 Primary optic atrophy, bilateral
H47.219 Primary optic atrophy, unspecified eye
H47.22 Hereditary optic atrophy
Leber's optic atrophy
+ H47.23 Glaucomatous optic atrophy
H47.231 Glaucomatous optic atrophy, right eye
H47.232 Glaucomatous optic atrophy, left eye
H47.233 Glaucomatous optic atrophy, bilateral
H47.239 Glaucomatous optic atrophy, unspecified eye
+ H47.29 Other optic atrophy
Temporal pallor of optic disc
H47.291 Other optic atrophy, right eye
H47.292 Other optic atrophy, left eye
H47.293 Other optic atrophy, bilateral
H47.299 Other optic atrophy, unspecified eye
+ H47.3 Other disorders of optic disc
+ H47.31 Coloboma of optic disc
H47.311 Coloboma of optic disc, right eye
H47.312 Coloboma of optic disc, left eye
H47.313 Coloboma of optic disc, bilateral
H47.319 Coloboma of optic disc, unspecified eye
+ H47.32 Drusen of optic disc
H47.321 Drusen of optic disc, right eye
H47.322 Drusen of optic disc, left eye
H47.323 Drusen of optic disc, bilateral
H47.329 Drusen of optic disc, unspecified eye
+ H47.33 Pseudopapilledema of optic disc
H47.331 Pseudopapilledema of optic disc, right eye
H47.332 Pseudopapilledema of optic disc, left eye
H47.333 Pseudopapilledema of optic disc, bilateral
H47.339 Pseudopapilledema of optic disc, unspecified eye
+ H47.39 Other disorders of optic disc
H47.391 Other disorders of optic disc, right eye
H47.392 Other disorders of optic disc, left eye
H47.393 Other disorders of optic disc, bilateral
H47.399 Other disorders of optic disc, unspecified eye
+ H47.4 Disorders of optic chiasm
Code also underlying condition
CC H47.41 Disorders of optic chiasm in (due to) inflammatory disorders
CC Exclusion see Appendix A PDX collection 0635
CC H47.42 Disorders of optic chiasm in (due to) neoplasm
CC Exclusion see Appendix A PDX collection 0635
CC H47.43 Disorders of optic chiasm in (due to) vascular disorders
CC Exclusion see Appendix A PDX collection 0635
CC H47.49 Disorders of optic chiasm in (due to) other disorders
CC Exclusion see Appendix A PDX collection 0635

+ H47.5 Disorders of other visual pathways
Disorders of optic tracts, geniculate nuclei and optic radiations
Code also underlying condition
+ H47.51 Disorders of visual pathways in (due to) inflammatory disorders
CC H47.511 Disorders of visual pathways in (due to) inflammatory disorders, right side
CC Exclusion see Appendix A PDX collection 0635
CC H47.512 Disorders of visual pathways in (due to) inflammatory disorders, left side
CC Exclusion see Appendix A PDX collection 0635
CC H47.519 Disorders of visual pathways in (due to) inflammatory disorders, unspecified side
CC Exclusion see Appendix A PDX collection 0635
+ H47.52 Disorders of visual pathways in (due to) neoplasm
CC H47.521 Disorders of visual pathways in (due to) neoplasm, right side
CC Exclusion see Appendix A PDX collection 0635
CC H47.522 Disorders of visual pathways in (due to) neoplasm, left side
CC Exclusion see Appendix A PDX collection 0635
CC H47.529 Disorders of visual pathways in (due to) neoplasm, unspecified side
CC Exclusion see Appendix A PDX collection 0635
+ H47.53 Disorders of visual pathways in (due to) vascular disorders
CC H47.531 Disorders of visual pathways in (due to) vascular disorders, right side
CC Exclusion see Appendix A PDX collection 0635
CC H47.532 Disorders of visual pathways in (due to) vascular disorders, left side
CC Exclusion see Appendix A PDX collection 0635
CC H47.539 Disorders of visual pathways in (due to) vascular disorders, unspecified side
CC Exclusion see Appendix A PDX collection 0635
+ H47.6 Disorders of visual cortex
Code also underlying condition
Excludes1: *injury to visual cortex S04.04*
+ H47.61 Cortical blindness
H47.611 Cortical blindness, right side of brain
H47.612 Cortical blindness, left side of brain
H47.619 Cortical blindness, unspecified side of brain
+ H47.62 Disorders of visual cortex in (due to) inflammatory disorders
CC H47.621 Disorders of visual cortex in (due to) inflammatory disorders, right side of brain
CC Exclusion see Appendix A PDX collection 0636
CC H47.622 Disorders of visual cortex in (due to) inflammatory disorders, left side of brain
CC Exclusion see Appendix A PDX collection 0636
CC H47.629 Disorders of visual cortex in (due to) inflammatory disorders, unspecified side of brain
CC Exclusion see Appendix A PDX collection 0636
+ H47.63 Disorders of visual cortex in (due to) neoplasm
CC H47.631 Disorders of visual cortex in (due to) neoplasm, right side of brain
CC Exclusion see Appendix A PDX collection 0636
CC H47.632 Disorders of visual cortex in (due to) neoplasm, left side of brain
CC Exclusion see Appendix A PDX collection 0636
CC H47.639 Disorders of visual cortex in (due to) neoplasm, unspecified side of brain
CC Exclusion see Appendix A PDX collection 0636
+ H47.64 Disorders of visual cortex in (due to) vascular disorders
CC H47.641 Disorders of visual cortex in (due to) vascular disorders, right side of brain
CC Exclusion see Appendix A PDX collection 0636
CC H47.642 Disorders of visual cortex in (due to) vascular disorders, left side of brain
CC Exclusion see Appendix A PDX collection 063
CC H47.649 Disorders of visual cortex in (due to) vascular disorders, unspecified side of brain
CC Exclusion see Appendix A PDX collection 063
H47.9 Unspecified disorder of visual pathways

Disorders of ocular muscles, binocular movement, accommodation and refraction (H49-H52)

Excludes2: *nystagmus and other irregular eye movements (H55)*

H49 Paralytic strabismus

Excludes2: *internal ophthalmoplegia (H52.51-)*
internuclear ophthalmoplegia (H51.2-)
progressive supranuclear ophthalmoplegia (G23.1)

+ H49.0 Third [oculomotor] nerve palsy
H49.00 Third [oculomotor] nerve palsy, unspecified eye
H49.01 Third [oculomotor] nerve palsy, right eye
H49.02 Third [oculomotor] nerve palsy, left eye
H49.03 Third [oculomotor] nerve palsy, bilateral
+ H49.1 Fourth [trochlear] nerve palsy
H49.10 Fourth [trochlear] nerve palsy, unspecified eye
H49.11 Fourth [trochlear] nerve palsy, right eye
H49.12 Fourth [trochlear] nerve palsy, left eye
H49.13 Fourth [trochlear] nerve palsy, bilateral
+ H49.2 Sixth [abducent] nerve palsy
H49.20 Sixth [abducent] nerve palsy, unspecified eye
H49.21 Sixth [abducent] nerve palsy, right eye
H49.22 Sixth [abducent] nerve palsy, left eye
H49.23 Sixth [abducent] nerve palsy, bilateral
+ H49.3 Total (external) ophthalmoplegia
H49.30 Total (external) ophthalmoplegia, unspecified eye
H49.31 Total (external) ophthalmoplegia, right eye
H49.32 Total (external) ophthalmoplegia, left eye
H49.33 Total (external) ophthalmoplegia, bilateral
+ H49.4 Progressive external ophthalmoplegia
Excludes1: *Kearns-Sayre syndrome (H49.81-)*
H49.40 Progressive external ophthalmoplegia, unspecified eye
H49.41 Progressive external ophthalmoplegia, right eye
H49.42 Progressive external ophthalmoplegia, left eye
H49.43 Progressive external ophthalmoplegia, bilateral
+ H49.8 Other paralytic strabismus
+ H49.81 Kearns-Sayre syndrome
Progressive external ophthalmoplegia with pigmentary retinopathy
Use additional code for other manifestation, such as: heart block (I45.9)
CC H49.811 Kearns-Sayre syndrome, right eye
CC Exclusion see Appendix A PDX collection 0545
CC H49.812 Kearns-Sayre syndrome, left eye
CC Exclusion see Appendix A PDX collection 0545
CC H49.813 Kearns-Sayre syndrome, bilateral
CC Exclusion see Appendix A PDX collection 0545
CC H49.819 Kearns-Sayre syndrome, unspecified eye
CC Exclusion see Appendix A PDX collection 0545
+ H49.88 Other paralytic strabismus
External ophthalmoplegia NOS
H49.881 Other paralytic strabismus, right eye
H49.882 Other paralytic strabismus, left eye
H49.883 Other paralytic strabismus, bilateral
H49.889 Other paralytic strabismus, unspecified ey
H49.9 Unspecified paralytic strabismus

H50 Other strabismus

+ H50.0 Esotropia
Convergent concomitant strabismus
Excludes1: *intermittent esotropia (H50.31-, H50.32)*
H50.00 Unspecified esotropia
+ H50.01 Monocular esotropia
H50.011 Monocular esotropia, right eye
H50.012 Monocular esotropia, left eye

+ **H50.02 Monocular esotropia with A pattern**
H50.021 Monocular esotropia with A pattern, right eye
H50.022 Monocular esotropia with A pattern, left eye
+ **H50.03 Monocular esotropia with V pattern**
H50.031 Monocular esotropia with V pattern, right eye
H50.032 Monocular esotropia with V pattern, left eye
+ **H50.04 Monocular esotropia with other noncomitancies**
H50.041 Monocular esotropia with other noncomitancies, right eye
H50.042 Monocular esotropia with other noncomitancies, left eye
H50.05 Alternating esotropia
H50.06 Alternating esotropia with A pattern
H50.07 Alternating esotropia with V pattern
H50.08 Alternating esotropia with other noncomitancies
+ **H50.1 Exotropia**
Divergent concomitant strabismus
Excludes1: *intermittent exotropia (H50.33-, H50.34)*
H50.10 Unspecified exotropia
+ **H50.11 Monocular exotropia**
H50.111 Monocular exotropia, right eye
H50.112 Monocular exotropia, left eye
+ **H50.12 Monocular exotropia with A pattern**
H50.121 Monocular exotropia with A pattern, right eye
H50.122 Monocular exotropia with A pattern, left eye
+ **H50.13 Monocular exotropia with V pattern**
H50.131 Monocular exotropia with V pattern, right eye
H50.132 Monocular exotropia with V pattern, left eye
+ **H50.14 Monocular exotropia with other noncomitancies**
H50.141 Monocular exotropia with other noncomitancies, right eye
H50.142 Monocular exotropia with other noncomitancies, left eye
H50.15 Alternating exotropia
H50.16 Alternating exotropia with A pattern
H50.17 Alternating exotropia with V pattern
H50.18 Alternating exotropia with other noncomitancies
+ **H50.2 Vertical strabismus**
Hypertropia
H50.21 Vertical strabismus, right eye
H50.22 Vertical strabismus, left eye
+ **H50.3 Intermittent heterotropia**
H50.30 Unspecified intermittent heterotropia
+ **H50.31 Intermittent monocular esotropia**
H50.311 Intermittent monocular esotropia, right eye
H50.312 Intermittent monocular esotropia, left eye
H50.32 Intermittent alternating esotropia
+ **H50.33 Intermittent monocular exotropia**
H50.331 Intermittent monocular exotropia, right eye
H50.332 Intermittent monocular exotropia, left eye
H50.34 Intermittent alternating exotropia
+ **H50.4 Other and unspecified heterotropia**
H50.40 Unspecified heterotropia
+ **H50.41 Cyclotropia**
H50.411 Cyclotropia, right eye
H50.412 Cyclotropia, left eye
H50.42 Monofixation syndrome
H50.43 Accommodative component in esotropia
+ **H50.5 Heterophoria**
H50.50 Unspecified heterophoria
H50.51 Esophoria
H50.52 Exophoria
H50.53 Vertical heterophoria
H50.54 Cyclophoria
H50.55 Alternating heterophoria
+ **H50.6 Mechanical strabismus**
H50.60 Mechanical strabismus, unspecified
+ **H50.61 Brown's sheath syndrome**
H50.611 Brown's sheath syndrome, right eye
H50.612 Brown's sheath syndrome, left eye
H50.69 Other mechanical strabismus
Strabismus due to adhesions
Traumatic limitation of duction of eye muscle
+ **H50.8 Other specified strabismus**
+ **H50.81 Duane's syndrome**
H50.811 Duane's syndrome, right eye
H50.812 Duane's syndrome, left eye
H50.89 Other specified strabismus
H50.9 Unspecified strabismus

H51 Other disorders of binocular movement

H51.0 Palsy (spasm) of conjugate gaze
+ **H51.1 Convergence insufficiency and excess**
H51.11 Convergence insufficiency
H51.12 Convergence excess
+ **H51.2 Internuclear ophthalmoplegia**
H51.20 Internuclear ophthalmoplegia, unspecified eye
H51.21 Internuclear ophthalmoplegia, right eye
H51.22 Internuclear ophthalmoplegia, left eye
H51.23 Internuclear ophthalmoplegia, bilateral
H51.8 Other specified disorders of binocular movement
H51.9 Unspecified disorder of binocular movement

H52 Disorders of refraction and accommodation

+ **H52.0 Hypermetropia**
H52.00 Hypermetropia, unspecified eye
H52.01 Hypermetropia, right eye
H52.02 Hypermetropia, left eye
H52.03 Hypermetropia, bilateral
+ **H52.1 Myopia**
Excludes1: *degenerative myopia (H44.2-)*
H52.10 Myopia, unspecified eye
H52.11 Myopia, right eye
H52.12 Myopia, left eye
H52.13 Myopia, bilateral
+ **H52.2 Astigmatism**
+ **H52.20 Unspecified astigmatism**
H52.201 Unspecified astigmatism, right eye
H52.202 Unspecified astigmatism, left eye
H52.203 Unspecified astigmatism, bilateral
H52.209 Unspecified astigmatism, unspecified eye
+ **H52.21 Irregular astigmatism**
H52.211 Irregular astigmatism, right eye
H52.212 Irregular astigmatism, left eye
H52.213 Irregular astigmatism, bilateral
H52.219 Irregular astigmatism, unspecified eye
+ **H52.22 Regular astigmatism**
H52.221 Regular astigmatism, right eye
H52.222 Regular astigmatism, left eye
H52.223 Regular astigmatism, bilateral
H52.229 Regular astigmatism, unspecified eye
+ **H52.3 Anisometropia and aniseikonia**
H52.31 Anisometropia
H52.32 Aniseikonia
H52.4 Presbyopia
+ **H52.5 Disorders of accommodation**
+ **H52.51 Internal ophthalmoplegia (complete) (total)**
H52.511 Internal ophthalmoplegia (complete) (total), right eye
H52.512 Internal ophthalmoplegia (complete) (total), left eye
H52.513 Internal ophthalmoplegia (complete) (total), bilateral
H52.519 Internal ophthalmoplegia (complete) (total), unspecified eye
+ **H52.52 Paresis of accommodation**
H52.521 Paresis of accommodation, right eye
H52.522 Paresis of accommodation, left eye
H52.523 Paresis of accommodation, bilateral
H52.529 Paresis of accommodation, unspecified eye
+ **H52.53 Spasm of accommodation**
H52.531 Spasm of accommodation, right eye
H52.532 Spasm of accommodation, left eye
H52.533 Spasm of accommodation, bilateral
H52.539 Spasm of accommodation, unspecified eye
H52.6 Other disorders of refraction
H52.7 Unspecified disorder of refraction

Visual disturbances and blindness (H53-H54)

H53 Visual disturbances

+ **H53.0 Amblyopia ex anopsia**
  Excludes1: amblyopia due to vitamin A deficiency (E50.5)
  + **H53.00 Unspecified amblyopia**
    H53.001 Unspecified amblyopia, right eye
    H53.002 Unspecified amblyopia, left eye
    H53.003 Unspecified amblyopia, bilateral
    H53.009 Unspecified amblyopia, unspecified eye
  + **H53.01 Deprivation amblyopia**
    H53.011 Deprivation amblyopia, right eye
    H53.012 Deprivation amblyopia, left eye
    H53.013 Deprivation amblyopia, bilateral
    H53.019 Deprivation amblyopia, unspecified eye
  + **H53.02 Refractive amblyopia**
    H53.021 Refractive amblyopia, right eye
    H53.022 Refractive amblyopia, left eye
    H53.023 Refractive amblyopia, bilateral
    H53.029 Refractive amblyopia, unspecified eye
  + **H53.03 Strabismic amblyopia**
    Excludes1: strabismus (H50.-)
    H53.031 Strabismic amblyopia, right eye
    H53.032 Strabismic amblyopia, left eye
    H53.033 Strabismic amblyopia, bilateral
    H53.039 Strabismic amblyopia, unspecified eye
  + **H53.04 Amblyopia suspect**
    AHA CC: 4Q, 2016, 22-23
    H53.041 Amblyopia suspect, right eye
    H53.042 Amblyopia suspect, left eye
    H53.043 Amblyopia suspect, bilateral
    H53.049 Amblyopia suspect, unspecified eye
+ **H53.1 Subjective visual disturbances**
  Excludes1: subjective visual disturbances due to vitamin A deficiency (E50.5)
  visual hallucinations (R44.1)
  H53.10 Unspecified subjective visual disturbances
  H53.11 Day blindness
    Hemeralopia
  + **H53.12 Transient visual loss**
    Scintillating scotoma
    Excludes1: amaurosis fugax (G45.3-)
    transient retinal artery occlusion (H34.0-)
    CC **H53.121 Transient visual loss, right eye**
      CC Exclusion see Appendix A PDX collection 0637
    CC **H53.122 Transient visual loss, left eye**
      CC Exclusion see Appendix A PDX collection 0637
    CC **H53.123 Transient visual loss, bilateral**
      CC Exclusion see Appendix A PDX collection 0637
    CC **H53.129 Transient visual loss, unspecified eye**
      CC Exclusion see Appendix A PDX collection 0637
  + **H53.13 Sudden visual loss**
    CC **H53.131 Sudden visual loss, right eye**
      CC Exclusion see Appendix A PDX collection 0637
    CC **H53.132 Sudden visual loss, left eye**
      CC Exclusion see Appendix A PDX collection 0637
    CC **H53.133 Sudden visual loss, bilateral**
      CC Exclusion see Appendix A PDX collection 0637
    CC **H53.139 Sudden visual loss, unspecified eye**
      CC Exclusion see Appendix A PDX collection 0637
  + **H53.14 Visual discomfort**
    Asthenopia
    Photophobia
    H53.141 Visual discomfort, right eye
    H53.142 Visual discomfort, left eye
    H53.143 Visual discomfort, bilateral
    H53.149 Visual discomfort, unspecified
  H53.15 Visual distortions of shape and size
    Metamorphopsia
  H53.16 Psychophysical visual disturbances
  H53.19 Other subjective visual disturbances
    Visual halos
H53.2 Diplopia
  Double vision
+ **H53.3 Other and unspecified disorders of binocular vision**
  H53.30 Unspecified disorder of binocular vision
  H53.31 Abnormal retinal correspondence
  H53.32 Fusion with defective stereopsis
  H53.33 Simultaneous visual perception without fusion
  H53.34 Suppression of binocular vision
+ **H53.4 Visual field defects**
  H53.40 Unspecified visual field defects
  + **H53.41 Scotoma involving central area**
    Central scotoma
    H53.411 Scotoma involving central area, right eye
    H53.412 Scotoma involving central area, left eye
    H53.413 Scotoma involving central area, bilateral
    H53.419 Scotoma involving central area, unspecified eye
  + **H53.42 Scotoma of blind spot area**
    Enlarged blind spot
    H53.421 Scotoma of blind spot area, right eye
    H53.422 Scotoma of blind spot area, left eye
    H53.423 Scotoma of blind spot area, bilateral
    H53.429 Scotoma of blind spot area, unspecified eye
  + **H53.43 Sector or arcuate defects**
    Arcuate scotoma
    Bjerrum scotoma
    H53.431 Sector or arcuate defects, right eye
    H53.432 Sector or arcuate defects, left eye
    H53.433 Sector or arcuate defects, bilateral
    H53.439 Sector or arcuate defects, unspecified eye
  + **H53.45 Other localized visual field defect**
    Peripheral visual field defect
    Ring scotoma NOS
    Scotoma NOS
    H53.451 Other localized visual field defect, right eye
    H53.452 Other localized visual field defect, left eye
    H53.453 Other localized visual field defect, bilater
    H53.459 Other localized visual field defect, unspecified eye
  + **H53.46 Homonymous bilateral field defects**
    Homonymous hemianopsia
    Quadrant anopia
    Quadrant anopsia
    H53.461 Homonymous bilateral field defects, right side
    H53.462 Homonymous bilateral field defects, left side
    H53.469 Homonymous bilateral field defects, unspecified side
      Homonymous bilateral field defects NOS
  H53.47 Heteronymous bilateral field defects
    Heteronymous hemianop(s)ia
  + **H53.48 Generalized contraction of visual field**
    H53.481 Generalized contraction of visual field, right eye
    H53.482 Generalized contraction of visual field, left eye
    H53.483 Generalized contraction of visual field, bilateral
    H53.489 Generalized contraction of visual field, unspecified eye
+ **H53.5 Color vision deficiencies**
  Color blindness
  Excludes2: day blindness (H53.11)
  H53.50 Unspecified color vision deficiencies
    Color blindness NOS
  H53.51 Achromatopsia
  H53.52 Acquired color vision deficiency
  H53.53 Deuteranomaly
    Deuteranopia
  H53.54 Protanomaly
    Protanopia
  H53.55 Tritanomaly
    Tritanopia
  H53.59 Other color vision deficiencies
+ **H53.6 Night blindness**
  Excludes1: night blindness due to vitamin A deficiency (E50.
  H53.60 Unspecified night blindness
  H53.61 Abnormal dark adaptation curve

H53.62 Acquired night blindness
H53.63 Congenital night blindness
H53.69 Other night blindness
+ H53.7 Vision sensitivity deficiencies
H53.71 Glare sensitivity
H53.72 Impaired contrast sensitivity
H53.8 Other visual disturbances
H53.9 Unspecified visual disturbance

H54 Blindness and low vision

NOTE For definition of visual impairment categories see table below
Code first any associated underlying cause of the blindness
Excludes1: *amaurosis fugax (G45.3)*

+ **H54.0 Blindness, both eyes**
Visual impairment categories 3, 4, 5 in both eyes.
H54.0X Blindness, both eyes, different category levels
+ **H54.0X3 Blindness right eye, category 3**
H54.0X33 Blindness right eye category 3, blindness left eye category 3
H54.0X34 Blindness right eye category 3, blindness left eye category 4
H54.0X35 Blindness right eye category 3, blindness left eye category 5
+ **H54.0X4 Blindness right eye, category 4**
H54.0X43 Blindness right eye category 4, blindness left eye category 3
H54.0X44 Blindness right eye category 4, blindness left eye category 4
H54.0X45 Blindness right eye category 4, blindness left eye category 5
+ **H54.0X5 Blindness right eye, category 5**
H54.0X53 Blindness right eye category 5, blindness left eye category 3
H54.0X54 Blindness right eye category 5, blindness left eye category 4
H54.0X55 Blindness right eye category 5, blindness left eye category 5

+ **H54.1 Blindness, one eye, low vision other eye**
Visual impairment categories 3, 4, 5 in one eye, with categories 1 or 2 in the other eye.
H54.10 Blindness, one eye, low vision other eye, unspecified eyes
+ **H54.11 Blindness, right eye, low vision left eye**
+ **H54.113 Blindness right eye category 3, low vision left eye**
H54.1131 Blindness right eye category 3, low vision left eye category 1
H54.1132 Blindness right eye category 3, low vision left eye category 2
+ **H54.114 Blindness right eye category 4, low vision left eye**
H54.1141 Blindness right eye category 4, low vision left eye category 1
H54.1142 Blindness right eye category 4, low vision left eye category 2
+ **H54.115 Blindness right eye category 5, low vision left eye**
H54.1151 Blindness right eye category 5, low vision left eye category 1
H54.1152 Blindness right eye category 5, low vision left eye category 2
+ **H54.12 Blindness, left eye, low vision right eye**
+ **H54.121 Low vision right eye category 1, blindness left eye**
H54.1213 Low vision right eye category 1, blindness left eye category 3
H54.1214 Low vision right eye category 1, blindness left eye category 4
H54.1215 Low vision right eye category 1, blindness left eye category 5
+ **H54.122 Low vision right eye category 2, blindness left eye**
H54.1223 Low vision right eye category 2, blindness left eye category 3
H54.1224 Low vision right eye category 2, blindness left eye category 4
H54.1225 Low vision right eye category 2, blindness left eye category 5

+ **H54.2 Low vision, both eyes**
Visual impairment categories 1 or 2 in both eyes.
+ **H54.2X Low vision, both eyes, different category levels**
+ **H54.2X1 Low vision, right eye, category 1**
H54.2X11 Low vision, right eye, category 1, low vision left eye category 1
H54.2X12 Low vision, right eye, category 1, low vision left eye category 2
+ **H54.2X2 Low vision, right eye, category 2**
H54.2X21 Low vision, right eye, category 2, low vision left eye category 1
H54.2X22 Low vision, right eye, category 2, low vision left eye category 2

H54.3 Unqualified visual loss, both eyes
Visual impairment category 9 in both eyes.
Review coding guideline C.7.b

+ **H54.4 Blindness, one eye**
Visual impairment categories 3, 4, 5 in one eye [normal vision in other eye]
H54.40 Blindness, one eye, unspecified eye
+ **H54.41 Blindness, right eye, normal vision left eye**
+ **H54.413 Blindness, right eye, category 3**
H54.413A Blindness right eye category 3, normal vision left eye
+ **H54.414 Blindness, right eye, category 4**
H54.414A Blindness right eye category 4, normal vision left eye
+ **H54.415 Blindness, right eye, category 5**
H54.415A Blindness right eye category 5, normal vision left eye
+ **H54.42 Blindness, left eye, normal vision right eye**
+ **H54.42A Blindness, left eye, category 3-5**
H54.42A3 Blindness left eye category 3, normal vision right eye
H54.42A4 Blindness left eye category 4, normal vision right eye
H54.42A5 Blindness left eye category 5, normal vision right eye

+ **H54.5 Low vision, one eye**
Visual impairment categories 1 or 2 in one eye [normal vision in other eye].
H54.50 Low vision, one eye, unspecified eye
+ **H54.51 Low vision, right eye, normal vision left eye**
+ **H54.511 Low vision, right eye, category 1-2**
H54.511A Low vision right eye category 1, normal vision left eye
H54.512A Low vision right eye category 2, normal vision left eye
+ **H54.52 Low vision, left eye, normal vision right eye**
+ **H54.52A Low vision, left eye, category 1-2**
H54.52A1 Low vision left eye category 1, normal vision right eye
H54.52A2 Low vision left eye category 2, normal vision right eye

+ **H54.6 Unqualified visual loss, one eye**
Visual impairment category 9 in one eye [normal vision in other eye].
Review coding guideline C.7.b
H54.60 Unqualified visual loss, one eye, unspecified
H54.61 Unqualified visual loss, right eye, normal vision left eye
H54.62 Unqualified visual loss, left eye, normal vision right eye

H54.7 Unspecified visual loss
Visual impairment category 9 NOS
Review coding guideline C.7.b

H54.8 Legal blindness, as defined in USA
Blindness NOS according to USA definition
Excludes1: *legal blindness with specification of impairment level (H54.0-H54.7)*

NOTE The table below gives a classification of severity of visual impairment recommended by a WHO Study Group on the Prevention of Blindness, Geneva, 6-10 November 1972.
The term 'low vision' in category H54 comprises categories 1 and 2 of the table, the term 'blindness' categories 3, 4 and 5, and the term 'unqualified visual loss' category 9.
If the extent of the visual field is taken into account, patients with a field no greater than 10 but greater than 5 around central fixation should be placed in category 3 and patients with a field no greater than 5 around central fixation should be placed in category 4, even if the central acuity is not impaired.

Category of visual impairment	Visual acuity with best possible correction	
	Maximum less than:	Minimum equal to or better than:
	6/18	6/60
3/10(0.3)	1/10(0.1)	
20/70	20/200	
	6/60	3/60
1/10(0.1)	1/20(0.05)	
20/200	20/400	
	3/60	1/60(finger counting at one meter)
1/20(0.05)	1/50(0.02)	
20/400	5/300(20/1200)	
	1/60(finger counting at one meter)	Light perception
1/50(0.02)		
5/300		
	No light perception	
	Undetermined or unspecified	

Note: Document 508 compliance requires all cells in the above table to be filled.

Other disorders of eye and adnexa (H55-H57)

H55 Nystagmus and other irregular eye movements

+ H55.0 Nystagmus
H55.00 Unspecified nystagmus
H55.01 Congenital nystagmus
H55.02 Latent nystagmus
H55.03 Visual deprivation nystagmus
H55.04 Dissociated nystagmus
H55.09 Other forms of nystagmus
+ H55.8 Other irregular eye movements
H55.81 Saccadic eye movements
H55.89 Other irregular eye movements

H57 Other disorders of eye and adnexa

+ H57.0 Anomalies of pupillary function
H57.00 Unspecified anomaly of pupillary function
H57.01 Argyll Robertson pupil, atypical
Excludes1: *syphilitic Argyll Robertson pupil (A52.19)*
H57.02 Anisocoria
H57.03 Miosis
H57.04 Mydriasis
+ H57.05 Tonic pupil
H57.051 Tonic pupil, right eye
H57.052 Tonic pupil, left eye
H57.053 Tonic pupil, bilateral
H57.059 Tonic pupil, unspecified eye
H57.09 Other anomalies of pupillary function
+ H57.1 Ocular pain
H57.10 Ocular pain, unspecified eye
H57.11 Ocular pain, right eye
H57.12 Ocular pain, left eye
H57.13 Ocular pain, bilateral
H57.8 Other specified disorders of eye and adnexa
H57.9 Unspecified disorder of eye and adnexa

Intraoperative and postprocedural complications and disorders of eye and adnexa, not elsewhere classified (H59)

H59 Intraoperative and postprocedural complications and disorders of eye and adnexa, not elsewhere classified

Excludes1: *mechanical complication of intraocular lens (T85.2)*
mechanical complication of other ocular prosthetic devices, implants and grafts (T85.3)
pseudophakia (Z96.1)
secondary cataracts (H26.4-)

+ H59.0 Disorders of the eye following cataract surgery
+ H59.01 Keratopathy (bullous aphakic) following cataract surgery
Vitreal corneal syndrome
Vitreous (touch) syndrome
CC **H59.011 Keratopathy (bullous aphakic) following cataract surgery, right eye**
CC Exclusion see Appendix A PDX collection 0638
CC **H59.012 Keratopathy (bullous aphakic) following cataract surgery, left eye**
CC Exclusion see Appendix A PDX collection 0638
CC **H59.013 Keratopathy (bullous aphakic) following cataract surgery, bilateral**
CC Exclusion see Appendix A PDX collection 0638
CC **H59.019 Keratopathy (bullous aphakic) following cataract surgery, unspecified eye**
CC Exclusion see Appendix A PDX collection 0638
+ H59.02 Cataract (lens) fragments in eye following cataract surgery
H59.021 Cataract (lens) fragments in eye following cataract surgery, right eye
H59.022 Cataract (lens) fragments in eye following cataract surgery, left eye
H59.023 Cataract (lens) fragments in eye following cataract surgery, bilateral
H59.029 Cataract (lens) fragments in eye following cataract surgery, unspecified eye
+ H59.03 Cystoid macular edema following cataract surgery
CC **H59.031 Cystoid macular edema following cataract surgery, right eye**
CC Exclusion see Appendix A PDX collection 0638
CC **H59.032 Cystoid macular edema following cataract surgery, left eye**
CC Exclusion see Appendix A PDX collection 0638
CC **H59.033 Cystoid macular edema following cataract surgery, bilateral**
CC Exclusion see Appendix A PDX collection 0638
CC **H59.039 Cystoid macular edema following cataract surgery, unspecified eye**
CC Exclusion see Appendix A PDX collection 0638
+ H59.09 Other disorders of the eye following cataract surgery
CC **H59.091 Other disorders of the right eye following cataract surgery**
CC Exclusion see Appendix A PDX collection 0638
CC **H59.092 Other disorders of the left eye following cataract surgery**
CC Exclusion see Appendix A PDX collection 0638
CC **H59.093 Other disorders of the eye following cataract surgery, bilateral**
CC Exclusion see Appendix A PDX collection 0638
CC **H59.099 Other disorders of unspecified eye following cataract surgery**
CC Exclusion see Appendix A PDX collection 0638
+ H59.1 Intraoperative hemorrhage and hematoma of eye and adnexa complicating a procedure
Excludes1: *intraoperative hemorrhage and hematoma of eye and adnexa due to accidental puncture or laceration during a procedure (H59.2-)*
+ H59.11 Intraoperative hemorrhage and hematoma of eye and adnexa complicating an ophthalmic procedure
CC **H59.111 Intraoperative hemorrhage and hematoma of right eye and adnexa complicating an ophthalmic procedure**
CC Exclusion see Appendix A PDX collection 0639
CC **H59.112 Intraoperative hemorrhage and hematoma of left eye and adnexa complicating an ophthalmic procedure**
CC Exclusion see Appendix A PDX collection 0639

CC **H59.113** **Intraoperative hemorrhage and hematoma of eye and adnexa complicating an ophthalmic procedure, bilateral**
CC Exclusion see Appendix A PDX collection 0639

CC **H59.119** **Intraoperative hemorrhage and hematoma of unspecified eye and adnexa complicating an ophthalmic procedure**
CC Exclusion see Appendix A PDX collection 0639

\+ **H59.12** **Intraoperative hemorrhage and hematoma of eye and adnexa complicating other procedure**

CC **H59.121** **Intraoperative hemorrhage and hematoma of right eye and adnexa complicating other procedure**
CC Exclusion see Appendix A PDX collection 0639

CC **H59.122** **Intraoperative hemorrhage and hematoma of left eye and adnexa complicating other procedure**
CC Exclusion see Appendix A PDX collection 0639

CC **H59.123** **Intraoperative hemorrhage and hematoma of eye and adnexa complicating other procedure, bilateral**
CC Exclusion see Appendix A PDX collection 0639

CC **H59.129** **Intraoperative hemorrhage and hematoma of unspecified eye and adnexa complicating other procedure**
CC Exclusion see Appendix A PDX collection 0639

\+ **H59.2** **Accidental puncture and laceration of eye and adnexa during a procedure**

\+ **H59.21** **Accidental puncture and laceration of eye and adnexa during an ophthalmic procedure**

CC **H59.211** **Accidental puncture and laceration of right eye and adnexa during an ophthalmic procedure**
CC Exclusion see Appendix A PDX collection 0509

CC **H59.212** **Accidental puncture and laceration of left eye and adnexa during an ophthalmic procedure**
CC Exclusion see Appendix A PDX collection 0509

CC **H59.213** **Accidental puncture and laceration of eye and adnexa during an ophthalmic procedure, bilateral**
CC Exclusion see Appendix A PDX collection 0509

CC **H59.219** **Accidental puncture and laceration of unspecified eye and adnexa during an ophthalmic procedure**
CC Exclusion see Appendix A PDX collection 0509

\+ **H59.22** **Accidental puncture and laceration of eye and adnexa during other procedure**

CC **H59.221** **Accidental puncture and laceration of right eye and adnexa during other procedure**
CC Exclusion see Appendix A PDX collection 0509

CC **H59.222** **Accidental puncture and laceration of left eye and adnexa during other procedure**
CC Exclusion see Appendix A PDX collection 0509

CC **H59.223** **Accidental puncture and laceration of eye and adnexa during other procedure, bilateral**
CC Exclusion see Appendix A PDX collection 0509

CC **H59.229** **Accidental puncture and laceration of unspecified eye and adnexa during other procedure**
CC Exclusion see Appendix A PDX collection 0509

\+ **H59.3** **Postprocedural hemorrhage, hematoma and seroma of eye and adnexa following a procedure**
AHA CC: 4Q, 2016, 9-10

\+ **H59.31** **Postprocedural hemorrhage of eye and adnexa following an ophthalmic procedure**

CC **H59.311** **Postprocedural hemorrhage of right eye and adnexa following an ophthalmic procedure**
CC Exclusion see Appendix A PDX collection 0639

CC **H59.312** **Postprocedural hemorrhage of left eye and adnexa following an ophthalmic procedure**
CC Exclusion see Appendix A PDX collection 0639

CC **H59.313** **Postprocedural hemorrhage of eye and adnexa following an ophthalmic procedure, bilateral**
CC Exclusion see Appendix A PDX collection 0639

CC **H59.319** **Postprocedural hemorrhage of unspecified eye and adnexa following an ophthalmic procedure**
CC Exclusion see Appendix A PDX collection 0639

\+ **H59.32** **Postprocedural hemorrhage of eye and adnexa following other procedure**

CC **H59.321** **Postprocedural hemorrhage of right eye and adnexa following other procedure**
CC Exclusion see Appendix A PDX collection 0639

CC **H59.322** **Postprocedural hemorrhage of left eye and adnexa following other procedure**
CC Exclusion see Appendix A PDX collection 0639

CC **H59.323** **Postprocedural hemorrhage of eye and adnexa following other procedure, bilateral**
CC Exclusion see Appendix A PDX collection 0639

CC **H59.329** **Postprocedural hemorrhage of unspecified eye and adnexa following other procedure**
CC Exclusion see Appendix A PDX collection 0639

\+ **H59.33** **Postprocedural hematoma of eye and adnexa following an ophthalmic procedure**

CC **H59.331** **Postprocedural hematoma of right eye and adnexa following an ophthalmic procedure**
CC Exclusion see Appendix A PDX collection 0639

CC **H59.332** **Postprocedural hematoma of left eye and adnexa following an ophthalmic procedure**
CC Exclusion see Appendix A PDX collection 0639

CC **H59.333** **Postprocedural hematoma of eye and adnexa following an ophthalmic procedure, bilateral**
CC Exclusion see Appendix A PDX collection 0639

CC **H59.339** **Postprocedural hematoma of unspecified eye and adnexa following an ophthalmic procedure**
CC Exclusion see Appendix A PDX collection 0639

\+ **H59.34** **Postprocedural hematoma of eye and adnexa following other procedure**

CC **H59.341** **Postprocedural hematoma of right eye and adnexa following other procedure**
CC Exclusion see Appendix A PDX collection 0639

CC **H59.342** **Postprocedural hematoma of left eye and adnexa following other procedure**
CC Exclusion see Appendix A PDX collection 0639

CC **H59.343** **Postprocedural hematoma of eye and adnexa following other procedure, bilateral**
CC Exclusion see Appendix A PDX collection 0639

CC **H59.349** **Postprocedural hematoma of unspecified eye and adnexa following other procedure**
CC Exclusion see Appendix A PDX collection 0639

\+ **H59.35** **Postprocedural seroma of eye and adnexa following an ophthalmic procedure**

CC **H59.351** **Postprocedural seroma of right eye and adnexa following an ophthalmic procedure**
CC Exclusion see Appendix A PDX collection 0639

CC **H59.352** **Postprocedural seroma of left eye and adnexa following an ophthalmic procedure**
CC Exclusion see Appendix A PDX collection 0639

CC **H59.353 Postprocedural seroma of eye and adnexa following an ophthalmic procedure, bilateral**
CC Exclusion see Appendix A PDX collection 0639

CC **H59.359 Postprocedural seroma of unspecified eye and adnexa following an ophthalmic procedure**
CC Exclusion see Appendix A PDX collection 0639

\+ **H59.36 Postprocedural seroma of eye and adnexa following other procedure**

CC **H59.361 Postprocedural seroma of right eye and adnexa following other procedure**
CC Exclusion see Appendix A PDX collection 0639

CC **H59.362 Postprocedural seroma of left eye and adnexa following other procedure**
CC Exclusion see Appendix A PDX collection 0639

CC **H59.363 Postprocedural seroma of eye and adnexa following other procedure, bilateral**
CC Exclusion see Appendix A PDX collection 0639

CC **H59.369 Postprocedural seroma of unspecified eye and adnexa following other procedure**
CC Exclusion see Appendix A PDX collection 0639

\+ **H59.4 Inflammation (infection) of postprocedural bleb**
Postprocedural blebitis
Excludes1: *filtering (vitreous) bleb after glaucoma surgery status (Z98.83)*

H59.40 Inflammation (infection) of postprocedural bleb, unspecified

H59.41 Inflammation (infection) of postprocedural bleb, stage 1

H59.42 Inflammation (infection) of postprocedural bleb, stage 2

H59.43 Inflammation (infection) of postprocedural bleb, stage 3
Bleb endophthalmitis

\+ **H59.8 Other intraoperative and postprocedural complications and disorders of eye and adnexa, not elsewhere classified**

\+ **H59.81 Chorioretinal scars after surgery for detachment**

CC **H59.811 Chorioretinal scars after surgery for detachment, right eye**
CC Exclusion see Appendix A PDX collection 0638

CC **H59.812 Chorioretinal scars after surgery for detachment, left eye**
CC Exclusion see Appendix A PDX collection 0638

CC **H59.813 Chorioretinal scars after surgery for detachment, bilateral**
CC Exclusion see Appendix A PDX collection 0638

CC **H59.819 Chorioretinal scars after surgery for detachment, unspecified eye**
CC Exclusion see Appendix A PDX collection 0638

CC **H59.88 Other intraoperative complications of eye and adnexa, not elsewhere classified**
CC Exclusion see Appendix A PDX collection 0638

CC **H59.89 Other postprocedural complications and disorders eye and adnexa, not elsewhere classified**
CC Exclusion see Appendix A PDX collection 0638
One of the following 7th characters is to be assigned code H40.10 to designate the stage of glaucoma

Chapter 8: Diseases of the Ear and Mastoid Process (H60-H95)

NOTE Use an external cause code following the code for the ear condition, if applicable, to identify the cause of the ear condition

Excludes2: *certain conditions originating in the perinatal period (P04-P96)*
certain infectious and parasitic diseases (A00-B99)
complications of pregnancy, childbirth and the puerperium (O00-O9A)
congenital malformations, deformations and chromosomal abnormalities (Q00-Q99)
endocrine, nutritional and metabolic diseases (E00-E88)
injury, poisoning and certain other consequences of external causes (S00-T88)
neoplasms (C00-D49)
symptoms, signs and abnormal clinical and laboratory findings, not elsewhere classified (R00-R94)

This chapter contains the following category blocks:

H60-H62	Diseases of external ear
H65-H75	Diseases of middle ear and mastoid
H80-H83	Diseases of inner ear
H90-H94	Other disorders of ear
H95	Intraoperative and postprocedural complications and disorders of ear and mastoid process, not elsewhere classified

C. Chapter-Specific Coding Guidelines

In addition to general coding guidelines, there are guidelines for specific diagnoses and/or conditions in the classification. Unless otherwise indicated, these guidelines apply to all health care settings. Please refer to Section II for guidelines on the selection of principal diagnosis.

8. Chapter 8: Diseases of the Ear and Mastoid Process (H60-H95)

Reserved for future guideline expansion

Ear

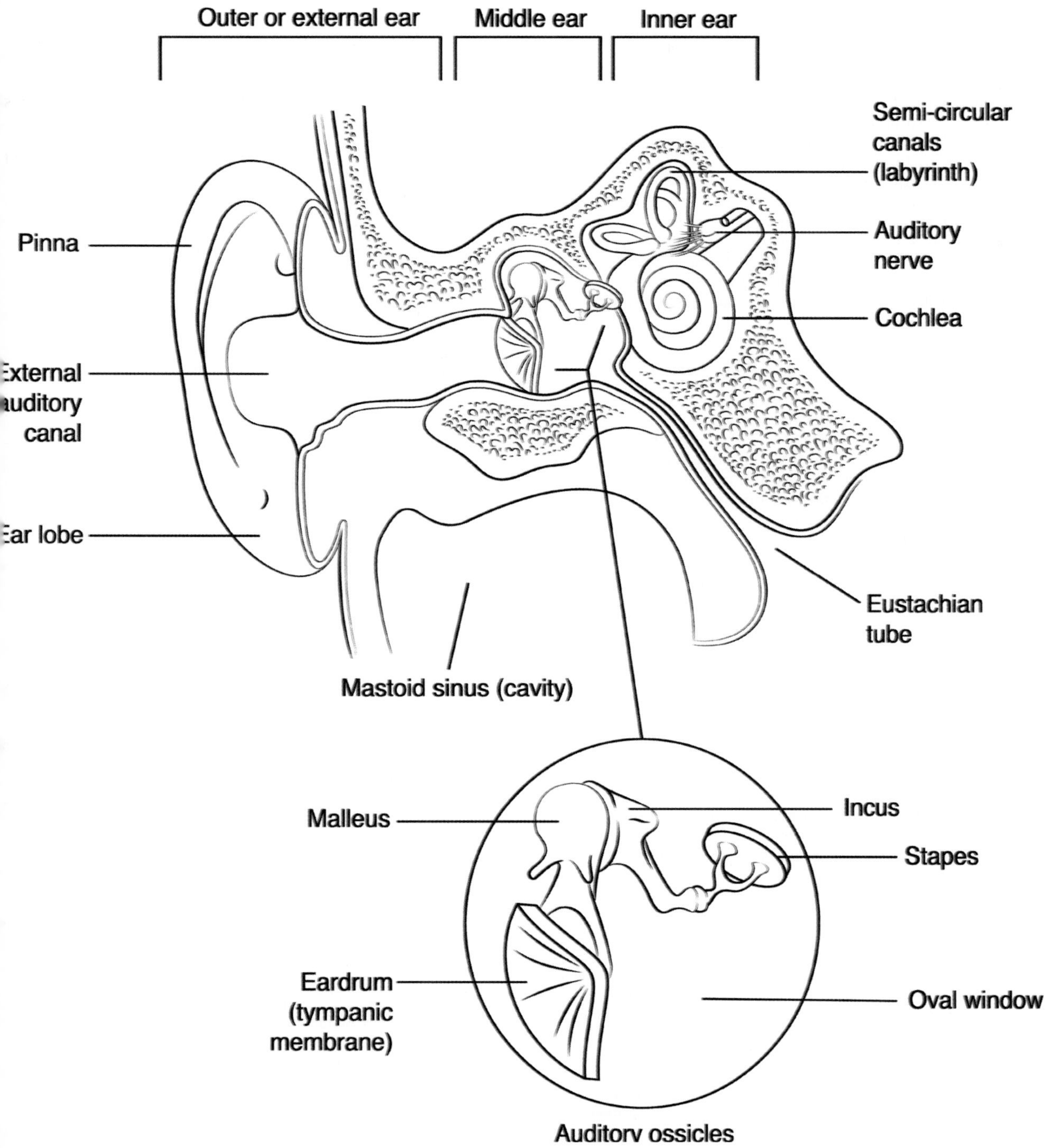

Diseases of external ear (H60-H62)

H60 Otitis externa

+ **H60.0 Abscess of external ear**
  Boil of external ear
  Carbuncle of auricle or external auditory canal
  Furuncle of external ear
  H60.00 Abscess of external ear, unspecified ear
  H60.01 Abscess of right external ear
  H60.02 Abscess of left external ear
  H60.03 Abscess of external ear, bilateral
+ **H60.1 Cellulitis of external ear**
  Cellulitis of auricle
  Cellulitis of external auditory canal
  H60.10 Cellulitis of external ear, unspecified ear
  H60.11 Cellulitis of right external ear
  H60.12 Cellulitis of left external ear
  H60.13 Cellulitis of external ear, bilateral
+ **H60.2 Malignant otitis externa**
  CC **H60.20 Malignant otitis externa, unspecified ear**
  CC Exclusion see Appendix A PDX collection 0640
  CC **H60.21 Malignant otitis externa, right ear**
  CC Exclusion see Appendix A PDX collection 0640
  CC **H60.22 Malignant otitis externa, left ear**
  CC Exclusion see Appendix A PDX collection 0640
  CC **H60.23 Malignant otitis externa, bilateral**
  CC Exclusion see Appendix A PDX collection 0640
+ **H60.3 Other infective otitis externa**
  + **H60.31 Diffuse otitis externa**
    H60.311 Diffuse otitis externa, right ear
    H60.312 Diffuse otitis externa, left ear
    H60.313 Diffuse otitis externa, bilateral
    H60.319 Diffuse otitis externa, unspecified ear
  + **H60.32 Hemorrhagic otitis externa**
    H60.321 Hemorrhagic otitis externa, right ear
    H60.322 Hemorrhagic otitis externa, left ear
    H60.323 Hemorrhagic otitis externa, bilateral
    H60.329 Hemorrhagic otitis externa, unspecified ear
  + **H60.33 Swimmer's ear**
    H60.331 Swimmer's ear, right ear
    H60.332 Swimmer's ear, left ear
    H60.333 Swimmer's ear, bilateral
    H60.339 Swimmer's ear, unspecified ear
  + **H60.39 Other infective otitis externa**
    H60.391 Other infective otitis externa, right ear
    H60.392 Other infective otitis externa, left ear
    H60.393 Other infective otitis externa, bilateral
    H60.399 Other infective otitis externa, unspecified ear
+ **H60.4 Cholesteatoma of external ear**
  Keratosis obturans of external ear (canal)
  Excludes2: *cholesteatoma of middle ear (H71.-)*
  recurrent cholesteatoma of postmastoidectomy cavity (H95.0-)
  H60.40 Cholesteatoma of external ear, unspecified ear
  H60.41 Cholesteatoma of right external ear
  H60.42 Cholesteatoma of left external ear
  H60.43 Cholesteatoma of external ear, bilateral
+ **H60.5 Acute noninfective otitis externa**
  + **H60.50 Unspecified acute noninfective otitis externa**
    Acute otitis externa NOS
    H60.501 Unspecified acute noninfective otitis externa, right ear
    H60.502 Unspecified acute noninfective otitis externa, left ear
    H60.503 Unspecified acute noninfective otitis externa, bilateral
    H60.509 Unspecified acute noninfective otitis externa, unspecified ear
  + **H60.51 Acute actinic otitis externa**
    H60.511 Acute actinic otitis externa, right ear
    H60.512 Acute actinic otitis externa, left ear
    H60.513 Acute actinic otitis externa, bilateral
    H60.519 Acute actinic otitis externa, unspecified ear
  + **H60.52 Acute chemical otitis externa**
    H60.521 Acute chemical otitis externa, right ear
    H60.522 Acute chemical otitis externa, left ear
    H60.523 Acute chemical otitis externa, bilateral
    H60.529 Acute chemical otitis externa, unspecified ear
  + **H60.53 Acute contact otitis externa**
    H60.531 Acute contact otitis externa, right ear
    H60.532 Acute contact otitis externa, left ear
    H60.533 Acute contact otitis externa, bilateral
    H60.539 Acute contact otitis externa, unspecified ear
  + **H60.54 Acute eczematoid otitis externa**
    H60.541 Acute eczematoid otitis externa, right ear
    H60.542 Acute eczematoid otitis externa, left ear
    H60.543 Acute eczematoid otitis externa, bilateral
    H60.549 Acute eczematoid otitis externa, unspecified ear
  + **H60.55 Acute reactive otitis externa**
    H60.551 Acute reactive otitis externa, right ear
    H60.552 Acute reactive otitis externa, left ear
    H60.553 Acute reactive otitis externa, bilateral
    H60.559 Acute reactive otitis externa, unspecified ear
  + **H60.59 Other noninfective acute otitis externa**
    H60.591 Other noninfective acute otitis externa, right ear
    H60.592 Other noninfective acute otitis externa, left ear
    H60.593 Other noninfective acute otitis externa, bilateral
    H60.599 Other noninfective acute otitis externa, unspecified ear
+ **H60.6 Unspecified chronic otitis externa**
  H60.60 Unspecified chronic otitis externa, unspecified ear
  H60.61 Unspecified chronic otitis externa, right ear
  H60.62 Unspecified chronic otitis externa, left ear
  H60.63 Unspecified chronic otitis externa, bilateral
+ **H60.8 Other otitis externa**
  + **H60.8X Other otitis externa**
    H60.8X1 Other otitis externa, right ear
    H60.8X2 Other otitis externa, left ear
    H60.8X3 Other otitis externa, bilateral
    H60.8X9 Other otitis externa, unspecified ear
+ **H60.9 Unspecified otitis externa**
  H60.90 Unspecified otitis externa, unspecified ear
  H60.91 Unspecified otitis externa, right ear
  H60.92 Unspecified otitis externa, left ear
  H60.93 Unspecified otitis externa, bilateral

H61 Other disorders of external ear

+ **H61.0 Chondritis and perichondritis of external ear**
  Chondrodermatitis nodularis chronica helicis
  Perichondritis of auricle
  Perichondritis of pinna
  + **H61.00 Unspecified perichondritis of external ear**
    H61.001 Unspecified perichondritis of right external ear
    H61.002 Unspecified perichondritis of left external ear
    H61.003 Unspecified perichondritis of external ear, bilateral
    H61.009 Unspecified perichondritis of external ear, unspecified ear
  + **H61.01 Acute perichondritis of external ear**
    H61.011 Acute perichondritis of right external ear
    H61.012 Acute perichondritis of left external ear
    H61.013 Acute perichondritis of external ear, bilateral
    H61.019 Acute perichondritis of external ear, unspecified ear
  + **H61.02 Chronic perichondritis of external ear**
    H61.021 Chronic perichondritis of right external ear
    H61.022 Chronic perichondritis of left external ear
    H61.023 Chronic perichondritis of external ear, bilateral
    H61.029 Chronic perichondritis of external ear, unspecified ear
  + **H61.03 Chondritis of external ear**
    Chondritis of auricle
    Chondritis of pinna
    H61.031 Chondritis of right external ear
    H61.032 Chondritis of left external ear
    AHA CC: 1Q, 2015, 18-19
    H61.033 Chondritis of external ear, bilateral
    H61.039 Chondritis of external ear, unspecified ear

+ **H61.1 Noninfective disorders of pinna**
Excludes2: *cauliflower ear (M95.1-)*
gouty tophi of ear (M1A.-)
+ **H61.10 Unspecified noninfective disorders of pinna**
Disorder of pinna NOS
H61.101 Unspecified noninfective disorders of pinna, right ear
H61.102 Unspecified noninfective disorders of pinna, left ear
H61.103 Unspecified noninfective disorders of pinna, bilateral
H61.109 Unspecified noninfective disorders of pinna, unspecified ear
+ **H61.11 Acquired deformity of pinna**
Acquired deformity of auricle
Excludes2: *cauliflower ear (M95.1-)*
H61.111 Acquired deformity of pinna, right ear
H61.112 Acquired deformity of pinna, left ear
H61.113 Acquired deformity of pinna, bilateral
H61.119 Acquired deformity of pinna, unspecified ear
+ **H61.12 Hematoma of pinna**
Hematoma of auricle
H61.121 Hematoma of pinna, right ear
H61.122 Hematoma of pinna, left ear
H61.123 Hematoma of pinna, bilateral
H61.129 Hematoma of pinna, unspecified ear
+ **H61.19 Other noninfective disorders of pinna**
H61.191 Noninfective disorders of pinna, right ear
H61.192 Noninfective disorders of pinna, left ear
H61.193 Noninfective disorders of pinna, bilateral
H61.199 Noninfective disorders of pinna, unspecified ear
+ **H61.2 Impacted cerumen**
Wax in ear
H61.20 Impacted cerumen, unspecified ear
H61.21 Impacted cerumen, right ear
H61.22 Impacted cerumen, left ear
H61.23 Impacted cerumen, bilateral
+ **H61.3 Acquired stenosis of external ear canal**
Collapse of external ear canal
Excludes1: *postprocedural stenosis of external ear canal (H95.81-)*
+ **H61.30 Acquired stenosis of external ear canal, unspecified**
H61.301 Acquired stenosis of right external ear canal, unspecified
H61.302 Acquired stenosis of left external ear canal, unspecified
H61.303 Acquired stenosis of external ear canal, unspecified, bilateral
H61.309 Acquired stenosis of external ear canal, unspecified, unspecified ear
+ **H61.31 Acquired stenosis of external ear canal secondary to trauma**
H61.311 Acquired stenosis of right external ear canal secondary to trauma
H61.312 Acquired stenosis of left external ear canal secondary to trauma
H61.313 Acquired stenosis of external ear canal secondary to trauma, bilateral
H61.319 Acquired stenosis of external ear canal secondary to trauma, unspecified ear
+ **H61.32 Acquired stenosis of external ear canal secondary to inflammation and infection**
H61.321 Acquired stenosis of right external ear canal secondary to inflammation and infection
H61.322 Acquired stenosis of left external ear canal secondary to inflammation and infection
H61.323 Acquired stenosis of external ear canal secondary to inflammation and infection, bilateral
H61.329 Acquired stenosis of external ear canal secondary to inflammation and infection, unspecified ear
+ **H61.39 Other acquired stenosis of external ear canal**
H61.391 Other acquired stenosis of right external ear canal
H61.392 Other acquired stenosis of left external ear canal
H61.393 Other acquired stenosis of external ear canal, bilateral
H61.399 Other acquired stenosis of external ear canal, unspecified ear
+ **H61.8 Other specified disorders of external ear**
+ **H61.81 Exostosis of external canal**
H61.811 Exostosis of right external canal
H61.812 Exostosis of left external canal
H61.813 Exostosis of external canal, bilateral
H61.819 Exostosis of external canal, unspecified ear
+ **H61.89 Other specified disorders of external ear**
H61.891 Other specified disorders of right external ear
H61.892 Other specified disorders of left external ear
H61.893 Other specified disorders of external ear, bilateral
H61.899 Other specified disorders of external ear, unspecified ear
+ **H61.9 Disorder of external ear, unspecified**
H61.90 Disorder of external ear, unspecified, unspecified ear
H61.91 Disorder of right external ear, unspecified
H61.92 Disorder of left external ear, unspecified
H61.93 Disorder of external ear, unspecified, bilateral

H62 Disorders of external ear in diseases classified elsewhere

+ **H62.4 Otitis externa in other diseases classified elsewhere**
Code first underlying disease, such as:
erysipelas (A46)
impetigo (L01.0)
Excludes1: *otitis externa (in):*
candidiasis (B37.84)
herpes viral [herpes simplex] (B00.1)
herpes zoster (B02.8)
H62.40 Otitis externa in other diseases classified elsewhere, unspecified ear
H62.41 Otitis externa in other diseases classified elsewhere, right ear
H62.42 Otitis externa in other diseases classified elsewhere, left ear
H62.43 Otitis externa in other diseases classified elsewhere, bilateral
+ **H62.8 Other disorders of external ear in diseases classified elsewhere**
Code first underlying disease, such as:
gout (M1A.-, M10.-)
+ **H62.8X Other disorders of external ear in diseases classified elsewhere**
H62.8X1 Other disorders of right external ear in diseases classified elsewhere
H62.8X2 Other disorders of left external ear in diseases classified elsewhere
H62.8X3 Other disorders of external ear in diseases classified elsewhere, bilateral
H62.8X9 Other disorders of external ear in diseases classified elsewhere, unspecified ear

Diseases of middle ear and mastoid (H65-H75)

H65 Nonsuppurative otitis media

Includes: nonsuppurative otitis media with myringitis
Use additional code for any associated perforated tympanic membrane (H72.-)

Use additional code to identify:
exposure to environmental tobacco smoke (Z77.22)
exposure to tobacco smoke in the perinatal period (P96.81)
history of tobacco dependence (Z87.891)
occupational exposure to environmental tobacco smoke (Z57.31)
tobacco dependence (F17.-)
tobacco use (Z72.0)
+ **H65.0 Acute serous otitis media**
Acute and subacute secretory otitis
H65.00 Acute serous otitis media, unspecified ear
H65.01 Acute serous otitis media, right ear
H65.02 Acute serous otitis media, left ear
H65.03 Acute serous otitis media, bilateral
H65.04 Acute serous otitis media, recurrent, right ear
H65.05 Acute serous otitis media, recurrent, left ear
H65.06 Acute serous otitis media, recurrent, bilateral
H65.07 Acute serous otitis media, recurrent, unspecified ear

+ **H65.1 Other acute nonsuppurative otitis media**
  Excludes1: *otitic barotrauma (T70.0)*
  otitis media (acute) NOS (H66.9)
  + **H65.11 Acute and subacute allergic otitis media (mucoid) (sanguinous) (serous)**
    H65.111 Acute and subacute allergic otitis media (mucoid) (sanguinous) (serous), right ear
    H65.112 Acute and subacute allergic otitis media (mucoid) (sanguinous) (serous), left ear
    H65.113 Acute and subacute allergic otitis media (mucoid) (sanguinous) (serous), bilateral
    H65.114 Acute and subacute allergic otitis media (mucoid) (sanguinous) (serous), recurrent, right ear
    H65.115 Acute and subacute allergic otitis media (mucoid) (sanguinous) (serous), recurrent, left ear
    H65.116 Acute and subacute allergic otitis media (mucoid) (sanguinous) (serous), recurrent, bilateral
    H65.117 Acute and subacute allergic otitis media (mucoid) (sanguinous) (serous), recurrent, unspecified ear
    H65.119 Acute and subacute allergic otitis media (mucoid) (sanguinous) (serous), unspecified ear
  + **H65.19 Other acute nonsuppurative otitis media**
    Acute and subacute mucoid otitis media
    Acute and subacute nonsuppurative otitis media NOS
    Acute and subacute sanguinous otitis media
    Acute and subacute seromucinous otitis media
    H65.191 Other acute nonsuppurative otitis media, right ear
    H65.192 Other acute nonsuppurative otitis media, left ear
    H65.193 Other acute nonsuppurative otitis media, bilateral
    H65.194 Other acute nonsuppurative otitis media, recurrent, right ear
    H65.195 Other acute nonsuppurative otitis media, recurrent, left ear
    H65.196 Other acute nonsuppurative otitis media, recurrent, bilateral
    H65.197 Other acute nonsuppurative otitis media recurrent, unspecified ear
    H65.199 Other acute nonsuppurative otitis media, unspecified ear

+ **H65.2 Chronic serous otitis media**
  Chronic tubotympanal catarrh
  H65.20 Chronic serous otitis media, unspecified ear
  H65.21 Chronic serous otitis media, right ear
  H65.22 Chronic serous otitis media, left ear
  H65.23 Chronic serous otitis media, bilateral

+ **H65.3 Chronic mucoid otitis media**
  Chronic mucinous otitis media
  Chronic secretory otitis media
  Chronic transudative otitis media
  Glue ear
  Excludes1: *adhesive middle ear disease (H74.1)*
  H65.30 Chronic mucoid otitis media, unspecified ear
  H65.31 Chronic mucoid otitis media, right ear
  H65.32 Chronic mucoid otitis media, left ear
  H65.33 Chronic mucoid otitis media, bilateral

+ **H65.4 Other chronic nonsuppurative otitis media**
  + **H65.41 Chronic allergic otitis media**
    H65.411 Chronic allergic otitis media, right ear
    H65.412 Chronic allergic otitis media, left ear
    H65.413 Chronic allergic otitis media, bilateral
    H65.419 Chronic allergic otitis media, unspecified ear
  + **H65.49 Other chronic nonsuppurative otitis media**
    Chronic exudative otitis media
    Chronic nonsuppurative otitis media NOS
    Chronic otitis media with effusion (nonpurulent)
    Chronic seromucinous otitis media
    H65.491 Other chronic nonsuppurative otitis media, right ear
    H65.492 Other chronic nonsuppurative otitis media, left ear
    H65.493 Other chronic nonsuppurative otitis med[ia,] bilateral
    H65.499 Other chronic nonsuppurative otitis med[ia,] unspecified ear

+ **H65.9 Unspecified nonsuppurative otitis media**
  Allergic otitis media NOS
  Catarrhal otitis media NOS
  Exudative otitis media NOS
  Mucoid otitis media NOS
  Otitis media with effusion (nonpurulent) NOS
  Secretory otitis media NOS
  Seromucinous otitis media NOS
  Serous otitis media NOS
  Transudative otitis media NOS
  H65.90 Unspecified nonsuppurative otitis media, unspecified ear
  H65.91 Unspecified nonsuppurative otitis media, right ear
  H65.92 Unspecified nonsuppurative otitis media, left ear
  H65.93 Unspecified nonsuppurative otitis media, bilateral

H66 Suppurative and unspecified otitis media

Includes: suppurative and unspecified otitis media with myringitis
Use additional code to identify:
exposure to environmental tobacco smoke (Z77.22)
exposure to tobacco smoke in the perinatal period (P96.81)
history of tobacco dependence (Z87.891)
occupational exposure to environmental tobacco smoke (Z57.31)
tobacco dependence (F17.-)
tobacco use (Z72.0)

+ **H66.0 Acute suppurative otitis media**
  + **H66.00 Acute suppurative otitis media without spontaneou[s] rupture of ear drum**
    H66.001 Acute suppurative otitis media without spontaneous rupture of ear drum, right e[ar]
    H66.002 Acute suppurative otitis media without spontaneous rupture of ear drum, left ea[r]
    H66.003 Acute suppurative otitis media without spontaneous rupture of ear drum, bilateral
    H66.004 Acute suppurative otitis media without spontaneous rupture of ear drum, recurrent, right ear
    H66.005 Acute suppurative otitis media without spontaneous rupture of ear drum, recurrent, left ear
    H66.006 Acute suppurative otitis media without spontaneous rupture of ear drum, recurrent, bilateral
    H66.007 Acute suppurative otitis media without spontaneous rupture of ear drum, recurrent, unspecified ear
    H66.009 Acute suppurative otitis media without spontaneous rupture of ear drum, unspecified ear
  + **H66.01 Acute suppurative otitis media with spontaneous rupture of ear drum**
    H66.011 Acute suppurative otitis media with spontaneous rupture of ear drum, right e[ar]
    H66.012 Acute suppurative otitis media with spontaneous rupture of ear drum, left ea[r]
    H66.013 Acute suppurative otitis media with spontaneous rupture of ear drum, bilateral
    H66.014 Acute suppurative otitis media with spontaneous rupture of ear drum, recurrent, right ear
    H66.015 Acute suppurative otitis media with spontaneous rupture of ear drum, recurrent, left ear
    H66.016 Acute suppurative otitis media with spontaneous rupture of ear drum, recurrent, bilateral
    H66.017 Acute suppurative otitis media with spontaneous rupture of ear drum, recurrent, unspecified ear
    H66.019 Acute suppurative otitis media with spontaneous rupture of ear drum, unspecified ear

+ **H66.1 Chronic tubotympanic suppurative otitis media**
Benign chronic suppurative otitis media
Chronic tubotympanic disease
Use additional code for any associated perforated tympanic membrane (H72.-)
H66.10 Chronic tubotympanic suppurative otitis media, unspecified
H66.11 Chronic tubotympanic suppurative otitis media, right ear
H66.12 Chronic tubotympanic suppurative otitis media, left ear
H66.13 Chronic tubotympanic suppurative otitis media, bilateral

+ **H66.2 Chronic atticoantral suppurative otitis media**
Chronic atticoantral disease
Use additional code for any associated perforated tympanic membrane (H72.-)
H66.20 Chronic atticoantral suppurative otitis media, unspecified ear
H66.21 Chronic atticoantral suppurative otitis media, right ear
H66.22 Chronic atticoantral suppurative otitis media, left ear
H66.23 Chronic atticoantral suppurative otitis media, bilateral

+ **H66.3 Other chronic suppurative otitis media**
Chronic suppurative otitis media NOS
Use additional code for any associated perforated tympanic membrane (H72.-)
Excludes1: *tuberculous otitis media (A18.6)*
+ **H66.3X Other chronic suppurative otitis media**
H66.3X1 Other chronic suppurative otitis media, right ear
H66.3X2 Other chronic suppurative otitis media, left ear
H66.3X3 Other chronic suppurative otitis media, bilateral
H66.3X9 Other chronic suppurative otitis media, unspecified ear

+ **H66.4 Suppurative otitis media, unspecified**
Purulent otitis media NOS
Use additional code for any associated perforated tympanic membrane (H72.-)
H66.40 Suppurative otitis media, unspecified, unspecified ear
H66.41 Suppurative otitis media, unspecified, right ear
H66.42 Suppurative otitis media, unspecified, left ear
H66.43 Suppurative otitis media, unspecified, bilateral

+ **H66.9 Otitis media, unspecified**
Otitis media NOS
Acute otitis media NOS
Chronic otitis media NOS
Use additional code for any associated perforated tympanic membrane (H72.-)
H66.90 Otitis media, unspecified, unspecified ear
H66.91 Otitis media, unspecified, right ear
H66.92 Otitis media, unspecified, left ear
H66.93 Otitis media, unspecified, bilateral

H67 Otitis media in diseases classified elsewhere

Code first underlying disease, such as:
viral disease NEC (B00-B34)

Use additional code for any associated perforated tympanic membrane (H72.-)

Excludes1: *otitis media in:*
influenza (J09.X9, J10.83, J11.83)
measles (B05.3)
scarlet fever (A38.0)
tuberculosis (A18.6)

H67.1 Otitis media in diseases classified elsewhere, right ear
H67.2 Otitis media in diseases classified elsewhere, left ear
H67.3 Otitis media in diseases classified elsewhere, bilateral
H67.9 Otitis media in diseases classified elsewhere, unspecified ear

H68 Eustachian salpingitis and obstruction

+ **H68.0 Eustachian salpingitis**
+ **H68.00 Unspecified Eustachian salpingitis**
H68.001 Unspecified Eustachian salpingitis, right ear
H68.002 Unspecified Eustachian salpingitis, left ear
H68.003 Unspecified Eustachian salpingitis, bilateral
H68.009 Unspecified Eustachian salpingitis, unspecified ear
+ **H68.01 Acute Eustachian salpingitis**
H68.011 Acute Eustachian salpingitis, right ear
H68.012 Acute Eustachian salpingitis, left ear
H68.013 Acute Eustachian salpingitis, bilateral
H68.019 Acute Eustachian salpingitis, unspecified ear
+ **H68.02 Chronic Eustachian salpingitis**
H68.021 Chronic Eustachian salpingitis, right ear
H68.022 Chronic Eustachian salpingitis, left ear
H68.023 Chronic Eustachian salpingitis, bilateral
H68.029 Chronic Eustachian salpingitis, unspecified ear

+ **H68.1 Obstruction of Eustachian tube**
Stenosis of Eustachian tube
Stricture of Eustachian tube
+ **H68.10 Unspecified obstruction of Eustachian tube**
H68.101 Unspecified obstruction of Eustachian tube, right ear
H68.102 Unspecified obstruction of Eustachian tube, left ear
H68.103 Unspecified obstruction of Eustachian tube, bilateral
H68.109 Unspecified obstruction of Eustachian tube, unspecified ear
+ **H68.11 Osseous obstruction of Eustachian tube**
H68.111 Osseous obstruction of Eustachian tube, right ear
H68.112 Osseous obstruction of Eustachian tube, left ear
H68.113 Osseous obstruction of Eustachian tube, bilateral
H68.119 Osseous obstruction of Eustachian tube, unspecified ear
+ **H68.12 Intrinsic cartilagenous obstruction of Eustachian tube**
H68.121 Intrinsic cartilagenous obstruction of Eustachian tube, right ear
H68.122 Intrinsic cartilagenous obstruction of Eustachian tube, left ear
H68.123 Intrinsic cartilagenous obstruction of Eustachian tube, bilateral
H68.129 Intrinsic cartilagenous obstruction of Eustachian tube, unspecified ear
+ **H68.13 Extrinsic cartilagenous obstruction of Eustachian tube**
Compression of Eustachian tube
H68.131 Extrinsic cartilagenous obstruction of Eustachian tube, right ear
H68.132 Extrinsic cartilagenous obstruction of Eustachian tube, left ear
H68.133 Extrinsic cartilagenous obstruction of Eustachian tube, bilateral
H68.139 Extrinsic cartilagenous obstruction of Eustachian tube, unspecified ear

H69 Other and unspecified disorders of Eustachian tube

+ **H69.0 Patulous Eustachian tube**
H69.00 Patulous Eustachian tube, unspecified ear
H69.01 Patulous Eustachian tube, right ear
H69.02 Patulous Eustachian tube, left ear
H69.03 Patulous Eustachian tube, bilateral
+ **H69.8 Other specified disorders of Eustachian tube**
H69.80 Other specified disorders of Eustachian tube, unspecified ear
H69.81 Other specified disorders of Eustachian tube, right ear
H69.82 Other specified disorders of Eustachian tube, left ear
H69.83 Other specified disorders of Eustachian tube, bilateral
+ **H69.9 Unspecified Eustachian tube disorder**
H69.90 Unspecified Eustachian tube disorder, unspecified ear
H69.91 Unspecified Eustachian tube disorder, right ear
H69.92 Unspecified Eustachian tube disorder, left ear
H69.93 Unspecified Eustachian tube disorder, bilateral

H70 Mastoiditis and related conditions

+ **H70.0 Acute mastoiditis**
  Abscess of mastoid
  Empyema of mastoid
  + **H70.00 Acute mastoiditis without complications**
    CC **H70.001 Acute mastoiditis without complications, right ear**
      CC Exclusion see Appendix A PDX collection 0641
    CC **H70.002 Acute mastoiditis without complications, left ear**
      CC Exclusion see Appendix A PDX collection 0641
    CC **H70.003 Acute mastoiditis without complications, bilateral**
      CC Exclusion see Appendix A PDX collection 0641
    CC **H70.009 Acute mastoiditis without complications, unspecified ear**
      CC Exclusion see Appendix A PDX collection 0641
  + **H70.01 Subperiosteal abscess of mastoid**
    CC **H70.011 Subperiosteal abscess of mastoid, right ear**
      CC Exclusion see Appendix A PDX collection 0641
    CC **H70.012 Subperiosteal abscess of mastoid, left ear**
      CC Exclusion see Appendix A PDX collection 0641
    CC **H70.013 Subperiosteal abscess of mastoid, bilateral**
      CC Exclusion see Appendix A PDX collection 0641
    CC **H70.019 Subperiosteal abscess of mastoid, unspecified ear**
      CC Exclusion see Appendix A PDX collection 0641
  + **H70.09 Acute mastoiditis with other complications**
    CC **H70.091 Acute mastoiditis with other complications, right ear**
      CC Exclusion see Appendix A PDX collection 0641
    CC **H70.092 Acute mastoiditis with other complications, left ear**
      CC Exclusion see Appendix A PDX collection 0641
    CC **H70.093 Acute mastoiditis with other complications, bilateral**
      CC Exclusion see Appendix A PDX collection 0641
    CC **H70.099 Acute mastoiditis with other complications, unspecified ear**
      CC Exclusion see Appendix A PDX collection 0641
+ **H70.1 Chronic mastoiditis**
  Caries of mastoid
  Fistula of mastoid
  Excludes1: *tuberculous mastoiditis (A18.03)*
  H70.10 Chronic mastoiditis, unspecified ear
  H70.11 Chronic mastoiditis, right ear
  H70.12 Chronic mastoiditis, left ear
  H70.13 Chronic mastoiditis, bilateral
+ **H70.2 Petrositis**
  Inflammation of petrous bone
  + **H70.20 Unspecified petrositis**
    H70.201 Unspecified petrositis, right ear
    H70.202 Unspecified petrositis, left ear
    H70.203 Unspecified petrositis, bilateral
    H70.209 Unspecified petrositis, unspecified ear
  + **H70.21 Acute petrositis**
    H70.211 Acute petrositis, right ear
    H70.212 Acute petrositis, left ear
    H70.213 Acute petrositis, bilateral
    H70.219 Acute petrositis, unspecified ear
  + **H70.22 Chronic petrositis**
    H70.221 Chronic petrositis, right ear
    H70.222 Chronic petrositis, left ear
    H70.223 Chronic petrositis, bilateral
    H70.229 Chronic petrositis, unspecified ear
+ **H70.8 Other mastoiditis and related conditions**
  Excludes1: *preauricular sinus and cyst (Q18.1)*
  sinus, fistula, and cyst of branchial cleft (Q18.0)
  + **H70.81 Postauricular fistula**
    H70.811 Postauricular fistula, right ear
    H70.812 Postauricular fistula, left ear
    H70.813 Postauricular fistula, bilateral
    H70.819 Postauricular fistula, unspecified ear
  + **H70.89 Other mastoiditis and related conditions**
    H70.891 Other mastoiditis and related conditions, right ear
    H70.892 Other mastoiditis and related conditions, left ear
    H70.893 Other mastoiditis and related conditions, bilateral
    H70.899 Other mastoiditis and related conditions, unspecified ear
+ **H70.9 Unspecified mastoiditis**
  H70.90 Unspecified mastoiditis, unspecified ear
  H70.91 Unspecified mastoiditis, right ear
  H70.92 Unspecified mastoiditis, left ear
  H70.93 Unspecified mastoiditis, bilateral

H71 Cholesteatoma of middle ear

Excludes2: *cholesteatoma of external ear (H60.4-)*
recurrent cholesteatoma of postmastoidectomy cavity (H95.0-)

+ **H71.0 Cholesteatoma of attic**
  H71.00 Cholesteatoma of attic, unspecified ear
  H71.01 Cholesteatoma of attic, right ear
  H71.02 Cholesteatoma of attic, left ear
  H71.03 Cholesteatoma of attic, bilateral
+ **H71.1 Cholesteatoma of tympanum**
  H71.10 Cholesteatoma of tympanum, unspecified ear
  H71.11 Cholesteatoma of tympanum, right ear
  H71.12 Cholesteatoma of tympanum, left ear
  H71.13 Cholesteatoma of tympanum, bilateral
+ **H71.2 Cholesteatoma of mastoid**
  H71.20 Cholesteatoma of mastoid, unspecified ear
  H71.21 Cholesteatoma of mastoid, right ear
  H71.22 Cholesteatoma of mastoid, left ear
  H71.23 Cholesteatoma of mastoid, bilateral
+ **H71.3 Diffuse cholesteatosis**
  H71.30 Diffuse cholesteatosis, unspecified ear
  H71.31 Diffuse cholesteatosis, right ear
  H71.32 Diffuse cholesteatosis, left ear
  H71.33 Diffuse cholesteatosis, bilateral
+ **H71.9 Unspecified cholesteatoma**
  H71.90 Unspecified cholesteatoma, unspecified ear
  H71.91 Unspecified cholesteatoma, right ear
  H71.92 Unspecified cholesteatoma, left ear
  H71.93 Unspecified cholesteatoma, bilateral

H72 Perforation of tympanic membrane

Includes: persistent post-traumatic perforation of ear drum
postinflammatory perforation of ear drum

Code first any associated otitis media (H65.-, H66.1-, H66.2-, H66.3-, H66.4-, H66.9-, H67.-)

Excludes1: *acute suppurative otitis media with rupture of the tympani membrane (H66.01-)*
traumatic rupture of ear drum (S09.2-)

+ **H72.0 Central perforation of tympanic membrane**
  H72.00 Central perforation of tympanic membrane, unspecified ear
  H72.01 Central perforation of tympanic membrane, right ear
  H72.02 Central perforation of tympanic membrane, left ear
  H72.03 Central perforation of tympanic membrane, bilateral
+ **H72.1 Attic perforation of tympanic membrane**
  Perforation of pars flaccida
  H72.10 Attic perforation of tympanic membrane, unspecified ear
  H72.11 Attic perforation of tympanic membrane, right ear
  H72.12 Attic perforation of tympanic membrane, left ear
  H72.13 Attic perforation of tympanic membrane, bilateral
+ **H72.2 Other marginal perforations of tympanic membrane**
  + **H72.2X Other marginal perforations of tympanic membran**
    H72.2X1 Other marginal perforations of tympanic membrane, right ear
    H72.2X2 Other marginal perforations of tympanic membrane, left ear
    H72.2X3 Other marginal perforations of tympanic membrane, bilateral
    H72.2X9 Other marginal perforations of tympanic membrane, unspecified ear

+ H72.8 Other perforations of tympanic membrane
+ H72.81 Multiple perforations of tympanic membrane
H72.811 Multiple perforations of tympanic membrane, right ear
H72.812 Multiple perforations of tympanic membrane, left ear
H72.813 Multiple perforations of tympanic membrane, bilateral
H72.819 Multiple perforations of tympanic membrane, unspecified ear
+ H72.82 Total perforations of tympanic membrane
H72.821 Total perforations of tympanic membrane, right ear
H72.822 Total perforations of tympanic membrane, left ear
H72.823 Total perforations of tympanic membrane, bilateral
H72.829 Total perforations of tympanic membrane, unspecified ear
+ H72.9 Unspecified perforation of tympanic membrane
H72.90 Unspecified perforation of tympanic membrane, unspecified ear
H72.91 Unspecified perforation of tympanic membrane, right ear
H72.92 Unspecified perforation of tympanic membrane, left ear
H72.93 Unspecified perforation of tympanic membrane, bilateral

H73 Other disorders of tympanic membrane

+ H73.0 Acute myringitis
Excludes1: *acute myringitis with otitis media (H65, H66)*
+ H73.00 Unspecified acute myringitis
Acute tympanitis NOS
H73.001 Acute myringitis, right ear
H73.002 Acute myringitis, left ear
H73.003 Acute myringitis, bilateral
H73.009 Acute myringitis, unspecified ear
+ H73.01 Bullous myringitis
H73.011 Bullous myringitis, right ear
H73.012 Bullous myringitis, left ear
H73.013 Bullous myringitis, bilateral
H73.019 Bullous myringitis, unspecified ear
+ H73.09 Other acute myringitis
H73.091 Other acute myringitis, right ear
H73.092 Other acute myringitis, left ear
H73.093 Other acute myringitis, bilateral
H73.099 Other acute myringitis, unspecified ear
+ H73.1 Chronic myringitis
Chronic tympanitis
Excludes1: *chronic myringitis with otitis media (H65, H66)*
H73.10 Chronic myringitis, unspecified ear
H73.11 Chronic myringitis, right ear
H73.12 Chronic myringitis, left ear
H73.13 Chronic myringitis, bilateral
+ H73.2 Unspecified myringitis
H73.20 Unspecified myringitis, unspecified ear
H73.21 Unspecified myringitis, right ear
H73.22 Unspecified myringitis, left ear
H73.23 Unspecified myringitis, bilateral
+ H73.8 Other specified disorders of tympanic membrane
+ H73.81 Atrophic flaccid tympanic membrane
H73.811 Atrophic flaccid tympanic membrane, right ear
H73.812 Atrophic flaccid tympanic membrane, left ear
H73.813 Atrophic flaccid tympanic membrane, bilateral
H73.819 Atrophic flaccid tympanic membrane, unspecified ear
+ H73.82 Atrophic nonflaccid tympanic membrane
H73.821 Atrophic nonflaccid tympanic membrane, right ear
H73.822 Atrophic nonflaccid tympanic membrane, left ear
H73.823 Atrophic nonflaccid tympanic membrane, bilateral
H73.829 Atrophic nonflaccid tympanic membrane, unspecified ear
+ H73.89 Other specified disorders of tympanic membrane
H73.891 Other specified disorders of tympanic membrane, right ear
H73.892 Other specified disorders of tympanic membrane, left ear
H73.893 Other specified disorders of tympanic membrane, bilateral
H73.899 Other specified disorders of tympanic membrane, unspecified ear
+ H73.9 Unspecified disorder of tympanic membrane
H73.90 Unspecified disorder of tympanic membrane, unspecified ear
H73.91 Unspecified disorder of tympanic membrane, right ear
H73.92 Unspecified disorder of tympanic membrane, left ear
H73.93 Unspecified disorder of tympanic membrane, bilateral

H74 Other disorders of middle ear mastoid

Excludes2: *mastoiditis (H70.-)*
+ H74.0 Tympanosclerosis
H74.01 Tympanosclerosis, right ear
H74.02 Tympanosclerosis, left ear
H74.03 Tympanosclerosis, bilateral
H74.09 Tympanosclerosis, unspecified ear
+ H74.1 Adhesive middle ear disease
Adhesive otitis
Excludes1: *glue ear (H65.3-)*
H74.11 Adhesive right middle ear disease
H74.12 Adhesive left middle ear disease
H74.13 Adhesive middle ear disease, bilateral
H74.19 Adhesive middle ear disease, unspecified ear
+ H74.2 Discontinuity and dislocation of ear ossicles
H74.20 Discontinuity and dislocation of ear ossicles, unspecified ear
H74.21 Discontinuity and dislocation of right ear ossicles
H74.22 Discontinuity and dislocation of left ear ossicles
H74.23 Discontinuity and dislocation of ear ossicles, bilateral
+ H74.3 Other acquired abnormalities of ear ossicles
+ H74.31 Ankylosis of ear ossicles
H74.311 Ankylosis of ear ossicles, right ear
H74.312 Ankylosis of ear ossicles, left ear
H74.313 Ankylosis of ear ossicles, bilateral
H74.319 Ankylosis of ear ossicles, unspecified ear
+ H74.32 Partial loss of ear ossicles
H74.321 Partial loss of ear ossicles, right ear
H74.322 Partial loss of ear ossicles, left ear
H74.323 Partial loss of ear ossicles, bilateral
H74.329 Partial loss of ear ossicles, unspecified ear
+ H74.39 Other acquired abnormalities of ear ossicles
H74.391 Other acquired abnormalities of right ear ossicles
H74.392 Other acquired abnormalities of left ear ossicles
H74.393 Other acquired abnormalities of ear ossicles, bilateral
H74.399 Other acquired abnormalities of ear ossicles, unspecified ear
+ H74.4 Polyp of middle ear
H74.40 Polyp of middle ear, unspecified ear
H74.41 Polyp of right middle ear
H74.42 Polyp of left middle ear
H74.43 Polyp of middle ear, bilateral
+ H74.8 Other specified disorders of middle ear and mastoid
+ H74.8X Other specified disorders of middle ear and mastoid
H74.8X1 Other specified disorders of right middle ear and mastoid
H74.8X2 Other specified disorders of left middle ear and mastoid
H74.8X3 Other specified disorders of middle ear and mastoid, bilateral
H74.8X9 Other specified disorders of middle ear and mastoid, unspecified ear
+ H74.9 Unspecified disorder of middle ear and mastoid
H74.90 Unspecified disorder of middle ear and mastoid, unspecified ear
H74.91 Unspecified disorder of right middle ear and mastoid
H74.92 Unspecified disorder of left middle ear and mastoid
H74.93 Unspecified disorder of middle ear and mastoid, bilateral

H75 Other disorders of middle ear and mastoid in diseases classified elsewhere

Code first underlying disease

+ **H75.0 Mastoiditis in infectious and parasitic diseases classified elsewhere**
  - ***Excludes1:*** *mastoiditis (in):*
    - *syphilis (A52.77)*
    - *tuberculosis (A18.03)*
  - **H75.00 Mastoiditis in infectious and parasitic diseases classified elsewhere, unspecified ear**
  - **H75.01 Mastoiditis in infectious and parasitic diseases classified elsewhere, right ear**
  - **H75.02 Mastoiditis in infectious and parasitic diseases classified elsewhere, left ear**
  - **H75.03 Mastoiditis in infectious and parasitic diseases classified elsewhere, bilateral**
+ **H75.8 Other specified disorders of middle ear and mastoid in diseases classified elsewhere**
  - **H75.80 Other specified disorders of middle ear and mastoid in diseases classified elsewhere, unspecified ear**
  - **H75.81 Other specified disorders of right middle ear and mastoid in diseases classified elsewhere**
  - **H75.82 Other specified disorders of left middle ear and mastoid in diseases classified elsewhere**
  - **H75.83 Other specified disorders of middle ear and mastoid in diseases classified elsewhere, bilateral**

Diseases of inner ear (H80-H83)

H80 Otosclerosis

Includes: Otospongiosis

+ **H80.0 Otosclerosis involving oval window, nonobliterative**
  - **H80.00 Otosclerosis involving oval window, nonobliterative, unspecified ear**
  - **H80.01 Otosclerosis involving oval window, nonobliterative, right ear**
  - **H80.02 Otosclerosis involving oval window, nonobliterative, left ear**
  - **H80.03 Otosclerosis involving oval window, nonobliterative, bilateral**
+ **H80.1 Otosclerosis involving oval window, obliterative**
  - **H80.10 Otosclerosis involving oval window, obliterative, unspecified ear**
  - **H80.11 Otosclerosis involving oval window, obliterative, right ear**
  - **H80.12 Otosclerosis involving oval window, obliterative, left ear**
  - **H80.13 Otosclerosis involving oval window, obliterative, bilateral**
+ **H80.2 Cochlear otosclerosis**
  - Otosclerosis involving otic capsule
  - Otosclerosis involving round window
  - **H80.20 Cochlear otosclerosis, unspecified ear**
  - **H80.21 Cochlear otosclerosis, right ear**
  - **H80.22 Cochlear otosclerosis, left ear**
  - **H80.23 Cochlear otosclerosis, bilateral**
+ **H80.8 Other otosclerosis**
  - **H80.80 Other otosclerosis, unspecified ear**
  - **H80.81 Other otosclerosis, right ear**
  - **H80.82 Other otosclerosis, left ear**
  - **H80.83 Other otosclerosis, bilateral**
+ **H80.9 Unspecified otosclerosis**
  - **H80.90 Unspecified otosclerosis, unspecified ear**
  - **H80.91 Unspecified otosclerosis, right ear**
  - **H80.92 Unspecified otosclerosis, left ear**
  - **H80.93 Unspecified otosclerosis, bilateral**

H81 Disorders of vestibular function

Excludes1: *epidemic vertigo (A88.1)*
vertigo NOS (R42)

+ **H81.0 Ménière's disease**
  - Labyrinthine hydrops
  - Ménière's syndrome or vertigo
  - **H81.01 Ménière's disease, right ear**
  - **H81.02 Ménière's disease, left ear**
  - **H81.03 Ménière's disease, bilateral**
  - **H81.09 Ménière's disease, unspecified ear**
+ **H81.1 Benign paroxysmal vertigo**
  - **H81.10 Benign paroxysmal vertigo, unspecified ear**
  - **H81.11 Benign paroxysmal vertigo, right ear**
  - **H81.12 Benign paroxysmal vertigo, left ear**
  - **H81.13 Benign paroxysmal vertigo, bilateral**
+ **H81.2 Vestibular neuronitis**
  - **H81.20 Vestibular neuronitis, unspecified ear**
  - **H81.21 Vestibular neuronitis, right ear**
  - **H81.22 Vestibular neuronitis, left ear**
  - **H81.23 Vestibular neuronitis, bilateral**
+ **H81.3 Other peripheral vertigo**
  + **H81.31 Aural vertigo**
    - **H81.311 Aural vertigo, right ear**
    - **H81.312 Aural vertigo, left ear**
    - **H81.313 Aural vertigo, bilateral**
    - **H81.319 Aural vertigo, unspecified ear**
  + **H81.39 Other peripheral vertigo**
    - Lermoyez' syndrome
    - Otogenic vertigo
    - Peripheral vertigo NOS
    - **H81.391 Other peripheral vertigo, right ear**
    - **H81.392 Other peripheral vertigo, left ear**
    - **H81.393 Other peripheral vertigo, bilateral**
    - **H81.399 Other peripheral vertigo, unspecified ear**
+ **H81.4 Vertigo of central origin**
  - Central positional nystagmus
  - **H81.41 Vertigo of central origin, right ear**
  - **H81.42 Vertigo of central origin, left ear**
  - **H81.43 Vertigo of central origin, bilateral**
  - **H81.49 Vertigo of central origin, unspecified ear**
+ **H81.8 Other disorders of vestibular function**
  + **H81.8X Other disorders of vestibular function**
    - **H81.8X1 Other disorders of vestibular function, right ear**
    - **H81.8X2 Other disorders of vestibular function, left ear**
    - **H81.8X3 Other disorders of vestibular function, bilateral**
    - **H81.8X9 Other disorders of vestibular function, unspecified ear**
+ **H81.9 Unspecified disorder of vestibular function**
  - Vertiginous syndrome NOS
  - **H81.90 Unspecified disorder of vestibular function, unspecified ear**
  - **H81.91 Unspecified disorder of vestibular function, right ea**
  - **H81.92 Unspecified disorder of vestibular function, left ear**
  - **H81.93 Unspecified disorder of vestibular function, bilatera**

H82 Vertiginous syndromes in diseases classified elsewhere

Code first underlying disease

Excludes1: *epidemic vertigo (A88.1)*

- **H82.1 Vertiginous syndromes in diseases classified elsewhere, right ear**
- **H82.2 Vertiginous syndromes in diseases classified elsewhere, left ea**
- **H82.3 Vertiginous syndromes in diseases classified elsewhere, bilateral**
- **H82.9 Vertiginous syndromes in diseases classified elsewhere, unspecified ear**

H83 Other diseases of inner ear

+ **H83.0 Labyrinthitis**
  - **H83.01 Labyrinthitis, right ear**
  - **H83.02 Labyrinthitis, left ear**
  - **H83.03 Labyrinthitis, bilateral**
  - **H83.09 Labyrinthitis, unspecified ear**
+ **H83.1 Labyrinthine fistula**
  - **H83.11 Labyrinthine fistula, right ear**
  - **H83.12 Labyrinthine fistula, left ear**
  - **H83.13 Labyrinthine fistula, bilateral**
  - **H83.19 Labyrinthine fistula, unspecified ear**
+ **H83.2 Labyrinthine dysfunction**
  - Labyrinthine hypersensitivity
  - Labyrinthine hypofunction
  - Labyrinthine loss of function
  + **H83.2X Labyrinthine dysfunction**
    - **H83.2X1 Labyrinthine dysfunction, right ear**
    - **H83.2X2 Labyrinthine dysfunction, left ear**
    - **H83.2X3 Labyrinthine dysfunction, bilateral**
    - **H83.2X9 Labyrinthine dysfunction, unspecified ear**
+ **H83.3 Noise effects on inner ear**
  - Acoustic trauma of inner ear
  - Noise-induced hearing loss of inner ear

+ H83.3X Noise effects on inner ear
H83.3X1 Noise effects on right inner ear
H83.3X2 Noise effects on left inner ear
H83.3X3 Noise effects on inner ear, bilateral
H83.3X9 Noise effects on inner ear, unspecified ear
+ H83.8 Other specified diseases of inner ear
+ H83.8X Other specified diseases of inner ear
H83.8X1 Other specified diseases of right inner ear
H83.8X2 Other specified diseases of left inner ear
H83.8X3 Other specified diseases of inner ear, bilateral
H83.8X9 Other specified diseases of inner ear, unspecified ear
+ H83.9 Unspecified disease of inner ear
H83.90 Unspecified disease of inner ear, unspecified ear
H83.91 Unspecified disease of right inner ear
H83.92 Unspecified disease of left inner ear
H83.93 Unspecified disease of inner ear, bilateral

Other disorders of ear (H90-H94)

H90 Conductive and sensorineural hearing loss

Excludes1: *deaf nonspeaking NEC (H91.3)*
deafness NOS (H91.9-)
hearing loss NOS (H91.9-)
noise-induced hearing loss (H83.3-)
ototoxic hearing loss (H91.0-)
sudden (idiopathic) hearing loss (H91.2-)

H90.0 Conductive hearing loss, bilateral
+ H90.1 Conductive hearing loss, unilateral with unrestricted hearing on the contralateral side
H90.11 Conductive hearing loss, unilateral, right ear, with unrestricted hearing on the contralateral side
H90.12 Conductive hearing loss, unilateral, left ear, with unrestricted hearing on the contralateral side
H90.2 Conductive hearing loss, unspecified
Conductive deafness NOS
H90.3 Sensorineural hearing loss, bilateral
+ H90.4 Sensorineural hearing loss, unilateral with unrestricted hearing on the contralateral side
H90.41 Sensorineural hearing loss, unilateral, right ear, with unrestricted hearing on the contralateral side
H90.42 Sensorineural hearing loss, unilateral, left ear, with unrestricted hearing on the contralateral side
H90.5 Unspecified sensorineural hearing loss
Central hearing loss NOS
Congenital deafness NOS
Neural hearing loss NOS
Perceptive hearing loss NOS
Sensorineural deafness NOS
Sensory hearing loss NOS
Excludes1: *abnormal auditory perception (H93.2-)*
psychogenic deafness (F44.6)
H90.6 Mixed conductive and sensorineural hearing loss, bilateral
AHA CC: 2Q, 2015, 7
+ H90.7 Mixed conductive and sensorineural hearing loss, unilateral with unrestricted hearing on the contralateral side
H90.71 Mixed conductive and sensorineural hearing loss, unilateral, right ear, with unrestricted hearing on the contralateral side
H90.72 Mixed conductive and sensorineural hearing loss, unilateral, left ear, with unrestricted hearing on the contralateral side
H90.8 Mixed conductive and sensorineural hearing loss, unspecified
+ H90.A Conductive and sensorineural hearing loss with restricted hearing on the contralateral side
AHA CC: 4Q, 2016, 23-24
+ H90.A1 Conductive hearing loss, unilateral, with restricted hearing on the contralateral side
H90.A11 Conductive hearing loss, unilateral, right ear with restricted hearing on the contralateral side
H90.A12 Conductive hearing loss, unilateral, left ear with restricted hearing on the contralateral side
AHA CC: 4Q, 2016, 24-25
+ H90.A2 Sensorineural hearing loss, unilateral, with restricted hearing on the contralateral side
H90.A21 Sensorineural hearing loss, unilateral, right ear, with restricted hearing on the contralateral side
AHA CC: 4Q, 2016, 24-25
H90.A22 Sensorineural hearing loss, unilateral, left ear, with restricted hearing on the contralateral side
+ H90.A3 Mixed conductive and sensorineural hearing loss, unilateral with restricted hearing on the contralateral side
H90.A31 Mixed conductive and sensorineural hearing loss, unilateral, right ear with restricted hearing on the contralateral side
H90.A32 Mixed conductive and sensorineural hearing, unilateral, left ear with restricted hearing on the contralateral side

H91 Other and unspecified hearing loss

Excludes1: *abnormal auditory perception (H93.2-)*
hearing loss as classified in H90.-
impacted cerumen (H61.2-)
noise-induced hearing loss (H83.3-)
psychogenic deafness (F44.6)
transient ischemic deafness (H93.01-)

+ H91.0 Ototoxic hearing loss
Code first poisoning due to drug or toxin, if applicable (T36-T65 with fifth or sixth character 1-4 or 6)
Use additional code for adverse effect, if applicable, to identify drug (T36-T50 with fifth or sixth character 5)
H91.01 Ototoxic hearing loss, right ear
H91.02 Ototoxic hearing loss, left ear
H91.03 Ototoxic hearing loss, bilateral
H91.09 Ototoxic hearing loss, unspecified ear
+ H91.1 Presbycusis
Presbyacusia
H91.10 Presbycusis, unspecified ear
H91.11 Presbycusis, right ear
H91.12 Presbycusis, left ear
H91.13 Presbycusis, bilateral
+ H91.2 Sudden idiopathic hearing loss
Sudden hearing loss NOS
H91.20 Sudden idiopathic hearing loss, unspecified ear
H91.21 Sudden idiopathic hearing loss, right ear
H91.22 Sudden idiopathic hearing loss, left ear
H91.23 Sudden idiopathic hearing loss, bilateral
H91.3 Deaf nonspeaking, not elsewhere classified
+ H91.8 Other specified hearing loss
+ H91.8X Other specified hearing loss
H91.8X1 Other specified hearing loss, right ear
H91.8X2 Other specified hearing loss, left ear
H91.8X3 Other specified hearing loss, bilateral
H91.8X9 Other specified hearing loss, unspecified ear
+ H91.9 Unspecified hearing loss
Deafness NOS
High frequency deafness
Low frequency deafness
H91.90 Unspecified hearing loss, unspecified ear
H91.91 Unspecified hearing loss, right ear
H91.92 Unspecified hearing loss, left ear
H91.93 Unspecified hearing loss, bilateral

H92 Otalgia and effusion of ear

+ H92.0 Otalgia
H92.01 Otalgia, right ear
H92.02 Otalgia, left ear
H92.03 Otalgia, bilateral
H92.09 Otalgia, unspecified ear
+ H92.1 Otorrhea
Excludes1: *leakage of cerebrospinal fluid through ear (G96.0)*
H92.10 Otorrhea, unspecified ear
H92.11 Otorrhea, right ear
H92.12 Otorrhea, left ear
H92.13 Otorrhea, bilateral
+ H92.2 Otorrhagia
Excludes1: *traumatic otorrhagia - code to injury*
H92.20 Otorrhagia, unspecified ear
H92.21 Otorrhagia, right ear
H92.22 Otorrhagia, left ear
H92.23 Otorrhagia, bilateral

H93 Other disorders of ear, not elsewhere classified

+ **H93.0 Degenerative and vascular disorders of ear**
  Excludes1: *presbycusis (H91.1)*
  + **H93.01 Transient ischemic deafness**
    - **H93.011 Transient ischemic deafness, right ear**
    - **H93.012 Transient ischemic deafness, left ear**
    - **H93.013 Transient ischemic deafness, bilateral**
    - **H93.019 Transient ischemic deafness, unspecified ear**
  + **H93.09 Unspecified degenerative and vascular disorders of ear**
    - **H93.091 Unspecified degenerative and vascular disorders of right ear**
    - **H93.092 Unspecified degenerative and vascular disorders of left ear**
    - **H93.093 Unspecified degenerative and vascular disorders of ear, bilateral**
    - **H93.099 Unspecified degenerative and vascular disorders of unspecified ear**

+ **H93.1 Tinnitus**
  - **H93.11 Tinnitus, right ear**
  - **H93.12 Tinnitus, left ear**
  - **H93.13 Tinnitus, bilateral**
  - **H93.19 Tinnitus, unspecified ear**

+ **H93.A Pulsatile tinnitus**
  AHA CC: 4Q, 2016, 25-26
  - **H93.A1 Pulsatile tinnitus, right ear**
    AHA CC: 4Q, 2016, 26
  - **H93.A2 Pulsatile tinnitus, left ear**
  - **H93.A3 Pulsatile tinnitus, bilateral**
  - **H93.A9 Pulsatile tinnitus, unspecified ear**

+ **H93.2 Other abnormal auditory perceptions**
  Excludes2: *auditory hallucinations (R44.0)*
  + **H93.21 Auditory recruitment**
    - **H93.211 Auditory recruitment, right ear**
    - **H93.212 Auditory recruitment, left ear**
    - **H93.213 Auditory recruitment, bilateral**
    - **H93.219 Auditory recruitment, unspecified ear**
  + **H93.22 Diplacusis**
    - **H93.221 Diplacusis, right ear**
    - **H93.222 Diplacusis, left ear**
    - **H93.223 Diplacusis, bilateral**
    - **H93.229 Diplacusis, unspecified ear**
  + **H93.23 Hyperacusis**
    - **H93.231 Hyperacusis, right ear**
    - **H93.232 Hyperacusis, left ear**
    - **H93.233 Hyperacusis, bilateral**
    - **H93.239 Hyperacusis, unspecified ear**
  + **H93.24 Temporary auditory threshold shift**
    - **H93.241 Temporary auditory threshold shift, right ear**
    - **H93.242 Temporary auditory threshold shift, left ear**
    - **H93.243 Temporary auditory threshold shift, bilateral**
    - **H93.249 Temporary auditory threshold shift, unspecified ear**
  - **H93.25 Central auditory processing disorder**
    Congenital auditory imperception
    Word deafness
    Excludes1: *mixed receptive-expressive language disorder (F80.2)*
  + **H93.29 Other abnormal auditory perceptions**
    - **H93.291 Other abnormal auditory perceptions, right ear**
    - **H93.292 Other abnormal auditory perceptions, left ear**
    - **H93.293 Other abnormal auditory perceptions, bilateral**
    - **H93.299 Other abnormal auditory perceptions, unspecified ear**

+ **H93.3 Disorders of acoustic nerve**
  Disorder of 8th cranial nerve
  Excludes1: *acoustic neuroma (D33.3)*
  syphilitic acoustic neuritis (A52.15)
  + **H93.3X Disorders of acoustic nerve**
    - **H93.3X1 Disorders of right acoustic nerve**
    - **H93.3X2 Disorders of left acoustic nerve**
    - **H93.3X3 Disorders of bilateral acoustic nerves**
    - **H93.3X9 Disorders of unspecified acoustic nerve**

+ **H93.8 Other specified disorders of ear**
  + **H93.8X Other specified disorders of ear**
    - **H93.8X1 Other specified disorders of right ear**
    - **H93.8X2 Other specified disorders of left ear**
    - **H93.8X3 Other specified disorders of ear, bilateral**
    - **H93.8X9 Other specified disorders of ear, unspecified ear**

+ **H93.9 Unspecified disorder of ear**
  - **H93.90 Unspecified disorder of ear, unspecified ear**
  - **H93.91 Unspecified disorder of right ear**
  - **H93.92 Unspecified disorder of left ear**
  - **H93.93 Unspecified disorder of ear, bilateral**

H94 Other disorders of ear in diseases classified elsewhere

+ **H94.0 Acoustic neuritis in infectious and parasitic diseases classified elsewhere**
  Code first underlying disease, such as:
  parasitic disease (B65-B89)
  Excludes1: *acoustic neuritis (in):*
  herpes zoster (B02.29)
  syphilis (A52.15)
  - **H94.00 Acoustic neuritis in infectious and parasitic diseases classified elsewhere, unspecified ear**
  - **H94.01 Acoustic neuritis in infectious and parasitic diseases classified elsewhere, right ear**
  - **H94.02 Acoustic neuritis in infectious and parasitic diseases classified elsewhere, left ear**
  - **H94.03 Acoustic neuritis in infectious and parasitic diseases classified elsewhere, bilateral**

+ **H94.8 Other specified disorders of ear in diseases classified elsewhere**
  Code first underlying disease, such as:
  congenital syphilis (A50.0)
  Excludes1: *aural myiasis (B87.4)*
  syphilitic labyrinthitis (A52.79)
  - **H94.80 Other specified disorders of ear in diseases classified elsewhere, unspecified ear**
  - **H94.81 Other specified disorders of right ear in diseases classified elsewhere**
  - **H94.82 Other specified disorders of left ear in diseases classified elsewhere**
  - **H94.83 Other specified disorders of ear in diseases classified elsewhere, bilateral**

Intraoperative and postprocedural complications and disorders of ear and mastoid process, not elsewhere classified (H95)

H95 Intraoperative and postprocedural complications and disorders of ear and mastoid process, not elsewhere classified
AHA CC: 4Q, 2016, 9-10

+ **H95.0 Recurrent cholesteatoma of postmastoidectomy cavity**
  - **H95.00 Recurrent cholesteatoma of postmastoidectomy cavity, unspecified ear**
  - **H95.01 Recurrent cholesteatoma of postmastoidectomy cavity, right ear**
  - **H95.02 Recurrent cholesteatoma of postmastoidectomy cavity, left ear**
  - **H95.03 Recurrent cholesteatoma of postmastoidectomy cavity, bilateral ears**

+ **H95.1 Other disorders of ear and mastoid process following mastoidectomy**
  + **H95.11 Chronic inflammation of postmastoidectomy cavity**
    - **H95.111 Chronic inflammation of postmastoidectomy cavity, right ear**
    - **H95.112 Chronic inflammation of postmastoidectomy cavity, left ear**
    - **H95.113 Chronic inflammation of postmastoidectomy cavity, bilateral ears**
    - **H95.119 Chronic inflammation of postmastoidectomy cavity, unspecified ear**
  + **H95.12 Granulation of postmastoidectomy cavity**
    - **H95.121 Granulation of postmastoidectomy cavity, right ear**
    - **H95.122 Granulation of postmastoidectomy cavity, left ear**
    - **H95.123 Granulation of postmastoidectomy cavity, bilateral ears**
    - **H95.129 Granulation of postmastoidectomy cavity, unspecified ear**

+ H95.13 Mucosal cyst of postmastoidectomy cavity
  - H95.131 Mucosal cyst of postmastoidectomy cavity, right ear
  - H95.132 Mucosal cyst of postmastoidectomy cavity, left ear
  - H95.133 Mucosal cyst of postmastoidectomy cavity, bilateral ears
  - H95.139 Mucosal cyst of postmastoidectomy cavity, unspecified ear

+ H95.19 Other disorders following mastoidectomy
  - H95.191 Other disorders following mastoidectomy, right ear
  - H95.192 Other disorders following mastoidectomy, left ear
  - H95.193 Other disorders following mastoidectomy, bilateral ears
  - H95.199 Other disorders following mastoidectomy, unspecified ear

+ H95.2 Intraoperative hemorrhage and hematoma of ear and mastoid process complicating a procedure

Excludes1: *intraoperative hemorrhage and hematoma of ear and mastoid process due to accidental puncture or laceration during a procedure (H95.3-)*

CC H95.21 Intraoperative hemorrhage and hematoma of ear and mastoid process complicating a procedure on the ear and mastoid process
CC Exclusion see Appendix A PDX collection 0642

CC H95.22 Intraoperative hemorrhage and hematoma of ear and mastoid process complicating other procedure
CC Exclusion see Appendix A PDX collection 0642

+ H95.3 Accidental puncture and laceration of ear and mastoid process during a procedure

CC H95.31 Accidental puncture and laceration of the ear and mastoid process during a procedure on the ear and mastoid process
CC Exclusion see Appendix A PDX collection 0509

CC H95.32 Accidental puncture and laceration of the ear and mastoid process during other procedure
CC Exclusion see Appendix A PDX collection 0509

+ H95.4 Postprocedural hemorrhage of ear and mastoid process following a procedure

CC H95.41 Postprocedural hemorrhage of ear and mastoid process following a procedure on the ear and mastoid process
CC Exclusion see Appendix A PDX collection 0642

CC H95.42 Postprocedural hemorrhage of ear and mastoid process following other procedure
CC Exclusion see Appendix A PDX collection 0642

+ H95.5 Postprocedural hematoma and seroma of ear and mastoid process following a procedure

CC H95.51 Postprocedural hematoma of ear and mastoid process following a procedure on the ear and mastoid process
CC Exclusion see Appendix A PDX collection 0642

CC H95.52 Postprocedural hematoma of ear and mastoid process following other procedure
CC Exclusion see Appendix A PDX collection 0642

CC H95.53 Postprocedureal seroma of ear and mastoid process following a procedure on the ear and mastoid process
CC Exclusion see Appendix A PDX collection 0642

CC H95.54 Postprocedureal seroma of ear and mastoid process following other procedure
CC Exclusion see Appendix A PDX collection 0642

+ H95.8 Other intraoperative and postprocedural complications and disorders of the ear and mastoid process, not elsewhere classified

Excludes2: *postprocedural complications and disorders following mastoidectomy (H95.0-, H95.1-)*

+ H95.81 Postprocedural stenosis of external ear canal

CC H95.811 Postprocedural stenosis of right external ear canal
CC Exclusion see Appendix A PDX collection 0643

CC H95.812 Postprocedural stenosis of left external ear canal
CC Exclusion see Appendix A PDX collection 0643

CC H95.813 Postprocedural stenosis of external ear canal, bilateral
CC Exclusion see Appendix A PDX collection 0643

CC H95.819 Postprocedural stenosis of unspecified external ear canal
CC Exclusion see Appendix A PDX collection 0643

CC H95.88 Other intraoperative complications and disorders of the ear and mastoid process, not elsewhere classified
Use additional code, if applicable, to further specify disorder
CC Exclusion see Appendix A PDX collection 0643

CC H95.89 Other postprocedural complications and disorders of the ear and mastoid process, not elsewhere classified
Use additional code, if applicable, to further specify disorder
CC Exclusion see Appendix A PDX collection 0643

Chapter 9: Diseases of the Circulatory System (I00-I99)

Excludes2: *certain conditions originating in the perinatal period (P04-P96)*
certain infectious and parasitic diseases (A00-B99)
complications of pregnancy, childbirth and the puerperium (O00-O9A)
congenital malformations, deformations, and chromosomal abnormalities (Q00-Q99)
endocrine, nutritional and metabolic diseases (E00-E88)
injury, poisoning and certain other consequences of external causes (S00-T88)
neoplasms (C00-D49)
symptoms, signs and abnormal clinical and laboratory findings, not elsewhere classified (R00-R94)
systemic connective tissue disorders (M30-M36)
transient cerebral ischemic attacks and related syndromes (G45.-)

This chapter contains the following category blocks:

I00-I02 Acute rheumatic fever
I05-I09 Chronic rheumatic heart diseases
I10-I16 Hypertensive diseases
I20-I25 Ischemic heart diseases
I26-I28 Pulmonary heart disease and diseases of pulmonary circulation
I30-I52 Other forms of heart disease
I60-I69 Cerebrovascular diseases
I70-I79 Diseases of arteries, arterioles and capillaries
I80-I89 Diseases of veins, lymphatic vessels and lymph nodes, not elsewhere classified
I95-I99 Other and unspecified disorders of the circulatory system

C. Chapter-Specific Coding Guidelines

In addition to general coding guidelines, there are guidelines for specific diagnoses and/or conditions in the classification. Unless otherwise indicated, these guidelines apply to all health care settings. Please refer to Section II for guidelines on the selection of principal diagnosis.

9. Chapter 9: Diseases of the Circulatory System (I00-I99)

a. Hypertension

The classification presumes a causal relationship between hypertension and heart involvement and between hypertension and kidney involvement, as the two conditions are linked by the term "with" in the Alphabetic Index. These conditions should be coded as related even in the absence of provider documentation explicitly linking them, unless the documentation clearly states the conditions are unrelated.

For hypertension and conditions not specifically linked by relational terms such as "with," "associated with" or "due to" in the classification, provider documentation must link the conditions in order to code them as related.

1) Hypertension with Heart Disease

Hypertension with heart conditions classified to I50.- or I51.4-I51.9, are assigned to, a code from category I11, Hypertensive heart disease. Use an additional code**(s)** from category I50, Heart failure, to identify the type**(s)** of heart failure in those patients with heart failure.

The same heart conditions (I50.-, I51.4-I51.9) with hypertension are coded separately if the provider has specifically documented a different cause. Sequence according to the circumstances of the admission/encounter.

2) Hypertensive Chronic Kidney Disease

Assign codes from category I12, Hypertensive chronic kidney disease, when both hypertension and a condition classifiable to category N18, Chronic kidney disease (CKD), are present. CKD should not be coded as hypertensive if the physician has specifically documented a different cause.

The appropriate code from category N18 should be used as a secondary code with a code from category I12 to identify the stage of chronic kidney disease.

See Section I.C.14. Chronic kidney disease.

If a patient has hypertensive chronic kidney disease and acute renal failure, an additional code for the acute renal failure is required.

3) Hypertensive Heart and Chronic Kidney Disease

Assign codes from combination category I13, Hypertensive heart and chronic kidney disease, when there is hypertension with both heart and kidney involvement. If heart failure is present, assign an additional code from category I50 to identify the type of heart failure.

The appropriate code from category N18, Chronic kidney disease, should be used as a secondary code with a code from category I13 to identify the stage of chronic kidney disease.

See Section I.C.14. Chronic kidney disease.

The codes in category I13, Hypertensive heart and chronic kidney disease, are combination codes that include hypertension, heart disease and chronic kidney disease. The Includes note at I13 specifies that the conditions included at I11 and I12 are included together in I13. If a patient has hypertension, heart disease and chronic kidney disease then a code from I13 should be used, not individual codes for hypertension, heart disease and chronic kidney disease, or codes from I11 or I12.

For patients with both acute renal failure and chronic kidney disease an additional code for acute renal failure is required.

4) Hypertensive Cerebrovascular Disease

For hypertensive cerebrovascular disease, first assign the appropriate code from categories I60-I69, followed by the appropriate hypertension code.

5) Hypertensive Retinopathy

Subcategory H35.0, Background retinopathy and retinal vascular changes should be used with a code from category I10 – I15, Hypertensive disease to include the systemic hypertension. The sequencing is based on the reason for the encounter.

6) Hypertension, Secondary

Secondary hypertension is due to an underlying condition. Two codes are required: one to identify the underlying etiology and one from category I15 to identify the hypertension. Sequencing of codes is determined by the reason for admission/encounter.

7) Hypertension, Transient

Assign code R03.0, Elevated blood pressure reading without diagnosis of hypertension, unless patient has an established diagnosis of hypertension. Assign code O13.-, Gestational [pregnancy-induced] hypertension without significant proteinuria, or O14.-, Pre-eclampsia, for transient hypertension of pregnancy.

8) Hypertension, Controlled

This diagnostic statement usually refers to an existing state of hypertension under control by therapy. Assign the appropriate code from categories I10-I15, Hypertensive diseases.

9) Hypertension, Uncontrolled

Uncontrolled hypertension may refer to untreated hypertension or hypertension not responding to current therapeutic regimen. In either case, assign the appropriate code from categories I10-I15, Hypertensive diseases.

10) Hypertensive Crisis

Assign a code from category I16, Hypertensive crisis, for documented hypertensive urgency, hypertensive emergency or unspecified hypertensive crisis. Code also any identified hypertensive disease (I10-I15). The sequencing is based on the reason for the encounter.

11) Pulmonary Hypertension

Pulmonary hypertension is classified to category I27, Other pulmonary heart diseases. For secondary pulmonary hypertension (I27.1, I27.2-) code also any associated conditions or adverse effects of drugs or toxins. The sequencing is based on the reason for the encounter.

b. Atherosclerotic Coronary Artery Disease and Angina

ICD-10-CM has combination codes for atherosclerotic heart disease with angina pectoris. The subcategories for these codes are I25.11, Atherosclerotic heart disease of native coronary artery with angina pectoris and I25.7, Atherosclerosis of coronary artery bypass graft(s) and coronary artery of transplanted heart with angina pectoris.

When using one of these combination codes it is not necessary to use an additional code for angina pectoris. A causal relationship can be assumed in a patient with both atherosclerosis and angina pectoris, unless the documentation indicates the angina is due to something other than the atherosclerosis.

If a patient with coronary artery disease is admitted due to an acute myocardial infarction (AMI), the AMI should be sequenced before the coronary artery disease.

See Section I.C.9. Acute myocardial infarction (AMI)

c. Intraoperative and Postprocedural Cerebrovascular Accident

Medical record documentation should clearly specify the cause- and-effect relationship between the medical intervention and the cerebrovascular accident in order to assign a code for intraoperative or postprocedural cerebrovascular accident.

Proper code assignment depends on whether it was an infarction or hemorrhage and whether it occurred intraoperatively or postoperatively. If it was a cerebral hemorrhage, code assignment depends on the type of procedure performed.

d. Sequelae of Cerebrovascular Disease

1) Category I69, Sequelae of Cerebrovascular disease

Category I69 is used to indicate conditions classifiable to categories I60-I67 as the causes of sequela (neurologic deficits), themselves classified elsewhere. These "late effects" include neurologic deficits that persist after initial onset of conditions classifiable to categories I60-I67. The neurologic deficits caused by cerebrovascular disease may be present from the onset or may arise at any time after the onset of the condition classifiable to categories I60-I67.

Codes from category I69, Sequelae of cerebrovascular disease, that specify hemiplegia, hemiparesis and monoplegia identify whether the dominant or nondominant side is affected. Should the affected side be documented, but not specified as dominant or nondominant, and the classification system does not indicate a default, code selection is as follows:

- For ambidextrous patients, the default should be dominant.
- If the left side is affected, the default is non-dominant.
- If the right side is affected, the default is dominant.

2) Codes from category I69 with codes from I60-I67

Codes from category I69 may be assigned on a health care record with codes from I60-I67, if the patient has a current cerebrovascular disease and deficits from an old cerebrovascular disease.

3) Codes from category I69 and Personal history of transient ischemic attack (TIA) and cerebral infarction (Z86.73)

Codes from category I69 should not be assigned if the patient does not have neurologic deficits.

See Section I.C.21. 4. History (of) for use of personal history codes

e. Acute myocardial infarction (AMI)

1) ST elevation myocardial infarction (STEMI) and non ST elevation myocardial infarction (NSTEMI)

The ICD-10-CM codes for **type 1** acute myocardial infarction (AMI) identify the site, such as anterolateral wall or true posterior wall. Subcategories I21.0-I21.2 and code I21.3 are used for **type 1** ST elevation myocardial infarction (STEMI). Code I21.4, Non-ST elevation (NSTEMI) myocardial infarction, is used for **type 1** non ST elevation myocardial infarction (NSTEMI) and nontransmural MIs.

If **a type 1** NSTEMI evolves to STEMI, assign the STEMI code. If **a type 1** STEMI converts to NSTEMI due to thrombolytic therapy, it is still coded as STEMI.

For encounters occurring while the myocardial infarction is equal to, or less than, four weeks old, including transfers to another acute setting or a postacute setting, and the myocardial infarction meets the definition for "other diagnoses" (see Section III, Reporting Additional Diagnoses), codes from category I21 may continue to be reported. For encounters after the 4 week time frame and the patient is still receiving care related to the myocardial infarction, the appropriate aftercare code should be assigned, rather than a code from category I21. For old or healed myocardial infarctions not requiring further care, code I25.2, Old myocardial infarction, may be assigned.

2) Acute myocardial infarction, unspecified

Code **I21.9, Acute myocardial infarction, unspecified**, is the default for unspecified acute myocardial infarction **or unspecified type**. If only **type 1** STEMI or transmural MI without the site is documented, assign code I21.3, **ST elevation (STEMI) myocardial infarction of unspecified site.**

3) AMI documented as nontransmural or subendocardial but site provided

If an AMI is documented as nontransmural or subendocardial, but the site is provided, it is still coded as a subendocardial AMI.

See Section I.C.21.3 for information on coding status post administration of tPA in a different facility within the last 24 hours.

4) Subsequent acute myocardial infarction

A code from category I22, Subsequent ST elevation (STEMI) and non ST elevation (NSTEMI) myocardial infarction, is to be used when a patient who has suffered **a type 1 or unspecified** AMI has a new AMI within the 4 week time frame of the initial AMI. A code from category I22 must be used in conjunction with a code from category I21. The sequencing of the I22 and I21 codes depends on the circumstances of the encounter.

Do not assign code I22 for subsequent myocardial infarctions other than type 1 or unspecified. For subsequent type 2 AMI assign only code I21.A1. For subsequent type 4 or type 5 AMI, assign only code I21.A9.

5) Other Types of Myocardial Infarction

The ICD-10-CM provides codes for different types of myocardial infarction. Type 1 myocardial infarctions are assigned to codes I21.0-I21.4.

Type 2 myocardial infarctions, and myocardial infarction due to demand ischemia or secondary to ischemic balance, is assigned to code I21.A1, Myocardial infarction type 2 with a code for the underlying cause. Do not assign code I24.8, Other forms of acute ischemic heart disease for the demand ischemia. Sequencing of type 2 AMI or the underlying cause is dependent on the circumstances of admission. When a type 2 AMI code is described as NSTEMI or STEMI, only assign code I21.A1. Codes I21.0-I21.4 should only be assigned for type 1 AMIs.

Acute myocardial infarctions type 3, 4a, 4b, 4c and 5 are assigned to code I21.A9, Other myocardial infarction type.

The "Code also" and "Code first" notes should be followed related to complications, and for coding of postprocedural myocardial infarctions during or following cardiac surgery.

Heart

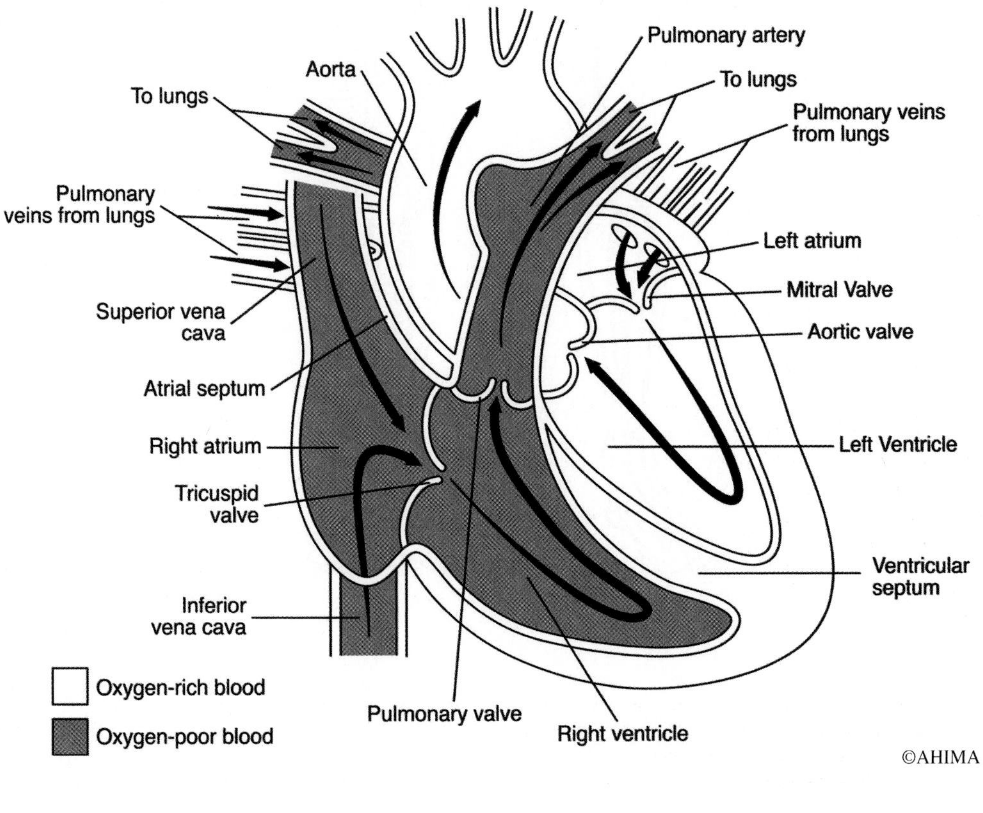

Veins

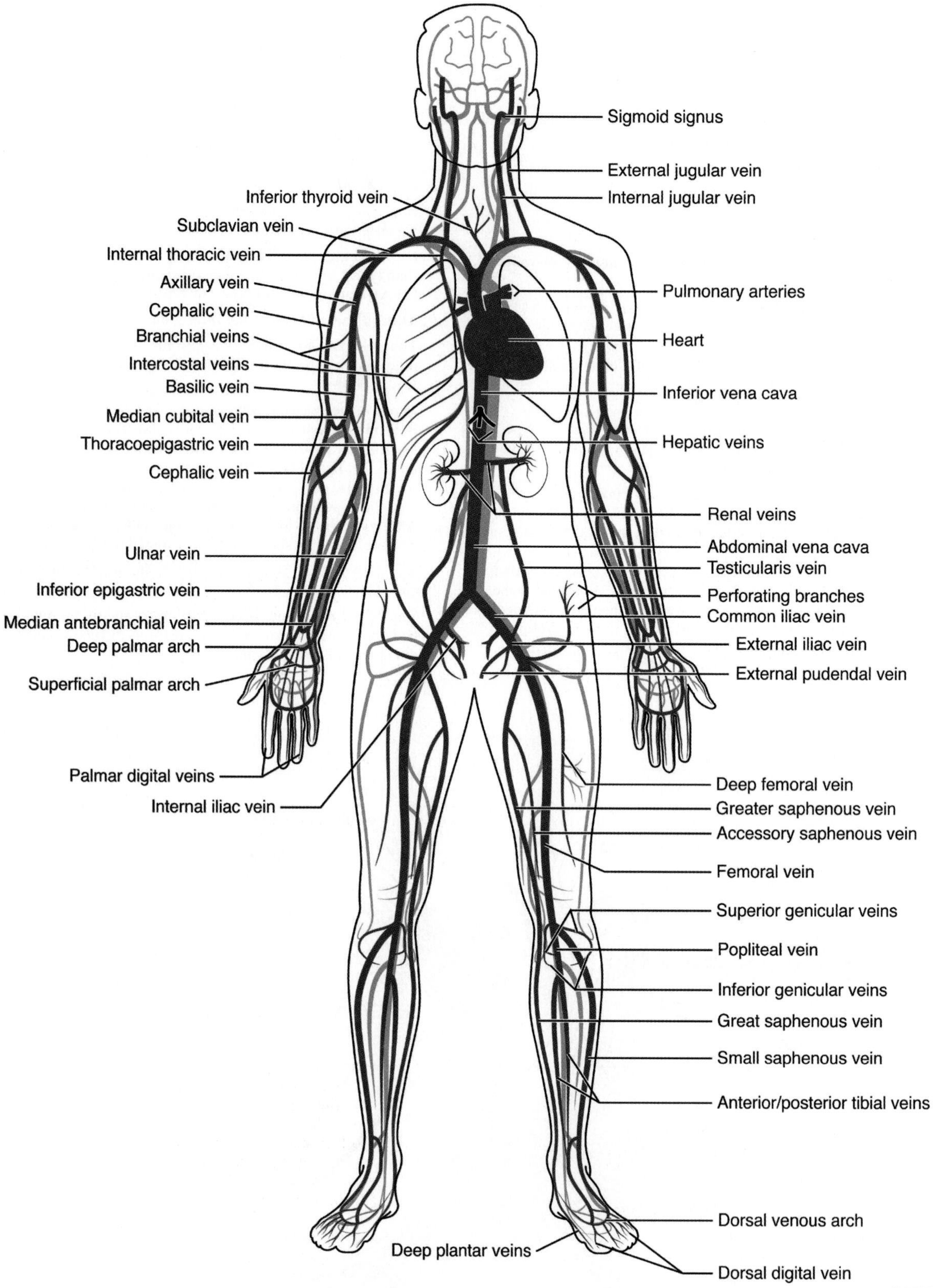
Sigmoid signus
External jugular vein
Internal jugular vein
Inferior thyroid vein
Subclavian vein
Internal thoracic vein
Axillary vein
Cephalic vein
Branchial veins
Intercostal veins
Basilic vein
Median cubital vein
Thoracoepigastric vein
Cephalic vein
Pulmonary arteries
Heart
Inferior vena cava
Hepatic veins
Renal veins
Abdominal vena cava
Testicularis vein
Ulnar vein
Inferior epigastric vein
Median antebranchial vein
Deep palmar arch
Superficial palmar arch
Perforating branches
Common iliac vein
External iliac vein
External pudendal vein
Palmar digital veins
Internal iliac vein
Deep femoral vein
Greater saphenous vein
Accessory saphenous vein
Femoral vein
Superior genicular veins
Popliteal vein
Inferior genicular veins
Great saphenous vein
Small saphenous vein
Anterior/posterior tibial veins
Dorsal venous arch
Deep plantar veins
Dorsal digital vein

Arteries

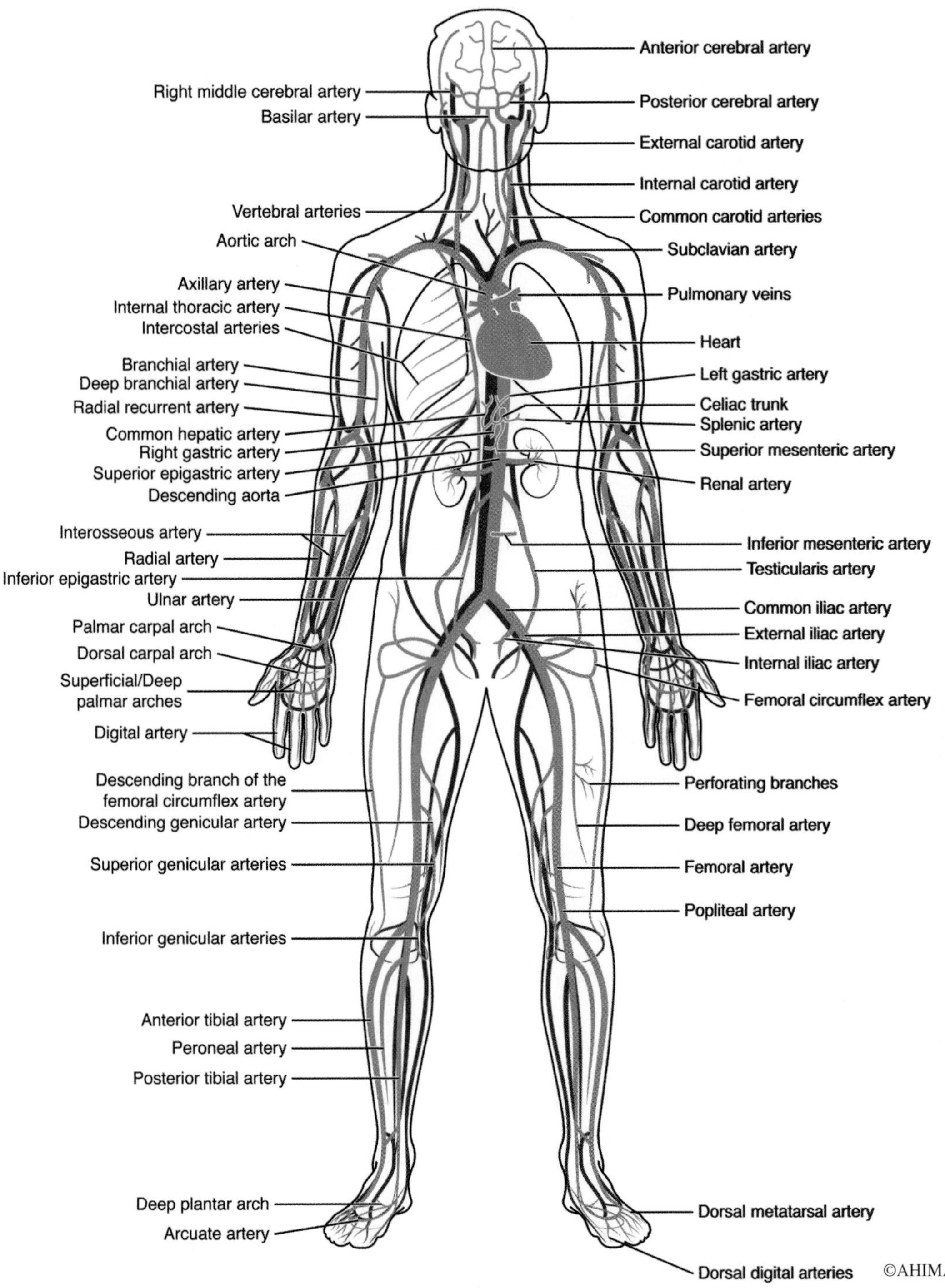

Acute rheumatic fever (I00-I02)

I00 Rheumatic fever without heart involvement

Includes: arthritis, rheumatic, acute or subacute
Excludes1: *rheumatic fever with heart involvement (I01.0-I01.9)*
Valid 3-character code, no further characters required

I01 Rheumatic fever with heart involvement

Excludes1: *chronic diseases of rheumatic origin (I05-I09) unless rheumatic fever is also present or there is evidence of reactivation or activity of the rheumatic process.*

CC **I01.0 Acute rheumatic pericarditis**
Any condition in I00 with pericarditis
Rheumatic pericarditis (acute)
Excludes1: *acute pericarditis not specified as rheumatic (I30.-)*
CC Exclusion see Appendix A PDX collection 0188

CC **I01.1 Acute rheumatic endocarditis**
Any condition in I00 with endocarditis or valvulitis
Acute rheumatic valvulitis
CC Exclusion see Appendix A PDX collection 0644

CC **I01.2 Acute rheumatic myocarditis**
Any condition in I00 with myocarditis
CC Exclusion see Appendix A PDX collection 0186

CC **I01.8 Other acute rheumatic heart disease**
Any condition in I00 with other or multiple types of heart involvement
Acute rheumatic pancarditis
CC Exclusion see Appendix A PDX collection 0645

CC **I01.9 Acute rheumatic heart disease, unspecified**
Any condition in I00 with unspecified type of heart involvement
Rheumatic carditis, acute
Rheumatic heart disease, active or acute
CC Exclusion see Appendix A PDX collection 0646

I02 Rheumatic chorea

Includes: Sydenham's chorea
Excludes1: *chorea NOS (G25.5)*
Huntington's chorea (G10)

CC **I02.0 Rheumatic chorea with heart involvement**
Chorea NOS with heart involvement
Rheumatic chorea with heart involvement of any type classifiable under I01.-
CC Exclusion see Appendix A PDX collection 0645

CC **I02.9 Rheumatic chorea without heart involvement**
Rheumatic chorea NOS
CC Exclusion see Appendix A PDX collection 0646

Chronic rheumatic heart diseases (I05-I09)

I05 Rheumatic mitral valve diseases

Includes: conditions classifiable to both I05.0 and I05.2-I05.9, whether specified as rheumatic or not
Excludes1: *mitral valve disease specified as nonrheumatic (I34.-)*
mitral valve disease with aortic and/or tricuspid valve involvement (I08.-)

I05.0 Rheumatic mitral stenosis
Mitral (valve) obstruction (rheumatic)

I05.1 Rheumatic mitral insufficiency
Rheumatic mitral incompetence
Rheumatic mitral regurgitation
Excludes1: *mitral insufficiency not specified as rheumatic (I34.0)*

I05.2 Rheumatic mitral stenosis with insufficiency
Rheumatic mitral stenosis with incompetence or regurgitation

I05.8 Other rheumatic mitral valve diseases
Rheumatic mitral (valve) failure

I05.9 Rheumatic mitral valve disease, unspecified
Rheumatic mitral (valve) disorder (chronic) NOS

I06 Rheumatic aortic valve diseases

Excludes1: *aortic valve disease not specified as rheumatic (I35.-)*
aortic valve disease with mitral and/or tricuspid valve involvement (I08.-)

I06.0 Rheumatic aortic stenosis
Rheumatic aortic (valve) obstruction

I06.1 Rheumatic aortic insufficiency
Rheumatic aortic incompetence
Rheumatic aortic regurgitation

I06.2 Rheumatic aortic stenosis with insufficiency
Rheumatic aortic stenosis with incompetence or regurgitation

I06.8 Other rheumatic aortic valve diseases

I06.9 Rheumatic aortic valve disease, unspecified
Rheumatic aortic (valve) disease NOS

I07 Rheumatic tricuspid valve diseases

Includes: rheumatic tricuspid valve diseases specified as rheumatic or unspecified
Excludes1: *tricuspid valve disease specified as nonrheumatic (I36.-)*
tricuspid valve disease with aortic and/or mitral valve involvement (I08.-)

I07.0 Rheumatic tricuspid stenosis
Tricuspid (valve) stenosis (rheumatic)

I07.1 Rheumatic tricuspid insufficiency
Tricuspid (valve) insufficiency (rheumatic)

I07.2 Rheumatic tricuspid stenosis and insufficiency

I07.8 Other rheumatic tricuspid valve diseases

I07.9 Rheumatic tricuspid valve disease, unspecified
Rheumatic tricuspid valve disorder NOS

I08 Multiple valve diseases

Includes: multiple valve diseases specified as rheumatic or unspecified
Excludes1: *endocarditis, valve unspecified (I38)*
multiple valve disease specified a nonrheumatic (I34.-, I35.-, I36.-, I37.-, I38.-, Q22.-, Q23.-, Q24.8-)
rheumatic valve disease NOS (I09.1)

I08.0 Rheumatic disorders of both mitral and aortic valves
Involvement of both mitral and aortic valves specified as rheumatic or unspecified

I08.1 Rheumatic disorders of both mitral and tricuspid valves

I08.2 Rheumatic disorders of both aortic and tricuspid valves

I08.3 Combined rheumatic disorders of mitral, aortic and tricuspid valves

I08.8 Other rheumatic multiple valve diseases

I08.9 Rheumatic multiple valve disease, unspecified

I09 Other rheumatic heart diseases

CC **I09.0 Rheumatic myocarditis**
Excludes1: *myocarditis not specified as rheumatic (I51.4)*
CC Exclusion see Appendix A PDX collection 0647

I09.1 Rheumatic diseases of endocardium, valve unspecified
Rheumatic endocarditis (chronic)
Rheumatic valvulitis (chronic)
Excludes1: *endocarditis, valve unspecified (I38)*

CC **I09.2 Chronic rheumatic pericarditis**
Adherent pericardium, rheumatic
Chronic rheumatic mediastinopericarditis
Chronic rheumatic myopericarditis
Excludes1: *chronic pericarditis not specified as rheumatic (I31.-)*
CC Exclusion see Appendix A PDX collection 0188

+ **I09.8 Other specified rheumatic heart diseases**

CC **I09.81 Rheumatic heart failure**
Use additional code to identify type of heart failure (I50.-)
CC Exclusion see Appendix A PDX collection 0648

I09.89 Other specified rheumatic heart diseases
Rheumatic disease of pulmonary valve

I09.9 Rheumatic heart disease, unspecified
Rheumatic carditis
Excludes1: *rheumatoid carditis (M05.31)*

Hypertensive diseases (I10-I16)

Use additional code to identify:
exposure to environmental tobacco smoke (Z77.22)
history of tobacco dependence (Z87.891)
occupational exposure to environmental tobacco smoke (Z57.31)
tobacco dependence (F17.-)
tobacco use (Z72.0)

Excludes1: *neonatal hypertension (P29.2)*
primary pulmonary hypertension (I27.0)

Excludes2: *hypertensive disease complicating pregnancy, childbirth and the puerperium (O10-O11, O13-O16)*

Review coding guidelines C.9, C.9.a.5, C.9.a.8 and C.9.a.9

I10 Essential (primary) hypertension

Includes: high blood pressure
hypertension (arterial) (benign) (essential) (malignant) (primary) (systemic)
Excludes1: *hypertensive disease complicating pregnancy, childbirth and the puerperium (O10-O11, O13-O16)*
Excludes2: *essential (primary) hypertension involving vessels of brain (I60-I69)*
essential (primary) hypertension involving vessels of eye (H35.0-)
AHA CC: 4Q, 2013, 128; 4Q, 2016, 27-28
Valid 3-character code, no further characters required

I11 Hypertensive heart disease

Includes: any condition in I50.-, I51.4-I51.9 due to hypertension
Review coding guidelines C.9.a.1 and C.9.a.3

I11.0 Hypertensive heart disease with heart failure
Hypertensive heart failure
Use additional code to identify type of heart failure (I50.-)
AHA CC: 1Q, 2017, 47

I11.9 Hypertensive heart disease without heart failure
Hypertensive heart disease NOS

I12 Hypertensive chronic kidney disease

Includes: any condition in N18 and N26 - due to hypertension
arteriosclerosis of kidney
arteriosclerotic nephritis (chronic) (interstitial)
hypertensive nephropathy
nephrosclerosis
Excludes1: *hypertension due to kidney disease (I15.0, I15.1)*
renovascular hypertension (I15.0)
secondary hypertension (I15.-)
Excludes2: *acute kidney failure (N17.-)*
Review coding guidelines C.9.a.2 and C.9.a.3

CC **I12.0 Hypertensive chronic kidney disease with stage 5 chronic kidney disease or end stage renal disease**
Use additional code to identify the stage of chronic kidney disease (N18.5, N18.6)
CC Exclusion see Appendix A PDX collection 0649

I12.9 Hypertensive chronic kidney disease with stage 1 through stage 4 chronic kidney disease, or unspecified chronic kidney disease
Hypertensive chronic kidney disease NOS
Hypertensive renal disease NOS
Use additional code to identify the stage of chronic kidney disease (N18.1-N18.4, N18.9)

I13 Hypertensive heart and chronic kidney disease

Includes: any condition in I11.- with any condition in I12.-
cardiorenal disease
cardiovascular renal disease

Review coding guideline C.9.a.3

CC **I13.0 Hypertensive heart and chronic kidney disease with heart failure and stage 1 through stage 4 chronic kidney disease, or unspecified chronic kidney disease**

Use additional code to identify type of heart failure (I50.-)

Use additional code to identify stage of chronic kidney disease (N18.1-N18.4, N18.9)

CC Exclusion see Appendix A PDX collection 0650

\+ **I13.1 Hypertensive heart and chronic kidney disease without heart failure**

I13.10 Hypertensive heart and chronic kidney disease without heart failure, with stage 1 through stage 4 chronic kidney disease, or unspecified chronic kidney disease

Hypertensive heart disease and hypertensive chronic kidney disease NOS

Use additional code to identify the stage of chronic kidney disease (N18.1-N18.4, N18.9)

CC **I13.11 Hypertensive heart and chronic kidney disease without heart failure, with stage 5 chronic kidney disease, or end stage renal disease**

Use additional code to identify the stage of chronic kidney disease (N18.5, N18.6)

CC Exclusion see Appendix A PDX collection 0650

CC **I13.2 Hypertensive heart and chronic kidney disease with heart failure and with stage 5 chronic kidney disease, or end stage renal disease**

Use additional code to identify type of heart failure (I50.-)

Use additional code to identify the stage of chronic kidney disease (N18.5, N18.6)

CC Exclusion see Appendix A PDX collection 0650

I15 Secondary hypertension

Code also underlying condition

Excludes1: *postprocedural hypertension (I97.3)*

Excludes2: *secondary hypertension involving vessels of brain (I60-I69)*
secondary hypertension involving vessels of eye (H35.0-)

Review coding guideline C.9.a.6

I15.0 Renovascular hypertension

I15.1 Hypertension secondary to other renal disorders

AHA CC: 3Q, 2016, 22-23

I15.2 Hypertension secondary to endocrine disorders

I15.8 Other secondary hypertension

I15.9 Secondary hypertension, unspecified

I16 Hypertensive crisis

Code also any identified hypertensive disease (I10-I15)

Review coding guideline C.9.a.10

AHA CC: 4Q, 2016, 26-28

I16.0 Hypertensive urgency

AHA CC: 4Q, 2016, 27-28

CC **I16.1 Hypertensive emergency**

No CC Exclusions

AHA CC: 4Q, 2016, 27-28

CC **I16.9 Hypertensive crisis, unspecified**

No CC Exclusions

schemic heart diseases (I20-I25)

Jse additional code to identify presence of hypertension (I10-I16)

I20 Angina pectoris

Use additional code to identify:
exposure to environmental tobacco smoke (Z77.22)
history of tobacco dependence (Z87.891)
occupational exposure to environmental tobacco smoke (Z57.31)
tobacco dependence (F17.-)
tobacco use (Z72.0)

Excludes1: *angina pectoris with atherosclerotic heart disease of native coronary arteries (I25.1-)*
atherosclerosis of coronary artery bypass graft(s) and coronary artery of transplanted heart with angina pectoris (I25.7-)
postinfarction angina (I23.7)

CC **I20.0 Unstable angina**

Accelerated angina
Crescendo angina
De novo effort angina
Intermediate coronary syndrome
Preinfarction syndrome
Worsening effort angina

CC Exclusion see Appendix A PDX collection 0651

CC **I20.1 Angina pectoris with documented spasm**

Angiospastic angina
Prinzmetal angina
Spasm-induced angina
Variant angina

CC Exclusion see Appendix A PDX collection 0652

I20.8 Other forms of angina pectoris

Angina equivalent
Angina of effort
Coronary slow flow syndrome
Stable angina
Stenocardia

Use additional code(s) for symptoms associated with angina equivalent

I20.9 Angina pectoris, unspecified

Angina NOS
Anginal syndrome
Cardiac angina
Ischemic chest pain

I21 Acute myocardial infarction

Includes: cardiac infarction
coronary (artery) embolism
coronary (artery) occlusion
coronary (artery) rupture
coronary (artery) thrombosis
infarction of heart, myocardium, or ventricle
myocardial infarction specified as acute or with a stated duration of 4 weeks (28 days) or less from onset

Use additional code, if applicable, to identify:
exposure to environmental tobacco smoke (Z77.22)
history of tobacco dependence (Z87.891)
occupational exposure to environmental tobacco smoke (Z57.31)
status post administration of tPA (rtPA) in a different facility within the last 24 hours prior to admission to current facility (Z92.82)
tobacco dependence (F17.-)
tobacco use (Z72.0)

Excludes2: *old myocardial infarction (I25.2)*
postmyocardial infarction syndrome (I24.1)
subsequent type 1 myocardial infarction (I22.-)

AHA CC: 1Q, 2013, 25; 4Q, 2016, 140

\+ **I21.0 ST elevation (STEMI) myocardial infarction of anterior wall**

Type 1 ST elevation myocardial infarction of anterior wall

Review coding guideline C.9.e.1

MCC **I21.01 ST elevation (STEMI) myocardial infarction involving left main coronary artery**

MCC Exclusion see Appendix A PDX collection 0653

MCC **I21.02 ST elevation (STEMI) myocardial infarction involving left anterior descending coronary artery**

ST elevation (STEMI) myocardial infarction involving diagonal coronary artery

MCC Exclusion see Appendix A PDX collection 0653

AHA CC: 1Q, 2013, 25-26

MCC **I21.09 ST elevation (STEMI) myocardial infarction involving other coronary artery of anterior wall**

Acute transmural myocardial infarction of anterior wall
Anteroapical transmural (Q wave) infarction (acute)
Anterolateral transmural (Q wave) infarction (acute)
Anteroseptal transmural (Q wave) infarction (acute)
Transmural (Q wave) infarction (acute) (of) anterior (wall) NOS

MCC Exclusion see Appendix A PDX collection 0653

AHA CC: 4Q, 2012, 102-104

\+ **I21.1 ST elevation (STEMI) myocardial infarction of inferior wall**

Type 1 ST elevation myocardial infarction of inferior wall

Review coding guideline C.9.e.1

MCC **I21.11 ST elevation (STEMI) myocardial infarction involving right coronary artery**

Inferoposterior transmural (Q wave) infarction (acute)

MCC Exclusion see Appendix A PDX collection 0653

MCC **I21.19 ST elevation (STEMI) myocardial infarction involving other coronary artery of inferior wall**

Acute transmural myocardial infarction of inferior wall
Inferolateral transmural (Q wave) infarction (acute)
Transmural (Q wave) infarction (acute) (of) diaphragmatic wall
Transmural (Q wave) infarction (acute) (of) inferior (wall) NOS

Excludes2: *ST elevation (STEMI) myocardial infarction involving left circumflex coronary artery (I21.21)*
MCC Exclusion see Appendix A PDX collection 0653
AHA CC: 4Q, 2012, 97

+ **I21.2 ST elevation (STEMI) myocardial infarction of other sites**
Type 1 ST elevation myocardial infarction of other sites
Review coding guideline C.9.e.1

MCC **I21.21 ST elevation (STEMI) myocardial infarction involving left circumflex coronary artery**
ST elevation (STEMI) myocardial infarction involving oblique marginal coronary artery
MCC Exclusion see Appendix A PDX collection 0653

MCC **I21.29 ST elevation (STEMI) myocardial infarction involving other sites**
Acute transmural myocardial infarction of other sites
Apical-lateral transmural (Q wave) infarction (acute)
Basal-lateral transmural (Q wave) infarction (acute)
High lateral transmural (Q wave) infarction (acute)
Lateral (wall) NOS transmural (Q wave) infarction (acute)
Posterior (true) transmural (Q wave) infarction (acute)
Posterobasal transmural (Q wave) infarction (acute)
Posterolateral transmural (Q wave) infarction (acute)
Posteroseptal transmural (Q wave) infarction (acute)
Septal transmural (Q wave) infarction (acute) NOS
MCC Exclusion see Appendix A PDX collection 0653

MCC **I21.3 ST elevation (STEMI) myocardial infarction of unspecified site**
Acute transmural myocardial infarction of unspecified site
Transmural (Q wave) myocardial infarction NOS
Type 1 ST elevation myocardial infarction of unspecified site
MCC Exclusion see Appendix A PDX collection 0653
Review coding guidelines C.9.e.1 and C.9.e.2

MCC **I21.4 Non-ST elevation (NSTEMI) myocardial infarction**
Acute subendocardial myocardial infarction
Non-Q wave myocardial infarction NOS
Nontransmural myocardial infarction NOS
Type 1 non-ST elevation myocardial infarction
MCC Exclusion see Appendix A PDX collection 0653
Review coding guideline C.9.e.1
AHA CC: 2Q, 2015, 16-17; 1Q, 2017, 44-45

MCC **I21.9 Acute myocardial infarction, unspecified**
Myocardial infarction (acute) NOS
MCC Exclusion see Appendix A PDX collection 0653
Review coding guideline C.9.e.5

+ **I21.A Other type of myocardial infarction**

MCC **I21.A1 Myocardial infarction type 2**
Myocardial infarction due to demand ischemia
Myocardial infarction secondary to ischemic imbalance
Code also the underlying cause, if known and applicable, such as:
anemia (D50.0-D64.9)
chronic obstructive pulmonary disease (J44.-)
heart failure (I50.-)
paroxysmal tachycardia (I47.0-I47.9)
renal failure (N17.0-N19)
shock (R57.0-R57.9)
MCC Exclusion see Appendix A PDX collection 0653

MCC **I21.A9 Other myocardial infarction type**
Myocardial infarction associated with revascularization procedure
Myocardial infarction type 3
Myocardial infarction type 4a
Myocardial infarction type 4b
Myocardial infarction type 4c
Myocardial infarction type 5
Code first, if applicable, postprocedural myocardial infarction following cardiac surgery (I97.190), or postprocedural myocardial infarction during cardiac surgery (I97.790)
Code also complication, if known and applicable, such as:
(acute) stent occlusion (T82.897-)
(acute) stent stenosis (T82.857-)
(acute) stent thrombosis (T82.867-)
cardiac arrest due to underlying cardiac condition (I46.2)
complication of percutaneous coronary intervention (PCI) (I97.89)
occlusion of coronary artery bypass graft (T82.218-)
MCC Exclusion see Appendix A PDX collection 0653

I22 Subsequent ST elevation (STEMI) and non-ST elevation (NSTEMI) myocardial infarction

Includes: acute myocardial infarction occurring within four weeks (28 days) of a previous acute myocardial infarction, regardless of site
cardiac infarction
coronary (artery) embolism
coronary (artery) occlusion
coronary (artery) rupture
coronary (artery) thrombosis
infarction of heart, myocardium, or ventricle
recurrent myocardial infarction
reinfarction of myocardium
rupture of heart, myocardium, or ventricle
subsequent type 1 myocardial infarction

Use additional code, if applicable, to identify:
exposure to environmental tobacco smoke (Z77.22)
history of tobacco dependence (Z87.891)
occupational exposure to environmental tobacco smoke (Z57.31)
status post administration of tPA (rtPA) in a different facility within the last 24 hours prior to admission to current facility (Z92.82)
tobacco dependence (F17.-)
tobacco use (Z72.0)

Excludes1: *subsequent myocardial infarction, type 2 (I21.A1)*
subsequent myocardial infarction of other type (type 3) (type 4) (type 5) (I21.A9)
Review coding guideline C.9.e.4
AHA CC: 1Q, 2013, 25

MCC **I22.0 Subsequent ST elevation (STEMI) myocardial infarction of anterior wall**
Subsequent acute transmural myocardial infarction of anterior wall
Subsequent transmural (Q wave) infarction (acute)(of) anterior (wall) NOS
Subsequent anteroapical transmural (Q wave) infarction (acute)
Subsequent anterolateral transmural (Q wave) infarction (acute)
Subsequent anteroseptal transmural (Q wave) infarction (acute)
MCC Exclusion see Appendix A PDX collection 0653

MCC **I22.1 Subsequent ST elevation (STEMI) myocardial infarction of inferior wall**
Subsequent acute transmural myocardial infarction of inferior wall
Subsequent transmural (Q wave) infarction (acute)(of) diaphragmatic wall
Subsequent transmural (Q wave) infarction (acute)(of) inferior (wall) NOS
Subsequent inferolateral transmural (Q wave) infarction (acute)
Subsequent inferoposterior transmural (Q wave) infarction (acute)
MCC Exclusion see Appendix A PDX collection 0653
AHA CC: 4Q, 2012, 102-104

MCC **I22.2 Subsequent non-ST elevation (NSTEMI) myocardial infarction**
Subsequent acute subendocardial myocardial infarction
Subsequent non-Q wave myocardial infarction NOS
Subsequent nontransmural myocardial infarction NOS
MCC Exclusion see Appendix A PDX collection 0653

MCC **I22.8 Subsequent ST elevation (STEMI) myocardial infarction of other sites**
Subsequent acute transmural myocardial infarction of other sites
Subsequent apical-lateral transmural (Q wave) myocardial infarction (acute)
Subsequent basal-lateral transmural (Q wave) myocardial infarction (acute)
Subsequent high lateral transmural (Q wave) myocardial infarction (acute)
Subsequent transmural (Q wave) myocardial infarction (acute) (of) lateral (wall) NOS
Subsequent posterior (true)transmural (Q wave) myocardial infarction (acute)
Subsequent posterobasal transmural (Q wave) myocardial infarction (acute)
Subsequent posterolateral transmural (Q wave) myocardial infarction (acute)
Subsequent posteroseptal transmural (Q wave) myocardial infarction (acute)
Subsequent septal NOS transmural (Q wave) myocardial infarction (acute)
MCC Exclusion see Appendix A PDX collection 0653

MCC **I22.9 Subsequent ST elevation (STEMI) myocardial infarction of unspecified site**
Subsequent acute myocardial infarction of unspecified site
Subsequent myocardial infarction (acute) NOS
MCC Exclusion see Appendix A PDX collection 0653

Great Vessels of the Heart

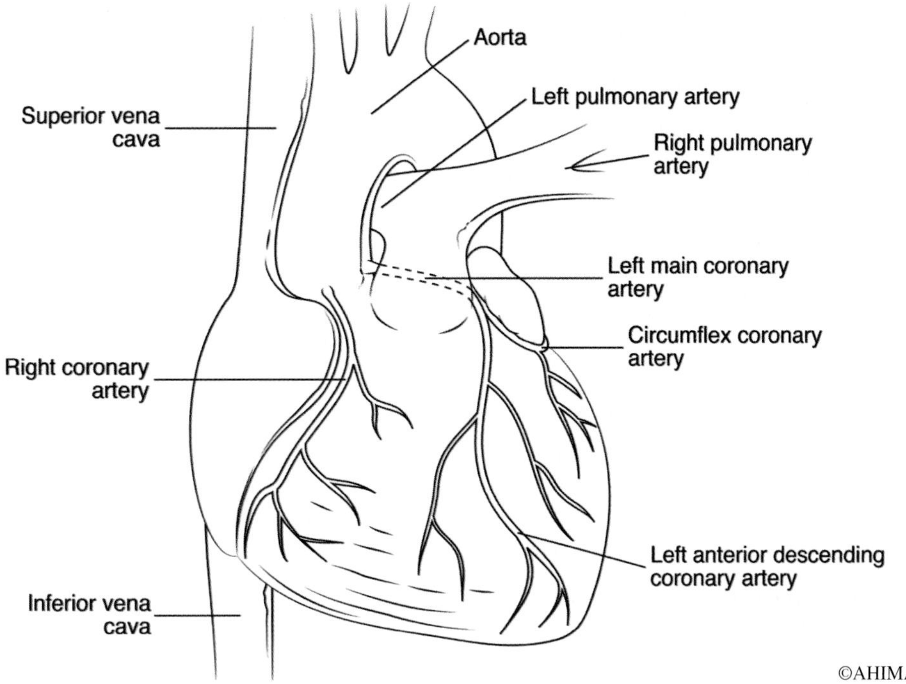

I23 Certain current complications following ST elevation (STEMI) and non-ST elevation (NSTEMI) myocardial infarction (within the 28 day period)

• CC **I23.0** **Hemopericardium as current complication following acute myocardial infarction**
Excludes1: *hemopericardium not specified as current complication following acute myocardial infarction (I31.2)*
CC Exclusion see Appendix A PDX collection 0654

• CC **I23.1** **Atrial septal defect as current complication following acute myocardial infarction**
Excludes1: *acquired atrial septal defect not specified as current complication following acute myocardial infarction (I51.0)*
CC Exclusion see Appendix A PDX collection 0654

• CC **I23.2** **Ventricular septal defect as current complication following acute myocardial infarction**
Excludes1: *acquired ventricular septal defect not specified as current complication following acute myocardial infarction (I51.0)*
CC Exclusion see Appendix A PDX collection 0654

• CC **I23.3** **Rupture of cardiac wall without hemopericardium as current complication following acute myocardial infarction**
CC Exclusion see Appendix A PDX collection 0654
AHA CC: 2Q, 2017, 11-12

MCC **I23.4** **Rupture of chordae tendineae as current complication following acute myocardial infarction**
Excludes1: *rupture of chordae tendineae not specified as current complication following acute myocardial infarction (I51.1)*
MCC Exclusion see Appendix A PDX collection 0655

MCC **I23.5** **Rupture of papillary muscle as current complication following acute myocardial infarction**
Excludes1: *rupture of papillary muscle not specified as current complication following acute myocardial infarction (I51.2)*
MCC Exclusion see Appendix A PDX collection 0656

• CC **I23.6** **Thrombosis of atrium, auricular appendage, and ventricle as current complications following acute myocardial infarction**
Excludes1: *thrombosis of atrium, auricular appendage, and ventricle not specified as current complication following acute myocardial infarction (I51.3)*
CC Exclusion see Appendix A PDX collection 0654

• CC **I23.7** **Postinfarction angina**
CC Exclusion see Appendix A PDX collection 0654
AHA CC: 2Q, 2015, 16-17

• CC **I23.8** **Other current complications following acute myocardial infarction**
CC Exclusion see Appendix A PDX collection 0654

I24 Other acute ischemic heart diseases
Excludes1: *angina pectoris (I20.-)*
transient myocardial ischemia in newborn (P29.4)

CC **I24.0** **Acute coronary thrombosis not resulting in myocardial infarction**
Acute coronary (artery) (vein) embolism not resulting in myocardial infarction
Acute coronary (artery) (vein) occlusion not resulting in myocardial infarction
Acute coronary (artery) (vein) thromboembolism not resulting in myocardial infarction
Excludes1: *atherosclerotic heart disease (I25.1-)*
CC Exclusion see Appendix A PDX collection 0657

CC **I24.1** **Dressler's syndrome**
Postmyocardial infarction syndrome
Excludes1: *postinfarction angina (I23.7)*
CC Exclusion see Appendix A PDX collection 0658

CC **I24.8** **Other forms of acute ischemic heart disease**
CC Exclusion see Appendix A PDX collection 0657
Excludes1: *myocardial infarction due to demand ischemia (I21.A1)*

CC **I24.9** **Acute ischemic heart disease, unspecified**
Excludes1: *ischemic heart disease (chronic) NOS (I25.9)*
CC Exclusion see Appendix A PDX collection 0657

I25 Chronic ischemic heart disease
Use additional code to identify:
chronic total occlusion of coronary artery (I25.82)
exposure to environmental tobacco smoke (Z77.22)
history of tobacco dependence (Z87.891)
occupational exposure to environmental tobacco smoke (Z57.31)
tobacco dependence (F17.-)
tobacco use (Z72.0)

+ **I25.1** **Atherosclerotic heart disease of native coronary artery**
Atherosclerotic cardiovascular disease
Coronary (artery) atheroma
Coronary (artery) atherosclerosis
Coronary (artery) disease
Coronary (artery) sclerosis
Use additional code, if applicable, to identify:
coronary atherosclerosis due to calcified coronary lesion (I25.84)
coronary atherosclerosis due to lipid rich plaque (I25.83)
Excludes2: *atheroembolism (I75.-)*
atherosclerosis of coronary artery bypass graft(s) and transplanted heart (I25.7-)

• **I25.10** **Atherosclerotic heart disease of native coronary artery without angina pectoris**
Atherosclerotic heart disease NOS
AHA CC: 4Q, 2012, 92-92; 4Q, 2013, 128

+ I25.11 **Atherosclerotic heart disease of native coronary artery with angina pectoris**
Review coding guideline C.9.b

• CC I25.110 **Atherosclerotic heart disease of native coronary artery with unstable angina pectoris**
Excludes1: *unstable angina without atheroscleroticheartdisease (I20.0)*
CC Exclusion see Appendix A PDX collection 0651

• I25.111 **Atherosclerotic heart disease of native coronary artery with angina pectoris with documented spasm**
Excludes1: *angina pectoris with documented spasm without atheroscleroticheartdisease (I20.1)*

• I25.118 **Atherosclerotic heart disease of native coronary artery with other forms of angina pectoris**
Excludes1: *other forms of angina pectoris withoutatheroscleroticheart disease (I20.8)*
AHA CC: 2Q, 2015, 16-17

• I25.119 **Atherosclerotic heart disease of native coronary artery with unspecified angina pectoris**
Atherosclerotic heart disease with angina NOS
Atherosclerotic heart disease with ischemic chest pain
Excludes1: *unspecified angina pectoris withoutatheroscleroticheart disease (I20.9)*

I25.2 **Old myocardial infarction**
Healed myocardial infarction
Past myocardial infarction diagnosed by ECG or other investigation, but currently presenting no symptoms

CC I25.3 **Aneurysm of heart**
Mural aneurysm
Ventricular aneurysm
CC Exclusion see Appendix A PDX collection 0659

+ I25.4 **Coronary artery aneurysm and dissection**

I25.41 **Coronary artery aneurysm**
Coronary arteriovenous fistula, acquired
Excludes1: *congenital coronary (artery) aneurysm (Q24.5)*

MCC I25.42 **Coronary artery dissection**
MCC Exclusion see Appendix A PDX collection 0660

I25.5 **Ischemic cardiomyopathy**
Excludes2: *coronary atherosclerosis (I25.1-, I25.7-)*

I25.6 **Silent myocardial ischemia**

+ I25.7 **Atherosclerosis of coronary artery bypass graft(s) and coronary artery of transplanted heart with angina pectoris**
Use additional code, if applicable, to identify:
coronary atherosclerosis due to calcified coronary lesion (I25.84)
coronary atherosclerosis due to lipid rich plaque (I25.83)
Excludes1: *atherosclerosis of bypass graft(s) of transplanted heart without angina pectoris (I25.812)*
atherosclerosis of coronary artery bypass graft(s) without angina pectoris (I25.810)
atherosclerosis of native coronary artery of transplanted heart without angina pectoris (I25.811)
Review coding guideline C.9.b

+ I25.70 **Atherosclerosis of coronary artery bypass graft(s), unspecified, with angina pectoris**

• CC I25.700 **Atherosclerosis of coronary artery bypass graft(s), unspecified, with unstable angina pectoris**
Excludes1: *unstable angina pectoris without atherosclerosis of coronary artery bypass graft (I20.0)*
CC Exclusion see Appendix A PDX collection 0651

• I25.701 **Atherosclerosis of coronary artery bypass graft(s), unspecified, with angina pectoris with documented spasm**
Excludes1: *angina pectoris with documented spasm without atherosclerosis of coronary artery bypass graft (I20.1)*

• I25.708 **Atherosclerosis of coronary artery bypass graft(s), unspecified, with other forms of angina pectoris**
Excludes1: *other forms of angina pectoris without atherosclerosis of coronary artery bypass graft (I20.8)*

• I25.709 **Atherosclerosis of coronary artery bypass graft(s), unspecified, with unspecified angina pectoris**
Excludes1: *unspecified angina pectoris without atherosclerosis of coronary artery bypass graft (I20.9)*

+ I25.71 **Atherosclerosis of autologous vein coronary artery bypass graft(s) with angina pectoris**

• CC I25.710 **Atherosclerosis of autologous vein coronary artery bypass graft(s) with unstable angina pectoris**
Excludes1: *unstable angina without atherosclerosisofautologous vein coronary artery bypass graft(s) (I20.0)*
Excludes2: *embolism or thrombus of coronary artery bypass graft(s) (T82.8-)*
CC Exclusion see Appendix A PDX collection 0661

• CC I25.711 **Atherosclerosis of autologous vein coronary artery bypass graft(s) with angina pectoris with documented spasm**
Excludes1: *angina pectoris with documented spasm without atherosclerosisofautologous vein coronary artery bypass graft(s) (I20.1)*
CC Exclusion see Appendix A PDX collection 0662

• CC I25.718 **Atherosclerosis of autologous vein coronary artery bypass graft(s) with other forms of angina pectoris**
Excludes1: *other forms of angina pectoris without atherosclerosis of autologous vein coronary arterybypassgraft(s)(I20.8)*
CC Exclusion see Appendix A PDX collection 0662

• CC I25.719 **Atherosclerosis of autologous vein coronary artery bypass graft(s) with unspecified angina pectoris**
Excludes1: *unspecified angina pectoris without atherosclerosis of autologous vein coronary arterybypassgraft(s)(I20.9)*
CC Exclusion see Appendix A PDX collection 0662

+ I25.72 **Atherosclerosis of autologous artery coronary artery bypass graft(s) with angina pectoris**
Atherosclerosis of internal mammary artery graft with angina pectoris

• CC I25.720 **Atherosclerosis of autologous artery coronary artery bypass graft(s) with unstable angina pectoris**
Excludes1: *unstable angina without atherosclerosisofautologous arterycoronaryarterybypass graft(s) (I20.0)*
CC Exclusion see Appendix A PDX collection 0661

• CC **I25.721** **Atherosclerosis of autologous artery coronary artery bypass graft(s) with angina pectoris with documented spasm**
Excludes1: *angina pectoris with documented spasm without atherosclerosisofautologous arterycoronaryarterybypass graft(s) (I20.1)*
CC Exclusion see Appendix A PDX collection 0662

• CC **I25.728** **Atherosclerosis of autologous artery coronary artery bypass graft(s) with other forms of angina pectoris**
Excludes1: *other forms of angina pectoris without atherosclerosis of autologous artery coronary arterybypassgraft(s)(I20.8)*
CC Exclusion see Appendix A PDX collection 0662

• CC **I25.729** **Atherosclerosis of autologous artery coronary artery bypass graft(s) with unspecified angina pectoris**
Excludes1: *unspecified angina pectoris without atherosclerosis of autologous artery coronary arterybypassgraft(s)(I20.9)*
CC Exclusion see Appendix A PDX collection 0662

+ **I25.73** **Atherosclerosis of nonautologous biological coronary artery bypass graft(s) with angina pectoris**

• CC **I25.730** **Atherosclerosis of nonautologous biological coronary artery bypass graft(s) with unstable angina pectoris**
Excludes1: *unstable angina without atherosclerosis of nonautologous biological coronary artery bypass graft(s) (I20.0)*
CC Exclusion see Appendix A PDX collection 0661

• CC **I25.731** **Atherosclerosis of nonautologous biological coronary artery bypass graft(s) with angina pectoris with documented spasm**
Excludes1: *angina pectoris with documented spasm without atherosclerosis of nonautologous biological coronary artery bypass graft(s) (I20.1)*
CC Exclusion see Appendix A PDX collection 0662

• CC **I25.738** **Atherosclerosis of nonautologous biological coronary artery bypass graft(s) with other forms of angina pectoris**
Excludes1: *other forms of angina pectoris without atherosclerosis of nonautologous biological coronary artery bypass graft(s) (I20.8)*
CC Exclusion see Appendix A PDX collection 0662

• CC **I25.739** **Atherosclerosis of nonautologous biological coronary artery bypass graft(s) with unspecified angina pectoris**
Excludes1: *unspecified angina pectoris without atherosclerosis of nonautologous biological coronary artery bypass graft(s) (I20.9)*
CC Exclusion see Appendix A PDX collection 0662

+ **I25.75** **Atherosclerosis of native coronary artery of transplanted heart with angina pectoris**
Excludes1: *atherosclerosis of native coronary artery of transplanted heart without angina pectoris (I25.811)*

CC **I25.750** **Atherosclerosis of native coronary artery of transplanted heart with unstable angina**
CC Exclusion see Appendix A PDX collection 0663

CC **I25.751** **Atherosclerosis of native coronary artery of transplanted heart with angina pectoris with documented spasm**
CC Exclusion see Appendix A PDX collection 0664

CC **I25.758** **Atherosclerosis of native coronary artery of transplanted heart with other forms of angina pectoris**
CC Exclusion see Appendix A PDX collection 0664

CC **I25.759** **Atherosclerosis of native coronary artery of transplanted heart with unspecified angina pectoris**
CC Exclusion see Appendix A PDX collection 0664

+ **I25.76** **Atherosclerosis of bypass graft of coronary artery of transplanted heart with angina pectoris**
Excludes1: *atherosclerosis of bypass graft of coronary artery of transplanted heart without angina pectoris (I25.812)*

• CC **I25.760** **Atherosclerosis of bypass graft of coronary artery of transplanted heart with unstable angina**
CC Exclusion see Appendix A PDX collection 0665

• CC **I25.761** **Atherosclerosis of bypass graft of coronary artery of transplanted heart with angina pectoris with documented spasm**
CC Exclusion see Appendix A PDX collection 0666

• CC **I25.768** **Atherosclerosis of bypass graft of coronary artery of transplanted heart with other forms of angina pectoris**
CC Exclusion see Appendix A PDX collection 0666

• CC **I25.769** **Atherosclerosis of bypass graft of coronary artery of transplanted heart with unspecified angina pectoris**
CC Exclusion see Appendix A PDX collection 0666

+ **I25.79** **Atherosclerosis of other coronary artery bypass graft(s) with angina pectoris**

• CC **I25.790** **Atherosclerosis of other coronary artery bypass graft(s) with unstable angina pectoris**
Excludes1: *unstable angina without atherosclerosis of other coronary artery bypass graft(s) (I20.0)*
CC Exclusion see Appendix A PDX collection 0651

• CC **I25.791** **Atherosclerosis of other coronary artery bypass graft(s) with angina pectoris with documented spasm**
Excludes1: *angina pectoris with documented spasm without atherosclerosis of other coronary artery bypass graft(s) (I20.1)*
No CC Exclusions

• CC **I25.798** **Atherosclerosis of other coronary artery bypass graft(s) with other forms of angina pectoris**
Excludes1: *other forms of angina pectoris without atherosclerosis of othercoronaryarterybypass graft(s) (I20.8)*
No CC Exclusions

• CC **I25.799** **Atherosclerosis of other coronary artery bypass graft(s) with unspecified angina pectoris**
Excludes1: *unspecified angina pectoris without atherosclerosis of othercoronaryarterybypass graft(s) (I20.9)*
No CC Exclusions

+ **I25.8 Other forms of chronic ischemic heart disease**

+ **I25.81 Atherosclerosis of other coronary vessels without angina pectoris**

Use additional code, if applicable, to identify:
coronary atherosclerosis due to calcified coronary lesion (I25.84)
coronary atherosclerosis due to lipid rich plaque (I25.83)

Excludes1: *atherosclerotic heart disease of native coronary artery without angina pectoris (I25.10)*

• CC **I25.810 Atherosclerosis of coronary artery bypass graft(s) without angina pectoris**

Atherosclerosis of coronary artery bypass graft NOS

Excludes1: *atherosclerosis of coronary bypass graft(s) with angina pectoris (I25.70-I25.73-, I25.79-)*

No CC Exclusions

CC **I25.811 Atherosclerosis of native coronary artery of transplanted heart without angina pectoris**

Atherosclerosis of native coronary artery of transplanted heart NOS

Excludes1: *atherosclerosis of native coronary artery of transplanted heart with angina pectoris (I25.75-)*

CC Exclusion see Appendix A PDX collection 0664

• CC **I25.812 Atherosclerosis of bypass graft of coronary artery of transplanted heart without angina pectoris**

Atherosclerosis of bypass graft of transplanted heart NOS

Excludes1: *atherosclerosis of bypass graft of transplanted heart with angina pectoris (I25.76)*

CC Exclusion see Appendix A PDX collection 0666

I25.82 Chronic total occlusion of coronary artery

Complete occlusion of coronary artery
Total occlusion of coronary artery
Code first coronary atherosclerosis (I25.1-, I25.7-, I25.81-)

Excludes1: *acute coronary occulsion with myocardial infarction (I21.0-I21.9, I22.-)*
acute coronary occulsion without myocardial infarction (I24.0)

• **I25.83 Coronary atherosclerosis due to lipid rich plaque**

Code first coronary atherosclerosis (I25.1-, I25.7-, I25.81-)

I25.84 Coronary atherosclerosis due to calcified coronary lesion

Coronary atherosclerosis due to severely calcified coronary lesion
Code first coronary atherosclerosis (I25.1-, I25.7-, I25.81-)

I25.89 Other forms of chronic ischemic heart disease

I25.9 Chronic ischemic heart disease, unspecified

Ischemic heart disease (chronic) NOS

Pulmonary heart disease and diseases of pulmonary circulation (I26-I28)

I26 Pulmonary embolism

Includes: pulmonary (acute) (artery)(vein) infarction
pulmonary (acute) (artery)(vein) thromboembolism
pulmonary (acute) (artery)(vein) thrombosis

Excludes2: *chronic pulmonary embolism (I27.82)*
personal history of pulmonary embolism (Z86.711)
pulmonary embolism due to trauma (T79.0, T79.1)
pulmonary embolism due to complications of surgical and medical care (T80.0, T81.7-, T82.8-)
pulmonary embolism complicating abortion, ectopic or molar pregnancy (O00-O07, O08.2)
pulmonary embolism complicating pregnancy, childbirth and the puerperium (O88.-)
septic (non-pulmonary) arterial embolism (I76)

+ **I26.0 Pulmonary embolism with acute cor pulmonale**

MCC **I26.01 Septic pulmonary embolism with acute cor pulmonale**

Code first underlying infection

MCC **I26.02 Saddle embolus of pulmonary artery with acute cor pulmonale**

MCC Exclusion see Appendix A PDX collection 0667

HAC *see Appendix B for HAC conditional logic*

MCC **I26.09 Other pulmonary embolism with acute cor pulmonale**

Acute cor pulmonale NOS

MCC Exclusion see Appendix A PDX collection 0667

HAC *see Appendix B for HAC conditional logic*

+ **I26.9 Pulmonary embolism without acute cor pulmonale**

MCC **I26.90 Septic pulmonary embolism without acute cor pulmonale**

Code first underlying infection

MCC Exclusion see Appendix A PDX collection 0668

MCC **I26.92 Saddle embolus of pulmonary artery without acute cor pulmonale**

MCC Exclusion see Appendix A PDX collection 0669

HAC *see Appendix B for HAC conditional logic*

MCC **I26.99 Other pulmonary embolism without acute cor pulmonale**

Acute pulmonary embolism NOS
Pulmonary embolism NOS

MCC Exclusion see Appendix A PDX collection 0670

HAC *see Appendix B for HAC conditional logic*

I27 Other pulmonary heart diseases

Review coding guideline C.9.a.11

CC **I27.0 Primary pulmonary hypertension**

Heritable pulmonary arterial hypertension
Idiopathic pulmonary arterial hypertension
Primary group 1 pulmonary hypertension
Primary pulmonary arterial hypertension

Excludes1: *persistent pulmonary hypertension of newborn (P29.30)*
pulmonary hypertension NOS (I27.20)
secondary pulmonary arterial hypertension (I27.21)
secondary pulmonary hypertension (I27.29)

CC Exclusion see Appendix A PDX collection 0671

CC **I27.1 Kyphoscoliotic heart disease**

CC Exclusion see Appendix A PDX collection 0533

+ **I27.2 Other secondary pulmonary hypertension**

Code also associated underlying condition

Excludes1: *Eisenmenger's syndrome (I27.83)*

AHA CC: 4Q, 2014, 21-22; 2Q, 2016, 8

I27.20 Pulmonary hypertension, unspecified

Pulmonary hypertension NOS

I27.21 Secondary pulmonary arterial hypertension

(Associated) (drug-induced) (toxin-induced) pulmonary arterial hypertension NOS
(Associated) (drug-induced) (toxin-induced) (secondary) group 1 pulmonary hypertension
Code also associated conditions if applicable, or adverse effects of drugs or toxins, such as:
adverse effect of appetite depressants (T50.5X5)
congenital heart disease (Q20-Q28)
human immunodeficiency virus [HIV] disease (B20)
polymyositis (M33.2-)
portal hypertension (K76.6)
rheumatoid arthritis (M05.-)
schistosomiasis (B65.-)
Sjögren syndrome (M35.0-)
systemic sclerosis (M34.-)

I27.22 **Pulmonary hypertension due to left heart disease**
Group 2 pulmonary hypertension
Code also associated left heart disease, if known, such as:
multiple valve disease (I08.-)
rheumatic mitral valve diseases (I05.-)
rheumatic aortic valve diseases (I06.-)

I27.23 **Pulmonary hypertension due to lung diseases and hypoxia**
Group 3 pulmonary hypertension
Code also associated lung disease, if known, such as:
bronchiectasis (J47.-)
cystic fibrosis with pulmonary manifestations (E84.0)
interstitial lung disease (J84.-)
pleural effusion (J90)
sleep apnea (G47.3-)

I27.24 **Chronic thromboembolic pulmonary hypertension**
Group 4 pulmonary hypertension
Code also associated pulmonary embolism, if applicable (I26.-, I27.82)

I27.29 **Other secondary pulmonary hypertension**
Group 5 pulmonary hypertension
Pulmonary hypertension with unclear multifactorial mechanisms
Pulmonary hypertension due to hematologic disorders
Pulmonary hypertension due to metabolic disorders
Pulmonary hypertension due to other systemic disorders
Code also other associated disorders, if known, such as:
chronic myeloid leukemia (C92.10-C92.22)
essential thrombocythemia (D47.3)
Gaucher disease (E75.22)
hypertensive chronic kidney disease with end stage renal disease (I12.0, I12.11, I13.2)
hyperthyroidism (E05.-)
hypothyroidism (E00-E03)
polycythemia vera (D45)
sarcoidosis (D86.-)

+ I27.8 **Other specified pulmonary heart diseases**

I27.81 **Cor pulmonale (chronic)**
Cor pulmonale NOS
Excludes1: *acute cor pulmonale (I26.0-)*
AHA CC: 4Q, 2014, 21-22

CC I27.82 **Chronic pulmonary embolism**
Use additional code, if applicable, for associated long-term (current) use of anticoagulants (Z79.01)
Excludes1: *personal history of pulmonary embolism (Z86.711)*
CC Exclusion see Appendix A PDX collection 0669

I27.83 **Eisenmenger's syndrome**
Eisenmenger's complex
(Irreversible) Eisenmenger's disease
Pulmonary hypertension with right to left shunt related to congenital heart disease
Code also underlying heart defect, if known, such as:
atrial septal defect (Q21.1)
Eisenmenger's defect (Q21.8)
patent ductus arteriosus (Q25.0)
ventricular septal defect (Q21.0)

I27.89 **Other specified pulmonary heart diseases**

I27.9 **Pulmonary heart disease, unspecified**
Chronic cardiopulmonary disease

I28 **Other diseases of pulmonary vessels**

CC I28.0 **Arteriovenous fistula of pulmonary vessels**
Excludes1: *congenital arteriovenous fistula (Q25.72)*
CC Exclusion see Appendix A PDX collection 0672

CC I28.1 **Aneurysm of pulmonary artery**
Excludes1: *congenital aneurysm (Q25.79)*
congenital arteriovenous aneurysm (Q25.72)
CC Exclusion see Appendix A PDX collection 0672

I28.8 **Other diseases of pulmonary vessels**
Pulmonary arteritis
Pulmonary endarteritis
Rupture of pulmonary vessels
Stenosis of pulmonary vessels
Stricture of pulmonary vessels

I28.9 **Disease of pulmonary vessels, unspecified**

Other forms of heart disease (I30-I52)

I30 **Acute pericarditis**

Includes: acute mediastinopericarditis
acute myopericarditis
acute pericardial effusion
acute pleuropericarditis
acute pneumopericarditis
Excludes1: *Dressler's syndrome (I24.1)*
rheumatic pericarditis (acute) (I01.0)
viral pericarditis due to Coxsakie virus (B33.23)

CC I30.0 **Acute nonspecific idiopathic pericarditis**
CC Exclusion see Appendix A PDX collection 0673

CC I30.1 **Infective pericarditis**
Pneumococcal pericarditis
Pneumopyopericardium
Purulent pericarditis
Pyopericarditis
Pyopericardium
Pyopneumopericardium
Staphylococcal pericarditis
Streptococcal pericarditis
Suppurative pericarditis
Viral pericarditis
Use additional code (B95-B97) to identify infectious agent
CC Exclusion see Appendix A PDX collection 0673

CC I30.8 **Other forms of acute pericarditis**
CC Exclusion see Appendix A PDX collection 0673

CC I30.9 **Acute pericarditis, unspecified**
CC Exclusion see Appendix A PDX collection 0673

I31 **Other diseases of pericardium**

Excludes1: *diseases of pericardium specified as rheumatic (I09.2)*
postcardiotomy syndrome (I97.0)
traumatic injury to pericardium (S26.-)

CC I31.0 **Chronic adhesive pericarditis**
Accretio cordis
Adherent pericardium
Adhesive mediastinopericarditis
CC Exclusion see Appendix A PDX collection 0674

CC I31.1 **Chronic constrictive pericarditis**
Concretio cordis
Pericardial calcification
CC Exclusion see Appendix A PDX collection 0674

CC I31.2 **Hemopericardium, not elsewhere classified**
Excludes1: *hemopericardium as current complication following acute myocardial infarction (I23.0)*
CC Exclusion see Appendix A PDX collection 0674

CC I31.3 **Pericardial effusion (noninflammatory)**
Chylopericardium
Excludes1: *acute pericardial effusion (I30.9)*
CC Exclusion see Appendix A PDX collection 0188

CC I31.4 **Cardiac tamponade**
Code first underlying cause
CC Exclusion see Appendix A PDX collection 0188

CC I31.8 **Other specified diseases of pericardium**
Epicardial plaques
Focal pericardial adhesions
CC Exclusion see Appendix A PDX collection 0188

CC I31.9 **Disease of pericardium, unspecified**
Pericarditis (chronic) NOS
CC Exclusion see Appendix A PDX collection 0188

CC I32 **Pericarditis in diseases classified elsewhere**

Code first underlying disease
Excludes1: *pericarditis (in):*
coxsackie (virus) (B33.23)
gonococcal (A54.83)
meningococcal (A39.53)
rheumatoid (arthritis) (M05.31)
syphilitic (A52.06)
systemic lupus erythematosus (M32.12)
tuberculosis (A18.84)
CC Exclusion see Appendix A PDX collection 0673
Valid 3-character code, no further characters required

I33 Acute and subacute endocarditis

Excludes1: *acute rheumatic endocarditis (I01.1)*
endocarditis NOS (I38)

MCC **I33.0 Acute and subacute infective endocarditis**
Bacterial endocarditis (acute) (subacute)
Infective endocarditis (acute) (subacute) NOS
Endocarditis lenta (acute) (subacute)
Malignant endocarditis (acute) (subacute)
Purulent endocarditis (acute) (subacute)
Septic endocarditis (acute) (subacute)
Ulcerative endocarditis (acute) (subacute)
Vegetative endocarditis (acute) (subacute)
Use additional code (B95-B97) to identify infectious agent
MCC Exclusion see Appendix A PDX collection 0675

MCC **I33.9 Acute and subacute endocarditis, unspecified**
Acute endocarditis NOS
Acute myoendocarditis NOS
Acute periendocarditis NOS
Subacute endocarditis NOS
Subacute myoendocarditis NOS
Subacute periendocarditis NOS
MCC Exclusion see Appendix A PDX collection 0675

I34 Nonrheumatic mitral valve disorders

Excludes1: *mitral valve disease (I05.9)*
mitral valve failure (I05.8)
mitral valve stenosis (I05.0)
mitral valve disorder of unspecified cause with diseases of aortic and/or tricuspid valve(s) (I08.-)
mitral valve disorder of unspecified cause with mitral stenosis or obstruction (I05.0)
mitral valve disorder specified as congenital (Q23.2, Q23.9)
mitral valve disorder specified as rheumatic (I05.-)

I34.0 Nonrheumatic mitral (valve) insufficiency
Nonrheumatic mitral (valve) incompetence NOS
Nonrheumatic mitral (valve) regurgitation NOS

I34.1 Nonrheumatic mitral (valve) prolapse
Floppy nonrheumatic mitral valve syndrome
Excludes1: *Marfan's syndrome (Q87.4-)*

I34.2 Nonrheumatic mitral (valve) stenosis

I34.8 Other nonrheumatic mitral valve disorders

I34.9 Nonrheumatic mitral valve disorder, unspecified

I35 Nonrheumatic aortic valve disorders

Excludes1: *aortic valve disorder of unspecified cause but with diseases of mitral and/or tricuspid valve(s) (I08.-)*
aortic valve disorder specified as congenital (Q23.0, Q23.1)
aortic valve disorder specified as rheumatic (I06.-)
hypertrophic subaortic stenosis (I42.1)

I35.0 Nonrheumatic aortic (valve) stenosis

I35.1 Nonrheumatic aortic (valve) insufficiency
Nonrheumatic aortic (valve) incompetence NOS
Nonrheumatic aortic (valve) regurgitation NOS

I35.2 Nonrheumatic aortic (valve) stenosis with insufficiency

I35.8 Other nonrheumatic aortic valve disorders

I35.9 Nonrheumatic aortic valve disorder, unspecified

I36 Nonrheumatic tricuspid valve disorders

Excludes1: *tricuspid valve disorders of unspecified cause (I07.-)*
tricuspid valve disorders specified as congenital (Q22.4, Q22.8, Q22.9)
tricuspid valve disorders specified as rheumatic (I07.-)
tricuspid valve disorders with aortic and/or mitral valve involvement (I08.-)

I36.0 Nonrheumatic tricuspid (valve) stenosis

I36.1 Nonrheumatic tricuspid (valve) insufficiency
Nonrheumatic tricuspid (valve) incompetence
Nonrheumatic tricuspid (valve) regurgitation

I36.2 Nonrheumatic tricuspid (valve) stenosis with insufficiency

I36.8 Other nonrheumatic tricuspid valve disorders

I36.9 Nonrheumatic tricuspid valve disorder, unspecified

I37 Nonrheumatic pulmonary valve disorders

Excludes1: *pulmonary valve disorder specified as congenital (Q22.1, Q22.2, Q22.3)*
pulmonary valve disorder specified as rheumatic (I09.89)

I37.0 Nonrheumatic pulmonary valve stenosis

I37.1 Nonrheumatic pulmonary valve insufficiency
Nonrheumatic pulmonary valve incompetence
Nonrheumatic pulmonary valve regurgitation

I37.2 Nonrheumatic pulmonary valve stenosis with insufficiency

I37.8 Other nonrheumatic pulmonary valve disorders

I37.9 Nonrheumatic pulmonary valve disorder, unspecified

CC **I38 Endocarditis, valve unspecified**

Includes: endocarditis (chronic) NOS
valvular incompetence NOS
valvular insufficiency NOS
valvular regurgitation NOS
valvular stenosis NOS
valvulitis (chronic) NOS

Excludes1: *congenital insufficiency of cardiac valve NOS (Q24.8)*
congenital stenosis of cardiac valve NOS (Q24.8)
endocardial fibroelastosis (I42.4)
endocarditis specified as rheumatic (I09.1)

CC Exclusion see Appendix A PDX collection 0676
Valid 3-character code, no further characters required

CC **I39 Endocarditis and heart valve disorders in diseases classified elsewhere**

Code first underlying disease, such as:
Q fever (A78)

Excludes1: *endocardial involvement in:*
candidiasis (B37.6)
gonococcal infection (A54.83)
Libman-Sacks disease (M32.11)
listerosis (A32.82)
meningococcal infection (A39.51)
rheumatoid arthritis (M05.31)
syphilis (A52.03)
tuberculosis (A18.84)
typhoid fever (A01.02)

CC Exclusion see Appendix A PDX collection 0676
Valid 3-character code, no further characters required

I40 Acute myocarditis

Includes: subacute myocarditis
Excludes1: *acute rheumatic myocarditis (I01.2)*

MCC **I40.0 Infective myocarditis**
Septic myocarditis
Use additional code (B95-B97) to identify infectious agent
MCC Exclusion see Appendix A PDX collection 0677

MCC **I40.1 Isolated myocarditis**
Fiedler's myocarditis
Giant cell myocarditis
Idiopathic myocarditis
MCC Exclusion see Appendix A PDX collection 0677

MCC **I40.8 Other acute myocarditis**
MCC Exclusion see Appendix A PDX collection 0677

MCC **I40.9 Acute myocarditis, unspecified**
MCC Exclusion see Appendix A PDX collection 0677

MCC **I41 Myocarditis in diseases classified elsewhere**

Code first underlying disease, such as:
typhus (A75.0-A75.9)

Excludes1: *myocarditis (in):*
Chagas' disease (chronic) (B57.2)
acute (B57.0)
coxsackie (virus) infection (B33.22)
diphtheritic (A36.81)
gonococcal (A54.83)
influenzal (J09.X9, J10.82, J11.82)
meningococcal (A39.52)
mumps (B26.82)
rheumatoid arthritis (M05.31)
sarcoid (D86.85)
syphilis (A52.06)
toxoplasmosis (B58.81)
tuberculous (A18.84)

MCC Exclusion see Appendix A PDX collection 0677
Valid 3-character code, no further characters required

I42 Cardiomyopathy

Includes: myocardiopathy
Code first pre-existing cardiomyopathy complicating pregnancy and puerperium (O99.4)

Excludes2: *ischemic cardiomyopathy (I25.5)*
peripartum cardiomyopathy (O90.3)
ventricular hypertrophy (I51.7)

CC **I42.0 Dilated cardiomyopathy**
Congestive cardiomyopathy
CC Exclusion see Appendix A PDX collection 0678

CC **I42.1** **Obstructive hypertrophic cardiomyopathy**
Hypertrophic subaortic stenosis (idiopathic)
CC Exclusion see Appendix A PDX collection 0678

CC **I42.2** **Other hypertrophic cardiomyopathy**
Nonobstructive hypertrophic cardiomyopathy
CC Exclusion see Appendix A PDX collection 0678

CC **I42.3** **Endomyocardial (eosinophilic) disease**
Endomyocardial (tropical) fibrosis
Löffler's endocarditis
CC Exclusion see Appendix A PDX collection 0678

CC **I42.4** **Endocardial fibroelastosis**
Congenital cardiomyopathy
Elastomyofibrosis
CC Exclusion see Appendix A PDX collection 0678

CC **I42.5** **Other restrictive cardiomyopathy**
Constrictive cardiomyopathy NOS
CC Exclusion see Appendix A PDX collection 0678

CC **I42.6** **Alcoholic cardiomyopathy**
Code also presence of alcoholism (F10.-)
CC Exclusion see Appendix A PDX collection 0678

CC **I42.7** **Cardiomyopathy due to drug and external agent**
Code first poisoning due to drug or toxin, if applicable (T36-T65 with fifth or sixth character 1-4 or 6)

Use additional code for adverse effect, if appv licable, to identify drug (T36-T50 with fifth or sixth character 5)
CC Exclusion see Appendix A PDX collection 0678

CC **I42.8** **Other cardiomyopathies**
CC Exclusion see Appendix A PDX collection 0678

CC **I42.9** **Cardiomyopathy, unspecified**
Cardiomyopathy (primary) (secondary) NOS
CC Exclusion see Appendix A PDX collection 0678

CC **I43** **Cardiomyopathy in diseases classified elsewhere**
Code first underlying disease, such as:
amyloidosis (E85.-)
glycogen storage disease (E74.0)
gout (M10.0-)
thyrotoxicosis (E05.0-E05.9-)
Excludes1: *cardiomyopathy (in):*
coxsackie (virus) (B33.24)
diphtheria (A36.81)
sarcoidosis (D86.85)
tuberculosis (A18.84)
CC Exclusion see Appendix A PDX collection 0678
Valid 3-character code, no further characters required

I44 **Atrioventricular and left bundle-branch block**

I44.0 **Atrioventricular block, first degree**

I44.1 **Atrioventricular block, second degree**
Atrioventricular block, type I and II
Möbitz block block, type I and II
Second degree block, type I and II
Wenckebach's block

CC **I44.2** **Atrioventricular block, complete**
Complete heart block NOS
Third degree block
CC Exclusion see Appendix A PDX collection 0679

\+ **I44.3** **Other and unspecified atrioventricular block**
Atrioventricular block NOS
I44.30 **Unspecified atrioventricular block**
I44.39 **Other atrioventricular block**

I44.4 **Left anterior fascicular block**

I44.5 **Left posterior fascicular block**

\+ **I44.6** **Other and unspecified fascicular block**
I44.60 **Unspecified fascicular block**
Left bundle-branch hemiblock NOS
I44.69 **Other fascicular block**

I44.7 **Left bundle-branch block, unspecified**

I45 **Other conduction disorders**

I45.0 **Right fascicular block**

\+ **I45.1** **Other and unspecified right bundle-branch block**
I45.10 **Unspecified right bundle-branch block**
Right bundle-branch block NOS
I45.19 **Other right bundle-branch block**

CC **I45.2** **Bifascicular block**
CC Exclusion see Appendix A PDX collection 0679

CC **I45.3** **Trifascicular block**
CC Exclusion see Appendix A PDX collection 0679

I45.4 **Nonspecific intraventricular block**
Bundle-branch block NOS

I45.5 **Other specified heart block**
Sinoatrial block
Sinoauricular block
Excludes1: *heart block NOS (I45.9)*

I45.6 **Pre-excitation syndrome**
Accelerated atrioventricular conduction
Accessory atrioventricular conduction
Anomalous atrioventricular excitation
Lown-Ganong-Levine syndrome
Pre-excitation atrioventricular conduction
Wolff-Parkinson-White syndrome

\+ **I45.8** **Other specified conduction disorders**
I45.81 **Long QT syndrome**
CC **I45.89** **Other specified conduction disorders**
Atrioventricular [AV] dissociation
Interference dissociation
Isorhythmic dissociation
Nonparoxysmal AV nodal tachycardia
CC Exclusion see Appendix A PDX collection 0679
AHA CC: 2Q, 2013, 31-32

I45.9 **Conduction disorder, unspecified**
Heart block NOS
Stokes-Adams syndrome

I46 **Cardiac arrest**
Excludes1: *cardiogenic shock (R57.0)*

MCC **I46.2** **Cardiac arrest due to underlying cardiac condition**
Code first underlying cardiac condition
MCC Exclusion see Appendix A PDX collection 0680

MCC **I46.8** **Cardiac arrest due to other underlying condition**
Code first underlying condition
MCC Exclusion see Appendix A PDX collection 0680

MCC **I46.9** **Cardiac arrest, cause unspecified**
MCC Exclusion see Appendix A PDX collection 0680

I47 **Paroxysmal tachycardia**
Code first tachycardia complicating:
abortion or ectopic or molar pregnancy (O00-O07, O08.8)
obstetric surgery and procedures (O75.4)
Excludes1: *tachycardia NOS (R00.0)*
sinoauricular tachycardia NOS (R00.0)
sinus [sinusal] tachycardia NOS (R00.0)

CC **I47.0** **Re-entry ventricular arrhythmia**
CC Exclusion see Appendix A PDX collection 0679

CC **I47.1** **Supraventricular tachycardia**
Atrial (paroxysmal) tachycardia
Atrioventricular [AV] (paroxysmal) tachycardia
Atrioventricular re-entrant (nodal) tachycardia [AVNRT] [AVRT]
Junctional (paroxysmal) tachycardia
Nodal (paroxysmal) tachycardia
CC Exclusion see Appendix A PDX collection 0679

CC **I47.2** **Ventricular tachycardia**
CC Exclusion see Appendix A PDX collection 0679
AHA CC: 3Q, 2013, 23-24

I47.9 **Paroxysmal tachycardia, unspecified**
Bouveret (-Hoffman) syndrome

I48 **Atrial fibrillation and flutter**

I48.0 **Paroxysmal atrial fibrillation**

CC **I48.1** **Persistent atrial fibrillation**
CC Exclusion see Appendix A PDX collection 0679

I48.2 **Chronic atrial fibrillation**
Permanent atrial fibrillation
AHA CC: 4Q, 2013, 128

CC **I48.3** **Typical atrial flutter**
Type I atrial flutter
CC Exclusion see Appendix A PDX collection 0679

CC **I48.4** **Atypical atrial flutter**
Type II atrial flutter
CC Exclusion see Appendix A PDX collection 0679

\+ **I48.9** **Unspecified atrial fibrillation and atrial flutter**
I48.91 **Unspecified atrial fibrillation**
CC **I48.92** **Unspecified atrial flutter**
CC Exclusion see Appendix A PDX collection 0679

I49 Other cardiac arrhythmias

Code first cardiac arrhythmia complicating:
abortion or ectopic or molar pregnancy (O00-O07, O08.8)
obstetric surgery and procedures (O75.4)

Excludes1: *neonatal dysrhythmia (P29.1-)*
sinoatrial bradycardia (R00.1)
sinus bradycardia (R00.1)
vagal bradycardia (R00.1)

Excludes2: *bradycardia NOS (R00.1)*

+ **I49.0 Ventricular fibrillation and flutter**
  - MCC **I49.01 Ventricular fibrillation**
    MCC Exclusion see Appendix A PDX collection 0679
  - MCC **I49.02 Ventricular flutter**
    MCC Exclusion see Appendix A PDX collection 0679

I49.1 Atrial premature depolarization
Atrial premature beats

CC **I49.2 Junctional premature depolarization**
CC Exclusion see Appendix A PDX collection 0679

I49.3 Ventricular premature depolarization

+ **I49.4 Other and unspecified premature depolarization**
  - **I49.40 Unspecified premature depolarization**
    Premature beats NOS
  - **I49.49 Other premature depolarization**
    Ectopic beats
    Extrasystoles
    Extrasystolic arrhythmias
    Premature contractions

I49.5 Sick sinus syndrome
Tachycardia-bradycardia syndrome

I49.8 Other specified cardiac arrhythmias
Brugada syndrome
Coronary sinus rhythm disorder
Ectopic rhythm disorder
Nodal rhythm disorder

I49.9 Cardiac arrhythmia, unspecified
Arrhythmia (cardiac) NOS

I50 Heart failure

Code first heart failure complicating abortion or ectopic or molar pregnancy (O00-O07, O08.8)
heart failure following surgery (I97.13-)
heart failure due to hypertension (I11.0)
heart failure due to hypertension with chronic kidney disease (I13.-)
obstetric surgery and procedures (O75.4)
rheumatic heart failure (I09.81)

Excludes1: *neonatal cardiac failure (P29.0)*

Excludes2: *cardiac arrest (I46.-)*

Review coding guidelines C.9.a.1 and C.9.a.3

AHA CC: 1Q, 2017, 47

CC **I50.1 Left ventricular failure, unspecified**
Cardiac asthma
Edema of lung with heart disease NOS
Edema of lung with heart failure
Left heart failure
Pulmonary edema with heart disease NOS
Pulmonary edema with heart failure
Excludes1: *edema of lung without heart disease or heart failure (J81.-)*
pulmonary edema without heart disease or failure (J81.-)
CC Exclusion see Appendix A PDX collection 0681

+ **I50.2 Systolic (congestive) heart failure**
Heart failure with reduced ejection fraction [HFrEF]
Systolic left ventricular heart failure
Code also end stage heart failure, if applicable (I50.84)
Excludes1: *combined systolic (congestive) and diastolic (congestive) heart failure (I50.4-)*
  - CC **I50.20 Unspecified systolic (congestive) heart failure**
    CC Exclusion see Appendix A PDX collection 0682
  - MCC **I50.21 Acute systolic (congestive) heart failure**
    MCC Exclusion see Appendix A PDX collection 0682
  - CC **I50.22 Chronic systolic (congestive) heart failure**
    CC Exclusion see Appendix A PDX collection 0682
  - MCC **I50.23 Acute on chronic systolic (congestive) heart failure**
    MCC Exclusion see Appendix A PDX collection 0682
    AHA CC: 2Q, 2013, 33

+ **I50.3 Diastolic (congestive) heart failure**
Diastolic left ventricular heart failure
Heart failure with normal ejection fraction
Heart failure with preserved ejection fraction [HFpEF]
Code also end stage heart failure, if applicable (I50.84)
Excludes1: *combined systolic (congestive) and diastolic (congestive) heart failure (I50.4-)*
  - CC **I50.30 Unspecified diastolic (congestive) heart failure**
    CC Exclusion see Appendix A PDX collection 0682
  - MCC **I50.31 Acute diastolic (congestive) heart failure**
    MCC Exclusion see Appendix A PDX collection 0682
    AHA CC: 1Q, 2017, 46
  - CC **I50.32 Chronic diastolic (congestive) heart failure**
    CC Exclusion see Appendix A PDX collection 0682
  - MCC **I50.33 Acute on chronic diastolic (congestive) heart failure**
    MCC Exclusion see Appendix A PDX collection 0682

+ **I50.4 Combined systolic (congestive) and diastolic (congestive) hear failure**
Combined systolic and diastolic left ventricular heart failure
Heart failure with reduced ejection fraction and diastolic dysfunction
Code also end stage heart failure, if applicable (I50.84)
  - CC **I50.40 Unspecified combined systolic (congestive) and diastolic (congestive) heart failure**
    CC Exclusion see Appendix A PDX collection 0682
  - MCC **I50.41 Acute combined systolic (congestive) and diastolic (congestive) heart failure**
    MCC Exclusion see Appendix A PDX collection 0682
  - CC **I50.42 Chronic combined systolic (congestive) and diastoli (congestive) heart failure**
    CC Exclusion see Appendix A PDX collection 0682
  - MCC **I50.43 Acute on chronic combined systolic (congestive) an diastolic (congestive) heart failure**
    MCC Exclusion see Appendix A PDX collection 0682

+ **I50.8 Other heart failure**
  - + **I50.81 Right heart failure**
    Right ventricular failure
    - **I50.810 Right heart failure, unspecified**
      Right heart failure without mention of left heart failure
      Right ventricular failure NOS
    - **I50.811 Acute right heart failure**
      Acute isolated right heart failure
      Acute (isolated) right ventricular failure
    - **I50.812 Chronic right heart failure**
      Chronic isolated right heart failure
      Chronic (isolated) right ventricular failure
    - **I50.813 Acute on chronic right heart failure**
      Acute on chronic isolated right heart failur
      Acute on chronic (isolated) right ventricula failure
      Acute decompensation of chronic (isolated right ventricular failure
      Acute exacerbation of chronic (isolated) right ventricular failure
    - **I50.814 Right heart failure, unspecified**
      Right ventricular failure secondary to left ventricular failure
      Code also the type of left ventricular failur if known (I50.2-I50.43)
      Excludes1: *right heart failure with but not due to left heart failure (I50.82)*
  - **I50.82 Biventricular heart failure**
    Code also the type of left ventricular failure as systoli diastolic, or combined, if known (I50.2-I50.43)
  - **I50.83 High output heart failure**
  - **I50.84 End stage heart failure**
    Stage D heart failure
    Code also the type of heart failure as systolic, diastoli or combined, if known (I50.2-I50.43)
  - **I50.89 Heart failure, unspecified**

I50.9 Heart failure, unspecified
Cardiac, heart or myocardial failure NOS
Congestive heart disease
Congestive heart failure NOS
Excludes2: *fluid overload (E87.70)*
AHA CC: 4Q, 2012, 92-93; 4Q, 2014, 21-22; 1Q, 2017, 46

I51 Complications and ill-defined descriptions of heart disease

Excludes1: *any condition in I51.4-I51.9 due to hypertension (I11.-)*
any condition in I51.4-I51.9 due to hypertension and chronic kidney disease (I13.-)
heart disease specified as rheumatic (I00-I09)

● CC **I51.0 Cardiac septal defect, acquired**
Acquired septal atrial defect (old)
Acquired septal auricular defect (old)
Acquired septal ventricular defect (old)
Excludes1: *cardiac septal defect as current complication following acute myocardial infarction (I23.1, I23.2)*
CC Exclusion see Appendix A PDX collection 0654

MCC **I51.1 Rupture of chordae tendineae, not elsewhere classified**
Excludes1: *rupture of chordae tendineae as current complication following acute myocardial infarction (I23.4)*
MCC Exclusion see Appendix A PDX collection 0655

MCC **I51.2 Rupture of papillary muscle, not elsewhere classified**
Excludes1: *rupture of papillary muscle as current complication following acute myocardial infarction (I23.5)*
MCC Exclusion see Appendix A PDX collection 0656

I51.3 Intracardiac thrombosis, not elsewhere classified
Apical thrombosis (old)
Atrial thrombosis (old)
Auricular thrombosis (old)
Mural thrombosis (old)
Ventricular thrombosis (old)
Excludes1: *intracardiac thrombosis as current complication following acute myocardial infarction (I23.6)*
AHA CC: 1Q, 2013, 24

I51.4 Myocarditis, unspecified
Chronic (interstitial) myocarditis
Myocardial fibrosis
Myocarditis NOS
Excludes1: *acute or subacute myocarditis (I40.-)*
Review coding guideline C.9.a.1

I51.5 Myocardial degeneration
Fatty degeneration of heart or myocardium
Myocardial disease
Senile degeneration of heart or myocardium
Review coding guideline C.9.a.1

I51.7 Cardiomegaly
Cardiac dilatation
Cardiac hypertrophy
Ventricular dilatation
Review coding guideline C.9.a.1

\+ **I51.8 Other ill-defined heart diseases**
Review coding guideline C.9.a.1

CC **I51.81 Takotsubo syndrome**
Reversible left ventricular dysfunction following sudden emotional stress
Stress induced cardiomyopathy
Takotsubo cardiomyopathy
Transient left ventricular apical ballooning syndrome
CC Exclusion see Appendix A PDX collection 0683

I51.89 Other ill-defined heart diseases
Carditis (acute)(chronic)
Pancarditis (acute)(chronic)

I51.9 Heart disease, unspecified
Review coding guideline C.9.a.1

I52 Other heart disorders in diseases classified elsewhere

Code first underlying disease, such as:
congenital syphilis (A50.5)
mucopolysaccharidosis (E76.3)
schistosomiasis (B65.0-B65.9)

Excludes1: *heart disease (in):*
gonococcal infection (A54.83)
meningococcal infection (A39.50)
rheumatoid arthritis (M05.31)
syphilis (A52.06)

Valid 3-character code, no further characters required

Cerebrovascular diseases (I60-I69)

Use additional code to identify presence of:
alcohol abuse and dependence (F10.-)
exposure to environmental tobacco smoke (Z77.22)
history of tobacco dependence (Z87.891)
hypertension (I10-I15)
occupational exposure to environmental tobacco smoke (Z57.31)
tobacco dependence (F17.-)
tobacco use (Z72.0)

Excludes1: *traumatic intracranial hemorrhage (S06.-)*

Review coding guidelines C.9.a.4 and C.9.d

I60 Nontraumatic subarachnoid hemorrhage

Excludes1: *syphilitic ruptured cerebral aneurysm (A52.05)*
Excludes2: *sequelae of subarachnoid hemorrhage (I69.0-)*

\+ **I60.0 Nontraumatic subarachnoid hemorrhage from carotid siphon and bifurcation**

MCC **I60.00 Nontraumatic subarachnoid hemorrhage from unspecified carotid siphon and bifurcation**
MCC Exclusion see Appendix A PDX collection 0684

MCC **I60.01 Nontraumatic subarachnoid hemorrhage from right carotid siphon and bifurcation**
MCC Exclusion see Appendix A PDX collection 0684

MCC **I60.02 Nontraumatic subarachnoid hemorrhage from left carotid siphon and bifurcation**
MCC Exclusion see Appendix A PDX collection 0684

\+ **I60.1 Nontraumatic subarachnoid hemorrhage from middle cerebral artery**

MCC **I60.10 Nontraumatic subarachnoid hemorrhage from unspecified middle cerebral artery**
MCC Exclusion see Appendix A PDX collection 0684

MCC **I60.11 Nontraumatic subarachnoid hemorrhage from right middle cerebral artery**
MCC Exclusion see Appendix A PDX collection 0684

MCC **I60.12 Nontraumatic subarachnoid hemorrhage from left middle cerebral artery**
MCC Exclusion see Appendix A PDX collection 0684

MCC **I60.2 Nontraumatic subarachnoid hemorrhage from anterior communicating artery**
MCC Exclusion see Appendix A PDX collection 0684

\+ **I60.3 Nontraumatic subarachnoid hemorrhage from posterior communicating artery**

MCC **I60.30 Nontraumatic subarachnoid hemorrhage from unspecified posterior communicating artery**
MCC Exclusion see Appendix A PDX collection 0684

MCC **I60.31 Nontraumatic subarachnoid hemorrhage from right posterior communicating artery**
MCC Exclusion see Appendix A PDX collection 0684

MCC **I60.32 Nontraumatic subarachnoid hemorrhage from left posterior communicating artery**
MCC Exclusion see Appendix A PDX collection 0684

MCC **I60.4 Nontraumatic subarachnoid hemorrhage from basilar artery**
MCC Exclusion see Appendix A PDX collection 0684

\+ **I60.5 Nontraumatic subarachnoid hemorrhage from vertebral artery**

MCC **I60.50 Nontraumatic subarachnoid hemorrhage from unspecified vertebral artery**
MCC Exclusion see Appendix A PDX collection 0684

MCC **I60.51 Nontraumatic subarachnoid hemorrhage from right vertebral artery**
MCC Exclusion see Appendix A PDX collection 0684

MCC **I60.52 Nontraumatic subarachnoid hemorrhage from left vertebral artery**
MCC Exclusion see Appendix A PDX collection 0684

MCC **I60.6 Nontraumatic subarachnoid hemorrhage from other intracranial arteries**
MCC Exclusion see Appendix A PDX collection 0684

MCC **I60.7 Nontraumatic subarachnoid hemorrhage from unspecified intracranial artery**
Ruptured (congenital) berry aneurysm
Ruptured (congenital) cerebral aneurysm
Subarachnoid hemorrhage (nontraumatic) from cerebral artery NOS
Subarachnoid hemorrhage (nontraumatic) from communicating artery NOS
Excludes1: *berry aneurysm, nonruptured (I67.1)*
MCC Exclusion see Appendix A PDX collection 0684

MCC **I60.8 Other nontraumatic subarachnoid hemorrhage**
Meningeal hemorrhage
Rupture of cerebral arteriovenous malformation
MCC Exclusion see Appendix A PDX collection 0684

MCC **I60.9 Nontraumatic subarachnoid hemorrhage, unspecified**
MCC Exclusion see Appendix A PDX collection 0684

I61 Nontraumatic intracerebral hemorrhage

Excludes2: *sequelae of intracerebral hemorrhage (I69.1-)*

AHA CC: 2Q, 2017, 10

MCC **I61.0** **Nontraumatic intracerebral hemorrhage in hemisphere, subcortical**

Deep intracerebral hemorrhage (nontraumatic)

MCC Exclusion see Appendix A PDX collection 0684

MCC **I61.1** **Nontraumatic intracerebral hemorrhage in hemisphere, cortical**

Cerebral lobe hemorrhage (nontraumatic)

Superficial intracerebral hemorrhage (nontraumatic)

MCC Exclusion see Appendix A PDX collection 0684

MCC **I61.2** **Nontraumatic intracerebral hemorrhage in hemisphere, unspecified**

MCC Exclusion see Appendix A PDX collection 0684

MCC **I61.3** **Nontraumatic intracerebral hemorrhage in brain stem**

MCC Exclusion see Appendix A PDX collection 0684

MCC **I61.4** **Nontraumatic intracerebral hemorrhage in cerebellum**

MCC Exclusion see Appendix A PDX collection 0684

MCC **I61.5** **Nontraumatic intracerebral hemorrhage, intraventricular**

MCC Exclusion see Appendix A PDX collection 0684

MCC **I61.6** **Nontraumatic intracerebral hemorrhage, multiple localized**

MCC Exclusion see Appendix A PDX collection 0684

MCC **I61.8** **Other nontraumatic intracerebral hemorrhage**

MCC Exclusion see Appendix A PDX collection 0684

MCC **I61.9** **Nontraumatic intracerebral hemorrhage, unspecified**

MCC Exclusion see Appendix A PDX collection 0684

I62 Other and unspecified nontraumatic intracranial hemorrhage

Excludes2: *sequelae of intracranial hemorrhage (I69.2)*

+ **I62.0** **Nontraumatic subdural hemorrhage**

MCC **I62.00** **Nontraumatic subdural hemorrhage, unspecified**

MCC Exclusion see Appendix A PDX collection 0684

MCC **I62.01** **Nontraumatic acute subdural hemorrhage**

MCC Exclusion see Appendix A PDX collection 0684

MCC **I62.02** **Nontraumatic subacute subdural hemorrhage**

MCC Exclusion see Appendix A PDX collection 0684

MCC **I62.03** **Nontraumatic chronic subdural hemorrhage**

MCC Exclusion see Appendix A PDX collection 0684

MCC **I62.1** **Nontraumatic extradural hemorrhage**

Nontraumatic epidural hemorrhage

MCC Exclusion see Appendix A PDX collection 0684

CC **I62.9** **Nontraumatic intracranial hemorrhage, unspecified**

CC Exclusion see Appendix A PDX collection 0684

I63 Cerebral infarction

Includes: occlusion and stenosis of cerebral and precerebral arteries, resulting in cerebral infarction

Use additional code, if applicable, to identify status post administration of tPA (rtPA) in a different facility within the last 24 hours prior to admission to current facility (Z92.82)

Use additional code, if known, to indicate National Institutes of Health Stroke Scale (NIHSS) score (R29.7-)

Excludes2: *sequelae of cerebral infarction (I69.3-)*

AHA CC: 4Q, 2016, 28

+ **I63.0** **Cerebral infarction due to thrombosis of precerebral arteries**

MCC **I63.00** **Cerebral infarction due to thrombosis of unspecified precerebral artery**

MCC Exclusion see Appendix A PDX collection 0685

+ **I63.01** **Cerebral infarction due to thrombosis of vertebral artery**

MCC **I63.011** **Cerebral infarction due to thrombosis of right vertebral artery**

MCC Exclusion see Appendix A PDX collection 0686

MCC **I63.012** **Cerebral infarction due to thrombosis of left vertebral artery**

MCC Exclusion see Appendix A PDX collection 0686

MCC **I63.013** **Cerebral infarction due to thrombosis of bilateral vertebral arteries**

MCC Exclusion see Appendix A PDX collection 0686

MCC **I63.019** **Cerebral infarction due to thrombosis of unspecified vertebral artery**

MCC Exclusion see Appendix A PDX collection 0686

MCC **I63.02** **Cerebral infarction due to thrombosis of basilar artery**

MCC Exclusion see Appendix A PDX collection 0685

+ **I63.03** **Cerebral infarction due to thrombosis of carotid artery**

MCC **I63.031** **Cerebral infarction due to thrombosis of right carotid artery**

MCC Exclusion see Appendix A PDX collection 0687

MCC **I63.032** **Cerebral infarction due to thrombosis of left carotid artery**

MCC Exclusion see Appendix A PDX collection 0687

MCC **I63.033** **Cerebral infarction due to thrombosis of bilateral carotid arteries**

MCC Exclusion see Appendix A PDX collection 0687

MCC **I63.039** **Cerebral infarction due to thrombosis of unspecified carotid artery**

MCC Exclusion see Appendix A PDX collection 0687

MCC **I63.09** **Cerebral infarction due to thrombosis of other precerebral artery**

MCC Exclusion see Appendix A PDX collection 0685

+ **I63.1** **Cerebral infarction due to embolism of precerebral arteries**

MCC **I63.10** **Cerebral infarction due to embolism of unspecified precerebral artery**

MCC Exclusion see Appendix A PDX collection 0685

+ **I63.11** **Cerebral infarction due to embolism of vertebral artery**

MCC **I63.111** **Cerebral infarction due to embolism of right vertebral artery**

MCC Exclusion see Appendix A PDX collection 0686

MCC **I63.112** **Cerebral infarction due to embolism of left vertebral artery**

MCC Exclusion see Appendix A PDX collection 0686

MCC **I63.113** **Cerebral infarction due to embolism of bilateral vertebral arteries**

MCC Exclusion see Appendix A PDX collection 0686

MCC **I63.119** **Cerebral infarction due to embolism of unspecified vertebral artery**

MCC Exclusion see Appendix A PDX collection 0686

MCC **I63.12** **Cerebral infarction due to embolism of basilar artery**

MCC Exclusion see Appendix A PDX collection 0685

+ **I63.13** **Cerebral infarction due to embolism of carotid artery**

MCC **I63.131** **Cerebral infarction due to embolism of right carotid artery**

MCC Exclusion see Appendix A PDX collection 0687

MCC **I63.132** **Cerebral infarction due to embolism of left carotid artery**

MCC Exclusion see Appendix A PDX collection 0687

MCC **I63.133** **Cerebral infarction due to embolism of bilateral carotid arteries**

MCC Exclusion see Appendix A PDX collection 0687

MCC **I63.139** **Cerebral infarction due to embolism of unspecified carotid artery**

MCC Exclusion see Appendix A PDX collection 0687

MCC **I63.19** **Cerebral infarction due to embolism of other precerebral artery**

MCC Exclusion see Appendix A PDX collection 0685

+ **I63.2** **Cerebral infarction due to unspecified occlusion or stenosis of precerebral arteries**

MCC **I63.20** **Cerebral infarction due to unspecified occlusion or stenosis of unspecified precerebral arteries**

MCC Exclusion see Appendix A PDX collection 0685

+ **I63.21** **Cerebral infarction due to unspecified occlusion or stenosis of vertebral arteries**

MCC **I63.211** **Cerebral infarction due to unspecified occlusion or stenosis of right vertebral artery**

MCC Exclusion see Appendix A PDX collection 0686

MCC **I63.212** **Cerebral infarction due to unspecified occlusion or stenosis of left vertebral artery**

MCC Exclusion see Appendix A PDX collection 0686

MCC **I63.213** **Cerebral infarction due to unspecified occlusion or stenosis of bilateral vertebral arteries**

MCC Exclusion see Appendix A PDX collection 0686

MCC **I63.219** **Cerebral infarction due to unspecified occlusion or stenosis of unspecified vertebral arteries**

MCC Exclusion see Appendix A PDX collection 0686

MCC **I63.22** Cerebral infarction due to unspecified occlusion or stenosis of basilar artery
MCC Exclusion see Appendix A PDX collection 0685

+ **I63.23** Cerebral infarction due to unspecified occlusion or stenosis of carotid arteries

MCC **I63.231** Cerebral infarction due to unspecified occlusion or stenosis of right carotid arteries
MCC Exclusion see Appendix A PDX collection 0687

MCC **I63.232** Cerebral infarction due to unspecified occlusion or stenosis of left carotid arteries
MCC Exclusion see Appendix A PDX collection 0687

MCC **I63.233** Cerebral infarction due to unspecified occlusion or stenosis of bilateral carotid arteries
MCC Exclusion see Appendix A PDX collection 0687

MCC **I63.239** Cerebral infarction due to unspecified occlusion or stenosis of unspecified carotid arteries
MCC Exclusion see Appendix A PDX collection 0687

MCC **I63.29** Cerebral infarction due to unspecified occlusion or stenosis of other precerebral arteries
MCC Exclusion see Appendix A PDX collection 0685

+ **I63.3** Cerebral infarction due to thrombosis of cerebral arteries

MCC **I63.30** Cerebral infarction due to thrombosis of unspecified cerebral artery
MCC Exclusion see Appendix A PDX collection 0688

+ **I63.31** Cerebral infarction due to thrombosis of middle cerebral artery

MCC **I63.311** Cerebral infarction due to thrombosis of right middle cerebral artery
MCC Exclusion see Appendix A PDX collection 0688

MCC **I63.312** Cerebral infarction due to thrombosis of left middle cerebral artery
MCC Exclusion see Appendix A PDX collection 0688

MCC **I63.313** Cerebral infarction due to thrombosis of bilateral middle cerebral arteries
MCC Exclusion see Appendix A PDX collection 0688

MCC **I63.319** Cerebral infarction due to thrombosis of unspecified middle cerebral artery
MCC Exclusion see Appendix A PDX collection 0688

+ **I63.32** Cerebral infarction due to thrombosis of anterior cerebral artery

MCC **I63.321** Cerebral infarction due to thrombosis of right anterior cerebral artery
MCC Exclusion see Appendix A PDX collection 0688

MCC **I63.322** Cerebral infarction due to thrombosis of left anterior cerebral artery
MCC Exclusion see Appendix A PDX collection 0688

MCC **I63.323** Cerebral infarction due to thrombosis of bilateral anterior cerebral arteries
MCC Exclusion see Appendix A PDX collection 0688

MCC **I63.329** Cerebral infarction due to thrombosis of unspecified anterior cerebral artery
MCC Exclusion see Appendix A PDX collection 0688

+ **I63.33** Cerebral infarction due to thrombosis of posterior cerebral artery

MCC **I63.331** Cerebral infarction due to thrombosis of right posterior cerebral artery
MCC Exclusion see Appendix A PDX collection 0688

MCC **I63.332** Cerebral infarction due to thrombosis of left posterior cerebral artery
MCC Exclusion see Appendix A PDX collection 0688

MCC **I63.333** Cerebral infarction to thrombosis of bilateral posterior cerebral arteries
MCC Exclusion see Appendix A PDX collection 0688

MCC **I63.339** Cerebral infarction due to thrombosis of unspecified posterior cerebral artery
MCC Exclusion see Appendix A PDX collection 0688

+ **I63.34** Cerebral infarction due to thrombosis of cerebellar artery

MCC **I63.341** Cerebral infarction due to thrombosis of right cerebellar artery
MCC Exclusion see Appendix A PDX collection 0688

MCC **I63.342** Cerebral infarction due to thrombosis of left cerebellar artery
MCC Exclusion see Appendix A PDX collection 0688

MCC **I63.343** Cerebral infarction to thrombosis of bilateral cerebellar arteries
MCC Exclusion see Appendix A PDX collection 0688

MCC **I63.349** Cerebral infarction due to thrombosis of unspecified cerebellar artery
MCC Exclusion see Appendix A PDX collection 0688

MCC **I63.39** Cerebral infarction due to thrombosis of other cerebral artery
MCC Exclusion see Appendix A PDX collection 0688

+ **I63.4** Cerebral infarction due to embolism of cerebral arteries

MCC **I63.40** Cerebral infarction due to embolism of unspecified cerebral artery
MCC Exclusion see Appendix A PDX collection 0688

+ **I63.41** Cerebral infarction due to embolism of middle cerebral artery

MCC **I63.411** Cerebral infarction due to embolism of right middle cerebral artery
MCC Exclusion see Appendix A PDX collection 0688

MCC **I63.412** Cerebral infarction due to embolism of left middle cerebral artery
MCC Exclusion see Appendix A PDX collection 0688

MCC **I63.413** Cerebral infarction due to embolism of bilateral middle cerebral arteries
MCC Exclusion see Appendix A PDX collection 0688

MCC **I63.419** Cerebral infarction due to embolism of unspecified middle cerebral artery
MCC Exclusion see Appendix A PDX collection 0688

+ **I63.42** Cerebral infarction due to embolism of anterior cerebral artery

MCC **I63.421** Cerebral infarction due to embolism of right anterior cerebral artery
MCC Exclusion see Appendix A PDX collection 0688

MCC **I63.422** Cerebral infarction due to embolism of left anterior cerebral artery
MCC Exclusion see Appendix A PDX collection 0688

MCC **I63.423** Cerebral infarction due to embolism of bilateral anterior cerebral arteries
MCC Exclusion see Appendix A PDX collection 0688

MCC **I63.429** Cerebral infarction due to embolism of unspecified anterior cerebral artery
MCC Exclusion see Appendix A PDX collection 0688

+ **I63.43** Cerebral infarction due to embolism of posterior cerebral artery

MCC **I63.431** Cerebral infarction due to embolism of right posterior cerebral artery
MCC Exclusion see Appendix A PDX collection 0688

MCC **I63.432** Cerebral infarction due to embolism of left posterior cerebral artery
MCC Exclusion see Appendix A PDX collection 0688

MCC **I63.433** Cerebral infarction due to embolism of bilateral posterior cerebral arteries
MCC Exclusion see Appendix A PDX collection 0688

MCC **I63.439** Cerebral infarction due to embolism of unspecified posterior cerebral artery
MCC Exclusion see Appendix A PDX collection 0688

+ **I63.44** Cerebral infarction due to embolism of cerebellar artery

MCC **I63.441** Cerebral infarction due to embolism of right cerebellar artery
MCC Exclusion see Appendix A PDX collection 0688

MCC **I63.442** **Cerebral infarction due to embolism of left cerebellar artery**
MCC Exclusion see Appendix A PDX collection 0688

MCC **I64.443** **Cerebral infarction due to embolism of bilateral cerebellar arteries**
MCC Exclusion see Appendix A PDX collection 0688

MCC **I63.449** **Cerebral infarction due to embolism of unspecified cerebellar artery**
MCC Exclusion see Appendix A PDX collection 0688

MCC **I63.49** **Cerebral infarction due to embolism of other cerebral artery**
MCC Exclusion see Appendix A PDX collection 0688

+ **I63.5** **Cerebral infarction due to unspecified occlusion or stenosis of cerebral arteries**

MCC **I63.50** **Cerebral infarction due to unspecified occlusion or stenosis of unspecified cerebral artery**
MCC Exclusion see Appendix A PDX collection 0688

+ **I63.51** **Cerebral infarction due to unspecified occlusion or stenosis of middle cerebral artery**

MCC **I63.511** **Cerebral infarction due to unspecified occlusion or stenosis of right middle cerebral artery**
MCC Exclusion see Appendix A PDX collection 0688

MCC **I63.512** **Cerebral infarction due to unspecified occlusion or stenosis of left middle cerebral artery**
MCC Exclusion see Appendix A PDX collection 0688

MCC **I63.513** **Cerebral infarction due to unspecified occlusion or stenosis of bilateral middle cerebral arteries**
MCC Exclusion see Appendix A PDX collection 0688

MCC **I63.519** **Cerebral infarction due to unspecified occlusion or stenosis of unspecified middle cerebral artery**
MCC Exclusion see Appendix A PDX collection 0688

+ **I63.52** **Cerebral infarction due to unspecified occlusion or stenosis of anterior cerebral artery**

MCC **I63.521** **Cerebral infarction due to unspecified occlusion or stenosis of right anterior cerebral artery**
MCC Exclusion see Appendix A PDX collection 0688

MCC **I63.522** **Cerebral infarction due to unspecified occlusion or stenosis of left anterior cerebral artery**
MCC Exclusion see Appendix A PDX collection 0688

MCC **I63.523** **Cerebral infarction due to unspecified occlusion or stenosis of bilateral anterior cerebral arteries**
MCC Exclusion see Appendix A PDX collection 0688

MCC **I63.529** **Cerebral infarction due to unspecified occlusion or stenosis of unspecified anterior cerebral artery**
MCC Exclusion see Appendix A PDX collection 0688

+ **I63.53** **Cerebral infarction due to unspecified occlusion or stenosis of posterior cerebral artery**

MCC **I63.531** **Cerebral infarction due to unspecified occlusion or stenosis of right posterior cerebral artery**
MCC Exclusion see Appendix A PDX collection 0688

MCC **I63.532** **Cerebral infarction due to unspecified occlusion or stenosis of left posterior cerebral artery**
MCC Exclusion see Appendix A PDX collection 0688
AHA CC: 2Q, 2017, 10

MCC **I63.533** **Cerebral infarction due to unspecified occlusion or stenosis of bilateral posterior cerebral arteries**
MCC Exclusion see Appendix A PDX collection 0688

MCC **I63.539** **Cerebral infarction due to unspecified occlusion or stenosis of unspecified posterior cerebral artery**
MCC Exclusion see Appendix A PDX collection 0688

+ **I63.54** **Cerebral infarction due to unspecified occlusion or stenosis of cerebellar artery**

MCC **I63.541** **Cerebral infarction due to unspecified occlusion or stenosis of right cerebellar artery**
MCC Exclusion see Appendix A PDX collection 0688

MCC **I63.542** **Cerebral infarction due to unspecified occlusion or stenosis of left cerebellar artery**
MCC Exclusion see Appendix A PDX collection 0688

MCC **I63.543** **Cerebral infarction due to unspecified occlusion or stenosis of bilateral cerebellar arteries**
MCC Exclusion see Appendix A PDX collection 0688

MCC **I63.549** **Cerebral infarction due to unspecified occlusion or stenosis of unspecified cerebellar artery**
MCC Exclusion see Appendix A PDX collection 0688

MCC **I63.59** **Cerebral infarction due to unspecified occlusion or stenosis of other cerebral artery**
MCC Exclusion see Appendix A PDX collection 0688

MCC **I63.6** **Cerebral infarction due to cerebral venous thrombosis, nonpyogenic**
MCC Exclusion see Appendix A PDX collection 0688

MCC **I63.8** **Other cerebral infarction**
MCC Exclusion see Appendix A PDX collection 0688
AHA CC: 2Q, 2017, 9-10

MCC **I63.9** **Cerebral infarction, unspecified**
Stroke NOS
Excludes2: *transient cerebral ischemic attacks and related syndromes (G45.-)*
MCC Exclusion see Appendix A PDX collection 0688
AHA CC: 1Q, 2015, 26; 4Q, 2016, 61-62

I65 **Occlusion and stenosis of precerebral arteries, not resulting in cerebral infarction**

Includes: embolism of precerebral artery
narrowing of precerebral artery
obstruction (complete) (partial) of precerebral artery
thrombosis of precerebral artery

Excludes1: *insufficiency, NOS, of precerebral artery (G45.-)*
insufficiency of precerebral arteries causing cerebral infarction (I63.0-I63.2)

+ **I65.0** **Occlusion and stenosis of vertebral artery**
I65.01 **Occlusion and stenosis of right vertebral artery**
I65.02 **Occlusion and stenosis of left vertebral artery**
I65.03 **Occlusion and stenosis of bilateral vertebral arteries**
I65.09 **Occlusion and stenosis of unspecified vertebral artery**

I65.1 **Occlusion and stenosis of basilar artery**

+ **I65.2** **Occlusion and stenosis of carotid artery**
I65.21 **Occlusion and stenosis of right carotid artery**
I65.22 **Occlusion and stenosis of left carotid artery**
I65.23 **Occlusion and stenosis of bilateral carotid arteries**
I65.29 **Occlusion and stenosis of unspecified carotid artery**

I65.8 **Occlusion and stenosis of other precerebral arteries**

I65.9 **Occlusion and stenosis of unspecified precerebral artery**
Occlusion and stenosis of precerebral artery NOS

I66 **Occlusion and stenosis of cerebral arteries, not resulting in cerebral infarction**

Includes: embolism of cerebral artery
narrowing of cerebral artery
obstruction (complete) (partial) of cerebral artery
thrombosis of cerebral artery

Excludes1: *Occlusion and stenosis of cerebral artery causing cerebral infarction (I63.3-I63.5)*

+ **I66.0** **Occlusion and stenosis of middle cerebral artery**
I66.01 **Occlusion and stenosis of right middle cerebral artery**
I66.02 **Occlusion and stenosis of left middle cerebral artery**

I66.03 **Occlusion and stenosis of bilateral middle cerebral arteries**
I66.09 **Occlusion and stenosis of unspecified middle cerebral artery**

+ I66.1 **Occlusion and stenosis of anterior cerebral artery**
I66.11 **Occlusion and stenosis of right anterior cerebral artery**
I66.12 **Occlusion and stenosis of left anterior cerebral artery**
I66.13 **Occlusion and stenosis of bilateral anterior cerebral arteries**
I66.19 **Occlusion and stenosis of unspecified anterior cerebral artery**

+ I66.2 **Occlusion and stenosis of posterior cerebral artery**
I66.21 **Occlusion and stenosis of right posterior cerebral artery**
I66.22 **Occlusion and stenosis of left posterior cerebral artery**
I66.23 **Occlusion and stenosis of bilateral posterior cerebral arteries**
I66.29 **Occlusion and stenosis of unspecified posterior cerebral artery**

I66.3 **Occlusion and stenosis of cerebellar arteries**
I66.8 **Occlusion and stenosis of other cerebral arteries**
Occlusion and stenosis of perforating arteries
I66.9 **Occlusion and stenosis of unspecified cerebral artery**

I67 Other cerebrovascular diseases

Excludes2: *sequelae of the listed conditions (I69.8)*

MCC I67.0 **Dissection of cerebral arteries, nonruptured**
Excludes1: *ruptured cerebral arteries (I60.7)*
MCC Exclusion see Appendix A PDX collection 0689

I67.1 **Cerebral aneurysm, nonruptured**
Cerebral aneurysm NOS
Cerebral arteriovenous fistula, acquired
Internal carotid artery aneurysm, intracranial portion
Internal carotid artery aneurysm, NOS
Excludes1: *congenital cerebral aneurysm, nonruptured (Q28.-)*
ruptured cerebral aneurysm (I60.7)

• I67.2 **Cerebral atherosclerosis**
Atheroma of cerebral and precerebral arteries

CC I67.3 **Progressive vascular leukoencephalopathy**
Binswanger's disease
CC Exclusion see Appendix A PDX collection 0133

CC I67.4 **Hypertensive encephalopathy**
Excludes2: *insufficiency, NOS, of precerebral arteries (G45.2)*
CC Exclusion see Appendix A PDX collection 0690

CC I67.5 **Moyamoya disease**
CC Exclusion see Appendix A PDX collection 0691

CC I67.6 **Nonpyogenic thrombosis of intracranial venous system**
Nonpyogenic thrombosis of cerebral vein
Nonpyogenic thrombosis of intracranial venous sinus
Excludes1: *nonpyogenic thrombosis of intracranial venous system causing infarction (I63.6)*
CC Exclusion see Appendix A PDX collection 0692

CC I67.7 **Cerebral arteritis, not elsewhere classified**
Granulomatous angiitis of the nervous system
Excludes1: *allergic granulomatous angiitis (M30.1)*
CC Exclusion see Appendix A PDX collection 0693

+ I67.8 **Other specified cerebrovascular diseases**
CC I67.81 **Acute cerebrovascular insufficiency**
Acute cerebrovascular insufficiency unspecified as to location or reversibility
CC Exclusion see Appendix A PDX collection 0694
CC I67.82 **Cerebral ischemia**
Chronic cerebral ischemia
CC Exclusion see Appendix A PDX collection 0694
MCC I67.83 **Posterior reversible encephalopathy syndrome**
PRES
MCC Exclusion see Appendix A PDX collection 0610
+ I67.84 **Cerebral vasospasm and vasoconstriction**
CC I67.841 **Reversible cerebrovascular vasoconstriction syndrome**
Call-Fleming syndrome
Code first underlying condition, if applicable, such as eclampsia (O15.00-O15.9)
CC Exclusion see Appendix A PDX collection 0586
CC I67.848 **Other cerebrovascular vasospasm and vasoconstriction**
CC Exclusion see Appendix A PDX collection 0586
CC I67.89 **Other cerebrovascular disease**
CC Exclusion see Appendix A PDX collection 0694

I67.9 **Cerebrovascular disease, unspecified**

I68 Cerebrovascular disorders in diseases classified elsewhere

I68.0 **Cerebral amyloid angiopathy**
Code first underlying amyloidosis (E85.-)

CC I68.2 **Cerebral arteritis in other diseases classified elsewhere**
Code first underlying disease
Excludes1: *cerebral arteritis (in):*
listerosis (A32.89)
systemic lupus erythematosus (M32.19)
syphilis (A52.04)
tuberculosis (A18.89)
CC Exclusion see Appendix A PDX collection 0693

I68.8 **Other cerebrovascular disorders in diseases classified elsewhere**
Code first underlying disease
Excludes1: *syphilitic cerebral aneurysm (A52.05)*

I69 Sequelae of cerebrovascular disease

NOTE Category I69 is to be used to indicate conditions in I60-I67 as the cause of sequelae. The 'sequelae' include conditions specified as such or as residuals which may occur at any time after the onset of the causal condition

Excludes1: *personal history of cerebral infarction without residual deficit (Z86.73)*
personal history of prolonged reversible ischemic neurologic deficit (PRIND) (Z86.73)
personal history of reversible ischemic neurologcial deficit (RIND) (Z86.73)
sequelae of traumatic intracranial injury (S06.-)

Review coding guideline C.9.d
AHA CC: 4Q, 2016, 28

+ I69.0 **Sequelae of nontraumatic subarachnoid hemorrhage**
I69.00 **Unspecified sequelae of nontraumatic subarachnoid hemorrhage**
+ I69.01 **Cognitive deficits following nontraumatic subarachnoid hemorrhage**
I69.010 **Attention and concentration deficit following nontraumatic subarachnoid hemorrhage**
I69.011 **Memory deficit following nontraumatic subarachnoid hemorrhage**
I69.012 **Visuospatial deficit and spatial neglect following nontraumatic subarachnoid hemorrhage**
I69.013 **Psychomotor deficit following nontraumatic subarachnoid hemorrhage**
I69.014 **Frontal lobe and executive function deficit following nontraumatic subarachnoid hemorrhage**
I69.015 **Cognitive social or emotional deficit following nontraumatic subarachnoid hemorrhage**
I69.018 **Other symptoms and signs involving cognitive functions following nontraumatic subarachnoid hemorrhage**
I69.019 **Unspecified symptoms and signs involving cognitive functions following nontraumatic subarachnoid hemorrhage**
+ I69.02 **Speech and language deficits following nontraumatic subarachnoid hemorrhage**
I69.020 **Aphasia following nontraumatic subarachnoid hemorrhage**
I69.021 **Dysphasia following nontraumatic subarachnoid hemorrhage**
I69.022 **Dysarthria following nontraumatic subarachnoid hemorrhage**
I69.023 **Fluency disorder following nontraumatic subarachnoid hemorrhage**
Stuttering following nontraumatic subarachnoid hemorrhage
I69.028 **Other speech and language deficits following nontraumatic subarachnoid hemorrhage**
+ I69.03 **Monoplegia of upper limb following nontraumatic subarachnoid hemorrhage**
I69.031 **Monoplegia of upper limb following nontraumatic subarachnoid hemorrhage affecting right dominant side**

I69.032 Monoplegia of upper limb following nontraumatic subarachnoid hemorrhage affecting left dominant side
I69.033 Monoplegia of upper limb following nontraumatic subarachnoid hemorrhage affecting right non-dominant side
I69.034 Monoplegia of upper limb following nontraumatic subarachnoid hemorrhage affecting left non-dominant side
I69.039 Monoplegia of upper limb following nontraumatic subarachnoid hemorrhage affecting unspecified side

+ I69.04 Monoplegia of lower limb following nontraumatic subarachnoid hemorrhage

I69.041 Monoplegia of lower limb following nontraumatic subarachnoid hemorrhage affecting right dominant side
I69.042 Monoplegia of lower limb following nontraumatic subarachnoid hemorrhage affecting left dominant side
I69.043 Monoplegia of lower limb following nontraumatic subarachnoid hemorrhage affecting right non-dominant side
I69.044 Monoplegia of lower limb following nontraumatic subarachnoid hemorrhage affecting left non-dominant side
I69.049 Monoplegia of lower limb following nontraumatic subarachnoid hemorrhage affecting unspecified side

+ I69.05 Hemiplegia and hemiparesis following nontraumatic subarachnoid hemorrhage

CC I69.051 Hemiplegia and hemiparesis following nontraumatic subarachnoid hemorrhage affecting right dominant side
CC Exclusion see Appendix A PDX collection 0695

CC I69.052 Hemiplegia and hemiparesis following nontraumatic subarachnoid hemorrhage affecting left dominant side
CC Exclusion see Appendix A PDX collection 0695

CC I69.053 Hemiplegia and hemiparesis following nontraumatic subarachnoid hemorrhage affecting right non-dominant side
CC Exclusion see Appendix A PDX collection 0696

CC I69.054 Hemiplegia and hemiparesis following nontraumatic subarachnoid hemorrhage affecting left non-dominant side
CC Exclusion see Appendix A PDX collection 0696

CC I69.059 Hemiplegia and hemiparesis following nontraumatic subarachnoid hemorrhage affecting unspecified side
CC Exclusion see Appendix A PDX collection 0697

+ I69.06 Other paralytic syndrome following nontraumatic subarachnoid hemorrhage

Use additional code to identify type of paralytic syndrome, such as:
locked-in state (G83.5)
quadriplegia (G82.5-)

Excludes1: *hemiplegia/hemiparesis following nontraumatic subarachnoid hemorrhage (I69.05-)*
monoplegia of lower limb following nontraumatic subarachnoid hemorrhage (I69.04-)
monoplegia of upper limb following nontraumatic subarachnoid hemorrhage (I69.03-)

I69.061 Other paralytic syndrome following nontraumatic subarachnoid hemorrhage affecting right dominant side
I69.062 Other paralytic syndrome following nontraumatic subarachnoid hemorrhage affecting left dominant side
I69.063 Other paralytic syndrome following nontraumatic subarachnoid hemorrhage affecting right non-dominant side
I69.064 Other paralytic syndrome following nontraumatic subarachnoid hemorrhage affecting left non-dominant side
I69.065 Other paralytic syndrome following nontraumatic subarachnoid hemorrhage, bilateral
I69.069 Other paralytic syndrome following nontraumatic subarachnoid hemorrhage affecting unspecified side

+ I69.09 Other sequelae of nontraumatic subarachnoid hemorrhage

I69.090 Apraxia following nontraumatic subarachnoid hemorrhage
I69.091 Dysphagia following nontraumatic subarachnoid hemorrhage
Use additional code to identify the type of dysphagia, if known (R13.1-)

I69.092 Facial weakness following nontraumatic subarachnoid hemorrhage
Facial droop following nontraumatic subarachnoid hemorrhage

I69.093 Ataxia following nontraumatic subarachnoid hemorrhage
I69.098 Other sequelae following nontraumatic subarachnoid hemorrhage
Alterations of sensation following nontraumatic subarachnoid hemorrhage
Disturbance of vision following nontraumatic subarachnoid hemorrhage
Use additional code to identify the sequelae

+ I69.1 Sequelae of nontraumatic intracerebral hemorrhage

I69.10 Unspecified sequelae of nontraumatic intracerebral hemorrhage

+ I69.11 Cognitive deficits following nontraumatic intracerebral hemorrhage

I69.110 Attention and concentration deficit following nontraumatic intracerebral hemorrhage
I69.111 Memory deficit following nontraumatic intracerebral hemorrhage
I69.112 Visuospatial deficit and spatial neglect following nontraumatic intracerebral hemorrhage
I69.113 Psychomotor deficit following nontraumatic intracerebral hemorrhage
I69.114 Frontal lobe and executive function deficit following nontraumatic intracerebral hemorrhage
I69.115 Cognitive social or emotional deficit following nontraumatic intracerebral hemorrhage
I69.118 Other symptoms and signs involving cognitive functions following nontraumati intracerebral hemorrhage
I69.119 Unspecified symptoms and signs involving cognitive functions following nontraumati intracerebral hemorrhage

+ I69.12 Speech and language deficits following nontraumati intracerebral hemorrhage

I69.120 Aphasia following nontraumatic intracerebral hemorrhage
I69.121 Dysphasia following nontraumatic intracerebral hemorrhage
I69.122 Dysarthria following nontraumatic intracerebral hemorrhage
I69.123 Fluency disorder following nontraumatic intracerebral hemorrhage
Stuttering following nontraumatic intracerebral hemorrhage

I69.128 Other speech and language deficits following nontraumatic intracerebral hemorrhage

+ I69.13 Monoplegia of upper limb following nontraumatic intracerebral hemorrhage

I69.131 Monoplegia of upper limb following nontraumatic intracerebral hemorrhage affecting right dominant side

I69.132 Monoplegia of upper limb following nontraumatic intracerebral hemorrhage affecting left dominant side

I69.133 Monoplegia of upper limb following nontraumatic intracerebral hemorrhage affecting right non-dominant side

I69.134 Monoplegia of upper limb following nontraumatic intracerebral hemorrhage affecting left non-dominant side

I69.139 Monoplegia of upper limb following nontraumatic intracerebral hemorrhage affecting unspecified side

+ I69.14 Monoplegia of lower limb following nontraumatic intracerebral hemorrhage

I69.141 Monoplegia of lower limb following nontraumatic intracerebral hemorrhage affecting right dominant side

I69.142 Monoplegia of lower limb following nontraumatic intracerebral hemorrhage affecting left dominant side

I69.143 Monoplegia of lower limb following nontraumatic intracerebral hemorrhage affecting right non-dominant side

I69.144 Monoplegia of lower limb following nontraumatic intracerebral hemorrhage affecting left non-dominant side

I69.149 Monoplegia of lower limb following nontraumatic intracerebral hemorrhage affecting unspecified side

+ I69.15 Hemiplegia and hemiparesis following nontraumatic intracerebral hemorrhage

CC I69.151 Hemiplegia and hemiparesis following nontraumatic intracerebral hemorrhage affecting right dominant side
CC Exclusion see Appendix A PDX collection 0695

CC I69.152 Hemiplegia and hemiparesis following nontraumatic intracerebral hemorrhage affecting left dominant side
CC Exclusion see Appendix A PDX collection 0695

CC I69.153 Hemiplegia and hemiparesis following nontraumatic intracerebral hemorrhage affecting right non-dominant side
CC Exclusion see Appendix A PDX collection 0696

CC I69.154 Hemiplegia and hemiparesis following nontraumatic intracerebral hemorrhage affecting left non-dominant side
CC Exclusion see Appendix A PDX collection 0696

CC I69.159 Hemiplegia and hemiparesis following nontraumatic intracerebral hemorrhage affecting unspecified side
CC Exclusion see Appendix A PDX collection 0697

+ I69.16 Other paralytic syndrome following nontraumatic intracerebral hemorrhage

Use additional code to identify type of paralytic syndrome, such as:
locked-in state (G83.5)
quadriplegia (G82.5-)

Excludes1: *hemiplegia/hemiparesis following nontraumatic intracerebral hemorrhage (I69.15-)*
monoplegia of lower limb following nontraumatic intracerebral hemorrhage (I69.14-)
monoplegia of upper limb following nontraumatic intracerebral hemorrhage (I69.13-)

I69.161 Other paralytic syndrome following nontraumatic intracerebral hemorrhage affecting right dominant side

I69.162 Other paralytic syndrome following nontraumatic intracerebral hemorrhage affecting left dominant side

I69.163 Other paralytic syndrome following nontraumatic intracerebral hemorrhage affecting right non-dominant side

I69.164 Other paralytic syndrome following nontraumatic intracerebral hemorrhage affecting left non-dominant side

I69.165 Other paralytic syndrome following nontraumatic intracerebral hemorrhage, bilateral

I69.169 Other paralytic syndrome following nontraumatic intracerebral hemorrhage affecting unspecified side

+ I69.19 Other sequelae of nontraumatic intracerebral hemorrhage

I69.190 Apraxia following nontraumatic intracerebral hemorrhage

I69.191 Dysphagia following nontraumatic intracerebral hemorrhage
Use additional code to identify the type of dysphagia, if known (R13.1-)

I69.192 Facial weakness following nontraumatic intracerebral hemorrhage
Facial droop following nontraumatic intracerebral hemorrhage

I69.193 Ataxia following nontraumatic intracerebral hemorrhage

I69.198 Other sequelae of nontraumatic intracerebral hemorrhage
Alteration of sensations following nontraumatic intracerebral hemorrhage
Disturbance of vision following nontraumatic intracerebral hemorrhage
Use additional code to identify the sequelae

+ I69.2 Sequelae of other nontraumatic intracranial hemorrhage

I69.20 Unspecified sequelae of other nontraumatic intracranial hemorrhage

+ I69.21 Cognitive deficits following other nontraumatic intracranial hemorrhage

I69.210 Attention and concentration deficit following other nontraumatic intracranial hemorrhage

I69.211 Memory deficit following other nontraumatic intracranial hemorrhage

I69.212 Visuospatial deficit and spatial neglect following other nontraumatic intracranial hemorrhage

I69.213 Psychomotor deficit following other nontraumatic intracranial hemorrhage

I69.214 Frontal lobe and executive function deficit following other nontraumatic intracranial hemorrhage

I69.215 Cognitive social or emotional deficit following other nontraumatic intracranial hemorrhage

I69.218 Other symptoms and signs involving cognitive functions following other nontraumatic intracranial hemorrhage

I69.219 Unspecified symptoms and signs involving cognitive functions following other nontraumatic intracranial hemorrhage

+ I69.22 Speech and language deficits following other nontraumatic intracranial hemorrhage

I69.220 Aphasia following other nontraumatic intracranial hemorrhage

I69.221 Dysphasia following other nontraumatic intracranial hemorrhage

I69.222 Dysarthria following other nontraumatic intracranial hemorrhage

I69.223 Fluency disorder following other nontraumatic intracranial hemorrhage
Stuttering following other nontraumatic intracranial hemorrhage

I69.228 Other speech and language deficits following other nontraumatic intracranial hemorrhage

+ I69.23 Monoplegia of upper limb following other nontraumatic intracranial hemorrhage

I69.231 Monoplegia of upper limb following other nontraumatic intracranial hemorrhage affecting right dominant side

I69.232 Monoplegia of upper limb following other nontraumatic intracranial hemorrhage affecting left dominant side

I69.233 Monoplegia of upper limb following other nontraumatic intracranial hemorrhage affecting right non-dominant side
I69.234 Monoplegia of upper limb following other nontraumatic intracranial hemorrhage affecting left non-dominant side
I69.239 Monoplegia of upper limb following other nontraumatic intracranial hemorrhage affecting unspecified side

+ I69.24 Monoplegia of lower limb following other nontraumatic intracranial hemorrhage
I69.241 Monoplegia of lower limb following other nontraumatic intracranial hemorrhage affecting right dominant side
I69.242 Monoplegia of lower limb following other nontraumatic intracranial hemorrhage affecting left dominant side
I69.243 Monoplegia of lower limb following other nontraumatic intracranial hemorrhage affecting right non-dominant side
I69.244 Monoplegia of lower limb following other nontraumatic intracranial hemorrhage affecting left non-dominant side
I69.249 Monoplegia of lower limb following other nontraumatic intracranial hemorrhage affecting unspecified side

+ I69.25 Hemiplegia and hemiparesis following other nontraumatic intracranial hemorrhage
CC I69.251 Hemiplegia and hemiparesis following other nontraumatic intracranial hemorrhage affecting right dominant side
CC Exclusion see Appendix A PDX collection 0695
CC I69.252 Hemiplegia and hemiparesis following other nontraumatic intracranial hemorrhage affecting left dominant side
CC Exclusion see Appendix A PDX collection 0695
CC I69.253 Hemiplegia and hemiparesis following other nontraumatic intracranial hemorrhage affecting right non-dominant side
CC Exclusion see Appendix A PDX collection 0696
CC I69.254 Hemiplegia and hemiparesis following other nontraumatic intracranial hemorrhage affecting left non-dominant side
CC Exclusion see Appendix A PDX collection 0696
CC I69.259 Hemiplegia and hemiparesis following other nontraumatic intracranial hemorrhage affecting unspecified side
CC Exclusion see Appendix A PDX collection 0697

+ I69.26 Other paralytic syndrome following other nontraumatic intracranial hemorrhage
Use additional code to identify type of paralytic syndrome, such as:
locked-in state (G83.5)
quadriplegia (G82.5-)
Excludes1: *hemiplegia/hemiparesis following other nontraumatic intracranial hemorrhage (I69.25-)*
monoplegia of lower limb following other nontraumatic intracranial hemorrhage (I69.24-)
monoplegia of upper limb following other nontraumatic intracranial hemorrhage (I69.23-)
I69.261 Other paralytic syndrome following other nontraumatic intracranial hemorrhage affecting right dominant side
I69.262 Other paralytic syndrome following other nontraumatic intracranial hemorrhage affecting left dominant side
I69.263 Other paralytic syndrome following other nontraumatic intracranial hemorrhage affecting right non-dominant side
I69.264 Other paralytic syndrome following other nontraumatic intracranial hemorrhage affecting left non-dominant side
I69.265 Other paralytic syndrome following other nontraumatic intracranial hemorrhage, bilateral
I69.269 Other paralytic syndrome following other nontraumatic intracranial hemorrhage affecting unspecified side

+ I69.29 Other sequelae of other nontraumatic intracranial hemorrhage
I69.290 Apraxia following other nontraumatic intracranial hemorrhage
I69.291 Dysphagia following other nontraumatic intracranial hemorrhage
Use additional code to identify the type of dysphagia, if known (R13.1-)
I69.292 Facial weakness following other nontraumatic intracranial hemorrhage
Facial droop following other nontraumatic intracranial hemorrhage
I69.293 Ataxia following other nontraumatic intracranial hemorrhage
I69.298 Other sequelae of other nontraumatic intracranial hemorrhage
Alteration of sensation following other nontraumatic intracranial hemorrhage
Disturbance of vision following other nontraumatic intracranial hemorrhage
Use additional code to identify the sequelae

+ I69.3 Sequelae of cerebral infarction
Sequelae of stroke NOS
AHA CC: 4Q, 2012, 95; 4Q, 2013, 127-128
I69.30 Unspecified sequelae of cerebral infarction

+ I69.31 Cognitive deficits following cerebral infarction
I69.310 Attention and concentration deficit following cerebral infarction
I69.311 Memory deficit following cerebral infarction
I69.312 Visuospatial deficit and spatial neglect following cerebral infarction
I69.313 Psychomotor deficit following cerebral infarction
I69.314 Frontal lobe and executive function deficit following cerebral infarction
I69.315 Cognitive social or emotional deficit following cerebral infarction
I69.318 Other symptoms and signs involving cognitive functions following cerebral infarction
I69.319 Unspecified symptoms and signs involving cognitive functions following cerebral infarction

+ I69.32 Speech and language deficits following cerebral infarction
I69.320 Aphasia following cerebral infarction
AHA CC: 4Q, 2013, 128
I69.321 Dysphasia following cerebral infarction
AHA CC: 4Q, 2012, 91
I69.322 Dysarthria following cerebral infarction
Excludes2: *transient ischemic attach (TIA) (G45.9)*
I69.323 Fluency disorder following cerebral infarction
Stuttering following cerebral hemorrhage
I69.328 Other speech and language deficits following cerebral infarction

+ I69.33 Monoplegia of upper limb following cerebral infarction
AHA CC: 1Q, 2017, 47-48
I69.331 Monoplegia of upper limb following cerebral infarction affecting right dominant side
I69.332 Monoplegia of upper limb following cerebral infarction affecting left dominant side
I69.333 Monoplegia of upper limb following cerebral infarction affecting right non-dominant side
I69.334 Monoplegia of upper limb following cerebral infarction affecting left non-dominant side
I69.339 Monoplegia of upper limb following cerebral infarction affecting unspecified side

+ I69.34 **Monoplegia of lower limb following cerebral infarction**

AHA CC: 1Q, 2017, 47-48

I69.341 **Monoplegia of lower limb following cerebral infarction affecting right dominant side**

I69.342 **Monoplegia of lower limb following cerebral infarction affecting left dominant side**

I69.343 **Monoplegia of lower limb following cerebral infarction affecting right non-dominant side**

I69.344 **Monoplegia of lower limb following cerebral infarction affecting left non-dominant side**

I69.349 **Monoplegia of lower limb following cerebral infarction affecting unspecified side**

+ I69.35 **Hemiplegia and hemiparesis following cerebral infarction**

CC I69.351 **Hemiplegia and hemiparesis following cerebral infarction affecting right dominant side**

Excludes2: *transient ischemic attach (TIA) (G45.9)*

CC Exclusion see Appendix A PDX collection 0695

AHA CC: 4Q, 2013, 128; 1Q, 2015, 25

CC I69.352 **Hemiplegia and hemiparesis following cerebral infarction affecting left dominant side**

CC Exclusion see Appendix A PDX collection 0695

CC I69.353 **Hemiplegia and hemiparesis following cerebral infarction affecting right non-dominant side**

CC Exclusion see Appendix A PDX collection 0696

CC I69.354 **Hemiplegia and hemiparesis following cerebral infarction affecting left non-dominant side**

CC Exclusion see Appendix A PDX collection 0696

AHA CC: 4Q, 2012, 91

CC I69.359 **Hemiplegia and hemiparesis following cerebral infarction affecting unspecified side**

CC Exclusion see Appendix A PDX collection 0697

+ I69.36 **Other paralytic syndrome following cerebral infarction**

Use additional code to identify type of paralytic syndrome, such as:
locked-in state (G83.5)
quadriplegia (G82.5-)

Excludes1: *hemiplegia/hemiparesis following cerebral infarction (I69.35-)*
monoplegia of lower limb following cerebral infarction (I69.34-)
monoplegia of upper limb following cerebral infarction (I69.33-)

I69.361 **Other paralytic syndrome following cerebral infarction affecting right dominant side**

I69.362 **Other paralytic syndrome following cerebral infarction affecting left dominant side**

I69.363 **Other paralytic syndrome following cerebral infarction affecting right non-dominant side**

I69.364 **Other paralytic syndrome following cerebral infarction affecting left non-dominant side**

I69.365 **Other paralytic syndrome following cerebral infarction, bilateral**

I69.369 **Other paralytic syndrome following cerebral infarction affecting unspecified side**

+ I69.39 **Other sequelae of cerebral infarction**

I69.390 **Apraxia following cerebral infarction**

I69.391 **Dysphagia following cerebral infarction**

Use additional code to identify the type of dysphagia, if known (R13.1-)

I69.392 **Facial weakness following cerebral infarction**

Facial droop following cerebral infarction

I69.393 **Ataxia following cerebral infarction**

I69.398 **Other sequelae of cerebral infarction**

Alteration of sensation following cerebral infarction

Disturbance of vision following cerebral infarction

Use additional code to identify the sequelae

+ I69.8 **Sequelae of other cerebrovascular diseases**

Excludes1: *sequelae of traumatic intracranial injury (S06.-)*

I69.80 **Unspecified sequelae of other cerebrovascular disease**

+ I69.81 **Cognitive deficits following other cerebrovascular disease**

I69.810 **Attention and concentration deficit following other cerebrovascular disease**

I69.811 **Memory deficit following other cerebrovascular disease**

I69.812 **Visuospatial deficit and spatial neglect following other cerebrovascular disease**

I69.813 **Psychomotor deficit following other cerebrovascular disease**

I69.814 **Frontal lobe and executive function deficit following other cerebrovascular disease**

I69.815 **Cognitive social or emotional deficit following other cerebrovascular disease**

I69.818 **Other symptoms and signs involving cognitive functions following other cerebrovascular disease**

I69.819 **Unspecified symptoms and signs involving cognitive functions following other cerebrovascular disease**

+ I69.82 **Speech and language deficits following other cerebrovascular disease**

I69.820 **Aphasia following other cerebrovascular disease**

I69.821 **Dysphasia following other cerebrovascular disease**

I69.822 **Dysarthria following other cerebrovascular disease**

I69.823 **Fluency disorder following other cerebrovascular disease**

Stuttering following other cerebrovascular disease hemorrhage

I69.828 **Other speech and language deficits following other cerebrovascular disease**

+ I69.83 **Monoplegia of upper limb following other cerebrovascular disease**

I69.831 **Monoplegia of upper limb following other cerebrovascular disease affecting right dominant side**

I69.832 **Monoplegia of upper limb following other cerebrovascular disease affecting left dominant side**

I69.833 **Monoplegia of upper limb following other cerebrovascular disease affecting right non-dominant side**

I69.834 **Monoplegia of upper limb following other cerebrovascular disease affecting left non-dominant side**

I69.839 **Monoplegia of upper limb following other cerebrovascular disease affecting unspecified side**

+ I69.84 **Monoplegia of lower limb following other cerebrovascular disease**

I69.841 **Monoplegia of lower limb following other cerebrovascular disease affecting right dominant side**

I69.842 **Monoplegia of lower limb following other cerebrovascular disease affecting left dominant side**

I69.843 **Monoplegia of lower limb following other cerebrovascular disease affecting right non-dominant side**

I69.844 **Monoplegia of lower limb following other cerebrovascular disease affecting left non-dominant side**

I69.849 **Monoplegia of lower limb following other cerebrovascular disease affecting unspecified side**

\+ **I69.85 Hemiplegia and hemiparesis following other cerebrovascular disease**

CC I69.851 **Hemiplegia and hemiparesis following other cerebrovascular disease affecting right dominant side**

CC Exclusion see Appendix A PDX collection 0695

CC I69.852 **Hemiplegia and hemiparesis following other cerebrovascular disease affecting left dominant side**

CC Exclusion see Appendix A PDX collection 0695

CC I69.853 **Hemiplegia and hemiparesis following other cerebrovascular disease affecting right non-dominant side**

CC Exclusion see Appendix A PDX collection 0696

CC I69.854 **Hemiplegia and hemiparesis following other cerebrovascular disease affecting left non-dominant side**

CC Exclusion see Appendix A PDX collection 0696

CC I69.859 **Hemiplegia and hemiparesis following other cerebrovascular disease affecting unspecified side**

CC Exclusion see Appendix A PDX collection 0697

\+ **I69.86 Other paralytic syndrome following other cerebrovascular disease**

Use additional code to identify type of paralytic syndrome, such as:
locked-in state (G83.5)
quadriplegia (G82.5-)

Excludes1: *hemiplegia/hemiparesis following other cerebrovascular disease (I69.85-)*
monoplegia of lower limb following other cerebrovascular disease (I69.84-)
monoplegia of upper limb following other cerebrovascular disease (I69.83-)

I69.861 **Other paralytic syndrome following other cerebrovascular disease affecting right dominant side**

I69.862 **Other paralytic syndrome following other cerebrovascular disease affecting left dominant side**

I69.863 **Other paralytic syndrome following other cerebrovascular disease affecting right non-dominant side**

I69.864 **Other paralytic syndrome following other cerebrovascular disease affecting left non-dominant side**

I69.865 **Other paralytic syndrome following other cerebrovascular disease, bilateral**

I69.869 **Other paralytic syndrome following other cerebrovascular disease affecting unspecified side**

\+ **I69.89 Other sequelae of other cerebrovascular disease**

I69.890 **Apraxia following other cerebrovascular disease**

I69.891 **Dysphagia following other cerebrovascular disease**

Use additional code to identify the type of dysphagia, if known (R13.1-)

I69.892 **Facial weakness following other cerebrovascular disease**

Facial droop following other cerebrovascular disease

I69.893 **Ataxia following other cerebrovascular disease**

I69.898 **Other sequelae of other cerebrovascular disease**

Alteration of sensation following other cerebrovascular disease
Disturbance of vision following other cerebrovascular disease
Use additional code to identify the sequelae

\+ **I69.9 Sequelae of unspecified cerebrovascular diseases**

Excludes1: *sequelae of stroke (I69.3)*
sequelae of traumatic intracranial injury (S06.-)

I69.90 Unspecified sequelae of unspecified cerebrovascular disease

\+ **I69.91 Cognitive deficits following unspecified cerebrovascular disease**

I69.910 **Attention and concentration deficit following unspecified cerebrovascular disease**

I69.911 **Memory deficit following unspecified cerebrovascular disease**

I69.912 **Visuospatial deficit and spatial neglect following unspecified cerebrovascular disease**

I69.913 **Psychomotor deficit following unspecified cerebrovascular disease**

I69.914 **Frontal lobe and executive function deficit following unspecified cerebrovascular disease**

I69.915 **Cognitive social or emotional deficit following unspecified cerebrovascular disease**

I69.918 **Other symptoms and signs involving cognitive functions following unspecified cerebrovascular disease**

I69.919 **Unspecified symptoms and signs involving cognitive functions following unspecified cerebrovascular disease**

\+ **I69.92 Speech and language deficits following unspecified cerebrovascular disease**

I69.920 **Aphasia following unspecified cerebrovascular disease**

I69.921 **Dysphasia following unspecified cerebrovascular disease**

I69.922 **Dysarthria following unspecified cerebrovascular disease**

I69.923 **Fluency disorder following unspecified cerebrovascular disease**

Stuttering following unspecified cerebrovascular disease

I69.928 **Other speech and language deficits following unspecified cerebrovascular disease**

\+ **I69.93 Monoplegia of upper limb following unspecified cerebrovascular disease**

I69.931 **Monoplegia of upper limb following unspecified cerebrovascular disease affecting right dominant side**

I69.932 **Monoplegia of upper limb following unspecified cerebrovascular disease affecting left dominant side**

I69.933 **Monoplegia of upper limb following unspecified cerebrovascular disease affecting right non-dominant side**

I69.934 **Monoplegia of upper limb following unspecified cerebrovascular disease affecting left non-dominant side**

I69.939 **Monoplegia of upper limb following unspecified cerebrovascular disease affecting unspecified side**

\+ **I69.94 Monoplegia of lower limb following unspecified cerebrovascular disease**

I69.941 **Monoplegia of lower limb following unspecified cerebrovascular disease affecting right dominant side**

I69.942 **Monoplegia of lower limb following unspecified cerebrovascular disease affecting left dominant side**

I69.943 **Monoplegia of lower limb following unspecified cerebrovascular disease affecting right non-dominant side**

I69.944 Monoplegia of lower limb following unspecified cerebrovascular disease affecting left non-dominant side

I69.949 Monoplegia of lower limb following unspecified cerebrovascular disease affecting unspecified side

+ I69.95 Hemiplegia and hemiparesis following unspecified cerebrovascular disease

CC I69.951 Hemiplegia and hemiparesis following unspecified cerebrovascular disease affecting right dominant side
CC Exclusion see Appendix A PDX collection 0695

CC I69.952 Hemiplegia and hemiparesis following unspecified cerebrovascular disease affecting left dominant side
CC Exclusion see Appendix A PDX collection 0695

CC I69.953 Hemiplegia and hemiparesis following unspecified cerebrovascular disease affecting right non-dominant side
CC Exclusion see Appendix A PDX collection 0696

CC I69.954 Hemiplegia and hemiparesis following unspecified cerebrovascular disease affecting left non-dominant side
CC Exclusion see Appendix A PDX collection 0696

CC I69.959 Hemiplegia and hemiparesis following unspecified cerebrovascular disease affecting unspecified side
CC Exclusion see Appendix A PDX collection 0697

+ I69.96 Other paralytic syndrome following unspecified cerebrovascular disease

Use additional code to identify type of paralytic syndrome, such as:
locked-in state (G83.5)
quadriplegia (G82.5-)

Excludes1: *hemiplegia/hemiparesis following unspecified cerebrovascular disease (I69.95-)*
monoplegia of lower limb following unspecified cerebrovascular disease (I69.94-)
monoplegia of upper limb following unspecified cerebrovascular disease (I69.93-)

I69.961 Other paralytic syndrome following unspecified cerebrovascular disease affecting right dominant side

I69.962 Other paralytic syndrome following unspecified cerebrovascular disease affecting left dominant side

I69.963 Other paralytic syndrome following unspecified cerebrovascular disease affecting right non-dominant side

I69.964 Other paralytic syndrome following unspecified cerebrovascular disease affecting left non-dominant side

I69.965 Other paralytic syndrome following unspecified cerebrovascular disease, bilateral

I69.969 Other paralytic syndrome following unspecified cerebrovascular disease affecting unspecified side

+ I69.99 Other sequelae of unspecified cerebrovascular disease

I69.990 Apraxia following unspecified cerebrovascular disease

I69.991 Dysphagia following unspecified cerebrovascular disease
Use additional code to identify the type of dysphagia, if known (R13.1-)

I69.992 Facial weakness following unspecified cerebrovascular disease
Facial droop following unspecified cerebrovascular disease

I69.993 Ataxia following unspecified cerebrovascular disease

I69.998 Other sequelae following unspecified cerebrovascular disease
Alteration in sensation following unspecified cerebrovascular disease
Disturbance of vision following unspecified cerebrovascular disease
Use additional code to identify the sequelae

Diseases of arteries, arterioles and capillaries (I70-I79)

I70 Atherosclerosis

Includes: arteriolosclerosis
arterial degeneration
arteriosclerosis
arteriosclerotic vascular disease
arteriovascular degeneration
atheroma
endarteritis deformans or obliterans
senile arteritis
senile endarteritis
vascular degeneration

Use additional code to identify:
exposure to environmental tobacco smoke (Z77.22)
history of tobacco dependence (Z87.891)
occupational exposure to environmental tobacco smoke (Z57.31)
tobacco dependence (F17.-)
tobacco use (Z72.0)

Excludes2: *arteriosclerotic cardiovascular disease (I25.1-)*
arteriosclerotic heart disease (I25.1-)
atheroembolism (I75.-)
cerebral atherosclerosis (I67.2)
coronary atherosclerosis (I25.1-)
mesenteric atherosclerosis (K55.1)
precerebral atherosclerosis (I67.2)
primary pulmonary atherosclerosis (I27.0)

• I70.0 Atherosclerosis of aorta

• I70.1 Atherosclerosis of renal artery
Goldblatt's kidney
Excludes2: *atherosclerosis of renal arterioles (I12.-)*

+ I70.2 Atherosclerosis of native arteries of the extremities
Mönckeberg's (medial) sclerosis
Use additional code, if applicable, to identify chronic total occlusion of artery of extremity (I70.92)
Excludes2: *atherosclerosis of bypass graft of extremities (I70.30-I70.79)*

+ I70.20 Unspecified atherosclerosis of native arteries of extremities

• I70.201 Unspecified atherosclerosis of native arteries of extremities, right leg

• I70.202 Unspecified atherosclerosis of native arteries of extremities, left leg

• I70.203 Unspecified atherosclerosis of native arteries of extremities, bilateral legs

• I70.208 Unspecified atherosclerosis of native arteries of extremities, other extremity

• I70.209 Unspecified atherosclerosis of native arteries of extremities, unspecified extremity

+ I70.21 Atherosclerosis of native arteries of extremities with intermittent claudication

• I70.211 Atherosclerosis of native arteries of extremities with intermittent claudication, right leg

• I70.212 Atherosclerosis of native arteries of extremities with intermittent claudication, left leg

• I70.213 Atherosclerosis of native arteries of extremities with intermittent claudication, bilateral legs

• I70.218 Atherosclerosis of native arteries of extremities with intermittent claudication, other extremity

• I70.219 Atherosclerosis of native arteries of extremities with intermittent claudication, unspecified extremity

+ I70.22 Atherosclerosis of native arteries of extremities with rest pain
Includes: any condition classifiable to I70.21-

• I70.221 Atherosclerosis of native arteries of extremities with rest pain, right leg

• I70.222 Atherosclerosis of native arteries of extremities with rest pain, left leg

• I70.223 Atherosclerosis of native arteries of extremities with rest pain, bilateral legs

• I70.228 Atherosclerosis of native arteries of extremities with rest pain, other extremity

• I70.229 Atherosclerosis of native arteries of extremities with rest pain, unspecified extremity

+ **I70.23 Atherosclerosis of native arteries of right leg with ulceration**
  Includes: any condition classifiable to I70.211 and I70.221
  Use additional code to identify severity of ulcer (L97.-)
  - **I70.231 Atherosclerosis of native arteries of right leg with ulceration of thigh**
  - **I70.232 Atherosclerosis of native arteries of right leg with ulceration of calf**
  - **I70.233 Atherosclerosis of native arteries of right leg with ulceration of ankle**
  - **I70.234 Atherosclerosis of native arteries of right leg with ulceration of heel and midfoot**
    Atherosclerosis of native arteries of right leg with ulceration of plantar surface of midfoot
  - **I70.235 Atherosclerosis of native arteries of right leg with ulceration of other part of foot**
    Atherosclerosis of native arteries of right leg extremities with ulceration of toe
  - **I70.238 Atherosclerosis of native arteries of right leg with ulceration of other part of lower right leg**
  - **I70.239 Atherosclerosis of native arteries of right leg with ulceration of unspecified site**

+ **I70.24 Atherosclerosis of native arteries of left leg with ulceration**
  Includes: any condition classifiable to I70.212 and I70.222
  Use additional code to identify severity of ulcer (L97.-)
  - **I70.241 Atherosclerosis of native arteries of left leg with ulceration of thigh**
  - **I70.242 Atherosclerosis of native arteries of left leg with ulceration of calf**
  - **I70.243 Atherosclerosis of native arteries of left leg with ulceration of ankle**
  - **I70.244 Atherosclerosis of native arteries of left leg with ulceration of heel and midfoot**
    Atherosclerosis of native arteries of left leg with ulceration of plantar surface of midfoot
  - **I70.245 Atherosclerosis of native arteries of left leg with ulceration of other part of foot**
    Atherosclerosis of native arteries of left leg extremities with ulceration of toe
  - **I70.248 Atherosclerosis of native arteries of left leg with ulceration of other part of lower left leg**
  - **I70.249 Atherosclerosis of native arteries of left leg with ulceration of unspecified site**

- **I70.25 Atherosclerosis of native arteries of other extremities with ulceration**
  Includes: any condition classifiable to I70.218 and I70.228
  Use additional code to identify the severity of the ulcer (L98.49-)

+ **I70.26 Atherosclerosis of native arteries of extremities with gangrene**
  Includes: any condition classifiable to I70.21-, I70.22-, I70.23-, I70.24-, and I70.25-
  Use additional code to identify the severity of any ulcer (L97.-, L98.49-), if applicable
  - CC **I70.261 Atherosclerosis of native arteries of extremities with gangrene, right leg**
    CC Exclusion see Appendix A PDX collection 0519
  - CC **I70.262 Atherosclerosis of native arteries of extremities with gangrene, left leg**
    CC Exclusion see Appendix A PDX collection 0519
  - CC **I70.263 Atherosclerosis of native arteries of extremities with gangrene, bilateral legs**
    CC Exclusion see Appendix A PDX collection 0519
  - CC **I70.268 Atherosclerosis of native arteries of extremities with gangrene, other extremity**
    CC Exclusion see Appendix A PDX collection 0519
  - CC **I70.269 Atherosclerosis of native arteries of extremities with gangrene, unspecified extremity**
    CC Exclusion see Appendix A PDX collection 0519

+ **I70.29 Other atherosclerosis of native arteries of extremities**
  - **I70.291 Other atherosclerosis of native arteries of extremities, right leg**
  - **I70.292 Other atherosclerosis of native arteries of extremities, left leg**
  - **I70.293 Other atherosclerosis of native arteries of extremities, bilateral legs**
  - **I70.298 Other atherosclerosis of native arteries of extremities, other extremity**
  - **I70.299 Other atherosclerosis of native arteries of extremities, unspecified extremity**

+ **I70.3 Atherosclerosis of unspecified type of bypass graft(s) of the extremities**
  Use additional code, if applicable, to identify chronic total occlusion of artery of extremity (I70.92)
  Excludes1: *embolism or thrombus of bypass graft(s) of extremities (T82.8-)*

+ **I70.30 Unspecified atherosclerosis of unspecified type of bypass graft(s) of the extremities**
  - **I70.301 Unspecified atherosclerosis of unspecified type of bypass graft(s) of the extremities, right leg**
  - **I70.302 Unspecified atherosclerosis of unspecified type of bypass graft(s) of the extremities, left leg**
  - **I70.303 Unspecified atherosclerosis of unspecified type of bypass graft(s) of the extremities, bilateral legs**
  - **I70.308 Unspecified atherosclerosis of unspecified type of bypass graft(s) of the extremities, other extremity**
  - **I70.309 Unspecified atherosclerosis of unspecified type of bypass graft(s) of the extremities, unspecified extremity**

+ **I70.31 Atherosclerosis of unspecified type of bypass graft(s) of the extremities with intermittent claudication**
  - **I70.311 Atherosclerosis of unspecified type of bypass graft(s) of the extremities with intermittent claudication, right leg**
  - **I70.312 Atherosclerosis of unspecified type of bypass graft(s) of the extremities with intermittent claudication, left leg**
  - **I70.313 Atherosclerosis of unspecified type of bypass graft(s) of the extremities with intermittent claudication, bilateral legs**
  - **I70.318 Atherosclerosis of unspecified type of bypass graft(s) of the extremities with intermittent claudication, other extremity**
  - **I70.319 Atherosclerosis of unspecified type of bypass graft(s) of the extremities with intermittent claudication, unspecified extremity**

+ **I70.32 Atherosclerosis of unspecified type of bypass graft(s) of the extremities with rest pain**
  Includes: any condition classifiable to I70.31-
  - **I70.321 Atherosclerosis of unspecified type of bypass graft(s) of the extremities with rest pain, right leg**
  - **I70.322 Atherosclerosis of unspecified type of bypass graft(s) of the extremities with rest pain, left leg**
  - **I70.323 Atherosclerosis of unspecified type of bypass graft(s) of the extremities with rest pain, bilateral legs**
  - **I70.328 Atherosclerosis of unspecified type of bypass graft(s) of the extremities with rest pain, other extremity**
  - **I70.329 Atherosclerosis of unspecified type of bypass graft(s) of the extremities with rest pain, unspecified extremity**

+ **I70.33 Atherosclerosis of unspecified type of bypass graft(s) of the right leg with ulceration**
  Includes: any condition classifiable to I70.311 and I70.321
  Use additional code to identify severity of ulcer (L97.-)
  - CC **I70.331 Atherosclerosis of unspecified type of bypass graft(s) of the right leg with ulceration of thigh**
    CC Exclusion see Appendix A PDX collection 0698

• CC **I70.332** **Atherosclerosis of unspecified type of bypass graft(s) of the right leg with ulceration of calf**
CC Exclusion see Appendix A PDX collection 0698

• CC **I70.333** **Atherosclerosis of unspecified type of bypass graft(s) of the right leg with ulceration of ankle**
CC Exclusion see Appendix A PDX collection 0698

• CC **I70.334** **Atherosclerosis of unspecified type of bypass graft(s) of the right leg with ulceration of heel and midfoot**
Atherosclerosis of unspecified type of bypass graft(s) of right leg with ulceration of plantar surface of midfoot
CC Exclusion see Appendix A PDX collection 0698

• **I70.335** **Atherosclerosis of unspecified type of bypass graft(s) of the right leg with ulceration of other part of foot**
Atherosclerosis of unspecified type of bypass graft(s) of the right leg with ulceration of toe

• CC **I70.338** **Atherosclerosis of unspecified type of bypass graft(s) of the right leg with ulceration of other part of lower leg**
CC Exclusion see Appendix A PDX collection 0698

• CC **I70.339** **Atherosclerosis of unspecified type of bypass graft(s) of the right leg with ulceration of unspecified site**
CC Exclusion see Appendix A PDX collection 0698

+ **I70.34** **Atherosclerosis of unspecified type of bypass graft(s) of the left leg with ulceration**
Includes: any condition classifiable to I70.312 and I70.322
Use additional code to identify severity of ulcer (L97.-)

• CC **I70.341** **Atherosclerosis of unspecified type of bypass graft(s) of the left leg with ulceration of thigh**
CC Exclusion see Appendix A PDX collection 0698

• CC **I70.342** **Atherosclerosis of unspecified type of bypass graft(s) of the left leg with ulceration of calf**
CC Exclusion see Appendix A PDX collection 0698

• CC **I70.343** **Atherosclerosis of unspecified type of bypass graft(s) of the left leg with ulceration of ankle**
CC Exclusion see Appendix A PDX collection 0698

• CC **I70.344** **Atherosclerosis of unspecified type of bypass graft(s) of the left leg with ulceration of heel and midfoot**
Atherosclerosis of unspecified type of bypass graft(s) of left leg with ulceration of plantar surface of midfoot
CC Exclusion see Appendix A PDX collection 0698

• **I70.345** **Atherosclerosis of unspecified type of bypass graft(s) of the left leg with ulceration of other part of foot**
Atherosclerosis of unspecified type of bypass graft(s) of the left leg with ulceration of toe

• CC **I70.348** **Atherosclerosis of unspecified type of bypass graft(s) of the left leg with ulceration of other part of lower leg**
CC Exclusion see Appendix A PDX collection 0698

• CC **I70.349** **Atherosclerosis of unspecified type of bypass graft(s) of the left leg with ulceration of unspecified site**
CC Exclusion see Appendix A PDX collection 0698

• **I70.35** **Atherosclerosis of unspecified type of bypass graft(s) of other extremity with ulceration**
Includes: any condition classifiable to I70.318 and I70.328
Use additional code to identify severity of ulcer (L98.49-)

+ **I70.36** **Atherosclerosis of unspecified type of bypass graft(s) of the extremities with gangrene**
Includes: any condition classifiable to I70.31-, I70.32-, I70.33-, I70.34-, I70.35
Use additional code to identify the severity of any ulcer (L97.-, L98.49-), if applicable

• CC **I70.361** **Atherosclerosis of unspecified type of bypass graft(s) of the extremities with gangrene, right leg**
CC Exclusion see Appendix A PDX collection 0519

• CC **I70.362** **Atherosclerosis of unspecified type of bypass graft(s) of the extremities with gangrene, left leg**
CC Exclusion see Appendix A PDX collection 0519

• CC **I70.363** **Atherosclerosis of unspecified type of bypass graft(s) of the extremities with gangrene, bilateral legs**
CC Exclusion see Appendix A PDX collection 0519

• CC **I70.368** **Atherosclerosis of unspecified type of bypass graft(s) of the extremities with gangrene, other extremity**
CC Exclusion see Appendix A PDX collection 0519

• CC **I70.369** **Atherosclerosis of unspecified type of bypass graft(s) of the extremities with gangrene, unspecified extremity**
CC Exclusion see Appendix A PDX collection 0519

+ **I70.39** **Other atherosclerosis of unspecified type of bypass graft(s) of the extremities**

• **I70.391** **Other atherosclerosis of unspecified type of bypass graft(s) of the extremities, right leg**

• **I70.392** **Other atherosclerosis of unspecified type of bypass graft(s) of the extremities, left leg**

• **I70.393** **Other atherosclerosis of unspecified type of bypass graft(s) of the extremities, bilateral legs**

• **I70.398** **Other atherosclerosis of unspecified type of bypass graft(s) of the extremities, other extremity**

• **I70.399** **Other atherosclerosis of unspecified type of bypass graft(s) of the extremities, unspecified extremity**

+ **I70.4** **Atherosclerosis of autologous vein bypass graft(s) of the extremities**
Use additional code, if applicable, to identify chronic total occlusion of artery of extremity (I70.92)

+ **I70.40** **Unspecified atherosclerosis of autologous vein bypass graft(s) of the extremities**

• **I70.401** **Unspecified atherosclerosis of autologous vein bypass graft(s) of the extremities, right leg**

• **I70.402** **Unspecified atherosclerosis of autologous vein bypass graft(s) of the extremities, left leg**

• **I70.403** **Unspecified atherosclerosis of autologous vein bypass graft(s) of the extremities, bilateral legs**

• **I70.408** **Unspecified atherosclerosis of autologous vein bypass graft(s) of the extremities, other extremity**

• **I70.409** **Unspecified atherosclerosis of autologous vein bypass graft(s) of the extremities, unspecified extremity**

+ **I70.41** **Atherosclerosis of autologous vein bypass graft(s) of the extremities with intermittent claudication**

• **I70.411** **Atherosclerosis of autologous vein bypass graft(s) of the extremities with intermittent claudication, right leg**

• **I70.412** **Atherosclerosis of autologous vein bypass graft(s) of the extremities with intermittent claudication, left leg**

- **I70.413** **Atherosclerosis of autologous vein bypass graft(s) of the extremities with intermittent claudication, bilateral legs**
- **I70.418** **Atherosclerosis of autologous vein bypass graft(s) of the extremities with intermittent claudication, other extremity**
- **I70.419** **Atherosclerosis of autologous vein bypass graft(s) of the extremities with intermittent claudication, unspecified extremity**

+ **I70.42** **Atherosclerosis of autologous vein bypass graft(s) of the extremities with rest pain**
  Includes: any condition classifiable to I70.41-
- **I70.421** **Atherosclerosis of autologous vein bypass graft(s) of the extremities with rest pain, right leg**
- **I70.422** **Atherosclerosis of autologous vein bypass graft(s) of the extremities with rest pain, left leg**
- **I70.423** **Atherosclerosis of autologous vein bypass graft(s) of the extremities with rest pain, bilateral legs**
- **I70.428** **Atherosclerosis of autologous vein bypass graft(s) of the extremities with rest pain, other extremity**
- **I70.429** **Atherosclerosis of autologous vein bypass graft(s) of the extremities with rest pain, unspecified extremity**

+ **I70.43** **Atherosclerosis of autologous vein bypass graft(s) of the right leg with ulceration**
  Includes: any condition classifiable to I70.411 and I70.421
  Use additional code to identify severity of ulcer (L97.-)
- CC **I70.431** **Atherosclerosis of autologous vein bypass graft(s) of the right leg with ulceration of thigh**
  CC Exclusion see Appendix A PDX collection 0698
- CC **I70.432** **Atherosclerosis of autologous vein bypass graft(s) of the right leg with ulceration of calf**
  CC Exclusion see Appendix A PDX collection 0698
- CC **I70.433** **Atherosclerosis of autologous vein bypass graft(s) of the right leg with ulceration of ankle**
  CC Exclusion see Appendix A PDX collection 0698
- CC **I70.434** **Atherosclerosis of autologous vein bypass graft(s) of the right leg with ulceration of heel and midfoot**
  CC Exclusion see Appendix A PDX collection 0698
  Atherosclerosis of autologous vein bypass graft(s) of right leg with ulceration of plantar surface of midfoot
- **I70.435** **Atherosclerosis of autologous vein bypass graft(s) of the right leg with ulceration of other part of foot**
  Atherosclerosis of autologous vein bypass graft(s) of right leg with ulceration of toe
- CC **I70.438** **Atherosclerosis of autologous vein bypass graft(s) of the right leg with ulceration of other part of lower leg**
  CC Exclusion see Appendix A PDX collection 0698
- CC **I70.439** **Atherosclerosis of autologous vein bypass graft(s) of the right leg with ulceration of unspecified site**
  CC Exclusion see Appendix A PDX collection 0698

+ **I70.44** **Atherosclerosis of autologous vein bypass graft(s) of the left leg with ulceration**
  Includes: any condition classifiable to I70.412 and I70.422
  Use additional code to identify severity of ulcer (L97.-)
- CC **I70.441** **Atherosclerosis of autologous vein bypass graft(s) of the left leg with ulceration of thigh**
  CC Exclusion see Appendix A PDX collection 0698
- CC **I70.442** **Atherosclerosis of autologous vein bypass graft(s) of the left leg with ulceration of ca**
  CC Exclusion see Appendix A PDX collection 0698
- CC **I70.443** **Atherosclerosis of autologous vein bypass graft(s) of the left leg with ulceration of ankle**
  CC Exclusion see Appendix A PDX collection 0698
- CC **I70.444** **Atherosclerosis of autologous vein bypass graft(s) of the left leg with ulceration of heel and midfoot**
  Atherosclerosis of autologous vein bypass graft(s) of left leg with ulceration of plantar surface of midfoot
  CC Exclusion see Appendix A PDX collection 0698
- **I70.445** **Atherosclerosis of autologous vein bypass graft(s) of the left leg with ulceration of other part of foot**
  Atherosclerosis of autologous vein bypass graft(s) of left leg with ulceration of toe
- CC **I70.448** **Atherosclerosis of autologous vein bypass graft(s) of the left leg with ulceration of other part of lower leg**
  CC Exclusion see Appendix A PDX collection 0698
- CC **I70.449** **Atherosclerosis of autologous vein bypass graft(s) of the left leg with ulceration of unspecified site**
  CC Exclusion see Appendix A PDX collection 0698

- **I70.45** **Atherosclerosis of autologous vein bypass graft(s) of other extremity with ulceration**
  Includes: any condition classifiable to I70.418, I70.428, and I70.438
  Use additional code to identify severity of ulcer (L98.4

+ **I70.46** **Atherosclerosis of autologous vein bypass graft(s) of the extremities with gangrene**
  Includes: any condition classifiable to I70.41-, I70.4, and I70.43-, I70.44-, I70.45
  Use additional code to identify the severity of any ulcer (L97.-, L98.49-), if applicable
- CC **I70.461** **Atherosclerosis of autologous vein bypass graft(s) of the extremities with gangrene, right leg**
  CC Exclusion see Appendix A PDX collection 0519
- CC **I70.462** **Atherosclerosis of autologous vein bypass graft(s) of the extremities with gangrene, left leg**
  CC Exclusion see Appendix A PDX collection 0519
- CC **I70.463** **Atherosclerosis of autologous vein bypass graft(s) of the extremities with gangrene, bilateral legs**
  CC Exclusion see Appendix A PDX collection 0519
- CC **I70.468** **Atherosclerosis of autologous vein bypass graft(s) of the extremities with gangrene, other extremity**
  CC Exclusion see Appendix A PDX collection 0519
- CC **I70.469** **Atherosclerosis of autologous vein bypass graft(s) of the extremities with gangrene, unspecified extremity**
  CC Exclusion see Appendix A PDX collection 0519

+ **I70.49** **Other atherosclerosis of autologous vein bypass graft(s) of the extremities**
- **I70.491** **Other atherosclerosis of autologous vein bypass graft(s) of the extremities, right leg**
- **I70.492** **Other atherosclerosis of autologous vein bypass graft(s) of the extremities, left leg**
- **I70.493** **Other atherosclerosis of autologous vein bypass graft(s) of the extremities, bilateral legs**
- **I70.498** **Other atherosclerosis of autologous vein bypass graft(s) of the extremities, other extremity**
- **I70.499** **Other atherosclerosis of autologous vein bypass graft(s) of the extremities, unspecified extremity**

+ I70.5 **Atherosclerosis of nonautologous biological bypass graft(s) of the extremities**
Use additional code, if applicable, to identify chronic total occlusion of artery of extremity (I70.92)

+ I70.50 **Unspecified atherosclerosis of nonautologous biological bypass graft(s) of the extremities**

• I70.501 **Unspecified atherosclerosis of nonautologous biological bypass graft(s) of the extremities, right leg**

• I70.502 **Unspecified atherosclerosis of nonautologous biological bypass graft(s) of the extremities, left leg**

• I70.503 **Unspecified atherosclerosis of nonautologous biological bypass graft(s) of the extremities, bilateral legs**

• I70.508 **Unspecified atherosclerosis of nonautologous biological bypass graft(s) of the extremities, other extremity**

• I70.509 **Unspecified atherosclerosis of nonautologous biological bypass graft(s) of the extremities, unspecified extremity**

+ I70.51 **Atherosclerosis of nonautologous biological bypass graft(s) of the extremities intermittent claudication**

• I70.511 **Atherosclerosis of nonautologous biological bypass graft(s) of the extremities with intermittent claudication, right leg**

• I70.512 **Atherosclerosis of nonautologous biological bypass graft(s) of the extremities with intermittent claudication, left leg**

• I70.513 **Atherosclerosis of nonautologous biological bypass graft(s) of the extremities with intermittent claudication, bilateral legs**

• I70.518 **Atherosclerosis of nonautologous biological bypass graft(s) of the extremities with intermittent claudication, other extremity**

• I70.519 **Atherosclerosis of nonautologous biological bypass graft(s) of the extremities with intermittent claudication, unspecified extremity**

+ I70.52 **Atherosclerosis of nonautologous biological bypass graft(s) of the extremities with rest pain**
Includes: any condition classifiable to I70.51-

• I70.521 **Atherosclerosis of nonautologous biological bypass graft(s) of the extremities with rest pain, right leg**

• I70.522 **Atherosclerosis of nonautologous biological bypass graft(s) of the extremities with rest pain, left leg**

• I70.523 **Atherosclerosis of nonautologous biological bypass graft(s) of the extremities with rest pain, bilateral legs**

• I70.528 **Atherosclerosis of nonautologous biological bypass graft(s) of the extremities with rest pain, other extremity**

• I70.529 **Atherosclerosis of nonautologous biological bypass graft(s) of the extremities with rest pain, unspecified extremity**

+ I70.53 **Atherosclerosis of nonautologous biological bypass graft(s) of the right leg with ulceration**
Includes: *any condition classifiable to I70.511 and I70.521*
Use additional code to identify severity of ulcer (L97.-)

• CC I70.531 **Atherosclerosis of nonautologous biological bypass graft(s) of the right leg with ulceration of thigh**
CC Exclusion see Appendix A PDX collection 0698

• CC I70.532 **Atherosclerosis of nonautologous biological bypass graft(s) of the right leg with ulceration of calf**
CC Exclusion see Appendix A PDX collection 0698

• CC I70.533 **Atherosclerosis of nonautologous biological bypass graft(s) of the right leg with ulceration of ankle**
CC Exclusion see Appendix A PDX collection 0698

• CC I70.534 **Atherosclerosis of nonautologous biological bypass graft(s) of the right leg with ulceration of heel and midfoot**
Atherosclerosis of nonautologous biological bypass graft(s) of right leg with ulceration of plantar surface of midfoot
CC Exclusion see Appendix A PDX collection 0698

• I70.535 **Atherosclerosis of nonautologous biological bypass graft(s) of the right leg with ulceration of other part of foot**
Atherosclerosis of nonautologous biological bypass graft(s) of the right leg with ulceration of toe

• CC I70.538 **Atherosclerosis of nonautologous biological bypass graft(s) of the right leg with ulceration of other part of lower leg**
CC Exclusion see Appendix A PDX collection 0698

• CC I70.539 **Atherosclerosis of nonautologous biological bypass graft(s) of the right leg with ulceration of unspecified site**
CC Exclusion see Appendix A PDX collection 0698

+ I70.54 **Atherosclerosis of nonautologous biological bypass graft(s) of the left leg with ulceration**
Includes: any condition classifiable to I70.512 and I70.522
Use additional code to identify severity of ulcer (L97.-)

• CC I70.541 **Atherosclerosis of nonautologous biological bypass graft(s) of the left leg with ulceration of thigh**
CC Exclusion see Appendix A PDX collection 0698

• CC I70.542 **Atherosclerosis of nonautologous biological bypass graft(s) of the left leg with ulceration of calf**
CC Exclusion see Appendix A PDX collection 0698

• CC I70.543 **Atherosclerosis of nonautologous biological bypass graft(s) of the left leg with ulceration of ankle**
CC Exclusion see Appendix A PDX collection 0698

• CC I70.544 **Atherosclerosis of nonautologous biological bypass graft(s) of the left leg with ulceration of heel and midfoot**
Atherosclerosis of nonautologous biological bypass graft(s) of left leg with ulceration of plantar surface of midfoot
CC Exclusion see Appendix A PDX collection 0698

• I70.545 **Atherosclerosis of nonautologous biological bypass graft(s) of the left leg with ulceration of other part of foot**
Atherosclerosis of nonautologous biological bypass graft(s) of the left leg with ulceration of toe

• CC I70.548 **Atherosclerosis of nonautologous biological bypass graft(s) of the left leg with ulceration of other part of lower leg**
CC Exclusion see Appendix A PDX collection 0698

• CC I70.549 **Atherosclerosis of nonautologous biological bypass graft(s) of the left leg with ulceration of unspecified site**
CC Exclusion see Appendix A PDX collection 0698

• I70.55 **Atherosclerosis of nonautologous biological bypass graft(s) of other extremity with ulceration**
Includes: any condition classifiable to I70.518, I70.528, and I70.538
Use additional code to identify severity of ulcer (L98.49)

+ I70.56 **Atherosclerosis of nonautologous biological bypass graft(s) of the extremities with gangrene**
Includes: any condition classifiable to I70.51-, I70.52-, and I70.53-, I70.54-, I70.55
Use additional code to identify the severity of any ulcer (L97.-, L98.49-), if applicable
- CC I70.561 **Atherosclerosis of nonautologous biological bypass graft(s) of the extremities with gangrene, right leg**
CC Exclusion see Appendix A PDX collection 0519
- CC I70.562 **Atherosclerosis of nonautologous biological bypass graft(s) of the extremities with gangrene, left leg**
CC Exclusion see Appendix A PDX collection 0519
- CC I70.563 **Atherosclerosis of nonautologous biological bypass graft(s) of the extremities with gangrene, bilateral legs**
CC Exclusion see Appendix A PDX collection 0519
- CC I70.568 **Atherosclerosis of nonautologous biological bypass graft(s) of the extremities with gangrene, other extremity**
CC Exclusion see Appendix A PDX collection 0519
- CC I70.569 **Atherosclerosis of nonautologous biological bypass graft(s) of the extremities with gangrene, unspecified extremity**
CC Exclusion see Appendix A PDX collection 0519

+ I70.59 **Other atherosclerosis of nonautologous biological bypass graft(s) of the extremities**
- I70.591 **Other atherosclerosis of nonautologous biological bypass graft(s) of the extremities, right leg**
- I70.592 **Other atherosclerosis of nonautologous biological bypass graft(s) of the extremities, left leg**
- I70.593 **Other atherosclerosis of nonautologous biological bypass graft(s) of the extremities, bilateral legs**
- I70.598 **Other atherosclerosis of nonautologous biological bypass graft(s) of the extremities, other extremity**
- I70.599 **Other atherosclerosis of nonautologous biological bypass graft(s) of the extremities, unspecified extremity**

+ I70.6 **Atherosclerosis of nonbiological bypass graft(s) of the extremities**
Use additional code, if applicable, to identify chronic total occlusion of artery of extremity (I70.92)

+ I70.60 **Unspecified atherosclerosis of nonbiological bypass graft(s) of the extremities**
- I70.601 **Unspecified atherosclerosis of nonbiological bypass graft(s) of the extremities, right leg**
- I70.602 **Unspecified atherosclerosis of nonbiological bypass graft(s) of the extremities, left leg**
- I70.603 **Unspecified atherosclerosis of nonbiological bypass graft(s) of the extremities, bilateral legs**
- I70.608 **Unspecified atherosclerosis of nonbiological bypass graft(s) of the extremities, other extremity**
- I70.609 **Unspecified atherosclerosis of nonbiological bypass graft(s) of the extremities, unspecified extremity**

+ I70.61 **Atherosclerosis of nonbiological bypass graft(s) of the extremities with intermittent claudication**
- I70.611 **Atherosclerosis of nonbiological bypass graft(s) of the extremities with intermittent claudication, right leg**
- I70.612 **Atherosclerosis of nonbiological bypass graft(s) of the extremities with intermittent claudication, left leg**
- I70.613 **Atherosclerosis of nonbiological bypass graft(s) of the extremities with intermittent claudication, bilateral legs**
- I70.618 **Atherosclerosis of nonbiological bypass graft(s) of the extremities with intermittent claudication, other extremity**
- I70.619 **Atherosclerosis of nonbiological bypass graft(s) of the extremities with intermittent claudication, unspecified extremity**

+ I70.62 **Atherosclerosis of nonbiological bypass graft(s) of the extremities with rest pain**
Includes: any condition classifiable to I70.61-
- I70.621 **Atherosclerosis of nonbiological bypass graft(s) of the extremities with rest pain, right leg**
- I70.622 **Atherosclerosis of nonbiological bypass graft(s) of the extremities with rest pain, left leg**
- I70.623 **Atherosclerosis of nonbiological bypass graft(s) of the extremities with rest pain, bilateral legs**
- I70.628 **Atherosclerosis of nonbiological bypass graft(s) of the extremities with rest pain, other extremity**
- I70.629 **Atherosclerosis of nonbiological bypass graft(s) of the extremities with rest pain, unspecified extremity**

+ I70.63 **Atherosclerosis of nonbiological bypass graft(s) of the right leg with ulceration**
Includes: any condition classifiable to I70.611 and I70.621
Use additional code to identify severity of ulcer (L97.-)
- CC I70.631 **Atherosclerosis of nonbiological bypass graft(s) of the right leg with ulceration of thigh**
CC Exclusion see Appendix A PDX collection 0698
- CC I70.632 **Atherosclerosis of nonbiological bypass graft(s) of the right leg with ulceration of calf**
CC Exclusion see Appendix A PDX collection 0698
- CC I70.633 **Atherosclerosis of nonbiological bypass graft(s) of the right leg with ulceration of ankle**
CC Exclusion see Appendix A PDX collection 0698
- CC I70.634 **Atherosclerosis of nonbiological bypass graft(s) of the right leg with ulceration of heel and midfoot**
Atherosclerosis of nonbiological bypass graft(s) of right leg with ulceration of plantar surface of midfoot
CC Exclusion see Appendix A PDX collection 0698
- I70.635 **Atherosclerosis of nonbiological bypass graft(s) of the right leg with ulceration of other part of foot**
Atherosclerosis of nonbiological bypass graft(s) of the right leg with ulceration of toe
- CC I70.638 **Atherosclerosis of nonbiological bypass graft(s) of the right leg with ulceration of other part of lower leg**
CC Exclusion see Appendix A PDX collection 0698
- CC I70.639 **Atherosclerosis of nonbiological bypass graft(s) of the right leg with ulceration of unspecified site**
CC Exclusion see Appendix A PDX collection 0698

+ I70.64 **Atherosclerosis of nonbiological bypass graft(s) of the left leg with ulceration**
Includes: any condition classifiable to I70.612 and I70.622
Use additional code to identify severity of ulcer (L97.-)
- CC I70.641 **Atherosclerosis of nonbiological bypass graft(s) of the left leg with ulceration of thigh**
CC Exclusion see Appendix A PDX collection 0698
- CC I70.642 **Atherosclerosis of nonbiological bypass graft(s) of the left leg with ulceration of calf**
CC Exclusion see Appendix A PDX collection 0698

• CC **I70.643** **Atherosclerosis of nonbiological bypass graft(s) of the left leg with ulceration of ankle**
CC Exclusion see Appendix A PDX collection 0698

• CC **I70.644** **Atherosclerosis of nonbiological bypass graft(s) of the left leg with ulceration of heel and midfoot**
Atherosclerosis of nonbiological bypass graft(s) of left leg with ulceration of plantar surface of midfoot
CC Exclusion see Appendix A PDX collection 0698

• **I70.645** **Atherosclerosis of nonbiological bypass graft(s) of the left leg with ulceration of other part of foot**
Atherosclerosis of nonbiological bypass graft(s) of the left leg with ulceration of toe

• CC **I70.648** **Atherosclerosis of nonbiological bypass graft(s) of the left leg with ulceration of other part of lower leg**
CC Exclusion see Appendix A PDX collection 0698

• CC **I70.649** **Atherosclerosis of nonbiological bypass graft(s) of the left leg with ulceration of unspecified site**
CC Exclusion see Appendix A PDX collection 0698

• **I70.65** **Atherosclerosis of nonbiological bypass graft(s) of other extremity with ulceration**
Includes: any condition classifiable to I70.618 and I70.628
Use additional code to identify severity of ulcer (L98.49)

+ **I70.66** **Atherosclerosis of nonbiological bypass graft(s) of the extremities with gangrene**
Includes: any condition classifiable to I70.61-, I70.62-, I70.63-, I70.64-, I70.65
Use additional code to identify the severity of any ulcer (L97.-, L98.49-), if applicable

• CC **I70.661** **Atherosclerosis of nonbiological bypass graft(s) of the extremities with gangrene, right leg**
CC Exclusion see Appendix A PDX collection 0519

• CC **I70.662** **Atherosclerosis of nonbiological bypass graft(s) of the extremities with gangrene, left leg**
CC Exclusion see Appendix A PDX collection 0519

• CC **I70.663** **Atherosclerosis of nonbiological bypass graft(s) of the extremities with gangrene, bilateral legs**
CC Exclusion see Appendix A PDX collection 0519

• CC **I70.668** **Atherosclerosis of nonbiological bypass graft(s) of the extremities with gangrene, other extremity**
CC Exclusion see Appendix A PDX collection 0519

• CC **I70.669** **Atherosclerosis of nonbiological bypass graft(s) of the extremities with gangrene, unspecified extremity**
CC Exclusion see Appendix A PDX collection 0519

+ **I70.69** **Other atherosclerosis of nonbiological bypass graft(s) of the extremities**

• **I70.691** **Other atherosclerosis of nonbiological bypass graft(s) of the extremities, right leg**

• **I70.692** **Other atherosclerosis of nonbiological bypass graft(s) of the extremities, left leg**

• **I70.693** **Other atherosclerosis of nonbiological bypass graft(s) of the extremities, bilateral legs**

• **I70.698** **Other atherosclerosis of nonbiological bypass graft(s) of the extremities, other extremity**

• **I70.699** **Other atherosclerosis of nonbiological bypass graft(s) of the extremities, unspecified extremity**

+ **I70.7** **Atherosclerosis of other type of bypass graft(s) of the extremities**
Use additional code, if applicable, to identify chronic total occlusion of artery of extremity (I70.92)

+ **I70.70** **Unspecified atherosclerosis of other type of bypass graft(s) of the extremities**

• **I70.701** **Unspecified atherosclerosis of other type of bypass graft(s) of the extremities, right leg**

• **I70.702** **Unspecified atherosclerosis of other type of bypass graft(s) of the extremities, left leg**

• **I70.703** **Unspecified atherosclerosis of other type of bypass graft(s) of the extremities, bilateral legs**

• **I70.708** **Unspecified atherosclerosis of other type of bypass graft(s) of the extremities, other extremity**

• **I70.709** **Unspecified atherosclerosis of other type of bypass graft(s) of the extremities, unspecified extremity**

+ **I70.71** **Atherosclerosis of other type of bypass graft(s) of the extremities with intermittent claudication**

• **I70.711** **Atherosclerosis of other type of bypass graft(s) of the extremities with intermittent claudication, right leg**

• **I70.712** **Atherosclerosis of other type of bypass graft(s) of the extremities with intermittent claudication, left leg**

• **I70.713** **Atherosclerosis of other type of bypass graft(s) of the extremities with intermittent claudication, bilateral legs**

• **I70.718** **Atherosclerosis of other type of bypass graft(s) of the extremities with intermittent claudication, other extremity**

• **I70.719** **Atherosclerosis of other type of bypass graft(s) of the extremities with intermittent claudication, unspecified extremity**

+ **I70.72** **Atherosclerosis of other type of bypass graft(s) of the extremities with rest pain**
Includes: any condition classifiable to I70.71-

• **I70.721** **Atherosclerosis of other type of bypass graft(s) of the extremities with rest pain, right leg**

• **I70.722** **Atherosclerosis of other type of bypass graft(s) of the extremities with rest pain, left leg**

• **I70.723** **Atherosclerosis of other type of bypass graft(s) of the extremities with rest pain, bilateral legs**

• **I70.728** **Atherosclerosis of other type of bypass graft(s) of the extremities with rest pain, other extremity**

• **I70.729** **Atherosclerosis of other type of bypass graft(s) of the extremities with rest pain, unspecified extremity**

+ **I70.73** **Atherosclerosis of other type of bypass graft(s) of the right leg with ulceration**
Includes: any condition classifiable to I70.711 and I70.721
Use additional code to identify severity of ulcer (L97.-)

• CC **I70.731** **Atherosclerosis of other type of bypass graft(s) of the right leg with ulceration of thigh**
CC Exclusion see Appendix A PDX collection 0698

• CC **I70.732** **Atherosclerosis of other type of bypass graft(s) of the right leg with ulceration of calf**
CC Exclusion see Appendix A PDX collection 0698

• CC **I70.733** **Atherosclerosis of other type of bypass graft(s) of the right leg with ulceration of ankle**
CC Exclusion see Appendix A PDX collection 0698

• CC **I70.734** **Atherosclerosis of other type of bypass graft(s) of the right leg with ulceration of heel and midfoot**
Atherosclerosis of other type of bypass graft(s) of right leg with ulceration of plantar surface of midfoot
CC Exclusion see Appendix A PDX collection 0698

• I70.735 **Atherosclerosis of other type of bypass graft(s) of the right leg with ulceration of other part of foot**
Atherosclerosis of other type of bypass graft(s) of right leg with ulceration of toe

• CC I70.738 **Atherosclerosis of other type of bypass graft(s) of the right leg with ulceration of other part of lower leg**
CC Exclusion see Appendix A PDX collection 0698

• CC I70.739 **Atherosclerosis of other type of bypass graft(s) of the right leg with ulceration of unspecified site**
CC Exclusion see Appendix A PDX collection 0698

+ I70.74 **Atherosclerosis of other type of bypass graft(s) of the left leg with ulceration**
Includes: any condition classifiable to I70.712 and I70.722
Use additional code to identify severity of ulcer (L97.-)

• CC I70.741 **Atherosclerosis of other type of bypass graft(s) of the left leg with ulceration of thigh**
CC Exclusion see Appendix A PDX collection 0698

• CC I70.742 **Atherosclerosis of other type of bypass graft(s) of the left leg with ulceration of calf**
CC Exclusion see Appendix A PDX collection 0698

• CC I70.743 **Atherosclerosis of other type of bypass graft(s) of the left leg with ulceration of ankle**
CC Exclusion see Appendix A PDX collection 0698

• CC I70.744 **Atherosclerosis of other type of bypass graft(s) of the left leg with ulceration of heel and midfoot**
Atherosclerosis of other type of bypass graft(s) of left leg with ulceration of plantar surface of midfoot
CC Exclusion see Appendix A PDX collection 0698

• I70.745 **Atherosclerosis of other type of bypass graft(s) of the left leg with ulceration of other part of foot**
Atherosclerosis of other type of bypass graft(s) of left leg with ulceration of toe

• CC I70.748 **Atherosclerosis of other type of bypass graft(s) of the left leg with ulceration of other part of lower leg**
CC Exclusion see Appendix A PDX collection 0698

• CC I70.749 **Atherosclerosis of other type of bypass graft(s) of the left leg with ulceration of unspecified site**
CC Exclusion see Appendix A PDX collection 0698

• I70.75 **Atherosclerosis of other type of bypass graft(s) of other extremity with ulceration**
Includes: any condition classifiable to I70.718 and I70.728
Use additional code to identify severity of ulcer (L98.49)

+ I70.76 **Atherosclerosis of other type of bypass graft(s) of the extremities with gangrene**
Includes: any condition classifiable to I70.71-, I70.72-, I70.73-, I70.74-, I70.75
Use additional code to identify the severity of any ulcer (L97.-, L98.49-), if applicable

• CC I70.761 **Atherosclerosis of other type of bypass graft(s) of the extremities with gangrene, right leg**
CC Exclusion see Appendix A PDX collection 0519

• CC I70.762 **Atherosclerosis of other type of bypass graft(s) of the extremities with gangrene, left leg**
CC Exclusion see Appendix A PDX collection 0519

• CC I70.763 **Atherosclerosis of other type of bypass graft(s) of the extremities with gangrene, bilateral legs**
CC Exclusion see Appendix A PDX collection 0519

• CC I70.768 **Atherosclerosis of other type of bypass graft(s) of the extremities with gangrene, other extremity**
CC Exclusion see Appendix A PDX collection 0519

• CC I70.769 **Atherosclerosis of other type of bypass graft(s) of the extremities with gangrene, unspecified extremity**
CC Exclusion see Appendix A PDX collection 0519

+ I70.79 **Other atherosclerosis of other type of bypass graft(s) of the extremities**

• I70.791 **Other atherosclerosis of other type of bypass graft(s) of the extremities, right leg**

• I70.792 **Other atherosclerosis of other type of bypass graft(s) of the extremities, left leg**

• I70.793 **Other atherosclerosis of other type of bypass graft(s) of the extremities, bilateral legs**

• I70.798 **Other atherosclerosis of other type of bypass graft(s) of the extremities, other extremity**

• I70.799 **Other atherosclerosis of other type of bypass graft(s) of the extremities, unspecified extremity**

• I70.8 **Atherosclerosis of other arteries**

+ I70.9 **Other and unspecified atherosclerosis**

• I70.90 **Unspecified atherosclerosis**

• I70.91 **Generalized atherosclerosis**

• CC I70.92 **Chronic total occlusion of artery of the extremities**
Complete occlusion of artery of the extremities
Total occlusion of artery of the extremities
Code first atherosclerosis of arteries of the extremities (I70.2-, I70.3-, I70.4-, I70.5-, I70.6-, I70.7-)
CC Exclusion see Appendix A PDX collection 0699

I71 Aortic aneurysm and dissection

Excludes1: *aortic ectasia (I77.81-)*
syphilitic aortic aneurysm (A52.01)
traumatic aortic aneurysm (S25.09, S35.09)

+ I71.0 **Dissection of aorta**

MCC I71.00 **Dissection of unspecified site of aorta**
MCC Exclusion see Appendix A PDX collection 0700

MCC I71.01 **Dissection of thoracic aorta**
MCC Exclusion see Appendix A PDX collection 0700

MCC I71.02 **Dissection of abdominal aorta**
MCC Exclusion see Appendix A PDX collection 0700

MCC I71.03 **Dissection of thoracoabdominal aorta**
MCC Exclusion see Appendix A PDX collection 0700

MCC I71.1 **Thoracic aortic aneurysm, ruptured**
MCC Exclusion see Appendix A PDX collection 0700

I71.2 **Thoracic aortic aneurysm, without rupture**

MCC I71.3 **Abdominal aortic aneurysm, ruptured**
MCC Exclusion see Appendix A PDX collection 0700

I71.4 **Abdominal aortic aneurysm, without rupture**

MCC I71.5 **Thoracoabdominal aortic aneurysm, ruptured**
MCC Exclusion see Appendix A PDX collection 0700

I71.6 **Thoracoabdominal aortic aneurysm, without rupture**

MCC I71.8 **Aortic aneurysm of unspecified site, ruptured**
Rupture of aorta NOS
MCC Exclusion see Appendix A PDX collection 0700

I71.9 **Aortic aneurysm of unspecified site, without rupture**
Aneurysm of aorta
Dilatation of aorta
Hyaline necrosis of aorta

I72 Other aneurysm

Includes: aneurysm (cirsoid) (false) (ruptured)
Excludes2: *acquired aneurysm (I77.0)*
aneurysm (of) aorta (I71.-)
aneurysm (of) arteriovenous NOS (Q27.3-)
carotid artery dissection (I77.71)
cerebral (nonruptured) aneurysm (I67.1)
coronary aneurysm (I25.4)
coronary artery dissection (I25.42)
dissection of artery NEC (I77.79)
dissection of precerebral artery, congenital (nonruptured) (Q28.1)
heart aneurysm (I25.3)
iliac artery dissection (I77.72)
precerebral artery, congenital (nonruptured) (Q28.1)
pulmonary artery aneurysm (I28.1)
renal artery dissection (I77.73)
retinal aneurysm (H35.0)
ruptured cerebral aneurysm (I60.7)
varicose aneurysm (I77.0)
vertebral artery dissection (I77.74)

I72.0 Aneurysm of carotid artery
Aneurysm of common carotid artery
Aneurysm of external carotid artery
Aneurysm of internal carotid artery, extracranial portion
Excludes1: *aneurysm of internal carotid artery, intracranial portion (I67.1)*
aneurysm of internal carotid artery NOS (I67.1)

I72.1 Aneurysm of artery of upper extremity
I72.2 Aneurysm of renal artery
I72.3 Aneurysm of iliac artery
I72.4 Aneurysm of artery of lower extremity
I72.5 Aneurysm of other precerebral arteries
Aneurysm of basilar artery (trunk)
Excludes2: *aneurysm of carotid artery (I72.0)*
aneurysm of vertebral artery (I72.6)
dissection of carotid artery (I77.71)
dissection of other precerebral arteries (I77.75)
dissection of vertebral artery (I77.74)
AHA CC: 4Q, 2016, 28-29

I72.6 Aneurysm of vertebral artery
Excludes2: *dissection of vertebral artery (I77.74)*
AHA CC: 4Q, 2016, 28-29

I72.8 Aneurysm of other specified arteries
I72.9 Aneurysm of unspecified site

I73 Other peripheral vascular diseases

Excludes2: *chilblains (T69.1)*
frostbite (T33-T34)
immersion hand or foot (T69.0-)
spasm of cerebral artery (G45.9)

\+ **I73.0 Raynaud's syndrome**
Raynaud's disease
Raynaud's phenomenon (secondary)
I73.00 Raynaud's syndrome without gangrene
CC **I73.01 Raynaud's syndrome with gangrene**
CC Exclusion see Appendix A PDX collection 0519

I73.1 Thromboangiitis obliterans [Buerger's disease]
\+ **I73.8 Other specified peripheral vascular diseases**
Excludes1: *diabetic (peripheral) angiopathy (E08-E13 with .51-.52)*
I73.81 Erythromelalgia
I73.89 Other specified peripheral vascular diseases
Acrocyanosis
Erythrocyanosis
Simple acroparesthesia [Schultze's type]
Vasomotor acroparesthesia [Nothnagel's type]

I73.9 Peripheral vascular disease, unspecified
Intermittent claudication
Peripheral angiopathy NOS
Spasm of artery
Excludes1: *atherosclerosis of the extremities (I70.2--I70.7-)*

I74 Arterial embolism and thrombosis

Includes: embolic infarction
embolic occlusion
thrombotic infarction
thrombotic occlusion
Code first embolism and thrombosis complicating abortion or ectopic or molar pregnancy (O00-O07, O08.2)
embolism and thrombosis complicating pregnancy, childbirth and the puerperium (O88.-)
Excludes2: *atheroembolism (I75.-)*
basilar embolism and thrombosis (I63.0-I63.2, I65.1)
carotid embolism and thrombosis (I63.0-I63.2, I65.2)
cerebral embolism and thrombosis (I63.3-I63.5, I66.-)
coronary embolism and thrombosis (I21-I25)
mesenteric embolism and thrombosis (K55.0-)
ophthalmic embolism and thrombosis (H34.-)
precerebral embolism and thrombosis NOS (I63.0-I63.2, I65.9)
pulmonary embolism and thrombosis (I26.-)
renal embolism and thrombosis (N28.0)
retinal embolism and thrombosis (H34.-)
septic embolism and thrombosis (I76)
vertebral embolism and thrombosis (I63.0-I63.2, I65.0)

\+ **I74.0 Embolism and thrombosis of abdominal aorta**
MCC **I74.01 Saddle embolus of abdominal aorta**
MCC Exclusion see Appendix A PDX collection 0669
CC **I74.09 Other arterial embolism and thrombosis of abdominal aorta**
Aortic bifurcation syndrome
Aortoiliac obstruction
Leriche's syndrome
CC Exclusion see Appendix A PDX collection 0669

\+ **I74.1 Embolism and thrombosis of other and unspecified parts of aorta**
CC **I74.10 Embolism and thrombosis of unspecified parts of aorta**
CC Exclusion see Appendix A PDX collection 0669
CC **I74.11 Embolism and thrombosis of thoracic aorta**
CC Exclusion see Appendix A PDX collection 0701
CC **I74.19 Embolism and thrombosis of other parts of aorta**
CC Exclusion see Appendix A PDX collection 0669

CC **I74.2 Embolism and thrombosis of arteries of the upper extremities**
CC Exclusion see Appendix A PDX collection 0702
CC **I74.3 Embolism and thrombosis of arteries of the lower extremities**
CC Exclusion see Appendix A PDX collection 0703
CC **I74.4 Embolism and thrombosis of arteries of extremities, unspecified**
Peripheral arterial embolism NOS
CC Exclusion see Appendix A PDX collection 0703
CC **I74.5 Embolism and thrombosis of iliac artery**
CC Exclusion see Appendix A PDX collection 0704
CC **I74.8 Embolism and thrombosis of other arteries**
CC Exclusion see Appendix A PDX collection 0705
CC **I74.9 Embolism and thrombosis of unspecified artery**
CC Exclusion see Appendix A PDX collection 0705

I75 Atheroembolism

Includes: atherothrombotic microembolism
cholesterol embolism

\+ **I75.0 Atheroembolism of extremities**
\+ **I75.01 Atheroembolism of upper extremity**
CC **I75.011 Atheroembolism of right upper extremity**
CC Exclusion see Appendix A PDX collection 0706
CC **I75.012 Atheroembolism of left upper extremity**
CC Exclusion see Appendix A PDX collection 0706
CC **I75.013 Atheroembolism of bilateral upper extremities**
CC Exclusion see Appendix A PDX collection 0706
CC **I75.019 Atheroembolism of unspecified upper extremity**
CC Exclusion see Appendix A PDX collection 0706
\+ **I75.02 Atheroembolism of lower extremity**
CC **I75.021 Atheroembolism of right lower extremity**
CC Exclusion see Appendix A PDX collection 0707
CC **I75.022 Atheroembolism of left lower extremity**
CC Exclusion see Appendix A PDX collection 0707

CC **I75.023 Atheroembolism of bilateral lower extremities**
CC Exclusion see Appendix A PDX collection 0707

CC **I75.029 Atheroembolism of unspecified lower extremity**
CC Exclusion see Appendix A PDX collection 0707

+ **I75.8 Atheroembolism of other sites**

CC **I75.81 Atheroembolism of kidney**
Use additional code for any associated acute kidney failure and chronic kidney disease (N17.-, N18.-)
CC Exclusion see Appendix A PDX collection 0708

CC **I75.89 Atheroembolism of other site**
CC Exclusion see Appendix A PDX collection 0709

CC **I76 Septic arterial embolism**
Code first underlying infection, such as:
infective endocarditis (I33.0)
lung abscess (J85.-)

Use additional code to identify the site of the embolism (I74.-)
Excludes2: *septic pulmonary embolism (I26.01, I26.90)*
CC Exclusion see Appendix A PDX collection 0705
Valid 3-character code, no further characters required

I77 Other disorders of arteries and arterioles
Excludes2: *collagen (vascular) diseases (M30-M36)*
hypersensitivity angiitis (M31.0)
pulmonary artery (I28.-)

I77.0 Arteriovenous fistula, acquired
Aneurysmal varix
Arteriovenous aneurysm, acquired
Excludes1: *arteriovenous aneurysm NOS (Q27.3-)*
presence of arteriovenous shunt (fistula) for dialysis (Z99.2)
traumatic - see injury of blood vessel by body region
Excludes2: *cerebral (I67.1)*
coronary (I25.4)

I77.1 Stricture of artery
Narrowing of artery

CC **I77.2 Rupture of artery**
Erosion of artery
Fistula of artery
Ulcer of artery
Excludes1: *traumatic rupture of artery - see injury of blood vessel by body region*
CC Exclusion see Appendix A PDX collection 0710

I77.3 Arterial fibromuscular dysplasia
Fibromuscular hyperplasia (of) carotid artery
Fibromuscular hyperplasia (of) renal artery

CC **I77.4 Celiac artery compression syndrome**
CC Exclusion see Appendix A PDX collection 0711

CC **I77.5 Necrosis of artery**
CC Exclusion see Appendix A PDX collection 0712

I77.6 Arteritis, unspecified
Aortitis NOS
Endarteritis NOS
Excludes1: *arteritis or endarteritis:*
aortic arch (M31.4)
cerebral NEC (I67.7)
coronary (I25.89)
deformans (I70.-)
giant cell (M31.5, M31.6)
obliterans (I70.-)
senile (I70.-)

+ **I77.7 Other arterial dissection**
Excludes2: *dissection of aorta (I71.0-)*
dissection of coronary artery (I25.42)

MCC **I77.70 Dissection of unspecified artery**
MCC Exclusion see Appendix A PDX collection 0689
AHA CC: 4Q, 2016, 28-29

MCC **I77.71 Dissection of carotid artery**
MCC Exclusion see Appendix A PDX collection 0689

MCC **I77.72 Dissection of iliac artery**
MCC Exclusion see Appendix A PDX collection 0689

MCC **I77.73 Dissection of renal artery**
MCC Exclusion see Appendix A PDX collection 0689

MCC **I77.74 Dissection of vertebral artery**
Excludes2: *aneurysm of vertebral artery (I72.6)*
MCC Exclusion see Appendix A PDX collection 0689

MCC **I77.75 Dissection of other precerebral arteries**
Dissection of basilar artery (trunk)
Excludes2: *aneurysm of carotid artery (I72.0)*
aneurysm of other precerebral arteries (I72.5)
aneurysm of vertebral artery (I72.6)
dissection of carotid artery (I77.71)
dissection of vertebral artery (I77.74)
MCC Exclusion see Appendix A PDX collection 0689
AHA CC: 4Q, 2016, 28-29

MCC **I77.76 Dissection of artery of upper extremity**
MCC Exclusion see Appendix A PDX collection 0689
AHA CC: 4Q, 2016, 28-29

MCC **I77.77 Dissection of artery of lower extremity**
MCC Exclusion see Appendix A PDX collection 0689
AHA CC: 4Q, 2016, 28-29

MCC **I77.79 Dissection of other specified artery**
MCC Exclusion see Appendix A PDX collection 0689

+ **I77.8 Other specified disorders of arteries and arterioles**

+ **I77.81 Aortic ectasia**
Ectasis aorta
Excludes1: *aortic aneurysm and dissection (I71.0-)*

I77.810 Thoracic aortic ectasia

I77.811 Abdominal aortic ectasia

I77.812 Thoracoabdominal aortic ectasia

I77.819 Aortic ectasia, unspecified site

I77.89 Other specified disorders of arteries and arterioles

I77.9 Disorder of arteries and arterioles, unspecified

I78 Diseases of capillaries

I78.0 Hereditary hemorrhagic telangiectasia
Rendu-Osler-Weber disease

I78.1 Nevus, non-neoplastic
Araneus nevus
Senile nevus
Spider nevus
Stellar nevus
Excludes1: *nevus NOS (D22.-)*
vascular NOS (Q82.5)
Excludes2: *blue nevus (D22.-)*
flammeus nevus (Q82.5)
hairy nevus (D22.-)
melanocytic nevus (D22.-)
pigmented nevus (D22.-)
portwine nevus (Q82.5)
sanguineous nevus (Q82.5)
strawberry nevus (Q82.5)
verrucous nevus (Q82.5)

I78.8 Other diseases of capillaries

I78.9 Disease of capillaries, unspecified

I79 Disorders of arteries, arterioles and capillaries in diseases classified elsewhere

I79.0 Aneurysm of aorta in diseases classified elsewhere
Code first underlying disease
Excludes1: *syphilitic aneurysm (A52.01)*

I79.1 Aortitis in diseases classified elsewhere
Code first underlying disease
Excludes1: *syphilitic aortitis (A52.02)*

I79.8 Other disorders of arteries, arterioles and capillaries in diseases classified elsewhere
Code first underlying disease, such as:
amyloidosis (E85.-)
Excludes1: *diabetic (peripheral) angiopathy (E08-E13 with .51-.52)*
syphilitic endarteritis (A52.09)
tuberculous endarteritis (A18.89)

Diseases of veins, lymphatic vessels and lymph nodes, not elsewhere classified (I80-I89)

I80 Phlebitis and thrombophlebitis

Includes: endophlebitis
inflammation, vein
periphlebitis
suppurative phlebitis

Code first phlebitis and thrombophlebitis complicating abortion, ectopic or molar pregnancy (O00-O07, O08.7)
phlebitis and thrombophlebitis complicating pregnancy, childbirth and the puerperium (O22.-, O87.-)

Excludes1: *venous embolism and thrombosis of lower extremities (I82.4-, I82.5-, I82.81-)*

+ **I80.0 Phlebitis and thrombophlebitis of superficial vessels of lower extremities**
  Phlebitis and thrombophlebitis of femoropopliteal vein
  I80.00 Phlebitis and thrombophlebitis of superficial vessels of unspecified lower extremity
  I80.01 Phlebitis and thrombophlebitis of superficial vessels of right lower extremity
  I80.02 Phlebitis and thrombophlebitis of superficial vessels of left lower extremity
  I80.03 Phlebitis and thrombophlebitis of superficial vessels of lower extremities, bilateral
+ **I80.1 Phlebitis and thrombophlebitis of femoral vein**
  CC **I80.10 Phlebitis and thrombophlebitis of unspecified femoral vein**
  CC Exclusion see Appendix A PDX collection 0713
  CC **I80.11 Phlebitis and thrombophlebitis of right femoral vein**
  CC Exclusion see Appendix A PDX collection 0713
  CC **I80.12 Phlebitis and thrombophlebitis of left femoral vein**
  CC Exclusion see Appendix A PDX collection 0713
  CC **I80.13 Phlebitis and thrombophlebitis of femoral vein, bilateral**
  CC Exclusion see Appendix A PDX collection 0713
+ **I80.2 Phlebitis and thrombophlebitis of other and unspecified deep vessels of lower extremities**
  + **I80.20 Phlebitis and thrombophlebitis of unspecified deep vessels of lower extremities**
    CC **I80.201 Phlebitis and thrombophlebitis of unspecified deep vessels of right lower extremity**
    CC Exclusion see Appendix A PDX collection 0713
    CC **I80.202 Phlebitis and thrombophlebitis of unspecified deep vessels of left lower extremity**
    CC Exclusion see Appendix A PDX collection 0713
    CC **I80.203 Phlebitis and thrombophlebitis of unspecified deep vessels of lower extremities, bilateral**
    CC Exclusion see Appendix A PDX collection 0713
    CC **I80.209 Phlebitis and thrombophlebitis of unspecified deep vessels of unspecified lower extremity**
    CC Exclusion see Appendix A PDX collection 0713
  + **I80.21 Phlebitis and thrombophlebitis of iliac vein**
    CC **I80.211 Phlebitis and thrombophlebitis of right iliac vein**
    CC Exclusion see Appendix A PDX collection 0713
    CC **I80.212 Phlebitis and thrombophlebitis of left iliac vein**
    CC Exclusion see Appendix A PDX collection 0713
    CC **I80.213 Phlebitis and thrombophlebitis of iliac vein, bilateral**
    CC Exclusion see Appendix A PDX collection 0713
    CC **I80.219 Phlebitis and thrombophlebitis of unspecified iliac vein**
    CC Exclusion see Appendix A PDX collection 0713
  + **I80.22 Phlebitis and thrombophlebitis of popliteal vein**
    CC **I80.221 Phlebitis and thrombophlebitis of right popliteal vein**
    CC Exclusion see Appendix A PDX collection 0713
    CC **I80.222 Phlebitis and thrombophlebitis of left popliteal vein**
    CC Exclusion see Appendix A PDX collection 0713
    CC **I80.223 Phlebitis and thrombophlebitis of popliteal vein, bilateral**
    CC Exclusion see Appendix A PDX collection 0713
    CC **I80.229 Phlebitis and thrombophlebitis of unspecified popliteal vein**
    CC Exclusion see Appendix A PDX collection 0713
  + **I80.23 Phlebitis and thrombophlebitis of tibial vein**
    CC **I80.231 Phlebitis and thrombophlebitis of right tibial vein**
    CC Exclusion see Appendix A PDX collection 0713
    CC **I80.232 Phlebitis and thrombophlebitis of left tibial vein**
    CC Exclusion see Appendix A PDX collection 0713
    CC **I80.233 Phlebitis and thrombophlebitis of tibial vein, bilateral**
    CC Exclusion see Appendix A PDX collection 0713
    CC **I80.239 Phlebitis and thrombophlebitis of unspecified tibial vein**
    CC Exclusion see Appendix A PDX collection 0713
  + **I80.29 Phlebitis and thrombophlebitis of other deep vessels of lower extremities**
    CC **I80.291 Phlebitis and thrombophlebitis of other deep vessels of right lower extremity**
    CC Exclusion see Appendix A PDX collection 0713
    CC **I80.292 Phlebitis and thrombophlebitis of other deep vessels of left lower extremity**
    CC Exclusion see Appendix A PDX collection 0713
    CC **I80.293 Phlebitis and thrombophlebitis of other deep vessels of lower extremity, bilateral**
    CC Exclusion see Appendix A PDX collection 0713
    CC **I80.299 Phlebitis and thrombophlebitis of other deep vessels of unspecified lower extremity**
    CC Exclusion see Appendix A PDX collection 0713

I80.3 Phlebitis and thrombophlebitis of lower extremities, unspecified
I80.8 Phlebitis and thrombophlebitis of other sites
I80.9 Phlebitis and thrombophlebitis of unspecified site

MCC **I81 Portal vein thrombosis**

Portal (vein) obstruction

Excludes2: *hepatic vein thrombosis (I82.0)*
phlebitis of portal vein (K75.1)

MCC Exclusion see Appendix A PDX collection 0714
Valid 3-character code, no further characters required

I82 Other venous embolism and thrombosis

Code first venous embolism and thrombosis complicating:
abortion, ectopic or molar pregnancy (O00-O07, O08.7)
pregnancy, childbirth and the puerperium (O22.-, O87.-)

Excludes2: *venous embolism and thrombosis (of):*
cerebral (I63.6, I67.6)
coronary (I21-I25)
intracranial and intraspinal, septic or NOS (G08)
intracranial, nonpyogenic (I67.6)
intraspinal, nonpyogenic (G95.1)
mesenteric (K55.0-)
portal (I81)
pulmonary (I26.-)

MCC **I82.0 Budd-Chiari syndrome**
Hepatic vein thrombosis
MCC Exclusion see Appendix A PDX collection 0715

CC **I82.1 Thrombophlebitis migrans**
CC Exclusion see Appendix A PDX collection 0716

+ **I82.2 Embolism and thrombosis of vena cava and other thoracic veins**
  + **I82.21 Embolism and thrombosis of superior vena cava**
    CC **I82.210 Acute embolism and thrombosis of superior vena cava**
    Embolism and thrombosis of superior vena cava NOS
    CC Exclusion see Appendix A PDX collection 0717
    CC **I82.211 Chronic embolism and thrombosis of superior vena cava**
    CC Exclusion see Appendix A PDX collection 0717

+ I82.22 **Embolism and thrombosis of inferior vena cava**

MCC **I82.220 Acute embolism and thrombosis of inferior vena cava**

Embolism and thrombosis of inferior vena cava NOS

MCC Exclusion see Appendix A PDX collection 0718

MCC **I82.221 Chronic embolism and thrombosis of inferior vena cava**

MCC Exclusion see Appendix A PDX collection 0718

+ I82.29 **Embolism and thrombosis of other thoracic veins**

Embolism and thrombosis of brachiocephalic (innominate) vein

CC **I82.290 Acute embolism and thrombosis of other thoracic veins**

CC Exclusion see Appendix A PDX collection 0717

CC **I82.291 Chronic embolism and thrombosis of other thoracic veins**

CC Exclusion see Appendix A PDX collection 0717

CC **I82.3 Embolism and thrombosis of renal vein**

CC Exclusion see Appendix A PDX collection 0719

+ I82.4 **Acute embolism and thrombosis of deep veins of lower extremity**

+ I82.40 **Acute embolism and thrombosis of unspecified deep veins of lower extremity**

Deep vein thrombosis NOS

DVT NOS

Excludes1: *acute embolism and thrombosis of unspecified deep veins of distal lower extremity (I82.4Z-)*

acute embolism and thrombosis of unspecified deep veins of proximal lower extremity (I82.4Y-)

CC **I82.401 Acute embolism and thrombosis of unspecified deep veins of right lower extremity**

CC Exclusion see Appendix A PDX collection 0717

HAC see Appendix B for HAC conditional logic

CC **I82.402 Acute embolism and thrombosis of unspecified deep veins of left lower extremity**

CC Exclusion see Appendix A PDX collection 0717

HAC see Appendix B for HAC conditional logic

CC **I82.403 Acute embolism and thrombosis of unspecified deep veins of lower extremity, bilateral**

CC Exclusion see Appendix A PDX collection 0717

HAC see Appendix B for HAC conditional logic

CC **I82.409 Acute embolism and thrombosis of unspecified deep veins of unspecified lower extremity**

CC Exclusion see Appendix A PDX collection 0717

HAC see Appendix B for HAC conditional logic

+ I82.41 **Acute embolism and thrombosis of femoral vein**

CC **I82.411 Acute embolism and thrombosis of right femoral vein**

CC Exclusion see Appendix A PDX collection 0717

HAC see Appendix B for HAC conditional logic

CC **I82.412 Acute embolism and thrombosis of left femoral vein**

CC Exclusion see Appendix A PDX collection 0717

HAC see Appendix B for HAC conditional logic

CC **I82.413 Acute embolism and thrombosis of femoral vein, bilateral**

CC Exclusion see Appendix A PDX collection 0717

HAC see Appendix B for HAC conditional logic

CC **I82.419 Acute embolism and thrombosis of unspecified femoral vein**

CC Exclusion see Appendix A PDX collection 0717

HAC see Appendix B for HAC conditional logic

+ I82.42 **Acute embolism and thrombosis of iliac vein**

CC **I82.421 Acute embolism and thrombosis of right iliac vein**

CC Exclusion see Appendix A PDX collection 0717

HAC see Appendix B for HAC conditional logic

CC **I82.422 Acute embolism and thrombosis of left iliac vein**

CC Exclusion see Appendix A PDX collection 0717

HAC see Appendix B for HAC conditional logic

CC **I82.423 Acute embolism and thrombosis of iliac vein, bilateral**

CC Exclusion see Appendix A PDX collection 0717

HAC see Appendix B for HAC conditional logic

CC **I82.429 Acute embolism and thrombosis of unspecified iliac vein**

CC Exclusion see Appendix A PDX collection 0717

HAC see Appendix B for HAC conditional logic

+ I82.43 **Acute embolism and thrombosis of popliteal vein**

CC **I82.431 Acute embolism and thrombosis of right popliteal vein**

CC Exclusion see Appendix A PDX collection 0717

HAC see Appendix B for HAC conditional logic

CC **I82.432 Acute embolism and thrombosis of left popliteal vein**

CC Exclusion see Appendix A PDX collection 0717

HAC see Appendix B for HAC conditional logic

CC **I82.433 Acute embolism and thrombosis of popliteal vein, bilateral**

CC Exclusion see Appendix A PDX collection 0717

HAC see Appendix B for HAC conditional logic

CC **I82.439 Acute embolism and thrombosis of unspecified popliteal vein**

CC Exclusion see Appendix A PDX collection 0717

HAC see Appendix B for HAC conditional logic

+ I82.44 **Acute embolism and thrombosis of tibial vein**

CC **I82.441 Acute embolism and thrombosis of right tibial vein**

CC Exclusion see Appendix A PDX collection 0717

HAC see Appendix B for HAC conditional logic

CC **I82.442 Acute embolism and thrombosis of left tibial vein**

CC Exclusion see Appendix A PDX collection 0717

HAC see Appendix B for HAC conditional logic

CC **I82.443 Acute embolism and thrombosis of tibial vein, bilateral**

CC Exclusion see Appendix A PDX collection 0717

HAC see Appendix B for HAC conditional logic

CC **I82.449 Acute embolism and thrombosis of unspecified tibial vein**

CC Exclusion see Appendix A PDX collection 0717

HAC see Appendix B for HAC conditional logic

+ I82.49 **Acute embolism and thrombosis of other specified deep vein of lower extremity**

CC **I82.491 Acute embolism and thrombosis of other specified deep vein of right lower extremity**

CC Exclusion see Appendix A PDX collection 0717

HAC see Appendix B for HAC conditional logic

CC **I82.492 Acute embolism and thrombosis of other specified deep vein of left lower extremity**

CC Exclusion see Appendix A PDX collection 0717

HAC see Appendix B for HAC conditional logic

CC **I82.493 Acute embolism and thrombosis of other specified deep vein of lower extremity, bilateral**

CC Exclusion see Appendix A PDX collection 0717

HAC see Appendix B for HAC conditional logic

CC **I82.499 Acute embolism and thrombosis of other specified deep vein of unspecified lower extremity**

CC Exclusion see Appendix A PDX collection 0717

HAC see Appendix B for HAC conditional logic

+ I82.4Y **Acute embolism and thrombosis of unspecified deep veins of proximal lower extremity**
  Acute embolism and thrombosis of deep vein of thigh NOS
  Acute embolism and thrombosis of deep vein of upper leg NOS
  CC **I82.4Y1 Acute embolism and thrombosis of unspecified deep veins of right proximal lower extremity**
  CC Exclusion see Appendix A PDX collection 0717
  HAC see Appendix B for HAC conditional logic
  CC **I82.4Y2 Acute embolism and thrombosis of unspecified deep veins of left proximal lower extremity**
  CC Exclusion see Appendix A PDX collection 0717
  HAC see Appendix B for HAC conditional logic
  CC **I82.4Y3 Acute embolism and thrombosis of unspecified deep veins of proximal lower extremity, bilateral**
  CC Exclusion see Appendix A PDX collection 0717
  HAC see Appendix B for HAC conditional logic
  CC **I82.4Y9 Acute embolism and thrombosis of unspecified deep veins of unspecified proximal lower extremity**
  CC Exclusion see Appendix A PDX collection 0717
  HAC see Appendix B for HAC conditional logic

+ I82.4Z **Acute embolism and thrombosis of unspecified deep veins of distal lower extremity**
  Acute embolism and thrombosis of deep vein of calf NOS
  Acute embolism and thrombosis of deep vein of lower leg NOS
  CC **I82.4Z1 Acute embolism and thrombosis of unspecified deep veins of right distal lower extremity**
  CC Exclusion see Appendix A PDX collection 0717
  HAC see Appendix B for HAC conditional logic
  CC **I82.4Z2 Acute embolism and thrombosis of unspecified deep veins of left distal lower extremity**
  CC Exclusion see Appendix A PDX collection 0717
  HAC see Appendix B for HAC conditional logic
  CC **I82.4Z3 Acute embolism and thrombosis of unspecified deep veins of distal lower extremity, bilateral**
  CC Exclusion see Appendix A PDX collection 0717
  HAC see Appendix B for HAC conditional logic
  CC **I82.4Z9 Acute embolism and thrombosis of unspecified deep veins of unspecified distal lower extremity**
  CC Exclusion see Appendix A PDX collection 0717
  HAC see Appendix B for HAC conditional logic

+ **I82.5 Chronic embolism and thrombosis of deep veins of lower extremity**
  Use additional code, if applicable, for associated long-term (current) use of anticoagulants (Z79.01)
  Excludes1: *personal history of venous embolism and thrombosis (Z86.718)*

+ **I82.50 Chronic embolism and thrombosis of unspecified deep veins of lower extremity**
  Excludes1: *chronic embolism and thrombosis of unspecified deep veins of distal lower extremity (I82.5Z-)*
  chronic embolism and thrombosis of unspecified deep veins of proximal lower extremity (I82.5Y-)
  CC **I82.501 Chronic embolism and thrombosis of unspecified deep veins of right lower extremity**
  CC Exclusion see Appendix A PDX collection 0717
  CC **I82.502 Chronic embolism and thrombosis of unspecified deep veins of left lower extremity**
  CC Exclusion see Appendix A PDX collection 0717
  CC **I82.503 Chronic embolism and thrombosis of unspecified deep veins of lower extremity, bilateral**
  CC Exclusion see Appendix A PDX collection 0717
  CC **I82.509 Chronic embolism and thrombosis of unspecified deep veins of unspecified lower extremity**
  CC Exclusion see Appendix A PDX collection 0717

+ **I82.51 Chronic embolism and thrombosis of femoral vein**
  CC **I82.511 Chronic embolism and thrombosis of right femoral vein**
  CC Exclusion see Appendix A PDX collection 0717
  CC **I82.512 Chronic embolism and thrombosis of left femoral vein**
  CC Exclusion see Appendix A PDX collection 0717
  CC **I82.513 Chronic embolism and thrombosis of femoral vein, bilateral**
  CC Exclusion see Appendix A PDX collection 0717
  CC **I82.519 Chronic embolism and thrombosis of unspecified femoral vein**
  CC Exclusion see Appendix A PDX collection 0717

+ **I82.52 Chronic embolism and thrombosis of iliac vein**
  CC **I82.521 Chronic embolism and thrombosis of right iliac vein**
  CC Exclusion see Appendix A PDX collection 0717
  CC **I82.522 Chronic embolism and thrombosis of left iliac vein**
  CC Exclusion see Appendix A PDX collection 0717
  CC **I82.523 Chronic embolism and thrombosis of iliac vein, bilateral**
  CC Exclusion see Appendix A PDX collection 0717
  CC **I82.529 Chronic embolism and thrombosis of unspecified iliac vein**
  CC Exclusion see Appendix A PDX collection 0717

+ **I82.53 Chronic embolism and thrombosis of popliteal vein**
  CC **I82.531 Chronic embolism and thrombosis of right popliteal vein**
  CC Exclusion see Appendix A PDX collection 0717
  CC **I82.532 Chronic embolism and thrombosis of left popliteal vein**
  CC Exclusion see Appendix A PDX collection 0717
  CC **I82.533 Chronic embolism and thrombosis of popliteal vein, bilateral**
  CC Exclusion see Appendix A PDX collection 0717
  CC **I82.539 Chronic embolism and thrombosis of unspecified popliteal vein**
  CC Exclusion see Appendix A PDX collection 0717

+ **I82.54 Chronic embolism and thrombosis of tibial vein**
  CC **I82.541 Chronic embolism and thrombosis of right tibial vein**
  CC Exclusion see Appendix A PDX collection 0717
  CC **I82.542 Chronic embolism and thrombosis of left tibial vein**
  CC Exclusion see Appendix A PDX collection 0717
  CC **I82.543 Chronic embolism and thrombosis of tibial vein, bilateral**
  CC Exclusion see Appendix A PDX collection 0717
  CC **I82.549 Chronic embolism and thrombosis of unspecified tibial vein**
  CC Exclusion see Appendix A PDX collection 0717

+ **I82.59 Chronic embolism and thrombosis of other specified deep vein of lower extremity**
  CC **I82.591 Chronic embolism and thrombosis of other specified deep vein of right lower extremity**
  CC Exclusion see Appendix A PDX collection 0717

CC **I82.592** **Chronic embolism and thrombosis of other specified deep vein of left lower extremity**
CC Exclusion see Appendix A PDX collection 0717

CC **I82.593** **Chronic embolism and thrombosis of other specified deep vein of lower extremity, bilateral**
CC Exclusion see Appendix A PDX collection 0717

CC **I82.599** **Chronic embolism and thrombosis of other specified deep vein of unspecified lower extremity**
CC Exclusion see Appendix A PDX collection 0717

+ **I82.5Y** **Chronic embolism and thrombosis of unspecified deep veins of proximal lower extremity**
Chronic embolism and thrombosis of deep veins of thigh NOS
Chronic embolism and thrombosis of deep veins of upper leg NOS

CC **I82.5Y1** **Chronic embolism and thrombosis of unspecified deep veins of right proximal lower extremity**
CC Exclusion see Appendix A PDX collection 0717

CC **I82.5Y2** **Chronic embolism and thrombosis of unspecified deep veins of left proximal lower extremity**
CC Exclusion see Appendix A PDX collection 0717

CC **I82.5Y3** **Chronic embolism and thrombosis of unspecified deep veins of proximal lower extremity, bilateral**
CC Exclusion see Appendix A PDX collection 0717

CC **I82.5Y9** **Chronic embolism and thrombosis of unspecified deep veins of unspecified proximal lower extremity**
CC Exclusion see Appendix A PDX collection 0717

+ **I82.5Z** **Chronic embolism and thrombosis of unspecified deep veins of distal lower extremity**
Chronic embolism and thrombosis of deep veins of calf NOS
Chronic embolism and thrombosis of deep veins of lower leg NOS

CC **I82.5Z1** **Chronic embolism and thrombosis of unspecified deep veins of right distal lower extremity**
CC Exclusion see Appendix A PDX collection 0717

CC **I82.5Z2** **Chronic embolism and thrombosis of unspecified deep veins of left distal lower extremity**
CC Exclusion see Appendix A PDX collection 0717

CC **I82.5Z3** **Chronic embolism and thrombosis of unspecified deep veins of distal lower extremity, bilateral**
CC Exclusion see Appendix A PDX collection 0717

CC **I82.5Z9** **Chronic embolism and thrombosis of unspecified deep veins of unspecified distal lower extremity**
CC Exclusion see Appendix A PDX collection 0717

+ **I82.6** **Acute embolism and thrombosis of veins of upper extremity**

+ **I82.60** **Acute embolism and thrombosis of unspecified veins of upper extremity**

CC **I82.601** **Acute embolism and thrombosis of unspecified veins of right upper extremity**
CC Exclusion see Appendix A PDX collection 0717

CC **I82.602** **Acute embolism and thrombosis of unspecified veins of left upper extremity**
CC Exclusion see Appendix A PDX collection 0717

CC **I82.603** **Acute embolism and thrombosis of unspecified veins of upper extremity, bilateral**
CC Exclusion see Appendix A PDX collection 0717

CC **I82.609** **Acute embolism and thrombosis of unspecified veins of unspecified upper extremity**
CC Exclusion see Appendix A PDX collection 0717

+ **I82.61** **Acute embolism and thrombosis of superficial veins of upper extremity**
Acute embolism and thrombosis of antecubital vein
Acute embolism and thrombosis of basilic vein
Acute embolism and thrombosis of cephalic vein

CC **I82.611** **Acute embolism and thrombosis of superficial veins of right upper extremity**
CC Exclusion see Appendix A PDX collection 0717

CC **I82.612** **Acute embolism and thrombosis of superficial veins of left upper extremity**
CC Exclusion see Appendix A PDX collection 0717

CC **I82.613** **Acute embolism and thrombosis of superficial veins of upper extremity, bilateral**
CC Exclusion see Appendix A PDX collection 0717

CC **I82.619** **Acute embolism and thrombosis of superficial veins of unspecified upper extremity**
CC Exclusion see Appendix A PDX collection 0717

+ **I82.62** **Acute embolism and thrombosis of deep veins of upper extremity**
Acute embolism and thrombosis of brachial vein
Acute embolism and thrombosis of radial vein
Acute embolism and thrombosis of ulnar vein

CC **I82.621** **Acute embolism and thrombosis of deep veins of right upper extremity**
CC Exclusion see Appendix A PDX collection 0717

CC **I82.622** **Acute embolism and thrombosis of deep veins of left upper extremity**
CC Exclusion see Appendix A PDX collection 0717

CC **I82.623** **Acute embolism and thrombosis of deep veins of upper extremity, bilateral**
CC Exclusion see Appendix A PDX collection 0717

CC **I82.629** **Acute embolism and thrombosis of deep veins of unspecified upper extremity**
CC Exclusion see Appendix A PDX collection 0717

+ **I82.7** **Chronic embolism and thrombosis of veins of upper extremity**
Use additional code, if applicable, for associated long-term (current) use of anticoagulants (Z79.01)
Excludes1: *personal history of venous embolism and thrombosis (Z86.718)*

+ **I82.70** **Chronic embolism and thrombosis of unspecified veins of upper extremity**

CC **I82.701** **Chronic embolism and thrombosis of unspecified veins of right upper extremity**
CC Exclusion see Appendix A PDX collection 0717

CC **I82.702** **Chronic embolism and thrombosis of unspecified veins of left upper extremity**
CC Exclusion see Appendix A PDX collection 0717

CC **I82.703** **Chronic embolism and thrombosis of unspecified veins of upper extremity, bilateral**
CC Exclusion see Appendix A PDX collection 0717

CC **I82.709** **Chronic embolism and thrombosis of unspecified veins of unspecified upper extremity**
CC Exclusion see Appendix A PDX collection 0717

+ **I82.71** **Chronic embolism and thrombosis of superficial veins of upper extremity**
Chronic embolism and thrombosis of antecubital vein
Chronic embolism and thrombosis of basilic vein
Chronic embolism and thrombosis of cephalic vein

CC **I82.711** **Chronic embolism and thrombosis of superficial veins of right upper extremity**
CC Exclusion see Appendix A PDX collection 0717

CC I82.712 **Chronic embolism and thrombosis of superficial veins of left upper extremity**
CC Exclusion see Appendix A PDX collection 0717

CC I82.713 **Chronic embolism and thrombosis of superficial veins of upper extremity, bilateral**
CC Exclusion see Appendix A PDX collection 0717

CC I82.719 **Chronic embolism and thrombosis of superficial veins of unspecified upper extremity**
CC Exclusion see Appendix A PDX collection 0717

\+ I82.72 **Chronic embolism and thrombosis of deep veins of upper extremity**
Chronic embolism and thrombosis of brachial vein
Chronic embolism and thrombosis of radial vein
Chronic embolism and thrombosis of ulnar vein

CC I82.721 **Chronic embolism and thrombosis of deep veins of right upper extremity**
CC Exclusion see Appendix A PDX collection 0717

CC I82.722 **Chronic embolism and thrombosis of deep veins of left upper extremity**
CC Exclusion see Appendix A PDX collection 0717

CC I82.723 **Chronic embolism and thrombosis of deep veins of upper extremity, bilateral**
CC Exclusion see Appendix A PDX collection 0717

CC I82.729 **Chronic embolism and thrombosis of deep veins of unspecified upper extremity**
CC Exclusion see Appendix A PDX collection 0717

\+ I82.A **Embolism and thrombosis of axillary vein**

\+ I82.A1 **Acute embolism and thrombosis of axillary vein**

CC I82.A11 **Acute embolism and thrombosis of right axillary vein**
CC Exclusion see Appendix A PDX collection 0717

CC I82.A12 **Acute embolism and thrombosis of left axillary vein**
CC Exclusion see Appendix A PDX collection 0717

CC I82.A13 **Acute embolism and thrombosis of axillary vein, bilateral**
CC Exclusion see Appendix A PDX collection 0717

CC I82.A19 **Acute embolism and thrombosis of unspecified axillary vein**
CC Exclusion see Appendix A PDX collection 0717

\+ I82.A2 **Chronic embolism and thrombosis of axillary vein**

CC I82.A21 **Chronic embolism and thrombosis of right axillary vein**
CC Exclusion see Appendix A PDX collection 0717

CC I82.A22 **Chronic embolism and thrombosis of left axillary vein**
CC Exclusion see Appendix A PDX collection 0717

CC I82.A23 **Chronic embolism and thrombosis of axillary vein, bilateral**
CC Exclusion see Appendix A PDX collection 0717

CC I82.A29 **Chronic embolism and thrombosis of unspecified axillary vein**
CC Exclusion see Appendix A PDX collection 0717

\+ I82.B **Embolism and thrombosis of subclavian vein**

\+ I82.B1 **Acute embolism and thrombosis of subclavian≈vein**

CC I82.B11 **Acute embolism and thrombosis of right subclavian vein**
CC Exclusion see Appendix A PDX collection 0717

CC I82.B12 **Acute embolism and thrombosis of left subclavian vein**
CC Exclusion see Appendix A PDX collection 0717

CC I82.B13 **Acute embolism and thrombosis of subclavian vein, bilateral**
CC Exclusion see Appendix A PDX collection 0717

CC I82.B19 **Acute embolism and thrombosis of unspecified subclavian vein**
CC Exclusion see Appendix A PDX collection 0717

\+ I82.B2 **Chronic embolism and thrombosis of subclavian vein**

CC I82.B21 **Chronic embolism and thrombosis of right subclavian vein**
CC Exclusion see Appendix A PDX collection 0717

CC I82.B22 **Chronic embolism and thrombosis of left subclavian vein**
CC Exclusion see Appendix A PDX collection 0717

CC I82.B23 **Chronic embolism and thrombosis of subclavian vein, bilateral**
CC Exclusion see Appendix A PDX collection 0717

CC I82.B29 **Chronic embolism and thrombosis of unspecified subclavian vein**
CC Exclusion see Appendix A PDX collection 0717

\+ I82.C **Embolism and thrombosis of internal jugular vein**

\+ I82.C1 **Acute embolism and thrombosis of internal jugular vein**

CC I82.C11 **Acute embolism and thrombosis of right internal jugular vein**
CC Exclusion see Appendix A PDX collection 0717

CC I82.C12 **Acute embolism and thrombosis of left internal jugular vein**
CC Exclusion see Appendix A PDX collection 0717

CC I82.C13 **Acute embolism and thrombosis of internal jugular vein, bilateral**
CC Exclusion see Appendix A PDX collection 0717

CC I82.C19 **Acute embolism and thrombosis of unspecified internal jugular vein**
CC Exclusion see Appendix A PDX collection 0717

\+ I82.C2 **Chronic embolism and thrombosis of internal jugular vein**

CC I82.C21 **Chronic embolism and thrombosis of right internal jugular vein**
CC Exclusion see Appendix A PDX collection 0717

CC I82.C22 **Chronic embolism and thrombosis of left internal jugular vein**
CC Exclusion see Appendix A PDX collection 0717

CC I82.C23 **Chronic embolism and thrombosis of internal jugular vein, bilateral**
CC Exclusion see Appendix A PDX collection 0717

CC I82.C29 **Chronic embolism and thrombosis of unspecified internal jugular vein**
CC Exclusion see Appendix A PDX collection 0717

\+ I82.8 **Embolism and thrombosis of other specified veins**
Use additional code, if applicable, for associated long-term (current) use of anticoagulants (Z79.01)

\+ I82.81 **Embolism and thrombosis of superficial veins of lower extremities**
Embolism and thrombosis of saphenous vein (greater) (lesser)

CC I82.811 **Embolism and thrombosis of superficial veins of right lower extremity**
CC Exclusion see Appendix A PDX collection 0717

CC I82.812 **Embolism and thrombosis of superficial veins of left lower extremity**
CC Exclusion see Appendix A PDX collection 0717

CC I82.813 **Embolism and thrombosis of superficial veins of lower extremities, bilateral**
CC Exclusion see Appendix A PDX collection 0717

CC I82.819 **Embolism and thrombosis of superficial veins of unspecified lower extremity**
CC Exclusion see Appendix A PDX collection 0717

+ I82.89 Embolism and thrombosis of other specified veins

CC I82.890 **Acute embolism and thrombosis of other specified veins**
CC Exclusion see Appendix A PDX collection 0717

CC I82.891 **Chronic embolism and thrombosis of other specified veins**
CC Exclusion see Appendix A PDX collection 0717

+ I82.9 **Embolism and thrombosis of unspecified vein**

CC I82.90 **Acute embolism and thrombosis of unspecified vein**
Embolism of vein NOS
Thrombosis (vein) NOS
CC Exclusion see Appendix A PDX collection 0717

CC I82.91 **Chronic embolism and thrombosis of unspecified vein**
CC Exclusion see Appendix A PDX collection 0717

I83 Varicose veins of lower extremities

Excludes1: *varicose veins complicating pregnancy (O22.0-)*
varicose veins complicating the puerperium (O87.4)

+ I83.0 **Varicose veins of lower extremities with ulcer**
Use additional code to identify severity of ulcer (L97.-)

+ I83.00 **Varicose veins of unspecified lower extremity with ulcer**

• I83.001 **Varicose veins of unspecified lower extremity with ulcer of thigh**

• I83.002 **Varicose veins of unspecified lower extremity with ulcer of calf**

• I83.003 **Varicose veins of unspecified lower extremity with ulcer of ankle**

• I83.004 **Varicose veins of unspecified lower extremity with ulcer of heel and midfoot**
Varicose veins of unspecified lower extremity with ulcer of plantar surface of midfoot

• I83.005 **Varicose veins of unspecified lower extremity with ulcer other part of foot**
Varicose veins of unspecified lower extremity with ulcer of toe

• I83.008 **Varicose veins of unspecified lower extremity with ulcer other part of lower leg**

• I83.009 **Varicose veins of unspecified lower extremity with ulcer of unspecified site**

+ I83.01 **Varicose veins of right lower extremity with ulcer**

• I83.011 **Varicose veins of right lower extremity with ulcer of thigh**

• I83.012 **Varicose veins of right lower extremity with ulcer of calf**

• I83.013 **Varicose veins of right lower extremity with ulcer of ankle**

• I83.014 **Varicose veins of right lower extremity with ulcer of heel and midfoot**
Varicose veins of right lower extremity with ulcer of plantar surface of midfoot

• I83.015 **Varicose veins of right lower extremity with ulcer other part of foot**
Varicose veins of right lower extremity with ulcer of toe

• I83.018 **Varicose veins of right lower extremity with ulcer other part of lower leg**

• I83.019 **Varicose veins of right lower extremity with ulcer of unspecified site**

+ I83.02 **Varicose veins of left lower extremity with ulcer**

• I83.021 **Varicose veins of left lower extremity with ulcer of thigh**

• I83.022 **Varicose veins of left lower extremity with ulcer of calf**

• I83.023 **Varicose veins of left lower extremity with ulcer of ankle**

• I83.024 **Varicose veins of left lower extremity with ulcer of heel and midfoot**
Varicose veins of left lower extremity with ulcer of plantar surface of midfoot

• I83.025 **Varicose veins of left lower extremity with ulcer other part of foot**
Varicose veins of left lower extremity with ulcer of toe

• I83.028 **Varicose veins of left lower extremity with ulcer other part of lower leg**

• I83.029 **Varicose veins of left lower extremity with ulcer of unspecified site**

+ I83.1 **Varicose veins of lower extremities with inflammation**

• I83.10 **Varicose veins of unspecified lower extremity with inflammation**

• I83.11 **Varicose veins of right lower extremity with inflammation**

• I83.12 **Varicose veins of left lower extremity with inflammation**

+ I83.2 **Varicose veins of lower extremities with both ulcer and inflammation**
Use additional code to identify severity of ulcer (L97.-)

+ I83.20 **Varicose veins of unspecified lower extremity with both ulcer and inflammation**

• CC I83.201 **Varicose veins of unspecified lower extremity with both ulcer of thigh and inflammation**
CC Exclusion see Appendix A PDX collection 0720

• CC I83.202 **Varicose veins of unspecified lower extremity with both ulcer of calf and inflammation**
CC Exclusion see Appendix A PDX collection 0720

• CC I83.203 **Varicose veins of unspecified lower extremity with both ulcer of ankle and inflammation**
CC Exclusion see Appendix A PDX collection 0720

• CC I83.204 **Varicose veins of unspecified lower extremity with both ulcer of heel and midfoot and inflammation**
Varicose veins of unspecified lower extremity with both ulcer of plantar surface of midfoot and inflammation
CC Exclusion see Appendix A PDX collection 0720

• CC I83.205 **Varicose veins of unspecified lower extremity with both ulcer other part of foot and inflammation**
Varicose veins of unspecified lower extremity with both ulcer of toe and inflammation
CC Exclusion see Appendix A PDX collection 0720

• CC I83.208 **Varicose veins of unspecified lower extremity with both ulcer of other part of lower extremity and inflammation**
CC Exclusion see Appendix A PDX collection 0720

• CC I83.209 **Varicose veins of unspecified lower extremity with both ulcer of unspecified site and inflammation**
CC Exclusion see Appendix A PDX collection 0720

+ I83.21 **Varicose veins of right lower extremity with both ulcer and inflammation**

• CC I83.211 **Varicose veins of right lower extremity with both ulcer of thigh and inflammation**
CC Exclusion see Appendix A PDX collection 0720

• CC I83.212 **Varicose veins of right lower extremity with both ulcer of calf and inflammation**
CC Exclusion see Appendix A PDX collection 0720

• CC I83.213 **Varicose veins of right lower extremity with both ulcer of ankle and inflammation**
CC Exclusion see Appendix A PDX collection 0720

• CC I83.214 **Varicose veins of right lower extremity with both ulcer of heel and midfoot and inflammation**
Varicose veins of right lower extremity with both ulcer of plantar surface of midfoot and inflammation
CC Exclusion see Appendix A PDX collection 0720

• CC I83.215 **Varicose veins of right lower extremity with both ulcer other part of foot and inflammation**
Varicose veins of right lower extremity with both ulcer of toe and inflammation
CC Exclusion see Appendix A PDX collection 0720

● CC **I83.218** **Varicose veins of right lower extremity with both ulcer of other part of lower extremity and inflammation**
CC Exclusion see Appendix A PDX collection 0720

● CC **I83.219** **Varicose veins of right lower extremity with both ulcer of unspecified site and inflammation**
CC Exclusion see Appendix A PDX collection 0720

+ **I83.22** **Varicose veins of left lower extremity with both ulcer and inflammation**

● CC **I83.221** **Varicose veins of left lower extremity with both ulcer of thigh and inflammation**
CC Exclusion see Appendix A PDX collection 0720

● CC **I83.222** **Varicose veins of left lower extremity with both ulcer of calf and inflammation**
CC Exclusion see Appendix A PDX collection 0720

● CC **I83.223** **Varicose veins of left lower extremity with both ulcer of ankle and inflammation**
CC Exclusion see Appendix A PDX collection 0720

● CC **I83.224** **Varicose veins of left lower extremity with both ulcer of heel and midfoot and inflammation**
Varicose veins of left lower extremity with both ulcer of plantar surface of midfoot and inflammation
CC Exclusion see Appendix A PDX collection 0720

● CC **I83.225** **Varicose veins of left lower extremity with both ulcer other part of foot and inflammation**
Varicose veins of left lower extremity with both ulcer of toe and inflammation
CC Exclusion see Appendix A PDX collection 0720

● CC **I83.228** **Varicose veins of left lower extremity with both ulcer of other part of lower extremity and inflammation**
CC Exclusion see Appendix A PDX collection 0720

● CC **I83.229** **Varicose veins of left lower extremity with both ulcer of unspecified site and inflammation**
CC Exclusion see Appendix A PDX collection 0720

+ **I83.8** **Varicose veins of lower extremities with other complications**

+ **I83.81** **Varicose veins of lower extremities with pain**

● **I83.811** **Varicose veins of right lower extremity with pain**

● **I83.812** **Varicose veins of left lower extremity with pain**

● **I83.813** **Varicose veins of bilateral lower extremities with pain**

● **I83.819** **Varicose veins of unspecified lower extremity with pain**

+ **I83.89** **Varicose veins of lower extremities with other complications**
Varicose veins of lower extremities with edema
Varicose veins of lower extremities with swelling

● **I83.891** **Varicose veins of right lower extremity with other complications**

● **I83.892** **Varicose veins of left lower extremity with other complications**

● **I83.893** **Varicose veins of bilateral lower extremities with other complications**

● **I83.899** **Varicose veins of unspecified lower extremity with other complications**

+ **I83.9** **Asymptomatic varicose veins of lower extremities**
Phlebectasia of lower extremities
Varicose veins of lower extremities
Varix of lower extremities

● **I83.90** **Asymptomatic varicose veins of unspecified lower extremity**
Varicose veins NOS

● **I83.91** **Asymptomatic varicose veins of right lower extremity**

● **I83.92** **Asymptomatic varicose veins of left lower extremity**

● **I83.93** **Asymptomatic varicose veins of bilateral lower extremities**

I85 Esophageal varices

Use additional code to identify:
alcohol abuse and dependence (F10.-)

+ **I85.0** **Esophageal varices**
Idiopathic esophageal varices
Primary esophageal varices

CC **I85.00** **Esophageal varices without bleeding**
Esophageal varices NOS
CC Exclusion see Appendix A PDX collection 0721

MCC **I85.01** **Esophageal varices with bleeding**
MCC Exclusion see Appendix A PDX collection 0722

+ **I85.1** **Secondary esophageal varices**
Esophageal varices secondary to alcoholic liver disease
Esophageal varices secondary to cirrhosis of liver
Esophageal varices secondary to schistosomiasis
Esophageal varices secondary to toxic liver disease
Code first underlying disease

CC **I85.10** **Secondary esophageal varices without bleeding**
CC Exclusion see Appendix A PDX collection 0723

MCC **I85.11** **Secondary esophageal varices with bleeding**
MCC Exclusion see Appendix A PDX collection 0724

I86 Varicose veins of other sites

Excludes1: *varicose veins of unspecified site (I83.9-)*
Excludes2: *retinal varices (H35.0-)*

I86.0 **Sublingual varices**

♂ **I86.1** **Scrotal varices**
Varicocele

I86.2 **Pelvic varices**

♀ **I86.3** **Vulval varices**
Excludes1: *vulval varices complicating childbirth and the puerperium (O87.8)*
vulval varices complicating pregnancy (O22.1-)

I86.4 **Gastric varices**

● **I86.8** **Varicose veins of other specified sites**
Varicose ulcer of nasal septum

I87 Other disorders of veins

+ **I87.0** **Postthrombotic syndrome**
Chronic venous hypertension due to deep vein thrombosis
Postphlebitic syndrome
Excludes1: *chronic venous hypertension without deep vein thrombosis (I87.3-)*

+ **I87.00** **Postthrombotic syndrome without complications**
Asymptomatic Postthrombotic syndrome

I87.001 **Postthrombotic syndrome without complications of right lower extremity**

I87.002 **Postthrombotic syndrome without complications of left lower extremity**

I87.003 **Postthrombotic syndrome without complications of bilateral lower extremity**

I87.009 **Postthrombotic syndrome without complications of unspecified extremity**
Postthrombotic syndrome NOS

+ **I87.01** **Postthrombotic syndrome with ulcer**
Use additional code to specify site and severity of ulcer (L97.-)

CC **I87.011** **Postthrombotic syndrome with ulcer of right lower extremity**
CC Exclusion see Appendix A PDX collection 0725

CC **I87.012** **Postthrombotic syndrome with ulcer of left lower extremity**
CC Exclusion see Appendix A PDX collection 0725

CC **I87.013** **Postthrombotic syndrome with ulcer of bilateral lower extremity**
CC Exclusion see Appendix A PDX collection 0725

CC **I87.019** **Postthrombotic syndrome with ulcer of unspecified lower extremity**
CC Exclusion see Appendix A PDX collection 0725

+ **I87.02** **Postthrombotic syndrome with inflammation**

I87.021 **Postthrombotic syndrome with inflammation of right lower extremity**

I87.022 **Postthrombotic syndrome with inflammation of left lower extremity**

I87.023 **Postthrombotic syndrome with inflammation of bilateral lower extremity**

I87.029 **Postthrombotic syndrome with inflammation of unspecified lower extremity**

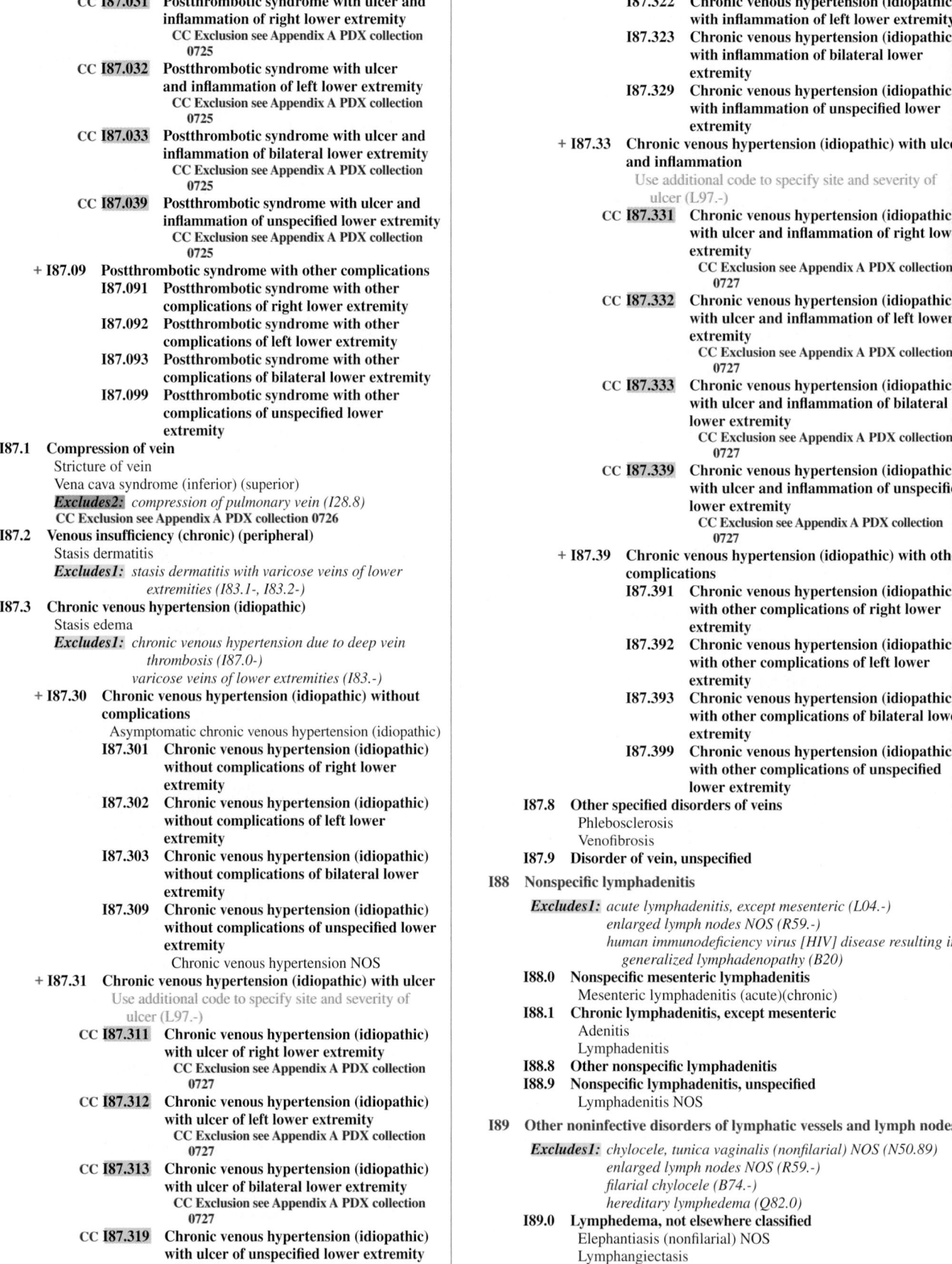

+ I87.03 **Postthrombotic syndrome with ulcer and inflammation**
Use additional code to specify site and severity of ulcer (L97.-)
CC I87.031 **Postthrombotic syndrome with ulcer and inflammation of right lower extremity**
CC Exclusion see Appendix A PDX collection 0725
CC I87.032 **Postthrombotic syndrome with ulcer and inflammation of left lower extremity**
CC Exclusion see Appendix A PDX collection 0725
CC I87.033 **Postthrombotic syndrome with ulcer and inflammation of bilateral lower extremity**
CC Exclusion see Appendix A PDX collection 0725
CC I87.039 **Postthrombotic syndrome with ulcer and inflammation of unspecified lower extremity**
CC Exclusion see Appendix A PDX collection 0725
+ I87.09 **Postthrombotic syndrome with other complications**
I87.091 **Postthrombotic syndrome with other complications of right lower extremity**
I87.092 **Postthrombotic syndrome with other complications of left lower extremity**
I87.093 **Postthrombotic syndrome with other complications of bilateral lower extremity**
I87.099 **Postthrombotic syndrome with other complications of unspecified lower extremity**
CC I87.1 **Compression of vein**
Stricture of vein
Vena cava syndrome (inferior) (superior)
Excludes2: *compression of pulmonary vein (I28.8)*
CC Exclusion see Appendix A PDX collection 0726
I87.2 **Venous insufficiency (chronic) (peripheral)**
Stasis dermatitis
Excludes1: *stasis dermatitis with varicose veins of lower extremities (I83.1-, I83.2-)*
+ I87.3 **Chronic venous hypertension (idiopathic)**
Stasis edema
Excludes1: *chronic venous hypertension due to deep vein thrombosis (I87.0-)*
varicose veins of lower extremities (I83.-)
+ I87.30 **Chronic venous hypertension (idiopathic) without complications**
Asymptomatic chronic venous hypertension (idiopathic)
I87.301 **Chronic venous hypertension (idiopathic) without complications of right lower extremity**
I87.302 **Chronic venous hypertension (idiopathic) without complications of left lower extremity**
I87.303 **Chronic venous hypertension (idiopathic) without complications of bilateral lower extremity**
I87.309 **Chronic venous hypertension (idiopathic) without complications of unspecified lower extremity**
Chronic venous hypertension NOS
+ I87.31 **Chronic venous hypertension (idiopathic) with ulcer**
Use additional code to specify site and severity of ulcer (L97.-)
CC I87.311 **Chronic venous hypertension (idiopathic) with ulcer of right lower extremity**
CC Exclusion see Appendix A PDX collection 0727
CC I87.312 **Chronic venous hypertension (idiopathic) with ulcer of left lower extremity**
CC Exclusion see Appendix A PDX collection 0727
CC I87.313 **Chronic venous hypertension (idiopathic) with ulcer of bilateral lower extremity**
CC Exclusion see Appendix A PDX collection 0727
CC I87.319 **Chronic venous hypertension (idiopathic) with ulcer of unspecified lower extremity**
CC Exclusion see Appendix A PDX collection 0727
+ I87.32 **Chronic venous hypertension (idiopathic) with inflammation**
I87.321 **Chronic venous hypertension (idiopathic) with inflammation of right lower extremity**
I87.322 **Chronic venous hypertension (idiopathic) with inflammation of left lower extremity**
I87.323 **Chronic venous hypertension (idiopathic) with inflammation of bilateral lower extremity**
I87.329 **Chronic venous hypertension (idiopathic) with inflammation of unspecified lower extremity**
+ I87.33 **Chronic venous hypertension (idiopathic) with ulcer and inflammation**
Use additional code to specify site and severity of ulcer (L97.-)
CC I87.331 **Chronic venous hypertension (idiopathic) with ulcer and inflammation of right lower extremity**
CC Exclusion see Appendix A PDX collection 0727
CC I87.332 **Chronic venous hypertension (idiopathic) with ulcer and inflammation of left lower extremity**
CC Exclusion see Appendix A PDX collection 0727
CC I87.333 **Chronic venous hypertension (idiopathic) with ulcer and inflammation of bilateral lower extremity**
CC Exclusion see Appendix A PDX collection 0727
CC I87.339 **Chronic venous hypertension (idiopathic) with ulcer and inflammation of unspecified lower extremity**
CC Exclusion see Appendix A PDX collection 0727
+ I87.39 **Chronic venous hypertension (idiopathic) with other complications**
I87.391 **Chronic venous hypertension (idiopathic) with other complications of right lower extremity**
I87.392 **Chronic venous hypertension (idiopathic) with other complications of left lower extremity**
I87.393 **Chronic venous hypertension (idiopathic) with other complications of bilateral lower extremity**
I87.399 **Chronic venous hypertension (idiopathic) with other complications of unspecified lower extremity**
I87.8 **Other specified disorders of veins**
Phlebosclerosis
Venofibrosis
I87.9 **Disorder of vein, unspecified**

I88 Nonspecific lymphadenitis

Excludes1: *acute lymphadenitis, except mesenteric (L04.-)*
enlarged lymph nodes NOS (R59.-)
human immunodeficiency virus [HIV] disease resulting in generalized lymphadenopathy (B20)
I88.0 **Nonspecific mesenteric lymphadenitis**
Mesenteric lymphadenitis (acute)(chronic)
I88.1 **Chronic lymphadenitis, except mesenteric**
Adenitis
Lymphadenitis
I88.8 **Other nonspecific lymphadenitis**
I88.9 **Nonspecific lymphadenitis, unspecified**
Lymphadenitis NOS

I89 Other noninfective disorders of lymphatic vessels and lymph nodes

Excludes1: *chylocele, tunica vaginalis (nonfilarial) NOS (N50.89)*
enlarged lymph nodes NOS (R59.-)
filarial chylocele (B74.-)
hereditary lymphedema (Q82.0)
I89.0 **Lymphedema, not elsewhere classified**
Elephantiasis (nonfilarial) NOS
Lymphangiectasis
Obliteration, lymphatic vessel
Praecox lymphedema
Secondary lymphedema
Excludes1: *postmastectomy lymphedema (I97.2)*

I89.1 **Lymphangitis**
Chronic lymphangitis
Lymphangitis NOS
Subacute lymphangitis
Excludes1: *acute lymphangitis (L03.-)*

I89.8 **Other specified noninfective disorders of lymphatic vessels and lymph nodes**
Chylocele (nonfilarial)
Chylous ascites
Chylous cyst
Lipomelanotic reticulosis
Lymph node or vessel fistula
Lymph node or vessel infarction
Lymph node or vessel rupture

I89.9 **Noninfective disorder of lymphatic vessels and lymph nodes, unspecified**
Disease of lymphatic vessels NOS

ther and unspecified disorders of the circulatory system 95-I99)

I95 Hypotension
Excludes1: *cardiovascular collapse (R57.9)*
maternal hypotension syndrome (O26.5-)
nonspecific low blood pressure reading NOS (R03.1)

I95.0 **Idiopathic hypotension**
I95.1 **Orthostatic hypotension**
Hypotension, postural
Excludes1: *neurogenic orthostatic hypotension [Shy-Drager] (G90.3)*
orthostatic hypotension due to drugs (I95.2)
I95.2 **Hypotension due to drugs**
Orthostatic hypotension due to drugs
Use additional code for adverse effect, if applicable, to identify drug (T36-T50 with fifth or sixth character 5)
I95.3 **Hypotension of hemodialysis**
Intra-dialytic hypotension
I95.8 **Other hypotension**
I95.81 **Postprocedural hypotension**
I95.89 **Other hypotension**
Chronic hypotension
I95.9 **Hypotension, unspecified**

I96 Gangrene, not elsewhere classified
Gangrenous cellulitis
Excludes1: *gangrene in atherosclerosis of native arteries of the extremities (I70.26)*
gangrene in hernia (K40.1, K40.4, K41.1, K41.4, K42.1, K43.1-, K44.1, K45.1, K46.1)
gangrene in other peripheral vascular diseases (I73.-)
gangrene of certain specified sites - see Alphabetical Index
gas gangrene (A48.0)
pyoderma gangrenosum (L88)
Excludes2: *gangrene in diabetes mellitus (E08-E13 with .52)*
CC Exclusion see Appendix A PDX collection 0519
AHA CC: Q2, 2013, 34-35
Valid 3-character code, no further characters required

I97 Intraoperative and postprocedural complications and disorders of circulatory system, not elsewhere classified
Excludes2: *postprocedural shock (T81.1-)*

I97.0 **Postcardiotomy syndrome**
+ I97.1 **Other postprocedural cardiac functional disturbances**
Excludes2: *acute pulmonary insufficiency following thoracic surgery (J95.1)*
intraoperative cardiac functional disturbances (I97.7-)
+ I97.11 **Postprocedural cardiac insufficiency**
CC I97.110 **Postprocedural cardiac insufficiency following cardiac surgery**
CC Exclusion see Appendix A PDX collection 0728
CC I97.111 **Postprocedural cardiac insufficiency following other surgery**
CC Exclusion see Appendix A PDX collection 0728
+ I97.12 **Postprocedural cardiac arrest**
CC I97.120 **Postprocedural cardiac arrest following cardiac surgery**
CC Exclusion see Appendix A PDX collection 0728
CC I97.121 **Postprocedural cardiac arrest following other surgery**
CC Exclusion see Appendix A PDX collection 0728
+ I97.13 **Postprocedural heart failure**
Use additional code to identify the heart failure (I50.-)
CC I97.130 **Postprocedural heart failure following cardiac surgery**
CC Exclusion see Appendix A PDX collection 0728
CC I97.131 **Postprocedural heart failure following other surgery**
CC Exclusion see Appendix A PDX collection 0728
+ I97.19 **Other postprocedural cardiac functional disturbances**
Use additional code, if applicable, to further specify disorder
CC I97.190 **Other postprocedural cardiac functional disturbances following cardiac surgery**
Use additional code, if applicable, for type 4 or type 5 myocardial infarction, to further specify disorder
CC Exclusion see Appendix A PDX collection 0728
CC I97.191 **Other postprocedural cardiac functional disturbances following other surgery**
CC Exclusion see Appendix A PDX collection 0728

• I97.2 **Postmastectomy lymphedema syndrome**
Elephantiasis due to mastectomy
Obliteration of lymphatic vessels
I97.3 **Postprocedural hypertension**
+ I97.4 **Intraoperative hemorrhage and hematoma of a circulatory system organ or structure complicating a procedure**
Excludes1: *intraoperative hemorrhage and hematoma of a circulatory system organ or structure due to accidental puncture and laceration during a procedure (I97.5-)*
Excludes2: *intraoperative cerebrovascular hemorrhage complicating a procedure (G97.3-)*
+ I97.41 **Intraoperative hemorrhage and hematoma of a circulatory system organ or structure complicating a circulatory system procedure**
CC I97.410 **Intraoperative hemorrhage and hematoma of a circulatory system organ or structure complicating a cardiac catheterization**
CC Exclusion see Appendix A PDX collection 0729
CC I97.411 **Intraoperative hemorrhage and hematoma of a circulatory system organ or structure complicating a cardiac bypass**
CC Exclusion see Appendix A PDX collection 0729
CC I97.418 **Intraoperative hemorrhage and hematoma of a circulatory system organ or structure complicating other circulatory system procedure**
CC Exclusion see Appendix A PDX collection 0729
CC I97.42 **Intraoperative hemorrhage and hematoma of a circulatory system organ or structure complicating other procedure**
CC Exclusion see Appendix A PDX collection 0729
AHA CC: 4Q, 2016, 100-101
+ I97.5 **Accidental puncture and laceration of a circulatory system organ or structure during a procedure**
Excludes2: *accidental puncture and laceration of brain during a procedure (G97.4-)*
CC I97.51 **Accidental puncture and laceration of a circulatory system organ or structure during a circulatory system procedure**
CC Exclusion see Appendix A PDX collection 0509
CC I97.52 **Accidental puncture and laceration of a circulatory system organ or structure during other procedure**
CC Exclusion see Appendix A PDX collection 0509

+ **I97.6 Postprocedural hemorrhage, hematoma and seroma of a circulatory system organ or structure following a procedure**
 Excludes2: *postprocedural cerebrovascular hemorrhage complicating a procedure (G97.5-)*
 AHA CC: 4Q, 2016, 9-10

+ **I97.61 Postprocedural hemorrhage of a circulatory system organ or structure following a circulatory system procedure**
 CC **I97.610 Postprocedural hemorrhage of a circulatory system organ or structure following a cardiac catheterization**
 CC Exclusion see Appendix A PDX collection 0729
 CC **I97.611 Postprocedural hemorrhage of a circulatory system organ or structure following cardiac bypass**
 CC Exclusion see Appendix A PDX collection 0729
 CC **I97.618 Postprocedural hemorrhage of a circulatory system organ or structure following other circulatory system procedure**
 CC Exclusion see Appendix A PDX collection 0729

+ **I97.62 Postprocedural hemorrhage, hematoma and seroma of a circulatory system organ or structure following other procedure**
 CC **I97.620 Postprocedural hemorrhage of a circulatory system organ or structure following other procedure**
 CC Exclusion see Appendix A PDX collection 0729
 CC **I97.621 Postprocedural hematoma of a circulatory system organ or structure following other procedure**
 CC Exclusion see Appendix A PDX collection 0729
 CC **I97.622 Postprocedural seroma of a circulatory system organ or structure following other procedure**
 CC Exclusion see Appendix A PDX collection 0729

+ **I97.63 Postprocedural hematoma of a circulatory system organ or structure following a circulatory system procedure**
 CC **I97.630 Postprocedural hematoma of a circulatory system organ or structure following a cardiac catheterization**
 CC Exclusion see Appendix A PDX collection 0729
 CC **I97.631 Postprocedural hematoma of a circulatory system organ or structure following cardiac bypass**
 CC Exclusion see Appendix A PDX collection 0729
 CC **I97.638 Postprocedural hematoma of a circulatory system organ or structure following other circulatory system procedure**
 CC Exclusion see Appendix A PDX collection 0729

I97.64 Postprocedural seroma of a circulatory system organ or structure following a circulatory system procedure
 CC **I97.640 Postprocedural seroma of a circulatory system organ or structure following a cardiac catheterization**
 CC Exclusion see Appendix A PDX collection 0729
 CC **I97.641 Postprocedural seroma of a circulatory system organ or structure following cardiac bypass**
 CC Exclusion see Appendix A PDX collection 0729
 CC **I97.648 Postprocedural seroma of a circulatory system organ or structure following other circulatory system procedure**
 CC Exclusion see Appendix A PDX collection 0729

+ **I97.7 Intraoperative cardiac functional disturbances**
 Excludes2: *acute pulmonary insufficiency following thoracic surgery (J95.1)*
 postprocedural cardiac functional disturbances (I97.1-)

+ **I97.71 Intraoperative cardiac arrest**
 CC **I97.710 Intraoperative cardiac arrest during cardiac surgery**
 CC Exclusion see Appendix A PDX collection 0728
 CC **I97.711 Intraoperative cardiac arrest during other surgery**
 CC Exclusion see Appendix A PDX collection 0728

+ **I97.79 Other intraoperative cardiac functional disturbances**
 Use additional code, if applicable, to further specify disorder
 CC **I97.790 Other intraoperative cardiac functional disturbances during cardiac surgery**
 CC Exclusion see Appendix A PDX collection 0728
 CC **I97.791 Other intraoperative cardiac functional disturbances during other surgery**
 CC Exclusion see Appendix A PDX collection 0728

+ **I97.8 Other intraoperative and postprocedural complications and disorders of the circulatory system, not elsewhere classified**
 Use additional code, if applicable, to further specify disorder

+ **I97.81 Intraoperative cerebrovascular infarction**
 CC **I97.810 Intraoperative cerebrovascular infarction during cardiac surgery**
 CC Exclusion see Appendix A PDX collection 0617
 CC **I97.811 Intraoperative cerebrovascular infarction during other surgery**
 CC Exclusion see Appendix A PDX collection 0617

+ **I97.82 Postprocedural cerebrovascular infarction**
 CC **I97.820 Postprocedural cerebrovascular infarction following cardiac surgery**
 CC Exclusion see Appendix A PDX collection 0617
 CC **I97.821 Postprocedural cerebrovascular infarction following other surgery**
 CC Exclusion see Appendix A PDX collection 0617

CC **I97.88 Other intraoperative complications of the circulatory system, not elsewhere classified**
 CC Exclusion see Appendix A PDX collection 0728

CC **I97.89 Other postprocedural complications and disorders of the circulatory system, not elsewhere classified**
 CC Exclusion see Appendix A PDX collection 0728

I99 Other and unspecified disorders of circulatory system

I99.8 Other disorder of circulatory system

I99.9 Unspecified disorder of circulatory system

hapter 10: Diseases of the Respiratory System 00-J99)

OTE When a respiratory condition is described as occurring in more than one site and is not specifically indexed, it should be classified to the lower anatomic site (e.g. tracheobronchitis to bronchitis in J40).

e additional code, where applicable, to identify:
exposure to environmental tobacco smoke (Z77.22)
exposure to tobacco smoke in the perinatal period (P96.81)
history of tobacco dependence (Z87.891)
occupational exposure to environmental tobacco smoke (Z57.31)
tobacco dependence (F17.-)
tobacco use (Z72.0)

cludes2: *certain conditions originating in the perinatal period (P04-P96)*
certain infectious and parasitic diseases (A00-B99)
complications of pregnancy, childbirth and the puerperium (O00-O9A)
congenital malformations, deformations and chromosomal abnormalities (Q00-Q99)
endocrine, nutritional and metabolic diseases (E00-E88)
injury, poisoning and certain other consequences of external causes (S00-T88)
neoplasms (C00-D49)
smoke inhalation (T59.81-)
symptoms, signs and abnormal clinical and laboratory findings, not elsewhere classified (R00-R94)

is chapter contains the following category blocks:

J00-J06	Acute upper respiratory infections
J09-J18	Influenza and pneumonia
J20-J22	Other acute lower respiratory infections
J30-J39	Other diseases of upper respiratory tract
J40-J47	Chronic lower respiratory diseases
J60-J70	Lung diseases due to external agents
J80-J84	Other respiratory diseases principally affecting the interstitium
J85-J86	Suppurative and necrotic conditions of the lower respiratory tract
J90-J94	Other diseases of the pleura
J95	Intraoperative and postprocedural complications and disorders of respiratory system, not elsewhere classified
J96-J99	Other diseases of the respiratory system

Chapter-Specific Coding Guidelines

addition to general coding guidelines, there are guidelines for specific diagnoses d/or conditions in the classification. Unless otherwise indicated, these guidelines ply to all health care settings. Please refer to Section II for guidelines on the ection of principal diagnosis.

. Chapter 10: Diseases of the Respiratory System (J00-J99)

a. Chronic Obstructive Pulmonary Disease [COPD] and Asthma

1) Acute exacerbation of chronic obstructive bronchitis and asthma

The codes in categories J44 and J45 distinguish between uncomplicated cases and those in acute exacerbation. An acute exacerbation is a worsening or a decompensation of a chronic condition. An acute exacerbation is not equivalent to an infection superimposed on a chronic condition, though an exacerbation may be triggered by an infection.

b. Acute Respiratory Failure

1) Acute respiratory failure as principal diagnosis

A code from subcategory J96.0, Acute respiratory failure, or subcategory J96.2, Acute and chronic respiratory failure, may be assigned as a principal diagnosis when it is the condition established after study to be chiefly responsible for occasioning the admission to the hospital, and the selection is supported by the Alphabetic Index and Tabular List. However, chapter-specific coding guidelines (such as obstetrics, poisoning, HIV, newborn) that provide sequencing direction take precedence.

2) Acute respiratory failure as secondary diagnosis

Respiratory failure may be listed as a secondary diagnosis if it occurs after admission, or if it is present on admission, but does not meet the definition of principal diagnosis.

3) Sequencing of acute respiratory failure and another acute condition

When a patient is admitted with respiratory failure and another acute condition, (e.g., myocardial infarction, cerebrovascular accident, aspiration pneumonia), the principal diagnosis will not be the same in every situation. This applies whether the other acute condition is a respiratory or nonrespiratory condition. Selection of the principal diagnosis will be dependent on the circumstances of admission. If both the respiratory failure and the other acute condition are equally responsible for occasioning the admission to the hospital, and there are no chapter-specific sequencing rules, the guideline regarding two or more diagnoses that equally meet the definition for principal diagnosis *(Section II, C.)* may be applied in these situations.

If the documentation is not clear as to whether acute respiratory failure and another condition are equally responsible for occasioning the admission, query the provider for clarification.

c. Influenza due to certain identified influenza viruses

Code only confirmed cases of influenza due to certain identified influenza viruses (category J09), and due to other identified influenza virus (category J10). This is an exception to the hospital inpatient guideline Section II, H. (Uncertain Diagnosis).

In this context, "confirmation" does not require documentation of positive laboratory testing specific for avian or other novel influenza A or other identified influenza virus. However, coding should be based on the provider's diagnostic statement that the patient has avian influenza, or other novel influenza A, for category J09, or has another particular identified strain of influenza, such as H1N1 or H3N2, but not identified as novel or variant, for category J10.

If the provider records "suspected" or "possible" or "probable" avian influenza, or novel influenza, or other identified influenza, then the appropriate influenza code from category J11, Influenza due to unidentified influenza virus, should be assigned. A code from category J09, Influenza due to certain identified influenza viruses, should not be assigned nor should a code from category J10, Influenza due to other identified influenza virus.

d. Ventilator associated Pneumonia

1) Documentation of Ventilator associated Pneumonia

As with all procedural or postprocedural complications, code assignment is based on the provider's documentation of the relationship between the condition and the procedure.

Code J95.851, Ventilator associated pneumonia, should be assigned only when the provider has documented ventilator associated pneumonia (VAP). An additional code to identify the organism (e.g., Pseudomonas aeruginosa, code B96.5) should also be assigned. Do not assign an additional code from categories J12-J18 to identify the type of pneumonia.

Code J95.851 should not be assigned for cases where the patient has pneumonia and is on a mechanical ventilator and the provider has not specifically stated that the pneumonia is ventilator-associated pneumonia. If the documentation is unclear as to whether the patient has a pneumonia that is a complication attributable to the mechanical ventilator, query the provider.

2) Ventilator associated Pneumonia Develops after Admission

A patient may be admitted with one type of pneumonia (e.g., code J13, Pneumonia due to Streptococcus pneumonia) and subsequently develop VAP. In this instance, the principal diagnosis would be the appropriate code from categories J12- J18 for the pneumonia diagnosed at the time of admission. Code J95.851, Ventilator associated pneumonia, would be assigned as an additional diagnosis when the provider has also documented the presence of ventilator associated pneumonia.

Acute upper respiratory infections (J00-J06)

Excludes1: *chronic obstructive pulmonary disease with acute lower respiratory infection (J44.0)*
influenza virus with other respiratory manifestations (J09.X2, J10.1, J11.1)

J00 Acute nasopharyngitis [common cold]

Acute rhinitis
Coryza (acute)
Infective nasopharyngitis NOS
Infective rhinitis
Nasal catarrh, acute
Nasopharyngitis NOS

Excludes1: *acute pharyngitis (J02.-)*
acute sore throat NOS (J02.9)
pharyngitis NOS (J02.9)
rhinitis NOS (J31.0)
sore throat NOS (J02.9)

Excludes2: *allergic rhinitis (J30.1-J30.9)*
chronic pharyngitis (J31.2)
chronic rhinitis (J31.0)
chronic sore throat (J31.2)
nasopharyngitis, chronic (J31.1)
vasomotor rhinitis (J30.0)

Valid 3-character code, no further characters required

Nose and Sinus

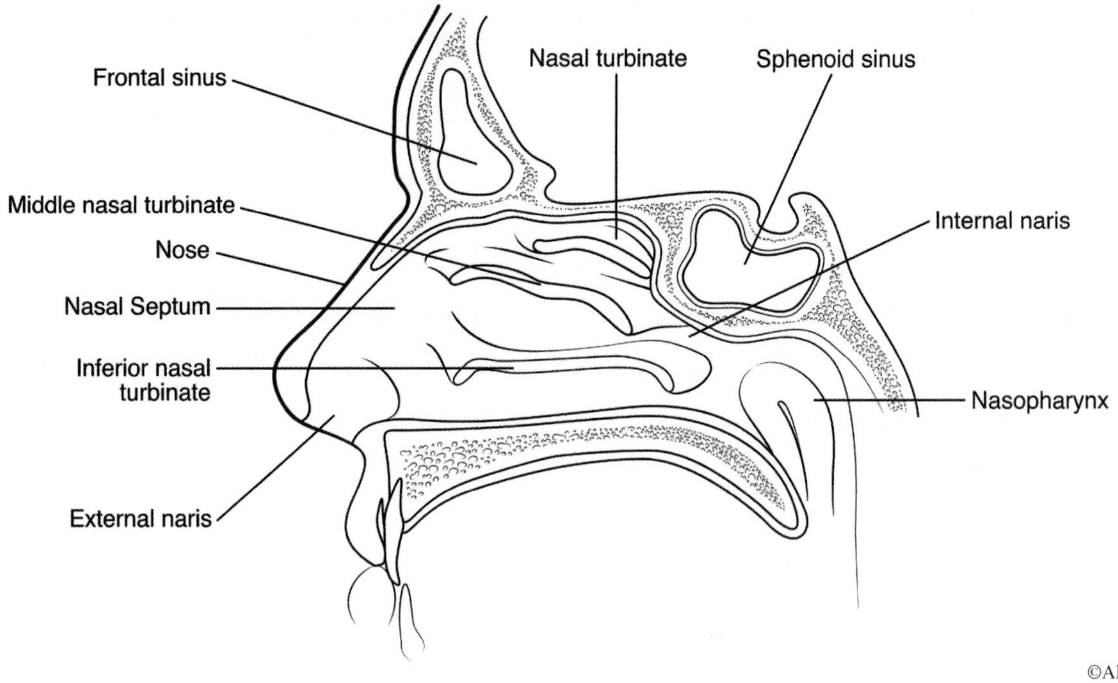

©AHIMA

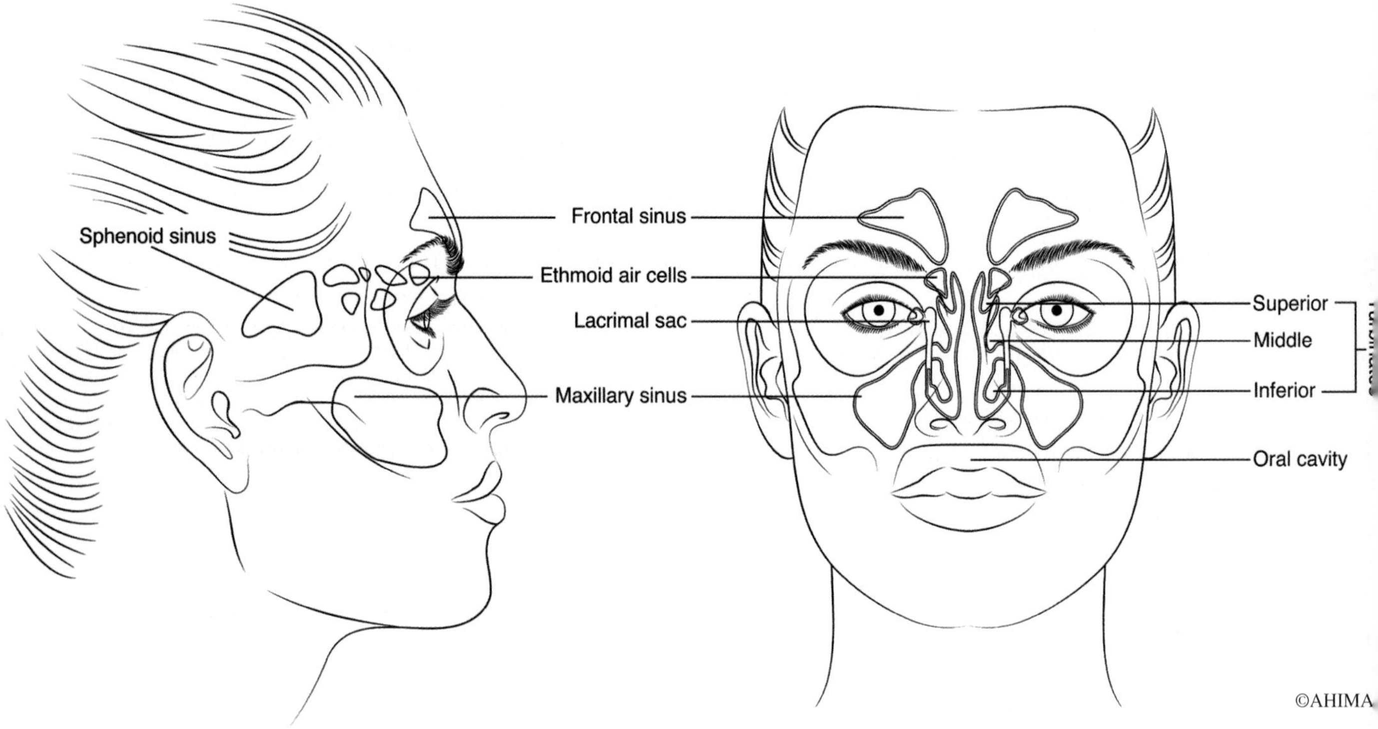

©AHIMA

J01 Acute sinusitis

Includes: acute abscess of sinus
acute empyema of sinus
acute infection of sinus
acute inflammation of sinus
acute suppuration of sinus

Use additional code (B95-B97) to identify infectious agent

Excludes1: *sinusitis NOS (J32.9)*

Excludes2: *chronic sinusitis (J32.0-J32.8)*

\+ **J01.0 Acute maxillary sinusitis**
Acute antritis
J01.00 Acute maxillary sinusitis, unspecified
J01.01 Acute recurrent maxillary sinusitis

\+ **J01.1 Acute frontal sinusitis**
J01.10 Acute frontal sinusitis, unspecified
J01.11 Acute recurrent frontal sinusitis

\+ **J01.2 Acute ethmoidal sinusitis**
J01.20 Acute ethmoidal sinusitis, unspecified
J01.21 Acute recurrent ethmoidal sinusitis

\+ **J01.3 Acute sphenoidal sinusitis**
J01.30 Acute sphenoidal sinusitis, unspecified
J01.31 Acute recurrent sphenoidal sinusitis

\+ **J01.4 Acute pansinusitis**
J01.40 Acute pansinusitis, unspecified
J01.41 Acute recurrent pansinusitis

\+ **J01.8 Other acute sinusitis**
J01.80 Other acute sinusitis
Acute sinusitis involving more than one sinus but not pansinusitis
J01.81 Other acute recurrent sinusitis
Acute recurrent sinusitis involving more than one sinus but not pansinusitis

+ **J01.9 Acute sinusitis, unspecified**
J01.90 Acute sinusitis, unspecified
J01.91 Acute recurrent sinusitis, unspecified

J02 Acute pharyngitis
Includes: acute sore throat
Excludes1: *acute laryngopharyngitis (J06.0)*
peritonsillar abscess (J36)
pharyngeal abscess (J39.1)
retropharyngeal abscess (J39.0)
Excludes2: *chronic pharyngitis (J31.2)*

J02.0 Streptococcal pharyngitis
Septic pharyngitis
Streptococcal sore throat
Excludes2: *scarlet fever (A38.-)*

J02.8 Acute pharyngitis due to other specified organisms
Use additional code (B95-B97) to identify infectious agent
Excludes1: *acute pharyngitis due to coxsackie virus (B08.5)*
acute pharyngitis due to gonococcus (A54.5)
acute pharyngitis due to herpes [simplex] virus (B00.2)
acute pharyngitis due to infectious mononucleosis (B27.-)
enteroviral vesicular pharyngitis (B08.5)

J02.9 Acute pharyngitis, unspecified
Gangrenous pharyngitis (acute)
Infective pharyngitis (acute) NOS
Pharyngitis (acute) NOS
Sore throat (acute) NOS
Suppurative pharyngitis (acute)
Ulcerative pharyngitis (acute)

J03 Acute tonsillitis
Excludes1: *acute sore throat (J02.-)*
hypertrophy of tonsils (J35.1)
peritonsillar abscess (J36)
sore throat NOS (J02.9)
streptococcal sore throat (J02.0)
Excludes2: *chronic tonsillitis (J35.0)*

+ **J03.0 Streptococcal tonsillitis**
J03.00 Acute streptococcal tonsillitis, unspecified
J03.01 Acute recurrent streptococcal tonsillitis

+ **J03.8 Acute tonsillitis due to other specified organisms**
Use additional code (B95-B97) to identify infectious agent
Excludes1: *diphtheritic tonsillitis (A36.0)*
herpesviral pharyngotonsillitis (B00.2)
streptococcal tonsillitis (J03.0)
tuberculous tonsillitis (A15.8)
Vincent's tonsillitis (A69.1)
J03.80 Acute tonsillitis due to other specified organisms
J03.81 Acute recurrent tonsillitis due to other specified organisms

+ **J03.9 Acute tonsillitis, unspecified**
Follicular tonsillitis (acute)
Gangrenous tonsillitis (acute)
Infective tonsillitis (acute)
Tonsillitis (acute) NOS
Ulcerative tonsillitis (acute)
J03.90 Acute tonsillitis, unspecified
J03.91 Acute recurrent tonsillitis, unspecified

J04 Acute laryngitis and tracheitis
Use additional code (B95-B97) to identify infectious agent
Excludes1: *acute obstructive laryngitis [croup] and epiglottitis (J05.-)*
Excludes2: *laryngismus (stridulus) (J38.5)*

J04.0 Acute laryngitis
Edematous laryngitis (acute)
Laryngitis (acute) NOS
Subglottic laryngitis (acute)
Suppurative laryngitis (acute)
Ulcerative laryngitis (acute)
Excludes1: *acute obstructive laryngitis (J05.0)*
Excludes2: *chronic laryngitis (J37.0)*

+ **J04.1 Acute tracheitis**
Acute viral tracheitis
Catarrhal tracheitis (acute)
Tracheitis (acute) NOS
Excludes2: *chronic tracheitis (J42)*
J04.10 Acute tracheitis without obstruction
MCC **J04.11 Acute tracheitis with obstruction**
MCC Exclusion see Appendix A PDX collection 0730

J04.2 Acute laryngotracheitis
Laryngotracheitis NOS
Tracheitis (acute) with laryngitis (acute)
Excludes1: *acute obstructive laryngotracheitis (J05.0)*
Excludes2: *chronic laryngotracheitis (J37.1)*

+ **J04.3 Supraglottitis, unspecified**
J04.30 Supraglottitis, unspecified, without obstruction
MCC **J04.31 Supraglottitis, unspecified, with obstruction**
MCC Exclusion see Appendix A PDX collection 0731

J05 Acute obstructive laryngitis [croup] and epiglottitis
Use additional code (B95-B97) to identify infectious agent

J05.0 Acute obstructive laryngitis [croup]
Obstructive laryngitis (acute) NOS
Obstructive laryngotracheitis NOS

+ **J05.1 Acute epiglottitis**
Excludes2: *epiglottitis, chronic (J37.0)*
CC **J05.10 Acute epiglottitis without obstruction**
Epiglottitis NOS
CC Exclusion see Appendix A PDX collection 0732
MCC **J05.11 Acute epiglottitis with obstruction**
MCC Exclusion see Appendix A PDX collection 0730

J06 Acute upper respiratory infections of multiple and unspecified sites
Excludes1: *acute respiratory infection NOS (J22)*
streptococcal pharyngitis (J02.0)

J06.0 Acute laryngopharyngitis

J06.9 Acute upper respiratory infection, unspecified
Upper respiratory disease, acute
Upper respiratory infection NOS

Influenza and pneumonia (J09-J18)

Excludes2: *allergic or eosinophilic pneumonia (J82)*
aspiration pneumonia NOS (J69.0)
meconium pneumonia (P24.01)
neonatal aspiration pneumonia (P24.-)
pneumonia due to solids and liquids (J69-)
congenital pneumonia (P23.9)
lipid pneumonia (J69.1)
rheumatic pneumonia (I00)
ventilator associated pneumonia (J95.851)

J09 Influenza due to certain identified influenza viruses
Excludes1: *influenza A/H1N1 (J10.-)*
influenza due to other identified influenza virus (J10.-)
influenza due to unidentified influenza virus (J11.-)
seasonal influenza due to other identified influenza virus (J10.-)
seasonal influenza due to unidentified influenza virus (J11.-)
Review coding guideline C.10.c

+ **J09.X Influenza due to identified novel influenza A virus**
Avian influenza
Bird influenza
Influenza A/H5N1
Influenza of other animal origin, not bird or swine
Swine influenza virus (viruses that normally cause infections in pigs)

MCC **J09.X1 Influenza due to identified novel influenza A virus with pneumonia**
Code also if applicable, associated:
lung abscess (J85.1)
other specified type of pneumonia
MCC Exclusion see Appendix A PDX collection 0110

J09.X2 Influenza due to identified novel influenza A virus with other respiratory manifestations
Influenza due to identified novel influenza A virus NOS
Influenza due to identified novel influenza A virus with laryngitis
Influenza due to identified novel influenza A virus with pharyngitis
Influenza due to identified novel influenza A virus with upper respiratory symptoms
Use additional code, if applicable, for associated:
pleural effusion (J91.8)
sinusitis (J01.-)

J09.X3 Influenza due to identified novel influenza A virus with gastrointestinal manifestations
Influenza due to identified novel influenza A virus gastroenteritis
Excludes1: *'intestinal flu' [viral gastroenteritis] (A08.-)*

Lungs

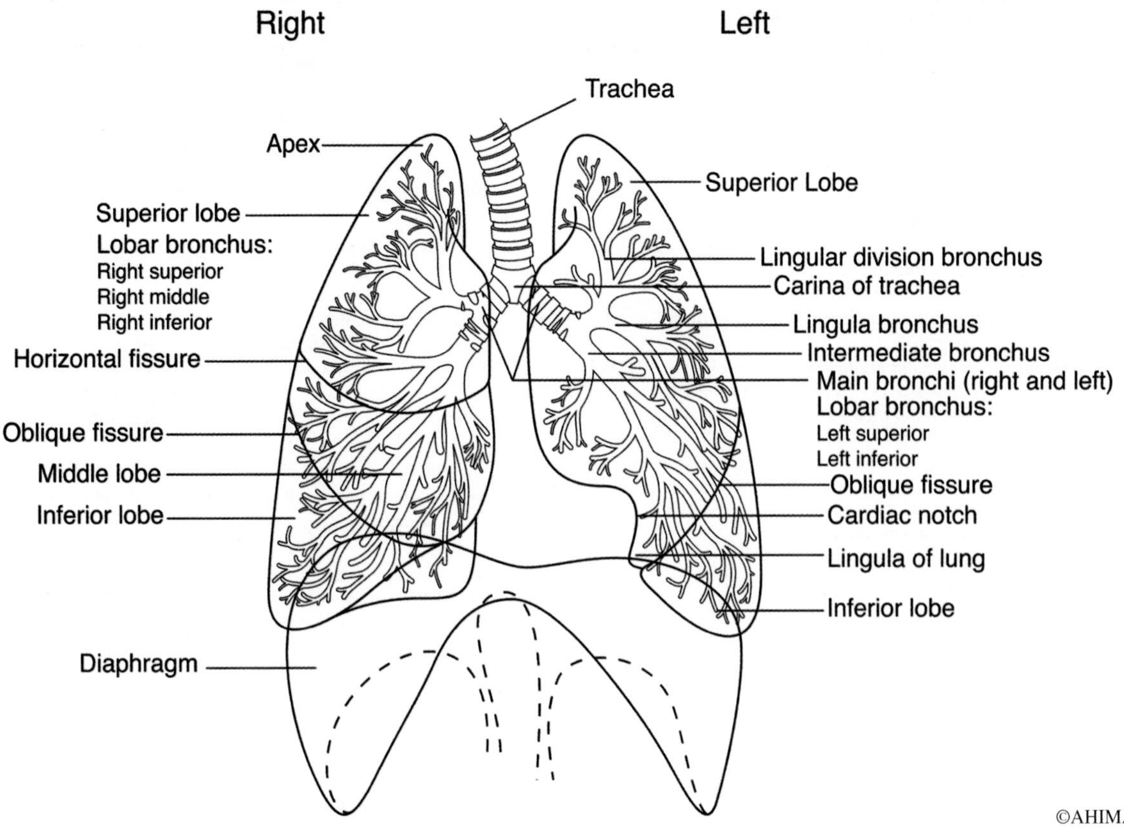

©AHIMA

J09.X9 Influenza due to identified novel influenza A virus with other manifestations
Influenza due to identified novel influenza A virus with encephalopathy
Influenza due to identified novel influenza A virus with myocarditis
Influenza due to identified novel influenza A virus with otitis media
Use additional code to identify manifestation

J10 Influenza due to other identified influenza virus

Excludes1: *influenza due to avian influenza virus (J09.X-)*
influenza due to swine flu (J09.X-)
influenza due to unidentifed influenza virus (J11.-)

Review coding guideline C.10.c

\+ **J10.0 Influenza due to other identified influenza virus with pneumonia**
Code also associated lung abscess, if applicable (J85.1)

MCC **J10.00 Influenza due to other identified influenza virus with unspecified type of pneumonia**
MCC Exclusion see Appendix A PDX collection 0110

MCC **J10.01 Influenza due to other identified influenza virus with the same other identified influenza virus pneumonia**
MCC Exclusion see Appendix A PDX collection 0110

MCC **J10.08 Influenza due to other identified influenza virus with other specified pneumonia**
Code also other specified type of pneumonia
MCC Exclusion see Appendix A PDX collection 0733

J10.1 Influenza due to other identified influenza virus with other respiratory manifestations
Influenza due to other identified influenza virus NOS
Influenza due to other identified influenza virus with laryngitis
Influenza due to other identified influenza virus with pharyngitis
Influenza due to other identified influenza virus with upper respiratory symptoms
Use additional code for associated pleural effusion, if applicable (J91.8)
Use additional code for associated sinusitis, if applicable (J01.-)
AHA CC: 3Q, 2016, 10-11

J10.2 Influenza due to other identified influenza virus with gastrointestinal manifestations
Influenza due to other identified influenza virus gastroenteritis
Excludes1: *'intestinal flu' [viral gastroenteritis] (A08.-)*

\+ **J10.8 Influenza due to other identified influenza virus with other manifestations**

J10.81 Influenza due to other identified influenza virus wi encephalopathy

J10.82 Influenza due to other identified influenza virus wi myocarditis

J10.83 Influenza due to other identified influenza virus wi otitis media
Use additional code for any associated perforated tympanic membrane (H72.-)

J10.89 Influenza due to other identified influenza virus wi other manifestations
Use additional codes to identify the manifestations

J11 Influenza due to unidentified influenza virus

\+ **J11.0 Influenza due to unidentified influenza virus with pneumoni**
Code also associated lung abscess, if applicable (J85.1)

MCC **J11.00 Influenza due to unidentified influenza virus with unspecified type of pneumonia**
Influenza with pneumonia NOS
MCC Exclusion see Appendix A PDX collection 0110
AHA CC: 3Q, 2016, 11-12

MCC **J11.08 Influenza due to unidentified influenza virus with specified pneumonia**
Code also other specified type of pneumonia
MCC Exclusion see Appendix A PDX collection 0110

J11.1 Influenza due to unidentified influenza virus with other respiratory manifestations
Influenza NOS
Influenzal laryngitis NOS
Influenzal pharyngitis NOS
Influenza with upper respiratory symptoms NOS
Use additional code for associated pleural effusion, if applicable (J91.8)

Use additional code for associated sinusitis, if applicable (J01

J11.2 Influenza due to unidentified influenza virus with gastrointestinal manifestations
Influenza gastroenteritis NOS
Excludes1: 'intestinal flu' [viral gastroenteritis] (A08.-)

\+ **J11.8 Influenza due to unidentified influenza virus with other manifestations**

J11.81 Influenza due to unidentified influenza virus with encephalopathy
Influenzal encephalopathy NOS

J11.82 **Influenza due to unidentified influenza virus with myocarditis**
Influenzal myocarditis NOS

J11.83 **Influenza due to unidentified influenza virus with otitis media**
Influenzal otitis media NOS
Use additional code for any associated perforated tympanic membrane (H72.-)

J11.89 **Influenza due to unidentified influenza virus with other manifestations**
Use additional codes to identify the manifestations

J12 Viral pneumonia, not elsewhere classified

Includes: bronchopneumonia due to viruses other than influenza viruses
Code first associated influenza, if applicable (J09.X1, J10.0-, J11.0-)

Code also associated abscess, if applicable (J85.1)
Excludes1: *aspiration pneumonia due to anesthesia during labor and delivery (O74.0)*
aspiration pneumonia due to anesthesia during pregnancy (O29)
aspiration pneumonia due to anesthesia during puerperium (O89.0)
aspiration pneumonia due to solids and liquids (J69.-)
aspiration pneumonia NOS (J69.0)
congenital pneumonia (P23.0)
congenital rubella pneumonitis (P35.0)
interstitial pneumonia NOS (J84.9)
lipid pneumonia (J69.1)
neonatal aspiration pneumonia (P24.-)

MCC **J12.0 Adenoviral pneumonia**
MCC Exclusion see Appendix A PDX collection 0734

MCC **J12.1 Respiratory syncytial virus pneumonia**
MCC Exclusion see Appendix A PDX collection 0734

MCC **J12.2 Parainfluenza virus pneumonia**
MCC Exclusion see Appendix A PDX collection 0734

MCC **J12.3 Human metapneumovirus pneumonia**
MCC Exclusion see Appendix A PDX collection 0734

+ **J12.8 Other viral pneumonia**

MCC **J12.81 Pneumonia due to SARS-associated coronavirus**
Severe acute respiratory syndrome NOS
MCC Exclusion see Appendix A PDX collection 0735

MCC **J12.89 Other viral pneumonia**
MCC Exclusion see Appendix A PDX collection 0734

MCC **J12.9 Viral pneumonia, unspecified**
MCC Exclusion see Appendix A PDX collection 0734

J13 Pneumonia due to Streptococcus pneumoniae

Bronchopneumonia due to S. pneumoniae
Code first associated influenza, if applicable (J09.X1, J10.0-, J11.0-)

Code also associated abscess, if applicable (J85.1)
Excludes1: *congenital pneumonia due to S. pneumoniae (P23.6)*
lobar pneumonia, unspecified organism (J18.1)
pneumonia due to other streptococci (J15.3-J15.4)
MCC Exclusion see Appendix A PDX collection 0110
Valid 3-character code, no further characters required

J14 Pneumonia due to Hemophilus influenzae

Bronchopneumonia due to H. influenzae
Code first associated influenza, if applicable (J09.X1, J10.0-, J11.0-)

Code also associated abscess, if applicable (J85.1)
Excludes1: *congenital pneumonia due to H. influenzae (P23.6)*
MCC Exclusion see Appendix A PDX collection 0110
Valid 3-character code, no further characters required

J15 Bacterial pneumonia, not elsewhere classified

Includes: bronchopneumonia due to bacteria other than S. pneumoniae and H. influenzae
Code first associated influenza, if applicable (J09.X1, J10.0-, J11.0-)

Code also associated abscess, if applicable (J85.1)
Excludes1: *chlamydial pneumonia (J16.0)*
congenital pneumonia (P23.-)
Legionnaires' disease (A48.1)
spirochetal pneumonia (A69.8)

MCC **J15.0 Pneumonia due to Klebsiella pneumoniae**
MCC Exclusion see Appendix A PDX collection 0110

MCC **J15.1 Pneumonia due to Pseudomonas**
MCC Exclusion see Appendix A PDX collection 0110

+ **J15.2 Pneumonia due to staphylococcus**

MCC **J15.20 Pneumonia due to staphylococcus, unspecified**
MCC Exclusion see Appendix A PDX collection 0110

+ **J15.21 Pneumonia due to staphylococcus aureus**

MCC **J15.211 Pneumonia due to Methicillin susceptible Staphylococcus aureus**
MSSA pneumonia
Pneumonia due to Staphylococcus aureus NOS
MCC Exclusion see Appendix A PDX collection 0110

MCC **J15.212 Pneumonia due to Methicillin resistant Staphylococcus aureus**
MCC Exclusion see Appendix A PDX collection 0110
Review coding guideline C.1.e.1.a

MCC **J15.29 Pneumonia due to other staphylococcus**
MCC Exclusion see Appendix A PDX collection 0110

MCC **J15.3 Pneumonia due to streptococcus, group B**
MCC Exclusion see Appendix A PDX collection 0110

MCC **J15.4 Pneumonia due to other streptococci**
Excludes1: *pneumonia due to streptococcus, group B (J15.3)*
pneumonia due to Streptococcus pneumoniae (J13)
MCC Exclusion see Appendix A PDX collection 0110

MCC **J15.5 Pneumonia due to Escherichia coli**
MCC Exclusion see Appendix A PDX collection 0110

MCC **J15.6 Pneumonia due to other Gram-negative bacteria**
Pneumonia due to other aerobic Gram-negative bacteria
Pneumonia due to Serratia marcescens
MCC Exclusion see Appendix A PDX collection 0110

MCC **J15.7 Pneumonia due to Mycoplasma pneumoniae**

MCC **J15.8 Pneumonia due to other specified bacteria**
MCC Exclusion see Appendix A PDX collection 0110

MCC **J15.9 Unspecified bacterial pneumonia**
Pneumonia due to gram-positive bacteria
MCC Exclusion see Appendix A PDX collection 0110

J16 Pneumonia due to other infectious organisms, not elsewhere classified

Code first associated influenza, if applicable (J09.X1, J10.0-, J11.0-)

Code also associated abscess, if applicable (J85.1)
Excludes1: *congenital pneumonia (P23.-)*
ornithosis (A70)
pneumocystosis (B59)
pneumonia NOS (J18.9)

MCC **J16.0 Chlamydial pneumonia**
MCC Exclusion see Appendix A PDX collection 0110

MCC **J16.8 Pneumonia due to other specified infectious organisms**
MCC Exclusion see Appendix A PDX collection 0110

MCC **J17 Pneumonia in diseases classified elsewhere**

Code first underlying disease, such as:
Q fever (A78)
rheumatic fever (I00)
schistosomiasis (B65.0-B65.9)
Excludes1: *candidial pneumonia (B37.1)*
chlamydial pneumonia (J16.0)
gonorrheal pneumonia (A54.84)
histoplasmosis pneumonia (B39.0-B39.2)
measles pneumonia (B05.2)
nocardiosis pneumonia (A43.0)
pneumocystosis (B59)
pneumonia due to Pneumocystis carinii (B59)
pneumonia due to Pneumocystis jiroveci (B59)
pneumonia in actinomycosis (A42.0)
pneumonia in anthrax (A22.1)
pneumonia in ascariasis (B77.81)
pneumonia in aspergillosis (B44.0-B44.1)
pneumonia in coccidioidomycosis (B38.0-B38.2)
pneumonia in cytomegalovirus disease(B25.0)
pneumonia in toxoplasmosis (B58.3)
rubella pneumonia (B06.81)
salmonella pneumonia (A02.22)
spirochetal infection NEC with pneumonia (A69.8)
tularemia pneumonia (A21.2)
typhoid fever with pneumonia (A01.03)
varicella pneumonia (B01.2)
whooping cough with pneumonia (A37 with fifth-character 1)
MCC Exclusion see Appendix A PDX collection 0110
Valid 3-character code, no further characters required

J18 Pneumonia, unspecified organism

Code first associated influenza, if applicable (J09.X1, J10.0-, J11.0-)

Excludes1: *abscess of lung with pneumonia (J85.1)*
aspiration pneumonia due to anesthesia during labor and delivery (O74.0)
aspiration pneumonia due to anesthesia during pregnancy (O29)
aspiration pneumonia due to anesthesia during puerperium (O89.0)
aspiration pneumonia due to solids and liquids (J69.-)
aspiration pneumonia NOS (J69.0)
congenital pneumonia (P23.0)
drug-induced interstitial lung disorder (J70.2-J70.4)
interstitial pneumonia NOS (J84.9)
lipid pneumonia (J69.1)
neonatal aspiration pneumonia (P24.-)
pneumonitis due to external agents (J67-J70)
pneumonitis due to fumes and vapors (J68.0)
usual interstitial pneumonia (J84.17)

MCC **J18.0 Bronchopneumonia, unspecified organism**
Excludes1: *hypostatic bronchopneumonia (J18.2)*
lipid pneumonia (J69.1)
Excludes2: *acute bronchiolitis (J21.-)*
chronic bronchiolitis (J44.9)
MCC Exclusion see Appendix A PDX collection 0110

MCC **J18.1 Lobar pneumonia, unspecified organism**
MCC Exclusion see Appendix A PDX collection 0110
AHA CC: 3Q, 2016, 15

CC **J18.2 Hypostatic pneumonia, unspecified organism**
Hypostatic bronchopneumonia
Passive pneumonia
CC Exclusion see Appendix A PDX collection 0736

MCC **J18.8 Other pneumonia, unspecified organism**
MCC Exclusion see Appendix A PDX collection 0110

MCC **J18.9 Pneumonia, unspecified organism**
MCC Exclusion see Appendix A PDX collection 0110
AHA CC: 4Q, 2012, 94; 3Q, 2014, 4; 3Q, 2016, 15-16

Other acute lower respiratory infections (J20-J22)

Excludes2: *chronic obstructive pulmonary disease with acute lower respiratory infection (J44.0)*

J20 Acute bronchitis

Includes: acute and subacute bronchitis (with) bronchospasm
acute and subacute bronchitis (with) tracheitis
acute and subacute bronchitis (with) tracheobronchitis, acute
acute and subacute fibrinous bronchitis
acute and subacute membranous bronchitis
acute and subacute purulent bronchitis
acute and subacute septic bronchitis

Excludes1: *bronchitis NOS (J40)*
tracheobronchitis NOS (J40)

Excludes2: *acute bronchitis with bronchiectasis (J47.0)*
acute bronchitis with chronic obstructive asthma (J44.0)
acute bronchitis with chronic obstructive pulmonary disease (J44.0)
allergic bronchitis NOS (J45.909-)
bronchitis due to chemicals, fumes and vapors (J68.0)
chronic bronchitis NOS (J42)
chronic mucopurulent bronchitis (J41.1)
chronic obstructive bronchitis (J44.-)
chronic obstructive tracheobronchitis (J44.-)
chronic simple bronchitis (J41.0)
chronic tracheobronchitis (J42)

J20.0 Acute bronchitis due to Mycoplasma pneumoniae
J20.1 Acute bronchitis due to Hemophilus influenzae
J20.2 Acute bronchitis due to streptococcus
J20.3 Acute bronchitis due to coxsackievirus
J20.4 Acute bronchitis due to parainfluenza virus
J20.5 Acute bronchitis due to respiratory syncytial virus
J20.6 Acute bronchitis due to rhinovirus
AHA CC: 3Q, 2016, 10
J20.7 Acute bronchitis due to echovirus
J20.8 Acute bronchitis due to other specified organisms
AHA CC: 3Q, 2016, 10-11
J20.9 Acute bronchitis, unspecified
AHA CC: 3Q, 2016, 16

J21 Acute bronchiolitis

Includes: *acute bronchiolitis with bronchospasm*
Excludes2: *respiratory bronchiolitis interstitial lung disease (J84.11)*

CC **J21.0 Acute bronchiolitis due to respiratory syncytial virus**
CC Exclusion see Appendix A PDX collection 0737

CC **J21.1 Acute bronchiolitis due to human metapneumovirus**
CC Exclusion see Appendix A PDX collection 0738

CC **J21.8 Acute bronchiolitis due to other specified organisms**
CC Exclusion see Appendix A PDX collection 0738

CC **J21.9 Acute bronchiolitis, unspecified**
Bronchiolitis (acute)
Excludes1: *chronic bronchiolitis (J44.-)*
CC Exclusion see Appendix A PDX collection 0738

J22 Unspecified acute lower respiratory infection

Acute (lower) respiratory (tract) infection NOS
Excludes1: *upper respiratory infection (acute) (J06.9)*
Valid 3-character code, no further characters required

Other diseases of upper respiratory tract (J30-J39)

J30 Vasomotor and allergic rhinitis

Includes: spasmodic rhinorrhea
Excludes1: *allergic rhinitis with asthma (bronchial) (J45.909)*
rhinitis NOS (J31.0)

J30.0 Vasomotor rhinitis
J30.1 Allergic rhinitis due to pollen
Allergy NOS due to pollen
Hay fever
Pollinosis
J30.2 Other seasonal allergic rhinitis
J30.5 Allergic rhinitis due to food
\+ **J30.8 Other allergic rhinitis**
J30.81 Allergic rhinitis due to animal (cat) (dog) hair and dander
J30.89 Other allergic rhinitis
Perennial allergic rhinitis
J30.9 Allergic rhinitis, unspecified

J31 Chronic rhinitis, nasopharyngitis and pharyngitis

Use additional code to identify:
exposure to environmental tobacco smoke (Z77.22)
exposure to tobacco smoke in the perinatal period (P96.81)
history of tobacco dependence (Z87.891)
occupational exposure to environmental tobacco smoke (Z57.31)
tobacco dependence (F17.-)
tobacco use (Z72.0)

J31.0 Chronic rhinitis
Atrophic rhinitis (chronic)
Granulomatous rhinitis (chronic)
Hypertrophic rhinitis (chronic)
Obstructive rhinitis (chronic)
Ozena
Purulent rhinitis (chronic)
Rhinitis (chronic) NOS
Ulcerative rhinitis (chronic)
Excludes1: *allergic rhinitis (J30.1-J30.9)*
vasomotor rhinitis (J30.0)

J31.1 Chronic nasopharyngitis
Excludes2: *acute nasopharyngitis (J00)*

J31.2 Chronic pharyngitis
Chronic sore throat
Atrophic pharyngitis (chronic)
Granular pharyngitis (chronic)
Hypertrophic pharyngitis (chronic)
Excludes2: *acute pharyngitis (J02.9)*

J32 Chronic sinusitis

Includes: sinus abscess
sinus empyema
sinus infection
sinus suppuration

Use additional code to identify:
exposure to environmental tobacco smoke (Z77.22)
exposure to tobacco smoke in the perinatal period (P96.81)
history of tobacco dependence (Z87.891)
infectious agent (B95-B97)
occupational exposure to environmental tobacco smoke (Z57.31)
tobacco dependence (F17.-)
tobacco use (Z72.0)

Excludes2: *acute sinusitis (J01.-)*

J32.0 Chronic maxillary sinusitis
Antritis (chronic)
Maxillary sinusitis NOS

J32.1 Chronic frontal sinusitis
Frontal sinusitis NOS

J32.2 Chronic ethmoidal sinusitis
Ethmoidal sinusitis NOS
Excludes1: *Woakes' ethmoiditis (J33.1)*

J32.3 Chronic sphenoidal sinusitis
Sphenoidal sinusitis NOS

J32.4 Chronic pansinusitis
Pansinusitis NOS

J32.8 Other chronic sinusitis
Sinusitis (chronic) involving more than one sinus but not pansinusitis

J32.9 Chronic sinusitis, unspecified
Sinusitis (chronic) NOS

J33 Nasal polyp

Use additional code to identify:
exposure to environmental tobacco smoke (Z77.22)
exposure to tobacco smoke in the perinatal period (P96.81)
history of tobacco dependence (Z87.891)
occupational exposure to environmental tobacco smoke (Z57.31)
tobacco dependence (F17.-)
tobacco use (Z72.0)

Excludes1: *adenomatous polyps (D14.0)*

J33.0 Polyp of nasal cavity
Choanal polyp
Nasopharyngeal polyp

J33.1 Polypoid sinus degeneration
Woakes' syndrome or ethmoiditis

J33.8 Other polyp of sinus
Accessory polyp of sinus
Ethmoidal polyp of sinus
Maxillary polyp of sinus
Sphenoidal polyp of sinus

J33.9 Nasal polyp, unspecified

J34 Other and unspecified disorders of nose and nasal sinuses

Excludes2: *varicose ulcer of nasal septum (I86.8)*

J34.0 Abscess, furuncle and carbuncle of nose
Cellulitis of nose
Necrosis of nose
Ulceration of nose

J34.1 Cyst and mucocele of nose and nasal sinus

J34.2 Deviated nasal septum
Deflection or deviation of septum (nasal) (acquired)
Excludes1: *congenital deviated nasal septum (Q67.4)*

J34.3 Hypertrophy of nasal turbinates

\+ **J34.8 Other specified disorders of nose and nasal sinuses**

J34.81 Nasal mucositis (ulcerative)
Code also type of associated therapy, such as:
antineoplastic and immunosuppressive drugs (T45.1X-)
radiological procedure and radiotherapy (Y84.2)
Excludes2: *gastrointestinal mucositis (ulcerative) (K92.81)*
mucositis (ulcerative) of vagina and vulva (N76.81)
oral mucositis (ulcerative) (K12.3-)

J34.89 Other specified disorders of nose and nasal sinuses
Perforation of nasal septum NOS
Rhinolith

J34.9 Unspecified disorder of nose and nasal sinuses

J35 Chronic diseases of tonsils and adenoids

Use additional code to identify:
exposure to environmental tobacco smoke (Z77.22)
exposure to tobacco smoke in the perinatal period (P96.81)
history of tobacco dependence (Z87.891)
occupational exposure to environmental tobacco smoke (Z57.31)
tobacco dependence (F17.-)
tobacco use (Z72.0)

\+ **J35.0 Chronic tonsillitis and adenoiditis**
Excludes2: *acute tonsillitis (J03.-)*

J35.01 Chronic tonsillitis

J35.02 Chronic adenoiditis

J35.03 Chronic tonsillitis and adenoiditis

J35.1 Hypertrophy of tonsils
Enlargement of tonsils
Excludes1: *hypertrophy of tonsils with tonsillitis (J35.0-)*

J35.2 Hypertrophy of adenoids
Enlargement of adenoids
Excludes1: *hypertrophy of adenoids with adenoiditis (J35.0-)*

J35.3 Hypertrophy of tonsils with hypertrophy of adenoids
Excludes1: *hypertrophy of tonsils and adenoids with tonsillitis and adenoiditis (J35.03)*

J35.8 Other chronic diseases of tonsils and adenoids
Adenoid vegetations
Amygdalolith
Calculus, tonsil
Cicatrix of tonsil (and adenoid)
Tonsillar tag
Ulcer of tonsil

J35.9 Chronic disease of tonsils and adenoids, unspecified
Disease (chronic) of tonsils and adenoids NOS

CC **J36 Peritonsillar abscess**

Includes: abscess of tonsil
peritonsillar cellulitis
quinsy

Use additional code (B95-B97) to identify infectious agent

Excludes1: *acute tonsillitis (J03.-)*
chronic tonsillitis (J35.0)
retropharyngeal abscess (J39.0)
tonsillitis NOS (J03.9-)

CC Exclusion see Appendix A PDX collection 0739
Valid 3-character code, no further characters required

J37 Chronic laryngitis and laryngotracheitis

Use additional code to identify:
exposure to environmental tobacco smoke (Z77.22)
exposure to tobacco smoke in the perinatal period (P96.81)
history of tobacco dependence (Z87.891)
infectious agent (B95-B97)
occupational exposure to environmental tobacco smoke (Z57.31)
tobacco dependence (F17.-)
tobacco use (Z72.0)

J37.0 Chronic laryngitis
Catarrhal laryngitis
Hypertrophic laryngitis
Sicca laryngitis
Excludes2: *acute laryngitis (J04.0)*
obstructive (acute) laryngitis (J05.0)

J37.1 Chronic laryngotracheitis
Laryngitis, chronic, with tracheitis (chronic)
Tracheitis, chronic, with laryngitis
Excludes1: *chronic tracheitis (J42)*
Excludes2: *acute laryngotracheitis (J04.2)*
acute tracheitis (J04.1)

J38 Diseases of vocal cords and larynx, not elsewhere classified

Use additional code to identify:
exposure to environmental tobacco smoke (Z77.22)
exposure to tobacco smoke in the perinatal period (P96.81)
history of tobacco dependence (Z87.891)
occupational exposure to environmental tobacco smoke (Z57.31)
tobacco dependence (F17.-)
tobacco use (Z72.0)

Excludes1: *congenital laryngeal stridor (P28.89)*
obstructive laryngitis (acute) (J05.0)
postprocedural subglottic stenosis (J95.5)
stridor (R06.1)
ulcerative laryngitis (J04.0)

+ **J38.0 Paralysis of vocal cords and larynx**
Laryngoplegia
Paralysis of glottis
J38.00 Paralysis of vocal cords and larynx, unspecified
J38.01 Paralysis of vocal cords and larynx, unilateral
J38.02 Paralysis of vocal cords and larynx, bilateral

J38.1 Polyp of vocal cord and larynx
Excludes1: *adenomatous polyps (D14.1)*

J38.2 Nodules of vocal cords
Chorditis (fibrinous)(nodosa)(tuberosa)
Singer's nodes
Teacher's nodes

J38.3 Other diseases of vocal cords
Abscess of vocal cords
Cellulitis of vocal cords
Granuloma of vocal cords
Leukokeratosis of vocal cords
Leukoplakia of vocal cords

J38.4 Edema of larynx
Edema (of) glottis
Subglottic edema
Supraglottic edema
Excludes1: *acute obstructive laryngitis [croup] (J05.0)*
edematous laryngitis (J04.0)

J38.5 Laryngeal spasm
Laryngismus (stridulus)

J38.6 Stenosis of larynx

J38.7 Other diseases of larynx
Abscess of larynx
Cellulitis of larynx
Disease of larynx NOS
Necrosis of larynx
Pachyderma of larynx
Perichondritis of larynx
Ulcer of larynx

J39 Other diseases of upper respiratory tract

Excludes1: *acute respiratory infection NOS (J22)*
acute upper respiratory infection (J06.9)
upper respiratory inflammation due to chemicals, gases, fumes or vapors (J68.2)

CC **J39.0 Retropharyngeal and parapharyngeal abscess**
Peripharyngeal abscess
Excludes1: *peritonsillar abscess (J36)*
CC Exclusion see Appendix A PDX collection 0740

CC **J39.1 Other abscess of pharynx**
Cellulitis of pharynx
Nasopharyngeal abscess
CC Exclusion see Appendix A PDX collection 0740

J39.2 Other diseases of pharynx
Cyst of pharynx
Edema of pharynx
Excludes2: *chronic pharyngitis (J31.2)*
ulcerative pharyngitis (J02.9)

J39.3 Upper respiratory tract hypersensitivity reaction, site unspecified
Excludes1: *hypersensitivity reaction of upper respiratory tract, such as:*
extrinsic allergic alveolitis (J67.9)
pneumoconiosis (J60-J67.9)

J39.8 Other specified diseases of upper respiratory tract

J39.9 Disease of upper respiratory tract, unspecified

Chronic lower respiratory diseases (J40-J47)

Excludes1: *bronchitis due to chemicals, gases, fumes and vapors (J68.0)*

Excludes2: *cystic fibrosis (E84.-)*

J40 Bronchitis, not specified as acute or chronic

Bronchitis NOS
Bronchitis with tracheitis NOS
Catarrhal bronchitis
Tracheobronchitis NOS
Use additional code to identify:
exposure to environmental tobacco smoke (Z77.22)
exposure to tobacco smoke in the perinatal period (P96.81)
history of tobacco dependence (Z87.891)
occupational exposure to environmental tobacco smoke (Z57.31)
tobacco dependence (F17.-)
tobacco use (Z72.0)
Excludes1: *allergic bronchitis NOS (J45.909-)*
asthmatic bronchitis NOS (J45.9-)
acute bronchitis (J20.-)
bronchitis due to chemicals, gases, fumes and vapors (J68
Valid 3-character code, no further characters required

J41 Simple and mucopurulent chronic bronchitis

Use additional code to identify:
exposure to environmental tobacco smoke (Z77.22)
exposure to tobacco smoke in the perinatal period (P96.81)
history of tobacco dependence (Z87.891)
occupational exposure to environmental tobacco smoke (Z57.31)
tobacco dependence (F17.-)
tobacco use (Z72.0)
Excludes1: *chronic bronchitis NOS (J42)*
chronic obstructive bronchitis (J44.-)

J41.0 Simple chronic bronchitis
J41.1 Mucopurulent chronic bronchitis
J41.8 Mixed simple and mucopurulent chronic bronchitis

J42 Unspecified chronic bronchitis

Chronic bronchitis NOS
Chronic tracheitis
Chronic tracheobronchitis
Use additional code to identify:
exposure to environmental tobacco smoke (Z77.22)
exposure to tobacco smoke in the perinatal period (P96.81)
history of tobacco dependence (Z87.891)
occupational exposure to environmental tobacco smoke (Z57.31)
tobacco dependence (F17.-)
tobacco use (Z72.0)
Excludes1: *chronic asthmatic bronchitis (J44.-)*
chronic bronchitis with airways obstruction (J44.-)
chronic emphysematous bronchitis (J44.-)
chronic obstructive pulmonary disease NOS (J44.9)
simple and mucopurulent chronic bronchitis (J41.-)
Valid 3-character code, no further characters required

J43 Emphysema

Use additional code to identify:
exposure to environmental tobacco smoke (Z77.22)
history of tobacco dependence (Z87.891)
occupational exposure to environmental tobacco smoke (Z57.31)
tobacco dependence (F17.-)
tobacco use (Z72.0)
Excludes1: *compensatory emphysema (J98.3)*
emphysema due to inhalation of chemicals, gases, fumes vapors (J68.4)
emphysema with chronic (obstructive) bronchitis (J44.-)
emphysematous (obstructive) bronchitis (J44.-)
interstitial emphysema (J98.2)
mediastinal emphysema (J98.2)
neonatal interstitial emphysema (P25.0)
surgical (subcutaneous) emphysema (T81.82)
traumatic subcutaneous emphysema (T79.7)

J43.0 Unilateral pulmonary emphysema [MacLeod's syndrome]
Swyer-James syndrome
Unilateral emphysema
Unilateral hyperlucent lung
Unilateral pulmonary artery functional hypoplasia
Unilateral transparency of lung

J43.1 Panlobular emphysema
Panacinar emphysema

J43.2 Centrilobular emphysema

J43.8 Other emphysema

J43.9 Emphysema, unspecified
Bullous emphysema (lung)(pulmonary)
Emphysema (lung)(pulmonary) NOS
Emphysematous bleb
Vesicular emphysema (lung)(pulmonary)

J44 Other chronic obstructive pulmonary disease

Includes: asthma with chronic obstructive pulmonary disease
chronic asthmatic (obstructive) bronchitis
chronic bronchitis with airways obstruction
chronic bronchitis with emphysema
chronic emphysematous bronchitis
chronic obstructive asthma
chronic obstructive bronchitis
chronic obstructive tracheobronchitis
Code also type of asthma, if applicable (J45.-)

Use additional code to identify:
exposure to environmental tobacco smoke (Z77.22)
history of tobacco dependence (Z87.891)
occupational exposure to environmental tobacco smoke (Z57.31)
tobacco dependence (F17.-)
tobacco use (Z72.0)

Excludes1: *bronchiectasis (J47.-)*
chronic bronchitis NOS (J42)
chronic simple and mucopurulent bronchitis (J41.-)
chronic tracheitis (J42)
chronic tracheobronchitis (J42)
emphysema without chronic bronchitis (J43.-)

Review coding guideline C.10.a.1

CC **J44.0 Chronic obstructive pulmonary disease with acute lower respiratory infection**
Code also to identify the infection
CC Exclusion see Appendix A PDX collection 0741
AHA CC: 3Q, 2016, 15-16

CC **J44.1 Chronic obstructive pulmonary disease with (acute) exacerbation**
Decompensated COPD
Decompensated COPD with (acute) exacerbation
Excludes2: *chronic obstructive pulmonary disease [COPD] with acute bronchitis (J44.0)*
lung diseases due to external agents (J60-J70)
CC Exclusion see Appendix A PDX collection 0741
AHA CC: 1Q, 2016, 36; 3Q, 2016, 15-16, 26; 1Q, 2017, 26

J44.9 Chronic obstructive pulmonary disease, unspecified
Chronic obstructive airway disease NOS
Chronic obstructive lung disease NOS
Excludes2: *lung diseases due to external agents (J60-J70)*
AHA CC: 4Q, 2013, 109, 129; 4Q, 2014, 21-22; 1Q, 2016, 36-37; 1Q, 2017, 24-25

J45 Asthma

Includes: allergic (predominantly) asthma
allergic bronchitis NOS
allergic rhinitis with asthma
atopic asthma
extrinsic allergic asthma
hay fever with asthma
idiosyncratic asthma
intrinsic nonallergic asthma
nonallergic asthma

Use additional code to identify:
exposure to environmental tobacco smoke (Z77.22)
exposure to tobacco smoke in the perinatal period (P96.81)
history of tobacco dependence (Z87.891)
occupational exposure to environmental tobacco smoke (Z57.31)
tobacco dependence (F17.-)
tobacco use (Z72.0)

Excludes1: *detergent asthma (J69.8)*
eosinophilic asthma (J82)
miner's asthma (J60)
wheezing NOS (R06.2)
wood asthma (J67.8)

Excludes2: *asthma with chronic obstructive pulmonary disease (J44.9)*
chronic asthmatic (obstructive) bronchitis (J44.9)
chronic obstructive asthma (J44.9)

Review coding guideline C.10.a.1

+ **J45.2 Mild intermittent asthma**

J45.20 Mild intermittent asthma, uncomplicated
Mild intermittent asthma NOS

CC **J45.21 Mild intermittent asthma with (acute) exacerbation**
CC Exclusion see Appendix A PDX collection 0742

CC **J45.22 Mild intermittent asthma with status asthmaticus**
CC Exclusion see Appendix A PDX collection 0742

+ **J45.3 Mild persistent asthma**

J45.30 Mild persistent asthma, uncomplicated
Mild persistent asthma NOS

CC **J45.31 Mild persistent asthma with (acute) exacerbation**
CC Exclusion see Appendix A PDX collection 0742
AHA CC: 1Q, 2016, 35

CC **J45.32 Mild persistent asthma with status asthmaticus**
CC Exclusion see Appendix A PDX collection 0742

+ **J45.4 Moderate persistent asthma**

J45.40 Moderate persistent asthma, uncomplicated
Moderate persistent asthma NOS

CC **J45.41 Moderate persistent asthma with (acute) exacerbation**
CC Exclusion see Appendix A PDX collection 0742
AHA CC: 1Q, 2017, 26

CC **J45.42 Moderate persistent asthma with status asthmaticus**
CC Exclusion see Appendix A PDX collection 0742

+ **J45.5 Severe persistent asthma**

J45.50 Severe persistent asthma, uncomplicated
Severe persistent asthma NOS

CC **J45.51 Severe persistent asthma with (acute) exacerbation**
CC Exclusion see Appendix A PDX collection 0742

CC **J45.52 Severe persistent asthma with status asthmaticus**
CC Exclusion see Appendix A PDX collection 0742

+ **J45.9 Other and unspecified asthma**

+ **J45.90 Unspecified asthma**
Asthmatic bronchitis NOS
Childhood asthma NOS
Late onset asthma

CC **J45.901 Unspecified asthma with (acute) exacerbation**
CC Exclusion see Appendix A PDX collection 0742

CC **J45.902 Unspecified asthma with status asthmaticus**
CC Exclusion see Appendix A PDX collection 0742

J45.909 Unspecified asthma, uncomplicated
Asthma NOS
Excludes2: *lung diseases due to external agents (J60-J70)*

+ **J45.99 Other asthma**

J45.990 Exercise induced bronchospasm

J45.991 Cough variant asthma

J45.998 Other asthma

J47 Bronchiectasis

Includes: bronchiolectasis
Use additional code to identify:
exposure to environmental tobacco smoke (Z77.22)
exposure to tobacco smoke in the perinatal period (P96.81)
history of tobacco dependence (Z87.891)
occupational exposure to environmental tobacco smoke (Z57.31)
tobacco dependence (F17.-)
tobacco use (Z72.0)

Excludes1: *congenital bronchiectasis (Q33.4)*
tuberculous bronchiectasis (current disease) (A15.0)

CC **J47.0 Bronchiectasis with acute lower respiratory infection**
Bronchiectasis with acute bronchitis
Use additional code to identify the infection
CC Exclusion see Appendix A PDX collection 0743

CC **J47.1 Bronchiectasis with (acute) exacerbation**
CC Exclusion see Appendix A PDX collection 0743

J47.9 Bronchiectasis, uncomplicated
Bronchiectasis NOS

Lung diseases due to external agents (J60-J70)

Excludes2: *asthma (J45.-)*
malignant neoplasm of bronchus and lung (C34.-)

• **J60 Coalworker's pneumoconiosis**
Anthracosilicosis
Anthracosis
Black lung disease
Coalworker's lung
Excludes1: *coalworker pneumoconiosis with tuberculosis, any type in A15 (J65)*
Valid 3-character code, no further characters required

• **J61 Pneumoconiosis due to asbestos and other mineral fibers**
Asbestosis
Excludes1: *pleural plaque with asbestosis (J92.0)*
pneumoconiosis with tuberculosis, any type in A15 (J65)
Valid 3-character code, no further characters required

J62 Pneumoconiosis due to dust containing silica
Includes: silicotic fibrosis (massive) of lung
Excludes1: *pneumoconiosis with tuberculosis, any type in A15 (J65)*
J62.0 Pneumoconiosis due to talc dust
J62.8 Pneumoconiosis due to other dust containing silica
Silicosis NOS

J63 Pneumoconiosis due to other inorganic dusts
Excludes1: *pneumoconiosis with tuberculosis, any type in A15 (J65)*
J63.0 Aluminosis (of lung)
J63.1 Bauxite fibrosis (of lung)
J63.2 Berylliosis
J63.3 Graphite fibrosis (of lung)
J63.4 Siderosis
J63.5 Stannosis
J63.6 Pneumoconiosis due to other specified inorganic dusts

J64 Unspecified pneumoconiosis
Excludes1: *pneumonoconiosis with tuberculosis, any type in A15 (J65)*
Valid 3-character code, no further characters required

J65 Pneumoconiosis associated with tuberculosis
Any condition in J60-J64 with tuberculosis, any type in A15
Silicotuberculosis
Valid 3-character code, no further characters required

J66 Airway disease due to specific organic dust
Excludes2: *allergic alveolitis (J67.-)*
asbestosis (J61)
bagassosis (J67.1)
farmer's lung (J67.0)
hypersensitivity pneumonitis due to organic dust (J67.-)
reactive airways dysfunction syndrome (J68.3)
J66.0 Byssinosis
Airway disease due to cotton dust
J66.1 Flax-dressers' disease
J66.2 Cannabinosis
J66.8 Airway disease due to other specific organic dusts

J67 Hypersensitivity pneumonitis due to organic dust
Includes: allergic alveolitis and pneumonitis due to inhaled organic dust and particles of fungal, actinomycetic or other origin
Excludes1: *pneumonitis due to inhalation of chemicals, gases, fumes or vapors (J68.0)*
J67.0 Farmer's lung
Harvester's lung
Haymaker's lung
Moldy hay disease
J67.1 Bagassosis
Bagasse disease
Bagasse pneumonitis
J67.2 Bird fancier's lung
Budgerigar fancier's disease or lung
Pigeon fancier's disease or lung
J67.3 Suberosis
Corkhandler's disease or lung
Corkworker's disease or lung
J67.4 Maltworker's lung
Alveolitis due to Aspergillus clavatus
J67.5 Mushroom-worker's lung
J67.6 Maple-bark-stripper's lung
Alveolitis due to Cryptostroma corticale
Cryptostromosis

CC **J67.7 Air conditioner and humidifier lung**
Allergic alveolitis due to fungal, thermophilic actinomycetes and other organisms growing in ventilation [air conditionin systems
CC Exclusion see Appendix A PDX collection 0110

CC **J67.8 Hypersensitivity pneumonitis due to other organic dusts**
Cheese-washer's lung
Coffee-worker's lung
Fish-meal worker's lung
Furrier's lung
Sequoiosis
CC Exclusion see Appendix A PDX collection 0110

CC **J67.9 Hypersensitivity pneumonitis due to unspecified organic dus**
Allergic alveolitis (extrinsic) NOS
Hypersensitivity pneumonitis NOS
CC Exclusion see Appendix A PDX collection 0110

J68 Respiratory conditions due to inhalation of chemicals, gases, fume and vapors
Code first (T51-T65) to identify cause
Use additional code to identify associated respiratory conditions, suc as:
acute respiratory failure (J96.0-)

CC **J68.0 Bronchitis and pneumonitis due to chemicals, gases, fumes a vapors**
Chemical bronchitis (acute)
CC Exclusion see Appendix A PDX collection 0110

MCC **J68.1 Pulmonary edema due to chemicals, gases, fumes and vapor**
Chemical pulmonary edema (acute) (chronic)
Excludes1: *pulmonary edema (acute) (chronic) NOS (J81.-)*
MCC Exclusion see Appendix A PDX collection 0110

J68.2 Upper respiratory inflammation due to chemicals, gases, fu and vapors, not elsewhere classified
J68.3 Other acute and subacute respiratory conditions due to chemicals, gases, fumes and vapors
Reactive airways dysfunction syndrome
J68.4 Chronic respiratory conditions due to chemicals, gases, fum and vapors
Emphysema (diffuse) (chronic) due to inhalation of chemical gases, fumes and vapors
Obliterative bronchiolitis (chronic) (subacute) due to inhalati of chemicals, gases, fumes and vapors
Pulmonary fibrosis (chronic) due to inhalation of chemicals, gases, fumes and vapors
Excludes1: *chronic pulmonary edema due to chemicals, gas fumes and vapors (J68.1)*
J68.8 Other respiratory conditions due to chemicals, gases, fumes and vapors
J68.9 Unspecified respiratory condition due to chemicals, gases, fumes and vapors

J69 Pneumonitis due to solids and liquids
Excludes1: *neonatal aspiration syndromes (P24.-)*
postprocedural pneumonitis (J95.4)

MCC **J69.0 Pneumonitis due to inhalation of food and vomit**
Aspiration pneumonia NOS
Aspiration pneumonia (due to) food (regurgitated)
Aspiration pneumonia (due to) gastric secretions
Aspiration pneumonia (due to) milk
Aspiration pneumonia (due to) vomit
Code also any associated foreign body in respiratory tract (T17.-)
Excludes1: *chemical pneumonitis due to anesthesia (J95.4)*
obstetric aspiration pneumonitis (O74.0)
MCC Exclusion see Appendix A PDX collection 0110
AHA CC: 1Q, 2017, 24

MCC **J69.1 Pneumonitis due to inhalation of oils and essences**
Exogenous lipoid pneumonia
Lipid pneumonia NOS
Code first (T51-T65) to identify substance
Excludes1: *endogenous lipoid pneumonia (J84.89)*
MCC Exclusion see Appendix A PDX collection 0110

MCC **J69.8 Pneumonitis due to inhalation of other solids and liquids**
Pneumonitis due to aspiration of blood
Pneumonitis due to aspiration of detergent
Code first (T51-T65) to identify substance
MCC Exclusion see Appendix A PDX collection 0110

J70 Respiratory conditions due to other external agents

CC **J70.0 Acute pulmonary manifestations due to radiation**
Radiation pneumonitis
Use additional code (W88-W90, X39.0-) to identify the external cause
CC Exclusion see Appendix A PDX collection 0110

CC **J70.1 Chronic and other pulmonary manifestations due to radiation**
Fibrosis of lung following radiation
Use additional code (W88-W90, X39.0-) to identify the external cause
CC Exclusion see Appendix A PDX collection 0110

J70.2 Acute drug-induced interstitial lung disorders
Use additional code for adverse effect, if applicable, to identify drug (T36-T50 with fifth or sixth character 5)
Excludes1: *interstitial pneumonia NOS (J84.9)*
lymphoid interstitial pneumonia (J84.2)

J70.3 Chronic drug-induced interstitial lung disorders
Use additional code for adverse effect, if applicable, to identify drug (T36-T50 with fifth or sixth character 5)
Excludes1: *interstitial pneumonia NOS (J84.9)*
lymphoid interstitial pneumonia (J84.2)

J70.4 Drug-induced interstitial lung disorders, unspecified
Use additional code for adverse effect, if applicable, to identify drug (T36-T50 with fifth or sixth character 5)
Excludes1: *interstitial pneumonia NOS (J84.9)*
lymphoid interstitial pneumonia (J84.2)

J70.5 Respiratory conditions due to smoke inhalation
Smoke inhalation NOS
Excludes1: *smoke inhalation due to chemicals, gases, fumes and vapors (J68.9)*

J70.8 Respiratory conditions due to other specified external agents
Code first (T51-T65) to identify the external agent

J70.9 Respiratory conditions due to unspecified external agent
Code first (T51-T65) to identify the external agent

her respiratory diseases principally affecting the erstitium (J80-J84)

J80 Acute respiratory distress syndrome

Acute respiratory distress syndrome in adult or child
Adult hyaline membrane disease
Excludes1: *respiratory distress syndrome in newborn (perinatal) (P22.0)*
CC Exclusion see Appendix A PDX collection 0744
AHA CC: 1Q, 2017, 26-27
Valid 3-character code, no further characters required

J81 Pulmonary edema

Use additional code to identify:
exposure to environmental tobacco smoke (Z77.22)
history of tobacco dependence (Z87.891)
occupational exposure to environmental tobacco smoke (Z57.31)
tobacco dependence (F17.-)
tobacco use (Z72.0)
Excludes1: *chemical (acute) pulmonary edema (J68.1)*
hypostatic pneumonia (J18.2)
passive pneumonia (J18.2)
pulmonary edema due to external agents (J60-J70)
pulmonary edema with heart disease NOS (I50.1)
pulmonary edema with heart failure (I50.1)

MCC **J81.0 Acute pulmonary edema**
Acute edema of lung
MCC Exclusion see Appendix A PDX collection 0745

CC **J81.1 Chronic pulmonary edema**
Pulmonary congestion (chronic) (passive)
Pulmonary edema NOS
CC Exclusion see Appendix A PDX collection 0736

CC **J82 Pulmonary eosinophilia, not elsewhere classified**

Allergic pneumonia
Eosinophilic asthma
Eosinophilic pneumonia
Löffler's pneumonia
Tropical (pulmonary) eosinophilia NOS
Excludes1: *pulmonary eosinophilia due to aspergillosis (B44.-)*
pulmonary eosinophilia due to drugs (J70.2-J70.4)
pulmonary eosinophilia due to specified parasitic infection (B50-B83)
pulmonary eosinophilia due to systemic connective tissue disorders (M30-M36)
pulmonary infiltrate NOS (R91.8)
CC Exclusion see Appendix A PDX collection 0746
Valid 3-character code, no further characters required

J84 Other interstitial pulmonary diseases

Excludes1: *drug-induced interstitial lung disorders (J70.2-J70.4)*
interstitial emphysema (J98.2)
Excludes2: *lung diseases due to external agents (J60-J70)*

\+ **J84.0 Alveolar and parieto-alveolar conditions**

CC **J84.01 Alveolar proteinosis**
CC Exclusion see Appendix A PDX collection 0747

CC **J84.02 Pulmonary alveolar microlithiasis**
CC Exclusion see Appendix A PDX collection 0747

CC **J84.03 Idiopathic pulmonary hemosiderosis**
Essential brown induration of lung
Code first underlying disease, such as:
disorders of iron metabolism (E83.1-)
Excludes1: *acute idiopathic pulmonary hemorrhage in infants [AIPHI] (R04.81)*
CC Exclusion see Appendix A PDX collection 0747

CC **J84.09 Other alveolar and parieto-alveolar conditions**
CC Exclusion see Appendix A PDX collection 0747

\+ **J84.1 Other interstitial pulmonary diseases with fibrosis**
Excludes1: *pulmonary fibrosis (chronic) due to inhalation of chemicals, gases, fumes or vapors (J68.4)*
pulmonary fibrosis (chronic) following radiation (J70.1)

J84.10 Pulmonary fibrosis, unspecified
Capillary fibrosis of lung
Cirrhosis of lung (chronic) NOS
Fibrosis of lung (atrophic) (chronic) (confluent) (massive) (perialveolar) (peribronchial) NOS
Induration of lung (chronic) NOS
Postinflammatory pulmonary fibrosis

\+ **J84.11 Idiopathic interstitial pneumonia**
Excludes1: *lymphoid interstitial pneumonia (J84.2)*
pneumocystis pneumonia (B59)

J84.111 Idiopathic interstitial pneumonia, not otherwise specified

J84.112 Idiopathic pulmonary fibrosis
Cryptogenic fibrosing alveolitis
Idiopathic fibrosing alveolitis

J84.113 Idiopathic non-specific interstitial pneumonitis
Excludes1: *non-specific interstitial pneumonia NOS, or due to known underlying cause (J84.89)*

CC **J84.114 Acute interstitial pneumonitis**
Hamman-Rich syndrome
Excludes1: *pneumocystis pneumonia (B59)*
CC Exclusion see Appendix A PDX collection 0747

J84.115 Respiratory bronchiolitis interstitial lung disease

CC **J84.116 Cryptogenic organizing pneumonia**
Excludes1: *organizing pneumonia NOS, or due to known underlying cause (J84.89)*
CC Exclusion see Appendix A PDX collection 0747

CC **J84.117 Desquamative interstitial pneumonia**
CC Exclusion see Appendix A PDX collection 0747

J84.17 Other interstitial pulmonary diseases with fibrosis in diseases classified elsewhere
Interstitial pneumonia (nonspecific) (usual) due to collagen vascular disease
Interstitial pneumonia (nonspecific) (usual) in diseases classified elsewhere
Organizing pneumonia due to collagen vascular disease
Organizing pneumonia in diseases classified elsewhere
Code first underlying disease, such as:
progressive systemic sclerosis (M34.0)
rheumatoid arthritis (M05.00-M06.9)
systemic lupus erythematosis (M32.0-M32.9)

CC **J84.2 Lymphoid interstitial pneumonia**
Lymphoid interstitial pneumonitis
CC Exclusion see Appendix A PDX collection 0747

+ **J84.8 Other specified interstitial pulmonary diseases**
Excludes1: *exogenous lipoid pneumonia (J69.1)*
unspecified lipoid pneumonia (J69.1)

MCC **J84.81 Lymphangioleiomyomatosis**
Lymphangiomyomatosis
MCC Exclusion see Appendix A PDX collection 0747

• CC **J84.82 Adult pulmonary Langerhans cell histiocytosis**
Adult PLCH
CC Exclusion see Appendix A PDX collection 0747

MCC **J84.83 Surfactant mutations of the lung**
MCC Exclusion see Appendix A PDX collection 0748

+ **J84.84 Other interstitial lung diseases of childhood**

MCC **J84.841 Neuroendocrine cell hyperplasia of infancy**
MCC Exclusion see Appendix A PDX collection 0748

MCC **J84.842 Pulmonary interstitial glycogenosis**
MCC Exclusion see Appendix A PDX collection 0748

MCC **J84.843 Alveolar capillary dysplasia with vein misalignment**
MCC Exclusion see Appendix A PDX collection 0748

MCC **J84.848 Other interstitial lung diseases of childhood**
MCC Exclusion see Appendix A PDX collection 0748

J84.89 Other specified interstitial pulmonary diseases
Endogenous lipoid pneumonia
Interstitial pneumonitis
Non-specific interstitial pneumonitis NOS
Organizing pneumonia NOS
Code first if applicable:
poisoning due to drug or toxin (T51-T65 with fifth or sixth character to indicate intent), for toxic pneumonopathy
underlying cause of pneumonopathy, if known

Use additional code, for adverse effect, to identify drug (T36-T50 with fifth or sixth character 5), if drug-induced
Excludes1: *cryptogenic organizing pneumonia (J84.116)*
idiopathic non-specific interstitial pneumonitis (J84.113)
lipoid pneumonia, exogenous or unspecified (J69.1)
lymphoid interstitial pneumonia (J84.2)

CC **J84.9 Interstitial pulmonary disease, unspecified**
Interstitial pneumonia NOS
CC Exclusion see Appendix A PDX collection 0747

Suppurative and necrotic conditions of the lower respiratory tract (J85-J86)

J85 Abscess of lung and mediastinum
Use additional code (B95-B97) to identify infectious agent

MCC **J85.0 Gangrene and necrosis of lung**
MCC Exclusion see Appendix A PDX collection 0749

MCC **J85.1 Abscess of lung with pneumonia**
Code also the type of pneumonia
MCC Exclusion see Appendix A PDX collection 0749

MCC **J85.2 Abscess of lung without pneumonia**
Abscess of lung NOS
MCC Exclusion see Appendix A PDX collection 0749

MCC **J85.3 Abscess of mediastinum**
MCC Exclusion see Appendix A PDX collection 0750

J86 Pyothorax
Use additional code (B95-B97) to identify infectious agent
Excludes1: *abscess of lung (J85.-)*
pyothorax due to tuberculosis (A15.6)

MCC **J86.0 Pyothorax with fistula**
Bronchocutaneous fistula
Bronchopleural fistula
Hepatopleural fistula
Mediastinal fistula
Pleural fistula
Thoracic fistula
Any condition classifiable to J86.9 with fistula
MCC Exclusion see Appendix A PDX collection 0751

MCC **J86.9 Pyothorax without fistula**
Abscess of pleura
Abscess of thorax
Empyema (chest) (lung) (pleura)
Fibrinopurulent pleurisy
Purulent pleurisy
Pyopneumothorax
Septic pleurisy
Seropurulent pleurisy
Suppurative pleurisy
MCC Exclusion see Appendix A PDX collection 0751

Other diseases of the pleura (J90-J94)

CC **J90 Pleural effusion, not elsewhere classified**
Encysted pleurisy
Pleural effusion NOS
Pleurisy with effusion (exudative) (serous)
Excludes1: *chylous (pleural) effusion (J94.0)*
malignant pleural effusion (J91.0)
pleurisy NOS (R09.1)
tuberculous pleural effusion (A15.6)
CC Exclusion see Appendix A PDX collection 0752
Valid 3-character code, no further characters required

J91 Pleural effusion in conditions classified elsewhere
Excludes2: *pleural effusion in heart failure (I50.-)*
pleural effusion in systemic lupus erythematosus (M32.1

CC **J91.0 Malignant pleural effusion**
Code first underlying neoplasm
CC Exclusion see Appendix A PDX collection 0753

CC **J91.8 Pleural effusion in other conditions classified elsewhere**
Code first underlying disease, such as:
filariasis (B74.0-B74.9)
influenza (J09.X2, J10.1, J11.1)
CC Exclusion see Appendix A PDX collection 0752
AHA CC: 2Q, 2015, 15-16

J92 Pleural plaque
Includes: pleural thickening
J92.0 Pleural plaque with presence of asbestos
J92.9 Pleural plaque without asbestos
Pleural plaque NOS

J93 Pneumothorax and air leak
Excludes1: *congenital or perinatal pneumothorax (P25.1)*
postprocedural air leak (J95.812)
postprocedural pneumothorax (J95.811)
traumatic pneumothorax (S27.0)
tuberculous (current disease) pneumothorax (A15.-)
pyopneumothorax (J86.-)

MCC **J93.0 Spontaneous tension pneumothorax**
MCC Exclusion see Appendix A PDX collection 0754

+ **J93.1 Other spontaneous pneumothorax**

CC **J93.11 Primary spontaneous pneumothorax**
CC Exclusion see Appendix A PDX collection 0754

CC **J93.12 Secondary spontaneous pneumothorax**
Code first underlying condition, such as:
catamenial pneumothorax due to endometriosis (N80.8)
cystic fibrosis (E84.-)
eosinophilic pneumonia (J82)
lymphangioleiomyomatosis (J84.81)
malignant neoplasm of bronchus and lung (C34.-)
Marfan's syndrome (Q87.4)
pneumonia due to Pneumocystis carinii (B59)
secondary malignant neoplasm of lung (C78.0-)
spontaneous rupture of the esophagus (K22.3)
CC Exclusion see Appendix A PDX collection 0754

+ **J93.8 Other pneumothorax and air leak**
  CC **J93.81 Chronic pneumothorax**
  CC Exclusion see Appendix A PDX collection 0754
  CC **J93.82 Other air leak**
  Persistent air leak
  CC Exclusion see Appendix A PDX collection 0754
  CC **J93.83 Other pneumothorax**
  Acute pneumothorax
  Spontaneous pneumothorax NOS
  CC Exclusion see Appendix A PDX collection 0754
CC **J93.9 Pneumothorax, unspecified**
Pneumothorax NOS
CC Exclusion see Appendix A PDX collection 0754

J94 Other pleural conditions
Excludes1: *pleurisy NOS (R09.1)*
traumatic hemopneumothorax (S27.2)
traumatic hemothorax (S27.1)
tuberculous pleural conditions (current disease) (A15.-)
CC **J94.0 Chylous effusion**
Chyliform effusion
CC Exclusion see Appendix A PDX collection 0752
J94.1 Fibrothorax
CC **J94.2 Hemothorax**
Hemopneumothorax
CC Exclusion see Appendix A PDX collection 0752
CC **J94.8 Other specified pleural conditions**
Hydropneumothorax
Hydrothorax
No CC Exclusions
J94.9 Pleural condition, unspecified

ntraoperative and postprocedural complications and isorders of respiratory system, not elsewhere classified (J95)

J95 Intraoperative and postprocedural complications and disorders of respiratory system, not elsewhere classified
Excludes2: *aspiration pneumonia (J69.-)*
emphysema (subcutaneous) resulting from a procedure (T81.82)
hypostatic pneumonia (J18.2)
pulmonary manifestations due to radiation (J70.0-J70.1)
+ **J95.0 Tracheostomy complications**
  CC **J95.00 Unspecified tracheostomy complication**
  CC Exclusion see Appendix A PDX collection 0755
  CC **J95.01 Hemorrhage from tracheostomy stoma**
  CC Exclusion see Appendix A PDX collection 0755
  CC **J95.02 Infection of tracheostomy stoma**
  Use additional code to identify type of infection, such as:
  cellulitis of neck (L03.221)
  sepsis (A40, A41.-)
  CC Exclusion see Appendix A PDX collection 0755
  CC **J95.03 Malfunction of tracheostomy stoma**
  Mechanical complication of tracheostomy stoma
  Obstruction of tracheostomy airway
  Tracheal stenosis due to tracheostomy
  CC Exclusion see Appendix A PDX collection 0755
  CC **J95.04 Tracheo-esophageal fistula following tracheostomy**
  CC Exclusion see Appendix A PDX collection 0755
  CC **J95.09 Other tracheostomy complication**
  CC Exclusion see Appendix A PDX collection 0755
MCC **J95.1 Acute pulmonary insufficiency following thoracic surgery**
Excludes2: *Functional disturbances following cardiac surgery (I97.0, I97.1-)*
MCC Exclusion see Appendix A PDX collection 0756
MCC **J95.2 Acute pulmonary insufficiency following nonthoracic surgery**
Excludes2: *Functional disturbances following cardiac surgery (I97.0, I97.1-)*
MCC Exclusion see Appendix A PDX collection 0756
MCC **J95.3 Chronic pulmonary insufficiency following surgery**
Excludes2: *Functional disturbances following cardiac surgery (I97.0, I97.1-)*
MCC Exclusion see Appendix A PDX collection 0756
CC **J95.4 Chemical pneumonitis due to anesthesia**
Mendelson's syndrome
Postprocedural aspiration pneumonia
Use additional code for adverse effect, if applicable, to identify drug (T41.- with fifth or sixth character 5)
Excludes1: *aspiration pneumonitis due to anesthesia complicating labor and delivery (O74.0)*
aspiration pneumonitis due to anesthesia complicating pregnancy (O29)
aspiration pneumonitis due to anesthesia complicating the puerperium (O89.01)
CC Exclusion see Appendix A PDX collection 0757
CC **J95.5 Postprocedural subglottic stenosis**
CC Exclusion see Appendix A PDX collection 0757
+ **J95.6 Intraoperative hemorrhage and hematoma of a respiratory system organ or structure complicating a procedure**
Excludes1: *intraoperative hemorrhage and hematoma of a respiratory system organ or structure due to accidental puncture and laceration during procedure (J95.7-)*
  CC **J95.61 Intraoperative hemorrhage and hematoma of a respiratory system organ or structure complicating a respiratory system procedure**
  CC Exclusion see Appendix A PDX collection 0758
  CC **J95.62 Intraoperative hemorrhage and hematoma of a respiratory system organ or structure complicating other procedure**
  CC Exclusion see Appendix A PDX collection 0758
+ **J95.7 Accidental puncture and laceration of a respiratory system organ or structure during a procedure**
Excludes2: *postprocedural pneumothorax (J95.811)*
  CC **J95.71 Accidental puncture and laceration of a respiratory system organ or structure during a respiratory system procedure**
  CC Exclusion see Appendix A PDX collection 0509
  CC **J95.72 Accidental puncture and laceration of a respiratory system organ or structure during other procedure**
  CC Exclusion see Appendix A PDX collection 0509
+ **J95.8 Other intraoperative and postprocedural complications and disorders of respiratory system, not elsewhere classified**
AHA CC: 4Q, 2016, 9-10
  + **J95.81 Postprocedural pneumothorax and air leak**
    CC **J95.811 Postprocedural pneumothorax**
    CC Exclusion see Appendix A PDX collection 0754
    HAC see Appendix B for HAC conditional logic
    CC **J95.812 Postprocedural air leak**
    CC Exclusion see Appendix A PDX collection 0754
  + **J95.82 Postprocedural respiratory failure**
  Excludes1: *Respiratory failure in other conditions (J96.-)*
    MCC **J95.821 Acute postprocedural respiratory failure**
    Postprocedural respiratory failure NOS
    MCC Exclusion see Appendix A PDX collection 0756
    MCC **J95.822 Acute and chronic postprocedural respiratory failure**
    MCC Exclusion see Appendix A PDX collection 0756
  + **J95.83 Postprocedural hemorrhage of a respiratory system organ or structure following a procedure**
    CC **J95.830 Postprocedural hemorrhage of a respiratory system organ or structure following a respiratory system procedure**
    CC Exclusion see Appendix A PDX collection 0758
    CC **J95.831 Postprocedural hemorrhage of a respiratory system organ or structure following other procedure**
    CC Exclusion see Appendix A PDX collection 0758
  CC **J95.84 Transfusion-related acute lung injury (TRALI)**
  CC Exclusion see Appendix A PDX collection 0757
  + **J95.85 Complication of respirator [ventilator]**
    CC **J95.850 Mechanical complication of respirator**
    Excludes1: *encounter for respirator [ventilator] dependence duringpowerfailure(Z99.12)*
    CC Exclusion see Appendix A PDX collection 0759

CC **J95.851** **Ventilator associated pneumonia**
Ventilator associated pneumonitis
Use additional code to identify the organism, if known (B95.-, B96.-, B97.-)
Excludes1: *ventilator lung in newborn (P27.8)*
CC Exclusion see Appendix A PDX collection 0757
Review coding guideline C.10.d.1
AHA CC: 1Q, 2017, 25

CC **J95.859** **Other complication of respirator [ventilator]**
CC Exclusion see Appendix A PDX collection 0757

\+ **J95.86** **Postprocedural hematoma and seroma of a respiratory system organ or structure following a procedure**

CC **J95.860** **Postprocedural hematoma of a respiratory system organ or structure following a respiratory system procedure**
CC Exclusion see Appendix A PDX collection 0758

CC **J95.861** **Postprocedural hematoma of a respiratory system organ or structure following other procedure**
CC Exclusion see Appendix A PDX collection 0758

CC **J95.862** **Postprocedural seroma of a respiratory system organ or structure following a respiratory system procedure**
CC Exclusion see Appendix A PDX collection 0758

CC **J95.863** **Postprocedural seroma of a respiratory system organ or structure following other procedure**
CC Exclusion see Appendix A PDX collection 0758

CC **J95.88** **Other intraoperative complications of respiratory system, not elsewhere classified**
CC Exclusion see Appendix A PDX collection 0757

CC **J95.89** **Other postprocedural complications and disorders of respiratory system, not elsewhere classified**
Use additional code to identify disorder, such as:
aspiration pneumonia (J69.-)
bacterial or viral pneumonia (J12-J18)
Excludes2: *acute pulmonary insufficiency following thoracic surgery (J95.1)*
postprocedural subglottic stenosis (J95.5)
CC Exclusion see Appendix A PDX collection 0757

Other diseases of the respiratory system (J96-J99)

J96 **Respiratory failure, not elsewhere classified**

Excludes1: *acute respiratory distress syndrome (J80)*
cardiorespiratory failure (R09.2)
newborn respiratory distress syndrome (P22.0)
postprocedural respiratory failure (J95.82-)
respiratory arrest (R09.2)
respiratory arrest of newborn (P28.81)
respiratory failure of newborn (P28.5)

\+ **J96.0** **Acute respiratory failure**
Review coding guideline C.10.b

MCC **J96.00** **Acute respiratory failure, unspecified whether with hypoxia or hypercapnia**
MCC Exclusion see Appendix A PDX collection 0744
AHA CC: 4Q, 2013, 121; 3Q, 2016, 14

MCC **J96.01** **Acute respiratory failure with hypoxia**
MCC Exclusion see Appendix A PDX collection 0744

MCC **J96.02** **Acute respiratory failure with hypercapnia**
MCC Exclusion see Appendix A PDX collection 0744

\+ **J96.1** **Chronic respiratory failure**

CC **J96.10** **Chronic respiratory failure, unspecified whether with hypoxia or hypercapnia**
CC Exclusion see Appendix A PDX collection 0744
AHA CC: 1Q, 2015, 21

CC **J96.11** **Chronic respiratory failure with hypoxia**
CC Exclusion see Appendix A PDX collection 0744
AHA CC: 4Q, 2013, 129

CC **J96.12** **Chronic respiratory failure with hypercapnia**
CC Exclusion see Appendix A PDX collection 0744

\+ **J96.2** **Acute and chronic respiratory failure**
Acute on chronic respiratory failure
Review coding guideline C.10.b

MCC **J96.20** **Acute and chronic respiratory failure, unspecified whether with hypoxia or hypercapnia**
MCC Exclusion see Appendix A PDX collection 0744

MCC **J96.21** **Acute and chronic respiratory failure with hypoxia**
MCC Exclusion see Appendix A PDX collection 0744

MCC **J96.22** **Acute and chronic respiratory failure with hypercapnia**
MCC Exclusion see Appendix A PDX collection 0744

\+ **J96.9** **Respiratory failure, unspecified**

MCC **J96.90** **Respiratory failure, unspecified, unspecified whethe with hypoxia or hypercapnia**
MCC Exclusion see Appendix A PDX collection 0744

MCC **J96.91** **Respiratory failure, unspecified with hypoxia**
MCC Exclusion see Appendix A PDX collection 0744

MCC **J96.92** **Respiratory failure, unspecified with hypercapnia**
MCC Exclusion see Appendix A PDX collection 0744

J98 **Other respiratory disorders**

Use additional code to identify:
exposure to environmental tobacco smoke (Z77.22)
exposure to tobacco smoke in the perinatal period (P96.81)
history of tobacco dependence (Z87.891)
occupational exposure to environmental tobacco smoke (Z57.31)
tobacco dependence (F17.-)
tobacco use (Z72.0)
Excludes1: *newborn apnea (P28.4)*
newborn sleep apnea (P28.3)
Excludes2: *apnea NOS (R06.81)*
sleep apnea (G47.3-)

\+ **J98.0** **Diseases of bronchus, not elsewhere classified**

J98.01 **Acute bronchospasm**
Excludes1: *acute bronchiolitis with bronchospasm (J21.-)*
acute bronchitis with bronchospasm (J20.-)
asthma (J45.-)
exercise induced bronchospasm (J45.990)

J98.09 **Other diseases of bronchus, not elsewhere classified**
Broncholithiasis
Calcification of bronchus
Stenosis of bronchus
Tracheobronchial collapse
Tracheobronchial dyskinesia
Ulcer of bronchus

\+ **J98.1** **Pulmonary collapse**
Excludes1: *therapeutic collapse of lung status (Z98.3)*

CC **J98.11** **Atelectasis**
Excludes1: *newborn atelectasis tuberculous atelectasis (current disease) (A15)*
CC Exclusion see Appendix A PDX collection 0760

CC **J98.19** **Other pulmonary collapse**
CC Exclusion see Appendix A PDX collection 0760

J98.2 **Interstitial emphysema**
Mediastinal emphysema
Excludes1: *emphysema NOS (J43.9)*
emphysema in newborn (P25.0)
surgical emphysema (subcutaneous) (T81.82)
traumatic subcutaneous emphysema (T79.7)

J98.3 **Compensatory emphysema**

J98.4 **Other disorders of lung**
Calcification of lung
Cystic lung disease (acquired)
Lung disease NOS
Pulmolithiasis
Excludes1: *acute interstitial pneumonitis (J84.114)*
pulmonary insufficiency following surgery (J95.1-J95.2)

\+ **J98.5** **Diseases of mediastinum, not elsewhere classified**
Excludes2: *abscess of mediastinum (J85.3)*
AHA CC: 4Q, 2016, 29

MCC **J98.51** **Mediastinitis**
Code first underlying condition, if applicable, such as postoperative mediastinitis (T81.-)
No MCC Exclusions

MCC **J98.59** **Other diseases of mediastinum, not elsewhere classified**
Fibrosis of mediastinum
Hernia of mediastinum
Retraction of mediastinum
No MCC Exclusions

J98.6 Disorders of diaphragm
Diaphragmatitis
Paralysis of diaphragm
Relaxation of diaphragm
Excludes1: *congenital malformation of diaphragm NEC (Q79.1)*
congenital diaphragmatic hernia (Q79.0)
Excludes2: *diaphragmatic hernia (K44.-)*

J98.8 Other specified respiratory disorders

J98.9 Respiratory disorder, unspecified
Respiratory disease (chronic) NOS

J99 Respiratory disorders in diseases classified elsewhere
Code first underlying disease, such as:
amyloidosis (E85.-)
ankylosing spondylitis (M45)
congenital syphilis (A50.5)
cryoglobulinemia (D89.1)
early congenital syphilis (A50.0)
schistosomiasis (B65.0-B65.9)
Excludes1: *respiratory disorders in:*
amebiasis (A06.5)
blastomycosis (B40.0-B40.2)
candidiasis (B37.1)
coccidioidomycosis (B38.0-B38.2)
cystic fibrosis with pulmonary manifestations (E84.0)
dermatomyositis (M33.01, M33.11)
histoplasmosis (B39.0-B39.2)
late syphilis (A52.72, A52.73)
polymyositis (M33.21)
sicca syndrome (M35.02)
systemic lupus erythematosus (M32.13)
systemic sclerosis (M34.81)
Wegener's granulomatosis (M31.30-M31.31)
Valid 3-character code, no further characters required

Chapter 11: Diseases of the Digestive System (K00-K95)

Excludes2: *certain conditions originating in the perinatal period (P04-P96)*
certain infectious and parasitic diseases (A00-B99)
complications of pregnancy, childbirth and the puerperium (O00-O9A)
congenital malformations, deformations and chromosomal abnormalities (Q00-Q99)
endocrine, nutritional and metabolic diseases (E00-E88)
injury, poisoning and certain other consequences of external causes (S00-T88)
neoplasms (C00-D49)
symptoms, signs and abnormal clinical and laboratory findings, not elsewhere classified (R00-R94)

This chapter contains the following category blocks:

K00-K14 Diseases of oral cavity and salivary glands
K20-K31 Diseases of esophagus, stomach and duodenum
K35-K38 Diseases of appendix
K40-K46 Hernia
K50-K52 Noninfective enteritis and colitis
K55-K64 Other diseases of intestines
K65-K68 Diseases of peritoneum and retroperitoneum
K70-K77 Diseases of liver
K80-K87 Disorders of gallbladder, biliary tract and pancreas
K90-K95 Other diseases of the digestive system

C. Chapter-Specific Coding Guidelines

In addition to general coding guidelines, there are guidelines for specific diagnoses and/or conditions in the classification. Unless otherwise indicated, these guidelines apply to all health care settings. Please refer to Section II for guidelines on the selection of principal diagnosis.

11. Chapter 11: Diseases of the Digestive System (K00-K95)

Reserved for future guideline expansion

Diseases of oral cavity and salivary glands (K00-K14)

K00 Disorders of tooth development and eruption

Excludes2: *embedded and impacted teeth (K01.-)*

K00.0 Anodontia
Hypodontia
Oligodontia
Excludes1: *acquired absence of teeth (K08.1-)*

K00.1 Supernumerary teeth
Distomolar
Fourth molar
Mesiodens
Paramolar
Supplementary teeth
Excludes2: *supernumerary roots (K00.2)*

K00.2 Abnormalities of size and form of teeth
Concrescence of teeth
Fusion of teeth
Gemination of teeth
Dens evaginatus
Dens in dente
Dens invaginatus
Enamel pearls
Macrodontia
Microdontia
Peg-shaped [conical] teeth
Supernumerary roots
Taurodontism
Tuberculum paramolare
Excludes1: *abnormalities of teeth due to congenital syphilis (A50.5)*
tuberculum Carabelli, which is regarded as a normal variation and should not be coded

K00.3 Mottled teeth
Dental fluorosis
Mottling of enamel
Nonfluoride enamel opacities
Excludes2: *deposits [accretions] on teeth (K03.6)*

K00.4 Disturbances in tooth formation
Aplasia and hypoplasia of cementum
Dilaceration of tooth
Enamel hypoplasia (neonatal) (postnatal) (prenatal)
Regional odontodysplasia
Turner's tooth
Excludes1: *Hutchinson's teeth and mulberry molars in congenital syphilis (A50.5)*
Excludes2: *mottled teeth (K00.3)*

K00.5 Hereditary disturbances in tooth structure, not elsewhere classified
Amelogenesis imperfecta
Dentinogenesis imperfecta
Odontogenesis imperfecta
Dentinal dysplasia
Shell teeth

Oral Cavity

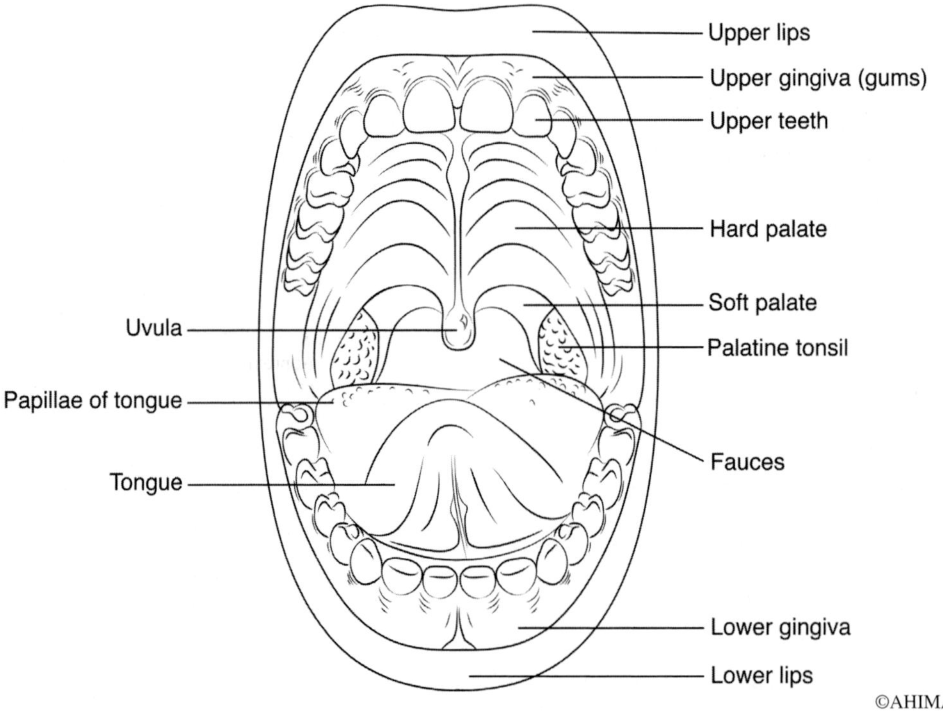

Glands of the Oral Cavity

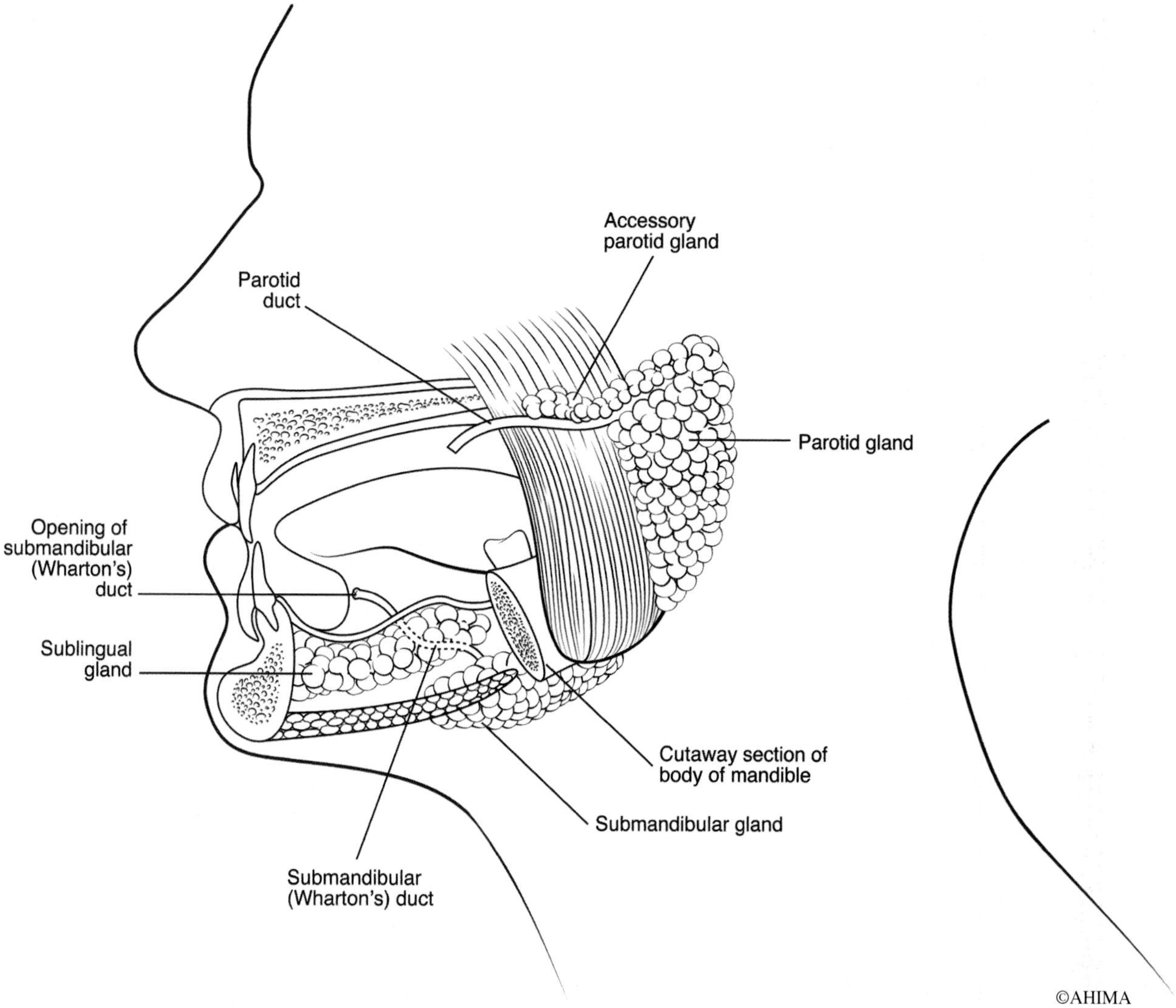

K00.6 Disturbances in tooth eruption
Dentia praecox
Natal tooth
Neonatal tooth
Premature eruption of tooth
Premature shedding of primary [deciduous] tooth
Prenatal teeth
Retained [persistent] primary tooth
Excludes2: *embedded and impacted teeth (K01.-)*

K00.7 Teething syndrome

K00.8 Other disorders of tooth development
Color changes during tooth formation
Intrinsic staining of teeth NOS
Excludes2: *posteruptive color changes (K03.7)*

K00.9 Disorder of tooth development, unspecified
Disorder of odontogenesis NOS

K01 Embedded and impacted teeth

Excludes1: *abnormal position of fully erupted teeth (M26.3-)*

K01.0 Embedded teeth

K01.1 Impacted teeth

K02 Dental caries

Includes: caries of dentine
dental cavities
early childhood caries
pre-eruptive caries
recurrent caries (dentino enamel junction) (enamel) (to the pulp)
tooth decay

K02.3 Arrested dental caries
Arrested coronal and root caries

+ **K02.5 Dental caries on pit and fissure surface**
Dental caries on chewing surface of tooth

K02.51 Dental caries on pit and fissure surface limited to enamel
White spot lesions [initial caries] on pit and fissure surface of tooth

K02.52 Dental caries on pit and fissure surface penetrating into dentin
Primary dental caries, cervical origin

K02.53 Dental caries on pit and fissure surface penetrating into pulp

+ **K02.6 Dental caries on smooth surface**

K02.61 Dental caries on smooth surface limited to enamel
White spot lesions [initial caries] on smooth surface of tooth

K02.62 Dental caries on smooth surface penetrating into dentin

K02.63 Dental caries on smooth surface penetrating into pulp

K02.7 Dental root caries

K02.9 Dental caries, unspecified

K03 Other diseases of hard tissues of teeth

Excludes2: *bruxism (F45.8)*
dental caries (K02.-)
teeth-grinding NOS (F45.8)

K03.0 Excessive attrition of teeth
Approximal wear of teeth
Occlusal wear of teeth

K03.1 Abrasion of teeth
Dentifrice abrasion of teeth
Habitual abrasion of teeth
Occupational abrasion of teeth
Ritual abrasion of teeth
Traditional abrasion of teeth
Wedge defect NOS

K03.2 Erosion of teeth
Erosion of teeth due to diet
Erosion of teeth due to drugs and medicaments
Erosion of teeth due to persistent vomiting
Erosion of teeth NOS
Idiopathic erosion of teeth
Occupational erosion of teeth

K03.3 Pathological resorption of teeth
Internal granuloma of pulp
Resorption of teeth (external)
K03.4 Hypercementosis
Cementation hyperplasia
K03.5 Ankylosis of teeth
K03.6 Deposits [accretions] on teeth
Betel deposits [accretions] on teeth
Black deposits [accretions] on teeth
Extrinsic staining of teeth NOS
Green deposits [accretions] on teeth
Materia alba deposits [accretions] on teeth
Orange deposits [accretions] on teeth
Staining of teeth NOS
Subgingival dental calculus
Supragingival dental calculus
Tobacco deposits [accretions] on teeth
K03.7 Posteruptive color changes of dental hard tissues
Excludes2: *deposits [accretions] on teeth (K03.6)*
+ **K03.8 Other specified diseases of hard tissues of teeth**
K03.81 Cracked tooth
Excludes1: *asymptomatic craze lines in enamel - omit code*
broken or fractured tooth due to trauma (S02.5)
K03.89 Other specified diseases of hard tissues of teeth
K03.9 Disease of hard tissues of teeth, unspecified

K04 Diseases of pulp and periapical tissues

AHA CC: 4Q, 2016, 29-30

+ **K04.0 Pulpitis**
Acute pulpitis
Chronic (hyperplastic) (ulcerative) pulpitis
CC **K04.01 Reversible pulpitis**
CC Exclusion see Appendix A PDX collection 0761
CC **K04.02 Irreversible pulpitis**
CC Exclusion see Appendix A PDX collection 0761
K04.1 Necrosis of pulp
Pulpal gangrene
K04.2 Pulp degeneration
Denticles
Pulpal calcifications
Pulpal stones
K04.3 Abnormal hard tissue formation in pulp
Secondary or irregular dentine
CC **K04.4 Acute apical periodontitis of pulpal origin**
Acute apical periodontitis NOS
Excludes1: *acute periodontitis (K05.2-)*
CC Exclusion see Appendix A PDX collection 0761
K04.5 Chronic apical periodontitis
Apical or periapical granuloma
Apical periodontitis NOS
Excludes1: *chronic periodontitis (K05.3-)*
K04.6 Periapical abscess with sinus
Dental abscess with sinus
Dentoalveolar abscess with sinus
K04.7 Periapical abscess without sinus
Dental abscess without sinus
Dentoalveolar abscess without sinus
K04.8 Radicular cyst
Apical (periodontal) cyst
Periapical cyst
Residual radicular cyst
Excludes2: *lateral periodontal cyst (K09.0)*
+ **K04.9 Other and unspecified diseases of pulp and periapical tissues**
K04.90 Unspecified diseases of pulp and periapical tissues
K04.99 Other diseases of pulp and periapical tissues

K05 Gingivitis and periodontal diseases

Use additional code to identify:
alcohol abuse and dependence (F10.-)
exposure to environmental tobacco smoke (Z77.22)
exposure to tobacco smoke in the perinatal period (P96.81)
history of tobacco dependence (Z87.891)
occupational exposure to environmental tobacco smoke (Z57.31)
tobacco dependence (F17.-)
tobacco use (Z72.0)
AHA CC: 4Q, 2016, 29-30

+ **K05.0 Acute gingivitis**
Excludes1: *acute necrotizing ulcerative gingivitis (A69.1)*
herpesviral [herpes simplex] gingivostomatitis (B00.
K05.00 Acute gingivitis, plaque induced
Acute gingivitis NOS
Plaque induced gingival disease
K05.01 Acute gingivitis, non-plaque induced
+ **K05.1 Chronic gingivitis**
Desquamative gingivitis (chronic)
Gingivitis (chronic) NOS
Hyperplastic gingivitis (chronic)
Pregnancy associated gingivitis
Simple marginal gingivitis (chronic)
Ulcerative gingivitis (chronic)
Code first, if applicable, diseases of the digestive system complicating pregnancy (O99.61-)
K05.10 Chronic gingivitis, plaque induced
Chronic gingivitis NOS
Gingivitis NOS
K05.11 Chronic gingivitis, non-plaque induced
+ **K05.2 Aggressive periodontitis**
Acute pericoronitis
Excludes1: *acute apical periodontitis (K04.4)*
periapical abscess (K04.7)
periapical abscess with sinus (K04.6)
K05.20 Aggressive periodontitis, unspecified
+ **K05.21 Aggressive periodontitis, localized**
Periodontal abscess
K05.211 Aggressive periodontitis, localized, slight
K05.212 Aggressive periodontitis, localized, moderate
K05.213 Aggressive periodontitis, localized, severe
K05.219 Aggressive periodontitis, localized, unspecified severity
+ **K05.22 Aggressive periodontitis, generalized**
K05.221 Aggressive periodontitis, generalized, slig
K05.222 Aggressive periodontitis, generalized, moderate
K05.223 Aggressive periodontitis, generalized, severe
K05.229 Aggressive periodontitis, generalized, unspecified severity
+ **K05.3 Chronic periodontitis**
Chronic pericoronitis
Complex periodontitis
Periodontitis NOS
Simplex periodontitis
Excludes1: *chronic apical periodontitis (K04.5)*
K05.30 Chronic periodontitis, unspecified
+ **K05.31 Chronic periodontitis, localized**
K05.311 Chronic periodontitis, localized, slight
K05.312 Chronic periodontitis, localized, moderate
K05.313 Chronic periodontitis, localized, severe
K05.319 Chronic periodontitis, localized, unspecified severity
+ **K05.32 Chronic periodontitis, generalized**
K05.321 Chronic periodontitis, generalized, slight
K05.322 Chronic periodontitis, generalized, modera
K05.323 Chronic periodontitis, generalized, severe
K05.329 Chronic periodontitis, generalized, unspecified severity
K05.4 Periodontosis
Juvenile periodontosis
K05.5 Other periodontal diseases
Combined periodontic-endodontic lesion
Narrow gingival width (of periodontal soft tissue)
Excludes2: *leukoplakia of gingiva (K13.21)*
K05.6 Periodontal disease, unspecified

K06 Other disorders of gingiva and edentulous alveolar ridge

Excludes2: *acute gingivitis (K05.0)*
atrophy of edentulous alveolar ridge (K08.2)
chronic gingivitis (K05.1)
gingivitis NOS (K05.1)
AHA CC: 4Q, 2016, 29-30
K06.0 Gingival recession
Gingival recession (postinfective) (postprocedural)
+ **K06.01 Gingival recession, localized**
K06.010 Localized gingival recession, unspecified
Localized gingival recession, NOS
K06.011 Localized gingival recession, minimal

K06.012 Localized gingival recession, moderate
K06.013 Localized gingival recession, severe
+ **K06.02 Gingival recession, generalized**
K06.020 Generalized gingival recession, unspecified
Generalized gingival recession, NOS
K06.021 Generalized gingival recession, minimal
K06.022 Generalized gingival recession, moderate
K06.023 Generalized gingival recession, severe

K06.1 Gingival enlargement
Gingival fibromatosis

K06.2 Gingival and edentulous alveolar ridge lesions associated with trauma
Irritative hyperplasia of edentulous ridge [denture hyperplasia]
Use additional code (Chapter 20) to identify external cause or denture status (Z97.2)

K06.3 Horizontal alveolar bone loss

K06.8 Other specified disorders of gingiva and edentulous alveolar ridge
Fibrous epulis
Flabby alveolar ridge
Giant cell epulis
Peripheral giant cell granuloma of gingiva
Pyogenic granuloma of gingiva
Vertical ridge deficiency
Excludes2: *gingival cyst (K09.0)*

K06.9 Disorder of gingiva and edentulous alveolar ridge, unspecified

K08 Other disorders of teeth and supporting structures
Excludes2: *dentofacial anomalies [including malocclusion] (M26.-)*
disorders of jaw (M27.-)
AHA CC: 4Q, 2016, 29-30

K08.0 Exfoliation of teeth due to systemic causes
Code also underlying systemic condition

+ **K08.1 Complete loss of teeth**
Acquired loss of teeth, complete
Excludes1: *congenital absence of teeth (K00.0)*
exfoliation of teeth due to systemic causes (K08.0)
partial loss of teeth (K08.4-)

+ **K08.10 Complete loss of teeth, unspecified cause**
K08.101 Complete loss of teeth, unspecified cause, class I
K08.102 Complete loss of teeth, unspecified cause, class II
K08.103 Complete loss of teeth, unspecified cause, class III
K08.104 Complete loss of teeth, unspecified cause, class IV
K08.109 Complete loss of teeth, unspecified cause, unspecified class
Edentulism NOS

+ **K08.11 Complete loss of teeth due to trauma**
K08.111 Complete loss of teeth due to trauma, class I
K08.112 Complete loss of teeth due to trauma, class II
K08.113 Complete loss of teeth due to trauma, class III
K08.114 Complete loss of teeth due to trauma, class IV
K08.119 Complete loss of teeth due to trauma, unspecified class

+ **K08.12 Complete loss of teeth due to periodontal diseases**
K08.121 Complete loss of teeth due to periodontal diseases, class I
K08.122 Complete loss of teeth due to periodontal diseases, class II
K08.123 Complete loss of teeth due to periodontal diseases, class III
K08.124 Complete loss of teeth due to periodontal diseases, class IV
K08.129 Complete loss of teeth due to periodontal diseases, unspecified class

+ **K08.13 Complete loss of teeth due to caries**
K08.131 Complete loss of teeth due to caries, class I
K08.132 Complete loss of teeth due to caries, class II
K08.133 Complete loss of teeth due to caries, class III
K08.134 Complete loss of teeth due to caries, class IV
K08.139 Complete loss of teeth due to caries, unspecified class

+ **K08.19 Complete loss of teeth due to other specified cause**
K08.191 Complete loss of teeth due to other specified cause, class I
K08.192 Complete loss of teeth due to other specified cause, class II
K08.193 Complete loss of teeth due to other specified cause, class III
K08.194 Complete loss of teeth due to other specified cause, class IV
K08.199 Complete loss of teeth due to other specified cause, unspecified class

+ **K08.2 Atrophy of edentulous alveolar ridge**
K08.20 Unspecified atrophy of edentulous alveolar ridge
Atrophy of the mandible NOS
Atrophy of the maxilla NOS
K08.21 Minimal atrophy of the mandible
Minimal atrophy of the edentulous mandible
K08.22 Moderate atrophy of the mandible
Moderate atrophy of the edentulous mandible
K08.23 Severe atrophy of the mandible
Severe atrophy of the edentulous mandible
K08.24 Minimal atrophy of maxilla
Minimal atrophy of the edentulous maxilla
K08.25 Moderate atrophy of the maxilla
Moderate atrophy of the edentulous maxilla
K08.26 Severe atrophy of the maxilla
Severe atrophy of the edentulous maxilla

K08.3 Retained dental root

+ **K08.4 Partial loss of teeth**
Acquired loss of teeth, partial
Excludes1: *complete loss of teeth (K08.1-)*
congenital absence of teeth (K00.0)
Excludes2: *exfoliation of teeth due to systemic causes (K08.0)*

+ **K08.40 Partial loss of teeth, unspecified cause**
K08.401 Partial loss of teeth, unspecified cause, class I
K08.402 Partial loss of teeth, unspecified cause, class II
K08.403 Partial loss of teeth, unspecified cause, class III
K08.404 Partial loss of teeth, unspecified cause, class IV
K08.409 Partial loss of teeth, unspecified cause, unspecified class
Tooth extraction status NOS

+ **K08.41 Partial loss of teeth due to trauma**
K08.411 Partial loss of teeth due to trauma, class I
K08.412 Partial loss of teeth due to trauma, class II
K08.413 Partial loss of teeth due to trauma, class III
K08.414 Partial loss of teeth due to trauma, class IV
K08.419 Partial loss of teeth due to trauma, unspecified class

+ **K08.42 Partial loss of teeth due to periodontal diseases**
K08.421 Partial loss of teeth due to periodontal diseases, class I
K08.422 Partial loss of teeth due to periodontal diseases, class II
K08.423 Partial loss of teeth due to periodontal diseases, class III
K08.424 Partial loss of teeth due to periodontal diseases, class IV
K08.429 Partial loss of teeth due to periodontal diseases, unspecified class

+ **K08.43 Partial loss of teeth due to caries**
K08.431 Partial loss of teeth due to caries, class I
K08.432 Partial loss of teeth due to caries, class II
K08.433 Partial loss of teeth due to caries, class III
K08.434 Partial loss of teeth due to caries, class IV
K08.439 Partial loss of teeth due to caries, unspecified class

+ **K08.49 Partial loss of teeth due to other specified cause**
K08.491 Partial loss of teeth due to other specified cause, class I
K08.492 Partial loss of teeth due to other specified cause, class II
K08.493 Partial loss of teeth due to other specified cause, class III
K08.494 Partial loss of teeth due to other specified cause, class IV
K08.499 Partial loss of teeth due to other specified cause, unspecified class

+ **K08.5 Unsatisfactory restoration of tooth**
Defective bridge, crown, filling
Defective dental restoration
Excludes1: *dental restoration status (Z98.811)*
Excludes2: *endosseous dental implant failure (M27.6-)*
unsatisfactory endodontic treatment (M27.5-)
K08.50 Unsatisfactory restoration of tooth, unspecified
Defective dental restoration NOS

K08.51 **Open restoration margins of tooth**
Dental restoration failure of marginal integrity
Open margin on tooth restoration
Poor gingival margin to tooth restoration

K08.52 **Unrepairable overhanging of dental restorative materials**
Overhanging of tooth restoration

\+ K08.53 **Fractured dental restorative material**
Excludes1: *cracked tooth (K03.81)*
traumatic fracture of tooth (S02.5)

K08.530 **Fractured dental restorative material without loss of material**

K08.531 **Fractured dental restorative material with loss of material**

K08.539 **Fractured dental restorative material, unspecified**

K08.54 **Contour of existing restoration of tooth biologically incompatible with oral health**
Dental restoration failure of periodontal anatomical integrity
Unacceptable contours of existing restoration of tooth
Unacceptable morphology of existing restoration of tooth

K08.55 **Allergy to existing dental restorative material**
Use additional code to identify the specific type of allergy

K08.56 **Poor aesthetic of existing restoration of tooth**
Dental restoration aesthetically inadequate or displeasing

K08.59 **Other unsatisfactory restoration of tooth**
Other defective dental restoration

\+ K08.8 **Other specified disorders of teeth and supporting structures**

K08.81 **Primary occlusal trauma**

K08.82 **Secondary occlusal trauma**

K08.89 **Other specified disorders of teeth and supporting structures**
Enlargement of alveolar ridge NOS
Insufficient anatomic crown height
Insufficient clinical crown length
Irregular alveolar process
Toothache NOS

K08.9 **Disorder of teeth and supporting structures, unspecified**

K09 Cysts of oral region, not elsewhere classified

Includes: lesions showing histological features both of aneurysmal cyst and of another fibro-osseous lesion
Excludes2: *cysts of jaw (M27.0-, M27.4-)*
radicular cyst (K04.8)

K09.0 **Developmental odontogenic cysts**
Dentigerous cyst
Eruption cyst
Follicular cyst
Gingival cyst
Lateral periodontal cyst
Primordial cyst
Excludes2: *keratocysts (D16.4, D16.5)*
odontogenic keratocystic tumors (D16.4, D16.5)

K09.1 **Developmental (nonodontogenic) cysts of oral region**
Cyst (of) incisive canal
Cyst (of) palatine of papilla
Globulomaxillary cyst
Median palatal cyst
Nasoalveolar cyst
Nasolabial cyst
Nasopalatine duct cyst

K09.8 **Other cysts of oral region, not elsewhere classified**
Dermoid cyst
Epidermoid cyst
Lymphoepithelial cyst
Epstein's pearl

K09.9 **Cyst of oral region, unspecified**

K11 Diseases of salivary glands

Use additional code to identify:
alcohol abuse and dependence (F10.-)
exposure to environmental tobacco smoke (Z77.22)
exposure to tobacco smoke in the perinatal period (P96.81)
history of tobacco dependence (Z87.891)
occupational exposure to environmental tobacco smoke (Z57.31)
tobacco dependence (F17.-)
tobacco use (Z72.0)

K11.0 **Atrophy of salivary gland**

K11.1 **Hypertrophy of salivary gland**

\+ K11.2 **Sialoadenitis**
Parotitis
Excludes1: *epidemic parotitis (B26.-)*
mumps (B26.-)
uveoparotid fever [Heerfordt] (D86.89)

K11.20 **Sialoadenitis, unspecified**

K11.21 **Acute sialoadenitis**
Excludes1: *acute recurrent sialoadenitis (K11.22)*

K11.22 **Acute recurrent sialoadenitis**

K11.23 **Chronic sialoadenitis**

CC K11.3 **Abscess of salivary gland**
CC Exclusion see Appendix A PDX collection 0762

CC K11.4 **Fistula of salivary gland**
Excludes1: *congenital fistula of salivary gland (Q38.4)*
CC Exclusion see Appendix A PDX collection 0762

K11.5 **Sialolithiasis**
Calculus of salivary gland or duct
Stone of salivary gland or duct

K11.6 **Mucocele of salivary gland**
Mucous extravasation cyst of salivary gland
Mucous retention cyst of salivary gland
Ranula

K11.7 **Disturbances of salivary secretion**
Hypoptyalism
Ptyalism
Xerostomia
Excludes2: *dry mouth NOS (R68.2)*

K11.8 **Other diseases of salivary glands**
Benign lymphoepithelial lesion of salivary gland
Mikulicz' disease
Necrotizing sialometaplasia
Sialectasia
Stenosis of salivary duct
Stricture of salivary duct
Excludes1: *sicca syndrome [Sjögren] (M35.0-)*

K11.9 **Disease of salivary gland, unspecified**
Sialoadenopathy NOS

K12 Stomatitis and related lesions

Use additional code to identify:
alcohol abuse and dependence (F10.-)
exposure to environmental tobacco smoke (Z77.22)
exposure to tobacco smoke in the perinatal period (P96.81)
history of tobacco dependence (Z87.891)
occupational exposure to environmental tobacco smoke (Z57.31)
tobacco dependence (F17.-)
tobacco use (Z72.0)
Excludes1: *cancrum oris (A69.0)*
cheilitis (K13.0)
gangrenous stomatitis (A69.0)
herpesviral [herpes simplex] gingivostomatitis (B00.2)
noma (A69.0)

K12.0 **Recurrent oral aphthae**
Aphthous stomatitis (major) (minor)
Bednar's aphthae
Periadenitis mucosa necrotica recurrens
Recurrent aphthous ulcer
Stomatitis herpetiformis

K12.1 **Other forms of stomatitis**
Stomatitis NOS
Denture stomatitis
Ulcerative stomatitis
Vesicular stomatitis
Excludes1: *acute necrotizing ulcerative stomatitis (A69.1)*
Vincent's stomatitis (A69.1)

CC K12.2 **Cellulitis and abscess of mouth**
Cellulitis of mouth (floor)
Submandibular abscess
Excludes2: *abscess of salivary gland (K11.3)*
abscess of tongue (K14.0)
periapical abscess (K04.6-K04.7)
periodontal abscess (K05.21)
peritonsillar abscess (J36)
CC Exclusion see Appendix A PDX collection 0763

\+ K12.3 **Oral mucositis (ulcerative)**
Mucositis (oral) (oropharyneal)
Excludes2: *gastrointestinal mucositis (ulcerative) (K92.81)*
mucositis (ulcerative) of vagina and vulva (N76.81)
nasal mucositis (ulcerative) (J34.81)

K12.30 **Oral mucositis (ulcerative), unspecified**

K12.31 Oral mucositis (ulcerative) due to antineoplastic therapy
Use additional code for adverse effect, if applicable, to identify antineoplastic and immunosuppressive drugs (T45.1X5)
Use additional code for other antineoplastic therapy, such as: radiological procedure and radiotherapy (Y84.2)
K12.32 Oral mucositis (ulcerative) due to other drugs
Use additional code for adverse effect, if applicable, to identify drug (T36-T50 with fifth or sixth character 5)
K12.33 Oral mucositis (ulcerative) due to radiation
Use additional external cause code (W88-W90, X39.0-) to identify cause
K12.39 Other oral mucositis (ulcerative)
Viral oral mucositis (ulcerative)

K13 Other diseases of lip and oral mucosa
Includes: epithelial disturbances of tongue
Use additional code to identify:
alcohol abuse and dependence (F10.-)
exposure to environmental tobacco smoke (Z77.22)
exposure to tobacco smoke in the perinatal period (P96.81)
history of tobacco dependence (Z87.891)
occupational exposure to environmental tobacco smoke (Z57.31)
tobacco dependence (F17.-)
tobacco use (Z72.0)
Excludes2: *certain disorders of gingiva and edentulous alveolar ridge (K05-K06)*
cysts of oral region (K09.-)
diseases of tongue (K14.-)
stomatitis and related lesions (K12.-)
K13.0 Diseases of lips
Abscess of lips
Angular cheilitis
Cellulitis of lips
Cheilitis NOS
Cheilodynia
Cheilosis
Exfoliative cheilitis
Fistula of lips
Glandular cheilitis
Hypertrophy of lips
Perlèche NEC
Excludes1: *ariboflavinosis (E53.0)*
cheilitis due to radiation-related disorders (L55-L59)
congenital fistula of lips (Q38.0)
congenital hypertrophy of lips (Q18.6)
Perlèche due to candidiasis (B37.83)
Perlèche due to riboflavin deficiency (E53.0)
K13.1 Cheek and lip biting
+ **K13.2 Leukoplakia and other disturbances of oral epithelium, including tongue**
Excludes1: *carcinoma in situ of oral epithelium (D00.0-)*
hairy leukoplakia (K13.3)
K13.21 Leukoplakia of oral mucosa, including tongue
Leukokeratosis of oral mucosa
Leukoplakia of gingiva, lips, tongue
Excludes1: *hairy leukoplakia (K13.3)*
leukokeratosis nicotina palati (K13.24)
K13.22 Minimal keratinized residual ridge mucosa
Minimal keratinization of alveolar ridge mucosa
K13.23 Excessive keratinized residual ridge mucosa
Excessive keratinization of alveolar ridge mucosa
K13.24 Leukokeratosis nicotina palati
Smoker's palate
K13.29 Other disturbances of oral epithelium, including tongue
Erythroplakia of mouth or tongue
Focal epithelial hyperplasia of mouth or tongue
Leukoedema of mouth or tongue
Other oral epithelium disturbances
K13.3 Hairy leukoplakia
K13.4 Granuloma and granuloma-like lesions of oral mucosa
Eosinophilic granuloma
Granuloma pyogenicum
Verrucous xanthoma
K13.5 Oral submucous fibrosis
Submucous fibrosis of tongue
K13.6 Irritative hyperplasia of oral mucosa
Excludes2: *irritative hyperplasia of edentulous ridge [denture hyperplasia] (K06.2)*
+ **K13.7 Other and unspecified lesions of oral mucosa**
K13.70 Unspecified lesions of oral mucosa
K13.79 Other lesions of oral mucosa
Focal oral mucinosis

K14 Diseases of tongue
Use additional code to identify:
alcohol abuse and dependence (F10.-)
exposure to environmental tobacco smoke (Z77.22)
history of tobacco dependence (Z87.891)
occupational exposure to environmental tobacco smoke (Z57.31)
tobacco dependence (F17.-)
tobacco use (Z72.0)
Excludes2: *erythroplakia (K13.29)*
focal epithelial hyperplasia (K13.29)
leukedema of tongue (K13.29)
leukoplakia of tongue (K13.21)
hairy leukoplakia (K13.3)
macroglossia (congenital) (Q38.2)
submucous fibrosis of tongue (K13.5)
K14.0 Glossitis
Abscess of tongue
Ulceration (traumatic) of tongue
Excludes1: *atrophic glossitis (K14.4)*
K14.1 Geographic tongue
Benign migratory glossitis
Glossitis areata exfoliativa
K14.2 Median rhomboid glossitis
K14.3 Hypertrophy of tongue papillae
Black hairy tongue
Coated tongue
Hypertrophy of foliate papillae
Lingua villosa nigra
K14.4 Atrophy of tongue papillae
Atrophic glossitis
K14.5 Plicated tongue
Fissured tongue
Furrowed tongue
Scrotal tongue
Excludes1: *fissured tongue, congenital (Q38.3)*
K14.6 Glossodynia
Glossopyrosis
Painful tongue
K14.8 Other diseases of tongue
Atrophy of tongue
Crenated tongue
Enlargement of tongue
Glossocele
Glossoptosis
Hypertrophy of tongue
K14.9 Disease of tongue, unspecified
Glossopathy NOS

Diseases of esophagus, stomach and duodenum (K20-K31)

Excludes2: *hiatus hernia (K44.-)*

K20 Esophagitis
Use additional code to identify:
alcohol abuse and dependence (F10.-)
Excludes1: *erosion of esophagus (K22.1-)*
esophagitis with gastro-esophageal reflux disease (K21.0)
reflux esophagitis (K21.0)
ulcerative esophagitis (K22.1-)
Excludes2: *eosinophilic gastritis or gastroenteritis (K52.81)*
K20.0 Eosinophilic esophagitis
K20.8 Other esophagitis
Abscess of esophagus
K20.9 Esophagitis, unspecified Esophagitis NOS

K21 Gastro-esophageal reflux disease
Excludes1: *newborn esophageal reflux (P78.83)*
K21.0 Gastro-esophageal reflux disease with esophagitis
Reflux esophagitis
K21.9 Gastro-esophageal reflux disease without esophagitis
Esophageal reflux NOS
CC AHA: 1Q, 2016, 18

K22 Other diseases of esophagus
Excludes2: *esophageal varices (I85.-)*
K22.0 Achalasia of cardia
Achalasia NOS
Cardiospasm
Excludes1: *congenital cardiospasm (Q39.5)*

Gastrointestinal System Side View

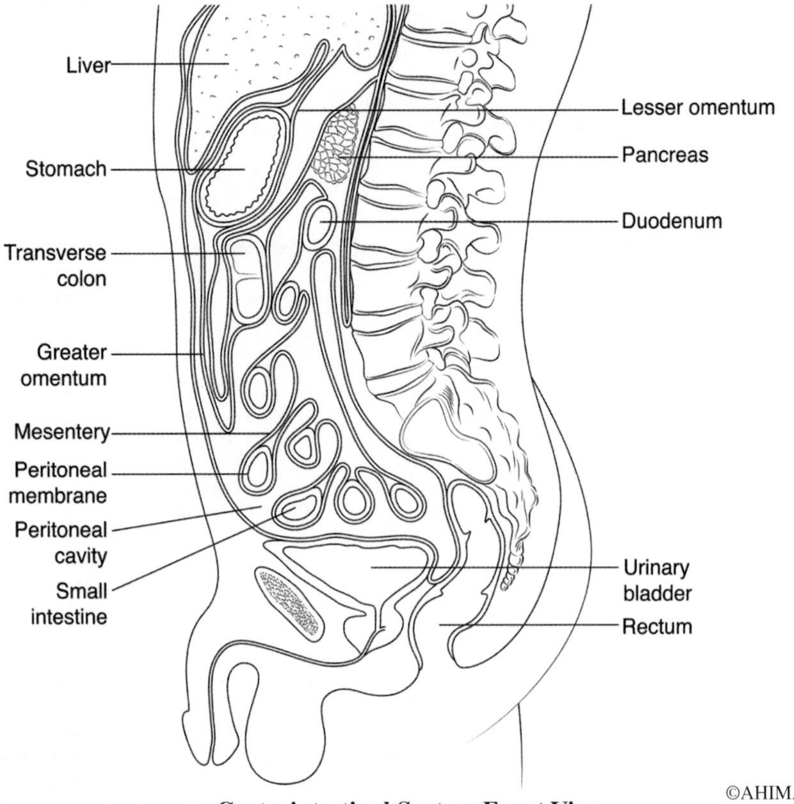

©AHIMA

Gastrointestinal System Front View

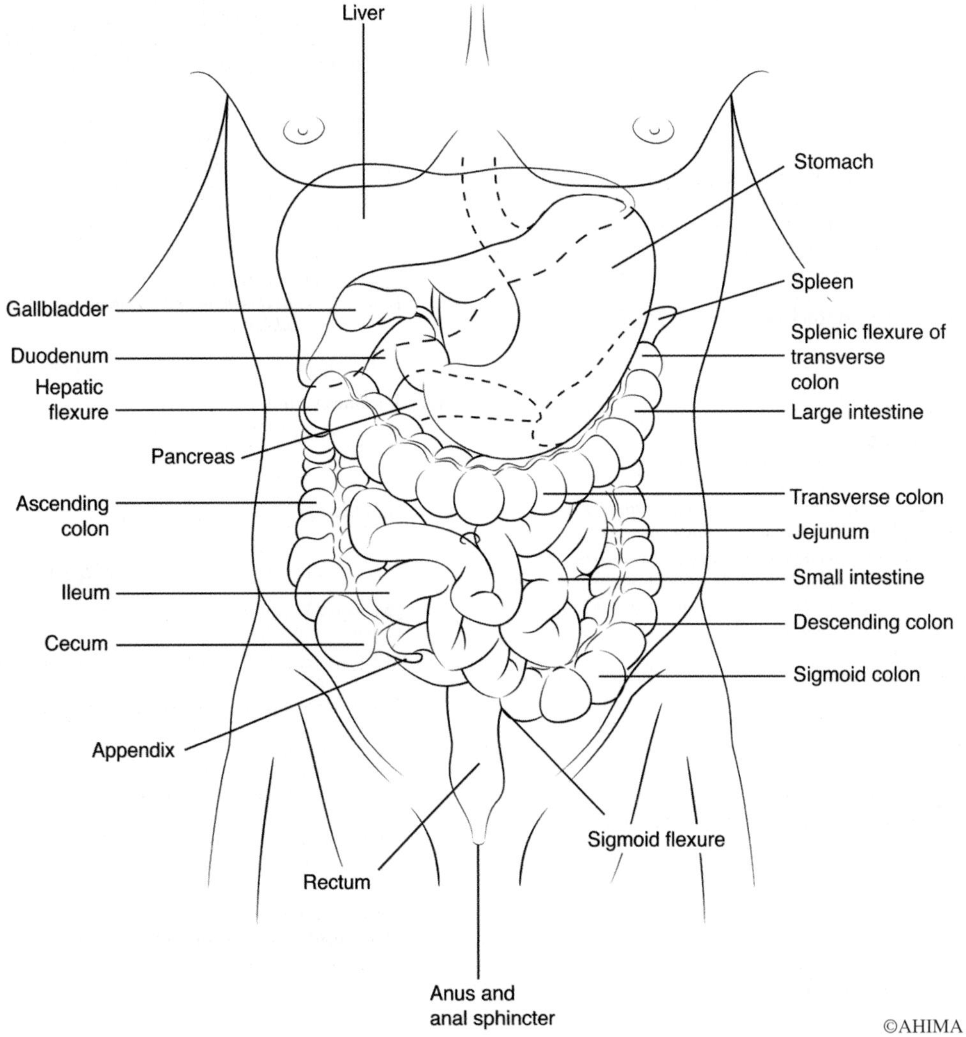

©AHIMA

Upper Gastrointestinal System

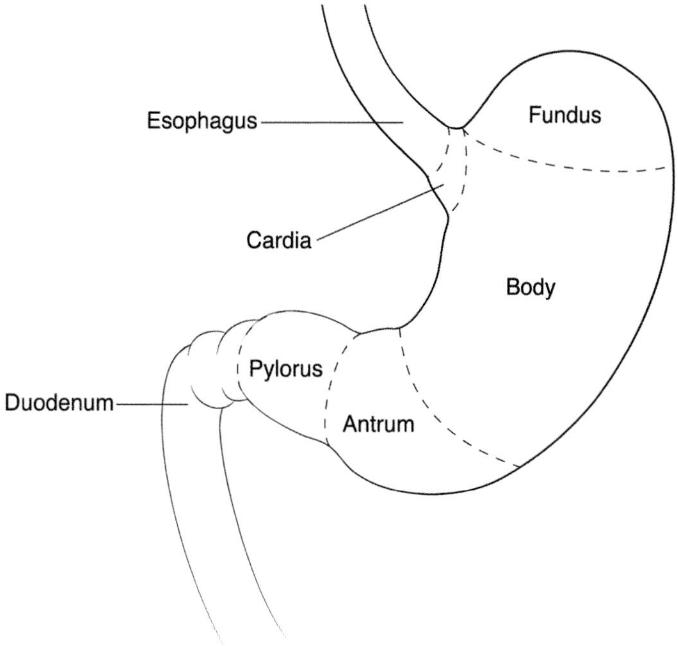

+ **K22.1 Ulcer of esophagus**
  Barrett's ulcer
  Erosion of esophagus
  Fungal ulcer of esophagus
  Peptic ulcer of esophagus
  Ulcer of esophagus due to ingestion of chemicals
  Ulcer of esophagus due to ingestion of drugs and medicaments
  Ulcerative esophagitis
  Code first poisoning due to drug or toxin, if applicable (T36-T65 with fifth or sixth character 1-4 or 6)

  Use additional code for adverse effect, if applicable, to identify drug (T36-T50 with fifth or sixth character 5)
  Excludes1: *Barrett's esophagus (K22.7-)*

CC **K22.10 Ulcer of esophagus without bleeding**
  Ulcer of esophagus NOS
  CC Exclusion see Appendix A PDX collection 0764

MCC **K22.11 Ulcer of esophagus with bleeding**
  Excludes2: *bleeding esophageal varices (I85.01, I85.11)*
  MCC Exclusion see Appendix A PDX collection 0765

K22.2 Esophageal obstruction
  Compression of esophagus
  Constriction of esophagus
  Stenosis of esophagus
  Stricture of esophagus
  Excludes1: *congenital stenosis or stricture of esophagus (Q39.3)*

MCC **K22.3 Perforation of esophagus**
  Rupture of esophagus
  Excludes1: *traumatic perforation of (thoracic) esophagus (S27.8-)*
  MCC Exclusion see Appendix A PDX collection 0766

K22.4 Dyskinesia of esophagus
  Corkscrew esophagus
  Diffuse esophageal spasm
  Spasm of esophagus
  Excludes1: *cardiospasm (K22.0)*

K22.5 Diverticulum of esophagus, acquired
  Esophageal pouch, acquired
  Excludes1: *diverticulum of esophagus (congenital) (Q39.6)*

MCC **K22.6 Gastro-esophageal laceration-hemorrhage syndrome**
  Mallory-Weiss syndrome
  MCC Exclusion see Appendix A PDX collection 0767

+ **K22.7 Barrett's esophagus**
  Barrett's disease
  Barrett's syndrome
  Excludes1: *Barrett's ulcer (K22.1)*
  malignant neoplasm of esophagus (C15.-)

K22.70 Barrett's esophagus without dysplasia
  Barrett's esophagus NOS

+ **K22.71 Barrett's esophagus with dysplasia**
  K22.710 Barrett's esophagus with low grade dysplasia
  K22.711 Barrett's esophagus with high grade dysplasia
  K22.719 Barrett's esophagus with dysplasia, unspecified

K22.8 Other specified diseases of esophagus
  Hemorrhage of esophagus NOS
  Excludes2: *esophageal varices (I85.-)*
  Paterson-Kelly syndrome (D50.1)

K22.9 Disease of esophagus, unspecified

K23 Disorders of esophagus in diseases classified elsewhere
  Code first underlying disease, such as:
  congenital syphilis (A50.5)
  Excludes1: *late syphilis (A52.79)*
  megaesophagus due to Chagas' disease (B57.31)
  tuberculosis (A18.83)
  Valid 3-character code, no further characters required

K25 Gastric ulcer
  Includes: erosion (acute) of stomach
  pylorus ulcer (peptic)
  stomach ulcer (peptic)
  Use additional code to identify:
  alcohol abuse and dependence (F10.-)
  Excludes1: *acute gastritis (K29.0-)*
  peptic ulcer NOS (K27.-)

MCC **K25.0 Acute gastric ulcer with hemorrhage**
  MCC Exclusion see Appendix A PDX collection 0765

MCC **K25.1 Acute gastric ulcer with perforation**
  MCC Exclusion see Appendix A PDX collection 0765

MCC **K25.2 Acute gastric ulcer with both hemorrhage and perforation**
  MCC Exclusion see Appendix A PDX collection 0765

CC **K25.3 Acute gastric ulcer without hemorrhage or perforation**
  CC Exclusion see Appendix A PDX collection 0765

MCC **K25.4 Chronic or unspecified gastric ulcer with hemorrhage**
  MCC Exclusion see Appendix A PDX collection 0765

MCC **K25.5 Chronic or unspecified gastric ulcer with perforation**
  MCC Exclusion see Appendix A PDX collection 0765

MCC **K25.6 Chronic or unspecified gastric ulcer with both hemorrhage and perforation**
  MCC Exclusion see Appendix A PDX collection 0765

K25.7 Chronic gastric ulcer without hemorrhage or perforation

K25.9 Gastric ulcer, unspecified as acute or chronic, without hemorrhage or perforation

K26 Duodenal ulcer

Includes: erosion (acute) of duodenum
duodenum ulcer (peptic)
postpyloric ulcer (peptic)

Use additional code to identify:
alcohol abuse and dependence (F10.-)

Excludes1: *peptic ulcer NOS (K27.-)*

MCC **K26.0 Acute duodenal ulcer with hemorrhage**
MCC Exclusion see Appendix A PDX collection 0768

K26.1 Acute duodenal ulcer with perforation
MCC Exclusion see Appendix A PDX collection 0768

K26.2 Acute duodenal ulcer with both hemorrhage and perforation
MCC Exclusion see Appendix A PDX collection 0768

CC **K26.3 Acute duodenal ulcer without hemorrhage or perforation**
CC Exclusion see Appendix A PDX collection 0769

MCC **K26.4 Chronic or unspecified duodenal ulcer with hemorrhage**
MCC Exclusion see Appendix A PDX collection 0768
CC AHA: 1Q, 2016, 14

MCC **K26.5 Chronic or unspecified duodenal ulcer with perforation**
MCC Exclusion see Appendix A PDX collection 0768

MCC **K26.6 Chronic or unspecified duodenal ulcer with both hemorrhage and perforation**
MCC Exclusion see Appendix A PDX collection 0768

K26.7 Chronic duodenal ulcer without hemorrhage or perforation

K26.9 Duodenal ulcer, unspecified as acute or chronic, without hemorrhage or perforation

K27 Peptic ulcer, site unspecified

Includes: gastroduodenal ulcer NOS
peptic ulcer NOS

Use additional code to identify:
alcohol abuse and dependence (F10.-)

Excludes1: *peptic ulcer of newborn (P78.82)*

MCC **K27.0 Acute peptic ulcer, site unspecified, with hemorrhage**
MCC Exclusion see Appendix A PDX collection 0768

MCC **K27.1 Acute peptic ulcer, site unspecified, with perforation**
MCC Exclusion see Appendix A PDX collection 0768

K27.2 Acute peptic ulcer, site unspecified, with both hemorrhage and perforation
MCC Exclusion see Appendix A PDX collection 0768

CC **K27.3 Acute peptic ulcer, site unspecified, without hemorrhage or perforation**
CC Exclusion see Appendix A PDX collection 0768

MCC **K27.4 Chronic or unspecified peptic ulcer, site unspecified, with hemorrhage**
MCC Exclusion see Appendix A PDX collection 0768

MCC **K27.5 Chronic or unspecified peptic ulcer, site unspecified, with perforation**
MCC Exclusion see Appendix A PDX collection 0768

MCC **K27.6 Chronic or unspecified peptic ulcer, site unspecified, with both hemorrhage and perforation**
MCC Exclusion see Appendix A PDX collection 0768

K27.7 Chronic peptic ulcer, site unspecified, without hemorrhage or perforation

K27.9 Peptic ulcer, site unspecified, unspecified as acute or chronic, without hemorrhage or perforation

K28 Gastrojejunal ulcer

Includes: anastomotic ulcer (peptic) or erosion
gastrocolic ulcer (peptic) or erosion
gastrointestinal ulcer (peptic) or erosion
gastrojejunal ulcer (peptic) or erosion
jejunal ulcer (peptic) or erosion
marginal ulcer (peptic) or erosion
stomal ulcer (peptic) or erosion

Use additional code to identify:
alcohol abuse and dependence (F10.-)

Excludes1: *primary ulcer of small intestine (K63.3)*

MCC **K28.0 Acute gastrojejunal ulcer with hemorrhage**
MCC Exclusion see Appendix A PDX collection 0765

MCC **K28.1 Acute gastrojejunal ulcer with perforation**
MCC Exclusion see Appendix A PDX collection 0765

MCC **K28.2 Acute gastrojejunal ulcer with both hemorrhage and perforation**
MCC Exclusion see Appendix A PDX collection 0765

CC **K28.3 Acute gastrojejunal ulcer without hemorrhage or perforation**
CC Exclusion see Appendix A PDX collection 0765

MCC **K28.4 Chronic or unspecified gastrojejunal ulcer with hemorrhage**
MCC Exclusion see Appendix A PDX collection 0765

MCC **K28.5 Chronic or unspecified gastrojejunal ulcer with perforation**
MCC Exclusion see Appendix A PDX collection 0765

MCC **K28.6 Chronic or unspecified gastrojejunal ulcer with both hemorrhage and perforation**
MCC Exclusion see Appendix A PDX collection 0765

K28.7 Chronic gastrojejunal ulcer without hemorrhage or perforatio

K28.9 Gastrojejunal ulcer, unspecified as acute or chronic, without hemorrhage or perforation

K29 Gastritis and duodenitis

Excludes1: *eosinophilic gastritis or gastroenteritis (K52.81)*
Zollinger-Ellison syndrome (E16.4)

\+ **K29.0 Acute gastritis**

Use additional code to identify:
alcohol abuse and dependence (F10.-)

Excludes1: *erosion (acute) of stomach (K25.-)*

K29.00 Acute gastritis without bleeding

MCC **K29.01 Acute gastritis with bleeding**
MCC Exclusion see Appendix A PDX collection 0770

\+ **K29.2 Alcoholic gastritis**

Use additional code to identify:
alcohol abuse and dependence (F10.-)

K29.20 Alcoholic gastritis without bleeding

MCC **K29.21 Alcoholic gastritis with bleeding**
MCC Exclusion see Appendix A PDX collection 0770

\+ **K29.3 Chronic superficial gastritis**

K29.30 Chronic superficial gastritis without bleeding

MCC **K29.31 Chronic superficial gastritis with bleeding**
MCC Exclusion see Appendix A PDX collection 0770

\+ **K29.4 Chronic atrophic gastritis**

Gastric atrophy

K29.40 Chronic atrophic gastritis without bleeding

MCC **K29.41 Chronic atrophic gastritis with bleeding**
MCC Exclusion see Appendix A PDX collection 0770

\+ **K29.5 Unspecified chronic gastritis**

Chronic antral gastritis
Chronic fundal gastritis

K29.50 Unspecified chronic gastritis without bleeding

MCC **K29.51 Unspecified chronic gastritis with bleeding**
MCC Exclusion see Appendix A PDX collection 0770

\+ **K29.6 Other gastritis**

Giant hypertrophic gastritis
Granulomatous gastritis
Ménétrier's disease

K29.60 Other gastritis without bleeding

MCC **K29.61 Other gastritis with bleeding**
MCC Exclusion see Appendix A PDX collection 0770

\+ **K29.7 Gastritis, unspecified**

K29.70 Gastritis, unspecified, without bleeding

MCC **K29.71 Gastritis, unspecified, with bleeding**
MCC Exclusion see Appendix A PDX collection 0770

\+ **K29.8 Duodenitis**

K29.80 Duodenitis without bleeding

MCC **K29.81 Duodenitis with bleeding**
MCC Exclusion see Appendix A PDX collection 0770

\+ **K29.9 Gastroduodenitis, unspecified**

K29.90 Gastroduodenitis, unspecified, without bleeding

MCC **K29.91 Gastroduodenitis, unspecified, with bleeding**
MCC Exclusion see Appendix A PDX collection 0770

K30 Functional dyspepsia

Indigestion

Excludes1: *dyspepsia NOS (R10.13)*
heartburn (R12)
nervous dyspepsia (F45.8)
neurotic dyspepsia (F45.8)
psychogenic dyspepsia (F45.8)

Valid 3-character code, no further characters required

K31 Other diseases of stomach and duodenum

Includes: functional disorders of stomach

Excludes2: *diabetic gastroparesis (E08.43, E09.43, E10.43, E11.43, E13.43)*
diverticulum of duodenum (K57.00-K57.13)

CC **K31.0 Acute dilatation of stomach**
Acute distention of stomach
CC Exclusion see Appendix A PDX collection 0771

• CC **K31.1 Adult hypertrophic pyloric stenosis**
Pyloric stenosis NOS

Excludes1: *congenital or infantile pyloric stenosis (Q40.0)*

CC Exclusion see Appendix A PDX collection 0772

K31.2 Hourglass stricture and stenosis of stomach

Excludes1: *congenital hourglass stomach (Q40.2)*
hourglass contraction of stomach (K31.89)

K31.3 Pylorospasm, not elsewhere classified

Excludes1: *congenital or infantile pylorospasm (Q40.0)*
neurotic pylorospasm (F45.8)
psychogenic pylorospasm (F45.8)v

K31.4 Gastric diverticulum
Excludes1: congenital diverticulum of stomach (Q40.2)

CC **K31.5 Obstruction of duodenum**
Constriction of duodenum
Duodenal ileus (chronic)
Stenosis of duodenum
Stricture of duodenum
Volvulus of duodenum
Excludes1: congenital stenosis of duodenum (Q41.0)
CC Exclusion see Appendix A PDX collection 0773

CC **K31.6 Fistula of stomach and duodenum**
Gastrocolic fistula
Gastrojejunocolic fistula
CC Exclusion see Appendix A PDX collection 0774

K31.7 Polyp of stomach and duodenum
Excludes1: adenomatous polyp of stomach (D13.1)

+ **K31.8 Other specified diseases of stomach and duodenum**

+ **K31.81 Angiodysplasia of stomach and duodenum**

MCC **K31.811 Angiodysplasia of stomach and duodenum with bleeding**
MCC Exclusion see Appendix A PDX collection 0770

K31.819 Angiodysplasia of stomach and duodenum without bleeding
Angiodysplasia of stomach and duodenum NOS

MCC **K31.82 Dieulafoy lesion (hemorrhagic) of stomach and duodenum**
Excludes2: Dieulafoy lesion of intestine (K63.81)
MCC Exclusion see Appendix A PDX collection 0775

K31.83 Achlorhydria

K31.84 Gastroparesis
Gastroparalysis
Code first underlying disease, if known, such as:
anorexia nervosa (F50.0-)
diabetes mellitus (E08.43, E09.43, E10.43, E11.43, E13.43)
scleroderma (M34.-)
AHA CC: 4Q, 2013, 114-115

K31.89 Other diseases of stomach and duodenum
AHA CC: 1Q, 2017, 28

K31.9 Disease of stomach and duodenum, unspecified

Diseases of appendix (K35-K38)

K35 Acute appendicitis

MCC **K35.2 Acute appendicitis with generalized peritonitis**
Appendicitis (acute) with generalized (diffuse) peritonitis following rupture or perforation of appendix
Perforated appendix NOS
Ruptured appendix NOS
MCC Exclusion see Appendix A PDX collection 0776

MCC **K35.3 Acute appendicitis with localized peritonitis**
Acute appendicitis with or without perforation or rupture with peritonitis NOS
Acute appendicitis with or without perforation or rupture with localized peritonitis
Acute appendicitis with peritoneal abscess
MCC Exclusion see Appendix A PDX collection 0776

+ **K35.8 Other and unspecified acute appendicitis**

CC **K35.80 Unspecified acute appendicitis**
Acute appendicitis NOS
Acute appendicitis without (localized) (generalized) peritonitis
CC Exclusion see Appendix A PDX collection 0776

CC **K35.89 Other acute appendicitis**
CC Exclusion see Appendix A PDX collection 0776

K36 Other appendicitis

Chronic appendicitis
Recurrent appendicitis
Valid 3-character code, no further characters required

K37 Unspecified appendicitis

Excludes1: ~~unspecified appendicitis with peritonitis (K35.2-K35.3)~~
Valid 3-character code, no further characters required

K38 Other diseases of appendix

K38.0 Hyperplasia of appendix

K38.1 Appendicular concretions
Fecalith of appendix
Stercolith of appendix

K38.2 Diverticulum of appendix

K38.3 Fistula of appendix

K38.8 Other specified diseases of appendix
Intussusception of appendix

K38.9 Disease of appendix, unspecified

Hernia (K40-K46)

NOTE Hernia with both gangrene and obstruction is classified to hernia with gangrene.

Includes: acquired hernia
congenital [except diaphragmatic or hiatus] hernia
recurrent hernia

K40 Inguinal hernia

Includes: bubonocele
direct inguinal hernia
double inguinal hernia
indirect inguinal hernia
inguinal hernia NOS
oblique inguinal hernia
scrotal hernia

+ **K40.0 Bilateral inguinal hernia, with obstruction, without gangrene**
Inguinal hernia (bilateral) causing obstruction without gangrene
Incarcerated inguinal hernia (bilateral) without gangrene
Irreducible inguinal hernia (bilateral) without gangrene
Strangulated inguinal hernia (bilateral) without gangrene

CC **K40.00 Bilateral inguinal hernia, with obstruction, without gangrene, not specified as recurrent**
Bilateral inguinal hernia, with obstruction, without gangrene NOS
CC Exclusion see Appendix A PDX collection 0777

CC **K40.01 Bilateral inguinal hernia, with obstruction, without gangrene, recurrent**
CC Exclusion see Appendix A PDX collection 0777

+ **K40.1 Bilateral inguinal hernia, with gangrene**

MCC **K40.10 Bilateral inguinal hernia, with gangrene, not specified as recurrent**
Bilateral inguinal hernia, with gangrene NOS
MCC Exclusion see Appendix A PDX collection 0777

MCC **K40.11 Bilateral inguinal hernia, with gangrene, recurrent**
MCC Exclusion see Appendix A PDX collection 0777

+ **K40.2 Bilateral inguinal hernia, without obstruction or gangrene**

K40.20 Bilateral inguinal hernia, without obstruction or gangrene, not specified as recurrent
Bilateral inguinal hernia NOS

K40.21 Bilateral inguinal hernia, without obstruction or gangrene, recurrent

+ **K40.3 Unilateral inguinal hernia, with obstruction, without gangrene**
Inguinal hernia (unilateral) causing obstruction without gangrene
Incarcerated inguinal hernia (unilateral) without gangrene
Irreducible inguinal hernia (unilateral) without gangrene
Strangulated inguinal hernia (unilateral) without gangrene

CC **K40.30 Unilateral inguinal hernia, with obstruction, without gangrene, not specified as recurrent**
Inguinal hernia, with obstruction NOS
Unilateral inguinal hernia, with obstruction, without gangrene NOS
CC Exclusion see Appendix A PDX collection 0777

CC **K40.31 Unilateral inguinal hernia, with obstruction, without gangrene, recurrent**
CC Exclusion see Appendix A PDX collection 0777

+ **K40.4 Unilateral inguinal hernia, with gangrene**

MCC **K40.40 Unilateral inguinal hernia, with gangrene, not specified as recurrent**
Inguinal hernia with gangrene NOS
Unilateral inguinal hernia with gangrene NOS
MCC Exclusion see Appendix A PDX collection 0777

MCC **K40.41 Unilateral inguinal hernia, with gangrene, recurrent**
MCC Exclusion see Appendix A PDX collection 0777

+ **K40.9 Unilateral inguinal hernia, without obstruction or gangrene**

K40.90 Unilateral inguinal hernia, without obstruction or gangrene, not specified as recurrent
Inguinal hernia NOS
Unilateral inguinal hernia NOS

K40.91 Unilateral inguinal hernia, without obstruction or gangrene, recurrent

K41 Femoral hernia

+ **K41.0 Bilateral femoral hernia, with obstruction, without gangrene**
Femoral hernia (bilateral) causing obstruction, without gangrene
Incarcerated femoral hernia (bilateral), without gangrene
Irreducible femoral hernia (bilateral), without gangrene
Strangulated femoral hernia (bilateral), without gangrene

CC **K41.00 Bilateral femoral hernia, with obstruction, without gangrene, not specified as recurrent**
Bilateral femoral hernia, with obstruction, without gangrene NOS
CC Exclusion see Appendix A PDX collection 0778

CC **K41.01 Bilateral femoral hernia, with obstruction, without gangrene, recurrent**
CC Exclusion see Appendix A PDX collection 0778

\+ **K41.1 Bilateral femoral hernia, with gangrene**

MCC **K41.10 Bilateral femoral hernia, with gangrene, not specified as recurrent**
Bilateral femoral hernia, with gangrene NOS
MCC Exclusion see Appendix A PDX collection 0779

MCC **K41.11 Bilateral femoral hernia, with gangrene, recurrent**
MCC Exclusion see Appendix A PDX collection 0779

\+ **K41.2 Bilateral femoral hernia, without obstruction or gangrene**

K41.20 Bilateral femoral hernia, without obstruction or gangrene, not specified as recurrent
Bilateral femoral hernia NOS

K41.21 Bilateral femoral hernia, without obstruction or gangrene, recurrent

\+ **K41.3 Unilateral femoral hernia, with obstruction, without gangrene**
Femoral hernia (unilateral) causing obstruction, without gangrene
Incarcerated femoral hernia (unilateral), without gangrene
Irreducible femoral hernia (unilateral), without gangrene
Strangulated femoral hernia (unilateral), without gangrene

CC **K41.30 Unilateral femoral hernia, with obstruction, without gangrene, not specified as recurrent**
Femoral hernia, with obstruction NOS
Unilateral femoral hernia, with obstruction NOS
CC Exclusion see Appendix A PDX collection 0778

CC **K41.31 Unilateral femoral hernia, with obstruction, without gangrene, recurrent**
CC Exclusion see Appendix A PDX collection 0778

\+ **K41.4 Unilateral femoral hernia, with gangrene**

MCC **K41.40 Unilateral femoral hernia, with gangrene, not specified as recurrent**
Femoral hernia, with gangrene NOS
Unilateral femoral hernia, with gangrene NOS
MCC Exclusion see Appendix A PDX collection 0779

MCC **K41.41 Unilateral femoral hernia, with gangrene, recurrent**
MCC Exclusion see Appendix A PDX collection 0779

\+ **K41.9 Unilateral femoral hernia, without obstruction or gangrene**

K41.90 Unilateral femoral hernia, without obstruction or gangrene, not specified as recurrent
Femoral hernia NOS
Unilateral femoral hernia NOS

K41.91 Unilateral femoral hernia, without obstruction or gangrene, recurrent

K42 Umbilical hernia

Includes: paraumbilical hernia
Excludes1: *omphalocele (Q79.2)*

CC **K42.0 Umbilical hernia with obstruction, without gangrene**
Umbilical hernia causing obstruction, without gangrene
Incarcerated umbilical hernia, without gangrene
Irreducible umbilical hernia, without gangrene
Strangulated umbilical hernia, without gangrene
CC Exclusion see Appendix A PDX collection 0780

MCC **K42.1 Umbilical hernia with gangrene**
Gangrenous umbilical hernia
MCC Exclusion see Appendix A PDX collection 0781

K42.9 Umbilical hernia without obstruction or gangrene
Umbilical hernia NOS

K43 Ventral hernia

CC **K43.0 Incisional hernia with obstruction, without gangrene**
Incisional hernia causing obstruction, without gangrene
Incarcerated incisional hernia, without gangrene
Irreducible incisional hernia, without gangrene
Strangulated incisional hernia, without gangrene
CC Exclusion see Appendix A PDX collection 0780

MCC **K43.1 Incisional hernia with gangrene**
Gangrenous incisional hernia
MCC Exclusion see Appendix A PDX collection 0781

K43.2 Incisional hernia without obstruction or gangrene
Incisional hernia NOS

CC **K43.3 Parastomal hernia with obstruction, without gangrene**
Incarcerated parastomal hernia, without gangrene
Irreducible parastomal hernia, without gangrene
Parastomal hernia causing obstruction, without gangrene
Strangulated parastomal hernia, without gangrene
CC Exclusion see Appendix A PDX collection 0780

MCC **K43.4 Parastomal hernia with gangrene**
Gangrenous parastomal hernia
MCC Exclusion see Appendix A PDX collection 0781

K43.5 Parastomal hernia without obstruction or gangrene
Parastomal hernia NOS

CC **K43.6 Other and unspecified ventral hernia with obstruction, without gangrene**
Epigastric hernia causing obstruction, without gangrene
Hypogastric hernia causing obstruction, without gangrene
Incarcerated epigastric hernia without gangrene
Incarcerated hypogastric hernia without gangrene
Incarcerated midline hernia without gangrene
Incarcerated spigelian hernia without gangrene
Incarcerated subxiphoid hernia without gangrene
Irreducible epigastric hernia without gangrene
Irreducible hypogastric hernia without gangrene
Irreducible midline hernia without gangrene
Irreducible spigelian hernia without gangrene
Irreducible subxiphoid hernia without gangrene
Midline hernia causing obstruction, without gangrene
Spigelian hernia causing obstruction, without gangrene
Strangulated epigastric hernia without gangrene
Strangulated hypogastric hernia without gangrene
Strangulated midline hernia without gangrene
Strangulated spigelian hernia without gangrene
Strangulated subxiphoid hernia without gangrene
Subxiphoid hernia causing obstruction, without gangrene
CC Exclusion see Appendix A PDX collection 0780

MCC **K43.7 Other and unspecified ventral hernia with gangrene**
Any condition listed under K43.6 specified as gangrenous
MCC Exclusion see Appendix A PDX collection 0781

K43.9 Ventral hernia without obstruction or gangrene
Epigastric hernia
Ventral hernia NOS

K44 Diaphragmatic hernia

Includes: hiatus hernia (esophageal) (sliding)
paraesophageal hernia
Excludes1: *congenital diaphragmatic hernia (Q79.0)*
congenital hiatus hernia (Q40.1)

CC **K44.0 Diaphragmatic hernia with obstruction, without gangrene**
Diaphragmatic hernia causing obstruction
Incarcerated diaphragmatic hernia
Irreducible diaphragmatic hernia
Strangulated diaphragmatic hernia
CC Exclusion see Appendix A PDX collection 0782

MCC **K44.1 Diaphragmatic hernia with gangrene**
Gangrenous diaphragmatic hernia
MCC Exclusion see Appendix A PDX collection 0782

K44.9 Diaphragmatic hernia without obstruction or gangrene
Diaphragmatic hernia NOS

K45 Other abdominal hernia

Includes: abdominal hernia, specified site NEC
lumbar hernia
obturator hernia
pudendal hernia
retroperitoneal hernia
sciatic hernia

CC **K45.0 Other specified abdominal hernia with obstruction, without gangrene**
Other specified abdominal hernia causing obstruction
Other specified incarcerated abdominal hernia
Other specified irreducible abdominal hernia
Other specified strangulated abdominal hernia
CC Exclusion see Appendix A PDX collection 0783

MCC **K45.1 Other specified abdominal hernia with gangrene**
Any condition listed under K45 specified as gangrenous
MCC Exclusion see Appendix A PDX collection 0784

K45.8 Other specified abdominal hernia without obstruction or gangrene

K46 Unspecified abdominal hernia

Includes: enterocele
epiplocele
hernia NOS
interstitial hernia
intestinal hernia
intra-abdominal hernia

Excludes1: *vaginal enterocele (N81.5)*

CC **K46.0 Unspecified abdominal hernia with obstruction, without gangrene**
Unspecified abdominal hernia causing obstruction
Unspecified incarcerated abdominal hernia
Unspecified irreducible abdominal hernia
Unspecified strangulated abdominal hernia
CC Exclusion see Appendix A PDX collection 0783

MCC **K46.1 Unspecified abdominal hernia with gangrene**
Any condition listed under K46 specified as gangrenous
MCC Exclusion see Appendix A PDX collection 0784

K46.9 Unspecified abdominal hernia without obstruction or gangrene
Abdominal hernia NOS

Noninfective enteritis and colitis (K50-K52)

Includes: noninfective inflammatory bowel disease

Excludes1: *irritable bowel syndrome (K58.-)*
megacolon (K59.3-)

K50 Crohn's disease [regional enteritis]

Includes: granulomatous enteritis
Use additional code to identify manifestations, such as:
pyoderma gangrenosum (L88)

Excludes1: *ulcerative colitis (K51.-)*

\+ **K50.0 Crohn's disease of small intestine**
Crohn's disease [regional enteritis] of duodenum
Crohn's disease [regional enteritis] of ileum
Crohn's disease [regional enteritis] of jejunum
Regional ileitis
Terminal ileitis
Excludes1: *Crohn's disease of both small and large intestine (K50.8-)*

CC **K50.00 Crohn's disease of small intestine without complications**
CC Exclusion see Appendix A PDX collection 0785

\+ **K50.01 Crohn's disease of small intestine with complications**

CC **K50.011 Crohn's disease of small intestine with rectal bleeding**
CC Exclusion see Appendix A PDX collection 0785

CC **K50.012 Crohn's disease of small intestine with intestinal obstruction**
CC Exclusion see Appendix A PDX collection 0785

CC **K50.013 Crohn's disease of small intestine with fistula**
CC Exclusion see Appendix A PDX collection 0785

CC **K50.014 Crohn's disease of small intestine with abscess**
CC Exclusion see Appendix A PDX collection 0785
AHA CC: 4Q, 2012, 104

CC **K50.018 Crohn's disease of small intestine with other complication**
CC Exclusion see Appendix A PDX collection 0785

CC **K50.019 Crohn's disease of small intestine with unspecified complications**
CC Exclusion see Appendix A PDX collection 0785

\+ **K50.1 Crohn's disease of large intestine**
Crohn's disease [regional enteritis] of colon
Crohn's disease [regional enteritis] of large bowel
Crohn's disease [regional enteritis] of rectum
Granulomatous colitis
Regional colitis
Excludes1: *Crohn's disease of both small and large intestine (K50.8)*

CC **K50.10 Crohn's disease of large intestine without complications**
CC Exclusion see Appendix A PDX collection 0785

\+ **K50.11 Crohn's disease of large intestine with complications**

CC **K50.111 Crohn's disease of large intestine with rectal bleeding**
CC Exclusion see Appendix A PDX collection 0785

CC **K50.112 Crohn's disease of large intestine with intestinal obstruction**
CC Exclusion see Appendix A PDX collection 0785

CC **K50.113 Crohn's disease of large intestine with fistula**
CC Exclusion see Appendix A PDX collection 0785

CC **K50.114 Crohn's disease of large intestine with abscess**
CC Exclusion see Appendix A PDX collection 0785
AHA CC: 4Q, 2012, 104

CC **K50.118 Crohn's disease of large intestine with other complication**
CC Exclusion see Appendix A PDX collection 0785

CC **K50.119 Crohn's disease of large intestine with unspecified complications**
CC Exclusion see Appendix A PDX collection 0785

\+ **K50.8 Crohn's disease of both small and large intestine**

CC **K50.80 Crohn's disease of both small and large intestine without complications**
CC Exclusion see Appendix A PDX collection 0785

\+ **K50.81 Crohn's disease of both small and large intestine with complications**

CC **K50.811 Crohn's disease of both small and large intestine with rectal bleeding**
CC Exclusion see Appendix A PDX collection 0785

CC **K50.812 Crohn's disease of both small and large intestine with intestinal obstruction**
CC Exclusion see Appendix A PDX collection 0785

CC **K50.813 Crohn's disease of both small and large intestine with fistula**
CC Exclusion see Appendix A PDX collection 0785

CC **K50.814 Crohn's disease of both small and large intestine with abscess**
CC Exclusion see Appendix A PDX collection 0785

CC **K50.818 Crohn's disease of both small and large intestine with other complication**
CC Exclusion see Appendix A PDX collection 0785

CC **K50.819 Crohn's disease of both small and large intestine with unspecified complications**
CC Exclusion see Appendix A PDX collection 0785

\+ **K50.9 Crohn's disease, unspecified**

CC **K50.90 Crohn's disease, unspecified, without complications**
Crohn's disease NOS
Regional enteritis NOS
CC Exclusion see Appendix A PDX collection 0786

\+ **K50.91 Crohn's disease, unspecified, with complications**

CC **K50.911 Crohn's disease, unspecified, with rectal bleeding**
CC Exclusion see Appendix A PDX collection 0786

CC **K50.912 Crohn's disease, unspecified, with intestinal obstruction**
CC Exclusion see Appendix A PDX collection 0786

CC **K50.913 Crohn's disease, unspecified, with fistula**
CC Exclusion see Appendix A PDX collection 0786

CC **K50.914 Crohn's disease, unspecified, with abscess**
CC Exclusion see Appendix A PDX collection 0786

CC **K50.918 Crohn's disease, unspecified, with other complication**
CC Exclusion see Appendix A PDX collection 0786

CC **K50.919 Crohn's disease, unspecified, with unspecified complications**
CC Exclusion see Appendix A PDX collection 0786

K51 Ulcerative colitis
Use additional code to identify manifestations, such as:
pyoderma gangrenosum (L88)
Excludes1: *Crohn's disease [regional enteritis] (K50.-)*

+ **K51.0 Ulcerative (chronic) pancolitis**
Backwash ileitis
CC **K51.00 Ulcerative (chronic) pancolitis without complications**
Ulcerative (chronic) pancolitis NOS
CC Exclusion see Appendix A PDX collection 0785
+ **K51.01 Ulcerative (chronic) pancolitis with complications**
CC **K51.011 Ulcerative (chronic) pancolitis with rectal bleeding**
CC Exclusion see Appendix A PDX collection 0785
CC **K51.012 Ulcerative (chronic) pancolitis with intestinal obstruction**
CC Exclusion see Appendix A PDX collection 0785
CC **K51.013 Ulcerative (chronic) pancolitis with fistula**
CC Exclusion see Appendix A PDX collection 0785
CC **K51.014 Ulcerative (chronic) pancolitis with abscess**
CC Exclusion see Appendix A PDX collection 0785
CC **K51.018 Ulcerative (chronic) pancolitis with other complication**
CC Exclusion see Appendix A PDX collection 0785
CC **K51.019 Ulcerative (chronic) pancolitis with unspecified complications**
CC Exclusion see Appendix A PDX collection 0785

+ **K51.2 Ulcerative (chronic) proctitis**
CC **K51.20 Ulcerative (chronic) proctitis without complications**
Ulcerative (chronic) proctitis NOS
CC Exclusion see Appendix A PDX collection 0785
+ **K51.21 Ulcerative (chronic) proctitis with complications**
CC **K51.211 Ulcerative (chronic) proctitis with rectal bleeding**
CC Exclusion see Appendix A PDX collection 0785
CC **K51.212 Ulcerative (chronic) proctitis with intestinal obstruction**
CC Exclusion see Appendix A PDX collection 0785
CC **K51.213 Ulcerative (chronic) proctitis with fistula**
CC Exclusion see Appendix A PDX collection 0785
CC **K51.214 Ulcerative (chronic) proctitis with abscess**
CC Exclusion see Appendix A PDX collection 0785
CC **K51.218 Ulcerative (chronic) proctitis with other complication**
CC Exclusion see Appendix A PDX collection 0785
CC **K51.219 Ulcerative (chronic) proctitis with unspecified complications**
CC Exclusion see Appendix A PDX collection 0785

+ **K51.3 Ulcerative (chronic) rectosigmoiditis**
CC **K51.30 Ulcerative (chronic) rectosigmoiditis without complications**
Ulcerative (chronic) rectosigmoiditis NOS
CC Exclusion see Appendix A PDX collection 0785
+ **K51.31 Ulcerative (chronic) rectosigmoiditis with complications**
CC **K51.311 Ulcerative (chronic) rectosigmoiditis with rectal bleeding**
CC Exclusion see Appendix A PDX collection 0785
CC **K51.312 Ulcerative (chronic) rectosigmoiditis with intestinal obstruction**
CC Exclusion see Appendix A PDX collection 0785
CC **K51.313 Ulcerative (chronic) rectosigmoiditis with fistula**
CC Exclusion see Appendix A PDX collection 0785
CC **K51.314 Ulcerative (chronic) rectosigmoiditis with abscess**
CC Exclusion see Appendix A PDX collection 0785
CC **K51.318 Ulcerative (chronic) rectosigmoiditis with other complication**
CC Exclusion see Appendix A PDX collection 0785
CC **K51.319 Ulcerative (chronic) rectosigmoiditis with unspecified complications**
CC Exclusion see Appendix A PDX collection 0785

+ **K51.4 Inflammatory polyps of colon**
Excludes1: *adenomatous polyp of colon (D12.6)*
polyposis of colon (D12.6)
polyps of colon NOS (K63.5)
CC **K51.40 Inflammatory polyps of colon without complications**
Inflammatory polyps of colon NOS
CC Exclusion see Appendix A PDX collection 0785
+ **K51.41 Inflammatory polyps of colon with complications**
CC **K51.411 Inflammatory polyps of colon with rectal bleeding**
CC Exclusion see Appendix A PDX collection 0785
CC **K51.412 Inflammatory polyps of colon with intestinal obstruction**
CC Exclusion see Appendix A PDX collection 0785
CC **K51.413 Inflammatory polyps of colon with fistula**
CC Exclusion see Appendix A PDX collection 0785
CC **K51.414 Inflammatory polyps of colon with abscess**
CC Exclusion see Appendix A PDX collection 0785
CC **K51.418 Inflammatory polyps of colon with other complication**
CC Exclusion see Appendix A PDX collection 0785
CC **K51.419 Inflammatory polyps of colon with unspecified complications**
CC Exclusion see Appendix A PDX collection 0785

+ **K51.5 Left sided colitis**
Left hemicolitis
CC **K51.50 Left sided colitis without complications**
Left sided colitis NOS
CC Exclusion see Appendix A PDX collection 0785
+ **K51.51 Left sided colitis with complications**
CC **K51.511 Left sided colitis with rectal bleeding**
CC Exclusion see Appendix A PDX collection 0785
CC **K51.512 Left sided colitis with intestinal obstruction**
CC Exclusion see Appendix A PDX collection 0785
CC **K51.513 Left sided colitis with fistula**
CC Exclusion see Appendix A PDX collection 0785
CC **K51.514 Left sided colitis with abscess**
CC Exclusion see Appendix A PDX collection 0785
CC **K51.518 Left sided colitis with other complication**
CC Exclusion see Appendix A PDX collection 0785
CC **K51.519 Left sided colitis with unspecified complications**
CC Exclusion see Appendix A PDX collection 0785

+ **K51.8 Other ulcerative colitis**
CC **K51.80 Other ulcerative colitis without complications**
CC Exclusion see Appendix A PDX collection 0785
+ **K51.81 Other ulcerative colitis with complications**
CC **K51.811 Other ulcerative colitis with rectal bleeding**
CC Exclusion see Appendix A PDX collection 0785
CC **K51.812 Other ulcerative colitis with intestinal obstruction**
CC Exclusion see Appendix A PDX collection 0785
CC **K51.813 Other ulcerative colitis with fistula**
CC Exclusion see Appendix A PDX collection 0785
CC **K51.814 Other ulcerative colitis with abscess**
CC Exclusion see Appendix A PDX collection 0785
CC **K51.818 Other ulcerative colitis with other complication**
CC Exclusion see Appendix A PDX collection 0785

CC **K51.819 Other ulcerative colitis with unspecified complications**
CC Exclusion see Appendix A PDX collection 0785

\+ **K51.9 Ulcerative colitis, unspecified**

CC **K51.90 Ulcerative colitis, unspecified, without complications**
CC Exclusion see Appendix A PDX collection 0787

\+ **K51.91 Ulcerative colitis, unspecified, with complications**

CC **K51.911 Ulcerative colitis, unspecified with rectal bleeding**
CC Exclusion see Appendix A PDX collection 0787

CC **K51.912 Ulcerative colitis, unspecified with intestinal obstruction**
CC Exclusion see Appendix A PDX collection 0787

CC **K51.913 Ulcerative colitis, unspecified with fistula**
CC Exclusion see Appendix A PDX collection 0787

CC **K51.914 Ulcerative colitis, unspecified with abscess**
CC Exclusion see Appendix A PDX collection 0787

CC **K51.918 Ulcerative colitis, unspecified with other complication**
CC Exclusion see Appendix A PDX collection 0787

CC **K51.919 Ulcerative colitis, unspecified with unspecified complications**
CC Exclusion see Appendix A PDX collection 0787

K52 Other and unspecified noninfective gastroenteritis and colitis

AHA CC: 4Q, 2016, 30-31

CC **K52.0 Gastroenteritis and colitis due to radiation**
CC Exclusion see Appendix A PDX collection 0788

CC **K52.1 Toxic gastroenteritis and colitis**
CC Exclusion see Appendix A PDX collection 0789
Drug-induced gastroenteritis and colitis
Code first (T51-T65) to identify toxic agent

Use additional code for adverse effect, if applicable, to identify drug (T36-T50 with fifth or sixth character 5)

\+ **K52.2 Allergic and dietetic gastroenteritis and colitis**
Food hypersensitivity gastroenteritis or colitis
Use additional code to identify type of food allergy (Z91.01-, Z91.02-)
Excludes2: *allergic eosinophilic colitis (K52.82)*
allergic eosinophilic esophagitis (K20.0)
allergic eosinophilic gastritis (K52.81)
allergic eosinophilic gastroenteritis (K52.81)
food protein-induced proctocolitis (K52.82)

K52.21 Food protein-induced enterocolitis syndrome
Use additional code for hypovolemic shock, if present (R57.1)

K52.22 Food protein-induced enteropathy

K52.29 Other allergic and dietetic gastroenteritis and colitis
Food hypersensitivity gastroenteritis or colitis
Immediate gastrointestinal hypersensitivity

K52.3 Indeterminate colitis
Colonic inflammatory bowel disease unclassified (IBDU)
Excludes1: *unspecified colitis (K52.9)*

\+ **K52.8 Other specified noninfective gastroenteritis and colitis**

K52.81 Eosinophilic gastritis or gastroenteritis
Eosinophilic enteritis
Excludes2: *eosinophilic esophagitis (K20.0)*

K52.82 Eosinophilic colitis
Allergic proctocolitis
Food-induced eosinophilic proctocolitis
Food protein-induced proctocolitis
Milk protein-induced proctocolitis

\+ **K52.83 Microscopic colitis**

K52.831 Collagenous colitis

K52.832 Lymphocytic colitis

K52.838 Other microscopic colitis

K52.839 Microscopic colitis, unspecified

K52.89 Other specified noninfective gastroenteritis and colitis

K52.9 Noninfective gastroenteritis and colitis, unspecified
Colitis NOS
Enteritis NOS
Gastroenteritis NOS
Ileitis NOS
Jejunitis NOS
Sigmoiditis NOS
Excludes1: *diarrhea NOS (R19.7)*
functional diarrhea (K59.1)
infectious gastroenteritis and colitis NOS (A09)
neonatal diarrhea (noninfective) (P78.3)
psychogenic diarrhea (F45.8)

Other diseases of intestines (K55-K64)

K55 Vascular disorders of intestine

Excludes1: *necrotizing enterocolitis of newborn (P77.-)*
AHA CC: 4Q, 2016, 32-33

\+ **K55.0 Acute vascular disorders of intestine**
Infarction of appendices epiploicae
Mesenteric (artery) (vein) embolism
Mesenteric (artery) (vein) infarction
Mesenteric (artery) (vein) thrombosis

\+ **K55.01 Acute (reversible) ischemia of small intestine**

MCC **K55.011 Focal (segmental) acute (reversible) ischemia of small intestine**
MCC Exclusion see Appendix A PDX collection 0790

MCC **K55.012 Diffuse acute (reversible) ischemia of small intestine**
MCC Exclusion see Appendix A PDX collection 0790

MCC **K55.019 Acute (reversible) ischemia of small intestine, extent unspecified**
MCC Exclusion see Appendix A PDX collection 0790

\+ **K55.02 Acute infarction of small intestine**
Gangrene of small intestine
Necrosis of small intestine

MCC **K55.021 Focal (segmental) acute infarction of small intestine**
MCC Exclusion see Appendix A PDX collection 0790

MCC **K55.022 Diffuse acute infarction of small intestine**
MCC Exclusion see Appendix A PDX collection 0790

MCC **K55.029 Acute infarction of small intestine, extent unspecified**
MCC Exclusion see Appendix A PDX collection 0790

\+ **K55.03 Acute (reversible) ischemia of large intestine**
Acute fulminant ischemic colitis
Subacute ischemic colitis

MCC **K55.031 Focal (segmental) acute (reversible) ischemia of large intestine**
MCC Exclusion see Appendix A PDX collection 0790

MCC **K55.032 Diffuse acute (reversible) ischemia of large intestine**
MCC Exclusion see Appendix A PDX collection 0790

MCC **K55.039 Acute (reversible) ischemia of large intestine, extent unspecified**
MCC Exclusion see Appendix A PDX collection 0790

\+ **K55.04 Acute infarction of large intestine**
Gangrene of large intestine
Necrosis of large intestine

MCC **K55.041 Focal (segmental) acute infarction of large intestine**
MCC Exclusion see Appendix A PDX collection 0790

MCC **K55.042 Diffuse acute infarction of large intestine**
MCC Exclusion see Appendix A PDX collection 0790

MCC **K55.049 Acute infarction of large intestine, extent unspecified**
MCC Exclusion see Appendix A PDX collection 0790

\+ **K55.05 Acute (reversible) ischemia of intestine, part unspecified**

MCC **K55.051 Focal (segmental) acute (reversible) ischemia of intestine, part unspecified**
MCC Exclusion see Appendix A PDX collection 0790

MCC **K55.052 Diffuse acute (reversible) ischemia of intestine, part unspecified**
MCC Exclusion see Appendix A PDX collection 0790

MCC **K55.059 Acute (reversible) ischemia of intestine, part and extent unspecified**
MCC Exclusion see Appendix A PDX collection 0790

+ **K55.06 Acute infarction of intestine, part unspecified**
  Acute intestinal infarction
  Gangrene of intestine
  Necrosis of intestine
  MCC **K55.061 Focal (segmental) acute infarction of intestine, part unspecified**
  MCC Exclusion see Appendix A PDX collection 0790
  MCC **K55.062 Diffuse acute infarction of intestine, part unspecified**
  MCC Exclusion see Appendix A PDX collection 0790
  MCC **K55.069 Acute infarction of intestine, part and extent unspecified**
  MCC Exclusion see Appendix A PDX collection 0790

CC **K55.1 Chronic vascular disorders of intestine**
  Chronic ischemic colitis
  Chronic ischemic enteritis
  Chronic ischemic enterocolitis
  Ischemic stricture of intestine
  Mesenteric atherosclerosis
  Mesenteric vascular insufficiency
  CC Exclusion see Appendix A PDX collection 0791

+ **K55.2 Angiodysplasia of colon**
  K55.20 Angiodysplasia of colon without hemorrhage
  MCC **K55.21 Angiodysplasia of colon with hemorrhage**
  MCC Exclusion see Appendix A PDX collection 0770

+ **K55.3 Necrotizing enterocolitis**
  Excludes1: *necrotizing enterocolitis of newborn (P77.-)*
  Excludes2: *necrotizing enterocolitis due to Clostridium difficile (A04.7-)*
  MCC **K55.30 Necrotizing enterocolitis, unspecified**
  Necrotizing enterocolitis, NOS
  MCC Exclusion see Appendix A PDX collection 0790
  MCC **K55.31 Stage 1 necrotizing enterocolitis**
  Necrotizing enterocolitis without pneumatosis, without perforation
  MCC Exclusion see Appendix A PDX collection 0790
  MCC **K55.32 Stage 2 necrotizing enterocolitis**
  Necrotizing enterocolitis with pneumatosis, without perforation
  MCC Exclusion see Appendix A PDX collection 0790
  MCC **K55.33 Stage 3 necrotizing enterocolitis**
  Necrotizing enterocolitis with perforation
  Necrotizing enterocolitis with pneumatosis and perforation
  MCC Exclusion see Appendix A PDX collection 0790

CC **K55.8 Other vascular disorders of intestine**
  CC Exclusion see Appendix A PDX collection 0791

CC **K55.9 Vascular disorder of intestine, unspecified**
  Ischemic colitis
  Ischemic enteritis
  Ischemic enterocolitis
  CC Exclusion see Appendix A PDX collection 0791

K56 Paralytic ileus and intestinal obstruction without hernia

Excludes1: *congenital stricture or stenosis of intestine (Q41-Q42)*
cystic fibrosis with meconium ileus (E84.11)
ischemic stricture of intestine (K55.1)
meconium ileus NOS (P76.0)
neonatal intestinal obstructions classifiable to P76.-
obstruction of duodenum (K31.5)
postprocedural intestinal obstruction (K91.3-)
stenosis of anus or rectum (K62.4)

CC **K56.0 Paralytic ileus**
  Paralysis of bowel
  Paralysis of colon
  Paralysis of intestine
  Excludes1: *gallstone ileus (K56.3)*
  ileus NOS (K56.7)
  obstructive ileus NOS (K56.69-)
  CC Exclusion see Appendix A PDX collection 0792

CC **K56.1 Intussusception**
  Intussusception or invagination of bowel
  Intussusception or invagination of colon
  Intussusception or invagination of intestine
  Intussusception or invagination of rectum
  Excludes2: *intussusception of appendix (K38.8)*
  CC Exclusion see Appendix A PDX collection 0792

MCC **K56.2 Volvulus**
  Strangulation of colon or intestine
  Torsion of colon or intestine
  Twist of colon or intestine
  Excludes2: *volvulus of duodenum (K31.5)*
  MCC Exclusion see Appendix A PDX collection 0792

K56.3 Gallstone ileus
  Obstruction of intestine by gallstone
  CC Exclusion see Appendix A PDX collection 0792

+ **K56.4 Other impaction of intestine**
  K56.41 Fecal impaction
  Excludes1: *constipation (K59.0-)*
  incomplete defecation (R15.0)
  CC **K56.49 Other impaction of intestine**
  CC Exclusion see Appendix A PDX collection 0792

+ **K56.5 Intestinal adhesions [bands] with obstruction (postinfection)**
  Abdominal hernia due to adhesions with obstruction
  Peritoneal adhesions [bands] with intestinal obstruction (postinfection)
  CC **K56.50 Intestinal adhesions [bands], unspecified as to partial versus complete obstruction**
  Intestinal adhesions with obstruction NOS
  CC Exclusion see Appendix A PDX collection 0792
  CC **K56.51 Intestinal adhesions [bands], with partial obstruction**
  Intestinal adhesions with incomplete obstruction
  CC Exclusion see Appendix A PDX collection 0792
  CC **K56.52 Intestinal adhesions [bands] with complete obstruction**
  CC Exclusion see Appendix A PDX collection 0792

+ **K56.6 Other and unspecified intestinal obstruction**
  + **K56.60 Unspecified intestinal obstruction**
  Excludes1: *intestinal obstruction due to specified condition-code to condition*
  CC **K56.600 Partial intestinal obstruction, unspecified as to cause**
  Incomplete intestinal obstruction, NOS
  CC Exclusion see Appendix A PDX collection 0792
  CC **K56.601 Complete intestinal obstruction, unspecified as to cause**
  CC Exclusion see Appendix A PDX collection 0792
  CC **K56.609 Unspecified intestinal obstruction, unspecified as to partial versus complete obstruction**
  Intestinal obstruction NOS
  CC Exclusion see Appendix A PDX collection 0792
  + **K56.69 Other intestinal obstruction**
  Enterostenosis NOS
  Obstructive ileus NOS
  Occlusion of colon or intestine NOS
  Stenosis of colon or intestine NOS
  Stricture of colon or intestine NOS
  Excludes1: *intestinal obstruction due to specified condition-code to condition*
  CC **K56.690 Other partial intestinal obstruction**
  Other incomplete intestinal obstruction
  CC Exclusion see Appendix A PDX collection 0792
  CC **K56.691 Other complete intestinal obstruction**
  CC Exclusion see Appendix A PDX collection 0792
  CC **K56.699 Other intestinal obstruction unspecified as to partial versus complete obstruction**
  Other intestinal obstruction, NEC
  CC Exclusion see Appendix A PDX collection 0792

CC **K56.7 Ileus, unspecified**
  Excludes1: *obstructive ileus (K56.69-)*
  Excludes2: *intestinal obstruction with hernia (K40-K46)*
  CC Exclusion see Appendix A PDX collection 0792
  AHA CC: 1Q, 2017, 40-41

K57 Diverticular disease of intestine

Excludes1: *congenital diverticulum of intestine (Q43.8)*
Meckel's diverticulum (Q43.0)
Excludes2: *diverticulum of appendix (K38.2)*

+ **K57.0 Diverticulitis of small intestine with perforation and abscess**
  Diverticulitis of small intestine with peritonitis
  Excludes1: *diverticulitis of both small and large intestine with perforation and abscess (K57.4-)*

CC **K57.00 Diverticulitis of small intestine with perforation and abscess without bleeding**
CC Exclusion see Appendix A PDX collection 0793

MCC **K57.01 Diverticulitis of small intestine with perforation and abscess with bleeding**
MCC Exclusion see Appendix A PDX collection 0770

+ **K57.1 Diverticular disease of small intestine without perforation or abscess**
Excludes1: *diverticular disease of both small and large intestine without perforation or abscess (K57.5-)*

K57.10 Diverticulosis of small intestine without perforation or abscess without bleeding
Diverticular disease of small intestine NOS

MCC **K57.11 Diverticulosis of small intestine without perforation or abscess with bleeding**
MCC Exclusion see Appendix A PDX collection 0770

CC **K57.12 Diverticulitis of small intestine without perforation or abscess without bleeding**
CC Exclusion see Appendix A PDX collection 0793

MCC **K57.13 Diverticulitis of small intestine without perforation or abscess with bleeding**
MCC Exclusion see Appendix A PDX collection 0770

+ **K57.2 Diverticulitis of large intestine with perforation and abscess**
Diverticulitis of colon with peritonitis
Excludes1: *diverticulitis of both small and large intestine with perforation and abscess (K57.4-)*

CC **K57.20 Diverticulitis of large intestine with perforation and abscess without bleeding**
CC Exclusion see Appendix A PDX collection 0794

MCC **K57.21 Diverticulitis of large intestine with perforation and abscess with bleeding**
MCC Exclusion see Appendix A PDX collection 0770

+ **K57.3 Diverticular disease of large intestine without perforation or abscess**
Excludes1: *diverticular disease of both small and large intestine without perforation or abscess (K57.5-)*

K57.30 Diverticulosis of large intestine without perforation or abscess without bleeding
Diverticular disease of colon NOS

MCC **K57.31 Diverticulosis of large intestine without perforation or abscess with bleeding**
MCC Exclusion see Appendix A PDX collection 0770

CC **K57.32 Diverticulitis of large intestine without perforation or abscess without bleeding**
CC Exclusion see Appendix A PDX collection 0794

MCC **K57.33 Diverticulitis of large intestine without perforation or abscess with bleeding**
MCC Exclusion see Appendix A PDX collection 0770

+ **K57.4 Diverticulitis of both small and large intestine with perforation and abscess**
Diverticulitis of both small and large intestine with peritonitis

CC **K57.40 Diverticulitis of both small and large intestine with perforation and abscess without bleeding**
CC Exclusion see Appendix A PDX collection 0794

MCC **K57.41 Diverticulitis of both small and large intestine with perforation and abscess with bleeding**
MCC Exclusion see Appendix A PDX collection 0770

+ **K57.5 Diverticular disease of both small and large intestine without perforation or abscess**

K57.50 Diverticulosis of both small and large intestine without perforation or abscess without bleeding
Diverticular disease of both small and large intestine NOS

MCC **K57.51 Diverticulosis of both small and large intestine without perforation or abscess with bleeding**
MCC Exclusion see Appendix A PDX collection 0770

CC **K57.52 Diverticulitis of both small and large intestine without perforation or abscess without bleeding**
CC Exclusion see Appendix A PDX collection 0794

MCC **K57.53 Diverticulitis of both small and large intestine without perforation or abscess with bleeding**
MCC Exclusion see Appendix A PDX collection 0770

+ **K57.8 Diverticulitis of intestine, part unspecified, with perforation and abscess**
Diverticulitis of intestine NOS with peritonitis

CC **K57.80 Diverticulitis of intestine, part unspecified, with perforation and abscess without bleeding**
CC Exclusion see Appendix A PDX collection 0794

MCC **K57.81 Diverticulitis of intestine, part unspecified, with perforation and abscess with bleeding**
MCC Exclusion see Appendix A PDX collection 0770

+ **K57.9 Diverticular disease of intestine, part unspecified, without perforation or abscess**

K57.90 Diverticulosis of intestine, part unspecified, without perforation or abscess without bleeding
Diverticular disease of intestine NOS

MCC **K57.91 Diverticulosis of intestine, part unspecified, without perforation or abscess with bleeding**
MCC Exclusion see Appendix A PDX collection 0770

CC **K57.92 Diverticulitis of intestine, part unspecified, without perforation or abscess without bleeding**
CC Exclusion see Appendix A PDX collection 0794

MCC **K57.93 Diverticulitis of intestine, part unspecified, without perforation or abscess with bleeding**
MCC Exclusion see Appendix A PDX collection 0770

K58 Irritable bowel syndrome

Includes: irritable colon
spastic colon

K58.0 Irritable bowel syndrome with diarrhea

K58.1 Irritable bowel syndrome with constipation
AHA CC: 4Q, 2016, 32-33

K58.2 Mixed irritable bowel syndrome
AHA CC: 4Q, 2016, 32-33

K58.8 Other irritable bowel syndrome
AHA CC: 4Q, 2016, 32-33

K58.9 Irritable bowel syndrome without diarrhea
Irritable bowel syndrome NOS

K59 Other functional intestinal disorders

Excludes1: *change in bowel habit NOS (R19.4)*
intestinal malabsorption (K90.-)
psychogenic intestinal disorders (F45.8)
Excludes2: *functional disorders of stomach (K31.-)*

+ **K59.0 Constipation**
Use additional code for adverse effect, if applicable, to identify drug (T36-T50 with fifth or sixth character 5)
Excludes1: *fecal impaction (K56.41)*
incomplete defecation (R15.0)

K59.00 Constipation, unspecified

K59.01 Slow transit constipation

K59.02 Outlet dysfunction constipation

K59.03 Drug induced constipation
Use additional code for adverse effect, if applicable, to identify drug (T36-T50 with fifth or sixth character 5)
AHA CC: 4Q, 2016, 33

K59.04 Chronic idiopathic constipation
Functional constipation
AHA CC: 4Q, 2016, 33

K59.09 Other constipation
Chronic constipation

K59.1 Functional diarrhea
Excludes1: *diarrhea NOS (R19.7)*
irritable bowel syndrome with diarrhea (K58.0)

CC **K59.2 Neurogenic bowel, not elsewhere classified**
CC Exclusion see Appendix A PDX collection 0795

+ **K59.3 Megacolon, not elsewhere classified**
Dilatation of colon
Code first, if applicable (T51-T65) to identify toxic agent
Excludes1: *congenital megacolon (aganglionic) (Q43.1)*
megacolon (due to) (in) Chagas' disease (B57.32)
megacolon (due to) (in) Clostridium difficile (A04.7-)
megacolon (due to) (in) Hirschsprung's disease (Q43.1)
AHA CC: 4Q, 2016, 33-34

CC **K59.31 Toxic megacolon**
CC Exclusion see Appendix A PDX collection 0795

CC **K59.39 Other megacolon**
Megacolon NOS
CC Exclusion see Appendix A PDX collection 0795

K59.4 Anal spasm
Proctalgia fugax

K59.8 Other specified functional intestinal disorders
Atony of colon
Pseudo-obstruction (acute) (chronic) of intestine

K59.9 Functional intestinal disorder, unspecified

K60 Fissure and fistula of anal and rectal regions

Excludes1: *fissure and fistula of anal and rectal regions with abscess or cellulitis (K61.-)*
Excludes2: *anal sphincter tear (healed) (nontraumatic) (old) (K62.81)*

K60.0 Acute anal fissure

K60.1 Chronic anal fissure
K60.2 Anal fissure, unspecified
K60.3 Anal fistula
K60.4 Rectal fistula
Fistula of rectum to skin
Excludes1: *rectovaginal fistula (N82.3)*
vesicorectal fistual (N32.1)
K60.5 Anorectal fistula

K61 Abscess of anal and rectal regions

Includes: abscess of anal and rectal regions
cellulitis of anal and rectal regions

CC **K61.0 Anal abscess**
Perianal abscess
Excludes1: *intrasphincteric abscess (K61.4)*
CC Exclusion see Appendix A PDX collection 0796

CC **K61.1 Rectal abscess**
Perirectal abscess
Excludes1: *ischiorectal abscess (K61.3)*
CC Exclusion see Appendix A PDX collection 0796

CC **K61.2 Anorectal abscess**
CC Exclusion see Appendix A PDX collection 0796

+ **K61.3 Ischiorectal abscess**
Abscess of ischiorectal fossa

CC **K61.31 Horseshoe abscess**
CC Exclusion see Appendix A PDX collection 0796

CC **K61.32 Ischiorectal abscess, NOS**
CC Exclusion see Appendix A PDX collection 0796

CC **K61.4 Intrasphincteric abscess**
CC Exclusion see Appendix A PDX collection 0796

CC **K61.5 Supralevator abscess**
CC Exclusion see Appendix A PDX collection 0796

K62 Other diseases of anus and rectum

Includes: anal canal
Excludes2: *colostomy and enterostomy malfunction (K94.0-, K94.1-)*
fecal incontinence (R15.-)
hemorrhoids (K64.-)

K62.0 Anal polyp
K62.1 Rectal polyp
Excludes1: *adenomatous polyp (D12.8)*
K62.2 Anal prolapse
Prolapse of anal canal
K62.3 Rectal prolapse
Prolapse of rectal mucosa
K62.4 Stenosis of anus and rectum
Stricture of anus (sphincter)

CC **K62.5 Hemorrhage of anus and rectum**
Excludes1: *gastrointestinal bleeding NOS (K92.2)*
melena (K92.1)
neonatal rectal hemorrhage (P54.2)
CC Exclusion see Appendix A PDX collection 0770

CC **K62.6 Ulcer of anus and rectum**
Solitary ulcer of anus and rectum
Stercoral ulcer of anus and rectum
Excludes1: *fissure and fistula of anus and rectum (K60.-)*
ulcerative colitis (K51.-)
CC Exclusion see Appendix A PDX collection 0797

K62.7 Radiation proctitis
Use additional code to identify the type of radiation (W90.-)

+ **K62.8 Other specified diseases of anus and rectum**
Excludes2: *ulcerative proctitis (K51.2)*

K62.81 Anal sphincter tear (healed) (nontraumatic) (old)
Tear of anus, nontraumatic
Use additional code for any associated fecal incontinence (R15.-)
Excludes2: *anal fissure (K60.-)*
anal sphincter tear (healed) (old) complicating delivery (O34.7-)
traumatic tear of anal sphincter (S31.831

K62.82 Dysplasia of anus
Anal intraepithelial neoplasia I and II (AIN I and II) (histologically confirmed)
Dysplasia of anus NOS
Mild and moderate dysplasia of anus (histologically confirmed)
Excludes1: *abnormal results from anal cytologic examination without histologic confirmation (R85.61-)*
anal intraepithelial neoplasia III (D01.3)
carcinoma in situ of anus (D01.3)
HGSIL of anus (R85.613)
severe dysplasia of anus (D01.3)

K62.89 Other specified diseases of anus and rectum
Proctitis NOS
Use additional code for any associated fecal incontinence (R15.-)

K62.9 Disease of anus and rectum, unspecified

K63 Other diseases of intestine

CC **K63.0 Abscess of intestine**
Excludes1: *abscess of intestine with Crohn's disease (K50.014 K50.114, K50.814, K50.914,)*
abscess of intestine with diverticular disease (K57.0, K57.2, K57.4, K57.8)
abscess of intestine with ulcerative colitis (K51.014, K51.214, K51.314, K51.414, K51.514, K51.814, K51.914)
Excludes2: *abscess of anal and rectal regions (K61.-)*
abscess of appendix (K35.3)
CC Exclusion see Appendix A PDX collection 0798

Hepatobiliary System and Pancreas

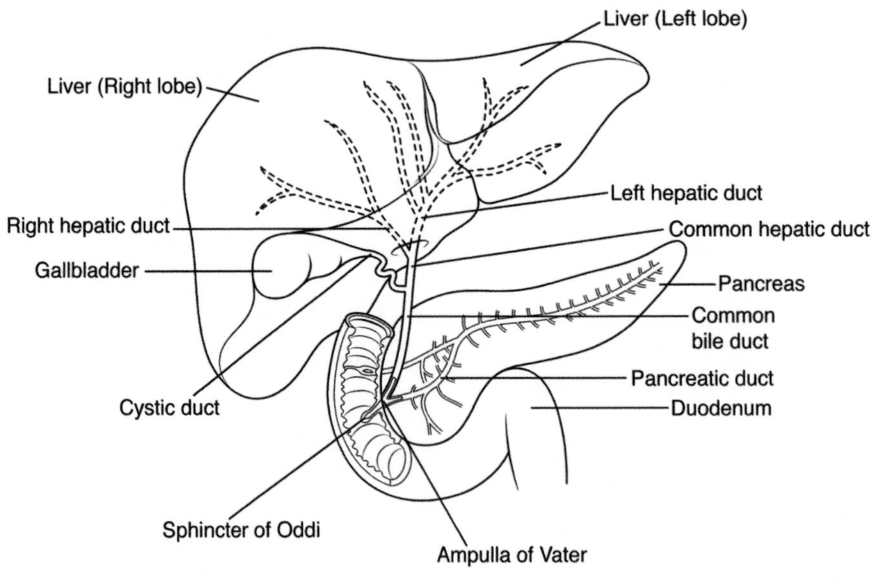

©AHIMA

MCC **K63.1 Perforation of intestine (nontraumatic)**
Perforation (nontraumatic) of rectum
Excludes1: *perforation (nontraumatic) of duodenum (K26.-)*
perforation (nontraumatic) of intestine with diverticular disease (K57.0, K57.2, K57.4, K57.8)
Excludes2: *perforation (nontraumatic) of appendix (K35.2, K35.3)*
MCC Exclusion see Appendix A PDX collection 0799

CC **K63.2 Fistula of intestine**
Excludes1: *fistula of duodenum (K31.6)*
fistula of intestine with Crohn's disease (K50.013, K50.113, K50.813, K50.913,)
fistula of intestine with ulcerative colitis (K51.013, K51.213, K51.313, K51.413, K51.513, K51.813, K51.913)
Excludes2: *fistula of anal and rectal regions (K60.-)*
fistula of appendix (K38.3)
intestinal-genital fistula, female (N82.2-N82.4)
vesicointestinal fistula (N32.1)
CC Exclusion see Appendix A PDX collection 0800

CC **K63.3 Ulcer of intestine**
Primary ulcer of small intestine
Excludes1: *duodenal ulcer (K26.-)*
gastrointestinal ulcer (K28.-)
gastrojejunal ulcer (K28.-)
jejunal ulcer (K28.-)
peptic ulcer, site unspecified (K27.-)
ulcer of intestine with perforation (K63.1)
ulcer of anus or rectum (K62.6)
ulcerative colitis (K51.-)
CC Exclusion see Appendix A PDX collection 0801

CC **K63.4 Enteroptosis**
CC Exclusion see Appendix A PDX collection 0803

K63.5 Polyp of colon
Excludes1: *adenomatous polyp of colon (D12.6)*
inflammatory polyp of colon (K51.4-)
polyposis of colon (D12.6)
AHA CC: 2Q, 2015, 14; 1Q, 2017, 15-16

\+ **K63.8 Other specified diseases of intestine**

MCC **K63.81 Dieulafoy lesion of intestine**
Excludes2: *Dieulafoy lesion of stomach and duodenum (K31.82)*
MCC Exclusion see Appendix A PDX collection 0802

K63.89 Other specified diseases of intestine

K63.9 Disease of intestine, unspecified

K64 Hemorrhoids and perianal venous thrombosis

Includes: piles
Excludes1: *hemorrhoids complicating childbirth and the puerperium (O87.2)*
hemorrhoids complicating pregnancy (O22.4)

K64.0 First degree hemorrhoids
Grade/stage I hemorrhoids
Hemorrhoids (bleeding) without prolapse outside of anal canal

K64.1 Second degree hemorrhoids
Grade/stage II hemorrhoids
Hemorrhoids (bleeding) that prolapse with straining, but retract spontaneously

K64.2 Third degree hemorrhoids
Grade/stage III hemorrhoids
Hemorrhoids (bleeding) that prolapse with straining and require manual replacement back inside anal canal

K64.3 Fourth degree hemorrhoids
Grade/stage IV hemorrhoids
Hemorrhoids (bleeding) with prolapsed tissue that cannot be manually replaced

K64.4 Residual hemorrhoidal skin tags
External hemorrhoids, NOS
Skin tags of anus

K64.5 Perianal venous thrombosis
External hemorrhoids with thrombosis
Perianal hematoma
Thrombosed hemorrhoids NOS

K64.8 Other hemorrhoids
Internal hemorrhoids, without mention of degree
Prolapsed hemorrhoids, degree not specified

K64.9 Unspecified hemorrhoids
Hemorrhoids (bleeding) NOS
Hemorrhoids (bleeding) without mention of degree

Diseases of peritoneum and retroperitoneum (K65-K68)

K65 Peritonitis

Use additional code (B95-B97), to identify infectious agent
Excludes1: *acute appendicitis with generalized peritonitis (K35.2)*
aseptic peritonitis (T81.6)
benign paroxysmal peritonitis (E85.0)
chemical peritonitis (T81.6)
diverticulitis of both small and large intestine with peritonitis (K57.4-)
diverticulitis of colon with peritonitis (K57.2-)
diverticulitis of intestine, NOS, with peritonitis (K57.8-)
diverticulitis of small intestine with peritonitis (K57.0-)
gonococcal peritonitis (A54.85)
neonatal peritonitis (P78.0-P78.1)
pelvic peritonitis, female (N73.3-N73.5)
periodic familial peritonitis (E85.0)
peritonitis due to talc or other foreign substance (T81.6)
peritonitis in chlamydia (A74.81)
peritonitis in diphtheria (A36.89)
peritonitis in syphilis (late) (A52.74)
peritonitis in tuberculosis (A18.31)
peritonitis with or following abortion or ectopic or molar pregnancy (O00-O07, O08.0)
peritonitis with or following appendicitis (K35.-)
peritonitis with or following diverticular disease of intestine (K57.-)
puerperal peritonitis (O85)
retroperitoneal infections (K68.-)

MCC **K65.0 Generalized (acute) peritonitis**
Pelvic peritonitis (acute), male
Subphrenic peritonitis (acute)
Suppurative peritonitis (acute)
MCC Exclusion see Appendix A PDX collection 0803

MCC **K65.1 Peritoneal abscess**
Abdominopelvic abscess
Abscess (of) omentum
Abscess (of) peritoneum
Mesenteric abscess
Retrocecal abscess
Subdiaphragmatic abscess
Subhepatic abscess
Subphrenic abscess
MCC Exclusion see Appendix A PDX collection 0803

MCC **K65.2 Spontaneous bacterial peritonitis**
Excludes1: *bacterial peritonitis NOS (K65.9)*
MCC Exclusion see Appendix A PDX collection 0803

MCC **K65.3 Choleperitonitis**
Peritonitis due to bile
MCC Exclusion see Appendix A PDX collection 0803

CC **K65.4 Sclerosing mesenteritis**
Fat necrosis of peritoneum
(Idiopathic) sclerosing mesenteric fibrosis
Mesenteric lipodystrophy
Mesenteric panniculitis
Retractile mesenteritis
CC Exclusion see Appendix A PDX collection 0803

MCC **K65.8 Other peritonitis**
Chronic proliferative peritonitis
Peritonitis due to urine
MCC Exclusion see Appendix A PDX collection 0803

MCC **K65.9 Peritonitis, unspecified**
Bacterial peritonitis NOS
MCC Exclusion see Appendix A PDX collection 0803
AHA CC: 2Q, 2013, 31

K66 Other disorders of peritoneum

Excludes2: *ascites (R18.-)*
peritoneal effusion (chronic) (R18.8)

K66.0 Peritoneal adhesions (postprocedural) (postinfection)
Adhesions (of) abdominal (wall)
Adhesions (of) diaphragm
Adhesions (of) intestine
Adhesions (of) male pelvis
Adhesions (of) omentum
Adhesions (of) stomach
Adhesive bands
Mesenteric adhesions
Excludes1: *female pelvic adhesions [bands] (N73.6)*
peritoneal adhesions with intestinal obstruction (K56.5-)

MCC **K66.1 Hemoperitoneum**

Excludes1: *traumatic hemoperitoneum (S36.8-)*

MCC Exclusion see Appendix A PDX collection 0804

K66.8 Other specified disorders of peritoneum

K66.9 Disorder of peritoneum, unspecified

MCC K67 Disorders of peritoneum in infectious diseases classified elsewhere

Code first underlying disease, such as :
congenital syphilis (A50.0)
helminthiasis (B65.0-B83.9)

Excludes1: *peritonitis in chlamydia (A74.81)*
peritonitis in diphtheria (A36.89)
peritonitis in gonococcal (A54.85)
peritonitis in syphilis (late) (A52.74)
peritonitis in tuberculosis (A18.31)

MCC Exclusion see Appendix A PDX collection 0803

Valid 3-character code, no further characters required

K68 Disorders of retroperitoneum

\+ **K68.1 Retroperitoneal abscess**

CC **K68.11 Postprocedural retroperitoneal abscess**

CC Exclusion see Appendix A PDX collection 0805

HAC see Appendix B for HAC conditional logic

MCC **K68.12 Psoas muscle abscess**

MCC Exclusion see Appendix A PDX collection 0806

MCC **K68.19 Other retroperitoneal abscess**

MCC Exclusion see Appendix A PDX collection 0803

MCC **K68.9 Other disorders of retroperitoneum**

MCC Exclusion see Appendix A PDX collection 0803

Diseases of liver (K70-K77)

Excludes1: *jaundice NOS (R17)*

Excludes2: *hemochromatosis (E83.11-)*
Reye's syndrome (G93.7)
viral hepatitis (B15-B19)
Wilson's disease (E83.0)

K70 Alcoholic liver disease

Use additional code to identify:
alcohol abuse and dependence (F10.-)

• **K70.0 Alcoholic fatty liver**

\+ **K70.1 Alcoholic hepatitis**

• **K70.10 Alcoholic hepatitis without ascites**

• **K70.11 Alcoholic hepatitis with ascites**

• **K70.2 Alcoholic fibrosis and sclerosis of liver**

\+ **K70.3 Alcoholic cirrhosis of liver**

Alcoholic cirrhosis NOS

• **K70.30 Alcoholic cirrhosis of liver without ascites**

• **K70.31 Alcoholic cirrhosis of liver with ascites**

\+ **K70.4 Alcoholic hepatic failure**

Acute alcoholic hepatic failure
Alcoholic hepatic failure NOS
Chronic alcoholic hepatic failure
Subacute alcoholic hepatic failure

• **K70.40 Alcoholic hepatic failure without coma**

• MCC **K70.41 Alcoholic hepatic failure with coma**

MCC Exclusion see Appendix A PDX collection 0807

• **K70.9 Alcoholic liver disease, unspecified**

K71 Toxic liver disease

Includes: drug-induced idiosyncratic (unpredictable) liver disease
drug-induced toxic (predictable) liver disease

Code first poisoning due to drug or toxin, if applicable (T36-T65 with fifth or sixth character 1-4 or 6)

Use additional code for adverse effect, if applicable, to identify drug (T36-T50 with fifth or sixth character 5)

Excludes2: *alcoholic liver disease (K70.-)*
Budd-Chiari syndrome (I82.0)

K71.0 Toxic liver disease with cholestasis

Cholestasis with hepatocyte injury
'Pure' cholestasis

\+ **K71.1 Toxic liver disease with hepatic necrosis**

Hepatic failure (acute) (chronic) due to drugs

K71.10 Toxic liver disease with hepatic necrosis, without coma

MCC **K71.11 Toxic liver disease with hepatic necrosis, with coma**

MCC Exclusion see Appendix A PDX collection 0807

K71.2 Toxic liver disease with acute hepatitis

K71.3 Toxic liver disease with chronic persistent hepatitis

K71.4 Toxic liver disease with chronic lobular hepatitis

\+ **K71.5 Toxic liver disease with chronic active hepatitis**

Toxic liver disease with lupoid hepatitis

K71.50 Toxic liver disease with chronic active hepatitis without ascites

K71.51 Toxic liver disease with chronic active hepatitis with ascites

K71.6 Toxic liver disease with hepatitis, not elsewhere classified

K71.7 Toxic liver disease with fibrosis and cirrhosis of liver

K71.8 Toxic liver disease with other disorders of liver

Toxic liver disease with focal nodular hyperplasia
Toxic liver disease with hepatic granulomas
Toxic liver disease with peliosis hepatis
Toxic liver disease with veno-occlusive disease of liver

K71.9 Toxic liver disease, unspecified

K72 Hepatic failure, not elsewhere classified

Includes: fulminant hepatitis NEC, with hepatic failure
hepatic encephalopathy NOS
liver (cell) necrosis with hepatic failure
malignant hepatitis NEC, with hepatic failure
yellow liver atrophy or dystrophy

Excludes1: *alcoholic hepatic failure (K70.4)*
hepatic failure with toxic liver disease (K71.1-)
icterus of newborn (P55-P59)
postprocedural hepatic failure (K91.82)

Excludes2: *hepatic failure complicating abortion or ectopic or molar pregnancy (O00-O07, O08.8)*
hepatic failure complicating pregnancy, childbirth and the puerperium (O26.6-)
viral hepatitis with hepatic coma (B15-B19)

\+ **K72.0 Acute and subacute hepatic failure**

Acute non-viral hepatitis NOS

AHA CC: 2Q, 2014, 13

MCC **K72.00 Acute and subacute hepatic failure without coma**

MCC Exclusion see Appendix A PDX collection 0808

MCC **K72.01 Acute and subacute hepatic failure with coma**

MCC Exclusion see Appendix A PDX collection 0808

\+ **K72.1 Chronic hepatic failure**

K72.10 Chronic hepatic failure without coma

AHA CC: 1Q, 2017, 41

MCC **K72.11 Chronic hepatic failure with coma**

MCC Exclusion see Appendix A PDX collection 0807

\+ **K72.9 Hepatic failure, unspecified**

K72.90 Hepatic failure, unspecified without coma

AHA CC: 2Q, 2016, 35

MCC **K72.91 Hepatic failure, unspecified with coma**

Hepatic coma NOS

MCC Exclusion see Appendix A PDX collection 0807

K73 Chronic hepatitis, not elsewhere classified

Excludes1: *alcoholic hepatitis (chronic) (K70.1-)*
drug-induced hepatitis (chronic) (K71.-)
granulomatous hepatitis (chronic) NEC (K75.3)
reactive, nonspecific hepatitis (chronic) (K75.2)
viral hepatitis (chronic) (B15-B19)

K73.0 Chronic persistent hepatitis, not elsewhere classified

K73.1 Chronic lobular hepatitis, not elsewhere classified

K73.2 Chronic active hepatitis, not elsewhere classified

K73.8 Other chronic hepatitis, not elsewhere classified

K73.9 Chronic hepatitis, unspecified

K74 Fibrosis and cirrhosis of liver

Code also, if applicable, viral hepatitis (acute) (chronic) (B15-B19)

Excludes1: *alcoholic cirrhosis (of liver) (K70.3)*
alcoholic fibrosis of liver (K70.2)
cardiac sclerosis of liver (K76.1)
cirrhosis (of liver) with toxic liver disease (K71.7)
congenital cirrhosis (of liver) (P78.81)
pigmentary cirrhosis (of liver) (E83.110)

K74.0 Hepatic fibrosis

K74.1 Hepatic sclerosis

K74.2 Hepatic fibrosis with hepatic sclerosis

K74.3 Primary biliary cirrhosis

Chronic nonsuppurative destructive cholangitis

K74.4 Secondary biliary cirrhosis

K74.5 Biliary cirrhosis, unspecified

\+ **K74.6 Other and unspecified cirrhosis of liver**

K74.60 Unspecified cirrhosis of liver

Cirrhosis (of liver) NOS

K74.69 Other cirrhosis of liver

Cryptogenic cirrhosis (of liver)
Macronodular cirrhosis (of liver)
Micronodular cirrhosis (of liver)
Mixed type cirrhosis (of liver)
Portal cirrhosis (of liver)
Postnecrotic cirrhosis (of liver)

K75 Other inflammatory liver diseases

Excludes2: *toxic liver disease (K71.-)*

MCC **K75.0 Abscess of liver**
Cholangitic hepatic abscess
Hematogenic hepatic abscess
Hepatic abscess NOS
Lymphogenic hepatic abscess
Pylephlebitic hepatic abscess
Excludes1: *amebic liver abscess (A06.4)*
cholangitis without liver abscess (K83.0)
pylephlebitis without liver abscess (K75.1)
Excludes2: *acute or subacute hepatitis NOS (B17.9)*
acute or subacute non-viral hepatitis (K72.0)
chronic hepatitis NEC (K73.8)
MCC Exclusion see Appendix A PDX collection 0809

MCC **K75.1 Phlebitis of portal vein**
Pylephlebitis
Excludes1: *pylephlebitic liver abscess (K75.0)*
MCC Exclusion see Appendix A PDX collection 0809

K75.2 Nonspecific reactive hepatitis
Excludes1: *acute or subacute hepatitis (K72.0-)*
chronic hepatitis NEC (K73.-)
viral hepatitis (B15-B19)

K75.3 Granulomatous hepatitis, not elsewhere classified
Excludes1: *acute or subacute hepatitis (K72.0-)*
chronic hepatitis NEC (K73.-)
viral hepatitis (B15-B19)

K75.4 Autoimmune hepatitis
Lupoid hepatitis NEC

\+ **K75.8 Other specified inflammatory liver diseases**
K75.81 Nonalcoholic steatohepatitis (NASH)
K75.89 Other specified inflammatory liver diseases

K75.9 Inflammatory liver disease, unspecified
Hepatitis NOS
Excludes1: *acute or subacute hepatitis (K72.0-)*
chronic hepatitis NEC (K73.-)
viral hepatitis (B15-B19)

K76 Other diseases of liver

Excludes2: *alcoholic liver disease (K70.-)*
amyloid degeneration of liver (E85.-)
cystic disease of liver (congenital) (Q44.6)
hepatic vein thrombosis (I82.0)
hepatomegaly NOS (R16.0)
pigmentary cirrhosis (of liver) (E83.110)
portal vein thrombosis (I81)
toxic liver disease (K71.-)

K76.0 Fatty (change of) liver, not elsewhere classified
Nonalcoholic fatty liver disease (NAFLD)
Excludes1: *nonalcoholic steatohepatitis (NASH) (K75.81)*

K76.1 Chronic passive congestion of liver
Cardiac cirrhosis
Cardiac sclerosis

MCC **K76.2 Central hemorrhagic necrosis of liver**
Excludes1: *liver necrosis with hepatic failure (K72.-)*
MCC Exclusion see Appendix A PDX collection 0808

MCC **K76.3 Infarction of liver**
MCC Exclusion see Appendix A PDX collection 0808

K76.4 Peliosis hepatis
Hepatic angiomatosis

K76.5 Hepatic veno-occlusive disease
Excludes1: *Budd-Chiari syndrome (I82.0)*

CC **K76.6 Portal hypertension**
Use additional code for any associated complications, such as:
portal hypertensive gastropathy (K31.89)
CC Exclusion see Appendix A PDX collection 0810

MCC **K76.7 Hepatorenal syndrome**
Excludes1: *hepatorenal syndrome following labor and delivery (O90.4)*
postprocedural hepatorenal syndrome (K91.83)
MCC Exclusion see Appendix A PDX collection 0811

\+ **K76.8 Other specified diseases of liver**
K76.81 Hepatopulmonary syndrome
Code first underlying liver disease, such as:
alcoholic cirrhosis of liver (K70.3-)
cirrhosis of liver without mention of alcohol (K74.6-)
K76.89 Other specified diseases of liver
Cyst (simple) of liver
Focal nodular hyperplasia of liver
Hepatoptosis

K76.9 Liver disease, unspecified

CC **K77 Liver disorders in diseases classified elsewhere**
Code first underlying disease, such as:
amyloidosis (E85.-)
congenital syphilis (A50.0, A50.5)
congenital toxoplasmosis (P37.1)
schistosomiasis (B65.0-B65.9)
Excludes1: *alcoholic hepatitis (K70.1-)*
alcoholic liver disease (K70.-)
cytomegaloviral hepatitis (B25.1)
herpesviral [herpes simplex] hepatitis (B00.81)
infectious mononucleosis with liver disease (B27.0-B27.9 with .9)
mumps hepatitis (B26.81)
sarcoidosis with liver disease (D86.89)
secondary syphilis with liver disease (A51.45)
syphilis (late) with liver disease (A52.74)
toxoplasmosis (acquired) hepatitis (B58.1)
tuberculosis with liver disease (A18.83)
No CC Exclusions
Valid 3-character code, no further characters required

Disorders of gallbladder, biliary tract and pancreas (K80-K87)

K80 Cholelithiasis

Excludes1: *retained cholelithiasis following cholecystectomy (K91.86)*

\+ **K80.0 Calculus of gallbladder with acute cholecystitis**
Any condition listed in K80.2 with acute cholecystitis
CC **K80.00 Calculus of gallbladder with acute cholecystitis without obstruction**
CC Exclusion see Appendix A PDX collection 0812
CC **K80.01 Calculus of gallbladder with acute cholecystitis with obstruction**
CC Exclusion see Appendix A PDX collection 0813

\+ **K80.1 Calculus of gallbladder with other cholecystitis**
CC **K80.10 Calculus of gallbladder with chronic cholecystitis without obstruction**
Cholelithiasis with cholecystitis NOS
CC Exclusion see Appendix A PDX collection 0813
CC **K80.11 Calculus of gallbladder with chronic cholecystitis with obstruction**
CC Exclusion see Appendix A PDX collection 0813
CC **K80.12 Calculus of gallbladder with acute and chronic cholecystitis without obstruction**
CC Exclusion see Appendix A PDX collection 0812
CC **K80.13 Calculus of gallbladder with acute and chronic cholecystitis with obstruction**
CC Exclusion see Appendix A PDX collection 0813
CC **K80.18 Calculus of gallbladder with other cholecystitis without obstruction**
CC Exclusion see Appendix A PDX collection 0813
CC **K80.19 Calculus of gallbladder with other cholecystitis with obstruction**
CC Exclusion see Appendix A PDX collection 0813

\+ **K80.2 Calculus of gallbladder without cholecystitis**
Cholecystolithiasis without cholecystitis
Cholelithiasis (without cholecystitis)
Colic (recurrent) of gallbladder (without cholecystitis)
Gallstone (impacted) of cystic duct (without cholecystitis)
Gallstone (impacted) of gallbladder (without cholecystitis)
K80.20 Calculus of gallbladder without cholecystitis without obstruction
CC **K80.21 Calculus of gallbladder without cholecystitis with obstruction**
CC Exclusion see Appendix A PDX collection 0813

\+ **K80.3 Calculus of bile duct with cholangitis**
Any condition listed in K80.5 with cholangitis
CC **K80.30 Calculus of bile duct with cholangitis, unspecified, without obstruction**
CC Exclusion see Appendix A PDX collection 0814
CC **K80.31 Calculus of bile duct with cholangitis, unspecified, with obstruction**
CC Exclusion see Appendix A PDX collection 0815
CC **K80.32 Calculus of bile duct with acute cholangitis without obstruction**
CC Exclusion see Appendix A PDX collection 0814
CC **K80.33 Calculus of bile duct with acute cholangitis with obstruction**
CC Exclusion see Appendix A PDX collection 0815
CC **K80.34 Calculus of bile duct with chronic cholangitis without obstruction**
CC Exclusion see Appendix A PDX collection 0814

CC **K80.35 Calculus of bile duct with chronic cholangitis with obstruction**
CC Exclusion see Appendix A PDX collection 0815

CC **K80.36 Calculus of bile duct with acute and chronic cholangitis without obstruction**
CC Exclusion see Appendix A PDX collection 0814

CC **K80.37 Calculus of bile duct with acute and chronic cholangitis with obstruction**
CC Exclusion see Appendix A PDX collection 0815

\+ **K80.4 Calculus of bile duct with cholecystitis**
Any condition listed in K80.5 with cholecystitis (with cholangitis)

CC **K80.40 Calculus of bile duct with cholecystitis, unspecified, without obstruction**
CC Exclusion see Appendix A PDX collection 0815

CC **K80.41 Calculus of bile duct with cholecystitis, unspecified, with obstruction**
CC Exclusion see Appendix A PDX collection 0815

CC **K80.42 Calculus of bile duct with acute cholecystitis without obstruction**
CC Exclusion see Appendix A PDX collection 0815

CC **K80.43 Calculus of bile duct with acute cholecystitis with obstruction**
CC Exclusion see Appendix A PDX collection 0815

CC **K80.44 Calculus of bile duct with chronic cholecystitis without obstruction**
CC Exclusion see Appendix A PDX collection 0815

CC **K80.45 Calculus of bile duct with chronic cholecystitis with obstruction**
CC Exclusion see Appendix A PDX collection 0815

CC **K80.46 Calculus of bile duct with acute and chronic cholecystitis without obstruction**
CC Exclusion see Appendix A PDX collection 0815

CC **K80.47 Calculus of bile duct with acute and chronic cholecystitis with obstruction**
CC Exclusion see Appendix A PDX collection 0815

\+ **K80.5 Calculus of bile duct without cholangitis or cholecystitis**
Choledocholithiasis (without cholangitis or cholecystitis)
Gallstone (impacted) of bile duct NOS (without cholangitis or cholecystitis)
Gallstone (impacted) of common duct (without cholangitis or cholecystitis)
Gallstone (impacted) of hepatic duct (without cholangitis or cholecystitis)
Hepatic cholelithiasis (without cholangitis or cholecystitis)
Hepatic colic (recurrent) (without cholangitis or cholecystitis)

K80.50 Calculus of bile duct without cholangitis or cholecystitis without obstruction

CC **K80.51 Calculus of bile duct without cholangitis or cholecystitis with obstruction**
CC Exclusion see Appendix A PDX collection 0815

\+ **K80.6 Calculus of gallbladder and bile duct with cholecystitis**

CC **K80.60 Calculus of gallbladder and bile duct with cholecystitis, unspecified, without obstruction**
CC Exclusion see Appendix A PDX collection 0815

CC **K80.61 Calculus of gallbladder and bile duct with cholecystitis, unspecified, with obstruction**
CC Exclusion see Appendix A PDX collection 0815

CC **K80.62 Calculus of gallbladder and bile duct with acute cholecystitis without obstruction**
CC Exclusion see Appendix A PDX collection 0816

CC **K80.63 Calculus of gallbladder and bile duct with acute cholecystitis with obstruction**
CC Exclusion see Appendix A PDX collection 0816

CC **K80.64 Calculus of gallbladder and bile duct with chronic cholecystitis without obstruction**
CC Exclusion see Appendix A PDX collection 0815

CC **K80.65 Calculus of gallbladder and bile duct with chronic cholecystitis with obstruction**
CC Exclusion see Appendix A PDX collection 0815

CC **K80.66 Calculus of gallbladder and bile duct with acute and chronic cholecystitis without obstruction**
CC Exclusion see Appendix A PDX collection 0817

MCC **K80.67 Calculus of gallbladder and bile duct with acute and chronic cholecystitis with obstruction**
MCC Exclusion see Appendix A PDX collection 0817

\+ **K80.7 Calculus of gallbladder and bile duct without cholecystitis**

K80.70 Calculus of gallbladder and bile duct without cholecystitis without obstruction

CC **K80.71 Calculus of gallbladder and bile duct without cholecystitis with obstruction**
CC Exclusion see Appendix A PDX collection 0815

\+ **K80.8 Other cholelithiasis**

K80.80 Other cholelithiasis without obstruction

CC **K80.81 Other cholelithiasis with obstruction**
CC Exclusion see Appendix A PDX collection 0815

K81 Cholecystitis

Excludes1: *cholecystitis with cholelithiasis (K80.-)*

K81.0 Acute cholecystitis
Abscess of gallbladder
Angiocholecystitis
Emphysematous (acute) cholecystitis
Empyema of gallbladder
Gangrene of gallbladder
Gangrenous cholecystitis
Suppurative cholecystitis

K81.1 Chronic cholecystitis

CC **K81.2 Acute cholecystitis with chronic cholecystitis**
CC Exclusion see Appendix A PDX collection 0819

K81.9 Cholecystitis, unspecified

K82 Other diseases of gallbladder

Excludes1: *nonvisualization of gallbladder (R93.2)*
postcholecystectomy syndrome (K91.5)

CC **K82.0 Obstruction of gallbladder**
Occlusion of cystic duct or gallbladder without cholelithiasis
Stenosis of cystic duct or gallbladder without cholelithiasis
Stricture of cystic duct or gallbladder without cholelithiasis
Excludes1: *obstruction of gallbladder with cholelithiasis (K80.-)*
CC Exclusion see Appendix A PDX collection 0820

CC **K82.1 Hydrops of gallbladder**
Mucocele of gallbladder
CC Exclusion see Appendix A PDX collection 0820

MCC **K82.2 Perforation of gallbladder**
Rupture of cystic duct or gallbladder
MCC Exclusion see Appendix A PDX collection 0820

CC **K82.3 Fistula of gallbladder**
Cholecystocolic fistula
Cholecystoduodenal fistula
CC Exclusion see Appendix A PDX collection 0820

K82.4 Cholesterolosis of gallbladder
Strawberry gallbladder
Excludes1: *cholesterolosis of gallbladder with cholecystitis (K81.-)*
cholesterolosis of gallbladder with cholelithiasis (K80.-)

K82.8 Other specified diseases of gallbladder
Adhesions of cystic duct or gallbladder
Atrophy of cystic duct or gallbladder
Cyst of cystic duct or gallbladder
Dyskinesia of cystic duct or gallbladder
Hypertrophy of cystic duct or gallbladder
Nonfunctioning of cystic duct or gallbladder
Ulcer of cystic duct or gallbladder

K82.9 Disease of gallbladder, unspecified

K83 Other diseases of biliary tract

Excludes1: *postcholecystectomy syndrome (K91.5)*
Excludes2: *conditions involving the gallbladder (K81-K82)*
conditions involving the cystic duct (K81-K82)

CC **K83.0 Cholangitis**
Ascending cholangitis
Cholangitis NOS
Primary cholangitis
Recurrent cholangitis
Sclerosing cholangitis
Secondary cholangitis
Stenosing cholangitis
Suppurative cholangitis
Excludes1: *cholangitic liver abscess (K75.0)*
cholangitis with choledocholithiasis (K80.3-, K80.4-)
chronic nonsuppurative destructive cholangitis (K74.3)
CC Exclusion see Appendix A PDX collection 0814

MCC **K83.1 Obstruction of bile duct**
Occlusion of bile duct without cholelithiasis
Stenosis of bile duct without cholelithiasis
Stricture of bile duct without cholelithiasis
Excludes1: *congenital obstruction of bile duct (Q44.3)*
obstruction of bile duct with cholelithiasis (K80.-)
MCC Exclusion see Appendix A PDX collection 0821
CC AHA: 1Q, 2016, 18-19

MCC **K83.2 Perforation of bile duct**
Rupture of bile duct
MCC Exclusion see Appendix A PDX collection 0822

CC **K83.3 Fistula of bile duct**
Choledochoduodenal fistula
CC Exclusion see Appendix A PDX collection 0822

K83.4 Spasm of sphincter of Oddi

K83.5 Biliary cyst

K83.8 Other specified diseases of biliary tract
Adhesions of biliary tract
Atrophy of biliary tract
Hypertrophy of biliary tract
Ulcer of biliary tract

K83.9 Disease of biliary tract, unspecified

K85 Acute pancreatitis

Includes: acute (recurrent) pancreatitis
subacute pancreatitis
AHA CC: 4Q, 2016, 34

\+ **K85.0 Idiopathic acute pancreatitis**

MCC **K85.00 Idiopathic acute pancreatitis without necrosis or infection**
MCC Exclusion see Appendix A PDX collection 0177

MCC **K85.01 Idiopathic acute pancreatitis with uninfected necrosis**
MCC Exclusion see Appendix A PDX collection 0177

MCC **K85.02 Idiopathic acute pancreatitis with infected necrosis**
MCC Exclusion see Appendix A PDX collection 0177

\+ **K85.1 Biliary acute pancreatitis**
Gallstone pancreatitis

MCC **K85.10 Biliary acute pancreatitis without necrosis or infection**
MCC Exclusion see Appendix A PDX collection 0177

MCC **K85.11 Biliary acute pancreatitis with uninfected necrosis**
MCC Exclusion see Appendix A PDX collection 0177

MCC **K85.12 Biliary acute pancreatitis with infected necrosis**
MCC Exclusion see Appendix A PDX collection 0177

\+ **K85.2 Alcohol induced acute pancreatitis**
Excludes2: *alcohol induced chronic pancreatitis (K86.0)*

MCC **K85.20 Alcohol induced acute pancreatitis without necrosis or infection**
MCC Exclusion see Appendix A PDX collection 0177

MCC **K85.21 Alcohol induced acute pancreatitis with uninfected necrosis**
MCC Exclusion see Appendix A PDX collection 0177

MCC **K85.22 Alcohol induced acute pancreatitis with infected necrosis**
MCC Exclusion see Appendix A PDX collection 0177

\+ **K85.3 Drug induced acute pancreatitis**
Use additional code for adverse effect, if applicable, to identify drug (T36-T50 with fifth or sixth character 5)

Use additional code to identify drug abuse and dependence (F11.-F17.-)

MCC **K85.30 Drug induced acute pancreatitis without necrosis or infection**
MCC Exclusion see Appendix A PDX collection 0177

MCC **K85.31 Drug induced acute pancreatitis with uninfected necrosis**
MCC Exclusion see Appendix A PDX collection 0177

MCC **K85.32 Drug induced acute pancreatitis with infected necrosis**
MCC Exclusion see Appendix A PDX collection 0177

\+ **K85.8 Other acute pancreatitis**

MCC **K85.80 Other acute pancreatitis without necrosis or infection**
MCC Exclusion see Appendix A PDX collection 0177

MCC **K85.81 Other acute pancreatitis with uninfected necrosis**
MCC Exclusion see Appendix A PDX collection 0177

MCC **K85.82 Other acute pancreatitis with infected necrosis**
MCC Exclusion see Appendix A PDX collection 0177

\+ **K85.9 Acute pancreatitis, unspecified**
Pancreatitis NOS

MCC **K85.90 Acute pancreatitis without necrosis or infection, unspecified**
MCC Exclusion see Appendix A PDX collection 0177

MCC **K85.91 Acute pancreatitis with uninfected necrosis, unspecified**
MCC Exclusion see Appendix A PDX collection 0177

MCC **K85.92 Acute pancreatitis with infected necrosis, unspecified**
MCC Exclusion see Appendix A PDX collection 0177

K86 Other diseases of pancreas

Excludes2: *fibrocystic disease of pancreas (E84.-)*
islet cell tumor (of pancreas) (D13.7)
pancreatic steatorrhea (K90.3)

CC **K86.0 Alcohol-induced chronic pancreatitis**
Use additional code to identify:
alcohol abuse and dependence (F10.-)

Code also exocrine pancreatic insufficiency (K86.81)
Excludes2: *alcohol induced acute pancreatitis (K85.2-)*
CC Exclusion see Appendix A PDX collection 0823

CC **K86.1 Other chronic pancreatitis**
Chronic pancreatitis NOS
Infectious chronic pancreatitis
Recurrent chronic pancreatitis
Relapsing chronic pancreatitis
Code also exocrine pancreatic insufficiency (K86.81)
CC Exclusion see Appendix A PDX collection 0823

CC **K86.2 Cyst of pancreas**
CC Exclusion see Appendix A PDX collection 0824

CC **K86.3 Pseudocyst of pancreas**
CC Exclusion see Appendix A PDX collection 0824

\+ **K86.8 Other specified diseases of pancreas**
AHA CC: 4Q, 2016, 33

K86.81 Exocrine pancreatic insufficiency

K86.89 Other specified diseases of pancreas
Aseptic pancreatic necrosis, unrelated to acute pancreatitis
Atrophy of pancreas
Calculus of pancreas
Cirrhosis of pancreas
Fibrosis of pancreas
Pancreatic fat necrosis, unrelated to acute pancreatitis
Pancreatic infantilism
Pancreatic necrosis NOS, unrelated to acute pancreatitis

K86.9 Disease of pancreas, unspecified

K87 Disorders of gallbladder, biliary tract and pancreas in diseases classified elsewhere

Code first underlying disease
Excludes1: *cytomegaloviral pancreatitis(B25.2)*
mumps pancreatitis (B26.3)
syphilitic gallbladder (A52.74)
syphilitic pancreas (A52.74)
tuberculosis of gallbladder (A18.83)
tuberculosis of pancreas (A18.83)
Valid 3-character code, no further characters required

Other diseases of the digestive system (K90-K95)

K90 Intestinal malabsorption

Excludes1: *intestinal malabsorption following gastrointestinal surgery (K91.2)*

K90.0 Celiac disease
Celiac disease with steatorrhea
Celiac gluten-sensitive enteropathy
Nontropical sprue
Code also exocrine pancreatic insufficiency (K86.81)

Use additional code for associated disorders including:
dermatitis herpetiformis (L13.0)
gluten ataxia (G32.81)

CC **K90.1 Tropical sprue**
Sprue NOS
Tropical steatorrhea
CC Exclusion see Appendix A PDX collection 0825

CC **K90.2 Blind loop syndrome, not elsewhere classified**
Blind loop syndrome NOS
Excludes1: *congenital blind loop syndrome (Q43.8)*
postsurgical blind loop syndrome (K91.2)
CC Exclusion see Appendix A PDX collection 0825

CC **K90.3 Pancreatic steatorrhea**
CC Exclusion see Appendix A PDX collection 0825

\+ **K90.4 Other malabsorption due to intolerance**
Excludes2: *celiac gluten-sensitive enteropathy (K90.0)*
lactose intolerance (E73.-)

CC **K90.41 Non-celiac gluten sensitivity**
Gluten sensitivity NOS
Non-celiac gluten sensitive enteropathy
CC Exclusion see Appendix A PDX collection 0825
AHA CC: 4Q, 2016, 35-36

CC **K90.49 Malabsorption due to intolerance, not elsewhere classified**
Malabsorption due to intolerance to carbohydrate
Malabsorption due to intolerance to fat
Malabsorption due to intolerance to protein
Malabsorption due to intolerance to starch
CC Exclusion see Appendix A PDX collection 0825

\+ **K90.8 Other intestinal malabsorption**
CC **K90.81 Whipple's disease**
CC Exclusion see Appendix A PDX collection 0826
CC **K90.89 Other intestinal malabsorption**
CC Exclusion see Appendix A PDX collection 0825
CC **K90.9 Intestinal malabsorption, unspecified**
CC Exclusion see Appendix A PDX collection 0825

K91 Intraoperative and postprocedural complications and disorders of digestive system, not elsewhere classified

Excludes2: *complications of artificial opening of digestive system (K94.-)*
complications of bariatric procedures (K95.-)
gastrojejunal ulcer (K28.-)
postprocedural (radiation) retroperitoneal abscess (K68.11)
radiation colitis (K52.0)
radiation gastroenteritis (K52.0)
radiation proctitis (K62.7)
AHA CC: 4Q, 2016, 9-10

K91.0 Vomiting following gastrointestinal surgery
K91.1 Postgastric surgery syndromes
Dumping syndrome
Postgastrectomy syndrome
Postvagotomy syndrome
CC **K91.2 Postsurgical malabsorption, not elsewhere classified**
Postsurgical blind loop syndrome
Excludes1: *malabsorption osteomalacia in adults (M83.2)*
malabsorption osteoporosis, postsurgical (M80.8-, M81.8)
CC Exclusion see Appendix A PDX collection 0827

\+ **K91.3 Postprocedural intestinal obstruction**
CC **K91.30 Postprocedural intestinal obstruction, unspecified as to partial versus complete**
Postprocedural intestinal obstruction NOS
CC Exclusion see Appendix A PDX collection 0828
CC **K91.31 Postprocedural partial intestinal obstruction**
Postprocedural incomplete intestinal obstruction
CC Exclusion see Appendix A PDX collection 0828
CC **K91.32 Postprocedural complete intestinal obstruction**
CC Exclusion see Appendix A PDX collection 0828

K91.5 Postcholecystectomy syndrome

\+ **K91.6 Intraoperative hemorrhage and hematoma of a digestive system organ or structure complicating a procedure**
Excludes1: *intraoperative hemorrhage and hematoma of a digestive system organ or structure due to accidental puncture and laceration during a procedure (K91.7-)*
CC **K91.61 Intraoperative hemorrhage and hematoma of a digestive system organ or structure complicating a digestive sytem procedure**
CC Exclusion see Appendix A PDX collection 0829
CC **K91.62 Intraoperative hemorrhage and hematoma of a digestive system organ or structure complicating other procedure**
CC Exclusion see Appendix A PDX collection 0829

\+ **K91.7 Accidental puncture and laceration of a digestive system organ or structure during a procedure**
CC **K91.71 Accidental puncture and laceration of a digestive system organ or structure during a digestive system procedure**
CC Exclusion see Appendix A PDX collection 0509
CC **K91.72 Accidental puncture and laceration of a digestive system organ or structure during other procedure**
CC Exclusion see Appendix A PDX collection 0509

\+ **K91.8 Other intraoperative and postprocedural complications and disorders of digestive system**
CC **K91.81 Other intraoperative complications of digestive system**
CC Exclusion see Appendix A PDX collection 0828
CC **K91.82 Postprocedural hepatic failure**
CC Exclusion see Appendix A PDX collection 0828
CC **K91.83 Postprocedural hepatorenal syndrome**
CC Exclusion see Appendix A PDX collection 0828

\+ **K91.84 Postprocedural hemorrhage of a digestive system organ or structure following a procedure**
CC **K91.840 Postprocedural hemorrhage of a digestive system organ or structure following a digestive system procedure**
CC Exclusion see Appendix A PDX collection 0829
AHA CC: 1Q, 2016, 15
CC **K91.841 Postprocedural hemorrhage of a digestive system organ or structure following other procedure**
CC Exclusion see Appendix A PDX collection 0829

\+ **K91.85 Complications of intestinal pouch**
CC **K91.850 Pouchitis**
Inflammation of internal ileoanal pouch
CC Exclusion see Appendix A PDX collection 0828
CC **K91.858 Other complications of intestinal pouch**
CC Exclusion see Appendix A PDX collection 0828

CC **K91.86 Retained cholelithiasis following cholecystectomy**
CC Exclusion see Appendix A PDX collection 0828

\+ **K91.87 Postprocedural hematoma and seroma of a digestive system organ or structure following a procedure**
CC **K91.870 Postprocedural hematoma of a digestive system organ or structure following a digestive system procedure**
CC Exclusion see Appendix A PDX collection 0829
CC **K91.871 Postprocedural hematoma of a digestive system organ or structure following other procedure**
CC Exclusion see Appendix A PDX collection 0829
CC **K91.872 Postprocedural seroma of a digestive system organ or structure following a digestive system procedure**
CC Exclusion see Appendix A PDX collection 0829
CC **K91.873 Postprocedural seroma of a digestive system organ or structure following other procedure**
CC Exclusion see Appendix A PDX collection 0829

CC **K91.89 Other postprocedural complications and disorders of digestive system**
Use additional code, if applicable, to further specify disorder
Excludes2: *postprocedural retroperitoneal abscess (K68.11)*
CC Exclusion see Appendix A PDX collection 0828
AHA CC: 1Q, 2017, 40-41

K92 Other diseases of digestive system

Excludes1: *neonatal gastrointestinal hemorrhage (P54.0-P54.3)*

CC **K92.0 Hematemesis**
CC Exclusion see Appendix A PDX collection 0770
CC **K92.1 Melena**
Excludes1: *occult blood in feces (R19.5)*
CC Exclusion see Appendix A PDX collection 0770
CC **K92.2 Gastrointestinal hemorrhage, unspecified**
Gastric hemorrhage NOS
Intestinal hemorrhage NOS
Excludes1: *acute hemorrhagic gastritis (K29.01)*
hemorrhage of anus and rectum (K62.5)
angiodysplasia of stomach with hemorrhage (K31.811)
diverticular disease with hemorrhage (K57.-)
gastritis and duodenitis with hemorrhage (K29.-)
peptic ulcer with hemorrhage (K25-K28)
CC Exclusion see Appendix A PDX collection 0770

\+ **K92.8 Other specified diseases of the digestive system**
CC **K92.81 Gastrointestinal mucositis (ulcerative)**
Code also type of associated therapy, such as:
antineoplastic and immunosuppressive drugs (T45.1X-)
radiological procedure and radiotherapy (Y84.2)
Excludes2: *mucositis (ulcerative) of vagina and vulva (N76.81)*
nasal mucositis (ulcerative) (J34.81)
oral mucositis (ulcerative) (K12.3-)
CC Exclusion see Appendix A PDX collection 0765

K92.89 Other specified diseases of the digestive system

K92.9 Disease of digestive system, unspecified

K94 Complications of artificial openings of the digestive system

+ **K94.0 Colostomy complications**
  - **K94.00 Colostomy complication, unspecified**
  - CC **K94.01 Colostomy hemorrhage**
    CC Exclusion see Appendix A PDX collection 0830
  - CC **K94.02 Colostomy infection**
    Use additional code to specify type of infection, such as:
    cellulitis of abdominal wall (L03.311)
    sepsis (A40.-, A41.-)
    CC Exclusion see Appendix A PDX collection 0830
  - CC **K94.03 Colostomy malfunction**
    Mechanical complication of colostomy
    CC Exclusion see Appendix A PDX collection 0831
  - **K94.09 Other complications of colostomy**
    CC Exclusion see Appendix A PDX collection 0830

+ **K94.1 Enterostomy complications**
  - **K94.10 Enterostomy complication, unspecified**
  - CC **K94.11 Enterostomy hemorrhage**
    CC Exclusion see Appendix A PDX collection 0830
  - CC **K94.12 Enterostomy infection**
    Use additional code to specify type of infection, such as:
    cellulitis of abdominal wall (L03.311)
    sepsis (A40.-, A41.-)
    CC Exclusion see Appendix A PDX collection 0830
  - CC **K94.13 Enterostomy malfunction**
    Mechanical complication of enterostomy
    CC Exclusion see Appendix A PDX collection 0831
  - CC **K94.19 Other complications of enterostomy**
    CC Exclusion see Appendix A PDX collection 0830

+ **K94.2 Gastrostomy complications**
  - **K94.20 Gastrostomy complication, unspecified**
  - **K94.21 Gastrostomy hemorrhage**
  - CC **K94.22 Gastrostomy infection**
    Use additional code to specify type of infection, such as:
    cellulitis of abdominal wall (L03.311)
    sepsis (A40.-, A41.-)
    CC Exclusion see Appendix A PDX collection 0828
  - CC **K94.23 Gastrostomy malfunction**
    Mechanical complication of gastrostomy
    CC Exclusion see Appendix A PDX collection 0828
  - **K94.29 Other complications of gastrostomy**

+ **K94.3 Esophagostomy complications**
  - CC **K94.30 Esophagostomy complications, unspecified**
    CC Exclusion see Appendix A PDX collection 0828
  - CC **K94.31 Esophagostomy hemorrhage**
    CC Exclusion see Appendix A PDX collection 0828
  - CC **K94.32 Esophagostomy infection**
    Use additional code to identify the infection
    CC Exclusion see Appendix A PDX collection 0828
  - CC **K94.33 Esophagostomy malfunction**
    Mechanical complication of esophagostomy
    CC Exclusion see Appendix A PDX collection 0828
  - CC **K94.39 Other complications of esophagostomy**
    CC Exclusion see Appendix A PDX collection 0828

+ K95 Complications of bariatric procedures

+ **K95.0 Complications of gastric band procedure**
  - CC **K95.01 Infection due to gastric band procedure**
    Use additional code to specify type of infection or organism, such as:
    bacterial and viral infectious agents (B95.-, B96.-)
    cellulitis of abdominal wall (L03.311)
    sepsis (A40.-, A41.-)
    CC Exclusion see Appendix A PDX collection 0828
    HAC see Appendix B for HAC conditional logic
  - CC **K95.09 Other complications of gastric band procedure**
    Use additional code, if applicable, to further specify complication
    CC Exclusion see Appendix A PDX collection 0828

+ **K95.8 Complications of other bariatric procedure**
  Excludes1: *complications of gastric band surgery (K95.0-)*
  - CC **K95.81 Infection due to other bariatric procedure**
    Use additional code to specify type of infection or organism, such as:
    bacterial and viral infectious agents (B95.-, B96.-)
    cellulitis of abdominal wall (L03.311)
    sepsis (A40.-, A41.-)
    CC Exclusion see Appendix A PDX collection 0828
    HAC see Appendix B for HAC conditional logic
  - CC **K95.89 Other complications of other bariatric procedure**
    Use additional code, if applicable, to further specify complication
    CC Exclusion see Appendix A PDX collection 0828

Chapter 12: Diseases of the Skin and Subcutaneous Tissue (L00-L99)

Excludes2: certain conditions originating in the perinatal period (P04-P96)
certain infectious and parasitic diseases (A00-B99)
complications of pregnancy, childbirth and the puerperium (O00-O9A)
congenital malformations, deformations, and chromosomal abnormalities (Q00-Q99)
endocrine, nutritional and metabolic diseases (E00-E88)
lipomelanotic reticulosis (I89.8)
neoplasms (C00-D49)
symptoms, signs and abnormal clinical and laboratory findings, not elsewhere classified (R00-R94)
systemic connective tissue disorders (M30-M36)
viral warts (B07.-)

This chapter contains the following category blocks:

L00-L08	Infections of the skin and subcutaneous tissue
L10-L14	Bullous disorders
L20-L30	Dermatitis and eczema
L40-L45	Papulosquamous disorders
L49-L54	Urticaria and erythema
L55-L59	Radiation-related disorders of the skin and subcutaneous tissue
L60-L75	Disorders of skin appendages
L76	Intraoperative and postprocedural complications of skin and subcutaneous tissue
L80-L99	Other disorders of the skin and subcutaneous tissue

C. Chapter-Specific Coding Guidelines

In addition to general coding guidelines, there are guidelines for specific diagnoses and/or conditions in the classification. Unless otherwise indicated, these guidelines apply to all health care settings. Please refer to Section II for guidelines on the selection of principal diagnosis.

12. Chapter 12: Diseases of the Skin and Subcutaneous Tissue (L00-L99)

a. Pressure ulcer stage codes

1) Pressure ulcer stages

Codes from category L89, Pressure ulcer, are combination codes that identify the site of the pressure ulcer as well as the stage of the ulcer.

The ICD-10-CM classifies pressure ulcer stages based on severity, which is designated by stages 1-4, unspecified stage and unstageable.

Assign as many codes from category L89 as needed to identify all the pressure ulcers the patient has, if applicable.

2) Unstageable pressure ulcers

Assignment of the code for unstageable pressure ulcer (L89.--0) should be based on the clinical documentation. These codes are used for pressure ulcers whose stage cannot be clinically determined (e.g., the ulcer is covered by eschar or has been treated with a skin or muscle graft) and pressure ulcers that are documented as deep tissue injury but not documented as due to trauma. This code should not be confused with the codes for unspecified stage (L89.--9). When there is no documentation regarding the stage of the pressure ulcer, assign the appropriate code for unspecified stage (L89.--9).

3) Documented pressure ulcer stage

Assignment of the pressure ulcer stage code should be guided by clinical documentation of the stage or documentation of the terms found in the Alphabetic Index. For clinical terms describing the stage that are not found in the Alphabetic Index, and there is no documentation of the stage, the provider should be queried.

4) Patients admitted with pressure ulcers documented as healed

No code is assigned if the documentation states that the pressure ulcer is completely healed.

5) Patients admitted with pressure ulcers documented as healing

Pressure ulcers described as healing should be assigned the appropriate pressure ulcer stage code based on the documentation in the medical record. If the documentation does not provide information about the stage of the healing pressure ulcer, assign the appropriate code for unspecified stage.

If the documentation is unclear as to whether the patient has a current (new) pressure ulcer or if the patient is being treated for a healing pressure ulcer, query the provider.

For ulcers that were present on admission but healed at the time of discharge, assign the code for the site and stage of the pressure ulcer at the time of admission.

6) Patient admitted with pressure ulcer evolving into another stage during the admission

If a patient is admitted **to an inpatient hospital** with a pressure ulcer at one stage and it progresses to a higher stage, two separate codes should be assigned: one code for the site and stage of the ulcer on admission and a second code for the same ulcer site and the highest stage reported during the stay.

b. Non-Pressure Chronic Ulcers

1) Patients admitted with non-pressure ulcers documented as healed

No code is assigned if the documentation states that the non-pressure ulcer is completely healed.

2) Patients admitted with non-pressure ulcers documented as healing

Non-pressure ulcers described as healing should be assigned the appropriate non-pressure ulcer code based on the documentation in the medical record. If the documentation does not provide information about the severity of the healing non-pressure ulcer, assign the appropriate code unspecified severity.

If the documentation is unclear as to whether the patient has a current (new) non-pressure ulcer or if the patient is being treated for a healing non-pressure ulcer, query the provider.

For ulcers that were present on admission but healed at the time of discharge, assign the code for the site and severity of the non-pressure ulcer at the time of admission.

3) Patient admitted with non-pressure ulcer that progresses to another severity level during the admission

If a patient is admitted to an inpatient hospital with a non-pressure ulcer at one severity level and it progresses to a higher severity level, two separate codes should be assigned; one code for the site and severity level of the ulcer on admission and a second code for the same ulcer site and the highest severity level reported during the stay.

Skin and Subcutaneous Tissue

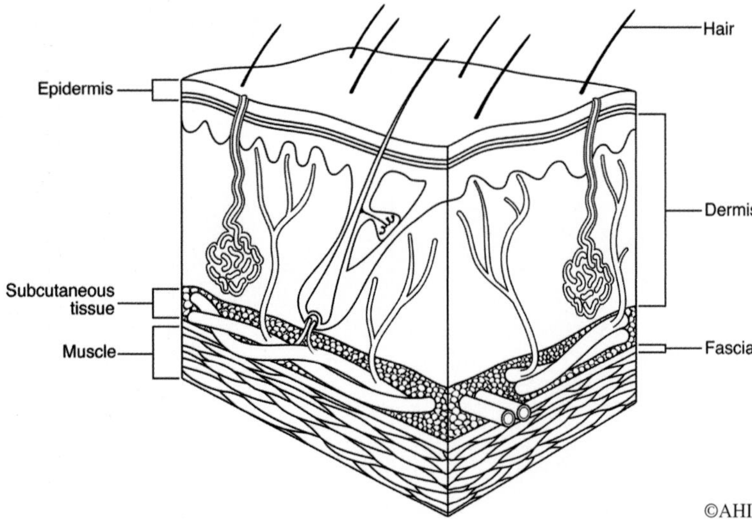

Infections of the skin and subcutaneous tissue (L00-L08)

Use additional code (B95-B97) to identify infectious agent

Excludes2: *hordeolum (H00.0)*
infective dermatitis (L30.3)
local infections of skin classified in Chapter 1
lupus panniculitis (L93.2)
panniculitis NOS (M79.3)
panniculitis of neck and back (M54.0-)
Perlèche NOS (K13.0)
Perlèche due to candidiasis (B37.0)
Perlèche due to riboflavin deficiency (E53.0)
pyogenic granuloma (L98.0)
relapsing panniculitis [Weber-Christian] (M35.6)
viral warts (B07.-)
zoster (B02.-)

L00 Staphylococcal scalded skin syndrome
Ritter's disease
Use additional code to identify percentage of skin exfoliation (L49.-)
Excludes1: *bullous impetigo (L01.03)*
pemphigus neonatorum (L01.03)
toxic epidermal necrolysis [Lyell] (L51.2)
Valid 3-character code, no further characters required

L01 Impetigo
Excludes1: *impetigo herpetiformis (L40.1)*
+ **L01.0 Impetigo**
Impetigo contagiosa
Impetigo vulgaris
L01.00 Impetigo, unspecified
Impetigo NOS
L01.01 Non-bullous impetigo
L01.02 Bockhart's impetigo
Impetigo follicularis
Perifolliculitis NOS
Superficial pustular perifolliculitis
L01.03 Bullous impetigo
Impetigo neonatorum
Pemphigus neonatorum
L01.09 Other impetigo
Ulcerative impetigo
L01.1 Impetiginization of other dermatoses

L02 Cutaneous abscess, furuncle and carbuncle
Use additional code to identify organism (B95-B96)
Excludes2: *abscess of anus and rectal regions (K61.-)*
abscess of female genital organs (external) (N76.4)
abscess of male genital organs (external) (N48.2, N49.-)
+ **L02.0 Cutaneous abscess, furuncle and carbuncle of face**
Excludes2: *abscess of ear, external (H60.0)*
abscess of eyelid (H00.0)
abscess of head [any part, except face] (L02.8)
abscess of lacrimal gland (H04.0)
abscess of lacrimal passages (H04.3)
abscess of mouth (K12.2)
abscess of nose (J34.0)
abscess of orbit (H05.0)
submandibular abscess (K12.2)
CC **L02.01 Cutaneous abscess of face**
No CC Exclusions
L02.02 Furuncle of face
Boil of face
Folliculitis of face
L02.03 Carbuncle of face
+ **L02.1 Cutaneous abscess, furuncle and carbuncle of neck**
CC **L02.11 Cutaneous abscess of neck**
CC Exclusion see Appendix A PDX collection 0832
L02.12 Furuncle of neck
Boil of neck
Folliculitis of neck
L02.13 Carbuncle of neck
+ **L02.2 Cutaneous abscess, furuncle and carbuncle of trunk**
Excludes1: *non-newborn omphalitis (L08.82)*
omphalitis of newborn (P38.-)
Excludes2: *abscess of breast (N61.1)*
abscess of buttocks (L02.3)
abscess of female external genital organs (N76.4)
abscess of male external genital organs (N48.2, N49.-)
abscess of hip (L02.4)
CC **L02.21 Cutaneous abscess of trunk**
CC **L02.211 Cutaneous abscess of abdominal wall**
CC Exclusion see Appendix A PDX collection 0833
CC **L02.212 Cutaneous abscess of back [any part, except buttock]**
CC Exclusion see Appendix A PDX collection 0833
CC **L02.213 Cutaneous abscess of chest wall**
CC Exclusion see Appendix A PDX collection 0833
CC **L02.214 Cutaneous abscess of groin**
CC Exclusion see Appendix A PDX collection 0833
CC **L02.215 Cutaneous abscess of perineum**
CC Exclusion see Appendix A PDX collection 0833
CC **L02.216 Cutaneous abscess of umbilicus**
CC Exclusion see Appendix A PDX collection 0833
CC **L02.219 Cutaneous abscess of trunk, unspecified**
CC Exclusion see Appendix A PDX collection 0833
+ **L02.22 Furuncle of trunk**
Boil of trunk
Folliculitis of trunk
L02.221 Furuncle of abdominal wall
L02.222 Furuncle of back [any part, except buttock]
L02.223 Furuncle of chest wall
L02.224 Furuncle of groin
L02.225 Furuncle of perineum
L02.226 Furuncle of umbilicus
L02.229 Furuncle of trunk, unspecified
+ **L02.23 Carbuncle of trunk**
L02.231 Carbuncle of abdominal wall
L02.232 Carbuncle of back [any part, except buttock]
L02.233 Carbuncle of chest wall
L02.234 Carbuncle of groin
L02.235 Carbuncle of perineum
L02.236 Carbuncle of umbilicus
L02.239 Carbuncle of trunk, unspecified
+ **L02.3 Cutaneous abscess, furuncle and carbuncle of buttock**
Excludes1: *pilonidal cyst with abscess (L05.01)*
CC **L02.31 Cutaneous abscess of buttock**
Cutaneous abscess of gluteal region
CC Exclusion see Appendix A PDX collection 0834
L02.32 Furuncle of buttock
Boil of buttock
Folliculitis of buttock
Furuncle of gluteal region
L02.33 Carbuncle of buttock
Carbuncle of gluteal region
+ **L02.4 Cutaneous abscess, furuncle and carbuncle of limb**
Excludes2: *Cutaneous abscess, furuncle and carbuncle of groin (L02.214, L02.224, L02.234)*
Cutaneous abscess, furuncle and carbuncle of hand (L02.5-)
Cutaneous abscess, furuncle and carbuncle of foot (L02.6-)
+ **L02.41 Cutaneous abscess of limb**
CC **L02.411 Cutaneous abscess of right axilla**
CC Exclusion see Appendix A PDX collection 0835
CC **L02.412 Cutaneous abscess of left axilla**
CC Exclusion see Appendix A PDX collection 0835
CC **L02.413 Cutaneous abscess of right upper limb**
CC Exclusion see Appendix A PDX collection 0835
CC **L02.414 Cutaneous abscess of left upper limb**
CC Exclusion see Appendix A PDX collection 0835

CC **L02.415 Cutaneous abscess of right lower limb**
CC Exclusion see Appendix A PDX collection 0836

CC **L02.416 Cutaneous abscess of left lower limb**
CC Exclusion see Appendix A PDX collection 0836

CC **L02.419 Cutaneous abscess of limb, unspecified**
CC Exclusion see Appendix A PDX collection 0836

\+ **L02.42 Furuncle of limb**
Boil of limb
Folliculitis of limb

L02.421 Furuncle of right axilla
L02.422 Furuncle of left axilla
L02.423 Furuncle of right upper limb
L02.424 Furuncle of left upper limb
L02.425 Furuncle of right lower limb
L02.426 Furuncle of left lower limb
L02.429 Furuncle of limb, unspecified

\+ **L02.43 Carbuncle of limb**
L02.431 Carbuncle of right axilla
L02.432 Carbuncle of left axilla
L02.433 Carbuncle of right upper limb
L02.434 Carbuncle of left upper limb
L02.435 Carbuncle of right lower limb
L02.436 Carbuncle of left lower limb
L02.439 Carbuncle of limb, unspecified

\+ **L02.5 Cutaneous abscess, furuncle and carbuncle of hand**

\+ **L02.51 Cutaneous abscess of hand**

CC **L02.511 Cutaneous abscess of right hand**
CC Exclusion see Appendix A PDX collection 0837

CC **L02.512 Cutaneous abscess of left hand**
CC Exclusion see Appendix A PDX collection 0837

CC **L02.519 Cutaneous abscess of unspecified hand**
CC Exclusion see Appendix A PDX collection 0837

\+ **L02.52 Furuncle hand**
Boil of hand
Folliculitis of hand

L02.521 Furuncle right hand
L02.522 Furuncle left hand
L02.529 Furuncle unspecified hand

\+ **L02.53 Carbuncle of hand**
L02.531 Carbuncle of right hand
L02.532 Carbuncle of left hand
L02.539 Carbuncle of unspecified hand

\+ **L02.6 Cutaneous abscess, furuncle and carbuncle of foot**

\+ **L02.61 Cutaneous abscess of foot**

CC **L02.611 Cutaneous abscess of right foot**
CC Exclusion see Appendix A PDX collection 0838

CC **L02.612 Cutaneous abscess of left foot**
CC Exclusion see Appendix A PDX collection 0838

CC **L02.619 Cutaneous abscess of unspecified foot**
CC Exclusion see Appendix A PDX collection 0838

\+ **L02.62 Furuncle of foot**
Boil of foot
Folliculitis of foot

L02.621 Furuncle of right foot
L02.622 Furuncle of left foot
L02.629 Furuncle of unspecified foot

\+ **L02.63 Carbuncle of foot**
L02.631 Carbuncle of right foot
L02.632 Carbuncle of left foot
L02.639 Carbuncle of unspecified foot

\+ **L02.8 Cutaneous abscess, furuncle and carbuncle of other sites**

\+ **L02.81 Cutaneous abscess of other sites**

CC **L02.811 Cutaneous abscess of head [any part, except face]**
CC Exclusion see Appendix A PDX collection 0839

CC **L02.818 Cutaneous abscess of other sites**
CC Exclusion see Appendix A PDX collection 0839

\+ **L02.82 Furuncle of other sites**
Boil of other sites
Folliculitis of other sites

L02.821 Furuncle of head [any part, except face]
L02.828 Furuncle of other sites

\+ **L02.83 Carbuncle of other sites**
L02.831 Carbuncle of head [any part, except face]
L02.838 Carbuncle of other sites

\+ **L02.9 Cutaneous abscess, furuncle and carbuncle, unspecified**

CC **L02.91 Cutaneous abscess, unspecified**
CC Exclusion see Appendix A PDX collection 0839

L02.92 Furuncle, unspecified
Boil NOS
Furunculosis NOS

L02.93 Carbuncle, unspecified

L03 Cellulitis and acute lymphangitis

Excludes2: *cellulitis of anal and rectal region (K61.-)*
cellulitis of external auditory canal (H60.1)
cellulitis of eyelid (H00.0)
cellulitis of female external genital organs (N76.4)
cellulitis of lacrimal apparatus (H04.3)
cellulitis of male external genital organs (N48.2, N49.-)
cellulitis of mouth (K12.2)
cellulitis of nose (J34.0)
eosinophilic cellulitis [Wells] (L98.3)
febrile neutrophilic dermatosis [Sweet] (L98.2)
lymphangitis (chronic) (subacute) (I89.1)

\+ **L03.0 Cellulitis and acute lymphangitis of finger and toe**
Infection of nail
Onychia
Paronychia
Perionychia

\+ **L03.01 Cellulitis of finger**
Felon
Whitlow
Excludes1: herpetic whitlow (B00.89)

L03.011 Cellulitis of right finger
L03.012 Cellulitis of left finger
L03.019 Cellulitis of unspecified finger

\+ **L03.02 Acute lymphangitis of finger**
Hangnail with lymphangitis of finger

L03.021 Acute lymphangitis of right finger
L03.022 Acute lymphangitis of left finger
L03.029 Acute lymphangitis of unspecified finger

\+ **L03.03 Cellulitis of toe**
L03.031 Cellulitis of right toe
L03.032 Cellulitis of left toe
L03.039 Cellulitis of unspecified toe

\+ **L03.04 Acute lymphangitis of toe**
Hangnail with lymphangitis of toe

L03.041 Acute lymphangitis of right toe
L03.042 Acute lymphangitis of left toe
L03.049 Acute lymphangitis of unspecified toe

\+ **L03.1 Cellulitis and acute lymphangitis of other parts of limb**

\+ **L03.11 Cellulitis of other parts of limb**
Excludes2: *cellulitis of fingers (L03.01-)*
cellulitis of toes (L03.03-)
groin (L03.314)

CC **L03.111 Cellulitis of right axilla**
CC Exclusion see Appendix A PDX collection 0835

CC **L03.112 Cellulitis of left axilla**
CC Exclusion see Appendix A PDX collection 0835

CC **L03.113 Cellulitis of right upper limb**
CC Exclusion see Appendix A PDX collection 0835

CC **L03.114 Cellulitis of left upper limb**
CC Exclusion see Appendix A PDX collection 0835

CC **L03.115 Cellulitis of right lower limb**
CC Exclusion see Appendix A PDX collection 0836

CC **L03.116 Cellulitis of left lower limb**
CC Exclusion see Appendix A PDX collection 0836

CC **L03.119 Cellulitis of unspecified part of limb**
CC Exclusion see Appendix A PDX collection 0836

\+ **L03.12 Acute lymphangitis of other parts of limb**
Excludes2: *acute lymphangitis of fingers (L03.2-)*
acute lymphangitis of toes (L03.04-)
acute lymphangitis of groin (L03.324)

CC **L03.121 Acute lymphangitis of right axilla**
CC Exclusion see Appendix A PDX collection 0835

CC **L03.122 Acute lymphangitis of left axilla**
CC Exclusion see Appendix A PDX collection 0835

CC **L03.123 Acute lymphangitis of right upper limb**
CC Exclusion see Appendix A PDX collection 0835

CC **L03.124 Acute lymphangitis of left upper limb**
CC Exclusion see Appendix A PDX collection 0835

CC **L03.125 Acute lymphangitis of right lower limb**
CC Exclusion see Appendix A PDX collection 0836

CC **L03.126 Acute lymphangitis of left lower limb**
CC Exclusion see Appendix A PDX collection 0836

CC **L03.129 Acute lymphangitis of unspecified part of limb**
CC Exclusion see Appendix A PDX collection 0836

+ **L03.2 Cellulitis and acute lymphangitis of face and neck**

+ **L03.21 Cellulitis and acute lymphangitis of face**

CC **L03.211 Cellulitis of face**
Excludes2: *abscess of orbit (H05.01-)*
cellulitis of ear (H60.1-)
cellulitis of eyelid (H00.0-)
cellulitis of head (L03.81)
cellulitis of lacrimal apparatus (H04.3)
cellulitis of lip (K13.0)
cellulitis of mouth (K12.2)
cellulitis of nose (internal) (J34.0)
cellulitis of orbit (H05.01-)
cellulitis of scalp (L03.81)
CC Exclusion see Appendix A PDX collection 0840
AHA CC: 4Q, 2013, 123

CC **L03.212 Acute lymphangitis of face**
No CC Exclusions

CC **L03.213 Periorbital cellulitis**
Preseptal cellulitis
CC Exclusion see Appendix A PDX collection 0840
AHA CC: 4Q, 2016, 36

+ **L03.22 Cellulitis and acute lymphangitis of neck**

CC **L03.221 Cellulitis of neck**
CC Exclusion see Appendix A PDX collection 0832

CC **L03.222 Acute lymphangitis of neck**
CC Exclusion see Appendix A PDX collection 0832

+ **L03.3 Cellulitis and acute lymphangitis of trunk**

+ **L03.31 Cellulitis of trunk**
Excludes2: *cellulitis of anal and rectal regions (K61.-)*
cellulitis of breast NOS (N61.0)
cellulitis of female external genital organs (N76.4)
cellulitis of male external genital organs (N48.2, N49.-)
omphalitis of newborn (P38.-)
puerperal cellulitis of breast (O91.2)

CC **L03.311 Cellulitis of abdominal wall**
Excludes2: *cellulitis of umbilicus (L03.316)*
cellulitis of groin (L03.314)
CC Exclusion see Appendix A PDX collection 0833

CC **L03.312 Cellulitis of back [any part except buttock]**
CC Exclusion see Appendix A PDX collection 0833

CC **L03.313 Cellulitis of chest wall**
CC Exclusion see Appendix A PDX collection 0833

CC **L03.314 Cellulitis of groin**
CC Exclusion see Appendix A PDX collection 0833

CC **L03.315 Cellulitis of perineum**
CC Exclusion see Appendix A PDX collection 0833

CC **L03.316 Cellulitis of umbilicus**
CC Exclusion see Appendix A PDX collection 0833

CC **L03.317 Cellulitis of buttock**
CC Exclusion see Appendix A PDX collection 0834

CC **L03.319 Cellulitis of trunk, unspecified**
CC Exclusion see Appendix A PDX collection 0833

+ **L03.32 Acute lymphangitis of trunk**

CC **L03.321 Acute lymphangitis of abdominal wall**
CC Exclusion see Appendix A PDX collection 0833

CC **L03.322 Acute lymphangitis of back [any part except buttock]**
CC Exclusion see Appendix A PDX collection 0833

CC **L03.323 Acute lymphangitis of chest wall**
CC Exclusion see Appendix A PDX collection 0833

CC **L03.324 Acute lymphangitis of groin**
CC Exclusion see Appendix A PDX collection 0833

CC **L03.325 Acute lymphangitis of perineum**
CC Exclusion see Appendix A PDX collection 0833

CC **L03.326 Acute lymphangitis of umbilicus**
CC Exclusion see Appendix A PDX collection 0833

CC **L03.327 Acute lymphangitis of buttock**
CC Exclusion see Appendix A PDX collection 0834

CC **L03.329 Acute lymphangitis of trunk, unspecified**
CC Exclusion see Appendix A PDX collection 0833

+ **L03.8 Cellulitis and acute lymphangitis of other sites**

+ **L03.81 Cellulitis of other sites**

CC **L03.811 Cellulitis of head [any part, except face]**
Cellulitis of scalp
Excludes2: *cellulitis of face (L03.211)*
CC Exclusion see Appendix A PDX collection 0839

CC **L03.818 Cellulitis of other sites**
CC Exclusion see Appendix A PDX collection 0839

+ **L03.89 Acute lymphangitis of other sites**

CC **L03.891 Acute lymphangitis of head [any part, except face]**
CC Exclusion see Appendix A PDX collection 0839

CC **L03.898 Acute lymphangitis of other sites**
CC Exclusion see Appendix A PDX collection 0839

+ **L03.9 Cellulitis and acute lymphangitis, unspecified**

CC **L03.90 Cellulitis, unspecified**
CC Exclusion see Appendix A PDX collection 0839

CC **L03.91 Acute lymphangitis, unspecified**
Excludes1: *lymphangitis NOS (I89.1)*
CC Exclusion see Appendix A PDX collection 0839

L04 Acute lymphadenitis

Includes: abscess (acute) of lymph nodes, except mesenteric
acute lymphadenitis, except mesenteric

Excludes1: *chronic or subacute lymphadenitis, except mesenteric (I88.1)*
enlarged lymph nodes (R59.-)
human immunodeficiency virus [HIV] disease resulting in generalized lymphadenopathy (B20)
lymphadenitis NOS (I88.9)
nonspecific mesenteric lymphadenitis (I88.0)

L04.0 Acute lymphadenitis of face, head and neck

L04.1 Acute lymphadenitis of trunk

L04.2 Acute lymphadenitis of upper limb
Acute lymphadenitis of axilla
Acute lymphadenitis of shoulder

L04.3 Acute lymphadenitis of lower limb
Acute lymphadenitis of hip
Excludes2: *acute lymphadenitis of groin (L04.1)*

L04.8 Acute lymphadenitis of other sites

L04.9 Acute lymphadenitis, unspecified

L05 Pilonidal cyst and sinus

+ **L05.0 Pilonidal cyst and sinus with abscess**

CC **L05.01 Pilonidal cyst with abscess**
Pilonidal abscess
Pilonidal dimple with abscess
Postanal dimple with abscess
Excludes2: *congenital sacral dimple (Q82.6)*
parasacral dimple (Q82.6)
CC Exclusion see Appendix A PDX collection 0841

CC **L05.02 Pilonidal sinus with abscess**
Coccygeal fistula with abscess
Coccygeal sinus with abscess
Pilonidal fistula with abscess
CC Exclusion see Appendix A PDX collection 0841

+ L05.9 **Pilonidal cyst and sinus without abscess**

L05.91 **Pilonidal cyst without abscess**
Pilonidal dimple
Postanal dimple
Pilonidal cyst NOS
Excludes2: *congenital sacral dimple (Q82.6)*
parasacral dimple (Q82.6)

L05.92 **Pilonidal sinus without abscess**
Coccygeal fistula
Coccygeal sinus without abscess
Pilonidal fistula

L08 Other local infections of skin and subcutaneous tissue

L08.0 **Pyoderma**
Dermatitis gangrenosa
Purulent dermatitis
Septic dermatitis
Suppurative dermatitis
Excludes1: *pyoderma gangrenosum (L88)*
pyoderma vegetans (L08.81)

CC L08.1 **Erythrasma**
CC Exclusion see Appendix A PDX collection 0107

+ L08.8 **Other specified local infections of the skin and subcutaneous tissue**

L08.81 **Pyoderma vegetans**
Excludes1: *pyoderma gangrenosum (L88)*
pyoderma NOS (L08.0)

L08.82 **Omphalitis not of newborn**
Excludes1: *omphalitis of newborn (P38.-)*

L08.89 **Other specified local infections of the skin and subcutaneous tissue**

L08.9 **Local infection of the skin and subcutaneous tissue, unspecified**

Bullous disorders (L10-L14)

Excludes1: *benign familial pemphigus [Hailey-Hailey] (Q82.8)*
staphylococcal scalded skin syndrome (L00)
toxic epidermal necrolysis [Lyell] (L51.2)

L10 Pemphigus

Excludes1: *pemphigus neonatorum (L01.03)*

CC L10.0 **Pemphigus vulgaris**
CC Exclusion see Appendix A PDX collection 0842

CC L10.1 **Pemphigus vegetans**
CC Exclusion see Appendix A PDX collection 0842

CC L10.2 **Pemphigus foliaceous**
CC Exclusion see Appendix A PDX collection 0842

CC L10.3 **Brazilian pemphigus [fogo selvagem]**
CC Exclusion see Appendix A PDX collection 0842

CC L10.4 **Pemphigus erythematosus**
Senear-Usher syndrome
CC Exclusion see Appendix A PDX collection 0842

CC L10.5 **Drug-induced pemphigus**
Use additional code for adverse effect, if applicable, to identify drug (T36-T50 with fifth or sixth character 5)
CC Exclusion see Appendix A PDX collection 0842

+ L10.8 **Other pemphigus**

CC L10.81 **Paraneoplastic pemphigus**
CC Exclusion see Appendix A PDX collection 0842

CC L10.89 **Other pemphigus**
CC Exclusion see Appendix A PDX collection 0842

CC L10.9 **Pemphigus, unspecified**
CC Exclusion see Appendix A PDX collection 0842

L11 Other acantholytic disorders

L11.0 **Acquired keratosis follicularis**
Excludes1: *keratosis follicularis (congenital) [Darier-White] (Q82.8)*

L11.1 **Transient acantholytic dermatosis [Grover]**

L11.8 **Other specified acantholytic disorders**

L11.9 **Acantholytic disorder, unspecified**

L12 Pemphigoid

Excludes1: *herpes gestationis (O26.4-)*
impetigo herpetiformis (L40.1)

CC L12.0 **Bullous pemphigoid**
CC Exclusion see Appendix A PDX collection 0842

L12.1 **Cicatricial pemphigoid**
Benign mucous membrane pemphigoid

• L12.2 **Chronic bullous disease of childhood**
Juvenile dermatitis herpetiformis

+ L12.3 **Acquired epidermolysis bullosa**
Excludes1: *epidermolysis bullosa (congenital) (Q81.-)*

CC L12.30 **Acquired epidermolysis bullosa, unspecified**
CC Exclusion see Appendix A PDX collection 0843

CC L12.31 **Epidermolysis bullosa due to drug**
Use additional code for adverse effect, if applicable, to identify drug (T36-T50 with fifth or sixth character 5)
CC Exclusion see Appendix A PDX collection 0843

CC L12.35 **Other acquired epidermolysis bullosa**
CC Exclusion see Appendix A PDX collection 0843

CC L12.8 **Other pemphigoid**
CC Exclusion see Appendix A PDX collection 0842

CC L12.9 **Pemphigoid, unspecified**
CC Exclusion see Appendix A PDX collection 0842

L13 Other bullous disorders

L13.0 **Dermatitis herpetiformis**
Duhring's disease
Hydroa herpetiformis
Excludes1: *juvenile dermatitis herpetiformis (L12.2)*
senile dermatitis herpetiformis (L12.0)

L13.1 **Subcorneal pustular dermatitis**
Sneddon-Wilkinson disease

L13.8 **Other specified bullous disorders**

L13.9 **Bullous disorder, unspecified**

L14 Bullous disorders in diseases classified elsewhere

Code first underlying disease
Valid 3-character code, no further characters required

Dermatitis and eczema (L20-L30)

NOTE In this block the terms dermatitis and eczema are used synonymously and interchangeably.

Excludes2: *chronic (childhood) granulomatous disease (D71)*
dermatitis gangrenosa (L08.0)
dermatitis herpetiformis (L13.0)
dry skin dermatitis (L85.3)
factitial dermatitis (L98.1)
perioral dermatitis (L71.0)
radiation-related disorders of the skin and subcutaneous tissue (L55-L59)
stasis dermatitis (I87.2)

L20 Atopic dermatitis

L20.0 **Besnier's prurigo**

+ L20.8 **Other atopic dermatitis**
Excludes2: *circumscribed neurodermatitis (L28.0)*

L20.81 **Atopic neurodermatitis**
Diffuse neurodermatitis

L20.82 **Flexural eczema**

• L20.83 **Infantile (acute) (chronic) eczema**

L20.84 **Intrinsic (allergic) eczema**

L20.89 **Other atopic dermatitis**

L20.9 **Atopic dermatitis, unspecified**

L21 Seborrheic dermatitis

Excludes2: *infective dermatitis (L30.3)*
seborrheic keratosis (L82.-)

L21.0 **Seborrhea capitis**
Cradle cap

• L21.1 **Seborrheic infantile dermatitis**

L21.8 **Other seborrheic dermatitis**

L21.9 **Seborrheic dermatitis, unspecified**
Seborrhea NOS

L22 Diaper dermatitis

Diaper erythema
Diaper rash
Psoriasiform diaper rash
Valid 3-character code, no further characters required

L23 Allergic contact dermatitis

Excludes1: *allergy NOS (T78.40)*
contact dermatitis NOS (L25.9)
dermatitis NOS (L30.9)
Excludes2: *dermatitis due to substances taken internally (L27.-)*
dermatitis of eyelid (H01.1-)
diaper dermatitis (L22)
eczema of external ear (H60.5-)
irritant contact dermatitis (L24.-)
perioral dermatitis (L71.0)
radiation-related disorders of the skin and subcutaneous tissue (L55-L59)

L23.0 Allergic contact dermatitis due to metals
Allergic contact dermatitis due to chromium
Allergic contact dermatitis due to nickel
L23.1 Allergic contact dermatitis due to adhesives
L23.2 Allergic contact dermatitis due to cosmetics
L23.3 Allergic contact dermatitis due to drugs in contact with skin
Use additional code for adverse effect, if applicable, to identify drug (T36-T50 with fifth or sixth character 5)
Excludes2: *dermatitis due to ingested drugs and medicaments (L27.0-L27.1)*
L23.4 Allergic contact dermatitis due to dyes
L23.5 Allergic contact dermatitis due to other chemical products
Allergic contact dermatitis due to cement
Allergic contact dermatitis due to insecticide
Allergic contact dermatitis due to plastic
Allergic contact dermatitis due to rubber
L23.6 Allergic contact dermatitis due to food in contact with the skin
Excludes2: *dermatitis due to ingested food (L27.2)*
L23.7 Allergic contact dermatitis due to plants, except food
Excludes2: *allergy NOS due to pollen (J30.1)*
\+ **L23.8 Allergic contact dermatitis due to other agents**
L23.81 Allergic contact dermatitis due to animal (cat) (dog) dander
Allergic contact dermatitis due to animal (cat) (dog) hair
L23.89 Allergic contact dermatitis due to other agents
L23.9 Allergic contact dermatitis, unspecified cause
Allergic contact eczema NOS

L24 Irritant contact dermatitis

Excludes1: *allergy NOS (T78.40)*
contact dermatitis NOS (L25.9)
dermatitis NOS (L30.9)
Excludes2: *allergic contact dermatitis (L23.-)*
dermatitis due to substances taken internally (L27.-)
dermatitis of eyelid (H01.1-)
diaper dermatitis (L22)
eczema of external ear (H60.5-)
perioral dermatitis (L71.0)
radiation-related disorders of the skin and subcutaneous tissue (L55-L59)

L24.0 Irritant contact dermatitis due to detergents
L24.1 Irritant contact dermatitis due to oils and greases
L24.2 Irritant contact dermatitis due to solvents
Irritant contact dermatitis due to chlorocompound
Irritant contact dermatitis due to cyclohexane
Irritant contact dermatitis due to ester
Irritant contact dermatitis due to glycol
Irritant contact dermatitis due to hydrocarbon
Irritant contact dermatitis due to ketone
L24.3 Irritant contact dermatitis due to cosmetics
L24.4 Irritant contact dermatitis due to drugs in contact with skin
Use additional code for adverse effect, if applicable, to identify drug (T36-T50 with fifth or sixth character 5)
L24.5 Irritant contact dermatitis due to other chemical products
Irritant contact dermatitis due to cement
Irritant contact dermatitis due to insecticide
Irritant contact dermatitis due to plastic
Irritant contact dermatitis due to rubber
L24.6 Irritant contact dermatitis due to food in contact with skin
Excludes2: *dermatitis due to ingested food (L27.2)*
L24.7 Irritant contact dermatitis due to plants, except food
Excludes2: *allergy NOS to pollen (J30.1)*
\+ **L24.8 Irritant contact dermatitis due to other agents**
L24.81 Irritant contact dermatitis due to metals
Irritant contact dermatitis due to chromium
Irritant contact dermatitis due to nickel
L24.89 Irritant contact dermatitis due to other agents
Irritant contact dermatitis due to dyes
L24.9 Irritant contact dermatitis, unspecified cause
Irritant contact eczema NOS

L25 Unspecified contact dermatitis

Excludes1: *allergic contact dermatitis (L23.-)*
allergy NOS (T78.40)
dermatitis NOS (L30.9)
irritant contact dermatitis (L24.-)
Excludes2: *dermatitis due to ingested substances (L27.-)*
dermatitis of eyelid (H01.1-)
eczema of external ear (H60.5-)
perioral dermatitis (L71.0)
radiation-related disorders of the skin and subcutaneous tissue (L55-L59)

L25.0 Unspecified contact dermatitis due to cosmetics
L25.1 Unspecified contact dermatitis due to drugs in contact with skin
Use additional code for adverse effect, if applicable, to identify drug (T36-T50 with fifth or sixth character 5)
Excludes2: *dermatitis due to ingested drugs and medicaments (L27.0-L27.1)*
L25.2 Unspecified contact dermatitis due to dyes
L25.3 Unspecified contact dermatitis due to other chemical products
Unspecified contact dermatitis due to cement
Unspecified contact dermatitis due to insecticide
L25.4 Unspecified contact dermatitis due to food in contact with skin
Excludes2: *dermatitis due to ingested food (L27.2)*
L25.5 Unspecified contact dermatitis due to plants, except food
Excludes1: *nettle rash (L50.9)*
Excludes2: *allergy NOS due to pollen (J30.1)*
L25.8 Unspecified contact dermatitis due to other agents
L25.9 Unspecified contact dermatitis, unspecified cause
Contact dermatitis (occupational) NOS
Contact eczema (occupational) NOS

L26 Exfoliative dermatitis

Hebra's pityriasis
Excludes1: *Ritter's disease (L00)*
Valid 3-character code, no further characters required

L27 Dermatitis due to substances taken internally

Excludes1: *allergy NOS (T78.40)*
Excludes2: *adverse food reaction, except dermatitis (T78.0-T78.1)*
contact dermatitis (L23-L25)
drug photoallergic response (L56.1)
drug phototoxic response (L56.0)
urticaria (L50.-)

L27.0 Generalized skin eruption due to drugs and medicaments taken internally
Use additional code for adverse effect, if applicable, to identify drug (T36-T50 with fifth or sixth character 5)
L27.1 Localized skin eruption due to drugs and medicaments taken internally
Use additional code for adverse effect, if applicable, to identify drug (T36-T50 with fifth or sixth character 5)
L27.2 Dermatitis due to ingested food
Excludes2: *dermatitis due to food in contact with skin (L23.6, L24.6, L25.4)*
L27.8 Dermatitis due to other substances taken internally
L27.9 Dermatitis due to unspecified substance taken internally

L28 Lichen simplex chronicus and prurigo

L28.0 Lichen simplex chronicus
Circumscribed neurodermatitis
Lichen NOS
L28.1 Prurigo nodularis
L28.2 Other prurigo
Prurigo NOS
Prurigo Hebra
Prurigo mitis
Urticaria papulosa

L29 Pruritus

Excludes1: *neurotic excoriation (L98.1)*
psychogenic pruritus (F45.8)

L29.0 Pruritus ani
♂ **L29.1 Pruritus scroti**
♀ **L29.2 Pruritus vulvae**
L29.3 Anogenital pruritus, unspecified
L29.8 Other pruritus
L29.9 Pruritus, unspecified
Itch NOS

L30 Other and unspecified dermatitis

Excludes2: *contact dermatitis (L23-L25)*
dry skin dermatitis (L85.3)
small plaque parapsoriasis (L41.3)
stasis dermatitis (I87.2)

L30.0 Nummular dermatitis
L30.1 Dyshidrosis [pompholyx]
L30.2 Cutaneous autosensitization
Candidid [levurid]
Dermatophytid
Eczematid
L30.3 Infective dermatitis
Infectious eczematoid dermatitis
L30.4 Erythema intertrigo
L30.5 Pityriasis alba
L30.8 Other specified dermatitis
L30.9 Dermatitis, unspecified
Eczema NOS

Papulosquamous disorders (L40-L45)

L40 Psoriasis

L40.0 Psoriasis vulgaris
Nummular psoriasis
Plaque psoriasis
L40.1 Generalized pustular psoriasis
Impetigo herpetiformis
Von Zumbusch's disease
L40.2 Acrodermatitis continua
L40.3 Pustulosis palmaris et plantaris
L40.4 Guttate psoriasis
+ **L40.5 Arthropathic psoriasis**
L40.50 Arthropathic psoriasis, unspecified
L40.51 Distal interphalangeal psoriatic arthropathy
L40.52 Psoriatic arthritis mutilans
L40.53 Psoriatic spondylitis
L40.54 Psoriatic juvenile arthropathy
L40.59 Other psoriatic arthropathy
L40.8 Other psoriasis
Flexural psoriasis
L40.9 Psoriasis, unspecified

L41 Parapsoriasis

Excludes1: *poikiloderma vasculare atrophicans (L94.5)*

L41.0 Pityriasis lichenoides et varioliformis acuta
Mucha-Habermann disease
L41.1 Pityriasis lichenoides chronica
L41.3 Small plaque parapsoriasis
L41.4 Large plaque parapsoriasis
L41.5 Retiform parapsoriasis
L41.8 Other parapsoriasis
L41.9 Parapsoriasis, unspecified

L42 Pityriasis rosea

Valid 3-character code, no further characters required

L43 Lichen planus

Excludes1: *lichen planopilaris (L66.1)*

L43.0 Hypertrophic lichen planus
L43.1 Bullous lichen planus
L43.2 Lichenoid drug reaction
Use additional code for adverse effect, if applicable, to identify drug (T36-T50 with fifth or sixth character 5)
L43.3 Subacute (active) lichen planus
Lichen planus tropicus
L43.8 Other lichen planus
L43.9 Lichen planus, unspecified

L44 Other papulosquamous disorders

L44.0 Pityriasis rubra pilaris
L44.1 Lichen nitidus
L44.2 Lichen striatus
L44.3 Lichen ruber moniliformis
• **L44.4 Infantile papular acrodermatitis [Gianotti-Crosti]**
L44.8 Other specified papulosquamous disorders
L44.9 Papulosquamous disorder, unspecified

L45 Papulosquamous disorders in diseases classified elsewhere

Code first underlying disease.
Valid 3-character code, no further characters required

Urticaria and erythema (L49-L54)

Excludes1: *Lyme disease (A69.2-)*
rosacea (L71.-)

L49 Exfoliation due to erythematous conditions according to extent of body surface involved

Code first erythematous condition causing exfoliation, such as:
Ritter's disease (L00)
(Staphylococcal) scalded skin syndrom (L00)
Stevens-Johnson syndrome (L51.1)
Stevens-Johnson syndrome-toxic epidermal necrolysis overlap syndrome (L51.3)
Toxic epidermal necrolysis (L51.2)

L49.0 Exfoliation due to erythematous condition involving less than 10 percent of body surface
Exfoliation due to erythematous condition NOS
L49.1 Exfoliation due to erythematous condition involving 10-19 percent of body surface
L49.2 Exfoliation due to erythematous condition involving 20-29 percent of body surface
CC **L49.3 Exfoliation due to erythematous condition involving 30-39 percent of body surface**
CC Exclusion see Appendix A PDX collection 0844
CC **L49.4 Exfoliation due to erythematous condition involving 40-49 percent of body surface**
CC Exclusion see Appendix A PDX collection 0845
CC **L49.5 Exfoliation due to erythematous condition involving 50-59 percent of body surface**
CC Exclusion see Appendix A PDX collection 0846
CC **L49.6 Exfoliation due to erythematous condition involving 60-69 percent of body surface**
CC Exclusion see Appendix A PDX collection 0847
CC **L49.7 Exfoliation due to erythematous condition involving 70-79 percent of body surface**
CC Exclusion see Appendix A PDX collection 0848
CC **L49.8 Exfoliation due to erythematous condition involving 80-89 percent of body surface**
CC Exclusion see Appendix A PDX collection 0849
CC **L49.9 Exfoliation due to erythematous condition involving 90 or more percent of body surface**
CC Exclusion see Appendix A PDX collection 0850

L50 Urticaria

Excludes1: *allergic contact dermatitis (L23.-)*
angioneurotic edema (T78.3)
giant urticaria (T78.3)
hereditary angio-edema (D84.1)
Quincke's edema (T78.3)
serum urticaria (T80.6-)
solar urticaria (L56.3)
urticaria neonatorum (P83.8)
urticaria papulosa (L28.2)
urticaria pigmentosa (Q82.2)

L50.0 Allergic urticaria
L50.1 Idiopathic urticaria
L50.2 Urticaria due to cold and heat
Excludes2: *familial cold urticaria (M04.2)*
L50.3 Dermatographic urticaria
L50.4 Vibratory urticaria
L50.5 Cholinergic urticaria
L50.6 Contact urticaria
L50.8 Other urticaria
Chronic urticaria
Recurrent periodic urticaria
L50.9 Urticaria, unspecified

L51 Erythema multiforme

Use additional code for adverse effect, if applicable, to identify drug (T36-T50 with fifth or sixth character 5)

Use additional code to identify associated manifestations, such as:
- arthropathy associated with dermatological disorders (M14.8-)
- conjunctival edema (H11.42)
- conjunctivitis (H10.22-)
- corneal scars and opacities (H17.-)
- corneal ulcer (H16.0-)
- edema of eyelid (H02.84)
- inflammation of eyelid (H01.8)
- keratoconjunctivitis sicca (H16.22-)
- mechanical lagophthalmos (H02.22-)
- stomatitis (K12.-)
- symblepharon (H11.23-)

Use additional code to identify percentage of skin exfoliation (L49.-)

Excludes1: *staphylococcal scalded skin syndrome (L00)*
Ritter's disease (L00)

L51.0 Nonbullous erythema multiforme

CC **L51.1 Stevens-Johnson syndrome**
CC Exclusion see Appendix A PDX collection 0843

CC **L51.2 Toxic epidermal necrolysis [Lyell]**
CC Exclusion see Appendix A PDX collection 0843

CC **L51.3 Stevens-Johnson syndrome-toxic epidermal necrolysis overlap syndrome**
SJS-TEN overlap syndrome
CC Exclusion see Appendix A PDX collection 0843

L51.8 Other erythema multiforme

L51.9 Erythema multiforme, unspecified
Erythema iris
Erythema multiforme major NOS
Erythema multiforme minor NOS
Herpes iris

L52 Erythema nodosum

Excludes1: *tuberculous erythema nodosum (A18.4)*
Valid 3-character code, no further characters required

L53 Other erythematous conditions

Excludes1: *erythema ab igne (L59.0)*
erythema due to external agents in contact with skin (L23-L25)
erythema intertrigo (L30.4)

CC **L53.0 Toxic erythema**
Code first poisoning due to drug or toxin, if applicable (T36-T65 with fifth or sixth character 1-4 or 6)

Use additional code for adverse effect, if applicable, to identify drug (T36-T50 with fifth or sixth character 5)
Excludes1: *neonatal erythema toxicum (P83.1)*
CC Exclusion see Appendix A PDX collection 0851

CC **L53.1 Erythema annulare centrifugum**
CC Exclusion see Appendix A PDX collection 0851

CC **L53.2 Erythema marginatum**
CC Exclusion see Appendix A PDX collection 0851

CC **L53.3 Other chronic figurate erythema**
CC Exclusion see Appendix A PDX collection 0851

L53.8 Other specified erythematous conditions

L53.9 Erythematous condition, unspecified
Erythema NOS
Erythroderma NOS

L54 Erythema in diseases classified elsewhere

Code first underlying disease
Valid 3-character code, no further characters required

Radiation-related disorders of the skin and subcutaneous tissue (L55-L59)

L55 Sunburn

L55.0 Sunburn of first degree
L55.1 Sunburn of second degree
L55.2 Sunburn of third degree
L55.9 Sunburn, unspecified

L56 Other acute skin changes due to ultraviolet radiation

Use additional code to identify the source of the ultraviolet radiation (W89, X32)

L56.0 Drug phototoxic response
Use additional code for adverse effect, if applicable, to identify drug (T36-T50 with fifth or sixth character 5)

L56.1 Drug photoallergic response
Use additional code for adverse effect, if applicable, to identify drug (T36-T50 with fifth or sixth character 5)

L56.2 Photocontact dermatitis [berloque dermatitis]
L56.3 Solar urticaria
L56.4 Polymorphous light eruption
L56.5 Disseminated superficial actinic porokeratosis (DSAP)
L56.8 Other specified acute skin changes due to ultraviolet radiation
L56.9 Acute skin change due to ultraviolet radiation, unspecified

L57 Skin changes due to chronic exposure to nonionizing radiation

Use additional code to identify the source of the ultraviolet radiation (W89)

L57.0 Actinic keratosis
Keratosis NOS
Senile keratosis
Solar keratosis

L57.1 Actinic reticuloid
L57.2 Cutis rhomboidalis nuchae
L57.3 Poikiloderma of Civatte
L57.4 Cutis laxa senilis
Elastosis senilis
L57.5 Actinic granuloma
L57.8 Other skin changes due to chronic exposure to nonionizing radiation
Farmer's skin
Sailor's skin
Solar dermatitis
L57.9 Skin changes due to chronic exposure to nonionizing radiation, unspecified

L58 Radiodermatitis

Use additional code to identify the source of the radiation (W88, W90)

L58.0 Acute radiodermatitis
L58.1 Chronic radiodermatitis
L58.9 Radiodermatitis, unspecified

L59 Other disorders of skin and subcutaneous tissue related to radiation

L59.0 Erythema ab igne [dermatitis ab igne]
L59.8 Other specified disorders of the skin and subcutaneous tissue related to radiation
AHA CC: 1Q, 2017, 33-34
L59.9 Disorder of the skin and subcutaneous tissue related to radiation, unspecified

Disorders of skin appendages (L60-L75)

Excludes1: *congenital malformations of integument (Q84.-)*

L60 Nail disorders

Excludes2: *clubbing of nails (R68.3)*
onychia and paronychia (L03.0-)

L60.0 Ingrowing nail
L60.1 Onycholysis
L60.2 Onychogryphosis
L60.3 Nail dystrophy
L60.4 Beau's lines
L60.5 Yellow nail syndrome
L60.8 Other nail disorders
L60.9 Nail disorder, unspecified

L62 Nail disorders in diseases classified elsewhere

Code first underlying disease, such as:
pachydermoperiostosis (M89.4-)
Valid 3-character code, no further characters required

L63 Alopecia areata

L63.0 Alopecia (capitis) totalis
L63.1 Alopecia universalis
L63.2 Ophiasis
L63.8 Other alopecia areata
L63.9 Alopecia areata, unspecified

L64 Androgenic alopecia

Includes: male-pattern baldness

L64.0 Drug-induced androgenic alopecia
Use additional code for adverse effect, if applicable, to identify drug (T36-T50 with fifth or sixth character 5)
L64.8 Other androgenic alopecia
L64.9 Androgenic alopecia, unspecified

L65 Other nonscarring hair loss

Use additional code for adverse effect, if applicable, to identify drug (T36-T50 with fifth or sixth character 5)

Excludes1: *trichotillomania (F63.3)*

L65.0 Telogen effluvium
L65.1 Anagen effluvium
L65.2 Alopecia mucinosa
L65.8 Other specified nonscarring hair loss
L65.9 Nonscarring hair loss, unspecified
Alopecia NOS

L66 Cicatricial alopecia [scarring hair loss]

L66.0 Pseudopelade
L66.1 Lichen planopilaris
Follicular lichen planus
L66.2 Folliculitis decalvans
L66.3 Perifolliculitis capitis abscedens
L66.4 Folliculitis ulerythematosa reticulata
L66.8 Other cicatricial alopecia
AHA CC: 1Q, 2015, 19
L66.9 Cicatricial alopecia, unspecified

L67 Hair color and hair shaft abnormalities

Excludes1: *monilethrix (Q84.1)*
pili annulati (Q84.1)
telogen effluvium (L65.0)

L67.0 Trichorrhexis nodosa
L67.1 Variations in hair color
Canities
Greyness, hair (premature)
Heterochromia of hair
Poliosis circumscripta, acquired
Poliosis NOS
L67.8 Other hair color and hair shaft abnormalities
Fragilitas crinium
L67.9 Hair color and hair shaft abnormality, unspecified

L68 Hypertrichosis

Includes: excess hair
Excludes1: *congenital hypertrichosis (Q84.2)*
persistent lanugo (Q84.2)

L68.0 Hirsutism
L68.1 Acquired hypertrichosis lanuginosa
L68.2 Localized hypertrichosis
L68.3 Polytrichia
L68.8 Other hypertrichosis
L68.9 Hypertrichosis, unspecified

L70 Acne

Excludes2: *acne keloid (L73.0)*

L70.0 Acne vulgaris
L70.1 Acne conglobata
L70.2 Acne varioliformis
Acne necrotica miliaris
L70.3 Acne tropica
• **L70.4 Infantile acne**
L70.5 Acné excoriée
Acné exocoriée des jeunes filles
Picker's acne
L70.8 Other acne
L70.9 Acne, unspecified

L71 Rosacea

Use additional code for adverse effect, if applicable, to identify drug (T36-T50 with fifth or sixth character 5)

L71.0 Perioral dermatitis
L71.1 Rhinophyma
L71.8 Other rosacea
L71.9 Rosacea, unspecified

L72 Follicular cysts of skin and subcutaneous tissue

L72.0 Epidermal cyst
+ **L72.1 Pilar and trichodermal cyst**
L72.11 Pilar cyst
L72.12 Trichodermal cyst
Trichilemmal (proliferating) cyst
L72.2 Steatocystoma multiplex
L72.3 Sebaceous cyst
Excludes2: *pilar cyst (L72.11)*
trichilemmal (proliferating) cyst (L72.12)
L72.8 Other follicular cysts of the skin and subcutaneous tissue
L72.9 Follicular cyst of the skin and subcutaneous tissue, unspecified

L73 Other follicular disorders

L73.0 Acne keloid
L73.1 Pseudofolliculitis barbae
L73.2 Hidradenitis suppurativa
L73.8 Other specified follicular disorders
Sycosis barbae
L73.9 Follicular disorder, unspecified

L74 Eccrine sweat disorders

Excludes2: *generalized hyperhidrosis (R61)*

L74.0 Miliaria rubra
L74.1 Miliaria crystallina
L74.2 Miliaria profunda
Miliaria tropicalis
L74.3 Miliaria, unspecified
L74.4 Anhidrosis
Hypohidrosis
+ **L74.5 Focal hyperhidrosis**
+ **L74.51 Primary focal hyperhidrosis**
L74.510 Primary focal hyperhidrosis, axilla
L74.511 Primary focal hyperhidrosis, face
L74.512 Primary focal hyperhidrosis, palms
L74.513 Primary focal hyperhidrosis, soles
L74.519 Primary focal hyperhidrosis, unspecified
L74.52 Secondary focal hyperhidrosis
Frey's syndrome
L74.8 Other eccrine sweat disorders
L74.9 Eccrine sweat disorder, unspecified
Sweat gland disorder NOS

L75 Apocrine sweat disorders

Excludes1: *dyshidrosis (L30.1)*
hidradenitis suppurativa (L73.2)

L75.0 Bromhidrosis
L75.1 Chromhidrosis
L75.2 Apocrine miliaria
Fox-Fordyce disease
L75.8 Other apocrine sweat disorders
L75.9 Apocrine sweat disorder, unspecified

Intraoperative and postprocedural complications of skin and subcutaneous tissue (L76)

L76 Intraoperative and postprocedural complications of skin and subcutaneous tissue

AHA CC: 4Q, 2016, 9-10

+ **L76.0 Intraoperative hemorrhage and hematoma of skin and subcutaneous tissue complicating a procedure**
Excludes1: *intraoperative hemorrhage and hematoma of skin and subcutaneous tissue due to accidental puncture and laceration during a procedure (L76.1-)*
CC **L76.01 Intraoperative hemorrhage and hematoma of skin and subcutaneous tissue complicating a dermatologic procedure**
CC Exclusion see Appendix A PDX collection 0852
CC **L76.02 Intraoperative hemorrhage and hematoma of skin and subcutaneous tissue complicating other procedure**
CC Exclusion see Appendix A PDX collection 0852
+ **L76.1 Accidental puncture and laceration of skin and subcutaneous tissue during a procedure**
CC **L76.11 Accidental puncture and laceration of skin and subcutaneous tissue during a dermatologic procedure**
CC Exclusion see Appendix A PDX collection 0509
CC **L76.12 Accidental puncture and laceration of skin and subcutaneous tissue during other procedure**
CC Exclusion see Appendix A PDX collection 0509
+ **L76.2 Postprocedural hemorrhage of skin and subcutaneous tissue following a procedure**
CC **L76.21 Postprocedural hemorrhage of skin and subcutaneous tissue following a dermatologic procedure**
CC Exclusion see Appendix A PDX collection 0852
CC **L76.22 Postprocedural hemorrhage of skin and subcutaneous tissue following other procedure**
CC Exclusion see Appendix A PDX collection 0852
+ **L76.3 Postprocedural hematoma and seroma of skin and subcutaneous issue following a procedure**
CC **L76.31 Postprocedural hematoma of skin and subcutaneous tissue following a dermatologic procedure**
CC Exclusion see Appendix A PDX collection 0852

CC **L76.32 Postprocedural hematoma of skin and subcutaneous tissue following other procedure**
CC Exclusion see Appendix A PDX collection 0852

CC **L76.33 Postprocedural seroma of skin and subcutaneous tissue following a dermatologic procedure**
CC Exclusion see Appendix A PDX collection 0852

CC **L76.34 Postprocedural seroma of skin and subcutaneous tissue following other procedure**
CC Exclusion see Appendix A PDX collection 0852

\+ **L76.8 Other intraoperative and postprocedural complications of skin and subcutaneous tissue**
Use additional code, if applicable, to further specify disorder

L76.81 Other intraoperative complications of skin and subcutaneous tissue

L76.82 Other postprocedural complications of skin and subcutaneous tissue

Other disorders of the skin and subcutaneous tissue (L80-L99)

L80 Vitiligo

Excludes2: *vitiligo of eyelids (H02.73-)*
vitiligo of vulva (N90.89)
Valid 3-character code, no further characters required

L81 Other disorders of pigmentation

Excludes1: *birthmark NOS (Q82.5)*
Peutz-Jeghers syndrome (Q85.8)
Excludes2: *nevus - see Alphabetical Index*

L81.0 Postinflammatory hyperpigmentation

L81.1 Chloasma

L81.2 Freckles

L81.3 Café au lait spots

L81.4 Other melanin hyperpigmentation
Lentigo

L81.5 Leukoderma, not elsewhere classified

L81.6 Other disorders of diminished melanin formation

L81.7 Pigmented purpuric dermatosis
Angioma serpiginosum

L81.8 Other specified disorders of pigmentation
Iron pigmentation
Tattoo pigmentation

L81.9 Disorder of pigmentation, unspecified

L82 Seborrheic keratosis

Includes: basal cell papilloma
dermatosis papulosa nigra
Leser-Trélat disease
Excludes2: *seborrheic dermatitis (L21.-)*

L82.0 Inflamed seborrheic keratosis

L82.1 Other seborrheic keratosis
Seborrheic keratosis NOS

L83 Acanthosis nigricans

Confluent and reticulated papillomatosis
Valid 3-character code, no further characters required

L84 Corns and callosities

Callus
Clavus
Valid 3-character code, no further characters required

L85 Other epidermal thickening

Excludes2: *hypertrophic disorders of the skin (L91.-)*

L85.0 Acquired ichthyosis
Excludes1: *congenital ichthyosis (Q80.-)*

L85.1 Acquired keratosis [keratoderma] palmaris et plantaris
Excludes1: *inherited keratosis palmaris et plantaris (Q82.8)*

L85.2 Keratosis punctata (palmaris et plantaris)

L85.3 Xerosis cutis
Dry skin dermatitis

L85.8 Other specified epidermal thickening
Cutaneous horn

L85.9 Epidermal thickening, unspecified

L86 Keratoderma in diseases classified elsewhere

Code first underlying disease, such as:
Reiter's disease (M02.3-)
Excludes1: *gonococcal keratoderma (A54.89)*
gonococcal keratosis (A54.89)
keratoderma due to vitamin A deficiency (E50.8)
keratosis due to vitamin A deficiency (E50.8)
xeroderma due to vitamin A deficiency (E50.8)
Valid 3-character code, no further characters required

L87 Transepidermal elimination disorders

Excludes1: *granuloma annulare (perforating) (L92.0)*

L87.0 Keratosis follicularis et parafollicularis in cutem penetrans
Kyrle disease
Hyperkeratosis follicularis penetrans

L87.1 Reactive perforating collagenosis

L87.2 Elastosis perforans serpiginosa

L87.8 Other transepidermal elimination disorders

L87.9 Transepidermal elimination disorder, unspecified

CC **L88 Pyoderma gangrenosum**

Phagedenic pyoderma
Excludes1: *dermatitis gangrenosa (L08.0)*
CC Exclusion see Appendix A PDX collection 0853
Valid 3-character code, no further characters required

L89 Pressure ulcer

Includes: bed sore
decubitus ulcer
plaster ulcer
pressure area
pressure sore
Code first any associated gangrene (I96)
Excludes2: *decubitus (trophic) ulcer of cervix (uteri) (N86)*
diabetic ulcers (E08.621, E08.622, E09.621, E09.622, E10.621, E10.622, E11.621, E11.622, E13.621, E13.622)
non-pressure chronic ulcer of skin (L97.-)
skin infections (L00-L08)
varicose ulcer (I83.0, I83.2)
Review coding guideline C.12.a

\+ **L89.0 Pressure ulcer of elbow**

\+ **L89.00 Pressure ulcer of unspecified elbow**

L89.000 Pressure ulcer of unspecified elbow, unstageable

L89.001 Pressure ulcer of unspecified elbow, stage 1
Healing pressure ulcer of unspecified elbow, stage 1
Pressure pre-ulcer skin changes limited to persistent focal edema, unspecified elbow

L89.002 Pressure ulcer of unspecified elbow, stage 2
Healing pressure ulcer of unspecified elbow, stage 2
Pressure ulcer with abrasion, blister, partial thickness skin loss involving epidermis and/or dermis, unspecified elbow

MCC **L89.003 Pressure ulcer of unspecified elbow, stage 3**
Healing pressure ulcer of unspecified elbow, stage 3
Pressure ulcer with full thickness skin loss involving damage or necrosis of subcutaneous tissue, unspecified elbow
MCC Exclusion see Appendix A PDX collection 0854
HAC see Appendix B for HAC conditional logic

MCC **L89.004 Pressure ulcer of unspecified elbow, stage 4**
Healing pressure ulcer of unspecified elbow, stage 4
Pressure ulcer with necrosis of soft tissues through to underlying muscle, tendon, or bone, unspecified elbow
MCC Exclusion see Appendix A PDX collection 0854
HAC see Appendix B for HAC conditional logic

L89.009 Pressure ulcer of unspecified elbow, unspecified stage
Healing pressure ulcer of elbow NOS
Healing pressure ulcer of unspecified elbow, unspecified stage

\+ **L89.01 Pressure ulcer of right elbow**

L89.010 Pressure ulcer of right elbow, unstageable

L89.011 Pressure ulcer of right elbow, stage 1
Healing pressure ulcer of right elbow, stage 1
Pressure pre-ulcer skin changes limited to persistent focal edema, right elbow

L89.012 Pressure ulcer of right elbow, stage 2
Healing pressure ulcer of right elbow, stage 2
Pressure ulcer with abrasion, blister, partial thickness skin loss involving epidermis and/or dermis, right elbow

MCC **L89.013 Pressure ulcer of right elbow, stage 3**
Healing pressure ulcer of right elbow, stage 3
Pressure ulcer with full thickness skin loss involving damage or necrosis of subcutaneous tissue, right elbow
MCC Exclusion see Appendix A PDX collection 0854
HAC see Appendix B for HAC conditional logic

MCC **L89.014 Pressure ulcer of right elbow, stage 4**
Healing pressure ulcer of right elbow, stage 4
Pressure ulcer with necrosis of soft tissues through to underlying muscle, tendon, or bone, right elbow
MCC Exclusion see Appendix A PDX collection 0854
HAC see Appendix B for HAC conditional logic

L89.019 Pressure ulcer of right elbow, unspecified stage
Healing pressure right of elbow NOS
Healing pressure ulcer of right elbow, unspecified stage

+ L89.02 Pressure ulcer of left elbow

L89.020 Pressure ulcer of left elbow, unstageable

L89.021 Pressure ulcer of left elbow, stage 1
Healing pressure ulcer of left elbow, stage 1
Pressure pre-ulcer skin changes limited to persistent focal edema, left elbow

L89.022 Pressure ulcer of left elbow, stage 2
Healing pressure ulcer of left elbow, stage 2
Pressure ulcer with abrasion, blister, partial thickness skin loss involving epidermis and/or dermis, left elbow

MCC **L89.023 Pressure ulcer of left elbow, stage 3**
Healing pressure ulcer of left elbow, stage 3
Pressure ulcer with full thickness skin loss involving damage or necrosis of subcutaneous tissue, left elbow
MCC Exclusion see Appendix A PDX collection 0854
HAC see Appendix B for HAC conditional logic

MCC **L89.024 Pressure ulcer of left elbow, stage 4**
Healing pressure ulcer of left elbow, stage 4
Pressure ulcer with necrosis of soft tissues through to underlying muscle, tendon, or bone, left elbow
MCC Exclusion see Appendix A PDX collection 0854
HAC see Appendix B for HAC conditional logic

L89.029 Pressure ulcer of left elbow, unspecified stage
Healing pressure ulcer of left of elbow NOS
Healing pressure ulcer of left elbow, unspecified stage

+ L89.1 Pressure ulcer of back

+ L89.10 Pressure ulcer of unspecified part of back

L89.100 Pressure ulcer of unspecified part of back, unstageable

L89.101 Pressure ulcer of unspecified part of back, stage 1
Healing pressure ulcer of unspecified part of back, stage 1
Pressure pre-ulcer skin changes limited to persistent focal edema, unspecified part of back

L89.102 Pressure ulcer of unspecified part of back, stage 2
Healing pressure ulcer of unspecified part of back, stage 2
Pressure ulcer with abrasion, blister, partial thickness skin loss involving epidermis and/or dermis, unspecified part of back

MCC **L89.103 Pressure ulcer of unspecified part of back, stage 3**
Healing pressure ulcer of unspecified part of back, stage 3
Pressure ulcer with full thickness skin loss involving damage or necrosis of subcutaneous tissue, unspecified part of back
MCC Exclusion see Appendix A PDX collection 0854
HAC see Appendix B for HAC conditional logic

MCC **L89.104 Pressure ulcer of unspecified part of back, stage 4**
Healing pressure ulcer of unspecified part of back, stage 4
Pressure ulcer with necrosis of soft tissues through to underlying muscle, tendon, or bone, unspecified part of back
MCC Exclusion see Appendix A PDX collection 0854
HAC see Appendix B for HAC conditional logic

L89.109 Pressure ulcer of unspecified part of back, unspecified stage
Healing pressure ulcer of unspecified part of back NOS
Healing pressure ulcer of unspecified part of back, unspecified stage

+ L89.11 Pressure ulcer of right upper back
Pressure ulcer of right shoulder blade

L89.110 Pressure ulcer of right upper back, unstageable

L89.111 Pressure ulcer of right upper back, stage 1
Healing pressure ulcer of right upper back, stage 1
Pressure pre-ulcer skin changes limited to persistent focal edema, right upper back

L89.112 Pressure ulcer of right upper back, stage 2
Healing pressure ulcer of right upper back, stage 2
Pressure ulcer with abrasion, blister, partial thickness skin loss involving epidermis and/or dermis, right upper back

MCC **L89.113 Pressure ulcer of right upper back, stage 3**
Healing pressure ulcer of right upper back, stage 3
Pressure ulcer with full thickness skin loss involving damage or necrosis of subcutaneous tissue, right upper back
MCC Exclusion see Appendix A PDX collection 0854
HAC see Appendix B for HAC conditional logic

MCC **L89.114 Pressure ulcer of right upper back, stage 4**
Healing pressure ulcer of right upper back, stage 4
Pressure ulcer with necrosis of soft tissues through to underlying muscle, tendon, or bone, right upper back
MCC Exclusion see Appendix A PDX collection 0854
HAC see Appendix B for HAC conditional logic

L89.119 Pressure ulcer of right upper back, unspecified stage
Healing pressure ulcer of right upper back NOS
Healing pressure ulcer of right upper back, unspecified stage

+ L89.12 Pressure ulcer of left upper back
Pressure ulcer of left shoulder blade

L89.120 Pressure ulcer of left upper back, unstageable

L89.121 Pressure ulcer of left upper back, stage 1
Healing pressure ulcer of left upper back, stage 1
Pressure pre-ulcer skin changes limited to persistent focal edema, left upper back

L89.122 Pressure ulcer of left upper back, stage 2
Healing pressure ulcer of left upper back, stage 2
Pressure ulcer with abrasion, blister, partial thickness skin loss involving epidermis and/or dermis, left upper back

MCC **L89.123 Pressure ulcer of left upper back, stage 3**
Healing pressure ulcer of left upper back, stage 3
Pressure ulcer with full thickness skin loss involving damage or necrosis of subcutaneous tissue, left upper back
MCC Exclusion see Appendix A PDX collection 0854
HAC see Appendix B for HAC conditional logic

MCC **L89.124** **Pressure ulcer of left upper back, stage 4**
Healing pressure ulcer of left upper back, stage 4
Pressure ulcer with necrosis of soft tissues through to underlying muscle, tendon, or bone, left upper back
MCC Exclusion see Appendix A PDX collection 0854
HAC see Appendix B for HAC conditional logic

L89.129 **Pressure ulcer of left upper back, unspecified stage**
Healing pressure ulcer of left upper back NOS
Healing pressure ulcer of left upper back, unspecified stage

+ **L89.13** **Pressure ulcer of right lower back**

L89.130 **Pressure ulcer of right lower back, unstageable**

L89.131 **Pressure ulcer of right lower back, stage 1**
Healing pressure ulcer of right lower back, stage 1
Pressure pre-ulcer skin changes limited to persistent focal edema, right lower back

L89.132 **Pressure ulcer of right lower back, stage 2**
Healing pressure ulcer of right lower back, stage 2
Pressure ulcer with abrasion, blister, partial thickness skin loss involving epidermis and/or dermis, right lower back

MCC **L89.133** **Pressure ulcer of right lower back, stage 3**
Healing pressure ulcer of right lower back, stage 3
Pressure ulcer with full thickness skin loss involving damage or necrosis of subcutaneous tissue, right lower back
MCC Exclusion see Appendix A PDX collection 0854
HAC see Appendix B for HAC conditional logic

MCC **L89.134** **Pressure ulcer of right lower back, stage 4**
Healing pressure ulcer of right lower back, stage 4
Pressure ulcer with necrosis of soft tissues through to underlying muscle, tendon, or bone, right lower back
MCC Exclusion see Appendix A PDX collection 0854
HAC see Appendix B for HAC conditional logic

L89.139 **Pressure ulcer of right lower back, unspecified stage**
Healing pressure ulcer of right lower back NOS
Healing pressure ulcer of right lower back, unspecified stage

+ **L89.14** **Pressure ulcer of left lower back**

L89.140 **Pressure ulcer of left lower back, unstageable**

L89.141 **Pressure ulcer of left lower back, stage 1**
Healing pressure ulcer of left lower back, stage 1
Pressure pre-ulcer skin changes limited to persistent focal edema, left lower back

L89.142 **Pressure ulcer of left lower back, stage 2**
Healing pressure ulcer of left lower back, stage 2
Pressure ulcer with abrasion, blister, partial thickness skin loss involving epidermis and/or dermis, left lower back

MCC **L89.143** **Pressure ulcer of left lower back, stage 3**
Healing pressure ulcer of left lower back, stage 3
Pressure ulcer with full thickness skin loss involving damage or necrosis of subcutaneous tissue, left lower back
MCC Exclusion see Appendix A PDX collection 0854
HAC see Appendix B for HAC conditional logic

MCC **L89.144** **Pressure ulcer of left lower back, stage 4**
Healing pressure ulcer of left lower back, stage 4
Pressure ulcer with necrosis of soft tissues through to underlying muscle, tendon, or bone, left lower back
MCC Exclusion see Appendix A PDX collection 0854
HAC see Appendix B for HAC conditional logic

L89.149 **Pressure ulcer of left lower back, unspecified stage**
Healing pressure ulcer of left lower back NOS
Healing pressure ulcer of left lower back, unspecified stage

+ **L89.15** **Pressure ulcer of sacral region**
Pressure ulcer of coccyx
Pressure ulcer of tailbone

L89.150 **Pressure ulcer of sacral region, unstageable**

L89.151 **Pressure ulcer of sacral region, stage 1**
Healing pressure ulcer of sacral region, stage 1
Pressure pre-ulcer skin changes limited to persistent focal edema, sacral region

L89.152 **Pressure ulcer of sacral region, stage 2**
Healing pressure ulcer of sacral region, stage 2
Pressure ulcer with abrasion, blister, partial thickness skin loss involving epidermis and/or dermis, sacral region

MCC **L89.153** **Pressure ulcer of sacral region, stage 3**
Healing pressure ulcer of sacral region, stage 3
Pressure ulcer with full thickness skin loss involving damage or necrosis of subcutaneous tissue, sacral region
MCC Exclusion see Appendix A PDX collection 0854
HAC see Appendix B for HAC conditional logic

MCC **L89.154** **Pressure ulcer of sacral region, stage 4**
Healing pressure ulcer of sacral region, stage 4
Pressure ulcer with necrosis of soft tissues through to underlying muscle, tendon, or bone, sacral region
MCC Exclusion see Appendix A PDX collection 0854
HAC see Appendix B for HAC conditional logic

L89.159 **Pressure ulcer of sacral region, unspecified stage**
Healing pressure ulcer of sacral region NOS
Healing pressure ulcer of sacral region, unspecified stage

+ **L89.2** **Pressure ulcer of hip**

+ **L89.20** **Pressure ulcer of unspecified hip**

L89.200 **Pressure ulcer of unspecified hip, unstageable**

L89.201 **Pressure ulcer of unspecified hip, stage 1**
Healing pressure ulcer of unspecified hip back, stage 1
Pressure pre-ulcer skin changes limited to persistent focal edema, unspecified hip

L89.202 **Pressure ulcer of unspecified hip, stage 2**
Healing pressure ulcer of unspecified hip, stage 2
Pressure ulcer with abrasion, blister, partial thickness skin loss involving epidermis and/or dermis, unspecified hip

MCC **L89.203** **Pressure ulcer of unspecified hip, stage 3**
Healing pressure ulcer of unspecified hip, stage 3
Pressure ulcer with full thickness skin loss involving damage or necrosis of subcutaneous tissue, unspecified hip
MCC Exclusion see Appendix A PDX collection 0854
HAC see Appendix B for HAC conditional logic

MCC **L89.204 Pressure ulcer of unspecified hip, stage 4**
Healing pressure ulcer of unspecified hip, stage 4
Pressure ulcer with necrosis of soft tissues through to underlying muscle, tendon, or bone, unspecified hip
MCC Exclusion see Appendix A PDX collection 0854
HAC see Appendix B for HAC conditional logic

L89.209 Pressure ulcer of unspecified hip, unspecified stage
Healing pressure ulcer of unspecified hip NOS
Healing pressure ulcer of unspecified hip, unspecified stage

+ **L89.21 Pressure ulcer of right hip**

L89.210 Pressure ulcer of right hip, unstageable

L89.211 Pressure ulcer of right hip, stage 1
Healing pressure ulcer of right hip back, stage 1
Pressure pre-ulcer skin changes limited to persistent focal edema, right hip

L89.212 Pressure ulcer of right hip, stage 2
Healing pressure ulcer of right hip, stage 2
Pressure ulcer with abrasion, blister, partial thickness skin loss involving epidermis and/or dermis, right hip

MCC **L89.213 Pressure ulcer of right hip, stage 3**
Healing pressure ulcer of right hip, stage 3
Pressure ulcer with full thickness skin loss involving damage or necrosis of subcutaneous tissue, right hip
MCC Exclusion see Appendix A PDX collection 0854
HAC see Appendix B for HAC conditional logic

MCC **L89.214 Pressure ulcer of right hip, stage 4**
Healing pressure ulcer of right hip, stage 4
Pressure ulcer with necrosis of soft tissues through to underlying muscle, tendon, or bone, right hip
MCC Exclusion see Appendix A PDX collection 0854
HAC see Appendix B for HAC conditional logic

L89.219 Pressure ulcer of right hip, unspecified stage
Healing pressure ulcer of right hip NOS
Healing pressure ulcer of right hip, unspecified stage

+ **L89.22 Pressure ulcer of left hip**

L89.220 Pressure ulcer of left hip, unstageable

L89.221 Pressure ulcer of left hip, stage 1
Healing pressure ulcer of left hip back, stage 1
Pressure pre-ulcer skin changes limited to persistent focal edema, left hip

L89.222 Pressure ulcer of left hip, stage 2
Healing pressure ulcer of left hip, stage 2
Pressure ulcer with abrasion, blister, partial thickness skin loss involving epidermis and/or dermis, left hip

MCC **L89.223 Pressure ulcer of left hip, stage 3**
Healing pressure ulcer of left hip, stage 3
Pressure ulcer with full thickness skin loss involving damage or necrosis of subcutaneous tissue, left hip
MCC Exclusion see Appendix A PDX collection 0854
HAC see Appendix B for HAC conditional logic

MCC **L89.224 Pressure ulcer of left hip, stage 4**
Healing pressure ulcer of left hip, stage 4
Pressure ulcer with necrosis of soft tissues through to underlying muscle, tendon, or bone, left hip
MCC Exclusion see Appendix A PDX collection 0854
HAC see Appendix B for HAC conditional logic

L89.229 Pressure ulcer of left hip, unspecified stage
Healing pressure ulcer of left hip NOS
Healing pressure ulcer of left hip, unspecified stage

+ **L89.3 Pressure ulcer of buttock**

+ **L89.30 Pressure ulcer of unspecified buttock**

L89.300 Pressure ulcer of unspecified buttock, unstageable

L89.301 Pressure ulcer of unspecified buttock, stage 1
Healing pressure ulcer of unspecified buttock, stage 1
Pressure pre-ulcer skin changes limited to persistent focal edema, unspecified buttock

L89.302 Pressure ulcer of unspecified buttock, stage 2
Healing pressure ulcer of unspecified buttock, stage 2
Pressure ulcer with abrasion, blister, partial thickness skin loss involving epidermis and/or dermis, unspecified buttock

MCC **L89.303 Pressure ulcer of unspecified buttock, stage 3**
Healing pressure ulcer of unspecified buttock, stage 3
Pressure ulcer with full thickness skin loss involving damage or necrosis of subcutaneous tissue, unspecified buttock
MCC Exclusion see Appendix A PDX collectio 0854
HAC see Appendix B for HAC conditional logi

MCC **L89.304 Pressure ulcer of unspecified buttock, stage 4**
Healing pressure ulcer of unspecified buttock, stage 4
Pressure ulcer with necrosis of soft tissues through to underlying muscle, tendon, or bone, unspecified buttock
MCC Exclusion see Appendix A PDX collectio 0854
HAC see Appendix B for HAC conditional logi

L89.309 Pressure ulcer of unspecified buttock, unspecified stage
Healing pressure ulcer of unspecified buttock NOS
Healing pressure ulcer of unspecified buttock, unspecified stage

+ **L89.31 Pressure ulcer of right buttock**

L89.310 Pressure ulcer of right buttock, unstageable

L89.311 Pressure ulcer of right buttock, stage 1
Healing pressure ulcer of right buttock, stage 1
Pressure pre-ulcer skin changes limited to persistent focal edema, right buttock

L89.312 Pressure ulcer of right buttock, stage 2
Healing pressure ulcer of right buttock, stage 2
Pressure ulcer with abrasion, blister, partial thickness skin loss involving epidermis and/or dermis, right buttock

MCC **L89.313 Pressure ulcer of right buttock, stage 3**
Healing pressure ulcer of right buttock, stage 3
Pressure ulcer with full thickness skin loss involving damage or necrosis of subcutaneous tissue, right buttock
MCC Exclusion see Appendix A PDX collection 0854
HAC see Appendix B for HAC conditional logi

MCC **L89.314 Pressure ulcer of right buttock, stage 4**
Healing pressure ulcer of right buttock, stage 4
Pressure ulcer with necrosis of soft tissues through to underlying muscle, tendon, or bone, right buttock
MCC Exclusion see Appendix A PDX collectio 0854
HAC see Appendix B for HAC conditional logi

L89.319 Pressure ulcer of right buttock, unspecifie stage
Healing pressure ulcer of right buttock NO
Healing pressure ulcer of right buttock, unspecified stage

+ L89.32 **Pressure ulcer of left buttock**
L89.320 **Pressure ulcer of left buttock, unstageable**
L89.321 **Pressure ulcer of left buttock, stage 1**
Healing pressure ulcer of left buttock, stage 1
Pressure pre-ulcer skin changes limited to persistent focal edema, left buttock
L89.322 **Pressure ulcer of left buttock, stage 2**
Healing pressure ulcer of left buttock, stage 2
Pressure ulcer with abrasion, blister, partial thickness skin loss involving epidermis and/or dermis, left buttock
MCC L89.323 **Pressure ulcer of left buttock, stage 3**
Healing pressure ulcer of left buttock, stage 3
Pressure ulcer with full thickness skin loss involving damage or necrosis of subcutaneous tissue, left buttock
MCC Exclusion see Appendix A PDX collection 0854
HAC see Appendix B for HAC conditional logic
MCC L89.324 **Pressure ulcer of left buttock, stage 4**
Healing pressure ulcer of left buttock, stage 4
Pressure ulcer with necrosis of soft tissues through to underlying muscle, tendon, or bone, left buttock
MCC Exclusion see Appendix A PDX collection 0854
HAC see Appendix B for HAC conditional logic
L89.329 **Pressure ulcer of left buttock, unspecified stage**
Healing pressure ulcer of left buttock NOS
Healing pressure ulcer of left buttock, unspecified stage
+ L89.4 **Pressure ulcer of contiguous site of back, buttock and hip**
L89.40 **Pressure ulcer of contiguous site of back, buttock and hip, unspecified stage**
Healing pressure ulcer of contiguous site of back, buttock and hip NOS
Healing pressure ulcer of contiguous site of back, buttock and hip, unspecified stage
L89.41 **Pressure ulcer of contiguous site of back, buttock and hip, stage 1**
Healing pressure ulcer of contiguous site of back, buttock and hip, stage 1
Pressure pre-ulcer skin changes limited to persistent focal edema, contiguous site of back, buttock and hip
L89.42 **Pressure ulcer of contiguous site of back, buttock and hip, stage 2**
Healing pressure ulcer of contiguous site of back, buttock and hip, stage 2
Pressure ulcer with abrasion, blister, partial thickness skin loss involving epidermis and/or dermis, contiguous site of back, buttock and hip
MCC L89.43 **Pressure ulcer of contiguous site of back, buttock and hip, stage 3**
Healing pressure ulcer of contiguous site of back, buttock and hip, stage 3
Pressure ulcer with full thickness skin loss involving damage or necrosis of subcutaneous tissue, contiguous site of back, buttock and hip
MCC Exclusion see Appendix A PDX collection 0854
HAC see Appendix B for HAC conditional logic
MCC L89.44 **Pressure ulcer of contiguous site of back, buttock and hip, stage 4**
Healing pressure ulcer of contiguous site of back, buttock and hip, stage 4
Pressure ulcer with necrosis of soft tissues through to underlying muscle, tendon, or bone, contiguous site of back, buttock and hip
MCC Exclusion see Appendix A PDX collection 0854
HAC see Appendix B for HAC conditional logic
L89.45 **Pressure ulcer of contiguous site of back, buttock and hip, unstageable**
+ L89.5 **Pressure ulcer of ankle**
+ L89.50 **Pressure ulcer of unspecified ankle**
L89.500 **Pressure ulcer of unspecified ankle, unstageable**
L89.501 **Pressure ulcer of unspecified ankle, stage 1**
Healing pressure ulcer of unspecified ankle, stage 1
Pressure pre-ulcer skin changes limited to persistent focal edema, unspecified ankle
L89.502 **Pressure ulcer of unspecified ankle, stage 2**
Healing pressure ulcer of unspecified ankle, stage 2
Pressure ulcer with abrasion, blister, partial thickness skin loss involving epidermis and/or dermis, unspecified ankle
MCC L89.503 **Pressure ulcer of unspecified ankle, stage 3**
Healing pressure ulcer of unspecified ankle, stage 3
Pressure ulcer with full thickness skin loss involving damage or necrosis of subcutaneous tissue, unspecified ankle
MCC Exclusion see Appendix A PDX collection 0854
HAC see Appendix B for HAC conditional logic
MCC L89.504 **Pressure ulcer of unspecified ankle, stage 4**
Healing pressure ulcer of unspecified ankle, stage 4
Pressure ulcer with necrosis of soft tissues through to underlying muscle, tendon, or bone, unspecified ankle
MCC Exclusion see Appendix A PDX collection 0854
HAC see Appendix B for HAC conditional logic
L89.509 **Pressure ulcer of unspecified ankle, unspecified stage**
Healing pressure ulcer of unspecified ankle NOS
Healing pressure ulcer of unspecified ankle, unspecified stage
+ L89.51 **Pressure ulcer of right ankle**
L89.510 **Pressure ulcer of right ankle, unstageable**
L89.511 **Pressure ulcer of right ankle, stage 1**
Healing pressure ulcer of right ankle, stage 1
Pressure pre-ulcer skin changes limited to persistent focal edema, right ankle
L89.512 **Pressure ulcer of right ankle, stage 2**
Healing pressure ulcer of right ankle, stage 2
Pressure ulcer with abrasion, blister, partial thickness skin loss involving epidermis and/or dermis, right ankle
MCC L89.513 **Pressure ulcer of right ankle, stage 3**
Healing pressure ulcer of right ankle, stage 3
Pressure ulcer with full thickness skin loss involving damage or necrosis of subcutaneous tissue, right ankle
MCC Exclusion see Appendix A PDX collection 0854
HAC see Appendix B for HAC conditional logic
MCC L89.514 **Pressure ulcer of right ankle, stage 4**
Healing pressure ulcer of right ankle, stage 4
Pressure ulcer with necrosis of soft tissues through to underlying muscle, tendon, or bone, right ankle
MCC Exclusion see Appendix A PDX collection 0854
HAC see Appendix B for HAC conditional logic
L89.519 **Pressure ulcer of right ankle, unspecified stage**
Healing pressure ulcer of right ankle NOS
Healing pressure ulcer of right ankle, unspecified stage
+ L89.52 **Pressure ulcer of left ankle**
L89.520 **Pressure ulcer of left ankle, unstageable**
L89.521 **Pressure ulcer of left ankle, stage 1**
Healing pressure ulcer of left ankle, stage 1
Pressure pre-ulcer skin changes limited to persistent focal edema, left ankle
L89.522 **Pressure ulcer of left ankle, stage 2**
Healing pressure ulcer of left ankle, stage 2
Pressure ulcer with abrasion, blister, partial thickness skin loss involving epidermis and/or dermis, left ankle

MCC **L89.523 Pressure ulcer of left ankle, stage 3**
Healing pressure ulcer of left ankle, stage 3
Pressure ulcer with full thickness skin loss involving damage or necrosis of subcutaneous tissue, left ankle
MCC Exclusion see Appendix A PDX collection 0854
HAC see Appendix B for HAC conditional logic

MCC **L89.524 Pressure ulcer of left ankle, stage 4**
Healing pressure ulcer of left ankle, stage 4
Pressure ulcer with necrosis of soft tissues through to underlying muscle, tendon, or bone, left ankle
MCC Exclusion see Appendix A PDX collection 0854
HAC see Appendix B for HAC conditional logic

L89.529 Pressure ulcer of left ankle, unspecified stage
Healing pressure ulcer of left ankle NOS
Healing pressure ulcer of left ankle, unspecified stage

+ L89.6 Pressure ulcer of heel

+ L89.60 Pressure ulcer of unspecified heel

L89.600 Pressure ulcer of unspecified heel, unstageable

L89.601 Pressure ulcer of unspecified heel, stage 1
Healing pressure ulcer of unspecified heel, stage 1
Pressure pre-ulcer skin changes limited to persistent focal edema, unspecified heel

L89.602 Pressure ulcer of unspecified heel, stage 2
Healing pressure ulcer of unspecified heel, stage 2
Pressure ulcer with abrasion, blister, partial thickness skin loss involving epidermis and/or dermis, unspecified heel

MCC **L89.603 Pressure ulcer of unspecified heel, stage 3**
Healing pressure ulcer of unspecified heel, stage 3
Pressure ulcer with full thickness skin loss involving damage or necrosis of subcutaneous tissue, unspecified heel
MCC Exclusion see Appendix A PDX collection 0854
HAC see Appendix B for HAC conditional logic

MCC **L89.604 Pressure ulcer of unspecified heel, stage 4**
Healing pressure ulcer of unspecified heel, stage 4
Pressure ulcer with necrosis of soft tissues through to underlying muscle, tendon, or bone, unspecified heel
MCC Exclusion see Appendix A PDX collection 0854
HAC see Appendix B for HAC conditional logic

L89.609 Pressure ulcer of unspecified heel, unspecified stage
Healing pressure ulcer of unspecified heel NOS
Healing pressure ulcer of unspecified heel, unspecified stage

+ L89.61 Pressure ulcer of right heel

L89.610 Pressure ulcer of right heel, unstageable

L89.611 Pressure ulcer of right heel, stage 1
Healing pressure ulcer of right heel, stage 1
Pressure pre-ulcer skin changes limited to persistent focal edema, right heel

L89.612 Pressure ulcer of right heel, stage 2
Healing pressure ulcer of right heel, stage 2
Pressure ulcer with abrasion, blister, partial thickness skin loss involving epidermis and/or dermis, right heel

MCC **L89.613 Pressure ulcer of right heel, stage 3**
Healing pressure ulcer of right heel, stage 3
Pressure ulcer with full thickness skin loss involving damage or necrosis of subcutaneous tissue, right heel
MCC Exclusion see Appendix A PDX collection 0854
HAC see Appendix B for HAC conditional logic

MCC **L89.614 Pressure ulcer of right heel, stage 4**
Healing pressure ulcer of right heel, stage
Pressure ulcer with necrosis of soft tissues through to underlying muscle, tendon, o bone, right heel
MCC Exclusion see Appendix A PDX collecti 0854
HAC see Appendix B for HAC conditional log

L89.619 Pressure ulcer of right heel, unspecified stage
Healing pressure ulcer of right heel NOS
Healing pressure ulcer of right heel, unspecified stage

+ L89.62 Pressure ulcer of left heel

L89.620 Pressure ulcer of left heel, unstageable

L89.621 Pressure ulcer of left heel, stage 1
Healing pressure ulcer of left heel, stage 1
Pressure pre-ulcer skin changes limited to persistent focal edema, left heel

L89.622 Pressure ulcer of left heel, stage 2
Healing pressure ulcer of left heel, stage 2
Pressure ulcer with abrasion, blister, partia thickness skin loss involving epidermis and/or dermis, left heel
AHA CC: 4Q, 2016, 144

MCC **L89.623 Pressure ulcer of left heel, stage 3**
Healing pressure ulcer of left heel, stage 3
Pressure ulcer with full thickness skin loss involving damage or necrosis of subcutaneous tissue, left heel
MCC Exclusion see Appendix A PDX collecti 0854
AHA CC: 4Q, 2016, 144
HAC see Appendix B for HAC conditional log

MCC **L89.624 Pressure ulcer of left heel, stage 4**
Healing pressure ulcer of left heel, stage 4
Pressure ulcer with necrosis of soft tissues through to underlying muscle, tendon, o bone, left heel
MCC Exclusion see Appendix A PDX collecti 0854
HAC see Appendix B for HAC conditional log

L89.629 Pressure ulcer of left heel, unspecified sta
Healing pressure ulcer of left heel NOS
Healing pressure ulcer of left heel, unspecified stage

+ L89.8 Pressure ulcer of other site

+ L89.81 Pressure ulcer of head
Pressure ulcer of face

L89.810 Pressure ulcer of head, unstageable

L89.811 Pressure ulcer of head, stage 1
Healing pressure ulcer of head, stage 1
Pressure pre-ulcer skin changes limited to persistent focal edema, head

L89.812 Pressure ulcer of head, stage 2
Healing pressure ulcer of head, stage 2
Pressure ulcer with abrasion, blister, partia thickness skin loss involving epidermis and/or dermis, head

MCC **L89.813 Pressure ulcer of head, stage 3**
Healing pressure ulcer of head, stage 3
Pressure ulcer with full thickness skin loss involving damage or necrosis of subcutaneous tissue, head
MCC Exclusion see Appendix A PDX collecti 0854
HAC see Appendix B for HAC conditional log

MCC **L89.814 Pressure ulcer of head, stage 4**
Healing pressure ulcer of head, stage 4
Pressure ulcer with necrosis of soft tissues through to underlying muscle, tendon, c bone, head
MCC Exclusion see Appendix A PDX collecti 0854
HAC see Appendix B for HAC conditional log

L89.819 Pressure ulcer of head, unspecified stage
Healing pressure ulcer of head NOS
Healing pressure ulcer of head, unspecifie stage

+ **L89.89 Pressure ulcer of other site**

L89.890 Pressure ulcer of other site, unstageable

L89.891 Pressure ulcer of other site, stage 1

Healing pressure ulcer of other site, stage 1
Pressure pre-ulcer skin changes limited to persistent focal edema, other site

L89.892 Pressure ulcer of other site, stage 2

Healing pressure ulcer of other site, stage 2
Pressure ulcer with abrasion, blister, partial thickness skin loss involving epidermis and/or dermis, other site

MCC **L89.893 Pressure ulcer of other site, stage 3**

Healing pressure ulcer of other site, stage 3
Pressure ulcer with full thickness skin loss involving damage or necrosis of subcutaneous tissue, other site
MCC Exclusion see Appendix A PDX collection 0854
HAC see Appendix B for HAC conditional logic

MCC **L89.894 Pressure ulcer of other site, stage 4**

Healing pressure ulcer of other site, stage 4
Pressure ulcer with necrosis of soft tissues through to underlying muscle, tendon, or bone, other site
MCC Exclusion see Appendix A PDX collection 0854
HAC see Appendix B for HAC conditional logic

L89.899 Pressure ulcer of other site, unspecified stage

Healing pressure ulcer of other site NOS
Healing pressure ulcer of other site, unspecified stage

+ **L89.9 Pressure ulcer of unspecified site**

L89.90 Pressure ulcer of unspecified site, unspecified stage

Healing pressure ulcer of unspecified site NOS
Healing pressure ulcer of unspecified site, unspecified stage

L89.91 Pressure ulcer of unspecified site, stage 1

Healing pressure ulcer of unspecified site, stage 1
Pressure pre-ulcer skin changes limited to persistent focal edema, unspecified site

L89.92 Pressure ulcer of unspecified site, stage 2

Healing pressure ulcer of unspecified site, stage 2
Pressure ulcer with abrasion, blister, partial thickness skin loss involving epidermis and/or dermis, unspecified site

MCC **L89.93 Pressure ulcer of unspecified site, stage 3**

Healing pressure ulcer of unspecified site, stage 3
Pressure ulcer with full thickness skin loss involving damage or necrosis of subcutaneous tissue, unspecified site
MCC Exclusion see Appendix A PDX collection 0854
HAC see Appendix B for HAC conditional logic

MCC **L89.94 Pressure ulcer of unspecified site, stage 4**

Healing pressure ulcer of unspecified site, stage 4
Pressure ulcer with necrosis of soft tissues through to underlying muscle, tendon, or bone, unspecified site
MCC Exclusion see Appendix A PDX collection 0854
HAC see Appendix B for HAC conditional logic

L89.95 Pressure ulcer of unspecified site, unstageable

L90 Atrophic disorders of skin

L90.0 Lichen sclerosus et atrophicus

Excludes2: *lichen sclerosus of external female genital organs (N90.4)*
lichen sclerosus of external male genital organs (N48.0)

L90.1 Anetoderma of Schweninger-Buzzi
L90.2 Anetoderma of Jadassohn-Pellizzari
L90.3 Atrophoderma of Pasini and Pierini
L90.4 Acrodermatitis chronica atrophicans
L90.5 Scar conditions and fibrosis of skin

Adherent scar (skin)
Cicatrix
Disfigurement of skin due to scar
Fibrosis of skin NOS
Scar NOS
Excludes2: *hypertrophic scar (L91.0)*
keloid scar (L91.0)
AHA CC: 1Q, 2015, 19; 2Q, 2016, 5

L90.6 Striae atrophicae
L90.8 Other atrophic disorders of skin
L90.9 Atrophic disorder of skin, unspecified

L91 Hypertrophic disorders of skin

L91.0 Hypertrophic scar

Keloid
Keloid scar
Excludes2: *acne keloid (L73.0)*
scar NOS (L90.5)

L91.8 Other hypertrophic disorders of the skin
L91.9 Hypertrophic disorder of the skin, unspecified

L92 Granulomatous disorders of skin and subcutaneous tissue

Excludes2: *actinic granuloma (L57.5)*

L92.0 Granuloma annulare

Perforating granuloma annulare

L92.1 Necrobiosis lipoidica, not elsewhere classified

Excludes1: *necrobiosis lipoidica associated with diabetes mellitus (E08-E13 with .620)*

L92.2 Granuloma faciale [eosinophilic granuloma of skin]
L92.3 Foreign body granuloma of the skin and subcutaneous tissue

Use additional code to identify the type of retained foreign body (Z18.-)

L92.8 Other granulomatous disorders of the skin and subcutaneous tissue
L92.9 Granulomatous disorder of the skin and subcutaneous tissue, unspecified

Excludes2: *umbilical granuloma (P83.81)*

L93 Lupus erythematosus

Use additional code for adverse effect, if applicable, to identify drug (T36-T50 with fifth or sixth character 5)
Excludes1: *lupus exedens (A18.4)*
lupus vulgaris (A18.4)
scleroderma (M34.-)
systemic lupus erythematosus (M32.-)

L93.0 Discoid lupus erythematosus

Lupus erythematosus NOS

L93.1 Subacute cutaneous lupus erythematosus
L93.2 Other local lupus erythematosus

Lupus erythematosus profundus
Lupus panniculitis

L94 Other localized connective tissue disorders

Excludes1: *systemic connective tissue disorders (M30-M36)*

L94.0 Localized scleroderma [morphea]

Circumscribed scleroderma

L94.1 Linear scleroderma

En coup de sabre lesion

L94.2 Calcinosis cutis
L94.3 Sclerodactyly
L94.4 Gottron's papules
L94.5 Poikiloderma vasculare atrophicans
L94.6 Ainhum
L94.8 Other specified localized connective tissue disorders
L94.9 Localized connective tissue disorder, unspecified

L95 Vasculitis limited to skin, not elsewhere classified

Excludes1: *angioma serpiginosum (L81.7)*
Henoch(-Schönlein) purpura (D69.0)
hypersensitivity angiitis (M31.0)
lupus panniculitis (L93.2)
panniculitis NOS (M79.3)
panniculitis of neck and back (M54.0-)
polyarteritis nodosa (M30.0)
relapsing panniculitis (M35.6)
rheumatoid vasculitis (M05.2)
serum sickness (T80.6-)
urticaria (L50.-)
Wegener's granulomatosis (M31.3-)

L95.0 Livedoid vasculitis

Atrophie blanche (en plaque)

L95.1 Erythema elevatum diutinum
L95.8 Other vasculitis limited to the skin
L95.9 Vasculitis limited to the skin, unspecified

L97 Non-pressure chronic ulcer of lower limb, not elsewhere classified

Includes: chronic ulcer of skin of lower limb NOS
non-healing ulcer of skin
non-infected sinus of skin
trophic ulcer NOS
tropical ulcer NOS
ulcer of skin of lower limb NOS

Code first any associated underlying condition, such as:
any associated gangrene (I96)
atherosclerosis of the lower extremities (I70.23-, I70.24-, I70.33-, I70.34-, I70.43-, I70.44-, I70.53-, I70.54-, I70.63-, I70.64-, I70.73-, I70.74-)
chronic venous hypertension (I87.31-, I87.33-)
diabetic ulcers (E08.621, E08.622, E09.621, E09.622, E10.621, E10.622, E11.621, E11.622, E13.621, E13.622)
postphlebitic syndrome (I87.01-, I87.03-)
postthrombotic syndrome (I87.01-, I87.03-)
varicose ulcer (I83.0-, I83.2-)

Excludes2: *pressure ulcer (pressure area) (L89.-)*
skin infections (L00-L08)
specific infections classified to A00-B99

Review coding guideline C.12.b

+ L97.1 Non-pressure chronic ulcer of thigh

+ L97.10 Non-pressure chronic ulcer of unspecified thigh

CC **L97.101 Non-pressure chronic ulcer of unspecified thigh limited to breakdown of skin**
CC Exclusion see Appendix A PDX collection 0698

CC **L97.102 Non-pressure chronic ulcer of unspecified thigh with fat layer exposed**
CC Exclusion see Appendix A PDX collection 0698

CC **L97.103 Non-pressure chronic ulcer of unspecified thigh with necrosis of muscle**
CC Exclusion see Appendix A PDX collection 0698

CC **L97.104 Non-pressure chronic ulcer of unspecified thigh with necrosis of bone**
CC Exclusion see Appendix A PDX collection 0698

CC **L97.105 Non-pressure chronic ulcer of unspecified thigh with muscle involvement without evidence of necrosis**
CC Exclusion see Appendix A PDX collection 0698

CC **L97.106 Non-pressure chronic ulcer of unspecified thigh with bone involvement without evidence of necrosis**
CC Exclusion see Appendix A PDX collection 0698

CC **L97.108 Non-pressure chronic ulcer of unspecified thigh with other specified severity**
CC Exclusion see Appendix A PDX collection 0698

CC **L97.109 Non-pressure chronic ulcer of unspecified thigh with unspecified severity**
CC Exclusion see Appendix A PDX collection 0698

+ L97.11 Non-pressure chronic ulcer of right thigh

CC **L97.111 Non-pressure chronic ulcer of right thigh limited to breakdown of skin**
CC Exclusion see Appendix A PDX collection 0698

CC **L97.112 Non-pressure chronic ulcer of right thigh with fat layer exposed**
CC Exclusion see Appendix A PDX collection 0698

CC **L97.113 Non-pressure chronic ulcer of right thigh with necrosis of muscle**
CC Exclusion see Appendix A PDX collection 0698

CC **L97.114 Non-pressure chronic ulcer of right thigh with necrosis of bone**
CC Exclusion see Appendix A PDX collection 0698

CC **L97.115 Non-pressure chronic ulcer of right thigh with muscle involvement without evidence of necrosis**
CC Exclusion see Appendix A PDX collection 0698

CC **L97.116 Non-pressure chronic ulcer of right thigh with bone involvement without evidence of necrosis**
CC Exclusion see Appendix A PDX collection 0698

CC **L97.118 Non-pressure chronic ulcer of right thigh with other specified severity**
CC Exclusion see Appendix A PDX collection 0698

CC **L97.119 Non-pressure chronic ulcer of right thigh with unspecified severity**
CC Exclusion see Appendix A PDX collection 0698

+ L97.12 Non-pressure chronic ulcer of left thigh

CC **L97.121 Non-pressure chronic ulcer of left thigh limited to breakdown of skin**
CC Exclusion see Appendix A PDX collection 0698

CC **L97.122 Non-pressure chronic ulcer of left thigh with fat layer exposed**
CC Exclusion see Appendix A PDX collection 0698

CC **L97.123 Non-pressure chronic ulcer of left thigh with necrosis of muscle**
CC Exclusion see Appendix A PDX collection 0698

CC **L97.124 Non-pressure chronic ulcer of left thigh with necrosis of bone**
CC Exclusion see Appendix A PDX collection 0698

CC **L97.125 Non-pressure chronic ulcer of left thigh with muscle involvement without evidence of necrosis**
CC Exclusion see Appendix A PDX collection 0698

CC **L97.126 Non-pressure chronic ulcer of left thigh with bone involvement without evidence of necrosis**
CC Exclusion see Appendix A PDX collection 0698

CC **L97.128 Non-pressure chronic ulcer of left thigh with other specified severity**
CC Exclusion see Appendix A PDX collection 0698

CC **L97.129 Non-pressure chronic ulcer of left thigh with unspecified severity**
CC Exclusion see Appendix A PDX collection 0698

+ L97.2 Non-pressure chronic ulcer of calf

+ L97.20 Non-pressure chronic ulcer of unspecified calf

CC **L97.201 Non-pressure chronic ulcer of unspecified calf limited to breakdown of skin**
CC Exclusion see Appendix A PDX collection 0698

CC **L97.202 Non-pressure chronic ulcer of unspecified calf with fat layer exposed**
CC Exclusion see Appendix A PDX collection 0698

CC **L97.203 Non-pressure chronic ulcer of unspecified calf with necrosis of muscle**
CC Exclusion see Appendix A PDX collection 0698

CC **L97.204 Non-pressure chronic ulcer of unspecified calf with necrosis of bone**
CC Exclusion see Appendix A PDX collection 0698

CC **L97.205 Non-pressure chronic ulcer of unspecified calf with muscle involvement without evidence of necrosis**
CC Exclusion see Appendix A PDX collection 0698

CC **L97.206 Non-pressure chronic ulcer of unspecified calf with bone involvement without evidence of necrosis**
CC Exclusion see Appendix A PDX collection 0698

CC **L97.208 Non-pressure chronic ulcer of unspecified calf with other specified severity**
CC Exclusion see Appendix A PDX collection 0698

CC **L97.209 Non-pressure chronic ulcer of unspecified calf with unspecified severity**
CC Exclusion see Appendix A PDX collection 0698

+ L97.21 Non-pressure chronic ulcer of right calf
 - CC L97.211 Non-pressure chronic ulcer of right calf limited to breakdown of skin
 CC Exclusion see Appendix A PDX collection 0698
 - CC L97.212 Non-pressure chronic ulcer of right calf with fat layer exposed
 CC Exclusion see Appendix A PDX collection 0698
 - CC L97.213 Non-pressure chronic ulcer of right calf with necrosis of muscle
 CC Exclusion see Appendix A PDX collection 0698
 - CC L97.214 Non-pressure chronic ulcer of right calf with necrosis of bone
 CC Exclusion see Appendix A PDX collection 0698
 - CC L97.215 Non-pressure chronic ulcer of right calf with muscle involvement without evidence of necrosis
 CC Exclusion see Appendix A PDX collection 0698
 - CC L97.216 Non-pressure chronic ulcer of right calf with bone involvement without evidence of necrosis
 CC Exclusion see Appendix A PDX collection 0698
 - CC L97.218 Non-pressure chronic ulcer of right calf with other specified severity
 CC Exclusion see Appendix A PDX collection 0698
 - CC L97.219 Non-pressure chronic ulcer of right calf with unspecified severity
 CC Exclusion see Appendix A PDX collection 0698

+ L97.22 Non-pressure chronic ulcer of left calf
 - CC L97.221 Non-pressure chronic ulcer of left calf limited to breakdown of skin
 CC Exclusion see Appendix A PDX collection 0698
 - CC L97.222 Non-pressure chronic ulcer of left calf with fat layer exposed
 CC Exclusion see Appendix A PDX collection 0698
 AHA CC: 1Q, 2016, 12-13
 - CC L97.223 Non-pressure chronic ulcer of left calf with necrosis of muscle
 CC Exclusion see Appendix A PDX collection 0698
 - CC L97.224 Non-pressure chronic ulcer of left calf with necrosis of bone
 CC Exclusion see Appendix A PDX collection 0698
 - CC L97.225 Non-pressure chronic ulcer of left calf with muscle involvement without evidence of necrosis
 CC Exclusion see Appendix A PDX collection 0698
 - CC L97.226 Non-pressure chronic ulcer of left calf with bone involvement without evidence of necrosis
 CC Exclusion see Appendix A PDX collection 0698
 - CC L97.228 Non-pressure chronic ulcer of left calf with other specified severity
 CC Exclusion see Appendix A PDX collection 0698
 - CC L97.229 Non-pressure chronic ulcer of left calf with unspecified severity
 CC Exclusion see Appendix A PDX collection 0698

+ L97.3 Non-pressure chronic ulcer of ankle

+ L97.30 Non-pressure chronic ulcer of unspecified ankle
 - CC L97.301 Non-pressure chronic ulcer of unspecified ankle limited to breakdown of skin
 CC Exclusion see Appendix A PDX collection 0698
 - CC L97.302 Non-pressure chronic ulcer of unspecified ankle with fat layer exposed
 CC Exclusion see Appendix A PDX collection 0698
 - CC L97.303 Non-pressure chronic ulcer of unspecified ankle with necrosis of muscle
 CC Exclusion see Appendix A PDX collection 0698
 - CC L97.304 Non-pressure chronic ulcer of unspecified ankle with necrosis of bone
 CC Exclusion see Appendix A PDX collection 0698
 - CC L97.305 Non-pressure chronic ulcer of unspecified ankle with muscle involvement without evidence of necrosis
 CC Exclusion see Appendix A PDX collection 0698
 - CC L97.306 Non-pressure chronic ulcer of unspecified ankle with bone involvement without evidence of necrosis
 CC Exclusion see Appendix A PDX collection 0698
 - CC L97.308 Non-pressure chronic ulcer of unspecified ankle with other specified severity
 CC Exclusion see Appendix A PDX collection 0698
 - CC L97.309 Non-pressure chronic ulcer of unspecified ankle with unspecified severity
 CC Exclusion see Appendix A PDX collection 0698

+ L97.31 Non-pressure chronic ulcer of right ankle
 - CC L97.311 Non-pressure chronic ulcer of right ankle limited to breakdown of skin
 CC Exclusion see Appendix A PDX collection 0698
 - CC L97.312 Non-pressure chronic ulcer of right ankle with fat layer exposed
 CC Exclusion see Appendix A PDX collection 0698
 - CC L97.313 Non-pressure chronic ulcer of right ankle with necrosis of muscle
 CC Exclusion see Appendix A PDX collection 0698
 - CC L97.314 Non-pressure chronic ulcer of right ankle with necrosis of bone
 CC Exclusion see Appendix A PDX collection 0698
 - CC L97.315 Non-pressure chronic ulcer of right ankle with muscle involvement without evidence of necrosis
 CC Exclusion see Appendix A PDX collection 0698
 - CC L97.316 Non-pressure chronic ulcer of right ankle with bone involvement without evidence of necrosis
 CC Exclusion see Appendix A PDX collection 0698
 - CC L97.318 Non-pressure chronic ulcer of right ankle with other specified severity
 CC Exclusion see Appendix A PDX collection 0698
 - CC L97.319 Non-pressure chronic ulcer of right ankle with unspecified severity
 CC Exclusion see Appendix A PDX collection 0698

+ L97.32 Non-pressure chronic ulcer of left ankle
 - CC L97.321 Non-pressure chronic ulcer of left ankle limited to breakdown of skin
 CC Exclusion see Appendix A PDX collection 0698
 - CC L97.322 Non-pressure chronic ulcer of left ankle with fat layer exposed
 CC Exclusion see Appendix A PDX collection 0698
 - CC L97.323 Non-pressure chronic ulcer of left ankle with necrosis of muscle
 CC Exclusion see Appendix A PDX collection 0698
 - CC L97.324 Non-pressure chronic ulcer of left ankle with necrosis of bone
 CC Exclusion see Appendix A PDX collection 0698
 - CC L97.325 Non-pressure chronic ulcer of left ankle with muscle involvement without evidence of necrosis
 CC Exclusion see Appendix A PDX collection 0698
 - CC L97.326 Non-pressure chronic ulcer of left ankle with bone involvement without evidence of necrosis
 CC Exclusion see Appendix A PDX collection 0698

CC L97.328 Non-pressure chronic ulcer of left ankle with other specified severity
CC Exclusion see Appendix A PDX collection 0698

CC L97.329 Non-pressure chronic ulcer of left ankle with unspecified severity
CC Exclusion see Appendix A PDX collection 0698

+ L97.4 Non-pressure chronic ulcer of heel and midfoot
Non-pressure chronic ulcer of plantar surface of midfoot

+ L97.40 Non-pressure chronic ulcer of unspecified heel and midfoot

CC L97.401 Non-pressure chronic ulcer of unspecified heel and midfoot limited to breakdown of skin
CC Exclusion see Appendix A PDX collection 0698

CC L97.402 Non-pressure chronic ulcer of unspecified heel and midfoot with fat layer exposed
CC Exclusion see Appendix A PDX collection 0698

CC L97.403 Non-pressure chronic ulcer of unspecified heel and midfoot with necrosis of muscle
CC Exclusion see Appendix A PDX collection 0698

CC L97.404 Non-pressure chronic ulcer of unspecified heel and midfoot with necrosis of bone
CC Exclusion see Appendix A PDX collection 0698

CC L97.405 Non-pressure chronic ulcer of unspecified heel and midfoot with muscle involvement without evidence of necrosis
CC Exclusion see Appendix A PDX collection 0698

CC L97.406 Non-pressure chronic ulcer of unspecified heel and midfoot with bone involvement without evidence of necrosis
CC Exclusion see Appendix A PDX collection 0698

CC L97.408 Non-pressure chronic ulcer of unspecified heel and midfoot with other specified severity
CC Exclusion see Appendix A PDX collection 0698

CC L97.409 Non-pressure chronic ulcer of unspecified heel and midfoot with unspecified severity
CC Exclusion see Appendix A PDX collection 0698

+ L97.41 Non-pressure chronic ulcer of right heel and midfoot

CC L97.411 Non-pressure chronic ulcer of right heel and midfoot limited to breakdown of skin
CC Exclusion see Appendix A PDX collection 0698

CC L97.412 Non-pressure chronic ulcer of right heel and midfoot with fat layer exposed
CC Exclusion see Appendix A PDX collection 0698

CC L97.413 Non-pressure chronic ulcer of right heel and midfoot with necrosis of muscle
CC Exclusion see Appendix A PDX collection 0698

CC L97.414 Non-pressure chronic ulcer of right heel and midfoot with necrosis of bone
CC Exclusion see Appendix A PDX collection 0698

CC L97.415 Non-pressure chronic ulcer of right heel and midfoot with muscle involvement without evidence of necrosis
CC Exclusion see Appendix A PDX collection 0698

CC L97.416 Non-pressure chronic ulcer of right heel and midfoot with bone involvement without evidence of necrosis
CC Exclusion see Appendix A PDX collection 0698

CC L97.418 Non-pressure chronic ulcer of right heel and midfoot with other specified severity
CC Exclusion see Appendix A PDX collection 0698

CC L97.419 Non-pressure chronic ulcer of right heel and midfoot with unspecified severity
CC Exclusion see Appendix A PDX collection 0698

+ L97.42 Non-pressure chronic ulcer of left heel and midfoot

CC L97.421 Non-pressure chronic ulcer of left heel and midfoot limited to breakdown of skin
CC Exclusion see Appendix A PDX collection 0698

CC L97.422 Non-pressure chronic ulcer of left heel and midfoot with fat layer exposed
CC Exclusion see Appendix A PDX collection 0698

CC L97.423 Non-pressure chronic ulcer of left heel and midfoot with necrosis of muscle
CC Exclusion see Appendix A PDX collection 0698

CC L97.424 Non-pressure chronic ulcer of left heel and midfoot with necrosis of bone
CC Exclusion see Appendix A PDX collection 06

CC L97.425 Non-pressure chronic ulcer of left heel and midfoot with muscle involvement without evidence of necrosis
CC Exclusion see Appendix A PDX collection 06

CC L97.426 Non-pressure chronic ulcer of left heel and midfoot with bone involvement without evidence of necrosis
CC Exclusion see Appendix A PDX collection 06

CC L97.428 Non-pressure chronic ulcer of left heel and midfoot with other specified severity
CC Exclusion see Appendix A PDX collection 06

CC L97.429 Non-pressure chronic ulcer of left heel and midfoot with unspecified severity
CC Exclusion see Appendix A PDX collection 06

+ L97.5 Non-pressure chronic ulcer of other part of foot
Non-pressure chronic ulcer of toe

+ L97.50 Non-pressure chronic ulcer of other part of unspecified foot

L97.501 Non-pressure chronic ulcer of other part of unspecified foot limited to breakdown of skin

L97.502 Non-pressure chronic ulcer of other part of unspecified foot with fat layer exposed

L97.503 Non-pressure chronic ulcer of other part of unspecified foot with necrosis of muscle

L97.504 Non-pressure chronic ulcer of other part of unspecified foot with necrosis of bone

CC L97.505 Non-pressure chronic ulcer of other part of unspecified foot with muscle involvement without evidence of necrosis
CC Exclusion see Appendix A PDX collection 06

CC L97.506 Non-pressure chronic ulcer of other part of unspecified foot with bone involvement without evidence of necrosis
CC Exclusion see Appendix A PDX collection 06

CC L97.508 Non-pressure chronic ulcer of other part of unspecified foot with other specified severity
CC Exclusion see Appendix A PDX collection 06

L97.509 Non-pressure chronic ulcer of other part of unspecified foot with unspecified severity

+ L97.51 Non-pressure chronic ulcer of other part of right foot

L97.511 Non-pressure chronic ulcer of other part of right foot limited to breakdown of skin

L97.512 Non-pressure chronic ulcer of other part of right foot with fat layer exposed

L97.513 Non-pressure chronic ulcer of other part of right foot with necrosis of muscle

L97.514 Non-pressure chronic ulcer of other part of right foot with necrosis of bone

CC L97.515 Non-pressure chronic ulcer of other part of right foot with muscle involvement without evidence of necrosis
CC Exclusion see Appendix A PDX collection 06

CC L97.516 Non-pressure chronic ulcer of other part of right foot with bone involvement without evidence of necrosis
CC Exclusion see Appendix A PDX collection 06

CC L97.518 Non-pressure chronic ulcer of other part of right foot with other specified severity
CC Exclusion see Appendix A PDX collection 06

L97.519 Non-pressure chronic ulcer of other part of right foot with unspecified severity

+ L97.52 Non-pressure chronic ulcer of other part of left foot

L97.521 Non-pressure chronic ulcer of other part of left foot limited to breakdown of skin

L97.522 Non-pressure chronic ulcer of other part of left foot with fat layer exposed

L97.523 Non-pressure chronic ulcer of other part of left foot with necrosis of muscle

L97.524 Non-pressure chronic ulcer of other part of left foot with necrosis of bone

CC L97.525 Non-pressure chronic ulcer of other part of left foot with muscle involvement without evidence of necrosis
CC Exclusion see Appendix A PDX collection 0698

CC L97.526 Non-pressure chronic ulcer of other part of left foot with bone involvement without evidence of necrosis
CC Exclusion see Appendix A PDX collection 0698

CC L97.528 Non-pressure chronic ulcer of other part of left foot with other specified severity
CC Exclusion see Appendix A PDX collection 0698

L97.529 Non-pressure chronic ulcer of other part of left foot with unspecified severity

+ L97.8 Non-pressure chronic ulcer of other part of lower leg

+ L97.80 Non-pressure chronic ulcer of other part of unspecified lower leg

CC L97.801 Non-pressure chronic ulcer of other part of unspecified lower leg limited to breakdown of skin
CC Exclusion see Appendix A PDX collection 0698

CC L97.802 Non-pressure chronic ulcer of other part of unspecified lower leg with fat layer exposed
CC Exclusion see Appendix A PDX collection 0698

CC L97.803 Non-pressure chronic ulcer of other part of unspecified lower leg with necrosis of muscle
CC Exclusion see Appendix A PDX collection 0698

CC L97.804 Non-pressure chronic ulcer of other part of unspecified lower leg with necrosis of bone
CC Exclusion see Appendix A PDX collection 0698

CC L97.805 Non-pressure chronic ulcer of other part of unspecified lower leg with muscle involvement without evidence of necrosis
CC Exclusion see Appendix A PDX collection 0698

CC L97.806 Non-pressure chronic ulcer of other part of unspecified lower leg with bone involvement without evidence of necrosis
CC Exclusion see Appendix A PDX collection 0698

CC L97.808 Non-pressure chronic ulcer of other part of unspecified lower leg with other specified severity
CC Exclusion see Appendix A PDX collection 0698

CC L97.809 Non-pressure chronic ulcer of other part of unspecified lower leg with unspecified severity
CC Exclusion see Appendix A PDX collection 0698

+ L97.81 Non-pressure chronic ulcer of other part of right lower leg

CC L97.811 Non-pressure chronic ulcer of other part of right lower leg limited to breakdown of skin
CC Exclusion see Appendix A PDX collection 0698

CC L97.812 Non-pressure chronic ulcer of other part of right lower leg with fat layer exposed
CC Exclusion see Appendix A PDX collection 0698

CC L97.813 Non-pressure chronic ulcer of other part of right lower leg with necrosis of muscle
CC Exclusion see Appendix A PDX collection 0698

CC L97.814 Non-pressure chronic ulcer of other part of right lower leg with necrosis of bone
CC Exclusion see Appendix A PDX collection 0698

CC L97.815 Non-pressure chronic ulcer of other part of right lower leg with muscle involvement without evidence of necrosis
CC Exclusion see Appendix A PDX collection 0698

CC L97.816 Non-pressure chronic ulcer of other part of right lower leg with bone involvement without evidence of necrosis
CC Exclusion see Appendix A PDX collection 0698

CC L97.818 Non-pressure chronic ulcer of other part of right lower leg with other specified severity
CC Exclusion see Appendix A PDX collection 0698

CC L97.819 Non-pressure chronic ulcer of other part of right lower leg with unspecified severity
CC Exclusion see Appendix A PDX collection 0698

+ L97.82 Non-pressure chronic ulcer of other part of left lower leg

CC L97.821 Non-pressure chronic ulcer of other part of left lower leg limited to breakdown of skin
CC Exclusion see Appendix A PDX collection 0698

CC L97.822 Non-pressure chronic ulcer of other part of left lower leg with fat layer exposed
CC Exclusion see Appendix A PDX collection 0698

CC L97.823 Non-pressure chronic ulcer of other part of left lower leg with necrosis of muscle
CC Exclusion see Appendix A PDX collection 0698

CC L97.824 Non-pressure chronic ulcer of other part of left lower leg with necrosis of bone
CC Exclusion see Appendix A PDX collection 0698

CC L97.825 Non-pressure chronic ulcer of other part of left lower leg with muscle involvement without evidence of necrosis
CC Exclusion see Appendix A PDX collection 0698

CC L97.826 Non-pressure chronic ulcer of other part of left lower leg with bone involvement without evidence of necrosis
CC Exclusion see Appendix A PDX collection 0698

CC L97.828 Non-pressure chronic ulcer of other part of left lower leg with other specified severity
CC Exclusion see Appendix A PDX collection 0698

CC L97.829 Non-pressure chronic ulcer of other part of left lower leg with unspecified severity
CC Exclusion see Appendix A PDX collection 0698

+ L97.9 Non-pressure chronic ulcer of unspecified part of lower leg

+ L97.90 Non-pressure chronic ulcer of unspecified part of unspecified lower leg

CC L97.901 Non-pressure chronic ulcer of unspecified part of unspecified lower leg limited to breakdown of skin
CC Exclusion see Appendix A PDX collection 0698

CC L97.902 Non-pressure chronic ulcer of unspecified part of unspecified lower leg with fat layer exposed
CC Exclusion see Appendix A PDX collection 0698

CC L97.903 Non-pressure chronic ulcer of unspecified part of unspecified lower leg with necrosis of muscle
CC Exclusion see Appendix A PDX collection 0698

CC L97.904 Non-pressure chronic ulcer of unspecified part of unspecified lower leg with necrosis of bone
CC Exclusion see Appendix A PDX collection 0698

CC L97.905 Non-pressure chronic ulcer of unspecified part of unspecified lower leg with muscle involvement without evidence of necrosis
CC Exclusion see Appendix A PDX collection 0698

CC L97.906 Non-pressure chronic ulcer of unspecified part of unspecified lower leg with bone involvement without evidence of necrosis
CC Exclusion see Appendix A PDX collection 0698

CC L97.908 Non-pressure chronic ulcer of unspecified part of unspecified lower leg with other specified severity
CC Exclusion see Appendix A PDX collection 0698

CC L97.909 Non-pressure chronic ulcer of unspecified part of unspecified lower leg with unspecified severity
CC Exclusion see Appendix A PDX collection 0698

+ L97.91 Non-pressure chronic ulcer of unspecified part of right lower leg

CC L97.911 Non-pressure chronic ulcer of unspecified part of right lower leg limited to breakdown of skin
CC Exclusion see Appendix A PDX collection 0698

CC L97.912 Non-pressure chronic ulcer of unspecified part of right lower leg with fat layer exposed
CC Exclusion see Appendix A PDX collection 0698

CC L97.913 Non-pressure chronic ulcer of unspecified part of right lower leg with necrosis of muscle
CC Exclusion see Appendix A PDX collection 0698

CC L97.914 Non-pressure chronic ulcer of unspecified part of right lower leg with necrosis of bone
CC Exclusion see Appendix A PDX collection 0698

CC L97.915 Non-pressure chronic ulcer of unspecified part of right lower leg with muscle involvement without evidence of necrosis
CC Exclusion see Appendix A PDX collection 0698

CC L97.916 Non-pressure chronic ulcer of unspecified part of right lower leg with bone involvement without evidence of necrosis
CC Exclusion see Appendix A PDX collection 0698

CC L97.918 Non-pressure chronic ulcer of unspecified part of right lower leg with other specified severity
CC Exclusion see Appendix A PDX collection 0698

CC L97.919 Non-pressure chronic ulcer of unspecified part of right lower leg with unspecified severity
CC Exclusion see Appendix A PDX collection 0698

+ L97.92 Non-pressure chronic ulcer of unspecified part of left lower leg

CC L97.921 Non-pressure chronic ulcer of unspecified part of left lower leg limited to breakdown of skin
CC Exclusion see Appendix A PDX collection 0698

CC L97.922 Non-pressure chronic ulcer of unspecified part of left lower leg with fat layer exposed
CC Exclusion see Appendix A PDX collection 0698

CC L97.923 Non-pressure chronic ulcer of unspecified part of left lower leg with necrosis of muscle
CC Exclusion see Appendix A PDX collection 0698

CC L97.924 Non-pressure chronic ulcer of unspecified part of left lower leg with necrosis of bone
CC Exclusion see Appendix A PDX collection 0698

CC L97.925 Non-pressure chronic ulcer of unspecified part of left lower leg with muscle involvement without evidence of necrosis
CC Exclusion see Appendix A PDX collection 0698

CC L97.926 Non-pressure chronic ulcer of unspecified part of left lower leg with bone involveme
without evidence of necrosis
CC Exclusion see Appendix A PDX collection 06

CC L97.928 Non-pressure chronic ulcer of unspecified part of left lower leg with other specified severity
CC Exclusion see Appendix A PDX collection 06

CC L97.929 Non-pressure chronic ulcer of unspecified part of left lower leg with unspecified severity
CC Exclusion see Appendix A PDX collection 06

L98 Other disorders of skin and subcutaneous tissue, not elsewhere classified

L98.0 Pyogenic granuloma
Excludes2: *pyogenic granuloma of gingiva (K06.8)*
pyogenic granuloma of maxillary alveolar ridge (K04.5)
pyogenic granuloma of oral mucosa (K13.4)

L98.1 Factitial dermatitis
Neurotic excoriation
Excludes1: *Excoriation (skin-picking) disorder (F42.4)*

L98.2 Febrile neutrophilic dermatosis [Sweet]

CC **L98.3 Eosinophilic cellulitis [Wells]**
CC Exclusion see Appendix A PDX collection 0839

+ **L98.4 Non-pressure chronic ulcer of skin, not elsewhere classified**
Chronic ulcer of skin NOS
Tropical ulcer NOS
Ulcer of skin NOS
Excludes2: *pressure ulcer (pressure area) (L89.-)*
gangrene (I96)
skin infections (L00-L08)
specific infections classified to A00-B99
ulcer of lower limb NEC (L97.-)
varicose ulcer (I83.0-I82.2)

+ L98.41 Non-pressure chronic ulcer of buttock

L98.411 Non-pressure chronic ulcer of buttock limited to breakdown of skin

L98.412 Non-pressure chronic ulcer of buttock wit fat layer exposed

L98.413 Non-pressure chronic ulcer of buttock wit necrosis of muscle

L98.414 Non-pressure chronic ulcer of buttock wit necrosis of bone

CC L98.415 Non-pressure chronic ulcer of buttock wit muscle involvement without evidence of necrosis
CC Exclusion see Appendix A PDX collection 06

CC L98.416 Non-pressure chronic ulcer of buttock with bone involvement without evidence o necrosis
CC Exclusion see Appendix A PDX collection 06

CC L98.418 Non-pressure chronic ulcer of buttock wit other specified severity
CC Exclusion see Appendix A PDX collection 06

L98.419 Non-pressure chronic ulcer of buttock wit unspecified severity

+ L98.42 Non-pressure chronic ulcer of back

L98.421 Non-pressure chronic ulcer of back limite to breakdown of skin

L98.422 Non-pressure chronic ulcer of back with fat layer exposed

L98.423 Non-pressure chronic ulcer of back with necrosis of muscle

L98.424 Non-pressure chronic ulcer of back with necrosis of bone

CC L98.425 Non-pressure chronic ulcer of back with muscle involvement without evidence of necrosis
CC Exclusion see Appendix A PDX collection 06

CC L98.426 Non-pressure chronic ulcer of back with bone involvement without evidence of necrosis
CC Exclusion see Appendix A PDX collection 06

CC L98.428 Non-pressure chronic ulcer of back with other specified severity
CC Exclusion see Appendix A PDX collection 06

L98.429 Non-pressure chronic ulcer of back with unspecified severity

+ **L98.49 Non-pressure chronic ulcer of skin of other sites**
Non-pressure chronic ulcer of skin NOS
L98.491 Non-pressure chronic ulcer of skin of other sites limited to breakdown of skin
L98.492 Non-pressure chronic ulcer of skin of other sites with fat layer exposed
L98.493 Non-pressure chronic ulcer of skin of other sites with necrosis of muscle
L98.494 Non-pressure chronic ulcer of skin of other sites with necrosis of bone
CC **L98.495 Non-pressure chronic ulcer of other sites with muscle involvement without evidence of necrosis**
CC Exclusion see Appendix A PDX collection 0698
CC **L98.496 Non-pressure chronic ulcer of other sites with bone involvement without evidence of necrosis**
CC Exclusion see Appendix A PDX collection 0698
CC **L98.498 Non-pressure chronic ulcer of other sites with other specified severity**
CC Exclusion see Appendix A PDX collection 0698
L98.499 Non-pressure chronic ulcer of skin of other sites with unspecified severity

L98.5 Mucinosis of the skin
Focal mucinosis
Lichen myxedematosus
Reticular erythematous mucinosis
Excludes1: *focal oral mucinosis (K13.79)*
myxedema (E03.9)

L98.6 Other infiltrative disorders of the skin and subcutaneous tissue
Excludes1: *hyalinosis cutis et mucosae (E78.89)*

L98.7 Excessive and redundant skin and subcutaneous tissue
Loose or sagging skin following bariatric surgery weight loss
Loose or sagging skin following dietary weight loss
Loose or sagging skin, NOS
Excludes2: *acquired excess or redundant skin of eyelid (H02.3-)*
congenital excess or redundant skin or eyelid (Q10.3)
skin changes due to chronic exposure to nonionizing radiation (L57.-)
AHA CC: 4Q, 2016, 36

L98.8 Other specified disorders of the skin and subcutaneous tissue
AHA CC: 2Q, 2013, 32-33

L98.9 Disorder of the skin and subcutaneous tissue, unspecified

L99 Other disorders of skin and subcutaneous tissue in diseases classified elsewhere
Code first underlying disease, such as:
amyloidosis (E85.-)
Excludes1: *skin disorders in diabetes (E08-E13 with .62)*
skin disorders in gonorrhea (A54.89)
skin disorders in syphilis (A51.31, A52.79)
Valid 3-character code, no further characters required

Intervertebral Joint

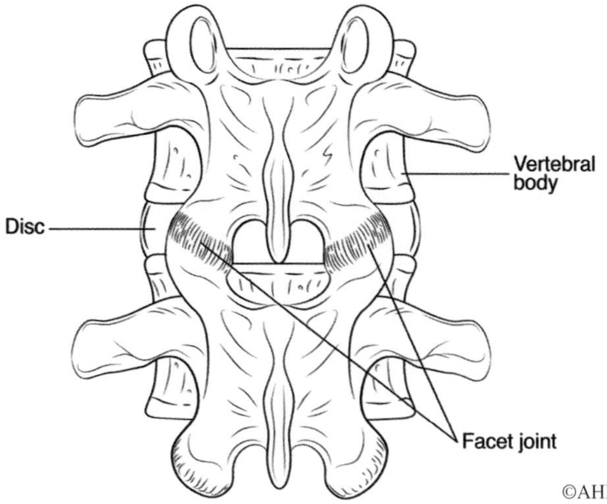

Shoulder Joint

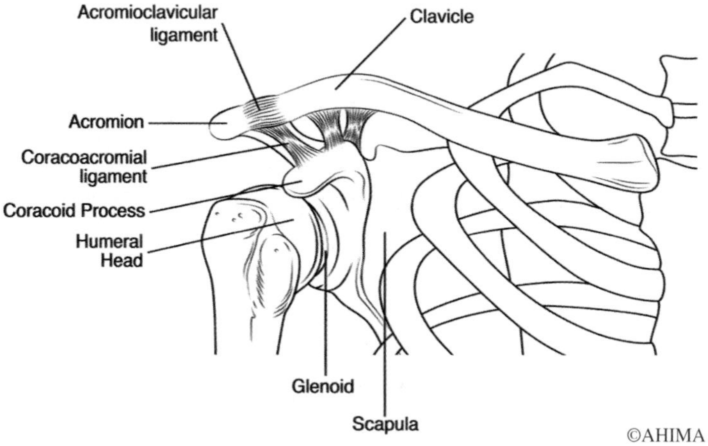

Elbow

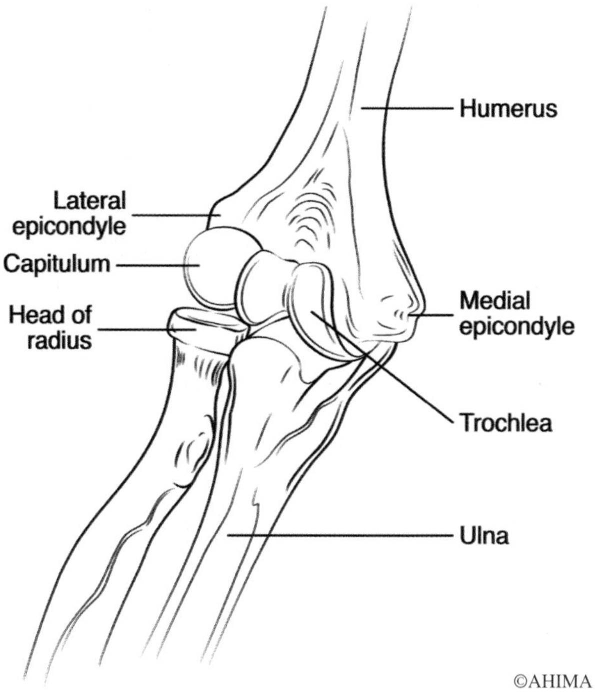

Wrist

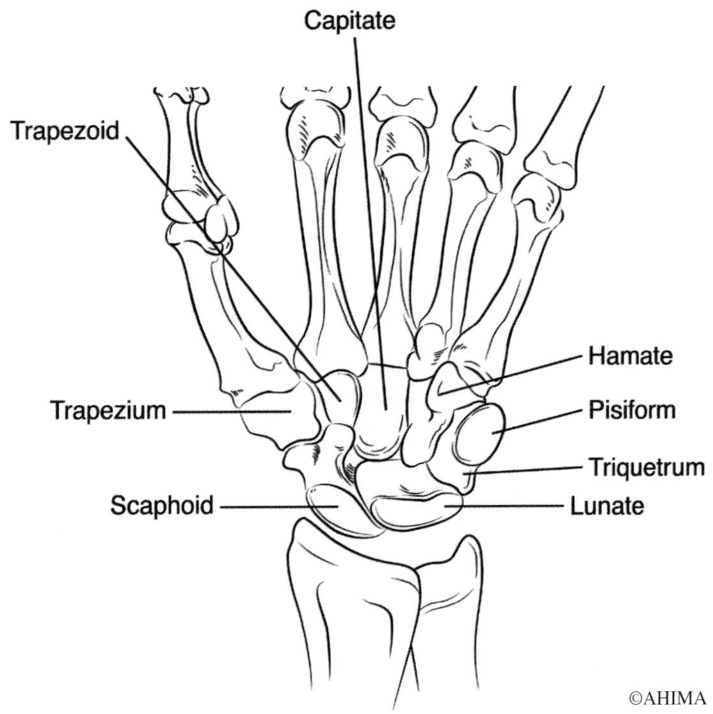

Capitate
Trapezoid
Hamate
Trapezium
Pisiform
Triquetrum
Scaphoid
Lunate
©AHIMA

Hip Joint

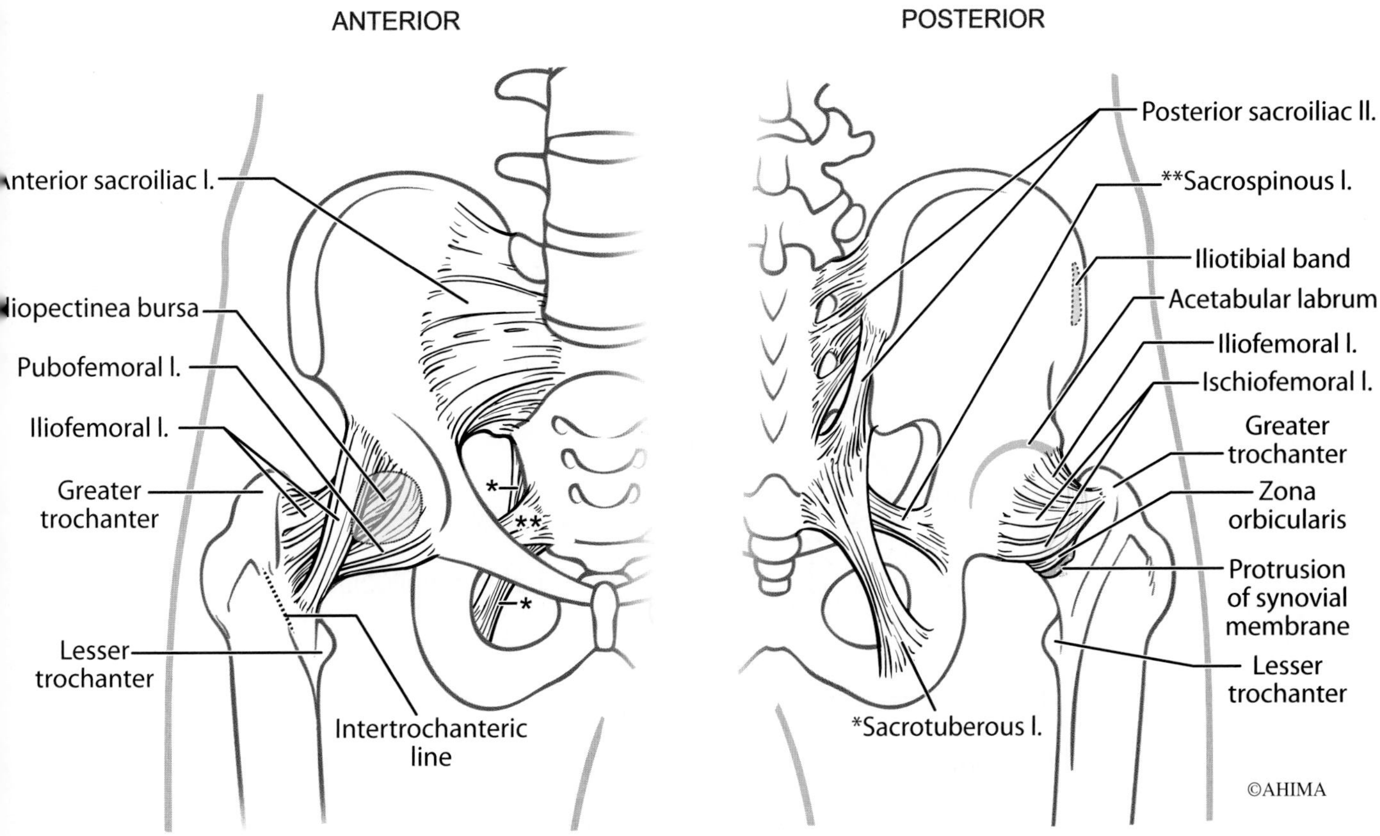

ANTERIOR
POSTERIOR
nterior sacroiliac l.
iopectinea bursa
Pubofemoral l.
Iliofemoral l.
Greater trochanter
Lesser trochanter
Intertrochanteric line
*
**
*
Posterior sacroiliac ll.
**Sacrospinous l.
Iliotibial band
Acetabular labrum
Iliofemoral l.
Ischiofemoral l.
Greater trochanter
Zona orbicularis
Protrusion of synovial membrane
Lesser trochanter
*Sacrotuberous l.
©AHIMA

Knee Joint

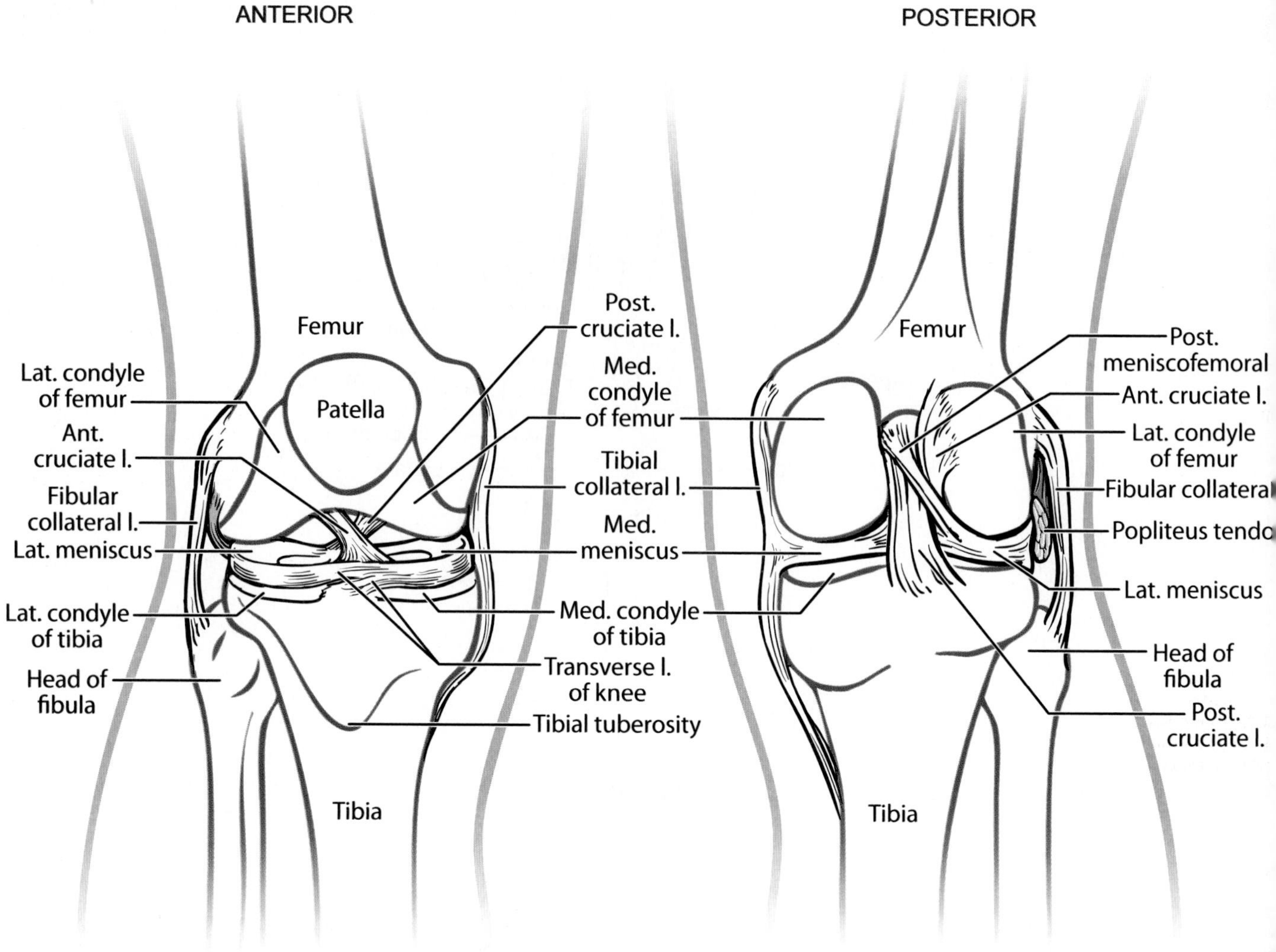
ANTERIOR
POSTERIOR
Femur
Patella
Lat. condyle of femur
Ant. cruciate l.
Fibular collateral l.
Lat. meniscus
Lat. condyle of tibia
Head of fibula
Post. cruciate l.
Med. condyle of femur
Tibial collateral l.
Med. meniscus
Med. condyle of tibia
Transverse l. of knee
Tibial tuberosity
Tibia
Femur
Post. meniscofemoral
Ant. cruciate l.
Lat. condyle of femur
Fibular collateral
Popliteus tendo
Lat. meniscus
Head of fibula
Post. cruciate l.
Tibia

Ankle

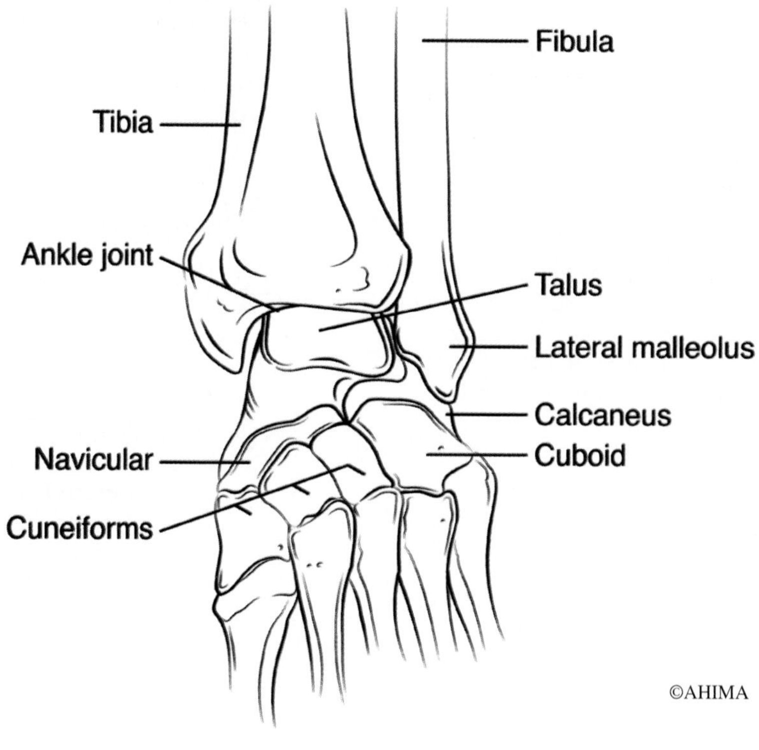
Fibula
Tibia
Ankle joint
Talus
Lateral malleolus
Calcaneus
Navicular
Cuboid
Cuneiforms

Chapter 13: Diseases of the Musculoskeletal System and Connective Tissue (M00-M99)

NOTE Use an external cause code following the code for the musculoskeletal condition, if applicable, to identify the cause of the musculoskeletal condition

Excludes2: *arthropathic psoriasis (L40.5-)*
certain conditions originating in the perinatal period (P04-P96)
certain infectious and parasitic diseases (A00-B99)
compartment syndrome (traumatic) (T79.A-)
complications of pregnancy, childbirth and the puerperium (O00-O9A)
congenital malformations, deformations, and chromosomal abnormalities (Q00-Q99)
endocrine, nutritional and metabolic diseases (E00-E88)
injury, poisoning and certain other consequences of external causes (S00-T88)
neoplasms (C00-D49)
symptoms, signs and abnormal clinical and laboratory findings, not elsewhere classified (R00-R94)

This chapter contains the following category blocks:

M00-M02	Infectious arthropathies
M05-M14	Inflammatory polyarthropathies
M15-M19	Osteoarthritis
M20-M25	Other joint disorders
M26-M27	Dentofacial anomalies [including malocclusion] and other disorders of jaw
M30-M36	Systemic connective tissue disorders
M40-M43	Deforming dorsopathies
M45-M49	Spondylopathies
M50-M54	Other dorsopathies
M60-M63	Disorders of muscles
M65-M67	Disorders of synovium and tendon
M70-M79	Other soft tissue disorders
M80-M85	Disorders of bone density and structure
M86-M90	Other osteopathies
M91-M94	Chondropathies
M95	Other disorders of the musculoskeletal system and connective tissue
M96	Intraoperative and postprocedural complications and disorders of musculoskeletal system, not elsewhere classified
M99	Biomechanical lesions, not elsewhere classified

I. Chapter-Specific Coding Guidelines

In addition to general coding guidelines, there are guidelines for specific diagnoses and/or conditions in the classification. Unless otherwise indicated, these guidelines apply to all health care settings. Please refer to Section II for guidelines on the selection of principal diagnosis.

13. Chapter 13: Diseases of the Musculoskeletal System and Connective Tissue (M00-M99)

a. Site and laterality

Most of the codes within Chapter 13 have site and laterality designations. The site represents the bone, joint or the muscle involved. For some conditions where more than one bone, joint or muscle is usually involved, such as osteoarthritis, there is a "multiple sites" code available. For categories where no multiple site code is provided and more than one bone, joint or muscle is involved, multiple codes should be used to indicate the different sites involved.

1) Bone versus joint

For certain conditions, the bone may be affected at the upper or lower end, (e.g., avascular necrosis of bone, M87, Osteoporosis, M80, M81). Though the portion of the bone affected may be at the joint, the site designation will be the bone, not the joint.

b. Acute traumatic versus chronic or recurrent musculoskeletal conditions

Many musculoskeletal conditions are a result of previous injury or trauma to a site, or are recurrent conditions. Bone, joint or muscle conditions that are the result of a healed injury are usually found in chapter 13. Recurrent bone, joint or muscle conditions are also usually found in chapter 13. Any current, acute injury should be coded to the appropriate injury code from chapter 19. Chronic or recurrent conditions should generally be coded with a code from chapter 13. If it is difficult to determine from the documentation in the record which code is best to describe a condition, query the provider.

c. Coding of Pathologic Fractures

7th character A is for use as long as the patient is receiving active treatment for the fracture. While the patient may be seen by a new or different provider over the course of treatment for a pathological fracture, assignment of the 7th character is based on whether the patient is undergoing active treatment and not whether the provider is seeing the patient for the first time.

7th character, D is to be used for encounters after the patient has completed active treatment **for the fracture and is receiving routine care for the fracture during the healing or recovery phase**. The other 7th characters, listed under each subcategory in the Tabular List, are to be used for subsequent encounters for routine care of fractures during the healing and recovery phase as well as treatment of problems associated with the healing, such as malunions, nonunions, and sequelae.

Care for complications of surgical treatment for fracture repairs during the healing or recovery phase should be coded with the appropriate complication codes.

See Section I.C.19. Coding of traumatic fractures.

d. Osteoporosis

Osteoporosis is a systemic condition, meaning that all bones of the musculoskeletal system are affected. Therefore, site is not a component of the codes under category M81, Osteoporosis without current pathological fracture. The site codes under category M80, Osteoporosis with current pathological fracture, identify the site of the fracture, not the osteoporosis.

1) Osteoporosis without pathological fracture

Category M81, Osteoporosis without current pathological fracture, is for use for patients with osteoporosis who do not currently have a pathologic fracture due to the osteoporosis, even if they have had a fracture in the past. For patients with a history of osteoporosis fractures, status code Z87.310, Personal history of (healed) osteoporosis fracture, should follow the code from M81.

2) Osteoporosis with current pathological fracture

Category M80, Osteoporosis with current pathological fracture, is for patients who have a current pathologic fracture at the time of an encounter. The codes under M80 identify the site of the fracture. A code from category M80, not a traumatic fracture code, should be used for any patient with known osteoporosis who suffers a fracture, even if the patient had a minor fall or trauma, if that fall or trauma would not usually break a normal, healthy bone.

ARTHROPATHIES (M00-M25)

Includes: Disorders affecting predominantly peripheral (limb) joints

Infectious arthropathies (M00-M02)

NOTE This block comprises arthropathies due to microbiological agents. Distinction is made between the following types of etiological relationship:
a) direct infection of joint, where organisms invade synovial tissue and microbial antigen is present in the joint;
b) indirect infection, which may be of two types: a reactive arthropathy, where microbial infection of the body is established but neither organisms nor antigens can be identified in the joint, and a postinfective arthropathy, where microbial antigen is present but recovery of an organism is inconstant and evidence of local multiplication is lacking.

M00 Pyogenic arthritis

\+ **M00.0 Staphylococcal arthritis and polyarthritis**
Use additional code (B95.61-B95.8) to identify bacterial agent
Excludes2: *infection and inflammatory reaction due to internal joint prosthesis (T84.5-)*

CC **M00.00 Staphylococcal arthritis, unspecified joint**
CC Exclusion see Appendix A PDX collection 0855

\+ **M00.01 Staphylococcal arthritis, shoulder**
M00.011 Staphylococcal arthritis, right shoulder
M00.012 Staphylococcal arthritis, left shoulder
CC **M00.019 Staphylococcal arthritis, unspecified shoulder**
CC Exclusion see Appendix A PDX collection 0856

\+ **M00.02 Staphylococcal arthritis, elbow**
M00.021 Staphylococcal arthritis, right elbow
M00.022 Staphylococcal arthritis, left elbow
CC **M00.029 Staphylococcal arthritis, unspecified elbow**
CC Exclusion see Appendix A PDX collection 0857

\+ **M00.03 Staphylococcal arthritis, wrist**
Staphylococcal arthritis of carpal bones
M00.031 Staphylococcal arthritis, right wrist
M00.032 Staphylococcal arthritis, left wrist
CC **M00.039 Staphylococcal arthritis, unspecified wrist**
CC Exclusion see Appendix A PDX collection 0858

+ M00.04 **Staphylococcal arthritis, hand**
Staphylococcal arthritis of metacarpus and phalanges
M00.041 **Staphylococcal arthritis, right hand**
M00.042 **Staphylococcal arthritis, left hand**
CC M00.049 **Staphylococcal arthritis, unspecified hand**
CC Exclusion see Appendix A PDX collection 0859
+ M00.05 **Staphylococcal arthritis, hip**
M00.051 **Staphylococcal arthritis, right hip**
M00.052 **Staphylococcal arthritis, left hip**
CC M00.059 **Staphylococcal arthritis, unspecified hip**
CC Exclusion see Appendix A PDX collection 0860
+ M00.06 **Staphylococcal arthritis, knee**
M00.061 **Staphylococcal arthritis, right knee**
M00.062 **Staphylococcal arthritis, left knee**
CC M00.069 **Staphylococcal arthritis, unspecified knee**
CC Exclusion see Appendix A PDX collection 0861
+ M00.07 **Staphylococcal arthritis, ankle and foot**
Staphylococcal arthritis, tarsus, metatarsus and phalanges
M00.071 **Staphylococcal arthritis, right ankle and foot**
M00.072 **Staphylococcal arthritis, left ankle and foot**
CC M00.079 **Staphylococcal arthritis, unspecified ankle and foot**
CC Exclusion see Appendix A PDX collection 0862
CC M00.08 **Staphylococcal arthritis, vertebrae**
CC Exclusion see Appendix A PDX collection 0855
CC M00.09 **Staphylococcal polyarthritis**
CC Exclusion see Appendix A PDX collection 0855
+ M00.1 **Pneumococcal arthritis and polyarthritis**
CC M00.10 **Pneumococcal arthritis, unspecified joint**
CC Exclusion see Appendix A PDX collection 0855
+ M00.11 **Pneumococcal arthritis, shoulder**
CC M00.111 **Pneumococcal arthritis, right shoulder**
CC Exclusion see Appendix A PDX collection 0856
CC M00.112 **Pneumococcal arthritis, left shoulder**
CC Exclusion see Appendix A PDX collection 0856
CC M00.119 **Pneumococcal arthritis, unspecified shoulder**
CC Exclusion see Appendix A PDX collection 0856
+ M00.12 **Pneumococcal arthritis, elbow**
CC M00.121 **Pneumococcal arthritis, right elbow**
CC Exclusion see Appendix A PDX collection 0857
CC M00.122 **Pneumococcal arthritis, left elbow**
CC Exclusion see Appendix A PDX collection 0857
CC M00.129 **Pneumococcal arthritis, unspecified elbow**
CC Exclusion see Appendix A PDX collection 0857
+ M00.13 **Pneumococcal arthritis, wrist**
Pneumococcal arthritis of carpal bones
CC M00.131 **Pneumococcal arthritis, right wrist**
CC Exclusion see Appendix A PDX collection 0858
CC M00.132 **Pneumococcal arthritis, left wrist**
CC Exclusion see Appendix A PDX collection 0858
CC M00.139 **Pneumococcal arthritis, unspecified wrist**
CC Exclusion see Appendix A PDX collection 0858
+ M00.14 **Pneumococcal arthritis, hand**
Pneumococcal arthritis of metacarpus and phalanges
CC M00.141 **Pneumococcal arthritis, right hand**
CC Exclusion see Appendix A PDX collection 0859
CC M00.142 **Pneumococcal arthritis, left hand**
CC Exclusion see Appendix A PDX collection 0859
CC M00.149 **Pneumococcal arthritis, unspecified hand**
CC Exclusion see Appendix A PDX collection 0859
+ M00.15 **Pneumococcal arthritis, hip**
CC M00.151 **Pneumococcal arthritis, right hip**
CC Exclusion see Appendix A PDX collection 0860
CC M00.152 **Pneumococcal arthritis, left hip**
CC Exclusion see Appendix A PDX collection 0860
CC M00.159 **Pneumococcal arthritis, unspecified hip**
CC Exclusion see Appendix A PDX collection 0860
+ M00.16 **Pneumococcal arthritis, knee**
CC M00.161 **Pneumococcal arthritis, right knee**
CC Exclusion see Appendix A PDX collection 0861
CC M00.162 **Pneumococcal arthritis, left knee**
CC Exclusion see Appendix A PDX collection 0861
CC M00.169 **Pneumococcal arthritis, unspecified knee**
CC Exclusion see Appendix A PDX collection 0861
+ M00.17 **Pneumococcal arthritis, ankle and foot**
Pneumococcal arthritis, tarsus, metatarsus and phalanges
CC M00.171 **Pneumococcal arthritis, right ankle and foo**
CC Exclusion see Appendix A PDX collection 0862
CC M00.172 **Pneumococcal arthritis, left ankle and foo**
CC Exclusion see Appendix A PDX collection 0862
CC M00.179 **Pneumococcal arthritis, unspecified ankle and foot**
CC Exclusion see Appendix A PDX collection 0862
CC M00.18 **Pneumococcal arthritis, vertebrae**
CC Exclusion see Appendix A PDX collection 0855
CC M00.19 **Pneumococcal polyarthritis**
CC Exclusion see Appendix A PDX collection 0855
+ M00.2 **Other streptococcal arthritis and polyarthritis**
Use additional code (B95.0-B95.2, B95.4-B95.5) to identify bacterial agent
CC M00.20 **Other streptococcal arthritis, unspecified joint**
CC Exclusion see Appendix A PDX collection 0855
+ M00.21 **Other streptococcal arthritis, shoulder**
CC M00.211 **Other streptococcal arthritis, right shoulde**
CC Exclusion see Appendix A PDX collection 0856
CC M00.212 **Other streptococcal arthritis, left shoulder**
CC Exclusion see Appendix A PDX collection 0856
CC M00.219 **Other streptococcal arthritis, unspecified shoulder**
CC Exclusion see Appendix A PDX collection 0856
+ M00.22 **Other streptococcal arthritis, elbow**
CC M00.221 **Other streptococcal arthritis, right elbow**
CC Exclusion see Appendix A PDX collection 0857
CC M00.222 **Other streptococcal arthritis, left elbow**
CC Exclusion see Appendix A PDX collection 0857
CC M00.229 **Other streptococcal arthritis, unspecified elbow**
CC Exclusion see Appendix A PDX collection 0857
+ M00.23 **Other streptococcal arthritis, wrist**
Other streptococcal arthritis of carpal bones
CC M00.231 **Other streptococcal arthritis, right wrist**
CC Exclusion see Appendix A PDX collection 0858
CC M00.232 **Other streptococcal arthritis, left wrist**
CC Exclusion see Appendix A PDX collection 0858
CC M00.239 **Other streptococcal arthritis, unspecified wrist**
CC Exclusion see Appendix A PDX collection 0858
+ M00.24 **Other streptococcal arthritis, hand**
Other streptococcal arthritis metacarpus and phalange
CC M00.241 **Other streptococcal arthritis, right hand**
CC Exclusion see Appendix A PDX collection 0859
CC M00.242 **Other streptococcal arthritis, left hand**
CC Exclusion see Appendix A PDX collection 0859
CC M00.249 **Other streptococcal arthritis, unspecified hand**
CC Exclusion see Appendix A PDX collection 0859
+ M00.25 **Other streptococcal arthritis, hip**
CC M00.251 **Other streptococcal arthritis, right hip**
CC Exclusion see Appendix A PDX collection 0860

CC **M00.252 Other streptococcal arthritis, left hip**
CC Exclusion see Appendix A PDX collection 0860

CC **M00.259 Other streptococcal arthritis, unspecified hip**
CC Exclusion see Appendix A PDX collection 0860

+ **M00.26 Other streptococcal arthritis, knee**

CC **M00.261 Other streptococcal arthritis, right knee**
CC Exclusion see Appendix A PDX collection 0861

CC **M00.262 Other streptococcal arthritis, left knee**
CC Exclusion see Appendix A PDX collection 0861

CC **M00.269 Other streptococcal arthritis, unspecified knee**
CC Exclusion see Appendix A PDX collection 0861

+ **M00.27 Other streptococcal arthritis, ankle and foot**
Other streptococcal arthritis, tarsus, metatarsus and phalanges

CC **M00.271 Other streptococcal arthritis, right ankle and foot**
CC Exclusion see Appendix A PDX collection 0862

CC **M00.272 Other streptococcal arthritis, left ankle and foot**
CC Exclusion see Appendix A PDX collection 0862

CC **M00.279 Other streptococcal arthritis, unspecified ankle and foot**
CC Exclusion see Appendix A PDX collection 0862

CC **M00.28 Other streptococcal arthritis, vertebrae**
CC Exclusion see Appendix A PDX collection 0855

CC **M00.29 Other streptococcal polyarthritis**
CC Exclusion see Appendix A PDX collection 0855

+ **M00.8 Arthritis and polyarthritis due to other bacteria**
Use additional code (B96) to identify bacteria

CC **M00.80 Arthritis due to other bacteria, unspecified joint**
CC Exclusion see Appendix A PDX collection 0855

+ **M00.81 Arthritis due to other bacteria, shoulder**

CC **M00.811 Arthritis due to other bacteria, right shoulder**
CC Exclusion see Appendix A PDX collection 0856

CC **M00.812 Arthritis due to other bacteria, left shoulder**
CC Exclusion see Appendix A PDX collection 0856

CC **M00.819 Arthritis due to other bacteria, unspecified shoulder**
CC Exclusion see Appendix A PDX collection 0856

+ **M00.82 Arthritis due to other bacteria, elbow**

CC **M00.821 Arthritis due to other bacteria, right elbow**
CC Exclusion see Appendix A PDX collection 0857

CC **M00.822 Arthritis due to other bacteria, left elbow**
CC Exclusion see Appendix A PDX collection 0857

CC **M00.829 Arthritis due to other bacteria, unspecified elbow**
CC Exclusion see Appendix A PDX collection 0857

+ **M00.83 Arthritis due to other bacteria, wrist**
Arthritis due to other bacteria, carpal bones

CC **M00.831 Arthritis due to other bacteria, right wrist**
CC Exclusion see Appendix A PDX collection 0858

CC **M00.832 Arthritis due to other bacteria, left wrist**
CC Exclusion see Appendix A PDX collection 0858

CC **M00.839 Arthritis due to other bacteria, unspecified wrist**
CC Exclusion see Appendix A PDX collection 0858

+ **M00.84 Arthritis due to other bacteria, hand**
Arthritis due to other bacteria, metacarpus and phalanges

CC **M00.841 Arthritis due to other bacteria, right hand**
CC Exclusion see Appendix A PDX collection 0859

CC **M00.842 Arthritis due to other bacteria, left hand**
CC Exclusion see Appendix A PDX collection 0859

CC **M00.849 Arthritis due to other bacteria, unspecified hand**
CC Exclusion see Appendix A PDX collection 0859

+ **M00.85 Arthritis due to other bacteria, hip**

CC **M00.851 Arthritis due to other bacteria, right hip**
CC Exclusion see Appendix A PDX collection 0860

CC **M00.852 Arthritis due to other bacteria, left hip**
CC Exclusion see Appendix A PDX collection 0860

CC **M00.859 Arthritis due to other bacteria, unspecified hip**
CC Exclusion see Appendix A PDX collection 0860

+ **M00.86 Arthritis due to other bacteria, knee**

CC **M00.861 Arthritis due to other bacteria, right knee**
CC Exclusion see Appendix A PDX collection 0861

CC **M00.862 Arthritis due to other bacteria, left knee**
CC Exclusion see Appendix A PDX collection 0861

CC **M00.869 Arthritis due to other bacteria, unspecified knee**
CC Exclusion see Appendix A PDX collection 0861

+ **M00.87 Arthritis due to other bacteria, ankle and foot**
Arthritis due to other bacteria, tarsus, metatarsus, and phalanges

CC **M00.871 Arthritis due to other bacteria, right ankle and foot**
CC Exclusion see Appendix A PDX collection 0862

CC **M00.872 Arthritis due to other bacteria, left ankle and foot**
CC Exclusion see Appendix A PDX collection 0862

CC **M00.879 Arthritis due to other bacteria, unspecified ankle and foot**
CC Exclusion see Appendix A PDX collection 0862

CC **M00.88 Arthritis due to other bacteria, vertebrae**
CC Exclusion see Appendix A PDX collection 0855

CC **M00.89 Polyarthritis due to other bacteria**
CC Exclusion see Appendix A PDX collection 0855

CC **M00.9 Pyogenic arthritis, unspecified**
Infective arthritis NOS
CC Exclusion see Appendix A PDX collection 0855

M01 Direct infections of joint in infectious and parasitic diseases classified elsewhere

Code first underlying disease, such as:
leprosy [Hansen's disease] (A30.-)
mycoses (B35-B49)
O'nyong-nyong fever (A92.1)
paratyphoid fever (A01.1-A01.4)

Excludes1: *arthropathy in Lyme disease (A69.23)*
gonococcal arthritis (A54.42)
meningococcal arthritis (A39.83)
mumps arthritis (B26.85)
postinfective arthropathy (M02.-)
postmeningococcal arthritis (39.84)
reactive arthritis (M02.3)
rubella arthritis (B06.82)
sarcoidosis arthritis (D86.86)
tuberculosis arthritis (A18.01-A18.02)
typhoid fever arthritis (A01.04)

+ **M01.X Direct infection of joint in infectious and parasitic diseases classified elsewhere**

CC **M01.X0 Direct infection of unspecified joint in infectious and parasitic diseases classified elsewhere**
CC Exclusion see Appendix A PDX collection 0863

+ **M01.X1 Direct infection of shoulder joint in infectious and parasitic diseases classified elsewhere**

CC **M01.X11 Direct infection of right shoulder in infectious and parasitic diseases classified elsewhere**
CC Exclusion see Appendix A PDX collection 0864

CC **M01.X12 Direct infection of left shoulder in infectious and parasitic diseases classified elsewhere**
CC Exclusion see Appendix A PDX collection 0864

CC **M01.X19 Direct infection of unspecified shoulder in infectious and parasitic diseases classified elsewhere**
CC Exclusion see Appendix A PDX collection 0864

+ **M01.X2 Direct infection of elbow in infectious and parasitic diseases classified elsewhere**

CC **M01.X21 Direct infection of right elbow in infectious and parasitic diseases classified elsewhere**
CC Exclusion see Appendix A PDX collection 0863

CC **M01.X22 Direct infection of left elbow in infectious and parasitic diseases classified elsewhere**
CC Exclusion see Appendix A PDX collection 0863

CC **M01.X29 Direct infection of unspecified elbow in infectious and parasitic diseases classified elsewhere**
CC Exclusion see Appendix A PDX collection 0863

+ **M01.X3 Direct infection of wrist in infectious and parasitic diseases classified elsewhere**
Direct infection of carpal bones in infectious and parasitic diseases classified elsewhere

CC **M01.X31 Direct infection of right wrist in infectious and parasitic diseases classified elsewhere**
CC Exclusion see Appendix A PDX collection 0863

CC **M01.X32 Direct infection of left wrist in infectious and parasitic diseases classified elsewhere**
CC Exclusion see Appendix A PDX collection 0863

CC **M01.X39 Direct infection of unspecified wrist in infectious and parasitic diseases classified elsewhere**
CC Exclusion see Appendix A PDX collection 0863

+ **M01.X4 Direct infection of hand in infectious and parasitic diseases classified elsewhere**
Direct infection of metacarpus and phalanges in infectious and parasitic diseases classified elsewhere

CC **M01.X41 Direct infection of right hand in infectious and parasitic diseases classified elsewhere**
CC Exclusion see Appendix A PDX collection 0863

CC **M01.X42 Direct infection of left hand in infectious and parasitic diseases classified elsewhere**
CC Exclusion see Appendix A PDX collection 0863

CC **M01.X49 Direct infection of unspecified hand in infectious and parasitic diseases classified elsewhere**
CC Exclusion see Appendix A PDX collection 0863

+ **M01.X5 Direct infection of hip in infectious and parasitic diseases classified elsewhere**

CC **M01.X51 Direct infection of right hip in infectious and parasitic diseases classified elsewhere**
CC Exclusion see Appendix A PDX collection 0863

CC **M01.X52 Direct infection of left hip in infectious and parasitic diseases classified elsewhere**
CC Exclusion see Appendix A PDX collection 0863

CC **M01.X59 Direct infection of unspecified hip in infectious and parasitic diseases classified elsewhere**
CC Exclusion see Appendix A PDX collection 0863

+ **M01.X6 Direct infection of knee in infectious and parasitic diseases classified elsewhere**

CC **M01.X61 Direct infection of right knee in infectious and parasitic diseases classified elsewhere**
CC Exclusion see Appendix A PDX collection 0863

CC **M01.X62 Direct infection of left knee in infectious and parasitic diseases classified elsewhere**
CC Exclusion see Appendix A PDX collection 0863

CC **M01.X69 Direct infection of unspecified knee in infectious and parasitic diseases classified elsewhere**
CC Exclusion see Appendix A PDX collection 0863

+ **M01.X7 Direct infection of ankle and foot in infectious and parasitic diseases classified elsewhere**
Direct infection of tarsus, metatarsus and phalanges in infectious and parasitic diseases classified elsewhere

CC **M01.X71 Direct infection of right ankle and foot in infectious and parasitic diseases classified elsewhere**
CC Exclusion see Appendix A PDX collection 0863

CC **M01.X72 Direct infection of left ankle and foot in infectious and parasitic diseases classified elsewhere**
CC Exclusion see Appendix A PDX collection 0863

CC **M01.X79 Direct infection of unspecified ankle and foot in infectious and parasitic diseases classified elsewhere**
CC Exclusion see Appendix A PDX collection 0863

CC **M01.X8 Direct infection of vertebrae in infectious and parasitic diseases classified elsewhere**
CC Exclusion see Appendix A PDX collection 0863

CC **M01.X9 Direct infection of multiple joints in infectious and parasitic diseases classified elsewhere**
CC Exclusion see Appendix A PDX collection 0863

M02 Postinfective and reactive arthropathies

Code first underlying disease, such as:
congenital syphilis [Clutton's joints] (A50.5)
enteritis due to Yersinia enterocolitica (A04.6)
infective endocarditis (I33.0)
viral hepatitis (B15-B19)

Excludes1: *Behçet's disease (M35.2)*
direct infections of joint in infectious and parasitic diseases classified elsewhere (M01.-)
postmeningcoccal arthritis (A39.84)
mumps arthritis (B26.85)
rubella arthritis (B06.82)
syphilis arthritis (late) (A52.77)
rheumatic fever (I00)
tabetic arthropathy [Charcôt's] (A52.16)

+ **M02.0 Arthropathy following intestinal bypass**

M02.00 Arthropathy following intestinal bypass, unspecified site

+ **M02.01 Arthropathy following intestinal bypass, shoulder**

M02.011 Arthropathy following intestinal bypass, right shoulder

M02.012 Arthropathy following intestinal bypass, left shoulder

M02.019 Arthropathy following intestinal bypass, unspecified shoulder

+ **M02.02 Arthropathy following intestinal bypass, elbow**

M02.021 Arthropathy following intestinal bypass, right elbow

M02.022 Arthropathy following intestinal bypass, left elbow

M02.029 Arthropathy following intestinal bypass, unspecified elbow

+ **M02.03 Arthropathy following intestinal bypass, wrist**
Arthropathy following intestinal bypass, carpal bones

M02.031 Arthropathy following intestinal bypass, right wrist

M02.032 Arthropathy following intestinal bypass, left wrist

M02.039 Arthropathy following intestinal bypass, unspecified wrist

+ **M02.04 Arthropathy following intestinal bypass, hand**
Arthropathy following intestinal bypass, metacarpals and phalanges

M02.041 Arthropathy following intestinal bypass, right hand

M02.042 Arthropathy following intestinal bypass, left hand

M02.049 Arthropathy following intestinal bypass, unspecified hand

+ M02.05 Arthropathy following intestinal bypass, hip
M02.051 Arthropathy following intestinal bypass, right hip
M02.052 Arthropathy following intestinal bypass, left hip
M02.059 Arthropathy following intestinal bypass, unspecified hip
+ M02.06 Arthropathy following intestinal bypass, knee
M02.061 Arthropathy following intestinal bypass, right knee
M02.062 Arthropathy following intestinal bypass, left knee
M02.069 Arthropathy following intestinal bypass, unspecified knee
+ M02.07 Arthropathy following intestinal bypass, ankle and foot
Arthropathy following intestinal bypass, tarsus, metatarsus and phalanges
M02.071 Arthropathy following intestinal bypass, right ankle and foot
M02.072 Arthropathy following intestinal bypass, left ankle and foot
M02.079 Arthropathy following intestinal bypass, unspecified ankle and foot
M02.08 Arthropathy following intestinal bypass, vertebrae
M02.09 Arthropathy following intestinal bypass, multiple sites
+ M02.1 Postdysenteric arthropathy
CC M02.10 Postdysenteric arthropathy, unspecified site
CC Exclusion see Appendix A PDX collection 0863
+ M02.11 Postdysenteric arthropathy, shoulder
CC M02.111 Postdysenteric arthropathy, right shoulder
CC Exclusion see Appendix A PDX collection 0863
CC M02.112 Postdysenteric arthropathy, left shoulder
CC Exclusion see Appendix A PDX collection 0863
CC M02.119 Postdysenteric arthropathy, unspecified shoulder
CC Exclusion see Appendix A PDX collection 0863
+ M02.12 Postdysenteric arthropathy, elbow
CC M02.121 Postdysenteric arthropathy, right elbow
CC Exclusion see Appendix A PDX collection 0863
CC M02.122 Postdysenteric arthropathy, left elbow
CC Exclusion see Appendix A PDX collection 0863
CC M02.129 Postdysenteric arthropathy, unspecified elbow
CC Exclusion see Appendix A PDX collection 0863
+ M02.13 Postdysenteric arthropathy, wrist
Postdysenteric arthropathy, carpal bones
CC M02.131 Postdysenteric arthropathy, right wrist
CC Exclusion see Appendix A PDX collection 0863
CC M02.132 Postdysenteric arthropathy, left wrist
CC Exclusion see Appendix A PDX collection 0863
CC M02.139 Postdysenteric arthropathy, unspecified wrist
CC Exclusion see Appendix A PDX collection 0863
+ M02.14 Postdysenteric arthropathy, hand
Postdysenteric arthropathy, metacarpus and phalanges
CC M02.141 Postdysenteric arthropathy, right hand
CC Exclusion see Appendix A PDX collection 0863
CC M02.142 Postdysenteric arthropathy, left hand
CC Exclusion see Appendix A PDX collection 0863
CC M02.149 Postdysenteric arthropathy, unspecified hand
CC Exclusion see Appendix A PDX collection 0863
+ M02.15 Postdysenteric arthropathy, hip
CC M02.151 Postdysenteric arthropathy, right hip
CC Exclusion see Appendix A PDX collection 0863
CC M02.152 Postdysenteric arthropathy, left hip
CC Exclusion see Appendix A PDX collection 0863
CC M02.159 Postdysenteric arthropathy, unspecified hip
CC Exclusion see Appendix A PDX collection 0863
+ M02.16 Postdysenteric arthropathy, knee
CC M02.161 Postdysenteric arthropathy, right knee
CC Exclusion see Appendix A PDX collection 0865
CC M02.162 Postdysenteric arthropathy, left knee
CC Exclusion see Appendix A PDX collection 0865
CC M02.169 Postdysenteric arthropathy, unspecified knee
CC Exclusion see Appendix A PDX collection 0865
+ M02.17 Postdysenteric arthropathy, ankle and foot
Postdysenteric arthropathy, tarsus, metatarsus and phalanges
CC M02.171 Postdysenteric arthropathy, right ankle and foot
CC Exclusion see Appendix A PDX collection 0863
CC M02.172 Postdysenteric arthropathy, left ankle and foot
CC Exclusion see Appendix A PDX collection 0863
CC M02.179 Postdysenteric arthropathy, unspecified ankle and foot
CC Exclusion see Appendix A PDX collection 0863
CC M02.18 Postdysenteric arthropathy, vertebrae
CC Exclusion see Appendix A PDX collection 0866
CC M02.19 Postdysenteric arthropathy, multiple sites
CC Exclusion see Appendix A PDX collection 0863
+ M02.2 Postimmunization arthropathy
M02.20 Postimmunization arthropathy, unspecified site
+ M02.21 Postimmunization arthropathy, shoulder
M02.211 Postimmunization arthropathy, right shoulder
M02.212 Postimmunization arthropathy, left shoulder
M02.219 Postimmunization arthropathy, unspecified shoulder
+ M02.22 Postimmunization arthropathy, elbow
M02.221 Postimmunization arthropathy, right elbow
M02.222 Postimmunization arthropathy, left elbow
M02.229 Postimmunization arthropathy, unspecified elbow
+ M02.23 Postimmunization arthropathy, wrist
Postimmunization arthropathy, carpal bones
M02.231 Postimmunization arthropathy, right wrist
M02.232 Postimmunization arthropathy, left wrist
M02.239 Postimmunization arthropathy, unspecified wrist
+ M02.24 Postimmunization arthropathy, hand
Postimmunization arthropathy, metacarpus and phalanges
M02.241 Postimmunization arthropathy, right hand
M02.242 Postimmunization arthropathy, left hand
M02.249 Postimmunization arthropathy, unspecified hand
+ M02.25 Postimmunization arthropathy, hip
M02.251 Postimmunization arthropathy, right hip
M02.252 Postimmunization arthropathy, left hip
M02.259 Postimmunization arthropathy, unspecified hip
+ M02.26 Postimmunization arthropathy, knee
M02.261 Postimmunization arthropathy, right knee
M02.262 Postimmunization arthropathy, left knee
M02.269 Postimmunization arthropathy, unspecified knee
+ M02.27 Postimmunization arthropathy, ankle and foot
Postimmunization arthropathy, tarsus, metatarsus and phalanges
M02.271 Postimmunization arthropathy, right ankle and foot
M02.272 Postimmunization arthropathy, left ankle and foot
M02.279 Postimmunization arthropathy, unspecified ankle and foot
M02.28 Postimmunization arthropathy, vertebrae
M02.29 Postimmunization arthropathy, multiple sites

+ **M02.3 Reiter's disease**
Reactive arthritis
CC **M02.30 Reiter's disease, unspecified site**
CC Exclusion see Appendix A PDX collection 0863
+ **M02.31 Reiter's disease, shoulder**
CC **M02.311 Reiter's disease, right shoulder**
CC Exclusion see Appendix A PDX collection 0863
CC **M02.312 Reiter's disease, left shoulder**
CC Exclusion see Appendix A PDX collection 0863
CC **M02.319 Reiter's disease, unspecified shoulder**
CC Exclusion see Appendix A PDX collection 0863
+ **M02.32 Reiter's disease, elbow**
CC **M02.321 Reiter's disease, right elbow**
CC Exclusion see Appendix A PDX collection 0863
CC **M02.322 Reiter's disease, left elbow**
CC Exclusion see Appendix A PDX collection 0863
CC **M02.329 Reiter's disease, unspecified elbow**
CC Exclusion see Appendix A PDX collection 0863
+ **M02.33 Reiter's disease, wrist**
Reiter's disease, carpal bones
CC **M02.331 Reiter's disease, right wrist**
CC Exclusion see Appendix A PDX collection 0863
CC **M02.332 Reiter's disease, left wrist**
CC Exclusion see Appendix A PDX collection 0863
CC **M02.339 Reiter's disease, unspecified wrist**
CC Exclusion see Appendix A PDX collection 0863
+ **M02.34 Reiter's disease, hand**
Reiter's disease, metacarpus and phalanges
CC **M02.341 Reiter's disease, right hand**
CC Exclusion see Appendix A PDX collection 0863
CC **M02.342 Reiter's disease, left hand**
CC Exclusion see Appendix A PDX collection 0863
CC **M02.349 Reiter's disease, unspecified hand**
CC Exclusion see Appendix A PDX collection 0863
+ **M02.35 Reiter's disease, hip**
CC **M02.351 Reiter's disease, right hip**
CC Exclusion see Appendix A PDX collection 0863
CC **M02.352 Reiter's disease, left hip**
CC Exclusion see Appendix A PDX collection 0863
CC **M02.359 Reiter's disease, unspecified hip**
CC Exclusion see Appendix A PDX collection 0863
+ **M02.36 Reiter's disease, knee**
CC **M02.361 Reiter's disease, right knee**
CC Exclusion see Appendix A PDX collection 0863
CC **M02.362 Reiter's disease, left knee**
CC Exclusion see Appendix A PDX collection 0863
CC **M02.369 Reiter's disease, unspecified knee**
CC Exclusion see Appendix A PDX collection 0863
+ **M02.37 Reiter's disease, ankle and foot**
Reiter's disease, tarsus, metatarsus and phalanges
CC **M02.371 Reiter's disease, right ankle and foot**
CC Exclusion see Appendix A PDX collection 0863
CC **M02.372 Reiter's disease, left ankle and foot**
CC Exclusion see Appendix A PDX collection 0863
CC **M02.379 Reiter's disease, unspecified ankle and foot**
CC Exclusion see Appendix A PDX collection 0863
CC **M02.38 Reiter's disease, vertebrae**
CC Exclusion see Appendix A PDX collection 0863
CC **M02.39 Reiter's disease, multiple sites**
CC Exclusion see Appendix A PDX collection 0863
+ **M02.8 Other reactive arthropathies**
CC **M02.80 Other reactive arthropathies, unspecified site**
CC Exclusion see Appendix A PDX collection 0863
+ **M02.81 Other reactive arthropathies, shoulder**
CC **M02.811 Other reactive arthropathies, right should**
CC Exclusion see Appendix A PDX collection 0864
CC **M02.812 Other reactive arthropathies, left should**
CC Exclusion see Appendix A PDX collection 0864
CC **M02.819 Other reactive arthropathies, unspecified shoulder**
CC Exclusion see Appendix A PDX collection 0864
+ **M02.82 Other reactive arthropathies, elbow**
CC **M02.821 Other reactive arthropathies, right elbow**
CC Exclusion see Appendix A PDX collection 0863
CC **M02.822 Other reactive arthropathies, left elbow**
CC Exclusion see Appendix A PDX collection 0863
CC **M02.829 Other reactive arthropathies, unspecified elbow**
CC Exclusion see Appendix A PDX collection 0863
+ **M02.83 Other reactive arthropathies, wrist**
Other reactive arthropathies, carpal bones
CC **M02.831 Other reactive arthropathies, right wrist**
CC Exclusion see Appendix A PDX collection 0863
CC **M02.832 Other reactive arthropathies, left wrist**
CC Exclusion see Appendix A PDX collection 0863
CC **M02.839 Other reactive arthropathies, unspecified wrist**
CC Exclusion see Appendix A PDX collection 0863
+ **M02.84 Other reactive arthropathies, hand**
Other reactive arthropathies, metacarpus and phalan
CC **M02.841 Other reactive arthropathies, right hand**
CC Exclusion see Appendix A PDX collection 0863
CC **M02.842 Other reactive arthropathies, left hand**
CC Exclusion see Appendix A PDX collection 0863
CC **M02.849 Other reactive arthropathies, unspecified hand**
CC Exclusion see Appendix A PDX collection 0863
+ **M02.85 Other reactive arthropathies, hip**
CC **M02.851 Other reactive arthropathies, right hip**
CC Exclusion see Appendix A PDX collection 0863
CC **M02.852 Other reactive arthropathies, left hip**
CC Exclusion see Appendix A PDX collection 0863
CC **M02.859 Other reactive arthropathies, unspecified h**
CC Exclusion see Appendix A PDX collection 0863
+ **M02.86 Other reactive arthropathies, knee**
CC **M02.861 Other reactive arthropathies, right knee**
CC Exclusion see Appendix A PDX collection 0863
CC **M02.862 Other reactive arthropathies, left knee**
CC Exclusion see Appendix A PDX collection 0863
CC **M02.869 Other reactive arthropathies, unspecified knee**
CC Exclusion see Appendix A PDX collection 0863
+ **M02.87 Other reactive arthropathies, ankle and foot**
Other reactive arthropathies, tarsus, metatarsus and phalanges
CC **M02.871 Other reactive arthropathies, right ankle and foot**
CC Exclusion see Appendix A PDX collection 0863
CC **M02.872 Other reactive arthropathies, left ankle and foot**
CC Exclusion see Appendix A PDX collection 0863
CC **M02.879 Other reactive arthropathies, unspecified ankle and foot**
CC Exclusion see Appendix A PDX collection 08
CC **M02.88 Other reactive arthropathies, vertebrae**
CC Exclusion see Appendix A PDX collection 0863
CC **M02.89 Other reactive arthropathies, multiple sites**
CC Exclusion see Appendix A PDX collection 0863
M02.9 Reactive arthropathy, unspecified

utoinflammatory syndromes (M04)

M04 Autoinflammatory syndromes

Excludes2: Crohn's disease (K50.-)
AHA CC: 4Q, 2016, 37

M04.1 Periodic fever syndromes
Familial Mediterranean fever
Hyperimmunoglobin D syndrome
Mevalonate kinase deficiency
Tumor necrosis factor receptor associated periodic syndrome [TRAPS]

M04.2 Cryopyrin-associated periodic syndromes
Chronic infantile neurological, cutaneous and articular syndrome [CINCA]
Familial cold autoinflammatory syndrome
Familial cold urticaria
Muckle-Wells syndrome
Neonatal onset multisystemic inflammatory disorder [NOMID]

M04.8 Other autoinflammatory syndromes
Blau syndrome
Deficiency of interleukin 1 receptor antagonist [DIRA]
Majeed syndrome
Periodic fever, aphthous stomatitis, pharyngitis, and adenopathy syndrome [PFAPA]
Pyogenic arthritis, pyoderma gangrenosum, and acne syndrome [PAPA]

M04.9 Autoinflammatory syndrome, unspecified

nflammatory polyarthropathies (M05-M14)

M05 Rheumatoid arthritis with rheumatoid factor

Excludes1: rheumatic fever (I00)
juvenile rheumatoid arthritis (M08.-)
rheumatoid arthritis of spine (M45.-)

+ **M05.0 Felty's syndrome**
Rheumatoid arthritis with splenoadenomegaly and leukopenia
M05.00 Felty's syndrome, unspecified site
+ **M05.01 Felty's syndrome, shoulder**
M05.011 Felty's syndrome, right shoulder
M05.012 Felty's syndrome, left shoulder
M05.019 Felty's syndrome, unspecified shoulder
+ **M05.02 Felty's syndrome, elbow**
M05.021 Felty's syndrome, right elbow
M05.022 Felty's syndrome, left elbow
M05.029 Felty's syndrome, unspecified elbow
+ **M05.03 Felty's syndrome, wrist**
Felty's syndrome, carpal bones
M05.031 Felty's syndrome, right wrist
M05.032 Felty's syndrome, left wrist
M05.039 Felty's syndrome, unspecified wrist
+ **M05.04 Felty's syndrome, hand**
Felty's syndrome, metacarpus and phalanges
M05.041 Felty's syndrome, right hand
M05.042 Felty's syndrome, left hand
M05.049 Felty's syndrome, unspecified hand
+ **M05.05 Felty's syndrome, hip**
M05.051 Felty's syndrome, right hip
M05.052 Felty's syndrome, left hip
M05.059 Felty's syndrome, unspecified hip
+ **M05.06 Felty's syndrome, knee**
M05.061 Felty's syndrome, right knee
M05.062 Felty's syndrome, left knee
M05.069 Felty's syndrome, unspecified knee
+ **M05.07 Felty's syndrome, ankle and foot**
Felty's syndrome, tarsus, metatarsus and phalanges
M05.071 Felty's syndrome, right ankle and foot
M05.072 Felty's syndrome, left ankle and foot
M05.079 Felty's syndrome, unspecified ankle and foot
M05.09 Felty's syndrome, multiple sites
+ **M05.1 Rheumatoid lung disease with rheumatoid arthritis**
M05.10 Rheumatoid lung disease with rheumatoid arthritis of unspecified site
+ **M05.11 Rheumatoid lung disease with rheumatoid arthritis of shoulder**
M05.111 Rheumatoid lung disease with rheumatoid arthritis of right shoulder
M05.112 Rheumatoid lung disease with rheumatoid arthritis of left shoulder
M05.119 Rheumatoid lung disease with rheumatoid arthritis of unspecified shoulder
+ **M05.12 Rheumatoid lung disease with rheumatoid arthritis of elbow**
M05.121 Rheumatoid lung disease with rheumatoid arthritis of right elbow
M05.122 Rheumatoid lung disease with rheumatoid arthritis of left elbow
M05.129 Rheumatoid lung disease with rheumatoid arthritis of unspecified elbow
+ **M05.13 Rheumatoid lung disease with rheumatoid arthritis of wrist**
Rheumatoid lung disease with rheumatoid arthritis, carpal bones
M05.131 Rheumatoid lung disease with rheumatoid arthritis of right wrist
M05.132 Rheumatoid lung disease with rheumatoid arthritis of left wrist
M05.139 Rheumatoid lung disease with rheumatoid arthritis of unspecified wrist
+ **M05.14 Rheumatoid lung disease with rheumatoid arthritis of hand**
Rheumatoid lung disease with rheumatoid arthritis, metacarpus and phalanges
M05.141 Rheumatoid lung disease with rheumatoid arthritis of right hand
M05.142 Rheumatoid lung disease with rheumatoid arthritis of left hand
M05.149 Rheumatoid lung disease with rheumatoid arthritis of unspecified hand
+ **M05.15 Rheumatoid lung disease with rheumatoid arthritis of hip**
M05.151 Rheumatoid lung disease with rheumatoid arthritis of right hip
M05.152 Rheumatoid lung disease with rheumatoid arthritis of left hip
M05.159 Rheumatoid lung disease with rheumatoid arthritis of unspecified hip
+ **M05.16 Rheumatoid lung disease with rheumatoid arthritis of knee**
M05.161 Rheumatoid lung disease with rheumatoid arthritis of right knee
M05.162 Rheumatoid lung disease with rheumatoid arthritis of left knee
M05.169 Rheumatoid lung disease with rheumatoid arthritis of unspecified knee
+ **M05.17 Rheumatoid lung disease with rheumatoid arthritis of ankle and foot**
Rheumatoid lung disease with rheumatoid arthritis, tarsus, metatarsus and phalanges
M05.171 Rheumatoid lung disease with rheumatoid arthritis of right ankle and foot
M05.172 Rheumatoid lung disease with rheumatoid arthritis of left ankle and foot
M05.179 Rheumatoid lung disease with rheumatoid arthritis of unspecified ankle and foot
M05.19 Rheumatoid lung disease with rheumatoid arthritis of multiple sites
+ **M05.2 Rheumatoid vasculitis with rheumatoid arthritis**
M05.20 Rheumatoid vasculitis with rheumatoid arthritis of unspecified site
+ **M05.21 Rheumatoid vasculitis with rheumatoid arthritis of shoulder**
M05.211 Rheumatoid vasculitis with rheumatoid arthritis of right shoulder
M05.212 Rheumatoid vasculitis with rheumatoid arthritis of left shoulder
M05.219 Rheumatoid vasculitis with rheumatoid arthritis of unspecified shoulder
+ **M05.22 Rheumatoid vasculitis with rheumatoid arthritis of elbow**
M05.221 Rheumatoid vasculitis with rheumatoid arthritis of right elbow
M05.222 Rheumatoid vasculitis with rheumatoid arthritis of left elbow
M05.229 Rheumatoid vasculitis with rheumatoid arthritis of unspecified elbow

+ **M05.23 Rheumatoid vasculitis with rheumatoid arthritis of wrist**
  Rheumatoid vasculitis with rheumatoid arthritis, carpal bones
  - **M05.231 Rheumatoid vasculitis with rheumatoid arthritis of right wrist**
  - **M05.232 Rheumatoid vasculitis with rheumatoid arthritis of left wrist**
  - **M05.239 Rheumatoid vasculitis with rheumatoid arthritis of unspecified wrist**

+ **M05.24 Rheumatoid vasculitis with rheumatoid arthritis of hand**
  Rheumatoid vasculitis with rheumatoid arthritis, metacarpus and phalanges
  - **M05.241 Rheumatoid vasculitis with rheumatoid arthritis of right hand**
  - **M05.242 Rheumatoid vasculitis with rheumatoid arthritis of left hand**
  - **M05.249 Rheumatoid vasculitis with rheumatoid arthritis of unspecified hand**

+ **M05.25 Rheumatoid vasculitis with rheumatoid arthritis of hip**
  - **M05.251 Rheumatoid vasculitis with rheumatoid arthritis of right hip**
  - **M05.252 Rheumatoid vasculitis with rheumatoid arthritis of left hip**
  - **M05.259 Rheumatoid vasculitis with rheumatoid arthritis of unspecified hip**

+ **M05.26 Rheumatoid vasculitis with rheumatoid arthritis of knee**
  - **M05.261 Rheumatoid vasculitis with rheumatoid arthritis of right knee**
  - **M05.262 Rheumatoid vasculitis with rheumatoid arthritis of left knee**
  - **M05.269 Rheumatoid vasculitis with rheumatoid arthritis of unspecified knee**

+ **M05.27 Rheumatoid vasculitis with rheumatoid arthritis of ankle and foot**
  Rheumatoid vasculitis with rheumatoid arthritis, tarsus, metatarsus and phalanges
  - **M05.271 Rheumatoid vasculitis with rheumatoid arthritis of right ankle and foot**
  - **M05.272 Rheumatoid vasculitis with rheumatoid arthritis of left ankle and foot**
  - **M05.279 Rheumatoid vasculitis with rheumatoid arthritis of unspecified ankle and foot**

M05.29 Rheumatoid vasculitis with rheumatoid arthritis of multiple sites

+ **M05.3 Rheumatoid heart disease with rheumatoid arthritis**
  Rheumatoid carditis
  Rheumatoid endocarditis
  Rheumatoid myocarditis
  Rheumatoid pericarditis

M05.30 Rheumatoid heart disease with rheumatoid arthritis of unspecified site

+ **M05.31 Rheumatoid heart disease with rheumatoid arthritis of shoulder**
  - **M05.311 Rheumatoid heart disease with rheumatoid arthritis of right shoulder**
  - **M05.312 Rheumatoid heart disease with rheumatoid arthritis of left shoulder**
  - **M05.319 Rheumatoid heart disease with rheumatoid arthritis of unspecified shoulder**

+ **M05.32 Rheumatoid heart disease with rheumatoid arthritis of elbow**
  - **M05.321 Rheumatoid heart disease with rheumatoid arthritis of right elbow**
  - **M05.322 Rheumatoid heart disease with rheumatoid arthritis of left elbow**
  - **M05.329 Rheumatoid heart disease with rheumatoid arthritis of unspecified elbow**

+ **M05.33 Rheumatoid heart disease with rheumatoid arthritis of wrist**
  Rheumatoid heart disease with rheumatoid arthritis, carpal bones
  - **M05.331 Rheumatoid heart disease with rheumatoid arthritis of right wrist**
  - **M05.332 Rheumatoid heart disease with rheumatoid arthritis of left wrist**
  - **M05.339 Rheumatoid heart disease with rheumatoid arthritis of unspecified wrist**

+ **M05.34 Rheumatoid heart disease with rheumatoid arthriti of hand**
  Rheumatoid heart disease with rheumatoid arthritis, metacarpus and phalanges
  - **M05.341 Rheumatoid heart disease with rheumato arthritis of right hand**
  - **M05.342 Rheumatoid heart disease with rheumato arthritis of left hand**
  - **M05.349 Rheumatoid heart disease with rheumato arthritis of unspecified hand**

+ **M05.35 Rheumatoid heart disease with rheumatoid arthriti of hip**
  - **M05.351 Rheumatoid heart disease with rheumato arthritis of right hip**
  - **M05.352 Rheumatoid heart disease with rheumato arthritis of left hip**
  - **M05.359 Rheumatoid heart disease with rheumato arthritis of unspecified hip**

+ **M05.36 Rheumatoid heart disease with rheumatoid arthriti of knee**
  - **M05.361 Rheumatoid heart disease with rheumato arthritis of right knee**
  - **M05.362 Rheumatoid heart disease with rheumato arthritis of left knee**
  - **M05.369 Rheumatoid heart disease with rheumato arthritis of unspecified knee**

+ **M05.37 Rheumatoid heart disease with rheumatoid arthriti of ankle and foot**
  Rheumatoid heart disease with rheumatoid arthritis, tarsus, metatarsus and phalanges
  - **M05.371 Rheumatoid heart disease with rheumato arthritis of right ankle and foot**
  - **M05.372 Rheumatoid heart disease with rheumato arthritis of left ankle and foot**
  - **M05.379 Rheumatoid heart disease with rheumato arthritis of unspecified ankle and foot**

M05.39 Rheumatoid heart disease with rheumatoid arthriti of multiple sites

+ **M05.4 Rheumatoid myopathy with rheumatoid arthritis**

CC **M05.40 Rheumatoid myopathy with rheumatoid arthritis o unspecified site**
  CC Exclusion see Appendix A PDX collection 0867

+ **M05.41 Rheumatoid myopathy with rheumatoid arthritis of shoulder**
  - CC **M05.411 Rheumatoid myopathy with rheumatoid arthritis of right shoulder**
    CC Exclusion see Appendix A PDX collection 08
  - CC **M05.412 Rheumatoid myopathy with rheumatoid arthritis of left shoulder**
    CC Exclusion see Appendix A PDX collection 08
  - CC **M05.419 Rheumatoid myopathy with rheumatoid arthritis of unspecified shoulder**
    CC Exclusion see Appendix A PDX collection 0867

+ **M05.42 Rheumatoid myopathy with rheumatoid arthritis of elbow**
  - CC **M05.421 Rheumatoid myopathy with rheumatoid arthritis of right elbow**
    CC Exclusion see Appendix A PDX collection 0867
  - CC **M05.422 Rheumatoid myopathy with rheumatoid arthritis of left elbow**
    CC Exclusion see Appendix A PDX collection 0867
  - CC **M05.429 Rheumatoid myopathy with rheumatoid arthritis of unspecified elbow**
    CC Exclusion see Appendix A PDX collection 0867

+ **M05.43 Rheumatoid myopathy with rheumatoid arthritis of wrist**
  Rheumatoid myopathy with rheumatoid arthritis, carpal bones
  - CC **M05.431 Rheumatoid myopathy with rheumatoid arthritis of right wrist**
    CC Exclusion see Appendix A PDX collection 0867
  - CC **M05.432 Rheumatoid myopathy with rheumatoid arthritis of left wrist**
    CC Exclusion see Appendix A PDX collection 0867

CC M05.439 Rheumatoid myopathy with rheumatoid arthritis of unspecified wrist
CC Exclusion see Appendix A PDX collection 0867

+ M05.44 Rheumatoid myopathy with rheumatoid arthritis of hand
Rheumatoid myopathy with rheumatoid arthritis, metacarpus and phalanges

CC M05.441 Rheumatoid myopathy with rheumatoid arthritis of right hand
CC Exclusion see Appendix A PDX collection 0867

CC M05.442 Rheumatoid myopathy with rheumatoid arthritis of left hand
CC Exclusion see Appendix A PDX collection 0867

CC M05.449 Rheumatoid myopathy with rheumatoid arthritis of unspecified hand
CC Exclusion see Appendix A PDX collection 0867

+ M05.45 Rheumatoid myopathy with rheumatoid arthritis of hip

CC M05.451 Rheumatoid myopathy with rheumatoid arthritis of right hip
CC Exclusion see Appendix A PDX collection 0867

CC M05.452 Rheumatoid myopathy with rheumatoid arthritis of left hip
CC Exclusion see Appendix A PDX collection 0867

CC M05.459 Rheumatoid myopathy with rheumatoid arthritis of unspecified hip
CC Exclusion see Appendix A PDX collection 0867

+ M05.46 Rheumatoid myopathy with rheumatoid arthritis of knee

CC M05.461 Rheumatoid myopathy with rheumatoid arthritis of right knee
CC Exclusion see Appendix A PDX collection 0867

CC M05.462 Rheumatoid myopathy with rheumatoid arthritis of left knee
CC Exclusion see Appendix A PDX collection 0867

CC M05.469 Rheumatoid myopathy with rheumatoid arthritis of unspecified knee
CC Exclusion see Appendix A PDX collection 0867

+ M05.47 Rheumatoid myopathy with rheumatoid arthritis of ankle and foot
Rheumatoid myopathy with rheumatoid arthritis, tarsus, metatarsus and phalanges

CC M05.471 Rheumatoid myopathy with rheumatoid arthritis of right ankle and foot
CC Exclusion see Appendix A PDX collection 0867

CC M05.472 Rheumatoid myopathy with rheumatoid arthritis of left ankle and foot
CC Exclusion see Appendix A PDX collection 0867

CC M05.479 Rheumatoid myopathy with rheumatoid arthritis of unspecified ankle and foot
CC Exclusion see Appendix A PDX collection 0867

CC M05.49 Rheumatoid myopathy with rheumatoid arthritis of multiple sites
CC Exclusion see Appendix A PDX collection 0867

+ M05.5 Rheumatoid polyneuropathy with rheumatoid arthritis

M05.50 Rheumatoid polyneuropathy with rheumatoid arthritis of unspecified site

+ M05.51 Rheumatoid polyneuropathy with rheumatoid arthritis of shoulder

M05.511 Rheumatoid polyneuropathy with rheumatoid arthritis of right shoulder

M05.512 Rheumatoid polyneuropathy with rheumatoid arthritis of left shoulder

M05.519 Rheumatoid polyneuropathy with rheumatoid arthritis of unspecified shoulder

+ M05.52 Rheumatoid polyneuropathy with rheumatoid arthritis of elbow

M05.521 Rheumatoid polyneuropathy with rheumatoid arthritis of right elbow

M05.522 Rheumatoid polyneuropathy with rheumatoid arthritis of left elbow

M05.529 Rheumatoid polyneuropathy with rheumatoid arthritis of unspecified elbow

+ M05.53 Rheumatoid polyneuropathy with rheumatoid arthritis of wrist
Rheumatoid polyneuropathy with rheumatoid arthritis, carpal bones

M05.531 Rheumatoid polyneuropathy with rheumatoid arthritis of right wrist

M05.532 Rheumatoid polyneuropathy with rheumatoid arthritis of left wrist

M05.539 Rheumatoid polyneuropathy with rheumatoid arthritis of unspecified wrist

+ M05.54 Rheumatoid polyneuropathy with rheumatoid arthritis of hand
Rheumatoid polyneuropathy with rheumatoid arthritis, metacarpus and phalanges

M05.541 Rheumatoid polyneuropathy with rheumatoid arthritis of right hand

M05.542 Rheumatoid polyneuropathy with rheumatoid arthritis of left hand

M05.549 Rheumatoid polyneuropathy with rheumatoid arthritis of unspecified hand

+ M05.55 Rheumatoid polyneuropathy with rheumatoid arthritis of hip

M05.551 Rheumatoid polyneuropathy with rheumatoid arthritis of right hip

M05.552 Rheumatoid polyneuropathy with rheumatoid arthritis of left hip

M05.559 Rheumatoid polyneuropathy with rheumatoid arthritis of unspecified hip

+ M05.56 Rheumatoid polyneuropathy with rheumatoid arthritis of knee

M05.561 Rheumatoid polyneuropathy with rheumatoid arthritis of right knee

M05.562 Rheumatoid polyneuropathy with rheumatoid arthritis of left knee

M05.569 Rheumatoid polyneuropathy with rheumatoid arthritis of unspecified knee

+ M05.57 Rheumatoid polyneuropathy with rheumatoid arthritis of ankle and foot
Rheumatoid polyneuropathy with rheumatoid arthritis, tarsus, metatarsus and phalanges

M05.571 Rheumatoid polyneuropathy with rheumatoid arthritis of right ankle and foot

M05.572 Rheumatoid polyneuropathy with rheumatoid arthritis of left ankle and foot

M05.579 Rheumatoid polyneuropathy with rheumatoid arthritis of unspecified ankle and foot

M05.59 Rheumatoid polyneuropathy with rheumatoid arthritis of multiple sites

+ M05.6 Rheumatoid arthritis with involvement of other organs and systems

M05.60 Rheumatoid arthritis of unspecified site with involvement of other organs and systems

+ M05.61 Rheumatoid arthritis of shoulder with involvement of other organs and systems

M05.611 Rheumatoid arthritis of right shoulder with involvement of other organs and systems

M05.612 Rheumatoid arthritis of left shoulder with involvement of other organs and systems

M05.619 Rheumatoid arthritis of unspecified shoulder with involvement of other organs and systems

+ M05.62 Rheumatoid arthritis of elbow with involvement of other organs and systems

M05.621 Rheumatoid arthritis of right elbow with involvement of other organs and systems

M05.622 Rheumatoid arthritis of left elbow with involvement of other organs and systems

M05.629 Rheumatoid arthritis of unspecified elbow with involvement of other organs and systems

+ M05.63 Rheumatoid arthritis of wrist with involvement of other organs and systems
Rheumatoid arthritis of carpal bones with involvement of other organs and systems

M05.631 Rheumatoid arthritis of right wrist with involvement of other organs and systems

M05.632 **Rheumatoid arthritis of left wrist with involvement of other organs and systems**

M05.639 **Rheumatoid arthritis of unspecified wrist with involvement of other organs and systems**

+ M05.64 **Rheumatoid arthritis of hand with involvement of other organs and systems**

Rheumatoid arthritis of metacarpus and phalanges with involvement of other organs and systems

M05.641 **Rheumatoid arthritis of right hand with involvement of other organs and systems**

M05.642 **Rheumatoid arthritis of left hand with involvement of other organs and systems**

M05.649 **Rheumatoid arthritis of unspecified hand with involvement of other organs and systems**

+ M05.65 **Rheumatoid arthritis of hip with involvement of other organs and systems**

M05.651 **Rheumatoid arthritis of right hip with involvement of other organs and systems**

M05.652 **Rheumatoid arthritis of left hip with involvement of other organs and systems**

M05.659 **Rheumatoid arthritis of unspecified hip with involvement of other organs and systems**

+ M05.66 **Rheumatoid arthritis of knee with involvement of other organs and systems**

M05.661 **Rheumatoid arthritis of right knee with involvement of other organs and systems**

M05.662 **Rheumatoid arthritis of left knee with involvement of other organs and systems**

M05.669 **Rheumatoid arthritis of unspecified knee with involvement of other organs and systems**

+ M05.67 **Rheumatoid arthritis of ankle and foot with involvement of other organs and systems**

Rheumatoid arthritis of tarsus, metatarsus and phalanges with involvement of other organs and systems

M05.671 **Rheumatoid arthritis of right ankle and foot with involvement of other organs and systems**

M05.672 **Rheumatoid arthritis of left ankle and foot with involvement of other organs and systems**

M05.679 **Rheumatoid arthritis of unspecified ankle and foot with involvement of other organs and systems**

M05.69 **Rheumatoid arthritis of multiple sites with involvement of other organs and systems**

+ M05.7 **Rheumatoid arthritis with rheumatoid factor without organ or systems involvement**

M05.70 **Rheumatoid arthritis with rheumatoid factor of unspecified site without organ or systems involvement**

+ M05.71 **Rheumatoid arthritis with rheumatoid factor of shoulder without organ or systems involvement**

M05.711 **Rheumatoid arthritis with rheumatoid factor of right shoulder without organ or systems involvement**

M05.712 **Rheumatoid arthritis with rheumatoid factor of left shoulder without organ or systems involvement**

M05.719 **Rheumatoid arthritis with rheumatoid factor of unspecified shoulder without organ or systems involvement**

+ M05.72 **Rheumatoid arthritis with rheumatoid factor of elbow without organ or systems involvement**

M05.721 **Rheumatoid arthritis with rheumatoid factor of right elbow without organ or systems involvement**

M05.722 **Rheumatoid arthritis with rheumatoid factor of left elbow without organ or systems involvement**

M05.729 **Rheumatoid arthritis with rheumatoid factor of unspecified elbow without organ or systems involvement**

+ M05.73 **Rheumatoid arthritis with rheumatoid factor of wrist without organ or systems involvement**

M05.731 **Rheumatoid arthritis with rheumatoid factor of right wrist without organ or systems involvement**

M05.732 **Rheumatoid arthritis with rheumatoid factor of left wrist without organ or systems involvement**

M05.739 **Rheumatoid arthritis with rheumatoid factor of unspecified wrist without organ or systems involvement**

+ M05.74 **Rheumatoid arthritis with rheumatoid factor of hand without organ or systems involvement**

M05.741 **Rheumatoid arthritis with rheumatoid factor of right hand without organ or systems involvement**

M05.742 **Rheumatoid arthritis with rheumatoid factor of left hand without organ or systems involvement**

M05.749 **Rheumatoid arthritis with rheumatoid factor of unspecified hand without organ or systems involvement**

+ M05.75 **Rheumatoid arthritis with rheumatoid factor of hip without organ or systems involvement**

M05.751 **Rheumatoid arthritis with rheumatoid factor of right hip without organ or systems involvement**

M05.752 **Rheumatoid arthritis with rheumatoid factor of left hip without organ or systems involvement**

M05.759 **Rheumatoid arthritis with rheumatoid factor of unspecified hip without organ or systems involvement**

+ M05.76 **Rheumatoid arthritis with rheumatoid factor of knee without organ or systems involvement**

M05.761 **Rheumatoid arthritis with rheumatoid factor of right knee without organ or systems involvement**

M05.762 **Rheumatoid arthritis with rheumatoid factor of left knee without organ or systems involvement**

M05.769 **Rheumatoid arthritis with rheumatoid factor of unspecified knee without organ or systems involvement**

+ M05.77 **Rheumatoid arthritis with rheumatoid factor of ankle and foot without organ or systems involvement**

M05.771 **Rheumatoid arthritis with rheumatoid factor of right ankle and foot without organ or systems involvement**

M05.772 **Rheumatoid arthritis with rheumatoid factor of left ankle and foot without organ or systems involvement**

M05.779 **Rheumatoid arthritis with rheumatoid factor of unspecified ankle and foot without organ or systems involvement**

M05.79 **Rheumatoid arthritis with rheumatoid factor of multiple sites without organ or systems involvement**

+ M05.8 **Other rheumatoid arthritis with rheumatoid factor**

M05.80 **Other rheumatoid arthritis with rheumatoid factor of unspecified site**

+ M05.81 **Other rheumatoid arthritis with rheumatoid factor of shoulder**

M05.811 **Other rheumatoid arthritis with rheumatoid factor of right shoulder**

M05.812 **Other rheumatoid arthritis with rheumatoid factor of left shoulder**

M05.819 **Other rheumatoid arthritis with rheumatoid factor of unspecified shoulder**

+ M05.82 **Other rheumatoid arthritis with rheumatoid factor of elbow**

M05.821 **Other rheumatoid arthritis with rheumatoid factor of right elbow**

M05.822 **Other rheumatoid arthritis with rheumatoid factor of left elbow**

M05.829 **Other rheumatoid arthritis with rheumatoid factor of unspecified elbow**

+ M05.83 **Other rheumatoid arthritis with rheumatoid factor of wrist**

M05.831 **Other rheumatoid arthritis with rheumatoid factor of right wrist**

M05.832 **Other rheumatoid arthritis with rheumatoid factor of left wrist**

M05.839 **Other rheumatoid arthritis with rheumatoid factor of unspecified wrist**

+ M05.84 Other rheumatoid arthritis with rheumatoid factor of hand
M05.841 Other rheumatoid arthritis with rheumatoid factor of right hand
M05.842 Other rheumatoid arthritis with rheumatoid factor of left hand
M05.849 Other rheumatoid arthritis with rheumatoid factor of unspecified hand
+ M05.85 Other rheumatoid arthritis with rheumatoid factor of hip
M05.851 Other rheumatoid arthritis with rheumatoid factor of right hip
M05.852 Other rheumatoid arthritis with rheumatoid factor of left hip
M05.859 Other rheumatoid arthritis with rheumatoid factor of unspecified hip
+ M05.86 Other rheumatoid arthritis with rheumatoid factor of knee
M05.861 Other rheumatoid arthritis with rheumatoid factor of right knee
M05.862 Other rheumatoid arthritis with rheumatoid factor of left knee
M05.869 Other rheumatoid arthritis with rheumatoid factor of unspecified knee
+ M05.87 Other rheumatoid arthritis with rheumatoid factor of ankle and foot
M05.871 Other rheumatoid arthritis with rheumatoid factor of right ankle and foot
M05.872 Other rheumatoid arthritis with rheumatoid factor of left ankle and foot
M05.879 Other rheumatoid arthritis with rheumatoid factor of unspecified ankle and foot
M05.89 Other rheumatoid arthritis with rheumatoid factor of multiple sites
M05.9 Rheumatoid arthritis with rheumatoid factor, unspecified

M06 Other rheumatoid arthritis

+ M06.0 Rheumatoid arthritis without rheumatoid factor
M06.00 Rheumatoid arthritis without rheumatoid factor, unspecified site
+ M06.01 Rheumatoid arthritis without rheumatoid factor, shoulder
M06.011 Rheumatoid arthritis without rheumatoid factor, right shoulder
M06.012 Rheumatoid arthritis without rheumatoid factor, left shoulder
M06.019 Rheumatoid arthritis without rheumatoid factor, unspecified shoulder
+ M06.02 Rheumatoid arthritis without rheumatoid factor, elbow
M06.021 Rheumatoid arthritis without rheumatoid factor, right elbow
M06.022 Rheumatoid arthritis without rheumatoid factor, left elbow
M06.029 Rheumatoid arthritis without rheumatoid factor, unspecified elbow
+ M06.03 Rheumatoid arthritis without rheumatoid factor, wrist
M06.031 Rheumatoid arthritis without rheumatoid factor, right wrist
M06.032 Rheumatoid arthritis without rheumatoid factor, left wrist
M06.039 Rheumatoid arthritis without rheumatoid factor, unspecified wrist
+ M06.04 Rheumatoid arthritis without rheumatoid factor, hand
M06.041 Rheumatoid arthritis without rheumatoid factor, right hand
M06.042 Rheumatoid arthritis without rheumatoid factor, left hand
M06.049 Rheumatoid arthritis without rheumatoid factor, unspecified hand
+ M06.05 Rheumatoid arthritis without rheumatoid factor, hip
M06.051 Rheumatoid arthritis without rheumatoid factor, right hip
M06.052 Rheumatoid arthritis without rheumatoid factor, left hip
M06.059 Rheumatoid arthritis without rheumatoid factor, unspecified hip
+ M06.06 Rheumatoid arthritis without rheumatoid factor, knee
M06.061 Rheumatoid arthritis without rheumatoid factor, right knee
M06.062 Rheumatoid arthritis without rheumatoid factor, left knee
M06.069 Rheumatoid arthritis without rheumatoid factor, unspecified knee
+ M06.07 Rheumatoid arthritis without rheumatoid factor, ankle and foot
M06.071 Rheumatoid arthritis without rheumatoid factor, right ankle and foot
M06.072 Rheumatoid arthritis without rheumatoid factor, left ankle and foot
M06.079 Rheumatoid arthritis without rheumatoid factor, unspecified ankle and foot
M06.08 Rheumatoid arthritis without rheumatoid factor, vertebrae
M06.09 Rheumatoid arthritis without rheumatoid factor, multiple sites
• M06.1 Adult-onset Still's disease
Excludes1: *Still's disease NOS (M08.2-)*
+ M06.2 Rheumatoid bursitis
M06.20 Rheumatoid bursitis, unspecified site
+ M06.21 Rheumatoid bursitis, shoulder
M06.211 Rheumatoid bursitis, right shoulder
M06.212 Rheumatoid bursitis, left shoulder
M06.219 Rheumatoid bursitis, unspecified shoulder
+ M06.22 Rheumatoid bursitis, elbow
M06.221 Rheumatoid bursitis, right elbow
M06.222 Rheumatoid bursitis, left elbow
M06.229 Rheumatoid bursitis, unspecified elbow
+ M06.23 Rheumatoid bursitis, wrist
M06.231 Rheumatoid bursitis, right wrist
M06.232 Rheumatoid bursitis, left wrist
M06.239 Rheumatoid bursitis, unspecified wrist
+ M06.24 Rheumatoid bursitis, hand
M06.241 Rheumatoid bursitis, right hand
M06.242 Rheumatoid bursitis, left hand
M06.249 Rheumatoid bursitis, unspecified hand
+ M06.25 Rheumatoid bursitis, hip
M06.251 Rheumatoid bursitis, right hip
M06.252 Rheumatoid bursitis, left hip
M06.259 Rheumatoid bursitis, unspecified hip
+ M06.26 Rheumatoid bursitis, knee
M06.261 Rheumatoid bursitis, right knee
M06.262 Rheumatoid bursitis, left knee
M06.269 Rheumatoid bursitis, unspecified knee
+ M06.27 Rheumatoid bursitis, ankle and foot
M06.271 Rheumatoid bursitis, right ankle and foot
M06.272 Rheumatoid bursitis, left ankle and foot
M06.279 Rheumatoid bursitis, unspecified ankle and foot
M06.28 Rheumatoid bursitis, vertebrae
M06.29 Rheumatoid bursitis, multiple sites
+ M06.3 Rheumatoid nodule
M06.30 Rheumatoid nodule, unspecified site
+ M06.31 Rheumatoid nodule, shoulder
M06.311 Rheumatoid nodule, right shoulder
M06.312 Rheumatoid nodule, left shoulder
M06.319 Rheumatoid nodule, unspecified shoulder
+ M06.32 Rheumatoid nodule, elbow
M06.321 Rheumatoid nodule, right elbow
M06.322 Rheumatoid nodule, left elbow
M06.329 Rheumatoid nodule, unspecified elbow
+ M06.33 Rheumatoid nodule, wrist
M06.331 Rheumatoid nodule, right wrist
M06.332 Rheumatoid nodule, left wrist
M06.339 Rheumatoid nodule, unspecified wrist
+ M06.34 Rheumatoid nodule, hand
M06.341 Rheumatoid nodule, right hand
M06.342 Rheumatoid nodule, left hand
M06.349 Rheumatoid nodule, unspecified hand
+ M06.35 Rheumatoid nodule, hip
M06.351 Rheumatoid nodule, right hip
M06.352 Rheumatoid nodule, left hip
M06.359 Rheumatoid nodule, unspecified hip

+ **M06.36 Rheumatoid nodule, knee**
  - **M06.361 Rheumatoid nodule, right knee**
  - **M06.362 Rheumatoid nodule, left knee**
  - **M06.369 Rheumatoid nodule, unspecified knee**

+ **M06.37 Rheumatoid nodule, ankle and foot**
  - **M06.371 Rheumatoid nodule, right ankle and foot**
  - **M06.372 Rheumatoid nodule, left ankle and foot**
  - **M06.379 Rheumatoid nodule, unspecified ankle and foot**

M06.38 Rheumatoid nodule, vertebrae

M06.39 Rheumatoid nodule, multiple sites

M06.4 Inflammatory polyarthropathy

Excludes1: *polyarthritis NOS (M13.0)*

+ **M06.8 Other specified rheumatoid arthritis**
  - **M06.80 Other specified rheumatoid arthritis, unspecified site**

+ **M06.81 Other specified rheumatoid arthritis, shoulder**
  - **M06.811 Other specified rheumatoid arthritis, right shoulder**
  - **M06.812 Other specified rheumatoid arthritis, left shoulder**
  - **M06.819 Other specified rheumatoid arthritis, unspecified shoulder**

+ **M06.82 Other specified rheumatoid arthritis, elbow**
  - **M06.821 Other specified rheumatoid arthritis, right elbow**
  - **M06.822 Other specified rheumatoid arthritis, left elbow**
  - **M06.829 Other specified rheumatoid arthritis, unspecified elbow**

+ **M06.83 Other specified rheumatoid arthritis, wrist**
  - **M06.831 Other specified rheumatoid arthritis, right wrist**
  - **M06.832 Other specified rheumatoid arthritis, left wrist**
  - **M06.839 Other specified rheumatoid arthritis, unspecified wrist**

+ **M06.84 Other specified rheumatoid arthritis, hand**
  - **M06.841 Other specified rheumatoid arthritis, right hand**
  - **M06.842 Other specified rheumatoid arthritis, left hand**
  - **M06.849 Other specified rheumatoid arthritis, unspecified hand**

+ **M06.85 Other specified rheumatoid arthritis, hip**
  - **M06.851 Other specified rheumatoid arthritis, right hip**
  - **M06.852 Other specified rheumatoid arthritis, left hip**
  - **M06.859 Other specified rheumatoid arthritis, unspecified hip**

+ **M06.86 Other specified rheumatoid arthritis, knee**
  - **M06.861 Other specified rheumatoid arthritis, right knee**
  - **M06.862 Other specified rheumatoid arthritis, left knee**
  - **M06.869 Other specified rheumatoid arthritis, unspecified knee**

+ **M06.87 Other specified rheumatoid arthritis, ankle and foot**
  - **M06.871 Other specified rheumatoid arthritis, right ankle and foot**
  - **M06.872 Other specified rheumatoid arthritis, left ankle and foot**
  - **M06.879 Other specified rheumatoid arthritis, unspecified ankle and foot**

M06.88 Other specified rheumatoid arthritis, vertebrae

M06.89 Other specified rheumatoid arthritis, multiple sites

M06.9 Rheumatoid arthritis, unspecified

M07 Enteropathic arthropathies

Code also associated enteropathy, such as:
regional enteritis [Crohn's disease] (K50.-)
ulcerative colitis (K51.-)

Excludes1: *psoriatic arthropathies (L40.5-)*

+ **M07.6 Enteropathic arthropathies**
  - **M07.60 Enteropathic arthropathies, unspecified site**

+ **M07.61 Enteropathic arthropathies, shoulder**
  - **M07.611 Enteropathic arthropathies, right shoulder**
  - **M07.612 Enteropathic arthropathies, left shoulder**
  - **M07.619 Enteropathic arthropathies, unspecified shoulder**

+ **M07.62 Enteropathic arthropathies, elbow**
  - **M07.621 Enteropathic arthropathies, right elbow**
  - **M07.622 Enteropathic arthropathies, left elbow**
  - **M07.629 Enteropathic arthropathies, unspecified elbow**

+ **M07.63 Enteropathic arthropathies, wrist**
  - **M07.631 Enteropathic arthropathies, right wrist**
  - **M07.632 Enteropathic arthropathies, left wrist**
  - **M07.639 Enteropathic arthropathies, unspecified wrist**

+ **M07.64 Enteropathic arthropathies, hand**
  - **M07.641 Enteropathic arthropathies, right hand**
  - **M07.642 Enteropathic arthropathies, lefthand**
  - **M07.649 Enteropathic arthropathies, unspecified hand**

+ **M07.65 Enteropathic arthropathies, hip**
  - **M07.651 Enteropathic arthropathies, right hip**
  - **M07.652 Enteropathic arthropathies, left hip**
  - **M07.659 Enteropathic arthropathies, unspecified h**

+ **M07.66 Enteropathic arthropathies, knee**
  - **M07.661 Enteropathic arthropathies, right knee**
  - **M07.662 Enteropathic arthropathies, left knee**
  - **M07.669 Enteropathic arthropathies, unspecified knee**

+ **M07.67 Enteropathic arthropathies, ankle and foot**
  - **M07.671 Enteropathic arthropathies, right ankle and foot**
  - **M07.672 Enteropathic arthropathies, left ankle an foot**
  - **M07.679 Enteropathic arthropathies, unspecified ankle and foot**

M07.68 Enteropathic arthropathies, vertebrae

M07.69 Enteropathic arthropathies, multiple sites

M08 Juvenile arthritis

Code also any associated underlying condition, such as:
regional enteritis [Crohn's disease] (K50.-)
ulcerative colitis (K51.-)

Excludes1: *arthropathy in Whipple's disease (M14.8)*
Felty's syndrome (M05.0)
juvenile dermatomyositis (M33.0-)
psoriatic juvenile arthropathy (L40.54)

+ **M08.0 Unspecified juvenile rheumatoid arthritis**

Juvenile rheumatoid arthritis with or without rheumatoid fact

  - **M08.00 Unspecified juvenile rheumatoid arthritis of unspecified site**

+ **M08.01 Unspecified juvenile rheumatoid arthritis, shoulde**
  - **M08.011 Unspecified juvenile rheumatoid arthriti right shoulder**
  - **M08.012 Unspecified juvenile rheumatoid arthriti left shoulder**
  - **M08.019 Unspecified juvenile rheumatoid arthriti unspecified shoulder**

+ **M08.02 Unspecified juvenile rheumatoid arthritis of elbow**
  - **M08.021 Unspecified juvenile rheumatoid arthriti right elbow**
  - **M08.022 Unspecified juvenile rheumatoid arthriti left elbow**
  - **M08.029 Unspecified juvenile rheumatoid arthriti unspecified elbow**

+ **M08.03 Unspecified juvenile rheumatoid arthritis, wrist**
  - **M08.031 Unspecified juvenile rheumatoid arthriti right wrist**
  - **M08.032 Unspecified juvenile rheumatoid arthriti left wrist**
  - **M08.039 Unspecified juvenile rheumatoid arthriti unspecified wrist**

+ **M08.04 Unspecified juvenile rheumatoid arthritis, hand**
  - **M08.041 Unspecified juvenile rheumatoid arthriti right hand**
  - **M08.042 Unspecified juvenile rheumatoid arthriti left hand**
  - **M08.049 Unspecified juvenile rheumatoid arthriti unspecified hand**

+ **M08.05 Unspecified juvenile rheumatoid arthritis, hip**
  - **M08.051 Unspecified juvenile rheumatoid arthriti right hip**
  - **M08.052 Unspecified juvenile rheumatoid arthriti left hip**
  - **M08.059 Unspecified juvenile rheumatoid arthriti unspecified hip**

+ M08.06 Unspecified juvenile rheumatoid arthritis, knee
M08.061 Unspecified juvenile rheumatoid arthritis, right knee
M08.062 Unspecified juvenile rheumatoid arthritis, left knee
M08.069 Unspecified juvenile rheumatoid arthritis, unspecified knee
+ M08.07 Unspecified juvenile rheumatoid arthritis, ankle and foot
M08.071 Unspecified juvenile rheumatoid arthritis, right ankle and foot
M08.072 Unspecified juvenile rheumatoid arthritis, left ankle and foot
M08.079 Unspecified juvenile rheumatoid arthritis, unspecified ankle and foot
M08.08 Unspecified juvenile rheumatoid arthritis, vertebrae
M08.09 Unspecified juvenile rheumatoid arthritis, multiple sites
M08.1 Juvenile ankylosing spondylitis
Excludes1: *ankylosing spondylitis in adults (M45.0-)*
+ M08.2 Juvenile rheumatoid arthritis with systemic onset
Still's disease NOS
Excludes1: *adult-onset Still's disease (M06.1-)*
M08.20 Juvenile rheumatoid arthritis with systemic onset, unspecified site
+ M08.21 Juvenile rheumatoid arthritis with systemic onset, shoulder
M08.211 Juvenile rheumatoid arthritis with systemic onset, right shoulder
M08.212 Juvenile rheumatoid arthritis with systemic onset, left shoulder
M08.219 Juvenile rheumatoid arthritis with systemic onset, unspecified shoulder
+ M08.22 Juvenile rheumatoid arthritis with systemic onset, elbow
M08.221 Juvenile rheumatoid arthritis with systemic onset, right elbow
M08.222 Juvenile rheumatoid arthritis with systemic onset, left elbow
M08.229 Juvenile rheumatoid arthritis with systemic onset, unspecified elbow
+ M08.23 Juvenile rheumatoid arthritis with systemic onset, wrist
M08.231 Juvenile rheumatoid arthritis with systemic onset, right wrist
M08.232 Juvenile rheumatoid arthritis with systemic onset, left wrist
M08.239 Juvenile rheumatoid arthritis with systemic onset, unspecified wrist
+ M08.24 Juvenile rheumatoid arthritis with systemic onset, hand
M08.241 Juvenile rheumatoid arthritis with systemic onset, right hand
M08.242 Juvenile rheumatoid arthritis with systemic onset, left hand
M08.249 Juvenile rheumatoid arthritis with systemic onset, unspecified hand
+ M08.25 Juvenile rheumatoid arthritis with systemic onset, hip
M08.251 Juvenile rheumatoid arthritis with systemic onset, right hip
M08.252 Juvenile rheumatoid arthritis with systemic onset, left hip
M08.259 Juvenile rheumatoid arthritis with systemic onset, unspecified hip
+ M08.26 Juvenile rheumatoid arthritis with systemic onset, knee
M08.261 Juvenile rheumatoid arthritis with systemic onset, right knee
M08.262 Juvenile rheumatoid arthritis with systemic onset, left knee
M08.269 Juvenile rheumatoid arthritis with systemic onset, unspecified knee
+ M08.27 Juvenile rheumatoid arthritis with systemic onset, ankle and foot
M08.271 Juvenile rheumatoid arthritis with systemic onset, right ankle and foot
M08.272 Juvenile rheumatoid arthritis with systemic onset, left ankle and foot
M08.279 Juvenile rheumatoid arthritis with systemic onset, unspecified ankle and foot
M08.28 Juvenile rheumatoid arthritis with systemic onset, vertebrae
M08.29 Juvenile rheumatoid arthritis with systemic onset, multiple sites
M08.3 Juvenile rheumatoid polyarthritis (seronegative)
+ M08.4 Pauciarticular juvenile rheumatoid arthritis
M08.40 Pauciarticular juvenile rheumatoid arthritis, unspecified site
+ M08.41 Pauciarticular juvenile rheumatoid arthritis, shoulder
M08.411 Pauciarticular juvenile rheumatoid arthritis, right shoulder
M08.412 Pauciarticular juvenile rheumatoid arthritis, left shoulder
M08.419 Pauciarticular juvenile rheumatoid arthritis, unspecified shoulder
+ M08.42 Pauciarticular juvenile rheumatoid arthritis, elbow
M08.421 Pauciarticular juvenile rheumatoid arthritis, right elbow
M08.422 Pauciarticular juvenile rheumatoid arthritis, left elbow
M08.429 Pauciarticular juvenile rheumatoid arthritis, unspecified elbow
+ M08.43 Pauciarticular juvenile rheumatoid arthritis, wrist
M08.431 Pauciarticular juvenile rheumatoid arthritis, right wrist
M08.432 Pauciarticular juvenile rheumatoid arthritis, left wrist
M08.439 Pauciarticular juvenile rheumatoid arthritis, unspecified wrist
+ M08.44 Pauciarticular juvenile rheumatoid arthritis, hand
M08.441 Pauciarticular juvenile rheumatoid arthritis, right hand
M08.442 Pauciarticular juvenile rheumatoid arthritis, left hand
M08.449 Pauciarticular juvenile rheumatoid arthritis, unspecified hand
+ M08.45 Pauciarticular juvenile rheumatoid arthritis, hip
M08.451 Pauciarticular juvenile rheumatoid arthritis, right hip
M08.452 Pauciarticular juvenile rheumatoid arthritis, left hip
M08.459 Pauciarticular juvenile rheumatoid arthritis, unspecified hip
+ M08.46 Pauciarticular juvenile rheumatoid arthritis, knee
M08.461 Pauciarticular juvenile rheumatoid arthritis, right knee
M08.462 Pauciarticular juvenile rheumatoid arthritis, left knee
M08.469 Pauciarticular juvenile rheumatoid arthritis, unspecified knee
+ M08.47 Pauciarticular juvenile rheumatoid arthritis, ankle and foot
M08.471 Pauciarticular juvenile rheumatoid arthritis, right ankle and foot
M08.472 Pauciarticular juvenile rheumatoid arthritis, left ankle and foot
M08.479 Pauciarticular juvenile rheumatoid arthritis, unspecified ankle and foot
M08.48 Pauciarticular juvenile rheumatoid arthritis, vertebrae
+ M08.8 Other juvenile arthritis
M08.80 Other juvenile arthritis, unspecified site
+ M08.81 Other juvenile arthritis, shoulder
M08.811 Other juvenile arthritis, right shoulder
M08.812 Other juvenile arthritis, left shoulder
M08.819 Other juvenile arthritis, unspecified shoulder
+ M08.82 Other juvenile arthritis, elbow
M08.821 Other juvenile arthritis, right elbow
M08.822 Other juvenile arthritis, left elbow
M08.829 Other juvenile arthritis, unspecified elbow
+ M08.83 Other juvenile arthritis, wrist
M08.831 Other juvenile arthritis, right wrist
M08.832 Other juvenile arthritis, left wrist
M08.839 Other juvenile arthritis, unspecified wrist
+ M08.84 Other juvenile arthritis, hand
M08.841 Other juvenile arthritis, right hand
M08.842 Other juvenile arthritis, left hand
M08.849 Other juvenile arthritis, unspecified hand

+ M08.85 **Other juvenile arthritis, hip**
  - M08.851 **Other juvenile arthritis, right hip**
  - M08.852 **Other juvenile arthritis, left hip**
  - M08.859 **Other juvenile arthritis, unspecified hip**
+ M08.86 **Other juvenile arthritis, knee**
  - M08.861 **Other juvenile arthritis, right knee**
  - M08.862 **Other juvenile arthritis, left knee**
  - M08.869 **Other juvenile arthritis, unspecified knee**
+ M08.87 **Other juvenile arthritis, ankle and foot**
  - M08.871 **Other juvenile arthritis, right ankle and foot**
  - M08.872 **Other juvenile arthritis, left ankle and foot**
  - M08.879 **Other juvenile arthritis, unspecified ankle and foot**

M08.88 **Other juvenile arthritis, other specified site**
Other juvenile arthritis, vertebrae

M08.89 **Other juvenile arthritis, multiple sites**

+ M08.9 **Juvenile arthritis, unspecified**
Excludes1: juvenile rheumatoid arthritis, unspecified (M08.0-)

M08.90 **Juvenile arthritis, unspecified, unspecified site**

+ M08.91 **Juvenile arthritis, unspecified, shoulder**
  - M08.911 **Juvenile arthritis, unspecified, right shoulder**
  - M08.912 **Juvenile arthritis, unspecified, left shoulder**
  - M08.919 **Juvenile arthritis, unspecified, unspecified shoulder**
+ M08.92 **Juvenile arthritis, unspecified, elbow**
  - M08.921 **Juvenile arthritis, unspecified, right elbow**
  - M08.922 **Juvenile arthritis, unspecified, left elbow**
  - M08.929 **Juvenile arthritis, unspecified, unspecified elbow**
+ M08.93 **Juvenile arthritis, unspecified, wrist**
  - M08.931 **Juvenile arthritis, unspecified, right wrist**
  - M08.932 **Juvenile arthritis, unspecified, left wrist**
  - M08.939 **Juvenile arthritis, unspecified, unspecified wrist**
+ M08.94 **Juvenile arthritis, unspecified, hand**
  - M08.941 **Juvenile arthritis, unspecified, right hand**
  - M08.942 **Juvenile arthritis, unspecified, left hand**
  - M08.949 **Juvenile arthritis, unspecified, unspecified hand**
+ M08.95 **Juvenile arthritis, unspecified, hip**
  - M08.951 **Juvenile arthritis, unspecified, right hip**
  - M08.952 **Juvenile arthritis, unspecified, left hip**
  - M08.959 **Juvenile arthritis, unspecified, unspecified hip**
+ M08.96 **Juvenile arthritis, unspecified, knee**
  - M08.961 **Juvenile arthritis, unspecified, right knee**
  - M08.962 **Juvenile arthritis, unspecified, left knee**
  - M08.969 **Juvenile arthritis, unspecified, unspecified knee**
+ M08.97 **Juvenile arthritis, unspecified, ankle and foot**
  - M08.971 **Juvenile arthritis, unspecified, right ankle and foot**
  - M08.972 **Juvenile arthritis, unspecified, left ankle and foot**
  - M08.979 **Juvenile arthritis, unspecified, unspecified ankle and foot**

M08.98 **Juvenile arthritis, unspecified, vertebrae**

M08.99 **Juvenile arthritis, unspecified, multiple sites**

M1A Chronic gout

Use additional code to identify:
Autonomic neuropathy in diseases classified elsewhere (G99.0)
Calculus of urinary tract in diseases classified elsewhere (N22)
Cardiomyopathy in diseases classified elsewhere (I43)
Disorders of external ear in diseases classified elsewhere (H61.1-, H62.8-)
Disorders of iris and ciliary body in diseases classified elsewhere (H22)
Glomerular disorders in diseases classified elsewhere (N08)

Excludes1: gout NOS (M10.-)
Excludes2: acute gout (M10.-)

The appropriate 7th character is to be added to each code from category M1A
0 without tophus (tophi)
1 with tophus (tophi)

+ M1A.0 **Idiopathic chronic gout**
Chronic gouty bursitis
Primary chronic gout

X+7th M1A.00 **Idiopathic chronic gout, unspecified site**

+ M1A.01 **Idiopathic chronic gout, shoulder**
  - +7th M1A.011 **Idiopathic chronic gout, right shoulder**
  - +7th M1A.012 **Idiopathic chronic gout, left shoulder**
  - +7th M1A.019 **Idiopathic chronic gout, unspecified shoulder**
+ M1A.02 **Idiopathic chronic gout, elbow**
  - +7th M1A.021 **Idiopathic chronic gout, right elbow**
  - +7th M1A.022 **Idiopathic chronic gout, left elbow**
  - +7th M1A.029 **Idiopathic chronic gout, unspecified elbow**
+ M1A.03 **Idiopathic chronic gout, wrist**
  - +7th M1A.031 **Idiopathic chronic gout, right wrist**
  - +7th M1A.032 **Idiopathic chronic gout, left wrist**
  - +7th M1A.039 **Idiopathic chronic gout, unspecified wrist**
+ M1A.04 **Idiopathic chronic gout, hand**
  - +7th M1A.041 **Idiopathic chronic gout, right hand**
  - +7th M1A.042 **Idiopathic chronic gout, left hand**
  - +7th M1A.049 **Idiopathic chronic gout, unspecified hand**
+ M1A.05 **Idiopathic chronic gout, hip**
  - +7th M1A.051 **Idiopathic chronic gout, right hip**
  - +7th M1A.052 **Idiopathic chronic gout, left hip**
  - +7th M1A.059 **Idiopathic chronic gout, unspecified hip**
+ M1A.06 **Idiopathic chronic gout, knee**
  - +7th M1A.061 **Idiopathic chronic gout, right knee**
  - +7th M1A.062 **Idiopathic chronic gout, left knee**
  - +7th M1A.069 **Idiopathic chronic gout, unspecified knee**
+ M1A.07 **Idiopathic chronic gout, ankle and foot**
  - +7th M1A.071 **Idiopathic chronic gout, right ankle and foot**
  - +7th M1A.072 **Idiopathic chronic gout, left ankle and foot**
  - +7th M1A.079 **Idiopathic chronic gout, unspecified ankle and foot**

X+7th M1A.08 **Idiopathic chronic gout, vertebrae**

M1A.09 **Idiopathic chronic gout, multiple sites**

+ M1A.1 **Lead-induced chronic gout**
Code first toxic effects of lead and its compounds (T56.0-)

X+7th M1A.10 **Lead-induced chronic gout, unspecified site**

+ M1A.11 **Lead-induced chronic gout, shoulder**
  - +7th M1A.111 **Lead-induced chronic gout, right shoulder**
  - +7th M1A.112 **Lead-induced chronic gout, left shoulder**
  - +7th M1A.119 **Lead-induced chronic gout, unspecified shoulder**
+ M1A.12 **Lead-induced chronic gout, elbow**
  - +7th M1A.121 **Lead-induced chronic gout, right elbow**
  - +7th M1A.122 **Lead-induced chronic gout, left elbow**
  - +7th M1A.129 **Lead-induced chronic gout, unspecified elbow**
+ M1A.13 **Lead-induced chronic gout, wrist**
  - +7th M1A.131 **Lead-induced chronic gout, right wrist**
  - +7th M1A.132 **Lead-induced chronic gout, left wrist**
  - +7th M1A.139 **Lead-induced chronic gout, unspecified wrist**
+ M1A.14 **Lead-induced chronic gout, hand**
  - +7th M1A.141 **Lead-induced chronic gout, right hand**
  - +7th M1A.142 **Lead-induced chronic gout, left hand**
  - +7th M1A.149 **Lead-induced chronic gout, unspecified hand**
+ M1A.15 **Lead-induced chronic gout, hip**
  - +7th M1A.151 **Lead-induced chronic gout, right hip**
  - +7th M1A.152 **Lead-induced chronic gout, left hip**
  - +7th M1A.159 **Lead-induced chronic gout, unspecified hip**
+ M1A.16 **Lead-induced chronic gout, knee**
  - +7th M1A.161 **Lead-induced chronic gout, right knee**
  - +7th M1A.162 **Lead-induced chronic gout, left knee**
  - +7th M1A.169 **Lead-induced chronic gout, unspecified knee**
+ M1A.17 **Lead-induced chronic gout, ankle and foot**
  - +7th M1A.171 **Lead-induced chronic gout, right ankle and foot**
  - +7th M1A.172 **Lead-induced chronic gout, left ankle and foot**
  - +7th M1A.179 **Lead-induced chronic gout, unspecified ankle and foot**

X+7th M1A.18 **Lead-induced chronic gout, vertebrae**

X+7th M1A.19 **Lead-induced chronic gout, multiple sites**

+ M1A.2 **Drug-induced chronic gout**
Use additional code for adverse effect, if applicable, to identify drug (T36-T50 with fifth or sixth character 5)

X+7th M1A.20 **Drug-induced chronic gout, unspecified site**

+ M1A.21 Drug-induced chronic gout, shoulder
+7th M1A.211 Drug-induced chronic gout, right shoulder
+7th M1A.212 Drug-induced chronic gout, left shoulder
+7th M1A.219 Drug-induced chronic gout, unspecified shoulder
+ M1A.22 Drug-induced chronic gout, elbow
+7th M1A.221 Drug-induced chronic gout, right elbow
+7th M1A.222 Drug-induced chronic gout, left elbow
+7th M1A.229 Drug-induced chronic gout, unspecified elbow
+ M1A.23 Drug-induced chronic gout, wrist
+7th M1A.231 Drug-induced chronic gout, right wrist
+7th M1A.232 Drug-induced chronic gout, left wrist
+7th M1A.239 Drug-induced chronic gout, unspecified wrist
+ M1A.24 Drug-induced chronic gout, hand
+7th M1A.241 Drug-induced chronic gout, right hand
+7th M1A.242 Drug-induced chronic gout, left hand
+7th M1A.249 Drug-induced chronic gout, unspecified hand
+ M1A.25 Drug-induced chronic gout, hip
+7th M1A.251 Drug-induced chronic gout, right hip
+7th M1A.252 Drug-induced chronic gout, left hip
+7th M1A.259 Drug-induced chronic gout, unspecified hip
+ M1A.26 Drug-induced chronic gout, knee
+7th M1A.261 Drug-induced chronic gout, right knee
+7th M1A.262 Drug-induced chronic gout, left knee
+7th M1A.269 Drug-induced chronic gout, unspecified knee
+ M1A.27 Drug-induced chronic gout, ankle and foot
+7th M1A.271 Drug-induced chronic gout, right ankle and foot
+7th M1A.272 Drug-induced chronic gout, left ankle and foot
+7th M1A.279 Drug-induced chronic gout, unspecified ankle and foot
X+7th M1A.28 Drug-induced chronic gout, vertebrae
X+7th M1A.29 Drug-induced chronic gout, multiple sites
+ M1A.3 Chronic gout due to renal impairment
Code first associated renal disease
X+7th M1A.30 Chronic gout due to renal impairment, unspecified site
+ M1A.31 Chronic gout due to renal impairment, shoulder
+7th M1A.311 Chronic gout due to renal impairment, right shoulder
+7th M1A.312 Chronic gout due to renal impairment, left shoulder
+7th M1A.319 Chronic gout due to renal impairment, unspecified shoulder
+ M1A.32 Chronic gout due to renal impairment, elbow
+7th M1A.321 Chronic gout due to renal impairment, right elbow
+7th M1A.322 Chronic gout due to renal impairment, left elbow
+7th M1A.329 Chronic gout due to renal impairment, unspecified elbow
+ M1A.33 Chronic gout due to renal impairment, wrist
+7th M1A.331 Chronic gout due to renal impairment, right wrist
+7th M1A.332 Chronic gout due to renal impairment, left wrist
+7th M1A.339 Chronic gout due to renal impairment, unspecified wrist
+ M1A.34 Chronic gout due to renal impairment, hand
+7th M1A.341 Chronic gout due to renal impairment, right hand
+7th M1A.342 Chronic gout due to renal impairment, left hand
+7th M1A.349 Chronic gout due to renal impairment, unspecified hand
+ M1A.35 Chronic gout due to renal impairment, hip
+7th M1A.351 Chronic gout due to renal impairment, right hip
+7th M1A.352 Chronic gout due to renal impairment, left hip
+7th M1A.359 Chronic gout due to renal impairment, unspecified hip
+ M1A.36 Chronic gout due to renal impairment, knee
+7th M1A.361 Chronic gout due to renal impairment, right knee
+7th M1A.362 Chronic gout due to renal impairment, left knee
+7th M1A.369 Chronic gout due to renal impairment, unspecified knee
+ M1A.37 Chronic gout due to renal impairment, ankle and foot
+7th M1A.371 Chronic gout due to renal impairment, right ankle and foot
+7th M1A.372 Chronic gout due to renal impairment, left ankle and foot
+7th M1A.379 Chronic gout due to renal impairment, unspecified ankle and foot
X+7th M1A.38 Chronic gout due to renal impairment, vertebrae
X+7th M1A.39 Chronic gout due to renal impairment, multiple sites
+ M1A.4 Other secondary chronic gout
Code first associated condition
X+7th M1A.40 Other secondary chronic gout, unspecified site
+ M1A.41 Other secondary chronic gout, shoulder
+7th M1A.411 Other secondary chronic gout, right shoulder
+7th M1A.412 Other secondary chronic gout, left shoulder
+7th M1A.419 Other secondary chronic gout, unspecified shoulder
+ M1A.42 Other secondary chronic gout, elbow
+7th M1A.421 Other secondary chronic gout, right elbow
+7th M1A.422 Other secondary chronic gout, left elbow
+7th M1A.429 Other secondary chronic gout, unspecified elbow
+ M1A.43 Other secondary chronic gout, wrist
+7th M1A.431 Other secondary chronic gout, right wrist
+7th M1A.432 Other secondary chronic gout, left wrist
+7th M1A.439 Other secondary chronic gout, unspecified wrist
+ M1A.44 Other secondary chronic gout, hand
+7th M1A.441 Other secondary chronic gout, right hand
+7th M1A.442 Other secondary chronic gout, left hand
+7th M1A.449 Other secondary chronic gout, unspecified hand
+ M1A.45 Other secondary chronic gout, hip
+7th M1A.451 Other secondary chronic gout, right hip
+7th M1A.452 Other secondary chronic gout, left hip
+7th M1A.459 Other secondary chronic gout, unspecified hip
+ M1A.46 Other secondary chronic gout, knee
+7th M1A.461 Other secondary chronic gout, right knee
+7th M1A.462 Other secondary chronic gout, left knee
+7th M1A.469 Other secondary chronic gout, unspecified knee
+ M1A.47 Other secondary chronic gout, ankle and foot
+7th M1A.471 Other secondary chronic gout, right ankle and foot
+7th M1A.472 Other secondary chronic gout, left ankle and foot
+7th M1A.479 Other secondary chronic gout, unspecified ankle and foot
X+7th M1A.48 Other secondary chronic gout, vertebrae
X+7th M1A.49 Other secondary chronic gout, multiple sites
X+7th M1A.9 Chronic gout, unspecified

M10 Gout

Acute gout
Gout attack
Gout flare
Podagra
Use additional code to identify:
Autonomic neuropathy in diseases classified elsewhere (G99.0)
Calculus of urinary tract in diseases classified elsewhere (N22)
Cardiomyopathy in diseases classified elsewhere (I43)
Disorders of external ear in diseases classified elsewhere (H61.1-, H62.8-)
Disorders of iris and ciliary body in diseases classified elsewhere (H22)
Glomerular disorders in diseases classified elsewhere (N08)
Excludes2: *chronic gout (M1A.-)*

+ M10.0 Idiopathic gout
Gouty bursitis
Primary gout
M10.00 Idiopathic gout, unspecified site

+ **M10.01 Idiopathic gout, shoulder**
  - **M10.011 Idiopathic gout, right shoulder**
  - **M10.012 Idiopathic gout, left shoulder**
  - **M10.019 Idiopathic gout, unspecified shoulder**
+ **M10.02 Idiopathic gout, elbow**
  - **M10.021 Idiopathic gout, right elbow**
  - **M10.022 Idiopathic gout, left elbow**
  - **M10.029 Idiopathic gout, unspecified elbow**
+ **M10.03 Idiopathic gout, wrist**
  - **M10.031 Idiopathic gout, right wrist**
  - **M10.032 Idiopathic gout, left wrist**
  - **M10.039 Idiopathic gout, unspecified wrist**
+ **M10.04 Idiopathic gout, hand**
  - **M10.041 Idiopathic gout, right hand**
  - **M10.042 Idiopathic gout, left hand**
  - **M10.049 Idiopathic gout, unspecified hand**
+ **M10.05 Idiopathic gout, hip**
  - **M10.051 Idiopathic gout, right hip**
  - **M10.052 Idiopathic gout, left hip**
  - **M10.059 Idiopathic gout, unspecified hip**
+ **M10.06 Idiopathic gout, knee**
  - **M10.061 Idiopathic gout, right knee**
  - **M10.062 Idiopathic gout, left knee**
  - **M10.069 Idiopathic gout, unspecified knee**
+ **M10.07 Idiopathic gout, ankle and foot**
  - **M10.071 Idiopathic gout, right ankle and foot**
  - **M10.072 Idiopathic gout, left ankle and foot**
  - **M10.079 Idiopathic gout, unspecified ankle and foot**

M10.08 Idiopathic gout, vertebrae

M10.09 Idiopathic gout, multiple sites

+ **M10.1 Lead-induced gout**

Code first toxic effects of lead and its compounds (T56.0-)

M10.10 Lead-induced gout, unspecified site

+ **M10.11 Lead-induced gout, shoulder**
  - **M10.111 Lead-induced gout, right shoulder**
  - **M10.112 Lead-induced gout, left shoulder**
  - **M10.119 Lead-induced gout, unspecified shoulder**
+ **M10.12 Lead-induced gout, elbow**
  - **M10.121 Lead-induced gout, right elbow**
  - **M10.122 Lead-induced gout, left elbow**
  - **M10.129 Lead-induced gout, unspecified elbow**
+ **M10.13 Lead-induced gout, wrist**
  - **M10.131 Lead-induced gout, right wrist**
  - **M10.132 Lead-induced gout, left wrist**
  - **M10.139 Lead-induced gout, unspecified wrist**
+ **M10.14 Lead-induced gout, hand**
  - **M10.141 Lead-induced gout, right hand**
  - **M10.142 Lead-induced gout, left hand**
  - **M10.149 Lead-induced gout, unspecified hand**
+ **M10.15 Lead-induced gout, hip**
  - **M10.151 Lead-induced gout, right hip**
  - **M10.152 Lead-induced gout, left hip**
  - **M10.159 Lead-induced gout, unspecified hip**
+ **M10.16 Lead-induced gout, knee**
  - **M10.161 Lead-induced gout, right knee**
  - **M10.162 Lead-induced gout, left knee**
  - **M10.169 Lead-induced gout, unspecified knee**
+ **M10.17 Lead-induced gout, ankle and foot**
  - **M10.171 Lead-induced gout, right ankle and foot**
  - **M10.172 Lead-induced gout, left ankle and foot**
  - **M10.179 Lead-induced gout, unspecified ankle and foot**

M10.18 Lead-induced gout, vertebrae

M10.19 Lead-induced gout, multiple sites

+ **M10.2 Drug-induced gout**

Use additional code for adverse effect, if applicable, to identify drug (T36-T50 with fifth or sixth character 5)

M10.20 Drug-induced gout, unspecified site

+ **M10.21 Drug-induced gout, shoulder**
  - **M10.211 Drug-induced gout, right shoulder**
  - **M10.212 Drug-induced gout, left shoulder**
  - **M10.219 Drug-induced gout, unspecified shoulder**
+ **M10.22 Drug-induced gout, elbow**
  - **M10.221 Drug-induced gout, right elbow**
  - **M10.222 Drug-induced gout, left elbow**
  - **M10.229 Drug-induced gout, unspecified elbow**
+ **M10.23 Drug-induced gout, wrist**
  - **M10.231 Drug-induced gout, right wrist**
  - **M10.232 Drug-induced gout, left wrist**
  - **M10.239 Drug-induced gout, unspecified wrist**
+ **M10.24 Drug-induced gout, hand**
  - **M10.241 Drug-induced gout, right hand**
  - **M10.242 Drug-induced gout, left hand**
  - **M10.249 Drug-induced gout, unspecified hand**
+ **M10.25 Drug-induced gout, hip**
  - **M10.251 Drug-induced gout, right hip**
  - **M10.252 Drug-induced gout, left hip**
  - **M10.259 Drug-induced gout, unspecified hip**
+ **M10.26 Drug-induced gout, knee**
  - **M10.261 Drug-induced gout, right knee**
  - **M10.262 Drug-induced gout, left knee**
  - **M10.269 Drug-induced gout, unspecified knee**
+ **M10.27 Drug-induced gout, ankle and foot**
  - **M10.271 Drug-induced gout, right ankle and foot**
  - **M10.272 Drug-induced gout, left ankle and foot**
  - **M10.279 Drug-induced gout, unspecified ankle and foot**

M10.28 Drug-induced gout, vertebrae

M10.29 Drug-induced gout, multiple sites

+ **M10.3 Gout due to renal impairment**

Code first associated renal disease

M10.30 Gout due to renal impairment, unspecified site

+ **M10.31 Gout due to renal impairment, shoulder**
  - **M10.311 Gout due to renal impairment, right shoulder**
  - **M10.312 Gout due to renal impairment, left shoulder**
  - **M10.319 Gout due to renal impairment, unspecified shoulder**
+ **M10.32 Gout due to renal impairment, elbow**
  - **M10.321 Gout due to renal impairment, right elbow**
  - **M10.322 Gout due to renal impairment, left elbow**
  - **M10.329 Gout due to renal impairment, unspecified elbow**
+ **M10.33 Gout due to renal impairment, wrist**
  - **M10.331 Gout due to renal impairment, right wrist**
  - **M10.332 Gout due to renal impairment, left wrist**
  - **M10.339 Gout due to renal impairment, unspecified wrist**
+ **M10.34 Gout due to renal impairment, hand**
  - **M10.341 Gout due to renal impairment, right hand**
  - **M10.342 Gout due to renal impairment, left hand**
  - **M10.349 Gout due to renal impairment, unspecified hand**
+ **M10.35 Gout due to renal impairment, hip**
  - **M10.351 Gout due to renal impairment, right hip**
  - **M10.352 Gout due to renal impairment, left hip**
  - **M10.359 Gout due to renal impairment, unspecified hip**
+ **M10.36 Gout due to renal impairment, knee**
  - **M10.361 Gout due to renal impairment, right knee**
  - **M10.362 Gout due to renal impairment, left knee**
  - **M10.369 Gout due to renal impairment, unspecified knee**
+ **M10.37 Gout due to renal impairment, ankle and foot**
  - **M10.371 Gout due to renal impairment, right ankle and foot**
  - **M10.372 Gout due to renal impairment, left ankle and foot**
  - **M10.379 Gout due to renal impairment, unspecified ankle and foot**

M10.38 Gout due to renal impairment, vertebrae

M10.39 Gout due to renal impairment, multiple sites

+ **M10.4 Other secondary gout**

Code first associated condition

M10.40 Other secondary gout, unspecified site

+ **M10.41 Other secondary gout, shoulder**
  - **M10.411 Other secondary gout, right shoulder**
  - **M10.412 Other secondary gout, left shoulder**
  - **M10.419 Other secondary gout, unspecified shoulder**
+ **M10.42 Other secondary gout, elbow**
  - **M10.421 Other secondary gout, right elbow**
  - **M10.422 Other secondary gout, left elbow**
  - **M10.429 Other secondary gout, unspecified elbow**
+ **M10.43 Other secondary gout, wrist**
  - **M10.431 Other secondary gout, right wrist**
  - **M10.432 Other secondary gout, left wrist**
  - **M10.439 Other secondary gout, unspecified wrist**

+ M10.44 Other secondary gout, hand
M10.441 Other secondary gout, right hand
M10.442 Other secondary gout, left hand
M10.449 Other secondary gout, unspecified hand
+ M10.45 Other secondary gout, hip
M10.451 Other secondary gout, right hip
M10.452 Other secondary gout, left hip
M10.459 Other secondary gout, unspecified hip
+ M10.46 Other secondary gout, knee
M10.461 Other secondary gout, right knee
M10.462 Other secondary gout, left knee
M10.469 Other secondary gout, unspecified knee
+ M10.47 Other secondary gout, ankle and foot
M10.471 Other secondary gout, right ankle and foot
M10.472 Other secondary gout, left ankle and foot
M10.479 Other secondary gout, unspecified ankle and foot
M10.48 Other secondary gout, vertebrae
M10.49 Other secondary gout, multiple sites
M10.9 Gout, unspecified
Gout NOS

M11 Other crystal arthropathies

+ M11.0 Hydroxyapatite deposition disease
M11.00 Hydroxyapatite deposition disease, unspecified site
+ M11.01 Hydroxyapatite deposition disease, shoulder
M11.011 Hydroxyapatite deposition disease, right shoulder
M11.012 Hydroxyapatite deposition disease, left shoulder
M11.019 Hydroxyapatite deposition disease, unspecified shoulder
+ M11.02 Hydroxyapatite deposition disease, elbow
M11.021 Hydroxyapatite deposition disease, right elbow
M11.022 Hydroxyapatite deposition disease, left elbow
M11.029 Hydroxyapatite deposition disease, unspecified elbow
+ M11.03 Hydroxyapatite deposition disease, wrist
M11.031 Hydroxyapatite deposition disease, right wrist
M11.032 Hydroxyapatite deposition disease, left wrist
M11.039 Hydroxyapatite deposition disease, unspecified wrist
+ M11.04 Hydroxyapatite deposition disease, hand
M11.041 Hydroxyapatite deposition disease, right hand
M11.042 Hydroxyapatite deposition disease, left hand
M11.049 Hydroxyapatite deposition disease, unspecified hand
+ M11.05 Hydroxyapatite deposition disease, hip
M11.051 Hydroxyapatite deposition disease, right hip
M11.052 Hydroxyapatite deposition disease, left hip
M11.059 Hydroxyapatite deposition disease, unspecified hip
+ M11.06 Hydroxyapatite deposition disease, knee
M11.061 Hydroxyapatite deposition disease, right knee
M11.062 Hydroxyapatite deposition disease, left knee
M11.069 Hydroxyapatite deposition disease, unspecified knee
+ M11.07 Hydroxyapatite deposition disease, ankle and foot
M11.071 Hydroxyapatite deposition disease, right ankle and foot
M11.072 Hydroxyapatite deposition disease, left ankle and foot
M11.079 Hydroxyapatite deposition disease, unspecified ankle and foot
M11.08 Hydroxyapatite deposition disease, vertebrae
M11.09 Hydroxyapatite deposition disease, multiple sites
+ M11.1 Familial chondrocalcinosis
M11.10 Familial chondrocalcinosis, unspecified site
+ M11.11 Familial chondrocalcinosis, shoulder
M11.111 Familial chondrocalcinosis, right shoulder
M11.112 Familial chondrocalcinosis, left shoulder
M11.119 Familial chondrocalcinosis, unspecified shoulder
+ M11.12 Familial chondrocalcinosis, elbow
M11.121 Familial chondrocalcinosis, right elbow
M11.122 Familial chondrocalcinosis, left elbow
M11.129 Familial chondrocalcinosis, unspecified elbow
+ M11.13 Familial chondrocalcinosis, wrist
M11.131 Familial chondrocalcinosis, right wrist
M11.132 Familial chondrocalcinosis, left wrist
M11.139 Familial chondrocalcinosis, unspecified wrist
+ M11.14 Familial chondrocalcinosis, hand
M11.141 Familial chondrocalcinosis, right hand
M11.142 Familial chondrocalcinosis, left hand
M11.149 Familial chondrocalcinosis, unspecified hand
+ M11.15 Familial chondrocalcinosis, hip
M11.151 Familial chondrocalcinosis, right hip
M11.152 Familial chondrocalcinosis, left hip
M11.159 Familial chondrocalcinosis, unspecified hip
+ M11.16 Familial chondrocalcinosis, knee
M11.161 Familial chondrocalcinosis, right knee
M11.162 Familial chondrocalcinosis, left knee
M11.169 Familial chondrocalcinosis, unspecified knee
+ M11.17 Familial chondrocalcinosis, ankle and foot
M11.171 Familial chondrocalcinosis, right ankle and foot
M11.172 Familial chondrocalcinosis, left ankle and foot
M11.179 Familial chondrocalcinosis, unspecified ankle and foot
M11.18 Familial chondrocalcinosis, vertebrae
M11.19 Familial chondrocalcinosis, multiple sites
+ M11.2 Other chondrocalcinosis
Chondrocalcinosis NOS
M11.20 Other chondrocalcinosis, unspecified site
+ M11.21 Other chondrocalcinosis, shoulder
M11.211 Other chondrocalcinosis, right shoulder
M11.212 Other chondrocalcinosis, left shoulder
M11.219 Other chondrocalcinosis, unspecified shoulder
+ M11.22 Other chondrocalcinosis, elbow
M11.221 Other chondrocalcinosis, right elbow
M11.222 Other chondrocalcinosis, left elbow
M11.229 Other chondrocalcinosis, unspecified elbow
+ M11.23 Other chondrocalcinosis, wrist
M11.231 Other chondrocalcinosis, right wrist
M11.232 Other chondrocalcinosis, left wrist
M11.239 Other chondrocalcinosis, unspecified wrist
+ M11.24 Other chondrocalcinosis, hand
M11.241 Other chondrocalcinosis, right hand
M11.242 Other chondrocalcinosis, left hand
M11.249 Other chondrocalcinosis, unspecified hand
+ M11.25 Other chondrocalcinosis, hip
M11.251 Other chondrocalcinosis, right hip
M11.252 Other chondrocalcinosis, left hip
M11.259 Other chondrocalcinosis, unspecified hip
+ M11.26 Other chondrocalcinosis, knee
M11.261 Other chondrocalcinosis, right knee
M11.262 Other chondrocalcinosis, left knee
M11.269 Other chondrocalcinosis, unspecified knee
+ M11.27 Other chondrocalcinosis, ankle and foot
M11.271 Other chondrocalcinosis, right ankle and foot
M11.272 Other chondrocalcinosis, left ankle and foot
M11.279 Other chondrocalcinosis, unspecified ankle and foot
M11.28 Other chondrocalcinosis, vertebrae
M11.29 Other chondrocalcinosis, multiple sites
+ M11.8 Other specified crystal arthropathies
M11.80 Other specified crystal arthropathies, unspecified site
+ M11.81 Other specified crystal arthropathies, shoulder
M11.811 Other specified crystal arthropathies, right shoulder
M11.812 Other specified crystal arthropathies, left shoulder
M11.819 Other specified crystal arthropathies, unspecified shoulder

+ **M11.82 Other specified crystal arthropathies, elbow**
  - **M11.821 Other specified crystal arthropathies, right elbow**
  - **M11.822 Other specified crystal arthropathies, left elbow**
  - **M11.829 Other specified crystal arthropathies, unspecified elbow**

+ **M11.83 Other specified crystal arthropathies, wrist**
  - **M11.831 Other specified crystal arthropathies, right wrist**
  - **M11.832 Other specified crystal arthropathies, left wrist**
  - **M11.839 Other specified crystal arthropathies, unspecified wrist**

+ **M11.84 Other specified crystal arthropathies, hand**
  - **M11.841 Other specified crystal arthropathies, right hand**
  - **M11.842 Other specified crystal arthropathies, left hand**
  - **M11.849 Other specified crystal arthropathies, unspecified hand**

+ **M11.85 Other specified crystal arthropathies, hip**
  - **M11.851 Other specified crystal arthropathies, right hip**
  - **M11.852 Other specified crystal arthropathies, left hip**
  - **M11.859 Other specified crystal arthropathies, unspecified hip**

+ **M11.86 Other specified crystal arthropathies, knee**
  - **M11.861 Other specified crystal arthropathies, right knee**
  - **M11.862 Other specified crystal arthropathies, left knee**
  - **M11.869 Other specified crystal arthropathies, unspecified knee**

+ **M11.87 Other specified crystal arthropathies, ankle and foot**
  - **M11.871 Other specified crystal arthropathies, right ankle and foot**
  - **M11.872 Other specified crystal arthropathies, left ankle and foot**
  - **M11.879 Other specified crystal arthropathies, unspecified ankle and foot**

M11.88 Other specified crystal arthropathies, vertebrae

M11.89 Other specified crystal arthropathies, multiple sites

M11.9 Crystal arthropathy, unspecified

M12 Other and unspecified arthropathy

Excludes1: *arthrosis (M15-M19)*
cricoarytenoid arthropathy (J38.7)

+ **M12.0 Chronic postrheumatic arthropathy [Jaccoud]**
  - **M12.00 Chronic postrheumatic arthropathy [Jaccoud], unspecified site**
  - + **M12.01 Chronic postrheumatic arthropathy [Jaccoud], shoulder**
    - **M12.011 Chronic postrheumatic arthropathy [Jaccoud], right shoulder**
    - **M12.012 Chronic postrheumatic arthropathy [Jaccoud], left shoulder**
    - **M12.019 Chronic postrheumatic arthropathy [Jaccoud], unspecified shoulder**
  - + **M12.02 Chronic postrheumatic arthropathy [Jaccoud], elbow**
    - **M12.021 Chronic postrheumatic arthropathy [Jaccoud], right elbow**
    - **M12.022 Chronic postrheumatic arthropathy [Jaccoud], left elbow**
    - **M12.029 Chronic postrheumatic arthropathy [Jaccoud], unspecified elbow**
  - + **M12.03 Chronic postrheumatic arthropathy [Jaccoud], wrist**
    - **M12.031 Chronic postrheumatic arthropathy [Jaccoud], right wrist**
    - **M12.032 Chronic postrheumatic arthropathy [Jaccoud], left wrist**
    - **M12.039 Chronic postrheumatic arthropathy [Jaccoud], unspecified wrist**
  - + **M12.04 Chronic postrheumatic arthropathy [Jaccoud], hand**
    - **M12.041 Chronic postrheumatic arthropathy [Jaccoud], right hand**
    - **M12.042 Chronic postrheumatic arthropathy [Jaccoud], left hand**
    - **M12.049 Chronic postrheumatic arthropathy [Jaccoud], unspecified hand**
  - + **M12.05 Chronic postrheumatic arthropathy [Jaccoud], hip**
    - **M12.051 Chronic postrheumatic arthropathy [Jaccoud], right hip**
    - **M12.052 Chronic postrheumatic arthropathy [Jaccoud], left hip**
    - **M12.059 Chronic postrheumatic arthropathy [Jaccoud], unspecified hip**
  - + **M12.06 Chronic postrheumatic arthropathy [Jaccoud], knee**
    - **M12.061 Chronic postrheumatic arthropathy [Jaccoud], right knee**
    - **M12.062 Chronic postrheumatic arthropathy [Jaccoud], left knee**
    - **M12.069 Chronic postrheumatic arthropathy [Jaccoud], unspecified knee**
  - + **M12.07 Chronic postrheumatic arthropathy [Jaccoud], ankle and foot**
    - **M12.071 Chronic postrheumatic arthropathy [Jaccoud], right ankle and foot**
    - **M12.072 Chronic postrheumatic arthropathy [Jaccoud], left ankle and foot**
    - **M12.079 Chronic postrheumatic arthropathy [Jaccoud], unspecified ankle and foot**
  - **M12.08 Chronic postrheumatic arthropathy [Jaccoud], other specified site**
    Chronic postrheumatic arthropathy [Jaccoud], vertebrae
  - **M12.09 Chronic postrheumatic arthropathy [Jaccoud], multiple sites**

+ **M12.1 Kaschin-Beck disease**
  Osteochondroarthrosis deformans endemica
  - **M12.10 Kaschin-Beck disease, unspecified site**
  - + **M12.11 Kaschin-Beck disease, shoulder**
    - **M12.111 Kaschin-Beck disease, right shoulder**
    - **M12.112 Kaschin-Beck disease, left shoulder**
    - **M12.119 Kaschin-Beck disease, unspecified shoulder**
  - + **M12.12 Kaschin-Beck disease, elbow**
    - **M12.121 Kaschin-Beck disease, right elbow**
    - **M12.122 Kaschin-Beck disease, left elbow**
    - **M12.129 Kaschin-Beck disease, unspecified elbow**
  - + **M12.13 Kaschin-Beck disease, wrist**
    - **M12.131 Kaschin-Beck disease, right wrist**
    - **M12.132 Kaschin-Beck disease, left wrist**
    - **M12.139 Kaschin-Beck disease, unspecified wrist**
  - + **M12.14 Kaschin-Beck disease, hand**
    - **M12.141 Kaschin-Beck disease, right hand**
    - **M12.142 Kaschin-Beck disease, left hand**
    - **M12.149 Kaschin-Beck disease, unspecified hand**
  - + **M12.15 Kaschin-Beck disease, hip**
    - **M12.151 Kaschin-Beck disease, right hip**
    - **M12.152 Kaschin-Beck disease, left hip**
    - **M12.159 Kaschin-Beck disease, unspecified hip**
  - + **M12.16 Kaschin-Beck disease, knee**
    - **M12.161 Kaschin-Beck disease, right knee**
    - **M12.162 Kaschin-Beck disease, left knee**
    - **M12.169 Kaschin-Beck disease, unspecified knee**
  - + **M12.17 Kaschin-Beck disease, ankle and foot**
    - **M12.171 Kaschin-Beck disease, right ankle and foot**
    - **M12.172 Kaschin-Beck disease, left ankle and foot**
    - **M12.179 Kaschin-Beck disease, unspecified ankle and foot**
  - **M12.18 Kaschin-Beck disease, vertebrae**
  - **M12.19 Kaschin-Beck disease, multiple sites**

+ **M12.2 Villonodular synovitis (pigmented)**
  - **M12.20 Villonodular synovitis (pigmented), unspecified site**
  - + **M12.21 Villonodular synovitis (pigmented), shoulder**
    - **M12.211 Villonodular synovitis (pigmented), right shoulder**
    - **M12.212 Villonodular synovitis (pigmented), left shoulder**
    - **M12.219 Villonodular synovitis (pigmented), unspecified shoulder**
  - + **M12.22 Villonodular synovitis (pigmented), elbow**
    - **M12.221 Villonodular synovitis (pigmented), right elbow**
    - **M12.222 Villonodular synovitis (pigmented), left elbow**
    - **M12.229 Villonodular synovitis (pigmented), unspecified elbow**

+ M12.23 Villonodular synovitis (pigmented), wrist
M12.231 Villonodular synovitis (pigmented), right wrist
M12.232 Villonodular synovitis (pigmented), left wrist
M12.239 Villonodular synovitis (pigmented), unspecified wrist
+ M12.24 Villonodular synovitis (pigmented), hand
M12.241 Villonodular synovitis (pigmented), right hand
M12.242 Villonodular synovitis (pigmented), left hand
M12.249 Villonodular synovitis (pigmented), unspecified hand
+ M12.25 Villonodular synovitis (pigmented), hip
M12.251 Villonodular synovitis (pigmented), right hip
M12.252 Villonodular synovitis (pigmented), left hip
M12.259 Villonodular synovitis (pigmented), unspecified hip
+ M12.26 Villonodular synovitis (pigmented), knee
M12.261 Villonodular synovitis (pigmented), right knee
M12.262 Villonodular synovitis (pigmented), left knee
M12.269 Villonodular synovitis (pigmented), unspecified knee
+ M12.27 Villonodular synovitis (pigmented), ankle and foot
M12.271 Villonodular synovitis (pigmented), right ankle and foot
M12.272 Villonodular synovitis (pigmented), left ankle and foot
M12.279 Villonodular synovitis (pigmented), unspecified ankle and foot
M12.28 Villonodular synovitis (pigmented), other specified site
Villonodular synovitis (pigmented), vertebrae
M12.29 Villonodular synovitis (pigmented), multiple sites
+ M12.3 Palindromic rheumatism
M12.30 Palindromic rheumatism, unspecified site
+ M12.31 Palindromic rheumatism, shoulder
M12.311 Palindromic rheumatism, right shoulder
M12.312 Palindromic rheumatism, left shoulder
M12.319 Palindromic rheumatism, unspecified shoulder
+ M12.32 Palindromic rheumatism, elbow
M12.321 Palindromic rheumatism, right elbow
M12.322 Palindromic rheumatism, left elbow
M12.329 Palindromic rheumatism, unspecified elbow
+ M12.33 Palindromic rheumatism, wrist
M12.331 Palindromic rheumatism, right wrist
M12.332 Palindromic rheumatism, left wrist
M12.339 Palindromic rheumatism, unspecified wrist
+ M12.34 Palindromic rheumatism, hand
M12.341 Palindromic rheumatism, right hand
M12.342 Palindromic rheumatism, left hand
M12.349 Palindromic rheumatism, unspecified hand
+ M12.35 Palindromic rheumatism, hip
M12.351 Palindromic rheumatism, right hip
M12.352 Palindromic rheumatism, left hip
M12.359 Palindromic rheumatism, unspecified hip
+ M12.36 Palindromic rheumatism, knee
M12.361 Palindromic rheumatism, right knee
M12.362 Palindromic rheumatism, left knee
M12.369 Palindromic rheumatism, unspecified knee
+ M12.37 Palindromic rheumatism, ankle and foot
M12.371 Palindromic rheumatism, right ankle and foot
M12.372 Palindromic rheumatism, left ankle and foot
M12.379 Palindromic rheumatism, unspecified ankle and foot
M12.38 Palindromic rheumatism, other specified site
Palindromic rheumatism, vertebrae
M12.39 Palindromic rheumatism, multiple sites
+ M12.4 Intermittent hydrarthrosis
M12.40 Intermittent hydrarthrosis, unspecified site
+ M12.41 Intermittent hydrarthrosis, shoulder
M12.411 Intermittent hydrarthrosis, right shoulder
M12.412 Intermittent hydrarthrosis, left shoulder
M12.419 Intermittent hydrarthrosis, unspecified shoulder
+ M12.42 Intermittent hydrarthrosis, elbow
M12.421 Intermittent hydrarthrosis, right elbow
M12.422 Intermittent hydrarthrosis, left elbow
M12.429 Intermittent hydrarthrosis, unspecified elbow
+ M12.43 Intermittent hydrarthrosis, wrist
M12.431 Intermittent hydrarthrosis, right wrist
M12.432 Intermittent hydrarthrosis, left wrist
M12.439 Intermittent hydrarthrosis, unspecified wrist
+ M12.44 Intermittent hydrarthrosis, hand
M12.441 Intermittent hydrarthrosis, right hand
M12.442 Intermittent hydrarthrosis, left hand
M12.449 Intermittent hydrarthrosis, unspecified hand
+ M12.45 Intermittent hydrarthrosis, hip
M12.451 Intermittent hydrarthrosis, right hip
M12.452 Intermittent hydrarthrosis, left hip
M12.459 Intermittent hydrarthrosis, unspecified hip
+ M12.46 Intermittent hydrarthrosis, knee
M12.461 Intermittent hydrarthrosis, right knee
M12.462 Intermittent hydrarthrosis, left knee
M12.469 Intermittent hydrarthrosis, unspecified knee
+ M12.47 Intermittent hydrarthrosis, ankle and foot
M12.471 Intermittent hydrarthrosis, right ankle and foot
M12.472 Intermittent hydrarthrosis, left ankle and foot
M12.479 Intermittent hydrarthrosis, unspecified ankle and foot
M12.48 Intermittent hydrarthrosis, other site
M12.49 Intermittent hydrarthrosis, multiple sites
+ M12.5 Traumatic arthropathy
Excludes1: *current injury-see Alphabetic Index*
post-traumatic osteoarthritis of first carpometacarpal joint (M18.2-M18.3)
post-traumatic osteoarthritis of hip (M16.4-M16.5)
post-traumatic osteoarthritis of knee (M17.2-M17.3)
post-traumatic osteoarthritis NOS (M19.1-)
post-traumatic osteoarthritis of other single joints (M19.1-)
M12.50 Traumatic arthropathy, unspecified site
+ M12.51 Traumatic arthropathy, shoulder
M12.511 Traumatic arthropathy, right shoulder
M12.512 Traumatic arthropathy, left shoulder
M12.519 Traumatic arthropathy, unspecified shoulder
+ M12.52 Traumatic arthropathy, elbow
M12.521 Traumatic arthropathy, right elbow
M12.522 Traumatic arthropathy, left elbow
M12.529 Traumatic arthropathy, unspecified elbow
+ M12.53 Traumatic arthropathy, wrist
M12.531 Traumatic arthropathy, right wrist
M12.532 Traumatic arthropathy, left wrist
M12.539 Traumatic arthropathy, unspecified wrist
+ M12.54 Traumatic arthropathy, hand
M12.541 Traumatic arthropathy, right hand
M12.542 Traumatic arthropathy, left hand
M12.549 Traumatic arthropathy, unspecified hand
+ M12.55 Traumatic arthropathy, hip
M12.551 Traumatic arthropathy, right hip
M12.552 Traumatic arthropathy, left hip
AHA CC: 1Q, 2015, 17-18
M12.559 Traumatic arthropathy, unspecified hip
+ M12.56 Traumatic arthropathy, knee
M12.561 Traumatic arthropathy, right knee
M12.562 Traumatic arthropathy, left knee
M12.569 Traumatic arthropathy, unspecified knee
+ M12.57 Traumatic arthropathy, ankle and foot
M12.571 Traumatic arthropathy, right ankle and foot
M12.572 Traumatic arthropathy, left ankle and foot
M12.579 Traumatic arthropathy, unspecified ankle and foot

M12.58 Traumatic arthropathy, other specified site
Traumatic arthropathy, vertebrae
M12.59 Traumatic arthropathy, multiple sites
+ M12.8 Other specific arthropathies, not elsewhere classified
Transient arthropathy
M12.80 Other specific arthropathies, not elsewhere classified, unspecified site
+ M12.81 Other specific arthropathies, not elsewhere classified, shoulder
M12.811 Other specific arthropathies, not elsewhere classified, right shoulder
M12.812 Other specific arthropathies, not elsewhere classified, left shoulder
M12.819 Other specific arthropathies, not elsewhere classified, unspecified shoulder
+ M12.82 Other specific arthropathies, not elsewhere classified, elbow
M12.821 Other specific arthropathies, not elsewhere classified, right elbow
M12.822 Other specific arthropathies, not elsewhere classified, left elbow
M12.829 Other specific arthropathies, not elsewhere classified, unspecified elbow
+ M12.83 Other specific arthropathies, not elsewhere classified, wrist
M12.831 Other specific arthropathies, not elsewhere classified, right wrist
M12.832 Other specific arthropathies, not elsewhere classified, left wrist
M12.839 Other specific arthropathies, not elsewhere classified, unspecified wrist
+ M12.84 Other specific arthropathies, not elsewhere classified, hand
M12.841 Other specific arthropathies, not elsewhere classified, right hand
M12.842 Other specific arthropathies, not elsewhere classified, left hand
M12.849 Other specific arthropathies, not elsewhere classified, unspecified hand
+ M12.85 Other specific arthropathies, not elsewhere classified, hip
M12.851 Other specific arthropathies, not elsewhere classified, right hip
M12.852 Other specific arthropathies, not elsewhere classified, left hip
M12.859 Other specific arthropathies, not elsewhere classified, unspecified hip
+ M12.86 Other specific arthropathies, not elsewhere classified, knee
M12.861 Other specific arthropathies, not elsewhere classified, right knee
M12.862 Other specific arthropathies, not elsewhere classified, left knee
M12.869 Other specific arthropathies, not elsewhere classified, unspecified knee
+ M12.87 Other specific arthropathies, not elsewhere classified, ankle and foot
M12.871 Other specific arthropathies, not elsewhere classified, right ankle and foot
M12.872 Other specific arthropathies, not elsewhere classified, left ankle and foot
M12.879 Other specific arthropathies, not elsewhere classified, unspecified ankle and foot
M12.88 Other specific arthropathies, not elsewhere classified, other specified site
Other specific arthropathies, not elsewhere classified, vertebrae
M12.89 Other specific arthropathies, not elsewhere classified, multiple sites
M12.9 Arthropathy, unspecified

M13 Other arthritis

Excludes1: *arthrosis (M15-M19)*
osteoarthritis (M15-M19)

M13.0 Polyarthritis, unspecified
+ M13.1 Monoarthritis, not elsewhere classified
M13.10 Monoarthritis, not elsewhere classified, unspecified site
+ M13.11 Monoarthritis, not elsewhere classified, shoulder
M13.111 Monoarthritis, not elsewhere classified, right shoulder
M13.112 Monoarthritis, not elsewhere classified, left shoulder
M13.119 Monoarthritis, not elsewhere classified, unspecified shoulder
+ M13.12 Monoarthritis, not elsewhere classified, elbow
M13.121 Monoarthritis, not elsewhere classified, right elbow
M13.122 Monoarthritis, not elsewhere classified, left elbow
M13.129 Monoarthritis, not elsewhere classified, unspecified elbow
+ M13.13 Monoarthritis, not elsewhere classified, wrist
M13.131 Monoarthritis, not elsewhere classified, right wrist
M13.132 Monoarthritis, not elsewhere classified, left wrist
M13.139 Monoarthritis, not elsewhere classified, unspecified wrist
+ M13.14 Monoarthritis, not elsewhere classified, hand
M13.141 Monoarthritis, not elsewhere classified, right hand
M13.142 Monoarthritis, not elsewhere classified, left hand
M13.149 Monoarthritis, not elsewhere classified, unspecified hand
+ M13.15 Monoarthritis, not elsewhere classified, hip
M13.151 Monoarthritis, not elsewhere classified, right hip
M13.152 Monoarthritis, not elsewhere classified, left hip
M13.159 Monoarthritis, not elsewhere classified, unspecified hip
+ M13.16 Monoarthritis, not elsewhere classified, knee
M13.161 Monoarthritis, not elsewhere classified, right knee
M13.162 Monoarthritis, not elsewhere classified, left knee
M13.169 Monoarthritis, not elsewhere classified, unspecified knee
+ M13.17 Monoarthritis, not elsewhere classified, ankle and foot
M13.171 Monoarthritis, not elsewhere classified, right ankle and foot
M13.172 Monoarthritis, not elsewhere classified, left ankle and foot
M13.179 Monoarthritis, not elsewhere classified, unspecified ankle and foot
+ M13.8 Other specified arthritis
Allergic arthritis
Excludes1: *osteoarthritis (M15-M19)*
M13.80 Other specified arthritis, unspecified site
+ M13.81 Other specified arthritis, shoulder
M13.811 Other specified arthritis, right shoulder
M13.812 Other specified arthritis, left shoulder
M13.819 Other specified arthritis, unspecified shoulder
+ M13.82 Other specified arthritis, elbow
M13.821 Other specified arthritis, right elbow
M13.822 Other specified arthritis, left elbow
M13.829 Other specified arthritis, unspecified elbow
+ M13.83 Other specified arthritis, wrist
M13.831 Other specified arthritis, right wrist
M13.832 Other specified arthritis, left wrist
M13.839 Other specified arthritis, unspecified wrist
+ M13.84 Other specified arthritis, hand
M13.841 Other specified arthritis, right hand
M13.842 Other specified arthritis, left hand
M13.849 Other specified arthritis, unspecified hand
+ M13.85 Other specified arthritis, hip
M13.851 Other specified arthritis, right hip
M13.852 Other specified arthritis, left hip
M13.859 Other specified arthritis, unspecified hip
+ M13.86 Other specified arthritis, knee
M13.861 Other specified arthritis, right knee
M13.862 Other specified arthritis, left knee
M13.869 Other specified arthritis, unspecified knee
+ M13.87 Other specified arthritis, ankle and foot
M13.871 Other specified arthritis, right ankle and foot

M13.872 Other specified arthritis, left ankle and foot
M13.879 Other specified arthritis, unspecified ankle and foot
M13.88 Other specified arthritis, other site
M13.89 Other specified arthritis, multiple sites

M14 Arthropathies in other diseases classified elsewhere

Excludes1: *arthropathy in:*
diabetes mellitus (E08-E13 with .61-)
hematological disorders (M36.2-M36.3)
hypersensitivity reactions (M36.4)
neoplastic disease (M36.1)
neurosyphillis (A52.16)
sarcoidosis (D86.86)
enteropathic arthropathies (M07.-)
juvenile psoriatic arthropathy (L40.54)
lipoid dermatoarthritis (E78.81)

+ M14.6 Charcôt's joint
Neuropathic arthropathy
Excludes1: *Charcôt's joint in diabetes mellitus (E08-E13 with .610)*
Charcôt's joint in tabes dorsalis (A52.16)
M14.60 Charcôt's joint, unspecified site
+ M14.61 Charcôt's joint, shoulder
M14.611 Charcôt's joint, right shoulder
M14.612 Charcôt's joint, left shoulder
M14.619 Charcôt's joint, unspecified shoulder
+ M14.62 Charcôt's joint, elbow
M14.621 Charcôt's joint, right elbow
M14.622 Charcôt's joint, left elbow
M14.629 Charcôt's joint, unspecified elbow
+ M14.63 Charcôt's joint, wrist
M14.631 Charcôt's joint, right wrist
M14.632 Charcôt's joint, left wrist
M14.639 Charcôt's joint, unspecified wrist
+ M14.64 Charcôt's joint, hand
M14.641 Charcôt's joint, right hand
M14.642 Charcôt's joint, left hand
M14.649 Charcôt's joint, unspecified hand
+ M14.65 Charcôt's joint, hip
M14.651 Charcôt's joint, right hip
M14.652 Charcôt's joint, left hip
M14.659 Charcôt's joint, unspecified hip
+ M14.66 Charcôt's joint, knee
M14.661 Charcôt's joint, right knee
M14.662 Charcôt's joint, left knee
M14.669 Charcôt's joint, unspecified knee
+ M14.67 Charcôt's joint, ankle and foot
M14.671 Charcôt's joint, right ankle and foot
M14.672 Charcôt's joint, left ankle and foot
M14.679 Charcôt's joint, unspecified ankle and foot
M14.68 Charcôt's joint, vertebrae
M14.69 Charcôt's joint, multiple sites

+ M14.8 Arthropathies in other specified diseases classified elsewhere
Code first underlying disease, such as:
amyloidosis (E85.-)
erythema multiforme (L51.-)
erythema nodosum (L52)
hemochromatosis (E83.11-)
hyperparathyroidism (E21.-)
hypothyroidism (E00-E03)
sickle-cell disorders (D57.-)
thyrotoxicosis [hyperthyroidism] (E05.-)
Whipple's disease (K90.81)
M14.80 Arthropathies in other specified diseases classified elsewhere, unspecified site
+ M14.81 Arthropathies in other specified diseases classified elsewhere, shoulder
M14.811 Arthropathies in other specified diseases classified elsewhere, right shoulder
M14.812 Arthropathies in other specified diseases classified elsewhere, left shoulder
M14.819 Arthropathies in other specified diseases classified elsewhere, unspecified shoulder
+ M14.82 Arthropathies in other specified diseases classified elsewhere, elbow
M14.821 Arthropathies in other specified diseases classified elsewhere, right elbow
M14.822 Arthropathies in other specified diseases classified elsewhere, left elbow
M14.829 Arthropathies in other specified diseases classified elsewhere, unspecified elbow
+ M14.83 Arthropathies in other specified diseases classified elsewhere, wrist
M14.831 Arthropathies in other specified diseases classified elsewhere, right wrist
M14.832 Arthropathies in other specified diseases classified elsewhere, left wrist
M14.839 Arthropathies in other specified diseases classified elsewhere, unspecified wrist
+ M14.84 Arthropathies in other specified diseases classified elsewhere, hand
M14.841 Arthropathies in other specified diseases classified elsewhere, right hand
M14.842 Arthropathies in other specified diseases classified elsewhere, left hand
M14.849 Arthropathies in other specified diseases classified elsewhere, unspecified hand
+ M14.85 Arthropathies in other specified diseases classified elsewhere, hip
M14.851 Arthropathies in other specified diseases classified elsewhere, right hip
M14.852 Arthropathies in other specified diseases classified elsewhere, left hip
M14.859 Arthropathies in other specified diseases classified elsewhere, unspecified hip
+ M14.86 Arthropathies in other specified diseases classified elsewhere, knee
M14.861 Arthropathies in other specified diseases classified elsewhere, right knee
M14.862 Arthropathies in other specified diseases classified elsewhere, left knee
M14.869 Arthropathies in other specified diseases classified elsewhere, unspecified knee
+ M14.87 Arthropathies in other specified diseases classified elsewhere, ankle and foot
M14.871 Arthropathies in other specified diseases classified elsewhere, right ankle and foot
M14.872 Arthropathies in other specified diseases classified elsewhere, left ankle and foot
M14.879 Arthropathies in other specified diseases classified elsewhere, unspecified ankle and foot
M14.88 Arthropathies in other specified diseases classified elsewhere, vertebrae
M14.89 Arthropathies in other specified diseases classified elsewhere, multiple sites

Osteoarthritis (M15-M19)

Excludes2: *osteoarthritis of spine (M47.-)*

M15 Polyosteoarthritis

Includes: arthritis of multiple sites
Excludes1: *bilateral involvement of single joint (M16-M19)*
M15.0 Primary generalized (osteo)arthritis
M15.1 Heberden's nodes (with arthropathy)
Interphalangeal distal osteoarthritis
M15.2 Bouchard's nodes (with arthropathy)
Juxtaphalangeal distal osteoarthritis
M15.3 Secondary multiple arthritis
Post-traumatic polyosteoarthritis
M15.4 Erosive (osteo)arthritis
M15.8 Other polyosteoarthritis
M15.9 Polyosteoarthritis, unspecified
Generalized osteoarthritis NOS

M16 Osteoarthritis of hip

M16.0 Bilateral primary osteoarthritis of hip
AHA CC: 4Q, 2016, 146
+ M16.1 Unilateral primary osteoarthritis of hip
Primary osteoarthritis of hip NOS
M16.10 Unilateral primary osteoarthritis, unspecified hip
M16.11 Unilateral primary osteoarthritis, right hip
M16.12 Unilateral primary osteoarthritis, left hip
M16.2 Bilateral osteoarthritis resulting from hip dysplasia
+ M16.3 Unilateral osteoarthritis resulting from hip dysplasia
Dysplastic osteoarthritis of hip NOS
M16.30 Unilateral osteoarthritis resulting from hip dysplasia, unspecified hip

M16.31 Unilateral osteoarthritis resulting from hip dysplasia, right hip
M16.32 Unilateral osteoarthritis resulting from hip dysplasia, left hip
M16.4 Bilateral post-traumatic osteoarthritis of hip
+ M16.5 Unilateral post-traumatic osteoarthritis of hip
Post-traumatic osteoarthritis of hip NOS
M16.50 Unilateral post-traumatic osteoarthritis, unspecified hip
M16.51 Unilateral post-traumatic osteoarthritis, right hip
M16.52 Unilateral post-traumatic osteoarthritis, left hip
M16.6 Other bilateral secondary osteoarthritis of hip
M16.7 Other unilateral secondary osteoarthritis of hip
Secondary osteoarthritis of hip NOS
M16.9 Osteoarthritis of hip, unspecified

M17 Osteoarthritis of knee

M17.0 Bilateral primary osteoarthritis of knee
+ M17.1 Unilateral primary osteoarthritis of knee
Primary osteoarthritis of knee NOS
M17.10 Unilateral primary osteoarthritis, unspecified knee
AHA CC: 4Q, 2016, 147
M17.11 Unilateral primary osteoarthritis, right knee
M17.12 Unilateral primary osteoarthritis, left knee
AHA CC: 4Q, 2016, 146
M17.2 Bilateral post-traumatic osteoarthritis of knee
+ M17.3 Unilateral post-traumatic osteoarthritis of knee
Post-traumatic osteoarthritis of knee NOS
M17.30 Unilateral post-traumatic osteoarthritis, unspecified knee
M17.31 Unilateral post-traumatic osteoarthritis, right knee
M17.32 Unilateral post-traumatic osteoarthritis, left knee
M17.4 Other bilateral secondary osteoarthritis of knee
M17.5 Other unilateral secondary osteoarthritis of knee
Secondary osteoarthritis of knee NOS
M17.9 Osteoarthritis of knee, unspecified

M18 Osteoarthritis of first carpometacarpal joint

M18.0 Bilateral primary osteoarthritis of first carpometacarpal joints
+ M18.1 Unilateravl primary osteoarthritis of first carpometacarpal joint
Primary osteoarthritis of first carpometacarpal joint NOS
M18.10 Unilateral primary osteoarthritis of first carpometacarpal joint, unspecified hand
M18.11 Unilateral primary osteoarthritis of first carpometacarpal joint, right hand
M18.12 Unilateral primary osteoarthritis of first carpometacarpal joint, left hand
M18.2 Bilateral post-traumatic osteoarthritis of first carpometacarpal joints
+ M18.3 Unilateral post-traumatic osteoarthritis of first carpometacarpal joint
Post-traumatic osteoarthritis of first carpometacarpal joint NOS
M18.30 Unilateral post-traumatic osteoarthritis of first carpometacarpal joint, unspecified hand
M18.31 Unilateral post-traumatic osteoarthritis of first carpometacarpal joint, right hand
M18.32 Unilateral post-traumatic osteoarthritis of first carpometacarpal joint, left hand
M18.4 Other bilateral secondary osteoarthritis of first carpometacarpal joints
+ M18.5 Other unilateral secondary osteoarthritis of first carpometacarpal joint
Secondary osteoarthritis of first carpometacarpal joint NOS
M18.50 Other unilateral secondary osteoarthritis of first carpometacarpal joint, unspecified hand
M18.51 Other unilateral secondary osteoarthritis of first carpometacarpal joint, right hand
M18.52 Other unilateral secondary osteoarthritis of first carpometacarpal joint, left hand
M18.9 Osteoarthritis of first carpometacarpal joint, unspecified

M19 Other and unspecified osteoarthritis

Excludes1: *polyarthritis (M15.-)*
Excludes2: *arthrosis of spine (M47.-)*
hallux rigidus (M20.2)
osteoarthritis of spine (M47.-)

+ M19.0 Primary osteoarthritis of other joints
+ M19.01 Primary osteoarthritis, shoulder
M19.011 Primary osteoarthritis, right shoulder
AHA CC: 4Q, 2016, 145
M19.012 Primary osteoarthritis, left shoulder
M19.019 Primary osteoarthritis, unspecified shoulder
+ M19.02 Primary osteoarthritis, elbow
M19.021 Primary osteoarthritis, right elbow
M19.022 Primary osteoarthritis, left elbow
M19.029 Primary osteoarthritis, unspecified elbow
+ M19.03 Primary osteoarthritis, wrist
M19.031 Primary osteoarthritis, right wrist
M19.032 Primary osteoarthritis, left wrist
M19.039 Primary osteoarthritis, unspecified wrist
+ M19.04 Primary osteoarthritis, hand
Excludes2: *primary osteoarthritis of first carpometacarpaljoint(M18.0-,M18.1-)*
M19.041 Primary osteoarthritis, right hand
M19.042 Primary osteoarthritis, left hand
M19.049 Primary osteoarthritis, unspecified hand
+ M19.07 Primary osteoarthritis ankle and foot
M19.071 Primary osteoarthritis, right ankle and foot
M19.072 Primary osteoarthritis, left ankle and foot
M19.079 Primary osteoarthritis, unspecified ankle and foot
+ M19.1 Post-traumatic osteoarthritis of other joints
+ M19.11 Post-traumatic osteoarthritis, shoulder
M19.111 Post-traumatic osteoarthritis, right shoulde
M19.112 Post-traumatic osteoarthritis, left shoulde
M19.119 Post-traumatic osteoarthritis, unspecified shoulder
+ M19.12 Post-traumatic osteoarthritis, elbow
M19.121 Post-traumatic osteoarthritis, right elbow
M19.122 Post-traumatic osteoarthritis, left elbow
M19.129 Post-traumatic osteoarthritis, unspecified elbow
+ M19.13 Post-traumatic osteoarthritis, wrist
M19.131 Post-traumatic osteoarthritis, right wrist
M19.132 Post-traumatic osteoarthritis, left wrist
M19.139 Post-traumatic osteoarthritis, unspecified wrist
+ M19.14 Post-traumatic osteoarthritis, hand
Excludes2: *post-traumatic osteoarthritis of first carpometacarpaljoint(M18.2-,M18.3-)*
M19.141 Post-traumatic osteoarthritis, right hand
M19.142 Post-traumatic osteoarthritis, left hand
M19.149 Post-traumatic osteoarthritis, unspecified hand
+ M19.17 Post-traumatic osteoarthritis, ankle and foot
M19.171 Post-traumatic osteoarthritis, right ankle and foot
M19.172 Post-traumatic osteoarthritis, left ankle and foot
M19.179 Post-traumatic osteoarthritis, unspecified ankle and foot
+ M19.2 Secondary osteoarthritis of other joints
+ M19.21 Secondary osteoarthritis, shoulder
M19.211 Secondary osteoarthritis, right shoulder
M19.212 Secondary osteoarthritis, left shoulder
M19.219 Secondary osteoarthritis, unspecified shoulder
+ M19.22 Secondary osteoarthritis, elbow
M19.221 Secondary osteoarthritis, right elbow
M19.222 Secondary osteoarthritis, left elbow
M19.229 Secondary osteoarthritis, unspecified elbo
+ M19.23 Secondary osteoarthritis, wrist
M19.231 Secondary osteoarthritis, right wrist
M19.232 Secondary osteoarthritis, left wrist
M19.239 Secondary osteoarthritis, unspecified wris
+ M19.24 Secondary osteoarthritis, hand
M19.241 Secondary osteoarthritis, right hand
M19.242 Secondary osteoarthritis, left hand
M19.249 Secondary osteoarthritis, unspecified han
+ M19.27 Secondary osteoarthritis, ankle and foot
M19.271 Secondary osteoarthritis, right ankle and foot
M19.272 Secondary osteoarthritis, left ankle and fo
M19.279 Secondary osteoarthritis, unspecified ank and foot
+ M19.9 Osteoarthritis, unspecified site
M19.90 Unspecified osteoarthritis, unspecified site
Arthrosis NOS
Arthritis NOS
Osteoarthritis NOS
AHA CC: 4Q, 2016, 147

M19.91 Primary osteoarthritis, unspecified site
Primary osteoarthritis NOS
M19.92 Post-traumatic osteoarthritis, unspecified site
Post-traumatic osteoarthritis NOS
M19.93 Secondary osteoarthritis, unspecified site
Secondary osteoarthritis NOS

Other joint disorders (M20-M25)

Excludes2: *joints of the spine (M40-M54)*

M20 Acquired deformities of fingers and toes
Excludes1: *acquired absence of fingers and toes (Z89.-)*
congenital absence of fingers and toes (Q71.3-, Q72.3-)
congenital deformities and malformations of fingers and toes (Q66.-, Q68-Q70, Q74.-)

\+ **M20.0 Deformity of finger(s)**
Excludes1: *clubbing of fingers (R68.3)*
palmar fascial fibromatosis [Dupuytren] (M72.0)
trigger finger (M65.3)
\+ **M20.00 Unspecified deformity of finger(s)**
M20.001 Unspecified deformity of right finger(s)
M20.002 Unspecified deformity of left finger(s)
M20.009 Unspecified deformity of unspecified finger(s)
\+ **M20.01 Mallet finger**
M20.011 Mallet finger of right finger(s)
M20.012 Mallet finger of left finger(s)
M20.019 Mallet finger of unspecified finger(s)
\+ **M20.02 Boutonnière deformity**
M20.021 Boutonnière deformity of right finger(s)
M20.022 Boutonnière deformity of left finger(s)
M20.029 Boutonnière deformity of unspecified finger(s)
\+ **M20.03 Swan-neck deformity**
M20.031 Swan-neck deformity of right finger(s)
M20.032 Swan-neck deformity of left finger(s)
M20.039 Swan-neck deformity of unspecified finger(s)
\+ **M20.09 Other deformity of finger(s)**
M20.091 Other deformity of right finger(s)
M20.092 Other deformity of left finger(s)
M20.099 Other deformity of finger(s), unspecified finger(s)
\+ **M20.1 Hallux valgus (acquired)**
Excludes2: *bunion (M21.6-)*
M20.10 Hallux valgus (acquired), unspecified foot
M20.11 Hallux valgus (acquired), right foot
M20.12 Hallux valgus (acquired), left foot
\+ **M20.2 Hallux rigidus**
M20.20 Hallux rigidus, unspecified foot
M20.21 Hallux rigidus, right foot
M20.22 Hallux rigidus, left foot
\+ **M20.3 Hallux varus (acquired)**
M20.30 Hallux varus (acquired), unspecified foot
M20.31 Hallux varus (acquired), right foot
M20.32 Hallux varus (acquired), left foot
\+ **M20.4 Other hammer toe(s) (acquired)**
M20.40 Other hammer toe(s) (acquired), unspecified foot
M20.41 Other hammer toe(s) (acquired), right foot
M20.42 Other hammer toe(s) (acquired), left foot
\+ **M20.5 Other deformities of toe(s) (acquired)**
\+ **M20.5X Other deformities of toe(s) (acquired)**
M20.5X1 Other deformities of toe(s) (acquired), right foot
M20.5X2 Other deformities of toe(s) (acquired), left foot
M20.5X9 Other deformities of toe(s) (acquired), unspecified foot
\+ **M20.6 Acquired deformities of toe(s), unspecified**
M20.60 Acquired deformities of toe(s), unspecified, unspecified foot
M20.61 Acquired deformities of toe(s), unspecified, right foot
M20.62 Acquired deformities of toe(s), unspecified, left foot

M21 Other acquired deformities of limbs
Excludes1: *acquired absence of limb (Z89.-)*
congenital absence of limbs (Q71-Q73)
congenital deformities and malformations of limbs (Q65-Q66, Q68-Q74)
Excludes2: *acquired deformities of fingers or toes (M20.-)*
coxa plana (M91.2)

\+ **M21.0 Valgus deformity, not elsewhere classified**
Excludes1: *metatarsus valgus (Q66.6)*
talipes calcaneovalgus (Q66.4)
M21.00 Valgus deformity, not elsewhere classified, unspecified site
\+ **M21.02 Valgus deformity, not elsewhere classified, elbow**
Cubitus valgus
M21.021 Valgus deformity, not elsewhere classified, right elbow
M21.022 Valgus deformity, not elsewhere classified, left elbow
M21.029 Valgus deformity, not elsewhere classified, unspecified elbow
\+ **M21.05 Valgus deformity, not elsewhere classified, hip**
M21.051 Valgus deformity, not elsewhere classified, right hip
M21.052 Valgus deformity, not elsewhere classified, left hip
M21.059 Valgus deformity, not elsewhere classified, unspecified hip
\+ **M21.06 Valgus deformity, not elsewhere classified, knee**
Genu valgum
Knock knee
M21.061 Valgus deformity, not elsewhere classified, right knee
M21.062 Valgus deformity, not elsewhere classified, left knee
M21.069 Valgus deformity, not elsewhere classified, unspecified knee
\+ **M21.07 Valgus deformity, not elsewhere classified, ankle**
M21.071 Valgus deformity, not elsewhere classified, right ankle
M21.072 Valgus deformity, not elsewhere classified, left ankle
M21.079 Valgus deformity, not elsewhere classified, unspecified ankle
\+ **M21.1 Varus deformity, not elsewhere classified**
Excludes1: *metatarsus varus (Q66.22)*
tibia vara (M92.5)
M21.10 Varus deformity, not elsewhere classified, unspecified site
\+ **M21.12 Varus deformity, not elsewhere classified, elbow**
Cubitus varus, elbow
M21.121 Varus deformity, not elsewhere classified, right elbow
M21.122 Varus deformity, not elsewhere classified, left elbow
M21.129 Varus deformity, not elsewhere classified, unspecified elbow
\+ **M21.15 Varus deformity, not elsewhere classified, hip**
M21.151 Varus deformity, not elsewhere classified, right hip
M21.152 Varus deformity, not elsewhere classified, left hip
M21.159 Varus deformity, not elsewhere classified, unspecified
\+ **M21.16 Varus deformity, not elsewhere classified, knee**
Bow leg
Genu varum
M21.161 Varus deformity, not elsewhere classified, right knee
M21.162 Varus deformity, not elsewhere classified, left knee
M21.169 Varus deformity, not elsewhere classified, unspecified knee
\+ **M21.17 Varus deformity, not elsewhere classified, ankle**
M21.171 Varus deformity, not elsewhere classified, right ankle
M21.172 Varus deformity, not elsewhere classified, left ankle
M21.179 Varus deformity, not elsewhere classified, unspecified ankle
\+ **M21.2 Flexion deformity**
M21.20 Flexion deformity, unspecified site
\+ **M21.21 Flexion deformity, shoulder**
M21.211 Flexion deformity, right shoulder
M21.212 Flexion deformity, left shoulder
M21.219 Flexion deformity, unspecified shoulder
\+ **M21.22 Flexion deformity, elbow**
M21.221 Flexion deformity, right elbow

M21.222 Flexion deformity, left elbow
M21.229 Flexion deformity, unspecified elbow
+ M21.23 Flexion deformity, wrist
M21.231 Flexion deformity, right wrist
M21.232 Flexion deformity, left wrist
M21.239 Flexion deformity, unspecified wrist
+ M21.24 Flexion deformity, finger joints
M21.241 Flexion deformity, right finger joints
M21.242 Flexion deformity, left finger joints
M21.249 Flexion deformity, unspecified finger joints
+ M21.25 Flexion deformity, hip
M21.251 Flexion deformity, right hip
M21.252 Flexion deformity, left hip
M21.259 Flexion deformity, unspecified hip
+ M21.26 Flexion deformity, knee
M21.261 Flexion deformity, right knee
M21.262 Flexion deformity, left knee
M21.269 Flexion deformity, unspecified knee
+ M21.27 Flexion deformity, ankle and toes
M21.271 Flexion deformity, right ankle and toes
M21.272 Flexion deformity, left ankle and toes
M21.279 Flexion deformity, unspecified ankle and toes
+ M21.3 Wrist or foot drop (acquired)
+ M21.33 Wrist drop (acquired)
M21.331 Wrist drop, right wrist
M21.332 Wrist drop, left wrist
M21.339 Wrist drop, unspecified wrist
+ M21.37 Foot drop (acquired)
M21.371 Foot drop, right foot
M21.372 Foot drop, left foot
M21.379 Foot drop, unspecified foot
+ M21.4 Flat foot [pes planus] (acquired)
Excludes1: *congenital pes planus (Q66.5-)*
M21.40 Flat foot [pes planus] (acquired), unspecified foot
M21.41 Flat foot [pes planus] (acquired), right foot
M21.42 Flat foot [pes planus] (acquired), left foot
+ M21.5 Acquired clawhand, clubhand, clawfoot and clubfoot
Excludes1: *clubfoot, not specified as acquired (Q66.89)*
+ M21.51 Acquired clawhand
M21.511 Acquired clawhand, right hand
M21.512 Acquired clawhand, left hand
M21.519 Acquired clawhand, unspecified hand
+ M21.52 Acquired clubhand
M21.521 Acquired clubhand, right hand
M21.522 Acquired clubhand, left hand
M21.529 Acquired clubhand, unspecified hand
+ M21.53 Acquired clawfoot
M21.531 Acquired clawfoot, right foot
M21.532 Acquired clawfoot, left foot
M21.539 Acquired clawfoot, unspecified foot
+ M21.54 Acquired clubfoot
M21.541 Acquired clubfoot, right foot
M21.542 Acquired clubfoot, left foot
M21.549 Acquired clubfoot, unspecified foot
+ M21.6 Other acquired deformities of foot
Excludes2: *deformities of toe (acquired) (M20.1-M20.6-)*
AHA CC: 4Q, 2016, 38
+ M21.61 Bunion
M21.611 Bunion of right foot
M21.612 Bunion of left foot
M21.619 Bunion of unspecified foot
+ M21.62 Bunionette
M21.621 Bunionette of right foot
M21.622 Bunionette of left foot
M21.629 Bunionette of unspecified foot
+ M21.6X Other acquired deformities of foot
M21.6X1 Other acquired deformities of right foot
M21.6X2 Other acquired deformities of left foot
M21.6X9 Other acquired deformities of unspecified foot
+ M21.7 Unequal limb length (acquired)
NOTE The site used should correspond to the shorter limb
M21.70 Unequal limb length (acquired), unspecified site
+ M21.72 Unequal limb length (acquired), humerus
M21.721 Unequal limb length (acquired), right humerus
M21.722 Unequal limb length (acquired), left humerus
M21.729 Unequal limb length (acquired), unspecified humerus
+ M21.73 Unequal limb length (acquired), ulna and radius
M21.731 Unequal limb length (acquired), right ulna
M21.732 Unequal limb length (acquired), left ulna
M21.733 Unequal limb length (acquired), right radius
M21.734 Unequal limb length (acquired), left radius
M21.739 Unequal limb length (acquired), unspecified ulna and radius
+ M21.75 Unequal limb length (acquired), femur
M21.751 Unequal limb length (acquired), right femur
M21.752 Unequal limb length (acquired), left femur
M21.759 Unequal limb length (acquired), unspecified femur
+ M21.76 Unequal limb length (acquired), tibia and fibula
M21.761 Unequal limb length (acquired), right tibia
M21.762 Unequal limb length (acquired), left tibia
M21.763 Unequal limb length (acquired), right fibula
M21.764 Unequal limb length (acquired), left fibula
M21.769 Unequal limb length (acquired), unspecified tibia and fibula
+ M21.8 Other specified acquired deformities of limbs
Excludes2: *coxa plana (M91.2)*
M21.80 Other specified acquired deformities of unspecified limb
+ M21.82 Other specified acquired deformities of upper arm
M21.821 Other specified acquired deformities of right upper arm
M21.822 Other specified acquired deformities of left upper arm
M21.829 Other specified acquired deformities of unspecified upper arm
+ M21.83 Other specified acquired deformities of forearm
M21.831 Other specified acquired deformities of right forearm
M21.832 Other specified acquired deformities of left forearm
M21.839 Other specified acquired deformities of unspecified forearm
+ M21.85 Other specified acquired deformities of thigh
M21.851 Other specified acquired deformities of right thigh
M21.852 Other specified acquired deformities of left thigh
M21.859 Other specified acquired deformities of unspecified thigh
+ M21.86 Other specified acquired deformities of lower leg
M21.861 Other specified acquired deformities of right lower leg
M21.862 Other specified acquired deformities of left lower leg
M21.869 Other specified acquired deformities of unspecified lower leg
+ M21.9 Unspecified acquired deformity of limb and hand
M21.90 Unspecified acquired deformity of unspecified limb
+ M21.92 Unspecified acquired deformity of upper arm
M21.921 Unspecified acquired deformity of right upper arm
M21.922 Unspecified acquired deformity of left upper arm
M21.929 Unspecified acquired deformity of unspecified upper arm
+ M21.93 Unspecified acquired deformity of forearm
M21.931 Unspecified acquired deformity of right forearm
M21.932 Unspecified acquired deformity of left forearm
M21.939 Unspecified acquired deformity of unspecified forearm
+ M21.94 Unspecified acquired deformity of hand
M21.941 Unspecified acquired deformity of hand, right hand
M21.942 Unspecified acquired deformity of hand, left hand
M21.949 Unspecified acquired deformity of hand, unspecified hand
+ M21.95 Unspecified acquired deformity of thigh
M21.951 Unspecified acquired deformity of right thigh
M21.952 Unspecified acquired deformity of left thigh
M21.959 Unspecified acquired deformity of unspecified thigh

+ **M21.96 Unspecified acquired deformity of lower leg**
M21.961 Unspecified acquired deformity of right lower leg
M21.962 Unspecified acquired deformity of left lower leg
M21.969 Unspecified acquired deformity of unspecified lower leg

M22 Disorder of patella

Excludes1: *traumatic dislocation of patella (S83.0-)*

+ **M22.0 Recurrent dislocation of patella**
M22.00 Recurrent dislocation of patella, unspecified knee
M22.01 Recurrent dislocation of patella, right knee
M22.02 Recurrent dislocation of patella, left knee
+ **M22.1 Recurrent subluxation of patella**
Incomplete dislocation of patella
M22.10 Recurrent subluxation of patella, unspecified knee
M22.11 Recurrent subluxation of patella, right knee
M22.12 Recurrent subluxation of patella, left knee
+ **M22.2 Patellofemoral disorders**
+ **M22.2X Patellofemoral disorders**
M22.2X1 Patellofemoral disorders, right knee
M22.2X2 Patellofemoral disorders, left knee
M22.2X9 Patellofemoral disorders, unspecified knee
+ **M22.3 Other derangements of patella**
+ **M22.3X Other derangements of patella**
M22.3X1 Other derangements of patella, right knee
M22.3X2 Other derangements of patella, left knee
M22.3X9 Other derangements of patella, unspecified knee
+ **M22.4 Chondromalacia patellae**
M22.40 Chondromalacia patellae, unspecified knee
M22.41 Chondromalacia patellae, right knee
M22.42 Chondromalacia patellae, left knee
+ **M22.8 Other disorders of patella**
+ **M22.8X Other disorders of patella**
M22.8X1 Other disorders of patella, right knee
M22.8X2 Other disorders of patella, left knee
M22.8X9 Other disorders of patella, unspecified knee
+ **M22.9 Unspecified disorder of patella**
M22.90 Unspecified disorder of patella, unspecified knee
M22.91 Unspecified disorder of patella, right knee
M22.92 Unspecified disorder of patella, left knee

M23 Internal derangement of knee

Excludes1: *ankylosis (M24.66)*
current injury - see injury of knee and lower leg (S80-S89)
deformity of knee (M21.-)
osteochondritis dissecans (M93.2)
recurrent dislocation or subluxation of joints (M24.4)
recurrent dislocation or subluxation of patella (M22.0-M22.1)

+ **M23.0 Cystic meniscus**
+ **M23.00 Cystic meniscus, unspecified meniscus**
Cystic meniscus, unspecified lateral meniscus
Cystic meniscus, unspecified medial meniscus
M23.000 Cystic meniscus, unspecified lateral meniscus, right knee
M23.001 Cystic meniscus, unspecified lateral meniscus, left knee
M23.002 Cystic meniscus, unspecified lateral meniscus, unspecified knee
M23.003 Cystic meniscus, unspecified medial meniscus, right knee
M23.004 Cystic meniscus, unspecified medial meniscus, left knee
M23.005 Cystic meniscus, unspecified medial meniscus, unspecified knee
M23.006 Cystic meniscus, unspecified meniscus, right knee
M23.007 Cystic meniscus, unspecified meniscus, left knee
M23.009 Cystic meniscus, unspecified meniscus, unspecified knee
+ **M23.01 Cystic meniscus, anterior horn of medial meniscus**
M23.011 Cystic meniscus, anterior horn of medial meniscus, right knee
M23.012 Cystic meniscus, anterior horn of medial meniscus, left knee
M23.019 Cystic meniscus, anterior horn of medial meniscus, unspecified knee
+ **M23.02 Cystic meniscus, posterior horn of medial meniscus**
M23.021 Cystic meniscus, posterior horn of medial meniscus, right knee
M23.022 Cystic meniscus, posterior horn of medial meniscus, left knee
M23.029 Cystic meniscus, posterior horn of medial meniscus, unspecified knee
+ **M23.03 Cystic meniscus, other medial meniscus**
M23.031 Cystic meniscus, other medial meniscus, right knee
M23.032 Cystic meniscus, other medial meniscus, left knee
M23.039 Cystic meniscus, other medial meniscus, unspecified knee
+ **M23.04 Cystic meniscus, anterior horn of lateral meniscus**
M23.041 Cystic meniscus, anterior horn of lateral meniscus, right knee
M23.042 Cystic meniscus, anterior horn of lateral meniscus, left knee
M23.049 Cystic meniscus, anterior horn of lateral meniscus, unspecified knee
+ **M23.05 Cystic meniscus, posterior horn of lateral meniscus**
M23.051 Cystic meniscus, posterior horn of lateral meniscus, right knee
M23.052 Cystic meniscus, posterior horn of lateral meniscus, left knee
M23.059 Cystic meniscus, posterior horn of lateral meniscus, unspecified knee
+ **M23.06 Cystic meniscus, other lateral meniscus**
M23.061 Cystic meniscus, other lateral meniscus, right knee
M23.062 Cystic meniscus, other lateral meniscus, left knee
M23.069 Cystic meniscus, other lateral meniscus, unspecified knee
+ **M23.2 Derangement of meniscus due to old tear or injury**
Old bucket-handle tear
+ **M23.20 Derangement of unspecified meniscus due to old tear or injury**
Derangement of unspecified lateral meniscus due to old tear or injury
Derangement of unspecified medial meniscus due to old tear or injury
M23.200 Derangement of unspecified lateral meniscus due to old tear or injury, right knee
M23.201 Derangement of unspecified lateral meniscus due to old tear or injury, left knee
M23.202 Derangement of unspecified lateral meniscus due to old tear or injury, unspecified knee
M23.203 Derangement of unspecified medial meniscus due to old tear or injury, right knee
M23.204 Derangement of unspecified medial meniscus due to old tear or injury, left knee
M23.205 Derangement of unspecified medial meniscus due to old tear or injury, unspecified knee
M23.206 Derangement of unspecified meniscus due to old tear or injury, right knee
M23.207 Derangement of unspecified meniscus due to old tear or injury, left knee
M23.209 Derangement of unspecified meniscus due to old tear or injury, unspecified knee
+ **M23.21 Derangement of anterior horn of medial meniscus due to old tear or injury**
M23.211 Derangement of anterior horn of medial meniscus due to old tear or injury, right knee
M23.212 Derangement of anterior horn of medial meniscus due to old tear or injury, left knee
M23.219 Derangement of anterior horn of medial meniscus due to old tear or injury, unspecified knee

+ **M23.22** **Derangement of posterior horn of medial meniscus due to old tear or injury**
  - **M23.221** **Derangement of posterior horn of medial meniscus due to old tear or injury, right knee**
  - **M23.222** **Derangement of posterior horn of medial meniscus due to old tear or injury, left knee**
  - **M23.229** **Derangement of posterior horn of medial meniscus due to old tear or injury, unspecified knee**

+ **M23.23** **Derangement of other medial meniscus due to old tear or injury**
  - **M23.231** **Derangement of other medial meniscus due to old tear or injury, right knee**
  - **M23.232** **Derangement of other medial meniscus due to old tear or injury, left knee**
  - **M23.239** **Derangement of other medial meniscus due to old tear or injury, unspecified knee**

+ **M23.24** **Derangement of anterior horn of lateral meniscus due to old tear or injury**
  - **M23.241** **Derangement of anterior horn of lateral meniscus due to old tear or injury, right knee**
  - **M23.242** **Derangement of anterior horn of lateral meniscus due to old tear or injury, left knee**
  - **M23.249** **Derangement of anterior horn of lateral meniscus due to old tear or injury, unspecified knee**

+ **M23.25** **Derangement of posterior horn of lateral meniscus due to old tear or injury**
  - **M23.251** **Derangement of posterior horn of lateral meniscus due to old tear or injury, right knee**
  - **M23.252** **Derangement of posterior horn of lateral meniscus due to old tear or injury, left knee**
  - **M23.259** **Derangement of posterior horn of lateral meniscus due to old tear or injury, unspecified knee**

+ **M23.26** **Derangement of other lateral meniscus due to old tear or injury**
  - **M23.261** **Derangement of other lateral meniscus due to old tear or injury, right knee**
  - **M23.262** **Derangement of other lateral meniscus due to old tear or injury, left knee**
  - **M23.269** **Derangement of other lateral meniscus due to old tear or injury, unspecified knee**

+ **M23.3** **Other meniscus derangements**

  Degenerate meniscus
  Detached meniscus
  Retained meniscus

+ **M23.30** **Other meniscus derangements, unspecified meniscus**

  Other meniscus derangements, unspecified lateral meniscus
  Other meniscus derangements, unspecified medial meniscus

  - **M23.300** **Other meniscus derangements, unspecified lateral meniscus, right knee**
  - **M23.301** **Other meniscus derangements, unspecified lateral meniscus, left knee**
  - **M23.302** **Other meniscus derangements, unspecified lateral meniscus, unspecified knee**
  - **M23.303** **Other meniscus derangements, unspecified medial meniscus, right knee**
  - **M23.304** **Other meniscus derangements, unspecified medial meniscus, left knee**
  - **M23.305** **Other meniscus derangements, unspecified medial meniscus, unspecified knee**
  - **M23.306** **Other meniscus derangements, unspecified meniscus, right knee**
  - **M23.307** **Other meniscus derangements, unspecified meniscus, left knee**
  - **M23.309** **Other meniscus derangements, unspecified meniscus, unspecified knee**

+ **M23.31** **Other meniscus derangements, anterior horn of medial meniscus**
  - **M23.311** **Other meniscus derangements, anterior horn of medial meniscus, right knee**
  - **M23.312** **Other meniscus derangements, anterior horn of medial meniscus, left knee**
  - **M23.319** **Other meniscus derangements, anterior horn of medial meniscus, unspecified knee**

+ **M23.32** **Other meniscus derangements, posterior horn of medial meniscus**
  - **M23.321** **Other meniscus derangements, posterior horn of medial meniscus, right knee**
  - **M23.322** **Other meniscus derangements, posterior horn of medial meniscus, left knee**
  - **M23.329** **Other meniscus derangements, posterior horn of medial meniscus, unspecified knee**

+ **M23.33** **Other meniscus derangements, other medial meniscus**
  - **M23.331** **Other meniscus derangements, other medial meniscus, right knee**
  - **M23.332** **Other meniscus derangements, other medial meniscus, left knee**
  - **M23.339** **Other meniscus derangements, other medial meniscus, unspecified knee**

+ **M23.34** **Other meniscus derangements, anterior horn of lateral meniscus**
  - **M23.341** **Other meniscus derangements, anterior horn of lateral meniscus, right knee**
  - **M23.342** **Other meniscus derangements, anterior horn of lateral meniscus, left knee**
  - **M23.349** **Other meniscus derangements, anterior horn of lateral meniscus, unspecified knee**

+ **M23.35** **Other meniscus derangements, posterior horn of lateral meniscus**
  - **M23.351** **Other meniscus derangements, posterior horn of lateral meniscus, right knee**
  - **M23.352** **Other meniscus derangements, posterior horn of lateral meniscus, left knee**
  - **M23.359** **Other meniscus derangements, posterior horn of lateral meniscus, unspecified knee**

+ **M23.36** **Other meniscus derangements, other lateral meniscus**
  - **M23.361** **Other meniscus derangements, other lateral meniscus, right knee**
  - **M23.362** **Other meniscus derangements, other lateral meniscus, left knee**
  - **M23.369** **Other meniscus derangements, other lateral meniscus, unspecified knee**

+ **M23.4** **Loose body in knee**
  - **M23.40** **Loose body in knee, unspecified knee**
  - **M23.41** **Loose body in knee, right knee**
  - **M23.42** **Loose body in knee, left knee**

+ **M23.5** **Chronic instability of knee**
  - **M23.50** **Chronic instability of knee, unspecified knee**
  - **M23.51** **Chronic instability of knee, right knee**
  - **M23.52** **Chronic instability of knee, left knee**

+ **M23.6** **Other spontaneous disruption of ligament(s) of knee**

+ **M23.60** **Other spontaneous disruption of unspecified ligament of knee**
  - **M23.601** **Other spontaneous disruption of unspecified ligament of right knee**
  - **M23.602** **Other spontaneous disruption of unspecified ligament of left knee**
  - **M23.609** **Other spontaneous disruption of unspecified ligament of unspecified knee**

+ **M23.61** **Other spontaneous disruption of anterior cruciate ligament of knee**
  - **M23.611** **Other spontaneous disruption of anterior cruciate ligament of right knee**
  - **M23.612** **Other spontaneous disruption of anterior cruciate ligament of left knee**
  - **M23.619** **Other spontaneous disruption of anterior cruciate ligament of unspecified knee**

+ **M23.62** **Other spontaneous disruption of posterior cruciate ligament of knee**
  - **M23.621** **Other spontaneous disruption of posterior cruciate ligament of right knee**
  - **M23.622** **Other spontaneous disruption of posterior cruciate ligament of left knee**
  - **M23.629** **Other spontaneous disruption of posterior cruciate ligament of unspecified knee**

+ M23.63 Other spontaneous disruption of medial collateral ligament of knee
M23.631 Other spontaneous disruption of medial collateral ligament of right knee
M23.632 Other spontaneous disruption of medial collateral ligament of left knee
M23.639 Other spontaneous disruption of medial collateral ligament of unspecified knee
+ M23.64 Other spontaneous disruption of lateral collateral ligament of knee
M23.641 Other spontaneous disruption of lateral collateral ligament of right knee
M23.642 Other spontaneous disruption of lateral collateral ligament of left knee
M23.649 Other spontaneous disruption of lateral collateral ligament of unspecified knee
+ M23.67 Other spontaneous disruption of capsular ligament of knee
M23.671 Other spontaneous disruption of capsular ligament of right knee
M23.672 Other spontaneous disruption of capsular ligament of left knee
M23.679 Other spontaneous disruption of capsular ligament of unspecified knee
+ M23.8 Other internal derangements of knee
Laxity of ligament of knee
Snapping knee
+ M23.8X Other internal derangements of knee
M23.8X1 Other internal derangements of right knee
M23.8X2 Other internal derangements of left knee
M23.8X9 Other internal derangements of unspecified knee
+ M23.9 Unspecified internal derangement of knee
M23.90 Unspecified internal derangement of unspecified knee
M23.91 Unspecified internal derangement of right knee
M23.92 Unspecified internal derangement of left knee

M24 Other specific joint derangements

Excludes1: *current injury - see injury of joint by body region*
Excludes2: *ganglion (M67.4)*
snapping knee (M23.8-)
temporomandibular joint disorders (M26.6-)

+ M24.0 Loose body in joint
Excludes2: *loose body in knee (M23.4)*
M24.00 Loose body in unspecified joint
+ M24.01 Loose body in shoulder
M24.011 Loose body in right shoulder
M24.012 Loose body in left shoulder
M24.019 Loose body in unspecified shoulder
+ M24.02 Loose body in elbow
M24.021 Loose body in right elbow
M24.022 Loose body in left elbow
M24.029 Loose body in unspecified elbow
+ M24.03 Loose body in wrist
M24.031 Loose body in right wrist
M24.032 Loose body in left wrist
M24.039 Loose body in unspecified wrist
+ M24.04 Loose body in finger joints
M24.041 Loose body in right finger joint(s)
M24.042 Loose body in left finger joint(s)
M24.049 Loose body in unspecified finger joint(s)
+ M24.05 Loose body in hip
M24.051 Loose body in right hip
M24.052 Loose body in left hip
M24.059 Loose body in unspecified hip
+ M24.07 Loose body in ankle and toe joints
M24.071 Loose body in right ankle
M24.072 Loose body in left ankle
M24.073 Loose body in unspecified ankle
M24.074 Loose body in right toe joint(s)
M24.075 Loose body in left toe joint(s)
M24.076 Loose body in unspecified toe joints
M24.08 Loose body, other site
+ M24.1 Other articular cartilage disorders
Excludes2: *chondrocalcinosis (M11.1, M11.2-)*
internal derangement of knee (M23.-)
metastatic calcification (E83.5)
ochronosis (E70.2)
M24.10 Other articular cartilage disorders, unspecified site
+ M24.11 Other articular cartilage disorders, shoulder
M24.111 Other articular cartilage disorders, right shoulder
M24.112 Other articular cartilage disorders, left shoulder
M24.119 Other articular cartilage disorders, unspecified shoulder
+ M24.12 Other articular cartilage disorders, elbow
M24.121 Other articular cartilage disorders, right elbow
M24.122 Other articular cartilage disorders, left elbow
M24.129 Other articular cartilage disorders, unspecified elbow
+ M24.13 Other articular cartilage disorders, wrist
M24.131 Other articular cartilage disorders, right wrist
M24.132 Other articular cartilage disorders, left wrist
M24.139 Other articular cartilage disorders, unspecified wrist
+ M24.14 Other articular cartilage disorders, hand
M24.141 Other articular cartilage disorders, right hand
M24.142 Other articular cartilage disorders, left hand
M24.149 Other articular cartilage disorders, unspecified hand
+ M24.15 Other articular cartilage disorders, hip
M24.151 Other articular cartilage disorders, right hip
M24.152 Other articular cartilage disorders, left hip
M24.159 Other articular cartilage disorders, unspecified hip
+ M24.17 Other articular cartilage disorders, ankle and foot
M24.171 Other articular cartilage disorders, right ankle
M24.172 Other articular cartilage disorders, left ankle
M24.173 Other articular cartilage disorders, unspecified ankle
M24.174 Other articular cartilage disorders, right foot
M24.175 Other articular cartilage disorders, left foot
M24.176 Other articular cartilage disorders, unspecified foot
+ M24.2 Disorder of ligament
Instability secondary to old ligament injury
Ligamentous laxity NOS
Excludes1: *familial ligamentous laxity (M35.7)*
Excludes2: *internal derangement of knee (M23.5-M23.89)*
M24.20 Disorder of ligament, unspecified site
+ M24.21 Disorder of ligament, shoulder
M24.211 Disorder of ligament, right shoulder
M24.212 Disorder of ligament, left shoulder
M24.219 Disorder of ligament, unspecified shoulder
+ M24.22 Disorder of ligament, elbow
M24.221 Disorder of ligament, right elbow
M24.222 Disorder of ligament, left elbow
M24.229 Disorder of ligament, unspecified elbow
+ M24.23 Disorder of ligament, wrist
M24.231 Disorder of ligament, right wrist
M24.232 Disorder of ligament, left wrist
M24.239 Disorder of ligament, unspecified wrist
+ M24.24 Disorder of ligament, hand
M24.241 Disorder of ligament, right hand
M24.242 Disorder of ligament, left hand
M24.249 Disorder of ligament, unspecified hand
+ M24.25 Disorder of ligament, hip
M24.251 Disorder of ligament, right hip
M24.252 Disorder of ligament, left hip
M24.259 Disorder of ligament, unspecified hip
+ M24.27 Disorder of ligament, ankle and foot
M24.271 Disorder of ligament, right ankle
M24.272 Disorder of ligament, left ankle
M24.273 Disorder of ligament, unspecified ankle
M24.274 Disorder of ligament, right foot
M24.275 Disorder of ligament, left foot
M24.276 Disorder of ligament, unspecifiedfoot
M24.28 Disorder of ligament, vertebrae

+ **M24.3 Pathological dislocation of joint, not elsewhere classified**
  Excludes1: *congenital dislocation or displacement of joint- see congenital malformations and deformations of the musculoskeletal system (Q65-Q79)*
  current injury - see injury of joints and ligaments by body region
  recurrent dislocation of joint (M24.4-)
  M24.30 Pathological dislocation of unspecified joint, not elsewhere classified
  + **M24.31 Pathological dislocation of shoulder, not elsewhere classified**
    M24.311 Pathological dislocation of right shoulder, not elsewhere classified
    M24.312 Pathological dislocation of left shoulder, not elsewhere classified
    M24.319 Pathological dislocation of unspecified shoulder, not elsewhere classified
  + **M24.32 Pathological dislocation of elbow, not elsewhere classified**
    M24.321 Pathological dislocation of right elbow, not elsewhere classified
    M24.322 Pathological dislocation of left elbow, not elsewhere classified
    M24.329 Pathological dislocation of unspecified elbow, not elsewhere classified
  + **M24.33 Pathological dislocation of wrist, not elsewhere classified**
    M24.331 Pathological dislocation of right wrist, not elsewhere classified
    M24.332 Pathological dislocation of left wrist, not elsewhere classified
    M24.339 Pathological dislocation of unspecified wrist, not elsewhere classified
  + **M24.34 Pathological dislocation of hand, not elsewhere classified**
    M24.341 Pathological dislocation of right hand, not elsewhere classified
    M24.342 Pathological dislocation of left hand, not elsewhere classified
    M24.349 Pathological dislocation of unspecified hand, not elsewhere classified
  + **M24.35 Pathological dislocation of hip, not elsewhere classified**
    M24.351 Pathological dislocation of right hip, not elsewhere classified
    M24.352 Pathological dislocation of left hip, not elsewhere classified
    M24.359 Pathological dislocation of unspecified hip, not elsewhere classified
  + **M24.36 Pathological dislocation of knee, not elsewhere classified**
    M24.361 Pathological dislocation of right knee, not elsewhere classified
    M24.362 Pathological dislocation of left knee, not elsewhere classified
    M24.369 Pathological dislocation of unspecified knee, not elsewhere classified
  + **M24.37 Pathological dislocation of ankle and foot, not elsewhere classified**
    M24.371 Pathological dislocation of right ankle, not elsewhere classified
    M24.372 Pathological dislocation of left ankle, not elsewhere classified
    M24.373 Pathological dislocation of unspecified ankle, not elsewhere classified
    M24.374 Pathological dislocation of right foot, not elsewhere classified
    M24.375 Pathological dislocation of left foot, not elsewhere classified
    M24.376 Pathological dislocation of unspecified foot, not elsewhere classified

+ **M24.4 Recurrent dislocation of joint**
  Recurrent subluxation of joint
  Excludes2: *recurrent dislocation of patella (M22.0-M22.1)*
  recurrent vertebral dislocation (M43.3-, M43.4, M43.5-)
  M24.40 Recurrent dislocation, unspecified joint
  + **M24.41 Recurrent dislocation, shoulder**
    M24.411 Recurrent dislocation, right shoulder
    M24.412 Recurrent dislocation, left shoulder
    M24.419 Recurrent dislocation, unspecified shoulder
  + **M24.42 Recurrent dislocation, elbow**
    M24.421 Recurrent dislocation, right elbow
    M24.422 Recurrent dislocation, left elbow
    M24.429 Recurrent dislocation, unspecified elbow
  + **M24.43 Recurrent dislocation, wrist**
    M24.431 Recurrent dislocation, right wrist
    M24.432 Recurrent dislocation, left wrist
    M24.439 Recurrent dislocation, unspecified wrist
  + **M24.44 Recurrent dislocation, hand and finger(s)**
    M24.441 Recurrent dislocation, right hand
    M24.442 Recurrent dislocation, left hand
    M24.443 Recurrent dislocation, unspecified hand
    M24.444 Recurrent dislocation, right finger
    M24.445 Recurrent dislocation, left finger
    M24.446 Recurrent dislocation, unspecified finger
  + **M24.45 Recurrent dislocation, hip**
    M24.451 Recurrent dislocation, right hip
    M24.452 Recurrent dislocation, left hip
    M24.459 Recurrent dislocation, unspecified hip
  + **M24.46 Recurrent dislocation, knee**
    M24.461 Recurrent dislocation, right knee
    M24.462 Recurrent dislocation, left knee
    M24.469 Recurrent dislocation, unspecified knee
  + **M24.47 Recurrent dislocation, ankle, foot and toes**
    M24.471 Recurrent dislocation, right ankle
    M24.472 Recurrent dislocation, left ankle
    M24.473 Recurrent dislocation, unspecified ankle
    M24.474 Recurrent dislocation, right foot
    M24.475 Recurrent dislocation, left foot
    M24.476 Recurrent dislocation, unspecified foot
    M24.477 Recurrent dislocation, right toe(s)
    M24.478 Recurrent dislocation, left toe(s)
    M24.479 Recurrent dislocation, unspecified toe(s)

+ **M24.5 Contracture of joint**
  Excludes1: *contracture of muscle without contracture of joint (M62.4-)*
  contracture of tendon (sheath) without contracture of joint (M62.4-)
  Dupuytren's contracture (M72.0)
  Excludes2: *acquired deformities of limbs (M20-M21)*
  AHA CC: 2Q, 2016, 6
  M24.50 Contracture, unspecified joint
  + **M24.51 Contracture, shoulder**
    M24.511 Contracture, right shoulder
    M24.512 Contracture, left shoulder
    M24.519 Contracture, unspecified shoulder
  + **M24.52 Contracture, elbow**
    M24.521 Contracture, right elbow
    M24.522 Contracture, left elbow
    M24.529 Contracture, unspecified elbow
  + **M24.53 Contracture, wrist**
    M24.531 Contracture, right wrist
    M24.532 Contracture, left wrist
    M24.539 Contracture, unspecified wrist
  + **M24.54 Contracture, hand**
    M24.541 Contracture, right hand
    M24.542 Contracture, left hand
    M24.549 Contracture, unspecified hand
  + **M24.55 Contracture, hip**
    M24.551 Contracture, right hip
    M24.552 Contracture, left hip
    M24.559 Contracture, unspecified hip
  + **M24.56 Contracture, knee**
    M24.561 Contracture, right knee
    M24.562 Contracture, left knee
    M24.569 Contracture, unspecified knee
  + **M24.57 Contracture, ankle and foot**
    M24.571 Contracture, right ankle
    M24.572 Contracture, left ankle
    M24.573 Contracture, unspecified ankle
    M24.574 Contracture, right foot
    M24.575 Contracture, left foot
    M24.576 Contracture, unspecified foot

+ **M24.6 Ankylosis of joint**
  Excludes1: *stiffness of joint without ankylosis (M25.6-)*
  Excludes2: *spine (M43.2-)*
  M24.60 Ankylosis, unspecified joint
  + **M24.61 Ankylosis, shoulder**
    M24.611 Ankylosis, right shoulder
    M24.612 Ankylosis, left shoulder
    M24.619 Ankylosis, unspecified shoulder

+ M24.62 Ankylosis, elbow
M24.621 Ankylosis, right elbow
M24.622 Ankylosis, left elbow
M24.629 Ankylosis, unspecified elbow
+ M24.63 Ankylosis, wrist
M24.631 Ankylosis, right wrist
M24.632 Ankylosis, left wrist
M24.639 Ankylosis, unspecified wrist
+ M24.64 Ankylosis, hand
M24.641 Ankylosis, right hand
M24.642 Ankylosis, left hand
M24.649 Ankylosis, unspecified hand
+ M24.65 Ankylosis, hip
M24.651 Ankylosis, right hip
M24.652 Ankylosis, left hip
M24.659 Ankylosis, unspecified hip
+ M24.66 Ankylosis, knee
M24.661 Ankylosis, right knee
M24.662 Ankylosis, left knee
M24.669 Ankylosis, unspecified knee
+ M24.67 Ankylosis, ankle and foot
M24.671 Ankylosis, right ankle
M24.672 Ankylosis, left ankle
M24.673 Ankylosis, unspecified ankle
M24.674 Ankylosis, right foot
M24.675 Ankylosis, left foot
M24.676 Ankylosis, unspecified foot
M24.7 Protrusio acetabuli
+ M24.8 Other specific joint derangements, not elsewhere classified
Excludes2: *iliotibial band syndrome (M76.3)*
M24.80 Other specific joint derangements of unspecified joint, not elsewhere classified
+ M24.81 Other specific joint derangements of shoulder, not elsewhere classified
M24.811 Other specific joint derangements of right shoulder, not elsewhere classified
M24.812 Other specific joint derangements of left shoulder, not elsewhere classified
M24.819 Other specific joint derangements of unspecified shoulder, not elsewhere classified
+ M24.82 Other specific joint derangements of elbow, not elsewhere classified
M24.821 Other specific joint derangements of right elbow, not elsewhere classified
M24.822 Other specific joint derangements of left elbow, not elsewhere classified
M24.829 Other specific joint derangements of unspecified elbow, not elsewhere classified
+ M24.83 Other specific joint derangements of wrist, not elsewhere classified
M24.831 Other specific joint derangements of right wrist, not elsewhere classified
M24.832 Other specific joint derangements of left wrist, not elsewhere classified
M24.839 Other specific joint derangements of unspecified wrist, not elsewhere classified
+ M24.84 Other specific joint derangements of hand, not elsewhere classified
M24.841 Other specific joint derangements of right hand, not elsewhere classified
M24.842 Other specific joint derangements of left hand, not elsewhere classified
M24.849 Other specific joint derangements of unspecified hand, not elsewhere classified
+ M24.85 Other specific joint derangements of hip, not elsewhere classified
Irritable hip
M24.851 Other specific joint derangements of right hip, not elsewhere classified
M24.852 Other specific joint derangements of left hip, not elsewhere classified
M24.859 Other specific joint derangements of unspecified hip, not elsewhere classified
+ M24.87 Other specific joint derangements of ankle and foot, not elsewhere classified
M24.871 Other specific joint derangements of right ankle, not elsewhere classified
M24.872 Other specific joint derangements of left ankle, not elsewhere classified
M24.873 Other specific joint derangements of unspecified ankle, not elsewhere classified
M24.874 Other specific joint derangements of right foot, not elsewhere classified
M24.875 Other specific joint derangements left foot, not elsewhere classified
M24.876 Other specific joint derangements of unspecified foot, not elsewhere classified
M24.9 Joint derangement, unspecified

M25 Other joint disorder, not elsewhere classified

Excludes2: *abnormality of gait and mobility (R26.-)*
acquired deformities of limb (M20-M21)
calcification of bursa (M71.4-)
calcification of shoulder (joint) (M75.3)
calcification of tendon (M65.2-)
difficulty in walking (R26.2)
temporomandibular joint disorder (M26.6-)
+ M25.0 Hemarthrosis
Excludes1: *current injury - see injury of joint by body region*
hemophilic arthropathy (M36.2)
CC M25.00 Hemarthrosis, unspecified joint
CC Exclusion see Appendix A PDX collection 0868
+ M25.01 Hemarthrosis, shoulder
CC M25.011 Hemarthrosis, right shoulder
CC Exclusion see Appendix A PDX collection 0869
CC M25.012 Hemarthrosis, left shoulder
CC Exclusion see Appendix A PDX collection 0869
CC M25.019 Hemarthrosis, unspecified shoulder
CC Exclusion see Appendix A PDX collection 0869
+ M25.02 Hemarthrosis, elbow
CC M25.021 Hemarthrosis, right elbow
CC Exclusion see Appendix A PDX collection 0870
CC M25.022 Hemarthrosis, left elbow
CC Exclusion see Appendix A PDX collection 0870
CC M25.029 Hemarthrosis, unspecified elbow
CC Exclusion see Appendix A PDX collection 0870
+ M25.03 Hemarthrosis, wrist
CC M25.031 Hemarthrosis, right wrist
CC Exclusion see Appendix A PDX collection 0871
CC M25.032 Hemarthrosis, left wrist
CC Exclusion see Appendix A PDX collection 0871
CC M25.039 Hemarthrosis, unspecified wrist
CC Exclusion see Appendix A PDX collection 0871
+ M25.04 Hemarthrosis, hand
CC M25.041 Hemarthrosis, right hand
CC Exclusion see Appendix A PDX collection 0872
CC M25.042 Hemarthrosis, left hand
CC Exclusion see Appendix A PDX collection 0872
CC M25.049 Hemarthrosis, unspecified hand
CC Exclusion see Appendix A PDX collection 0872
+ M25.05 Hemarthrosis, hip
CC M25.051 Hemarthrosis, right hip
CC Exclusion see Appendix A PDX collection 0868
CC M25.052 Hemarthrosis, left hip
CC Exclusion see Appendix A PDX collection 0868
CC M25.059 Hemarthrosis, unspecified hip
CC Exclusion see Appendix A PDX collection 0868
+ M25.06 Hemarthrosis, knee
CC M25.061 Hemarthrosis, right knee
CC Exclusion see Appendix A PDX collection 0873
CC M25.062 Hemarthrosis, left knee
CC Exclusion see Appendix A PDX collection 0873
CC M25.069 Hemarthrosis, unspecified knee
CC Exclusion see Appendix A PDX collection 0873

+ **M25.07 Hemarthrosis, ankle and foot**
  - CC **M25.071 Hemarthrosis, right ankle**
    - CC Exclusion see Appendix A PDX collection 0873
  - CC **M25.072 Hemarthrosis, left ankle**
    - CC Exclusion see Appendix A PDX collection 0873
  - CC **M25.073 Hemarthrosis, unspecified ankle**
    - CC Exclusion see Appendix A PDX collection 0873
  - CC **M25.074 Hemarthrosis, right foot**
    - CC Exclusion see Appendix A PDX collection 0873
  - CC **M25.075 Hemarthrosis, left foot**
    - CC Exclusion see Appendix A PDX collection 0873
  - CC **M25.076 Hemarthrosis, unspecified foot**
    - CC Exclusion see Appendix A PDX collection 0873

CC **M25.08 Hemarthrosis, other specified site**
Hemarthrosis, vertebrae
CC Exclusion see Appendix A PDX collection 0868

+ **M25.1 Fistula of joint**
M25.10 Fistula, unspecified joint
+ **M25.11 Fistula, shoulder**
M25.111 Fistula, right shoulder
M25.112 Fistula, left shoulder
M25.119 Fistula, unspecified shoulder
+ **M25.12 Fistula, elbow**
M25.121 Fistula, right elbow
M25.122 Fistula, left elbow
M25.129 Fistula, unspecified elbow
+ **M25.13 Fistula, wrist**
M25.131 Fistula, right wrist
M25.132 Fistula, left wrist
M25.139 Fistula, unspecified wrist
+ **M25.14 Fistula, hand**
M25.141 Fistula, right hand
M25.142 Fistula, left hand
M25.149 Fistula, unspecified hand
+ **M25.15 Fistula, hip**
M25.151 Fistula, right hip
M25.152 Fistula, left hip
M25.159 Fistula, unspecified hip
+ **M25.16 Fistula, knee**
M25.161 Fistula, right knee
M25.162 Fistula, left knee
M25.169 Fistula, unspecified knee
+ **M25.17 Fistula, ankle and foot**
M25.171 Fistula, right ankle
M25.172 Fistula, left ankle
M25.173 Fistula, unspecified ankle
M25.174 Fistula, right foot
M25.175 Fistula, left foot
M25.176 Fistula, unspecified foot
M25.18 Fistula, other specified site
Fistula, vertebrae

+ **M25.2 Flail joint**
M25.20 Flail joint, unspecified joint
+ **M25.21 Flail joint, shoulder**
M25.211 Flail joint, right shoulder
M25.212 Flail joint, left shoulder
M25.219 Flail joint, unspecified shoulder
+ **M25.22 Flail joint, elbow**
M25.221 Flail joint, right elbow
M25.222 Flail joint, left elbow
M25.229 Flail joint, unspecified elbow
+ **M25.23 Flail joint, wrist**
M25.231 Flail joint, right wrist
M25.232 Flail joint, left wrist
M25.239 Flail joint, unspecified wrist
+ **M25.24 Flail joint, hand**
M25.241 Flail joint, right hand
M25.242 Flail joint, left hand
M25.249 Flail joint, unspecified hand
+ **M25.25 Flail joint, hip**
M25.251 Flail joint, right hip
M25.252 Flail joint, left hip
M25.259 Flail joint, unspecified hip
+ **M25.26 Flail joint, knee**
M25.261 Flail joint, right knee
M25.262 Flail joint, left knee
M25.269 Flail joint, unspecified knee
+ **M25.27 Flail joint, ankle and foot**
M25.271 Flail joint, right ankle and foot
M25.272 Flail joint, left ankle and foot
M25.279 Flail joint, unspecified ankle and foot
M25.28 Flail joint, other site

+ **M25.3 Other instability of joint**
Excludes1: *instability of joint secondary to old ligament injury (M24.2-)*
instability of joint secondary to removal of joint prosthesis (M96.8-)
Excludes2: *spinal instabilities (M53.2-)*
M25.30 Other instability, unspecified joint
+ **M25.31 Other instability, shoulder**
M25.311 Other instability, right shoulder
M25.312 Other instability, left shoulder
M25.319 Other instability, unspecified shoulder
+ **M25.32 Other instability, elbow**
M25.321 Other instability, right elbow
M25.322 Other instability, left elbow
M25.329 Other instability, unspecified elbow
+ **M25.33 Other instability, wrist**
M25.331 Other instability, right wrist
M25.332 Other instability, left wrist
M25.339 Other instability, unspecified wrist
+ **M25.34 Other instability, hand**
M25.341 Other instability, right hand
M25.342 Other instability, left hand
M25.349 Other instability, unspecified hand
+ **M25.35 Other instability, hip**
M25.351 Other instability, right hip
M25.352 Other instability, left hip
M25.359 Other instability, unspecified hip
+ **M25.36 Other instability, knee**
M25.361 Other instability, right knee
M25.362 Other instability, left knee
M25.369 Other instability, unspecified knee
+ **M25.37 Other instability, ankle and foot**
M25.371 Other instability, right ankle
M25.372 Other instability, left ankle
M25.373 Other instability, unspecified ankle
M25.374 Other instability, right foot
M25.375 Other instability, left foot
M25.376 Other instability, unspecified foot

+ **M25.4 Effusion of joint**
Excludes1: *hydrarthrosis in yaws (A66.6)*
intermittent hydrarthrosis (M12.4-)
other infective (teno)synovitis (M65.1-)
M25.40 Effusion, unspecified joint
+ **M25.41 Effusion, shoulder**
M25.411 Effusion, right shoulder
M25.412 Effusion, left shoulder
M25.419 Effusion, unspecified shoulder
+ **M25.42 Effusion, elbow**
M25.421 Effusion, right elbow
M25.422 Effusion, left elbow
M25.429 Effusion, unspecified elbow
+ **M25.43 Effusion, wrist**
M25.431 Effusion, right wrist
M25.432 Effusion, left wrist
M25.439 Effusion, unspecified wrist
+ **M25.44 Effusion, hand**
M25.441 Effusion, right hand
M25.442 Effusion, left hand
M25.449 Effusion, unspecified hand
+ **M25.45 Effusion, hip**
M25.451 Effusion, right hip
M25.452 Effusion, left hip
M25.459 Effusion, unspecified hip
+ **M25.46 Effusion, knee**
M25.461 Effusion, right knee
M25.462 Effusion, left knee
M25.469 Effusion, unspecified knee
+ **M25.47 Effusion, ankle and foot**
M25.471 Effusion, right ankle
M25.472 Effusion, left ankle
M25.473 Effusion, unspecified ankle

M25.474 Effusion, right foot
M25.475 Effusion, left foot
M25.476 Effusion, unspecified foot
M25.48 Effusion, other site
+ M25.5 Pain in joint
Excludes2: *pain in hand (M79.64-)*
pain in fingers (M79.64-)
pain in foot (M79.67-)
pain in limb (M79.6-)
pain in toes (M79.67-)
AHA CC: 4Q, 2016, 38
M25.50 Pain in unspecified joint
+ M25.51 Pain in shoulder
M25.511 Pain in right shoulder
M25.512 Pain in left shoulder
M25.519 Pain in unspecified shoulder
+ M25.52 Pain in elbow
M25.521 Pain in right elbow
M25.522 Pain in left elbow
M25.529 Pain in unspecified elbow
+ M25.53 Pain in wrist
M25.531 Pain in right wrist
M25.532 Pain in left wrist
M25.539 Pain in unspecified wrist
+ M25.54 Pain in joints of hand
M25.541 Pain in joints of right hand
M25.542 Pain in joints of left hand
M25.549 Pain in joints of unspecified hand
Pain in joints of hand NOS
+ M25.55 Pain in hip
M25.551 Pain in right hip
M25.552 Pain in left hip
M25.559 Pain in unspecified hip
+ M25.56 Pain in knee
M25.561 Pain in right knee
M25.562 Pain in left knee
M25.569 Pain in unspecified knee
+ M25.57 Pain in ankle and joints of foot
M25.571 Pain in right ankle and joints of right foot
M25.572 Pain in left ankle and joints of left foot
M25.579 Pain in unspecified ankle and joints of unspecified foot
+ M25.6 Stiffness of joint, not elsewhere classified
Excludes1: *ankylosis of joint (M24.6-)*
contracture of joint (M24.5-)
M25.60 Stiffness of unspecified joint, not elsewhere classified
+ M25.61 Stiffness of shoulder, not elsewhere classified
M25.611 Stiffness of right shoulder, not elsewhere classified
M25.612 Stiffness of left shoulder, not elsewhere classified
M25.619 Stiffness of unspecified shoulder, not elsewhere classified
+ M25.62 Stiffness of elbow, not elsewhere classified
M25.621 Stiffness of right elbow, not elsewhere classified
M25.622 Stiffness of left elbow, not elsewhere classified
M25.629 Stiffness of unspecified elbow, not elsewhere classified
+ M25.63 Stiffness of wrist, not elsewhere classified
M25.631 Stiffness of right wrist, not elsewhere classified
M25.632 Stiffness of left wrist, not elsewhere classified
M25.639 Stiffness of unspecified wrist, not elsewhere classified
+ M25.64 Stiffness of hand, not elsewhere classified
M25.641 Stiffness of right hand, not elsewhere classified
M25.642 Stiffness of left hand, not elsewhere classified
M25.649 Stiffness of unspecified hand, not elsewhere classified
+ M25.65 Stiffness of hip, not elsewhere classified
M25.651 Stiffness of right hip, not elsewhere classified
M25.652 Stiffness of left hip, not elsewhere classified
M25.659 Stiffness of unspecified hip, not elsewhere classified
+ M25.66 Stiffness of knee, not elsewhere classified
M25.661 Stiffness of right knee, not elsewhere classified
M25.662 Stiffness of left knee, not elsewhere classified
M25.669 Stiffness of unspecified knee, not elsewhere classified
+ M25.67 Stiffness of ankle and foot, not elsewhere classified
M25.671 Stiffness of right ankle, not elsewhere classified
M25.672 Stiffness of left ankle, not elsewhere classified
M25.673 Stiffness of unspecified ankle, not elsewhere classified
M25.674 Stiffness of right foot, not elsewhere classified
M25.675 Stiffness of left foot, not elsewhere classified
M25.676 Stiffness of unspecified foot, not elsewhere classified
+ M25.7 Osteophyte
M25.70 Osteophyte, unspecified joint
+ M25.71 Osteophyte, shoulder
M25.711 Osteophyte, right shoulder
M25.712 Osteophyte, left shoulder
M25.719 Osteophyte, unspecified shoulder
+ M25.72 Osteophyte, elbow
M25.721 Osteophyte, right elbow
M25.722 Osteophyte, left elbow
M25.729 Osteophyte, unspecified elbow
+ M25.73 Osteophyte, wrist
M25.731 Osteophyte, right wrist
M25.732 Osteophyte, left wrist
M25.739 Osteophyte, unspecified wrist
+ M25.74 Osteophyte, hand
M25.741 Osteophyte, right hand
M25.742 Osteophyte, left hand
M25.749 Osteophyte, unspecified hand
+ M25.75 Osteophyte, hip
M25.751 Osteophyte, right hip
M25.752 Osteophyte, left hip
M25.759 Osteophyte, unspecified hip
+ M25.76 Osteophyte, knee
M25.761 Osteophyte, right knee
M25.762 Osteophyte, left knee
M25.769 Osteophyte, unspecified knee
+ M25.77 Osteophyte, ankle and foot
M25.771 Osteophyte, right ankle
M25.772 Osteophyte, left ankle
M25.773 Osteophyte, unspecified ankle
M25.774 Osteophyte, right foot
M25.775 Osteophyte, left foot
M25.776 Osteophyte, unspecified foot
M25.78 Osteophyte, vertebrae
+ M25.8 Other specified joint disorders
M25.80 Other specified joint disorders, unspecified joint
+ M25.81 Other specified joint disorders, shoulder
M25.811 Other specified joint disorders, right shoulder
M25.812 Other specified joint disorders, left shoulder
M25.819 Other specified joint disorders, unspecified shoulder
+ M25.82 Other specified joint disorders, elbow
M25.821 Other specified joint disorders, right elbow
M25.822 Other specified joint disorders, left elbow
M25.829 Other specified joint disorders, unspecified elbow
+ M25.83 Other specified joint disorders, wrist
M25.831 Other specified joint disorders, right wrist
M25.832 Other specified joint disorders, left wrist
M25.839 Other specified joint disorders, unspecified wrist
+ M25.84 Other specified joint disorders, hand
M25.841 Other specified joint disorders, right hand
M25.842 Other specified joint disorders, left hand
M25.849 Other specified joint disorders, unspecified hand

+ **M25.85 Other specified joint disorders, hip**
  - **M25.851 Other specified joint disorders, right hip**
  - **M25.852 Other specified joint disorders, left hip**
    AHA CC: 4Q, 2014, 25
  - **M25.859 Other specified joint disorders, unspecified hip**
+ **M25.86 Other specified joint disorders, knee**
  - **M25.861 Other specified joint disorders, right knee**
  - **M25.862 Other specified joint disorders, left knee**
  - **M25.869 Other specified joint disorders, unspecified knee**
+ **M25.87 Other specified joint disorders, ankle and foot**
  - **M25.871 Other specified joint disorders, right ankle and foot**
  - **M25.872 Other specified joint disorders, left ankle and foot**
  - **M25.879 Other specified joint disorders, unspecified ankle and foot**

M25.9 Joint disorder, unspecified

Dentofacial anomalies [including malocclusion] and other disorders of jaw (M26-M27)

Excludes1: *hemifacial atrophy or hypertrophy (Q67.4)*
unilateral condylar hyperplasia or hypoplasia (M27.8)

M26 Dentofacial anomalies [including malocclusion]

+ **M26.0 Major anomalies of jaw size**
  Excludes1: *acromegaly (E22.0)*
  Robin's syndrome (Q87.0)
  - **M26.00 Unspecified anomaly of jaw size**
  - **M26.01 Maxillary hyperplasia**
  - **M26.02 Maxillary hypoplasia**
    AHA CC: 3Q, 2014, 23-24
  - **M26.03 Mandibular hyperplasia**
  - **M26.04 Mandibular hypoplasia**
  - **M26.05 Macrogenia**
  - **M26.06 Microgenia**
  - **M26.07 Excessive tuberosity of jaw**
    Entire maxillary tuberosity
  - **M26.09 Other specified anomalies of jaw size**
+ **M26.1 Anomalies of jaw-cranial base relationship**
  - **M26.10 Unspecified anomaly of jaw-cranial base relationship**
  - **M26.11 Maxillary asymmetry**
  - **M26.12 Other jaw asymmetry**
  - **M26.19 Other specified anomalies of jaw-cranial base relationship**
+ **M26.2 Anomalies of dental arch relationship**
  - **M26.20 Unspecified anomaly of dental arch relationship**
  - + **M26.21 Malocclusion, Angle's class**
    - **M26.211 Malocclusion, Angle's class I**
      Neutro-occlusion
    - **M26.212 Malocclusion, Angle's class II**
      Disto-occlusion Division I
      Disto-occlusion Division II
    - **M26.213 Malocclusion, Angle's class III**
      Mesio-occlusion
    - **M26.219 Malocclusion, Angle's class, unspecified**
  - + **M26.22 Open occlusal relationship**
    - **M26.220 Open anterior occlusal relationship**
      Anterior openbite
    - **M26.221 Open posterior occlusal relationship**
      Posterior openbite
  - **M26.23 Excessive horizontal overlap**
    Excessive horizontal overjet
  - **M26.24 Reverse articulation**
    Crossbite (anterior) (posterior)
  - **M26.25 Anomalies of interarch distance**
  - **M26.29 Other anomalies of dental arch relationship**
    Midline deviation of dental arch
    Overbite (excessive) deep
    Overbite (excessive) horizontal
    Overbite (excessive) vertical
    Posterior lingual occlusion of mandibular teeth
+ **M26.3 Anomalies of tooth position of fully erupted tooth or teeth**
  Excludes2: *embedded and impacted teeth (K01.-)*
  - **M26.30 Unspecified anomaly of tooth position of fully erupted tooth or teeth**
    Abnormal spacing of fully erupted tooth or teeth NOS
    Displacement of fully erupted tooth or teeth NOS
    Transposition of fully erupted tooth or teeth NOS
  - **M26.31 Crowding of fully erupted teeth**
  - **M26.32 Excessive spacing of fully erupted teeth**
    Diastema of fully erupted tooth or teeth NOS
  - **M26.33 Horizontal displacement of fully erupted tooth or teeth**
    Tipped tooth or teeth
    Tipping of fully erupted tooth
  - **M26.34 Vertical displacement of fully erupted tooth or teeth**
    Extruded tooth
    Infraeruption of tooth or teeth
    Supraeruption of tooth or teeth
  - **M26.35 Rotation of fully erupted tooth or teeth**
  - **M26.36 Insufficient interocclusal distance of fully erupted teeth (ridge)**
    Lack of adequate intermaxillary vertical dimension of fully erupted teeth
  - **M26.37 Excessive interocclusal distance of fully erupted teeth**
    Excessive intermaxillary vertical dimension of fully erupted teeth
    Loss of occlusal vertical dimension of fully erupted teeth
  - **M26.39 Other anomalies of tooth position of fully erupted tooth or teeth**

M26.4 Malocclusion, unspecified

+ **M26.5 Dentofacial functional abnormalities**
  Excludes1: *bruxism (F45.8)*
  teeth-grinding NOS (F45.8)
  - **M26.50 Dentofacial functional abnormalities, unspecified**
  - **M26.51 Abnormal jaw closure**
  - **M26.52 Limited mandibular range of motion**
  - **M26.53 Deviation in opening and closing of the mandible**
  - **M26.54 Insufficient anterior guidance**
    Insufficient anterior occlusal guidance
  - **M26.55 Centric occlusion maximum intercuspation discrepancy**
    Excludes1: *centric occlusion NOS (M26.59)*
  - **M26.56 Non-working side interference**
    Balancing side interference
  - **M26.57 Lack of posterior occlusal support**
  - **M26.59 Other dentofacial functional abnormalities**
    Centric occlusion (of teeth) NOS
    Malocclusion due to abnormal swallowing
    Malocclusion due to mouth breathing
    Malocclusion due to tongue, lip or finger habits
+ **M26.6 Temporomandibular joint disorders**
  Excludes2: *current temporomandibular joint dislocation (S03.0)*
  current temporomandibular joint sprain (S03.4)
  AHA CC: 4Q, 2016, 38-39
  - + **M26.60 Temporomandibular joint disorder, unspecified**
    - **M26.601 Right temporomandibular joint disorder, unspecified**
    - **M26.602 Left temporomandibular joint disorder, unspecified**
    - **M26.603 Bilateral temporomandibular joint disorder, unspecified**
    - **M26.609 Unspecified temporomandibular joint disorder, unspecified side**
      Temporomandibular joint disorder NOS
  - + **M26.61 Adhesions and ankylosis of temporomandibular joint**
    - **M26.611 Adhesions and ankylosis of right temporomandibular joint**
    - **M26.612 Adhesions and ankylosis of left temporomandibular joint**
    - **M26.613 Adhesions and ankylosis of bilateral temporomandibular joint**
    - **M26.619 Adhesions and ankylosis of temporomandibular joint, unspecified side**
  - + **M26.62 Arthralgia of temporomandibular joint**
    - **M26.621 Arthralgia of right temporomandibular joint**
    - **M26.622 Arthralgia of left temporomandibular joint**
    - **M26.623 Arthralgia of bilateral temporomandibular joint**
    - **M26.629 Arthralgia of temporomandibular joint, unspecified side**
  - + **M26.63 Articular disc disorder of temporomandibular joint**
    - **M26.631 Articular disc disorder of right temporomandibular joint**
    - **M26.632 Articular disc disorder of left temporomandibular joint**

M26.633 **Articular disc disorder of bilateral temporomandibular joint**
M26.639 **Articular disc disorder of temporomandibular joint, unspecified side**
M26.69 **Other specified disorders of temporomandibular joint**
+ M26.7 **Dental alveolar anomalies**
M26.70 **Unspecified alveolar anomaly**
M26.71 **Alveolar maxillary hyperplasia**
M26.72 **Alveolar mandibular hyperplasia**
M26.73 **Alveolar maxillary hypoplasia**
M26.74 **Alveolar mandibular hypoplasia**
M26.79 **Other specified alveolar anomalies**
+ M26.8 **Other dentofacial anomalies**
M26.81 **Anterior soft tissue impingement**
Anterior soft tissue impingement on teeth
M26.82 **Posterior soft tissue impingement**
Posterior soft tissue impingement on teeth
M26.89 **Other dentofacial anomalies**
M26.9 **Dentofacial anomaly, unspecified**

M27 Other diseases of jaws

M27.0 **Developmental disorders of jaws**
Latent bone cyst of jaw
Stafne's cyst
Torus mandibularis
Torus palatinus
M27.1 **Giant cell granuloma, central**
Giant cell granuloma NOS
Excludes1: *peripheral giant cell granuloma (K06.8)*
M27.2 **Inflammatory conditions of jaws**
Osteitis of jaw(s)
Osteomyelitis (neonatal) jaw(s)
Osteoradionecrosis jaw(s)
Periostitis jaw(s)
Sequestrum of jaw bone
Use additional code (W88-W90, X39.0) to identify radiation, if radiation-induced
Excludes2: *osteonecrosis of jaw due to drug (M87.180)*
M27.3 **Alveolitis of jaws**
Alveolar osteitis
Dry socket
+ M27.4 **Other and unspecified cysts of jaw**
Excludes1: *cysts of oral region (K09.-)*
latent bone cyst of jaw (M27.0)
Stafne's cyst (M27.0)
M27.40 **Unspecified cyst of jaw**
Cyst of jaw NOS
M27.49 **Other cysts of jaw**
Aneurysmal cyst of jaw
Hemorrhagic cyst of jaw
Traumatic cyst of jaw
+ M27.5 **Periradicular pathology associated with previous endodontic treatment**
M27.51 **Perforation of root canal space due to endodontic treatment**
M27.52 **Endodontic overfill**
M27.53 **Endodontic underfill**
M27.59 **Other periradicular pathology associated with previous endodontic treatment**
+ M27.6 **Endosseous dental implant failure**
M27.61 **Osseointegration failure of dental implant**
Hemorrhagic complications of dental implant placement
Iatrogenic osseointegration failure of dental implant
Osseointegration failure of dental implant due to complications of systemic disease
Osseointegration failure of dental implant due to poor bone quality
Pre-integration failure of dental implant NOS
Pre-osseointegration failure of dental implant
M27.62 **Post-osseointegration biological failure of dental implant**
Failure of dental implant due to lack of attached gingiva
Failure of dental implant due to occlusal trauma (caused by poor prosthetic design)
Failure of dental implant due to parafunctional habits
Failure of dental implant due to periodontal infection (peri-implantitis)
Failure of dental implant due to poor oral hygiene
Iatrogenic post-osseointegration failure of dental implant
Post-osseointegration failure of dental implant due to complications of systemic disease
M27.63 **Post-osseointegration mechanical failure of dental implant**
Failure of dental prosthesis causing loss of dental implant
Fracture of dental implant
Excludes2: *cracked tooth (K03.81)*
fractured dental restorative material with loss of material (K08.531)
fractured dental restorative material without loss of material (K08.530)
fractured tooth (S02.5)
M27.69 **Other endosseous dental implant failure**
Dental implant failure NOS
M27.8 **Other specified diseases of jaws**
Cherubism
Exostosis
Fibrous dysplasia
Unilateral condylar hyperplasia
Unilateral condylar hypoplasia
Excludes1: *jaw pain (R68.84)*
M27.9 **Disease of jaws, unspecified**

Systemic connective tissue disorders (M30-M36)

Includes: autoimmune disease NOS
collagen (vascular) disease NOS
systemic autoimmune disease
systemic collagen (vascular) disease

Excludes1: *autoimmune disease, single organ or single cell-type -code to relevant condition category*

M30 Polyarteritis nodosa and related conditions

Excludes1: *microscopic polyarteritis (M31.7)*
CC M30.0 **Polyarteritis nodosa**
CC Exclusion see Appendix A PDX collection 0874
CC M30.1 **Polyarteritis with lung involvement [Churg-Strauss]**
Allergic granulomatous angiitis
CC Exclusion see Appendix A PDX collection 0874
CC M30.2 **Juvenile polyarteritis**
CC Exclusion see Appendix A PDX collection 0874
CC M30.3 **Mucocutaneous lymph node syndrome [Kawasaki]**
CC Exclusion see Appendix A PDX collection 0875
CC M30.8 **Other conditions related to polyarteritis nodosa**
Polyangiitis overlap syndrome
CC Exclusion see Appendix A PDX collection 0874

M31 Other necrotizing vasculopathies

CC M31.0 **Hypersensitivity angiitis**
Goodpasture's syndrome
CC Exclusion see Appendix A PDX collection 0874
MCC M31.1 **Thrombotic microangiopathy**
Thrombotic thrombocytopenic purpura
MCC Exclusion see Appendix A PDX collection 0874
CC M31.2 **Lethal midline granuloma**
CC Exclusion see Appendix A PDX collection 0874
+ M31.3 **Wegener's granulomatosis**
Necrotizing respiratory granulomatosis
CC M31.30 **Wegener's granulomatosis without renal involvement**
Wegener's granulomatosis NOS
CC Exclusion see Appendix A PDX collection 0874
CC M31.31 **Wegener's granulomatosis with renal involvement**
CC Exclusion see Appendix A PDX collection 0874
CC M31.4 **Aortic arch syndrome [Takayasu]**
CC Exclusion see Appendix A PDX collection 0874
M31.5 **Giant cell arteritis with polymyalgia rheumatica**
M31.6 **Other giant cell arteritis**
CC M31.7 **Microscopic polyangiitis**
Microscopic polyarteritis
Excludes1: *polyarteritis nodosa (M30.0)*
CC Exclusion see Appendix A PDX collection 0874
CC M31.8 **Other specified necrotizing vasculopathies**
Hypocomplementemic vasculitis
Septic vasculitis
CC Exclusion see Appendix A PDX collection 0712
CC M31.9 **Necrotizing vasculopathy, unspecified**
CC Exclusion see Appendix A PDX collection 0712

M32 Systemic lupus erythematosus (SLE)

Excludes1: *lupus erythematosus (discoid) (NOS) (L93.0)*

M32.0 Drug-induced systemic lupus erythematosus
Use additional code for adverse effect, if applicable, to identify drug (T36-T50 with fifth or sixth character 5)

+ **M32.1 Systemic lupus erythematosus with organ or system involvement**

M32.10 Systemic lupus erythematosus, organ or system involvement unspecified

CC **M32.11 Endocarditis in systemic lupus erythematosus**
Libman-Sacks disease
CC Exclusion see Appendix A PDX collection 0676

CC **M32.12 Pericarditis in systemic lupus erythematosus**
Lupus pericarditis
CC Exclusion see Appendix A PDX collection 0673

M32.13 Lung involvement in systemic lupus erythematosus
Pleural effusion due to systemic lupus erythematosus

M32.14 Glomerular disease in systemic lupus erythematosus
Lupus renal disease NOS
AHA CC: 4Q, 2013, 125

M32.15 Tubulo-interstitial nephropathy in systemic lupus erythematosus

M32.19 Other organ or system involvement in systemic lupus erythematosus

M32.8 Other forms of systemic lupus erythematosus

M32.9 Systemic lupus erythematosus, unspecified
SLE NOS
Systemic lupus erythematosus NOS
Systemic lupus erythematosus without organ involvement

M33 Dermatopolymyositis

+ **M33.0 Juvenile dermatomyositis**

CC **M33.00 Juvenile dermatomyositis, organ involvement unspecified**
CC Exclusion see Appendix A PDX collection 0876

CC **M33.01 Juvenile dermatomyositis with respiratory involvement**
CC Exclusion see Appendix A PDX collection 0876

CC **M33.02 Juvenile dermatomyositis with myopathy**
CC Exclusion see Appendix A PDX collection 0877

CC **M33.03 Juvenile dermatomyositis without myopathy**
CC Exclusion see Appendix A PDX collection 0877

CC **M33.09 Juvenile dermatomyositis with other organ involvement**
CC Exclusion see Appendix A PDX collection 0876

+ **M33.1 Other dermatomyositis**
Adult dematomyositis

CC **M33.10 Other dermatomyositis, organ involvement unspecified**
CC Exclusion see Appendix A PDX collection 0876

CC **M33.11 Other dermatomyositis with respiratory involvement**
CC Exclusion see Appendix A PDX collection 0876

CC **M33.12 Other dermatomyositis with myopathy**
CC Exclusion see Appendix A PDX collection 0877

CC **M33.13 Other dermatomyositis without myopathy**
Dermatomyositis NOS
CC Exclusion see Appendix A PDX collection 0877

CC **M33.19 Other dermatomyositis with other organ involvement**
CC Exclusion see Appendix A PDX collection 0876

+ **M33.2 Polymyositis**

CC **M33.20 Polymyositis, organ involvement unspecified**
CC Exclusion see Appendix A PDX collection 0878

CC **M33.21 Polymyositis with respiratory involvement**
CC Exclusion see Appendix A PDX collection 0878

CC **M33.22 Polymyositis with myopathy**
CC Exclusion see Appendix A PDX collection 0879

CC **M33.29 Polymyositis with other organ involvement**
CC Exclusion see Appendix A PDX collection 0878

+ **M33.9 Dermatopolymyositis, unspecified**

CC **M33.90 Dermatopolymyositis, unspecified, organ involvement unspecified**
CC Exclusion see Appendix A PDX collection 0876

CC **M33.91 Dermatopolymyositis, unspecified with respiratory involvement**
CC Exclusion see Appendix A PDX collection 0876

CC **M33.92 Dermatopolymyositis, unspecified with myopathy**
CC Exclusion see Appendix A PDX collection 0877

CC **M33.93 Dermatopolymyositis, unspecified without myopathy**
CC Exclusion see Appendix A PDX collection 0877

CC **M33.99 Dermatopolymyositis, unspecified with other organ involvement**
CC Exclusion see Appendix A PDX collection 0876

M34 Systemic sclerosis [scleroderma]

Excludes1: *circumscribed scleroderma (L94.0)*
neonatal scleroderma (P83.8)

M34.0 Progressive systemic sclerosis

M34.1 CR(E)ST syndrome
Combination of calcinosis, Raynaud's phenomenon, esophageal dysfunction, sclerodactyly, telangiectasia

M34.2 Systemic sclerosis induced by drug and chemical
Code first poisoning due to drug or toxin, if applicable (T36-T65 with fifth or sixth character 1-4 or 6)

Use additional code for adverse effect, if applicable, to identify drug (T36-T50 with fifth or sixth character 5)

+ **M34.8 Other forms of systemic sclerosis**

CC **M34.81 Systemic sclerosis with lung involvement**
No CC Exclusions

CC **M34.82 Systemic sclerosis with myopathy**
CC Exclusion see Appendix A PDX collection 0867

M34.83 Systemic sclerosis with polyneuropathy

M34.89 Other systemic sclerosis

M34.9 Systemic sclerosis, unspecified

M35 Other systemic involvement of connective tissue

Excludes1: *reactive perforating collagenosis (L87.1)*

+ **M35.0 Sicca syndrome [Sjögren]**

M35.00 Sicca syndrome, unspecified

M35.01 Sicca syndrome with keratoconjunctivitis

M35.02 Sicca syndrome with lung involvement

CC **M35.03 Sicca syndrome with myopathy**
CC Exclusion see Appendix A PDX collection 0867

M35.04 Sicca syndrome with tubulo-interstitial nephropathy
Renal tubular acidosis in sicca syndrome

M35.09 Sicca syndrome with other organ involvement

CC **M35.1 Other overlap syndromes**
Mixed connective tissue disease
Excludes1: *polyangiitis overlap syndrome (M30.8)*
CC Exclusion see Appendix A PDX collection 0880

CC **M35.2 Behçet's disease**
CC Exclusion see Appendix A PDX collection 0863

M35.3 Polymyalgia rheumatica
Excludes1: *polymyalgia rheumatica with giant cell arteritis (M31.5)*

M35.4 Diffuse (eosinophilic) fasciitis

CC **M35.5 Multifocal fibrosclerosis**
CC Exclusion see Appendix A PDX collection 0880

M35.6 Relapsing panniculitis [Weber-Christian]
Excludes1: *lupus panniculitis (L93.2)*
panniculitis NOS (M79.3-)

M35.7 Hypermobility syndrome
Familial ligamentous laxity
Excludes1: *Ehlers-Danlos syndrome (Q79.6)*
ligamentous laxity, NOS (M24.2-)

CC **M35.8 Other specified systemic involvement of connective tissue**
CC Exclusion see Appendix A PDX collection 0880

M35.9 Systemic involvement of connective tissue, unspecified
Autoimmune disease (systemic) NOS
Collagen (vascular) disease NOS

M36 Systemic disorders of connective tissue in diseases classified elsewhere

Excludes2: *arthropathies in diseases classified elsewhere (M14.-)*

CC **M36.0 Dermato(poly)myositis in neoplastic disease**
Code first underlying neoplasm (C00-D49)
CC Exclusion see Appendix A PDX collection 0876

M36.1 Arthropathy in neoplastic disease
Code first underlying neoplasm, such as:
leukemia (C91-C95)
malignant histiocytosis (C96.A)
multiple myeloma (C90.0)

M36.2 Hemophilic arthropathy
Hemarthrosis in hemophilic arthropathy
Code first underlying disease, such as:
factor VIII deficiency (D66)
with vascular defect (D68.0)
factor IX deficiency (D67)
hemophilia (classical) (D66)
hemophilia B (D67)
hemophilia C (D68.1)

M36.3 Arthropathy in other blood disorders

M36.4 Arthropathy in hypersensitivity reactions classified elsewhere
Code first underlying disease, such as:
Henoch (-Schönlein) purpura (D69.0)
serum sickness (T80.6-)

M36.8 **Systemic disorders of connective tissue in other diseases classified elsewhere**
Code first underlying disease, such as:
alkaptonuria (E70.2)
hypogammaglobulinemia (D80.-)
ochronosis (E70.2)

DORSOPATHIES (M40-M54)

Deforming dorsopathies (M40-M43)

M40 Kyphosis and lordosis

Excludes1: *congenital kyphosis and lordosis (Q76.4)*
kyphoscoliosis (M41.-)
postprocedural kyphosis and lordosis (M96.-)

\+ **M40.0 Postural kyphosis**
Excludes1: *osteochondrosis of spine (M42.-)*
M40.00 Postural kyphosis, site unspecified
M40.03 Postural kyphosis, cervicothoracic region
M40.04 Postural kyphosis, thoracic region
M40.05 Postural kyphosis, thoracolumbar region

\+ **M40.1 Other secondary kyphosis**
M40.10 Other secondary kyphosis, site unspecified
M40.12 Other secondary kyphosis, cervical region
M40.13 Other secondary kyphosis, cervicothoracic region
M40.14 Other secondary kyphosis, thoracic region
M40.15 Other secondary kyphosis, thoracolumbar region

\+ **M40.2 Other and unspecified kyphosis**
\+ **M40.20 Unspecified kyphosis**
M40.202 Unspecified kyphosis, cervical region
M40.203 Unspecified kyphosis, cervicothoracic region
M40.204 Unspecified kyphosis, thoracic region
M40.205 Unspecified kyphosis, thoracolumbar region
M40.209 Unspecified kyphosis, site unspecified
\+ **M40.29 Other kyphosis**
M40.292 Other kyphosis, cervical region
M40.293 Other kyphosis, cervicothoracic region
M40.294 Other kyphosis, thoracic region
M40.295 Other kyphosis, thoracolumbar region
M40.299 Other kyphosis, site unspecified

\+ **M40.3 Flatback syndrome**
M40.30 Flatback syndrome, site unspecified
M40.35 Flatback syndrome, thoracolumbar region
M40.36 Flatback syndrome, lumbar region
M40.37 Flatback syndrome, lumbosacral region

\+ **M40.4 Postural lordosis**
Acquired lordosis
M40.40 Postural lordosis, site unspecified
M40.45 Postural lordosis, thoracolumbar region
M40.46 Postural lordosis, lumbar region
M40.47 Postural lordosis, lumbosacral region

\+ **M40.5 Lordosis, unspecified**
M40.50 Lordosis, unspecified, site unspecified
M40.55 Lordosis, unspecified, thoracolumbar region
M40.56 Lordosis, unspecified, lumbar region
M40.57 Lordosis, unspecified, lumbosacral region

M41 Scoliosis

Includes: kyphoscoliosis
Excludes1: *congenital scoliosis NOS (Q67.5)*
congenital scoliosis due to bony malformation (Q76.3)
postural congenital scoliosis (Q67.5)
kyphoscoliotic heart disease (I27.1)
postprocedural scoliosis (M96.-)

\+ **M41.0 Infantile idiopathic scoliosis**
M41.00 Infantile idiopathic scoliosis, site unspecified
M41.02 Infantile idiopathic scoliosis, cervical region
M41.03 Infantile idiopathic scoliosis, cervicothoracic region
M41.04 Infantile idiopathic scoliosis, thoracic region
AHA CC: 4Q, 2014, 26-27
M41.05 Infantile idiopathic scoliosis, thoracolumbar region
M41.06 Infantile idiopathic scoliosis, lumbar region
M41.07 Infantile idiopathic scoliosis, lumbosacral region
M41.08 Infantile idiopathic scoliosis, sacral and sacrococcygeal region

\+ **M41.1 Juvenile and adolescent idiopathic scoliosis**
\+ **M41.11 Juvenile idiopathic scoliosis**
M41.112 Juvenile idiopathic scoliosis, cervical region
M41.113 Juvenile idiopathic scoliosis, cervicothoracic region
M41.114 Juvenile idiopathic scoliosis, thoracic region
M41.115 Juvenile idiopathic scoliosis, thoracolumbar region
M41.116 Juvenile idiopathic scoliosis, lumbar region
M41.117 Juvenile idiopathic scoliosis, lumbosacral region
M41.119 Juvenile idiopathic scoliosis, site unspecified
AHA CC: 4Q, 2014, 28-29
\+ **M41.12 Adolescent scoliosis**
M41.122 Adolescent idiopathic scoliosis, cervical region
M41.123 Adolescent idiopathic scoliosis, cervicothoracic region
M41.124 Adolescent idiopathic scoliosis, thoracic region
M41.125 Adolescent idiopathic scoliosis, thoracolumbar region
M41.126 Adolescent idiopathic scoliosis, lumbar region
M41.127 Adolescent idiopathic scoliosis, lumbosacral region
M41.129 Adolescent idiopathic scoliosis, site unspecified

\+ **M41.2 Other idiopathic scoliosis**
M41.20 Other idiopathic scoliosis, site unspecified
M41.22 Other idiopathic scoliosis, cervical region
M41.23 Other idiopathic scoliosis, cervicothoracic region
M41.24 Other idiopathic scoliosis, thoracic region
M41.25 Other idiopathic scoliosis, thoracolumbar region
M41.26 Other idiopathic scoliosis, lumbar region
M41.27 Other idiopathic scoliosis, lumbosacral region

\+ **M41.3 Thoracogenic scoliosis**
M41.30 Thoracogenic scoliosis, site unspecified
M41.34 Thoracogenic scoliosis, thoracic region
M41.35 Thoracogenic scoliosis, thoracolumbar region

\+ **M41.4 Neuromuscular scoliosis**
Scoliosis secondary to cerebral palsy, Friedreich's ataxia, poliomyelitis and other neuromuscular disorders
Code also underlying condition
M41.40 Neuromuscular scoliosis, site unspecified
M41.41 Neuromuscular scoliosis, occipito-atlanto-axial region
M41.42 Neuromuscular scoliosis, cervical region
M41.43 Neuromuscular scoliosis, cervicothoracic region
M41.44 Neuromuscular scoliosis, thoracic region
M41.45 Neuromuscular scoliosis, thoracolumbar region
AHA CC: 4Q, 2014, 27-28
M41.46 Neuromuscular scoliosis, lumbar region
M41.47 Neuromuscular scoliosis, lumbosacral region

\+ **M41.5 Other secondary scoliosis**
M41.50 Other secondary scoliosis, site unspecified
M41.52 Other secondary scoliosis, cervical region
M41.53 Other secondary scoliosis, cervicothoracic region
M41.54 Other secondary scoliosis, thoracic region
M41.55 Other secondary scoliosis, thoracolumbar region
M41.56 Other secondary scoliosis, lumbar region
M41.57 Other secondary scoliosis, lumbosacral region

\+ **M41.8 Other forms of scoliosis**
M41.80 Other forms of scoliosis, site unspecified
M41.82 Other forms of scoliosis, cervical region
M41.83 Other forms of scoliosis, cervicothoracic region
M41.84 Other forms of scoliosis, thoracic region
M41.85 Other forms of scoliosis, thoracolumbar region
M41.86 Other forms of scoliosis, lumbar region
M41.87 Other forms of scoliosis, lumbosacral region

M41.9 Scoliosis, unspecified

M42 Spinal osteochondrosis

\+ **M42.0 Juvenile osteochondrosis of spine**
Calvé's disease
Scheuermann's disease
Excludes1: *postural kyphosis (M40.0)*
M42.00 Juvenile osteochondrosis of spine, site unspecified
M42.01 Juvenile osteochondrosis of spine, occipito-atlanto-axial region
M42.02 Juvenile osteochondrosis of spine, cervical region

M42.03 Juvenile osteochondrosis of spine, cervicothoracic region
M42.04 Juvenile osteochondrosis of spine, thoracic region
M42.05 Juvenile osteochondrosis of spine, thoracolumbar region
M42.06 Juvenile osteochondrosis of spine, lumbar region
M42.07 Juvenile osteochondrosis of spine, lumbosacral region
M42.08 Juvenile osteochondrosis of spine, sacral and sacrococcygeal region
M42.09 Juvenile osteochondrosis of spine, multiple sites in spine

\+ **M42.1 Adult osteochondrosis of spine**
- M42.10 Adult osteochondrosis of spine, site unspecified
- M42.11 Adult osteochondrosis of spine, occipito-atlanto-axial region
- M42.12 Adult osteochondrosis of spine, cervical region
- M42.13 Adult osteochondrosis of spine, cervicothoracic region
- M42.14 Adult osteochondrosis of spine, thoracic region
- M42.15 Adult osteochondrosis of spine, thoracolumbar region
- M42.16 Adult osteochondrosis of spine, lumbar region
- M42.17 Adult osteochondrosis of spine, lumbosacral region
- M42.18 Adult osteochondrosis of spine, sacral and sacrococcygeal region
- M42.19 Adult osteochondrosis of spine, multiple sites in spine

M42.9 Spinal osteochondrosis, unspecified

M43 Other deforming dorsopathies

Excludes1: *congenital spondylolysis and spondylolisthesis (Q76.2)*
hemivertebra (Q76.3-Q76.4)
Klippel-Feil syndrome (Q76.1)
lumbarization and sacralization (Q76.4)
platyspondylisis (Q76.4)
spina bifida occulta (Q76.0)
spinal curvature in osteoporosis (M80.-)
spinal curvature in Paget's disease of bone [osteitis deformans] (M88.-)

\+ **M43.0 Spondylolysis**
Excludes1: *congenital spondylolysis (Q76.2)*
spondylolisthesis (M43.1)
M43.00 Spondylolysis, site unspecified
M43.01 Spondylolysis, occipito-atlanto-axial region
M43.02 Spondylolysis, cervical region
M43.03 Spondylolysis, cervicothoracic region
M43.04 Spondylolysis, thoracic region
M43.05 Spondylolysis, thoracolumbar region
M43.06 Spondylolysis, lumbar region
M43.07 Spondylolysis, lumbosacral region
M43.08 Spondylolysis, sacral and sacrococcygeal region
M43.09 Spondylolysis, multiple sites in spine

\+ **M43.1 Spondylolisthesis**
Excludes1: *acute traumatic of lumbosacral region (S33.1)*
acute traumatic of sites other than lumbosacral- code to Fracture, vertebra, by region
congenital spondylolisthesis (Q76.2)
M43.10 Spondylolisthesis, site unspecified
M43.11 Spondylolisthesis, occipito-atlanto-axial region
M43.12 Spondylolisthesis, cervical region
M43.13 Spondylolisthesis, cervicothoracic region
M43.14 Spondylolisthesis, thoracic region
M43.15 Spondylolisthesis, thoracolumbar region
M43.16 Spondylolisthesis, lumbar region
M43.17 Spondylolisthesis, lumbosacral region
M43.18 Spondylolisthesis, sacral and sacrococcygeal region
M43.19 Spondylolisthesis, multiple sites in spine

\+ **M43.2 Fusion of spine**
Ankylosis of spinal joint
Excludes1: *ankylosing spondylitis (M45.0-)*
congenital fusion of spine (Q76.4)
Excludes2: *arthrodesis status (Z98.1)*
pseudoarthrosis after fusion or arthrodesis (M96.0)
M43.20 Fusion of spine, site unspecified
M43.21 Fusion of spine, occipito-atlanto-axial region
M43.22 Fusion of spine, cervical region
M43.23 Fusion of spine, cervicothoracic region
M43.24 Fusion of spine, thoracic region
M43.25 Fusion of spine, thoracolumbar region
M43.26 Fusion of spine, lumbar region
M43.27 Fusion of spine, lumbosacral region
M43.28 Fusion of spine, sacral and sacrococcygeal region

M43.3 Recurrent atlantoaxial dislocation with myelopathy
M43.4 Other recurrent atlantoaxial dislocation
\+ **M43.5 Other recurrent vertebral dislocation**
Excludes1: *biomechanical lesions NEC (M99.-)*
\+ **M43.5X Other recurrent vertebral dislocation**
M43.5X2 Other recurrent vertebral dislocation, cervical region
M43.5X3 Other recurrent vertebral dislocation, cervicothoracic region
M43.5X4 Other recurrent vertebral dislocation, thoracic region
M43.5X5 Other recurrent vertebral dislocation, thoracolumbar region
M43.5X6 Other recurrent vertebral dislocation, lumbar region
M43.5X7 Other recurrent vertebral dislocation, lumbosacral region
M43.5X8 Other recurrent vertebral dislocation, sacral and sacrococcygeal region
M43.5X9 Other recurrent vertebral dislocation, site unspecified

M43.6 Torticollis
Excludes1: *congenital (sternomastoid) torticollis (Q68.0)*
current injury - see Injury, of spine, by body region
ocular torticollis (R29.891)
psychogenic torticollis (F45.8)
spasmodic torticollis (G24.3)
torticollis due to birth injury (P15.2)

\+ **M43.8 Other specified deforming dorsopathies**
Excludes2: *kyphosis and lordosis (M40.-)*
scoliosis (M41.-)
\+ **M43.8X Other specified deforming dorsopathies**
M43.8X1 Other specified deforming dorsopathies, occipito-atlanto-axial region
M43.8X2 Other specified deforming dorsopathies, cervical region
M43.8X3 Other specified deforming dorsopathies, cervicothoracic region
M43.8X4 Other specified deforming dorsopathies, thoracic region
M43.8X5 Other specified deforming dorsopathies, thoracolumbar region
M43.8X6 Other specified deforming dorsopathies, lumbar region
M43.8X7 Other specified deforming dorsopathies, lumbosacral region
M43.8X8 Other specified deforming dorsopathies, sacral and sacrococcygeal region
M43.8X9 Other specified deforming dorsopathies, site unspecified

M43.9 Deforming dorsopathy, unspecified
Curvature of spine NOS

Spondylopathies (M45-M49)

M45 Ankylosing spondylitis

Rheumatoid arthritis of spine
Excludes1: *arthropathy in Reiter's disease (M02.3-)*
juvenile (ankylosing) spondylitis (M08.1)
Excludes2: *Behçet's disease (M35.2)*
M45.0 Ankylosing spondylitis of multiple sites in spine
M45.1 Ankylosing spondylitis of occipito-atlanto-axial region
M45.2 Ankylosing spondylitis of cervical region
M45.3 Ankylosing spondylitis of cervicothoracic region
M45.4 Ankylosing spondylitis of thoracic region
M45.5 Ankylosing spondylitis of thoracolumbar region
M45.6 Ankylosing spondylitis lumbar region
M45.7 Ankylosing spondylitis of lumbosacral region
M45.8 Ankylosing spondylitis sacral and sacrococcygeal region
M45.9 Ankylosing spondylitis of unspecified sites in spine

M46 Other inflammatory spondylopathies

\+ **M46.0 Spinal enthesopathy**
Disorder of ligamentous or muscular attachments of spine
M46.00 Spinal enthesopathy, site unspecified
M46.01 Spinal enthesopathy, occipito-atlanto-axial region
M46.02 Spinal enthesopathy, cervical region
M46.03 Spinal enthesopathy, cervicothoracic region
M46.04 Spinal enthesopathy, thoracic region
M46.05 Spinal enthesopathy, thoracolumbar region
M46.06 Spinal enthesopathy, lumbar region

M46.07 Spinal enthesopathy, lumbosacral region
M46.08 Spinal enthesopathy, sacral and sacrococcygeal region
M46.09 Spinal enthesopathy, multiple sites in spine
M46.1 Sacroiliitis, not elsewhere classified
+ M46.2 Osteomyelitis of vertebra
CC M46.20 Osteomyelitis of vertebra, site unspecified
CC Exclusion see Appendix A PDX collection 0881
CC M46.21 Osteomyelitis of vertebra, occipito-atlanto-axial region
CC Exclusion see Appendix A PDX collection 0881
CC M46.22 Osteomyelitis of vertebra, cervical region
CC Exclusion see Appendix A PDX collection 0881
CC M46.23 Osteomyelitis of vertebra, cervicothoracic region
CC Exclusion see Appendix A PDX collection 0881
CC M46.24 Osteomyelitis of vertebra, thoracic region
CC Exclusion see Appendix A PDX collection 0881
CC M46.25 Osteomyelitis of vertebra, thoracolumbar region
CC Exclusion see Appendix A PDX collection 0881
CC M46.26 Osteomyelitis of vertebra, lumbar region
CC Exclusion see Appendix A PDX collection 0881
CC M46.27 Osteomyelitis of vertebra, lumbosacral region
CC Exclusion see Appendix A PDX collection 0881
CC M46.28 Osteomyelitis of vertebra, sacral and sacrococcygeal region
CC Exclusion see Appendix A PDX collection 0881
+ M46.3 Infection of intervertebral disc (pyogenic)
Use additional code (B95-B97) to identify infectious agent
CC M46.30 Infection of intervertebral disc (pyogenic), site unspecified
CC Exclusion see Appendix A PDX collection 0882
CC M46.31 Infection of intervertebral disc (pyogenic), occipito-atlanto-axial region
CC Exclusion see Appendix A PDX collection 0882
CC M46.32 Infection of intervertebral disc (pyogenic), cervical region
CC Exclusion see Appendix A PDX collection 0882
CC M46.33 Infection of intervertebral disc (pyogenic), cervicothoracic region
CC Exclusion see Appendix A PDX collection 0882
CC M46.34 Infection of intervertebral disc (pyogenic), thoracic region
CC Exclusion see Appendix A PDX collection 0882
CC M46.35 Infection of intervertebral disc (pyogenic), thoracolumbar region
CC Exclusion see Appendix A PDX collection 0882
CC M46.36 Infection of intervertebral disc (pyogenic), lumbar region
CC Exclusion see Appendix A PDX collection 0882
CC M46.37 Infection of intervertebral disc (pyogenic), lumbosacral region
CC Exclusion see Appendix A PDX collection 0882
CC M46.38 Infection of intervertebral disc (pyogenic), sacral and sacrococcygeal region
CC Exclusion see Appendix A PDX collection 0882
CC M46.39 Infection of intervertebral disc (pyogenic), multiple sites in spine
CC Exclusion see Appendix A PDX collection 0882
+ M46.4 Discitis, unspecified
M46.40 Discitis, unspecified, site unspecified
M46.41 Discitis, unspecified, occipito-atlanto-axial region
M46.42 Discitis, unspecified, cervical region
M46.43 Discitis, unspecified, cervicothoracic region
M46.44 Discitis, unspecified, thoracic region
M46.45 Discitis, unspecified, thoracolumbar region
M46.46 Discitis, unspecified, lumbar region
M46.47 Discitis, unspecified, lumbosacral region
M46.48 Discitis, unspecified, sacral and sacrococcygeal region
M46.49 Discitis, unspecified, multiple sites in spine
+ M46.5 Other infective spondylopathies
M46.50 Other infective spondylopathies, site unspecified
M46.51 Other infective spondylopathies, occipito-atlanto-axial region
M46.52 Other infective spondylopathies, cervical region
M46.53 Other infective spondylopathies, cervicothoracic region
M46.54 Other infective spondylopathies, thoracic region
M46.55 Other infective spondylopathies, thoracolumbar region
M46.56 Other infective spondylopathies, lumbar region
M46.57 Other infective spondylopathies, lumbosacral region
M46.58 Other infective spondylopathies, sacral and sacrococcygeal region
M46.59 Other infective spondylopathies, multiple sites in spine
+ M46.8 Other specified inflammatory spondylopathies
M46.80 Other specified inflammatory spondylopathies, site unspecified
M46.81 Other specified inflammatory spondylopathies, occipito-atlanto-axial region
M46.82 Other specified inflammatory spondylopathies, cervical region
M46.83 Other specified inflammatory spondylopathies, cervicothoracic region
M46.84 Other specified inflammatory spondylopathies, thoracic region
M46.85 Other specified inflammatory spondylopathies, thoracolumbar region
M46.86 Other specified inflammatory spondylopathies, lumbar region
M46.87 Other specified inflammatory spondylopathies, lumbosacral region
M46.88 Other specified inflammatory spondylopathies, sacral and sacrococcygeal region
M46.89 Other specified inflammatory spondylopathies, multiple sites in spine
+ M46.9 Unspecified inflammatory spondylopathy
M46.90 Unspecified inflammatory spondylopathy, site unspecified
M46.91 Unspecified inflammatory spondylopathy, occipito-atlanto-axial region
M46.92 Unspecified inflammatory spondylopathy, cervical region
M46.93 Unspecified inflammatory spondylopathy, cervicothoracic region
M46.94 Unspecified inflammatory spondylopathy, thoracic region
M46.95 Unspecified inflammatory spondylopathy, thoracolumbar region
M46.96 Unspecified inflammatory spondylopathy, lumbar region
M46.97 Unspecified inflammatory spondylopathy, lumbosacral region
M46.98 Unspecified inflammatory spondylopathy, sacral and sacrococcygeal region
M46.99 Unspecified inflammatory spondylopathy, multiple sites in spine

M47 Spondylosis

Includes: arthrosis or osteoarthritis of spine
degeneration of facet joints
+ M47.0 Anterior spinal and vertebral artery compression syndromes
+ M47.01 Anterior spinal artery compression syndromes
CC M47.011 Anterior spinal artery compression syndromes, occipito-atlanto-axial region
CC Exclusion see Appendix A PDX collection 0883
CC M47.012 Anterior spinal artery compression syndromes, cervical region
CC Exclusion see Appendix A PDX collection 0883
CC M47.013 Anterior spinal artery compression syndromes, cervicothoracic region
CC Exclusion see Appendix A PDX collection 0883
CC M47.014 Anterior spinal artery compression syndromes, thoracic region
CC Exclusion see Appendix A PDX collection 0883
CC M47.015 Anterior spinal artery compression syndromes, thoracolumbar region
CC Exclusion see Appendix A PDX collection 0883
CC M47.016 Anterior spinal artery compression syndromes, lumbar region
CC Exclusion see Appendix A PDX collection 0883
CC M47.019 Anterior spinal artery compression syndromes, site unspecified
CC Exclusion see Appendix A PDX collection 0883
+ M47.02 Vertebral artery compression syndromes
CC M47.021 Vertebral artery compression syndromes, occipito-atlanto-axial region
CC Exclusion see Appendix A PDX collection 0883
CC M47.022 Vertebral artery compression syndromes, cervical region
CC Exclusion see Appendix A PDX collection 0883
CC M47.029 Vertebral artery compression syndromes, site unspecified
CC Exclusion see Appendix A PDX collection 0883

+ **M47.1 Other spondylosis with myelopathy**
  Spondylogenic compression of spinal cord
  Excludes1: *vertebral subluxation (M43.3-M43.59)*
CC **M47.10 Other spondylosis with myelopathy, site unspecified**
  CC Exclusion see Appendix A PDX collection 0884
CC **M47.11 Other spondylosis with myelopathy, occipito-atlanto-axial region**
  CC Exclusion see Appendix A PDX collection 0883
CC **M47.12 Other spondylosis with myelopathy, cervical region**
  CC Exclusion see Appendix A PDX collection 0883
CC **M47.13 Other spondylosis with myelopathy, cervicothoracic region**
  CC Exclusion see Appendix A PDX collection 0883
CC **M47.14 Other spondylosis with myelopathy, thoracic region**
  CC Exclusion see Appendix A PDX collection 0885
CC **M47.15 Other spondylosis with myelopathy, thoracolumbar region**
  CC Exclusion see Appendix A PDX collection 0885
CC **M47.16 Other spondylosis with myelopathy, lumbar region**
  CC Exclusion see Appendix A PDX collection 0886
+ **M47.2 Other spondylosis with radiculopathy**
  M47.20 Other spondylosis with radiculopathy, site unspecified
  M47.21 Other spondylosis with radiculopathy, occipito-atlanto-axial region
  M47.22 Other spondylosis with radiculopathy, cervical region
  M47.23 Other spondylosis with radiculopathy, cervicothoracic region
  M47.24 Other spondylosis with radiculopathy, thoracic region
  M47.25 Other spondylosis with radiculopathy, thoracolumbar region
  M47.26 Other spondylosis with radiculopathy, lumbar region
  M47.27 Other spondylosis with radiculopathy, lumbosacral region
  M47.28 Other spondylosis with radiculopathy, sacral and sacrococcygeal region
+ **M47.8 Other spondylosis**
+ **M47.81 Spondylosis without myelopathy or radiculopathy**
  M47.811 Spondylosis without myelopathy or radiculopathy, occipito-atlanto-axial region
  M47.812 Spondylosis without myelopathy or radiculopathy, cervical region
  M47.813 Spondylosis without myelopathy or radiculopathy, cervicothoracic region
  M47.814 Spondylosis without myelopathy or radiculopathy, thoracic region
  M47.815 Spondylosis without myelopathy or radiculopathy, thoracolumbar region
  M47.816 Spondylosis without myelopathy or radiculopathy, lumbar region
  M47.817 Spondylosis without myelopathy or radiculopathy, lumbosacral region
  M47.818 Spondylosis without myelopathy or radiculopathy, sacral and sacrococcygeal region
  M47.819 Spondylosis without myelopathy or radiculopathy, site unspecified
+ **M47.89 Other spondylosis**
  M47.891 Other spondylosis, occipito-atlanto-axial region
  M47.892 Other spondylosis, cervical region
  M47.893 Other spondylosis, cervicothoracic region
  M47.894 Other spondylosis, thoracic region
  M47.895 Other spondylosis, thoracolumbar region
  M47.896 Other spondylosis, lumbar region
  M47.897 Other spondylosis, lumbosacral region
  M47.898 Other spondylosis, sacral and sacrococcygeal region
  M47.899 Other spondylosis, site unspecified
M47.9 Spondylosis, unspecified

M48 Other spondylopathies

+ **M48.0 Spinal stenosis**
  Caudal stenosis
  M48.00 Spinal stenosis, site unspecified
  M48.01 Spinal stenosis, occipito-atlanto-axial region
  M48.02 Spinal stenosis, cervical region
  M48.03 Spinal stenosis, cervicothoracic region
  M48.04 Spinal stenosis, thoracic region
  M48.05 Spinal stenosis, thoracolumbar region
+ **M48.06 Spinal stenosis, lumbar region**
  M48.061 Spinal stenosis, lumbar region without neurogenic claudication
  Spinal stenosis. lumbar region NOS
  M48.062 Spinal stenosis, lumbar region with neurogenic claudication
  M48.07 Spinal stenosis, lumbosacral region
  M48.08 Spinal stenosis, sacral and sacrococcygeal region
+ **M48.1 Ankylosing hyperostosis [Forestier]**
  Diffuse idiopathic skeletal hyperostosis [DISH]
  M48.10 Ankylosing hyperostosis [Forestier], site unspecified
  M48.11 Ankylosing hyperostosis [Forestier], occipito-atlanto-axial region
  M48.12 Ankylosing hyperostosis [Forestier], cervical region
  M48.13 Ankylosing hyperostosis [Forestier], cervicothoracic region
  M48.14 Ankylosing hyperostosis [Forestier], thoracic region
  M48.15 Ankylosing hyperostosis [Forestier], thoracolumbar region
  M48.16 Ankylosing hyperostosis [Forestier], lumbar region
  M48.17 Ankylosing hyperostosis [Forestier], lumbosacral regio
  M48.18 Ankylosing hyperostosis [Forestier], sacral and sacrococcygeal region
  M48.19 Ankylosing hyperostosis [Forestier], multiple sites in spine
+ **M48.2 Kissing spine**
  M48.20 Kissing spine, site unspecified
  M48.21 Kissing spine, occipito-atlanto-axial region
  M48.22 Kissing spine, cervical region
  M48.23 Kissing spine, cervicothoracic region
  M48.24 Kissing spine, thoracic region
  M48.25 Kissing spine, thoracolumbar region
  M48.26 Kissing spine, lumbar region
  M48.27 Kissing spine, lumbosacral region
+ **M48.3 Traumatic spondylopathy**
CC **M48.30 Traumatic spondylopathy, site unspecified**
  CC Exclusion see Appendix A PDX collection 0887
CC **M48.31 Traumatic spondylopathy, occipito-atlanto-axial regio**
  CC Exclusion see Appendix A PDX collection 0887
CC **M48.32 Traumatic spondylopathy, cervical region**
  CC Exclusion see Appendix A PDX collection 0887
CC **M48.33 Traumatic spondylopathy, cervicothoracic region**
  CC Exclusion see Appendix A PDX collection 0887
CC **M48.34 Traumatic spondylopathy, thoracic region**
  CC Exclusion see Appendix A PDX collection 0887
CC **M48.35 Traumatic spondylopathy, thoracolumbar region**
  CC Exclusion see Appendix A PDX collection 0887
CC **M48.36 Traumatic spondylopathy, lumbar region**
  CC Exclusion see Appendix A PDX collection 0887
CC **M48.37 Traumatic spondylopathy, lumbosacral region**
  CC Exclusion see Appendix A PDX collection 0887
CC **M48.38 Traumatic spondylopathy, sacral and sacrococcyge. region**
  CC Exclusion see Appendix A PDX collection 0887
+ **M48.4 Fatigue fracture of vertebra**
  Stress fracture of vertebra
  Excludes1: *pathological fracture NOS (M84.4-)*
  pathological fracture of vertebra due to neoplasm (M84.58)
  pathological fracture of vertebra due to other diagnosis (M84.68)
  pathological fracture of vertebra due to osteoporosis (M80.-)
  traumatic fracture of vertebrae (S12.0-S12.3-, S22.0-, S32.0-)

The appropriate 7th character is to be added to each code from subcategory **M48.4**:
A initial encounter for fracture
D subsequent encounter for fracture with routine healing
G subsequent encounter for fracture with delayed healing
S sequela of fracture

X+7th **M48.40 Fatigue fracture of vertebra, site unspecified**
X+7th **M48.41 Fatigue fracture of vertebra, occipito-atlanto-axial region**
X+7th **M48.42 Fatigue fracture of vertebra, cervical region**
X+7th **M48.43 Fatigue fracture of vertebra, cervicothoracic region**
X+7th **M48.44 Fatigue fracture of vertebra, thoracic region**
X+7th **M48.45 Fatigue fracture of vertebra, thoracolumbar region**
X+7th **M48.46 Fatigue fracture of vertebra, lumbar region**

X+7th **M48.47 Fatigue fracture of vertebra, lumbosacral region**
X+7th **M48.48 Fatigue fracture of vertebra, sacral and sacrococcygeal region**

+ **M48.5 Collapsed vertebra, not elsewhere classified**
Collapsed vertebra NOS
Compression fracture of vertebra NOS
Wedging of vertebra NOS
Excludes1: *current injury - see Injury of spine, by body region*
fatigue fracture of vertebra (M48.4)
pathological fracture of vertebra due to neoplasm (M84.58)
pathological fracture of vertebra due to other diagnosis (M84.68)
pathological fracture of vertebra due to osteoporosis (M80.-)
pathological fracture NOS (M84.4-)
stress fracture of vertebra (M48.4-)
traumatic fracture of vertebra (S12.-, S22.-, S32.-)

The appropriate 7th character is to be added to each code from subcategory **M48.5**:
A initial encounter for fracture
D subsequent encounter for fracture with routine healing
G subsequent encounter for fracture with delayed healing
S sequela of fracture

CC X+7th **M48.50 Collapsed vertebra, not elsewhere classified, site unspecified**
CC Exclusion 7th character A see Appendix A PDX collection 0888
CC X+7th **M48.51 Collapsed vertebra, not elsewhere classified, occipito-atlanto-axial region**
CC Exclusion 7th character A see Appendix A PDX collection 0888
CC X+7th **M48.52 Collapsed vertebra, not elsewhere classified, cervical region**
CC Exclusion 7th character A see Appendix A PDX collection 0888
CC X+7th **M48.53 Collapsed vertebra, not elsewhere classified, cervicothoracic region**
CC Exclusion 7th character A see Appendix A PDX collection 0888
CC X+7th **M48.54 Collapsed vertebra, not elsewhere classified, thoracic region**
CC Exclusion 7th character A see Appendix A PDX collection 0888
CC X+7th **M48.55 Collapsed vertebra, not elsewhere classified, thoracolumbar region**
CC Exclusion 7th character A see Appendix A PDX collection 0888
CC X+7th **M48.56 Collapsed vertebra, not elsewhere classified, lumbar region**
CC Exclusion 7th character A see Appendix A PDX collection 0888
CC X+7th **M48.57 Collapsed vertebra, not elsewhere classified, lumbosacral region**
CC Exclusion 7th character A see Appendix A PDX collection 0888
CC X+7th **M48.58 Collapsed vertebra, not elsewhere classified, sacral and sacrococcygeal region**
CC Exclusion 7th character A see Appendix A PDX collection 0888

+ **M48.8 Other specified spondylopathies**
Ossification of posterior longitudinal ligament
+ **M48.8X Other specified spondylopathies**
M48.8X1 Other specified spondylopathies, occipito-atlanto-axial region
M48.8X2 Other specified spondylopathies, cervical region
M48.8X3 Other specified spondylopathies, cervicothoracic region
M48.8X4 Other specified spondylopathies, thoracic region
M48.8X5 Other specified spondylopathies, thoracolumbar region
M48.8X6 Other specified spondylopathies, lumbar region
M48.8X7 Other specified spondylopathies, lumbosacral region
M48.8X8 Other specified spondylopathies, sacral and sacrococcygeal region
M48.8X9 Other specified spondylopathies, site unspecified

M48.9 Spondylopathy, unspecified

M49 Spondylopathies in diseases classified elsewhere
Includes: curvature of spine in diseases classified elsewhere
deformity of spine in diseases classified elsewhere
kyphosis in diseases classified elsewhere
scoliosis in diseases classified elsewhere
spondylopathy in diseases classified elsewhere
Code first *underlying disease, such as:*
brucellosis (A23.-)
Charcot-Marie-Tooth disease (G60.0)
enterobacterial infections (A01-A04)
osteitis fibrosa cystica (E21.0)
Excludes1: *curvature of spine in tuberculosis [Pott's] (A18.01)*
enteropathic arthropathies (M07.-)
gonococcal spondylitis (A54.41)
neuropathic [tabes dorsalis] spondylitis (A52.11)
neuropathic spondylopathy in syringomyelia (G95.0)
neuropathic spondylopathy in tabes dorsalis (A52.11)
nonsyphilitic neuropathic spondylopathy NEC (G98.0)
spondylitis in syphilis (acquired) (A52.77)
tuberculous spondylitis (A18.01)
typhoid fever spondylitis (A01.05)

+ **M49.8 Spondylopathy in diseases classified elsewhere**
M49.80 Spondylopathy in diseases classified elsewhere, site unspecified
M49.81 Spondylopathy in diseases classified elsewhere, occipito-atlanto-axial region
M49.82 Spondylopathy in diseases classified elsewhere, cervical region
M49.83 Spondylopathy in diseases classified elsewhere, cervicothoracic region
M49.84 Spondylopathy in diseases classified elsewhere, thoracic region
M49.85 Spondylopathy in diseases classified elsewhere, thoracolumbar region
M49.86 Spondylopathy in diseases classified elsewhere, lumbar region
M49.87 Spondylopathy in diseases classified elsewhere, lumbosacral region
M49.88 Spondylopathy in diseases classified elsewhere, sacral and sacrococcygeal region
M49.89 Spondylopathy in diseases classified elsewhere, multiple sites in spine

Other dorsopathies (M50-M54)

Excludes1: *current injury - see injury of spine by body region*
discitis NOS (M46.4-)

M50 Cervical disc disorders
NOTE code to the most superior level of disorder
Includes: cervicothoracic disc disorders with cervicalgia
cervicothoracic disc disorders

+ **M50.0 Cervical disc disorder with myelopathy**
CC **M50.00 Cervical disc disorder with myelopathy, unspecified cervical region**
CC Exclusion see Appendix A PDX collection 0889
CC **M50.01 Cervical disc disorder with myelopathy, high cervical region**
C2-C3 disc disorder with myelopathy
C3-C4 disc disorder with myelopathy
CC Exclusion see Appendix A PDX collection 0889
AHA CC: 1Q, 2016, 17
+ **M50.02 Cervical disc disorder with myelopathy, mid-cervical region**
AHA CC: 4Q, 2016, 39-40
CC **M50.020 Cervical disc disorder with myelopathy, mid-cervical region, unspecified level**
CC Exclusion see Appendix A PDX collection 0889
CC **M50.021 Cervical disc disorder at C4-C5 level with myelopathy**
C4-C5 disc disorder with myelopathy
CC Exclusion see Appendix A PDX collection 0889
CC **M50.022 Cervical disc disorder at C5-C6 level with myelopathy**
C5-C6 disc disorder with myelopathy
CC Exclusion see Appendix A PDX collection 0889
CC **M50.023 Cervical disc disorder at C6-C7 level with myelopathy**
C6-C7 disc disorder with myelopathy
CC Exclusion see Appendix A PDX collection 0889

CC **M50.03 Cervical disc disorder with myelopathy, cervicothoracic region**
C7-T1 disc disorder with myelopathy
CC Exclusion see Appendix A PDX collection 0889

+ **M50.1 Cervical disc disorder with radiculopathy**
Excludes2: *brachial radiculitis NOS (M54.13)*

M50.10 Cervical disc disorder with radiculopathy, unspecified cervical region

M50.11 Cervical disc disorder with radiculopathy, high cervical region
C2-C3 disc disorder with radiculopathy
C3 radiculopathy due to disc disorder
C3-C4 disc disorder with radiculopathy
C4 radiculopathy due to disc disorder

+ **M50.12 Cervical disc disorder with radiculopathy, mid-cervical region**
AHA CC: 4Q, 2016, 39-40

M50.120 Mid-cervical disc disorder, unspecified

M50.121 Cervical disc disorder at C4-C5 level with radiculopathy
C4-C5 disc disorder with radiculopathy
C5 radiculopathy due to disc disorder

M50.122 Cervical disc disorder at C5-C6 level with radiculopathy
C5-C6 disc disorder with radiculopathy
C6 radiculopathy due to disc disorder

M50.123 Cervical disc disorder at C6-C7 level with radiculopathy
C6-C7 disc disorder with radiculopathy
C7 radiculopathy due to disc disorder

M50.13 Cervical disc disorder with radiculopathy, cervicothoracic region
C7-T1 disc disorder with radiculopathy
C8 radiculopathy due to disc disorder

+ **M50.2 Other cervical disc displacement**

M50.20 Other cervical disc displacement, unspecified cervical region

M50.21 Other cervical disc displacement, high cervical region
Other C2-C3 cervical disc displacement
Other C3-C4 cervical disc displacement

+ **M50.22 Other cervical disc displacement, mid-cervical region**

M50.220 Other cervical disc displacement, mid-cervical region, unspecified level

M50.221 Other cervical disc displacement at C4-C5 level
Other C4-C5 cervical disc displacement

M50.222 Other cervical disc displacement at C5-C6 level
Other C5-C6 cervical disc displacement

M50.223 Other cervical disc displacement at C6-C7 level
Other C6-C7 cervical disc displacement

+ **M50.23 Other cervical disc displacement, cervicothoracic region**
Other C7-T1 cervical disc displacement

+ **M50.3 Other cervical disc degeneration**

M50.30 Other cervical disc degeneration, unspecified cervical region

M50.31 Other cervical disc degeneration, high cervical region
Other C2-C3 cervical disc degeneration
Other C3-C4 cervical disc degeneration

+ **M50.32 Other cervical disc degeneration, mid-cervical region**

M50.320 Other cervical disc degeneration, mid-cervical region, unspecified level

M50.321 Other cervical disc degeneration at C4-C5 level
Other C4-C5 cervical disc degeneration

M50.322 Other cervical disc degeneration at C5-C6 level
Other C5-C6 cervical disc degeneration

M50.323 Other cervical disc degeneration at C6-C7 level
Other C6-C7 cervical disc degeneration

M50.33 Other cervical disc degeneration, cervicothoracic region
Other C7-T1 cervical disc degeneration

+ **M50.8 Other cervical disc disorders**

M50.80 Other cervical disc disorders, unspecified cervical region

M50.81 Other cervical disc disorders, high cervical region
Other C2-C3 cervical disc disorders
Other C3-C4 cervical disc disorders

+ **M50.82 Other cervical disc disorders, mid-cervical region**

M50.820 Other cervical disc disorders, mid-cervical region, unspecified level

M50.821 Other cervical disc disorders at C4-C5 level
Other C4-C5 cervical disc disorders

M50.822 Other cervical disc disorders at C5-C6 level
Other C5-C6 cervical disc disorders

M50.823 Other cervical disc disorders at C6-C7 level
Other C6-C7 cervical disc disorders

M50.83 Other cervical disc disorders, cervicothoracic region
Other C7-T1 cervical disc disorders

+ **M50.9 Cervical disc disorder, unspecified**

M50.90 Cervical disc disorder, unspecified, unspecified cervical region

M50.91 Cervical disc disorder, unspecified, high cervical region
Other C2-C3 cervical disc disorder, unspecified
Other C3-C4 cervical disc disorder, unspecified

+ **M50.92 Cervical disc disorder, unspecified, mid-cervical region**

M50.920 Unspecified cervical disc disorder, mid-cervical region, unspecified level

M50.921 Unspecified cervical disc disorder at C4-C5 level
Unspecified C4-C5 cervical disc disorder

M50.922 Unspecified cervical disc disorder at C5-C6 level
Unspecified C5-C6 cervical disc disorder

M50.923 Unspecified cervical disc disorder at C6-C7 level
Unspecified C6-C7 cervical disc disorder

M50.93 Cervical disc disorder, unspecified, cervicothoracic region
Other C7-T1 cervical disc disorder, unspecified

M51 Thoracic, thoracolumbar, and lumbosacral intervertebral disc disorders

Excludes2: *cervical and cervicothoracic disc disorders (M50.-)*
sacral and sacrococcygeal disorders (M53.3)

+ **M51.0 Thoracic, thoracolumbar and lumbosacral intervertebral disc disorders with myelopathy**

CC **M51.04 Intervertebral disc disorders with myelopathy, thoracic region**
CC Exclusion see Appendix A PDX collection 0890

CC **M51.05 Intervertebral disc disorders with myelopathy, thoracolumbar region**
CC Exclusion see Appendix A PDX collection 0890

CC **M51.06 Intervertebral disc disorders with myelopathy, lumbar region**
CC Exclusion see Appendix A PDX collection 0891

+ **M51.1 Thoracic, thoracolumbar and lumbosacral intervertebral disc disorders with radiculopathy**
Sciatica due to intervertebral disc disorder
Excludes1: *lumbar radiculitis NOS (M54.16)*
sciatica NOS (M54.3)

M51.14 Intervertebral disc disorders with radiculopathy, thoracic region

M51.15 Intervertebral disc disorders with radiculopathy, thoracolumbar region

M51.16 Intervertebral disc disorders with radiculopathy, lumbar region

M51.17 Intervertebral disc disorders with radiculopathy, lumbosacral region

+ **M51.2 Other thoracic, thoracolumbar and lumbosacral intervertebral disc displacement**
Lumbago due to displacement of intervertebral disc

M51.24 Other intervertebral disc displacement, thoracic region

M51.25 Other intervertebral disc displacement, thoracolumbar region

M51.26 **Other intervertebral disc displacement, lumbar region**
M51.27 **Other intervertebral disc displacement, lumbosacral region**

+ **M51.3 Other thoracic, thoracolumbar and lumbosacral intervertebral disc degeneration**
M51.34 **Other intervertebral disc degeneration, thoracic region**
M51.35 **Other intervertebral disc degeneration, thoracolumbar region**
M51.36 **Other intervertebral disc degeneration, lumbar region**
M51.37 **Other intervertebral disc degeneration, lumbosacral region**

+ **M51.4 Schmorl's nodes**
M51.44 **Schmorl's nodes, thoracic region**
M51.45 **Schmorl's nodes, thoracolumbar region**
M51.46 **Schmorl's nodes, lumbar region**
M51.47 **Schmorl's nodes, lumbosacral region**

+ **M51.8 Other thoracic, thoracolumbar and lumbosacral intervertebral disc disorders**
M51.84 **Other intervertebral disc disorders, thoracic region**
M51.85 **Other intervertebral disc disorders, thoracolumbar region**
M51.86 **Other intervertebral disc disorders, lumbar region**
M51.87 **Other intervertebral disc disorders, lumbosacral region**

M51.9 Unspecified thoracic, thoracolumbar and lumbosacral intervertebral disc disorder

M53 Other and unspecified dorsopathies, not elsewhere classified

M53.0 Cervicocranial syndrome
Posterior cervical sympathetic syndrome

M53.1 Cervicobrachial syndrome
Excludes2: *cervical disc disorder (M50.-)*
thoracic outlet syndrome (G54.0)

+ **M53.2 Spinal instabilities**
+ **M53.2X Spinal instabilities**
M53.2X1 **Spinal instabilities, occipito-atlanto-axial region**
M53.2X2 **Spinal instabilities, cervical region**
M53.2X3 **Spinal instabilities, cervicothoracic region**
M53.2X4 **Spinal instabilities, thoracic region**
M53.2X5 **Spinal instabilities, thoracolumbar region**
M53.2X6 **Spinal instabilities, lumbar region**
M53.2X7 **Spinal instabilities, lumbosacral region**
M53.2X8 **Spinal instabilities, sacral and sacrococcygeal region**
M53.2X9 **Spinal instabilities, site unspecified**

M53.3 Sacrococcygeal disorders, not elsewhere classified
Coccygodynia

+ **M53.8 Other specified dorsopathies**
M53.80 **Other specified dorsopathies, site unspecified**
M53.81 **Other specified dorsopathies, occipito-atlanto-axial region**
M53.82 **Other specified dorsopathies, cervical region**
M53.83 **Other specified dorsopathies, cervicothoracic region**
M53.84 **Other specified dorsopathies, thoracic region**
M53.85 **Other specified dorsopathies, thoracolumbar region**
M53.86 **Other specified dorsopathies, lumbar region**
M53.87 **Other specified dorsopathies, lumbosacral region**
M53.88 **Other specified dorsopathies, sacral and sacrococcygeal region**

M53.9 Dorsopathy, unspecified

M54 Dorsalgia

Excludes1: *psychogenic dorsalgia (F45.41)*

+ **M54.0 Panniculitis affecting regions of neck and back**
Excludes1: *lupus panniculitis (L93.2)*
panniculitis NOS (M79.3)
relapsing [Weber-Christian] panniculitis (M35.6)
M54.00 **Panniculitis affecting regions of neck and back, site unspecified**
M54.01 **Panniculitis affecting regions of neck and back, occipito-atlanto-axial region**
M54.02 **Panniculitis affecting regions of neck and back, cervical region**
M54.03 **Panniculitis affecting regions of neck and back, cervicothoracic region**
M54.04 **Panniculitis affecting regions of neck and back, thoracic region**
M54.05 **Panniculitis affecting regions of neck and back, thoracolumbar region**
M54.06 **Panniculitis affecting regions of neck and back, lumbar region**
M54.07 **Panniculitis affecting regions of neck and back, lumbosacral region**
M54.08 **Panniculitis affecting regions of neck and back, sacral and sacrococcygeal region**
M54.09 **Panniculitis affecting regions, neck and back, multiple sites in spine**

+ **M54.1 Radiculopathy**
Brachial neuritis or radiculitis NOS
Lumbar neuritis or radiculitis NOS
Lumbosacral neuritis or radiculitis NOS
Thoracic neuritis or radiculitis NOS
Radiculitis NOS
Excludes1: *neuralgia and neuritis NOS (M79.2)*
radiculopathy with cervical disc disorder (M50.1)
radiculopathy with lumbar and other intervertebral disc disorder (M51.1-)
radiculopathy with spondylosis (M47.2-)
M54.10 **Radiculopathy, site unspecified**
M54.11 **Radiculopathy, occipito-atlanto-axial region**
M54.12 **Radiculopathy, cervical region**
M54.13 **Radiculopathy, cervicothoracic region**
M54.14 **Radiculopathy, thoracic region**
M54.15 **Radiculopathy, thoracolumbar region**
M54.16 **Radiculopathy, lumbar region**
M54.17 **Radiculopathy, lumbosacral region**
M54.18 **Radiculopathy, sacral and sacrococcygeal region**

M54.2 Cervicalgia
Excludes1: *cervicalgia due to intervertebral cervical disc disorder (M50.-)*

+ **M54.3 Sciatica**
Excludes1: *lesion of sciatic nerve (G57.0)*
sciatica due to intervertebral disc disorder (M51.1-)
sciatica with lumbago (M54.4-)
M54.30 **Sciatica, unspecified side**
M54.31 **Sciatica, right side**
M54.32 **Sciatica, left side**

+ **M54.4 Lumbago with sciatica**
Excludes1: *lumbago with sciatica due to intervertebral disc disorder (M51.1-)*
M54.40 **Lumbago with sciatica, unspecified side**
M54.41 **Lumbago with sciatica, right side**
M54.42 **Lumbago with sciatica, left side**
AHA CC: 2Q, 2016, 7

M54.5 Low back pain
Loin pain
Lumbago NOS
Excludes1: *low back strain (S39.012)*
lumbago due to intervertebral disc displacement (M51.2-)
lumbago with sciatica (M54.4-)

M54.6 Pain in thoracic spine
Excludes1: *pain in thoracic spine due to intervertebral disc disorder (M51.-)*

+ **M54.8 Other dorsalgia**
Excludes1: *dorsalgia in thoracic region (M54.6)*
low back pain (M54.5)
M54.81 **Occipital neuralgia**
M54.89 **Other dorsalgia**

M54.9 Dorsalgia, unspecified
Backache NOS
Back pain NOS

SOFT TISSUE DISORDERS (M60-M79)

Disorders of muscles (M60-M63)

Excludes1: *dermatopolymyositis (M33.-)*
muscular dystrophies and myopathies (G71-G72)
myopathy in amyloidosis (E85.-)
myopathy in polyarteritis nodosa (M30.0)
myopathy in rheumatoid arthritis (M05.32)
myopathy in scleroderma (M34.-)
myopathy in Sjögren's syndrome (M35.03)
myopathy in systemic lupus erythematosus (M32.-)

M60 Myositis

Excludes2: *inclusion body myositis [IBM] (G72.41)*

+ **M60.0 Infective myositis**
Tropical pyomyositis
Use additional code (B95-B97) to identify infectious agent

+ **M60.00 Infective myositis, unspecified site**
CC **M60.000 Infective myositis, unspecified right arm**
Infective myositis, right upper limb NOS
CC Exclusion see Appendix A PDX collection 0806
CC **M60.001 Infective myositis, unspecified left arm**
Infective myositis, left upper limb NOS
CC Exclusion see Appendix A PDX collection 0806
CC **M60.002 Infective myositis, unspecified arm**
Infective myositis, upper limb NOS
CC Exclusion see Appendix A PDX collection 0806
CC **M60.003 Infective myositis, unspecified right leg**
Infective myositis, right lower limb NOS
CC Exclusion see Appendix A PDX collection 0806
CC **M60.004 Infective myositis, unspecified left leg**
Infective myositis, left lower limb NOS
CC Exclusion see Appendix A PDX collection 0806
CC **M60.005 Infective myositis, unspecified leg**
Infective myositis, lower limb NOS
CC Exclusion see Appendix A PDX collection 0806
CC **M60.009 Infective myositis, unspecified site**
CC Exclusion see Appendix A PDX collection 0806

+ **M60.01 Infective myositis, shoulder**
CC **M60.011 Infective myositis, right shoulder**
CC Exclusion see Appendix A PDX collection 0806
CC **M60.012 Infective myositis, left shoulder**
CC Exclusion see Appendix A PDX collection 0806
CC **M60.019 Infective myositis, unspecified shoulder**
CC Exclusion see Appendix A PDX collection 0806

+ **M60.02 Infective myositis, upper arm**
CC **M60.021 Infective myositis, right upper arm**
CC Exclusion see Appendix A PDX collection 0806
CC **M60.022 Infective myositis, left upper arm**
CC Exclusion see Appendix A PDX collection 0806
CC **M60.029 Infective myositis, unspecified upper arm**
CC Exclusion see Appendix A PDX collection 0806

+ **M60.03 Infective myositis, forearm**
CC **M60.031 Infective myositis, right forearm**
CC Exclusion see Appendix A PDX collection 0806
CC **M60.032 Infective myositis, left forearm**
CC Exclusion see Appendix A PDX collection 0806
CC **M60.039 Infective myositis, unspecified forearm**
CC Exclusion see Appendix A PDX collection 0806

+ **M60.04 Infective myositis, hand and fingers**
CC **M60.041 Infective myositis, right hand**
CC Exclusion see Appendix A PDX collection 0806
CC **M60.042 Infective myositis, left hand**
CC Exclusion see Appendix A PDX collection 0806
CC **M60.043 Infective myositis, unspecified hand**
CC Exclusion see Appendix A PDX collection 0806
CC **M60.044 Infective myositis, right finger(s)**
CC Exclusion see Appendix A PDX collection 0806
CC **M60.045 Infective myositis, left finger(s)**
CC Exclusion see Appendix A PDX collection 0806
CC **M60.046 Infective myositis, unspecified finger(s)**
CC Exclusion see Appendix A PDX collection 0806

+ **M60.05 Infective myositis, thigh**
CC **M60.051 Infective myositis, right thigh**
CC Exclusion see Appendix A PDX collection 0806
CC **M60.052 Infective myositis, left thigh**
CC Exclusion see Appendix A PDX collection 0806
CC **M60.059 Infective myositis, unspecified thigh**
CC Exclusion see Appendix A PDX collection 0806

+ **M60.06 Infective myositis, lower leg**
CC **M60.061 Infective myositis, right lower leg**
CC Exclusion see Appendix A PDX collection 080
CC **M60.062 Infective myositis, left lower leg**
CC Exclusion see Appendix A PDX collection 080
CC **M60.069 Infective myositis, unspecified lower leg**
CC Exclusion see Appendix A PDX collection 080

+ **M60.07 Infective myositis, ankle, foot and toes**
CC **M60.070 Infective myositis, right ankle**
CC Exclusion see Appendix A PDX collection 080
CC **M60.071 Infective myositis, left ankle**
CC Exclusion see Appendix A PDX collection 080
CC **M60.072 Infective myositis, unspecified ankle**
CC Exclusion see Appendix A PDX collection 080
CC **M60.073 Infective myositis, right foot**
CC Exclusion see Appendix A PDX collection 080
CC **M60.074 Infective myositis, left foot**
CC Exclusion see Appendix A PDX collection 080
CC **M60.075 Infective myositis, unspecified foot**
CC Exclusion see Appendix A PDX collection 080
CC **M60.076 Infective myositis, right toe(s)**
CC Exclusion see Appendix A PDX collection 080
CC **M60.077 Infective myositis, left toe(s)**
CC Exclusion see Appendix A PDX collection 080
CC **M60.078 Infective myositis, unspecified toe(s)**
CC Exclusion see Appendix A PDX collection 080

CC **M60.08 Infective myositis, other site**
CC Exclusion see Appendix A PDX collection 0806
CC **M60.09 Infective myositis, multiple sites**
CC Exclusion see Appendix A PDX collection 0806

+ **M60.1 Interstitial myositis**
M60.10 Interstitial myositis of unspecified site

+ **M60.11 Interstitial myositis, shoulder**
M60.111 Interstitial myositis, right shoulder
M60.112 Interstitial myositis, left shoulder
M60.119 Interstitial myositis, unspecified shoulder

+ **M60.12 Interstitial myositis, upper arm**
M60.121 Interstitial myositis, right upper arm
M60.122 Interstitial myositis, left upper arm
M60.129 Interstitial myositis, unspecified upper arm

+ **M60.13 Interstitial myositis, forearm**
M60.131 Interstitial myositis, right forearm
M60.132 Interstitial myositis, left forearm
M60.139 Interstitial myositis, unspecified forearm

+ **M60.14 Interstitial myositis, hand**
M60.141 Interstitial myositis, right hand
M60.142 Interstitial myositis, left hand
M60.149 Interstitial myositis, unspecifiedhand

+ **M60.15 Interstitial myositis, thigh**
M60.151 Interstitial myositis, right thigh
M60.152 Interstitial myositis, left thigh
M60.159 Interstitial myositis, unspecifiedthigh

+ **M60.16 Interstitial myositis, lower leg**
M60.161 Interstitial myositis, right lower leg
M60.162 Interstitial myositis, left lower leg
M60.169 Interstitial myositis, unspecified lower leg

+ **M60.17 Interstitial myositis, ankle and foot**
M60.171 Interstitial myositis, right ankle and foot
M60.172 Interstitial myositis, left ankle and foot
M60.179 Interstitial myositis, unspecified ankle and foot

M60.18 Interstitial myositis, other site
M60.19 Interstitial myositis, multiple sites

+ **M60.2 Foreign body granuloma of soft tissue, not elsewhere classified**
Use additional code to identify the type of retained foreign body (Z18.-)
Excludes1: *foreign body granuloma of skin and subcutaneous tissue (L92.3)*

M60.20 Foreign body granuloma of soft tissue, not elsewhere classified, unspecified site

+ **M60.21 Foreign body granuloma of soft tissue, not elsewhere classified, shoulder**
M60.211 Foreign body granuloma of soft tissue, not elsewhere classified, right shoulder
M60.212 Foreign body granuloma of soft tissue, not elsewhere classified, left shoulder
M60.219 Foreign body granuloma of soft tissue, not elsewhere classified, unspecified shoulder

+ **M60.22 Foreign body granuloma of soft tissue, not elsewhere classified, upper arm**
M60.221 Foreign body granuloma of soft tissue, not elsewhere classified, right upper arm

M60.222 Foreign body granuloma of soft tissue, not elsewhere classified, left upper arm
M60.229 Foreign body granuloma of soft tissue, not elsewhere classified, unspecified upper arm
+ M60.23 Foreign body granuloma of soft tissue, not elsewhere classified, forearm
M60.231 Foreign body granuloma of soft tissue, not elsewhere classified, right forearm
M60.232 Foreign body granuloma of soft tissue, not elsewhere classified, left forearm
M60.239 Foreign body granuloma of soft tissue, not elsewhere classified, unspecified forearm
+ M60.24 Foreign body granuloma of soft tissue, not elsewhere classified, hand
M60.241 Foreign body granuloma of soft tissue, not elsewhere classified, right hand
M60.242 Foreign body granuloma of soft tissue, not elsewhere classified, left hand
M60.249 Foreign body granuloma of soft tissue, not elsewhere classified, unspecified hand
+ M60.25 Foreign body granuloma of soft tissue, not elsewhere classified, thigh
M60.251 Foreign body granuloma of soft tissue, not elsewhere classified, right thigh
M60.252 Foreign body granuloma of soft tissue, not elsewhere classified, left thigh
M60.259 Foreign body granuloma of soft tissue, not elsewhere classified, unspecified thigh
+ M60.26 Foreign body granuloma of soft tissue, not elsewhere classified, lower leg
M60.261 Foreign body granuloma of soft tissue, not elsewhere classified, right lower leg
M60.262 Foreign body granuloma of soft tissue, not elsewhere classified, left lower leg
M60.269 Foreign body granuloma of soft tissue, not elsewhere classified, unspecified lower leg
+ M60.27 Foreign body granuloma of soft tissue, not elsewhere classified, ankle and foot
M60.271 Foreign body granuloma of soft tissue, not elsewhere classified, right ankle and foot
M60.272 Foreign body granuloma of soft tissue, not elsewhere classified, left ankle and foot
M60.279 Foreign body granuloma of soft tissue, not elsewhere classified, unspecified ankle and foot
M60.28 Foreign body granuloma of soft tissue, not elsewhere classified, other site
+ M60.8 Other myositis
M60.80 Other myositis, unspecified site
+ M60.81 Other myositis shoulder
M60.811 Other myositis, right shoulder
M60.812 Other myositis, left shoulder
M60.819 Other myositis, unspecified shoulder
+ M60.82 Other myositis, upper arm
M60.821 Other myositis, right upper arm
M60.822 Other myositis, left upper arm
M60.829 Other myositis, unspecified upper arm
+ M60.83 Other myositis, forearm
M60.831 Other myositis, right forearm
M60.832 Other myositis, left forearm
M60.839 Other myositis, unspecified forearm
+ M60.84 Other myositis, hand
M60.841 Other myositis, right hand
M60.842 Other myositis, left hand
M60.849 Other myositis, unspecified hand
+ M60.85 Other myositis, thigh
M60.851 Other myositis, right thigh
M60.852 Other myositis, left thigh
M60.859 Other myositis, unspecified thigh
+ M60.86 Other myositis, lower leg
M60.861 Other myositis, right lower leg
M60.862 Other myositis, left lower leg
M60.869 Other myositis, unspecified lower leg
+ M60.87 Other myositis, ankle and foot
M60.871 Other myositis, right ankle and foot
M60.872 Other myositis, left ankle and foot
M60.879 Other myositis, unspecified ankle and foot
M60.88 Other myositis, other site
M60.89 Other myositis, multiple sites
M60.9 Myositis, unspecified

M61 Calcification and ossification of muscle
+ M61.0 Myositis ossificans traumatica
M61.00 Myositis ossificans traumatica, unspecified site
+ M61.01 Myositis ossificans traumatica, shoulder
M61.011 Myositis ossificans traumatica, right shoulder
M61.012 Myositis ossificans traumatica, left shoulder
M61.019 Myositis ossificans traumatica, unspecified shoulder
+ M61.02 Myositis ossificans traumatica, upper arm
M61.021 Myositis ossificans traumatica, right upper arm
M61.022 Myositis ossificans traumatica, left upper arm
M61.029 Myositis ossificans traumatica, unspecified upper arm
+ M61.03 Myositis ossificans traumatica, forearm
M61.031 Myositis ossificans traumatica, right forearm
M61.032 Myositis ossificans traumatica, left forearm
M61.039 Myositis ossificans traumatica, unspecified forearm
+ M61.04 Myositis ossificans traumatica, hand
M61.041 Myositis ossificans traumatica, right hand
M61.042 Myositis ossificans traumatica, left hand
M61.049 Myositis ossificans traumatica, unspecified hand
+ M61.05 Myositis ossificans traumatica, thigh
M61.051 Myositis ossificans traumatica, right thigh
M61.052 Myositis ossificans traumatica, left thigh
M61.059 Myositis ossificans traumatica, unspecified thigh
+ M61.06 Myositis ossificans traumatica, lower leg
M61.061 Myositis ossificans traumatica, right lower leg
M61.062 Myositis ossificans traumatica, left lower leg
M61.069 Myositis ossificans traumatica, unspecified lower leg
+ M61.07 Myositis ossificans traumatica, ankle and foot
M61.071 Myositis ossificans traumatica, right ankle and foot
M61.072 Myositis ossificans traumatica, left ankle and foot
M61.079 Myositis ossificans traumatica, unspecified ankle and foot
M61.08 Myositis ossificans traumatica, other site
M61.09 Myositis ossificans traumatica, multiple sites
+ M61.1 Myositis ossificans progressiva
Fibrodysplasia ossificans progressiva
M61.10 Myositis ossificans progressiva, unspecified site
+ M61.11 Myositis ossificans progressiva, shoulder
M61.111 Myositis ossificans progressiva, right shoulder
M61.112 Myositis ossificans progressiva, left shoulder
M61.119 Myositis ossificans progressiva, unspecified shoulder
+ M61.12 Myositis ossificans progressiva, upper arm
M61.121 Myositis ossificans progressiva, right upper arm
M61.122 Myositis ossificans progressiva, left upper arm
M61.129 Myositis ossificans progressiva, unspecified arm
+ M61.13 Myositis ossificans progressiva, forearm
M61.131 Myositis ossificans progressiva, right forearm
M61.132 Myositis ossificans progressiva, left forearm
M61.139 Myositis ossificans progressiva, unspecified forearm
+ M61.14 Myositis ossificans progressiva, hand and finger(s)
M61.141 Myositis ossificans progressiva, right hand
M61.142 Myositis ossificans progressiva, left hand
M61.143 Myositis ossificans progressiva, unspecified hand
M61.144 Myositis ossificans progressiva, right finger(s)

M61.145 Myositis ossificans progressiva, left finger(s)
M61.146 Myositis ossificans progressiva, unspecified finger(s)
+ M61.15 Myositis ossificans progressiva, thigh
M61.151 Myositis ossificans progressiva, right thigh
M61.152 Myositis ossificans progressiva, left thigh
M61.159 Myositis ossificans progressiva, unspecified thigh
+ M61.16 Myositis ossificans progressiva, lower leg
M61.161 Myositis ossificans progressiva, right lower leg
M61.162 Myositis ossificans progressiva, left lower leg
M61.169 Myositis ossificans progressiva, unspecified lower leg
+ M61.17 Myositis ossificans progressiva, ankle, foot and toe(s)
M61.171 Myositis ossificans progressiva, right ankle
M61.172 Myositis ossificans progressiva, left ankle
M61.173 Myositis ossificans progressiva, unspecified ankle
M61.174 Myositis ossificans progressiva, right foot
M61.175 Myositis ossificans progressiva, left foot
M61.176 Myositis ossificans progressiva, unspecified foot
M61.177 Myositis ossificans progressiva, right toe(s)
M61.178 Myositis ossificans progressiva, left toe(s)
M61.179 Myositis ossificans progressiva, unspecified toe(s)
M61.18 Myositis ossificans progressiva, other site
M61.19 Myositis ossificans progressiva, multiple sites
+ M61.2 Paralytic calcification and ossification of muscle
Myositis ossificans associated with quadriplegia or paraplegia
M61.20 Paralytic calcification and ossification of muscle, unspecified site
+ M61.21 Paralytic calcification and ossification of muscle, shoulder
M61.211 Paralytic calcification and ossification of muscle, right shoulder
M61.212 Paralytic calcification and ossification of muscle, left shoulder
M61.219 Paralytic calcification and ossification of muscle, unspecified shoulder
+ M61.22 Paralytic calcification and ossification of muscle, upper arm
M61.221 Paralytic calcification and ossification of muscle, right upper arm
M61.222 Paralytic calcification and ossification of muscle, left upper arm
M61.229 Paralytic calcification and ossification of muscle, unspecified upper arm
+ M61.23 Paralytic calcification and ossification of muscle, forearm
M61.231 Paralytic calcification and ossification of muscle, right forearm
M61.232 Paralytic calcification and ossification of muscle, left forearm
M61.239 Paralytic calcification and ossification of muscle, unspecified forearm
+ M61.24 Paralytic calcification and ossification of muscle, hand
M61.241 Paralytic calcification and ossification of muscle, right hand
M61.242 Paralytic calcification and ossification of muscle, left hand
M61.249 Paralytic calcification and ossification of muscle, unspecified hand
+ M61.25 Paralytic calcification and ossification of muscle, thigh
M61.251 Paralytic calcification and ossification of muscle, right thigh
M61.252 Paralytic calcification and ossification of muscle, left thigh
M61.259 Paralytic calcification and ossification of muscle, unspecified thigh
+ M61.26 Paralytic calcification and ossification of muscle, lower leg
M61.261 Paralytic calcification and ossification of muscle, right lower leg
M61.262 Paralytic calcification and ossification of muscle, left lower leg
M61.269 Paralytic calcification and ossification of muscle, unspecified lower leg
+ M61.27 Paralytic calcification and ossification of muscle, ankle and foot
M61.271 Paralytic calcification and ossification of muscle, right ankle and foot
M61.272 Paralytic calcification and ossification of muscle, left ankle and foot
M61.279 Paralytic calcification and ossification of muscle, unspecified ankle and foot
M61.28 Paralytic calcification and ossification of muscle, other site
M61.29 Paralytic calcification and ossification of muscle, multiple sites
+ M61.3 Calcification and ossification of muscles associated with burns
Myositis ossificans associated with burns
M61.30 Calcification and ossification of muscles associated with burns, unspecified site
+ M61.31 Calcification and ossification of muscles associated with burns, shoulder
M61.311 Calcification and ossification of muscles associated with burns, right shoulder
M61.312 Calcification and ossification of muscles associated with burns, left shoulder
M61.319 Calcification and ossification of muscles associated with burns, unspecified shoulder
+ M61.32 Calcification and ossification of muscles associated with burns, upper arm
M61.321 Calcification and ossification of muscles associated with burns, right upper arm
M61.322 Calcification and ossification of muscles associated with burns, left upper arm
M61.329 Calcification and ossification of muscles associated with burns, unspecified upper arm
+ M61.33 Calcification and ossification of muscles associated with burns, forearm
M61.331 Calcification and ossification of muscles associated with burns, right forearm
M61.332 Calcification and ossification of muscles associated with burns, left forearm
M61.339 Calcification and ossification of muscles associated with burns, unspecified forearm
+ M61.34 Calcification and ossification of muscles associated with burns, hand
M61.341 Calcification and ossification of muscles associated with burns, right hand
M61.342 Calcification and ossification of muscles associated with burns, left hand
M61.349 Calcification and ossification of muscles associated with burns, unspecified hand
+ M61.35 Calcification and ossification of muscles associated with burns, thigh
M61.351 Calcification and ossification of muscles associated with burns, right thigh
M61.352 Calcification and ossification of muscles associated with burns, left thigh
M61.359 Calcification and ossification of muscles associated with burns, unspecified thigh
+ M61.36 Calcification and ossification of muscles associated with burns, lower leg
M61.361 Calcification and ossification of muscles associated with burns, right lower leg
M61.362 Calcification and ossification of muscles associated with burns, left lower leg
M61.369 Calcification and ossification of muscles associated with burns, unspecified lower leg
+ M61.37 Calcification and ossification of muscles associated with burns, ankle and foot
M61.371 Calcification and ossification of muscles associated with burns, right ankle and foot
M61.372 Calcification and ossification of muscles associated with burns, left ankle and foot
M61.379 Calcification and ossification of muscles associated with burns, unspecified ankle and foot

M61.38 Calcification and ossification of muscles associated with burns, other site
M61.39 Calcification and ossification of muscles associated with burns, multiple sites
+ M61.4 Other calcification of muscle
Excludes1: *calcific tendinitis NOS (M65.2-)*
calcific tendinitis of shoulder (M75.3)
M61.40 Other calcification of muscle, unspecified site
+ M61.41 Other calcification of muscle, shoulder
M61.411 Other calcification of muscle, right shoulder
M61.412 Other calcification of muscle, left shoulder
M61.419 Other calcification of muscle, unspecified shoulder
+ M61.42 Other calcification of muscle, upper arm
M61.421 Other calcification of muscle, right upper arm
M61.422 Other calcification of muscle, left upper arm
M61.429 Other calcification of muscle, unspecified upper arm
+ M61.43 Other calcification of muscle, forearm
M61.431 Other calcification of muscle, right forearm
M61.432 Other calcification of muscle, left forearm
M61.439 Other calcification of muscle, unspecified forearm
+ M61.44 Other calcification of muscle, hand
M61.441 Other calcification of muscle, right hand
M61.442 Other calcification of muscle, left hand
M61.449 Other calcification of muscle, unspecified hand
+ M61.45 Other calcification of muscle, thigh
M61.451 Other calcification of muscle, right thigh
M61.452 Other calcification of muscle, left thigh
M61.459 Other calcification of muscle, unspecified thigh
+ M61.46 Other calcification of muscle, lower leg
M61.461 Other calcification of muscle, right lower leg
M61.462 Other calcification of muscle, left lower leg
M61.469 Other calcification of muscle, unspecified lower leg
+ M61.47 Other calcification of muscle, ankle and foot
M61.471 Other calcification of muscle, right ankle and foot
M61.472 Other calcification of muscle, left ankle and foot
M61.479 Other calcification of muscle, unspecified ankle and foot
M61.48 Other calcification of muscle, other site
M61.49 Other calcification of muscle, multiple sites
+ M61.5 Other ossification of muscle
M61.50 Other ossification of muscle, unspecified site
+ M61.51 Other ossification of muscle, shoulder
M61.511 Other ossification of muscle, right shoulder
M61.512 Other ossification of muscle, left shoulder
M61.519 Other ossification of muscle, unspecified shoulder
+ M61.52 Other ossification of muscle, upper arm
M61.521 Other ossification of muscle, right upper arm
M61.522 Other ossification of muscle, left upper arm
M61.529 Other ossification of muscle, unspecified upper arm
+ M61.53 Other ossification of muscle, forearm
M61.531 Other ossification of muscle, right forearm
M61.532 Other ossification of muscle, left forearm
M61.539 Other ossification of muscle, unspecified forearm
+ M61.54 Other ossification of muscle, hand
M61.541 Other ossification of muscle, right hand
M61.542 Other ossification of muscle, left hand
M61.549 Other ossification of muscle, unspecified hand
+ M61.55 Other ossification of muscle, thigh
M61.551 Other ossification of muscle, right thigh
M61.552 Other ossification of muscle, left thigh
M61.559 Other ossification of muscle, unspecified thigh
+ M61.56 Other ossification of muscle, lower leg
M61.561 Other ossification of muscle, right lower leg
M61.562 Other ossification of muscle, left lower leg
M61.569 Other ossification of muscle, unspecified lower leg
+ M61.57 Other ossification of muscle, ankle and foot
M61.571 Other ossification of muscle, right ankle and foot
M61.572 Other ossification of muscle, left ankle and foot
M61.579 Other ossification of muscle, unspecified ankle and foot
M61.58 Other ossification of muscle, other site
M61.59 Other ossification of muscle, multiple sites
M61.9 Calcification and ossification of muscle, unspecified

M62 Other disorders of muscle

Excludes1: *alcoholic myopathy (G72.1)*
cramp and spasm (R25.2)
drug-induced myopathy (G72.0)
myalgia (M79.1)
stiff-man syndrome (G25.82)
Excludes2: *nontraumatic hematoma of muscle (M79.81)*
+ M62.0 Separation of muscle (nontraumatic)
Diastasis of muscle
Excludes1: *diastasis recti complicating pregnancy, labor and delivery (O71.8)*
traumatic separation of muscle- see strain of muscle by body region
M62.00 Separation of muscle (nontraumatic), unspecified site
+ M62.01 Separation of muscle (nontraumatic), shoulder
M62.011 Separation of muscle (nontraumatic), right shoulder
M62.012 Separation of muscle (nontraumatic), left shoulder
M62.019 Separation of muscle (nontraumatic), unspecified shoulder
+ M62.02 Separation of muscle (nontraumatic), upper arm
M62.021 Separation of muscle (nontraumatic), right upper arm
M62.022 Separation of muscle (nontraumatic), left upper arm
M62.029 Separation of muscle (nontraumatic), unspecified upper arm
+ M62.03 Separation of muscle (nontraumatic), forearm
M62.031 Separation of muscle (nontraumatic), right forearm
M62.032 Separation of muscle (nontraumatic), left forearm
M62.039 Separation of muscle (nontraumatic), unspecified forearm
+ M62.04 Separation of muscle (nontraumatic), hand
M62.041 Separation of muscle (nontraumatic), right hand
M62.042 Separation of muscle (nontraumatic), left hand
M62.049 Separation of muscle (nontraumatic), unspecified hand
+ M62.05 Separation of muscle (nontraumatic), thigh
M62.051 Separation of muscle (nontraumatic), right thigh
M62.052 Separation of muscle (nontraumatic), left thigh
M62.059 Separation of muscle (nontraumatic), unspecified thigh
+ M62.06 Separation of muscle (nontraumatic), lower leg
M62.061 Separation of muscle (nontraumatic), right lower leg
M62.062 Separation of muscle (nontraumatic), left lower leg
M62.069 Separation of muscle (nontraumatic), unspecified lower leg
+ M62.07 Separation of muscle (nontraumatic), ankle and foot
M62.071 Separation of muscle (nontraumatic), right ankle and foot
M62.072 Separation of muscle (nontraumatic), left ankle and foot
M62.079 Separation of muscle (nontraumatic), unspecified ankle and foot
M62.08 Separation of muscle (nontraumatic), other site

+ **M62.1 Other rupture of muscle (nontraumatic)**
  Excludes1: *traumatic rupture of muscle - see strain of muscle by body region*
  Excludes2: *rupture of tendon (M66.-)*
  M62.10 Other rupture of muscle (nontraumatic), unspecified site
  + **M62.11 Other rupture of muscle (nontraumatic), shoulder**
    M62.111 Other rupture of muscle (nontraumatic), right shoulder
    M62.112 Other rupture of muscle (nontraumatic), left shoulder
    M62.119 Other rupture of muscle (nontraumatic), unspecified shoulder
  + **M62.12 Other rupture of muscle (nontraumatic), upper arm**
    M62.121 Other rupture of muscle (nontraumatic), right upper arm
    M62.122 Other rupture of muscle (nontraumatic), left upper arm
    M62.129 Other rupture of muscle (nontraumatic), unspecified upper arm
  + **M62.13 Other rupture of muscle (nontraumatic), forearm**
    M62.131 Other rupture of muscle (nontraumatic), right forearm
    M62.132 Other rupture of muscle (nontraumatic), left forearm
    M62.139 Other rupture of muscle (nontraumatic), unspecified forearm
  + **M62.14 Other rupture of muscle (nontraumatic), hand**
    M62.141 Other rupture of muscle (nontraumatic), right hand
    M62.142 Other rupture of muscle (nontraumatic), left hand
    M62.149 Other rupture of muscle (nontraumatic), unspecified hand
  + **M62.15 Other rupture of muscle (nontraumatic), thigh**
    M62.151 Other rupture of muscle (nontraumatic), right thigh
    M62.152 Other rupture of muscle (nontraumatic), left thigh
    M62.159 Other rupture of muscle (nontraumatic), unspecified thigh
  + **M62.16 Other rupture of muscle (nontraumatic), lower leg**
    M62.161 Other rupture of muscle (nontraumatic), right lower leg
    M62.162 Other rupture of muscle (nontraumatic), left lower leg
    M62.169 Other rupture of muscle (nontraumatic), unspecified lower leg
  + **M62.17 Other rupture of muscle (nontraumatic), ankle and foot**
    M62.171 Other rupture of muscle (nontraumatic), right ankle and foot
    M62.172 Other rupture of muscle (nontraumatic), left ankle and foot
    M62.179 Other rupture of muscle (nontraumatic), unspecified ankle and foot
  M62.18 Other rupture of muscle (nontraumatic), other site

+ **M62.2 Nontraumatic ischemic infarction of muscle**
  Excludes1: *compartment syndrome (traumatic) (T79.A-)*
  nontraumatic compartment syndrome (M79.A-)
  traumatic ischemia of muscle (T79.6)
  rhabdomyolysis (M62.82)
  Volkmann's ischemic contracture (T79.6)
  M62.20 Nontraumatic ischemic infarction of muscle, unspecified site
  + **M62.21 Nontraumatic ischemic infarction of muscle, shoulder**
    M62.211 Nontraumatic ischemic infarction of muscle, right shoulder
    M62.212 Nontraumatic ischemic infarction of muscle, left shoulder
    M62.219 Nontraumatic ischemic infarction of muscle, unspecified shoulder
  + **M62.22 Nontraumatic ischemic infarction of muscle, upper arm**
    M62.221 Nontraumatic ischemic infarction of muscle, right upper arm
    M62.222 Nontraumatic ischemic infarction of muscle, left upper arm
    M62.229 Nontraumatic ischemic infarction of muscle, unspecified upper arm
  + **M62.23 Nontraumatic ischemic infarction of muscle, forear**
    M62.231 Nontraumatic ischemic infarction of muscle, right forearm
    M62.232 Nontraumatic ischemic infarction of muscle, left forearm
    M62.239 Nontraumatic ischemic infarction of muscle, unspecified forearm
  + **M62.24 Nontraumatic ischemic infarction of muscle, hand**
    M62.241 Nontraumatic ischemic infarction of muscle, right hand
    M62.242 Nontraumatic ischemic infarction of muscle, left hand
    M62.249 Nontraumatic ischemic infarction of muscle, unspecified hand
  + **M62.25 Nontraumatic ischemic infarction of muscle, thigh**
    M62.251 Nontraumatic ischemic infarction of muscle, right thigh
    M62.252 Nontraumatic ischemic infarction of muscle, left thigh
    M62.259 Nontraumatic ischemic infarction of muscle, unspecified thigh
  + **M62.26 Nontraumatic ischemic infarction of muscle, lower leg**
    M62.261 Nontraumatic ischemic infarction of muscle, right lower leg
    M62.262 Nontraumatic ischemic infarction of muscle, left lower leg
    M62.269 Nontraumatic ischemic infarction of muscle, unspecified lower leg
  + **M62.27 Nontraumatic ischemic infarction of muscle, ankle and foot**
    M62.271 Nontraumatic ischemic infarction of muscle, right ankle and foot
    M62.272 Nontraumatic ischemic infarction of muscle, left ankle and foot
    M62.279 Nontraumatic ischemic infarction of muscle, unspecified ankle and foot
  M62.28 Nontraumatic ischemic infarction of muscle, other site

M62.3 Immobility syndrome (paraplegic)

+ **M62.4 Contracture of muscle**
  Contracture of tendon (sheath)
  Excludes1: *contracture of joint (M24.5-)*
  M62.40 Contracture of muscle, unspecified site
  + **M62.41 Contracture of muscle, shoulder**
    M62.411 Contracture of muscle, right shoulder
    M62.412 Contracture of muscle, left shoulder
    M62.419 Contracture of muscle, unspecified shoulder
  + **M62.42 Contracture of muscle, upper arm**
    M62.421 Contracture of muscle, right upper arm
    M62.422 Contracture of muscle, left upper arm
    M62.429 Contracture of muscle, unspecified upper arm
  + **M62.43 Contracture of muscle, forearm**
    M62.431 Contracture of muscle, right forearm
    M62.432 Contracture of muscle, left forearm
    M62.439 Contracture of muscle, unspecified forear
  + **M62.44 Contracture of muscle, hand**
    M62.441 Contracture of muscle, right hand
    M62.442 Contracture of muscle, left hand
    M62.449 Contracture of muscle, unspecified hand
  + **M62.45 Contracture of muscle, thigh**
    M62.451 Contracture of muscle, right thigh
    M62.452 Contracture of muscle, left thigh
    M62.459 Contracture of muscle, unspecified thigh
  + **M62.46 Contracture of muscle, lower leg**
    M62.461 Contracture of muscle, right lower leg
    M62.462 Contracture of muscle, left lower leg
    M62.469 Contracture of muscle, unspecified lower leg
  + **M62.47 Contracture of muscle, ankle and foot**
    M62.471 Contracture of muscle, right ankle and fo
    M62.472 Contracture of muscle, left ankle and foot
    M62.479 Contracture of muscle, unspecified ankle and foot
  M62.48 Contracture of muscle, other site
  M62.49 Contracture of muscle, multiple sites

+ **M62.5 Muscle wasting and atrophy, not elsewhere classified**
Disuse atrophy NEC
Excludes1: *neuralgic amyotrophy (G54.5)*
progressive muscular atrophy (G12.21)
sarcopenia (M62.84)
Excludes2: *pelvic muscle wasting (N81.84)*
M62.50 Muscle wasting and atrophy, not elsewhere classified, unspecified site
+ **M62.51 Muscle wasting and atrophy, not elsewhere classified, shoulder**
M62.511 Muscle wasting and atrophy, not elsewhere classified, right shoulder
M62.512 Muscle wasting and atrophy, not elsewhere classified, left shoulder
M62.519 Muscle wasting and atrophy, not elsewhere classified, unspecified shoulder
+ **M62.52 Muscle wasting and atrophy, not elsewhere classified, upper arm**
M62.521 Muscle wasting and atrophy, not elsewhere classified, right upper arm
M62.522 Muscle wasting and atrophy, not elsewhere classified, left upper arm
M62.529 Muscle wasting and atrophy, not elsewhere classified, unspecified upper arm
+ **M62.53 Muscle wasting and atrophy, not elsewhere classified, forearm**
M62.531 Muscle wasting and atrophy, not elsewhere classified, right forearm
M62.532 Muscle wasting and atrophy, not elsewhere classified, left forearm
M62.539 Muscle wasting and atrophy, not elsewhere classified, unspecified forearm
+ **M62.54 Muscle wasting and atrophy, not elsewhere classified, hand**
M62.541 Muscle wasting and atrophy, not elsewhere classified, right hand
M62.542 Muscle wasting and atrophy, not elsewhere classified, left hand
M62.549 Muscle wasting and atrophy, not elsewhere classified, unspecified hand
+ **M62.55 Muscle wasting and atrophy, not elsewhere classified, thigh**
M62.551 Muscle wasting and atrophy, not elsewhere classified, right thigh
M62.552 Muscle wasting and atrophy, not elsewhere classified, left thigh
M62.559 Muscle wasting and atrophy, not elsewhere classified, unspecified thigh
+ **M62.56 Muscle wasting and atrophy, not elsewhere classified, lower leg**
M62.561 Muscle wasting and atrophy, not elsewhere classified, right lower leg
M62.562 Muscle wasting and atrophy, not elsewhere classified, left lower leg
M62.569 Muscle wasting and atrophy, not elsewhere classified, unspecified lower leg
+ **M62.57 Muscle wasting and atrophy, not elsewhere classified, ankle and foot**
M62.571 Muscle wasting and atrophy, not elsewhere classified, right ankle and foot
M62.572 Muscle wasting and atrophy, not elsewhere classified, left ankle and foot
M62.579 Muscle wasting and atrophy, not elsewhere classified, unspecified ankle and foot
M62.58 Muscle wasting and atrophy, not elsewhere classified, other site
M62.59 Muscle wasting and atrophy, not elsewhere classified, multiple sites
+ **M62.8 Other specified disorders of muscle**
Excludes2: *nontraumatic hematoma of muscle (M79.81)*
M62.81 Muscle weakness (generalized)
Excludes1: *muscle weakness in sarcopenia (M62.84)*
CC **M62.82 Rhabdomyolysis**
Excludes1: *traumatic rhabdomyolysis (T79.6)*
CC Exclusion see Appendix A PDX collection 0892
+ **M62.83 Muscle spasm**
M62.830 Muscle spasm of back
M62.831 Muscle spasm of calf
Charley-horse
M62.838 Other muscle spasm
M62.84 Sarcopenia
Age-related sarcopenia
Code first underlying disease, if applicable, such as:
disorders of myoneural junction and muscle disease in diseases classified elsewhere (G73.-)
other and unspecified myopathies (G72.-)
primary disorders of muscles (G71.-)
AHA CC: 4Q, 2016, 41
M62.89 Other specified disorders of muscle
Muscle (sheath) hernia
M62.9 Disorder of muscle, unspecified

M63 Disorders of muscle in diseases classified elsewhere

Code first underlying disease, such as:
leprosy (A30.-)
neoplasm (C49.-, C79.89, D21.-, D48.1)
schistosomiasis (B65.-)
trichinellosis (B75)
Excludes1: *myopathy in cysticercosis (B69.81)*
myopathy in endocrine diseases (G73.7)
myopathy in metabolic diseases (G73.7)
myopathy in sarcoidosis (D86.87)
myopathy in secondary syphilis (A51.49)
myopathy in syphilis (late) (A52.78)
myopathy in toxoplasmosis (B58.82)
myopathy in tuberculosis (A18.09)
+ **M63.8 Disorders of muscle in diseases classified elsewhere**
M63.80 Disorders of muscle in diseases classified elsewhere, unspecified site
+ **M63.81 Disorders of muscle in diseases classified elsewhere, shoulder**
M63.811 Disorders of muscle in diseases classified elsewhere, right shoulder
M63.812 Disorders of muscle in diseases classified elsewhere, left shoulder
M63.819 Disorders of muscle in diseases classified elsewhere, unspecified shoulder
+ **M63.82 Disorders of muscle in diseases classified elsewhere, upper arm**
M63.821 Disorders of muscle in diseases classified elsewhere, right upper arm
M63.822 Disorders of muscle in diseases classified elsewhere, left upper arm
M63.829 Disorders of muscle in diseases classified elsewhere, unspecified upper arm
+ **M63.83 Disorders of muscle in diseases classified elsewhere, forearm**
M63.831 Disorders of muscle in diseases classified elsewhere, right forearm
M63.832 Disorders of muscle in diseases classified elsewhere, left forearm
M63.839 Disorders of muscle in diseases classified elsewhere, unspecified forearm
+ **M63.84 Disorders of muscle in diseases classified elsewhere, hand**
M63.841 Disorders of muscle in diseases classified elsewhere, right hand
M63.842 Disorders of muscle in diseases classified elsewhere, left hand
M63.849 Disorders of muscle in diseases classified elsewhere, unspecified hand
+ **M63.85 Disorders of muscle in diseases classified elsewhere, thigh**
M63.851 Disorders of muscle in diseases classified elsewhere, right thigh
M63.852 Disorders of muscle in diseases classified elsewhere, left thigh
M63.859 Disorders of muscle in diseases classified elsewhere, unspecified thigh
+ **M63.86 Disorders of muscle in diseases classified elsewhere, lower leg**
M63.861 Disorders of muscle in diseases classified elsewhere, right lower leg
M63.862 Disorders of muscle in diseases classified elsewhere, left lower leg
M63.869 Disorders of muscle in diseases classified elsewhere, unspecified lower leg

+ M63.87 Disorders of muscle in diseases classified elsewhere, ankle and foot
M63.871 Disorders of muscle in diseases classified elsewhere, right ankle and foot
M63.872 Disorders of muscle in diseases classified elsewhere, left ankle and foot
M63.879 Disorders of muscle in diseases classified elsewhere, unspecified ankle and foot
M63.88 Disorders of muscle in diseases classified elsewhere, other site
M63.89 Disorders of muscle in diseases classified elsewhere, multiple sites

Disorders of synovium and tendon (M65-M67)

M65 Synovitis and tenosynovitis

Excludes1: *chronic crepitant synovitis of hand and wrist (M70.0-)*
current injury - see injury of ligament or tendon by body region
soft tissue disorders related to use, overuse and pressure (M70.-)

+ M65.0 Abscess of tendon sheath
Use additional code (B95-B96) to identify bacterial agent
M65.00 Abscess of tendon sheath, unspecified site
+ M65.01 Abscess of tendon sheath, shoulder
M65.011 Abscess of tendon sheath, right shoulder
M65.012 Abscess of tendon sheath, left shoulder
M65.019 Abscess of tendon sheath, unspecified shoulder
+ M65.02 Abscess of tendon sheath, upper arm
M65.021 Abscess of tendon sheath, right upper arm
M65.022 Abscess of tendon sheath, left upper arm
M65.029 Abscess of tendon sheath, unspecified upper arm
+ M65.03 Abscess of tendon sheath, forearm
M65.031 Abscess of tendon sheath, right forearm
M65.032 Abscess of tendon sheath, left forearm
M65.039 Abscess of tendon sheath, unspecified forearm
+ M65.04 Abscess of tendon sheath, hand
M65.041 Abscess of tendon sheath, right hand
M65.042 Abscess of tendon sheath, left hand
M65.049 Abscess of tendon sheath, unspecified hand
+ M65.05 Abscess of tendon sheath, thigh
M65.051 Abscess of tendon sheath, right thigh
M65.052 Abscess of tendon sheath, left thigh
M65.059 Abscess of tendon sheath, unspecified thigh
+ M65.06 Abscess of tendon sheath, lower leg
M65.061 Abscess of tendon sheath, right lower leg
M65.062 Abscess of tendon sheath, left lower leg
M65.069 Abscess of tendon sheath, unspecified lower leg
+ M65.07 Abscess of tendon sheath, ankle and foot
M65.071 Abscess of tendon sheath, right ankle and foot
M65.072 Abscess of tendon sheath, left ankle and foot
M65.079 Abscess of tendon sheath, unspecified ankle and foot
M65.08 Abscess of tendon sheath, other site
+ M65.1 Other infective (teno)synovitis
M65.10 Other infective (teno)synovitis, unspecified site
+ M65.11 Other infective (teno)synovitis, shoulder
M65.111 Other infective (teno)synovitis, right shoulder
M65.112 Other infective (teno)synovitis, left shoulder
M65.119 Other infective (teno)synovitis, unspecified shoulder
+ M65.12 Other infective (teno)synovitis, elbow
M65.121 Other infective (teno)synovitis, right elbow
M65.122 Other infective (teno)synovitis, left elbow
M65.129 Other infective (teno)synovitis, unspecified elbow
+ M65.13 Other infective (teno)synovitis, wrist
M65.131 Other infective (teno)synovitis, right wrist
M65.132 Other infective (teno)synovitis, left wrist
M65.139 Other infective (teno)synovitis, unspecified wrist
+ M65.14 Other infective (teno)synovitis, hand
M65.141 Other infective (teno)synovitis, right hand
M65.142 Other infective (teno)synovitis, left hand
M65.149 Other infective (teno)synovitis, unspecified hand
+ M65.15 Other infective (teno)synovitis, hip
M65.151 Other infective (teno)synovitis, right hip
M65.152 Other infective (teno)synovitis, left hip
M65.159 Other infective (teno)synovitis, unspecified hip
+ M65.16 Other infective (teno)synovitis, knee
M65.161 Other infective (teno)synovitis, right knee
M65.162 Other infective (teno)synovitis, left knee
M65.169 Other infective (teno)synovitis, unspecified knee
+ M65.17 Other infective (teno)synovitis, ankle and foot
M65.171 Other infective (teno)synovitis, right ankle and foot
M65.172 Other infective (teno)synovitis, left ankle and foot
M65.179 Other infective (teno)synovitis, unspecified ankle and foot
M65.18 Other infective (teno)synovitis, other site
M65.19 Other infective (teno)synovitis, multiple sites
+ M65.2 Calcific tendinitis
Excludes1: *tendinitis as classified in M75-M77*
calcified tendinitis of shoulder (M75.3)
M65.20 Calcific tendinitis, unspecified site
+ M65.22 Calcific tendinitis, upper arm
M65.221 Calcific tendinitis, right upper arm
M65.222 Calcific tendinitis, left upper arm
M65.229 Calcific tendinitis, unspecified upper arm
+ M65.23 Calcific tendinitis, forearm
M65.231 Calcific tendinitis, right forearm
M65.232 Calcific tendinitis, left forearm
M65.239 Calcific tendinitis, unspecified forearm
+ M65.24 Calcific tendinitis, hand
M65.241 Calcific tendinitis, right hand
M65.242 Calcific tendinitis, left hand
M65.249 Calcific tendinitis, unspecified hand
+ M65.25 Calcific tendinitis, thigh
M65.251 Calcific tendinitis, right thigh
M65.252 Calcific tendinitis, left thigh
M65.259 Calcific tendinitis, unspecified thigh
+ M65.26 Calcific tendinitis, lower leg
M65.261 Calcific tendinitis, right lower leg
M65.262 Calcific tendinitis, left lower leg
M65.269 Calcific tendinitis, unspecified lower leg
+ M65.27 Calcific tendinitis, ankle and foot
M65.271 Calcific tendinitis, right ankle and foot
M65.272 Calcific tendinitis, left ankle and foot
M65.279 Calcific tendinitis, unspecified ankle and foot
M65.28 Calcific tendinitis, other site
M65.29 Calcific tendinitis, multiple sites
+ M65.3 Trigger finger
Nodular tendinous disease
M65.30 Trigger finger, unspecified finger
+ M65.31 Trigger thumb
M65.311 Trigger thumb, right thumb
M65.312 Trigger thumb, left thumb
M65.319 Trigger thumb, unspecified thumb
+ M65.32 Trigger finger, index finger
M65.321 Trigger finger, right index finger
M65.322 Trigger finger, left index finger
M65.329 Trigger finger, unspecified index finger
+ M65.33 Trigger finger, middle finger
M65.331 Trigger finger, right middle finger
M65.332 Trigger finger, left middle finger
M65.339 Trigger finger, unspecified middle finger
+ M65.34 Trigger finger, ring finger
M65.341 Trigger finger, right ring finger
M65.342 Trigger finger, left ring finger
M65.349 Trigger finger, unspecified ring finger
+ M65.35 Trigger finger, little finger
M65.351 Trigger finger, right little finger
M65.352 Trigger finger, left little finger
M65.359 Trigger finger, unspecified little finger
M65.4 Radial styloid tenosynovitis [de Quervain]

+ M65.8 Other synovitis and tenosynovitis
M65.80 Other synovitis and tenosynovitis, unspecified site
+ M65.81 Other synovitis and tenosynovitis, shoulder
M65.811 Other synovitis and tenosynovitis, right shoulder
M65.812 Other synovitis and tenosynovitis, left shoulder
M65.819 Other synovitis and tenosynovitis, unspecified shoulder
+ M65.82 Other synovitis and tenosynovitis, upper arm
M65.821 Other synovitis and tenosynovitis, right upper arm
M65.822 Other synovitis and tenosynovitis, left upper arm
M65.829 Other synovitis and tenosynovitis, unspecified upper arm
+ M65.83 Other synovitis and tenosynovitis, forearm
M65.831 Other synovitis and tenosynovitis, right forearm
M65.832 Other synovitis and tenosynovitis, left forearm
M65.839 Other synovitis and tenosynovitis, unspecified forearm
+ M65.84 Other synovitis and tenosynovitis, hand
M65.841 Other synovitis and tenosynovitis, right hand
M65.842 Other synovitis and tenosynovitis, left hand
M65.849 Other synovitis and tenosynovitis, unspecified hand
+ M65.85 Other synovitis and tenosynovitis, thigh
M65.851 Other synovitis and tenosynovitis, right thigh
M65.852 Other synovitis and tenosynovitis, left thigh
M65.859 Other synovitis and tenosynovitis, unspecified thigh
+ M65.86 Other synovitis and tenosynovitis, lower leg
M65.861 Other synovitis and tenosynovitis, right lower leg
M65.862 Other synovitis and tenosynovitis, left lower leg
M65.869 Other synovitis and tenosynovitis, unspecified lower leg
+ M65.87 Other synovitis and tenosynovitis, ankle and foot
M65.871 Other synovitis and tenosynovitis, right ankle and foot
M65.872 Other synovitis and tenosynovitis, left ankle and foot
M65.879 Other synovitis and tenosynovitis, unspecified ankle and foot
M65.88 Other synovitis and tenosynovitis, other site
M65.89 Other synovitis and tenosynovitis, multiple sites
M65.9 Synovitis and tenosynovitis, unspecified

M66 Spontaneous rupture of synovium and tendon

Includes: rupture that occurs when a normal force is applied to tissues that are inferred to have less than normal strength
Excludes2: *rotator cuff syndrome (M75.1-)*
rupture where an abnormal force is applied to normal tissue - see injury of tendon by body region

M66.0 Rupture of popliteal cyst
+ M66.1 Rupture of synovium
Rupture of synovial cyst
Excludes2: *rupture of popliteal cyst (M66.0)*
M66.10 Rupture of synovium, unspecified joint
+ M66.11 Rupture of synovium, shoulder
M66.111 Rupture of synovium, right shoulder
M66.112 Rupture of synovium, left shoulder
M66.119 Rupture of synovium, unspecified shoulder
+ M66.12 Rupture of synovium, elbow
M66.121 Rupture of synovium, right elbow
M66.122 Rupture of synovium, left elbow
M66.129 Rupture of synovium, unspecified elbow
+ M66.13 Rupture of synovium, wrist
M66.131 Rupture of synovium, right wrist
M66.132 Rupture of synovium, left wrist
M66.139 Rupture of synovium, unspecified wrist
+ M66.14 Rupture of synovium, hand and fingers
M66.141 Rupture of synovium, right hand
M66.142 Rupture of synovium, left hand
M66.143 Rupture of synovium, unspecified hand
M66.144 Rupture of synovium, right finger(s)
M66.145 Rupture of synovium, left finger(s)
M66.146 Rupture of synovium, unspecified finger(s)
+ M66.15 Rupture of synovium, hip
M66.151 Rupture of synovium, right hip
M66.152 Rupture of synovium, left hip
M66.159 Rupture of synovium, unspecified hip
+ M66.17 Rupture of synovium, ankle, foot and toes
M66.171 Rupture of synovium, right ankle
M66.172 Rupture of synovium, left ankle
M66.173 Rupture of synovium, unspecified ankle
M66.174 Rupture of synovium, right foot
M66.175 Rupture of synovium, left foot
M66.176 Rupture of synovium, unspecified foot
M66.177 Rupture of synovium, right toe(s)
M66.178 Rupture of synovium, left toe(s)
M66.179 Rupture of synovium, unspecified toe(s)
M66.18 Rupture of synovium, other site
+ M66.2 Spontaneous rupture of extensor tendons
M66.20 Spontaneous rupture of extensor tendons, unspecified site
+ M66.21 Spontaneous rupture of extensor tendons, shoulder
M66.211 Spontaneous rupture of extensor tendons, right shoulder
M66.212 Spontaneous rupture of extensor tendons, left shoulder
M66.219 Spontaneous rupture of extensor tendons, unspecified shoulder
+ M66.22 Spontaneous rupture of extensor tendons, upper arm
M66.221 Spontaneous rupture of extensor tendons, right upper arm
M66.222 Spontaneous rupture of extensor tendons, left upper arm
M66.229 Spontaneous rupture of extensor tendons, unspecified upper arm
+ M66.23 Spontaneous rupture of extensor tendons, forearm
M66.231 Spontaneous rupture of extensor tendons, right forearm
M66.232 Spontaneous rupture of extensor tendons, left forearm
M66.239 Spontaneous rupture of extensor tendons, unspecified forearm
+ M66.24 Spontaneous rupture of extensor tendons, hand
M66.241 Spontaneous rupture of extensor tendons, right hand
M66.242 Spontaneous rupture of extensor tendons, left hand
M66.249 Spontaneous rupture of extensor tendons, unspecified hand
+ M66.25 Spontaneous rupture of extensor tendons, thigh
M66.251 Spontaneous rupture of extensor tendons, right thigh
M66.252 Spontaneous rupture of extensor tendons, left thigh
M66.259 Spontaneous rupture of extensor tendons, unspecified thigh
+ M66.26 Spontaneous rupture of extensor tendons, lower leg
M66.261 Spontaneous rupture of extensor tendons, right lower leg
M66.262 Spontaneous rupture of extensor tendons, left lower leg
M66.269 Spontaneous rupture of extensor tendons, unspecified lower leg
+ M66.27 Spontaneous rupture of extensor tendons, ankle and foot
M66.271 Spontaneous rupture of extensor tendons, right ankle and foot
M66.272 Spontaneous rupture of extensor tendons, left ankle and foot
M66.279 Spontaneous rupture of extensor tendons, unspecified ankle and foot
M66.28 Spontaneous rupture of extensor tendons, other site
M66.29 Spontaneous rupture of extensor tendons, multiple sites
+ M66.3 Spontaneous rupture of flexor tendons
M66.30 Spontaneous rupture of flexor tendons, unspecified site
+ M66.31 Spontaneous rupture of flexor tendons, shoulder
M66.311 Spontaneous rupture of flexor tendons, right shoulder

M66.312 Spontaneous rupture of flexor tendons, left shoulder
M66.319 Spontaneous rupture of flexor tendons, unspecified shoulder
+ **M66.32** Spontaneous rupture of flexor tendons, upper arm
M66.321 Spontaneous rupture of flexor tendons, right upper arm
M66.322 Spontaneous rupture of flexor tendons, left upper arm
M66.329 Spontaneous rupture of flexor tendons, unspecified upper arm
+ **M66.33** Spontaneous rupture of flexor tendons, forearm
M66.331 Spontaneous rupture of flexor tendons, right forearm
M66.332 Spontaneous rupture of flexor tendons, left forearm
M66.339 Spontaneous rupture of flexor tendons, unspecified forearm
+ **M66.34** Spontaneous rupture of flexor tendons, hand
M66.341 Spontaneous rupture of flexor tendons, right hand
M66.342 Spontaneous rupture of flexor tendons, left hand
M66.349 Spontaneous rupture of flexor tendons, unspecified hand
+ **M66.35** Spontaneous rupture of flexor tendons, thigh
M66.351 Spontaneous rupture of flexor tendons, right thigh
M66.352 Spontaneous rupture of flexor tendons, left thigh
M66.359 Spontaneous rupture of flexor tendons, unspecified thigh
+ **M66.36** Spontaneous rupture of flexor tendons, lower leg
M66.361 Spontaneous rupture of flexor tendons, right lower leg
M66.362 Spontaneous rupture of flexor tendons, left lower leg
M66.369 Spontaneous rupture of flexor tendons, unspecified lower leg
+ **M66.37** Spontaneous rupture of flexor tendons, ankle and foot
M66.371 Spontaneous rupture of flexor tendons, right ankle and foot
M66.372 Spontaneous rupture of flexor tendons, left ankle and foot
M66.379 Spontaneous rupture of flexor tendons, unspecified ankle and foot
M66.38 Spontaneous rupture of flexor tendons, other site
M66.39 Spontaneous rupture of flexor tendons, multiple sites
+ **M66.8** Spontaneous rupture of other tendons
M66.80 Spontaneous rupture of other tendons, unspecified site
+ **M66.81** Spontaneous rupture of other tendons, shoulder
M66.811 Spontaneous rupture of other tendons, right shoulder
M66.812 Spontaneous rupture of other tendons, left shoulder
M66.819 Spontaneous rupture of other tendons, unspecified shoulder
+ **M66.82** Spontaneous rupture of other tendons, upper arm
M66.821 Spontaneous rupture of other tendons, right upper arm
M66.822 Spontaneous rupture of other tendons, left upper arm
M66.829 Spontaneous rupture of other tendons, unspecified upper arm
+ **M66.83** Spontaneous rupture of other tendons, forearm
M66.831 Spontaneous rupture of other tendons, right forearm
M66.832 Spontaneous rupture of other tendons, left forearm
M66.839 Spontaneous rupture of other tendons, unspecified forearm
+ **M66.84** Spontaneous rupture of other tendons, hand
M66.841 Spontaneous rupture of other tendons, right hand
M66.842 Spontaneous rupture of other tendons, left hand
M66.849 Spontaneous rupture of other tendons, unspecified hand
+ **M66.85** Spontaneous rupture of other tendons, thigh
M66.851 Spontaneous rupture of other tendons, right thigh
M66.852 Spontaneous rupture of other tendons, left thigh
M66.859 Spontaneous rupture of other tendons, unspecified thigh
+ **M66.86** Spontaneous rupture of other tendons, lower leg
M66.861 Spontaneous rupture of other tendons, right lower leg
M66.862 Spontaneous rupture of other tendons, left lower leg
M66.869 Spontaneous rupture of other tendons, unspecified lower leg
+ **M66.87** Spontaneous rupture of other tendons, ankle and foot
M66.871 Spontaneous rupture of other tendons, right ankle and foot
M66.872 Spontaneous rupture of other tendons, left ankle and foot
M66.879 Spontaneous rupture of other tendons, unspecified ankle and foot
M66.88 Spontaneous rupture of other tendons, other
M66.89 Spontaneous rupture of other tendons, multiple sites
M66.9 Spontaneous rupture of unspecified tendon
Rupture at musculotendinous junction, nontraumatic

M67 Other disorders of synovium and tendon

Excludes1: *palmar fascial fibromatosis [Dupuytren] (M72.0)*
tendinitis NOS (M77.9-)
xanthomatosis localized to tendons (E78.2)

+ **M67.0** Short Achilles tendon (acquired)
M67.00 Short Achilles tendon (acquired), unspecified ankle
M67.01 Short Achilles tendon (acquired), right ankle
M67.02 Short Achilles tendon (acquired), left ankle
+ **M67.2** Synovial hypertrophy, not elsewhere classified
Excludes1: *villonodular synovitis (pigmented) (M12.2-)*
M67.20 Synovial hypertrophy, not elsewhere classified, unspecified site
+ **M67.21** Synovial hypertrophy, not elsewhere classified, shoulder
M67.211 Synovial hypertrophy, not elsewhere classified, right shoulder
M67.212 Synovial hypertrophy, not elsewhere classified, left shoulder
M67.219 Synovial hypertrophy, not elsewhere classified, unspecified shoulder
+ **M67.22** Synovial hypertrophy, not elsewhere classified, upper arm
M67.221 Synovial hypertrophy, not elsewhere classified, right upper arm
M67.222 Synovial hypertrophy, not elsewhere classified, left upper arm
M67.229 Synovial hypertrophy, not elsewhere classified, unspecified upper arm
+ **M67.23** Synovial hypertrophy, not elsewhere classified, forearm
M67.231 Synovial hypertrophy, not elsewhere classified, right forearm
M67.232 Synovial hypertrophy, not elsewhere classified, left forearm
M67.239 Synovial hypertrophy, not elsewhere classified, unspecified forearm
+ **M67.24** Synovial hypertrophy, not elsewhere classified, hand
M67.241 Synovial hypertrophy, not elsewhere classified, right hand
M67.242 Synovial hypertrophy, not elsewhere classified, left hand
M67.249 Synovial hypertrophy, not elsewhere classified, unspecified hand
+ **M67.25** Synovial hypertrophy, not elsewhere classified, thigh
M67.251 Synovial hypertrophy, not elsewhere classified, right thigh
M67.252 Synovial hypertrophy, not elsewhere classified, left thigh
M67.259 Synovial hypertrophy, not elsewhere classified, unspecified thigh

+ **M67.26** **Synovial hypertrophy, not elsewhere classified, lower leg**
  - **M67.261** **Synovial hypertrophy, not elsewhere classified, right lower leg**
  - **M67.262** **Synovial hypertrophy, not elsewhere classified, left lower leg**
  - **M67.269** **Synovial hypertrophy, not elsewhere classified, unspecified lower leg**

+ **M67.27** **Synovial hypertrophy, not elsewhere classified, ankle and foot**
  - **M67.271** **Synovial hypertrophy, not elsewhere classified, right ankle and foot**
  - **M67.272** **Synovial hypertrophy, not elsewhere classified, left ankle and foot**
  - **M67.279** **Synovial hypertrophy, not elsewhere classified, unspecified ankle and foot**

M67.28 **Synovial hypertrophy, not elsewhere classified, other site**

M67.29 **Synovial hypertrophy, not elsewhere classified, multiple sites**

+ **M67.3** **Transient synovitis**

Toxic synovitis

Excludes1: *palindromic rheumatism (M12.3-)*

M67.30 **Transient synovitis, unspecified site**

+ **M67.31** **Transient synovitis, shoulder**
  - **M67.311** **Transient synovitis, right shoulder**
  - **M67.312** **Transient synovitis, left shoulder**
  - **M67.319** **Transient synovitis, unspecified shoulder**

+ **M67.32** **Transient synovitis, elbow**
  - **M67.321** **Transient synovitis, right elbow**
  - **M67.322** **Transient synovitis, left elbow**
  - **M67.329** **Transient synovitis, unspecified elbow**

+ **M67.33** **Transient synovitis, wrist**
  - **M67.331** **Transient synovitis, right wrist**
  - **M67.332** **Transient synovitis, left wrist**
  - **M67.339** **Transient synovitis, unspecified wrist**

+ **M67.34** **Transient synovitis, hand**
  - **M67.341** **Transient synovitis, right hand**
  - **M67.342** **Transient synovitis, left hand**
  - **M67.349** **Transient synovitis, unspecified hand**

+ **M67.35** **Transient synovitis, hip**
  - **M67.351** **Transient synovitis, right hip**
  - **M67.352** **Transient synovitis, left hip**
  - **M67.359** **Transient synovitis, unspecified hip**

+ **M67.36** **Transient synovitis, knee**
  - **M67.361** **Transient synovitis, right knee**
  - **M67.362** **Transient synovitis, left knee**
  - **M67.369** **Transient synovitis, unspecified knee**

+ **M67.37** **Transient synovitis, ankle and foot**
  - **M67.371** **Transient synovitis, right ankle and foot**
  - **M67.372** **Transient synovitis, left ankle and foot**
  - **M67.379** **Transient synovitis, unspecified ankle and foot**

M67.38 **Transient synovitis, other site**

M67.39 **Transient synovitis, multiple sites**

+ **M67.4** **Ganglion**

Ganglion of joint or tendon (sheath)

Excludes1: *ganglion in yaws (A66.6)*

Excludes2: *cyst of bursa (M71.2-M71.3)*
cyst of synovium (M71.2-M71.3)

M67.40 **Ganglion, unspecified site**

+ **M67.41** **Ganglion, shoulder**
  - **M67.411** **Ganglion, right shoulder**
  - **M67.412** **Ganglion, left shoulder**
  - **M67.419** **Ganglion, unspecified shoulder**

+ **M67.42** **Ganglion, elbow**
  - **M67.421** **Ganglion, right elbow**
  - **M67.422** **Ganglion, left elbow**
  - **M67.429** **Ganglion, unspecified elbow**

+ **M67.43** **Ganglion, wrist**
  - **M67.431** **Ganglion, right wrist**
  - **M67.432** **Ganglion, left wrist**
  - **M67.439** **Ganglion, unspecified wrist**

+ **M67.44** **Ganglion, hand**
  - **M67.441** **Ganglion, right hand**
  - **M67.442** **Ganglion, left hand**
  - **M67.449** **Ganglion, unspecified hand**

+ **M67.45** **Ganglion, hip**
  - **M67.451** **Ganglion, right hip**
  - **M67.452** **Ganglion, left hip**
  - **M67.459** **Ganglion, unspecified hip**

+ **M67.46** **Ganglion, knee**
  - **M67.461** **Ganglion, right knee**
  - **M67.462** **Ganglion, left knee**
  - **M67.469** **Ganglion, unspecified knee**

+ **M67.47** **Ganglion, ankle and foot**
  - **M67.471** **Ganglion, right ankle and foot**
  - **M67.472** **Ganglion, left ankle and foot**
  - **M67.479** **Ganglion, unspecified ankle and foot**

M67.48 **Ganglion, other site**

M67.49 **Ganglion, multiple sites**

+ **M67.5** **Plica syndrome**

Plica knee

M67.50 **Plica syndrome, unspecified knee**

M67.51 **Plica syndrome, right knee**

M67.52 **Plica syndrome, left knee**

+ **M67.8** **Other specified disorders of synovium and tendon**

M67.80 **Other specified disorders of synovium and tendon, unspecified site**

+ **M67.81** **Other specified disorders of synovium and tendon, shoulder**
  - **M67.811** **Other specified disorders of synovium, right shoulder**
  - **M67.812** **Other specified disorders of synovium, left shoulder**
  - **M67.813** **Other specified disorders of tendon, right shoulder**
  - **M67.814** **Other specified disorders of tendon, left shoulder**
  - **M67.819** **Other specified disorders of synovium and tendon, unspecified shoulder**

+ **M67.82** **Other specified disorders of synovium and tendon, elbow**
  - **M67.821** **Other specified disorders of synovium, right elbow**
  - **M67.822** **Other specified disorders of synovium, left elbow**
  - **M67.823** **Other specified disorders of tendon, right elbow**
  - **M67.824** **Other specified disorders of tendon, left elbow**
  - **M67.829** **Other specified disorders of synovium and tendon, unspecified elbow**

+ **M67.83** **Other specified disorders of synovium and tendon, wrist**
  - **M67.831** **Other specified disorders of synovium, right wrist**
  - **M67.832** **Other specified disorders of synovium, left wrist**
  - **M67.833** **Other specified disorders of tendon, right wrist**
  - **M67.834** **Other specified disorders of tendon, left wrist**
  - **M67.839** **Other specified disorders of synovium and tendon, unspecified forearm**

+ **M67.84** **Other specified disorders of synovium and tendon, hand**
  - **M67.841** **Other specified disorders of synovium, right hand**
  - **M67.842** **Other specified disorders of synovium, left hand**
  - **M67.843** **Other specified disorders of tendon, right hand**
  - **M67.844** **Other specified disorders of tendon, left hand**
  - **M67.849** **Other specified disorders of synovium and tendon, unspecified hand**

+ **M67.85** **Other specified disorders of synovium and tendon, hip**
  - **M67.851** **Other specified disorders of synovium, right hip**
  - **M67.852** **Other specified disorders of synovium, left hip**
  - **M67.853** **Other specified disorders of tendon, right hip**
  - **M67.854** **Other specified disorders of tendon, left hip**
  - **M67.859** **Other specified disorders of synovium and tendon, unspecified hip**

+ M67.86 Other specified disorders of synovium and tendon, knee
  - M67.861 Other specified disorders of synovium, right knee
  - M67.862 Other specified disorders of synovium, left knee
  - M67.863 Other specified disorders of tendon, right knee
  - M67.864 Other specified disorders of tendon, left knee
  - M67.869 Other specified disorders of synovium and tendon, unspecified knee

+ M67.87 Other specified disorders of synovium and tendon, ankle and foot
  - M67.871 Other specified disorders of synovium, right ankle and foot
  - M67.872 Other specified disorders of synovium, left ankle and foot
  - M67.873 Other specified disorders of tendon, right ankle and foot
  - M67.874 Other specified disorders of tendon, left ankle and foot
  - M67.879 Other specified disorders of synovium and tendon, unspecified ankle and foot

M67.88 Other specified disorders of synovium and tendon, other site

M67.89 Other specified disorders of synovium and tendon, multiple sites

+ M67.9 Unspecified disorder of synovium and tendon

M67.90 Unspecified disorder of synovium and tendon, unspecified site

+ M67.91 Unspecified disorder of synovium and tendon, shoulder
  - M67.911 Unspecified disorder of synovium and tendon, right shoulder
  - M67.912 Unspecified disorder of synovium and tendon, left shoulder
  - M67.919 Unspecified disorder of synovium and tendon, unspecified shoulder

+ M67.92 Unspecified disorder of synovium and tendon, upper arm
  - M67.921 Unspecified disorder of synovium and tendon, right upper arm
  - M67.922 Unspecified disorder of synovium and tendon, left upper arm
  - M67.929 Unspecified disorder of synovium and tendon, unspecified upper arm

+ M67.93 Unspecified disorder of synovium and tendon, forearm
  - M67.931 Unspecified disorder of synovium and tendon, right forearm
  - M67.932 Unspecified disorder of synovium and tendon, left forearm
  - M67.939 Unspecified disorder of synovium and tendon, unspecified forearm

+ M67.94 Unspecified disorder of synovium and tendon, hand
  - M67.941 Unspecified disorder of synovium and tendon, right hand
  - M67.942 Unspecified disorder of synovium and tendon, left hand
  - M67.949 Unspecified disorder of synovium and tendon, unspecified hand

+ M67.95 Unspecified disorder of synovium and tendon, thigh
  - M67.951 Unspecified disorder of synovium and tendon, right thigh
  - M67.952 Unspecified disorder of synovium and tendon, left thigh
  - M67.959 Unspecified disorder of synovium and tendon, unspecified thigh

+ M67.96 Unspecified disorder of synovium and tendon, lower leg
  - M67.961 Unspecified disorder of synovium and tendon, right lower leg
  - M67.962 Unspecified disorder of synovium and tendon, left lower leg
  - M67.969 Unspecified disorder of synovium and tendon, unspecified lower leg

+ M67.97 Unspecified disorder of synovium and tendon, ankle and foot
  - M67.971 Unspecified disorder of synovium and tendon, right ankle and foot
  - M67.972 Unspecified disorder of synovium and tendon, left ankle and foot
  - M67.979 Unspecified disorder of synovium and tendon, unspecified ankle and foot

M67.98 Unspecified disorder of synovium and tendon, other site

M67.99 Unspecified disorder of synovium and tendon, multiple sites

Other soft tissue disorders (M70-M79)

M70 Soft tissue disorders related to use, overuse and pressure

Includes: soft tissue disorders of occupational origin

Use additional external cause code to identify activity causing disorder (Y93.-)

Excludes1: *bursitis NOS (M71.9-)*

Excludes2: *bursitis of shoulder (M75.5)*
enthesopathies (M76-M77)
pressure ulcer (pressure area) (L89.-)

+ M70.0 Crepitant synovitis (acute) (chronic) of hand and wrist

+ M70.03 Crepitant synovitis (acute) (chronic), wrist
  - M70.031 Crepitant synovitis (acute) (chronic), right wrist
  - M70.032 Crepitant synovitis (acute) (chronic), left wrist
  - M70.039 Crepitant synovitis (acute) (chronic), unspecified wrist

+ M70.04 Crepitant synovitis (acute) (chronic), hand
  - M70.041 Crepitant synovitis (acute) (chronic), right hand
  - M70.042 Crepitant synovitis (acute) (chronic), left hand
  - M70.049 Crepitant synovitis (acute) (chronic), unspecified hand

+ M70.1 Bursitis of hand
  - M70.10 Bursitis, unspecified hand
  - M70.11 Bursitis, right hand
  - M70.12 Bursitis, left hand

+ M70.2 Olecranon bursitis
  - M70.20 Olecranon bursitis, unspecified elbow
  - M70.21 Olecranon bursitis, right elbow
  - M70.22 Olecranon bursitis, left elbow

+ M70.3 Other bursitis of elbow
  - M70.30 Other bursitis of elbow, unspecified elbow
  - M70.31 Other bursitis of elbow, right elbow
  - M70.32 Other bursitis of elbow, left elbow

+ M70.4 Prepatellar bursitis
  - M70.40 Prepatellar bursitis, unspecified knee
  - M70.41 Prepatellar bursitis, right knee
  - M70.42 Prepatellar bursitis, left knee

+ M70.5 Other bursitis of knee
  - M70.50 Other bursitis of knee, unspecified knee
  - M70.51 Other bursitis of knee, right knee
  - M70.52 Other bursitis of knee, left knee

+ M70.6 Trochanteric bursitis

Trochanteric tendinitis
  - M70.60 Trochanteric bursitis, unspecified hip
  - M70.61 Trochanteric bursitis, right hip
  - M70.62 Trochanteric bursitis, left hip

+ M70.7 Other bursitis of hip

Ischial bursitis
  - M70.70 Other bursitis of hip, unspecified hip
  - M70.71 Other bursitis of hip, right hip
  - M70.72 Other bursitis of hip, left hip

+ M70.8 Other soft tissue disorders related to use, overuse and pressure

M70.80 Other soft tissue disorders related to use, overuse and pressure of unspecified site

+ M70.81 Other soft tissue disorders related to use, overuse and pressure of shoulder
  - M70.811 Other soft tissue disorders related to use, overuse and pressure, right shoulder
  - M70.812 Other soft tissue disorders related to use, overuse and pressure, left shoulder
  - M70.819 Other soft tissue disorders related to use, overuse and pressure, unspecified shoulder

+ M70.82 Other soft tissue disorders related to use, overuse and pressure of upper arm
M70.821 Other soft tissue disorders related to use, overuse and pressure, right upper arm
M70.822 Other soft tissue disorders related to use, overuse and pressure, left upper arm
M70.829 Other soft tissue disorders related to use, overuse and pressure, unspecified upper arms
+ M70.83 Other soft tissue disorders related to use, overuse and pressure of forearm
M70.831 Other soft tissue disorders related to use, overuse and pressure, right forearm
M70.832 Other soft tissue disorders related to use, overuse and pressure, left forearm
M70.839 Other soft tissue disorders related to use, overuse and pressure, unspecified forearm
+ M70.84 Other soft tissue disorders related to use, overuse and pressure of hand
M70.841 Other soft tissue disorders related to use, overuse and pressure, right hand
M70.842 Other soft tissue disorders related to use, overuse and pressure, left hand
M70.849 Other soft tissue disorders related to use, overuse and pressure, unspecified hand
+ M70.85 Other soft tissue disorders related to use, overuse and pressure of thigh
M70.851 Other soft tissue disorders related to use, overuse and pressure, right thigh
M70.852 Other soft tissue disorders related to use, overuse and pressure, left thigh
M70.859 Other soft tissue disorders related to use, overuse and pressure, unspecified thigh
+ M70.86 Other soft tissue disorders related to use, overuse and pressure lower leg
M70.861 Other soft tissue disorders related to use, overuse and pressure, right lower leg
M70.862 Other soft tissue disorders related to use, overuse and pressure, left lower leg
M70.869 Other soft tissue disorders related to use, overuse and pressure, unspecified leg
+ M70.87 Other soft tissue disorders related to use, overuse and pressure of ankle and foot
M70.871 Other soft tissue disorders related to use, overuse and pressure, right ankle and foot
M70.872 Other soft tissue disorders related to use, overuse and pressure, left ankle and foot
M70.879 Other soft tissue disorders related to use, overuse and pressure, unspecified ankle and foot
M70.88 Other soft tissue disorders related to use, overuse and pressure other site
M70.89 Other soft tissue disorders related to use, overuse and pressure multiple sites
+ M70.9 Unspecified soft tissue disorder related to use, overuse and pressure
M70.90 Unspecified soft tissue disorder related to use, overuse and pressure of unspecified site
+ M70.91 Unspecified soft tissue disorder related to use, overuse and pressure of shoulder
M70.911 Unspecified soft tissue disorder related to use, overuse and pressure, right shoulder
M70.912 Unspecified soft tissue disorder related to use, overuse and pressure, left shoulder
M70.919 Unspecified soft tissue disorder related to use, overuse and pressure, unspecified shoulder
+ M70.92 Unspecified soft tissue disorder related to use, overuse and pressure of upper arm
M70.921 Unspecified soft tissue disorder related to use, overuse and pressure, right upper arm
M70.922 Unspecified soft tissue disorder related to use, overuse and pressure, left upper arm
M70.929 Unspecified soft tissue disorder related to use, overuse and pressure, unspecified upper arm
+ M70.93 Unspecified soft tissue disorder related to use, overuse and pressure of forearm
M70.931 Unspecified soft tissue disorder related to use, overuse and pressure, right forearm
M70.932 Unspecified soft tissue disorder related to use, overuse and pressure, left forearm
M70.939 Unspecified soft tissue disorder related to use, overuse and pressure, unspecified forearm
+ M70.94 Unspecified soft tissue disorder related to use, overuse and pressure of hand
M70.941 Unspecified soft tissue disorder related to use, overuse and pressure, right hand
M70.942 Unspecified soft tissue disorder related to use, overuse and pressure, left hand
M70.949 Unspecified soft tissue disorder related to use, overuse and pressure, unspecified hand
+ M70.95 Unspecified soft tissue disorder related to use, overuse and pressure of thigh
M70.951 Unspecified soft tissue disorder related to use, overuse and pressure, right thigh
M70.952 Unspecified soft tissue disorder related to use, overuse and pressure, left thigh
M70.959 Unspecified soft tissue disorder related to use, overuse and pressure, unspecified thigh
+ M70.96 Unspecified soft tissue disorder related to use, overuse and pressure lower leg
M70.961 Unspecified soft tissue disorder related to use, overuse and pressure, right lower leg
M70.962 Unspecified soft tissue disorder related to use, overuse and pressure, left lower leg
M70.969 Unspecified soft tissue disorder related to use, overuse and pressure, unspecified lower leg
+ M70.97 Unspecified soft tissue disorder related to use, overuse and pressure of ankle and foot
M70.971 Unspecified soft tissue disorder related to use, overuse and pressure, right ankle and foot
M70.972 Unspecified soft tissue disorder related to use, overuse and pressure, left ankle and foot
M70.979 Unspecified soft tissue disorder related to use, overuse and pressure, unspecified ankle and foot
M70.98 Unspecified soft tissue disorder related to use, overuse and pressure other
M70.99 Unspecified soft tissue disorder related to use, overuse and pressure multiple sites

M71 Other bursopathies

Excludes1: *bunion (M20.1)*
bursitis related to use, overuse or pressure (M70.-)
enthesopathies (M76-M77)

+ M71.0 Abscess of bursa
Use additional code (B95.-, B96.-) to identify causative organism
M71.00 Abscess of bursa, unspecified site
+ M71.01 Abscess of bursa, shoulder
M71.011 Abscess of bursa, right shoulder
M71.012 Abscess of bursa, left shoulder
M71.019 Abscess of bursa, unspecified shoulder
+ M71.02 Abscess of bursa, elbow
M71.021 Abscess of bursa, right elbow
M71.022 Abscess of bursa, left elbow
M71.029 Abscess of bursa, unspecified elbow
+ M71.03 Abscess of bursa, wrist
M71.031 Abscess of bursa, right wrist
M71.032 Abscess of bursa, left wrist
M71.039 Abscess of bursa, unspecified wrist
+ M71.04 Abscess of bursa, hand
M71.041 Abscess of bursa, right hand
M71.042 Abscess of bursa, left hand
M71.049 Abscess of bursa, unspecified hand
+ M71.05 Abscess of bursa, hip
M71.051 Abscess of bursa, right hip
M71.052 Abscess of bursa, left hip
M71.059 Abscess of bursa, unspecified hip
+ M71.06 Abscess of bursa, knee
M71.061 Abscess of bursa, right knee
M71.062 Abscess of bursa, left knee
M71.069 Abscess of bursa, unspecified knee
+ M71.07 Abscess of bursa, ankle and foot
M71.071 Abscess of bursa, right ankle and foot

M71.072 Abscess of bursa, left ankle and foot
M71.079 Abscess of bursa, unspecified ankle and foot
M71.08 Abscess of bursa, other site
M71.09 Abscess of bursa, multiple sites
+ M71.1 Other infective bursitis
Use additional code (B95.-, B96.-) to identify causative organism
M71.10 Other infective bursitis, unspecified site
+ M71.11 Other infective bursitis, shoulder
M71.111 Other infective bursitis, right shoulder
M71.112 Other infective bursitis, left shoulder
M71.119 Other infective bursitis, unspecified shoulder
+ M71.12 Other infective bursitis, elbow
M71.121 Other infective bursitis, right elbow
M71.122 Other infective bursitis, left elbow
M71.129 Other infective bursitis, unspecified elbow
+ M71.13 Other infective bursitis, wrist
M71.131 Other infective bursitis, right wrist
M71.132 Other infective bursitis, left wrist
M71.139 Other infective bursitis, unspecified wrist
+ M71.14 Other infective bursitis, hand
M71.141 Other infective bursitis, right hand
M71.142 Other infective bursitis, left hand
M71.149 Other infective bursitis, unspecified hand
+ M71.15 Other infective bursitis, hip
M71.151 Other infective bursitis, right hip
M71.152 Other infective bursitis, left hip
M71.159 Other infective bursitis, unspecified hip
+ M71.16 Other infective bursitis, knee
M71.161 Other infective bursitis, right knee
M71.162 Other infective bursitis, left knee
M71.169 Other infective bursitis, unspecified knee
+ M71.17 Other infective bursitis, ankle and foot
M71.171 Other infective bursitis, right ankle and foot
M71.172 Other infective bursitis, left ankle and foot
M71.179 Other infective bursitis, unspecified ankle and foot
M71.18 Other infective bursitis, other site
M71.19 Other infective bursitis, multiple sites
+ M71.2 Synovial cyst of popliteal space [Baker]
Excludes1: *synovial cyst of popliteal space with rupture (M66.0)*
M71.20 Synovial cyst of popliteal space [Baker], unspecified knee
M71.21 Synovial cyst of popliteal space [Baker], right knee
M71.22 Synovial cyst of popliteal space [Baker], left knee
+ M71.3 Other bursal cyst
Synovial cyst NOS
Excludes1: *synovial cyst with rupture (M66.1-)*
M71.30 Other bursal cyst, unspecified site
+ M71.31 Other bursal cyst, shoulder
M71.311 Other bursal cyst, right shoulder
M71.312 Other bursal cyst, left shoulder
M71.319 Other bursal cyst, unspecified shoulder
+ M71.32 Other bursal cyst, elbow
M71.321 Other bursal cyst, right elbow
M71.322 Other bursal cyst, left elbow
M71.329 Other bursal cyst, unspecified elbow
+ M71.33 Other bursal cyst, wrist
M71.331 Other bursal cyst, right wrist
M71.332 Other bursal cyst, left wrist
M71.339 Other bursal cyst, unspecified wrist
+ M71.34 Other bursal cyst, hand
M71.341 Other bursal cyst, right hand
M71.342 Other bursal cyst, left hand
M71.349 Other bursal cyst, unspecified hand
+ M71.35 Other bursal cyst, hip
M71.351 Other bursal cyst, right hip
M71.352 Other bursal cyst, left hip
M71.359 Other bursal cyst, unspecified hip
+ M71.37 Other bursal cyst, ankle and foot
M71.371 Other bursal cyst, right ankle and foot
M71.372 Other bursal cyst, left ankle and foot
M71.379 Other bursal cyst, unspecified ankle and foot
M71.38 Other bursal cyst, other site
M71.39 Other bursal cyst, multiple sites
+ M71.4 Calcium deposit in bursa
Excludes2: *calcium deposit in bursa of shoulder (M75.3)*
M71.40 Calcium deposit in bursa, unspecified site
+ M71.42 Calcium deposit in bursa, elbow
M71.421 Calcium deposit in bursa, right elbow
M71.422 Calcium deposit in bursa, left elbow
M71.429 Calcium deposit in bursa, unspecified elbow
+ M71.43 Calcium deposit in bursa, wrist
M71.431 Calcium deposit in bursa, right wrist
M71.432 Calcium deposit in bursa, left wrist
M71.439 Calcium deposit in bursa, unspecified wrist
+ M71.44 Calcium deposit in bursa, hand
M71.441 Calcium deposit in bursa, right hand
M71.442 Calcium deposit in bursa, left hand
M71.449 Calcium deposit in bursa, unspecified hand
+ M71.45 Calcium deposit in bursa, hip
M71.451 Calcium deposit in bursa, right hip
M71.452 Calcium deposit in bursa, left hip
M71.459 Calcium deposit in bursa, unspecified hip
+ M71.46 Calcium deposit in bursa, knee
M71.461 Calcium deposit in bursa, right knee
M71.462 Calcium deposit in bursa, left knee
M71.469 Calcium deposit in bursa, unspecified knee
+ M71.47 Calcium deposit in bursa, ankle and foot
M71.471 Calcium deposit in bursa, right ankle and foot
M71.472 Calcium deposit in bursa, left ankle and foot
M71.479 Calcium deposit in bursa, unspecified ankle and foot
M71.48 Calcium deposit in bursa, other site
M71.49 Calcium deposit in bursa, multiple sites
+ M71.5 Other bursitis, not elsewhere classified
Excludes1: *bursitis NOS (M71.9-)*
Excludes2: *bursitis of shoulder (M75.5)*
bursitis of tibial collateral [Pellegrini-Stieda] (M76.4-)
M71.50 Other bursitis, not elsewhere classified, unspecified site
+ M71.52 Other bursitis, not elsewhere classified, elbow
M71.521 Other bursitis, not elsewhere classified, right elbow
M71.522 Other bursitis, not elsewhere classified, left elbow
M71.529 Other bursitis, not elsewhere classified, unspecified elbow
+ M71.53 Other bursitis, not elsewhere classified, wrist
M71.531 Other bursitis, not elsewhere classified, right wrist
M71.532 Other bursitis, not elsewhere classified, left wrist
M71.539 Other bursitis, not elsewhere classified, unspecified wrist
+ M71.54 Other bursitis, not elsewhere classified, hand
M71.541 Other bursitis, not elsewhere classified, right hand
M71.542 Other bursitis, not elsewhere classified, left hand
M71.549 Other bursitis, not elsewhere classified, unspecified hand
+ M71.55 Other bursitis, not elsewhere classified, hip
M71.551 Other bursitis, not elsewhere classified, right hip
M71.552 Other bursitis, not elsewhere classified, left hip
M71.559 Other bursitis, not elsewhere classified, unspecified hip
+ M71.56 Other bursitis, not elsewhere classified, knee
M71.561 Other bursitis, not elsewhere classified, right knee
M71.562 Other bursitis, not elsewhere classified, left knee
M71.569 Other bursitis, not elsewhere classified, unspecified knee
+ M71.57 Other bursitis, not elsewhere classified, ankle and foot
M71.571 Other bursitis, not elsewhere classified, right ankle and foot

M71.572 Other bursitis, not elsewhere classified, left ankle and foot
M71.579 Other bursitis, not elsewhere classified, unspecified ankle and foot
M71.58 Other bursitis, not elsewhere classified, other site
+ M71.8 Other specified bursopathies
M71.80 Other specified bursopathies, unspecified site
+ M71.81 Other specified bursopathies, shoulder
M71.811 Other specified bursopathies, right shoulder
M71.812 Other specified bursopathies, left shoulder
M71.819 Other specified bursopathies, unspecified shoulder
+ M71.82 Other specified bursopathies, elbow
M71.821 Other specified bursopathies, right elbow
M71.822 Other specified bursopathies, left elbow
M71.829 Other specified bursopathies, unspecified elbow
+ M71.83 Other specified bursopathies, wrist
M71.831 Other specified bursopathies, right wrist
M71.832 Other specified bursopathies, left wrist
M71.839 Other specified bursopathies, unspecified wrist
+ M71.84 Other specified bursopathies, hand
M71.841 Other specified bursopathies, right hand
M71.842 Other specified bursopathies, left hand
M71.849 Other specified bursopathies, unspecified hand
+ M71.85 Other specified bursopathies, hip
M71.851 Other specified bursopathies, right hip
M71.852 Other specified bursopathies, left hip
M71.859 Other specified bursopathies, unspecified hip
+ M71.86 Other specified bursopathies, knee
M71.861 Other specified bursopathies, right knee
M71.862 Other specified bursopathies, left knee
M71.869 Other specified bursopathies, unspecified knee
+ M71.87 Other specified bursopathies, ankle and foot
M71.871 Other specified bursopathies, right ankle and foot
M71.872 Other specified bursopathies, left ankle and foot
M71.879 Other specified bursopathies, unspecified ankle and foot
M71.88 Other specified bursopathies, other site
M71.89 Other specified bursopathies, multiple sites
M71.9 Bursopathy, unspecified
Bursitis NOS

M72 Fibroblastic disorders

Excludes2: *retroperitoneal fibromatosis (D48.3)*
• M72.0 Palmar fascial fibromatosis [Dupuytren]
M72.1 Knuckle pads
M72.2 Plantar fascial fibromatosis
Plantar fasciitis
M72.4 Pseudosarcomatous fibromatosis
Nodular fasciitis
MCC M72.6 Necrotizing fasciitis
Use additional code (B95.-, B96.-) to identify causative organism
MCC Exclusion see Appendix A PDX collection 0806
M72.8 Other fibroblastic disorders
Abscess of fascia
Fasciitis NEC
Other infective fasciitis
Use additional code to (B95.-, B96.-) identify causative organism
Excludes1: *diffuse (eosinophilic) fasciitis (M35.4)*
necrotizing fasciitis (M72.6)
nodular fasciitis (M72.4)
perirenal fasciitis NOS (N13.5)
perirenal fasciitis with infection (N13.6)
plantar fasciitis (M72.2)
M72.9 Fibroblastic disorder, unspecified
Fasciitis NOS
Fibromatosis NOS

M75 Shoulder lesions

Excludes2: *shoulder-hand syndrome (M89.0-)*
+ M75.0 Adhesive capsulitis of shoulder
Frozen shoulder
Periarthritis of shoulder
M75.00 Adhesive capsulitis of unspecified shoulder
M75.01 Adhesive capsulitis of right shoulder
M75.02 Adhesive capsulitis of left shoulder
+ M75.1 Rotator cuff tear or rupture, not specified as traumatic
Rotator cuff syndrome
Supraspinatus tear or rupture, not specified as traumatic
Supraspinatus syndrome
Excludes1: *tear of rotator cuff, traumatic (S46.01-)*
+ M75.10 Unspecified rotator cuff tear or rupture, not specified as traumatic
M75.100 Unspecified rotator cuff tear or rupture of unspecified shoulder, not specified as traumatic
M75.101 Unspecified rotator cuff tear or rupture of right shoulder, not specified as traumatic
M75.102 Unspecified rotator cuff tear or rupture of left shoulder, not specified as traumatic
+ M75.11 Incomplete rotator cuff tear or rupture not specified as traumatic
M75.110 Incomplete rotator cuff tear or rupture of unspecified shoulder, not specified as traumatic
M75.111 Incomplete rotator cuff tear or rupture of right shoulder, not specified as traumatic
M75.112 Incomplete rotator cuff tear or rupture of left shoulder, not specified as traumatic
+ M75.12 Complete rotator cuff tear or rupture not specified as traumatic
M75.120 Complete rotator cuff tear or rupture of unspecified shoulder, not specified as traumatic
M75.121 Complete rotator cuff tear or rupture of right shoulder, not specified as traumatic
M75.122 Complete rotator cuff tear or rupture of left shoulder, not specified as traumatic
+ M75.2 Bicipital tendinitis
M75.20 Bicipital tendinitis, unspecified shoulder
M75.21 Bicipital tendinitis, right shoulder
M75.22 Bicipital tendinitis, left shoulder
+ M75.3 Calcific tendinitis of shoulder
Calcified bursa of shoulder
M75.30 Calcific tendinitis of unspecified shoulder
M75.31 Calcific tendinitis of right shoulder
M75.32 Calcific tendinitis of left shoulder
+ M75.4 Impingement syndrome of shoulder
M75.40 Impingement syndrome of unspecified shoulder
M75.41 Impingement syndrome of right shoulder
M75.42 Impingement syndrome of left shoulder
+ M75.5 Bursitis of shoulder
M75.50 Bursitis of unspecified shoulder
M75.51 Bursitis of right shoulder
M75.52 Bursitis of left shoulder
+ M75.8 Other shoulder lesions
M75.80 Other shoulder lesions, unspecified shoulder
M75.81 Other shoulder lesions, right shoulder
M75.82 Other shoulder lesions, left shoulder
+ M75.9 Shoulder lesion, unspecified
M75.90 Shoulder lesion, unspecified, unspecified shoulder
M75.91 Shoulder lesion, unspecified, right shoulder
M75.92 Shoulder lesion, unspecified, left shoulder

M76 Enthesopathies, lower limb, excluding foot

Excludes2: *bursitis due to use, overuse and pressure (M70.-)*
enthesopathies of ankle and foot (M77.5-)
+ M76.0 Gluteal tendinitis
M76.00 Gluteal tendinitis, unspecified hip
M76.01 Gluteal tendinitis, right hip
M76.02 Gluteal tendinitis, left hip
+ M76.1 Psoas tendinitis
M76.10 Psoas tendinitis, unspecified hip
M76.11 Psoas tendinitis, right hip
M76.12 Psoas tendinitis, left hip
+ M76.2 Iliac crest spur
M76.20 Iliac crest spur, unspecified hip
M76.21 Iliac crest spur, right hip
M76.22 Iliac crest spur, left hip

+ **M76.3 Iliotibial band syndrome**
  - **M76.30 Iliotibial band syndrome, unspecified leg**
  - **M76.31 Iliotibial band syndrome, right leg**
  - **M76.32 Iliotibial band syndrome, left leg**
+ **M76.4 Tibial collateral bursitis [Pellegrini-Stieda]**
  - **M76.40 Tibial collateral bursitis [Pellegrini-Stieda], unspecified leg**
  - **M76.41 Tibial collateral bursitis [Pellegrini-Stieda], right leg**
  - **M76.42 Tibial collateral bursitis [Pellegrini-Stieda], left leg**
+ **M76.5 Patellar tendinitis**
  - **M76.50 Patellar tendinitis, unspecified knee**
  - **M76.51 Patellar tendinitis, right knee**
  - **M76.52 Patellar tendinitis, left knee**
+ **M76.6 Achilles tendinitis**
  Achilles bursitis
  - **M76.60 Achilles tendinitis, unspecified leg**
  - **M76.61 Achilles tendinitis, right leg**
  - **M76.62 Achilles tendinitis, left leg**
+ **M76.7 Peroneal tendinitis**
  - **M76.70 Peroneal tendinitis, unspecified leg**
  - **M76.71 Peroneal tendinitis, right leg**
  - **M76.72 Peroneal tendinitis, left leg**
+ **M76.8 Other specified enthesopathies of lower limb, excluding foot**
  + **M76.81 Anterior tibial syndrome**
    - **M76.811 Anterior tibial syndrome, right leg**
    - **M76.812 Anterior tibial syndrome, left leg**
    - **M76.819 Anterior tibial syndrome, unspecified leg**
  + **M76.82 Posterior tibial tendinitis**
    - **M76.821 Posterior tibial tendinitis, right leg**
    - **M76.822 Posterior tibial tendinitis, left leg**
    - **M76.829 Posterior tibial tendinitis, unspecified leg**
  + **M76.89 Other specified enthesopathies of lower limb, excluding foot**
    - **M76.891 Other specified enthesopathies of right lower limb, excluding foot**
    - **M76.892 Other specified enthesopathies of left lower limb, excluding foot**
    - **M76.899 Other specified enthesopathies of unspecified lower limb, excluding foot**

M76.9 Unspecified enthesopathy, lower limb, excluding foot

M77 Other enthesopathies

Excludes1: *bursitis NOS (M71.9-)*
Excludes2: *bursitis due to use, overuse and pressure (M70.-)*
osteophyte (M25.7)
spinal enthesopathy (M46.0-)

+ **M77.0 Medial epicondylitis**
  - **M77.00 Medial epicondylitis, unspecified elbow**
  - **M77.01 Medial epicondylitis, right elbow**
  - **M77.02 Medial epicondylitis, left elbow**
+ **M77.1 Lateral epicondylitis**
  Tennis elbow
  - **M77.10 Lateral epicondylitis, unspecified elbow**
  - **M77.11 Lateral epicondylitis, right elbow**
  - **M77.12 Lateral epicondylitis, left elbow**
+ **M77.2 Periarthritis of wrist**
  - **M77.20 Periarthritis, unspecified wrist**
  - **M77.21 Periarthritis, right wrist**
  - **M77.22 Periarthritis, left wrist**
+ **M77.3 Calcaneal spur**
  - **M77.30 Calcaneal spur, unspecified foot**
  - **M77.31 Calcaneal spur, right foot**
  - **M77.32 Calcaneal spur, left foot**
+ **M77.4 Metatarsalgia**
  Excludes1: *Morton's metatarsalgia (G57.6)*
  - **M77.40 Metatarsalgia, unspecified foot**
  - **M77.41 Metatarsalgia, right foot**
  - **M77.42 Metatarsalgia, left foot**
+ **M77.5 Other enthesopathy of foot**
  - **M77.50 Other enthesopathy of unspecified foot**
  - **M77.51 Other enthesopathy of right foot**
  - **M77.52 Other enthesopathy of left foot**

M77.8 Other enthesopathies, not elsewhere classified

M77.9 Enthesopathy, unspecified
Bone spur NOS
Capsulitis NOS
Periarthritis NOS
Tendinitis NOS

M79 Other and unspecified soft tissue disorders, not elsewhere classified

Excludes1: *psychogenic rheumatism (F45.8)*
soft tissue pain, psychogenic (F45.41)

M79.0 Rheumatism, unspecified
Excludes1: *fibromyalgia (M79.7)*
palindromic rheumatism (M12.3-)

M79.1 Myalgia
Myofascial pain syndrome
Excludes1: *fibromyalgia (M79.7)*
myositis (M60.-)

M79.2 Neuralgia and neuritis, unspecified
Excludes1: *brachial radiculitis NOS (M54.1)*
lumbosacral radiculitis NOS (M54.1)
mononeuropathies (G56-G58)
radiculitis NOS (M54.1)
sciatica (M54.3-M54.4)

M79.3 Panniculitis, unspecified
Excludes1: *lupus panniculitis (L93.2)*
neck and back panniculitis (M54.0-)
relapsing [Weber-Christian] panniculitis (M35.6)

M79.4 Hypertrophy of (infrapatellar) fat pad

M79.5 Residual foreign body in soft tissue
Excludes1: *foreign body granuloma of skin and subcutaneous tissue (L92.3)*
foreign body granuloma of soft tissue (M60.2-)

+ **M79.6 Pain in limb, hand, foot, fingers and toes**
  Excludes2: *pain in joint (M25.5-)*
  + **M79.60 Pain in limb, unspecified**
    - **M79.601 Pain in right arm**
      Pain in right upper limb NOS
    - **M79.602 Pain in left arm**
      Pain in left upper limb NOS
    - **M79.603 Pain in arm, unspecified**
      Pain in upper limb NOS
    - **M79.604 Pain in right leg**
      Pain in right lower limb NOS
    - **M79.605 Pain in left leg**
      Pain in left lower limb NOS
    - **M79.606 Pain in leg, unspecified**
      Pain in lower limb NOS
    - **M79.609 Pain in unspecified limb**
      Pain in limb NOS
  + **M79.62 Pain in upper arm**
    Pain in axillary region
    - **M79.621 Pain in right upper arm**
    - **M79.622 Pain in left upper arm**
    - **M79.629 Pain in unspecified upper arm**
  + **M79.63 Pain in forearm**
    - **M79.631 Pain in right forearm**
    - **M79.632 Pain in left forearm**
    - **M79.639 Pain in unspecified forearm**
  + **M79.64 Pain in hand and fingers**
    - **M79.641 Pain in right hand**
    - **M79.642 Pain in left hand**
    - **M79.643 Pain in unspecified hand**
    - **M79.644 Pain in right finger(s)**
    - **M79.645 Pain in left finger(s)**
    - **M79.646 Pain in unspecified finger(s)**
  + **M79.65 Pain in thigh**
    - **M79.651 Pain in right thigh**
    - **M79.652 Pain in left thigh**
    - **M79.659 Pain in unspecified thigh**
  + **M79.66 Pain in lower leg**
    - **M79.661 Pain in right lower leg**
    - **M79.662 Pain in left lower leg**
    - **M79.669 Pain in unspecified lower leg**
  + **M79.67 Pain in foot and toes**
    - **M79.671 Pain in right foot**
    - **M79.672 Pain in left foot**
    - **M79.673 Pain in unspecified foot**
    - **M79.674 Pain in right toe(s)**
    - **M79.675 Pain in left toe(s)**
    - **M79.676 Pain in unspecified toe(s)**

M79.7 Fibromyalgia
Fibromyositis
Fibrositis
Myofibrositis

+ **M79.A Nontraumatic compartment syndrome**
  Code first if applicable, associated postprocedural complication
  Excludes1: *compartment syndrome NOS (T79.A-)*
  fibromyalgia (M79.7)
  nontraumatic ischemic infarction of muscle (M62.2-)
  traumatic compartment syndrome (T79.A-)
+ **M79.A1 Nontraumatic compartment syndrome of upper extremity**
  Nontraumatic compartment syndrome of shoulder, arm, forearm, wrist, hand, and fingers
CC **M79.A11 Nontraumatic compartment syndrome of right upper extremity**
  CC Exclusion see Appendix A PDX collection 0893
CC **M79.A12 Nontraumatic compartment syndrome of left upper extremity**
  CC Exclusion see Appendix A PDX collection 0893
CC **M79.A19 Nontraumatic compartment syndrome of unspecified upper extremity**
  CC Exclusion see Appendix A PDX collection 0893
+ **M79.A2 Nontraumatic compartment syndrome of lower extremity**
  Nontraumatic compartment syndrome of hip, buttock, thigh, leg, foot, and toes
CC **M79.A21 Nontraumatic compartment syndrome of right lower extremity**
  CC Exclusion see Appendix A PDX collection 0894
CC **M79.A22 Nontraumatic compartment syndrome of left lower extremity**
  CC Exclusion see Appendix A PDX collection 0894
CC **M79.A29 Nontraumatic compartment syndrome of unspecified lower extremity**
  CC Exclusion see Appendix A PDX collection 0894
CC **M79.A3 Nontraumatic compartment syndrome of abdomen**
  CC Exclusion see Appendix A PDX collection 0895
CC **M79.A9 Nontraumatic compartment syndrome of other sites**
  CC Exclusion see Appendix A PDX collection 0896
+ **M79.8 Other specified soft tissue disorders**
M79.81 Nontraumatic hematoma of soft tissue
  Nontraumatic hematoma of muscle
  Nontraumatic seroma of muscle and soft tissue
M79.89 Other specified soft tissue disorders
  Polyalgia
M79.9 Soft tissue disorder, unspecified

OSTEOPATHIES AND CHONDROPATHIES (M80-M94)

isorders of bone density and structure (M80-M85)

M80 Osteoporosis with current pathological fracture
  Includes: osteoporosis with current fragility fracture
  Use additional code to identify major osseous defect, if applicable (M89.7-)
  Excludes1: *collapsed vertebra NOS (M48.5)*
  pathological fracture NOS (M84.4)
  wedging of vertebra NOS (M48.5)
  Excludes2: *personal history of (healed) osteoporosis fracture (Z87.310)*

The appropriate 7th character is to be added to each code from category M80:
A initial encounter for fracture
D subsequent encounter for fracture with routine healing
G subsequent encounter for fracture with delayed healing
K subsequent encounter for fracture with nonunion
P subsequent encounter for fracture with malunion
S sequela

Review coding guideline C.13.c
Review coding guideline C.19.c.1

+ **M80.0 Age-related osteoporosis with current pathological fracture**
  Involutional osteoporosis with current pathological fracture
  Osteoporosis NOS with current pathological fracture
  Postmenopausal osteoporosis with current pathological fracture
  Senile osteoporosis with current pathological fracture
• CC X+7th **M80.00 Age-related osteoporosis with current pathological fracture, unspecified site**
  CC Exclusion 7th character A see Appendix A PDX collection 0888
  CC Exclusion 7th characters K & P see Appendix A PDX collection 0897
+ **M80.01 Age-related osteoporosis with current pathological fracture, shoulder**
• CC +7th **M80.011 Age-related osteoporosis with current pathological fracture, right shoulder**
  CC Exclusion 7th character A see Appendix A PDX collection 0888
  CC Exclusion 7th characters K & P see Appendix A PDX collection 0897
• CC +7th **M80.012 Age-related osteoporosis with current pathological fracture, left shoulder**
  CC Exclusion 7th character A see Appendix A PDX collection 0888
  CC Exclusion 7th characters K & P see Appendix A PDX collection 0897
• CC +7th **M80.019 Age-related osteoporosis with current pathological fracture, unspecified shoulder**
  CC Exclusion 7th character A see Appendix A PDX collection 0888
  CC Exclusion 7th characters K & P see Appendix A PDX collection 0897
+ **M80.02 Age-related osteoporosis with current pathological fracture, humerus**
• CC +7th **M80.021 Age-related osteoporosis with current pathological fracture, right humerus**
  CC Exclusion 7th character A see Appendix A PDX collection 0888
  CC Exclusion 7th characters K & P see Appendix A PDX collection 0897
• CC +7th **M80.022 Age-related osteoporosis with current pathological fracture, left humerus**
  CC Exclusion 7th character A see Appendix A PDX collection 0888
  CC Exclusion 7th characters K & P see Appendix A PDX collection 0897
• CC +7th **M80.029 Age-related osteoporosis with current pathological fracture, unspecified humerus**
  CC Exclusion 7th character A see Appendix A PDX collection 0888
  CC Exclusion 7th characters K & P see Appendix A PDX collection 0897
+ **M80.03 Age-related osteoporosis with current pathological fracture, forearm**
  Age-related osteoporosis with current pathological fracture of wrist
• CC +7th **M80.031 Age-related osteoporosis with current pathological fracture, right forearm**
  CC Exclusion 7th character A see Appendix A PDX collection 0888
  CC Exclusion 7th characters K & P see Appendix A PDX collection 0897
• CC +7th **M80.032 Age-related osteoporosis with current pathological fracture, left forearm**
  CC Exclusion 7th character A see Appendix A PDX collection 0888
  CC Exclusion 7th characters K & P see Appendix A PDX collection 0897
• CC +7th **M80.039 Age-related osteoporosis with current pathological fracture, unspecified forearm**
  CC Exclusion 7th character A see Appendix A PDX collection 0888
  CC Exclusion 7th characters K & P see Appendix A PDX collection 0897
+ **M80.04 Age-related osteoporosis with current pathological fracture, hand**
• CC +7th **M80.041 Age-related osteoporosis with current pathological fracture, right hand**
  CC Exclusion 7th character A see Appendix A PDX collection 0888
  CC Exclusion 7th characters K & P see Appendix A PDX collection 0897
• CC +7th **M80.042 Age-related osteoporosis with current pathological fracture, left hand**
  CC Exclusion 7th character A see Appendix A PDX collection 0888
  CC Exclusion 7th characters K & P see Appendix A PDX collection 0897

• CC +7th **M80.049** **Age-related osteoporosis with current pathological fracture, unspecified hand**
CC Exclusion 7th character A see Appendix A PDX collection 0888
CC Exclusion 7th characters K & P see Appendix A PDX collection 0897

\+ **M80.05** **Age-related osteoporosis with current pathological fracture, femur**
Age-related osteoporosis with current pathological fracture of hip

• CC +7th **M80.051** **Age-related osteoporosis with current pathological fracture, right femur**
CC Exclusion 7th character A see Appendix A PDX collection 0888
CC Exclusion 7th characters K & P see Appendix A PDX collection 0897

• CC +7th **M80.052** **Age-related osteoporosis with current pathological fracture, left femur**
CC Exclusion 7th character A see Appendix A PDX collection 0888
CC Exclusion 7th characters K & P see Appendix A PDX collection 0897

• CC +7th **M80.059** **Age-related osteoporosis with current pathological fracture, unspecified femur**
CC Exclusion 7th character A see Appendix A PDX collection 0888
CC Exclusion 7th characters K & P see Appendix A PDX collection 0897

\+ **M80.06** **Age-related osteoporosis with current pathological fracture, lower leg**

• CC +7th **M80.061** **Age-related osteoporosis with current pathological fracture, right lower leg**
CC Exclusion 7th character A see Appendix A PDX collection 0888
CC Exclusion 7th characters K & P see Appendix A PDX collection 0897

• CC +7th **M80.062** **Age-related osteoporosis with current pathological fracture, left lower leg**
CC Exclusion 7th character A see Appendix A PDX collection 0888
CC Exclusion 7th characters K & P see Appendix A PDX collection 0897

• CC +7th **M80.069** **Age-related osteoporosis with current pathological fracture, unspecified lower leg**
CC Exclusion 7th character A see Appendix A PDX collection 0888
CC Exclusion 7th characters K & P see Appendix A PDX collection 0897

\+ **M80.07** **Age-related osteoporosis with current pathological fracture, ankle and foot**

• CC +7th **M80.071** **Age-related osteoporosis with current pathological fracture, right ankle and foot**
CC Exclusion 7th character A see Appendix A PDX collection 0888
CC Exclusion 7th characters K & P see Appendix A PDX collection 0897

• CC +7th **M80.072** **Age-related osteoporosis with current pathological fracture, left ankle and foot**
CC Exclusion 7th character A see Appendix A PDX collection 0888
CC Exclusion 7th characters K & P see Appendix A PDX collection 0897

• CC +7th **M80.079** **Age-related osteoporosis with current pathological fracture, unspecified ankle and foot**
CC Exclusion 7th character A see Appendix A PDX collection 0888
CC Exclusion 7th characters K & P see Appendix A PDX collection 0897

• CC +7th **M80.08** **Age-related osteoporosis with current pathological fracture, vertebra(e)**
CC Exclusion 7th character A see Appendix A PDX collection 0888
CC Exclusion 7th characters K & P see Appendix A PDX collection 0897

\+ **M80.8** **Other osteoporosis with current pathological fracture**
Drug-induced osteoporosis with current pathological fracture
Idiopathic osteoporosis with current pathological fracture
Osteoporosis of disuse with current pathological fracture
Postoophorectomy osteoporosis with current pathological fracture
Postsurgical malabsorption osteoporosis with current pathological fracture
Post-traumatic osteoporosis with current pathological fracture
Use additional code for adverse effect, if applicable, to identify drug (T36-T50 with fifth or sixth character 5)

CC X+7th **M80.80** **Other osteoporosis with current pathological fracture, unspecified site**
CC Exclusion 7th character A see Appendix A PDX collection 0888
CC Exclusion 7th characters K & P see Appendix A PDX collection 0897

\+ **M80.81** **Other osteoporosis with pathological fracture, shoulder**

CC +7th **M80.811** **Other osteoporosis with current pathological fracture, right shoulder**
CC Exclusion 7th character A see Appendix A PDX collection 0888
CC Exclusion 7th characters K & P see Appendix A PDX collection 0897

CC +7th **M80.812** **Other osteoporosis with current pathological fracture, left shoulder**
CC Exclusion 7th character A see Appendix A PDX collection 0888
CC Exclusion 7th characters K & P see Appendix A PDX collection 0897

CC +7th **M80.819** **Other osteoporosis with current pathological fracture, unspecified shoulder**
CC Exclusion 7th character A see Appendix A PDX collection 0888
CC Exclusion 7th characters K & P see Appendix A PDX collection 0897

\+ **M80.82** **Other osteoporosis with current pathological fracture, humerus**

CC +7th **M80.821** **Other osteoporosis with current pathological fracture, right humerus**
CC Exclusion 7th character A see Appendix A PDX collection 0888
CC Exclusion 7th characters K & P see Appendix A PDX collection 0897

CC +7th **M80.822** **Other osteoporosis with current pathological fracture, left humerus**
CC Exclusion 7th character A see Appendix A PDX collection 0888
CC Exclusion 7th characters K & P see Appendix A PDX collection 0897

CC +7th **M80.829** **Other osteoporosis with current pathological fracture, unspecified humeru**
CC Exclusion 7th character A see Appendix A PDX collection 0888
CC Exclusion 7th characters K & P see Appendix A PDX collection 0897

\+ **M80.83** **Other osteoporosis with current pathological fracture, forearm**
Other osteoporosis with current pathological fracture of wrist

CC +7th **M80.831** **Other osteoporosis with current pathological fracture, right forearm**
CC Exclusion 7th character A see Appendix A PDX collection 0888
CC Exclusion 7th characters K & P see Appendix A PDX collection 0897

CC +7th **M80.832** **Other osteoporosis with current pathological fracture, left forearm**
CC Exclusion 7th character A see Appendix A PDX collection 0888
CC Exclusion 7th characters K & P see Appendix A PDX collection 0897

CC +7th **M80.839** **Other osteoporosis with current pathological fracture, unspecified forearm**
CC Exclusion 7th character A see Appendix A PDX collection 0888
CC Exclusion 7th characters K & P see Appendix A PDX collection 0897

\+ **M80.84** **Other osteoporosis with current pathological fracture, hand**

CC +7th **M80.841** **Other osteoporosis with current pathological fracture, right hand**
CC Exclusion 7th character A see Appendix A PDX collection 0888
CC Exclusion 7th characters K & P see Appendix A PDX collection 0897

CC +7th **M80.842** **Other osteoporosis with current pathological fracture, left hand**
CC Exclusion 7th character A see Appendix A PDX collection 0888
CC Exclusion 7th characters K & P see Appendix A PDX collection 0897

CC +7th **M80.849** **Other osteoporosis with current pathological fracture, unspecified hand**
CC Exclusion 7th character A see Appendix A PDX collection 0888
CC Exclusion 7th characters K & P see Appendix A PDX collection 0897

+ **M80.85 Other osteoporosis with current pathological fracture, femur**
Other osteoporosis with current pathological fracture of hip

CC +7th **M80.851** **Other osteoporosis with current pathological fracture, right femur**
CC Exclusion 7th character A see Appendix A PDX collection 0888
CC Exclusion 7th characters K & P see Appendix A PDX collection 0897

CC +7th **M80.852** **Other osteoporosis with current pathological fracture, left femur**
CC Exclusion 7th character A see Appendix A PDX collection 0888
CC Exclusion 7th characters K & P see Appendix A PDX collection 0897

CC +7th **M80.859** **Other osteoporosis with current pathological fracture, unspecified femur**
CC Exclusion 7th character A see Appendix A PDX collection 0888
CC Exclusion 7th characters K & P see Appendix A PDX collection 0897

+ **M80.86 Other osteoporosis with current pathological fracture, lower leg**

CC +7th **M80.861** **Other osteoporosis with current pathological fracture, right lower leg**
CC Exclusion 7th character A see Appendix A PDX collection 0888
CC Exclusion 7th characters K & P see Appendix A PDX collection 0897

CC +7th **M80.862** **Other osteoporosis with current pathological fracture, left lower leg**
CC Exclusion 7th character A see Appendix A PDX collection 0888
CC Exclusion 7th characters K & P see Appendix A PDX collection 0897

CC +7th **M80.869** **Other osteoporosis with current pathological fracture, unspecified lower leg**
CC Exclusion 7th character A see Appendix A PDX collection 0888
CC Exclusion 7th characters K & P see Appendix A PDX collection 0897

+ **M80.87 Other osteoporosis with current pathological fracture, ankle and foot**

CC +7th **M80.871** **Other osteoporosis with current pathological fracture, right ankle and foot**
CC Exclusion 7th character A see Appendix A PDX collection 0888
CC Exclusion 7th characters K & P see Appendix A PDX collection 0897

CC +7th **M80.872** **Other osteoporosis with current pathological fracture, left ankle and foot**
CC Exclusion 7th character A see Appendix A PDX collection 0888
CC Exclusion 7th characters K & P see Appendix A PDX collection 0897

CC +7th **M80.879** **Other osteoporosis with current pathological fracture, unspecified ankle and foot**
CC Exclusion 7th character A see Appendix A PDX collection 0888
CC Exclusion 7th characters K & P see Appendix A PDX collection 0897

CC X+7th **M80.88** **Other osteoporosis with current pathological fracture, vertebra(e)**
CC Exclusion 7th character A see Appendix A PDX collection 0888
CC Exclusion 7th characters K & P see Appendix A PDX collection 0897

M81 Osteoporosis without current pathological fracture

Use additional code to identify:
major osseous defect, if applicable (M89.7-)
personal history of (healed) osteoporosis fracture, if applicable (Z87.310)

Excludes1: *osteoporosis with current pathological fracture (M80.-)*
Sudeck's atrophy (M89.0)

Review coding guideline C.13.d

• **M81.0** **Age-related osteoporosis without current pathological fracture**
Involutional osteoporosis without current pathological fracture
Osteoporosis NOS
Postmenopausal osteoporosis without current pathological fracture
Senile osteoporosis without current pathological fracture

M81.6 **Localized osteoporosis [Lequesne]**
Excludes1: *Sudeck's atrophy (M89.0)*

M81.8 **Other osteoporosis without current pathological fracture**
Drug-induced osteoporosis without current pathological fracture
Idiopathic osteoporosis without current pathological fracture
Osteoporosis of disuse without current pathological fracture
Postoophorectomy osteoporosis without current pathological fracture
Postsurgical malabsorption osteoporosis without current pathological fracture
Post-traumatic osteoporosis without current pathological fracture
Use additional code for adverse effect, if applicable, to identify drug (T36-T50 with fifth or sixth character 5)

M83 Adult osteomalacia

Excludes1: *infantile and juvenile osteomalacia (E55.0)*
renal osteodystrophy (N25.0)
rickets (active) (E55.0)
rickets (active) sequelae (E64.3)
vitamin D-resistant osteomalacia (E83.3)
vitamin D-resistant rickets (active) (E83.3)

• ♀ **M83.0** **Puerperal osteomalacia**
• **M83.1** **Senile osteomalacia**
• **M83.2** **Adult osteomalacia due to malabsorption**
Postsurgical malabsorption osteomalacia in adults
• **M83.3** **Adult osteomalacia due to malnutrition**
M83.4 **Aluminum bone disease**
• **M83.5** **Other drug-induced osteomalacia in adults**
Use additional code for adverse effect, if applicable, to identify drug (T36-T50 with fifth or sixth character 5)
• **M83.8** **Other adult osteomalacia**
• **M83.9** **Adult osteomalacia, unspecified**

M84 Disorder of continuity of bone

Excludes2: *traumatic fracture of bone-see fracture, by site*

+ **M84.3 Stress fracture**
Fatigue fracture
March fracture
Stress fracture NOS
Stress reaction
external cause code(s) to identify the cause of the stress fracture

Excludes1: *pathological fracture NOS (M84.4.-)*
pathological fracture due to osteoporosis (M80.-)
traumatic fracture (S12.-, S22.-, S32.-, S42.-, S52.-, S62.-, S72.-, S82.-, S92.-)

Excludes2: *personal history of (healed) stress (fatigue) fracture (Z87.312)*
stress fracture of vertebra (M48.4-)

The appropriate 7th character is to be added to each code from subcategory **M84.3**:
A initial encounter for fracture
D subsequent encounter for fracture with routine healing
G subsequent encounter for fracture with delayed healing
K subsequent encounter for fracture with nonunion
P subsequent encounter for fracture with malunion
S sequela

CC X+7th **M84.30 Stress fracture, unspecified site**
CC Exclusion 7th characters K & P see Appendix A PDX collection 0897

+ **M84.31 Stress fracture, shoulder**

CC +7th **M84.311 Stress fracture, right shoulder**
CC Exclusion 7th characters K & P see Appendix A PDX collection 0897

CC +7th M84.312 Stress fracture, left shoulder
CC Exclusion 7th characters K & P see Appendix A PDX collection 0897

CC +7th M84.319 Stress fracture, unspecified shoulder
CC Exclusion 7th characters K & P see Appendix A PDX collection 0897

+ M84.32 Stress fracture, humerus

CC +7th M84.321 Stress fracture, right humerus
CC Exclusion 7th characters K & P see Appendix A PDX collection 0897

CC +7th M84.322 Stress fracture, left humerus
CC Exclusion 7th characters K & P see Appendix A PDX collection 0897

CC +7th M84.329 Stress fracture, unspecified humerus
CC Exclusion 7th characters K & P see Appendix A PDX collection 0897

+ M84.33 Stress fracture, ulna and radius

CC +7th M84.331 Stress fracture, right ulna
CC Exclusion 7th characters K & P see Appendix A PDX collection 0897

CC +7th M84.332 Stress fracture, left ulna
CC Exclusion 7th characters K & P see Appendix A PDX collection 0897

CC +7th M84.333 Stress fracture, right radius
CC Exclusion 7th characters K & P see Appendix A PDX collection 0897

CC +7th M84.334 Stress fracture, left radius
CC Exclusion 7th characters K & P see Appendix A PDX collection 0897

CC +7th M84.339 Stress fracture, unspecified ulna and radius
CC Exclusion 7th characters K & P see Appendix A PDX collection 0897

+ M84.34 Stress fracture, hand and fingers

CC +7th M84.341 Stress fracture, right hand
CC Exclusion 7th characters K & P see Appendix A PDX collection 0897

CC +7th M84.342 Stress fracture, left hand
CC Exclusion 7th characters K & P see Appendix A PDX collection 0897

CC +7th M84.343 Stress fracture, unspecified hand
CC Exclusion 7th characters K & P see Appendix A PDX collection 0897

CC +7th M84.344 Stress fracture, right finger(s)
CC Exclusion 7th characters K & P see Appendix A PDX collection 0897

CC +7th M84.345 Stress fracture, left finger(s)
CC Exclusion 7th characters K & P see Appendix A PDX collection 0897

CC +7th M84.346 Stress fracture, unspecified finger(s)
CC Exclusion 7th characters K & P see Appendix A PDX collection 0897

+ M84.35 Stress fracture, pelvis and femur
Stress fracture, hip

CC +7th M84.350 Stress fracture, pelvis
CC Exclusion 7th characters K & P see Appendix A PDX collection 0897

CC +7th M84.351 Stress fracture, right femur
CC Exclusion 7th characters K & P see Appendix A PDX collection 0897

CC +7th M84.352 Stress fracture, left femur
CC Exclusion 7th characters K & P see Appendix A PDX collection 0897

CC +7th M84.353 Stress fracture, unspecified femur
CC Exclusion 7th characters K & P see Appendix A PDX collection 0897

CC +7th M84.359 Stress fracture, hip, unspecified
CC Exclusion 7th characters K & P see Appendix A PDX collection 0897

+ M84.36 Stress fracture, tibia and fibula

CC +7th M84.361 Stress fracture, right tibia
CC Exclusion 7th characters K & P see Appendix A PDX collection 0897

CC +7th M84.362 Stress fracture, left tibia
CC Exclusion 7th characters K & P see Appendix A PDX collection 0897

CC +7th M84.363 Stress fracture, right fibula
CC Exclusion 7th characters K & P see Appendix A PDX collection 0897

CC +7th M84.364 Stress fracture, left fibula
CC Exclusion 7th characters K & P see Appendix A PDX collection 0897

CC +7th M84.369 Stress fracture, unspecified tibia and fibula
CC Exclusion 7th characters K & P see Appendix A PDX collection 0897

+ M84.37 Stress fracture, ankle, foot and toes

CC +7th M84.371 Stress fracture, right ankle
CC Exclusion 7th characters K & P see Appendix A PDX collection 0897

CC +7th M84.372 Stress fracture, left ankle
CC Exclusion 7th characters K & P see Appendix A PDX collection 0897

CC +7th M84.373 Stress fracture, unspecified ankle
CC Exclusion 7th characters K & P see Appendix A PDX collection 0897

CC +7th M84.374 Stress fracture, right foot
CC Exclusion 7th characters K & P see Appendix A PDX collection 0897

CC +7th M84.375 Stress fracture, left foot
CC Exclusion 7th characters K & P see Appendix A PDX collection 0897

CC +7th M84.376 Stress fracture, unspecified foot
CC Exclusion 7th characters K & P see Appendix A PDX collection 0897

CC +7th M84.377 Stress fracture, right toe(s)
CC Exclusion 7th characters K & P see Appendix A PDX collection 0897

CC +7th M84.378 Stress fracture, left toe(s)
CC Exclusion 7th characters K & P see Appendix A PDX collection 0897

CC +7th M84.379 Stress fracture, unspecified toe(s)
CC Exclusion 7th characters K & P see Appendix A PDX collection 0897

CC X+7th M84.38 Stress fracture, other site
Excludes2: *stress fracture of vertebra (M48.4-)*
CC Exclusion 7th characters K & P see Appendix A PDX collection 0897

+ M84.4 Pathological fracture, not elsewhere classified
Chronic fracture
Pathological fracture NOS
Excludes1: *collapsed vertebra NEC (M48.5)*
pathological fracture in neoplastic disease (M84.5
pathological fracture in osteoporosis (M80.-)
pathological fracture in other disease (M84.6-)
stress fracture (M84.3-)
traumatic fracture (S12.-, S22.-, S32.-, S42.-, S52.- S62.-, S72.-, S82.-, S92.-)
Excludes2: *personal history of (healed) pathological fracture (Z87.311)*

The appropriate 7th character is to be added to each code from subcategory **M84.4**:
A initial encounter for fracture
D subsequent encounter for fracture with routine healing
G subsequent encounter for fracture with delayed healing
K subsequent encounter for fracture with nonunion
P subsequent encounter for fracture with malunion
S sequela

CC X+7th M84.40 Pathological fracture, unspecified site
CC Exclusion 7th character A see Appendix A PDX collection 0888
CC Exclusion 7th characters K & P see Appendix A PDX collection 0897

+ M84.41 Pathological fracture, shoulder

CC +7th M84.411 Pathological fracture, right shoulder
CC Exclusion 7th character A see Appendix A PDX collection 0888
CC Exclusion 7th characters K & P see Appendix A PDX collection 0897

CC +7th M84.412 Pathological fracture, left shoulder
CC Exclusion 7th character A see Appendix A PDX collection 0888
CC Exclusion 7th characters K & P see Appendix A PDX collection 0897

CC +7th M84.419 Pathological fracture, unspecified shoulde
CC Exclusion 7th character A see Appendix A PDX collection 0888
CC Exclusion 7th characters K & P see Appendix A PDX collection 0897

+ M84.42 Pathological fracture, humerus

CC +7th M84.421 Pathological fracture, right humerus
CC Exclusion 7th character A see Appendix A PDX collection 0888
CC Exclusion 7th characters K & P see Appendix A PDX collection 0897

CC +7th M84.422 Pathological fracture, left humerus
CC Exclusion 7th character A see Appendix A PDX collection 0888
CC Exclusion 7th characters K & P see Appendix A PDX collection 0897

CC +7th M84.429 **Pathological fracture, unspecified humerus**
CC Exclusion 7th character A see Appendix A PDX collection 0888
CC Exclusion 7th characters K & P see Appendix A PDX collection 0897

\+ M84.43 **Pathological fracture, ulna and radius**

CC +7th M84.431 **Pathological fracture, right ulna**
CC Exclusion 7th character A see Appendix A PDX collection 0888
CC Exclusion 7th characters K & P see Appendix A PDX collection 0897

CC +7th M84.432 **Pathological fracture, left ulna**
CC Exclusion 7th character A see Appendix A PDX collection 0888
CC Exclusion 7th characters K & P see Appendix A PDX collection 0897

CC +7th M84.433 **Pathological fracture, right radius**
CC Exclusion 7th character A see Appendix A PDX collection 0888
CC Exclusion 7th characters K & P see Appendix A PDX collection 0897

CC +7th M84.434 **Pathological fracture, left radius**
CC Exclusion 7th character A see Appendix A PDX collection 0888
CC Exclusion 7th characters K & P see Appendix A PDX collection 0897

CC +7th M84.439 **Pathological fracture, unspecified ulna and radius**
CC Exclusion 7th character A see Appendix A PDX collection 0888
CC Exclusion 7th characters K & P see Appendix A PDX collection 0897

\+ M84.44 **Pathological fracture, hand and fingers**

CC +7th M84.441 **Pathological fracture, right hand**
CC Exclusion 7th character A see Appendix A PDX collection 0888
CC Exclusion 7th characters K & P see Appendix A PDX collection 0897

CC +7th M84.442 **Pathological fracture, left hand**
CC Exclusion 7th character A see Appendix A PDX collection 0888
CC Exclusion 7th characters K & P see Appendix A PDX collection 0897

CC +7th M84.443 **Pathological fracture, unspecified hand**
CC Exclusion 7th character A see Appendix A PDX collection 0888
CC Exclusion 7th characters K & P see Appendix A PDX collection 0897

CC +7th M84.444 **Pathological fracture, right finger(s)**
CC Exclusion 7th character A see Appendix A PDX collection 0888
CC Exclusion 7th characters K & P see Appendix A PDX collection 0897

CC +7th M84.445 **Pathological fracture, left finger(s)**
CC Exclusion 7th character A see Appendix A PDX collection 0888
CC Exclusion 7th characters K & P see Appendix A PDX collection 0897

CC +7th M84.446 **Pathological fracture, unspecified finger(s)**
CC Exclusion 7th character A see Appendix A PDX collection 0888
CC Exclusion 7th characters K & P see Appendix A PDX collection 0897

\+ M84.45 **Pathological fracture, femur and pelvis**

CC +7th M84.451 **Pathological fracture, right femur**
CC Exclusion 7th character A see Appendix A PDX collection 0888
CC Exclusion 7th characters K & P see Appendix A PDX collection 0897

CC +7th M84.452 **Pathological fracture, left femur**
CC Exclusion 7th character A see Appendix A PDX collection 0888
CC Exclusion 7th characters K & P see Appendix A PDX collection 0897

CC +7th M84.453 **Pathological fracture, unspecified femur**
CC Exclusion 7th character A see Appendix A PDX collection 0888
CC Exclusion 7th characters K & P see Appendix A PDX collection 0897

CC +7th M84.454 **Pathological fracture, pelvis**
CC Exclusion 7th character A see Appendix A PDX collection 0888
CC Exclusion 7th characters K & P see Appendix A PDX collection 0897
AHA CC: 4Q, 2016, 42-43

CC +7th M84.459 **Pathological fracture, hip, unspecified**
CC Exclusion 7th character A see Appendix A PDX collection 0888
CC Exclusion 7th characters K & P see Appendix A PDX collection 0897

\+ M84.46 **Pathological fracture, tibia and fibula**

CC +7th M84.461 **Pathological fracture, right tibia**
CC Exclusion 7th character A see Appendix A PDX collection 0888
CC Exclusion 7th characters K & P see Appendix A PDX collection 0897

CC +7th M84.462 **Pathological fracture, left tibia**
CC Exclusion 7th character A see Appendix A PDX collection 0888
CC Exclusion 7th characters K & P see Appendix A PDX collection 0897

CC +7th M84.463 **Pathological fracture, right fibula**
CC Exclusion 7th character A see Appendix A PDX collection 0888
CC Exclusion 7th characters K & P see Appendix A PDX collection 0897

CC +7th M84.464 **Pathological fracture, left fibula**
CC Exclusion 7th character A see Appendix A PDX collection 0888
CC Exclusion 7th characters K & P see Appendix A PDX collection 0897

CC +7th M84.469 **Pathological fracture, unspecified tibia and fibula**
CC Exclusion 7th character A see Appendix A PDX collection 0888
CC Exclusion 7th characters K & P see Appendix A PDX collection 0897

\+ M84.47 **Pathological fracture, ankle, foot and toes**

CC +7th M84.471 **Pathological fracture, right ankle**
CC Exclusion 7th character A see Appendix A PDX collection 0888
CC Exclusion 7th characters K & P see Appendix A PDX collection 0897

CC +7th M84.472 **Pathological fracture, left ankle**
CC Exclusion 7th character A see Appendix A PDX collection 0888
CC Exclusion 7th characters K & P see Appendix A PDX collection 0897

CC +7th M84.473 **Pathological fracture, unspecified ankle**
CC Exclusion 7th character A see Appendix A PDX collection 0888
CC Exclusion 7th characters K & P see Appendix A PDX collection 0897

CC +7th M84.474 **Pathological fracture, right foot**
CC Exclusion 7th character A see Appendix A PDX collection 0888
CC Exclusion 7th characters K & P see Appendix A PDX collection 0897

CC +7th M84.475 **Pathological fracture, left foot**
CC Exclusion 7th character A see Appendix A PDX collection 0888
CC Exclusion 7th characters K & P see Appendix A PDX collection 0897

CC +7th M84.476 **Pathological fracture, unspecified foot**
CC Exclusion 7th character A see Appendix A PDX collection 0888
CC Exclusion 7th characters K & P see Appendix A PDX collection 0897

CC +7th M84.477 **Pathological fracture, right toe(s)**
CC Exclusion 7th character A see Appendix A PDX collection 0888
CC Exclusion 7th characters K & P see Appendix A PDX collection 0897

CC +7th M84.478 **Pathological fracture, left toe(s)**
CC Exclusion 7th character A see Appendix A PDX collection 0888
CC Exclusion 7th characters K & P see Appendix A PDX collection 0897

CC +7th M84.479 **Pathological fracture, unspecified toe(s)**
CC Exclusion 7th character A see Appendix A PDX collection 0888
CC Exclusion 7th characters K & P see Appendix A PDX collection 0897

CC X+7th M84.48 **Pathological fracture, other site**
CC Exclusion 7th character A see Appendix A PDX collection 0888
CC Exclusion 7th characters K & P see Appendix A PDX collection 0897

+ **M84.5 Pathological fracture in neoplastic disease**
Code also underlying neoplasm

The appropriate 7th character is to be added to each code from subcategory **M84.5**:
A initial encounter for fracture
D subsequent encounter for fracture with routine healing
G subsequent encounter for fracture with delayed healing
K subsequent encounter for fracture with nonunion
P subsequent encounter for fracture with malunion
S sequela

Review coding guideline C.2.l.6

CC X+7th **M84.50 Pathological fracture in neoplastic disease, unspecified site**
CC Exclusion 7th character A see Appendix A PDX collection 0888
CC Exclusion 7th characters K & P see Appendix A PDX collection 0897

+ **M84.51 Pathological fracture in neoplastic disease, shoulder**

CC +7th **M84.511 Pathological fracture in neoplastic disease, right shoulder**
CC Exclusion 7th character A see Appendix A PDX collection 0888
CC Exclusion 7th characters K & P see Appendix A PDX collection 0897

CC +7th **M84.512 Pathological fracture in neoplastic disease, left shoulder**
CC Exclusion 7th character A see Appendix A PDX collection 0888
CC Exclusion 7th characters K & P see Appendix A PDX collection 0897

CC +7th **M84.519 Pathological fracture in neoplastic disease, unspecified shoulder**
CC Exclusion 7th character A see Appendix A PDX collection 0888
CC Exclusion 7th characters K & P see Appendix A PDX collection 0897

+ **M84.52 Pathological fracture in neoplastic disease, humerus**

CC +7th **M84.521 Pathological fracture in neoplastic disease, right humerus**
CC Exclusion 7th character A see Appendix A PDX collection 0888
CC Exclusion 7th characters K & P see Appendix A PDX collection 0897

CC +7th **M84.522 Pathological fracture in neoplastic disease, left humerus**
CC Exclusion 7th character A see Appendix A PDX collection 0888
CC Exclusion 7th characters K & P see Appendix A PDX collection 0897

CC +7th **M84.529 Pathological fracture in neoplastic disease, unspecified humerus**
CC Exclusion 7th character A see Appendix A PDX collection 0888
CC Exclusion 7th characters K & P see Appendix A PDX collection 0897

+ **M84.53 Pathological fracture in neoplastic disease, ulna and radius**

CC +7th **M84.531 Pathological fracture in neoplastic disease, right ulna**
CC Exclusion 7th character A see Appendix A PDX collection 0888
CC Exclusion 7th characters K & P see Appendix A PDX collection 0897

CC +7th **M84.532 Pathological fracture in neoplastic disease, left ulna**
CC Exclusion 7th character A see Appendix A PDX collection 0888
CC Exclusion 7th characters K & P see Appendix A PDX collection 0897

CC +7th **M84.533 Pathological fracture in neoplastic disease, right radius**
CC Exclusion 7th character A see Appendix A PDX collection 0888
CC Exclusion 7th characters K & P see Appendix A PDX collection 0897

CC +7th **M84.534 Pathological fracture in neoplastic disease, left radius**
CC Exclusion 7th character A see Appendix A PDX collection 0888
CC Exclusion 7th characters K & P see Appendix A PDX collection 0897

CC +7th **M84.539 Pathological fracture in neoplastic disea unspecified ulna and radius**
CC Exclusion 7th character A see Appendix PDX collection 0888
CC Exclusion 7th characters K & P see Appendix A PDX collection 0897

+ **M84.54 Pathological fracture in neoplastic disease, hand**

CC +7th **M84.541 Pathological fracture in neoplastic disea right hand**
CC Exclusion 7th character A see Appendix PDX collection 0888
CC Exclusion 7th characters K & P see Appendix A PDX collection 0897

CC +7th **M84.542 Pathological fracture in neoplastic disea left hand**
CC Exclusion 7th character A see Appendix PDX collection 0888
CC Exclusion 7th characters K & P see Appendix A PDX collection 0897

CC +7th **M84.549 Pathological fracture in neoplastic disea unspecified hand**
CC Exclusion 7th character A see Appendix PDX collection 0888
CC Exclusion 7th characters K & P see Appendix A PDX collection 0897

+ **M84.55 Pathological fracture in neoplastic disease, pelvis and femur**

CC +7th **M84.550 Pathological fracture in neoplastic disea pelvis**
CC Exclusion 7th character A see Appendix PDX collection 0888
CC Exclusion 7th characters K & P see Appendix A PDX collection 0897

CC +7th **M84.551 Pathological fracture in neoplastic disea right femur**
CC Exclusion 7th character A see Appendix PDX collection 0888
CC Exclusion 7th characters K & P see Appendix A PDX collection 0897

CC +7th **M84.552 Pathological fracture in neoplastic disea left femur**
CC Exclusion 7th character A see Appendix PDX collection 0888
CC Exclusion 7th characters K & P see Appendix A PDX collection 0897

CC +7th **M84.553 Pathological fracture in neoplastic disea unspecified femur**
CC Exclusion 7th character A see Appendix PDX collection 0888
CC Exclusion 7th characters K & P see Appendix A PDX collection 0897

CC +7th **M84.559 Pathological fracture in neoplastic disea hip, unspecified**
CC Exclusion 7th character A see Appendix PDX collection 0888
CC Exclusion 7th characters K & P see Appendix A PDX collection 0897

+ **M84.56 Pathological fracture in neoplastic disease, tibia a fibula**

CC +7th **M84.561 Pathological fracture in neoplastic disea right tibia**
CC Exclusion 7th character A see Appendix PDX collection 0888
CC Exclusion 7th characters K & P see Appendix A PDX collection 0897

CC +7th **M84.562 Pathological fracture in neoplastic disea left tibia**
CC Exclusion 7th character A see Appendix PDX collection 0888
CC Exclusion 7th characters K & P see Appendix A PDX collection 089

CC +7th **M84.563 Pathological fracture in neoplastic disea right fibula**
CC Exclusion 7th character A see Appendix PDX collection 0888
CC Exclusion 7th characters K & P see Appendix A PDX collection 089

CC +7th **M84.564 Pathological fracture in neoplastic disea left fibula**
CC Exclusion 7th character A see Appendix PDX collection 0888
CC Exclusion 7th characters K & P see Appendix A PDX collection 089

CC +7th **M84.569** **Pathological fracture in neoplastic disease, unspecified tibia and fibula**
CC Exclusion 7th character A see Appendix A PDX collection 0888
CC Exclusion 7th characters K & P see Appendix A PDX collection 0897

\+ **M84.57** **Pathological fracture in neoplastic disease, ankle and foot**

CC +7th **M84.571** **Pathological fracture in neoplastic disease, right ankle**
CC Exclusion 7th character A see Appendix A PDX collection 0888
CC Exclusion 7th characters K & P see Appendix A PDX collection 0897

CC +7th **M84.572** **Pathological fracture in neoplastic disease, left ankle**
CC Exclusion 7th character A see Appendix A PDX collection 0888
CC Exclusion 7th characters K & P see Appendix A PDX collection 0897

CC +7th **M84.573** **Pathological fracture in neoplastic disease, unspecified ankle**
CC Exclusion 7th character A see Appendix A PDX collection 0888
CC Exclusion 7th characters K & P see Appendix A PDX collection 0897

CC +7th **M84.574** **Pathological fracture in neoplastic disease, right foot**
CC Exclusion 7th character A see Appendix A PDX collection 0888
CC Exclusion 7th characters K & P see Appendix A PDX collection 0897

CC +7th **M84.575** **Pathological fracture in neoplastic disease, left foot**
CC Exclusion 7th character A see Appendix A PDX collection 0888
CC Exclusion 7th characters K & P see Appendix A PDX collection 0897

CC +7th **M84.576** **Pathological fracture in neoplastic disease, unspecified foot**
CC Exclusion 7th character A see Appendix A PDX collection 0888
CC Exclusion 7th characters K & P see Appendix A PDX collection 0897

CC X+7th **M84.58** **Pathological fracture in neoplastic disease, other specified site**
Pathological fracture in neoplastic disease, vertebrae
CC Exclusion 7th character A see Appendix A PDX collection 0888
CC Exclusion 7th characters K & P see Appendix A PDX collection 0897

\+ **M84.6** **Pathological fracture in other disease**
Code also underlying condition
Excludes1: *pathological fracture in osteoporosis (M80.-)*

The appropriate 7th character is to be added to each code from subcategory **M84.6**:
A initial encounter for fracture
D subsequent encounter for fracture with routine healing
G subsequent encounter for fracture with delayed healing
K subsequent encounter for fracture with nonunion
P subsequent encounter for fracture with malunion
S sequela

CC X+7th **M84.60** **Pathological fracture in other disease, unspecified site**
CC Exclusion 7th character A see Appendix A PDX collection 0888
CC Exclusion 7th characters K & P see Appendix A PDX collection 0897

\+ **M84.61** **Pathological fracture in other disease, shoulder**

CC +7th **M84.611** **Pathological fracture in other disease, right shoulder**
CC Exclusion 7th character A see Appendix A PDX collection 0888
CC Exclusion 7th characters K & P see Appendix A PDX collection 0897

CC +7th **M84.612** **Pathological fracture in other disease, left shoulder**
CC Exclusion 7th character A see Appendix A PDX collection 0888
CC Exclusion 7th characters K & P see Appendix A PDX collection 0897

CC +7th **M84.619** **Pathological fracture in other disease, unspecified shoulder**
CC Exclusion 7th character A see Appendix A PDX collection 0888
CC Exclusion 7th characters K & P see Appendix A PDX collection 0897

\+ **M84.62** **Pathological fracture in other disease, humerus**

CC +7th **M84.621** **Pathological fracture in other disease, right humerus**
CC Exclusion 7th character A see Appendix A PDX collection 0888
CC Exclusion 7th characters K & P see Appendix A PDX collection 0897

CC +7th **M84.622** **Pathological fracture in other disease, left humerus**
CC Exclusion 7th character A see Appendix A PDX collection 0888
CC Exclusion 7th characters K & P see Appendix A PDX collection 0897

CC +7th **M84.629** **Pathological fracture in other disease, unspecified humerus**
CC Exclusion 7th character A see Appendix A PDX collection 0888
CC Exclusion 7th characters K & P see Appendix A PDX collection 0897

\+ **M84.63** **Pathological fracture in other disease, ulna and radius**

CC +7th **M84.631** **Pathological fracture in other disease, right ulna**
CC Exclusion 7th character A see Appendix A PDX collection 0888
CC Exclusion 7th characters K & P see Appendix A PDX collection 0897

CC +7th **M84.632** **Pathological fracture in other disease, left ulna**
CC Exclusion 7th character A see Appendix A PDX collection 0888
CC Exclusion 7th characters K & P see Appendix A PDX collection 0897

CC +7th **M84.633** **Pathological fracture in other disease, right radius**
CC Exclusion 7th character A see Appendix A PDX collection 0888
CC Exclusion 7th characters K & P see Appendix A PDX collection 0897

CC +7th **M84.634** **Pathological fracture in other disease, left radius**
CC Exclusion 7th character A see Appendix A PDX collection 0888
CC Exclusion 7th characters K & P see Appendix A PDX collection 0897

CC +7th **M84.639** **Pathological fracture in other disease, unspecified ulna and radius**
CC Exclusion 7th character A see Appendix A PDX collection 0888
CC Exclusion 7th characters K & P see Appendix A PDX collection 0897

\+ **M84.64** **Pathological fracture in other disease, hand**

CC +7th **M84.641** **Pathological fracture in other disease, right hand**
CC Exclusion 7th character A see Appendix A PDX collection 0888
CC Exclusion 7th characters K & P see Appendix A PDX collection 0897

CC +7th **M84.642** **Pathological fracture in other disease, left hand**
CC Exclusion 7th character A see Appendix A PDX collection 0888
CC Exclusion 7th characters K & P see Appendix A PDX collection 0897

CC +7th **M84.649** **Pathological fracture in other disease, unspecified hand**
CC Exclusion 7th character A see Appendix A PDX collection 0888
CC Exclusion 7th characters K & P see Appendix A PDX collection 0897

\+ **M84.65** **Pathological fracture in other disease, pelvis and femur**

M84.650 **Pathological fracture in other disease, pelvis**

CC +7th **M84.651** **Pathological fracture in other disease, right femur**
CC Exclusion 7th character A see Appendix A PDX collection 0888
CC Exclusion 7th characters K & P see Appendix A PDX collection 0897

CC +7th **M84.652** **Pathological fracture in other disease, left femur**
CC Exclusion 7th character A see Appendix A PDX collection 0888
CC Exclusion 7th characters K & P see Appendix A PDX collection 0897

CC +7th **M84.653** **Pathological fracture in other disease, unspecified femur**
CC Exclusion 7th character A see Appendix A PDX collection 0888
CC Exclusion 7th characters K & P see Appendix A PDX collection 0897

CC +7th **M84.659** **Pathological fracture in other disease, hip, unspecified**
CC Exclusion 7th character A see Appendix A PDX collection 0888
CC Exclusion 7th characters K & P see Appendix A PDX collection 0897

+ **M84.66** **Pathological fracture in other disease, tibia and fibula**

CC +7th **M84.661** **Pathological fracture in other disease, right tibia**
CC Exclusion 7th character A see Appendix A PDX collection 0888
CC Exclusion 7th characters K & P see Appendix A PDX collection 0897

CC +7th **M84.662** **Pathological fracture in other disease, left tibia**
CC Exclusion 7th character A see Appendix A PDX collection 0888
CC Exclusion 7th characters K & P see Appendix A PDX collection 0897

CC +7th **M84.663** **Pathological fracture in other disease, right fibula**
CC Exclusion 7th character A see Appendix A PDX collection 0888
CC Exclusion 7th characters K & P see Appendix A PDX collection 0897

CC +7th **M84.664** **Pathological fracture in other disease, left fibula**
CC Exclusion 7th character A see Appendix A PDX collection 0888
CC Exclusion 7th characters K & P see Appendix A PDX collection 0897

CC +7th **M84.669** **Pathological fracture in other disease, unspecified tibia and fibula**
CC Exclusion 7th character A see Appendix A PDX collection 0888
CC Exclusion 7th characters K & P see Appendix A PDX collection 0897

+ **M84.67** **Pathological fracture in other disease, ankle and foot**

CC +7th **M84.671** **Pathological fracture in other disease, right ankle**
CC Exclusion 7th character A see Appendix A PDX collection 0888
CC Exclusion 7th characters K & P see Appendix A PDX collection 0897

CC +7th **M84.672** **Pathological fracture in other disease, left ankle**
CC Exclusion 7th character A see Appendix A PDX collection 0888
CC Exclusion 7th characters K & P see Appendix A PDX collection 0897

CC +7th **M84.673** **Pathological fracture in other disease, unspecified ankle**
CC Exclusion 7th character A see Appendix A PDX collection 0888
CC Exclusion 7th characters K & P see Appendix A PDX collection 0897

CC +7th **M84.674** **Pathological fracture in other disease, right foot**
CC Exclusion 7th character A see Appendix A PDX collection 0888
CC Exclusion 7th characters K & P see Appendix A PDX collection 0897

CC +7th **M84.675** **Pathological fracture in other disease, left foot**
CC Exclusion 7th character A see Appendix A PDX collection 0888
CC Exclusion 7th characters K & P see Appendix A PDX collection 0897

CC +7th **M84.676** **Pathological fracture in other disease, unspecified foot**
CC Exclusion 7th character A see Appendix A PDX collection 0888
CC Exclusion 7th characters K & P see Appendix A PDX collection 0897

CC X+7th **M84.68** **Pathological fracture in other disease, other site**
CC Exclusion 7th character A see Appendix A PDX collection 0888
CC Exclusion 7th characters K & P see Appendix A PDX collection 0897

+ **M84.7** **Nontraumatic fracture, not elsewhere classified**

+ **M84.75** **Atypical femoral fracture**
AHA CC: 4Q, 2016, 41-42

The appropriate 7th character is to be added to each code from subcategory **M84.75**:
A initial encounter for fracture
D subsequent encounter for fracture with routine healing
G subsequent encounter for fracture with delayed healing
K subsequent encounter for fracture with nonunion
P subsequent encounter for fracture with malunion
S sequela

CC +7th **M84.750** **Atypical femoral fracture, unspecified**
CC Exclusion 7th character A see Appendix A PDX collection 0888
CC Exclusion 7th character K & P see Appen A PDX collection 0897

CC +7th **M84.751** **Incomplete atypical femoral fracture, rig leg**
CC Exclusion 7th character A see Appendix A PDX collection 0888
CC Exclusion 7th character K & P see Appen A PDX collection 0897

CC +7th **M84.752** **Incomplete atypical femoral fracture, lef leg**
CC Exclusion 7th character A see Appendix A PDX collection 0888
CC Exclusion 7th character K & P see Appen A PDX collection 0897

CC +7th **M84.753** **Incomplete atypical femoral fracture, unspecified leg**
CC Exclusion 7th character A see Appendix A PDX collection 0888
CC Exclusion 7th character K & P see Appen A PDX collection 0897

CC +7th **M84.754** **Complete transverse atypical femoral fracture, right leg**
CC Exclusion 7th character A see Appendix A PDX collection 0888
CC Exclusion 7th character K & P see Appen A PDX collection 0897

CC +7th **M84.755** **Complete transverse atypical femoral fracture, left leg**
CC Exclusion 7th character A see Appendix A PDX collection 0888
CC Exclusion 7th character K & P see Appen A PDX collection 0897

CC +7th **M84.756** **Complete transverse atypical femoral fracture, unspecified leg**
CC Exclusion 7th character A see Appendix A PDX collection 0888
CC Exclusion 7th character K & P see Appen A PDX collection 0897

CC +7th **M84.757** **Complete oblique atypical femoral fracture, right leg**
CC Exclusion 7th character A see Appendix A PDX collection 0888
CC Exclusion 7th character K & P see Appen A PDX collection 0897

CC +7th **M84.758** **Complete oblique atypical femoral fracture, left leg**
CC Exclusion 7th character A see Appendix A PDX collection 0888
CC Exclusion 7th character K & P see Appen A PDX collection 0897

CC +7th **M84.759** **Complete oblique atypical femoral fracture, unspecified leg**
CC Exclusion 7th character A see Appendix A PDX collection 0888
CC Exclusion 7th character K & P see Appen A PDX collection 0897

+ **M84.8** **Other disorders of continuity of bone**

M84.80 **Other disorders of continuity of bone, unspecified si**

+ **M84.81** **Other disorders of continuity of bone, shoulder**

M84.811 **Other disorders of continuity of bone, rig shoulder**

M84.812 **Other disorders of continuity of bone, lef shoulder**

M84.819 **Other disorders of continuity of bone, unspecified shoulder**

+ M84.82 Other disorders of continuity of bone, humerus
M84.821 Other disorders of continuity of bone, right humerus
M84.822 Other disorders of continuity of bone, left humerus
M84.829 Other disorders of continuity of bone, unspecified humerus
+ M84.83 Other disorders of continuity of bone, ulna and radius
M84.831 Other disorders of continuity of bone, right ulna
M84.832 Other disorders of continuity of bone, left ulna
M84.833 Other disorders of continuity of bone, right radius
M84.834 Other disorders of continuity of bone, left radius
M84.839 Other disorders of continuity of bone, unspecified ulna and radius
+ M84.84 Other disorders of continuity of bone, hand
M84.841 Other disorders of continuity of bone, right hand
M84.842 Other disorders of continuity of bone, left hand
M84.849 Other disorders of continuity of bone, unspecified hand
+ M84.85 Other disorders of continuity of bone, pelvic region and thigh
M84.851 Other disorders of continuity of bone, right pelvic region and thigh
M84.852 Other disorders of continuity of bone, left pelvic region and thigh
M84.859 Other disorders of continuity of bone, unspecified pelvic region and thigh
+ M84.86 Other disorders of continuity of bone, tibia and fibula
M84.861 Other disorders of continuity of bone, right tibia
M84.862 Other disorders of continuity of bone, left tibia
M84.863 Other disorders of continuity of bone, right fibula
M84.864 Other disorders of continuity of bone, left fibula
M84.869 Other disorders of continuity of bone, unspecified tibia and fibula
+ M84.87 Other disorders of continuity of bone, ankle and foot
M84.871 Other disorders of continuity of bone, right ankle and foot
M84.872 Other disorders of continuity of bone, left ankle and foot
M84.879 Other disorders of continuity of bone, unspecified ankle and foot
M84.88 Other disorders of continuity of bone, other site
M84.9 Disorder of continuity of bone, unspecified

M85 Other disorders of bone density and structure

Excludes1: *osteogenesis imperfecta (Q78.0)*
osteopetrosis (Q78.2)
osteopoikilosis (Q78.8)
polyostotic fibrous dysplasia (Q78.1)

+ M85.0 Fibrous dysplasia (monostotic)
Excludes2: *fibrous dysplasia of jaw (M27.8)*
M85.00 Fibrous dysplasia (monostotic), unspecified site
+ M85.01 Fibrous dysplasia (monostotic), shoulder
M85.011 Fibrous dysplasia (monostotic), right shoulder
M85.012 Fibrous dysplasia (monostotic), left shoulder
M85.019 Fibrous dysplasia (monostotic), unspecified shoulder
+ M85.02 Fibrous dysplasia (monostotic), upper arm
M85.021 Fibrous dysplasia (monostotic), right upper arm
M85.022 Fibrous dysplasia (monostotic), left upper arm
M85.029 Fibrous dysplasia (monostotic), unspecified upper arm
+ M85.03 Fibrous dysplasia (monostotic), forearm
M85.031 Fibrous dysplasia (monostotic), right forearm
M85.032 Fibrous dysplasia (monostotic), left forearm
M85.039 Fibrous dysplasia (monostotic), unspecified forearm
+ M85.04 Fibrous dysplasia (monostotic), hand
M85.041 Fibrous dysplasia (monostotic), right hand
M85.042 Fibrous dysplasia (monostotic), left hand
M85.049 Fibrous dysplasia (monostotic), unspecified hand
+ M85.05 Fibrous dysplasia (monostotic), thigh
M85.051 Fibrous dysplasia (monostotic), right thigh
M85.052 Fibrous dysplasia (monostotic), left thigh
M85.059 Fibrous dysplasia (monostotic), unspecified thigh
+ M85.06 Fibrous dysplasia (monostotic), lower leg
M85.061 Fibrous dysplasia (monostotic), right lower leg
M85.062 Fibrous dysplasia (monostotic), left lower leg
M85.069 Fibrous dysplasia (monostotic), unspecified lower leg
+ M85.07 Fibrous dysplasia (monostotic), ankle and foot
M85.071 Fibrous dysplasia (monostotic), right ankle and foot
M85.072 Fibrous dysplasia (monostotic), left ankle and foot
M85.079 Fibrous dysplasia (monostotic), unspecified ankle and foot
M85.08 Fibrous dysplasia (monostotic), other site
M85.09 Fibrous dysplasia (monostotic), multiple sites
+ M85.1 Skeletal fluorosis
M85.10 Skeletal fluorosis, unspecified site
+ M85.11 Skeletal fluorosis, shoulder
M85.111 Skeletal fluorosis, right shoulder
M85.112 Skeletal fluorosis, left shoulder
M85.119 Skeletal fluorosis, unspecified shoulder
+ M85.12 Skeletal fluorosis, upper arm
M85.121 Skeletal fluorosis, right upper arm
M85.122 Skeletal fluorosis, left upper arm
M85.129 Skeletal fluorosis, unspecified upper arm
+ M85.13 Skeletal fluorosis, forearm
M85.131 Skeletal fluorosis, right forearm
M85.132 Skeletal fluorosis, left forearm
M85.139 Skeletal fluorosis, unspecified forearm
+ M85.14 Skeletal fluorosis, hand
M85.141 Skeletal fluorosis, right hand
M85.142 Skeletal fluorosis, left hand
M85.149 Skeletal fluorosis, unspecified hand
+ M85.15 Skeletal fluorosis, thigh
M85.151 Skeletal fluorosis, right thigh
M85.152 Skeletal fluorosis, left thigh
M85.159 Skeletal fluorosis, unspecified thigh
+ M85.16 Skeletal fluorosis, lower leg
M85.161 Skeletal fluorosis, right lower leg
M85.162 Skeletal fluorosis, left lower leg
M85.169 Skeletal fluorosis, unspecified lower leg
+ M85.17 Skeletal fluorosis, ankle and foot
M85.171 Skeletal fluorosis, right ankle and foot
M85.172 Skeletal fluorosis, left ankle and foot
M85.179 Skeletal fluorosis, unspecified ankle and foot
M85.18 Skeletal fluorosis, other site
M85.19 Skeletal fluorosis, multiple sites
M85.2 Hyperostosis of skull
+ M85.3 Osteitis condensans
M85.30 Osteitis condensans, unspecified site
+ M85.31 Osteitis condensans, shoulder
M85.311 Osteitis condensans, right shoulder
M85.312 Osteitis condensans, left shoulder
M85.319 Osteitis condensans, unspecified shoulder
+ M85.32 Osteitis condensans, upper arm
M85.321 Osteitis condensans, right upper arm
M85.322 Osteitis condensans, left upper arm
M85.329 Osteitis condensans, unspecified upper arm
+ M85.33 Osteitis condensans, forearm
M85.331 Osteitis condensans, right forearm
M85.332 Osteitis condensans, left forearm
M85.339 Osteitis condensans, unspecified forearm
+ M85.34 Osteitis condensans, hand
M85.341 Osteitis condensans, right hand
M85.342 Osteitis condensans, left hand
M85.349 Osteitis condensans, unspecified hand
+ M85.35 Osteitis condensans, thigh
M85.351 Osteitis condensans, right thigh
M85.352 Osteitis condensans, left thigh
M85.359 Osteitis condensans, unspecified thigh

+ **M85.36 Osteitis condensans, lower leg**
  - **M85.361 Osteitis condensans, right lower leg**
  - **M85.362 Osteitis condensans, left lower leg**
  - **M85.369 Osteitis condensans, unspecified lower leg**

+ **M85.37 Osteitis condensans, ankle and foot**
  - **M85.371 Osteitis condensans, right ankle and foot**
  - **M85.372 Osteitis condensans, left ankle and foot**
  - **M85.379 Osteitis condensans, unspecified ankle and foot**

M85.38 Osteitis condensans, other site

M85.39 Osteitis condensans, multiple sites

+ **M85.4 Solitary bone cyst**

Excludes2: *solitary cyst of jaw (M27.4)*

M85.40 Solitary bone cyst, unspecified site

+ **M85.41 Solitary bone cyst, shoulder**
  - **M85.411 Solitary bone cyst, right shoulder**
  - **M85.412 Solitary bone cyst, left shoulder**
  - **M85.419 Solitary bone cyst, unspecified shoulder**

+ **M85.42 Solitary bone cyst, humerus**
  - **M85.421 Solitary bone cyst, right humerus**
  - **M85.422 Solitary bone cyst, left humerus**
  - **M85.429 Solitary bone cyst, unspecified humerus**

+ **M85.43 Solitary bone cyst, ulna and radius**
  - **M85.431 Solitary bone cyst, right ulna and radius**
  - **M85.432 Solitary bone cyst, left ulna and radius**
  - **M85.439 Solitary bone cyst, unspecified ulna and radius**

+ **M85.44 Solitary bone cyst, hand**
  - **M85.441 Solitary bone cyst, right hand**
  - **M85.442 Solitary bone cyst, left hand**
  - **M85.449 Solitary bone cyst, unspecified hand**

+ **M85.45 Solitary bone cyst, pelvis**
  - **M85.451 Solitary bone cyst, right pelvis**
  - **M85.452 Solitary bone cyst, left pelvis**
  - **M85.459 Solitary bone cyst, unspecified pelvis**

+ **M85.46 Solitary bone cyst, tibia and fibula**
  - **M85.461 Solitary bone cyst, right tibia and fibula**
  - **M85.462 Solitary bone cyst, left tibia and fibula**
  - **M85.469 Solitary bone cyst, unspecified tibia and fibula**

+ **M85.47 Solitary bone cyst, ankle and foot**
  - **M85.471 Solitary bone cyst, right ankle and foot**
  - **M85.472 Solitary bone cyst, left ankle and foot**
  - **M85.479 Solitary bone cyst, unspecified ankle and foot**

M85.48 Solitary bone cyst, other site

+ **M85.5 Aneurysmal bone cyst**

Excludes2: *aneurysmal cyst of jaw (M27.4)*

M85.50 Aneurysmal bone cyst, unspecified site

+ **M85.51 Aneurysmal bone cyst, shoulder**
  - **M85.511 Aneurysmal bone cyst, right shoulder**
  - **M85.512 Aneurysmal bone cyst, left shoulder**
  - **M85.519 Aneurysmal bone cyst, unspecified shoulder**

+ **M85.52 Aneurysmal bone cyst, upper arm**
  - **M85.521 Aneurysmal bone cyst, right upper arm**
  - **M85.522 Aneurysmal bone cyst, left upper arm**
  - **M85.529 Aneurysmal bone cyst, unspecified upper arm**

+ **M85.53 Aneurysmal bone cyst, forearm**
  - **M85.531 Aneurysmal bone cyst, right forearm**
  - **M85.532 Aneurysmal bone cyst, left forearm**
  - **M85.539 Aneurysmal bone cyst, unspecified forearm**

+ **M85.54 Aneurysmal bone cyst, hand**
  - **M85.541 Aneurysmal bone cyst, right hand**
  - **M85.542 Aneurysmal bone cyst, left hand**
  - **M85.549 Aneurysmal bone cyst, unspecified hand**

+ **M85.55 Aneurysmal bone cyst, thigh**
  - **M85.551 Aneurysmal bone cyst, right thigh**
  - **M85.552 Aneurysmal bone cyst, left thigh**
  - **M85.559 Aneurysmal bone cyst, unspecified thigh**

+ **M85.56 Aneurysmal bone cyst, lower leg**
  - **M85.561 Aneurysmal bone cyst, right lower leg**
  - **M85.562 Aneurysmal bone cyst, left lower leg**
  - **M85.569 Aneurysmal bone cyst, unspecified lower leg**

+ **M85.57 Aneurysmal bone cyst, ankle and foot**
  - **M85.571 Aneurysmal bone cyst, right ankle and foot**
  - **M85.572 Aneurysmal bone cyst, left ankle and foot**
  - **M85.579 Aneurysmal bone cyst, unspecified ankle and foot**

M85.58 Aneurysmal bone cyst, other site

M85.59 Aneurysmal bone cyst, multiple sites

+ **M85.6 Other cyst of bone**

Excludes1: *cyst of jaw NEC (M27.4)*
osteitis fibrosa cystica generalisata [von Recklinghausen's disease of bone] (E21.0)

M85.60 Other cyst of bone, unspecified site

+ **M85.61 Other cyst of bone, shoulder**
  - **M85.611 Other cyst of bone, right shoulder**
  - **M85.612 Other cyst of bone, left shoulder**
  - **M85.619 Other cyst of bone, unspecified shoulder**

+ **M85.62 Other cyst of bone, upper arm**
  - **M85.621 Other cyst of bone, right upper arm**
  - **M85.622 Other cyst of bone, left upper arm**
  - **M85.629 Other cyst of bone, unspecified upper arm**

+ **M85.63 Other cyst of bone, forearm**
  - **M85.631 Other cyst of bone, right forearm**
  - **M85.632 Other cyst of bone, left forearm**
  - **M85.639 Other cyst of bone, unspecified forearm**

+ **M85.64 Other cyst of bone, hand**
  - **M85.641 Other cyst of bone, right hand**
  - **M85.642 Other cyst of bone, left hand**
  - **M85.649 Other cyst of bone, unspecified hand**

+ **M85.65 Other cyst of bone, thigh**
  - **M85.651 Other cyst of bone, right thigh**
  - **M85.652 Other cyst of bone, left thigh**
  - **M85.659 Other cyst of bone, unspecified thigh**

+ **M85.66 Other cyst of bone, lower leg**
  - **M85.661 Other cyst of bone, right lower leg**
  - **M85.662 Other cyst of bone, left lower leg**
  - **M85.669 Other cyst of bone, unspecified lower leg**

+ **M85.67 Other cyst of bone, ankle and foot**
  - **M85.671 Other cyst of bone, right ankle and foot**
  - **M85.672 Other cyst of bone, left ankle and foot**
  - **M85.679 Other cyst of bone, unspecified ankle and foot**

M85.68 Other cyst of bone, other site

M85.69 Other cyst of bone, multiple sites

+ **M85.8 Other specified disorders of bone density and structure**

Hyperostosis of bones, except skull
Osteosclerosis, acquired

Excludes1: *diffuse idiopathic skeletal hyperostosis [DISH] (M48.1)*
osteosclerosis congenita (Q77.4)
osteosclerosis fragilitas (generalista) (Q78.2)
osteosclerosis myelofibrosis (D75.81)

M85.80 Other specified disorders of bone density and structure, unspecified site

+ **M85.81 Other specified disorders of bone density and structure, shoulder**
  - **M85.811 Other specified disorders of bone density and structure, right shoulder**
  - **M85.812 Other specified disorders of bone density and structure, left shoulder**
  - **M85.819 Other specified disorders of bone density and structure, unspecified shoulder**

+ **M85.82 Other specified disorders of bone density and structure, upper arm**
  - **M85.821 Other specified disorders of bone density and structure, right upper arm**
  - **M85.822 Other specified disorders of bone density and structure, left upper arm**
  - **M85.829 Other specified disorders of bone density and structure, unspecified upper arm**

+ **M85.83 Other specified disorders of bone density and structure, forearm**
  - **M85.831 Other specified disorders of bone density and structure, right forearm**
  - **M85.832 Other specified disorders of bone density and structure, left forearm**
  - **M85.839 Other specified disorders of bone density and structure, unspecified forearm**

+ **M85.84 Other specified disorders of bone density and structure, hand**
  - **M85.841 Other specified disorders of bone density and structure, right hand**
  - **M85.842 Other specified disorders of bone density and structure, left hand**
  - **M85.849 Other specified disorders of bone density and structure, unspecified hand**

+ **M85.85 Other specified disorders of bone density and structure, thigh**
  - **M85.851 Other specified disorders of bone density and structure, right thigh**
  - **M85.852 Other specified disorders of bone density and structure, left thigh**
  - **M85.859 Other specified disorders of bone density and structure, unspecified thigh**

+ **M85.86 Other specified disorders of bone density and structure, lower leg**
  - **M85.861 Other specified disorders of bone density and structure, right lower leg**
  - **M85.862 Other specified disorders of bone density and structure, left lower leg**
  - **M85.869 Other specified disorders of bone density and structure, unspecified lower leg**

+ **M85.87 Other specified disorders of bone density and structure, ankle and foot**
  - **M85.871 Other specified disorders of bone density and structure, right ankle and foot**
  - **M85.872 Other specified disorders of bone density and structure, left ankle and foot**
  - **M85.879 Other specified disorders of bone density and structure, unspecified ankle and foot**

M85.88 Other specified disorders of bone density and structure, other site

M85.89 Other specified disorders of bone density and structure, multiple sites

M85.9 Disorder of bone density and structure, unspecified

ther osteopathies (M86-M90)

cludes1: *postprocedural osteopathies (M96.-)*

M86 Osteomyelitis

Use additional code (B95-B97) to identify infectious agent

Use additional code to identify major osseous defect, if applicable (M89.7-)

Excludes1: *osteomyelitis due to:*
echinococcus (B67.2)
gonococcus (A54.43)
salmonella (A02.24)

Excludes2: *ostemyelitis of:*
orbit (H05.0-)
petrous bone (H70.2-)
vertebra (M46.2-)

+ **M86.0 Acute hematogenous osteomyelitis**
  - CC **M86.00 Acute hematogenous osteomyelitis, unspecifiedsite**
    CC Exclusion see Appendix A PDX collection 0898

+ **M86.01 Acute hematogenous osteomyelitis, shoulder**
  - CC **M86.011 Acute hematogenous osteomyelitis, right shoulder**
    CC Exclusion see Appendix A PDX collection 0899
  - CC **M86.012 Acute hematogenous osteomyelitis, left shoulder**
    CC Exclusion see Appendix A PDX collection 0899
  - CC **M86.019 Acute hematogenous osteomyelitis, unspecified shoulder**
    CC Exclusion see Appendix A PDX collection 0899

+ **M86.02 Acute hematogenous osteomyelitis, humerus**
  - CC **M86.021 Acute hematogenous osteomyelitis, right humerus**
    CC Exclusion see Appendix A PDX collection 0900
  - CC **M86.022 Acute hematogenous osteomyelitis, left humerus**
    CC Exclusion see Appendix A PDX collection 0900
  - CC **M86.029 Acute hematogenous osteomyelitis, unspecified humerus**
    CC Exclusion see Appendix A PDX collection 0900

+ **M86.03 Acute hematogenous osteomyelitis, radius and ulna**
  - CC **M86.031 Acute hematogenous osteomyelitis, right radius and ulna**
    CC Exclusion see Appendix A PDX collection 0901
  - CC **M86.032 Acute hematogenous osteomyelitis, left radius and ulna**
    CC Exclusion see Appendix A PDX collection 0901
  - CC **M86.039 Acute hematogenous osteomyelitis, unspecified radius and ulna**
    CC Exclusion see Appendix A PDX collection 0901

+ **M86.04 Acute hematogenous osteomyelitis, hand**
  - CC **M86.041 Acute hematogenous osteomyelitis, right hand**
    CC Exclusion see Appendix A PDX collection 0902
  - CC **M86.042 Acute hematogenous osteomyelitis, left hand**
    CC Exclusion see Appendix A PDX collection 0902
  - CC **M86.049 Acute hematogenous osteomyelitis, unspecified hand**
    CC Exclusion see Appendix A PDX collection 0902

+ **M86.05 Acute hematogenous osteomyelitis, femur**
  - CC **M86.051 Acute hematogenous osteomyelitis, right femur**
    CC Exclusion see Appendix A PDX collection 0903
  - CC **M86.052 Acute hematogenous osteomyelitis, left femur**
    CC Exclusion see Appendix A PDX collection 0903
  - CC **M86.059 Acute hematogenous osteomyelitis, unspecified femur**
    CC Exclusion see Appendix A PDX collection 0903

+ **M86.06 Acute hematogenous osteomyelitis, tibia and fibula**
  - CC **M86.061 Acute hematogenous osteomyelitis, right tibia and fibula**
    CC Exclusion see Appendix A PDX collection 0904
  - CC **M86.062 Acute hematogenous osteomyelitis, left tibia and fibula**
    CC Exclusion see Appendix A PDX collection 0904
  - CC **M86.069 Acute hematogenous osteomyelitis, unspecified tibia and fibula**
    CC Exclusion see Appendix A PDX collection 0904

+ **M86.07 Acute hematogenous osteomyelitis, ankle and foot**
  - CC **M86.071 Acute hematogenous osteomyelitis, right ankle and foot**
    CC Exclusion see Appendix A PDX collection 0905
  - CC **M86.072 Acute hematogenous osteomyelitis, left ankle and foot**
    CC Exclusion see Appendix A PDX collection 0905
  - CC **M86.079 Acute hematogenous osteomyelitis, unspecified ankle and foot**
    CC Exclusion see Appendix A PDX collection 0905

CC **M86.08 Acute hematogenous osteomyelitis, other sites**
CC Exclusion see Appendix A PDX collection 0882

CC **M86.09 Acute hematogenous osteomyelitis, multiple sites**
CC Exclusion see Appendix A PDX collection 0898

+ **M86.1 Other acute osteomyelitis**
  - CC **M86.10 Other acute osteomyelitis, unspecified site**
    CC Exclusion see Appendix A PDX collection 0898

+ **M86.11 Other acute osteomyelitis, shoulder**
  - CC **M86.111 Other acute osteomyelitis, right shoulder**
    CC Exclusion see Appendix A PDX collection 0899
  - CC **M86.112 Other acute osteomyelitis, left shoulder**
    CC Exclusion see Appendix A PDX collection 0899
  - CC **M86.119 Other acute osteomyelitis, unspecified shoulder**
    CC Exclusion see Appendix A PDX collection 0899

+ **M86.12 Other acute osteomyelitis, humerus**
  - CC **M86.121 Other acute osteomyelitis, right humerus**
    CC Exclusion see Appendix A PDX collection 0900
  - CC **M86.122 Other acute osteomyelitis, left humerus**
    CC Exclusion see Appendix A PDX collection 0900
  - CC **M86.129 Other acute osteomyelitis, unspecified humerus**
    CC Exclusion see Appendix A PDX collection 0900

+ **M86.13 Other acute osteomyelitis, radius and ulna**
  - CC **M86.131 Other acute osteomyelitis, right radius and ulna**
    CC Exclusion see Appendix A PDX collection 0901
  - CC **M86.132 Other acute osteomyelitis, left radius and ulna**
    CC Exclusion see Appendix A PDX collection 0901
  - CC **M86.139 Other acute osteomyelitis, unspecified radius and ulna**
    CC Exclusion see Appendix A PDX collection 0901

+ **M86.14 Other acute osteomyelitis, hand**
  - CC **M86.141 Other acute osteomyelitis, righthand**
    CC Exclusion see Appendix A PDX collection 0902

CC **M86.142 Other acute osteomyelitis, left hand**
CC Exclusion see Appendix A PDX collection 0902

CC **M86.149 Other acute osteomyelitis, unspecified hand**
CC Exclusion see Appendix A PDX collection 0902

\+ **M86.15 Other acute osteomyelitis, femur**

CC **M86.151 Other acute osteomyelitis, right femur**
CC Exclusion see Appendix A PDX collection 0903

CC **M86.152 Other acute osteomyelitis, left femur**
CC Exclusion see Appendix A PDX collection 0903

CC **M86.159 Other acute osteomyelitis, unspecified femur**
CC Exclusion see Appendix A PDX collection 0903

\+ **M86.16 Other acute osteomyelitis, tibia and fibula**

CC **M86.161 Other acute osteomyelitis, right tibia and fibula**
CC Exclusion see Appendix A PDX collection 0904

CC **M86.162 Other acute osteomyelitis, left tibia and fibula**
CC Exclusion see Appendix A PDX collection 0904

CC **M86.169 Other acute osteomyelitis, unspecified tibia and fibula**
CC Exclusion see Appendix A PDX collection 0904

\+ **M86.17 Other acute osteomyelitis, ankle and foot**

CC **M86.171 Other acute osteomyelitis, right ankle and foot**
CC Exclusion see Appendix A PDX collection 0905

CC **M86.172 Other acute osteomyelitis, left ankle and foot**
CC Exclusion see Appendix A PDX collection 0905

CC **M86.179 Other acute osteomyelitis, unspecified ankle and foot**
CC Exclusion see Appendix A PDX collection 0905

CC **M86.18 Other acute osteomyelitis, other site**
CC Exclusion see Appendix A PDX collection 0882

CC **M86.19 Other acute osteomyelitis, multiple sites**
CC Exclusion see Appendix A PDX collection 0898

\+ **M86.2 Subacute osteomyelitis**

CC **M86.20 Subacute osteomyelitis, unspecified site**
CC Exclusion see Appendix A PDX collection 0898

\+ **M86.21 Subacute osteomyelitis, shoulder**

CC **M86.211 Subacute osteomyelitis, right shoulder**
CC Exclusion see Appendix A PDX collection 0899

CC **M86.212 Subacute osteomyelitis, left shoulder**
CC Exclusion see Appendix A PDX collection 0899

CC **M86.219 Subacute osteomyelitis, unspecified shoulder**
CC Exclusion see Appendix A PDX collection 0899

\+ **M86.22 Subacute osteomyelitis, humerus**

CC **M86.221 Subacute osteomyelitis, right humerus**
CC Exclusion see Appendix A PDX collection 0900

CC **M86.222 Subacute osteomyelitis, left humerus**
CC Exclusion see Appendix A PDX collection 0900

CC **M86.229 Subacute osteomyelitis, unspecified humerus**
CC Exclusion see Appendix A PDX collection 0900

\+ **M86.23 Subacute osteomyelitis, radius and ulna**

CC **M86.231 Subacute osteomyelitis, right radius and ulna**
CC Exclusion see Appendix A PDX collection 0901

CC **M86.232 Subacute osteomyelitis, left radius and ulna**
CC Exclusion see Appendix A PDX collection 0901

CC **M86.239 Subacute osteomyelitis, unspecified radius and ulna**
CC Exclusion see Appendix A PDX collection 0901

\+ **M86.24 Subacute osteomyelitis, hand**

CC **M86.241 Subacute osteomyelitis, right hand**
CC Exclusion see Appendix A PDX collection 0902

CC **M86.242 Subacute osteomyelitis, left hand**
CC Exclusion see Appendix A PDX collection 0902

CC **M86.249 Subacute osteomyelitis, unspecified hand**
CC Exclusion see Appendix A PDX collection 0902

\+ **M86.25 Subacute osteomyelitis, femur**

CC **M86.251 Subacute osteomyelitis, right femur**
CC Exclusion see Appendix A PDX collection 0903

CC **M86.252 Subacute osteomyelitis, left femur**
CC Exclusion see Appendix A PDX collection 0903

CC **M86.259 Subacute osteomyelitis, unspecified femur**
CC Exclusion see Appendix A PDX collection 0903

\+ **M86.26 Subacute osteomyelitis, tibia and fibula**

CC **M86.261 Subacute osteomyelitis, right tibia and fibula**
CC Exclusion see Appendix A PDX collection 0904

CC **M86.262 Subacute osteomyelitis, left tibia and fibula**
CC Exclusion see Appendix A PDX collection 0904

CC **M86.269 Subacute osteomyelitis, unspecified tibia and fibula**
CC Exclusion see Appendix A PDX collection 0904

\+ **M86.27 Subacute osteomyelitis, ankle and foot**

CC **M86.271 Subacute osteomyelitis, right ankle and foot**
CC Exclusion see Appendix A PDX collection 0905

CC **M86.272 Subacute osteomyelitis, left ankle and foot**
CC Exclusion see Appendix A PDX collection 0905

CC **M86.279 Subacute osteomyelitis, unspecified ankle and foot**
CC Exclusion see Appendix A PDX collection 0905

CC **M86.28 Subacute osteomyelitis, other site**
CC Exclusion see Appendix A PDX collection 0882

CC **M86.29 Subacute osteomyelitis, multiple sites**
CC Exclusion see Appendix A PDX collection 0898

\+ **M86.3 Chronic multifocal osteomyelitis**

CC **M86.30 Chronic multifocal osteomyelitis, unspecified site**
CC Exclusion see Appendix A PDX collection 0906

\+ **M86.31 Chronic multifocal osteomyelitis, shoulder**

CC **M86.311 Chronic multifocal osteomyelitis, right shoulder**
CC Exclusion see Appendix A PDX collection 0881

CC **M86.312 Chronic multifocal osteomyelitis, left shoulder**
CC Exclusion see Appendix A PDX collection 0881

CC **M86.319 Chronic multifocal osteomyelitis, unspecified shoulder**
CC Exclusion see Appendix A PDX collection 0881

\+ **M86.32 Chronic multifocal osteomyelitis, humerus**

CC **M86.321 Chronic multifocal osteomyelitis, right humerus**
CC Exclusion see Appendix A PDX collection 0881

CC **M86.322 Chronic multifocal osteomyelitis, left humerus**
CC Exclusion see Appendix A PDX collection 0881

CC **M86.329 Chronic multifocal osteomyelitis, unspecified humerus**
CC Exclusion see Appendix A PDX collection 0881

\+ **M86.33 Chronic multifocal osteomyelitis, radius and ulna**

CC **M86.331 Chronic multifocal osteomyelitis, right radius and ulna**
CC Exclusion see Appendix A PDX collection 0881

CC **M86.332 Chronic multifocal osteomyelitis, left radius and ulna**
CC Exclusion see Appendix A PDX collection 0881

CC **M86.339** Chronic multifocal osteomyelitis, unspecified radius and ulna
CC Exclusion see Appendix A PDX collection 0881

+ **M86.34** Chronic multifocal osteomyelitis, hand

CC **M86.341** Chronic multifocal osteomyelitis, right hand
CC Exclusion see Appendix A PDX collection 0881

CC **M86.342** Chronic multifocal osteomyelitis, left hand
CC Exclusion see Appendix A PDX collection 0881

CC **M86.349** Chronic multifocal osteomyelitis, unspecified hand
CC Exclusion see Appendix A PDX collection 0881

+ **M86.35** Chronic multifocal osteomyelitis, femur

CC **M86.351** Chronic multifocal osteomyelitis, right femur
CC Exclusion see Appendix A PDX collection 0881

CC **M86.352** Chronic multifocal osteomyelitis, left femur
CC Exclusion see Appendix A PDX collection 0881

CC **M86.359** Chronic multifocal osteomyelitis, unspecified femur
CC Exclusion see Appendix A PDX collection 0881

+ **M86.36** Chronic multifocal osteomyelitis, tibia and fibula

CC **M86.361** Chronic multifocal osteomyelitis, right tibia and fibula
CC Exclusion see Appendix A PDX collection 0881

CC **M86.362** Chronic multifocal osteomyelitis, left tibia and fibula
CC Exclusion see Appendix A PDX collection 0881

CC **M86.369** Chronic multifocal osteomyelitis, unspecified tibia and fibula
CC Exclusion see Appendix A PDX collection 0881

+ **M86.37** Chronic multifocal osteomyelitis, ankle and foot

CC **M86.371** Chronic multifocal osteomyelitis, right ankle and foot
CC Exclusion see Appendix A PDX collection 0881

CC **M86.372** Chronic multifocal osteomyelitis, left ankle and foot
CC Exclusion see Appendix A PDX collection 0881

CC **M86.379** Chronic multifocal osteomyelitis, unspecified ankle and foot
CC Exclusion see Appendix A PDX collection 0881

CC **M86.38** Chronic multifocal osteomyelitis, other site
CC Exclusion see Appendix A PDX collection 0881

CC **M86.39** Chronic multifocal osteomyelitis, multiple sites
CC Exclusion see Appendix A PDX collection 0881

+ **M86.4** Chronic osteomyelitis with draining sinus

CC **M86.40** Chronic osteomyelitis with draining sinus, unspecified site
CC Exclusion see Appendix A PDX collection 0906

+ **M86.41** Chronic osteomyelitis with draining sinus, shoulder

CC **M86.411** Chronic osteomyelitis with draining sinus, right shoulder
CC Exclusion see Appendix A PDX collection 0881

CC **M86.412** Chronic osteomyelitis with draining sinus, left shoulder
CC Exclusion see Appendix A PDX collection 0881

CC **M86.419** Chronic osteomyelitis with draining sinus, unspecified shoulder
CC Exclusion see Appendix A PDX collection 0881

+ **M86.42** Chronic osteomyelitis with draining sinus, humerus

CC **M86.421** Chronic osteomyelitis with draining sinus, right humerus
CC Exclusion see Appendix A PDX collection 0881

CC **M86.422** Chronic osteomyelitis with draining sinus, left humerus
CC Exclusion see Appendix A PDX collection 0881

CC **M86.429** Chronic osteomyelitis with draining sinus, unspecified humerus
CC Exclusion see Appendix A PDX collection 0881

+ **M86.43** Chronic osteomyelitis with draining sinus, radius and ulna

CC **M86.431** Chronic osteomyelitis with draining sinus, right radius and ulna
CC Exclusion see Appendix A PDX collection 0881

CC **M86.432** Chronic osteomyelitis with draining sinus, left radius and ulna
CC Exclusion see Appendix A PDX collection 0881

CC **M86.439** Chronic osteomyelitis with draining sinus, unspecified radius and ulna
CC Exclusion see Appendix A PDX collection 0881

+ **M86.44** Chronic osteomyelitis with draining sinus, hand

CC **M86.441** Chronic osteomyelitis with draining sinus, right hand
CC Exclusion see Appendix A PDX collection 0881

CC **M86.442** Chronic osteomyelitis with draining sinus, left hand
CC Exclusion see Appendix A PDX collection 0881

CC **M86.449** Chronic osteomyelitis with draining sinus, unspecified hand
CC Exclusion see Appendix A PDX collection 0881

+ **M86.45** Chronic osteomyelitis with draining sinus, femur

CC **M86.451** Chronic osteomyelitis with draining sinus, right femur
CC Exclusion see Appendix A PDX collection 0881

CC **M86.452** Chronic osteomyelitis with draining sinus, left femur
CC Exclusion see Appendix A PDX collection 0881

CC **M86.459** Chronic osteomyelitis with draining sinus, unspecified femur
CC Exclusion see Appendix A PDX collection 0881

+ **M86.46** Chronic osteomyelitis with draining sinus, tibia and fibula

CC **M86.461** Chronic osteomyelitis with draining sinus, right tibia and fibula
CC Exclusion see Appendix A PDX collection 0881

CC **M86.462** Chronic osteomyelitis with draining sinus, left tibia and fibula
CC Exclusion see Appendix A PDX collection 0881

CC **M86.469** Chronic osteomyelitis with draining sinus, unspecified tibia and fibula
CC Exclusion see Appendix A PDX collection 0881

+ **M86.47** Chronic osteomyelitis with draining sinus, ankle and foot

CC **M86.471** Chronic osteomyelitis with draining sinus, right ankle and foot
CC Exclusion see Appendix A PDX collection 0881

CC **M86.472** Chronic osteomyelitis with draining sinus, left ankle and foot
CC Exclusion see Appendix A PDX collection 0881

CC **M86.479** Chronic osteomyelitis with draining sinus, unspecified ankle and foot
CC Exclusion see Appendix A PDX collection 0881

CC **M86.48** Chronic osteomyelitis with draining sinus, other site
CC Exclusion see Appendix A PDX collection 0881

CC **M86.49** Chronic osteomyelitis with draining sinus, multiple sites
CC Exclusion see Appendix A PDX collection 0881

+ M86.5 Other chronic hematogenous osteomyelitis
CC M86.50 Other chronic hematogenous osteomyelitis, unspecified site
CC Exclusion see Appendix A PDX collection 0906
+ M86.51 Other chronic hematogenous osteomyelitis, shoulder
CC M86.511 Other chronic hematogenous osteomyelitis, right shoulder
CC Exclusion see Appendix A PDX collection 0881
CC M86.512 Other chronic hematogenous osteomyelitis, left shoulder
CC Exclusion see Appendix A PDX collection 0881
CC M86.519 Other chronic hematogenous osteomyelitis, unspecified shoulder
CC Exclusion see Appendix A PDX collection 0881
+ M86.52 Other chronic hematogenous osteomyelitis, humerus
CC M86.521 Other chronic hematogenous osteomyelitis, right humerus
CC Exclusion see Appendix A PDX collection 0881
CC M86.522 Other chronic hematogenous osteomyelitis, left humerus
CC Exclusion see Appendix A PDX collection 0881
CC M86.529 Other chronic hematogenous osteomyelitis, unspecified humerus
CC Exclusion see Appendix A PDX collection 0881
+ M86.53 Other chronic hematogenous osteomyelitis, radius and ulna
CC M86.531 Other chronic hematogenous osteomyelitis, right radius and ulna
CC Exclusion see Appendix A PDX collection 0881
CC M86.532 Other chronic hematogenous osteomyelitis, left radius and ulna
CC Exclusion see Appendix A PDX collection 0881
CC M86.539 Other chronic hematogenous osteomyelitis, unspecified radius and ulna
CC Exclusion see Appendix A PDX collection 0881
+ M86.54 Other chronic hematogenous osteomyelitis, hand
CC M86.541 Other chronic hematogenous osteomyelitis, right hand
CC Exclusion see Appendix A PDX collection 0881
CC M86.542 Other chronic hematogenous osteomyelitis, left hand
CC Exclusion see Appendix A PDX collection 0881
CC M86.549 Other chronic hematogenous osteomyelitis, unspecified hand
CC Exclusion see Appendix A PDX collection 0881
+ M86.55 Other chronic hematogenous osteomyelitis, femur
CC M86.551 Other chronic hematogenous osteomyelitis, right femur
CC Exclusion see Appendix A PDX collection 0881
CC M86.552 Other chronic hematogenous osteomyelitis, left femur
CC Exclusion see Appendix A PDX collection 0881
CC M86.559 Other chronic hematogenous osteomyelitis, unspecified femur
CC Exclusion see Appendix A PDX collection 0881
+ M86.56 Other chronic hematogenous osteomyelitis, tibia and fibula
CC M86.561 Other chronic hematogenous osteomyelitis, right tibia and fibula
CC Exclusion see Appendix A PDX collection 0881
CC M86.562 Other chronic hematogenous osteomyelitis, left tibia and fibula
CC Exclusion see Appendix A PDX collection 0881
CC M86.569 Other chronic hematogenous osteomyelitis, unspecified tibia and fibula
CC Exclusion see Appendix A PDX collection 0881
+ M86.57 Other chronic hematogenous osteomyelitis, ankle and foot
CC M86.571 Other chronic hematogenous osteomyelit right ankle and foot
CC Exclusion see Appendix A PDX collection 0881
CC M86.572 Other chronic hematogenous osteomyelit left ankle and foot
CC Exclusion see Appendix A PDX collection 0881
CC M86.579 Other chronic hematogenous osteomyelit unspecified ankle and foot
CC Exclusion see Appendix A PDX collection 0881
CC M86.58 Other chronic hematogenous osteomyelitis, other s
CC Exclusion see Appendix A PDX collection 0881
CC M86.59 Other chronic hematogenous osteomyelitis, multip sites
CC Exclusion see Appendix A PDX collection 0881
+ M86.6 Other chronic osteomyelitis
CC M86.60 Other chronic osteomyelitis, unspecified site
CC Exclusion see Appendix A PDX collection 0906
+ M86.61 Other chronic osteomyelitis, shoulder
CC M86.611 Other chronic osteomyelitis, right should
CC Exclusion see Appendix A PDX collection 0881
CC M86.612 Other chronic osteomyelitis, left shoulder
CC Exclusion see Appendix A PDX collection 0881
CC M86.619 Other chronic osteomyelitis, unspecified shoulder
CC Exclusion see Appendix A PDX collection 0881
+ M86.62 Other chronic osteomyelitis, humerus
CC M86.621 Other chronic osteomyelitis, right humer
CC Exclusion see Appendix A PDX collection 0881
CC M86.622 Other chronic osteomyelitis, left humerus
CC Exclusion see Appendix A PDX collection 0881
CC M86.629 Other chronic osteomyelitis, unspecified humerus
CC Exclusion see Appendix A PDX collection 0881
+ M86.63 Other chronic osteomyelitis, radius and ulna
CC M86.631 Other chronic osteomyelitis, right radius and ulna
CC Exclusion see Appendix A PDX collection 0881
CC M86.632 Other chronic osteomyelitis, left radius and ulna
CC Exclusion see Appendix A PDX collection 0881
CC M86.639 Other chronic osteomyelitis, unspecified radius and ulna
CC Exclusion see Appendix A PDX collection 0881
+ M86.64 Other chronic osteomyelitis, hand
CC M86.641 Other chronic osteomyelitis, right hand
CC Exclusion see Appendix A PDX collection 0881
CC M86.642 Other chronic osteomyelitis, left hand
CC Exclusion see Appendix A PDX collection 0881
CC M86.649 Other chronic osteomyelitis, unspecified hand
CC Exclusion see Appendix A PDX collection 0881
+ M86.65 Other chronic osteomyelitis, thigh
CC M86.651 Other chronic osteomyelitis, right thigh
CC Exclusion see Appendix A PDX collection 0881
CC M86.652 Other chronic osteomyelitis, left thigh
CC Exclusion see Appendix A PDX collection 0881
CC M86.659 Other chronic osteomyelitis, unspecified thigh
CC Exclusion see Appendix A PDX collection 0881
+ M86.66 Other chronic osteomyelitis, tibia and fibula
CC M86.661 Other chronic osteomyelitis, right tibia and fibula
CC Exclusion see Appendix A PDX collection 0881

CC M86.662 Other chronic osteomyelitis, left tibia and fibula
CC Exclusion see Appendix A PDX collection 0881

CC M86.669 Other chronic osteomyelitis, unspecified tibia and fibula
CC Exclusion see Appendix A PDX collection 0881

+ M86.67 Other chronic osteomyelitis, ankle and foot

CC M86.671 Other chronic osteomyelitis, right ankle and foot
CC Exclusion see Appendix A PDX collection 0881
AHA CC: 1Q, 2016, 13

CC M86.672 Other chronic osteomyelitis, left ankle and foot
CC Exclusion see Appendix A PDX collection 0881

CC M86.679 Other chronic osteomyelitis, unspecified ankle and foot
CC Exclusion see Appendix A PDX collection 0881

CC M86.68 Other chronic osteomyelitis, other site
CC Exclusion see Appendix A PDX collection 0881

CC M86.69 Other chronic osteomyelitis, multiple sites
CC Exclusion see Appendix A PDX collection 0881

+ M86.8 Other osteomyelitis
Brodie's abscess

+ M86.8X Other osteomyelitis

CC M86.8X0 Other osteomyelitis, multiple sites
CC Exclusion see Appendix A PDX collection 0881

CC M86.8X1 Other osteomyelitis, shoulder
CC Exclusion see Appendix A PDX collection 0881

CC M86.8X2 Other osteomyelitis, upper arm
CC Exclusion see Appendix A PDX collection 0881

CC M86.8X3 Other osteomyelitis, forearm
CC Exclusion see Appendix A PDX collection 0881

CC M86.8X4 Other osteomyelitis, hand
CC Exclusion see Appendix A PDX collection 0881

CC M86.8X5 Other osteomyelitis, thigh
CC Exclusion see Appendix A PDX collection 0881

CC M86.8X6 Other osteomyelitis, lower leg
CC Exclusion see Appendix A PDX collection 0881

CC M86.8X7 Other osteomyelitis, ankle and foot
CC Exclusion see Appendix A PDX collection 0881

CC M86.8X8 Other osteomyelitis, other site
CC Exclusion see Appendix A PDX collection 0881

CC M86.8X9 Other osteomyelitis, unspecified sites
CC Exclusion see Appendix A PDX collection 0906

CC M86.9 Osteomyelitis, unspecified
Infection of bone NOS
Periostitis without osteomyelitis
CC Exclusion see Appendix A PDX collection 0906

M87 Osteonecrosis

Includes: avascular necrosis of bone
Use additional code to identify major osseous defect, if applicable (M89.7-)
Excludes1: *juvenile osteonecrosis (M91-M92)*
osteochondropathies (M90-M93)

+ M87.0 Idiopathic aseptic necrosis of bone

CC M87.00 Idiopathic aseptic necrosis of unspecifiedbone
CC Exclusion see Appendix A PDX collection 0907

+ M87.01 Idiopathic aseptic necrosis of shoulder
Idiopathic aseptic necrosis of clavicle and scapula

CC M87.011 Idiopathic aseptic necrosis of right shoulder
CC Exclusion see Appendix A PDX collection 0908

CC M87.012 Idiopathic aseptic necrosis of left shoulder
CC Exclusion see Appendix A PDX collection 0908

CC M87.019 Idiopathic aseptic necrosis of unspecified shoulder
CC Exclusion see Appendix A PDX collection 0908

+ M87.02 Idiopathic aseptic necrosis of humerus

CC M87.021 Idiopathic aseptic necrosis of right humerus
CC Exclusion see Appendix A PDX collection 0908

CC M87.022 Idiopathic aseptic necrosis of left humerus
CC Exclusion see Appendix A PDX collection 0908

CC M87.029 Idiopathic aseptic necrosis of unspecified humerus
CC Exclusion see Appendix A PDX collection 0908

+ M87.03 Idiopathic aseptic necrosis of radius, ulna and carpus

CC M87.031 Idiopathic aseptic necrosis of right radius
CC Exclusion see Appendix A PDX collection 0907

CC M87.032 Idiopathic aseptic necrosis of left radius
CC Exclusion see Appendix A PDX collection 0907

CC M87.033 Idiopathic aseptic necrosis of unspecified radius
CC Exclusion see Appendix A PDX collection 0907

CC M87.034 Idiopathic aseptic necrosis of right ulna
CC Exclusion see Appendix A PDX collection 0907

CC M87.035 Idiopathic aseptic necrosis of left ulna
CC Exclusion see Appendix A PDX collection 0907

CC M87.036 Idiopathic aseptic necrosis of unspecified ulna
CC Exclusion see Appendix A PDX collection 0907

CC M87.037 Idiopathic aseptic necrosis of right carpus
CC Exclusion see Appendix A PDX collection 0907

CC M87.038 Idiopathic aseptic necrosis of left carpus
CC Exclusion see Appendix A PDX collection 0907

CC M87.039 Idiopathic aseptic necrosis of unspecified carpus
CC Exclusion see Appendix A PDX collection 0907

+ M87.04 Idiopathic aseptic necrosis of hand and fingers
Idiopathic aseptic necrosis of metacarpals and phalanges of hands

CC M87.041 Idiopathic aseptic necrosis of right hand
CC Exclusion see Appendix A PDX collection 0907

CC M87.042 Idiopathic aseptic necrosis of left hand
CC Exclusion see Appendix A PDX collection 0907

CC M87.043 Idiopathic aseptic necrosis of unspecified hand
CC Exclusion see Appendix A PDX collection 0907

CC M87.044 Idiopathic aseptic necrosis of right finger(s)
CC Exclusion see Appendix A PDX collection 0907

CC M87.045 Idiopathic aseptic necrosis of left finger(s)
CC Exclusion see Appendix A PDX collection 0907

CC M87.046 Idiopathic aseptic necrosis of unspecified finger(s)
CC Exclusion see Appendix A PDX collection 0907

+ M87.05 Idiopathic aseptic necrosis of pelvis and femur

CC M87.050 Idiopathic aseptic necrosis of pelvis
CC Exclusion see Appendix A PDX collection 0907

CC M87.051 Idiopathic aseptic necrosis of right femur
CC Exclusion see Appendix A PDX collection 0909

CC M87.052 Idiopathic aseptic necrosis of left femur
CC Exclusion see Appendix A PDX collection 0909

CC M87.059 Idiopathic aseptic necrosis of unspecified femur
Idiopathic aseptic necrosis of hip NOS
CC Exclusion see Appendix A PDX collection 0909

+ M87.06 **Idiopathic aseptic necrosis of tibia and fibula**
  - CC **M87.061** **Idiopathic aseptic necrosis of right tibia**
    CC Exclusion see Appendix A PDX collection 0907
  - CC **M87.062** **Idiopathic aseptic necrosis of left tibia**
    CC Exclusion see Appendix A PDX collection 0907
  - CC **M87.063** **Idiopathic aseptic necrosis of unspecified tibia**
    CC Exclusion see Appendix A PDX collection 0907
  - CC **M87.064** **Idiopathic aseptic necrosis of right fibula**
    CC Exclusion see Appendix A PDX collection 0907
  - CC **M87.065** **Idiopathic aseptic necrosis of left fibula**
    CC Exclusion see Appendix A PDX collection 0907
  - CC **M87.066** **Idiopathic aseptic necrosis of unspecified fibula**
    CC Exclusion see Appendix A PDX collection 0907

+ M87.07 **Idiopathic aseptic necrosis of ankle, foot and toes**
  Idiopathic aseptic necrosis of metatarsus, tarsus, and phalanges of toes
  - CC **M87.071** **Idiopathic aseptic necrosis of right ankle**
    CC Exclusion see Appendix A PDX collection 0907
  - CC **M87.072** **Idiopathic aseptic necrosis of left ankle**
    CC Exclusion see Appendix A PDX collection 0907
  - CC **M87.073** **Idiopathic aseptic necrosis of unspecified ankle**
    CC Exclusion see Appendix A PDX collection 0907
  - CC **M87.074** **Idiopathic aseptic necrosis of right foot**
    CC Exclusion see Appendix A PDX collection 0910
  - CC **M87.075** **Idiopathic aseptic necrosis of left foot**
    CC Exclusion see Appendix A PDX collection 0910
  - CC **M87.076** **Idiopathic aseptic necrosis of unspecified foot**
    CC Exclusion see Appendix A PDX collection 0910
  - CC **M87.077** **Idiopathic aseptic necrosis of right toe(s)**
    CC Exclusion see Appendix A PDX collection 0907
  - CC **M87.078** **Idiopathic aseptic necrosis of left toe(s)**
    CC Exclusion see Appendix A PDX collection 0907
  - CC **M87.079** **Idiopathic aseptic necrosis of unspecified toe(s)**
    CC Exclusion see Appendix A PDX collection 0907

CC **M87.08** **Idiopathic aseptic necrosis of bone, other site**
CC Exclusion see Appendix A PDX collection 0907

CC **M87.09** **Idiopathic aseptic necrosis of bone, multiple sites**
CC Exclusion see Appendix A PDX collection 0907

+ M87.1 **Osteonecrosis due to drugs**
Use additional code for adverse effect, if applicable, to identify drug (T36-T50 with fifth or sixth character 5)

CC **M87.10** **Osteonecrosis due to drugs, unspecified bone**
CC Exclusion see Appendix A PDX collection 0907

+ M87.11 **Osteonecrosis due to drugs, shoulder**
  - CC **M87.111** **Osteonecrosis due to drugs, right shoulder**
    CC Exclusion see Appendix A PDX collection 0907
  - CC **M87.112** **Osteonecrosis due to drugs, left shoulder**
    CC Exclusion see Appendix A PDX collection 0907
  - CC **M87.119** **Osteonecrosis due to drugs, unspecified shoulder**
    CC Exclusion see Appendix A PDX collection 0907

+ M87.12 **Osteonecrosis due to drugs, humerus**
  - CC **M87.121** **Osteonecrosis due to drugs, right humerus**
    CC Exclusion see Appendix A PDX collection 0908
  - CC **M87.122** **Osteonecrosis due to drugs, left humerus**
    CC Exclusion see Appendix A PDX collection 0908
  - CC **M87.129** **Osteonecrosis due to drugs, unspecified humerus**
    CC Exclusion see Appendix A PDX collection 0908

+ M87.13 **Osteonecrosis due to drugs of radius, ulna and carpus**
  - CC **M87.131** **Osteonecrosis due to drugs of right radius**
    CC Exclusion see Appendix A PDX collection 0907
  - CC **M87.132** **Osteonecrosis due to drugs of left radius**
    CC Exclusion see Appendix A PDX collection 0907
  - CC **M87.133** **Osteonecrosis due to drugs of unspecified radius**
    CC Exclusion see Appendix A PDX collection 0907
  - CC **M87.134** **Osteonecrosis due to drugs of right ulna**
    CC Exclusion see Appendix A PDX collection 0907
  - CC **M87.135** **Osteonecrosis due to drugs of left ulna**
    CC Exclusion see Appendix A PDX collection 0907
  - CC **M87.136** **Osteonecrosis due to drugs of unspecified ulna**
    CC Exclusion see Appendix A PDX collection 0907
  - CC **M87.137** **Osteonecrosis due to drugs of right carpus**
    CC Exclusion see Appendix A PDX collection 0907
  - CC **M87.138** **Osteonecrosis due to drugs of left carpus**
    CC Exclusion see Appendix A PDX collection 0907
  - CC **M87.139** **Osteonecrosis due to drugs of unspecified carpus**
    CC Exclusion see Appendix A PDX collection 0907

+ M87.14 **Osteonecrosis due to drugs, hand and fingers**
  - CC **M87.141** **Osteonecrosis due to drugs, right hand**
    CC Exclusion see Appendix A PDX collection 0907
  - CC **M87.142** **Osteonecrosis due to drugs, left hand**
    CC Exclusion see Appendix A PDX collection 0907
  - CC **M87.143** **Osteonecrosis due to drugs, unspecified hand**
    CC Exclusion see Appendix A PDX collection 0907
  - CC **M87.144** **Osteonecrosis due to drugs, right finger(s)**
    CC Exclusion see Appendix A PDX collection 0907
  - CC **M87.145** **Osteonecrosis due to drugs, left finger(s)**
    CC Exclusion see Appendix A PDX collection 0907
  - CC **M87.146** **Osteonecrosis due to drugs, unspecified finger(s)**
    CC Exclusion see Appendix A PDX collection 0907

+ M87.15 **Osteonecrosis due to drugs, pelvis and femur**
  - CC **M87.150** **Osteonecrosis due to drugs, pelvis**
    CC Exclusion see Appendix A PDX collection 0909
  - CC **M87.151** **Osteonecrosis due to drugs, right femur**
    CC Exclusion see Appendix A PDX collection 0909
  - CC **M87.152** **Osteonecrosis due to drugs, left femur**
    CC Exclusion see Appendix A PDX collection 0909
  - CC **M87.159** **Osteonecrosis due to drugs, unspecified femur**
    CC Exclusion see Appendix A PDX collection 0909

+ M87.16 **Osteonecrosis due to drugs, tibia and fibula**
  - CC **M87.161** **Osteonecrosis due to drugs, right tibia**
    CC Exclusion see Appendix A PDX collection 0907
  - CC **M87.162** **Osteonecrosis due to drugs, left tibia**
    CC Exclusion see Appendix A PDX collection 0907
  - CC **M87.163** **Osteonecrosis due to drugs, unspecified tibia**
    CC Exclusion see Appendix A PDX collection 0907
  - CC **M87.164** **Osteonecrosis due to drugs, right fibula**
    CC Exclusion see Appendix A PDX collection 0907

CC M87.165 Osteonecrosis due to drugs, left fibula
CC Exclusion see Appendix A PDX collection 0907

CC M87.166 Osteonecrosis due to drugs, unspecified fibula
CC Exclusion see Appendix A PDX collection 0907

+ M87.17 Osteonecrosis due to drugs, ankle, foot and toes

CC M87.171 Osteonecrosis due to drugs, right ankle
CC Exclusion see Appendix A PDX collection 0907

CC M87.172 Osteonecrosis due to drugs, left ankle
CC Exclusion see Appendix A PDX collection 0907

CC M87.173 Osteonecrosis due to drugs, unspecified ankle
CC Exclusion see Appendix A PDX collection 0907

CC M87.174 Osteonecrosis due to drugs, right foot
CC Exclusion see Appendix A PDX collection 0910

CC M87.175 Osteonecrosis due to drugs, left foot
CC Exclusion see Appendix A PDX collection 0910

CC M87.176 Osteonecrosis due to drugs, unspecified foot
CC Exclusion see Appendix A PDX collection 0910

CC M87.177 Osteonecrosis due to drugs, right toe(s)
CC Exclusion see Appendix A PDX collection 0907

CC M87.178 Osteonecrosis due to drugs, left toe(s)
CC Exclusion see Appendix A PDX collection 0907

CC M87.179 Osteonecrosis due to drugs, unspecified toe(s)
CC Exclusion see Appendix A PDX collection 0907

+ M87.18 Osteonecrosis due to drugs, other site

CC M87.180 Osteonecrosis due to drugs, jaw
CC Exclusion see Appendix A PDX collection 0907

CC M87.188 Osteonecrosis due to drugs, other site
CC Exclusion see Appendix A PDX collection 0907

CC M87.19 Osteonecrosis due to drugs, multiple sites
CC Exclusion see Appendix A PDX collection 0907

+ M87.2 Osteonecrosis due to previous trauma

CC M87.20 Osteonecrosis due to previous trauma, unspecified bone
CC Exclusion see Appendix A PDX collection 0907

+ M87.21 Osteonecrosis due to previous trauma, shoulder

CC M87.211 Osteonecrosis due to previous trauma, right shoulder
CC Exclusion see Appendix A PDX collection 0907

CC M87.212 Osteonecrosis due to previous trauma, left shoulder
CC Exclusion see Appendix A PDX collection 0907

CC M87.219 Osteonecrosis due to previous trauma, unspecified shoulder
CC Exclusion see Appendix A PDX collection 0907

+ M87.22 Osteonecrosis due to previous trauma, humerus

CC M87.221 Osteonecrosis due to previous trauma, right humerus
CC Exclusion see Appendix A PDX collection 0908

CC M87.222 Osteonecrosis due to previous trauma, left humerus
CC Exclusion see Appendix A PDX collection 0908

CC M87.229 Osteonecrosis due to previous trauma, unspecified humerus
CC Exclusion see Appendix A PDX collection 0908

+ M87.23 Osteonecrosis due to previous trauma of radius, ulna and carpus

CC M87.231 Osteonecrosis due to previous trauma of right radius
CC Exclusion see Appendix A PDX collection 0907

CC M87.232 Osteonecrosis due to previous trauma of left radius
CC Exclusion see Appendix A PDX collection 0907

CC M87.233 Osteonecrosis due to previous trauma of unspecified radius
CC Exclusion see Appendix A PDX collection 0907

CC M87.234 Osteonecrosis due to previous trauma of right ulna
CC Exclusion see Appendix A PDX collection 0907

CC M87.235 Osteonecrosis due to previous trauma of left ulna
CC Exclusion see Appendix A PDX collection 0907

CC M87.236 Osteonecrosis due to previous trauma of unspecified ulna
CC Exclusion see Appendix A PDX collection 0907

CC M87.237 Osteonecrosis due to previous trauma of right carpus
CC Exclusion see Appendix A PDX collection 0907

CC M87.238 Osteonecrosis due to previous trauma of left carpus
CC Exclusion see Appendix A PDX collection 0907

CC M87.239 Osteonecrosis due to previous trauma of unspecified carpus
CC Exclusion see Appendix A PDX collection 0907

+ M87.24 Osteonecrosis due to previous trauma, hand and fingers

CC M87.241 Osteonecrosis due to previous trauma, right hand
CC Exclusion see Appendix A PDX collection 0907

CC M87.242 Osteonecrosis due to previous trauma, left hand
CC Exclusion see Appendix A PDX collection 0907

CC M87.243 Osteonecrosis due to previous trauma, unspecified hand
CC Exclusion see Appendix A PDX collection 0907

CC M87.244 Osteonecrosis due to previous trauma, right finger(s)
CC Exclusion see Appendix A PDX collection 0907

CC M87.245 Osteonecrosis due to previous trauma, left finger(s)
CC Exclusion see Appendix A PDX collection 0907

CC M87.246 Osteonecrosis due to previous trauma, unspecified finger(s)
CC Exclusion see Appendix A PDX collection 0907

+ M87.25 Osteonecrosis due to previous trauma, pelvis and femur

CC M87.250 Osteonecrosis due to previous trauma, pelvis
CC Exclusion see Appendix A PDX collection 0907

CC M87.251 Osteonecrosis due to previous trauma, right femur
CC Exclusion see Appendix A PDX collection 0909

CC M87.252 Osteonecrosis due to previous trauma, left femur
CC Exclusion see Appendix A PDX collection 0909

CC M87.256 Osteonecrosis due to previous trauma, unspecified femur
CC Exclusion see Appendix A PDX collection 0909

+ M87.26 Osteonecrosis due to previous trauma, tibia and fibula

CC M87.261 Osteonecrosis due to previous trauma, right tibia
CC Exclusion see Appendix A PDX collection 0907

CC M87.262 Osteonecrosis due to previous trauma, left tibia
CC Exclusion see Appendix A PDX collection 0907

CC **M87.263** **Osteonecrosis due to previous trauma, unspecified tibia**
CC Exclusion see Appendix A PDX collection 0907

CC **M87.264** **Osteonecrosis due to previous trauma, right fibula**
CC Exclusion see Appendix A PDX collection 0907

CC **M87.265** **Osteonecrosis due to previous trauma, left fibula**
CC Exclusion see Appendix A PDX collection 0907

CC **M87.266** **Osteonecrosis due to previous trauma, unspecified fibula**
CC Exclusion see Appendix A PDX collection 0907

\+ **M87.27** **Osteonecrosis due to previous trauma, ankle, foot and toes**

CC **M87.271** **Osteonecrosis due to previous trauma, right ankle**
CC Exclusion see Appendix A PDX collection 0907

CC **M87.272** **Osteonecrosis due to previous trauma, left ankle**
CC Exclusion see Appendix A PDX collection 0907

CC **M87.273** **Osteonecrosis due to previous trauma, unspecified ankle**
CC Exclusion see Appendix A PDX collection 0907

CC **M87.274** **Osteonecrosis due to previous trauma, right foot**
CC Exclusion see Appendix A PDX collection 0910

CC **M87.275** **Osteonecrosis due to previous trauma, left foot**
CC Exclusion see Appendix A PDX collection 0910

CC **M87.276** **Osteonecrosis due to previous trauma, unspecified foot**
CC Exclusion see Appendix A PDX collection 0910

CC **M87.277** **Osteonecrosis due to previous trauma, right toe(s)**
CC Exclusion see Appendix A PDX collection 0907

CC **M87.278** **Osteonecrosis due to previous trauma, left toe(s)**
CC Exclusion see Appendix A PDX collection 0907

CC **M87.279** **Osteonecrosis due to previous trauma, unspecified toe(s)**
CC Exclusion see Appendix A PDX collection 0907

CC **M87.28** **Osteonecrosis due to previous trauma, other site**
CC Exclusion see Appendix A PDX collection 0907

CC **M87.29** **Osteonecrosis due to previous trauma, multiple sites**
CC Exclusion see Appendix A PDX collection 0907

\+ **M87.3** **Other secondary osteonecrosis**

CC **M87.30** **Other secondary osteonecrosis, unspecified bone**
CC Exclusion see Appendix A PDX collection 0907

\+ **M87.31** **Other secondary osteonecrosis, shoulder**

CC **M87.311** **Other secondary osteonecrosis, right shoulder**
CC Exclusion see Appendix A PDX collection 0907

CC **M87.312** **Other secondary osteonecrosis, left shoulder**
CC Exclusion see Appendix A PDX collection 0907

CC **M87.319** **Other secondary osteonecrosis, unspecified shoulder**
CC Exclusion see Appendix A PDX collection 0907

\+ **M87.32** **Other secondary osteonecrosis, humerus**

CC **M87.321** **Other secondary osteonecrosis, right humerus**
CC Exclusion see Appendix A PDX collection 0908

CC **M87.322** **Other secondary osteonecrosis, left humerus**
CC Exclusion see Appendix A PDX collection 0908

CC **M87.329** **Other secondary osteonecrosis, unspecifi humerus**
CC Exclusion see Appendix A PDX collection 0908

\+ **M87.33** **Other secondary osteonecrosis of radius, ulna and carpus**

CC **M87.331** **Other secondary osteonecrosis of right radius**
CC Exclusion see Appendix A PDX collection 0907

CC **M87.332** **Other secondary osteonecrosis of left radius**
CC Exclusion see Appendix A PDX collection 0907

CC **M87.333** **Other secondary osteonecrosis of unspecified radius**
CC Exclusion see Appendix A PDX collection 0907

CC **M87.334** **Other secondary osteonecrosis of right ulna**
CC Exclusion see Appendix A PDX collection 0907

CC **M87.335** **Other secondary osteonecrosis of left uln**
CC Exclusion see Appendix A PDX collection 0907

CC **M87.336** **Other secondary osteonecrosis of unspecified ulna**
CC Exclusion see Appendix A PDX collection 0907

CC **M87.337** **Other secondary osteonecrosis of right carpus**
CC Exclusion see Appendix A PDX collection 0907

CC **M87.338** **Other secondary osteonecrosis of left carpus**
CC Exclusion see Appendix A PDX collection 0907

CC **M87.339** **Other secondary osteonecrosis of unspecified carpus**
CC Exclusion see Appendix A PDX collection 0907

\+ **M87.34** **Other secondary osteonecrosis, hand and fingers**

CC **M87.341** **Other secondary osteonecrosis, right han**
CC Exclusion see Appendix A PDX collection 0907

CC **M87.342** **Other secondary osteonecrosis, left hand**
CC Exclusion see Appendix A PDX collection 0907

CC **M87.343** **Other secondary osteonecrosis, unspecified hand**
CC Exclusion see Appendix A PDX collection 0907

CC **M87.344** **Other secondary osteonecrosis, right finger(s)**
CC Exclusion see Appendix A PDX collection 0907

CC **M87.345** **Other secondary osteonecrosis, left finger(s)**
CC Exclusion see Appendix A PDX collection 0907

CC **M87.346** **Other secondary osteonecrosis, unspecified finger(s)**
CC Exclusion see Appendix A PDX collection 0907

\+ **M87.35** **Other secondary osteonecrosis, pelvis and femur**

CC **M87.350** **Other secondary osteonecrosis, pelvis**
CC Exclusion see Appendix A PDX collection 0909

CC **M87.351** **Other secondary osteonecrosis, right fem**
CC Exclusion see Appendix A PDX collection 0909

CC **M87.352** **Other secondary osteonecrosis, left femu**
CC Exclusion see Appendix A PDX collection 0909

CC **M87.353** **Other secondary osteonecrosis, unspecified femur**
CC Exclusion see Appendix A PDX collection 0909

\+ **M87.36** **Other secondary osteonecrosis, tibia and fibula**

CC **M87.361** **Other secondary osteonecrosis, right tibi**
CC Exclusion see Appendix A PDX collection 0907

CC **M87.362** **Other secondary osteonecrosis, left tibia**
CC Exclusion see Appendix A PDX collection 0907

CC M87.363 Other secondary osteonecrosis, unspecified tibia
CC Exclusion see Appendix A PDX collection 0907

CC M87.364 Other secondary osteonecrosis, right fibula
CC Exclusion see Appendix A PDX collection 0907

CC M87.365 Other secondary osteonecrosis, left fibula
CC Exclusion see Appendix A PDX collection 0907

CC M87.366 Other secondary osteonecrosis, unspecified fibula
CC Exclusion see Appendix A PDX collection 0907

+ M87.37 Other secondary osteonecrosis, ankle and foot

CC M87.371 Other secondary osteonecrosis, right ankle
CC Exclusion see Appendix A PDX collection 0907

CC M87.372 Other secondary osteonecrosis, left ankle
CC Exclusion see Appendix A PDX collection 0907

CC M87.373 Other secondary osteonecrosis, unspecified ankle
CC Exclusion see Appendix A PDX collection 0907

CC M87.374 Other secondary osteonecrosis, right foot
CC Exclusion see Appendix A PDX collection 0910

CC M87.375 Other secondary osteonecrosis, left foot
CC Exclusion see Appendix A PDX collection 0910

CC M87.376 Other secondary osteonecrosis, unspecified foot
CC Exclusion see Appendix A PDX collection 0910

CC M87.377 Other secondary osteonecrosis, right toe(s)
CC Exclusion see Appendix A PDX collection 0907

CC M87.378 Other secondary osteonecrosis, left toe(s)
CC Exclusion see Appendix A PDX collection 0907

CC M87.379 Other secondary osteonecrosis, unspecified toe(s)
CC Exclusion see Appendix A PDX collection 0907

CC M87.38 Other secondary osteonecrosis, other site
CC Exclusion see Appendix A PDX collection 0907

CC M87.39 Other secondary osteonecrosis, multiple sites
CC Exclusion see Appendix A PDX collection 0907

+ M87.8 Other osteonecrosis

CC M87.80 Other osteonecrosis, unspecified bone
CC Exclusion see Appendix A PDX collection 0907

+ M87.81 Other osteonecrosis, shoulder

CC M87.811 Other osteonecrosis, right shoulder
CC Exclusion see Appendix A PDX collection 0907

CC M87.812 Other osteonecrosis, left shoulder
CC Exclusion see Appendix A PDX collection 0907

CC M87.819 Other osteonecrosis, unspecified shoulder
CC Exclusion see Appendix A PDX collection 0907

+ M87.82 Other osteonecrosis, humerus

CC M87.821 Other osteonecrosis, right humerus
CC Exclusion see Appendix A PDX collection 0908

CC M87.822 Other osteonecrosis, left humerus
CC Exclusion see Appendix A PDX collection 0908

CC M87.829 Other osteonecrosis, unspecified humerus
CC Exclusion see Appendix A PDX collection 0908

+ M87.83 Other osteonecrosis of radius, ulna and carpus

CC M87.831 Other osteonecrosis of right radius
CC Exclusion see Appendix A PDX collection 0907

CC M87.832 Other osteonecrosis of left radius
CC Exclusion see Appendix A PDX collection 0907

CC M87.833 Other osteonecrosis of unspecified radius
CC Exclusion see Appendix A PDX collection 0907

CC M87.834 Other osteonecrosis of right ulna
CC Exclusion see Appendix A PDX collection 0907

CC M87.835 Other osteonecrosis of left ulna
CC Exclusion see Appendix A PDX collection 0907

CC M87.836 Other osteonecrosis of unspecified ulna
CC Exclusion see Appendix A PDX collection 0907

CC M87.837 Other osteonecrosis of right carpus
CC Exclusion see Appendix A PDX collection 0907

CC M87.838 Other osteonecrosis of left carpus
CC Exclusion see Appendix A PDX collection 0907

CC M87.839 Other osteonecrosis of unspecified carpus
CC Exclusion see Appendix A PDX collection 0907

+ M87.84 Other osteonecrosis, hand and fingers

CC M87.841 Other osteonecrosis, right hand
CC Exclusion see Appendix A PDX collection 0907

CC M87.842 Other osteonecrosis, left hand
CC Exclusion see Appendix A PDX collection 0907

CC M87.843 Other osteonecrosis, unspecified hand
CC Exclusion see Appendix A PDX collection 0907

CC M87.844 Other osteonecrosis, right finger(s)
CC Exclusion see Appendix A PDX collection 0907

CC M87.845 Other osteonecrosis, left finger(s)
CC Exclusion see Appendix A PDX collection 0907

CC M87.849 Other osteonecrosis, unspecified finger(s)
CC Exclusion see Appendix A PDX collection 0907

+ M87.85 Other osteonecrosis, pelvis and femur

CC M87.850 Other osteonecrosis, pelvis
CC Exclusion see Appendix A PDX collection 0909

CC M87.851 Other osteonecrosis, right femur
CC Exclusion see Appendix A PDX collection 0909

CC M87.852 Other osteonecrosis, left femur
CC Exclusion see Appendix A PDX collection 0909

CC M87.859 Other osteonecrosis, unspecified femur
CC Exclusion see Appendix A PDX collection 0909

+ M87.86 Other osteonecrosis, tibia and fibula

CC M87.861 Other osteonecrosis, right tibia
CC Exclusion see Appendix A PDX collection 0907

CC M87.862 Other osteonecrosis, left tibia
CC Exclusion see Appendix A PDX collection 0907

CC M87.863 Other osteonecrosis, unspecified tibia
CC Exclusion see Appendix A PDX collection 0907

CC M87.864 Other osteonecrosis, right fibula
CC Exclusion see Appendix A PDX collection 0907

CC M87.865 Other osteonecrosis, left fibula
CC Exclusion see Appendix A PDX collection 0907

CC M87.869 Other osteonecrosis, unspecified fibula
CC Exclusion see Appendix A PDX collection 0907

+ M87.87 Other osteonecrosis, ankle, foot and toes

CC M87.871 Other osteonecrosis, right ankle
CC Exclusion see Appendix A PDX collection 0907

CC M87.872 Other osteonecrosis, left ankle
CC Exclusion see Appendix A PDX collection 0907

CC M87.873 Other osteonecrosis, unspecified ankle
CC Exclusion see Appendix A PDX collection 0907

CC M87.874 Other osteonecrosis, right foot
CC Exclusion see Appendix A PDX collection 0910

CC M87.875 Other osteonecrosis, left foot
CC Exclusion see Appendix A PDX collection 0910

CC M87.876 Other osteonecrosis, unspecified foot
CC Exclusion see Appendix A PDX collection 0910

CC **M87.877 Other osteonecrosis, right toe(s)**
CC Exclusion see Appendix A PDX collection 0907

CC **M87.878 Other osteonecrosis, left toe(s)**
CC Exclusion see Appendix A PDX collection 0907

CC **M87.879 Other osteonecrosis, unspecified toe(s)**
CC Exclusion see Appendix A PDX collection 0907

CC **M87.88 Other osteonecrosis, other site**
CC Exclusion see Appendix A PDX collection 0907

CC **M87.89 Other osteonecrosis, multiple sites**
CC Exclusion see Appendix A PDX collection 0907

CC **M87.9 Osteonecrosis, unspecified**
Necrosis of bone NOS
CC Exclusion see Appendix A PDX collection 0907

M88 Osteitis deformans [Paget's disease of bone]

Excludes1: *osteitis deformans in neoplastic disease (M90.6)*

M88.0 Osteitis deformans of skull
M88.1 Osteitis deformans of vertebrae
\+ **M88.8 Osteitis deformans of other bones**
\+ **M88.81 Osteitis deformans of shoulder**
M88.811 Osteitis deformans of right shoulder
M88.812 Osteitis deformans of left shoulder
M88.819 Osteitis deformans of unspecified shoulder
\+ **M88.82 Osteitis deformans of upper arm**
M88.821 Osteitis deformans of right upper arm
M88.822 Osteitis deformans of left upper arm
M88.829 Osteitis deformans of unspecified upper arm
\+ **M88.83 Osteitis deformans of forearm**
M88.831 Osteitis deformans of right forearm
M88.832 Osteitis deformans of left forearm
M88.839 Osteitis deformans of unspecified forearm
\+ **M88.84 Osteitis deformans of hand**
M88.841 Osteitis deformans of right hand
M88.842 Osteitis deformans of left hand
M88.849 Osteitis deformans of unspecified hand
\+ **M88.85 Osteitis deformans of thigh**
M88.851 Osteitis deformans of right thigh
M88.852 Osteitis deformans of left thigh
M88.859 Osteitis deformans of unspecified thigh
\+ **M88.86 Osteitis deformans of lower leg**
M88.861 Osteitis deformans of right lower leg
M88.862 Osteitis deformans of left lower leg
M88.869 Osteitis deformans of unspecified lower leg
\+ **M88.87 Osteitis deformans of ankle and foot**
M88.871 Osteitis deformans of right ankle and foot
M88.872 Osteitis deformans of left ankle and foot
M88.879 Osteitis deformans of unspecified ankle and foot
M88.88 Osteitis deformans of other bones
Excludes2: *osteitis deformans of skull (M88.0)*
osteitis deformans of vertebrae (M88.1)
M88.89 Osteitis deformans of multiple sites
M88.9 Osteitis deformans of unspecified bone

M89 Other disorders of bone

\+ **M89.0 Algoneurodystrophy**
Shoulder-hand syndrome
Sudeck's atrophy
Excludes1: *causalgia, lower limb (G57.7-)*
causalgia, upper limb (G56.4-)
complex regional pain syndrome II, lower limb (G57.7-)
complex regional pain syndrome II, upper limb (G56.4-)
reflex sympathetic dystrophy (G90.5-)
M89.00 Algoneurodystrophy, unspecified site
\+ **M89.01 Algoneurodystrophy, shoulder**
M89.011 Algoneurodystrophy, right shoulder
M89.012 Algoneurodystrophy, left shoulder
M89.019 Algoneurodystrophy, unspecified shoulder
\+ **M89.02 Algoneurodystrophy, upper arm**
M89.021 Algoneurodystrophy, right upper arm
M89.022 Algoneurodystrophy, left upper arm
M89.029 Algoneurodystrophy, unspecified upper arm
\+ **M89.03 Algoneurodystrophy, forearm**
M89.031 Algoneurodystrophy, right forearm
M89.032 Algoneurodystrophy, left forearm
M89.039 Algoneurodystrophy, unspecified forearm
\+ **M89.04 Algoneurodystrophy, hand**
M89.041 Algoneurodystrophy, right≈hand
M89.042 Algoneurodystrophy, left hand
M89.049 Algoneurodystrophy, unspecified hand
\+ **M89.05 Algoneurodystrophy, thigh**
M89.051 Algoneurodystrophy, right thigh
M89.052 Algoneurodystrophy, left thigh
M89.059 Algoneurodystrophy, unspecified thigh
\+ **M89.06 Algoneurodystrophy, lower leg**
M89.061 Algoneurodystrophy, right lower leg
M89.062 Algoneurodystrophy, left lower leg
M89.069 Algoneurodystrophy, unspecified lower
\+ **M89.07 Algoneurodystrophy, ankle and foot**
M89.071 Algoneurodystrophy, right ankle and foo
M89.072 Algoneurodystrophy, left ankle and foot
M89.079 Algoneurodystrophy, unspecified ankle a foot
M89.08 Algoneurodystrophy, other site
M89.09 Algoneurodystrophy, multiple sites
\+ **M89.1 Physeal arrest**
Arrest of growth plate
Epiphyseal arrest
Growth plate arrest
\+ **M89.12 Physeal arrest, humerus**
M89.121 Complete physeal arrest, right proximal humerus
M89.122 Complete physeal arrest, left proximal humerus
M89.123 Partial physeal arrest, right proximal humerus
M89.124 Partial physeal arrest, left proximal humerus
M89.125 Complete physeal arrest, right distal humerus
M89.126 Complete physeal arrest, left distal humerus
M89.127 Partial physeal arrest, right distal hume
M89.128 Partial physeal arrest, left distal humeru
M89.129 Physeal arrest, humerus, unspecified
\+ **M89.13 Physeal arrest, forearm**
M89.131 Complete physeal arrest, right distal radius
M89.132 Complete physeal arrest, left distal radiu
M89.133 Partial physeal arrest, right distal radius
M89.134 Partial physeal arrest, left distal radius
M89.138 Other physeal arrest of forearm
M89.139 Physeal arrest, forearm, unspecified
\+ **M89.15 Physeal arrest, femur**
M89.151 Complete physeal arrest, right proximal femur
M89.152 Complete physeal arrest, left proximal femur
M89.153 Partial physeal arrest, right proximal femur
M89.154 Partial physeal arrest, left proximal fem
M89.155 Complete physeal arrest, right distal fen
M89.156 Complete physeal arrest, left distal femu
M89.157 Partial physeal arrest, right distal femur
M89.158 Partial physeal arrest, left distal femur
M89.159 Physeal arrest, femur, unspecified
\+ **M89.16 Physeal arrest, lower leg**
M89.160 Complete physeal arrest, right proximal tibia
M89.161 Complete physeal arrest, left proximal tibia
M89.162 Partial physeal arrest, right proximal tib
M89.163 Partial physeal arrest, left proximal tibia
M89.164 Complete physeal arrest, right distal tib
M89.165 Complete physeal arrest, left distal tibia
M89.166 Partial physeal arrest, right distal tibia
M89.167 Partial physeal arrest, left distal tibia
M89.168 Other physeal arrest of lower leg
M89.169 Physeal arrest, lower leg, unspecified
M89.18 Physeal arrest, other site
\+ **M89.2 Other disorders of bone development and growth**
M89.20 Other disorders of bone development and growth, unspecified site
\+ **M89.21 Other disorders of bone development and growth, shoulder**
M89.211 Other disorders of bone development an growth, right shoulder

M89.212 Other disorders of bone development and growth, left shoulder
M89.219 Other disorders of bone development and growth, unspecified shoulder
+ M89.22 Other disorders of bone development and growth, humerus
M89.221 Other disorders of bone development and growth, right humerus
M89.222 Other disorders of bone development and growth, left humerus
M89.229 Other disorders of bone development and growth, unspecified humerus
+ M89.23 Other disorders of bone development and growth, ulna and radius
M89.231 Other disorders of bone development and growth, right ulna
M89.232 Other disorders of bone development and growth, left ulna
M89.233 Other disorders of bone development and growth, right radius
M89.234 Other disorders of bone development and growth, left radius
M89.239 Other disorders of bone development and growth, unspecified ulna and radius
+ M89.24 Other disorders of bone development and growth, hand
M89.241 Other disorders of bone development and growth, right hand
M89.242 Other disorders of bone development and growth, left hand
M89.249 Other disorders of bone development and growth, unspecified hand
+ M89.25 Other disorders of bone development and growth, femur
M89.251 Other disorders of bone development and growth, right femur
M89.252 Other disorders of bone development and growth, left femur
M89.259 Other disorders of bone development and growth, unspecified femur
+ M89.26 Other disorders of bone development and growth, tibia and fibula
M89.261 Other disorders of bone development and growth, right tibia
M89.262 Other disorders of bone development and growth, left tibia
M89.263 Other disorders of bone development and growth, right fibula
M89.264 Other disorders of bone development and growth, left fibula
M89.269 Other disorders of bone development and growth, unspecified lower leg
+ M89.27 Other disorders of bone development and growth, ankle and foot
M89.271 Other disorders of bone development and growth, right ankle and foot
M89.272 Other disorders of bone development and growth, left ankle and foot
M89.279 Other disorders of bone development and growth, unspecified ankle and foot
M89.28 Other disorders of bone development and growth, other site
M89.29 Other disorders of bone development and growth, multiple sites
+ M89.3 Hypertrophy of bone
M89.30 Hypertrophy of bone, unspecified site
+ M89.31 Hypertrophy of bone, shoulder
M89.311 Hypertrophy of bone, right shoulder
M89.312 Hypertrophy of bone, left shoulder
M89.319 Hypertrophy of bone, unspecified shoulder
+ M89.32 Hypertrophy of bone, humerus
M89.321 Hypertrophy of bone, right humerus
M89.322 Hypertrophy of bone, left humerus
M89.329 Hypertrophy of bone, unspecified humerus
+ M89.33 Hypertrophy of bone, ulna and radius
M89.331 Hypertrophy of bone, right ulna
M89.332 Hypertrophy of bone, left ulna
M89.333 Hypertrophy of bone, right radius
M89.334 Hypertrophy of bone, left radius
M89.339 Hypertrophy of bone, unspecified ulna and radius
+ M89.34 Hypertrophy of bone, hand
M89.341 Hypertrophy of bone, right hand
M89.342 Hypertrophy of bone, left hand
M89.349 Hypertrophy of bone, unspecified hand
+ M89.35 Hypertrophy of bone, femur
M89.351 Hypertrophy of bone, right femur
M89.352 Hypertrophy of bone, left femur
M89.359 Hypertrophy of bone, unspecified femur
+ M89.36 Hypertrophy of bone, tibia and fibula
M89.361 Hypertrophy of bone, right tibia
M89.362 Hypertrophy of bone, left tibia
M89.363 Hypertrophy of bone, right fibula
M89.364 Hypertrophy of bone, left fibula
M89.369 Hypertrophy of bone, unspecified tibia and fibula
+ M89.37 Hypertrophy of bone, ankle and foot
M89.371 Hypertrophy of bone, right ankle and foot
M89.372 Hypertrophy of bone, left ankle and foot
M89.379 Hypertrophy of bone, unspecified ankle and foot
M89.38 Hypertrophy of bone, other site
M89.39 Hypertrophy of bone, multiple sites
+ M89.4 Other hypertrophic osteoarthropathy
Marie-Bamberger disease
Pachydermoperiostosis
M89.40 Other hypertrophic osteoarthropathy, unspecified site
+ M89.41 Other hypertrophic osteoarthropathy, shoulder
M89.411 Other hypertrophic osteoarthropathy, right shoulder
M89.412 Other hypertrophic osteoarthropathy, left shoulder
M89.419 Other hypertrophic osteoarthropathy, unspecified shoulder
+ M89.42 Other hypertrophic osteoarthropathy, upper arm
M89.421 Other hypertrophic osteoarthropathy, right upper arm
M89.422 Other hypertrophic osteoarthropathy, left upper arm
M89.429 Other hypertrophic osteoarthropathy, unspecified upper arm
+ M89.43 Other hypertrophic osteoarthropathy, forearm
M89.431 Other hypertrophic osteoarthropathy, right forearm
M89.432 Other hypertrophic osteoarthropathy, left forearm
M89.439 Other hypertrophic osteoarthropathy, unspecified forearm
+ M89.44 Other hypertrophic osteoarthropathy, hand
M89.441 Other hypertrophic osteoarthropathy, right hand
M89.442 Other hypertrophic osteoarthropathy, left hand
M89.449 Other hypertrophic osteoarthropathy, unspecified hand
+ M89.45 Other hypertrophic osteoarthropathy, thigh
M89.451 Other hypertrophic osteoarthropathy, right thigh
M89.452 Other hypertrophic osteoarthropathy, left thigh
M89.459 Other hypertrophic osteoarthropathy, unspecified thigh
+ M89.46 Other hypertrophic osteoarthropathy, lower leg
M89.461 Other hypertrophic osteoarthropathy, right lower leg
M89.462 Other hypertrophic osteoarthropathy, left lower leg
M89.469 Other hypertrophic osteoarthropathy, unspecified lower leg
+ M89.47 Other hypertrophic osteoarthropathy, ankle and foot
M89.471 Other hypertrophic osteoarthropathy, right ankle and foot
M89.472 Other hypertrophic osteoarthropathy, left ankle and foot
M89.479 Other hypertrophic osteoarthropathy, unspecified ankle and foot
M89.48 Other hypertrophic osteoarthropathy, other site
M89.49 Other hypertrophic osteoarthropathy, multiple sites

+ **M89.5 Osteolysis**
  Use additional code to identify major osseous defect, if applicable (M89.7-)
  Excludes2: *periprosthetic osteolysis of internal prosthetic joint (T84.05-)*
  M89.50 Osteolysis, unspecified site
  + **M89.51 Osteolysis, shoulder**
    M89.511 Osteolysis, right shoulder
    M89.512 Osteolysis, left shoulder
    M89.519 Osteolysis, unspecified shoulder
  + **M89.52 Osteolysis, upper arm**
    M89.521 Osteolysis, right upper arm
    M89.522 Osteolysis, left upper arm
    M89.529 Osteolysis, unspecified upper arm
  + **M89.53 Osteolysis, forearm**
    M89.531 Osteolysis, right forearm
    M89.532 Osteolysis, left forearm
    M89.539 Osteolysis, unspecified forearm
  + **M89.54 Osteolysis, hand**
    M89.541 Osteolysis, right hand
    M89.542 Osteolysis, left hand
    M89.549 Osteolysis, unspecified hand
  + **M89.55 Osteolysis, thigh**
    M89.551 Osteolysis, right thigh
    M89.552 Osteolysis, left thigh
    M89.559 Osteolysis, unspecified thigh
  + **M89.56 Osteolysis, lower leg**
    M89.561 Osteolysis, right lower leg
    M89.562 Osteolysis, left lower leg
    M89.569 Osteolysis, unspecified lower leg
  + **M89.57 Osteolysis, ankle and foot**
    M89.571 Osteolysis, right ankle and foot
    M89.572 Osteolysis, left ankle and foot
    M89.579 Osteolysis, unspecified ankle and foot
  M89.58 Osteolysis, other site
  M89.59 Osteolysis, multiple sites

+ **M89.6 Osteopathy after poliomyelitis**
  Use additional code (B91) to identify previous poliomyelitis
  Excludes1: *postpolio syndrome (G14)*
  M89.60 Osteopathy after poliomyelitis, unspecified site
  + **M89.61 Osteopathy after poliomyelitis, shoulder**
    M89.611 Osteopathy after poliomyelitis, right shoulder
    M89.612 Osteopathy after poliomyelitis, left shoulder
    M89.619 Osteopathy after poliomyelitis, unspecified shoulder
  + **M89.62 Osteopathy after poliomyelitis, upper arm**
    M89.621 Osteopathy after poliomyelitis, right upper arm
    M89.622 Osteopathy after poliomyelitis, left upper arm
    M89.629 Osteopathy after poliomyelitis, unspecified upper arm
  + **M89.63 Osteopathy after poliomyelitis, forearm**
    M89.631 Osteopathy after poliomyelitis, right forearm
    M89.632 Osteopathy after poliomyelitis, left forearm
    M89.639 Osteopathy after poliomyelitis, unspecified forearm
  + **M89.64 Osteopathy after poliomyelitis, hand**
    M89.641 Osteopathy after poliomyelitis, right hand
    M89.642 Osteopathy after poliomyelitis, left hand
    M89.649 Osteopathy after poliomyelitis, unspecified hand
  + **M89.65 Osteopathy after poliomyelitis, thigh**
    M89.651 Osteopathy after poliomyelitis, right thigh
    M89.652 Osteopathy after poliomyelitis, left thigh
    M89.659 Osteopathy after poliomyelitis, unspecified thigh
  + **M89.66 Osteopathy after poliomyelitis, lower leg**
    M89.661 Osteopathy after poliomyelitis, right lower leg
    M89.662 Osteopathy after poliomyelitis, left lower leg
    M89.669 Osteopathy after poliomyelitis, unspecified lower leg
  + **M89.67 Osteopathy after poliomyelitis, ankle and foot**
    M89.671 Osteopathy after poliomyelitis, right ankle and foot
    M89.672 Osteopathy after poliomyelitis, left ankle and foot
    M89.679 Osteopathy after poliomyelitis, unspecified ankle and foot
  M89.68 Osteopathy after poliomyelitis, other site
  M89.69 Osteopathy after poliomyelitis, multiple sites

+ **M89.7 Major osseous defect**
  Code first underlying disease, if known, such as:
    aseptic necrosis of bone (M87.-)
    malignant neoplasm of bone (C40.-)
    osteolysis (M89.5)
    osteomyelitis (M86.-)
    osteonecrosis (M87.-)
    osteoporosis (M80.-, M81.-)
    periprosthetic osteolysis (T84.05-)
  M89.70 Major osseous defect, unspecified site
  + **M89.71 Major osseous defect, shoulder region**
    Major osseous defect clavicle or scapula
    M89.711 Major osseous defect, right shoulder region
    M89.712 Major osseous defect, left shoulder region
    M89.719 Major osseous defect, unspecified shoulder region
  + **M89.72 Major osseous defect, humerus**
    M89.721 Major osseous defect, right humerus
    M89.722 Major osseous defect, left humerus
    M89.729 Major osseous defect, unspecified humerus
  + **M89.73 Major osseous defect, forearm**
    Major osseous defect of radius and ulna
    M89.731 Major osseous defect, right forearm
    M89.732 Major osseous defect, left forearm
    M89.739 Major osseous defect, unspecified forearm
  + **M89.74 Major osseous defect, hand**
    Major osseous defect of carpus, fingers, metacarpus
    M89.741 Major osseous defect, right hand
    M89.742 Major osseous defect, left hand
    M89.749 Major osseous defect, unspecified hand
  + **M89.75 Major osseous defect, pelvic region and thigh**
    Major osseous defect of femur and pelvis
    M89.751 Major osseous defect, right pelvic region and thigh
    M89.752 Major osseous defect, left pelvic region and thigh
    M89.759 Major osseous defect, unspecified pelvic region and thigh
  + **M89.76 Major osseous defect, lower leg**
    Major osseous defect of fibula and tibia
    M89.761 Major osseous defect, right lower leg
    M89.762 Major osseous defect, left lower leg
    M89.769 Major osseous defect, unspecified lower leg
  + **M89.77 Major osseous defect, ankle and foot**
    Major osseous defect of metatarsus, tarsus, toes
    M89.771 Major osseous defect, right ankle and foot
    M89.772 Major osseous defect, left ankle and foot
    M89.779 Major osseous defect, unspecified ankle and foot
  M89.78 Major osseous defect, other site
  M89.79 Major osseous defect, multiple sites

+ **M89.8 Other specified disorders of bone**
  Infantile cortical hyperostoses
  Post-traumatic subperiosteal ossification
  + **M89.8X Other specified disorders of bone**
    M89.8X0 Other specified disorders of bone, multiple sites
    M89.8X1 Other specified disorders of bone, shoulder
    M89.8X2 Other specified disorders of bone, upper arm
    M89.8X3 Other specified disorders of bone, forearm
    M89.8X4 Other specified disorders of bone, hand
    M89.8X5 Other specified disorders of bone, thigh
    M89.8X6 Other specified disorders of bone, lower leg
    M89.8X7 Other specified disorders of bone, ankle and foot
    M89.8X8 Other specified disorders of bone, other site
    M89.8X9 Other specified disorders of bone, unspecified site

M89.9 Disorder of bone, unspecified

M90 Osteopathies in diseases classified elsewhere

Excludes1: *osteochondritis, osteomyelitis, and osteopathy (in):*
cryptococcosis (B45.3)
diabetes mellitus (E08-E13 with .69-)
gonococcal (A54.43)
neurogenic syphilis (A52.11)
renal osteodystrophy (N25.0)
salmonellosis (A02.24)
secondary syphilis (A51.46)
syphilis (late) (A52.77)

\+ **M90.5 Osteonecrosis in diseases classified elsewhere**
Code first underlying disease, such as:
caisson disease (T70.3)
hemoglobinopathy (D50-D64)

CC **M90.50 Osteonecrosis in diseases classified elsewhere, unspecified site**
CC Exclusion see Appendix A PDX collection 0907

\+ **M90.51 Osteonecrosis in diseases classified elsewhere, shoulder**

CC **M90.511 Osteonecrosis in diseasesclassified elsewhere, rightshoulder**
CC Exclusion see Appendix A PDX collection 0908

CC **M90.512 Osteonecrosis in diseases classified elsewhere, left shoulder**
CC Exclusion see Appendix A PDX collection 0908

CC **M90.519 Osteonecrosis in diseases classified elsewhere, unspecified shoulder**
CC Exclusion see Appendix A PDX collection 0908

\+ **M90.52 Osteonecrosis in diseases classified elsewhere, upper arm**

CC **M90.521 Osteonecrosis in diseases classified elsewhere, right upper arm**
CC Exclusion see Appendix A PDX collection 0907

CC **M90.522 Osteonecrosis in diseases classified elsewhere, left upper arm**
CC Exclusion see Appendix A PDX collection 0907

CC **M90.529 Osteonecrosis in diseases classified elsewhere, unspecified upper arm**
CC Exclusion see Appendix A PDX collection 0907

\+ **M90.53 Osteonecrosis in diseases classified elsewhere, forearm**

CC **M90.531 Osteonecrosis in diseases classified elsewhere, right forearm**
CC Exclusion see Appendix A PDX collection 0907

CC **M90.532 Osteonecrosis in diseases classified elsewhere, left forearm**
CC Exclusion see Appendix A PDX collection 0907

CC **M90.539 Osteonecrosis in diseases classified elsewhere, unspecified forearm**
CC Exclusion see Appendix A PDX collection 0907

\+ **M90.54 Osteonecrosis in diseases classified elsewhere, hand**

CC **M90.541 Osteonecrosis in diseases classified elsewhere, right hand**
CC Exclusion see Appendix A PDX collection 0907

CC **M90.542 Osteonecrosis in diseases classified elsewhere, left hand**
CC Exclusion see Appendix A PDX collection 0907

CC **M90.549 Osteonecrosis in diseases classified elsewhere, unspecified hand**
CC Exclusion see Appendix A PDX collection 0907

\+ **M90.55 Osteonecrosis in diseases classified elsewhere, thigh**

CC **M90.551 Osteonecrosis in diseases classified elsewhere, right thigh**
CC Exclusion see Appendix A PDX collection 0909

CC **M90.552 Osteonecrosis in diseases classified elsewhere, left thigh**
CC Exclusion see Appendix A PDX collection 0909

CC **M90.559 Osteonecrosis in diseases classified elsewhere, unspecified thigh**
CC Exclusion see Appendix A PDX collection 0909

\+ **M90.56 Osteonecrosis in diseases classified elsewhere, lower leg**

CC **M90.561 Osteonecrosis in diseases classified elsewhere, right lower leg**
CC Exclusion see Appendix A PDX collection 0907

CC **M90.562 Osteonecrosis in diseases classified elsewhere, left lower leg**
CC Exclusion see Appendix A PDX collection 0907

CC **M90.569 Osteonecrosis in diseases classified elsewhere, unspecified lower leg**
CC Exclusion see Appendix A PDX collection 0907

\+ **M90.57 Osteonecrosis in diseases classified elsewhere, ankle and foot**

CC **M90.571 Osteonecrosis in diseases classified elsewhere, right ankle and foot**
CC Exclusion see Appendix A PDX collection 0907

CC **M90.572 Osteonecrosis in diseases classified elsewhere, left ankle and foot**
CC Exclusion see Appendix A PDX collection 0907

CC **M90.579 Osteonecrosis in diseases classified elsewhere, unspecified ankle and foot**
CC Exclusion see Appendix A PDX collection 0907

CC **M90.58 Osteonecrosis in diseases classified elsewhere, other site**
CC Exclusion see Appendix A PDX collection 0907

CC **M90.59 Osteonecrosis in diseases classified elsewhere, multiple sites**
CC Exclusion see Appendix A PDX collection 0907

\+ **M90.6 Osteitis deformans in neoplastic diseases**
Osteitis deformans in malignant neoplasm of bone
Code first the neoplasm (C40.-, C41.-)
Excludes1: *osteitis deformans [Paget's disease of bone] (M88.-)*

M90.60 Osteitis deformans in neoplastic diseases, unspecified site

\+ **M90.61 Osteitis deformans in neoplastic diseases, shoulder**

M90.611 Osteitis deformans in neoplastic diseases, right shoulder

M90.612 Osteitis deformans in neoplastic diseases, left shoulder

M90.619 Osteitis deformans in neoplastic diseases, unspecified shoulder

\+ **M90.62 Osteitis deformans in neoplastic diseases, upper arm**

M90.621 Osteitis deformans in neoplastic diseases, right upper arm

M90.622 Osteitis deformans in neoplastic diseases, left upper arm

M90.629 Osteitis deformans in neoplastic diseases, unspecified upper arm

\+ **M90.63 Osteitis deformans in neoplastic diseases, forearm**

M90.631 Osteitis deformans in neoplastic diseases, right forearm

M90.632 Osteitis deformans in neoplastic diseases, left forearm

M90.639 Osteitis deformans in neoplastic diseases, unspecified forearm

\+ **M90.64 Osteitis deformans in neoplastic diseases, hand**

M90.641 Osteitis deformans in neoplastic diseases, right hand

M90.642 Osteitis deformans in neoplastic diseases, left hand

M90.649 Osteitis deformans in neoplastic diseases, unspecified hand

\+ **M90.65 Osteitis deformans in neoplastic diseases, thigh**

M90.651 Osteitis deformans in neoplastic diseases, right thigh

M90.652 Osteitis deformans in neoplastic diseases, left thigh

M90.659 Osteitis deformans in neoplastic diseases, unspecified thigh

+ **M90.66 Osteitis deformans in neoplastic diseases, lower leg**
  - **M90.661 Osteitis deformans in neoplastic diseases, right lower leg**
  - **M90.662 Osteitis deformans in neoplastic diseases, left lower leg**
  - **M90.669 Osteitis deformans in neoplastic diseases, unspecified lower leg**

+ **M90.67 Osteitis deformans in neoplastic diseases, ankle and foot**
  - **M90.671 Osteitis deformans in neoplastic diseases, right ankle and foot**
  - **M90.672 Osteitis deformans in neoplastic diseases, left ankle and foot**
  - **M90.679 Osteitis deformans in neoplastic diseases, unspecified ankle and foot**

M90.68 Osteitis deformans in neoplastic diseases, other site

M90.69 Osteitis deformans in neoplastic diseases, multiple sites

+ **M90.8 Osteopathy in diseases classified elsewhere**

Code first underlying disease, such as:
rickets (E55.0)
vitamin-D-resistant rickets (E83.3)

M90.80 Osteopathy in diseases classified elsewhere, unspecified site

+ **M90.81 Osteopathy in diseases classified elsewhere, shoulder**
  - **M90.811 Osteopathy in diseases classified elsewhere, right shoulder**
  - **M90.812 Osteopathy in diseases classified elsewhere, left shoulder**
  - **M90.819 Osteopathy in diseases classified elsewhere, unspecified shoulder**

+ **M90.82 Osteopathy in diseases classified elsewhere, upper arm**
  - **M90.821 Osteopathy in diseases classified elsewhere, right upper arm**
  - **M90.822 Osteopathy in diseases classified elsewhere, left upper arm**
  - **M90.829 Osteopathy in diseases classified elsewhere, unspecified upper arm**

+ **M90.83 Osteopathy in diseases classified elsewhere, forearm**
  - **M90.831 Osteopathy in diseases classified elsewhere, right forearm**
  - **M90.832 Osteopathy in diseases classified elsewhere, left forearm**
  - **M90.839 Osteopathy in diseases classified elsewhere, unspecified forearm**

+ **M90.84 Osteopathy in diseases classified elsewhere, hand**
  - **M90.841 Osteopathy in diseases classified elsewhere, right hand**
  - **M90.842 Osteopathy in diseases classified elsewhere, left hand**
  - **M90.849 Osteopathy in diseases classified elsewhere, unspecified hand**

+ **M90.85 Osteopathy in diseases classified elsewhere, thigh**
  - **M90.851 Osteopathy in diseases classified elsewhere, right thigh**
  - **M90.852 Osteopathy in diseases classified elsewhere, left thigh**
  - **M90.859 Osteopathy in diseases classified elsewhere, unspecified thigh**

+ **M90.86 Osteopathy in diseases classified elsewhere, lower leg**
  - **M90.861 Osteopathy in diseases classified elsewhere, right lower leg**
  - **M90.862 Osteopathy in diseases classified elsewhere, left lower leg**
  - **M90.869 Osteopathy in diseases classified elsewhere, unspecified lower leg**

+ **M90.87 Osteopathy in diseases classified elsewhere, ankle and foot**
  - **M90.871 Osteopathy in diseases classified elsewhere, right ankle and foot**
  - **M90.872 Osteopathy in diseases classified elsewhere, left ankle and foot**
  - **M90.879 Osteopathy in diseases classified elsewhere, unspecified ankle and foot**

M90.88 Osteopathy in diseases classified elsewhere, other site

M90.89 Osteopathy in diseases classified elsewhere, multiple sites

Chondropathies (M91-M94)

Excludes1: *postprocedural chondropathies (M96.-)*

M91 Juvenile osteochondrosis of hip and pelvis

Excludes1: *slipped upper femoral epiphysis (nontraumatic) (M93.0)*

M91.0 Juvenile osteochondrosis of pelvis

Osteochondrosis (juvenile) of acetabulum
Osteochondrosis (juvenile) of iliac crest [Buchanan]
Osteochondrosis (juvenile) of ischiopubic synchondrosis [van Neck]
Osteochondrosis (juvenile) of symphysis pubis [Pierson]

+ **M91.1 Juvenile osteochondrosis of head of femur [Legg-Calvé-Perthes]**
  - **M91.10 Juvenile osteochondrosis of head of femur [Legg-Calvé-Perthes], unspecified leg**
  - **M91.11 Juvenile osteochondrosis of head of femur [Legg-Calvé-Perthes], right leg**
  - **M91.12 Juvenile osteochondrosis of head of femur [Legg-Calvé-Perthes], left leg**

+ **M91.2 Coxa plana**

  Hip deformity due to previous juvenile osteochondrosis
  - **M91.20 Coxa plana, unspecified hip**
  - **M91.21 Coxa plana, right hip**
  - **M91.22 Coxa plana, left hip**

+ **M91.3 Pseudocoxalgia**
  - **M91.30 Pseudocoxalgia, unspecified hip**
  - **M91.31 Pseudocoxalgia, right hip**
  - **M91.32 Pseudocoxalgia, left hip**

+ **M91.4 Coxa magna**
  - **M91.40 Coxa magna, unspecified hip**
  - **M91.41 Coxa magna, right hip**
  - **M91.42 Coxa magna, left hip**

+ **M91.8 Other juvenile osteochondrosis of hip and pelvis**

  Juvenile osteochondrosis after reduction of congenital dislocation of hip
  - **M91.80 Other juvenile osteochondrosis of hip and pelvis, unspecified leg**
  - **M91.81 Other juvenile osteochondrosis of hip and pelvis, right leg**
  - **M91.82 Other juvenile osteochondrosis of hip and pelvis, left leg**

+ **M91.9 Juvenile osteochondrosis of hip and pelvis, unspecified**
  - **M91.90 Juvenile osteochondrosis of hip and pelvis, unspecified, unspecified leg**
  - **M91.91 Juvenile osteochondrosis of hip and pelvis, unspecified, right leg**
  - **M91.92 Juvenile osteochondrosis of hip and pelvis, unspecified, left leg**

M92 Other juvenile osteochondrosis

+ **M92.0 Juvenile osteochondrosis of humerus**

  Osteochondrosis (juvenile) of capitulum of humerus [Panner]
  Osteochondrosis (juvenile) of head of humerus [Haas]
  - **M92.00 Juvenile osteochondrosis of humerus, unspecified arm**
  - **M92.01 Juvenile osteochondrosis of humerus, right arm**
  - **M92.02 Juvenile osteochondrosis of humerus, left arm**

+ **M92.1 Juvenile osteochondrosis of radius and ulna**

  Osteochondrosis (juvenile) of lower ulna [Burns]
  Osteochondrosis (juvenile) of radial head [Brailsford]
  - **M92.10 Juvenile osteochondrosis of radius and ulna, unspecified arm**
  - **M92.11 Juvenile osteochondrosis of radius and ulna, right arm**
  - **M92.12 Juvenile osteochondrosis of radius and ulna, left ar**

+ **M92.2 Juvenile osteochondrosis, hand**
  + **M92.20 Unspecified juvenile osteochondrosis, hand**
    - **M92.201 Unspecified juvenile osteochondrosis, right hand**
    - **M92.202 Unspecified juvenile osteochondrosis, left hand**
    - **M92.209 Unspecified juvenile osteochondrosis, unspecified hand**
  + **M92.21 Osteochondrosis (juvenile) of carpal lunate [Kienböck]**
    - **M92.211 Osteochondrosis (juvenile) of carpal luna [Kienböck], right hand**
    - **M92.212 Osteochondrosis (juvenile) of carpal luna [Kienböck], left hand**
    - **M92.219 Osteochondrosis (juvenile) of carpal luna [Kienböck], unspecified hand**

+ M92.22 Osteochondrosis (juvenile) of metacarpal heads [Mauclaire]
  - M92.221 Osteochondrosis (juvenile) of metacarpal heads [Mauclaire], right hand
  - M92.222 Osteochondrosis (juvenile) of metacarpal heads [Mauclaire], left hand
  - M92.229 Osteochondrosis (juvenile) of metacarpal heads [Mauclaire], unspecified hand

+ M92.29 Other juvenile osteochondrosis, hand
  - M92.291 Other juvenile osteochondrosis, right hand
  - M92.292 Other juvenile osteochondrosis, left hand
  - M92.299 Other juvenile osteochondrosis, unspecified hand

+ M92.3 Other juvenile osteochondrosis, upper limb
  - M92.30 Other juvenile osteochondrosis, unspecified upper limb
  - M92.31 Other juvenile osteochondrosis, right upper limb
  - M92.32 Other juvenile osteochondrosis, left upper limb

+ M92.4 Juvenile osteochondrosis of patella

Osteochondrosis (juvenile) of primary patellar center [Köhler]
Osteochondrosis (juvenile) of secondary patellar centre [Sinding Larsen]

  - M92.40 Juvenile osteochondrosis of patella, unspecified knee
  - M92.41 Juvenile osteochondrosis of patella, right knee
  - M92.42 Juvenile osteochondrosis of patella, left knee

+ M92.5 Juvenile osteochondrosis of tibia and fibula

Osteochondrosis (juvenile) of proximal tibia [Blount]
Osteochondrosis (juvenile) of tibial tubercle [Osgood-Schlatter]
Tibia vara

  - M92.50 Juvenile osteochondrosis of tibia and fibula, unspecified leg
  - M92.51 Juvenile osteochondrosis of tibia and fibula, right leg
  - M92.52 Juvenile osteochondrosis of tibia and fibula, left leg

+ M92.6 Juvenile osteochondrosis of tarsus

Osteochondrosis (juvenile) of calcaneum [Sever]
Osteochondrosis (juvenile) of os tibiale externum [Haglund]
Osteochondrosis (juvenile) of talus [Diaz]
Osteochondrosis (juvenile) of tarsal navicular [Köhler]

  - M92.60 Juvenile osteochondrosis of tarsus, unspecified ankle
  - M92.61 Juvenile osteochondrosis of tarsus, right ankle
  - M92.62 Juvenile osteochondrosis of tarsus, left ankle

+ M92.7 Juvenile osteochondrosis of metatarsus

Osteochondrosis (juvenile) of fifth metatarsus [Iselin]
Osteochondrosis (juvenile) of second metatarsus [Freiberg]

  - M92.70 Juvenile osteochondrosis of metatarsus, unspecified foot
  - M92.71 Juvenile osteochondrosis of metatarsus, right foot
  - M92.72 Juvenile osteochondrosis of metatarsus, left foot

M92.8 Other specified juvenile osteochondrosis

Calcaneal apophysitis

M92.9 Juvenile osteochondrosis, unspecified

Juvenile apophysitis NOS
Juvenile epiphysitis NOS
Juvenile osteochondritis NOS
Juvenile osteochondrosis NOS

M93 Other osteochondropathies

Excludes2: *osteochondrosis of spine (M42.-)*

+ M93.0 Slipped upper femoral epiphysis (nontraumatic)

Use additional code for associated chondrolysis (M94.3)

+ M93.00 Unspecified slipped upper femoral epiphysis (nontraumatic)
  - M93.001 Unspecified slipped upper femoral epiphysis (nontraumatic), right hip
  - M93.002 Unspecified slipped upper femoral epiphysis (nontraumatic), left hip
  - M93.003 Unspecified slipped upper femoral epiphysis (nontraumatic), unspecified hip

+ M93.01 Acute slipped upper femoral epiphysis (nontraumatic)
  - M93.011 Acute slipped upper femoral epiphysis (nontraumatic), right hip
  - M93.012 Acute slipped upper femoral epiphysis (nontraumatic), left hip
  - M93.013 Acute slipped upper femoral epiphysis (nontraumatic), unspecified hip

+ M93.02 Chronic slipped upper femoral epiphysis (nontraumatic)
  - M93.021 Chronic slipped upper femoral epiphysis (nontraumatic), right hip
  - M93.022 Chronic slipped upper femoral epiphysis (nontraumatic), left hip
  - M93.023 Chronic slipped upper femoral epiphysis (nontraumatic), unspecified hip

+ M93.03 Acute on chronic slipped upper femoral epiphysis (nontraumatic)
  - M93.031 Acute on chronic slipped upper femoral epiphysis (nontraumatic), right hip
  - M93.032 Acute on chronic slipped upper femoral epiphysis (nontraumatic), left hip
  - M93.033 Acute on chronic slipped upper femoral epiphysis (nontraumatic), unspecified hip

• M93.1 Kienböck's disease of adults

Adult osteochondrosis of carpal lunates

+ M93.2 Osteochondritis dissecans
  - M93.20 Osteochondritis dissecans of unspecified site

+ M93.21 Osteochondritis dissecans of shoulder
  - M93.211 Osteochondritis dissecans, right shoulder
  - M93.212 Osteochondritis dissecans, left shoulder
  - M93.219 Osteochondritis dissecans, unspecified shoulder

+ M93.22 Osteochondritis dissecans of elbow
  - M93.221 Osteochondritis dissecans, right elbow
  - M93.222 Osteochondritis dissecans, left elbow
  - M93.229 Osteochondritis dissecans, unspecified elbow

+ M93.23 Osteochondritis dissecans of wrist
  - M93.231 Osteochondritis dissecans, right wrist
  - M93.232 Osteochondritis dissecans, left wrist
  - M93.239 Osteochondritis dissecans, unspecified wrist

+ M93.24 Osteochondritis dissecans of joints of hand
  - M93.241 Osteochondritis dissecans, joints of right hand
  - M93.242 Osteochondritis dissecans, joints of left hand
  - M93.249 Osteochondritis dissecans, joints of unspecified hand

+ M93.25 Osteochondritis dissecans of hip
  - M93.251 Osteochondritis dissecans, right hip
  - M93.252 Osteochondritis dissecans, left hip
  - M93.259 Osteochondritis dissecans, unspecified hip

+ M93.26 Osteochondritis dissecans knee
  - M93.261 Osteochondritis dissecans, right knee
  - M93.262 Osteochondritis dissecans, left knee
  - M93.269 Osteochondritis dissecans, unspecified knee

+ M93.27 Osteochondritis dissecans of ankle and joints of foot
  - M93.271 Osteochondritis dissecans, right ankle and joints of right foot
  - M93.272 Osteochondritis dissecans, left ankle and joints of left foot
  - M93.279 Osteochondritis dissecans, unspecified ankle and joints of foot

M93.28 Osteochondritis dissecans other site
M93.29 Osteochondritis dissecans multiple sites

+ M93.8 Other specified osteochondropathies
  - M93.80 Other specified osteochondropathies of unspecified site

+ M93.81 Other specified osteochondropathies of shoulder
  - M93.811 Other specified osteochondropathies, right shoulder
  - M93.812 Other specified osteochondropathies, left shoulder
  - M93.819 Other specified osteochondropathies, unspecified shoulder

+ M93.82 Other specified osteochondropathies of upper arm
  - M93.821 Other specified osteochondropathies, right upper arm
  - M93.822 Other specified osteochondropathies, left upper arm
  - M93.829 Other specified osteochondropathies, unspecified upper arm

+ M93.83 Other specified osteochondropathies of forearm
  - M93.831 Other specified osteochondropathies, right forearm
  - M93.832 Other specified osteochondropathies, left forearm
  - M93.839 Other specified osteochondropathies, unspecified forearm

+ M93.84 Other specified osteochondropathies of hand
  - M93.841 Other specified osteochondropathies, right hand
  - M93.842 Other specified osteochondropathies, left hand
  - M93.849 Other specified osteochondropathies, unspecified hand
+ M93.85 Other specified osteochondropathies of thigh
  - M93.851 Other specified osteochondropathies, right thigh
  - M93.852 Other specified osteochondropathies, left thigh
  - M93.859 Other specified osteochondropathies, unspecified thigh
+ M93.86 Other specified osteochondropathies lower leg
  - M93.861 Other specified osteochondropathies, right lower leg
  - M93.862 Other specified osteochondropathies, left lower leg
  - M93.869 Other specified osteochondropathies, unspecified lower leg
+ M93.87 Other specified osteochondropathies of ankle and foot
  - M93.871 Other specified osteochondropathies, right ankle and foot
  - M93.872 Other specified osteochondropathies, left ankle and foot
  - M93.879 Other specified osteochondropathies, unspecified ankle and foot

M93.88 Other specified osteochondropathies other

M93.89 Other specified osteochondropathies multiple sites

+ M93.9 Osteochondropathy, unspecified

Apophysitis NOS
Epiphysitis NOS
Osteochondritis NOS
Osteochondrosis NOS

M93.90 Osteochondropathy, unspecified of unspecified site

+ M93.91 Osteochondropathy, unspecified of shoulder
  - M93.911 Osteochondropathy, unspecified, right shoulder
  - M93.912 Osteochondropathy, unspecified, left shoulder
  - M93.919 Osteochondropathy, unspecified, unspecified shoulder
+ M93.92 Osteochondropathy, unspecified of upper arm
  - M93.921 Osteochondropathy, unspecified, right upper arm
  - M93.922 Osteochondropathy, unspecified, left upper arm
  - M93.929 Osteochondropathy, unspecified, unspecified upper arm
+ M93.93 Osteochondropathy, unspecified of forearm
  - M93.931 Osteochondropathy, unspecified, right forearm
  - M93.932 Osteochondropathy, unspecified, left forearm
  - M93.939 Osteochondropathy, unspecified, unspecified forearm
+ M93.94 Osteochondropathy, unspecified of hand
  - M93.941 Osteochondropathy, unspecified, right hand
  - M93.942 Osteochondropathy, unspecified, left hand
  - M93.949 Osteochondropathy, unspecified, unspecified hand
+ M93.95 Osteochondropathy, unspecified of thigh
  - M93.951 Osteochondropathy, unspecified, right thigh
  - M93.952 Osteochondropathy, unspecified, left thigh
  - M93.959 Osteochondropathy, unspecified, unspecified thigh
+ M93.96 Osteochondropathy, unspecified lower leg
  - M93.961 Osteochondropathy, unspecified, right lower leg
  - M93.962 Osteochondropathy, unspecified, left lower leg
  - M93.969 Osteochondropathy, unspecified, unspecified lower leg
+ M93.97 Osteochondropathy, unspecified of ankle and foot
  - M93.971 Osteochondropathy, unspecified, right ankle and foot
  - M93.972 Osteochondropathy, unspecified, left ankle and foot
  - M93.979 Osteochondropathy, unspecified, unspecified ankle and foot

M93.98 Osteochondropathy, unspecified other

M93.99 Osteochondropathy, unspecified multiple sites

M94 Other disorders of cartilage

M94.0 Chondrocostal junction syndrome [Tietze]

Costochondritis

M94.1 Relapsing polychondritis

+ M94.2 Chondromalacia

Excludes1: *chondromalacia patellae (M22.4)*

M94.20 Chondromalacia, unspecified site

+ M94.21 Chondromalacia, shoulder
  - M94.211 Chondromalacia, right shoulder
  - M94.212 Chondromalacia, left shoulder
  - M94.219 Chondromalacia, unspecified shoulder
+ M94.22 Chondromalacia, elbow
  - M94.221 Chondromalacia, right elbow
  - M94.222 Chondromalacia, left elbow
  - M94.229 Chondromalacia, unspecified elbow
+ M94.23 Chondromalacia, wrist
  - M94.231 Chondromalacia, right wrist
  - M94.232 Chondromalacia, left wrist
  - M94.239 Chondromalacia, unspecified wrist
+ M94.24 Chondromalacia, joints of hand
  - M94.241 Chondromalacia, joints of right hand
  - M94.242 Chondromalacia, joints of left hand
  - M94.249 Chondromalacia, joints of unspecified hand
+ M94.25 Chondromalacia, hip
  - M94.251 Chondromalacia, right hip
  - M94.252 Chondromalacia, left hip
  - M94.259 Chondromalacia, unspecified hip
+ M94.26 Chondromalacia, knee
  - M94.261 Chondromalacia, right knee
  - M94.262 Chondromalacia, left knee
  - M94.269 Chondromalacia, unspecified knee
+ M94.27 Chondromalacia, ankle and joints of foot
  - M94.271 Chondromalacia, right ankle and joints of right foot
  - M94.272 Chondromalacia, left ankle and joints of left foot
  - M94.279 Chondromalacia, unspecified ankle and joints of foot

M94.28 Chondromalacia, other site

M94.29 Chondromalacia, multiple sites

+ M94.3 Chondrolysis

Code first any associated slipped upper femoral epiphysis (nontraumatic) (M93.0-)

+ M94.35 Chondrolysis, hip
  - M94.351 Chondrolysis, right hip
  - M94.352 Chondrolysis, left hip
  - M94.359 Chondrolysis, unspecified hip

+ M94.8 Other specified disorders of cartilage

+ M94.8X Other specified disorders of cartilage
  - M94.8X0 Other specified disorders of cartilage, multiple sites
  - M94.8X1 Other specified disorders of cartilage, shoulder
  - M94.8X2 Other specified disorders of cartilage, upper arm
  - M94.8X3 Other specified disorders of cartilage, forearm
  - M94.8X4 Other specified disorders of cartilage, han
  - M94.8X5 Other specified disorders of cartilage, thig
  - M94.8X6 Other specified disorders of cartilage, lower leg
  - M94.8X7 Other specified disorders of cartilage, ankle and foot
  - M94.8X8 Other specified disorders of cartilage, other site
  - M94.8X9 Other specified disorders of cartilage, unspecified sites

M94.9 Disorder of cartilage, unspecified

Other disorders of the musculoskeletal system and connective tissue (M95)

M95 Other acquired deformities of musculoskeletal system and connective tissue

Excludes2: *acquired absence of limbs and organs (Z89-Z90)*
acquired deformities of limbs (M20-M21)
congenital malformations and deformations of the musculoskeletal system (Q65-Q79)
deforming dorsopathies (M40-M43)
dentofacial anomalies [including malocclusion] (M26.-)
postprocedural musculoskeletal disorders (M96.-)

M95.0 Acquired deformity of nose
Excludes2: *deviated nasal septum (J34.2)*

\+ **M95.1 Cauliflower ear**
Excludes2: *other acquired deformities of ear (H61.1)*
M95.10 Cauliflower ear, unspecified ear
M95.11 Cauliflower ear, right ear
M95.12 Cauliflower ear, left ear

M95.2 Other acquired deformity of head
M95.3 Acquired deformity of neck
M95.4 Acquired deformity of chest and rib
AHA CC: 4Q, 2014, 26-27
M95.5 Acquired deformity of pelvis
Excludes1: *maternal care for known or suspected disproportion (O33.-)*
M95.8 Other specified acquired deformities of musculoskeletal system
M95.9 Acquired deformity of musculoskeletal system, unspecified

Intraoperative and postprocedural complications and disorders of musculoskeletal system, not elsewhere classified (M96)

M96 Intraoperative and postprocedural complications and disorders of musculoskeletal system, not elsewhere classified

Excludes2: *arthropathy following intestinal bypass (M02.0-)*
complications of internal orthopedic prosthetic devices, implants and grafts (T84.-)
disorders associated with osteoporosis (M80)
periprosthetic fracture around internal prosthetic joint (M97.-)
presence of functional implants and other devices (Z96-Z97)

CC **M96.0 Pseudarthrosis after fusion or arthrodesis**
There are no CC exclusions for this code
M96.1 Postlaminectomy syndrome, not elsewhere classified
M96.2 Postradiation kyphosis
M96.3 Postlaminectomy kyphosis
M96.4 Postsurgical lordosis
M96.5 Postradiation scoliosis

\+ **M96.6 Fracture of bone following insertion of orthopedic implant, joint prosthesis, or bone plate**
Intraoperative fracture of bone during insertion of orthopedic implant, joint prosthesis, or bone plate
Excludes2: *complication of internal orthopedic devices, implants or grafts (T84.-)*

\+ **M96.62 Fracture of humerus following insertion of orthopedic implant, joint prosthesis, or bone plate**
CC **M96.621 Fracture of humerus following insertion of orthopedic implant, joint prosthesis, or bone plate, right arm**
CC Exclusion see Appendix A PDX collection 0911
CC **M96.622 Fracture of humerus following insertion of orthopedic implant, joint prosthesis, or bone plate, left arm**
CC Exclusion see Appendix A PDX collection 0911
CC **M96.629 Fracture of humerus following insertion of orthopedic implant, joint prosthesis, or bone plate, unspecified arm**
CC Exclusion see Appendix A PDX collection 0911

\+ **M96.63 Fracture of radius or ulna following insertion of orthopedic implant, joint prosthesis, or bone plate**
CC **M96.631 Fracture of radius or ulna following insertion of orthopedic implant, joint prosthesis, or bone plate, right arm**
CC Exclusion see Appendix A PDX collection 0911
CC **M96.632 Fracture of radius or ulna following insertion of orthopedic implant, joint prosthesis, or bone plate, left arm**
CC Exclusion see Appendix A PDX collection 0911
CC **M96.639 Fracture of radius or ulna following insertion of orthopedic implant, joint prosthesis, or bone plate, unspecified arm**
CC Exclusion see Appendix A PDX collection 0911

CC **M96.65 Fracture of pelvis following insertion of orthopedic implant, joint prosthesis, or bone plate**
CC Exclusion see Appendix A PDX collection 0911

\+ **M96.66 Fracture of femur following insertion of orthopedic implant, joint prosthesis, or bone plate**
CC **M96.661 Fracture of femur following insertion of orthopedic implant, joint prosthesis, or bone plate, right leg**
CC Exclusion see Appendix A PDX collection 0911
CC **M96.662 Fracture of femur following insertion of orthopedic implant, joint prosthesis, or bone plate, left leg**
CC Exclusion see Appendix A PDX collection 0911
CC **M96.669 Fracture of femur following insertion of orthopedic implant, joint prosthesis, or bone plate, unspecified leg**
CC Exclusion see Appendix A PDX collection 0911

\+ **M96.67 Fracture of tibia or fibula following insertion of orthopedic implant, joint prosthesis, or bone plate**
CC **M96.671 Fracture of tibia or fibula following insertion of orthopedic implant, joint prosthesis, or bone plate, right leg**
CC Exclusion see Appendix A PDX collection 0911
CC **M96.672 Fracture of tibia or fibula following insertion of orthopedic implant, joint prosthesis, or bone plate, left leg**
CC Exclusion see Appendix A PDX collection 0911
CC **M96.679 Fracture of tibia or fibula following insertion of orthopedic implant, joint prosthesis, or bone plate, unspecified leg**
CC Exclusion see Appendix A PDX collection 0911

CC **M96.69 Fracture of other bone following insertion of orthopedic implant, joint prosthesis, or bone plate**
CC Exclusion see Appendix A PDX collection 0911

\+ **M96.8 Other intraoperative and postprocedural complications and disorders of musculoskeletal system, not elsewhere classified**
AHA CC: 4Q, 2016, 9-10

\+ **M96.81 Intraoperative hemorrhage and hematoma of a musculoskeletal structure complicating a procedure**
Excludes1: *intraoperative hemorrhage and hematoma of a musculoskeletal structure due to accidental puncture and laceration during a procedure (M96.82)*
CC **M96.810 Intraoperative hemorrhage and hematoma of a musculoskeletal structure complicating a musculoskeletal system procedure**
CC Exclusion see Appendix A PDX collection 0912
CC **M96.811 Intraoperative hemorrhage and hematoma of a musculoskeletal structure complicating other procedure**
CC Exclusion see Appendix A PDX collection 0912

\+ **M96.82 Accidental puncture and laceration of a musculoskeletal structure during a procedure**
CC **M96.820 Accidental puncture and laceration of a musculoskeletal structure during a musculoskeletal system procedure**
CC Exclusion see Appendix A PDX collection 0509
CC **M96.821 Accidental puncture and laceration of a musculoskeletal structure during other procedure**
CC Exclusion see Appendix A PDX collection 0509

+ **M96.83 Postprocedural hemorrhage of a musculoskeletal structure following a procedure**
  - CC **M96.830 Postprocedural hemorrhage of a musculoskeletal structure following a musculoskeletal system procedure**
    CC Exclusion see Appendix A PDX collection 0912
  - CC **M96.831 Postprocedural hemorrhage of a musculoskeletal structure following other procedure**
    CC Exclusion see Appendix A PDX collection 0912

+ **M96.84 Postprocedural hematoma and seroma of a musculoskeletal structure following a procedure**
  - CC **M96.840 Postprocedural hematoma of a musculoskeletal structure following a musculoskeletal system procedure**
    CC Exclusion see Appendix A PDX collection 0912
  - CC **M96.841 Postprocedural hematoma of a musculoskeletal structure following other procedure**
    CC Exclusion see Appendix A PDX collection 0912
    AHA CC: 4Q, 2016, 9-10
  - CC **M96.842 Postprocedural seroma of a musculoskeletal structure following a musculoskeletal system procedure**
    CC Exclusion see Appendix A PDX collection 0912
  - CC **M96.843 Postprocedural seroma of a musculoskeletal structure following other procedure**
    CC Exclusion see Appendix A PDX collection 0912

+ CC **M96.89 Other intraoperative and postprocedural complications and disorders of the musculoskeletal system**
  Instability of joint secondary to removal of joint prosthesis
  Use additional code, if applicable, to further specify disorder
  CC Exclusion see Appendix A PDX collection 0643

Periprosthetic fracture around internal prosthetic joint (M97)

M97 Periprosthetic fracture around internal prosthetic joint

Excludes2: *fracture of bone following insertion of orthopedic implant, joint prosthesis or bone plate (M96.6-)*
breakage (fracture) of prosthetic joint (T84.01-)
AHA CC: 4Q, 2016, 42-43

The appropriate 7th character is to be added to each code from category M97:
A initial encounter
D subsequent encounter
S sequela

+ **M97.0 Periprosthetic fracture around internal prosthetic hip joint**
  - CC X+7th **M97.01 Periprosthetic fracture around internal prosthetic right hip joint**
    CC Exclusion 7th character A see Appendix A PDX collection 0911
    AHA CC: 4Q, 2016, 42-43
  - CC X+7th **M97.02 Periprosthetic fracture around internal prosthetic left hip joint**
    CC Exclusion 7th character A see Appendix A PDX collection 0911

+ **M97.1 Periprosthetic fracture around internal prosthetic knee joint**
  - CC X+7th **M97.11 Periprosthetic fracture around internal prosthetic right knee joint**
    CC Exclusion 7th character A see Appendix A PDX collection 0911
  - CC X+7th **M97.12 Periprosthetic fracture around internal prosthetic left knee joint**
    CC Exclusion 7th character A see Appendix A PDX collection 0911

+ **M97.2 Periprosthetic fracture around internal prosthetic ankle joint**
  - CC X+7th **M97.21 Periprosthetic fracture around internal prosthetic right ankle joint**
    CC Exclusion 7th character A see Appendix A PDX collection 0911
  - CC X+7th **M97.22 Periprosthetic fracture around internal prosthetic left ankle joint**
    CC Exclusion 7th character A see Appendix A PDX collection 0911

+ **M97.3 Periprosthetic fracture around internal prosthetic shoulder joint**
  - CC X+7th **M97.31 Periprosthetic fracture around internal prosthetic right shoulder joint**
    CC Exclusion 7th character A see Appendix A PDX collection 0911
  - CC X+7th **M97.32 Periprosthetic fracture around internal prosthetic left shoulder joint**
    CC Exclusion 7th character A see Appendix A PDX collection 0911

+ **M97.4 Periprosthetic fracture around internal prosthetic elbow joint**
  - CC X+7th **M97.41 Periprosthetic fracture around internal prosthetic right elbow joint**
    CC Exclusion 7th character A see Appendix A PDX collection 0911
  - CC X+7th **M97.42 Periprosthetic fracture around internal prosthetic left elbow joint**
    CC Exclusion 7th character A see Appendix A PDX collection 0911

CC X+7th **M97.8 Periprosthetic fracture around other internal prosthetic joint**
Periprosthetic fracture around internal prosthetic finger joint
Periprosthetic fracture around internal prosthetic spinal joint
Periprosthetic fracture around internal prosthetic toe joint
Periprosthetic fracture around internal prosthetic wrist joint
Use additional code to identify the joint (Z96.6-)
CC Exclusion 7th character A see Appendix A PDX collection 0911

CC X+7th **M97.9 Periprosthetic fracture around unspecified internal prosthetic joint**
CC Exclusion 7th character A see Appendix A PDX collection 0911

Biomechanical lesions, not elsewhere classified (M99)

M99 Biomechanical lesions, not elsewhere classified

NOTE This category should not be used if the condition can be classified elsewhere.

+ **M99.0 Segmental and somatic dysfunction**
  - **M99.00 Segmental and somatic dysfunction of head region**
  - **M99.01 Segmental and somatic dysfunction of cervical region**
  - **M99.02 Segmental and somatic dysfunction of thoracic region**
  - **M99.03 Segmental and somatic dysfunction of lumbar regio**
  - **M99.04 Segmental and somatic dysfunction of sacral region**
  - **M99.05 Segmental and somatic dysfunction of pelvic region**
  - **M99.06 Segmental and somatic dysfunction of lower extremity**
  - **M99.07 Segmental and somatic dysfunction of upper extremity**
  - **M99.08 Segmental and somatic dysfunction of rib cage**
  - **M99.09 Segmental and somatic dysfunction of abdomen and other regions**

+ **M99.1 Subluxation complex (vertebral)**
  - CC **M99.10 Subluxation complex (vertebral) of head region**
    CC Exclusion see Appendix A PDX collection 0913
    HAC see Appendix B for HAC conditional logic
  - CC **M99.11 Subluxation complex (vertebral) of cervical region**
    CC Exclusion see Appendix A PDX collection 0913
    HAC see Appendix B for HAC conditional logic
  - **M99.12 Subluxation complex (vertebral) of thoracic region**
  - **M99.13 Subluxation complex (vertebral) of lumbar region**
  - **M99.14 Subluxation complex (vertebral) of sacral region**
  - **M99.15 Subluxation complex (vertebral) of pelvic region**
  - **M99.16 Subluxation complex (vertebral) of lower extremity**
  - **M99.17 Subluxation complex (vertebral) of upper extremity**
  - CC **M99.18 Subluxation complex (vertebral) of rib cage**
    CC Exclusion see Appendix A PDX collection 0914
    HAC see Appendix B for HAC conditional logic
  - **M99.19 Subluxation complex (vertebral) of abdomen and other regions**

+ **M99.2 Subluxation stenosis of neural canal**
  - **M99.20 Subluxation stenosis of neural canal of head region**
  - **M99.21 Subluxation stenosis of neural canal of cervical region**
  - **M99.22 Subluxation stenosis of neural canal of thoracic regi**
  - **M99.23 Subluxation stenosis of neural canal of lumbar regi**
  - **M99.24 Subluxation stenosis of neural canal of sacral regio**
  - **M99.25 Subluxation stenosis of neural canal of pelvic regio**
  - **M99.26 Subluxation stenosis of neural canal of lower extremity**
  - **M99.27 Subluxation stenosis of neural canal of upper extremity**

M99.28 Subluxation stenosis of neural canal of rib cage
M99.29 Subluxation stenosis of neural canal of abdomen and other regions

+ M99.3 Osseous stenosis of neural canal
M99.30 Osseous stenosis of neural canal of head region
M99.31 Osseous stenosis of neural canal of cervical region
M99.32 Osseous stenosis of neural canal of thoracic region
M99.33 Osseous stenosis of neural canal of lumbar region
M99.34 Osseous stenosis of neural canal of sacral region
M99.35 Osseous stenosis of neural canal of pelvic region
M99.36 Osseous stenosis of neural canal of lower extremity
M99.37 Osseous stenosis of neural canal of upper extremity
M99.38 Osseous stenosis of neural canal of rib cage
M99.39 Osseous stenosis of neural canal of abdomen and other regions

+ M99.4 Connective tissue stenosis of neural canal
M99.40 Connective tissue stenosis of neural canal of head region
M99.41 Connective tissue stenosis of neural canal of cervical region
M99.42 Connective tissue stenosis of neural canal of thoracic region
M99.43 Connective tissue stenosis of neural canal of lumbar region
M99.44 Connective tissue stenosis of neural canal of sacral region
M99.45 Connective tissue stenosis of neural canal of pelvic region
M99.46 Connective tissue stenosis of neural canal of lower extremity
M99.47 Connective tissue stenosis of neural canal of upper extremity
M99.48 Connective tissue stenosis of neural canal of rib cage
M99.49 Connective tissue stenosis of neural canal of abdomen and other regions

+ M99.5 Intervertebral disc stenosis of neural canal
M99.50 Intervertebral disc stenosis of neural canal of head region
M99.51 Intervertebral disc stenosis of neural canal of cervical region
M99.52 Intervertebral disc stenosis of neural canal of thoracic region
M99.53 Intervertebral disc stenosis of neural canal of lumbar region
M99.54 Intervertebral disc stenosis of neural canal of sacral region
M99.55 Intervertebral disc stenosis of neural canal of pelvic region
M99.56 Intervertebral disc stenosis of neural canal of lower extremity
M99.57 Intervertebral disc stenosis of neural canal of upper extremity
M99.58 Intervertebral disc stenosis of neural canal of rib cage
M99.59 Intervertebral disc stenosis of neural canal of abdomen and other regions

+ M99.6 Osseous and subluxation stenosis of intervertebral foramina
M99.60 Osseous and subluxation stenosis of intervertebral foramina of head region
M99.61 Osseous and subluxation stenosis of intervertebral foramina of cervical region
M99.62 Osseous and subluxation stenosis of intervertebral foramina of thoracic region
M99.63 Osseous and subluxation stenosis of intervertebral foramina of lumbar region
M99.64 Osseous and subluxation stenosis of intervertebral foramina of sacral region
M99.65 Osseous and subluxation stenosis of intervertebral foramina of pelvic region
M99.66 Osseous and subluxation stenosis of intervertebral foramina of lower extremity
M99.67 Osseous and subluxation stenosis of intervertebral foramina of upper extremity
M99.68 Osseous and subluxation stenosis of intervertebral foramina of rib cage
M99.69 Osseous and subluxation stenosis of intervertebral foramina of abdomen and other regions

+ M99.7 Connective tissue and disc stenosis of intervertebral foramina
M99.70 Connective tissue and disc stenosis of intervertebral foramina of head region
M99.71 Connective tissue and disc stenosis of intervertebral foramina of cervical region
M99.72 Connective tissue and disc stenosis of intervertebral foramina of thoracic region
M99.73 Connective tissue and disc stenosis of intervertebral foramina of lumbar region
M99.74 Connective tissue and disc stenosis of intervertebral foramina of sacral region
M99.75 Connective tissue and disc stenosis of intervertebral foramina of pelvic region
M99.76 Connective tissue and disc stenosis of intervertebral foramina of lower extremity
M99.77 Connective tissue and disc stenosis of intervertebral foramina of upper extremity
M99.78 Connective tissue and disc stenosis of intervertebral foramina of rib cage
M99.79 Connective tissue and disc stenosis of intervertebral foramina of abdomen and other regions

+ M99.8 Other biomechanical lesions
M99.80 Other biomechanical lesions of head region
M99.81 Other biomechanical lesions of cervical region
M99.82 Other biomechanical lesions of thoracic region
M99.83 Other biomechanical lesions of lumbar region
M99.84 Other biomechanical lesions of sacral region
M99.85 Other biomechanical lesions of pelvic region
M99.86 Other biomechanical lesions of lower extremity
M99.87 Other biomechanical lesions of upper extremity
M99.88 Other biomechanical lesions of rib cage
M99.89 Other biomechanical lesions of abdomen and other regions

M99.9 Biomechanical lesion, unspecified

Chapter 14: Diseases of the Genitourinary System (N00-N99)

Excludes2: *certain conditions originating in the perinatal period (P04-P96)*
certain infectious and parasitic diseases (A00-B99)
complications of pregnancy, childbirth and the puerperium (O00-O9A)
congenital malformations, deformations and chromosomal abnormalities (Q00-Q99)
endocrine, nutritional and metabolic diseases (E00-E88)
injury, poisoning and certain other consequences of external causes (S00-T88)
neoplasms (C00-D49)
symptoms, signs and abnormal clinical and laboratory findings, not elsewhere classified (R00-R94)

This chapter contains the following category blocks:

- N00-N08 Glomerular diseases
- N10-N16 Renal tubulo-interstitial diseases
- N17-N19 Acute kidney failure and chronic kidney disease
- N20-N23 Urolithiasis
- N25-N29 Other disorders of kidney and ureter
- N30-N39 Other diseases of the urinary system
- N40-N53 Diseases of male genital organs
- N60-N65 Disorders of breast
- N70-N77 Inflammatory diseases of female pelvic organs
- N80-N98 Noninflammatory disorders of female genital tract
- N99 Intraoperative and postprocedural complications and disorders of genitourinary system, not elsewhere classified

C. Chapter-Specific Coding Guidelines

In addition to general coding guidelines, there are guidelines for specific diagnoses and/or conditions in the classification. Unless otherwise indicated, these guidelines apply to all health care settings. Please refer to Section II for guidelines on th selection of principal diagnosis.

14. Chapter 14: Diseases of the Genitourinary System (N00-N99)

a. Chronic kidney disease

1) Stages of chronic kidney disease (CKD)

The ICD-10-CM classifies CKD based on severity. The severity of CKD i designated by stages 1-5. Stage 2, code N18.2, equates to mild CKD; stag 3, code N18.3, equates to moderate CKD; and stage 4, code N18.4, equate to severe CKD. Code N18.6, End stage renal disease (ESRD), is assigne when the provider has documented end-stage-renal disease (ESRD).

If both a stage of CKD and ESRD are documented, assign code N18.6 onl

2) Chronic kidney disease and kidney transplant status

Patients who have undergone kidney transplant may still have some for of chronic kidney disease (CKD) because the kidney transplant may n fully restore kidney function. Therefore, the presence of CKD alone doe not constitute a transplant complication. Assign the appropriate N18 coc for the patient's stage of CKD and code Z94.0, Kidney transplant statu If a transplant complication such as failure or rejection or other transpla complication is documented, see section I.C.19.g for information on codin complications of a kidney transplant. If the documentation is unclear as t whether the patient has a complication of the transplant, query the provide

3) Chronic kidney disease with other conditions

Patients with CKD may also suffer from other serious conditions, mo commonly diabetes mellitus and hypertension. The sequencing of th CKD code in relationship to codes for other contributing conditions based on the conventions in the Tabular List.

See I.C.9. Hypertensive chronic kidney disease.

See I.C.19. Chronic kidney disease and kidney transplant complications.

Urinary System

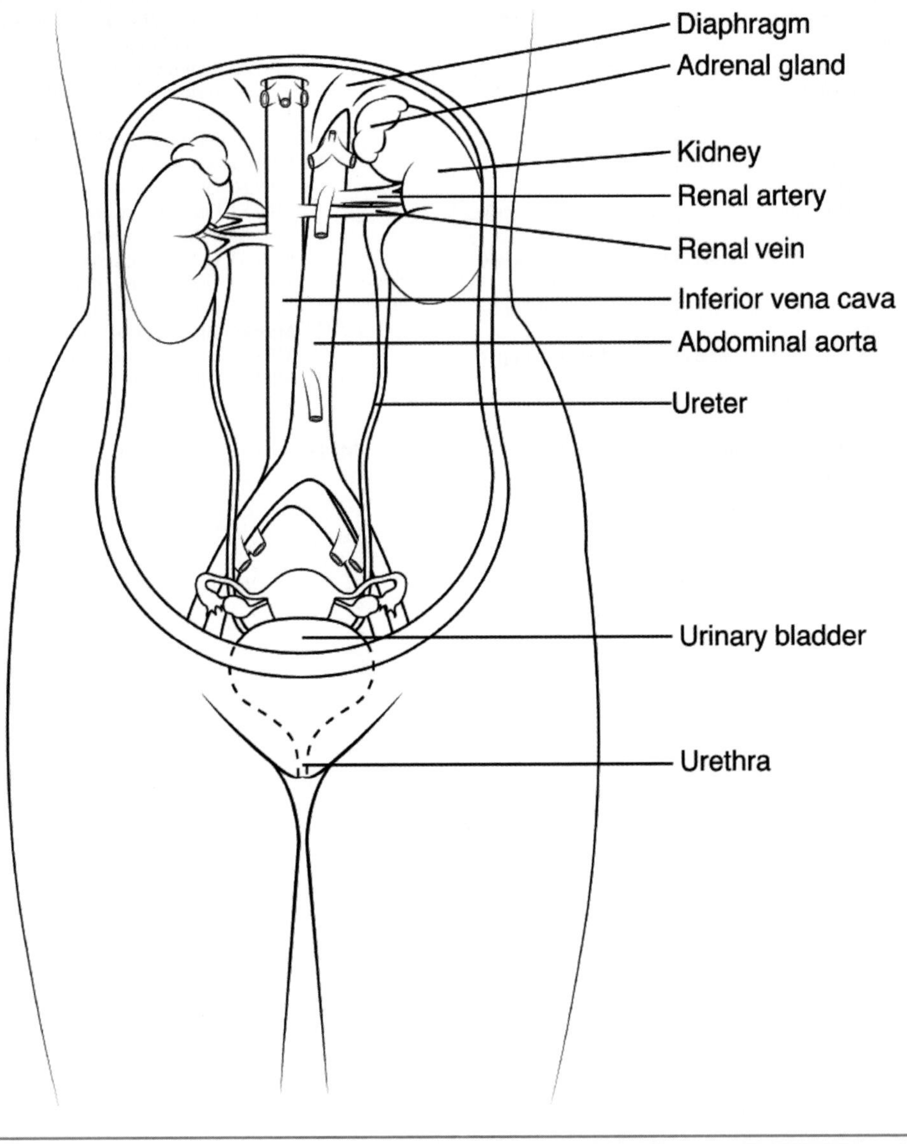

Kidney

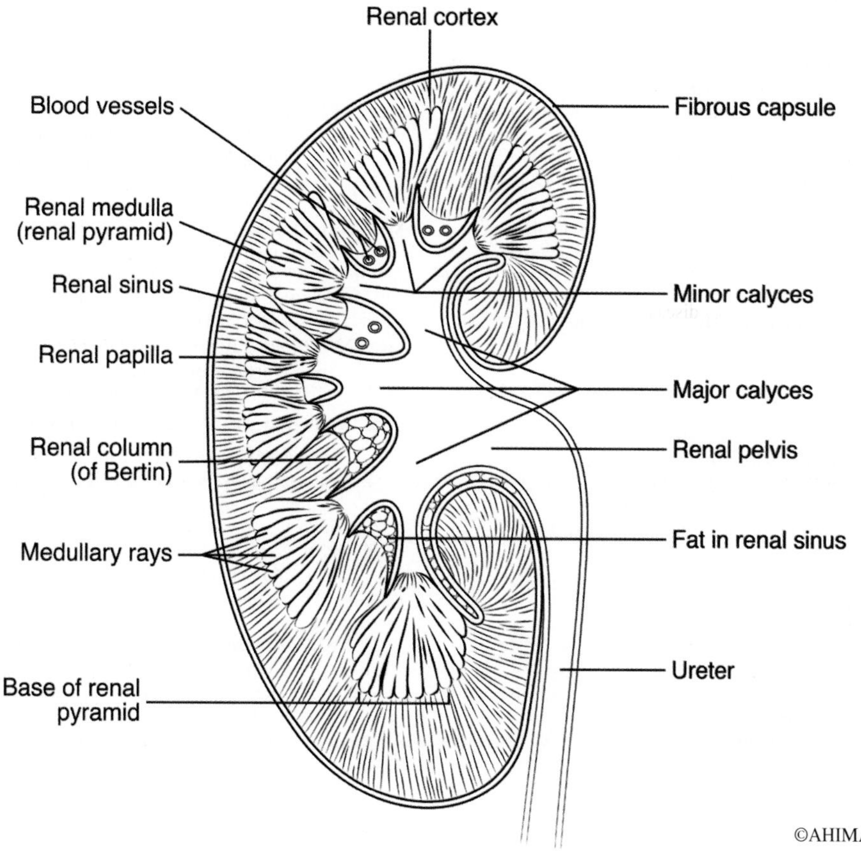

Renal cortex
Blood vessels
Fibrous capsule
Renal medulla
(renal pyramid)
Renal sinus
Minor calyces
Renal papilla
Major calyces
Renal column
(of Bertin)
Renal pelvis
Medullary rays
Fat in renal sinus
Ureter
Base of renal
pyramid

©AHIMA

Lower Urinary Tract

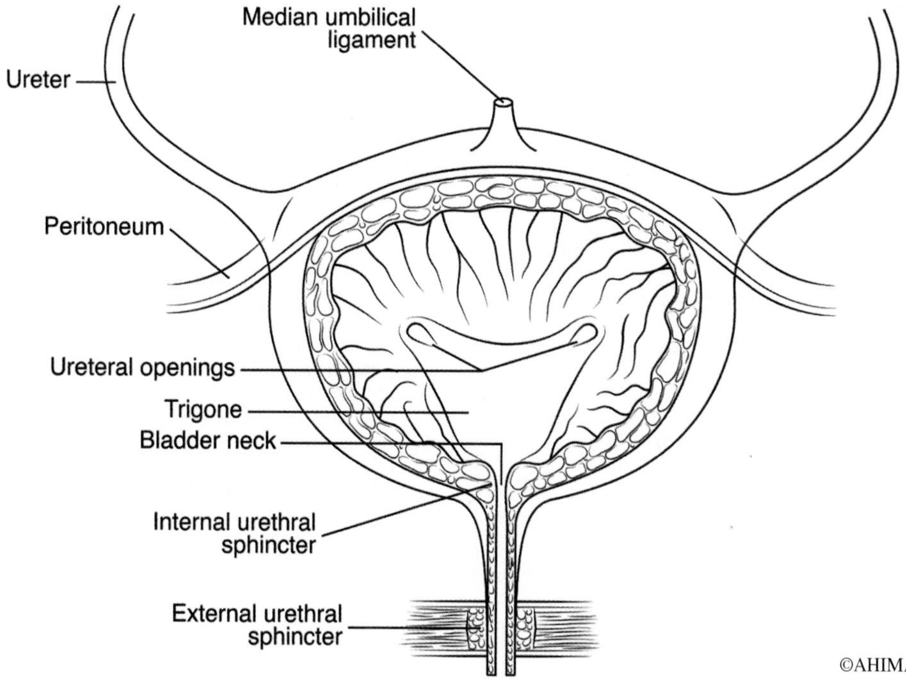

Median umbilical
ligament
Ureter
Peritoneum
Ureteral openings
Trigone
Bladder neck
Internal urethral
sphincter
External urethral
sphincter

©AHIMA

Glomerular diseases (N00-N08)

Code also any associated kidney failure (N17-N19)

Excludes1: *hypertensive chronic kidney disease (I12.-)*

N00 Acute nephritic syndrome

Includes: acute glomerular disease
acute glomerulonephritis
acute nephritis

Excludes1: *acute tubulo-interstitial nephritis (N10)*
nephritic syndrome NOS (N05.-)

MCC **N00.0 Acute nephritic syndrome with minor glomerular abnormality**
Acute nephritic syndrome with minimal change lesion
MCC Exclusion see Appendix A PDX collection 0915

MCC **N00.1 Acute nephritic syndrome with focal and segmental glomerular lesions**
Acute nephritic syndrome with focal and segmental hyalinosis
Acute nephritic syndrome with focal and segmental sclerosis
Acute nephritic syndrome with focal glomerulonephritis
MCC Exclusion see Appendix A PDX collection 0915

MCC **N00.2 Acute nephritic syndrome with diffuse membranous glomerulonephritis**
MCC Exclusion see Appendix A PDX collection 0915

MCC **N00.3 Acute nephritic syndrome with diffuse mesangial proliferative glomerulonephritis**
MCC Exclusion see Appendix A PDX collection 0915

MCC **N00.4 Acute nephritic syndrome with diffuse endocapillary proliferative glomerulonephritis**
MCC Exclusion see Appendix A PDX collection 0915

MCC **N00.5 Acute nephritic syndrome with diffuse mesangiocapillary glomerulonephritis**
Acute nephritic syndrome with membranoproliferative glomerulonephritis, types 1 and 3, or NOS
MCC Exclusion see Appendix A PDX collection 0915

MCC **N00.6 Acute nephritic syndrome with dense deposit disease**
Acute nephritic syndrome with membranoproliferative glomerulonephritis, type 2
MCC Exclusion see Appendix A PDX collection 0915

MCC **N00.7 Acute nephritic syndrome with diffuse crescentic glomerulonephritis**
Acute nephritic syndrome with extracapillary glomerulonephritis
MCC Exclusion see Appendix A PDX collection 0915

MCC **N00.8 Acute nephritic syndrome with other morphologic changes**
Acute nephritic syndrome with proliferative glomerulonephritis NOS
MCC Exclusion see Appendix A PDX collection 0916

MCC **N00.9 Acute nephritic syndrome with unspecified morphologic changes**
MCC Exclusion see Appendix A PDX collection 0915

N01 Rapidly progressive nephritic syndrome

Includes: rapidly progressive glomerular disease
rapidly progressive glomerulonephritis
rapidly progressive nephritis

Excludes1: *nephritic syndrome NOS (N05.-)*

MCC **N01.0 Rapidly progressive nephritic syndrome with minor glomerular abnormality**
Rapidly progressive nephritic syndrome with minimal change lesion
MCC Exclusion see Appendix A PDX collection 0915

MCC **N01.1 Rapidly progressive nephritic syndrome with focal and segmental glomerular lesions**
Rapidly progressive nephritic syndrome with focal and segmental hyalinosis
Rapidly progressive nephritic syndrome with focal and segmental sclerosis
Rapidly progressive nephritic syndrome with focal glomerulonephritis
MCC Exclusion see Appendix A PDX collection 0915

MCC **N01.2 Rapidly progressive nephritic syndrome with diffuse membranous glomerulonephritis**
MCC Exclusion see Appendix A PDX collection 0915

MCC **N01.3 Rapidly progressive nephritic syndrome with diffuse mesangial proliferative glomerulonephritis**
MCC Exclusion see Appendix A PDX collection 0915

MCC **N01.4 Rapidly progressive nephritic syndrome with diffuse endocapillary proliferative glomerulonephritis**
MCC Exclusion see Appendix A PDX collection 0915

MCC **N01.5 Rapidly progressive nephritic syndrome with diffuse mesangiocapillary glomerulonephritis**
Rapidly progressive nephritic syndrome with membranoproliferative glomerulonephritis, types 1 and 3, or NOS
MCC Exclusion see Appendix A PDX collection 0915

MCC **N01.6 Rapidly progressive nephritic syndrome with dense deposit disease**
Rapidly progressive nephritic syndrome with membranoproliferative glomerulonephritis, type 2
MCC Exclusion see Appendix A PDX collection 0915

MCC **N01.7 Rapidly progressive nephritic syndrome with diffuse crescentic glomerulonephritis**
Rapidly progressive nephritic syndrome with extracapillary glomerulonephritis
MCC Exclusion see Appendix A PDX collection 0915

MCC **N01.8 Rapidly progressive nephritic syndrome with other morphologic changes**
Rapidly progressive nephritic syndrome with proliferative glomerulonephritis NOS
MCC Exclusion see Appendix A PDX collection 0915

MCC **N01.9 Rapidly progressive nephritic syndrome with unspecified morphologic changes**
MCC Exclusion see Appendix A PDX collection 0915

N02 Recurrent and persistent hematuria

Excludes1: *acute cystitis with hematuria (N30.01)*
hematuria NOS (R31.9)
hematuria not associated with specified morphologic lesions (R31.-)

CC **N02.0 Recurrent and persistent hematuria with minor glomerular abnormality**
Recurrent and persistent hematuria with minimal change lesion
CC Exclusion see Appendix A PDX collection 0917

CC **N02.1 Recurrent and persistent hematuria with focal and segmental glomerular lesions**
Recurrent and persistent hematuria with focal and segmental hyalinosis
Recurrent and persistent hematuria with focal and segmental sclerosis
Recurrent and persistent hematuria with focal glomerulonephritis
CC Exclusion see Appendix A PDX collection 0917

CC **N02.2 Recurrent and persistent hematuria with diffuse membranous glomerulonephritis**
CC Exclusion see Appendix A PDX collection 0917

CC **N02.3 Recurrent and persistent hematuria with diffuse mesangial proliferative glomerulonephritis**
CC Exclusion see Appendix A PDX collection 0917

CC **N02.4 Recurrent and persistent hematuria with diffuse endocapillary proliferative glomerulonephritis**
CC Exclusion see Appendix A PDX collection 0917

CC **N02.5 Recurrent and persistent hematuria with diffuse mesangiocapillary glomerulonephritis**
Recurrent and persistent hematuria with membranoproliferative glomerulonephritis, types 1 and 3, or NOS
CC Exclusion see Appendix A PDX collection 0917

CC **N02.6 Recurrent and persistent hematuria with dense deposit disease**
Recurrent and persistent hematuria with membranoproliferative glomerulonephritis, type 2
CC Exclusion see Appendix A PDX collection 0917

CC **N02.7 Recurrent and persistent hematuria with diffuse crescentic glomerulonephritis**
Recurrent and persistent hematuria with extracapillary glomerulonephritis
CC Exclusion see Appendix A PDX collection 0917

CC **N02.8 Recurrent and persistent hematuria with other morphologic changes**
Recurrent and persistent hematuria with proliferative glomerulonephritis NOS
CC Exclusion see Appendix A PDX collection 0915

CC **N02.9 Recurrent and persistent hematuria with unspecified morphologic changes**
CC Exclusion see Appendix A PDX collection 0915
AHA CC: 2Q, 2017, 5

N03 Chronic nephritic syndrome

Includes: chronic glomerular disease
chronic glomerulonephritis
chronic nephritis

Excludes1: *chronic tubulo-interstitial nephritis (N11.-)*
diffuse sclerosing glomerulonephritis (N05.8-)
nephritic syndrome NOS (N05.-)

CC **N03.0 Chronic nephritic syndrome with minor glomerular abnormality**
Chronic nephritic syndrome with minimal change lesion
CC Exclusion see Appendix A PDX collection 0918

CC **N03.1 Chronic nephritic syndrome with focal and segmental glomerular lesions**
Chronic nephritic syndrome with focal and segmental hyalinosis
Chronic nephritic syndrome with focal and segmental sclerosis
Chronic nephritic syndrome with focal glomerulonephritis
CC Exclusion see Appendix A PDX collection 0918

CC **N03.2 Chronic nephritic syndrome with diffuse membranous glomerulonephritis**
CC Exclusion see Appendix A PDX collection 0918

CC **N03.3 Chronic nephritic syndrome with diffuse mesangial proliferative glomerulonephritis**
CC Exclusion see Appendix A PDX collection 0918

CC **N03.4 Chronic nephritic syndrome with diffuse endocapillary proliferative glomerulonephritis**
CC Exclusion see Appendix A PDX collection 0918

CC **N03.5 Chronic nephritic syndrome with diffuse mesangiocapillary glomerulonephritis**
Chronic nephritic syndrome with membranoproliferative glomerulonephritis, types 1 and 3, or NOS
CC Exclusion see Appendix A PDX collection 0918

CC **N03.6 Chronic nephritic syndrome with dense deposit disease**
Chronic nephritic syndrome with membranoproliferative glomerulonephritis, type 2
CC Exclusion see Appendix A PDX collection 0918

CC **N03.7 Chronic nephritic syndrome with diffuse crescentic glomerulonephritis**
Chronic nephritic syndrome with extracapillary glomerulonephritis
CC Exclusion see Appendix A PDX collection 0918

CC **N03.8 Chronic nephritic syndrome with other morphologic changes**
Chronic nephritic syndrome with proliferative glomerulonephritis NOS
CC Exclusion see Appendix A PDX collection 0918

CC **N03.9 Chronic nephritic syndrome with unspecified morphologic changes**
CC Exclusion see Appendix A PDX collection 0918

N04 Nephrotic syndrome

Includes: congenital nephrotic syndrome
lipoid nephrosis

CC **N04.0 Nephrotic syndrome with minor glomerular abnormality**
Nephrotic syndrome with minimal change lesion
CC Exclusion see Appendix A PDX collection 0917

CC **N04.1 Nephrotic syndrome with focal and segmental glomerular lesions**
Nephrotic syndrome with focal and segmental hyalinosis
Nephrotic syndrome with focal and segmental sclerosis
Nephrotic syndrome with focal glomerulonephritis
CC Exclusion see Appendix A PDX collection 0917

CC **N04.2 Nephrotic syndrome with diffuse membranous glomerulonephritis**
CC Exclusion see Appendix A PDX collection 0917

CC **N04.3 Nephrotic syndrome with diffuse mesangial proliferative glomerulonephritis**
CC Exclusion see Appendix A PDX collection 0917

CC **N04.4 Nephrotic syndrome with diffuse endocapillary proliferative glomerulonephritis**
CC Exclusion see Appendix A PDX collection 0917

CC **N04.5 Nephrotic syndrome with diffuse mesangiocapillary glomerulonephritis**
Nephrotic syndrome with membranoproliferative glomerulonephritis, types 1 and 3, or NOS
CC Exclusion see Appendix A PDX collection 0917

CC **N04.6 Nephrotic syndrome with dense deposit disease**
Nephrotic syndrome with membranoproliferative glomerulonephritis, type 2
CC Exclusion see Appendix A PDX collection 0917

CC **N04.7 Nephrotic syndrome with diffuse crescentic glomerulonephritis**
Nephrotic syndrome with extracapillary glomerulonephritis
CC Exclusion see Appendix A PDX collection 0915

CC **N04.8 Nephrotic syndrome with other morphologic changes**
Nephrotic syndrome with proliferative glomerulonephritis NOS
CC Exclusion see Appendix A PDX collection 0915

CC **N04.9 Nephrotic syndrome with unspecified morphologic changes**
CC Exclusion see Appendix A PDX collection 0915

N05 Unspecified nephritic syndrome

Includes: glomerular disease NOS
glomerulonephritis NOS
nephritis NOS
nephropathy NOS and renal disease NOS with morphological lesion specified in .0-.8

Excludes1: *nephropathy NOS with no stated morphological lesion (N28.9)*
renal disease NOS with no stated morphological lesion (N28.9)
tubulo-interstitial nephritis NOS (N12)

N05.0 Unspecified nephritic syndrome with minor glomerular abnormality
Unspecified nephritic syndrome with minimal change lesion

N05.1 Unspecified nephritic syndrome with focal and segmental glomerular lesions
Unspecified nephritic syndrome with focal and segmental hyalinosis
Unspecified nephritic syndrome with focal and segmental sclerosis
Unspecified nephritic syndrome with focal glomerulonephritis

CC **N05.2 Unspecified nephritic syndrome with diffuse membranous glomerulonephritis**
CC Exclusion see Appendix A PDX collection 0918

CC **N05.3 Unspecified nephritic syndrome with diffuse mesangial proliferative glomerulonephritis**
CC Exclusion see Appendix A PDX collection 0918

CC **N05.4 Unspecified nephritic syndrome with diffuse endocapillary proliferative glomerulonephritis**
CC Exclusion see Appendix A PDX collection 0918

CC **N05.5 Unspecified nephritic syndrome with diffuse mesangiocapillary glomerulonephritis**
Unspecified nephritic syndrome with membranoproliferative glomerulonephritis, types 1 and 3, or NOS
CC Exclusion see Appendix A PDX collection 0918

N05.6 Unspecified nephritic syndrome with dense deposit disease
Unspecified nephritic syndrome with membranoproliferative glomerulonephritis, type 2

N05.7 Unspecified nephritic syndrome with diffuse crescentic glomerulonephritis
Unspecified nephritic syndrome with extracapillary glomerulonephritis

N05.8 Unspecified nephritic syndrome with other morphologic changes
Unspecified nephritic syndrome with proliferative glomerulonephritis NOS

N05.9 Unspecified nephritic syndrome with unspecified morphologic changes

N06 Isolated proteinuria with specified morphological lesion

Excludes1: *Proteinuria not associated with specific morphologic lesions (R80.0)*

N06.0 Isolated proteinuria with minor glomerular abnormality
Isolated proteinuria with minimal change lesion

N06.1 Isolated proteinuria with focal and segmental glomerular lesions
Isolated proteinuria with focal and segmental hyalinosis
Isolated proteinuria with focal and segmental sclerosis
Isolated proteinuria with focal glomerulonephritis

CC **N06.2 Isolated proteinuria with diffuse membranous glomerulonephritis**
CC Exclusion see Appendix A PDX collection 0918

CC **N06.3 Isolated proteinuria with diffuse mesangial proliferative glomerulonephritis**
CC Exclusion see Appendix A PDX collection 0918

CC **N06.4 Isolated proteinuria with diffuse endocapillary proliferative glomerulonephritis**
CC Exclusion see Appendix A PDX collection 0918

CC **N06.5 Isolated proteinuria with diffuse mesangiocapillary glomerulonephritis**
Isolated proteinuria with membranoproliferative glomerulonephritis, types 1 and 3, or NOS
CC Exclusion see Appendix A PDX collection 0918

N06.6 Isolated proteinuria with dense deposit disease
Isolated proteinuria with membranoproliferative glomerulonephritis, type 2

N06.7 Isolated proteinuria with diffuse crescentic glomerulonephritis
Isolated proteinuria with extracapillary glomerulonephritis

N06.8 Isolated proteinuria with other morphologic lesion
Isolated proteinuria with proliferative glomerulonephritis NOS

N06.9 Isolated proteinuria with unspecified morphologic lesion

N07 Hereditary nephropathy, not elsewhere classified

Excludes2: *Alport's syndrome (Q87.81-)*
hereditary amyloid nephropathy (E85.-)
nail patella syndrome (Q87.2)
non-neuropathic heredofamilial amyloidosis (E85.-)

N07.0 Hereditary nephropathy, not elsewhere classified with minor glomerular abnormality
Hereditary nephropathy, not elsewhere classified with minimal change lesion

N07.1 Hereditary nephropathy, not elsewhere classified with focal and segmental glomerular lesions
Hereditary nephropathy, not elsewhere classified with focal and segmental hyalinosis
Hereditary nephropathy, not elsewhere classified with focal and segmental sclerosis
Hereditary nephropathy, not elsewhere classified with focal glomerulonephritis

CC **N07.2 Hereditary nephropathy, not elsewhere classified with diffuse membranous glomerulonephritis**
CC Exclusion see Appendix A PDX collection 0918

CC **N07.3 Hereditary nephropathy, not elsewhere classified with diffuse mesangial proliferative glomerulonephritis**
CC Exclusion see Appendix A PDX collection 0918

CC **N07.4 Hereditary nephropathy, not elsewhere classified with diffuse endocapillary proliferative glomerulonephritis**
CC Exclusion see Appendix A PDX collection 0918

CC **N07.5 Hereditary nephropathy, not elsewhere classified with diffuse mesangiocapillary glomerulonephritis**
Hereditary nephropathy, not elsewhere classified with membranoproliferative glomerulonephritis, types 1 and 3, or NOS
CC Exclusion see Appendix A PDX collection 0918

N07.6 Hereditary nephropathy, not elsewhere classified with dense deposit disease
Hereditary nephropathy, not elsewhere classified with membranoproliferative glomerulonephritis, type 2

N07.7 Hereditary nephropathy, not elsewhere classified with diffuse crescentic glomerulonephritis
Hereditary nephropathy, not elsewhere classified with extracapillary glomerulonephritis

N07.8 Hereditary nephropathy, not elsewhere classified with other morphologic lesions
Hereditary nephropathy, not elsewhere classified with proliferative glomerulonephritis NOS

N07.9 Hereditary nephropathy, not elsewhere classified with unspecified morphologic lesions

N08 Glomerular disorders in diseases classified elsewhere

Glomerulonephritis
Nephritis
Nephropathy
Code first underlying disease, such as:
amyloidosis (E85.-)
congenital syphilis (A50.5)
cryoglobulinemia (D89.1)
disseminated intravascular coagulation (D65)
gout (M1A.-, M10.-)
microscopic polyangiitis (M31.7)
multiple myeloma (C90.0-)
sepsis (A40.0-A41.9)
sickle-cell disease (D57.0-D57.8)

Excludes1: *glomerulonephritis, nephritis and nephropathy (in):*
antiglomerular basement membrane disease (M31.0)
diabetes (E08-E13 with .21)
gonococcal (A54.21)
Goodpasture's syndrome (M31.0)
hemolytic-uremic syndrome (D59.3)
lupus (M32.14)
mumps (B26.83)
syphilis (A52.75)
systemic lupus erythematosus (M32.14)
Wegener's granulomatosis (M31.31)
pyelonephritis in diseases classified elsewhere (N16)
renal tubulo-interstitial disorders classified elsewhere (N16)

Valid 3-character code, no further characters required

Renal tubulo-interstitial diseases (N10-N16)

Includes: pyelonephritis

Excludes1: *pyeloureteritis cystica (N28.85)*

CC **N10 Acute pyelonephritis**

Acute infectious interstitial nephritis
Acute pyelitis
Acute tubulo-interstitial nephritis
Hemoglobin nephrosis
Myoglobin nephrosis
Use additional code (B95-B97), to identify infectious agent
CC Exclusion see Appendix A PDX collection 0919
HAC see Appendix B for HAC conditional logic
Valid 3-character code, no further characters required

N11 Chronic tubulo-interstitial nephritis

Includes: chronic infectious interstitial nephritis
chronic pyelitis
chronic pyelonephritis
Use additional code (B95-B97), to identify infectious agent

N11.0 Nonobstructive reflux-associated chronic pyelonephritis
Pyelonephritis (chronic) associated with (vesicoureteral) reflux
Excludes1: *vesicoureteral reflux NOS (N13.70)*

CC **N11.1 Chronic obstructive pyelonephritis**
Pyelonephritis (chronic) associated with anomaly of pelviureteric junction
Pyelonephritis (chronic) associated with anomaly of pyeloureteric junction
Pyelonephritis (chronic) associated with crossing of vessel
Pyelonephritis (chronic) associated with kinking of ureter
Pyelonephritis (chronic) associated with obstruction of ureter
Pyelonephritis (chronic) associated with stricture of pelviureteric junction
Pyelonephritis (chronic) associated with stricture of ureter
Excludes1: *calculous pyelonephritis (N20.9)*
obstructive uropathy (N13.-)
CC Exclusion see Appendix A PDX collection 0920

CC **N11.8 Other chronic tubulo-interstitial nephritis**
Nonobstructive chronic pyelonephritis NOS
CC Exclusion see Appendix A PDX collection 0921

CC **N11.9 Chronic tubulo-interstitial nephritis, unspecified**
Chronic interstitial nephritis NOS
Chronic pyelitis NOS
Chronic pyelonephritis NOS
CC Exclusion see Appendix A PDX collection 0922
HAC see Appendix B for HAC conditional logic

CC **N12 Tubulo-interstitial nephritis, not specified as acute or chronic**

Interstitial nephritis NOS
Pyelitis NOS
Pyelonephritis NOS
Excludes1: *calculous pyelonephritis (N20.9)*
CC Exclusion see Appendix A PDX collection 0922
HAC see Appendix B for HAC conditional logic
Valid 3-character code, no further characters required

N13 Obstructive and reflux uropathy

Excludes2: *calculus of kidney and ureter without hydronephrosis (N20.-)*
congenital obstructive defects of renal pelvis and ureter (Q62.0-Q62.3)
hydronephrosis with ureteropelvic junction obstruction (Q62.11)
obstructive pyelonephritis (N11.1)

CC **N13.0 Hydronephrosis with ureteropelvic junction obstruction**
Hydronephrosis due to acquired occlusion of ureteropelvic junction
Excludes2: *Hydronephrosis with ureteropelvic junction obstruction due to calculus (N13.2)*
CC Exclusion see Appendix A PDX collection 0922
AHA CC: 4Q, 2016, 43

CC **N13.1 Hydronephrosis with ureteral stricture, not elsewhere classified**
Excludes1: *hydronephrosis with ureteral stricture with infection (N13.6)*
CC Exclusion see Appendix A PDX collection 0922

N13.2 Hydronephrosis with renal and ureteral calculous obstruction
Excludes1: *hydronephrosis with renal and ureteral calculous obstruction with infection (N13.6)*
CC Exclusion see Appendix A PDX collection 0922

\+ **N13.3 Other and unspecified hydronephrosis**
Excludes1: *hydronephrosis with infection (N13.6)*

CC **N13.30 Unspecified hydronephrosis**
CC Exclusion see Appendix A PDX collection 0922

CC **N13.39 Other hydronephrosis**
CC Exclusion see Appendix A PDX collection 0922

CC N13.4 **Hydroureter**
Excludes1: *congenital hydroureter (Q62.3-)*
hydroureter with infection (N13.6)
vesicoureteral-reflux with hydroureter (N13.73-)
CC Exclusion see Appendix A PDX collection 0923

N13.5 **Crossing vessel and stricture of ureter without hydronephrosis**
Kinking and stricture of ureter without hydronephrosis
Excludes1: *Crossing vessel and stricture of ureter without hydronephrosis with infection (N13.6)*

CC N13.6 **Pyonephrosis**
Conditions in N13.0-N13.5 with infection
Obstructive uropathy with infection
CC Exclusion see Appendix A PDX collection 0922
Use additional code (B95-B97), to identify infectious agent
HAC see Appendix B for HAC conditional logic

\+ N13.7 **Vesicoureteral-reflux**
Excludes1: *reflux-associated pyelonephritis (N11.0)*

N13.70 **Vesicoureteral-reflux, unspecified**
Vesicoureteral-reflux NOS

N13.71 **Vesicoureteral-reflux without reflux nephropathy**

\+ N13.72 **Vesicoureteral-reflux with reflux nephropathy without hydroureter**

N13.721 **Vesicoureteral-reflux with reflux nephropathy without hydroureter, unilateral**

N13.722 **Vesicoureteral-reflux with reflux nephropathy without hydroureter, bilateral**

N13.729 **Vesicoureteral-reflux with reflux nephropathy without hydroureter, unspecified**

\+ N13.73 **Vesicoureteral-reflux with reflux nephropathy with hydroureter**

N13.731 **Vesicoureteral-reflux with reflux nephropathy with hydroureter, unilateral**

N13.732 **Vesicoureteral-reflux with reflux nephropathy with hydroureter, bilateral**

N13.739 **Vesicoureteral-reflux with reflux nephropathy with hydroureter, unspecified**

CC N13.8 **Other obstructive and reflux uropathy**
Urinary tract obstruction due to specified cause
Code first, if applicable, any causal condition, such as:
enlarged prostate (N40.1)
CC Exclusion see Appendix A PDX collection 0920

N13.9 **Obstructive and reflux uropathy, unspecified**
Urinary tract obstruction NOS

N14 **Drug- and heavy-metal-induced tubulo-interstitial and tubular conditions**

Code first poisoning due to drug or toxin, if applicable (T36-T65 with fifth or sixth character 1-4 or 6)

Use additional code for adverse effect, if applicable, to identify drug (T36-T50 with fifth or sixth character 5)

N14.0 **Analgesic nephropathy**

N14.1 **Nephropathy induced by other drugs, medicaments and biological substances**

N14.2 **Nephropathy induced by unspecified drug, medicament or biological substance**

N14.3 **Nephropathy induced by heavy metals**

N14.4 **Toxic nephropathy, not elsewhere classified**

N15 **Other renal tubulo-interstitial diseases**

N15.0 **Balkan nephropathy**
Balkan endemic nephropathy

MCC N15.1 **Renal and perinephric abscess**
MCC Exclusion see Appendix A PDX collection 0919
HAC see Appendix B for HAC conditional logic

N15.8 **Other specified renal tubulo-interstitial diseases**

N15.9 **Renal tubulo-interstitial disease, unspecified**
Infection of kidney NOS
Excludes1: *urinary tract infection NOS (N39.0)*

N16 **Renal tubulo-interstitial disorders in diseases classified elsewhere**
Pyelonephritis
Tubulo-interstitial nephritis
Code first underlying disease, such as:
brucellosis (A23.0-A23.9)
cryoglobulinemia (D89.1)
glycogen storage disease (E74.0)
leukemia (C91-C95)
lymphoma (C81.0-C85.9, C96.0-C96.9)
multiple myeloma (C90.0-)
sepsis (A40.0-A41.9)
Wilson's disease (E83.0)
Excludes1: *diphtheritic pyelonephritis and tubulo-interstitial nephritis (A36.84)*
pyelonephritis and tubulo-interstitial nephritis in candidiasis (B37.49)
pyelonephritis and tubulo-interstitial nephritis in cystinosis (E72.04)
pyelonephritis and tubulo-interstitial nephritis in salmonella infection (A02.25)
pyelonephritis and tubulo-interstitial nephritis in sarcoidosis (D86.84)
pyelonephritis and tubulo-interstitial nephritis in sicca syndrome [Sjogren's] (M35.04)
pyelonephritis and tubulo-interstitial nephritis in systemic lupus erythematosus (M32.15)
pyelonephritis and tubulo-interstitial nephritis in toxoplasmosis (B58.83)
renal tubular degeneration in diabetes (E08-E13 with .29)
syphilitic pyelonephritis and tubulo-interstitial nephritis (A52.75)
Valid 3-character code, no further characters required

Acute kidney failure and chronic kidney disease (N17-N19)

Excludes2: *congenital renal failure (P96.0)*
drug- and heavy-metal-induced tubulo-interstitial and tubular conditions (N14.-)
extrarenal uremia (R39.2)
hemolytic-uremic syndrome (D59.3)
hepatorenal syndrome (K76.7)
postpartum hepatorenal syndrome (O90.4)
posttraumatic renal failure (T79.5)
prerenal uremia (R39.2)
renal failure complicating abortion or ectopic or molar pregnancy (O00-O07, O08.4)
renal failure following labor and delivery (O90.4)
renal failure postprocedural (N99.0)

N17 **Acute kidney failure**
Code also associated underlying condition
Excludes1: *posttraumatic renal failure (T79.5)*

MCC N17.0 **Acute kidney failure with tubular necrosis**
Acute tubular necrosis
Renal tubular necrosis
Tubular necrosis NOS
MCC Exclusion see Appendix A PDX collection 0924

MCC N17.1 **Acute kidney failure with acute cortical necrosis**
Acute cortical necrosis
Cortical necrosis NOS
Renal cortical necrosis
MCC Exclusion see Appendix A PDX collection 0924

N17.2 **Acute kidney failure with medullary necrosis**
Medullary [papillary] necrosis NOS
Acute medullary [papillary] necrosis
Renal medullary [papillary] necrosis
MCC Exclusion see Appendix A PDX collection 0924

CC N17.8 **Other acute kidney failure**
CC Exclusion see Appendix A PDX collection 0925

CC N17.9 **Acute kidney failure, unspecified**
Acute kidney injury (nontraumatic)
Excludes2: *traumatic kidney injury (S37.0-)*
CC Exclusion see Appendix A PDX collection 0924

N18 Chronic kidney disease (CKD)

Code first any associated:
diabetic chronic kidney disease (E08.22, E09.22, E10.22, E11.22, E13.22)
hypertensive chronic kidney disease (I12.-, I13.-)

Use additional code to identify kidney transplant status, if applicable, (Z94.0)

Review coding guidelines C.9.a.2 and C.9.a.3
Review coding guidelines C.14.a.1 and C.14.a.2

N18.1 Chronic kidney disease, stage 1
N18.2 Chronic kidney disease, stage 2 (mild)
N18.3 Chronic kidney disease, stage 3 (moderate)
CC **N18.4 Chronic kidney disease, stage 4 (severe)**
CC Exclusion see Appendix A PDX collection 0926
CC **N18.5 Chronic kidney disease, stage 5**
Excludes1: *chronic kidney disease, stage 5 requiring chronic dialysis (N18.6)*
CC Exclusion see Appendix A PDX collection 0926
MCC **N18.6 End stage renal disease**
Chronic kidney disease requiring chronic dialysis
Use additional code to identify dialysis status (Z99.2)
MCC Exclusion see Appendix A PDX collection 0927
AHA CC: 4Q, 2013, 125; 3Q, 2016, 22-23
N18.9 Chronic kidney disease, unspecified
Chronic renal disease
Chronic renal failure NOS
Chronic renal insufficiency
Chronic uremia NOS
Diffuse sclerosing glomerulonephritis NOS

N19 Unspecified kidney failure
Uremia NOS
Excludes1: *acute kidney failure (N17.-)*
chronic kidney disease (N18.-)
chronic uremia (N18.9)
extrarenal uremia (R39.2)
prerenal uremia (R39.2)
renal insufficiency (acute) (N28.9)
uremia of newborn (P96.0)
Valid 3-character code, no further characters required

Urolithiasis (N20-N23)

N20 Calculus of kidney and ureter
Calculous pyelonephritis
Excludes1: *nephrocalcinosis (E83.5)*
that with hydronephrosis (N13.2)
N20.0 Calculus of kidney
Nephrolithiasis NOS
Renal calculus
Renal stone
Staghorn calculus
Stone in kidney
AHA CC: 1Q, 2017, 5
CC **N20.1 Calculus of ureter**
Ureteric stone
CC Exclusion see Appendix A PDX collection 0928
AHA CC: 3Q, 2016, 23-24
CC **N20.2 Calculus of kidney with calculus of ureter**
CC Exclusion see Appendix A PDX collection 0928
AHA CC: 2Q, 2015, 8-9
N20.9 Urinary calculus, unspecified

N21 Calculus of lower urinary tract
Includes: calculus of lower urinary tract with cystitis and urethritis
N21.0 Calculus in bladder
Calculus in diverticulum of bladder
Urinary bladder stone
Excludes2: *staghorn calculus (N20.0)*
N21.1 Calculus in urethra
Excludes2: *calculus of prostate (N42.0)*
N21.8 Other lower urinary tract calculus
N21.9 Calculus of lower urinary tract, unspecified
Excludes1: *calculus of urinary tract NOS (N20.9)*

N22 Calculus of urinary tract in diseases classified elsewhere
Code first underlying disease, such as:
gout (M1A.-, M10.-)
schistosomiasis (B65.0-B65.9)
Valid 3-character code, no further characters required

N23 Unspecified renal colic
Valid 3-character code, no further characters required

Other disorders of kidney and ureter (N25-N29)

Excludes2: *disorders of kidney and ureter with urolithiasis (N20-N23)*

N25 Disorders resulting from impaired renal tubular function
N25.0 Renal osteodystrophy
Azotemic osteodystrophy
Phosphate-losing tubular disorders
Renal rickets
Renal short stature
Excludes2: metabolic disorders classifiable to E70-E88
CC **N25.1 Nephrogenic diabetes insipidus**
Excludes1: *diabetes insipidus NOS (E23.2)*
CC Exclusion see Appendix A PDX collection 0929
\+ **N25.8 Other disorders resulting from impaired renal tubular function**
CC **N25.81 Secondary hyperparathyroidism of renal origin**
Excludes1: *secondary hyperparathyroidism, non-renal (E21.1)*
CC Exclusion see Appendix A PDX collection 0930
Excludes2: *metabolic disorders classifiable to E70-E88*
N25.89 Other disorders resulting from impaired renal tubular function
Hypokalemic nephropathy
Lightwood-Albright syndrome
Renal tubular acidosis NOS
N25.9 Disorder resulting from impaired renal tubular function, unspecified

N26 Unspecified contracted kidney
Excludes1: *contracted kidney due to hypertension (I12.-)*
diffuse sclerosing glomerulonephritis (N05.8.-)
hypertensive nephrosclerosis (arteriolar) (arteriosclerotic) (I12.-)
small kidney of unknown cause (N27.-)
N26.1 Atrophy of kidney (terminal)
N26.2 Page kidney
N26.9 Renal sclerosis, unspecified

N27 Small kidney of unknown cause
Includes: oligonephronia
N27.0 Small kidney, unilateral
N27.1 Small kidney, bilateral
N27.9 Small kidney, unspecified

N28 Other disorders of kidney and ureter, not elsewhere classified
CC **N28.0 Ischemia and infarction of kidney**
Renal artery embolism
Renal artery obstruction
Renal artery occlusion
Renal artery thrombosis
Renal infarct
Excludes1: *atherosclerosis of renal artery (extrarenal part) (I70.1)*
congenital stenosis of renal artery (Q27.1)
Goldblatt's kidney (I70.1)
CC Exclusion see Appendix A PDX collection 0931
N28.1 Cyst of kidney, acquired
Cyst (multiple) (solitary) of kidney (acquired)
Excludes1: *cystic kidney disease (congenital) (Q61.-)*
\+ **N28.8 Other specified disorders of kidney and ureter**
Excludes1: *hydroureter (N13.4)*
ureteric stricture with hydronephrosis (N13.1)
ureteric stricture without hydronephrosis (N13.5)
N28.81 Hypertrophy of kidney
N28.82 Megaloureter
N28.83 Nephroptosis
CC **N28.84 Pyelitis cystica**
CC Exclusion see Appendix A PDX collection 0922
HAC see Appendix B for HAC conditional logic
CC **N28.85 Pyeloureteritis cystica**
CC Exclusion see Appendix A PDX collection 0922
HAC see Appendix B for HAC conditional logic
CC **N28.86 Ureteritis cystica**
CC Exclusion see Appendix A PDX collection 0922
HAC see Appendix B for HAC conditional logic
N28.89 Other specified disorders of kidney and ureter
N28.9 Disorder of kidney and ureter, unspecified
Nephropathy NOS
Renal disease (acute) NOS
Renal insufficiency (acute)
Excludes1: *chronic renal insufficiency (N18.9)*
unspecified nephritic syndrome (N05.-)
AHA CC: 1Q, 2016, 13

N29 Other disorders of kidney and ureter in diseases classified elsewhere

Code first underlying disease, such as:
amyloidosis (E85.-)
nephrocalcinosis (E83.5)
schistosomiasis (B65.0-B65.9)

Excludes1: *disorders of kidney and ureter in:*
cystinosis (E72.0)
gonorrhea (A54.21)
syphilis (A52.75)
tuberculosis (A18.11)

Valid 3-character code, no further characters required

Other diseases of the urinary system (N30-N39)

Excludes1: *urinary infection (complicating):*
abortion or ectopic or molar pregnancy (O00-O07, O08.8)
pregnancy, childbirth and the puerperium (O23.-, O75.3, O86.2-)

N30 Cystitis

Use additional code to identify infectious agent (B95-B97)

Excludes1: *prostatocystitis (N41.3)*

+ **N30.0 Acute cystitis**
  Excludes1: *irradiation cystitis (N30.4-)*
  trigonitis (N30.3-)
  - CC **N30.00 Acute cystitis without hematuria**
    CC Exclusion see Appendix A PDX collection 0932
    HAC see Appendix B for HAC conditional logic
  - CC **N30.01 Acute cystitis with hematuria**
    CC Exclusion see Appendix A PDX collection 0932
    HAC see Appendix B for HAC conditional logic
+ **N30.1 Interstitial cystitis (chronic)**
  - **N30.10 Interstitial cystitis (chronic) without hematuria**
  - **N30.11 Interstitial cystitis (chronic) with hematuria**
+ **N30.2 Other chronic cystitis**
  - **N30.20 Other chronic cystitis without hematuria**
  - **N30.21 Other chronic cystitis with hematuria**
+ **N30.3 Trigonitis**
  Urethrotrigonitis
  - **N30.30 Trigonitis without hematuria**
  - **N30.31 Trigonitis with hematuria**
+ **N30.4 Irradiation cystitis**
  - CC **N30.40 Irradiation cystitis without hematuria**
    CC Exclusion see Appendix A PDX collection 0932
  - CC **N30.41 Irradiation cystitis with hematuria**
    CC Exclusion see Appendix A PDX collection 0932
+ **N30.8 Other cystitis**
  Abscess of bladder
  - **N30.80 Other cystitis without hematuria**
  - **N30.81 Other cystitis with hematuria**
+ **N30.9 Cystitis, unspecified**
  - **N30.90 Cystitis, unspecified without hematuria**
  - **N30.91 Cystitis, unspecified with hematuria**

N31 Neuromuscular dysfunction of bladder, not elsewhere classified

Use additional code to identify any associated urinary incontinence (N39.3-N39.4-)

Excludes1: *cord bladder NOS (G95.89)*
neurogenic bladder due to cauda equina syndrome (G83.4)
neuromuscular dysfunction due to spinal cord lesion (G95.89)

N31.0 Uninhibited neuropathic bladder, not elsewhere classified
N31.1 Reflex neuropathic bladder, not elsewhere classified
N31.2 Flaccid neuropathic bladder, not elsewhere classified
Atonic (motor) (sensory) neuropathic bladder
Autonomous neuropathic bladder
Nonreflex neuropathic bladder
N31.8 Other neuromuscular dysfunction of bladder
N31.9 Neuromuscular dysfunction of bladder, unspecified
Neurogenic bladder dysfunction NOS

N32 Other disorders of bladder

Excludes2: *calculus of bladder (N21.0)*
cystocele (N81.1-)
hernia or prolapse of bladder, female (N81.1-)

N32.0 Bladder-neck obstruction
Bladder-neck stenosis (acquired)
Excludes1: *congenital bladder-neck obstruction (Q64.3-)*

CC **N32.1 Vesicointestinal fistula**
Vesicorectal fistula
CC Exclusion see Appendix A PDX collection 0933

CC **N32.2 Vesical fistula, not elsewhere classified**
Excludes1: *fistula between bladder and female genital tract (N82.0-N82.1)*
CC Exclusion see Appendix A PDX collection 0933

N32.3 Diverticulum of bladder
Excludes1: *congenital diverticulum of bladder (Q64.6)*
diverticulitis of bladder (N30.8-)

+ **N32.8 Other specified disorders of bladder**
  - **N32.81 Overactive bladder**
    Detrusor muscle hyperactivity
    Excludes1: *frequent urination due to specified bladder condition- code to condition*
  - **N32.89 Other specified disorders of bladder**
    Bladder hemorrhage
    Bladder hypertrophy
    Calcified bladder
    Contracted bladder

N32.9 Bladder disorder, unspecified

N33 Bladder disorders in diseases classified elsewhere

Code first underlying disease, such as:
schistosomiasis (B65.0-B65.9)

Excludes1: *bladder disorder in syphilis (A52.76)*
bladder disorder in tuberculosis (A18.12)
candidal cystitis (B37.41)
chlamydial cystitis (A56.01)
cystitis in gonorrhea (A54.01)
cystitis in neurogenic bladder (N31.-)
diphtheritic cystitis (A36.85)
syphilitic cystitis (A52.76)
trichomonal cystitis (A59.03)

Valid 3-character code, no further characters required

N34 Urethritis and urethral syndrome

Use additional code (B95-B97), to identify infectious agent.

Excludes2: *Reiter's disease (M02.3-)*
urethritis in diseases with a predominantly sexual mode of transmission (A50-A64)
urethrotrigonitis (N30.3-)

CC **N34.0 Urethral abscess**
Abscess (of) Cowper's gland
Abscess (of) Littré's gland
Abscess (of) urethral (gland)
Periurethral abscess
Excludes1: *urethral caruncle (N36.2)*
CC Exclusion see Appendix A PDX collection 0934
HAC see Appendix B for HAC conditional logic

N34.1 Nonspecific urethritis
Nongonococcal urethritis
Nonvenereal urethritis

N34.2 Other urethritis
Meatitis, urethral
Postmenopausal urethritis
Ulcer of urethra (meatus)
Urethritis NOS

N34.3 Urethral syndrome, unspecified

N35 Urethral stricture

Excludes1: *congenital urethral stricture (Q64.3-)*
postprocedural urethral stricture (N99.1-)

+ **N35.0 Post-traumatic urethral stricture**
  Urethral stricture due to injury
  Excludes1: *postprocedural urethral stricture (N99.1-)*
  + **N35.01 Post-traumatic urethral stricture, male**
    - ♂ **N35.010 Post-traumatic urethral stricture, male, meatal**
    - ♂ **N35.011 Post-traumatic bulbous urethral stricture**
    - ♂ **N35.012 Post-traumatic membranous urethral stricture**
    - ♂ **N35.013 Post-traumatic anterior urethral stricture**
    - ♂ **N35.014 Post-traumatic urethral stricture, male, unspecified**
  + **N35.02 Post-traumatic urethral stricture, female**
    - ♀ **N35.021 Urethral stricture due to childbirth**
    - ♀ **N35.028 Other post-traumatic urethral stricture, female**
+ **N35.1 Postinfective urethral stricture, not elsewhere classified**
  Excludes1: *urethral stricture associated with schistosomiasis (B65.-, N29)*
  gonococcal urethral stricture (A54.01)
  syphilitic urethral stricture (A52.76)

+ **N35.11 Postinfective urethral stricture, not elsewhere classified, male**
    - ♂ **N35.111 Postinfective urethral stricture, not elsewhere classified, male, meatal**
    - ♂ **N35.112 Postinfective bulbous urethral stricture, not elsewhere classified, male**
    - ♂ **N35.113 Postinfective membranous urethral stricture, not elsewhere classified, male**
    - ♂ **N35.114 Postinfective anterior urethral stricture, not elsewhere classified, male**
    - ♂ **N35.119 Postinfective urethral stricture, not elsewhere classified, male, unspecified**

♀ **N35.12 Postinfective urethral stricture, not elsewhere classified, female**

N35.8 Other urethral stricture
Excludes1: *postprocedural urethral stricture (N99.1-)*

N35.9 Urethral stricture, unspecified

N36 Other disorders of urethra

CC **N36.0 Urethral fistula**
Urethroperineal fistula
Urethrorectal fistula
Urinary fistula NOS
Excludes1: *urethroscrotal fistula (N50.89)*
urethrovaginal fistula (N82.1)
urethrovesicovaginal fistula (N82.1)
CC Exclusion see Appendix A PDX collection 0935

N36.1 Urethral diverticulum

N36.2 Urethral caruncle

+ **N36.4 Urethral functional and muscular disorders**
Use additional code to identify associated urinary stress incontinence (N39.3)
- **N36.41 Hypermobility of urethra**
- **N36.42 Intrinsic sphincter deficiency (ISD)**
- **N36.43 Combined hypermobility of urethra and intrinsic sphincter deficiency**
- **N36.44 Muscular disorders of urethra**
  Bladder sphincter dyssynergy

N36.5 Urethral false passage

N36.8 Other specified disorders of urethra
Excludes1: *congenital urethrocele (Q64.7)*
female urethrocele (N81.0)

N36.9 Urethral disorder, unspecified

N37 Urethral disorders in diseases classified elsewhere

Code first underlying disease
Excludes1: *urethritis (in):*
candidal infection (B37.41)
chlamydial (A56.01)
gonorrhea (A54.01)
syphilis (A52.76)
trichomonal infection (A59.03)
tuberculosis (A18.13)
Valid 3-character code, no further characters required

N39 Other disorders of urinary system

Excludes2: *hematuria NOS (R31.-)*
recurrent or persistent hematuria (N02.-)
recurrent or persistent hematuria with specified morphological lesion (N02.-)
proteinuria NOS (R80.-)

CC **N39.0 Urinary tract infection, site not specified**
Use additional code (B95-B97), to identify infectious agent
Excludes1: *candidiasis of urinary tract (B37.4-)*
neonatal urinary tract infection (P39.3)
urinary tract infection of specified site, such as:
cystitis (N30.-)
urethritis (N34.-)
CC Exclusion see Appendix A PDX collection 0936
HAC see Appendix B for HAC conditional logic
AHA CC: 4Q, 2012, 94

N39.3 Stress incontinence (female) (male)
Code also any associated overactive bladder (N32.81)
Excludes1: *mixed incontinence (N39.46)*

+ **N39.4 Other specified urinary incontinence**
Code also any associated overactive bladder (N32.81)
Excludes1: *enuresis NOS (R32)*
functional urinary incontinence (R39.81)
urinary incontinence associated with cognitive impairment (R39.81)
urinary incontinence NOS (R32)
urinary incontinence of nonorganic origin (F98.0)

- **N39.41 Urge incontinence**
  Excludes1: *mixed incontinence (N39.46)*
- **N39.42 Incontinence without sensory awareness**
  Insensible (urinary) incontinence
- **N39.43 Post-void dribbling**
- **N39.44 Nocturnal enuresis**
- **N39.45 Continuous leakage**
- **N39.46 Mixed incontinence**
  Urge and stress incontinence
- + **N39.49 Other specified urinary incontinence**
  AHA CC: 4Q, 2016, 44
    - **N39.490 Overflow incontinence**
    - **N39.491 Coital incontinence**
    - **N39.492 Postural (urinary) incontinence**
    - **N39.498 Other specified urinary incontinence**
      Reflex incontinence
      Total incontinence

N39.8 Other specified disorders of urinary system

N39.9 Disorder of urinary system, unspecified

Diseases of male genital organs (N40-N53)

N40 Benign prostatic hyperplasia

Includes: adenofibromatous hypertrophy of prostate
benign hypertrophy of the prostate
benign prostatic hypertrophy
BPH
enlarged prostate
nodular prostate
polyp of prostate
Excludes1: *benign neoplasms of prostate (adenoma, benign) (fibroadenoma) (fibroma) (myoma) (D29.1)*
Excludes2: *malignant neoplasm of prostate (C61)*

● ♂ **N40.0 Benign prostatic hyperplasia without lower urinary tract symptoms**
Enlarged prostate without LUTS
Enlarged prostate NOS

● ♂ **N40.1 Benign prostatic hyperplasia with lower urinary tract symptoms**
Enlarged prostate with LUTS
Use additional code for associated symptoms, when specified:
incomplete bladder emptying (R39.14)
nocturia (R35.1)
straining on urination (R39.16)
urinary frequency (R35.0)
urinary hesitancy (R39.11)
urinary incontinence (N39.4-)
urinary obstruction (N13.8)
urinary retention (R33.8)
urinary urgency (R39.15)
weak urinary stream (R39.12)

● ♂ **N40.2 Nodular prostate without lower urinary tract symptoms**
Nodular prostate without LUTS

● ♂ **N40.3 Nodular prostate with lower urinary tract symptoms**
Use additional code for associated symptoms, when specified:
incomplete bladder emptying (R39.14)
nocturia (R35.1)
straining on urination (R39.16)
urinary frequency (R35.0)
urinary hesitancy (R39.11)
urinary incontinence (N39.4-)
urinary obstruction (N13.8)
urinary retention (R33.8)
urinary urgency (R39.15)
weak urinary stream (R39.12)

N41 Inflammatory diseases of prostate

Use additional code (B95-B97), to identify infectious agent

● ♂ CC **N41.0 Acute prostatitis**
CC Exclusion see Appendix A PDX collection 0937

● ♂ **N41.1 Chronic prostatitis**

● ♂ CC **N41.2 Abscess of prostate**
CC Exclusion see Appendix A PDX collection 0937

● ♂ **N41.3 Prostatocystitis**

● ♂ **N41.4 Granulomatous prostatitis**

● ♂ **N41.8 Other inflammatory diseases of prostate**

● ♂ **N41.9 Inflammatory disease of prostate, unspecified**
Prostatitis NOS

Male Reproductive System

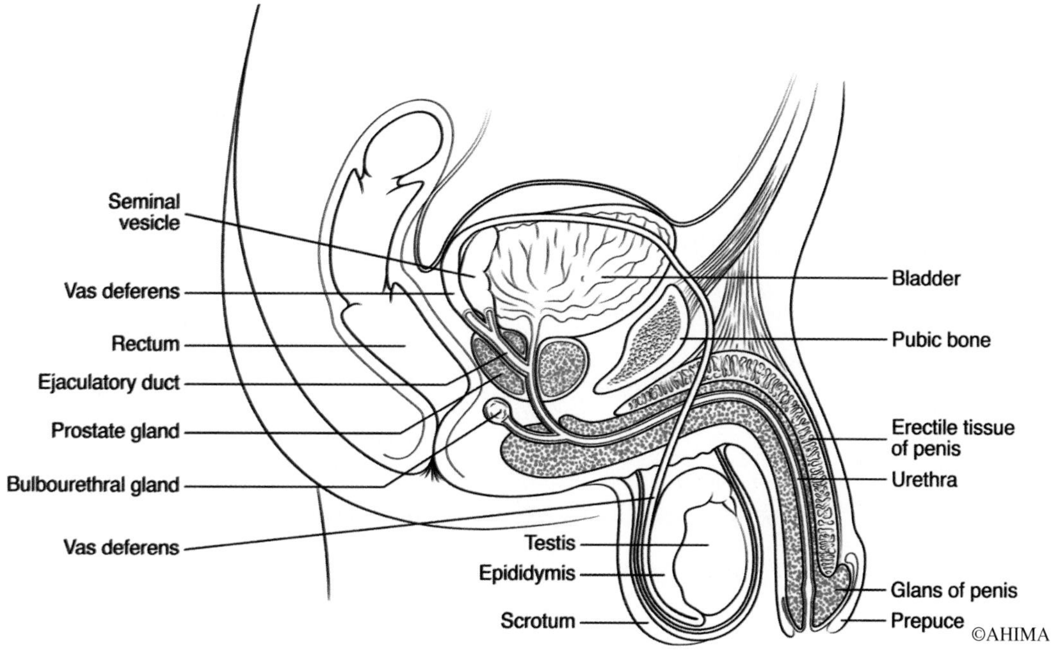
Seminal vesicle
Vas deferens
Rectum
Ejaculatory duct
Prostate gland
Bulbourethral gland
Vas deferens
Bladder
Pubic bone
Erectile tissue of penis
Urethra
Testis
Epididymis
Scrotum
Glans of penis
Prepuce

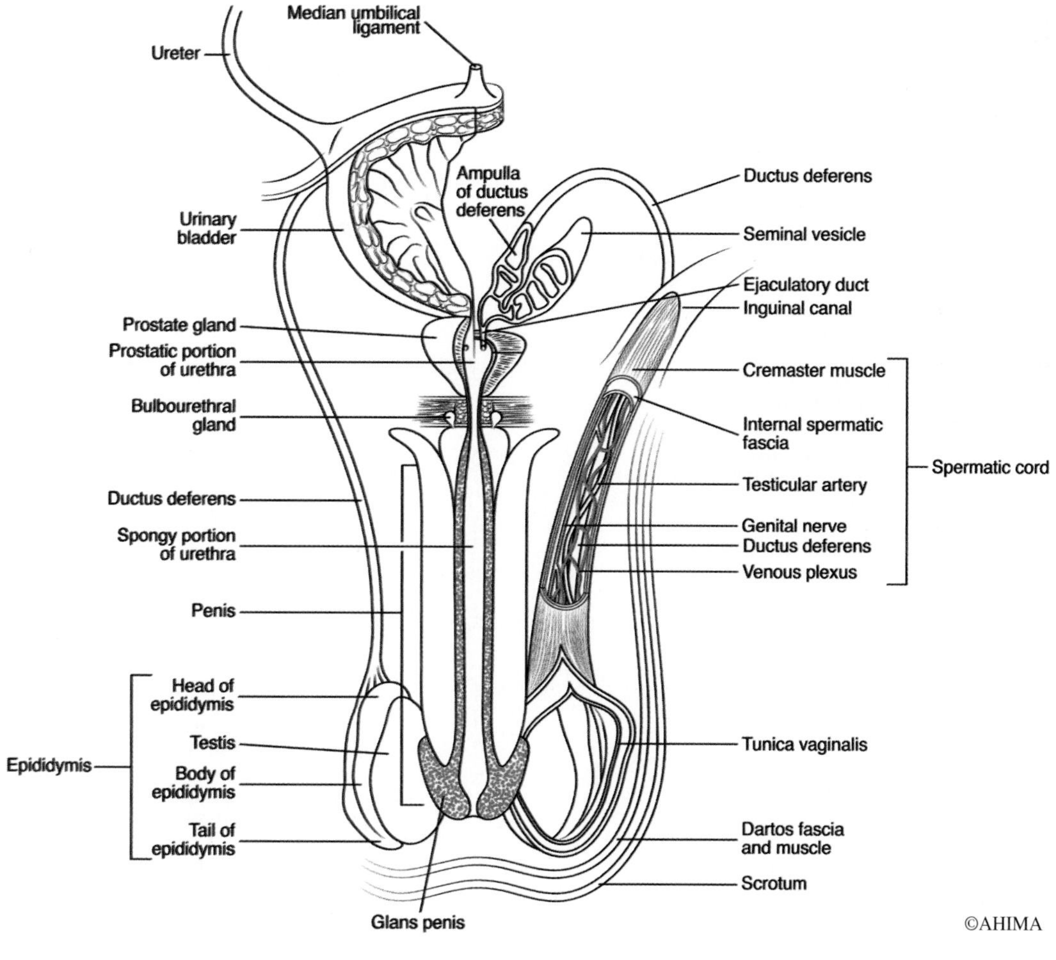
Median umbilical ligament
Ureter
Urinary bladder
Ampulla of ductus deferens
Ductus deferens
Seminal vesicle
Ejaculatory duct
Inguinal canal
Prostate gland
Prostatic portion of urethra
Cremaster muscle
Bulbourethral gland
Internal spermatic fascia
Spermatic cord
Testicular artery
Ductus deferens
Spongy portion of urethra
Genital nerve
Ductus deferens
Venous plexus
Penis
Head of epididymis
Epididymis
Testis
Body of epididymis
Tunica vaginalis
Tail of epididymis
Dartos fascia and muscle
Scrotum
Glans penis

N42 Other and unspecified disorders of prostate

• ♂ **N42.0 Calculus of prostate**
Prostatic stone

• ♂ **N42.1 Congestion and hemorrhage of prostate**
Excludes1: *enlarged prostate (N40.-)*
hematuria (R31.-)
hyperplasia of prostate (N40.-)
inflammatory diseases of prostate (N41.-)

\+ **N42.3 Dysplasia of prostate**
AHA CC: 4Q, 2016, 44

♂ **N42.30 Unspecified dysplasia of prostate**

♂ **N42.31 Prostatic intraepithelial neoplasia**
PIN
Prostatic intraepithelial neoplasia I (PIN I)
Prostatic intraepithelial neoplasia II (PIN II)
Exlcudes1: *prostatic intraepithelial neoplasia III (PIN III) (D07.5)*

♂ **N42.32 Atypical small acinar proliferation of prostate**

♂ **N42.39 Other dysplasia of prostate**

\+ **N42.8 Other specified disorders of prostate**

• ♂ **N42.81 Prostatodynia syndrome**
Painful prostate syndrome

• ♂ **N42.82 Prostatosis syndrome**

• ♂ **N42.83 Cyst of prostate**

• ♂ **N42.89 Other specified disorders of prostate**

• ♂ **N42.9 Disorder of prostate, unspecified**

N43 Hydrocele and spermatocele

Includes: hydrocele of spermatic cord, testis or tunica vaginalis
Excludes1: *congenital hydrocele (P83.5)*

♂ **N43.0 Encysted hydrocele**

CC ♂ **N43.1 Infected hydrocele**
CC Exclusion see Appendix A PDX collection 0938
Use additional code (B95-B97), to identify infectious agent

♂ **N43.2 Other hydrocele**

♂ **N43.3 Hydrocele, unspecified**

\+ **N43.4 Spermatocele of epididymis**
Spermatic cyst

♂ **N43.40 Spermatocele of epididymis, unspecified**

♂ **N43.41 Spermatocele of epididymis, single**

♂ **N43.42 Spermatocele of epididymis, multiple**

N44 Noninflammatory disorders of testis

\+ **N44.0 Torsion of testis**

CC ♂ **N44.00 Torsion of testis, unspecified**
CC Exclusion see Appendix A PDX collection 0939

CC ♂ **N44.01 Extravaginal torsion of spermatic cord**
CC Exclusion see Appendix A PDX collection 0939

CC ♂ **N44.02 Intravaginal torsion of spermatic cord**
Torsion of spermatic cord NOS
CC Exclusion see Appendix A PDX collection 0939

CC ♂ **N44.03 Torsion of appendix testis**
CC Exclusion see Appendix A PDX collection 0939

CC ♂ **N44.04 Torsion of appendix epididymis**
CC Exclusion see Appendix A PDX collection 0939

♂ **N44.1 Cyst of tunica albuginea testis**

♂ **N44.2 Benign cyst of testis**

♂ **N44.8 Other noninflammatory disorders of the testis**

N45 Orchitis and epididymitis

Use additional code (B95-B97), to identify infectious agent

♂ **N45.1 Epididymitis**

♂ **N45.2 Orchitis**

♂ **N45.3 Epididymo-orchitis**

CC ♂ **N45.4 Abscess of epididymis or testis**
CC Exclusion see Appendix A PDX collection 0940

N46 Male infertility

Excludes1: *vasectomy status (Z98.52)*

\+ **N46.0 Azoospermia**
Absolute male infertility
Male infertility due to germinal (cell) aplasia
Male infertility due to spermatogenic arrest (complete)

• ♂ **N46.01 Organic azoospermia**
Azoospermia NOS

\+ **N46.02 Azoospermia due to extratesticular causes**
Code also associated cause

• ♂ **N46.021 Azoospermia due to drug therapy**

• ♂ **N46.022 Azoospermia due to infection**

• ♂ **N46.023 Azoospermia due to obstruction of efferent ducts**

• ♂ **N46.024 Azoospermia due to radiation**

• ♂ **N46.025 Azoospermia due to systemic disease**

• ♂ **N46.029 Azoospermia due to other extratesticular causes**

\+ **N46.1 Oligospermia**
Male infertility due to germinal cell desquamation
Male infertility due to hypospermatogenesis
Male infertility due to incomplete spermatogenic arrest

• ♂ **N46.11 Organic oligospermia**
Oligospermia NOS

\+ **N46.12 Oligospermia due to extratesticular causes**
Code also associated cause

• ♂ **N46.121 Oligospermia due to drug therapy**

• ♂ **N46.122 Oligospermia due to infection**

• ♂ **N46.123 Oligospermia due to obstruction of efferent ducts**

• ♂ **N46.124 Oligospermia due to radiation**

• ♂ **N46.125 Oligospermia due to systemic disease**

• ♂ **N46.129 Oligospermia due to other extratesticular causes**

• ♂ **N46.8 Other male infertility**

• ♂ **N46.9 Male infertility, unspecified**

N47 Disorders of prepuce

• ♂ **N47.0 Adherent prepuce, newborn**

♂ **N47.1 Phimosis**

♂ **N47.2 Paraphimosis**

♂ **N47.3 Deficient foreskin**

♂ **N47.4 Benign cyst of prepuce**

♂ **N47.5 Adhesions of prepuce and glans penis**

♂ **N47.6 Balanoposthitis**
Use additional code (B95-B97), to identify infectious agent
Excludes1: *balanitis (N48.1)*

♂ **N47.7 Other inflammatory diseases of prepuce**
Use additional code (B95-B97), to identify infectious agent

♂ **N47.8 Other disorders of prepuce**

N48 Other disorders of penis

♂ **N48.0 Leukoplakia of penis**
Balanitis xerotica obliterans
Kraurosis of penis
Lichen sclerosus of external male genital organs
Excludes1: *carcinoma in situ of penis (D07.4)*

♂ **N48.1 Balanitis**
Use additional code (B95-B97), to identify infectious agent
Excludes1: *amebic balanitis (A06.8)*
balanitis xerotica obliterans (N48.0)
candidal balanitis (B37.42)
gonococcal balanitis (A54.23)
herpesviral [herpes simplex] balanitis (A60.01)

\+ **N48.2 Other inflammatory disorders of penis**
Use additional code (B95-B97), to identify infectious agent
Excludes1: *balanitis (N48.1)*
balanitis xerotica obliterans (N48.0)
balanoposthitis (N47.6)

♂ **N48.21 Abscess of corpus cavernosum and penis**

♂ **N48.22 Cellulitis of corpus cavernosum and penis**

♂ **N48.29 Other inflammatory disorders of penis**

\+ **N48.3 Priapism**
Painful erection
Code first underlying cause

CC ♂ **N48.30 Priapism, unspecified**
CC Exclusion see Appendix A PDX collection 0941

CC ♂ **N48.31 Priapism due to trauma**
CC Exclusion see Appendix A PDX collection 0941

CC ♂ **N48.32 Priapism due to disease classified elsewhere**
CC Exclusion see Appendix A PDX collection 0941

CC ♂ **N48.33 Priapism, drug-induced**
CC Exclusion see Appendix A PDX collection 0941

CC ♂ **N48.39 Other priapism**
CC Exclusion see Appendix A PDX collection 0941

♂ **N48.5 Ulcer of penis**

♂ **N48.6 Induration penis plastica**
Peyronie's disease
Plastic induration of penis

\+ **N48.8 Other specified disorders of penis**

♂ **N48.81 Thrombosis of superficial vein of penis**

♂ **N48.82 Acquired torsion of penis**
Acquired torsion of penis NOS
Excludes1: *congenital torsion of penis (Q55.63)*

♂ **N48.83 Acquired buried penis**
Excludes1: *congenital hidden penis (Q55.64)*
♂ **N48.89 Other specified disorders of penis**
♂ **N48.9 Disorder of penis, unspecified**

N49 Inflammatory disorders of male genital organs, not elsewhere classified
Use additional code (B95-B97), to identify infectious agent
Excludes1: *inflammation of penis (N48.1, N48.2-)*
orchitis and epididymitis (N45.-)
♂ **N49.0 Inflammatory disorders of seminal vesicle**
Vesiculitis NOS
♂ **N49.1 Inflammatory disorders of spermatic cord, tunica vaginalis and vas deferens**
Vasitis
♂ **N49.2 Inflammatory disorders of scrotum**
♂ **N49.3 Fournier gangrene**
♂ **N49.8 Inflammatory disorders of other specified male genital organs**
Inflammation of multiple sites in male genital organs
♂ **N49.9 Inflammatory disorder of unspecified male genital organ**
Abscess of unspecified male genital organ
Boil of unspecified male genital organ
Carbuncle of unspecified male genital organ
Cellulitis of unspecified male genital organ

N50 Other and unspecified disorders of male genital organs
Excludes2: *torsion of testis (N44.0-)*
♂ **N50.0 Atrophy of testis**
♂ **N50.1 Vascular disorders of male genital organs**
Hematocele, NOS, of male genital organs
Hemorrhage of male genital organs
Thrombosis of male genital organs
♂ **N50.3 Cyst of epididymis**
+ **N50.8 Other specified disorders of male genital organs**
AHA CC: 4Q, 2016, 45
+ **N50.81 Testicular pain**
♂ **N50.811 Right testicular pain**
♂ **N50.812 Left testicular pain**
♂ **N50.819 Testicular pain, unspecified**
♂ **N50.82 Scrotal pain**
♂ **N50.89 Other specified disorders of the male genital organs**
Atrophy of scrotum, seminal vesicle, spermatic cord, tunica vaginalis and vas deferens
Chylocele, tunica vaginalis (nonfilarial) NOS
Edema of scrotum, seminal vesicle, spermatic cord, tunica vaginalis and vas deferens
Hypertrophy of scrotum, seminal vesicle, spermatic cord, tunica vaginalis and vas deferens
Stricture of spermatic cord, tunical vaginalis, and vas deferens
Ulcer of scrotum, seminal vesicle, spermatic cord, testis, tunica vaginalis and vas deferens
Urethroscrotal fistula
♂ **N50.9 Disorder of male genital organs, unspecified**

♂ **N51 Disorders of male genital organs in diseases classified elsewhere**
Code first underlying disease, such as:
filariasis (B74.0-B74.9)
Excludes1: *amebic balanitis (A06.8)*
candidal balanitis (B37.42)
gonococcal balanitis (A54.23)
gonococcal prostatitis (A54.22)
herpesviral [herpes simplex] balanitis (A60.01)
trichomonal prostatitis (A59.02)
tuberculous prostatitis (A18.14)
Valid 3-character code, no further characters required

N52 Male erectile dysfunction
Excludes1: *psychogenic impotence (F52.21)*
+ **N52.0 Vasculogenic erectile dysfunction**
● ♂ **N52.01 Erectile dysfunction due to arterial insufficiency**
● ♂ **N52.02 Corporo-venous occlusive erectile dysfunction**
● ♂ **N52.03 Combined arterial insufficiency and corporo-venous occlusive erectile dysfunction**
● ♂ CC **N52.1 Erectile dysfunction due to diseases classified elsewhere**
Code first underlying disease
● ♂ CC **N52.2 Drug-induced erectile dysfunction**
+ **N52.3 Postprocedural erectile dysfunction**
AHA CC: 4Q, 2016, 45
● ♂ **N52.31 Erectile dysfunction following radical prostatectomy**
● ♂ **N52.32 Erectile dysfunction following radical cystectomy**
● ♂ **N52.33 Erectile dysfunction following urethral surgery**
● ♂ **N52.34 Erectile dysfunction following simple prostatectomy**
● ♂ **N52.35 Erectile dysfunction following radiation therapy**
● ♂ **N52.36 Erectile dysfunction following interstitial seed therapy**
● ♂ **N52.37 Erectile dysfunction following prostate ablative therapy**
Erectile dysfunction following cryotherapy
Erectile dysfunction following other prostate ablative therapies
Erectile dysfunction following ultrasound ablative therapies
● ♂ **N52.39 Other and unspecified postprocedural erectile dysfunction**
● ♂ **N52.8 Other male erectile dysfunction**
● ♂ **N52.9 Male erectile dysfunction, unspecified**
Impotence NOS

N53 Other male sexual dysfunction
Excludes1: *psychogenic sexual dysfunction (F52.-)*
+ **N53.1 Ejaculatory dysfunction**
Excludes1: *premature ejaculation (F52.4)*
♂ **N53.11 Retarded ejaculation**
♂ **N53.12 Painful ejaculation**
♂ **N53.13 Anejaculatory orgasm**
♂ **N53.14 Retrograde ejaculation**
♂ **N53.19 Other ejaculatory dysfunction**
Ejaculatory dysfunction NOS
♂ **N53.8 Other male sexual dysfunction**
♂ **N53.9 Unspecified male sexual dysfunction**

Disorders of breast (N60-N65)

Excludes1: *disorders of breast associated with childbirth (O91-O92)*

N60 Benign mammary dysplasia
Includes: fibrocystic mastopathy
+ **N60.0 Solitary cyst of breast**
Cyst of breast
N60.01 Solitary cyst of right breast
N60.02 Solitary cyst of left breast
N60.09 Solitary cyst of unspecified breast
+ **N60.1 Diffuse cystic mastopathy**
Cystic breast
Fibrocystic disease of breast
Excludes1: *diffuse cystic mastopathy with epithelial proliferation (N60.3-)*
● **N60.11 Diffuse cystic mastopathy of right breast**
● **N60.12 Diffuse cystic mastopathy of left breast**
● **N60.19 Diffuse cystic mastopathy of unspecified breast**
+ **N60.2 Fibroadenosis of breast**
Adenofibrosis of breast
Excludes2: *fibroadenoma of breast (D24.-)*
N60.21 Fibroadenosis of right breast
N60.22 Fibroadenosis of left breast
N60.29 Fibroadenosis of unspecified breast
+ **N60.3 Fibrosclerosis of breast**
Cystic mastopathy with epithelial proliferation
N60.31 Fibrosclerosis of right breast
N60.32 Fibrosclerosis of left breast
N60.39 Fibrosclerosis of unspecified breast
+ **N60.4 Mammary duct ectasia**
N60.41 Mammary duct ectasia of right breast
N60.42 Mammary duct ectasia of left breast
N60.49 Mammary duct ectasia of unspecified breast
+ **N60.8 Other benign mammary dysplasias**
N60.81 Other benign mammary dysplasias of right breast
N60.82 Other benign mammary dysplasias of left breast
N60.89 Other benign mammary dysplasias of unspecified breast
+ **N60.9 Unspecified benign mammary dysplasia**
N60.91 Unspecified benign mammary dysplasia of right breast
N60.92 Unspecified benign mammary dysplasia of left breast
N60.99 Unspecified benign mammary dysplasia of unspecified breast

N61 Inflammatory disorders of breast
Excludes1: *inflammatory carcinoma of breast (C50.9)*
inflammatory disorder of breast associated with childbirth (O91.-)
neonatal infective mastitis (P39.0)
thrombophlebitis of breast [Mondor's disease] (I80.8)
N61.0 Mastitis without abscess
Infective mastitis (acute) (nonpuerperal) (subacute)
Mastitis (acute) (nonpuerperal) (subacute) NOS
Cellulitis (acute) (nonpuerperal) (subacute) of breast NOS
Cellulitis (acute) (nonpuerperal) (subacute) of nipple NOS

Breast

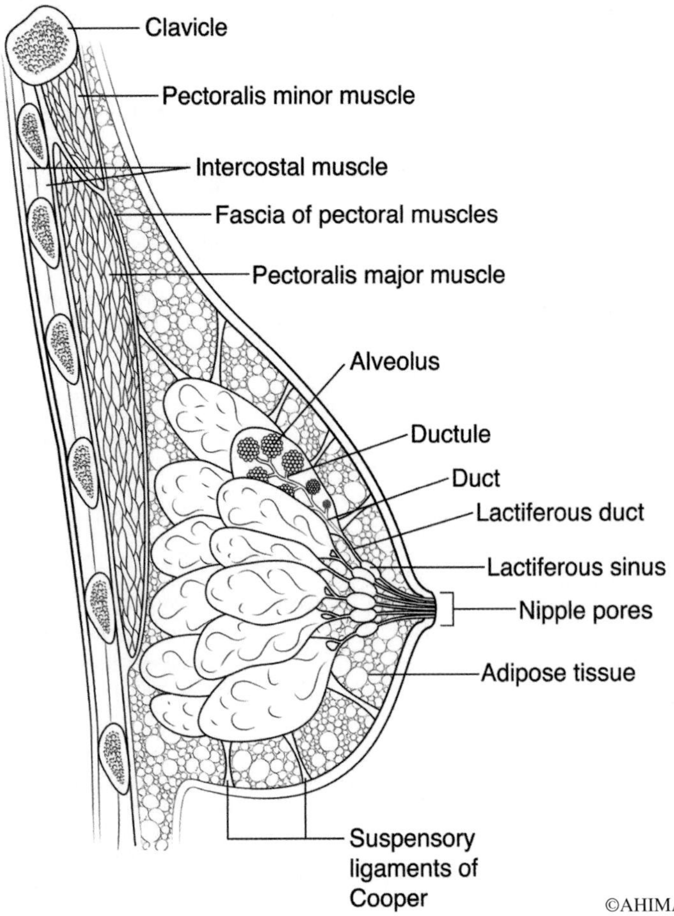

N61.1 Abscess of the breast and nipple
Abscess (acute) (chronic) (nonpuerperal) of areola
Abscess (acute) (chronic) (nonpuerperal) of breast
Carbuncle of breast
Mastitis with abscess

N62 Hypertrophy of breast
Gynecomastia
Hypertrophy of breast NOS
Massive pubertal hypertrophy of breast
Excludes1: *breast engorgement of newborn (P83.4)*
disproportion of reconstructed breast (N65.1)
Valid 3-character code, no further characters required

N63 Unspecified lump in breast
Nodule(s) NOS in breast
N63.0 Unspecified lump in unspecified breast
+ **N63.1 Unspecified lump in the right breast**
N63.10 Unspecified lump in the right breast, unspecified quadrant
N63.11 Unspecified lump in the right breast, upper outer quadrant
N63.12 Unspecified lump in the right breast, upper inner quadrant
N63.13 Unspecified lump in the right breast, lower outer quadrant
N63.14 Unspecified lump in the right breast, lower inner quadrant
+ **N63.2 Unspecified lump in the left breast**
N63.20 Unspecified lump in the left breast, unspecified quadrant
N63.21 Unspecified lump in the left breast, upper outer quadrant
N63.22 Unspecified lump in the left breast, upper inner quadrant
N63.23 Unspecified lump in the left breast, lower outer quadrant
N63.24 Unspecified lump in the left breast, lower inner quadrant
+ **N63.3 Unspecified lump in axillary tail**
N63.31 Unspecified lump in axillary tail of the right breast
N63.32 Unspecified lump in axillary tail of the left breast
+ **N63.4 Unspecified lump in breast, subareolar**
N63.41 Unspecified lump in right breast, subareolar
N63.42 Unspecified lump in left breast, subareolar

N64 Other disorders of breast
Excludes2: *mechanical complication of breast prosthesis and implant (T85.4-)*
N64.0 Fissure and fistula of nipple
N64.1 Fat necrosis of breast
Fat necrosis (segmental) of breast
Code first breast necrosis due to breast graft (T85.898)
N64.2 Atrophy of breast
N64.3 Galactorrhea not associated with childbirth
N64.4 Mastodynia
+ **N64.5 Other signs and symptoms in breast**
Excludes2: *abnormal findings on diagnostic imaging of breast (R92.-)*
N64.51 Induration of breast
N64.52 Nipple discharge
Excludes1: *abnormal findings in nipple discharge (R89.-)*
N64.53 Retraction of nipple
N64.59 Other signs and symptoms in breast
+ **N64.8 Other specified disorders of breast**
• **N64.81 Ptosis of breast**
Excludes1: *ptosis of native breast in relation to reconstructed breast (N65.1)*
• **N64.82 Hypoplasia of breast**
Micromastia
Excludes1: *congenital absence of breast (Q83.0)*
hypoplasia of native breast in relation to reconstructed breast (N65.1)
N64.89 Other specified disorders of breast
Galactocele
Subinvolution of breast (postlactational)
N64.9 Disorder of breast, unspecified

Female Reproductive System

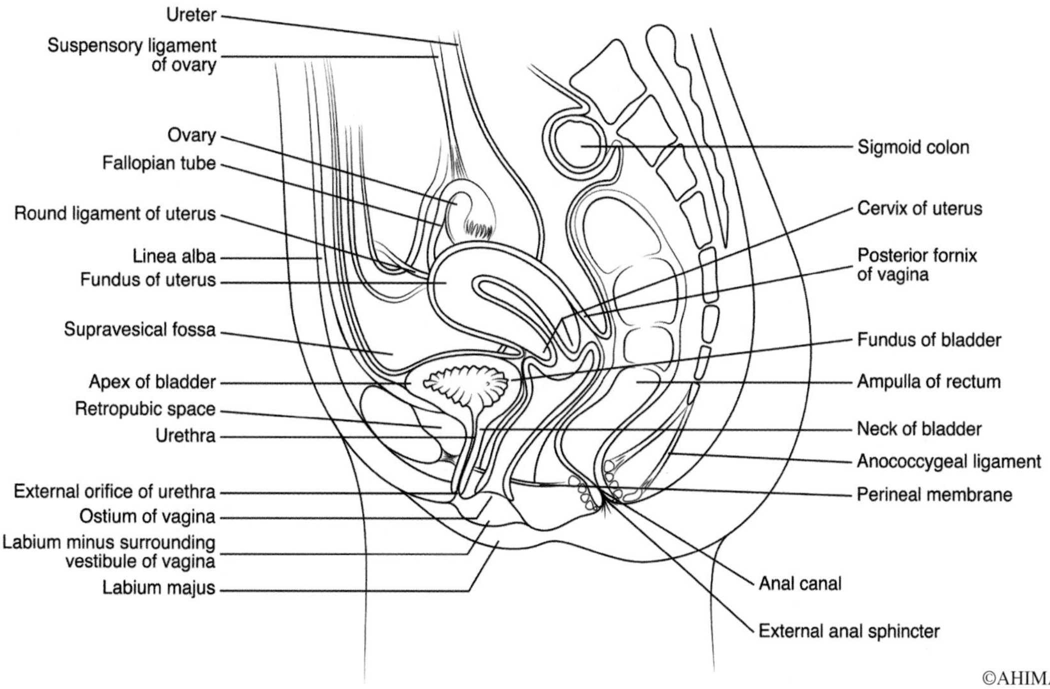

Ureter
Suspensory ligament of ovary
Ovary
Fallopian tube
Round ligament of uterus
Linea alba
Fundus of uterus
Supravesical fossa
Apex of bladder
Retropubic space
Urethra
External orifice of urethra
Ostium of vagina
Labium minus surrounding vestibule of vagina
Labium majus
Sigmoid colon
Cervix of uterus
Posterior fornix of vagina
Fundus of bladder
Ampulla of rectum
Neck of bladder
Anococcygeal ligament
Perineal membrane
Anal canal
External anal sphincter

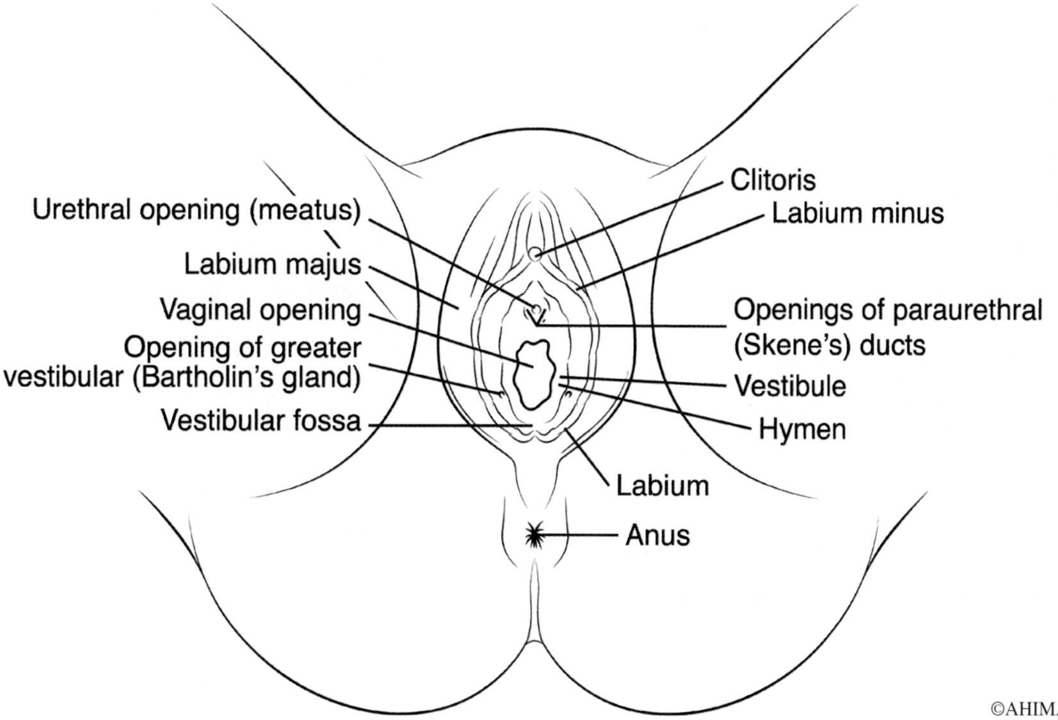

Urethral opening (meatus)
Labium majus
Vaginal opening
Opening of greater vestibular (Bartholin's gland)
Vestibular fossa
Clitoris
Labium minus
Openings of paraurethral (Skene's) ducts
Vestibule
Hymen
Labium
Anus

N65 **Deformity and disproportion of reconstructed breast**

• **N65.0 Deformity of reconstructed breast**
Contour irregularity in reconstructed breast
Excess tissue in reconstructed breast
Misshapen reconstructed breast

• **N65.1 Disproportion of reconstructed breast**
Breast asymmetry between native breast and reconstructed breast
Disproportion between native breast and reconstructed breast

Inflammatory diseases of female pelvic organs (N70-N77)

Excludes1: *inflammatory diseases of female pelvic organs complicating:*
abortion or ectopic or molar pregnancy (O00-O07, O08.0)
pregnancy, childbirth and the puerperium (O23.-, O75.3, O85, O86.-)

N70 Salpingitis and oophoritis

Includes: abscess (of) fallopian tube
abscess (of) ovary
pyosalpinx
salpingo-oophoritis
tubo-ovarian abscess
tubo-ovarian inflammatory disease

Use additional code (B95-B97), to identify infectious agent

Excludes1: *gonococcal infection (A54.24)*
tuberculous infection (A18.17)

\+ **N70.0 Acute salpingitis and oophoritis**
♀ CC **N70.01 Acute salpingitis**
CC Exclusion see Appendix A PDX collection 0942
♀ CC **N70.02 Acute oophoritis**
CC Exclusion see Appendix A PDX collection 0942
♀ CC **N70.03 Acute salpingitis and oophoritis**
CC Exclusion see Appendix A PDX collection 0942

\+ **N70.1 Chronic salpingitis and oophoritis**
Hydrosalpinx
♀ **N70.11 Chronic salpingitis**
♀ **N70.12 Chronic oophoritis**
♀ **N70.13 Chronic salpingitis and oophoritis**

\+ **N70.9 Salpingitis and oophoritis, unspecified**
♀ **N70.91 Salpingitis, unspecified**
♀ **N70.92 Oophoritis, unspecified**
♀ **N70.93 Salpingitis and oophoritis, unspecified**

N71 Inflammatory disease of uterus, except cervix

Includes: endo (myo) metritis
metritis
myometritis
pyometra
uterine abscess

Use additional code (B95-B97), to identify infectious agent

Excludes1: *hyperplastic endometritis (N85.0-)*
infection of uterus following delivery (O85, O86.-)

♀ CC **N71.0 Acute inflammatory disease of uterus**
CC Exclusion see Appendix A PDX collection 0943
♀ **N71.1 Chronic inflammatory disease of uterus**
♀ **N71.9 Inflammatory disease of uterus, unspecified**

♀ **N72 Inflammatory disease of cervix uteri**

Includes: cervicitis (with or without erosion or ectropion)
endocervicitis (with or without erosion or ectropion)
exocervicitis (with or without erosion or ectropion)

Use additional code (B95-B97), to identify infectious agent

Excludes1: *erosion and ectropion of cervix without cervicitis (N86)*

Valid 3-character code, no further characters required

N73 Other female pelvic inflammatory diseases

Use additional code (B95-B97), to identify infectious agent

♀ CC **N73.0 Acute parametritis and pelvic cellulitis**
Abscess of broad ligament
Abscess of parametrium
Pelvic cellulitis, female
CC Exclusion see Appendix A PDX collection 0942

♀ **N73.1 Chronic parametritis and pelvic cellulitis**
Any condition in N73.0 specified as chronic
Excludes1: *tuberculous parametritis and pelvic cellultis (A18.17)*

♀ **N73.2 Unspecified parametritis and pelvic cellulitis**
Any condition in N73.0 unspecified whether acute or chronic

♀ MCC **N73.3 Female acute pelvic peritonitis**
MCC Exclusion see Appendix A PDX collection 0942

♀ CC **N73.4 Female chronic pelvic peritonitis**
Excludes1: *tuberculous pelvic (female) peritonitis (A18.17)*
CC Exclusion see Appendix A PDX collection 0942

♀ **N73.5 Female pelvic peritonitis, unspecified**

♀ **N73.6 Female pelvic peritoneal adhesions (postinfective)**
Excludes2: *postprocedural pelvic peritoneal adhesions (N99.4)*
AHA CC: 1Q, 2014, 6

♀ **N73.8 Other specified female pelvic inflammatory diseases**

♀ **N73.9 Female pelvic inflammatory disease, unspecified**
Female pelvic infection or inflammation NOS

♀ **N74 Female pelvic inflammatory disorders in diseases classified elsewhere**

Code first underlying disease

Excludes1: *chlamydial cervicitis (A56.02)*
chlamydial pelvic inflammatory disease (A56.11)
gonococcal cervicitis (A54.03)
gonococcal pelvic inflammatory disease (A54.24)
herpesviral [herpes simplex] cervicitis (A60.03)
herpesviral [herpes simplex] pelvic inflammatory disease (A60.09)
syphilitic cervicitis (A52.76)
syphilitic pelvic inflammatory disease (A52.76)
trichomonal cervicitis (A59.09)
tuberculous cervicitis (A18.16)
tuberculous pelvic inflammatory disease (A18.17)

Valid 3-character code, no further characters required

N75 Diseases of Bartholin's gland

♀ **N75.0 Cyst of Bartholin's gland**
♀ CC **N75.1 Abscess of Bartholin's gland**
♀ **N75.8 Other diseases of Bartholin's gland**
Bartholinitis
CC Exclusion see Appendix A PDX collection 0944
♀ **N75.9 Disease of Bartholin's gland, unspecified**

N76 Other inflammation of vagina and vulva

Use additional code (B95-B97), to identify infectious agent

Excludes2: *senile (atrophic) vaginitis (N95.2)*
vulvar vestibulitis (N94.810)

♀ **N76.0 Acute vaginitis**
Acute vulvovaginitis
Vaginitis NOS
Vulvovaginitis NOS

♀ **N76.1 Subacute and chronic vaginitis**
Chronic vulvovaginitis
Subacute vulvovaginitis

♀ **N76.2 Acute vulvitis**
Vulvitis NOS

♀ **N76.3 Subacute and chronic vulvitis**

♀ CC **N76.4 Abscess of vulva**
Furuncle of vulva
CC Exclusion see Appendix A PDX collection 0944

♀ **N76.5 Ulceration of vagina**
♀ **N76.6 Ulceration of vulva**

\+ **N76.8 Other specified inflammation of vagina and vulva**
♀ CC **N76.81 Mucositis (ulcerative) of vagina and vulva**
Code also type of associated therapy, such as:
antineoplastic and immunosuppressive drugs (T45.1X-)
radiological procedure and radiotherapy (Y84.2)
Excludes2: *gastrointestinal mucositis (ulcerative) (K92.81)*
nasal mucositis (ulcerative) (J34.81)
oral mucositis (ulcerative) (K12.3-)
CC Exclusion see Appendix A PDX collection 0945
♀ **N76.89 Other specified inflammation of vagina and vulva**

N77 Vulvovaginal ulceration and inflammation in diseases classified elsewhere

♀ **N77.0 Ulceration of vulva in diseases classified elsewhere**
Code first underlying disease, such as:
Behçet's disease (M35.2)
Excludes1: *ulceration of vulva in gonococcal infection (A54.02)*
ulceration of vulva in herpesviral [herpes simplex] infection (A60.04)
ulceration of vulva in syphilis (A51.0)
ulceration of vulva in tuberculosis (A18.18)

♀ **N77.1 Vaginitis, vulvitis and vulvovaginitis in diseases classified elsewhere**
Code first underlying disease, such as:
pinworm (B80)
Excludes1: *candidal vulvovaginitis (B37.3)*
chlamydial vulvovaginitis (A56.02)
gonococcal vulvovaginitis (A54.02)
herpesviral [herpes simplex] vulvovaginitis (A60.04)
trichomonal vulvovaginitis (A59.01)
tuberculous vulvovaginitis (A18.18)
vulvovaginitis in early syphilis (A51.0)
vulvovaginitis in late syphilis (A52.76)

Noninflammatory disorders of female genital tract (N80-N98)

N80 Endometriosis

♀ **N80.0 Endometriosis of uterus**
Adenomyosis
Excludes1: *stromal endometriosis (D39.0)*
♀ **N80.1 Endometriosis of ovary**
♀ **N80.2 Endometriosis of fallopian tube**
♀ **N80.3 Endometriosis of pelvic peritoneum**
♀ **N80.4 Endometriosis of rectovaginal septum and vagina**
♀ **N80.5 Endometriosis of intestine**
♀ **N80.6 Endometriosis in cutaneous scar**
♀ **N80.8 Other endometriosis**
Endometriosis of thorax
♀ **N80.9 Endometriosis, unspecified**

N81 Female genital prolapse

Excludes1: *genital prolapse complicating pregnancy, labor or delivery (O34.5-)*
prolapse and hernia of ovary and fallopian tube (N83.4-)
prolapse of vaginal vault after hysterectomy (N99.3)

♀ **N81.0 Urethrocele**
Excludes1: *urethrocele with cystocele (N81.1-)*
urethrocele with prolapse of uterus (N81.2-N81.4)
\+ **N81.1 Cystocele**
Cystocele with urethrocele
Cystourethrocele
Excludes1: *cystocele with prolapse of uterus (N81.2-N81.4)*
♀ **N81.10 Cystocele, unspecified**
Prolapse of (anterior) vaginal wall NOS
♀ **N81.11 Cystocele, midline**
♀ **N81.12 Cystocele, lateral**
Paravaginal cystocele
♀ **N81.2 Incomplete uterovaginal prolapse**
First degree uterine prolapse
Prolapse of cervix NOS
Second degree uterine prolapse
Excludes1: *cervical stump prolapse (N81.85)*
♀ **N81.3 Complete uterovaginal prolapse**
Procidentia (uteri) NOS
Third degree uterine prolapse
♀ **N81.4 Uterovaginal prolapse, unspecified**
Prolapse of uterus NOS
♀ **N81.5 Vaginal enterocele**
Excludes1: *enterocele with prolapse of uterus (N81.2-N81.4)*
♀ **N81.6 Rectocele**
Prolapse of posterior vaginal wall
Use additional code for any associated fecal incontinence, if applicable (R15.-)
Excludes2: *perineocele (N81.81)*
rectal prolapse (K62.3)
rectocele with prolapse of uterus (N81.2-N81.4)
\+ **N81.8 Other female genital prolapse**
♀ **N81.81 Perineocele**
♀ **N81.82 Incompetence or weakening of pubocervical tissue**
♀ **N81.83 Incompetence or weakening of rectovaginal tissue**
♀ **N81.84 Pelvic muscle wasting**
Disuse atrophy of pelvic muscles and anal sphincter
♀ **N81.85 Cervical stump prolapse**
♀ **N81.89 Other female genital prolapse**
Deficient perineum
Old laceration of muscles of pelvic floor
♀ **N81.9 Female genital prolapse, unspecified**

N82 Fistulae involving female genital tract

Excludes1: *vesicointestinal fistulae (N32.1)*

♀ CC **N82.0 Vesicovaginal fistula**
CC Exclusion see Appendix A PDX collection 0946
♀ CC **N82.1 Other female urinary-genital tract fistulae**
Cervicovesical fistula
Ureterovaginal fistula
Urethrovaginal fistula
Uteroureteric fistula
Uterovesical fistula
CC Exclusion see Appendix A PDX collection 0946
♀ CC **N82.2 Fistula of vagina to small intestine**
CC Exclusion see Appendix A PDX collection 0946
♀ CC **N82.3 Fistula of vagina to large intestine**
Rectovaginal fistula
CC Exclusion see Appendix A PDX collection 0946
♀ CC **N82.4 Other female intestinal-genital tract fistulae**
Intestinouterine fistula
CC Exclusion see Appendix A PDX collection 0946
♀ CC **N82.5 Female genital tract-skin fistulae**
Uterus to abdominal wall fistula
Vaginoperineal fistula
CC Exclusion see Appendix A PDX collection 0946
♀ CC **N82.8 Other female genital tract fistulae**
CC Exclusion see Appendix A PDX collection 0946
♀ CC **N82.9 Female genital tract fistula, unspecified**
CC Exclusion see Appendix A PDX collection 0946

N83 Noninflammatory disorders of ovary, fallopian tube and broad ligament

Excludes2: *hydrosalpinx (N70.1-)*
AHA CC: 4Q, 2016, 46

\+ **N83.0 Follicular cyst of ovary**
Cyst of graafian follicle
Hemorrhagic follicular cyst (of ovary)
♀ **N83.00 Follicular cyst of ovary, unspecified side**
♀ **N83.01 Follicular cyst of right ovary**
♀ **N83.02 Follicular cyst of left ovary**
\+ **N83.1 Corpus luteum cyst**
Hemorrhagic corpus luteum cyst
♀ **N83.10 Corpus luteum cyst of ovary, unspecified side**
♀ **N83.11 Corpus luteum cyst of right ovary**
♀ **N83.12 Corpus luteum cyst of left ovary**
\+ **N83.2 Other and unspecified ovarian cysts**
Excludes1: *developmental ovarian cyst (Q50.1)*
neoplastic ovarian cyst (D27.-)
polycystic ovarian syndrome (E28.2)
Stein-Leventhal syndrome (E28.2)
\+ **N83.20 Unspecified ovarian cysts**
♀ **N83.201 Unspecified ovarian cyst, right side**
♀ **N83.202 Unspecified ovarian cyst, left side**
♀ **N83.209 Unspecified ovarian cyst, unspecified side**
Ovarian cyst, NOS
\+ **N83.29 Other ovarian cysts**
Retention cyst of ovary
Simple cyst of ovary
♀ **N83.291 Other ovarian cyst, right side**
♀ **N83.292 Other ovarian cyst, left side**
♀ **N83.299 Other ovarian cyst, unspecified side**
\+ **N83.3 Acquired atrophy of ovary and fallopian tube**
\+ **N83.31 Acquired atrophy of ovary**
♀ **N83.311 Acquired atrophy of right ovary**
♀ **N83.312 Acquired atrophy of left ovary**
♀ **N83.319 Acquired atrophy of ovary, unspecified side**
Acquired atrophy of ovary, NOS
\+ **N83.32 Acquired atrophy of fallopian tube**
♀ **N83.321 Acquired atrophy of right fallopian tube**
♀ **N83.322 Acquired atrophy of left fallopian tube**
♀ **N83.329 Acquired atrophy of fallopian tube, unspecified side**
Acquired atrophy of fallopian tube, NOS
\+ **N83.33 Acquired atrophy of ovary and fallopian tube**
♀ **N83.331 Acquired atrophy of right ovary and fallopian tube**
♀ **N83.332 Acquired atrophy of left ovary and fallopian tube**
♀ **N83.339 Acquired atrophy of ovary and fallopian tube, unspecified side**
Acquired atrophy of ovary and fallopian tube, NOS
\+ **N83.4 Prolapse and hernia of ovary and fallopian tube**
♀ **N83.40 Prolapse and hernia of ovary and fallopian tube, unspecified side**
Prolapse and hernia of ovary and fallopian tube, NOS
♀ **N83.41 Prolapse and hernia of right ovary and fallopian tube**
♀ **N83.42 Prolapse and hernia of left ovary and fallopian tube**

+ **N83.5 Torsion of ovary, ovarian pedicle and fallopian tube**
  Torsion of accessory tube
  + **N83.51 Torsion of ovary and ovarian pedicle**
    ♀ CC **N83.511 Torsion of right ovary and ovarian pedicle**
    CC Exclusion see Appendix A PDX collection 0947
    ♀ CC **N83.512 Torsion of left ovary and ovarian pedicle**
    CC Exclusion see Appendix A PDX collection 0947
    ♀ CC **N83.519 Torsion of ovary and ovarian pedicle, unspecified side**
    Torsion of ovary and ovarian pedicle, NOS
    CC Exclusion see Appendix A PDX collection 0947
  + **N83.52 Torsion of fallopian tube**
    Torsion of hydatid of Morgagni
    ♀ CC **N83.521 Torsion of right fallopian tube**
    CC Exclusion see Appendix A PDX collection 0947
    ♀ CC **N83.522 Torsion of left fallopian tube**
    CC Exclusion see Appendix A PDX collection 0947
    ♀ CC **N83.529 Torsion of fallopian tube, unspecified side**
    Torsion of fallopian tube, NOS
    CC Exclusion see Appendix A PDX collection 0947
  ♀ CC **N83.53 Torsion of ovary, ovarian pedicle and fallopian tube**
  CC Exclusion see Appendix A PDX collection 0947

♀ **N83.6 Hematosalpinx**
Excludes1: *hematosalpinx (with) (in):*
hematocolpos (N89.7)
hematometra (N85.7)
tubal pregnancy (O00.1-)

♀ **N83.7 Hematoma of broad ligament**

♀ **N83.8 Other noninflammatory disorders of ovary, fallopian tube and broad ligament**
Broad ligament laceration syndrome [Allen-Masters]

♀ **N83.9 Noninflammatory disorder of ovary, fallopian tube and broad ligament, unspecified**

N84 Polyp of female genital tract

Excludes1: *adenomatous polyp (D28.-)*
placental polyp (O90.89)

♀ **N84.0 Polyp of corpus uteri**
Polyp of endometrium
Polyp of uterus NOS
Excludes1: *polypoid endometrial hyperplasia (N85.0-)*

♀ **N84.1 Polyp of cervix uteri**
Mucous polyp of cervix

♀ **N84.2 Polyp of vagina**

♀ **N84.3 Polyp of vulva**
Polyp of labia

♀ **N84.8 Polyp of other parts of female genital tract**

♀ **N84.9 Polyp of female genital tract, unspecified**

N85 Other noninflammatory disorders of uterus, except cervix

Excludes1: *endometriosis (N80.-)*
inflammatory diseases of uterus (N71.-)
noninflammatory disorders of cervix, except malposition (N86-N88)
polyp of corpus uteri (N84.0)
uterine prolapse (N81.-)

+ **N85.0 Endometrial hyperplasia**
  ♀ **N85.00 Endometrial hyperplasia, unspecified**
  Hyperplasia (adenomatous) (cystic) (glandular) of endometrium
  Hyperplastic endometritis
  ♀ **N85.01 Benign endometrial hyperplasia**
  Endometrial hyperplasia (complex) (simple) without atypia
  ♀ **N85.02 Endometrial intraepithelial neoplasia [EIN]**
  Endometrial hyperplasia with atypia
  Excludes1: *malignant neoplasm of endometrium (with endometrial intraepithelial neoplasia [EIN]) (C54.1)*

♀ **N85.2 Hypertrophy of uterus**
Bulky or enlarged uterus
Excludes1: *puerperal hypertrophy of uterus (O90.89)*

♀ **N85.3 Subinvolution of uterus**
Excludes1: *puerperal subinvolution of uterus (O90.89)*

♀ **N85.4 Malposition of uterus**
Anteversion of uterus
Retroflexion of uterus
Retroversion of uterus
Excludes1: *malposition of uterus complicating pregnancy, labor or delivery (O34.5-, O65.5)*

♀ **N85.5 Inversion of uterus**
Excludes1: *current obstetric trauma (O71.2)*
postpartum inversion of uterus (O71.2)

♀ **N85.6 Intrauterine synechiae**

♀ **N85.7 Hematometra**
Hematosalpinx with hematometra
Excludes1: *hematometra with hematocolpos (N89.7)*

♀ **N85.8 Other specified noninflammatory disorders of uterus**
Atrophy of uterus, acquired
Fibrosis of uterus NOS

♀ **N85.9 Noninflammatory disorder of uterus, unspecified**
Disorder of uterus NOS

♀ N86 Erosion and ectropion of cervix uteri

Decubitus (trophic) ulcer of cervix
Eversion of cervix
Excludes1: *erosion and ectropion of cervix with cervicitis (N72)*
Valid 3-character code, no further characters required

N87 Dysplasia of cervix uteri

Excludes1: *abnormal results from cervical cytologic examination without histologic confirmation (R87.61-)*
carcinoma in situ of cervix uteri (D06.-)
cervical intraepithelial neoplasia III [CIN III] (D06.-)
HGSIL of cervix (R87.613)
severe dysplasia of cervix uteri (D06.-)

♀ **N87.0 Mild cervical dysplasia**
Cervical intraepithelial neoplasia I [CIN I]

♀ **N87.1 Moderate cervical dysplasia**
Cervical intraepithelial neoplasia II [CIN II]

♀ **N87.9 Dysplasia of cervix uteri, unspecified**
Anaplasia of cervix
Cervical atypism
Cervical dysplasia NOS

N88 Other noninflammatory disorders of cervix uteri

Excludes2: *inflammatory disease of cervix (N72)*
polyp of cervix (N84.1)

♀ **N88.0 Leukoplakia of cervix uteri**

♀ **N88.1 Old laceration of cervix uteri**
Adhesions of cervix
Excludes1: *current obstetric trauma (O71.3)*

♀ **N88.2 Stricture and stenosis of cervix uteri**
Excludes1: *stricture and stenosis of cervix uteri complicating labor (O65.5)*

♀ **N88.3 Incompetence of cervix uteri**
Investigation and management of (suspected) cervical incompetence in a nonpregnant woman
Excludes1: *cervical incompetence complicating pregnancy (O34.3-)*

♀ **N88.4 Hypertrophic elongation of cervix uteri**

♀ **N88.8 Other specified noninflammatory disorders of cervix uteri**
Excludes1: *current obstetric trauma (O71.3)*

♀ **N88.9 Noninflammatory disorder of cervix uteri, unspecified**

N89 Other noninflammatory disorders of vagina

Excludes1: *abnormal results from vaginal cytologic examination without histologic confirmation (R87.62-)*
carcinoma in situ of vagina (D07.2)
HGSIL of vagina (R87.623)
inflammation of vagina (N76.-)
senile (atrophic) vaginitis (N95.2)
severe dysplasia of vagina (D07.2)
trichomonal leukorrhea (A59.00)
vaginal intraepithelial neoplasia [VAIN], grade III (D07.2

♀ **N89.0 Mild vaginal dysplasia**
Vaginal intraepithelial neoplasia [VAIN], grade I

♀ **N89.1 Moderate vaginal dysplasia**
Vaginal intraepithelial neoplasia [VAIN], grade II

♀ **N89.3 Dysplasia of vagina, unspecified**

♀ **N89.4 Leukoplakia of vagina**

♀ **N89.5 Stricture and atresia of vagina**
Vaginal adhesions
Vaginal stenosis
Excludes1: *congenital atresia or stricture (Q52.4)*
postprocedural adhesions of vagina (N99.2)

♀ **N89.6 Tight hymenal ring**
Rigid hymen
Tight introitus
Excludes1: *imperforate hymen (Q52.3)*

♀ **N89.7 Hematocolpos**
Hematocolpos with hematometra or hematosalpinx
AHA CC: 4Q, 2016, 58-59

♀ **N89.8 Other specified noninflammatory disorders of vagina**
Leukorrhea NOS
Old vaginal laceration
Pessary ulcer of vagina
Excludes1: *current obstetric trauma (O70.-, O71.4, O71.7-O71.8)*
old laceration involving muscles of pelvic floor (N81.8)

♀ **N89.9 Noninflammatory disorder of vagina, unspecified**

N90 Other noninflammatory disorders of vulva and perineum
Excludes1: *anogenital (venereal) warts (A63.0)*
carcinoma in situ of vulva (D07.1)
condyloma acuminatum (A63.0)
current obstetric trauma (O70.-, O71.7-O71.8)
inflammation of vulva (N76.-)
severe dysplasia of vulva (D07.1)
vulvar intraepithelial neoplasm III [VIN III] (D07.1)

♀ **N90.0 Mild vulvar dysplasia**
Vulvar intraepithelial neoplasia [VIN], grade I

♀ **N90.1 Moderate vulvar dysplasia**
Vulvar intraepithelial neoplasia [VIN], grade II

♀ **N90.3 Dysplasia of vulva, unspecified**

♀ **N90.4 Leukoplakia of vulva**
Dystrophy of vulva
Kraurosis of vulva
Lichen sclerosus of external female genital organs

♀ **N90.5 Atrophy of vulva**
Stenosis of vulva

\+ **N90.6 Hypertrophy of vulva**
AHA CC: 4Q, 2016, 46

♀ **N90.60 Unspecified hypertrophy of vulva**
Unspecified hypertrophy of labia

♀ **N90.61 Childhood asymmetric labium majus enlargement**
CALME

♀ **N90.69 Other specified hypertrophy of vulva**
Other specified hypertrophy of labia

♀ **N90.7 Vulvar cyst**

\+ **N90.8 Other specified noninflammatory disorders of vulva and perineum**

\+ **N90.81 Female genital mutilation status**
Female genital cutting status

♀ **N90.810 Female genital mutilation status, unspecified**
Female genital cutting status, unspecified
Female genital mutilation status NOS

♀ **N90.811 Female genital mutilation Type I status**
Clitorectomy status
Female genital cutting Type I status

♀ **N90.812 Female genital mutilation Type II status**
Clitorectomy with excision of labia minora status
Female genital cutting Type II status

♀ **N90.813 Female genital mutilation Type III status**
Female genital cutting Type III status
Infibulation status

♀ **N90.818 Other female genital mutilation status**
Female genital cutting Type IV status
Female genital mutilation Type IV status
Other female genital cutting status

♀ **N90.89 Other specified noninflammatory disorders of vulva and perineum**
Adhesions of vulva
Hypertrophy of clitoris

♀ **N90.9 Noninflammatory disorder of vulva and perineum, unspecified**

N91 Absent, scanty and rare menstruation
Excludes1: *ovarian dysfunction (E28.-)*

♀ **N91.0 Primary amenorrhea**
♀ **N91.1 Secondary amenorrhea**
♀ **N91.2 Amenorrhea, unspecified**
♀ **N91.3 Primary oligomenorrhea**
♀ **N91.4 Secondary oligomenorrhea**
♀ **N91.5 Oligomenorrhea, unspecified**
Hypomenorrhea NOS

N92 Excessive, frequent and irregular menstruation
Excludes1: *postmenopausal bleeding (N95.0)*
precocious puberty (menstruation) (E30.1)

♀ **N92.0 Excessive and frequent menstruation with regular cycle**
Heavy periods NOS
Menorrhagia NOS
Polymenorrhea

♀ **N92.1 Excessive and frequent menstruation with irregular cycle**
Irregular intermenstrual bleeding
Irregular, shortened intervals between menstrual bleeding
Menometrorrhagia
Metrorrhagia

● ♀ **N92.2 Excessive menstruation at puberty**
Excessive bleeding associated with onset of menstrual periods
Pubertal menorrhagia
Puberty bleeding

♀ **N92.3 Ovulation bleeding**
Regular intermenstrual bleeding

♀ **N92.4 Excessive bleeding in the premenopausal period**
Climacteric menorrhagia or metrorrhagia
Menopausal menorrhagia or metrorrhagia
Preclimacteric menorrhagia or metrorrhagia
Premenopausal menorrhagia or metrorrhagia

♀ **N92.5 Other specified irregular menstruation**

♀ **N92.6 Irregular menstruation, unspecified**
Irregular bleeding NOS
Irregular periods NOS
Excludes1: *irregular menstruation with:*
lengthened intervals or scanty bleeding (N91.3-N91.5)
shortened intervals or excessive bleeding (N92.1)

N93 Other abnormal uterine and vaginal bleeding
Excludes1: *neonatal vaginal hemorrhage (P54.6)*
precocious puberty (menstruation) (E30.1)
pseudomenses (P54.6)

♀ **N93.0 Postcoital and contact bleeding**

♀ **N93.1 Pre-pubertal vaginal bleeding**
AHA CC: 4Q, 2016, 47

♀ **N93.8 Other specified abnormal uterine and vaginal bleeding**
Dysfunctional or functional uterine or vaginal bleeding NOS

♀ **N93.9 Abnormal uterine and vaginal bleeding,unspecified**

N94 Pain and other conditions associated with female genital organs and menstrual cycle

♀ **N94.0 Mittelschmerz**

\+ **N94.1 Dyspareunia**
Excludes1: *psychogenic dyspareunia (F52.6)*
AHA CC: 4Q, 2016, 47

♀ **N94.10 Unspecified dyspareunia**
♀ **N94.11 Superficial (introital) dyspareunia**
♀ **N94.12 Deep dyspareunia**
♀ **N94.19 Other specified dyspareunia**

♀ **N94.2 Vaginismus**
Excludes1: *psychogenic vaginismus (F52.5)*

♀ **N94.3 Premenstrual tension syndrome**
Code also associated menstrual migraine (G43.82-, G43.83-)
Excludes1: *Premenstrual dysphoric disorder (F32.81)*

♀ **N94.4 Primary dysmenorrhea**
♀ **N94.5 Secondary dysmenorrhea**
♀ **N94.6 Dysmenorrhea, unspecified**
Excludes1: *psychogenic dysmenorrhea (F45.8)*

\+ **N94.8 Other specified conditions associated with female genital organs and menstrual cycle**

\+ **N94.81 Vulvodynia**

♀ **N94.810 Vulvar vestibulitis**
♀ **N94.818 Other vulvodynia**
♀ **N94.819 Vulvodynia, unspecified**
Vulvodynia NOS

♀ **N94.89 Other specified conditions associated with female genital organs and menstrual cycle**

♀ **N94.9 Unspecified condition associated with female genital organs and menstrual cycle**

N95 Menopausal and other perimenopausal disorders

Menopausal and other perimenopausal disorders due to naturally occurring (age-related) menopause and perimenopause

Excludes1: *excessive bleeding in the premenopausal period (N92.4)*
menopausal and perimenopausal disorders due to artificial or premature menopause (E89.4-, E28.31-)
premature menopause (E28.31-)

Excludes2: *postmenopausal osteoporosis (M81.0-)*
postmenopausal osteoporosis with current pathological fracture (M80.0-)
postmenopausal urethritis (N34.2)

♀ **N95.0 Postmenopausal bleeding**

♀ **N95.1 Menopausal and female climacteric states**

Symptoms such as flushing, sleeplessness, headache, lack of concentration, associated with natural (age-related) menopause

Use additional code for associated symptoms

Excludes1: *asymptomatic menopausal state (Z78.0)*
symptoms associated with artificial menopause (E89.41)
symptoms associated with premature menopause (E28.310)

♀ **N95.2 Postmenopausal atrophic vaginitis**

Senile (atrophic) vaginitis

♀ **N95.8 Other specified menopausal and perimenopausal disorders**

♀ **N95.9 Unspecified menopausal and perimenopausal disorder**

♀ **N96 Recurrent pregnancy loss**

Investigation or care in a nonpregnant woman with history of recurrent pregnancy loss

Excludes1: *recurrent pregancy loss with current pregnancy (O26.2-)*

Valid 3-character code, no further characters required

N97 Female infertility

Includes: inability to achieve a pregnancy
sterility, female NOS

Excludes1: *female infertility associated with:*
hypopituitarism (E23.0)
Stein-Leventhal syndrome (E28.2)

Excludes2: *incompetence of cervix uteri (N88.3)*

♀ **N97.0 Female infertility associated with anovulation**

♀ **N97.1 Female infertility of tubal origin**

Female infertility associated with congenital anomaly of tube
Female infertility due to tubal block
Female infertility due to tubal occlusion
Female infertility due to tubal stenosis

♀ **N97.2 Female infertility of uterine origin**

Female infertility associated with congenital anomaly of uterus
Female infertility due to nonimplantation of ovum

♀ **N97.8 Female infertility of other origin**

♀ **N97.9 Female infertility, unspecified**

N98 Complications associated with artificial fertilization

♀ CC **N98.0 Infection associated with artificial insemination**
CC Exclusion see Appendix A PDX collection 0948

♀ CC **N98.1 Hyperstimulation of ovaries**

Hyperstimulation of ovaries NOS
Hyperstimulation of ovaries associated with induced ovulation
CC Exclusion see Appendix A PDX collection 0643

♀ CC **N98.2 Complications of attempted introduction of fertilized ovum following in vitro fertilization**
CC Exclusion see Appendix A PDX collection 0643

♀ CC **N98.3 Complications of attempted introduction of embryo in embryo transfer**
CC Exclusion see Appendix A PDX collection 0643

♀ CC **N98.8 Other complications associated with artificial fertilization**
CC Exclusion see Appendix A PDX collection 0643

♀ **N98.9 Complication associated with artificial fertilization, unspecified**
CC Exclusion see Appendix A PDX collection 0643

Intraoperative and postprocedural complications and disorders of genitourinary system, not elsewhere classified (N99)

N99 Intraoperative and postprocedural complications and disorders of genitourinary system, not elsewhere classified

Excludes2: *irradiation cystitis (N30.4-)*
postoophorectomy osteoporosis with current pathological fracture (M80.8-)
postoophorectomy osteoporosis without current pathological fracture (M81.8)

N99.0 Postprocedural (acute) (chronic) kidney failure

Use additional code to type of kidney disease

\+ **N99.1 Postprocedural urethral stricture**

Postcatheterization urethral stricture

\+ **N99.11 Postprocedural urethral stricture, male**

♂ **N99.110 Postprocedural urethral stricture, male, meatal**

♂ **N99.111 Postprocedural bulbous urethral stricture, male**

♂ **N99.112 Postprocedural membranous urethral stricture, male**

♂ **N99.113 Postprocedural anterior bulbous urethral stricture, male**

AHA CC: 4Q, 2016, 47-48

♂ **N99.114 Postprocedural urethral stricture, male, unspecified**

♂ **N99.115 Postprocedural fossa navicularis urethral stricture**

AHA CC: 4Q, 2016, 47-48

♀ **N99.12 Postprocedural urethral stricture, female**

♀ **N99.2 Postprocedural adhesions of vagina**

♀ **N99.3 Prolapse of vaginal vault after hysterectomy**

N99.4 Postprocedural pelvic peritoneal adhesions

Excludes2: *pelvic peritoneal adhesions NOS (N73.6)*
postinfective pelvic peritoneal adhesions (N73.6)

\+ **N99.5 Complications of stoma of urinary tract**

Excludes2: *mechanical complication of urinary catheter (T83.0-)*

AHA CC: 4Q, 2016, 48

\+ **N99.51 Complication of cystostomy**

CC **N99.510 Cystostomy hemorrhage**
CC Exclusion see Appendix A PDX collection 0949

CC **N99.511 Cystostomy infection**
CC Exclusion see Appendix A PDX collection 0950

CC **N99.512 Cystostomy malfunction**
CC Exclusion see Appendix A PDX collection 0951

CC **N99.518 Other cystostomy complication**
CC Exclusion see Appendix A PDX collection 0949

\+ **N99.52 Complication of incontinent external stoma of urinary tract**

N99.520 Hemorrhage of incontinent external stoma of urinary tract

N99.521 Infection of incontinent external stoma of urinary tract

AHA CC: 4Q, 2016, 48

N99.522 Malfunction of incontinent external stoma of urinary tract

N99.523 Herniation of incontinent stoma of urinary tract

N99.524 Stenosis of incontinent stoma of urinary tract

N99.528 Other complication of incontinent external stoma of urinary tract

\+ **N99.53 Complication of continent stoma of urinary tract**

N99.530 Hemorrhage of continent stoma of urinary tract

N99.531 Infection of continent stoma of urinary tract

N99.532 Malfunction of continent stoma of urinary tract

N99.533 Herniation of continent stoma of urinary tract

N99.534 Stenosis of continent stoma of urinary tract

N99.538 Other complication of continent stoma of urinary tract

\+ **N99.6 Intraoperative hemorrhage and hematoma of a genitourinary system organ or structure complicating a procedure**

Excludes1: *intraoperative hemorrhage and hematoma of a genitourinary system organ or structure due to accidental puncture or laceration during a procedure (N99.7-)*

N99.61 Intraoperative hemorrhage and hematoma of a genitourinary system organ or structure complicating a genitourinary system procedure
CC Exclusion see Appendix A PDX collection 0952

CC **N99.62 Intraoperative hemorrhage and hematoma of a genitourinary system organ or structure complicating other procedure**
CC Exclusion see Appendix A PDX collection 0952

\+ **N99.7 Accidental puncture and laceration of a genitourinary system organ or structure during a procedure**

CC **N99.71 Accidental puncture and laceration of a genitourinary system organ or structure during a genitourinary system procedure**
CC Exclusion see Appendix A PDX collection 0509

CC N99.72 Accidental puncture and laceration of a genitourinary system organ or structure during other procedure
CC Exclusion see Appendix A PDX collection 0509

+ N99.8 Other intraoperative and postprocedural complications and disorders of genitourinary system
AHA CC: 4Q, 2016, 9-10

N99.81 Other intraoperative complications of genitourinary system

+ N99.82 Postprocedural hemorrhage of a genitourinary system organ or structure following a procedure

CC N99.820 Postprocedural hemorrhage of a genitourinary system organ or structure following a genitourinary system procedure
CC Exclusion see Appendix A PDX collection 0952

CC N99.821 Postprocedural hemorrhage of a genitourinary system organ or structure following other procedure
CC Exclusion see Appendix A PDX collection 0952

♀ N99.83 Residual ovary syndrome

+ N99.84 Postprocedural hematoma and seroma of a genitourinary system organ or structure following a procedure

CC N99.840 Postprocedural hematoma of a genitourinary system organ or structure following a genitourinary system procedure
CC Exclusion see Appendix A PDX collection 0952

CC N99.841 Postprocedural hematoma of a genitourinary system organ or structure following other procedure
CC Exclusion see Appendix A PDX collection 0952

CC N99.842 Postprocedural seroma of a genitourinary system organ or structure following a genitourinary system procedure
CC Exclusion see Appendix A PDX collection 0952

CC N99.843 Postprocedural seroma of a genitourinary system organ or structure following other procedure
CC Exclusion see Appendix A PDX collection 0952

N99.89 Other postprocedural complications and disorders of genitourinary system

Chapter 15: Pregnancy, Childbirth and the Puerperium (O00-O9A)

NOTE Codes from this chapter are for use only on maternal records, never on newborn records
Codes from this chapter are for use for conditions related to or aggravated by the pregnancy, childbirth, or by the puerperium (maternal causes or obstetric causes)

NOTE Trimesters are counted from the first day of the last menstrual period. They are defined as follows:
1st trimester- less than 14 weeks 0 days
2nd trimester- 14 weeks 0 days to less than 28 weeks 0 days
3rd trimester- 28 weeks 0 days until delivery

Use additional code from category Z3A, Weeks of gestation, to identify the specific week of the pregnancy, if known

Excludes1: *supervision of normal pregnancy (Z34.-)*

Excludes2: *mental and behavioral disorders associated with the puerperium (F53)*
obstetrical tetanus (A34)
postpartum necrosis of pituitary gland (E23.0)
puerperal osteomalacia (M83.0)

This chapter contains the following category blocks:

O00-O08	Pregnancy with abortive outcome
O09	Supervision of high risk pregnancy
O10-O16	Edema, proteinuria and hypertensive disorders in pregnancy, childbirth and the puerperium
O20-O29	Other maternal disorders predominantly related to pregnancy
O30-O48	Maternal care related to the fetus and amniotic cavity and possible delivery problems
O60-O77	Complications of labor and delivery
O80-O82	Encounter for delivery
O85-O92	Complications predominantly related to the puerperium
O94-O9A	Other obstetric conditions, not elsewhere classified

C. Chapter-Specific Coding Guidelines

In addition to general coding guidelines, there are guidelines for specific diagnoses and/or conditions in the classification. Unless otherwise indicated, these guidelines apply to all health care settings. Please refer to Section II for guidelines on the selection of principal diagnosis.

15. Chapter 15: Pregnancy, Childbirth and the Puerperium (O00-O9A)

a. General Rules for Obstetric Cases

1) Codes from chapter 15 and sequencing priority

Obstetric cases require codes from chapter 15, codes in the range O00-O9A, Pregnancy, Childbirth, and the Puerperium. Chapter 15 codes have sequencing priority over codes from other chapters. Additional codes from other chapters may be used in conjunction with chapter 15 codes to further specify conditions. Should the provider document that the pregnancy is incidental to the encounter, then code Z33.1, Pregnant state, incidental, should be used in place of any chapter 15 codes. It is the provider's responsibility to state that the condition being treated is not affecting the pregnancy.

2) Chapter 15 codes used only on the maternal record

Chapter 15 codes are to be used only on the maternal record, never on the record of the newborn.

3) Final character for trimester

The majority of codes in Chapter 15 have a final character indicating the trimester of pregnancy. The timeframes for the trimesters are indicated at the beginning of the chapter. If trimester is not a component of a code it is because the condition always occurs in a specific trimester, or the concept of trimester of pregnancy is not applicable. Certain codes have characters for only certain trimesters because the condition does not occur in all trimesters, but it may occur in more than just one.

Assignment of the final character for trimester should be based on the provider's documentation of the trimester (or number of weeks) for the current admission/encounter. This applies to the assignment of trimester for pre-existing conditions as well as those that develop during or are due to the pregnancy. The provider's documentation of the number of weeks may be used to assign the appropriate code identifying the trimester.

Whenever delivery occurs during the current admission, and there is an "in childbirth" option for the obstetric complication being coded, the "in childbirth" code should be assigned.

4) Selection of trimester for inpatient admissions that encompass more than one trimester

In instances when a patient is admitted to a hospital for complications of pregnancy during one trimester and remains in the hospital into a subsequent trimester, the trimester character for the antepartum complication code should be assigned on the basis of the trimester when the complication developed, not the trimester of the discharge. If the condition developed prior to the current admission/encounter or represents a pre-existing condition, the trimester character for the trimester at the time of the admission/encounter should be assigned.

5) Unspecified trimester

Each category that includes codes for trimester has a code for "unspecified trimester." The "unspecified trimester" code should rarely be used, such as when the documentation in the record is insufficient to determine the trimester and it is not possible to obtain clarification.

6) 7th character for Fetus Identification

Where applicable, a 7th character is to be assigned for certain categories (O31, O32, O33.3 - O33.6, O35, O36, O40, O41, O60.1, O60.2, O64, and O69) to identify the fetus for which the complication code applies.

Assign 7th character "0":

- For single gestations
- When the documentation in the record is insufficient to determine the fetus affected and it is not possible to obtain clarification.
- When it is not possible to clinically determine which fetus is affected.

b. Selection of OB Principal or First-listed Diagnosis

1) Routine outpatient prenatal visits

For routine outpatient prenatal visits when no complications are present, a code from category Z34, Encounter for supervision of normal pregnancy, should be used as the first-listed diagnosis. These codes should not be used in conjunction with chapter 15 codes.

2) Supervision of High-Risk Pregnancy

Codes from category O09, Supervision of high-risk pregnancy, are intended for use only during the prenatal period. For complications during the labor or delivery episode as a result of a high-risk pregnancy, assign the applicable complication codes from Chapter 15. If there are no complications during the labor or delivery episode, assign code O80, Encounter for full-term uncomplicated delivery.

For routine prenatal outpatient visits for patients with high-risk pregnancies, a code from category O09, Supervision of high-risk pregnancy, should be used as the first-listed diagnosis. Secondary chapter 15 codes may be used in conjunction with these codes if appropriate.

3) Episodes when no delivery occurs

In episodes when no delivery occurs, the principal diagnosis should correspond to the principal complication of the pregnancy which necessitated the encounter. Should more than one complication exist, all of which are treated or monitored, any of the complications codes may be sequenced first.

4) When a delivery occurs

When an obstetric patient is admitted and delivers during that admission, the condition that prompted the admission should be sequenced as the principal diagnosis. If multiple conditions prompted the admission, sequence the one most related to the delivery as the principal diagnosis. A code for any complication of the delivery should be assigned as an additional diagnosis. In cases of cesarean delivery, if the patient was admitted with a condition that resulted in the performance of a cesarean procedure, that condition should be selected as the principal diagnosis. If the reason for the admission was unrelated to the condition resulting in the cesarean delivery, the condition related to the reason for the admission should be selected as the principal diagnosis.

5) Outcome of delivery

A code from category Z37, Outcome of delivery, should be included on every maternal record when a delivery has occurred. These codes are not to be used on subsequent records or on the newborn record.

c. Pre-existing conditions versus conditions due to the pregnancy

Certain categories in Chapter 15 distinguish between conditions of the mother that existed prior to pregnancy (pre-existing) and those that are a direct result of pregnancy. When assigning codes from Chapter 15, it is important to assess if a condition was pre-existing prior to pregnancy or developed during or due to the pregnancy in order to assign the correct code.

Categories that do not distinguish between pre-existing and pregnancy- related conditions may be used for either. It is acceptable to use codes specifically for the puerperium with codes complicating pregnancy and childbirth if a condition arises postpartum during the delivery encounter.

d. Pre-existing hypertension in pregnancy

Category O10, Pre-existing hypertension complicating pregnancy, childbirth and the puerperium, includes codes for hypertensive heart and hypertensive chronic kidney disease. When assigning one of the O10 codes that includes hypertensive heart disease or hypertensive chronic kidney disease, it is necessary to add a secondary code from the appropriate hypertension category to specify the type of heart failure or chronic kidney disease.

See Section I.C.9. Hypertension.

e. Fetal Conditions Affecting the Management of the Mother

1) Codes from categories O35 and O36

Codes from categories O35, Maternal care for known or suspected fetal abnormality and damage, and O36, Maternal care for other fetal problems, are assigned only when the fetal condition is actually responsible for modifying the management of the mother, i.e., by requiring diagnostic studies, additional observation, special care, or termination of pregnancy. The fact that the fetal condition exists does not justify assigning a code from this series to the mother's record.

2) In utero surgery

In cases when surgery is performed on the fetus, a diagnosis code from category O35, Maternal care for known or suspected fetal abnormality and damage, should be assigned identifying the fetal condition. Assign the appropriate procedure code for the procedure performed.

No code from Chapter 16, the perinatal codes, should be used on the mother's record to identify fetal conditions. Surgery performed in utero on a fetus is still to be coded as an obstetric encounter.

f. HIV Infection in Pregnancy, Childbirth and the Puerperium

During pregnancy, childbirth or the puerperium, a patient admitted because of an HIV-related illness should receive a principal diagnosis from subcategory O98.7-, Human immunodeficiency [HIV] disease complicating pregnancy, childbirth and the puerperium, followed by the code(s) for the HIV-related illness(es).

Patients with asymptomatic HIV infection status admitted during pregnancy, childbirth, or the puerperium should receive codes of O98.7- and Z21, Asymptomatic human immunodeficiency virus [HIV] infection status.

g. Diabetes mellitus in pregnancy

Diabetes mellitus is a significant complicating factor in pregnancy. Pregnant women who are diabetic should be assigned a code from category O24, Diabetes mellitus in pregnancy, childbirth, and the puerperium, first, followed by the appropriate diabetes code(s) (E08- E13) from Chapter 4.

h. Long term use of insulin and oral hypoglycemics

See section I.C.4.a.3 for information on the long term use of insulin and oral hypoglycemic.

i. Gestational (pregnancy induced) diabetes

Gestational (pregnancy induced) diabetes can occur during the second and third trimester of pregnancy in women who were not diabetic prior to pregnancy. Gestational diabetes can cause complications in the pregnancy similar to those of pre-existing diabetes mellitus. It also puts the woman at greater risk of developing diabetes after the pregnancy. Codes for gestational diabetes are in subcategory O24.4, Gestational diabetes mellitus. No other code from category O24, Diabetes mellitus in pregnancy, childbirth, and the puerperium, should be used with a code from O24.4

The codes under subcategory O24.4 include diet controlled, insulin controlled, and controlled by oral hypoglycemic drugs. If a patient with gestational diabetes is treated with both diet and insulin, only the code for insulin-controlled is required. If a patient with gestational diabetes is treated with both diet and oral hypoglycemic medications, only the code for "controlled by oral hypoglycemic drugs" is required.

Code Z79.4, Long-term (current) use of insulin or code Z79.84, Long-term (current) use of oral hypoglycemic drugs, should not be assigned with codes from subcategory O24.4.

An abnormal glucose tolerance in pregnancy is assigned a code from subcategory O99.81, Abnormal glucose complicating pregnancy, childbirth, and the puerperium.

j. Sepsis and septic shock complicating abortion, pregnancy, childbirth and the puerperium

When assigning a chapter 15 code for sepsis complicating abortion, pregnancy, childbirth, and the puerperium, a code for the specific type of infection should be assigned as an additional diagnosis. If severe sepsis is present, a code from subcategory R65.2, Severe sepsis, and code(s) for associated organ dysfunction(s) should also be assigned as additional diagnoses.

k. Puerperal sepsis

Code O85, Puerperal sepsis, should be assigned with a secondary code to identify the causal organism (e.g., for a bacterial infection, assign a code from category B95-B96, Bacterial infections in conditions classified elsewhere). A code from category A40, Streptococcal sepsis, or A41, Other sepsis, should not be used for puerperal sepsis. If applicable, use additional codes to identify severe sepsis (R65.2-) and any associated acute organ dysfunction.

l. Alcohol and tobacco use during pregnancy, childbirth and the puerperium

1) Alcohol use during pregnancy, childbirth and the puerperium

Codes under subcategory O99.31, Alcohol use complicating pregnancy, childbirth, and the puerperium, should be assigned for any pregnancy case when a mother uses alcohol during the pregnancy or postpartum. A secondary code from category F10, Alcohol related disorders, should also be assigned to identify manifestations of the alcohol use.

2) Tobacco use during pregnancy, childbirth and the puerperium

Codes under subcategory O99.33, Smoking (tobacco) complicating pregnancy, childbirth, and the puerperium, should be assigned for any pregnancy case when a mother uses any type of tobacco product during the pregnancy or postpartum. A secondary code from category F17, Nicotine dependence, should also be assigned to identify the type of nicotine dependence.

m. Poisoning, toxic effects, adverse effects and underdosing in a pregnant patient

A code from subcategory O9A.2, Injury, poisoning and certain other consequences of external causes complicating pregnancy, childbirth, and the puerperium, should be sequenced first, followed by the appropriate injury, poisoning, toxic effect, adverse effect or underdosing code, and then the additional code(s) that specifies the condition caused by the poisoning, toxic effect, adverse effect or underdosing.

See Section I.C.19. Adverse effects, poisoning, underdosing and toxic effects.

n. Normal Delivery, Code O80

1) Encounter for full term uncomplicated delivery

Code O80 should be assigned when a woman is admitted for a full-term normal delivery and delivers a single, healthy infant without any complications antepartum, during the delivery, or postpartum during the delivery episode. Code O80 is always a principal diagnosis. It is not to be used if any other code from chapter 15 is needed to describe a current complication of the antenatal, delivery, or perinatal period. Additional codes from other chapters may be used with code O80 if they are not related to or are in any way complicating the pregnancy.

2) Uncomplicated delivery with resolved antepartum complication

Code O80 may be used if the patient had a complication at some point during the pregnancy, but the complication is not present at the time of the admission for delivery.

3) Outcome of delivery for O80

Z37.0, Single live birth, is the only outcome of delivery code appropriate for use with O80.

o. The Peripartum and Postpartum Periods

1) Peripartum and Postpartum periods

The postpartum period begins immediately after delivery and continues for six weeks following delivery. The peripartum period is defined as the last month of pregnancy to five months postpartum.

2) Peripartum and postpartum complication

A postpartum complication is any complication occurring within the six-week period.

3) Pregnancy-related complications after 6 week period

Chapter 15 codes may also be used to describe pregnancy-related complications after the peripartum or postpartum period if the provider documents that a condition is pregnancy related.

4) Admission for routine postpartum care following delivery outside hospital

When the mother delivers outside the hospital prior to admission and is admitted for routine postpartum care and no complications are noted, code Z39.0, Encounter for care and examination of mother immediately after delivery, should be assigned as the principal diagnosis.

5) Pregnancy associated cardiomyopathy

Pregnancy associated cardiomyopathy, code O90.3, is unique in that it may be diagnosed in the third trimester of pregnancy but may continue to progress months after delivery. For this reason, it is referred to as peripartum cardiomyopathy. Code O90.3 is only for use when the cardiomyopathy develops as a result of pregnancy in a woman who did not have pre-existing heart disease.

p. Code O94, Sequelae of complication of pregnancy, childbirth, and the puerperium

1) Code O94

Code O94, Sequelae of complication of pregnancy, childbirth, and the puerperium, is for use in those cases when an initial complication of a pregnancy develops a sequelae requiring care or treatment at a future date.

2) After the initial postpartum period

This code may be used at any time after the initial postpartum period.

3) Sequencing of Code O94

This code, like all sequela codes, is to be sequenced following the code describing the sequelae of the complication.

q. Termination of Pregnancy and Spontaneous abortions

1) Abortion with Liveborn Fetus

When an attempted termination of pregnancy results in a liveborn fetus, assign code Z33.2, Encounter for elective termination of pregnancy and a code from category Z37, Outcome of Delivery.

2) Retained Products of Conception following an abortion

Subsequent encounters for retained products of conception following a spontaneous abortion or elective termination of pregnancy, **without complications** are assigned O03**.4, Incomplete spontaneous,** abortion **without complication,** or codes O07.4, Failed attempted termination of pregnancy without complication. This advice is appropriate even when the patient was discharged previously with a discharge diagnosis of complete abortion. **If the patient has a specific complication associated with the spontaneous abortion or elective termination of pregnancy in addition to retained products of conception, assign the appropriate complication in category O03 or O07 instead of code O03.4 or O07.4.**

3) Complications leading to abortion

Codes from Chapter 15 may be used as additional codes to identify any documented complications of the pregnancy in conjunction with codes in categories in **O04,** O07 and O08.

r. Abuse in a pregnant patient

For suspected or confirmed cases of abuse of a pregnant patient, a code(s) from subcategories O9A.3, Physical abuse complicating pregnancy, childbirth, and the puerperium, O9A.4, Sexual abuse complicating pregnancy, childbirth, and the puerperium, and O9A.5, Psychological abuse complicating pregnancy, childbirth, and the puerperium, should be sequenced first, followed by the appropriate codes (if applicable) to identify any associated current injury due to physical abuse, sexual abuse, and the perpetrator of abuse.

See Section I.C.19. Adult and child abuse, neglect and other maltreatment.

Pregnancy with abortive outcome (O00-O08)

Excludes1: *continuing pregnancy in multiple gestation after abortion of one fetus or more (O31.1-, O31.3-)*

O00 Ectopic pregnancy

Includes: ruptured ectopic pregnancy

Use additional code from category O08 to identify any associated complication

AHA CC: 4Q, 2016, 48-50

+ **O00.0 Abdominal pregnancy**
  - **Excludes1:** *maternal care for viable fetus in abdominal pregnancy (O36.7-)*
- • ♀ CC **O00.00 Abdominal pregnancy without intrauterine pregnancy**
  - Abdominal pregnancy NOS
  - **CC Exclusion see Appendix A PDX collection 0953**
- • ♀ CC **O00.01 Abdominal pregnancy with intrauterine pregnancy**
  - **CC Exclusion see Appendix A PDX collection 0953**

+ **O00.1 Tubal pregnancy**
  - Fallopian pregnancy
  - Rupture of (fallopian) tube due to pregnancy
  - Tubal abortion
- + **O00.10 Tubal pregnancy without intrauterine pregnancy**
  - Tubal pregnancy NOS
  - • ♀ CC **O00.101 Right tubal pregnancy without intrauterine pregnancy**
    - **CC Exclusion see Appendix A PDX collection 0953**
  - • ♀ CC **O00.102 Left tubal pregnancy without intrauterine pregnancy**
    - **CC Exclusion see Appendix A PDX collection 0953**
  - • ♀ CC **O00.109 Unspecified tubal pregnancy without intrauterine pregnancy**
    - **CC Exclusion see Appendix A PDX collection 0953**
- + **O00.11 Tubal pregnancy with intrauterine pregnancy**
  - • ♀ CC **O00.111 Right tubal pregnancy with intrauterine pregnancy**
    - **CC Exclusion see Appendix A PDX collection 0953**
  - • ♀ CC **O00.112 Left tubal pregnancy with intrauterine pregnancy**
    - **CC Exclusion see Appendix A PDX collection 0953**
  - • ♀ CC **O00.119 Unspecified tubal pregnancy with intrauterine pregnancy**
    - **CC Exclusion see Appendix A PDX collection 0953**

+ **O00.2 Ovarian pregnancy**
- + **O00.20 Ovarian pregnancy without intrauterine pregnancy**
  - Ovarian pregnancy NOS
  - • ♀ CC **O00.201 Right ovarian pregnancy without intrauterine pregnancy**
    - **CC Exclusion see Appendix A PDX collection 0953**
  - • ♀ CC **O00.202 Left ovarian pregnancy without intrauterine pregnancy**
    - **CC Exclusion see Appendix A PDX collection 0953**
  - • ♀ CC **O00.209 Unspecified ovarian pregnancy without intrauterine pregnancy**
    - **CC Exclusion see Appendix A PDX collection 0953**
- + **O00.21 Ovarian pregnancy with intrauterine pregnancy**
  - • ♀ CC **O00.211 Right ovarian pregnancy with intrauterine pregnancy**
    - **CC Exclusion see Appendix A PDX collection 0953**
  - • ♀ CC **O00.212 Left ovarian pregnancy with intrauterine pregnancy**
    - **CC Exclusion see Appendix A PDX collection 0953**
  - • ♀ CC **O00.219 Unspecified ovarian pregnancy with intrauterine pregnancy**
    - **CC Exclusion see Appendix A PDX collection 0953**

+ **O00.8 Other ectopic pregnancy**
  - Cervical pregnancy
  - Cornual pregnancy
  - Intraligamentous pregnancy
  - Mural pregnancy
- • ♀ CC **O00.80 Other ectopic pregnancy without intrauterine pregnancy**
  - Other ectopic pregnancy NOS
  - **CC Exclusion see Appendix A PDX collection 0953**
- • ♀ CC **O00.81 Other ectopic pregnancy with intrauterine pregnancy**
  - **CC Exclusion see Appendix A PDX collection 0953**

+ **O00.9 Ectopic pregnancy, unspecified**
- • ♀ CC **O00.90 Unspecified ectopic pregnancy without intrauterine pregnancy**
  - Ectopic pregnancy NOS
  - **CC Exclusion see Appendix A PDX collection 0953**
- • ♀ CC **O00.91 Unspecified ectopic pregnancy with intrauterine pregnancy**
  - **CC Exclusion see Appendix A PDX collection 0953**

O01 Hydatidiform mole

Use additional code from category O08 to identify any associated complication

Excludes1: *chorioadenoma (destruens) (D39.2)*
malignant hydatidiform mole (D39.2)

- • ♀ **O01.0 Classical hydatidiform mole**
  - Complete hydatidiform mole
- • ♀ **O01.1 Incomplete and partial hydatidiform mole**
- • ♀ **O01.9 Hydatidiform mole, unspecified**
  - Trophoblastic disease NOS
  - Vesicular mole NOS

O02 Other abnormal products of conception

Use additional code from category O08 to identify any associated complication

Excludes1: *papyraceous fetus (O31.0-)*

- • ♀ **O02.0 Blighted ovum and nonhydatidiform mole**
  - Carneous mole
  - Fleshy mole
  - Intrauterine mole NOS
  - Molar pregnancy NEC
  - Pathological ovum

• ♀ O02.1 **Missed abortion**
Early fetal death, before completion of 20 weeks of gestation, with retention of dead fetus
Excludes1: *failed induced abortion (O07.-)*
fetal death (intrauterine) (late) (O36.4)
missed abortion with blighted ovum (O02.0)
missed abortion with hydatidiform mole (O01.-)
missed abortion with nonhydatidiform (O02.0)
missed abortion with other abnormal products of conception (O02.8-)
missed delivery (O36.4)
stillbirth (P95)

+ O02.8 **Other specified abnormal products of conception**
Excludes1: *abnormal products of conception with blighted ovum (O02.0)*
abnormal products of conception with hydatidiform mole (O01.-)
abnormal products of conception with nonhydatidiform mole (O02.0)

• ♀ O02.81 **Inappropriate change in quantitative human chorionic gonadotropin (hCG) in early pregnancy**
Biochemical pregnancy
Chemical pregnancy
Inappropriate level of quantitative human chorionic gonadotropin (hCG) for gestational age in early pregnancy

• ♀ O02.89 **Other abnormal products of conception**

• ♀ O02.9 **Abnormal product of conception, unspecified**

O03 Spontaneous abortion

NOTE Incomplete abortion includes retained products of conception following spontaneous abortion
Includes: miscarriage
Review coding guideline C.15.q.2

• ♀ CC O03.0 **Genital tract and pelvic infection following incomplete spontaneous abortion**
Endometritis following incomplete spontaneous abortion
Oophoritis following incomplete spontaneous abortion
Parametritis following incomplete spontaneous abortion
Pelvic peritonitis following incomplete spontaneous abortion
Salpingitis following incomplete spontaneous abortion
Salpingo-oophoritis following incomplete spontaneous abortion
Excludes1: *sepsis following incomplete spontaneous abortion (O03.37)*
urinary tract infection following incomplete spontaneous abortion (O03.38)
CC Exclusion see Appendix A PDX collection 0954

• ♀ O03.1 **Delayed or excessive hemorrhage following incomplete spontaneous abortion**
Afibrinogenemia following incomplete spontaneous abortion
Defibrination syndrome following incomplete spontaneous abortion
Hemolysis following incomplete spontaneous abortion
Intravascular coagulation following incomplete spontaneous abortion

♀ MCC O03.2 **Embolism following incomplete spontaneous abortion**
Air embolism following incomplete spontaneous abortion
Amniotic fluid embolism following incomplete spontaneous abortion
Blood-clot embolism following incomplete spontaneous abortion
Embolism NOS following incomplete spontaneous abortion
Fat embolism following incomplete spontaneous abortion
Pulmonary embolism following incomplete spontaneous abortion
Pyemic embolism following incomplete spontaneous abortion
Septic or septicopyemic embolism following incomplete spontaneous abortion
Soap embolism following incomplete spontaneous abortion
MCC Exclusion see Appendix A PDX collection 0954
Review coding guideline C.15.j

+ O03.3 **Other and unspecified complications following incomplete spontaneous abortion**

• ♀ CC O03.30 **Unspecified complication following incomplete spontaneous abortion**
CC Exclusion see Appendix A PDX collection 0954

• ♀ MCC O03.31 **Shock following incomplete spontaneous abortion**
Circulatory collapse following incomplete spontaneous abortion
Shock (postprocedural) following incomplete spontaneous abortion
Excludes1: *shock due to infection following incomplete spontaneous abortion (O03.37)*
MCC Exclusion see Appendix A PDX collection 0954

• ♀ MCC O03.32 **Renal failure following incomplete spontaneous abortion**
Kidney failure (acute) following incomplete spontaneous abortion
Oliguria following incomplete spontaneous abortion
Renal shutdown following incomplete spontaneous abortion
Renal tubular necrosis following incomplete spontaneous abortion
Uremia following incomplete spontaneous abortion
MCC Exclusion see Appendix A PDX collection 0954

• ♀ CC O03.33 **Metabolic disorder following incomplete spontaneous abortion**
CC Exclusion see Appendix A PDX collection 0954

• ♀ CC O03.34 **Damage to pelvic organs following incomplete spontaneous abortion**
Laceration, perforation, tear or chemical damage of bladder following incomplete spontaneous abortion
Laceration, perforation, tear or chemical damage of bowel following incomplete spontaneous abortion
Laceration, perforation, tear or chemical damage of broad ligament following incomplete spontaneous abortion
Laceration, perforation, tear or chemical damage of cervix following incomplete spontaneous abortion
Laceration, perforation, tear or chemical damage of periurethral tissue following incomplete spontaneous abortion
Laceration, perforation, tear or chemical damage of uterus following incomplete spontaneous abortion
Laceration, perforation, tear or chemical damage of vagina following incomplete spontaneous abortion
CC Exclusion see Appendix A PDX collection 0954

• ♀ CC O03.35 **Other venous complications following incomplete spontaneous abortion**
CC Exclusion see Appendix A PDX collection 0954

• ♀ CC O03.36 **Cardiac arrest following incomplete spontaneous abortion**
CC Exclusion see Appendix A PDX collection 0954

• ♀ CC O03.37 **Sepsis following incomplete spontaneous abortion**
Use additional code to identify infectious agent (B95-B97)
Use additional code to identify severe sepsis, if applicable (R65.2-)
Excludes1: *septic or septicopyemic embolism following incomplete spontaneous abortion (O03.2)*
CC Exclusion see Appendix A PDX collection 0954
Review coding guideline C.15.j

• ♀ CC O03.38 **Urinary tract infection following incomplete spontaneous abortion**
Cystitis following incomplete spontaneous abortion
CC Exclusion see Appendix A PDX collection 0954

• ♀ CC O03.39 **Incomplete spontaneous abortion with other complications**
CC Exclusion see Appendix A PDX collection 0954

• ♀ O03.4 **Incomplete spontaneous abortion without complication**

• ♀ CC O03.5 **Genital tract and pelvic infection following complete or unspecified spontaneous abortion**
Endometritis following complete or unspecified spontaneous abortion
Oophoritis following complete or unspecified spontaneous abortion
Parametritis following complete or unspecified spontaneous abortion
Pelvic peritonitis following complete or unspecified spontaneous abortion
Salpingitis following complete or unspecified spontaneous abortion
Salpingo-oophoritis following complete or unspecified spontaneous abortion
Excludes1: *sepsis following complete or unspecified spontaneous abortion (O03.87)*
urinary tract infection following complete or unspecified spontaneous abortion (O03.88)
CC Exclusion see Appendix A PDX collection 0954

• ♀ O03.6 **Delayed or excessive hemorrhage following complete or unspecified spontaneous abortion**
Afibrinogenemia following complete or unspecified spontaneous abortion
Defibrination syndrome following complete or unspecified spontaneous abortion

Hemolysis following complete or unspecified spontaneous abortion
Intravascular coagulation following complete or unspecified spontaneous abortion

● ♀ CC **O03.7 Embolism following complete or unspecified spontaneous abortion**
Air embolism following complete or unspecified spontaneous abortion
Amniotic fluid embolism following complete or unspecified spontaneous abortion
Blood-clot embolism following complete or unspecified spontaneous abortion
Embolism NOS following complete or unspecified spontaneous abortion
Fat embolism following complete or unspecified spontaneous abortion
Pulmonary embolism following complete or unspecified spontaneous abortion
Pyemic embolism following complete or unspecified spontaneous abortion
Septic or septicopyemic embolism following complete or unspecified spontaneous abortion
Soap embolism following complete or unspecified spontaneous abortion
CC Exclusion see Appendix A PDX collection 0954

\+ **O03.8 Other and unspecified complications following complete or unspecified spontaneous abortion**

● ♀ CC **O03.80 Unspecified complication following complete or unspecified spontaneous abortion**
CC Exclusion see Appendix A PDX collection 0954

● ♀ MCC **O03.81 Shock following complete or unspecified spontaneous abortion**
Circulatory collapse following complete or unspecified spontaneous abortion
Shock (postprocedural) following complete or unspecified spontaneous abortion
Excludes1: *shock due to infection following complete or unspecified spontaneous abortion (O03.87)*
MCC Exclusion see Appendix A PDX collection 0954

● ♀ MCC **O03.82 Renal failure following complete or unspecified spontaneous abortion**
Kidney failure (acute) following complete or unspecified spontaneous abortion
Oliguria following complete or unspecified spontaneous abortion
Renal shutdown following complete or unspecified spontaneous abortion
Renal tubular necrosis following complete or unspecified spontaneous abortion
Uremia following complete or unspecified spontaneous abortion
MCC Exclusion see Appendix A PDX collection 0954

● ♀ CC **O03.83 Metabolic disorder following complete or unspecified spontaneous abortion**
CC Exclusion see Appendix A PDX collection 0954

● ♀ CC **O03.84 Damage to pelvic organs following complete or unspecified spontaneous abortion**
Laceration, perforation, tear or chemical damage of bladder following complete or unspecified spontaneous abortion
Laceration, perforation, tear or chemical damage of bowel following complete or unspecified spontaneous abortion
Laceration, perforation, tear or chemical damage of broad ligament following complete or unspecified spontaneous abortion
Laceration, perforation, tear or chemical damage of cervix following complete or unspecified spontaneous abortion
Laceration, perforation, tear or chemical damage of periurethral tissue following complete or unspecified spontaneous abortion
Laceration, perforation, tear or chemical damage of uterus following complete or unspecified spontaneous abortion
Laceration, perforation, tear or chemical damage of vagina following complete or unspecified spontaneous abortion
CC Exclusion see Appendix A PDX collection 0954

● ♀ CC **O03.85 Other venous complications following complete or unspecified spontaneous abortion**
CC Exclusion see Appendix A PDX collection 0954

● ♀ CC **O03.86 Cardiac arrest following complete or unspecified spontaneous abortion**

● ♀ CC **O03.87 Sepsis following complete or unspecified spontaneo abortion**
Use additional code to identify infectious agent (B95-B97)
Use additional code to identify severe sepsis, if applicable (R65.2-)
Excludes1: *septic or septicopyemic embolism following complete or unspecified spontaneous abortion (O03.7)*
CC Exclusion see Appendix A PDX collection 0954
Review coding guideline C.15.j

● ♀ CC **O03.88 Urinary tract infection following complete or unspecified spontaneous abortion**
Cystitis following complete or unspecified spontaneous abortion
CC Exclusion see Appendix A PDX collection 0954

● ♀ CC **O03.89 Complete or unspecified spontaneous abortion witl other complications**
CC Exclusion see Appendix A PDX collection 0954

● ♀ **O03.9 Complete or unspecified spontaneous abortion without complication**
Miscarriage NOS
Spontaneous abortion NOS

O04 Complications following (induced) termination of pregnancy

Includes: complications following (induced) termination of pregnanc
Excludes1: *encounter for elective termination of pregnancy, uncomplicated (Z33.2)*
failed attempted termination of pregnancy (O07.-)

● ♀ CC **O04.5 Genital tract and pelvic infection following (induced) termination of pregnancy**
Endometritis following (induced) termination of pregnancy
Oophoritis following (induced) termination of pregnancy
Parametritis following (induced) termination of pregnancy
Pelvic peritonitis following (induced) termination of pregnanc
Salpingitis following (induced) termination of pregnancy
Salpingo-oophoritis following (induced) termination of pregnan
Excludes1: *sepsis following (induced) termination of pregnancy (O04.87)*
urinary tract infection following (induced) termination of pregnancy (O04.88)
CC Exclusion see Appendix A PDX collection 0954

● ♀ **O04.6 Delayed or excessive hemorrhage following (induced) termination of pregnancy**
Afibrinogenemia following (induced) termination of pregnanc
Defibrination syndrome following (induced) termination of pregnancy
Hemolysis following (induced) termination of pregnancy
Intravascular coagulation following (induced) termination of pregnancy

● ♀ MCC **O04.7 Embolism following (induced) termination of pregnancy**
Air embolism following (induced) termination of pregnancy
Amniotic fluid embolism following (induced) termination of pregnancy
Blood-clot embolism following (induced) termination of pregnan
Embolism NOS following (induced) termination of pregnancy
Fat embolism following (induced) termination of pregnancy
Pulmonary embolism following (induced) termination of pregnancy
Pyemic embolism following (induced) termination of pregnan
Septic or septicopyemic embolism following (induced) termination of pregnancy
Soap embolism following (induced) termination of pregnancy
MCC Exclusion see Appendix A PDX collection 0954

\+ **O04.8 (Induced) termination of pregnancy with other and unspecifi complications**

● ♀ CC **O04.80 (Induced) termination of pregnancy with unspecific complications**
CC Exclusion see Appendix A PDX collection 0954

● ♀ MCC **O04.81 Shock following (induced) termination of pregnanc**
Circulatory collapse following (induced) termination of pregnancy
Shock (postprocedural) following (induced) termination of pregnancy
Excludes1: *shock due to infection following (induce termination of pregnancy (O04.87)*
MCC Exclusion see Appendix A PDX collection 0954

• ♀ MCC **O04.82 Renal failure following (induced) termination of pregnancy**
Kidney failure (acute) following (induced) termination of pregnancy
Oliguria following (induced) termination of pregnancy
Renal shutdown following (induced) termination of pregnancy
Renal tubular necrosis following (induced) termination of pregnancy
Uremia following (induced) termination of pregnancy
MCC Exclusion see Appendix A PDX collection 0954

• ♀ CC **O04.83 Metabolic disorder following (induced) termination of pregnancy**
CC Exclusion see Appendix A PDX collection 0954

• ♀ CC **O04.84 Damage to pelvic organs following (induced) termination of pregnancy**
Laceration, perforation, tear or chemical damage of bladder following (induced) termination of pregnancy
Laceration, perforation, tear or chemical damage of bowel following (induced) termination of pregnancy
Laceration, perforation, tear or chemical damage of broad ligament following (induced) termination of pregnancy
Laceration, perforation, tear or chemical damage of cervix following (induced) termination of pregnancy
Laceration, perforation, tear or chemical damage of periurethral tissue following (induced) termination of pregnancy
Laceration, perforation, tear or chemical damage of uterus following (induced) termination of pregnancy
Laceration, perforation, tear or chemical damage of vagina following (induced) termination of pregnancy
CC Exclusion see Appendix A PDX collection 0954

• ♀ CC **O04.85 Other venous complications following (induced) termination of pregnancy**
CC Exclusion see Appendix A PDX collection 0954

• ♀ CC **O04.86 Cardiac arrest following (induced) termination of pregnancy**
CC Exclusion see Appendix A PDX collection 0954

• ♀ CC **O04.87 Sepsis following (induced) termination of pregnancy**
Use additional code to identify infectious agent (B95-B97)

Use additional code to identify severe sepsis, if applicable (R65.2-)
Excludes1: *septic or septicopyemic embolism following (induced) termination of pregnancy (O04.7)*
CC Exclusion see Appendix A PDX collection 0954
Review coding guideline C.15.j

• ♀ CC **O04.88 Urinary tract infection following (induced) termination of pregnancy**
Cystitis following (induced) termination of pregnancy
CC Exclusion see Appendix A PDX collection 0954

• ♀ CC **O04.89 (Induced) termination of pregnancy with other complications**
CC Exclusion see Appendix A PDX collection 0954

O07 Failed attempted termination of pregnancy
Includes: failure of attempted induction of termination of pregnancy
incomplete elective abortion
Excludes1: *incomplete spontaneous abortion (O03.0-)*

• ♀ CC **O07.0 Genital tract and pelvic infection following failed attempted termination of pregnancy**
Endometritis following failed attempted termination of pregnancy
Oophoritis following failed attempted termination of pregnancy
Parametritis following failed attempted termination of pregnancy
Pelvic peritonitis following failed attempted termination of pregnancy
Salpingitis following failed attempted termination of pregnancy
Salpingo-oophoritis following failed attempted termination of pregnancy
Excludes1: *sepsis following failed attempted termination of pregnancy (O07.37)*
urinary tract infection following failed attempted termination of pregnancy (O07.38)
CC Exclusion see Appendix A PDX collection 0956

• ♀ CC **O07.1 Delayed or excessive hemorrhage following failed attempted termination of pregnancy**
Afibrinogenemia following failed attempted termination of pregnancy
Defibrination syndrome following failed attempted termination of pregnancy
Hemolysis following failed attempted termination of pregnancy
Intravascular coagulation following failed attempted termination of pregnancy
CC Exclusion see Appendix A PDX collection 0957

• ♀ MCC **O07.2 Embolism following failed attempted termination of pregnancy**
Air embolism following failed attempted termination of pregnancy
Amniotic fluid embolism following failed attempted termination of pregnancy
Blood-clot embolism following failed attempted termination of pregnancy
Embolism NOS following failed attempted termination of pregnancy
Fat embolism following failed attempted termination of pregnancy
Pulmonary embolism following failed attempted termination of pregnancy
Pyemic embolism following failed attempted termination of pregnancy
Septic or septicopyemic embolism following failed attempted termination of pregnancy
Soap embolism following failed attempted termination of pregnancy
MCC Exclusion see Appendix A PDX collection 0958

\+ **O07.3 Failed attempted termination of pregnancy with other and unspecified complications**

• ♀ CC **O07.30 Failed attempted termination of pregnancy with unspecified complications**
CC Exclusion see Appendix A PDX collection 0954

• ♀ MCC **O07.31 Shock following failed attempted termination of pregnancy**
Circulatory collapse following failed attempted termination of pregnancy
Shock (postprocedural) following failed attempted termination of pregnancy
Excludes1: *shock due to infection following failed attempted termination of pregnancy (O07.37)*
MCC Exclusion see Appendix A PDX collection 0959

• ♀ MCC **O07.32 Renal failure following failed attempted termination of pregnancy**
Kidney failure (acute) following failed attempted termination of pregnancy
Oliguria following failed attempted termination of pregnancy
Renal shutdown following failed attempted termination of pregnancy
Renal tubular necrosis following failed attempted termination of pregnancy
Uremia following failed attempted termination of pregnancy
MCC Exclusion see Appendix A PDX collection 0960

• ♀ CC **O07.33 Metabolic disorder following failed attempted termination of pregnancy**
CC Exclusion see Appendix A PDX collection 0954

• ♀ CC **O07.34 Damage to pelvic organs following failed attempted termination of pregnancy**
Laceration, perforation, tear or chemical damage of bladder following failed attempted termination of pregnancy
Laceration, perforation, tear or chemical damage of bowel following failed attempted termination of pregnancy
Laceration, perforation, tear or chemical damage of broad ligament following failed attempted termination of pregnancy
Laceration, perforation, tear or chemical damage of cervix following failed attempted termination of pregnancy
Laceration, perforation, tear or chemical damage of periurethral tissue following failed attempted termination of pregnancy
Laceration, perforation, tear or chemical damage of uterus following failed attempted termination of pregnancy

Laceration, perforation, tear or chemical damage of vagina following failed attempted termination of pregnancy
CC Exclusion see Appendix A PDX collection 0961

● ♀ CC **O07.35 Other venous complications following failed attempted termination of pregnancy**
CC Exclusion see Appendix A PDX collection 0954

● ♀ CC **O07.36 Cardiac arrest following failed attempted termination of pregnancy**
CC Exclusion see Appendix A PDX collection 0954

● ♀ CC **O07.37 Sepsis following failed attempted termination of pregnancy**
Use additional code (B95-B97), to identify infectious agent

Use additional code (R65.2-) to identify severe sepsis, if applicable

Excludes1: *septic or septicopyemic embolism following failed attempted termination of pregnancy (O07.2)*

CC Exclusion see Appendix A PDX collection 0956
Review coding guideline C.15.j

● ♀ CC **O07.38 Urinary tract infection following failed attempted termination of pregnancy**
Cystitis following failed attempted termination of pregnancy
CC Exclusion see Appendix A PDX collection 0954

● ♀ CC **O07.39 Failed attempted termination of pregnancy with other complications**
CC Exclusion see Appendix A PDX collection 0954

● ♀ CC **O07.4 Failed attempted termination of pregnancy without complication**
Review coding guideline C.15.q.2

O08 Complications following ectopic and molar pregnancy

This category is for use with categories O00-O02 to identify any associated complications

● ♀ CC **O08.0 Genital tract and pelvic infection following ectopic and molar pregnancy**
Endometritis following ectopic and molar pregnancy
Oophoritis following ectopic and molar pregnancy
Parametritis following ectopic and molar pregnancy
Pelvic peritonitis following ectopic and molar pregnancy
Salpingitis following ectopic and molar pregnancy
Salpingo-oophoritis following ectopic and molar pregnancy
Excludes1: *sepsis following ectopic and molar pregnancy (O08.82)*
urinary tract infection (O08.83)
CC Exclusion see Appendix A PDX collection 0085

● ♀ CC **O08.1 Delayed or excessive hemorrhage following ectopic and molar pregnancy**
Afibrinogenemia following ectopic and molar pregnancy
Defibrination syndrome following ectopic and molar pregnancy
Hemolysis following ectopic and molar pregnancy
Intravascular coagulation following ectopic and molar pregnancy
Excludes1: *delayed or excessive hemorrhage due to incomplete abortion (O03.1)*
CC Exclusion see Appendix A PDX collection 0962

● ♀ MCC **O08.2 Embolism following ectopic and molar pregnancy**
Air embolism following ectopic and molar pregnancy
Amniotic fluid embolism following ectopic and molar pregnancy
Blood-clot embolism following ectopic and molar pregnancy
Embolism NOS following ectopic and molar pregnancy
Fat embolism following ectopic and molar pregnancy
Pulmonary embolism following ectopic and molar pregnancy
Pyemic embolism following ectopic and molar pregnancy
Septic or septicopyemic embolism following ectopic and molar pregnancy
Soap embolism following ectopic and molar pregnancy
MCC Exclusion see Appendix A PDX collection 0963

● ♀ MCC **O08.3 Shock following ectopic and molar pregnancy**
Circulatory collapse following ectopic and molar pregnancy
Shock (postprocedural) following ectopic and molar pregnancy
Excludes1: *shock due to infection following ectopic and molar pregnancy (O08.82)*
MCC Exclusion see Appendix A PDX collection 0963

● ♀ MCC **O08.4 Renal failure following ectopic and molar pregnancy**
Kidney failure (acute) following ectopic and molar pregnancy
Oliguria following ectopic and molar pregnancy
Renal shutdown following ectopic and molar pregnancy
Renal tubular necrosis following ectopic and molar pregnancy
Uremia following ectopic and molar pregnancy
MCC Exclusion see Appendix A PDX collection 0963

● ♀ CC **O08.5 Metabolic disorders following an ectopic and molar pregnancy**
CC Exclusion see Appendix A PDX collection 0963

● ♀ CC **O08.6 Damage to pelvic organs and tissues following an ectopic and molar pregnancy**
Laceration, perforation, tear or chemical damage of bladder following an ectopic and molar pregnancy
Laceration, perforation, tear or chemical damage of bowel following an ectopic and molar pregnancy
Laceration, perforation, tear or chemical damage of broad ligament following an ectopic and molar pregnancy
Laceration, perforation, tear or chemical damage of cervix following an ectopic and molar pregnancy
Laceration, perforation, tear or chemical damage of periurethral tissue following an ectopic and molar pregnancy
Laceration, perforation, tear or chemical damage of uterus following an ectopic and molar pregnancy
Laceration, perforation, tear or chemical damage of vagina following an ectopic and molar pregnancy
CC Exclusion see Appendix A PDX collection 0963

● ♀ CC **O08.7 Other venous complications following an ectopic and molar pregnancy**
CC Exclusion see Appendix A PDX collection 0963

+ **O08.8 Other complications following an ectopic and molar pregnancy**

● ♀ CC **O08.81 Cardiac arrest following an ectopic and molar pregnancy**
CC Exclusion see Appendix A PDX collection 0963

● ♀ CC **O08.82 Sepsis following ectopic and molar pregnancy**
Use additional code (B95-B97), to identify infectious agent

Use additional code (R65.2-) to identify severe sepsis, if applicable

Excludes1: *septic or septicopyemic embolism following ectopic and molar pregnancy (O08.2)*

CC Exclusion see Appendix A PDX collection 0085
Review coding guideline C.15.j

● ♀ CC **O08.83 Urinary tract infection following an ectopic and molar pregnancy**
Cystitis following an ectopic and molar pregnancy
CC Exclusion see Appendix A PDX collection 0963

● ♀ CC **O08.89 Other complications following an ectopic and molar pregnancy**
CC Exclusion see Appendix A PDX collection 0963

● ♀ CC **O08.9 Unspecified complication following an ectopic and molar pregnancy**
CC Exclusion see Appendix A PDX collection 0963

Supervision of high risk pregnancy (O09)

O09 Supervision of high risk pregnancy
Review coding guideline C.15.b.2
AHA CC: 4Q, 2016, 48-50

+ **O09.0 Supervision of pregnancy with history of infertility**

● ♀ **O09.00 Supervision of pregnancy with history of infertility, unspecified trimester**

● ♀ **O09.01 Supervision of pregnancy with history of infertility, first trimester**

● ♀ **O09.02 Supervision of pregnancy with history of infertility, second trimester**

● ♀ **O09.03 Supervision of pregnancy with history of infertility, third trimester**

+ **O09.1 Supervision of pregnancy with history of ectopic pregnancy**

● ♀ **O09.10 Supervision of pregnancy with history of ectopic pregnancy, unspecified trimester**

● ♀ **O09.11 Supervision of pregnancy with history of ectopic pregnancy, first trimester**

● ♀ **O09.12 Supervision of pregnancy with history of ectopic pregnancy, second trimester**

● ♀ **O09.13 Supervision of pregnancy with history of ectopic pregnancy, third trimester**

+ **O09.A Supervision of pregnancy with history of molar pregnancy**

● ♀ **O09.A0 Supervision of pregnancy with history of molar pregnancy, unspecified trimester**

● ♀ **O09.A1 Supervision of pregnancy with history of molar pregnancy, first trimester**

● ♀ **O09.A2 Supervision of pregnancy with history of molar pregnancy, second trimester**

• ♀ O09.A3 Supervision of pregnancy with history of molar pregnancy, third trimester

+ O09.2 Supervision of pregnancy with other poor reproductive or obstetric history

Excludes2: *pregnancy care for patient with history of recurrent pregnancy loss (O26.2-)*

+ O09.21 Supervision of pregnancy with history of pre-term labor

• ♀ O09.211 Supervision of pregnancy with history of pre-term labor, first trimester

• ♀ O09.212 Supervision of pregnancy with history of pre-term labor, second trimester

• ♀ O09.213 Supervision of pregnancy with history of pre-term labor, third trimester

• ♀ O09.219 Supervision of pregnancy with history of pre-term labor, unspecified trimester

+ O09.29 Supervision of pregnancy with other poor reproductive or obstetric history

Supervision of pregnancy with history of neonatal death

Supervision of pregnancy with history of stillbirth

• ♀ O09.291 Supervision of pregnancy with other poor reproductive or obstetric history, first trimester

• ♀ O09.292 Supervision of pregnancy with other poor reproductive or obstetric history, second trimester

• ♀ O09.293 Supervision of pregnancy with other poor reproductive or obstetric history, third trimester

• ♀ O09.299 Supervision of pregnancy with other poor reproductive or obstetric history, unspecified trimester

+ O09.3 Supervision of pregnancy with insufficient antenatal care

Supervision of concealed pregnancy

Supervision of hidden pregnancy

• ♀ O09.30 Supervision of pregnancy with insufficient antenatal care, unspecified trimester

• ♀ O09.31 Supervision of pregnancy with insufficient antenatal care, first trimester

• ♀ O09.32 Supervision of pregnancy with insufficient antenatal care, second trimester

• ♀ O09.33 Supervision of pregnancy with insufficient antenatal care, third trimester

+ O09.4 Supervision of pregnancy with grand multiparity

• ♀ O09.40 Supervision of pregnancy with grand multiparity, unspecified trimester

• ♀ O09.41 Supervision of pregnancy with grand multiparity, first trimester

• ♀ O09.42 Supervision of pregnancy with grand multiparity, second trimester

• ♀ O09.43 Supervision of pregnancy with grand multiparity, third trimester

+ O09.5 Supervision of elderly primigravida and multigravida

Pregnancy for a female 35 years and older at expected date of delivery

+ O09.51 Supervision of elderly primigravida

• ♀ O09.511 Supervision of elderly primigravida, first trimester

• ♀ O09.512 Supervision of elderly primigravida, second trimester

• ♀ O09.513 Supervision of elderly primigravida, third trimester

• ♀ O09.519 Supervision of elderly primigravida, unspecified trimester

+ O09.52 Supervision of elderly multigravida

• ♀ O09.521 Supervision of elderly multigravida, first trimester

• ♀ O09.522 Supervision of elderly multigravida, second trimester

• ♀ O09.523 Supervision of elderly multigravida, third trimester

• ♀ O09.529 Supervision of elderly multigravida, unspecified trimester

+ O09.6 Supervision of young primigravida and multigravida

Supervision of pregnancy for a female less than 16 years old at expected date of delivery

+ O09.61 Supervision of young primigravida

• ♀ O09.611 Supervision of young primigravida, first trimester

• ♀ O09.612 Supervision of young primigravida, second trimester

• ♀ O09.613 Supervision of young primigravida, third trimester

• ♀ O09.619 Supervision of young primigravida, unspecified trimester

+ O09.62 Supervision of young multigravida

• ♀ O09.621 Supervision of young multigravida, first trimester

• ♀ O09.622 Supervision of young multigravida, second trimester

• ♀ O09.623 Supervision of young multigravida, third trimester

• ♀ O09.629 Supervision of young multigravida, unspecified trimester

+ O09.7 Supervision of high risk pregnancy due to social problems

• ♀ O09.70 Supervision of high risk pregnancy due to social problems, unspecified trimester

• ♀ O09.71 Supervision of high risk pregnancy due to social problems, first trimester

• ♀ O09.72 Supervision of high risk pregnancy due to social problems, second trimester

• ♀ O09.73 Supervision of high risk pregnancy due to social problems, third trimester

+ O09.8 Supervision of other high risk pregnancies

+ O09.81 Supervision of pregnancy resulting from assisted reproductive technology

Supervision of pregnancy resulting from in-vitro fertilization

Excludes2: *gestational carrier status (Z33.3)*

• ♀ O09.811 Supervision of pregnancy resulting from assisted reproductive technology, first trimester

• ♀ O09.812 Supervision of pregnancy resulting from assisted reproductive technology, second trimester

• ♀ O09.813 Supervision of pregnancy resulting from assisted reproductive technology, third trimester

• ♀ O09.819 Supervision of pregnancy resulting from assisted reproductive technology, unspecified trimester

+ O09.82 Supervision of pregnancy with history of in utero procedure during previous pregnancy

• ♀ O09.821 Supervision of pregnancy with history of in utero procedure during previous pregnancy, first trimester

• ♀ O09.822 Supervision of pregnancy with history of in utero procedure during previous pregnancy, second trimester

• ♀ O09.823 Supervision of pregnancy with history of in utero procedure during previous pregnancy, third trimester

• ♀ O09.829 Supervision of pregnancy with history of in utero procedure during previous pregnancy, unspecified trimester

Excludes1: *supervision of pregnancy affectedbyinuteroprocedure during current pregnancy (O35.7)*

+ O09.89 Supervision of other high risk pregnancies

• ♀ O09.891 Supervision of other high risk pregnancies, first trimester

• ♀ O09.892 Supervision of other high risk pregnancies, second trimester

• ♀ O09.893 Supervision of other high risk pregnancies, third trimester

• ♀ O09.899 Supervision of other high risk pregnancies, unspecified trimester

+ O09.9 Supervision of high risk pregnancy, unspecified

• ♀ O09.90 Supervision of high risk pregnancy, unspecified, unspecified trimester

• ♀ O09.91 Supervision of high risk pregnancy, unspecified, first trimester

• ♀ O09.92 Supervision of high risk pregnancy, unspecified, second trimester

• ♀ O09.93 Supervision of high risk pregnancy, unspecified, third trimester

Edema, proteinuria and hypertensive disorders in pregnancy, childbirth and the puerperium (O10-O16)

O10 Pre-existing hypertension complicating pregnancy, childbirth and the puerperium

Includes: pre-existing hypertension with pre-existing proteinuria complicating pregnancy, childbirth and the puerperium

Excludes2: *pre-existing hypertension with superimposed pre-eclampsia complicating pregnancy, childbirth and the puerperium (O11.-)*

Review coding guideline C.15.d

+ **O10.0 Pre-existing essential hypertension complicating pregnancy, childbirth and the puerperium**
  Any condition in I10 specified as a reason for obstetric care during pregnancy, childbirth or the puerperium
  + **O10.01 Pre-existing essential hypertension complicating pregnancy,**
    - ● ♀ CC **O10.011 Pre-existing essential hypertension complicating pregnancy, first trimester**
      CC Exclusion see Appendix A PDX collection 0964
    - ● ♀ CC **O10.012 Pre-existing essential hypertension complicating pregnancy, second trimester**
      CC Exclusion see Appendix A PDX collection 0964
    - ● ♀ CC **O10.013 Pre-existing essential hypertension complicating pregnancy, third trimester**
      CC Exclusion see Appendix A PDX collection 0964
    - ● ♀ **O10.019 Pre-existing essential hypertension complicating pregnancy, unspecified trimester**
  - ● ♀ CC **O10.02 Pre-existing essential hypertension complicating childbirth**
    CC Exclusion see Appendix A PDX collection 0964
  - ● ♀ **O10.03 Pre-existing essential hypertension complicating the puerperium**
+ **O10.1 Pre-existing hypertensive heart disease complicating pregnancy, childbirth and the puerperium**
  Any condition in I11 specified as a reason for obstetric care during pregnancy, childbirth or the puerperium
  Use additional code from I11 to identify the type of hypertensive heart disease
  + **O10.11 Pre-existing hypertensive heart disease complicating pregnancy**
    - ● ♀ **O10.111 Pre-existing hypertensive heart disease complicating pregnancy, first trimester**
    - ● ♀ **O10.112 Pre-existing hypertensive heart disease complicating pregnancy, second trimester**
    - ● ♀ **O10.113 Pre-existing hypertensive heart disease complicating pregnancy, third trimester**
    - ● ♀ **O10.119 Pre-existing hypertensive heart disease complicating pregnancy, unspecified trimester**
  - ● ♀ **O10.12 Pre-existing hypertensive heart disease complicating childbirth**
  - ● ♀ **O10.13 Pre-existing hypertensive heart disease complicating the puerperium**
+ **O10.2 Pre-existing hypertensive chronic kidney disease complicating pregnancy, childbirth and the puerperium**
  Any condition in I12 specified as a reason for obstetric care during pregnancy, childbirth or the puerperium
  Use additional code from I12 to identify the type of hypertensive chronic kidney disease
  + **O10.21 Pre-existing hypertensive chronic kidney disease complicating pregnancy**
    - ● ♀ **O10.211 Pre-existing hypertensive chronic kidney disease complicating pregnancy, first trimester**
    - ● ♀ **O10.212 Pre-existing hypertensive chronic kidney disease complicating pregnancy, second trimester**
    - ● ♀ **O10.213 Pre-existing hypertensive chronic kidney disease complicating pregnancy, third trimester**
    - ● ♀ **O10.219 Pre-existing hypertensive chronic kidney disease complicating pregnancy, unspecified trimester**
  - ● ♀ **O10.22 Pre-existing hypertensive chronic kidney disease complicating childbirth**
  - ● ♀ **O10.23 Pre-existing hypertensive chronic kidney disease complicating the puerperium**
+ **O10.3 Pre-existing hypertensive heart and chronic kidney disease complicating pregnancy, childbirth and the puerperium**
  Any condition in I13 specified as a reason for obstetric care during pregnancy, childbirth or the puerperium
  Use additional code from I13 to identify the type of hypertensive heart and chronic kidney disease
  + **O10.31 Pre-existing hypertensive heart and chronic kidney disease complicating pregnancy**
    - ● ♀ **O10.311 Pre-existing hypertensive heart and chronic kidney disease complicating pregnancy, first trimester**
    - ● ♀ **O10.312 Pre-existing hypertensive heart and chronic kidney disease complicating pregnancy, second trimester**
    - ● ♀ **O10.313 Pre-existing hypertensive heart and chronic kidney disease complicating pregnancy, third trimester**
    - ● ♀ **O10.319 Pre-existing hypertensive heart and chronic kidney disease complicating pregnancy, unspecified trimester**
  - ● ♀ **O10.32 Pre-existing hypertensive heart and chronic kidney disease complicating childbirth**
  - ● ♀ **O10.33 Pre-existing hypertensive heart and chronic kidney disease complicating the puerperium**
+ **O10.4 Pre-existing secondary hypertension complicating pregnancy, childbirth and the puerperium**
  Any condition in I15 specified as a reason for obstetric care during pregnancy, childbirth or the puerperium
  Use additional code from I15 to identify the type of secondary hypertension
  + **O10.41 Pre-existing secondary hypertension complicating pregnancy**
    - ● ♀ CC **O10.411 Pre-existing secondary hypertension complicating pregnancy, first trimester**
      CC Exclusion see Appendix A PDX collection 0964
    - ● ♀ CC **O10.412 Pre-existing secondary hypertension complicating pregnancy, second trimester**
      CC Exclusion see Appendix A PDX collection 0964
    - ● ♀ CC **O10.413 Pre-existing secondary hypertension complicating pregnancy, third trimester**
      CC Exclusion see Appendix A PDX collection 0964
    - ● ♀ **O10.419 Pre-existing secondary hypertension complicating pregnancy, unspecified trimester**
  - ● ♀ MCC **O10.42 Pre-existing secondary hypertension complicating childbirth**
    MCC Exclusion see Appendix A PDX collection 0964
  - ● ♀ CC **O10.43 Pre-existing secondary hypertension complicating the puerperium**
    CC Exclusion see Appendix A PDX collection 0964
+ **O10.9 Unspecified pre-existing hypertension complicating pregnanc childbirth and the puerperium**
  + **O10.91 Unspecified pre-existing hypertension complicating pregnancy**
    - ● ♀ CC **O10.911 Unspecified pre-existing hypertension complicating pregnancy, first trimester**
      CC Exclusion see Appendix A PDX collection 09
    - ● ♀ CC **O10.912 Unspecified pre-existing hypertension complicating pregnancy, second trimester**
      CC Exclusion see Appendix A PDX collection 09
    - ● ♀ CC **O10.913 Unspecified pre-existing hypertension complicating pregnancy, third trimester**
      CC Exclusion see Appendix A PDX collection 09
    - ● ♀ **O10.919 Unspecified pre-existing hypertension complicating pregnancy, unspecified trimester**
  - ● ♀ CC **O10.92 Unspecified pre-existing hypertension complicating childbirth**
    CC Exclusion see Appendix A PDX collection 0964
  - ● ♀ **O10.93 Unspecified pre-existing hypertension complicating the puerperium**

O11 Pre-existing hypertension with pre-eclampsia

Includes: conditions in O10 complicated by pre-eclampsia
pre-eclampsia superimposed pre-existing hypertension

Use additional code from O10 to identify the type of hypertension

AHA CC: 4Q, 2016, 50

♀ MCC **O11.1 Pre-existing hypertension with pre-eclampsia, first trimester**
MCC Exclusion see Appendix A PDX collection 0964

♀ MCC **O11.2 Pre-existing hypertension with pre-eclampsia, second trimester**
MCC Exclusion see Appendix A PDX collection 0964

♀ MCC **O11.3 Pre-existing hypertension with pre-eclampsia, third trimester**
MCC Exclusion see Appendix A PDX collection 0964

● ♀ **O11.4 Pre-existing hypertension with pre-eclampsia, complicating childbirth**

● ♀ **O11.5 Pre-existing hypertension with pre-eclampsia, complicating the puerperium**

● ♀ **O11.9 Pre-existing hypertension with pre-eclampsia, unspecified trimester**

O12 Gestational [pregnancy-induced] edema and proteinuria without hypertension

AHA CC: 4Q, 2016, 50

\+ **O12.0 Gestational edema**

● ♀ **O12.00 Gestational edema, unspecified trimester**

● ♀ **O12.01 Gestational edema, first trimester**

● ♀ **O12.02 Gestational edema, second trimester**

● ♀ **O12.03 Gestational edema, third trimester**

● ♀ **O12.04 Gestational edema, complicating childbirth**

● ♀ **O12.05 Gestational edema, complicating the puerperium**

\+ **O12.1 Gestational proteinuria**

● ♀ **O12.10 Gestational proteinuria, unspecified trimester**

● ♀ CC **O12.11 Gestational proteinuria, first trimester**
CC Exclusion see Appendix A PDX collection 0965

● ♀ CC **O12.12 Gestational proteinuria, second trimester**
CC Exclusion see Appendix A PDX collection 0965

● ♀ CC **O12.13 Gestational proteinuria, third trimester**
CC Exclusion see Appendix A PDX collection 0965

● ♀ **O12.14 Gestational proteinuria, complicating childbirth**

● ♀ **O12.15 Gestational proteinuria, complicating the puerperium**

\+ **O12.2 Gestational edema with proteinuria**

● ♀ **O12.20 Gestational edema with proteinuria, unspecified trimester**

● ♀ CC **O12.21 Gestational edema with proteinuria, first trimester**
CC Exclusion see Appendix A PDX collection 0965

● ♀ CC **O12.22 Gestational edema with proteinuria, second trimester**
CC Exclusion see Appendix A PDX collection 0965

● ♀ CC **O12.23 Gestational edema with proteinuria, third trimester**
CC Exclusion see Appendix A PDX collection 0965

● ♀ **O12.24 Gestational edema with proteinuria, complicating childbirth**

● ♀ **O12.25 Gestational edema with proteinuria, complicating the puerperium**

O13 Gestational [pregnancy-induced] hypertension without significant proteinuria

Includes: gestational hypertension NOS
transient hypertension of pregnancy

Review coding guideline C.9.a.7

AHA CC: 4Q, 2016, 50

● ♀ **O13.1 Gestational [pregnancy-induced] hypertension without significant proteinuria, first trimester**

● ♀ **O13.2 Gestational [pregnancy-induced] hypertension without significant proteinuria, second trimester**

● ♀ **O13.3 Gestational [pregnancy-induced] hypertension without significant proteinuria, third trimester**

● ♀ **O13.4 Gestational [pregnancy-induced] hypertension without significant proteinuria, complicating childbirth**

● ♀ **O13.5 Gestational [pregnancy-induced] hypertension without significant proteinuria, complicating the puerperium**

● ♀ **O13.9 Gestational [pregnancy-induced] hypertension without significant proteinuria, unspecified trimester**

O14 Pre-eclampsia

Excludes1: *pre-existing hypertension with pre-eclampsia (O11)*

Review coding guideline C.9.a.7

AHA CC: 4Q, 2016, 50

\+ **O14.0 Mild to moderate pre-eclampsia**

● ♀ **O14.00 Mild to moderate pre-eclampsia, unspecified trimester**

● ♀ CC **O14.02 Mild to moderate pre-eclampsia, second trimester**
CC Exclusion see Appendix A PDX collection 0964

● ♀ CC **O14.03 Mild to moderate pre-eclampsia, third trimester**
CC Exclusion see Appendix A PDX collection 0964

● ♀ **O14.04 Mild to moderate pre-eclampsia, complicating childbirth**

● ♀ **O14.05 Mild to moderate pre-eclampsia, complicating the puerperium**

\+ **O14.1 Severe pre-eclampsia**

Excludes1: *HELLP syndrome (O14.2-)*

● ♀ **O14.10 Severe pre-eclampsia, unspecified trimester**

● ♀ MCC **O14.12 Severe pre-eclampsia, second trimester**
MCC Exclusion see Appendix A PDX collection 0964

● ♀ MCC **O14.13 Severe pre-eclampsia, third trimester**
MCC Exclusion see Appendix A PDX collection 0964

● ♀ **O14.14 Severe pre-eclampsia complicating childbirth**

● ♀ **O14.15 Severe pre-eclampsia, complicating the puerperium**

\+ **O14.2 HELLP syndrome**

Severe pre-eclampsia with hemolysis, elevated liver enzymes and low platelet count (HELLP)

● ♀ **O14.20 HELLP syndrome (HELLP), unspecified trimester**

● ♀ MCC **O14.22 HELLP syndrome (HELLP), second trimester**
MCC Exclusion see Appendix A PDX collection 0964

● ♀ MCC **O14.23 HELLP syndrome (HELLP), third trimester**
MCC Exclusion see Appendix A PDX collection 0964

● ♀ **O14.24 HELLP syndrome, complicating childbirth**

● ♀ **O14.25 HELLP syndrome, complicating the puerperium**

\+ **O14.9 Unspecified pre-eclampsia**

● ♀ **O14.90 Unspecified pre-eclampsia, unspecified trimester**

● ♀ CC **O14.92 Unspecified pre-eclampsia, second trimester**
CC Exclusion see Appendix A PDX collection 0964

● ♀ CC **O14.93 Unspecified pre-eclampsia, third trimester**
CC Exclusion see Appendix A PDX collection 0964

● ♀ **O14.94 Unspecified pre-eclampsia, complicating childbirth**

● ♀ **O14.95 Unspecified pre-eclampsia, complicating the puerperium**

O15 Eclampsia

Includes: convulsions following conditions in O10-O14 and O16

\+ **O15.0 Eclampsia complicating pregnancy**

AHA CC: 4Q, 2016, 50

● ♀ **O15.00 Eclampsia complicating pregnancy, unspecified trimester**

● ♀ MCC **O15.02 Eclampsia complicating pregnancy, second trimester**
MCC Exclusion see Appendix A PDX collection 0964

● ♀ MCC **O15.03 Eclampsia complicating pregnancy, third trimester**
MCC Exclusion see Appendix A PDX collection 0964

● ♀ MCC **O15.1 Eclampsia complicating labor**
MCC Exclusion see Appendix A PDX collection 0964

● ♀ MCC **O15.2 Eclampsia complicating the puerperium**
MCC Exclusion see Appendix A PDX collection 0964

● ♀ **O15.9 Eclampsia, unspecified as to time period**
Eclampsia NOS

O16 Unspecified maternal hypertension

AHA CC: 4Q, 2016, 50

● ♀ CC **O16.1 Unspecified maternal hypertension, first trimester**
CC Exclusion see Appendix A PDX collection 0964

● ♀ CC **O16.2 Unspecified maternal hypertension, second trimester**
CC Exclusion see Appendix A PDX collection 0964

● ♀ CC **O16.3 Unspecified maternal hypertension, third trimester**
CC Exclusion see Appendix A PDX collection 0964

● ♀ **O16.4 Unspecified maternal hypertension, complicating childbirth**

● ♀ **O16.5 Unspecified maternal hypertension, complicating the puerperium**

● ♀ **O16.9 Unspecified maternal hypertension, unspecified trimester**

Other maternal disorders predominantly related to pregnancy (O20-O29)

Excludes2: *maternal care related to the fetus and amniotic cavity and possible delivery problems (O30-O48)*
maternal diseases classifiable elsewhere but complicating pregnancy, labor and delivery, and the puerperium (O98-O99)

O20 Hemorrhage in early pregnancy

Includes: hemorrhage before completion of 20 weeks gestation

Excludes1: *pregnancy with abortive outcome (O00-O08)*

● ♀ CC **O20.0 Threatened abortion**
Hemorrhage specified as due to threatened abortion
CC Exclusion see Appendix A PDX collection 0966

● ♀ **O20.8 Other hemorrhage in early pregnancy**

● ♀ CC **O20.9 Hemorrhage in early pregnancy, unspecified**
CC Exclusion see Appendix A PDX collection 0966

O21 Excessive vomiting in pregnancy

● ♀ **O21.0 Mild hyperemesis gravidarum**
Hyperemesis gravidarum, mild or unspecified, starting before the end of the 20th week of gestation

• ♀ **O21.1 Hyperemesis gravidarum with metabolic disturbance**
Hyperemesis gravidarum, starting before the end of the 20th week of gestation, with metabolic disturbance such as carbohydrate depletion
Hyperemesis gravidarum, starting before the end of the 20th week of gestation, with metabolic disturbance such as dehydration
Hyperemesis gravidarum, starting before the end of the 20th week of gestation, with metabolic disturbance such as electrolyte imbalance

• ♀ **O21.2 Late vomiting of pregnancy**
Excessive vomiting starting after 20 completed weeks of gestation

• ♀ **O21.8 Other vomiting complicating pregnancy**
Vomiting due to diseases classified elsewhere, complicating pregnancy
Use additional code, to identify cause.

• ♀ **O21.9 Vomiting of pregnancy, unspecified**

O22 Venous complications and hemorrhoids in pregnancy

Excludes1: *venous complications of:*
abortion NOS (O03.9)
ectopic or molar pregnancy (O08.7)
failed attempted abortion (O07.35)
induced abortion (O04.85)
spontaneous abortion (O03.89)

Excludes2: *obstetric pulmonary embolism (O88.-)*
venous complications and hemorrhoids of childbirth and the puerperium (O87.-)

\+ **O22.0 Varicose veins of lower extremity in pregnancy**
Varicose veins NOS in pregnancy
• ♀ **O22.00 Varicose veins of lower extremity in pregnancy, unspecified trimester**
• ♀ **O22.01 Varicose veins of lower extremity in pregnancy, first trimester**
• ♀ **O22.02 Varicose veins of lower extremity in pregnancy, second trimester**
• ♀ **O22.03 Varicose veins of lower extremity in pregnancy, third trimester**

\+ **O22.1 Genital varices in pregnancy**
Perineal varices in pregnancy
Vaginal varices in pregnancy
Vulval varices in pregnancy
• ♀ **O22.10 Genital varices in pregnancy, unspecified trimester**
• ♀ **O22.11 Genital varices in pregnancy, first trimester**
• ♀ **O22.12 Genital varices in pregnancy, second trimester**
• ♀ **O22.13 Genital varices in pregnancy, third trimester**

\+ **O22.2 Superficial thrombophlebitis in pregnancy**
Phlebitis in pregnancy NOS
Thrombophlebitis of legs in pregnancy
Thrombosis in pregnancy NOS
Use additional code to identify the superficial thrombophlebitis (I80.0-)
• ♀ CC **O22.20 Superficial thrombophlebitis in pregnancy, unspecified trimester**
CC Exclusion see Appendix A PDX collection 0967
• ♀ CC **O22.21 Superficial thrombophlebitis in pregnancy, first trimester**
CC Exclusion see Appendix A PDX collection 0967
• ♀ CC **O22.22 Superficial thrombophlebitis in pregnancy, second trimester**
CC Exclusion see Appendix A PDX collection 0967
• ♀ CC **O22.23 Superficial thrombophlebitis in pregnancy, third trimester**
CC Exclusion see Appendix A PDX collection 0967

\+ **O22.3 Deep phlebothrombosis in pregnancy**
Deep vein thrombosis, antepartum
Use additional code to identify the deep vein thrombosis (I82.4-, I82.5-, I82.62-. I82.72-)

Use additional code, if applicable, for associated long-term (current) use of anticoagulants (Z79.01)
• ♀ CC **O22.30 Deep phlebothrombosis in pregnancy, unspecified trimester**
CC Exclusion see Appendix A PDX collection 0967
• ♀ MCC **O22.31 Deep phlebothrombosis in pregnancy, first trimester**
MCC Exclusion see Appendix A PDX collection 0967
• ♀ MCC **O22.32 Deep phlebothrombosis in pregnancy, second trimester**
MCC Exclusion see Appendix A PDX collection 0967
• ♀ MCC **O22.33 Deep phlebothrombosis in pregnancy, third trimester**
MCC Exclusion see Appendix A PDX collection 0967

\+ **O22.4 Hemorrhoids in pregnancy**
• ♀ CC **O22.40 Hemorrhoids in pregnancy, unspecified trimester**
CC Exclusion see Appendix A PDX collection 0967
• ♀ CC **O22.41 Hemorrhoids in pregnancy, first trimester**
CC Exclusion see Appendix A PDX collection 0967
• ♀ CC **O22.42 Hemorrhoids in pregnancy, second trimester**
CC Exclusion see Appendix A PDX collection 0967
• ♀ CC **O22.43 Hemorrhoids in pregnancy, third trimester**
CC Exclusion see Appendix A PDX collection 0967

\+ **O22.5 Cerebral venous thrombosis in pregnancy**
Cerebrovenous sinus thrombosis in pregnancy
• ♀ CC **O22.50 Cerebral venous thrombosis in pregnancy, unspecified trimester**
CC Exclusion see Appendix A PDX collection 0967
• ♀ CC **O22.51 Cerebral venous thrombosis in pregnancy, first trimester**
CC Exclusion see Appendix A PDX collection 0967
• ♀ CC **O22.52 Cerebral venous thrombosis in pregnancy, second trimester**
CC Exclusion see Appendix A PDX collection 0967
• ♀ CC **O22.53 Cerebral venous thrombosis in pregnancy, third trimester**
CC Exclusion see Appendix A PDX collection 0967

\+ **O22.8 Other venous complications in pregnancy**
\+ **O22.8X Other venous complications in pregnancy**
• ♀ CC **O22.8X1 Other venous complications in pregnancy, first trimester**
CC Exclusion see Appendix A PDX collection 096
• ♀ CC **O22.8X2 Other venous complications in pregnancy, second trimester**
CC Exclusion see Appendix A PDX collection 096
• ♀ CC **O22.8X3 Other venous complications in pregnancy, third trimester**
CC Exclusion see Appendix A PDX collection 09
• ♀ CC **O22.8X9 Other venous complications in pregnancy, unspecified trimester**
CC Exclusion see Appendix A PDX collection 0967

\+ **O22.9 Venous complication in pregnancy, unspecified**
Gestational phlebitis NOS
Gestational phlebopathy NOS
Gestational thrombosis NOS
• ♀ CC **O22.90 Venous complication in pregnancy, unspecified, unspecified trimester**
CC Exclusion see Appendix A PDX collection 0967
• ♀ **O22.91 Venous complication in pregnancy, unspecified, first trimester**
• ♀ **O22.92 Venous complication in pregnancy, unspecified, second trimester**
• ♀ **O22.93 Venous complication in pregnancy, unspecified, thir trimester**

O23 Infections of genitourinary tract in pregnancy

Use additional code to identify organism (B95.-, B96.-)

Excludes2: *gonococcal infections complicating pregnancy, childbirth and the puerperium (O98.2)*
infections with a predominantly sexual mode of transmission NOS complicating pregnancy, childbirth and the puerperium (O98.3)
syphilis complicating pregnancy, childbirth and the puerperium (O98.1)
tuberculosis of genitourinary system complicating pregnancy, childbirth and the puerperium (O98.0)
venereal disease NOS complicating pregnancy, childbirth and the puerperium (O98.3)

\+ **O23.0 Infections of kidney in pregnancy**
Pyelonephritis in pregnancy
• ♀ **O23.00 Infections of kidney in pregnancy, unspecified trimest**
• ♀ CC **O23.01 Infections of kidney in pregnancy, first trimester**
CC Exclusion see Appendix A PDX collection 0968
• ♀ CC **O23.02 Infections of kidney in pregnancy, second trimester**
CC Exclusion see Appendix A PDX collection 0968
• ♀ CC **O23.03 Infections of kidney in pregnancy, third trimester**
CC Exclusion see Appendix A PDX collection 0968

\+ **O23.1 Infections of bladder in pregnancy**
• ♀ **O23.10 Infections of bladder in pregnancy, unspecified trimester**
• ♀ CC **O23.11 Infections of bladder in pregnancy, first trimester**
CC Exclusion see Appendix A PDX collection 0968

• ♀ CC **O23.12 Infections of bladder in pregnancy, second trimester**
CC Exclusion see Appendix A PDX collection 0968
• ♀ CC **O23.13 Infections of bladder in pregnancy, third trimester**
CC Exclusion see Appendix A PDX collection 0968
+ **O23.2 Infections of urethra in pregnancy**
• ♀ **O23.20 Infections of urethra in pregnancy, unspecified trimester**
• ♀ CC **O23.21 Infections of urethra in pregnancy, first trimester**
CC Exclusion see Appendix A PDX collection 0968
• ♀ CC **O23.22 Infections of urethra in pregnancy, second trimester**
CC Exclusion see Appendix A PDX collection 0968
• ♀ CC **O23.23 Infections of urethra in pregnancy, third trimester**
CC Exclusion see Appendix A PDX collection 0968
+ **O23.3 Infections of other parts of urinary tract in pregnancy**
• ♀ **O23.30 Infections of other parts of urinary tract in pregnancy, unspecified trimester**
• ♀ CC **O23.31 Infections of other parts of urinary tract in pregnancy, first trimester**
CC Exclusion see Appendix A PDX collection 0968
• ♀ CC **O23.32 Infections of other parts of urinary tract in pregnancy, second trimester**
CC Exclusion see Appendix A PDX collection 0968
• ♀ CC **O23.33 Infections of other parts of urinary tract in pregnancy, third trimester**
CC Exclusion see Appendix A PDX collection 0968
+ **O23.4 Unspecified infection of urinary tract in pregnancy**
• ♀ **O23.40 Unspecified infection of urinary tract in pregnancy, unspecified trimester**
• ♀ CC **O23.41 Unspecified infection of urinary tract in pregnancy, first trimester**
CC Exclusion see Appendix A PDX collection 0968
• ♀ CC **O23.42 Unspecified infection of urinary tract in pregnancy, second trimester**
CC Exclusion see Appendix A PDX collection 0968
• ♀ CC **O23.43 Unspecified infection of urinary tract in pregnancy, third trimester**
CC Exclusion see Appendix A PDX collection 0968
+ **O23.5 Infections of the genital tract in pregnancy**
+ **O23.51 Infection of cervix in pregnancy**
• ♀ CC **O23.511 Infections of cervix in pregnancy, first trimester**
CC Exclusion see Appendix A PDX collection 0968
• ♀ CC **O23.512 Infections of cervix in pregnancy, second trimester**
CC Exclusion see Appendix A PDX collection 0968
• ♀ CC **O23.513 Infections of cervix in pregnancy, third trimester**
CC Exclusion see Appendix A PDX collection 0968
• ♀ **O23.519 Infections of cervix in pregnancy, unspecified trimester**
+ **O23.52 Salpingo-oophoritis in pregnancy**
Oophoritis in pregnancy
Salpingitis in pregnancy
• ♀ CC **O23.521 Salpingo-oophoritis in pregnancy, first trimester**
CC Exclusion see Appendix A PDX collection 0968
• ♀ CC **O23.522 Salpingo-oophoritis in pregnancy, second trimester**
CC Exclusion see Appendix A PDX collection 0968
• ♀ CC **O23.523 Salpingo-oophoritis in pregnancy, third trimester**
CC Exclusion see Appendix A PDX collection 0968
• ♀ **O23.529 Salpingo-oophoritis in pregnancy, unspecified trimester**
+ **O23.59 Infection of other part of genital tract in pregnancy**
• ♀ CC **O23.591 Infection of other part of genital tract in pregnancy, first trimester**
CC Exclusion see Appendix A PDX collection 0968
• ♀ CC **O23.592 Infection of other part of genital tract in pregnancy, second trimester**
CC Exclusion see Appendix A PDX collection 0968
• ♀ CC **O23.593 Infection of other part of genital tract in pregnancy, third trimester**
CC Exclusion see Appendix A PDX collection 0968
• ♀ **O23.599 Infection of other part of genital tract in pregnancy, unspecified trimester**
+ **O23.9 Unspecified genitourinary tract infection in pregnancy**
Genitourinary tract infection in pregnancy NOS
• ♀ **O23.90 Unspecified genitourinary tract infection in pregnancy, unspecified trimester**
• ♀ CC **O23.91 Unspecified genitourinary tract infection in pregnancy, first trimester**
CC Exclusion see Appendix A PDX collection 0968
• ♀ CC **O23.92 Unspecified genitourinary tract infection in pregnancy, second trimester**
CC Exclusion see Appendix A PDX collection 0968
• ♀ CC **O23.93 Unspecified genitourinary tract infection in pregnancy, third trimester**
CC Exclusion see Appendix A PDX collection 0968

O24 Diabetes mellitus in pregnancy, childbirth, and the puerperium
Review coding guideline C.15.g
+ **O24.0 Pre-existing type 1 diabetes mellitus, in pregnancy, childbirth and the puerperium**
Juvenile onset diabetes mellitus, in pregnancy, childbirth and the puerperium
Ketosis-prone diabetes mellitus in pregnancy, childbirth and the puerperium
Use additional code from category E10 to further identify any manifestations
+ **O24.01 Pre-existing type 1 diabetes mellitus, in pregnancy**
• ♀ CC **O24.011 Pre-existing type 1 diabetes mellitus, in pregnancy, first trimester**
CC Exclusion see Appendix A PDX collection 0969
• ♀ CC **O24.012 Pre-existing type 1 diabetes mellitus, in pregnancy, second trimester**
CC Exclusion see Appendix A PDX collection 0969
• ♀ CC **O24.013 Pre-existing type 1 diabetes mellitus, in pregnancy, third trimester**
CC Exclusion see Appendix A PDX collection 0969
• ♀ CC **O24.019 Pre-existing type 1 diabetes mellitus, in pregnancy, unspecified trimester**
CC Exclusion see Appendix A PDX collection 0969
• ♀ MCC **O24.02 Pre-existing type 1 diabetes mellitus, in childbirth**
MCC Exclusion see Appendix A PDX collection 0969
• ♀ CC **O24.03 Pre-existing type 1 diabetes mellitus, in the puerperium**
CC Exclusion see Appendix A PDX collection 0969
+ **O24.1 Pre-existing type 2 diabetes mellitus, in pregnancy, childbirth and the puerperium**
Insulin-resistant diabetes mellitus in pregnancy, childbirth and the puerperium
Use additional code (for):
from category E11 to further identify any manifestations
long-term (current) use of insulin (Z79.4)
+ **O24.11 Pre-existing type 2 diabetes mellitus, in pregnancy**
• ♀ CC **O24.111 Pre-existing type 2 diabetes mellitus, in pregnancy, first trimester**
CC Exclusion see Appendix A PDX collection 0969
• ♀ CC **O24.112 Pre-existing type 2 diabetes mellitus, in pregnancy, second trimester**
CC Exclusion see Appendix A PDX collection 0969
• ♀ CC **O24.113 Pre-existing type 2 diabetes mellitus, in pregnancy, third trimester**
CC Exclusion see Appendix A PDX collection 0969
• ♀ CC **O24.119 Pre-existing type 2 diabetes mellitus, in pregnancy, unspecified trimester**
CC Exclusion see Appendix A PDX collection 0969
• ♀ MCC **O24.12 Pre-existing type 2 diabetes mellitus, in childbirth**
MCC Exclusion see Appendix A PDX collection 0969
• ♀ CC **O24.13 Pre-existing type 2 diabetes mellitus, in the puerperium**
CC Exclusion see Appendix A PDX collection 0969
+ **O24.3 Unspecified pre-existing diabetes mellitus in pregnancy, childbirth and the puerperium**
Use additional code (for):
from category E11 to further identify any manifestation
long-term (current) use of insulin (Z79.4)
+ **O24.31 Unspecified pre-existing diabetes mellitus in pregnancy**
• ♀ CC **O24.311 Unspecified pre-existing diabetes mellitus in pregnancy, first trimester**
CC Exclusion see Appendix A PDX collection 0969
• ♀ CC **O24.312 Unspecified pre-existing diabetes mellitus in pregnancy, second trimester**
CC Exclusion see Appendix A PDX collection 0969
• ♀ CC **O24.313 Unspecified pre-existing diabetes mellitus in pregnancy, third trimester**
CC Exclusion see Appendix A PDX collection 0969

• ♀ CC **O24.319 Unspecified pre-existing diabetes mellitus in pregnancy, unspecified trimester**
CC Exclusion see Appendix A PDX collection 0969

• ♀ MCC **O24.32 Unspecified pre-existing diabetes mellitus in childbirth**
MCC Exclusion see Appendix A PDX collection 0969

• ♀ CC **O24.33 Unspecified pre-existing diabetes mellitus in the puerperium**
CC Exclusion see Appendix A PDX collection 0969

\+ **O24.4 Gestational diabetes mellitus**
Diabetes mellitus arising in pregnancy
Gestational diabetes mellitus NOS
Review coding guideline C.15.i
AHA CC: 4Q, 2016, 50

\+ **O24.41 Gestational diabetes mellitus in pregnancy**

• ♀ **O24.410 Gestational diabetes mellitus in pregnancy, diet controlled**

• ♀ **O24.414 Gestational diabetes mellitus in pregnancy, insulin controlled**

• ♀ **O24.415 Gestational diabetes mellitus in pregnancy, controlled by oral hypoglycemic drugs**
Gestational diabetes mellitus in pregnancy, controlled by oral antidiabetic drugs

• ♀ **O24.419 Gestational diabetes mellitus in pregnancy, unspecified control**
AHA CC: 4Q, 2015, 34

\+ **O24.42 Gestational diabetes mellitus in childbirth**

• ♀ **O24.420 Gestational diabetes mellitus in childbirth, diet controlled**

• ♀ **O24.424 Gestational diabetes mellitus in childbirth, insulin controlled**

• ♀ **O24.425 Gestational diabetes mellitus in childbirth, controlled by oral hypoglycemic drugs**
Gestational diabetes mellitus in childbirth, controlled by oral antidiabetic drugs

• ♀ **O24.429 Gestational diabetes mellitus in childbirth, unspecified control**

\+ **O24.43 Gestational diabetes mellitus in the puerperium**

• ♀ **O24.430 Gestational diabetes mellitus in the puerperium, diet controlled**

• ♀ **O24.434 Gestational diabetes mellitus in the puerperium, insulin controlled**

• ♀ **O24.435 Gestational diabetes mellitus in puerperium, controlled by oral hypoglycemic drugs**
Gestational diabetes mellitus in puerperium, controlled by oral antidiabetic drugs

• ♀ **O24.439 Gestational diabetes mellitus in the puerperium, unspecified control**

\+ **O24.8 Other pre-existing diabetes mellitus in pregnancy, childbirth, and the puerperium**
Use additional code (for):
from categories E08, E09 and E13 to further identify any manifestation
long-term (current) use of insulin (Z79.4)

\+ **O24.81 Other pre-existing diabetes mellitus in pregnancy**

• ♀ CC **O24.811 Other pre-existing diabetes mellitus in pregnancy, first trimester**
CC Exclusion see Appendix A PDX collection 0969

• ♀ CC **O24.812 Other pre-existing diabetes mellitus in pregnancy, second trimester**
CC Exclusion see Appendix A PDX collection 0969

• ♀ CC **O24.813 Other pre-existing diabetes mellitus in pregnancy, third trimester**
CC Exclusion see Appendix A PDX collection 0969

• ♀ CC **O24.819 Other pre-existing diabetes mellitus in pregnancy, unspecified trimester**
CC Exclusion see Appendix A PDX collection 0969

• ♀ MCC **O24.82 Other pre-existing diabetes mellitus in childbirth**
MCC Exclusion see Appendix A PDX collection 0969

• ♀ CC **O24.83 Other pre-existing diabetes mellitus in the puerperium**
CC Exclusion see Appendix A PDX collection 0969

\+ **O24.9 Unspecified diabetes mellitus in pregnancy, childbirth and the puerperium**
Use additional code for long-term (current) use of insulin (Z79.4)

\+ **O24.91 Unspecified diabetes mellitus in pregnancy**

• ♀ CC **O24.911 Unspecified diabetes mellitus in pregnancy, first trimester**
CC Exclusion see Appendix A PDX collection 0969

• ♀ CC **O24.912 Unspecified diabetes mellitus in pregnancy, second trimester**
CC Exclusion see Appendix A PDX collection 0969

• ♀ CC **O24.913 Unspecified diabetes mellitus in pregnancy, third trimester**
CC Exclusion see Appendix A PDX collection 0969

• ♀ CC **O24.919 Unspecified diabetes mellitus in pregnancy, unspecified trimester**
CC Exclusion see Appendix A PDX collection 0969

• ♀ **O24.92 Unspecified diabetes mellitus in childbirth**

• ♀ CC **O24.93 Unspecified diabetes mellitus in the puerperium**
CC Exclusion see Appendix A PDX collection 0969

O25 Malnutrition in pregnancy, childbirth and the puerperium

\+ **O25.1 Malnutrition in pregnancy**

• ♀ **O25.10 Malnutrition in pregnancy, unspecified trimester**

• ♀ **O25.11 Malnutrition in pregnancy, first trimester**

• ♀ **O25.12 Malnutrition in pregnancy, second trimester**

• ♀ **O25.13 Malnutrition in pregnancy, third trimester**

• ♀ **O25.2 Malnutrition in childbirth**

• ♀ **O25.3 Malnutrition in the puerperium**

O26 Maternal care for other conditions predominantly related to pregnancy

\+ **O26.0 Excessive weight gain in pregnancy**
Excludes2: *gestational edema (O12.0, O12.2)*

• ♀ **O26.00 Excessive weight gain in pregnancy, unspecified trimester**

• ♀ **O26.01 Excessive weight gain in pregnancy, first trimester**

• ♀ **O26.02 Excessive weight gain in pregnancy, second trimeste**

• ♀ **O26.03 Excessive weight gain in pregnancy, third trimester**

\+ **O26.1 Low weight gain in pregnancy**

• ♀ **O26.10 Low weight gain in pregnancy, unspecified trimeste**

• ♀ **O26.11 Low weight gain in pregnancy, first trimester**

• ♀ **O26.12 Low weight gain in pregnancy, second trimester**

• ♀ **O26.13 Low weight gain in pregnancy, third trimester**

\+ **O26.2 Pregnancy care for patient with recurrent pregnancy loss**

• ♀ **O26.20 Pregnancy care for patient with recurrent pregnanc loss, unspecified trimester**

• ♀ **O26.21 Pregnancy care for patient with recurrent pregnanc loss, first trimester**

• ♀ **O26.22 Pregnancy care for patient with recurrent pregnanc loss, second trimester**

• ♀ **O26.23 Pregnancy care for patient with recurrent pregnanc loss, third trimester**

\+ **O26.3 Retained intrauterine contraceptive device in pregnancy**

• ♀ **O26.30 Retained intrauterine contraceptive device in pregnancy, unspecified trimester**

• ♀ **O26.31 Retained intrauterine contraceptive device in pregnancy, first trimester**

• ♀ **O26.32 Retained intrauterine contraceptive device in pregnancy, second trimester**

• ♀ **O26.33 Retained intrauterine contraceptive device in pregnancy, third trimester**

\+ **O26.4 Herpes gestationis**

• ♀ **O26.40 Herpes gestationis, unspecified trimester**

• ♀ **O26.41 Herpes gestationis, first trimester**

• ♀ **O26.42 Herpes gestationis, second trimester**

• ♀ **O26.43 Herpes gestationis, third trimester**

\+ **O26.5 Maternal hypotension syndrome**
Supine hypotensive syndrome

• ♀ **O26.50 Maternal hypotension syndrome, unspecified trimester**

• ♀ **O26.51 Maternal hypotension syndrome, first trimester**

• ♀ **O26.52 Maternal hypotension syndrome, second trimester**

• ♀ **O26.53 Maternal hypotension syndrome, third trimester**

\+ **O26.6 Liver and biliary tract disorders in pregnancy, childbirth and the puerperium**
Use additional code to identify the specific disorder
Excludes2: *hepatorenal syndrome following labor and deliver (O90.4)*

\+ **O26.61 Liver and biliary tract disorders in pregnancy**

• ♀ CC **O26.611 Liver and biliary tract disorders in pregnancy, first trimester**
CC Exclusion see Appendix A PDX collection 0972
• ♀ CC **O26.612 Liver and biliary tract disorders in pregnancy, second trimester**
CC Exclusion see Appendix A PDX collection 0972
• ♀ CC **O26.613 Liver and biliary tract disorders in pregnancy, third trimester**
CC Exclusion see Appendix A PDX collection 0972
• ♀ **O26.619 Liver and biliary tract disorders in pregnancy, unspecified trimester**
• ♀ CC **O26.62 Liver and biliary tract disorders in childbirth**
CC Exclusion see Appendix A PDX collection 0972
• ♀ **O26.63 Liver and biliary tract disorders in the puerperium**
+ **O26.7 Subluxation of symphysis (pubis) in pregnancy, childbirth and the puerperium**
Excludes1: *traumatic separation of symphysis (pubis) during childbirth (O71.6)*
+ **O26.71 Subluxation of symphysis (pubis) in pregnancy**
• ♀ **O26.711 Subluxation of symphysis (pubis) in pregnancy, first trimester**
• ♀ **O26.712 Subluxation of symphysis (pubis) in pregnancy, second trimester**
• ♀ **O26.713 Subluxation of symphysis (pubis) in pregnancy, third trimester**
• ♀ **O26.719 Subluxation of symphysis (pubis) in pregnancy, unspecified trimester**
• ♀ **O26.72 Subluxation of symphysis (pubis) in childbirth**
• ♀ **O26.73 Subluxation of symphysis (pubis) in the puerperium**
+ **O26.8 Other specified pregnancy related conditions**
+ **O26.81 Pregnancy related exhaustion and fatigue**
• ♀ **O26.811 Pregnancy related exhaustion and fatigue, first trimester**
• ♀ **O26.812 Pregnancy related exhaustion and fatigue, second trimester**
• ♀ **O26.813 Pregnancy related exhaustion and fatigue, third trimester**
• ♀ **O26.819 Pregnancy related exhaustion and fatigue, unspecified trimester**
+ **O26.82 Pregnancy related peripheral neuritis**
• ♀ **O26.821 Pregnancy related peripheral neuritis, first trimester**
• ♀ **O26.822 Pregnancy related peripheral neuritis, second trimester**
• ♀ **O26.823 Pregnancy related peripheral neuritis, third trimester**
• ♀ **O26.829 Pregnancy related peripheral neuritis, unspecified trimester**
+ **O26.83 Pregnancy related renal disease**
Use additional code to identify the specific disorder
• ♀ CC **O26.831 Pregnancy related renal disease, first trimester**
CC Exclusion see Appendix A PDX collection 0965
• ♀ CC **O26.832 Pregnancy related renal disease, second trimester**
CC Exclusion see Appendix A PDX collection 0965
• ♀ CC **O26.833 Pregnancy related renal disease, third trimester**
CC Exclusion see Appendix A PDX collection 0965
• ♀ **O26.839 Pregnancy related renal disease, unspecified trimester**
+ **O26.84 Uterine size-date discrepancy complicating pregnancy**
Excludes1: *encounter for suspected problem with fetal growth ruled out (Z03.74)*
• ♀ **O26.841 Uterine size-date discrepancy, first trimester**
• ♀ **O26.842 Uterine size-date discrepancy, second trimester**
• ♀ **O26.843 Uterine size-date discrepancy, third trimester**
• ♀ **O26.849 Uterine size-date discrepancy, unspecified trimester**
+ **O26.85 Spotting complicating pregnancy**
• ♀ **O26.851 Spotting complicating pregnancy, first trimester**
• ♀ **O26.852 Spotting complicating pregnancy, second trimester**
• ♀ **O26.853 Spotting complicating pregnancy, third trimester**
• ♀ **O26.859 Spotting complicating pregnancy, unspecified trimester**
• ♀ **O26.86 Pruritic urticarial papules and plaques of pregnancy (PUPPP)**
Polymorphic eruption of pregnancy
+ **O26.87 Cervical shortening**
Excludes1: *encounter for suspected cervical shortening ruled out (Z03.75)*
• ♀ CC **O26.872 Cervical shortening, second trimester**
CC Exclusion see Appendix A PDX collection 0973
• ♀ CC **O26.873 Cervical shortening, third trimester**
CC Exclusion see Appendix A PDX collection 0973
• ♀ CC **O26.879 Cervical shortening, unspecified trimester**
CC Exclusion see Appendix A PDX collection 0973
+ **O26.89 Other specified pregnancy related conditions**
• ♀ **O26.891 Other specified pregnancy related conditions, first trimester**
• ♀ **O26.892 Other specified pregnancy related conditions, second trimester**
• ♀ **O26.893 Other specified pregnancy related conditions, third trimester**
AHA CC: 3Q, 2015, 40
• ♀ **O26.899 Other specified pregnancy related conditions, unspecified trimester**
+ **O26.9 Pregnancy related conditions, unspecified**
• ♀ **O26.90 Pregnancy related conditions, unspecified, unspecified trimester**
• ♀ **O26.91 Pregnancy related conditions, unspecified, first trimester**
• ♀ **O26.92 Pregnancy related conditions, unspecified, second trimester**
• ♀ **O26.93 Pregnancy related conditions, unspecified, third trimester**

O28 Abnormal findings on antenatal screening of mother

Excludes1: *diagnostic findings classified elsewhere - see Alphabetical Index*
• ♀ **O28.0 Abnormal hematological finding on antenatal screening of mother**
• ♀ **O28.1 Abnormal biochemical finding on antenatal screening of mother**
• ♀ **O28.2 Abnormal cytological finding on antenatal screening of mother**
• ♀ **O28.3 Abnormal ultrasonic finding on antenatal screening of mother**
AHA CC: 4Q, 2016, 4-7
• ♀ **O28.4 Abnormal radiological finding on antenatal screening of mother**
• ♀ **O28.5 Abnormal chromosomal and genetic finding on antenatal screening of mother**
• ♀ **O28.8 Other abnormal findings on antenatal screening of mother**
• ♀ **O28.9 Unspecified abnormal findings on antenatal screening of mother**

O29 Complications of anesthesia during pregnancy

Includes: maternal complications arising from the administration of a general, regional or local anesthetic, analgesic or other sedation during pregnancy
Use additional code, if necessary, to identify the complication
Excludes2: *complications of anesthesia during labor and delivery (O74.-)*
complications of anesthesia during the puerperium (O89.-)
+ **O29.0 Pulmonary complications of anesthesia during pregnancy**
+ **O29.01 Aspiration pneumonitis due to anesthesia during pregnancy**
Inhalation of stomach contents or secretions NOS due to anesthesia during pregnancy
Mendelson's syndrome due to anesthesia during pregnancy
• ♀ **O29.011 Aspiration pneumonitis due to anesthesia during pregnancy, first trimester**
• ♀ **O29.012 Aspiration pneumonitis due to anesthesia during pregnancy, second trimester**

• ♀ O29.013 Aspiration pneumonitis due to anesthesia during pregnancy, third trimester
• ♀ O29.019 Aspiration pneumonitis due to anesthesia during pregnancy, unspecified trimester
+ O29.02 Pressure collapse of lung due to anesthesia during pregnancy
• ♀ O29.021 Pressure collapse of lung due to anesthesia during pregnancy, first trimester
• ♀ O29.022 Pressure collapse of lung due to anesthesia during pregnancy, second trimester
• ♀ O29.023 Pressure collapse of lung due to anesthesia during pregnancy, third trimester
• ♀ O29.029 Pressure collapse of lung due to anesthesia during pregnancy, unspecified trimester
+ O29.09 Other pulmonary complications of anesthesia during pregnancy
• ♀ O29.091 Other pulmonary complications of anesthesia during pregnancy, first trimester
• ♀ O29.092 Other pulmonary complications of anesthesia during pregnancy, second trimester
• ♀ O29.093 Other pulmonary complications of anesthesia during pregnancy, third trimester
• ♀ O29.099 Other pulmonary complications of anesthesia during pregnancy, unspecified trimester
+ O29.1 Cardiac complications of anesthesia during pregnancy
+ O29.11 Cardiac arrest due to anesthesia during pregnancy
• ♀ O29.111 Cardiac arrest due to anesthesia during pregnancy, first trimester
• ♀ O29.112 Cardiac arrest due to anesthesia during pregnancy, second trimester
• ♀ O29.113 Cardiac arrest due to anesthesia during pregnancy, third trimester
• ♀ O29.119 Cardiac arrest due to anesthesia during pregnancy, unspecified trimester
+ O29.12 Cardiac failure due to anesthesia during pregnancy
• ♀ O29.121 Cardiac failure due to anesthesia during pregnancy, first trimester
• ♀ O29.122 Cardiac failure due to anesthesia during pregnancy, second trimester
• ♀ O29.123 Cardiac failure due to anesthesia during pregnancy, third trimester
• ♀ O29.129 Cardiac failure due to anesthesia during pregnancy, unspecified trimester
+ O29.19 Other cardiac complications of anesthesia during pregnancy
• ♀ O29.191 Other cardiac complications of anesthesia during pregnancy, first trimester
• ♀ O29.192 Other cardiac complications of anesthesia during pregnancy, second trimester
• ♀ O29.193 Other cardiac complications of anesthesia during pregnancy, third trimester
• ♀ O29.199 Other cardiac complications of anesthesia during pregnancy, unspecified trimester
+ O29.2 Central nervous system complications of anesthesia during pregnancy
+ O29.21 Cerebral anoxia due to anesthesia during pregnancy
• ♀ O29.211 Cerebral anoxia due to anesthesia during pregnancy, first trimester
• ♀ O29.212 Cerebral anoxia due to anesthesia during pregnancy, second trimester
• ♀ O29.213 Cerebral anoxia due to anesthesia during pregnancy, third trimester
• ♀ O29.219 Cerebral anoxia due to anesthesia during pregnancy, unspecified trimester
+ O29.29 Other central nervous system complications of anesthesia during pregnancy
• ♀ O29.291 Other central nervous system complications of anesthesia during pregnancy, first trimester
• ♀ O29.292 Other central nervous system complications of anesthesia during pregnancy, second trimester
• ♀ O29.293 Other central nervous system complications of anesthesia during pregnancy, third trimester
• ♀ O29.299 Other central nervous system complications of anesthesia during pregnancy, unspecified trimester
+ O29.3 Toxic reaction to local anesthesia during pregnancy
+ O29.3X Toxic reaction to local anesthesia during pregnancy
• ♀ O29.3X1 Toxic reaction to local anesthesia during pregnancy, first trimester
• ♀ O29.3X2 Toxic reaction to local anesthesia during pregnancy, second trimester
• ♀ O29.3X3 Toxic reaction to local anesthesia during pregnancy, third trimester
• ♀ O29.3X9 Toxic reaction to local anesthesia during pregnancy, unspecified trimester
+ O29.4 Spinal and epidural anesthesia induced headache during pregnancy
• ♀ O29.40 Spinal and epidural anesthesia induced headache during pregnancy, unspecified trimester
• ♀ O29.41 Spinal and epidural anesthesia induced headache during pregnancy, first trimester
• ♀ O29.42 Spinal and epidural anesthesia induced headache during pregnancy, second trimester
• ♀ O29.43 Spinal and epidural anesthesia induced headache during pregnancy, third trimester
+ O29.5 Other complications of spinal and epidural anesthesia during pregnancy
+ O29.5X Other complications of spinal and epidural anesthesia during pregnancy
• ♀ O29.5X1 Other complications of spinal and epidural anesthesia during pregnancy, fir[st] trimester
• ♀ O29.5X2 Other complications of spinal and epidura[l] anesthesia during pregnancy, second trimester
• ♀ O29.5X3 Other complications of spinal and epidur[al] anesthesia during pregnancy, third trimester
• ♀ O29.5X9 Other complications of spinal and epidural anesthesia during pregnancy, unspecified trimester
+ O29.6 Failed or difficult intubation for anesthesia during pregnancy
• ♀ O29.60 Failed or difficult intubation for anesthesia during pregnancy, unspecified trimester
• ♀ O29.61 Failed or difficult intubation for anesthesia during pregnancy, first trimester
• ♀ O29.62 Failed or difficult intubation for anesthesia during pregnancy, second trimester
• ♀ O29.63 Failed or difficult intubation for anesthesia during pregnancy, third trimester
+ O29.8 Other complications of anesthesia during pregnancy
+ O29.8X Other complications of anesthesia during pregnanc[y]
• ♀ O29.8X1 Other complications of anesthesia during pregnancy, first trimester
• ♀ O29.8X2 Other complications of anesthesia during pregnancy, second trimester
• ♀ O29.8X3 Other complications of anesthesia during pregnancy, third trimester
• ♀ O29.8X9 Other complications of anesthesia during pregnancy, unspecified trimester
+ O29.9 Unspecified complication of anesthesia during pregnancy
• ♀ O29.90 Unspecified complication of anesthesia during pregnancy, unspecified trimester
• ♀ O29.91 Unspecified complication of anesthesia during pregnancy, first trimester
• ♀ O29.92 Unspecified complication of anesthesia during pregnancy, second trimester
• ♀ O29.93 Unspecified complication of anesthesia during pregnancy, third trimester

Maternal care related to the fetus and amniotic cavity and possible delivery problems (O30-O48)

O30 Multiple gestation

Code also any complications specific to multiple gestation

+ O30.0 Twin pregnancy
+ O30.00 Twin pregnancy, unspecified number of placenta a[nd] unspecified number of amniotic sacs
• ♀ O30.001 Twin pregnancy, unspecified number of placenta and unspecified number of amniotic sacs, first trimester

• ♀ O30.002 Twin pregnancy, unspecified number of placenta and unspecified number of amniotic sacs, second trimester
• ♀ O30.003 Twin pregnancy, unspecified number of placenta and unspecified number of amniotic sacs, third trimester
• ♀ O30.009 Twin pregnancy, unspecified number of placenta and unspecified number of amniotic sacs, unspecified trimester

+ O30.01 Twin pregnancy, monochorionic/monoamniotic
Twin pregnancy, one placenta, one amniotic sac
Excludes1: *conjoined twins (O30.02-)*
• ♀ O30.011 Twin pregnancy, monochorionic/monoamniotic, first trimester
• ♀ O30.012 Twin pregnancy, monochorionic/monoamniotic, second trimester
• ♀ O30.013 Twin pregnancy, monochorionic/monoamniotic, third trimester
• ♀ O30.019 Twin pregnancy, monochorionic/monoamniotic, unspecified trimester

+ O30.02 Conjoined twin pregnancy
• ♀ O30.021 Conjoined twin pregnancy, first trimester
• ♀ O30.022 Conjoined twin pregnancy, second trimester
• ♀ O30.023 Conjoined twin pregnancy, third trimester
• ♀ O30.029 Conjoined twin pregnancy, unspecified trimester

+ O30.03 Twin pregnancy, monochorionic/diamniotic
Twin pregnancy, one placenta, two amniotic sacs
• ♀ O30.031 Twin pregnancy, monochorionic/diamniotic, first trimester
• ♀ O30.032 Twin pregnancy, monochorionic/diamniotic, second trimester
• ♀ O30.033 Twin pregnancy, monochorionic/diamniotic, third trimester
• ♀ O30.039 Twin pregnancy, monochorionic/diamniotic, unspecified trimester

+ O30.04 Twin pregnancy, dichorionic/diamniotic
Twin pregnancy, two placentae, two amniotic sacs
• ♀ O30.041 Twin pregnancy, dichorionic/diamniotic, first trimester
• ♀ O30.042 Twin pregnancy, dichorionic/diamniotic, second trimester
• ♀ O30.043 Twin pregnancy, dichorionic/diamniotic, third trimester
• ♀ O30.049 Twin pregnancy, dichorionic/diamniotic, unspecified trimester

+ O30.09 Twin pregnancy, unable to determine number of placenta and number of amniotic sacs
• ♀ O30.091 Twin pregnancy, unable to determine number of placenta and number of amniotic sacs, first trimester
• ♀ O30.092 Twin pregnancy, unable to determine number of placenta and number of amniotic sacs, second trimester
• ♀ O30.093 Twin pregnancy, unable to determine number of placenta and number of amniotic sacs, third trimester
• ♀ O30.099 Twin pregnancy, unable to determine number of placenta and number of amniotic sacs, unspecified trimester

+ O30.1 Triplet pregnancy

+ O30.10 Triplet pregnancy, unspecified number of placenta and unspecified number of amniotic sacs
• ♀ CC O30.101 Triplet pregnancy, unspecified number of placenta and unspecified number of amniotic sacs, first trimester
CC Exclusion see Appendix A PDX collection 0976
• ♀ CC O30.102 Triplet pregnancy, unspecified number of placenta and unspecified number of amniotic sacs, second trimester
CC Exclusion see Appendix A PDX collection 0976
• ♀ CC O30.103 Triplet pregnancy, unspecified number of placenta and unspecified number of amniotic sacs, third trimester
CC Exclusion see Appendix A PDX collection 0976
AHA CC: 2Q, 2016, 8
• ♀ O30.109 Triplet pregnancy, unspecified number of placenta and unspecified number of amniotic sacs, unspecified trimester

+ O30.11 Triplet pregnancy with two or more monochorionic fetuses
• ♀ CC O30.111 Triplet pregnancy with two or more monochorionic fetuses, first trimester
CC Exclusion see Appendix A PDX collection 0976
• ♀ CC O30.112 Triplet pregnancy with two or more monochorionic fetuses, second trimester
CC Exclusion see Appendix A PDX collection 0976
• ♀ CC O30.113 Triplet pregnancy with two or more monochorionic fetuses, third trimester
CC Exclusion see Appendix A PDX collection 0976
• ♀ O30.119 Triplet pregnancy with two or more monochorionic fetuses, unspecified trimester

+ O30.12 Triplet pregnancy with two or more monoamniotic fetuses
• ♀ CC O30.121 Triplet pregnancy with two or more monoamniotic fetuses, first trimester
CC Exclusion see Appendix A PDX collection 0976
• ♀ CC O30.122 Triplet pregnancy with two or more monoamniotic fetuses, second trimester
CC Exclusion see Appendix A PDX collection 0976
• ♀ CC O30.123 Triplet pregnancy with two or more monoamniotic fetuses, third trimester
CC Exclusion see Appendix A PDX collection 0976
• ♀ O30.129 Triplet pregnancy with two or more monoamniotic fetuses, unspecified trimester

+ O30.19 Triplet pregnancy, unable to determine number of placenta and number of amniotic sacs
• ♀ CC O30.191 Triplet pregnancy, unable to determine number of placenta and number of amniotic sacs, first trimester
CC Exclusion see Appendix A PDX collection 0976
• ♀ CC O30.192 Triplet pregnancy, unable to determine number of placenta and number of amniotic sacs, second trimester
CC Exclusion see Appendix A PDX collection 0976
• ♀ CC O30.193 Triplet pregnancy, unable to determine number of placenta and number of amniotic sacs, third trimester
CC Exclusion see Appendix A PDX collection 0976
• ♀ O30.199 Triplet pregnancy, unable to determine number of placenta and number of amniotic sacs, unspecified trimester

+ O30.2 Quadruplet pregnancy

+ O30.20 Quadruplet pregnancy, unspecified number of placenta and unspecified number of amniotic sacs
• ♀ CC O30.201 Quadruplet pregnancy, unspecified number of placenta and unspecified number of amniotic sacs, first trimester
CC Exclusion see Appendix A PDX collection 0976
• ♀ CC O30.202 Quadruplet pregnancy, unspecified number of placenta and unspecified number of amniotic sacs, second trimester
CC Exclusion see Appendix A PDX collection 0976
• ♀ CC O30.203 Quadruplet pregnancy, unspecified number of placenta and unspecified number of amniotic sacs, third trimester
CC Exclusion see Appendix A PDX collection 0976
• ♀ O30.209 Quadruplet pregnancy, unspecified number of placenta and unspecified number of amniotic sacs, unspecified trimester

+ O30.21 Quadruplet pregnancy with two or more monochorionic fetuses
• ♀ CC O30.211 Quadruplet pregnancy with two or more monochorionic fetuses, first trimester
CC Exclusion see Appendix A PDX collection 0976
• ♀ CC O30.212 Quadruplet pregnancy with two or more monochorionic fetuses, second trimester
CC Exclusion see Appendix A PDX collection 0976
• ♀ CC O30.213 Quadruplet pregnancy with two or more monochorionic fetuses, third trimester
CC Exclusion see Appendix A PDX collection 0976
• ♀ O30.219 Quadruplet pregnancy with two or more monochorionic fetuses, unspecified trimester

+ **O30.22 Quadruplet pregnancy with two or more monoamniotic fetuses**
  - ● ♀ CC **O30.221 Quadruplet pregnancy with two or more monoamniotic fetuses, first trimester**
    CC Exclusion see Appendix A PDX collection 0976
  - ● ♀ CC **O30.222 Quadruplet pregnancy with two or more monoamniotic fetuses, second trimester**
    CC Exclusion see Appendix A PDX collection 0976
  - ● ♀ CC **O30.223 Quadruplet pregnancy with two or more monoamniotic fetuses, third trimester**
    CC Exclusion see Appendix A PDX collection 0976
  - ● ♀ **O30.229 Quadruplet pregnancy with two or more monoamniotic fetuses, unspecified trimester**

+ **O30.29 Quadruplet pregnancy, unable to determine number of placenta and number of amniotic sacs**
  - ● ♀ CC **O30.291 Quadruplet pregnancy, unable to determine number of placenta and number of amniotic sacs, first trimester**
    CC Exclusion see Appendix A PDX collection 0976
  - ● ♀ CC **O30.292 Quadruplet pregnancy, unable to determine number of placenta and number of amniotic sacs, second trimester**
    CC Exclusion see Appendix A PDX collection 0976
  - ● ♀ CC **O30.293 Quadruplet pregnancy, unable to determine number of placenta and number of amniotic sacs, third trimester**
    CC Exclusion see Appendix A PDX collection 0976
  - ● ♀ **O30.299 Quadruplet pregnancy, unable to determine number of placenta and number of amniotic sacs, unspecified trimester**

+ **O30.8 Other specified multiple gestation**
  Multiple gestation pregnancy greater then quadruplets

+ **O30.80 Other specified multiple gestation, unspecified number of placenta and unspecified number of amniotic sacs**
  - ● ♀ CC **O30.801 Other specified multiple gestation, unspecified number of placenta and unspecified number of amniotic sacs, first trimester**
    CC Exclusion see Appendix A PDX collection 0976
  - ● ♀ CC **O30.802 Other specified multiple gestation, unspecified number of placenta and unspecified number of amniotic sacs, second trimester**
    CC Exclusion see Appendix A PDX collection 0976
  - ● ♀ CC **O30.803 Other specified multiple gestation, unspecified number of placenta and unspecified number of amniotic sacs, third trimester**
    CC Exclusion see Appendix A PDX collection 0976
  - ● ♀ **O30.809 Other specified multiple gestation, unspecified number of placenta and unspecified number of amniotic sacs, unspecified trimester**

+ **O30.81 Other specified multiple gestation with two or more monochorionic fetuses**
  - ● ♀ CC **O30.811 Other specified multiple gestation with two or more monochorionic fetuses, first trimester**
    CC Exclusion see Appendix A PDX collection 0976
  - ● ♀ CC **O30.812 Other specified multiple gestation with two or more monochorionic fetuses, second trimester**
    CC Exclusion see Appendix A PDX collection 0976
  - ● ♀ CC **O30.813 Other specified multiple gestation with two or more monochorionic fetuses, third trimester**
    CC Exclusion see Appendix A PDX collection 0976
  - ● ♀ **O30.819 Other specified multiple gestation with two or more monochorionic fetuses, unspecified trimester**

+ **O30.82 Other specified multiple gestation with two or more monoamniotic fetuses**
  - ● ♀ CC **O30.821 Other specified multiple gestation with two or more monoamniotic fetuses, first trimester**
    CC Exclusion see Appendix A PDX collection 0976
  - ● ♀ CC **O30.822 Other specified multiple gestation with two or more monoamniotic fetuses, second trimester**
    CC Exclusion see Appendix A PDX collection 0976
  - ● ♀ CC **O30.823 Other specified multiple gestation with two or more monoamniotic fetuses, third trimester**
    CC Exclusion see Appendix A PDX collection 0976
  - ● ♀ **O30.829 Other specified multiple gestation with two or more monoamniotic fetuses, unspecified trimester**

+ **O30.89 Other specified multiple gestation, unable to determine number of placenta and number of amniotic sacs**
  - ● ♀ CC **O30.891 Other specified multiple gestation, unable to determine number of placenta and number of amniotic sacs, first trimester**
    CC Exclusion see Appendix A PDX collection 0976
  - ● ♀ CC **O30.892 Other specified multiple gestation, unable to determine number of placenta and number of amniotic sacs, second trimester**
    CC Exclusion see Appendix A PDX collection 0976
  - ● ♀ CC **O30.893 Other specified multiple gestation, unable to determine number of placenta and number of amniotic sacs, third trimester**
    CC Exclusion see Appendix A PDX collection 0976
  - ● ♀ **O30.899 Other specified multiple gestation, unable to determine number of placenta and number of amniotic sacs, unspecified trimester**

+ **O30.9 Multiple gestation, unspecified**
  Multiple pregnancy NOS
  - ● ♀ **O30.90 Multiple gestation, unspecified, unspecified trimester**
  - ● ♀ **O30.91 Multiple gestation, unspecified, first trimester**
  - ● ♀ **O30.92 Multiple gestation, unspecified, second trimester**
  - ● ♀ **O30.93 Multiple gestation, unspecified, third trimester**

O31 Complications specific to multiple gestation

Excludes2: *delayed delivery of second twin, triplet, etc. (O63.2)*
malpresentation of one fetus or more (O32.9)
placental transfusion syndromes (O43.0-)

One of the following 7th characters is to be assigned to each code under category O31. 7th character 0 is for single gestations and multiple gestations where the fetus is unspecified. 7th characters 1 through 9 are for cases of multiple gestations to identify the fetus for which the code applies. The appropriate code from category O30, Multiple gestation, must also be assigned when assigning a code from category O31 that has a 7th character of 1 through 9.

0 - not applicable or unspecified
1 - fetus 1
2 - fetus 2
3 - fetus 3
4 - fetus 4
5 - fetus 5
9 - other fetus

+ **O31.0 Papyraceous fetus**
  Fetus compressus
  - ● ♀ X+7th **O31.00 Papyraceous fetus, unspecified trimester**
  - ● ♀ X+7th **O31.01 Papyraceous fetus, first trimester**
  - ● ♀ X+7th **O31.02 Papyraceous fetus, second trimester**
  - ● ♀ X+7th **O31.03 Papyraceous fetus, third trimester**

+ **O31.1 Continuing pregnancy after spontaneous abortion of one fetu or more**
  - ● ♀ X+7th **O31.10 Continuing pregnancy after spontaneous abortion of one fetus or more, unspecified trimester**
  - ● ♀ X+7th **O31.11 Continuing pregnancy after spontaneous abortion o one fetus or more, first trimester**
  - ● ♀ X+7th **O31.12 Continuing pregnancy after spontaneous abortion o one fetus or more, second trimester**
  - ● ♀ X+7th **O31.13 Continuing pregnancy after spontaneous abortion o one fetus or more, third trimester**

+ **O31.2 Continuing pregnancy after intrauterine death of one fetus or more**
  - ● ♀ X+7th **O31.20 Continuing pregnancy after intrauterine death of one fetus or more, unspecified trimester**

• ♀ X+7th **O31.21 Continuing pregnancy after intrauterine death of one fetus or more, first trimester**
• ♀ X+7th **O31.22 Continuing pregnancy after intrauterine death of one fetus or more, second trimester**
• ♀ X+7th **O31.23 Continuing pregnancy after intrauterine death of one fetus or more, third trimester**
+ **O31.3 Continuing pregnancy after elective fetal reduction of one fetus or more**
Continuing pregnancy after selective termination of one fetus or more
• ♀ X+7th **O31.30 Continuing pregnancy after elective fetal reduction of one fetus or more, unspecified trimester**
• ♀ X+7th **O31.31 Continuing pregnancy after elective fetal reduction of one fetus or more, first trimester**
• ♀ X+7th **O31.32 Continuing pregnancy after elective fetal reduction of one fetus or more, second trimester**
• ♀ X+7th **O31.33 Continuing pregnancy after elective fetal reduction of one fetus or more, third trimester**
+ **O31.8 Other complications specific to multiple gestation**
+ **O31.8X Other complications specific to multiple gestation**
• ♀ CC +7th **O31.8X1 Other complications specific to multiple gestation, first trimester**
CC Exclusion for all 7th characters see Appendix A PDX collection 0976
• ♀ +7th **O31.8X2 Other complications specific to multiple gestation, second trimester**
• ♀ +7th **O31.8X3 Other complications specific to multiple gestation, third trimester**
• ♀ +7th **O31.8X9 Other complications specific to multiple gestation, unspecified trimester**

O32 Maternal care for malpresentation of fetus

Includes: the listed conditions as a reason for observation, hospitalization or other obstetric care of the mother, or for cesarean delivery before onset of labor
Excludes1: *malpresentation of fetus with obstructed labor (O64.-)*

One of the following 7th characters is to be assigned to each code under category O32. 7th character 0 is for single gestations and multiple gestations where the fetus is unspecified. 7th characters 1 through 9 are for cases of multiple gestations to identify the fetus for which the code applies. The appropriate code from category O30, Multiple gestation, must also be assigned when assigning a code from category O32 that has a 7th character of 1 through 9.
0 - not applicable or unspecified
1 - fetus 1
2 - fetus 2
3 - fetus 3
4 - fetus 4
5 - fetus 5
9 - other fetus

♀ X+7th **O32.0 Maternal care for unstable lie**
♀ X+7th **O32.1 Maternal care for breech presentation**
Maternal care for buttocks presentation
Maternal care for complete breech
Maternal care for frank breech
Excludes1: *footling presentation (O32.8)*
incomplete breech (O32.8)
♀ X+7th **O32.2 Maternal care for transverse and oblique lie**
Maternal care for oblique presentation
Maternal care for transverse presentation
♀ X+7th **O32.3 Maternal care for face, brow and chin presentation**
♀ X+7th **O32.4 Maternal care for high head at term**
Maternal care for failure of head to enter pelvic brim
♀ X+7th **O32.6 Maternal care for compound presentation**
♀ X+7th **O32.8 Maternal care for other malpresentation of fetus**
Maternal care for footling presentation
Maternal care for incomplete breech
♀ X+7th **O32.9 Maternal care for malpresentation of fetus, unspecified**

O33 Maternal care for disproportion

Includes: the listed conditions as a reason for observation, hospitalization or other obstetric care of the mother, or for cesarean delivery before onset of labor
Excludes1: *disproportion with obstructed labor (O65-O66)*

• ♀ CC **O33.0 Maternal care for disproportion due to deformity of maternal pelvic bones**
Maternal care for disproportion due to pelvic deformity causing disproportion NOS
CC Exclusion see Appendix A PDX collection 0977
• ♀ **O33.1 Maternal care for disproportion due to generally contracted pelvis**
Maternal care for disproportion due to contracted pelvis NOS causing disproportion
• ♀ **O33.2 Maternal care for disproportion due to inlet contraction of pelvis**
Maternal care for disproportion due to inlet contraction (pelvis) causing disproportion
• ♀ +7th **O33.3 Maternal care for disproportion due to outlet contraction of pelvis**
Maternal care for disproportion due to mid-cavity contraction (pelvis)
Maternal care for disproportion due to outlet contraction (pelvis)

One of the following 7th characters is to be assigned to code **O33.3.** 7th character 0 is for single gestations and multiple gestations where the fetus is unspecified. 7th characters 1 through 9 are for cases of multiple gestations to identify the fetus for which the code applies. The appropriate code from category O30, Multiple gestation, must also be assigned when assigning code O33.3 with a 7th character of 1 through 9.
0 - not applicable or unspecified
1 - fetus 1
2 - fetus 2
3 - fetus 3
4 - fetus 4
5 - fetus 5
9 - other fetus

• ♀ X+7th **O33.4 Maternal care for disproportion of mixed maternal and fetal origin**

One of the following 7th characters is to be assigned to code **O33.4.** 7th character 0 is for single gestations and multiple gestations where the fetus is unspecified. 7th characters 1 through 9 are for cases of multiple gestations to identify the fetus for which the code applies. The appropriate code from category O30, Multiple gestation, must also be assigned when assigning code O33.4 with a 7th character of 1 through 9.
0 - not applicable or unspecified
1 - fetus 1
2 - fetus 2
3 - fetus 3
4 - fetus 4
5 - fetus 5
9 - other fetus

• ♀ X+7th **O33.5 Maternal care for disproportion due to unusually large fetus**
Maternal care for disproportion due to disproportion of fetal origin with normally formed fetus
Maternal care for disproportion due to fetal disproportion NOS

One of the following 7th characters is to be assigned to code **O33.5.** 7th character 0 is for single gestations and multiple gestations where the fetus is unspecified. 7th characters 1 through 9 are for cases of multiple gestations to identify the fetus for which the code applies. The appropriate code from category O30, Multiple gestation, must also be assigned when assigning code O33.5 with a 7th character of 1 through 9.
0 - not applicable or unspecified
1 - fetus 1
2 - fetus 2
3 - fetus 3
4 - fetus 4
5 - fetus 5
9 - other fetus

• ♀ X+7th **O33.6 Maternal care for disproportion due to hydrocephalic fetus**

One of the following 7th characters is to be assigned to code **O33.6.** 7th character 0 is for single gestations and multiple gestations where the fetus is unspecified. 7th characters 1 through 9 are for cases of multiple gestations to identify the fetus for which the code applies. The appropriate code from category O30, Multiple gestation, must also be assigned when assigning code O33.6 with a 7th character of 1 through 9.
0 - not applicable or unspecified
1 - fetus 1
2 - fetus 2
3 - fetus 3
4 - fetus 4
5 - fetus 5
9 - other fetus

• ♀ X+7th **O33.7 Maternal care for disproportion due to other fetal deformities**
Maternal care for disproportion due to fetal ascites
Maternal care for disproportion due to fetal hydrops
Maternal care for disproportion due to fetal meningomyelocele
Maternal care for disproportion due to fetal sacral teratoma
Maternal care for disproportion due to fetal tumor
Excludes1: *obstructed labor due to other fetal deformities (O66.3)*
AHA CC: 4Q, 2016, 51

One of the following 7th characters is to be assigned to code **O33.7.** 7th character 0 is for single gestations and multiple gestations where the fetus is unspecified. 7th characters 1 through 9 are for cases of multiple gestations to identify the fetus for which the code applies. The appropriate code from category O30, Multiple gestation, must also be assigned when assigning code O33.7 with a 7th character of 1 through 9.
0 - not applicable or unspecified
1 - fetus 1
2 - fetus 2
3 - fetus 3
4 - fetus 4
5 - fetus 5
9 - other fetus

• ♀ **O33.8 Maternal care for disproportion of other origin**
• ♀ **O33.9 Maternal care for disproportion, unspecified**
Maternal care for disproportion due to cephalopelvic disproportion NOS
Maternal care for disproportion due to fetopelvic disproportion NOS

O34 Maternal care for abnormality of pelvic organs
Includes: the listed conditions as a reason for hospitalization or other obstetric care of the mother, or for cesarean delivery before onset of labor
Code first any associated obstructed labor (O65.5)

Use additional code for specific condition
+ **O34.0 Maternal care for congenital malformation of uterus**
Maternal care for double uterus
Maternal care for uterus bicornis
• ♀ **O34.00 Maternal care for unspecified congenital malformation of uterus, unspecified trimester**
• ♀ **O34.01 Maternal care for unspecified congenital malformation of uterus, first trimester**
• ♀ **O34.02 Maternal care for unspecified congenital malformation of uterus, second trimester**
• ♀ **O34.03 Maternal care for unspecified congenital malformation of uterus, third trimester**
+ **O34.1 Maternal care for benign tumor of corpus uteri**
Excludes2: *maternal care for benign tumor of cervix (O34.4-)*
maternal care for malignant neoplasm of uterus (O9A.1-)
• ♀ **O34.10 Maternal care for benign tumor of corpus uteri, unspecified trimester**
• ♀ **O34.11 Maternal care for benign tumor of corpus uteri, first trimester**
• ♀ **O34.12 Maternal care for benign tumor of corpus uteri, second trimester**
• ♀ **O34.13 Maternal care for benign tumor of corpus uteri, third trimester**
+ **O34.2 Maternal care due to uterine scar from previous surgery**
+ **O34.21 Maternal care for scar from previous cesarean delivery**
AHA CC: 4Q, 2016, 51-52
• ♀ **O34.211 Maternal care for low transverse scar from previous cesarean delivery**
• ♀ **O34.212 Maternal care for vertical scar from previous cesarean delivery**
Maternal care for classical scar from previous cesarean delivery
• ♀ **O34.219 Maternal care for unspecified type scar from previous cesarean delivery**
• ♀ **O34.29 Maternal care due to uterine scar from other previous surgery**
Maternal care due to uterine scar from other transmural uterine
+ **O34.3 Maternal care for cervical incompetence**
Maternal care for cerclage with or without cervical incompetence
Maternal care for Shirodkar suture with or without cervical incompetence

• ♀ **O34.30 Maternal care for cervical incompetence, unspecified trimester**
• ♀ MCC **O34.31 Maternal care for cervical incompetence, first trimester**
MCC Exclusion see Appendix A PDX collection 0973
• ♀ MCC **O34.32 Maternal care for cervical incompetence, second trimester**
MCC Exclusion see Appendix A PDX collection 0973
• ♀ MCC **O34.33 Maternal care for cervical incompetence, third trimester**
MCC Exclusion see Appendix A PDX collection 0973
+ **O34.4 Maternal care for other abnormalities of cervix**
• ♀ **O34.40 Maternal care for other abnormalities of cervix, unspecified trimester**
• ♀ **O34.41 Maternal care for other abnormalities of cervix, first trimester**
• ♀ **O34.42 Maternal care for other abnormalities of cervix, second trimester**
• ♀ **O34.43 Maternal care for other abnormalities of cervix, third trimester**
+ **O34.5 Maternal care for other abnormalities of gravid uterus**
+ **O34.51 Maternal care for incarceration of gravid uterus**
• ♀ **O34.511 Maternal care for incarceration of gravid uterus, first trimester**
• ♀ **O34.512 Maternal care for incarceration of gravid uterus, second trimester**
• ♀ **O34.513 Maternal care for incarceration of gravid uterus, third trimester**
• ♀ **O34.519 Maternal care for incarceration of gravid uterus, unspecified trimester**
+ **O34.52 Maternal care for prolapse of gravid uterus**
• ♀ **O34.521 Maternal care for prolapse of gravid uterus, first trimester**
• ♀ **O34.522 Maternal care for prolapse of gravid uterus, second trimester**
• ♀ **O34.523 Maternal care for prolapse of gravid uterus, third trimester**
• ♀ **O34.529 Maternal care for prolapse of gravid uterus, unspecified trimester**
+ **O34.53 Maternal care for retroversion of gravid uterus**
• ♀ **O34.531 Maternal care for retroversion of gravid uterus, first trimester**
• ♀ **O34.532 Maternal care for retroversion of gravid uterus, second trimester**
• ♀ **O34.533 Maternal care for retroversion of gravid uterus, third trimester**
• ♀ **O34.539 Maternal care for retroversion of gravid uterus, unspecified trimester**
+ **O34.59 Maternal care for other abnormalities of gravid uterus**
• ♀ **O34.591 Maternal care for other abnormalities of gravid uterus, first trimester**
• ♀ **O34.592 Maternal care for other abnormalities of gravid uterus, second trimester**
• ♀ **O34.593 Maternal care for other abnormalities of gravid uterus, third trimester**
• ♀ **O34.599 Maternal care for other abnormalities of gravid uterus, unspecified trimester**
O34.6 Maternal care for abnormality of vagina
Excludes2: *maternal care for vaginal varices in pregnancy (O22.1-)*
• ♀ **O34.60 Maternal care for abnormality of vagina, unspecified trimester**
• ♀ **O34.61 Maternal care for abnormality of vagina, first trimester**
• ♀ **O34.62 Maternal care for abnormality of vagina, second trimester**
• ♀ **O34.63 Maternal care for abnormality of vagina, third trimester**
+ **O34.7 Maternal care for abnormality of vulva and perineum**
Excludes2: *maternal care for perineal and vulval varices in pregnancy (O22.1-)*
• ♀ **O34.70 Maternal care for abnormality of vulva and perineum, unspecified trimester**
• ♀ **O34.71 Maternal care for abnormality of vulva and perineum, first trimester**
• ♀ **O34.72 Maternal care for abnormality of vulva and perineum, second trimester**
• ♀ **O34.73 Maternal care for abnormality of vulva and perineum, third trimester**
+ **O34.8 Maternal care for other abnormalities of pelvic organs**

• ♀ O34.80 **Maternal care for other abnormalities of pelvic organs, unspecified trimester**
• ♀ O34.81 **Maternal care for other abnormalities of pelvic organs, first trimester**
• ♀ O34.82 **Maternal care for other abnormalities of pelvic organs, second trimester**
• ♀ O34.83 **Maternal care for other abnormalities of pelvic organs, third trimester**
+ O34.9 **Maternal care for abnormality of pelvic organ, unspecified**
• ♀ O34.90 **Maternal care for abnormality of pelvic organ, unspecified, unspecified trimester**
• ♀ O34.91 **Maternal care for abnormality of pelvic organ, unspecified, first trimester**
• ♀ O34.92 **Maternal care for abnormality of pelvic organ, unspecified, second trimester**
• ♀ O34.93 **Maternal care for abnormality of pelvic organ, unspecified, third trimester**

O35 Maternal care for known or suspected fetal abnormality and damage

Includes: the listed conditions in the fetus as a reason for hospitalization or other obstetric care to the mother, or for termination of pregnancy

Code also any associated maternal condition

Excludes1: *encounter for suspected maternal and fetal conditions ruled out (Z03.7-)*

One of the following 7th characters is to be assigned to each code under category O35. 7th character 0 is for single gestations and multiple gestations where the fetus is unspecified. 7th characters 1 through 9 are for cases of multiple gestations to identify the fetus for which the code applies. The appropriate code from category O30, Multiple gestation, must also be assigned when assigning a code from category O35 that has a 7th character of 1 through 9.

0 - not applicable or unspecified
1 - fetus 1
2 - fetus 2
3 - fetus 3
4 - fetus 4
5 - fetus 5
9 - other fetus

Review coding guideline C.15.e

♀ X+7th O35.0 **Maternal care for (suspected) central nervous system malformation in fetus**
Maternal care for fetal anencephaly
Maternal care for fetal hydrocephalus
Maternal care for fetal spina bifida
Excludes2: *chromosomal abnormality in fetus (O35.1)*

♀ X+7th O35.1 **Maternal care for (suspected) chromosomal abnormality in fetus**

♀ X+7th O35.2 **Maternal care for (suspected) hereditary disease in fetus**
Excludes2: *chromosomal abnormality in fetus (O35.1)*

♀ X+7th O35.3 **Maternal care for (suspected) damage to fetus from viral disease in mother**
Maternal care for damage to fetus from maternal cytomegalovirus infection
Maternal care for damage to fetus from maternal rubella
AHA CC: 4Q, 2016, 4-7

♀ X+7th O35.4 **Maternal care for (suspected) damage to fetus from alcohol**

♀ X+7th O35.5 **Maternal care for (suspected) damage to fetus by drugs**
Maternal care for damage to fetus from drug addiction

♀ X+7th O35.6 **Maternal care for (suspected) damage to fetus by radiation**

♀ X+7th O35.7 **Maternal care for (suspected) damage to fetus by other medical procedures**
Maternal care for damage to fetus by amniocentesis
Maternal care for damage to fetus by biopsy procedures
Maternal care for damage to fetus by hematological investigation
Maternal care for damage to fetus by intrauterine contraceptive device
Maternal care for damage to fetus by intrauterine surgery

♀ X+7th O35.8 **Maternal care for other (suspected) fetal abnormality and damage**
Maternal care for damage to fetus from maternal listeriosis
Maternal care for damage to fetus from maternal toxoplasmosis

♀ X+7th O35.9 **Maternal care for (suspected) fetal abnormality and damage, unspecified**

O36 Maternal care for other fetal problems

Includes: the listed conditions in the fetus as a reason for hospitalization or other obstetric care of the mother, or for termination of pregnancy

Excludes1: *encounter for suspected maternal and fetal conditions ruled out (Z03.7-)*
placental transfusion syndromes (O43.0-)

Excludes2: *labor and delivery complicated by fetal stress (O77.-)*

One of the following 7th characters is to be assigned to each code under category O36. 7th character 0 is for single gestations and multiple gestations where the fetus is unspecified. 7th characters 1 through 9 are for cases of multiple gestations to identify the fetus for which the code applies. The appropriate code from category O30, Multiple gestation, must also be assigned when assigning a code from category O36 that has a 7th character of 1 through 9.

0 - not applicable or unspecified
1 - fetus 1
2 - fetus 2
3 - fetus 3
4 - fetus 4
5 - fetus 5
9 - other fetus

Review coding guideline C.15.e

+ O36.0 **Maternal care for rhesus isoimmunization**
Maternal care for Rh incompatibility (with hydrops fetalis)

+ O36.01 **Maternal care for anti-D [Rh] antibodies**
• ♀ CC +7th O36.011 **Maternal care for anti-D [Rh] antibodies, first trimester**
CC Exclusion for all 7th characters see Appendix A PDX collection 0978
• ♀ CC +7th O36.012 **Maternal care for anti-D [Rh] antibodies, second trimester**
CC Exclusion for all 7th characters see Appendix A PDX collection 0978
• ♀ CC +7th O36.013 **Maternal care for anti-D [Rh] antibodies, third trimester**
CC Exclusion for all 7th characters see Appendix A PDX collection 0978
AHA CC: 4Q, 2014, 17-18
• ♀ +7th O36.019 **Maternal care for anti-D [Rh] antibodies, unspecified trimester**

+ O36.09 **Maternal care for other rhesus isoimmunization**
• ♀ CC +7th O36.091 **Maternal care for other rhesus isoimmunization, first trimester**
CC Exclusion for all 7th characters see Appendix A PDX collection 0978
• ♀ CC +7th O36.092 **Maternal care for other rhesus isoimmunization, second trimester**
CC Exclusion for all 7th characters see Appendix A PDX collection 0978
• ♀ CC +7th O36.093 **Maternal care for other rhesus isoimmunization, third trimester**
CC Exclusion for all 7th characters see Appendix A PDX collection 0978
• ♀ +7th O36.099 **Maternal care for other rhesus isoimmunization, unspecified trimester**

+ O36.1 **Maternal care for other isoimmunization**
Maternal care for ABO isoimmunization

+ O36.11 **Maternal care for Anti-A sensitization**
Maternal care for isoimmunization NOS (with hydrops fetalis)
• ♀ +7th O36.111 **Maternal care for Anti-A sensitization, first trimester**
• ♀ +7th O36.112 **Maternal care for Anti-A sensitization, second trimester**
• ♀ +7th O36.113 **Maternal care for Anti-A sensitization, third trimester**
• ♀ +7th O36.119 **Maternal care for Anti-A sensitization, unspecified trimester**

+ O36.19 **Maternal care for other isoimmunization**
Maternal care for Anti-B sensitization
• ♀ +7th O36.191 **Maternal care for other isoimmunization, first trimester**
• ♀ +7th O36.192 **Maternal care for other isoimmunization, second trimester**
• ♀ +7th O36.193 **Maternal care for other isoimmunization, third trimester**
• ♀ +7th O36.199 **Maternal care for other isoimmunization, unspecified trimester**

+ **O36.2 Maternal care for hydrops fetalis**
Maternal care for hydrops fetalis NOS
Maternal care for hydrops fetalis not associated with isoimmunization
Excludes1: *hydrops fetalis associated with ABO isoimmunization (O36.1-)*
hydrops fetalis associated with rhesus isoimmunization (O36.0-)
• ♀ X+7th **O36.20 Maternal care for hydrops fetalis, unspecified trimester**
• ♀ X+7th **O36.21 Maternal care for hydrops fetalis, first trimester**
• ♀ X+7th **O36.22 Maternal care for hydrops fetalis, second trimester**
• ♀ X+7th **O36.23 Maternal care for hydrops fetalis, third trimester**
• ♀ CC X+7th **O36.4 Maternal care for intrauterine death**
Maternal care for intrauterine fetal death NOS
Maternal care for intrauterine fetal death after completion of 20 weeks of gestation
Maternal care for late fetal death
Maternal care for missed delivery
Excludes1: *missed abortion (O02.1)stillbirth (P95)*
CC Exclusion for all 7th characters see Appendix A PDX collection 0979
+ **O36.5 Maternal care for known or suspected poor fetal growth**
+ **O36.51 Maternal care for known or suspected placental insufficiency**
• ♀ +7th **O36.511 Maternal care for known or suspected placental insufficiency, first trimester**
• ♀ +7th **O36.512 Maternal care for known or suspected placental insufficiency, second trimester**
• ♀ +7th **O36.513 Maternal care for known or suspected placental insufficiency, third trimester**
• ♀ +7th **O36.519 Maternal care for known or suspected placental insufficiency, unspecified trimester**
+ **O36.59 Maternal care for other known or suspected poor fetal growth**
Maternal care for known or suspected light-for-dates NOS
Maternal care for known or suspected small-for-dates NOS
• ♀ +7th **O36.591 Maternal care for other known or suspected poor fetal growth, first trimester**
• ♀ +7th **O36.592 Maternal care for other known or suspected poor fetal growth, second trimester**
• ♀ +7th **O36.593 Maternal care for other known or suspected poor fetal growth, third trimester**
• ♀ +7th **O36.599 Maternal care for other known or suspected poor fetal growth, unspecified trimester**
+ **O36.6 Maternal care for excessive fetal growth**
Maternal care for known or suspected large-for-dates
• ♀ X+7th **O36.60 Maternal care for excessive fetal growth, unspecified trimester**
• ♀ X+7th **O36.61 Maternal care for excessive fetal growth, first trimester**
• ♀ X+7th **O36.62 Maternal care for excessive fetal growth, second trimester**
• ♀ X+7th **O36.63 Maternal care for excessive fetal growth, third trimester**
+ **O36.7 Maternal care for viable fetus in abdominal pregnancy**
• ♀ X+7th **O36.70 Maternal care for viable fetus in abdominal pregnancy, unspecified trimester**
• ♀ X+7th **O36.71 Maternal care for viable fetus in abdominal pregnancy, first trimester**
• ♀ X+7th **O36.72 Maternal care for viable fetus in abdominal pregnancy, second trimester**
• ♀ X+7th **O36.73 Maternal care for viable fetus in abdominal pregnancy, third trimester**
+ **O36.8 Maternal care for other specified fetal problems**
• ♀ X+7th **O36.80 Pregnancy with inconclusive fetal viability**
Encounter to determine fetal viability of pregnancy
+ **O36.81 Decreased fetal movements**
• ♀ +7th **O36.812 Decreased fetal movements, second trimester**
• ♀ +7th **O36.813 Decreased fetal movements, third trimester**
• ♀ +7th **O36.819 Decreased fetal movements, unspecified trimester**
+ **O36.82 Fetal anemia and thrombocytopenia**
• ♀ +7th **O36.821 Fetal anemia and thrombocytopenia, first trimester**
• ♀ +7th **O36.822 Fetal anemia and thrombocytopenia, second trimester**
• ♀ +7th **O36.823 Fetal anemia and thrombocytopenia, third trimester**
• ♀ +7th **O36.829 Fetal anemia and thrombocytopenia, unspecified trimester**
+ **O36.83 Maternal care for abnormalities of the fetal heart rate or rhythm**
• ♀ +7th **O36.831 Maternal care for abnormalities of the fetal heart rate or rhythm, first trimester**
• ♀ +7th **O36.832 Maternal care for abnormalities of the fetal heart rate or rhythm, second trimester**
• ♀ +7th **O36.833 Maternal care for abnormalities of the fetal heart rate or rhythm, third trimester**
• ♀ +7th **O36.839 Maternal care for abnormalities of the fetal heart rate or rhythm, unspecified trimester**
+ **O36.89 Maternal care for other specified fetal problems**
• ♀ +7th **O36.891 Maternal care for other specified fetal problems, first trimester**
• ♀ +7th **O36.892 Maternal care for other specified fetal problems, second trimester**
• ♀ +7th **O36.893 Maternal care for other specified fetal problems, third trimester**
• ♀ +7th **O36.899 Maternal care for other specified fetal problems, unspecified trimester**
+ **O36.9 Maternal care for fetal problem, unspecified**
• ♀ X+7th **O36.90 Maternal care for fetal problem, unspecified, unspecified trimester**
• ♀ X+7th **O36.91 Maternal care for fetal problem, unspecified, first trimester**
• ♀ X+7th **O36.92 Maternal care for fetal problem, unspecified, second trimester**
• ♀ X+7th **O36.93 Maternal care for fetal problem, unspecified, third trimester**

O40 Polyhydramnios

Includes: hydramnios
Excludes1: *encounter for suspected maternal and fetal conditions ruled out (Z03.7-)*

One of the following 7th characters is to be assigned to each code under category O40. 7th character 0 is for single gestations and multiple gestations where the fetus is unspecified. 7th characters 1 through 9 are for cases of multiple gestations to identify the fetus for which the code applies. The appropriate code from category O30, Multiple gestation, must also be assigned when assigning a code from category O40 that has a 7th character of 1 through 9.
0 - not applicable or unspecified
1 - fetus 1
2 - fetus 2
3 - fetus 3
4 - fetus 4
5 - fetus 5
9 - other fetus

• ♀ X+7th **O40.1 Polyhydramnios, first trimester**
• ♀ X+7th **O40.2 Polyhydramnios, second trimester**
• ♀ X+7th **O40.3 Polyhydramnios, third trimester**
• ♀ X+7th **O40.9 Polyhydramnios, unspecified trimester**

O41 Other disorders of amniotic fluid and membranes

Excludes1: *encounter for suspected maternal and fetal conditions ruled out (Z03.7-)*

One of the following 7th characters is to be assigned to each code under category O41. 7th character 0 is for single gestations and multiple gestations where the fetus is unspecified. 7th characters 1 through 9 are for cases of multiple gestations to identify the fetus for which the code applies. The appropriate code from category O30, Multiple gestation, must also be assigned when assigning a code from category O41 that has a 7th character of 1 through 9.
0 - not applicable or unspecified
1 - fetus 1
2 - fetus 2
3 - fetus 3
4 - fetus 4
5 - fetus 5
9 - other fetus

\+ O41.0 **Oligohydramnios**
Oligohydramnios without rupture of membranes
● ♀ X+7th **O41.00 Oligohydramnios, unspecified trimester**
● ♀ CC X+7th **O41.01 Oligohydramnios, first trimester**
CC Exclusion for all 7th characters see Appendix A PDX collection 0982
● ♀ CC X+7th **O41.02 Oligohydramnios, second trimester**
CC Exclusion for all 7th characters see Appendix A PDX collection 0982
● ♀ CC X+7th **O41.03 Oligohydramnios, third trimester**
CC Exclusion for all 7th characters see Appendix A PDX collection 0982
\+ **O41.1 Infection of amniotic sac and membranes**
\+ **O41.10 Infection of amniotic sac and membranes, unspecified**
● ♀ MCC +7th **O41.101 Infection of amniotic sac and membranes, unspecified, first trimester**
MCC Exclusion for all 7th characters see Appendix A PDX collection 0983
● ♀ MCC +7th **O41.102 Infection of amniotic sac and membranes, unspecified, second trimester**
MCC Exclusion for all 7th characters see Appendix A PDX collection 0983
● ♀ MCC +7th **O41.103 Infection of amniotic sac and membranes, unspecified, third trimester**
MCC Exclusion for all 7th characters see Appendix A PDX collection 0983
● ♀ +7th **O41.109 Infection of amniotic sac and membranes, unspecified, unspecified trimester**
\+ **O41.12 Chorioamnionitis**
● ♀ MCC +7th **O41.121 Chorioamnionitis, first trimester**
MCC Exclusion for all 7th characters see Appendix A PDX collection 0983
● ♀ MCC +7th **O41.122 Chorioamnionitis, second trimester**
MCC Exclusion for all 7th characters see Appendix A PDX collection 0983
● ♀ MCC +7th **O41.123 Chorioamnionitis, third trimester**
MCC Exclusion for all 7th characters see Appendix A PDX collection 0983
● ♀ +7th **O41.129 Chorioamnionitis, unspecified trimester**
\+ **O41.14 Placentitis**
● ♀ MCC +7th **O41.141 Placentitis, first trimester**
MCC Exclusion for all 7th characters see Appendix A PDX collection 0983
● ♀ MCC +7th **O41.142 Placentitis, second trimester**
MCC Exclusion for all 7th characters see Appendix A PDX collection 0983
● ♀ MCC +7th **O41.143 Placentitis, third trimester**
MCC Exclusion for all 7th characters see Appendix A PDX collection 0983
● ♀ +7th **O41.149 Placentitis, unspecified trimester**
\+ **O41.8 Other specified disorders of amniotic fluid and membranes**
\+ **O41.8X Other specified disorders of amniotic fluid and membranes**
● ♀ +7th **O41.8X1 Other specified disorders of amniotic fluid and membranes, first trimester**
● ♀ +7th **O41.8X2 Other specified disorders of amniotic fluid and membranes, second trimester**
● ♀ +7th **O41.8X3 Other specified disorders of amniotic fluid and membranes, third trimester**
● ♀ +7th **O41.8X9 Other specified disorders of amniotic fluid and membranes, unspecified trimester**
\+ **O41.9 Disorder of amniotic fluid and membranes, unspecified**
● ♀ X+7th **O41.90 Disorder of amniotic fluid and membranes, unspecified, unspecified trimester**
● ♀ X+7th **O41.91 Disorder of amniotic fluid and membranes, unspecified, first trimester**
● ♀ X+7th **O41.92 Disorder of amniotic fluid and membranes, unspecified, second trimester**
● ♀ X+7th **O41.93 Disorder of amniotic fluid and membranes, unspecified, third trimester**

O42 Premature rupture of membranes

\+ **O42.0 Premature rupture of membranes, onset of labor within 24 hours of rupture**
● ♀ **O42.00 Premature rupture of membranes, onset of labor within 24 hours of rupture, unspecified weeks of gestation**
\+ **O42.01 Preterm premature rupture of membranes, onset of labor within 24 hours of rupture**
Premature rupture of membranes before 37 completed weeks of gestation, onset of labor within 24 hours of rupture
● ♀ **O42.011 Preterm premature rupture of membranes, onset of labor within 24 hours of rupture, first trimester**
● ♀ **O42.012 Preterm premature rupture of membranes, onset of labor within 24 hours of rupture, second trimester**
● ♀ **O42.013 Preterm premature rupture of membranes, onset of labor within 24 hours of rupture, third trimester**
● ♀ **O42.019 Preterm premature rupture of membranes, onset of labor within 24 hours of rupture, unspecified trimester**
● ♀ **O42.02 Full-term premature rupture of membranes, onset of labor within 24 hours of rupture**
Premature rupture of membranes at or after 37 completed weeks of gestation, onset of labor within 24 hours of rupture
\+ **O42.1 Premature rupture of membranes, onset of labor more than 24 hours following rupture**
● ♀ **O42.10 Premature rupture of membranes, onset of labor more than 24 hours following rupture, unspecified weeks of gestation**
\+ **O42.11 Preterm premature rupture of membranes, onset of labor more than 24 hours following rupture**
Premature rupture of membranes before 37 completed weeks of gestation
● ♀ **O42.111 Preterm premature rupture of membranes, onset of labor more than 24 hours following rupture, first trimester**
● ♀ **O42.112 Preterm premature rupture of membranes, onset of labor more than 24 hours following rupture, second trimester**
● ♀ **O42.113 Preterm premature rupture of membranes, onset of labor more than 24 hours following rupture, third trimester**
● ♀ **O42.119 Preterm premature rupture of membranes, onset of labor more than 24 hours following rupture, unspecified trimester**
● ♀ **O42.12 Full-term premature rupture of membranes, onset of labor more than 24 hours following rupture**
Premature rupture of membranes at or after 37 completed weeks of gestation, onset of labor more than 24 hours following rupture
\+ **O42.9 Premature rupture of membranes, unspecified as to length of time between rupture and onset of labor**
● ♀ **O42.90 Premature rupture of membranes, unspecified as to length of time between rupture and onset of labor, unspecified weeks of gestation**
\+ **O42.91 Preterm premature rupture of membranes, unspecified as to length of time between rupture and onset of labor**
Premature rupture of membranes before 37 completed weeks of gestation
● ♀ **O42.911 Preterm premature rupture of membranes, unspecified as to length of time between rupture and onset of labor, first trimester**
● ♀ **O42.912 Preterm premature rupture of membranes, unspecified as to length of time between rupture and onset of labor, second trimester**
● ♀ **O42.913 Preterm premature rupture of membranes, unspecified as to length of time between rupture and onset of labor, third trimester**
● ♀ **O42.919 Preterm premature rupture of membranes, unspecified as to length of time between rupture and onset of labor, unspecified trimester**
● ♀ **O42.92 Full-term premature rupture of membranes, unspecified as to length of time between rupture and onset of labor**
Premature rupture of membranes at or after 37 completed weeks of gestation, unspecified as to length of time between rupture and onset of labor

O43 Placental disorders

Excludes2: *maternal care for poor fetal growth due to placental insufficiency (O36.5-)*
placenta previa (O44.-)
placental polyp (O90.89)
placentitis (O41.14-)
premature separation of placenta [abruptio placentae] (O45.-)

+ **O43.0 Placental transfusion syndromes**
  + **O43.01 Fetomaternal placental transfusion syndrome**
    Maternofetal placental transfusion syndrome
    - ♀ **O43.011 Fetomaternal placental transfusion syndrome, first trimester**
    - ♀ **O43.012 Fetomaternal placental transfusion syndrome, second trimester**
    - ♀ **O43.013 Fetomaternal placental transfusion syndrome, third trimester**
    - ♀ **O43.019 Fetomaternal placental transfusion syndrome, unspecified trimester**
  + **O43.02 Fetus-to-fetus placental transfusion syndrome**
    - ♀ **O43.021 Fetus-to-fetus placental transfusion syndrome, first trimester**
    - ♀ **O43.022 Fetus-to-fetus placental transfusion syndrome, second trimester**
    - ♀ **O43.023 Fetus-to-fetus placental transfusion syndrome, third trimester**
    - ♀ **O43.029 Fetus-to-fetus placental transfusion syndrome, unspecified trimester**

+ **O43.1 Malformation of placenta**
  + **O43.10 Malformation of placenta, unspecified**
    Abnormal placenta NOS
    - ♀ **O43.101 Malformation of placenta, unspecified, first trimester**
    - ♀ **O43.102 Malformation of placenta, unspecified, second trimester**
    - ♀ **O43.103 Malformation of placenta, unspecified, third trimester**
    - ♀ **O43.109 Malformation of placenta, unspecified, unspecified trimester**
  + **O43.11 Circumvallate placenta**
    - ♀ **O43.111 Circumvallate placenta, first trimester**
    - ♀ **O43.112 Circumvallate placenta, second trimester**
    - ♀ **O43.113 Circumvallate placenta, third trimester**
    - ♀ **O43.119 Circumvallate placenta, unspecified trimester**
  + **O43.12 Velamentous insertion of umbilical cord**
    - ♀ **O43.121 Velamentous insertion of umbilical cord, first trimester**
    - ♀ **O43.122 Velamentous insertion of umbilical cord, second trimester**
    - ♀ **O43.123 Velamentous insertion of umbilical cord, third trimester**
    - ♀ **O43.129 Velamentous insertion of umbilical cord, unspecified trimester**
  + **O43.19 Other malformation of placenta**
    - ♀ **O43.191 Other malformation of placenta, first trimester**
    - ♀ **O43.192 Other malformation of placenta, second trimester**
    - ♀ **O43.193 Other malformation of placenta, third trimester**
    - ♀ **O43.199 Other malformation of placenta, unspecified trimester**

+ **O43.2 Morbidly adherent placenta**
  Code also associated third stage postpartum hemorrhage, if applicable (O72.0)
  MCC *Excludes1:* *retained placenta (O73.-)*
  + **O43.21 Placenta accreta**
    - ♀ **O43.211 Placenta accreta, first trimester**
    - MCC ♀ **O43.212 Placenta accreta, second trimester**
    - ♀ **O43.213 Placenta accreta, third trimester**
    - ♀ **O43.219 accreta, unspecified trimester**
  + **O43.22 Placenta increta**
    - ♀ **O43.221 Placenta increta, first trimester**
    - ♀ **O43.222 Placenta increta, second trimester**
    - ♀ **O43.223 Placenta increta, third trimester**
    - ♀ **O43.229 Placenta increta, unspecified trimester**
  + **O43.23 Placenta percreta**
    - ♀ **O43.231 Placenta percreta, first trimester**
    - ♀ **O43.232 Placenta percreta, second trimester**
    - ♀ **O43.233 Placenta percreta, third trimester**
    - ♀ **O43.239 Placenta percreta, unspecified trimester**

+ **O43.8 Other placental disorders**
  + **O43.81 Placental infarction**
    - ♀ **O43.811 Placental infarction, first trimester**
    - ♀ **O43.812 Placental infarction, second trimester**
    - ♀ **O43.813 Placental infarction, third trimester**
    - ♀ **O43.819 Placental infarction, unspecified trimeste**
  + **O43.89 Other placental disorders**
    Placental dysfunction
    - ♀ **O43.891 Other placental disorders, first trimester**
    - ♀ **O43.892 Other placental disorders, second trimest**
    - ♀ **O43.893 Other placental disorders, third trimeste**
    - ♀ **O43.899 Other placental disorders, unspecified trimester**

+ **O43.9 Unspecified placental disorder**
  - ♀ **O43.90 Unspecified placental disorder, unspecified trimeste**
  - ♀ **O43.91 Unspecified placental disorder, first trimester**
  - ♀ **O43.92 Unspecified placental disorder, second trimester**
  - ♀ **O43.93 Unspecified placental disorder, third trimester**

O44 Placenta previa

AHA CC: 4Q, 2016, 52-53

+ **O44.0 Complete placenta previa NOS or without hemorrhage**
  Placenta previa NOS
  - ♀ **O44.00 Complete placenta previa NOS or without hemorrhage, unspecified trimester**
  - ♀ CC **O44.01 Complete placenta previa NOS or without hemorrhage, first trimester**
    CC Exclusion see Appendix A PDX collection 0966
  - ♀ CC **O44.02 Complete placenta previa NOS or without hemorrhage, second trimester**
    CC Exclusion see Appendix A PDX collection 0966
  - ♀ CC **O44.03 Complete placenta previa NOS or without hemorrhage, third trimester**
    CC Exclusion see Appendix A PDX collection 0966

+ **O44.1 Complete placenta previa with hemorrhage**
  Excludes1: *labor and delivery complicated by hemorrhage from vasa previa (O69.4)*
  - ♀ **O44.10 Complete placenta previa with hemorrhage, unspecified trimester**
  - ♀ MCC **O44.11 Complete placenta previa with hemorrhage, first trimester**
    MCC Exclusion see Appendix A PDX collection 0966
  - ♀ MCC **O44.12 Complete placenta previa with hemorrhage, seconc trimester**
    MCC Exclusion see Appendix A PDX collection 0966
  - ♀ MCC **O44.13 Complete placenta previa with hemorrhage, third trimester**
    MCC Exclusion see Appendix A PDX collection 0966

+ **O44.2 Partial placenta previa without hemorrhage**
  Marginal placenta previa, NOS or without hemorrhage
  - ♀ **O44.20 Partial placenta previa NOS or without hemorrhag unspecified trimester**
  - ♀ CC **O44.21 Partial placenta previa NOS or without hemorrhag first trimester**
    CC Exclusion see Appendix A PDX collection 0966
  - ♀ CC **O44.22 Partial placenta previa NOS or without hemorrhag second trimester**
    CC Exclusion see Appendix A PDX collection 0966
  - ♀ CC **O44.23 Partial placenta previa NOS or without hemorrhag third trimester**
    CC Exclusion see Appendix A PDX collection 0966

+ **O44.3 Partial placenta previa with hemorrhage**
  Marginal placenta previa with hemorrhage
  - ♀ **O44.30 Partial placenta previa with hemorrhage, unspecifi trimester**
  - ♀ MCC **O44.31 Partial placenta previa with hemorrhage, first trimester**
    MCC Exclusion see Appendix A PDX collection 0966
  - ♀ MCC **O44.32 Partial placenta previa with hemorrhage, second trimester**
    MCC Exclusion see Appendix A PDX collection 0966
  - ♀ MCC **O44.33 Partial placenta previa with hemorrhage, third trimester**
    MCC Exclusion see Appendix A PDX collection 0966

+ **O44.4 Low lying placenta NOS or without hemorrhage**
  Low implantation of placenta NOS or without hemorrhage
  - ♀ **O44.40 Low lying placenta NOS or without hemorrhage, unspecified trimester**

● ♀ CC **O44.41 Low lying placenta NOS or without hemorrhage, first trimester**
CC Exclusion see Appendix A PDX collection 0966
● ♀ CC **O44.42 Low lying placenta NOS or without hemorrhage, second trimester**
CC Exclusion see Appendix A PDX collection 0966
● ♀ CC **O44.43 Low lying placenta NOS or without hemorrhage, third trimester**
CC Exclusion see Appendix A PDX collection 0966
\+ **O44.5 Low lying placenta with hemorrhage**
Low implantation of placenta with hemorrhage
● ♀ **O44.50 Low lying placenta with hemorrhage, unspecified trimester**
● ♀ MCC **O44.51 Low lying placenta with hemorrhage, first trimester**
MCC Exclusion see Appendix A PDX collection 0966
● ♀ MCC **O44.52 Low lying placenta with hemorrhage, second trimester**
MCC Exclusion see Appendix A PDX collection 0966
● ♀ MCC **O44.53 Low lying placenta with hemorrhage, third trimester**
MCC Exclusion see Appendix A PDX collection 0966

O45 Premature separation of placenta [abruptio placentae]

\+ **O45.0 Premature separation of placenta with coagulation defect**
\+ **O45.00 Premature separation of placenta with coagulation defect, unspecified**
● ♀ MCC **O45.001 Premature separation of placenta with coagulation defect, unspecified, first trimester**
MCC Exclusion see Appendix A PDX collection 0985
● ♀ MCC **O45.002 Premature separation of placenta with coagulation defect, unspecified, second trimester**
MCC Exclusion see Appendix A PDX collection 0985
● ♀ MCC **O45.003 Premature separation of placenta with coagulation defect, unspecified, third trimester**
MCC Exclusion see Appendix A PDX collection 0985
● ♀ **O45.009 Premature separation of placenta with coagulation defect, unspecified, unspecified trimester**
\+ **O45.01 Premature separation of placenta with afibrinogenemia**
Premature separation of placenta with hypofibrinogenemia
● ♀ MCC **O45.011 Premature separation of placenta with afibrinogenemia, first trimester**
MCC Exclusion see Appendix A PDX collection 0985
● ♀ MCC **O45.012 Premature separation of placenta with afibrinogenemia, second trimester**
MCC Exclusion see Appendix A PDX collection 0985
● ♀ MCC **O45.013 Premature separation of placenta with afibrinogenemia, third trimester**
MCC Exclusion see Appendix A PDX collection 0985
● ♀ **O45.019 Premature separation of placenta with afibrinogenemia, unspecified trimester**
\+ **O45.02 Premature separation of placenta with disseminated intravascular coagulation**
● ♀ MCC **O45.021 Premature separation of placenta with disseminated intravascular coagulation, first trimester**
MCC Exclusion see Appendix A PDX collection 0985
● ♀ MCC **O45.022 Premature separation of placenta with disseminated intravascular coagulation, second trimester**
MCC Exclusion see Appendix A PDX collection 0985
● ♀ MCC **O45.023 Premature separation of placenta with disseminated intravascular coagulation, third trimester**
MCC Exclusion see Appendix A PDX collection 0985
● ♀ **O45.029 Premature separation of placenta with disseminated intravascular coagulation, unspecified trimester**
O45.09 Premature separation of placenta with other coagulation defect
● ♀ MCC **O45.091 Premature separation of placenta with other coagulation defect, first trimester**
MCC Exclusion see Appendix A PDX collection 0985
● ♀ MCC **O45.092 Premature separation of placenta with other coagulation defect, second trimester**
MCC Exclusion see Appendix A PDX collection 0985
● ♀ MCC **O45.093 Premature separation of placenta with other coagulation defect, third trimester**
MCC Exclusion see Appendix A PDX collection 0985
● ♀ **O45.099 Premature separation of placenta with other coagulation defect, unspecified trimester**
\+ **O45.8 Other premature separation of placenta**
\+ **O45.8X Other premature separation of placenta**
● ♀ MCC **O45.8X1 Other premature separation of placenta, first trimester**
MCC Exclusion see Appendix A PDX collection 0986
● ♀ MCC **O45.8X2 Other premature separation of placenta, second trimester**
MCC Exclusion see Appendix A PDX collection 0986
● ♀ MCC **O45.8X3 Other premature separation of placenta, third trimester**
MCC Exclusion see Appendix A PDX collection 0986
● ♀ **O45.8X9 Other premature separation of placenta, unspecified trimester**
\+ **O45.9 Premature separation of placenta, unspecified**
Abruptio placentae NOS
● ♀ **O45.90 Premature separation of placenta, unspecified, unspecified trimester**
● ♀ MCC **O45.91 Premature separation of placenta, unspecified, first trimester**
MCC Exclusion see Appendix A PDX collection 0986
● ♀ MCC **O45.92 Premature separation of placenta, unspecified, second trimester**
MCC Exclusion see Appendix A PDX collection 0986
● ♀ MCC **O45.93 Premature separation of placenta, unspecified, third trimester**
MCC Exclusion see Appendix A PDX collection 0986

O46 Antepartum hemorrhage, not elsewhere classified

Excludes1: *hemorrhage in early pregnancy (O20.-)*
intrapartum hemorrhage NEC (O67.-)
placenta previa (O44.-)
premature separation of placenta [abruptio placentae] (O45.-)

\+ **O46.0 Antepartum hemorrhage with coagulation defect**
\+ **O46.00 Antepartum hemorrhage with coagulation defect, unspecified**
● ♀ MCC **O46.001 Antepartum hemorrhage with coagulation defect, unspecified, first trimester**
MCC Exclusion see Appendix A PDX collection 0985
● ♀ MCC **O46.002 Antepartum hemorrhage with coagulation defect, unspecified, second trimester**
MCC Exclusion see Appendix A PDX collection 0985
● ♀ MCC **O46.003 Antepartum hemorrhage with coagulation defect, unspecified, third trimester**
MCC Exclusion see Appendix A PDX collection 0985
● ♀ **O46.009 Antepartum hemorrhage with coagulation defect, unspecified, unspecified trimester**
\+ **O46.01 Antepartum hemorrhage with afibrinogenemia**
Antepartum hemorrhage with hypofibrinogenemia
● ♀ MCC **O46.011 Antepartum hemorrhage with afibrinogenemia, first trimester**
MCC Exclusion see Appendix A PDX collection 0985
● ♀ MCC **O46.012 Antepartum hemorrhage with afibrinogenemia, second trimester**
MCC Exclusion see Appendix A PDX collection 0985

• ♀ MCC **O46.013 Antepartum hemorrhage with afibrinogenemia, third trimester**
MCC Exclusion see Appendix A PDX collection 0985

• ♀ **O46.019 Antepartum hemorrhage with afibrinogenemia, unspecified trimester**

\+ **O46.02 Antepartum hemorrhage with disseminated intravascular coagulation**

• ♀ MCC **O46.021 Antepartum hemorrhage with disseminated intravascular coagulation, first trimester**
MCC Exclusion see Appendix A PDX collection 0985

• ♀ MCC **O46.022 Antepartum hemorrhage with disseminated intravascular coagulation, second trimester**
MCC Exclusion see Appendix A PDX collection 0985

• ♀ MCC **O46.023 Antepartum hemorrhage with disseminated intravascular coagulation, third trimester**
MCC Exclusion see Appendix A PDX collection 0985

• ♀ **O46.029 Antepartum hemorrhage with disseminated intravascular coagulation, unspecified trimester**

\+ **O46.09 Antepartum hemorrhage with other coagulation defect**

• ♀ MCC **O46.091 Antepartum hemorrhage with other coagulation defect, first trimester**
MCC Exclusion see Appendix A PDX collection 0985

• ♀ MCC **O46.092 Antepartum hemorrhage with other coagulation defect, second trimester**
MCC Exclusion see Appendix A PDX collection 0985

• ♀ MCC **O46.093 Antepartum hemorrhage with other coagulation defect, third trimester**
MCC Exclusion see Appendix A PDX collection 0985

• ♀ **O46.099 Antepartum hemorrhage with other coagulation defect, unspecified trimester**

\+ **O46.8 Other antepartum hemorrhage**

\+ **O46.8X Other antepartum hemorrhage**

• ♀ **O46.8X1 Other antepartum hemorrhage, first trimester**

• ♀ **O46.8X2 Other antepartum hemorrhage, second trimester**

• ♀ **O46.8X3 Other antepartum hemorrhage, third trimester**

• ♀ **O46.8X9 Other antepartum hemorrhage, unspecified trimester**

\+ **O46.9 Antepartum hemorrhage, unspecified**

• ♀ **O46.90 Antepartum hemorrhage, unspecified, unspecified trimester**

• ♀ **O46.91 Antepartum hemorrhage, unspecified, first trimester**

• ♀ **O46.92 Antepartum hemorrhage, unspecified, second trimester**

• ♀ **O46.93 Antepartum hemorrhage, unspecified, third trimester**

O47 False labor

Includes: Braxton Hicks contractions
threatened labor

Excludes1: *preterm labor (O60.-)*

\+ **O47.0 False labor before 37 completed weeks of gestation**

• ♀ **O47.00 False labor before 37 completed weeks of gestation, unspecified trimester**

• ♀ CC **O47.02 False labor before 37 completed weeks of gestation, second trimester**
CC Exclusion see Appendix A PDX collection 0987

• ♀ CC **O47.03 False labor before 37 completed weeks of gestation, third trimester**
CC Exclusion see Appendix A PDX collection 0987

• ♀ CC **O47.1 False labor at or after 37 completed weeks of gestation**
CC Exclusion see Appendix A PDX collection 0987

• ♀ **O47.9 False labor, unspecified**

O48 Late pregnancy

• ♀ **O48.0 Post-term pregnancy**
Pregnancy over 40 completed weeks to 42 completed weeks gestation

• ♀ **O48.1 Prolonged pregnancy**
Pregnancy which has advanced beyond 42 completed weeks gestation

Complications of labor and delivery (O60-O77)

O60 Preterm labor

Includes: onset (spontaneous) of labor before 37 completed weeks of gestation

Excludes1: *false labor (O47.0-)*
threatened labor NOS (O47.0-)

\+ **O60.0 Preterm labor without delivery**

• ♀ **O60.00 Preterm labor without delivery, unspecified trimester**

• ♀ MCC **O60.02 Preterm labor without delivery, second trimester**
MCC Exclusion see Appendix A PDX collection 0987

• ♀ MCC **O60.03 Preterm labor without delivery, third trimester**
MCC Exclusion see Appendix A PDX collection 0987

\+ **O60.1 Preterm labor with preterm delivery**

One of the following 7th characters is to be assigned to each code under subcategory **O60.1.** 7th character 0 is for single gestations and multiple gestations where the fetus is unspecified. 7th characters 1 through 9 are for cases of multiple gestations to identify the fetus for which the code applies. The appropriate code from category O30, Multiple gestation, must also be assigned when assigning a code from subcategory O60.1 that has a 7th character of 1 through 9.

0 - not applicable or unspecified
1 - fetus 1
2 - fetus 2
3 - fetus 3
4 - fetus 4
5 - fetus 5
9 - other fetus

• ♀ CC X+7th **O60.10 Preterm labor with preterm delivery, unspecified trimester**
Preterm labor with delivery NOS
CC Exclusion for all 7th characters see Appendix A PDX collection 0987

• ♀ MCC X+7th **O60.12 Preterm labor second trimester with preterm delivery second trimester**
MCC Exclusion for all 7th characters see Appendix A PDX collection 0987

• ♀ MCC X+7th **O60.13 Preterm labor second trimester with preterm delivery third trimester**
MCC Exclusion for all 7th characters see Appendix A PDX collection 0987

• ♀ MCC X+7th **O60.14 Preterm labor third trimester with preterm delivery third trimester**
MCC Exclusion for all 7th characters see Appendix A PDX collection 0987
AHA CC: 2Q, 2016, 10-11

\+ **O60.2 Term delivery with preterm labor**

One of the following 7th characters is to be assigned to each code under subcategory **O60.2.** 7th character 0 is for single gestations and multiple gestations where the fetus is unspecified. 7th characters 1 through 9 are for cases of multiple gestations to identify the fetus for which the code applies. The appropriate code from category O30, Multiple gestation, must also be assigned when assigning a code from subcategory O60.2 that has a 7th character of 1 through 9.

0 - not applicable or unspecified
1 - fetus 1
2 - fetus 2
3 - fetus 3
4 - fetus 4
5 - fetus 5
9 - other fetus

• ♀ CC X+7th **O60.20 Term delivery with preterm labor, unspecified trimester**
CC Exclusion for all 7th characters see Appendix A PDX collection 0987

• ♀ MCC X+7th **O60.22 Term delivery with preterm labor, second trimester**
MCC Exclusion for all 7th characters see Appendix A PDX collection 0987

• ♀ MCC X+7th **O60.23 Term delivery with preterm labor, third trimester**
MCC Exclusion for all 7th characters see Appendix A PDX collection 0987

O61 Failed induction of labor

• ♀ **O61.0 Failed medical induction of labor**
Failed induction (of labor) by oxytocin
Failed induction (of labor) by prostaglandins

• ♀ **O61.1 Failed instrumental induction of labor**
Failed mechanical induction (of labor)
Failed surgical induction (of labor)

• ♀ **O61.8 Other failed induction of labor**

• ♀ **O61.9 Failed induction of labor, unspecified**

O62 Abnormalities of forces of labor

• ♀ **O62.0 Primary inadequate contractions**
Failure of cervical dilatation
Primary hypotonic uterine dysfunction
Uterine inertia during latent phase of labor

• ♀ **O62.1 Secondary uterine inertia**
Arrested active phase of labor
Secondary hypotonic uterine dysfunction

• ♀ **O62.2 Other uterine inertia**
Atony of uterus without hemorrhage
Atony of uterus NOS
Desultory labor
Hypotonic uterine dysfunction NOS
Irregular labor
Poor contractions
Slow slope active phase of labor
Uterine inertia NOS
Excludes1: *atony of uterus with hemorrhage (postpartum) (O72.1)*
postpartum atony of uterus without hemorrhage (O75.89)

• ♀ **O62.3 Precipitate labor**

• ♀ **O62.4 Hypertonic, incoordinate, and prolonged uterine contractions**
Cervical spasm
Contraction ring dystocia
Dyscoordinate labor
Hour-glass contraction of uterus
Hypertonic uterine dysfunction
Incoordinate uterine action
Tetanic contractions
Uterine dystocia NOS
Uterine spasm
Excludes1: *dystocia (fetal) (maternal) NOS (O66.9)*

• ♀ **O62.8 Other abnormalities of forces of labor**

• ♀ **O62.9 Abnormality of forces of labor, unspecified**

O63 Long labor

• ♀ **O63.0 Prolonged first stage (of labor)**

• ♀ **O63.1 Prolonged second stage (of labor)**

• ♀ **O63.2 Delayed delivery of second twin, triplet, etc.**

• ♀ CC **O63.9 Long labor, unspecified**
Prolonged labor NOS
CC Exclusion see Appendix A PDX collection 0988

O64 Obstructed labor due to malposition and malpresentation of fetus

One of the following 7th characters is to be assigned to each code under category O64. 7th character 0 is for single gestations and multiple gestations where the fetus is unspecified. 7th characters 1 through 9 are for cases of multiple gestations to identify the fetus for which the code applies. The appropriate code from category O30, Multiple gestation, must also be assigned when assigning a code from category O64 that has a 7th character of 1 through 9.
0 - not applicable or unspecified
1 - fetus 1
2 - fetus 2
3 - fetus 3
4 - fetus 4
5 - fetus 5
9 - other fetus

♀ X+7th **O64.0 Obstructed labor due to incomplete rotation of fetal head**
Deep transverse arrest
Obstructed labor due to persistent occipitoiliac (position)
Obstructed labor due to persistent occipitoposterior (position)
Obstructed labor due to persistent occipitosacral (position)
Obstructed labor due to persistent occipitotransverse (position)

• ♀ X+7th **O64.1 Obstructed labor due to breech presentation**
Obstructed labor due to buttocks presentation
Obstructed labor due to complete breech presentation
Obstructed labor due to frank breech presentation

• ♀ X+7th **O64.2 Obstructed labor due to face presentation**
Obstructed labor due to chin presentation

• ♀ X+7th **O64.3 Obstructed labor due to brow presentation**

• ♀ X+7th **O64.4 Obstructed labor due to shoulder presentation**
Prolapsed arm
Excludes1: *impacted shoulders (O66.0)*
shoulder dystocia (O66.0)

• ♀ X+7th **O64.5 Obstructed labor due to compound presentation**

• ♀ X+7th **O64.8 Obstructed labor due to other malposition and malpresentation**
Obstructed labor due to footling presentation
Obstructed labor due to incomplete breech presentation

• ♀ X+7th **O64.9 Obstructed labor due to malposition and malpresentation, unspecified**

O65 Obstructed labor due to maternal pelvic abnormality

• ♀ **O65.0 Obstructed labor due to deformed pelvis**

• ♀ **O65.1 Obstructed labor due to generally contracted pelvis**

• ♀ **O65.2 Obstructed labor due to pelvic inlet contraction**

• ♀ **O65.3 Obstructed labor due to pelvic outlet and mid-cavity contraction**

• ♀ **O65.4 Obstructed labor due to fetopelvic disproportion, unspecified**
Excludes1: *dystocia due to abnormality of fetus (O66.2-O66.3)*

• ♀ **O65.5 Obstructed labor due to abnormality of maternal pelvic organs**
Obstructed labor due to conditions listed in O34.-
Use additional code to identify abnormality of pelvic organs O34.-

• ♀ **O65.8 Obstructed labor due to other maternal pelvic abnormalities**

• ♀ **O65.9 Obstructed labor due to maternal pelvic abnormality, unspecified**

O66 Other obstructed labor

• ♀ **O66.0 Obstructed labor due to shoulder dystocia**
Impacted shoulders

• ♀ **O66.1 Obstructed labor due to locked twins**

• ♀ **O66.2 Obstructed labor due to unusually large fetus**

• ♀ **O66.3 Obstructed labor due to other abnormalities of fetus**
Dystocia due to fetal ascites
Dystocia due to fetal hydrops
Dystocia due to fetal meningomyelocele
Dystocia due to fetal sacral teratoma
Dystocia due to fetal tumor
Dystocia due to hydrocephalic fetus
Use additional code to identify cause of obstruction

\+ **O66.4 Failed trial of labor**

• ♀ **O66.40 Failed trial of labor, unspecified**

• ♀ **O66.41 Failed attempted vaginal birth after previous cesarean delivery**
Code first rupture of uterus, if applicable (O71.0-, O71.1)

• ♀ **O66.5 Attempted application of vacuum extractor and forceps**
Attempted application of vacuum or forceps, with subsequent delivery by forceps or cesarean delivery

• ♀ **O66.6 Obstructed labor due to other multiple fetuses**

• ♀ **O66.8 Other specified obstructed labor**
Use additional code to identify cause of obstruction

• ♀ **O66.9 Obstructed labor, unspecified**
Dystocia NOS
Fetal dystocia NOS
Maternal dystocia NOS

O67 Labor and delivery complicated by intrapartum hemorrhage, not elsewhere classified

Excludes1: *antepartum hemorrhage NEC (O46.-)*
placenta previa (O44.-)
premature separation of placenta [abruptio placentae] (O45.-)
Excludes2: *postpartum hemorrhage (O72.-)*

• ♀ MCC **O67.0 Intrapartum hemorrhage with coagulation defect**
Intrapartum hemorrhage (excessive) associated with afibrinogenemia
Intrapartum hemorrhage (excessive) associated with disseminated intravascular coagulation
Intrapartum hemorrhage (excessive) associated with hyperfibrinolysis
Intrapartum hemorrhage (excessive) associated with hypofibrinogenemia
MCC Exclusion see Appendix A PDX collection 0985

• ♀ **O67.8 Other intrapartum hemorrhage**
Excessive intrapartum hemorrhage

• ♀ **O67.9 Intrapartum hemorrhage, unspecified**

• ♀ CC **O68 Labor and delivery complicated by abnormality of fetal acid-base balance**
Fetal acidemia complicating labor and delivery
Fetal acidosis complicating labor and delivery
Fetal alkalosis complicating labor and delivery
Fetal metabolic acidemia complicating labor and delivery
Excludes1: *fetal stress NOS (O77.9)*
labor and delivery complicated by electrocardiographic evidence of fetal stress (O77.8)
labor and delivery complicated by ultrasonic evidence of fetal stress (O77.8)
Excludes2: *abnormality in fetal heart rate or rhythm (O76)*
labor and delivery complicated by meconium in amniotic fluid (O77.0)
CC Exclusion see Appendix A PDX collection 0989
Valid 3-character code, no further characters required

O69 Labor and delivery complicated by umbilical cord complications

One of the following 7th characters is to be assigned to each code under category O69. 7th character 0 is for single gestations and multiple gestations where the fetus is unspecified. 7th characters 1 through 9 are for cases of multiple gestations to identify the fetus for which the code applies. The appropriate code from category O30, Multiple gestation, must also be assigned when assigning a code from category O69 that has a 7th character of 1 through 9.
0 - not applicable or unspecified
1 - fetus 1
2 - fetus 2
3 - fetus 3
4 - fetus 4
5 - fetus 5
9 - other fetus

• ♀ X+7th **O69.0 Labor and delivery complicated by prolapse of cord**

• ♀ X+7th **O69.1 Labor and delivery complicated by cord around neck, with compression**
Excludes1: *labor and delivery complicated by cord around neck, without compression (O69.81)*

• ♀ X+7th **O69.2 Labor and delivery complicated by other cord entanglement, with compression**
Labor and delivery complicated by compression of cord NOS
Labor and delivery complicated by entanglement of cords of twins in monoamniotic sac
Labor and delivery complicated by knot in cord
Excludes1: *labor and delivery complicated by other cord entanglement, without compression (O69.82)*

• ♀ X+7th **O69.3 Labor and delivery complicated by short cord**

• ♀ X+7th **O69.4 Labor and delivery complicated by vasa previa**
Labor and delivery complicated by hemorrhage from vasa previa

• ♀ X+7th **O69.5 Labor and delivery complicated by vascular lesion of cord**
Labor and delivery complicated by cord bruising
Labor and delivery complicated by cord hematoma
Labor and delivery complicated by thrombosis of umbilical vessels

X+7th **O69.8 Labor and delivery complicated by other cord complications**

• ♀ X+7th **O69.81 Labor and delivery complicated by cord around neck, without compression**

• ♀ X+7th **O69.82 Labor and delivery complicated by other cord entanglement, without compression**

• ♀ X+7th **O69.89 Labor and delivery complicated by other cord complications**

• ♀ X+7th **O69.9 Labor and delivery complicated by cord complication, unspecified**

O70 Perineal laceration during delivery

Includes: episiotomy extended by laceration
Excludes1: *obstetric high vaginal laceration alone (O71.4)*

• ♀ **O70.0 First degree perineal laceration during delivery**
Perineal laceration, rupture or tear involving fourchette during delivery
Perineal laceration, rupture or tear involving labia during delivery
Perineal laceration, rupture or tear involving skin during delivery
Perineal laceration, rupture or tear involving vagina during delivery
Perineal laceration, rupture or tear involving vulva during delivery
Slight perineal laceration, rupture or tear during delivery

• ♀ **O70.1 Second degree perineal laceration during delivery**
Perineal laceration, rupture or tear during delivery as in O70.0, also involving pelvic floor
Perineal laceration, rupture or tear during delivery as in O70.0 also involving perineal muscles
Perineal laceration, rupture or tear during delivery as in O70.0 also involving vaginal muscles
Excludes1: *perineal laceration involving anal sphincter (O70.2)*
AHA CC: 2Q, 2016, 34

\+ **O70.2 Third degree perineal laceration during delivery**
Perineal laceration, rupture or tear during delivery as in O70.1 also involving anal sphincter
Perineal laceration, rupture or tear during delivery as in O70.1 also involving rectovaginal septum
Perineal laceration, rupture or tear during delivery as in O70.1 also involving sphincter NOS
Excludes1: *anal sphincter tear during delivery without third degree perineal laceration (O70.4)*
perineal laceration involving anal or rectal muco (O70.3)
AHA CC: 4Q, 2016, 53-54

• ♀ CC **O70.20 Third degree perineal laceration during delivery, unspecified**
CC Exclusion see Appendix A PDX collection 0990

• ♀ CC **O70.21 Third degree perineal laceration during delivery, II**
Third degree perineal laceration during delivery with less than 50% of external anal sphincter (EAS) thickness torn
CC Exclusion see Appendix A PDX collection 0990

• ♀ CC **O70.22 Third degree perineal laceration during delivery, II**
Third degree perineal laceration during delivery with more than 50% of external anal sphincter (EAS) thickness torn
CC Exclusion see Appendix A PDX collection 0990

• ♀ CC **O70.23 Third degree perineal laceration during delivery, IIIc**
Third degree perineal laceration during delivery with both external anal sphincter (EAS) and internal an sphincter (IAS) torn
CC Exclusion see Appendix A PDX collection 0990

• ♀ CC **O70.3 Fourth degree perineal laceration during delivery**
Perineal laceration, rupture or tear during delivery as in O70.2 also involving anal mucosa
Perineal laceration, rupture or tear during delivery as in O70.2 also involving rectal mucosa
CC Exclusion see Appendix A PDX collection 0991

• ♀ CC **O70.4 Anal sphincter tear complicating delivery, not associated wit third degree laceration**
Excludes1: *anal sphincter tear with third degree perineal laceration (O70.2)*
CC Exclusion see Appendix A PDX collection 0992

• ♀ **O70.9 Perineal laceration during delivery, unspecified**

O71 Other obstetric trauma

Includes: obstetric damage from instruments

\+ **O71.0 Rupture of uterus (spontaneous) before onset of labor**
Excludes1: *disruption of (current) cesarean delivery wound (O90.0)*
laceration of uterus, NEC (O71.81)

• ♀ **O71.00 Rupture of uterus before onset of labor, unspecified trimester**

• ♀ MCC **O71.02 Rupture of uterus before onset of labor, second trimes**
MCC Exclusion see Appendix A PDX collection 0993

• ♀ MCC **O71.03 Rupture of uterus before onset of labor, third trimester**
MCC Exclusion see Appendix A PDX collection 0993

• ♀ MCC **O71.1 Rupture of uterus during labor**
Rupture of uterus not stated as occurring before onset of labor
Excludes1: *disruption of cesarean delivery wound (O90.0)*
laceration of uterus, NEC (O71.81)
MCC Exclusion see Appendix A PDX collection 0993

• ♀ CC **O71.2 Postpartum inversion of uterus**
CC Exclusion see Appendix A PDX collection 0994

• ♀ CC **O71.3 Obstetric laceration of cervix**
Annular detachment of cervix
CC Exclusion see Appendix A PDX collection 0995

• ♀ CC **O71.4 Obstetric high vaginal laceration alone**
Laceration of vaginal wall without perineal laceration
Excludes1: *obstetric high vaginal laceration with perineal laceration (O70.-)*
CC Exclusion see Appendix A PDX collection 0996

• ♀ CC **O71.5 Other obstetric injury to pelvic organs**
Obstetric injury to bladder
Obstetric injury to urethra
Excludes2: *obstetric periurethral trauma (O71.82)*
CC Exclusion see Appendix A PDX collection 0993

• ♀ CC **O71.6 Obstetric damage to pelvic joints and ligaments**
Obstetric avulsion of inner symphyseal cartilage
Obstetric damage to coccyx
CC Exclusion see Appendix A PDX collection 0997
Obstetric traumatic separation of symphysis (pubis)

• ♀ CC **O71.7 Obstetric hematoma of pelvis**
Obstetric hematoma of perineum
Obstetric hematoma of vagina
Obstetric hematoma of vulva
CC Exclusion see Appendix A PDX collection 0998

\+ **O71.8 Other specified obstetric trauma**

• ♀ **O71.81 Laceration of uterus, not elsewhere classified**

• ♀ **O71.82 Other specified trauma to perineum and vulva**
Obstetric periurethral trauma
AHA CC: 4Q, 2014, 18-19

• ♀ **O71.89 Other specified obstetric trauma**

• ♀ **O71.9 Obstetric trauma, unspecified**

O72 Postpartum hemorrhage

Includes: hemorrhage after delivery of fetus or infant

• ♀ CC **O72.0 Third-stage hemorrhage**
Hemorrhage associated with retained, trapped or adherent placenta
Retained placenta NOS
Code also type of adherent placenta (O43.2-)
CC Exclusion see Appendix A PDX collection 0999

• ♀ CC **O72.1 Other immediate postpartum hemorrhage**
Hemorrhage following delivery of placenta
Postpartum hemorrhage (atonic) NOS
Uterine atony with hemorrhage
Excludes1: *uterine atony NOS (O62.2)*
uterine atony without hemorrhage (O62.2)
postpartum atony of uterus without hemorrhage (O75.89)
CC Exclusion see Appendix A PDX collection 1000

• ♀ CC **O72.2 Delayed and secondary postpartum hemorrhage**
Hemorrhage associated with retained portions of placenta or membranes after the first 24 hours following delivery of placenta
Retained products of conception NOS, following delivery
CC Exclusion see Appendix A PDX collection 1001

• ♀ **O72.3 Postpartum coagulation defects**
Postpartum afibrinogenemia
Postpartum fibrinolysis

O73 Retained placenta and membranes, without hemorrhage

Excludes1: *placenta accreta (O43.21-)*
placenta increta (O43.22-)
placenta percreta (O43.23-)

• ♀ **O73.0 Retained placenta without hemorrhage**
Adherent placenta, without hemorrhage
Trapped placenta without hemorrhage

• ♀ **O73.1 Retained portions of placenta and membranes, without hemorrhage**
Retained products of conception following delivery, without hemorrhage

O74 Complications of anesthesia during labor and delivery

Includes: maternal complications arising from the administration of a general, regional or local anesthetic, analgesic or other sedation during labor and delivery
Use additional code, if applicable, to identify specific complication

• ♀ **O74.0 Aspiration pneumonitis due to anesthesia during labor and delivery**
Inhalation of stomach contents or secretions NOS due to anesthesia during labor and delivery
Mendelson's syndrome due to anesthesia during labor and delivery

• ♀ **O74.1 Other pulmonary complications of anesthesia during labor and delivery**

• ♀ **O74.2 Cardiac complications of anesthesia during labor and delivery**

• ♀ **O74.3 Central nervous system complications of anesthesia during labor and delivery**

• ♀ **O74.4 Toxic reaction to local anesthesia during labor and delivery**

• ♀ **O74.5 Spinal and epidural anesthesia-induced headache during labor and delivery**

• ♀ **O74.6 Other complications of spinal and epidural anesthesia during labor and delivery**

• ♀ **O74.7 Failed or difficult intubation for anesthesia during labor and delivery**

• ♀ **O74.8 Other complications of anesthesia during labor and delivery**

• ♀ **O74.9 Complication of anesthesia during labor and delivery, unspecified**

O75 Other complications of labor and delivery, not elsewhere classified

Excludes2: *puerperal (postpartum) infection (O86.-)*
puerperal (postpartum) sepsis (O85)

• ♀ **O75.0 Maternal distress during labor and delivery**

• ♀ MCC **O75.1 Shock during or following labor and delivery**
Obstetric shock following labor and delivery
MCC Exclusion see Appendix A PDX collection 1002

• ♀ CC **O75.2 Pyrexia during labor, not elsewhere classified**
CC Exclusion see Appendix A PDX collection 1003

• ♀ MCC **O75.3 Other infection during labor**
Sepsis during labor
Use additional code (B95-B97), to identify infectious agent
MCC Exclusion see Appendix A PDX collection 1004
Review coding guideline C.15.j

• ♀ **O75.4 Other complications of obstetric surgery and procedures**
Cardiac arrest following obstetric surgery or procedures
Cardiac failure following obstetric surgery or procedures
Cerebral anoxia following obstetric surgery or procedures
Pulmonary edema following obstetric surgery or procedures
Use additional code to identify specific complication
Excludes2: *complications of anesthesia during labor and delivery (O74.-)*
disruption of obstetrical (surgical) wound (O90.0-O90.1)
hematoma of obstetrical (surgical) wound (O90.2)
infection of obstetrical (surgical) wound (O86.0)

• ♀ **O75.5 Delayed delivery after artificial rupture of membranes**

\+ **O75.8 Other specified complications of labor and delivery**

• ♀ **O75.81 Maternal exhaustion complicating labor and delivery**

• ♀ **O75.82 Onset (spontaneous) of labor after 37 completed weeks of gestation but before 39 completed weeks gestation, with delivery by (planned) cesarean section**
Delivery by (planned) cesarean section occurring after 37 completed weeks of gestation but before 39 completed weeks gestation due to (spontaneous) onset of labor
Code first to specify reason for planned cesarean section such as:
cephalopelvic disproportion (normally formed fetus) (O33.9)
previous cesarean delivery (O34.21)

• ♀ **O75.89 Other specified complications of labor and delivery**

• ♀ **O75.9 Complication of labor and delivery, unspecified**

• ♀ **O76 Abnormality in fetal heart rate and rhythm complicating labor and delivery**

Depressed fetal heart rate tones complicating labor and delivery
Fetal bradycardia complicating labor and delivery
Fetal heart rate decelerations complicating labor and delivery
Fetal heart rate irregularity complicating labor and delivery
Fetal heart rate abnormal variability complicating labor and delivery
Fetal tachycardia complicating labor and delivery
Non-reassuring fetal heart rate or rhythm complicating labor and delivery
Excludes1: *fetal stress NOS (O77.9)*
labor and delivery complicated by electrocardiographic evidence of fetal stress (O77.8)
labor and delivery complicated by ultrasonic evidence of fetal stress (O77.8)
Excludes2: *fetal metabolic acidemia (O68)*
other fetal stress (O77.0-O77.1)
AHA CC: 4Q, 2013, 118
Valid 3-character code, no further characters required

O77 Other fetal stress complicating labor and delivery

• ♀ **O77.0 Labor and delivery complicated by meconium in amniotic fluid**
AHA CC: 4Q, 2013, 118

- ♀ **O77.1 Fetal stress in labor or delivery due to drug administration**
- ♀ **O77.8 Labor and delivery complicated by other evidence of fetal stress**
  Labor and delivery complicated by electrocardiographic evidence of fetal stress
  Labor and delivery complicated by ultrasonic evidence of fetal stress
  Excludes1: *abnormality of fetal acid-base balance (O68)*
  abnormality in fetal heart rate or rhythm (O76)
  fetal metabolic acidemia (O68)
- ♀ **O77.9 Labor and delivery complicated by fetal stress, unspecified**
  Excludes1: *abnormality of fetal acid-base balance (O68)*
  abnormality in fetal heart rate or rhythm (O76)
  fetal metabolic acidemia (O68)

Encounter for delivery (O80-O82)

- ♀ **O80 Encounter for full-term uncomplicated delivery**
  Delivery requiring minimal or no assistance, with or without episiotomy, without fetal manipulation [e.g., rotation version] or instrumentation [forceps] of a spontaneous, cephalic, vaginal, full-term, single, live-born infant. This code is for use as a single diagnosis code and is not to be used with any other code from chapter 15.
  Use additional code to indicate outcome of delivery (Z37.0)
  AHA CC: 2Q, 2014, 9; 4Q, 2016, 150
  Review coding guideline C.15.n
  Valid 3-character code, no further characters required
- ♀ **O82 Encounter for cesarean delivery without indication**
  Use additional code to indicate outcome of delivery (Z37.0)
  Valid 3-character code, no further characters required

Complications predominantly related to the puerperium (O85-O92)

Excludes2: *mental and behavioral disorders associated with the puerperium (F53)*
obstetrical tetanus (A34)
puerperal osteomalacia (M83.0)

O85 Puerperal sepsis
MCC ♀
Postpartum sepsis
Puerperal peritonitis
Puerperal pyemia
Use additional code (B95-B97), to identify infectious agent
Use additional code (R65.2-) to identify severe sepsis, if applicable
Excludes1: *fever of unknown origin following delivery (O86.4)*
genital tract infection following delivery (O86.1-)
obstetric pyemic and septic embolism (O88.3-)
puerperal septic thrombophlebitis (O86.81)
urinary tract infection following delivery (O86.2-)
Excludes2: *sepsis during labor (O75.3)*
Review coding guideline C.15.k
MCC Exclusion see Appendix A PDX collection 1005
Valid 3-character code, no further characters required

O86 Other puerperal infections
Use additional code (B95-B97), to identify infectious agent
Excludes2: *infection during labor (O75.3)*
obstetrical tetanus (A34)

- ♀ **O86.0 Infection of obstetric surgical wound**
  Infected cesarean delivery wound following delivery
  Infected perineal repair following delivery
  Review coding guideline C.1.d.5
- \+ **O86.1 Other infection of genital tract following delivery**
  - ♀ CC **O86.11 Cervicitis following delivery**
    CC Exclusion see Appendix A PDX collection 0968
  - ♀ CC **O86.12 Endometritis following delivery**
    CC Exclusion see Appendix A PDX collection 1005
  - ♀ CC **O86.13 Vaginitis following delivery**
    CC Exclusion see Appendix A PDX collection 0968
  - ♀ CC **O86.19 Other infection of genital tract following delivery**
    CC Exclusion see Appendix A PDX collection 0968
- \+ **O86.2 Urinary tract infection following delivery**
  - ♀ CC **O86.20 Urinary tract infection following delivery, unspecified**
    Puerperal urinary tract infection NOS
    CC Exclusion see Appendix A PDX collection 0968
  - ♀ CC **O86.21 Infection of kidney following delivery**
    CC Exclusion see Appendix A PDX collection 0968
  - ♀ CC **O86.22 Infection of bladder following delivery**
    Infection of urethra following delivery
    CC Exclusion see Appendix A PDX collection 0968
  - ♀ CC **O86.29 Other urinary tract infection following delivery**
    CC Exclusion see Appendix A PDX collection 0968
- ♀ CC **O86.4 Pyrexia of unknown origin following delivery**
  Puerperal infection NOS following delivery
  Puerperal pyrexia NOS following delivery
  Excludes2: *pyrexia during labor (O75.2)*
  CC Exclusion see Appendix A PDX collection 1006
- \+ **O86.8 Other specified puerperal infections**
  - ♀ MCC **O86.81 Puerperal septic thrombophlebitis**
    MCC Exclusion see Appendix A PDX collection 1005
  - ♀ MCC **O86.89 Other specified puerperal infections**
    MCC Exclusion see Appendix A PDX collection 1005

O87 Venous complications and hemorrhoids in the puerperium
Includes: venous complications in labor, delivery and the puerperium
Excludes2: *obstetric embolism (O88.-)*
puerperal septic thrombophlebitis (O86.81)
venous complications in pregnancy (O22.-)

- ♀ CC **O87.0 Superficial thrombophlebitis in the puerperium**
  Puerperal phlebitis NOS
  Puerperal thrombosis NOS
  CC Exclusion see Appendix A PDX collection 0967
- ♀ MCC **O87.1 Deep phlebothrombosis in the puerperium**
  Deep vein thrombosis, postpartum
  Pelvic thrombophlebitis, postpartum
  Use additional code to identify the deep vein thrombosis (I82.4-, I82.5-, I82.62-, I82.72-)
  Use additional code, if applicable, for associated long-term (current) use of anticoagulants (Z79.01)
  MCC Exclusion see Appendix A PDX collection 0967
- ♀ CC **O87.2 Hemorrhoids in the puerperium**
  CC Exclusion see Appendix A PDX collection 0967
- ♀ CC **O87.3 Cerebral venous thrombosis in the puerperium**
  Cerebrovenous sinus thrombosis in the puerperium
  CC Exclusion see Appendix A PDX collection 0967
- ♀ **O87.4 Varicose veins of lower extremity in the puerperium**
- ♀ CC **O87.8 Other venous complications in the puerperium**
  Genital varices in the puerperium
  CC Exclusion see Appendix A PDX collection 0967
- ♀ **O87.9 Venous complication in the puerperium, unspecified**
  Puerperal phlebopathy NOS

O88 Obstetric embolism
Excludes1: *embolism complicating abortion NOS (O03.2)*
embolism complicating ectopic or molar pregnancy (O08.2)
embolism complicating failed attempted abortion (O07.2)
embolism complicating induced abortion (O04.7)
embolism complicating spontaneous abortion (O03.2, O03.7)

- \+ **O88.0 Obstetric air embolism**
  - \+ **O88.01 Obstetric air embolism in pregnancy**
    - ♀ MCC **O88.011 Air embolism in pregnancy, first trimester**
      MCC Exclusion see Appendix A PDX collection 1007
    - ♀ MCC **O88.012 Air embolism in pregnancy, second trimester**
      MCC Exclusion see Appendix A PDX collection 1007
    - ♀ MCC **O88.013 Air embolism in pregnancy, third trimester**
      MCC Exclusion see Appendix A PDX collection 1007
    - ♀ **O88.019 Air embolism in pregnancy, unspecified trimester**
  - ♀ MCC **O88.02 Air embolism in childbirth**
    MCC Exclusion see Appendix A PDX collection 1007
  - ♀ MCC **O88.03 Air embolism in the puerperium**
    MCC Exclusion see Appendix A PDX collection 1007
- \+ **O88.1 Amniotic fluid embolism**
  Anaphylactoid syndrome in pregnancy
  - \+ **O88.11 Amniotic fluid embolism in pregnancy**
    - ♀ MCC **O88.111 Amniotic fluid embolism in pregnancy, first trimester**
      MCC Exclusion see Appendix A PDX collection 1007

• ♀ MCC **O88.112 Amniotic fluid embolism in pregnancy, second trimester**
MCC Exclusion see Appendix A PDX collection 1007
• ♀ MCC **O88.113 Amniotic fluid embolism in pregnancy, third trimester**
MCC Exclusion see Appendix A PDX collection 1007
• ♀ **O88.119 Amniotic fluid embolism in pregnancy, unspecified trimester**
• ♀ MCC **O88.12 Amniotic fluid embolism in childbirth**
MCC Exclusion see Appendix A PDX collection 1007
• ♀ MCC **O88.13 Amniotic fluid embolism in the puerperium**
MCC Exclusion see Appendix A PDX collection 1007
+ **O88.2 Obstetric thromboembolism**
+ **O88.21 Thromboembolism in pregnancy**
Obstetric (pulmonary) embolism NOS
• ♀ MCC **O88.211 Thromboembolism in pregnancy, first trimester**
MCC Exclusion see Appendix A PDX collection 1007
• ♀ MCC **O88.212 Thromboembolism in pregnancy, second trimester**
MCC Exclusion see Appendix A PDX collection 1007
• ♀ MCC **O88.213 Thromboembolism in pregnancy, third trimester**
MCC Exclusion see Appendix A PDX collection 1007
• ♀ **O88.219 Thromboembolism in pregnancy, unspecified trimester**
• ♀ MCC **O88.22 Thromboembolism in childbirth**
MCC Exclusion see Appendix A PDX collection 1007
• ♀ MCC **O88.23 Thromboembolism in the puerperium**
Puerperal (pulmonary) embolism NOS
MCC Exclusion see Appendix A PDX collection 1007
+ **O88.3 Obstetric pyemic and septic embolism**
+ **O88.31 Pyemic and septic embolism in pregnancy**
• ♀ MCC **O88.311 Pyemic and septic embolism in pregnancy, first trimester**
MCC Exclusion see Appendix A PDX collection 1007
• ♀ MCC **O88.312 Pyemic and septic embolism in pregnancy, second trimester**
MCC Exclusion see Appendix A PDX collection 1007
• ♀ MCC **O88.313 Pyemic and septic embolism in pregnancy, third trimester**
MCC Exclusion see Appendix A PDX collection 1007
• ♀ **O88.319 Pyemic and septic embolism in pregnancy, unspecified trimester**
• ♀ MCC **O88.32 Pyemic and septic embolism in childbirth**
MCC Exclusion see Appendix A PDX collection 1007
• ♀ MCC **O88.33 Pyemic and septic embolism in the puerperium**
MCC Exclusion see Appendix A PDX collection 1007
+ **O88.8 Other obstetric embolism**
Obstetric fat embolism
+ **O88.81 Other embolism in pregnancy**
• ♀ MCC **O88.811 Other embolism in pregnancy, first trimester**
MCC Exclusion see Appendix A PDX collection 1007
• ♀ MCC **O88.812 Other embolism in pregnancy, second trimester**
MCC Exclusion see Appendix A PDX collection 1007
• ♀ MCC **O88.813 Other embolism in pregnancy, third trimester**
MCC Exclusion see Appendix A PDX collection 1007
• ♀ CC **O88.819 Other embolism in pregnancy, unspecified trimester**
CC Exclusion see Appendix A PDX collection 1007
• ♀ MCC **O88.82 Other embolism in childbirth**
MCC Exclusion see Appendix A PDX collection 1007
• ♀ MCC **O88.83 Other embolism in the puerperium**
MCC Exclusion see Appendix A PDX collection 1007

O89 Complications of anesthesia during the puerperium

Includes: maternal complications arising from the administration of a general, regional or local anesthetic, analgesic or other sedation during the puerperium
Use additional code, if applicable, to identify specific complication
+ **O89.0 Pulmonary complications of anesthesia during the puerperium**
• ♀ **O89.01 Aspiration pneumonitis due to anesthesia during the puerperium**
Inhalation of stomach contents or secretions NOS due to anesthesia during the puerperium
Mendelson's syndrome due to anesthesia during the puerperium
• ♀ **O89.09 Other pulmonary complications of anesthesia during the puerperium**
• ♀ **O89.1 Cardiac complications of anesthesia during the puerperium**
• ♀ **O89.2 Central nervous system complications of anesthesia during the puerperium**
• ♀ **O89.3 Toxic reaction to local anesthesia during the puerperium**
• ♀ **O89.4 Spinal and epidural anesthesia-induced headache during the puerperium**
• ♀ **O89.5 Other complications of spinal and epidural anesthesia during the puerperium**
• ♀ **O89.6 Failed or difficult intubation for anesthesia during the puerperium**
• ♀ **O89.8 Other complications of anesthesia during the puerperium**
• ♀ **O89.9 Complication of anesthesia during the puerperium, unspecified**

O90 Complications of the puerperium, not elsewhere classified

• ♀ **O90.0 Disruption of cesarean delivery wound**
Dehiscence of cesarean delivery wound
Excludes1: *rupture of uterus (spontaneous) before onset of labor (O71.0-)*
rupture of uterus during labor (O71.1)
• ♀ **O90.1 Disruption of perineal obstetric wound**
Disruption of wound of episiotomy
Disruption of wound of perineal laceration
Secondary perineal tear
• ♀ **O90.2 Hematoma of obstetric wound**
• ♀ MCC **O90.3 Peripartum cardiomyopathy**
Conditions in I42.- arising during pregnancy and the puerperium
Excludes1: *pre-existing heart disease complicating pregnancy and the puerperium (O99.4-)*
MCC Exclusion see Appendix A PDX collection 1008
Review coding guideline C.15.o.5
• ♀ MCC **O90.4 Postpartum acute kidney failure**
Hepatorenal syndrome following labor and delivery
MCC Exclusion see Appendix A PDX collection 1009
• ♀ **O90.5 Postpartum thyroiditis**
• ♀ **O90.6 Postpartum mood disturbance**
Postpartum blues
Postpartum dysphoria
Postpartum sadness
Excludes1: *postpartum depression (F53)*
puerperal psychosis (F53)
+ **O90.8 Other complications of the puerperium, not elsewhere classified**
• ♀ **O90.81 Anemia of the puerperium**
Postpartum anemia NOS
Excludes1: *pre-existing anemia complicating the puerperium (O99.03)*
• ♀ **O90.89 Other complications of the puerperium, not elsewhere classified**
Placental polyp
• ♀ **O90.9 Complication of the puerperium, unspecified**

O91 Infections of breast associated with pregnancy, the puerperium and lactation

Use additional code to identify infection
+ **O91.0 Infection of nipple associated with pregnancy, the puerperium and lactation**
+ **O91.01 Infection of nipple associated with pregnancy**
Gestational abscess of nipple
• ♀ **O91.011 Infection of nipple associated with pregnancy, first trimester**
• ♀ **O91.012 Infection of nipple associated with pregnancy, second trimester**
• ♀ **O91.013 Infection of nipple associated with pregnancy, third trimester**
• ♀ **O91.019 Infection of nipple associated with pregnancy, unspecified trimester**
• ♀ **O91.02 Infection of nipple associated with the puerperium**
Puerperal abscess of nipple

• ♀ **O91.03 Infection of nipple associated with lactation**
Abscess of nipple associated with lactation

\+ **O91.1 Abscess of breast associated with pregnancy, the puerperium and lactation**

\+ **O91.11 Abscess of breast associated with pregnancy**
Gestational mammary abscess
Gestational purulent mastitis
Gestational subareolar abscess

• ♀ **O91.111 Abscess of breast associated with pregnancy, first trimester**

• ♀ **O91.112 Abscess of breast associated with pregnancy, second trimester**

• ♀ **O91.113 Abscess of breast associated with pregnancy, third trimester**

• ♀ **O91.119 Abscess of breast associated with pregnancy, unspecified trimester**

• ♀ **O91.12 Abscess of breast associated with the puerperium**
Puerperal mammary abscess
Puerperal purulent mastitis
Puerperal subareolar abscess

• ♀ **O91.13 Abscess of breast associated with lactation**
Mammary abscess associated with lactation
Purulent mastitis associated with lactation
Subareolar abscess associated with lactation

\+ **O91.2 Nonpurulent mastitis associated with pregnancy, the puerperium and lactation**

\+ **O91.21 Nonpurulent mastitis associated with pregnancy**
Gestational interstitial mastitis
Gestational lymphangitis of breast
Gestational mastitis NOS
Gestational parenchymatous mastitis

• ♀ **O91.211 Nonpurulent mastitis associated with pregnancy, first trimester**

• ♀ **O91.212 Nonpurulent mastitis associated with pregnancy, second trimester**

• ♀ **O91.213 Nonpurulent mastitis associated with pregnancy, third trimester**

• ♀ **O91.219 Nonpurulent mastitis associated with pregnancy, unspecified trimester**

• ♀ **O91.22 Nonpurulent mastitis associated with the puerperium**
Puerperal interstitial mastitis
Puerperal lymphangitis of breast
Puerperal mastitis NOS
Puerperal parenchymatous mastitis

• ♀ **O91.23 Nonpurulent mastitis associated with lactation**
Interstitial mastitis associated with lactation
Lymphangitis of breast associated with lactation
Mastitis NOS associated with lactation
Parenchymatous mastitis associated with lactation

O92 Other disorders of breast and disorders of lactation associated with pregnancy and the puerperium

\+ **O92.0 Retracted nipple associated with pregnancy, the puerperium, and lactation**

\+ **O92.01 Retracted nipple associated with pregnancy**

• ♀ **O92.011 Retracted nipple associated with pregnancy, first trimester**

• ♀ **O92.012 Retracted nipple associated with pregnancy, second trimester**

• ♀ **O92.013 Retracted nipple associated with pregnancy, third trimester**

• ♀ **O92.019 Retracted nipple associated with pregnancy, unspecified trimester**

• ♀ **O92.02 Retracted nipple associated with the puerperium**

• ♀ **O92.03 Retracted nipple associated with lactation**

\+ **O92.1 Cracked nipple associated with pregnancy, the puerperium, and lactation**
Fissure of nipple, gestational or puerperal

\+ **O92.11 Cracked nipple associated with pregnancy**

• ♀ **O92.111 Cracked nipple associated with pregnancy, first trimester**

• ♀ **O92.112 Cracked nipple associated with pregnancy, second trimester**

• ♀ **O92.113 Cracked nipple associated with pregnancy, third trimester**

• ♀ **O92.119 Cracked nipple associated with pregnancy, unspecified trimester**

• ♀ **O92.12 Cracked nipple associated with the puerperium**

• ♀ **O92.13 Cracked nipple associated with lactation**

\+ **O92.2 Other and unspecified disorders of breast associated with pregnancy and the puerperium**

• ♀ **O92.20 Unspecified disorder of breast associated with pregnancy and the puerperium**

• ♀ **O92.29 Other disorders of breast associated with pregnanc and the puerperium**

• ♀ **O92.3 Agalactia**
Primary agalactia
Excludes1: *Elective agalactia (O92.5)*
Secondary agalactia (O92.5)
Therapeutic agalactia (O92.5)

• ♀ **O92.4 Hypogalactia**

• ♀ **O92.5 Suppressed lactation**
Elective agalactia
Secondary agalactia
Therapeutic agalactia
Excludes1: *primary agalactia (O92.3)*

• ♀ **O92.6 Galactorrhea**

\+ **O92.7 Other and unspecified disorders of lactation**

• ♀ **O92.70 Unspecified disorders of lactation**

• ♀ **O92.79 Other disorders of lactation**
Puerperal galactocele

Other obstetric conditions, not elsewhere classified (O94-O9A)

• ♀ **O94 Sequelae of complication of pregnancy, childbirth, and the puerperium**

NOTE This category is to be used to indicate conditions in O00-O77.-, O85-O94 and O98-O9A.- as the cause of late effects. The sequelae include conditions specified as such, or late effects, which may occur at any time after the puerperium

Code first condition resulting from (sequela) of complication of pregnancy, childbirth, and the puerperium
Review coding guideline C.15.p
Valid 3-character code, no further characters required

O98 Maternal infectious and parasitic diseases classifiable elsewhere bu complicating pregnancy, childbirth and the puerperium

Includes: the listed conditions when complicating the pregnant state, when aggravated by the pregnancy, or as a reason for obstetric care

Use additional code (Chapter 1), to identify specific infectious or parasitic disease

Excludes2: *herpes gestationis (O26.4-)*
infectious carrier state (O99.82-, O99.83-)
obstetrical tetanus (A34)
puerperal infection (O86.-)
puerperal sepsis (O85)
when the reason for maternal care is that the disease is known or suspected to have affected the fetus (O35-O36)

\+ **O98.0 Tuberculosis complicating pregnancy, childbirth and the puerperium**
Conditions in A15-A19

\+ **O98.01 Tuberculosis complicating pregnancy**

• ♀ CC **O98.011 Tuberculosis complicating pregnancy, firs trimester**
CC Exclusion see Appendix A PDX collection 1(

• ♀ CC **O98.012 Tuberculosis complicating pregnancy, second trimester**
CC Exclusion see Appendix A PDX collection 1011

• ♀ CC **O98.013 Tuberculosis complicating pregnancy, thi trimester**
CC Exclusion see Appendix A PDX collection 1011

• ♀ **O98.019 Tuberculosis complicating pregnancy, unspecified trimester**

• ♀ CC **O98.02 Tuberculosis complicating childbirth**
CC Exclusion see Appendix A PDX collection 1011

• ♀ CC **O98.03 Tuberculosis complicating the puerperium**
CC Exclusion see Appendix A PDX collection 1011

\+ **O98.1 Syphilis complicating pregnancy, childbirth and the puerperiu**
Conditions in A50-A53

\+ **O98.11 Syphilis complicating pregnancy**

• ♀ CC **O98.111 Syphilis complicating pregnancy, first trimester**
CC Exclusion see Appendix A PDX collection 1012

• ♀ CC **O98.112 Syphilis complicating pregnancy, second trimester**
CC Exclusion see Appendix A PDX collection 1012

• ♀ CC **O98.113 Syphilis complicating pregnancy, third trimester**
CC Exclusion see Appendix A PDX collection 1012
• ♀ **O98.119 Syphilis complicating pregnancy, unspecified trimester**
• ♀ CC **O98.12 Syphilis complicating childbirth**
CC Exclusion see Appendix A PDX collection 1012
• ♀ CC **O98.13 Syphilis complicating the puerperium**
CC Exclusion see Appendix A PDX collection 1012
+ **O98.2 Gonorrhea complicating pregnancy, childbirth and the puerperium**
Conditions in A54.-
+ **O98.21 Gonorrhea complicating pregnancy**
• ♀ CC **O98.211 Gonorrhea complicating pregnancy, first trimester**
CC Exclusion see Appendix A PDX collection 1012
• ♀ CC **O98.212 Gonorrhea complicating pregnancy, second trimester**
CC Exclusion see Appendix A PDX collection 1012
• ♀ CC **O98.213 Gonorrhea complicating pregnancy, third trimester**
CC Exclusion see Appendix A PDX collection 1012
• ♀ **O98.219 Gonorrhea complicating pregnancy, unspecified trimester**
• ♀ CC **O98.22 Gonorrhea complicating childbirth**
CC Exclusion see Appendix A PDX collection 1012
• ♀ CC **O98.23 Gonorrhea complicating the puerperium**
CC Exclusion see Appendix A PDX collection 1012
+ **O98.3 Other infections with a predominantly sexual mode of transmission complicating pregnancy, childbirth and the puerperium**
Conditions in A55-A64
+ **O98.31 Other infections with a predominantly sexual mode of transmission complicating pregnancy**
• ♀ CC **O98.311 Other infections with a predominantly sexual mode of transmission complicating pregnancy, first trimester**
CC Exclusion see Appendix A PDX collection 1012
• ♀ CC **O98.312 Other infections with a predominantly sexual mode of transmission complicating pregnancy, second trimester**
CC Exclusion see Appendix A PDX collection 1012
• ♀ CC **O98.313 Other infections with a predominantly sexual mode of transmission complicating pregnancy, third trimester**
CC Exclusion see Appendix A PDX collection 1012
• ♀ **O98.319 Other infections with a predominantly sexual mode of transmission complicating pregnancy, unspecified trimester**
• ♀ CC **O98.32 Other infections with a predominantly sexual mode of transmission complicating childbirth**
CC Exclusion see Appendix A PDX collection 1012
• ♀ CC **O98.33 Other infections with a predominantly sexual mode of transmission complicating the puerperium**
CC Exclusion see Appendix A PDX collection 1012
+ **O98.4 Viral hepatitis complicating pregnancy, childbirth and the puerperium**
Conditions in B15-B19
+ **O98.41 Viral hepatitis complicating pregnancy**
• ♀ CC **O98.411 Viral hepatitis complicating pregnancy, first trimester**
CC Exclusion see Appendix A PDX collection 1013
• ♀ CC **O98.412 Viral hepatitis complicating pregnancy, second trimester**
CC Exclusion see Appendix A PDX collection 1013
• ♀ CC **O98.413 Viral hepatitis complicating pregnancy, third trimester**
CC Exclusion see Appendix A PDX collection 1013
• ♀ **O98.419 Viral hepatitis complicating pregnancy, unspecified trimester**
• ♀ CC **O98.42 Viral hepatitis complicating childbirth**
CC Exclusion see Appendix A PDX collection 1013
• ♀ CC **O98.43 Viral hepatitis complicating the puerperium**
CC Exclusion see Appendix A PDX collection 1013
+ **O98.5 Other viral diseases complicating pregnancy, childbirth and the puerperium**
Conditions in A80-B09, B25-B34, R87.81-, R87.82-
Excludes1: *human immunodeficiency virus [HIV] disease complicating pregnancy, childbirth and the puerperium (O98.7-)*
+ **O98.51 Other viral diseases complicating pregnancy**
• ♀ CC **O98.511 Other viral diseases complicating pregnancy, first trimester**
CC Exclusion see Appendix A PDX collection 1013
• ♀ CC **O98.512 Other viral diseases complicating pregnancy, second trimester**
CC Exclusion see Appendix A PDX collection 1013
AHA CC: 4Q, 2016, 4-7
• ♀ CC **O98.513 Other viral diseases complicating pregnancy, third trimester**
CC Exclusion see Appendix A PDX collection 1013
AHA CC: 4Q, 2016, 4-7
• ♀ **O98.519 Other viral diseases complicating pregnancy, unspecified trimester**
• ♀ CC **O98.52 Other viral diseases complicating childbirth**
CC Exclusion see Appendix A PDX collection 1013
• ♀ CC **O98.53 Other viral diseases complicating the puerperium**
CC Exclusion see Appendix A PDX collection 1013
+ **O98.6 Protozoal diseases complicating pregnancy, childbirth and the puerperium**
Conditions in B50-B64
+ **O98.61 Protozoal diseases complicating pregnancy**
• ♀ CC **O98.611 Protozoal diseases complicating pregnancy, first trimester**
CC Exclusion see Appendix A PDX collection 1014
• ♀ CC **O98.612 Protozoal diseases complicating pregnancy, second trimester**
CC Exclusion see Appendix A PDX collection 1014
• ♀ CC **O98.613 Protozoal diseases complicating pregnancy, third trimester**
CC Exclusion see Appendix A PDX collection 1014
• ♀ **O98.619 Protozoal diseases complicating pregnancy, unspecified trimester**
• ♀ CC **O98.62 Protozoal diseases complicating childbirth**
CC Exclusion see Appendix A PDX collection 1015
• ♀ CC **O98.63 Protozoal diseases complicating the puerperium**
CC Exclusion see Appendix A PDX collection 1015
+ **O98.7 Human immunodeficiency virus [HIV] disease complicating pregnancy, childbirth and the puerperium**
Use additional code to identify the type of HIV disease:
Acquired immune deficiency syndrome (AIDS) (B20)
Asymptomatic HIV status (Z21)
HIV positive NOS (Z21)
Symptomatic HIV disease (B20)
Review coding guideline C.1.a.2.g
Review coding guideline C.15.f
+ **O98.71 Human immunodeficiency virus [HIV] disease complicating pregnancy**
• ♀ CC **O98.711 Human immunodeficiency virus [HIV] disease complicating pregnancy, first trimester**
CC Exclusion see Appendix A PDX collection 1013
• ♀ CC **O98.712 Human immunodeficiency virus [HIV] disease complicating pregnancy, second trimester**
CC Exclusion see Appendix A PDX collection 1013
• ♀ CC **O98.713 Human immunodeficiency virus [HIV] disease complicating pregnancy, third trimester**
CC Exclusion see Appendix A PDX collection 1013
• ♀ **O98.719 Human immunodeficiency virus [HIV] disease complicating pregnancy, unspecified trimester**

• ♀ CC **O98.72 Human immunodeficiency virus [HIV] disease complicating childbirth**
CC Exclusion see Appendix A PDX collection 1013

• ♀ CC **O98.73 Human immunodeficiency virus [HIV] disease complicating the puerperium**
CC Exclusion see Appendix A PDX collection 1013

+ **O98.8 Other maternal infectious and parasitic diseases complicating pregnancy, childbirth and the puerperium**

+ **O98.81 Other maternal infectious and parasitic diseases complicating pregnancy**

• ♀ CC **O98.811 Other maternal infectious and parasitic diseases complicating pregnancy, first trimester**
CC Exclusion see Appendix A PDX collection 1013

• ♀ CC **O98.812 Other maternal infectious and parasitic diseases complicating pregnancy, second trimester**
CC Exclusion see Appendix A PDX collection 1013

• ♀ CC **O98.813 Other maternal infectious and parasitic diseases complicating pregnancy, third trimester**
CC Exclusion see Appendix A PDX collection 1013

• ♀ **O98.819 Other maternal infectious and parasitic diseases complicating pregnancy, unspecified trimester**

• ♀ CC **O98.82 Other maternal infectious and parasitic diseases complicating childbirth**
CC Exclusion see Appendix A PDX collection 1013

• ♀ CC **O98.83 Other maternal infectious and parasitic diseases complicating the puerperium**
CC Exclusion see Appendix A PDX collection 1013

+ **O98.9 Unspecified maternal infectious and parasitic disease complicating pregnancy, childbirth and the puerperium**

+ **O98.91 Unspecified maternal infectious and parasitic disease complicating pregnancy**

• ♀ CC **O98.911 Unspecified maternal infectious and parasitic disease complicating pregnancy, first trimester**
CC Exclusion see Appendix A PDX collection 1013

• ♀ CC **O98.912 Unspecified maternal infectious and parasitic disease complicating pregnancy, second trimester**
CC Exclusion see Appendix A PDX collection 1013

• ♀ CC **O98.913 Unspecified maternal infectious and parasitic disease complicating pregnancy, third trimester**
CC Exclusion see Appendix A PDX collection 1013

• ♀ **O98.919 Unspecified maternal infectious and parasitic disease complicating pregnancy, unspecified trimester**

• ♀ CC **O98.92 Unspecified maternal infectious and parasitic disease complicating childbirth**
CC Exclusion see Appendix A PDX collection 1013

• ♀ CC **O98.93 Unspecified maternal infectious and parasitic disease complicating the puerperium**
CC Exclusion see Appendix A PDX collection 1013

O99 Other maternal diseases classifiable elsewhere but complicating pregnancy, childbirth and the puerperium

Includes: conditions which complicate the pregnant state, are aggravated by the pregnancy or are a main reason for obstetric care

Use additional code to identify specific condition

Excludes2: *when the reason for maternal care is that the condition is known or suspected to have affected the fetus (O35-O36)*

+ **O99.0 Anemia complicating pregnancy, childbirth and the puerperium**
Conditions in D50-D64
Excludes1: *anemia arising in the puerperium (O90.81)*
postpartum anemia NOS (O90.81)

+ **O99.01 Anemia complicating pregnancy**

• ♀ **O99.011 Anemia complicating pregnancy, first trimester**

• ♀ **O99.012 Anemia complicating pregnancy, second trimester**

• ♀ **O99.013 Anemia complicating pregnancy, third trimester**

• ♀ **O99.019 Anemia complicating pregnancy, unspecified trimester**

• ♀ **O99.02 Anemia complicating childbirth**

• ♀ **O99.03 Anemia complicating the puerperium**
Excludes1: *postpartum anemia not pre-existing prior to delivery (O90.81)*

+ **O99.1 Other diseases of the blood and blood-forming organs and certain disorders involving the immune mechanism complicating pregnancy, childbirth and the puerperium**
Conditions in D65-D89
Excludes1: *hemorrhage with coagulation defects (O45.-, O46.0-, O67.0, O72.3)*

+ **O99.11 Other diseases of the blood and blood-forming organs and certain disorders involving the immune mechanism complicating pregnancy**

• ♀ CC **O99.111 Other diseases of the blood and blood-forming organs and certain disorders involving the immune mechanism complicating pregnancy, first trimester**
CC Exclusion see Appendix A PDX collection 1016

• ♀ CC **O99.112 Other diseases of the blood and blood-forming organs and certain disorders involving the immune mechanism complicating pregnancy, second trimester**
CC Exclusion see Appendix A PDX collection 1016

• ♀ CC **O99.113 Other diseases of the blood and blood-forming organs and certain disorders involving the immune mechanism complicating pregnancy, third trimester**
CC Exclusion see Appendix A PDX collection 1016

• ♀ CC **O99.119 Other diseases of the blood and blood-forming organs and certain disorders involving the immune mechanism complicating pregnancy, unspecified trimester**
CC Exclusion see Appendix A PDX collection 1017

• ♀ CC **O99.12 Other diseases of the blood and blood-forming organs and certain disorders involving the immune mechanism complicating childbirth**
CC Exclusion see Appendix A PDX collection 1016

• ♀ CC **O99.13 Other diseases of the blood and blood-forming organs and certain disorders involving the immune mechanism complicating the puerperium**
CC Exclusion see Appendix A PDX collection 1016

+ **O99.2 Endocrine, nutritional and metabolic diseases complicating pregnancy, childbirth and the puerperium**
Conditions in E00-E88
Excludes2: *diabetes mellitus (O24.-)*
malnutrition (O25.-)
postpartum thyroiditis (O90.5)

+ **O99.21 Obesity complicating pregnancy, childbirth, and the puerperium**
Use additional code to identify the type of obesity (E66.-)

• ♀ **O99.210 Obesity complicating pregnancy, unspecified trimester**

• ♀ **O99.211 Obesity complicating pregnancy, first trimester**

• ♀ **O99.212 Obesity complicating pregnancy, second trimester**

• ♀ **O99.213 Obesity complicating pregnancy, third trimester**

• ♀ **O99.214 Obesity complicating childbirth**

• ♀ **O99.215 Obesity complicating the puerperium**

+ **O99.28 Other endocrine, nutritional and metabolic diseases complicating pregnancy, childbirth and the puerperium**

• ♀ **O99.280 Endocrine, nutritional and metabolic diseases complicating pregnancy, unspecified trimester**

• ♀ **O99.281 Endocrine, nutritional and metabolic diseases complicating pregnancy, first trimester**

- • ♀ O99.282 **Endocrine, nutritional and metabolic diseases complicating pregnancy, second trimester**
- • ♀ O99.283 **Endocrine, nutritional and metabolic diseases complicating pregnancy, third trimester**
- • ♀ O99.284 **Endocrine, nutritional and metabolic diseases complicating childbirth**
- • ♀ O99.285 **Endocrine, nutritional and metabolic diseases complicating the puerperium**

\+ O99.3 **Mental disorders and diseases of the nervous system complicating pregnancy, childbirth and the puerperium**

\+ O99.31 **Alcohol use complicating pregnancy, childbirth, and the puerperium**
Use additional code(s) from F10 to identify manifestations of the alcohol use
Review coding guideline C.15.l.1

- • ♀ O99.310 **Alcohol use complicating pregnancy, unspecified trimester**
- • ♀ O99.311 **Alcohol use complicating pregnancy, first trimester**
- • ♀ O99.312 **Alcohol use complicating pregnancy, second trimester**
- • ♀ O99.313 **Alcohol use complicating pregnancy, third trimester**
- • ♀ O99.314 **Alcohol use complicating childbirth**
- • ♀ O99.315 **Alcohol use complicating the puerperium**

\+ O99.32 **Drug use complicating pregnancy, childbirth, and the puerperium**
Use additional code(s) from F11-F16 and F18-F19 to identify manifestations of the drug use

- • ♀ O99.320 **Drug use complicating pregnancy, unspecified trimester**
- • ♀ CC O99.321 **Drug use complicating pregnancy, first trimester**
  CC Exclusion see Appendix A PDX collection 1018
- • ♀ CC O99.322 **Drug use complicating pregnancy, second trimester**
  CC Exclusion see Appendix A PDX collection 1018
- • ♀ CC O99.323 **Drug use complicating pregnancy, third trimester**
  CC Exclusion see Appendix A PDX collection 1018
- • ♀ CC O99.324 **Drug use complicating childbirth**
  CC Exclusion see Appendix A PDX collection 1018
- • ♀ CC O99.325 **Drug use complicating the puerperium**
  CC Exclusion see Appendix A PDX collection 1018

\+ O99.33 **Tobacco use disorder complicating pregnancy, childbirth, and the puerperium**
Smoking complicating pregnancy, childbirth, and the puerperium
Use additional code from category F17 to identify type of tobacco nicotine dependence
Review coding guideline C.15.l.2

- • ♀ O99.330 **Smoking (tobacco) complicating pregnancy, unspecified trimester**
- • ♀ O99.331 **Smoking (tobacco) complicating pregnancy, first trimester**
- • ♀ O99.332 **Smoking (tobacco) complicating pregnancy, second trimester**
- • ♀ O99.333 **Smoking (tobacco) complicating pregnancy, third trimester**
- • ♀ O99.334 **Smoking (tobacco) complicating childbirth**
- • ♀ O99.335 **Smoking (tobacco) complicating the puerperium**

\+ O99.34 **Other mental disorders complicating pregnancy, childbirth, and the puerperium**
Conditions in F01-F09 and F20-F99
Excludes2: *postpartum mood disturbance (O90.6)*
postnatal psychosis (F53)
puerperal psychosis (F53)

- • ♀ O99.340 **Other mental disorders complicating pregnancy, unspecified trimester**
- • ♀ O99.341 **Other mental disorders complicating pregnancy, first trimester**
- • ♀ O99.342 **Other mental disorders complicating pregnancy, second trimester**
- • ♀ O99.343 **Other mental disorders complicating pregnancy, third trimester**
- • ♀ O99.344 **Other mental disorders complicating childbirth**
- • ♀ O99.345 **Other mental disorders complicating the puerperium**

\+ O99.35 **Diseases of the nervous system complicating pregnancy, childbirth, and the puerperium**
Conditions in G00-G99
Excludes2: *pregnancy related peripheral neuritis (O26.8-)*

- • ♀ O99.350 **Diseases of the nervous system complicating pregnancy, unspecified trimester**
- • ♀ O99.351 **Diseases of the nervous system complicating pregnancy, first trimester**
- • ♀ O99.352 **Diseases of the nervous system complicating pregnancy, second trimester**
- • ♀ O99.353 **Diseases of the nervous system complicating pregnancy, third trimester**
- • ♀ CC O99.354 **Diseases of the nervous system complicating childbirth**
  CC Exclusion see Appendix A PDX collection 1016
- • ♀ CC O99.355 **Diseases of the nervous system complicating the puerperium**
  CC Exclusion see Appendix A PDX collection 1016

\+ O99.4 **Diseases of the circulatory system complicating pregnancy, childbirth and the puerperium**
Conditions in I00-I99
Excludes1: *peripartum cardiomyopathy (O90.3)*
Excludes2: *hypertensive disorders (O10-O16)*
obstetric embolism (O88.-)
venous complications and cerebrovenous sinus thrombosis in labor, childbirth and the puerperium (O87.-)
venous complications and cerebrovenous sinus thrombosis in pregnancy (O22.-)

\+ O99.41 **Diseases of the circulatory system complicating pregnancy**
AHA CC: 2Q, 2016, 8

- • ♀ CC O99.411 **Diseases of the circulatory system complicating pregnancy, first trimester**
  CC Exclusion see Appendix A PDX collection 1019
- • ♀ CC O99.412 **Diseases of the circulatory system complicating pregnancy, second trimester**
  CC Exclusion see Appendix A PDX collection 1019
- • ♀ CC O99.413 **Diseases of the circulatory system complicating pregnancy, third trimester**
  CC Exclusion see Appendix A PDX collection 1019
- • ♀ O99.419 **Diseases of the circulatory system complicating pregnancy, unspecified trimester**

• ♀ MCC O99.42 **Diseases of the circulatory system complicating childbirth**
MCC Exclusion see Appendix A PDX collection 1008

• ♀ CC O99.43 **Diseases of the circulatory system complicating the puerperium**
CC Exclusion see Appendix A PDX collection 1019

\+ O99.5 **Diseases of the respiratory system complicating pregnancy, childbirth and the puerperium**
Conditions in J00-J99

\+ O99.51 **Diseases of the respiratory system complicating pregnancy**

- • ♀ O99.511 **Diseases of the respiratory system complicating pregnancy, first trimester**
- • ♀ O99.512 **Diseases of the respiratory system complicating pregnancy, second trimester**
- • ♀ O99.513 **Diseases of the respiratory system complicating pregnancy, third trimester**
- • ♀ O99.519 **Diseases of the respiratory system complicating pregnancy, unspecified trimester**

• ♀ O99.52 **Diseases of the respiratory system complicating childbirth**

• ♀ O99.53 **Diseases of the respiratory system complicating the puerperium**

+ **O99.6 Diseases of the digestive system complicating pregnancy, childbirth and the puerperium**
Conditions in K00-K93
Excludes2: *liver and biliary tract disorders in pregnancy, childbirth and the puerperium (O26.6-)*
hemorrhoids in pregnancy (O22.4-)
+ **O99.61 Diseases of the digestive system complicating pregnancy**
• ♀ **O99.611 Diseases of the digestive system complicating pregnancy, first trimester**
• ♀ **O99.612 Diseases of the digestive system complicating pregnancy, second trimester**
• ♀ **O99.613 Diseases of the digestive system complicating pregnancy, third trimester**
• ♀ **O99.619 Diseases of the digestive system complicating pregnancy, unspecified trimester**
• ♀ **O99.62 Diseases of the digestive system complicating childbirth**
• ♀ **O99.63 Diseases of the digestive system complicating the puerperium**
+ **O99.7 Diseases of the skin and subcutaneous tissue complicating pregnancy, childbirth and the puerperium**
Conditions in L00-L99
Excludes2: *herpes gestationis (O26.4)*
pruritic urticarial papules and plaques of pregnancy (PUPPP) (O26.86)
+ **O99.71 Diseases of the skin and subcutaneous tissue complicating pregnancy**
• ♀ **O99.711 Diseases of the skin and subcutaneous tissue complicating pregnancy, first trimester**
• ♀ **O99.712 Diseases of the skin and subcutaneous tissue complicating pregnancy, second trimester**
• ♀ **O99.713 Diseases of the skin and subcutaneous tissue complicating pregnancy, third trimester**
• ♀ **O99.719 Diseases of the skin and subcutaneous tissue complicating pregnancy, unspecified trimester**
• ♀ **O99.72 Diseases of the skin and subcutaneous tissue complicating childbirth**
• ♀ **O99.73 Diseases of the skin and subcutaneous tissue complicating the puerperium**
+ **O99.8 Other specified diseases and conditions complicating pregnancy, childbirth and the puerperium**
Conditions in D00-D48, H00-H95, M00-N99, and Q00-Q99
Use additional code to identify condition
Excludes2: *genitourinary infections in pregnancy (O23.-)*
infection of genitourinary tract following delivery (O86.1-O86.3)
malignant neoplasm complicating pregnancy, childbirth and the puerperium (O9A.1-)
maternal care for known or suspected abnormality of maternal pelvic organs (O34.-)
postpartum acute kidney failure (O90.4)
traumatic injuries in pregnancy (O9A.2-)
+ **O99.81 Abnormal glucose complicating pregnancy, childbirth and the puerperium**
Excludes1: *gestational diabetes (O24.4-)*
Review coding guideline C.15.i
• ♀ **O99.810 Abnormal glucose complicating pregnancy**
• ♀ **O99.814 Abnormal glucose complicating childbirth**
• ♀ **O99.815 Abnormal glucose complicating the puerperium**
+ **O99.82 Streptococcus B carrier state complicating pregnancy, childbirth and the puerperium**
Excludes1: *Carrier of streptococcus group B (GBS) in a nonpregnant woman (Z22.330)*
• ♀ **O99.820 Streptococcus B carrier state complicating pregnancy**
• ♀ **O99.824 Streptococcus B carrier state complicating childbirth**
• ♀ **O99.825 Streptococcus B carrier state complicating the puerperium**
+ **O99.83 Other infection carrier state complicating pregnancy, childbirth and the puerperium**
Use additional code to identify the carrier state (Z22.-)
• ♀ CC **O99.830 Other infection carrier state complicatin pregnancy**
CC Exclusion see Appendix A PDX collection 1013
• ♀ CC **O99.834 Other infection carrier state complicatin childbirth**
CC Exclusion see Appendix A PDX collection 1013
• ♀ CC **O99.835 Other infection carrier state complicatin the puerperium**
CC Exclusion see Appendix A PDX collection 1013
+ **O99.84 Bariatric surgery status complicating pregnancy, childbirth and the puerperium**
Gastric banding status complicating pregnancy, childbirth and the puerperium
Gastric bypass status for obesity complicating pregnancy, childbirth and the puerperium
Obesity surgery status complicating pregnancy, childbirth and the puerperium
• ♀ **O99.840 Bariatric surgery status complicating pregnancy, unspecified trimester**
• ♀ **O99.841 Bariatric surgery status complicating pregnancy, first trimester**
• ♀ **O99.842 Bariatric surgery status complicating pregnancy, second trimester**
• ♀ **O99.843 Bariatric surgery status complicating pregnancy, third trimester**
• ♀ **O99.844 Bariatric surgery status complicating childbirth**
• ♀ **O99.845 Bariatric surgery status complicating the puerperium**
• ♀ **O99.89 Other specified diseases and conditions complicati pregnancy, childbirth and the puerperium**

O9A Maternal malignant neoplasms, traumatic injuries and abuse classifiable elsewhere but complicating pregnancy, childbirth and the puerperium

+ **O9A.1 Malignant neoplasm complicating pregnancy, childbirth and the puerperium**
Conditions in C00-C96
Use additional code to identify neoplasm
Excludes2: *maternal care for benign tumor of corpus uteri (O34.1-)*
maternal care for benign tumor of cervix (O34.4
Review coding guideline C.2.l.3
+ **O9A.11 Malignant neoplasm complicating pregnancy**
• ♀ **O9A.111 Malignant neoplasm complicating pregnancy, first trimester**
• ♀ **O9A.112 Malignant neoplasm complicating pregnancy, second trimester**
• ♀ **O9A.113 Malignant neoplasm complicating pregnancy, third trimester**
• ♀ **O9A.119 Malignant neoplasm complicating pregnancy, unspecified trimester**
• ♀ **O9A.12 Malignant neoplasm complicating childbirth**
• ♀ **O9A.13 Malignant neoplasm complicating the puerperium**
AHA CC: 3Q, 2015, 19-20
+ **O9A.2 Injury, poisoning and certain other consequences of externa causes complicating pregnancy, childbirth and the puerperi**
Conditions in S00-T88, except T74 and T76
Use additional code(s) to identify the injury or poisoning
Excludes2: *physical, sexual and psychological abuse complicating pregnancy, childbirth and the puerperium (O9A.3-, O9A.4-, O9A.5-)*
Review coding guideline C.15.m
+ **O9A.21 Injury, poisoning and certain other consequences external causes complicating pregnancy**
• ♀ **O9A.211 Injury, poisoning and certain other consequences of external causes complicating pregnancy, first trimester**
• ♀ **O9A.212 Injury, poisoning and certain other consequences of external causes complicating pregnancy, second trimeste**
• ♀ **O9A.213 Injury, poisoning and certain other consequences of external causes complicating pregnancy, third trimester**
• ♀ **O9A.219 Injury, poisoning and certain other consequences of external causes complicating pregnancy, unspecified trimester**

- ● ♀ **O9A.22 Injury, poisoning and certain other consequences of external causes complicating childbirth**
- ● ♀ **O9A.23 Injury, poisoning and certain other consequences of external causes complicating the puerperium**

+ **O9A.3 Physical abuse complicating pregnancy, childbirth and the puerperium**
  Conditions in T74.11 or T76.11
  Use additional code (if applicable):
  to identify any associated current injury due to physical abuse
  to identify the perpetrator of abuse (Y07.-)
  Excludes2: *sexual abuse complicating pregnancy, childbirth and the puerperium (O9A.4)*
  Review coding guideline C.15.r
  + **O9A.31 Physical abuse complicating pregnancy**
    - ● ♀ **O9A.311 Physical abuse complicating pregnancy, first trimester**
    - ● ♀ **O9A.312 Physical abuse complicating pregnancy, second trimester**
    - ● ♀ **O9A.313 Physical abuse complicating pregnancy, third trimester**
    - ● ♀ **O9A.319 Physical abuse complicating pregnancy, unspecified trimester**
  - ● ♀ **O9A.32 Physical abuse complicating childbirth**
  - ● ♀ **O9A.33 Physical abuse complicating the puerperium**

+ **O9A.4 Sexual abuse complicating pregnancy, childbirth and the puerperium**
  Conditions in T74.21 or T76.21
  Use additional code (if applicable):
  to identify any associated current injury due to sexual abuse
  to identify the perpetrator of abuse (Y07.-)
  Review coding guideline C.15.r
  + **O9A.41 Sexual abuse complicating pregnancy**
    - ● ♀ **O9A.411 Sexual abuse complicating pregnancy, first trimester**
    - ● ♀ **O9A.412 Sexual abuse complicating pregnancy, second trimester**
    - ● ♀ **O9A.413 Sexual abuse complicating pregnancy, third trimester**
    - ● ♀ **O9A.419 Sexual abuse complicating pregnancy, unspecified trimester**
  - ● ♀ **O9A.42 Sexual abuse complicating childbirth**
  - ● ♀ **O9A.43 Sexual abuse complicating the puerperium**

+ **O9A.5 Psychological abuse complicating pregnancy, childbirth and the puerperium**
  Conditions in T74.31 or T76.31
  Use additional code to identify the perpetrator of abuse (Y07.-)
  Review coding guideline C.15.r
  + **O9A.51 Psychological abuse complicating pregnancy**
    - ● ♀ **O9A.511 Psychological abuse complicating pregnancy, first trimester**
    - ● ♀ **O9A.512 Psychological abuse complicating pregnancy, second trimester**
    - ● ♀ **O9A.513 Psychological abuse complicating pregnancy, third trimester**
    - ● ♀ **O9A.519 Psychological abuse complicating pregnancy, unspecified trimester**
  - ● ♀ **O9A.52 Psychological abuse complicating childbirth**
  - ● ♀ **O9A.53 Psychological abuse complicating the puerperium**

Chapter 16: Certain Conditions Originating in the Perinatal Period (P00-P96)

NOTE Codes from this chapter are for use on newborn records only, never on maternal records

Includes: conditions that have their origin in the fetal or perinatal period (before birth through the first 28 days after birth) even if morbidity occurs later

Excludes2: *congenital malformations, deformations and chromosomal abnormalities (Q00-Q99)*
endocrine, nutritional and metabolic diseases (E00-E88)
injury, poisoning and certain other consequences of external causes (S00-T88)
neoplasms (C00-D49)
tetanus neonatorum (A33)

This chapter contains the following category blocks:

- P00-P04 Newborn affected by maternal factors and by complications of pregnancy, labor, and delivery
- P05-P08 Disorders of newborn related to length of gestation and fetal growth
- P09 Abnormal findings on neonatal screening
- P10-P15 Birth trauma
- P19-P29 Respiratory and cardiovascular disorders specific to the perinatal period
- P35-P39 Infections specific to the perinatal period
- P50-P61 Hemorrhagic and hematological disorders of newborn
- P70-P74 Transitory endocrine and metabolic disorders specific to newborn
- P76-P78 Digestive system disorders of newborn
- P80-P83 Conditions involving the integument and temperature regulation of newborn
- P84 Other problems with newborn
- P90-P96 Other disorders originating in the perinatal period

C. Chapter-Specific Coding Guidelines

In addition to general coding guidelines, there are guidelines for specific diagnoses and/or conditions in the classification. Unless otherwise indicated, these guidelines apply to all health care settings. Please refer to Section II for guidelines on the selection of principal diagnosis.

16. Chapter 16: Certain Conditions Originating in the Perinatal Period (P00-P96)

For coding and reporting purposes the perinatal period is defined as before birth through the 28th day following birth. The following guidelines are provided for reporting purposes

a. General Perinatal Rules

1) Use of Chapter 16 Codes

Codes in this chapter are <u>never</u> for use on the maternal record. Codes from Chapter 15, the obstetric chapter, are never permitted on the newborn record. Chapter 16 codes may be used throughout the life of the patient if the condition is still present.

2) Principal Diagnosis for Birth Record

When coding the birth episode in a newborn record, assign a code from category Z38, Liveborn infants according to place of birth and type of delivery, as the principal diagnosis. A code from category Z38 is assigned only once, to a newborn at the time of birth. If a newborn is transferred to another institution, a code from category Z38 should not be used at the receiving hospital.

A code from category Z38 is used only on the newborn record, not on the mother's record.

3) Use of Codes from other Chapters with Codes from Chapter 16

Codes from other chapters may be used with codes from chapter 16 if the codes from the other chapters provide more specific detail. Codes for signs and symptoms may be assigned when a definitive diagnosis has not been established. If the reason for the encounter is a perinatal condition, the code from chapter 16 should be sequenced first.

4) Use of Chapter 16 Codes after the Perinatal Period

Should a condition originate in the perinatal period, and continue throughout the life of the patient, the perinatal code should continue to be used regardless of the patient's age.

5) Birth process or community acquired conditions

If a newborn has a condition that may be either due to the birth process or community acquired and the documentation does not indicate which it is, the default is due to the birth process and the code from Chapter 16 should be used. If the condition is community-acquired, a code from Chapter 16 should not be assigned.

6) Code all clinically significant conditions

All clinically significant conditions noted on routine newborn examinatio should be coded. A condition is clinically significant if it requires:

- clinical evaluation; or
- therapeutic treatment; or
- diagnostic procedures; or
- extended length of hospital stay; or
- increased nursing care and/or monitoring; or
- has implications for future health care needs

Note: The perinatal guidelines listed above are the same as the gener coding guidelines for "additional diagnoses", except for the final poi regarding implications for future health care needs. Codes should b assigned for conditions that have been specified by the provider as havir implications for future health care needs.

b. Observation and Evaluation of Newborns for Suspected Conditions n Found

1) ***Use of Z05 codes***

Assign a code from category Z05, Observation and evaluation of newbor and infants for suspected conditions ruled out, to identify those instances whe a healthy newborn is evaluated for a suspected condition that is determine after study not to be present. Do not use a code from category Z05 when t patient has identified signs or symptoms of a suspected problem; in suc cases code the sign or symptom.

2) ***Z05 on Other than the Birth Record***

A code from category Z05 may also be assigned as a principal or first-liste code for readmissions or encounters when the code from category Z38 co no longer applies. Codes from category Z05 are fur use only for healt newborns and infants for which no condition after study is found to be prese

3) Z05 on a birth record

A code from category Z05 is to be used as a secondary code after the co from category Z38, Liveborn infants according to place of birth and ty of delivery.

c. Coding Additional Perinatal Diagnoses

1) Assigning codes for conditions that require treatment

Assign codes for conditions that require treatment or further investigatic prolong the length of stay, or require resource utilization.

2) Codes for conditions specified as having implications for future heal care needs

Assign codes for conditions that have been specified by the provider having implications for future health care needs.

Note: This guideline should not be used for adult patients.

d. Prematurity and Fetal Growth Retardation

Providers utilize different criteria in determining prematurity. A code prematurity should not be assigned unless it is documented. Assignment codes in categories P05, Disorders of newborn related to slow fetal grow and fetal malnutrition, and P07, Disorders of newborn related to sh gestation and low birth weight, not elsewhere classified, should be based the recorded birth weight and estimated gestational age.

When both birth weight and gestational age are available, two codes fro category P07 should be assigned, with the code for birth weight sequenc before the code for gestational age.

e. Low birth weight and immaturity status

Codes from category P07, Disorders of newborn related to short gestation a low birth weight, not elsewhere classified, are for use for a child or adult w was premature or had a low birth weight as a newborn and this is affecting patient's current health status.

See Section I.C.21. Factors influencing health status and contact with hea services, Status.

f. Bacterial Sepsis of Newborn

Category P36, Bacterial sepsis of newborn, includes congenital sepsis. I perinate is documented as having sepsis without documentation of congeni or community acquired, the default is congenital and a code from catego P36 should be assigned. If the P36 code includes the causal organism, additional code from category B95, Streptococcus, Staphylococcus, a Enterococcus as the cause of diseases classified elsewhere, or B96, Ot bacterial agents as the cause of diseases classified elsewhere, should not assigned. If the P36 code does not include the causal organism, assign additional code from category B96. If applicable, use additional codes identify severe sepsis (R65.2-) and any associated acute organ dysfunction

g. Stillbirth

Code P95, Stillbirth, is only for use in institutions that maintain separ records for stillbirths. No other code should be used with P95. Code P should not be used on the mother's record.

Newborn affected by maternal factors and by complications of pregnancy, labor, and delivery (P00-P04)

NOTE These codes are for use when the listed maternal conditions are specified as the cause of confirmed morbidity or potential morbidity which have their origin in the perinatal period (before birth through the first 28 days after birth).

AHA CC: 4Q, 2016, 54-55

P00 Newborn affected by maternal conditions that may be unrelated to present pregnancy

Code first any current condition in newborn

Excludes2: *encounter for observation for newborn for suspected diseases and conditions ruled out (Z05.-)*
newborn affected by maternal complications of pregnancy (P01.-)
newborn affected by maternal endocrine and metabolic disorders (P70-P74)
newborn affected by noxious substances transmitted via placenta or breast milk (P04.-)

P00.0 Newborn affected by maternal hypertensive disorders
Newborn affected by maternal conditions classifiable to O10-O11, O13-O16

P00.1 Newborn affected by maternal renal and urinary tract diseases
Newborn affected by maternal conditions classifiable to N00-N39

P00.2 Newborn affected by maternal infectious and parasitic diseases
Newborn affected by maternal infectious disease classifiable to A00-B99, J09 and J10
Excludes1: *maternal genital tract or other localized infections (P00.8)*
Excludes2: *infections specific to the perinatal period (P35-P39)*
AHA CC: 3Q, 2015, 20

P00.3 Newborn affected by other maternal circulatory and respiratory diseases
Newborn affected by maternal conditions classifiable to I00-I99, J00-J99, Q20-Q34 and not included in P00.0, P00.2

P00.4 Newborn affected by maternal nutritional disorders
Newborn affected by maternal disorders classifiable to E40-E64
Maternal malnutrition NOS

P00.5 Newborn affected by maternal injury
Newborn affected by maternal conditions classifiable to O9A.2-

P00.6 Newborn affected by surgical procedure on mother
Newborn affected by amniocentesis
Excludes1: *Cesarean delivery for present delivery (P03.4)*
damage to placenta from amniocentesis, Cesarean delivery or surgical induction (P02.1)
previous surgery to uterus or pelvic organs (P03.89)
Excludes2: *newborn affected by complication of (fetal) intrauterine procedure (P96.5)*

P00.7 Newborn affected by other medical procedures on mother, not elsewhere classified
Newborn affected by radiation to mother
Excludes1: *damage to placenta from amniocentesis, cesarean delivery or surgical induction (P02.1)*
newborn affected by other complications of labor and delivery (P03.-)

+ **P00.8 Newborn affected by other maternal conditions**
P00.81 Newborn affected by periodontal disease in mother
P00.89 Newborn affected by other maternal conditions
Newborn affected by conditions classifiable to T80-T88
Newborn affected by maternal genital tract or other localized infections
Newborn affected by maternal systemic lupus erythematosus

P00.9 Newborn affected by unspecified maternal condition

P01 Newborn affected by maternal complications of pregnancy

Code first any current condition in newborn

Excludes2: *encounter for observation of newborn for suspected diseases and conditions ruled out (Z05.-)*

P01.0 Newborn affected by incompetent cervix

P01.1 Newborn affected by premature rupture of membranes

P01.2 Newborn affected by oligohydramnios
Excludes1: *oligohydramnios due to premature rupture of membranes (P01.1)*

P01.3 Newborn affected by polyhydramnios
Newborn affected by hydramnios

P01.4 Newborn affected by ectopic pregnancy
Newborn affected by abdominal pregnancy

P01.5 Newborn affected by multiple pregnancy
Newborn affected by triplet (pregnancy)
Newborn affected by twin (pregnancy)

P01.6 Newborn affected by maternal death

P01.7 Newborn affected by malpresentation before labor
Newborn affected by breech presentation before labor
Newborn affected by external version before labor
Newborn affected by face presentation before labor
Newborn affected by transverse lie before labor
Newborn affected by unstable lie before labor

P01.8 Newborn affected by other maternal complications of pregnancy

P01.9 Newborn affected by maternal complication of pregnancy, unspecified

P02 Newborn affected by complications of placenta, cord and membranes

Code first any current condition in newborn

Excludes2: *encounter for observation of newborn for suspected diseases and conditions ruled out (Z05.-)*

P02.0 Newborn affected by placenta previa

P02.1 Newborn affected by other forms of placental separation and hemorrhage
Newborn affected by abruptio placenta
Newborn affected by accidental hemorrhage
Newborn affected by antepartum hemorrhage
Newborn affected by damage to placenta from amniocentesis, cesarean delivery or surgical induction
Newborn affected by maternal blood loss
Newborn affected by premature separation of placenta

+ **P02.2 Newborn affected by other and unspecified morphological and functional abnormalities of placenta**
P02.20 Newborn affected by unspecified morphological and functional abnormalities of placenta
P02.29 Newborn affected by other morphological and functional abnormalities of placenta
Newborn affected by placental dysfunction
Newborn affected by placental infarction
Newborn affected by placental insufficiency

P02.3 Newborn affected by placental transfusion syndromes
Newborn affected by placental and cord abnormalities resulting in twin-to-twin or other transplacental transfusion

P02.4 Newborn affected by prolapsed cord

P02.5 Newborn affected by other compression of umbilical cord
Newborn affected by umbilical cord (tightly) around neck
Newborn affected by entanglement of umbilical cord
Newborn affected by knot in umbilical cord

+ **P02.6 Newborn affected by other and unspecified conditions of umbilical cord**
P02.60 Newborn affected by unspecified conditions of umbilical cord
P02.69 Newborn affected by other conditions of umbilical cord
Newborn affected by short umbilical cord
Newborn affected by vasa previa
Excludes1: *newborn affected by single umbilical artery (Q27.0)*

P02.7 Newborn affected by chorioamnionitis
Newborn affected by amnionitis
Newborn affected by membranitis
Newborn affected by placentitis

P02.8 Newborn affected by other abnormalities of membranes

P02.9 Newborn affected by abnormality of membranes, unspecified

P03 Newborn affected by other complications of labor and delivery

Code first any current condition in newborn

Excludes2: *encounter for observation of newborn for suspected diseases and conditions ruled out (Z05.-)*

P03.0 Newborn affected by breech delivery and extraction

P03.1 Newborn affected by other malpresentation, malposition and disproportion during labor and delivery

Newborn affected by contracted pelvis
Newborn affected by conditions classifiable to O64-O66
Newborn affected by persistent occipitoposterior
Newborn affected by transverse lie

P03.2 Newborn affected by forceps delivery

P03.3 Newborn affected by delivery by vacuum extractor [ventouse]

P03.4 Newborn affected by Cesarean delivery

P03.5 Newborn affected by precipitate delivery

Newborn affected by rapid second stage

P03.6 Newborn affected by abnormal uterine contractions

Newborn affected by conditions classifiable to O62.-, except O62.3
Newborn affected by hypertonic labor
Newborn affected by uterine inertia

\+ **P03.8 Newborn affected by other specified complications of labor and delivery**

\+ **P03.81 Newborn affected by abnormality in fetal (intrauterine) heart rate or rhythm**

Excludes1: *neonatal cardiac dysrhythmia (P29.1-)*

P03.810 Newborn affected by abnormality in fetal (intrauterine) heart rate or rhythm before the onset of labor

P03.811 Newborn affected by abnormality in fetal (intrauterine) heart rate or rhythm during labor

P03.819 Newborn affected by abnormality in fetal (intrauterine) heart rate or rhythm, unspecified as to time of onset

P03.82 Meconium passage during delivery

Excludes1: *meconium aspiration (P24.00, P24.01)*
meconium staining (P96.83)

P03.89 Newborn affected by other specified complications of labor and delivery

Newborn affected by abnormality of maternal soft tissues
Newborn affected by conditions classifiable to O60-O75 and by procedures used in labor and delivery not included in P02.- and P03.0-P03.6
Newborn affected by induction of labor

P03.9 Newborn affected by complication of labor and delivery, unspecified

P04 Newborn affected by noxious substances transmitted via placenta or breast milk

Includes: nonteratogenic effects of substances transmitted via placenta

Excludes2: *congenital malformations (Q00-Q99)*
encounter for observation of newborn for suspected diseases and conditions ruled out (Z05.-)
neonatal jaundice from excessive hemolysis due to drugs or toxins transmitted from mother (P58.4)
newborn in contact with and (suspected) exposures hazardous to health not transmitted via placenta or breast milk (Z77.-)

P04.0 Newborn affected by maternal anesthesia and analgesia in pregnancy, labor and delivery

Newborn affected by reactions and intoxications from maternal opiates and tranquilizers administered during labor and delivery

P04.1 Newborn affected by other maternal medication

Newborn affected by cancer chemotherapy
Newborn affected by cytotoxic drugs

Excludes1: *dysmorphism due to warfarin (Q86.2)*
fetal hydantoin syndrome (Q86.1)
maternal use of drugs of addiction (P04.4-)

AHA CC: 4Q, 2016, 54-55

P04.2 Newborn affected by maternal use of tobacco

Newborn affected by exposure in utero to tobacco smoke

Excludes2: *newborn exposure to environmental tobacco smoke (P96.81)*

P04.3 Newborn affected by maternal use of alcohol

Excludes1: *fetal alcohol syndrome (Q86.0)*

\+ **P04.4 Newborn affected by maternal use of drugs of addiction**

P04.41 Newborn affected by maternal use of cocaine

'Crack baby'

P04.49 Newborn affected by maternal use of other drugs of addiction

Excludes2: *newborn affected by maternal anesthesia and analgesia (P04.0)*
withdrawal symptoms from maternal use of drugs of addiction (P96.1)

P04.5 Newborn affected by maternal use of nutritional chemical substances

P04.6 Newborn affected by maternal exposure to environmental chemical substances

P04.8 Newborn affected by other maternal noxious substances

P04.9 Newborn affected by maternal noxious substance, unspecified

Disorders of newborn related to length of gestation and fetal growth (P05-P08)

P05 Disorders of newborn related to slow fetal growth and fetal malnutrition

Review coding guideline C.16.d

\+ **P05.0 Newborn light for gestational age**

Newborn light-for-dates
Weight below but length above 10th percentile for gestational age

P05.00 Newborn light for gestational age, unspecified weight

P05.01 Newborn light for gestational age, less than 500 grams

P05.02 Newborn light for gestational age, 500-749 grams

P05.03 Newborn light for gestational age, 750-999 grams

P05.04 Newborn light for gestational age, 1000-1249 grams

P05.05 Newborn light for gestational age, 1250-1499 grams

P05.06 Newborn light for gestational age, 1500-1749 grams

P05.07 Newborn light for gestational age, 1750-1999 grams

P05.08 Newborn light for gestational age, 2000-2499 grams

P05.09 Newborn light for gestational age, 2500 grams and over

Newborn light for gestational age, other

AHA CC: 4Q, 2016, 55-56

\+ **P05.1 Newborn small for gestational age**

Newborn small-and-light-for-dates
Newborn small-for-dates
Weight and length below 10th percentile for gestational age

P05.10 Newborn small for gestational age, unspecified weight

P05.11 Newborn small for gestational age, less than 500 grams

P05.12 Newborn small for gestational age, 500-749 grams

P05.13 Newborn small for gestational age, 750-999 grams

P05.14 Newborn small for gestational age, 1000-1249 grams

P05.15 Newborn small for gestational age, 1250-1499 grams

P05.16 Newborn small for gestational age, 1500-1749 grams

P05.17 Newborn small for gestational age, 1750-1999 grams

P05.18 Newborn small for gestational age, 2000-2499 grams

P05.19 Newborn small for gestational age, other

Newborn small for gestational age, 2500 grams and over

AHA CC: 4Q, 2016, 55-56

P05.2 Newborn affected by fetal (intrauterine) malnutrition not light or small for gestational age
Infant, not light or small for gestational age, showing signs of fetal malnutrition, such as dry, peeling skin and loss of subcutaneous tissue
Excludes1: *newborn affected by fetal malnutrition with light for gestational age (P05.0-)*
newborn affected by fetal malnutrition with small for gestational age (P05.1-)

P05.9 Newborn affected by slow intrauterine growth, unspecified
Newborn affected by fetal growth retardation NOS

P07 Disorders of newborn related to short gestation and low birth weight, not elsewhere classified

NOTE When both birth weight and gestational age of the newborn are available, both should be coded with birth weight sequenced before gestational age

Includes: the listed conditions, without further specification, as the cause of morbidity or additional care, in newborn

Review coding guidelines C.16.d and C.16.e

\+ **P07.0 Extremely low birth weight newborn**
Newborn birth weight 999 g. or less
Excludes1: low birth weight due to slow fetal growth and fetal malnutrition (P05.-)

P07.00 Extremely low birth weight newborn, unspecified weight
P07.01 Extremely low birth weight newborn, less than 500 grams
P07.02 Extremely low birth weight newborn, 500-749 grams
P07.03 Extremely low birth weight newborn, 750-999 grams

\+ **P07.1 Other low birth weight newborn**
Newborn birth weight 1000-2499 g.
Excludes1: low birth weight due to slow fetal growth and fetal malnutrition (P05.-)

P07.10 Other low birth weight newborn, unspecified weight
P07.14 Other low birth weight newborn, 1000-1249 grams
P07.15 Other low birth weight newborn, 1250-1499 grams
P07.16 Other low birth weight newborn, 1500-1749 grams
P07.17 Other low birth weight newborn, 1750-1999 grams
P07.18 Other low birth weight newborn, 2000-2499 grams

\+ **P07.2 Extreme immaturity of newborn**
Less than 28 completed weeks (less than 196 completed days) of gestation.

P07.20 Extreme immaturity of newborn, unspecified weeks of gestation
Gestational age less than 28 completed weeks NOS

P07.21 Extreme immaturity of newborn, gestational age less than 23 completed weeks
Extreme immaturity of newborn, gestational age less than 23 weeks, 0 days

P07.22 Extreme immaturity of newborn, gestational age 23 completed weeks
Extreme immaturity of newborn, gestational age 23 weeks, 0 days through 23 weeks, 6 days

P07.23 Extreme immaturity of newborn, gestational age 24 completed weeks
Extreme immaturity of newborn, gestational age 24 weeks, 0 days through 24 weeks, 6 days

P07.24 Extreme immaturity of newborn, gestational age 25 completed weeks
Extreme immaturity of newborn, gestational age 25 weeks, 0 days through 25 weeks, 6 days

P07.25 Extreme immaturity of newborn, gestational age 26 completed weeks
Extreme immaturity of newborn, gestational age 26 weeks, 0 days through 26 weeks, 6 days

P07.26 Extreme immaturity of newborn, gestational age 27 completed weeks
Extreme immaturity of newborn, gestational age 27 weeks, 0 days through 27 weeks, 6 days

\+ **P07.3 Preterm [premature] newborn [other]**
28 completed weeks or more but less than 37 completed weeks (196 completed days but less than 259 completed days) of gestation.
Prematurity NOS

P07.30 Preterm newborn, unspecified weeks of gestation
P07.31 Preterm newborn, gestational age 28 completed weeks
Preterm newborn, gestational age 28 weeks, 0 days through 28 weeks, 6 days

P07.32 Preterm newborn, gestational age 29 completed weeks
Preterm newborn, gestational age 29 weeks, 0 days through 29 weeks, 6 days

P07.33 Preterm newborn, gestational age 30 completed weeks
Preterm newborn, gestational age 30 weeks, 0 days through 30 weeks, 6 days

P07.34 Preterm newborn, gestational age 31 completed weeks
Preterm newborn, gestational age 31 weeks, 0 days through 31 weeks, 6 days

P07.35 Preterm newborn, gestational age 32 completed weeks
Preterm newborn, gestational age 32 weeks, 0 days through 32 weeks, 6 days

P07.36 Preterm newborn, gestational age 33 completed weeks
Preterm newborn, gestational age 33 weeks, 0 days through 33 weeks, 6 days

P07.37 Preterm newborn, gestational age 34 completed weeks
Preterm newborn, gestational age 34 weeks, 0 days through 34 weeks, 6 days
AHA CC: 2Q, 2017, 7

P07.38 Preterm newborn, gestational age 35 completed weeks
Preterm newborn, gestational age 35 weeks, 0 days through 35 weeks, 6 days

P07.39 Preterm newborn, gestational age 36 completed weeks
Preterm newborn, gestational age 36 weeks, 0 days through 36 weeks, 6 days

P08 Disorders of newborn related to long gestation and high birth weight

NOTE When both birth weight and gestational age of the newborn are available, priority of assignment should be given to birth weight

Includes: the listed conditions, without further specification, as causes of morbidity or additional care, in newborn

P08.0 Exceptionally large newborn baby
Usually implies a birth weight of 4500 g. or more
Excludes1: *syndrome of infant of diabetic mother (P70.1)*
syndrome of infant of mother with gestational diabetes (P70.0)

P08.1 Other heavy for gestational age newborn
Other newborn heavy- or large-for-dates regardless of period of gestation
Usually implies a birth weight of 4000 g. to 4499 g.
Excludes1: *newborn with a birth weight of 4500 or more (P08.0)*
syndrome of infant of diabetic mother (P70.1)
syndrome of infant of mother with gestational diabetes (P70.0).

\+ **P08.2 Late newborn, not heavy for gestational age**

P08.21 Post-term newborn
Newborn with gestation period over 40 completed weeks to 42 completed weeks
AHA CC: 1Q, 2014, 14

P08.22 Prolonged gestation of newborn
Newborn with gestation period over 42 completed weeks (294 days or more), not heavy- or large-for-dates.
Postmaturity NOS
AHA CC: 1Q, 2014, 14

Abnormal findings on neonatal screening (P09)

P09 Abnormal findings on neonatal screening

Use additional code to identify signs, symptoms and conditions associated with the screening

Excludes2: *nonspecific serologic evidence of human immunodeficiency virus [HIV] (R75)*

Valid 3-character code, no further characters required

Birth trauma (P10-P15)

P10 Intracranial laceration and hemorrhage due to birth injury

Excludes1: *intracranial hemorrhage of newborn NOS (P52.9)*
intracranial hemorrhage of newborn due to anoxia or hypoxia (P52.-)
nontraumatic intracranial hemorrhage of newborn (P52.-)

MCC **P10.0 Subdural hemorrhage due to birth injury**
Subdural hematoma (localized) due to birth injury
Excludes1: *subdural hemorrhage accompanying tentorial tear (P10.4)*
MCC Exclusion see Appendix A PDX collection 1020

MCC **P10.1 Cerebral hemorrhage due to birth injury**
MCC Exclusion see Appendix A PDX collection 1020

CC **P10.2 Intraventricular hemorrhage due to birth injury**
CC Exclusion see Appendix A PDX collection 1021

MCC **P10.3 Subarachnoid hemorrhage due to birth injury**
MCC Exclusion see Appendix A PDX collection 1022

MCC **P10.4 Tentorial tear due to birth injury**
MCC Exclusion see Appendix A PDX collection 1020

MCC **P10.8 Other intracranial lacerations and hemorrhages due to birth injury**
MCC Exclusion see Appendix A PDX collection 1020

MCC **P10.9 Unspecified intracranial laceration and hemorrhage due to birth injury**
MCC Exclusion see Appendix A PDX collection 1020

P11 Other birth injuries to central nervous system

MCC **P11.0 Cerebral edema due to birth injury**
MCC Exclusion see Appendix A PDX collection 1020

P11.1 Other specified brain damage due to birth injury

MCC **P11.2 Unspecified brain damage due to birth injury**
MCC Exclusion see Appendix A PDX collection 1020

P11.3 Birth injury to facial nerve
Facial palsy due to birth injury

P11.4 Birth injury to other cranial nerves

P11.5 Birth injury to spine and spinal cord
Fracture of spine due to birth injury

MCC **P11.9 Birth injury to central nervous system, unspecified**
MCC Exclusion see Appendix A PDX collection 1020

P12 Birth injury to scalp

P12.0 Cephalhematoma due to birth injury

P12.1 Chignon (from vacuum extraction) due to birth injury

CC **P12.2 Epicranial subaponeurotic hemorrhage due to birth injury**
Subgaleal hemorrhage
CC Exclusion see Appendix A PDX collection 1023

P12.3 Bruising of scalp due to birth injury

P12.4 Injury of scalp of newborn due to monitoring equipment
Sampling incision of scalp of newborn
Scalp clip (electrode) injury of newborn

\+ **P12.8 Other birth injuries to scalp**
P12.81 Caput succedaneum
P12.89 Other birth injuries to scalp

P12.9 Birth injury to scalp, unspecified

P13 Birth injury to skeleton

Excludes2: *birth injury to spine (P11.5)*

P13.0 Fracture of skull due to birth injury

P13.1 Other birth injuries to skull
Excludes1: *cephalhematoma (P12.0)*

P13.2 Birth injury to femur

P13.3 Birth injury to other long bones

P13.4 Fracture of clavicle due to birth injury

P13.8 Birth injuries to other parts of skeleton

P13.9 Birth injury to skeleton, unspecified

P14 Birth injury to peripheral nervous system

P14.0 Erb's paralysis due to birth injury
P14.1 Klumpke's paralysis due to birth injury
P14.2 Phrenic nerve paralysis due to birth injury
P14.3 Other brachial plexus birth injuries
P14.8 Birth injuries to other parts of peripheral nervous system
P14.9 Birth injury to peripheral nervous system, unspecified

P15 Other birth injuries

P15.0 Birth injury to liver
Rupture of liver due to birth injury

P15.1 Birth injury to spleen
Rupture of spleen due to birth injury

P15.2 Sternomastoid injury due to birth injury

P15.3 Birth injury to eye
Subconjunctival hemorrhage due to birth injury
Traumatic glaucoma due to birth injury

P15.4 Birth injury to face
Facial congestion due to birth injury

P15.5 Birth injury to external genitalia
P15.6 Subcutaneous fat necrosis due to birth injury
P15.8 Other specified birth injuries
P15.9 Birth injury, unspecified

Respiratory and cardiovascular disorders specific to the perinatal period (P19-P29)

P19 Metabolic acidemia in newborn

Includes: metabolic acidemia in newborn

P19.0 Metabolic acidemia in newborn first noted before onset of labor
P19.1 Metabolic acidemia in newborn first noted during labor
P19.2 Metabolic acidemia noted at birth
P19.9 Metabolic acidemia, unspecified

P22 Respiratory distress of newborn

Excludes1: *respiratory arrest of newborn (P28.81)*
respiratory failure of newborn NOS (P28.5)

MCC **P22.0 Respiratory distress syndrome of newborn**
Cardiorespiratory distress syndrome of newborn
Hyaline membrane disease
Idiopathic respiratory distress syndrome [IRDS or RDS] of newborn
Pulmonary hypoperfusion syndrome
Respiratory distress syndrome, type I
MCC Exclusion see Appendix A PDX collection 0748

P22.1 Transient tachypnea of newborn
Idiopathic tachypnea of newborn
Respiratory distress syndrome, type II
Wet lung syndrome

P22.8 Other respiratory distress of newborn
P22.9 Respiratory distress of newborn, unspecified

P23 Congenital pneumonia

Includes: infective pneumonia acquired in utero or during birth
Excludes1: *neonatal pneumonia resulting from aspiration (P24.-)*

MCC **P23.0 Congenital pneumonia due to viral agent**
Use additional code (B97) to identify organism
Excludes1: *congenital rubella pneumonitis (P35.0)*
MCC Exclusion see Appendix A PDX collection 0748

MCC **P23.1 Congenital pneumonia due to Chlamydia**
MCC Exclusion see Appendix A PDX collection 0748

MCC **P23.2 Congenital pneumonia due to staphylococcus**
MCC Exclusion see Appendix A PDX collection 0748

MCC **P23.3 Congenital pneumonia due to streptococcus, group B**
MCC Exclusion see Appendix A PDX collection 0748

MCC **P23.4 Congenital pneumonia due to Escherichia coli**
MCC Exclusion see Appendix A PDX collection 0748

P23.5 Congenital pneumonia due to Pseudomonas

MCC **P23.6 Congenital pneumonia due to other bacterial agents**
Congenital pneumonia due to Hemophilus influenzae
Congenital pneumonia due to Klebsiella pneumoniae
Congenital pneumonia due to Mycoplasma
Congenital pneumonia due to Streptococcus, except group B
Use additional code (B95-B96) to identify organism
MCC Exclusion see Appendix A PDX collection 0748

MCC **P23.8 Congenital pneumonia due to other organisms**
MCC Exclusion see Appendix A PDX collection 0748

MCC **P23.9 Congenital pneumonia, unspecified**
MCC Exclusion see Appendix A PDX collection 0748

P24 Neonatal aspiration

Includes: aspiration in utero and during delivery

\+ **P24.0 Meconium aspiration**

Excludes1: *meconium passage (without aspiration) during delivery (P03.82)*
meconium staining (P96.83)

P24.00 Meconium aspiration without respiratory symptoms
Meconium aspiration NOS

MCC **P24.01 Meconium aspiration with respiratory symptoms**
Meconium aspiration pneumonia
Meconium aspiration pneumonitis
Meconium aspiration syndrome NOS
Use additional code to identify any secondary pulmonary hypertension, if applicable (I27.2-)
MCC Exclusion see Appendix A PDX collection 0748

\+ **P24.1 Neonatal aspiration of (clear) amniotic fluid and mucus**
Neonatal aspiration of liquor (amnii)

P24.10 Neonatal aspiration of (clear) amniotic fluid and mucus without respiratory symptoms
Neonatal aspiration of amniotic fluid and mucus NOS

MCC **P24.11 Neonatal aspiration of (clear) amniotic fluid and mucus with respiratory symptoms**
Neonatal aspiration of amniotic fluid and mucus with pneumonia
Neonatal aspiration of amniotic fluid and mucus with pneumonitis
Use additional code to identify any secondary pulmonary hypertension, if applicable (I27.2-)
MCC Exclusion see Appendix A PDX collection 0748

\+ **P24.2 Neonatal aspiration of blood**

P24.20 Neonatal aspiration of blood without respiratory symptoms
Neonatal aspiration of blood NOS

MCC **P24.21 Neonatal aspiration of blood with respiratory symptoms**
Neonatal aspiration of blood with pneumonia
Neonatal aspiration of blood with pneumonitis
Use additional code to identify any secondary pulmonary hypertension, if applicable (I27.2-)
MCC Exclusion see Appendix A PDX collection 0748

\+ **P24.3 Neonatal aspiration of milk and regurgitated food**
Neonatal aspiration of stomach contents

P24.30 Neonatal aspiration of milk and regurgitated food without respiratory symptoms
Neonatal aspiration of milk and regurgitated food NOS

MCC **P24.31 Neonatal aspiration of milk and regurgitated food with respiratory symptoms**
Neonatal aspiration of milk and regurgitated food with pneumonia
Neonatal aspiration of milk and regurgitated food with pneumonitis
Use additional code to identify any secondary pulmonary hypertension, if applicable (I27.2-)
MCC Exclusion see Appendix A PDX collection 0748

\+ **P24.8 Other neonatal aspiration**

P24.80 Other neonatal aspiration without respiratory symptoms
Neonatal aspiration NEC

MCC **P24.81 Other neonatal aspiration with respiratory symptoms**
Neonatal aspiration pneumonia NEC
Neonatal aspiration with pneumonitis NEC
Neonatal aspiration with pneumonia NOS
Neonatal aspiration with pneumonitis NOS
Use additional code to identify any secondary pulmonary hypertension, if applicable (I27.2-)
MCC Exclusion see Appendix A PDX collection 0748

P24.9 Neonatal aspiration, unspecified

P25 Interstitial emphysema and related conditions originating in the perinatal period

MCC **P25.0 Interstitial emphysema originating in the perinatal period**
MCC Exclusion see Appendix A PDX collection 0748

MCC **P25.1 Pneumothorax originating in the perinatal period**
MCC Exclusion see Appendix A PDX collection 0748

MCC **P25.2 Pneumomediastinum originating in the perinatal period**
MCC Exclusion see Appendix A PDX collection 0748

MCC **P25.3 Pneumopericardium originating in the perinatal period**
MCC Exclusion see Appendix A PDX collection 0748

MCC **P25.8 Other conditions related to interstitial emphysema originating in the perinatal period**
MCC Exclusion see Appendix A PDX collection 0748

P26 Pulmonary hemorrhage originating in the perinatal period

Excludes1: *acute idiopathic hemorrhage in infants over 28 days old (R04.81)*

MCC **P26.0 Tracheobronchial hemorrhage originating in the perinatal period**
MCC Exclusion see Appendix A PDX collection 0748

MCC **P26.1 Massive pulmonary hemorrhage originating in the perinatal period**
MCC Exclusion see Appendix A PDX collection 0748

MCC **P26.8 Other pulmonary hemorrhages originating in the perinatal period**
MCC Exclusion see Appendix A PDX collection 0748

MCC **P26.9 Unspecified pulmonary hemorrhage originating in the perinatal period**
MCC Exclusion see Appendix A PDX collection 0748

P27 Chronic respiratory disease originating in the perinatal period

Excludes2: *respiratory distress of newborn (P22.0-P22.9)*

MCC **P27.0 Wilson-Mikity syndrome**
Pulmonary dysmaturity
MCC Exclusion see Appendix A PDX collection 0748

MCC **P27.1 Bronchopulmonary dysplasia originating in the perinatal period**
MCC Exclusion see Appendix A PDX collection 0748

MCC **P27.8 Other chronic respiratory diseases originating in the perinatal period**
Congenital pulmonary fibrosis
Ventilator lung in newborn
MCC Exclusion see Appendix A PDX collection 0748

MCC **P27.9 Unspecified chronic respiratory disease originating in the perinatal period**
MCC Exclusion see Appendix A PDX collection 0748

P28 Other respiratory conditions originating in the perinatal period

Excludes1: *congenital malformations of the respiratory system (Q30-Q34)*

CC **P28.0 Primary atelectasis of newborn**
Primary failure to expand terminal respiratory units
Pulmonary hypoplasia associated with short gestation
Pulmonary immaturity NOS
CC Exclusion see Appendix A PDX collection 0748

\+ **P28.1 Other and unspecified atelectasis of newborn**

CC **P28.10 Unspecified atelectasis of newborn**
Atelectasis of newborn NOS
CC Exclusion see Appendix A PDX collection 0748

CC **P28.11 Resorption atelectasis without respiratory distress syndrome**
Excludes1: *resorption atelectasis with respiratory distress syndrome (P22.0)*
CC Exclusion see Appendix A PDX collection 0748

CC **P28.19 Other atelectasis of newborn**
Partial atelectasis of newborn
Secondary atelectasis of newborn
CC Exclusion see Appendix A PDX collection 0748

CC **P28.2 Cyanotic attacks of newborn**
Excludes1: *apnea of newborn (P28.3-P28.4)*
CC Exclusion see Appendix A PDX collection 1024

CC **P28.3 Primary sleep apnea of newborn**
Central sleep apnea of newborn
Obstructive sleep apnea of newborn
Sleep apnea of newborn NOS
CC Exclusion see Appendix A PDX collection 1025

CC **P28.4 Other apnea of newborn**
Apnea of prematurity
Obstructive apnea of newborn
Excludes1: *obstructive sleep apnea of newborn (P28.3)*
CC Exclusion see Appendix A PDX collection 1026

MCC **P28.5 Respiratory failure of newborn**
Excludes1: *respiratory arrest of newborn (P28.81)*
respiratory distress of newborn (P22.0-)
MCC Exclusion see Appendix A PDX collection 0748

+ **P28.8 Other specified respiratory conditions of newborn**
  - MCC **P28.81 Respiratory arrest of newborn**
    - **MCC Exclusion see Appendix A PDX collection 1027**
    - *AHA CC: 2Q, 2017, 6-7*
  - **P28.89 Other specified respiratory conditions of newborn**
    - Congenital laryngeal stridor
    - Sniffles in newborn
    - Snuffles in newborn
    - ***Excludes1:*** *early congenital syphilitic rhinitis (A50.05)*
- **P28.9 Respiratory condition of newborn, unspecified**
  - Respiratory depression in newborn

P29 Cardiovascular disorders originating in the perinatal period

Excludes1: *congenital malformations of the circulatory system (Q20-Q28)*

- **P29.0 Neonatal cardiac failure**
- + **P29.1 Neonatal cardiac dysrhythmia**
  - **P29.11 Neonatal tachycardia**
  - **P29.12 Neonatal bradycardia**
- **P29.2 Neonatal hypertension**
- + **P29.3 Persistent fetal circulation**
  - MCC **P29.30 Pulmonary hypertension of newborn**
    - Persistent pulmonary hypertension of newborn
    - **MCC Exclusion see Appendix A PDX collection 1028**
  - MCC **P29.38 Other persistent fetal circulation**
    - Delayed closure of ductus arteriosus
    - **MCC Exclusion see Appendix A PDX collection 1028**
- **P29.4 Transient myocardial ischemia in newborn**
- + **P29.8 Other cardiovascular disorders originating in the perinatal period**
  - MCC **P29.81 Cardiac arrest of newborn**
    - **MCC Exclusion see Appendix A PDX collection 1029**
  - **P29.89 Other cardiovascular disorders originating in the perinatal period**
    - *AHA CC: 4Q, 2014, 23*
- **P29.9 Cardiovascular disorder originating in the perinatal period, unspecified**

Infections specific to the perinatal period (P35-P39)

Infections acquired in utero, during birth via the umbilicus, or during the first 28 days after birth

Excludes2: *asymptomatic human immunodeficiency virus [HIV] infection status (Z21)*
congenital gonococcal infection (A54.-)
congenital pneumonia (P23.-)
congenital syphilis (A50.-)
human immunodeficiency virus [HIV] disease (B20)
infant botulism (A48.51)
infectious diseases not specific to the perinatal period (A00-B99, J09, J10.-)
intestinal infectious disease (A00-A09)
laboratory evidence of human immunodeficiency virus [HIV] (R75)
tetanus neonatorum (A33)

P35 Congenital viral diseases

Includes: infections acquired in utero or during birth

- CC **P35.0 Congenital rubella syndrome**
  - Congenital rubella pneumonitis
  - **CC Exclusion see Appendix A PDX collection 1030**
- MCC **P35.1 Congenital cytomegalovirus infection**
  - **MCC Exclusion see Appendix A PDX collection 1030**
- MCC **P35.2 Congenital herpesviral [herpes simplex] infection**
  - **MCC Exclusion see Appendix A PDX collection 0562**
- MCC **P35.3 Congenital viral hepatitis**
  - **MCC Exclusion see Appendix A PDX collection 0562**
- MCC **P35.8 Other congenital viral diseases**
  - Congenital varicella [chickenpox]
  - **MCC Exclusion see Appendix A PDX collection 0562**
  - *AHA CC: 4Q, 2016, 4-7*
- MCC **P35.9 Congenital viral disease, unspecified**
  - **MCC Exclusion see Appendix A PDX collection 0562**

P36 Bacterial sepsis of newborn

Includes: congenital sepsis

Use additional code(s), if applicable, to identify severe sepsis (R65.2-) and associated acute organ dysfunction(s)

Review coding guideline C.1.d and C.16.f

- MCC **P36.0 Sepsis of newborn due to streptococcus, group B**
  - **MCC Exclusion see Appendix A PDX collection 1031**
- + **P36.1 Sepsis of newborn due to other and unspecified streptococci**
  - MCC **P36.10 Sepsis of newborn due to unspecified streptococci**
    - **MCC Exclusion see Appendix A PDX collection 1031**
  - MCC **P36.19 Sepsis of newborn due to other streptococci**
    - **MCC Exclusion see Appendix A PDX collection 1031**
- MCC **P36.2 Sepsis of newborn due to Staphylococcus aureus**
  - **MCC Exclusion see Appendix A PDX collection 1031**
- + **P36.3 Sepsis of newborn due to other and unspecified staphylococci**
  - MCC **P36.30 Sepsis of newborn due to unspecified staphylococci**
    - **MCC Exclusion see Appendix A PDX collection 1031**
  - MCC **P36.39 Sepsis of newborn due to other staphylococci**
    - **MCC Exclusion see Appendix A PDX collection 1031**
- MCC **P36.4 Sepsis of newborn due to Escherichia coli**
  - **MCC Exclusion see Appendix A PDX collection 1031**
- MCC **P36.5 Sepsis of newborn due to anaerobes**
  - **MCC Exclusion see Appendix A PDX collection 1031**
- MCC **P36.8 Other bacterial sepsis of newborn**
  - Use additional code from category B96 to identify organism
  - **MCC Exclusion see Appendix A PDX collection 1031**
- MCC **P36.9 Bacterial sepsis of newborn, unspecified**
  - **MCC Exclusion see Appendix A PDX collection 1031**

P37 Other congenital infectious and parasitic diseases

Excludes2: *congenital syphilis (A50.-)*
infectious neonatal diarrhea (A00-A09)
necrotizing enterocolitis in newborn (P77.-)
noninfectious neonatal diarrhea (P78.3)
ophthalmia neonatorum due to gonococcus (A54.31)
tetanus neonatorum (A33)

- MCC **P37.0 Congenital tuberculosis**
  - **MCC Exclusion see Appendix A PDX collection 0562**
- MCC **P37.1 Congenital toxoplasmosis**
  - Hydrocephalus due to congenital toxoplasmosis
  - **MCC Exclusion see Appendix A PDX collection 0562**
- MCC **P37.2 Neonatal (disseminated) listeriosis**
  - **MCC Exclusion see Appendix A PDX collection 0562**
- MCC **P37.3 Congenital falciparum malaria**
  - **MCC Exclusion see Appendix A PDX collection 0562**
- MCC **P37.4 Other congenital malaria**
  - **MCC Exclusion see Appendix A PDX collection 0562**
- **P37.5 Neonatal candidiasis**
- MCC **P37.8 Other specified congenital infectious and parasitic diseases**
  - **MCC Exclusion see Appendix A PDX collection 0562**
- MCC **P37.9 Congenital infectious or parasitic disease, unspecified**
  - **MCC Exclusion see Appendix A PDX collection 0562**

P38 Omphalitis of newborn

Excludes1: *omphalitis not of newborn (L08.82)*
tetanus omphalitis (A33)
umbilical hemorrhage of newborn (P51.-)

- CC **P38.1 Omphalitis with mild hemorrhage**
  - **CC Exclusion see Appendix A PDX collection 1032**
- CC **P38.9 Omphalitis without hemorrhage**
  - Omphalitis of newborn NOS
  - **CC Exclusion see Appendix A PDX collection 1032**

P39 Other infections specific to the perinatal period

Use additional code to identify organism or specific infection

- CC **P39.0 Neonatal infective mastitis**
  - ***Excludes1:*** *breast engorgement of newborn (P83.4)*
    noninfective mastitis of newborn (P83.4)
  - **CC Exclusion see Appendix A PDX collection 1032**
- **P39.1 Neonatal conjunctivitis and dacryocystitis**
  - Neonatal chlamydial conjunctivitis
  - Ophthalmia neonatorum NOS
  - ***Excludes1:*** *gonococcal conjunctivitis (A54.31)*
- CC **P39.2 Intra-amniotic infection affecting newborn, not elsewhere classified**
  - **CC Exclusion see Appendix A PDX collection 1034**
- CC **P39.3 Neonatal urinary tract infection**
  - **CC Exclusion see Appendix A PDX collection 1033**
- CC **P39.4 Neonatal skin infection**
  - Neonatal pyoderma
  - ***Excludes1:*** *pemphigus neonatorum (L00)*
    staphylococcal scalded skin syndrome (L00)
  - **CC Exclusion see Appendix A PDX collection 1033**
- CC **P39.8 Other specified infections specific to the perinatal period**
  - **CC Exclusion see Appendix A PDX collection 1033**
- CC **P39.9 Infection specific to the perinatal period, unspecified**
  - **CC Exclusion see Appendix A PDX collection 1033**

Hemorrhagic and hematological disorders of newborn (P50-P61)

Excludes1: *congenital stenosis and stricture of bile ducts (Q44.3)*
Crigler-Najjar syndrome (E80.5)
Dubin-Johnson syndrome (E80.6)
Gilbert syndrome (E80.4)
hereditary hemolytic anemias (D55-D58)

P50 Newborn affected by intrauterine (fetal) blood loss

Excludes1: *congenital anemia from intrauterine (fetal) blood loss (P61.3)*

P50.0 Newborn affected by intrauterine (fetal) blood loss from vasa previa
P50.1 Newborn affected by intrauterine (fetal) blood loss from ruptured cord
P50.2 Newborn affected by intrauterine (fetal) blood loss from placenta
P50.3 Newborn affected by hemorrhage into co-twin
P50.4 Newborn affected by hemorrhage into maternal circulation
P50.5 Newborn affected by intrauterine (fetal) blood loss from cut end of co-twin's cord
P50.8 Newborn affected by other intrauterine (fetal) blood loss
P50.9 Newborn affected by intrauterine (fetal) blood loss, unspecified
Newborn affected by fetal hemorrhage NOS

P51 Umbilical hemorrhage of newborn

Excludes1: *omphalitis with mild hemorrhage (P38.1)*
umbilical hemorrhage from cut end of co-twins cord (P50.5)

P51.0 Massive umbilical hemorrhage of newborn
P51.8 Other umbilical hemorrhages of newborn
Slipped umbilical ligature NOS
P51.9 Umbilical hemorrhage of newborn, unspecified

P52 Intracranial nontraumatic hemorrhage of newborn

Includes: intracranial hemorrhage due to anoxia or hypoxia
Excludes1: *intracranial hemorrhage due to birth injury (P10.-)*
intracranial hemorrhage due to other injury (S06.-)

CC **P52.0 Intraventricular (nontraumatic) hemorrhage, grade 1, of newborn**
Subependymal hemorrhage (without intraventricular extension)
Bleeding into germinal matrix
CC Exclusion see Appendix A PDX collection 1021

CC **P52.1 Intraventricular (nontraumatic) hemorrhage, grade 2, of newborn**
Subependymal hemorrhage with intraventricular extension
Bleeding into ventricle
CC Exclusion see Appendix A PDX collection 1021

\+ **P52.2 Intraventricular (nontraumatic) hemorrhage, grade 3 and grade 4, of newborn**

MCC **P52.21 Intraventricular (nontraumatic) hemorrhage, grade 3, of newborn**
Subependymal hemorrhage with intraventricular extension with enlargement of ventricle
MCC Exclusion see Appendix A PDX collection 1021

MCC **P52.22 Intraventricular (nontraumatic) hemorrhage, grade 4, of newborn**
Bleeding into cerebral cortex
Subependymal hemorrhage with intracerebral extension
MCC Exclusion see Appendix A PDX collection 1021

CC **P52.3 Unspecified intraventricular (nontraumatic) hemorrhage of newborn**
CC Exclusion see Appendix A PDX collection 1021

MCC **P52.4 Intracerebral (nontraumatic) hemorrhage of newborn**
MCC Exclusion see Appendix A PDX collection 1020

MCC **P52.5 Subarachnoid (nontraumatic) hemorrhage of newborn**
MCC Exclusion see Appendix A PDX collection 1022

MCC **P52.6 Cerebellar (nontraumatic) and posterior fossa hemorrhage of newborn**
MCC Exclusion see Appendix A PDX collection 1020

MCC **P52.8 Other intracranial (nontraumatic) hemorrhages of newborn**
MCC Exclusion see Appendix A PDX collection 1020

MCC **P52.9 Intracranial (nontraumatic) hemorrhage of newborn, unspecified**
MCC Exclusion see Appendix A PDX collection 1020

CC **P53 Hemorrhagic disease of newborn**

Vitamin K deficiency of newborn
CC Exclusion see Appendix A PDX collection 1035
Valid 3-character code, no further characters required

P54 Other neonatal hemorrhages

Excludes1: *newborn affected by (intrauterine) blood loss (P50.-)*
pulmonary hemorrhage originating in the perinatal period (P26.-)

P54.0 Neonatal hematemesis
Excludes1: *neonatal hematemesis due to swallowed maternal blood (P78.2)*

MCC **P54.1 Neonatal melena**
Excludes1: *neonatal melena due to swallowed maternal blood (P78.2)*
MCC Exclusion see Appendix A PDX collection 1036

MCC **P54.2 Neonatal rectal hemorrhage**
MCC Exclusion see Appendix A PDX collection 1036

MCC **P54.3 Other neonatal gastrointestinal hemorrhage**
MCC Exclusion see Appendix A PDX collection 1036

CC **P54.4 Neonatal adrenal hemorrhage**
CC Exclusion see Appendix A PDX collection 1036

P54.5 Neonatal cutaneous hemorrhage
Neonatal bruising
Neonatal ecchymoses
Neonatal petechiae
Neonatal superficial hematomata
Excludes2: *bruising of scalp due to birth injury (P12.3)*
cephalhematoma due to birth injury (P12.0)

♀ **P54.6 Neonatal vaginal hemorrhage**
Neonatal pseudomenses

P54.8 Other specified neonatal hemorrhages
P54.9 Neonatal hemorrhage, unspecified

P55 Hemolytic disease of newborn

P55.0 Rh isoimmunization of newborn
P55.1 ABO isoimmunization of newborn
AHA CC: 3Q, 2015, 20
P55.8 Other hemolytic diseases of newborn
P55.9 Hemolytic disease of newborn, unspecified

P56 Hydrops fetalis due to hemolytic disease

Excludes1: *hydrops fetalis NOS (P83.2)*

MCC **P56.0 Hydrops fetalis due to isoimmunization**
MCC Exclusion see Appendix A PDX collection 1037

\+ **P56.9 Hydrops fetalis due to other and unspecified hemolytic disease**

MCC **P56.90 Hydrops fetalis due to unspecified hemolytic disease**
MCC Exclusion see Appendix A PDX collection 1037

MCC **P56.99 Hydrops fetalis due to other hemolytic disease**
MCC Exclusion see Appendix A PDX collection 1037

P57 Kernicterus

MCC **P57.0 Kernicterus due to isoimmunization**
MCC Exclusion see Appendix A PDX collection 1037

MCC **P57.8 Other specified kernicterus**
Excludes1: *Crigler-Najjar syndrome (E80.5)*
MCC Exclusion see Appendix A PDX collection 1038

MCC **P57.9 Kernicterus, unspecified**
MCC Exclusion see Appendix A PDX collection 1038

P58 Neonatal jaundice due to other excessive hemolysis

Excludes1: *jaundice due to isoimmunization (P55-P57)*

P58.0 Neonatal jaundice due to bruising
P58.1 Neonatal jaundice due to bleeding
P58.2 Neonatal jaundice due to infection
P58.3 Neonatal jaundice due to polycythemia

\+ **P58.4 Neonatal jaundice due to drugs or toxins transmitted from mother or given to newborn**
Code first poisoning due to drug or toxin, if applicable (T36-T65 with fifth or sixth character 1-4 or 6)

Use additional code for adverse effect, if applicable, to identify drug (T36-T50 with fifth or sixth character 5)

P58.41 Neonatal jaundice due to drugs or toxins transmitted from mother
P58.42 Neonatal jaundice due to drugs or toxins given to newborn

P58.5 Neonatal jaundice due to swallowed maternal blood
P58.8 Neonatal jaundice due to other specified excessive hemolysis
P58.9 Neonatal jaundice due to excessive hemolysis, unspecified

P59 Neonatal jaundice from other and unspecified causes

Excludes1: *jaundice due to inborn errors of metabolism (E70-E88)*
kernicterus (P57.-)

P59.0 Neonatal jaundice associated with preterm delivery
Hyperbilirubinemia of prematurity
Jaundice due to delayed conjugation associated with preterm delivery

MCC **P59.1 Inspissated bile syndrome**
MCC Exclusion see Appendix A PDX collection 1038

+ **P59.2 Neonatal jaundice from other and unspecified hepatocellular damage**
Excludes1: *congenital viral hepatitis (P35.3)*

MCC **P59.20 Neonatal jaundice from unspecified hepatocellular damage**
MCC Exclusion see Appendix A PDX collection 1038

MCC **P59.29 Neonatal jaundice from other hepatocellular damage**
Neonatal giant cell hepatitis
Neonatal (idiopathic) hepatitis
MCC Exclusion see Appendix A PDX collection 1038

P59.3 Neonatal jaundice from breast milk inhibitor

P59.8 Neonatal jaundice from other specified causes

P59.9 Neonatal jaundice, unspecified
Neonatal physiological jaundice (intense)(prolonged) NOS
AHA CC: 3Q, 2015, 20

P60 Disseminated intravascular coagulation of newborn
MCC
Defibrination syndrome of newborn
MCC Exclusion see Appendix A PDX collection 1035
Valid 3-character code, no further characters required

P61 Other perinatal hematological disorders

Excludes1: *transient hypogammaglobulinemia of infancy (D80.7)*

MCC **P61.0 Transient neonatal thrombocytopenia**
Neonatal thrombocytopenia due to exchange transfusion
Neonatal thrombocytopenia due to idiopathic maternal thrombocytopenia
Neonatal thrombocytopenia due to isoimmunization
MCC Exclusion see Appendix A PDX collection 1035

P61.1 Polycythemia neonatorum

CC **P61.2 Anemia of prematurity**
CC Exclusion see Appendix A PDX collection 1039

CC **P61.3 Congenital anemia from fetal blood loss**
CC Exclusion see Appendix A PDX collection 1039

CC **P61.4 Other congenital anemias, not elsewhere classified**
Congenital anemia NOS
CC Exclusion see Appendix A PDX collection 1039

MCC **P61.5 Transient neonatal neutropenia**
Excludes1: *congenital neutropenia (nontransient) (D70.0)*
MCC Exclusion see Appendix A PDX collection 1040

CC **P61.6 Other transient neonatal disorders of coagulation**
CC Exclusion see Appendix A PDX collection 1035

P61.8 Other specified perinatal hematological disorders

P61.9 Perinatal hematological disorder, unspecified

Transitory endocrine and metabolic disorders specific to newborn (P70-P74)

Includes: transitory endocrine and metabolic disturbances caused by the infant's response to maternal endocrine and metabolic factors, or its adjustment to extrauterine environment

P70 Transitory disorders of carbohydrate metabolism specific to newborn

P70.0 Syndrome of infant of mother with gestational diabetes
Newborn (with hypoglycemia) affected by maternal gestational diabetes
Excludes1: *newborn (with hypoglycemia) affected by maternal (pre-existing) diabetes mellitus (P70.1)*
syndrome of infant of a diabetic mother (P70.1)

P70.1 Syndrome of infant of a diabetic mother
Newborn (with hypoglycemia) affected by maternal (pre-existing) diabetes mellitus
Excludes1: *newborn (with hypoglycemia) affected by maternal gestational diabetes (P70.0)*
syndrome of infant of mother with gestational diabetes (P70.0)

CC **P70.2 Neonatal diabetes mellitus**
CC Exclusion see Appendix A PDX collection 1041

P70.3 Iatrogenic neonatal hypoglycemia

P70.4 Other neonatal hypoglycemia
Transitory neonatal hypoglycemia

CC **P70.8 Other transitory disorders of carbohydrate metabolism of newborn**
CC Exclusion see Appendix A PDX collection 1042

P70.9 Transitory disorder of carbohydrate metabolism of newborn, unspecified

P71 Transitory neonatal disorders of calcium and magnesium metabolism

CC **P71.0 Cow's milk hypocalcemia in newborn**
CC Exclusion see Appendix A PDX collection 1041

CC **P71.1 Other neonatal hypocalcemia**
Excludes1: *neonatal hypoparathyroidism (P71.4)*
CC Exclusion see Appendix A PDX collection 1041

CC **P71.2 Neonatal hypomagnesemia**
CC Exclusion see Appendix A PDX collection 1041

CC **P71.3 Neonatal tetany without calcium or magnesium deficiency**
Neonatal tetany NOS
CC Exclusion see Appendix A PDX collection 1041

CC **P71.4 Transitory neonatal hypoparathyroidism**
CC Exclusion see Appendix A PDX collection 1041

CC **P71.8 Other transitory neonatal disorders of calcium and magnesium metabolism**
CC Exclusion see Appendix A PDX collection 1041
AHA CC: 4Q, 2016, 54-55

CC **P71.9 Transitory neonatal disorder of calcium and magnesium metabolism, unspecified**
CC Exclusion see Appendix A PDX collection 1041

P72 Other transitory neonatal endocrine disorders

Excludes1: *congenital hypothyroidism with or without goiter (E03.0-E03.1)*
dyshormogenetic goiter (E07.1)
Pendred's syndrome (E07.1)

CC **P72.0 Neonatal goiter, not elsewhere classified**
Transitory congenital goiter with normal functioning
CC Exclusion see Appendix A PDX collection 1042

CC **P72.1 Transitory neonatal hyperthyroidism**
Neonatal thyrotoxicosis
CC Exclusion see Appendix A PDX collection 1041

CC **P72.2 Other transitory neonatal disorders of thyroid function, not elsewhere classified**
Transitory neonatal hypothyroidism
CC Exclusion see Appendix A PDX collection 1042

CC **P72.8 Other specified transitory neonatal endocrine disorders**
CC Exclusion see Appendix A PDX collection 1042

P72.9 Transitory neonatal endocrine disorder, unspecified

P74 Other transitory neonatal electrolyte and metabolic disturbances

MCC **P74.0 Late metabolic acidosis of newborn**
Excludes1: *(fetal) metabolic acidosis of newborn (P19)*
MCC Exclusion see Appendix A PDX collection 1041

P74.1 Dehydration of newborn

P74.2 Disturbances of sodium balance of newborn

P74.3 Disturbances of potassium balance of newborn

P74.4 Other transitory electrolyte disturbances of newborn

CC **P74.5 Transitory tyrosinemia of newborn**
CC Exclusion see Appendix A PDX collection 1042

CC **P74.6 Transitory hyperammonemia of newborn**
CC Exclusion see Appendix A PDX collection 1042

CC **P74.8 Other transitory metabolic disturbances of newborn**
Amino-acid metabolic disorders described as transitory
CC Exclusion see Appendix A PDX collection 1042

P74.9 Transitory metabolic disturbance of newborn, unspecified

Digestive system disorders of newborn (P76-P78)

P76 Other intestinal obstruction of newborn

P76.0 Meconium plug syndrome
Meconium ileus NOS
Excludes1: *meconium ileus in cystic fibrosis (E84.11)*

CC **P76.1 Transitory ileus of newborn**
Excludes1: *Hirschsprung's disease (Q43.1)*
CC Exclusion see Appendix A PDX collection 1043

P76.2 Intestinal obstruction due to inspissated milk

P76.8 Other specified intestinal obstruction of newborn
Excludes1: *intestinal obstruction classifiable to K56.-*

P76.9 Intestinal obstruction of newborn, unspecified

P77 Necrotizing enterocolitis of newborn

MCC **P77.1 Stage 1 necrotizing enterocolitis in newborn**
Necrotizing enterocolitis without pneumatosis, without perforation
MCC Exclusion see Appendix A PDX collection 1044

MCC **P77.2 Stage 2 necrotizing enterocolitis in newborn**
Necrotizing enterocolitis with pneumatosis, without perforation
MCC Exclusion see Appendix A PDX collection 1044

MCC **P77.3 Stage 3 necrotizing enterocolitis in newborn**
Necrotizing enterocolitis with perforation
Necrotizing enterocolitis with pneumatosis and perforation
MCC Exclusion see Appendix A PDX collection 1044

MCC **P77.9 Necrotizing enterocolitis in newborn, unspecified**
Necrotizing enterocolitis in newborn, NOS
MCC Exclusion see Appendix A PDX collection 1044

P78 Other perinatal digestive system disorders

Excludes1: *cystic fibrosis (E84.0-E84.9)*
neonatal gastrointestinal hemorrhages (P54.0-P54.3)

MCC **P78.0 Perinatal intestinal perforation**
Meconium peritonitis
MCC Exclusion see Appendix A PDX collection 1044

P78.1 Other neonatal peritonitis
Neonatal peritonitis NOS

P78.2 Neonatal hematemesis and melena due to swallowed maternal blood

P78.3 Noninfective neonatal diarrhea
Neonatal diarrhea NOS

\+ **P78.8 Other specified perinatal digestive system disorders**

P78.81 Congenital cirrhosis (of liver)

P78.82 Peptic ulcer of newborn

P78.83 Newborn esophageal reflux
Neonatal esophageal reflux

P78.84 Gestational alloimmune liver disease
GALD
Neonatal hemochromatosis
Excludes1: *hemochromatosis (E83.11-)*

P78.89 Other specified perinatal digestive system disorders

P78.9 Perinatal digestive system disorder, unspecified

Conditions involving the integument and temperature regulation of newborn (P80-P83)

P80 Hypothermia of newborn

P80.0 Cold injury syndrome
Severe and usually chronic hypothermia associated with a pink flushed appearance, edema and neurological and biochemical abnormalities.
Excludes1: *mild hypothermia of newborn (P80.8)*

P80.8 Other hypothermia of newborn
Mild hypothermia of newborn

P80.9 Hypothermia of newborn, unspecified

P81 Other disturbances of temperature regulation of newborn

P81.0 Environmental hyperthermia of newborn

P81.8 Other specified disturbances of temperature regulation of newborn

P81.9 Disturbance of temperature regulation of newborn, unspecified
Fever of newborn NOS

P83 Other conditions of integument specific to newborn

Excludes1: *congenital malformations of skin and integument (Q80-Q84)*
hydrops fetalis due to hemolytic disease (P56.-)
neonatal skin infection (P39.4)
staphylococcal scalded skin syndrome (L00)
Excludes2: *cradle cap (L21.0)*
diaper [napkin] dermatitis (L22)

CC **P83.0 Sclerema neonatorum**
CC Exclusion see Appendix A PDX collection 1045

P83.1 Neonatal erythema toxicum

MCC **P83.2 Hydrops fetalis not due to hemolytic disease**
Hydrops fetalis NOS
MCC Exclusion see Appendix A PDX collection 1046

\+ **P83.3 Other and unspecified edema specific to newborn**

CC **P83.30 Unspecified edema specific to newborn**
CC Exclusion see Appendix A PDX collection 1047

CC **P83.39 Other edema specific to newborn**
CC Exclusion see Appendix A PDX collection 1047

P83.4 Breast engorgement of newborn
Noninfective mastitis of newborn

♂ **P83.5 Congenital hydrocele**

P83.6 Umbilical polyp of newborn

\+ **P83.8 Other specified conditions of integument specific to newborn**

P83.81 Umbilical granuloma
Excludes2: *granulomatous disorder of the skin and subcutaneous tissue, unspecified (L92.9)*

P83.88 Other specified conditions of integument specific to newborn
Bronze baby syndrome
Neonatal scleroderma
Urticaria neonatorum

P83.9 Condition of the integument specific to newborn, unspecified

Other problems with newborn (P84)

P84 Other problems with newborn

Acidemia of newborn
Acidosis of newborn
Anoxia of newborn NOS
Asphyxia of newborn NOS
Hypercapnia of newborn
Hypoxemia of newborn
Hypoxia of newborn NOS
Mixed metabolic and respiratory acidosis of newborn
Excludes1: *intracranial hemorrhage due to anoxia or hypoxia (P52.-)*
hypoxic ischemic encephalopathy [HIE] (P91.6-)
late metabolic acidosis of newborn (P74.0)
Valid 3-character code, no further characters required

Other disorders originating in the perinatal period (P90-P96)

MCC **P90 Convulsions of newborn**

Excludes1: *benign myoclonic epilepsy in infancy (G40.3-)*
benign neonatal convulsions (familial) (G40.3-)
MCC Exclusion see Appendix A PDX collection 1048
Valid 3-character code, no further characters required

P91 Other disturbances of cerebral status of newborn

MCC **P91.0 Neonatal cerebral ischemia**
MCC Exclusion see Appendix A PDX collection 1049

MCC **P91.1 Acquired periventricular cysts of newborn**
MCC Exclusion see Appendix A PDX collection 1049

MCC **P91.2 Neonatal cerebral leukomalacia**
Periventricular leukomalacia
MCC Exclusion see Appendix A PDX collection 1022

MCC **P91.3 Neonatal cerebral irritability**
MCC Exclusion see Appendix A PDX collection 1049

MCC **P91.4 Neonatal cerebral depression**
MCC Exclusion see Appendix A PDX collection 1049

MCC **P91.5 Neonatal coma**
MCC Exclusion see Appendix A PDX collection 1049

\+ **P91.6 Hypoxic ischemic encephalopathy [HIE]**
Excludes1: *neonatal cerebral depression (P91.4)*
neonatal cerebral irritability (P91.3)
neonatal coma (P91.5)

CC **P91.60 Hypoxic ischemic encephalopathy [HIE], unspecified**
CC Exclusion see Appendix A PDX collection 1050

CC **P91.61 Mild hypoxic ischemic encephalopathy [HIE]**
CC Exclusion see Appendix A PDX collection 1050

P91.62 Moderate hypoxic ischemic encephalopathy [HIE]

MCC **P91.63 Severe hypoxic ischemic encephalopathy [HIE]**
MCC Exclusion see Appendix A PDX collection 1050

\+ **P91.8 Other specified disturbances of cerebral status of newborn**

\+ **P91.81 Neonatal encephalopathy**

P91.811 Neonatal encephalopathy in diseases classified elsewhere
Code first underlying condition, if known, such as:
congenital cirrhosis (of liver) (P78.71)
intracranial nontraumatic hemorrhage of newborn (P52.-)
kernicterus (P57.-)

P91.819 Neonatal encephalopathy, unspecified

P91.88 Other specified disturbances of cerebral status of newborn

P91.9 Disturbance of cerebral status of newborn, unspecified

P92 Feeding problems of newborn

Excludes1: *eating disorders (F50.-)*
feeding problems in child over 28 days old (R63.3)

+ **P92.0 Vomiting of newborn**
  Excludes1: *vomiting of child over 28 days old (R11.-)*
  MCC **P92.01 Bilious vomiting of newborn**
    Excludes1: *bilious vomiting in child over 28 days old (R11.14)*
    MCC Exclusion see Appendix A PDX collection 1051
  P92.09 Other vomiting of newborn
    Excludes1: *regurgitation of food in newborn (P92.1)*
P92.1 Regurgitation and rumination of newborn
P92.2 Slow feeding of newborn
P92.3 Underfeeding of newborn
P92.4 Overfeeding of newborn
P92.5 Neonatal difficulty in feeding at breast
  AHA CC: 3Q, 2016, 19; 1Q, 2017, 28-29
P92.6 Failure to thrive in newborn
  Excludes1: *failure to thrive in child over 28 days old (R62.51)*
P92.8 Other feeding problems of newborn
P92.9 Feeding problem of newborn, unspecified

P93 Reactions and intoxications due to drugs administered to newborn

Includes: reactions and intoxications due to drugs administered to fetus affecting newborn
Excludes1: *jaundice due to drugs or toxins transmitted from mother or given to newborn (P58.4-)*
reactions and intoxications from maternal opiates, tranquilizers and other medication (P04.0-P04.1, P04.4)
withdrawal symptoms from maternal use of drugs of addiction (P96.1)
withdrawal symptoms from therapeutic use of drugs in newborn (P96.2)

CC **P93.0 Grey baby syndrome**
  Grey syndrome from chloramphenicol administration in newborn
  CC Exclusion see Appendix A PDX collection 1052
CC **P93.8 Other reactions and intoxications due to drugs administered to newborn**
  Use additional code for adverse effect, if applicable, to identify drug (T36-T50 with fifth or sixth character 5)
  CC Exclusion see Appendix A PDX collection 1052

P94 Disorders of muscle tone of newborn

CC **P94.0 Transient neonatal myasthenia gravis**
  Excludes1: *myasthenia gravis (G70.0)*
  CC Exclusion see Appendix A PDX collection 1041
P94.1 Congenital hypertonia
P94.2 Congenital hypotonia
  Floppy baby syndrome, unspecified
P94.8 Other disorders of muscle tone of newborn
P94.9 Disorder of muscle tone of newborn,unspecified

P95 Stillbirth

Deadborn fetus NOS
Fetal death of unspecified cause
Stillbirth NOS
Excludes1: *maternal care for intrauterine death (O36.4)*
missed abortion (O02.1)
outcome of delivery, stillbirth (Z37.1, Z37.3, Z37.4, Z37.7)
Review coding guideline C.16.g
Valid 3-character code, no further characters required

P96 Other conditions originating in the perinatal period

P96.0 Congenital renal failure
  Uremia of newborn
CC **P96.1 Neonatal withdrawal symptoms from maternal use of drugs of addiction**
  Drug withdrawal syndrome in infant of dependent mother
  Neonatal abstinence syndrome
  Excludes1: *reactions and intoxications from maternal opiates and tranquilizers administered during labor and delivery (P04.0)*
  CC Exclusion see Appendix A PDX collection 1052
CC **P96.2 Withdrawal symptoms from therapeutic use of drugs in newborn**
  CC Exclusion see Appendix A PDX collection 1052
P96.3 Wide cranial sutures of newborn
  Neonatal craniotabes
P96.5 Complication to newborn due to (fetal) intrauterine procedure
  Excludes2: *newborn affected by amniocentesis (P00.6)*
+ **P96.8 Other specified conditions originating in the perinatal period**
  P96.81 Exposure to (parental) (environmental) tobacco smoke in the perinatal period
    Excludes2: *newborn affected by in utero exposure to tobacco (P04.2)*
    exposure to environmental tobacco smoke after the perinatal period (Z77.22)
  P96.82 Delayed separation of umbilical cord
  P96.83 Meconium staining
    Excludes1: *meconium aspiration (P24.00, P24.01)*
    meconium passage during delivery (P03.82)
  P96.89 Other specified conditions originating in the perinatal period
    Use additional code to specify condition
P96.9 Condition originating in the perinatal period, unspecified
  Congenital debility NOS

Chapter 17: Congenital Malformations, Deformations and Chromosomal Abnormalities (Q00-Q99)

NOTE Codes from this chapter are not for use on maternal or fetal records

Excludes2: *inborn errors of metabolism (E70-E88)*

This chapter contains the following category blocks:

- Q00-Q07 Congenital malformations of the nervous system
- Q10-Q18 Congenital malformations of eye, ear, face and neck
- Q20-Q28 Congenital malformations of the circulatory system
- Q30-Q34 Congenital malformations of the respiratory system
- Q35-Q37 Cleft lip and cleft palate
- Q38-Q45 Other congenital malformations of the digestive system
- Q50-Q56 Congenital malformations of genital organs
- Q60-Q64 Congenital malformations of the urinary system
- Q65-Q79 Congenital malformations and deformations of the musculoskeletal system
- Q80-Q89 Other congenital malformations
- Q90-Q99 Chromosomal abnormalities, not elsewhere classified

C. Chapter-Specific Coding Guidelines

In addition to general coding guidelines, there are guidelines for specific diagnoses and/or conditions in the classification. Unless otherwise indicated, these guidelines apply to all health care settings. Please refer to Section II for guidelines on the selection of principal diagnosis.

17. Chapter 17: Congenital Malformations, Deformations and Chromosomal Abnormalities (Q00-Q99)

Assign an appropriate code(s) from categories Q00-Q99, Congenital malformations, deformations, and chromosomal abnormalities when a malformation/deformation or chromosomal abnormality is documented. A malformation/deformation or chromosomal abnormality may be the principal/first-listed diagnosis on a record or a secondary diagnosis.

When a malformation/deformation or chromosomal abnormality does not have a unique code assignment, assign additional code(s) for any manifestations that may be present.

When the code assignment specifically identifies the malformation/deformation/ or chromosomal abnormality, manifestations that are an inherent component of the anomaly should not be coded separately. Additional codes should be assigned for manifestations that are not an inherent component.

Codes from Chapter 17 may be used throughout the life of the patient. If a congenital malformation or deformity has been corrected, a personal history code should be used to identify the history of the malformation or deformity. Although present at birth, malformation/deformation or chromosomal abnormality may not be identified until later in life. Whenever the condition is diagnosed by the physician, it is appropriate to assign a code from codes Q00-Q99. For the birth admission, the appropriate code from category Z38, Liveborn infants, according to place of birth and type of delivery, should be sequenced as the principal diagnosis, followed by any congenital anomaly codes, Q00-Q99.

Congenital malformations of the nervous system (Q00-Q07)

Q00 Anencephaly and similar malformations

MCC **Q00.0 Anencephaly**
Acephaly
Acrania
Amyelencephaly
Hemianencephaly
Hemicephaly
MCC Exclusion see Appendix A PDX collection 1053

MCC **Q00.1 Craniorachischisis**
MCC Exclusion see Appendix A PDX collection 1053

MCC **Q00.2 Iniencephaly**
MCC Exclusion see Appendix A PDX collection 1053

Q01 Encephalocele

Includes: Arnold-Chiari syndrome, type III
encephalocystocele
encephalomyelocele
hydroencephalocele
hydromeningocele, cranial
meningocele, cerebral
meningoencephalocele

Excludes1: *Meckel-Gruber syndrome (Q61.9)*

CC **Q01.0 Frontal encephalocele**
CC Exclusion see Appendix A PDX collection 1054

CC **Q01.1 Nasofrontal encephalocele**
CC Exclusion see Appendix A PDX collection 1054

CC **Q01.2 Occipital encephalocele**
CC Exclusion see Appendix A PDX collection 1054

CC **Q01.8 Encephalocele of other sites**
CC Exclusion see Appendix A PDX collection 1054

CC **Q01.9 Encephalocele, unspecified**
CC Exclusion see Appendix A PDX collection 1054

Q02 Microcephaly

Includes: hydromicrocephaly
micrencephalon

Excludes1: *Meckel-Gruber syndrome (Q61.9)*

AHA CC: 4Q, 2016, 4-7

Valid 3-character code, no further characters required

Q03 Congenital hydrocephalus

Includes: hydrocephalus in newborn

Excludes1: *Arnold-Chiari syndrome, type II (Q07.0-)*
acquired hydrocephalus (G91.-)
hydrocephalus due to congenital toxoplasmosis (P37.1)
hydrocephalus with spina bifida (Q05.0-Q05.4)

Q03.0 Malformations of aqueduct of Sylvius
Anomaly of aqueduct of Sylvius
Obstruction of aqueduct of Sylvius, congenital
Stenosis of aqueduct of Sylvius

Q03.1 Atresia of foramina of Magendie and Luschka
Dandy-Walker syndrome

Q03.8 Other congenital hydrocephalus

Q03.9 Congenital hydrocephalus, unspecified

Q04 Other congenital malformations of brain

Excludes1: *cyclopia (Q87.0)*
macrocephaly (Q75.3)

MCC **Q04.0 Congenital malformations of corpus callosum**
Agenesis of corpus callosum
MCC Exclusion see Appendix A PDX collection 1054

MCC **Q04.1 Arhinencephaly**
MCC Exclusion see Appendix A PDX collection 1054

MCC **Q04.2 Holoprosencephaly**
MCC Exclusion see Appendix A PDX collection 1054

MCC **Q04.3 Other reduction deformities of brain**
Absence of part of brain
Agenesis of part of brain
Agyria
Aplasia of part of brain
Hydranencephaly
Hypoplasia of part of brain
Lissencephaly
Microgyria
Pachygyria
Excludes1: *congenital malformations of corpus callosum (Q04.0)*
MCC Exclusion see Appendix A PDX collection 1054

CC **Q04.4 Septo-optic dysplasia of brain**
CC Exclusion see Appendix A PDX collection 1055

CC **Q04.5 Megalencephaly**
CC Exclusion see Appendix A PDX collection 1055

CC **Q04.6 Congenital cerebral cysts**
Porencephaly
Schizencephaly
Excludes1: *acquired porencephalic cyst (G93.0)*
CC Exclusion see Appendix A PDX collection 1055

CC **Q04.8 Other specified congenital malformations of brain**
Arnold-Chiari syndrome, type IV
Macrogyria
CC Exclusion see Appendix A PDX collection 1055

Q04.9 Congenital malformation of brain, unspecified
Congenital anomaly NOS of brain
Congenital deformity NOS of brain
Congenital disease or lesion NOS of brain
Multiple anomalies NOS of brain, congenital

Q05 Spina bifida

Includes: hydromeningocele (spinal)
meningocele (spinal)
meningomyelocele
myelocele
myelomeningocele
rachischisis
spina bifida (aperta)(cystica)
syringomyelocele

Use additional code for any associated paraplegia (paraparesis) (G82.2-)

Excludes1: *Arnold-Chiari syndrome, type II (Q07.0-)*
spina bifida occulta (Q76.0)

CC **Q05.0 Cervical spina bifida with hydrocephalus**
CC Exclusion see Appendix A PDX collection 1056

CC **Q05.1 Thoracic spina bifida with hydrocephalus**
Dorsal spina bifida with hydrocephalus
Thoracolumbar spina bifida with hydrocephalus
CC Exclusion see Appendix A PDX collection 1056

CC **Q05.2 Lumbar spina bifida with hydrocephalus**
CC Exclusion see Appendix A PDX collection 1056
Lumbosacral spina bifida with hydrocephalus
CC Exclusion see Appendix A PDX collection 1056

CC **Q05.3 Sacral spina bifida with hydrocephalus**
CC Exclusion see Appendix A PDX collection 1056

CC **Q05.4 Unspecified spina bifida with hydrocephalus**
CC Exclusion see Appendix A PDX collection 1056

Q05.5 Cervical spina bifida without hydrocephalus

Q05.6 Thoracic spina bifida without hydrocephalus
Dorsal spina bifida NOS
Thoracolumbar spina bifida NOS

Q05.7 Lumbar spina bifida without hydrocephalus
Lumbosacral spina bifida NOS

Q05.8 Sacral spina bifida without hydrocephalus

Q05.9 Spina bifida, unspecified

Q06 Other congenital malformations of spinal cord

Q06.0 Amyelia

Q06.1 Hypoplasia and dysplasia of spinal cord
Atelomyelia
Myelatelia
Myelodysplasia of spinal cord

Q06.2 Diastematomyelia

Q06.3 Other congenital cauda equina malformations

Q06.4 Hydromyelia
Hydrorachis

Q06.8 Other specified congenital malformations of spinal cord

Q06.9 Congenital malformation of spinal cord, unspecified
Congenital anomaly NOS of spinal cord
Congenital deformity NOS of spinal cord
Congenital disease or lesion NOS of spinal cord

Q07 Other congenital malformations of nervous system

Excludes2: *congenital central alveolar hypoventilation syndrome (G47.35)*
familial dysautonomia [Riley-Day] (G90.1)
neurofibromatosis (nonmalignant) (Q85.0-)

\+ **Q07.0 Arnold-Chiari syndrome**
Arnold-Chiari syndrome, type II
Excludes1: *Arnold-Chiari syndrome, type III (Q01.-)*
Arnold-Chiari syndrome, type IV (Q04.8)

Q07.00 Arnold-Chiari syndrome without spina bifida or hydrocephalus

Q07.01 Arnold-Chiari syndrome with spina bifida

CC **Q07.02 Arnold-Chiari syndrome with hydrocephalus**
CC Exclusion see Appendix A PDX collection 1056

CC **Q07.03 Arnold-Chiari syndrome with spina bifida and hydrocephalus**
CC Exclusion see Appendix A PDX collection 1056

Q07.8 Other specified congenital malformations of nervous system
Agenesis of nerve
Displacement of brachial plexus
Jaw-winking syndrome
Marcus Gunn's syndrome

Q07.9 Congenital malformation of nervous system, unspecified
Congenital anomaly NOS of nervous system
Congenital deformity NOS of nervous system
Congenital disease or lesion NOS of nervous system

Congenital malformations of eye, ear, face and neck (Q10-Q18)

Excludes2: *cleft lip and cleft palate (Q35-Q37)*
congenital malformation of cervical spine (Q05.0, Q05.5, Q67.5, Q76.0-Q76.4)
congenital malformation of larynx (Q31.-)
congenital malformation of lip NEC (Q38.0)
congenital malformation of nose (Q30.-)
congenital malformation of parathyroid gland (Q89.2)
congenital malformation of thyroid gland (Q89.2)

Q10 Congenital malformations of eyelid, lacrimal apparatus and orbit

Excludes1: *cryptophthalmos NOS (Q11.2)*
cryptophthalmos syndrome (Q87.0)

Q10.0 Congenital ptosis

Q10.1 Congenital ectropion

Q10.2 Congenital entropion

Q10.3 Other congenital malformations of eyelid
Ablepharon
Blepharophimosis, congenital
Coloboma of eyelid
Congenital absence or agenesis of cilia
Congenital absence or agenesis of eyelid
Congenital accessory eyelid
Congenital accessory eye muscle
Congenital malformation of eyelid NOS

Q10.4 Absence and agenesis of lacrimal apparatus
Congenital absence of punctum lacrimale

Q10.5 Congenital stenosis and stricture of lacrimal duct

Q10.6 Other congenital malformations of lacrimal apparatus
Congenital malformation of lacrimal apparatus NOS

Q10.7 Congenital malformation of orbit

Q11 Anophthalmos, microphthalmos and macrophthalmos

Q11.0 Cystic eyeball

Q11.1 Other anophthalmos
Anophthalmos NOS
Agenesis of eye
Aplasia of eye

Q11.2 Microphthalmos
Cryptophthalmos NOS
Dysplasia of eye
Hypoplasia of eye
Rudimentary eye
Excludes1: *cryptophthalmos syndrome (Q87.0)*

Q11.3 Macrophthalmos
Excludes1: *macrophthalmos in congenital glaucoma (Q15.0)*

Q12 Congenital lens malformations

CC **Q12.0 Congenital cataract**
CC Exclusion see Appendix A PDX collection 1057

CC **Q12.1 Congenital displaced lens**
CC Exclusion see Appendix A PDX collection 1058

CC **Q12.2 Coloboma of lens**
CC Exclusion see Appendix A PDX collection 1057

Q12.3 Congenital aphakia

Q12.4 Spherophakia

Q12.8 Other congenital lens malformations
Microphakia

Q12.9 Congenital lens malformation, unspecified

Q13 Congenital malformations of anterior segment of eye

Q13.0 Coloboma of iris
Coloboma NOS

Q13.1 Absence of iris
Aniridia
Use additional code for associated glaucoma (H42)

Q13.2 Other congenital malformations of iris
Anisocoria, congenital
Atresia of pupil
Congenital malformation of iris NOS
Corectopia

Q13.3 Congenital corneal opacity

Q13.4 Other congenital corneal malformations
Congenital malformation of cornea NOS
Microcornea
Peter's anomaly

Q13.5 Blue sclera

Q13.8 Other congenital malformations of anterior segment of eye

Q13.81 Rieger's anomaly
Use additional code for associated glaucoma (H42)

Q13.89 Other congenital malformations of anterior segment of eye

Q13.9 Congenital malformation of anterior segment of eye, unspecified

Q14 Congenital malformations of posterior segment of eye

Excludes2: *optic nerve hypoplasia (H47.03-)*

Q14.0 Congenital malformation of vitreous humor
Congenital vitreous opacity

Q14.1 Congenital malformation of retina
Congenital retinal aneurysm

Q14.2 Congenital malformation of optic disc
Coloboma of optic disc

Q14.3 Congenital malformation of choroid

Q14.8 Other congenital malformations of posterior segment of eye
Coloboma of the fundus

Q14.9 Congenital malformation of posterior segment of eye, unspecified

Q15 Other congenital malformations of eye

Excludes1: *congenital nystagmus (H55.01)*
ocular albinism (E70.31-)
optic nerve hypoplasia (H47.03-)
retinitis pigmentosa (H35.52)

Q15.0 Congenital glaucoma
Axenfeld's anomaly
Buphthalmos
Glaucoma of childhood
Glaucoma of newborn
Hydrophthalmos
Keratoglobus, congenital, with glaucoma
Macrocornea with glaucoma
Macrophthalmos in congenital glaucoma
Megalocornea with glaucoma

Q15.8 Other specified congenital malformations of eye

Q15.9 Congenital malformation of eye, unspecified
Congenital anomaly of eye
Congenital deformity of eye

Q16 Congenital malformations of ear causing impairment of hearing

Excludes1: *congenital deafness (H90.-)*

Q16.0 Congenital absence of (ear) auricle

Q16.1 Congenital absence, atresia and stricture of auditory canal (external)
Congenital atresia or stricture of osseous meatus

Q16.2 Absence of eustachian tube

Q16.3 Congenital malformation of ear ossicles
Congenital fusion of ear ossicles

Q16.4 Other congenital malformations of middle ear
Congenital malformation of middle ear NOS

Q16.5 Congenital malformation of inner ear
Congenital anomaly of membranous labyrinth
Congenital anomaly of organ of Corti

Q16.9 Congenital malformation of ear causing impairment of hearing, unspecified
Congenital absence of ear NOS

Q17 Other congenital malformations of ear

Excludes1: *congenital malformations of ear with impairment of hearing (Q16.0-Q16.9)*
preauricular sinus (Q18.1)

Q17.0 Accessory auricle
Accessory tragus
Polyotia
Preauricular appendage or tag
Supernumerary ear
Supernumerary lobule

Q17.1 Macrotia

Q17.2 Microtia

Q17.3 Other misshapen ear
Pointed ear

Q17.4 Misplaced ear
Low-set ears
Excludes1: *cervical auricle (Q18.2)*

Q17.5 Prominent ear
Bat ear

Q17.8 Other specified congenital malformations of ear
Congenital absence of lobe of ear

Q17.9 Congenital malformation of ear, unspecified
Congenital anomaly of ear NOS

Q18 Other congenital malformations of face and neck

Excludes1: *cleft lip and cleft palate (Q35-Q37)*
conditions classified to (Q67.0-Q67.4)
congenital malformations of skull and face bones (Q75.-)
cyclopia (Q87.0)
dentofacial anomalies [including malocclusion] (M26.-)
malformation syndromes affecting facial appearance (Q87.0)
persistent thyroglossal duct (Q89.2)

Q18.0 Sinus, fistula and cyst of branchial cleft
Branchial vestige

Q18.1 Preauricular sinus and cyst
Fistula of auricle, congenital
Cervicoaural fistula

Q18.2 Other branchial cleft malformations
Branchial cleft malformation NOS
Cervical auricle
Otocephaly

Q18.3 Webbing of neck
Pterygium colli

Q18.4 Macrostomia

Q18.5 Microstomia

Q18.6 Macrocheilia
Hypertrophy of lip, congenital

Q18.7 Microcheilia

Q18.8 Other specified congenital malformations of face and neck
Medial cyst of face and neck
Medial fistula of face and neck
Medial sinus of face and neck

Q18.9 Congenital malformation of face and neck, unspecified
Congenital anomaly NOS of face and neck

Congenital malformations of the circulatory system (Q20-Q28)

Q20 Congenital malformations of cardiac chambers and connections

Excludes1: *dextrocardia with situs inversus (Q89.3)*
mirror-image atrial arrangement with situs inversus (Q89.3)

MCC **Q20.0 Common arterial trunk**
Persistent truncus arteriosus
Excludes1: *aortic septal defect (Q21.4)*
MCC Exclusion see Appendix A PDX collection 1057

MCC **Q20.1 Double outlet right ventricle**
Taussig-Bing syndrome
MCC Exclusion see Appendix A PDX collection 1057

MCC **Q20.2 Double outlet left ventricle**
MCC Exclusion see Appendix A PDX collection 1057

MCC **Q20.3 Discordant ventriculoarterial connection**
Dextrotransposition of aorta
Transposition of great vessels (complete)
MCC Exclusion see Appendix A PDX collection 1057

MCC **Q20.4 Double inlet ventricle**
Common ventricle
Cor triloculare biatriatum
Single ventricle
MCC Exclusion see Appendix A PDX collection 1057

CC **Q20.5 Discordant atrioventricular connection**
Corrected transposition
Levotransposition
Ventricular inversion
CC Exclusion see Appendix A PDX collection 1057

Q20.6 Isomerism of atrial appendages
Isomerism of atrial appendages with asplenia or polysplenia

Q20.8 Other congenital malformations of cardiac chambers and connections
Cor binoculare

Q20.9 Congenital malformation of cardiac chambers and connections, unspecified

Q21 Congenital malformations of cardiac septa

Excludes1: *acquired cardiac septal defect (I51.0)*

Q21.0 Ventricular septal defect
Roger's disease

Q21.1 Atrial septal defect
Coronary sinus defect
Patent or persistent foramen ovale
Patent or persistent ostium secundum defect (type II)
Patent or persistent sinus venosus defect

Q21.2 Atrioventricular septal defect
Common atrioventricular canal
Endocardial cushion defect
Ostium primum atrial septal defect (type I)

MCC **Q21.3 Tetralogy of Fallot**
Ventricular septal defect with pulmonary stenosis or atresia, dextroposition of aorta and hypertrophy of right ventricle.
MCC Exclusion see Appendix A PDX collection 1057
AHA CC: 3Q, 2014, 16-17

Q21.4 Aortopulmonary septal defect
Aortic septal defect
Aortopulmonary window

Q21.8 Other congenital malformations of cardiac septa
Eisenmenger's defect
Pentalogy of Fallot
Code also if applicable:
Eisenmenger's complex (I27.83)
Eisenmenger's syndrome (I27.83)

Q21.9 Congenital malformation of cardiac septum, unspecified
Septal (heart) defect NOS

Q22 Congenital malformations of pulmonary and tricuspid valves

MCC **Q22.0 Pulmonary valve atresia**
MCC Exclusion see Appendix A PDX collection 1059

CC **Q22.1 Congenital pulmonary valve stenosis**
CC Exclusion see Appendix A PDX collection 1060

CC **Q22.2 Congenital pulmonary valve insufficiency**
Congenital pulmonary valve regurgitation
CC Exclusion see Appendix A PDX collection 1060

CC **Q22.3 Other congenital malformations of pulmonary valve**
Congenital malformation of pulmonary valve NOS
Supernumerary cusps of pulmonary valve
CC Exclusion see Appendix A PDX collection 1060

MCC **Q22.4 Congenital tricuspid stenosis**
Congenital tricuspid atresia
MCC Exclusion see Appendix A PDX collection 1061

MCC **Q22.5 Ebstein's anomaly**
MCC Exclusion see Appendix A PDX collection 1061

MCC **Q22.6 Hypoplastic right heart syndrome**
MCC Exclusion see Appendix A PDX collection 1061

MCC **Q22.8 Other congenital malformations of tricuspid valve**
MCC Exclusion see Appendix A PDX collection 1061

MCC **Q22.9 Congenital malformation of tricuspid valve, unspecified**
MCC Exclusion see Appendix A PDX collection 1061

Q23 Congenital malformations of aortic and mitral valves

CC **Q23.0 Congenital stenosis of aortic valve**
Congenital aortic atresia
Congenital aortic stenosis NOS
Excludes1: *congenital stenosis of aortic valve in hypoplastic left heart syndrome (Q23.4)*
congenital subaortic stenosis (Q24.4)
supravalvular aortic stenosis (congenital) (Q25.3)
CC Exclusion see Appendix A PDX collection 1061

CC **Q23.1 Congenital insufficiency of aortic valve**
Bicuspid aortic valve
Congenital aortic insufficiency
CC Exclusion see Appendix A PDX collection 1061

CC **Q23.2 Congenital mitral stenosis**
Congenital mitral atresia
CC Exclusion see Appendix A PDX collection 1061

CC **Q23.3 Congenital mitral insufficiency**
CC Exclusion see Appendix A PDX collection 1061

MCC **Q23.4 Hypoplastic left heart syndrome**
MCC Exclusion see Appendix A PDX collection 1063

CC **Q23.8 Other congenital malformations of aortic and mitral valves**

CC **Q23.9 Congenital malformation of aortic and mitral valves, unspecified**

Q24 Other congenital malformations of heart

Excludes1: *endocardial fibroelastosis (I42.4)*

CC **Q24.0 Dextrocardia**
Excludes1: *dextrocardia with situs inversus (Q89.3)*
isomerism of atrial appendages (with asplenia or polysplenia) (Q20.6)
mirror-image atrial arrangement with situs inversus (Q89.3)
CC Exclusion see Appendix A PDX collection 1062

CC **Q24.1 Levocardia**
CC Exclusion see Appendix A PDX collection 1062

MCC **Q24.2 Cor triatriatum**
MCC Exclusion see Appendix A PDX collection 1063

CC **Q24.3 Pulmonary infundibular stenosis**
Subvalvular pulmonic stenosis
CC Exclusion see Appendix A PDX collection 1063

MCC **Q24.4 Congenital subaortic stenosis**
MCC Exclusion see Appendix A PDX collection 1063

CC **Q24.5 Malformation of coronary vessels**
Congenital coronary (artery) aneurysm
CC Exclusion see Appendix A PDX collection 1064

MCC **Q24.6 Congenital heart block**
MCC Exclusion see Appendix A PDX collection 1065

Q24.8 Other specified congenital malformations of heart
Congenital diverticulum of left ventricle
Congenital malformation of myocardium
Congenital malformation of pericardium
Malposition of heart
Uhl's disease

Q24.9 Congenital malformation of heart, unspecified
Congenital anomaly of heart
Congenital disease of heart

Q25 Congenital malformations of great arteries

CC **Q25.0 Patent ductus arteriosus**
Patent ductus Botallo
Persistent ductus arteriosus
CC Exclusion see Appendix A PDX collection 1066

CC **Q25.1 Coarctation of aorta**
Coarctation of aorta (preductal) (postductal)
Stenosis of aorta
CC Exclusion see Appendix A PDX collection 1067
AHA CC: 4Q, 2016, 56-57

\+ **Q25.2 Atresia of aorta**
AHA CC: 4Q, 2016, 56-57

CC **Q25.21 Interruption of aortic arch**
Atresia of aortic arch
CC Exclusion see Appendix A PDX collection 1068

CC **Q25.29 Other atresia of aorta**
Atresia of aorta
CC Exclusion see Appendix A PDX collection 1068

CC **Q25.3 Supravalvular aortic stenosis**
Excludes1: *congenital aortic stenosis NOS (Q23.0)*
congenital stenosis of aortic valve (Q23.0)
CC Exclusion see Appendix A PDX collection 1068

\+ **Q25.4 Other congenital malformations of aorta**
Excludes1: *hypoplasia of aorta in hypoplastic left heart syndrome (Q23.4)*
AHA CC: 4Q, 2016, 57

CC **Q25.40 Congenital malformation of aorta unspecified**
CC Exclusion see Appendix A PDX collection 1069

CC **Q25.41 Absence and aplasia of aorta**
CC Exclusion see Appendix A PDX collection 1069

CC **Q25.42 Hypoplasia of aorta**
CC Exclusion see Appendix A PDX collection 1069

CC **Q25.43 Congenital aneurysm of aorta**
Congenital aneurysm of aortic root
Congenital aneurysm of aortic sinus
CC Exclusion see Appendix A PDX collection 1069

CC **Q25.44 Congenital dilation of aorta**
CC Exclusion see Appendix A PDX collection 1069

CC **Q25.45 Double aortic arch**
Vascular ring of aorta
CC Exclusion see Appendix A PDX collection 1069

CC **Q25.46 Tortuous aortic arch**
Persistent convolutions of aortic arch
CC Exclusion see Appendix A PDX collection 1069

CC **Q25.47 Right aortic arch**
Persistent right aortic arch
CC Exclusion see Appendix A PDX collection 1069

CC **Q25.48 Anomalous origin of subclavian artery**
CC Exclusion see Appendix A PDX collection 1069

CC **Q25.49 Other congenital malformations of aorta**
Aortic arch
Bovine arch
CC Exclusion see Appendix A PDX collection 1069

MCC **Q25.5 Atresia of pulmonary artery**
MCC Exclusion see Appendix A PDX collection 1070

MCC **Q25.6 Stenosis of pulmonary artery**
Supravalvular pulmonary stenosis
MCC Exclusion see Appendix A PDX collection 1070

\+ **Q25.7 Other congenital malformations of pulmonary artery**

MCC **Q25.71 Coarctation of pulmonary artery**
MCC Exclusion see Appendix A PDX collection 1070

MCC **Q25.72 Congenital pulmonary arteriovenous malformation**
Congenital pulmonary arteriovenous aneurysm
MCC Exclusion see Appendix A PDX collection 1070

MCC Q25.79 **Other congenital malformations of pulmonary artery**
Aberrant pulmonary artery
Agenesis of pulmonary artery
Congenital aneurysm of pulmonary artery
Congenital anomaly of pulmonary artery
Hypoplasia of pulmonary artery
MCC Exclusion see Appendix A PDX collection 1070

Q25.8 Other congenital malformations of other great arteries
CC Exclusion see Appendix A PDX collection 1069

CC **Q25.9 Congenital malformation of great arteries, unspecified**
CC Exclusion see Appendix A PDX collection 1069

Q26 Congenital malformations of great veins

CC **Q26.0 Congenital stenosis of vena cava**
Congenital stenosis of vena cava (inferior)(superior)
CC Exclusion see Appendix A PDX collection 1071

CC **Q26.1 Persistent left superior vena cava**
CC Exclusion see Appendix A PDX collection 1071

CC **Q26.2 Total anomalous pulmonary venous connection**
Total anomalous pulmonary venous return [TAPVR], subdiaphragmatic
Total anomalous pulmonary venous return [TAPVR], supradiaphragmatic
CC Exclusion see Appendix A PDX collection 1072

CC **Q26.3 Partial anomalous pulmonary venous connection**
Partial anomalous pulmonary venous return
CC Exclusion see Appendix A PDX collection 1073

CC **Q26.4 Anomalous pulmonary venous connection, unspecified**
CC Exclusion see Appendix A PDX collection 1073

Q26.5 Anomalous portal venous connection

Q26.6 Portal vein-hepatic artery fistula

CC **Q26.8 Other congenital malformations of great veins**
Absence of vena cava (inferior) (superior)
Azygos continuation of inferior vena cava
Persistent left posterior cardinal vein
Scimitar syndrome
CC Exclusion see Appendix A PDX collection 1071

CC **Q26.9 Congenital malformation of great vein, unspecified**
Congenital anomaly of vena cava (inferior) (superior) NOS
CC Exclusion see Appendix A PDX collection 1074

Q27 Other congenital malformations of peripheral vascular system

Excludes2: *anomalies of cerebral and precerebral vessels (Q28.0-Q28.3)*
anomalies of coronary vessels (Q24.5)
anomalies of pulmonary artery (Q25.5-Q25.7)
congenital retinal aneurysm (Q14.1)
hemangioma and lymphangioma (D18.-)

Q27.0 Congenital absence and hypoplasia of umbilical artery
Single umbilical artery

Q27.1 Congenital renal artery stenosis

Q27.2 Other congenital malformations of renal artery
Congenital malformation of renal artery NOS
Multiple renal arteries

+ **Q27.3 Arteriovenous malformation (peripheral)**
Arteriovenous aneurysm
Excludes1: *acquired arteriovenous aneurysm (I77.0)*
Excludes2: *arteriovenous malformation of cerebral vessels (Q28.2)*
arteriovenous malformation of precerebral vessels (Q28.0)

CC **Q27.30 Arteriovenous malformation, site unspecified**
CC Exclusion see Appendix A PDX collection 1075

Q27.31 Arteriovenous malformation of vessel of upper limb

Q27.32 Arteriovenous malformation of vessel of lower limb

Q27.33 Arteriovenous malformation of digestive system vessel

Q27.34 Arteriovenous malformation of renal vessel

Q27.39 Arteriovenous malformation, other site

CC **Q27.4 Congenital phlebectasia**
CC Exclusion see Appendix A PDX collection 1075

Q27.8 Other specified congenital malformations of peripheral vascular system
Absence of peripheral vascular system
Atresia of peripheral vascular system
Congenital aneurysm (peripheral)
Congenital stricture, artery
Congenital varix
Excludes1: *arteriovenous malformation (Q27.3-)*

Q27.9 Congenital malformation of peripheral vascular system, unspecified
Anomaly of artery or vein NOS

Q28 Other congenital malformations of circulatory system

Excludes1: *congenital aneurysm NOS (Q27.8)*
congenital coronary aneurysm (Q24.5)
ruptured cerebral arteriovenous malformation (I60.8)
ruptured malformation of precerebral vessels (I72.0)
Excludes2: *congenital peripheral aneurysm (Q27.8)*
congenital pulmonary aneurysm (Q25.79)
congenital retinal aneurysm (Q14.1)

CC **Q28.0 Arteriovenous malformation of precerebral vessels**
Congenital arteriovenous precerebral aneurysm (nonruptured)
CC Exclusion see Appendix A PDX collection 1075

CC **Q28.1 Other malformations of precerebral vessels**
Congenital malformation of precerebral vessels NOS
Congenital precerebral aneurysm (nonruptured)
CC Exclusion see Appendix A PDX collection 1075

MCC **Q28.2 Arteriovenous malformation of cerebral vessels**
Arteriovenous malformation of brain NOS
Congenital arteriovenous cerebral aneurysm (nonruptured)
MCC Exclusion see Appendix A PDX collection 1076

MCC **Q28.3 Other malformations of cerebral vessels**
Congenital cerebral aneurysm (nonruptured)
Congenital malformation of cerebral vessels NOS
Developmental venous anomaly
MCC Exclusion see Appendix A PDX collection 1076

CC **Q28.8 Other specified congenital malformations of circulatory system**
Congenital aneurysm, specified site NEC
Spinal vessel anomaly
CC Exclusion see Appendix A PDX collection 1075

CC **Q28.9 Congenital malformation of circulatory system, unspecified**
CC Exclusion see Appendix A PDX collection 1077

Congenital malformations of the respiratory system (Q30-Q34)

Q30 Congenital malformations of nose

Excludes1: *congenital deviation of nasal septum (Q67.4)*

Q30.0 Choanal atresia
Atresia of nares (anterior) (posterior)
Congenital stenosis of nares (anterior) (posterior)

Q30.1 Agenesis and underdevelopment of nose
Congenital absent of nose

Q30.2 Fissured, notched and cleft nose

Q30.3 Congenital perforated nasal septum

Q30.8 Other congenital malformations of nose
Accessory nose
Congenital anomaly of nasal sinus wall

Q30.9 Congenital malformation of nose, unspecified

Q31 Congenital malformations of larynx

Excludes1: *congenital laryngeal stridor NOS (P28.89)*

Q31.0 Web of larynx
Glottic web of larynx
Subglottic web of larynx
Web of larynx NOS

CC **Q31.1 Congenital subglottic stenosis**
CC Exclusion see Appendix A PDX collection 1078

CC **Q31.2 Laryngeal hypoplasia**
CC Exclusion see Appendix A PDX collection 1078

CC **Q31.3 Laryngocele**
CC Exclusion see Appendix A PDX collection 1078

CC **Q31.5 Congenital laryngomalacia**
CC Exclusion see Appendix A PDX collection 1078

CC **Q31.8 Other congenital malformations of larynx**
Absence of larynx
Agenesis of larynx
Atresia of larynx
Congenital cleft thyroid cartilage
Congenital fissure of epiglottis
Congenital stenosis of larynx NEC
Posterior cleft of cricoid cartilage
CC Exclusion see Appendix A PDX collection 1078

CC **Q31.9 Congenital malformation of larynx, unspecified**
CC Exclusion see Appendix A PDX collection 1078

Q32 Congenital malformations of trachea and bronchus

Excludes1: *congenital bronchiectasis (Q33.4)*

CC **Q32.0 Congenital tracheomalacia**
CC Exclusion see Appendix A PDX collection 1078

CC **Q32.1 Other congenital malformations of trachea**
Atresia of trachea
Congenital anomaly of tracheal cartilage
Congenital dilatation of trachea
Congenital malformation of trachea
Congenital stenosis of trachea
Congenital tracheocele
CC Exclusion see Appendix A PDX collection 1078

CC **Q32.2 Congenital bronchomalacia**
CC Exclusion see Appendix A PDX collection 1078

CC **Q32.3 Congenital stenosis of bronchus**
CC Exclusion see Appendix A PDX collection 1078

CC **Q32.4 Other congenital malformations of bronchus**
Absence of bronchus
Agenesis of bronchus
Atresia of bronchus
Congenital diverticulum of bronchus
Congenital malformation of bronchus NOS
CC Exclusion see Appendix A PDX collection 1078

Q33 Congenital malformations of lung

CC **Q33.0 Congenital cystic lung**
Congenital cystic lung disease
Congenital honeycomb lung
Congenital polycystic lung disease
Excludes1: *cystic fibrosis (E84.0)*
cystic lung disease, acquired or unspecified (J98.4)
CC Exclusion see Appendix A PDX collection 1079

Q33.1 Accessory lobe of lung
Azygos lobe (fissured), lung

MCC **Q33.2 Sequestration of lung**
MCC Exclusion see Appendix A PDX collection 1079

MCC **Q33.3 Agenesis of lung**
Congenital absence of lung (lobe)
MCC Exclusion see Appendix A PDX collection 1079

CC **Q33.4 Congenital bronchiectasis**
CC Exclusion see Appendix A PDX collection 1080

Q33.5 Ectopic tissue in lung

MCC **Q33.6 Congenital hypoplasia and dysplasia of lung**
Excludes1: *pulmonary hypoplasia associated with short gestation (P28.0)*
MCC Exclusion see Appendix A PDX collection 1079

Q33.8 Other congenital malformations of lung

Q33.9 Congenital malformation of lung, unspecified

Q34 Other congenital malformations of respiratory system

Excludes2: *congenital central alveolar hypoventilation syndrome (G47.35)*

Q34.0 Anomaly of pleura

Q34.1 Congenital cyst of mediastinum

Q34.8 Other specified congenital malformations of respiratory system
Atresia of nasopharynx

Q34.9 Congenital malformation of respiratory system, unspecified
Congenital absence of respiratory system
Congenital anomaly of respiratory system NOS

Cleft lip and cleft palate (Q35-Q37)

Use additional code to identify associated malformation of the nose (Q30.2)

Excludes1: *Robin's syndrome (Q87.0)*

Q35 Cleft palate

Includes: fissure of palate
palatoschisis
Excludes1: *cleft palate with cleft lip (Q37.-)*

Q35.1 Cleft hard palate

Q35.3 Cleft soft palate

Q35.5 Cleft hard palate with cleft soft palate

Q35.7 Cleft uvula

Q35.9 Cleft palate, unspecified
Cleft palate NOS

Q36 Cleft lip

Includes: cheiloschisis
congenital fissure of lip
harelip
labium leporinum
Excludes1: *cleft lip with cleft palate (Q37.-)*

Q36.0 Cleft lip, bilateral

Q36.1 Cleft lip, median

Q36.9 Cleft lip, unilateral
Cleft lip NOS

Q37 Cleft palate with cleft lip

Includes: cheilopalatoschisis

Q37.0 Cleft hard palate with bilateral cleft lip

Q37.1 Cleft hard palate with unilateral cleft lip
Cleft hard palate with cleft lip NOS

Q37.2 Cleft soft palate with bilateral cleft lip

Q37.3 Cleft soft palate with unilateral cleft lip
Cleft soft palate with cleft lip NOS

Q37.4 Cleft hard and soft palate with bilateral cleft lip

Q37.5 Cleft hard and soft palate with unilateral cleft lip
Cleft hard and soft palate with cleft lip NOS

Q37.8 Unspecified cleft palate with bilateral cleft lip

Q37.9 Unspecified cleft palate with unilateral cleft lip
Cleft palate with cleft lip NOS

Other congenital malformations of the digestive system (Q38-Q45)

Q38 Other congenital malformations of tongue, mouth and pharynx

Excludes1: *dentofacial anomalies (M26.-)*
macrostomia (Q18.4)
microstomia (Q18.5)

Q38.0 Congenital malformations of lips, not elsewhere classified
Congenital fistula of lip
Congenital malformation of lip NOS
Van der Woude's syndrome
Excludes1: *cleft lip (Q36.-)*
cleft lip with cleft palate (Q37.-)
macrocheilia (Q18.6)
microcheilia (Q18.7)

Q38.1 Ankyloglossia
Tongue tie

Q38.2 Macroglossia
Congenital hypertrophy of tongue

Q38.3 Other congenital malformations of tongue
Aglossia
Bifid tongue
Congenital adhesion of tongue
Congenital fissure of tongue
Congenital malformation of tongue NOS
Double tongue
Hypoglossia
Hypoplasia of tongue
Microglossia

Q38.4 Congenital malformations of salivary glands and ducts
Atresia of salivary glands and ducts
Congenital absence of salivary glands and ducts
Congenital accessory salivary glands and ducts
Congenital fistula of salivary gland

Q38.5 Congenital malformations of palate, not elsewhere classified
Congenital absence of uvula
Congenital malformation of palate NOS
Congenital high arched palate
Excludes1: *cleft palate (Q35.-)*
cleft palate with cleft lip (Q37.-)

Q38.6 Other congenital malformations of mouth
Congenital malformation of mouth NOS

Q38.7 Congenital pharyngeal pouch
Congenital diverticulum of pharynx
Excludes1: *pharyngeal pouch syndrome (D82.1)*

Q38.8 Other congenital malformations of pharynx
Congenital malformation of pharynx NOS
Imperforate pharynx

Q39 Congenital malformations of esophagus

MCC **Q39.0 Atresia of esophagus without fistula**
Atresia of esophagus NOS
MCC Exclusion see Appendix A PDX collection 1081

MCC **Q39.1 Atresia of esophagus with tracheo-esophageal fistula**
Atresia of esophagus with broncho-esophageal fistula
MCC Exclusion see Appendix A PDX collection 1081

MCC **Q39.2 Congenital tracheo-esophageal fistula without atresia**
Congenital tracheo-esophageal fistula NOS
MCC Exclusion see Appendix A PDX collection 1081

MCC **Q39.3 Congenital stenosis and stricture of esophagus**
MCC Exclusion see Appendix A PDX collection 1081

MCC **Q39.4 Esophageal web**
MCC Exclusion see Appendix A PDX collection 1081

CC **Q39.5 Congenital dilatation of esophagus**
Congenital cardiospasm
CC Exclusion see Appendix A PDX collection 1082

CC **Q39.6 Congenital diverticulum of esophagus**
Congenital esophageal pouch
CC Exclusion see Appendix A PDX collection 1082

CC **Q39.8 Other congenital malformations of esophagus**
Congenital absence of esophagus
Congenital displacement of esophagus
Congenital duplication of esophagus
CC Exclusion see Appendix A PDX collection 1082

CC **Q39.9 Congenital malformation of esophagus, unspecified**
CC Exclusion see Appendix A PDX collection 1082

Q40 Other congenital malformations of upper alimentary tract

Q40.0 Congenital hypertrophic pyloric stenosis
Congenital or infantile constriction
Congenital or infantile hypertrophy
Congenital or infantile spasm
Congenital or infantile stenosis
Congenital or infantile stricture

Q40.1 Congenital hiatus hernia
Congenital displacement of cardia through esophageal hiatus
Excludes1: *congenital diaphragmatic hernia (Q79.0)*

Q40.2 Other specified congenital malformations of stomach
Congenital displacement of stomach
Congenital diverticulum of stomach
Congenital hourglass stomach
Congenital duplication of stomach
Megalogastria
Microgastria

Q40.3 Congenital malformation of stomach, unspecified

Q40.8 Other specified congenital malformations of upper alimentary tract

Q40.9 Congenital malformation of upper alimentary tract, unspecified
Congenital anomaly of upper alimentary tract
Congenital deformity of upper alimentary tract

Q41 Congenital absence, atresia and stenosis of small intestine

Includes: congenital obstruction, occlusion or stricture of small intestine or intestine NOS
Excludes1: *cystic fibrosis with intestinal manifestation (E84.11)*
meconium ileus NOS (without cystic fibrosis) (P76.0)

CC **Q41.0 Congenital absence, atresia and stenosis of duodenum**
CC Exclusion see Appendix A PDX collection 1083

CC **Q41.1 Congenital absence, atresia and stenosis of jejunum**
Apple peel syndrome
Imperforate jejunum
CC Exclusion see Appendix A PDX collection 1083

CC **Q41.2 Congenital absence, atresia and stenosis of ileum**
CC Exclusion see Appendix A PDX collection 1083

CC **Q41.8 Congenital absence, atresia and stenosis of other specified parts of small intestine**
CC Exclusion see Appendix A PDX collection 1083

CC **Q41.9 Congenital absence, atresia and stenosis of small intestine, part unspecified**
Congenital absence, atresia and stenosis of intestine NOS
CC Exclusion see Appendix A PDX collection 1083

Q42 Congenital absence, atresia and stenosis of large intestine

Includes: congenital obstruction, occlusion and stricture of large intestine

CC **Q42.0 Congenital absence, atresia and stenosis of rectum with fistula**
CC Exclusion see Appendix A PDX collection 1084

CC **Q42.1 Congenital absence, atresia and stenosis of rectum without fistula**
Imperforate rectum
CC Exclusion see Appendix A PDX collection 1084

CC **Q42.2 Congenital absence, atresia and stenosis of anus with fistula**
CC Exclusion see Appendix A PDX collection 1084

CC **Q42.3 Congenital absence, atresia and stenosis of anus without fistula**
Imperforate anus
CC Exclusion see Appendix A PDX collection 1084

CC **Q42.8 Congenital absence, atresia and stenosis of other parts of large intestine**
CC Exclusion see Appendix A PDX collection 1084

CC **Q42.9 Congenital absence, atresia and stenosis of large intestine, part unspecified**
CC Exclusion see Appendix A PDX collection 1084

Q43 Other congenital malformations of intestine

Q43.0 Meckel's diverticulum (displaced) (hypertrophic)
Persistent omphalomesenteric duct
Persistent vitelline duct

CC **Q43.1 Hirschsprung's disease**
Aganglionosis
Congenital (aganglionic) megacolon
CC Exclusion see Appendix A PDX collection 1085

CC **Q43.2 Other congenital functional disorders of colon**
Congenital dilatation of colon
CC Exclusion see Appendix A PDX collection 1085

CC **Q43.3 Congenital malformations of intestinal fixation**
Congenital omental, anomalous adhesions [bands]
Congenital peritoneal adhesions [bands]
Incomplete rotation of cecum and colon
Insufficient rotation of cecum and colon
Jackson's membrane
Malrotation of colon
Rotation failure of cecum and colon
Universal mesentery
CC Exclusion see Appendix A PDX collection 1086

CC **Q43.4 Duplication of intestine**
CC Exclusion see Appendix A PDX collection 1087

CC **Q43.5 Ectopic anus**
CC Exclusion see Appendix A PDX collection 1087

CC **Q43.6 Congenital fistula of rectum and anus**
Excludes1: *congenital fistula of anus with absence, atresia and stenosis (Q42.2)*
congenital fistula of rectum with absence, atresia and stenosis (Q42.0)
congenital rectovaginal fistula (Q52.2)
congenital urethrorectal fistula (Q64.73)
pilonidal fistula or sinus (L05.-)
CC Exclusion see Appendix A PDX collection 1087

CC **Q43.7 Persistent cloaca**
Cloaca NOS
CC Exclusion see Appendix A PDX collection 1087

CC **Q43.8 Other specified congenital malformations of intestine**
Congenital blind loop syndrome
Congenital diverticulitis, colon
Congenital diverticulum, intestine
Dolichocolon
Megaloappendix
Megaloduodenum
Microcolon
Transposition of appendix
Transposition of colon
Transposition of intestine
CC Exclusion see Appendix A PDX collection 1087
AHA CC: 2Q, 2013, 31

CC **Q43.9 Congenital malformation of intestine, unspecified**
CC Exclusion see Appendix A PDX collection 1087

Q44 Congenital malformations of gallbladder, bile ducts and liver

CC **Q44.0 Agenesis, aplasia and hypoplasia of gallbladder**
Congenital absence of gallbladder
CC Exclusion see Appendix A PDX collection 1088

CC **Q44.1 Other congenital malformations of gallbladder**
Congenital malformation of gallbladder NOS
Intrahepatic gallbladder
CC Exclusion see Appendix A PDX collection 1088

MCC **Q44.2 Atresia of bile ducts**
MCC Exclusion see Appendix A PDX collection 1089

MCC **Q44.3 Congenital stenosis and stricture of bile ducts**
MCC Exclusion see Appendix A PDX collection 1089

CC **Q44.4 Choledochal cyst**
CC Exclusion see Appendix A PDX collection 1088

CC **Q44.5 Other congenital malformations of bile ducts**
Accessory hepatic duct
Biliary duct duplication
Congenital malformation of bile duct NOS
Cystic duct duplication
CC Exclusion see Appendix A PDX collection 1088

CC **Q44.6 Cystic disease of liver**
Fibrocystic disease of liver
CC Exclusion see Appendix A PDX collection 1090

CC **Q44.7 Other congenital malformations of liver**
Accessory liver
Alagille's syndrome
Congenital absence of liver
Congenital hepatomegaly
Congenital malformation of liver NOS
CC Exclusion see Appendix A PDX collection 1088

Q45 Other congenital malformations of digestive system

Excludes2: *congenital diaphragmatic hernia (Q79.0)*
congenital hiatus hernia (Q40.1)

CC **Q45.0 Agenesis, aplasia and hypoplasia of pancreas**
Congenital absence of pancreas
CC Exclusion see Appendix A PDX collection 1091

CC **Q45.1 Annular pancreas**
CC Exclusion see Appendix A PDX collection 1091

CC **Q45.2 Congenital pancreatic cyst**
CC Exclusion see Appendix A PDX collection 1091

Q45.3 Other congenital malformations of pancreas and pancreatic duct
Accessory pancreas
Congenital malformation of pancreas or pancreatic duct NOS
Excludes1: *congenital diabetes mellitus (E10.-)*
cystic fibrosis (E84.0-E84.9)
fibrocystic disease of pancreas (E84.-)
neonatal diabetes mellitus (P70.2)
CC Exclusion see Appendix A PDX collection 1091

Q45.8 Other specified congenital malformations of digestive system
Absence (complete) (partial) of alimentary tract NOS
Duplication of digestive system
Malposition, congenital of digestive system

Q45.9 Congenital malformation of digestive system, unspecified
Congenital anomaly of digestive system
Congenital deformity of digestive system

Congenital malformations of genital organs (Q50-Q56)

Excludes1: *androgen insensitivity syndrome (E34.5-)*
syndromes associated with anomalies in the number and form of chromosomes (Q90-Q99)

Q50 Congenital malformations of ovaries, fallopian tubes and broad ligaments

\+ **Q50.0 Congenital absence of ovary**
Excludes1: *Turner's syndrome (Q96.-)*
♀ **Q50.01 Congenital absence of ovary, unilateral**
♀ **Q50.02 Congenital absence of ovary, bilateral**

♀ **Q50.1 Developmental ovarian cyst**

♀ **Q50.2 Congenital torsion of ovary**

\+ **Q50.3 Other congenital malformations of ovary**
♀ **Q50.31 Accessory ovary**
♀ **Q50.32 Ovarian streak**
46, XX with streak gonads
♀ **Q50.39 Other congenital malformation of ovary**
Congenital malformation of ovary NOS

♀ **Q50.4 Embryonic cyst of fallopian tube**
Fimbrial cyst

♀ **Q50.5 Embryonic cyst of broad ligament**
Epoophoron cyst
Parovarian cyst

♀ **Q50.6 Other congenital malformations of fallopian tube and broad ligament**
Absence of fallopian tube and broad ligament
Accessory fallopian tube and broad ligament
Atresia of fallopian tube and broad ligament
Congenital malformation of fallopian tube or broad ligament NOS

Q51 Congenital malformations of uterus and cervix

♀ **Q51.0 Agenesis and aplasia of uterus**
Congenital absence of uterus

\+ **Q51.1 Doubling of uterus with doubling of cervix and vagina**
♀ **Q51.10 Doubling of uterus with doubling of cervix and vagina without obstruction**
Doubling of uterus with doubling of cervix and vagina NOS
♀ **Q51.11 Doubling of uterus with doubling of cervix and vagina with obstruction**

♀ **Q51.2 Other doubling of uterus**
Doubling of uterus NOS
Septate uterus, complete or partial

♀ **Q51.3 Bicornate uterus**
Bicornate uterus, complete or partial

♀ **Q51.4 Unicornate uterus**
Unicornate uterus with or without a separate uterine horn
Uterus with only one functioning horn

♀ **Q51.5 Agenesis and aplasia of cervix**
Congenital absence of cervix

♀ **Q51.6 Embryonic cyst of cervix**

♀ **Q51.7 Congenital fistulae between uterus and digestive and urinary tracts**

\+ **Q51.8 Other congenital malformations of uterus and cervix**
\+ **Q51.81 Other congenital malformations of uterus**
♀ **Q51.810 Arcuate uterus**
Arcuatus uterus
♀ **Q51.811 Hypoplasia of uterus**
♀ **Q51.818 Other congenital malformations of uterus**
Müllerian anomaly of uterus NEC
\+ **Q51.82 Other congenital malformations of cervix**
♀ **Q51.820 Cervical duplication**
♀ **Q51.821 Hypoplasia of cervix**
♀ **Q51.828 Other congenital malformations of cervix**

♀ **Q51.9 Congenital malformation of uterus and cervix, unspecified**

Q52 Other congenital malformations of female genitalia

♀ **Q52.0 Congenital absence of vagina**
Vaginal agenesis, total or partial

\+ **Q52.1 Doubling of vagina**
Excludes1: *doubling of vagina with doubling of uterus and cervix (Q51.1-)*
♀ **Q52.10 Doubling of vagina, unspecified**
Septate vagina NOS
♀ **Q52.11 Transverse vaginal septum**
\+ **Q52.12 Longitudinal vaginal septum**
AHA CC: 4Q, 2016, 58-59
♀ **Q52.120 Longitudinal vaginal septum, nonobstructing**
♀ **Q52.121 Longitudinal vaginal septum, obstructing, right side**
♀ **Q52.122 Longitudinal vaginal septum, obstructing, left side**
♀ **Q52.123 Longitudinal vaginal septum, microperforate, right side**
♀ **Q52.124 Longitudinal vaginal septum, microperforate, left side**
AHA CC: 4Q, 2016, 58-59
♀ **Q52.129 Other and unspecified longitudinal vaginal septum**

♀ **Q52.2 Congenital rectovaginal fistula**
Excludes1: *cloaca (Q43.7)*

♀ **Q52.3 Imperforate hymen**

♀ **Q52.4 Other congenital malformations of vagina**
Canal of Nuck cyst, congenital
Congenital malformation of vagina NOS
Embryonic vaginal cyst
Gartner's duct cyst

♀ **Q52.5 Fusion of labia**

♀ **Q52.6 Congenital malformation of clitoris**

\+ **Q52.7 Other and unspecified congenital malformations of vulva**
♀ **Q52.70 Unspecified congenital malformations of vulva**
Congenital malformation of vulva NOS
♀ **Q52.71 Congenital absence of vulva**
♀ **Q52.79 Other congenital malformations of vulva**
Congenital cyst of vulva

♀ **Q52.8 Other specified congenital malformations of female genitalia**

♀ **Q52.9 Congenital malformation of female genitalia, unspecified**

Q53 Undescended and ectopic testicle

\+ **Q53.0 Ectopic testis**
♂ **Q53.00 Ectopic testis, unspecified**
♂ **Q53.01 Ectopic testis, unilateral**
♂ **Q53.02 Ectopic testes, bilateral**

\+ **Q53.1 Undescended testicle, unilateral**
♂ **Q53.10 Unspecified undescended testicle, unilateral**
\+ **Q53.11 Abdominal testis, unilateral**
♂ **Q53.111 Unilateral intraabdominal testis**
♂ **Q53.112 Unilateral inguinal testis**
♂ **Q53.12 Ectopic perineal testis, unilateral**
♂ **Q53.13 Unilateral high scrotal testis**

\+ **Q53.2 Undescended testicle, bilateral**
♂ **Q53.20 Undescended testicle, unspecified, bilateral**
\+ **Q53.21 Abdominal testis, bilateral**
♂ **Q53.211 Bilateral intraabdominal testes**
♂ **Q53.212 Bilateral inguinal testes**
♂ **Q53.22 Ectopic perineal testis, bilateral**
♂ **Q53.23 Bilateral high scrotal testes**

♂ **Q53.9 Undescended testicle, unspecified**
Cryptorchism NOS

Q54 Hypospadias

Excludes1: epispadias (Q64.0)

♂ **Q54.0 Hypospadias, balanic**
Hypospadias, coronal
Hypospadias, glandular

♂ **Q54.1 Hypospadias, penile**

♂ **Q54.2 Hypospadias, penoscrotal**

♂ **Q54.3 Hypospadias, perineal**

♂ **Q54.4 Congenital chordee**
Chordee without hypospadias

♂ **Q54.8 Other hypospadias**
Hypospadias with intersex state

♂ **Q54.9 Hypospadias, unspecified**

Q55 Other congenital malformations of male genital organs

Excludes1: congenital hydrocele (P83.5)
hypospadias (Q54.-)

♂ **Q55.0 Absence and aplasia of testis**
Monorchism

♂ **Q55.1 Hypoplasia of testis and scrotum**
Fusion of testes

\+ **Q55.2 Other and unspecified congenital malformations of testis and scrotum**

♂ **Q55.20 Unspecified congenital malformations of testis and scrotum**
Congenital malformation of testis or scrotum NOS

♂ **Q55.21 Polyorchism**

♂ **Q55.22 Retractile testis**

♂ **Q55.23 Scrotal transposition**

♂ **Q55.29 Other congenital malformations of testis and scrotum**

♂ **Q55.3 Atresia of vas deferens**
Code first any associated cystic fibrosis (E84.-)

♂ **Q55.4 Other congenital malformations of vas deferens, epididymis, seminal vesicles and prostate**
Absence or aplasia of prostate
Absence or aplasia of spermatic cord
Congenital malformation of vas deferens, epididymis, seminal vesicles or prostate NOS

♂ **Q55.5 Congenital absence and aplasia of penis**

\+ **Q55.6 Other congenital malformations of penis**

♂ **Q55.61 Curvature of penis (lateral)**

♂ **Q55.62 Hypoplasia of penis**
Micropenis

♂ **Q55.63 Congenital torsion of penis**
Excludes1: acquired torsion of penis (N48.82)

♂ **Q55.64 Hidden penis**
Buried penis
Concealed penis
Excludes1: acquired buried penis (N48.83)

♂ **Q55.69 Other congenital malformation of penis**
Congenital malformation of penis NOS

♂ **Q55.7 Congenital vasocutaneous fistula**

♂ **Q55.8 Other specified congenital malformations of male genital organs**

♂ **Q55.9 Congenital malformation of male genital organ, unspecified**
Congenital anomaly of male genital organ
Congenital deformity of male genital organ

Q56 Indeterminate sex and pseudohermaphroditism

Excludes1: 46,XX true hermaphrodite (Q99.1)
androgen insensitivity syndrome (E34.5-)
chimera 46,XX/46,XY true hermaphrodite (Q99.0)
female pseudohermaphroditism with adrenocortical disorder (E25.-)
pseudohermaphroditism with specified chromosomal anomaly (Q96-Q99)
pure gonadal dysgenesis (Q99.1)

Q56.0 Hermaphroditism, not elsewhere classified
Ovotestis

♂ **Q56.1 Male pseudohermaphroditism, not elsewhere classified**
46, XY with streak gonads
Male pseudohermaphroditism NOS

♀ **Q56.2 Female pseudohermaphroditism, not elsewhere classified**
Female pseudohermaphroditism NOS

Q56.3 Pseudohermaphroditism, unspecified

Q56.4 Indeterminate sex, unspecified
Ambiguous genitalia

Congenital malformations of the urinary system (Q60-Q64)

Q60 Renal agenesis and other reduction defects of kidney

Includes: congenital absence of kidney
congenital atrophy of kidney
infantile atrophy of kidney

CC **Q60.0 Renal agenesis, unilateral**
CC Exclusion see Appendix A PDX collection 1092

CC **Q60.1 Renal agenesis, bilateral**
CC Exclusion see Appendix A PDX collection 1092

CC **Q60.2 Renal agenesis, unspecified**
CC Exclusion see Appendix A PDX collection 1092

CC **Q60.3 Renal hypoplasia, unilateral**
CC Exclusion see Appendix A PDX collection 1092

CC **Q60.4 Renal hypoplasia, bilateral**
CC Exclusion see Appendix A PDX collection 1092

CC **Q60.5 Renal hypoplasia, unspecified**
CC Exclusion see Appendix A PDX collection 1092

CC **Q60.6 Potter's syndrome**
CC Exclusion see Appendix A PDX collection 1092

Q61 Cystic kidney disease

Excludes1: acquired cyst of kidney (N28.1)
Potter's syndrome (Q60.6)

\+ **Q61.0 Congenital renal cyst**

CC **Q61.00 Congenital renal cyst, unspecified**
Cyst of kidney NOS (congenital)
CC Exclusion see Appendix A PDX collection 1093

CC **Q61.01 Congenital single renal cyst**
CC Exclusion see Appendix A PDX collection 1094

CC **Q61.02 Congenital multiple renal cysts**
CC Exclusion see Appendix A PDX collection 1095

\+ **Q61.1 Polycystic kidney, infantile type**
Polycystic kidney, autosomal recessive

CC **Q61.11 Cystic dilatation of collecting ducts**
CC Exclusion see Appendix A PDX collection 1096

CC **Q61.19 Other polycystic kidney, infantile type**
CC Exclusion see Appendix A PDX collection 1096

CC **Q61.2 Polycystic kidney, adult type**
Polycystic kidney, autosomal dominant
CC Exclusion see Appendix A PDX collection 1096

CC **Q61.3 Polycystic kidney, unspecified**
CC Exclusion see Appendix A PDX collection 1096
AHA CC: 3Q, 2016, 22-23

CC **Q61.4 Renal dysplasia**
Multicystic dysplastic kidney
Multicystic kidney (development)
Multicystic kidney disease
Multicystic renal dysplasia
Excludes1: polycystic kidney disease (Q61.11-Q61.3)
CC Exclusion see Appendix A PDX collection 1097

CC **Q61.5 Medullary cystic kidney**
Nephronopthisis
Sponge kidney NOS
CC Exclusion see Appendix A PDX collection 1095

CC **Q61.8 Other cystic kidney diseases**
Fibrocystic kidney
Fibrocystic renal degeneration or disease
CC Exclusion see Appendix A PDX collection 1095

CC **Q61.9 Cystic kidney disease, unspecified**
Meckel-Gruber syndrome
CC Exclusion see Appendix A PDX collection 1093

Q62 Congenital obstructive defects of renal pelvis and congenital malformations of ureter

CC **Q62.0 Congenital hydronephrosis**
CC Exclusion see Appendix A PDX collection 1098

\+ **Q62.1 Congenital occlusion of ureter**
Atresia and stenosis of ureter

CC **Q62.10 Congenital occlusion of ureter, unspecified**
CC Exclusion see Appendix A PDX collection 1098

CC **Q62.11 Congenital occlusion of ureteropelvic junction**
CC Exclusion see Appendix A PDX collection 1098

CC **Q62.12 Congenital occlusion of ureterovesical orifice**
CC Exclusion see Appendix A PDX collection 1098

Q62.2 Congenital megaureter
Congenital dilatation of ureter
CC Exclusion see Appendix A PDX collection 1098

\+ **Q62.3 Other obstructive defects of renal pelvis and ureter**

CC **Q62.31 Congenital ureterocele, orthotopic**
CC Exclusion see Appendix A PDX collection 1098

CC **Q62.32 Cecoureterocele**
Ectopic ureterocele
CC Exclusion see Appendix A PDX collection 1098

CC **Q62.39 Other obstructive defects of renal pelvis and ureter**
Ureteropelvic junction obstruction NOS
CC Exclusion see Appendix A PDX collection 1098

Q62.4 Agenesis of ureter
Congenital absence ureter

Q62.5 Duplication of ureter
Accessory ureter
Double ureter

\+ **Q62.6 Malposition of ureter**
Q62.60 Malposition of ureter, unspecified
Q62.61 Deviation of ureter
Q62.62 Displacement of ureter
Q62.63 Anomalous implantation of ureter
Ectopia of ureter
Ectopic ureter
Q62.69 Other malposition of ureter

Q62.7 Congenital vesico-uretero-renal reflux

Q62.8 Other congenital malformations of ureter
Anomaly of ureter NOS

Q63 Other congenital malformations of kidney

Excludes1: *congenital nephrotic syndrome (N04.-)*

Q63.0 Accessory kidney
Q63.1 Lobulated, fused and horseshoe kidney
Q63.2 Ectopic kidney
Congenital displaced kidney
Malrotation of kidney
Q63.3 Hyperplastic and giant kidney
Compensatory hypertrophy of kidney
Q63.8 Other specified congenital malformations of kidney
Congenital renal calculi
Q63.9 Congenital malformation of kidney, unspecified

Q64 Other congenital malformations of urinary system

Q64.0 Epispadias
Excludes1: *hypospadias (Q54.-)*

\+ **Q64.1 Exstrophy of urinary bladder**
CC **Q64.10 Exstrophy of urinary bladder, unspecified**
Ectopia vesicae
CC Exclusion see Appendix A PDX collection 1099
CC **Q64.11 Supravesical fissure of urinary bladder**
CC Exclusion see Appendix A PDX collection 1099
CC **Q64.12 Cloacal exstrophy of urinary bladder**
CC Exclusion see Appendix A PDX collection 1099
CC **Q64.19 Other exstrophy of urinary bladder**
Extroversion of bladder
CC Exclusion see Appendix A PDX collection 1099

CC **Q64.2 Congenital posterior urethral valves**
CC Exclusion see Appendix A PDX collection 1100

\+ **Q64.3 Other atresia and stenosis of urethra and bladder neck**
CC **Q64.31 Congenital bladder neck obstruction**
Congenital obstruction of vesicourethral orifice
CC Exclusion see Appendix A PDX collection 1100
CC **Q64.32 Congenital stricture of urethra**
CC Exclusion see Appendix A PDX collection 1100
CC **Q64.33 Congenital stricture of urinary meatus**
CC Exclusion see Appendix A PDX collection 1100
CC **Q64.39 Other atresia and stenosis of urethra and bladder neck**
Atresia and stenosis of urethra and bladder neck NOS
CC Exclusion see Appendix A PDX collection 1100

Q64.4 Malformation of urachus
Cyst of urachus
Patent urachus
Prolapse of urachus

Q64.5 Congenital absence of bladder and urethra
Q64.6 Congenital diverticulum of bladder

\+ **Q64.7 Other and unspecified congenital malformations of bladder and urethra**
Excludes1: *congenital prolapse of bladder (mucosa) (Q79.4)*
Q64.70 Unspecified congenital malformation of bladder and urethra
Malformation of bladder or urethra NOS
Q64.71 Congenital prolapse of urethra
Q64.72 Congenital prolapse of urinary meatus
Q64.73 Congenital urethrorectal fistula
Q64.74 Double urethra
Q64.75 Double urinary meatus
Q64.79 Other congenital malformations of bladder and urethra

Q64.8 Other specified congenital malformations of urinary system

Q64.9 Congenital malformation of urinary system, unspecified
Congenital anomaly NOS of urinary system
Congenital deformity NOS of urinary system

Congenital malformations and deformations of the musculoskeletal system (Q65-Q79)

Q65 Congenital deformities of hip

Excludes1: *clicking hip (R29.4)*

\+ **Q65.0 Congenital dislocation of hip, unilateral**
Q65.00 Congenital dislocation of unspecified hip, unilateral
Q65.01 Congenital dislocation of right hip, unilateral
Q65.02 Congenital dislocation of left hip, unilateral
Q65.1 Congenital dislocation of hip, bilateral
Q65.2 Congenital dislocation of hip, unspecified
\+ **Q65.3 Congenital partial dislocation of hip, unilateral**
Q65.30 Congenital partial dislocation of unspecified hip, unilateral
Q65.31 Congenital partial dislocation of right hip, unilateral
Q65.32 Congenital partial dislocation of left hip, unilateral
Q65.4 Congenital partial dislocation of hip, bilateral
Q65.5 Congenital partial dislocation of hip, unspecified
Q65.6 Congenital unstable hip
Congenital dislocatable hip
\+ **Q65.8 Other congenital deformities of hip**
Q65.81 Congenital coxa valga
Q65.82 Congenital coxa vara
Q65.89 Other specified congenital deformities of hip
Anteversion of femoral neck
Congenital acetabular dysplasia
Q65.9 Congenital deformity of hip, unspecified

Q66 Congenital deformities of feet

Excludes1: *reduction defects of feet (Q72.-)*
valgus deformities (acquired) (M21.0-)
varus deformities (acquired) (M21.1-)

Q66.0 Congenital talipes equinovarus
Q66.1 Congenital talipes calcaneovarus
\+ **Q66.2 Congenital metatarsus (primus) varus**
AHA CC: 4Q, 2016, 59
Q66.21 Congenital metatarsus primus varus
Q66.22 Congenital metatarsus adductus
Congenital metatarsus varus
Q66.3 Other congenital varus deformities of feet
Hallux varus, congenital
Q66.4 Congenital talipes calcaneovalgus
\+ **Q66.5 Congenital pes planus**
Congenital flat foot
Congenital rigid flat foot
Congenital spastic (everted) flat foot
Excludes1: *pes planus, acquired (M21.4)*
Q66.50 Congenital pes planus, unspecified foot
Q66.51 Congenital pes planus, right foot
Q66.52 Congenital pes planus, left foot
Q66.6 Other congenital valgus deformities of feet
Congenital metatarsus valgus
Q66.7 Congenital pes cavus
\+ **Q66.8 Other congenital deformities of feet**
Q66.80 Congenital vertical talus deformity, unspecified foot
Q66.81 Congenital vertical talus deformity, right foot
Q66.82 Congenital vertical talus deformity, left foot
Q66.89 Other specified congenital deformities of feet
Congenital asymmetric talipes
Congenital clubfoot NOS
Congenital talipes NOS
Congenital tarsal coalition
Hammer toe, congenital
Q66.9 Congenital deformity of feet, unspecified

Q67 Congenital musculoskeletal deformities of head, face, spine and ches

Excludes1: *congenital malformation syndromes classified to Q87.-*
Potter's syndrome (Q60.6)

Q67.0 Congenital facial asymmetry
Q67.1 Congenital compression facies
Q67.2 Dolichocephaly
Q67.3 Plagiocephaly

Q67.4 Other congenital deformities of skull, face and jaw
Congenital depressions in skull
Congenital hemifacial atrophy or hypertrophy
Deviation of nasal septum, congenital
Squashed or bent nose, congenital
Excludes1: *dentofacial anomalies [including malocclusion] (M26.-)*
syphilitic saddle nose (A50.5)

CC **Q67.5 Congenital deformity of spine**
Congenital postural scoliosis
Congenital scoliosis NOS
Excludes1: *infantile idiopathic scoliosis (M41.0)*
scoliosis due to congenital bony malformation (Q76.3)
CC Exclusion see Appendix A PDX collection 1101
AHA CC: 4Q, 2014, 26

Q67.6 Pectus excavatum
Congenital funnel chest

Q67.7 Pectus carinatum
Congenital pigeon chest

CC **Q67.8 Other congenital deformities of chest**
Congenital deformity of chest wall NOS
CC Exclusion see Appendix A PDX collection 1102

Q68 Other congenital musculoskeletal deformities

Excludes1: *reduction defects of limb(s) (Q71-Q73)*
Excludes2: *congenital myotonic chondrodystrophy (G71.13)*

Q68.0 Congenital deformity of sternocleidomastoid muscle
Congenital contracture of sternocleidomastoid (muscle)
Congenital (sternomastoid) torticollis
Sternomastoid tumor (congenital)

CC **Q68.1 Congenital deformity of finger(s) and hand**
Congenital clubfinger
Spade-like hand (congenital)
CC Exclusion see Appendix A PDX collection 1102

Q68.2 Congenital deformity of knee
Congenital dislocation of knee
Congenital genu recurvatum

Q68.3 Congenital bowing of femur
Excludes1: *anteversion of femur (neck) (Q65.89)*

Q68.4 Congenital bowing of tibia and fibula
Q68.5 Congenital bowing of long bones of leg, unspecified
Q68.6 Discoid meniscus
Q68.8 Other specified congenital musculoskeletal deformities
Congenital deformity of clavicle
Congenital deformity of elbow
Congenital deformity of forearm
Congenital deformity of scapula
Congenital deformity of wrist
Congenital dislocation of elbow
Congenital dislocation of shoulder
Congenital dislocation of wrist

Q69 Polydactyly

Q69.0 Accessory finger(s)
Q69.1 Accessory thumb(s)
Q69.2 Accessory toe(s)
Accessory hallux
Q69.9 Polydactyly, unspecified
Supernumerary digit(s) NOS

Q70 Syndactyly

+ **Q70.0 Fused fingers**
Complex syndactyly of fingers with synostosis
Q70.00 Fused fingers, unspecified hand
Q70.01 Fused fingers, right hand
Q70.02 Fused fingers, left hand
Q70.03 Fused fingers, bilateral

+ **Q70.1 Webbed fingers**
Simple syndactyly of fingers without synostosis
Q70.10 Webbed fingers, unspecified hand
Q70.11 Webbed fingers, right hand
Q70.12 Webbed fingers, left hand
Q70.13 Webbed fingers, bilateral

+ **Q70.2 Fused toes**
Complex syndactyly of toes with synostosis
Q70.20 Fused toes, unspecified foot
Q70.21 Fused toes, right foot
Q70.22 Fused toes, left foot
Q70.23 Fused toes, bilateral

+ **Q70.3 Webbed toes**
Simple syndactyly of toes without synostosis
Q70.30 Webbed toes, unspecified foot
Q70.31 Webbed toes, right foot
Q70.32 Webbed toes, left foot
Q70.33 Webbed toes, bilateral

Q70.4 Polysyndactyly, unspecified
Excludes1: *specified syndactyly of hand and feet - code to specified conditions (Q70.0-Q70.3-)*

Q70.9 Syndactyly, unspecified
Symphalangy NOS

Q71 Reduction defects of upper limb

+ **Q71.0 Congenital complete absence of upper limb**
Q71.00 Congenital complete absence of unspecified upper limb
Q71.01 Congenital complete absence of right upper limb
Q71.02 Congenital complete absence of left upper limb
Q71.03 Congenital complete absence of upper limb, bilateral

+ **Q71.1 Congenital absence of upper arm and forearm with hand present**
Q71.10 Congenital absence of unspecified upper arm and forearm with hand present
Q71.11 Congenital absence of right upper arm and forearm with hand present
Q71.12 Congenital absence of left upper arm and forearm with hand present
Q71.13 Congenital absence of upper arm and forearm with hand present, bilateral

+ **Q71.2 Congenital absence of both forearm and hand**
Q71.20 Congenital absence of both forearm and hand, unspecified upper limb
Q71.21 Congenital absence of both forearm and hand, right upper limb
Q71.22 Congenital absence of both forearm and hand, left upper limb
Q71.23 Congenital absence of both forearm and hand, bilateral

+ **Q71.3 Congenital absence of hand and finger**
Q71.30 Congenital absence of unspecified hand and finger
Q71.31 Congenital absence of right hand and finger
Q71.32 Congenital absence of left hand and finger
Q71.33 Congenital absence of hand and finger, bilateral

+ **Q71.4 Longitudinal reduction defect of radius**
Clubhand (congenital)
Radial clubhand
Q71.40 Longitudinal reduction defect of unspecified radius
Q71.41 Longitudinal reduction defect of right radius
Q71.42 Longitudinal reduction defect of left radius
Q71.43 Longitudinal reduction defect of radius, bilateral

+ **Q71.5 Longitudinal reduction defect of ulna**
Q71.50 Longitudinal reduction defect of unspecified ulna
Q71.51 Longitudinal reduction defect of right ulna
Q71.52 Longitudinal reduction defect of left ulna
Q71.53 Longitudinal reduction defect of ulna, bilateral

+ **Q71.6 Lobster-claw hand**
Q71.60 Lobster-claw hand, unspecified hand
Q71.61 Lobster-claw right hand
Q71.62 Lobster-claw left hand
Q71.63 Lobster-claw hand, bilateral

+ **Q71.8 Other reduction defects of upper limb**
+ **Q71.81 Congenital shortening of upper limb**
Q71.811 Congenital shortening of right upper limb
Q71.812 Congenital shortening of left upper limb
Q71.813 Congenital shortening of upper limb, bilateral
Q71.819 Congenital shortening of unspecified upper limb
+ **Q71.89 Other reduction defects of upper limb**
Q71.891 Other reduction defects of right upper limb
Q71.892 Other reduction defects of left upper limb
Q71.893 Other reduction defects of upper limb, bilateral
Q71.899 Other reduction defects of unspecified upper limb

+ **Q71.9 Unspecified reduction defect of upper limb**
Q71.90 Unspecified reduction defect of unspecified upper limb
Q71.91 Unspecified reduction defect of right upper limb
Q71.92 Unspecified reduction defect of left upper limb
Q71.93 Unspecified reduction defect of upper limb, bilateral

Q72 Reduction defects of lower limb

+ **Q72.0 Congenital complete absence of lower limb**
  - **Q72.00 Congenital complete absence of unspecified lower limb**
  - **Q72.01 Congenital complete absence of right lower limb**
  - **Q72.02 Congenital complete absence of left lower limb**
  - **Q72.03 Congenital complete absence of lower limb, bilateral**

+ **Q72.1 Congenital absence of thigh and lower leg with foot present**
  - **Q72.10 Congenital absence of unspecified thigh and lower leg with foot present**
  - **Q72.11 Congenital absence of right thigh and lower leg with foot present**
  - **Q72.12 Congenital absence of left thigh and lower leg with foot present**
  - **Q72.13 Congenital absence of thigh and lower leg with foot present, bilateral**

+ **Q72.2 Congenital absence of both lower leg and foot**
  - **Q72.20 Congenital absence of both lower leg and foot, unspecified lower limb**
  - **Q72.21 Congenital absence of both lower leg and foot, right lower limb**
  - **Q72.22 Congenital absence of both lower leg and foot, left lower limb**
  - **Q72.23 Congenital absence of both lower leg and foot, bilateral**

+ **Q72.3 Congenital absence of foot and toe(s)**
  - **Q72.30 Congenital absence of unspecified foot and toe(s)**
  - **Q72.31 Congenital absence of right foot and toe(s)**
  - **Q72.32 Congenital absence of left foot and toe(s)**
  - **Q72.33 Congenital absence of foot and toe(s), bilateral**

+ **Q72.4 Longitudinal reduction defect of femur**
  Proximal femoral focal deficiency
  - **Q72.40 Longitudinal reduction defect of unspecified femur**
  - **Q72.41 Longitudinal reduction defect of right femur**
  - **Q72.42 Longitudinal reduction defect of left femur**
  - **Q72.43 Longitudinal reduction defect of femur, bilateral**

+ **Q72.5 Longitudinal reduction defect of tibia**
  - **Q72.50 Longitudinal reduction defect of unspecified tibia**
  - **Q72.51 Longitudinal reduction defect of right tibia**
  - **Q72.52 Longitudinal reduction defect of left tibia**
  - **Q72.53 Longitudinal reduction defect of tibia, bilateral**

+ **Q72.6 Longitudinal reduction defect of fibula**
  - **Q72.60 Longitudinal reduction defect of unspecified fibula**
  - **Q72.61 Longitudinal reduction defect of right fibula**
  - **Q72.62 Longitudinal reduction defect of left fibula**
  - **Q72.63 Longitudinal reduction defect of fibula, bilateral**

+ **Q72.7 Split foot**
  - **Q72.70 Split foot, unspecified lower limb**
  - **Q72.71 Split foot, right lower limb**
  - **Q72.72 Split foot, left lower limb**
  - **Q72.73 Split foot, bilateral**

+ **Q72.8 Other reduction defects of lower limb**
  + **Q72.81 Congenital shortening of lower limb**
    - **Q72.811 Congenital shortening of right lower limb**
    - **Q72.812 Congenital shortening of left lower limb**
    - **Q72.813 Congenital shortening of lower limb, bilateral**
    - **Q72.819 Congenital shortening of unspecified lower limb**
  + **Q72.89 Other reduction defects of lower limb**
    - **Q72.891 Other reduction defects of right lower limb**
    - **Q72.892 Other reduction defects of left lower limb**
    - **Q72.893 Other reduction defects of lower limb, bilateral**
    - **Q72.899 Other reduction defects of unspecified lower limb**

+ **Q72.9 Unspecified reduction defect of lower limb**
  - **Q72.90 Unspecified reduction defect of unspecified lower limb**
  - **Q72.91 Unspecified reduction defect of right lower limb**
  - **Q72.92 Unspecified reduction defect of left lower limb**
  - **Q72.93 Unspecified reduction defect of lower limb, bilateral**

Q73 Reduction defects of unspecified limb

Q73.0 Congenital absence of unspecified limb(s)
Amelia NOS

Q73.1 Phocomelia, unspecified limb(s)
Phocomelia NOS

Q73.8 Other reduction defects of unspecified limb(s)
Longitudinal reduction deformity of unspecified limb(s)
Ectromelia of limb NOS
Hemimelia of limb NOS
Reduction defect of limb NOS

Q74 Other congenital malformations of limb(s)

Excludes1: *polydactyly (Q69.-)*
reduction defect of limb (Q71-Q73)
syndactyly (Q70.-)

Q74.0 Other congenital malformations of upper limb(s), including shoulder girdle
Accessory carpal bones
Cleidocranial dysostosis
Congenital pseudarthrosis of clavicle
Macrodactylia (fingers)
Madelung's deformity
Radioulnar synostosis
Sprengel's deformity
Triphalangeal thumb

Q74.1 Congenital malformation of knee
Congenital absence of patella
Congenital dislocation of patella
Congenital genu valgum
Congenital genu varum
Rudimentary patella
Excludes1: *congenital dislocation of knee (Q68.2)*
congenital genu recurvatum (Q68.2)
nail patella syndrome (Q87.2)

Q74.2 Other congenital malformations of lower limb(s), including pelvic girdle
Congenital fusion of sacroiliac joint
Congenital malformation of ankle joint
Congenital malformation of sacroiliac joint
Excludes1: *anteversion of femur (neck) (Q65.89)*

CC **Q74.3 Arthrogryposis multiplex congenita**
CC Exclusion see Appendix A PDX collection 1102

Q74.8 Other specified congenital malformations of limb(s)

Q74.9 Unspecified congenital malformation of limb(s)
Congenital anomaly of limb(s) NOS

Q75 Other congenital malformations of skull and face bones

Excludes1: *congenital malformation of face NOS (Q18.-)*
congenital malformation syndromes classified to (Q87.-)
dentofacial anomalies [including malocclusion] (M26.-)
musculoskeletal deformities of head and face (Q67.0-Q67.4)
skull defects associated with congenital anomalies of brain such as:
anencephaly (Q00.0)
encephalocele (Q01.-)
hydrocephalus (Q03.-)
microcephaly (Q02)

Q75.0 Craniosynostosis
Acrocephaly
Imperfect fusion of skull
Oxycephaly
Trigonocephaly

Q75.1 Craniofacial dysostosis
Crouzon's disease

Q75.2 Hypertelorism

Q75.3 Macrocephaly

Q75.4 Mandibulofacial dysostosis
Franceschetti syndrome
Treacher Collins syndrome

Q75.5 Oculomandibular dysostosis

Q75.8 Other specified congenital malformations of skull and face bones
Absence of skull bone, congenital
Congenital deformity of forehead
Platybasia

Q75.9 Congenital malformation of skull and face bones, unspecified
Congenital anomaly of face bones NOS
Congenital anomaly of skull NOS

Q76 Congenital malformations of spine and bony thorax

Excludes1: *congenital musculoskeletal deformities of spine and chest (Q67.5-Q67.8)*

Q76.0 Spina bifida occulta
Excludes1: *meningocele (spinal) (Q05.-)*
spina bifida (aperta) (cystica) (Q05.-)

Q76.1 Klippel-Feil syndrome
Cervical fusion syndrome

Q76.2 Congenital spondylolisthesis
Congenital spondylolysis
Excludes1: *spondylolisthesis (acquired) (M43.1-)*
spondylolysis (acquired) (M43.0-)

CC **Q76.3 Congenital scoliosis due to congenital bony malformation**
Hemivertebra fusion or failure of segmentation with scoliosis
CC Exclusion see Appendix A PDX collection 1101

\+ **Q76.4 Other congenital malformations of spine, not associated with scoliosis**

\+ **Q76.41 Congenital kyphosis**

Q76.411 Congenital kyphosis, occipito-atlanto-axial region
Q76.412 Congenital kyphosis, cervical region
Q76.413 Congenital kyphosis, cervicothoracic region
Q76.414 Congenital kyphosis, thoracic region
Q76.415 Congenital kyphosis, thoracolumbar region
Q76.419 Congenital kyphosis, unspecified region

\+ **Q76.42 Congenital lordosis**

CC **Q76.425 Congenital lordosis, thoracolumbar region**
CC Exclusion see Appendix A PDX collection 1101
CC **Q76.426 Congenital lordosis, lumbar region**
CC Exclusion see Appendix A PDX collection 1101
CC **Q76.427 Congenital lordosis, lumbosacral region**
CC Exclusion see Appendix A PDX collection 1101
CC **Q76.428 Congenital lordosis, sacral and sacrococcygeal region**
CC Exclusion see Appendix A PDX collection 1101
CC **Q76.429 Congenital lordosis, unspecified region**
CC Exclusion see Appendix A PDX collection 1101

Q76.49 Other congenital malformations of spine, not associated with scoliosis
Congenital absence of vertebra NOS
Congenital fusion of spine NOS
Congenital malformation of lumbosacral (joint) (region) NOS
Congenital malformation of spine NOS
Hemivertebra NOS
Malformation of spine NOS
Platyspondylisis NOS
Supernumerary vertebra NOS

Q76.5 Cervical rib
Supernumerary rib in cervical region

CC **Q76.6 Other congenital malformations of ribs**
Accessory rib
Congenital absence of rib
Congenital fusion of ribs
Congenital malformation of ribs NOS
Excludes1: *short rib syndrome (Q77.2)*
CC Exclusion see Appendix A PDX collection 1103

CC **Q76.7 Congenital malformation of sternum**
Congenital absence of sternum
Sternum bifidum
CC Exclusion see Appendix A PDX collection 1103

CC **Q76.8 Other congenital malformations of bony thorax**
CC Exclusion see Appendix A PDX collection 1103

CC **Q76.9 Congenital malformation of bony thorax, unspecified**
CC Exclusion see Appendix A PDX collection 1103

Q77 Osteochondrodysplasia with defects of growth of tubular bones and spine

Excludes1: *mucopolysaccharidosis (E76.0-E76.3)*
Excludes2: *congenital myotonic chondrodystrophy (G71.13)*

Q77.0 Achondrogenesis
Hypochondrogenesis
Q77.1 Thanatophoric short stature
CC **Q77.2 Short rib syndrome**
Asphyxiating thoracic dysplasia [Jeune]
CC Exclusion see Appendix A PDX collection 1103
Q77.3 Chondrodysplasia punctata
Excludes1: *Rhizomelic chondrodysplasia punctata (E71.43)*
Q77.4 Achondroplasia
Hypochondroplasia
Osteosclerosis congenita
Q77.5 Diastrophic dysplasia
Q77.6 Chondroectodermal dysplasia
Ellis-van Creveld syndrome
Q77.7 Spondyloepiphyseal dysplasia
Q77.8 Other osteochondrodysplasia with defects of growth of tubular bones and spine
Q77.9 Osteochondrodysplasia with defects of growth of tubular bones and spine, unspecified

Q78 Other osteochondrodysplasias

Excludes2: *congenital myotonic chondrodystrophy (G71.13)*

CC **Q78.0 Osteogenesis imperfecta**
Fragilitas ossium
Osteopsathyrosis
CC Exclusion see Appendix A PDX collection 1104
Q78.1 Polyostotic fibrous dysplasia
Albright(-McCune)(-Sternberg) syndrome
CC **Q78.2 Osteopetrosis**
Albers-Schönberg syndrome
Osteosclerosis NOS
CC Exclusion see Appendix A PDX collection 1104
Q78.3 Progressive diaphyseal dysplasia
Camurati-Engelmann syndrome
Q78.4 Enchondromatosis
Maffucci's syndrome
Ollier's disease
Q78.5 Metaphyseal dysplasia
Pyle's syndrome
Q78.6 Multiple congenital exostoses
Diaphyseal aclasis
Q78.8 Other specified osteochondrodysplasias
Osteopoikilosis
Q78.9 Osteochondrodysplasia, unspecified
Chondrodystrophy NOS
Osteodystrophy NOS

Q79 Congenital malformations of musculoskeletal system, not elsewhere classified

Excludes2: *congenital (sternomastoid) torticollis (Q68.0)*

MCC **Q79.0 Congenital diaphragmatic hernia**
Excludes1: *congenital hiatus hernia (Q40.1)*
MCC Exclusion see Appendix A PDX collection 1105
MCC **Q79.1 Other congenital malformations of diaphragm**
Absence of diaphragm
Congenital malformation of diaphragm NOS
Eventration of diaphragm
MCC Exclusion see Appendix A PDX collection 1105
MCC **Q79.2 Exomphalos**
Omphalocele
Excludes1: *umbilical hernia (K42.-)*
MCC Exclusion see Appendix A PDX collection 1106
MCC **Q79.3 Gastroschisis**
MCC Exclusion see Appendix A PDX collection 1106
MCC **Q79.4 Prune belly syndrome**
Congenital prolapse of bladder mucosa
Eagle-Barrett syndrome
MCC Exclusion see Appendix A PDX collection 1106
\+ **Q79.5 Other congenital malformations of abdominal wall**
Excludes1: *umbilical hernia (K42.-)*
MCC **Q79.51 Congenital hernia of bladder**
MCC Exclusion see Appendix A PDX collection 1106
MCC **Q79.59 Other congenital malformations of abdominal wall**
MCC Exclusion see Appendix A PDX collection 1106
CC **Q79.6 Ehlers-Danlos syndrome**
CC Exclusion see Appendix A PDX collection 1107
Q79.8 Other congenital malformations of musculoskeletal system
Absence of muscle
Absence of tendon
Accessory muscle
Amyotrophia congenita
Congenital constricting bands
Congenital shortening of tendon
Poland syndrome
Q79.9 Congenital malformation of musculoskeletal system, unspecified
Congenital anomaly of musculoskeletal system NOS
Congenital deformity of musculoskeletal system NOS

Other congenital malformations (Q80-Q89)

Q80 Congenital ichthyosis

Excludes1: *Refsum's disease (G60.1)*

Q80.0 Ichthyosis vulgaris
Q80.1 X-linked ichthyosis
Q80.2 Lamellar ichthyosis
Collodion baby
Q80.3 Congenital bullous ichthyosiform erythroderma
Q80.4 Harlequin fetus
Q80.8 Other congenital ichthyosis
Q80.9 Congenital ichthyosis, unspecified

Q81 Epidermolysis bullosa

Q81.0 Epidermolysis bullosa simplex
Excludes1: *Cockayne's syndrome (Q87.1)*

Q81.1 Epidermolysis bullosa letalis
Herlitz' syndrome

Q81.2 Epidermolysis bullosa dystrophica

Q81.8 Other epidermolysis bullosa

Q81.9 Epidermolysis bullosa, unspecified

Q82 Other congenital malformations of skin

Excludes1: *acrodermatitis enteropathica (E83.2)*
congenital erythropoietic porphyria (E80.0)
pilonidal cyst or sinus (L05.-)
Sturge-Weber (-Dimitri) syndrome (Q85.8)

Q82.0 Hereditary lymphedema

Q82.1 Xeroderma pigmentosum

Q82.2 Congenital cutaneous mastocytosis
Congenital diffuse cutaneous mastocytosis
Congenital maculopapular cutaneous mastocytosis
Congenital urticaria pigmentosa
Excludes1: *cutaneous mastocytosis NOS (D47.01)*
diffuse cutaneous mastocytosis (with onset after newborn period) (D47.01)
malignant mastocytosis (C96.2-)
systemic mastocytosis (D47.02)
urticaria pigmentosa (non-congenital) (with onset after newborn period) (D47.01)

Q82.3 Incontinentia pigmenti

Q82.4 Ectodermal dysplasia (anhidrotic)
Excludes1: *Ellis-van Creveld syndrome (Q77.6)*

Q82.5 Congenital non-neoplastic nevus
Birthmark NOS
Flammeus Nevus
Portwine Nevus
Sanguineous Nevus
Strawberry Nevus
Vascular Nevus NOS
Verrucous Nevus
Excludes2: *Café au lait spots (L81.3)*
lentigo (L81.4)
nevus NOS (D22.-)
araneus nevus (I78.1)
melanocytic nevus (D22.-)
pigmented nevus (D22.-)
spider nevus (I78.1)
stellar nevus (I78.1)

Q82.6 Congenital sacral dimple
Parasacral dimple
Excludes2: *pilonidal cyst with abscess (L05.01)*
pilonidal cyst without abscess (L05.91)
AHA CC: 4Q, 2016, 60

Q82.8 Other specified congenital malformations of skin
Abnormal palmar creases
Accessory skin tags
Benign familial pemphigus [Hailey-Hailey]
Congenital poikiloderma
Cutis laxa (hyperelastica)
Dermatoglyphic anomalies
Inherited keratosis palmaris et plantaris
Keratosis follicularis [Darier-White]
Excludes1: *Ehlers-Danlos syndrome (Q79.6)*
AHA CC: 1Q, 2016, 17

Q82.9 Congenital malformation of skin, unspecified

Q83 Congenital malformations of breast

Excludes2: *absence of pectoral muscle (Q79.8)*
hypoplasia of breast (N64.82)
micromastia (N64.82)

Q83.0 Congenital absence of breast with absent nipple

Q83.1 Accessory breast
Supernumerary breast

Q83.2 Absent nipple

Q83.3 Accessory nipple
Supernumerary nipple

Q83.8 Other congenital malformations of breast

Q83.9 Congenital malformation of breast, unspecified

Q84 Other congenital malformations of integument

Q84.0 Congenital alopecia
Congenital atrichosis

Q84.1 Congenital morphological disturbances of hair, not elsewhere classified
Beaded hair
Monilethrix
Pili annulati
Excludes1: *Menkes' kinky hair syndrome (E83.0)*

Q84.2 Other congenital malformations of hair
Congenital hypertrichosis
Congenital malformation of hair NOS
Persistent lanugo

Q84.3 Anonychia
Excludes1: *nail patella syndrome (Q87.2)*

Q84.4 Congenital leukonychia

Q84.5 Enlarged and hypertrophic nails
Congenital onychauxis
Pachyonychia

Q84.6 Other congenital malformations of nails
Congenital clubnail
Congenital koilonychia
Congenital malformation of nail NOS

Q84.8 Other specified congenital malformations of integument
Aplasia cutis congenita

Q84.9 Congenital malformation of integument, unspecified
Congenital anomaly of integument NOS
Congenital deformity of integument NOS

Q85 Phakomatoses, not elsewhere classified

Excludes1: *ataxia telangiectasia [Louis-Bar] (G11.3)*
familial dysautonomia [Riley-Day] (G90.1)

\+ **Q85.0 Neurofibromatosis (nonmalignant)**

Q85.00 Neurofibromatosis, unspecified

Q85.01 Neurofibromatosis, type 1
Von Recklinghausen disease

Q85.02 Neurofibromatosis, type 2
Acoustic neurofibromatosis

Q85.03 Schwannomatosis

Q85.09 Other neurofibromatosis

CC **Q85.1 Tuberous sclerosis**
Bourneville's disease
Epiloia
CC Exclusion see Appendix A PDX collection 1108

CC **Q85.8 Other phakomatoses, not elsewhere classified**
Peutz-Jeghers Syndrome
Sturge-Weber(-Dimitri) syndrome
von Hippel-Lindau syndrome
Excludes1: *Meckel-Gruber syndrome (Q61.9)*
CC Exclusion see Appendix A PDX collection 1109

CC **Q85.9 Phakomatosis, unspecified**
Hamartosis NOS
CC Exclusion see Appendix A PDX collection 1109

Q86 Congenital malformation syndromes due to known exogenous causes, not elsewhere classified

Excludes2: *iodine-deficiency-related hypothyroidism (E00-E02)*
nonteratogenic effects of substances transmitted via placenta or breast milk (P04.-)

Q86.0 Fetal alcohol syndrome (dysmorphic)

Q86.1 Fetal hydantoin syndrome
Meadow's syndrome

Q86.2 Dysmorphism due to warfarin

Q86.8 Other congenital malformation syndromes due to known exogenous causes

Q87 Other specified congenital malformation syndromes affecting multiple systems

Use additional code(s) to identify all associated manifestations

Q87.0 Congenital malformation syndromes predominantly affecting facial appearance
Acrocephalopolysyndactyly
Acrocephalosyndactyly [Apert]
Cryptophthalmos syndrome
Cyclopia
Goldenhar syndrome
Moebius syndrome
Oro-facial-digital syndrome
Robin syndrome
Whistling face

CC **Q87.1 Congenital malformation syndromes predominantly associated with short stature**
Aarskog syndrome
Cockayne syndrome
De Lange syndrome
Dubowitz syndrome
Noonan syndrome
Prader-Willi syndrome
Robinow-Silverman-Smith syndrome
Russell-Silver syndrome
Seckel syndrome
Excludes1: *Ellis-van Creveld syndrome (Q77.6)*
Smith-Lemli-Opitz syndrome (E78.72)
CC Exclusion see Appendix A PDX collection 1110

CC **Q87.2 Congenital malformation syndromes predominantly involving limbs**
Holt-Oram syndrome
Klippel-Trenaunay-Weber syndrome
Nail patella syndrome
Rubinstein-Taybi syndrome
Sirenomelia syndrome
Thrombocytopenia with absent radius [TAR] syndrome
VATER syndrome
CC Exclusion see Appendix A PDX collection 0540

CC **Q87.3 Congenital malformation syndromes involving early overgrowth**
Beckwith-Wiedemann syndrome
Sotos syndrome
Weaver syndrome
CC Exclusion see Appendix A PDX collection 0540

\+ **Q87.4 Marfan's syndrome**
CC **Q87.40 Marfan's syndrome, unspecified**
CC Exclusion see Appendix A PDX collection 1110
\+ **Q87.41 Marfan's syndrome with cardiovascular manifestations**
CC **Q87.410 Marfan's syndrome with aortic dilation**
CC Exclusion see Appendix A PDX collection 1110
CC **Q87.418 Marfan's syndrome with other cardiovascular manifestations**
CC Exclusion see Appendix A PDX collection 1110
CC **Q87.42 Marfan's syndrome with ocular manifestations**
CC Exclusion see Appendix A PDX collection 1110
CC **Q87.43 Marfan's syndrome with skeletal manifestation**
CC Exclusion see Appendix A PDX collection 1110

CC **Q87.5 Other congenital malformation syndromes with other skeletal changes**
CC Exclusion see Appendix A PDX collection 0540

\+ **Q87.8 Other specified congenital malformation syndromes, not elsewhere classified**
Excludes1: *Zellweger syndrome (E71.510)*
CC **Q87.81 Alport syndrome**
Use additional code to identify stage of chronic kidney disease (N18.1-N18.6)
CC Exclusion see Appendix A PDX collection 0540
CC **Q87.82 Arterial tortuosity syndrome**
CC Exclusion see Appendix A PDX collection 0540
AHA CC: 4Q, 2016, 60-61
CC **Q87.89 Other specified congenital malformation syndromes, not elsewhere classified**
Laurence-Moon (-Bardet)-Biedl syndrome
CC Exclusion see Appendix A PDX collection 0540

Q89 Other congenital malformations, not elsewhere classified

\+ **Q89.0 Congenital absence and malformations of spleen**
Excludes1: *isomerism of atrial appendages (with asplenia or polysplenia) (Q20.6)*
CC **Q89.01 Asplenia (congenital)**
CC Exclusion see Appendix A PDX collection 1111
CC **Q89.09 Congenital malformations of spleen**
Congenital splenomegaly
CC Exclusion see Appendix A PDX collection 1111

Q89.1 Congenital malformations of adrenal gland
Excludes1: *adrenogenital disorders (E25.-)*
congenital adrenal hyperplasia (E25.0)

Q89.2 Congenital malformations of other endocrine glands
Congenital malformation of parathyroid or thyroid gland
Persistent thyroglossal duct
Thyroglossal cyst
Excludes1: *congenital goiter (E03.0)*
congenital hypothyroidism (E03.1)

CC **Q89.3 Situs inversus**
Dextrocardia with situs inversus
Mirror-image atrial arrangement with situs inversus
Situs inversus or transversus abdominalis
Situs inversus or transversus thoracis
Transposition of abdominal viscera
Transposition of thoracic viscera
Excludes1: *dextrocardia NOS (Q24.0)*
CC Exclusion see Appendix A PDX collection 1112

MCC **Q89.4 Conjoined twins**
Craniopagus
Dicephaly
Pygopagus
Thoracopagus
MCC Exclusion see Appendix A PDX collection 1113

CC **Q89.7 Multiple congenital malformations, not elsewhere classified**
Multiple congenital anomalies NOS
Multiple congenital deformities NOS
Excludes1: *congenital malformation syndromes affecting multiple systems (Q87.-)*
CC Exclusion see Appendix A PDX collection 1112

CC **Q89.8 Other specified congenital malformations**
Use additional code(s) to identify all associated manifestations
CC Exclusion see Appendix A PDX collection 0540

Q89.9 Congenital malformation, unspecified
Congenital anomaly NOS
Congenital deformity NOS

Chromosomal abnormalities, not elsewhere classified (Q90-Q99)

Excludes2: *mitochondrial metabolic disorders (E88.4-)*

Q90 Down syndrome
Use additional code(s) to identify any associated physical conditions and degree of intellectual disabilities (F70-F79)
Q90.0 Trisomy 21, nonmosaicism (meiotic nondisjunction)
Q90.1 Trisomy 21, mosaicism (mitotic nondisjunction)
Q90.2 Trisomy 21, translocation
Q90.9 Down syndrome, unspecified
Trisomy 21 NOS

Q91 Trisomy 18 and Trisomy 13
CC **Q91.0 Trisomy 18, nonmosaicism (meiotic nondisjunction)**
CC Exclusion see Appendix A PDX collection 1114
CC **Q91.1 Trisomy 18, mosaicism (mitotic nondisjunction)**
CC Exclusion see Appendix A PDX collection 1114
CC **Q91.2 Trisomy 18, translocation**
CC Exclusion see Appendix A PDX collection 1114
CC **Q91.3 Trisomy 18, unspecified**
CC Exclusion see Appendix A PDX collection 1114
CC **Q91.4 Trisomy 13, nonmosaicism (meiotic nondisjunction)**
CC Exclusion see Appendix A PDX collection 1114
CC **Q91.5 Trisomy 13, mosaicism (mitotic nondisjunction)**
CC Exclusion see Appendix A PDX collection 1114
CC **Q91.6 Trisomy 13, translocation**
CC Exclusion see Appendix A PDX collection 1114
CC **Q91.7 Trisomy 13, unspecified**
CC Exclusion see Appendix A PDX collection 1114

Q92 Other trisomies and partial trisomies of the autosomes, not elsewhere classified
Includes: unbalanced translocations and insertions
Excludes1: *trisomies of chromosomes 13, 18, 21 (Q90-Q91)*
Q92.0 Whole chromosome trisomy, nonmosaicism (meiotic nondisjunction)
Q92.1 Whole chromosome trisomy, mosaicism (mitotic nondisjunction)
Q92.2 Partial trisomy
Less than whole arm duplicated
Whole arm or more duplicated
Excludes1: *partial trisomy due to unbalanced translocation (Q92.5)*
Q92.5 Duplications with other complex rearrangements
Partial trisomy due to unbalanced translocations
Code also any associated deletions due to unbalanced translocations, inversions and insertions (Q93.7)
\+ **Q92.6 Marker chromosomes**
Trisomies due to dicentrics
Trisomies due to extra rings
Trisomies due to isochromosomes
Individual with marker heterochromatin

Q92.61 Marker chromosomes in normal individual
Q92.62 Marker chromosomes in abnormal individual
Q92.7 Triploidy and polyploidy
Q92.8 Other specified trisomies and partial trisomies of autosomes
Duplications identified by fluorescence in situ hybridization (FISH)
Duplications identified by in situ hybridization (ISH)
Duplications seen only at prometaphase
Q92.9 Trisomy and partial trisomy of autosomes, unspecified

Q93 Monosomies and deletions from the autosomes, not elsewhere classified

Q93.0 Whole chromosome monosomy, nonmosaicism (meiotic nondisjunction)
Q93.1 Whole chromosome monosomy, mosaicism (mitotic nondisjunction)
Q93.2 Chromosome replaced with ring, dicentric or isochromosome
CC **Q93.3 Deletion of short arm of chromosome 4**
Wolff-Hirschorn syndrome
CC Exclusion see Appendix A PDX collection 1115
CC **Q93.4 Deletion of short arm of chromosome 5**
Cri-du-chat syndrome
CC Exclusion see Appendix A PDX collection 1116
CC **Q93.5 Other deletions of part of a chromosome**
Angelman syndrome
CC Exclusion see Appendix A PDX collection 1115
CC **Q93.7 Deletions with other complex rearrangements**
Deletions due to unbalanced translocations, inversions and insertions
Code also any associated duplications due to unbalanced translocations, inversions and insertions (Q92.5)
CC Exclusion see Appendix A PDX collection 1115
+ **Q93.8 Other deletions from the autosomes**
MCC **Q93.81 Velo-cardio-facial syndrome**
Deletion 22q11.2
MCC Exclusion see Appendix A PDX collection 1117
CC **Q93.88 Other microdeletions**
Miller-Dieker syndrome
Smith-Magenis syndrome
CC Exclusion see Appendix A PDX collection 1118
CC **Q93.89 Other deletions from the autosomes**
Deletions identified by fluorescence in situ hybridization (FISH)
Deletions identified by in situ hybridization (ISH)
Deletions seen only at prometaphase
CC Exclusion see Appendix A PDX collection 1115
CC **Q93.9 Deletion from autosomes, unspecified**
CC Exclusion see Appendix A PDX collection 1115

Q95 Balanced rearrangements and structural markers, not elsewhere classified

Includes: Robertsonian and balanced reciprocal translocations and insertions
Q95.0 Balanced translocation and insertion in normal individual
Q95.1 Chromosome inversion in normal individual
Q95.2 Balanced autosomal rearrangement in abnormal individual
Q95.3 Balanced sex/autosomal rearrangement in abnormal individual
Q95.5 Individual with autosomal fragile site
Q95.8 Other balanced rearrangements and structural markers
Q95.9 Balanced rearrangement and structural marker, unspecified

Q96 Turner's syndrome

Excludes1: *Noonan syndrome (Q87.1)*
♀ **Q96.0 Karyotype 45, X**
♀ **Q96.1 Karyotype 46, X iso (Xq)**
Karyotype 46, isochromosome Xq
♀ **Q96.2 Karyotype 46, X with abnormal sex chromosome, except iso (Xq)**
Karyotype 46, X with abnormal sex chromosome, except isochromosome Xq
♀ **Q96.3 Mosaicism, 45, X/46, XX or XY**
♀ **Q96.4 Mosaicism, 45, X/other cell line(s) with abnormal sex chromosome**
♀ **Q96.8 Other variants of Turner's syndrome**
♀ **Q96.9 Turner's syndrome, unspecified**

Q97 Other sex chromosome abnormalities, female phenotype, not elsewhere classified

Excludes1: *Turner's syndrome (Q96.-)*
♀ **Q97.0 Karyotype 47, XXX**
♀ **Q97.1 Female with more than three X chromosomes**
♀ **Q97.2 Mosaicism, lines with various numbers of X chromosomes**
♀ **Q97.3 Female with 46, XY karyotype**
♀ **Q97.8 Other specified sex chromosome abnormalities, female phenotype**
♀ **Q97.9 Sex chromosome abnormality, female phenotype, unspecified**

Q98 Other sex chromosome abnormalities, male phenotype, not elsewhere classified

♂ **Q98.0 Klinefelter syndrome karyotype 47, XXY**
♂ **Q98.1 Klinefelter syndrome, male with more than two X chromosomes**
♂ **Q98.3 Other male with 46, XX karyotype**
♂ **Q98.4 Klinefelter syndrome, unspecified**
Q98.5 Karyotype 47, XYY
♂ **Q98.6 Male with structurally abnormal sex chromosome**
♂ **Q98.7 Male with sex chromosome mosaicism**
♂ **Q98.8 Other specified sex chromosome abnormalities, male phenotype**
♂ **Q98.9 Sex chromosome abnormality, male phenotype, unspecified**

Q99 Other chromosome abnormalities, not elsewhere classified

Q99.0 Chimera 46, XX/46, XY
Chimera 46, XX/46, XY true hermaphrodite
Q99.1 46, XX true hermaphrodite
46, XX with streak gonads
46, XY with streak gonads
Pure gonadal dysgenesis
Q99.2 Fragile X chromosome
Fragile X syndrome
Q99.8 Other specified chromosome abnormalities
Q99.9 Chromosomal abnormality, unspecified

Chapter 18: Symptoms, Signs and Abnormal Clinical and Laboratory Findings, Not Elsewhere Classified (R00-R99)

OTE This chapter includes symptoms, signs, abnormal results of clinical or other investigative procedures, and ill-defined conditions regarding which no diagnosis classifiable elsewhere is recorded.

Signs and symptoms that point rather definitely to a given diagnosis have been assigned to a category in other chapters of the classification. In general, categories in this chapter include the less well-defined conditions and symptoms that, without the necessary study of the case to establish a final diagnosis, point perhaps equally to two or more diseases or to two or more systems of the body. Practically all categories in the chapter could be designated 'not otherwise specified', 'unknown etiology' or 'transient'. The Alphabetical Index should be consulted to determine which symptoms and signs are to be allocated here and which to other chapters. The residual subcategories, numbered .8, are generally provided for other relevant symptoms that cannot be allocated elsewhere in the classification.

The conditions and signs or symptoms included in categories R00-R94 consist of:

(a) cases for which no more specific diagnosis can be made even after all the facts bearing on the case have been investigated;

(b) signs or symptoms existing at the time of initial encounter that proved to be transient and whose causes could not be determined;

(c) provisional diagnosis in a patient who failed to return for further investigation or care;

(d) cases referred elsewhere for investigation or treatment before the diagnosis was made;

(e) cases in which a more precise diagnosis was not available for any other reason;

(f) certain symptoms, for which supplementary information is provided, that represent important problems in medical care in their own right.

xcludes2: *abnormal findings on antenatal screening of mother (O28.-)*
certain conditions originating in the perinatal period (P04-P96)
signs and symptoms classified in the body system chapters
signs and symptoms of breast (N63, N64.5)

his chapter contains the following category blocks:

R00-R09	Symptoms and signs involving the circulatory and respiratory systems
R10-R19	Symptoms and signs involving the digestive system and abdomen
R20-R23	Symptoms and signs involving the skin and subcutaneous tissue
R25-R29	Symptoms and signs involving the nervous and musculoskeletal systems
R30-R39	Symptoms and signs involving the genitourinary system
R40-R46	Symptoms and signs involving cognition, perception, emotional state and behavior
R47-R49	Symptoms and signs involving speech and voice
R50-R69	General symptoms and signs
R70-R79	Abnormal findings on examination of blood, without diagnosis
R80-R82	Abnormal findings on examination of urine, without diagnosis
R83-R89	Abnormal findings on examination of other body fluids, substances and tissues, without diagnosis
R90-R94	Abnormal findings on diagnostic imaging and in function studies, without diagnosis
R97	Abnormal tumor markers
R99	Ill-defined and unknown cause of mortality

. Chapter-Specific Coding Guidelines

addition to general coding guidelines, there are guidelines for specific diagnoses d/or conditions in the classification. Unless otherwise indicated, these guidelines ply to all health care settings. Please refer to Section II for guidelines on the lection of principal diagnosis.

. Chapter 18: Symptoms, Signs, and Abnormal Clinical and Laboratory Findings, Not Elsewhere Classified (R00-R99)

Chapter 18 includes symptoms, signs, abnormal results of clinical or other investigative procedures, and ill-defined conditions regarding which no diagnosis classifiable elsewhere is recorded. Signs and symptoms that point to a specific diagnosis have been assigned to a category in other chapters of the classification.

a. Use of symptom codes

Codes that describe symptoms and signs are acceptable for reporting purposes when a related definitive diagnosis has not been established (confirmed) by the provider.

b. Use of a symptom code with a definitive diagnosis code

Codes for signs and symptoms may be reported in addition to a related definitive diagnosis when the sign or symptom is not routinely associated with that diagnosis, such as the various signs and symptoms associated with complex syndromes. The definitive diagnosis code should be sequenced before the symptom code.

Signs or symptoms that are associated routinely with a disease process should not be assigned as additional codes, unless otherwise instructed by the classification.

c. Combination codes that include symptoms

ICD-10-CM contains a number of combination codes that identify both the definitive diagnosis and common symptoms of that diagnosis. When using one of these combination codes, an additional code should not be assigned for the symptom.

d. Repeated falls

Code R29.6, Repeated falls, is for use for encounters when a patient has recently fallen and the reason for the fall is being investigated.

Code Z91.81, History of falling, is for use when a patient has fallen in the past and is at risk for future falls. When appropriate, both codes R29.6 and Z91.81 may be assigned together.

e. Coma scale

The coma scale codes (R40.2-) can be used in conjunction with traumatic brain injury codes, acute cerebrovascular disease or sequelae of cerebrovascular disease codes. These codes are primarily for use by trauma registries, but they may be used in any setting where this information is collected. The coma scale may also be used to assess the status of the central nervous system for other non-trauma conditions, such as monitoring patients in the intensive care unit regardless of medical conditions. The coma scale codes should be sequenced after the diagnosis code(s).

These codes, one from each subcategory, are needed to complete the scale. The 7th character indicates when the scale was recorded. The 7th character should match for all three codes.

At a minimum, report the initial score documented on presentation at your facility. This may be a score from the emergency medicine technician (EMT) or in the emergency department. If desired, a facility may choose to capture multiple coma scale scores.

Assign code R40.24, Glasgow coma scale, total score, when only the total score is documented in the medical record and not the individual score(s).

f. Functional quadriplegia

GUIDELINE HAS BEEN DELETED EFFECTIVE OCTOBER 1, 2017

g. SIRS due to Non-Infectious Process

The systemic inflammatory response syndrome (SIRS) can develop as a result of certain non-infectious disease processes, such as trauma, malignant neoplasm, or pancreatitis. When SIRS is documented with a noninfectious condition, and no subsequent infection is documented, the code for the underlying condition, such as an injury, should be assigned, followed by code R65.10, Systemic inflammatory response syndrome (SIRS) of non-infectious origin without acute organ dysfunction, or code R65.11, Systemic inflammatory response syndrome (SIRS) of non-infectious origin with acute organ dysfunction. If an associated acute organ dysfunction is documented, the appropriate code(s) for the specific type of organ dysfunction(s) should be assigned in addition to code R65.11. If acute organ dysfunction is documented, but it cannot be determined if the acute organ dysfunction is associated with SIRS or due to another condition (e.g., directly due to the trauma), the provider should be queried.

h. Death NOS

Code R99, Ill-defined and unknown cause of mortality, is only for use in the very limited circumstance when a patient who has already died is brought into an emergency department or other healthcare facility and is pronounced dead upon arrival. It does not represent the discharge disposition of death.

i. NIHSS Stroke Scale

The NIH stroke scale (NIHSS) codes (R29.7--) can be used in conjunction with acute stroke codes (I63) to identify the patient's neurological status and the severity of the stroke. The stroke scale codes should be sequenced after the acute stroke diagnosis code(s).

At a minimum, report the initial score documented. If desired, a facility may choose to capture multiple stroke scale scores.

See Section I.B.14 for information concerning the medical record documentations that may be used for assignment of the NIHSS codes.

Symptoms and signs involving the circulatory and respiratory systems (R00-R09)

R00 Abnormalities of heart beat

Excludes1: *abnormalities originating in the perinatal period (P29.1-)*
Excludes2: *specified arrhythmias (I47-I49)*

R00.0 Tachycardia, unspecified
Rapid heart beat
Sinoauricular tachycardia NOS
Sinus [sinusal] tachycardia NOS
Excludes1: *neonatal tachycardia (P29.11)*
paroxysmal tachycardia (I47.-)

R00.1 Bradycardia, unspecified
Sinoatrial bradycardia
Sinus bradycardia
Slow heart beat
Systolic murmur NOS
Vagal bradycardia
Use additional code for adverse effect, if applicable, to identify drug (T36-T50 with fifth or sixth character 5)
Excludes1: *neonatal bradycardia (P29.12)*

R00.2 Palpitations
Awareness of heart beat

R00.8 Other abnormalities of heart beat

R00.9 Unspecified abnormalities of heart beat

R01 Cardiac murmurs and other cardiac sounds

Excludes1: *cardiac murmurs and sounds originating in the perinatal period (P29.8)*

R01.0 Benign and innocent cardiac murmurs
Functional cardiac murmur

R01.1 Cardiac murmur, unspecified
Cardiac bruit NOS
Heart murmur NOS
Systolic murmur NOS

R01.2 Other cardiac sounds
Cardiac dullness, increased or decreased
Precordial friction

R03 Abnormal blood-pressure reading, without diagnosis

R03.0 Elevated blood-pressure reading, without diagnosis of hypertension
NOTE This category is to be used to record an episode of elevated blood pressure in a patient in whom no formal diagnosis of hypertension has been made, or as an isolated incidental finding.
Review coding guideline C.9.a.7

R03.1 Nonspecific low blood-pressure reading
Excludes1: *hypotension (I95.-)*
maternal hypotension syndrome (O26.5-)
neurogenic orthostatic hypotension (G90.3)

R04 Hemorrhage from respiratory passages

R04.0 Epistaxis
Hemorrhage from nose
Nosebleed

R04.1 Hemorrhage from throat
Excludes2: *hemoptysis (R04.2)*

CC **R04.2 Hemoptysis**
Blood-stained sputum
Cough with hemorrhage
CC Exclusion see Appendix A PDX collection 1119
AHA CC: 4Q, 2013, 118

\+ **R04.8 Hemorrhage from other sites in respiratory passages**

• CC **R04.81 Acute idiopathic pulmonary hemorrhage in infants**
AIPHI
Acute idiopathic hemorrhage in infants over 28 days old
Excludes1: *perinatal pulmonary hemorrhage (P26.-)*
von Willebrand's disease (D68.0)
CC Exclusion see Appendix A PDX collection 1119

CC **R04.89 Hemorrhage from other sites in respiratory passages**
Pulmonary hemorrhage NOS
CC Exclusion see Appendix A PDX collection 1119

CC **R04.9 Hemorrhage from respiratory passages, unspecified**
CC Exclusion see Appendix A PDX collection 1119

R05 Cough

Excludes1: *cough with hemorrhage (R04.2)*
smoker's cough (J41.0)
AHA CC: 2Q, 2016, 34
Valid 3-character code, no further characters required

R06 Abnormalities of breathing

Excludes1: *acute respiratory distress syndrome (J80)*
respiratory arrest (R09.2)
respiratory arrest of newborn (P28.81)
respiratory distress syndrome of newborn (P22.-)
respiratory failure (J96.-)
respiratory failure of newborn (P28.5)

\+ **R06.0 Dyspnea**
Excludes1: *tachypnea NOS (R06.82)*
transient tachypnea of newborn (P22.1)

R06.00 Dyspnea, unspecified
AHA CC: 1Q, 2017, 26-27

R06.01 Orthopnea

R06.02 Shortness of breath

R06.03 Acute respiratory distress

R06.09 Other forms of dyspnea

R06.1 Stridor
Excludes1: *congenital laryngeal stridor (P28.89)*
laryngismus (stridulus) (J38.5)

R06.2 Wheezing
Excludes1: *Asthma (J45.-)*
AHA CC: 2Q, 2016, 34

CC **R06.3 Periodic breathing**
Cheyne-Stokes breathing
CC Exclusion see Appendix A PDX collection 1120

R06.4 Hyperventilation
Excludes1: *psychogenic hyperventilation (F45.8)*

R06.5 Mouth breathing
Excludes2: *dry mouth NOS (R68.2)*

R06.6 Hiccough
Excludes1: *psychogenic hiccough (F45.8)*

R06.7 Sneezing

\+ **R06.8 Other abnormalities of breathing**

R06.81 Apnea, not elsewhere classified
Apnea NOS
Excludes1: *apnea (of) newborn (P28.4)*
sleep apnea (G47.3-)
sleep apnea of newborn (primary) (P28.3

R06.82 Tachypnea, not elsewhere classified
Tachypnea NOS
Excludes1: *transitory tachypnea of newborn (P22.1)*

R06.83 Snoring

R06.89 Other abnormalities of breathing
Breath-holding (spells)
Sighing

R06.9 Unspecified abnormalities of breathing

R07 Pain in throat and chest

Excludes1: *epidemic myalgia (B33.0)*
Excludes2: *jaw pain (R68.84)*
pain in breast (N64.4)

R07.0 Pain in throat
Excludes1: *chronic sore throat (J31.2)*
sore throat (acute) NOS (J02.9)
Excludes2: *dysphagia (R13.1-)*
pain in neck (M54.2)

R07.1 Chest pain on breathing
Painful respiration

R07.2 Precordial pain

\+ **R07.8 Other chest pain**

R07.81 Pleurodynia
Pleurodynia NOS
Excludes1: *epidemic pleurodynia (B33.0)*

R07.82 Intercostal pain

R07.89 Other chest pain
Anterior chest-wall pain NOS

R07.9 Chest pain, unspecified

R09 Other symptoms and signs involving the circulatory and respiratory system

Excludes1: *acute respiratory distress syndrome (J80)*
respiratory arrest of newborn (P28.81)
respiratory distress syndrome of newborn (P22.0)
respiratory failure (J96.-)
respiratory failure of newborn (P28.5)

+ **R09.0 Asphyxia and hypoxemia**
Excludes1: *asphyxia due to carbon monoxide (T58.-)*
asphyxia due to foreign body in respiratory tract (T17.-)
birth (intrauterine) asphyxia (P84)
hyperventilation (R06.4)
traumatic asphyxia (T71-)
Excludes2: *hypercapnia (R06.89)*

CC **R09.01 Asphyxia**
CC Exclusion see Appendix A PDX collection 1121

R09.02 Hypoxemia

R09.1 Pleurisy
Excludes1: *pleurisy with effusion (J90)*

MCC **R09.2 Respiratory arrest**
Cardiorespiratory failure
Excludes1: *cardiac arrest (I46.-)*
respiratory arrest of newborn (P28.81)
respiratory distress of newborn (P22.0)
respiratory failure (J96.-)
respiratory failure of newborn (P28.5)
respiratory insufficiency (R06.89)
respiratory insufficiency of newborn (P28.5)
MCC Exclusion see Appendix A PDX collection 1121

R09.3 Abnormal sputum
Abnormal amount of sputum
Abnormal color of sputum
Abnormal odor of sputum
Excessive sputum
Excludes1: *blood-stained sputum (R04.2)*

+ **R09.8 Other specified symptoms and signs involving the circulatory and respiratory systems**
R09.81 Nasal congestion
R09.82 Postnasal drip
R09.89 Other specified symptoms and signs involving the circulatory and respiratory systems
Bruit (arterial)
Abnormal chest percussion
Feeling of foreign body in throat
Friction sounds in chest
Chest tympany
Choking sensation
Rales
Weak pulse
Excludes2: *foreign body in throat (T17.2-)*
wheezing (R06.2)

Symptoms and signs involving the digestive system and abdomen (R10-R19)

Excludes2: *congenital or infantile pylorospasm (Q40.0)*
gastrointestinal hemorrhage (K92.0-K92.2)
intestinal obstruction (K56.-)
newborn gastrointestinal hemorrhage (P54.0-P54.3)
newborn intestinal obstruction (P76.-)
pylorospasm (K31.3)
signs and symptoms involving the urinary system (R30-R39)
symptoms referable to female genital organs (N94.-)
symptoms referable to male genital organs male (N48-N50)

R10 Abdominal and pelvic pain

Excludes1: *renal colic (N23)*
Excludes2: *dorsalgia (M54.-)*
flatulence and related conditions (R14.-)

R10.0 Acute abdomen
Severe abdominal pain (generalized) (with abdominal rigidity)
Excludes1: *abdominal rigidity NOS (R19.3)*
generalized abdominal pain NOS (R10.84)
localized abdominal pain (R10.1-R10.3-)

+ **R10.1 Pain localized to upper abdomen**
R10.10 Upper abdominal pain, unspecified
R10.11 Right upper quadrant pain
R10.12 Left upper quadrant pain
R10.13 Epigastric pain
Dyspepsia
Excludes1: *functional dyspepsia (K30)*

R10.2 Pelvic and perineal pain
Excludes1: *vulvodynia (N94.81)*

+ **R10.3 Pain localized to other parts of lower abdomen**
R10.30 Lower abdominal pain, unspecified
R10.31 Right lower quadrant pain
R10.32 Left lower quadrant pain
R10.33 Periumbilical pain

+ **R10.8 Other abdominal pain**
+ **R10.81 Abdominal tenderness**
Abdominal tenderness NOS
R10.811 Right upper quadrant abdominal tenderness
R10.812 Left upper quadrant abdominal tenderness
R10.813 Right lower quadrant abdominal tenderness
R10.814 Left lower quadrant abdominal tenderness
R10.815 Periumbilic abdominal tenderness
R10.816 Epigastric abdominal tenderness
R10.817 Generalized abdominal tenderness
R10.819 Abdominal tenderness, unspecified site
+ **R10.82 Rebound abdominal tenderness**
R10.821 Right upper quadrant rebound abdominal tenderness
R10.822 Left upper quadrant rebound abdominal tenderness
R10.823 Right lower quadrant rebound abdominal tenderness
R10.824 Left lower quadrant rebound abdominal tenderness
R10.825 Periumbilic rebound abdominal tenderness
R10.826 Epigastric rebound abdominal tenderness
R10.827 Generalized rebound abdominal tenderness
R10.829 Rebound abdominal tenderness, unspecified site
• **R10.83 Colic**
Colic NOS
Infantile colic
Excludes1: *colic in adult and child over 12 months old (R10.84)*
R10.84 Generalized abdominal pain
Excludes1: *generalized abdominal pain associated with acute abdomen (R10.0)*

R10.9 Unspecified abdominal pain

R11 Nausea and vomiting

Excludes1: *cyclical vomiting associated with migraine (G43.A-)*
excessive vomiting in pregnancy (O21.-)
hematemesis (K92.0)
neonatal hematemesis (P54.0)
newborn vomiting (P92.0-)
psychogenic vomiting (F50.89)
vomiting associated with bulimia nervosa (F50.2)
vomiting following gastrointestinal surgery (K91.0)
AHA CC: 1Q, 2017, 28

R11.0 Nausea
Nausea NOS
Nausea without vomiting

+ **R11.1 Vomiting**
R11.10 Vomiting, unspecified
Vomiting NOS
R11.11 Vomiting without nausea
R11.12 Projectile vomiting
R11.13 Vomiting of fecal matter
R11.14 Bilious vomiting
Bilious emesis

R11.2 Nausea with vomiting, unspecified
Persistent nausea with vomiting NOS

R12 Heartburn

Excludes1: *dyspepsia NOS (R10.13)*
functional dyspepsia (K30)
Valid 3-character code, no further characters required

R13 Aphagia and dysphagia

R13.0 Aphagia
Inability to swallow
Excludes1: *psychogenic aphagia (F50.9)*

+ **R13.1 Dysphagia**
Code first if applicable, dysphagia following cerebrovascular disease (I69. with final characters -91)
Excludes1: *psychogenic dysphagia (F45.8)*

R13.10 Dysphagia, unspecified
Difficulty in swallowing NOS
R13.11 Dysphagia, oral phase
R13.12 Dysphagia, oropharyngeal phase
R13.13 Dysphagia, pharyngeal phase
R13.14 Dysphagia, pharyngoesophageal phase
R13.19 Other dysphagia
Cervical dysphagia
Neurogenic dysphagia

R14 Flatulence and related conditions

Excludes1: *psychogenic aerophagy (F45.8)*

R14.0 Abdominal distension (gaseous)
Bloating
Tympanites (abdominal) (intestinal)
R14.1 Gas pain
R14.2 Eructation
R14.3 Flatulence

R15 Fecal incontinence

Includes: encopresis NOS
Excludes1: *fecal incontinence of nonorganic origin (F98.1)*

R15.0 Incomplete defecation
Excludes1: *constipation (K59.0-)*
fecal impaction (K56.41)
R15.1 Fecal smearing
Fecal soiling
R15.2 Fecal urgency
R15.9 Full incontinence of feces
Fecal incontinence NOS

R16 Hepatomegaly and splenomegaly, not elsewhere classified

R16.0 Hepatomegaly, not elsewhere classified
Hepatomegaly NOS
R16.1 Splenomegaly, not elsewhere classified
Splenomegaly NOS
R16.2 Hepatomegaly with splenomegaly, not elsewhere classified
Hepatosplenomegaly NOS

R17 Unspecified jaundice

Excludes1: *neonatal jaundice (P55, P57-P59)*
CC Exclusion see Appendix A PDX collection 1122
Valid 3-character code, no further characters required

CC **R18 Ascites**

Includes: fluid in peritoneal cavity
Excludes1: *ascites in alcoholic cirrhosis (K70.31)*
ascites in alcoholic hepatitis (K70.11)
ascites in toxic liver disease with chronic active hepatitis (K71.51)
CC Exclusion see Appendix A PDX collection 1123

CC **R18.0 Malignant ascites**
Code first malignancy, such as:
malignant neoplasm of ovary (C56.-)
secondary malignant neoplasm of retroperitoneum and peritoneum (C78.6)
CC Exclusion see Appendix A PDX collection 1123

CC **R18.8 Other ascites**
Ascites NOS
Peritoneal effusion (chronic)
CC Exclusion see Appendix A PDX collection 1123

R19 Other symptoms and signs involving the digestive system and abdomen

Excludes1: *acute abdomen (R10.0)*

+ **R19.0 Intra-abdominal and pelvic swelling, mass and lump**
Excludes1: *abdominal distension (gaseous) (R14.-)*
ascites (R18.-)

R19.00 Intra-abdominal and pelvic swelling, mass and lump, unspecified site
R19.01 Right upper quadrant abdominal swelling, mass and lump
R19.02 Left upper quadrant abdominal swelling, mass and lump
R19.03 Right lower quadrant abdominal swelling, mass and lump
R19.04 Left lower quadrant abdominal swelling, mass and lump
R19.05 Periumbilic swelling, mass or lump
Diffuse or generalized umbilical swelling or mass
R19.06 Epigastric swelling, mass or lump
R19.07 Generalized intra-abdominal and pelvic swelling, mass and lump
Diffuse or generalized intra-abdominal swelling or mass NOS
Diffuse or generalized pelvic swelling or mass NOS
R19.09 Other intra-abdominal and pelvic swelling, mass and lump

+ **R19.1 Abnormal bowel sounds**
R19.11 Absent bowel sounds
R19.12 Hyperactive bowel sounds
R19.15 Other abnormal bowel sounds
Abnormal bowel sounds NOS

R19.2 Visible peristalsis
Hyperperistalsis

+ **R19.3 Abdominal rigidity**
Excludes1: *abdominal rigidity with severe abdominal pain (R10.0)*

R19.30 Abdominal rigidity, unspecified site
R19.31 Right upper quadrant abdominal rigidity
R19.32 Left upper quadrant abdominal rigidity
R19.33 Right lower quadrant abdominal rigidity
R19.34 Left lower quadrant abdominal rigidity
R19.35 Periumbilic abdominal rigidity
R19.36 Epigastric abdominal rigidity
R19.37 Generalized abdominal rigidity

R19.4 Change in bowel habit
Excludes1: *constipation (K59.0-)*
functional diarrhea (K59.1)

R19.5 Other fecal abnormalities
Abnormal stool color
Bulky stools
Mucus in stools
Occult blood in feces
Occult blood in stools
Excludes1: *melena (K92.1)*
neonatal melena (P54.1)

R19.6 Halitosis

R19.7 Diarrhea, unspecified
Diarrhea NOS
Excludes1: *functional diarrhea (K59.1)*
neonatal diarrhea (P78.3)
psychogenic diarrhea (F45.8)

R19.8 Other specified symptoms and signs involving the digestive system and abdomen

Symptoms and signs involving the skin and subcutaneous tissue (R20-R23)

Excludes2: *symptoms relating to breast (N64.4-N64.5)*

R20 Disturbances of skin sensation

Excludes1: *dissociative anesthesia and sensory loss (F44.6)*
psychogenic disturbances (F45.8)

R20.0 Anesthesia of skin
R20.1 Hypoesthesia of skin
R20.2 Paresthesia of skin
Formication
Pins and needles
Tingling skin
Excludes1: *acroparesthesia (I73.8)*
R20.3 Hyperesthesia
R20.8 Other disturbances of skin sensation
R20.9 Unspecified disturbances of skin sensation

R21 Rash and other nonspecific skin eruption

Includes: rash NOS
Excludes1: *specified type of rash- code to condition vesicular eruption (R23.8)*
Valid 3-character code, no further characters required

R22 Localized swelling, mass and lump of skin and subcutaneous tissue

Includes: subcutaneous nodules (localized)(superficial)

Excludes1: *abnormal findings on diagnostic imaging (R90-R93)*
edema (R60.-)
enlarged lymph nodes (R59.-)
localized adiposity (E65)
swelling of joint (M25.4-)

R22.0 Localized swelling, mass and lump, head
R22.1 Localized swelling, mass and lump, neck
R22.2 Localized swelling, mass and lump, trunk
Excludes1: *intra-abdominal or pelvic mass and lump (R19.0-)*
intra-abdominal or pelvic swelling (R19.0-)
Excludes2: *breast mass and lump (N63)*
\+ **R22.3 Localized swelling, mass and lump, upper limb**
R22.30 Localized swelling, mass and lump, unspecified upper limb
R22.31 Localized swelling, mass and lump, right upper limb
R22.32 Localized swelling, mass and lump, left upper limb
R22.33 Localized swelling, mass and lump, upper limb, bilateral
\+ **R22.4 Localized swelling, mass and lump, lower limb**
R22.40 Localized swelling, mass and lump, unspecified lower limb
R22.41 Localized swelling, mass and lump, right lower limb
R22.42 Localized swelling, mass and lump, left lower limb
R22.43 Localized swelling, mass and lump, lower limb, bilateral
R22.9 Localized swelling, mass and lump, unspecified

R23 Other skin changes

R23.0 Cyanosis
Excludes1: *acrocyanosis (I73.8)*
cyanotic attacks of newborn (P28.2)
R23.1 Pallor
Clammy skin
R23.2 Flushing
Excessive blushing
Code first, if applicable, menopausal and female climacteric states (N95.1)
R23.3 Spontaneous ecchymoses
Petechiae
Excludes1: *ecchymoses of newborn (P54.5)*
purpura (D69.-)
R23.4 Changes in skin texture
Desquamation of skin
Induration of skin
Scaling of skin
Excludes1: *epidermal thickening NOS (L85.9)*
R23.8 Other skin changes
R23.9 Unspecified skin changes

;ymptoms and signs involving the nervous and musculoskeletal systems (R25-R29)

R25 Abnormal involuntary movements

Excludes1: *specific movement disorders (G20-G26)*
stereotyped movement disorders (F98.4)
tic disorders (F95.-)

R25.0 Abnormal head movements
R25.1 Tremor, unspecified
Excludes1: *chorea NOS (G25.5)*
essential tremor (G25.0)
hysterical tremor (F44.4)
intention tremor (G25.2)
R25.2 Cramp and spasm
Excludes2: *carpopedal spasm (R29.0)*
charley-horse (M62.831)
infantile spasms (G40.4-)
muscle spasm of back (M62.830)
muscle spasm of calf (M62.831)
R25.3 Fasciculation
Twitching NOS
R25.8 Other abnormal involuntary movements
R25.9 Unspecified abnormal involuntary movements

R26 Abnormalities of gait and mobility

Excludes1: *ataxia NOS (R27.0)*
hereditary ataxia (G11.-)
locomotor (syphilitic) ataxia (A52.11)
immobility syndrome (paraplegic) (M62.3)

R26.0 Ataxic gait
Staggering gait
R26.1 Paralytic gait
Spastic gait
R26.2 Difficulty in walking, not elsewhere classified
Excludes1: *falling (R29.6)*
unsteadiness on feet (R26.81)
AHA CC: 2Q, 2016, 7
R26.8 Other abnormalities of gait and mobility
R26.81 Unsteadiness on feet
R26.89 Other abnormalities of gait and mobility
R26.9 Unspecified abnormalities of gait and mobility

R27 Other lack of coordination

Excludes1: *ataxic gait (R26.0)*
hereditary ataxia (G11.-)
vertigo NOS (R42)

R27.0 Ataxia, unspecified
Excludes1: *ataxia following cerebrovascular disease (I69. with final characters -93)*
R27.8 Other lack of coordination
R27.9 Unspecified lack of coordination

R29 Other symptoms and signs involving the nervous and musculoskeletal systems

CC **R29.0 Tetany**
Carpopedal spasm
Excludes1: *hysterical tetany (F44.5)*
neonatal tetany (P71.3)
parathyroid tetany (E20.9)
post-thyroidectomy tetany (E89.2)
CC Exclusion see Appendix A PDX collection 1124
CC **R29.1 Meningismus**
CC Exclusion see Appendix A PDX collection 1125
R29.2 Abnormal reflex
Excludes2: *abnormal pupillary reflex (H57.0)*
hyperactive gag reflex (J39.2)
vasovagal reaction or syncope (R55)
R29.3 Abnormal posture
R29.4 Clicking hip
Excludes1: *congenital deformities of hip (Q65.-)*
CC **R29.5 Transient paralysis**
Code first any associated spinal cord injury (S14.0, S14.1-, S24.0, S24.1-, S34.0-, S34.1-)
Excludes1: *transient ischemic attack (G45.9)*
CC Exclusion see Appendix A PDX collection 1126
R29.6 Repeated falls
Falling
Tendency to fall
Excludes2: *at risk for falling (Z91.81)*
history of falling (Z91.81)
Review coding guideline C.18.d
AHA CC: 2Q, 2016, 6-7
\+ **R29.7 National Institutes of Health Stroke Scale (NIHSS) score**
Code first the type of cerebral infarction (I63-)
Review coding guideline C.18.i
AHA CC: 4Q, 2016, 61-62
\+ **R29.70 NIHSS score 0-9**
R29.700 NIHSS score 0
R29.701 NIHSS score 1
R29.702 NIHSS score 2
R29.703 NIHSS score 3
R29.704 NIHSS score 4
R29.705 NIHSS score 5
R29.706 NIHSS score 6
R29.707 NIHSS score 7
R29.708 NIHSS score 8
R29.709 NIHSS score 9
\+ **R29.71 NIHSS score 10-19**
R29.710 NIHSS score 10
R29.711 NIHSS score 11
R29.712 NIHSS score 12
R29.713 NIHSS score 13
R29.714 NIHSS score 14
R29.715 NIHSS score 15
R29.716 NIHSS score 16
R29.717 NIHSS score 17
R29.718 NIHSS score 18
R29.719 NIHSS score 19

+ **R29.72 NIHSS score 20-29**
R29.720 NIHSS score 20
R29.721 NIHSS score 21
R29.722 NIHSS score 22
R29.723 NIHSS score 23
R29.724 NIHSS score 24
R29.725 NIHSS score 25
R29.726 NIHSS score 26
R29.727 NIHSS score 27
R29.728 NIHSS score 28
R29.729 NIHSS score 29
+ **R29.73 NIHSS score 30-39**
R29.730 NIHSS score 30
AHA CC: 4Q, 2016, 61-62
R29.731 NIHSS score 31
R29.732 NIHSS score 32
R29.733 NIHSS score 33
R29.734 NIHSS score 34
R29.735 NIHSS score 35
R29.736 NIHSS score 36
R29.737 NIHSS score 37
R29.738 NIHSS score 38
R29.739 NIHSS score 39
+ **R29.74 NIHSS score 40-42**
R29.740 NIHSS score 40
R29.741 NIHSS score 41
R29.742 NIHSS score 42
+ **R29.8 Other symptoms and signs involving the nervous and musculoskeletal systems**
+ **R29.81 Other symptoms and signs involving the nervous system**
R29.810 Facial weakness
Facial droop
Excludes1: *Bell's palsy (G51.0)*
facial weakness following cerebrovascular disease (I69. with final characters -92)
R29.818 Other symptoms and signs involving the nervous system
+ **R29.89 Other symptoms and signs involving the musculoskeletal system**
Excludes2: *pain in limb (M79.6-)*
R29.890 Loss of height
Excludes1: *osteoporosis (M80-M81)*
R29.891 Ocular torticollis
Excludes1: *congenital (sternomastoid) torticollis (Q68.0)*
psychogenic torticollis (F45.8)
spasmodic torticollis (G24.3)
torticollis due to birth injury (P15.8)
torticollis NOS (M43.6)
R29.898 Other symptoms and signs involving the musculoskeletal system
+ **R29.9 Unspecified symptoms and signs involving the nervous and musculoskeletal systems**
R29.90 Unspecified symptoms and signs involving the nervous system
R29.91 Unspecified symptoms and signs involving the musculoskeletal system

Symptoms and signs involving the genitourinary system (R30-R39)

R30 Pain associated with micturition
Excludes1: *psychogenic pain associated with micturition (F45.8)*
R30.0 Dysuria
Strangury
R30.1 Vesical tenesmus
R30.9 Painful micturition, unspecified
Painful urination NOS

R31 Hematuria
Excludes1: *hematuria included with underlying conditions, such as:*
acute cystitis with hematuria (N30.01)
recurrent and persistent hematuria in glomerular diseases (N02.-)
R31.0 Gross hematuria
AHA CC: 1Q, 2017, 17-18
R31.1 Benign essential microscopic hematuria
+ **R31.2 Other microscopic hematuria**
AHA CC: 4Q, 2016, 62
R31.21 Asymptomatic microscopic hematuria
AMH
AHA CC: 4Q, 2016, 62
R31.29 Other microscopic hematuria
R31.9 Hematuria, unspecified
AHA CC: 1Q, 2017, 6

R32 Unspecified urinary incontinence
Enuresis NOS
Excludes1: *functional urinary incontinence (R39.81)*
nonorganic enuresis (F98.0)
stress incontinence and other specified urinary incontinence (N39.3-N39.4-)
urinary incontinence associated with cognitive impairment (R39.81)
Valid 3-character code, no further characters required

R33 Retention of urine
Excludes1: *psychogenic retention of urine (F45.8)*
R33.0 Drug induced retention of urine
Use additional code for adverse effect, if applicable, to identify drug (T36-T50 with fifth or sixth character 5)
R33.8 Other retention of urine
Code first if applicable, any causal condition, such as:
enlarged prostate (N40.1)
R33.9 Retention of urine, unspecified

R34 Anuria and oliguria
Excludes1: *anuria and oliguria complicating abortion or ectopic or molar pregnancy (O00-O07, O08.4)*
anuria and oliguria complicating pregnancy (O26.83-)
anuria and oliguria complicating the puerperium (O90.4)
Valid 3-character code, no further characters required

R35 Polyuria
Code first if applicable, any causal condition, such as:
enlarged prostate (N40.1)
Excludes1: *psychogenic polyuria (F45.8)*
R35.0 Frequency of micturition
R35.1 Nocturia
R35.8 Other polyuria
Polyuria NOS

R36 Urethral discharge
R36.0 Urethral discharge without blood
♂ **R36.1 Hematospermia**
R36.9 Urethral discharge, unspecified
Penile discharge NOS
Urethrorrhea

R37 Sexual dysfunction, unspecified
Valid 3-character code, no further characters required

R39 Other and unspecified symptoms and signs involving the genitourinary system
CC **R39.0 Extravasation of urine**
CC Exclusion see Appendix A PDX collection 1127
+ **R39.1 Other difficulties with micturition**
Code first if applicable, any causal condition, such as:
enlarged prostate (N40.1)
R39.11 Hesitancy of micturition
R39.12 Poor urinary stream
Weak urinary steam
R39.13 Splitting of urinary stream
R39.14 Feeling of incomplete bladder emptying
R39.15 Urgency of urination
Excludes1: *urge incontinence (N39.41, N39.46)*
R39.16 Straining to void
+ **R39.19 Other difficulties with micturition**
AHA CC: 4Q, 2016, 63
R39.191 Need to immediately re-void
R39.192 Position dependent micturition
R39.198 Other difficulties with micturition

R39.2 **Extrarenal uremia**
Prerenal uremia
Excludes1: *uremia NOS (N19)*

\+ R39.8 **Other symptoms and signs involving the genitourinary system**
AHA CC: 4Q, 2016, 64

R39.81 **Functional urinary incontinence**
Urinary incontinence due to cognitive impairment, or severe physical disability or immobility
Excludes1: *stress incontinence and other specified urinary incontinence (N39.3-N39.4-)*
urinary incontinence NOS (R32)

R39.82 **Chronic bladder pain**
AHA CC: 4Q, 2016, 64

♂ R39.83 **Unilateral non-palpable testicle**

♂ R39.84 **Bilateral non-palpable testicles**

R39.89 **Other symptoms and signs involving the genitourinary system**

R39.9 **Unspecified symptoms and signs involving the genitourinary system**

Symptoms and signs involving cognition, perception, emotional state and behavior (R40-R46)

Excludes2: *symptoms and signs constituting part of a pattern of mental disorder (F01-F99)*

R40 **Somnolence, stupor and coma**
Excludes1: *neonatal coma (P91.5)*
somnolence, stupor and coma in diabetes (E08-E13)
somnolence, stupor and coma in hepatic failure (K72.-)
somnolence, stupor and coma in hypoglycemia (nondiabetic) (E15)

R40.0 **Somnolence**
Drowsiness
Excludes1: *coma (R40.2-)*

R40.1 **Stupor**
Catatonic stupor
Semicoma
Excludes1: *catatonic schizophrenia (F20.2)*
coma (R40.2-)
depressive stupor (F31-F33)
dissociative stupor (F44.2)
manic stupor (F30.2)

\+ R40.2 **Coma**
Code first any associated:
fracture of skull (S02.-)
intracranial injury (S06.-)
NOTE One code from each subcategory, R40.21-R40.23, is required to complete the coma scale
Review coding guideline C.18.e
AHA CC: 1Q, 2014, 19-20; 2Q, 2015, 17-18

MCC X+7th R40.20 **Unspecified coma**
Coma NOS
Unconsciousness NOS
MCC Exclusion see Appendix A PDX collection 0515

\+ R40.21 **Coma scale, eyes open**

The appropriate 7th character is to be added to each code from subcategory **R40.21-**:
0 unspecified time
1 in the field [EMT or ambulance]
2 at arrival to emergency department
3 at hospital admission
4 24 hours or more after hospital admission

MCC +7th R40.211 **Coma scale, eyes open, never**
MCC Exclusion for all 7th characters see Appendix A PDX collection 0515

MCC +7th R40.212 **Coma scale, eyes open, to pain**
MCC Exclusion for all 7th characters see Appendix A PDX collection 0515

+7th R40.213 **Coma scale, eyes open, to sound**

+7th R40.214 **Coma scale, eyes open, spontaneous**

\+ R40.22 **Coma scale, best verbal response**

The appropriate 7th character is to be added to each code from subcategory **R40.22-**:
0 unspecified time
1 in the field [EMT or ambulance]
2 at arrival to emergency department
3 at hospital admission
4 24 hours or more after hospital admission

MCC +7th R40.221 **Coma scale, best verbal response, none**
MCC Exclusion for all 7th characters see Appendix A PDX collection 0515

MCC +7th R40.222 **Coma scale, best verbal response, incomprehensible words**
Incomprehensible sounds (2-5 years of age)
Moans/grunts to pain (<2 years of age)
MCC Exclusion for all 7th characters see Appendix A PDX collection 0515

+7th R40.223 **Coma scale, best verbal response, inappropriate words**
Inappropriate crying or screaming (<2 years of age)
Screaming (2-5 years of age)

+7th R40.224 **Coma scale, best verbal response, confused conversation**
Inappropriate words (2-5 years of age)
Irritable cries (<2 years of age)

+7th R40.225 **Coma scale, best verbal response, oriented**
Cooing or babbling or crying appropriately (<2 years of age)
Uses appropriate words (2-5 years of age)

\+ R40.23 **Coma scale, best motor response**

The appropriate 7th character is to be added to each code from subcategory **R40.23-**:
0 unspecified time
1 in the field [EMT or ambulance]
2 at arrival to emergency department
3 at hospital admission
4 24 hours or more after hospital admission

MCC +7th R40.231 **Coma scale, best motor response, none**
MCC Exclusion for all 7th characters see Appendix A PDX collection 0515

MCC +7th R40.232 **Coma scale, best motor response, extension**
Abnormal extensor posturing to pain or noxious stimuli (<2 years of age)
Extensor posturing to pain or noxious stimuli (2-5 years of age)
MCC Exclusion for all 7th characters see Appendix A PDX collection 0515

+7th R40.233 **Coma scale, best motor response, abnormal**
Abnormal flexure posturing to pain or noxious stimuli (0-5 years of age)
Flexion/decorticate posturing (<2 years of age)

MCC +7th R40.234 **Coma scale, best motor response, flexion withdrawal**
Withdraws from pain or noxious stimuli (0-5 years of age)
MCC Exclusion for all 7th characters see Appendix A PDX collection 0515

+7th R40.235 **Coma scale, best motor response, localizes pain**
Localizes pain (2-5 years of age)
Withdraws to touch (<2 years of age)

+7th R40.236 **Coma scale, best motor response, obeys commands**
Normal or spontaneous movement (<2 years of age)
Obeys commands (2-5 years of age)

\+ R40.24 **Glasgow coma scale, total score**
NOTE Assign a code from subcategory R40.24, when only the total coma score is documented.
AHA CC: 4Q, 2016, 64-65

The appropriate 7th character is to be added to each code from subcategory **R40.24-**:
0 unspecified time
1 in the field [EMT or ambulance]
2 at arrival to emergency department
3 at hospital admission
4 24 hours or more after hospital admission

+7th R40.241 **Glasgow coma scale score 13-15**

+7th R40.242 **Glasgow coma scale score 9-12**

+7th R40.243 **Glasgow coma scale score 3-8**

+7th R40.244 **Other coma, without documented Glasgow coma scale score, or with partial score reported**

CC R40.3 **Persistent vegetative state**
CC Exclusion see Appendix A PDX collection 0515

R40.4 **Transient alteration of awareness**

R41 Other symptoms and signs involving cognitive functions and awareness

Excludes1: *dissociative [conversion] disorders (F44.-)*
mild cognitive impairment, so stated (G31.84)

R41.0 Disorientation, unspecified
Confusion NOS
Delirium NOS
AHA CC: 4Q, 2016, 74-76

R41.1 Anterograde amnesia

R41.2 Retrograde amnesia

R41.3 Other amnesia
Amnesia NOS
Memory loss NOS
Excludes1: *amnestic disorder due to known physiologic condition (F04)*
amnestic syndrome due to psychoactive substance use (F10-F19 with 5th character .6)
mild memory disturbance due to known physiological condition (F06.8)
transient global amnesia (G45.4)

CC **R41.4 Neurologic neglect syndrome**
Asomatognosia
Hemi-akinesia
Hemi-inattention
Hemispatial neglect
Left-sided neglect
Sensory neglect
Visuospatial neglect
Excludes1: *visuospatial deficit (R41.842)*
CC Exclusion see Appendix A PDX collection 1128

\+ **R41.8 Other symptoms and signs involving cognitive functions and awareness**

• **R41.81 Age-related cognitive decline**
Senility NOS

R41.82 Altered mental status, unspecified
Change in mental status NOS
Excludes1: *altered level of consciousness (R40.-)*
altered mental status due to known condition - code to condition delirium NOS (R41.0)
AHA CC: 4Q, 2012, 98

R41.83 Borderline intellectual functioning
IQ level 71 to 84
Excludes1: *intellectual disabilities (F70-F79)*

\+ **R41.84 Other specified cognitive deficit**
Excludes1: *cognitive deficits as sequelae of cerebrovascular disease (I69.01-, I69.11-, I19.21-, I69.31-, I59.81-, I69.91-)*

R41.840 Attention and concentration deficit
Excludes1: *attention-deficit hyperactivity disorders (F90.-)*

R41.841 Cognitive communication deficit

R41.842 Visuospatial deficit

R41.843 Psychomotor deficit

R41.844 Frontal lobe and executive function deficit

R41.89 Other symptoms and signs involving cognitive functions and awareness
Anosognosia

R41.9 Unspecified symptoms and signs involving cognitive functions and awareness
Unspecified neurocognitive disorder

R42 Dizziness and giddiness

Light-headedness
Vertigo NOS
Excludes1: *vertiginous syndromes (H81.-)*
vertigo from infrasound (T75.23)
Valid 3-character code, no further characters required

R43 Disturbances of smell and taste

R43.0 Anosmia

R43.1 Parosmia

R43.2 Parageusia

R43.8 Other disturbances of smell and taste
Mixed disturbance of smell and taste

R43.9 Unspecified disturbances of smell and taste

R44 Other symptoms and signs involving general sensations and perceptions

Excludes1: *alcoholic hallucinations (F1.5)*
hallucinations in drug psychosis (F11-F19 with .5)
hallucinations in mood disorders with psychotic symptoms (F30.2, F31.5, F32.3, F33.3)
hallucinations in schizophrenia, schizotypal and delusional disorders (F20-F29)
Excludes2: *disturbances of skin sensation (R20.-)*

CC **R44.0 Auditory hallucinations**
CC Exclusion see Appendix A PDX collection 1129

R44.1 Visual hallucinations

CC **R44.2 Other hallucinations**
CC Exclusion see Appendix A PDX collection 1129

CC **R44.3 Hallucinations, unspecified**
CC Exclusion see Appendix A PDX collection 1129

R44.8 Other symptoms and signs involving general sensations and perceptions

R44.9 Unspecified symptoms and signs involving general sensations and perceptions

R45 Symptoms and signs involving emotional state

R45.0 Nervousness
Nervous tension

R45.1 Restlessness and agitation

R45.2 Unhappiness

R45.3 Demoralization and apathy
Excludes1: *anhedonia (R45.84)*

R45.4 Irritability and anger

R45.5 Hostility

R45.6 Violent behavior

R45.7 State of emotional shock and stress, unspecified

\+ **R45.8 Other symptoms and signs involving emotional state**

R45.81 Low self-esteem

R45.82 Worries

R45.83 Excessive crying of child, adolescent or adult
Excludes1: *excessive crying of infant (baby) (R68.11)*

R45.84 Anhedonia

\+ **R45.85 Homicidal and suicidal ideations**
Excludes1: *suicide attempt (T14.91)*

R45.850 Homicidal ideations

CC **R45.851 Suicidal ideations**
CC Exclusion see Appendix A PDX collection 113

R45.86 Emotional lability

R45.87 Impulsiveness

R45.89 Other symptoms and signs involving emotional state

R46 Symptoms and signs involving appearance and behavior

Excludes1: *appearance and behavior in schizophrenia, schizotypal and delusional disorders (F20-F29)*
mental and behavioral disorders (F01-F99)

R46.0 Very low level of personal hygiene

R46.1 Bizarre personal appearance

R46.2 Strange and inexplicable behavior

R46.3 Overactivity

R46.4 Slowness and poor responsiveness
Excludes1: *stupor (R40.1)*

R46.5 Suspiciousness and marked evasiveness

R46.6 Undue concern and preoccupation with stressful events

R46.7 Verbosity and circumstantial detail obscuring reason for contact

\+ **R46.8 Other symptoms and signs involving appearance and behavior**

R46.81 Obsessive-compulsive behavior
Excludes1: *obsessive-compulsive disorder (F42.-)*

R46.89 Other symptoms and signs involving appearance and behavior

ymptoms and signs involving speech and voice (R47-R49)

R47 Speech disturbances, not elsewhere classified

Excludes1: *autism (F84.0)*
cluttering (F80.81)
specific developmental disorders of speech and language (F80.-)
stuttering (F80.81)

\+ **R47.0 Dysphasia and aphasia**

CC **R47.01 Aphasia**

Excludes1: *aphasia following cerebrovascular disease (I69. with final characters -20)*
progressive isolated aphasia (G31.01)

CC Exclusion see Appendix A PDX collection 1131

R47.02 Dysphasia

Excludes1: *dysphasia following cerebrovascular disease (I69. with final characters -21)*

R47.1 Dysarthria and anarthria

Excludes1: *dysarthria following cerebrovascular disease (I69. with final characters -22)*

\+ **R47.8 Other speech disturbances**

Excludes1: *dysarthria following cerebrovascular disease (I69. with final characters -28)*

R47.81 Slurred speech

R47.82 Fluency disorder in conditions classified elsewhere

Stuttering in conditions classified elsewhere

Code first underlying disease or condition, such as:
Parkinson's disease (G20)

Excludes1: *adult onset fluency disorder (F98.5)*
childhood onset fluency disorder (F80.81)
fluency disorder (stuttering) following cerebrovascular disease (I69. with final characters -23)

R47.89 Other speech disturbances

R47.9 Unspecified speech disturbances

R48 Dyslexia and other symbolic dysfunctions, not elsewhere classified

Excludes1: *specific developmental disorders of scholastic skills (F81.-)*

R48.0 Dyslexia and alexia

R48.1 Agnosia

Astereognosia (astereognosis)
Autotopagnosia

Excludes1: *visual object agnosia (R48.3)*

R48.2 Apraxia

Excludes1: *apraxia following cerebrovascular disease (I69. with final characters -90)*

R48.3 Visual agnosia

Prosopagnosia
Simultanagnosia (asimultagnosia)

R48.8 Other symbolic dysfunctions

Acalculia
Agraphia

AHA CC: 1Q, 2017, 27-28

R48.9 Unspecified symbolic dysfunctions

R49 Voice and resonance disorders

Excludes1: *psychogenic voice and resonance disorders (F44.4)*

R49.0 Dysphonia

Hoarseness

R49.1 Aphonia

Loss of voice

\+ **R49.2 Hypernasality and hyponasality**

R49.21 Hypernasality

R49.22 Hyponasality

R49.8 Other voice and resonance disorders

R49.9 Unspecified voice and resonance disorder

Change in voice NOS
Resonance disorder NOS

eneral symptoms and signs (R50-R69)

R50 Fever of other and unknown origin

Excludes1: *chills without fever (R68.83)*
febrile convulsions (R56.0-)
fever of unknown origin during labor (O75.2)
fever of unknown origin in newborn (P81.9)
hypothermia due to illness (R68.0)
malignant hyperthermia due to anesthesia (T88.3)
puerperal pyrexia NOS (O86.4)

R50.2 Drug induced fever

Use additional code for adverse effect, if applicable, to identify drug (T36-T50 with fifth or sixth character 5)

Excludes1: *postvaccination (postimmunization) fever (R50.83)*

\+ **R50.8 Other specified fever**

R50.81 Fever presenting with conditions classified elsewhere

Code first underlying condition when associated fever is present, such as with:
leukemia (C91-C95)
neutropenia (D70.-)
sickle-cell disease (D57.-)

AHA CC: 4Q, 2014, 22-23

R50.82 Postprocedural fever

Excludes1: *postprocedural infection (T81.4-)*
posttransfusion fever (R50.84)
postvaccination (postimmunization) fever (R50.83)

R50.83 Postvaccination fever

Postimmunization fever

R50.84 Febrile nonhemolytic transfusion reaction

FNHTR
Posttransfusion fever

R50.9 Fever, unspecified

Fever NOS
Fever of unknown origin [FUO]
Fever with chills
Fever with rigors
Hyperpyrexia NOS
Persistent fever
Pyrexia NOS

R51 Headache

Facial pain NOS

Excludes1: *atypical face pain (G50.1)*
migraine and other headache syndromes (G43-G44)
trigeminal neuralgia (G50.0)

Valid 3-character code, no further characters required

R52 Pain, unspecified

Acute pain NOS
Generalized pain NOS
Pain NOS

Excludes1: *acute and chronic pain, not elsewhere classified (G89.-)*
localized pain, unspecified type - code to pain by site, such as:
abdomen pain (R10.-)
back pain (M54.9)
breast pain (N64.4)
chest pain (R07.1-R07.9)
ear pain (H92.0-)
eye pain (H57.1)
headache (R51)
joint pain (M25.5-)
limb pain (M79.6-)
lumbar region pain (M54.5)
pelvic and perineal pain (R10.2)
shoulder pain (M25.51-)
spine pain (M54.-)
throat pain (R07.0)
tongue pain (K14.6)
tooth pain (K08.8)
renal colic (N23)
pain disorders exclusively related to psychological factors (F45.41)

Valid 3-character code, no further characters required

R53 Malaise and fatigue

R53.0 Neoplastic (malignant) related fatigue

Code first associated neoplasm

R53.1 Weakness

Asthenia NOS

Excludes1: *age-related weakness (R54)*
muscle weakness (M62.8-)
sarcopenia (M62.84)
senile asthenia (R54)

AHA CC: 1Q, 2017, 7

MCC **R53.2 Functional quadriplegia**

Complete immobility due to severe physical disability or frailty

Excludes1: *frailty NOS (R54)*
hysterical paralysis (F44.4)
immobility syndrome (M62.3)
neurologic quadriplegia (G82.5-)
quadriplegia (G82.50)

MCC Exclusion see Appendix A PDX collection 0595
Review coding guideline C.18.f

AHA CC: 2Q, 2016, 6

+ **R53.8 Other malaise and fatigue**
Excludes1: *combat exhaustion and fatigue (F43.0)*
congenital debility (P96.9)
exhaustion and fatigue due to excessive exertion (T73.3)
exhaustion and fatigue due to exposure (T73.2)
exhaustion and fatigue due to heat (T67.-)
exhaustion and fatigue due to pregnancy (O26.8-)
exhaustion and fatigue due to recurrent depressive episode (F33)
exhaustion and fatigue due to senile debility (R54)

R53.81 Other malaise
Chronic debility
Debility NOS
General physical deterioration
Malaise NOS
Nervous debility
Excludes1: *age-related physical debility (R54)*

R53.82 Chronic fatigue, unspecified
Chronic fatigue syndrome NOS
Excludes1: *postviral fatigue syndrome (G93.3)*

R53.83 Other fatigue
Fatigue NOS
Lack of energy
Lethargy
Tiredness
Excludes2: *exhaustion and fatigue due to depressive episode (F32.-)*
AHA CC: 1Q, 2017, 7

• **R54 Age-related physical debility**
Frailty
Old age
Senescence
Senile asthenia
Senile debility
Excludes1: *age-related cognitive decline (R41.81)*
sarcopenia (M62.84)
senile psychosis (F03)
senility NOS (R41.81)
Valid 3-character code, no further characters required

R55 Syncope and collapse
Blackout
Fainting
Vasovagal attack
Excludes1: *cardiogenic shock (R57.0)*
carotid sinus syncope (G90.01)
heat syncope (T67.1)
neurocirculatory asthenia (F45.8)
neurogenic orthostatic hypotension (G90.3)
orthostatic hypotension (I95.1)
postprocedural shock (T81.1-)
psychogenic syncope (F48.8)
shock NOS (R57.9)
shock complicating or following abortion or ectopic or molar pregnancy (O00-O07, O08.3)
shock complicating or following labor and delivery (O75.1)
Stokes-Adams attack (I45.9)
unconsciousness NOS (R40.2-)
Valid 3-character code, no further characters required

R56 Convulsions, not elsewhere classified
Excludes1: *dissociative convulsions and seizures (F44.5)*
epileptic convulsions and seizures (G40.-)
newborn convulsions and seizures (P90)

+ **R56.0 Febrile convulsions**

CC **R56.00 Simple febrile convulsions**
Febrile convulsion NOS
Febrile seizure NOS
CC Exclusion see Appendix A PDX collection 1132

CC **R56.01 Complex febrile convulsions**
Atypical febrile seizure
Complex febrile seizure
Complicated febrile seizure
Excludes1: *status epilepticus (G40.901)*
CC Exclusion see Appendix A PDX collection 1132

CC **R56.1 Post traumatic seizures**
Excludes1: *post traumatic epilepsy (G40.-)*
CC Exclusion see Appendix A PDX collection 0582

R56.9 Unspecified convulsions
Convulsion disorder
Fit NOS
Recurrent convulsions
Seizure(s) (convulsive) NOS

R57 Shock, not elsewhere classified
Excludes1: *anaphylactic shock NOS (T78.2)*
anaphylactic reaction or shock due to adverse food reaction (T78.0-)
anaphylactic shock due to adverse effect of correct drug or medicament properly administered (T88.6)
anaphylactic shock due to serum (T80.5-)
anesthetic shock (T88.3)
electric shock (T75.4)
obstetric shock (O75.1)
postprocedural shock (T81.1-)
psychic shock (F43.0)
shock complicating or following ectopic or molar pregnancy (O00-O07, O08.3)
shock due to lightning (T75.01)
traumatic shock (T79.4)
toxic shock syndrome (A48.3)

MCC **R57.0 Cardiogenic shock**
Excludes2: *septic shock (R65.21)*
MCC Exclusion see Appendix A PDX collection 1133

MCC **R57.1 Hypovolemic shock**
MCC Exclusion see Appendix A PDX collection 1133

MCC **R57.8 Other shock**
MCC Exclusion see Appendix A PDX collection 1133

CC **R57.9 Shock, unspecified**
Failure of peripheral circulation NOS
CC Exclusion see Appendix A PDX collection 1133

R58 Hemorrhage, not elsewhere classified
Hemorrhage NOS
Excludes1: *hemorrhage included with underlying conditions, such as:*
acute duodenal ulcer with hemorrhage (K26.0)
acute gastritis with bleeding (K29.01)
ulcerative enterocolitis with rectal bleeding (K51.01)
Valid 3-character code, no further characters required

R59 Enlarged lymph nodes
Includes: swollen glands
Excludes1: *lymphadenitis NOS (I88.9)*
acute lymphadenitis (L04.-)
chronic lymphadenitis (I88.1)
mesenteric (acute) (chronic) lymphadenitis (I88.0)

R59.0 Localized enlarged lymph nodes

R59.1 Generalized enlarged lymph nodes
Lymphadenopathy NOS

R59.9 Enlarged lymph nodes, unspecified

R60 Edema, not elsewhere classified
Excludes1: *angioneurotic edema (T78.3)*
ascites (R18.-)
cerebral edema (G93.6)
cerebral edema due to birth injury (P11.0)
edema of larynx (J38.4)
edema of nasopharynx (J39.2)
edema of pharynx (J39.2)
gestational edema (O12.0-)
hereditary edema (Q82.0)
hydrops fetalis NOS (P83.2)
hydrothorax (J94.8)
hydrops fetalis NOS (P83.2)
newborn edema (P83.3)
pulmonary edema (J81.-)

R60.0 Localized edema

R60.1 Generalized edema
Excludes2: *nutritional edema (E40-E46)*

R60.9 Edema, unspecified
Fluid retention NOS

R61 Generalized hyperhidrosis
Excessive sweating
Night sweats
Secondary hyperhidrosis
Code first if applicable, menopausal and female climacteric states (N95.
Excludes1: *focal (primary) (secondary) hyperhidrosis (L74.5-)*
Frey's syndrome (L74.52)
localized (primary) (secondary) hyperhidrosis (L74.5-)
Valid 3-character code, no further characters required

R62 Lack of expected normal physiological development in childhood and adults

Excludes1: *delayed puberty (E30.0)*
gonadal dysgenesis (Q99.1)
hypopituitarism (E23.0)

● **R62.0 Delayed milestone in childhood**
Delayed attainment of expected physiological developmental stage
Late talker
Late walker

+ **R62.5 Other and unspecified lack of expected normal physiological development in childhood**
Excludes1: *HIV disease resulting in failure to thrive (B20)*
physical retardation due to malnutrition (E45)

R62.50 Unspecified lack of expected normal physiological development in childhood
Infantilism NOS

● **R62.51 Failure to thrive (child)**
Failure to gain weight
Excludes1: *failure to thrive in child under 28 days old (P92.6)*

R62.52 Short stature (child)
Lack of growth
Physical retardation
Short stature NOS
Excludes1: *short stature due to endocrine disorder (E34.3)*

R62.59 Other lack of expected normal physiological development in childhood

● **R62.7 Adult failure to thrive**

R63 Symptoms and signs concerning food and fluid intake

Excludes1: *bulimia NOS (F50.2)*
eating disorders of nonorganic origin (F50.-)
malnutrition (E40-E46)

R63.0 Anorexia
Loss of appetite
Excludes1: *anorexia nervosa (F50.0-)*
loss of appetite of nonorganic origin (F50.89)

R63.1 Polydipsia
Excessive thirst

R63.2 Polyphagia
Excessive eating
Hyperalimentation NOS

R63.3 Feeding difficulties
Feeding problem (elderly) (infant) NOS
Picky eater
Excludes1: *eating disorders (F50.-)*
feeding problems of newborn (P92.-)
infant feeding disorder of nonorganic origin (F98.2-)

R63.4 Abnormal weight loss

R63.5 Abnormal weight gain
Excludes1: *excessive weight gain in pregnancy (O26.0-)*
obesity (E66.-)

R63.6 Underweight
Use additional code to identify body mass index (BMI), if known (Z68.-)
Excludes1: *abnormal weight loss (R63.4)*
anorexia nervosa (F50.0-)
malnutrition (E40-E46)

R63.8 Other symptoms and signs concerning food and fluid intake

C **R64 Cachexia**

Wasting syndrome
Code first underlying condition, if known
Excludes1: *abnormal weight loss (R63.4)*
nutritional marasmus (E41)
CC Exclusion see Appendix A PDX collection 1134
Valid 3-character code, no further characters required

R65 Symptoms and signs specifically associated with systemic inflammation and infection

+ **R65.1 Systemic inflammatory response syndrome (SIRS) of non-infectious origin**
Code first underlying condition, such as:
heatstroke (T67.0)
injury and trauma (S00-T88)
Excludes1: *sepsis- code to infection*
severe sepsis (R65.2)

CC **R65.10 Systemic inflammatory response syndrome (SIRS) of non-infectious origin without acute organ dysfunction**
Systemic inflammatory response syndrome (SIRS) NOS
CC Exclusion see Appendix A PDX collection 0071
Review coding guideline C.18.g

MCC **R65.11 Systemic inflammatory response syndrome (SIRS) of non-infectious origin with acute organ dysfunction**
Use additional code to identify specific acute organ dysfunction, such as:
acute kidney failure (N17.-)
acute respiratory failure (J96.0-)
critical illness myopathy (G72.81)
critical illness polyneuropathy (G62.81)
disseminated intravascular coagulopathy [DIC] (D65)
encephalopathy (metabolic) (septic) (G93.41)
hepatic failure (K72.0-)
MCC Exclusion see Appendix A PDX collection 0071
Review coding guideline C.18.g

+ **R65.2 Severe sepsis**
Infection with associated acute organ dysfunction
Sepsis with acute organ dysfunction
Sepsis with multiple organ dysfunction
Systemic inflammatory response syndrome due to infectious process with acute organ dysfunction
Code first underlying infection, such as:
infection following a procedure (T81.4-)
infections following infusion, transfusion and therapeutic injection (T80.2-)
puerperal sepsis (O85)
sepsis following complete or unspecified spontaneous abortion (O03.87)
sepsis following ectopic and molar pregnancy (O08.82)
sepsis following incomplete spontaneous abortion (O03.37)
sepsis following (induced) termination of pregnancy (O04.87)
sepsis NOS (A41.9)

Use additional code to identify specific acute organ dysfunction, such as:
acute kidney failure (N17.-)
acute respiratory failure (J96.0-)
critical illness myopathy (G72.81)
critical illness polyneuropathy (G62.81)
disseminated intravascular coagulopathy [DIC] (D65)
encephalopathy (metabolic) (septic) (G93.41)
hepatic failure (K72.0-)
Review coding guideline C.1.d

MCC **R65.20 Severe sepsis without septic shock**
Severe sepsis NOS
MCC Exclusion see Appendix A PDX collection 0071
AHA CC: 3Q, 2016, 14

MCC **R65.21 Severe sepsis with septic shock**
MCC Exclusion see Appendix A PDX collection 1133
Review coding guideline C.1.d.2

R68 Other general symptoms and signs

R68.0 Hypothermia, not associated with low environmental temperature
Excludes1: *hypothermia NOS (accidental) (T68)*
hypothermia due to anesthesia (T88.51)
hypothermia due to low environmental temperature (T68)
newborn hypothermia (P80.-)

+ **R68.1 Nonspecific symptoms peculiar to infancy**
Excludes1: *colic, infantile (R10.83)*
neonatal cerebral irritability (P91.3)
teething syndrome (K00.7)

● **R68.11 Excessive crying of infant (baby)**
Excludes1: *excessive crying of child, adolescent, or adult (R45.83)*

● **R68.12 Fussy infant (baby)**
Irritable infant

- • **R68.13 Apparent life threatening event in infant (ALTE)**
  Apparent life threatening event in newborn
  Brief resolved unexplained event (BRUE)
  Code first confirmed diagnosis, if known
  Use additional code(s) for associated signs and symptoms if no confirmed diagnosis established, or if signs and symptoms are not associated routinely with confirmed diagnosis, or provide additional information for cause of ALTE
- • **R68.19 Other nonspecific symptoms peculiar to infancy**

R68.2 Dry mouth, unspecified
Excludes1: *dry mouth due to dehydration (E86.0)*
dry mouth due to sicca syndrome [Sjögren] (M35.0-)
salivary gland hyposecretion (K11.7)

R68.3 Clubbing of fingers
Clubbing of nails
Excludes1: *congenital clubfinger (Q68.1)*

\+ **R68.8 Other general symptoms and signs**
R68.81 Early satiety
• **R68.82 Decreased libido**
Decreased sexual desire
R68.83 Chills (without fever)
Chills NOS
Excludes1: *chills with fever (R50.9)*
R68.84 Jaw pain
Mandibular pain
Maxilla pain
Excludes1: *temporomandibular joint arthralgia (M26.62-)*
R68.89 Other general symptoms and signs

R69 Illness, unspecified
Unknown and unspecified cases of morbidity
Valid 3-character code, no further characters required

Abnormal findings on examination of blood, without diagnosis (R70-R79)

Excludes2: *abnormal findings on antenatal screening of mother (O28.-)*
abnormalities of lipids (E78.-)
abnormalities of platelets and thrombocytes (D69.-)
abnormalities of white blood cells classified elsewhere (D70-D72)
coagulation hemorrhagic disorders (D65-D68)
diagnostic abnormal findings classified elsewhere - see Alphabetic Index
hemorrhagic and hematological disorders of newborn (P50-P61)

R70 Elevated erythrocyte sedimentation rate and abnormality of plasma viscosity
R70.0 Elevated erythrocyte sedimentation rate
R70.1 Abnormal plasma viscosity

R71 Abnormality of red blood cells
Excludes1: *anemias (D50-D64)*
anemia of premature infant (P61.2)
benign (familial) polycythemia (D75.0)
congenital anemias (P61.2-P61.4)
newborn anemia due to isoimmunization (P55.-)
polycythemia neonatorum (P61.1)
polycythemia NOS (D75.1)
polycythemia vera (D45)
secondary polycythemia (D75.1)
CC **R71.0 Precipitous drop in hematocrit**
Drop (precipitous) in hemoglobin
Drop in hematocrit
CC Exclusion see Appendix A PDX collection 1135
R71.8 Other abnormality of red blood cells
Abnormal red-cell morphology NOS
Abnormal red-cell volume NOS
Anisocytosis
Poikilocytosis

R73 Elevated blood glucose level
Excludes1: *diabetes mellitus (E08-E13)*
diabetes mellitus in pregnancy, childbirth and the puerperium (O24.-)
neonatal disorders (P70.0-P70.2)
postsurgical hypoinsulinemia (E89.1)

\+ **R73.0 Abnormal glucose**
Excludes1: *abnormal glucose in pregnancy (O99.81-)*
diabetes mellitus (E08-E13)
dysmetabolic syndrome X (E88.81)
gestational diabetes (O24.4-)
glycosuria (R81)
hypoglycemia (E16.2)
R73.01 Impaired fasting glucose
Elevated fasting glucose
R73.02 Impaired glucose tolerance (oral)
Elevated glucose tolerance
R73.03 Prediabetes
Latent diabetes
AHA CC: 4Q, 2016, 65
R73.09 Other abnormal glucose
Abnormal glucose NOS
Abnormal non-fasting glucose tolerance
R73.9 Hyperglycemia, unspecified

R74 Abnormal serum enzyme levels
R74.0 Nonspecific elevation of levels of transaminase and lactic acid dehydrogenase [LDH]
R74.8 Abnormal levels of other serum enzymes
Abnormal level of acid phosphatase
Abnormal level of alkaline phosphatase
Abnormal level of amylase
Abnormal level of lipase [triacylglycerol lipase]
R74.9 Abnormal serum enzyme level, unspecified

R75 Inconclusive laboratory evidence of human immunodeficiency virus [HIV]
Nonconclusive HIV-test finding in infants
Excludes1: *asymptomatic human immunodeficiency virus [HIV] infection status (Z21)*
human immunodeficiency virus [HIV] disease (B20)
Review coding guidelines C.1.a.2.e and C.1.a.2.f
Valid 3-character code, no further characters required

R76 Other abnormal immunological findings in serum
R76.0 Raised antibody titer
Excludes1: *isoimmunization in pregnancy (O36.0-O36.1)*
isoimmunization affecting newborn (P55.-)
\+ **R76.1 Nonspecific reaction to test for tuberculosis**
R76.11 Nonspecific reaction to tuberculin skin test without active tuberculosis
Abnormal result of Mantoux test
PPD positive
Tuberculin (skin test) positive
Tuberculin (skin test) reactor
Excludes1: *nonspecific reaction to cell mediated immunity measurement of gamma interferon antigen response without active tuberculosis (R76.12)*
R76.12 Nonspecific reaction to cell mediated immunity measurement of gamma interferon antigen respons[e] without active tuberculosis
Nonspecific reaction to QuantiFERON-TB test (QFT) without active tuberculosis
Excludes1: *nonspecific reaction to tuberculin skin te[st] without active tuberculosis (R76.11)*
positive tuberculin skin test (R76.11)
R76.8 Other specified abnormal immunological findings in serum
Raised level of immunoglobulins NOS
R76.9 Abnormal immunological finding in serum, unspecified

R77 Other abnormalities of plasma proteins
Excludes1: *disorders of plasma-protein metabolism (E88.0)*
R77.0 Abnormality of albumin
R77.1 Abnormality of globulin
Hyperglobulinemia NOS
R77.2 Abnormality of alphafetoprotein
R77.8 Other specified abnormalities of plasma proteins
R77.9 Abnormality of plasma protein, unspecified

R78 Findings of drugs and other substances, not normally found in blood

Use additional code to identify the any retained foreign body, if applicable (Z18.-)

Excludes1: *mental or behavioral disorders due to psychoactive substance use (F10-F19)*

R78.0 Finding of alcohol in blood

external cause code (Y90.-), for detail regarding alcohol level.

R78.1 Finding of opiate drug in blood

R78.2 Finding of cocaine in blood

R78.3 Finding of hallucinogen in blood

R78.4 Finding of other drugs of addictive potential in blood

R78.5 Finding of other psychotropic drug in blood

R78.6 Finding of steroid agent in blood

\+ **R78.7 Finding of abnormal level of heavy metals in blood**

R78.71 Abnormal lead level in blood

Excludes1: *lead poisoning (T56.0-)*

R78.79 Finding of abnormal level of heavy metals in blood

\+ **R78.8 Finding of other specified substances, not normally found in blood**

CC **R78.81 Bacteremia**

Excludes1: *sepsis-code to specified infection*

CC Exclusion see Appendix A PDX collection 1136

R78.89 Finding of other specified substances, not normally found in blood

Finding of abnormal level of lithium in blood

R78.9 Finding of unspecified substance, not normally found in blood

R79 Other abnormal findings of blood chemistry

Use additional code to identify any retained foreign body, if applicable (Z18.-)

Excludes1: *asymptomatic hyperuricemia (E79.0)*
hyperglycemia NOS (R73.9)
hypoglycemia NOS (E16.2)
neonatal hypoglycemia (P70.3-P70.4)
specific findings indicating disorder of amino-acid metabolism (E70-E72)
specific findings indicating disorder of carbohydrate metabolism (E73-E74)
specific findings indicating disorder of lipid metabolism (E75.-)

R79.0 Abnormal level of blood mineral

Abnormal blood level of cobalt
Abnormal blood level of copper
Abnormal blood level of iron
Abnormal blood level of magnesium
Abnormal blood level of mineral NEC
Abnormal blood level of zinc

Excludes1: *abnormal level of lithium (R78.89)*
disorders of mineral metabolism (E83.-)
neonatal hypomagnesemia (P71.2)
nutritional mineral deficiency (E58-E61)

R79.1 Abnormal coagulation profile

Abnormal or prolonged bleeding time
Abnormal or prolonged coagulation time
Abnormal or prolonged partial thromboplastin time [PTT]
Abnormal or prolonged prothrombin time [PT]

Excludes2: *abnormality of fluid, electrolyte or acid-base balance (E86-E87)*
coagulation defects (D68.-)

\+ **R79.8 Other specified abnormal findings of blood chemistry**

R79.81 Abnormal blood-gas level

R79.82 Elevated C-reactive protein (CRP)

R79.89 Other specified abnormal findings of blood chemistry

R79.9 Abnormal finding of blood chemistry, unspecified

bnormal findings on examination of urine, without diagnosis 80-R82)

cludes1: *abnormal findings on antenatal screening of mother (O28.-)*
diagnostic abnormal findings classified elsewhere - see Alphabetical Index
specific findings indicating disorder of amino-acid metabolism (E70-E72)
specific findings indicating disorder of carbohydrate metabolism (E73-E74)

R80 Proteinuria

Excludes1: *gestational proteinuria (O12.1-)*

R80.0 Isolated proteinuria

Idiopathic proteinuria

Excludes1: *isolated proteinuria with specific morphological lesion (N06.-)*

R80.1 Persistent proteinuria, unspecified

R80.2 Orthostatic proteinuria, unspecified

Postural proteinuria

R80.3 Bence Jones proteinuria

R80.8 Other proteinuria

R80.9 Proteinuria, unspecified

Albuminuria NOS

R81 Glycosuria

Excludes1: *renal glycosuria (E74.8)*

Valid 3-character code, no further characters required

R82 Other and unspecified abnormal findings in urine

Includes: chromoabnormalities in urine

Use additional code to identify any retained foreign body, if applicable (Z18.-)

Excludes2: *hematuria (R31.-)*

CC **R82.0 Chyluria**

Excludes1: *filarial chyluria (B74.-)*

CC Exclusion see Appendix A PDX collection 1137

CC **R82.1 Myoglobinuria**

CC Exclusion see Appendix A PDX collection 1138

R82.2 Biliuria

R82.3 Hemoglobinuria

Excludes1: *hemoglobinuria due to hemolysis from external causes NEC (D59.6)*
hemoglobinuria due to paroxysmal nocturnal [Marchiafava-Micheli] (D59.5)

R82.4 Acetonuria

Ketonuria

R82.5 Elevated urine levels of drugs, medicaments and biological substances

Elevated urine levels of catecholamines
Elevated urine levels of indoleacetic acid
Elevated urine levels of 17-ketosteroids
Elevated urine levels of steroids

R82.6 Abnormal urine levels of substances chiefly nonmedicinal as to source

Abnormal urine level of heavy metals

\+ **R82.7 Abnormal findings on microbiological examination of urine**

Excludes1: *colonization status (Z22.-)*

AHA CC: 4Q, 2016, 65

R82.71 Bacteriuria

R82.79 Other abnormal findings on microbiological examination of urine

Positive culture findings of urine

R82.8 Abnormal findings on cytological and histological examination of urine

\+ **R82.9 Other and unspecified abnormal findings in urine**

R82.90 Unspecified abnormal findings in urine

R82.91 Other chromoabnormalities of urine

Chromoconversion (dipstick)
Idiopathic dipstick converts positive for blood with no cellular forms in sediment

Excludes1: *hemoglobinuria (R82.3)*
myoglobinuria (R82.1)

R82.99 Other abnormal findings in urine

Cells and casts in urine
Crystalluria
Melanuria

Abnormal findings on examination of other body fluids, substances and tissues, without diagnosis (R83-R89)

Excludes1: *abnormal findings on antenatal screening of mother (O28.-)*
diagnostic abnormal findings classified elsewhere - see Alphabetical Index

Excludes2: *abnormal findings on examination of blood, without diagnosis (R70-R79)*
abnormal findings on examination of urine, without diagnosis (R80-R82)
abnormal tumor markers (R97.-)

R83 Abnormal findings in cerebrospinal fluid

R83.0 Abnormal level of enzymes in cerebrospinal fluid

R83.1 Abnormal level of hormones in cerebrospinal fluid

R83.2 Abnormal level of other drugs, medicaments and biological substances in cerebrospinal fluid

R83.3 Abnormal level of substances chiefly nonmedicinal as to source in cerebrospinal fluid

R83.4 Abnormal immunological findings in cerebrospinal fluid

R83.5 Abnormal microbiological findings in cerebrospinal fluid

Positive culture findings in cerebrospinal fluid

Excludes1: *colonization status (Z22.-)*

R83.6 Abnormal cytological findings in cerebrospinal fluid
R83.8 Other abnormal findings in cerebrospinal fluid
Abnormal chromosomal findings in cerebrospinal fluid
R83.9 Unspecified abnormal finding in cerebrospinal fluid

R84 Abnormal findings in specimens from respiratory organs and thorax

Includes: abnormal findings in bronchial washings
abnormal findings in nasal secretions
abnormal findings in pleural fluid
abnormal findings in sputum
abnormal findings in throat scrapings
Excludes1: *blood-stained sputum (R04.2)*

R84.0 Abnormal level of enzymes in specimens from respiratory organs and thorax
R84.1 Abnormal level of hormones in specimens from respiratory organs and thorax
R84.2 Abnormal level of other drugs, medicaments and biological substances in specimens from respiratory organs and thorax
R84.3 Abnormal level of substances chiefly nonmedicinal as to source in specimens from respiratory organs and thorax
R84.4 Abnormal immunological findings in specimens from respiratory organs and thorax
R84.5 Abnormal microbiological findings in specimens from respiratory organs and thorax
Positive culture findings in specimens from respiratory organs and thorax
Excludes1: *colonization status (Z22.-)*
R84.6 Abnormal cytological findings in specimens from respiratory organs and thorax
R84.7 Abnormal histological findings in specimens from respiratory organs and thorax
R84.8 Other abnormal findings in specimens from respiratory organs and thorax
Abnormal chromosomal findings in specimens from respiratory organs and thorax
R84.9 Unspecified abnormal finding in specimens from respiratory organs and thorax

R85 Abnormal findings in specimens from digestive organs and abdominal cavity

Includes: abnormal findings in peritoneal fluid
abnormal findings in saliva
Excludes1: *cloudy peritoneal dialysis effluent (R88.0)*
fecal abnormalities (R19.5)

R85.0 Abnormal level of enzymes in specimens from digestive organs and abdominal cavity
R85.1 Abnormal level of hormones in specimens from digestive organs and abdominal cavity
R85.2 Abnormal level of other drugs, medicaments and biological substances in specimens from digestive organs and abdominal cavity
R85.3 Abnormal level of substances chiefly nonmedicinal as to source in specimens from digestive organs and abdominal cavity
R85.4 Abnormal immunological findings in specimens from digestive organs and abdominal cavity
R85.5 Abnormal microbiological findings in specimens from digestive organs and abdominal cavity
Positive culture findings in specimens from digestive organs and abdominal cavity
Excludes1: *colonization status (Z22.-)*
+ **R85.6 Abnormal cytological findings in specimens from digestive organs and abdominal cavity**
+ **R85.61 Abnormal cytologic smear of anus**
Excludes1: *abnormal cytological findings in specimens from other digestive organs and abdominal cavity (R85.69)*
carcinoma in situ of anus (histologically confirmed) (D01.3)
anal intraepithelial neoplasia I [AIN I] (K62.82)
anal intraepithelial neoplasia II [AIN II] (K62.82)
anal intraepithelial neoplasia III [AIN III] (D01.3)
dysplasia (mild) (moderate) of anus (histologically confirmed) (K62.82)
severe dysplasia of anus (histologically confirmed) (D01.3)
Excludes2: *anal high risk human papillomavirus (HPV) DNA test positive (R85.81)*
anal low risk human papillomavirus (HPV) DNA test positive (R85.82)

R85.610 Atypical squamous cells of undetermined significance on cytologic smear of anus (ASC-US)
R85.611 Atypical squamous cells cannot exclude high grade squamous intraepithelial lesion on cytologic smear of anus (ASC-H)
R85.612 Low grade squamous intraepithelial lesion on cytologic smear of anus (LGSIL)
R85.613 High grade squamous intraepithelial lesion on cytologic smear of anus (HGSIL)
R85.614 Cytologic evidence of malignancy on smear of anus
R85.615 Unsatisfactory cytologic smear of anus
Inadequate sample of cytologic smear of anus
R85.616 Satisfactory anal smear but lacking transformation zone
R85.618 Other abnormal cytological findings on specimens from anus
R85.619 Unspecified abnormal cytological findings in specimens from anus
Abnormal anal cytology NOS
Atypical glandular cells of anus NOS
R85.69 Abnormal cytological findings in specimens from other digestive organs and abdominal cavity
R85.7 Abnormal histological findings in specimens from digestive organs and abdominal cavity
+ **R85.8 Other abnormal findings in specimens from digestive organs and abdominal cavity**
R85.81 Anal high risk human papillomavirus (HPV) DNA test positive
Excludes1: *anogenital warts due to human papillomavirus (HPV) (A63.0)*
condyloma acuminatum (A63.0)
R85.82 Anal low risk human papillomavirus (HPV) DNA test positive
Use additional code for associated human papillomavirus (B97.7)
R85.89 Other abnormal findings in specimens from digestive organs and abdominal cavity
Abnormal chromosomal findings in specimens from digestive organs and abdominal cavity
R85.9 Unspecified abnormal finding in specimens from digestive organs and abdominal cavity

R86 Abnormal findings in specimens from male genital organs

Includes: abnormal findings in prostatic secretions
abnormal findings in semen, seminal fluid
abnormal spermatozoa
Excludes1: *azoospermia (N46.0-)*
oligospermia (N46.1-)

♂ **R86.0 Abnormal level of enzymes in specimens from male genital organs**
♂ **R86.1 Abnormal level of hormones in specimens from male genital organs**
♂ **R86.2 Abnormal level of other drugs, medicaments and biological substances in specimens from male genital organs**
♂ **R86.3 Abnormal level of substances chiefly nonmedicinal as to source in specimens from male genital organs**
♂ **R86.4 Abnormal immunological findings in specimens from male genital organs**
♂ **R86.5 Abnormal microbiological findings in specimens from male genital organs**
Positive culture findings in specimens from male genital organs
Excludes1: *colonization status (Z22.-)*
♂ **R86.6 Abnormal cytological findings in specimens from male genital organs**
♂ **R86.7 Abnormal histological findings in specimens from male genital organs**
♂ **R86.8 Other abnormal findings in specimens from male genital organs**
Abnormal chromosomal findings in specimens from male genital organs
♂ **R86.9 Unspecified abnormal finding in specimens from male genital organs**

R87 Abnormal findings in specimens from female genital organs

Includes: abnormal findings in secretion and smears from cervix uteri
abnormal findings in secretion and smears from vagina
abnormal findings in secretion and smears from vulva

♀ **R87.0 Abnormal level of enzymes in specimens from female genital organs**

♀ **R87.1 Abnormal level of hormones in specimens from female genital organs**

♀ **R87.2 Abnormal level of other drugs, medicaments and biological substances in specimens from female genital organs**

♀ **R87.3 Abnormal level of substances chiefly nonmedicinal as to source in specimens from female genital organs**

♀ **R87.4 Abnormal immunological findings in specimens from female genital organs**

♀ **R87.5 Abnormal microbiological findings in specimens from female genital organs**

Positive culture findings in specimens from female genital organs

Excludes1: *colonization status (Z22.-)*

\+ **R87.6 Abnormal cytological findings in specimens from female genital organs**

\+ **R87.61 Abnormal cytological findings in specimens from cervix uteri**

Excludes1: *abnormal cytological findings in specimens from other female genital organs (R87.69)*
abnormal cytological findings in specimens from vagina (R87.62-)
carcinoma in situ of cervix uteri (histologically confirmed) (D06.-)
cervical intraepithelial neoplasia I [CIN I] (N87.0)
cervical intraepithelial neoplasia II [CIN II] (N87.1)
cervical intraepithelial neoplasia III [CIN III] (D06.-)
dysplasia (mild) (moderate) of cervix uteri (histologically confirmed) (N87.-)
severe dysplasia of cervix uteri (histologically confirmed) (D06.-)

Excludes2: *cervical high risk human papillomavirus (HPV) DNA test positive (R87.810)*
cervical low risk human papillomavirus (HPV) DNA test positive (R87.820)

♀ **R87.610 Atypical squamous cells of undetermined significance on cytologic smear of cervix (ASC-US)**

♀ **R87.611 Atypical squamous cells cannot exclude high grade squamous intraepithelial lesion on cytologic smear of cervix (ASC-H)**

♀ **R87.612 Low grade squamous intraepithelial lesion on cytologic smear of cervix (LGSIL)**

♀ **R87.613 High grade squamous intraepithelial lesion on cytologic smear of cervix (HGSIL)**

♀ **R87.614 Cytologic evidence of malignancy on smear of cervix**

♀ **R87.615 Unsatisfactory cytologic smear of cervix**

Inadequate sample of cytologic smear of cervix

♀ **R87.616 Satisfactory cervical smear but lacking transformation zone**

♀ **R87.618 Other abnormal cytological findings on specimens from cervix uteri**

♀ **R87.619 Unspecified abnormal cytological findings in specimens from cervix uteri**

Abnormal cervical cytology NOS
Abnormal Papanicolaou smear of cervix NOS
Abnormal thin preparation smear of cervix NOS
Atypical endocervial cells of cervix NOS
Atypical endometrial cells of cervix NOS
Atypical glandular cells of cervix NOS

\+ **R87.62 Abnormal cytological findings in specimens from vagina**

Use additional code to identify acquired absence of uterus and cervix, if applicable (Z90.71-)

Excludes1: *abnormal cytological findings in specimens from cervix uteri (R87.61-)*
abnormal cytological findings in specimens from other female genital organs (R87.69)
carcinoma in situ of vagina (histologically confirmed) (D07.2)
vaginal intraepithelial neoplasia I [VAIN I] (N89.0)
vaginal intraepithelial neoplasia II [VAIN II] (N89.1)
vaginal intraepithelial neoplasia III [VAIN III] (D07.2)
dysplasia (mild) (moderate) of vagina (histologically confirmed) (N89.-)
severe dysplasia of vagina (histologically confirmed) (D07.2)

Excludes2: *vaginal high risk human papillomavirus (HPV) DNA test positive (R87.811)*
vaginal low risk human papillomavirus (HPV) DNA test positive (R87.821)

♀ **R87.620 Atypical squamous cells of undetermined significance on cytologic smear of vagina (ASC-US)**

♀ **R87.621 Atypical squamous cells cannot exclude high grade squamous intraepithelial lesion on cytologic smear of vagina (ASC-H)**

♀ **R87.622 Low grade squamous intraepithelial lesion on cytologic smear of vagina (LGSIL)**

♀ **R87.623 High grade squamous intraepithelial lesion on cytologic smear of vagina (HGSIL)**

♀ **R87.624 Cytologic evidence of malignancy on smear of vagina**

♀ **R87.625 Unsatisfactory cytologic smear of vagina**

Inadequate sample of cytologic smear of vagina

♀ **R87.628 Other abnormal cytological findings on specimens from vagina**

♀ **R87.629 Unspecified abnormal cytological findings in specimens from vagina**

Abnormal Papanicolaou smear of vagina NOS
Abnormal thin preparation smear of vagina NOS
Abnormal vaginal cytology NOS
Atypical endocervical cells of vagina NOS
Atypical endometrial cells of vagina NOS
Atypical glandular cells of vagina NOS

♀ **R87.69 Abnormal cytological findings in specimens from other female genital organs**

Abnormal cytological findings in specimens from female genital organs NOS

Excludes1: *dysplasia of vulva (histologically confirmed) (N90.0-N90.3)*

♀ **R87.7 Abnormal histological findings in specimens from female genital organs**

Excludes1: *carcinoma in situ (histologically confirmed) of female genital organs (D06-D07.3)*
cervical intraepithelial neoplasia I [CIN I] (N87.0)
cervical intraepithelial neoplasia II [CIN II] (N87.1)
cervical intraepithelial neoplasia III [CIN III] (D06.-)
dysplasia (mild) (moderate) of cervix uteri (histologically confirmed) (N87.-)
dysplasia (mild) (moderate) of vagina (histologically confirmed) (N89.-)
vaginal intraepithelial neoplasia I [VAIN I] (N89.0)
vaginal intraepithelial neoplasia II [VAIN II] (N89.1)
vaginal intraepithelial neoplasia III [VAIN III] (D07.2)
severe dysplasia of cervix uteri (histologically confirmed) (D06.-)
severe dysplasia of vagina (histologically confirmed) (D07.2)

+ **R87.8 Other abnormal findings in specimens from female genital organs**
  + **R87.81 High risk human papillomavirus (HPV) DNA test positive from female genital organs**
    Excludes1: *anogenital warts due to human papillomavirus (HPV) (A63.0)*
    condyloma acuminatum (A63.0)
    ♀ **R87.810 Cervical high risk human papillomavirus (HPV) DNA test positive**
    ♀ **R87.811 Vaginal high risk human papillomavirus (HPV) DNA test positive**
  + **R87.82 Low risk human papillomavirus (HPV) DNA test positive from female genital organs**
    Use additional code for associated human papillomavirus (B97.7)
    ♀ **R87.820 Cervical low risk human papillomavirus (HPV) DNA test positive**
    ♀ **R87.821 Vaginal low risk human papillomavirus (HPV) DNA test positive**
  ♀ **R87.89 Other abnormal findings in specimens from female genital organs**
    Abnormal chromosomal findings in specimens from female genital organs

♀ **R87.9 Unspecified abnormal finding in specimens from female genital organs**

R88 Abnormal findings in other body fluids and substances

R88.0 Cloudy (hemodialysis) (peritoneal) dialysis effluent
R88.8 Abnormal findings in other body fluids and substances

R89 Abnormal findings in specimens from other organs, systems and tissues

Includes: abnormal findings in nipple discharge
abnormal findings in synovial fluid
abnormal findings in wound secretions

R89.0 Abnormal level of enzymes in specimens from other organs, systems and tissues
R89.1 Abnormal level of hormones in specimens from other organs, systems and tissues
R89.2 Abnormal level of other drugs, medicaments and biological substances in specimens from other organs, systems and tissues
R89.3 Abnormal level of substances chiefly nonmedicinal as to source in specimens from other organs, systems and tissues
R89.4 Abnormal immunological findings in specimens from other organs, systems and tissues
R89.5 Abnormal microbiological findings in specimens from other organs, systems and tissues
Positive culture findings in specimens from other organs, systems and tissues
Excludes1: *colonization status (Z22.-)*
R89.6 Abnormal cytological findings in specimens from other organs, systems and tissues
R89.7 Abnormal histological findings in specimens from other organs, systems and tissues
R89.8 Other abnormal findings in specimens from other organs, systems and tissues
Abnormal chromosomal findings in specimens from other organs, systems and tissues
R89.9 Unspecified abnormal finding in specimens from other organs, systems and tissues

Abnormal findings on diagnostic imaging and in function studies, without diagnosis (R90-R94)

Includes: nonspecific abnormal findings on diagnostic imaging by computerized axial tomography [CAT scan]
nonspecific abnormal findings on diagnostic imaging by magnetic resonance imaging [MRI][NMR]
nonspecific abnormal findings on diagnostic imaging by positron emission tomography [PET scan]
nonspecific abnormal findings on diagnostic imaging by thermography
nonspecific abnormal findings on diagnostic imaging by ultrasound [echogram]
nonspecific abnormal findings on diagnostic imaging by X-ray examination

Excludes1: *abnormal findings on antenatal screening of mother (O28.-)*
diagnostic abnormal findings classified elsewhere - see Alphabetical Index

R90 Abnormal findings on diagnostic imaging of central nervous system

R90.0 Intracranial space-occupying lesion found on diagnostic imaging of central nervous system
+ **R90.8 Other abnormal findings on diagnostic imaging of central nervous system**
  R90.81 Abnormal echoencephalogram
  R90.82 White matter disease, unspecified
  R90.89 Other abnormal findings on diagnostic imaging of central nervous system
  Other cerebrovascular abnormality found on diagnostic imaging of central nervous system

R91 Abnormal findings on diagnostic imaging of lung

R91.1 Solitary pulmonary nodule
Coin lesion lung
Solitary pulmonary nodule, subsegmental branch of the bronchial tree
R91.8 Other nonspecific abnormal finding of lung field
Lung mass NOS found on diagnostic imaging of lung
Pulmonary infiltrate NOS
Shadow, lung

R92 Abnormal and inconclusive findings on diagnostic imaging of breast

R92.0 Mammographic microcalcification found on diagnostic imaging of breast
Excludes2: *mammographic calcification (calculus) found on diagnostic imaging of breast (R92.1)*
R92.1 Mammographic calcification found on diagnostic imaging of breast
Mammographic calculus found on diagnostic imaging of breast
R92.2 Inconclusive mammogram
Dense breasts NOS
Inconclusive mammogram NEC
Inconclusive mammography due to dense breasts
Inconclusive mammography NEC
AHA CC: 1Q, 2015, 24
R92.8 Other abnormal and inconclusive findings on diagnostic imaging of breast

R93 Abnormal findings on diagnostic imaging of other body structures

R93.0 Abnormal findings on diagnostic imaging of skull and head, not elsewhere classified
Excludes1: *intracranial space-occupying lesion found on diagnostic imaging (R90.0)*
R93.1 Abnormal findings on diagnostic imaging of heart and coronary circulation
Abnormal echocardiogram NOS
Abnormal heart shadow
R93.2 Abnormal findings on diagnostic imaging of liver and biliary tract
Nonvisualization of gallbladder
R93.3 Abnormal findings on diagnostic imaging of other parts of digestive tract
+ **R93.4 Abnormal findings on diagnostic imaging of urinary organs**
  Excludes2: *hypertrophy of kidney (N28.81)*
  AHA CC: 4Q, 2016, 66
  R93.41 Abnormal radiologic findings on diagnostic imaging of renal pelvis, ureter, or bladder
  Filling defect of bladder found on diagnostic imaging
  Filling defect of renal pelvis found on diagnostic imaging
  Filling defect of ureter found on diagnostic imaging
  + **R93.42 Abnormal radiologic findings on diagnostic imaging of kidney**
    R93.421 Abnormal radiologic findings on diagnostic imaging of right kidney
    R93.422 Abnormal radiologic findings on diagnostic imaging of left kidney
    R93.429 Abnormal radiologic findings on diagnostic imaging of unspecified kidney
  R93.49 Abnormal radiologic findings on diagnostic imaging of other urinary organs

R93.5 Abnormal findings on diagnostic imaging of other abdominal regions, including retroperitoneum
R93.6 Abnormal findings on diagnostic imaging of limbs
Excludes2: *abnormal finding in skin and subcutaneous tissue (R93.8)*
R93.7 Abnormal findings on diagnostic imaging of other parts of musculoskeletal system
Excludes2: *abnormal findings on diagnostic imaging of skull (R93.0)*

R93.8 **Abnormal findings on diagnostic imaging of other specified body structures**
Abnormal finding by radioisotope localization of placenta
Abnormal radiological finding in skin and subcutaneous tissue
Mediastinal shift

R93.9 **Diagnostic imaging inconclusive due to excess body fat of patient**

R94 Abnormal results of function studies

Includes: abnormal results of radionuclide [radioisotope] uptake studies
abnormal results of scintigraphy

+ **R94.0 Abnormal results of function studies of central nervous system**
R94.01 Abnormal electroencephalogram [EEG]
R94.02 Abnormal brain scan
R94.09 Abnormal results of other function studies of central nervous system

+ **R94.1 Abnormal results of function studies of peripheral nervous system and special senses**
+ **R94.11 Abnormal results of function studies of eye**
R94.110 Abnormal electro-oculogram [EOG]
R94.111 Abnormal electroretinogram [ERG]
Abnormal retinal function study
R94.112 Abnormal visually evoked potential [VEP]
R94.113 Abnormal oculomotor study
R94.118 Abnormal results of other function studies of eye
+ **R94.12 Abnormal results of function studies of ear and other special senses**
R94.120 Abnormal auditory function study
AHA CC: 3Q, 2016, 17
R94.121 Abnormal vestibular function study
R94.128 Abnormal results of other function studies of ear and other special senses
+ **R94.13 Abnormal results of function studies of peripheral nervous system**
R94.130 Abnormal response to nerve stimulation, unspecified
R94.131 Abnormal electromyogram [EMG]
Excludes1: *electromyogram of eye (R94.113)*
R94.138 Abnormal results of other function studies of peripheral nervous system

R94.2 Abnormal results of pulmonary function studies
Reduced ventilatory capacity
Reduced vital capacity

+ **R94.3 Abnormal results of cardiovascular function studies**
R94.30 Abnormal result of cardiovascular function study, unspecified
R94.31 Abnormal electrocardiogram [ECG] [EKG]
Excludes1: *long QT syndrome (I45.81)*
R94.39 Abnormal result of other cardiovascular function study
Abnormal electrophysiological intracardiac studies
Abnormal phonocardiogram
Abnormal vectorcardiogram

R94.4 Abnormal results of kidney function studies
Abnormal renal function test

R94.5 Abnormal results of liver function studies

R94.6 Abnormal results of thyroid function studies

R94.7 Abnormal results of other endocrine function studies
Excludes2: *abnormal glucose (R73.0-)*

R94.8 Abnormal results of function studies of other organs and systems
Abnormal basal metabolic rate [BMR]
Abnormal bladder function test
Abnormal splenic function test

Abnormal tumor markers (R97)

R97 Abnormal tumor markers

Elevated tumor associated antigens [TAA]
Elevated tumor specific antigens [TSA]

R97.0 Elevated carcinoembryonic antigen [CEA]

R97.1 Elevated cancer antigen 125 [CA 125]

+ **R97.2 Elevated prostate specific antigen [PSA]**
AHA CC: 4Q, 2016, 66
• ♂ **R97.20 Elevated prostate specific antigen [PSA]**
• ♂ **R97.21 Rising PSA following treatment for malignant neoplasm of prostate**

R97.8 Other abnormal tumor markers

Ill-defined and unknown cause of mortality (R99)

R99 Ill-defined and unknown cause of mortality

Death (unexplained) NOS
Unspecified cause of mortality
Review coding guideline C.18.h
Valid 3-character code, no further characters required

Muscles

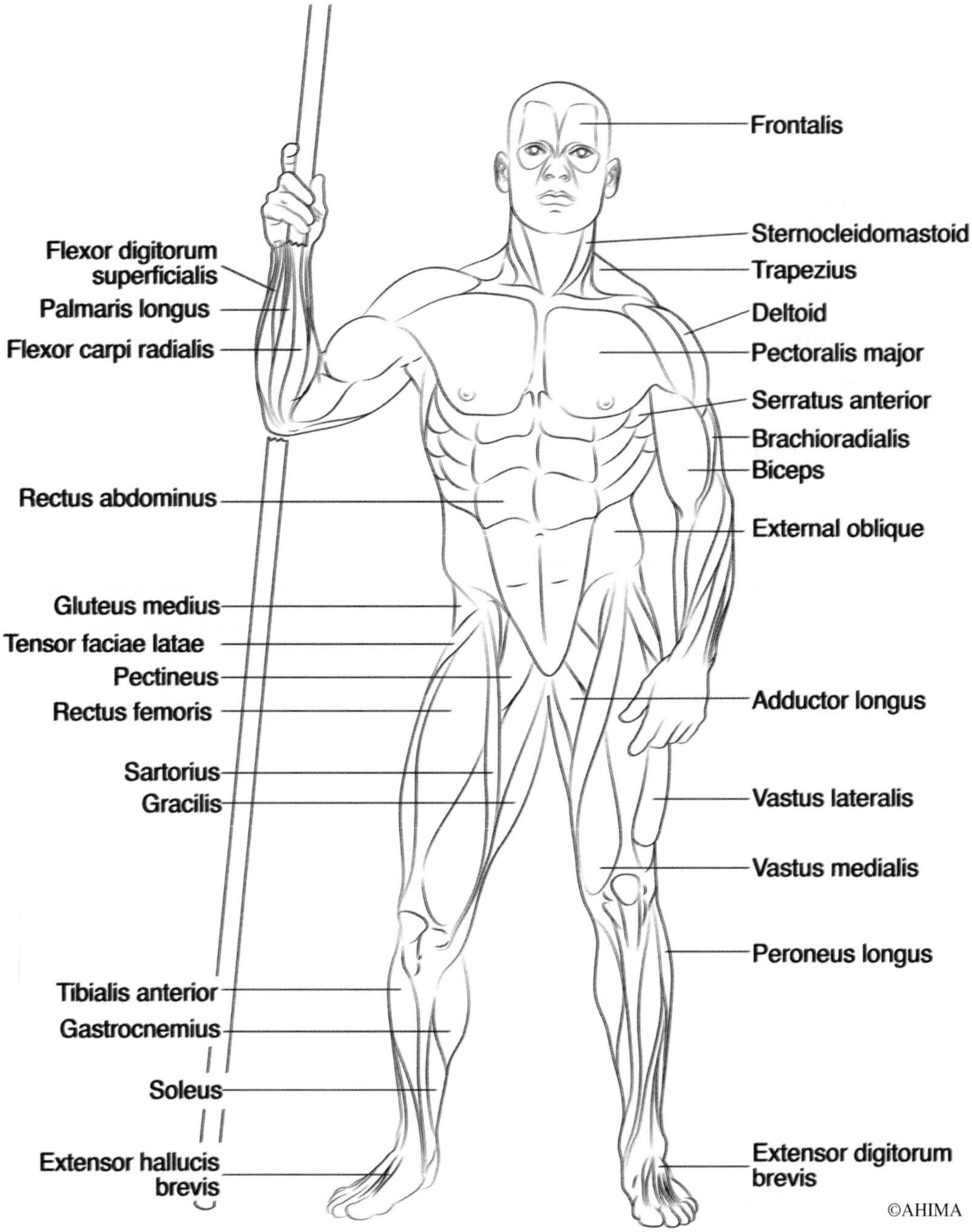
Frontalis
Flexor digitorum superficialis
Sternocleidomastoid
Trapezius
Palmaris longus
Deltoid
Flexor carpi radialis
Pectoralis major
Serratus anterior
Brachioradialis
Biceps
Rectus abdominus
External oblique
Gluteus medius
Tensor faciae latae
Pectineus
Adductor longus
Rectus femoris
Sartorius
Vastus lateralis
Gracilis
Vastus medialis
Peroneus longus
Tibialis anterior
Gastrocnemius
Soleus
Extensor hallucis brevis
Extensor digitorum brevis
©AHIMA

Skeleton - Front and Side Views

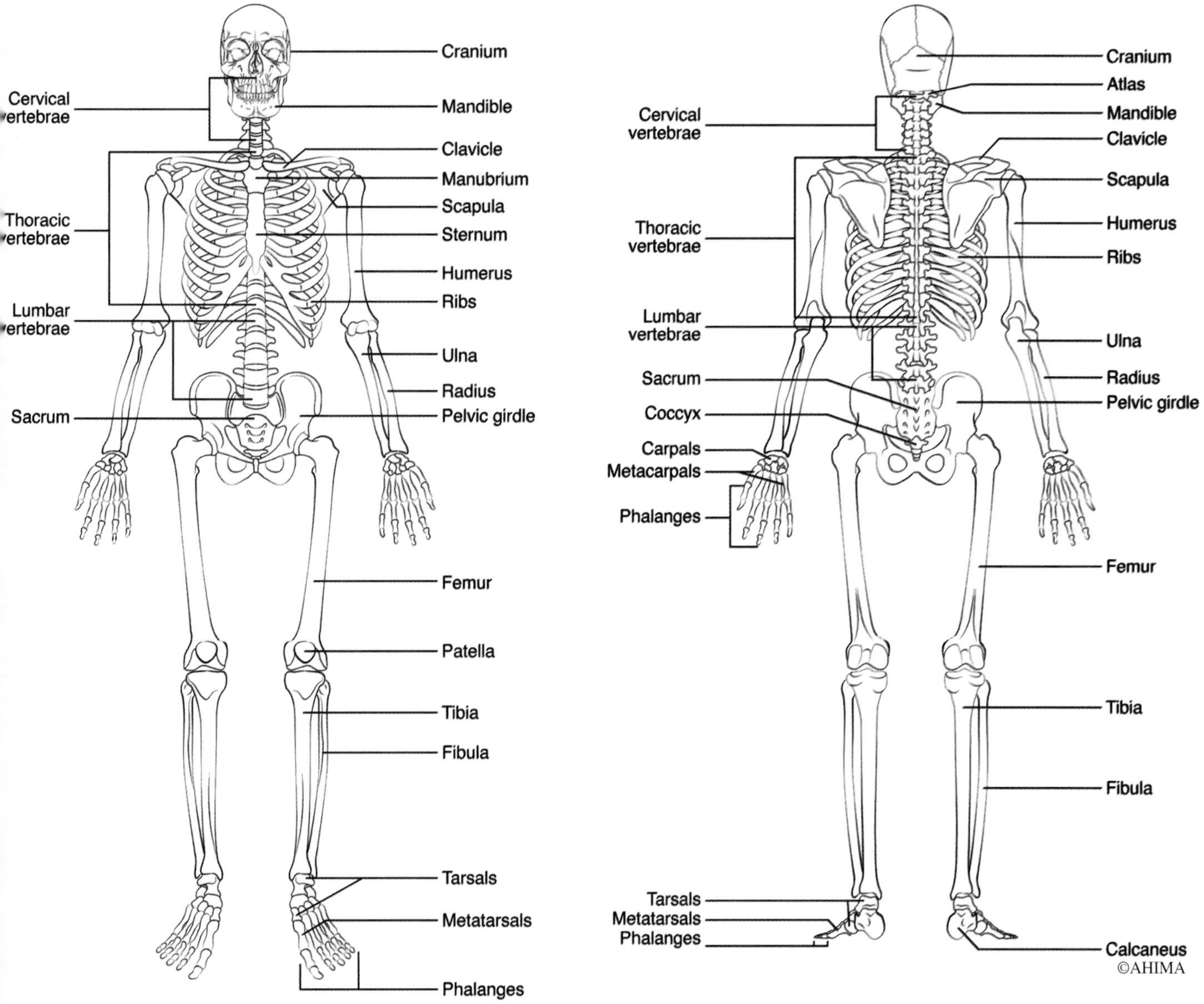

Chapter 19: Injury, Poisoning and Certain Other Consequences of External Causes (S00-T88)

NOTE Use secondary code(s) from Chapter 20, External causes of morbidity, to indicate cause of injury. Codes within the T-section that include the external cause do not require an additional external cause code

Use additional code to identify any retained foreign body, if applicable (Z18.-)

Excludes1: *birth trauma (P10-P15)*
obstetric trauma (O70-O71)

NOTE The chapter uses the S-section for coding different types of injuries related to single body regions and the T-section to cover injuries to unspecified body regions as well as poisoning and certain other consequences of external causes.
AHA CC: 1Q, 2015, 3-21

This chapter contains the following category blocks:

- S00-S09 Injuries to the head
- S10-S19 Injuries to the neck
- S20-S29 Injuries to the thorax
- S30-S39 Injuries to the abdomen, lower back, lumbar spine, pelvis and external genitals
- S40-S49 Injuries to the shoulder and upper arm
- S50-S59 Injuries to the elbow and forearm
- S60-S69 Injuries to the wrist, hand and fingers
- S70-S79 Injuries to the hip and thigh
- S80-S89 Injuries to the knee and lower leg
- S90-S99 Injuries to the ankle and foot
- T07 Injuries involving multiple body regions
- T14 Injury of unspecified body region
- T15-T19 Effects of foreign body entering through natural orifice
- T20-T25 Burns and corrosions of external body surface, specified by site
- T26-T28 Burns and corrosions confined to eye and internal organs
- T30-T32 Burns and corrosions of multiple and unspecified body regions
- T33-T34 Frostbite
- T36-T50 Poisoning by, adverse effect of and underdosing of drugs, medicaments and biological substances
- T51-T65 Toxic effects of substances chiefly nonmedicinal as to source
- T66-T78 Other and unspecified effects of external causes
- T79 Certain early complications of trauma
- T80-T88 Complications of surgical and medical care, not elsewhere classified

C. Chapter-Specific Coding Guidelines

In addition to general coding guidelines, there are guidelines for specific diagnoses and/or conditions in the classification. Unless otherwise indicated, these guidelines apply to all health care settings. Please refer to Section II for guidelines on the selection of principal diagnosis.

19. Chapter 19: Injury, Poisoning and Certain Other Consequences of External Causes (S00-T88)

a. Application of 7th Characters in Chapter 19

Most categories in chapter 19 have a 7th character requirement for each applicable code. Most categories in this chapter have three 7th character values (with the exception of fractures): A, initial encounter, D, subsequent encounter and S, sequela. Categories for traumatic fractures have additional 7th character values. While the patient may be seen by a new or different provider over the course of treatment for an injury, assignment of the 7th character is based on whether the patient is undergoing active treatment and not whether the provider is seeing the patient for the first time.

For complication codes, active treatment refers to treatment for the condition described by the code, even though it may be related to an earlier precipitating problem. For example, code T84.50XA, Infection and inflammatory reaction due to unspecified internal joint prosthesis, initial encounter, is used when active treatment is provided for the infection, even though the condition relates to the prosthetic device, implant or graft that was placed at a previous encounter.

7th character "A", initial encounter is used for each encounter where the patient is receiving active treatment for the condition.

7th character "D" subsequent encounter is used for encounters after the patient has completed active treatment of the condition and is receiving routine care for the condition during the healing or recovery phase.

The aftercare Z codes should not be used for aftercare for conditions such as injuries or poisonings, where 7th characters are provided to identify subsequent care. For example, for aftercare of an injury, assign the acute injury code with the 7th character "D" (subsequent encounter).

7th character "S", sequela, is for use for complications or conditions that arise as a direct result of a condition, such as scar formation after a burn. The scars are sequelae of the burn. When using 7th character "S", it is necessary to use both the injury code that precipitated the sequela and the code for the sequela itself. The "S" is added only to the injury code, not the sequela code. The 7th character "S" identifies the injury responsible for the sequela. The specifi type of sequela (e.g. scar) is sequenced first, followed by the injury code.

See Section I.B.10 Sequela (Late Effects)

b. Coding of Injuries

When coding injuries, assign separate codes for each injury unless a combinatio code is provided, in which case the combination code is assigned. **Codes fror category** T07, Unspecified multiple injuries should not be assigned in th inpatient setting unless information for a more specific code is not availabl Traumatic injury codes (S00-T14.9) are not to be used for normal, healin surgical wounds or to identify complications of surgical wounds.

The code for the most serious injury, as determined by the provider and th focus of treatment, is sequenced first.

1) Superficial injuries

Superficial injuries such as abrasions or contusions are not coded whe associated with more severe injuries of the same site.

2) Primary injury with damage to nerves/blood vessels

When a primary injury results in minor damage to peripheral nerves c blood vessels, the primary injury is sequenced first with additional code(s for injuries to nerves and spinal cord (such as category S04), and/or injur to blood vessels (such as category S15). When the primary injury is to th blood vessels or nerves, that injury should be sequenced first.

c. Coding of Traumatic Fractures

The principles of multiple coding of injuries should be followed in codin fractures. Fractures of specified sites are coded individually by site in accordanc with both the provisions within categories S02, S12, S22, S32, S42, S49, S5 S59, S62, S72, S79, S82, S89, S92 and the level of detail furnished by medic record content.

A fracture not indicated as open or closed should be coded to closed. A fractur not indicated whether displaced or not displaced should be coded to displace

More specific guidelines are as follows:

1) Initial vs. Subsequent Encounter for Fractures

Traumatic fractures are coded using the appropriate 7th character for initi encounter (A, B, C) for each encounter where the patient is receivin active treatment for the fracture. The appropriate 7th character for initi encounter should also be assigned for a patient who delayed seekin treatment for the fracture or nonunion.

Fractures are coded using the appropriate 7th character for subsequer care for encounters after the patient has completed active treatment of th fracture and is receiving routine care for the fracture during the healing c recovery phase.

Care for complications of surgical treatment for fracture repairs durin the healing or recovery phase should be coded with the appropria complication codes.

Care of complications of fractures, such as malunion and nonunion, shoul be reported with the appropriate 7th character for subsequent care wit nonunion (K, M, N,) or subsequent care with malunion (P, Q, R).

Malunion/nonunion: The appropriate 7th character for initial encounte should also be assigned for a patient who delayed seeking treatment for th fracture or nonunion.

The open fracture designations in the assignment of the 7th character f fractures of the forearm, femur and lower leg, including ankle are based c the Gustilo open fracture classification. When the Gustilo classificatic type is not specified for an open fracture, the 7th character for open fractu type I or II should be assigned (B, E, H, M, Q).

A code from category M80, not a traumatic fracture code, should be use for any patient with known osteoporosis who suffers a fracture, even if th patient had a minor fall or trauma, if that fall or trauma would not usual break a normal, healthy bone.

See Section I.C.13. Osteoporosis.

The aftercare Z codes should not be used for aftercare for traumati fractures. For aftercare of a traumatic fracture, assign the acute fractur code with the appropriate 7th character.

2) Multiple fractures sequencing

Multiple fractures are sequenced in accordance with the severity of th fracture.

d. Coding of Burns and Corrosions

The ICD-10-CM makes a distinction between burns and corrosions. The bu codes are for thermal burns, except sunburns, that come from a heat sourc such as a fire or hot appliance. The burn codes are also for burns resultin from electricity and radiation. Corrosions are burns due to chemicals. Th guidelines are the same for burns and corrosions.

Current burns (T20-T25) are classified by depth, extent and by agent (code). Burns are classified by depth as first degree (erythema), second degre (blistering), and third degree (full-thickness involvement). Burns of the ey and internal organs (T26-T28) are classified by site, but not by degree.

1) **Sequencing of burn and related condition codes**

Sequence first the code that reflects the highest degree of burn when more than one burn is present.

a. When the reason for the admission or encounter is for treatment of external multiple burns, sequence first the code that reflects the burn of the highest degree.

b. When a patient has both internal and external burns, the circumstances of admission govern the selection of the principal diagnosis or first-listed diagnosis.

c. When a patient is admitted for burn injuries and other related conditions such as smoke inhalation and/or respiratory failure, the circumstances of admission govern the selection of the principal or first-listed diagnosis.

2) **Burns of the same local site**

Classify burns of the same local site (three-character category level, T20-T28) but of different degrees to the subcategory identifying the highest degree recorded in the diagnosis.

3) **Non-healing burns**

Non-healing burns are coded as acute burns.

Necrosis of burned skin should be coded as a non-healed burn.

4) **Infected Burn**

For any documented infected burn site, use an additional code for the infection.

5) **Assign separate codes for each burn site**

When coding burns, assign separate codes for each burn site. Category T30, Burn and corrosion, body region unspecified is extremely vague and should rarely be used.

6) **Burns and Corrosions Classified According to Extent of Body Surface Involved**

Assign codes from category T31, Burns classified according to extent of body surface involved, or T32, Corrosions classified according to extent of body surface involved, when the site of the burn is not specified or when there is a need for additional data. It is advisable to use category T31 as additional coding when needed to provide data for evaluating burn mortality, such as that needed by burn units. It is also advisable to use category T31 as an additional code for reporting purposes when there is mention of a third-degree burn involving 20 percent or more of the body surface.

Categories T31 and T32 are based on the classic "rule of nines" in estimating body surface involved: head and neck are assigned nine percent, each arm nine percent, each leg 18 percent, the anterior trunk 18 percent, posterior trunk 18 percent, and genitalia one percent. Providers may change these percentage assignments where necessary to accommodate infants and children who have proportionately larger heads than adults, and patients who have large buttocks, thighs, or abdomen that involve burns.

7) **Encounters for treatment of sequela of burns**

Encounters for the treatment of the late effects of burns or corrosions (i.e., scars or joint contractures) should be coded with a burn or corrosion code with the 7th character "S" for sequela.

8) **Sequelae with a late effect code and current burn**

When appropriate, both a code for a current burn or corrosion with 7th character "A" or "D" and a burn or corrosion code with 7th character "S" may be assigned on the same record (when both a current burn and sequelae of an old burn exist). Burns and corrosions do not heal at the same rate and a current healing wound may still exist with sequela of a healed burn or corrosion. *See Section I.B.10 Sequela (Late Effects)*

9) **Use of an external cause code with burns and corrosions**

An external cause code should be used with burns and corrosions to identify the source and intent of the burn, as well as the place where it occurred.

e. Adverse Effects, Poisoning, Underdosing and Toxic Effects

Codes in categories T36-T65 are combination codes that include the substance that was taken as well as the intent. No additional external cause code is required for poisonings, toxic effects, adverse effects and underdosing codes.

1) **Do not code directly from the Table of Drugs**

Do not code directly from the Table of Drugs and Chemicals. Always refer back to the Tabular List.

2) **Use as many codes as necessary to describe**

Use as many codes as necessary to describe completely all drugs, medicinal or biological substances.

3) **If the same code would describe the causative agent**

If the same code would describe the causative agent for more than one adverse reaction, poisoning, toxic effect or underdosing, assign the code only once.

4) **If two or more drugs, medicinal or biological substances**

If two or more drugs, medicinal or biological substances are reported, code each individually unless a combination code is listed in the Table of Drugs and Chemicals.

5) **The occurrence of drug toxicity is classified in ICD-10-CM as follows:**

(a) Adverse Effect

When coding an adverse effect of a drug that has been correctly prescribed and properly administered, assign the appropriate code for the nature of the adverse effect followed by the appropriate code for the adverse effect of the drug (T36-T50). The code for the drug should have a 5th or 6th character "5" (for example T36.0X5-) Examples of the nature of an adverse effect are tachycardia, delirium, gastrointestinal hemorrhaging, vomiting, hypokalemia, hepatitis, renal failure, or respiratory failure.

(b) Poisoning

When coding a poisoning or reaction to the improper use of a medication (e.g., overdose, wrong substance given or taken in error, wrong route of administration), first assign the appropriate code from categories T36-T50. The poisoning codes have an associated intent as their 5th or 6th character (accidental, intentional self-harm, assault and undetermined.) If the intent of the poisoning is unknown or unspecified, code the intent as accidental intent. The undetermined intent is only for use if the documentation in the record specifies that the intent cannot be determined. Use additional code(s) for all manifestations of poisonings.

If there is also a diagnosis of abuse or dependence of the substance, the abuse or dependence is assigned as an additional code.

Examples of poisoning include:

(i) Error was made in drug prescription

Errors made in drug prescription or in the administration of the drug by provider, nurse, patient, or other person.

(ii) Overdose of a drug intentionally taken

If an overdose of a drug was intentionally taken or administered and resulted in drug toxicity, it would be coded as a poisoning.

(iii) Nonprescribed drug taken with correctly prescribed and properly administered drug

If a nonprescribed drug or medicinal agent was taken in combination with a correctly prescribed and properly administered drug, any drug toxicity or other reaction resulting from the interaction of the two drugs would be classified as a poisoning.

(iv) Interaction of drug(s) and alcohol

When a reaction results from the interaction of a drug(s) and alcohol, this would be classified as poisoning.

See Section I.C.4. if poisoning is the result of insulin pump malfunctions.

(c) Underdosing

Underdosing refers to taking less of a medication than is prescribed by a provider or a manufacturer's instruction. For underdosing, assign the code from categories T36-T50 (fifth or sixth character "6").

Codes for underdosing should never be assigned as principal or first-listed codes. If a patient has a relapse or exacerbation of the medical condition for which the drug is prescribed because of the reduction in dose, then the medical condition itself should be coded.

Noncompliance (Z91.12-, Z91.13-) or complication of care (Y63.6-Y63.9) codes are to be used with an underdosing code to indicate intent, if known.

(d) Toxic Effects

When a harmful substance is ingested or comes in contact with a person, this is classified as a toxic effect. The toxic effect codes are in categories T51-T65.

Toxic effect codes have an associated intent: accidental, intentional self-harm, assault and undetermined.

f. Adult and child abuse, neglect and other maltreatment

Sequence first the appropriate code from categories T74.- (Adult and child abuse, neglect and other maltreatment, confirmed) or T76.- (Adult and child abuse, neglect and other maltreatment, suspected) for abuse, neglect and other maltreatment, followed by any accompanying mental health or injury code(s).

If the documentation in the medical record states abuse or neglect it is coded as confirmed (T74.-). It is coded as suspected if it is documented as suspected (T76.-).

For cases of confirmed abuse or neglect an external cause code from the assault section (X92-Y09) should be added to identify the cause of any physical injuries. A perpetrator code (Y07) should be added when the perpetrator of the abuse is known. For suspected cases of abuse or neglect, do not report external cause or perpetrator code.

If a suspected case of abuse, neglect or mistreatment is ruled out during an encounter code Z04.71, Encounter for examination and observation following alleged physical adult abuse, ruled out, or code Z04.72, Encounter for examination and observation following alleged child physical abuse, ruled out, should be used, not a code from T76.

If a suspected case of alleged rape or sexual abuse is ruled out during an encounter code Z04.41, Encounter for examination and observation following alleged adult rape or code Z04.42, Encounter for examination and observation following alleged child rape, should be used, not a code from T76.

See Section I.C.15. Abuse in a pregnant patient.

g. Complications of care

1) General guidelines for complications of care

(a) Documentation of complications of care

See Section I.B.16. for information on documentation of complications of care.

2) Pain due to medical devices

Pain associated with devices, implants or grafts left in a surgical site (for example painful hip prosthesis) is assigned to the appropriate code(s) found in Chapter 19, Injury, poisoning, and certain other consequences of external causes. Specific codes for pain due to medical devices are found in the T code section of the ICD-10-CM. Use additional code(s) from category G89 to identify acute or chronic pain due to presence of the device, implant or graft (G89.18 or G89.28).

3) Transplant complications

(a) Transplant complications other than kidney

Codes under category T86, Complications of transplanted organs and tissues, are for use for both complications and rejection of transplanted organs. A transplant complication code is only assigned if the complication affects the function of the transplanted organ. Two codes are required to fully describe a transplant complication: the appropriate code from category T86 and a secondary code that identifies the complication.

Pre-existing conditions or conditions that develop after the transplant are not coded as complications unless they affect the function of the transplanted organs.

See I.C.21. for transplant organ removal status.

See I.C.2. for malignant neoplasm associated with transplanted organ.

(b) Kidney transplant complications

Patients who have undergone kidney transplant may still have some form of chronic kidney disease (CKD) because the kidney transplant may not fully restore kidney function. Code T86.1- should be assigned for documented complications of a kidney transplant, such as transplant failure or rejection or other transplant complication. Code T86.1- should not be assigned for post kidney transplant patients who have chronic kidney (CKD) unless a transplant complication such as transplant failure or rejection is documented. If the documentation is unclear as to whether the patient has a complication of the transplant, query the provider.

Conditions that affect the function of the transplanted kidney, other than CKD, should be assigned a code from subcategory T86.1, Complications of transplanted organ, Kidney, and a secondary code that identifies the complication.

For patients with CKD following a kidney transplant, but who do not have a complication such as failure or rejection, *see section I.C.14. Chronic kidney disease and kidney transplant status.*

4) Complication codes that include the external cause

As with certain other T codes, some of the complications of care codes have the external cause included in the code. The code includes the nature of the complication as well as the type of procedure that caused the complication. No external cause code indicating the type of procedure is necessary for these codes.

5) Complications of care codes within the body system chapters

Intraoperative and postprocedural complication codes are found within the body system chapters with codes specific to the organs and structures of that body system. These codes should be sequenced first, followed by a code(s) for the specific complication, if applicable.

Injuries to the head (S00-S09)

Includes: *injuries of ear*
injuries of eye
injuries of face [any part]
injuries of gum
injuries of jaw
injuries of oral cavity
injuries of palate
injuries of periocular area
injuries of scalp
injuries of temporomandibular joint area
injuries of tongue
injuries of tooth

Code also for any associated infection

Excludes2: *burns and corrosions (T20-T32)*
effects of foreign body in ear (T16)
effects of foreign body in larynx (T17.3)
effects of foreign body in mouth NOS (T18.0)
effects of foreign body in nose (T17.0-T17.1)
effects of foreign body in pharynx (T17.2)
effects of foreign body on external eye (T15.-)
frostbite (T33-T34)
insect bite or sting, venomous (T63.4)

S00 Superficial injury of head

Excludes1: *diffuse cerebral contusion (S06.2-)*
focal cerebral contusion (S06.3-)
injury of eye and orbit (S05.-)
open wound of head (S01.-)

The appropriate 7th character is to be added to each code from category S00
A initial encounter
D subsequent encounter
S sequela

+ **S00.0 Superficial injury of scalp**
  - X+7th **S00.00 Unspecified superficial injury of scalp**
  - X+7th **S00.01 Abrasion of scalp**
  - X+7th **S00.02 Blister (nonthermal) of scalp**
  - X+7th **S00.03 Contusion of scalp**
    Bruise of scalp
    Hematoma of scalp
  - X+7th **S00.04 External constriction of part of scalp**
  - X+7th **S00.05 Superficial foreign body of scalp**
    Splinter in the scalp
  - X+7th **S00.06 Insect bite (nonvenomous) of scalp**
  - X+7th **S00.07 Other superficial bite of scalp**
    Excludes1: *open bite of scalp (S01.05)*

+ **S00.1 Contusion of eyelid and periocular area**
  Black eye
  Excludes2: *contusion of eyeball and orbital tissues (S05.1)*
  - X+7th **S00.10 Contusion of unspecified eyelid and periocular area**
  - X+7th **S00.11 Contusion of right eyelid and periocular area**
  - X+7th **S00.12 Contusion of left eyelid and periocular area**

+ **S00.2 Other and unspecified superficial injuries of eyelid and periocular area**
  Excludes2: *superficial injury of conjunctiva and cornea (S05.0-)*
  - + **S00.20 Unspecified superficial injury of eyelid and periocular area**
    - +7th **S00.201 Unspecified superficial injury of right eyelid and periocular area**
    - +7th **S00.202 Unspecified superficial injury of left eyelid and periocular area**
    - +7th **S00.209 Unspecified superficial injury of unspecified eyelid and periocular area**
  - + **S00.21 Abrasion of eyelid and periocular area**
    - +7th **S00.211 Abrasion of right eyelid and periocular area**
    - +7th **S00.212 Abrasion of left eyelid and periocular area**
    - +7th **S00.219 Abrasion of unspecified eyelid and periocular area**
  - + **S00.22 Blister (nonthermal) of eyelid and periocular area**
    - +7th **S00.221 Blister (nonthermal) of right eyelid and periocular area**
    - +7th **S00.222 Blister (nonthermal) of left eyelid and periocular area**
    - +7th **S00.229 Blister (nonthermal) of unspecified eyelid and periocular area**

+ **S00.24** **External constriction of eyelid and periocular area**
+7th **S00.241** **External constriction of right eyelid and periocular area**
+7th **S00.242** **External constriction of left eyelid and periocular area**
+7th **S00.249** **External constriction of unspecified eyelid and periocular area**
+ **S00.25** **Superficial foreign body of eyelid and periocular area**
Splinter of eyelid and periocular area
Excludes2: *retained foreign body in eyelid (H02.81-)*
+7th **S00.251** **Superficial foreign body of right eyelid and periocular area**
+7th **S00.252** **Superficial foreign body of left eyelid and periocular area**
+7th **S00.259** **Superficial foreign body of unspecified eyelid and periocular area**
+ **S00.26** **Insect bite (nonvenomous) of eyelid and periocular area**
+7th **S00.261** **Insect bite (nonvenomous) of right eyelid and periocular area**
+7th **S00.262** **Insect bite (nonvenomous) of left eyelid and periocular area**
+7th **S00.269** **Insect bite (nonvenomous) of unspecified eyelid and periocular area**
+ **S00.27** **Other superficial bite of eyelid and periocular area**
Excludes1: *open bite of eyelid and periocular area (S01.15)*
+7th **S00.271** **Other superficial bite of right eyelid and periocular area**
+7th **S00.272** **Other superficial bite of left eyelid and periocular area**
+7th **S00.279** **Other superficial bite of unspecified eyelid and periocular area**
+ **S00.3** **Superficial injury of nose**
X+7th **S00.30** **Unspecified superficial injury of nose**
X+7th **S00.31** **Abrasion of nose**
X+7th **S00.32** **Blister (nonthermal) of nose**
X+7th **S00.33** **Contusion of nose**
Bruise of nose
Hematoma of nose
X+7th **S00.34** **External constriction of nose**
X+7th **S00.35** **Superficial foreign body of nose**
Splinter in the nose
X+7th **S00.36** **Insect bite (nonvenomous) of nose**
X+7th **S00.37** **Other superficial bite of nose**
Excludes1: *open bite of nose (S01.25)*
+ **S00.4** **Superficial injury of ear**
+ **S00.40** **Unspecified superficial injury of ear**
+7th **S00.401** **Unspecified superficial injury of right ear**
+7th **S00.402** **Unspecified superficial injury of left ear**
+7th **S00.409** **Unspecified superficial injury of unspecified ear**
+ **S00.41** **Abrasion of ear**
+7th **S00.411** **Abrasion of right ear**
+7th **S00.412** **Abrasion of left ear**
+7th **S00.419** **Abrasion of unspecified ear**
+ **S00.42** **Blister (nonthermal) of ear**
+7th **S00.421** **Blister (nonthermal) of right ear**
+7th **S00.422** **Blister (nonthermal) of left ear**
+7th **S00.429** **Blister (nonthermal) of unspecified ear**
+ **S00.43** **Contusion of ear**
Bruise of ear
Hematoma of ear
+7th **S00.431** **Contusion of right ear**
+7th **S00.432** **Contusion of left ear**
+7th **S00.439** **Contusion of unspecified ear**
+ **S00.44** **External constriction of ear**
+7th **S00.441** **External constriction of right ear**
+7th **S00.442** **External constriction of left ear**
+7th **S00.449** **External constriction of unspecified ear**
+ **S00.45** **Superficial foreign body of ear**
Splinter in the ear
+7th **S00.451** **Superficial foreign body of right ear**
+7th **S00.452** **Superficial foreign body of left ear**
+7th **S00.459** **Superficial foreign body of unspecified ear**
+ **S00.46** **Insect bite (nonvenomous) of ear**
+7th **S00.461** **Insect bite (nonvenomous) of right ear**
+7th **S00.462** **Insect bite (nonvenomous) of left ear**
+7th **S00.469** **Insect bite (nonvenomous) of unspecified ear**
+ **S00.47** **Other superficial bite of ear**
Excludes1: *open bite of ear (S01.35)*
+7th **S00.471** **Other superficial bite of right ear**
+7th **S00.472** **Other superficial bite of left ear**
+7th **S00.479** **Other superficial bite of unspecified ear**
+ **S00.5** **Superficial injury of lip and oral cavity**
+ **S00.50** **Unspecified superficial injury of lip and oral cavity**
+7th **S00.501** **Unspecified superficial injury of lip**
+7th **S00.502** **Unspecified superficial injury of oral cavity**
+ **S00.51** **Abrasion of lip and oral cavity**
+7th **S00.511** **Abrasion of lip**
+7th **S00.512** **Abrasion of oral cavity**
+ **S00.52** **Blister (nonthermal) of lip and oral cavity**
+7th **S00.521** **Blister (nonthermal) of lip**
+7th **S00.522** **Blister (nonthermal) of oral cavity**
+ **S00.53** **Contusion of lip and oral cavity**
+7th **S00.531** **Contusion of lip**
Bruise of lip
Hematoma of lip
+7th **S00.532** **Contusion of oral cavity**
Bruise of oral cavity
Hematoma of oral cavity
+ **S00.54** **External constriction of lip and oral cavity**
+7th **S00.541** **External constriction of lip**
+7th **S00.542** **External constriction of oral cavity**
+ **S00.55** **Superficial foreign body of lip and oral cavity**
+7th **S00.551** **Superficial foreign body of lip**
Splinter of lip and oral cavity
+7th **S00.552** **Superficial foreign body of oral cavity**
Splinter of lip and oral cavity
+ **S00.56** **Insect bite (nonvenomous) of lip and oral cavity**
+7th **S00.561** **Insect bite (nonvenomous) of lip**
+7th **S00.562** **Insect bite (nonvenomous) of oral cavity**
+ **S00.57** **Other superficial bite of lip and oral cavity**
+7th **S00.571** **Other superficial bite of lip**
Excludes1: *open bite of lip (S01.551)*
+7th **S00.572** **Other superficial bite of oral cavity**
Excludes1: *open bite of oral cavity (S01.552)*
+ **S00.8** **Superficial injury of other parts of head**
Superficial injuries of face [any part]
X+7th **S00.80** **Unspecified superficial injury of other part of head**
X+7th **S00.81** **Abrasion of other part of head**
X+7th **S00.82** **Blister (nonthermal) of other part of head**
X+7th **S00.83** **Contusion of other part of head**
Bruise of other part of head
Hematoma of other part of head
X+7th **S00.84** **External constriction of other part of head**
X+7th **S00.85** **Superficial foreign body of other part of head**
Splinter in other part of head
X+7th **S00.86** **Insect bite (nonvenomous) of other part of head**
X+7th **S00.87** **Other superficial bite of other part of head**
Excludes1: *open bite of other part of head (S01.85)*
+ **S00.9** **Superficial injury of unspecified part of head**
X+7th **S00.90** **Unspecified superficial injury of unspecified part of head**
X+7th **S00.91** **Abrasion of unspecified part of head**
X+7th **S00.92** **Blister (nonthermal) of unspecified part of head**
X+7th **S00.93** **Contusion of unspecified part of head**
Bruise of head
Hematoma of head
X+7th **S00.94** **External constriction of unspecified part of head**
X+7th **S00.95** **Superficial foreign body of unspecified part of head**
Splinter of head
X+7th **S00.96** **Insect bite (nonvenomous) of unspecified part of head**
X+7th **S00.97** **Other superficial bite of unspecified part of head**
Excludes1: *open bite of head (S01.95)*

S01 Open wound of head

Code also any associated:
injury of cranial nerve (S04.-)
injury of muscle and tendon of head (S09.1-)
intracranial injury (S06.-)
wound infection

Excludes1: *open skull fracture (S02.- with 7th character B)*
Excludes2: *injury of eye and orbit (S05.-)*
traumatic amputation of part of head (S08.-)

The appropriate 7th character is to be added to each code from category S01
A initial encounter
D subsequent encounter
S sequela

+ **S01.0 Open wound of scalp**
Excludes1: *avulsion of scalp (S08.0)*
X+7th **S01.00 Unspecified open wound of scalp**
X+7th **S01.01 Laceration without foreign body of scalp**
X+7th **S01.02 Laceration with foreign body of scalp**
AHA CC: 1Q, 2015, 3-21
X+7th **S01.03 Puncture wound without foreign body of scalp**
X+7th **S01.04 Puncture wound with foreign body of scalp**
X+7th **S01.05 Open bite of scalp**
Bite of scalp NOS
Excludes1: *superficial bite of scalp (S00.06, S00.07-)*

+ **S01.1 Open wound of eyelid and periocular area**
Open wound of eyelid and periocular area with or without involvement of lacrimal passages
+ **S01.10 Unspecified open wound of eyelid and periocular area**
CC +7th **S01.101 Unspecified open wound of right eyelid and periocular area**
CC Exclusion 7th character A see Appendix A PDX collection 1139
CC +7th **S01.102 Unspecified open wound of left eyelid and periocular area**
CC Exclusion 7th character A see Appendix A PDX collection 1139
CC +7th **S01.109 Unspecified open wound of unspecified eyelid and periocular area**
CC Exclusion 7th character A see Appendix A PDX collection 1139
+ **S01.11 Laceration without foreign body of eyelid and periocular area**
+7th **S01.111 Laceration without foreign body of right eyelid and periocular area**
+7th **S01.112 Laceration without foreign body of left eyelid and periocular area**
+7th **S01.119 Laceration without foreign body of unspecified eyelid and periocular area**
+ **S01.12 Laceration with foreign body of eyelid and periocular area**
+7th **S01.121 Laceration with foreign body of right eyelid and periocular area**
+7th **S01.122 Laceration with foreign body of left eyelid and periocular area**
+7th **S01.129 Laceration with foreign body of unspecified eyelid and periocular area**
+ **S01.13 Puncture wound without foreign body of eyelid and periocular area**
+7th **S01.131 Puncture wound without foreign body of right eyelid and periocular area**
+7th **S01.132 Puncture wound without foreign body of left eyelid and periocular area**
+7th **S01.139 Puncture wound without foreign body of unspecified eyelid and periocular area**
+ **S01.14 Puncture wound with foreign body of eyelid and periocular area**
+7th **S01.141 Puncture wound with foreign body of right eyelid and periocular area**
+7th **S01.142 Puncture wound with foreign body of left eyelid and periocular area**
+7th **S01.149 Puncture wound with foreign body of unspecified eyelid and periocular area**
+ **S01.15 Open bite of eyelid and periocular area**
Bite of eyelid and periocular area NOS
Excludes1: *superficial bite of eyelid and periocular area (S00.26, S00.27)*
+7th **S01.151 Open bite of right eyelid and periocular area**
+7th **S01.152 Open bite of left eyelid and periocular are**
+7th **S01.159 Open bite of unspecified eyelid and periocular area**

+ **S01.2 Open wound of nose**
X+7th **S01.20 Unspecified open wound of nose**
X+7th **S01.21 Laceration without foreign body of nose**
AHA CC: 1Q, 2015, 3-21
X+7th **S01.22 Laceration with foreign body of nose**
X+7th **S01.23 Puncture wound without foreign body of nose**
X+7th **S01.24 Puncture wound with foreign body of nose**
X+7th **S01.25 Open bite of nose**
Bite of nose NOS
Excludes1: *superficial bite of nose (S00.36, S00.37)*

+ **S01.3 Open wound of ear**
+ **S01.30 Unspecified open wound of ear**
+7th **S01.301 Unspecified open wound of right ear**
+7th **S01.302 Unspecified open wound of left ear**
+7th **S01.309 Unspecified open wound of unspecified ea**
+ **S01.31 Laceration without foreign body of ear**
+7th **S01.311 Laceration without foreign body of right ear**
+7th **S01.312 Laceration without foreign body of left ea**
+7th **S01.319 Laceration without foreign body of unspecified ear**
+ **S01.32 Laceration with foreign body of ear**
+7th **S01.321 Laceration with foreign body of right ear**
+7th **S01.322 Laceration with foreign body of left ear**
+7th **S01.329 Laceration with foreign body of unspecified ear**
+ **S01.33 Puncture wound without foreign body of ear**
+7th **S01.331 Puncture wound without foreign body of right ear**
+7th **S01.332 Puncture wound without foreign body of left ear**
+7th **S01.339 Puncture wound without foreign body of unspecified ear**
+ **S01.34 Puncture wound with foreign body of ear**
+7th **S01.341 Puncture wound with foreign body of right ear**
+7th **S01.342 Puncture wound with foreign body of left ear**
+7th **S01.349 Puncture wound with foreign body of unspecified ear**
+ **S01.35 Open bite of ear**
Bite of ear NOS
Excludes1: *superficial bite of ear (S00.46, S00.47)*
+7th **S01.351 Open bite of right ear**
+7th **S01.352 Open bite of left ear**
+7th **S01.359 Open bite of unspecified ear**

+ **S01.4 Open wound of cheek and temporomandibular area**
+ **S01.40 Unspecified open wound of cheek and temporomandibular area**
+7th **S01.401 Unspecified open wound of right cheek ar temporomandibular area**
+7th **S01.402 Unspecified open wound of left cheek and temporomandibular area**
+7th **S01.409 Unspecified open wound of unspecified cheek and temporomandibular area**
+ **S01.41 Laceration without foreign body of cheek and temporomandibular area**
+7th **S01.411 Laceration without foreign body of right cheek and temporomandibular area**
AHA CC: 1Q, 2015, 3-21
+7th **S01.412 Laceration without foreign body of left cheek and temporomandibular area**
+7th **S01.419 Laceration without foreign body of unspecified cheek and temporomandibula area**
+ **S01.42 Laceration with foreign body of cheek and temporomandibular area**
+7th **S01.421 Laceration with foreign body of right cheek and temporomandibular area**
+7th **S01.422 Laceration with foreign body of left cheek and temporomandibular area**
+7th **S01.429 Laceration with foreign body of unspecified cheek and temporomandibula area**

+ **S01.43 Puncture wound without foreign body of cheek and temporomandibular area**
  - +7th **S01.431 Puncture wound without foreign body of right cheek and temporomandibular area**
  - +7th **S01.432 Puncture wound without foreign body of left cheek and temporomandibular area**
  - +7th **S01.439 Puncture wound without foreign body of unspecified cheek and temporomandibular area**
+ **S01.44 Puncture wound with foreign body of cheek and temporomandibular area**
  - +7th **S01.441 Puncture wound with foreign body of right cheek and temporomandibular area**
  - +7th **S01.442 Puncture wound with foreign body of left cheek and temporomandibular area**
  - +7th **S01.449 Puncture wound with foreign body of unspecified cheek and temporomandibular area**
+ **S01.45 Open bite of cheek and temporomandibular area**
  Bite of cheek and temporomandibular area NOS
  Excludes2: *superficial bite of cheek and temporomandibular area (S00.86, S00.87)*
  - +7th **S01.451 Open bite of right cheek and temporomandibular area**
  - +7th **S01.452 Open bite of left cheek and temporomandibular area**
  - +7th **S01.459 Open bite of unspecified cheek and temporomandibular area**

+ **S01.5 Open wound of lip and oral cavity**
  Excludes2: *tooth dislocation (S03.2)*
  tooth fracture (S02.5)
  + **S01.50 Unspecified open wound of lip and oral cavity**
    - +7th **S01.501 Unspecified open wound of lip**
    - +7th **S01.502 Unspecified open wound of oral cavity**
  + **S01.51 Laceration of lip and oral cavity without foreign body**
    - +7th **S01.511 Laceration without foreign body of lip**
    - +7th **S01.512 Laceration without foreign body of oral cavity**
  + **S01.52 Laceration of lip and oral cavity with foreign body**
    - +7th **S01.521 Laceration with foreign body of lip**
    - +7th **S01.522 Laceration with foreign body of oral cavity**
  + **S01.53 Puncture wound of lip and oral cavity without foreign body**
    - +7th **S01.531 Puncture wound without foreign body of lip**
    - +7th **S01.532 Puncture wound without foreign body of oral cavity**
  + **S01.54 Puncture wound of lip and oral cavity with foreign body**
    - +7th **S01.541 Puncture wound with foreign body of lip**
    - +7th **S01.542 Puncture wound with foreign body of oral cavity**
  + **S01.55 Open bite of lip and oral cavity**
    - +7th **S01.551 Open bite of lip**
      Bite of lip NOS
      Excludes1: *superficial bite of lip (S00.571)*
    - +7th **S01.552 Open bite of oral cavity**
      Bite of oral cavity NOS
      Excludes1: *superficial bite of oral cavity (S00.572)*

+ **S01.8 Open wound of other parts of head**
  - X+7th **S01.80 Unspecified open wound of other part of head**
  - X+7th **S01.81 Laceration without foreign body of other part of head**
  - X+7th **S01.82 Laceration with foreign body of other part of head**
  - X+7th **S01.83 Puncture wound without foreign body of other part of head**
  - X+7th **S01.84 Puncture wound with foreign body of other part of head**
  - X+7th **S01.85 Open bite of other part of head**
    Bite of other part of head NOS
    Excludes1: *superficial bite of other part of head (S00.87)*

+ **S01.9 Open wound of unspecified part of head**
  - X+7th **S01.90 Unspecified open wound of unspecified part of head**
  - X+7th **S01.91 Laceration without foreign body of unspecified part of head**
  - X+7th **S01.92 Laceration with foreign body of unspecified part of head**
  - X+7th **S01.93 Puncture wound without foreign body of unspecified part of head**
  - X+7th **S01.94 Puncture wound with foreign body of unspecified part of head**
  - X+7th **S01.95 Open bite of unspecified part of head**
    Bite of head NOS
    Excludes1: *superficial bite of head NOS (S00.97)*

S02 Fracture of skull and facial bones

NOTE A fracture not indicated as open or closed should be coded to closed

Code also any associated intracranial injury (S06.-)

Review coding guideline C.19.c

AHA CC: 4Q, 2016, 66-67

The appropriate 7th character is to be added to each code from category S02
- A initial encounter for closed fracture
- B initial encounter for open fracture
- D subsequent encounter for fracture with routine healing
- G subsequent encounter for fracture with delayed healing
- K subsequent encounter for fracture with nonunion
- S sequela

CC MCC X+7th **S02.0 Fracture of vault of skull**
Fracture of frontal bone
Fracture of parietal bone
CC Exclusion 7th character A see Appendix A PDX collection 1140
CC Exclusion 7th character K see Appendix A PDX collection 0897
MCC Exclusion 7th character B see Appendix A PDX collection 1140
HAC 7th characters A & B see Appendix B for HAC conditional logic

+ **S02.1 Fracture of base of skull**
  Excludes1: *orbit NOS (S02.8)*
  Excludes2: *orbital floor (S02.3-)*
  + **S02.10 Unspecified fracture of base of skull**
    - CC MCC +7th **S02.101 Fracture of base of skull, right side**
      CC Exclusion 7th character A see Appendix A PDX collection 1140
      CC Exclusion 7th character K see Appendix A PDX collection 0897
      MCC Exclusion 7th character B see Appendix A PDX collection 1140
      HAC 7th characters A & B see Appendix B for HAC conditional logic
    - CC MCC +7th **S02.102 Fracture of base of skull, left side**
      CC Exclusion 7th character A see Appendix A PDX collection 1140
      CC Exclusion 7th character K see Appendix A PDX collection 0897
      MCC Exclusion 7th character B see Appendix A PDX collection 1140
      HAC 7th characters A & B see Appendix B for HAC conditional logic
    - CC MCC +7th **S02.109 Fracture of base of skull, unspecified side**
      CC Exclusion 7th character A see Appendix A PDX collection 1140
      CC Exclusion 7th character K see Appendix A PDX collection 0897
      MCC Exclusion 7th character B see Appendix A PDX collection 1140
      HAC 7th characters A & B see Appendix B for HAC conditional logic
  + **S02.11 Fracture of occiput**
    - CC MCC +7th **S02.110 Type I occipital condyle fracture, unspecified side**
      CC Exclusion 7th character A see Appendix A PDX collection 1140
      CC Exclusion 7th character K see Appendix A PDX collection 0897
      MCC Exclusion 7th character B see Appendix A PDX collection 1140
      HAC 7th characters A & B see Appendix B for HAC conditional logic
    - CC MCC +7th **S02.111 Type II occipital condyle fracture, unspecified side**
      CC Exclusion 7th character A see Appendix A PDX collection 1140
      CC Exclusion 7th character K see Appendix A PDX collection 0897
      MCC Exclusion 7th character B see Appendix A PDX collection 1140
      HAC 7th characters A & B see Appendix B for HAC conditional logic

Head and Facial Bones - Side View

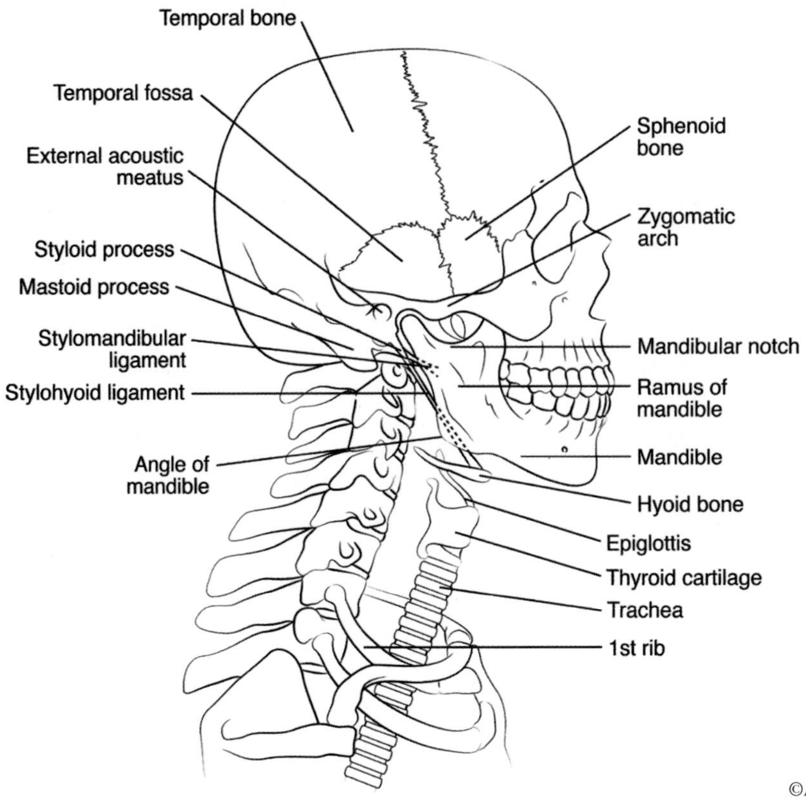
Temporal bone
Temporal fossa
External acoustic meatus
Styloid process
Mastoid process
Stylomandibular ligament
Stylohyoid ligament
Angle of mandible
Sphenoid bone
Zygomatic arch
Mandibular notch
Ramus of mandible
Mandible
Hyoid bone
Epiglottis
Thyroid cartilage
Trachea
1st rib

Head and Facial Bones - Side View

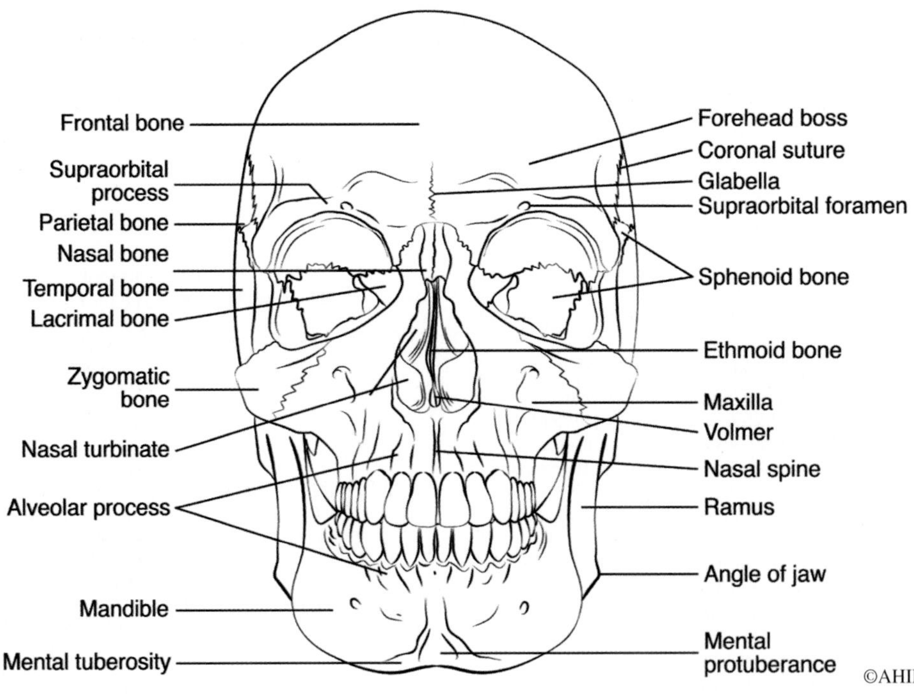
Frontal bone
Supraorbital process
Parietal bone
Nasal bone
Temporal bone
Lacrimal bone
Zygomatic bone
Nasal turbinate
Alveolar process
Mandible
Mental tuberosity
Forehead boss
Coronal suture
Glabella
Supraorbital foramen
Sphenoid bone
Ethmoid bone
Maxilla
Volmer
Nasal spine
Ramus
Angle of jaw
Mental protuberance

CC MCC +7th **S02.112** **Type III occipital condyle fracture, unspecified side**
CC Exclusion 7th character A see Appendix A PDX collection 1140
CC Exclusion 7th character K see Appendix A PDX collection 0897
MCC Exclusion 7th character B see Appendix A PDX collection 1140
HAC 7th characters A & B see Appendix B for HAC conditional logic

CC MCC +7th **S02.113** **Unspecified occipital condyle fracture**
CC Exclusion 7th character A see Appendix A PDX collection 1140
CC Exclusion 7th character K see Appendix A PDX collection 0897
MCC Exclusion 7th character B see Appendix A PDX collection 1140
HAC 7th characters A & B see Appendix B for HAC conditional logic

CC MCC +7th **S02.118** **Other fracture of occiput, unspecified side**
CC Exclusion 7th character A see Appendix A PDX collection 1140
CC Exclusion 7th character K see Appendix A PDX collection 0897
MCC Exclusion 7th character B see Appendix A PDX collection 1140
HAC 7th characters A & B see Appendix B for HAC conditional logic

CC MCC +7th **S02.119** **Unspecified fracture of occiput**
CC Exclusion 7th character A see Appendix A PDX collection 1140
CC Exclusion 7th character K see Appendix A PDX collection 0897
MCC Exclusion 7th character B see Appendix A PDX collection 1140
HAC 7th characters A & B see Appendix B for HAC conditional logic

CC MCC +7th **S02.11A** **Type I occipital condyle fracture, right side**
CC Exclusion 7th character A see Appendix A PDX collection 1140
CC Exclusion 7th character K see Appendix A PDX collection 0897
MCC Exclusion 7th character B see Appendix A PDX collection 1140
HAC 7th characters A & B see Appendix B for HAC conditional logic

CC MCC +7th **S02.11B** **Type I occipital condyle fracture, left side**
CC Exclusion 7th character A see Appendix A PDX collection 1140
CC Exclusion 7th character K see Appendix A PDX collection 0897
MCC Exclusion 7th character B see Appendix A PDX collection 1140
HAC 7th characters A & B see Appendix B for HAC conditional logic

CC MCC +7th **S02.11C** **Type II occipital condyle fracture, right side**
CC Exclusion 7th character A see Appendix A PDX collection 1140
CC Exclusion 7th character K see Appendix A PDX collection 0897
MCC Exclusion 7th character B see Appendix A PDX collection 1140
HAC 7th characters A & B see Appendix B for HAC conditional logic

CC MCC +7th **S02.11D** **Type II occipital condyle fracture, left side**
CC Exclusion 7th character A see Appendix A PDX collection 1140
CC Exclusion 7th character K see Appendix A PDX collection 0897
MCC Exclusion 7th character B see Appendix A PDX collection 1140
HAC 7th characters A & B see Appendix B for HAC conditional logic

CC MCC +7th **S02.11E** **Type III occipital condyle fracture, right side**
CC Exclusion 7th character A see Appendix A PDX collection 1140
CC Exclusion 7th character K see Appendix A PDX collection 0897
MCC Exclusion 7th character B see Appendix A PDX collection 1140
HAC 7th characters A & B see Appendix B for HAC conditional logic

CC MCC +7th **S02.11F** **Type III occipital condyle fracture, left side**
CC Exclusion 7th character A see Appendix A PDX collection 1140
CC Exclusion 7th character K see Appendix A PDX collection 0897
MCC Exclusion 7th character B see Appendix A PDX collection 1140
HAC 7th characters A & B see Appendix B for HAC conditional logic

CC MCC +7th **S02.11G** **Other fracture or occiput, right side**
CC Exclusion 7th character A see Appendix A PDX collection 1140
CC Exclusion 7th character K see Appendix A PDX collection 0897
MCC Exclusion 7th character B see Appendix A PDX collection 1140
HAC 7th characters A & B see Appendix B for HAC conditional logic

CC MCC +7th **S02.11H** **Other fracture or occiput, left side**
CC Exclusion 7th character A see Appendix A PDX collection 1140
CC Exclusion 7th character K see Appendix A PDX collection 0897
MCC Exclusion 7th character B see Appendix A PDX collection 1140
HAC 7th characters A & B see Appendix B for HAC conditional logic

CC MCC X+7th **S02.19** **Other fracture of base of skull**
Fracture of anterior fossa of base of skull
Fracture of ethmoid sinus
Fracture of frontal sinus
Fracture of middle fossa of base of skull
Fracture of orbital roof
Fracture of posterior fossa of base of skull
Fracture of sphenoid
Fracture of temporal bone
CC Exclusion 7th character A see Appendix A PDX collection 1140
CC Exclusion 7th character K see Appendix A PDX collection 0897
MCC Exclusion 7th character B see Appendix A PDX collection 1140
HAC 7th characters A & B see Appendix B for HAC conditional logic

CC X+7th **S02.2** **Fracture of nasal bones**
CC Exclusion 7th character B see Appendix A PDX collection 1141
CC Exclusion 7th character K see Appendix A PDX collection 0897
HAC 7th character B see Appendix B for HAC conditional logic

\+ **S02.3** **Fracture of orbital floor**
Excludes1: *orbit NOS (S02.8)*
Excludes2: *orbital roof (S02.1-)*

CC X+7th **S02.30** **Fracture of orbital floor, unspecified side**
CC Exclusion 7th characters A & B see Appendix A PDX collection 1142
CC Exclusion 7th character K see Appendix A PDX collection 0897
HAC 7th characters A & B see Appendix B for HAC conditional logic

CC X+7th **S02.31** **Fracture of orbital floor, right side**
CC Exclusion 7th characters A & B see Appendix A PDX collection 1142
CC Exclusion 7th character K see Appendix A PDX collection 0897
HAC 7th characters A & B see Appendix B for HAC conditional logic

CC X+7th **S02.32** **Fracture of orbital floor, left side**
CC Exclusion 7th characters A & B see Appendix A PDX collection 1142
CC Exclusion 7th character K see Appendix A PDX collection 0897
HAC 7th characters A & B see Appendix B for HAC conditional logic

\+ **S02.4** **Fracture of malar, maxillary and zygoma bones**
Fracture of superior maxilla
Fracture of upper jaw (bone)
Fracture of zygomatic process of temporal bone

\+ **S02.40** **Fracture of malar, maxillary and zygoma bones, unspecified**

CC +7th **S02.400** **Malar fracture, unspecified side**
CC Exclusion 7th characters A & B see Appendix A PDX collection 1143
CC Exclusion 7th character K see Appendix A PDX collection 0897
HAC 7th characters A & B see Appendix B for HAC conditional logic

CC +7th **S02.401 Maxillary fracture, unspecified side**
CC Exclusion 7th characters A & B see Appendix A PDX collection 1143
CC Exclusion 7th character K see Appendix A PDX collection 0897
HAC 7th characters A & B see Appendix B for HAC conditional logic

CC +7th **S02.402 Zygomatic fracture, unspecified side**
CC Exclusion 7th characters A & B see Appendix A PDX collection 1143
CC Exclusion 7th character K see Appendix A PDX collection 0897
HAC 7th characters A & B see Appendix B for HAC conditional logic

CC +7th **S02.40A Malar fracture, right side**
CC Exclusion 7th characters A & B see Appendix A PDX collection 1143
CC Exclusion 7th character K see Appendix A PDX collection 0897
HAC 7th characters A & B see Appendix B for HAC conditional logic

CC +7th **S02.40B Malar fracture, left side**
CC Exclusion 7th characters A & B see Appendix A PDX collection 1143
CC Exclusion 7th character K see Appendix A PDX collection 0897
HAC 7th characters A & B see Appendix B for HAC conditional logic

CC +7th **S02.40C Maxillary fracture, right side**
CC Exclusion 7th characters A & B see Appendix A PDX collection 1143
CC Exclusion 7th character K see Appendix A PDX collection 0897
HAC 7th characters A & B see Appendix B for HAC conditional logic

CC +7th **S02.40D Maxillary fracture, left side**
CC Exclusion 7th characters A & B see Appendix A PDX collection 1143
CC Exclusion 7th character K see Appendix A PDX collection 0897
HAC 7th characters A & B see Appendix B for HAC conditional logic

CC +7th **S02.40E Zygomatic fracture, right side**
CC Exclusion 7th characters A & B see Appendix A PDX collection 1143
CC Exclusion 7th character K see Appendix A PDX collection 0897
HAC 7th characters A & B see Appendix B for HAC conditional logic

CC +7th **S02.40F Zygomatic fracture, left side**
CC Exclusion 7th characters A & B see Appendix A PDX collection 1143
CC Exclusion 7th character K see Appendix A PDX collection 0897
HAC 7th characters A & B see Appendix B for HAC conditional logic

\+ **S02.41 LeFort fracture**

CC +7th **S02.411 LeFort I fracture**
CC Exclusion 7th characters A & B see Appendix A PDX collection 1143
CC Exclusion 7th character K see Appendix A PDX collection 0897
HAC 7th characters A & B see Appendix B for HAC conditional logic

CC +7th **S02.412 LeFort II fracture**
CC Exclusion 7th characters A & B see Appendix A PDX collection 1143
CC Exclusion 7th character K see Appendix A PDX collection 0897
HAC 7th characters A & B see Appendix B for HAC conditional logic

CC +7th **S02.413 LeFort III fracture**
CC Exclusion 7th characters A & B see Appendix A PDX collection 1143
CC Exclusion 7th character K see Appendix A PDX collection 0897
HAC 7th characters A & B see Appendix B for HAC conditional logic

CC X+7th **S02.42 Fracture of alveolus of maxilla**
CC Exclusion 7th characters A & B see Appendix A PDX collection 1142
CC Exclusion 7th character K see Appendix A PDX collection 0897
HAC 7th characters A & B see Appendix B for HAC conditional logic

CC X+7th **S02.5 Fracture of tooth (traumatic)**
Broken tooth
Excludes1: *cracked tooth (nontraumatic) (K03.81)*
CC Exclusion 7th character K see Appendix A PDX collection 089

\+ **S02.6 Fracture of mandible**
Fracture of lower jaw (bone)

\+ **S02.60 Fracture of mandible, unspecified**

CC+7th **S02.600 Fracture of unspecified part of body of mandible, unspecified side**
CC Exclusion 7th characters A & B see Appendix A PDX collection 1143
CC Exclusion 7th character K see Appendix PDX collection 0897
HAC 7th characters A & B see Appendix B fc HAC conditional logic

CC +7th **S02.601 Fracture of unspecified part of body of right mandible**
CC Exclusion 7th characters A & B see Appendix A PDX collection 1143
CC Exclusion 7th character K see Appendix PDX collection 0897
HAC 7th characters A & B see Appendix B fc HAC conditional logic

CC +7th **S02.602 Fracture of unspecified part of body of l mandible**
CC Exclusion 7th characters A & B see Appendix A PDX collection 1143
CC Exclusion 7th character K see Appendix PDX collection 0897
HAC 7th characters A & B see Appendix B fc HAC conditional logic

CC X+7th **S02.609 Fracture of mandible, unspecified**
CC Exclusion 7th characters A & B see Appendix A PDX collection 1143
CC Exclusion 7th character K see Appendix PDX collection 0897
HAC 7th characters A & B see Appendix B f HAC conditional logic

\+ **S02.61 Fracture of condylar process of mandible**

CC +7th **S02.610 Fracture of condylar process of mandib unspecified side**
CC Exclusion 7th characters A & B see Appendix A PDX collection 1143
CC Exclusion 7th character K see Appendix PDX collection 0897
HAC 7th characters A & B see Appendix B f HAC conditional logic

CC +7th **S02.611 Fracture of condylar process of right mandible**
CC Exclusion 7th characters A & B see Appendix A PDX collection 1143
CC Exclusion 7th character K see Appendix PDX collection 0897
HAC 7th characters A & B see Appendix B f HAC conditional logic

CC +7th **S02.612 Fracture of condylar process of left mandible**
CC Exclusion 7th characters A & B see Appendix A PDX collection 1143
CC Exclusion 7th character K see Appendix PDX collection 0897
HAC 7th characters A & B see Appendix B f HAC conditional logic

\+ **S02.62 Fracture of subcondylar process of mandible**

CC +7th **S02.620 Fracture of subcondylar process of mandible, unspecified side**
CC Exclusion 7th characters A & B see Appendix A PDX collection 1143
CC Exclusion 7th character K see Appendix PDX collection 0897
HAC 7th characters A & B see Appendix B f HAC conditional logic

CC +7th **S02.621 Fracture of subcondylar process of righ mandible**
CC Exclusion 7th characters A & B see Appendix A PDX collection 1143
CC Exclusion 7th character K see Appendix PDX collection 0897
HAC 7th characters A & B see Appendix B f HAC conditional logic

CC +7th **S02.622 Fracture of subcondylar process of left mandible**
CC Exclusion 7th characters A & B see Appendix A PDX collection 1143
CC Exclusion 7th character K see Appendix PDX collection 0897
HAC 7th characters A & B see Appendix B f HAC conditional logic

+ S02.63 **Fracture of coronoid process of mandible**

CC +7th **S02.630** **Fracture of coronoid process of mandible, unspecified side**
CC Exclusion 7th characters A & B see Appendix A PDX collection 1143
CC Exclusion 7th character K see Appendix A PDX collection 0897
HAC 7th characters A & B see Appendix B for HAC conditional logic

CC +7th **S02.631** **Fracture of coronoid process of right mandible**
CC Exclusion 7th characters A & B see Appendix A PDX collection 1143
CC Exclusion 7th character K see Appendix A PDX collection 0897
HAC 7th characters A & B see Appendix B for HAC conditional logic

CC +7th **S02.632** **Fracture of coronoid process of left mandible**
CC Exclusion 7th characters A & B see Appendix A PDX collection 1143
CC Exclusion 7th character K see Appendix A PDX collection 0897
HAC 7th characters A & B see Appendix B for HAC conditional logic

+ S02.64 **Fracture of ramus of mandible**

CC +7th **S02.640** **Fracture of ramus of mandible, unspecified side**
CC Exclusion 7th characters A & B see Appendix A PDX collection 1143
CC Exclusion 7th character K see Appendix A PDX collection 0897
HAC 7th characters A & B see Appendix B for HAC conditional logic

CC +7th **S02.641** **Fracture of ramus of right mandible**
CC Exclusion 7th characters A & B see Appendix A PDX collection 1143
CC Exclusion 7th character K see Appendix A PDX collection 0897
HAC 7th characters A & B see Appendix B for HAC conditional logic

CC +7th **S02.642** **Fracture of ramus of left mandible**
CC Exclusion 7th characters A & B see Appendix A PDX collection 1143
CC Exclusion 7th character K see Appendix A PDX collection 0897
HAC 7th characters A & B see Appendix B for HAC conditional logic

+ S02.65 **Fracture of angle of mandible**

CC +7th **S02.650** **Fracture of angle of mandible, unspecified side**
CC Exclusion 7th characters A & B see Appendix A PDX collection 1143
CC Exclusion 7th character K see Appendix A PDX collection 0897
HAC 7th characters A & B see Appendix B for HAC conditional logic

CC +7th **S02.651** **Fracture of angle of right mandible**
CC Exclusion 7th characters A & B see Appendix A PDX collection 1143
CC Exclusion 7th character K see Appendix A PDX collection 0897
HAC 7th characters A & B see Appendix B for HAC conditional logic

CC +7th **S02.652** **Fracture of angle of left mandible**
CC Exclusion 7th characters A & B see Appendix A PDX collection 1143
CC Exclusion 7th character K see Appendix A PDX collection 0897
HAC 7th characters A & B see Appendix B for HAC conditional logic

CC X+7th **S02.66** **Fracture of symphysis of mandible**
CC Exclusion 7th characters A & B see Appendix A PDX collection 1143
CC Exclusion 7th character K see Appendix A PDX collection 0897
HAC 7th characters A & B see Appendix B for HAC conditional logic

+ S02.67 **Fracture of alveolus of mandible**

CC +7th **S02.670** **Fracture of alveolus of mandible, unspecified side**
CC Exclusion 7th characters A & B see Appendix A PDX collection 1143
CC Exclusion 7th character K see Appendix A PDX collection 0897
HAC 7th characters A & B see Appendix B for HAC conditional logic

CC +7th **S02.671** **Fracture of alveolus of right mandible**
CC Exclusion 7th characters A & B see Appendix A PDX collection 1143
CC Exclusion 7th character K see Appendix A PDX collection 0897
HAC 7th characters A & B see Appendix B for HAC conditional logic

CC +7th **S02.672** **Fracture of alveolus of left mandible**
CC Exclusion 7th characters A & B see Appendix A PDX collection 1143
CC Exclusion 7th character K see Appendix A PDX collection 0897
HAC 7th characters A & B see Appendix B for HAC conditional logic

CC X+7th **S02.69** **Fracture of mandible of other specified site**
CC Exclusion 7th characters A & B see Appendix A PDX collection 1143
CC Exclusion 7th character K see Appendix A PDX collection 0897
HAC 7th characters A & B see Appendix B for HAC conditional logic

+ S02.8 **Fractures of other specified skull and facial bones**
Fracture of orbit NOS
Fracture of palate
Excludes1: *fracture of orbital floor (S02.3-)*
fracture of orbital roof (S02.1-)

CC X+7th **S02.80** **Fracture of other specified skull and facial bones, unspecified side**
CC Exclusion 7th characters A & B see Appendix A PDX collection 1142
CC Exclusion 7th character K see Appendix A PDX collection 0897
HAC 7th characters A & B see Appendix B for HAC conditional logic

CC X+7th **S02.81** **Fracture of other specified skull and facial bones, right side**
CC Exclusion 7th characters A & B see Appendix A PDX collection 1142
CC Exclusion 7th character K see Appendix A PDX collection 0897
HAC 7th characters A & B see Appendix B for HAC conditional logic

CC X+7th **S02.82** **Fracture of other specified skull and facial bones, left side**
CC Exclusion 7th characters A & B see Appendix A PDX collection 1142
CC Exclusion 7th character K see Appendix A PDX collection 0897
HAC 7th characters A & B see Appendix B for HAC conditional logic

+ S02.9 **Fracture of unspecified skull and facial bones**

CC MCC X+7th **S02.91** **Unspecified fracture of skull**
CC Exclusion 7th character A see Appendix A PDX collection 1140
CC Exclusion 7th character K see Appendix A PDX collection 0897
MCC Exclusion 7th character B see Appendix A PDX collection 1140
HAC 7th characters A & B see Appendix B for HAC conditional logic

CC X+7th **S02.92** **Unspecified fracture of facial bones**
CC Exclusion 7th characters A & B see Appendix A PDX collection 1142
CC Exclusion 7th character K see Appendix A PDX collection 0897
HAC 7th characters A & B see Appendix B for HAC conditional logic

S03 Dislocation and sprain of joints and ligaments of head

Includes: avulsion of joint (capsule) or ligament of head
laceration of cartilage, joint (capsule) or ligament of head
sprain of cartilage, joint (capsule) or ligament of head
traumatic hemarthrosis of joint or ligament of head
traumatic rupture of joint or ligament of head
traumatic subluxation of joint or ligament of head
traumatic tear of joint or ligament of head

Code also any associated open wound

Excludes2: *Strain of muscle or tendon of head (S09.1)*

The appropriate 7th character is to be added to each code from category S03
A initial encounter
D subsequent encounter
S sequela

\+ **S03.0 Dislocation of jaw**
Dislocation of jaw (cartilage) (meniscus)
Dislocation of mandible
Dislocation of temporomandibular (joint)
AHA CC: 4Q, 2016, 67

X+7th **S03.00 Dislocation of jaw, unspecified side**
X+7th **S03.01 Dislocation of jaw, right side**
X+7th **S03.02 Dislocation of jaw, left side**
X+7th **S03.03 Dislocation of jaw, bilateral**
X+7th **S03.1 Dislocation of septal cartilage of nose**
X+7th **S03.2 Dislocation of tooth**

\+ **S03.4 Sprain of jaw**
Sprain of temporomandibular (joint) (ligament)
AHA CC: 4Q, 2016, 67

X+7th **S03.40 Sprain of jaw, unspecified side**
X+7th **S03.41 Sprain of jaw, right side**
X+7th **S03.42 Sprain of jaw, left side**
X+7th **S03.43 Sprain of jaw, bilateral**
X+7th **S03.8 Sprain of joints and ligaments of other parts of head**
X+7th **S03.9 Sprain of joints and ligaments of unspecified parts of head**

S04 Injury of cranial nerve

The selection of side should be based on the side of the body being affected

Code first any associated intracranial injury (S06.-)

Code also any associated:
open wound of head (S01.-)
skull fracture (S02.-)

The appropriate 7th character is to be added to each code from category S04
A initial encounter
D subsequent encounter
S sequela

\+ **S04.0 Injury of optic nerve and pathways**
Use additional code to identify any visual field defect or blindness (H53.4-, H54.-)

\+ **S04.01 Injury of optic nerve**
Injury of 2nd cranial nerve

CC +7th **S04.011 Injury of optic nerve, right eye**
CC Exclusion 7th character A see Appendix A PDX collection 1144

CC +7th **S04.012 Injury of optic nerve, left eye**
CC Exclusion 7th character A see Appendix A PDX collection 1144

CC +7th **S04.019 Injury of optic nerve, unspecified eye**
Injury of optic nerve NOS
CC Exclusion 7th character A see Appendix A PDX collection 1144

CC X+7th **S04.02 Injury of optic chiasm**
CC Exclusion 7th character A see Appendix A PDX collection 1144

\+ **S04.03 Injury of optic tract and pathways**
Injury of optic radiation

CC +7th **S04.031 Injury of optic tract and pathways, right side**
CC Exclusion 7th character A see Appendix A PDX collection 1144

CC +7th **S04.032 Injury of optic tract and pathways, left side**
CC Exclusion 7th character A see Appendix A PDX collection 1144

CC +7th **S04.039 Injury of optic tract and pathways, unspecified side**
Injury of optic tract and pathways NOS
CC Exclusion 7th character A see Appendix A PDX collection 1144

\+ **S04.04 Injury of visual cortex**

CC +7th **S04.041 Injury of visual cortex, right side**
CC Exclusion 7th character A see Appendix A PDX collection 1144

CC +7th **S04.042 Injury of visual cortex, left side**
CC Exclusion 7th character A see Appendix A PDX collection 1144

CC +7th **S04.049 Injury of visual cortex, unspecified side**
Injury of visual cortex NOS
CC Exclusion 7th character A see Appendix A PDX collection 1144

\+ **S04.1 Injury of oculomotor nerve**
Injury of 3rd cranial nerve

CC X+7th **S04.10 Injury of oculomotor nerve, unspecified side**
CC Exclusion 7th character A see Appendix A PDX collection 1145

CC X+7th **S04.11 Injury of oculomotor nerve, right side**
CC Exclusion 7th character A see Appendix A PDX collection 1145

CC X+7th **S04.12 Injury of oculomotor nerve, left side**
CC Exclusion 7th character A see Appendix A PDX collection 1145

\+ **S04.2 Injury of trochlear nerve**
Injury of 4th cranial nerve

CC X+7th **S04.20 Injury of trochlear nerve, unspecified side**
CC Exclusion 7th character A see Appendix A PDX collection 1146

CC X+7th **S04.21 Injury of trochlear nerve, right side**
CC Exclusion 7th character A see Appendix A PDX collection 1146

CC X+7th **S04.22 Injury of trochlear nerve, left side**
CC Exclusion 7th character A see Appendix A PDX collection 1146

\+ **S04.3 Injury of trigeminal nerve**
Injury of 5th cranial nerve

CC X+7th **S04.30 Injury of trigeminal nerve, unspecified side**
CC Exclusion 7th character A see Appendix A PDX collection 1147

CC X+7th **S04.31 Injury of trigeminal nerve, right side**
CC Exclusion 7th character A see Appendix A PDX collection 1147

CC X+7th **S04.32 Injury of trigeminal nerve, left side**
CC Exclusion 7th character A see Appendix A PDX collection 1147

\+ **S04.4 Injury of abducent nerve**
Injury of 6th cranial nerve

CC X+7th **S04.40 Injury of abducent nerve, unspecified side**
CC Exclusion 7th character A see Appendix A PDX collection 1148

CC X+7th **S04.41 Injury of abducent nerve, right side**
CC Exclusion 7th character A see Appendix A PDX collection 1148

CC X+7th **S04.42 Injury of abducent nerve, left side**
CC Exclusion 7th character A see Appendix A PDX collection 1148

\+ **S04.5 Injury of facial nerve**
Injury of 7th cranial nerve

CC X+7th **S04.50 Injury of facial nerve, unspecified side**
CC Exclusion 7th character A see Appendix A PDX collection 1149

CC X+7th **S04.51 Injury of facial nerve, right side**
CC Exclusion 7th character A see Appendix A PDX collection 1149

CC X+7th **S04.52 Injury of facial nerve, left side**
CC Exclusion 7th character A see Appendix A PDX collection 1149

\+ **S04.6 Injury of acoustic nerve**
Injury of auditory nerve
Injury of 8th cranial nerve

CC X+7th **S04.60 Injury of acoustic nerve, unspecified side**
CC Exclusion 7th character A see Appendix A PDX collection 1150

CC X+7th **S04.61 Injury of acoustic nerve, right side**
CC Exclusion 7th character A see Appendix A PDX collection 1150

CC X+7th **S04.62 Injury of acoustic nerve, left side**
CC Exclusion 7th character A see Appendix A PDX collection 1150

\+ **S04.7 Injury of accessory nerve**
Injury of 11th cranial nerve

CC X+7th **S04.70 Injury of accessory nerve, unspecified side**
CC Exclusion 7th character A see Appendix A PDX collection 1151

CC X+7th **S04.71 Injury of accessory nerve, right side**
CC Exclusion 7th character A see Appendix A PDX collection 1151

CC X+7th **S04.72 Injury of accessory nerve, left side**
CC Exclusion 7th character A see Appendix A PDX collection 1151

+ **S04.8 Injury of other cranial nerves**

+ **S04.81 Injury of olfactory [1st] nerve**

CC +7th **S04.811 Injury of olfactory [1st] nerve, right side**
CC Exclusion 7th character A see Appendix A PDX collection 1152

CC +7th **S04.812 Injury of olfactory [1st] nerve, left side**
CC Exclusion 7th character A see Appendix A PDX collection 1152

CC +7th **S04.819 Injury of olfactory [1st] nerve, unspecified side**
CC Exclusion 7th character A see Appendix A PDX collection 1152

+ **S04.89 Injury of other cranial nerves**
Injury of vagus [10th] nerve

CC +7th **S04.891 Injury of other cranial nerves, right side**
CC Exclusion 7th character A see Appendix A PDX collection 1152

CC +7th **S04.892 Injury of other cranial nerves, left side**
CC Exclusion 7th character A see Appendix A PDX collection 1152

CC +7th **S04.899 Injury of other cranial nerves, unspecified side**
CC Exclusion 7th character A see Appendix A PDX collection 1152

X+7th **S04.9 Injury of unspecified cranial nerve**
CC Exclusion 7th character A see Appendix A PDX collection 1152

S05 Injury of eye and orbit

Includes: open wound of eye and orbit
Excludes2: *2nd cranial [optic] nerve injury (S04.0-)*
3rd cranial [oculomotor] nerve injury (S04.1-)
open wound of eyelid and periocular area (S01.1-)
orbital bone fracture (S02.1-, S02.3-, S02.8-)
superficial injury of eyelid (S00.1-S00.2)

The appropriate 7th character is to be added to each code from category S05
A initial encounter
D subsequent encounter
S sequela

+ **S05.0 Injury of conjunctiva and corneal abrasion without foreign body**
Excludes1: *foreign body in conjunctival sac (T15.1)*
foreign body in cornea (T15.0)

X+7th **S05.00 Injury of conjunctiva and corneal abrasion without foreign body, unspecified eye**

X+7th **S05.01 Injury of conjunctiva and corneal abrasion without foreign body, right eye**

X+7th **S05.02 Injury of conjunctiva and corneal abrasion without foreign body, left eye**

+ **S05.1 Contusion of eyeball and orbital tissues**
Traumatic hyphema
Excludes2: *black eye NOS (S00.1)*
contusion of eyelid and periocular area (S00.1)

X+7th **S05.10 Contusion of eyeball and orbital tissues, unspecified eye**

X+7th **S05.11 Contusion of eyeball and orbital tissues, right eye**

X+7th **S05.12 Contusion of eyeball and orbital tissues, left eye**

+ **S05.2 Ocular laceration and rupture with prolapse or loss of intraocular tissue**

CC X+7th **S05.20 Ocular laceration and rupture with prolapse or loss of intraocular tissue, unspecified eye**
CC Exclusion 7th character A see Appendix A PDX collection 1139

CC X+7th **S05.21 Ocular laceration and rupture with prolapse or loss of intraocular tissue, right eye**
CC Exclusion 7th character A see Appendix A PDX collection 1139

CC X+7th **S05.22 Ocular laceration and rupture with prolapse or loss of intraocular tissue, left eye**
CC Exclusion 7th character A see Appendix A PDX collection 1139

+ **S05.3 Ocular laceration without prolapse or loss of intraocular tissue**
Laceration of eye NOS

CC X+7th **S05.30 Ocular laceration without prolapse or loss of intraocular tissue, unspecified eye**
CC Exclusion 7th character A see Appendix A PDX collection 1139

CC X+7th **S05.31 Ocular laceration without prolapse or loss of intraocular tissue, right eye**
CC Exclusion 7th character A see Appendix A PDX collection 1139

CC X+7th **S05.32 Ocular laceration without prolapse or loss of intraocular tissue, left eye**
CC Exclusion 7th character A see Appendix A PDX collection 1139

+ **S05.4 Penetrating wound of orbit with or without foreign body**
Excludes2: *retained (old) foreign body following penetrating wound in orbit (H05.5-)*

CC X+7th **S05.40 Penetrating wound of orbit with or without foreign body, unspecified eye**
CC Exclusion 7th character A see Appendix A PDX collection 1139

CC X+7th **S05.41 Penetrating wound of orbit with or without foreign body, right eye**
CC Exclusion 7th character A see Appendix A PDX collection 1139

CC X+7th **S05.42 Penetrating wound of orbit with or without foreign body, left eye**
CC Exclusion 7th character A see Appendix A PDX collection 1139

+ **S05.5 Penetrating wound with foreign body of eyeball**
Excludes2: *retained (old) intraocular foreign body (H44.6-, H44.7)*

CC X+7th **S05.50 Penetrating wound with foreign body of unspecified eyeball**
CC Exclusion 7th character A see Appendix A PDX collection 1153

CC X+7th **S05.51 Penetrating wound with foreign body of right eyeball**
CC Exclusion 7th character A see Appendix A PDX collection 1153

CC X+7th **S05.52 Penetrating wound with foreign body of left eyeball**
CC Exclusion 7th character A see Appendix A PDX collection 1153

+ **S05.6 Penetrating wound without foreign body of eyeball**
Ocular penetration NOS

X+7th **S05.60 Penetrating wound without foreign body of unspecified eyeball**

X+7th **S05.61 Penetrating wound without foreign body of right eyeball**

X+7th **S05.62 Penetrating wound without foreign body of left eyeball**

+ **S05.7 Avulsion of eye**
Traumatic enucleation

CC X+7th **S05.70 Avulsion of unspecified eye**
CC Exclusion 7th character A see Appendix A PDX collection 1139

CC X+7th **S05.71 Avulsion of right eye**
CC Exclusion 7th character A see Appendix A PDX collection 1139

CC X+7th **S05.72 Avulsion of left eye**
CC Exclusion 7th character A see Appendix A PDX collection 1139

CC + **S05.8 Other injuries of eye and orbit**
Lacrimal duct injury
CC Exclusion 7th character A see Appendix A PDX collection 1139

+ **S05.8X Other injuries of eye and orbit**

+7th **S05.8X1 Other injuries of right eye and orbit**

+7th **S05.8X2 Other injuries of left eye and orbit**

+7th **S05.8X9 Other injuries of unspecified eye and orbit**

+ **S05.9 Unspecified injury of eye and orbit**
Injury of eye NOS

X+7th **S05.90 Unspecified injury of unspecified eye and orbit**

CC X+7th **S05.91 Unspecified injury of right eye and orbit**
CC Exclusion 7th character A see Appendix A PDX collection 1139

CC X+7th **S05.92 Unspecified injury of left eye and orbit**
CC Exclusion 7th character A see Appendix A PDX collection 1139

S06 Intracranial injury

Includes: traumatic brain injury

Code also any associated:
open wound of head (S01.-)
skull fracture (S02.-)

Excludes1: *head injury NOS (S09.90)*

The appropriate 7th character is to be added to each code from category S06
A initial encounter
D subsequent encounter
S sequela

NOTE 7th characters D and S do not apply to codes in category S06 with 6th character 7 - death due to brain injury prior to regaining consciousness, or 8 - death due to other cause prior to regaining consciousness.

+ **S06.0 Concussion**
Commotio cerebri
Excludes1: *concussion with other intracranial injuries classified in category S06.1- to S06.6-, S06.81- and S06.82- code to specified intracranial injury*
AHA CC: 4Q, 2016, 67-68

+ **S06.0X Concussion**

CC +7th **S06.0X0 Concussion without loss of consciousness**
CC Exclusion 7th character A see Appendix A PDX collection 1154
HAC 7th character A see Appendix B for HAC conditional logic

CC +7th **S06.0X1 Concussion with loss of consciousness of 30 minutes or less**
CC Exclusion 7th character A see Appendix A PDX collection 1154
HAC 7th character A see Appendix B for HAC conditional logic

CC +7th **S06.0X9 Concussion with loss of consciousness of unspecified duration**
Concussion NOS
CC Exclusion 7th character A see Appendix A PDX collection 1154
HAC 7th character A see Appendix B for HAC conditional logic

+ **S06.1 Traumatic cerebral edema**
Diffuse traumatic cerebral edema
Focal traumatic cerebral edema

+ **S06.1X Traumatic cerebral edema**

MCC +7th **S06.1X0 Traumatic cerebral edema without loss of consciousness**
MCC Exclusion 7th character A see Appendix A PDX collection 0612
HAC 7th character A see Appendix B for HAC conditional logic
AHA CC: 1Q, 2015, 3-21

MCC +7th **S06.1X1 Traumatic cerebral edema with loss of consciousness of 30 minutes or less**
MCC Exclusion 7th character A see Appendix A PDX collection 1155
HAC 7th character A see Appendix B for HAC conditional logic

MCC +7th **S06.1X2 Traumatic cerebral edema with loss of consciousness of 31 minutes to 59 minutes**
MCC Exclusion 7th character A see Appendix A PDX collection 1155
HAC 7th character A see Appendix B for HAC conditional logic

MCC +7th **S06.1X3 Traumatic cerebral edema with loss of consciousness of 1 hour to 5 hours 59 minutes**
MCC Exclusion 7th character A see Appendix A PDX collection 1155
HAC 7th character A see Appendix B for HAC conditional logic

MCC +7th **S06.1X4 Traumatic cerebral edema with loss of consciousness of 6 hours to 24 hours**
MCC Exclusion 7th character A see Appendix A PDX collection 1155
HAC 7th character A see Appendix B for HAC conditional logic

MCC +7th **S06.1X5 Traumatic cerebral edema with loss of consciousness greater than 24 hours with return to pre-existing conscious level**
MCC Exclusion 7th character A see Appendix A PDX collection 1155
HAC 7th character A see Appendix B for HAC conditional logic

MCC +7th **S06.1X6 Traumatic cerebral edema with loss of consciousness greater than 24 hours without return to pre-existing conscious level with patient surviving**
MCC Exclusion 7th character A see Appendix PDX collection 1154
HAC 7th character A see Appendix B for HAC conditional logic

MCC +7th **S06.1X7 Traumatic cerebral edema with loss of consciousness of any duration with death due to brain injury prior to regaining consciousness**
MCC Exclusion 7th character A see Appendix PDX collection 1154
HAC 7th character A see Appendix B for HAC conditional logic

MCC +7th **S06.1X8 Traumatic cerebral edema with loss of consciousness of any duration with death due to other cause prior to regaining consciousness**
MCC Exclusion 7th character A see Appendix PDX collection 1154
HAC 7th character A see Appendix B for HAC conditional logic

MCC +7th **S06.1X9 Traumatic cerebral edema with loss of consciousness of unspecified duration**
Traumatic cerebral edema NOS
MCC Exclusion 7th character A see Appendix PDX collection 1155
HAC 7th character A see Appendix B for HAC conditional logic

CC + **S06.2 Diffuse traumatic brain injury**
Diffuse axonal brain injury
Excludes1: *traumatic diffuse cerebral edema (S06.1X-)*
CC Exclusion 7th character A see Appendix A PDX collection 1154

+ **S06.2X Diffuse traumatic brain injury**

+7th **S06.2X0 Diffuse traumatic brain injury without lo of consciousness**
HAC 7th character A see Appendix B for HAC conditional logic

+7th **S06.2X1 Diffuse traumatic brain injury with loss consciousness of 30 minutes or less**
HAC 7th character A see Appendix B for HAC conditional logic

+7th **S06.2X2 Diffuse traumatic brain injury with loss consciousness of 31 minutes to 59 minute**
HAC 7th character A see Appendix B for HAC conditional logic

+7th **S06.2X3 Diffuse traumatic brain injury with loss of consciousness of 1 hour to 5 hours 59 minutes**
HAC 7th character A see Appendix B for HAC conditional logic

+7th **S06.2X4 Diffuse traumatic brain injury with loss consciousness of 6 hours to 24 hours**
HAC 7th character A see Appendix B for HAC conditional logic

+7th **S06.2X5 Diffuse traumatic brain injury with loss consciousness greater than 24 hours with return to pre-existing conscious levels**
HAC 7th character A see Appendix B for HAC conditional logic

MCC +7th **S06.2X6 Diffuse traumatic brain injury with loss of consciousness greater than 24 hours without return to pre-existing conscious level with patient surviving**
MCC Exclusion 7th character A see Appendi PDX collection 1154
HAC 7th character A see Appendix B for HAC conditional logic

MCC +7th **S06.2X7 Diffuse traumatic brain injury with loss consciousness of any duration with death due to brain injury prior to regaining consciousness**
MCC Exclusion 7th character A see Appendi PDX collection 1154
HAC 7th character A see Appendix B for HAC conditional logic

MCC +7th **S06.2X8 Diffuse traumatic brain injury with loss of consciousness of any duration with death due to other cause prior to regaini consciousness**
MCC Exclusion 7th character A see Appendi PDX collection 1154
HAC 7th character A see Appendix B for HAC conditional logic

+7th **S06.2X9 Diffuse traumatic brain injury with loss of consciousness of unspecified duration**
Diffuse traumatic brain injury NOS
HAC 7th character A see Appendix B for HAC conditional logic

+ **S06.3 Focal traumatic brain injury**
Excludes1: *any condition classifiable to S06.4-S06.6*
focal cerebral edema (S06.1)

+ **S06.30 Unspecified focal traumatic brain injury**

+7th **S06.300 Unspecified focal traumatic brain injury without loss of consciousness**

CC +7th **S06.301 Unspecified focal traumatic brain injury with loss of consciousness of 30 minutes or less**
CC Exclusion 7th character A see Appendix A PDX collection 1154
HAC 7th character A see Appendix B for HAC conditional logic

CC +7th **S06.302 Unspecified focal traumatic brain injury with loss of consciousness of 31 minutes to 59 minutes**
CC Exclusion 7th character A see Appendix A PDX collection 1154
HAC 7th character A see Appendix B for HAC conditional logic

CC +7th **S06.303 Unspecified focal traumatic brain injury with loss of consciousness of 1 hour to 5 hours 59 minutes**
CC Exclusion 7th character A see Appendix A PDX collection 1154
HAC 7th character A see Appendix B for HAC conditional logic

CC +7th **S06.304 Unspecified focal traumatic brain injury with loss of consciousness of 6 hours to 24 hours**
CC Exclusion 7th character A see Appendix A PDX collection 1154
HAC 7th character A see Appendix B for HAC conditional logic

CC +7th **S06.305 Unspecified focal traumatic brain injury with loss of consciousness greater than 24 hours with return to pre-existing conscious level**
CC Exclusion 7th character A see Appendix A PDX collection 1154
HAC 7th character A see Appendix B for HAC conditional logic

MCC +7th **S06.306 Unspecified focal traumatic brain injury with loss of consciousness greater than 24 hours without return to pre-existing conscious level with patient surviving**
MCC Exclusion 7th character A see Appendix A PDX collection 1154
HAC 7th character A see Appendix B for HAC conditional logic

MCC +7th **S06.307 Unspecified focal traumatic brain injury with loss of consciousness of any duration with death due to brain injury prior to regaining consciousness**
MCC Exclusion 7th character A see Appendix A PDX collection 1154
HAC 7th character A see Appendix B for HAC conditional logic

MCC +7th **S06.308 Unspecified focal traumatic brain injury with loss of consciousness of any duration with death due to other cause prior to regaining consciousness**
MCC Exclusion 7th character A see Appendix A PDX collection 1154
HAC 7th character A see Appendix B for HAC conditional logic

CC +7th **S06.309 Unspecified focal traumatic brain injury with loss of consciousness of unspecified duration**
Unspecified focal traumatic brain injury NOS
CC Exclusion 7th character A see Appendix A PDX collection 1154
HAC 7th character A see Appendix B for HAC conditional logic

+ **S06.31 Contusion and laceration of right cerebrum**

MCC +7th **S06.310 Contusion and laceration of right cerebrum without loss of consciousness**
MCC Exclusion 7th character A see Appendix A PDX collection 1154
HAC 7th character A see Appendix B for HAC conditional logic

MCC +7th **S06.311 Contusion and laceration of right cerebrum with loss of consciousness of 30 minutes or less**
MCC Exclusion 7th character A see Appendix A PDX collection 1154
HAC 7th character A see Appendix B for HAC conditional logic

MCC +7th **S06.312 Contusion and laceration of right cerebrum with loss of consciousness of 31 minutes to 59 minutes**
MCC Exclusion 7th character A see Appendix A PDX collection 1154
HAC 7th character A see Appendix B for HAC conditional logic

MCC +7th **S06.313 Contusion and laceration of right cerebrum with loss of consciousness of 1 hour to 5 hours 59 minutes**
MCC Exclusion 7th character A see Appendix A PDX collection 1154
HAC 7th character A see Appendix B for HAC conditional logic

MCC +7th **S06.314 Contusion and laceration of right cerebrum with loss of consciousness of 6 hours to 24 hours**
MCC Exclusion 7th character A see Appendix A PDX collection 1154
HAC 7th character A see Appendix B for HAC conditional logic

MCC +7th **S06.315 Contusion and laceration of right cerebrum with loss of consciousness greater than 24 hours with return to pre-existing conscious level**
MCC Exclusion 7th character A see Appendix A PDX collection 1154
HAC 7th character A see Appendix B for HAC conditional logic

MCC +7th **S06.316 Contusion and laceration of right cerebrum with loss of consciousness greater than 24 hours without return to pre-existing conscious level with patient surviving**
MCC Exclusion 7th character A see Appendix A PDX collection 1154
HAC 7th character A see Appendix B for HAC conditional logic

MCC +7th **S06.317 Contusion and laceration of right cerebrum with loss of consciousness of any duration with death due to brain injury prior to regaining consciousness**
MCC Exclusion 7th character A see Appendix A PDX collection 1154
HAC 7th character A see Appendix B for HAC conditional logic

MCC +7th **S06.318 Contusion and laceration of right cerebrum with loss of consciousness of any duration with death due to other cause prior to regaining consciousness**
MCC Exclusion 7th character A see Appendix A PDX collection 1154
HAC 7th character A see Appendix B for HAC conditional logic

MCC +7th **S06.319 Contusion and laceration of right cerebrum with loss of consciousness of unspecified duration**
Contusion and laceration of right cerebrum NOS
MCC Exclusion 7th character A see Appendix A PDX collection 1154
HAC 7th character A see Appendix B for HAC conditional logic

+ **S06.32 Contusion and laceration of left cerebrum**

MCC +7th **S06.320 Contusion and laceration of left cerebrum without loss of consciousness**
MCC Exclusion 7th character A see Appendix A PDX collection 1154
HAC 7th character A see Appendix B for HAC conditional logic

MCC +7th **S06.321 Contusion and laceration of left cerebrum with loss of consciousness of 30 minutes or less**
MCC Exclusion 7th character A see Appendix A PDX collection 1154
HAC 7th character A see Appendix B for HAC conditional logic

MCC +7th **S06.322** **Contusion and laceration of left cerebrum with loss of consciousness of 31 minutes to 59 minutes**
MCC Exclusion 7th character A see Appendix A
PDX collection 1154
HAC 7th character A see Appendix B for HAC conditional logic

MCC +7th **S06.323** **Contusion and laceration of left cerebrum with loss of consciousness of 1 hour to 5 hours 59 minutes**
MCC Exclusion 7th character A see Appendix A
PDX collection 1154
HAC 7th character A see Appendix B for HAC conditional logic

MCC +7th **S06.324** **Contusion and laceration of left cerebrum with loss of consciousness of 6 hours to 24 hours**
MCC Exclusion 7th character A see Appendix A
PDX collection 1154
HAC 7th character A see Appendix B for HAC conditional logic

MCC +7th **S06.325** **Contusion and laceration of left cerebrum with loss of consciousness greater than 24 hours with return to pre-existing conscious level**
MCC Exclusion 7th character A see Appendix A
PDX collection 1154
HAC 7th character A see Appendix B for HAC conditional logic

MCC +7th **S06.326** **Contusion and laceration of left cerebrum with loss of consciousness greater than 24 hours without return to pre-existing conscious level with patient surviving**
MCC Exclusion 7th character A see Appendix A
PDX collection 1154
HAC 7th character A see Appendix B for HAC conditional logic

MCC +7th **S06.327** **Contusion and laceration of left cerebrum with loss of consciousness of any duration with death due to brain injury prior to regaining consciousness**
MCC Exclusion 7th character A see Appendix A
PDX collection 1154
HAC 7th character A see Appendix B for HAC conditional logic

MCC +7th **S06.328** **Contusion and laceration of left cerebrum with loss of consciousness of any duration with death due to other cause prior to regaining consciousness**
MCC Exclusion 7th character A see Appendix A
PDX collection 1154
HAC 7th character A see Appendix B for HAC conditional logic

MCC +7th **S06.329** **Contusion and laceration of left cerebrum with loss of consciousness of unspecified duration**
Contusion and laceration of left cerebrum NOS
MCC Exclusion 7th character A see Appendix A
PDX collection 1154
HAC 7th character A see Appendix B for HAC conditional logic

+ S06.33 Contusion and laceration of cerebrum, unspecified

MCC +7th **S06.330** **Contusion and laceration of cerebrum, unspecified, without loss of consciousness**
MCC Exclusion 7th character A see Appendix A
PDX collection 1154
HAC 7th character A see Appendix B for HAC conditional logic

MCC +7th **S06.331** **Contusion and laceration of cerebrum, unspecified, with loss of consciousness of 30 minutes or less**
MCC Exclusion 7th character A see Appendix A
PDX collection 1154
HAC 7th character A see Appendix B for HAC conditional logic

MCC +7th **S06.332** **Contusion and laceration of cerebrum, unspecified, with loss of consciousness of 31 minutes to 59 minutes**
MCC Exclusion 7th character A see Appendix A
PDX collection 1154
HAC 7th character A see Appendix B for HAC conditional logic

MCC +7th **S06.333** **Contusion and laceration of cerebrum, unspecified, with loss of consciousness of 1 hour to 5 hours 59 minutes**
MCC Exclusion 7th character A see Appendix
PDX collection 1154
HAC 7th character A see Appendix B for HAC conditional logic

MCC +7th **S06.334** **Contusion and laceration of cerebrum, unspecified, with loss of consciousness of 6 hours to 24 hours**
MCC Exclusion 7th character A see Appendix
PDX collection 1154
HAC 7th character A see Appendix B for HAC conditional logic

MCC +7th **S06.335** **Contusion and laceration of cerebrum, unspecified, with loss of consciousness greater than 24 hours with return to pre-existing conscious level**
MCC Exclusion 7th character A see Appendix
PDX collection 1154
HAC 7th character A see Appendix B for HAC conditional logic

MCC +7th **S06.336** **Contusion and laceration of cerebrum, unspecified, with loss of consciousness greater than 24 hours without return to pre-existing conscious level with patient surviving**
MCC Exclusion 7th character A see Appendix
PDX collection 1154
HAC 7th character A see Appendix B for HAC conditional logic

MCC +7th **S06.337** **Contusion and laceration of cerebrum, unspecified, with loss of consciousness of any duration with death due to brain injury prior to regaining consciousness**
MCC Exclusion 7th character A see Appendix
PDX collection 1154
HAC 7th character A see Appendix B for HAC conditional logic

MCC +7th **S06.338** **Contusion and laceration of cerebrum, unspecified, with loss of consciousness of any duration with death due to other cau prior to regaining consciousness**
MCC Exclusion 7th character A see Appendix
PDX collection 1154
HAC 7th character A see Appendix B for HAC conditional logic

MCC +7th **S06.339** **Contusion and laceration of cerebrum, unspecified, with loss of consciousness of unspecified duration**
Contusion and laceration of cerebrum NOS
MCC Exclusion 7th character A see Appendix
PDX collection 1154
HAC 7th character A see Appendix B for HAC conditional logic

+ S06.34 Traumatic hemorrhage of right cerebrum
Traumatic intracerebral hemorrhage and hematoma of right cerebrum

MCC +7th **S06.340** **Traumatic hemorrhage of right cerebrum without loss of consciousness**
MCC Exclusion 7th character A see Appendix
PDX collection 1154
HAC 7th character A see Appendix B for HAC conditional logic
AHA CC: 1Q, 2015, 3-21

MCC +7th **S06.341** **Traumatic hemorrhage of right cerebrum with loss of consciousness of 30 minutes or less**
MCC Exclusion 7th character A see Appendi
PDX collection 1154
HAC 7th character A see Appendix B for HAC conditional logic

MCC +7th **S06.342** **Traumatic hemorrhage of right cerebrum with loss of consciousness of 31 minutes to 59 minutes**
MCC Exclusion 7th character A see Appendi
PDX collection 1154
HAC 7th character A see Appendix B for HAC conditional logic

MCC +7th **S06.343** **Traumatic hemorrhage of right cerebrum with loss of consciousness of 1 hours to 5 hours 59 minutes**
MCC Exclusion 7th character A see Appendi
PDX collection 1154
HAC 7th character A see Appendix B for HAC conditional logic

MCC +7th **S06.344** **Traumatic hemorrhage of right cerebrum with loss of consciousness of 6 hours to 24 hours**
MCC Exclusion 7th character A see Appendix A PDX collection 1154
HAC 7th character A see Appendix B for HAC conditional logic

MCC +7th **S06.345** **Traumatic hemorrhage of right cerebrum with loss of consciousness greater than 24 hours with return to pre-existing conscious level**
MCC Exclusion 7th character A see Appendix A PDX collection 1154
HAC 7th character A see Appendix B for HAC conditional logic

MCC +7th **S06.346** **Traumatic hemorrhage of right cerebrum with loss of consciousness greater than 24 hours without return to pre-existing conscious level with patient surviving**
MCC Exclusion 7th character A see Appendix A PDX collection 1154
HAC 7th character A see Appendix B for HAC conditional logic

MCC +7th **S06.347** **Traumatic hemorrhage of right cerebrum with loss of consciousness of any duration with death due to brain injury prior to regaining consciousness**
MCC Exclusion 7th character A see Appendix A PDX collection 1154
HAC 7th character A see Appendix B for HAC conditional logic

MCC +7th **S06.348** **Traumatic hemorrhage of right cerebrum with loss of consciousness of any duration with death due to other cause prior to regaining consciousness**
MCC Exclusion 7th character A see Appendix A PDX collection 1154
HAC 7th character A see Appendix B for HAC conditional logic

MCC +7th **S06.349** **Traumatic hemorrhage of right cerebrum with loss of consciousness of unspecified duration**
Traumatic hemorrhage of right cerebrum NOS
MCC Exclusion 7th character A see Appendix A PDX collection 1154
HAC 7th character A see Appendix B for HAC conditional logic

\+ **S06.35** **Traumatic hemorrhage of left cerebrum**
Traumatic intracerebral hemorrhage and hematoma of left cerebrum

MCC +7th **S06.350** **Traumatic hemorrhage of left cerebrum without loss of consciousness**
MCC Exclusion 7th character A see Appendix A PDX collection 1154
HAC 7th character A see Appendix B for HAC conditional logic

MCC +7th **S06.351** **Traumatic hemorrhage of left cerebrum with loss of consciousness of 30 minutes or less**
MCC Exclusion 7th character A see Appendix A PDX collection 1154
HAC 7th character A see Appendix B for HAC conditional logic

MCC +7th **S06.352** **Traumatic hemorrhage of left cerebrum with loss of consciousness of 31 minutes to 59 minutes**
MCC Exclusion 7th character A see Appendix A PDX collection 1154
HAC 7th character A see Appendix B for HAC conditional logic

MCC +7th **S06.353** **Traumatic hemorrhage of left cerebrum with loss of consciousness of 1 hours to 5 hours 59 minutes**
MCC Exclusion 7th character A see Appendix A PDX collection 1154
HAC 7th character A see Appendix B for HAC conditional logic

MCC +7th **S06.354** **Traumatic hemorrhage of left cerebrum with loss of consciousness of 6 hours to 24 hours**
MCC Exclusion 7th character A see Appendix A PDX collection 1154
HAC 7th character A see Appendix B for HAC conditional logic

MCC +7th **S06.355** **Traumatic hemorrhage of left cerebrum with loss of consciousness greater than 24 hours with return to pre-existing conscious level**
MCC Exclusion 7th character A see Appendix A PDX collection 1154
HAC 7th character A see Appendix B for HAC conditional logic

MCC +7th **S06.356** **Traumatic hemorrhage of left cerebrum with loss of consciousness greater than 24 hours without return to pre-existing conscious level with patient surviving**
MCC Exclusion 7th character A see Appendix A PDX collection 1154
HAC 7th character A see Appendix B for HAC conditional logic

MCC +7th **S06.357** **Traumatic hemorrhage of left cerebrum with loss of consciousness of≈any duration with death due to brain injury prior to regaining consciousness**
MCC Exclusion 7th character A see Appendix A PDX collection 1154
HAC 7th character A see Appendix B for HAC conditional logic

MCC +7th **S06.358** **Traumatic hemorrhage of left cerebrum with loss of consciousness of any duration with death due to other cause prior to regaining consciousness**
MCC Exclusion 7th character A see Appendix A PDX collection 1154
HAC 7th character A see Appendix B for HAC conditional logic

MCC +7th **S06.359** **Traumatic hemorrhage of left cerebrum with loss of consciousness of unspecified duration**
Traumatic hemorrhage of left cerebrum NOS
MCC Exclusion 7th character A see Appendix A PDX collection 1154
HAC 7th character A see Appendix B for HAC conditional logic

\+ **S06.36** **Traumatic hemorrhage of cerebrum, unspecified**
Traumatic intracerebral hemorrhage and hematoma, unspecified

MCC +7th **S06.360** **Traumatic hemorrhage of cerebrum, unspecified, without loss of consciousness**
MCC Exclusion 7th character A see Appendix A PDX collection 1154
HAC 7th character A see Appendix B for HAC conditional logic

MCC +7th **S06.361** **Traumatic hemorrhage of cerebrum, unspecified, with loss of consciousness of 30 minutes or less**
MCC Exclusion 7th character A see Appendix A PDX collection 1154
HAC 7th character A see Appendix B for HAC conditional logic

MCC +7th **S06.362** **Traumatic hemorrhage of cerebrum, unspecified, with loss of consciousness of 31 minutes to 59 minutes**
MCC Exclusion 7th character A see Appendix A PDX collection 1154
HAC 7th character A see Appendix B for HAC conditional logic

MCC +7th **S06.363** **Traumatic hemorrhage of cerebrum, unspecified, with loss of consciousness of 1 hours to 5 hours 59 minutes**
MCC Exclusion 7th character A see Appendix A PDX collection 1154
HAC 7th character A see Appendix B for HAC conditional logic

MCC +7th **S06.364** **Traumatic hemorrhage of cerebrum, unspecified, with loss of consciousness of 6 hours to 24 hours**
MCC Exclusion 7th character A see Appendix A PDX collection 1154
HAC 7th character A see Appendix B for HAC conditional logic

MCC +7th **S06.365** **Traumatic hemorrhage of cerebrum, unspecified, with loss of consciousness greater than 24 hours with return to pre-existing conscious level**
MCC Exclusion 7th character A see Appendix A PDX collection 1154
HAC 7th character A see Appendix B for HAC conditional logic

MCC +7th **S06.366 Traumatic hemorrhage of cerebrum, unspecified, with loss of consciousness greater than 24 hours without return to pre-existing conscious level with patient surviving**
MCC Exclusion 7th character A see Appendix A
PDX collection 1154
HAC 7th character A see Appendix B for HAC conditional logic

MCC +7th **S06.367 Traumatic hemorrhage of cerebrum, unspecified, with loss of consciousness of any duration with death due to brain injury prior to regaining consciousness**
MCC Exclusion 7th character A see Appendix A
PDX collection 1154
HAC 7th character A see Appendix B for HAC conditional logic

MCC +7th **S06.368 Traumatic hemorrhage of cerebrum, unspecified, with loss of consciousness of any duration with death due to other cause prior to regaining consciousness**
MCC Exclusion 7th character A see Appendix A
PDX collection 1154
HAC 7th character A see Appendix B for HAC conditional logic

MCC +7th **S06.369 Traumatic hemorrhage of cerebrum, unspecified, with loss of consciousness of unspecified duration**
Traumatic hemorrhage of cerebrum NOS
MCC Exclusion 7th character A see Appendix A
PDX collection 1154
HAC 7th character A see Appendix B for HAC conditional logic

+ **S06.37 Contusion, laceration, and hemorrhage of cerebellum**

MCC +7th **S06.370 Contusion, laceration, and hemorrhage of cerebellum without loss of consciousness**
No MCC Exclusions
HAC 7th character A see Appendix B for HAC conditional logic

CC +7th **S06.371 Contusion, laceration, and hemorrhage of cerebellum with loss of consciousness of 30 minutes or less**
CC Exclusion 7th character A see Appendix A
PDX collection 1154
HAC 7th character A see Appendix B for HAC conditional logic

CC +7th **S06.372 Contusion, laceration, and hemorrhage of cerebellum with loss of consciousness of 31 minutes to 59 minutes**
CC Exclusion 7th character A see Appendix A
PDX collection 1154
HAC 7th character A see Appendix B for HAC conditional logic

CC +7th **S06.373 Contusion, laceration, and hemorrhage of cerebellum with loss of consciousness of 1 hour to 5 hours 59 minutes**
CC Exclusion 7th character A see Appendix A
PDX collection 1154
HAC 7th character A see Appendix B for HAC conditional logic

CC +7th **S06.374 Contusion, laceration, and hemorrhage of cerebellum with loss of consciousness of 6 hours to 24 hours**
CC Exclusion 7th character A see Appendix A
PDX collection 1154
HAC 7th character A see Appendix B for HAC conditional logic

CC +7th **S06.375 Contusion, laceration, and hemorrhage of cerebellum with loss of consciousness greater than 24 hours with return to pre-existing conscious level**
CC Exclusion 7th character A see Appendix A
PDX collection 1154
HAC 7th character A see Appendix B for HAC conditional logic

MCC +7th **S06.376 Contusion, laceration, and hemorrhage of cerebellum with loss of consciousness greater than 24 hours without return to pre-existing conscious level with patient surviving**
MCC Exclusion 7th character A see Appendix A
PDX collection 1154
HAC 7th character A see Appendix B for HAC conditional logic

MCC +7th **S06.377 Contusion, laceration, and hemorrhage of cerebellum with loss of consciousness of any duration with death due to brain injury prior to regaining consciousness**
MCC Exclusion 7th character A see Appendix
PDX collection 1154
HAC 7th character A see Appendix B for HAC conditional logic

MCC +7th **S06.378 Contusion, laceration, and hemorrhage of cerebellum with loss of consciousness of any duration with death due to other caus prior to regaining consciousness**
MCC Exclusion 7th character A see Appendix
PDX collection 1154
HAC 7th character A see Appendix B for HAC conditional logic

CC +7th **S06.379 Contusion, laceration, and hemorrhage of cerebellum with loss of consciousness of unspecified duration**
Contusion, laceration, and hemorrhage of cerebellum NOS
CC Exclusion 7th character A see Appendix A
PDX collection 1154
HAC 7th character A see Appendix B for HAC conditional logic

+ **S06.38 Contusion, laceration, and hemorrhage of brainste**

MCC +7th **S06.380 Contusion, laceration, and hemorrhage of brainstem without loss of consciousness**
No MCC Exclusions
HAC 7th character A see Appendix B for HAC conditional logic

CC +7th **S06.381 Contusion, laceration, and hemorrhage of brainstem with loss of consciousness of 30 minutes or less**
CC Exclusion 7th character A see Appendix A
PDX collection 1154
HAC 7th character A see Appendix B for HAC conditional logic

CC +7th **S06.382 Contusion, laceration, and hemorrhage of brainstem with loss of consciousness of 31 minutes to 59 minutes**
CC Exclusion 7th character A see Appendix A
PDX collection 1154
HAC 7th character A see Appendix B for HAC conditional logic

CC +7th **S06.383 Contusion, laceration, and hemorrhage of brainstem with loss of consciousness of 1 hour to 5 hours 59 minutes**
CC Exclusion 7th character A see Appendix A
PDX collection 1154
HAC 7th character A see Appendix B for HAC conditional logic

CC +7th **S06.384 Contusion, laceration, and hemorrhage of brainstem with loss of consciousness of 6 hours to 24 hours**
CC Exclusion 7th character A see Appendix A
PDX collection 1154
HAC 7th character A see Appendix B for HAC conditional logic

CC +7th **S06.385 Contusion, laceration, and hemorrhage of brainstem with loss of consciousness greater than 24 hours with return to pre-existing conscious level**
CC Exclusion 7th character A see Appendix A
PDX collection 1154
HAC 7th character A see Appendix B for HAC conditional logic

MCC +7th **S06.386 Contusion, laceration, and hemorrhage of brainstem with loss of consciousness greater than 24 hours without return to pre-existing conscious level with patient surviving**
MCC Exclusion 7th character A see Appendix
PDX collection 1154
HAC 7th character A see Appendix B for HAC conditional logic

MCC +7th **S06.387 Contusion, laceration, and hemorrhage of brainstem with loss of consciousness of any duration with death due to brain injury prior to regaining consciousness**
MCC Exclusion 7th character A see Appendix
PDX collection 1154
HAC 7th character A see Appendix B for HAC conditional logic

MCC +7th **S06.388 Contusion, laceration, and hemorrhage of brainstem with loss of consciousness of any duration with death due to other cause prior to regaining consciousness**
MCC Exclusion 7th character A see Appendix A
PDX collection 1154
HAC 7th character A see Appendix B for HAC conditional logic

CC +7th **S06.389 Contusion, laceration, and hemorrhage of brainstem with loss of consciousness of unspecified duration**
Contusion, laceration, and hemorrhage of brainstem NOS
CC Exclusion 7th character A see Appendix A
PDX collection 1154
HAC 7th character A see Appendix B for HAC conditional logic

+ **S06.4 Epidural hemorrhage**
Extradural hemorrhage NOS
Extradural hemorrhage (traumatic)

+ **S06.4X Epidural hemorrhage**

MCC +7th **S06.4X0 Epidural hemorrhage without loss of consciousness**
MCC Exclusion 7th character A see Appendix A
PDX collection 1154
HAC 7th character A see Appendix B for HAC conditional logic

MCC +7th **S06.4X1 Epidural hemorrhage with loss of consciousness of 30 minutes or less**
MCC Exclusion 7th character A see Appendix A
PDX collection 1154
HAC 7th character A see Appendix B for HAC conditional logic

MCC +7th **S06.4X2 Epidural hemorrhage with loss of consciousness of 31 minutes to 59 minutes**
MCC Exclusion 7th character A see Appendix A
PDX collection 1154
HAC 7th character A see Appendix B for HAC conditional logic

MCC +7th **S06.4X3 Epidural hemorrhage with loss of consciousness of 1 hour to 5 hours 59 minutes**
MCC Exclusion 7th character A see Appendix A
PDX collection 1154
HAC 7th character A see Appendix B for HAC conditional logic

MCC +7th **S06.4X4 Epidural hemorrhage with loss of consciousness of 6 hours to 24 hours**
MCC Exclusion 7th character A see Appendix A
PDX collection 1154
HAC 7th character A see Appendix B for HAC conditional logic

MCC +7th **S06.4X5 Epidural hemorrhage with loss of consciousness greater than 24 hours with return to pre-existing conscious level**
MCC Exclusion 7th character A see Appendix A
PDX collection 1154
HAC 7th character A see Appendix B for HAC conditional logic

MCC +7th **S06.4X6 Epidural hemorrhage with loss of consciousness greater than 24 hours without return to pre-existing conscious level with patient surviving**
MCC Exclusion 7th character A see Appendix A
PDX collection 1154
HAC 7th character A see Appendix B for HAC conditional logic

MCC +7th **S06.4X7 Epidural hemorrhage with loss of consciousness of any duration with death due to brain injury prior to regaining consciousness**
MCC Exclusion 7th character A see Appendix A
PDX collection 1154
HAC 7th character A see Appendix B for HAC conditional logic

MCC +7th **S06.4X8 Epidural hemorrhage with loss of consciousness of any duration with death due to other causes prior to regaining consciousness**
MCC Exclusion 7th character A see Appendix A
PDX collection 1154
HAC 7th character A see Appendix B for HAC conditional logic

MCC +7th **S06.4X9 Epidural hemorrhage with loss of consciousness of unspecified duration**
Epidural hemorrhage NOS
MCC Exclusion 7th character A see Appendix A
PDX collection 1154
HAC 7th character A see Appendix B for HAC conditional logic

+ **S06.5 Traumatic subdural hemorrhage**

+ **S06.5X Traumatic subdural hemorrhage**

MCC +7th **S06.5X0 Traumatic subdural hemorrhage without loss of consciousness**
MCC Exclusion 7th character A see Appendix A
PDX collection 1154
HAC 7th character A see Appendix B for HAC conditional logic
AHA CC: 3Q, 2015, 37

MCC +7th **S06.5X1 Traumatic subdural hemorrhage with loss of consciousness of 30 minutes or less**
MCC Exclusion 7th character A see Appendix A
PDX collection 1154
HAC 7th character A see Appendix B for HAC conditional logic

MCC +7th **S06.5X2 Traumatic subdural hemorrhage with loss of consciousness of 31 minutes to 59 minutes**
MCC Exclusion 7th character A see Appendix A
PDX collection 1154
HAC 7th character A see Appendix B for HAC conditional logic

MCC +7th **S06.5X3 Traumatic subdural hemorrhage with loss of consciousness of 1 hour to 5 hours 59 minutes**
MCC Exclusion 7th character A see Appendix A
PDX collection 1154
HAC 7th character A see Appendix B for HAC conditional logic

MCC +7th **S06.5X4 Traumatic subdural hemorrhage with loss of consciousness of 6 hours to 24 hours**
MCC Exclusion 7th character A see Appendix A
PDX collection 1154
HAC 7th character A see Appendix B for HAC conditional logic

MCC +7th **S06.5X5 Traumatic subdural hemorrhage with loss of consciousness greater than 24 hours with return to pre-existing conscious level**
MCC Exclusion 7th character A see Appendix A
PDX collection 1154
HAC 7th character A see Appendix B for HAC conditional logic

MCC +7th **S06.5X6 Traumatic subdural hemorrhage with loss of consciousness greater than 24 hours without return to pre-existing conscious level with patient surviving**
MCC Exclusion 7th character A see Appendix A
PDX collection 1154
HAC 7th character A see Appendix B for HAC conditional logic

MCC +7th **S06.5X7 Traumatic subdural hemorrhage with loss of consciousness of any duration with death due to brain injury before regaining consciousness**
MCC Exclusion 7th character A see Appendix A
PDX collection 1154
HAC 7th character A see Appendix B for HAC conditional logic

MCC +7th **S06.5X8 Traumatic subdural hemorrhage with loss of consciousness of any duration with death due to other cause before regaining consciousness**
MCC Exclusion 7th character A see Appendix A
PDX collection 1154
HAC 7th character A see Appendix B for HAC conditional logic

MCC +7th **S06.5X9 Traumatic subdural hemorrhage with loss of consciousness of unspecified duration**
Traumatic subdural hemorrhage NOS
MCC Exclusion 7th character A see Appendix A
PDX collection 1154
HAC 7th character A see Appendix B for HAC conditional logic

+ **S06.6 Traumatic subarachnoid hemorrhage**

+ **S06.6X Traumatic subarachnoid hemorrhage**

MCC +7th **S06.6X0 Traumatic subarachnoid hemorrhage without loss of consciousness**
MCC Exclusion 7th character A see Appendix A
PDX collection 1154
HAC 7th character A see Appendix B for HAC conditional logic
AHA CC: 3Q, 2015, 37

MCC +7th **S06.6X1** **Traumatic subarachnoid hemorrhage with loss of consciousness of 30 minutes or less**
MCC Exclusion 7th character A see Appendix A
PDX collection 1154
HAC 7th character A see Appendix B for HAC conditional logic

MCC +7th **S06.6X2** **Traumatic subarachnoid hemorrhage with loss of consciousness of 31 minutes to 59 minutes**
MCC Exclusion 7th character A see Appendix A
PDX collection 1154
HAC 7th character A see Appendix B for HAC conditional logic

MCC +7th **S06.6X3** **Traumatic subarachnoid hemorrhage with loss of consciousness of 1 hour to 5 hours 59 minutes**
MCC Exclusion 7th character A see Appendix A
PDX collection 1154
HAC 7th character A see Appendix B for HAC conditional logic

MCC +7th **S06.6X4** **Traumatic subarachnoid hemorrhage with loss of consciousness of 6 hours to 24 hours**
MCC Exclusion 7th character A see Appendix A
PDX collection 1154
HAC 7th character A see Appendix B for HAC conditional logic

MCC +7th **S06.6X5** **Traumatic subarachnoid hemorrhage with loss of consciousness greater than 24 hours with return to pre-existing conscious level**
MCC Exclusion 7th character A see Appendix A
PDX collection 1154
HAC 7th character A see Appendix B for HAC conditional logic

MCC +7th **S06.6X6** **Traumatic subarachnoid hemorrhage with loss of consciousness greater than 24 hours without return to pre-existing conscious level with patient surviving**
MCC Exclusion 7th character A see Appendix A
PDX collection 1154
HAC 7th character A see Appendix B for HAC conditional logic

MCC +7th **S06.6X7** **Traumatic subarachnoid hemorrhage with loss of consciousness of any duration with death due to brain injury prior to regaining consciousness**
MCC Exclusion 7th character A see Appendix A
PDX collection 1154
HAC 7th character A see Appendix B for HAC conditional logic

MCC +7th **S06.6X8** **Traumatic subarachnoid hemorrhage with loss of consciousness of any duration with death due to other cause prior to regaining consciousness**
MCC Exclusion 7th character A see Appendix A
PDX collection 1154
HAC 7th character A see Appendix B for HAC conditional logic

MCC +7th **S06.6X9** **Traumatic subarachnoid hemorrhage with loss of consciousness of unspecified duration**
Traumatic subarachnoid hemorrhage NOS
MCC Exclusion 7th character A see Appendix A
PDX collection 1154
HAC 7th character A see Appendix B for HAC conditional logic

+ S06.8 Other specified intracranial injuries

+ S06.81 Injury of right internal carotid artery, intracranial portion, not elsewhere classified

+7th **S06.810** **Injury of right internal carotid artery, intracranial portion, not elsewhere classified without loss of consciousness**

CC +7th **S06.811** **Injury of right internal carotid artery, intracranial portion, not elsewhere classified with loss of consciousness of 30 minutes or less**
CC Exclusion 7th character A see Appendix A
PDX collection 1154
HAC 7th character A see Appendix B for HAC conditional logic

CC +7th **S06.812** **Injury of right internal carotid artery, intracranial portion, not elsewhere classified with loss of consciousness of 31 minutes to 59 minutes**
CC Exclusion 7th character A see Appendix A
PDX collection 1154
HAC 7th character A see Appendix B for HAC conditional logic

CC +7th **S06.813** **Injury of right internal carotid artery, intracranial portion, not elsewhere classified with loss of consciousness of 1 hour to 5 hours 59 minutes**
CC Exclusion 7th character A see Appendix A
PDX collection 1154
HAC 7th character A see Appendix B for HAC conditional logic

CC +7th **S06.814** **Injury of right internal carotid artery, intracranial portion, not elsewhere classified with loss of consciousness of 6 hours to 24 hours**
CC Exclusion 7th character A see Appendix A
PDX collection 1154
HAC 7th character A see Appendix B for HAC conditional logic

CC +7th **S06.815** **Injury of right internal carotid artery, intracranial portion, not elsewhere classified with loss of consciousness greater than 24 hours with return to pre-existing conscious level**
CC Exclusion 7th character A see Appendix A
PDX collection 1154
HAC 7th character A see Appendix B for HAC conditional logic

MCC +7th **S06.816** **Injury of right internal carotid artery, intracranial portion, not elsewhere classified with loss of consciousness greater than 24 hours without return to pre-existing conscious level with patient surviving**
MCC Exclusion 7th character A see Appendix
PDX collection 1154
HAC 7th character A see Appendix B for HAC conditional logic

MCC +7th **S06.817** **Injury of right internal carotid artery, intracranial portion, not elsewhere classified with loss of consciousness of any duration with death due to brain injury prior to regaining consciousness**
MCC Exclusion 7th character A see Appendix
PDX collection 1154
HAC 7th character A see Appendix B for HAC conditional logic

MCC +7th **S06.818** **Injury of right internal carotid artery, intracranial portion, not elsewhere classified with loss of consciousness of any duration with death due to other cause prior to regaining consciousness**
MCC Exclusion 7th character A see Appendix
PDX collection 1154
HAC 7th character A see Appendix B for HAC conditional logic

CC +7th **S06.819** **Injury of right internal carotid artery, intracranial portion, not elsewhere classified with loss of consciousness of unspecified duration**
Injury of right internal carotid artery, intracranial portion, not elsewhere classified NOS
CC Exclusion 7th character A see Appendix A
PDX collection 1154
HAC 7th character A see Appendix B for HAC conditional logic

+ S06.82 Injury of left internal carotid artery, intracranial portion, not elsewhere classified

+7th **S06.820** **Injury of left internal carotid artery, intracranial portion, not elsewhere classified without loss of consciousness**

CC +7th **S06.821** **Injury of left internal carotid artery, intracranial portion, not elsewhere classified with loss of consciousness of 30 minutes or less**
CC Exclusion 7th character A see Appendix A
PDX collection 1154
HAC 7th character A see Appendix B for HAC conditional logic

CC +7th **S06.822** **Injury of left internal carotid artery, intracranial portion, not elsewhere classified with loss of consciousness of 31 minutes to 59 minutes**
CC Exclusion 7th character A see Appendix A
PDX collection 1154
HAC 7th character A see Appendix B for HAC conditional logic

CC +7th **S06.823** **Injury of left internal carotid artery, intracranial portion, not elsewhere classified with loss of consciousness of 1 hour to 5 hours 59 minutes**
CC Exclusion 7th character A see Appendix A PDX collection 1154
HAC 7th character A see Appendix B for HAC conditional logic

CC +7th **S06.824** **Injury of left internal carotid artery, intracranial portion, not elsewhere classified with loss of consciousness of 6 hours to 24 hours**
CC Exclusion 7th character A see Appendix A PDX collection 1154
HAC 7th character A see Appendix B for HAC conditional logic

CC +7th **S06.825** **Injury of left internal carotid artery, intracranial portion, not elsewhere classified with loss of consciousness greater than 24 hours with return to pre-existing conscious level**
CC Exclusion 7th character A see Appendix A PDX collection 1154
HAC 7th character A see Appendix B for HAC conditional logic

MCC +7th **S06.826** **Injury of left internal carotid artery, intracranial portion, not elsewhere classified with loss of consciousness greater than 24 hours without return to pre-existing conscious level with patient surviving**
MCC Exclusion 7th character A see Appendix A PDX collection 1154
HAC 7th character A see Appendix B for HAC conditional logic

MCC +7th **S06.827** **Injury of left internal carotid artery, intracranial portion, not elsewhere classified with loss of consciousness of any duration with death due to brain injury prior to regaining consciousness**
MCC Exclusion 7th character A see Appendix A PDX collection 1154
HAC 7th character A see Appendix B for HAC conditional logic

MCC +7th **S06.828** **Injury of left internal carotid artery, intracranial portion, not elsewhere classified with loss of consciousness of any duration with death due to other cause prior to regaining consciousness**
MCC Exclusion 7th character A see Appendix A PDX collection 1154
HAC 7th character A see Appendix B for HAC conditional logic

CC +7th **S06.829** **Injury of left internal carotid artery, intracranial portion, not elsewhere classified with loss of consciousness of unspecified duration**
Injury of left internal carotid artery, intracranial portion, not elsewhere classified NOS
CC Exclusion 7th character A see Appendix A PDX collection 1154
HAC 7th character A see Appendix B for HAC conditional logic

\+ **S06.89** **Other specified intracranial injury**
Excludes1: *concussion (S06.0X-)*

+7th **S06.890** **Other specified intracranial injury without loss of consciousness**

CC +7th **S06.891** **Other specified intracranial injury with loss of consciousness of 30 minutes or less**
CC Exclusion 7th character A see Appendix A PDX collection 1154
HAC 7th character A see Appendix B for HAC conditional logic

CC +7th **S06.892** **Other specified intracranial injury with loss of consciousness of 31 minutes to 59 minutes**
CC Exclusion 7th character A see Appendix A PDX collection 1154
HAC 7th character A see Appendix B for HAC conditional logic

CC +7th **S06.893** **Other specified intracranial injury with loss of consciousness of 1 hour to 5 hours 59 minutes**
CC Exclusion 7th character A see Appendix A PDX collection 1154
HAC 7th character A see Appendix B for HAC conditional logic

CC +7th **S06.894** **Other specified intracranial injury with loss of consciousness of 6 hours to 24 hours**
CC Exclusion 7th character A see Appendix A PDX collection 1154
HAC 7th character A see Appendix B for HAC conditional logic

CC +7th **S06.895** **Other specified intracranial injury with loss of consciousness greater than 24 hours with return to pre-existing conscious level**
CC Exclusion 7th character A see Appendix A PDX collection 1154
HAC 7th character A see Appendix B for HAC conditional logic

MCC +7th **S06.896** **Other specified intracranial injury with loss of consciousness greater than 24 hours without return to pre-existing conscious level with patient surviving**
MCC Exclusion 7th character A see Appendix A PDX collection 1154
HAC 7th character A see Appendix B for HAC conditional logic

MCC +7th **S06.897** **Other specified intracranial injury with loss of consciousness of any duration with death due to brain injury prior to regaining consciousness**
MCC Exclusion 7th character A see Appendix A PDX collection 1154
HAC 7th character A see Appendix B for HAC conditional logic

MCC +7th **S06.898** **Other specified intracranial injury with loss of consciousness of any duration with death due to other cause prior to regaining consciousness**
MCC Exclusion 7th character A see Appendix A PDX collection 1154
HAC 7th character A see Appendix B for HAC conditional logic

CC +7th **S06.899** **Other specified intracranial injury with loss of consciousness of unspecified duration**
CC Exclusion 7th character A see Appendix A PDX collection 1154
HAC 7th character A see Appendix B for HAC conditional logic

CC + **S06.9** **Unspecified intracranial injury**
Brain injury NOS
Head injury NOS with loss of consciousness
Traumatic brain injury NOS
Excludes1: *conditions classifiable to S06.0- to S06.8- code to specified intracranial injury*
head injury NOS (S09.90)
CC Exclusion 7th character A see Appendix A PDX collection 1154

\+ **S06.9X** **Unspecified intracranial injury**

+7th **S06.9X0** **Unspecified intracranial injury without loss of consciousness**
HAC 7th character A see Appendix B for HAC conditional logic

+7th **S06.9X1** **Unspecified intracranial injury with loss of consciousness of 30 minutes or less**
HAC 7th character A see Appendix B for HAC conditional logic

+7th **S06.9X2** **Unspecified intracranial injury with loss of consciousness of 31 minutes to 59 minutes**
HAC 7th character A see Appendix B for HAC conditional logic

+7th **S06.9X3** **Unspecified intracranial injury with loss of consciousness of 1 hour to 5 hours 59 minutes**
HAC 7th character A see Appendix B for HAC conditional logic

+7th **S06.9X4** **Unspecified intracranial injury with loss of consciousness of 6 hours to 24 hours**
HAC 7th character A see Appendix B for HAC conditional logic

+7th **S06.9X5** **Unspecified intracranial injury with loss of consciousness greater than 24 hours with return to pre-existing conscious level**
HAC 7th character A see Appendix B for HAC conditional logic

MCC +7th **S06.9X6** **Unspecified intracranial injury with loss of consciousness greater than 24 hours without return to pre-existing conscious level with patient surviving**
MCC Exclusion 7th character A see Appendix A PDX collection 1154
HAC 7th character A see Appendix B for HAC conditional logic

MCC +7th **S06.9X7** **Unspecified intracranial injury with loss of consciousness of any duration with death due to brain injury prior to regaining consciousness**
MCC Exclusion 7th character A see Appendix A PDX collection 1154
HAC 7th character A see Appendix B for HAC conditional logic

MCC +7th **S06.9X8** **Unspecified intracranial injury with loss of consciousness of any duration with death due to other cause prior to regaining consciousness**
MCC Exclusion 7th character A see Appendix A PDX collection 1154
HAC 7th character A see Appendix B for HAC conditional logic

+7th **S06.9X9** **Unspecified intracranial injury with loss of consciousness of unspecified duration**
HAC 7th character A see Appendix B for HAC conditional logic

S07 Crushing injury of head

Use additional code for all associated injuries, such as:
intracranial injuries (S06.-)
skull fractures (S02.-)

The appropriate 7th character is to be added to each code from category S07
A initial encounter
D subsequent encounter
S sequela

CC X+7th **S07.0** **Crushing injury of face**
CC Exclusion 7th character A see Appendix A PDX collection 1156
HAC 7th character A see Appendix B for HAC conditional logic

CC X+7th **S07.1** **Crushing injury of skull**
CC Exclusion 7th character A see Appendix A PDX collection 1156
HAC 7th character A see Appendix B for HAC conditional logic

CC X+7th **S07.8** **Crushing injury of other parts of head**
CC Exclusion 7th character A see Appendix A PDX collection 1156
HAC 7th character A see Appendix B for HAC conditional logic

CC X+7th **S07.9** **Crushing injury of head, part unspecified**
CC Exclusion 7th character A see Appendix A PDX collection 1156
HAC 7th character A see Appendix B for HAC conditional logic

S08 Avulsion and traumatic amputation of part of head

An amputation not identified as partial or complete should be coded to complete

The appropriate 7th character is to be added to each code from category S08
A initial encounter
D subsequent encounter
S sequela

X+7th **S08.0** **Avulsion of scalp**
\+ **S08.1** **Traumatic amputation of ear**
\+ **S08.11** **Complete traumatic amputation of ear**
+7th **S08.111** **Complete traumatic amputation of right ear**
+7th **S08.112** **Complete traumatic amputation of left ear**
+7th **S08.119** **Complete traumatic amputation of unspecified ear**
\+ **S08.12** **Partial traumatic amputation of ear**
+7th **S08.121** **Partial traumatic amputation of right ear**
+7th **S08.122** **Partial traumatic amputation of left ear**
+7th **S08.129** **Partial traumatic amputation of unspecified ear**
\+ **S08.8** **Traumatic amputation of other parts of head**
\+ **S08.81** **Traumatic amputation of nose**
+7th **S08.811** **Complete traumatic amputation of nose**
+7th **S08.812** **Partial traumatic amputation of nose**
X+7th **S08.89** **Traumatic amputation of other parts of head**

S09 Other and unspecified injuries of head

The appropriate 7th character is to be added to each code from category S09
A initial encounter
D subsequent encounter
S sequela

CC X+7th **S09.0** **Injury of blood vessels of head, not elsewhere classified**
Excludes1: *injury of cerebral blood vessels (S06.-)*
injury of precerebral blood vessels (S15.-)
CC Exclusion 7th character A see Appendix A PDX collection 1157

\+ **S09.1** **Injury of muscle and tendon of head**
Code also any associated open wound (S01.-)
Excludes2: *sprain to joints and ligament of head (S03.9)*
X+7th **S09.10** **Unspecified injury of muscle and tendon of head**
Injury of muscle and tendon of head NOS
X+7th **S09.11** **Strain of muscle and tendon of head**
X+7th **S09.12** **Laceration of muscle and tendon of head**
X+7th **S09.19** **Other specified injury of muscle and tendon of hea**

\+ **S09.2** **Traumatic rupture of ear drum**
Excludes1: *traumatic rupture of ear drum due to blast injury (S09.31-)*
CC X+7th **S09.20** **Traumatic rupture of unspecified ear drum**
CC Exclusion 7th character A see Appendix A PDX collection 1158
CC X+7th **S09.21** **Traumatic rupture of right ear drum**
CC Exclusion 7th character A see Appendix A PDX collection 1158
CC X+7th **S09.22** **Traumatic rupture of left ear drum**
CC Exclusion 7th character A see Appendix A PDX collection 1158

\+ **S09.3** **Other specified and unspecified injury of middle and inner ea**
Excludes1: *injury to ear NOS (S09.91-)*
Excludes2: *injury to external ear (S00.4-, S01.3-, S08.1-)*
\+ **S09.30** **Unspecified injury of middle and inner ear**
CC +7th **S09.301** **Unspecified injury of right middle and inner ear**
CC Exclusion 7th character A see Appendix A PDX collection 1158
CC +7th **S09.302** **Unspecified injury of left middle and inne ear**
CC Exclusion 7th character A see Appendix A PDX collection 1158
CC +7th **S09.309** **Unspecified injury of unspecified middle and inner ear**
CC Exclusion 7th character A see Appendix A PDX collection 1158
\+ **S09.31** **Primary blast injury of ear**
Blast injury of ear NOS
CC +7th **S09.311** **Primary blast injury of right ear**
CC Exclusion 7th character A see Appendix A PDX collection 1158
CC +7th **S09.312** **Primary blast injury of left ear**
CC Exclusion 7th character A see Appendix A PDX collection 1158
CC +7th **S09.313** **Primary blast injury of ear, bilateral**
CC Exclusion 7th character A see Appendix A PDX collection 1158
CC +7th **S09.319** **Primary blast injury of unspecified ear**
CC Exclusion 7th character A see Appendix A PDX collection 1158
\+ **S09.39** **Other specified injury of middle and inner ear**
Secondary blast injury to ear
CC +7th **S09.391** **Other specified injury of right middle an inner ear**
CC Exclusion 7th character A see Appendix A PDX collection 1158
CC +7th **S09.392** **Other specified injury of left middle and inner ear**
CC Exclusion 7th character A see Appendix A PDX collection 1158
CC +7th **S09.399** **Other specified injury of unspecified middle and inner ear**
CC Exclusion 7th character A see Appendix A PDX collection 1158

X+7th **S09.8** **Other specified injuries of head**
\+ **S09.9** **Unspecified injury of face and head**
X+7th **S09.90** **Unspecified injury of head**
Head injury NOS
Excludes1: *brain injury NOS (S06.9-)*
head injury NOS with loss of consciousness (S06.9-)
intracranial injury NOS (S06.9-)

X+7th **S09.91 Unspecified injury of ear**
Injury of ear NOS

X+7th **S09.92 Unspecified injury of nose**
Injury of nose NOS

X+7th **S09.93 Unspecified injury of face**
Injury of face NOS

Injuries to the neck (S10-S19)

Includes: injuries of nape
injuries of supraclavicular region
injuries of throat

Excludes2: *burns and corrosions (T20-T32)*
effects of foreign body in esophagus (T18.1)
effects of foreign body in larynx (T17.3)
effects of foreign body in pharynx (T17.2)
effects of foreign body in trachea (T17.4)
frostbite (T33-T34)
insect bite or sting, venomous (T63.4)

S10 Superficial injury of neck

The appropriate 7th character is to be added to each code from category S10
A initial encounter
D subsequent encounter
S sequela

X+7th **S10.0 Contusion of throat**
Contusion of cervical esophagus
Contusion of larynx
Contusion of pharynx
Contusion of trachea

\+ **S10.1 Other and unspecified superficial injuries of throat**

X+7th **S10.10 Unspecified superficial injuries of throat**

X+7th **S10.11 Abrasion of throat**

X+7th **S10.12 Blister (nonthermal) of throat**

X+7th **S10.14 External constriction of part of throat**

X+7th **S10.15 Superficial foreign body of throat**
Splinter in the throat

X+7th **S10.16 Insect bite (nonvenomous) of throat**

X+7th **S10.17 Other superficial bite of throat**
Excludes1: *open bite of throat (S11.85)*

\+ **S10.8 Superficial injury of other specified parts of neck**

X+7th **S10.80 Unspecified superficial injury of other specified part of neck**

X+7th **S10.81 Abrasion of other specified part of neck**

X+7th **S10.82 Blister (nonthermal) of other specified part of neck**

X+7th **S10.83 Contusion of other specified part of neck**

X+7th **S10.84 External constriction of other specified part of neck**

X+7th **S10.85 Superficial foreign body of other specified part of neck**
Splinter in other specified part of neck

X+7th **S10.86 Insect bite of other specified part of neck**

X+7th **S10.87 Other superficial bite of other specified part of neck**
Excludes1: *open bite of other specified parts of neck (S11.85)*

\+ **S10.9 Superficial injury of unspecified part of neck**

X+7th **S10.90 Unspecified superficial injury of unspecified part of neck**

X+7th **S10.91 Abrasion of unspecified part of neck**

X+7th **S10.92 Blister (nonthermal) of unspecified part of neck**

X+7th **S10.93 Contusion of unspecified part of neck**

X+7th **S10.94 External constriction of unspecified part of neck**

X+7th **S10.95 Superficial foreign body of unspecified part of neck**

X+7th **S10.96 Insect bite of unspecified part of neck**

X+7th **S10.97 Other superficial bite of unspecified part of neck**

Vertebrae

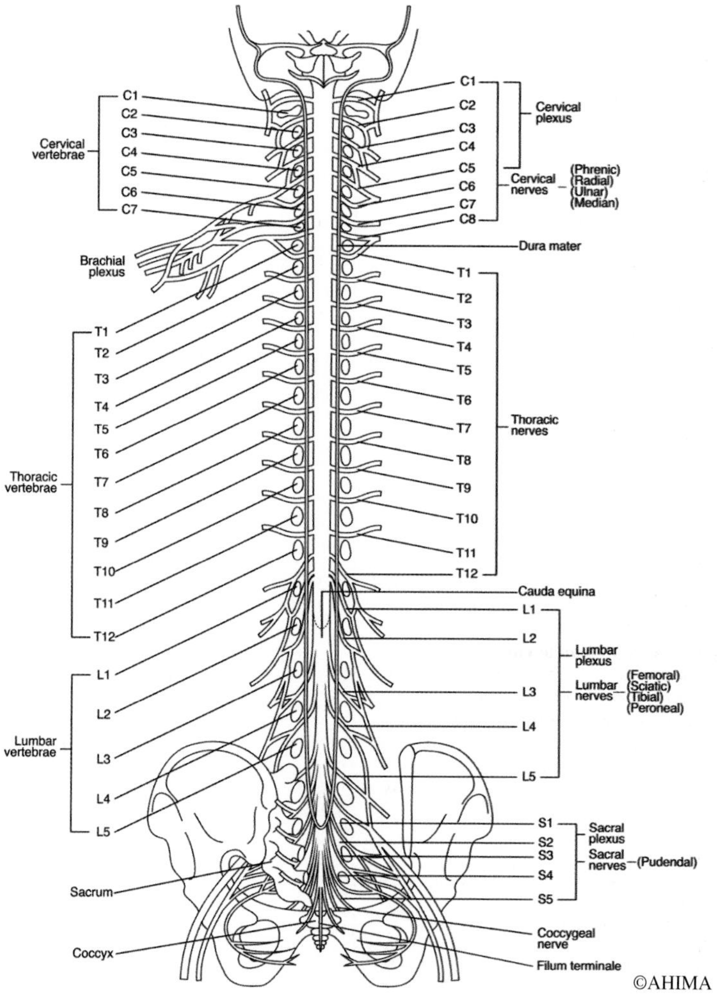

©AHIMA

S11 Open wound of neck

Code also any associated:
spinal cord injury (S14.0, S14.1-)
wound infection

Excludes2: *open fracture of vertebra (S12.- with 7th character B)*

The appropriate 7th character is to be added to each code from category S11
A initial encounter
D subsequent encounter
S sequela

+ **S11.0 Open wound of larynx and trachea**

+ **S11.01 Open wound of larynx**
Excludes2: *open wound of vocal cord (S11.03)*

MCC +7th **S11.011 Laceration without foreign body of larynx**
MCC Exclusion 7th character A see Appendix A PDX collection 1159

MCC +7th **S11.012 Laceration with foreign body of larynx**
MCC Exclusion 7th character A see Appendix A PDX collection 1159

MCC +7th **S11.013 Puncture wound without foreign body of larynx**
MCC Exclusion 7th character A see Appendix A PDX collection 1159

MCC +7th **S11.014 Puncture wound with foreign body of larynx**
MCC Exclusion 7th character A see Appendix A PDX collection 1159

MCC +7th **S11.015 Open bite of larynx**
Bite of larynx NOS
MCC Exclusion 7th character A see Appendix A PDX collection 1159

MCC +7th **S11.019 Unspecified open wound of larynx**
MCC Exclusion 7th character A see Appendix A PDX collection 1159

+ **S11.02 Open wound of trachea**
Open wound of cervical trachea
Open wound of trachea NOS
Excludes2: *open wound of thoracic trachea (S27.5-)*

MCC +7th **S11.021 Laceration without foreign body of trachea**
MCC Exclusion 7th character A see Appendix A PDX collection 1159

MCC +7th **S11.022 Laceration with foreign body of trachea**
MCC Exclusion 7th character A see Appendix A PDX collection 1159

MCC +7th **S11.023 Puncture wound without foreign body of trachea**
MCC Exclusion 7th character A see Appendix A PDX collection 1159

MCC +7th **S11.024 Puncture wound with foreign body of trachea**
MCC Exclusion 7th character A see Appendix A PDX collection 1159

MCC +7th **S11.025 Open bite of trachea**
Bite of trachea NOS
MCC Exclusion 7th character A see Appendix A PDX collection 1159

MCC +7th **S11.029 Unspecified open wound of trachea**
MCC Exclusion 7th character A see Appendix A PDX collection 1159

+ **S11.03 Open wound of vocal cord**

MCC +7th **S11.031 Laceration without foreign body of vocal cord**
MCC Exclusion 7th character A see Appendix A PDX collection 1159

MCC +7th **S11.032 Laceration with foreign body of vocal cord**
MCC Exclusion 7th character A see Appendix A PDX collection 1159

MCC +7th **S11.033 Puncture wound without foreign body of vocal cord**
MCC Exclusion 7th character A see Appendix A PDX collection 1159

MCC +7th **S11.034 Puncture wound with foreign body of vocal cord**
MCC Exclusion 7th character A see Appendix A PDX collection 1159

MCC +7th **S11.035 Open bite of vocal cord**
Bite of vocal cord NOS
MCC Exclusion 7th character A see Appendix A PDX collection 1159

MCC +7th **S11.039 Unspecified open wound of vocal cord**
MCC Exclusion 7th character A see Appendix A PDX collection 1159

+ **S11.1 Open wound of thyroid gland**

CC X+7th **S11.10 Unspecified open wound of thyroid gland**
CC Exclusion 7th character A see Appendix A PDX collection 1160

CC X+7th **S11.11 Laceration without foreign body of thyroid gland**
CC Exclusion 7th character A see Appendix A PDX collection 1160

CC X+7th **S11.12 Laceration with foreign body of thyroid gland**
CC Exclusion 7th character A see Appendix A PDX collection 1161

CC X+7th **S11.13 Puncture wound without foreign body of thyroid gland**
CC Exclusion 7th character A see Appendix A PDX collection 1160

CC X+7th **S11.14 Puncture wound with foreign body of thyroid gland**
CC Exclusion 7th character A see Appendix A PDX collection 1161

CC X+7th **S11.15 Open bite of thyroid gland**
Bite of thyroid gland NOS
CC Exclusion 7th character A see Appendix A PDX collection 1160

+ **S11.2 Open wound of pharynx and cervical esophagus**
Excludes1: *open wound of esophagus NOS (S27.8-)*

CC X+7th **S11.20 Unspecified open wound of pharynx and cervical esophagus**
CC Exclusion 7th character A see Appendix A PDX collection 1162

CC X+7th **S11.21 Laceration without foreign body of pharynx and cervical esophagus**
CC Exclusion 7th character A see Appendix A PDX collection 1162

CC X+7th **S11.22 Laceration with foreign body of pharynx and cervical esophagus**
CC Exclusion 7th character A see Appendix A PDX collection 1163

CC X+7th **S11.23 Puncture wound without foreign body of pharynx and cervical esophagus**
CC Exclusion 7th character A see Appendix A PDX collection 1162

CC X+7th **S11.24 Puncture wound with foreign body of pharynx and cervical esophagus**
CC Exclusion 7th character A see Appendix A PDX collection 1163

CC X+7th **S11.25 Open bite of pharynx and cervical esophagus**
Bite of pharynx and cervical esophagus NOS
CC Exclusion 7th character A see Appendix A PDX collection 1162

+ **S11.8 Open wound of other specified parts of neck**

X+7th **S11.80 Unspecified open wound of other specified part of neck**

X+7th **S11.81 Laceration without foreign body of other specified part of neck**

X+7th **S11.82 Laceration with foreign body of other specified part of neck**

X+7th **S11.83 Puncture wound without foreign body of other specified part of neck**

X+7th **S11.84 Puncture wound with foreign body of other specified part of neck**

X+7th **S11.85 Open bite of other specified part of neck**
Bite of other specified part of neck NOS
Excludes1: *superficial bite of other specified part of neck (S10.87)*

S11.89 Other open wound of other specified part of neck

+ **S11.9 Open wound of unspecified part of neck**

X+7th **S11.90 Unspecified open wound of unspecified part of neck**

X+7th **S11.91 Laceration without foreign body of unspecified part of neck**

X+7th **S11.92 Laceration with foreign body of unspecified part of neck**

X+7th **S11.93 Puncture wound without foreign body of unspecified part of neck**

X+7th **S11.94 Puncture wound with foreign body of unspecified part of neck**

X+7th **S11.95 Open bite of unspecified part of neck**
Bite of neck NOS
Excludes1: *superficial bite of neck (S10.97)*

S12 Fracture of cervical vertebra and other parts of neck

NOTE A fracture not indicated as displaced or nondisplaced should be coded to displaced

A fracture not indicated as open or closed should be coded to closed

Includes: fracture of cervical neural arch
fracture of cervical spine
fracture of cervical spinous process
fracture of cervical transverse process
fracture of cervical vertebral arch
fracture of neck

Code first any associated cervical spinal cord injury (S14.0, S14.1-)

The appropriate 7th character is to be added to all codes from subcategories **S12.0-S12.6**
- A initial encounter for closed fracture
- B initial encounter for open fracture
- D subsequent encounter for fracture with routine healing
- G subsequent encounter for fracture with delayed healing
- K subsequent encounter for fracture with nonunion
- S sequela

Review coding guideline C.19.c

+ **S12.0 Fracture of first cervical vertebra**
Atlas

+ **S12.00 Unspecified fracture of first cervical vertebra**

CC MCC +7th **S12.000 Unspecified displaced fracture of first cervical vertebra**
CC Exclusion 7th character A see Appendix A PDX collection 1164
CC Exclusion 7th character K see Appendix A PDX collection 0897
MCC Exclusion 7th character B see Appendix A PDX collection 1164
HAC 7th characters A & B see Appendix B for HAC conditional logic

CC MCC +7th **S12.001 Unspecified nondisplaced fracture of first cervical vertebra**
CC Exclusion 7th character A see Appendix A PDX collection 1164
CC Exclusion 7th character K see Appendix A PDX collection 0897
MCC Exclusion 7th character B see Appendix A PDX collection 1164
HAC 7th characters A & B see Appendix B for HAC conditional logic

CC MCC X+7th **S12.01 Stable burst fracture of first cervical vertebra**
CC Exclusion 7th character A see Appendix A PDX collection 1164
CC Exclusion 7th character K see Appendix A PDX collection 0897
MCC Exclusion 7th character B see Appendix A PDX collection 1164
HAC 7th characters A & B see Appendix B for HAC conditional logic

CC MCC X+7th **S12.02 Unstable burst fracture of first cervical vertebra**
CC Exclusion 7th character A see Appendix A PDX collection 1164
CC Exclusion 7th character K see Appendix A PDX collection 0897
MCC Exclusion 7th character B see Appendix A PDX collection 1164
HAC 7th characters A & B see Appendix B for HAC conditional logic

+ **S12.03 Posterior arch fracture of first cervical vertebra**

CC MCC +7th **S12.030 Displaced posterior arch fracture of first cervical vertebra**
CC Exclusion 7th character A see Appendix A PDX collection 1164
CC Exclusion 7th character K see Appendix A PDX collection 0897
MCC Exclusion 7th character B see Appendix A PDX collection 1164
HAC 7th characters A & B see Appendix B for HAC conditional logic

CC MCC +7th **S12.031 Nondisplaced posterior arch fracture of first cervical vertebra**
CC Exclusion 7th character A see Appendix A PDX collection 1164
CC Exclusion 7th character K see Appendix A PDX collection 0897
MCC Exclusion 7th character B see Appendix A PDX collection 1164
HAC 7th characters A & B see Appendix B for HAC conditional logic

+ **S12.04 Lateral mass fracture of first cervical vertebra**

CC MCC +7th **S12.040 Displaced lateral mass fracture of first cervical vertebra**
CC Exclusion 7th character A see Appendix A PDX collection 1164
CC Exclusion 7th character K see Appendix A PDX collection 0897
MCC Exclusion 7th character B see Appendix A PDX collection 1164
HAC 7th characters A & B see Appendix B for HAC conditional logic

CC MCC +7th **S12.041 Nondisplaced lateral mass fracture of first cervical vertebra**
CC Exclusion 7th character A see Appendix A PDX collection 1164
CC Exclusion 7th character K see Appendix A PDX collection 0897
MCC Exclusion 7th character B see Appendix A PDX collection 1164
HAC 7th characters A & B see Appendix B for HAC conditional logic

+ **S12.09 Other fracture of first cervical vertebra**

CC MCC +7th **S12.090 Other displaced fracture of first cervical vertebra**
CC Exclusion 7th character A see Appendix A PDX collection 1164
CC Exclusion 7th character K see Appendix A PDX collection 0897
MCC Exclusion 7th character B see Appendix A PDX collection 1164
HAC 7th characters A & B see Appendix B for HAC conditional logic

CC MCC +7th **S12.091 Other nondisplaced fracture of first cervical vertebra**
CC Exclusion 7th character A see Appendix A PDX collection 1164
CC Exclusion 7th character K see Appendix A PDX collection 0897
MCC Exclusion 7th character B see Appendix A PDX collection 1164
HAC 7th characters A & B see Appendix B for HAC conditional logic

+ **S12.1 Fracture of second cervical vertebra**
Axis

+ **S12.10 Unspecified fracture of second cervical vertebra**

CC MCC +7th **S12.100 Unspecified displaced fracture of second cervical vertebra**
CC Exclusion 7th character A see Appendix A PDX collection 1164
CC Exclusion 7th character K see Appendix A PDX collection 0897
MCC Exclusion 7th character B see Appendix A PDX collection 1164
HAC 7th characters A & B see Appendix B for HAC conditional logic

CC MCC +7th **S12.101 Unspecified nondisplaced fracture of second cervical vertebra**
CC Exclusion 7th character A see Appendix A PDX collection 1164
CC Exclusion 7th character K see Appendix A PDX collection 0897
MCC Exclusion 7th character B see Appendix A PDX collection 1164
HAC 7th characters A & B see Appendix B for HAC conditional logic

+ **S12.11 Type II dens fracture**

CC MCC +7th **S12.110 Anterior displaced Type II dens fracture**
CC Exclusion 7th character A see Appendix A PDX collection 1164
CC Exclusion 7th character K see Appendix A PDX collection 0897
MCC Exclusion 7th character B see Appendix A PDX collection 1164
HAC 7th characters A & B see Appendix B for HAC conditional logic

CC MCC +7th **S12.111 Posterior displaced Type II dens fracture**
CC Exclusion 7th character A see Appendix A PDX collection 1164
CC Exclusion 7th character K see Appendix A PDX collection 0897
MCC Exclusion 7th character B see Appendix A PDX collection 1164
HAC 7th characters A & B see Appendix B for HAC conditional logic

CC MCC +7th **S12.112** **Nondisplaced Type II dens fracture**
CC Exclusion 7th character A see Appendix A PDX collection 1164
CC Exclusion 7th character K see Appendix A PDX collection 0897
MCC Exclusion 7th character B see Appendix A PDX collection 1164
HAC 7th characters A & B see Appendix B for HAC conditional logic

+ **S12.12** **Other dens fracture**

CC MCC +7th **S12.120** **Other displaced dens fracture**
CC Exclusion 7th character A see Appendix A PDX collection 1164
CC Exclusion 7th character K see Appendix A PDX collection 0897
MCC Exclusion 7th character B see Appendix A PDX collection 1164
HAC 7th characters A & B see Appendix B for HAC conditional logic

CC MCC +7th **S12.121** **Other nondisplaced dens fracture**
CC Exclusion 7th character A see Appendix A PDX collection 1164
CC Exclusion 7th character K see Appendix A PDX collection 0897
MCC Exclusion 7th character B see Appendix A PDX collection 1164
HAC 7th characters A & B see Appendix B for HAC conditional logic

+ **S12.13** **Unspecified traumatic spondylolisthesis of second cervical vertebra**

CC MCC +7th **S12.130** **Unspecified traumatic displaced spondylolisthesis of second cervical vertebra**
CC Exclusion 7th character A see Appendix A PDX collection 1164
CC Exclusion 7th character K see Appendix A PDX collection 0897
MCC Exclusion 7th character B see Appendix A PDX collection 1164
HAC 7th characters A & B see Appendix B for HAC conditional logic

CC MCC +7th **S12.131** **Unspecified traumatic nondisplaced spondylolisthesis of second cervical vertebra**
CC Exclusion 7th character A see Appendix A PDX collection 1164
CC Exclusion 7th character K see Appendix A PDX collection 0897
MCC Exclusion 7th character B see Appendix A PDX collection 1164
HAC 7th characters A & B see Appendix B for HAC conditional logic

CC MCC X+7th **S12.14** **Type III traumatic spondylolisthesis of second cervical vertebra**
CC Exclusion 7th character A see Appendix A PDX collection 1164
CC Exclusion 7th character K see Appendix A PDX collection 0897
MCC Exclusion 7th character B see Appendix A PDX collection 1164
HAC 7th characters A & B see Appendix B for HAC conditional logic

+ **S12.15** **Other traumatic spondylolisthesis of second cervical vertebra**

CC MCC +7th **S12.150** **Other traumatic displaced spondylolisthesis of second cervical vertebra**
CC Exclusion 7th character A see Appendix A PDX collection 1164
CC Exclusion 7th character K see Appendix A PDX collection 0897
MCC Exclusion 7th character B see Appendix A PDX collection 1164
HAC 7th characters A & B see Appendix B for HAC conditional logic

CC MCC +7th **S12.151** **Other traumatic nondisplaced spondylolisthesis of second cervical vertebra**
CC Exclusion 7th character A see Appendix A PDX collection 1164
CC Exclusion 7th character K see Appendix A PDX collection 0897
MCC Exclusion 7th character B see Appendix A PDX collection 1164
HAC 7th characters A & B see Appendix B for HAC conditional logic

+ **S12.19** **Other fracture of second cervical vertebra**

CC MCC +7th **S12.190** **Other displaced fracture of second cervical vertebra**
CC Exclusion 7th character A see Appendix A PDX collection 1164
CC Exclusion 7th character K see Appendix A PDX collection 0897
MCC Exclusion 7th character B see Appendix A PDX collection 1164
HAC 7th characters A & B see Appendix B for HAC conditional logic

CC MCC +7th **S12.191** **Other nondisplaced fracture of second cervical vertebra**
CC Exclusion 7th character A see Appendix A PDX collection 1164
CC Exclusion 7th character K see Appendix A PDX collection 0897
MCC Exclusion 7th character B see Appendix A PDX collection 1164
HAC 7th characters A & B see Appendix B for HAC conditional logic

+ **S12.2** **Fracture of third cervical vertebra**

+ **S12.20** **Unspecified fracture of third cervical vertebra**

CC MCC +7th **S12.200** **Unspecified displaced fracture of third cervical vertebra**
CC Exclusion 7th character A see Appendix A PDX collection 1164
CC Exclusion 7th character K see Appendix A PDX collection 0897
MCC Exclusion 7th character B see Appendix A PDX collection 1164
HAC 7th characters A & B see Appendix B for HAC conditional logic

CC MCC +7th **S12.201** **Unspecified nondisplaced fracture of third cervical vertebra**
CC Exclusion 7th character A see Appendix A PDX collection 1164
CC Exclusion 7th character K see Appendix A PDX collection 0897
MCC Exclusion 7th character B see Appendix A PDX collection 1164
HAC 7th characters A & B see Appendix B for HAC conditional logic

+ **S12.23** **Unspecified traumatic spondylolisthesis of third cervical vertebra**

CC MCC +7th **S12.230** **Unspecified traumatic displaced spondylolisthesis of third cervical vertebra**
CC Exclusion 7th character A see Appendix A PDX collection 1164
CC Exclusion 7th character K see Appendix A PDX collection 0897
MCC Exclusion 7th character B see Appendix A PDX collection 1164
HAC 7th characters A & B see Appendix B for HAC conditional logic

CC MCC +7th **S12.231** **Unspecified traumatic nondisplaced spondylolisthesis of third cervical vertebra**
CC Exclusion 7th character A see Appendix A PDX collection 1164
CC Exclusion 7th character K see Appendix A PDX collection 0897
MCC Exclusion 7th character B see Appendix A PDX collection 1164
HAC 7th characters A & B see Appendix B for HAC conditional logic

CC MCC X+7th **S12.24** **Type III traumatic spondylolisthesis of third cervical vertebra**
CC Exclusion 7th character A see Appendix A PDX collection 1164
CC Exclusion 7th character K see Appendix A PDX collection 0897
MCC Exclusion 7th character B see Appendix A PDX collection 1164
HAC 7th characters A & B see Appendix B for HAC conditional logic

+ **S12.25** **Other traumatic spondylolisthesis of third cervical vertebra**

CC MCC +7th **S12.250** **Other traumatic displaced spondylolisthesis of third cervical vertebra**
CC Exclusion 7th character A see Appendix A PDX collection 1164
CC Exclusion 7th character K see Appendix A PDX collection 0897
MCC Exclusion 7th character B see Appendix PDX collection 1164
HAC 7th characters A & B see Appendix B for HAC conditional logic

CC MCC +7th **S12.251** **Other traumatic nondisplaced spondylolisthesis of third cervical vertebra**
CC Exclusion 7th character A see Appendix A PDX collection 1164
CC Exclusion 7th character K see Appendix A PDX collection 0897
MCC Exclusion 7th character B see Appendix A PDX collection 1164
HAC 7th characters A & B see Appendix B for HAC conditional logic

\+ **S12.29** **Other fracture of third cervical vertebra**

CC MCC +7th **S12.290** **Other displaced fracture of third cervical vertebra**
CC Exclusion 7th character A see Appendix A PDX collection 1164
CC Exclusion 7th character K see Appendix A PDX collection 0897
MCC Exclusion 7th character B see Appendix A PDX collection 1164
HAC 7th characters A & B see Appendix B for HAC conditional logic

CC MCC +7th **S12.291** **Other nondisplaced fracture of third cervical vertebra**
CC Exclusion 7th character A see Appendix A PDX collection 1164
CC Exclusion 7th character K see Appendix A PDX collection 0897
MCC Exclusion 7th character B see Appendix A PDX collection 1164
HAC 7th characters A & B see Appendix B for HAC conditional logic

\+ **S12.3** **Fracture of fourth cervical vertebra**

\+ **S12.30** **Unspecified fracture of fourth cervical vertebra**

CC MCC +7th **S12.300** **Unspecified displaced fracture of fourth cervical vertebra**
CC Exclusion 7th character A see Appendix A PDX collection 1164
CC Exclusion 7th character K see Appendix A PDX collection 0897
MCC Exclusion 7th character B see Appendix A PDX collection 1164
HAC 7th characters A & B see Appendix B for HAC conditional logic

CC MCC +7th **S12.301** **Unspecified nondisplaced fracture of fourth cervical vertebra**
CC Exclusion 7th character A see Appendix A PDX collection 1164
CC Exclusion 7th character K see Appendix A PDX collection 0897
MCC Exclusion 7th character B see Appendix A PDX collection 1164
HAC 7th characters A & B see Appendix B for HAC conditional logic

\+ **S12.33** **Unspecified traumatic spondylolisthesis of fourth cervical vertebra**

CC MCC +7th **S12.330** **Unspecified traumatic displaced spondylolisthesis of fourth cervical vertebra**
CC Exclusion 7th character A see Appendix A PDX collection 1164
CC Exclusion 7th character K see Appendix A PDX collection 0897
MCC Exclusion 7th character B see Appendix A PDX collection 1164
HAC 7th characters A & B see Appendix B for HAC conditional logic

CC MCC +7th **S12.331** **Unspecified traumatic nondisplaced spondylolisthesis of fourth cervical vertebra**
CC Exclusion 7th character A see Appendix A PDX collection 1164
CC Exclusion 7th character K see Appendix A PDX collection 0897
MCC Exclusion 7th character B see Appendix A PDX collection 1164
HAC 7th characters A & B see Appendix B for HAC conditional logic

CC MCC X+7th **S12.34** **Type III traumatic spondylolisthesis of fourth cervical vertebra**
CC Exclusion 7th character A see Appendix A PDX collection 1164
CC Exclusion 7th character K see Appendix A PDX collection 0897
MCC Exclusion 7th character B see Appendix A PDX collection 1164
HAC 7th characters A & B see Appendix B for HAC conditional logic

\+ **S12.35** **Other traumatic spondylolisthesis of fourth cervical vertebra**

CC MCC +7th **S12.350** **Other traumatic displaced spondylolisthesis of fourth cervical vertebra**
CC Exclusion 7th character A see Appendix A PDX collection 1164
CC Exclusion 7th character K see Appendix A PDX collection 0897
MCC Exclusion 7th character B see Appendix A PDX collection 1164
HAC 7th characters A & B see Appendix B for HAC conditional logic

CC MCC +7th **S12.351** **Other traumatic nondisplaced spondylolisthesis of fourth cervical vertebra**
CC Exclusion 7th character A see Appendix A PDX collection 1164
CC Exclusion 7th character K see Appendix A PDX collection 0897
MCC Exclusion 7th character B see Appendix A PDX collection 1164
HAC 7th characters A & B see Appendix B for HAC conditional logic

\+ **S12.39** **Other fracture of fourth cervical vertebra**

CC MCC +7th **S12.390** **Other displaced fracture of fourth cervical vertebra**
CC Exclusion 7th character A see Appendix A PDX collection 1164
CC Exclusion 7th character K see Appendix A PDX collection 0897
MCC Exclusion 7th character B see Appendix A PDX collection 1164
HAC 7th characters A & B see Appendix B for HAC conditional logic

CC MCC +7th **S12.391** **Other nondisplaced fracture of fourth cervical vertebra**
CC Exclusion 7th character A see Appendix A PDX collection 1164
CC Exclusion 7th character K see Appendix A PDX collection 0897
MCC Exclusion 7th character B see Appendix A PDX collection 1164
HAC 7th characters A & B see Appendix B for HAC conditional logic

\+ **S12.4** **Fracture of fifth cervical vertebra**

\+ **S12.40** **Unspecified fracture of fifth cervical vertebra**

CC MCC +7th **S12.400** **Unspecified displaced fracture of fifth cervical vertebra**
CC Exclusion 7th character A see Appendix A PDX collection 1164
CC Exclusion 7th character K see Appendix A PDX collection 0897
MCC Exclusion 7th character B see Appendix A PDX collection 1164
HAC 7th characters A & B see Appendix B for HAC conditional logic

CC MCC +7th **S12.401** **Unspecified nondisplaced fracture of fifth cervical vertebra**
CC Exclusion 7th character A see Appendix A PDX collection 1164
CC Exclusion 7th character K see Appendix A PDX collection 0897
MCC Exclusion 7th character B see Appendix A PDX collection 1164
HAC 7th characters A & B see Appendix B for HAC conditional logic

\+ **S12.43** **Unspecified traumatic spondylolisthesis of fifth cervical vertebra**

CC MCC +7th **S12.430** **Unspecified traumatic displaced spondylolisthesis of fifth cervical vertebra**
CC Exclusion 7th character A see Appendix A PDX collection 1164
CC Exclusion 7th character K see Appendix A PDX collection 0897
MCC Exclusion 7th character B see Appendix A PDX collection 1164
HAC 7th characters A & B see Appendix B for HAC conditional logic

CC MCC +7th **S12.431** **Unspecified traumatic nondisplaced spondylolisthesis of fifth cervical vertebra**
CC Exclusion 7th character A see Appendix A PDX collection 1164
CC Exclusion 7th character K see Appendix A PDX collection 0897
MCC Exclusion 7th character B see Appendix A PDX collection 1164
HAC 7th characters A & B see Appendix B for HAC conditional logic

CC MCC X+7th **S12.44** **Type III traumatic spondylolisthesis of fifth cervical vertebra**
CC Exclusion 7th character A see Appendix A PDX collection 1164
CC Exclusion 7th character K see Appendix A PDX collection 0897
MCC Exclusion 7th character B see Appendix A PDX collection 1164
HAC 7th characters A & B see Appendix B for HAC conditional logic

+ **S12.45** **Other traumatic spondylolisthesis of fifth cervical vertebra**

CC MCC +7th **S12.450** **Other traumatic displaced spondylolisthesis of fifth cervical vertebra**
CC Exclusion 7th character A see Appendix A PDX collection 1164
CC Exclusion 7th character K see Appendix A PDX collection 0897
MCC Exclusion 7th character B see Appendix A PDX collection 1164
HAC 7th characters A & B see Appendix B for HAC conditional logic

CC MCC +7th **S12.451** **Other traumatic nondisplaced spondylolisthesis of fifth cervical vertebra**
CC Exclusion 7th character A see Appendix A PDX collection 1164
CC Exclusion 7th character K see Appendix A PDX collection 0897
MCC Exclusion 7th character B see Appendix A PDX collection 1164
HAC 7th characters A & B see Appendix B for HAC conditional logic

+ **S12.49** **Other fracture of fifth cervical vertebra**

CC MCC +7th **S12.490** **Other displaced fracture of fifth cervical vertebra**
CC Exclusion 7th character A see Appendix A PDX collection 1164
CC Exclusion 7th character K see Appendix A PDX collection 0897
MCC Exclusion 7th character B see Appendix A PDX collection 1164
HAC 7th characters A & B see Appendix B for HAC conditional logic

CC MCC +7th **S12.491** **Other nondisplaced fracture of fifth cervical vertebra**
CC Exclusion 7th character A see Appendix A PDX collection 1164
CC Exclusion 7th character K see Appendix A PDX collection 0897
MCC Exclusion 7th character B see Appendix A PDX collection 1164
HAC 7th characters A & B see Appendix B for HAC conditional logic

+ **S12.5** **Fracture of sixth cervical vertebra**

+ **S12.50** **Unspecified fracture of sixth cervical vertebra**

CC MCC +7th **S12.500** **Unspecified displaced fracture of sixth cervical vertebra**
CC Exclusion 7th character A see Appendix A PDX collection 1164
CC Exclusion 7th character K see Appendix A PDX collection 0897
MCC Exclusion 7th character B see Appendix A PDX collection 1164
HAC 7th characters A & B see Appendix B for HAC conditional logic

CC MCC +7th **S12.501** **Unspecified nondisplaced fracture of sixth cervical vertebra**
CC Exclusion 7th character A see Appendix A PDX collection 1164
CC Exclusion 7th character K see Appendix A PDX collection 0897
MCC Exclusion 7th character B see Appendix A PDX collection 1164
HAC 7th characters A & B see Appendix B for HAC conditional logic

+ **S12.53** **Unspecified traumatic spondylolisthesis of sixth cervical vertebra**

CC MCC +7th **S12.530** **Unspecified traumatic displaced spondylolisthesis of sixth cervical vertebra**
CC Exclusion 7th character A see Appendix A PDX collection 1164
CC Exclusion 7th character K see Appendix A PDX collection 0897
MCC Exclusion 7th character B see Appendix A PDX collection 1164
HAC 7th characters A & B see Appendix B for HAC conditional logic

CC MCC +7th **S12.531** **Unspecified traumatic nondisplaced spondylolisthesis of sixth cervical vertebra**
CC Exclusion 7th character A see Appendix A PDX collection 1164
CC Exclusion 7th character K see Appendix A PDX collection 0897
MCC Exclusion 7th character B see Appendix A PDX collection 1164
HAC 7th characters A & B see Appendix B for HAC conditional logic

CC MCC X+7th **S12.54** **Type III traumatic spondylolisthesis of sixth cervical vertebra**
CC Exclusion 7th character A see Appendix A PDX collection 1164
CC Exclusion 7th character K see Appendix A PDX collection 0897
MCC Exclusion 7th character B see Appendix A PDX collection 1164
HAC 7th characters A & B see Appendix B for HAC conditional logic

+ **S12.55** **Other traumatic spondylolisthesis of sixth cervical vertebra**

CC MCC +7th **S12.550** **Other traumatic displaced spondylolisthesis of sixth cervical vertebra**
CC Exclusion 7th character A see Appendix A PDX collection 1164
CC Exclusion 7th character K see Appendix A PDX collection 0897
MCC Exclusion 7th character B see Appendix A PDX collection 1164
HAC 7th characters A & B see Appendix B for HAC conditional logic

CC MCC +7th **S12.551** **Other traumatic nondisplaced spondylolisthesis of sixth cervical vertebra**
CC Exclusion 7th character A see Appendix A PDX collection 1164
CC Exclusion 7th character K see Appendix A PDX collection 0897
MCC Exclusion 7th character B see Appendix A PDX collection 1164
HAC 7th characters A & B see Appendix B for HAC conditional logic

+ **S12.59** **Other fracture of sixth cervical vertebra**

CC MCC +7th **S12.590** **Other displaced fracture of sixth cervical vertebra**
CC Exclusion 7th character A see Appendix A PDX collection 1164
CC Exclusion 7th character K see Appendix A PDX collection 0897
MCC Exclusion 7th character B see Appendix A PDX collection 1164
HAC 7th characters A & B see Appendix B for HAC conditional logic

CC MCC +7th **S12.591** **Other nondisplaced fracture of sixth cervical vertebra**
CC Exclusion 7th character A see Appendix A PDX collection 1164
CC Exclusion 7th character K see Appendix A PDX collection 0897
MCC Exclusion 7th character B see Appendix A PDX collection 1164
HAC 7th characters A & B see Appendix B for HAC conditional logic

+ **S12.6** **Fracture of seventh cervical vertebra**

+ **S12.60** **Unspecified fracture of seventh cervical vertebra**

CC MCC +7th **S12.600** **Unspecified displaced fracture of seventh cervical vertebra**
CC Exclusion 7th character A see Appendix A PDX collection 1164
CC Exclusion 7th character K see Appendix A PDX collection 0897
MCC Exclusion 7th character B see Appendix A PDX collection 1164
HAC 7th characters A & B see Appendix B for HAC conditional logic

CC MCC +7th **S12.601** **Unspecified nondisplaced fracture of seventh cervical vertebra**
CC Exclusion 7th character A see Appendix A PDX collection 1164
CC Exclusion 7th character K see Appendix A PDX collection 0897
MCC Exclusion 7th character B see Appendix A PDX collection 1164
HAC 7th characters A & B see Appendix B for HAC conditional logic

+ **S12.63 Unspecified traumatic spondylolisthesis of seventh cervical vertebra**

CC MCC +7th **S12.630 Unspecified traumatic displaced spondylolisthesis of seventh cervical vertebra**
CC Exclusion 7th character A see Appendix A PDX collection 1164
CC Exclusion 7th character K see Appendix A PDX collection 0897
MCC Exclusion 7th character B see Appendix A PDX collection 1164
HAC 7th characters A & B see Appendix B for HAC conditional logic

CC MCC +7th **S12.631 Unspecified traumatic nondisplaced spondylolisthesis of seventh cervical vertebra**
CC Exclusion 7th character A see Appendix A PDX collection 1164
CC Exclusion 7th character K see Appendix A PDX collection 0897
MCC Exclusion 7th character B see Appendix A PDX collection 1164
HAC 7th characters A & B see Appendix B for HAC conditional logic

CC MCC X+7th **S12.64 Type III traumatic spondylolisthesis of seventh cervical vertebra**
CC Exclusion 7th character A see Appendix A PDX collection 1164
CC Exclusion 7th character K see Appendix A PDX collection 0897
MCC Exclusion 7th character B see Appendix A PDX collection 1164
HAC 7th characters A & B see Appendix B for HAC conditional logic

+ **S12.65 Other traumatic spondylolisthesis of seventh cervical vertebra**

CC MCC +7th **S12.650 Other traumatic displaced spondylolisthesis of seventh cervical vertebra**
CC Exclusion 7th character A see Appendix A PDX collection 1164
CC Exclusion 7th character A see Appendix A PDX collection 1164
MCC Exclusion 7th character B see Appendix A PDX collection 1164
HAC 7th characters A & B see Appendix B for HAC conditional logic

CC MCC +7th **S12.651 Other traumatic nondisplaced spondylolisthesis of seventh cervical vertebra**
CC Exclusion 7th character A see Appendix A PDX collection 1164
CC Exclusion 7th character K see Appendix A PDX collection 0897
MCC Exclusion 7th character B see Appendix A PDX collection 1164
HAC 7th characters A & B see Appendix B for HAC conditional logic

+ **S12.69 Other fracture of seventh cervical vertebra**

CC MCC +7th **S12.690 Other displaced fracture of seventh cervical vertebra**
CC Exclusion 7th character A see Appendix A PDX collection 1164
CC Exclusion 7th character K see Appendix A PDX collection 0897
MCC Exclusion 7th character B see Appendix A PDX collection 1164
HAC 7th characters A & B see Appendix B for HAC conditional logic

CC MCC +7th **S12.691 Other nondisplaced fracture of seventh cervical vertebra**
CC Exclusion 7th character A see Appendix A PDX collection 1164
CC Exclusion 7th character K see Appendix A PDX collection 0897
MCC Exclusion 7th character B see Appendix A PDX collection 1164
HAC 7th characters A & B see Appendix B for HAC conditional logic

X+7th MCC **S12.8 Fracture of other parts of neck**

The appropriate 7th character is to be added to code **S12.8**
A initial encounter
D subsequent encounter
S sequela

Hyoid bone
Larynx
Thyroid cartilage
Trachea
MCC Exclusion 7th character A see Appendix A PDX collection 1165
HAC 7th character A see Appendix B for HAC conditional logic

CC X+7th **S12.9 Fracture of neck, unspecified**

The appropriate 7th character is to be added to code **S12.9**
A initial encounter
D subsequent encounter
S sequela

Fracture of neck NOS
Fracture of cervical spine NOS
Fracture of cervical vertebra NOS
CC Exclusion 7th character A see Appendix A PDX collection 1164
HAC 7th character A see Appendix B for HAC conditional logic

S13 Dislocation and sprain of joints and ligaments at neck level

Includes: avulsion of joint or ligament at neck level
laceration of cartilage, joint or ligament at neck level
sprain of cartilage, joint or ligament at neck level
traumatic hemarthrosis of joint or ligament at neck level
traumatic rupture of joint or ligament at neck level
traumatic subluxation of joint or ligament at neck level
traumatic tear of joint or ligament at neck level

Code also any associated open wound

Excludes2: *strain of muscle or tendon at neck level (S16.1)*

The appropriate 7th character is to be added to each code from category S13
A initial encounter
D subsequent encounter
S sequela

CC X+7th **S13.0 Traumatic rupture of cervical intervertebral disc**
Excludes1: *rupture or displacement (nontraumatic) of cervical intervertebral disc NOS (M50.-)*
CC Exclusion 7th character A see Appendix A PDX collection 0913
HAC 7th character A see Appendix B for HAC conditional logic

+ **S13.1 Subluxation and dislocation of cervical vertebrae**
Code also any associated:
open wound of neck (S11.-)
spinal cord injury (S14.1-)
Excludes2: *fracture of cervical vertebrae (S12.0-S12.3-)*

+ **S13.10 Subluxation and dislocation of unspecified cervical vertebrae**

CC +7th **S13.100 Subluxation of unspecified cervical vertebrae**
CC Exclusion 7th character A see Appendix A PDX collection 0913
HAC 7th character A see Appendix B for HAC conditional logic

CC +7th **S13.101 Dislocation of unspecified cervical vertebrae**
CC Exclusion 7th character A see Appendix A PDX collection 0913
HAC 7th character A see Appendix B for HAC conditional logic

+ **S13.11 Subluxation and dislocation of C0/C1 cervical vertebrae**
Subluxation and dislocation of atlantooccipital joint
Subluxation and dislocation of atloidooccipital joint
Subluxation and dislocation of occipitoatloid joint

CC +7th **S13.110 Subluxation of C0/C1 cervical vertebrae**
CC Exclusion 7th character A see Appendix A PDX collection 0913
HAC 7th character A see Appendix B for HAC conditional logic

CC +7th **S13.111 Dislocation of C0/C1 cervical vertebrae**
CC Exclusion 7th character A see Appendix A PDX collection 0913
HAC 7th character A see Appendix B for HAC conditional logic

+ **S13.12 Subluxation and dislocation of C1/C2 cervical vertebrae**
  Subluxation and dislocation of atlantoaxial joint

CC +7th **S13.120 Subluxation of C1/C2 cervical vertebrae**
CC Exclusion 7th character A see Appendix A PDX collection 0913
HAC 7th character A see Appendix B for HAC conditional logic

CC +7th **S13.121 Dislocation of C1/C2 cervical vertebrae**
CC Exclusion 7th character A see Appendix A PDX collection 0913
HAC 7th character A see Appendix B for HAC conditional logic

+ **S13.13 Subluxation and dislocation of C2/C3 cervical vertebrae**

CC +7th **S13.130 Subluxation of C2/C3 cervical vertebrae**
CC Exclusion 7th character A see Appendix A PDX collection 0913
HAC 7th character A see Appendix B for HAC conditional logic

CC +7th **S13.131 Dislocation of C2/C3 cervical vertebrae**
CC Exclusion 7th character A see Appendix A PDX collection 0913
HAC 7th character A see Appendix B for HAC conditional logic

+ **S13.14 Subluxation and dislocation of C3/C4 cervical vertebrae**

CC +7th **S13.140 Subluxation of C3/C4 cervical vertebrae**
CC Exclusion 7th character A see Appendix A PDX collection 0913
HAC 7th character A see Appendix B for HAC conditional logic

CC +7th **S13.141 Dislocation of C3/C4 cervical vertebrae**
CC Exclusion 7th character A see Appendix A PDX collection 0913
HAC 7th character A see Appendix B for HAC conditional logic

+ **S13.15 Subluxation and dislocation of C4/C5 cervical vertebrae**

CC +7th **S13.150 Subluxation of C4/C5 cervical vertebrae**
CC Exclusion 7th character A see Appendix A PDX collection 0913
HAC 7th character A see Appendix B for HAC conditional logic

CC +7th **S13.151 Dislocation of C4/C5 cervical vertebrae**
CC Exclusion 7th character A see Appendix A PDX collection 0913
HAC 7th character A see Appendix B for HAC conditional logic

+ **S13.16 Subluxation and dislocation of C5/C6 cervical vertebrae**

CC +7th **S13.160 Subluxation of C5/C6 cervical vertebrae**
CC Exclusion 7th character A see Appendix A PDX collection 0913
HAC 7th character A see Appendix B for HAC conditional logic

CC +7th **S13.161 Dislocation of C5/C6 cervical vertebrae**
CC Exclusion 7th character A see Appendix A PDX collection 0913
HAC 7th character A see Appendix B for HAC conditional logic

+ **S13.17 Subluxation and dislocation of C6/C7 cervical vertebrae**

CC +7th **S13.170 Subluxation of C6/C7 cervical vertebrae**
CC Exclusion 7th character A see Appendix A PDX collection 0913
HAC 7th character A see Appendix B for HAC conditional logic

CC +7th **S13.171 Dislocation of C6/C7 cervical vertebrae**
CC Exclusion 7th character A see Appendix A PDX collection 0913
HAC 7th character A see Appendix B for HAC conditional logic

+ **S13.18 Subluxation and dislocation of C7/T1 cervical vertebrae**

CC +7th **S13.180 Subluxation of C7/T1 cervical vertebrae**
CC Exclusion 7th character A see Appendix A PDX collection 0913
HAC 7th character A see Appendix B for HAC conditional logic

CC +7th **S13.181 Dislocation of C7/T1 cervical vertebrae**
CC Exclusion 7th character A see Appendix A PDX collection 0913
HAC 7th character A see Appendix B for HAC conditional logic

+ **S13.2 Dislocation of other and unspecified parts of neck**

CC X+7th **S13.20 Dislocation of unspecified parts of neck**
CC Exclusion 7th character A see Appendix A PDX collection 0913
HAC 7th character A see Appendix B for HAC conditional logic

CC X+7th **S13.29 Dislocation of other parts of neck**
CC Exclusion 7th character A see Appendix A PDX collection 0913
HAC 7th character A see Appendix B for HAC conditional logic

X+7th **S13.4 Sprain of ligaments of cervical spine**
  Sprain of anterior longitudinal (ligament), cervical
  Sprain of atlanto-axial (joints)
  Sprain of atlanto-occipital (joints)
  Whiplash injury of cervical spine

X+7th **S13.5 Sprain of thyroid region**
  Sprain of cricoarytenoid (joint) (ligament)
  Sprain of cricothyroid (joint) (ligament)
  Sprain of thyroid cartilage

X+7th **S13.8 Sprain of joints and ligaments of other parts of neck**

X+7th **S13.9 Sprain of joints and ligaments of unspecified parts of neck**

S14 Injury of nerves and spinal cord at neck level

NOTE Code to highest level of cervical cord injury

Code also any associated:
  fracture of cervical vertebra (S12.0--S12.6.-)
  open wound of neck (S11.-)
  transient paralysis (R29.5)

The appropriate 7th character is to be added to each code from category S14
A initial encounter
D subsequent encounter
S sequela

MCC X+7th **S14.0 Concussion and edema of cervical spinal cord**
MCC Exclusion 7th character A see Appendix A PDX collection 1166

+ **S14.1 Other and unspecified injuries of cervical spinal cord**

+ **S14.10 Unspecified injury of cervical spinal cord**

MCC +7th **S14.101 Unspecified injury at C1 level of cervical spinal cord**
MCC Exclusion 7th character A see Appendix A PDX collection 1166
HAC 7th character A see Appendix B for HAC conditional logic

MCC +7th **S14.102 Unspecified injury at C2 level of cervical spinal cord**
MCC Exclusion 7th character A see Appendix A PDX collection 1166
HAC 7th character A see Appendix B for HAC conditional logic

MCC +7th **S14.103 Unspecified injury at C3 level of cervical spinal cord**
MCC Exclusion 7th character A see Appendix A PDX collection 1166
HAC 7th character A see Appendix B for HAC conditional logic

MCC +7th **S14.104 Unspecified injury at C4 level of cervical spinal cord**
MCC Exclusion 7th character A see Appendix A PDX collection 1166
HAC 7th character A see Appendix B for HAC conditional logic

MCC +7th **S14.105 Unspecified injury at C5 level of cervical spinal cord**
MCC Exclusion 7th character A see Appendix A PDX collection 1166
HAC 7th character A see Appendix B for HAC conditional logic

MCC +7th **S14.106 Unspecified injury at C6 level of cervical spinal cord**
MCC Exclusion 7th character A see Appendix A PDX collection 1166
HAC 7th character A see Appendix B for HAC conditional logic

MCC +7th **S14.107 Unspecified injury at C7 level of cervical spinal cord**
MCC Exclusion 7th character A see Appendix A PDX collection 1166
HAC 7th character A see Appendix B for HAC conditional logic

MCC +7th **S14.108** **Unspecified injury at C8 level of cervical spinal cord**
MCC Exclusion 7th character A see Appendix A
PDX collection 1166

+7th **S14.109** **Unspecified injury at unspecified level of cervical spinal cord**
Injury of cervical spinal cord NOS
HAC 7th character A see Appendix B for HAC conditional logic

+ **S14.11 Complete lesion of cervical spinal cord**

MCC +7th **S14.111** **Complete lesion at C1 level of cervical spinal cord**
MCC Exclusion 7th character A see Appendix A
PDX collection 1166
HAC 7th character A see Appendix B for HAC conditional logic

MCC +7th **S14.112** **Complete lesion at C2 level of cervical spinal cord**
MCC Exclusion 7th character A see Appendix A
PDX collection 1166
HAC 7th character A see Appendix B for HAC conditional logic

MCC +7th **S14.113** **Complete lesion at C3 level of cervical spinal cord**
MCC Exclusion 7th character A see Appendix A
PDX collection 1166
HAC 7th character A see Appendix B for HAC conditional logic

MCC +7th **S14.114** **Complete lesion at C4 level of cervical spinal cord**
MCC Exclusion 7th character A see Appendix A
PDX collection 1166
HAC 7th character A see Appendix B for HAC conditional logic

MCC +7th **S14.115** **Complete lesion at C5 level of cervical spinal cord**
MCC Exclusion 7th character A see Appendix A
PDX collection 1166
HAC 7th character A see Appendix B for HAC conditional logic

MCC +7th **S14.116** **Complete lesion at C6 level of cervical spinal cord**
MCC Exclusion 7th character A see Appendix A
PDX collection 1166
HAC 7th character A see Appendix B for HAC conditional logic

MCC +7th **S14.117** **Complete lesion at C7 level of cervical spinal cord**
MCC Exclusion 7th character A see Appendix A
PDX collection 1166
HAC 7th character A see Appendix B for HAC conditional logic

MCC +7th **S14.118** **Complete lesion at C8 level of cervical spinal cord**
MCC Exclusion 7th character A see Appendix A
PDX collection 1166

+7th **S14.119** **Complete lesion at unspecified level of cervical spinal cord**

+ **S14.12 Central cord syndrome of cervical spinal cord**

MCC +7th **S14.121** **Central cord syndrome at C1 level of cervical spinal cord**
MCC Exclusion 7th character A see Appendix A
PDX collection 1166
HAC 7th character A see Appendix B for HAC conditional logic

MCC +7th **S14.122** **Central cord syndrome at C2 level of cervical spinal cord**
MCC Exclusion 7th character A see Appendix A
PDX collection 1166
HAC 7th character A see Appendix B for HAC conditional logic

MCC +7th **S14.123** **Central cord syndrome at C3 level of cervical spinal cord**
MCC Exclusion 7th character A see Appendix A
PDX collection 1166
HAC 7th character A see Appendix B for HAC conditional logic

MCC +7th **S14.124** **Central cord syndrome at C4 level of cervical spinal cord**
MCC Exclusion 7th character A see Appendix A
PDX collection 1166
HAC 7th character A see Appendix B for HAC conditional logic

MCC +7th **S14.125** **Central cord syndrome at C5 level of cervical spinal cord**
MCC Exclusion 7th character A see Appendix A
PDX collection 1166
HAC 7th character A see Appendix B for HAC conditional logic

MCC +7th **S14.126** **Central cord syndrome at C6 level of cervical spinal cord**
MCC Exclusion 7th character A see Appendix A
PDX collection 1166
HAC 7th character A see Appendix B for HAC conditional logic

MCC +7th **S14.127** **Central cord syndrome at C7 level of cervical spinal cord**
MCC Exclusion 7th character A see Appendix A
PDX collection 1166
HAC 7th character A see Appendix B for HAC conditional logic

MCC +7th **S14.128** **Central cord syndrome at C8 level of cervical spinal cord**
MCC Exclusion 7th character A see Appendix A
PDX collection 1166

+7th **S14.129** **Central cord syndrome at unspecified level of cervical spinal cord**

+ **S14.13 Anterior cord syndrome of cervical spinal cord**

MCC +7th **S14.131** **Anterior cord syndrome at C1 level of cervical spinal cord**
MCC Exclusion 7th character A see Appendix A
PDX collection 1166
HAC 7th character A see Appendix B for HAC conditional logic

MCC +7th **S14.132** **Anterior cord syndrome at C2 level of cervical spinal cord**
MCC Exclusion 7th character A see Appendix A
PDX collection 1166
HAC 7th character A see Appendix B for HAC conditional logic

MCC +7th **S14.133** **Anterior cord syndrome at C3 level of cervical spinal cord**
MCC Exclusion 7th character A see Appendix A
PDX collection 1166
HAC 7th character A see Appendix B for HAC conditional logic

MCC +7th **S14.134** **Anterior cord syndrome at C4 level of cervical spinal cord**
MCC Exclusion 7th character A see Appendix A
PDX collection 1166
HAC 7th character A see Appendix B for HAC conditional logic

MCC +7th **S14.135** **Anterior cord syndrome at C5 level of cervical spinal cord**
MCC Exclusion 7th character A see Appendix A
PDX collection 1166
HAC 7th character A see Appendix B for HAC conditional logic

MCC +7th **S14.136** **Anterior cord syndrome at C6 level of cervical spinal cord**
MCC Exclusion 7th character A see Appendix A
PDX collection 1166
HAC 7th character A see Appendix B for HAC conditional logic

MCC +7th **S14.137** **Anterior cord syndrome at C7 level of cervical spinal cord**
MCC Exclusion 7th character A see Appendix A
PDX collection 1166
HAC 7th character A see Appendix B for HAC conditional logic

MCC +7th **S14.138** **Anterior cord syndrome at C8 level of cervical spinal cord**
MCC Exclusion 7th character A see Appendix A
PDX collection 1166

+7th **S14.139** **Anterior cord syndrome at unspecified level of cervical spinal cord**

+ **S14.14 Brown-Séquard syndrome of cervical spinal cord**

MCC +7th **S14.141 Brown-Séquard syndrome at C1 level of cervical spinal cord**
MCC Exclusion 7th character A see Appendix A
PDX collection 1166

MCC +7th **S14.142 Brown-Séquard syndrome at C2 level of cervical spinal cord**
MCC Exclusion 7th character A see Appendix A
PDX collection 1166

MCC +7th **S14.143 Brown-Séquard syndrome at C3 level of cervical spinal cord**
MCC Exclusion 7th character A see Appendix A
PDX collection 1166

MCC +7th **S14.144 Brown-Séquard syndrome at C4 level of cervical spinal cord**
MCC Exclusion 7th character A see Appendix A
PDX collection 1166

MCC +7th **S14.145 Brown-Séquard syndrome at C5 level of cervical spinal cord**
MCC Exclusion 7th character A see Appendix A
PDX collection 1166

MCC +7th **S14.146 Brown-Séquard syndrome at C6 level of cervical spinal cord**
MCC Exclusion 7th character A see Appendix A
PDX collection 1166

MCC +7th **S14.147 Brown-Séquard syndrome at C7 level of cervical spinal cord**
MCC Exclusion 7th character A see Appendix A
PDX collection 1166

MCC +7th **S14.148 Brown-Séquard syndrome at C8 level of cervical spinal cord**
MCC Exclusion 7th character A see Appendix A
PDX collection 1166

+7th **S14.149 Brown-Séquard syndrome at unspecified level of cervical spinal cord**

+ **S14.15 Other incomplete lesions of cervical spinal cord**
Incomplete lesion of cervical spinal cord NOS
Posterior cord syndrome of cervical spinal cord

MCC +7th **S14.151 Other incomplete lesion at C1 level of cervical spinal cord**
MCC Exclusion 7th character A see Appendix A
PDX collection 1166
HAC 7th character A see Appendix B for HAC conditional logic

MCC +7th **S14.152 Other incomplete lesion at C2 level of cervical spinal cord**
MCC Exclusion 7th character A see Appendix A
PDX collection 1166
HAC 7th character A see Appendix B for HAC conditional logic

MCC +7th **S14.153 Other incomplete lesion at C3 level of cervical spinal cord**
MCC Exclusion 7th character A see Appendix A
PDX collection 1166
HAC 7th character A see Appendix B for HAC conditional logic

MCC +7th **S14.154 Other incomplete lesion at C4 level of cervical spinal cord**
MCC Exclusion 7th character A see Appendix A
PDX collection 1166
HAC 7th character A see Appendix B for HAC conditional logic

MCC +7th **S14.155 Other incomplete lesion at C5 level of cervical spinal cord**
MCC Exclusion 7th character A see Appendix A
PDX collection 1166
HAC 7th character A see Appendix B for HAC conditional logic

MCC +7th **S14.156 Other incomplete lesion at C6 level of cervical spinal cord**
MCC Exclusion 7th character A see Appendix A
PDX collection 1166
HAC 7th character A see Appendix B for HAC conditional logic

MCC +7th **S14.157 Other incomplete lesion at C7 level of cervical spinal cord**
MCC Exclusion 7th character A see Appendix A
PDX collection 1166
HAC 7th character A see Appendix B for HAC conditional logic

MCC +7th **S14.158 Other incomplete lesion at C8 level of cervical spinal cord**
MCC Exclusion 7th character A see Appendix
PDX collection 1166

+7th **S14.159 Other incomplete lesion at unspecified lev of cervical spinal cord**

X+7th **S14.2 Injury of nerve root of cervical spine**

X+7th **S14.3 Injury of brachial plexus**

X+7th **S14.4 Injury of peripheral nerves of neck**

X+7th **S14.5 Injury of cervical sympathetic nerves**

X+7th **S14.8 Injury of other specified nerves of neck**

X+7th **S14.9 Injury of unspecified nerves of neck**

S15 Injury of blood vessels at neck level

Code also any associated open wound (S11.-)

The appropriate 7th character is to be added to each code from category S15
- A initial encounter
- D subsequent encounter
- S sequela

+ **S15.0 Injury of carotid artery of neck**
Injury of carotid artery (common) (external) (internal, extracranial portion)
Injury of carotid artery NOS
Excludes1: *injury of internal carotid artery, intracranial portion (S06.8)*

+ **S15.00 Unspecified injury of carotid artery**

CC +7th **S15.001 Unspecified injury of right carotid artery**
CC Exclusion 7th character A see Appendix A
PDX collection 1167

CC +7th **S15.002 Unspecified injury of left carotid artery**
CC Exclusion 7th character A see Appendix A
PDX collection 1167

CC +7th **S15.009 Unspecified injury of unspecified carotid artery**
CC Exclusion 7th character A see Appendix A
PDX collection 1167

+ **S15.01 Minor laceration of carotid artery**
Incomplete transection of carotid artery
Laceration of carotid artery NOS
Superficial laceration of carotid artery

CC +7th **S15.011 Minor laceration of right carotid artery**
CC Exclusion 7th character A see Appendix A
PDX collection 1167

CC +7th **S15.012 Minor laceration of left carotid artery**
CC Exclusion 7th character A see Appendix A
PDX collection 1167

CC +7th **S15.019 Minor laceration of unspecified carotid artery**
CC Exclusion 7th character A see Appendix A
PDX collection 1167

+ **S15.02 Major laceration of carotid artery**
Complete transection of carotid artery
Traumatic rupture of carotid artery

CC +7th **S15.021 Major laceration of right carotid artery**
CC Exclusion 7th character A see Appendix A
PDX collection 1167

CC +7th **S15.022 Major laceration of left carotid artery**
CC Exclusion 7th character A see Appendix A
PDX collection 1167

CC +7th **S15.029 Major laceration of unspecified carotid artery**
CC Exclusion 7th character A see Appendix A
PDX collection 1167

+ **S15.09 Other specified injury of carotid artery**

CC +7th **S15.091 Other specified injury of right carotid artery**
CC Exclusion 7th character A see Appendix A
PDX collection 1167

CC +7th **S15.092 Other specified injury of left carotid arte**
CC Exclusion 7th character A see Appendix A
PDX collection 1167

CC +7th **S15.099 Other specified injury of unspecified carotid artery**
CC Exclusion 7th character A see Appendix A
PDX collection 1167

+ **S15.1 Injury of vertebral artery**
+ **S15.10 Unspecified injury of vertebral artery**

CC +7th **S15.101 Unspecified injury of right vertebral artery**
CC Exclusion 7th character A see Appendix A
PDX collection 1157

CC +7th **S15.102 Unspecified injury of left vertebral artery**
CC Exclusion 7th character A see Appendix A
PDX collection 1157

CC +7th **S15.109 Unspecified injury of unspecified vertebral artery**
CC Exclusion 7th character A see Appendix A
PDX collection 1157

+ **S15.11 Minor laceration of vertebral artery**
Incomplete transection of vertebral artery
Laceration of vertebral artery NOS
Superficial laceration of vertebral artery

CC +7th **S15.111 Minor laceration of right vertebral artery**
CC Exclusion 7th character A see Appendix A
PDX collection 1157

CC +7th **S15.112 Minor laceration of left vertebral artery**
CC Exclusion 7th character A see Appendix A
PDX collection 1157

CC +7th **S15.119 Minor laceration of unspecified vertebral artery**
CC Exclusion 7th character A see Appendix A
PDX collection 1157

+ **S15.12 Major laceration of vertebral artery**
Complete transection of vertebral artery
Traumatic rupture of vertebral artery

CC +7th **S15.121 Major laceration of right vertebral artery**
CC Exclusion 7th character A see Appendix A
PDX collection 1157

CC +7th **S15.122 Major laceration of left vertebral artery**
CC Exclusion 7th character A see Appendix A
PDX collection 1157

CC +7th **S15.129 Major laceration of unspecified vertebral artery**
CC Exclusion 7th character A see Appendix A
PDX collection 1157

+ **S15.19 Other specified injury of vertebral artery**

CC +7th **S15.191 Other specified injury of right vertebral artery**
CC Exclusion 7th character A see Appendix A
PDX collection 1157

CC +7th **S15.192 Other specified injury of left vertebral artery**
CC Exclusion 7th character A see Appendix A
PDX collection 1157

CC +7th **S15.199 Other specified injury of unspecified vertebral artery**
CC Exclusion 7th character A see Appendix A
PDX collection 1157

+ **S15.2 Injury of external jugular vein**
+ **S15.20 Unspecified injury of external jugular vein**

CC +7th **S15.201 Unspecified injury of right external jugular vein**
CC Exclusion 7th character A see Appendix A
PDX collection 1157

CC +7th **S15.202 Unspecified injury of left external jugular vein**
CC Exclusion 7th character A see Appendix A
PDX collection 1157

CC +7th **S15.209 Unspecified injury of unspecified external jugular vein**
CC Exclusion 7th character A see Appendix A
PDX collection 1157

+ **S15.21 Minor laceration of external jugular vein**
Incomplete transection of external jugular vein
Laceration of external jugular vein NOS
Superficial laceration of external jugular vein

CC +7th **S15.211 Minor laceration of right external jugular vein**
CC Exclusion 7th character A see Appendix A
PDX collection 1157

CC +7th **S15.212 Minor laceration of left external jugular vein**
CC Exclusion 7th character A see Appendix A
PDX collection 1157

CC +7th **S15.219 Minor laceration of unspecified external jugular vein**
CC Exclusion 7th character A see Appendix A
PDX collection 1157

+ **S15.22 Major laceration of external jugular vein**
Complete transection of external jugular vein
Traumatic rupture of external jugular vein

CC +7th **S15.221 Major laceration of right external jugular vein**
CC Exclusion 7th character A see Appendix A
PDX collection 1157

CC +7th **S15.222 Major laceration of left external jugular vein**
CC Exclusion 7th character A see Appendix A
PDX collection 1157

CC +7th **S15.229 Major laceration of unspecified external jugular vein**
CC Exclusion 7th character A see Appendix A
PDX collection 1157

+ **S15.29 Other specified injury of external jugular vein**

CC +7th **S15.291 Other specified injury of right external jugular vein**
CC Exclusion 7th character A see Appendix A
PDX collection 1157

CC +7th **S15.292 Other specified injury of left external jugular vein**
CC Exclusion 7th character A see Appendix A
PDX collection 1157

CC +7th **S15.299 Other specified injury of unspecified external jugular vein**
CC Exclusion 7th character A see Appendix A
PDX collection 1157

+ **S15.3 Injury of internal jugular vein**
+ **S15.30 Unspecified injury of internal jugular vein**

CC +7th **S15.301 Unspecified injury of right internal jugular vein**
CC Exclusion 7th character A see Appendix A
PDX collection 1157

CC +7th **S15.302 Unspecified injury of left internal jugular vein**
CC Exclusion 7th character A see Appendix A
PDX collection 1157

CC +7th **S15.309 Unspecified injury of unspecified internal jugular vein**
CC Exclusion 7th character A see Appendix A
PDX collection 1157

+ **S15.31 Minor laceration of internal jugular vein**
Incomplete transection of internal jugular vein
Laceration of internal jugular vein NOS
Superficial laceration of internal jugular vein

CC +7th **S15.311 Minor laceration of right internal jugular vein**
CC Exclusion 7th character A see Appendix A
PDX collection 1157

CC +7th **S15.312 Minor laceration of left internal jugular vein**
CC Exclusion 7th character A see Appendix A
PDX collection 1157

CC +7th **S15.319 Minor laceration of unspecified internal jugular vein**
CC Exclusion 7th character A see Appendix A
PDX collection 1157

+ **S15.32 Major laceration of internal jugular vein**
Complete transection of internal jugular vein
Traumatic rupture of internal jugular vein

CC +7th **S15.321 Major laceration of right internal jugular vein**
CC Exclusion 7th character A see Appendix A
PDX collection 1157

CC +7th **S15.322 Major laceration of left internal jugular vein**
CC Exclusion 7th character A see Appendix A
PDX collection 1157

CC +7th **S15.329 Major laceration of unspecified internal jugular vein**
CC Exclusion 7th character A see Appendix A
PDX collection 1157

+ **S15.39 Other specified injury of internal jugular vein**
  - CC +7th **S15.391 Other specified injury of right internal jugular vein**
    CC Exclusion 7th character A see Appendix A PDX collection 1157
  - CC +7th **S15.392 Other specified injury of left internal jugular vein**
    CC Exclusion 7th character A see Appendix A PDX collection 1157
  - CC +7th **S15.399 Other specified injury of unspecified internal jugular vein**
    CC Exclusion 7th character A see Appendix A PDX collection 1157

CC X+7th **S15.8 Injury of other specified blood vessels at neck level**
CC Exclusion 7th character A see Appendix A PDX collection 1157

CC X+7th **S15.9 Injury of unspecified blood vessel at neck level**
CC Exclusion 7th character A see Appendix A PDX collection 1157

S16 Injury of muscle, fascia and tendon at neck level

Code also any associated open wound (S11.-)

Excludes2: *sprain of joint or ligament at neck level (S13.9)*

The appropriate 7th character is to be added to each code from category S16
A initial encounter
D subsequent encounter
S sequela

X+7th **S16.1 Strain of muscle, fascia and tendon at neck level**
X+7th **S16.2 Laceration of muscle, fascia and tendon at neck level**
X+7th **S16.8 Other specified injury of muscle, fascia and tendon at neck level**
X+7th **S16.9 Unspecified injury of muscle, fascia and tendon at neck level**

S17 Crushing injury of neck

Use additional code for all associated injuries, such as:
injury of blood vessels (S15.-)
open wound of neck (S11.-)
spinal cord injury (S14.0, S14.1-)
vertebral fracture (S12.0--S12.3-)

The appropriate 7th character is to be added to each code from category S17
A initial encounter
D subsequent encounter
S sequela

CC X+7th **S17.0 Crushing injury of larynx and trachea**
CC Exclusion 7th character A see Appendix A PDX collection 1156
HAC 7th character A see Appendix B for HAC conditional logic

CC X+7th **S17.8 Crushing injury of other specified parts of neck**
CC Exclusion 7th character A see Appendix A PDX collection 1156
HAC 7th character A see Appendix B for HAC conditional logic

CC X+7th **S17.9 Crushing injury of neck, part unspecified**
CC Exclusion 7th character A see Appendix A PDX collection 1156
HAC 7th character A see Appendix B for HAC conditional logic

S19 Other specified and unspecified injuries of neck

The appropriate 7th character is to be added to each code from category S19
A initial encounter
D subsequent encounter
S sequela

+ **S19.8 Other specified injuries of neck**
  - X+7th **S19.80 Other specified injuries of unspecified part of neck**
  - X+7th **S19.81 Other specified injuries of larynx**
  - X+7th **S19.82 Other specified injuries of cervical trachea**
    Excludes2: *other specified injury of thoracic trachea (S27.5-)*
  - X+7th **S19.83 Other specified injuries of vocal cord**
  - X+7th **S19.84 Other specified injuries of thyroid gland**
  - X+7th **S19.85 Other specified injuries of pharynx and cervical esophagus**
  - X+7th **S19.89 Other specified injuries of other specified part of neck**

X+7th **S19.9 Unspecified injury of neck**

Injuries to the thorax (S20-S29)

Includes: injuries of breast
injuries of chest (wall)
injuries of interscapular area

Excludes2: *burns and corrosions (T20-T32)*
effects of foreign body in bronchus (T17.5)
effects of foreign body in esophagus (T18.1)
effects of foreign body in lung (T17.8)
effects of foreign body in trachea (T17.4)
frostbite (T33-T34)
injuries of axilla
injuries of clavicle
injuries of scapular region
injuries of shoulder
insect bite or sting, venomous (T63.4)

S20 Superficial injury of thorax

The appropriate 7th character is to be added to each code from category S20
A initial encounter
D subsequent encounter
S sequela

+ **S20.0 Contusion of breast**
  - X+7th **S20.00 Contusion of breast, unspecified breast**
  - X+7th **S20.01 Contusion of right breast**
  - X+7th **S20.02 Contusion of left breast**
+ **S20.1 Other and unspecified superficial injuries of breast**
  + **S20.10 Unspecified superficial injuries of breast**
    - +7th **S20.101 Unspecified superficial injuries of breast, right breast**
    - +7th **S20.102 Unspecified superficial injuries of breast, left breast**
    - +7th **S20.109 Unspecified superficial injuries of breast, unspecified breast**
  + **S20.11 Abrasion of breast**
    - +7th **S20.111 Abrasion of breast, right breast**
    - +7th **S20.112 Abrasion of breast, left breast**
    - +7th **S20.119 Abrasion of breast, unspecified breast**
  + **S20.12 Blister (nonthermal) of breast**
    - +7th **S20.121 Blister (nonthermal) of breast, right breas**
    - +7th **S20.122 Blister (nonthermal) of breast, left breast**
    - +7th **S20.129 Blister (nonthermal) of breast, unspecifie breast**
  + **S20.14 External constriction of part of breast**
    - +7th **S20.141 External constriction of part of breast, right breast**
    - +7th **S20.142 External constriction of part of breast, le breast**
    - +7th **S20.149 External constriction of part of breast, unspecified breast**
  + **S20.15 Superficial foreign body of breast**
    Splinter in the breast
    - +7th **S20.151 Superficial foreign body of breast, right breast**
    - +7th **S20.152 Superficial foreign body of breast, left breast**
    - +7th **S20.159 Superficial foreign body of breast, unspecified breast**
  + **S20.16 Insect bite (nonvenomous) of breast**
    - +7th **S20.161 Insect bite (nonvenomous) of breast, righ breast**
    - +7th **S20.162 Insect bite (nonvenomous) of breast, left breast**
    - +7th **S20.169 Insect bite (nonvenomous) of breast, unspecified breast**
  + **S20.17 Other superficial bite of breast**
    Excludes1: *open bite of breast (S21.05-)*
    - +7th **S20.171 Other superficial bite of breast, right breast**
    - +7th **S20.172 Other superficial bite of breast, left breas**
    - +7th **S20.179 Other superficial bite of breast, unspecifi breast**
+ **S20.2 Contusion of thorax**
  - X+7th **S20.20 Contusion of thorax, unspecified**
  + **S20.21 Contusion of front wall of thorax**
    - +7th **S20.211 Contusion of right front wall of thorax**
    - +7th **S20.212 Contusion of left front wall of thorax**
    - +7th **S20.219 Contusion of unspecified front wall of thorax**

+ S20.22 Contusion of back wall of thorax
+7th S20.221 Contusion of right back wall of thorax
+7th S20.222 Contusion of left back wall of thorax
+7th S20.229 Contusion of unspecified back wall of thorax
+ S20.3 Other and unspecified superficial injuries of front wall of thorax
+ S20.30 Unspecified superficial injuries of front wall of thorax
+7th S20.301 Unspecified superficial injuries of right front wall of thorax
+7th S20.302 Unspecified superficial injuries of left front wall of thorax
+7th S20.309 Unspecified superficial injuries of unspecified front wall of thorax
+ S20.31 Abrasion of front wall of thorax
+7th S20.311 Abrasion of right front wall of thorax
+7th S20.312 Abrasion of left front wall of thorax
+7th S20.319 Abrasion of unspecified front wall of thorax
+ S20.32 Blister (nonthermal) of front wall of thorax
+7th S20.321 Blister (nonthermal) of right front wall of thorax
+7th S20.322 Blister (nonthermal) of left front wall of thorax
+7th S20.329 Blister (nonthermal) of unspecified front wall of thorax
+ S20.34 External constriction of front wall of thorax
+7th S20.341 External constriction of right front wall of thorax
+7th S20.342 External constriction of left front wall of thorax
+7th S20.349 External constriction of unspecified front wall of thorax
+ S20.35 Superficial foreign body of front wall of thorax
Splinter in front wall of thorax
+7th S20.351 Superficial foreign body of right front wall of thorax
+7th S20.352 Superficial foreign body of left front wall of thorax
+7th S20.359 Superficial foreign body of unspecified front wall of thorax
+ S20.36 Insect bite (nonvenomous) of front wall of thorax
+7th S20.361 Insect bite (nonvenomous) of right front wall of thorax
+7th S20.362 Insect bite (nonvenomous) of left front wall of thorax
+7th S20.369 Insect bite (nonvenomous) of unspecified front wall of thorax
+ S20.37 Other superficial bite of front wall of thorax
Excludes1: *open bite of front wall of thorax (S21.14)*
+7th S20.371 Other superficial bite of right front wall of thorax
+7th S20.372 Other superficial bite of left front wall of thorax
+7th S20.379 Other superficial bite of unspecified front wall of thorax
+ S20.4 Other and unspecified superficial injuries of back wall of thorax
+ S20.40 Unspecified superficial injuries of back wall of thorax
+7th S20.401 Unspecified superficial injuries of right back wall of thorax
+7th S20.402 Unspecified superficial injuries of left back wall of thorax
+7th S20.409 Unspecified superficial injuries of unspecified back wall of thorax
+ S20.41 Abrasion of back wall of thorax
+7th S20.411 Abrasion of right back wall of thorax
+7th S20.412 Abrasion of left back wall of thorax
+7th S20.419 Abrasion of unspecified back wall of thorax
+ S20.42 Blister (nonthermal) of back wall of thorax
+7th S20.421 Blister (nonthermal) of right back wall of thorax
+7th S20.422 Blister (nonthermal) of left back wall of thorax
+7th S20.429 Blister (nonthermal) of unspecified back wall of thorax
+ S20.44 External constriction of back wall of thorax
+7th S20.441 External constriction of right back wall of thorax
+7th S20.442 External constriction of left back wall of thorax
+7th S20.449 External constriction of unspecified back wall of thorax
+ S20.45 Superficial foreign body of back wall of thorax
Splinter of back wall of thorax
+7th S20.451 Superficial foreign body of right back wall of thorax
+7th S20.452 Superficial foreign body of left back wall of thorax
+7th S20.459 Superficial foreign body of unspecified back wall of thorax
+ S20.46 Insect bite (nonvenomous) of back wall of thorax
+7th S20.461 Insect bite (nonvenomous) of right back wall of thorax
+7th S20.462 Insect bite (nonvenomous) of left back wall of thorax
+7th S20.469 Insect bite (nonvenomous) of unspecified back wall of thorax
+ S20.47 Other superficial bite of back wall of thorax
Excludes1: *open bite of back wall of thorax (S21.24)*
+7th S20.471 Other superficial bite of right back wall of thorax
+7th S20.472 Other superficial bite of left back wall of thorax
+7th S20.479 Other superficial bite of unspecified back wall of thorax
+ S20.9 Superficial injury of unspecified parts of thorax
Excludes1: *contusion of thorax NOS (S20.20)*
X+7th S20.90 Unspecified superficial injury of unspecified parts of thorax
Superficial injury of thoracic wall NOS
X+7th S20.91 Abrasion of unspecified parts of thorax
X+7th S20.92 Blister (nonthermal) of unspecified parts of thorax
X+7th S20.94 External constriction of unspecified parts of thorax
X+7th S20.95 Superficial foreign body of unspecified parts of thorax
Splinter in thorax NOS
X+7th S20.96 Insect bite (nonvenomous) of unspecified parts of thorax
X+7th S20.97 Other superficial bite of unspecified parts of thorax
Excludes1: *open bite of thorax NOS (S21.95)*

S21 Open wound of thorax

Code also any associated injury, such as:
injury of heart (S26.-)
injury of intrathoracic organs (S27.-)
rib fracture (S22.3-, S22.4-)
spinal cord injury (S24.0-, S24.1-)
traumatic hemothorax (S27.1)
traumatic hemopneumothorax (S27.3)
traumatic pneumothorax (S27.0)
wound infection

Excludes1: *traumatic amputation (partial) of thorax (S28.1)*

The appropriate 7th character is to be added to each code from category S21
A initial encounter
D subsequent encounter
S sequela

+ S21.0 Open wound of breast
+ S21.00 Unspecified open wound of breast
+7th S21.001 Unspecified open wound of right breast
+7th S21.002 Unspecified open wound of left breast
+7th S21.009 Unspecified open wound of unspecified breast
+ S21.01 Laceration without foreign body of breast
+7th S21.011 Laceration without foreign body of right breast
+7th S21.012 Laceration without foreign body of left breast
+7th S21.019 Laceration without foreign body of unspecified breast
+ S21.02 Laceration with foreign body of breast
+7th S21.021 Laceration with foreign body of right breast
+7th S21.022 Laceration with foreign body of left breast
+7th S21.029 Laceration with foreign body of unspecified breast

+ **S21.03 Puncture wound without foreign body of breast**
  - +7th **S21.031 Puncture wound without foreign body of right breast**
  - +7th **S21.032 Puncture wound without foreign body of left breast**
  - +7th **S21.039 Puncture wound without foreign body of unspecified breast**

+ **S21.04 Puncture wound with foreign body of breast**
  - +7th **S21.041 Puncture wound with foreign body of right breast**
  - +7th **S21.042 Puncture wound with foreign body of left breast**
  - +7th **S21.049 Puncture wound with foreign body of unspecified breast**

+ **S21.05 Open bite of breast**
  Bite of breast NOS
  Excludes1: *superficial bite of breast (S20.17)*
  - **S21.051 Open bite of right breast**
  - **S21.052 Open bite of left breast**
  - **S21.059 Open bite of unspecified breast**

+ **S21.1 Open wound of front wall of thorax without penetration into thoracic cavity**
  Open wound of chest without penetration into thoracic cavity

+ **S21.10 Unspecified open wound of front wall of thorax without penetration into thoracic cavity**
  - CC +7th **S21.101 Unspecified open wound of right front wall of thorax without penetration into thoracic cavity**
    CC Exclusion 7th character A see Appendix A
    PDX collection 1168
  - CC +7th **S21.102 Unspecified open wound of left front wall of thorax without penetration into thoracic cavity**
    CC Exclusion 7th character A see Appendix A
    PDX collection 1168
  - CC +7th **S21.109 Unspecified open wound of unspecified front wall of thorax without penetration into thoracic cavity**
    CC Exclusion 7th character A see Appendix A
    PDX collection 1168

+ **S21.11 Laceration without foreign body of front wall of thorax without penetration into thoracic cavity**
  - CC +7th **S21.111 Laceration without foreign body of right front wall of thorax without penetration into thoracic cavity**
    CC Exclusion 7th character A see Appendix A
    PDX collection 1168
  - CC +7th **S21.112 Laceration without foreign body of left front wall of thorax without penetration into thoracic cavity**
    CC Exclusion 7th character A see Appendix A
    PDX collection 1168
  - CC +7th **S21.119 Laceration without foreign body of unspecified front wall of thorax without penetration into thoracic cavity**
    CC Exclusion 7th character A see Appendix A
    PDX collection 1168

+ **S21.12 Laceration with foreign body of front wall of thorax without penetration into thoracic cavity**
  - CC +7th **S21.121 Laceration with foreign body of right front wall of thorax without penetration into thoracic cavity**
    CC Exclusion 7th character A see Appendix A
    PDX collection 1168
  - CC +7th **S21.122 Laceration with foreign body of left front wall of thorax without penetration into thoracic cavity**
    CC Exclusion 7th character A see Appendix A
    PDX collection 1168
  - CC +7th **S21.129 Laceration with foreign body of unspecified front wall of thorax without penetration into thoracic cavity**
    CC Exclusion 7th character A see Appendix A
    PDX collection 1168

+ **S21.13 Puncture wound without foreign body of front wall of thorax without penetration into thoracic cavity**
  - CC +7th **S21.131 Puncture wound without foreign body of right front wall of thorax without penetration into thoracic cavity**
    CC Exclusion 7th character A see Appendix A
    PDX collection 1168
  - CC +7th **S21.132 Puncture wound without foreign body of left front wall of thorax without penetration into thoracic cavity**
    CC Exclusion 7th character A see Appendix A
    PDX collection 1168
  - CC +7th **S21.139 Puncture wound without foreign body of unspecified front wall of thorax without penetration into thoracic cavity**
    CC Exclusion 7th character A see Appendix A
    PDX collection 1168

+ **S21.14 Puncture wound with foreign body of front wall of thorax without penetration into thoracic cavity**
  - CC +7th **S21.141 Puncture wound with foreign body of right front wall of thorax without penetration into thoracic cavity**
    CC Exclusion 7th character A see Appendix A
    PDX collection 1168
  - CC +7th **S21.142 Puncture wound with foreign body of left front wall of thorax without penetration into thoracic cavity**
    CC Exclusion 7th character A see Appendix A
    PDX collection 1168
  - CC +7th **S21.149 Puncture wound with foreign body of unspecified front wall of thorax without penetration into thoracic cavity**
    CC Exclusion 7th character A see Appendix A
    PDX collection 1168

+ **S21.15 Open bite of front wall of thorax without penetration into thoracic cavity**
  Bite of front wall of thorax NOS
  Excludes1: *superficial bite of front wall of thorax (S20.37)*
  - CC +7th **S21.151 Open bite of right front wall of thorax without penetration into thoracic cavity**
    CC Exclusion 7th character A see Appendix A
    PDX collection 1168
  - CC +7th **S21.152 Open bite of left front wall of thorax without penetration into thoracic cavity**
    CC Exclusion 7th character A see Appendix A
    PDX collection 1168
  - CC +7th **S21.159 Open bite of unspecified front wall of thorax without penetration into thoracic cavity**
    CC Exclusion 7th character A see Appendix A
    PDX collection 1168

+ **S21.2 Open wound of back wall of thorax without penetration into thoracic cavity**

+ **S21.20 Unspecified open wound of back wall of thorax without penetration into thoracic cavity**
  - +7th **S21.201 Unspecified open wound of right back wall of thorax without penetration into thoracic cavity**
  - +7th **S21.202 Unspecified open wound of left back wall of thorax without penetration into thoracic cavity**
  - +7th **S21.209 Unspecified open wound of unspecified back wall of thorax without penetration into thoracic cavity**

+ **S21.21 Laceration without foreign body of back wall of thorax without penetration into thoracic cavity**
  - +7th **S21.211 Laceration without foreign body of right back wall of thorax without penetration into thoracic cavity**
  - +7th **S21.212 Laceration without foreign body of left back wall of thorax without penetration into thoracic cavity**
  - +7th **S21.219 Laceration without foreign body of unspecified back wall of thorax without penetration into thoracic cavity**

+ **S21.22 Laceration with foreign body of back wall of thorax without penetration into thoracic cavity**
  - +7th **S21.221 Laceration with foreign body of right back wall of thorax without penetration into thoracic cavity**
  - +7th **S21.222 Laceration with foreign body of left back wall of thorax without penetration into thoracic cavity**
  - +7th **S21.229 Laceration with foreign body of unspecified back wall of thorax without penetration into thoracic cavity**

+ S21.23 **Puncture wound without foreign body of back wall of thorax without penetration into thoracic cavity**
+7th S21.231 **Puncture wound without foreign body of right back wall of thorax without penetration into thoracic cavity**
+7th S21.232 **Puncture wound without foreign body of left back wall of thorax without penetration into thoracic cavity**
+7th S21.239 **Puncture wound without foreign body of unspecified back wall of thorax without penetration into thoracic cavity**
+ S21.24 **Puncture wound with foreign body of back wall of thorax without penetration into thoracic cavity**
+7th S21.241 **Puncture wound with foreign body of right back wall of thorax without penetration into thoracic cavity**
+7th S21.242 **Puncture wound with foreign body of left back wall of thorax without penetration into thoracic cavity**
+7th S21.249 **Puncture wound with foreign body of unspecified back wall of thorax without penetration into thoracic cavity**
+ S21.25 **Open bite of back wall of thorax without penetration into thoracic cavity**
Bite of back wall of thorax NOS
Excludes1: *superficial bite of back wall of thorax (S20.47)*
+7th S21.251 **Open bite of right back wall of thorax without penetration into thoracic cavity**
+7th S21.252 **Open bite of left back wall of thorax without penetration into thoracic cavity**
+7th S21.259 **Open bite of unspecified back wall of thorax without penetration into thoracic cavity**
+ S21.3 **Open wound of front wall of thorax with penetration into thoracic cavity**
Open wound of chest with penetration into thoracic cavity
+ S21.30 **Unspecified open wound of front wall of thorax with penetration into thoracic cavity**
MCC +7th S21.301 **Unspecified open wound of right front wall of thorax with penetration into thoracic cavity**
MCC Exclusion 7th character A see Appendix A PDX collection 1169
MCC +7th S21.302 **Unspecified open wound of left front wall of thorax with penetration into thoracic cavity**
MCC Exclusion 7th character A see Appendix A PDX collection 1169
MCC +7th S21.309 **Unspecified open wound of unspecified front wall of thorax with penetration into thoracic cavity**
MCC Exclusion 7th character A see Appendix A PDX collection 1170
+ S21.31 **Laceration without foreign body of front wall of thorax with penetration into thoracic cavity**
MCC +7th S21.311 **Laceration without foreign body of right front wall of thorax with penetration into thoracic cavity**
MCC Exclusion 7th character A see Appendix A PDX collection 1169
MCC +7th S21.312 **Laceration without foreign body of left front wall of thorax with penetration into thoracic cavity**
MCC Exclusion 7th character A see Appendix A PDX collection 1169
MCC +7th S21.319 **Laceration without foreign body of unspecified front wall of thorax with penetration into thoracic cavity**
MCC Exclusion 7th character A see Appendix A PDX collection 1169
+ S21.32 **Laceration with foreign body of front wall of thorax with penetration into thoracic cavity**
MCC +7th S21.321 **Laceration with foreign body of right front wall of thorax with penetration into thoracic cavity**
MCC Exclusion 7th character A see Appendix A PDX collection 1169
MCC +7th S21.322 **Laceration with foreign body of left front wall of thorax with penetration into thoracic cavity**
MCC Exclusion 7th character A see Appendix A PDX collection 1169
MCC +7th S21.329 **Laceration with foreign body of unspecified front wall of thorax with penetration into thoracic cavity**
MCC Exclusion 7th character A see Appendix A PDX collection 1169
+ S21.33 **Puncture wound without foreign body of front wall of thorax with penetration into thoracic cavity**
MCC +7th S21.331 **Puncture wound without foreign body of right front wall of thorax with penetration into thoracic cavity**
MCC Exclusion 7th character A see Appendix A PDX collection 1169
MCC +7th S21.332 **Puncture wound without foreign body of left front wall of thorax with penetration into thoracic cavity**
MCC Exclusion 7th character A see Appendix A PDX collection 1169
MCC +7th S21.339 **Puncture wound without foreign body of unspecified front wall of thorax with penetration into thoracic cavity**
MCC Exclusion 7th character A see Appendix A PDX collection 1169
+ S21.34 **Puncture wound with foreign body of front wall of thorax with penetration into thoracic cavity**
MCC +7th S21.341 **Puncture wound with foreign body of right front wall of thorax with penetration into thoracic cavity**
MCC Exclusion 7th character A see Appendix A PDX collection 1169
MCC +7th S21.342 **Puncture wound with foreign body of left front wall of thorax with penetration into thoracic cavity**
MCC Exclusion 7th character A see Appendix A PDX collection 1169
MCC +7th S21.349 **Puncture wound with foreign body of unspecified front wall of thorax with penetration into thoracic cavity**
MCC Exclusion 7th character A see Appendix A PDX collection 1169
+ S21.35 **Open bite of front wall of thorax with penetration into thoracic cavity**
Excludes1: *superficial bite of front wall of thorax (S20.37)*
MCC +7th S21.351 **Open bite of right front wall of thorax with penetration into thoracic cavity**
MCC Exclusion 7th character A see Appendix A PDX collection 1169
MCC +7th S21.352 **Open bite of left front wall of thorax with penetration into thoracic cavity**
MCC Exclusion 7th character A see Appendix A PDX collection 1169
MCC +7th S21.359 **Open bite of unspecified front wall of thorax with penetration into thoracic cavity**
MCC Exclusion 7th character A see Appendix A PDX collection 1169
+ S21.4 **Open wound of back wall of thorax with penetration into thoracic cavity**
+ S21.40 **Unspecified open wound of back wall of thorax with penetration into thoracic cavity**
MCC +7th S21.401 **Unspecified open wound of right back wall of thorax with penetration into thoracic cavity**
MCC Exclusion 7th character A see Appendix A PDX collection 1169
MCC +7th S21.402 **Unspecified open wound of left back wall of thorax with penetration into thoracic cavity**
MCC Exclusion 7th character A see Appendix A PDX collection 1169
MCC +7th S21.409 **Unspecified open wound of unspecified back wall of thorax with penetration into thoracic cavity**
MCC Exclusion 7th character A see Appendix A PDX collection 1169

+ **S21.41 Laceration without foreign body of back wall of thorax with penetration into thoracic cavity**

MCC +7th **S21.411 Laceration without foreign body of right back wall of thorax with penetration into thoracic cavity**
MCC Exclusion 7th character A see Appendix A PDX collection 1169

MCC +7th **S21.412 Laceration without foreign body of left back wall of thorax with penetration into thoracic cavity**
MCC Exclusion 7th character A see Appendix A PDX collection 1169

MCC +7th **S21.419 Laceration without foreign body of unspecified back wall of thorax with penetration into thoracic cavity**
MCC Exclusion 7th character A see Appendix A PDX collection 1169

+ **S21.42 Laceration with foreign body of back wall of thorax with penetration into thoracic cavity**

MCC +7th **S21.421 Laceration with foreign body of right back wall of thorax with penetration into thoracic cavity**
MCC Exclusion 7th character A see Appendix A PDX collection 1169

MCC +7th **S21.422 Laceration with foreign body of left back wall of thorax with penetration into thoracic cavity**
MCC Exclusion 7th character A see Appendix A PDX collection 1169

MCC +7th **S21.429 Laceration with foreign body of unspecified back wall of thorax with penetration into thoracic cavity**
MCC Exclusion 7th character A see Appendix A PDX collection 1169

+ **S21.43 Puncture wound without foreign body of back wall of thorax with penetration into thoracic cavity**

MCC +7th **S21.431 Puncture wound without foreign body of right back wall of thorax with penetration into thoracic cavity**
MCC Exclusion 7th character A see Appendix A PDX collection 1169

MCC +7th **S21.432 Puncture wound without foreign body of left back wall of thorax with penetration into thoracic cavity**
MCC Exclusion 7th character A see Appendix A PDX collection 1169

MCC +7th **S21.439 Puncture wound without foreign body of unspecified back wall of thorax with penetration into thoracic cavity**
MCC Exclusion 7th character A see Appendix A PDX collection 1169

+ **S21.44 Puncture wound with foreign body of back wall of thorax with penetration into thoracic cavity**

MCC +7th **S21.441 Puncture wound with foreign body of right back wall of thorax with penetration into thoracic cavity**
MCC Exclusion 7th character A see Appendix A PDX collection 1169

MCC +7th **S21.442 Puncture wound with foreign body of left back wall of thorax with penetration into thoracic cavity**
MCC Exclusion 7th character A see Appendix A PDX collection 1169

MCC +7th **S21.449 Puncture wound with foreign body of unspecified back wall of thorax with penetration into thoracic cavity**
MCC Exclusion 7th character A see Appendix A PDX collection 1169

+ **S21.45 Open bite of back wall of thorax with penetration into thoracic cavity**
Bite of back wall of thorax NOS
Excludes1: *superficial bite of back wall of thorax (S20.47)*

MCC +7th **S21.451 Open bite of right back wall of thorax with penetration into thoracic cavity**
MCC Exclusion 7th character A see Appendix A PDX collection 1169

MCC +7th **S21.452 Open bite of left back wall of thorax with penetration into thoracic cavity**
MCC Exclusion 7th character A see Appendix A PDX collection 1169

MCC +7th **S21.459 Open bite of unspecified back wall of thorax with penetration into thoracic cavity**
MCC Exclusion 7th character A see Appendix A PDX collection 1169

+ **S21.9 Open wound of unspecified part of thorax**
Open wound of thoracic wall NOS

CC X+7th **S21.90 Unspecified open wound of unspecified part of thorax**
CC Exclusion 7th character A see Appendix A PDX collection 1168

CC X+7th **S21.91 Laceration without foreign body of unspecified part of thorax**
CC Exclusion 7th character A see Appendix A PDX collection 1168

CC X+7th **S21.92 Laceration with foreign body of unspecified part of thorax**
CC Exclusion 7th character A see Appendix A PDX collection 1168

CC X+7th **S21.93 Puncture wound without foreign body of unspecified part of thorax**
CC Exclusion 7th character A see Appendix A PDX collection 1168

CC X+7th **S21.94 Puncture wound with foreign body of unspecified part of thorax**
CC Exclusion 7th character A see Appendix A PDX collection 1168

CC X+7th **S21.95 Open bite of unspecified part of thorax**
Excludes1: *superficial bite of thorax (S20.97)*
CC Exclusion 7th character A see Appendix A PDX collection 1168

See page 961 for Vertebrae Illustration.

S22 Fracture of rib(s), sternum and thoracic spine

NOTE A fracture not indicated as displaced or nondisplaced should be coded to displaced
A fracture not indicated as open or closed should be coded to closed

Includes: fracture of thoracic neural arch
fracture of thoracic spinous process
fracture of thoracic transverse process
fracture of thoracic vertebra
fracture of thoracic vertebral arch

Code first any associated:
injury of intrathoracic organ (S27.-)
spinal cord injury (S24.0-, S24.1-)

Excludes1: *transection of thorax (S28.1)*
Excludes2: *fracture of clavicle (S42.0-)*
fracture of scapula (S42.1-)

The appropriate 7th character is to be added to each code from category S22
A initial encounter for closed fracture
B initial encounter for open fracture
D subsequent encounter for fracture with routine healing
G subsequent encounter for fracture with delayed healing
K subsequent encounter for fracture with nonunion
S sequela

Review coding guideline C.19.c

+ **S22.0 Fracture of thoracic vertebra**

+ **S22.00 Fracture of unspecified thoracic vertebra**

CC MCC +7th **S22.000 Wedge compression fracture of unspecified thoracic vertebra**
CC Exclusion 7th character A see Appendix A PDX collection 1171
CC Exclusion 7th character K see Appendix A PDX collection 0897
MCC Exclusion 7th character B see Appendix A PDX collection 1171
HAC 7th characters A & B see Appendix B for HAC conditional logic

CC MCC +7th **S22.001 Stable burst fracture of unspecified thoracic vertebra**
CC Exclusion 7th character A see Appendix A PDX collection 1171
CC Exclusion 7th character K see Appendix A PDX collection 0897
MCC Exclusion 7th character B see Appendix A PDX collection 1171
HAC 7th characters A & B see Appendix B for HAC conditional logic

CC MCC +7th **S22.002** **Unstable burst fracture of unspecified thoracic vertebra**
CC Exclusion 7th character A see Appendix A PDX collection 1171
CC Exclusion 7th character K see Appendix A PDX collection 0897
MCC Exclusion 7th character B see Appendix A PDX collection 1171
HAC 7th characters A & B see Appendix B for HAC conditional logic

CC MCC +7th **S22.008** **Other fracture of unspecified thoracic vertebra**
CC Exclusion 7th character A see Appendix A PDX collection 1171
CC Exclusion 7th character K see Appendix A PDX collection 0897
MCC Exclusion 7th character B see Appendix A PDX collection 1171
HAC 7th characters A & B see Appendix B for HAC conditional logic

CC MCC +7th **S22.009** **Unspecified fracture of unspecified thoracic vertebra**
CC Exclusion 7th character A see Appendix A PDX collection 1171
CC Exclusion 7th character K see Appendix A PDX collection 0897
MCC Exclusion 7th character B see Appendix A PDX collection 1171
HAC 7th characters A & B see Appendix B for HAC conditional logic

+ **S22.01** **Fracture of first thoracic vertebra**

CC MCC +7th **S22.010** **Wedge compression fracture of first thoracic vertebra**
CC Exclusion 7th character A see Appendix A PDX collection 1171
CC Exclusion 7th character K see Appendix A PDX collection 0897
MCC Exclusion 7th character B see Appendix A PDX collection 1171
HAC 7th characters A & B see Appendix B for HAC conditional logic

CC MCC +7th **S22.011** **Stable burst fracture of first thoracic vertebra**
CC Exclusion 7th character A see Appendix A PDX collection 1171
CC Exclusion 7th character K see Appendix A PDX collection 0897
MCC Exclusion 7th character B see Appendix A PDX collection 1171
HAC 7th characters A & B see Appendix B for HAC conditional logic

CC MCC +7th **S22.012** **Unstable burst fracture of first thoracic vertebra**
CC Exclusion 7th character A see Appendix A PDX collection 1171
CC Exclusion 7th character K see Appendix A PDX collection 0897
MCC Exclusion 7th character B see Appendix A PDX collection 1171
HAC 7th characters A & B see Appendix B for HAC conditional logic

CC MCC +7th **S22.018** **Other fracture of first thoracic vertebra**
CC Exclusion 7th character A see Appendix A PDX collection 1171
CC Exclusion 7th character K see Appendix A PDX collection 0897
MCC Exclusion 7th character B see Appendix A PDX collection 1171
HAC 7th characters A & B see Appendix B for HAC conditional logic

CC MCC +7th **S22.019** **Unspecified fracture of first thoracic vertebra**
CC Exclusion 7th character A see Appendix A PDX collection 1171
CC Exclusion 7th character K see Appendix A PDX collection 0897
MCC Exclusion 7th character B see Appendix A PDX collection 1171
HAC 7th characters A & B see Appendix B for HAC conditional logic

+ **S22.02** **Fracture of second thoracic vertebra**

CC MCC +7th **S22.020** **Wedge compression fracture of second thoracic vertebra**
CC Exclusion 7th character A see Appendix A PDX collection 1171
CC Exclusion 7th character K see Appendix A PDX collection 0897
MCC Exclusion 7th character B see Appendix A PDX collection 1171
HAC 7th characters A & B see Appendix B for HAC conditional logic

CC MCC +7th **S22.021** **Stable burst fracture of second thoracic vertebra**
CC Exclusion 7th character A see Appendix A PDX collection 1171
CC Exclusion 7th character K see Appendix A PDX collection 0897
MCC Exclusion 7th character B see Appendix A PDX collection 1171
HAC 7th characters A & B see Appendix B for HAC conditional logic

CC MCC +7th **S22.022** **Unstable burst fracture of second thoracic vertebra**
CC Exclusion 7th character A see Appendix A PDX collection 1171
CC Exclusion 7th character K see Appendix A PDX collection 0897
MCC Exclusion 7th character B see Appendix A PDX collection 1171
HAC 7th characters A & B see Appendix B for HAC conditional logic

CC MCC +7th **S22.028** **Other fracture of second thoracic vertebra**
CC Exclusion 7th character A see Appendix A PDX collection 1171
CC Exclusion 7th character K see Appendix A PDX collection 0897
MCC Exclusion 7th character B see Appendix A PDX collection 1171
HAC 7th characters A & B see Appendix B for HAC conditional logic

CC MCC +7th **S22.029** **Unspecified fracture of second thoracic vertebra**
CC Exclusion 7th character A see Appendix A PDX collection 1171
CC Exclusion 7th character K see Appendix A PDX collection 0897
MCC Exclusion 7th character B see Appendix A PDX collection 1171
HAC 7th characters A & B see Appendix B for HAC conditional logic

+ **S22.03** **Fracture of third thoracic vertebra**

CC MCC +7th **S22.030** **Wedge compression fracture of third thoracic vertebra**
CC Exclusion 7th character A see Appendix A PDX collection 1171
CC Exclusion 7th character K see Appendix A PDX collection 0897
MCC Exclusion 7th character B see Appendix A PDX collection 1171
HAC 7th characters A & B see Appendix B for HAC conditional logic

CC MCC +7th **S22.031** **Stable burst fracture of third thoracic vertebra**
CC Exclusion 7th character A see Appendix A PDX collection 1171
CC Exclusion 7th character K see Appendix A PDX collection 0897
MCC Exclusion 7th character B see Appendix A PDX collection 1171
HAC 7th characters A & B see Appendix B for HAC conditional logic

CC MCC +7th **S22.032** **Unstable burst fracture of third thoracic vertebra**
CC Exclusion 7th character A see Appendix A PDX collection 1171
CC Exclusion 7th character K see Appendix A PDX collection 0897
MCC Exclusion 7th character B see Appendix A PDX collection 1171
HAC 7th characters A & B see Appendix B for HAC conditional logic

CC MCC +7th **S22.038** **Other fracture of third thoracic vertebra**
CC Exclusion 7th character A see Appendix A
PDX collection 1171
CC Exclusion 7th character K see Appendix A
PDX collection 0897
MCC Exclusion 7th character B see Appendix A
PDX collection 1171
HAC 7th characters A & B see Appendix B for HAC conditional logic

CC MCC +7th **S22.039** **Unspecified fracture of third thoracic vertebra**
CC Exclusion 7th character A see Appendix A
PDX collection 1171
CC Exclusion 7th character K see Appendix A
PDX collection 0897
MCC Exclusion 7th character B see Appendix A
PDX collection 1171
HAC 7th characters A & B see Appendix B for HAC conditional logic

\+ **S22.04** **Fracture of fourth thoracic vertebra**

CC MCC +7th **S22.040** **Wedge compression fracture of fourth thoracic vertebra**
CC Exclusion 7th character A see Appendix A
PDX collection 1171
CC Exclusion 7th character K see Appendix A
PDX collection 0897
MCC Exclusion 7th character B see Appendix A
PDX collection 1171
HAC 7th characters A & B see Appendix B for HAC conditional logic

CC MCC +7th **S22.041** **Stable burst fracture of fourth thoracic vertebra**
CC Exclusion 7th character A see Appendix A
PDX collection 1171
CC Exclusion 7th character K see Appendix A
PDX collection 0897
MCC Exclusion 7th character B see Appendix A
PDX collection 1171
HAC 7th characters A & B see Appendix B for HAC conditional logic

CC MCC +7th **S22.042** **Unstable burst fracture of fourth thoracic vertebra**
CC Exclusion 7th character A see Appendix A
PDX collection 1171
CC Exclusion 7th character K see Appendix A
PDX collection 0897
MCC Exclusion 7th character B see Appendix A
PDX collection 1171
HAC 7th characters A & B see Appendix B for HAC conditional logic

CC MCC +7th **S22.048** **Other fracture of fourth thoracic vertebra**
CC Exclusion 7th character A see Appendix A
PDX collection 1171
CC Exclusion 7th character K see Appendix A
PDX collection 0897
MCC Exclusion 7th character B see Appendix A
PDX collection 1171
HAC 7th characters A & B see Appendix B for HAC conditional logic

CC MCC +7th **S22.049** **Unspecified fracture of fourth thoracic vertebra**
CC Exclusion 7th character A see Appendix A
PDX collection 1171
CC Exclusion 7th character K see Appendix A
PDX collection 0897
MCC Exclusion 7th character B see Appendix A
PDX collection 1171
HAC 7th characters A & B see Appendix B for HAC conditional logic

\+ **S22.05** **Fracture of T5-T6 vertebra**

CC MCC +7th **S22.050** **Wedge compression fracture of T5-T6 vertebra**
CC Exclusion 7th character A see Appendix A
PDX collection 1171
CC Exclusion 7th character K see Appendix A
PDX collection 0897
MCC Exclusion 7th character B see Appendix A
PDX collection 1171
HAC 7th characters A & B see Appendix B for HAC conditional logic

CC MCC +7th **S22.051** **Stable burst fracture of T5-T6 vertebra**
CC Exclusion 7th character A see Appendix A
PDX collection 1171
CC Exclusion 7th character K see Appendix A
PDX collection 0897
MCC Exclusion 7th character B see Appendix A
PDX collection 1171
HAC 7th characters A & B see Appendix B for HAC conditional logic

CC MCC +7th **S22.052** **Unstable burst fracture of T5-T6 vertebra**
CC Exclusion 7th character A see Appendix A
PDX collection 1171
CC Exclusion 7th character K see Appendix A
PDX collection 0897
MCC Exclusion 7th character B see Appendix A
PDX collection 1171
HAC 7th characters A & B see Appendix B for HAC conditional logic

CC MCC +7th **S22.058** **Other fracture of T5-T6 vertebra**
CC Exclusion 7th character A see Appendix A
PDX collection 1171
CC Exclusion 7th character K see Appendix A
PDX collection 0897
MCC Exclusion 7th character B see Appendix A
PDX collection 1171
HAC 7th characters A & B see Appendix B for HAC conditional logic

CC MCC +7th **S22.059** **Unspecified fracture of T5-T6 vertebra**
CC Exclusion 7th character A see Appendix A
PDX collection 1171
CC Exclusion 7th character K see Appendix A
PDX collection 0897
MCC Exclusion 7th character B see Appendix A
PDX collection 1171
HAC 7th characters A & B see Appendix B for HAC conditional logic

\+ **S22.06** **Fracture of T7-T8 vertebra**

CC MCC +7th **S22.060** **Wedge compression fracture of T7-T8 vertebra**
CC Exclusion 7th character A see Appendix A
PDX collection 1171
CC Exclusion 7th character K see Appendix A
PDX collection 0897
MCC Exclusion 7th character B see Appendix A
PDX collection 1171
HAC 7th characters A & B see Appendix B for HAC conditional logic

CC MCC +7th **S22.061** **Stable burst fracture of T7-T8 vertebra**
CC Exclusion 7th character A see Appendix A
PDX collection 1171
CC Exclusion 7th character K see Appendix A
PDX collection 0897
MCC Exclusion 7th character B see Appendix A
PDX collection 1171
HAC 7th characters A & B see Appendix B for HAC conditional logic

CC MCC +7th **S22.062** **Unstable burst fracture of T7-T8 vertebra**
CC Exclusion 7th character A see Appendix A
PDX collection 1171
CC Exclusion 7th character K see Appendix A
PDX collection 0897
MCC Exclusion 7th character B see Appendix A
PDX collection 1171
HAC 7th characters A & B see Appendix B for HAC conditional logic

CC MCC +7th **S22.068** **Other fracture of T7-T8 thoracic vertebra**
CC Exclusion 7th character A see Appendix A
PDX collection 1171
CC Exclusion 7th character K see Appendix A
PDX collection 0897
MCC Exclusion 7th character B see Appendix A
PDX collection 1171
HAC 7th characters A & B see Appendix B for HAC conditional logic

CC MCC +7th **S22.069** **Unspecified fracture of T7-T8 vertebra**
CC Exclusion 7th character A see Appendix A
PDX collection 1171
CC Exclusion 7th character K see Appendix A
PDX collection 0897
MCC Exclusion 7th character B see Appendix A
PDX collection 1171
HAC 7th characters A & B see Appendix B for HAC conditional logic

\+ **S22.07** **Fracture of T9-T10 vertebra**

CC MCC +7th **S22.070** **Wedge compression fracture of T9-T10 vertebra**
CC Exclusion 7th character A see Appendix A
PDX collection 1171
CC Exclusion 7th character K see Appendix A
PDX collection 0897
MCC Exclusion 7th character B see Appendix A
PDX collection 1171
HAC 7th characters A & B see Appendix B for HAC conditional logic

CC MCC +7th **S22.071** **Stable burst fracture of T9-T10 vertebra**
CC Exclusion 7th character A see Appendix A PDX collection 1171
CC Exclusion 7th character K see Appendix A PDX collection 0897
MCC Exclusion 7th character B see Appendix A PDX collection 1171
HAC 7th characters A & B see Appendix B for HAC conditional logic

CC MCC +7th **S22.072** **Unstable burst fracture of T9-T10 vertebra**
CC Exclusion 7th character A see Appendix A PDX collection 1171
CC Exclusion 7th character K see Appendix A PDX collection 0897
MCC Exclusion 7th character B see Appendix A PDX collection 1171
HAC 7th characters A & B see Appendix B for HAC conditional logic

CC MCC +7th **S22.078** **Other fracture of T9-T10 vertebra**
CC Exclusion 7th character A see Appendix A PDX collection 1171
CC Exclusion 7th character K see Appendix A PDX collection 0897
MCC Exclusion 7th character B see Appendix A PDX collection 1171
HAC 7th characters A & B see Appendix B for HAC conditional logic

CC MCC +7th **S22.079** **Unspecified fracture of T9-T10 vertebra**
CC Exclusion 7th character A see Appendix A PDX collection 1171
CC Exclusion 7th character K see Appendix A PDX collection 0897
MCC Exclusion 7th character B see Appendix A PDX collection 1171
HAC 7th characters A & B see Appendix B for HAC conditional logic

\+ **S22.08** **Fracture of T11-T12 vertebra**

CC MCC +7th **S22.080** **Wedge compression fracture of T11-T12 vertebra**
CC Exclusion 7th character A see Appendix A PDX collection 1171
CC Exclusion 7th character K see Appendix A PDX collection 0897
MCC Exclusion 7th character B see Appendix A PDX collection 1171
HAC 7th characters A & B see Appendix B for HAC conditional logic

CC MCC +7th **S22.081** **Stable burst fracture of T11-T12 vertebra**
CC Exclusion 7th character A see Appendix A PDX collection 1171
CC Exclusion 7th character K see Appendix A PDX collection 0897
MCC Exclusion 7th character B see Appendix A PDX collection 1171
HAC 7th characters A & B see Appendix B for HAC conditional logic

CC MCC +7th **S22.082** **Unstable burst fracture of T11-T12 vertebra**
CC Exclusion 7th character A see Appendix A PDX collection 1171
CC Exclusion 7th character K see Appendix A PDX collection 0897
MCC Exclusion 7th character B see Appendix A PDX collection 1171
HAC 7th characters A & B see Appendix B for HAC conditional logic

CC MCC +7th **S22.088** **Other fracture of T11-T12 vertebra**
CC Exclusion 7th character A see Appendix A PDX collection 1171
CC Exclusion 7th character K see Appendix A PDX collection 0897
MCC Exclusion 7th character B see Appendix A PDX collection 1171
HAC 7th characters A & B see Appendix B for HAC conditional logic

CC MCC +7th **S22.089** **Unspecified fracture of T11-T12 vertebra**
CC Exclusion 7th character A see Appendix A PDX collection 1171
CC Exclusion 7th character K see Appendix A PDX collection 0897
MCC Exclusion 7th character B see Appendix A PDX collection 1171
HAC 7th characters A & B see Appendix B for HAC conditional logic

\+ **S22.2** **Fracture of sternum**

CC MCC X+7th **S22.20** **Unspecified fracture of sternum**
CC Exclusion 7th character A see Appendix A PDX collection 1172
CC Exclusion 7th character K see Appendix A PDX collection 0897
MCC Exclusion 7th character B see Appendix A PDX collection 1172
HAC 7th characters A & B see Appendix B for HAC conditional logic

CC MCC X+7th **S22.21** **Fracture of manubrium**
CC Exclusion 7th character A see Appendix A PDX collection 1172
CC Exclusion 7th character K see Appendix A PDX collection 0897
MCC Exclusion 7th character B see Appendix A PDX collection 1172
HAC 7th characters A & B see Appendix B for HAC conditional logic

CC MCC X+7th **S22.22** **Fracture of body of sternum**
CC Exclusion 7th character A see Appendix A PDX collection 1172
CC Exclusion 7th character K see Appendix A PDX collection 0897
MCC Exclusion 7th character B see Appendix A PDX collection 1172
HAC 7th characters A & B see Appendix B for HAC conditional logic

CC MCC X+7th **S22.23** **Sternal manubrial dissociation**
CC Exclusion 7th character A see Appendix A PDX collection 1172
CC Exclusion 7th character K see Appendix A PDX collection 0897
MCC Exclusion 7th character B see Appendix A PDX collection 1172
HAC 7th characters A & B see Appendix B for HAC conditional logic

CC MCC X+7th **S22.24** **Fracture of xiphoid process**
CC Exclusion 7th character A see Appendix A PDX collection 1172
CC Exclusion 7th character K see Appendix A PDX collection 0897
MCC Exclusion 7th character B see Appendix A PDX collection 1172
HAC 7th characters A & B see Appendix B for HAC conditional logic

\+ **S22.3** **Fracture of one rib**

CC MCC X+7th **S22.31** **Fracture of one rib, right side**
CC Exclusion 7th character A see Appendix A PDX collection 1173
CC Exclusion 7th character K see Appendix A PDX collection 0897
MCC Exclusion 7th character B see Appendix A PDX collection 1174
HAC 7th characters A & B see Appendix B for HAC conditional logic

CC MCC X+7th **S22.32** **Fracture of one rib, left side**
CC Exclusion 7th character A see Appendix A PDX collection 1173
CC Exclusion 7th character K see Appendix A PDX collection 0897
MCC Exclusion 7th character B see Appendix A PDX collection 1174
HAC 7th characters A & B see Appendix B for HAC conditional logic

CC MCC X+7th **S22.39** **Fracture of one rib, unspecified side**
CC Exclusion 7th character A see Appendix A PDX collection 1173
CC Exclusion 7th character K see Appendix A PDX collection 0897
MCC Exclusion 7th character B see Appendix A PDX collection 1174
HAC 7th characters A & B see Appendix B for HAC conditional logic

\+ **S22.4** **Multiple fractures of ribs**
Fractures of two or more ribs
Excludes1: *flail chest (S22.5-)*

CC MCC X+7th **S22.41** **Multiple fractures of ribs, right side**
CC Exclusion 7th character A see Appendix A PDX collection 1174
CC Exclusion 7th character K see Appendix A PDX collection 0897
MCC Exclusion 7th character B see Appendix A PDX collection 1174
HAC 7th characters A & B see Appendix B for HAC conditional logic

CC MCC X+7th **S22.42 Multiple fractures of ribs, left side**
CC Exclusion 7th character A see Appendix A PDX collection 1174
CC Exclusion 7th character K see Appendix A PDX collection 0897
MCC Exclusion 7th character B see Appendix A PDX collection 1174
HAC 7th characters A & B see Appendix B for HAC conditional logic

CC MCC X+7th **S22.43 Multiple fractures of ribs, bilateral**
CC Exclusion 7th character A see Appendix A PDX collection 1174
CC Exclusion 7th character K see Appendix A PDX collection 0897
MCC Exclusion 7th character B see Appendix A PDX collection 1174
HAC 7th characters A & B see Appendix B for HAC conditional logic

CC MCC X+7th **S22.49 Multiple fractures of ribs, unspecified side**
CC Exclusion 7th character A see Appendix A PDX collection 1174
CC Exclusion 7th character K see Appendix A PDX collection 0897
No MCC Exclusions
HAC 7th characters A & B see Appendix B for HAC conditional logic

X+7th **S22.5 Flail chest**
CC MCC
CC Exclusion 7th character K see Appendix A PDX collection 0897
MCC Exclusion 7th characters A & B see Appendix A PDX collection 1175
HAC 7th characters A & B see Appendix B for HAC conditional logic

X+7th **S22.9 Fracture of bony thorax, part unspecified**
CC MCC
CC Exclusion 7th character A see Appendix A PDX collection 1176
CC Exclusion 7th character K see Appendix A PDX collection 0897
MCC Exclusion 7th character B see Appendix A PDX collection 1176
HAC 7th characters A & B see Appendix B for HAC conditional logic

S23 Dislocation and sprain of joints and ligaments of thorax

Includes: avulsion of joint or ligament of thorax
laceration of cartilage, joint or ligament of thorax
sprain of cartilage, joint or ligament of thorax
traumatic hemarthrosis of joint or ligament of thorax
traumatic rupture of joint or ligament of thorax
traumatic subluxation of joint or ligament of thorax
traumatic tear of joint or ligament of thorax

Code also any associated open wound

Excludes2: *dislocation, sprain of sternoclavicular joint (S43.2, S43.6)*
strain of muscle or tendon of thorax (S29.01-)

The appropriate 7th character is to be added to each code from category S23
A initial encounter
D subsequent encounter
S sequela

X+7th **S23.0 Traumatic rupture of thoracic intervertebral disc**
Excludes1: *rupture or displacement (nontraumatic) of thoracic intervertebral disc NOS (M51.- with fifth character 4)*

\+ **S23.1 Subluxation and dislocation of thoracic vertebra**
Code also any associated
open wound of thorax (S21.-)
spinal cord injury (S24.0-, S24.1-)
Excludes2: *fracture of thoracic vertebrae (S22.0-)*

\+ **S23.10 Subluxation and dislocation of unspecified thoracic vertebra**
+7th **S23.100 Subluxation of unspecified thoracic vertebra**
+7th **S23.101 Dislocation of unspecified thoracic vertebra**

\+ **S23.11 Subluxation and dislocation of T1/T2 thoracic vertebra**
+7th **S23.110 Subluxation of T1/T2 thoracic vertebra**
+7th **S23.111 Dislocation of T1/T2 thoracic vertebra**

\+ **S23.12 Subluxation and dislocation of T2/T3-T3/T4 thoracic vertebra**
+7th **S23.120 Subluxation of T2/T3 thoracic vertebra**
+7th **S23.121 Dislocation of T2/T3 thoracic vertebra**
+7th **S23.122 Subluxation of T3/T4 thoracic vertebra**
+7th **S23.123 Dislocation of T3/T4 thoracic vertebra**

\+ **S23.13 Subluxation and dislocation of T4/T5-T5/T6 thoracic vertebra**
+7th **S23.130 Subluxation of T4/T5 thoracic vertebra**
+7th **S23.131 Dislocation of T4/T5 thoracic vertebra**
+7th **S23.132 Subluxation of T5/T6 thoracic vertebra**
+7th **S23.133 Dislocation of T5/T6 thoracic vertebra**

\+ **S23.14 Subluxation and dislocation of T6/T7-T7/T8 thoracic vertebra**
+7th **S23.140 Subluxation of T6/T7 thoracic vertebra**
+7th **S23.141 Dislocation of T6/T7 thoracic vertebra**
+7th **S23.142 Subluxation of T7/T8 thoracic vertebra**
+7th **S23.143 Dislocation of T7/T8 thoracic vertebra**

\+ **S23.15 Subluxation and dislocation of T8/T9-T9/T10 thoracic vertebra**
+7th **S23.150 Subluxation of T8/T9 thoracic vertebra**
+7th **S23.151 Dislocation of T8/T9 thoracic vertebra**
+7th **S23.152 Subluxation of T9/T10 thoracic vertebra**
+7th **S23.153 Dislocation of T9/T10 thoracic vertebra**

\+ **S23.16 Subluxation and dislocation of T10/T11-T11/T12 thoracic vertebra**
+7th **S23.160 Subluxation of T10/T11 thoracic vertebra**
+7th **S23.161 Dislocation of T10/T11 thoracic vertebra**
+7th **S23.162 Subluxation of T11/T12 thoracic vertebra**
+7th **S23.163 Dislocation of T11/T12 thoracic vertebra**

\+ **S23.17 Subluxation and dislocation of T12/L1 thoracic vertebra**
+7th **S23.170 Subluxation of T12/L1 thoracic vertebra**
+7th **S23.171 Dislocation of T12/L1 thoracic vertebra**

\+ **S23.2 Dislocation of other and unspecified parts of thorax**
X+7th **S23.20 Dislocation of unspecified part of thorax**
X+7th **S23.29 Dislocation of other parts of thorax**

X+7th **S23.3 Sprain of ligaments of thoracic spine**

\+ **S23.4 Sprain of ribs and sternum**
X+7th **S23.41 Sprain of ribs**
\+ **S23.42 Sprain of sternum**
+7th **S23.420 Sprain of sternoclavicular (joint) (ligament)**
+7th **S23.421 Sprain of chondrosternal joint**
+7th **S23.428 Other sprain of sternum**
+7th **S23.429 Unspecified sprain of sternum**

X+7th **S23.8 Sprain of other specified parts of thorax**
X+7th **S23.9 Sprain of unspecified parts of thorax**

S24 Injury of nerves and spinal cord at thorax level

NOTE Code to highest level of thoracic spinal cord injury
Injuries to the spinal cord (S24.0 and S24.1) refer to the cord level and not bone level injury, and can affect nerve roots at and below the level given.

Code also any associated:
fracture of thoracic vertebra (S22.0-)
open wound of thorax (S21.-)
transient paralysis (R29.5)

Excludes2: *injury of brachial plexus (S14.3)*

The appropriate 7th character is to be added to each code from category S24
A initial encounter
D subsequent encounter
S sequela

MCC X+7th **S24.0 Concussion and edema of thoracic spinal cord**
MCC Exclusion 7th character A see Appendix A PDX collection 1177

\+ **S24.1 Other and unspecified injuries of thoracic spinal cord**
\+ **S24.10 Unspecified injury of thoracic spinal cord**

MCC +7th **S24.101 Unspecified injury at T1 level of thoracic spinal cord**
MCC Exclusion 7th character A see Appendix A PDX collection 1177
HAC 7th character A see Appendix B for HAC conditional logic

MCC +7th **S24.102 Unspecified injury at T2-T6 level of thoracic spinal cord**
MCC Exclusion 7th character A see Appendix A PDX collection 1177
HAC 7th character A see Appendix B for HAC conditional logic

MCC +7th **S24.103 Unspecified injury at T7-T10 level of thoracic spinal cord**
MCC Exclusion 7th character A see Appendix A PDX collection 1177
HAC 7th character A see Appendix B for HAC conditional logic

MCC +7th **S24.104 Unspecified injury at T11-T12 level of thoracic spinal cord**
MCC Exclusion 7th character A see Appendix A PDX collection 1177
HAC 7th character A see Appendix B for HAC conditional logic

+7th **S24.109 Unspecified injury at unspecified level of thoracic spinal cord**
Injury of thoracic spinal cord NOS
HAC 7th character A see Appendix B for HAC conditional logic

+ **S24.11 Complete lesion of thoracic spinal cord**

MCC +7th **S24.111 Complete lesion at T1 level of thoracic spinal cord**
MCC Exclusion 7th character A see Appendix A PDX collection 1177
HAC 7th character A see Appendix B for HAC conditional logic

MCC +7th **S24.112 Complete lesion at T2-T6 level of thoracic spinal cord**
MCC Exclusion 7th character A see Appendix A PDX collection 1177
HAC 7th character A see Appendix B for HAC conditional logic

MCC +7th **S24.113 Complete lesion at T7-T10 level of thoracic spinal cord**
MCC Exclusion 7th character A see Appendix A PDX collection 1177
HAC 7th character A see Appendix B for HAC conditional logic

MCC +7th **S24.114 Complete lesion at T11-T12 level of thoracic spinal cord**
MCC Exclusion 7th character A see Appendix A PDX collection 1177
HAC 7th character A see Appendix B for HAC conditional logic

+7th **S24.119 Complete lesion at unspecified level of thoracic spinal cord**

+ **S24.13 Anterior cord syndrome of thoracic spinal cord**

MCC +7th **S24.131 Anterior cord syndrome at T1 level of thoracic spinal cord**
MCC Exclusion 7th character A see Appendix A PDX collection 1177
HAC 7th character A see Appendix B for HAC conditional logic

MCC +7th **S24.132 Anterior cord syndrome at T2-T6 level of thoracic spinal cord**
MCC Exclusion 7th character A see Appendix A PDX collection 1177
HAC 7th character A see Appendix B for HAC conditional logic

MCC +7th **S24.133 Anterior cord syndrome at T7-T10 level of thoracic spinal cord**
MCC Exclusion 7th character A see Appendix A PDX collection 1177
HAC 7th character A see Appendix B for HAC conditional logic

MCC +7th **S24.134 Anterior cord syndrome at T11-T12 level of thoracic spinal cord**
MCC Exclusion 7th character A see Appendix A PDX collection 1177
HAC 7th character A see Appendix B for HAC conditional logic

+7th **S24.139 Anterior cord syndrome at unspecified level of thoracic spinal cord**

+ **S24.14 Brown-Séquard syndrome of thoracic spinal cord**

MCC +7th **S24.141 Brown-Séquard syndrome at T1 level of thoracic spinal cord**
MCC Exclusion 7th character A see Appendix A PDX collection 1177

MCC +7th **S24.142 Brown-Séquard syndrome at T2-T6 level of thoracic spinal cord**
MCC Exclusion 7th character A see Appendix A PDX collection 1177

MCC +7th **S24.143 Brown-Séquard syndrome at T7-T10 level of thoracic spinal cord**
MCC Exclusion 7th character A see Appendix A PDX collection 1177

MCC +7th **S24.144 Brown-Séquard syndrome at T11-T12 level of thoracic spinal cord**
MCC Exclusion 7th character A see Appendix A PDX collection 1177

+7th **S24.149 Brown-Séquard syndrome at unspecified level of thoracic spinal cord**

+ **S24.15 Other incomplete lesions of thoracic spinal cord**
Incomplete lesion of thoracic spinal cord NOS
Posterior cord syndrome of thoracic spinal cord

MCC +7th **S24.151 Other incomplete lesion at T1 level of thoracic spinal cord**
MCC Exclusion 7th character A see Appendix A PDX collection 1177
HAC 7th character A see Appendix B for HAC conditional logic

MCC +7th **S24.152 Other incomplete lesion at T2-T6 level of thoracic spinal cord**
MCC Exclusion 7th character A see Appendix A PDX collection 1177
HAC 7th character A see Appendix B for HAC conditional logic

MCC +7th **S24.153 Other incomplete lesion at T7-T10 level of thoracic spinal cord**
MCC Exclusion 7th character A see Appendix A PDX collection 1177
HAC 7th character A see Appendix B for HAC conditional logic

MCC +7th **S24.154 Other incomplete lesion at T11-T12 level of thoracic spinal cord**
MCC Exclusion 7th character A see Appendix A PDX collection 1177
HAC 7th character A see Appendix B for HAC conditional logic

+7th **S24.159 Other incomplete lesion at unspecified level of thoracic spinal cord**

X+7th **S24.2 Injury of nerve root of thoracic spine**

X+7th **S24.3 Injury of peripheral nerves of thorax**

X+7th **S24.4 Injury of thoracic sympathetic nervous system**
Injury of cardiac plexus
Injury of esophageal plexus
Injury of pulmonary plexus
Injury of stellate ganglion
Injury of thoracic sympathetic ganglion

X+7th **S24.8 Injury of other specified nerves of thorax**

X+7th **S24.9 Injury of unspecified nerve of thorax**

S25 Injury of blood vessels of thorax

Code also any associated open wound (S21.-)

The appropriate 7th character is to be added to each code from category S25
A initial encounter
D subsequent encounter
S sequela

+ **S25.0 Injury of thoracic aorta**
Injury of aorta NOS

MCC X+7th **S25.00 Unspecified injury of thoracic aorta**
MCC Exclusion 7th character A see Appendix A PDX collection 1178

MCC X+7th **S25.01 Minor laceration of thoracic aorta**
Incomplete transection of thoracic aorta
Laceration of thoracic aorta NOS
Superficial laceration of thoracic aorta
MCC Exclusion 7th character A see Appendix A PDX collection 1178

MCC X+7th **S25.02 Major laceration of thoracic aorta**
Complete transection of thoracic aorta
Traumatic rupture of thoracic aorta
MCC Exclusion 7th character A see Appendix A PDX collection 1178

MCC X+7th **S25.09 Other specified injury of thoracic aorta**
MCC Exclusion 7th character A see Appendix A PDX collection 1178

+ **S25.1 Injury of innominate or subclavian artery**

+ **S25.10 Unspecified injury of innominate or subclavian artery**

MCC +7th **S25.101 Unspecified injury of right innominate or subclavian artery**
MCC Exclusion 7th character A see Appendix A PDX collection 1179

MCC +7th **S25.102 Unspecified injury of left innominate or subclavian artery**
MCC Exclusion 7th character A see Appendix A PDX collection 1179

MCC +7th **S25.109 Unspecified injury of unspecified innominate or subclavian artery**
MCC Exclusion 7th character A see Appendix A PDX collection 1179

+ **S25.11 Minor laceration of innominate or subclavian artery**
  Incomplete transection of innominate or subclavian artery
  Laceration of innominate or subclavian artery NOS
  Superficial laceration of innominate or subclavian artery

MCC +7th **S25.111 Minor laceration of right innominate or subclavian artery**
MCC Exclusion 7th character A see Appendix A PDX collection 1179

MCC +7th **S25.112 Minor laceration of left innominate or subclavian artery**
MCC Exclusion 7th character A see Appendix A PDX collection 1179

MCC +7th **S25.119 Minor laceration of unspecified innominate or subclavian artery**
MCC Exclusion 7th character A see Appendix A PDX collection 1179

+ **S25.12 Major laceration of innominate or subclavian artery**
  Complete transection of innominate or subclavian artery
  Traumatic rupture of innominate or subclavian artery

MCC +7th **S25.121 Major laceration of right innominate or subclavian artery**
MCC Exclusion 7th character A see Appendix A PDX collection 1179

MCC +7th **S25.122 Major laceration of left innominate or subclavian artery**
MCC Exclusion 7th character A see Appendix A PDX collection 1179

MCC +7th **S25.129 Major laceration of unspecified innominate or subclavian artery**
MCC Exclusion 7th character A see Appendix A PDX collection 1179

+ **S25.19 Other specified injury of innominate or subclavian artery**

MCC +7th **S25.191 Other specified injury of right innominate or subclavian artery**
MCC Exclusion 7th character A see Appendix A PDX collection 1179

MCC +7th **S25.192 Other specified injury of left innominate or subclavian artery**
MCC Exclusion 7th character A see Appendix A PDX collection 1179

MCC +7th **S25.199 Other specified injury of unspecified innominate or subclavian artery**
MCC Exclusion 7th character A see Appendix A PDX collection 1179

+ **S25.2 Injury of superior vena cava**
  Injury of vena cava NOS

MCC X+7th **S25.20 Unspecified injury of superior vena cava**
MCC Exclusion 7th character A see Appendix A PDX collection 1180

MCC X+7th **S25.21 Minor laceration of superior vena cava**
  Incomplete transection of superior vena cava
  Laceration of superior vena cava NOS
  Superficial laceration of superior vena cava
MCC Exclusion 7th character A see Appendix A PDX collection 1180

MCC X+7th **S25.22 Major laceration of superior vena cava**
  Complete transection of superior vena cava
  Traumatic rupture of superior vena cava
MCC Exclusion 7th character A see Appendix A PDX collection 1180

MCC X+7th **S25.29 Other specified injury of superior vena cava**
MCC Exclusion 7th character A see Appendix A PDX collection 1180

+ **S25.3 Injury of innominate or subclavian vein**

+ **S25.30 Unspecified injury of innominate or subclavian vein**

MCC +7th **S25.301 Unspecified injury of right innominate or subclavian vein**
MCC Exclusion 7th character A see Appendix A PDX collection 1181

MCC +7th **S25.302 Unspecified injury of left innominate or subclavian vein**
MCC Exclusion 7th character A see Appendix A PDX collection 1181

MCC +7th **S25.309 Unspecified injury of unspecified innominate or subclavian vein**
MCC Exclusion 7th character A see Appendix A PDX collection 1181

+ **S25.31 Minor laceration of innominate or subclavian vein**
  Incomplete transection of innominate or subclavian vein
  Laceration of innominate or subclavian vein NOS
  Superficial laceration of innominate or subclavian vein

MCC +7th **S25.311 Minor laceration of right innominate or subclavian vein**
MCC Exclusion 7th character A see Appendix A PDX collection 1181

MCC +7th **S25.312 Minor laceration of left innominate or subclavian vein**
MCC Exclusion 7th character A see Appendix A PDX collection 1181

MCC +7th **S25.319 Minor laceration of unspecified innominate or subclavian vein**
MCC Exclusion 7th character A see Appendix A PDX collection 1181

+ **S25.32 Major laceration of innominate or subclavian vein**
  Complete transection of innominate or subclavian vein
  Traumatic rupture of innominate or subclavian vein

MCC +7th **S25.321 Major laceration of right innominate or subclavian vein**
MCC Exclusion 7th character A see Appendix A PDX collection 1181

MCC +7th **S25.322 Major laceration of left innominate or subclavian vein**
MCC Exclusion 7th character A see Appendix A PDX collection 1181

MCC +7th **S25.329 Major laceration of unspecified innominate or subclavian vein**
MCC Exclusion 7th character A see Appendix A PDX collection 1181

+ **S25.39 Other specified injury of innominate or subclavian vein**

MCC +7th **S25.391 Other specified injury of right innominate or subclavian vein**
MCC Exclusion 7th character A see Appendix A PDX collection 1181

MCC +7th **S25.392 Other specified injury of left innominate or subclavian vein**
MCC Exclusion 7th character A see Appendix A PDX collection 1181

MCC +7th **S25.399 Other specified injury of unspecified innominate or subclavian vein**
MCC Exclusion 7th character A see Appendix A PDX collection 1181

+ **S25.4 Injury of pulmonary blood vessels**

+ **S25.40 Unspecified injury of pulmonary blood vessels**

MCC +7th **S25.401 Unspecified injury of right pulmonary blood vessels**
MCC Exclusion 7th character A see Appendix A PDX collection 1182

MCC +7th **S25.402 Unspecified injury of left pulmonary blood vessels**
MCC Exclusion 7th character A see Appendix A PDX collection 1182

MCC +7th **S25.409 Unspecified injury of unspecified pulmonary blood vessels**
MCC Exclusion 7th character A see Appendix A PDX collection 1182

+ **S25.41 Minor laceration of pulmonary blood vessels**
  Incomplete transection of pulmonary blood vessels
  Laceration of pulmonary blood vessels NOS
  Superficial laceration of pulmonary blood vessels

MCC +7th **S25.411 Minor laceration of right pulmonary blood vessels**
MCC Exclusion 7th character A see Appendix A PDX collection 1182

MCC +7th **S25.412 Minor laceration of left pulmonary blood vessels**
MCC Exclusion 7th character A see Appendix A PDX collection 1182

MCC +7th **S25.419 Minor laceration of unspecified pulmonary blood vessels**
MCC Exclusion 7th character A see Appendix A PDX collection 1182

+ **S25.42 Major laceration of pulmonary blood vessels**
  Complete transection of pulmonary blood vessels
  Traumatic rupture of pulmonary blood vessels

MCC +7th **S25.421 Major laceration of right pulmonary blood vessels**
MCC Exclusion 7th character A see Appendix A PDX collection 1183

MCC +7th **S25.422 Major laceration of left pulmonary blood vessels**
MCC Exclusion 7th character A see Appendix A PDX collection 1182

MCC +7th **S25.429 Major laceration of unspecified pulmonary blood vessels**
MCC Exclusion 7th character A see Appendix A PDX collection 1182

+ **S25.49 Other specified injury of pulmonary blood vessels**

MCC +7th **S25.491 Other specified injury of right pulmonary blood vessels**
MCC Exclusion 7th character A see Appendix A PDX collection 1182

MCC +7th **S25.492 Other specified injury of left pulmonary blood vessels**
MCC Exclusion 7th character A see Appendix A PDX collection 1182

MCC +7th **S25.499 Other specified injury of unspecified pulmonary blood vessels**
MCC Exclusion 7th character A see Appendix A PDX collection 1182

+ **S25.5 Injury of intercostal blood vessels**

+ **S25.50 Unspecified injury of intercostal blood vessels**

CC +7th **S25.501 Unspecified injury of intercostal blood vessels, right side**
CC Exclusion 7th character A see Appendix A PDX collection 1184

CC +7th **S25.502 Unspecified injury of intercostal blood vessels, left side**
CC Exclusion 7th character A see Appendix A PDX collection 1184

CC +7th **S25.509 Unspecified injury of intercostal blood vessels, unspecified side**
CC Exclusion 7th character A see Appendix A PDX collection 1184

+ **S25.51 Laceration of intercostal blood vessels**

CC +7th **S25.511 Laceration of intercostal blood vessels, right side**
CC Exclusion 7th character A see Appendix A PDX collection 1184

CC +7th **S25.512 Laceration of intercostal blood vessels, left side**
CC Exclusion 7th character A see Appendix A PDX collection 1184

CC +7th **S25.519 Laceration of intercostal blood vessels, unspecified side**
CC Exclusion 7th character A see Appendix A PDX collection 1184

+ **S25.59 Other specified injury of intercostal blood vessels**

CC +7th **S25.591 Other specified injury of intercostal blood vessels, right side**
CC Exclusion 7th character A see Appendix A PDX collection 1184

CC +7th **S25.592 Other specified injury of intercostal blood vessels, left side**
CC Exclusion 7th character A see Appendix A PDX collection 1184

CC +7th **S25.599 Other specified injury of intercostal blood vessels, unspecified side**
CC Exclusion 7th character A see Appendix A PDX collection 1184

+ **S25.8 Injury of other blood vessels of thorax**
Injury of azygos vein
Injury of mammary artery or vein

+ **S25.80 Unspecified injury of other blood vessels of thorax**

CC +7th **S25.801 Unspecified injury of other blood vessels of thorax, right side**
CC Exclusion 7th character A see Appendix A PDX collection 1185

CC +7th **S25.802 Unspecified injury of other blood vessels of thorax, left side**
CC Exclusion 7th character A see Appendix A PDX collection 1185

CC +7th **S25.809 Unspecified injury of other blood vessels of thorax, unspecified side**
CC Exclusion 7th character A see Appendix A PDX collection 1185

+ **S25.81 Laceration of other blood vessels of thorax**

CC +7th **S25.811 Laceration of other blood vessels of thorax, right side**
CC Exclusion 7th character A see Appendix A PDX collection 1185

CC +7th **S25.812 Laceration of other blood vessels of thorax, left side**
CC Exclusion 7th character A see Appendix A PDX collection 1185

CC +7th **S25.819 Laceration of other blood vessels of thorax, unspecified side**
CC Exclusion 7th character A see Appendix A PDX collection 1185

+ **S25.89 Other specified injury of other blood vessels of thorax**

CC +7th **S25.891 Other specified injury of other blood vessels of thorax, right side**
CC Exclusion 7th character A see Appendix A PDX collection 1185

CC +7th **S25.892 Other specified injury of other blood vessels of thorax, left side**
CC Exclusion 7th character A see Appendix A PDX collection 1185

CC +7th **S25.899 Other specified injury of other blood vessels of thorax, unspecified side**
CC Exclusion 7th character A see Appendix A PDX collection 1185

+ **S25.9 Injury of unspecified blood vessel of thorax**

CC X+7th **S25.90 Unspecified injury of unspecified blood vessel of thorax**
CC Exclusion 7th character A see Appendix A PDX collection 1185

CC X+7th **S25.91 Laceration of unspecified blood vessel of thorax**
CC Exclusion 7th character A see Appendix A PDX collection 1185

CC X+7th **S25.99 Other specified injury of unspecified blood vessel of thorax**
CC Exclusion 7th character A see Appendix A PDX collection 1185

S26 Injury of heart

Code also any associated:
open wound of thorax (S21.-)
traumatic hemopneumothorax (S27.2)
traumatic hemothorax (S27.1)
traumatic pneumothorax (S27.0)

The appropriate 7th character is to be added to each code from category S26
A initial encounter
D subsequent encounter
S sequela

+ **S26.0 Injury of heart with hemopericardium**

CC X+7th **S26.00 Unspecified injury of heart with hemopericardium**
CC Exclusion 7th character A see Appendix A PDX collection 1186

CC X+7th **S26.01 Contusion of heart with hemopericardium**
CC Exclusion 7th character A see Appendix A PDX collection 1187

+ **S26.02 Laceration of heart with hemopericardium**

MCC +7th **S26.020 Mild laceration of heart with hemopericardium**
Laceration of heart without penetration of heart chamber
MCC Exclusion 7th character A see Appendix A PDX collection 1187

MCC +7th **S26.021 Moderate laceration of heart with hemopericardium**
Laceration of heart with penetration of heart chamber
MCC Exclusion 7th character A see Appendix A PDX collection 1187

MCC +7th **S26.022 Major laceration of heart with hemopericardium**
Laceration of heart with penetration of multiple heart chambers
MCC Exclusion 7th character A see Appendix A PDX collection 1187

CC X+7th **S26.09 Other injury of heart with hemopericardium**
CC Exclusion 7th character A see Appendix A PDX collection 1186

+ **S26.1 Injury of heart without hemopericardium**

CC X+7th **S26.10 Unspecified injury of heart without hemopericardium**
CC Exclusion 7th character A see Appendix A PDX collection 1186

CC X+7th **S26.11 Contusion of heart without hemopericardium**
CC Exclusion 7th character A see Appendix A PDX collection 1187

MCC X+7th **S26.12 Laceration of heart without hemopericardium**
MCC Exclusion 7th character A see Appendix A PDX collection 1187

CC X+7th **S26.19 Other injury of heart without hemopericardium**
CC Exclusion 7th character A see Appendix A PDX collection 1186

+ **S26.9 Injury of heart, unspecified with or without hemopericardium**

CC X+7th **S26.90 Unspecified injury of heart, unspecified with or without hemopericardium**
CC Exclusion 7th character A see Appendix A PDX collection 1186

CC X+7th **S26.91 Contusion of heart, unspecified with or without hemopericardium**
CC Exclusion 7th character A see Appendix A PDX collection 1187

MCC X+7th **S26.92 Laceration of heart, unspecified with or without hemopericardium**
Laceration of heart NOS
MCC Exclusion 7th character A see Appendix A PDX collection 1187

CC X+7th **S26.99 Other injury of heart, unspecified with or without hemopericardium**
CC Exclusion 7th character A see Appendix A PDX collection 1186

S27 Injury of other and unspecified intrathoracic organs

Code also associated open wound of thorax (S21.-)

Excludes2: *injury of cervical esophagus (S10-S19)*
injury of trachea (cervical) (S10-S19)

The appropriate 7th character is to be added to each code from category S27
A initial encounter
D subsequent encounter
S sequela

CC X+7th **S27.0 Traumatic pneumothorax**
Excludes1: *spontaneous pneumothorax (J93.-)*
CC Exclusion 7th character A see Appendix A PDX collection 1188

MCC X+7th **S27.1 Traumatic hemothorax**
MCC Exclusion 7th character A see Appendix A PDX collection 1188

MCC X+7th **S27.2 Traumatic hemopneumothorax**
MCC Exclusion 7th character A see Appendix A PDX collection 1188

S27.3 Other and unspecified injuries of lung

+ **S27.30 Unspecified injury of lung**

CC +7th **S27.301 Unspecified injury of lung, unilateral**
CC Exclusion 7th character A see Appendix A PDX collection 1189

CC +7th **S27.302 Unspecified injury of lung, bilateral**
CC Exclusion 7th character A see Appendix A PDX collection 1189

CC +7th **S27.309 Unspecified injury of lung, unspecified**
CC Exclusion 7th character A see Appendix A PDX collection 1189

+ **S27.31 Primary blast injury of lung**
Blast injury of lung NOS

CC +7th **S27.311 Primary blast injury of lung, unilateral**
CC Exclusion 7th character A see Appendix A PDX collection 1189

CC +7th **S27.312 Primary blast injury of lung, bilateral**
CC Exclusion 7th character A see Appendix A PDX collection 1189

CC +7th **S27.319 Primary blast injury of lung, unspecified**
CC Exclusion 7th character A see Appendix A PDX collection 1189

+ **S27.32 Contusion of lung**

CC +7th **S27.321 Contusion of lung, unilateral**
CC Exclusion 7th character A see Appendix A PDX collection 1189

CC +7th **S27.322 Contusion of lung, bilateral**
CC Exclusion 7th character A see Appendix A PDX collection 1189

CC +7th **S27.329 Contusion of lung, unspecified**
CC Exclusion 7th character A see Appendix A PDX collection 1189

+ **S27.33 Laceration of lung**

MCC +7th **S27.331 Laceration of lung, unilateral**
MCC Exclusion 7th character A see Appendix A PDX collection 1190

MCC +7th **S27.332 Laceration of lung, bilateral**
MCC Exclusion 7th character A see Appendix A PDX collection 1190

MCC +7th **S27.339 Laceration of lung, unspecified**
MCC Exclusion 7th character A see Appendix A PDX collection 1190

+ **S27.39 Other injuries of lung**
Secondary blast injury of lung

CC +7th **S27.391 Other injuries of lung, unilateral**
CC Exclusion 7th character A see Appendix A PDX collection 1189

CC +7th **S27.392 Other injuries of lung, bilateral**
CC Exclusion 7th character A see Appendix A PDX collection 1189

CC +7th **S27.399 Other injuries of lung, unspecified**
CC Exclusion 7th character A see Appendix A PDX collection 1189

S27.4 Injury of bronchus

+ **S27.40 Unspecified injury of bronchus**

MCC +7th **S27.401 Unspecified injury of bronchus, unilateral**
MCC Exclusion 7th character A see Appendix A PDX collection 1191

MCC +7th **S27.402 Unspecified injury of bronchus, bilateral**
MCC Exclusion 7th character A see Appendix A PDX collection 1191

MCC +7th **S27.409 Unspecified injury of bronchus, unspecified**
MCC Exclusion 7th character A see Appendix A PDX collection 1191

+ **S27.41 Primary blast injury of bronchus**
Blast injury of bronchus NOS

MCC +7th **S27.411 Primary blast injury of bronchus, unilateral**
MCC Exclusion 7th character A see Appendix A PDX collection 1191

MCC +7th **S27.412 Primary blast injury of bronchus, bilateral**
MCC Exclusion 7th character A see Appendix A PDX collection 1191

MCC +7th **S27.419 Primary blast injury of bronchus, unspecified**
MCC Exclusion 7th character A see Appendix A PDX collection 1191

+ **S27.42 Contusion of bronchus**

MCC +7th **S27.421 Contusion of bronchus, unilateral**
MCC Exclusion 7th character A see Appendix A PDX collection 1191

MCC +7th **S27.422 Contusion of bronchus, bilateral**
MCC Exclusion 7th character A see Appendix A PDX collection 1191

MCC +7th **S27.429 Contusion of bronchus, unspecified**
MCC Exclusion 7th character A see Appendix A PDX collection 1191

+ **S27.43 Laceration of bronchus**

MCC +7th **S27.431 Laceration of bronchus, unilateral**
MCC Exclusion 7th character A see Appendix A PDX collection 1191

MCC +7th **S27.432 Laceration of bronchus, bilateral**
MCC Exclusion 7th character A see Appendix A PDX collection 1191

MCC +7th **S27.439 Laceration of bronchus, unspecified**
MCC Exclusion 7th character A see Appendix A PDX collection 1191

+ **S27.49 Other injury of bronchus**
Secondary blast injury of bronchus

MCC +7th **S27.491 Other injury of bronchus, unilateral**
MCC Exclusion 7th character A see Appendix A PDX collection 1191

MCC +7th **S27.492 Other injury of bronchus, bilateral**
MCC Exclusion 7th character A see Appendix A PDX collection 1191

MCC +7th **S27.499 Other injury of bronchus, unspecified**
MCC Exclusion 7th character A see Appendix A PDX collection 1191

+ **S27.5 Injury of thoracic trachea**

CC X+7th **S27.50 Unspecified injury of thoracic trachea**
CC Exclusion 7th character A see Appendix A PDX collection 1169

CC X+7th **S27.51 Primary blast injury of thoracic trachea**
Blast injury of thoracic trachea NOS
CC Exclusion 7th character A see Appendix A PDX collection 1169

CC X+7th **S27.52 Contusion of thoracic trachea**
CC Exclusion 7th character A see Appendix A PDX collection 1169

CC X+7th **S27.53 Laceration of thoracic trachea**
CC Exclusion 7th character A see Appendix A PDX collection 1169

CC X+7th **S27.59 Other injury of thoracic trachea**
Secondary blast injury of thoracic trachea
CC Exclusion 7th character A see Appendix A PDX collection 1169

+ S27.6 Injury of pleura
CC X+7th S27.60 Unspecified injury of pleura
CC Exclusion 7th character A see Appendix A PDX collection 1169
CC X+7th S27.63 Laceration of pleura
CC Exclusion 7th character A see Appendix A PDX collection 1169
CC X+7th S27.69 Other injury of pleura
CC Exclusion 7th character A see Appendix A PDX collection 1169
+ S27.8 Injury of other specified intrathoracic organs
+ S27.80 Injury of diaphragm
CC +7th S27.802 Contusion of diaphragm
CC Exclusion 7th character A see Appendix A PDX collection 1192
CC +7th S27.803 Laceration of diaphragm
CC Exclusion 7th character A see Appendix A PDX collection 1192
CC +7th S27.808 Other injury of diaphragm
CC Exclusion 7th character A see Appendix A PDX collection 1192
CC +7th S27.809 Unspecified injury of diaphragm
CC Exclusion 7th character A see Appendix A PDX collection 1192
+ S27.81 Injury of esophagus (thoracic part)
MCC +7th S27.812 Contusion of esophagus (thoracic part)
MCC Exclusion 7th character A see Appendix A PDX collection 1193
MCC +7th S27.813 Laceration of esophagus (thoracic part)
MCC Exclusion 7th character A see Appendix A PDX collection 1193
MCC +7th S27.818 Other injury of esophagus (thoracic part)
MCC Exclusion 7th character A see Appendix A PDX collection 1193
MCC +7th S27.819 Unspecified injury of esophagus (thoracic part)
MCC Exclusion 7th character A see Appendix A PDX collection 1193
+ S27.89 Injury of other specified intrathoracic organs
Injury of lymphatic thoracic duct
Injury of thymus gland
CC +7th S27.892 Contusion of other specified intrathoracic organs
CC Exclusion 7th character A see Appendix A PDX collection 1169
CC +7th S27.893 Laceration of other specified intrathoracic organs
CC Exclusion 7th character A see Appendix A PDX collection 1169
CC +7th S27.898 Other injury of other specified intrathoracic organs
CC Exclusion 7th character A see Appendix A PDX collection 1169
CC +7th S27.899 Unspecified injury of other specified intrathoracic organs
CC Exclusion 7th character A see Appendix A PDX collection 1169
CC X+7th S27.9 Injury of unspecified intrathoracic organ
CC Exclusion 7th character A see Appendix A PDX collection 1194

S28 Crushing injury of thorax, and traumatic amputation of part of thorax

The appropriate 7th character is to be added to each code from category S28
A initial encounter
D subsequent encounter
S sequela

X+7th S28.0 Crushed chest
Use additional code for all associated injuries
Excludes1: *flail chest (S22.5)*
CC X+7th S28.1 Traumatic amputation (partial) of part of thorax, except breast
CC Exclusion 7th character A see Appendix A PDX collection 1168
+ S28.2 Traumatic amputation of breast
+ S28.21 Complete traumatic amputation of breast
Traumatic amputation of breast NOS
+7th S28.211 Complete traumatic amputation of right breast
+7th S28.212 Complete traumatic amputation of left breast
+7th S28.219 Complete traumatic amputation of unspecified breast
+ S28.22 Partial traumatic amputation of breast
+7th S28.221 Partial traumatic amputation of right breast
+7th S28.222 Partial traumatic amputation of left breast
+7th S28.229 Partial traumatic amputation of unspecified breast

S29 Other and unspecified injuries of thorax
Code also any associated open wound (S21.-)

The appropriate 7th character is to be added to each code from category S29
A initial encounter
D subsequent encounter
S sequela

+ S29.0 Injury of muscle and tendon at thorax level
+ S29.00 Unspecified injury of muscle and tendon of thorax
+7th S29.001 Unspecified injury of muscle and tendon of front wall of thorax
+7th S29.002 Unspecified injury of muscle and tendon of back wall of thorax
+7th S29.009 Unspecified injury of muscle and tendon of unspecified wall of thorax
+ S29.01 Strain of muscle and tendon of thorax
+7th S29.011 Strain of muscle and tendon of front wall of thorax
+7th S29.012 Strain of muscle and tendon of back wall of thorax
+7th S29.019 Strain of muscle and tendon of unspecified wall of thorax
+ S29.02 Laceration of muscle and tendon of thorax
CC +7th S29.021 Laceration of muscle and tendon of front wall of thorax
CC Exclusion 7th character A see Appendix A PDX collection 1168
+7th S29.022 Laceration of muscle and tendon of back wall of thorax
CC +7th S29.029 Laceration of muscle and tendon of unspecified wall of thorax
CC Exclusion 7th character A see Appendix A PDX collection 1168
+ S29.09 Other injury of muscle and tendon of thorax
+7th S29.091 Other injury of muscle and tendon of front wall of thorax
+7th S29.092 Other injury of muscle and tendon of back wall of thorax
+7th S29.099 Other injury of muscle and tendon of unspecified wall of thorax
X+7th S29.8 Other specified injuries of thorax
X+7th S29.9 Unspecified injury of thorax

Injuries to the abdomen, lower back, lumbar spine, pelvis and external genitals (S30-S39)

Includes: injuries to the abdominal wall
injuries to the anus
injuries to the buttock
injuries to the external genitalia
injuries to the flank
injuries to the groin

Excludes2: *burns and corrosions (T20-T32)*
effects of foreign body in anus and rectum (T18.5)
effects of foreign body in genitourinary tract (T19.-)
effects of foreign body in stomach, small intestine and colon (T18.2-T18.4)
frostbite (T33-T34)
insect bite or sting, venomous (T63.4)

S30 Superficial injury of abdomen, lower back, pelvis and external genitals
Excludes2: *superficial injury of hip (S70.-)*

The appropriate 7th character is to be added to each code from category S30
A initial encounter
D subsequent encounter
S sequela

X+7th S30.0 Contusion of lower back and pelvis
Contusion of buttock
X+7th S30.1 Contusion of abdominal wall
Contusion of flank
Contusion of groin

+ **S30.2 Contusion of external genital organs**
+ **S30.20 Contusion of unspecified external genital organ**
♂ +7th **S30.201 Contusion of unspecified external genital organ, male**
♀ +7th **S30.202 Contusion of unspecified external genital organ, female**
♂ X+7th **S30.21 Contusion of penis**
♂ X+7th **S30.22 Contusion of scrotum and testes**
♀ X+7th **S30.23 Contusion of vagina and vulva**
X+7th **S30.3 Contusion of anus**
X+7th **S30.8 Other superficial injuries of abdomen, lower back, pelvis and external genitals**
+ **S30.81 Abrasion of abdomen, lower back, pelvis and external genitals**
+7th **S30.810 Abrasion of lower back and pelvis**
+7th **S30.811 Abrasion of abdominal wall**
♂ +7th **S30.812 Abrasion of penis**
♂ +7th **S30.813 Abrasion of scrotum and testes**
♀ +7th **S30.814 Abrasion of vagina and vulva**
♂ +7th **S30.815 Abrasion of unspecified external genital organs, male**
♀ +7th **S30.816 Abrasion of unspecified external genital organs, female**
+7th **S30.817 Abrasion of anus**
+ **S30.82 Blister (nonthermal) of abdomen, lower back, pelvis and external genitals**
+7th **S30.820 Blister (nonthermal) of lower back and pelvis**
+7th **S30.821 Blister (nonthermal) of abdominal wall**
♂ +7th **S30.822 Blister (nonthermal) of penis**
♂ +7th **S30.823 Blister (nonthermal) of scrotum and testes**
♀ +7th **S30.824 Blister (nonthermal) of vagina and vulva**
♂ +7th **S30.825 Blister (nonthermal) of unspecified external genital organs, male**
♀ +7th **S30.826 Blister (nonthermal) of unspecified external genital organs, female**
+7th **S30.827 Blister (nonthermal) of anus**
+ **S30.84 External constriction of abdomen, lower back, pelvis and external genitals**
+7th **S30.840 External constriction of lower back and pelvis**
+7th **S30.841 External constriction of abdominal wall**
♂ +7th **S30.842 External constriction of penis**
Hair tourniquet syndrome of penis
Use additional cause code to identify the constricting item (W49.0-)
♂ +7th **S30.843 External constriction of scrotum and testes**
♀ +7th **S30.844 External constriction of vagina and vulva**
♂ +7th **S30.845 External constriction of unspecified external genital organs, male**
♀ +7th **S30.846 External constriction of unspecified external genital organs, female**
+ **S30.85 Superficial foreign body of abdomen, lower back, pelvis and external genitals**
Splinter in the abdomen, lower back, pelvis and external genitals
+7th **S30.850 Superficial foreign body of lower back and pelvis**
+7th **S30.851 Superficial foreign body of abdominal wall**
♂ +7th **S30.852 Superficial foreign body of penis**
♂ +7th **S30.853 Superficial foreign body of scrotum and testes**
♀ +7th **S30.854 Superficial foreign body of vagina and vulva**
♂ +7th **S30.855 Superficial foreign body of unspecified external genital organs, male**
♀ +7th **S30.856 Superficial foreign body of unspecified external genital organs, female**
+7th **S30.857 Superficial foreign body of anus**
+ **S30.86 Insect bite (nonvenomous) of abdomen, lower back, pelvis and external genitals**
+7th **S30.860 Insect bite (nonvenomous) of lower back and pelvis**
+7th **S30.861 Insect bite (nonvenomous) of abdominal wall**
♂ +7th **S30.862 Insect bite (nonvenomous) of penis**
♂ +7th **S30.863 Insect bite (nonvenomous) of scrotum and testes**
♀ +7th **S30.864 Insect bite (nonvenomous) of vagina and vulva**
♂ +7th **S30.865 Insect bite (nonvenomous) of unspecified external genital organs, male**
♀ +7th **S30.866 Insect bite (nonvenomous) of unspecified external genital organs, female**
+7th **S30.867 Insect bite (nonvenomous) of anus**
+ **S30.87 Other superficial bite of abdomen, lower back, pelvis and external genitals**
Excludes1: *open bite of abdomen, lower back, pelvis and external genitals (S31.05, S31.15, S31.25, S31.35, S31.45, S31.55)*
+7th **S30.870 Other superficial bite of lower back and pelvis**
+7th **S30.871 Other superficial bite of abdominal wall**
♂ +7th **S30.872 Other superficial bite of penis**
♂ +7th **S30.873 Other superficial bite of scrotum and testes**
♀ +7th **S30.874 Other superficial bite of vagina and vulva**
♂ +7th **S30.875 Other superficial bite of unspecified external genital organs, male**
♀ +7th **S30.876 Other superficial bite of unspecified external genital organs, female**
+7th **S30.877 Other superficial bite of anus**
+ **S30.9 Unspecified superficial injury of abdomen, lower back, pelvis and external genitals**
X+7th **S30.91 Unspecified superficial injury of lower back and pelvis**
X+7th **S30.92 Unspecified superficial injury of abdominal wall**
♂ X+7th **S30.93 Unspecified superficial injury of penis**
♂ X+7th **S30.94 Unspecified superficial injury of scrotum and testes**
♀ X+7th **S30.95 Unspecified superficial injury of vagina and vulva**
♂ X+7th **S30.96 Unspecified superficial injury of unspecified external genital organs, male**
♀ X+7th **S30.97 Unspecified superficial injury of unspecified external genital organs, female**
X+7th **S30.98 Unspecified superficial injury of anus**

S31 Open wound of abdomen, lower back, pelvis and external genitals

Code also any associated:
spinal cord injury (S24.0, S24.1-, S34.0-, S34.1-)
wound infection

Excludes1: *traumatic amputation of part of abdomen, lower back and pelvis (S38.2-, S38.3)*
Excludes2: *open wound of hip (S71.00-S71.02)*
open fracture of pelvis (S32.1--S32.9 with 7th character B)

The appropriate 7th character is to be added to each code from category S31
A initial encounter
D subsequent encounter
S sequela

+ **S31.0 Open wound of lower back and pelvis**
+ **S31.00 Unspecified open wound of lower back and pelvis**
+7th **S31.000 Unspecified open wound of lower back and pelvis without penetration into retroperitoneum**
Unspecified open wound of lower back and pelvis NOS
MCC +7th **S31.001 Unspecified open wound of lower back and pelvis with penetration into retroperitoneum**
MCC Exclusion 7th character A see Appendix A PDX collection 1195
+ **S31.01 Laceration without foreign body of lower back and pelvis**
+7th **S31.010 Laceration without foreign body of lower back and pelvis without penetration into retroperitoneum**
Laceration without foreign body of lower back and pelvis NOS
MCC +7th **S31.011 Laceration without foreign body of lower back and pelvis with penetration into retroperitoneum**
MCC Exclusion 7th character A see Appendix A PDX collection 1195
+ **S31.02 Laceration with foreign body of lower back and pelvis**
+7th **S31.020 Laceration with foreign body of lower back and pelvis without penetration into retroperitoneum**
Laceration with foreign body of lower back and pelvis NOS

MCC +7th **S31.021 Laceration with foreign body of lower back and pelvis with penetration into retroperitoneum**
MCC Exclusion 7th character A see Appendix A PDX collection 1195

+ **S31.03 Puncture wound without foreign body of lower back and pelvis**

+7th **S31.030 Puncture wound without foreign body of lower back and pelvis without penetration into retroperitoneum**
Puncture wound without foreign body of lower back and pelvis NOS

MCC +7th **S31.031 Puncture wound without foreign body of lower back and pelvis with penetration into retroperitoneum**
MCC Exclusion 7th character A see Appendix A PDX collection 1195

+ **S31.04 Puncture wound with foreign body of lower back and pelvis**

+7th **S31.040 Puncture wound with foreign body of lower back and pelvis without penetration into retroperitoneum**
Puncture wound with foreign body of lower back and pelvis NOS

MCC +7th **S31.041 Puncture wound with foreign body of lower back and pelvis with penetration into retroperitoneum**
MCC Exclusion 7th character A see Appendix A PDX collection 1195

+ **S31.05 Open bite of lower back and pelvis**
Bite of lower back and pelvis NOS
Excludes1: *superficial bite of lower back and pelvis (S30.860, S30.870)*

+7th **S31.050 Open bite of lower back and pelvis without penetration into retroperitoneum**
Open bite of lower back and pelvis NOS

MCC +7th **S31.051 Open bite of lower back and pelvis with penetration into retroperitoneum**
MCC Exclusion 7th character A see Appendix A PDX collection 1195

+ **S31.1 Open wound of abdominal wall without penetration into peritoneal cavity**
Open wound of abdominal wall NOS
Excludes2: *open wound of abdominal wall with penetration into peritoneal cavity (S31.6-)*

+ **S31.10 Unspecified open wound of abdominal wall without penetration into peritoneal cavity**

+7th **S31.100 Unspecified open wound of abdominal wall, right upper quadrant without penetration into peritoneal cavity**

+7th **S31.101 Unspecified open wound of abdominal wall, left upper quadrant without penetration into peritoneal cavity**

+7th **S31.102 Unspecified open wound of abdominal wall, epigastric region without penetration into peritoneal cavity**

+7th **S31.103 Unspecified open wound of abdominal wall, right lower quadrant without penetration into peritoneal cavity**

+7th **S31.104 Unspecified open wound of abdominal wall, left lower quadrant without penetration into peritoneal cavity**

+7th **S31.105 Unspecified open wound of abdominal wall, periumbilic region without penetration into peritoneal cavity**

+7th **S31.109 Unspecified open wound of abdominal wall, unspecified quadrant without penetration into peritoneal cavity**
Unspecified open wound of abdominal wall NOS

+ **S31.11 Laceration without foreign body of abdominal wall without penetration into peritoneal cavity**

+7th **S31.110 Laceration without foreign body of abdominal wall, right upper quadrant without penetration into peritoneal cavity**

+7th **S31.111 Laceration without foreign body of abdominal wall, left upper quadrant without penetration into peritoneal cavity**

+7th **S31.112 Laceration without foreign body of abdominal wall, epigastric region without penetration into peritoneal cavity**

+7th **S31.113 Laceration without foreign body of abdominal wall, right lower quadrant without penetration into peritoneal cavity**

+7th **S31.114 Laceration without foreign body of abdominal wall, left lower quadrant without penetration into peritoneal cavity**

+7th **S31.115 Laceration without foreign body of abdominal wall, periumbilic region without penetration into peritoneal cavity**

+7th **S31.119 Laceration without foreign body of abdominal wall, unspecified quadrant without penetration into peritoneal cavity**

+ **S31.12 Laceration with foreign body of abdominal wall without penetration into peritoneal cavity**

+7th **S31.120 Laceration of abdominal wall with foreign body, right upper quadrant without penetration into peritoneal cavity**

+7th **S31.121 Laceration of abdominal wall with foreign body, left upper quadrant without penetration into peritoneal cavity**

+7th **S31.122 Laceration of abdominal wall with foreign body, epigastric region without penetration into peritoneal cavity**

+7th **S31.123 Laceration of abdominal wall with foreign body, right lower quadrant without penetration into peritoneal cavity**

+7th **S31.124 Laceration of abdominal wall with foreign body, left lower quadrant without penetration into peritoneal cavity**

+7th **S31.125 Laceration of abdominal wall with foreign body, periumbilic region without penetration into peritoneal cavity**

+7th **S31.129 Laceration of abdominal wall with foreign body, unspecified quadrant without penetration into peritoneal cavity**

+ **S31.13 Puncture wound of abdominal wall without foreign body without penetration into peritoneal cavity**

+7th **S31.130 Puncture wound of abdominal wall without foreign body, right upper quadrant without penetration into peritoneal cavity**

+7th **S31.131 Puncture wound of abdominal wall without foreign body, left upper quadrant without penetration into peritoneal cavity**

+7th **S31.132 Puncture wound of abdominal wall without foreign body, epigastric region without penetration into peritoneal cavity**

+7th **S31.133 Puncture wound of abdominal wall without foreign body, right lower quadrant without penetration into peritoneal cavity**

+7th **S31.134 Puncture wound of abdominal wall without foreign body, left lower quadrant without penetration into peritoneal cavity**

+7th **S31.135 Puncture wound of abdominal wall without foreign body, periumbilic region without penetration into peritoneal cavity**

+7th **S31.139 Puncture wound of abdominal wall without foreign body, unspecified quadrant without penetration into peritoneal cavity**

+ **S31.14 Puncture wound of abdominal wall with foreign body without penetration into peritoneal cavity**

+7th **S31.140 Puncture wound of abdominal wall with foreign body, right upper quadrant without penetration into peritoneal cavity**

+7th **S31.141 Puncture wound of abdominal wall with foreign body, left upper quadrant without penetration into peritoneal cavity**

+7th **S31.142 Puncture wound of abdominal wall with foreign body, epigastric region without penetration into peritoneal cavity**

+7th **S31.143 Puncture wound of abdominal wall with foreign body, right lower quadrant without penetration into peritoneal cavity**

+7th **S31.144 Puncture wound of abdominal wall with foreign body, left lower quadrant without penetration into peritoneal cavity**

+7th **S31.145 Puncture wound of abdominal wall with foreign body, periumbilic region without penetration into peritoneal cavity**

+7th **S31.149 Puncture wound of abdominal wall with foreign body, unspecified quadrant without penetration into peritoneal cavity**

+ **S31.15 Open bite of abdominal wall without penetration into peritoneal cavity**
  Bite of abdominal wall NOS
  Excludes1: *superficial bite of abdominal wall (S30.871)*
  +7th **S31.150 Open bite of abdominal wall, right upper quadrant without penetration into peritoneal cavity**
  +7th **S31.151 Open bite of abdominal wall, left upper quadrant without penetration into peritoneal cavity**
  +7th **S31.152 Open bite of abdominal wall, epigastric region without penetration into peritoneal cavity**
  +7th **S31.153 Open bite of abdominal wall, right lower quadrant without penetration into peritoneal cavity**
  +7th **S31.154 Open bite of abdominal wall, left lower quadrant without penetration into peritoneal cavity**
  +7th **S31.155 Open bite of abdominal wall, periumbilic region without penetration into peritoneal cavity**
  +7th **S31.159 Open bite of abdominal wall, unspecified quadrant without penetration into peritoneal cavity**

+ **S31.2 Open wound of penis**
  ♂ X+7th **S31.20 Unspecified open wound of penis**
  ♂ X+7th **S31.21 Laceration without foreign body of penis**
  ♂ X+7th **S31.22 Laceration with foreign body of penis**
  ♂ X+7th **S31.23 Puncture wound without foreign body of penis**
  ♂ X+7th **S31.24 Puncture wound with foreign body of penis**
  ♂ X+7th **S31.25 Open bite of penis**
  Bite of penis NOS
  Excludes1: *superficial bite of penis (S30.862, S30.872)*

+ **S31.3 Open wound of scrotum and testes**
  ♂ X+7th **S31.30 Unspecified open wound of scrotum and testes**
  ♂ X+7th **S31.31 Laceration without foreign body of scrotum and testes**
  ♂ X+7th **S31.32 Laceration with foreign body of scrotum and testes**
  ♂ X+7th **S31.33 Puncture wound without foreign body of scrotum and testes**
  ♂ X+7th **S31.34 Puncture wound with foreign body of scrotum and testes**
  ♂ X+7th **S31.35 Open bite of scrotum and testes**
  Bite of scrotum and testes NOS
  Excludes1: *superficial bite of scrotum and testes (S30.863, S30.873)*

+ **S31.4 Open wound of vagina and vulva**
  Excludes1: *injury to vagina and vulva during delivery (O70.-, O71.4)*
  ♀ X+7th **S31.40 Unspecified open wound of vagina and vulva**
  ♀ X+7th **S31.41 Laceration without foreign body of vagina and vulva**
  ♀ X+7th **S31.42 Laceration with foreign body of vagina and vulva**
  ♀ X+7th **S31.43 Puncture wound without foreign body of vagina and vulva**
  ♀ X+7th **S31.44 Puncture wound with foreign body of vagina and vulva**
  ♀ X+7th **S31.45 Open bite of vagina and vulva**
  Bite of vagina and vulva NOS
  Excludes1: *superficial bite of vagina and vulva (S30.864, S30.874)*

+ **S31.5 Open wound of unspecified external genital organs**
  Excludes1: *traumatic amputation of external genital organs (S38.21, S38.22)*
  + **S31.50 Unspecified open wound of unspecified external genital organs**
  ♂ +7th **S31.501 Unspecified open wound of unspecified external genital organs, male**
  ♀ +7th **S31.502 Unspecified open wound of unspecified external genital organs, female**
  + **S31.51 Laceration without foreign body of unspecified external genital organs**
  ♂ +7th **S31.511 Laceration without foreign body of unspecified external genital organs, male**
  ♀ +7th **S31.512 Laceration without foreign body of unspecified external genital organs, female**
  + **S31.52 Laceration with foreign body of unspecified external genital organs**
  ♂ +7th **S31.521 Laceration with foreign body of unspecified external genital organs, male**
  ♀ +7th **S31.522 Laceration with foreign body of unspecified external genital organs, female**
  + **S31.53 Puncture wound without foreign body of unspecified external genital organs**
  ♂ +7th **S31.531 Puncture wound without foreign body of unspecified external genital organs, male**
  ♀ +7th **S31.532 Puncture wound without foreign body of unspecified external genital organs, female**
  + **S31.54 Puncture wound with foreign body of unspecified external genital organs**
  ♂ +7th **S31.541 Puncture wound with foreign body of unspecified external genital organs, male**
  ♀ +7th **S31.542 Puncture wound with foreign body of unspecified external genital organs, female**
  + **S31.55 Open bite of unspecified external genital organs**
  Bite of unspecified external genital organs NOS
  Excludes1: *superficial bite of unspecified external genital organs (S30.865, S30.866, S30.875, S30.876)*
  ♂ +7th **S31.551 Open bite of unspecified external genital organs, male**
  ♀ +7th **S31.552 Open bite of unspecified external genital organs, female**

+ **S31.6 Open wound of abdominal wall with penetration into peritoneal cavity**
  + **S31.60 Unspecified open wound of abdominal wall with penetration into peritoneal cavity**
  MCC +7th **S31.600 Unspecified open wound of abdominal wall, right upper quadrant with penetration into peritoneal cavity**
  MCC Exclusion 7th character A see Appendix A PDX collection 1195
  MCC +7th **S31.601 Unspecified open wound of abdominal wall, left upper quadrant with penetration into peritoneal cavity**
  MCC Exclusion 7th character A see Appendix A PDX collection 1195
  MCC +7th **S31.602 Unspecified open wound of abdominal wall, epigastric region with penetration into peritoneal cavity**
  MCC Exclusion 7th character A see Appendix A PDX collection 1195
  MCC +7th **S31.603 Unspecified open wound of abdominal wall, right lower quadrant with penetration into peritoneal cavity**
  MCC Exclusion 7th character A see Appendix A PDX collection 1195
  MCC +7th **S31.604 Unspecified open wound of abdominal wall, left lower quadrant with penetration into peritoneal cavity**
  MCC Exclusion 7th character A see Appendix A PDX collection 1195
  MCC +7th **S31.605 Unspecified open wound of abdominal wall, periumbilic region with penetration into peritoneal cavity**
  MCC Exclusion 7th character A see Appendix A PDX collection 1195
  MCC +7th **S31.609 Unspecified open wound of abdominal wall, unspecified quadrant with penetration into peritoneal cavity**
  MCC Exclusion 7th character A see Appendix A PDX collection 1195
  + **S31.61 Laceration without foreign body of abdominal wall with penetration into peritoneal cavity**
  MCC +7th **S31.610 Laceration without foreign body of abdominal wall, right upper quadrant with penetration into peritoneal cavity**
  MCC Exclusion 7th character A see Appendix A PDX collection 1195
  MCC +7th **S31.611 Laceration without foreign body of abdominal wall, left upper quadrant with penetration into peritoneal cavity**
  MCC Exclusion 7th character A see Appendix A PDX collection 1195
  MCC +7th **S31.612 Laceration without foreign body of abdominal wall, epigastric region with penetration into peritoneal cavity**
  MCC Exclusion 7th character A see Appendix A PDX collection 1195

MCC +7th **S31.613 Laceration without foreign body of abdominal wall, right lower quadrant with penetration into peritoneal cavity**
MCC Exclusion 7th character A see Appendix A
PDX collection 1195
AHA CC: 4Q, 2015, 37-38

MCC +7th **S31.614 Laceration without foreign body of abdominal wall, left lower quadrant with penetration into peritoneal cavity**
MCC Exclusion 7th character A see Appendix A
PDX collection 1195

MCC +7th **S31.615 Laceration without foreign body of abdominal wall, periumbilic region with penetration into peritoneal cavity**
MCC Exclusion 7th character A see Appendix A
PDX collection 1195

MCC +7th **S31.619 Laceration without foreign body of abdominal wall, unspecified quadrant with penetration into peritoneal cavity**
MCC Exclusion 7th character A see Appendix A
PDX collection 1195

+ **S31.62 Laceration with foreign body of abdominal wall with penetration into peritoneal cavity**

MCC +7th **S31.620 Laceration with foreign body of abdominal wall, right upper quadrant with penetration into peritoneal cavity**
MCC Exclusion 7th character A see Appendix A
PDX collection 1195

MCC +7th **S31.621 Laceration with foreign body of abdominal wall, left upper quadrant with penetration into peritoneal cavity**
MCC Exclusion 7th character A see Appendix A
PDX collection 1195

MCC +7th **S31.622 Laceration with foreign body of abdominal wall, epigastric region with penetration into peritoneal cavity**
MCC Exclusion 7th character A see Appendix A
PDX collection 1195

MCC +7th **S31.623 Laceration with foreign body of abdominal wall, right lower quadrant with penetration into peritoneal cavity**
MCC Exclusion 7th character A see Appendix A
PDX collection 1195

MCC +7th **S31.624 Laceration with foreign body of abdominal wall, left lower quadrant with penetration into peritoneal cavity**
MCC Exclusion 7th character A see Appendix A
PDX collection 1195

MCC +7th **S31.625 Laceration with foreign body of abdominal wall, periumbilic region with penetration into peritoneal cavity**
MCC Exclusion 7th character A see Appendix A
PDX collection 1195

MCC +7th **S31.629 Laceration with foreign body of abdominal wall, unspecified quadrant with penetration into peritoneal cavity**
MCC Exclusion 7th character A see Appendix A
PDX collection 1195

+ **S31.63 Puncture wound without foreign body of abdominal wall with penetration into peritoneal cavity**

MCC +7th **S31.630 Puncture wound without foreign body of abdominal wall, right upper quadrant with penetration into peritoneal cavity**
MCC Exclusion 7th character A see Appendix A
PDX collection 1195

MCC +7th **S31.631 Puncture wound without foreign body of abdominal wall, left upper quadrant with penetration into peritoneal cavity**
MCC Exclusion 7th character A see Appendix A
PDX collection 1195

MCC +7th **S31.632 Puncture wound without foreign body of abdominal wall, epigastric region with penetration into peritoneal cavity**
MCC Exclusion 7th character A see Appendix A
PDX collection 1195

MCC +7th **S31.633 Puncture wound without foreign body of abdominal wall, right lower quadrant with penetration into peritoneal cavity**
MCC Exclusion 7th character A see Appendix A
PDX collection 1195

MCC +7th **S31.634 Puncture wound without foreign body of abdominal wall, left lower quadrant with penetration into peritoneal cavity**
MCC Exclusion 7th character A see Appendix A
PDX collection 1195

MCC +7th **S31.635 Puncture wound without foreign body of abdominal wall, periumbilic region with penetration into peritoneal cavity**
MCC Exclusion 7th character A see Appendix A
PDX collection 1195

MCC +7th **S31.639 Puncture wound without foreign body of abdominal wall, unspecified quadrant with penetration into peritoneal cavity**
MCC Exclusion 7th character A see Appendix A
PDX collection 1195

+ **S31.64 Puncture wound with foreign body of abdominal wall with penetration into peritoneal cavity**

MCC +7th **S31.640 Puncture wound with foreign body of abdominal wall, right upper quadrant with penetration into peritoneal cavity**
MCC Exclusion 7th character A see Appendix A
PDX collection 1195

MCC +7th **S31.641 Puncture wound with foreign body of abdominal wall, left upper quadrant with penetration into peritoneal cavity**
MCC Exclusion 7th character A see Appendix A
PDX collection 1195

MCC +7th **S31.642 Puncture wound with foreign body of abdominal wall, epigastric region with penetration into peritoneal cavity**
MCC Exclusion 7th character A see Appendix A
PDX collection 1195

MCC +7th **S31.643 Puncture wound with foreign body of abdominal wall, right lower quadrant with penetration into peritoneal cavity**
MCC Exclusion 7th character A see Appendix A
PDX collection 1195

MCC +7th **S31.644 Puncture wound with foreign body of abdominal wall, left lower quadrant with penetration into peritoneal cavity**
MCC Exclusion 7th character A see Appendix A
PDX collection 1195

MCC +7th **S31.645 Puncture wound with foreign body of abdominal wall, periumbilic region with penetration into peritoneal cavity**
MCC Exclusion 7th character A see Appendix A
PDX collection 1195

MCC +7th **S31.649 Puncture wound with foreign body of abdominal wall, unspecified quadrant with penetration into peritoneal cavity**
MCC Exclusion 7th character A see Appendix A
PDX collection 1195

+ **S31.65 Open bite of abdominal wall with penetration into peritoneal cavity**
Excludes1: *superficial bite of abdominal wall (S30.861, S30.871)*

MCC +7th **S31.650 Open bite of abdominal wall, right upper quadrant with penetration into peritoneal cavity**
MCC Exclusion 7th character A see Appendix A
PDX collection 1195

MCC +7th **S31.651 Open bite of abdominal wall, left upper quadrant with penetration into peritoneal cavity**
MCC Exclusion 7th character A see Appendix A
PDX collection 1195

MCC +7th **S31.652 Open bite of abdominal wall, epigastric region with penetration into peritoneal cavity**
MCC Exclusion 7th character A see Appendix A
PDX collection 1195

MCC +7th **S31.653 Open bite of abdominal wall, right lower quadrant with penetration into peritoneal cavity**
MCC Exclusion 7th character A see Appendix A
PDX collection 1195

MCC +7th **S31.654 Open bite of abdominal wall, left lower quadrant with penetration into peritoneal cavity**
MCC Exclusion 7th character A see Appendix A
PDX collection 1195

MCC +7th **S31.655 Open bite of abdominal wall, periumbilic region with penetration into peritoneal cavity**
MCC Exclusion 7th character A see Appendix A
PDX collection 1195

MCC +7th **S31.659 Open bite of abdominal wall, unspecified quadrant with penetration into peritoneal cavity**
MCC Exclusion 7th character A see Appendix A PDX collection 1195

+ **S31.8 Open wound of other parts of abdomen, lower back and pelvis**
+ **S31.80 Open wound of unspecified buttock**
+7th **S31.801 Laceration without foreign body of unspecified buttock**
+7th **S31.802 Laceration with foreign body of unspecified buttock**
+7th **S31.803 Puncture wound without foreign body of unspecified buttock**
+7th **S31.804 Puncture wound with foreign body of unspecified buttock**
+7th **S31.805 Open bite of unspecified buttock**
Bite of buttock NOS
Excludes1: *superficial bite of buttock (S30.870)*
S31.809 Unspecified open wound of unspecified buttock
+ **S31.81 Open wound of right buttock**
+7th **S31.811 Laceration without foreign body of right buttock**
+7th **S31.812 Laceration with foreign body of right buttock**
+7th **S31.813 Puncture wound without foreign body of right buttock**
+7th **S31.814 Puncture wound with foreign body of right buttock**
+7th **S31.815 Open bite of right buttock**
Bite of right buttock NOS
Excludes1: *superficial bite of buttock (S30.870)*
S31.819 Unspecified open wound of right buttock
+ **S31.82 Open wound of left buttock**
+7th **S31.821 Laceration without foreign body of left buttock**
+7th **S31.822 Laceration with foreign body of left buttock**
+7th **S31.823 Puncture wound without foreign body of left buttock**
+7th **S31.824 Puncture wound with foreign body of left buttock**
+7th **S31.825 Open bite of left buttock**
Bite of left buttock NOS
Excludes1: *superficial bite of buttock (S30.870)*
S31.829 Unspecified open wound of left buttock
+ **S31.83 Open wound of anus**
+7th **S31.831 Laceration without foreign body of anus**
+7th **S31.832 Laceration with foreign body of anus**
+7th **S31.833 Puncture wound without foreign body of anus**
+7th **S31.834 Puncture wound with foreign body of anus**
+7th **S31.835 Open bite of anus**
Bite of anus NOS
Excludes1: *superficial bite of anus (S30.877)*
+7th **S31.839 Unspecified open wound of anus**

See page 961 for Vertebrae Illustration.

S32 Fracture of lumbar spine and pelvis

NOTE A fracture not indicated as displaced or nondisplaced should be coded to displaced
A fracture not indicated as opened or closed should be coded to closed

Includes: fracture of lumbosacral neural arch
fracture of lumbosacral spinous process
fracture of lumbosacral transverse process
fracture of lumbosacral vertebra
fracture of lumbosacral vertebral arch

Code first any associated spinal cord and spinal nerve injury (S34.-)
Excludes1: *transection of abdomen (S38.3)*
Excludes2: *fracture of hip NOS (S72.0-)*

The appropriate 7th character is to be added to each code from category S32
A initial encounter for closed fracture
B initial encounter for open fracture
D subsequent encounter for fracture with routine healing
G subsequent encounter for fracture with delayed healing
K subsequent encounter for fracture with nonunion
S sequela

Review coding guideline C.19.c

+ **S32.0 Fracture of lumbar vertebra**
Fracture of lumbar spine NOS
+ **S32.00 Fracture of unspecified lumbar vertebra**

CC MCC +7th **S32.000 Wedge compression fracture of unspecified lumbar vertebra**
CC Exclusion 7th character A see Appendix A PDX collection 1196
CC Exclusion 7th character K see Appendix A PDX collection 0897
MCC Exclusion 7th character B see Appendix A PDX collection 1196
HAC 7th characters A & B see Appendix B for HAC conditional logic

CC MCC +7th **S32.001 Stable burst fracture of unspecified lumbar vertebra**
CC Exclusion 7th character A see Appendix A PDX collection 1196
CC Exclusion 7th character K see Appendix A PDX collection 0897
MCC Exclusion 7th character B see Appendix A PDX collection 1196
HAC 7th characters A & B see Appendix B for HAC conditional logic

CC MCC +7th **S32.002 Unstable burst fracture of unspecified lumbar vertebra**
CC Exclusion 7th character A see Appendix A PDX collection 1196
CC Exclusion 7th character K see Appendix A PDX collection 0897
MCC Exclusion 7th character B see Appendix A PDX collection 1196
HAC 7th characters A & B see Appendix B for HAC conditional logic

CC MCC +7th **S32.008 Other fracture of unspecified lumbar vertebra**
CC Exclusion 7th character A see Appendix A PDX collection 1196
CC Exclusion 7th character K see Appendix A PDX collection 0897
MCC Exclusion 7th character B see Appendix A PDX collection 1196
HAC 7th characters A & B see Appendix B for HAC conditional logic

CC MCC +7th **S32.009 Unspecified fracture of unspecified lumbar vertebra**
CC Exclusion 7th character A see Appendix A PDX collection 1196
CC Exclusion 7th character K see Appendix A PDX collection 0897
MCC Exclusion 7th character B see Appendix A PDX collection 1196
HAC 7th characters A & B see Appendix B for HAC conditional logic

+ **S32.01 Fracture of first lumbar vertebra**

CC MCC +7th **S32.010 Wedge compression fracture of first lumbar vertebra**
CC Exclusion 7th character A see Appendix A PDX collection 1196
CC Exclusion 7th character K see Appendix A PDX collection 0897
MCC Exclusion 7th character B see Appendix A PDX collection 1196
HAC 7th characters A & B see Appendix B for HAC conditional logic

CC MCC +7th **S32.011** **Stable burst fracture of first lumbar vertebra**
CC Exclusion 7th character A see Appendix A
PDX collection 1196
CC Exclusion 7th character K see Appendix A
PDX collection 0897
MCC Exclusion 7th character B see Appendix A
PDX collection 1196
HAC 7th characters A & B see Appendix B for HAC conditional logic

CC MCC +7th **S32.012** **Unstable burst fracture of first lumbar vertebra**
CC Exclusion 7th character A see Appendix A
PDX collection 1196
CC Exclusion 7th character K see Appendix A
PDX collection 0897
MCC Exclusion 7th character B see Appendix A
PDX collection 1196
HAC 7th characters A & B see Appendix B for HAC conditional logic

CC MCC +7th **S32.018** **Other fracture of first lumbar vertebra**
CC Exclusion 7th character A see Appendix A
PDX collection 1196
CC Exclusion 7th character K see Appendix A
PDX collection 0897
MCC Exclusion 7th character B see Appendix A
PDX collection 1196
HAC 7th characters A & B see Appendix B for HAC conditional logic

CC MCC +7th **S32.019** **Unspecified fracture of first lumbar vertebra**
CC Exclusion 7th character A see Appendix A
PDX collection 1196
CC Exclusion 7th character K see Appendix A
PDX collection 0897
MCC Exclusion 7th character B see Appendix A
PDX collection 1196
HAC 7th characters A & B see Appendix B for HAC conditional logic

+ **S32.02** **Fracture of second lumbar vertebra**

CC MCC +7th **S32.020** **Wedge compression fracture of second lumbar vertebra**
CC Exclusion 7th character A see Appendix A
PDX collection 1196
CC Exclusion 7th character K see Appendix A
PDX collection 0897
MCC Exclusion 7th character B see Appendix A
PDX collection 1196
HAC 7th characters A & B see Appendix B for HAC conditional logic

CC MCC +7th **S32.021** **Stable burst fracture of second lumbar vertebra**
CC Exclusion 7th character A see Appendix A
PDX collection 1196
CC Exclusion 7th character K see Appendix A
PDX collection 0897
MCC Exclusion 7th character B see Appendix A
PDX collection 1196
HAC 7th characters A & B see Appendix B for HAC conditional logic

CC MCC +7th **S32.022** **Unstable burst fracture of second lumbar vertebra**
CC Exclusion 7th character A see Appendix A
PDX collection 1196
CC Exclusion 7th character K see Appendix A
PDX collection 0897
MCC Exclusion 7th character B see Appendix A
PDX collection 1196
HAC 7th characters A & B see Appendix B for HAC conditional logic

CC MCC +7th **S32.028** **Other fracture of second lumbar vertebra**
CC Exclusion 7th character A see Appendix A
PDX collection 1196
CC Exclusion 7th character K see Appendix A
PDX collection 0897
MCC Exclusion 7th character B see Appendix A
PDX collection 1196
HAC 7th characters A & B see Appendix B for HAC conditional logic

CC MCC +7th **S32.029** **Unspecified fracture of second lumbar vertebra**
CC Exclusion 7th character A see Appendix A
PDX collection 1196
CC Exclusion 7th character K see Appendix A
PDX collection 0897
MCC Exclusion 7th character B see Appendix A
PDX collection 1196
HAC 7th characters A & B see Appendix B for HAC conditional logic

+ **S32.03** **Fracture of third lumbar vertebra**

CC MCC +7th **S32.030** **Wedge compression fracture of third lumbar vertebra**
CC Exclusion 7th character A see Appendix A
PDX collection 1196
CC Exclusion 7th character K see Appendix A
PDX collection 0897
MCC Exclusion 7th character B see Appendix A
PDX collection 1196
HAC 7th characters A & B see Appendix B for HAC conditional logic

CC MCC +7th **S32.031** **Stable burst fracture of third lumbar vertebra**
CC Exclusion 7th character A see Appendix A
PDX collection 1196
CC Exclusion 7th character K see Appendix A
PDX collection 0897
MCC Exclusion 7th character B see Appendix A
PDX collection 1196
HAC 7th characters A & B see Appendix B for HAC conditional logic

CC MCC +7th **S32.032** **Unstable burst fracture of third lumbar vertebra**
CC Exclusion 7th character A see Appendix A
PDX collection 1196
CC Exclusion 7th character K see Appendix A
PDX collection 0897
MCC Exclusion 7th character B see Appendix A
PDX collection 1196
HAC 7th characters A & B see Appendix B for HAC conditional logic

CC MCC +7th **S32.038** **Other fracture of third lumbar vertebra**
CC Exclusion 7th character A see Appendix A
PDX collection 1196
CC Exclusion 7th character K see Appendix A
PDX collection 0897
MCC Exclusion 7th character B see Appendix A
PDX collection 1196
HAC 7th characters A & B see Appendix B for HAC conditional logic

CC MCC +7th **S32.039** **Unspecified fracture of third lumbar vertebra**
CC Exclusion 7th character A see Appendix A
PDX collection 1196
CC Exclusion 7th character K see Appendix A
PDX collection 0897
MCC Exclusion 7th character B see Appendix A
PDX collection 1196
HAC 7th characters A & B see Appendix B for HAC conditional logic

+ **S32.04** **Fracture of fourth lumbar vertebra**

CC MCC +7th **S32.040** **Wedge compression fracture of fourth lumbar vertebra**
CC Exclusion 7th character A see Appendix A
PDX collection 1196
CC Exclusion 7th character K see Appendix A
PDX collection 0897
MCC Exclusion 7th character B see Appendix A
PDX collection 1196
HAC 7th characters A & B see Appendix B for HAC conditional logic

CC MCC +7th **S32.041** **Stable burst fracture of fourth lumbar vertebra**
CC Exclusion 7th character A see Appendix A
PDX collection 1196
CC Exclusion 7th character K see Appendix A
PDX collection 0897
MCC Exclusion 7th character B see Appendix A
PDX collection 1196
HAC 7th characters A & B see Appendix B for HAC conditional logic

CC MCC +7th **S32.042** **Unstable burst fracture of fourth lumbar vertebra**
CC Exclusion 7th character A see Appendix A
PDX collection 1196
CC Exclusion 7th character K see Appendix A
PDX collection 0897
MCC Exclusion 7th character B see Appendix A
PDX collection 1196
HAC 7th characters A & B see Appendix B for HAC conditional logic

CC MCC +7th **S32.048** **Other fracture of fourth lumbar vertebra**
CC Exclusion 7th character A see Appendix A PDX collection 1196
CC Exclusion 7th character K see Appendix A PDX collection 0897
MCC Exclusion 7th character B see Appendix A PDX collection 1196
HAC 7th characters A & B see Appendix B for HAC conditional logic

CC MCC +7th **S32.049** **Unspecified fracture of fourth lumbar vertebra**
CC Exclusion 7th character A see Appendix A PDX collection 1196
CC Exclusion 7th character K see Appendix A PDX collection 0897
MCC Exclusion 7th character B see Appendix A PDX collection 1196
HAC 7th characters A & B see Appendix B for HAC conditional logic

+ **S32.05** **Fracture of fifth lumbar vertebra**

CC MCC +7th **S32.050** **Wedge compression fracture of fifth lumbar vertebra**
CC Exclusion 7th character A see Appendix A PDX collection 1196
CC Exclusion 7th character K see Appendix A PDX collection 0897
MCC Exclusion 7th character B see Appendix A PDX collection 1196
HAC 7th characters A & B see Appendix B for HAC conditional logic

CC MCC +7th **S32.051** **Stable burst fracture of fifth lumbar vertebra**
CC Exclusion 7th character A see Appendix A PDX collection 1196
CC Exclusion 7th character K see Appendix A PDX collection 0897
MCC Exclusion 7th character B see Appendix A PDX collection 1196
HAC 7th characters A & B see Appendix B for HAC conditional logic

CC MCC +7th **S32.052** **Unstable burst fracture of fifth lumbar vertebra**
CC Exclusion 7th character A see Appendix A PDX collection 1196
CC Exclusion 7th character K see Appendix A PDX collection 0897
MCC Exclusion 7th character B see Appendix A PDX collection 1196
HAC 7th characters A & B see Appendix B for HAC conditional logic

CC MCC +7th **S32.058** **Other fracture of fifth lumbar vertebra**
CC Exclusion 7th character A see Appendix A PDX collection 1196
CC Exclusion 7th character K see Appendix A PDX collection 0897
MCC Exclusion 7th character B see Appendix A PDX collection 1196
HAC 7th characters A & B see Appendix B for HAC conditional logic

CC MCC +7th **S32.059** **Unspecified fracture of fifth lumbar vertebra**
CC Exclusion 7th character A see Appendix A PDX collection 1196
CC Exclusion 7th character K see Appendix A PDX collection 0897
MCC Exclusion 7th character B see Appendix A PDX collection 1196
HAC 7th characters A & B see Appendix B for HAC conditional logic

+ **S32.1** **Fracture of sacrum**
NOTE For vertical fractures, code to most medial fracture extension
Use two codes if both a vertical and transverse fracture are present

Code also any associated fracture of pelvic ring (S32.8-)

CC MCC X+7th **S32.10** **Unspecified fracture of sacrum**
CC Exclusion 7th character A see Appendix A PDX collection 1197
CC Exclusion 7th character K see Appendix A PDX collection 0897
MCC Exclusion 7th character B see Appendix A PDX collection 1197
HAC 7th characters A & B see Appendix B for HAC conditional logic

+ **S32.11** **Zone I fracture of sacrum**
Vertical sacral ala fracture of sacrum

CC MCC +7th **S32.110** **Nondisplaced Zone I fracture of sacrum**
CC Exclusion 7th character A see Appendix A PDX collection 1197
CC Exclusion 7th character K see Appendix A PDX collection 0897
MCC Exclusion 7th character B see Appendix A PDX collection 1197
HAC 7th characters A & B see Appendix B for HAC conditional logic

CC MCC +7th **S32.111** **Minimally displaced Zone I fracture of sacrum**
CC Exclusion 7th character A see Appendix A PDX collection 1197
CC Exclusion 7th character K see Appendix A PDX collection 0897
MCC Exclusion 7th character B see Appendix A PDX collection 1197
HAC 7th characters A & B see Appendix B for HAC conditional logic

CC MCC +7th **S32.112** **Severely displaced Zone I fracture of sacrum**
CC Exclusion 7th character A see Appendix A PDX collection 1197
CC Exclusion 7th character K see Appendix A PDX collection 0897
MCC Exclusion 7th character B see Appendix A PDX collection 1197
HAC 7th characters A & B see Appendix B for HAC conditional logic

CC MCC +7th **S32.119** **Unspecified Zone I fracture of sacrum**
CC Exclusion 7th character A see Appendix A PDX collection 1197
CC Exclusion 7th character K see Appendix A PDX collection 0897
MCC Exclusion 7th character B see Appendix A PDX collection 1197
HAC 7th characters A & B see Appendix B for HAC conditional logic

+ **S32.12** **Zone II fracture of sacrum**
Vertical foraminal region fracture of sacrum

CC MCC +7th **S32.120** **Nondisplaced Zone II fracture of sacrum**
CC Exclusion 7th character A see Appendix A PDX collection 1197
CC Exclusion 7th character K see Appendix A PDX collection 0897
MCC Exclusion 7th character B see Appendix A PDX collection 1197
HAC 7th characters A & B see Appendix B for HAC conditional logic

CC MCC +7th **S32.121** **Minimally displaced Zone II fracture of sacrum**
CC Exclusion 7th character A see Appendix A PDX collection 1197
CC Exclusion 7th character K see Appendix A PDX collection 0897
MCC Exclusion 7th character B see Appendix A PDX collection 1197
HAC 7th characters A & B see Appendix B for HAC conditional logic

CC MCC +7th **S32.122** **Severely displaced Zone II fracture of sacrum**
CC Exclusion 7th character A see Appendix A PDX collection 1197
CC Exclusion 7th character K see Appendix A PDX collection 0897
MCC Exclusion 7th character B see Appendix A PDX collection 1197
HAC 7th characters A & B see Appendix B for HAC conditional logic

CC MCC +7th **S32.129** **Unspecified Zone II fracture of sacrum**
CC Exclusion 7th character A see Appendix A PDX collection 1197
CC Exclusion 7th character K see Appendix A PDX collection 0897
MCC Exclusion 7th character B see Appendix A PDX collection 1197
HAC 7th characters A & B see Appendix B for HAC conditional logic

+ **S32.13 Zone III fracture of sacrum**
Vertical fracture into spinal canal region of sacrum

CC MCC +7th **S32.130 Nondisplaced Zone III fracture of sacrum**
CC Exclusion 7th character A see Appendix A PDX collection 1197
CC Exclusion 7th character K see Appendix A PDX collection 0897
MCC Exclusion 7th character B see Appendix A PDX collection 1197
HAC 7th characters A & B see Appendix B for HAC conditional logic

CC MCC +7th **S32.131 Minimally displaced Zone III fracture of sacrum**
CC Exclusion 7th character A see Appendix A PDX collection 1197
CC Exclusion 7th character K see Appendix A PDX collection 0897
MCC Exclusion 7th character B see Appendix A PDX collection 1197
HAC 7th characters A & B see Appendix B for HAC conditional logic

CC MCC +7th **S32.132 Severely displaced Zone III fracture of sacrum**
CC Exclusion 7th character A see Appendix A PDX collection 1197
CC Exclusion 7th character K see Appendix A PDX collection 0897
MCC Exclusion 7th character B see Appendix A PDX collection 1197
HAC 7th characters A & B see Appendix B for HAC conditional logic

CC MCC +7th **S32.139 Unspecified Zone III fracture of sacrum**
CC Exclusion 7th character A see Appendix A PDX collection 1197
CC Exclusion 7th character K see Appendix A PDX collection 0897
MCC Exclusion 7th character B see Appendix A PDX collection 1197
HAC 7th characters A & B see Appendix B for HAC conditional logic

CC MCC X+7th **S32.14 Type 1 fracture of sacrum**
Transverse flexion fracture of sacrum without displacement
CC Exclusion 7th character A see Appendix A PDX collection 1197
CC Exclusion 7th character K see Appendix A PDX collection 0897
MCC Exclusion 7th character B see Appendix A PDX collection 1197
HAC 7th characters A & B see Appendix B for HAC conditional logic

CC MCC X+7th **S32.15 Type 2 fracture of sacrum**
Transverse flexion fracture of sacrum with posterior displacement
CC Exclusion 7th character A see Appendix A PDX collection 1197
CC Exclusion 7th character K see Appendix A PDX collection 0897
MCC Exclusion 7th character B see Appendix A PDX collection 1197
HAC 7th characters A & B see Appendix B for HAC conditional logic

CC MCC X+7th **S32.16 Type 3 fracture of sacrum**
Transverse extension fracture of sacrum with anterior displacement
CC Exclusion 7th character A see Appendix A PDX collection 1197
CC Exclusion 7th character K see Appendix A PDX collection 0897
MCC Exclusion 7th character B see Appendix A PDX collection 1197
HAC 7th characters A & B see Appendix B for HAC conditional logic

CC MCC X+7th **S32.17 Type 4 fracture of sacrum**
Transverse segmental comminution of upper sacrum
CC Exclusion 7th character A see Appendix A PDX collection 1197
CC Exclusion 7th character K see Appendix A PDX collection 0897
MCC Exclusion 7th character B see Appendix A PDX collection 1197
HAC 7th characters A & B see Appendix B for HAC conditional logic

CC MCC X+7th **S32.19 Other fracture of sacrum**
CC Exclusion 7th character A see Appendix A PDX collection 1197
CC Exclusion 7th character K see Appendix A PDX collection 0897
MCC Exclusion 7th character B see Appendix A PDX collection 1197
HAC 7th characters A & B see Appendix B for HAC conditional logic

X+7th CC MCC **S32.2 Fracture of coccyx**
CC Exclusion 7th character A see Appendix A PDX collection 1197
CC Exclusion 7th character K see Appendix A PDX collection 0897
MCC Exclusion 7th character B see Appendix A PDX collection 1197
HAC 7th characters A & B see Appendix B for HAC conditional logic

+ **S32.3 Fracture of ilium**
Excludes1: *fracture of ilium with associated disruption of pelvic ring (S32.8-)*

+ **S32.30 Unspecified fracture of ilium**

CC MCC +7th **S32.301 Unspecified fracture of right ilium**
CC Exclusion 7th character A see Appendix A PDX collection 1176
CC Exclusion 7th character K see Appendix A PDX collection 0897
MCC Exclusion 7th character B see Appendix A PDX collection 1198
HAC 7th characters A & B see Appendix B for HAC conditional logic

CC MCC +7th **S32.302 Unspecified fracture of left ilium**
CC Exclusion 7th character A see Appendix A PDX collection 1176
CC Exclusion 7th character K see Appendix A PDX collection 0897
MCC Exclusion 7th character B see Appendix A PDX collection 1198
HAC 7th characters A & B see Appendix B for HAC conditional logic

CC MCC +7th **S32.309 Unspecified fracture of unspecified ilium**
CC Exclusion 7th character A see Appendix A PDX collection 1176
CC Exclusion 7th character K see Appendix A PDX collection 0897
MCC Exclusion 7th character B see Appendix A PDX collection 1198
HAC 7th characters A & B see Appendix B for HAC conditional logic

+ **S32.31 Avulsion fracture of ilium**

CC MCC +7th **S32.311 Displaced avulsion fracture of right ilium**
CC Exclusion 7th character A see Appendix A PDX collection 1176
CC Exclusion 7th character K see Appendix A PDX collection 0897
MCC Exclusion 7th character B see Appendix A PDX collection 1198
HAC 7th characters A & B see Appendix B for HAC conditional logic

CC MCC +7th **S32.312 Displaced avulsion fracture of left ilium**
CC Exclusion 7th character A see Appendix A PDX collection 1176
CC Exclusion 7th character K see Appendix A PDX collection 0897
MCC Exclusion 7th character B see Appendix A PDX collection 1198
HAC 7th characters A & B see Appendix B for HAC conditional logic

CC MCC +7th **S32.313 Displaced avulsion fracture of unspecified ilium**
CC Exclusion 7th character A see Appendix A PDX collection 1176
CC Exclusion 7th character K see Appendix A PDX collection 0897
MCC Exclusion 7th character B see Appendix A PDX collection 1198
HAC 7th characters A & B see Appendix B for HAC conditional logic

CC MCC +7th **S32.314 Nondisplaced avulsion fracture of right ilium**
CC Exclusion 7th character A see Appendix A PDX collection 1176
CC Exclusion 7th character K see Appendix A PDX collection 0897
MCC Exclusion 7th character B see Appendix A PDX collection 1198
HAC 7th characters A & B see Appendix B for HAC conditional logic

CC MCC +7th **S32.315** **Nondisplaced avulsion fracture of left ilium**
CC Exclusion 7th character A see Appendix A
PDX collection 1176
CC Exclusion 7th character K see Appendix A
PDX collection 0897
MCC Exclusion 7th character B see Appendix A
PDX collection 1198
HAC 7th characters A & B see Appendix B for HAC conditional logic

CC MCC +7th **S32.316** **Nondisplaced avulsion fracture of unspecified ilium**
CC Exclusion 7th character A see Appendix A
PDX collection 1176
CC Exclusion 7th character K see Appendix A
PDX collection 0897
MCC Exclusion 7th character B see Appendix A
PDX collection 1198
HAC 7th characters A & B see Appendix B for HAC conditional logic

+ **S32.39** **Other fracture of ilium**

CC MCC +7th **S32.391** **Other fracture of right ilium**
CC Exclusion 7th character A see Appendix A
PDX collection 1176
CC Exclusion 7th character K see Appendix A
PDX collection 0897
MCC Exclusion 7th character B see Appendix A
PDX collection 1198
HAC 7th characters A & B see Appendix B for HAC conditional logic

CC MCC +7th **S32.392** **Other fracture of left ilium**
CC Exclusion 7th character A see Appendix A
PDX collection 1176
CC Exclusion 7th character K see Appendix A
PDX collection 0897
MCC Exclusion 7th character B see Appendix A
PDX collection 1198
HAC 7th characters A & B see Appendix B for HAC conditional logic

CC MCC +7th **S32.399** **Other fracture of unspecified ilium**
CC Exclusion 7th character A see Appendix A
PDX collection 1176
CC Exclusion 7th character K see Appendix A
PDX collection 0897
MCC Exclusion 7th character B see Appendix A
PDX collection 1198
HAC 7th characters A & B see Appendix B for HAC conditional logic

+ **S32.4** **Fracture of acetabulum**
Code also any associated fracture of pelvic ring (S32.8-)

+ **S32.40** **Unspecified fracture of acetabulum**

CC MCC +7th **S32.401** **Unspecified fracture of right acetabulum**
CC Exclusion 7th character K see Appendix A
PDX collection 0897
MCC Exclusion 7th character A see Appendix A
PDX collection 1199
MCC Exclusion 7th character B see Appendix A
PDX collection 1200
HAC 7th characters A & B see Appendix B for HAC conditional logic

CC MCC +7th **S32.402** **Unspecified fracture of left acetabulum**
CC Exclusion 7th character K see Appendix A
PDX collection 0897
MCC Exclusion 7th character A see Appendix A
PDX collection 1199
MCC Exclusion 7th character B see Appendix A
PDX collection 1200
HAC 7th characters A & B see Appendix B for HAC conditional logic

CC MCC +7th **S32.409** **Unspecified fracture of unspecified acetabulum**
CC Exclusion 7th character K see Appendix A
PDX collection 0897
MCC Exclusion 7th character A see Appendix A
PDX collection 1199
MCC Exclusion 7th character B see Appendix A
PDX collection 1200
HAC 7th characters A & B see Appendix B for HAC conditional logic

S32.41 **Fracture of anterior wall of acetabulum**

CC MCC +7th **S32.411** **Displaced fracture of anterior wall of right acetabulum**
CC Exclusion 7th character K see Appendix A
PDX collection 0897
MCC Exclusion 7th character A see Appendix A
PDX collection 1199
MCC Exclusion 7th character B see Appendix A
PDX collection 1200
HAC 7th characters A & B see Appendix B for HAC conditional logic

CC MCC +7th **S32.412** **Displaced fracture of anterior wall of left acetabulum**
CC Exclusion 7th character K see Appendix A
PDX collection 0897
MCC Exclusion 7th character A see Appendix A
PDX collection 1199
MCC Exclusion 7th character B see Appendix A
PDX collection 1200
HAC 7th characters A & B see Appendix B for HAC conditional logic

CC MCC +7th **S32.413** **Displaced fracture of anterior wall of unspecified acetabulum**
CC Exclusion 7th character K see Appendix A
PDX collection 0897
MCC Exclusion 7th character A see Appendix A
PDX collection 1199
MCC Exclusion 7th character B see Appendix A
PDX collection 1200
HAC 7th characters A & B see Appendix B for HAC conditional logic

CC MCC +7th **S32.414** **Nondisplaced fracture of anterior wall of right acetabulum**
CC Exclusion 7th character K see Appendix A
PDX collection 0897
MCC Exclusion 7th character A see Appendix A
PDX collection 1199
MCC Exclusion 7th character B see Appendix A
PDX collection 1200
HAC 7th characters A & B see Appendix B for HAC conditional logic

CC MCC +7th **S32.415** **Nondisplaced fracture of anterior wall of left acetabulum**
CC Exclusion 7th character K see Appendix A
PDX collection 0897
MCC Exclusion 7th character A see Appendix A
PDX collection 1199
MCC Exclusion 7th character B see Appendix A
PDX collection 1200
HAC 7th characters A & B see Appendix B for HAC conditional logic

CC MCC +7th **S32.416** **Nondisplaced fracture of anterior wall of unspecified acetabulum**
CC Exclusion 7th character K see Appendix A
PDX collection 0897
MCC Exclusion 7th character A see Appendix A
PDX collection 1199
MCC Exclusion 7th character B see Appendix A
PDX collection 1200
HAC 7th characters A & B see Appendix B for HAC conditional logic

+ **S32.42** **Fracture of posterior wall of acetabulum**

CC MCC +7th **S32.421** **Displaced fracture of posterior wall of right acetabulum**
CC Exclusion 7th character K see Appendix A
PDX collection 0897
MCC Exclusion 7th character A see Appendix A
PDX collection 1199
MCC Exclusion 7th character B see Appendix A
PDX collection 1200
HAC 7th characters A & B see Appendix B for HAC conditional logic

CC MCC +7th **S32.422** **Displaced fracture of posterior wall of left acetabulum**
CC Exclusion 7th character K see Appendix A
PDX collection 0897
MCC Exclusion 7th character A see Appendix A
PDX collection 1199
MCC Exclusion 7th character B see Appendix A
PDX collection 1200
HAC 7th characters A & B see Appendix B for HAC conditional logic

CC MCC +7th **S32.423** **Displaced fracture of posterior wall of unspecified acetabulum**
CC Exclusion 7th character K see Appendix A
PDX collection 0897
MCC Exclusion 7th character A see Appendix A
PDX collection 1199
MCC Exclusion 7th character B see Appendix A
PDX collection 1200
HAC 7th characters A & B see Appendix B for HAC conditional logic

CC MCC +7th **S32.424** **Nondisplaced fracture of posterior wall of right acetabulum**
CC Exclusion 7th character K see Appendix A PDX collection 0897
MCC Exclusion 7th character A see Appendix A PDX collection 1199
MCC Exclusion 7th character B see Appendix A PDX collection 1200
HAC 7th characters A & B see Appendix B for HAC conditional logic

CC MCC +7th **S32.425** **Nondisplaced fracture of posterior wall of left acetabulum**
CC Exclusion 7th character K see Appendix A PDX collection 0897
MCC Exclusion 7th character A see Appendix A PDX collection 1199
MCC Exclusion 7th character B see Appendix A PDX collection 1200
HAC 7th characters A & B see Appendix B for HAC conditional logic

CC MCC +7th **S32.426** **Nondisplaced fracture of posterior wall of unspecified acetabulum**
CC Exclusion 7th character K see Appendix A PDX collection 0897
MCC Exclusion 7th character A see Appendix A PDX collection 1199
MCC Exclusion 7th character B see Appendix A PDX collection 1200
HAC 7th characters A & B see Appendix B for HAC conditional logic

+ **S32.43** **Fracture of anterior column [iliopubic] of acetabulum**

CC MCC +7th **S32.431** **Displaced fracture of anterior column [iliopubic] of right acetabulum**
CC Exclusion 7th character K see Appendix A PDX collection 0897
MCC Exclusion 7th character A see Appendix A PDX collection 1199
MCC Exclusion 7th character B see Appendix A PDX collection 1200
HAC 7th characters A & B see Appendix B for HAC conditional logic

CC MCC +7th **S32.432** **Displaced fracture of anterior column [iliopubic] of left acetabulum**
CC Exclusion 7th character K see Appendix A PDX collection 0897
MCC Exclusion 7th character A see Appendix A PDX collection 1199
MCC Exclusion 7th character B see Appendix A PDX collection 1200
HAC 7th characters A & B see Appendix B for HAC conditional logic

CC MCC +7th **S32.433** **Displaced fracture of anterior column [iliopubic] of unspecified acetabulum**
CC Exclusion 7th character K see Appendix A PDX collection 0897
MCC Exclusion 7th character A see Appendix A PDX collection 1199
MCC Exclusion 7th character B see Appendix A PDX collection 1200
HAC 7th characters A & B see Appendix B for HAC conditional logic

CC MCC +7th **S32.434** **Nondisplaced fracture of anterior column [iliopubic] of right acetabulum**
CC Exclusion 7th character K see Appendix A PDX collection 0897
MCC Exclusion 7th character A see Appendix A PDX collection 1199
MCC Exclusion 7th character B see Appendix A PDX collection 1200
HAC 7th characters A & B see Appendix B for HAC conditional logic

CC MCC +7th **S32.435** **Nondisplaced fracture of anterior column [iliopubic] of left acetabulum**
CC Exclusion 7th character K see Appendix A PDX collection 0897
MCC Exclusion 7th character A see Appendix A PDX collection 1199
MCC Exclusion 7th character B see Appendix A PDX collection 1200
HAC 7th characters A & B see Appendix B for HAC conditional logic

CC MCC +7th **S32.436** **Nondisplaced fracture of anterior column [iliopubic] of unspecified acetabulum**
CC Exclusion 7th character K see Appendix A PDX collection 0897
MCC Exclusion 7th character A see Appendix A PDX collection 1199
MCC Exclusion 7th character B see Appendix A PDX collection 1200
HAC 7th characters A & B see Appendix B for HAC conditional logic

+ **S32.44** **Fracture of posterior column [ilioischial] of acetabulum**

CC MCC +7th **S32.441** **Displaced fracture of posterior column [ilioischial] of right acetabulum**
CC Exclusion 7th character K see Appendix A PDX collection 0897
MCC Exclusion 7th character A see Appendix A PDX collection 1199
MCC Exclusion 7th character B see Appendix A PDX collection 1200
HAC 7th characters A & B see Appendix B for HAC conditional logic

CC MCC +7th **S32.442** **Displaced fracture of posterior column [ilioischial] of left acetabulum**
CC Exclusion 7th character K see Appendix A PDX collection 0897
MCC Exclusion 7th character A see Appendix A PDX collection 1199
MCC Exclusion 7th character B see Appendix A PDX collection 1200
HAC 7th characters A & B see Appendix B for HAC conditional logic

CC MCC +7th **S32.443** **Displaced fracture of posterior column [ilioischial] of unspecified acetabulum**
CC Exclusion 7th character K see Appendix A PDX collection 0897
MCC Exclusion 7th character A see Appendix A PDX collection 1199
MCC Exclusion 7th character B see Appendix A PDX collection 1200
HAC 7th characters A & B see Appendix B for HAC conditional logic

CC MCC +7th **S32.444** **Nondisplaced fracture of posterior column [ilioischial] of right acetabulum**
CC Exclusion 7th character K see Appendix A PDX collection 0897
MCC Exclusion 7th character A see Appendix A PDX collection 1199
MCC Exclusion 7th character B see Appendix A PDX collection 1200
HAC 7th characters A & B see Appendix B for HAC conditional logic

CC MCC +7th **S32.445** **Nondisplaced fracture of posterior column [ilioischial] of left acetabulum**
CC Exclusion 7th character K see Appendix A PDX collection 0897
MCC Exclusion 7th character A see Appendix A PDX collection 1199
MCC Exclusion 7th character B see Appendix A PDX collection 1200
HAC 7th characters A & B see Appendix B for HAC conditional logic

CC MCC +7th **S32.446** **Nondisplaced fracture of posterior column [ilioischial] of unspecified acetabulum**
CC Exclusion 7th character K see Appendix A PDX collection 0897
MCC Exclusion 7th character A see Appendix A PDX collection 1199
MCC Exclusion 7th character B see Appendix A PDX collection 1200
HAC 7th characters A & B see Appendix B for HAC conditional logic

+ **S32.45** **Transverse fracture of acetabulum**

CC MCC +7th **S32.451** **Displaced transverse fracture of right acetabulum**
CC Exclusion 7th character K see Appendix A PDX collection 0897
MCC Exclusion 7th character A see Appendix A PDX collection 1199
MCC Exclusion 7th character B see Appendix A PDX collection 1200
HAC 7th characters A & B see Appendix B for HAC conditional logic

CC MCC +7th **S32.452** **Displaced transverse fracture of left acetabulum**
CC Exclusion 7th character K see Appendix A PDX collection 0897
MCC Exclusion 7th character A see Appendix A PDX collection 1199
MCC Exclusion 7th character B see Appendix A PDX collection 1200
HAC 7th characters A & B see Appendix B for HAC conditional logic

CC MCC +7th **S32.453** **Displaced transverse fracture of unspecified acetabulum**
CC Exclusion 7th character K see Appendix A PDX collection 0897
MCC Exclusion 7th character A see Appendix A PDX collection 1199
MCC Exclusion 7th character B see Appendix A PDX collection 1200
HAC 7th characters A & B see Appendix B for HAC conditional logic

CC MCC +7th **S32.454** **Nondisplaced transverse fracture of right acetabulum**
CC Exclusion 7th character K see Appendix A PDX collection 0897
MCC Exclusion 7th character A see Appendix A PDX collection 1199
MCC Exclusion 7th character B see Appendix A PDX collection 1200
HAC 7th characters A & B see Appendix B for HAC conditional logic

CC MCC +7th **S32.455** **Nondisplaced transverse fracture of left acetabulum**
CC Exclusion 7th character K see Appendix A PDX collection 0897
MCC Exclusion 7th character A see Appendix A PDX collection 1199
MCC Exclusion 7th character B see Appendix A PDX collection 1200
HAC 7th characters A & B see Appendix B for HAC conditional logic

CC MCC +7th **S32.456** **Nondisplaced transverse fracture of unspecified acetabulum**
CC Exclusion 7th character K see Appendix A PDX collection 0897
MCC Exclusion 7th character A see Appendix A PDX collection 1199
MCC Exclusion 7th character B see Appendix A PDX collection 1200
HAC 7th characters A & B see Appendix B for HAC conditional logic

\+ **S32.46** **Associated transverse-posterior fracture of acetabulum**

CC MCC +7th **S32.461** **Displaced associated transverse-posterior fracture of right acetabulum**
CC Exclusion 7th character K see Appendix A PDX collection 0897
MCC Exclusion 7th character A see Appendix A PDX collection 1199
MCC Exclusion 7th character B see Appendix A PDX collection 1200
HAC 7th characters A & B see Appendix B for HAC conditional logic

CC MCC +7th **S32.462** **Displaced associated transverse-posterior fracture of left acetabulum**
CC Exclusion 7th character K see Appendix A PDX collection 0897
MCC Exclusion 7th character A see Appendix A PDX collection 1199
MCC Exclusion 7th character B see Appendix A PDX collection 1200
HAC 7th characters A & B see Appendix B for HAC conditional logic

CC MCC +7th **S32.463** **Displaced associated transverse-posterior fracture of unspecified acetabulum**
CC Exclusion 7th character K see Appendix A PDX collection 0897
MCC Exclusion 7th character A see Appendix A PDX collection 1199
MCC Exclusion 7th character B see Appendix A PDX collection 1200
HAC 7th characters A & B see Appendix B for HAC conditional logic

CC MCC +7th **S32.464** **Nondisplaced associated transverse-posterior fracture of right acetabulum**
CC Exclusion 7th character K see Appendix A PDX collection 0897
MCC Exclusion 7th character A see Appendix PDX collection 1199
MCC Exclusion 7th character B see Appendix PDX collection 1200
HAC 7th characters A & B see Appendix B for HAC conditional logic

CC MCC +7th **S32.465** **Nondisplaced associated transverse-posterior fracture of left acetabulum**
CC Exclusion 7th character K see Appendix A PDX collection 0897
MCC Exclusion 7th character A see Appendix PDX collection 1199
MCC Exclusion 7th character B see Appendix PDX collection 1200
HAC 7th characters A & B see Appendix B for HAC conditional logic

CC MCC +7th **S32.466** **Nondisplaced associated transverse-posterior fracture of unspecified acetabulum**
CC Exclusion 7th character K see Appendix A PDX collection 0897
MCC Exclusion 7th character A see Appendix PDX collection 1199
MCC Exclusion 7th character B see Appendix PDX collection 1200
HAC 7th characters A & B see Appendix B for HAC conditional logic

\+ **S32.47** **Fracture of medial wall of acetabulum**

CC MCC +7th **S32.471** **Displaced fracture of medial wall of right acetabulum**
CC Exclusion 7th character K see Appendix A PDX collection 0897
MCC Exclusion 7th character A see Appendix PDX collection 1199
MCC Exclusion 7th character B see Appendix PDX collection 1200
HAC 7th characters A & B see Appendix B for HAC conditional logic

CC MCC +7th **S32.472** **Displaced fracture of medial wall of left acetabulum**
CC Exclusion 7th character K see Appendix A PDX collection 0897
MCC Exclusion 7th character A see Appendix PDX collection 1199
MCC Exclusion 7th character B see Appendix PDX collection 1200
HAC 7th characters A & B see Appendix B for HAC conditional logic

CC MCC +7th **S32.473** **Displaced fracture of medial wall of unspecified acetabulum**
CC Exclusion 7th character K see Appendix A PDX collection 0897
MCC Exclusion 7th character A see Appendix PDX collection 1199
MCC Exclusion 7th character B see Appendix PDX collection 1200
HAC 7th characters A & B see Appendix B for HAC conditional logic

CC MCC +7th **S32.474** **Nondisplaced fracture of medial wall of right acetabulum**
CC Exclusion 7th character K see Appendix A PDX collection 0897
MCC Exclusion 7th character A see Appendix PDX collection 1199
MCC Exclusion 7th character B see Appendix PDX collection 1200
HAC 7th characters A & B see Appendix B for HAC conditional logic

CC MCC +7th **S32.475** **Nondisplaced fracture of medial wall of l acetabulum**
CC Exclusion 7th character K see Appendix A PDX collection 0897
MCC Exclusion 7th character A see Appendix PDX collection 1199
MCC Exclusion 7th character B see Appendix PDX collection 1200
HAC 7th characters A & B see Appendix B for HAC conditional logic

CC MCC +7th **S32.476** **Nondisplaced fracture of medial wall of unspecified acetabulum**
CC Exclusion 7th character K see Appendix A PDX collection 0897
MCC Exclusion 7th character A see Appendix A PDX collection 1199
MCC Exclusion 7th character B see Appendix A PDX collection 1200
HAC 7th characters A & B see Appendix B for HAC conditional logic

+ **S32.48 Dome fracture of acetabulum**

CC MCC +7th **S32.481** **Displaced dome fracture of right acetabulum**
CC Exclusion 7th character K see Appendix A PDX collection 0897
MCC Exclusion 7th character A see Appendix A PDX collection 1199
MCC Exclusion 7th character B see Appendix A PDX collection 1200
HAC 7th characters A & B see Appendix B for HAC conditional logic

CC MCC +7th **S32.482** **Displaced dome fracture of left acetabulum**
CC Exclusion 7th character K see Appendix A PDX collection 0897
MCC Exclusion 7th character A see Appendix A PDX collection 1199
MCC Exclusion 7th character B see Appendix A PDX collection 1200
HAC 7th characters A & B see Appendix B for HAC conditional logic

CC MCC +7th **S32.483** **Displaced dome fracture of unspecified acetabulum**
CC Exclusion 7th character K see Appendix A PDX collection 0897
MCC Exclusion 7th character A see Appendix A PDX collection 1199
MCC Exclusion 7th character B see Appendix A PDX collection 1200
HAC 7th characters A & B see Appendix B for HAC conditional logic

CC MCC +7th **S32.484** **Nondisplaced dome fracture of right acetabulum**
CC Exclusion 7th character K see Appendix A PDX collection 0897
MCC Exclusion 7th character A see Appendix A PDX collection 1199
MCC Exclusion 7th character B see Appendix A PDX collection 1200
HAC 7th characters A & B see Appendix B for HAC conditional logic

CC MCC +7th **S32.485** **Nondisplaced dome fracture of left acetabulum**
CC Exclusion 7th character K see Appendix A PDX collection 0897
MCC Exclusion 7th character A see Appendix A PDX collection 1199
MCC Exclusion 7th character B see Appendix A PDX collection 1200
HAC 7th characters A & B see Appendix B for HAC conditional logic

CC MCC +7th **S32.486** **Nondisplaced dome fracture of unspecified acetabulum**
CC Exclusion 7th character K see Appendix A PDX collection 0897
MCC Exclusion 7th character A see Appendix A PDX collection 1199
MCC Exclusion 7th character B see Appendix A PDX collection 1200
HAC 7th characters A & B see Appendix B for HAC conditional logic

+ **S32.49 Other specified fracture of acetabulum**

CC MCC +7th **S32.491** **Other specified fracture of right acetabulum**
CC Exclusion 7th character K see Appendix A PDX collection 0897
MCC Exclusion 7th character A see Appendix A PDX collection 1199
MCC Exclusion 7th character B see Appendix A PDX collection 1200
HAC 7th characters A & B see Appendix B for HAC conditional logic

CC MCC +7th **S32.492** **Other specified fracture of left acetabulum**
CC Exclusion 7th character K see Appendix A PDX collection 0897
MCC Exclusion 7th character A see Appendix A PDX collection 1199
MCC Exclusion 7th character B see Appendix A PDX collection 1200
HAC 7th characters A & B see Appendix B for HAC conditional logic

CC MCC +7th **S32.499** **Other specified fracture of unspecified acetabulum**
CC Exclusion 7th character K see Appendix A PDX collection 0897
MCC Exclusion 7th character A see Appendix A PDX collection 1199
MCC Exclusion 7th character B see Appendix A PDX collection 1200
HAC 7th characters A & B see Appendix B for HAC conditional logic

+ **S32.5 Fracture of pubis**
Excludes1: *fracture of pubis with associated disruption of pelvic ring (S32.8-)*

+ **S32.50 Unspecified fracture of pubis**

CC MCC +7th **S32.501** **Unspecified fracture of right pubis**
CC Exclusion 7th character A see Appendix A PDX collection 1201
CC Exclusion 7th character K see Appendix A PDX collection 0897
MCC Exclusion 7th character B see Appendix A PDX collection 1201
HAC 7th characters A & B see Appendix B for HAC conditional logic

CC MCC +7th **S32.502** **Unspecified fracture of left pubis**
CC Exclusion 7th character A see Appendix A PDX collection 1201
CC Exclusion 7th character K see Appendix A PDX collection 0897
MCC Exclusion 7th character B see Appendix A PDX collection 1201
HAC 7th characters A & B see Appendix B for HAC conditional logic

CC MCC +7th **S32.509** **Unspecified fracture of unspecified pubis**
CC Exclusion 7th character A see Appendix A PDX collection 1201
CC Exclusion 7th character K see Appendix A PDX collection 0897
MCC Exclusion 7th character B see Appendix A PDX collection 1201
HAC 7th characters A & B see Appendix B for HAC conditional logic

+ **S32.51 Fracture of superior rim of pubis**

CC MCC +7th **S32.511** **Fracture of superior rim of right pubis**
CC Exclusion 7th character A see Appendix A PDX collection 1201
CC Exclusion 7th character K see Appendix A PDX collection 0897
MCC Exclusion 7th character B see Appendix A PDX collection 1201
HAC 7th characters A & B see Appendix B for HAC conditional logic

CC MCC +7th **S32.512** **Fracture of superior rim of left pubis**
CC Exclusion 7th character A see Appendix A PDX collection 1201
CC Exclusion 7th character K see Appendix A PDX collection 0897
MCC Exclusion 7th character B see Appendix A PDX collection 1201
HAC 7th characters A & B see Appendix B for HAC conditional logic

CC MCC +7th **S32.519** **Fracture of superior rim of unspecified pubis**
CC Exclusion 7th character A see Appendix A PDX collection 1201
CC Exclusion 7th character K see Appendix A PDX collection 0897
MCC Exclusion 7th character B see Appendix A PDX collection 1201
HAC 7th characters A & B see Appendix B for HAC conditional logic

+ **S32.59 Other specified fracture of pubis**

CC MCC +7th **S32.591** **Other specified fracture of right pubis**
CC Exclusion 7th character A see Appendix A PDX collection 1201
CC Exclusion 7th character K see Appendix A PDX collection 0897
MCC Exclusion 7th character B see Appendix A PDX collection 1201
HAC 7th characters A & B see Appendix B for HAC conditional logic

CC MCC +7th **S32.592** **Other specified fracture of left pubis**
CC Exclusion 7th character A see Appendix A PDX collection 1201
CC Exclusion 7th character K see Appendix A PDX collection 0897
MCC Exclusion 7th character B see Appendix A PDX collection 1201
HAC 7th characters A & B see Appendix B for HAC conditional logic

CC MCC +7th **S32.599** **Other specified fracture of unspecified pubis**
CC Exclusion 7th character A see Appendix A PDX collection 1201
CC Exclusion 7th character K see Appendix A PDX collection 0897
MCC Exclusion 7th character B see Appendix A PDX collection 1201
HAC 7th characters A & B see Appendix B for HAC conditional logic

+ **S32.6 Fracture of ischium**
Excludes1: fracture of ischium with associated disruption of pelvic ring (S32.8-)

+ **S32.60 Unspecified fracture of ischium**

CC MCC +7th **S32.601** **Unspecified fracture of right ischium**
CC Exclusion 7th character A see Appendix A PDX collection 1202
CC Exclusion 7th character K see Appendix A PDX collection 0897
MCC Exclusion 7th character B see Appendix A PDX collection 1203
HAC 7th characters A & B see Appendix B for HAC conditional logic

CC MCC +7th **S32.602** **Unspecified fracture of left ischium**
CC Exclusion 7th character A see Appendix A PDX collection 1202
CC Exclusion 7th character K see Appendix A PDX collection 0897
MCC Exclusion 7th character B see Appendix A PDX collection 1203
HAC 7th characters A & B see Appendix B for HAC conditional logic

CC MCC +7th **S32.609** **Unspecified fracture of unspecified ischium**
CC Exclusion 7th character A see Appendix A PDX collection 1202
CC Exclusion 7th character K see Appendix A PDX collection 0897
MCC Exclusion 7th character B see Appendix A PDX collection 1203
HAC 7th characters A & B see Appendix B for HAC conditional logic

+ **S32.61 Avulsion fracture of ischium**

CC MCC +7th **S32.611** **Displaced avulsion fracture of right ischium**
CC Exclusion 7th character A see Appendix A PDX collection 1202
CC Exclusion 7th character K see Appendix A PDX collection 0897
MCC Exclusion 7th character B see Appendix A PDX collection 1203
HAC 7th characters A & B see Appendix B for HAC conditional logic

CC MCC +7th **S32.612** **Displaced avulsion fracture of left ischium**
CC Exclusion 7th character A see Appendix A PDX collection 1202
CC Exclusion 7th character K see Appendix A PDX collection 0897
MCC Exclusion 7th character B see Appendix A PDX collection 1203
HAC 7th characters A & B see Appendix B for HAC conditional logic

CC MCC +7th **S32.613** **Displaced avulsion fracture of unspecified ischium**
CC Exclusion 7th character A see Appendix A PDX collection 1202
CC Exclusion 7th character K see Appendix A PDX collection 0897
MCC Exclusion 7th character B see Appendix A PDX collection 1203
HAC 7th characters A & B see Appendix B for HAC conditional logic

CC MCC +7th **S32.614** **Nondisplaced avulsion fracture of right ischium**
CC Exclusion 7th character A see Appendix A PDX collection 1202
CC Exclusion 7th character K see Appendix A PDX collection 0897
MCC Exclusion 7th character B see Appendix A PDX collection 1203
HAC 7th characters A & B see Appendix B for HAC conditional logic

CC MCC +7th **S32.615** **Nondisplaced avulsion fracture of left ischium**
CC Exclusion 7th character A see Appendix A PDX collection 1202
CC Exclusion 7th character K see Appendix A PDX collection 0897
MCC Exclusion 7th character B see Appendix PDX collection 1203
HAC 7th characters A & B see Appendix B for HAC conditional logic

CC MCC +7th **S32.616** **Nondisplaced avulsion fracture of unspecified ischium**
CC Exclusion 7th character A see Appendix A PDX collection 1202
CC Exclusion 7th character K see Appendix A PDX collection 0897
MCC Exclusion 7th character B see Appendix PDX collection 1203
HAC 7th characters A & B see Appendix B for HAC conditional logic

+ **S32.69 Other specified fracture of ischium**

CC MCC +7th **S32.691** **Other specified fracture of right ischium**
CC Exclusion 7th character A see Appendix A PDX collection 1202
CC Exclusion 7th character K see Appendix A PDX collection 0897
MCC Exclusion 7th character B see Appendix PDX collection 1203
HAC 7th characters A & B see Appendix B for HAC conditional logic

CC MCC +7th **S32.692** **Other specified fracture of left ischium**
CC Exclusion 7th character A see Appendix A PDX collection 1202
CC Exclusion 7th character K see Appendix A PDX collection 0897
MCC Exclusion 7th character B see Appendix PDX collection 1203
HAC 7th characters A & B see Appendix B for HAC conditional logic

CC MCC +7th **S32.699** **Other specified fracture of unspecified ischium**
CC Exclusion 7th character A see Appendix A PDX collection 1202
CC Exclusion 7th character K see Appendix A PDX collection 0897
MCC Exclusion 7th character B see Appendi PDX collection 1203
HAC 7th characters A & B see Appendix B fo HAC conditional logic

+ **S32.8 Fracture of other parts of pelvis**
Code also any associated:
fracture of acetabulum (S32.4-)
sacral fracture (S32.1-)

+ **S32.81 Multiple fractures of pelvis with disruption of pelvic ring**
Multiple pelvic fractures with disruption of pelvic circ

CC MCC +7th **S32.810** **Multiple fractures of pelvis with stable disruption of pelvic ring**
CC Exclusion 7th character A see Appendix A PDX collection 1204
CC Exclusion 7th character K see Appendix PDX collection 0897
MCC Exclusion 7th character B see Appendi PDX collection 1204
HAC 7th characters A & B see Appendix B fo HAC conditional logic

CC MCC +7th **S32.811** **Multiple fractures of pelvis with unstable disruption of pelvic ring**
CC Exclusion 7th character A see Appendix A PDX collection 1204
CC Exclusion 7th character K see Appendix PDX collection 0897
MCC Exclusion 7th character B see Appendi PDX collection 1204
HAC 7th characters A & B see Appendix B fo HAC conditional logic

CC MCC X+7th **S32.82** **Multiple fractures of pelvis without disruption of pelvic ring**
Multiple pelvic fractures without disruption of pelvic circle
CC Exclusion 7th character A see Appendix A PDX collection 1205
CC Exclusion 7th character K see Appendix A PDX collection 0897
MCC Exclusion 7th character B see Appendix A PDX collection 1205
HAC 7th characters A & B see Appendix B for HAC conditional logic

CC MCC X+7th **S32.89 Fracture of other parts of pelvis**
CC Exclusion 7th character A see Appendix A PDX collection 1206
CC Exclusion 7th character K see Appendix A PDX collection 0897
MCC Exclusion 7th character B see Appendix A PDX collection 1206
HAC 7th characters A & B see Appendix B for HAC conditional logic

X+7th MCC CC **S32.9 Fracture of unspecified parts of lumbosacral spine and pelvis**
Fracture of lumbosacral spine NOS
Fracture of pelvis NOS
CC Exclusion 7th character A see Appendix A PDX collection 1204
CC Exclusion 7th character K see Appendix A PDX collection 0897
MCC Exclusion 7th character B see Appendix A PDX collection 1204
HAC 7th characters A & B see Appendix B for HAC conditional logic

S33 Dislocation and sprain of joints and ligaments of lumbar spine and pelvis

Includes: avulsion of joint or ligament of lumbar spine and pelvis
laceration of cartilage, joint or ligament of lumbar spine and pelvis
sprain of cartilage, joint or ligament of lumbar spine and pelvis
traumatic hemarthrosis of joint or ligament of lumbar spine and pelvis
traumatic rupture of joint or ligament of lumbar spine and pelvis
traumatic subluxation of joint or ligament of lumbar spine and pelvis
traumatic tear of joint or ligament of lumbar spine and pelvis

Code also any associated open wound

Excludes1: *nontraumatic rupture or displacement of lumbar intervertebral disc NOS (M51.-)*
obstetric damage to pelvic joints and ligaments (O71.6)

Excludes2: *dislocation and sprain of joints and ligaments of hip (S73.-)*
strain of muscle of lower back and pelvis (S39.01-)

The appropriate 7th character is to be added to each code from category S33
A initial encounter
D subsequent encounter
S sequela

X+7th **S33.0 Traumatic rupture of lumbar intervertebral disc**
Excludes1: *rupture or displacement (nontraumatic) of lumbar intervertebral disc NOS (M51.- with fifth character 6)*

\+ **S33.1 Subluxation and dislocation of lumbar vertebra**
Code also any associated:
open wound of abdomen, lower back and pelvis (S31)
spinal cord injury (S24.0, S24.1-, S34.0-, S34.1-)
Excludes2: *fracture of lumbar vertebrae (S32.0-)*

\+ **S33.10 Subluxation and dislocation of unspecified lumbar vertebra**
+7th **S33.100 Subluxation of unspecified lumbar vertebra**
+7th **S33.101 Dislocation of unspecified lumbar vertebra**

\+ **S33.11 Subluxation and dislocation of L1/L2 lumbar vertebra**
+7th **S33.110 Subluxation of L1/L2 lumbar vertebra**
+7th **S33.111 Dislocation of L1/L2 lumbar vertebra**

\+ **S33.12 Subluxation and dislocation of L2/L3 lumbar vertebra**
+7th **S33.120 Subluxation of L2/L3 lumbar vertebra**
+7th **S33.121 Dislocation of L2/L3 lumbar vertebra**

\+ **S33.13 Subluxation and dislocation of L3/L4 lumbar vertebra**
+7th **S33.130 Subluxation of L3/L4 lumbar vertebra**
+7th **S33.131 Dislocation of L3/L4 lumbar vertebra**

\+ **S33.14 Subluxation and dislocation of L4/L5 lumbar vertebra**
+7th **S33.140 Subluxation of L4/L5 lumbar vertebra**
+7th **S33.141 Dislocation of L4/L5 lumbar vertebra**

X+7th **S33.2 Dislocation of sacroiliac and sacrococcygeal joint**

\+ **S33.3 Dislocation of other and unspecified parts of lumbar spine and pelvis**
X+7th **S33.30 Dislocation of unspecified parts of lumbar spine and pelvis**
X+7th **S33.39 Dislocation of other parts of lumbar spine and pelvis**

X+7th **S33.4 Traumatic rupture of symphysis pubis**
X+7th **S33.5 Sprain of ligaments of lumbar spine**
X+7th **S33.6 Sprain of sacroiliac joint**
X+7th **S33.8 Sprain of other parts of lumbar spine and pelvis**
X+7th **S33.9 Sprain of unspecified parts of lumbar spine and pelvis**

S34 Injury of lumbar and sacral spinal cord and nerves at abdomen, lower back and pelvis level

NOTE Code to highest level of lumbar cord injury
Injuries to the spinal cord (S34.0 and S34.1) refer to the cord level and not bone level injury, and can affect nerve roots at and below the level given.

Code also any associated:
fracture of vertebra (S22.0-, S32.0-)
open wound of abdomen, lower back and pelvis (S31.-)
transient paralysis (R29.5)

The appropriate 7th character is to be added to each code from category S34
A initial encounter
D subsequent encounter
S sequela

\+ **S34.0 Concussion and edema of lumbar and sacral spinal cord**
MCC X+7th **S34.01 Concussion and edema of lumbar spinal cord**
MCC Exclusion 7th character A see Appendix A PDX collection 1207
MCC X+7th **S34.02 Concussion and edema of sacral spinal cord**
Concussion and edema of conus medullaris
MCC Exclusion 7th character A see Appendix A PDX collection 1208

\+ **S34.1 Other and unspecified injury of lumbar and sacral spinal cord**

\+ **S34.10 Unspecified injury to lumbar spinal cord**

MCC +7th **S34.101 Unspecified injury to L1 level of lumbar spinal cord**
Unspecified injury to lumbar spinal cord level 1
MCC Exclusion 7th character A see Appendix A PDX collection 1207
HAC 7th character A see Appendix B for HAC conditional logic

MCC +7th **S34.102 Unspecified injury to L2 level of lumbar spinal cord**
Unspecified injury to lumbar spinal cord level 2
MCC Exclusion 7th character A see Appendix A PDX collection 1207
HAC 7th character A see Appendix B for HAC conditional logic

MCC +7th **S34.103 Unspecified injury to L3 level of lumbar spinal cord**
Unspecified injury to lumbar spinal cord level 3
MCC Exclusion 7th character A see Appendix A PDX collection 1207
HAC 7th character A see Appendix B for HAC conditional logic

MCC +7th **S34.104 Unspecified injury to L4 level of lumbar spinal cord**
Unspecified injury to lumbar spinal cord level 4
MCC Exclusion 7th character A see Appendix A PDX collection 1207
HAC 7th character A see Appendix B for HAC conditional logic

MCC +7th **S34.105 Unspecified injury to L5 level of lumbar spinal cord**
Unspecified injury to lumbar spinal cord level 5
MCC Exclusion 7th character A see Appendix A PDX collection 1207
HAC 7th character A see Appendix B for HAC conditional logic

MCC +7th **S34.109 Unspecified injury to unspecified level of lumbar spinal cord**
MCC Exclusion 7th character A see Appendix A PDX collection 1207
HAC 7th character A see Appendix B for HAC conditional logic

\+ **S34.11 Complete lesion of lumbar spinal cord**

MCC +7th **S34.111 Complete lesion of L1 level of lumbar spinal cord**
Complete lesion of lumbar spinal cord level 1
MCC Exclusion 7th character A see Appendix A PDX collection 1207
HAC 7th character A see Appendix B for HAC conditional logic

MCC +7th **S34.112** **Complete lesion of L2 level of lumbar spinal cord**
Complete lesion of lumbar spinal cord level 2
MCC Exclusion 7th character A see Appendix A PDX collection 1207
HAC 7th character A see Appendix B for HAC conditional logic

MCC +7th **S34.113** **Complete lesion of L3 level of lumbar spinal cord**
Complete lesion of lumbar spinal cord level 3
MCC Exclusion 7th character A see Appendix A PDX collection 1207
HAC 7th character A see Appendix B for HAC conditional logic

MCC +7th **S34.114** **Complete lesion of L4 level of lumbar spinal cord**
Complete lesion of lumbar spinal cord level 4
MCC Exclusion 7th character A see Appendix A PDX collection 1207
HAC 7th character A see Appendix B for HAC conditional logic

MCC +7th **S34.115** **Complete lesion of L5 level of lumbar spinal cord**
Complete lesion of lumbar spinal cord level 5
MCC Exclusion 7th character A see Appendix A PDX collection 1207
HAC 7th character A see Appendix B for HAC conditional logic

MCC +7th **S34.119** **Complete lesion of unspecified level of lumbar spinal cord**
MCC Exclusion 7th character A see Appendix A PDX collection 1207
HAC 7th character A see Appendix B for HAC conditional logic

+ **S34.12** **Incomplete lesion of lumbar spinal cord**

MCC +7th **S34.121** **Incomplete lesion of L1 level of lumbar spinal cord**
Incomplete lesion of lumbar spinal cord level 1
MCC Exclusion 7th character A see Appendix A PDX collection 1207
HAC 7th character A see Appendix B for HAC conditional logic

MCC +7th **S34.122** **Incomplete lesion of L2 level of lumbar spinal cord**
Incomplete lesion of lumbar spinal cord level 2
MCC Exclusion 7th character A see Appendix A PDX collection 1207
HAC 7th character A see Appendix B for HAC conditional logic

MCC +7th **S34.123** **Incomplete lesion of L3 level of lumbar spinal cord**
Incomplete lesion of lumbar spinal cord level 3
MCC Exclusion 7th character A see Appendix A PDX collection 1207
HAC 7th character A see Appendix B for HAC conditional logic

MCC +7th **S34.124** **Incomplete lesion of L4 level of lumbar spinal cord**
Incomplete lesion of lumbar spinal cord level 4
MCC Exclusion 7th character A see Appendix A PDX collection 1207
HAC 7th character A see Appendix B for HAC conditional logic

MCC +7th **S34.125** **Incomplete lesion of L5 level of lumbar spinal cord**
Incomplete lesion of lumbar spinal cord level 5
MCC Exclusion 7th character A see Appendix A PDX collection 1207
HAC 7th character A see Appendix B for HAC conditional logic

MCC +7th **S34.129** **Incomplete lesion of unspecified level of lumbar spinal cord**
MCC Exclusion 7th character A see Appendix A PDX collection 1207
HAC 7th character A see Appendix B for HAC conditional logic

+ **S34.13** **Other and unspecified injury to sacral spinal cord**
Other injury to conus medullaris

MCC +7th **S34.131** **Complete lesion of sacral spinal cord**
Complete lesion of conus medullaris
MCC Exclusion 7th character A see Appendix A PDX collection 1208
HAC 7th character A see Appendix B for HAC conditional logic

MCC +7th **S34.132** **Incomplete lesion of sacral spinal cord**
Incomplete lesion of conus medullaris
MCC Exclusion 7th character A see Appendix A PDX collection 1208
HAC 7th character A see Appendix B for HAC conditional logic

MCC +7th **S34.139** **Unspecified injury to sacral spinal cord**
Unspecified injury of conus medullaris
MCC Exclusion 7th character A see Appendix A PDX collection 1208
HAC 7th character A see Appendix B for HAC conditional logic

+ **S34.2** **Injury of nerve root of lumbar and sacral spine**
X+7th **S34.21** **Injury of nerve root of lumbar spine**
X+7th **S34.22** **Injury of nerve root of sacral spine**

MCC X+7th **S34.3** **Injury of cauda equina**
MCC Exclusion 7th character A see Appendix A PDX collection 120
HAC 7th character A see Appendix B for HAC conditional logic

X+7th **S34.4** **Injury of lumbosacral plexus**

X+7th **S34.5** **Injury of lumbar, sacral and pelvic sympathetic nerves**
Injury of celiac ganglion or plexus
Injury of hypogastric plexus
Injury of mesenteric plexus (inferior) (superior)
Injury of splanchnic nerve

X+7th **S34.6** **Injury of peripheral nerve(s) at abdomen, lower back and pelvis level**

X+7th **S34.8** **Injury of other nerves at abdomen, lower back and pelvis leve**

X+7th **S34.9** **Injury of unspecified nerves at abdomen, lower back and pelvis level**

S35 Injury of blood vessels at abdomen, lower back and pelvis level

Code also any associated open wound (S31.-)

The appropriate 7th character is to be added to each code from category S35
A initial encounter
D subsequent encounter
S sequela

+ **S35.0** **Injury of abdominal aorta**
Excludes1: *injury of aorta NOS (S25.0)*

MCC X+7th **S35.00** **Unspecified injury of abdominal aorta**
MCC Exclusion 7th character A see Appendix A PDX collection 1209

MCC X+7th **S35.01** **Minor laceration of abdominal aorta**
Incomplete transection of abdominal aorta
Laceration of abdominal aorta NOS
Superficial laceration of abdominal aorta
MCC Exclusion 7th character A see Appendix A PDX collection 1209

MCC X+7th **S35.02** **Major laceration of abdominal aorta**
Complete transection of abdominal aorta
Traumatic rupture of abdominal aorta
MCC Exclusion 7th character A see Appendix A PDX collection 1209

MCC X+7th **S35.09** **Other injury of abdominal aorta**
MCC Exclusion 7th character A see Appendix A PDX collection 1209

+ **S35.1** **Injury of inferior vena cava**
Injury of hepatic vein
Excludes1: *injury of vena cava NOS (S25.2)*

MCC X+7th **S35.10** **Unspecified injury of inferior vena cava**
MCC Exclusion 7th character A see Appendix A PDX collection 1210

MCC X+7th **S35.11** **Minor laceration of inferior vena cava**
Incomplete transection of inferior vena cava
Laceration of inferior vena cava NOS
Superficial laceration of inferior vena cava
MCC Exclusion 7th character A see Appendix A PDX collection 1210

MCC X+7th **S35.12** **Major laceration of inferior vena cava**
Complete transection of inferior vena cava
Traumatic rupture of inferior vena cava
MCC Exclusion 7th character A see Appendix A PDX collection 1210

MCC X+7th **S35.19 Other injury of inferior vena cava**
MCC Exclusion 7th character A see Appendix A PDX collection 1210

\+ **S35.2 Injury of celiac or mesenteric artery and branches**

\+ **S35.21 Injury of celiac artery**

MCC +7th **S35.211 Minor laceration of celiac artery**
Incomplete transection of celiac artery
Laceration of celiac artery NOS
Superficial laceration of celiac artery
MCC Exclusion 7th character A see Appendix A PDX collection 1211

MCC +7th **S35.212 Major laceration of celiac artery**
Complete transection of celiac artery
Traumatic rupture of celiac artery
MCC Exclusion 7th character A see Appendix A PDX collection 1211

MCC +7th **S35.218 Other injury of celiac artery**
MCC Exclusion 7th character A see Appendix A PDX collection 1211

MCC +7th **S35.219 Unspecified injury of celiac artery**
MCC Exclusion 7th character A see Appendix A PDX collection 1211

\+ **S35.22 Injury of superior mesenteric artery**

MCC +7th **S35.221 Minor laceration of superior mesenteric artery**
Incomplete transection of superior mesenteric artery
Laceration of superior mesenteric artery NOS
Superficial laceration of superior mesenteric artery
MCC Exclusion 7th character A see Appendix A PDX collection 1212

MCC +7th **S35.222 Major laceration of superior mesenteric artery**
Complete transection of superior mesenteric artery
Traumatic rupture of superior mesenteric artery
MCC Exclusion 7th character A see Appendix A PDX collection 1212

MCC +7th **S35.228 Other injury of superior mesenteric artery**
MCC Exclusion 7th character A see Appendix A PDX collection 1212

MCC +7th **S35.229 Unspecified injury of superior mesenteric artery**
MCC Exclusion 7th character A see Appendix A PDX collection 1212

\+ **S35.23 Injury of inferior mesenteric artery**

MCC +7th **S35.231 Minor laceration of inferior mesenteric artery**
Incomplete transection of inferior mesenteric artery
Laceration of inferior mesenteric artery NOS
Superficial laceration of inferior mesenteric artery
MCC Exclusion 7th character A see Appendix A PDX collection 1213

MCC +7th **S35.232 Major laceration of inferior mesenteric artery**
Complete transection of inferior mesenteric artery
Traumatic rupture of inferior mesenteric artery
MCC Exclusion 7th character A see Appendix A PDX collection 1213

MCC +7th **S35.238 Other injury of inferior mesenteric artery**
MCC Exclusion 7th character A see Appendix A PDX collection 1213

MCC +7th **S35.239 Unspecified injury of inferior mesenteric artery**
MCC Exclusion 7th character A see Appendix A PDX collection 1213

\+ **S35.29 Injury of branches of celiac and mesenteric artery**
Injury of gastric artery
Injury of gastroduodenal artery
Injury of hepatic artery
Injury of splenic artery

MCC +7th **S35.291 Minor laceration of branches of celiac and mesenteric artery**
Incomplete transection of branches of celiac and mesenteric artery
Laceration of branches of celiac and mesenteric artery NOS
Superficial laceration of branches of celiac and mesenteric artery
MCC Exclusion 7th character A see Appendix A PDX collection 1214

MCC +7th **S35.292 Major laceration of branches of celiac and mesenteric artery**
Complete transection of branches of celiac and mesenteric artery
Traumatic rupture of branches of celiac and mesenteric artery
MCC Exclusion 7th character A see Appendix A PDX collection 1215

MCC +7th **S35.298 Other injury of branches of celiac and mesenteric artery**
MCC Exclusion 7th character A see Appendix A PDX collection 1215

MCC +7th **S35.299 Unspecified injury of branches of celiac and mesenteric artery**
MCC Exclusion 7th character A see Appendix A PDX collection 1216

\+ **S35.3 Injury of portal or splenic vein and branches**

\+ **S35.31 Injury of portal vein**

MCC +7th **S35.311 Laceration of portal vein**
MCC Exclusion 7th character A see Appendix A PDX collection 1217

MCC +7th **S35.318 Other specified injury of portal vein**
MCC Exclusion 7th character A see Appendix A PDX collection 1217

MCC +7th **S35.319 Unspecified injury of portal vein**
MCC Exclusion 7th character A see Appendix A PDX collection 1217

\+ **S35.32 Injury of splenic vein**

MCC +7th **S35.321 Laceration of splenic vein**
MCC Exclusion 7th character A see Appendix A PDX collection 1218

MCC +7th **S35.328 Other specified injury of splenic vein**
MCC Exclusion 7th character A see Appendix A PDX collection 1218

MCC +7th **S35.329 Unspecified injury of splenic vein**
MCC Exclusion 7th character A see Appendix A PDX collection 1218

\+ **S35.33 Injury of superior mesenteric vein**

MCC +7th **S35.331 Laceration of superior mesenteric vein**
MCC Exclusion 7th character A see Appendix A PDX collection 1219

MCC +7th **S35.338 Other specified injury of superior mesenteric vein**
MCC Exclusion 7th character A see Appendix A PDX collection 1219

MCC +7th **S35.339 Unspecified injury of superior mesenteric vein**
MCC Exclusion 7th character A see Appendix A PDX collection 1219

\+ **S35.34 Injury of inferior mesenteric vein**

MCC +7th **S35.341 Laceration of inferior mesenteric vein**
MCC Exclusion 7th character A see Appendix A PDX collection 1220

MCC +7th **S35.348 Other specified injury of inferior mesenteric vein**
MCC Exclusion 7th character A see Appendix A PDX collection 1220

MCC +7th **S35.349 Unspecified injury of inferior mesenteric vein**
MCC Exclusion 7th character A see Appendix A PDX collection 1220

\+ **S35.4 Injury of renal blood vessels**

\+ **S35.40 Unspecified injury of renal blood vessel**

MCC +7th **S35.401 Unspecified injury of right renal artery**
MCC Exclusion 7th character A see Appendix A PDX collection 1221

MCC +7th **S35.402 Unspecified injury of left renal artery**
MCC Exclusion 7th character A see Appendix A PDX collection 1221

MCC +7th **S35.403 Unspecified injury of unspecified renal artery**
MCC Exclusion 7th character A see Appendix A PDX collection 1221

MCC +7th **S35.404 Unspecified injury of right renal vein**
MCC Exclusion 7th character A see Appendix A PDX collection 1222

MCC +7th **S35.405 Unspecified injury of left renal vein**
MCC Exclusion 7th character A see Appendix A PDX collection 1222

MCC +7th **S35.406 Unspecified injury of unspecified renal vein**
MCC Exclusion 7th character A see Appendix A PDX collection 1222

+ **S35.41 Laceration of renal blood vessel**

MCC +7th **S35.411 Laceration of right renal artery**
MCC Exclusion 7th character A see Appendix A PDX collection 1221

MCC +7th **S35.412 Laceration of left renal artery**
MCC Exclusion 7th character A see Appendix A PDX collection 1221

MCC +7th **S35.413 Laceration of unspecified renal artery**
MCC Exclusion 7th character A see Appendix A PDX collection 1221

MCC +7th **S35.414 Laceration of right renal vein**
MCC Exclusion 7th character A see Appendix A PDX collection 1222

MCC +7th **S35.415 Laceration of left renal vein**
MCC Exclusion 7th character A see Appendix A PDX collection 1222

MCC +7th **S35.416 Laceration of unspecified renal vein**
MCC Exclusion 7th character A see Appendix A PDX collection 1222

+ **S35.49 Other specified injury of renal blood vessel**

MCC +7th **S35.491 Other specified injury of right renal artery**
MCC Exclusion 7th character A see Appendix A PDX collection 1221

MCC +7th **S35.492 Other specified injury of left renal artery**
MCC Exclusion 7th character A see Appendix A PDX collection 1221

MCC +7th **S35.493 Other specified injury of unspecified renal artery**
MCC Exclusion 7th character A see Appendix A PDX collection 1221

MCC +7th **S35.494 Other specified injury of right renal vein**
MCC Exclusion 7th character A see Appendix A PDX collection 1222

MCC +7th **S35.495 Other specified injury of left renal vein**
MCC Exclusion 7th character A see Appendix A PDX collection 1222

MCC +7th **S35.496 Other specified injury of unspecified renal vein**
MCC Exclusion 7th character A see Appendix A PDX collection 1222

+ **S35.5 Injury of iliac blood vessels**

MCC X+7th **S35.50 Injury of unspecified iliac blood vessel(s)**
MCC Exclusion 7th character A see Appendix A PDX collection 1223

+ **S35.51 Injury of iliac artery or vein**
Injury of hypogastric artery or vein

MCC +7th **S35.511 Injury of right iliac artery**
MCC Exclusion 7th character A see Appendix A PDX collection 1224

MCC +7th **S35.512 Injury of left iliac artery**
MCC Exclusion 7th character A see Appendix A PDX collection 1224

MCC +7th **S35.513 Injury of unspecified iliac artery**
MCC Exclusion 7th character A see Appendix A PDX collection 1224

MCC +7th **S35.514 Injury of right iliac vein**
MCC Exclusion 7th character A see Appendix A PDX collection 1225

MCC +7th **S35.515 Injury of left iliac vein**
MCC Exclusion 7th character A see Appendix A PDX collection 1225

MCC +7th **S35.516 Injury of unspecified iliac vein**
MCC Exclusion 7th character A see Appendix A PDX collection 1225

+ **S35.53 Injury of uterine artery or vein**

♀ CC +7th **S35.531 Injury of right uterine artery**
CC Exclusion 7th character A see Appendix A PDX collection 1226

♀ CC +7th **S35.532 Injury of left uterine artery**
CC Exclusion 7th character A see Appendix A PDX collection 1226

♀ CC +7th **S35.533 Injury of unspecified uterine artery**
CC Exclusion 7th character A see Appendix A PDX collection 1226

♀ CC +7th **S35.534 Injury of right uterine vein**
CC Exclusion 7th character A see Appendix A PDX collection 1227

♀ CC +7th **S35.535 Injury of left uterine vein**
CC Exclusion 7th character A see Appendix A PDX collection 1227

♀ CC +7th **S35.536 Injury of unspecified uterine vein**
CC Exclusion 7th character A see Appendix A PDX collection 1227

MCC X+7th **S35.59 Injury of other iliac blood vessels**
MCC Exclusion 7th character A see Appendix A PDX collection 1223

CC + **S35.8 Injury of other blood vessels at abdomen, lower back and pelvis level**
Injury of ovarian artery or vein
CC Exclusion 7th character A see Appendix A PDX collection 122

+ **S35.8X Injury of other blood vessels at abdomen, lower back and pelvis level**

+7th **S35.8X1 Laceration of other blood vessels at abdomen, lower back and pelvis level**

+7th **S35.8X8 Other specified injury of other blood vessels at abdomen, lower back and pelvis level**

+7th **S35.8X9 Unspecified injury of other blood vessels abdomen, lower back and pelvis level**

+ **S35.9 Injury of unspecified blood vessel at abdomen, lower back and pelvis level**

CC X+7th **S35.90 Unspecified injury of unspecified blood vessel at abdomen, lower back and pelvis level**
CC Exclusion 7th character A see Appendix A PDX collection 1229

CC X+7th **S35.91 Laceration of unspecified blood vessel at abdomen, lower back and pelvis level**
CC Exclusion 7th character A see Appendix A PDX collection 1229

CC X+7th **S35.99 Other specified injury of unspecified blood vessel at abdomen, lower back and pelvis level**
CC Exclusion 7th character A see Appendix A PDX collection 1229

S36 Injury of intra-abdominal organs

Code also any associated open wound (S31.-)

The appropriate 7th character is to be added to each code from category S36
A initial encounter
D subsequent encounter
S sequela

+ **S36.0 Injury of spleen**

CC X+7th **S36.00 Unspecified injury of spleen**
CC Exclusion 7th character A see Appendix A PDX collection 1230

+ **S36.02 Contusion of spleen**

CC +7th **S36.020 Minor contusion of spleen**
Contusion of spleen less than 2 cm
CC Exclusion 7th character A see Appendix PDX collection 1230

CC +7th **S36.021 Major contusion of spleen**
Contusion of spleen greater than 2 cm
CC Exclusion 7th character A see Appendix PDX collection 1230

CC +7th **S36.029 Unspecified contusion of spleen**
CC Exclusion 7th character A see Appendix PDX collection 1230

+ **S36.03 Laceration of spleen**

CC +7th **S36.030 Superficial (capsular) laceration of spleen**
Laceration of spleen less than 1 cm
Minor laceration of spleen
CC Exclusion 7th character A see Appendix PDX collection 1230
AHA CC: 1Q, 2015, 3-21

MCC +7th **S36.031 Moderate laceration of spleen**
Laceration of spleen 1 to 3 cm
MCC Exclusion 7th character A see Append PDX collection 1230
AHA CC: 1Q, 2015, 3-21

MCC +7th **S36.032 Major laceration of spleen**
Avulsion of spleen
Laceration of spleen greater than 3 cm
Massive laceration of spleen
Multiple moderate lacerations of spleen
Stellate laceration of spleen
MCC Exclusion 7th character A see Appendix A PDX collection 1230

CC +7th **S36.039 Unspecified laceration of spleen**
CC Exclusion 7th character A see Appendix A PDX collection 1230

CC X+7th **S36.09 Other injury of spleen**
CC Exclusion 7th character A see Appendix A PDX collection 1230

+ **S36.1 Injury of liver and gallbladder and bile duct**

+ **S36.11 Injury of liver**

CC +7th **S36.112 Contusion of liver**
CC Exclusion 7th character A see Appendix A PDX collection 1231

CC +7th **S36.113 Laceration of liver, unspecified degree**
CC Exclusion 7th character A see Appendix A PDX collection 1231

CC +7th **S36.114 Minor laceration of liver**
Laceration involving capsule only, or, without significant involvement of hepatic parenchyma [i.e., less than 1 cmdeep]
CC Exclusion 7th character A see Appendix A PDX collection 1231

MCC +7th **S36.115 Moderate laceration of liver**
Laceration involving parenchyma but without major disruption of parenchyma [i.e., less than 10 cm long and less than 3 cm deep]
MCC Exclusion 7th character A see Appendix A PDX collection 1231

MCC +7th **S36.116 Major laceration of liver**
Laceration with significant disruption of hepatic parenchyma [i.e., greater than 10 cm long and 3 cm deep]
Multiple moderate lacerations, with or without hematoma
Stellate laceration of liver
MCC Exclusion 7th character A see Appendix A PDX collection 1231

CC +7th **S36.118 Other injury of liver**
CC Exclusion 7th character A see Appendix A PDX collection 1231

CC +7th **S36.119 Unspecified injury of liver**
CC Exclusion 7th character A see Appendix A PDX collection 1231

+ **S36.12 Injury of gallbladder**

CC +7th **S36.122 Contusion of gallbladder**
CC Exclusion 7th character A see Appendix A PDX collection 1232

CC +7th **S36.123 Laceration of gallbladder**
CC Exclusion 7th character A see Appendix A PDX collection 1232

CC +7th **S36.128 Other injury of gallbladder**
CC Exclusion 7th character A see Appendix A PDX collection 1232

CC +7th **S36.129 Unspecified injury of gallbladder**
CC Exclusion 7th character A see Appendix A PDX collection 1232

CC X+7th **S36.13 Injury of bile duct**
CC Exclusion 7th character A see Appendix A PDX collection 1232

+ **S36.2 Injury of pancreas**

+ **S36.20 Unspecified injury of pancreas**

CC +7th **S36.200 Unspecified injury of head of pancreas**
CC Exclusion 7th character A see Appendix A PDX collection 1233

CC +7th **S36.201 Unspecified injury of body of pancreas**
CC Exclusion 7th character A see Appendix A PDX collection 1233

CC +7th **S36.202 Unspecified injury of tail of pancreas**
CC Exclusion 7th character A see Appendix A PDX collection 1233

CC +7th **S36.209 Unspecified injury of unspecified part of pancreas**
CC Exclusion 7th character A see Appendix A PDX collection 1233

+ **S36.22 Contusion of pancreas**

CC **S36.220 Contusion of head of pancreas**
CC Exclusion 7th character A see Appendix A PDX collection 1233

CC **S36.221 Contusion of body of pancreas**
CC Exclusion 7th character A see Appendix A PDX collection 1233

CC **S36.222 Contusion of tail of pancreas**
CC Exclusion 7th character A see Appendix A PDX collection 1233

CC **S36.229 Contusion of unspecified part of pancreas**
CC Exclusion 7th character A see Appendix A PDX collection 1233

+ **S36.23 Laceration of pancreas, unspecified degree**

CC +7th **S36.230 Laceration of head of pancreas, unspecified degree**
CC Exclusion 7th character A see Appendix A PDX collection 1233

CC +7th **S36.231 Laceration of body of pancreas, unspecified degree**
CC Exclusion 7th character A see Appendix A PDX collection 1233

CC +7th **S36.232 Laceration of tail of pancreas, unspecified degree**
CC Exclusion 7th character A see Appendix A PDX collection 1233

CC +7th **S36.239 Laceration of unspecified part of pancreas, unspecified degree**
CC Exclusion 7th character A see Appendix A PDX collection 1233

+ **S36.24 Minor laceration of pancreas**

CC +7th **S36.240 Minor laceration of head of pancreas**
CC Exclusion 7th character A see Appendix A PDX collection 1233

CC +7th **S36.241 Minor laceration of body of pancreas**
CC Exclusion 7th character A see Appendix A PDX collection 1233

CC +7th **S36.242 Minor laceration of tail of pancreas**
CC Exclusion 7th character A see Appendix A PDX collection 1233

CC +7th **S36.249 Minor laceration of unspecified part of pancreas**
CC Exclusion 7th character A see Appendix A PDX collection 1233

+ **S36.25 Moderate laceration of pancreas**

CC +7th **S36.250 Moderate laceration of head of pancreas**
CC Exclusion 7th character A see Appendix A PDX collection 1233

CC +7th **S36.251 Moderate laceration of body of pancreas**
CC Exclusion 7th character A see Appendix A PDX collection 1233

CC +7th **S36.252 Moderate laceration of tail of pancreas**
CC Exclusion 7th character A see Appendix A PDX collection 1233

CC +7th **S36.259 Moderate laceration of unspecified part of pancreas**
CC Exclusion 7th character A see Appendix A PDX collection 1233

+ **S36.26 Major laceration of pancreas**

CC +7th **S36.260 Major laceration of head of pancreas**
CC Exclusion 7th character A see Appendix A PDX collection 1233

CC +7th **S36.261 Major laceration of body of pancreas**
CC Exclusion 7th character A see Appendix A PDX collection 1233

CC +7th **S36.262 Major laceration of tail of pancreas**
CC Exclusion 7th character A see Appendix A PDX collection 1233

CC +7th **S36.269 Major laceration of unspecified part of pancreas**
CC Exclusion 7th character A see Appendix A PDX collection 1233

+ **S36.29 Other injury of pancreas**

CC +7th **S36.290 Other injury of head of pancreas**
CC Exclusion 7th character A see Appendix A PDX collection 1233

CC +7th **S36.291 Other injury of body of pancreas**
CC Exclusion 7th character A see Appendix A PDX collection 1233

CC +7th **S36.292 Other injury of tail of pancreas**
CC Exclusion 7th character A see Appendix A PDX collection 1233

CC +7th **S36.299 Other injury of unspecified part of pancreas**
CC Exclusion 7th character A see Appendix A PDX collection 1233

+ **S36.3 Injury of stomach**

CC X+7th **S36.30 Unspecified injury of stomach**
CC Exclusion 7th character A see Appendix A PDX collection 1234

CC X+7th **S36.32 Contusion of stomach**
CC Exclusion 7th character A see Appendix A PDX collection 1234

CC X+7th **S36.33 Laceration of stomach**
CC Exclusion 7th character A see Appendix A PDX collection 1234

CC X+7th **S36.39 Other injury of stomach**
CC Exclusion 7th character A see Appendix A PDX collection 1234

+ S36.4 Injury of small intestine

+ S36.40 Unspecified injury of small intestine

CC +7th **S36.400 Unspecified injury of duodenum**
CC Exclusion 7th character A see Appendix A PDX collection 1235

CC +7th **S36.408 Unspecified injury of other part of small intestine**
CC Exclusion 7th character A see Appendix A PDX collection 1235

CC +7th **S36.409 Unspecified injury of unspecified part of small intestine**
CC Exclusion 7th character A see Appendix A PDX collection 1235

+ S36.41 Primary blast injury of small intestine
Blast injury of small intestine NOS

CC +7th **S36.410 Primary blast injury of duodenum**
CC Exclusion 7th character A see Appendix A PDX collection 1235

CC +7th **S36.418 Primary blast injury of other part of small intestine**
CC Exclusion 7th character A see Appendix A PDX collection 1235

CC +7th **S36.419 Primary blast injury of unspecified part of small intestine**
CC Exclusion 7th character A see Appendix A PDX collection 1235

+ S36.42 Contusion of small intestine

CC +7th **S36.420 Contusion of duodenum**
CC Exclusion 7th character A see Appendix A PDX collection 1235

CC +7th **S36.428 Contusion of other part of small intestine**
CC Exclusion 7th character A see Appendix A PDX collection 1235

CC +7th **S36.429 Contusion of unspecified part of small intestine**
CC Exclusion 7th character A see Appendix A PDX collection 1235

+ S36.43 Laceration of small intestine

CC +7th **S36.430 Laceration of duodenum**
CC Exclusion 7th character A see Appendix A PDX collection 1235

CC +7th **S36.438 Laceration of other part of small intestine**
CC Exclusion 7th character A see Appendix A PDX collection 1235

CC +7th **S36.439 Laceration of unspecified part of small intestine**
CC Exclusion 7th character A see Appendix A PDX collection 1235

+ S36.49 Other injury of small intestine

CC +7th **S36.490 Other injury of duodenum**
CC Exclusion 7th character A see Appendix A PDX collection 1235

CC +7th **S36.498 Other injury of other part of small intestine**
CC Exclusion 7th character A see Appendix A PDX collection 1235

CC +7th **S36.499 Other injury of unspecified part of small intestine**
CC Exclusion 7th character A see Appendix A PDX collection 1235

S36.5 Injury of colon
Excludes2: *injury of rectum (S36.6-)*

+ S36.50 Unspecified injury of colon

CC +7th **S36.500 Unspecified injury of ascending [right] colon**
CC Exclusion 7th character A see Appendix A PDX collection 1236

CC +7th **S36.501 Unspecified injury of transverse colon**
CC Exclusion 7th character A see Appendix A PDX collection 1236

CC +7th **S36.502 Unspecified injury of descending [left] colon**
CC Exclusion 7th character A see Appendix A PDX collection 1236

CC +7th **S36.503 Unspecified injury of sigmoid colon**
CC Exclusion 7th character A see Appendix A PDX collection 1236

CC +7th **S36.508 Unspecified injury of other part of colon**
CC Exclusion 7th character A see Appendix A PDX collection 1236

CC +7th **S36.509 Unspecified injury of unspecified part of colon**
CC Exclusion 7th character A see Appendix A PDX collection 1236

+ S36.51 Primary blast injury of colon
Blast injury of colon NOS

CC +7th **S36.510 Primary blast injury of ascending [right] colon**
CC Exclusion 7th character A see Appendix A PDX collection 1236

CC +7th **S36.511 Primary blast injury of transverse colon**
CC Exclusion 7th character A see Appendix A PDX collection 1236

CC +7th **S36.512 Primary blast injury of descending [left] colon**
CC Exclusion 7th character A see Appendix A PDX collection 1236

CC +7th **S36.513 Primary blast injury of sigmoid colon**
CC Exclusion 7th character A see Appendix A PDX collection 1236

CC +7th **S36.518 Primary blast injury of other part of colo**
CC Exclusion 7th character A see Appendix A PDX collection 1236

CC +7th **S36.519 Primary blast injury of unspecified part (colon**
CC Exclusion 7th character A see Appendix A PDX collection 1236

+ S36.52 Contusion of colon

CC +7th **S36.520 Contusion of ascending [right] colon**
CC Exclusion 7th character A see Appendix A PDX collection 1236

CC +7th **S36.521 Contusion of transverse colon**
CC Exclusion 7th character A see Appendix A PDX collection 1236

CC +7th **S36.522 Contusion of descending [left] colon**
CC Exclusion 7th character A see Appendix A PDX collection 1236

CC +7th **S36.523 Contusion of sigmoid colon**
CC Exclusion 7th character A see Appendix A PDX collection 1236

CC +7th **S36.528 Contusion of other part of colon**
CC Exclusion 7th character A see Appendix A PDX collection 1236

CC +7th **S36.529 Contusion of unspecified part of colon**
CC Exclusion 7th character A see Appendix A PDX collection 1236

+ S36.53 Laceration of colon

CC +7th **S36.530 Laceration of ascending [right] colon**
CC Exclusion 7th character A see Appendix A PDX collection 1236

CC +7th **S36.531 Laceration of transverse colon**
CC Exclusion 7th character A see Appendix A PDX collection 1236

CC +7th **S36.532 Laceration of descending [left] colon**
CC Exclusion 7th character A see Appendix A PDX collection 1236

CC +7th **S36.533 Laceration of sigmoid colon**
CC Exclusion 7th character A see Appendix A PDX collection 1236

CC +7th **S36.538 Laceration of other part of colon**
CC Exclusion 7th character A see Appendix A PDX collection 1236

CC +7th **S36.539 Laceration of unspecified part of colon**
CC Exclusion 7th character A see Appendix A PDX collection 1236

+ S36.59 Other injury of colon
Secondary blast injury of colon

CC +7th **S36.590 Other injury of ascending [right] colon**
CC Exclusion 7th character A see Appendix A PDX collection 1236

CC +7th **S36.591 Other injury of transverse colon**
CC Exclusion 7th character A see Appendix A PDX collection 1236

CC +7th **S36.592 Other injury of descending [left] colon**
CC Exclusion 7th character A see Appendix A PDX collection 1236

CC +7th **S36.593 Other injury of sigmoid colon**
CC Exclusion 7th character A see Appendix A PDX collection 1236

CC +7th **S36.598 Other injury of other part of colon**
CC Exclusion 7th character A see Appendix A PDX collection 1236

CC +7th **S36.599 Other injury of unspecified part of colon**
CC Exclusion 7th character A see Appendix A PDX collection 1236

+ **S36.6 Injury of rectum**

CC X+7th **S36.60 Unspecified injury of rectum**
CC Exclusion 7th character A see Appendix A PDX collection 1236

CC X+7th **S36.61 Primary blast injury of rectum**
Blast injury of rectum NOS
CC Exclusion 7th character A see Appendix A PDX collection 1236

CC X+7th **S36.62 Contusion of rectum**
CC Exclusion 7th character A see Appendix A PDX collection 1236

CC X+7th **S36.63 Laceration of rectum**
CC Exclusion 7th character A see Appendix A PDX collection 1236

CC X+7th **S36.69 Other injury of rectum**
Secondary blast injury of rectum
CC Exclusion 7th character A see Appendix A PDX collection 1236

+ **S36.8 Injury of other intra-abdominal organs**

CC X+7th **S36.81 Injury of peritoneum**
CC Exclusion 7th character A see Appendix A PDX collection 1195

+ **S36.89 Injury of other intra-abdominal organs**
Injury of retroperitoneum

CC +7th **S36.892 Contusion of other intra-abdominal organs**
CC Exclusion 7th character A see Appendix A PDX collection 1195

CC +7th **S36.893 Laceration of other intra-abdominal organs**
CC Exclusion 7th character A see Appendix A PDX collection 1195

CC +7th **S36.898 Other injury of other intra-abdominal organs**
CC Exclusion 7th character A see Appendix A PDX collection 1195

CC +7th **S36.899 Unspecified injury of other intra-abdominal organs**
CC Exclusion 7th character A see Appendix A PDX collection 1195

+ **S36.9 Injury of unspecified intra-abdominal organ**

CC X+7th **S36.90 Unspecified injury of unspecified intra-abdominal organ**
CC Exclusion 7th character A see Appendix A PDX collection 1195

CC X+7th **S36.92 Contusion of unspecified intra-abdominal organ**
CC Exclusion 7th character A see Appendix A PDX collection 1195

CC X+7th **S36.93 Laceration of unspecified intra-abdominal organ**
CC Exclusion 7th character A see Appendix A PDX collection 1195

CC X+7th **S36.99 Other injury of unspecified intra-abdominal organ**
CC Exclusion 7th character A see Appendix A PDX collection 1195

S37 Injury of urinary and pelvic organs

Code also any associated open wound (S31.-)
Excludes1: *obstetric trauma to pelvic organs (O71.-)*
Excludes2: *injury of peritoneum (S36.81)*
injury of retroperitoneum (S36.89-)

The appropriate 7th character is to be added to each code from category S37
A initial encounter
D subsequent encounter
S sequela

+ **S37.0 Injury of kidney**
Excludes2: *acute kidney injury (nontraumatic) (N17.9)*

+ **S37.00 Unspecified injury of kidney**

CC +7th **S37.001 Unspecified injury of right kidney**
CC Exclusion 7th character A see Appendix A PDX collection 1237

CC +7th **S37.002 Unspecified injury of left kidney**
CC Exclusion 7th character A see Appendix A PDX collection 1237

CC +7th **S37.009 Unspecified injury of unspecified kidney**
CC Exclusion 7th character A see Appendix A PDX collection 1237

+ **S37.01 Minor contusion of kidney**
Contusion of kidney less than 2 cm
Contusion of kidney NOS

CC +7th **S37.011 Minor contusion of right kidney**
CC Exclusion 7th character A see Appendix A PDX collection 1237

CC +7th **S37.012 Minor contusion of left kidney**
CC Exclusion 7th character A see Appendix A PDX collection 1237

CC +7th **S37.019 Minor contusion of unspecified kidney**
CC Exclusion 7th character A see Appendix A PDX collection 1237

+ **S37.02 Major contusion of kidney**
Contusion of kidney greater than 2 cm

CC +7th **S37.021 Major contusion of right kidney**
CC Exclusion 7th character A see Appendix A PDX collection 1237

CC +7th **S37.022 Major contusion of left kidney**
CC Exclusion 7th character A see Appendix A PDX collection 1237

CC +7th **S37.029 Major contusion of unspecified kidney**
CC Exclusion 7th character A see Appendix A PDX collection 1237

+ **S37.03 Laceration of kidney, unspecified degree**

CC +7th **S37.031 Laceration of right kidney, unspecified degree**
CC Exclusion 7th character A see Appendix A PDX collection 1237

CC +7th **S37.032 Laceration of left kidney, unspecified degree**
CC Exclusion 7th character A see Appendix A PDX collection 1237

CC +7th **S37.039 Laceration of unspecified kidney, unspecified degree**
CC Exclusion 7th character A see Appendix A PDX collection 1237

+ **S37.04 Minor laceration of kidney**
Laceration of kidney less than 1 cm

CC +7th **S37.041 Minor laceration of right kidney**
CC Exclusion 7th character A see Appendix A PDX collection 1237

CC +7th **S37.042 Minor laceration of left kidney**
CC Exclusion 7th character A see Appendix A PDX collection 1237

CC +7th **S37.049 Minor laceration of unspecified kidney**
CC Exclusion 7th character A see Appendix A PDX collection 1237

+ **S37.05 Moderate laceration of kidney**
Laceration of kidney 1 to 3 cm

CC +7th **S37.051 Moderate laceration of right kidney**
CC Exclusion 7th character A see Appendix A PDX collection 1237

CC +7th **S37.052 Moderate laceration of left kidney**
CC Exclusion 7th character A see Appendix A PDX collection 1237

CC +7th **S37.059 Moderate laceration of unspecified kidney**
CC Exclusion 7th character A see Appendix A PDX collection 1237

+ **S37.06 Major laceration of kidney**
Avulsion of kidney
Laceration of kidney greater than 3 cm
Massive laceration of kidney
Multiple moderate lacerations of kidney
Stellate laceration of kidney

MCC +7th **S37.061 Major laceration of right kidney**
MCC Exclusion 7th character A see Appendix A PDX collection 1237

MCC +7th **S37.062 Major laceration of left kidney**
MCC Exclusion 7th character A see Appendix A PDX collection 1237

MCC +7th **S37.069 Major laceration of unspecified kidney**
MCC Exclusion 7th character A see Appendix A PDX collection 1237

+ **S37.09 Other injury of kidney**

MCC +7th **S37.091 Other injury of right kidney**
MCC Exclusion 7th character A see Appendix A PDX collection 1237

MCC +7th **S37.092 Other injury of left kidney**
MCC Exclusion 7th character A see Appendix A PDX collection 1237

MCC +7th **S37.099 Other injury of unspecified kidney**
MCC Exclusion 7th character A see Appendix A PDX collection 1237

Shoulder

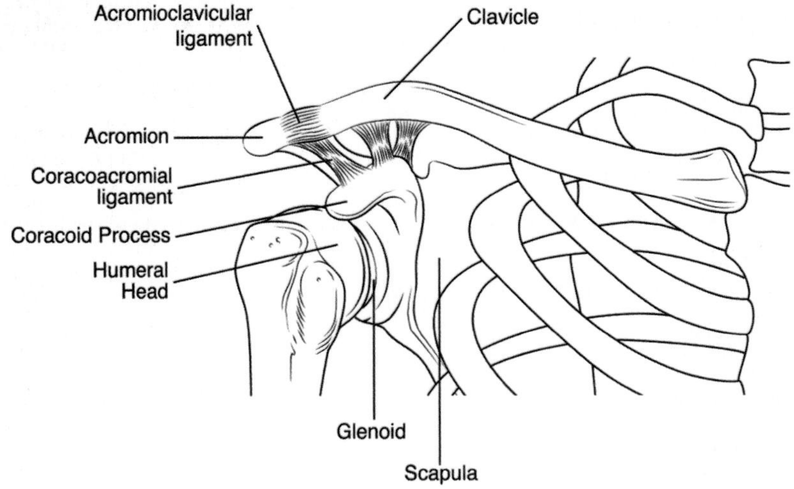

©AHIMA

Shoulder Tendons

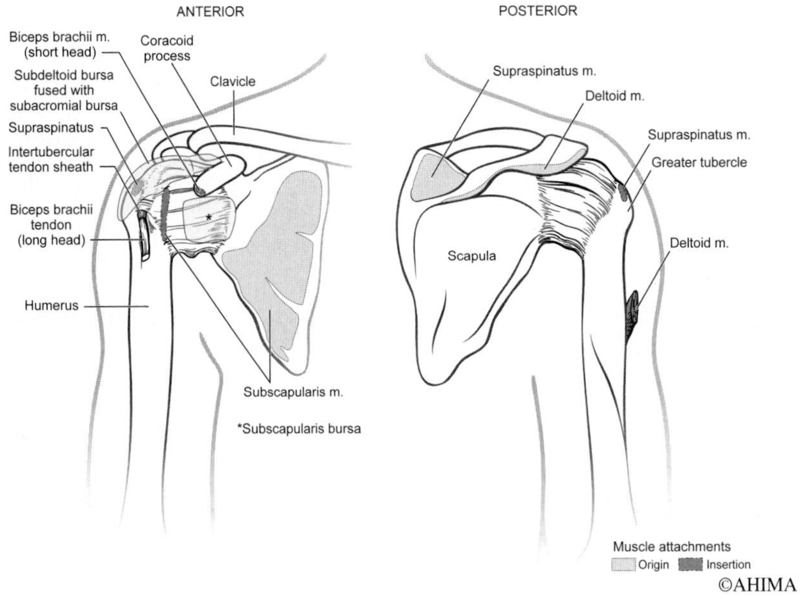

©AHIMA

Shoulder Ligaments

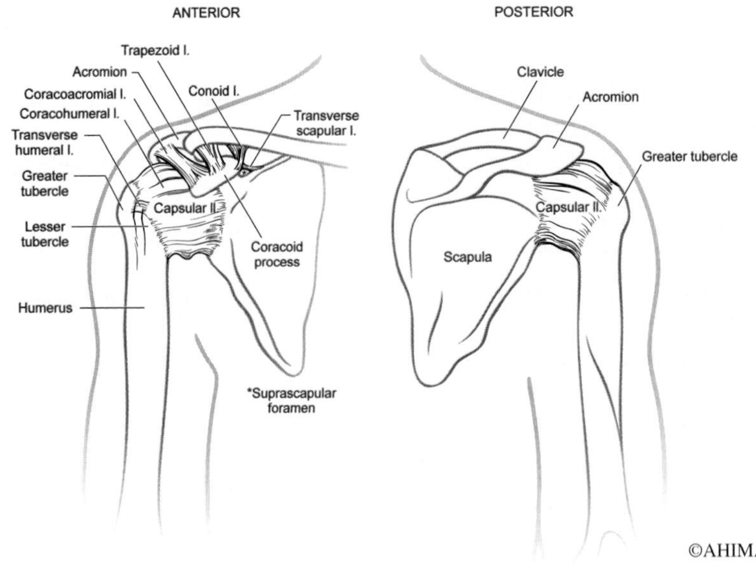

©AHIMA

+ S37.1 **Injury of ureter**
CC X+7th **S37.10 Unspecified injury of ureter**
CC Exclusion 7th character A see Appendix A PDX collection 1238
CC X+7th **S37.12 Contusion of ureter**
CC Exclusion 7th character A see Appendix A PDX collection 1238
CC X+7th **S37.13 Laceration of ureter**
CC Exclusion 7th character A see Appendix A PDX collection 1238
CC X+7th **S37.19 Other injury of ureter**
CC Exclusion 7th character A see Appendix A PDX collection 1238
+ S37.2 **Injury of bladder**
CC X+7th **S37.20 Unspecified injury of bladder**
CC Exclusion 7th character A see Appendix A PDX collection 1239
CC X+7th **S37.22 Contusion of bladder**
CC Exclusion 7th character A see Appendix A PDX collection 1239
CC X+7th **S37.23 Laceration of bladder**
CC Exclusion 7th character A see Appendix A PDX collection 1239
CC X+7th **S37.29 Other injury of bladder**
CC Exclusion 7th character A see Appendix A PDX collection 1239
+ S37.3 **Injury of urethra**
CC X+7th **S37.30 Unspecified injury of urethra**
CC Exclusion 7th character A see Appendix A PDX collection 1239
CC X+7th **S37.32 Contusion of urethra**
CC Exclusion 7th character A see Appendix A PDX collection 1239
CC X+7th **S37.33 Laceration of urethra**
CC Exclusion 7th character A see Appendix A PDX collection 1239
CC X+7th **S37.39 Other injury of urethra**
CC Exclusion 7th character A see Appendix A PDX collection 1239
+ S37.4 **Injury of ovary**
+ **S37.40 Unspecified injury of ovary**
♀ +7th **S37.401 Unspecified injury of ovary, unilateral**
♀ +7th **S37.402 Unspecified injury of ovary, bilateral**
♀ +7th **S37.409 Unspecified injury of ovary, unspecified**
+ **S37.42 Contusion of ovary**
♀ +7th **S37.421 Contusion of ovary, unilateral**
♀ +7th **S37.422 Contusion of ovary, bilateral**
♀ +7th **S37.429 Contusion of ovary, unspecified**
+ **S37.43 Laceration of ovary**
♀ +7th **S37.431 Laceration of ovary, unilateral**
♀ +7th **S37.432 Laceration of ovary, bilateral**
♀ +7th **S37.439 Laceration of ovary, unspecified**
+ **S37.49 Other injury of ovary**
♀ +7th **S37.491 Other injury of ovary, unilateral**
♀ +7th **S37.492 Other injury of ovary, bilateral**
♀ +7th **S37.499 Other injury of ovary, unspecified**
+ S37.5 **Injury of fallopian tube**
+ **S37.50 Unspecified injury of fallopian tube**
♀ +7th **S37.501 Unspecified injury of fallopian tube, unilateral**
♀ +7th **S37.502 Unspecified injury of fallopian tube, bilateral**
♀ +7th **S37.509 Unspecified injury of fallopian tube, unspecified**
+ **S37.51 Primary blast injury of fallopian tube**
Blast injury of fallopian tube NOS
♀ +7th **S37.511 Primary blast injury of fallopian tube, unilateral**
♀ +7th **S37.512 Primary blast injury of fallopian tube, bilateral**
♀ +7th **S37.519 Primary blast injury of fallopian tube, unspecified**
+ **S37.52 Contusion of fallopian tube**
♀ +7th **S37.521 Contusion of fallopian tube, unilateral**
♀ +7th **S37.522 Contusion of fallopian tube, bilateral**
♀ +7th **S37.529 Contusion of fallopian tube, unspecified**
+ **S37.53 Laceration of fallopian tube**
♀ +7th **S37.531 Laceration of fallopian tube, unilateral**
♀ +7th **S37.532 Laceration of fallopian tube, bilateral**
♀ +7th **S37.539 Laceration of fallopian tube, unspecified**
+ **S37.59 Other injury of fallopian tube**
Secondary blast injury of fallopian tube
♀ +7th **S37.591 Other injury of fallopian tube, unilateral**
♀ +7th **S37.592 Other injury of fallopian tube, bilateral**
♀ +7th **S37.599 Other injury of fallopian tube, unspecified**
+ S37.6 **Injury of uterus**
Excludes1: *injury to gravid uterus (O9A.2-)*
injury to uterus during delivery (O71.-)
♀ CC X+7th **S37.60 Unspecified injury of uterus**
CC Exclusion 7th character A see Appendix A PDX collection 1240
♀ CC X+7th **S37.62 Contusion of uterus**
CC Exclusion 7th character A see Appendix A PDX collection 1240
♀ CC X+7th **S37.63 Laceration of uterus**
CC Exclusion 7th character A see Appendix A PDX collection 1240
♀ CC X+7th **S37.69 Other injury of uterus**
CC Exclusion 7th character A see Appendix A PDX collection 1240
+ S37.8 **Injury of other urinary and pelvic organs**
+ **S37.81 Injury of adrenal gland**
CC +7th **S37.812 Contusion of adrenal gland**
CC Exclusion 7th character A see Appendix A PDX collection 1241
CC +7th **S37.813 Laceration of adrenal gland**
CC Exclusion 7th character A see Appendix A PDX collection 1241
CC +7th **S37.818 Other injury of adrenal gland**
CC Exclusion 7th character A see Appendix A PDX collection 1241
CC +7th **S37.819 Unspecified injury of adrenal gland**
CC Exclusion 7th character A see Appendix A PDX collection 1241
+ **S37.82 Injury of prostate**
♂ +7th **S37.822 Contusion of prostate**
♂ +7th **S37.823 Laceration of prostate**
♂ +7th **S37.828 Other injury of prostate**
♂ +7th **S37.829 Unspecified injury of prostate**
+ **S37.89 Injury of other urinary and pelvic organ**
CC +7th **S37.892 Contusion of other urinary and pelvic organ**
CC Exclusion 7th character A see Appendix A PDX collection 1242
CC +7th **S37.893 Laceration of other urinary and pelvic organ**
CC Exclusion 7th character A see Appendix A PDX collection 1242
CC +7th **S37.898 Other injury of other urinary and pelvic organ**
CC Exclusion 7th character A see Appendix A PDX collection 1242
CC +7th **S37.899 Unspecified injury of other urinary and pelvic organ**
CC Exclusion 7th character A see Appendix A PDX collection 1242
+ S37.9 **Injury of unspecified urinary and pelvic organ**
CC X+7th **S37.90 Unspecified injury of unspecified urinary and pelvic organ**
CC Exclusion 7th character A see Appendix A PDX collection 1242
CC X+7th **S37.92 Contusion of unspecified urinary and pelvic organ**
CC Exclusion 7th character A see Appendix A PDX collection 1242
CC X+7th **S37.93 Laceration of unspecified urinary and pelvic organ**
CC Exclusion 7th character A see Appendix A PDX collection 1242
CC X+7th **S37.99 Other injury of unspecified urinary and pelvic organ**
CC Exclusion 7th character A see Appendix A PDX collection 1242

S38 Crushing injury and traumatic amputation of abdomen, lower back, pelvis and external genitals

An amputation not identified as partial or complete should be coded to complete

The appropriate 7th character is to be added to each code from category S38
A initial encounter
D subsequent encounter
S sequela

+ **S38.0 Crushing injury of external genital organs**
  Use additional code for any associated injuries
  + **S38.00 Crushing injury of unspecified external genital organs**
    ♂ +7th **S38.001 Crushing injury of unspecified external genital organs, male**
    ♀ +7th **S38.002 Crushing injury of unspecified external genital organs, female**
  ♂ X+7th **S38.01 Crushing injury of penis**
  ♂ X+7th **S38.02 Crushing injury of scrotum and testis**
  ♀ X+7th **S38.03 Crushing injury of vulva**

X+7th **S38.1 Crushing injury of abdomen, lower back, and pelvis**
  Use additional code for all associated injuries, such as:
  fracture of thoracic or lumbar spine and pelvis (S22.0-, S32.-)
  injury to intra-abdominal organs (S36.-)
  injury to urinary and pelvic organs (S37.-)
  open wound of abdominal wall (S31.-)
  spinal cord injury (S34.0, S34.1-)
  Excludes2: *crushing injury of external genital organs (S38.0-)*

+ **S38.2 Traumatic amputation of external genital organs**
  + **S38.21 Traumatic amputation of female external genital organs**
    Traumatic amputation of clitoris
    Traumatic amputation of labium (majus) (minus)
    Traumatic amputation of vulva
    ♀ +7th **S38.211 Complete traumatic amputation of female external genital organs**
    ♀ +7th **S38.212 Partial traumatic amputation of female external genital organs**
  + **S38.22 Traumatic amputation of penis**
    ♂ +7th **S38.221 Complete traumatic amputation of penis**
    ♂ +7th **S38.222 Partial traumatic amputation of penis**
  + **S38.23 Traumatic amputation of scrotum and testis**
    ♂ +7th **S38.231 Complete traumatic amputation of scrotum and testis**
    ♂ +7th **S38.232 Partial traumatic amputation of scrotum and testis**

X+7th **S38.3 Transection (partial) of abdomen**

S39 Other and unspecified injuries of abdomen, lower back, pelvis and external genitals

Code also any associated open wound (S31.-)
Excludes2: *sprain of joints and ligaments of lumbar spine and pelvis (S33.-)*

The appropriate 7th character is to be added to each code from category S39
A initial encounter
D subsequent encounter
S sequela

+ **S39.0 Injury of muscle, fascia and tendon of abdomen, lower back and pelvis**
  + **S39.00 Unspecified injury of muscle, fascia and tendon of abdomen, lower back and pelvis**
    +7th **S39.001 Unspecified injury of muscle, fascia and tendon of abdomen**
    +7th **S39.002 Unspecified injury of muscle, fascia and tendon of lower back**
    +7th **S39.003 Unspecified injury of muscle, fascia and tendon of pelvis**
  + **S39.01 Strain of muscle, fascia and tendon of abdomen, lower back and pelvis**
    +7th **S39.011 Strain of muscle, fascia and tendon of abdomen**
    +7th **S39.012 Strain of muscle, fascia and tendon of lower back**
    AHA CC: 4Q, 2016, 73-74
    +7th **S39.013 Strain of muscle, fascia and tendon of pelvis**
  + **S39.02 Laceration of muscle, fascia and tendon of abdomen, lower back and pelvis**
    +7th **S39.021 Laceration of muscle, fascia and tendon of abdomen**
    +7th **S39.022 Laceration of muscle, fascia and tendon of lower back**
    +7th **S39.023 Laceration of muscle, fascia and tendon of pelvis**
  + **S39.09 Other injury of muscle, fascia and tendon of abdomen, lower back and pelvis**
    +7th **S39.091 Other injury of muscle, fascia and tendon of abdomen**
    +7th **S39.092 Other injury of muscle, fascia and tendon of lower back**
    +7th **S39.093 Other injury of muscle, fascia and tendon of pelvis**

+ **S39.8 Other specified injuries of abdomen, lower back, pelvis and external genitals**
  X+7th **S39.81 Other specified injuries of abdomen**
  X+7th **S39.82 Other specified injuries of lower back**
  X+7th **S39.83 Other specified injuries of pelvis**
  + **S39.84 Other specified injuries of external genitals**
    ♂ X+7th **S39.840 Fracture of corpus cavernosum penis**
    X+7th **S39.848 Other specified injuries of external genitals**

+ **S39.9 Unspecified injury of abdomen, lower back, pelvis and external genitals**
  X+7th **S39.91 Unspecified injury of abdomen**
  X+7th **S39.92 Unspecified injury of lower back**
  X+7th **S39.93 Unspecified injury of pelvis**
  X+7th **S39.94 Unspecified injury of external genitals**

Injuries to the shoulder and upper arm (S40-S49)

Includes: injuries of axilla
injuries of scapular region

Excludes2: *and corrosions (T20-T32)*
frostbite (T33-T34)
injuries of elbow (S50-S59)
insect bite or sting, venomous (T63.4)

S40 Superficial injury of shoulder and upper arm

The appropriate 7th character is to be added to each code from category S40
A initial encounter
D subsequent encounter
S sequela

+ **S40.0 Contusion of shoulder and upper arm**
  + **S40.01 Contusion of shoulder**
    +7th **S40.011 Contusion of right shoulder**
    +7th **S40.012 Contusion of left shoulder**
    +7th **S40.019 Contusion of unspecified shoulder**
  + **S40.02 Contusion of upper arm**
    +7th **S40.021 Contusion of right upper arm**
    +7th **S40.022 Contusion of left upper arm**
    +7th **S40.029 Contusion of unspecified upper arm**

+ **S40.2 Other superficial injuries of shoulder**
  + **S40.21 Abrasion of shoulder**
    +7th **S40.211 Abrasion of right shoulder**
    +7th **S40.212 Abrasion of left shoulder**
    +7th **S40.219 Abrasion of unspecified shoulder**
  + **S40.22 Blister (nonthermal) of shoulder**
    +7th **S40.221 Blister (nonthermal) of right shoulder**
    +7th **S40.222 Blister (nonthermal) of left shoulder**
    +7th **S40.229 Blister (nonthermal) of unspecified shoulder**
  + **S40.24 External constriction of shoulder**
    +7th **S40.241 External constriction of right shoulder**
    +7th **S40.242 External constriction of left shoulder**
    +7th **S40.249 External constriction of unspecified shoulder**
  + **S40.25 Superficial foreign body of shoulder**
    Splinter in the shoulder
    +7th **S40.251 Superficial foreign body of right shoulder**
    +7th **S40.252 Superficial foreign body of left shoulder**
    +7th **S40.259 Superficial foreign body of unspecified shoulder**

+ S40.26 Insect bite (nonvenomous) of shoulder
+7th S40.261 Insect bite (nonvenomous) of right shoulder
+7th S40.262 Insect bite (nonvenomous) of left shoulder
+7th S40.269 Insect bite (nonvenomous) of unspecified shoulder
+ S40.27 Other superficial bite of shoulder
Excludes1: open bite of shoulder (S41.05)
+7th S40.271 Other superficial bite of right shoulder
+7th S40.272 Other superficial bite of left shoulder
+7th S40.279 Other superficial bite of unspecified shoulder
+ S40.8 Other superficial injuries of upper arm
+ S40.81 Abrasion of upper arm
+7th S40.811 Abrasion of right upper arm
+7th S40.812 Abrasion of left upper arm
+7th S40.819 Abrasion of unspecified upper arm
+ S40.82 Blister (nonthermal) of upper arm
+7th S40.821 Blister (nonthermal) of right upper arm
+7th S40.822 Blister (nonthermal) of left upper arm
+7th S40.829 Blister (nonthermal) of unspecified upper arm
+ S40.84 External constriction of upper arm
+7th S40.841 External constriction of right upper arm
+7th S40.842 External constriction of left upper arm
+7th S40.849 External constriction of unspecified upper arm
+ S40.85 Superficial foreign body of upper arm
Splinter in the upper arm
+7th S40.851 Superficial foreign body of right upper arm
+7th S40.852 Superficial foreign body of left upper arm
+7th S40.859 Superficial foreign body of unspecified upper arm
+ S40.86 Insect bite (nonvenomous) of upper arm
+7th S40.861 Insect bite (nonvenomous) of right upper arm
+7th S40.862 Insect bite (nonvenomous) of left upper arm
+7th S40.869 Insect bite (nonvenomous) of unspecified upper arm
+ S40.87 Other superficial bite of upper arm
Excludes1: open bite of upper arm (S41.14)
Excludes2: other superficial bite of shoulder (S40.27-)
+7th S40.871 Other superficial bite of right upper arm
+7th S40.872 Other superficial bite of left upper arm
+7th S40.879 Other superficial bite of unspecified upper arm
+ S40.9 Unspecified superficial injury of shoulder and upper arm
+ S40.91 Unspecified superficial injury of shoulder
+7th S40.911 Unspecified superficial injury of right shoulder
+7th S40.912 Unspecified superficial injury of left shoulder
+7th S40.919 Unspecified superficial injury of unspecified shoulder
+ S40.92 Unspecified superficial injury of upper arm
+7th S40.921 Unspecified superficial injury of right upper arm
+7th S40.922 Unspecified superficial injury of left upper arm
+7th S40.929 Unspecified superficial injury of unspecified upper arm

S41 Open wound of shoulder and upper arm

Code also any associated wound infection
Excludes1: traumatic amputation of shoulder and upper arm (S48.-)
Excludes2: open fracture of shoulder and upper arm (S42.- with 7th character B or C)

The appropriate 7th character is to be added to each code from category S41
A initial encounter
D subsequent encounter
S sequela

+ S41.0 Open wound of shoulder
+ S41.00 Unspecified open wound of shoulder
+7th S41.001 Unspecified open wound of right shoulder
+7th S41.002 Unspecified open wound of left shoulder
+7th S41.009 Unspecified open wound of unspecified shoulder
+ S41.01 Laceration without foreign body of shoulder
+7th S41.011 Laceration without foreign body of right shoulder
+7th S41.012 Laceration without foreign body of left shoulder
+7th S41.019 Laceration without foreign body of unspecified shoulder
+ S41.02 Laceration with foreign body of shoulder
+7th S41.021 Laceration with foreign body of right shoulder
+7th S41.022 Laceration with foreign body of left shoulder
+7th S41.029 Laceration with foreign body of unspecified shoulder
+ S41.03 Puncture wound without foreign body of shoulder
+7th S41.031 Puncture wound without foreign body of right shoulder
+7th S41.032 Puncture wound without foreign body of left shoulder
+7th S41.039 Puncture wound without foreign body of unspecified shoulder
+ S41.04 Puncture wound with foreign body of shoulder
+7th S41.041 Puncture wound with foreign body of right shoulder
+7th S41.042 Puncture wound with foreign body of left shoulder
+7th S41.049 Puncture wound with foreign body of unspecified shoulder
+ S41.05 Open bite of shoulder
Bite of shoulder NOS
Excludes1: superficial bite of shoulder (S40.27)
+7th S41.051 Open bite of right shoulder
+7th S41.052 Open bite of left shoulder
+7th S41.059 Open bite of unspecified shoulder
+ S41.1 Open wound of upper arm
+ S41.10 Unspecified open wound of upper arm
+7th S41.101 Unspecified open wound of right upper arm
+7th S41.102 Unspecified open wound of left upper arm
+7th S41.109 Unspecified open wound of unspecified upper arm
+ S41.11 Laceration without foreign body of upper arm
S41.111 Laceration without foreign body of right upper arm
S41.112 Laceration without foreign body of left upper arm
S41.119 Laceration without foreign body of unspecified upper arm
+ S41.12 Laceration with foreign body of upper arm
+7th S41.121 Laceration with foreign body of right upper arm
+7th S41.122 Laceration with foreign body of left upper arm
+7th S41.129 Laceration with foreign body of unspecified upper arm
+ S41.13 Puncture wound without foreign body of upper arm
+7th S41.131 Puncture wound without foreign body of right upper arm
+7th S41.132 Puncture wound without foreign body of left upper arm
+7th S41.139 Puncture wound without foreign body of unspecified upper arm
+ S41.14 Puncture wound with foreign body of upper arm
+7th S41.141 Puncture wound with foreign body of right upper arm
+7th S41.142 Puncture wound with foreign body of left upper arm
+7th S41.149 Puncture wound with foreign body of unspecified upper arm
+ S41.15 Open bite of upper arm
Bite of upper arm NOS
Excludes1: superficial bite of upper arm (S40.87)
+7th S41.151 Open bite of right upper arm
+7th S41.152 Open bite of left upper arm
+7th S41.159 Open bite of unspecified upper arm

S42 Fracture of shoulder and upper arm

NOTE A fracture not indicated as displaced or nondisplaced should be coded to displaced

A fracture not indicated as open or closed should be coded to closed unless otherwise indicated.

Excludes1: *traumatic amputation of shoulder and upper arm (S48.-)*

The appropriate 7th character is to be added to all codes from category S42

- A initial encounter for closed fracture
- B initial encounter for open fracture
- D subsequent encounter for fracture with routine healing
- G subsequent encounter for fracture with delayed healing
- K subsequent encounter for fracture with nonunion
- P subsequent encounter for fracture with malunion
- S sequela

Review coding guideline C.19.c

+ S42.0 Fracture of clavicle

+ S42.00 Fracture of unspecified part of clavicle

CC +7th **S42.001 Fracture of unspecified part of right clavicle**
CC Exclusion 7th character B see Appendix A PDX collection 1243
CC Exclusion 7th characters K & P see Appendix A PDX collection 0897
HAC 7th character B see Appendix B for HAC conditional logic

CC +7th **S42.002 Fracture of unspecified part of left clavicle**
CC Exclusion 7th character B see Appendix A PDX collection 1243
CC Exclusion 7th characters K & P see Appendix A PDX collection 0897
HAC 7th character B see Appendix B for HAC conditional logic

CC +7th **S42.009 Fracture of unspecified part of unspecified clavicle**
CC Exclusion 7th character B see Appendix A PDX collection 1243
CC Exclusion 7th characters K & P see Appendix A PDX collection 0897
HAC 7th character B see Appendix B for HAC conditional logic

+ S42.01 Fracture of sternal end of clavicle

CC +7th **S42.011 Anterior displaced fracture of sternal end of right clavicle**
CC Exclusion 7th character B see Appendix A PDX collection 1243
CC Exclusion 7th characters K & P see Appendix A PDX collection 0897
HAC 7th character B see Appendix B for HAC conditional logic

CC +7th **S42.012 Anterior displaced fracture of sternal end of left clavicle**
CC Exclusion 7th character B see Appendix A PDX collection 1243
CC Exclusion 7th characters K & P see Appendix A PDX collection 0897
HAC 7th character B see Appendix B for HAC conditional logic

CC +7th **S42.013 Anterior displaced fracture of sternal end of unspecified clavicle**
Displaced fracture of sternal end of clavicle NOS
CC Exclusion 7th character B see Appendix A PDX collection 1243
CC Exclusion 7th characters K & P see Appendix A PDX collection 0897
HAC 7th character B see Appendix B for HAC conditional logic

CC +7th **S42.014 Posterior displaced fracture of sternal end of right clavicle**
CC Exclusion 7th character B see Appendix A PDX collection 1243
CC Exclusion 7th characters K & P see Appendix A PDX collection 0897
HAC 7th character B see Appendix B for HAC conditional logic

CC +7th **S42.015 Posterior displaced fracture of sternal end of left clavicle**
CC Exclusion 7th character B see Appendix A PDX collection 1243
CC Exclusion 7th characters K & P see Appendix A PDX collection 0897
HAC 7th character B see Appendix B for HAC conditional logic

CC +7th **S42.016 Posterior displaced fracture of sternal en of unspecified clavicle**
CC Exclusion 7th character B see Appendix A PDX collection 1243
CC Exclusion 7th characters K & P see Appendix A PDX collection 0897
HAC 7th character B see Appendix B for HAC conditional logic

CC +7th **S42.017 Nondisplaced fracture of sternal end of right clavicle**
CC Exclusion 7th character B see Appendix A PDX collection 1243
CC Exclusion 7th characters K & P see Appendix A PDX collection 0897
HAC 7th character B see Appendix B for HAC conditional logic

CC +7th **S42.018 Nondisplaced fracture of sternal end of l clavicle**
CC Exclusion 7th character B see Appendix A PDX collection 1243
CC Exclusion 7th characters K & P see Appendix A PDX collection 0897
HAC 7th character B see Appendix B for HAC conditional logic

CC +7th **S42.019 Nondisplaced fracture of sternal end of unspecified clavicle**
CC Exclusion 7th character B see Appendix A PDX collection 1243
CC Exclusion 7th characters K & P see Appendix A PDX collection 0897
HAC 7th character B see Appendix B for HAC conditional logic

+ S42.02 Fracture of shaft of clavicle

CC +7th **S42.021 Displaced fracture of shaft of right clavicle**
CC Exclusion 7th character B see Appendix PDX collection 1243
CC Exclusion 7th characters K & P see Appendix A PDX collection 0897
HAC 7th character B see Appendix B for HAC conditional logic

CC +7th **S42.022 Displaced fracture of shaft of left clavicle**
CC Exclusion 7th character B see Appendix PDX collection 1243
CC Exclusion 7th characters K & P see Appendix A PDX collection 0897
HAC 7th character B see Appendix B for HA conditional logic

CC +7th **S42.023 Displaced fracture of shaft of unspecifie clavicle**
CC Exclusion 7th character B see Appendix PDX collection 1243
CC Exclusion 7th characters K & P see Appendix A PDX collection 0897
HAC 7th character B see Appendix B for HA conditional logic

CC +7th **S42.024 Nondisplaced fracture of shaft of right clavicle**
CC Exclusion 7th character B see Appendix PDX collection 1243
CC Exclusion 7th characters K & P see Appendix A PDX collection 0897
HAC 7th character B see Appendix B for HA conditional logic

CC +7th **S42.025 Nondisplaced fracture of shaft of left clavicle**
CC Exclusion 7th character B see Appendix PDX collection 1243
CC Exclusion 7th characters K & P see Appendix A PDX collection 0897
HAC 7th character B see Appendix B for HA conditional logic

CC +7th **S42.026 Nondisplaced fracture of shaft of unspecified clavicle**
CC Exclusion 7th character B see Appendix PDX collection 1243
CC Exclusion 7th characters K & P see Appendix A PDX collection 0897
HAC 7th character B see Appendix B for HA conditional logic

+ S42.03 **Fracture of lateral end of clavicle**
Fracture of acromial end of clavicle

CC +7th **S42.031 Displaced fracture of lateral end of right clavicle**
CC Exclusion 7th character B see Appendix A PDX collection 1243
CC Exclusion 7th characters K & P see Appendix A PDX collection 0897
HAC 7th character B see Appendix B for HAC conditional logic

CC +7th **S42.032 Displaced fracture of lateral end of left clavicle**
CC Exclusion 7th character B see Appendix A PDX collection 1243
CC Exclusion 7th characters K & P see Appendix A PDX collection 0897
HAC 7th character B see Appendix B for HAC conditional logic

CC +7th **S42.033 Displaced fracture of lateral end of unspecified clavicle**
CC Exclusion 7th character B see Appendix A PDX collection 1243
CC Exclusion 7th characters K & P see Appendix A PDX collection 0897
HAC 7th character B see Appendix B for HAC conditional logic

CC +7th **S42.034 Nondisplaced fracture of lateral end of right clavicle**
CC Exclusion 7th character B see Appendix A PDX collection 1243
CC Exclusion 7th characters K & P see Appendix A PDX collection 0897
HAC 7th character B see Appendix B for HAC conditional logic

CC +7th **S42.035 Nondisplaced fracture of lateral end of left clavicle**
CC Exclusion 7th character B see Appendix A PDX collection 1243
CC Exclusion 7th characters K & P see Appendix A PDX collection 0897
HAC 7th character B see Appendix B for HAC conditional logic

CC +7th **S42.036 Nondisplaced fracture of lateral end of unspecified clavicle**
CC Exclusion 7th character B see Appendix A PDX collection 1243
CC Exclusion 7th characters K & P see Appendix A PDX collection 0897
HAC 7th character B see Appendix B for HAC conditional logic

+ **S42.1 Fracture of scapula**

+ **S42.10 Fracture of unspecified part of scapula**

CC +7th **S42.101 Fracture of unspecified part of scapula, right shoulder**
CC Exclusion 7th character B see Appendix A PDX collection 1244
CC Exclusion 7th characters K & P see Appendix A PDX collection 0897
HAC 7th character B see Appendix B for HAC conditional logic

CC +7th **S42.102 Fracture of unspecified part of scapula, left shoulder**
CC Exclusion 7th character B see Appendix A PDX collection 1244
CC Exclusion 7th characters K & P see Appendix A PDX collection 0897
HAC 7th character B see Appendix B for HAC conditional logic

CC +7th **S42.109 Fracture of unspecified part of scapula, unspecified shoulder**
CC Exclusion 7th character B see Appendix A PDX collection 1244
CC Exclusion 7th characters K & P see Appendix A PDX collection 0897
HAC 7th character B see Appendix B for HAC conditional logic

+ **S42.11 Fracture of body of scapula**

CC +7th **S42.111 Displaced fracture of body of scapula, right shoulder**
CC Exclusion 7th character B see Appendix A PDX collection 1244
CC Exclusion 7th characters K & P see Appendix A PDX collection 0897
HAC 7th character B see Appendix B for HAC conditional logic

CC +7th **S42.112 Displaced fracture of body of scapula, left shoulder**
CC Exclusion 7th character B see Appendix A PDX collection 1244
CC Exclusion 7th characters K & P see Appendix A PDX collection 0897
HAC 7th character B see Appendix B for HAC conditional logic

CC +7th **S42.113 Displaced fracture of body of scapula, unspecified shoulder**
CC Exclusion 7th character B see Appendix A PDX collection 1244
CC Exclusion 7th characters K & P see Appendix A PDX collection 0897
HAC 7th character B see Appendix B for HAC conditional logic

CC +7th **S42.114 Nondisplaced fracture of body of scapula, right shoulder**
CC Exclusion 7th character B see Appendix A PDX collection 1244
CC Exclusion 7th characters K & P see Appendix A PDX collection 0897
HAC 7th character B see Appendix B for HAC conditional logic

CC +7th **S42.115 Nondisplaced fracture of body of scapula, left shoulder**
CC Exclusion 7th character B see Appendix A PDX collection 1244
CC Exclusion 7th characters K & P see Appendix A PDX collection 0897
HAC 7th character B see Appendix B for HAC conditional logic

CC +7th **S42.116 Nondisplaced fracture of body of scapula, unspecified shoulder**
CC Exclusion 7th character B see Appendix A PDX collection 1244
CC Exclusion 7th characters K & P see Appendix A PDX collection 0897
HAC 7th character B see Appendix B for HAC conditional logic

+ **S42.12 Fracture of acromial process**

CC +7th **S42.121 Displaced fracture of acromial process, right shoulder**
CC Exclusion 7th character B see Appendix A PDX collection 1244
CC Exclusion 7th characters K & P see Appendix A PDX collection 0897
HAC 7th character B see Appendix B for HAC conditional logic

CC +7th **S42.122 Displaced fracture of acromial process, left shoulder**
CC Exclusion 7th character B see Appendix A PDX collection 1244
CC Exclusion 7th characters K & P see Appendix A PDX collection 0897
HAC 7th character B see Appendix B for HAC conditional logic

CC +7th **S42.123 Displaced fracture of acromial process, unspecified shoulder**
CC Exclusion 7th character B see Appendix A PDX collection 1244
CC Exclusion 7th characters K & P see Appendix A PDX collection 0897
HAC 7th character B see Appendix B for HAC conditional logic

CC +7th **S42.124 Nondisplaced fracture of acromial process, right shoulder**
CC Exclusion 7th character B see Appendix A PDX collection 1244
CC Exclusion 7th characters K & P see Appendix A PDX collection 0897
HAC 7th character B see Appendix B for HAC conditional logic

CC +7th **S42.125 Nondisplaced fracture of acromial process, left shoulder**
CC Exclusion 7th character B see Appendix A PDX collection 1244
CC Exclusion 7th characters K & P see Appendix A PDX collection 0897
HAC 7th character B see Appendix B for HAC conditional logic

CC +7th **S42.126 Nondisplaced fracture of acromial process, unspecified shoulder**
CC Exclusion 7th character B see Appendix A PDX collection 1244
CC Exclusion 7th characters K & P see Appendix A PDX collection 0897
HAC 7th character B see Appendix B for HAC conditional logic

+ S42.13 Fracture of coracoid process

CC +7th **S42.131 Displaced fracture of coracoid process, right shoulder**
CC Exclusion 7th character B see Appendix A PDX collection 1244
CC Exclusion 7th characters K & P see Appendix A PDX collection 0897
HAC 7th character B see Appendix B for HAC conditional logic

CC +7th **S42.132 Displaced fracture of coracoid process, left shoulder**
CC Exclusion 7th character B see Appendix A PDX collection 1244
CC Exclusion 7th characters K & P see Appendix A PDX collection 0897
HAC 7th character B see Appendix B for HAC conditional logic

CC +7th **S42.133 Displaced fracture of coracoid process, unspecified shoulder**
CC Exclusion 7th character B see Appendix A PDX collection 1244
CC Exclusion 7th characters K & P see Appendix A PDX collection 0897
HAC 7th character B see Appendix B for HAC conditional logic

CC +7th **S42.134 Nondisplaced fracture of coracoid process, right shoulder**
CC Exclusion 7th character B see Appendix A PDX collection 1244
CC Exclusion 7th characters K & P see Appendix A PDX collection 0897
HAC 7th character B see Appendix B for HAC conditional logic

CC +7th **S42.135 Nondisplaced fracture of coracoid process, left shoulder**
CC Exclusion 7th character B see Appendix A PDX collection 1244
CC Exclusion 7th characters K & P see Appendix A PDX collection 0897
HAC 7th character B see Appendix B for HAC conditional logic

CC +7th **S42.136 Nondisplaced fracture of coracoid process, unspecified shoulder**
CC Exclusion 7th character B see Appendix A PDX collection 1244
CC Exclusion 7th characters K & P see Appendix A PDX collection 0897
HAC 7th character B see Appendix B for HAC conditional logic

+ S42.14 Fracture of glenoid cavity of scapula

CC +7th **S42.141 Displaced fracture of glenoid cavity of scapula, right shoulder**
CC Exclusion 7th character B see Appendix A PDX collection 1244
CC Exclusion 7th characters K & P see Appendix A PDX collection 0897
HAC 7th character B see Appendix B for HAC conditional logic

CC +7th **S42.142 Displaced fracture of glenoid cavity of scapula, left shoulder**
CC Exclusion 7th character B see Appendix A PDX collection 1244
CC Exclusion 7th characters K & P see Appendix A PDX collection 0897
HAC 7th character B see Appendix B for HAC conditional logic

CC +7th **S42.143 Displaced fracture of glenoid cavity of scapula, unspecified shoulder**
CC Exclusion 7th character B see Appendix A PDX collection 1244
CC Exclusion 7th characters K & P see Appendix A PDX collection 0897
HAC 7th character B see Appendix B for HAC conditional logic

CC +7th **S42.144 Nondisplaced fracture of glenoid cavity of scapula, right shoulder**
CC Exclusion 7th character B see Appendix A PDX collection 1244
CC Exclusion 7th characters K & P see Appendix A PDX collection 0897
HAC 7th character B see Appendix B for HAC conditional logic

CC +7th **S42.145 Nondisplaced fracture of glenoid cavity of scapula, left shoulder**
CC Exclusion 7th character B see Appendix A PDX collection 1244
CC Exclusion 7th characters K & P see Appendix A PDX collection 0897
HAC 7th character B see Appendix B for HAC conditional logic

CC +7th **S42.146 Nondisplaced fracture of glenoid cavity o scapula, unspecified shoulder**
CC Exclusion 7th character B see Appendix A PDX collection 1244
CC Exclusion 7th characters K & P see Appendix A PDX collection 0897
HAC 7th character B see Appendix B for HAC conditional logic

+ S42.15 Fracture of neck of scapula

CC +7th **S42.151 Displaced fracture of neck of scapula, rig shoulder**
CC Exclusion 7th character B see Appendix A PDX collection 1244
CC Exclusion 7th characters K & P see Appendix A PDX collection 0897
HAC 7th character B see Appendix B for HAC conditional logic

CC +7th **S42.152 Displaced fracture of neck of scapula, left shoulder**
CC Exclusion 7th character B see Appendix A PDX collection 1244
CC Exclusion 7th characters K & P see Appendix A PDX collection 0897
HAC 7th character B see Appendix B for HAC conditional logic

CC +7th **S42.153 Displaced fracture of neck of scapula, unspecified shoulder**
CC Exclusion 7th character B see Appendix PDX collection 1244
CC Exclusion 7th characters K & P see Appendix A PDX collection 0897
HAC 7th character B see Appendix B for HAC conditional logic

CC +7th **S42.154 Nondisplaced fracture of neck of scapula right shoulder**
CC Exclusion 7th character B see Appendix PDX collection 1244
CC Exclusion 7th characters K & P see Appendix A PDX collection 0897
HAC 7th character B see Appendix B for HAC conditional logic

CC +7th **S42.155 Nondisplaced fracture of neck of scapula left shoulder**
CC Exclusion 7th character B see Appendix PDX collection 1244
CC Exclusion 7th characters K & P see Appendix A PDX collection 0897
HAC 7th character B see Appendix B for HAC conditional logic

CC +7th **S42.156 Nondisplaced fracture of neck of scapula unspecified shoulder**
CC Exclusion 7th character B see Appendix PDX collection 1244
CC Exclusion 7th characters K & P see Appendix A PDX collection 0897
HAC 7th character B see Appendix B for HAC conditional logic

+ S42.19 Fracture of other part of scapula

CC +7th **S42.191 Fracture of other part of scapula, right shoulder**
CC Exclusion 7th character B see Appendix PDX collection 1244
CC Exclusion 7th characters K & P see Appendix A PDX collection 0897
HAC 7th character B see Appendix B for HAC conditional logic

CC +7th **S42.192 Fracture of other part of scapula, left shoulder**
CC Exclusion 7th character B see Appendix PDX collection 1244
CC Exclusion 7th characters K & P see Appendix A PDX collection 0897
HAC 7th character B see Appendix B for HA conditional logic

CC +7th **S42.199 Fracture of other part of scapula, unspecified shoulder**
CC Exclusion 7th character B see Appendix PDX collection 1244
CC Exclusion 7th characters K & P see Appendix A PDX collection 0897
HAC 7th character B see Appendix B for HA conditional logic

+ **S42.2 Fracture of upper end of humerus**
Fracture of proximal end of humerus
Excludes2: *fracture of shaft of humerus (S42.3-)*
physeal fracture of upper end of humerus (S49.0-)

+ **S42.20 Unspecified fracture of upper end of humerus**

CC MCC +7th **S42.201 Unspecified fracture of upper end of right humerus**
CC Exclusion 7th character A see Appendix A PDX collection 1245
CC Exclusion 7th characters K & P see Appendix A PDX collection 0897
MCC Exclusion 7th character B see Appendix A PDX collection 1246
HAC 7th characters A & B see Appendix B for HAC conditional logic

CC MCC +7th **S42.202 Unspecified fracture of upper end of left humerus**
CC Exclusion 7th character A see Appendix A PDX collection 1247
CC Exclusion 7th characters K & P see Appendix A PDX collection 0897
MCC Exclusion 7th character B see Appendix A PDX collection 1246
HAC 7th characters A & B see Appendix B for HAC conditional logic

CC MCC +7th **S42.209 Unspecified fracture of upper end of unspecified humerus**
CC Exclusion 7th character A see Appendix A PDX collection 1248
CC Exclusion 7th characters K & P see Appendix A PDX collection 0897
MCC Exclusion 7th character B see Appendix A PDX collection 1246
HAC 7th characters A & B see Appendix B for HAC conditional logic

+ **S42.21 Unspecified fracture of surgical neck of humerus**
Fracture of neck of humerus NOS

CC MCC +7th **S42.211 Unspecified displaced fracture of surgical neck of right humerus**
CC Exclusion 7th character A see Appendix A PDX collection 1245
CC Exclusion 7th characters K & P see Appendix A PDX collection 0897
MCC Exclusion 7th character B see Appendix A PDX collection 1246
HAC 7th characters A & B see Appendix B for HAC conditional logic

CC MCC +7th **S42.212 Unspecified displaced fracture of surgical neck of left humerus**
CC Exclusion 7th character A see Appendix A PDX collection 1247
CC Exclusion 7th characters K & P see Appendix A PDX collection 0897
MCC Exclusion 7th character B see Appendix A PDX collection 1246

CC MCC +7th **S42.213 Unspecified displaced fracture of surgical neck of unspecified humerus**
CC Exclusion 7th character A see Appendix A PDX collection 1248
CC Exclusion 7th characters K & P see Appendix A PDX collection 0897
MCC Exclusion 7th character B see Appendix A PDX collection 1246
HAC 7th characters A & B see Appendix B for HAC conditional logic

CC MCC +7th **S42.214 Unspecified nondisplaced fracture of surgical neck of right humerus**
CC Exclusion 7th character A see Appendix A PDX collection 1245
CC Exclusion 7th characters K & P see Appendix A PDX collection 0897
MCC Exclusion 7th character B see Appendix A PDX collection 1246
HAC 7th characters A & B see Appendix B for HAC conditional logic

CC MCC +7th **S42.215 Unspecified nondisplaced fracture of surgical neck of left humerus**
CC Exclusion 7th character A see Appendix A PDX collection 1247
CC Exclusion 7th characters K & P see Appendix A PDX collection 0897
MCC Exclusion 7th character B see Appendix A PDX collection 1246
HAC 7th characters A & B see Appendix B for HAC conditional logic

CC MCC +7th **S42.216 Unspecified nondisplaced fracture of surgical neck of unspecified humerus**
CC Exclusion 7th character A see Appendix A PDX collection 1248
CC Exclusion 7th characters K & P see Appendix A PDX collection 0897
MCC Exclusion 7th character B see Appendix A PDX collection 1246
HAC 7th characters A & B see Appendix B for HAC conditional logic

+ **S42.22 2-part fracture of surgical neck of humerus**

CC MCC +7th **S42.221 2-part displaced fracture of surgical neck of right humerus**
CC Exclusion 7th character A see Appendix A PDX collection 1245
CC Exclusion 7th characters K & P see Appendix A PDX collection 0897
MCC Exclusion 7th character B see Appendix A PDX collection 1246
HAC 7th characters A & B see Appendix B for HAC conditional logic

CC MCC +7th **S42.222 2-part displaced fracture of surgical neck of left humerus**
CC Exclusion 7th character A see Appendix A PDX collection 1247
CC Exclusion 7th characters K & P see Appendix A PDX collection 0897
MCC Exclusion 7th character B see Appendix A PDX collection 1246
HAC 7th characters A & B see Appendix B for HAC conditional logic

CC MCC +7th **S42.223 2-part displaced fracture of surgical neck of unspecified humerus**
CC Exclusion 7th character A see Appendix A PDX collection 1248
CC Exclusion 7th characters K & P see Appendix A PDX collection 0897
MCC Exclusion 7th character B see Appendix A PDX collection 1246
HAC 7th characters A & B see Appendix B for HAC conditional logic

CC MCC +7th **S42.224 2-part nondisplaced fracture of surgical neck of right humerus**
CC Exclusion 7th character A see Appendix A PDX collection 1245
CC Exclusion 7th characters K & P see Appendix A PDX collection 0897
MCC Exclusion 7th character B see Appendix A PDX collection 1246
HAC 7th characters A & B see Appendix B for HAC conditional logic

CC MCC +7th **S42.225 2-part nondisplaced fracture of surgical neck of left humerus**
CC Exclusion 7th character A see Appendix A PDX collection 1247
CC Exclusion 7th characters K & P see Appendix A PDX collection 0897
MCC Exclusion 7th character B see Appendix A PDX collection 1246
HAC 7th characters A & B see Appendix B for HAC conditional logic

CC MCC +7th **S42.226 2-part nondisplaced fracture of surgical neck of unspecified humerus**
CC Exclusion 7th character A see Appendix A PDX collection 1248
CC Exclusion 7th characters K & P see Appendix A PDX collection 0897
MCC Exclusion 7th character B see Appendix A PDX collection 1246
HAC 7th characters A & B see Appendix B for HAC conditional logic

+ **S42.23 3-part fracture of surgical neck of humerus**

CC MCC +7th **S42.231 3-part fracture of surgical neck of right humerus**
CC Exclusion 7th character A see Appendix A PDX collection 1245
CC Exclusion 7th characters K & P see Appendix A PDX collection 0897
MCC Exclusion 7th character B see Appendix A PDX collection 1246
HAC 7th characters A & B see Appendix B for HAC conditional logic

CC MCC +7th **S42.232 3-part fracture of surgical neck of left humerus**
CC Exclusion 7th character A see Appendix A PDX collection 1247
CC Exclusion 7th characters K & P see Appendix A PDX collection 0897
MCC Exclusion 7th character B see Appendix A PDX collection 1246
HAC 7th characters A & B see Appendix B for HAC conditional logic

CC MCC +7th **S42.239 3-part fracture of surgical neck of unspecified humerus**
CC Exclusion 7th character A see Appendix A PDX collection 1248
CC Exclusion 7th characters K & P see Appendix A PDX collection 0897
MCC Exclusion 7th character B see Appendix A PDX collection 1246
HAC 7th characters A & B see Appendix B for HAC conditional logic

+ **S42.24 4-part fracture of surgical neck of humerus**

CC MCC +7th **S42.241 4-part fracture of surgical neck of right humerus**
CC Exclusion 7th character A see Appendix A PDX collection 1245
CC Exclusion 7th characters K & P see Appendix A PDX collection 0897
MCC Exclusion 7th character B see Appendix A PDX collection 1246
HAC 7th characters A & B see Appendix B for HAC conditional logic

CC MCC +7th **S42.242 4-part fracture of surgical neck of left humerus**
CC Exclusion 7th character A see Appendix A PDX collection 1247
CC Exclusion 7th characters K & P see Appendix A PDX collection 0897
MCC Exclusion 7th character B see Appendix A PDX collection 1246
HAC 7th characters A & B see Appendix B for HAC conditional logic

CC MCC +7th **S42.249 4-part fracture of surgical neck of unspecified humerus**
CC Exclusion 7th character A see Appendix A PDX collection 1248
CC Exclusion 7th characters K & P see Appendix A PDX collection 0897
MCC Exclusion 7th character B see Appendix A PDX collection 1246
HAC 7th characters A & B see Appendix B for HAC conditional logic

+ **S42.25 Fracture of greater tuberosity of humerus**

CC MCC +7th **S42.251 Displaced fracture of greater tuberosity of right humerus**
CC Exclusion 7th character A see Appendix A PDX collection 1245
CC Exclusion 7th characters K & P see Appendix A PDX collection 0897
MCC Exclusion 7th character B see Appendix A PDX collection 1246
HAC 7th characters A & B see Appendix B for HAC conditional logic

CC MCC +7th **S42.252 Displaced fracture of greater tuberosity of left humerus**
CC Exclusion 7th character A see Appendix A PDX collection 1247
CC Exclusion 7th characters K & P see Appendix A PDX collection 0897
MCC Exclusion 7th character B see Appendix A PDX collection 1246
HAC 7th characters A & B see Appendix B for HAC conditional logic

CC MCC +7th **S42.253 Displaced fracture of greater tuberosity of unspecified humerus**
CC Exclusion 7th character A see Appendix A PDX collection 1248
CC Exclusion 7th characters K & P see Appendix A PDX collection 0897
MCC Exclusion 7th character B see Appendix A PDX collection 1246
HAC 7th characters A & B see Appendix B for HAC conditional logic

CC MCC +7th **S42.254 Nondisplaced fracture of greater tuberosi of right humerus**
CC Exclusion 7th character A see Appendix A PDX collection 1245
CC Exclusion 7th characters K & P see Appendix A PDX collection 0897
MCC Exclusion 7th character B see Appendix PDX collection 1246
HAC 7th characters A & B see Appendix B for HAC conditional logic

CC MCC +7th **S42.255 Nondisplaced fracture of greater tuberosi of left humerus**
CC Exclusion 7th character A see Appendix A PDX collection 1247
CC Exclusion 7th characters K & P see Appendix A PDX collection 0897
MCC Exclusion 7th character B see Appendix PDX collection 1246
HAC 7th characters A & B see Appendix B for HAC conditional logic

CC MCC +7th **S42.256 Nondisplaced fracture of greater tuberos of unspecified humerus**
CC Exclusion 7th character A see Appendix A PDX collection 1248
CC Exclusion 7th characters K & P see Appendix A PDX collection 0897
MCC Exclusion 7th character B see Appendi PDX collection 1246
HAC 7th characters A & B see Appendix B fo HAC conditional logic

+ **S42.26 Fracture of lesser tuberosity of humerus**

CC MCC +7th **S42.261 Displaced fracture of lesser tuberosity of right humerus**
CC Exclusion 7th character A see Appendix PDX collection 1245
CC Exclusion 7th characters K & P see Appendix A PDX collection 0897
MCC Exclusion 7th character B see Appendi PDX collection 1246
HAC 7th characters A & B see Appendix B fo HAC conditional logic

CC MCC +7th **S42.262 Displaced fracture of lesser tuberosity of left humerus**
CC Exclusion 7th character A see Appendix PDX collection 1247
CC Exclusion 7th characters K & P see Appendix A PDX collection 0897
MCC Exclusion 7th character B see Appendi PDX collection 1246
HAC 7th characters A & B see Appendix B fo HAC conditional logic

CC MCC +7th **S42.263 Displaced fracture of lesser tuberosity of unspecified humerus**
CC Exclusion 7th character A see Appendix PDX collection 1248
CC Exclusion 7th characters K & P see Appendix A PDX collection 0897
MCC Exclusion 7th character B see Appendi PDX collection 1246
HAC 7th characters A & B see Appendix B fo HAC conditional logic

CC MCC +7th **S42.264 Nondisplaced fracture of lesser tuberosi of right humerus**
CC Exclusion 7th character A see Appendix PDX collection 1245
CC Exclusion 7th characters K & P see Appendix A PDX collection 0897
MCC Exclusion 7th character B see Appendi PDX collection 1246
HAC 7th characters A & B see Appendix B fo HAC conditional logic

CC MCC +7th **S42.265 Nondisplaced fracture of lesser tuberosi of left humerus**
CC Exclusion 7th character A see Appendix PDX collection 1247
CC Exclusion 7th characters K & P see Appendix A PDX collection 0897
MCC Exclusion 7th character B see Appendi PDX collection 1246
HAC 7th characters A & B see Appendix B f HAC conditional logic

CC MCC +7th **S42.266 Nondisplaced fracture of lesser tuberosity of unspecified humerus**
CC Exclusion 7th character A see Appendix A PDX collection 1248
CC Exclusion 7th characters K & P see Appendix A PDX collection 0897
MCC Exclusion 7th character B see Appendix A PDX collection 1246
HAC 7th characters A & B see Appendix B for HAC conditional logic

+ **S42.27 Torus fracture of upper end of humerus**

The appropriate 7th character is to be added to all codes in subcategory **S42.27**
A initial encounter for closed fracture
D subsequent encounter for fracture with routine healing
G subsequent encounter for fracture with delayed healing
K subsequent encounter for fracture with nonunion
P subsequent encounter for fracture with malunion
S sequela

CC +7th **S42.271 Torus fracture of upper end of right humerus**
CC Exclusion 7th character A see Appendix A PDX collection 1245
CC Exclusion 7th characters K & P see Appendix A PDX collection 0897
HAC 7th character A see Appendix B for HAC conditional logic

CC +7th **S42.272 Torus fracture of upper end of left humerus**
CC Exclusion 7th character A see Appendix A PDX collection 1247
CC Exclusion 7th characters K & P see Appendix A PDX collection 0897
HAC 7th character A see Appendix B for HAC conditional logic

CC +7th **S42.279 Torus fracture of upper end of unspecified humerus**
CC Exclusion 7th character A see Appendix A PDX collection 1248
CC Exclusion 7th characters K & P see Appendix A PDX collection 0897
HAC 7th character A see Appendix B for HAC conditional logic

+ **S42.29 Other fracture of upper end of humerus**
Fracture of anatomical neck of humerus
Fracture of articular head of humerus

CC MCC +7th **S42.291 Other displaced fracture of upper end of right humerus**
CC Exclusion 7th character A see Appendix A PDX collection 1245
CC Exclusion 7th characters K & P see Appendix A PDX collection 0897
MCC Exclusion 7th character B see Appendix A PDX collection 1246
HAC 7th characters A & B see Appendix B for HAC conditional logic

CC MCC +7th **S42.292 Other displaced fracture of upper end of left humerus**
CC Exclusion 7th character A see Appendix A PDX collection 1247
CC Exclusion 7th characters K & P see Appendix A PDX collection 0897
MCC Exclusion 7th character B see Appendix A PDX collection 1246
HAC 7th characters A & B see Appendix B for HAC conditional logic

CC MCC +7th **S42.293 Other displaced fracture of upper end of unspecified humerus**
CC Exclusion 7th character A see Appendix A PDX collection 1248
CC Exclusion 7th characters K & P see Appendix A PDX collection 0897
MCC Exclusion 7th character B see Appendix A PDX collection 1246
HAC 7th characters A & B see Appendix B for HAC conditional logic

CC MCC +7th **S42.294 Other nondisplaced fracture of upper end of right humerus**
CC Exclusion 7th character A see Appendix A PDX collection 1245
CC Exclusion 7th characters K & P see Appendix A PDX collection 0897
MCC Exclusion 7th character B see Appendix A PDX collection 1246
HAC 7th characters A & B see Appendix B for HAC conditional logic

CC MCC +7th **S42.295 Other nondisplaced fracture of upper end of left humerus**
CC Exclusion 7th character A see Appendix A PDX collection 1247
CC Exclusion 7th characters K & P see Appendix A PDX collection 0897
MCC Exclusion 7th character B see Appendix A PDX collection 1246
HAC 7th characters A & B see Appendix B for HAC conditional logic

CC MCC +7th **S42.296 Other nondisplaced fracture of upper end of unspecified humerus**
CC Exclusion 7th character A see Appendix A PDX collection 1248
CC Exclusion 7th characters K & P see Appendix A PDX collection 0897
MCC Exclusion 7th character B see Appendix A PDX collection 1246
HAC 7th characters A & B see Appendix B for HAC conditional logic

+ **S42.3 Fracture of shaft of humerus**
Fracture of humerus NOS
Fracture of upper arm NOS
Excludes2: *physeal fractures of upper end of humerus (S49.0-)*
physeal fractures of lower end of humerus (S49.1-)

+ **S42.30 Unspecified fracture of shaft of humerus**

CC MCC +7th **S42.301 Unspecified fracture of shaft of humerus, right arm**
CC Exclusion 7th character A see Appendix A PDX collection 1245
CC Exclusion 7th characters K & P see Appendix A PDX collection 0897
MCC Exclusion 7th character B see Appendix A PDX collection 1246
HAC 7th characters A & B see Appendix B for HAC conditional logic

CC MCC +7th **S42.302 Unspecified fracture of shaft of humerus, left arm**
CC Exclusion 7th character A see Appendix A PDX collection 1247
CC Exclusion 7th characters K & P see Appendix A PDX collection 0897
MCC Exclusion 7th character B see Appendix A PDX collection 1246
HAC 7th characters A & B see Appendix B for HAC conditional logic

CC MCC +7th **S42.309 Unspecified fracture of shaft of humerus, unspecified arm**
CC Exclusion 7th character A see Appendix A PDX collection 1248
CC Exclusion 7th characters K & P see Appendix A PDX collection 0897
MCC Exclusion 7th character B see Appendix A PDX collection 1246
HAC 7th characters A & B see Appendix B for HAC conditional logic

+ **S42.31 Greenstick fracture of shaft of humerus**

The appropriate 7th character is to be added to all codes in subcategory **S42.31**
A initial encounter for closed fracture
D subsequent encounter for fracture with routine healing
G subsequent encounter for fracture with delayed healing
K subsequent encounter for fracture with nonunion
P subsequent encounter for fracture with malunion
S sequela

CC +7th **S42.311 Greenstick fracture of shaft of humerus, right arm**
CC Exclusion 7th character A see AppendixA PDX collection 1249
CC Exclusion 7th characters K & P see Appendix A PDX collection 0897
HAC 7th character A see Appendix B for HAC conditional logic

CC +7th **S42.312 Greenstick fracture of shaft of humerus, left arm**
CC Exclusion 7th character A see Appendix A PDX collection 1250
CC Exclusion 7th characters K & P see Appendix A PDX collection 0897
HAC 7th character A see Appendix B for HAC conditional logic

CC +7th **S42.319 Greenstick fracture of shaft of humerus, unspecified arm**
CC Exclusion 7th character A see Appendix A PDX collection 1251
CC Exclusion 7th characters K & P see Appendix A PDX collection 0897
HAC 7th character A see Appendix B for HAC conditional logic

+ **S42.32 Transverse fracture of shaft of humerus**

CC MCC +7th **S42.321 Displaced transverse fracture of shaft of humerus, right arm**
CC Exclusion 7th character A see Appendix A PDX collection 1249
CC Exclusion 7th characters K & P see Appendix A PDX collection 0897
MCC Exclusion 7th character B see Appendix A PDX collection 1246
HAC 7th characters A & B see Appendix B for HAC conditional logic

CC MCC +7th **S42.322 Displaced transverse fracture of shaft of humerus, left arm**
CC Exclusion 7th character A see Appendix A PDX collection 1250
CC Exclusion 7th characters K & P see Appendix A PDX collection 0897
MCC Exclusion 7th character B see Appendix A PDX collection 1246
HAC 7th characters A & B see Appendix B for HAC conditional logic

CC MCC +7th **S42.323 Displaced transverse fracture of shaft of humerus, unspecified arm**
CC Exclusion 7th character A see Appendix A PDX collection 1251
CC Exclusion 7th characters K & P see Appendix A PDX collection 0897
MCC Exclusion 7th character B see Appendix A PDX collection 1246
HAC 7th characters A & B see Appendix B for HAC conditional logic

CC MCC +7th **S42.324 Nondisplaced transverse fracture of shaft of humerus, right arm**
CC Exclusion 7th character A see Appendix A PDX collection 1249
CC Exclusion 7th characters K & P see Appendix A PDX collection 0897
MCC Exclusion 7th character B see Appendix A PDX collection 1246
HAC 7th characters A & B see Appendix B for HAC conditional logic

CC MCC +7th **S42.325 Nondisplaced transverse fracture of shaft of humerus, left arm**
CC Exclusion 7th character A see Appendix A PDX collection 1250
CC Exclusion 7th characters K & P see Appendix A PDX collection 0897
MCC Exclusion 7th character B see Appendix A PDX collection 1246
HAC 7th characters A & B see Appendix B for HAC conditional logic

CC MCC +7th **S42.326 Nondisplaced transverse fracture of shaft of humerus, unspecified arm**
CC Exclusion 7th character A see Appendix A PDX collection 1251
CC Exclusion 7th characters K & P see Appendix A PDX collection 0897
MCC Exclusion 7th character B see Appendix A PDX collection 1246
HAC 7th characters A & B see Appendix B for HAC conditional logic

+ **S42.33 Oblique fracture of shaft of humerus**

CC MCC +7th **S42.331 Displaced oblique fracture of shaft of humerus, right arm**
CC Exclusion 7th character A see Appendix A PDX collection 1249
CC Exclusion 7th characters K & P see Appendix A PDX collection 0897
MCC Exclusion 7th character B see Appendix A PDX collection 1246
HAC 7th characters A & B see Appendix B for HAC conditional logic

CC MCC +7th **S42.332 Displaced oblique fracture of shaft of humerus, left arm**
CC Exclusion 7th character A see Appendix A PDX collection 1250
CC Exclusion 7th characters K & P see Appendix A PDX collection 0897
MCC Exclusion 7th character B see Appendix A PDX collection 1246
HAC 7th characters A & B see Appendix B for HAC conditional logic

CC MCC +7th **S42.333 Displaced oblique fracture of shaft of humerus, unspecified arm**
CC Exclusion 7th character A see Appendix A PDX collection 1251
CC Exclusion 7th characters K & P see Appendix A PDX collection 0897
MCC Exclusion 7th character B see Appendix A PDX collection 1246
HAC 7th characters A & B see Appendix B for HAC conditional logic

CC MCC +7th **S42.334 Nondisplaced oblique fracture of shaft of humerus, right arm**
CC Exclusion 7th character A see Appendix A PDX collection 1249
CC Exclusion 7th characters K & P see Appendix A PDX collection 0897
MCC Exclusion 7th character B see Appendix A PDX collection 1246
HAC 7th characters A & B see Appendix B for HAC conditional logic

CC MCC +7th **S42.335 Nondisplaced oblique fracture of shaft of humerus, left arm**
CC Exclusion 7th character A see Appendix A PDX collection 1250
CC Exclusion 7th characters K & P see Appendix A PDX collection 0897
MCC Exclusion 7th character B see Appendix A PDX collection 1246
HAC 7th characters A & B see Appendix B for HAC conditional logic

CC MCC +7th **S42.336 Nondisplaced oblique fracture of shaft of humerus, unspecified arm**
CC Exclusion 7th character A see Appendix A PDX collection 1251
CC Exclusion 7th characters K & P see Appendix A PDX collection 0897
MCC Exclusion 7th character B see Appendix A PDX collection 1246
HAC 7th characters A & B see Appendix B for HAC conditional logic

+ **S42.34 Spiral fracture of shaft of humerus**

CC MCC +7th **S42.341 Displaced spiral fracture of shaft of humerus, right arm**
CC Exclusion 7th character A see Appendix A PDX collection 1249
CC Exclusion 7th characters K & P see Appendix A PDX collection 0897
MCC Exclusion 7th character B see Appendix A PDX collection 1246
HAC 7th characters A & B see Appendix B for HAC conditional logic

CC MCC +7th **S42.342 Displaced spiral fracture of shaft of humerus, left arm**
CC Exclusion 7th character A see Appendix A PDX collection 1250
CC Exclusion 7th characters K & P see Appendix A PDX collection 0897
MCC Exclusion 7th character B see Appendix A PDX collection 1246
HAC 7th characters A & B see Appendix B for HAC conditional logic

CC MCC +7th **S42.343 Displaced spiral fracture of shaft of humerus, unspecified arm**
CC Exclusion 7th character A see Appendix A PDX collection 1251
CC Exclusion 7th characters K & P see Appendix A PDX collection 0897
MCC Exclusion 7th character B see Appendix A PDX collection 1246
HAC 7th characters A & B see Appendix B for HAC conditional logic

CC MCC +7th **S42.344 Nondisplaced spiral fracture of shaft of humerus, right arm**
CC Exclusion 7th character A see Appendix A PDX collection 1249
CC Exclusion 7th characters K & P see Appendix A PDX collection 0897
MCC Exclusion 7th character B see Appendix A PDX collection 1246
HAC 7th characters A & B see Appendix B for HAC conditional logic

CC MCC +7th **S42.345** **Nondisplaced spiral fracture of shaft of humerus, left arm**
CC Exclusion 7th character A see Appendix A PDX collection 1250
CC Exclusion 7th characters K & P see Appendix A PDX collection 0897
MCC Exclusion 7th character B see Appendix A PDX collection 1246
HAC 7th characters A & B see Appendix B for HAC conditional logic

CC MCC +7th **S42.346** **Nondisplaced spiral fracture of shaft of humerus, unspecified arm**
CC Exclusion 7th character A see Appendix A PDX collection 1251
CC Exclusion 7th characters K & P see Appendix A PDX collection 0897
MCC Exclusion 7th character B see Appendix A PDX collection 1246
HAC 7th characters A & B see Appendix B for HAC conditional logic

\+ **S42.35** **Comminuted fracture of shaft of humerus**

CC MCC +7th **S42.351** **Displaced comminuted fracture of shaft of humerus, right arm**
CC Exclusion 7th character A see Appendix A PDX collection 1249
CC Exclusion 7th characters K & P see Appendix A PDX collection 0897
MCC Exclusion 7th character B see Appendix A PDX collection 1246
HAC 7th characters A & B see Appendix B for HAC conditional logic

CC MCC +7th **S42.352** **Displaced comminuted fracture of shaft of humerus, left arm**
CC Exclusion 7th character A see Appendix A PDX collection 1250
CC Exclusion 7th characters K & P see Appendix A PDX collection 0897
MCC Exclusion 7th character B see Appendix A PDX collection 1246
HAC 7th characters A & B see Appendix B for HAC conditional logic

CC MCC +7th **S42.353** **Displaced comminuted fracture of shaft of humerus, unspecified arm**
CC Exclusion 7th character A see Appendix A PDX collection 1251
CC Exclusion 7th characters K & P see Appendix A PDX collection 0897
MCC Exclusion 7th character B see Appendix A PDX collection 1246
HAC 7th characters A & B see Appendix B for HAC conditional logic

CC MCC +7th **S42.354** **Nondisplaced comminuted fracture of shaft of humerus, right arm**
CC Exclusion 7th character A see Appendix A PDX collection 1249
CC Exclusion 7th characters K & P see Appendix A PDX collection 0897
MCC Exclusion 7th character B see Appendix A PDX collection 1246
HAC 7th characters A & B see Appendix B for HAC conditional logic

CC MCC +7th **S42.355** **Nondisplaced comminuted fracture of shaft of humerus, left arm**
CC Exclusion 7th character A see Appendix A PDX collection 1250
CC Exclusion 7th characters K & P see Appendix A PDX collection 0897
MCC Exclusion 7th character B see Appendix A PDX collection 1246
HAC 7th characters A & B see Appendix B for HAC conditional logic

CC MCC +7th **S42.356** **Nondisplaced comminuted fracture of shaft of humerus, unspecified arm**
CC Exclusion 7th character A see Appendix A PDX collection 1251
CC Exclusion 7th characters K & P see Appendix A PDX collection 0897
MCC Exclusion 7th character B see Appendix A PDX collection 1246
HAC 7th characters A & B see Appendix B for HAC conditional logic

\+ **S42.36** **Segmental fracture of shaft of humerus**

CC MCC +7th **S42.361** **Displaced segmental fracture of shaft of humerus, right arm**
CC Exclusion 7th character A see Appendix A PDX collection 1249
CC Exclusion 7th characters K & P see Appendix A PDX collection 0897
MCC Exclusion 7th character B see Appendix A PDX collection 1246
HAC 7th characters A & B see Appendix B for HAC conditional logic

CC MCC +7th **S42.362** **Displaced segmental fracture of shaft of humerus, left arm**
CC Exclusion 7th character A see Appendix A PDX collection 1250
CC Exclusion 7th characters K & P see Appendix A PDX collection 0897
MCC Exclusion 7th character B see Appendix A PDX collection 1246
HAC 7th characters A & B see Appendix B for HAC conditional logic

CC MCC +7th **S42.363** **Displaced segmental fracture of shaft of humerus, unspecified arm**
CC Exclusion 7th character A see Appendix A PDX collection 1251
CC Exclusion 7th characters K & P see Appendix A PDX collection 0897
MCC Exclusion 7th character B see Appendix A PDX collection 1246
HAC 7th characters A & B see Appendix B for HAC conditional logic

CC MCC +7th **S42.364** **Nondisplaced segmental fracture of shaft of humerus, right arm**
CC Exclusion 7th character A see Appendix A PDX collection 1249
CC Exclusion 7th characters K & P see Appendix A PDX collection 0897
MCC Exclusion 7th character B see Appendix A PDX collection 1246
HAC 7th characters A & B see Appendix B for HAC conditional logic

CC MCC +7th **S42.365** **Nondisplaced segmental fracture of shaft of humerus, left arm**
CC Exclusion 7th character A see Appendix A PDX collection 1250
CC Exclusion 7th characters K & P see Appendix A PDX collection 0897
MCC Exclusion 7th character B see Appendix A PDX collection 1246
HAC 7th characters A & B see Appendix B for HAC conditional logic

CC MCC +7th **S42.366** **Nondisplaced segmental fracture of shaft of humerus, unspecified arm**
CC Exclusion 7th character A see Appendix A PDX collection 1251
CC Exclusion 7th characters K & P see Appendix A PDX collection 0897
MCC Exclusion 7th character B see Appendix A PDX collection 1246
HAC 7th characters A & B see Appendix B for HAC conditional logic

\+ **S42.39** **Other fracture of shaft of humerus**

CC MCC +7th **S42.391** **Other fracture of shaft of right humerus**
CC Exclusion 7th character A see Appendix A PDX collection 1249
CC Exclusion 7th characters K & P see Appendix A PDX collection 0897
MCC Exclusion 7th character B see Appendix A PDX collection 1246
HAC 7th characters A & B see Appendix B for HAC conditional logic

CC MCC +7th **S42.392** **Other fracture of shaft of left humerus**
CC Exclusion 7th character A see Appendix A PDX collection 1250
CC Exclusion 7th characters K & P see Appendix A PDX collection 0897
MCC Exclusion 7th character B see Appendix A PDX collection 1246
HAC 7th characters A & B see Appendix B for HAC conditional logic

CC MCC +7th **S42.399** **Other fracture of shaft of unspecified humerus**
CC Exclusion 7th character A see Appendix A PDX collection 1251
CC Exclusion 7th characters K & P see Appendix A PDX collection 0897
MCC Exclusion 7th character B see Appendix A PDX collection 1246
HAC 7th characters A & B see Appendix B for HAC conditional logic

+ **S42.4 Fracture of lower end of humerus**
Fracture of distal end of humerus
Excludes2: *fracture of shaft of humerus (S42.3-)*
physeal fracture of lower end of humerus (S49.1-)

+ **S42.40 Unspecified fracture of lower end of humerus**
Fracture of elbow NOS

CC MCC +7th **S42.401 Unspecified fracture of lower end of right humerus**
CC Exclusion 7th character A see Appendix A PDX collection 1245
CC Exclusion 7th characters K & P see Appendix A PDX collection 0897
MCC Exclusion 7th character B see Appendix A PDX collection 1246
HAC 7th characters A & B see Appendix B for HAC conditional logic

CC MCC +7th **S42.402 Unspecified fracture of lower end of left humerus**
CC Exclusion 7th character A see Appendix A PDX collection 1247
CC Exclusion 7th characters K & P see Appendix A PDX collection 0897
MCC Exclusion 7th character B see Appendix A PDX collection 1246
HAC 7th characters A & B see Appendix B for HAC conditional logic

CC MCC +7th **S42.409 Unspecified fracture of lower end of unspecified humerus**
CC Exclusion 7th character A see Appendix A PDX collection 1248
CC Exclusion 7th characters K & P see Appendix A PDX collection 0897
MCC Exclusion 7th character B see Appendix A PDX collection 1246
HAC 7th characters A & B see Appendix B for HAC conditional logic

+ **S42.41 Simple supracondylar fracture without intercondylar fracture of humerus**

CC MCC +7th **S42.411 Displaced simple supracondylar fracture without intercondylar fracture of right humerus**
CC Exclusion 7th character A see Appendix A PDX collection 1245
CC Exclusion 7th characters K & P see Appendix A PDX collection 0897
MCC Exclusion 7th character B see Appendix A PDX collection 1246
HAC 7th characters A & B see Appendix B for HAC conditional logic

CC MCC +7th **S42.412 Displaced simple supracondylar fracture without intercondylar fracture of left humerus**
CC Exclusion 7th character A see Appendix A PDX collection 1247
CC Exclusion 7th characters K & P see Appendix A PDX collection 0897
MCC Exclusion 7th character B see Appendix A PDX collection 1246
HAC 7th characters A & B see Appendix B for HAC conditional logic

CC MCC +7th **S42.413 Displaced simple supracondylar fracture without intercondylar fracture of unspecified humerus**
CC Exclusion 7th character A see Appendix A PDX collection 1248
CC Exclusion 7th characters K & P see Appendix A PDX collection 0897
MCC Exclusion 7th character B see Appendix A PDX collection 1246
HAC 7th characters A & B see Appendix B for HAC conditional logic

CC MCC +7th **S42.414 Nondisplaced simple supracondylar fracture without intercondylar fracture of right humerus**
CC Exclusion 7th character A see Appendix A PDX collection 1245
CC Exclusion 7th characters K & P see Appendix A PDX collection 0897
MCC Exclusion 7th character B see Appendix A PDX collection 1246
HAC 7th characters A & B see Appendix B for HAC conditional logic

CC MCC +7th **S42.415 Nondisplaced simple supracondylar fracture without intercondylar fracture of left humerus**
CC Exclusion 7th character A see Appendix A PDX collection 1247
CC Exclusion 7th characters K & P see Appendix A PDX collection 0897
MCC Exclusion 7th character B see Appendix PDX collection 1246
HAC 7th characters A & B see Appendix B for HAC conditional logic

CC MCC +7th **S42.416 Nondisplaced simple supracondylar fracture without intercondylar fracture of unspecified humerus**
CC Exclusion 7th character A see Appendix A PDX collection 1248
CC Exclusion 7th characters K & P see Appendix A PDX collection 0897
MCC Exclusion 7th character B see Appendix PDX collection 1246
HAC 7th characters A & B see Appendix B for HAC conditional logic

+ **S42.42 Comminuted supracondylar fracture without intercondylar fracture of humerus**

CC MCC +7th **S42.421 Displaced comminuted supracondylar fracture without intercondylar fracture of right humerus**
CC Exclusion 7th character A see Appendix A PDX collection 1245
CC Exclusion 7th characters K & P see Appendix A PDX collection 0897
MCC Exclusion 7th character B see Appendix PDX collection 1246
HAC 7th characters A & B see Appendix B for HAC conditional logic

CC MCC +7th **S42.422 Displaced comminuted supracondylar fracture without intercondylar fracture of left humerus**
CC Exclusion 7th character A see Appendix A PDX collection 1247
CC Exclusion 7th characters K & P see Appendix A PDX collection 0897
MCC Exclusion 7th character B see Appendix PDX collection 1246
HAC 7th characters A & B see Appendix B for HAC conditional logic

CC MCC +7th **S42.423 Displaced comminuted supracondylar fracture without intercondylar fracture of unspecified humerus**
CC Exclusion 7th character A see Appendix A PDX collection 1248
CC Exclusion 7th characters K & P see Appendix A PDX collection 0897
MCC Exclusion 7th character B see Appendix PDX collection 1246
HAC 7th characters A & B see Appendix B for HAC conditional logic

CC MCC +7th **S42.424 Nondisplaced comminuted supracondylar fracture without intercondylar fracture of right humerus**
CC Exclusion 7th character A see Appendix A PDX collection 1245
CC Exclusion 7th characters K & P see Appendix A PDX collection 0897
MCC Exclusion 7th character B see Appendix PDX collection 1246
HAC 7th characters A & B see Appendix B for HAC conditional logic

CC MCC +7th **S42.425 Nondisplaced comminuted supracondylar fracture without intercondylar fracture of left humerus**
CC Exclusion 7th character A see Appendix A PDX collection 1247
CC Exclusion 7th characters K & P see Appendix A PDX collection 0897
MCC Exclusion 7th character B see Appendix PDX collection 1246
HAC 7th characters A & B see Appendix B for HAC conditional logic

CC MCC +7th **S42.426 Nondisplaced comminuted supracondylar fracture without intercondylar fracture of unspecified humerus**
CC Exclusion 7th character A see Appendix A PDX collection 1248
CC Exclusion 7th characters K & P see Appendix A PDX collection 0897
MCC Exclusion 7th character B see Appendix A PDX collection 1246
HAC 7th characters A & B see Appendix B for HAC conditional logic

\+ **S42.43 Fracture (avulsion) of lateral epicondyle of humerus**

CC MCC +7th **S42.431 Displaced fracture (avulsion) of lateral epicondyle of right humerus**
CC Exclusion 7th character A see Appendix A PDX collection 1245
CC Exclusion 7th characters K & P see Appendix A PDX collection 0897
MCC Exclusion 7th character B see Appendix A PDX collection 1246
HAC 7th characters A & B see Appendix B for HAC conditional logic

CC MCC +7th **S42.432 Displaced fracture (avulsion) of lateral epicondyle of left humerus**
CC Exclusion 7th character A see Appendix A PDX collection 1247
CC Exclusion 7th characters K & P see Appendix A PDX collection 0897
MCC Exclusion 7th character B see Appendix A PDX collection 1246
HAC 7th characters A & B see Appendix B for HAC conditional logic

CC MCC +7th **S42.433 Displaced fracture (avulsion) of lateral epicondyle of unspecified humerus**
CC Exclusion 7th character A see Appendix A PDX collection 1248
CC Exclusion 7th characters K & P see Appendix A PDX collection 0897
MCC Exclusion 7th character B see Appendix A PDX collection 1246
HAC 7th characters A & B see Appendix B for HAC conditional logic

CC MCC +7th **S42.434 Nondisplaced fracture (avulsion) of lateral epicondyle of right humerus**
CC Exclusion 7th character A see Appendix A PDX collection 1245
CC Exclusion 7th characters K & P see Appendix A PDX collection 0897
MCC Exclusion 7th character B see Appendix A PDX collection 1246
HAC 7th characters A & B see Appendix B for HAC conditional logic

CC MCC +7th **S42.435 Nondisplaced fracture (avulsion) of lateral epicondyle of left humerus**
CC Exclusion 7th character A see Appendix A PDX collection 1247
CC Exclusion 7th characters K & P see Appendix A PDX collection 0897
MCC Exclusion 7th character B see Appendix A PDX collection 1246
HAC 7th characters A & B see Appendix B for HAC conditional logic

CC MCC +7th **S42.436 Nondisplaced fracture (avulsion) of lateral epicondyle of unspecified humerus**
CC Exclusion 7th character A see Appendix A PDX collection 1248
CC Exclusion 7th characters K & P see Appendix A PDX collection 0897
MCC Exclusion 7th character B see Appendix A PDX collection 1246
HAC 7th characters A & B see Appendix B for HAC conditional logic

\+ **S42.44 Fracture (avulsion) of medial epicondyle of humerus**

CC MCC +7th **S42.441 Displaced fracture (avulsion) of medial epicondyle of right humerus**
CC Exclusion 7th character A see Appendix A PDX collection 1245
CC Exclusion 7th characters K & P see Appendix A PDX collection 0897
MCC Exclusion 7th character B see Appendix A PDX collection 1246
HAC 7th characters A & B see Appendix B for HAC conditional logic

CC MCC +7th **S42.442 Displaced fracture (avulsion) of medial epicondyle of left humerus**
CC Exclusion 7th character A see Appendix A PDX collection 1247
CC Exclusion 7th characters K & P see Appendix A PDX collection 0897
MCC Exclusion 7th character B see Appendix A PDX collection 1246
HAC 7th characters A & B see Appendix B for HAC conditional logic

CC MCC +7th **S42.443 Displaced fracture (avulsion) of medial epicondyle of unspecified humerus**
CC Exclusion 7th character A see Appendix A PDX collection 1248
CC Exclusion 7th characters K & P see Appendix A PDX collection 0897
MCC Exclusion 7th character B see Appendix A PDX collection 1246
HAC 7th characters A & B see Appendix B for HAC conditional logic

CC MCC +7th **S42.444 Nondisplaced fracture (avulsion) of medial epicondyle of right humerus**
CC Exclusion 7th character A see Appendix A PDX collection 1245
CC Exclusion 7th characters K & P see Appendix A PDX collection 0897
MCC Exclusion 7th character B see Appendix A PDX collection 1246
HAC 7th characters A & B see Appendix B for HAC conditional logic

CC MCC +7th **S42.445 Nondisplaced fracture (avulsion) of medial epicondyle of left humerus**
CC Exclusion 7th character A see Appendix A PDX collection 1247
CC Exclusion 7th characters K & P see Appendix A PDX collection 0897
MCC Exclusion 7th character B see Appendix A PDX collection 1246
HAC 7th characters A & B see Appendix B for HAC conditional logic

CC MCC +7th **S42.446 Nondisplaced fracture (avulsion) of medial epicondyle of unspecified humerus**
CC Exclusion 7th character A see Appendix A PDX collection 1248
CC Exclusion 7th characters K & P see Appendix A PDX collection 0897
MCC Exclusion 7th character B see Appendix A PDX collection 1246
HAC 7th characters A & B see Appendix B for HAC conditional logic

CC MCC +7th **S42.447 Incarcerated fracture (avulsion) of medial epicondyle of right humerus**
CC Exclusion 7th character A see Appendix A PDX collection 1245
CC Exclusion 7th characters K & P see Appendix A PDX collection 0897
MCC Exclusion 7th character B see Appendix A PDX collection 1246
HAC 7th characters A & B see Appendix B for HAC conditional logic

CC MCC +7th **S42.448 Incarcerated fracture (avulsion) of medial epicondyle of left humerus**
CC Exclusion 7th character A see Appendix A PDX collection 1247
CC Exclusion 7th characters K & P see Appendix A PDX collection 0897
MCC Exclusion 7th character B see Appendix A PDX collection 1246
HAC 7th characters A & B see Appendix B for HAC conditional logic

CC MCC +7th **S42.449 Incarcerated fracture (avulsion) of medial epicondyle of unspecified humerus**
CC Exclusion 7th character A see Appendix A PDX collection 1248
CC Exclusion 7th characters K & P see Appendix A PDX collection 0897
MCC Exclusion 7th character B see Appendix A PDX collection 1246
HAC 7th characters A & B see Appendix B for HAC conditional logic

+ S42.45 **Fracture of lateral condyle of humerus**
Fracture of capitellum of humerus

CC MCC +7th **S42.451 Displaced fracture of lateral condyle of right humerus**
CC Exclusion 7th character A see Appendix A PDX collection 1245
CC Exclusion 7th characters K & P see Appendix A PDX collection 0897
MCC Exclusion 7th character B see Appendix A PDX collection 1246
HAC 7th characters A & B see Appendix B for HAC conditional logic

CC MCC +7th **S42.452 Displaced fracture of lateral condyle of left humerus**
CC Exclusion 7th character A see Appendix A PDX collection 1247
CC Exclusion 7th characters K & P see Appendix A PDX collection 0897
MCC Exclusion 7th character B see Appendix A PDX collection 1246
HAC 7th characters A & B see Appendix B for HAC conditional logic

CC MCC +7th **S42.453 Displaced fracture of lateral condyle of unspecified humerus**
CC Exclusion 7th character A see Appendix A PDX collection 1248
CC Exclusion 7th characters K & P see Appendix A PDX collection 0897
MCC Exclusion 7th character B see Appendix A PDX collection 1246
HAC 7th characters A & B see Appendix B for HAC conditional logic

CC MCC +7th **S42.454 Nondisplaced fracture of lateral condyle of right humerus**
CC Exclusion 7th character A see Appendix A PDX collection 1245
CC Exclusion 7th characters K & P see Appendix A PDX collection 0897
MCC Exclusion 7th character B see Appendix A PDX collection 1246
HAC 7th characters A & B see Appendix B for HAC conditional logic

CC MCC +7th **S42.455 Nondisplaced fracture of lateral condyle of left humerus**
CC Exclusion 7th character A see Appendix A PDX collection 1247
CC Exclusion 7th characters K & P see Appendix A PDX collection 0897
MCC Exclusion 7th character B see Appendix A PDX collection 1246
HAC 7th characters A & B see Appendix B for HAC conditional logic

CC MCC +7th **S42.456 Nondisplaced fracture of lateral condyle of unspecified humerus**
CC Exclusion 7th character A see Appendix A PDX collection 1248
CC Exclusion 7th characters K & P see Appendix A PDX collection 0897
MCC Exclusion 7th character B see Appendix A PDX collection 1246
HAC 7th characters A & B see Appendix B for HAC conditional logic

+ S42.46 **Fracture of medial condyle of humerus**
Trochlea fracture of humerus

CC MCC +7th **S42.461 Displaced fracture of medial condyle of right humerus**
CC Exclusion 7th character A see Appendix A PDX collection 1245
CC Exclusion 7th characters K & P see Appendix A PDX collection 0897
MCC Exclusion 7th character B see Appendix A PDX collection 1246
HAC 7th characters A & B see Appendix B for HAC conditional logic

CC MCC +7th **S42.462 Displaced fracture of medial condyle of left humerus**
CC Exclusion 7th character A see Appendix A PDX collection 1247
CC Exclusion 7th characters K & P see Appendix A PDX collection 0897
MCC Exclusion 7th character B see Appendix A PDX collection 1246
HAC 7th characters A & B see Appendix B for HAC conditional logic

CC MCC +7th **S42.463 Displaced fracture of medial condyle of unspecified humerus**
CC Exclusion 7th character A see Appendix A PDX collection 1248
CC Exclusion 7th characters K & P see Appendix A PDX collection 0897
MCC Exclusion 7th character B see Appendix PDX collection 1246
HAC 7th characters A & B see Appendix B for HAC conditional logic

CC MCC +7th **S42.464 Nondisplaced fracture of medial condyle right humerus**
CC Exclusion 7th character A see Appendix A PDX collection 1245
CC Exclusion 7th characters K & P see Appendix A PDX collection 0897
MCC Exclusion 7th character B see Appendix PDX collection 1246
HAC 7th characters A & B see Appendix B for HAC conditional logic

CC MCC +7th **S42.465 Nondisplaced fracture of medial condyle left humerus**
CC Exclusion 7th character A see Appendix A PDX collection 1247
CC Exclusion 7th characters K & P see Appendix A PDX collection 0897
MCC Exclusion 7th character B see Appendix PDX collection 1246
HAC 7th characters A & B see Appendix B for HAC conditional logic

CC MCC +7th **S42.466 Nondisplaced fracture of medial condyle unspecified humerus**
CC Exclusion 7th character A see Appendix A PDX collection 1248
CC Exclusion 7th characters K & P see Appendix A PDX collection 0897
MCC Exclusion 7th character B see Appendix PDX collection 1246
HAC 7th characters A & B see Appendix B for HAC conditional logic

+ S42.47 **Transcondylar fracture of humerus**

CC MCC +7th **S42.471 Displaced transcondylar fracture of right humerus**
CC Exclusion 7th character A see Appendix A PDX collection 1245
CC Exclusion 7th characters K & P see Appendix A PDX collection 0897
MCC Exclusion 7th character B see Appendix PDX collection 1246
HAC 7th characters A & B see Appendix B for HAC conditional logic

CC MCC +7th **S42.472 Displaced transcondylar fracture of left humerus**
CC Exclusion 7th character A see Appendix A PDX collection 1247
CC Exclusion 7th characters K & P see Appendix A PDX collection 0897
MCC Exclusion 7th character B see Appendix PDX collection 1246
HAC 7th characters A & B see Appendix B for HAC conditional logic

CC MCC +7th **S42.473 Displaced transcondylar fracture of unspecified humerus**
CC Exclusion 7th character A see Appendix A PDX collection 1248
CC Exclusion 7th characters K & P see Appendix A PDX collection 0897
MCC Exclusion 7th character B see Appendix PDX collection 1246
HAC 7th characters A & B see Appendix B for HAC conditional logic

CC MCC +7th **S42.474 Nondisplaced transcondylar fracture of right humerus**
CC Exclusion 7th character A see Appendix A PDX collection 1245
CC Exclusion 7th characters K & P see Appendix A PDX collection 0897
MCC Exclusion 7th character B see Appendix PDX collection 1246
HAC 7th characters A & B see Appendix B for HAC conditional logic

CC MCC +7th **S42.475 Nondisplaced transcondylar fracture of left humerus**
CC Exclusion 7th character A see Appendix A PDX collection 1247
CC Exclusion 7th characters K & P see Appendix A PDX collection 0897
MCC Exclusion 7th character B see Appendix A PDX collection 1246
HAC 7th characters A & B see Appendix B for HAC conditional logic

CC MCC +7th **S42.476 Nondisplaced transcondylar fracture of unspecified humerus**
CC Exclusion 7th character A see Appendix A PDX collection 1248
CC Exclusion 7th characters K & P see Appendix A PDX collection 0897
MCC Exclusion 7th character B see Appendix A PDX collection 1246
HAC 7th characters A & B see Appendix B for HAC conditional logic

+ **S42.48 Torus fracture of lower end of humerus**

The appropriate 7th character is to be added to all codes in subcategory **S42.48**
A initial encounter for closed fracture
D subsequent encounter for fracture with routine healing
G subsequent encounter for fracture with delayed healing
K subsequent encounter for fracture with nonunion
P subsequent encounter for fracture with malunion
S sequela

CC +7th **S42.481 Torus fracture of lower end of right humerus**
CC Exclusion 7th character A see Appendix A PDX collection 1245
CC Exclusion 7th characters K & P see Appendix A PDX collection 0897
HAC 7th character A see Appendix B for HAC conditional logic

CC +7th **S42.482 Torus fracture of lower end of left humerus**
CC Exclusion 7th character A see Appendix A PDX collection 1247
CC Exclusion 7th characters K & P see Appendix A PDX collection 0897
HAC 7th character A see Appendix B for HAC conditional logic

CC +7th **S42.489 Torus fracture of lower end of unspecified humerus**
CC Exclusion 7th character A see Appendix A PDX collection 1248
CC Exclusion 7th characters K & P see Appendix A PDX collection 0897
HAC 7th character A see Appendix B for HAC conditional logic

+ **S42.49 Other fracture of lower end of humerus**

CC MCC +7th **S42.491 Other displaced fracture of lower end of right humerus**
CC Exclusion 7th character A see Appendix A PDX collection 1245
CC Exclusion 7th characters K & P see Appendix A PDX collection 0897
MCC Exclusion 7th character B see Appendix A PDX collection 1246
HAC 7th characters A & B see Appendix B for HAC conditional logic

CC MCC +7th **S42.492 Other displaced fracture of lower end of left humerus**
CC Exclusion 7th character A see Appendix A PDX collection 1247
CC Exclusion 7th characters K & P see Appendix A PDX collection 0897
MCC Exclusion 7th character B see Appendix A PDX collection 1246
HAC 7th characters A & B see Appendix B for HAC conditional logic

CC MCC +7th **S42.493 Other displaced fracture of lower end of unspecified humerus**
CC Exclusion 7th character A see Appendix A PDX collection 1248
CC Exclusion 7th characters K & P see Appendix A PDX collection 0897
MCC Exclusion 7th character B see Appendix A PDX collection 1246
HAC 7th characters A & B see Appendix B for HAC conditional logic

CC MCC +7th **S42.494 Other nondisplaced fracture of lower end of right humerus**
CC Exclusion 7th character A see Appendix A PDX collection 1245
CC Exclusion 7th characters K & P see Appendix A PDX collection 0897
MCC Exclusion 7th character B see Appendix A PDX collection 1246
HAC 7th characters A & B see Appendix B for HAC conditional logic

CC MCC +7th **S42.495 Other nondisplaced fracture of lower end of left humerus**
CC Exclusion 7th character A see Appendix A PDX collection 1247
CC Exclusion 7th characters K & P see Appendix A PDX collection 0897
MCC Exclusion 7th character B see Appendix A PDX collection 1246
HAC 7th characters A & B see Appendix B for HAC conditional logic

CC MCC +7th **S42.496 Other nondisplaced fracture of lower end of unspecified humerus**
CC Exclusion 7th character A see Appendix A PDX collection 1248
CC Exclusion 7th characters K & P see Appendix A PDX collection 0897
MCC Exclusion 7th character B see Appendix A PDX collection 1246
HAC 7th characters A & B see Appendix B for HAC conditional logic

+ **S42.9 Fracture of shoulder girdle, part unspecified**
Fracture of shoulder NOS

CC MCC X+7th **S42.90 Fracture of unspecified shoulder girdle, part unspecified**
CC Exclusion 7th character A see Appendix A PDX collection 1248
CC Exclusion 7th characters K & P see Appendix A PDX collection 0897
MCC Exclusion 7th character B see Appendix A PDX collection 1246
HAC 7th characters A & B see Appendix B for HAC conditional logic

CC MCC X+7th **S42.91 Fracture of right shoulder girdle, part unspecified**
CC Exclusion 7th character A see Appendix A PDX collection 1248
CC Exclusion 7th characters K & P see Appendix A PDX collection 0897
MCC Exclusion 7th character B see Appendix A PDX collection 1246
HAC 7th characters A & B see Appendix B for HAC conditional logic

CC MCC X+7th **S42.92 Fracture of left shoulder girdle, part unspecified**
CC Exclusion 7th character A see Appendix A PDX collection 1248
CC Exclusion 7th characters K & P see Appendix A PDX collection 0897
MCC Exclusion 7th character B see Appendix A PDX collection 1246
HAC 7th characters A & B see Appendix B for HAC conditional logic

S43 Dislocation and sprain of joints and ligaments of shoulder girdle

Includes: avulsion of joint or ligament of shoulder girdle
laceration of cartilage, joint or ligament of shoulder girdle
sprain of cartilage, joint or ligament of shoulder girdle
traumatic hemarthrosis of joint or ligament of shoulder girdle
traumatic rupture of joint or ligament of shoulder girdle
traumatic subluxation of joint or ligament of shoulder girdle
traumatic tear of joint or ligament of shoulder girdle

Code also any associated open wound

Excludes2: *strain of muscle, fascia and tendon of shoulder and upper arm (S46.-)*

The appropriate 7th character is to be added to each code from category S43
A initial encounter
D subsequent encounter
S sequela

+ **S43.0 Subluxation and dislocation of shoulder joint**
Dislocation of glenohumeral joint
Subluxation of glenohumeral joint

+ **S43.00 Unspecified subluxation and dislocation of shoulder joint**
Dislocation of humerus NOS
Subluxation of humerus NOS

+7th **S43.001 Unspecified subluxation of right shoulder joint**

+7th **S43.002** Unspecified subluxation of left shoulder joint
+7th **S43.003** Unspecified subluxation of unspecified shoulder joint
+7th **S43.004** Unspecified dislocation of right shoulder joint
+7th **S43.005** Unspecified dislocation of left shoulder joint
+7th **S43.006** Unspecified dislocation of unspecified shoulder joint

\+ **S43.01** Anterior subluxation and dislocation of humerus
+7th **S43.011** Anterior subluxation of right humerus
+7th **S43.012** Anterior subluxation of left humerus
+7th **S43.013** Anterior subluxation of unspecified humerus
+7th **S43.014** Anterior dislocation of right humerus
+7th **S43.015** Anterior dislocation of left humerus
+7th **S43.016** Anterior dislocation of unspecified humerus

\+ **S43.02** Posterior subluxation and dislocation of humerus
+7th **S43.021** Posterior subluxation of right humerus
+7th **S43.022** Posterior subluxation of left humerus
+7th **S43.023** Posterior subluxation of unspecified humerus
+7th **S43.024** Posterior dislocation of right humerus
+7th **S43.025** Posterior dislocation of left humerus
+7th **S43.026** Posterior dislocation of unspecified humerus

\+ **S43.03** Inferior subluxation and dislocation of humerus
+7th **S43.031** Inferior subluxation of right humerus
+7th **S43.032** Inferior subluxation of left humerus
+7th **S43.033** Inferior subluxation of unspecified humerus
+7th **S43.034** Inferior dislocation of right humerus
+7th **S43.035** Inferior dislocation of left humerus
+7th **S43.036** Inferior dislocation of unspecified humerus

\+ **S43.08** Other subluxation and dislocation of shoulder joint
+7th **S43.081** Other subluxation of right shoulder joint
+7th **S43.082** Other subluxation of left shoulder joint
+7th **S43.083** Other subluxation of unspecified shoulder joint
+7th **S43.084** Other dislocation of right shoulder joint
+7th **S43.085** Other dislocation of left shoulder joint
+7th **S43.086** Other dislocation of unspecified shoulder joint

\+ **S43.1** Subluxation and dislocation of acromioclavicular joint

\+ **S43.10** Unspecified dislocation of acromioclavicular joint
+7th **S43.101** Unspecified dislocation of right acromioclavicular joint
+7th **S43.102** Unspecified dislocation of left acromioclavicular joint
+7th **S43.109** Unspecified dislocation of unspecified acromioclavicular joint

\+ **S43.11** Subluxation of acromioclavicular joint
+7th **S43.111** Subluxation of right acromioclavicular joint
+7th **S43.112** Subluxation of left acromioclavicular joint
+7th **S43.119** Subluxation of unspecified acromioclavicular joint

\+ **S43.12** Dislocation of acromioclavicular joint, 100%-200% displacement
+7th **S43.121** Dislocation of right acromioclavicular joint, 100%-200% displacement
+7th **S43.122** Dislocation of left acromioclavicular joint, 100%-200% displacement
+7th **S43.129** Dislocation of unspecified acromioclavicular joint, 100%-200% displacement

\+ **S43.13** Dislocation of acromioclavicular joint, greater than 200% displacement
+7th **S43.131** Dislocation of right acromioclavicular joint, greater than 200% displacement
+7th **S43.132** Dislocation of left acromioclavicular joint, greater than 200% displacement
+7th **S43.139** Dislocation of unspecified acromioclavicular joint, greater than 200% displacement

\+ **S43.14** Inferior dislocation of acromioclavicular joint
+7th **S43.141** Inferior dislocation of right acromioclavicular joint
+7th **S43.142** Inferior dislocation of left acromioclavicular joint
+7th **S43.149** Inferior dislocation of unspecified acromioclavicular joint

\+ **S43.15** Posterior dislocation of acromioclavicular joint
+7th **S43.151** Posterior dislocation of right acromioclavicular joint
+7th **S43.152** Posterior dislocation of left acromioclavicular joint
+7th **S43.159** Posterior dislocation of unspecified acromioclavicular joint

\+ **S43.2** Subluxation and dislocation of sternoclavicular joint

\+ **S43.20** Unspecified subluxation and dislocation of sternoclavicular joint

CC +7th **S43.201** Unspecified subluxation of right sternoclavicular joint
CC Exclusion 7th character A see Appendix A PDX collection 1252
HAC 7th character A see Appendix B for HAC conditional logic

CC +7th **S43.202** Unspecified subluxation of left sternoclavicular joint
CC Exclusion 7th character A see Appendix A PDX collection 1253
HAC 7th character A see Appendix B for HAC conditional logic

CC +7th **S43.203** Unspecified subluxation of unspecified sternoclavicular joint
CC Exclusion 7th character A see Appendix A PDX collection 0914
HAC 7th character A see Appendix B for HAC conditional logic

CC +7th **S43.204** Unspecified dislocation of right sternoclavicular joint
CC Exclusion 7th character A see Appendix A PDX collection 1252
HAC 7th character A see Appendix B for HAC conditional logic

CC +7th **S43.205** Unspecified dislocation of left sternoclavicular joint
CC Exclusion 7th character A see Appendix A PDX collection 1253
HAC 7th character A see Appendix B for HAC conditional logic

CC +7th **S43.206** Unspecified dislocation of unspecified sternoclavicular joint
CC Exclusion 7th character A see Appendix A PDX collection 0914
HAC 7th character A see Appendix B for HAC conditional logic

\+ **S43.21** Anterior subluxation and dislocation of sternoclavicular joint

CC +7th **S43.211** Anterior subluxation of right sternoclavicular joint
CC Exclusion 7th character A see Appendix A PDX collection 1252
HAC 7th character A see Appendix B for HAC conditional logic

CC +7th **S43.212** Anterior subluxation of left sternoclavicular joint
CC Exclusion 7th character A see Appendix A PDX collection 1253
HAC 7th character A see Appendix B for HAC conditional logic

CC +7th **S43.213** Anterior subluxation of unspecified sternoclavicular joint
CC Exclusion 7th character A see Appendix A PDX collection 0914
HAC 7th character A see Appendix B for HAC conditional logic

CC +7th **S43.214** Anterior dislocation of right sternoclavicular joint
CC Exclusion 7th character A see Appendix A PDX collection 1252
HAC 7th character A see Appendix B for HAC conditional logic

CC +7th **S43.215** Anterior dislocation of left sternoclavicular joint
CC Exclusion 7th character A see Appendix A PDX collection 1253
HAC 7th character A see Appendix B for HAC conditional logic

CC +7th **S43.216** **Anterior dislocation of unspecified sternoclavicular joint**
CC Exclusion 7th character A see Appendix A PDX collection 0914
HAC 7th character A see Appendix B for HAC conditional logic

\+ **S43.22** **Posterior subluxation and dislocation of sternoclavicular joint**

CC +7th **S43.221** **Posterior subluxation of right sternoclavicular joint**
CC Exclusion 7th character A see Appendix A PDX collection 1252
HAC 7th character A see Appendix B for HAC conditional logic

CC +7th **S43.222** **Posterior subluxation of left sternoclavicular joint**
CC Exclusion 7th character A see Appendix A PDX collection 1253
HAC 7th character A see Appendix B for HAC conditional logic

CC +7th **S43.223** **Posterior subluxation of unspecified sternoclavicular joint**
CC Exclusion 7th character A see Appendix A PDX collection 0914
HAC 7th character A see Appendix B for HAC conditional logic

CC +7th **S43.224** **Posterior dislocation of right sternoclavicular joint**
CC Exclusion 7th character A see Appendix A PDX collection 1252
HAC 7th character A see Appendix B for HAC conditional logic

CC +7th **S43.225** **Posterior dislocation of left sternoclavicular joint**
CC Exclusion 7th character A see Appendix A PDX collection 1253
HAC 7th character A see Appendix B for HAC conditional logic

CC +7th **S43.226** **Posterior dislocation of unspecified sternoclavicular joint**
CC Exclusion 7th character A see Appendix A PDX collection 0914

\+ **S43.3** **Subluxation and dislocation of other and unspecified parts of shoulder girdle**

\+ **S43.30** **Subluxation and dislocation of unspecified parts of shoulder girdle**
Dislocation of shoulder girdle NOS
Subluxation of shoulder girdle NOS

+7th **S43.301** **Subluxation of unspecified parts of right shoulder girdle**
+7th **S43.302** **Subluxation of unspecified parts of left shoulder girdle**
+7th **S43.303** **Subluxation of unspecified parts of unspecified shoulder girdle**
+7th **S43.304** **Dislocation of unspecified parts of right shoulder girdle**
+7th **S43.305** **Dislocation of unspecified parts of left shoulder girdle**
+7th **S43.306** **Dislocation of unspecified parts of unspecified shoulder girdle**

\+ **S43.31** **Subluxation and dislocation of scapula**
+7th **S43.311** **Subluxation of right scapula**
+7th **S43.312** **Subluxation of left scapula**
+7th **S43.313** **Subluxation of unspecified scapula**
+7th **S43.314** **Dislocation of right scapula**
+7th **S43.315** **Dislocation of left scapula**
+7th **S43.316** **Dislocation of unspecified scapula**

\+ **S43.39** **Subluxation and dislocation of other parts of shoulder girdle**
+7th **S43.391** **Subluxation of other parts of right shoulder girdle**
+7th **S43.392** **Subluxation of other parts of left shoulder girdle**
+7th **S43.393** **Subluxation of other parts of unspecified shoulder girdle**
+7th **S43.394** **Dislocation of other parts of right shoulder girdle**
+7th **S43.395** **Dislocation of other parts of left shoulder girdle**
+7th **S43.396** **Dislocation of other parts of unspecified shoulder girdle**

\+ **S43.4** **Sprain of shoulder joint**

\+ **S43.40** **Unspecified sprain of shoulder joint**
+7th **S43.401** **Unspecified sprain of right shoulder joint**
+7th **S43.402** **Unspecified sprain of left shoulder joint**
+7th **S43.409** **Unspecified sprain of unspecified shoulder joint**

\+ **S43.41** **Sprain of coracohumeral (ligament)**
+7th **S43.411** **Sprain of right coracohumeral (ligament)**
+7th **S43.412** **Sprain of left coracohumeral (ligament)**
+7th **S43.419** **Sprain of unspecified coracohumeral (ligament)**

\+ **S43.42** **Sprain of rotator cuff capsule**
Excludes1: *rotator cuff syndrome (complete) (incomplete), not specified as traumatic (M75.1-)*
Excludes2: *injury of tendon of rotator cuff (S46.0-)*
+7th **S43.421** **Sprain of right rotator cuff capsule**
+7th **S43.422** **Sprain of left rotator cuff capsule**
+7th **S43.429** **Sprain of unspecified rotator cuff capsule**

\+ **S43.43** **Superior glenoid labrum lesion**
SLAP lesion
+7th **S43.431** **Superior glenoid labrum lesion of right shoulder**
+7th **S43.432** **Superior glenoid labrum lesion of left shoulder**
+7th **S43.439** **Superior glenoid labrum lesion of unspecified shoulder**

\+ **S43.49** **Other sprain of shoulder joint**
S43.491 **Other sprain of right shoulder joint**
S43.492 **Other sprain of left shoulder joint**
S43.499 **Other sprain of unspecified shoulder joint**

\+ **S43.5** **Sprain of acromioclavicular joint**
Sprain of acromioclavicular ligament
X+7th **S43.50** **Sprain of unspecified acromioclavicular joint**
X+7th **S43.51** **Sprain of right acromioclavicular joint**
X+7th **S43.52** **Sprain of left acromioclavicular joint**

\+ **S43.6** **Sprain of sternoclavicular joint**
X+7th **S43.60** **Sprain of unspecified sternoclavicular joint**
X+7th **S43.61** **Sprain of right sternoclavicular joint**
X+7th **S43.62** **Sprain of left sternoclavicular joint**

\+ **S43.8** **Sprain of other specified parts of shoulder girdle**
X+7th **S43.80** **Sprain of other specified parts of unspecified shoulder girdle**
X+7th **S43.81** **Sprain of other specified parts of right shoulder girdle**
X+7th **S43.82** **Sprain of other specified parts of left shoulder girdle**

\+ **S43.9** **Sprain of unspecified parts of shoulder girdle**
X+7th **S43.90** **Sprain of unspecified parts of unspecified shoulder girdle**
Sprain of shoulder girdle NOS
X+7th **S43.91** **Sprain of unspecified parts of right shoulder girdle**
X+7th **S43.92** **Sprain of unspecified parts of left shoulder girdle**

S44 Injury of nerves at shoulder and upper arm level

Code also any associated open wound (S41.-)
Excludes2: *injury of brachial plexus (S14.3-)*

The appropriate 7th character is to be added to each code from category S44
A initial encounter
D subsequent encounter
S sequela

\+ **S44.0** **Injury of ulnar nerve at upper arm level**
Excludes1: *ulnar nerve NOS (S54.0)*
X+7th **S44.00** **Injury of ulnar nerve at upper arm level, unspecified arm**
X+7th **S44.01** **Injury of ulnar nerve at upper arm level, right arm**
X+7th **S44.02** **Injury of ulnar nerve at upper arm level, left arm**

\+ **S44.1** **Injury of median nerve at upper arm level**
Excludes1: *median nerve NOS (S54.1)*
X+7th **S44.10** **Injury of median nerve at upper arm level, unspecified arm**
X+7th **S44.11** **Injury of median nerve at upper arm level, right arm**
X+7th **S44.12** **Injury of median nerve at upper arm level, left arm**

\+ **S44.2** **Injury of radial nerve at upper arm level**
Excludes1: *radial nerve NOS (S54.2)*
X+7th **S44.20** **Injury of radial nerve at upper arm level, unspecified arm**
X+7th **S44.21** **Injury of radial nerve at upper arm level, right arm**
X+7th **S44.22** **Injury of radial nerve at upper arm level, left arm**

\+ **S44.3 Injury of axillary nerve**
X+7th **S44.30 Injury of axillary nerve, unspecified arm**
X+7th **S44.31 Injury of axillary nerve, right arm**
X+7th **S44.32 Injury of axillary nerve, left arm**
\+ **S44.4 Injury of musculocutaneous nerve**
X+7th **S44.40 Injury of musculocutaneous nerve, unspecified arm**
X+7th **S44.41 Injury of musculocutaneous nerve, right arm**
X+7th **S44.42 Injury of musculocutaneous nerve, left arm**
\+ **S44.5 Injury of cutaneous sensory nerve at shoulder and upper arm level**
X+7th **S44.50 Injury of cutaneous sensory nerve at shoulder and upper arm level, unspecified arm**
X+7th **S44.51 Injury of cutaneous sensory nerve at shoulder and upper arm level, right arm**
X+7th **S44.52 Injury of cutaneous sensory nerve at shoulder and upper arm level, left arm**
\+ **S44.8 Injury of other nerves at shoulder and upper arm level**
\+ **S44.8X Injury of other nerves at shoulder and upper arm level**
+7th **S44.8X1 Injury of other nerves at shoulder and upper arm level, right arm**
+7th **S44.8X2 Injury of other nerves at shoulder and upper arm level, left arm**
+7th **S44.8X9 Injury of other nerves at shoulder and upper arm level, unspecified arm**
\+ **S44.9 Injury of unspecified nerve at shoulder and upper arm level**
X+7th **S44.90 Injury of unspecified nerve at shoulder and upper arm level, unspecified arm**
X+7th **S44.91 Injury of unspecified nerve at shoulder and upper arm level, right arm**
X+7th **S44.92 Injury of unspecified nerve at shoulder and upper arm level, left arm**

S45 Injury of blood vessels at shoulder and upper arm level

Code also any associated open wound (S41.-)
Excludes2: *injury of subclavian artery (S25.1)*
injury of subclavian vein (S25.3)

The appropriate 7th character is to be added to each code from category S45
A initial encounter
D subsequent encounter
S sequela

\+ **S45.0 Injury of axillary artery**
\+ **S45.00 Unspecified injury of axillary artery**
MCC +7th **S45.001 Unspecified injury of axillary artery, right side**
MCC Exclusion 7th character A see Appendix A
PDX collection 1254
MCC +7th **S45.002 Unspecified injury of axillary artery, left side**
MCC Exclusion 7th character A see Appendix A
PDX collection 1255
MCC +7th **S45.009 Unspecified injury of axillary artery, unspecified side**
MCC Exclusion 7th character A see Appendix A
PDX collection 1256
\+ **S45.01 Laceration of axillary artery**
MCC +7th **S45.011 Laceration of axillary artery, right side**
MCC Exclusion 7th character A see Appendix A
PDX collection 1254
MCC +7th **S45.012 Laceration of axillary artery, left side**
MCC Exclusion 7th character A see Appendix A
PDX collection 1255
MCC +7th **S45.019 Laceration of axillary artery, unspecified side**
MCC Exclusion 7th character A see Appendix A
PDX collection 1256
\+ **S45.09 Other specified injury of axillary artery**
MCC +7th **S45.091 Other specified injury of axillary artery, right side**
MCC Exclusion 7th character A see Appendix A
PDX collection 1254
MCC +7th **S45.092 Other specified injury of axillary artery, left side**
MCC Exclusion 7th character A see Appendix A
PDX collection 1255
MCC +7th **S45.099 Other specified injury of axillary artery, unspecified side**
MCC Exclusion 7th character A see Appendix A
PDX collection 1256

\+ **S45.1 Injury of brachial artery**
\+ **S45.10 Unspecified injury of brachial artery**
CC +7th **S45.101 Unspecified injury of brachial artery, right side**
CC Exclusion 7th character A see Appendix A
PDX collection 1257
CC +7th **S45.102 Unspecified injury of brachial artery, left side**
CC Exclusion 7th character A see Appendix A
PDX collection 1258
CC +7th **S45.109 Unspecified injury of brachial artery, unspecified side**
CC Exclusion 7th character A see Appendix A
PDX collection 1259
\+ **S45.11 Laceration of brachial artery**
CC +7th **S45.111 Laceration of brachial artery, right side**
CC Exclusion 7th character A see Appendix A
PDX collection 1257
CC +7th **S45.112 Laceration of brachial artery, left side**
CC Exclusion 7th character A see Appendix A
PDX collection 1258
CC +7th **S45.119 Laceration of brachial artery, unspecified side**
CC Exclusion 7th character A see Appendix A
PDX collection 1259
\+ **S45.19 Other specified injury of brachial artery**
CC +7th **S45.191 Other specified injury of brachial artery, right side**
CC Exclusion 7th character A see Appendix A
PDX collection 1257
CC +7th **S45.192 Other specified injury of brachial artery, left side**
CC Exclusion 7th character A see Appendix A
PDX collection 1258
CC +7th **S45.199 Other specified injury of brachial artery, unspecified side**
CC Exclusion 7th character A see Appendix A
PDX collection 1259
\+ **S45.2 Injury of axillary or brachial vein**
\+ **S45.20 Unspecified injury of axillary or brachial vein**
CC +7th **S45.201 Unspecified injury of axillary or brachial vein, right side**
CC Exclusion 7th character A see Appendix A
PDX collection 1257
CC +7th **S45.202 Unspecified injury of axillary or brachial vein, left side**
CC Exclusion 7th character A see Appendix A
PDX collection 1258
CC +7th **S45.209 Unspecified injury of axillary or brachial vein, unspecified side**
CC Exclusion 7th character A see Appendix A
PDX collection 1259
\+ **S45.21 Laceration of axillary or brachial vein**
CC +7th **S45.211 Laceration of axillary or brachial vein, right side**
CC Exclusion 7th character A see Appendix A
PDX collection 1257
CC +7th **S45.212 Laceration of axillary or brachial vein, left side**
CC Exclusion 7th character A see Appendix A
PDX collection 1258
CC +7th **S45.219 Laceration of axillary or brachial vein, unspecified side**
CC Exclusion 7th character A see Appendix A
PDX collection 1259
\+ **S45.29 Other specified injury of axillary or brachial vein**
CC +7th **S45.291 Other specified injury of axillary or brachial vein, right side**
CC Exclusion 7th character A see Appendix A
PDX collection 1257
CC +7th **S45.292 Other specified injury of axillary or brachial vein, left side**
CC Exclusion 7th character A see Appendix A
PDX collection 1258
CC +7th **S45.299 Other specified injury of axillary or brachial vein, unspecified side**
CC Exclusion 7th character A see Appendix A
PDX collection 1259

+ S45.3 Injury of superficial vein at shoulder and upper arm level
+ S45.30 Unspecified injury of superficial vein at shoulder and upper arm level
CC +7th S45.301 Unspecified injury of superficial vein at shoulder and upper arm level, right arm
CC Exclusion 7th character A see Appendix A
PDX collection 1260
CC +7th S45.302 Unspecified injury of superficial vein at shoulder and upper arm level, left arm
CC Exclusion 7th character A see Appendix A
PDX collection 1261
CC +7th S45.309 Unspecified injury of superficial vein at shoulder and upper arm level, unspecified arm
CC Exclusion 7th character A see Appendix A
PDX collection 1262
+ S45.31 Laceration of superficial vein at shoulder and upper arm level
CC +7th S45.311 Laceration of superficial vein at shoulder and upper arm level, right arm
CC Exclusion 7th character A see Appendix A
PDX collection 1260
CC +7th S45.312 Laceration of superficial vein at shoulder and upper arm level, left arm
CC Exclusion 7th character A see Appendix A
PDX collection 1261
CC +7th S45.319 Laceration of superficial vein at shoulder and upper arm level, unspecified arm
CC Exclusion 7th character A see Appendix A
PDX collection 1262
+ S45.39 Other specified injury of superficial vein at shoulder and upper arm level
CC +7th S45.391 Other specified injury of superficial vein at shoulder and upper arm level, right arm
CC Exclusion 7th character A see Appendix A
PDX collection 1260
CC +7th S45.392 Other specified injury of superficial vein at shoulder and upper arm level, left arm
CC Exclusion 7th character A see Appendix A
PDX collection 1261
CC +7th S45.399 Other specified injury of superficial vein at shoulder and upper arm level, unspecified arm
CC Exclusion 7th character A see Appendix A
PDX collection 1262
+ S45.8 Injury of other specified blood vessels at shoulder and upper arm level
+ S45.80 Unspecified injury of other specified blood vessels at shoulder and upper arm level
CC +7th S45.801 Unspecified injury of other specified blood vessels at shoulder and upper arm level, right arm
CC Exclusion 7th character A see Appendix A
PDX collection 1260
CC +7th S45.802 Unspecified injury of other specified blood vessels at shoulder and upper arm level, left arm
CC Exclusion 7th character A see Appendix A
PDX collection 1261
CC +7th S45.809 Unspecified injury of other specified blood vessels at shoulder and upper arm level, unspecified arm
CC Exclusion 7th character A see Appendix A
PDX collection 1262
+ S45.81 Laceration of other specified blood vessels at shoulder and upper arm level
CC +7th S45.811 Laceration of other specified blood vessels at shoulder and upper arm level, right arm
CC Exclusion 7th character A see Appendix A
PDX collection 1260
CC +7th S45.812 Laceration of other specified blood vessels at shoulder and upper arm level, left arm
CC Exclusion 7th character A see Appendix A
PDX collection 1261
CC +7th S45.819 Laceration of other specified blood vessels at shoulder and upper arm level, unspecified arm
CC Exclusion 7th character A see Appendix A
PDX collection 1262
+ S45.89 Other specified injury of other specified blood vessels at shoulder and upper arm level
CC +7th S45.891 Other specified injury of other specified blood vessels at shoulder and upper arm level, right arm
CC Exclusion 7th character A see Appendix A
PDX collection 1260
CC +7th S45.892 Other specified injury of other specified blood vessels at shoulder and upper arm level, left arm
CC Exclusion 7th character A see Appendix A
PDX collection 1261
CC +7th S45.899 Other specified injury of other specified blood vessels at shoulder and upper arm level, unspecified arm
CC Exclusion 7th character A see Appendix A
PDX collection 1262
+ S45.9 Injury of unspecified blood vessel at shoulder and upper arm level
+ S45.90 Unspecified injury of unspecified blood vessel at shoulder and upper arm level
CC +7th S45.901 Unspecified injury of unspecified blood vessel at shoulder and upper arm level, right arm
CC Exclusion 7th character A see Appendix A
PDX collection 1260
CC +7th S45.902 Unspecified injury of unspecified blood vessel at shoulder and upper arm level, left arm
CC Exclusion 7th character A see Appendix A
PDX collection 1261
CC +7th S45.909 Unspecified injury of unspecified blood vessel at shoulder and upper arm level, unspecified arm
CC Exclusion 7th character A see Appendix A
PDX collection 1262
+ S45.91 Laceration of unspecified blood vessel at shoulder and upper arm level
CC +7th S45.911 Laceration of unspecified blood vessel at shoulder and upper arm level, right arm
CC Exclusion 7th character A see Appendix A
PDX collection 1260
CC +7th S45.912 Laceration of unspecified blood vessel at shoulder and upper arm level, left arm
CC Exclusion 7th character A see Appendix A
PDX collection 1261
CC +7th S45.919 Laceration of unspecified blood vessel at shoulder and upper arm level, unspecified arm
CC Exclusion 7th character A see Appendix A
PDX collection 1262
+ S45.99 Other specified injury of unspecified blood vessel at shoulder and upper arm level
CC +7th S45.991 Other specified injury of unspecified blood vessel at shoulder and upper arm level, right arm
CC Exclusion 7th character A see Appendix A
PDX collection 1260
CC +7th S45.992 Other specified injury of unspecified blood vessel at shoulder and upper arm level, left arm
CC Exclusion 7th character A see Appendix A
PDX collection 1261
CC +7th S45.999 Other specified injury of unspecified blood vessel at shoulder and upper arm level, unspecified arm
CC Exclusion 7th character A see Appendix A
PDX collection 1262

S46 Injury of muscle, fascia and tendon at shoulder and upper arm level

Code also any associated open wound (S41.-)

Excludes2: *injury of muscle, fascia and tendon at elbow (S56.-)*
sprain of joints and ligaments of shoulder girdle (S43.9)

The appropriate 7th character is to be added to each code from category S46
A initial encounter
D subsequent encounter
S sequela

+ **S46.0 Injury of muscle(s) and tendon(s) of the rotator cuff of shoulder**
  + **S46.00 Unspecified injury of muscle(s) and tendon(s) of the rotator cuff of shoulder**
    - +7th **S46.001 Unspecified injury of muscle(s) and tendon(s) of the rotator cuff of right shoulder**
    - +7th **S46.002 Unspecified injury of muscle(s) and tendon(s) of the rotator cuff of left shoulder**
    - +7th **S46.009 Unspecified injury of muscle(s) and tendon(s) of the rotator cuff of unspecified shoulder**
  + **S46.01 Strain of muscle(s) and tendon(s) of the rotator cuff of shoulder**
    - +7th **S46.011 Strain of muscle(s) and tendon(s) of the rotator cuff of right shoulder**
    - +7th **S46.012 Strain of muscle(s) and tendon(s) of the rotator cuff of left shoulder**
    - +7th **S46.019 Strain of muscle(s) and tendon(s) of the rotator cuff of unspecified shoulder**
  + **S46.02 Laceration of muscle(s) and tendon(s) of the rotator cuff of shoulder**
    - CC +7th **S46.021 Laceration of muscle(s) and tendon(s) of the rotator cuff of right shoulder**
      CC Exclusion 7th character A see Appendix A PDX collection 1263
    - CC +7th **S46.022 Laceration of muscle(s) and tendon(s) of the rotator cuff of left shoulder**
      CC Exclusion 7th character A see Appendix A PDX collection 1264
    - CC +7th **S46.029 Laceration of muscle(s) and tendon(s) of the rotator cuff of unspecified shoulder**
      CC Exclusion 7th character A see Appendix A PDX collection 1265
  + **S46.09 Other injury of muscle(s) and tendon(s) of the rotator cuff of shoulder**
    - +7th **S46.091 Other injury of muscle(s) and tendon(s) of the rotator cuff of right shoulder**
    - +7th **S46.092 Other injury of muscle(s) and tendon(s) of the rotator cuff of left shoulder**
    - +7th **S46.099 Other injury of muscle(s) and tendon(s) of the rotator cuff of unspecified shoulder**

+ **S46.1 Injury of muscle, fascia and tendon of long head of biceps**
  + **S46.10 Unspecified injury of muscle, fascia and tendon of long head of biceps**
    - +7th **S46.101 Unspecified injury of muscle, fascia and tendon of long head of biceps, right arm**
    - +7th **S46.102 Unspecified injury of muscle, fascia and tendon of long head of biceps, left arm**
    - +7th **S46.109 Unspecified injury of muscle, fascia and tendon of long head of biceps, unspecified arm**
  + **S46.11 Strain of muscle, fascia and tendon of long head of biceps**
    - +7th **S46.111 Strain of muscle, fascia and tendon of long head of biceps, right arm**
    - +7th **S46.112 Strain of muscle, fascia and tendon of long head of biceps, left arm**
    - +7th **S46.119 Strain of muscle, fascia and tendon of long head of biceps, unspecified arm**
  + **S46.12 Laceration of muscle, fascia and tendon of long head of biceps**
    - CC +7th **S46.121 Laceration of muscle, fascia and tendon of long head of biceps, right arm**
      CC Exclusion 7th character A see Appendix A PDX collection 1263
    - CC +7th **S46.122 Laceration of muscle, fascia and tendon of long head of biceps, left arm**
      CC Exclusion 7th character A see Appendix A PDX collection 1264
    - CC +7th **S46.129 Laceration of muscle, fascia and tendon of long head of biceps, unspecified arm**
      CC Exclusion 7th character A see Appendix A PDX collection 1265
  + **S46.19 Other injury of muscle, fascia and tendon of long head of biceps**
    - +7th **S46.191 Other injury of muscle, fascia and tendon of long head of biceps, right arm**
    - +7th **S46.192 Other injury of muscle, fascia and tendon of long head of biceps, left arm**
    - +7th **S46.199 Other injury of muscle, fascia and tendon of long head of biceps, unspecified arm**

+ **S46.2 Injury of muscle, fascia and tendon of other parts of biceps**
  + **S46.20 Unspecified injury of muscle, fascia and tendon of other parts of biceps**
    - +7th **S46.201 Unspecified injury of muscle, fascia and tendon of other parts of biceps, right arm**
    - +7th **S46.202 Unspecified injury of muscle, fascia and tendon of other parts of biceps, left arm**
    - +7th **S46.209 Unspecified injury of muscle, fascia and tendon of other parts of biceps, unspecified arm**
  + **S46.21 Strain of muscle, fascia and tendon of other parts of biceps**
    - +7th **S46.211 Strain of muscle, fascia and tendon of other parts of biceps, right arm**
    - +7th **S46.212 Strain of muscle, fascia and tendon of other parts of biceps, left arm**
    - +7th **S46.219 Strain of muscle, fascia and tendon of other parts of biceps, unspecified arm**
  + **S46.22 Laceration of muscle, fascia and tendon of other parts of biceps**
    - CC +7th **S46.221 Laceration of muscle, fascia and tendon of other parts of biceps, right arm**
      CC Exclusion 7th character A see Appendix A PDX collection 1263
    - CC +7th **S46.222 Laceration of muscle, fascia and tendon of other parts of biceps, left arm**
      CC Exclusion 7th character A see Appendix A PDX collection 1264
    - CC +7th **S46.229 Laceration of muscle, fascia and tendon of other parts of biceps, unspecified arm**
      CC Exclusion 7th character A see Appendix A PDX collection 1265
  + **S46.29 Other injury of muscle, fascia and tendon of other parts of biceps**
    - +7th **S46.291 Other injury of muscle, fascia and tendon of other parts of biceps, right arm**
    - +7th **S46.292 Other injury of muscle, fascia and tendon of other parts of biceps, left arm**
    - +7th **S46.299 Other injury of muscle, fascia and tendon of other parts of biceps, unspecified arm**

+ **S46.3 Injury of muscle, fascia and tendon of triceps**
  + **S46.30 Unspecified injury of muscle, fascia and tendon of triceps**
    - +7th **S46.301 Unspecified injury of muscle, fascia and tendon of triceps, right arm**
    - +7th **S46.302 Unspecified injury of muscle, fascia and tendon of triceps, left arm**
    - +7th **S46.309 Unspecified injury of muscle, fascia and tendon of triceps, unspecified arm**
  + **S46.31 Strain of muscle, fascia and tendon of triceps**
    - +7th **S46.311 Strain of muscle, fascia and tendon of triceps, right arm**
    - +7th **S46.312 Strain of muscle, fascia and tendon of triceps, left arm**
    - +7th **S46.319 Strain of muscle, fascia and tendon of triceps, unspecified arm**
  + **S46.32 Laceration of muscle, fascia and tendon of triceps**
    - CC +7th **S46.321 Laceration of muscle, fascia and tendon of triceps, right arm**
      CC Exclusion 7th character A see Appendix A PDX collection 1263
    - CC +7th **S46.322 Laceration of muscle, fascia and tendon of triceps, left arm**
      CC Exclusion 7th character A see Appendix A PDX collection 1264
    - CC +7th **S46.329 Laceration of muscle, fascia and tendon of triceps, unspecified arm**
      CC Exclusion 7th character A see Appendix A PDX collection 1265

+ S46.39 Other injury of muscle, fascia and tendon of triceps
  - +7th S46.391 Other injury of muscle, fascia and tendon of triceps, right arm
  - +7th S46.392 Other injury of muscle, fascia and tendon of triceps, left arm
  - +7th S46.399 Other injury of muscle, fascia and tendon of triceps, unspecified arm

+ S46.8 Injury of other muscles, fascia and tendons at shoulder and upper arm level
  + S46.80 Unspecified injury of other muscles, fascia and tendons at shoulder and upper arm level
    - +7th S46.801 Unspecified injury of other muscles, fascia and tendons at shoulder and upper arm level, right arm
    - +7th S46.802 Unspecified injury of other muscles, fascia and tendons at shoulder and upper arm level, left arm
    - +7th S46.809 Unspecified injury of other muscles, fascia and tendons at shoulder and upper arm level, unspecified arm
  + S46.81 Strain of other muscles, fascia and tendons at shoulder and upper arm level
    - +7th S46.811 Strain of other muscles, fascia and tendons at shoulder and upper arm level, right arm
    - +7th S46.812 Strain of other muscles, fascia and tendons at shoulder and upper arm level, left arm
    - +7th S46.819 Strain of other muscles, fascia and tendons at shoulder and upper arm level, unspecified arm
  + S46.82 Laceration of other muscles, fascia and tendons at shoulder and upper arm level
    - CC +7th S46.821 Laceration of other muscles, fascia and tendons at shoulder and upper arm level, right arm
      CC Exclusion 7th character A see Appendix A PDX collection 1263
    - CC +7th S46.822 Laceration of other muscles, fascia and tendons at shoulder and upper arm level, left arm
      CC Exclusion 7th character A see Appendix A PDX collection 1264
    - CC +7th S46.829 Laceration of other muscles, fascia and tendons at shoulder and upper arm level, unspecified arm
      CC Exclusion 7th character A see Appendix A PDX collection 1265
  + S46.89 Other injury of other muscles, fascia and tendons at shoulder and upper arm level
    - +7th S46.891 Other injury of other muscles, fascia and tendons at shoulder and upper arm level, right arm
    - +7th S46.892 Other injury of other muscles, fascia and tendons at shoulder and upper arm level, left arm
    - +7th S46.899 Other injury of other muscles, fascia and tendons at shoulder and upper arm level, unspecified arm

+ S46.9 Injury of unspecified muscle, fascia and tendon at shoulder and upper arm level
  + S46.90 Unspecified injury of unspecified muscle, fascia and tendon at shoulder and upper arm level
    - +7th S46.901 Unspecified injury of unspecified muscle, fascia and tendon at shoulder and upper arm level, right arm
    - +7th S46.902 Unspecified injury of unspecified muscle, fascia and tendon at shoulder and upper arm level, left arm
    - +7th S46.909 Unspecified injury of unspecified muscle, fascia and tendon at shoulder and upper arm level, unspecified arm
  + S46.91 Strain of unspecified muscle, fascia and tendon at shoulder and upper arm level
    - +7th S46.911 Strain of unspecified muscle, fascia and tendon at shoulder and upper arm level, right arm
    - +7th S46.912 Strain of unspecified muscle, fascia and tendon at shoulder and upper arm level, left arm
    - +7th S46.919 Strain of unspecified muscle, fascia and tendon at shoulder and upper arm level, unspecified arm
  + S46.92 Laceration of unspecified muscle, fascia and tendon at shoulder and upper arm level
    - CC +7th S46.921 Laceration of unspecified muscle, fascia and tendon at shoulder and upper arm level, right arm
      CC Exclusion 7th character A see Appendix A PDX collection 1263
    - CC +7th S46.922 Laceration of unspecified muscle, fascia and tendon at shoulder and upper arm level, left arm
      CC Exclusion 7th character A see Appendix A PDX collection 1264
    - CC +7th S46.929 Laceration of unspecified muscle, fascia and tendon at shoulder and upper arm level, unspecified arm
      CC Exclusion 7th character A see Appendix A PDX collection 1265
  + S46.99 Other injury of unspecified muscle, fascia and tendon at shoulder and upper arm level
    - +7th S46.991 Other injury of unspecified muscle, fascia and tendon at shoulder and upper arm level, right arm
    - +7th S46.992 Other injury of unspecified muscle, fascia and tendon at shoulder and upper arm level, left arm
    - +7th S46.999 Other injury of unspecified muscle, fascia and tendon at shoulder and upper arm level, unspecified arm

S47 Crushing injury of shoulder and upper arm

Use additional code for all associated injuries

Excludes2: *crushing injury of elbow (S57.0-)*

The appropriate 7th character is to be added to each code from category S47
A initial encounter
D subsequent encounter
S sequela

- X+7th S47.1 Crushing injury of right shoulder and upper arm
- X+7th S47.2 Crushing injury of left shoulder and upper arm
- X+7th S47.9 Crushing injury of shoulder and upper arm, unspecified arm

S48 Traumatic amputation of shoulder and upper arm

An amputation not identified as partial or complete should be coded to complete

Excludes1: *traumatic amputation at elbow level (S58.0)*

The appropriate 7th character is to be added to each code from category S48
A initial encounter
D subsequent encounter
S sequela

+ S48.0 Traumatic amputation at shoulder joint
  + S48.01 Complete traumatic amputation at shoulder joint
    - CC +7th S48.011 Complete traumatic amputation at right shoulder joint
      CC Exclusion 7th character A see Appendix A PDX collection 1266
    - CC +7th S48.012 Complete traumatic amputation at left shoulder joint
      CC Exclusion 7th character A see Appendix A PDX collection 1267
    - CC +7th S48.019 Complete traumatic amputation at unspecified shoulder joint
      CC Exclusion 7th character A see Appendix A PDX collection 1268
  + S48.02 Partial traumatic amputation at shoulder joint
    - CC +7th S48.021 Partial traumatic amputation at right shoulder joint
      CC Exclusion 7th character A see Appendix A PDX collection 1266
    - CC +7th S48.022 Partial traumatic amputation at left shoulder joint
      CC Exclusion 7th character A see Appendix A PDX collection 1267
    - CC +7th S48.029 Partial traumatic amputation at unspecified shoulder joint
      CC Exclusion 7th character A see Appendix A PDX collection 1268

+ **S48.1 Traumatic amputation at level between shoulder and elbow**
  + **S48.11 Complete traumatic amputation at level between shoulder and elbow**
    - CC +7th **S48.111 Complete traumatic amputation at level between right shoulder and elbow**
      CC Exclusion 7th character A see Appendix A PDX collection 1266
    - CC +7th **S48.112 Complete traumatic amputation at level between left shoulder and elbow**
      CC Exclusion 7th character A see Appendix A PDX collection 1267
    - CC +7th **S48.119 Complete traumatic amputation at level between unspecified shoulder and elbow**
      CC Exclusion 7th character A see Appendix A PDX collection 1268
  + **S48.12 Partial traumatic amputation at level between shoulder and elbow**
    - CC +7th **S48.121 Partial traumatic amputation at level between right shoulder and elbow**
      CC Exclusion 7th character A see Appendix A PDX collection 1266
    - CC +7th **S48.122 Partial traumatic amputation at level between left shoulder and elbow**
      CC Exclusion 7th character A see Appendix A PDX collection 1267
    - CC +7th **S48.129 Partial traumatic amputation at level between unspecified shoulder and elbow**
      CC Exclusion 7th character A see Appendix A PDX collection 1268
+ **S48.9 Traumatic amputation of shoulder and upper arm, level unspecified**
  + **S48.91 Complete traumatic amputation of shoulder and upper arm, level unspecified**
    - CC +7th **S48.911 Complete traumatic amputation of right shoulder and upper arm, level unspecified**
      CC Exclusion 7th character A see Appendix A PDX collection 1266
    - CC +7th **S48.912 Complete traumatic amputation of left shoulder and upper arm, level unspecified**
      CC Exclusion 7th character A see Appendix A PDX collection 1267
    - CC +7th **S48.919 Complete traumatic amputation of unspecified shoulder and upper arm, level unspecified**
      CC Exclusion 7th character A see Appendix A PDX collection 1268
  + **S48.92 Partial traumatic amputation of shoulder and upper arm, level unspecified**
    - CC +7th **S48.921 Partial traumatic amputation of right shoulder and upper arm, level unspecified**
      CC Exclusion 7th character A see Appendix A PDX collection 1266
    - CC +7th **S48.922 Partial traumatic amputation of left shoulder and upper arm, level unspecified**
      CC Exclusion 7th character A see Appendix A PDX collection 1267
    - CC +7th **S48.929 Partial traumatic amputation of unspecified shoulder and upper arm, level unspecified**
      CC Exclusion 7th character A see Appendix A PDX collection 1268

S49 Other and unspecified injuries of shoulder and upper arm

The appropriate 7th character is to be added to each code from subcategories **S49.0** and **S49.1**
A initial encounter for closed fracture
D subsequent encounter for fracture with routine healing
G subsequent encounter for fracture with delayed healing
K subsequent encounter for fracture with nonunion
P subsequent encounter for fracture with malunion
S sequela

Review coding guideline C.19.c

+ **S49.0 Physeal fracture of upper end of humerus**
  + **S49.00 Unspecified physeal fracture of upper end of humerus**
    - CC +7th **S49.001 Unspecified physeal fracture of upper end of humerus, right arm**
      CC Exclusion 7th character A see Appendix A PDX collection 1245
      CC Exclusion 7th characters K & P see Appendix A PDX collection 0897
      HAC 7th character A see Appendix B for HAC conditional logic
    - CC +7th **S49.002 Unspecified physeal fracture of upper end of humerus, left arm**
      CC Exclusion 7th character A see Appendix A PDX collection 1247
      CC Exclusion 7th characters K & P see Appendix A PDX collection 0897
      HAC 7th character A see Appendix B for HAC conditional logic
    - CC +7th **S49.009 Unspecified physeal fracture of upper end of humerus, unspecified arm**
      CC Exclusion 7th character A see Appendix A PDX collection 1248
      CC Exclusion 7th characters K & P see Appendix A PDX collection 0897
      HAC 7th character A see Appendix B for HAC conditional logic
  + **S49.01 Salter-Harris Type I physeal fracture of upper end of humerus**
    - CC +7th **S49.011 Salter-Harris Type I physeal fracture of upper end of humerus, right arm**
      CC Exclusion 7th character A see Appendix A PDX collection 1245
      CC Exclusion 7th characters K & P see Appendix A PDX collection 0897
      HAC 7th character A see Appendix B for HAC conditional logic
    - CC +7th **S49.012 Salter-Harris Type I physeal fracture of upper end of humerus, left arm**
      CC Exclusion 7th character A see Appendix A PDX collection 1247
      CC Exclusion 7th characters K & P see Appendix A PDX collection 0897
      HAC 7th character A see Appendix B for HAC conditional logic
    - CC +7th **S49.019 Salter-Harris Type I physeal fracture of upper end of humerus, unspecified arm**
      CC Exclusion 7th character A see Appendix A PDX collection 1248
      CC Exclusion 7th characters K & P see Appendix A PDX collection 0897
      HAC 7th character A see Appendix B for HAC conditional logic
  + **S49.02 Salter-Harris Type II physeal fracture of upper end of humerus**
    - CC +7th **S49.021 Salter-Harris Type II physeal fracture of upper end of humerus, right arm**
      CC Exclusion 7th character A see Appendix A PDX collection 1245
      CC Exclusion 7th characters K & P see Appendix A PDX collection 0897
      HAC 7th character A see Appendix B for HAC conditional logic
    - CC +7th **S49.022 Salter-Harris Type II physeal fracture of upper end of humerus, left arm**
      CC Exclusion 7th character A see Appendix A PDX collection 1247
      CC Exclusion 7th characters K & P see Appendix A PDX collection 0897
      HAC 7th character A see Appendix B for HAC conditional logic

Elbow

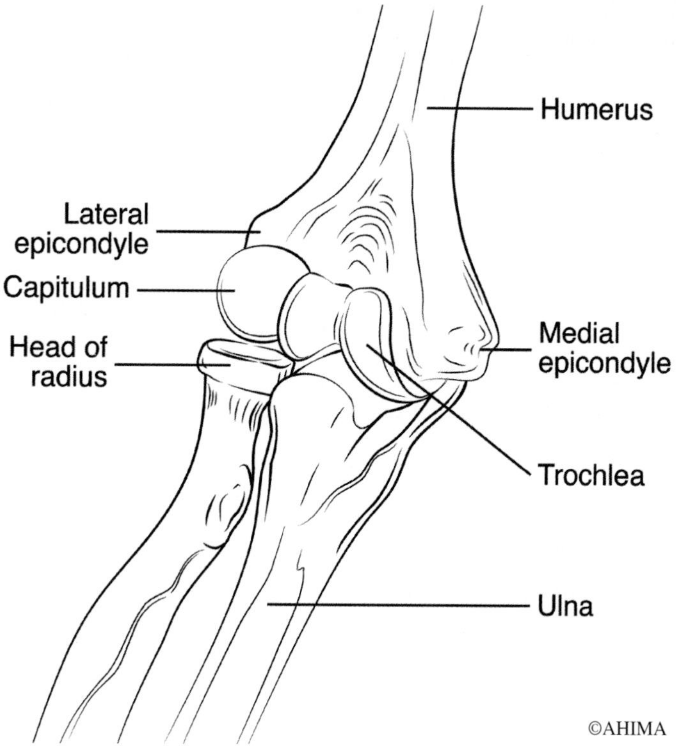

CC +7th **S49.029** **Salter-Harris Type II physeal fracture of upper end of humerus, unspecified arm**
CC Exclusion 7th character A see Appendix A PDX collection 1248
CC Exclusion 7th characters K & P see Appendix A PDX collection 0897
HAC 7th character A see Appendix B for HAC conditional logic

+ **S49.03** **Salter-Harris Type III physeal fracture of upper end of humerus**

CC +7th **S49.031** **Salter-Harris Type III physeal fracture of upper end of humerus, right arm**
CC Exclusion 7th character A see Appendix A PDX collection 1245
CC Exclusion 7th characters K & P see Appendix A PDX collection 0897
HAC 7th character A see Appendix B for HAC conditional logic

CC +7th **S49.032** **Salter-Harris Type III physeal fracture of upper end of humerus, left arm**
CC Exclusion 7th character A see Appendix A PDX collection 1247
CC Exclusion 7th characters K & P see Appendix A PDX collection 0897
HAC 7th character A see Appendix B for HAC conditional logic

CC +7th **S49.039** **Salter-Harris Type III physeal fracture of upper end of humerus, unspecified arm**
CC Exclusion 7th character A see Appendix A PDX collection 1248
CC Exclusion 7th characters K & P see Appendix A PDX collection 0897
HAC 7th character A see Appendix B for HAC conditional logic

+ **S49.04** **Salter-Harris Type IV physeal fracture of upper end of humerus**

CC +7th **S49.041** **Salter-Harris Type IV physeal fracture of upper end of humerus, right arm**
CC Exclusion 7th character A see Appendix A PDX collection 1245
CC Exclusion 7th characters K & P see Appendix A PDX collection 0897
HAC 7th character A see Appendix B for HAC conditional logic

CC +7th **S49.042** **Salter-Harris Type IV physeal fracture of upper end of humerus, left arm**
CC Exclusion 7th character A see Appendix A PDX collection 1247
CC Exclusion 7th characters K & P see Appendix A PDX collection 0897
HAC 7th character A see Appendix B for HAC conditional logic

CC +7th **S49.049** **Salter-Harris Type IV physeal fracture of upper end of humerus, unspecified arm**
CC Exclusion 7th character A see Appendix A PDX collection 1248
CC Exclusion 7th characters K & P see Appendix A PDX collection 0897
HAC 7th character A see Appendix B for HAC conditional logic

+ **S49.09** **Other physeal fracture of upper end of humerus**

CC +7th **S49.091** **Other physeal fracture of upper end of humerus, right arm**
CC Exclusion 7th character A see Appendix A PDX collection 1245
CC Exclusion 7th characters K & P see Appendix A PDX collection 0897
HAC 7th character A see Appendix B for HAC conditional logic

CC +7th **S49.092** **Other physeal fracture of upper end of humerus, left arm**
CC Exclusion 7th character A see Appendix A PDX collection 1247
CC Exclusion 7th characters K & P see Appendix A PDX collection 0897
HAC 7th character A see Appendix B for HAC conditional logic

CC +7th **S49.099** **Other physeal fracture of upper end of humerus, unspecified arm**
CC Exclusion 7th character A see Appendix A PDX collection 1248
CC Exclusion 7th characters K & P see Appendix A PDX collection 0897
HAC 7th character A see Appendix B for HAC conditional logic

\+ S49.1 Physeal fracture of lower end of humerus

\+ S49.10 Unspecified physeal fracture of lower end of humerus

CC +7th S49.101 Unspecified physeal fracture of lower end of humerus, right arm
CC Exclusion 7th character A see Appendix A PDX collection 1245
CC Exclusion 7th characters K & P see Appendix A PDX collection 0897
HAC 7th character A see Appendix B for HAC conditional logic

CC +7th S49.102 Unspecified physeal fracture of lower end of humerus, left arm
CC Exclusion 7th character A see Appendix A PDX collection 1247
CC Exclusion 7th characters K & P see Appendix A PDX collection 0897
HAC 7th character A see Appendix B for HAC conditional logic

CC +7th S49.109 Unspecified physeal fracture of lower end of humerus, unspecified arm
CC Exclusion 7th character A see Appendix A PDX collection 1248
CC Exclusion 7th characters K & P see Appendix A PDX collection 0897
HAC 7th character A see Appendix B for HAC conditional logic

\+ S49.11 Salter-Harris Type I physeal fracture of lower end of humerus

CC +7th S49.111 Salter-Harris Type I physeal fracture of lower end of humerus, right arm
CC Exclusion 7th character A see Appendix A PDX collection 1245
CC Exclusion 7th characters K & P see Appendix A PDX collection 0897
HAC 7th character A see Appendix B for HAC conditional logic

CC +7th S49.112 Salter-Harris Type I physeal fracture of lower end of humerus, left arm
CC Exclusion 7th character A see Appendix A PDX collection 1247
CC Exclusion 7th characters K & P see Appendix A PDX collection 0897
HAC 7th character A see Appendix B for HAC conditional logic

CC +7th S49.119 Salter-Harris Type I physeal fracture of lower end of humerus, unspecified arm
CC Exclusion 7th character A see Appendix A PDX collection 1248
CC Exclusion 7th characters K & P see Appendix A PDX collection 0897
HAC 7th character A see Appendix B for HAC conditional logic

\+ S49.12 Salter-Harris Type II physeal fracture of lower end of humerus

CC +7th S49.121 Salter-Harris Type II physeal fracture of lower end of humerus, right arm
CC Exclusion 7th character A see Appendix A PDX collection 1245
CC Exclusion 7th characters K & P see Appendix A PDX collection 0897
HAC 7th character A see Appendix B for HAC conditional logic

CC +7th S49.122 Salter-Harris Type II physeal fracture of lower end of humerus, left arm
CC Exclusion 7th character A see Appendix A PDX collection 1247
CC Exclusion 7th characters K & P see Appendix A PDX collection 0897
HAC 7th character A see Appendix B for HAC conditional logic

CC +7th S49.129 Salter-Harris Type II physeal fracture of lower end of humerus, unspecified arm
CC Exclusion 7th character A see Appendix A PDX collection 1248
CC Exclusion 7th characters K & P see Appendix A PDX collection 0897
HAC 7th character A see Appendix B for HAC conditional logic

\+ S49.13 Salter-Harris Type III physeal fracture of lower end of humerus

CC +7th S49.131 Salter-Harris Type III physeal fracture of lower end of humerus, right arm
CC Exclusion 7th character A see Appendix A PDX collection 1245
CC Exclusion 7th characters K & P see Appendix A PDX collection 0897
HAC 7th character A see Appendix B for HAC conditional logic

CC +7th S49.132 Salter-Harris Type III physeal fracture of lower end of humerus, left arm
CC Exclusion 7th character A see Appendix A PDX collection 1247
CC Exclusion 7th characters K & P see Appendix A PDX collection 0897
HAC 7th character A see Appendix B for HAC conditional logic

CC +7th S49.139 Salter-Harris Type III physeal fracture of lower end of humerus, unspecified arm
CC Exclusion 7th character A see Appendix A PDX collection 1248
CC Exclusion 7th characters K & P see Appendix A PDX collection 0897
HAC 7th character A see Appendix B for HAC conditional logic

\+ S49.14 Salter-Harris Type IV physeal fracture of lower end of humerus

CC +7th S49.141 Salter-Harris Type IV physeal fracture of lower end of humerus, right arm
CC Exclusion 7th character A see Appendix A PDX collection 1245
CC Exclusion 7th characters K & P see Appendix A PDX collection 0897
HAC 7th character A see Appendix B for HAC conditional logic

CC +7th S49.142 Salter-Harris Type IV physeal fracture of lower end of humerus, left arm
CC Exclusion 7th character A see Appendix A PDX collection 1247
CC Exclusion 7th characters K & P see Appendix A PDX collection 0897
HAC 7th character A see Appendix B for HAC conditional logic

CC +7th S49.149 Salter-Harris Type IV physeal fracture of lower end of humerus, unspecified arm
CC Exclusion 7th character A see Appendix A PDX collection 1248
CC Exclusion 7th characters K & P see Appendix A PDX collection 0897
HAC 7th character A see Appendix B for HAC conditional logic

\+ S49.19 Other physeal fracture of lower end of humerus

CC +7th S49.191 Other physeal fracture of lower end of humerus, right arm
CC Exclusion 7th character A see Appendix A PDX collection 1245
CC Exclusion 7th characters K & P see Appendix A PDX collection 0897
HAC 7th character A see Appendix B for HAC conditional logic

CC +7th S49.192 Other physeal fracture of lower end of humerus, left arm
CC Exclusion 7th character A see Appendix A PDX collection 1247
CC Exclusion 7th characters K & P see Appendix A PDX collection 0897
HAC 7th character A see Appendix B for HAC conditional logic

CC +7th S49.199 Other physeal fracture of lower end of humerus, unspecified arm
CC Exclusion 7th character A see Appendix A PDX collection 1248
CC Exclusion 7th characters K & P see Appendix A PDX collection 0897
HAC 7th character A see Appendix B for HAC conditional logic

\+ S49.8 Other specified injuries of shoulder and upper arm

The appropriate 7th character is to be added to each code in subcategory **S49.8**
A initial encounter
D subsequent encounter
S sequela

X+7th S49.80 Other specified injuries of shoulder and upper arm, unspecified arm

X+7th S49.81 Other specified injuries of right shoulder and upper arm

X+7th S49.82 Other specified injuries of left shoulder and upper arm

+ **S49.9 Unspecified injury of shoulder and upper arm**

The appropriate 7th character is to be added to each code in subcategory **S49.9**
A initial encounter
D subsequent encounter
S sequela

X+7th **S49.90 Unspecified injury of shoulder and upper arm, unspecified arm**
X+7th **S49.91 Unspecified injury of right shoulder and upper arm**
X+7th **S49.92 Unspecified injury of left shoulder and upper arm**

njuries to the elbow and forearm (S50-S59)

:xcludes2: *burns and corrosions (T20-T32)*
frostbite (T33-T34)
injuries of wrist and hand (S60-S69)
insect bite or sting, venomous (T63.4)

S50 Superficial injury of elbow and forearm

Excludes2: *superficial injury of wrist and hand (S60.-)*

The appropriate 7th character is to be added to each code from category S50
A initial encounter
D subsequent encounter
S sequela

+ **S50.0 Contusion of elbow**
X+7th **S50.00 Contusion of unspecified elbow**
X+7th **S50.01 Contusion of right elbow**
X+7th **S50.02 Contusion of left elbow**
+ **S50.1 Contusion of forearm**
X+7th **S50.10 Contusion of unspecified forearm**
X+7th **S50.11 Contusion of right forearm**
X+7th **S50.12 Contusion of left forearm**
+ **S50.3 Other superficial injuries of elbow**
+ **S50.31 Abrasion of elbow**
+7th **S50.311 Abrasion of right elbow**
+7th **S50.312 Abrasion of left elbow**
+7th **S50.319 Abrasion of unspecified elbow**
+ **S50.32 Blister (nonthermal) of elbow**
+7th **S50.321 Blister (nonthermal) of right elbow**
+7th **S50.322 Blister (nonthermal) of left elbow**
+7th **S50.329 Blister (nonthermal) of unspecified elbow**
+ **S50.34 External constriction of elbow**
+7th **S50.341 External constriction of right elbow**
+7th **S50.342 External constriction of left elbow**
+7th **S50.349 External constriction of unspecified elbow**
+ **S50.35 Superficial foreign body of elbow**
Splinter in the elbow
+7th **S50.351 Superficial foreign body of right elbow**
+7th **S50.352 Superficial foreign body of left elbow**
+7th **S50.359 Superficial foreign body of unspecified elbow**
+ **S50.36 Insect bite (nonvenomous) of elbow**
+7th **S50.361 Insect bite (nonvenomous) of right elbow**
+7th **S50.362 Insect bite (nonvenomous) of left elbow**
+7th **S50.369 Insect bite (nonvenomous) of unspecified elbow**
+ **S50.37 Other superficial bite of elbow**
Excludes1: *open bite of elbow (S51.04)*
+7th **S50.371 Other superficial bite of right elbow**
+7th **S50.372 Other superficial bite of left elbow**
+7th **S50.379 Other superficial bite of unspecified elbow**
+ **S50.8 Other superficial injuries of forearm**
+ **S50.81 Abrasion of forearm**
+7th **S50.811 Abrasion of right forearm**
+7th **S50.812 Abrasion of left forearm**
+7th **S50.819 Abrasion of unspecified forearm**
+ **S50.82 Blister (nonthermal) of forearm**
+7th **S50.821 Blister (nonthermal) of right forearm**
+7th **S50.822 Blister (nonthermal) of left forearm**
+7th **S50.829 Blister (nonthermal) of unspecified forearm**
+ **S50.84 External constriction of forearm**
+7th **S50.841 External constriction of right forearm**
+7th **S50.842 External constriction of left forearm**
+7th **S50.849 External constriction of unspecified forearm**
+ **S50.85 Superficial foreign body of forearm**
Splinter in the forearm
+7th **S50.851 Superficial foreign body of right forearm**
+7th **S50.852 Superficial foreign body of left forearm**
+7th **S50.859 Superficial foreign body of unspecified forearm**
+ **S50.86 Insect bite (nonvenomous) of forearm**
+7th **S50.861 Insect bite (nonvenomous) of right forearm**
+7th **S50.862 Insect bite (nonvenomous) of left forearm**
+7th **S50.869 Insect bite (nonvenomous) of unspecified forearm**
+ **S50.87 Other superficial bite of forearm**
Excludes1: *open bite of forearm (S51.84)*
+7th **S50.871 Other superficial bite of right forearm**
+7th **S50.872 Other superficial bite of left forearm**
+7th **S50.879 Other superficial bite of unspecified forearm**
+ **S50.9 Unspecified superficial injury of elbow and forearm**
+ **S50.90 Unspecified superficial injury of elbow**
+7th **S50.901 Unspecified superficial injury of right elbow**
+7th **S50.902 Unspecified superficial injury of left elbow**
+7th **S50.909 Unspecified superficial injury of unspecified elbow**
+ **S50.91 Unspecified superficial injury of forearm**
S50.911 Unspecified superficial injury of right forearm
S50.912 Unspecified superficial injury of left forearm
S50.919 Unspecified superficial injury of unspecified forearm

S51 Open wound of elbow and forearm

Code also any associated wound infection
Excludes1: *open fracture of elbow and forearm (S52.- with open fracture 7th character)*
traumatic amputation of elbow and forearm (S58.-)
Excludes2: *open wound of wrist and hand (S61.-)*

The appropriate 7th character is to be added to each code from category S51
A initial encounter
D subsequent encounter
S sequela

+ **S51.0 Open wound of elbow**
+ **S51.00 Unspecified open wound of elbow**
+7th **S51.001 Unspecified open wound of right elbow**
AHA CC: 4Q, 2012, 108
+7th **S51.002 Unspecified open wound of left elbow**
+7th **S51.009 Unspecified open wound of unspecified elbow**
Open wound of elbow NOS
+ **S51.01 Laceration without foreign body of elbow**
+7th **S51.011 Laceration without foreign body of right elbow**
+7th **S51.012 Laceration without foreign body of left elbow**
+7th **S51.019 Laceration without foreign body of unspecified elbow**
+ **S51.02 Laceration with foreign body of elbow**
+7th **S51.021 Laceration with foreign body of right elbow**
+7th **S51.022 Laceration with foreign body of left elbow**
+7th **S51.029 Laceration with foreign body of unspecified elbow**
+ **S51.03 Puncture wound without foreign body of elbow**
+7th **S51.031 Puncture wound without foreign body of right elbow**
+7th **S51.032 Puncture wound without foreign body of left elbow**
+7th **S51.039 Puncture wound without foreign body of unspecified elbow**
+ **S51.04 Puncture wound with foreign body of elbow**
+7th **S51.041 Puncture wound with foreign body of right elbow**
+7th **S51.042 Puncture wound with foreign body of left elbow**
+7th **S51.049 Puncture wound with foreign body of unspecified elbow**
+ **S51.05 Open bite of elbow**
Bite of elbow NOS
Excludes1: *superficial bite of elbow (S50.36, S50.37)*
+7th **S51.051 Open bite, right elbow**
+7th **S51.052 Open bite, left elbow**
+7th **S51.059 Open bite, unspecified elbow**

+ **S51.8 Open wound of forearm**
  Excludes2: *open wound of elbow (S51.0-)*
  + **S51.80 Unspecified open wound of forearm**
    +7th **S51.801 Unspecified open wound of right forearm**
    +7th **S51.802 Unspecified open wound of left forearm**
    +7th **S51.809 Unspecified open wound of unspecified forearm**
    Open wound of forearm NOS
  + **S51.81 Laceration without foreign body of forearm**
    +7th **S51.811 Laceration without foreign body of right forearm**
    +7th **S51.812 Laceration without foreign body of left forearm**
    +7th **S51.819 Laceration without foreign body of unspecified forearm**
  + **S51.82 Laceration with foreign body of forearm**
    +7th **S51.821 Laceration with foreign body of right forearm**
    +7th **S51.822 Laceration with foreign body of left forearm**
    +7th **S51.829 Laceration with foreign body of unspecified forearm**
  + **S51.83 Puncture wound without foreign body of forearm**
    +7th **S51.831 Puncture wound without foreign body of right forearm**
    +7th **S51.832 Puncture wound without foreign body of left forearm**
    +7th **S51.839 Puncture wound without foreign body of unspecified forearm**
  + **S51.84 Puncture wound with foreign body of forearm**
    +7th **S51.841 Puncture wound with foreign body of right forearm**
    +7th **S51.842 Puncture wound with foreign body of left forearm**
    +7th **S51.849 Puncture wound with foreign body of unspecified forearm**
  + **S51.85 Open bite of forearm**
    Bite of forearm NOS
    Excludes1: *superficial bite of forearm (S50.86, S50.87)*
    +7th **S51.851 Open bite of right forearm**
    +7th **S51.852 Open bite of left forearm**
    +7th **S51.859 Open bite of unspecified forearm**

S52 Fracture of forearm

NOTE A fracture not indicated as displaced or nondisplaced should be coded to displaced
A fracture not indicated as open or closed should be coded to closed
The open fracture designations are based on the Gustilo open fracture classification

Excludes1: *traumatic amputation of forearm (S58.-)*
Excludes2: *fracture at wrist and hand level (S62.-)*

The appropriate 7th character is to be added to all codes from category S52
- A initial encounter for closed fracture
- B initial encounter for open fracture type I or II initial encounter for open fracture NOS
- C initial encounter for open fracture type IIIA, IIIB, or IIIC
- D subsequent encounter for closed fracture with routine healing
- E subsequent encounter for open fracture type I or II with routine healing
- F subsequent encounter for open fracture type IIIA, IIIB, or IIIC with routine healing
- G subsequent encounter for closed fracture with delayed healing
- H subsequent encounter for open fracture type I or II with delayed healing
- J subsequent encounter for open fracture type IIIA, IIIB, or IIIC with delayed healing
- K subsequent encounter for closed fracture with nonunion
- M subsequent encounter for open fracture type I or II with nonunion
- N subsequent encounter for open fracture type IIIA, IIIB, or IIIC with nonunion
- P subsequent encounter for closed fracture with malunion
- Q subsequent encounter for open fracture type I or II with malunion
- R subsequent encounter for open fracture type IIIA, IIIB, or IIIC with malunion
- S sequela

Review coding guideline C.19.c

+ **S52.0 Fracture of upper end of ulna**
  Fracture of proximal end of ulna
  Excludes2: *fracture of elbow NOS (S42.40-)*
  fractures of shaft of ulna (S52.2-)
  + **S52.00 Unspecified fracture of upper end of ulna**
    CC MCC +7th **S52.001 Unspecified fracture of upper end of right ulna**
    CC Exclusion 7th characters K - R see Appendix A PDX collection 0897
    MCC Exclusion 7th characters B & C see Appendix A PDX collection 1269
    HAC 7th characters B & C see Appendix B for HAC conditional logic
    CC MCC +7th **S52.002 Unspecified fracture of upper end of left ulna**
    CC Exclusion 7th characters K - R see Appendix A PDX collection 0897
    MCC Exclusion 7th characters B & C see Appendix A PDX collection 1269
    HAC 7th characters B & C see Appendix B for HAC conditional logic
    CC MCC +7th **S52.009 Unspecified fracture of upper end of unspecified ulna**
    CC Exclusion 7th characters K - R see Appendix A PDX collection 0897
    MCC Exclusion 7th characters B & C see Appendix A PDX collection 1269
    HAC 7th characters B & C see Appendix B for HAC conditional logic
  + **S52.01 Torus fracture of upper end of ulna**

The appropriate 7th character is to be added to all codes in subcategory **S52.01**
- A initial encounter for closed fracture
- D subsequent encounter for fracture with routine healing
- G subsequent encounter for fracture with delayed healing
- K subsequent encounter for fracture with nonunion
- P - subsequent encounter for fracture with malunion
- S - sequela

    CC +7th **S52.011 Torus fracture of upper end of right ulna**
    CC Exclusion 7th character A see Appendix A PDX collection 1270
    CC Exclusion 7th characters K & P see Appendix A PDX collection 0897
    HAC 7th character A see Appendix B for HAC conditional logic
    CC +7th **S52.012 Torus fracture of upper end of left ulna**
    CC Exclusion 7th character A see Appendix A PDX collection 1271
    CC Exclusion 7th characters K & P see Appendix A PDX collection 0897
    HAC 7th character A see Appendix B for HAC conditional logic
    CC +7th **S52.019 Torus fracture of upper end of unspecified ulna**
    CC Exclusion 7th character A see Appendix A PDX collection 1272
    CC Exclusion 7th characters K & P see Appendix A PDX collection 0897
    HAC 7th character A see Appendix B for HAC conditional logic
  + **S52.02 Fracture of olecranon process without intraarticular extension of ulna**
    CC MCC +7th **S52.021 Displaced fracture of olecranon process without intraarticular extension of right ulna**
    CC Exclusion 7th characters K - R see Appendix A PDX collection 0897
    MCC Exclusion 7th characters B & C see Appendix A PDX collection 1273
    HAC 7th characters B & C see Appendix B for HAC conditional logic
    CC MCC +7th **S52.022 Displaced fracture of olecranon process without intraarticular extension of left ulna**
    CC Exclusion 7th characters K - R see Appendix A PDX collection 0897
    MCC Exclusion 7th characters B & C see Appendix A PDX collection 1273
    HAC 7th characters B & C see Appendix B for HAC conditional logic

CC MCC +7th **S52.023 Displaced fracture of olecranon process without intraarticular extension of unspecified ulna**
CC Exclusion 7th characters K - R see Appendix A PDX collection 0897
MCC Exclusion 7th characters B & C see Appendix A PDX collection 1273
HAC 7th characters B & C see Appendix B for HAC conditional logic

CC MCC +7th **S52.024 Nondisplaced fracture of olecranon process without intraarticular extension of right ulna**
CC Exclusion 7th characters K - R see Appendix A PDX collection 0897
MCC Exclusion 7th characters B & C see Appendix A PDX collection 1273
HAC 7th characters B & C see Appendix B for HAC conditional logic

CC MCC +7th **S52.025 Nondisplaced fracture of olecranon process without intraarticular extension of left ulna**
CC Exclusion 7th characters K - R see Appendix A PDX collection 0897
MCC Exclusion 7th characters B & C see Appendix A PDX collection 1273
HAC 7th characters B & C see Appendix B for HAC conditional logic

CC MCC +7th **S52.026 Nondisplaced fracture of olecranon process without intraarticular extension of unspecified ulna**
CC Exclusion 7th characters K - R see Appendix A PDX collection 0897
MCC Exclusion 7th characters B & C see Appendix A PDX collection 1273
HAC 7th characters B & C see Appendix B for HAC conditional logic

\+ **S52.03 Fracture of olecranon process with intraarticular extension of ulna**

CC MCC +7th **S52.031 Displaced fracture of olecranon process with intraarticular extension of right ulna**
CC Exclusion 7th characters K - R see Appendix A PDX collection 0897
MCC Exclusion 7th characters B & C see Appendix A PDX collection 1273
HAC 7th characters B & C see Appendix B for HAC conditional logic

CC MCC +7th **S52.032 Displaced fracture of olecranon process with intraarticular extension of left ulna**
CC Exclusion 7th characters K - R see Appendix A PDX collection 0897
MCC Exclusion 7th characters B & C see Appendix A PDX collection 1273
HAC 7th characters B & C see Appendix B for HAC conditional logic

CC MCC +7th **S52.033 Displaced fracture of olecranon process with intraarticular extension of unspecified ulna**
CC Exclusion 7th characters K - R see Appendix A PDX collection 0897
MCC Exclusion 7th characters B & C see Appendix A PDX collection 1273
HAC 7th characters B & C see Appendix B for HAC conditional logic

CC MCC +7th **S52.034 Nondisplaced fracture of olecranon process with intraarticular extension of right ulna**
CC Exclusion 7th characters K - R see Appendix A PDX collection 0897
MCC Exclusion 7th characters B & C see Appendix A PDX collection 1273
HAC 7th characters B & C see Appendix B for HAC conditional logic

CC MCC +7th **S52.035 Nondisplaced fracture of olecranon process with intraarticular extension of left ulna**
CC Exclusion 7th characters K - R see Appendix A PDX collection 0897
MCC Exclusion 7th characters B & C see Appendix A PDX collection 1273
HAC 7th characters B & C see Appendix B for HAC conditional logic

CC MCC +7th **S52.036 Nondisplaced fracture of olecranon process with intraarticular extension of unspecified ulna**
CC Exclusion 7th characters K - R see Appendix A PDX collection 0897
MCC Exclusion 7th characters B & C see Appendix A PDX collection 1273
HAC 7th characters B & C see Appendix B for HAC conditional logic

\+ **S52.04 Fracture of coronoid process of ulna**

CC MCC +7th **S52.041 Displaced fracture of coronoid process of right ulna**
CC Exclusion 7th characters K - R see Appendix A PDX collection 0897
MCC Exclusion 7th characters B & C see Appendix A PDX collection 1269
HAC 7th characters B & C see Appendix B for HAC conditional logic

CC MCC +7th **S52.042 Displaced fracture of coronoid process of left ulna**
CC Exclusion 7th characters K - R see Appendix A PDX collection 0897
MCC Exclusion 7th characters B & C see Appendix A PDX collection 1269
HAC 7th characters B & C see Appendix B for HAC conditional logic

CC MCC +7th **S52.043 Displaced fracture of coronoid process of unspecified ulna**
CC Exclusion 7th characters K - R see Appendix A PDX collection 0897
MCC Exclusion 7th characters B & C see Appendix A PDX collection 1269
HAC 7th characters B & C see Appendix B for HAC conditional logic

CC MCC +7th **S52.044 Nondisplaced fracture of coronoid process of right ulna**
CC Exclusion 7th characters K - R see Appendix A PDX collection 0897
MCC Exclusion 7th characters B & C see Appendix A PDX collection 1269
HAC 7th characters B & C see Appendix B for HAC conditional logic

CC MCC +7th **S52.045 Nondisplaced fracture of coronoid process of left ulna**
CC Exclusion 7th characters K - R see Appendix A PDX collection 0897
MCC Exclusion 7th characters B & C see Appendix A PDX collection 1269
HAC 7th characters B & C see Appendix B for HAC conditional logic

CC MCC +7th **S52.046 Nondisplaced fracture of coronoid process of unspecified ulna**
CC Exclusion 7th characters K - R see Appendix A PDX collection 0897
MCC Exclusion 7th characters B & C see Appendix A PDX collection 1269
HAC 7th characters B & C see Appendix B for HAC conditional logic

\+ **S52.09 Other fracture of upper end of ulna**

CC MCC +7th **S52.091 Other fracture of upper end of right ulna**
CC Exclusion 7th characters K - R see Appendix A PDX collection 0897
MCC Exclusion 7th characters B & C see Appendix A PDX collection 1269
HAC 7th characters B & C see Appendix B for HAC conditional logic

CC MCC +7th **S52.092 Other fracture of upper end of left ulna**
CC Exclusion 7th characters K - R see Appendix A PDX collection 0897
MCC Exclusion 7th characters B & C see Appendix A PDX collection 1269
HAC 7th characters B & C see Appendix B for HAC conditional logic

CC MCC +7th **S52.099 Other fracture of upper end of unspecified ulna**
CC Exclusion 7th characters K - R see Appendix A PDX collection 0897
MCC Exclusion 7th characters B & C see Appendix A PDX collection 1269
HAC 7th characters B & C see Appendix B for HAC conditional logic

\+ **S52.1 Fracture of upper end of radius**
Fracture of proximal end of radius
Excludes2: *physeal fractures of upper end of radius (S59.2-)*
fracture of shaft of radius (S52.3-)

\+ **S52.10 Unspecified fracture of upper end of radius**

CC MCC +7th **S52.101 Unspecified fracture of upper end of right radius**
CC Exclusion 7th characters K - R see Appendix A PDX collection 0897
MCC Exclusion 7th characters B & C see Appendix A PDX collection 1269
HAC 7th characters B & C see Appendix B for HAC conditional logic

CC MCC +7th **S52.102 Unspecified fracture of upper end of left radius**
CC Exclusion 7th characters K - R see Appendix A PDX collection 0897
MCC Exclusion 7th characters B & C see Appendix A PDX collection 1269
HAC 7th characters B & C see Appendix B for HAC conditional logic

CC MCC +7th **S52.109 Unspecified fracture of upper end of unspecified radius**
CC Exclusion 7th characters K - R see Appendix A PDX collection 0897
MCC Exclusion 7th characters B & C see Appendix A PDX collection 1269
HAC 7th characters B & C see Appendix B for HAC conditional logic

+ **S52.11 Torus fracture of upper end of radius**

The appropriate 7th character is to be added to all codes in subcategory **S52.11**
- A initial encounter for closed fracture
- D subsequent encounter for fracture with routine healing
- G subsequent encounter for fracture with delayed healing
- K subsequent encounter for fracture with nonunion
- P subsequent encounter for fracture with malunion
- S sequela

CC +7th **S52.111 Torus fracture of upper end of right radius**
CC Exclusion 7th character A see Appendix A PDX collection 1270
CC Exclusion 7th characters K & P see Appendix A PDX collection 0897
HAC 7th character A see Appendix B for HAC conditional logic

CC +7th **S52.112 Torus fracture of upper end of left radius**
CC Exclusion 7th character A see Appendix A PDX collection 1271
CC Exclusion 7th characters K & P see Appendix A PDX collection 0897
HAC 7th character A see Appendix B for HAC conditional logic

CC +7th **S52.119 Torus fracture of upper end of unspecified radius**
CC Exclusion 7th character A see Appendix A PDX collection 1272
CC Exclusion 7th characters K & P see Appendix A PDX collection 0897
HAC 7th character A see Appendix B for HAC conditional logic

+ **S52.12 Fracture of head of radius**

CC MCC +7th **S52.121 Displaced fracture of head of right radius**
CC Exclusion 7th characters K - R see Appendix A PDX collection 0897
MCC Exclusion 7th characters B & C see Appendix A PDX collection 1269
HAC 7th characters B & C see Appendix B for HAC conditional logic

CC MCC +7th **S52.122 Displaced fracture of head of left radius**
CC Exclusion 7th characters K - R see Appendix A PDX collection 0897
MCC Exclusion 7th characters B & C see Appendix A PDX collection 1269
HAC 7th characters B & C see Appendix B for HAC conditional logic

CC MCC +7th **S52.123 Displaced fracture of head of unspecified radius**
CC Exclusion 7th characters K - R see Appendix A PDX collection 0897
MCC Exclusion 7th characters B & C see Appendix A PDX collection 1269
HAC 7th characters B & C see Appendix B for HAC conditional logic

CC MCC +7th **S52.124 Nondisplaced fracture of head of right radius**
CC Exclusion 7th characters K - R see Appendix A PDX collection 0897
MCC Exclusion 7th characters B & C see Appendix A PDX collection 1269
HAC 7th characters B & C see Appendix B for HAC conditional logic

CC MCC +7th **S52.125 Nondisplaced fracture of head of left radius**
CC Exclusion 7th characters K - R see Appendix A PDX collection 0897
MCC Exclusion 7th characters B & C see Appendix A PDX collection 1269
HAC 7th characters B & C see Appendix B for HAC conditional logic

CC MCC +7th **S52.126 Nondisplaced fracture of head of unspecified radius**
CC Exclusion 7th characters K - R see Appendix A PDX collection 0897
MCC Exclusion 7th characters B & C see Appendix A PDX collection 1269
HAC 7th characters B & C see Appendix B for HAC conditional logic

+ **S52.13 Fracture of neck of radius**

CC MCC +7th **S52.131 Displaced fracture of neck of right radius**
CC Exclusion 7th characters K - R see Appendix A PDX collection 0897
MCC Exclusion 7th characters B & C see Appendix A PDX collection 1269
HAC 7th characters B & C see Appendix B for HAC conditional logic

CC MCC +7th **S52.132 Displaced fracture of neck of left radius**
CC Exclusion 7th characters K - R see Appendix A PDX collection 0897
MCC Exclusion 7th characters B & C see Appendix A PDX collection 1269
HAC 7th characters B & C see Appendix B for HAC conditional logic

CC MCC +7th **S52.133 Displaced fracture of neck of unspecified radius**
CC Exclusion 7th characters K - R see Appendix A PDX collection 0897
MCC Exclusion 7th characters B & C see Appendix A PDX collection 1269
HAC 7th characters B & C see Appendix B for HAC conditional logic

CC MCC +7th **S52.134 Nondisplaced fracture of neck of right radi**
CC Exclusion 7th characters K - R see Appendix A PDX collection 0897
MCC Exclusion 7th characters B & C see Appendix A PDX collection 1269
HAC 7th characters B & C see Appendix B for HAC conditional logic

CC MCC +7th **S52.135 Nondisplaced fracture of neck of left radiu**
CC Exclusion 7th characters K - R see Appendix A PDX collection 0897
MCC Exclusion 7th characters B & C see Appendix A PDX collection 1269
HAC 7th characters B & C see Appendix B for HAC conditional logic

CC MCC +7th **S52.136 Nondisplaced fracture of neck of unspecified radius**
CC Exclusion 7th characters K - R see Appendix A PDX collection 0897
MCC Exclusion 7th characters B & C see Appendix A PDX collection 1269
HAC 7th characters B & C see Appendix B for HAC conditional logic

+ **S52.18 Other fracture of upper end of radius**

CC MCC +7th **S52.181 Other fracture of upper end of right radi**
CC Exclusion 7th characters K - R see Appendix A PDX collection 0897
MCC Exclusion 7th characters B & C see Appendix A PDX collection 1269
HAC 7th characters B & C see Appendix B for HAC conditional logic

CC MCC +7th **S52.182 Other fracture of upper end of left radius**
CC Exclusion 7th characters K - R see Appendix A PDX collection 0897
MCC Exclusion 7th characters B & C see Appendix A PDX collection 1269
HAC 7th characters B & C see Appendix B for HAC conditional logic

CC MCC +7th **S52.189 Other fracture of upper end of unspecifie radius**
CC Exclusion 7th characters K - R see Appendix A PDX collection 0897
MCC Exclusion 7th characters B & C see Appendix A PDX collection 1269
HAC 7th characters B & C see Appendix B for HAC conditional logic

+ **S52.2 Fracture of shaft of ulna**

+ **S52.20 Unspecified fracture of shaft of ulna**
Fracture of ulna NOS

CC MCC +7th **S52.201 Unspecified fracture of shaft of right uln**
CC Exclusion 7th character A see Appendix A PDX collection 1270
CC Exclusion 7th characters K - R see Appendix A PDX collection 0897
MCC Exclusion 7th characters B & C see Appendix A PDX collection 1269
HAC 7th characters A - C see Appendix B for HAC conditional logic

CC MCC +7th **S52.202 Unspecified fracture of shaft of left ulna**
CC Exclusion 7th character A see Appendix A PDX collection 1271
CC Exclusion 7th characters K - R see Appendix A PDX collection 0897
MCC Exclusion 7th characters B & C see Appendix A PDX collection 1269
HAC 7th characters A - C see Appendix B for HAC conditional logic

CC MCC +7th **S52.209 Unspecified fracture of shaft of unspecified ulna**
CC Exclusion 7th character A see Appendix A PDX collection 1272
CC Exclusion 7th characters K - R see Appendix A PDX collection 0897
MCC Exclusion 7th characters B & C see Appendix A PDX collection 1269
HAC 7th characters A - C see Appendix B for HAC conditional logic

+ **S52.21 Greenstick fracture of shaft of ulna**

The appropriate 7th character is to be added to all codes in subcategory **S52.21**
A initial encounter for closed fracture
D subsequent encounter for fracture with routine healing
G subsequent encounter for fracture with delayed healing
K subsequent encounter for fracture with nonunion
P subsequent encounter for fracture with malunion
S sequela

CC +7th **S52.211 Greenstick fracture of shaft of right ulna**
CC Exclusion 7th character A see Appendix A PDX collection 1270
CC Exclusion 7th characters K - R see Appendix A PDX collection 0897
HAC 7th character A see Appendix B for HAC conditional logic

CC +7th **S52.212 Greenstick fracture of shaft of left ulna**
CC Exclusion 7th character A see Appendix A PDX collection 1271
CC Exclusion 7th characters K - R see Appendix A PDX collection 0897
HAC 7th character A see Appendix B for HAC conditional logic

CC +7th **S52.219 Greenstick fracture of shaft of unspecified ulna**
CC Exclusion 7th character A see Appendix A PDX collection 1272
CC Exclusion 7th characters K - R see Appendix A PDX collection 0897
HAC 7th character A see Appendix B for HAC conditional logic

+ **S52.22 Transverse fracture of shaft of ulna**

CC MCC +7th **S52.221 Displaced transverse fracture of shaft of right ulna**
CC Exclusion 7th character A see Appendix A PDX collection 1270
CC Exclusion 7th characters K - R see Appendix A PDX collection 0897
MCC Exclusion 7th characters B & C see Appendix A PDX collection 1269
HAC 7th characters A - C see Appendix B for HAC conditional logic

CC MCC +7th **S52.222 Displaced transverse fracture of shaft of left ulna**
CC Exclusion 7th character A see Appendix A PDX collection 1271
CC Exclusion 7th characters K - R see Appendix A PDX collection 0897
MCC Exclusion 7th characters B & C see Appendix A PDX collection 1269
HAC 7th characters A - C see Appendix B for HAC conditional logic

CC MCC +7th **S52.223 Displaced transverse fracture of shaft of unspecified ulna**
CC Exclusion 7th character A see Appendix A PDX collection 1272
CC Exclusion 7th characters K - R see Appendix A PDX collection 0897
MCC Exclusion 7th characters B & C see Appendix A PDX collection 1269
HAC 7th characters A - C see Appendix B for HAC conditional logic

CC MCC +7th **S52.224 Nondisplaced transverse fracture of shaft of right ulna**
CC Exclusion 7th character A see Appendix A PDX collection 1270
CC Exclusion 7th characters K - R see Appendix A PDX collection 0897
MCC Exclusion 7th characters B & C see Appendix A PDX collection 1269
HAC 7th characters A - C see Appendix B for HAC conditional logic

CC MCC +7th **S52.225 Nondisplaced transverse fracture of shaft of left ulna**
CC Exclusion 7th character A see Appendix A PDX collection 1271
CC Exclusion 7th characters K - R see Appendix A PDX collection 0897
MCC Exclusion 7th characters B & C see Appendix A PDX collection 1269
HAC 7th characters A - C see Appendix B for HAC conditional logic

CC MCC +7th **S52.226 Nondisplaced transverse fracture of shaft of unspecified ulna**
CC Exclusion 7th character A see Appendix A PDX collection 1272
CC Exclusion 7th characters K - R see Appendix A PDX collection 0897
MCC Exclusion 7th characters B & C see Appendix A PDX collection 1269
HAC 7th characters A - C see Appendix B for HAC conditional logic

+ **S52.23 Oblique fracture of shaft of ulna**

CC MCC +7th **S52.231 Displaced oblique fracture of shaft of right ulna**
CC Exclusion 7th character A see Appendix A PDX collection 1270
CC Exclusion 7th characters K - R see Appendix A PDX collection 0897
MCC Exclusion 7th characters B & C see Appendix A PDX collection 1269
HAC 7th characters A - C see Appendix B for HAC conditional logic

CC MCC +7th **S52.232 Displaced oblique fracture of shaft of left ulna**
CC Exclusion 7th character A see Appendix A PDX collection 1271
CC Exclusion 7th characters K - R see Appendix A PDX collection 0897
MCC Exclusion 7th characters B & C see Appendix A PDX collection 1269
HAC 7th characters A - C see Appendix B for HAC conditional logic

CC MCC +7th **S52.233 Displaced oblique fracture of shaft of unspecified ulna**
CC Exclusion 7th character A see Appendix A PDX collection 1272
CC Exclusion 7th characters K - R see Appendix A PDX collection 0897
MCC Exclusion 7th characters B & C see Appendix A PDX collection 1269
HAC 7th characters A - C see Appendix B for HAC conditional logic

CC MCC +7th **S52.234 Nondisplaced oblique fracture of shaft of right ulna**
CC Exclusion 7th character A see Appendix A PDX collection 1270
CC Exclusion 7th characters K - R see Appendix A PDX collection 0897
MCC Exclusion 7th characters B & C see Appendix A PDX collection 1269
HAC 7th characters A - C see Appendix B for HAC conditional logic

CC MCC +7th **S52.235 Nondisplaced oblique fracture of shaft of left ulna**
CC Exclusion 7th character A see Appendix A PDX collection 1271
CC Exclusion 7th characters K - R see Appendix A PDX collection 0897
MCC Exclusion 7th characters B & C see Appendix A PDX collection 1269
HAC 7th characters A - C see Appendix B for HAC conditional logic

CC MCC +7th **S52.236 Nondisplaced oblique fracture of shaft of unspecified ulna**
CC Exclusion 7th character A see Appendix A PDX collection 1272
CC Exclusion 7th characters K - R see Appendix A PDX collection 0897
MCC Exclusion 7th characters B & C see Appendix A PDX collection 1269
HAC 7th characters A - C see Appendix B for HAC conditional logic

\+ **S52.24 Spiral fracture of shaft of ulna**

CC MCC +7th **S52.241 Displaced spiral fracture of shaft of ulna, right arm**
CC Exclusion 7th character A see Appendix A PDX collection 1270
CC Exclusion 7th characters K - R see Appendix A PDX collection 0897
MCC Exclusion 7th characters B & C see Appendix A PDX collection 1269
HAC 7th characters A - C see Appendix B for HAC conditional logic

CC MCC +7th **S52.242 Displaced spiral fracture of shaft of ulna, left arm**
CC Exclusion 7th character A see Appendix A PDX collection 1271
CC Exclusion 7th characters K - R see Appendix A PDX collection 0897
MCC Exclusion 7th characters B & C see Appendix A PDX collection 1269
HAC 7th characters A - C see Appendix B for HAC conditional logic

CC MCC +7th **S52.243 Displaced spiral fracture of shaft of ulna, unspecified arm**
CC Exclusion 7th character A see Appendix A PDX collection 1272
CC Exclusion 7th characters K - R see Appendix A PDX collection 0897
MCC Exclusion 7th characters B & C see Appendix A PDX collection 1269
HAC 7th characters A - C see Appendix B for HAC conditional logic

CC MCC +7th **S52.244 Nondisplaced spiral fracture of shaft of ulna, right arm**
CC Exclusion 7th character A see Appendix A PDX collection 1270
CC Exclusion 7th characters K - R see Appendix A PDX collection 0897
MCC Exclusion 7th characters B & C see Appendix A PDX collection 1269
HAC 7th characters A - C see Appendix B for HAC conditional logic

CC MCC +7th **S52.245 Nondisplaced spiral fracture of shaft of ulna, left arm**
CC Exclusion 7th character A see Appendix A PDX collection 1271
CC Exclusion 7th characters K - R see Appendix A PDX collection 0897
MCC Exclusion 7th characters B & C see Appendix A PDX collection 1269
HAC 7th characters A - C see Appendix B for HAC conditional logic

CC MCC +7th **S52.246 Nondisplaced spiral fracture of shaft of ulna, unspecified arm**
CC Exclusion 7th character A see Appendix A PDX collection 1272
CC Exclusion 7th characters K - R see Appendix A PDX collection 0897
MCC Exclusion 7th characters B & C see Appendix A PDX collection 1269
HAC 7th characters A - C see Appendix B for HAC conditional logic

\+ **S52.25 Comminuted fracture of shaft of ulna**

CC MCC +7th **S52.251 Displaced comminuted fracture of shaft of ulna, right arm**
CC Exclusion 7th character A see Appendix A PDX collection 1270
CC Exclusion 7th characters K - R see Appendix A PDX collection 0897
MCC Exclusion 7th characters B & C see Appendix A PDX collection 1269
HAC 7th characters A - C see Appendix B for HAC conditional logic

CC MCC +7th **S52.252 Displaced comminuted fracture of shaft of ulna, left arm**
CC Exclusion 7th character A see Appendix A PDX collection 1271
CC Exclusion 7th characters K - R see Appendix A PDX collection 0897
MCC Exclusion 7th characters B & C see Appendix A PDX collection 1269
HAC 7th characters A - C see Appendix B for HAC conditional logic

CC MCC +7th **S52.253 Displaced comminuted fracture of shaft of ulna, unspecified arm**
CC Exclusion 7th character A see Appendix A PDX collection 1272
CC Exclusion 7th characters K - R see Appendix A PDX collection 0897
MCC Exclusion 7th characters B & C see Appendix A PDX collection 1269
HAC 7th characters A - C see Appendix B for HAC conditional logic

CC MCC +7th **S52.254 Nondisplaced comminuted fracture of shaft of ulna, right arm**
CC Exclusion 7th character A see Appendix A PDX collection 1270
CC Exclusion 7th characters K - R see Appendix A PDX collection 0897
MCC Exclusion 7th characters B & C see Appendix A PDX collection 1269
HAC 7th characters A - C see Appendix B for HAC conditional logic

CC MCC +7th **S52.255 Nondisplaced comminuted fracture of shaft of ulna, left arm**
CC Exclusion 7th character A see Appendix A PDX collection 1271
CC Exclusion 7th characters K - R see Appendix A PDX collection 0897
MCC Exclusion 7th characters B & C see Appendix A PDX collection 1269
HAC 7th characters A - C see Appendix B for HAC conditional logic

CC MCC +7th **S52.256 Nondisplaced comminuted fracture of shaft of ulna, unspecified arm**
CC Exclusion 7th character A see Appendix A PDX collection 1272
CC Exclusion 7th characters K - R see Appendix A PDX collection 0897
MCC Exclusion 7th characters B & C see Appendix A PDX collection 1269
HAC 7th characters A - C see Appendix B for HAC conditional logic

\+ **S52.26 Segmental fracture of shaft of ulna**

CC MCC +7th **S52.261 Displaced segmental fracture of shaft of ulna, right arm**
CC Exclusion 7th character A see Appendix A PDX collection 1270
CC Exclusion 7th characters K - R see Appendix A PDX collection 0897
MCC Exclusion 7th characters B & C see Appendix A PDX collection 1269
HAC 7th characters A - C see Appendix B for HAC conditional logic

CC MCC +7th **S52.262 Displaced segmental fracture of shaft of ulna, left arm**
CC Exclusion 7th character A see Appendix A PDX collection 1271
CC Exclusion 7th characters K - R see Appendix A PDX collection 0897
MCC Exclusion 7th characters B & C see Appendix A PDX collection 1269
HAC 7th characters A - C see Appendix B for HAC conditional logic

CC MCC +7th **S52.263 Displaced segmental fracture of shaft of ulna, unspecified arm**
CC Exclusion 7th character A see Appendix A PDX collection 1272
CC Exclusion 7th characters K - R see Appendix A PDX collection 0897
MCC Exclusion 7th characters B & C see Appendix A PDX collection 1269
HAC 7th characters A - C see Appendix B for HAC conditional logic

CC MCC +7th **S52.264 Nondisplaced segmental fracture of shaft of ulna, right arm**
CC Exclusion 7th character A see Appendix A PDX collection 1270
CC Exclusion 7th characters K - R see Appendix A PDX collection 0897
MCC Exclusion 7th characters B & C see Appendix A PDX collection 1269
HAC 7th characters A - C see Appendix B for HAC conditional logic

CC MCC +7th **S52.265 Nondisplaced segmental fracture of shaft of ulna, left arm**
CC Exclusion 7th character A see Appendix A PDX collection 1271
CC Exclusion 7th characters K - R see Appendix A PDX collection 0897
MCC Exclusion 7th characters B & C see Appendix A PDX collection 1269
HAC 7th characters A - C see Appendix B for HAC conditional logic

CC MCC +7th **S52.266 Nondisplaced segmental fracture of shaft of ulna, unspecified arm**
CC Exclusion 7th character A see Appendix A PDX collection 1272
CC Exclusion 7th characters K - R see Appendix A PDX collection 0897
MCC Exclusion 7th characters B & C see Appendix A PDX collection 1269
HAC 7th characters A - C see Appendix B for HAC conditional logic

+ **S52.27 Monteggia's fracture of ulna**
Fracture of upper shaft of ulna with dislocation of radial head

CC MCC +7th **S52.271 Monteggia's fracture of right ulna**
CC Exclusion 7th characters K - R see Appendix A PDX collection 0897
MCC Exclusion 7th characters B & C see Appendix A PDX collection 1269
HAC 7th characters B & C see Appendix B for HAC conditional logic

CC MCC +7th **S52.272 Monteggia's fracture of left ulna**
CC Exclusion 7th characters K - R see Appendix A PDX collection 0897
MCC Exclusion 7th characters B & C see Appendix A PDX collection 1269
HAC 7th characters B & C see Appendix B for HAC conditional logic

CC MCC +7th **S52.279 Monteggia's fracture of unspecified ulna**
CC Exclusion 7th characters K - R see Appendix A PDX collection 0897
MCC Exclusion 7th characters B & C see Appendix A PDX collection 1269
HAC 7th characters B & C see Appendix B for HAC conditional logic

+ **S52.28 Bent bone of ulna**

CC MCC +7th **S52.281 Bent bone of right ulna**
CC Exclusion 7th character A see Appendix A PDX collection 1270
CC Exclusion 7th characters K - R see Appendix A PDX collection 0897
MCC Exclusion 7th characters B & C see Appendix A PDX collection 1269
HAC 7th characters A - C see Appendix B for HAC conditional logic

CC MCC +7th **S52.282 Bent bone of left ulna**
CC Exclusion 7th character A see Appendix A PDX collection 1271
CC Exclusion 7th characters K - R see Appendix A PDX collection 0897
MCC Exclusion 7th characters B & C see Appendix A PDX collection 1269
HAC 7th characters A - C see Appendix B for HAC conditional logic

CC MCC +7th **S52.283 Bent bone of unspecified ulna**
CC Exclusion 7th character A see Appendix A PDX collection 1272
CC Exclusion 7th characters K - R see Appendix A PDX collection 0897
MCC Exclusion 7th characters B & C see Appendix A PDX collection 1269
HAC 7th characters A - C see Appendix B for HAC conditional logic

+ **S52.29 Other fracture of shaft of ulna**

CC MCC +7th **S52.291 Other fracture of shaft of right ulna**
CC Exclusion 7th character A see Appendix A PDX collection 1270
CC Exclusion 7th characters K - R see Appendix A PDX collection 0897
MCC Exclusion 7th characters B & C see Appendix A PDX collection 1269
HAC 7th characters A - C see Appendix B for HAC conditional logic

CC MCC +7th **S52.292 Other fracture of shaft of left ulna**
CC Exclusion 7th character A see Appendix A PDX collection 1271
CC Exclusion 7th characters K - R see Appendix A PDX collection 0897
MCC Exclusion 7th characters B & C see Appendix A PDX collection 1269
HAC 7th characters A - C see Appendix B for HAC conditional logic

CC MCC +7th **S52.299 Other fracture of shaft of unspecified ulna**
CC Exclusion 7th character A see Appendix A PDX collection 1272
CC Exclusion 7th characters K - R see Appendix A PDX collection 0897
MCC Exclusion 7th characters B & C see Appendix A PDX collection 1269
HAC 7th characters A - C see Appendix B for HAC conditional logic

+ **S52.3 Fracture of shaft of radius**

+ **S52.30 Unspecified fracture of shaft of radius**

CC MCC +7th **S52.301 Unspecified fracture of shaft of right radius**
CC Exclusion 7th character A see Appendix A PDX collection 1270
CC Exclusion 7th characters K - R see Appendix A PDX collection 0897
MCC Exclusion 7th characters B & C see Appendix A PDX collection 1269
HAC 7th characters A - C see Appendix B for HAC conditional logic

CC MCC +7th **S52.302 Unspecified fracture of shaft of left radius**
CC Exclusion 7th character A see Appendix A PDX collection 1271
CC Exclusion 7th characters K - R see Appendix A PDX collection 0897
MCC Exclusion 7th characters B & C see Appendix A PDX collection 1269
HAC 7th characters A - C see Appendix B for HAC conditional logic

CC MCC +7th **S52.309 Unspecified fracture of shaft of unspecified radius**
CC Exclusion 7th character A see Appendix A PDX collection 1272
CC Exclusion 7th characters K - R see Appendix A PDX collection 0897
MCC Exclusion 7th characters B & C see Appendix A PDX collection 1269
HAC 7th characters A - C see Appendix B for HAC conditional logic

+ **S52.31 Greenstick fracture of shaft of radius**

The appropriate 7th character is to be added to all codes in subcategory **S52.31**
A initial encounter for closed fracture
D subsequent encounter for fracture with routine healing
G subsequent encounter for fracture with delayed healing
K subsequent encounter for fracture with nonunion
P subsequent encounter for fracture with malunion
S sequela

CC +7th **S52.311 Greenstick fracture of shaft of radius, right arm**
CC Exclusion 7th character A see Appendix A PDX collection 1270
CC Exclusion 7th characters K - R see Appendix A PDX collection 0897
HAC 7th character A see Appendix B for HAC conditional logic

CC +7th **S52.312 Greenstick fracture of shaft of radius, left arm**
CC Exclusion 7th character A see Appendix A PDX collection 1271
CC Exclusion 7th characters K - R see Appendix A PDX collection 0897
HAC 7th character A see Appendix B for HAC conditional logic

CC +7th **S52.319 Greenstick fracture of shaft of radius, unspecified arm**
CC Exclusion 7th character A see Appendix A PDX collection 1272
CC Exclusion 7th characters K - R see Appendix A PDX collection 0897
HAC 7th character A see Appendix B for HAC conditional logic

+ **S52.32 Transverse fracture of shaft of radius**

CC MCC +7th **S52.321 Displaced transverse fracture of shaft of right radius**
CC Exclusion 7th character A see Appendix A PDX collection 1270
CC Exclusion 7th characters K - R see Appendix A PDX collection 0897
MCC Exclusion 7th characters B & C see Appendix A PDX collection 1269
HAC 7th characters A - C see Appendix B for HAC conditional logic

CC MCC +7th **S52.322 Displaced transverse fracture of shaft of left radius**
CC Exclusion 7th character A see Appendix A PDX collection 1271
CC Exclusion 7th characters K - R see Appendix A PDX collection 0897
MCC Exclusion 7th characters B & C see Appendix A PDX collection 1269
HAC 7th characters A - C see Appendix B for HAC conditional logic

CC MCC +7th **S52.323 Displaced transverse fracture of shaft of unspecified radius**
CC Exclusion 7th character A see Appendix A PDX collection 1272
CC Exclusion 7th characters K - R see Appendix A PDX collection 0897
MCC Exclusion 7th characters B & C see Appendix A PDX collection 1269
HAC 7th characters A - C see Appendix B for HAC conditional logic

CC MCC +7th **S52.324 Nondisplaced transverse fracture of shaft of right radius**
CC Exclusion 7th character A see Appendix A PDX collection 1270
CC Exclusion 7th characters K - R see Appendix A PDX collection 0897
MCC Exclusion 7th characters B & C see Appendix A PDX collection 1269
HAC 7th characters A - C see Appendix B for HAC conditional logic

CC MCC +7th **S52.325 Nondisplaced transverse fracture of shaft of left radius**
CC Exclusion 7th character A see Appendix A PDX collection 1271
CC Exclusion 7th characters K - R see Appendix A PDX collection 0897
MCC Exclusion 7th characters B & C see Appendix A PDX collection 1269
HAC 7th characters A - C see Appendix B for HAC conditional logic

CC MCC +7th **S52.326 Nondisplaced transverse fracture of shaft of unspecified radius**
CC Exclusion 7th character A see Appendix A PDX collection 1272
CC Exclusion 7th characters K - R see Appendix A PDX collection 0897
MCC Exclusion 7th characters B & C see Appendix A PDX collection 1269
HAC 7th characters A - C see Appendix B for HAC conditional logic

+ **S52.33 Oblique fracture of shaft of radius**

CC MCC +7th **S52.331 Displaced oblique fracture of shaft of right radius**
CC Exclusion 7th character A see Appendix A PDX collection 1270
CC Exclusion 7th characters K - R see Appendix A PDX collection 0897
MCC Exclusion 7th characters B & C see Appendix A PDX collection 1269
HAC 7th characters A - C see Appendix B for HAC conditional logic

CC MCC +7th **S52.332 Displaced oblique fracture of shaft of left radius**
CC Exclusion 7th character A see Appendix A PDX collection 1271
CC Exclusion 7th characters K - R see Appendix A PDX collection 0897
MCC Exclusion 7th characters B & C see Appendix A PDX collection 1269
HAC 7th characters A - C see Appendix B for HAC conditional logic

CC MCC +7th **S52.333 Displaced oblique fracture of shaft of unspecified radius**
CC Exclusion 7th character A see Appendix A PDX collection 1272
CC Exclusion 7th characters K - R see Appendix A PDX collection 0897
MCC Exclusion 7th characters B & C see Appendix A PDX collection 1269
HAC 7th characters A - C see Appendix B for HAC conditional logic

CC MCC +7th **S52.334 Nondisplaced oblique fracture of shaft of right radius**
CC Exclusion 7th character A see Appendix A PDX collection 1270
CC Exclusion 7th characters K - R see Appendix A PDX collection 0897
MCC Exclusion 7th characters B & C see Appendix A PDX collection 1269
HAC 7th characters A - C see Appendix B for HAC conditional logic

CC MCC +7th **S52.335 Nondisplaced oblique fracture of shaft of left radius**
CC Exclusion 7th character A see Appendix A PDX collection 1271
CC Exclusion 7th characters K - R see Appendix A PDX collection 0897
MCC Exclusion 7th characters B & C see Appendix A PDX collection 1269
HAC 7th characters A - C see Appendix B for HAC conditional logic

CC MCC +7th **S52.336 Nondisplaced oblique fracture of shaft of unspecified radius**
CC Exclusion 7th character A see Appendix A PDX collection 1272
CC Exclusion 7th characters K - R see Appendix A PDX collection 0897
MCC Exclusion 7th characters B & C see Appendix A PDX collection 1269
HAC 7th characters A - C see Appendix B for HAC conditional logic

+ **S52.34 Spiral fracture of shaft of radius**

CC MCC +7th **S52.341 Displaced spiral fracture of shaft of radius, right arm**
CC Exclusion 7th character A see Appendix A PDX collection 1270
CC Exclusion 7th characters K - R see Appendix A PDX collection 0897
MCC Exclusion 7th characters B & C see Appendix A PDX collection 1269
HAC 7th characters A - C see Appendix B for HAC conditional logic

CC MCC +7th **S52.342 Displaced spiral fracture of shaft of radius, left arm**
CC Exclusion 7th character A see Appendix A PDX collection 1271
CC Exclusion 7th characters K - R see Appendix A PDX collection 0897
MCC Exclusion 7th characters B & C see Appendix A PDX collection 1269
HAC 7th characters A - C see Appendix B for HAC conditional logic

CC MCC +7th **S52.343 Displaced spiral fracture of shaft of radius, unspecified arm**
CC Exclusion 7th character A see Appendix A PDX collection 1272
CC Exclusion 7th characters K - R see Appendix A PDX collection 0897
MCC Exclusion 7th characters B & C see Appendix A PDX collection 1269
HAC 7th characters A - C see Appendix B for HAC conditional logic

CC MCC +7th **S52.344 Nondisplaced spiral fracture of shaft of radius, right arm**
CC Exclusion 7th character A see Appendix A PDX collection 1270
CC Exclusion 7th characters K - R see Appendix A PDX collection 0897
MCC Exclusion 7th characters B & C see Appendix A PDX collection 1269
HAC 7th characters A - C see Appendix B for HAC conditional logic

CC MCC +7th **S52.345 Nondisplaced spiral fracture of shaft of radius, left arm**
CC Exclusion 7th character A see Appendix A PDX collection 1271
CC Exclusion 7th characters K - R see Appendix A PDX collection 0897
MCC Exclusion 7th characters B & C see Appendix A PDX collection 1269
HAC 7th characters A - C see Appendix B for HAC conditional logic

CC MCC +7th **S52.346 Nondisplaced spiral fracture of shaft of radius, unspecified arm**
CC Exclusion 7th character A see Appendix A PDX collection 1272
CC Exclusion 7th characters K - R see Appendix A PDX collection 0897
MCC Exclusion 7th characters B & C see Appendix A PDX collection 1269
HAC 7th characters A - C see Appendix B for HAC conditional logic

\+ **S52.35 Comminuted fracture of shaft of radius**

CC MCC +7th **S52.351 Displaced comminuted fracture of shaft of radius, right arm**
CC Exclusion 7th character A see Appendix A PDX collection 1270
CC Exclusion 7th characters K - R see Appendix A PDX collection 0897
MCC Exclusion 7th characters B & C see Appendix A PDX collection 1269
HAC 7th characters A - C see Appendix B for HAC conditional logic

CC MCC +7th **S52.352 Displaced comminuted fracture of shaft of radius, left arm**
CC Exclusion 7th character A see Appendix A PDX collection 1271
CC Exclusion 7th characters K - R see Appendix A PDX collection 0897
MCC Exclusion 7th characters B & C see Appendix A PDX collection 1269
HAC 7th characters A - C see Appendix B for HAC conditional logic

CC MCC +7th **S52.353 Displaced comminuted fracture of shaft of radius, unspecified arm**
CC Exclusion 7th character A see Appendix A PDX collection 1272
CC Exclusion 7th characters K - R see Appendix A PDX collection 0897
MCC Exclusion 7th characters B & C see Appendix A PDX collection 1269
HAC 7th characters A - C see Appendix B for HAC conditional logic

CC MCC +7th **S52.354 Nondisplaced comminuted fracture of shaft of radius, right arm**
CC Exclusion 7th character A see Appendix A PDX collection 1270
CC Exclusion 7th characters K - R see Appendix A PDX collection 0897
MCC Exclusion 7th characters B & C see Appendix A PDX collection 1269
HAC 7th characters A - C see Appendix B for HAC conditional logic

CC MCC +7th **S52.355 Nondisplaced comminuted fracture of shaft of radius, left arm**
CC Exclusion 7th character A see Appendix A PDX collection 1271
CC Exclusion 7th characters K - R see Appendix A PDX collection 0897
MCC Exclusion 7th characters B & C see Appendix A PDX collection 1269
HAC 7th characters A - C see Appendix B for HAC conditional logic

CC MCC +7th **S52.356 Nondisplaced comminuted fracture of shaft of radius, unspecified arm**
CC Exclusion 7th character A see Appendix A PDX collection 1272
CC Exclusion 7th characters K - R see Appendix A PDX collection 0897
MCC Exclusion 7th characters B & C see Appendix A PDX collection 1269
HAC 7th characters A - C see Appendix B for HAC conditional logic

\+ **S52.36 Segmental fracture of shaft of radius**

CC MCC +7th **S52.361 Displaced segmental fracture of shaft of radius, right arm**
CC Exclusion 7th character A see Appendix A PDX collection 1270
CC Exclusion 7th characters K - R see Appendix A PDX collection 0897
MCC Exclusion 7th characters B & C see Appendix A PDX collection 1269
HAC 7th characters A - C see Appendix B for HAC conditional logic

CC MCC +7th **S52.362 Displaced segmental fracture of shaft of radius, left arm**
CC Exclusion 7th character A see Appendix A PDX collection 1271
CC Exclusion 7th characters K - R see Appendix A PDX collection 0897
MCC Exclusion 7th characters B & C see Appendix A PDX collection 1269
HAC 7th characters A - C see Appendix B for HAC conditional logic

CC MCC +7th **S52.363 Displaced segmental fracture of shaft of radius, unspecified arm**
CC Exclusion 7th character A see Appendix A PDX collection 1272
CC Exclusion 7th characters K - R see Appendix A PDX collection 0897
MCC Exclusion 7th characters B & C see Appendix A PDX collection 1269
HAC 7th characters A - C see Appendix B for HAC conditional logic

CC MCC +7th **S52.364 Nondisplaced segmental fracture of shaft of radius, right arm**
CC Exclusion 7th character A see Appendix A PDX collection 1270
CC Exclusion 7th characters K - R see Appendix A PDX collection 0897
MCC Exclusion 7th characters B & C see Appendix A PDX collection 1269
HAC 7th characters A - C see Appendix B for HAC conditional logic

CC MCC +7th **S52.365 Nondisplaced segmental fracture of shaft of radius, left arm**
CC Exclusion 7th character A see Appendix A PDX collection 1271
CC Exclusion 7th characters K - R see Appendix A PDX collection 0897
MCC Exclusion 7th characters B & C see Appendix A PDX collection 1269
HAC 7th characters A - C see Appendix B for HAC conditional logic

CC MCC +7th **S52.366 Nondisplaced segmental fracture of shaft of radius, unspecified arm**
CC Exclusion 7th character A see Appendix A PDX collection 1272
CC Exclusion 7th characters K - R see Appendix A PDX collection 0897
MCC Exclusion 7th characters B & C see Appendix A PDX collection 1269
HAC 7th characters A - C see Appendix B for HAC conditional logic

\+ **S52.37 Galeazzi's fracture**
Fracture of lower shaft of radius with radioulnar joint dislocation

CC MCC +7th **S52.371 Galeazzi's fracture of right radius**
CC Exclusion 7th character A see Appendix A PDX collection 1270
CC Exclusion 7th characters K - R see Appendix A PDX collection 0897
MCC Exclusion 7th characters B & C see Appendix A PDX collection 1269
HAC 7th characters A - C see Appendix B for HAC conditional logic

CC MCC +7th **S52.372 Galeazzi's fracture of left radius**
CC Exclusion 7th character A see Appendix A PDX collection 1271
CC Exclusion 7th characters K - R see Appendix A PDX collection 0897
MCC Exclusion 7th characters B & C see Appendix A PDX collection 1269
HAC 7th characters A - C see Appendix B for HAC conditional logic

CC MCC +7th **S52.379 Galeazzi's fracture of unspecified radius**
CC Exclusion 7th character A see Appendix A PDX collection 1272
CC Exclusion 7th characters K - R see Appendix A PDX collection 0897
MCC Exclusion 7th characters B & C see Appendix A PDX collection 1269
HAC 7th characters A - C see Appendix B for HAC conditional logic

+ **S52.38 Bent bone of radius**

CC MCC +7th **S52.381 Bent bone of right radius**
CC Exclusion 7th character A see Appendix A PDX collection 1270
CC Exclusion 7th characters K - R see Appendix A PDX collection 0897
MCC Exclusion 7th characters B & C see Appendix A PDX collection 1269
HAC 7th characters A - C see Appendix B for HAC conditional logic

CC MCC +7th **S52.382 Bent bone of left radius**
CC Exclusion 7th character A see Appendix A PDX collection 1271
CC Exclusion 7th characters K - R see Appendix A PDX collection 0897
MCC Exclusion 7th characters B & C see Appendix A PDX collection 1269
HAC 7th characters A - C see Appendix B for HAC conditional logic

CC MCC +7th **S52.389 Bent bone of unspecified radius**
CC Exclusion 7th character A see Appendix A PDX collection 1272
CC Exclusion 7th characters K - R see Appendix A PDX collection 0897
MCC Exclusion 7th characters B & C see Appendix A PDX collection 1269
HAC 7th characters A - C see Appendix B for HAC conditional logic

+ **S52.39 Other fracture of shaft of radius**

CC MCC +7th **S52.391 Other fracture of shaft of radius, right arm**
CC Exclusion 7th character A see Appendix A PDX collection 1270
CC Exclusion 7th characters K - R see Appendix A PDX collection 0897
MCC Exclusion 7th characters B & C see Appendix A PDX collection 1269
HAC 7th characters A - C see Appendix B for HAC conditional logic

CC MCC +7th **S52.392 Other fracture of shaft of radius, left arm**
CC Exclusion 7th character A see Appendix A PDX collection 1271
CC Exclusion 7th characters K - R see Appendix A PDX collection 0897
MCC Exclusion 7th characters B & C see Appendix A PDX collection 1269
HAC 7th characters A - C see Appendix B for HAC conditional logic

CC MCC +7th **S52.399 Other fracture of shaft of radius, unspecified arm**
CC Exclusion 7th character A see Appendix A PDX collection 1272
CC Exclusion 7th characters K - R see Appendix A PDX collection 0897
MCC Exclusion 7th characters B & C see Appendix A PDX collection 1269
HAC 7th characters A - C see Appendix B for HAC conditional logic

+ **S52.5 Fracture of lower end of radius**
Fracture of distal end of radius
Excludes2: *physeal fractures of lower end of radius (S59.2-)*

+ **S52.50 Unspecified fracture of the lower end of radius**

CC MCC +7th **S52.501 Unspecified fracture of the lower end of right radius**
CC Exclusion 7th character A see Appendix A PDX collection 1270
CC Exclusion 7th characters K - R see Appendix A PDX collection 0897
MCC Exclusion 7th characters B & C see Appendix A PDX collection 1269
HAC 7th characters A - C see Appendix B for HAC conditional logic

CC MCC +7th **S52.502 Unspecified fracture of the lower end of left radius**
CC Exclusion 7th character A see Appendix A PDX collection 1271
CC Exclusion 7th characters K - R see Appendix A PDX collection 0897
MCC Exclusion 7th characters B & C see Appendix A PDX collection 1269
HAC 7th characters A - C see Appendix B for HAC conditional logic

CC MCC +7th **S52.509 Unspecified fracture of the lower end of unspecified radius**
CC Exclusion 7th character A see Appendix A PDX collection 1272
CC Exclusion 7th characters K - R see Appendix A PDX collection 0897
MCC Exclusion 7th characters B & C see Appendix A PDX collection 1269
HAC 7th characters A - C see Appendix B for HAC conditional logic

+ **S52.51 Fracture of radial styloid process**

CC MCC +7th **S52.511 Displaced fracture of right radial styloid process**
CC Exclusion 7th character A see Appendix A PDX collection 1270
CC Exclusion 7th characters K - R see Appendix A PDX collection 0897
MCC Exclusion 7th characters B & C see Appendix A PDX collection 1269
HAC 7th characters A - C see Appendix B for HAC conditional logic

CC MCC +7th **S52.512 Displaced fracture of left radial styloid process**
CC Exclusion 7th character A see Appendix A PDX collection 1271
CC Exclusion 7th characters K - R see Appendix A PDX collection 0897
MCC Exclusion 7th characters B & C see Appendix A PDX collection 1269
HAC 7th characters A - C see Appendix B for HAC conditional logic

CC MCC +7th **S52.513 Displaced fracture of unspecified radial styloid process**
CC Exclusion 7th character A see Appendix A PDX collection 1272
CC Exclusion 7th characters K - R see Appendix A PDX collection 0897
MCC Exclusion 7th characters B & C see Appendix A PDX collection 1269
HAC 7th characters A - C see Appendix B for HAC conditional logic

CC MCC +7th **S52.514 Nondisplaced fracture of right radial styloid process**
CC Exclusion 7th character A see Appendix A PDX collection 1270
CC Exclusion 7th characters K - R see Appendix A PDX collection 0897
MCC Exclusion 7th characters B & C see Appendix A PDX collection 1269
HAC 7th characters A - C see Appendix B for HAC conditional logic

CC MCC +7th **S52.515 Nondisplaced fracture of left radial styloid process**
CC Exclusion 7th character A see Appendix A PDX collection 1271
CC Exclusion 7th characters K - R see Appendix A PDX collection 0897
MCC Exclusion 7th characters B & C see Appendix A PDX collection 1269
HAC 7th characters A - C see Appendix B for HAC conditional logic

CC MCC +7th **S52.516 Nondisplaced fracture of unspecified radial styloid process**
CC Exclusion 7th character A see Appendix A PDX collection 1272
CC Exclusion 7th characters K - R see Appendix A PDX collection 0897
MCC Exclusion 7th characters B & C see Appendix A PDX collection 1269
HAC 7th characters A - C see Appendix B for HAC conditional logic

+ S52.52 Torus fracture of lower end of radius

The appropriate 7th character is to be added to all codes in subcategory **S52.52**
A initial encounter for closed fracture
D subsequent encounter for fracture with routine healing
G subsequent encounter for fracture with delayed healing
K subsequent encounter for fracture with nonunion
P subsequent encounter for fracture with malunion
S sequela

CC +7th **S52.521 Torus fracture of lower end of right radius**
CC Exclusion 7th character A see Appendix A PDX collection 1270
CC Exclusion 7th characters K - R see Appendix A PDX collection 0897
HAC 7th character A see Appendix B for HAC conditional logic

CC +7th **S52.522 Torus fracture of lower end of left radius**
CC Exclusion 7th character A see Appendix A PDX collection 1271
CC Exclusion 7th characters K - R see Appendix A PDX collection 0897
HAC 7th character A see Appendix B for HAC conditional logic

CC +7th **S52.529 Torus fracture of lower end of unspecified radius**
CC Exclusion 7th character A see Appendix A PDX collection 1272
CC Exclusion 7th characters K - R see Appendix A PDX collection 0897
HAC 7th character A see Appendix B for HAC conditional logic

+ S52.53 Colles' fracture

CC MCC +7th **S52.531 Colles' fracture of right radius**
CC Exclusion 7th character A see Appendix A PDX collection 1270
CC Exclusion 7th characters K - R see Appendix A PDX collection 0897
MCC Exclusion 7th characters B & C see Appendix A PDX collection 1269
HAC 7th characters A - C see Appendix B for HAC conditional logic

CC MCC +7th **S52.532 Colles' fracture of left radius**
CC Exclusion 7th character A see Appendix A PDX collection 1271
CC Exclusion 7th characters K - R see Appendix A PDX collection 0897
MCC Exclusion 7th characters B & C see Appendix A PDX collection 1269
AHA CC: 2Q, 2016, 4-5
HAC 7th characters A - C see Appendix B for HAC conditional logic

CC MCC +7th **S52.539 Colles' fracture of unspecified radius**
CC Exclusion 7th character A see Appendix A PDX collection 1272
CC Exclusion 7th characters K - R see Appendix A PDX collection 0897
MCC Exclusion 7th characters B & C see Appendix A PDX collection 1269
HAC 7th characters A - C see Appendix B for HAC conditional logic

+ S52.54 Smith's fracture

CC MCC +7th **S52.541 Smith's fracture of right radius**
CC Exclusion 7th character A see Appendix A PDX collection 1270
CC Exclusion 7th characters K - R see Appendix A PDX collection 0897
MCC Exclusion 7th characters B & C see Appendix A PDX collection 1269
HAC 7th characters A - C see Appendix B for HAC conditional logic

CC MCC +7th **S52.542 Smith's fracture of left radius**
CC Exclusion 7th character A see Appendix A PDX collection 1271
CC Exclusion 7th characters K - R see Appendix A PDX collection 0897
MCC Exclusion 7th characters B & C see Appendix A PDX collection 1269
HAC 7th characters A - C see Appendix B for HAC conditional logic

CC MCC +7th **S52.549 Smith's fracture of unspecified radius**
CC Exclusion 7th character A see Appendix A PDX collection 1272
CC Exclusion 7th characters K - R see Appendix A PDX collection 0897
MCC Exclusion 7th characters B & C see Appendix A PDX collection 1269
HAC 7th characters A - C see Appendix B for HAC conditional logic

+ S52.55 Other extraarticular fracture of lower end of radius

CC MCC +7th **S52.551 Other extraarticular fracture of lower end of right radius**
CC Exclusion 7th character A see Appendix A PDX collection 1270
CC Exclusion 7th characters K - R see Appendix A PDX collection 0897
MCC Exclusion 7th characters B & C see Appendix A PDX collection 1269
HAC 7th characters A - C see Appendix B for HAC conditional logic

CC MCC +7th **S52.552 Other extraarticular fracture of lower end of left radius**
CC Exclusion 7th character A see Appendix A PDX collection 1271
CC Exclusion 7th characters K - R see Appendix A PDX collection 0897
MCC Exclusion 7th characters B & C see Appendix A PDX collection 1269
HAC 7th characters A - C see Appendix B for HAC conditional logic

CC MCC +7th **S52.559 Other extraarticular fracture of lower end of unspecified radius**
CC Exclusion 7th character A see Appendix A PDX collection 1272
CC Exclusion 7th characters K - R see Appendix A PDX collection 0897
MCC Exclusion 7th characters B & C see Appendix A PDX collection 1269
HAC 7th characters A - C see Appendix B for HAC conditional logic

+ S52.56 Barton's fracture

CC MCC +7th **S52.561 Barton's fracture of right radius**
CC Exclusion 7th character A see Appendix A PDX collection 1270
CC Exclusion 7th characters K - R see Appendix A PDX collection 0897
MCC Exclusion 7th characters B & C see Appendix A PDX collection 1269
HAC 7th characters A - C see Appendix B for HAC conditional logic

CC MCC +7th **S52.562 Barton's fracture of left radius**
CC Exclusion 7th character A see Appendix A PDX collection 1271
CC Exclusion 7th characters K - R see Appendix A PDX collection 0897
MCC Exclusion 7th characters B & C see Appendix A PDX collection 1269
HAC 7th characters A - C see Appendix B for HAC conditional logic

CC MCC +7th **S52.569 Barton's fracture of unspecified radius**
CC Exclusion 7th character A see Appendix A PDX collection 1272
CC Exclusion 7th characters K - R see Appendix A PDX collection 0897
MCC Exclusion 7th characters B & C see Appendix A PDX collection 1269
HAC 7th characters A - C see Appendix B for HAC conditional logic

+ S52.57 Other intraarticular fracture of lower end of radius

CC MCC +7th **S52.571 Other intraarticular fracture of lower end of right radius**
CC Exclusion 7th character A see Appendix A PDX collection 1270
CC Exclusion 7th characters K - R see Appendix A PDX collection 0897
MCC Exclusion 7th characters B & C see Appendix A PDX collection 1269
HAC 7th characters A - C see Appendix B for HAC conditional logic

CC MCC +7th **S52.572 Other intraarticular fracture of lower end of left radius**
CC Exclusion 7th character A see Appendix A PDX collection 1271
CC Exclusion 7th characters K - R see Appendix A PDX collection 0897
MCC Exclusion 7th characters B & C see Appendix A PDX collection 1269
HAC 7th characters A - C see Appendix B for HAC conditional logic

CC MCC +7th **S52.579 Other intraarticular fracture of lower end of unspecified radius**
CC Exclusion 7th character A see Appendix A PDX collection 1272
CC Exclusion 7th characters K - R see Appendix A PDX collection 0897
MCC Exclusion 7th characters B & C see Appendix A PDX collection 1269
HAC 7th characters A - C see Appendix B for HAC conditional logic

+ **S52.59 Other fractures of lower end of radius**

CC MCC +7th **S52.591 Other fractures of lower end of right radius**
CC Exclusion 7th character A see Appendix A PDX collection 1270
CC Exclusion 7th characters K - R see Appendix A PDX collection 0897
MCC Exclusion 7th characters B & C see Appendix A PDX collection 1269
HAC 7th characters A - C see Appendix B for HAC conditional logic

CC MCC +7th **S52.592 Other fractures of lower end of left radius**
CC Exclusion 7th character A see Appendix A PDX collection 1271
CC Exclusion 7th characters K - R see Appendix A PDX collection 0897
MCC Exclusion 7th characters B & C see Appendix A PDX collection 1269
HAC 7th characters A - C see Appendix B for HAC conditional logic

CC MCC +7th **S52.599 Other fractures of lower end of unspecified radius**
CC Exclusion 7th character A see Appendix A PDX collection 1272
CC Exclusion 7th characters K - R see Appendix A PDX collection 0897
MCC Exclusion 7th characters B & C see Appendix A PDX collection 1269
HAC 7th characters A - C see Appendix B for HAC conditional logic

+ **S52.6 Fracture of lower end of ulna**

+ **S52.60 Unspecified fracture of lower end of ulna**

CC MCC +7th **S52.601 Unspecified fracture of lower end of right ulna**
CC Exclusion 7th character A see Appendix A PDX collection 1270
CC Exclusion 7th characters K - R see Appendix A PDX collection 0897
MCC Exclusion 7th characters B & C see Appendix A PDX collection 1269
HAC 7th characters A - C see Appendix B for HAC conditional logic

CC MCC +7th **S52.602 Unspecified fracture of lower end of left ulna**
CC Exclusion 7th character A see Appendix A PDX collection 1271
CC Exclusion 7th characters K - R see Appendix A PDX collection 0897
MCC Exclusion 7th characters B & C see Appendix A PDX collection 1269
HAC 7th characters A - C see Appendix B for HAC conditional logic

CC MCC +7th **S52.609 Unspecified fracture of lower end of unspecified ulna**
CC Exclusion 7th character A see Appendix A PDX collection 1272
CC Exclusion 7th characters K - R see Appendix A PDX collection 0897
MCC Exclusion 7th characters B & C see Appendix A PDX collection 1269
HAC 7th characters A - C see Appendix B for HAC conditional logic

+ **S52.61 Fracture of ulna styloid process**

CC MCC +7th **S52.611 Displaced fracture of right ulna styloid process**
CC Exclusion 7th character A see Appendix A PDX collection 1270
CC Exclusion 7th characters K - R see Appendix A PDX collection 0897
MCC Exclusion 7th characters B & C see Appendix A PDX collection 1269
HAC 7th characters A - C see Appendix B for HAC conditional logic

CC MCC +7th **S52.612 Displaced fracture of left ulna styloid process**
CC Exclusion 7th character A see Appendix A PDX collection 1271
CC Exclusion 7th characters K - R see Appendix A PDX collection 0897
MCC Exclusion 7th characters B & C see Appendix A PDX collection 1269
HAC 7th characters A - C see Appendix B for HAC conditional logic

CC MCC +7th **S52.613 Displaced fracture of unspecified ulna styloid process**
CC Exclusion 7th character A see Appendix A PDX collection 1272
CC Exclusion 7th characters K - R see Appendix A PDX collection 0897
MCC Exclusion 7th characters B & C see Appendix A PDX collection 1269
HAC 7th characters A - C see Appendix B for HAC conditional logic

CC MCC +7th **S52.614 Nondisplaced fracture of right ulna styloid process**
CC Exclusion 7th character A see Appendix A PDX collection 1270
CC Exclusion 7th characters K - R see Appendix A PDX collection 0897
MCC Exclusion 7th characters B & C see Appendix A PDX collection 1269
HAC 7th characters A - C see Appendix B for HAC conditional logic

CC MCC +7th **S52.615 Nondisplaced fracture of left ulna styloid process**
CC Exclusion 7th character A see Appendix A PDX collection 1271
CC Exclusion 7th characters K - R see Appendix A PDX collection 0897
MCC Exclusion 7th characters B & C see Appendix A PDX collection 1269
HAC 7th characters A - C see Appendix B for HAC conditional logic

CC MCC +7th **S52.616 Nondisplaced fracture of unspecified ulna styloid process**
CC Exclusion 7th character A see Appendix A PDX collection 1272
CC Exclusion 7th characters K - R see Appendix A PDX collection 0897
MCC Exclusion 7th characters B & C see Appendix A PDX collection 1269
HAC 7th characters A - C see Appendix B for HAC conditional logic

+ **S52.62 Torus fracture of lower end of ulna**

The appropriate 7th character is to be added to all codes in subcategory **S52.62**
A initial encounter for closed fracture
D subsequent encounter for fracture with routine healing
G subsequent encounter for fracture with delayed healing
K subsequent encounter for fracture with nonunion
P subsequent encounter for fracture with malunion
S sequela

CC +7th **S52.621 Torus fracture of lower end of right ulna**
CC Exclusion 7th character A see Appendix A PDX collection 1270
CC Exclusion 7th characters K - R see Appendix A PDX collection 0897
HAC 7th character A see Appendix B for HAC conditional logic

CC +7th **S52.622 Torus fracture of lower end of left ulna**
CC Exclusion 7th character A see Appendix A PDX collection 1271
CC Exclusion 7th characters K - R see Appendix A PDX collection 0897
HAC 7th character A see Appendix B for HAC conditional logic

CC +7th S52.629 **Torus fracture of lower end of unspecified ulna**
CC Exclusion 7th character A see Appendix A PDX collection 1272
CC Exclusion 7th characters K - R see Appendix A PDX collection 0897
HAC 7th character A see Appendix B for HAC conditional logic

\+ S52.69 **Other fracture of lower end of ulna**

CC MCC +7th S52.691 **Other fracture of lower end of right ulna**
CC Exclusion 7th character A see Appendix A PDX collection 1270
CC Exclusion 7th characters K - R see Appendix A PDX collection 0897
MCC Exclusion 7th characters B & C see Appendix A PDX collection 1269
HAC 7th characters A - C see Appendix B for HAC conditional logic

CC MCC +7th S52.692 **Other fracture of lower end of left ulna**
CC Exclusion 7th character A see Appendix A PDX collection 1271
CC Exclusion 7th characters K - R see Appendix A PDX collection 0897
MCC Exclusion 7th characters B & C see Appendix A PDX collection 1269
HAC 7th characters A - C see Appendix B for HAC conditional logic

CC MCC +7th S52.699 **Other fracture of lower end of unspecified ulna**
CC Exclusion 7th character A see Appendix A PDX collection 1272
CC Exclusion 7th characters K - R see Appendix A PDX collection 0897
MCC Exclusion 7th characters B & C see Appendix A PDX collection 1269
HAC 7th characters A - C see Appendix B for HAC conditional logic

\+ S52.9 **Unspecified fracture of forearm**

CC MCC X+7th S52.90 **Unspecified fracture of unspecified forearm**
CC Exclusion 7th character A see Appendix A PDX collection 1272
CC Exclusion 7th characters K - R see Appendix A PDX collection 0897
MCC Exclusion 7th characters B & C see Appendix A PDX collection 1269
HAC 7th characters A - C see Appendix B for HAC conditional logic

CC MCC X+7th S52.91 **Unspecified fracture of right forearm**
CC Exclusion 7th character A see Appendix A PDX collection 1272
CC Exclusion 7th characters K - R see Appendix A PDX collection 0897
MCC Exclusion 7th characters B & C see Appendix A PDX collection 1269
HAC 7th characters A - C see Appendix B for HAC conditional logic

CC MCC X+7th S52.92 **Unspecified fracture of left forearm**
CC Exclusion 7th character A see Appendix A PDX collection 1272
CC Exclusion 7th characters K - R see Appendix A PDX collection 0897
MCC Exclusion 7th characters B & C see Appendix A PDX collection 1269
HAC 7th characters A - C see Appendix B for HAC conditional logic

S53 Dislocation and sprain of joints and ligaments of elbow

Includes: avulsion of joint or ligament of elbow
laceration of cartilage, joint or ligament of elbow
sprain of cartilage, joint or ligament of elbow
traumatic hemarthrosis of joint or ligament of elbow
traumatic rupture of joint or ligament of elbow
traumatic subluxation of joint or ligament of elbow
traumatic tear of joint or ligament of elbow

Code also any associated open wound

Excludes2: *strain of muscle, fascia and tendon at forearm level (S56.-)*

The appropriate 7th character is to be added to each code from category S53
A initial encounter
D subsequent encounter
S sequela

\+ S53.0 **Subluxation and dislocation of radial head**
Dislocation of radiohumeral joint
Subluxation of radiohumeral joint
Excludes1: *Monteggia's fracture-dislocation (S52.27-)*

\+ S53.00 **Unspecified subluxation and dislocation of radial head**
+7th S53.001 **Unspecified subluxation of right radial head**
+7th S53.002 **Unspecified subluxation of left radial head**
+7th S53.003 **Unspecified subluxation of unspecified radial head**
+7th S53.004 **Unspecified dislocation of right radial head**
+7th S53.005 **Unspecified dislocation of left radial head**
+7th S53.006 **Unspecified dislocation of unspecified radial head**

\+ S53.01 **Anterior subluxation and dislocation of radial head**
Anteriomedial subluxation and dislocation of radial head
+7th S53.011 **Anterior subluxation of right radial head**
+7th S53.012 **Anterior subluxation of left radial head**
+7th S53.013 **Anterior subluxation of unspecified radial head**
+7th S53.014 **Anterior dislocation of right radial head**
+7th S53.015 **Anterior dislocation of left radial head**
+7th S53.016 **Anterior dislocation of unspecified radial head**

\+ S53.02 **Posterior subluxation and dislocation of radial head**
Posteriolateral subluxation and dislocation of radial head
+7th S53.021 **Posterior subluxation of right radial head**
+7th S53.022 **Posterior subluxation of left radial head**
+7th S53.023 **Posterior subluxation of unspecified radial head**
+7th S53.024 **Posterior dislocation of right radial head**
+7th S53.025 **Posterior dislocation of left radial head**
+7th S53.026 **Posterior dislocation of unspecified radial head**

\+ S53.03 **Nursemaid's elbow**
+7th S53.031 **Nursemaid's elbow, right elbow**
AHA CC: 1Q, 2015, 3-21
+7th S53.032 **Nursemaid's elbow, left elbow**
+7th S53.033 **Nursemaid's elbow, unspecified elbow**

\+ S53.09 **Other subluxation and dislocation of radial head**
+7th S53.091 **Other subluxation of right radial head**
+7th S53.092 **Other subluxation of left radial head**
+7th S53.093 **Other subluxation of unspecified radial head**
+7th S53.094 **Other dislocation of right radial head**
+7th S53.095 **Other dislocation of left radial head**
+7th S53.096 **Other dislocation of unspecified radial head**

\+ S53.1 **Subluxation and dislocation of ulnohumeral joint**
Subluxation and dislocation of elbow NOS
Excludes1: *dislocation of radial head alone (S53.0-)*

\+ S53.10 **Unspecified subluxation and dislocation of ulnohumeral joint**
+7th S53.101 **Unspecified subluxation of right ulnohumeral joint**
+7th S53.102 **Unspecified subluxation of left ulnohumeral joint**
+7th S53.103 **Unspecified subluxation of unspecified ulnohumeral joint**
+7th S53.104 **Unspecified dislocation of right ulnohumeral joint**
+7th S53.105 **Unspecified dislocation of left ulnohumeral joint**
+7th S53.106 **Unspecified dislocation of unspecified ulnohumeral joint**

\+ S53.11 **Anterior subluxation and dislocation of ulnohumeral joint**
+7th S53.111 **Anterior subluxation of right ulnohumeral joint**
+7th S53.112 **Anterior subluxation of left ulnohumeral joint**
+7th S53.113 **Anterior subluxation of unspecified ulnohumeral joint**
+7th S53.114 **Anterior dislocation of right ulnohumeral joint**
AHA CC: 4Q, 2012, 108
+7th S53.115 **Anterior dislocation of left ulnohumeral joint**
+7th S53.116 **Anterior dislocation of unspecified ulnohumeral joint**

+ **S53.12 Posterior subluxation and dislocation of ulnohumeral joint**
  - +7th **S53.121 Posterior subluxation of right ulnohumeral joint**
  - +7th **S53.122 Posterior subluxation of left ulnohumeral joint**
  - +7th **S53.123 Posterior subluxation of unspecified ulnohumeral joint**
  - +7th **S53.124 Posterior dislocation of right ulnohumeral joint**
  - +7th **S53.125 Posterior dislocation of left ulnohumeral joint**
  - +7th **S53.126 Posterior dislocation of unspecified ulnohumeral joint**
+ **S53.13 Medial subluxation and dislocation of ulnohumeral joint**
  - +7th **S53.131 Medial subluxation of right ulnohumeral joint**
  - +7th **S53.132 Medial subluxation of left ulnohumeral joint**
  - +7th **S53.133 Medial subluxation of unspecified ulnohumeral joint**
  - +7th **S53.134 Medial dislocation of right ulnohumeral joint**
  - +7th **S53.135 Medial dislocation of left ulnohumeral joint**
  - +7th **S53.136 Medial dislocation of unspecified ulnohumeral joint**
+ **S53.14 Lateral subluxation and dislocation of ulnohumeral joint**
  - +7th **S53.141 Lateral subluxation of right ulnohumeral joint**
  - +7th **S53.142 Lateral subluxation of left ulnohumeral joint**
  - +7th **S53.143 Lateral subluxation of unspecified ulnohumeral joint**
  - +7th **S53.144 Lateral dislocation of right ulnohumeral joint**
  - +7th **S53.145 Lateral dislocation of left ulnohumeral joint**
  - +7th **S53.146 Lateral dislocation of unspecified ulnohumeral joint**
+ **S53.19 Other subluxation and dislocation of ulnohumeral joint**
  - +7th **S53.191 Other subluxation of right ulnohumeral joint**
  - +7th **S53.192 Other subluxation of left ulnohumeral joint**
  - +7th **S53.193 Other subluxation of unspecified ulnohumeral joint**
  - +7th **S53.194 Other dislocation of right ulnohumeral joint**
  - +7th **S53.195 Other dislocation of left ulnohumeral joint**
  - +7th **S53.196 Other dislocation of unspecified ulnohumeral joint**

+ **S53.2 Traumatic rupture of radial collateral ligament**
  Excludes1: *sprain of radial collateral ligament NOS (S53.43-)*
  - X+7th **S53.20 Traumatic rupture of unspecified radial collateral ligament**
  - X+7th **S53.21 Traumatic rupture of right radial collateral ligament**
  - X+7th **S53.22 Traumatic rupture of left radial collateral ligament**
+ **S53.3 Traumatic rupture of ulnar collateral ligament**
  Excludes1: *sprain of ulnar collateral ligament (S53.44-)*
  - X+7th **S53.30 Traumatic rupture of unspecified ulnar collateral ligament**
  - X+7th **S53.31 Traumatic rupture of right ulnar collateral ligament**
  - X+7th **S53.32 Traumatic rupture of left ulnar collateral ligament**
+ **S53.4 Sprain of elbow**
  Excludes2: *traumatic rupture of radial collateral ligament (S53.2-)*
  traumatic rupture of ulnar collateral ligament (S53.3-)
  + **S53.40 Unspecified sprain of elbow**
    - +7th **S53.401 Unspecified sprain of right elbow**
    - +7th **S53.402 Unspecified sprain of left elbow**
    - +7th **S53.409 Unspecified sprain of unspecified elbow**
      Sprain of elbow NOS
  + **S53.41 Radiohumeral (joint) sprain**
    - +7th **S53.411 Radiohumeral (joint) sprain of right elbow**
    - +7th **S53.412 Radiohumeral (joint) sprain of left elbow**
    - +7th **S53.419 Radiohumeral (joint) sprain of unspecified elbow**
  + **S53.42 Ulnohumeral (joint) sprain**
    - +7th **S53.421 Ulnohumeral (joint) sprain of right elbow**
    - +7th **S53.422 Ulnohumeral (joint) sprain of left elbow**
    - +7th **S53.429 Ulnohumeral (joint) sprain of unspecified elbow**
  + **S53.43 Radial collateral ligament sprain**
    - +7th **S53.431 Radial collateral ligament sprain of right elbow**
    - +7th **S53.432 Radial collateral ligament sprain of left elbow**
    - +7th **S53.439 Radial collateral ligament sprain of unspecified elbow**
  + **S53.44 Ulnar collateral ligament sprain**
    - +7th **S53.441 Ulnar collateral ligament sprain of right elbow**
    - +7th **S53.442 Ulnar collateral ligament sprain of left elbow**
    - +7th **S53.449 Ulnar collateral ligament sprain of unspecified elbow**
  + **S53.49 Other sprain of elbow**
    - +7th **S53.491 Other sprain of right elbow**
    - +7th **S53.492 Other sprain of left elbow**
    - +7th **S53.499 Other sprain of unspecified elbow**

S54 Injury of nerves at forearm level

Code also any associated open wound (S51.-)

Excludes2: *injury of nerves at wrist and hand level (S64.-)*

The appropriate 7th character is to be added to each code from category S54
A initial encounter
D subsequent encounter
S sequela

+ **S54.0 Injury of ulnar nerve at forearm level**
  Injury of ulnar nerve NOS
  - X+7th **S54.00 Injury of ulnar nerve at forearm level, unspecified arm**
  - X+7th **S54.01 Injury of ulnar nerve at forearm level, right arm**
  - X+7th **S54.02 Injury of ulnar nerve at forearm level, left arm**
+ **S54.1 Injury of median nerve at forearm level**
  Injury of median nerve NOS
  - X+7th **S54.10 Injury of median nerve at forearm level, unspecified arm**
  - X+7th **S54.11 Injury of median nerve at forearm level, right arm**
  - X+7th **S54.12 Injury of median nerve at forearm level, left arm**
+ **S54.2 Injury of radial nerve at forearm level**
  Injury of radial nerve NOS
  - X+7th **S54.20 Injury of radial nerve at forearm level, unspecified arm**
  - X+7th **S54.21 Injury of radial nerve at forearm level, right arm**
  - X+7th **S54.22 Injury of radial nerve at forearm level, left arm**
+ **S54.3 Injury of cutaneous sensory nerve at forearm level**
  - X+7th **S54.30 Injury of cutaneous sensory nerve at forearm level, unspecified arm**
  - X+7th **S54.31 Injury of cutaneous sensory nerve at forearm level, right arm**
  - X+7th **S54.32 Injury of cutaneous sensory nerve at forearm level, left arm**
+ **S54.8 Injury of other nerves at forearm level**
  + **S54.8X Injury of other nerves at forearm level**
    - +7th **S54.8X1 Injury of other nerves at forearm level, right arm**
    - +7th **S54.8X2 Injury of other nerves at forearm level, left arm**
    - +7th **S54.8X9 Injury of other nerves at forearm level, unspecified arm**
+ **S54.9 Injury of unspecified nerve at forearm level**
  - X+7th **S54.90 Injury of unspecified nerve at forearm level, unspecified arm**
  - X+7th **S54.91 Injury of unspecified nerve at forearm level, right arm**
  - X+7th **S54.92 Injury of unspecified nerve at forearm level, left arm**

S55 Injury of blood vessels at forearm level

Code also any associated open wound (S51.-)

Excludes2: *injury of blood vessels at wrist and hand level (S65.-)*
injury of brachial vessels (S45.1-S45.2)

The appropriate 7th character is to be added to each code from category S55
A initial encounter
D subsequent encounter
S sequela

+ **S55.0 Injury of ulnar artery at forearm level**
  + **S55.00 Unspecified injury of ulnar artery at forearm level**
    - CC +7th **S55.001 Unspecified injury of ulnar artery at forearm level, right arm**
      CC Exclusion 7th character A see Appendix A
      PDX collection 1274
    - CC +7th **S55.002 Unspecified injury of ulnar artery at forearm level, left arm**
      CC Exclusion 7th character A see Appendix A
      PDX collection 1275
    - CC +7th **S55.009 Unspecified injury of ulnar artery at forearm level, unspecified arm**
      CC Exclusion 7th character A see Appendix A
      PDX collection 1276
  + **S55.01 Laceration of ulnar artery at forearm level**
    - CC +7th **S55.011 Laceration of ulnar artery at forearm level, right arm**
      CC Exclusion 7th character A see Appendix A
      PDX collection 1274
    - CC +7th **S55.012 Laceration of ulnar artery at forearm level, left arm**
      CC Exclusion 7th character A see Appendix A
      PDX collection 1275
    - CC +7th **S55.019 Laceration of ulnar artery at forearm level, unspecified arm**
      CC Exclusion 7th character A see Appendix A
      PDX collection 1276
  + **S55.09 Other specified injury of ulnar artery at forearm level**
    - CC +7th **S55.091 Other specified injury of ulnar artery at forearm level, right arm**
      CC Exclusion 7th character A see Appendix A
      PDX collection 1274
    - CC +7th **S55.092 Other specified injury of ulnar artery at forearm level, left arm**
      CC Exclusion 7th character A see Appendix A
      PDX collection 1275
    - CC +7th **S55.099 Other specified injury of ulnar artery at forearm level, unspecified arm**
      CC Exclusion 7th character A see Appendix A
      PDX collection 1276
+ **S55.1 Injury of radial artery at forearm level**
  + **S55.10 Unspecified injury of radial artery at forearm level**
    - CC +7th **S55.101 Unspecified injury of radial artery at forearm level, right arm**
      CC Exclusion 7th character A see Appendix A
      PDX collection 1277
    - CC +7th **S55.102 Unspecified injury of radial artery at forearm level, left arm**
      CC Exclusion 7th character A see Appendix A
      PDX collection 1278
    - CC +7th **S55.109 Unspecified injury of radial artery at forearm level, unspecified arm**
      CC Exclusion 7th character A see Appendix A
      PDX collection 1279
  + **S55.11 Laceration of radial artery at forearm level**
    - CC +7th **S55.111 Laceration of radial artery at forearm level, right arm**
      CC Exclusion 7th character A see Appendix A
      PDX collection 1277
    - CC +7th **S55.112 Laceration of radial artery at forearm level, left arm**
      CC Exclusion 7th character A see Appendix A
      PDX collection 1278
    - CC +7th **S55.119 Laceration of radial artery at forearm level, unspecified arm**
      CC Exclusion 7th character A see Appendix A
      PDX collection 1279
  + **S55.19 Other specified injury of radial artery at forearm level**
    - CC +7th **S55.191 Other specified injury of radial artery at forearm level, right arm**
      CC Exclusion 7th character A see Appendix A
      PDX collection 1277
    - CC +7th **S55.192 Other specified injury of radial artery at forearm level, left arm**
      CC Exclusion 7th character A see Appendix A
      PDX collection 1278
    - CC +7th **S55.199 Other specified injury of radial artery at forearm level, unspecified arm**
      CC Exclusion 7th character A see Appendix A
      PDX collection 1279
+ **S55.2 Injury of vein at forearm level**
  + **S55.20 Unspecified injury of vein at forearm level**
    - CC +7th **S55.201 Unspecified injury of vein at forearm level, right arm**
      CC Exclusion 7th character A see Appendix A
      PDX collection 1260
    - CC +7th **S55.202 Unspecified injury of vein at forearm level, left arm**
      CC Exclusion 7th character A see Appendix A
      PDX collection 1261
    - CC +7th **S55.209 Unspecified injury of vein at forearm level, unspecified arm**
      CC Exclusion 7th character A see Appendix A
      PDX collection 1262
  + **S55.21 Laceration of vein at forearm level**
    - CC +7th **S55.211 Laceration of vein at forearm level, right arm**
      CC Exclusion 7th character A see Appendix A
      PDX collection 1260
    - CC +7th **S55.212 Laceration of vein at forearm level, left arm**
      CC Exclusion 7th character A see Appendix A
      PDX collection 1261
    - CC +7th **S55.219 Laceration of vein at forearm level, unspecified arm**
      CC Exclusion 7th character A see Appendix A
      PDX collection 1262
  + **S55.29 Other specified injury of vein at forearm level**
    - CC +7th **S55.291 Other specified injury of vein at forearm level, right arm**
      CC Exclusion 7th character A see Appendix A
      PDX collection 1260
    - CC +7th **S55.292 Other specified injury of vein at forearm level, left arm**
      CC Exclusion 7th character A see Appendix A
      PDX collection 1261
    - CC +7th **S55.299 Other specified injury of vein at forearm level, unspecified arm**
      CC Exclusion 7th character A see Appendix A
      PDX collection 1262
+ **S55.8 Injury of other blood vessels at forearm level**
  + **S55.80 Unspecified injury of other blood vessels at forearm level**
    - CC +7th **S55.801 Unspecified injury of other blood vessels at forearm level, right arm**
      CC Exclusion 7th character A see Appendix A
      PDX collection 1260
    - CC +7th **S55.802 Unspecified injury of other blood vessels at forearm level, left arm**
      CC Exclusion 7th character A see Appendix A
      PDX collection 1261
    - CC +7th **S55.809 Unspecified injury of other blood vessels at forearm level, unspecified arm**
      CC Exclusion 7th character A see Appendix A
      PDX collection 1262
  + **S55.81 Laceration of other blood vessels at forearm level**
    - CC +7th **S55.811 Laceration of other blood vessels at forearm level, right arm**
      CC Exclusion 7th character A see Appendix A
      PDX collection 1260
    - CC +7th **S55.812 Laceration of other blood vessels at forearm level, left arm**
      CC Exclusion 7th character A see Appendix A
      PDX collection 1261
    - CC +7th **S55.819 Laceration of other blood vessels at forearm level, unspecified arm**
      CC Exclusion 7th character A see Appendix A
      PDX collection 1262
  + **S55.89 Other specified injury of other blood vessels at forearm level**
    - CC +7th **S55.891 Other specified injury of other blood vessels at forearm level, right arm**
      CC Exclusion 7th character A see Appendix A
      PDX collection 1260

CC +7th **S55.892** **Other specified injury of other blood vessels at forearm level, left arm**
CC Exclusion 7th character A see Appendix A PDX collection 1261

CC +7th **S55.899** **Other specified injury of other blood vessels at forearm level, unspecified arm**
CC Exclusion 7th character A see Appendix A PDX collection 1262

\+ **S55.9** **Injury of unspecified blood vessel at forearm level**

\+ **S55.90** **Unspecified injury of unspecified blood vessel at forearm level**

CC +7th **S55.901** **Unspecified injury of unspecified blood vessel at forearm level, right arm**
CC Exclusion 7th character A see Appendix A PDX collection 1260

CC +7th **S55.902** **Unspecified injury of unspecified blood vessel at forearm level, left arm**
CC Exclusion 7th character A see Appendix A PDX collection 1261

CC +7th **S55.909** **Unspecified injury of unspecified blood vessel at forearm level, unspecified arm**
CC Exclusion 7th character A see Appendix A PDX collection 1262

\+ **S55.91** **Laceration of unspecified blood vessel at forearm level**

CC +7th **S55.911** **Laceration of unspecified blood vessel at forearm level, right arm**
CC Exclusion 7th character A see Appendix A PDX collection 1260

CC +7th **S55.912** **Laceration of unspecified blood vessel at forearm level, left arm**
CC Exclusion 7th character A see Appendix A PDX collection 1261

CC +7th **S55.919** **Laceration of unspecified blood vessel at forearm level, unspecified arm**
CC Exclusion 7th character A see Appendix A PDX collection 1262

\+ **S55.99** **Other specified injury of unspecified blood vessel at forearm level**

CC +7th **S55.991** **Other specified injury of unspecified blood vessel at forearm level, right arm**
CC Exclusion 7th character A see Appendix A PDX collection 1260

CC +7th **S55.992** **Other specified injury of unspecified blood vessel at forearm level, left arm**
CC Exclusion 7th character A see Appendix A PDX collection 1261

CC +7th **S55.999** **Other specified injury of unspecified blood vessel at forearm level, unspecified arm**
CC Exclusion 7th character A see Appendix A PDX collection 1262

S56 **Injury of muscle, fascia and tendon at forearm level**

Code also any associated open wound (S51.-)

Excludes2: *injury of muscle, fascia and tendon at or below wrist (S66.-)*
sprain of joints and ligaments of elbow (S53.4-)

The appropriate 7th character is to be added to each code from category S56
A initial encounter
D subsequent encounter
S sequela

\+ **S56.0** **Injury of flexor muscle, fascia and tendon of thumb at forearm level**

\+ **S56.00** **Unspecified injury of flexor muscle, fascia and tendon of thumb at forearm level**

+7th **S56.001** **Unspecified injury of flexor muscle, fascia and tendon of right thumb at forearm level**

+7th **S56.002** **Unspecified injury of flexor muscle, fascia and tendon of left thumb at forearm level**

+7th **S56.009** **Unspecified injury of flexor muscle, fascia and tendon of unspecified thumb at forearm level**

\+ **S56.01** **Strain of flexor muscle, fascia and tendon of thumb at forearm level**

+7th **S56.011** **Strain of flexor muscle, fascia and tendon of right thumb at forearm level**

+7th **S56.012** **Strain of flexor muscle, fascia and tendon of left thumb at forearm level**

+7th **S56.019** **Strain of flexor muscle, fascia and tendon of unspecified thumb at forearm level**

\+ **S56.02** **Laceration of flexor muscle, fascia and tendon of thumb at forearm level**

CC +7th **S56.021** **Laceration of flexor muscle, fascia and tendon of right thumb at forearm level**
CC Exclusion 7th character A see Appendix A PDX collection 1280

CC +7th **S56.022** **Laceration of flexor muscle, fascia and tendon of left thumb at forearm level**
CC Exclusion 7th character A see Appendix A PDX collection 1281

CC +7th **S56.029** **Laceration of flexor muscle, fascia and tendon of unspecified thumb at forearm level**
CC Exclusion 7th character A see Appendix A PDX collection 1282

\+ **S56.09** **Other injury of flexor muscle, fascia and tendon of thumb at forearm level**

+7th **S56.091** **Other injury of flexor muscle, fascia and tendon of right thumb at forearm level**

+7th **S56.092** **Other injury of flexor muscle, fascia and tendon of left thumb at forearm level**

+7th **S56.099** **Other injury of flexor muscle, fascia and tendon of unspecified thumb at forearm level**

\+ **S56.1** **Injury of flexor muscle, fascia and tendon of other and unspecified finger at forearm level**

\+ **S56.10** **Unspecified injury of flexor muscle, fascia and tendon of other and unspecified finger at forearm level**

+7th **S56.101** **Unspecified injury of flexor muscle, fascia and tendon of right index finger at forearm level**

+7th **S56.102** **Unspecified injury of flexor muscle, fascia and tendon of left index finger at forearm level**

+7th **S56.103** **Unspecified injury of flexor muscle, fascia and tendon of right middle finger at forearm level**

+7th **S56.104** **Unspecified injury of flexor muscle, fascia and tendon of left middle finger at forearm level**

+7th **S56.105** **Unspecified injury of flexor muscle, fascia and tendon of right ring finger at forearm level**

+7th **S56.106** **Unspecified injury of flexor muscle, fascia and tendon of left ring finger at forearm level**

+7th **S56.107** **Unspecified injury of flexor muscle, fascia and tendon of right little finger at forearm level**

+7th **S56.108** **Unspecified injury of flexor muscle, fascia and tendon of left little finger at forearm level**

+7th **S56.109** **Unspecified injury of flexor muscle, fascia and tendon of unspecified finger at forearm level**

\+ **S56.11** **Strain of flexor muscle, fascia and tendon of other and unspecified finger at forearm level**

+7th **S56.111** **Strain of flexor muscle, fascia and tendon of right index finger at forearm level**

+7th **S56.112** **Strain of flexor muscle, fascia and tendon of left index finger at forearm level**

+7th **S56.113** **Strain of flexor muscle, fascia and tendon of right middle finger at forearm level**

+7th **S56.114** **Strain of flexor muscle, fascia and tendon of left middle finger at forearm level**

+7th **S56.115** **Strain of flexor muscle, fascia and tendon of right ring finger at forearm level**

+7th **S56.116** **Strain of flexor muscle, fascia and tendon of left ring finger at forearm level**

+7th **S56.117** **Strain of flexor muscle, fascia and tendon of right little finger at forearm level**

+7th **S56.118** **Strain of flexor muscle, fascia and tendon of left little finger at forearm level**

+7th **S56.119** **Strain of flexor muscle, fascia and tendon of finger of unspecified finger at forearm level**

\+ **S56.12** **Laceration of flexor muscle, fascia and tendon of other and unspecified finger at forearm level**

CC +7th **S56.121** Laceration of flexor muscle, fascia and tendon of right index finger at forearm level
CC Exclusion 7th character A see Appendix A PDX collection 1280

CC +7th **S56.122** Laceration of flexor muscle, fascia and tendon of left index finger at forearm level
CC Exclusion 7th character A see Appendix A PDX collection 1281

CC +7th **S56.123** Laceration of flexor muscle, fascia and tendon of right middle finger at forearm level
CC Exclusion 7th character A see Appendix A PDX collection 1280

CC +7th **S56.124** Laceration of flexor muscle, fascia and tendon of left middle finger at forearm level
CC Exclusion 7th character A see Appendix A PDX collection 1281

CC +7th **S56.125** Laceration of flexor muscle, fascia and tendon of right ring finger at forearm level
CC Exclusion 7th character A see Appendix A PDX collection 1280

CC +7th **S56.126** Laceration of flexor muscle, fascia and tendon of left ring finger at forearm level
CC Exclusion 7th character A see Appendix A PDX collection 1281

CC +7th **S56.127** Laceration of flexor muscle, fascia and tendon of right little finger at forearm level
CC Exclusion 7th character A see Appendix A PDX collection 1280

CC +7th **S56.128** Laceration of flexor muscle, fascia and tendon of left little finger at forearm level
CC Exclusion 7th character A see Appendix A PDX collection 1281

CC +7th **S56.129** Laceration of flexor muscle, fascia and tendon of unspecified finger at forearm level
CC Exclusion 7th character A see Appendix A PDX collection 1282

\+ **S56.19** Other injury of flexor muscle, fascia and tendon of other and unspecified finger at forearm level

+7th **S56.191** Other injury of flexor muscle, fascia and tendon of right index finger at forearm level

+7th **S56.192** Other injury of flexor muscle, fascia and tendon of left index finger at forearm level

+7th **S56.193** Other injury of flexor muscle, fascia and tendon of right middle finger at forearm level

+7th **S56.194** Other injury of flexor muscle, fascia and tendon of left middle finger at forearm level

+7th **S56.195** Other injury of flexor muscle, fascia and tendon of right ring finger at forearm level

+7th **S56.196** Other injury of flexor muscle, fascia and tendon of left ring finger at forearm level

+7th **S56.197** Other injury of flexor muscle, fascia and tendon of right little finger at forearm level

+7th **S56.198** Other injury of flexor muscle, fascia and tendon of left little finger at forearm level

+7th **S56.199** Other injury of flexor muscle, fascia and tendon of unspecified finger at forearm level

\+ **S56.2** Injury of other flexor muscle, fascia and tendon at forearm level

\+ **S56.20** Unspecified injury of other flexor muscle, fascia and tendon at forearm level

+7th **S56.201** Unspecified injury of other flexor muscle, fascia and tendon at forearm level, right arm

+7th **S56.202** Unspecified injury of other flexor muscle, fascia and tendon at forearm level, left arm

+7th **S56.209** Unspecified injury of other flexor muscle, fascia and tendon at forearm level, unspecified arm

\+ **S56.21** Strain of other flexor muscle, fascia and tendon at forearm level

+7th **S56.211** Strain of other flexor muscle, fascia and tendon at forearm level, right arm

+7th **S56.212** Strain of other flexor muscle, fascia and tendon at forearm level, left arm

+7th **S56.219** Strain of other flexor muscle, fascia and tendon at forearm level, unspecified arm

\+ **S56.22** Laceration of other flexor muscle, fascia and tendon at forearm level

CC +7th **S56.221** Laceration of other flexor muscle, fascia and tendon at forearm level, right arm
CC Exclusion 7th character A see Appendix A PDX collection 1280

CC +7th **S56.222** Laceration of other flexor muscle, fascia and tendon at forearm level, left arm
CC Exclusion 7th character A see Appendix A PDX collection 1281

CC +7th **S56.229** Laceration of other flexor muscle, fascia and tendon at forearm level, unspecified arm
CC Exclusion 7th character A see Appendix A PDX collection 1282

\+ **S56.29** Other injury of other flexor muscle, fascia and tendon at forearm level

+7th **S56.291** Other injury of other flexor muscle, fascia and tendon at forearm level, right arm

+7th **S56.292** Other injury of other flexor muscle, fascia and tendon at forearm level, left arm

+7th **S56.299** Other injury of other flexor muscle, fascia and tendon at forearm level, unspecified arm

\+ **S56.3** Injury of extensor or abductor muscles, fascia and tendons of thumb at forearm level

\+ **S56.30** Unspecified injury of extensor or abductor muscles, fascia and tendons of thumb at forearm level

+7th **S56.301** Unspecified injury of extensor or abductor muscles, fascia and tendons of right thumb at forearm level

+7th **S56.302** Unspecified injury of extensor or abductor muscles, fascia and tendons of left thumb at forearm level

+7th **S56.309** Unspecified injury of extensor or abductor muscles, fascia and tendons of unspecified thumb at forearm level

\+ **S56.31** Strain of extensor or abductor muscles, fascia and tendons of thumb at forearm level

+7th **S56.311** Strain of extensor or abductor muscles, fascia and tendons of right thumb at forearm level

+7th **S56.312** Strain of extensor or abductor muscles, fascia and tendons of left thumb at forearm level

+7th **S56.319** Strain of extensor or abductor muscles, fascia and tendons of unspecified thumb at forearm level

\+ **S56.32** Laceration of extensor or abductor muscles, fascia and tendons of thumb at forearm level

CC +7th **S56.321** Laceration of extensor or abductor muscles, fascia and tendons of right thumb at forearm level
CC Exclusion 7th character A see Appendix A PDX collection 1280

CC +7th **S56.322** Laceration of extensor or abductor muscles, fascia and tendons of left thumb at forearm level
CC Exclusion 7th character A see Appendix A PDX collection 1281

CC +7th **S56.329** Laceration of extensor or abductor muscles, fascia and tendons of unspecified thumb at forearm level
CC Exclusion 7th character A see Appendix A PDX collection 1282

\+ **S56.39** Other injury of extensor or abductor muscles, fascia and tendons of thumb at forearm level

+7th **S56.391** Other injury of extensor or abductor muscles, fascia and tendons of right thumb at forearm level

+7th **S56.392** Other injury of extensor or abductor muscles, fascia and tendons of left thumb at forearm level

+7th **S56.399** Other injury of extensor or abductor muscles, fascia and tendons of unspecified thumb at forearm level

+ **S56.4** Injury of extensor muscle, fascia and tendon of other and unspecified finger at forearm level
  + **S56.40** Unspecified injury of extensor muscle, fascia and tendon of other and unspecified finger at forearm level
    - +7th **S56.401** Unspecified injury of extensor muscle, fascia and tendon of right index finger at forearm level
    - +7th **S56.402** Unspecified injury of extensor muscle, fascia and tendon of left index finger at forearm level
    - +7th **S56.403** Unspecified injury of extensor muscle, fascia and tendon of right middle finger at forearm level
    - +7th **S56.404** Unspecified injury of extensor muscle, fascia and tendon of left middle finger at forearm level
    - +7th **S56.405** Unspecified injury of extensor muscle, fascia and tendon of right ring finger at forearm level
    - +7th **S56.406** Unspecified injury of extensor muscle, fascia and tendon of left ring finger at forearm level
    - +7th **S56.407** Unspecified injury of extensor muscle, fascia and tendon of right little finger at forearm level
    - +7th **S56.408** Unspecified injury of extensor muscle, fascia and tendon of left little finger at forearm level
    - +7th **S56.409** Unspecified injury of extensor muscle, fascia and tendon of unspecified finger at forearm level
  + **S56.41** Strain of extensor muscle, fascia and tendon of other and unspecified finger at forearm level
    - +7th **S56.411** Strain of extensor muscle, fascia and tendon of right index finger at forearm level
    - +7th **S56.412** Strain of extensor muscle, fascia and tendon of left index finger at forearm level
    - +7th **S56.413** Strain of extensor muscle, fascia and tendon of right middle finger at forearm level
    - +7th **S56.414** Strain of extensor muscle, fascia and tendon of left middle finger at forearm level
    - +7th **S56.415** Strain of extensor muscle, fascia and tendon of right ring finger at forearm level
    - +7th **S56.416** Strain of extensor muscle, fascia and tendon of left ring finger at forearm level
    - +7th **S56.417** Strain of extensor muscle, fascia and tendon of right little finger at forearm level
    - +7th **S56.418** Strain of extensor muscle, fascia and tendon of left little finger at forearm level
    - +7th **S56.419** Strain of extensor muscle, fascia and tendon of finger, unspecified finger at forearm level
  + **S56.42** Laceration of extensor muscle, fascia and tendon of other and unspecified finger at forearm level
    - CC +7th **S56.421** Laceration of extensor muscle, fascia and tendon of right index finger at forearm level
      CC Exclusion 7th character A see Appendix A PDX collection 1280
    - CC +7th **S56.422** Laceration of extensor muscle, fascia and tendon of left index finger at forearm level
      CC Exclusion 7th character A see Appendix A PDX collection 1281
    - CC +7th **S56.423** Laceration of extensor muscle, fascia and tendon of right middle finger at forearm level
      CC Exclusion 7th character A see Appendix A PDX collection 1280
    - CC +7th **S56.424** Laceration of extensor muscle, fascia and tendon of left middle finger at forearm level
      CC Exclusion 7th character A see Appendix A PDX collection 1281
    - CC +7th **S56.425** Laceration of extensor muscle, fascia and tendon of right ring finger at forearm level
      CC Exclusion 7th character A see Appendix A PDX collection 1280
    - CC +7th **S56.426** Laceration of extensor muscle, fascia and tendon of left ring finger at forearm level
      CC Exclusion 7th character A see Appendix A PDX collection 1281
    - CC +7th **S56.427** Laceration of extensor muscle, fascia and tendon of right little finger at forearm lev
      CC Exclusion 7th character A see Appendix A PDX collection 1280
    - CC +7th **S56.428** Laceration of extensor muscle, fascia and tendon of left little finger at forearm level
      CC Exclusion 7th character A see Appendix A PDX collection 1281
    - CC +7th **S56.429** Laceration of extensor muscle, fascia and tendon of unspecified finger at forearm level
      CC Exclusion 7th character A see Appendix A PDX collection 1282
  + **S56.49** Other injury of extensor muscle, fascia and tendon of other and unspecified finger at forearm level
    - +7th **S56.491** Other injury of extensor muscle, fascia and tendon of right index finger at forear level
    - +7th **S56.492** Other injury of extensor muscle, fascia an tendon of left index finger at forearm leve
    - +7th **S56.493** Other injury of extensor muscle, fascia an tendon of right middle finger at forearm level
    - +7th **S56.494** Other injury of extensor muscle, fascia and tendon of left middle finger at forear level
    - +7th **S56.495** Other injury of extensor muscle, fascia an tendon of right ring finger at forearm leve
    - +7th **S56.496** Other injury of extensor muscle, fascia an tendon of left ring finger at forearm level
    - +7th **S56.497** Other injury of extensor muscle, fascia an tendon of right little finger at forearm lev
    - +7th **S56.498** Other injury of extensor muscle, fascia an tendon of left little finger at forearm level
    - +7th **S56.499** Other injury of extensor muscle, fascia an tendon of unspecified finger at forearm level

+ **S56.5** Injury of other extensor muscle, fascia and tendon at forearm level
  + **S56.50** Unspecified injury of other extensor muscle, fascia and tendon at forearm level
    - +7th **S56.501** Unspecified injury of other extensor muscle, fascia and tendon at forearm leve right arm
    - +7th **S56.502** Unspecified injury of other extensor muscle, fascia and tendon at forearm leve left arm
    - +7th **S56.509** Unspecified injury of other extensor muscle, fascia and tendon at forearm leve unspecified arm
  + **S56.51** Strain of other extensor muscle, fascia and tendon forearm level
    - +7th **S56.511** Strain of other extensor muscle, fascia an tendon at forearm level, right arm
    - +7th **S56.512** Strain of other extensor muscle, fascia≈ar tendon at forearm level, left arm
    - +7th **S56.519** Strain of other extensor muscle, fascia an tendon at forearm level, unspecified arm
  + **S56.52** Laceration of other extensor muscle, fascia and tendon at forearm level
    - CC +7th **S56.521** Laceration of other extensor muscle, fasc and tendon at forearm level, right arm
      CC Exclusion 7th character A see Appendix A PDX collection 1280
    - CC +7th **S56.522** Laceration of other extensor muscle, fasc and tendon at forearm level, left arm
      CC Exclusion 7th character A see Appendix A PDX collection 1281
    - CC +7th **S56.529** Laceration of other extensor muscle, fasc and tendon at forearm level, unspecified arm
      CC Exclusion 7th character A see Appendix A PDX collection 1282
  + **S56.59** Other injury of other extensor muscle, fascia and tendon at forearm level
    - +7th **S56.591** Other injury of other extensor muscle, fascia and tendon at forearm leve right arm

+7th S56.592 Other injury of other extensor muscle, fascia and tendon at forearm level, left arm
+7th S56.599 Other injury of other extensor muscle, fascia and tendon at forearm level, unspecified arm
+ S56.8 Injury of other muscles, fascia and tendons at forearm level
+ S56.80 Unspecified injury of other muscles, fascia and tendons at forearm level
+7th S56.801 Unspecified injury of other muscles, fascia and tendons at forearm level, right arm
+7th S56.802 Unspecified injury of other muscles, fascia and tendons at forearm level, left arm
+7th S56.809 Unspecified injury of other muscles, fascia and tendons at forearm level, unspecified arm
+ S56.81 Strain of other muscles, fascia and tendons at forearm level
+7th S56.811 Strain of other muscles, fascia and tendons at forearm level, right arm
+7th S56.812 Strain of other muscles, fascia and tendons at forearm level, left arm
+7th S56.819 Strain of other muscles, fascia and tendons at forearm level, unspecified arm
+ S56.82 Laceration of other muscles, fascia and tendons at forearm level
CC +7th S56.821 Laceration of other muscles, fascia and tendons at forearm level, right arm
CC Exclusion 7th character A see Appendix A PDX collection 1280
CC +7th S56.822 Laceration of other muscles, fascia and tendons at forearm level, left arm
CC Exclusion 7th character A see Appendix A PDX collection 1281
CC +7th S56.829 Laceration of other muscles, fascia and tendons at forearm level, unspecified arm
CC Exclusion 7th character A see Appendix A PDX collection 1282
+ S56.89 Other injury of other muscles, fascia and tendons at forearm level
+7th S56.891 Other injury of other muscles, fascia and tendons at forearm level, right arm
+7th S56.892 Other injury of other muscles, fascia and tendons at forearm level, left arm
+7th S56.899 Other injury of other muscles, fascia and tendons at forearm level, unspecified arm
+ S56.9 Injury of unspecified muscles, fascia and tendons at forearm level
+ S56.90 Unspecified injury of unspecified muscles, fascia and tendons at forearm level
+7th S56.901 Unspecified injury of unspecified muscles, fascia and tendons at forearm level, right arm
+7th S56.902 Unspecified injury of unspecified muscles, fascia and tendons at forearm level, left arm
+7th S56.909 Unspecified injury of unspecified muscles, fascia and tendons at forearm level, unspecified arm
+ S56.91 Strain of unspecified muscles, fascia and tendons at forearm level
+7th S56.911 Strain of unspecified muscles, fascia and tendons at forearm level, right arm
+7th S56.912 Strain of unspecified muscles, fascia and tendons at forearm level, left arm
+7th S56.919 Strain of unspecified muscles, fascia and tendons at forearm level, unspecified arm
+ S56.92 Laceration of unspecified muscles, fascia and tendons at forearm level
CC +7th S56.921 Laceration of unspecified muscles, fascia and tendons at forearm level, right arm
CC Exclusion 7th character A see Appendix A PDX collection 1280
CC +7th S56.922 Laceration of unspecified muscles, fascia and tendons at forearm level, left arm
CC Exclusion 7th character A see Appendix A PDX collection 1281
CC +7th S56.929 Laceration of unspecified muscles, fascia and tendons at forearm level, unspecified arm
CC Exclusion 7th character A see Appendix A PDX collection 1282
+ S56.99 Other injury of unspecified muscles, fascia and tendons at forearm level
+7th S56.991 Other injury of unspecified muscles, fascia and tendons at forearm level, right arm
+7th S56.992 Other injury of unspecified muscles, fascia and tendons at forearm level, left arm
+7th S56.999 Other injury of unspecified muscles, fascia and tendons at forearm level, unspecified arm

S57 Crushing injury of elbow and forearm

Use additional code(s) for all associated injuries

Excludes2: *crushing injury of wrist and hand (S67.-)*

The appropriate 7th character is to be added to each code from category S57
A initial encounter
D subsequent encounter
S sequela

+ S57.0 Crushing injury of elbow
X+7th S57.00 Crushing injury of unspecified elbow
X+7th S57.01 Crushing injury of right elbow
X+7th S57.02 Crushing injury of left elbow
+ S57.8 Crushing injury of forearm
X+7th S57.80 Crushing injury of unspecified forearm
X+7th S57.81 Crushing injury of right forearm
X+7th S57.82 Crushing injury of left forearm

S58 Traumatic amputation of elbow and forearm

An amputation not identified as partial or complete should be coded to complete

Excludes1: *traumatic amputation of wrist and hand (S68.-)*

The appropriate 7th character is to be added to each code from category S58
A initial encounter
D subsequent encounter
S sequela

+ S58.0 Traumatic amputation at elbow level
+ S58.01 Complete traumatic amputation at elbow level
CC +7th S58.011 Complete traumatic amputation at elbow level, right arm
CC Exclusion 7th character A see Appendix A PDX collection 1266
CC +7th S58.012 Complete traumatic amputation at elbow level, left arm
CC Exclusion 7th character A see Appendix A PDX collection 1267
CC +7th S58.019 Complete traumatic amputation at elbow level, unspecified arm
CC Exclusion 7th character A see Appendix A PDX collection 1268
+ S58.02 Partial traumatic amputation at elbow level
CC +7th S58.021 Partial traumatic amputation at elbow level, right arm
CC Exclusion 7th character A see Appendix A PDX collection 1266
CC +7th S58.022 Partial traumatic amputation at elbow level, left arm
CC Exclusion 7th character A see Appendix A PDX collection 1267
CC +7th S58.029 Partial traumatic amputation at elbow level, unspecified arm
CC Exclusion 7th character A see Appendix A PDX collection 1268
+ S58.1 Traumatic amputation at level between elbow and wrist
+ S58.11 Complete traumatic amputation at level between elbow and wrist
CC +7th S58.111 Complete traumatic amputation at level between elbow and wrist, right arm
CC Exclusion 7th character A see Appendix A PDX collection 1266
CC +7th S58.112 Complete traumatic amputation at level between elbow and wrist, left arm
CC Exclusion 7th character A see Appendix A PDX collection 1267
CC +7th S58.119 Complete traumatic amputation at level between elbow and wrist, unspecified arm
CC Exclusion 7th character A see Appendix A PDX collection 1268

+ **S58.12 Partial traumatic amputation at level between elbow and wrist**
  - CC +7th **S58.121 Partial traumatic amputation at level between elbow and wrist, right arm**
    - CC Exclusion 7th character A see Appendix A PDX collection 1266
  - CC +7th **S58.122 Partial traumatic amputation at level between elbow and wrist, left arm**
    - CC Exclusion 7th character A see Appendix A PDX collection 1267
  - CC +7th **S58.129 Partial traumatic amputation at level between elbow and wrist, unspecified arm**
    - CC Exclusion 7th character A see Appendix A PDX collection 1268

+ **S58.9 Traumatic amputation of forearm, level unspecified**
  - ***Excludes1:*** *traumatic amputation of wrist (S68.-)*
+ **S58.91 Complete traumatic amputation of forearm, level unspecified**
  - CC +7th **S58.911 Complete traumatic amputation of right forearm, level unspecified**
    - CC Exclusion 7th character A see Appendix A PDX collection 1266
  - CC +7th **S58.912 Complete traumatic amputation of left forearm, level unspecified**
    - CC Exclusion 7th character A see Appendix A PDX collection 1267
  - CC +7th **S58.919 Complete traumatic amputation of unspecified forearm, level unspecified**
    - CC Exclusion 7th character A see Appendix A PDX collection 1268
+ **S58.92 Partial traumatic amputation of forearm, level unspecified**
  - CC +7th **S58.921 Partial traumatic amputation of right forearm, level unspecified**
    - CC Exclusion 7th character A see Appendix A PDX collection 1266
  - CC +7th **S58.922 Partial traumatic amputation of left forearm, level unspecified**
    - CC Exclusion 7th character A see Appendix A PDX collection 1267
  - CC +7th **S58.929 Partial traumatic amputation of unspecified forearm, level unspecified**
    - CC Exclusion 7th character A see Appendix A PDX collection 1268

S59 Other and unspecified injuries of elbow and forearm

Excludes2: *other and unspecified injuries of wrist and hand (S69.-)*

The appropriate 7th character is to be added to each code from subcategories **S59.0, S59.1,** and **S59.2**
A initial encounter for closed fracture
D subsequent encounter for fracture with routine healing
G subsequent encounter for fracture with delayed healing
K subsequent encounter for fracture with nonunion
P subsequent encounter for fracture with malunion
S sequela

Review coding guideline C.19.c

+ **S59.0 Physeal fracture of lower end of ulna**
+ **S59.00 Unspecified physeal fracture of lower end of ulna**
  - CC +7th **S59.001 Unspecified physeal fracture of lower end of ulna, right arm**
    - CC Exclusion 7th character A see Appendix A PDX collection 1270
    - CC Exclusion 7th characters K & P see Appendix A PDX collection 0897
    - HAC 7th character A see Appendix B for HAC conditional logic
  - CC +7th **S59.002 Unspecified physeal fracture of lower end of ulna, left arm**
    - CC Exclusion 7th character A see Appendix A PDX collection 1271
    - CC Exclusion 7th characters K & P see Appendix A PDX collection 0897
    - HAC 7th character A see Appendix B for HAC conditional logic
  - CC +7th **S59.009 Unspecified physeal fracture of lower end of ulna, unspecified arm**
    - CC Exclusion 7th character A see Appendix A PDX collection 1272
    - CC Exclusion 7th characters K & P see Appendix A PDX collection 0897
    - HAC 7th character A see Appendix B for HAC conditional logic

+ **S59.01 Salter-Harris Type I physeal fracture of lower end of ulna**
  - CC +7th **S59.011 Salter-Harris Type I physeal fracture of lower end of ulna, right arm**
    - CC Exclusion 7th character A see Appendix A PDX collection 1270
    - CC Exclusion 7th characters K & P see Appendix A PDX collection 0897
    - HAC 7th character A see Appendix B for HAC conditional logic
  - CC +7th **S59.012 Salter-Harris Type I physeal fracture of lower end of ulna, left arm**
    - CC Exclusion 7th character A see Appendix A PDX collection 1271
    - CC Exclusion 7th characters K & P see Appendix A PDX collection 0897
    - HAC 7th character A see Appendix B for HAC conditional logic
  - CC +7th **S59.019 Salter-Harris Type I physeal fracture of lower end of ulna, unspecified arm**
    - CC Exclusion 7th character A see Appendix A PDX collection 1272
    - CC Exclusion 7th characters K & P see Appendix A PDX collection 0897
    - HAC 7th character A see Appendix B for HAC conditional logic

+ **S59.02 Salter-Harris Type II physeal fracture of lower end of ulna**
  - CC +7th **S59.021 Salter-Harris Type II physeal fracture of lower end of ulna, right arm**
    - CC Exclusion 7th character A see Appendix A PDX collection 1270
    - CC Exclusion 7th characters K & P see Appendix A PDX collection 0897
    - HAC 7th character A see Appendix B for HAC conditional logic
  - CC +7th **S59.022 Salter-Harris Type II physeal fracture of lower end of ulna, left arm**
    - CC Exclusion 7th character A see Appendix A PDX collection 1271
    - CC Exclusion 7th characters K & P see Appendix A PDX collection 0897
    - HAC 7th character A see Appendix B for HAC conditional logic
  - CC +7th **S59.029 Salter-Harris Type II physeal fracture of lower end of ulna, unspecified arm**
    - CC Exclusion 7th character A see Appendix A PDX collection 1272
    - CC Exclusion 7th characters K & P see Appendix A PDX collection 0897
    - HAC 7th character A see Appendix B for HAC conditional logic

+ **S59.03 Salter-Harris Type III physeal fracture of lower end of ulna**
  - CC +7th **S59.031 Salter-Harris Type III physeal fracture of lower end of ulna, right arm**
    - CC Exclusion 7th character A see Appendix A PDX collection 1270
    - CC Exclusion 7th characters K & P see Appendix A PDX collection 0897
    - HAC 7th character A see Appendix B for HAC conditional logic
  - CC +7th **S59.032 Salter-Harris Type III physeal fracture of lower end of ulna, left arm**
    - CC Exclusion 7th character A see Appendix A PDX collection 1271
    - CC Exclusion 7th characters K & P see Appendix A PDX collection 0897
    - HAC 7th character A see Appendix B for HAC conditional logic
  - CC +7th **S59.039 Salter-Harris Type III physeal fracture of lower end of ulna, unspecified arm**
    - CC Exclusion 7th character A see Appendix A PDX collection 1272
    - CC Exclusion 7th characters K & P see Appendix A PDX collection 0897
    - HAC 7th character A see Appendix B for HAC conditional logic

+ **S59.04 Salter-Harris Type IV physeal fracture of lower end of ulna**
  - CC +7th **S59.041 Salter-Harris Type IV physeal fracture of lower end of ulna, right arm**
    - CC Exclusion 7th character A see Appendix A PDX collection 1270
    - CC Exclusion 7th characters K & P see Appendix A PDX collection 0897
    - HAC 7th character A see Appendix B for HAC conditional logic

CC +7th **S59.042** **Salter-Harris Type IV physeal fracture of lower end of ulna, left arm**
CC Exclusion 7th character A see Appendix A PDX collection 1271
CC Exclusion 7th characters K & P see Appendix A PDX collection 0897
HAC 7th character A see Appendix B for HAC conditional logic

CC +7th **S59.049** **Salter-Harris Type IV physeal fracture of lower end of ulna, unspecified arm**
CC Exclusion 7th character A see Appendix A PDX collection 1272
CC Exclusion 7th characters K & P see Appendix A PDX collection 0897
HAC 7th character A see Appendix B for HAC conditional logic

\+ **S59.09** **Other physeal fracture of lower end of ulna**

CC +7th **S59.091** **Other physeal fracture of lower end of ulna, right arm**
CC Exclusion 7th character A see Appendix A PDX collection 1270
CC Exclusion 7th characters K & P see Appendix A PDX collection 0897
HAC 7th character A see Appendix B for HAC conditional logic

CC +7th **S59.092** **Other physeal fracture of lower end of ulna, left arm**
CC Exclusion 7th character A see Appendix A PDX collection 1271
CC Exclusion 7th characters K & P see Appendix A PDX collection 0897
HAC 7th character A see Appendix B for HAC conditional logic

CC +7th **S59.099** **Other physeal fracture of lower end of ulna, unspecified arm**
CC Exclusion 7th character A see Appendix A PDX collection 1272
CC Exclusion 7th characters K & P see Appendix A PDX collection 0897
HAC 7th character A see Appendix B for HAC conditional logic

\+ **S59.1** **Physeal fracture of upper end of radius**

\+ **S59.10** **Unspecified physeal fracture of upper end of radius**

CC +7th **S59.101** **Unspecified physeal fracture of upper end of radius, right arm**
CC Exclusion 7th characters K & P see Appendix A PDX collection 0897

CC +7th **S59.102** **Unspecified physeal fracture of upper end of radius, left arm**
CC Exclusion 7th characters K & P see Appendix A PDX collection 0897

CC +7th **S59.109** **Unspecified physeal fracture of upper end of radius, unspecified arm**
CC Exclusion 7th characters K & P see Appendix A PDX collection 0897

\+ **S59.11** **Salter-Harris Type I physeal fracture of upper end of radius**

CC +7th **S59.111** **Salter-Harris Type I physeal fracture of upper end of radius, right arm**
CC Exclusion 7th characters K & P see Appendix A PDX collection 0897

CC +7th **S59.112** **Salter-Harris Type I physeal fracture of upper end of radius, left arm**
CC Exclusion 7th characters K & P see Appendix A PDX collection 0897

CC +7th **S59.119** **Salter-Harris Type I physeal fracture of upper end of radius, unspecified arm**
CC Exclusion 7th characters K & P see Appendix A PDX collection 0897

\+ **S59.12** **Salter-Harris Type II physeal fracture of upper end of radius**

CC +7th **S59.121** **Salter-Harris Type II physeal fracture of upper end of radius, right arm**
CC Exclusion 7th characters K & P see Appendix A PDX collection 0897

CC +7th **S59.122** **Salter-Harris Type II physeal fracture of upper end of radius, left arm**
CC Exclusion 7th characters K & P see Appendix A PDX collection 0897

CC +7th **S59.129** **Salter-Harris Type II physeal fracture of upper end of radius, unspecified arm**
CC Exclusion 7th characters K & P see Appendix A PDX collection 0897

\+ **S59.13** **Salter-Harris Type III physeal fracture of upper end of radius**

CC +7th **S59.131** **Salter-Harris Type III physeal fracture of upper end of radius, right arm**
CC Exclusion 7th characters K & P see Appendix A PDX collection 0897

CC +7th **S59.132** **Salter-Harris Type III physeal fracture of upper end of radius, left arm**
CC Exclusion 7th characters K & P see Appendix A PDX collection 0897

CC +7th **S59.139** **Salter-Harris Type III physeal fracture of upper end of radius, unspecified arm**
CC Exclusion 7th characters K & P see Appendix A PDX collection 0897

\+ **S59.14** **Salter-Harris Type IV physeal fracture of upper end of radius**

CC +7th **S59.141** **Salter-Harris Type IV physeal fracture of upper end of radius, right arm**
CC Exclusion 7th characters K & P see Appendix A PDX collection 0897

CC +7th **S59.142** **Salter-Harris Type IV physeal fracture of upper end of radius, left arm**
CC Exclusion 7th characters K & P see Appendix A PDX collection 0897

CC +7th **S59.149** **Salter-Harris Type IV physeal fracture of upper end of radius, unspecified arm**
CC Exclusion 7th characters K & P see Appendix A PDX collection 0897

\+ **S59.19** **Other physeal fracture of upper end of radius**

CC +7th **S59.191** **Other physeal fracture of upper end of radius, right arm**
CC Exclusion 7th characters K & P see Appendix A PDX collection 0897

CC +7th **S59.192** **Other physeal fracture of upper end of radius, left arm**
CC Exclusion 7th characters K & P see Appendix A PDX collection 0897

CC +7th **S59.199** **Other physeal fracture of upper end of radius, unspecified arm**
CC Exclusion 7th characters K & P see Appendix A PDX collection 0897

\+ **S59.2** **Physeal fracture of lower end of radius**

\+ **S59.20** **Unspecified physeal fracture of lower end of radius**

CC +7th **S59.201** **Unspecified physeal fracture of lower end of radius, right arm**
CC Exclusion 7th character A see Appendix A PDX collection 1270
CC Exclusion 7th characters K & P see Appendix A PDX collection 0897
HAC 7th character A see Appendix B for HAC conditional logic

CC +7th **S59.202** **Unspecified physeal fracture of lower end of radius, left arm**
CC Exclusion 7th character A see Appendix A PDX collection 1271
CC Exclusion 7th characters K & P see Appendix A PDX collection 0897
HAC 7th character A see Appendix B for HAC conditional logic

CC +7th **S59.209** **Unspecified physeal fracture of lower end of radius, unspecified arm**
CC Exclusion 7th character A see Appendix A PDX collection 1272
CC Exclusion 7th characters K & P see Appendix A PDX collection 0897
HAC 7th character A see Appendix B for HAC conditional logic

\+ **S59.21** **Salter-Harris Type I physeal fracture of lower end of radius**

CC +7th **S59.211** **Salter-Harris Type I physeal fracture of lower end of radius, right arm**
CC Exclusion 7th character A see Appendix A PDX collection 1270
CC Exclusion 7th characters K & P see Appendix A PDX collection 0897
HAC 7th character A see Appendix B for HAC conditional logic

CC +7th **S59.212** **Salter-Harris Type I physeal fracture of lower end of radius, left arm**
CC Exclusion 7th character A see Appendix A PDX collection 1271
CC Exclusion 7th characters K & P see Appendix A PDX collection 0897
HAC 7th character A see Appendix B for HAC conditional logic

CC +7th **S59.219 Salter-Harris Type I physeal fracture of lower end of radius, unspecified arm**
CC Exclusion 7th character A see Appendix A PDX collection 1272
CC Exclusion 7th characters K & P see Appendix A PDX collection 0897
HAC 7th character A see Appendix B for HAC conditional logic

\+ **S59.22 Salter-Harris Type II physeal fracture of lower end of radius**

CC +7th **S59.221 Salter-Harris Type II physeal fracture of lower end of radius, right arm**
CC Exclusion 7th character A see Appendix A PDX collection 1270
CC Exclusion 7th characters K & P see Appendix A PDX collection 0897
HAC 7th character A see Appendix B for HAC conditional logic

CC +7th **S59.222 Salter-Harris Type II physeal fracture of lower end of radius, left arm**
CC Exclusion 7th character A see Appendix A PDX collection 1271
CC Exclusion 7th characters K & P see Appendix A PDX collection 0897
HAC 7th character A see Appendix B for HAC conditional logic

CC +7th **S59.229 Salter-Harris Type II physeal fracture of lower end of radius, unspecified arm**
CC Exclusion 7th character A see Appendix A PDX collection 1272
CC Exclusion 7th characters K & P see Appendix A PDX collection 0897
HAC 7th character A see Appendix B for HAC conditional logic

\+ **S59.23 Salter-Harris Type III physeal fracture of lower end of radius**

CC +7th **S59.231 Salter-Harris Type III physeal fracture of lower end of radius, right arm**
CC Exclusion 7th character A see Appendix A PDX collection 1270
CC Exclusion 7th characters K & P see Appendix A PDX collection 0897
HAC 7th character A see Appendix B for HAC conditional logic

CC +7th **S59.232 Salter-Harris Type III physeal fracture of lower end of radius, left arm**
CC Exclusion 7th character A see Appendix A PDX collection 1271
CC Exclusion 7th characters K & P see Appendix A PDX collection 0897
HAC 7th character A see Appendix B for HAC conditional logic

CC +7th **S59.239 Salter-Harris Type III physeal fracture of lower end of radius, unspecified arm**
CC Exclusion 7th character A see Appendix A PDX collection 1272
CC Exclusion 7th characters K & P see Appendix A PDX collection 0897
HAC 7th character A see Appendix B for HAC conditional logic

\+ **S59.24 Salter-Harris Type IV physeal fracture of lower end of radius**

CC +7th **S59.241 Salter-Harris Type IV physeal fracture of lower end of radius, right arm**
CC Exclusion 7th character A see Appendix A PDX collection 1270
CC Exclusion 7th characters K & P see Appendix A PDX collection 0897
HAC 7th character A see Appendix B for HAC conditional logic

CC +7th **S59.242 Salter-Harris Type IV physeal fracture of lower end of radius, left arm**
CC Exclusion 7th character A see Appendix A PDX collection 1271
CC Exclusion 7th characters K & P see Appendix A PDX collection 0897
HAC 7th character A see Appendix B for HAC conditional logic

CC +7th **S59.249 Salter-Harris Type IV physeal fracture of lower end of radius, unspecified arm**
CC Exclusion 7th character A see Appendix A PDX collection 1272
CC Exclusion 7th characters K & P see Appendix A PDX collection 0897
HAC 7th character A see Appendix B for HAC conditional logic

\+ **S59.29 Other physeal fracture of lower end of radius**

CC +7th **S59.291 Other physeal fracture of lower end of radius, right arm**
CC Exclusion 7th character A see Appendix A PDX collection 1270
CC Exclusion 7th characters K & P see Appendix A PDX collection 0897
HAC 7th character A see Appendix B for HAC conditional logic

CC +7th **S59.292 Other physeal fracture of lower end of radius, left arm**
CC Exclusion 7th character A see Appendix A PDX collection 1271
CC Exclusion 7th characters K & P see Appendix A PDX collection 0897
HAC 7th character A see Appendix B for HAC conditional logic

CC +7th **S59.299 Other physeal fracture of lower end of radius, unspecified arm**
CC Exclusion 7th character A see Appendix A PDX collection 1272
CC Exclusion 7th characters K & P see Appendix A PDX collection 0897
HAC 7th character A see Appendix B for HAC conditional logic

\+ **S59.8 Other specified injuries of elbow and forearm**

The appropriate 7th character is to be added to each code in subcategory **S59.8**
A initial encounter
D subsequent encounter
S sequela

\+ **S59.80 Other specified injuries of elbow**
+7th **S59.801 Other specified injuries of right elbow**
+7th **S59.802 Other specified injuries of left elbow**
+7th **S59.809 Other specified injuries of unspecified elbow**

\+ **S59.81 Other specified injuries of forearm**
+7th **S59.811 Other specified injuries right forearm**
+7th **S59.812 Other specified injuries left forearm**
+7th **S59.819 Other specified injuries unspecified forearm**

\+ **S59.9 Unspecified injury of elbow and forearm**

The appropriate 7th character is to be added to each code in subcategory **S59.9**
A initial encounter
D subsequent encounter
S sequela

\+ **S59.90 Unspecified injury of elbow**
+7th **S59.901 Unspecified injury of right elbow**
+7th **S59.902 Unspecified injury of left elbow**
+7th **S59.909 Unspecified injury of unspecified elbow**

\+ **S59.91 Unspecified injury of forearm**
+7th **S59.911 Unspecified injury of right forearm**
+7th **S59.912 Unspecified injury of left forearm**
+7th **S59.919 Unspecified injury of unspecified forearm**

Injuries to the wrist, hand and fingers (S60-S69)

Excludes2: *burns and corrosions (T20-T32)*
frostbite (T33-T34)
insect bite or sting, venomous (T63.4)

S60 Superficial injury of wrist, hand and fingers

The appropriate 7th character is to be added to each code from category S60
A initial encounter
D subsequent encounter
S sequela

\+ **S60.0 Contusion of finger without damage to nail**
Excludes1: *contusion involving nail (matrix) (S60.1)*

X+7th **S60.00 Contusion of unspecified finger without damage to nail**
Contusion of finger(s) NOS

\+ **S60.01 Contusion of thumb without damage to nail**
+7th **S60.011 Contusion of right thumb without damage to nail**
+7th **S60.012 Contusion of left thumb without damage to nail**
+7th **S60.019 Contusion of unspecified thumb without damage to nail**

Wrist

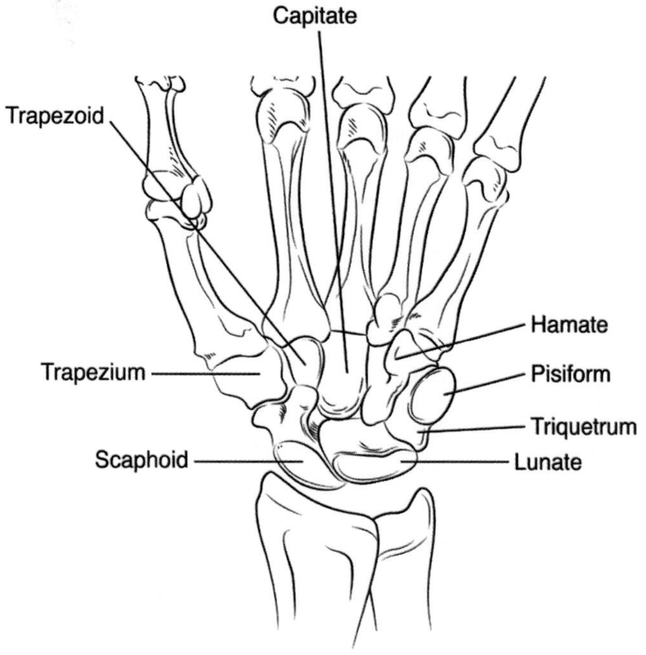
Capitate
Trapezoid
Hamate
Trapezium
Pisiform
Triquetrum
Scaphoid
Lunate

Bones of the Hand

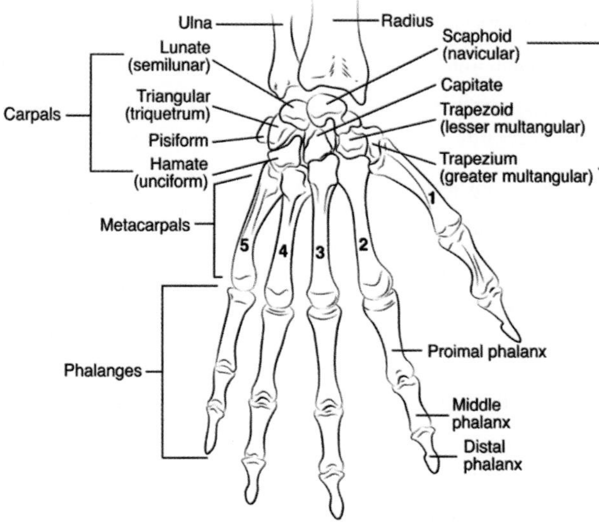
Ulna
Radius
Lunate
(semilunar)
Scaphoid
(navicular)
Capitate
Carpals
Triangular
(triquetrum)
Trapezoid
(lesser multangular)
Carpals
Pisiform
Hamate
(unciform)
Trapezium
(greater multangular)
1
Metacarpals
5
4
3
2
Phalanges
Proimal phalanx
Middle
phalanx
Distal
phalanx

Muscles of the Hand

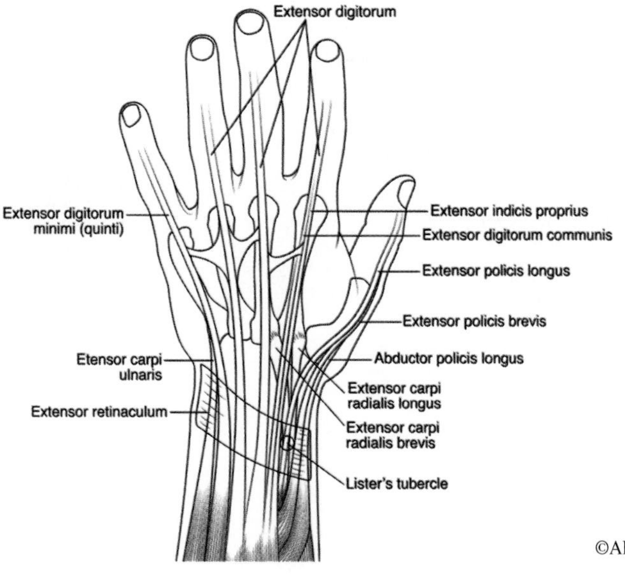
Extensor digitorum
Extensor digitorum
minimi (quinti)
Extensor indicis proprius
Extensor digitorum communis
Extensor policis longus
Extensor policis brevis
Etensor carpi
ulnaris
Abductor policis longus
Extensor retinaculum
Extensor carpi
radialis longus
Extensor carpi
radialis brevis
Lister's tubercle

+ S60.02 Contusion of index finger without damage to nail
    - +7th S60.021 Contusion of right index finger without damage to nail
    - +7th S60.022 Contusion of left index finger without damage to nail
    - +7th S60.029 Contusion of unspecified index finger without damage to nail
+ S60.03 Contusion of middle finger without damage to nail
    - +7th S60.031 Contusion of right middle finger without damage to nail
    - +7th S60.032 Contusion of left middle finger without damage to nail
    - +7th S60.039 Contusion of unspecified middle finger without damage to nail
+ S60.04 Contusion of ring finger without damage to nail
    - +7th S60.041 Contusion of right ring finger without damage to nail
    - +7th S60.042 Contusion of left ring finger without damage to nail
    - +7th S60.049 Contusion of unspecified ring finger without damage to nail
+ S60.05 Contusion of little finger without damage to nail
    - +7th S60.051 Contusion of right little finger without damage to nail
    - +7th S60.052 Contusion of left little finger without damage to nail
    - +7th S60.059 Contusion of unspecified little finger without damage to nail

+ S60.1 Contusion of finger with damage to nail
    - X+7th S60.10 Contusion of unspecified finger with damage to nail
    - + S60.11 Contusion of thumb with damage to nail
        - +7th S60.111 Contusion of right thumb with damage to nail
        - +7th S60.112 Contusion of left thumb with damage to nail
        - +7th S60.119 Contusion of unspecified thumb with damage to nail
    - + S60.12 Contusion of index finger with damage to nail
        - +7th S60.121 Contusion of right index finger with damage to nail
        - +7th S60.122 Contusion of left index finger with damage to nail
        - +7th S60.129 Contusion of unspecified index finger with damage to nail
    - + S60.13 Contusion of middle finger with damage to nail
        - +7th S60.131 Contusion of right middle finger with damage to nail
        - +7th S60.132 Contusion of left middle finger with damage to nail
        - +7th S60.139 Contusion of unspecified middle finger with damage to nail
    - + S60.14 Contusion of ring finger with damage to nail
        - +7th S60.141 Contusion of right ring finger with damage to nail
        - +7th S60.142 Contusion of left ring finger with damage to nail
        - +7th S60.149 Contusion of unspecified ring finger with damage to nail
    - + S60.15 Contusion of little finger with damage to nail
        - +7th S60.151 Contusion of right little finger with damage to nail
        - +7th S60.152 Contusion of left little finger with damage to nail
        - +7th S60.159 Contusion of unspecified little finger with damage to nail

+ S60.2 Contusion of wrist and hand
    Excludes2: *contusion of fingers (S60.0-, S60.1-)*
    - + S60.21 Contusion of wrist
        - +7th S60.211 Contusion of right wrist
        - +7th S60.212 Contusion of left wrist
        - +7th S60.219 Contusion of unspecified wrist
    - + S60.22 Contusion of hand
        - +7th S60.221 Contusion of right hand
        - +7th S60.222 Contusion of left hand
        - +7th S60.229 Contusion of unspecified hand

+ S60.3 Other superficial injuries of thumb
    - + S60.31 Abrasion of thumb
        - +7th S60.311 Abrasion of right thumb
        - +7th S60.312 Abrasion of left thumb
        - +7th S60.319 Abrasion of unspecified thumb
    - + S60.32 Blister (nonthermal) of thumb
        - +7th S60.321 Blister (nonthermal) of right thumb
        - +7th S60.322 Blister (nonthermal) of left thumb
        - +7th S60.329 Blister (nonthermal) of unspecified thumb
    - + S60.34 External constriction of thumb
        Hair tourniquet syndrome of thumb
        Use additional cause code to identify the constricting item (W49.0-)
        - +7th S60.341 External constriction of right thumb
        - +7th S60.342 External constriction of left thumb
        - +7th S60.349 External constriction of unspecified thumb
    - + S60.35 Superficial foreign body of thumb
        Splinter in the thumb
        - +7th S60.351 Superficial foreign body of right thumb
        - +7th S60.352 Superficial foreign body of left thumb
        - +7th S60.359 Superficial foreign body of unspecified thumb
    - + S60.36 Insect bite (nonvenomous) of thumb
        - +7th S60.361 Insect bite (nonvenomous) of right thumb
        - +7th S60.362 Insect bite (nonvenomous) of left thumb
        - +7th S60.369 Insect bite (nonvenomous) of unspecified thumb
    - + S60.37 Other superficial bite of thumb
        Excludes1: *open bite of thumb (S61.05-, S61.15-)*
        - +7th S60.371 Other superficial bite of right thumb
        - +7th S60.372 Other superficial bite of left thumb
        - +7th S60.379 Other superficial bite of unspecified thumb
    - + S60.39 Other superficial injuries of thumb
        - +7th S60.391 Other superficial injuries of right thumb
        - +7th S60.392 Other superficial injuries of left thumb
        - +7th S60.399 Other superficial injuries of unspecified thumb

+ S60.4 Other superficial injuries of other fingers
    - + S60.41 Abrasion of fingers
        - S60.410 Abrasion of right index finger
        - +7th S60.411 Abrasion of left index finger
        - +7th S60.412 Abrasion of right middle finger
        - +7th S60.413 Abrasion of left middle finger
        - +7th S60.414 Abrasion of right ring finger
        - +7th S60.415 Abrasion of left ring finger
        - +7th S60.416 Abrasion of right little finger
        - +7th S60.417 Abrasion of left little finger
        - +7th S60.418 Abrasion of other finger
            Abrasion of specified finger with unspecified laterality
        - +7th S60.419 Abrasion of unspecified finger
    - + S60.42 Blister (nonthermal) of fingers
        - S60.420 Blister (nonthermal) of right index finger
        - +7th S60.421 Blister (nonthermal) of left index finger
        - +7th S60.422 Blister (nonthermal) of right middle finger
        - +7th S60.423 Blister (nonthermal) of left middle finger
        - +7th S60.424 Blister (nonthermal) of right ring finger
        - +7th S60.425 Blister (nonthermal) of left ring finger
        - +7th S60.426 Blister (nonthermal) of right little finger
        - +7th S60.427 Blister (nonthermal) of left little finger
        - +7th S60.428 Blister (nonthermal) of other finger
            Blister (nonthermal) of specified finger with unspecified laterality
        - +7th S60.429 Blister (nonthermal) of unspecified finger
    - + S60.44 External constriction of fingers
        Hair tourniquet syndrome of finger
        Use additional cause code to identify the constricting item (W49.0-)
        - S60.440 External constriction of right index finger
        - +7th S60.441 External constriction of left index finger
        - +7th S60.442 External constriction of right middle finger
        - +7th S60.443 External constriction of left middle finger
        - +7th S60.444 External constriction of right ring finger
        - +7th S60.445 External constriction of left ring finger
        - +7th S60.446 External constriction of right little finger
        - +7th S60.447 External constriction of left little finger
        - +7th S60.448 External constriction of other finger
            External constriction of specified finger with unspecified laterality
        - +7th S60.449 External constriction of unspecified finger
    - + S60.45 Superficial foreign body of fingers
        Splinter in the finger(s)
        - S60.450 Superficial foreign body of right index finger
        - +7th S60.451 Superficial foreign body of left index finger
        - +7th S60.452 Superficial foreign body of right middle finger

+7th **S60.453 Superficial foreign body of left middle finger**
+7th **S60.454 Superficial foreign body of right ring finger**
+7th **S60.455 Superficial foreign body of left ring finger**
+7th **S60.456 Superficial foreign body of right little finger**
+7th **S60.457 Superficial foreign body of left little finger**
+7th **S60.458 Superficial foreign body of other finger**
Superficial foreign body of specified finger with unspecified laterality
+7th **S60.459 Superficial foreign body of unspecified finger**

\+ **S60.46 Insect bite (nonvenomous) of fingers**
S60.460 Insect bite (nonvenomous) of right index finger
+7th **S60.461 Insect bite (nonvenomous) of left index finger**
+7th **S60.462 Insect bite (nonvenomous) of right middle finger**
+7th **S60.463 Insect bite (nonvenomous) of left middle finger**
+7th **S60.464 Insect bite (nonvenomous) of right ring finger**
+7th **S60.465 Insect bite (nonvenomous) of left ring finger**
+7th **S60.466 Insect bite (nonvenomous) of right little finger**
+7th **S60.467 Insect bite (nonvenomous) of left little finger**
+7th **S60.468 Insect bite (nonvenomous) of other finger**
Insect bite (nonvenomous) of specified finger with unspecified laterality
+7th **S60.469 Insect bite (nonvenomous) of unspecified finger**

\+ **S60.47 Other superficial bite of fingers**
Excludes1: *open bite of fingers (S61.25-, S61.35-)*
S60.470 Other superficial bite of right index finger
+7th **S60.471 Other superficial bite of left index finger**
+7th **S60.472 Other superficial bite of right middle finger**
+7th **S60.473 Other superficial bite of left middle finger**
+7th **S60.474 Other superficial bite of right ring finger**
+7th **S60.475 Other superficial bite of left ring finger**
+7th **S60.476 Other superficial bite of right little finger**
+7th **S60.477 Other superficial bite of left little finger**
+7th **S60.478 Other superficial bite of other finger**
Other superficial bite of specified finger with unspecified laterality
+7th **S60.479 Other superficial bite of unspecified finger**

\+ **S60.5 Other superficial injuries of hand**
Excludes2: *superficial injuries of fingers (S60.3-, S60.4-)*

\+ **S60.51 Abrasion of hand**
+7th **S60.511 Abrasion of right hand**
+7th **S60.512 Abrasion of left hand**
+7th **S60.519 Abrasion of unspecified hand**

\+ **S60.52 Blister (nonthermal) of hand**
+7th **S60.521 Blister (nonthermal) of right hand**
+7th **S60.522 Blister (nonthermal) of left hand**
+7th **S60.529 Blister (nonthermal) of unspecified hand**

\+ **S60.54 External constriction of hand**
+7th **S60.541 External constriction of right hand**
+7th **S60.542 External constriction of left hand**
+7th **S60.549 External constriction of unspecified hand**

\+ **S60.55 Superficial foreign body of hand**
Splinter in the hand
+7th **S60.551 Superficial foreign body of right hand**
+7th **S60.552 Superficial foreign body of left hand**
+7th **S60.559 Superficial foreign body of unspecified hand**

\+ **S60.56 Insect bite (nonvenomous) of hand**
+7th **S60.561 Insect bite (nonvenomous) of right hand**
+7th **S60.562 Insect bite (nonvenomous) of left hand**
+7th **S60.569 Insect bite (nonvenomous) of unspecified hand**

\+ **S60.57 Other superficial bite of hand**
Excludes1: *open bite of hand (S61.45-)*
+7th **S60.571 Other superficial bite of hand of right hand**
+7th **S60.572 Other superficial bite of hand of left hand**
+7th **S60.579 Other superficial bite of hand of unspecified hand**

\+ **S60.8 Other superficial injuries of wrist**

\+ **S60.81 Abrasion of wrist**
+7th **S60.811 Abrasion of right wrist**
+7th **S60.812 Abrasion of left wrist**
+7th **S60.819 Abrasion of unspecified wrist**

\+ **S60.82 Blister (nonthermal) of wrist**
+7th **S60.821 Blister (nonthermal) of right wrist**
+7th **S60.822 Blister (nonthermal) of left wrist**
+7th **S60.829 Blister (nonthermal) of unspecified wrist**

\+ **S60.84 External constriction of wrist**
+7th **S60.841 External constriction of right wrist**
+7th **S60.842 External constriction of left wrist**
+7th **S60.849 External constriction of unspecified wrist**

\+ **S60.85 Superficial foreign body of wrist**
Splinter in the wrist
+7th **S60.851 Superficial foreign body of right wrist**
+7th **S60.852 Superficial foreign body of left wrist**
+7th **S60.859 Superficial foreign body of unspecified wrist**

\+ **S60.86 Insect bite (nonvenomous) of wrist**
+7th **S60.861 Insect bite (nonvenomous) of right wrist**
+7th **S60.862 Insect bite (nonvenomous) of left wrist**
+7th **S60.869 Insect bite (nonvenomous) of unspecified wrist**

\+ **S60.87 Other superficial bite of wrist**
Excludes1: *open bite of wrist (S61.55)*
+7th **S60.871 Other superficial bite of right wrist**
+7th **S60.872 Other superficial bite of left wrist**
+7th **S60.879 Other superficial bite of unspecified wrist**

\+ **S60.9 Unspecified superficial injury of wrist, hand and fingers**

\+ **S60.91 Unspecified superficial injury of wrist**
+7th **S60.911 Unspecified superficial injury of right wrist**
+7th **S60.912 Unspecified superficial injury of left wrist**
+7th **S60.919 Unspecified superficial injury of unspecified wrist**

\+ **S60.92 Unspecified superficial injury of hand**
+7th **S60.921 Unspecified superficial injury of right hand**
+7th **S60.922 Unspecified superficial injury of left hand**
+7th **S60.929 Unspecified superficial injury of unspecified hand**

\+ **S60.93 Unspecified superficial injury of thumb**
+7th **S60.931 Unspecified superficial injury of right thumb**
+7th **S60.932 Unspecified superficial injury of left thumb**
+7th **S60.939 Unspecified superficial injury of unspecified thumb**

\+ **S60.94 Unspecified superficial injury of other fingers**
S60.940 Unspecified superficial injury of right index finger
+7th **S60.941 Unspecified superficial injury of left index finger**
+7th **S60.942 Unspecified superficial injury of right middle finger**
+7th **S60.943 Unspecified superficial injury of left middle finger**
+7th **S60.944 Unspecified superficial injury of right ring finger**
+7th **S60.945 Unspecified superficial injury of left ring finger**
+7th **S60.946 Unspecified superficial injury of right little finger**
+7th **S60.947 Unspecified superficial injury of left little finger**
+7th **S60.948 Unspecified superficial injury of other finger**
Unspecified superficial injury of specified finger with unspecified laterality
+7th **S60.949 Unspecified superficial injury of unspecified finger**

S61 Open wound of wrist, hand and fingers

Code also any associated wound infection
Excludes1: *open fracture of wrist, hand and finger (S62.- with 7th character B)*
traumatic amputation of wrist and hand (S68.-)

The appropriate 7th character is to be added to each code from category S61
A initial encounter
D subsequent encounter
S sequela

+ **S61.0 Open wound of thumb without damage to nail**
Excludes1: *open wound of thumb with damage to nail (S61.1-)*
+ **S61.00 Unspecified open wound of thumb without damage to nail**
+7th **S61.001 Unspecified open wound of right thumb without damage to nail**
+7th **S61.002 Unspecified open wound of left thumb without damage to nail**
+7th **S61.009 Unspecified open wound of unspecified thumb without damage to nail**
+ **S61.01 Laceration without foreign body of thumb without damage to nail**
+7th **S61.011 Laceration without foreign body of right thumb without damage to nail**
+7th **S61.012 Laceration without foreign body of left thumb without damage to nail**
+7th **S61.019 Laceration without foreign body of unspecified thumb without damage to nail**
+ **S61.02 Laceration with foreign body of thumb without damage to nail**
+7th **S61.021 Laceration with foreign body of right thumb without damage to nail**
+7th **S61.022 Laceration with foreign body of left thumb without damage to nail**
+7th **S61.029 Laceration with foreign body of unspecified thumb without damage to nail**
+ **S61.03 Puncture wound without foreign body of thumb without damage to nail**
+7th **S61.031 Puncture wound without foreign body of right thumb without damage to nail**
+7th **S61.032 Puncture wound without foreign body of left thumb without damage to nail**
+7th **S61.039 Puncture wound without foreign body of unspecified thumb without damage to nail**
+ **S61.04 Puncture wound with foreign body of thumb without damage to nail**
+7th **S61.041 Puncture wound with foreign body of right thumb without damage to nail**
+7th **S61.042 Puncture wound with foreign body of left thumb without damage to nail**
+7th **S61.049 Puncture wound with foreign body of unspecified thumb without damage to nail**
+ **S61.05 Open bite of thumb without damage to nail**
Bite of thumb NOS
Excludes1: *superficial bite of thumb (S60.36-, S60.37-)*
+7th **S61.051 Open bite of right thumb without damage to nail**
+7th **S61.052 Open bite of left thumb without damage to nail**
+7th **S61.059 Open bite of unspecified thumb without damage to nail**
+ **S61.1 Open wound of thumb with damage to nail**
+ **S61.10 Unspecified open wound of thumb with damage to nail**
+7th **S61.101 Unspecified open wound of right thumb with damage to nail**
+7th **S61.102 Unspecified open wound of left thumb with damage to nail**
+7th **S61.109 Unspecified open wound of unspecified thumb with damage to nail**
+ **S61.11 Laceration without foreign body of thumb with damage to nail**
+7th **S61.111 Laceration without foreign body of right thumb with damage to nail**
+7th **S61.112 Laceration without foreign body of left thumb with damage to nail**
+7th **S61.119 Laceration without foreign body of unspecified thumb with damage to nail**
+ **S61.12 Laceration with foreign body of thumb with damage to nail**
+7th **S61.121 Laceration with foreign body of right thumb with damage to nail**
+7th **S61.122 Laceration with foreign body of left thumb with damage to nail**
+7th **S61.129 Laceration with foreign body of unspecified thumb with damage to nail**
+ **S61.13 Puncture wound without foreign body of thumb wit damage to nail**
+7th **S61.131 Puncture wound without foreign body of right thumb with damage to nail**
+7th **S61.132 Puncture wound without foreign body of left thumb with damage to nail**
+7th **S61.139 Puncture wound without foreign body of unspecified thumb with damage to nail**
+ **S61.14 Puncture wound with foreign body of thumb with damage to nail**
+7th **S61.141 Puncture wound with foreign body of righ thumb with damage to nail**
+7th **S61.142 Puncture wound with foreign body of left thumb with damage to nail**
+7th **S61.149 Puncture wound with foreign body of unspecified thumb with damage to nail**
+ **S61.15 Open bite of thumb with damage to nail**
Bite of thumb with damage to nail NOS
Excludes1: *superficial bite of thumb (S60.36-, S60.3)*
+7th **S61.151 Open bite of right thumb with damage to nail**
+7th **S61.152 Open bite of left thumb with damage to na**
+7th **S61.159 Open bite of unspecified thumb with damage to nail**
+ **S61.2 Open wound of other finger without damage to nail**
Excludes1: *open wound of finger involving nail (matrix) (S61.3-)*
Excludes2: *open wound of thumb without damage to nail (S61.0-)*
+ **S61.20 Unspecified open wound of other finger without damage to nail**
S61.200 Unspecified open wound of right index finger without damage to nail
+7th **S61.201 Unspecified open wound of left index fing without damage to nail**
+7th **S61.202 Unspecified open wound of right middle finger without damage to nail**
+7th **S61.203 Unspecified open wound of left middle finger without damage to nail**
+7th **S61.204 Unspecified open wound of right ring finger without damage to nail**
+7th **S61.205 Unspecified open wound of left ring finger without damage to nail**
+7th **S61.206 Unspecified open wound of right little finger without damage to nail**
+7th **S61.207 Unspecified open wound of left little finge without damage to nail**
+7th **S61.208 Unspecified open wound of other finger without damage to nail**
Unspecified open wound of specified finger with unspecified laterality without damage to nail
+7th **S61.209 Unspecified open wound of unspecified finger without damage to nail**
+ **S61.21 Laceration without foreign body of finger without damage to nail**
S61.210 Laceration without foreign body of right index finger without damage to nail
+7th **S61.211 Laceration without foreign body of left index finger without damage to nail**
+7th **S61.212 Laceration without foreign body of right middle finger without damage to na**
+7th **S61.213 Laceration without foreign body of left middle finger without damage to nail**
+7th **S61.214 Laceration without foreign body of right ring finger without damage to nail**
+7th **S61.215 Laceration without foreign body of left ring finger without damage to nail**
+7th **S61.216 Laceration without foreign body of right little finger without damage to nail**
+7th **S61.217 Laceration without foreign body of left little finger without damage to nail**
+7th **S61.218 Laceration without foreign body of other finger without damage to nail**
Laceration without foreign body of specifie finger with unspecified laterality withou damage to nail
+7th **S61.219 Laceration without foreign body of unspecified finger without damage to nail**

+ **S61.22 Laceration with foreign body of finger without damage to nail**
  - **S61.220 Laceration with foreign body of right index finger without damage to nail**
  - +7th **S61.221 Laceration with foreign body of left index finger without damage to nail**
  - +7th **S61.222 Laceration with foreign body of right middle finger without damage to nail**
  - +7th **S61.223 Laceration with foreign body of left middle finger without damage to nail**
  - +7th **S61.224 Laceration with foreign body of right ring finger without damage to nail**
  - +7th **S61.225 Laceration with foreign body of left ring finger without damage to nail**
  - +7th **S61.226 Laceration with foreign body of right little finger without damage to nail**
  - +7th **S61.227 Laceration with foreign body of left little finger without damage to nail**
  - +7th **S61.228 Laceration with foreign body of other finger without damage to nail**
    Laceration with foreign body of specified finger with unspecified laterality without damage to nail
  - +7th **S61.229 Laceration with foreign body of unspecified finger without damage to nail**

+ **S61.23 Puncture wound without foreign body of finger without damage to nail**
  - **S61.230 Puncture wound without foreign body of right index finger without damage to nail**
  - +7th **S61.231 Puncture wound without foreign body of left index finger without damage to nail**
  - +7th **S61.232 Puncture wound without foreign body of right middle finger without damage to nail**
  - +7th **S61.233 Puncture wound without foreign body of left middle finger without damage to nail**
  - +7th **S61.234 Puncture wound without foreign body of right ring finger without damage to nail**
  - +7th **S61.235 Puncture wound without foreign body of left ring finger without damage to nail**
  - +7th **S61.236 Puncture wound without foreign body of right little finger without damage to nail**
  - +7th **S61.237 Puncture wound without foreign body of left little finger without damage to nail**
  - +7th **S61.238 Puncture wound without foreign body of other finger without damage to nail**
    Puncture wound without foreign body of specified finger with unspecified laterality without damage to nail
  - +7th **S61.239 Puncture wound without foreign body of unspecified finger without damage to nail**

+ **S61.24 Puncture wound with foreign body of finger without damage to nail**
  - **S61.240 Puncture wound with foreign body of right index finger without damage to nail**
  - +7th **S61.241 Puncture wound with foreign body of left index finger without damage to nail**
  - +7th **S61.242 Puncture wound with foreign body of right middle finger without damage to nail**
  - +7th **S61.243 Puncture wound with foreign body of left middle finger without damage to nail**
  - +7th **S61.244 Puncture wound with foreign body of right ring finger without damage to nail**
  - +7th **S61.245 Puncture wound with foreign body of left ring finger without damage to nail**
  - +7th **S61.246 Puncture wound with foreign body of right little finger without damage to nail**
  - +7th **S61.247 Puncture wound with foreign body of left little finger without damage to nail**
  - +7th **S61.248 Puncture wound with foreign body of other finger without damage to nail**
    Puncture wound with foreign body of specified finger with unspecified laterality without damage to nail
  - +7th **S61.249 Puncture wound with foreign body of unspecified finger without damage to nail**

+ **S61.25 Open bite of finger without damage to nail**
  Bite of finger without damage to nail NOS
  Excludes1: *superficial bite of finger (S60.46-, S60.47-)*
  - **S61.250 Open bite of right index finger without damage to nail**
  - +7th **S61.251 Open bite of left index finger without damage to nail**
  - +7th **S61.252 Open bite of right middle finger without damage to nail**
  - +7th **S61.253 Open bite of left middle finger without damage to nail**
  - +7th **S61.254 Open bite of right ring finger without damage to nail**
  - +7th **S61.255 Open bite of left ring finger without damage to nail**
  - +7th **S61.256 Open bite of right little finger without damage to nail**
  - +7th **S61.257 Open bite of left little finger without damage to nail**
  - +7th **S61.258 Open bite of other finger without damage to nail**
    Open bite of specified finger with unspecified laterality without damage to nail
  - +7th **S61.259 Open bite of unspecified finger without damage to nail**

+ **S61.3 Open wound of other finger with damage to nail**

+ **S61.30 Unspecified open wound of finger with damage to nail**
  - **S61.300 Unspecified open wound of right index finger with damage to nail**
  - +7th **S61.301 Unspecified open wound of left index finger with damage to nail**
  - +7th **S61.302 Unspecified open wound of right middle finger with damage to nail**
  - +7th **S61.303 Unspecified open wound of left middle finger with damage to nail**
  - +7th **S61.304 Unspecified open wound of right ring finger with damage to nail**
  - +7th **S61.305 Unspecified open wound of left ring finger with damage to nail**
  - +7th **S61.306 Unspecified open wound of right little finger with damage to nail**
  - +7th **S61.307 Unspecified open wound of left little finger with damage to nail**
  - +7th **S61.308 Unspecified open wound of other finger with damage to nail**
    Unspecified open wound of specified finger with unspecified laterality with damage to nail
  - +7th **S61.309 Unspecified open wound of unspecified finger with damage to nail**

+ **S61.31 Laceration without foreign body of finger with damage to nail**
  - **S61.310 Laceration without foreign body of right index finger with damage to nail**
  - +7th **S61.311 Laceration without foreign body of left index finger with damage to nail**
  - +7th **S61.312 Laceration without foreign body of right middle finger with damage to nail**
  - +7th **S61.313 Laceration without foreign body of left middle finger with damage to nail**
  - +7th **S61.314 Laceration without foreign body of right ring finger with damage to nail**
  - +7th **S61.315 Laceration without foreign body of left ring finger with damage to nail**
  - +7th **S61.316 Laceration without foreign body of right little finger with damage to nail**
  - +7th **S61.317 Laceration without foreign body of left little finger with damage to nail**
  - +7th **S61.318 Laceration without foreign body of other finger with damage to nail**
    Laceration without foreign body of specified finger with unspecified laterality with damage to nail
  - +7th **S61.319 Laceration without foreign body of unspecified finger with damage to nail**

+ **S61.32 Laceration with foreign body of finger with damage to nail**
  - **S61.320 Laceration with foreign body of right index finger with damage to nail**
  - +7th **S61.321 Laceration with foreign body of left index finger with damage to nail**
  - +7th **S61.322 Laceration with foreign body of right middle finger with damage to nail**

+7th S61.323 **Laceration with foreign body of left middle finger with damage to nail**
+7th S61.324 **Laceration with foreign body of right ring finger with damage to nail**
+7th S61.325 **Laceration with foreign body of left ring finger with damage to nail**
+7th S61.326 **Laceration with foreign body of right little finger with damage to nail**
+7th S61.327 **Laceration with foreign body of left little finger with damage to nail**
+7th S61.328 **Laceration with foreign body of other finger with damage to nail**
Laceration with foreign body of specified finger with unspecified laterality with damage to nail
+7th S61.329 **Laceration with foreign body of unspecified finger with damage to nail**
+ **S61.33 Puncture wound without foreign body of finger with damage to nail**
S61.330 Puncture wound without foreign body of right index finger with damage to nail
+7th S61.331 **Puncture wound without foreign body of left index finger with damage to nail**
+7th S61.332 **Puncture wound without foreign body of right middle finger with damage to nail**
+7th S61.333 **Puncture wound without foreign body of left middle finger with damage to nail**
+7th S61.334 **Puncture wound without foreign body of right ring finger with damage to nail**
+7th S61.335 **Puncture wound without foreign body of left ring finger with damage to nail**
+7th S61.336 **Puncture wound without foreign body of right little finger with damage to nail**
+7th S61.337 **Puncture wound without foreign body of left little finger with damage to nail**
+7th S61.338 **Puncture wound without foreign body of other finger with damage to nail**
Puncture wound without foreign body of specified finger with unspecified laterality with damage to nail
+7th S61.339 **Puncture wound without foreign body of unspecified finger with damage to nail**
+ **S61.34 Puncture wound with foreign body of finger with damage to nail**
S61.340 Puncture wound with foreign body of right index finger with damage to nail
+7th S61.341 **Puncture wound with foreign body of left index finger with damage to nail**
+7th S61.342 **Puncture wound with foreign body of right middle finger with damage to nail**
+7th S61.343 **Puncture wound with foreign body of left middle finger with damage to nail**
+7th S61.344 **Puncture wound with foreign body of right ring finger with damage to nail**
+7th S61.345 **Puncture wound with foreign body of left ring finger with damage to nail**
+7th S61.346 **Puncture wound with foreign body of right little finger with damage to nail**
+7th S61.347 **Puncture wound with foreign body of left little finger with damage to nail**
+7th S61.348 **Puncture wound with foreign body of other finger with damage to nail**
Puncture wound with foreign body of specified finger with unspecified laterality with damage to nail
+7th S61.349 **Puncture wound with foreign body of unspecified finger with damage to nail**
+ **S61.35 Open bite of finger with damage to nail**
Bite of finger with damage to nail NOS
Excludes1: *superficial bite of finger (S60.46-, S60.47-)*
S61.350 Open bite of right index finger with damage to nail
+7th S61.351 **Open bite of left index finger with damage to nail**
+7th S61.352 **Open bite of right middle finger with damage to nail**
+7th S61.353 **Open bite of left middle finger with damage to nail**
+7th S61.354 **Open bite of right ring finger with damage to nail**
+7th S61.355 **Open bite of left ring finger with damage to nail**
+7th S61.356 **Open bite of right little finger with damage to nail**
+7th S61.357 **Open bite of left little finger with damage to nail**
+7th S61.358 **Open bite of other finger with damage to nail**
Open bite of specified finger with unspecified laterality with damage to nail
+7th S61.359 **Open bite of unspecified finger with damage to nail**
+ **S61.4 Open wound of hand**
+ **S61.40 Unspecified open wound of hand**
+7th S61.401 **Unspecified open wound of right hand**
+7th S61.402 **Unspecified open wound of left hand**
+7th S61.409 **Unspecified open wound of unspecified hand**
+ **S61.41 Laceration without foreign body of hand**
+7th S61.411 **Laceration without foreign body of right hand**
+7th S61.412 **Laceration without foreign body of left hand**
+7th S61.419 **Laceration without foreign body of unspecified hand**
+ **S61.42 Laceration with foreign body of hand**
+7th S61.421 **Laceration with foreign body of right hand**
+7th S61.422 **Laceration with foreign body of left hand**
+7th S61.429 **Laceration with foreign body of unspecified hand**
+ **S61.43 Puncture wound without foreign body of hand**
+7th S61.431 **Puncture wound without foreign body of right hand**
+7th S61.432 **Puncture wound without foreign body of left hand**
+7th S61.439 **Puncture wound without foreign body of unspecified hand**
+ **S61.44 Puncture wound with foreign body of hand**
+7th S61.441 **Puncture wound with foreign body of right hand**
+7th S61.442 **Puncture wound with foreign body of left hand**
+7th S61.449 **Puncture wound with foreign body of unspecified hand**
+ **S61.45 Open bite of hand**
Bite of hand NOS
Excludes1: *superficial bite of hand (S60.56-, S60.57-*
+7th S61.451 **Open bite of right hand**
+7th S61.452 **Open bite of left hand**
+7th S61.459 **Open bite of unspecified hand**
+ **S61.5 Open wound of wrist**
+ **S61.50 Unspecified open wound of wrist**
+7th S61.501 **Unspecified open wound of right wrist**
+7th S61.502 **Unspecified open wound of left wrist**
+7th S61.509 **Unspecified open wound of unspecified wrist**
+ **S61.51 Laceration without foreign body of wrist**
+7th S61.511 **Laceration without foreign body of right wrist**
+7th S61.512 **Laceration without foreign body of left wrist**
+7th S61.519 **Laceration without foreign body of unspecified wrist**
+ **S61.52 Laceration with foreign body of wrist**
+7th S61.521 **Laceration with foreign body of right wrist**
+7th S61.522 **Laceration with foreign body of left wrist**
+7th S61.529 **Laceration with foreign body of unspecified wrist**
+ **S61.53 Puncture wound without foreign body of wrist**
+7th S61.531 **Puncture wound without foreign body of right wrist**
+7th S61.532 **Puncture wound without foreign body of left wrist**
+7th S61.539 **Puncture wound without foreign body of unspecified wrist**
+ **S61.54 Puncture wound with foreign body of wrist**
+7th S61.541 **Puncture wound with foreign body of right wrist**

+7th **S61.542 Puncture wound with foreign body of left wrist**
+7th **S61.549 Puncture wound with foreign body of unspecified wrist**
+ **S61.55 Open bite of wrist**
Bite of wrist NOS
Excludes1: *superficial bite of wrist (S60.86-, S60.87-)*
+7th **S61.551 Open bite of right wrist**
+7th **S61.552 Open bite of left wrist**
+7th **S61.559 Open bite of unspecified wrist**

S62 Fracture at wrist and hand level

NOTE A fracture not indicated as displaced or nondisplaced should be coded to displaced
A fracture not indicated as open or closed should be coded to closed

Excludes1: *traumatic amputation of wrist and hand (S68.-)*
Excludes2: *fracture of distal parts of ulna and radius (S52.-)*

The appropriate 7th character is to be added to each code from category S62
A initial encounter for closed fracture
B initial encounter for open fracture
D subsequent encounter for fracture with routine healing
G subsequent encounter for fracture with delayed healing
K subsequent encounter for fracture with nonunion
P subsequent encounter for fracture with malunion
S sequela

Review coding guideline C.19.c

+ **S62.0 Fracture of navicular [scaphoid] bone of wrist**
+ **S62.00 Unspecified fracture of navicular [scaphoid] bone of wrist**

CC +7th **S62.001 Unspecified fracture of navicular [scaphoid] bone of right wrist**
CC Exclusion 7th character B see Appendix A PDX collection 1283
CC Exclusion 7th characters K & P see Appendix A PDX collection 0897
HAC 7th character B see Appendix B for HAC conditional logic

CC +7th **S62.002 Unspecified fracture of navicular [scaphoid] bone of left wrist**
CC Exclusion 7th character B see Appendix A PDX collection 1283
CC Exclusion 7th characters K & P see Appendix A PDX collection 0897
AHA CC: 4Q, 2012, 106
HAC 7th character B see Appendix B for HAC conditional logic

CC +7th **S62.009 Unspecified fracture of navicular [scaphoid] bone of unspecified wrist**
CC Exclusion 7th character B see Appendix A PDX collection 1283
CC Exclusion 7th characters K & P see Appendix A PDX collection 0897
HAC 7th character B see Appendix B for HAC conditional logic

+ **S62.01 Fracture of distal pole of navicular [scaphoid] bone of wrist**
Fracture of volar tuberosity of navicular [scaphoid] bone of wrist

CC +7th **S62.011 Displaced fracture of distal pole of navicular [scaphoid] bone of right wrist**
CC Exclusion 7th character B see Appendix A PDX collection 1283
CC Exclusion 7th characters K & P see Appendix A PDX collection 0897
HAC 7th character B see Appendix B for HAC conditional logic

CC +7th **S62.012 Displaced fracture of distal pole of navicular [scaphoid] bone of left wrist**
CC Exclusion 7th character B see Appendix A PDX collection 1283
CC Exclusion 7th characters K & P see Appendix A PDX collection 0897
HAC 7th character B see Appendix B for HAC conditional logic

CC +7th **S62.013 Displaced fracture of distal pole of navicular [scaphoid] bone of unspecified wrist**
CC Exclusion 7th character B see Appendix A PDX collection 1283
CC Exclusion 7th characters K & P see Appendix A PDX collection 0897
HAC 7th character B see Appendix B for HAC conditional logic

CC +7th **S62.014 Nondisplaced fracture of distal pole of navicular [scaphoid] bone of right wrist**
CC Exclusion 7th character B see Appendix A PDX collection 1283
CC Exclusion 7th characters K & P see Appendix A PDX collection 0897
HAC 7th character B see Appendix B for HAC conditional logic

CC +7th **S62.015 Nondisplaced fracture of distal pole of navicular [scaphoid] bone of left wrist**
CC Exclusion 7th character B see Appendix A PDX collection 1283
CC Exclusion 7th characters K & P see Appendix A PDX collection 0897
HAC 7th character B see Appendix B for HAC conditional logic

CC +7th **S62.016 Nondisplaced fracture of distal pole of navicular [scaphoid] bone of unspecified wrist**
CC Exclusion 7th character B see Appendix A PDX collection 1283
CC Exclusion 7th characters K & P see Appendix A PDX collection 0897
HAC 7th character B see Appendix B for HAC conditional logic

+ **S62.02 Fracture of middle third of navicular [scaphoid] bone of wrist**

CC +7th **S62.021 Displaced fracture of middle third of navicular [scaphoid] bone of right wrist**
CC Exclusion 7th character B see Appendix A PDX collection 1283
CC Exclusion 7th characters K & P see Appendix A PDX collection 0897
HAC 7th character B see Appendix B for HAC conditional logic

CC +7th **S62.022 Displaced fracture of middle third of navicular [scaphoid] bone of left wrist**
CC Exclusion 7th character B see Appendix A PDX collection 1283
CC Exclusion 7th characters K & P see Appendix A PDX collection 0897
HAC 7th character B see Appendix B for HAC conditional logic

CC +7th **S62.023 Displaced fracture of middle third of navicular [scaphoid] bone of unspecified wrist**
CC Exclusion 7th character B see Appendix A PDX collection 1283
CC Exclusion 7th characters K & P see Appendix A PDX collection 0897
HAC 7th character B see Appendix B for HAC conditional logic

CC +7th **S62.024 Nondisplaced fracture of middle third of navicular [scaphoid] bone of right wrist**
CC Exclusion 7th character B see Appendix A PDX collection 1283
CC Exclusion 7th characters K & P see Appendix A PDX collection 0897
HAC 7th character B see Appendix B for HAC conditional logic

CC +7th **S62.025 Nondisplaced fracture of middle third of navicular [scaphoid] bone of left wrist**
CC Exclusion 7th character B see Appendix A PDX collection 1283
CC Exclusion 7th characters K & P see Appendix A PDX collection 0897
HAC 7th character B see Appendix B for HAC conditional logic

CC +7th **S62.026 Nondisplaced fracture of middle third of navicular [scaphoid] bone of unspecified wrist**
CC Exclusion 7th character B see Appendix A PDX collection 1283
CC Exclusion 7th characters K & P see Appendix A PDX collection 0897
HAC 7th character B see Appendix B for HAC conditional logic

+ **S62.03 Fracture of proximal third of navicular [scaphoid] bone of wrist**

CC +7th **S62.031 Displaced fracture of proximal third of navicular [scaphoid] bone of right wrist**
CC Exclusion 7th character B see Appendix A PDX collection 1283
CC Exclusion 7th characters K & P see Appendix A PDX collection 0897
HAC 7th character B see Appendix B for HAC conditional logic

CC +7th **S62.032 Displaced fracture of proximal third of navicular [scaphoid] bone of left wrist**
CC Exclusion 7th character B see Appendix A PDX collection 1283
CC Exclusion 7th characters K & P see Appendix A PDX collection 0897
HAC 7th character B see Appendix B for HAC conditional logic

CC +7th **S62.033 Displaced fracture of proximal third of navicular [scaphoid] bone of unspecified wrist**
CC Exclusion 7th character B see Appendix A PDX collection 1283
CC Exclusion 7th characters K & P see Appendix A PDX collection 0897
HAC 7th character B see Appendix B for HAC conditional logic

CC +7th **S62.034 Nondisplaced fracture of proximal third of navicular [scaphoid] bone of right wrist**
CC Exclusion 7th character B see Appendix A PDX collection 1283
CC Exclusion 7th characters K & P see Appendix A PDX collection 0897
HAC 7th character B see Appendix B for HAC conditional logic

CC +7th **S62.035 Nondisplaced fracture of proximal third of navicular [scaphoid] bone of left wrist**
CC Exclusion 7th character B see Appendix A PDX collection 1283
CC Exclusion 7th characters K & P see Appendix A PDX collection 0897
HAC 7th character B see Appendix B for HAC conditional logic

CC +7th **S62.036 Nondisplaced fracture of proximal third of navicular [scaphoid] bone of unspecified wrist**
CC Exclusion 7th character B see Appendix A PDX collection 1283
CC Exclusion 7th characters K & P see Appendix A PDX collection 0897
HAC 7th character B see Appendix B for HAC conditional logic

\+ **S62.1 Fracture of other and unspecified carpal bone(s)**
Excludes2: *fracture of scaphoid of wrist (S62.0-)*

\+ **S62.10 Fracture of unspecified carpal bone**
Fracture of wrist NOS

CC +7th **S62.101 Fracture of unspecified carpal bone, right wrist**
CC Exclusion 7th character B see Appendix A PDX collection 1283
CC Exclusion 7th characters K & P see Appendix A PDX collection 0897
HAC 7th character B see Appendix B for HAC conditional logic

CC +7th **S62.102 Fracture of unspecified carpal bone, left wrist**
CC Exclusion 7th character B see Appendix A PDX collection 1283
CC Exclusion 7th characters K & P see Appendix A PDX collection 0897
AHA CC: 4Q, 2012, 95-96
HAC 7th character B see Appendix B for HAC conditional logic

CC +7th **S62.109 Fracture of unspecified carpal bone, unspecified wrist**
CC Exclusion 7th character B see Appendix A PDX collection 1283
CC Exclusion 7th characters K & P see Appendix A PDX collection 0897
HAC 7th character B see Appendix B for HAC conditional logic

\+ **S62.11 Fracture of triquetrum [cuneiform] bone of wrist**

CC +7th **S62.111 Displaced fracture of triquetrum [cuneiform] bone, right wrist**
CC Exclusion 7th character B see Appendix A PDX collection 1283
CC Exclusion 7th characters K & P see Appendix A PDX collection 0897
HAC 7th character B see Appendix B for HAC conditional logic

CC +7th **S62.112 Displaced fracture of triquetrum [cuneiform] bone, left wrist**
CC Exclusion 7th character B see Appendix A PDX collection 1283
CC Exclusion 7th characters K & P see Appendix A PDX collection 0897
HAC 7th character B see Appendix B for HAC conditional logic

CC +7th **S62.113 Displaced fracture of triquetrum [cuneiform] bone, unspecified wrist**
CC Exclusion 7th character B see Appendix A PDX collection 1283
CC Exclusion 7th characters K & P see Appendix A PDX collection 0897
HAC 7th character B see Appendix B for HAC conditional logic

CC +7th **S62.114 Nondisplaced fracture of triquetrum [cuneiform] bone, right wrist**
CC Exclusion 7th character B see Appendix A PDX collection 1283
CC Exclusion 7th characters K & P see Appendix A PDX collection 0897
HAC 7th character B see Appendix B for HAC conditional logic

CC +7th **S62.115 Nondisplaced fracture of triquetrum [cuneiform] bone, left wrist**
CC Exclusion 7th character B see Appendix A PDX collection 1283
CC Exclusion 7th characters K & P see Appendix A PDX collection 0897
HAC 7th character B see Appendix B for HAC conditional logic

CC +7th **S62.116 Nondisplaced fracture of triquetrum [cuneiform] bone, unspecified wrist**
CC Exclusion 7th character B see Appendix A PDX collection 1283
CC Exclusion 7th characters K & P see Appendix A PDX collection 0897
HAC 7th character B see Appendix B for HAC conditional logic

\+ **S62.12 Fracture of lunate [semilunar]**

CC +7th **S62.121 Displaced fracture of lunate [semilunar], right wrist**
CC Exclusion 7th character B see Appendix A PDX collection 1283
CC Exclusion 7th characters K & P see Appendix A PDX collection 0897
HAC 7th character B see Appendix B for HAC conditional logic

CC +7th **S62.122 Displaced fracture of lunate [semilunar], left wrist**
CC Exclusion 7th character B see Appendix A PDX collection 1283
CC Exclusion 7th characters K & P see Appendix A PDX collection 0897
HAC 7th character B see Appendix B for HAC conditional logic

CC +7th **S62.123 Displaced fracture of lunate [semilunar], unspecified wrist**
CC Exclusion 7th character B see Appendix A PDX collection 1283
CC Exclusion 7th characters K & P see Appendix A PDX collection 0897
HAC 7th character B see Appendix B for HAC conditional logic

CC +7th **S62.124 Nondisplaced fracture of lunate [semilunar], right wrist**
CC Exclusion 7th character B see Appendix A PDX collection 1283
CC Exclusion 7th characters K & P see Appendix A PDX collection 0897
HAC 7th character B see Appendix B for HAC conditional logic

CC +7th **S62.125 Nondisplaced fracture of lunate [semilunar], left wrist**
CC Exclusion 7th character B see Appendix A PDX collection 1283
CC Exclusion 7th characters K & P see Appendix A PDX collection 0897
HAC 7th character B see Appendix B for HAC conditional logic

CC +7th **S62.126 Nondisplaced fracture of lunate [semilunar], unspecified wrist**
CC Exclusion 7th character B see Appendix A PDX collection 1283
CC Exclusion 7th characters K & P see Appendix A PDX collection 0897
HAC 7th character B see Appendix B for HAC conditional logic

+ **S62.13 Fracture of capitate [os magnum] bone**

CC +7th **S62.131 Displaced fracture of capitate [os magnum] bone, right wrist**
CC Exclusion 7th character B see Appendix A PDX collection 1283
CC Exclusion 7th characters K & P see Appendix A PDX collection 0897
HAC 7th character B see Appendix B for HAC conditional logic

CC +7th **S62.132 Displaced fracture of capitate [os magnum] bone, left wrist**
CC Exclusion 7th character B see Appendix A PDX collection 1283
CC Exclusion 7th characters K & P see Appendix A PDX collection 0897
HAC 7th character B see Appendix B for HAC conditional logic

CC +7th **S62.133 Displaced fracture of capitate [os magnum] bone, unspecified wrist**
CC Exclusion 7th character B see Appendix A PDX collection 1283
CC Exclusion 7th characters K & P see Appendix A PDX collection 0897
HAC 7th character B see Appendix B for HAC conditional logic

CC +7th **S62.134 Nondisplaced fracture of capitate [os magnum] bone, right wrist**
CC Exclusion 7th character B see Appendix A PDX collection 1283
CC Exclusion 7th characters K & P see Appendix A PDX collection 0897
HAC 7th character B see Appendix B for HAC conditional logic

CC +7th **S62.135 Nondisplaced fracture of capitate [os magnum] bone, left wrist**
CC Exclusion 7th character B see Appendix A PDX collection 1283
CC Exclusion 7th characters K & P see Appendix A PDX collection 0897
HAC 7th character B see Appendix B for HAC conditional logic

CC +7th **S62.136 Nondisplaced fracture of capitate [os magnum] bone, unspecified wrist**
CC Exclusion 7th character B see Appendix A PDX collection 1283
CC Exclusion 7th characters K & P see Appendix A PDX collection 0897
HAC 7th character B see Appendix B for HAC conditional logic

+ **S62.14 Fracture of body of hamate [unciform] bone**
Fracture of hamate [unciform] bone NOS

CC +7th **S62.141 Displaced fracture of body of hamate [unciform] bone, right wrist**
CC Exclusion 7th character B see Appendix A PDX collection 1283
CC Exclusion 7th characters K & P see Appendix A PDX collection 0897
HAC 7th character B see Appendix B for HAC conditional logic

CC +7th **S62.142 Displaced fracture of body of hamate [unciform] bone, left wrist**
CC Exclusion 7th character B see Appendix A PDX collection 1283
CC Exclusion 7th characters K & P see Appendix A PDX collection 0897
HAC 7th character B see Appendix B for HAC conditional logic

CC +7th **S62.143 Displaced fracture of body of hamate [unciform] bone, unspecified wrist**
CC Exclusion 7th character B see Appendix A PDX collection 1283
CC Exclusion 7th characters K & P see Appendix A PDX collection 0897
HAC 7th character B see Appendix B for HAC conditional logic

CC +7th **S62.144 Nondisplaced fracture of body of hamate [unciform] bone, right wrist**
CC Exclusion 7th character B see Appendix A PDX collection 1283
CC Exclusion 7th characters K & P see Appendix A PDX collection 0897
HAC 7th character B see Appendix B for HAC conditional logic

CC +7th **S62.145 Nondisplaced fracture of body of hamate [unciform] bone, left wrist**
CC Exclusion 7th character B see Appendix A PDX collection 1283
CC Exclusion 7th characters K & P see Appendix A PDX collection 0897
HAC 7th character B see Appendix B for HAC conditional logic

CC +7th **S62.146 Nondisplaced fracture of body of hamate [unciform] bone, unspecified wrist**
CC Exclusion 7th character B see Appendix A PDX collection 1283
CC Exclusion 7th characters K & P see Appendix A PDX collection 0897
HAC 7th character B see Appendix B for HAC conditional logic

+ **S62.15 Fracture of hook process of hamate [unciform] bone**
Fracture of unciform process of hamate [unciform] bone

CC +7th **S62.151 Displaced fracture of hook process of hamate [unciform] bone, right wrist**
CC Exclusion 7th character B see Appendix A PDX collection 1283
CC Exclusion 7th characters K & P see Appendix A PDX collection 0897
HAC 7th character B see Appendix B for HAC conditional logic

CC +7th **S62.152 Displaced fracture of hook process of hamate [unciform] bone, left wrist**
CC Exclusion 7th character B see Appendix A PDX collection 1283
CC Exclusion 7th characters K & P see Appendix A PDX collection 0897
HAC 7th character B see Appendix B for HAC conditional logic

CC +7th **S62.153 Displaced fracture of hook process of hamate [unciform] bone, unspecified wrist**
CC Exclusion 7th character B see Appendix A PDX collection 1283
CC Exclusion 7th characters K & P see Appendix A PDX collection 0897
HAC 7th character B see Appendix B for HAC conditional logic

CC +7th **S62.154 Nondisplaced fracture of hook process of hamate [unciform] bone, right wrist**
CC Exclusion 7th character B see Appendix A PDX collection 1283
CC Exclusion 7th characters K & P see Appendix A PDX collection 0897
HAC 7th character B see Appendix B for HAC conditional logic

CC +7th **S62.155 Nondisplaced fracture of hook process of hamate [unciform] bone, left wrist**
CC Exclusion 7th character B see Appendix A PDX collection 1283
CC Exclusion 7th characters K & P see Appendix A PDX collection 0897
HAC 7th character B see Appendix B for HAC conditional logic

CC +7th **S62.156 Nondisplaced fracture of hook process of hamate [unciform] bone, unspecified wrist**
CC Exclusion 7th character B see Appendix A PDX collection 1283
CC Exclusion 7th characters K & P see Appendix A PDX collection 0897
HAC 7th character B see Appendix B for HAC conditional logic

+ **S62.16 Fracture of pisiform**

CC +7th **S62.161 Displaced fracture of pisiform, right wrist**
CC Exclusion 7th character B see Appendix A PDX collection 1283
CC Exclusion 7th characters K & P see Appendix A PDX collection 0897
HAC 7th character B see Appendix B for HAC conditional logic

CC +7th **S62.162 Displaced fracture of pisiform, left wrist**
CC Exclusion 7th character B see Appendix A PDX collection 1283
CC Exclusion 7th characters K & P see Appendix A PDX collection 0897
HAC 7th character B see Appendix B for HAC conditional logic

CC +7th **S62.163 Displaced fracture of pisiform, unspecified wrist**
CC Exclusion 7th character B see Appendix A PDX collection 1283
CC Exclusion 7th characters K & P see Appendix A PDX collection 0897
HAC 7th character B see Appendix B for HAC conditional logic

CC +7th **S62.164 Nondisplaced fracture of pisiform, right wrist**
CC Exclusion 7th character B see Appendix A PDX collection 1283
CC Exclusion 7th characters K & P see Appendix A PDX collection 0897
HAC 7th character B see Appendix B for HAC conditional logic

CC +7th **S62.165 Nondisplaced fracture of pisiform, left wrist**
CC Exclusion 7th character B see Appendix A PDX collection 1283
CC Exclusion 7th characters K & P see Appendix A PDX collection 0897
HAC 7th character B see Appendix B for HAC conditional logic

CC +7th **S62.166 Nondisplaced fracture of pisiform, unspecified wrist**
CC Exclusion 7th character B see Appendix A PDX collection 1283
CC Exclusion 7th characters K & P see Appendix A PDX collection 0897
HAC 7th character B see Appendix B for HAC conditional logic

\+ **S62.17 Fracture of trapezium [larger multangular]**

CC +7th **S62.171 Displaced fracture of trapezium [larger multangular], right wrist**
CC Exclusion 7th character B see Appendix A PDX collection 1283
CC Exclusion 7th characters K & P see Appendix A PDX collection 0897
HAC 7th character B see Appendix B for HAC conditional logic

CC +7th **S62.172 Displaced fracture of trapezium [larger multangular], left wrist**
CC Exclusion 7th character B see Appendix A PDX collection 1283
CC Exclusion 7th characters K & P see Appendix A PDX collection 0897
HAC 7th character B see Appendix B for HAC conditional logic

CC +7th **S62.173 Displaced fracture of trapezium [larger multangular], unspecified wrist**
CC Exclusion 7th character B see Appendix A PDX collection 1283
CC Exclusion 7th characters K & P see Appendix A PDX collection 0897
HAC 7th character B see Appendix B for HAC conditional logic

CC +7th **S62.174 Nondisplaced fracture of trapezium [larger multangular], right wrist**
CC Exclusion 7th character B see Appendix A PDX collection 1283
CC Exclusion 7th characters K & P see Appendix A PDX collection 0897
HAC 7th character B see Appendix B for HAC conditional logic

CC +7th **S62.175 Nondisplaced fracture of trapezium [larger multangular], left wrist**
CC Exclusion 7th character B see Appendix A PDX collection 1283
CC Exclusion 7th characters K & P see Appendix A PDX collection 0897
HAC 7th character B see Appendix B for HAC conditional logic

CC +7th **S62.176 Nondisplaced fracture of trapezium [larger multangular], unspecified wrist**
CC Exclusion 7th character B see Appendix A PDX collection 1283
CC Exclusion 7th characters K & P see Appendix A PDX collection 0897
HAC 7th character B see Appendix B for HAC conditional logic

\+ **S62.18 Fracture of trapezoid [smaller multangular]**

CC +7th **S62.181 Displaced fracture of trapezoid [smaller multangular], right wrist**
CC Exclusion 7th character B see Appendix A PDX collection 1283
CC Exclusion 7th characters K & P see Appendix A PDX collection 0897
HAC 7th character B see Appendix B for HAC conditional logic

CC +7th **S62.182 Displaced fracture of trapezoid [smaller multangular], left wrist**
CC Exclusion 7th character B see Appendix A PDX collection 1283
CC Exclusion 7th characters K & P see Appendix A PDX collection 0897
HAC 7th character B see Appendix B for HAC conditional logic

CC +7th **S62.183 Displaced fracture of trapezoid [smaller multangular], unspecified wrist**
CC Exclusion 7th character B see Appendix A PDX collection 1283
CC Exclusion 7th characters K & P see Appendix A PDX collection 0897
HAC 7th character B see Appendix B for HAC conditional logic

CC +7th **S62.184 Nondisplaced fracture of trapezoid [smaller multangular], right wrist**
CC Exclusion 7th character B see Appendix A PDX collection 1283
CC Exclusion 7th characters K & P see Appendix A PDX collection 0897
HAC 7th character B see Appendix B for HAC conditional logic

CC +7th **S62.185 Nondisplaced fracture of trapezoid [smaller multangular], left wrist**
CC Exclusion 7th character B see Appendix A PDX collection 1283
CC Exclusion 7th characters K & P see Appendix A PDX collection 0897
HAC 7th character B see Appendix B for HAC conditional logic

CC +7th **S62.186 Nondisplaced fracture of trapezoid [smaller multangular], unspecified wrist**
CC Exclusion 7th character B see Appendix A PDX collection 1283
CC Exclusion 7th characters K & P see Appendix A PDX collection 0897
HAC 7th character B see Appendix B for HAC conditional logic

\+ **S62.2 Fracture of first metacarpal bone**

\+ **S62.20 Unspecified fracture of first metacarpal bone**

CC +7th **S62.201 Unspecified fracture of first metacarpal bone, right hand**
CC Exclusion 7th character B see Appendix A PDX collection 1284
CC Exclusion 7th characters K & P see Appendix A PDX collection 0897
HAC 7th character B see Appendix B for HAC conditional logic

CC +7th **S62.202 Unspecified fracture of first metacarpal bone, left hand**
CC Exclusion 7th character B see Appendix A PDX collection 1284
CC Exclusion 7th characters K & P see Appendix A PDX collection 0897
HAC 7th character B see Appendix B for HAC conditional logic

CC +7th **S62.209 Unspecified fracture of first metacarpal bone, unspecified hand**
CC Exclusion 7th character B see Appendix A PDX collection 1284
CC Exclusion 7th characters K & P see Appendix A PDX collection 0897
HAC 7th character B see Appendix B for HAC conditional logic

\+ **S62.21 Bennett's fracture**

CC +7th **S62.211 Bennett's fracture, right hand**
CC Exclusion 7th character B see Appendix A PDX collection 1284
CC Exclusion 7th characters K & P see Appendix A PDX collection 0897
HAC 7th character B see Appendix B for HAC conditional logic

CC +7th **S62.212 Bennett's fracture, left hand**
CC Exclusion 7th character B see Appendix A PDX collection 1284
CC Exclusion 7th characters K & P see Appendix A PDX collection 0897
HAC 7th character B see Appendix B for HAC conditional logic

CC +7th **S62.213 Bennett's fracture, unspecified hand**
CC Exclusion 7th character B see Appendix A PDX collection 1284
CC Exclusion 7th characters K & P see Appendix A PDX collection 0897
HAC 7th character B see Appendix B for HAC conditional logic

+ **S62.22 Rolando's fracture**

CC +7th **S62.221 Displaced Rolando's fracture, right hand**
CC Exclusion 7th character B see Appendix A PDX collection 1284
CC Exclusion 7th characters K & P see Appendix A PDX collection 0897
HAC 7th character B see Appendix B for HAC conditional logic

CC +7th **S62.222 Displaced Rolando's fracture, left hand**
CC Exclusion 7th character B see Appendix A PDX collection 1284
CC Exclusion 7th characters K & P see Appendix A PDX collection 0897
HAC 7th character B see Appendix B for HAC conditional logic

CC +7th **S62.223 Displaced Rolando's fracture, unspecified hand**
CC Exclusion 7th character B see Appendix A PDX collection 1284
CC Exclusion 7th characters K & P see Appendix A PDX collection 0897
HAC 7th character B see Appendix B for HAC conditional logic

CC +7th **S62.224 Nondisplaced Rolando's fracture, right hand**
CC Exclusion 7th character B see Appendix A PDX collection 1284
CC Exclusion 7th characters K & P see Appendix A PDX collection 0897
HAC 7th character B see Appendix B for HAC conditional logic

CC +7th **S62.225 Nondisplaced Rolando's fracture, left hand**
CC Exclusion 7th character B see Appendix A PDX collection 1284
CC Exclusion 7th characters K & P see Appendix A PDX collection 0897
HAC 7th character B see Appendix B for HAC conditional logic

CC +7th **S62.226 Nondisplaced Rolando's fracture, unspecified hand**
CC Exclusion 7th character B see Appendix A PDX collection 1284
CC Exclusion 7th characters K & P see Appendix A PDX collection 0897
HAC 7th character B see Appendix B for HAC conditional logic

+ **S62.23 Other fracture of base of first metacarpal bone**

CC +7th **S62.231 Other displaced fracture of base of first metacarpal bone, right hand**
CC Exclusion 7th character B see Appendix A PDX collection 1284
CC Exclusion 7th characters K & P see Appendix A PDX collection 0897
HAC 7th character B see Appendix B for HAC conditional logic

CC +7th **S62.232 Other displaced fracture of base of first metacarpal bone, left hand**
CC Exclusion 7th character B see Appendix A PDX collection 1284
CC Exclusion 7th characters K & P see Appendix A PDX collection 0897
HAC 7th character B see Appendix B for HAC conditional logic

CC +7th **S62.233 Other displaced fracture of base of first metacarpal bone, unspecified hand**
CC Exclusion 7th character B see Appendix A PDX collection 1284
CC Exclusion 7th characters K & P see Appendix A PDX collection 0897
HAC 7th character B see Appendix B for HAC conditional logic

CC +7th **S62.234 Other nondisplaced fracture of base of first metacarpal bone, right hand**
CC Exclusion 7th character B see Appendix A PDX collection 1284
CC Exclusion 7th characters K & P see Appendix A PDX collection 0897
HAC 7th character B see Appendix B for HAC conditional logic

CC +7th **S62.235 Other nondisplaced fracture of base of first metacarpal bone, left hand**
CC Exclusion 7th character B see Appendix A PDX collection 1284
CC Exclusion 7th characters K & P see Appendix A PDX collection 0897
HAC 7th character B see Appendix B for HAC conditional logic

CC +7th **S62.236 Other nondisplaced fracture of base of first metacarpal bone, unspecified hand**
CC Exclusion 7th character B see Appendix A PDX collection 1284
CC Exclusion 7th characters K & P see Appendix A PDX collection 0897
HAC 7th character B see Appendix B for HAC conditional logic

+ **S62.24 Fracture of shaft of first metacarpal bone**

CC +7th **S62.241 Displaced fracture of shaft of first metacarpal bone, right hand**
CC Exclusion 7th character B see Appendix A PDX collection 1284
CC Exclusion 7th characters K & P see Appendix A PDX collection 0897
HAC 7th character B see Appendix B for HAC conditional logic

CC +7th **S62.242 Displaced fracture of shaft of first metacarpal bone, left hand**
CC Exclusion 7th character B see Appendix A PDX collection 1284
CC Exclusion 7th characters K & P see Appendix A PDX collection 0897
HAC 7th character B see Appendix B for HAC conditional logic

CC +7th **S62.243 Displaced fracture of shaft of first metacarpal bone, unspecified hand**
CC Exclusion 7th character B see Appendix A PDX collection 1284
CC Exclusion 7th characters K & P see Appendix A PDX collection 0897
HAC 7th character B see Appendix B for HAC conditional logic

CC +7th **S62.244 Nondisplaced fracture of shaft of first metacarpal bone, right hand**
CC Exclusion 7th character B see Appendix A PDX collection 1284
CC Exclusion 7th characters K & P see Appendix A PDX collection 0897
HAC 7th character B see Appendix B for HAC conditional logic

CC +7th **S62.245 Nondisplaced fracture of shaft of first metacarpal bone, left hand**
CC Exclusion 7th character B see Appendix A PDX collection 1284
CC Exclusion 7th characters K & P see Appendix A PDX collection 0897
HAC 7th character B see Appendix B for HAC conditional logic

CC +7th **S62.246 Nondisplaced fracture of shaft of first metacarpal bone, unspecified hand**
CC Exclusion 7th character B see Appendix A PDX collection 1284
CC Exclusion 7th characters K & P see Appendix A PDX collection 0897
HAC 7th character B see Appendix B for HAC conditional logic

+ **S62.25 Fracture of neck of first metacarpal bone**

CC +7th **S62.251 Displaced fracture of neck of first metacarpal bone, right hand**
CC Exclusion 7th character B see Appendix A PDX collection 1284
CC Exclusion 7th characters K & P see Appendix A PDX collection 0897
HAC 7th character B see Appendix B for HAC conditional logic

CC +7th **S62.252 Displaced fracture of neck of first metacarpal bone, left hand**
CC Exclusion 7th character B see Appendix A PDX collection 1284
CC Exclusion 7th characters K & P see Appendix A PDX collection 0897
HAC 7th character B see Appendix B for HAC conditional logic

CC +7th **S62.253 Displaced fracture of neck of first metacarpal bone, unspecified hand**
CC Exclusion 7th character B see Appendix A PDX collection 1284
CC Exclusion 7th characters K & P see Appendix A PDX collection 0897
HAC 7th character B see Appendix B for HAC conditional logic

CC +7th **S62.254 Nondisplaced fracture of neck of first metacarpal bone, right hand**
CC Exclusion 7th character B see Appendix A PDX collection 1284
CC Exclusion 7th characters K & P see Appendix A PDX collection 0897
HAC 7th character B see Appendix B for HAC conditional logic

CC +7th **S62.255 Nondisplaced fracture of neck of first metacarpal bone, left hand**
CC Exclusion 7th character B see Appendix A PDX collection 1284
CC Exclusion 7th characters K & P see Appendix A PDX collection 0897
HAC 7th character B see Appendix B for HAC conditional logic

CC +7th **S62.256 Nondisplaced fracture of neck of first metacarpal bone, unspecified hand**
CC Exclusion 7th character B see Appendix A PDX collection 1284
CC Exclusion 7th characters K & P see Appendix A PDX collection 0897
HAC 7th character B see Appendix B for HAC conditional logic

+ **S62.29 Other fracture of first metacarpal bone**

CC +7th **S62.291 Other fracture of first metacarpal bone, right hand**
CC Exclusion 7th character B see Appendix A PDX collection 1284
CC Exclusion 7th characters K & P see Appendix A PDX collection 0897
HAC 7th character B see Appendix B for HAC conditional logic

CC +7th **S62.292 Other fracture of first metacarpal bone, left hand**
CC Exclusion 7th character B see Appendix A PDX collection 1284
CC Exclusion 7th characters K & P see Appendix A PDX collection 0897
HAC 7th character B see Appendix B for HAC conditional logic

CC +7th **S62.299 Other fracture of first metacarpal bone, unspecified hand**
CC Exclusion 7th character B see Appendix A PDX collection 1284
CC Exclusion 7th characters K & P see Appendix A PDX collection 0897
HAC 7th character B see Appendix B for HAC conditional logic

+ **S62.3 Fracture of other and unspecified metacarpal bone**
Excludes2: *fracture of first metacarpal bone (S62.2-)*

+ **S62.30 Unspecified fracture of other metacarpal bone**

CC +7th **S62.300 Unspecified fracture of second metacarpal bone, right hand**
CC Exclusion 7th character B see Appendix A PDX collection 1284
CC Exclusion 7th characters K & P see Appendix A PDX collection 0897
HAC 7th character B see Appendix B for HAC conditional logic

CC +7th **S62.301 Unspecified fracture of second metacarpal bone, left hand**
CC Exclusion 7th character B see Appendix A PDX collection 1284
CC Exclusion 7th characters K & P see Appendix A PDX collection 0897
HAC 7th character B see Appendix B for HAC conditional logic

CC +7th **S62.302 Unspecified fracture of third metacarpal bone, right hand**
CC Exclusion 7th character B see Appendix A PDX collection 1284
CC Exclusion 7th characters K & P see Appendix A PDX collection 0897
HAC 7th character B see Appendix B for HAC conditional logic

CC +7th **S62.303 Unspecified fracture of third metacarpal bone, left hand**
CC Exclusion 7th character B see Appendix A PDX collection 1284
CC Exclusion 7th characters K & P see Appendix A PDX collection 0897
HAC 7th character B see Appendix B for HAC conditional logic

CC +7th **S62.304 Unspecified fracture of fourth metacarpal bone, right hand**
CC Exclusion 7th character B see Appendix A PDX collection 1284
CC Exclusion 7th characters K & P see Appendix A PDX collection 0897
HAC 7th character B see Appendix B for HAC conditional logic

CC +7th **S62.305 Unspecified fracture of fourth metacarpal bone, left hand**
CC Exclusion 7th character B see Appendix A PDX collection 1284
CC Exclusion 7th characters K & P see Appendix A PDX collection 0897
HAC 7th character B see Appendix B for HAC conditional logic

CC +7th **S62.306 Unspecified fracture of fifth metacarpal bone, right hand**
CC Exclusion 7th character B see Appendix A PDX collection 1284
CC Exclusion 7th characters K & P see Appendix A PDX collection 0897
HAC 7th character B see Appendix B for HAC conditional logic

CC +7th **S62.307 Unspecified fracture of fifth metacarpal bone, left hand**
CC Exclusion 7th character B see Appendix A PDX collection 1284
CC Exclusion 7th characters K & P see Appendix A PDX collection 0897
HAC 7th character B see Appendix B for HAC conditional logic

CC +7th **S62.308 Unspecified fracture of other metacarpal bone**
Unspecified fracture of specified metacarpa bone with unspecified laterality
CC Exclusion 7th character B see Appendix A PDX collection 1284
CC Exclusion 7th characters K & P see Appendix A PDX collection 0897
HAC 7th character B see Appendix B for HAC conditional logic

CC +7th **S62.309 Unspecified fracture of unspecified metacarpal bone**
CC Exclusion 7th character B see Appendix A PDX collection 1284
CC Exclusion 7th characters K & P see Appendix A PDX collection 0897
HAC 7th character B see Appendix B for HAC conditional logic

+ **S62.31 Displaced fracture of base of other metacarpal bone**

CC +7th **S62.310 Displaced fracture of base of second metacarpal bone, right hand**
CC Exclusion 7th character B see Appendix A PDX collection 1284
CC Exclusion 7th characters K & P see Appendix A PDX collection 0897
HAC 7th character B see Appendix B for HAC conditional logic

CC +7th **S62.311 Displaced fracture of base of second metacarpal bone, left hand**
CC Exclusion 7th character B see Appendix A PDX collection 1284
CC Exclusion 7th characters K & P see Appendix A PDX collection 0897
HAC 7th character B see Appendix B for HAC conditional logic

CC +7th **S62.312** **Displaced fracture of base of third metacarpal bone, right hand**
CC Exclusion 7th character B see Appendix A PDX collection 1284
CC Exclusion 7th characters K & P see Appendix A PDX collection 0897
HAC 7th character B see Appendix B for HAC conditional logic

CC +7th **S62.313** **Displaced fracture of base of third metacarpal bone, left hand**
CC Exclusion 7th character B see Appendix A PDX collection 1284
CC Exclusion 7th characters K & P see Appendix A PDX collection 0897
HAC 7th character B see Appendix B for HAC conditional logic

CC +7th **S62.314** **Displaced fracture of base of fourth metacarpal bone, right hand**
CC Exclusion 7th character B see Appendix A PDX collection 1284
CC Exclusion 7th characters K & P see Appendix A PDX collection 0897
HAC 7th character B see Appendix B for HAC conditional logic

CC +7th **S62.315** **Displaced fracture of base of fourth metacarpal bone, left hand**
CC Exclusion 7th character B see Appendix A PDX collection 1284
CC Exclusion 7th characters K & P see Appendix A PDX collection 0897
HAC 7th character B see Appendix B for HAC conditional logic

CC +7th **S62.316** **Displaced fracture of base of fifth metacarpal bone, right hand**
CC Exclusion 7th character B see Appendix A PDX collection 1284
CC Exclusion 7th characters K & P see Appendix A PDX collection 0897
HAC 7th character B see Appendix B for HAC conditional logic

CC +7th **S62.317** **Displaced fracture of base of fifth metacarpal bone, left hand**
CC Exclusion 7th character B see Appendix A PDX collection 1284
CC Exclusion 7th characters K & P see Appendix A PDX collection 0897
HAC 7th character B see Appendix B for HAC conditional logic

CC +7th **S62.318** **Displaced fracture of base of other metacarpal bone**
Displaced fracture of base of specified metacarpal bone with unspecified laterality
CC Exclusion 7th character B see Appendix A PDX collection 1284
CC Exclusion 7th characters K & P see Appendix A PDX collection 0897
HAC 7th character B see Appendix B for HAC conditional logic

CC +7th **S62.319** **Displaced fracture of base of unspecified metacarpal bone**
CC Exclusion 7th character B see Appendix A PDX collection 1284
CC Exclusion 7th characters K & P see Appendix A PDX collection 0897
HAC 7th character B see Appendix B for HAC conditional logic

\+ **S62.32** **Displaced fracture of shaft of other metacarpal bone**

CC +7th **S62.320** **Displaced fracture of shaft of second metacarpal bone, right hand**
CC Exclusion 7th character B see Appendix A PDX collection 1284
CC Exclusion 7th characters K & P see Appendix A PDX collection 0897
HAC 7th character B see Appendix B for HAC conditional logic

CC +7th **S62.321** **Displaced fracture of shaft of second metacarpal bone, left hand**
CC Exclusion 7th character B see Appendix A PDX collection 1284
CC Exclusion 7th characters K & P see Appendix A PDX collection 0897
HAC 7th character B see Appendix B for HAC conditional logic

CC +7th **S62.322** **Displaced fracture of shaft of third metacarpal bone, right hand**
CC Exclusion 7th character B see Appendix A PDX collection 1284
CC Exclusion 7th characters K & P see Appendix A PDX collection 0897
HAC 7th character B see Appendix B for HAC conditional logic

CC +7th **S62.323** **Displaced fracture of shaft of third metacarpal bone, left hand**
CC Exclusion 7th character B see Appendix A PDX collection 1284
CC Exclusion 7th characters K & P see Appendix A PDX collection 0897
HAC 7th character B see Appendix B for HAC conditional logic

CC +7th **S62.324** **Displaced fracture of shaft of fourth metacarpal bone, right hand**
CC Exclusion 7th character B see Appendix A PDX collection 1284
CC Exclusion 7th characters K & P see Appendix A PDX collection 0897
HAC 7th character B see Appendix B for HAC conditional logic

CC +7th **S62.325** **Displaced fracture of shaft of fourth metacarpal bone, left hand**
CC Exclusion 7th character B see Appendix A PDX collection 1284
CC Exclusion 7th characters K & P see Appendix A PDX collection 0897
HAC 7th character B see Appendix B for HAC conditional logic

CC +7th **S62.326** **Displaced fracture of shaft of fifth metacarpal bone, right hand**
CC Exclusion 7th character B see Appendix A PDX collection 1284
CC Exclusion 7th characters K & P see Appendix A PDX collection 0897
HAC 7th character B see Appendix B for HAC conditional logic

CC +7th **S62.327** **Displaced fracture of shaft of fifth metacarpal bone, left hand**
CC Exclusion 7th character B see Appendix A PDX collection 1284
CC Exclusion 7th characters K & P see Appendix A PDX collection 0897
HAC 7th character B see Appendix B for HAC conditional logic

CC +7th **S62.328** **Displaced fracture of shaft of other metacarpal bone**
Displaced fracture of shaft of specified metacarpal bone with unspecified laterality
CC Exclusion 7th character B see Appendix A PDX collection 1284
CC Exclusion 7th characters K & P see Appendix A PDX collection 0897
HAC 7th character B see Appendix B for HAC conditional logic

CC +7th **S62.329** **Displaced fracture of shaft of unspecified metacarpal bone**
CC Exclusion 7th character B see Appendix A PDX collection 1284
CC Exclusion 7th characters K & P see Appendix A PDX collection 0897
HAC 7th character B see Appendix B for HAC conditional logic

\+ **S62.33** **Displaced fracture of neck of other metacarpal bone**

CC +7th **S62.330** **Displaced fracture of neck of second metacarpal bone, right hand**
CC Exclusion 7th character B see Appendix A PDX collection 1284
CC Exclusion 7th characters K & P see Appendix A PDX collection 0897
HAC 7th character B see Appendix B for HAC conditional logic

CC +7th **S62.331** **Displaced fracture of neck of second metacarpal bone, left hand**
CC Exclusion 7th character B see Appendix A PDX collection 1284
CC Exclusion 7th characters K & P see Appendix A PDX collection 0897
HAC 7th character B see Appendix B for HAC conditional logic

CC +7th **S62.332** **Displaced fracture of neck of third metacarpal bone, right hand**
CC Exclusion 7th character B see Appendix A PDX collection 1284
CC Exclusion 7th characters K & P see Appendix A PDX collection 0897
HAC 7th character B see Appendix B for HAC conditional logic

CC +7th **S62.333** **Displaced fracture of neck of third metacarpal bone, left hand**
CC Exclusion 7th character B see Appendix A PDX collection 1284
CC Exclusion 7th characters K & P see Appendix A PDX collection 0897
HAC 7th character B see Appendix B for HAC conditional logic

CC +7th **S62.334** **Displaced fracture of neck of fourth metacarpal bone, right hand**
CC Exclusion 7th character B see Appendix A PDX collection 1284
CC Exclusion 7th characters K & P see Appendix A PDX collection 0897
HAC 7th character B see Appendix B for HAC conditional logic

CC +7th **S62.335** **Displaced fracture of neck of fourth metacarpal bone, left hand**
CC Exclusion 7th character B see Appendix A PDX collection 1284
CC Exclusion 7th characters K & P see Appendix A PDX collection 0897
HAC 7th character B see Appendix B for HAC conditional logic

CC +7th **S62.336** **Displaced fracture of neck of fifth metacarpal bone, right hand**
CC Exclusion 7th character B see Appendix A PDX collection 1284
CC Exclusion 7th characters K & P see Appendix A PDX collection 0897
HAC 7th character B see Appendix B for HAC conditional logic

CC +7th **S62.337** **Displaced fracture of neck of fifth metacarpal bone, left hand**
CC Exclusion 7th character B see Appendix A PDX collection 1284
CC Exclusion 7th characters K & P see Appendix A PDX collection 0897
HAC 7th character B see Appendix B for HAC conditional logic

CC +7th **S62.338** **Displaced fracture of neck of other metacarpal bone**
Displaced fracture of neck of specified metacarpal bone with unspecified laterality
CC Exclusion 7th character B see Appendix A PDX collection 1284
CC Exclusion 7th characters K & P see Appendix A PDX collection 0897
HAC 7th character B see Appendix B for HAC conditional logic

CC +7th **S62.339** **Displaced fracture of neck of unspecified metacarpal bone**
CC Exclusion 7th character B see Appendix A PDX collection 1284
CC Exclusion 7th characters K & P see Appendix A PDX collection 0897
HAC 7th character B see Appendix B for HAC conditional logic

+ **S62.34** **Nondisplaced fracture of base of other metacarpal bone**

CC +7th **S62.340** **Nondisplaced fracture of base of second metacarpal bone, right hand**
CC Exclusion 7th character B see Appendix A PDX collection 1284
CC Exclusion 7th characters K & P see Appendix A PDX collection 0897
HAC 7th character B see Appendix B for HAC conditional logic

CC +7th **S62.341** **Nondisplaced fracture of base of second metacarpal bone, left hand**
CC Exclusion 7th character B see Appendix A PDX collection 1284
CC Exclusion 7th characters K & P see Appendix A PDX collection 0897
HAC 7th character B see Appendix B for HAC conditional logic

CC +7th **S62.342** **Nondisplaced fracture of base of third metacarpal bone, right hand**
CC Exclusion 7th character B see Appendix A PDX collection 1284
CC Exclusion 7th characters K & P see Appendix A PDX collection 0897
HAC 7th character B see Appendix B for HAC conditional logic

CC +7th **S62.343** **Nondisplaced fracture of base of third metacarpal bone, left hand**
CC Exclusion 7th character B see Appendix A PDX collection 1284
CC Exclusion 7th characters K & P see Appendix A PDX collection 0897
HAC 7th character B see Appendix B for HAC conditional logic

CC +7th **S62.344** **Nondisplaced fracture of base of fourth metacarpal bone, right hand**
CC Exclusion 7th character B see Appendix A PDX collection 1284
CC Exclusion 7th characters K & P see Appendix A PDX collection 0897
HAC 7th character B see Appendix B for HAC conditional logic

CC +7th **S62.345** **Nondisplaced fracture of base of fourth metacarpal bone, left hand**
CC Exclusion 7th character B see Appendix A PDX collection 1284
CC Exclusion 7th characters K & P see Appendix A PDX collection 0897
HAC 7th character B see Appendix B for HAC conditional logic

CC +7th **S62.346** **Nondisplaced fracture of base of fifth metacarpal bone, right hand**
CC Exclusion 7th character B see Appendix A PDX collection 1284
CC Exclusion 7th characters K & P see Appendix A PDX collection 0897
HAC 7th character B see Appendix B for HAC conditional logic

CC +7th **S62.347** **Nondisplaced fracture of base of fifth metacarpal bone, left hand**
CC Exclusion 7th character B see Appendix A PDX collection 1284
CC Exclusion 7th characters K & P see Appendix A PDX collection 0897
HAC 7th character B see Appendix B for HAC conditional logic

CC +7th **S62.348** **Nondisplaced fracture of base of other metacarpal bone**
Nondisplaced fracture of base of specified metacarpal bone with unspecified laterality
CC Exclusion 7th character B see Appendix A PDX collection 1284
CC Exclusion 7th characters K & P see Appendix A PDX collection 0897
HAC 7th character B see Appendix B for HAC conditional logic

CC +7th **S62.349** **Nondisplaced fracture of base of unspecified metacarpal bone**
CC Exclusion 7th character B see Appendix A PDX collection 1284
CC Exclusion 7th characters K & P see Appendix A PDX collection 0897
HAC 7th character B see Appendix B for HAC conditional logic

+ **S62.35** **Nondisplaced fracture of shaft of other metacarpal bone**

CC +7th **S62.350** **Nondisplaced fracture of shaft of second metacarpal bone, right hand**
CC Exclusion 7th character B see Appendix A PDX collection 1284
CC Exclusion 7th characters K & P see Appendix A PDX collection 0897
HAC 7th character B see Appendix B for HAC conditional logic

CC +7th **S62.351** **Nondisplaced fracture of shaft of second metacarpal bone, left hand**
CC Exclusion 7th character B see Appendix A PDX collection 1284
CC Exclusion 7th characters K & P see Appendix A PDX collection 0897
HAC 7th character B see Appendix B for HAC conditional logic

CC +7th **S62.352 Nondisplaced fracture of shaft of third metacarpal bone, right hand**
CC Exclusion 7th character B see Appendix A PDX collection 1284
CC Exclusion 7th characters K & P see Appendix A PDX collection 0897
HAC 7th character B see Appendix B for HAC conditional logic

CC +7th **S62.353 Nondisplaced fracture of shaft of third metacarpal bone, left hand**
CC Exclusion 7th character B see Appendix A PDX collection 1284
CC Exclusion 7th characters K & P see Appendix A PDX collection 0897
HAC 7th character B see Appendix B for HAC conditional logic

CC +7th **S62.354 Nondisplaced fracture of shaft of fourth metacarpal bone, right hand**
CC Exclusion 7th character B see Appendix A PDX collection 1284
CC Exclusion 7th characters K & P see Appendix A PDX collection 0897
HAC 7th character B see Appendix B for HAC conditional logic

CC +7th **S62.355 Nondisplaced fracture of shaft of fourth metacarpal bone, left hand**
CC Exclusion 7th character B see Appendix A PDX collection 1284
CC Exclusion 7th characters K & P see Appendix A PDX collection 0897
HAC 7th character B see Appendix B for HAC conditional logic

CC +7th **S62.356 Nondisplaced fracture of shaft of fifth metacarpal bone, right hand**
CC Exclusion 7th character B see Appendix A PDX collection 1284
CC Exclusion 7th characters K & P see Appendix A PDX collection 0897
HAC 7th character B see Appendix B for HAC conditional logic

CC +7th **S62.357 Nondisplaced fracture of shaft of fifth metacarpal bone, left hand**
CC Exclusion 7th character B see Appendix A PDX collection 1284
CC Exclusion 7th characters K & P see Appendix A PDX collection 0897
HAC 7th character B see Appendix B for HAC conditional logic

CC +7th **S62.358 Nondisplaced fracture of shaft of other metacarpal bone**
Nondisplaced fracture of shaft of specified metacarpal bone with unspecified laterality
CC Exclusion 7th character B see Appendix A PDX collection 1284
CC Exclusion 7th characters K & P see Appendix A PDX collection 0897
HAC 7th character B see Appendix B for HAC conditional logic

CC +7th **S62.359 Nondisplaced fracture of shaft of unspecified metacarpal bone**
CC Exclusion 7th character B see Appendix A PDX collection 1284
CC Exclusion 7th characters K & P see Appendix A PDX collection 0897
HAC 7th character B see Appendix B for HAC conditional logic

+ **S62.36 Nondisplaced fracture of neck of other metacarpal bone**

CC +7th **S62.360 Nondisplaced fracture of neck of second metacarpal bone, right hand**
CC Exclusion 7th character B see Appendix A PDX collection 1284
CC Exclusion 7th characters K & P see Appendix A PDX collection 0897
HAC 7th character B see Appendix B for HAC conditional logic

CC +7th **S62.361 Nondisplaced fracture of neck of second metacarpal bone, left hand**
CC Exclusion 7th character B see Appendix A PDX collection 1284
CC Exclusion 7th characters K & P see Appendix A PDX collection 0897
HAC 7th character B see Appendix B for HAC conditional logic

CC +7th **S62.362 Nondisplaced fracture of neck of third metacarpal bone, right hand**
CC Exclusion 7th character B see Appendix A PDX collection 1284
CC Exclusion 7th characters K & P see Appendix A PDX collection 0897
HAC 7th character B see Appendix B for HAC conditional logic

CC +7th **S62.363 Nondisplaced fracture of neck of third metacarpal bone, left hand**
CC Exclusion 7th character B see Appendix A PDX collection 1284
CC Exclusion 7th characters K & P see Appendix A PDX collection 0897
HAC 7th character B see Appendix B for HAC conditional logic

CC +7th **S62.364 Nondisplaced fracture of neck of fourth metacarpal bone, right hand**
CC Exclusion 7th character B see Appendix A PDX collection 1284
CC Exclusion 7th characters K & P see Appendix A PDX collection 0897
HAC 7th character B see Appendix B for HAC conditional logic

CC +7th **S62.365 Nondisplaced fracture of neck of fourth metacarpal bone, left hand**
CC Exclusion 7th character B see Appendix A PDX collection 1284
CC Exclusion 7th characters K & P see Appendix A PDX collection 0897
HAC 7th character B see Appendix B for HAC conditional logic

CC +7th **S62.366 Nondisplaced fracture of neck of fifth metacarpal bone, right hand**
CC Exclusion 7th character B see Appendix A PDX collection 1284
CC Exclusion 7th characters K & P see Appendix A PDX collection 0897
HAC 7th character B see Appendix B for HAC conditional logic

CC +7th **S62.367 Nondisplaced fracture of neck of fifth metacarpal bone, left hand**
CC Exclusion 7th character B see Appendix A PDX collection 1284
CC Exclusion 7th characters K & P see Appendix A PDX collection 0897
HAC 7th character B see Appendix B for HAC conditional logic

CC +7th **S62.368 Nondisplaced fracture of neck of other metacarpal bone**
Nondisplaced fracture of neck of specified metacarpal bone with unspecified laterality
CC Exclusion 7th character B see Appendix A PDX collection 1284
CC Exclusion 7th characters K & P see Appendix A PDX collection 0897
HAC 7th character B see Appendix B for HAC conditional logic

CC +7th **S62.369 Nondisplaced fracture of neck of unspecified metacarpal bone**
CC Exclusion 7th character B see Appendix A PDX collection 1284
CC Exclusion 7th characters K & P see Appendix A PDX collection 0897
HAC 7th character B see Appendix B for HAC conditional logic

+ **S62.39 Other fracture of other metacarpal bone**

CC +7th **S62.390 Other fracture of second metacarpal bone, right hand**
CC Exclusion 7th character B see Appendix A PDX collection 1284
CC Exclusion 7th characters K & P see Appendix A PDX collection 0897
HAC 7th character B see Appendix B for HAC conditional logic

CC +7th **S62.391 Other fracture of second metacarpal bone, left hand**
CC Exclusion 7th character B see Appendix A PDX collection 1284
CC Exclusion 7th characters K & P see Appendix A PDX collection 0897
HAC 7th character B see Appendix B for HAC conditional logic

CC +7th **S62.392 Other fracture of third metacarpal bone, right hand**
CC Exclusion 7th character B see Appendix A PDX collection 1284
CC Exclusion 7th characters K & P see Appendix A PDX collection 0897
HAC 7th character B see Appendix B for HAC conditional logic

CC +7th **S62.393 Other fracture of third metacarpal bone, left hand**
CC Exclusion 7th character B see Appendix A PDX collection 1284
CC Exclusion 7th characters K & P see Appendix A PDX collection 0897
HAC 7th character B see Appendix B for HAC conditional logic

CC +7th **S62.394 Other fracture of fourth metacarpal bone, right hand**
CC Exclusion 7th character B see Appendix A PDX collection 1284
CC Exclusion 7th characters K & P see Appendix A PDX collection 0897
HAC 7th character B see Appendix B for HAC conditional logic

CC +7th **S62.395 Other fracture of fourth metacarpal bone, left hand**
CC Exclusion 7th character B see Appendix A PDX collection 1284
CC Exclusion 7th characters K & P see Appendix A PDX collection 0897
HAC 7th character B see Appendix B for HAC conditional logic

CC +7th **S62.396 Other fracture of fifth metacarpal bone, right hand**
CC Exclusion 7th character B see Appendix A PDX collection 1284
CC Exclusion 7th characters K & P see Appendix A PDX collection 0897
HAC 7th character B see Appendix B for HAC conditional logic

CC +7th **S62.397 Other fracture of fifth metacarpal bone, left hand**
CC Exclusion 7th character B see Appendix A PDX collection 1284
CC Exclusion 7th characters K & P see Appendix A PDX collection 0897
HAC 7th character B see Appendix B for HAC conditional logic

CC +7th **S62.398 Other fracture of other metacarpal bone**
Other fracture of specified metacarpal bone with unspecified laterality
CC Exclusion 7th character B see Appendix A PDX collection 1284
CC Exclusion 7th characters K & P see Appendix A PDX collection 0897
HAC 7th character B see Appendix B for HAC conditional logic

CC +7th **S62.399 Other fracture of unspecified metacarpal bone**
CC Exclusion 7th character B see Appendix A PDX collection 1284
CC Exclusion 7th characters K & P see Appendix A PDX collection 0897
HAC 7th character B see Appendix B for HAC conditional logic

\+ **S62.5 Fracture of thumb**

\+ **S62.50 Fracture of unspecified phalanx of thumb**

CC +7th **S62.501 Fracture of unspecified phalanx of right thumb**
CC Exclusion 7th character B see Appendix A PDX collection 1285
CC Exclusion 7th characters K & P see Appendix A PDX collection 0897
HAC 7th character B see Appendix B for HAC conditional logic

CC +7th **S62.502 Fracture of unspecified phalanx of left thumb**
CC Exclusion 7th character B see Appendix A PDX collection 1285
CC Exclusion 7th characters K & P see Appendix A PDX collection 0897
HAC 7th character B see Appendix B for HAC conditional logic

CC +7th **S62.509 Fracture of unspecified phalanx of unspecified thumb**
CC Exclusion 7th character B see Appendix A PDX collection 1285
CC Exclusion 7th characters K & P see Appendix A PDX collection 0897
HAC 7th character B see Appendix B for HAC conditional logic

\+ **S62.51 Fracture of proximal phalanx of thumb**

CC +7th **S62.511 Displaced fracture of proximal phalanx of right thumb**
CC Exclusion 7th character B see Appendix A PDX collection 1285
CC Exclusion 7th characters K & P see Appendix A PDX collection 0897
HAC 7th character B see Appendix B for HAC conditional logic

CC +7th **S62.512 Displaced fracture of proximal phalanx of left thumb**
CC Exclusion 7th character B see Appendix A PDX collection 1285
CC Exclusion 7th characters K & P see Appendix A PDX collection 0897
HAC 7th character B see Appendix B for HAC conditional logic

CC +7th **S62.513 Displaced fracture of proximal phalanx of unspecified thumb**
CC Exclusion 7th character B see Appendix A PDX collection 1285
CC Exclusion 7th characters K & P see Appendix A PDX collection 0897
HAC 7th character B see Appendix B for HAC conditional logic

CC +7th **S62.514 Nondisplaced fracture of proximal phalanx of right thumb**
CC Exclusion 7th character B see Appendix A PDX collection 1285
CC Exclusion 7th characters K & P see Appendix A PDX collection 0897
HAC 7th character B see Appendix B for HAC conditional logic

CC +7th **S62.515 Nondisplaced fracture of proximal phalanx of left thumb**
CC Exclusion 7th character B see Appendix A PDX collection 1285
CC Exclusion 7th characters K & P see Appendix A PDX collection 0897
HAC 7th character B see Appendix B for HAC conditional logic

CC +7th **S62.516 Nondisplaced fracture of proximal phalanx of unspecified thumb**
CC Exclusion 7th character B see Appendix A PDX collection 1285
CC Exclusion 7th characters K & P see Appendix A PDX collection 0897
HAC 7th character B see Appendix B for HAC conditional logic

\+ **S62.52 Fracture of distal phalanx of thumb**

CC +7th **S62.521 Displaced fracture of distal phalanx of right thumb**
CC Exclusion 7th character B see Appendix A PDX collection 1285
CC Exclusion 7th characters K & P see Appendix A PDX collection 0897
HAC 7th character B see Appendix B for HAC conditional logic

CC +7th **S62.522 Displaced fracture of distal phalanx of left thumb**
CC Exclusion 7th character B see Appendix A PDX collection 1285
CC Exclusion 7th characters K & P see Appendix A PDX collection 0897
HAC 7th character B see Appendix B for HAC conditional logic

CC +7th **S62.523 Displaced fracture of distal phalanx of unspecified thumb**
CC Exclusion 7th character B see Appendix A PDX collection 1285
CC Exclusion 7th characters K & P see Appendix A PDX collection 0897
HAC 7th character B see Appendix B for HAC conditional logic

CC +7th **S62.524 Nondisplaced fracture of distal phalanx of right thumb**
CC Exclusion 7th character B see Appendix A PDX collection 1285
CC Exclusion 7th characters K & P see Appendix A PDX collection 0897
HAC 7th character B see Appendix B for HAC conditional logic

CC +7th **S62.525 Nondisplaced fracture of distal phalanx of left thumb**
CC Exclusion 7th character B see Appendix A PDX collection 1285
CC Exclusion 7th characters K & P see Appendix A PDX collection 0897
HAC 7th character B see Appendix B for HAC conditional logic

CC +7th **S62.526 Nondisplaced fracture of distal phalanx of unspecified thumb**
CC Exclusion 7th character B see Appendix A PDX collection 1285
CC Exclusion 7th characters K & P see Appendix A PDX collection 0897
HAC 7th character B see Appendix B for HAC conditional logic

+ **S62.6 Fracture of other and unspecified finger(s)**
Excludes2: *fracture of thumb (S62.5-)*

+ **S62.60 Fracture of unspecified phalanx of finger**

CC +7th **S62.600 Fracture of unspecified phalanx of right index finger**
CC Exclusion 7th character B see Appendix A PDX collection 1285
CC Exclusion 7th characters K & P see Appendix A PDX collection 0897
HAC 7th character B see Appendix B for HAC conditional logic

CC +7th **S62.601 Fracture of unspecified phalanx of left index finger**
CC Exclusion 7th character B see Appendix A PDX collection 1285
CC Exclusion 7th characters K & P see Appendix A PDX collection 0897
HAC 7th character B see Appendix B for HAC conditional logic

CC +7th **S62.602 Fracture of unspecified phalanx of right middle finger**
CC Exclusion 7th character B see Appendix A PDX collection 1285
CC Exclusion 7th characters K & P see Appendix A PDX collection 0897
HAC 7th character B see Appendix B for HAC conditional logic

CC +7th **S62.603 Fracture of unspecified phalanx of left middle finger**
CC Exclusion 7th character B see Appendix A PDX collection 1285
CC Exclusion 7th characters K & P see Appendix A PDX collection 0897
HAC 7th character B see Appendix B for HAC conditional logic

CC +7th **S62.604 Fracture of unspecified phalanx of right ring finger**
CC Exclusion 7th character B see Appendix A PDX collection 1285
CC Exclusion 7th characters K & P see Appendix A PDX collection 0897
HAC 7th character B see Appendix B for HAC conditional logic

CC +7th **S62.605 Fracture of unspecified phalanx of left ring finger**
CC Exclusion 7th character B see Appendix A PDX collection 1285
CC Exclusion 7th characters K & P see Appendix A PDX collection 0897
HAC 7th character B see Appendix B for HAC conditional logic

CC +7th **S62.606 Fracture of unspecified phalanx of right little finger**
CC Exclusion 7th character B see Appendix A PDX collection 1285
CC Exclusion 7th characters K & P see Appendix A PDX collection 0897
HAC 7th character B see Appendix B for HAC conditional logic

CC +7th **S62.607 Fracture of unspecified phalanx of left little finger**
CC Exclusion 7th character B see Appendix A PDX collection 1285
CC Exclusion 7th characters K & P see Appendix A PDX collection 0897
HAC 7th character B see Appendix B for HAC conditional logic

CC +7th **S62.608 Fracture of unspecified phalanx of other finger**
Fracture of unspecified phalanx of specified finger with unspecified laterality
CC Exclusion 7th character B see Appendix A PDX collection 1285
CC Exclusion 7th characters K & P see Appendix A PDX collection 0897
HAC 7th character B see Appendix B for HAC conditional logic

CC +7th **S62.609 Fracture of unspecified phalanx of unspecified finger**
CC Exclusion 7th character B see Appendix A PDX collection 1285
CC Exclusion 7th characters K & P see Appendix A PDX collection 0897
HAC 7th character B see Appendix B for HAC conditional logic

+ **S62.61 Displaced fracture of proximal phalanx of finger**

CC +7th **S62.610 Displaced fracture of proximal phalanx of right index finger**
CC Exclusion 7th character B see Appendix A PDX collection 1285
CC Exclusion 7th characters K & P see Appendix A PDX collection 0897
HAC 7th character B see Appendix B for HAC conditional logic

CC +7th **S62.611 Displaced fracture of proximal phalanx of left index finger**
CC Exclusion 7th character B see Appendix A PDX collection 1285
CC Exclusion 7th characters K & P see Appendix A PDX collection 0897
HAC 7th character B see Appendix B for HAC conditional logic

CC +7th **S62.612 Displaced fracture of proximal phalanx of right middle finger**
CC Exclusion 7th character B see Appendix A PDX collection 1285
CC Exclusion 7th characters K & P see Appendix A PDX collection 0897
HAC 7th character B see Appendix B for HAC conditional logic

CC +7th **S62.613 Displaced fracture of proximal phalanx of left middle finger**
CC Exclusion 7th character B see Appendix A PDX collection 1285
CC Exclusion 7th characters K & P see Appendix A PDX collection 0897
HAC 7th character B see Appendix B for HAC conditional logic

CC +7th **S62.614 Displaced fracture of proximal phalanx of right ring finger**
CC Exclusion 7th character B see Appendix A PDX collection 1285
CC Exclusion 7th characters K & P see Appendix A PDX collection 0897
HAC 7th character B see Appendix B for HAC conditional logic

CC +7th **S62.615 Displaced fracture of proximal phalanx of left ring finger**
CC Exclusion 7th character B see Appendix A PDX collection 1285
CC Exclusion 7th characters K & P see Appendix A PDX collection 0897
HAC 7th character B see Appendix B for HAC conditional logic

CC +7th **S62.616 Displaced fracture of proximal phalanx of right little finger**
CC Exclusion 7th character B see Appendix A PDX collection 1285
CC Exclusion 7th characters K & P see Appendix A PDX collection 0897
HAC 7th character B see Appendix B for HAC conditional logic

CC +7th **S62.617 Displaced fracture of proximal phalanx of left little finger**
- **CC Exclusion 7th character B see Appendix A PDX collection 1285**
- **CC Exclusion 7th characters K & P see Appendix A PDX collection 0897**
- HAC 7th character B see Appendix B for HAC conditional logic

CC +7th **S62.618 Displaced fracture of proximal phalanx of other finger**
- Displaced fracture of proximal phalanx of specified finger with unspecified laterality
- **CC Exclusion 7th character B see Appendix A PDX collection 1285**
- **CC Exclusion 7th characters K & P see Appendix A PDX collection 0897**
- HAC 7th character B see Appendix B for HAC conditional logic

CC +7th **S62.619 Displaced fracture of proximal phalanx of unspecified finger**
- **CC Exclusion 7th character B see Appendix A PDX collection 1285**
- **CC Exclusion 7th characters K & P see Appendix A PDX collection 0897**
- HAC 7th character B see Appendix B for HAC conditional logic

\+ **S62.62 Displaced fracture of middle phalanx of finger**

CC +7th **S62.620 Displaced fracture of middle phalanx of right index finger**
- **CC Exclusion 7th character B see Appendix A PDX collection 1285**
- **CC Exclusion 7th characters K & P see Appendix A PDX collection 0897**
- HAC 7th character B see Appendix B for HAC conditional logic

CC +7th **S62.621 Displaced fracture of middle phalanx of left index finger**
- **CC Exclusion 7th character B see Appendix A PDX collection 1285**
- **CC Exclusion 7th characters K & P see Appendix A PDX collection 0897**
- HAC 7th character B see Appendix B for HAC conditional logic

CC +7th **S62.622 Displaced fracture of middle phalanx of right middle finger**
- **CC Exclusion 7th character B see Appendix A PDX collection 1285**
- **CC Exclusion 7th characters K & P see Appendix A PDX collection 0897**
- HAC 7th character B see Appendix B for HAC conditional logic

CC +7th **S62.623 Displaced fracture of middle phalanx of left middle finger**
- **CC Exclusion 7th character B see Appendix A PDX collection 1285**
- **CC Exclusion 7th characters K & P see Appendix A PDX collection 0897**
- HAC 7th character B see Appendix B for HAC conditional logic

CC +7th **S62.624 Displaced fracture of middle phalanx of right ring finger**
- **CC Exclusion 7th character B see Appendix A PDX collection 1285**
- **CC Exclusion 7th characters K & P see Appendix A PDX collection 0897**
- HAC 7th character B see Appendix B for HAC conditional logic

CC +7th **S62.625 Displaced fracture of middle phalanx of left ring finger**
- **CC Exclusion 7th character B see Appendix A PDX collection 1285**
- **CC Exclusion 7th characters K & P see Appendix A PDX collection 0897**
- HAC 7th character B see Appendix B for HAC conditional logic

CC +7th **S62.626 Displaced fracture of middle phalanx of right little finger**
- **CC Exclusion 7th character B see Appendix A PDX collection 1285**
- **CC Exclusion 7th characters K & P see Appendix A PDX collection 0897**
- HAC 7th character B see Appendix B for HAC conditional logic

CC +7th **S62.627 Displaced fracture of middle phalanx of left little finger**
- **CC Exclusion 7th character B see Appendix A PDX collection 1285**
- **CC Exclusion 7th characters K & P see Appendix A PDX collection 0897**
- HAC 7th character B see Appendix B for HAC conditional logic

CC +7th **S62.628 Displaced fracture of middle phalanx of other finger**
- Displaced fracture of middle phalanx of specified finger with unspecified laterality
- **CC Exclusion 7th character B see Appendix A PDX collection 1285**
- **CC Exclusion 7th characters K & P see Appendix A PDX collection 0897**
- HAC 7th character B see Appendix B for HAC conditional logic

CC +7th **S62.629 Displaced fracture of middle phalanx of unspecified finger**
- **CC Exclusion 7th character B see Appendix A PDX collection 1285**
- **CC Exclusion 7th characters K & P see Appendix A PDX collection 0897**
- HAC 7th character B see Appendix B for HAC conditional logic

\+ **S62.63 Displaced fracture of distal phalanx of finger**

CC +7th **S62.630 Displaced fracture of distal phalanx of right index finger**
- **CC Exclusion 7th character B see Appendix A PDX collection 1285**
- **CC Exclusion 7th characters K & P see Appendix A PDX collection 0897**
- HAC 7th character B see Appendix B for HAC conditional logic

CC +7th **S62.631 Displaced fracture of distal phalanx of left index finger**
- **CC Exclusion 7th character B see Appendix A PDX collection 1285**
- **CC Exclusion 7th characters K & P see Appendix A PDX collection 0897**
- HAC 7th character B see Appendix B for HAC conditional logic

CC +7th **S62.632 Displaced fracture of distal phalanx of right middle finger**
- **CC Exclusion 7th character B see Appendix A PDX collection 1285**
- **CC Exclusion 7th characters K & P see Appendix A PDX collection 0897**
- HAC 7th character B see Appendix B for HAC conditional logic

CC +7th **S62.633 Displaced fracture of distal phalanx of left middle finger**
- **CC Exclusion 7th character B see Appendix A PDX collection 1285**
- **CC Exclusion 7th characters K & P see Appendix A PDX collection 0897**
- HAC 7th character B see Appendix B for HAC conditional logic

CC +7th **S62.634 Displaced fracture of distal phalanx of right ring finger**
- **CC Exclusion 7th character B see Appendix A PDX collection 1285**
- **CC Exclusion 7th characters K & P see Appendix A PDX collection 0897**
- HAC 7th character B see Appendix B for HAC conditional logic

CC +7th **S62.635 Displaced fracture of distal phalanx of left ring finger**
- **CC Exclusion 7th character B see Appendix A PDX collection 1285**
- **CC Exclusion 7th characters K & P see Appendix A PDX collection 0897**
- HAC 7th character B see Appendix B for HAC conditional logic

CC +7th **S62.636 Displaced fracture of distal phalanx of right little finger**
- **CC Exclusion 7th character B see Appendix A PDX collection 1285**
- **CC Exclusion 7th characters K & P see Appendix A PDX collection 0897**
- HAC 7th character B see Appendix B for HAC conditional logic

CC +7th **S62.637 Displaced fracture of distal phalanx of left little finger**
CC Exclusion 7th character B see Appendix A PDX collection 1285
CC Exclusion 7th characters K & P see Appendix A PDX collection 0897
HAC 7th character B see Appendix B for HAC conditional logic

CC +7th **S62.638 Displaced fracture of distal phalanx of other finger**
Displaced fracture of distal phalanx of specified finger with unspecified laterality
CC Exclusion 7th character B see Appendix A PDX collection 1285
CC Exclusion 7th characters K & P see Appendix A PDX collection 0897
HAC 7th character B see Appendix B for HAC conditional logic

CC +7th **S62.639 Displaced fracture of distal phalanx of unspecified finger**
CC Exclusion 7th character B see Appendix A PDX collection 1285
CC Exclusion 7th characters K & P see Appendix A PDX collection 0897
HAC 7th character B see Appendix B for HAC conditional logic

+ **S62.64 Nondisplaced fracture of proximal phalanx of finger**

CC +7th **S62.640 Nondisplaced fracture of proximal phalanx of right index finger**
CC Exclusion 7th character B see Appendix A PDX collection 1285
CC Exclusion 7th characters K & P see Appendix A PDX collection 0897
HAC 7th character B see Appendix B for HAC conditional logic

CC +7th **S62.641 Nondisplaced fracture of proximal phalanx of left index finger**
CC Exclusion 7th character B see Appendix A PDX collection 1285
CC Exclusion 7th characters K & P see Appendix A PDX collection 0897
HAC 7th character B see Appendix B for HAC conditional logic

CC +7th **S62.642 Nondisplaced fracture of proximal phalanx of right middle finger**
CC Exclusion 7th character B see Appendix A PDX collection 1285
CC Exclusion 7th characters K & P see Appendix A PDX collection 0897
HAC 7th character B see Appendix B for HAC conditional logic

CC +7th **S62.643 Nondisplaced fracture of proximal phalanx of left middle finger**
CC Exclusion 7th character B see Appendix A PDX collection 1285
CC Exclusion 7th characters K & P see Appendix A PDX collection 0897
HAC 7th character B see Appendix B for HAC conditional logic

CC +7th **S62.644 Nondisplaced fracture of proximal phalanx of right ring finger**
CC Exclusion 7th character B see Appendix A PDX collection 1285
CC Exclusion 7th characters K & P see Appendix A PDX collection 0897
HAC 7th character B see Appendix B for HAC conditional logic

CC +7th **S62.645 Nondisplaced fracture of proximal phalanx of left ring finger**
CC Exclusion 7th character B see Appendix A PDX collection 1285
CC Exclusion 7th characters K & P see Appendix A PDX collection 0897
HAC 7th character B see Appendix B for HAC conditional logic

CC +7th **S62.646 Nondisplaced fracture of proximal phalanx of right little finger**
CC Exclusion 7th character B see Appendix A PDX collection 1285
CC Exclusion 7th characters K & P see Appendix A PDX collection 0897
HAC 7th character B see Appendix B for HAC conditional logic

CC +7th **S62.647 Nondisplaced fracture of proximal phalanx of left little finger**
CC Exclusion 7th character B see Appendix A PDX collection 1285
CC Exclusion 7th characters K & P see Appendix A PDX collection 0897
HAC 7th character B see Appendix B for HAC conditional logic

CC +7th **S62.648 Nondisplaced fracture of proximal phalanx of other finger**
Nondisplaced fracture of proximal phalanx of specified finger with unspecified laterality
CC Exclusion 7th character B see Appendix A PDX collection 1285
CC Exclusion 7th characters K & P see Appendix A PDX collection 0897
HAC 7th character B see Appendix B for HAC conditional logic

CC +7th **S62.649 Nondisplaced fracture of proximal phalanx of unspecified finger**
CC Exclusion 7th character B see Appendix A PDX collection 1285
CC Exclusion 7th characters K & P see Appendix A PDX collection 0897
HAC 7th character B see Appendix B for HAC conditional logic

+ **S62.65 Nondisplaced fracture of middle phalanx of finger**

CC +7th **S62.650 Nondisplaced fracture of middle phalanx of right index finger**
CC Exclusion 7th character B see Appendix A PDX collection 1285
CC Exclusion 7th characters K & P see Appendix A PDX collection 0897
HAC 7th character B see Appendix B for HAC conditional logic

CC +7th **S62.651 Nondisplaced fracture of middle phalanx of left index finger**
CC Exclusion 7th character B see Appendix A PDX collection 1285
CC Exclusion 7th characters K & P see Appendix A PDX collection 0897
HAC 7th character B see Appendix B for HAC conditional logic

CC +7th **S62.652 Nondisplaced fracture of middle phalanx of right middle finger**
CC Exclusion 7th character B see Appendix A PDX collection 1285
CC Exclusion 7th characters K & P see Appendix A PDX collection 0897
HAC 7th character B see Appendix B for HAC conditional logic

CC +7th **S62.653 Nondisplaced fracture of middle phalanx of left middle finger**
CC Exclusion 7th character B see Appendix A PDX collection 1285
CC Exclusion 7th characters K & P see Appendix A PDX collection 0897
HAC 7th character B see Appendix B for HAC conditional logic

CC +7th **S62.654 Nondisplaced fracture of middle phalanx of right ring finger**
CC Exclusion 7th character B see Appendix A PDX collection 1285
CC Exclusion 7th characters K & P see Appendix A PDX collection 0897
HAC 7th character B see Appendix B for HAC conditional logic

CC +7th **S62.655 Nondisplaced fracture of middle phalanx of left ring finger**
CC Exclusion 7th character B see Appendix A PDX collection 1285
CC Exclusion 7th characters K & P see Appendix A PDX collection 0897
HAC 7th character B see Appendix B for HAC conditional logic

CC +7th **S62.656 Nondisplaced fracture of middle phalanx of right little finger**
CC Exclusion 7th character B see Appendix A PDX collection 1285
CC Exclusion 7th characters K & P see Appendix A PDX collection 0897
HAC 7th character B see Appendix B for HAC conditional logic

CC +7th **S62.657 Nondisplaced fracture of middle phalanx of left little finger**
CC Exclusion 7th character B see Appendix A PDX collection 1285
CC Exclusion 7th characters K & P see Appendix A PDX collection 0897
HAC 7th character B see Appendix B for HAC conditional logic

CC +7th **S62.658 Nondisplaced fracture of middle phalanx of other finger**
Nondisplaced fracture of middle phalanx of specified finger with unspecified laterality
CC Exclusion 7th character B see Appendix A PDX collection 1285
CC Exclusion 7th characters K & P see Appendix A PDX collection 0897
HAC 7th character B see Appendix B for HAC conditional logic

CC +7th **S62.659 Nondisplaced fracture of middle phalanx of unspecified finger**
CC Exclusion 7th character B see Appendix A PDX collection 1285
CC Exclusion 7th characters K & P see Appendix A PDX collection 0897
HAC 7th character B see Appendix B for HAC conditional logic

+ **S62.66 Nondisplaced fracture of distal phalanx of finger**

CC +7th **S62.660 Nondisplaced fracture of distal phalanx of right index finger**
CC Exclusion 7th character B see Appendix A PDX collection 1285
CC Exclusion 7th characters K & P see Appendix A PDX collection 0897
HAC 7th character B see Appendix B for HAC conditional logic

CC +7th **S62.661 Nondisplaced fracture of distal phalanx of left index finger**
CC Exclusion 7th character B see Appendix A PDX collection 1285
CC Exclusion 7th characters K & P see Appendix A PDX collection 0897
HAC 7th character B see Appendix B for HAC conditional logic

CC +7th **S62.662 Nondisplaced fracture of distal phalanx of right middle finger**
CC Exclusion 7th character B see Appendix A PDX collection 1285
CC Exclusion 7th characters K & P see Appendix A PDX collection 0897
HAC 7th character B see Appendix B for HAC conditional logic

CC +7th **S62.663 Nondisplaced fracture of distal phalanx of left middle finger**
CC Exclusion 7th character B see Appendix A PDX collection 1285
CC Exclusion 7th characters K & P see Appendix A PDX collection 0897
HAC 7th character B see Appendix B for HAC conditional logic

CC +7th **S62.664 Nondisplaced fracture of distal phalanx of right ring finger**
CC Exclusion 7th character B see Appendix A PDX collection 1285
CC Exclusion 7th characters K & P see Appendix A PDX collection 0897
HAC 7th character B see Appendix B for HAC conditional logic

CC +7th **S62.665 Nondisplaced fracture of distal phalanx of left ring finger**
CC Exclusion 7th character B see Appendix A PDX collection 1285
CC Exclusion 7th characters K & P see Appendix A PDX collection 0897
HAC 7th character B see Appendix B for HAC conditional logic

CC +7th **S62.666 Nondisplaced fracture of distal phalanx of right little finger**
CC Exclusion 7th character B see Appendix A PDX collection 1285
CC Exclusion 7th characters K & P see Appendix A PDX collection 0897
HAC 7th character B see Appendix B for HAC conditional logic

CC +7th **S62.667 Nondisplaced fracture of distal phalanx of left little finger**
CC Exclusion 7th character B see Appendix A PDX collection 1285
CC Exclusion 7th characters K & P see Appendix A PDX collection 0897
HAC 7th character B see Appendix B for HAC conditional logic

CC +7th **S62.668 Nondisplaced fracture of distal phalanx of other finger**
Nondisplaced fracture of distal phalanx of specified finger with unspecified laterality
CC Exclusion 7th character B see Appendix A PDX collection 1285
CC Exclusion 7th characters K & P see Appendix A PDX collection 0897
HAC 7th character B see Appendix B for HAC conditional logic

CC +7th **S62.669 Nondisplaced fracture of distal phalanx of unspecified finger**
CC Exclusion 7th character B see Appendix A PDX collection 1285
CC Exclusion 7th characters K & P see Appendix A PDX collection 0897
HAC 7th character B see Appendix B for HAC conditional logic

+ **S62.9 Unspecified fracture of wrist and hand**

CC X+7th **S62.90 Unspecified fracture of unspecified wrist and hand**
CC Exclusion 7th character B see Appendix A PDX collection 1286
CC Exclusion 7th characters K & P see Appendix A PDX collection 0897
HAC 7th character B see Appendix B for HAC conditional logic

CC X+7th **S62.91 Unspecified fracture of right wrist and hand**
CC Exclusion 7th character B see Appendix A PDX collection 1287
CC Exclusion 7th characters K & P see Appendix A PDX collection 0897
HAC 7th character B see Appendix B for HAC conditional logic

CC X+7th **S62.92 Unspecified fracture of left wrist and hand**
CC Exclusion 7th character B see Appendix A PDX collection 1287
CC Exclusion 7th characters K & P see Appendix A PDX collection 0897
HAC 7th character B see Appendix B for HAC conditional logic

S63 Dislocation and sprain of joints and ligaments at wrist and hand level

Includes: avulsion of joint or ligament at wrist and hand level
laceration of cartilage, joint or ligament at wrist and hand level
sprain of cartilage, joint or ligament at wrist and hand level
traumatic hemarthrosis of joint or ligament at wrist and hand level
traumatic rupture of joint or ligament at wrist and hand level
traumatic subluxation of joint or ligament at wrist and hand level
traumatic tear of joint or ligament at wrist and hand level

Code also any associated open wound

Excludes2: *strain of muscle, fascia and tendon of wrist and hand (S66.*

The appropriate 7th character is to be added to each code from category S63
A initial encounter
D subsequent encounter
S sequela

+ **S63.0 Subluxation and dislocation of wrist and hand joints**

+ **S63.00 Unspecified subluxation and dislocation of wrist and hand**
Dislocation of carpal bone NOS
Dislocation of distal end of radius NOS
Subluxation of carpal bone NOS
Subluxation of distal end of radius NOS

+7th **S63.001 Unspecified subluxation of right wrist and hand**

+7th **S63.002 Unspecified subluxation of left wrist and hand**

+7th **S63.003 Unspecified subluxation of unspecified wrist and hand**

+7th **S63.004** Unspecified dislocation of right wrist and hand
+7th **S63.005** Unspecified dislocation of left wrist and hand
+7th **S63.006** Unspecified dislocation of unspecified wrist and hand
+ **S63.01** Subluxation and dislocation of distal radioulnar joint
+7th **S63.011** Subluxation of distal radioulnar joint of right wrist
+7th **S63.012** Subluxation of distal radioulnar joint of left wrist
+7th **S63.013** Subluxation of distal radioulnar joint of unspecified wrist
+7th **S63.014** Dislocation of distal radioulnar joint of right wrist
+7th **S63.015** Dislocation of distal radioulnar joint of left wrist
+7th **S63.016** Dislocation of distal radioulnar joint of unspecified wrist
+ **S63.02** Subluxation and dislocation of radiocarpal joint
+7th **S63.021** Subluxation of radiocarpal joint of right wrist
+7th **S63.022** Subluxation of radiocarpal joint of left wrist
+7th **S63.023** Subluxation of radiocarpal joint of unspecified wrist
+7th **S63.024** Dislocation of radiocarpal joint of right wrist
+7th **S63.025** Dislocation of radiocarpal joint of left wrist
+7th **S63.026** Dislocation of radiocarpal joint of unspecified wrist
+ **S63.03** Subluxation and dislocation of midcarpal joint
+7th **S63.031** Subluxation of midcarpal joint of right wrist
+7th **S63.032** Subluxation of midcarpal joint of left wrist
+7th **S63.033** Subluxation of midcarpal joint of unspecified wrist
+7th **S63.034** Dislocation of midcarpal joint of right wrist
+7th **S63.035** Dislocation of midcarpal joint of left wrist
+7th **S63.036** Dislocation of midcarpal joint of unspecified wrist
+ **S63.04** Subluxation and dislocation of carpometacarpal joint of thumb
Excludes2: *interphalangeal subluxation and dislocation of thumb (S63.1-)*
+7th **S63.041** Subluxation of carpometacarpal joint of right thumb
+7th **S63.042** Subluxation of carpometacarpal joint of left thumb
+7th **S63.043** Subluxation of carpometacarpal joint of unspecified thumb
+7th **S63.044** Dislocation of carpometacarpal joint of right thumb
+7th **S63.045** Dislocation of carpometacarpal joint of left thumb
+7th **S63.046** Dislocation of carpometacarpal joint of unspecified thumb
+ **S63.05** Subluxation and dislocation of other carpometacarpal joint
Excludes2: *subluxation and dislocation of carpometacarpal joint of thumb (S63.04-)*
+7th **S63.051** Subluxation of other carpometacarpal joint of right hand
+7th **S63.052** Subluxation of other carpometacarpal joint of left hand
+7th **S63.053** Subluxation of other carpometacarpal joint of unspecified hand
+7th **S63.054** Dislocation of other carpometacarpal joint of right hand
+7th **S63.055** Dislocation of other carpometacarpal joint of left hand
+7th **S63.056** Dislocation of other carpometacarpal joint of unspecified hand
+ **S63.06** Subluxation and dislocation of metacarpal (bone), proximal end
+7th **S63.061** Subluxation of metacarpal (bone), proximal end of right hand
+7th **S63.062** Subluxation of metacarpal (bone), proximal end of left hand
+7th **S63.063** Subluxation of metacarpal (bone), proximal end of unspecified hand
+7th **S63.064** Dislocation of metacarpal (bone), proximal end of right hand
+7th **S63.065** Dislocation of metacarpal (bone), proximal end of left hand
+7th **S63.066** Dislocation of metacarpal (bone), proximal end of unspecified hand
+ **S63.07** Subluxation and dislocation of distal end of ulna
+7th **S63.071** Subluxation of distal end of right ulna
+7th **S63.072** Subluxation of distal end of left ulna
+7th **S63.073** Subluxation of distal end of unspecified ulna
+7th **S63.074** Dislocation of distal end of right ulna
+7th **S63.075** Dislocation of distal end of left ulna
+7th **S63.076** Dislocation of distal end of unspecified ulna
+ **S63.09** Other subluxation and dislocation of wrist and hand
+7th **S63.091** Other subluxation of right wrist and hand
+7th **S63.092** Other subluxation of left wrist and hand
+7th **S63.093** Other subluxation of unspecified wrist and hand
+7th **S63.094** Other dislocation of right wrist and hand
+7th **S63.095** Other dislocation of left wrist and hand
+7th **S63.096** Other dislocation of unspecified wrist and hand
+ **S63.1** Subluxation and dislocation of thumb
+ **S63.10** Unspecified subluxation and dislocation of thumb
+7th **S63.101** Unspecified subluxation of right thumb
+7th **S63.102** Unspecified subluxation of left thumb
+7th **S63.103** Unspecified subluxation of unspecified thumb
+7th **S63.104** Unspecified dislocation of right thumb
+7th **S63.105** Unspecified dislocation of left thumb
+7th **S63.106** Unspecified dislocation of unspecified thumb
+ **S63.11** Subluxation and dislocation of metacarpophalangeal joint of thumb
+7th **S63.111** Subluxation of metacarpophalangeal joint of right thumb
+7th **S63.112** Subluxation of metacarpophalangeal joint of left thumb
+7th **S63.113** Subluxation of metacarpophalangeal joint of unspecified thumb
+7th **S63.114** Dislocation of metacarpophalangeal joint of right thumb
+7th **S63.115** Dislocation of metacarpophalangeal joint of left thumb
+7th **S63.116** Dislocation of metacarpophalangeal joint of unspecified thumb
+ **S63.12** Subluxation and dislocation of interphalangeal joint of thumb
+7th **S63.121** Subluxation of interphalangeal joint of right thumb
+7th **S63.122** Subluxation of interphalangeal joint of left thumb
+7th **S63.123** Subluxation of interphalangeal joint of unspecified thumb
+7th **S63.124** Dislocation of interphalangeal joint of right thumb
+7th **S63.125** Dislocation of interphalangeal joint of left thumb
+7th **S63.126** Dislocation of interphalangeal joint of unspecified thumb
+ **S63.2** Subluxation and dislocation of other finger(s)
Excludes2: *subluxation and dislocation of thumb (S63.1-)*
+ **S63.20** Unspecified subluxation of other finger
+7th **S63.200** Unspecified subluxation of right index finger
+7th **S63.201** Unspecified subluxation of left index finger
+7th **S63.202** Unspecified subluxation of right middle finger
+7th **S63.203** Unspecified subluxation of left middle finger
+7th **S63.204** Unspecified subluxation of right ring finger
+7th **S63.205** Unspecified subluxation of left ring finger
+7th **S63.206** Unspecified subluxation of right little finger

+7th **S63.207 Unspecified subluxation of left little finger**
+7th **S63.208 Unspecified subluxation of other finger**
Unspecified subluxation of specified finger with unspecified laterality
+7th **S63.209 Unspecified subluxation of unspecified finger**
\+ **S63.21 Subluxation of metacarpophalangeal joint of finger**
+7th **S63.210 Subluxation of metacarpophalangeal joint of right index finger**
+7th **S63.211 Subluxation of metacarpophalangeal joint of left index finger**
+7th **S63.212 Subluxation of metacarpophalangeal joint of right middle finger**
+7th **S63.213 Subluxation of metacarpophalangeal joint of left middle finger**
+7th **S63.214 Subluxation of metacarpophalangeal joint of right ring finger**
+7th **S63.215 Subluxation of metacarpophalangeal joint of left ring finger**
+7th **S63.216 Subluxation of metacarpophalangeal joint of right little finger**
+7th **S63.217 Subluxation of metacarpophalangeal joint of left little finger**
+7th **S63.218 Subluxation of metacarpophalangeal joint of other finger**
Subluxation of metacarpophalangeal joint of specified finger with unspecified laterality
+7th **S63.219 Subluxation of metacarpophalangeal joint of unspecified finger**
\+ **S63.22 Subluxation of unspecified interphalangeal joint of finger**
+7th **S63.220 Subluxation of unspecified interphalangeal joint of right index finger**
+7th **S63.221 Subluxation of unspecified interphalangeal joint of left index finger**
+7th **S63.222 Subluxation of unspecified interphalangeal joint of right middle finger**
+7th **S63.223 Subluxation of unspecified interphalangeal joint of left middle finger**
+7th **S63.224 Subluxation of unspecified interphalangeal joint of right ring finger**
+7th **S63.225 Subluxation of unspecified interphalangeal joint of left ring finger**
+7th **S63.226 Subluxation of unspecified interphalangeal joint of right little finger**
+7th **S63.227 Subluxation of unspecified interphalangeal joint of left little finger**
+7th **S63.228 Subluxation of unspecified interphalangeal joint of other finger**
Subluxation of unspecified interphalangeal joint of specified finger with unspecified laterality
+7th **S63.229 Subluxation of unspecified interphalangeal joint of unspecified finger**
\+ **S63.23 Subluxation of proximal interphalangeal joint of finger**
+7th **S63.230 Subluxation of proximal interphalangeal joint of right index finger**
+7th **S63.231 Subluxation of proximal interphalangeal joint of left index finger**
+7th **S63.232 Subluxation of proximal interphalangeal joint of right middle finger**
+7th **S63.233 Subluxation of proximal interphalangeal joint of left middle finger**
+7th **S63.234 Subluxation of proximal interphalangeal joint of right ring finger**
+7th **S63.235 Subluxation of proximal interphalangeal joint of left ring finger**
+7th **S63.236 Subluxation of proximal interphalangeal joint of right little finger**
+7th **S63.237 Subluxation of proximal interphalangeal joint of left little finger**
+7th **S63.238 Subluxation of proximal interphalangeal joint of other finger**
Subluxation of proximal interphalangeal joint of specified finger with unspecified laterality
+7th **S63.239 Subluxation of proximal interphalangeal joint of unspecified finger**
\+ **S63.24 Subluxation of distal interphalangeal joint of finger**
+7th **S63.240 Subluxation of distal interphalangeal joi of right index finger**
+7th **S63.241 Subluxation of distal interphalangeal joi of left index finger**
+7th **S63.242 Subluxation of distal interphalangeal joi of right middle finger**
+7th **S63.243 Subluxation of distal interphalangeal joi of left middle finger**
+7th **S63.244 Subluxation of distal interphalangeal joi of right ring finger**
+7th **S63.245 Subluxation of distal interphalangeal joi of left ring finger**
+7th **S63.246 Subluxation of distal interphalangeal joi of right little finger**
+7th **S63.247 Subluxation of distal interphalangeal joi of left little finger**
+7th **S63.248 Subluxation of distal interphalangeal joi of other finger**
Subluxation of distal interphalangeal joint of specified finger with unspecified laterality
+7th **S63.249 Subluxation of distal interphalangeal joi of unspecified finger**
\+ **S63.25 Unspecified dislocation of other finger**
+7th **S63.250 Unspecified dislocation of right index finger**
+7th **S63.251 Unspecified dislocation of left index finge**
+7th **S63.252 Unspecified dislocation of right middle finger**
+7th **S63.253 Unspecified dislocation of left middle finger**
+7th **S63.254 Unspecified dislocation of right ring fing**
+7th **S63.255 Unspecified dislocation of left ring finger**
+7th **S63.256 Unspecified dislocation of right little finger**
+7th **S63.257 Unspecified dislocation of left little finger**
+7th **S63.258 Unspecified dislocation of other finger**
Unspecified dislocation of specified finger with unspecified laterality
+7th **S63.259 Unspecified dislocation of unspecified finger**
Unspecified dislocation of unspecified fing with unspecified laterality
\+ **S63.26 Dislocation of metacarpophalangeal joint of finger**
+7th **S63.260 Dislocation of metacarpophalangeal join of right index finger**
+7th **S63.261 Dislocation of metacarpophalangeal join of left index finger**
+7th **S63.262 Dislocation of metacarpophalangeal join of right middle finger**
+7th **S63.263 Dislocation of metacarpophalangeal join of left middle finger**
+7th **S63.264 Dislocation of metacarpophalangeal join of right ring finger**
+7th **S63.265 Dislocation of metacarpophalangeal join of left ring finger**
+7th **S63.266 Dislocation of metacarpophalangeal join of right little finger**
+7th **S63.267 Dislocation of metacarpophalangeal join of left little finger**
+7th **S63.268 Dislocation of metacarpophalangeal join of other finger**
Dislocation of metacarpophalangeal joint of specified finger with unspecified laterality
+7th **S63.269 Dislocation of metacarpophalangeal join of unspecified finger**

+ **S63.27 Dislocation of unspecified interphalangeal joint of finger**
  +7th **S63.270 Dislocation of unspecified interphalangeal joint of right index finger**
  +7th **S63.271 Dislocation of unspecified interphalangeal joint of left index finger**
  +7th **S63.272 Dislocation of unspecified interphalangeal joint of right middle finger**
  +7th **S63.273 Dislocation of unspecified interphalangeal joint of left middle finger**
  +7th **S63.274 Dislocation of unspecified interphalangeal joint of right ring finger**
  +7th **S63.275 Dislocation of unspecified interphalangeal joint of left ring finger**
  +7th **S63.276 Dislocation of unspecified interphalangeal joint of right little finger**
  +7th **S63.277 Dislocation of unspecified interphalangeal joint of left little finger**
  +7th **S63.278 Dislocation of unspecified interphalangeal joint of other finger**
    Dislocation of unspecified interphalangeal joint of specified finger with unspecified laterality
  +7th **S63.279 Dislocation of unspecified interphalangeal joint of unspecified finger**
    Dislocation of unspecified interphalangeal joint of unspecified finger without specified laterality
+ **S63.28 Dislocation of proximal interphalangeal joint of finger**
  +7th **S63.280 Dislocation of proximal interphalangeal joint of right index finger**
  +7th **S63.281 Dislocation of proximal interphalangeal joint of left index finger**
  +7th **S63.282 Dislocation of proximal interphalangeal joint of right middle finger**
  +7th **S63.283 Dislocation of proximal interphalangeal joint of left middle finger**
  +7th **S63.284 Dislocation of proximal interphalangeal joint of right ring finger**
  +7th **S63.285 Dislocation of proximal interphalangeal joint of left ring finger**
  +7th **S63.286 Dislocation of proximal interphalangeal joint of right little finger**
  +7th **S63.287 Dislocation of proximal interphalangeal joint of left little finger**
  +7th **S63.288 Dislocation of proximal interphalangeal joint of other finger**
    Dislocation of proximal interphalangeal joint of specified finger with unspecified laterality
  +7th **S63.289 Dislocation of proximal interphalangeal joint of unspecified finger**
+ **S63.29 Dislocation of distal interphalangeal joint of finger**
  +7th **S63.290 Dislocation of distal interphalangeal joint of right index finger**
  +7th **S63.291 Dislocation of distal interphalangeal joint of left index finger**
  +7th **S63.292 Dislocation of distal interphalangeal joint of right middle finger**
  +7th **S63.293 Dislocation of distal interphalangeal joint of left middle finger**
  +7th **S63.294 Dislocation of distal interphalangeal joint of right ring finger**
  +7th **S63.295 Dislocation of distal interphalangeal joint of left ring finger**
  +7th **S63.296 Dislocation of distal interphalangeal joint of right little finger**
  +7th **S63.297 Dislocation of distal interphalangeal joint of left little finger**
  +7th **S63.298 Dislocation of distal interphalangeal joint of other finger**
    Dislocation of distal interphalangeal joint of specified finger with unspecified laterality
  +7th **S63.299 Dislocation of distal interphalangeal joint of unspecified finger**

+ **S63.3 Traumatic rupture of ligament of wrist**
+ **S63.30 Traumatic rupture of unspecified ligament of wrist**
  +7th **S63.301 Traumatic rupture of unspecified ligament of right wrist**
  +7th **S63.302 Traumatic rupture of unspecified ligament of left wrist**
  +7th **S63.309 Traumatic rupture of unspecified ligament of unspecified wrist**
+ **S63.31 Traumatic rupture of collateral ligament of wrist**
  +7th **S63.311 Traumatic rupture of collateral ligament of right wrist**
  +7th **S63.312 Traumatic rupture of collateral ligament of left wrist**
  +7th **S63.319 Traumatic rupture of collateral ligament of unspecified wrist**
+ **S63.32 Traumatic rupture of radiocarpal ligament**
  +7th **S63.321 Traumatic rupture of right radiocarpal ligament**
  +7th **S63.322 Traumatic rupture of left radiocarpal ligament**
  +7th **S63.329 Traumatic rupture of unspecified radiocarpal ligament**
+ **S63.33 Traumatic rupture of ulnocarpal (palmar) ligament**
  +7th **S63.331 Traumatic rupture of right ulnocarpal (palmar) ligament**
  +7th **S63.332 Traumatic rupture of left ulnocarpal (palmar) ligament**
  +7th **S63.339 Traumatic rupture of unspecified ulnocarpal (palmar) ligament**
+ **S63.39 Traumatic rupture of other ligament of wrist**
  +7th **S63.391 Traumatic rupture of other ligament of right wrist**
  +7th **S63.392 Traumatic rupture of other ligament of left wrist**
  +7th **S63.399 Traumatic rupture of other ligament of unspecified wrist**

+ **S63.4 Traumatic rupture of ligament of finger at metacarpophalangeal and interphalangeal joint(s)**
+ **S63.40 Traumatic rupture of unspecified ligament of finger at metacarpophalangeal and interphalangeal joint**
  +7th **S63.400 Traumatic rupture of unspecified ligament of right index finger at metacarpophalangeal and interphalangeal joint**
  +7th **S63.401 Traumatic rupture of unspecified ligament of left index finger at metacarpophalangeal and interphalangeal joint**
  +7th **S63.402 Traumatic rupture of unspecified ligament of right middle finger at metacarpophalangeal and interphalangeal joint**
  +7th **S63.403 Traumatic rupture of unspecified ligament of left middle finger at metacarpophalangeal and interphalangeal joint**
  +7th **S63.404 Traumatic rupture of unspecified ligament of right ring finger at metacarpophalangeal and interphalangeal joint**
  +7th **S63.405 Traumatic rupture of unspecified ligament of left ring finger at metacarpophalangeal and interphalangeal joint**
  +7th **S63.406 Traumatic rupture of unspecified ligament of right little finger at metacarpophalangeal and interphalangeal joint**
  +7th **S63.407 Traumatic rupture of unspecified ligament of left little finger at metacarpophalangeal and interphalangeal joint**
  +7th **S63.408 Traumatic rupture of unspecified ligament of other finger at metacarpophalangeal and interphalangeal joint**
    Traumatic rupture of unspecified ligament of specified finger with unspecified laterality at metacarpophalangeal and interphalangeal joint
  +7th **S63.409 Traumatic rupture of unspecified ligament of unspecified finger at metacarpophalangeal and interphalangeal joint**
+ **S63.41 Traumatic rupture of collateral ligament of finger at metacarpophalangeal and interphalangeal joint**
  +7th **S63.410 Traumatic rupture of collateral ligament of right index finger at metacarpophalangeal and interphalangeal joint**

+7th **S63.411 Traumatic rupture of collateral ligament of left index finger at metacarpophalangeal and interphalangeal joint**
+7th **S63.412 Traumatic rupture of collateral ligament of right middle finger at metacarpophalangeal and interphalangeal joint**
+7th **S63.413 Traumatic rupture of collateral ligament of left middle finger at metacarpophalangeal and interphalangeal joint**
+7th **S63.414 Traumatic rupture of collateral ligament of right ring finger at metacarpophalangeal and interphalangeal joint**
+7th **S63.415 Traumatic rupture of collateral ligament of left ring finger at metacarpophalangeal and interphalangeal joint**
+7th **S63.416 Traumatic rupture of collateral ligament of right little finger at metacarpophalangeal and interphalangeal joint**
+7th **S63.417 Traumatic rupture of collateral ligament of left little finger at metacarpophalangeal and interphalangeal joint**
+7th **S63.418 Traumatic rupture of collateral ligament of other finger at metacarpophalangeal and interphalangeal joint**
Traumatic rupture of collateral ligament of specified finger with unspecified laterality at metacarpophalangeal and interphalangeal joint
+7th **S63.419 Traumatic rupture of collateral ligament of unspecified finger at metacarpophalangeal and interphalangeal joint**

+ **S63.42 Traumatic rupture of palmar ligament of finger at metacarpophalangeal and interphalangeal joint**
+7th **S63.420 Traumatic rupture of palmarligament of right index finger at metacarpophalangeal and interphalangeal joint**
+7th **S63.421 Traumatic rupture of palmar ligament of left index finger at metacarpophalangeal and interphalangeal joint**
+7th **S63.422 Traumatic rupture of palmar ligament of right middle finger at metacarpophalangeal and interphalangeal joint**
+7th **S63.423 Traumatic rupture of palmar ligament of left middle finger at metacarpophalangeal and interphalangeal joint**
+7th **S63.424 Traumatic rupture of palmar ligament of right ring finger at metacarpophalangeal and interphalangeal joint**
+7th **S63.425 Traumatic rupture of palmar ligament of left ring finger at metacarpophalangeal and interphalangeal joint**
+7th **S63.426 Traumatic rupture of palmar ligament of right little finger at metacarpophalangeal and interphalangeal joint**
+7th **S63.427 Traumatic rupture of palmar ligament of left little finger at metacarpophalangeal and interphalangeal joint**
+7th **S63.428 Traumatic rupture of palmar ligament of other finger at metacarpophalangeal and interphalangeal joint**
Traumatic rupture of palmar ligament of specified finger with unspecified laterality at metacarpophalangeal and interphalangeal joint
+7th **S63.429 Traumatic rupture of palmar ligament of unspecified finger at metacarpophalangeal and interphalangeal joint**

+ **S63.43 Traumatic rupture of volar plate of finger at metacarpophalangeal and interphalangeal joint**
+7th **S63.430 Traumatic rupture of volar plate of right index finger at metacarpophalangeal and interphalangeal joint**
+7th **S63.431 Traumatic rupture of volar plate of left index finger at metacarpophalangeal and interphalangeal joint**
+7th **S63.432 Traumatic rupture of volar plate of right middle finger at metacarpophalangeal and interphalangeal joint**
+7th **S63.433 Traumatic rupture of volar plate of left middle finger at metacarpophalangeal and interphalangeal joint**
+7th **S63.434 Traumatic rupture of volar plate of right ring finger at metacarpophalangeal and interphalangeal joint**
+7th **S63.435 Traumatic rupture of volar plate of left ring finger at metacarpophalangeal and interphalangeal joint**
+7th **S63.436 Traumatic rupture of volar plate of right little finger at metacarpophalangeal and interphalangeal joint**
+7th **S63.437 Traumatic rupture of volar plate of left little finger at metacarpophalangeal and interphalangeal joint**
+7th **S63.438 Traumatic rupture of volar plate of other finger at metacarpophalangeal and interphalangeal joint**
Traumatic rupture of volar plate of specified finger with unspecified laterality at metacarpophalangeal and interphalangeal joint
+7th **S63.439 Traumatic rupture of volar plate of unspecified finger at metacarpophalangeal and interphalangeal joint**

+ **S63.49 Traumatic rupture of other ligament of finger at metacarpophalangeal and interphalangeal joint**
+7th **S63.490 Traumatic rupture of other ligament of right index finger at metacarpophalangeal and interphalangeal joint**
+7th **S63.491 Traumatic rupture of other ligament of left index finger at metacarpophalangeal and interphalangeal joint**
+7th **S63.492 Traumatic rupture of other ligament of right middle finger at metacarpophalangeal and interphalangeal joint**
+7th **S63.493 Traumatic rupture of other ligament of left middle finger at metacarpophalangeal and interphalangeal joint**
+7th **S63.494 Traumatic rupture of other ligament of right ring finger at metacarpophalangeal and interphalangeal joint**
+7th **S63.495 Traumatic rupture of other ligament of left ring finger at metacarpophalangeal and interphalangeal joint**
+7th **S63.496 Traumatic rupture of other ligament of right little finger at metacarpophalangeal and interphalangeal joint**
+7th **S63.497 Traumatic rupture of other ligament of left little finger at metacarpophalangeal and interphalangeal joint**
+7th **S63.498 Traumatic rupture of other ligament of other finger at metacarpophalangeal and interphalangeal joint**
Traumatic rupture of ligament of specified finger with unspecified laterality at metacarpophalangeal and interphalangeal joint
+7th **S63.499 Traumatic rupture of other ligament of unspecified finger at metacarpophalangeal and interphalangeal joint**

+ **S63.5 Other and unspecified sprain of wrist**
+ **S63.50 Unspecified sprain of wrist**
+7th **S63.501 Unspecified sprain of right wrist**
+7th **S63.502 Unspecified sprain of left wrist**
+7th **S63.509 Unspecified sprain of unspecified wrist**
+ **S63.51 Sprain of carpal (joint)**
+7th **S63.511 Sprain of carpal joint of right wrist**
+7th **S63.512 Sprain of carpal joint of left wrist**
+7th **S63.519 Sprain of carpal joint of unspecified wrist**
+ **S63.52 Sprain of radiocarpal joint**
Excludes1: *traumatic rupture of radiocarpal ligament (S63.32-)*
+7th **S63.521 Sprain of radiocarpal joint of right wrist**
+7th **S63.522 Sprain of radiocarpal joint of left wrist**
+7th **S63.529 Sprain of radiocarpal joint of unspecified wrist**

+ S63.59 Other specified sprain of wrist
  - +7th S63.591 Other specified sprain of right wrist
  - +7th S63.592 Other specified sprain of left wrist
  - +7th S63.599 Other specified sprain of unspecified wrist

+ S63.6 Other and unspecified sprain of finger(s)
  Excludes1: *traumatic rupture of ligament of finger at metacarpophalangeal and interphalangeal joint(s) (S63.4-)*

+ S63.60 Unspecified sprain of thumb
  - +7th S63.601 Unspecified sprain of right thumb
  - +7th S63.602 Unspecified sprain of left thumb
  - +7th S63.609 Unspecified sprain of unspecified thumb

+ S63.61 Unspecified sprain of other and unspecified finger(s)
  - +7th S63.610 Unspecified sprain of right index finger
  - +7th S63.611 Unspecified sprain of left index finger
  - +7th S63.612 Unspecified sprain of right middle finger
  - +7th S63.613 Unspecified sprain of left middle finger
  - +7th S63.614 Unspecified sprain of right ring finger
  - +7th S63.615 Unspecified sprain of left ring finger
  - +7th S63.616 Unspecified sprain of right little finger
  - +7th S63.617 Unspecified sprain of left little finger
  - +7th S63.618 Unspecified sprain of other finger
    Unspecified sprain of specified finger with unspecified laterality
  - +7th S63.619 Unspecified sprain of unspecified finger

+ S63.62 Sprain of interphalangeal joint of thumb
  - +7th S63.621 Sprain of interphalangeal joint of right thumb
  - +7th S63.622 Sprain of interphalangeal joint of left thumb
  - +7th S63.629 Sprain of interphalangeal joint of unspecified thumb

+ S63.63 Sprain of interphalangeal joint of other and unspecified finger(s)
  - +7th S63.630 Sprain of interphalangeal joint of right index finger
  - +7th S63.631 Sprain of interphalangeal joint of left index finger
  - +7th S63.632 Sprain of interphalangeal joint of right middle finger
  - +7th S63.633 Sprain of interphalangeal joint of left middle finger
  - +7th S63.634 Sprain of interphalangeal joint of right ring finger
  - +7th S63.635 Sprain of interphalangeal joint of left ring finger
  - +7th S63.636 Sprain of interphalangeal joint of right little finger
  - +7th S63.637 Sprain of interphalangeal joint of left little finger
  - +7th S63.638 Sprain of interphalangeal joint of other finger
  - +7th S63.639 Sprain of interphalangeal joint of unspecified finger

+ S63.64 Sprain of metacarpophalangeal joint of thumb
  - +7th S63.641 Sprain of metacarpophalangeal joint of right thumb
  - +7th S63.642 Sprain of metacarpophalangeal joint of left thumb
  - +7th S63.649 Sprain of metacarpophalangeal joint of unspecified thumb

+ S63.65 Sprain of metacarpophalangeal joint of other and unspecified finger(s)
  - +7th S63.650 Sprain of metacarpophalangeal joint of right index finger
  - +7th S63.651 Sprain of metacarpophalangeal joint of left index finger
  - +7th S63.652 Sprain of metacarpophalangeal joint of right middle finger
  - +7th S63.653 Sprain of metacarpophalangeal joint of left middle finger
  - +7th S63.654 Sprain of metacarpophalangeal joint of right ring finger
  - +7th S63.655 Sprain of metacarpophalangeal joint of left ring finger
  - +7th S63.656 Sprain of metacarpophalangeal joint of right little finger
  - +7th S63.657 Sprain of metacarpophalangeal joint of left little finger
  - +7th S63.658 Sprain of metacarpophalangeal joint of other finger
    Sprain of metacarpophalangeal joint of specified finger with unspecified laterality
  - +7th S63.659 Sprain of metacarpophalangeal joint of unspecified finger

+ S63.68 Other sprain of thumb
  - +7th S63.681 Other sprain of right thumb
  - +7th S63.682 Other sprain of left thumb
  - +7th S63.689 Other sprain of unspecified thumb

+ S63.69 Other sprain of other and unspecified finger(s)
  - +7th S63.690 Other sprain of right index finger
  - +7th S63.691 Other sprain of left index finger
  - +7th S63.692 Other sprain of right middle finger
  - +7th S63.693 Other sprain of left middle finger
  - +7th S63.694 Other sprain of right ring finger
  - +7th S63.695 Other sprain of left ring finger
  - +7th S63.696 Other sprain of right little finger
  - +7th S63.697 Other sprain of left little finger
  - +7th S63.698 Other sprain of other finger
    Other sprain of specified finger with unspecified laterality
  - +7th S63.699 Other sprain of unspecified finger

+ S63.8 Sprain of other part of wrist and hand
  + S63.8X Sprain of other part of wrist and hand
    - +7th S63.8X1 Sprain of other part of right wrist and hand
    - +7th S63.8X2 Sprain of other part of left wrist and hand
    - +7th S63.8X9 Sprain of other part of unspecified wrist and hand

+ S63.9 Sprain of unspecified part of wrist and hand
  - X+7th S63.90 Sprain of unspecified part of unspecified wrist and hand
  - X+7th S63.91 Sprain of unspecified part of right wrist and hand
  - X+7th S63.92 Sprain of unspecified part of left wrist and hand

S64 Injury of nerves at wrist and hand level

Code also any associated open wound (S61.-)

The appropriate 7th character is to be added to each code from category S64
A initial encounter
D subsequent encounter
S sequela

+ S64.0 Injury of ulnar nerve at wrist and hand level
  - X+7th S64.00 Injury of ulnar nerve at wrist and hand level of unspecified arm
  - X+7th S64.01 Injury of ulnar nerve at wrist and hand level of right arm
  - X+7th S64.02 Injury of ulnar nerve at wrist and hand level of left arm

+ S64.1 Injury of median nerve at wrist and hand level
  - X+7th S64.10 Injury of median nerve at wrist and hand level of unspecified arm
  - X+7th S64.11 Injury of median nerve at wrist and hand level of right arm
  - X+7th S64.12 Injury of median nerve at wrist and hand level of left arm

+ S64.2 Injury of radial nerve at wrist and hand level
  - X+7th S64.20 Injury of radial nerve at wrist and hand level of unspecified arm
  - X+7th S64.21 Injury of radial nerve at wrist and hand level of right arm
  - X+7th S64.22 Injury of radial nerve at wrist and hand level of left arm

+ S64.3 Injury of digital nerve of thumb
  - X+7th S64.30 Injury of digital nerve of unspecified thumb
  - X+7th S64.31 Injury of digital nerve of right thumb
  - X+7th S64.32 Injury of digital nerve of left thumb

+ S64.4 Injury of digital nerve of other and unspecified finger
  - X+7th S64.40 Injury of digital nerve of unspecified finger
  + S64.49 Injury of digital nerve of other finger
    - +7th S64.490 Injury of digital nerve of right index finger
    - +7th S64.491 Injury of digital nerve of left index finger
    - +7th S64.492 Injury of digital nerve of right middle finger
    - +7th S64.493 Injury of digital nerve of left middle finger
    - +7th S64.494 Injury of digital nerve of right ring finger
    - +7th S64.495 Injury of digital nerve of left ring finger
    - +7th S64.496 Injury of digital nerve of right little finger

+7th **S64.497** **Injury of digital nerve of left little finger**
+7th **S64.498** **Injury of digital nerve of other finger**
Injury of digital nerve of specified finger with unspecified laterality

\+ **S64.8** **Injury of other nerves at wrist and hand level**
\+ **S64.8X** **Injury of other nerves at wrist and hand level**
+7th **S64.8X1** **Injury of other nerves at wrist and hand level of right arm**
+7th **S64.8X2** **Injury of other nerves at wrist and hand level of left arm**
+7th **S64.8X9** **Injury of other nerves at wrist and hand level of unspecified arm**

\+ **S64.9** **Injury of unspecified nerve at wrist and hand level**
X+7th **S64.90** **Injury of unspecified nerve at wrist and hand level of unspecified arm**
X+7th **S64.91** **Injury of unspecified nerve at wrist and hand level of right arm**
X+7th **S64.92** **Injury of unspecified nerve at wrist and hand level of left arm**

S65 **Injury of blood vessels at wrist and hand level**
Code also any associated open wound (S61.-)

The appropriate 7th character is to be added to each code from category S65
A initial encounter
D subsequent encounter
S sequela

\+ **S65.0** **Injury of ulnar artery at wrist and hand level**
\+ **S65.00** **Unspecified injury of ulnar artery at wrist and hand level**
CC +7th **S65.001** **Unspecified injury of ulnar artery at wrist and hand level of right arm**
CC Exclusion 7th character A see Appendix A
PDX collection 1274
CC +7th **S65.002** **Unspecified injury of ulnar artery at wrist and hand level of left arm**
CC Exclusion 7th character A see Appendix A
PDX collection 1275
CC +7th **S65.009** **Unspecified injury of ulnar artery at wrist and hand level of unspecified arm**
CC Exclusion 7th character A see Appendix A
PDX collection 1276
\+ **S65.01** **Laceration of ulnar artery at wrist and hand level**
CC +7th **S65.011** **Laceration of ulnar artery at wrist and hand level of right arm**
CC Exclusion 7th character A see Appendix A
PDX collection 1274
CC +7th **S65.012** **Laceration of ulnar artery at wrist and hand level of left arm**
CC Exclusion 7th character A see Appendix A
PDX collection 1275
CC +7th **S65.019** **Laceration of ulnar artery at wrist and hand level of unspecified arm**
CC Exclusion 7th character A see Appendix A
PDX collection 1276
\+ **S65.09** **Other specified injury of ulnar artery at wrist and hand level**
CC +7th **S65.091** **Other specified injury of ulnar artery at wrist and hand level of right arm**
CC Exclusion 7th character A see Appendix A
PDX collection 1274
CC +7th **S65.092** **Other specified injury of ulnar artery at wrist and hand level of left arm**
CC Exclusion 7th character A see Appendix A
PDX collection 1275
CC +7th **S65.099** **Other specified injury of ulnar artery at wrist and hand level of unspecified arm**
CC Exclusion 7th character A see Appendix A
PDX collection 1276

\+ **S65.1** **Injury of radial artery at wrist and hand level**
\+ **S65.10** **Unspecified injury of radial artery at wrist and hand level**
CC +7th **S65.101** **Unspecified injury of radial artery at wrist and hand level of right arm**
CC Exclusion 7th character A see Appendix A
PDX collection 1277
CC +7th **S65.102** **Unspecified injury of radial artery at wrist and hand level of left arm**
CC Exclusion 7th character A see Appendix A
PDX collection 1278
CC +7th **S65.109** **Unspecified injury of radial artery at wri and hand level of unspecified arm**
CC Exclusion 7th character A see Appendix A
PDX collection 1279
\+ **S65.11** **Laceration of radial artery at wrist and hand level**
CC +7th **S65.111** **Laceration of radial artery at wrist and hand level of right arm**
CC Exclusion 7th character A see Appendix A
PDX collection 1277
CC +7th **S65.112** **Laceration of radial artery at wrist and hand level of left arm**
CC Exclusion 7th character A see Appendix A
PDX collection 1278
CC +7th **S65.119** **Laceration of radial artery at wrist and hand level of unspecified arm**
CC Exclusion 7th character A see Appendix A
PDX collection 1279
\+ **S65.19** **Other specified injury of radial artery at wrist and hand level**
CC +7th **S65.191** **Other specified injury of radial artery at wrist and hand level of right arm**
CC Exclusion 7th character A see Appendix A
PDX collection 1277
CC +7th **S65.192** **Other specified injury of radial artery at wrist and hand level of left arm**
CC Exclusion 7th character A see Appendix A
PDX collection 1278
CC +7th **S65.199** **Other specified injury of radial artery at wrist and hand level of unspecified arm**
CC Exclusion 7th character A see Appendix A
PDX collection 1279

\+ **S65.2** **Injury of superficial palmar arch**
\+ **S65.20** **Unspecified injury of superficial palmar arch**
CC +7th **S65.201** **Unspecified injury of superficial palmar arch of right hand**
CC Exclusion 7th character A see Appendix A
PDX collection 1288
CC +7th **S65.202** **Unspecified injury of superficial palmar arch of left hand**
CC Exclusion 7th character A see Appendix A
PDX collection 1289
CC +7th **S65.209** **Unspecified injury of superficial palmar arch of unspecified hand**
CC Exclusion 7th character A see Appendix A
PDX collection 1290
\+ **S65.21** **Laceration of superficial palmar arch**
CC +7th **S65.211** **Laceration of superficial palmar arch of right hand**
CC Exclusion 7th character A see Appendix A
PDX collection 1288
CC +7th **S65.212** **Laceration of superficial palmar arch of left hand**
CC Exclusion 7th character A see Appendix A
PDX collection 1289
CC +7th **S65.219** **Laceration of superficial palmar arch of unspecified hand**
CC Exclusion 7th character A see Appendix A
PDX collection 1290
\+ **S65.29** **Other specified injury of superficial palmar arch**
CC +7th **S65.291** **Other specified injury of superficial palmar arch of right hand**
CC Exclusion 7th character A see Appendix A
PDX collection 1288
CC +7th **S65.292** **Other specified injury of superficial palmar arch of left hand**
CC Exclusion 7th character A see Appendix A
PDX collection 1289
CC +7th **S65.299** **Other specified injury of superficial palmar arch of unspecified hand**
CC Exclusion 7th character A see Appendix A
PDX collection 1290

\+ **S65.3** **Injury of deep palmar arch**
\+ **S65.30** **Unspecified injury of deep palmar arch**
CC +7th **S65.301** **Unspecified injury of deep palmar arch o right hand**
CC Exclusion 7th character A see Appendix A
PDX collection 1288
CC +7th **S65.302** **Unspecified injury of deep palmar arch c left hand**
CC Exclusion 7th character A see Appendix A
PDX collection 1289

CC +7th **S65.309** **Unspecified injury of deep palmar arch of unspecified hand**
CC Exclusion 7th character A see Appendix A
PDX collection 1290

\+ **S65.31** **Laceration of deep palmar arch**

CC +7th **S65.311** **Laceration of deep palmar arch of right hand**
CC Exclusion 7th character A see Appendix A
PDX collection 1288

CC +7th **S65.312** **Laceration of deep palmar arch of left hand**
CC Exclusion 7th character A see Appendix A
PDX collection 1289

CC +7th **S65.319** **Laceration of deep palmar arch of unspecified hand**
CC Exclusion 7th character A see Appendix A
PDX collection 1290

\+ **S65.39** **Other specified injury of deep palmar arch**

CC +7th **S65.391** **Other specified injury of deep palmar arch of right hand**
CC Exclusion 7th character A see Appendix A
PDX collection 1288

CC +7th **S65.392** **Other specified injury of deep palmar arch of left hand**
CC Exclusion 7th character A see Appendix A
PDX collection 1289

CC +7th **S65.399** **Other specified injury of deep palmar arch of unspecified hand**
CC Exclusion 7th character A see Appendix A
PDX collection 1290

\+ **S65.4** **Injury of blood vessel of thumb**

\+ **S65.40** **Unspecified injury of blood vessel of thumb**

CC +7th **S65.401** **Unspecified injury of blood vessel of right thumb**
CC Exclusion 7th character A see Appendix A
PDX collection 1291

CC +7th **S65.402** **Unspecified injury of blood vessel of left thumb**
CC Exclusion 7th character A see Appendix A
PDX collection 1292

CC +7th **S65.409** **Unspecified injury of blood vessel of unspecified thumb**
CC Exclusion 7th character A see Appendix A
PDX collection 1293

\+ **S65.41** **Laceration of blood vessel of thumb**

CC +7th **S65.411** **Laceration of blood vessel of right thumb**
CC Exclusion 7th character A see Appendix A
PDX collection 1291

CC +7th **S65.412** **Laceration of blood vessel of left thumb**
CC Exclusion 7th character A see Appendix A
PDX collection 1292

CC +7th **S65.419** **Laceration of blood vessel of unspecified thumb**
CC Exclusion 7th character A see Appendix A
PDX collection 1293

\+ **S65.49** **Other specified injury of blood vessel of thumb**

CC +7th **S65.491** **Other specified injury of blood vessel of right thumb**
CC Exclusion 7th character A see Appendix A
PDX collection 1291

CC +7th **S65.492** **Other specified injury of blood vessel of left thumb**
CC Exclusion 7th character A see Appendix A
PDX collection 1292

CC +7th **S65.499** **Other specified injury of blood vessel of unspecified thumb**
CC Exclusion 7th character A see Appendix A
PDX collection 1293

\+ **S65.5** **Injury of blood vessel of other and unspecified finger**

\+ **S65.50** **Unspecified injury of blood vessel of other and unspecified finger**

CC +7th **S65.500** **Unspecified injury of blood vessel of right index finger**
CC Exclusion 7th character A see Appendix A
PDX collection 1291

CC +7th **S65.501** **Unspecified injury of blood vessel of left index finger**
CC Exclusion 7th character A see Appendix A
PDX collection 1292

CC +7th **S65.502** **Unspecified injury of blood vessel of right middle finger**
CC Exclusion 7th character A see Appendix A
PDX collection 1291

CC +7th **S65.503** **Unspecified injury of blood vessel of left middle finger**
CC Exclusion 7th character A see Appendix A
PDX collection 1292

CC +7th **S65.504** **Unspecified injury of blood vessel of right ring finger**
CC Exclusion 7th character A see Appendix A
PDX collection 1291

CC +7th **S65.505** **Unspecified injury of blood vessel of left ring finger**
CC Exclusion 7th character A see Appendix A
PDX collection 1292

CC +7th **S65.506** **Unspecified injury of blood vessel of right little finger**
CC Exclusion 7th character A see Appendix A
PDX collection 1291

CC +7th **S65.507** **Unspecified injury of blood vessel of left little finger**
CC Exclusion 7th character A see Appendix A
PDX collection 1292

CC +7th **S65.508** **Unspecified injury of blood vessel of other finger**
Unspecified injury of blood vessel of specified finger with unspecified laterality
CC Exclusion 7th character A see Appendix A
PDX collection 1293

CC +7th **S65.509** **Unspecified injury of blood vessel of unspecified finger**
CC Exclusion 7th character A see Appendix A
PDX collection 1293

\+ **S65.51** **Laceration of blood vessel of other and unspecified finger**

CC +7th **S65.510** **Laceration of blood vessel of right index finger**
CC Exclusion 7th character A see Appendix A
PDX collection 1291

CC +7th **S65.511** **Laceration of blood vessel of left index finger**
CC Exclusion 7th character A see Appendix A
PDX collection 1292

CC +7th **S65.512** **Laceration of blood vessel of right middle finger**
CC Exclusion 7th character A see Appendix A
PDX collection 1291

CC +7th **S65.513** **Laceration of blood vessel of left middle finger**
CC Exclusion 7th character A see Appendix A
PDX collection 1292

CC +7th **S65.514** **Laceration of blood vessel of right ring finger**
CC Exclusion 7th character A see Appendix A
PDX collection 1291

CC +7th **S65.515** **Laceration of blood vessel of left ring finger**
CC Exclusion 7th character A see Appendix A
PDX collection 1292

CC +7th **S65.516** **Laceration of blood vessel of right little finger**
CC Exclusion 7th character A see Appendix A
PDX collection 1291

CC +7th **S65.517** **Laceration of blood vessel of left little finger**
CC Exclusion 7th character A see Appendix A
PDX collection 1292

CC +7th **S65.518** **Laceration of blood vessel of other finger**
Laceration of blood vessel of specified finger with unspecified laterality
CC Exclusion 7th character A see Appendix A
PDX collection 1293

CC +7th **S65.519** **Laceration of blood vessel of unspecified finger**
CC Exclusion 7th character A see Appendix A
PDX collection 1293

\+ **S65.59** **Other specified injury of blood vessel of other and unspecified finger**

CC +7th **S65.590** **Other specified injury of blood vessel of right index finger**
CC Exclusion 7th character A see Appendix A
PDX collection 1291

CC +7th **S65.591** **Other specified injury of blood vessel of left index finger**
CC Exclusion 7th character A see Appendix A
PDX collection 1292

CC +7th **S65.592** **Other specified injury of blood vessel of right middle finger**
CC Exclusion 7th character A see Appendix A
PDX collection 1291

CC +7th **S65.593** **Other specified injury of blood vessel of left middle finger**
CC Exclusion 7th character A see Appendix A
PDX collection 1292

CC +7th **S65.594** **Other specified injury of blood vessel of right ring finger**
CC Exclusion 7th character A see Appendix A
PDX collection 1291

CC +7th **S65.595** **Other specified injury of blood vessel of left ring finger**
CC Exclusion 7th character A see Appendix A
PDX collection 1292

CC +7th **S65.596** **Other specified injury of blood vessel of right little finger**
CC Exclusion 7th character A see Appendix A
PDX collection 1291

CC +7th **S65.597** **Other specified injury of blood vessel of left little finger**
CC Exclusion 7th character A see Appendix A
PDX collection 1292

CC +7th **S65.598** **Other specified injury of blood vessel of other finger**
Other specified injury of blood vessel of specified finger with unspecified laterality
CC Exclusion 7th character A see Appendix A
PDX collection 1293

CC +7th **S65.599** **Other specified injury of blood vessel of unspecified finger**
CC Exclusion 7th character A see Appendix A
PDX collection 1293

\+ **S65.8** **Injury of other blood vessels at wrist and hand level**

\+ **S65.80** **Unspecified injury of other blood vessels at wrist and hand level**

CC +7th **S65.801** **Unspecified injury of other blood vessels at wrist and hand level of right arm**
CC Exclusion 7th character A see Appendix A
PDX collection 1260

CC +7th **S65.802** **Unspecified injury of other blood vessels at wrist and hand level of left arm**
CC Exclusion 7th character A see Appendix A
PDX collection 1261

CC +7th **S65.809** **Unspecified injury of other blood vessels at wrist and hand level of unspecified arm**
CC Exclusion 7th character A see Appendix A
PDX collection 1262

\+ **S65.81** **Laceration of other blood vessels at wrist and hand level**

CC +7th **S65.811** **Laceration of other blood vessels at wrist and hand level of right arm**
CC Exclusion 7th character A see Appendix A
PDX collection 1260

CC +7th **S65.812** **Laceration of other blood vessels at wrist and hand level of left arm**
CC Exclusion 7th character A see Appendix A
PDX collection 1261

CC +7th **S65.819** **Laceration of other blood vessels at wrist and hand level of unspecified arm**
CC Exclusion 7th character A see Appendix A
PDX collection 1262

\+ **S65.89** **Other specified injury of other blood vessels at wrist and hand level**

CC +7th **S65.891** **Other specified injury of other blood vessels at wrist and hand level of right arm**
CC Exclusion 7th character A see Appendix A
PDX collection 1260

CC +7th **S65.892** **Other specified injury of other blood vessels at wrist and hand level of left arm**
CC Exclusion 7th character A see Appendix A
PDX collection 1261

CC +7th **S65.899** **Other specified injury of other blood vessels at wrist and hand level of unspecified arm**
CC Exclusion 7th character A see Appendix A
PDX collection 1262

\+ **S65.9** **Injury of unspecified blood vessel at wrist and hand level**

\+ **S65.90** **Unspecified injury of unspecified blood vessel at wrist and hand level**

CC +7th **S65.901** **Unspecified injury of unspecified blood vessel at wrist and hand level of right arm**
CC Exclusion 7th character A see Appendix A
PDX collection 1260

CC +7th **S65.902** **Unspecified injury of unspecified blood vessel at wrist and hand level of left arm**
CC Exclusion 7th character A see Appendix A
PDX collection 1261

CC +7th **S65.909** **Unspecified injury of unspecified blood vessel at wrist and hand level of unspecifi arm**
CC Exclusion 7th character A see Appendix A
PDX collection 1262

\+ **S65.91** **Laceration of unspecified blood vessel at wrist and hand level**

CC +7th **S65.911** **Laceration of unspecified blood vessel at wrist and hand level of right arm**
CC Exclusion 7th character A see Appendix A
PDX collection 1260

CC +7th **S65.912** **Laceration of unspecified blood vessel at wrist and hand level of left arm**
CC Exclusion 7th character A see Appendix A
PDX collection 1261

CC +7th **S65.919** **Laceration of unspecified blood vessel at wrist and hand level of unspecified arm**
CC Exclusion 7th character A see Appendix A
PDX collection 1262

\+ **S65.99** **Other specified injury of unspecified blood vessel a wrist and hand level**

CC +7th **S65.991** **Other specified injury of unspecified bloo vessel at wrist and hand of right arm**
CC Exclusion 7th character A see Appendix A
PDX collection 1260

CC +7th **S65.992** **Other specified injury of unspecified bloo vessel at wrist and hand of left arm**
CC Exclusion 7th character A see Appendix A
PDX collection 1261

CC +7th **S65.999** **Other specified injury of unspecified bloo vessel at wrist and hand of unspecified ar**
CC Exclusion 7th character A see Appendix A
PDX collection 1262

S66 Injury of muscle, fascia and tendon at wrist and hand level

Code also any associated open wound (S61.-)

Excludes2: *sprain of joints and ligaments of wrist and hand (S63.-)*

The appropriate 7th character is to be added to each code from category S66
A initial encounter
D subsequent encounter
S sequela

\+ **S66.0** **Injury of long flexor muscle, fascia and tendon of thumb at wrist and hand level**

\+ **S66.00** **Unspecified injury of long flexor muscle, fascia and tendon of thumb at wrist and hand level**

+7th **S66.001** **Unspecified injury of long flexor muscle, fascia and tendon of right thumb at wrist and hand level**

+7th **S66.002** **Unspecified injury of long flexor muscle, fascia and tendon of left thumb at wrist and hand level**

+7th **S66.009** **Unspecified injury of long flexor muscle, fascia and tendon of unspecified thumb a wrist and hand level**

\+ **S66.01** **Strain of long flexor muscle, fascia and tendon of thumb at wrist and hand level**

+7th **S66.011** **Strain of long flexor muscle, fascia and tendon of right thumb at wrist and hand level**

+7th **S66.012** **Strain of long flexor muscle, fascia and tendon of left thumb at wrist and hand le**

+7th **S66.019** **Strain of long flexor muscle, fascia and tendon of unspecified thumb at wrist and hand level**

\+ **S66.02** **Laceration of long flexor muscle, fascia and tendo of thumb at wrist and hand level**

CC +7th **S66.021** **Laceration of long flexor muscle, fascia and tendon of right thumb at wrist and hand level**
CC Exclusion 7th character A see Appendix
PDX collection 1294

CC +7th **S66.022** **Laceration of long flexor muscle, fascia and tendon of left thumb at wrist and ha level**
CC Exclusion 7th character A see Appendix
PDX collection 1295

CC +7th **S66.029** **Laceration of long flexor muscle, fascia and tendon of unspecified thumb at wris and hand level**
CC Exclusion 7th character A see Appendix
PDX collection 1296

+ **S66.09** **Other specified injury of long flexor muscle, fascia and tendon of thumb at wrist and hand level**

+7th **S66.091** **Other specified injury of long flexor muscle, fascia and tendon of right thumb at wrist and hand level**

+7th **S66.092** **Other specified injury of long flexor muscle, fascia and tendon of left thumb at wrist and hand level**

+7th **S66.099** **Other specified injury of long flexor muscle, fascia and tendon of unspecified thumb at wrist and hand level**

+ **S66.1** **Injury of flexor muscle, fascia and tendon of other and unspecified finger at wrist and hand level**

Excludes2: *Injury of long flexor muscle, fascia and tendon of thumb at wrist and hand level (S66.0-)*

+ **S66.10** **Unspecified injury of flexor muscle, fascia and tendon of other and unspecified finger at wrist and hand level**

+7th **S66.100** **Unspecified injury of flexor muscle, fascia and tendon of right index finger at wrist and hand level**

+7th **S66.101** **Unspecified injury of flexor muscle, fascia and tendon of left index finger at wrist and hand level**

+7th **S66.102** **Unspecified injury of flexor muscle, fascia and tendon of right middle finger at wrist and hand level**

+7th **S66.103** **Unspecified injury of flexor muscle, fascia and tendon of left middle finger at wrist and hand level**

+7th **S66.104** **Unspecified injury of flexor muscle, fascia and tendon of right ring finger at wrist and hand level**

+7th **S66.105** **Unspecified injury of flexor muscle, fascia and tendon of left ring finger at wrist and hand level**

+7th **S66.106** **Unspecified injury of flexor muscle, fascia and tendon of right little finger at wrist and hand level**

+7th **S66.107** **Unspecified injury of flexor muscle, fascia and tendon of left little finger at wrist and hand level**

+7th **S66.108** **Unspecified injury of flexor muscle, fascia and tendon of other finger at wrist and hand level**

Unspecified injury of flexor muscle, fascia and tendon of specified finger with unspecified laterality at wrist and hand level

+7th **S66.109** **Unspecified injury of flexor muscle, fascia and tendon of unspecified finger at wrist and hand level**

+ **S66.11** **Strain of flexor muscle, fascia and tendon of other and unspecified finger at wrist and hand level**

+7th **S66.110** **Strain of flexor muscle, fascia and tendon of right index finger at wrist and hand level**

+7th **S66.111** **Strain of flexor muscle, fascia and tendon of left index finger at wrist and hand level**

+7th **S66.112** **Strain of flexor muscle, fascia and tendon of right middle finger at wrist and hand level**

+7th **S66.113** **Strain of flexor muscle, fascia and tendon of left middle finger at wrist and hand level**

+7th **S66.114** **Strain of flexor muscle, fascia and tendon of right ring finger at wrist and hand level**

+7th **S66.115** **Strain of flexor muscle, fascia and tendon of left ring finger at wrist and hand level**

+7th **S66.116** **Strain of flexor muscle, fascia and tendon of right little finger at wrist and hand level**

+7th **S66.117** **Strain of flexor muscle, fascia and tendon of left little finger at wrist and hand level**

+7th **S66.118** **Strain of flexor muscle, fascia and tendon of other finger at wrist and hand level**

Strain of flexor muscle, fascia and tendon of specified finger with unspecified laterality at wrist and hand level

+7th **S66.119** **Strain of flexor muscle, fascia and tendon of unspecified finger at wrist and hand level**

+ **S66.12** **Laceration of flexor muscle, fascia and tendon of other and unspecified finger at wrist and hand level**

CC +7th **S66.120** **Laceration of flexor muscle, fascia and tendon of right index finger at wrist and hand level**

CC Exclusion 7th character A see Appendix A
PDX collection 1294

CC +7th **S66.121** **Laceration of flexor muscle, fascia and tendon of left index finger at wrist and hand level**

CC Exclusion 7th character A see Appendix A
PDX collection 1295

CC +7th **S66.122** **Laceration of flexor muscle, fascia and tendon of right middle finger at wrist and hand level**

CC Exclusion 7th character A see Appendix A
PDX collection 1294

CC +7th **S66.123** **Laceration of flexor muscle, fascia and tendon of left middle finger at wrist and hand level**

CC Exclusion 7th character A see Appendix A
PDX collection 1295

CC +7th **S66.124** **Laceration of flexor muscle, fascia and tendon of right ring finger at wrist and hand level**

CC Exclusion 7th character A see Appendix A
PDX collection 1294

CC +7th **S66.125** **Laceration of flexor muscle, fascia and tendon of left ring finger at wrist and hand level**

CC Exclusion 7th character A see Appendix A
PDX collection 1295

CC +7th **S66.126** **Laceration of flexor muscle, fascia and tendon of right little finger at wrist and hand level**

CC Exclusion 7th character A see Appendix A
PDX collection 1294

CC +7th **S66.127** **Laceration of flexor muscle, fascia and tendon of left little finger at wrist and hand level**

CC Exclusion 7th character A see Appendix A
PDX collection 1295

CC +7th **S66.128** **Laceration of flexor muscle, fascia and tendon of other finger at wrist and hand level**

Laceration of flexor muscle, fascia and tendon of specified finger with unspecified laterality at wrist and hand level

CC Exclusion 7th character A see Appendix A
PDX collection 1296

CC +7th **S66.129** **Laceration of flexor muscle, fascia and tendon of unspecified finger at wrist and hand level**

CC Exclusion 7th character A see Appendix A
PDX collection 1296

+ **S66.19** **Other injury of flexor muscle, fascia and tendon of other and unspecified finger at wrist and hand level**

+7th **S66.190** **Other injury of flexor muscle, fascia and tendon of right index finger at wrist and hand level**

+7th **S66.191** **Other injury of flexor muscle, fascia and tendon of left index finger at wrist and hand level**

+7th **S66.192** **Other injury of flexor muscle, fascia and tendon of right middle finger at wrist and hand level**

+7th **S66.193** **Other injury of flexor muscle, fascia and tendon of left middle finger at wrist and hand level**

+7th **S66.194** **Other injury of flexor muscle, fascia and tendon of right ring finger at wrist and hand level**

+7th **S66.195** **Other injury of flexor muscle, fascia and tendon of left ring finger at wrist and hand level**

+7th **S66.196** **Other injury of flexor muscle, fascia and tendon of right little finger at wrist and hand level**

+7th **S66.197** **Other injury of flexor muscle, fascia and tendon of left little finger at wrist and hand level**

+7th **S66.198** **Other injury of flexor muscle, fascia and tendon of other finger at wrist and hand level**
Other injury of flexor muscle, fascia and tendon of specified finger with unspecified laterality at wrist and hand level

+7th **S66.199** **Other injury of flexor muscle, fascia and tendon of unspecified finger at wrist and hand level**

\+ **S66.2** **Injury of extensor muscle, fascia and tendon of thumb at wrist and hand level**

\+ **S66.20** **Unspecified injury of extensor muscle, fascia and tendon of thumb at wrist and hand level**

+7th **S66.201** **Unspecified injury of extensor muscle, fascia and tendon of right thumb at wrist and hand level**

+7th **S66.202** **Unspecified injury of extensor muscle, fascia and tendon of left thumb at wrist and hand level**

+7th **S66.209** **Unspecified injury of extensor muscle, fascia and tendon of unspecified thumb at wrist and hand level**

\+ **S66.21** **Strain of extensor muscle, fascia and tendon of thumb at wrist and hand level**

+7th **S66.211** **Strain of extensor muscle, fascia and tendon of right thumb at wrist and hand level**

+7th **S66.212** **Strain of extensor muscle, fascia and tendon of left thumb at wrist and hand level**

+7th **S66.219** **Strain of extensor muscle, fascia and tendon of unspecified thumb at wrist and hand level**

\+ **S66.22** **Laceration of extensor muscle, fascia and tendon of thumb at wrist and hand level**

CC +7th **S66.221** **Laceration of extensor muscle, fascia and tendon of right thumb at wrist and hand level**
CC Exclusion 7th character A see Appendix A PDX collection 1294

CC +7th **S66.222** **Laceration of extensor muscle, fascia and tendon of left thumb at wrist and hand level**
CC Exclusion 7th character A see Appendix A PDX collection 1295

CC +7th **S66.229** **Laceration of extensor muscle, fascia and tendon of unspecified thumb at wrist and hand level**
CC Exclusion 7th character A see Appendix A PDX collection 1296

\+ **S66.29** **Other specified injury of extensor muscle, fascia and tendon of thumb at wrist and hand level**

+7th **S66.291** **Other specified injury of extensor muscle, fascia and tendon of right thumb at wrist and hand level**

+7th **S66.292** **Other specified injury of extensor muscle, fascia and tendon of left thumb at wrist and hand level**

+7th **S66.299** **Other specified injury of extensor muscle, fascia and tendon of unspecified thumb at wrist and hand level**

\+ **S66.3** **Injury of extensor muscle, fascia and tendon of other and unspecified finger at wrist and hand level**
Excludes2: *Injury of extensor muscle, fascia and tendon of thumb at wrist and hand level (S66.2-)*

\+ **S66.30** **Unspecified injury of extensor muscle, fascia and tendon of other and unspecified finger at wrist and hand level**

+7th **S66.300** **Unspecified injury of extensor muscle, fascia and tendon of right index finger at wrist and hand level**

+7th **S66.301** **Unspecified injury of extensor muscle, fascia and tendon of left index finger at wrist and hand level**

+7th **S66.302** **Unspecified injury of extensor muscle, fascia and tendon of right middle finger at wrist and hand level**

+7th **S66.303** **Unspecified injury of extensor muscle, fascia and tendon of left middle finger at wrist and hand level**

+7th **S66.304** **Unspecified injury of extensor muscle, fascia and tendon of right ring finger at wrist and hand level**

+7th **S66.305** **Unspecified injury of extensor muscle, fascia and tendon of left ring finger at wri and hand level**

+7th **S66.306** **Unspecified injury of extensor muscle, fascia and tendon of right little finger at wrist and hand level**

+7th **S66.307** **Unspecified injury of extensor muscle, fascia and tendon of left little finger at wrist and hand level**

+7th **S66.308** **Unspecified injury of extensor muscle, fascia and tendon of other finger at wrist and hand level**
Unspecified injury of extensor muscle, fascia and tendon of specified finger wit unspecified laterality at wrist and hand level

+7th **S66.309** **Unspecified injury of extensor muscle, fascia and tendon of unspecified finger at wrist and hand level**

\+ **S66.31** **Strain of extensor muscle, fascia and tendon of other and unspecified finger at wrist and hand level**

+7th **S66.310** **Strain of extensor muscle, fascia and tendon of right index finger at wrist and hand level**

+7th **S66.311** **Strain of extensor muscle, fascia and tendon of left index finger at wrist and hand level**

+7th **S66.312** **Strain of extensor muscle, fascia and tendon of right middle finger at wrist and hand level**

+7th **S66.313** **Strain of extensor muscle, fascia and tendon of left middle finger at wrist and hand level**

+7th **S66.314** **Strain of extensor muscle, fascia and tendon of right ring finger at wrist and hand level**

+7th **S66.315** **Strain of extensor muscle, fascia and tendon of left ring finger at wrist and han level**

+7th **S66.316** **Strain of extensor muscle, fascia and tendon of right little finger at wrist and hand level**

+7th **S66.317** **Strain of extensor muscle, fascia and tendon of left little finger at wrist and ha level**

+7th **S66.318** **Strain of extensor muscle, fascia and tendon of other finger at wrist and hand level**
Strain of extensor muscle, fascia and tendo of specified finger with unspecified laterality at wrist and hand level

+7th **S66.319** **Strain of extensor muscle, fascia and tendon of unspecified finger at wrist and hand level**

\+ **S66.32** **Laceration of extensor muscle, fascia and tendon o other and unspecified finger at wrist and hand leve**

CC +7th **S66.320** **Laceration of extensor muscle, fascia and tendon of right index finger at wrist and hand level**
CC Exclusion 7th character A see Appendix A PDX collection 1294

CC +7th **S66.321** **Laceration of extensor muscle, fascia and tendon of left index finger at wrist and hand level**
CC Exclusion 7th character A see Appendix A PDX collection 1295

CC +7th **S66.322** **Laceration of extensor muscle, fascia and tendon of right middle finger at wrist and hand level**
CC Exclusion 7th character A see Appendix A PDX collection 1294

CC +7th **S66.323** **Laceration of extensor muscle, fascia and tendon of left middle finger at wrist and hand level**
CC Exclusion 7th character A see Appendix A PDX collection 1295

CC +7th **S66.324 Laceration of extensor muscle, fascia and tendon of right ring finger at wrist and hand level**
CC Exclusion 7th character A see Appendix A PDX collection 1294

CC +7th **S66.325 Laceration of extensor muscle, fascia and tendon of left ring finger at wrist and hand level**
CC Exclusion 7th character A see Appendix A PDX collection 1295

CC +7th **S66.326 Laceration of extensor muscle, fascia and tendon of right little finger at wrist and hand level**
CC Exclusion 7th character A see Appendix A PDX collection 1294

CC +7th **S66.327 Laceration of extensor muscle, fascia and tendon of left little finger at wrist and hand level**
CC Exclusion 7th character A see Appendix A PDX collection 1295

CC +7th **S66.328 Laceration of extensor muscle, fascia and tendon of other finger at wrist and hand level**
Laceration of extensor muscle, fascia and tendon of specified finger with unspecified laterality at wrist and hand level
CC Exclusion 7th character A see Appendix A PDX collection 1296

CC +7th **S66.329 Laceration of extensor muscle, fascia and tendon of unspecified finger at wrist and hand level**
CC Exclusion 7th character A see Appendix A PDX collection 1296

\+ **S66.39 Other injury of extensor muscle, fascia and tendon of other and unspecified finger at wrist and hand level**

+7th **S66.390 Other injury of extensor muscle, fascia and tendon of right index finger at wrist and hand level**

+7th **S66.391 Other injury of extensor muscle, fascia and tendon of left index finger at wrist and hand level**

+7th **S66.392 Other injury of extensor muscle, fascia and tendon of right middle finger at wrist and hand level**

+7th **S66.393 Other injury of extensor muscle, fascia and tendon of left middle finger at wrist and hand level**

+7th **S66.394 Other injury of extensor muscle, fascia and tendon of right ring finger at wrist and hand level**

+7th **S66.395 Other injury of extensor muscle, fascia and tendon of left ring finger at wrist and hand level**

+7th **S66.396 Other injury of extensor muscle, fascia and tendon of right little finger at wrist and hand level**

+7th **S66.397 Other injury of extensor muscle, fascia and tendon of left little finger at wrist and hand level**

+7th **S66.398 Other injury of extensor muscle, fascia and tendon of other finger at wrist and hand level**
Other injury of extensor muscle, fascia and tendon of specified finger with unspecified laterality at wrist and hand level

+7th **S66.399 Other injury of extensor muscle, fascia and tendon of unspecified finger at wrist and hand level**

\+ **S66.4 Injury of intrinsic muscle, fascia and tendon of thumb at wrist and hand level**

\+ **S66.40 Unspecified injury of intrinsic muscle, fascia and tendon of thumb at wrist and hand level**

+7th **S66.401 Unspecified injury of intrinsic muscle, fascia and tendon of right thumb at wrist and hand level**

+7th **S66.402 Unspecified injury of intrinsic muscle, fascia and tendon of left thumb at wrist and hand level**

+7th **S66.409 Unspecified injury of intrinsic muscle, fascia and tendon of unspecified thumb at wrist and hand level**

\+ **S66.41 Strain of intrinsic muscle, fascia and tendon of thumb at wrist and hand level**

+7th **S66.411 Strain of intrinsic muscle, fascia and tendon of right thumb at wrist and hand level**

+7th **S66.412 Strain of intrinsic muscle, fascia and tendon of left thumb at wrist and hand level**

+7th **S66.419 Strain of intrinsic muscle, fascia and tendon of unspecified thumb at wrist and hand level**

\+ **S66.42 Laceration of intrinsic muscle, fascia and tendon of thumb at wrist and hand level**

CC +7th **S66.421 Laceration of intrinsic muscle, fascia and tendon of right thumb at wrist and hand level**
CC Exclusion 7th character A see Appendix A PDX collection 1294

CC +7th **S66.422 Laceration of intrinsic muscle, fascia and tendon of left thumb at wrist and hand level**
CC Exclusion 7th character A see Appendix A PDX collection 1295

CC +7th **S66.429 Laceration of intrinsic muscle, fascia and tendon of unspecified thumb at wrist and hand level**
CC Exclusion 7th character A see Appendix A PDX collection 1296

\+ **S66.49 Other specified injury of intrinsic muscle, fascia and tendon of thumb at wrist and hand level**

+7th **S66.491 Other specified injury of intrinsic muscle, fascia and tendon of right thumb at wrist and hand level**

+7th **S66.492 Other specified injury of intrinsic muscle, fascia and tendon of left thumb at wrist and hand level**

+7th **S66.499 Other specified injury of intrinsic muscle, fascia and tendon of unspecified thumb at wrist and hand level**

\+ **S66.5 Injury of intrinsic muscle, fascia and tendon of other and unspecified finger at wrist and hand level**
Excludes2: *injury of intrinsic muscle, fascia and tendon of thumb at wrist and hand level (S66.4-)*

\+ **S66.50 Unspecified injury of intrinsic muscle, fascia and tendon of other and unspecified finger at wrist and hand level**

+7th **S66.500 Unspecified injury of intrinsic muscle, fascia and tendon of right index finger at wrist and hand level**

+7th **S66.501 Unspecified injury of intrinsic muscle, fascia and tendon of left index finger at wrist and hand level**

+7th **S66.502 Unspecified injury of intrinsic muscle, fascia and tendon of right middle finger at wrist and hand level**

+7th **S66.503 Unspecified injury of intrinsic muscle, fascia and tendon of left middle finger at wrist and hand level**

+7th **S66.504 Unspecified injury of intrinsic muscle, fascia and tendon of right ring finger at wrist and hand level**

+7th **S66.505 Unspecified injury of intrinsic muscle, fascia and tendon of left ring finger at wrist and hand level**

+7th **S66.506 Unspecified injury of intrinsic muscle, fascia and tendon of right little finger at wrist and hand level**

+7th **S66.507 Unspecified injury of intrinsic muscle, fascia and tendon of left little finger at wrist and hand level**

+7th **S66.508 Unspecified injury of intrinsic muscle, fascia and tendon of other finger at wrist and hand level**
Unspecified injury of intrinsic muscle, fascia and tendon of specified finger with unspecified laterality at wrist and hand level

+7th **S66.509 Unspecified injury of intrinsic muscle, fascia and tendon of unspecified finger at wrist and hand level**

\+ **S66.51 Strain of intrinsic muscle, fascia and tendon of other and unspecified finger at wrist and hand level**

+7th **S66.510 Strain of intrinsic muscle, fascia and tendon of right index finger at wrist and hand level**

+7th **S66.511** **Strain of intrinsic muscle, fascia and tendon of left index finger at wrist and hand level**

+7th **S66.512** **Strain of intrinsic muscle, fascia and tendon of right middle finger at wrist and hand level**

+7th **S66.513** **Strain of intrinsic muscle, fascia and tendon of left middle finger at wrist and hand level**

+7th **S66.514** **Strain of intrinsic muscle, fascia and tendon of right ring finger at wrist and hand level**

+7th **S66.515** **Strain of intrinsic muscle, fascia and tendon of left ring finger at wrist and hand level**

+7th **S66.516** **Strain of intrinsic muscle, fascia and tendon of right little finger at wrist and hand level**

+7th **S66.517** **Strain of intrinsic muscle, fascia and tendon of left little finger at wrist and hand level**

+7th **S66.518** **Strain of intrinsic muscle, fascia and tendon of other finger at wrist and hand level**

Strain of intrinsic muscle, fascia and tendon of specified finger with unspecified laterality at wrist and hand level

+7th **S66.519** **Strain of intrinsic muscle, fascia and tendon of unspecified finger at wrist and hand level**

\+ **S66.52** **Laceration of intrinsic muscle, fascia and tendon of other and unspecified finger at wrist and hand level**

CC +7th **S66.520** **Laceration of intrinsic muscle, fascia and tendon of right index finger at wrist and hand level**

CC Exclusion 7th character A see Appendix A PDX collection 1294

CC +7th **S66.521** **Laceration of intrinsic muscle, fascia and tendon of left index finger at wrist and hand level**

CC Exclusion 7th character A see Appendix A PDX collection 1295

CC +7th **S66.522** **Laceration of intrinsic muscle, fascia and tendon of right middle finger at wrist and hand level**

CC Exclusion 7th character A see Appendix A PDX collection 1294

CC +7th **S66.523** **Laceration of intrinsic muscle, fascia and tendon of left middle finger at wrist and hand level**

CC Exclusion 7th character A see Appendix A PDX collection 1295

CC +7th **S66.524** **Laceration of intrinsic muscle, fascia and tendon of right ring finger at wrist and hand level**

CC Exclusion 7th character A see Appendix A PDX collection 1294

CC +7th **S66.525** **Laceration of intrinsic muscle, fascia and tendon of left ring finger at wrist and hand level**

CC Exclusion 7th character A see Appendix A PDX collection 1295

CC +7th **S66.526** **Laceration of intrinsic muscle, fascia and tendon of right little finger at wrist and hand level**

CC Exclusion 7th character A see Appendix A PDX collection 1294

CC +7th **S66.527** **Laceration of intrinsic muscle, fascia and tendon of left little finger at wrist and hand level**

CC Exclusion 7th character A see Appendix A PDX collection 1295

CC +7th **S66.528** **Laceration of intrinsic muscle, fascia and tendon of other finger at wrist and hand level**

Laceration of intrinsic muscle, fascia and tendon of specified finger with unspecified laterality at wrist and hand level

CC Exclusion 7th character A see Appendix A PDX collection 1296

CC +7th **S66.529** **Laceration of intrinsic muscle, fascia an tendon of unspecified finger at wrist anc hand level**

CC Exclusion 7th character A see Appendix PDX collection 1296

\+ **S66.59** **Other injury of intrinsic muscle, fascia and tendo of other and unspecified finger at wrist and hand level**

+7th **S66.590** **Other injury of intrinsic muscle, fascia tendon of right index finger at wrist and hand level**

+7th **S66.591** **Other injury of intrinsic muscle, fascia and tendon of left index finger at wrist a hand level**

+7th **S66.592** **Other injury of intrinsic muscle, fascia tendon of right middle finger at wrist ar hand level**

+7th **S66.593** **Other injury of intrinsic muscle, fascia tendon of left middle finger at wrist and hand level**

+7th **S66.594** **Other injury of intrinsic muscle, fascia tendon of right ring finger at wrist and hand level**

+7th **S66.595** **Other injury of intrinsic muscle, fascia tendon of left ring finger at wrist and ha level**

+7th **S66.596** **Other injury of intrinsic muscle, fascia tendon of right little finger at wrist and hand level**

+7th **S66.597** **Other injury of intrinsic muscle, fascia tendon of left little finger at wrist and h level**

+7th **S66.598** **Other injury of intrinsic muscle, fascia tendon of other finger at wrist and hand level**

Other injury of intrinsic muscle, fascia ar tendon of specified finger with unspeci laterality at wrist and hand level

+7th **S66.599** **Other injury of intrinsic muscle, fascia tendon of unspecified finger at wrist anc hand level**

\+ **S66.8** **Injury of other specified muscles, fascia and tendons at wris and hand level**

\+ **S66.80** **Unspecified injury of other specified muscles, fasc and tendons at wrist and hand level**

+7th **S66.801** **Unspecified injury of other specified muscles, fascia and tendons at wrist and hand level, right hand**

+7th **S66.802** **Unspecified injury of other specified muscles, fascia and tendons at wrist and hand level, left hand**

+7th **S66.809** **Unspecified injury of other specified muscles, fascia and tendons at wrist and hand level, unspecified hand**

\+ **S66.81** **Strain of other specified muscles, fascia and tend at wrist and hand level**

+7th **S66.811** **Strain of other specified muscles, fascia tendons at wrist and hand level, right ha**

+7th **S66.812** **Strain of other specified muscles, fascia and tendons at wrist and hand level, left hand**

+7th **S66.819** **Strain of other specified muscles, fascia and tendons at wrist and hand level, unspecified hand**

\+ **S66.82** **Laceration of other specified muscles, fascia and tendons at wrist and hand level**

CC +7th **S66.821** **Laceration of other specified muscles, fascia and tendons at wrist and hand le right hand**

CC Exclusion 7th character A see Appendix PDX collection 1294

CC +7th **S66.822** **Laceration of other specified muscles, fascia and tendons at wrist and hand le left hand**

CC Exclusion 7th character A see Appendix PDX collection 1295

CC +7th **S66.829** **Laceration of other specified muscles, fascia and tendons at wrist and hand le unspecified hand**

CC Exclusion 7th character A see Appendix PDX collection 1296

+ S66.89 **Other injury of other specified muscles, fascia and tendons at wrist and hand level**
  - +7th S66.891 **Other injury of other specified muscles, fascia and tendons at wrist and hand level, right hand**
  - +7th S66.892 **Other injury of other specified muscles, fascia and tendons at wrist and hand level, left hand**
  - +7th S66.899 **Other injury of other specified muscles, fascia and tendons at wrist and hand level, unspecified hand**

+ S66.9 **Injury of unspecified muscle, fascia and tendon at wrist and hand level**
  - + S66.90 **Unspecified injury of unspecified muscle, fascia and tendon at wrist and hand level**
    - +7th S66.901 **Unspecified injury of unspecified muscle, fascia and tendon at wrist and hand level, right hand**
    - +7th S66.902 **Unspecified injury of unspecified muscle, fascia and tendon at wrist and hand level, left hand**
    - +7th S66.909 **Unspecified injury of unspecified muscle, fascia and tendon at wrist and hand level, unspecified hand**
  - + S66.91 **Strain of unspecified muscle, fascia and tendon at wrist and hand level**
    - +7th S66.911 **Strain of unspecified muscle, fascia and tendon at wrist and hand level, right hand**
    - +7th S66.912 **Strain of unspecified muscle, fascia and tendon at wrist and hand level, left hand**
    - +7th S66.919 **Strain of unspecified muscle, fascia and tendon at wrist and hand level, unspecified hand**
  - + S66.92 **Laceration of unspecified muscle, fascia and tendon at wrist and hand level**
    - CC +7th S66.921 **Laceration of unspecified muscle, fascia and tendon at wrist and hand level, right hand**
      CC Exclusion 7th character A see Appendix A PDX collection 1294
    - CC +7th S66.922 **Laceration of unspecified muscle, fascia and tendon at wrist and hand level, left hand**
      CC Exclusion 7th character A see Appendix A PDX collection 1295
    - CC +7th S66.929 **Laceration of unspecified muscle, fascia and tendon at wrist and hand level, unspecified hand**
      CC Exclusion 7th character A see Appendix A PDX collection 1296
  - + S66.99 **Other injury of unspecified muscle, fascia and tendon at wrist and hand level**
    - +7th S66.991 **Other injury of unspecified muscle, fascia and tendon at wrist and hand level, right hand**
    - +7th S66.992 **Other injury of unspecified muscle, fascia and tendon at wrist and hand level, left hand**
    - +7th S66.999 **Other injury of unspecified muscle, fascia and tendon at wrist and hand level, unspecified hand**

S67 Crushing injury of wrist, hand and fingers

Use additional code for all associated injuries, such as:
fracture of wrist and hand (S62.-)
open wound of wrist and hand (S61.-)

The appropriate 7th character is to be added to each code from category S67
A initial encounter
D subsequent encounter
S sequela

+ S67.0 **Crushing injury of thumb**
  - X+7th S67.00 **Crushing injury of unspecified thumb**
  - X+7th S67.01 **Crushing injury of right thumb**
  - X+7th S67.02 **Crushing injury of left thumb**

+ S67.1 **Crushing injury of other and unspecified finger(s)**
  Excludes2: *crushing injury of thumb (S67.0-)*
  - X+7th S67.10 **Crushing injury of unspecified finger(s)**
  - + S67.19 **Crushing injury of other finger(s)**
    - +7th S67.190 **Crushing injury of right index finger**
    - +7th S67.191 **Crushing injury of left index finger**
    - +7th S67.192 **Crushing injury of right middle finger**
    - +7th S67.193 **Crushing injury of left middle finger**
    - +7th S67.194 **Crushing injury of right ring finger**
    - +7th S67.195 **Crushing injury of left ring finger**
    - +7th S67.196 **Crushing injury of right little finger**
    - +7th S67.197 **Crushing injury of left little finger**
    - +7th S67.198 **Crushing injury of other finger**
      Crushing injury of specified finger with unspecified laterality

+ S67.2 **Crushing injury of hand**
  Excludes2: *crushing injury of fingers (S67.1-)*
  crushing injury of thumb (S67.0-)
  - X+7th S67.20 **Crushing injury of unspecified hand**
  - X+7th S67.21 **Crushing injury of right hand**
  - X+7th S67.22 **Crushing injury of left hand**

+ S67.3 **Crushing injury of wrist**
  - X+7th S67.30 **Crushing injury of unspecified wrist**
  - X+7th S67.31 **Crushing injury of right wrist**
  - X+7th S67.32 **Crushing injury of left wrist**

+ S67.4 **Crushing injury of wrist and hand**
  Excludes1: *crushing injury of hand alone (S67.2-)*
  crushing injury of wrist alone (S67.3-)
  Excludes2: *crushing injury of fingers (S67.1-)*
  crushing injury of thumb (S67.0-)
  - X+7th S67.40 **Crushing injury of unspecified wrist and hand**
  - X+7th S67.41 **Crushing injury of right wrist and hand**
  - X+7th S67.42 **Crushing injury of left wrist and hand**

+ S67.9 **Crushing injury of unspecified part(s) of wrist, hand and fingers**
  - X+7th S67.90 **Crushing injury of unspecified part(s) of unspecified wrist, hand and fingers**
  - X+7th S67.91 **Crushing injury of unspecified part(s) of right wrist, hand and fingers**
  - X+7th S67.92 **Crushing injury of unspecified part(s) of left wrist, hand and fingers**

S68 Traumatic amputation of wrist, hand and fingers

An amputation not identified as partial or complete should be coded to complete

The appropriate 7th character is to be added to each code from category S68
A initial encounter
D subsequent encounter
S sequela

+ S68.0 **Traumatic metacarpophalangeal amputation of thumb**
  Traumatic amputation of thumb NOS
  - + S68.01 **Complete traumatic metacarpophalangeal amputation of thumb**
    - +7th S68.011 **Complete traumatic metacarpophalangeal amputation of right thumb**
    - +7th S68.012 **Complete traumatic metacarpophalangeal amputation of left thumb**
    - +7th S68.019 **Complete traumatic metacarpophalangeal amputation of unspecified thumb**
  - + S68.02 **Partial traumatic metacarpophalangeal amputation of thumb**
    - +7th S68.021 **Partial traumatic metacarpophalangeal amputation of right thumb**
    - +7th S68.022 **Partial traumatic metacarpophalangeal amputation of left thumb**
    - +7th S68.029 **Partial traumatic metacarpophalangeal amputation of unspecified thumb**

+ S68.1 **Traumatic metacarpophalangeal amputation of other and unspecified finger**
  Traumatic amputation of finger NOS
  Excludes2: *traumatic metacarpophalangeal amputation of thumb (S68.0-)*
  - + S68.11 **Complete traumatic metacarpophalangeal amputation of other and unspecified finger**
    - +7th S68.110 **Complete traumatic metacarpophalangeal amputation of right index finger**
    - +7th S68.111 **Complete traumatic metacarpophalangeal amputation of left index finger**
    - +7th S68.112 **Complete traumatic metacarpophalangeal amputation of right middle finger**
    - +7th S68.113 **Complete traumatic metacarpophalangeal amputation of left middle finger**
    - +7th S68.114 **Complete traumatic metacarpophalangeal amputation of right ring finger**

+7th **S68.115** **Complete traumatic metacarpophalangeal amputation of left ring finger**

+7th **S68.116** **Complete traumatic metacarpophalangeal amputation of right little finger**

+7th **S68.117** **Complete traumatic metacarpophalangeal amputation of left little finger**

+7th **S68.118** **Complete traumatic metacarpophalangeal amputation of other finger**

Complete traumatic metacarpophalangeal amputation of specified finger with unspecified laterality

+7th **S68.119** **Complete traumatic metacarpophalangeal amputation of unspecified finger**

\+ **S68.12** **Partial traumatic metacarpophalangeal amputation of other and unspecified finger**

+7th **S68.120** **Partial traumatic metacarpophalangeal amputation of right index finger**

+7th **S68.121** **Partial traumatic metacarpophalangeal amputation of left index finger**

+7th **S68.122** **Partial traumatic metacarpophalangeal amputation of right middle finger**

+7th **S68.123** **Partial traumatic metacarpophalangeal amputation of left middle finger**

+7th **S68.124** **Partial traumatic metacarpophalangeal amputation of right ring finger**

+7th **S68.125** **Partial traumatic metacarpophalangeal amputation of left ring finger**

+7th **S68.126** **Partial traumatic metacarpophalangeal amputation of right little finger**

+7th **S68.127** **Partial traumatic metacarpophalangeal amputation of left little finger**

+7th **S68.128** **Partial traumatic metacarpophalangeal amputation of other finger**

Partial traumatic metacarpophalangeal amputation of specified finger with unspecified laterality

+7th **S68.129** **Partial traumatic metacarpophalangeal amputation of unspecified finger**

\+ **S68.4** **Traumatic amputation of hand at wrist level**

Traumatic amputation of hand NOS

Traumatic amputation of wrist

\+ **S68.41** **Complete traumatic amputation of hand at wrist level**

CC +7th **S68.411** **Complete traumatic amputation of right hand at wrist level**

CC Exclusion 7th character A see Appendix A PDX collection 1266

CC +7th **S68.412** **Complete traumatic amputation of left hand at wrist level**

CC Exclusion 7th character A see Appendix A PDX collection 1267

CC +7th **S68.419** **Complete traumatic amputation of unspecified hand at wrist level**

CC Exclusion 7th character A see Appendix A PDX collection 1268

\+ **S68.42** **Partial traumatic amputation of hand at wrist level**

CC +7th **S68.421** **Partial traumatic amputation of right hand at wrist level**

CC Exclusion 7th character A see Appendix A PDX collection 1266

CC +7th **S68.422** **Partial traumatic amputation of left hand at wrist level**

CC Exclusion 7th character A see Appendix A PDX collection 1267

CC +7th **S68.429** **Partial traumatic amputation of unspecified hand at wrist level**

CC Exclusion 7th character A see Appendix A PDX collection 1268

\+ **S68.5** **Traumatic transphalangeal amputation of thumb**

Traumatic interphalangeal joint amputation of thumb

\+ **S68.51** **Complete traumatic transphalangeal amputation of thumb**

+7th **S68.511** **Complete traumatic transphalangeal amputation of right thumb**

+7th **S68.512** **Complete traumatic transphalangeal amputation of left thumb**

+7th **S68.519** **Complete traumatic transphalangeal amputation of unspecified thumb**

\+ **S68.52** **Partial traumatic transphalangeal amputation of thumb**

+7th **S68.521** **Partial traumatic transphalangeal amputation of right thumb**

+7th **S68.522** **Partial traumatic transphalangeal amputation of left thumb**

+7th **S68.529** **Partial traumatic transphalangeal amputation of unspecified thumb**

\+ **S68.6** **Traumatic transphalangeal amputation of other and unspecified finger**

\+ **S68.61** **Complete traumatic transphalangeal amputation of other and unspecified finger(s)**

+7th **S68.610** **Complete traumatic transphalangeal amputation of right index finger**

+7th **S68.611** **Complete traumatic transphalangeal amputation of left index finger**

+7th **S68.612** **Complete traumatic transphalangeal amputation of right middle finger**

+7th **S68.613** **Complete traumatic transphalangeal amputation of left middle finger**

+7th **S68.614** **Complete traumatic transphalangeal amputation of right ring finger**

+7th **S68.615** **Complete traumatic transphalangeal amputation of left ring finger**

+7th **S68.616** **Complete traumatic transphalangeal amputation of right little finger**

+7th **S68.617** **Complete traumatic transphalangeal amputation of left little finger**

+7th **S68.618** **Complete traumatic transphalangeal amputation of other finger**

Complete traumatic transphalangeal amputation of specified finger with unspecified laterality

+7th **S68.619** **Complete traumatic transphalangeal amputation of unspecified finger**

\+ **S68.62** **Partial traumatic transphalangeal amputation of other and unspecified finger**

+7th **S68.620** **Partial traumatic transphalangeal amputation of right index finger**

+7th **S68.621** **Partial traumatic transphalangeal amputation of left index finger**

+7th **S68.622** **Partial traumatic transphalangeal amputation of right middle finger**

+7th **S68.623** **Partial traumatic transphalangeal amputation of left middle finger**

+7th **S68.624** **Partial traumatic transphalangeal amputation of right ring finger**

+7th **S68.625** **Partial traumatic transphalangeal amputation of left ring finger**

+7th **S68.626** **Partial traumatic transphalangeal amputation of right little finger**

+7th **S68.627** **Partial traumatic transphalangeal amputation of left little finger**

+7th **S68.628** **Partial traumatic transphalangeal amputation of other finger**

Partial traumatic transphalangeal amputation of specified finger with unspecified laterality

+7th **S68.629** **Partial traumatic transphalangeal amputation of unspecified finger**

\+ **S68.7** **Traumatic transmetacarpal amputation of hand**

\+ **S68.71** **Complete traumatic transmetacarpal amputation of hand**

CC +7th **S68.711** **Complete traumatic transmetacarpal amputation of right hand**

CC Exclusion 7th character A see Appendix A PDX collection 1266

CC +7th **S68.712** **Complete traumatic transmetacarpal amputation of left hand**

CC Exclusion 7th character A see Appendix A PDX collection 1267

CC +7th **S68.719** **Complete traumatic transmetacarpal amputation of unspecified hand**

CC Exclusion 7th character A see Appendix A PDX collection 1268

\+ **S68.72** **Partial traumatic transmetacarpal amputation of hand**

CC +7th **S68.721** **Partial traumatic transmetacarpal amputation of right hand**

CC Exclusion 7th character A see Appendix A PDX collection 1266

Hip Joint

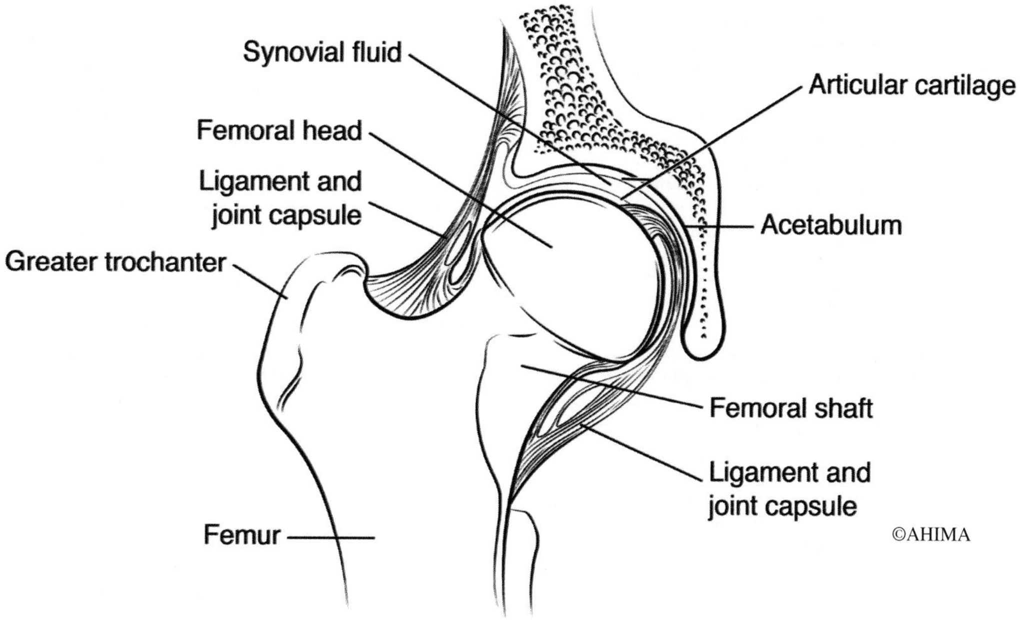

Hip Tendons and Ligaments

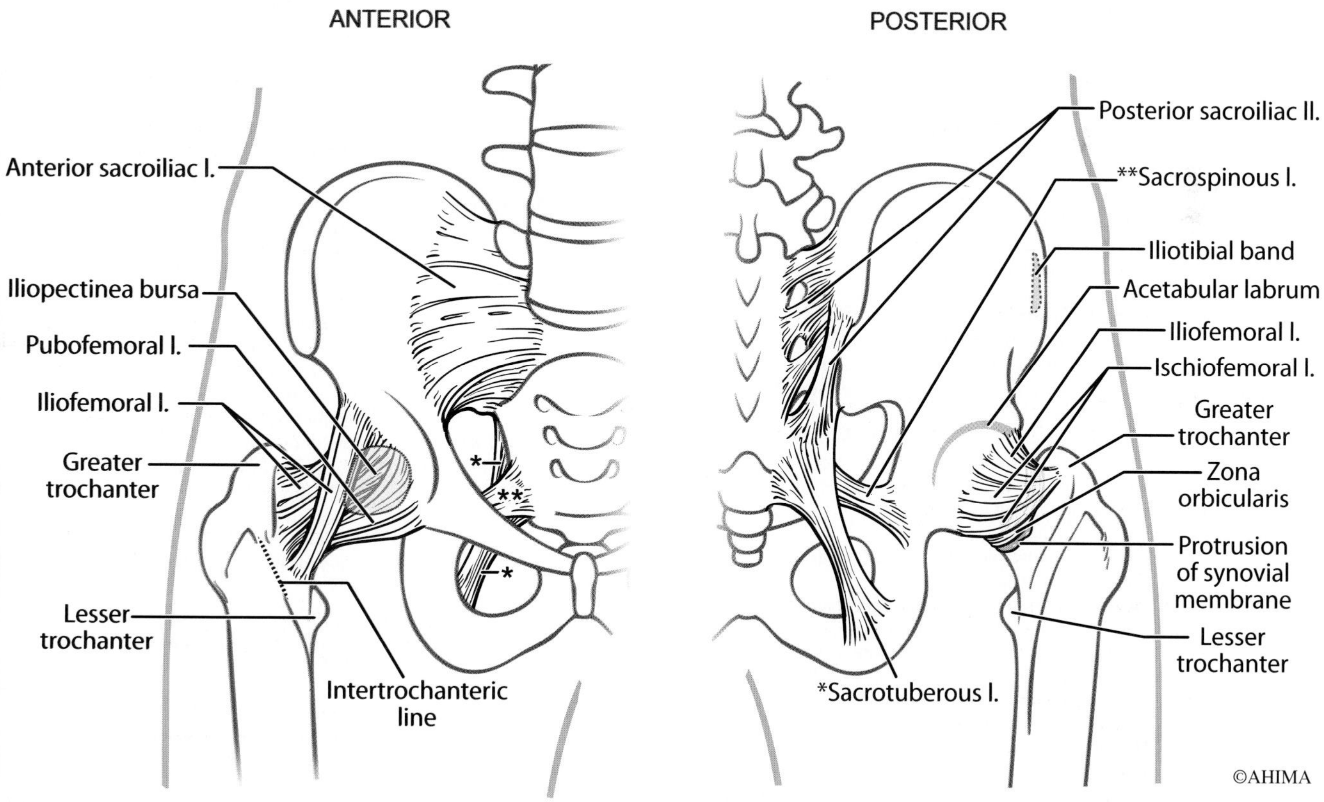

CC +7th **S68.722** **Partial traumatic transmetacarpal amputation of left hand**
CC Exclusion 7th character A see Appendix A
PDX collection 1267

CC +7th **S68.729** **Partial traumatic transmetacarpal amputation of unspecified hand**
CC Exclusion 7th character A see Appendix A
PDX collection 1268

S69 Other and unspecified injuries of wrist, hand and finger(s)

The appropriate 7th character is to be added to each code from category S69
A initial encounter
D subsequent encounter
S sequela

\+ **S69.8** **Other specified injuries of wrist, hand and finger(s)**
X+7th **S69.80** **Other specified injuries of unspecified wrist, hand and finger(s)**
X+7th **S69.81** **Other specified injuries of right wrist, hand and finger(s)**
X+7th **S69.82** **Other specified injuries of left wrist, hand and finger(s)**
\+ **S69.9** **Unspecified injury of wrist, hand and finger(s)**
X+7th **S69.90** **Unspecified injury of unspecified wrist, hand and finger(s)**
X+7th **S69.91** **Unspecified injury of right wrist, hand and finger(s)**
X+7th **S69.92** **Unspecified injury of left wrist, hand and finger(s)**

Injuries to the hip and thigh (S70-S79)

Excludes2: *burns and corrosions (T20-T32)*
frostbite (T33-T34)
snake bite (T63.0-)
venomous insect bite or sting (T63.4-)

S70 Superficial injury of hip and thigh

The appropriate 7th character is to be added to each code from category S70
A initial encounter
D subsequent encounter
S sequela

\+ **S70.0** **Contusion of hip**
X+7th **S70.00** **Contusion of unspecified hip**
X+7th **S70.01** **Contusion of right hip**
X+7th **S70.02** **Contusion of left hip**
\+ **S70.1** **Contusion of thigh**
X+7th **S70.10** **Contusion of unspecified thigh**
X+7th **S70.11** **Contusion of right thigh**
X+7th **S70.12** **Contusion of left thigh**
\+ **S70.2** **Other superficial injuries of hip**
\+ **S70.21** **Abrasion of hip**
+7th **S70.211** **Abrasion, right hip**
+7th **S70.212** **Abrasion, left hip**
+7th **S70.219** **Abrasion, unspecified hip**
\+ **S70.22** **Blister (nonthermal) of hip**
+7th **S70.221** **Blister (nonthermal), right hip**
+7th **S70.222** **Blister (nonthermal), left hip**
+7th **S70.229** **Blister (nonthermal), unspecified hip**
\+ **S70.24** **External constriction of hip**
+7th **S70.241** **External constriction, right hip**
+7th **S70.242** **External constriction, left hip**
+7th **S70.249** **External constriction, unspecified hip**
\+ **S70.25** **Superficial foreign body of hip**
Splinter in the hip
+7th **S70.251** **Superficial foreign body, right hip**
+7th **S70.252** **Superficial foreign body, left hip**
+7th **S70.259** **Superficial foreign body, unspecified hip**
\+ **S70.26** **Insect bite (nonvenomous) of hip**
+7th **S70.261** **Insect bite (nonvenomous), right hip**
+7th **S70.262** **Insect bite (nonvenomous), left hip**
+7th **S70.269** **Insect bite (nonvenomous), unspecified hip**
\+ **S70.27** **Other superficial bite of hip**
Excludes1: *open bite of hip (S71.05-)*
+7th **S70.271** **Other superficial bite of hip, right hip**
+7th **S70.272** **Other superficial bite of hip, left hip**
+7th **S70.279** **Other superficial bite of hip, unspecified hip**
\+ **S70.3** **Other superficial injuries of thigh**
\+ **S70.31** **Abrasion of thigh**
+7th **S70.311** **Abrasion, right thigh**
+7th **S70.312** **Abrasion, left thigh**
+7th **S70.319** **Abrasion, unspecified thigh**
\+ **S70.32** **Blister (nonthermal) of thigh**
+7th **S70.321** **Blister (nonthermal), right thigh**
+7th **S70.322** **Blister (nonthermal), left thigh**
+7th **S70.329** **Blister (nonthermal), unspecified thigh**
\+ **S70.34** **External constriction of thigh**
+7th **S70.341** **External constriction, right thigh**
+7th **S70.342** **External constriction, left thigh**
+7th **S70.349** **External constriction, unspecified thigh**
\+ **S70.35** **Superficial foreign body of thigh**
Splinter in the thigh
+7th **S70.351** **Superficial foreign body, right thigh**
+7th **S70.352** **Superficial foreign body, left thigh**
+7th **S70.359** **Superficial foreign body, unspecified thigh**
\+ **S70.36** **Insect bite (nonvenomous) of thigh**
+7th **S70.361** **Insect bite (nonvenomous), right thigh**
+7th **S70.362** **Insect bite (nonvenomous), left thigh**
+7th **S70.369** **Insect bite (nonvenomous), unspecified thigh**
\+ **S70.37** **Other superficial bite of thigh**
Excludes1: *open bite of thigh (S71.15)*
+7th **S70.371** **Other superficial bite of right thigh**
+7th **S70.372** **Other superficial bite of left thigh**
+7th **S70.379** **Other superficial bite of unspecified thigh**
\+ **S70.9** **Unspecified superficial injury of hip and thigh**
\+ **S70.91** **Unspecified superficial injury of hip**
+7th **S70.911** **Unspecified superficial injury of right hip**
+7th **S70.912** **Unspecified superficial injury of left hip**
+7th **S70.919** **Unspecified superficial injury of unspecified hip**
\+ **S70.92** **Unspecified superficial injury of thigh**
+7th **S70.921** **Unspecified superficial injury of right thig**
+7th **S70.922** **Unspecified superficial injury of left thigh**
+7th **S70.929** **Unspecified superficial injury of unspecified thigh**

S71 Open wound of hip and thigh

Code also any associated wound infection
Excludes1: *open fracture of hip and thigh (S72.-)*
traumatic amputation of hip and thigh (S78.-)
Excludes2: *bite of venomous animal (T63.-)*
open wound of ankle, foot and toes (S91.-)
open wound of knee and lower leg (S81.-)

The appropriate 7th character is to be added to each code from categor
S71
A initial encounter
D subsequent encounter
S sequela

\+ **S71.0** **Open wound of hip**
\+ **S71.00** **Unspecified open wound of hip**
+7th **S71.001** **Unspecified open wound, right hip**
+7th **S71.002** **Unspecified open wound, left hip**
+7th **S71.009** **Unspecified open wound, unspecified hip**
\+ **S71.01** **Laceration without foreign body of hip**
+7th **S71.011** **Laceration without foreign body, right hi**
+7th **S71.012** **Laceration without foreign body, left hip**
+7th **S71.019** **Laceration without foreign body, unspecified hip**
\+ **S71.02** **Laceration with foreign body of hip**
+7th **S71.021** **Laceration with foreign body, right hip**
+7th **S71.022** **Laceration with foreign body, left hip**
+7th **S71.029** **Laceration with foreign body, unspecified hip**
\+ **S71.03** **Puncture wound without foreign body of hip**
+7th **S71.031** **Puncture wound without foreign body, right hip**
+7th **S71.032** **Puncture wound without foreign body, lef hip**
+7th **S71.039** **Puncture wound without foreign body, unspecified hip**
\+ **S71.04** **Puncture wound with foreign body of hip**
+7th **S71.041** **Puncture wound with foreign body, right hip**
+7th **S71.042** **Puncture wound with foreign body, left hi**
+7th **S71.049** **Puncture wound with foreign body, unspecified hip**

+ **S71.05 Open bite of hip**
  Bite of hip NOS
  Excludes1: *superficial bite of hip (S70.26, S70.27)*
  +7th **S71.051 Open bite, right hip**
  +7th **S71.052 Open bite, left hip**
  +7th **S71.059 Open bite, unspecified hip**

+ **S71.1 Open wound of thigh**
  + **S71.10 Unspecified open wound of thigh**
    +7th **S71.101 Unspecified open wound, right thigh**
    +7th **S71.102 Unspecified open wound, left thigh**
    +7th **S71.109 Unspecified open wound, unspecified thigh**
  + **S71.11 Laceration without foreign body of thigh**
    +7th **S71.111 Laceration without foreign body, right thigh**
    +7th **S71.112 Laceration without foreign body, left thigh**
    +7th **S71.119 Laceration without foreign body, unspecified thigh**
  + **S71.12 Laceration with foreign body of thigh**
    +7th **S71.121 Laceration with foreign body, right thigh**
    +7th **S71.122 Laceration with foreign body, left thigh**
    +7th **S71.129 Laceration with foreign body, unspecified thigh**
  + **S71.13 Puncture wound without foreign body of thigh**
    +7th **S71.131 Puncture wound without foreign body, right thigh**
    +7th **S71.132 Puncture wound without foreign body, left thigh**
    +7th **S71.139 Puncture wound without foreign body, unspecified thigh**
  + **S71.14 Puncture wound with foreign body of thigh**
    +7th **S71.141 Puncture wound with foreign body, right thigh**
    +7th **S71.142 Puncture wound with foreign body, left thigh**
    +7th **S71.149 Puncture wound with foreign body, unspecified thigh**
  + **S71.15 Open bite of thigh**
    Bite of thigh NOS
    Excludes1: *superficial bite of thigh (S70.37-)*
    +7th **S71.151 Open bite, right thigh**
    +7th **S71.152 Open bite, left thigh**
    +7th **S71.159 Open bite, unspecified thigh**

S72 Fracture of femur

NOTE A fracture not indicated as displaced or nondisplaced should be coded to displaced
A fracture not indicated as open or closed should be coded to closed
The open fracture designations are based on the Gustilo open fracture classification

Excludes1: *traumatic amputation of hip and thigh (S78.-)*
Excludes2: *fracture of lower leg and ankle (S82.-)*
fracture of foot (S92.-)
periprosthetic fracture of prosthetic implant of hip (M97.0-)

The appropriate 7th character is to be added to all codes from category S72
- A initial encounter for closed fracture
- B initial encounter for open fracture type I or II
  initial encounter for open fracture NOS
- C initial encounter for open fracture type IIIA, IIIB, or IIIC
- D subsequent encounter for closed fracture with routine healing
- E subsequent encounter for open fracture type I or II with routine healing
- F subsequent encounter for open fracture type IIIA, IIIB, or IIIC with routine healing
- G subsequent encounter for closed fracture with delayed healing
- H subsequent encounter for open fracture type I or II with delayed healing
- J subsequent encounter for open fracture type IIIA, IIIB, or IIIC with delayed healing
- K subsequent encounter for closed fracture with nonunion
- M subsequent encounter for open fracture type I or II with nonunion
- N subsequent encounter for open fracture type IIIA, IIIB, or IIIC with nonunion
- P subsequent encounter for closed fracture with malunion
- Q subsequent encounter for open fracture type I or II with malunion
- R subsequent encounter for open fracture type IIIA, IIIB, or IIIC with malunion
- S sequela

Review coding guideline C.19.c

+ **S72.0 Fracture of head and neck of femur**
  Excludes2: *physeal fracture of upper end of femur (S79.0-)*
  + **S72.00 Fracture of unspecified part of neck of femur**
    Fracture of hip NOS
    Fracture of neck of femur NOS
    CC MCC +7th **S72.001 Fracture of unspecified part of neck of right femur**
      CC Exclusion 7th characters K - R see Appendix A PDX collection 0897
      MCC Exclusion 7th character A see Appendix A PDX collection 1297
      MCC Exclusion 7th characters B & C see Appendix A PDX collection 1298
      HAC 7th characters A - C see Appendix B for HAC conditional logic
    CC MCC +7th **S72.002 Fracture of unspecified part of neck of left femur**
      CC Exclusion 7th characters K - R see Appendix A PDX collection 0897
      MCC Exclusion 7th character A see Appendix A PDX collection 1299
      MCC Exclusion 7th characters B & C see Appendix A PDX collection 1298
      HAC 7th characters A - C see Appendix B for HAC conditional logic
      AHA CC: 1Q, 2015, 3-21; 4Q, 2015, 36-37
    CC MCC +7th **S72.009 Fracture of unspecified part of neck of unspecified femur**
      CC Exclusion 7th characters K - R see Appendix A PDX collection 0897
      MCC Exclusion 7th characters A - C see Appendix A PDX collection 1298
      HAC 7th characters A - C see Appendix B for HAC conditional logic
  + **S72.01 Unspecified intracapsular fracture of femur**
    Subcapital fracture of femur
    CC MCC +7th **S72.011 Unspecified intracapsular fracture of right femur**
      CC Exclusion 7th characters K - R see Appendix A PDX collection 0897
      MCC Exclusion 7th character A see Appendix A PDX collection 1297
      MCC Exclusion 7th characters B & C see Appendix A PDX collection 1298
      HAC 7th characters A - C see Appendix B for HAC conditional logic
    CC MCC +7th **S72.012 Unspecified intracapsular fracture of left femur**
      CC Exclusion 7th characters K - R see Appendix A PDX collection 0897
      MCC Exclusion 7th character A see Appendix A PDX collection 1299
      MCC Exclusion 7th characters B & C see Appendix A PDX collection 1298
      HAC 7th characters A - C see Appendix B for HAC conditional logic
    CC MCC +7th **S72.019 Unspecified intracapsular fracture of unspecified femur**
      CC Exclusion 7th characters K - R see Appendix A PDX collection 0897
      MCC Exclusion 7th characters A - C see Appendix A PDX collection 1298
      HAC 7th characters A - C see Appendix B for HAC conditional logic
  + **S72.02 Fracture of epiphysis (separation) (upper) of femur**
    Transepiphyseal fracture of femur
    Excludes1: *capital femoral epiphyseal fracture (pediatric) of femur (S79.01-)*
    Salter-Harris Type I physeal fracture of upper end of femur (S79.01-)
    CC MCC +7th **S72.021 Displaced fracture of epiphysis (separation) (upper) of right femur**
      CC Exclusion 7th characters K - R see Appendix A PDX collection 0897
      MCC Exclusion 7th character A see Appendix A PDX collection 1297
      MCC Exclusion 7th characters B & C see Appendix A PDX collection 1298
      HAC 7th characters A - C see Appendix B for HAC conditional logic

CC MCC +7th **S72.022** **Displaced fracture of epiphysis (separation) (upper) of left femur**
CC Exclusion 7th characters K - R see Appendix A PDX collection 0897
MCC Exclusion 7th character A see Appendix A PDX collection 1299
MCC Exclusion 7th characters B & C see Appendix A PDX collection 1298
HAC 7th characters A - C see Appendix B for HAC conditional logic

CC MCC +7th **S72.023** **Displaced fracture of epiphysis (separation) (upper) of unspecified femur**
CC Exclusion 7th characters K - R see Appendix A PDX collection 0897
MCC Exclusion 7th characters A - C see Appendix A PDX collection 1298
HAC 7th characters A - C see Appendix B for HAC conditional logic

CC MCC +7th **S72.024** **Nondisplaced fracture of epiphysis (separation) (upper) of right femur**
CC Exclusion 7th characters K - R see Appendix A PDX collection 0897
MCC Exclusion 7th character A see Appendix A PDX collection 1297
MCC Exclusion 7th characters B & C see Appendix A PDX collection 1298
HAC 7th characters A - C see Appendix B for HAC conditional logic

CC MCC +7th **S72.025** **Nondisplaced fracture of epiphysis (separation) (upper) of left femur**
CC Exclusion 7th characters K - R see Appendix A PDX collection 0897
MCC Exclusion 7th character A see Appendix A PDX collection 1299
MCC Exclusion 7th characters B & C see Appendix A PDX collection 1298
HAC 7th characters A - C see Appendix B for HAC conditional logic

CC MCC +7th **S72.026** **Nondisplaced fracture of epiphysis (separation) (upper) of unspecified femur**
CC Exclusion 7th characters K - R see Appendix A PDX collection 0897
MCC Exclusion 7th characters A - C see Appendix A PDX collection 1298
HAC 7th characters A - C see Appendix B for HAC conditional logic

\+ **S72.03** **Midcervical fracture of femur**
Transcervical fracture of femur NOS

CC MCC +7th **S72.031** **Displaced midcervical fracture of right femur**
CC Exclusion 7th characters K - R see Appendix A PDX collection 0897
MCC Exclusion 7th character A see Appendix A PDX collection 1297
MCC Exclusion 7th characters B & C see Appendix A PDX collection 1298
HAC 7th characters A - C see Appendix B for HAC conditional logic

CC MCC +7th **S72.032** **Displaced midcervical fracture of left femur**
CC Exclusion 7th characters K - R see Appendix A PDX collection 0897
MCC Exclusion 7th character A see Appendix A PDX collection 1299
MCC Exclusion 7th characters B & C see Appendix A PDX collection 1298
HAC 7th characters A - C see Appendix B for HAC conditional logic

CC MCC +7th **S72.033** **Displaced midcervical fracture of unspecified femur**
CC Exclusion 7th characters K - R see Appendix A PDX collection 0897
MCC Exclusion 7th characters A - C see Appendix A PDX collection 1298
HAC 7th characters A - C see Appendix B for HAC conditional logic

CC MCC +7th **S72.034** **Nondisplaced midcervical fracture of right femur**
CC Exclusion 7th characters K - R see Appendix A PDX collection 0897
MCC Exclusion 7th character A see Appendix A PDX collection 1297
MCC Exclusion 7th characters B & C see Appendix A PDX collection 1298
HAC 7th characters A - C see Appendix B for HAC conditional logic

CC MCC +7th **S72.035** **Nondisplaced midcervical fracture of left femur**
CC Exclusion 7th characters K - R see Appendix A PDX collection 0897
MCC Exclusion 7th character A see Appendix PDX collection 1299
MCC Exclusion 7th characters B & C see Appendix A PDX collection 1298
HAC 7th characters A - C see Appendix B for HAC conditional logic

CC MCC +7th **S72.036** **Nondisplaced midcervical fracture of unspecified femur**
CC Exclusion 7th characters K - R see Appendix A PDX collection 0897
MCC Exclusion 7th characters A - C see Appendix A PDX collection 1298
HAC 7th characters A - C see Appendix B for HAC conditional logic

\+ **S72.04** **Fracture of base of neck of femur**
Cervicotrochanteric fracture of femur

CC MCC +7th **S72.041** **Displaced fracture of base of neck of righ femur**
CC Exclusion 7th characters K - R see Appendix A PDX collection 0897
MCC Exclusion 7th character A see Appendix PDX collection 1297
MCC Exclusion 7th characters B & C see Appendix A PDX collection 1298
HAC 7th characters A - C see Appendix B for HAC conditional logic

CC MCC +7th **S72.042** **Displaced fracture of base of neck of left femur**
CC Exclusion 7th characters K - R see Appendix A PDX collection 0897
MCC Exclusion 7th character A see Appendi PDX collection 1299
MCC Exclusion 7th characters B & C see Appendix A PDX collection 1298
HAC 7th characters A - C see Appendix B for HAC conditional logic

CC MCC +7th **S72.043** **Displaced fracture of base of neck of unspecified femur**
CC Exclusion 7th characters K - R see Appendix A PDX collection 0897
MCC Exclusion 7th characters A - C see Appendix A PDX collection 1298
HAC 7th characters A - C see Appendix B for HAC conditional logic

CC MCC +7th **S72.044** **Nondisplaced fracture of base of neck of right femur**
CC Exclusion 7th characters K - R see Appendix A PDX collection 0897
MCC Exclusion 7th character A see Appendi PDX collection 1297
MCC Exclusion 7th characters B & C see Appendix A PDX collection 1298
HAC 7th characters A - C see Appendix B for HAC conditional logic

CC MCC +7th **S72.045** **Nondisplaced fracture of base of neck of left femur**
CC Exclusion 7th characters K - R see Appendix A PDX collection 0897
MCC Exclusion 7th character A see Appendi PDX collection 1299
MCC Exclusion 7th characters B & C see Appendix A PDX collection 1298
HAC 7th characters A - C see Appendix B for HAC conditional logic

CC MCC +7th **S72.046** **Nondisplaced fracture of base of neck of unspecified femur**
CC Exclusion 7th characters K - R see Appendix A PDX collection 0897
MCC Exclusion 7th characters A - C see Appendix A PDX collection 1298
HAC 7th characters A - C see Appendix B for HAC conditional logic

\+ **S72.05** **Unspecified fracture of head of femur**
Fracture of head of femur NOS

CC MCC +7th **S72.051** **Unspecified fracture of head of right fem**
CC Exclusion 7th characters K - R see Appendix A PDX collection 0897
MCC Exclusion 7th character A see Append PDX collection 1297
MCC Exclusion 7th characters B & C see Appendix A PDX collection 1298
HAC 7th characters A - C see Appendix B fo HAC conditional logic

CC MCC +7th **S72.052** **Unspecified fracture of head of left femur**
CC Exclusion 7th characters K - R see Appendix A PDX collection 0897
MCC Exclusion 7th character A see Appendix A PDX collection 1299
MCC Exclusion 7th characters B & C see Appendix A PDX collection 1298
HAC 7th characters A - C see Appendix B for HAC conditional logic

CC MCC +7th **S72.059** **Unspecified fracture of head of unspecified femur**
CC Exclusion 7th characters K - R see Appendix A PDX collection 0897
MCC Exclusion 7th characters A - C see Appendix A PDX collection 1298
HAC 7th characters A - C see Appendix B for HAC conditional logic

+ **S72.06 Articular fracture of head of femur**

CC MCC +7th **S72.061** **Displaced articular fracture of head of right femur**
CC Exclusion 7th characters K - R see Appendix A PDX collection 0897
MCC Exclusion 7th character A see Appendix A PDX collection 1297
MCC Exclusion 7th characters B & C see Appendix A PDX collection 1298
HAC 7th characters A - C see Appendix B for HAC conditional logic

CC MCC +7th **S72.062** **Displaced articular fracture of head of left femur**
CC Exclusion 7th characters K - R see Appendix A PDX collection 0897
MCC Exclusion 7th character A see Appendix A PDX collection 1299
MCC Exclusion 7th characters B & C see Appendix A PDX collection 1298
HAC 7th characters A - C see Appendix B for HAC conditional logic

CC MCC +7th **S72.063** **Displaced articular fracture of head of unspecified femur**
CC Exclusion 7th characters K - R see Appendix A PDX collection 0897
MCC Exclusion 7th characters A - C see Appendix A PDX collection 1298
HAC 7th characters A - C see Appendix B for HAC conditional logic

CC MCC +7th **S72.064** **Nondisplaced articular fracture of head of right femur**
CC Exclusion 7th characters K - R see Appendix A PDX collection 0897
MCC Exclusion 7th character A see Appendix A PDX collection 1297
MCC Exclusion 7th characters B & C see Appendix A PDX collection 1298
HAC 7th characters A - C see Appendix B for HAC conditional logic

CC MCC +7th **S72.065** **Nondisplaced articular fracture of head of left femur**
CC Exclusion 7th characters K - R see Appendix A PDX collection 0897
MCC Exclusion 7th character A see Appendix A PDX collection 1299
MCC Exclusion 7th characters B & C see Appendix A PDX collection 1298
HAC 7th characters A - C see Appendix B for HAC conditional logic

CC MCC +7th **S72.066** **Nondisplaced articular fracture of head of unspecified femur**
CC Exclusion 7th characters K - R see Appendix A PDX collection 0897
MCC Exclusion 7th characters A - C see Appendix A PDX collection 1298
HAC 7th characters A - C see Appendix B for HAC conditional logic

+ **S72.09 Other fracture of head and neck of femur**

CC MCC +7th **S72.091** **Other fracture of head and neck of right femur**
CC Exclusion 7th characters K - R see Appendix A PDX collection 0897
MCC Exclusion 7th character A see Appendix A PDX collection 1297
MCC Exclusion 7th characters B & C see Appendix A PDX collection 1298
HAC 7th characters A - C see Appendix B for HAC conditional logic

CC MCC +7th **S72.092** **Other fracture of head and neck of left femur**
CC Exclusion 7th characters K - R see Appendix A PDX collection 0897
MCC Exclusion 7th character A see Appendix A PDX collection 1299
MCC Exclusion 7th characters B & C see Appendix A PDX collection 1298
HAC 7th characters A - C see Appendix B for HAC conditional logic

CC MCC +7th **S72.099** **Other fracture of head and neck of unspecified femur**
CC Exclusion 7th characters K - R see Appendix A PDX collection 0897
MCC Exclusion 7th characters A - C see Appendix A PDX collection 1298
HAC 7th characters A - C see Appendix B for HAC conditional logic

+ **S72.1 Pertrochanteric fracture**

+ **S72.10 Unspecified trochanteric fracture of femur**
Fracture of trochanter NOS

CC MCC **S72.101** **Unspecified trochanteric fracture of right femur**
CC Exclusion 7th characters K - R see Appendix A PDX collection 0897
MCC Exclusion 7th character A see Appendix A PDX collection 1297
MCC Exclusion 7th characters B & C see Appendix A PDX collection 1298
HAC 7th characters A - C see Appendix B for HAC conditional logic

CC MCC **S72.102** **Unspecified trochanteric fracture of left femur**
CC Exclusion 7th characters K - R see Appendix A PDX collection 0897
MCC Exclusion 7th character A see Appendix A PDX collection 1299
MCC Exclusion 7th characters B & C see Appendix A PDX collection 1298
HAC 7th characters A - C see Appendix B for HAC conditional logic

CC MCC **S72.109** **Unspecified trochanteric fracture of unspecified femur**
CC Exclusion 7th characters K - R see Appendix A PDX collection 0897
MCC Exclusion 7th characters A - C see Appendix A PDX collection 1298
HAC 7th characters A - C see Appendix B for HAC conditional logic

+ **S72.11 Fracture of greater trochanter of femur**

CC MCC +7th **S72.111** **Displaced fracture of greater trochanter of right femur**
CC Exclusion 7th characters K - R see Appendix A PDX collection 0897
MCC Exclusion 7th character A see Appendix A PDX collection 1297
MCC Exclusion 7th characters B & C see Appendix A PDX collection 1298
HAC 7th characters A - C see Appendix B for HAC conditional logic

CC MCC +7th **S72.112** **Displaced fracture of greater trochanter of left femur**
CC Exclusion 7th characters K - R see Appendix A PDX collection 0897
MCC Exclusion 7th character A see Appendix A PDX collection 1299
MCC Exclusion 7th characters B & C see Appendix A PDX collection 1298
HAC 7th characters A - C see Appendix B for HAC conditional logic

CC MCC +7th **S72.113** **Displaced fracture of greater trochanter of unspecified femur**
CC Exclusion 7th characters K - R see Appendix A PDX collection 0897
MCC Exclusion 7th characters A - C see Appendix A PDX collection 1298
HAC 7th characters A - C see Appendix B for HAC conditional logic

CC MCC +7th **S72.114** **Nondisplaced fracture of greater trochanter of right femur**
CC Exclusion 7th characters K - R see Appendix A PDX collection 0897
MCC Exclusion 7th character A see Appendix A PDX collection 1297
MCC Exclusion 7th characters B & C see Appendix A PDX collection 1298
HAC 7th characters A - C see Appendix B for HAC conditional logic

CC MCC +7th **S72.115** **Nondisplaced fracture of greater trochanter of left femur**
CC Exclusion 7th characters K - R see Appendix A PDX collection 0897
MCC Exclusion 7th character A see Appendix A PDX collection 1299
MCC Exclusion 7th characters B & C see Appendix A PDX collection 1298
HAC 7th characters A - C see Appendix B for HAC conditional logic

CC MCC +7th **S72.116** **Nondisplaced fracture of greater trochanter of unspecified femur**
CC Exclusion 7th characters K - R see Appendix A PDX collection 0897
MCC Exclusion 7th characters A - C see Appendix A PDX collection 1298
HAC 7th characters A - C see Appendix B for HAC conditional logic

\+ **S72.12** **Fracture of lesser trochanter of femur**

CC MCC +7th **S72.121** **Displaced fracture of lesser trochanter of right femur**
CC Exclusion 7th characters K - R see Appendix A PDX collection 0897
MCC Exclusion 7th character A see Appendix A PDX collection 1297
MCC Exclusion 7th characters B & C see Appendix A PDX collection 1298
HAC 7th characters A - C see Appendix B for HAC conditional logic

CC MCC +7th **S72.122** **Displaced fracture of lesser trochanter of left femur**
CC Exclusion 7th characters K - R see Appendix A PDX collection 0897
MCC Exclusion 7th character A see Appendix A PDX collection 1299
MCC Exclusion 7th characters B & C see Appendix A PDX collection 1298
HAC 7th characters A - C see Appendix B for HAC conditional logic

CC MCC +7th **S72.123** **Displaced fracture of lesser trochanter of unspecified femur**
CC Exclusion 7th characters K - R see Appendix A PDX collection 0897
MCC Exclusion 7th characters A - C see Appendix A PDX collection 1298
HAC 7th characters A - C see Appendix B for HAC conditional logic

CC MCC +7th **S72.124** **Nondisplaced fracture of lesser trochanter of right femur**
CC Exclusion 7th characters K - R see Appendix A PDX collection 0897
MCC Exclusion 7th character A see Appendix A PDX collection 1297
MCC Exclusion 7th characters B & C see Appendix A PDX collection 1298
HAC 7th characters A - C see Appendix B for HAC conditional logic

CC MCC +7th **S72.125** **Nondisplaced fracture of lesser trochanter of left femur**
CC Exclusion 7th characters K - R see Appendix A PDX collection 0897
MCC Exclusion 7th character A see Appendix A PDX collection 1299
MCC Exclusion 7th characters B & C see Appendix A PDX collection 1298
HAC 7th characters A - C see Appendix B for HAC conditional logic

CC MCC +7th **S72.126** **Nondisplaced fracture of lesser trochanter of unspecified femur**
CC Exclusion 7th characters K - R see Appendix A PDX collection 0897
MCC Exclusion 7th characters A - C see Appendix A PDX collection 1298
HAC 7th characters A - C see Appendix B for HAC conditional logic

\+ **S72.13** **Apophyseal fracture of femur**
Excludes1: *chronic (nontraumatic) slipped upper femoral epiphysis (M93.0-)*

CC MCC +7th **S72.131** **Displaced apophyseal fracture of right femur**
CC Exclusion 7th characters K - R see Appendix A PDX collection 0897
MCC Exclusion 7th character A see Appendix A PDX collection 1297
MCC Exclusion 7th characters B & C see Appendix A PDX collection 1298
HAC 7th characters A - C see Appendix B for HAC conditional logic

CC MCC +7th **S72.132** **Displaced apophyseal fracture of left femur**
CC Exclusion 7th characters K - R see Appendix A PDX collection 0897
MCC Exclusion 7th character A see Appendix A PDX collection 1299
MCC Exclusion 7th characters B & C see Appendix A PDX collection 1298
HAC 7th characters A - C see Appendix B for HAC conditional logic

CC MCC +7th **S72.133** **Displaced apophyseal fracture of unspecified femur**
CC Exclusion 7th characters K - R see Appendix A PDX collection 0897
MCC Exclusion 7th characters A - C see Appendix A PDX collection 1298
HAC 7th characters A - C see Appendix B for HAC conditional logic

CC MCC +7th **S72.134** **Nondisplaced apophyseal fracture of right femur**
CC Exclusion 7th characters K - R see Appendix A PDX collection 0897
MCC Exclusion 7th character A see Appendix A PDX collection 1297
MCC Exclusion 7th characters B & C see Appendix A PDX collection 1298
HAC 7th characters A - C see Appendix B for HAC conditional logic

CC MCC +7th **S72.135** **Nondisplaced apophyseal fracture of left femur**
CC Exclusion 7th characters K - R see Appendix A PDX collection 0897
MCC Exclusion 7th character A see Appendix A PDX collection 1299
MCC Exclusion 7th characters B & C see Appendix A PDX collection 1298
HAC 7th characters A - C see Appendix B for HAC conditional logic

CC MCC +7th **S72.136** **Nondisplaced apophyseal fracture of unspecified femur**
CC Exclusion 7th characters K - R see Appendix A PDX collection 0897
MCC Exclusion 7th characters A - C see Appendix A PDX collection 1298
HAC 7th characters A - C see Appendix B for HAC conditional logic

\+ **S72.14** **Intertrochanteric fracture of femur**

CC MCC +7th **S72.141** **Displaced intertrochanteric fracture of right femur**
CC Exclusion 7th characters K - R see Appendix A PDX collection 0897
MCC Exclusion 7th character A see Appendix A PDX collection 1297
MCC Exclusion 7th characters B & C see Appendix A PDX collection 1298
AHA CC: 4Q, 2013, 128-129; 3Q, 2016, 16-17
HAC 7th characters A - C see Appendix B for HAC conditional logic

CC MCC +7th **S72.142** **Displaced intertrochanteric fracture of left femur**
CC Exclusion 7th characters K - R see Appendix A PDX collection 0897
MCC Exclusion 7th character A see Appendix A PDX collection 1299
MCC Exclusion 7th characters B & C see Appendix A PDX collection 1298
HAC 7th characters A - C see Appendix B for HAC conditional logic

CC MCC +7th **S72.143** **Displaced intertrochanteric fracture of unspecified femur**
CC Exclusion 7th characters K - R see Appendix A PDX collection 0897
MCC Exclusion 7th characters A - C see Appendix A PDX collection 1298
HAC 7th characters A - C see Appendix B for HAC conditional logic

CC MCC +7th **S72.144** **Nondisplaced intertrochanteric fracture of right femur**
CC Exclusion 7th characters K - R see Appendix A PDX collection 0897
MCC Exclusion 7th character A see Appendix A PDX collection 1297
MCC Exclusion 7th characters B & C see Appendix A PDX collection 1298
HAC 7th characters A - C see Appendix B for HAC conditional logic

CC MCC +7th **S72.145** **Nondisplaced intertrochanteric fracture of left femur**
CC Exclusion 7th characters K - R see Appendix A PDX collection 0897
MCC Exclusion 7th character A see Appendix A PDX collection 1299
MCC Exclusion 7th characters B & C see Appendix A PDX collection 1298
HAC 7th characters A - C see Appendix B for HAC conditional logic

CC MCC +7th **S72.146** **Nondisplaced intertrochanteric fracture of unspecified femur**
CC Exclusion 7th characters K - R see Appendix A PDX collection 0897
MCC Exclusion 7th characters A - C see Appendix A PDX collection 1298
HAC 7th characters A - C see Appendix B for HAC conditional logic

\+ S72.2 **Subtrochanteric fracture of femur**

CC MCC X+7th **S72.21** **Displaced subtrochanteric fracture of right femur**
CC Exclusion 7th characters K - R see Appendix A PDX collection 0897
MCC Exclusion 7th characters A - C see Appendix A PDX collection 1298
HAC 7th characters A - C see Appendix B for HAC conditional logic

CC MCC X+7th **S72.22** **Displaced subtrochanteric fracture of left femur**
CC Exclusion 7th characters K - R see Appendix A PDX collection 0897
MCC Exclusion 7th characters A - C see Appendix A PDX collection 1298
HAC 7th characters A - C see Appendix B for HAC conditional logic

CC MCC X+7th **S72.23** **Displaced subtrochanteric fracture of unspecified femur**
CC Exclusion 7th characters K - R see Appendix A PDX collection 0897
MCC Exclusion 7th characters A - C see Appendix A PDX collection 1298
HAC 7th characters A - C see Appendix B for HAC conditional logic

CC MCC X+7th **S72.24** **Nondisplaced subtrochanteric fracture of right femur**
CC Exclusion 7th characters K - R see Appendix A PDX collection 0897
MCC Exclusion 7th characters A - C see Appendix A PDX collection 1298
HAC 7th characters A - C see Appendix B for HAC conditional logic

CC MCC X+7th **S72.25** **Nondisplaced subtrochanteric fracture of left femur**
CC Exclusion 7th characters K - R see Appendix A PDX collection 0897
MCC Exclusion 7th characters A - C see Appendix A PDX collection 1298
HAC 7th characters A - C see Appendix B for HAC conditional logic

CC MCC X+7th **S72.26** **Nondisplaced subtrochanteric fracture of unspecified femur**
CC Exclusion 7th characters K - R see Appendix A PDX collection 0897
MCC Exclusion 7th characters A - C see Appendix A PDX collection 1298
HAC 7th characters A - C see Appendix B for HAC conditional logic

\+ S72.3 **Fracture of shaft of femur**

\+ S72.30 **Unspecified fracture of shaft of femur**

CC MCC +7th **S72.301** **Unspecified fracture of shaft of right femur**
CC Exclusion 7th characters K - R see Appendix A PDX collection 0897
MCC Exclusion 7th character A see Appendix A PDX collection 1297
MCC Exclusion 7th characters B & C see Appendix A PDX collection 1298
HAC 7th characters A - C see Appendix B for HAC conditional logic

CC MCC +7th **S72.302** **Unspecified fracture of shaft of left femur**
CC Exclusion 7th characters K - R see Appendix A PDX collection 0897
MCC Exclusion 7th character A see Appendix A PDX collection 1299
MCC Exclusion 7th characters B & C see Appendix A PDX collection 1298
HAC 7th characters A - C see Appendix B for HAC conditional logic

CC MCC +7th **S72.309** **Unspecified fracture of shaft of unspecified femur**
CC Exclusion 7th characters K - R see Appendix A PDX collection 0897
MCC Exclusion 7th characters A - C see Appendix A PDX collection 1298
HAC 7th characters A - C see Appendix B for HAC conditional logic

\+ S72.32 **Transverse fracture of shaft of femur**

CC MCC +7th **S72.321** **Displaced transverse fracture of shaft of right femur**
CC Exclusion 7th characters K - R see Appendix A PDX collection 0897
MCC Exclusion 7th character A see Appendix A PDX collection 1297
MCC Exclusion 7th characters B & C see Appendix A PDX collection 1298
HAC 7th characters A - C see Appendix B for HAC conditional logic

CC MCC +7th **S72.322** **Displaced transverse fracture of shaft of left femur**
CC Exclusion 7th characters K - R see Appendix A PDX collection 0897
MCC Exclusion 7th character A see Appendix A PDX collection 1299
MCC Exclusion 7th characters B & C see Appendix A PDX collection 1298
HAC 7th characters A - C see Appendix B for HAC conditional logic

CC MCC +7th **S72.323** **Displaced transverse fracture of shaft of unspecified femur**
CC Exclusion 7th characters K - R see Appendix A PDX collection 0897
MCC Exclusion 7th characters A - C see Appendix A PDX collection 1298
HAC 7th characters A - C see Appendix B for HAC conditional logic

CC MCC +7th **S72.324** **Nondisplaced transverse fracture of shaft of right femur**
CC Exclusion 7th characters K - R see Appendix A PDX collection 0897
MCC Exclusion 7th character A see Appendix A PDX collection 1297
MCC Exclusion 7th characters B & C see Appendix A PDX collection 1298
HAC 7th characters A - C see Appendix B for HAC conditional logic

CC MCC +7th **S72.325** **Nondisplaced transverse fracture of shaft of left femur**
CC Exclusion 7th characters K - R see Appendix A PDX collection 0897
MCC Exclusion 7th character A see Appendix A PDX collection 1299
MCC Exclusion 7th characters B & C see Appendix A PDX collection 1298
HAC 7th characters A - C see Appendix B for HAC conditional logic

CC MCC +7th **S72.326** **Nondisplaced transverse fracture of shaft of unspecified femur**
CC Exclusion 7th characters K - R see Appendix A PDX collection 0897
MCC Exclusion 7th characters A - C see Appendix A PDX collection 1298
HAC 7th characters A - C see Appendix B for HAC conditional logic

\+ S72.33 **Oblique fracture of shaft of femur**

CC MCC +7th **S72.331** **Displaced oblique fracture of shaft of right femur**
CC Exclusion 7th characters K - R see Appendix A PDX collection 0897
MCC Exclusion 7th character A see Appendix A PDX collection 1297
MCC Exclusion 7th characters B & C see Appendix A PDX collection 1298
HAC 7th characters A - C see Appendix B for HAC conditional logic

CC MCC +7th **S72.332** **Displaced oblique fracture of shaft of left femur**
CC Exclusion 7th characters K - R see Appendix A PDX collection 0897
MCC Exclusion 7th character A see Appendix A PDX collection 1299
MCC Exclusion 7th characters B & C see Appendix A PDX collection 1298
HAC 7th characters A - C see Appendix B for HAC conditional logic

CC MCC +7th **S72.333** **Displaced oblique fracture of shaft of unspecified femur**
CC Exclusion 7th characters K - R see Appendix A PDX collection 0897
MCC Exclusion 7th characters A - C see Appendix A PDX collection 1298
HAC 7th characters A - C see Appendix B for HAC conditional logic

CC MCC +7th **S72.334** **Nondisplaced oblique fracture of shaft of right femur**
CC Exclusion 7th characters K - R see Appendix A PDX collection 0897
MCC Exclusion 7th character A see Appendix A PDX collection 1297
MCC Exclusion 7th characters B & C see Appendix A PDX collection 1298
HAC 7th characters A - C see Appendix B for HAC conditional logic

CC MCC +7th **S72.335** **Nondisplaced oblique fracture of shaft of left femur**
CC Exclusion 7th characters K - R see Appendix A PDX collection 0897
MCC Exclusion 7th character A see Appendix A PDX collection 1299
MCC Exclusion 7th characters B & C see Appendix A PDX collection 1298
HAC 7th characters A - C see Appendix B for HAC conditional logic

CC MCC +7th **S72.336** **Nondisplaced oblique fracture of shaft of unspecified femur**
CC Exclusion 7th characters K - R see Appendix A PDX collection 0897
MCC Exclusion 7th characters A - C see Appendix A PDX collection 1298
HAC 7th characters A - C see Appendix B for HAC conditional logic

+ **S72.34** **Spiral fracture of shaft of femur**

CC MCC +7th **S72.341** **Displaced spiral fracture of shaft of right femur**
CC Exclusion 7th characters K - R see Appendix A PDX collection 0897
MCC Exclusion 7th character A see Appendix A PDX collection 1297
MCC Exclusion 7th characters B & C see Appendix A PDX collection 1298
HAC 7th characters A - C see Appendix B for HAC conditional logic

CC MCC +7th **S72.342** **Displaced spiral fracture of shaft of left femur**
CC Exclusion 7th characters K - R see Appendix A PDX collection 0897
MCC Exclusion 7th character A see Appendix A PDX collection 1299
MCC Exclusion 7th characters B & C see Appendix A PDX collection 1298
HAC 7th characters A - C see Appendix B for HAC conditional logic

CC MCC +7th **S72.343** **Displaced spiral fracture of shaft of unspecified femur**
CC Exclusion 7th characters K - R see Appendix A PDX collection 0897
MCC Exclusion 7th characters A - C see Appendix A PDX collection 1298
HAC 7th characters A - C see Appendix B for HAC conditional logic

CC MCC +7th **S72.344** **Nondisplaced spiral fracture of shaft of right femur**
CC Exclusion 7th characters K - R see Appendix A PDX collection 0897
MCC Exclusion 7th character A see Appendix A PDX collection 1297
MCC Exclusion 7th characters B & C see Appendix A PDX collection 1298
HAC 7th characters A - C see Appendix B for HAC conditional logic

CC MCC +7th **S72.345** **Nondisplaced spiral fracture of shaft of left femur**
CC Exclusion 7th characters K - R see Appendix A PDX collection 0897
MCC Exclusion 7th character A see Appendix A PDX collection 1299
MCC Exclusion 7th characters B & C see Appendix A PDX collection 1298
HAC 7th characters A - C see Appendix B for HAC conditional logic

CC MCC +7th **S72.346** **Nondisplaced spiral fracture of shaft of unspecified femur**
CC Exclusion 7th characters K - R see Appendix A PDX collection 0897
MCC Exclusion 7th characters A - C see Appendix A PDX collection 1298
HAC 7th characters A - C see Appendix B for HAC conditional logic

+ **S72.35** **Comminuted fracture of shaft of femur**

CC MCC +7th **S72.351** **Displaced comminuted fracture of shaft of right femur**
CC Exclusion 7th characters K - R see Appendix A PDX collection 0897
MCC Exclusion 7th character A see Appendix A PDX collection 1297
MCC Exclusion 7th characters B & C see Appendix A PDX collection 1298
HAC 7th characters A - C see Appendix B for HAC conditional logic

CC MCC +7th **S72.352** **Displaced comminuted fracture of shaft of left femur**
CC Exclusion 7th characters K - R see Appendix A PDX collection 0897
MCC Exclusion 7th character A see Appendix A PDX collection 1299
MCC Exclusion 7th characters B & C see Appendix A PDX collection 1298
HAC 7th characters A - C see Appendix B for HAC conditional logic

CC MCC +7th **S72.353** **Displaced comminuted fracture of shaft of unspecified femur**
CC Exclusion 7th characters K - R see Appendix A PDX collection 0897
MCC Exclusion 7th characters A - C see Appendix A PDX collection 1298
HAC 7th characters A - C see Appendix B for HAC conditional logic

CC MCC +7th **S72.354** **Nondisplaced comminuted fracture of shaft of right femur**
CC Exclusion 7th characters K - R see Appendix A PDX collection 0897
MCC Exclusion 7th character A see Appendix A PDX collection 1297
MCC Exclusion 7th characters B & C see Appendix A PDX collection 1298
HAC 7th characters A - C see Appendix B for HAC conditional logic

CC MCC +7th **S72.355** **Nondisplaced comminuted fracture of shaft of left femur**
CC Exclusion 7th characters K - R see Appendix A PDX collection 0897
MCC Exclusion 7th character A see Appendix A PDX collection 1299
MCC Exclusion 7th characters B & C see Appendix A PDX collection 1298
HAC 7th characters A - C see Appendix B for HAC conditional logic

CC MCC +7th **S72.356** **Nondisplaced comminuted fracture of shaft of unspecified femur**
CC Exclusion 7th characters K - R see Appendix A PDX collection 0897
MCC Exclusion 7th characters A - C see Appendix A PDX collection 1298
HAC 7th characters A - C see Appendix B for HAC conditional logic

+ **S72.36** **Segmental fracture of shaft of femur**

CC MCC +7th **S72.361** **Displaced segmental fracture of shaft of right femur**
CC Exclusion 7th characters K - R see Appendix A PDX collection 0897
MCC Exclusion 7th character A see Appendix A PDX collection 1297
MCC Exclusion 7th characters B & C see Appendix A PDX collection 1298
HAC 7th characters A - C see Appendix B for HAC conditional logic

CC MCC +7th **S72.362** **Displaced segmental fracture of shaft of left femur**
CC Exclusion 7th characters K - R see Appendix A PDX collection 0897
MCC Exclusion 7th character A see Appendix A PDX collection 1299
MCC Exclusion 7th characters B & C see Appendix A PDX collection 1298
HAC 7th characters A - C see Appendix B for HAC conditional logic

CC MCC +7th **S72.363** **Displaced segmental fracture of shaft of unspecified femur**
CC Exclusion 7th characters K - R see Appendix A PDX collection 0897
MCC Exclusion 7th characters A - C see Appendix A PDX collection 1298
HAC 7th characters A - C see Appendix B for HAC conditional logic

CC MCC +7th **S72.364** **Nondisplaced segmental fracture of shaft of right femur**
CC Exclusion 7th characters K - R see Appendix A PDX collection 0897
MCC Exclusion 7th character A see Appendix A PDX collection 1297
MCC Exclusion 7th characters B & C see Appendix A PDX collection 1298
HAC 7th characters A - C see Appendix B for HAC conditional logic

CC MCC +7th **S72.365** **Nondisplaced segmental fracture of shaft of left femur**
CC Exclusion 7th characters K - R see Appendix A PDX collection 0897
MCC Exclusion 7th character A see Appendix A PDX collection 1299
MCC Exclusion 7th characters B & C see Appendix A PDX collection 1298
HAC 7th characters A - C see Appendix B for HAC conditional logic

CC MCC +7th **S72.366** **Nondisplaced segmental fracture of shaft of unspecified femur**
CC Exclusion 7th characters K - R see Appendix A PDX collection 0897
MCC Exclusion 7th characters A - C see Appendix A PDX collection 1298
HAC 7th characters A - C see Appendix B for HAC conditional logic

\+ **S72.39** **Other fracture of shaft of femur**

CC MCC +7th **S72.391** **Other fracture of shaft of right femur**
CC Exclusion 7th characters K - R see Appendix A PDX collection 0897
MCC Exclusion 7th character A see Appendix A PDX collection 1297
MCC Exclusion 7th characters B & C see Appendix A PDX collection 1298
HAC 7th characters A - C see Appendix B for HAC conditional logic

CC MCC +7th **S72.392** **Other fracture of shaft of left femur**
CC Exclusion 7th characters K - R see Appendix A PDX collection 0897
MCC Exclusion 7th character A see Appendix A PDX collection 1299
MCC Exclusion 7th characters B & C see Appendix A PDX collection 1298
HAC 7th characters A - C see Appendix B for HAC conditional logic

CC MCC +7th **S72.399** **Other fracture of shaft of unspecified femur**
CC Exclusion 7th characters K - R see Appendix A PDX collection 0897
MCC Exclusion 7th characters A - C see Appendix A PDX collection 1298
HAC 7th characters A - C see Appendix B for HAC conditional logic

\+ **S72.4** **Fracture of lower end of femur**
Fracture of distal end of femur
Excludes2: *fracture of shaft of femur (S72.3-)*
physeal fracture of lower end of femur (S79.1-)

\+ **S72.40** **Unspecified fracture of lower end of femur**

CC MCC +7th **S72.401** **Unspecified fracture of lower end of right femur**
CC Exclusion 7th character A see Appendix A PDX collection 1300
CC Exclusion 7th characters K - R see Appendix A PDX collection 0897
MCC Exclusion 7th characters B & C see Appendix A PDX collection 1301
AHA CC: 4Q, 2016, 42-43
HAC 7th characters A - C see Appendix B for HAC conditional logic

CC MCC +7th **S72.402** **Unspecified fracture of lower end of left femur**
CC Exclusion 7th character A see Appendix A PDX collection 1302
CC Exclusion 7th characters K - R see Appendix A PDX collection 0897
MCC Exclusion 7th characters B & C see Appendix A PDX collection 1301
HAC 7th characters A - C see Appendix B for HAC conditional logic

CC MCC +7th **S72.409** **Unspecified fracture of lower end of unspecified femur**
CC Exclusion 7th character A see Appendix A PDX collection 1301
CC Exclusion 7th characters K - R see Appendix A PDX collection 0897
MCC Exclusion 7th characters B & C see Appendix A PDX collection 1301
HAC 7th characters A - C see Appendix B for HAC conditional logic

\+ **S72.41** **Unspecified condyle fracture of lower end of femur**
Condyle fracture of femur NOS

CC MCC +7th **S72.411** **Displaced unspecified condyle fracture of lower end of right femur**
CC Exclusion 7th character A see Appendix A PDX collection 1300
CC Exclusion 7th characters K - R see Appendix A PDX collection 0897
MCC Exclusion 7th characters B & C see Appendix A PDX collection 1301
HAC 7th characters A - C see Appendix B for HAC conditional logic

CC MCC +7th **S72.412** **Displaced unspecified condyle fracture of lower end of left femur**
CC Exclusion 7th character A see Appendix A PDX collection 1302
CC Exclusion 7th characters K - R see Appendix A PDX collection 0897
MCC Exclusion 7th characters B & C see Appendix A PDX collection 1301
HAC 7th characters A - C see Appendix B for HAC conditional logic

CC MCC +7th **S72.413** **Displaced unspecified condyle fracture of lower end of unspecified femur**
CC Exclusion 7th character A see Appendix A PDX collection 1301
CC Exclusion 7th characters K - R see Appendix A PDX collection 0897
MCC Exclusion 7th characters B & C see Appendix A PDX collection 1301
HAC 7th characters A - C see Appendix B for HAC conditional logic

CC MCC +7th **S72.414** **Nondisplaced unspecified condyle fracture of lower end of right femur**
CC Exclusion 7th character A see Appendix A PDX collection 1300
CC Exclusion 7th characters K - R see Appendix A PDX collection 0897
MCC Exclusion 7th characters B & C see Appendix A PDX collection 1301
HAC 7th characters A - C see Appendix B for HAC conditional logic

CC MCC +7th **S72.415** **Nondisplaced unspecified condyle fracture of lower end of left femur**
CC Exclusion 7th character A see Appendix A PDX collection 1302
CC Exclusion 7th characters K - R see Appendix A PDX collection 0897
MCC Exclusion 7th characters B & C see Appendix A PDX collection 1301
HAC 7th characters A - C see Appendix B for HAC conditional logic

CC MCC +7th **S72.416** **Nondisplaced unspecified condyle fracture of lower end of unspecified femur**
CC Exclusion 7th character A see Appendix A PDX collection 1301
CC Exclusion 7th characters K - R see Appendix A PDX collection 0897
MCC Exclusion 7th characters B & C see Appendix A PDX collection 1301
HAC 7th characters A - C see Appendix B for HAC conditional logic

\+ **S72.42** **Fracture of lateral condyle of femur**

CC MCC +7th **S72.421** **Displaced fracture of lateral condyle of right femur**
CC Exclusion 7th character A see Appendix A PDX collection 1300
CC Exclusion 7th characters K - R see Appendix A PDX collection 0897
MCC Exclusion 7th characters B & C see Appendix A PDX collection 1301
HAC 7th characters A - C see Appendix B for HAC conditional logic

CC MCC +7th **S72.422** **Displaced fracture of lateral condyle of left femur**
CC Exclusion 7th character A see Appendix A PDX collection 1302
CC Exclusion 7th characters K - R see Appendix A PDX collection 0897
MCC Exclusion 7th characters B & C see Appendix A PDX collection 1301
HAC 7th characters A - C see Appendix B for HAC conditional logic

CC MCC +7th **S72.423** **Displaced fracture of lateral condyle of unspecified femur**
CC Exclusion 7th character A see Appendix A PDX collection 1301
CC Exclusion 7th characters K - R see Appendix A PDX collection 0897
MCC Exclusion 7th characters B & C see Appendix A PDX collection 1301
HAC 7th characters A - C see Appendix B for HAC conditional logic

CC MCC +7th **S72.424** **Nondisplaced fracture of lateral condyle of right femur**
CC Exclusion 7th character A see Appendix A PDX collection 1300
CC Exclusion 7th characters K - R see Appendix A PDX collection 0897
MCC Exclusion 7th characters B & C see Appendix A PDX collection 1301
HAC 7th characters A - C see Appendix B for HAC conditional logic

CC MCC +7th **S72.425** **Nondisplaced fracture of lateral condyle of left femur**
CC Exclusion 7th character A see Appendix A PDX collection 1302
CC Exclusion 7th characters K - R see Appendix A PDX collection 0897
MCC Exclusion 7th characters B & C see Appendix A PDX collection 1301
HAC 7th characters A - C see Appendix B for HAC conditional logic

CC MCC +7th **S72.426** **Nondisplaced fracture of lateral condyle of unspecified femur**
CC Exclusion 7th character A see Appendix A PDX collection 1301
CC Exclusion 7th characters K - R see Appendix A PDX collection 0897
MCC Exclusion 7th characters B & C see Appendix A PDX collection 1301
HAC 7th characters A - C see Appendix B for HAC conditional logic

\+ **S72.43** **Fracture of medial condyle of femur**

CC MCC +7th **S72.431** **Displaced fracture of medial condyle of right femur**
CC Exclusion 7th character A see Appendix A PDX collection 1300
CC Exclusion 7th characters K - R see Appendix A PDX collection 0897
MCC Exclusion 7th characters B & C see Appendix A PDX collection 1301
HAC 7th characters A - C see Appendix B for HAC conditional logic

CC MCC +7th **S72.432** **Displaced fracture of medial condyle of left femur**
CC Exclusion 7th character A see Appendix A PDX collection 1302
CC Exclusion 7th characters K - R see Appendix A PDX collection 0897
MCC Exclusion 7th characters B & C see Appendix A PDX collection 1301
HAC 7th characters A - C see Appendix B for HAC conditional logic

CC MCC +7th **S72.433** **Displaced fracture of medial condyle of unspecified femur**
CC Exclusion 7th character A see Appendix A PDX collection 1301
CC Exclusion 7th characters K - R see Appendix A PDX collection 0897
MCC Exclusion 7th characters B & C see Appendix A PDX collection 1301
HAC 7th characters A - C see Appendix B for HAC conditional logic

CC MCC +7th **S72.434** **Nondisplaced fracture of medial condyle of right femur**
CC Exclusion 7th character A see Appendix A PDX collection 1300
CC Exclusion 7th characters K - R see Appendix A PDX collection 0897
MCC Exclusion 7th characters B & C see Appendix A PDX collection 1301
HAC 7th characters A - C see Appendix B for HAC conditional logic

CC MCC +7th **S72.435** **Nondisplaced fracture of medial condyle of left femur**
CC Exclusion 7th character A see Appendix A PDX collection 1302
CC Exclusion 7th characters K - R see Appendix A PDX collection 0897
MCC Exclusion 7th characters B & C see Appendix A PDX collection 1301
HAC 7th characters A - C see Appendix B for HAC conditional logic

CC MCC +7th **S72.436** **Nondisplaced fracture of medial condyle of unspecified femur**
CC Exclusion 7th character A see Appendix A PDX collection 1301
CC Exclusion 7th characters K - R see Appendix A PDX collection 0897
MCC Exclusion 7th characters B & C see Appendix A PDX collection 1301
HAC 7th characters A - C see Appendix B for HAC conditional logic

\+ **S72.44** **Fracture of lower epiphysis (separation) of femur**
Excludes1: *Salter-Harris Type I physeal fracture of lower end of femur (S79.11-)*

CC MCC +7th **S72.441** **Displaced fracture of lower epiphysis (separation) of right femur**
CC Exclusion 7th character A see Appendix A PDX collection 1300
CC Exclusion 7th characters K - R see Appendix A PDX collection 0897
MCC Exclusion 7th characters B & C see Appendix A PDX collection 1301
HAC 7th characters A - C see Appendix B for HAC conditional logic

CC MCC +7th **S72.442** **Displaced fracture of lower epiphysis (separation) of left femur**
CC Exclusion 7th character A see Appendix A PDX collection 1302
CC Exclusion 7th characters K - R see Appendix A PDX collection 0897
MCC Exclusion 7th characters B & C see Appendix A PDX collection 1301
HAC 7th characters A - C see Appendix B for HAC conditional logic

CC MCC +7th **S72.443** **Displaced fracture of lower epiphysis (separation) of unspecified femur**
CC Exclusion 7th character A see Appendix A PDX collection 1301
CC Exclusion 7th characters K - R see Appendix A PDX collection 0897
MCC Exclusion 7th characters B & C see Appendix A PDX collection 1301
HAC 7th characters A - C see Appendix B for HAC conditional logic

CC MCC +7th **S72.444** **Nondisplaced fracture of lower epiphysis (separation) of right femur**
CC Exclusion 7th character A see Appendix A PDX collection 1300
CC Exclusion 7th characters K - R see Appendix A PDX collection 0897
MCC Exclusion 7th characters B & C see Appendix A PDX collection 1301
HAC 7th characters A - C see Appendix B for HAC conditional logic

CC MCC +7th **S72.445** **Nondisplaced fracture of lower epiphysis (separation) of left femur**
CC Exclusion 7th character A see Appendix A PDX collection 1302
CC Exclusion 7th characters K - R see Appendix A PDX collection 0897
MCC Exclusion 7th characters B & C see Appendix A PDX collection 1301
HAC 7th characters A - C see Appendix B for HAC conditional logic

CC MCC +7th **S72.446** **Nondisplaced fracture of lower epiphysis (separation) of unspecified femur**
CC Exclusion 7th character A see Appendix A PDX collection 1303
CC Exclusion 7th characters K - R see Appendix A PDX collection 0897
MCC Exclusion 7th characters B & C see Appendix A PDX collection 1301
HAC 7th characters A - C see Appendix B for HAC conditional logic

+ S72.45 **Supracondylar fracture without intracondylar extension of lower end of femur**
Supracondylar fracture of lower end of femur NOS
Excludes1: *supracondylar fracture with intracondylar extension of lower end of femur (S72.46-)*

CC MCC +7th **S72.451** **Displaced supracondylar fracture without intracondylar extension of lower end of right femur**
CC Exclusion 7th character A see Appendix A PDX collection 1300
CC Exclusion 7th characters K - R see Appendix A PDX collection 0897
MCC Exclusion 7th characters B & C see Appendix A PDX collection 1301
HAC 7th characters A - C see Appendix B for HAC conditional logic

CC MCC +7th **S72.452** **Displaced supracondylar fracture without intracondylar extension of lower end of left femur**
CC Exclusion 7th character A see Appendix A PDX collection 1302
CC Exclusion 7th characters K - R see Appendix A PDX collection 0897
MCC Exclusion 7th characters B & C see Appendix A PDX collection 1301
HAC 7th characters A - C see Appendix B for HAC conditional logic

CC MCC +7th **S72.453** **Displaced supracondylar fracture without intracondylar extension of lower end of unspecified femur**
CC Exclusion 7th character A see Appendix A PDX collection 1301
CC Exclusion 7th characters K - R see Appendix A PDX collection 0897
MCC Exclusion 7th characters B & C see Appendix A PDX collection 1301
HAC 7th characters A - C see Appendix B for HAC conditional logic

CC MCC +7th **S72.454** **Nondisplaced supracondylar fracture without intracondylar extension of lower end of right femur**
CC Exclusion 7th character A see Appendix A PDX collection 1300
CC Exclusion 7th characters K - R see Appendix A PDX collection 0897
MCC Exclusion 7th characters B & C see Appendix A PDX collection 1301
HAC 7th characters A - C see Appendix B for HAC conditional logic

CC MCC +7th **S72.455** **Nondisplaced supracondylar fracture without intracondylar extension of lower end of left femur**
CC Exclusion 7th character A see Appendix A PDX collection 1302
CC Exclusion 7th characters K - R see Appendix A PDX collection 0897
MCC Exclusion 7th characters B & C see Appendix A PDX collection 1301
HAC 7th characters A - C see Appendix B for HAC conditional logic

CC MCC +7th **S72.456** **Nondisplaced supracondylar fracture without intracondylar extension of lower end of unspecified femur**
CC Exclusion 7th character A see Appendix A PDX collection 1301
CC Exclusion 7th characters K - R see Appendix A PDX collection 0897
MCC Exclusion 7th characters B & C see Appendix A PDX collection 1301
HAC 7th characters A - C see Appendix B for HAC conditional logic

+ S72.46 **Supracondylar fracture with intracondylar extension of lower end of femur**
Excludes1: *supracondylar fracture without intracondylar extension of lower end of femur (S72.45-)*

CC MCC +7th **S72.461** **Displaced supracondylar fracture with intracondylar extension of lower end of right femur**
CC Exclusion 7th character A see Appendix A PDX collection 1300
CC Exclusion 7th characters K - R see Appendix A PDX collection 0897
MCC Exclusion 7th characters B & C see Appendix A PDX collection 1301
HAC 7th characters A - C see Appendix B for HAC conditional logic

CC MCC +7th **S72.462** **Displaced supracondylar fracture with intracondylar extension of lower end of left femur**
CC Exclusion 7th character A see Appendix A PDX collection 1302
CC Exclusion 7th characters K - R see Appendix A PDX collection 0897
MCC Exclusion 7th characters B & C see Appendix A PDX collection 1301
HAC 7th characters A - C see Appendix B for HAC conditional logic

CC MCC +7th **S72.463** **Displaced supracondylar fracture with intracondylar extension of lower end of unspecified femur**
CC Exclusion 7th character A see Appendix A PDX collection 1301
CC Exclusion 7th characters K - R see Appendix A PDX collection 0897
MCC Exclusion 7th characters B & C see Appendix A PDX collection 1301
HAC 7th characters A - C see Appendix B for HAC conditional logic

CC MCC +7th **S72.464** **Nondisplaced supracondylar fracture with intracondylar extension of lower end of right femur**
CC Exclusion 7th character A see Appendix A PDX collection 1300
CC Exclusion 7th characters K - R see Appendix A PDX collection 0897
MCC Exclusion 7th characters B & C see Appendix A PDX collection 1301
HAC 7th characters A - C see Appendix B for HAC conditional logic

CC MCC +7th **S72.465** **Nondisplaced supracondylar fracture with intracondylar extension of lower end of left femur**
CC Exclusion 7th character A see Appendix A PDX collection 1302
CC Exclusion 7th characters K - R see Appendix A PDX collection 0897
MCC Exclusion 7th characters B & C see Appendix A PDX collection 1301
HAC 7th characters A - C see Appendix B for HAC conditional logic

CC MCC +7th **S72.466** **Nondisplaced supracondylar fracture with intracondylar extension of lower end of unspecified femur**
CC Exclusion 7th character A see Appendix A PDX collection 1301
CC Exclusion 7th characters K - R see Appendix A PDX collection 0897
MCC Exclusion 7th characters B & C see Appendix A PDX collection 1301
HAC 7th characters A - C see Appendix B for HAC conditional logic

+ S72.47 **Torus fracture of lower end of femur**

The appropriate 7th character is to be added to all codes in subcategory **S72.47**
A initial encounter for closed fracture
D subsequent encounter for fracture with routine healing
G subsequent encounter for fracture with delayed healing
K subsequent encounter for fracture with nonunion
P subsequent encounter for fracture with malunion
S sequela

CC +7th **S72.471** **Torus fracture of lower end of right femur**
CC Exclusion 7th character A see Appendix A PDX collection 1300
CC Exclusion 7th characters K - R see Appendix A PDX collection 0897
HAC 7th character A see Appendix B for HAC conditional logic

CC +7th **S72.472** **Torus fracture of lower end of left femur**
CC Exclusion 7th character A see Appendix A PDX collection 1302
CC Exclusion 7th characters K - R see Appendix A PDX collection 0897
HAC 7th character A see Appendix B for HAC conditional logic

CC +7th **S72.479** **Torus fracture of lower end of unspecified femur**
CC Exclusion 7th character A see Appendix A PDX collection 1301
CC Exclusion 7th characters K - R see Appendix A PDX collection 0897
HAC 7th character A see Appendix B for HAC conditional logic

\+ **S72.49** **Other fracture of lower end of femur**

CC MCC +7th **S72.491** **Other fracture of lower end of right femur**
CC Exclusion 7th character A see Appendix A PDX collection 1300
CC Exclusion 7th characters K - R see Appendix A PDX collection 0897
MCC Exclusion 7th characters B & C see Appendix A PDX collection 1303
HAC 7th characters A - C see Appendix B for HAC conditional logic

CC MCC +7th **S72.492** **Other fracture of lower end of left femur**
CC Exclusion 7th character A see Appendix A PDX collection 1302
CC Exclusion 7th characters K - R see Appendix A PDX collection 0897
MCC Exclusion 7th characters B & C see Appendix A PDX collection 1303
HAC 7th characters A - C see Appendix B for HAC conditional logic

CC MCC +7th **S72.499** **Other fracture of lower end of unspecified femur**
CC Exclusion 7th character A see Appendix A PDX collection 1301
CC Exclusion 7th characters K - R see Appendix A PDX collection 0897
MCC Exclusion 7th characters B & C see Appendix A PDX collection 1303
HAC 7th characters A - C see Appendix B for HAC conditional logic

MCC + CC **S72.8** **Other fracture of femur**
CC Exclusion 7th characters K - R see Appendix A PDX collection 0897
MCC Exclusion 7th characters A - C see Appendix A PDX collection 1298
HAC 7th characters A - C see Appendix B for HAC conditional logic

\+ **S72.8X** **Other fracture of femur**
+7th **S72.8X1** **Other fracture of right femur**
+7th **S72.8X2** **Other fracture of left femur**
+7th **S72.8X9** **Other fracture of unspecified femur**

\+ **S72.9** **Unspecified fracture of femur**
Fracture of thigh NOS
Fracture of upper leg NOS
Excludes1: *fracture of hip NOS (S72.00-, S72.01-)*

CC MCC X+7th **S72.90** **Unspecified fracture of unspecified femur**
CC Exclusion 7th characters K - R see Appendix A PDX collection 0897
MCC Exclusion 7th characters A - C see Appendix A PDX collection 1298
AHA CC: 4Q, 2012, 93-94
HAC 7th characters A - C see Appendix B for HAC conditional logic

CC MCC X+7th **S72.91** **Unspecified fracture of right femur**
CC Exclusion 7th characters K - R see Appendix A PDX collection 0897
MCC Exclusion 7th characters A - C see Appendix A PDX collection 1298
HAC 7th characters A - C see Appendix B for HAC conditional logic

CC MCC X+7th **S72.92** **Unspecified fracture of left femur**
CC Exclusion 7th characters K - R see Appendix A PDX collection 0897
MCC Exclusion 7th characters A - C see Appendix A PDX collection 1298
HAC 7th characters A - C see Appendix B for HAC conditional logic

S73 **Dislocation and sprain of joint and ligaments of hip**

Includes: avulsion of joint or ligament of hip
lacervw ation of cartilage, joint or ligament of hip
sprain of cartilage, joint or ligament of hip
traumatic hemarthrosis of joint or ligament of hip
traumatic rupture of joint or ligament of hip
traumatic subluxation of joint or ligament of hip
traumatic tear of joint or ligament of hip

Code also any associated open wound
Excludes2: *strain of muscle, fascia and tendon of hip and thigh (S76.-)*

The appropriate 7th character is to be added to each code from category S73
A initial encounter
D subsequent encounter
S sequela

\+ **S73.0** **Subluxation and dislocation of hip**
Excludes2: *dislocation and subluxation of hip prosthesis (T84.020, T84.021)*

\+ **S73.00** **Unspecified subluxation and dislocation of hip**
Dislocation of hip NOS
Subluxation of hip NOS

CC +7th **S73.001** **Unspecified subluxation of right hip**
CC Exclusion 7th character A see Appendix A PDX collection 1304
HAC 7th character A see Appendix B for HAC conditional logic

CC +7th **S73.002** **Unspecified subluxation of left hip**
CC Exclusion 7th character A see Appendix A PDX collection 1305
HAC 7th character A see Appendix B for HAC conditional logic

CC +7th **S73.003** **Unspecified subluxation of unspecified hip**
CC Exclusion 7th character A see Appendix A PDX collection 1306
HAC 7th character A see Appendix B for HAC conditional logic

CC +7th **S73.004** **Unspecified dislocation of right hip**
CC Exclusion 7th character A see Appendix A PDX collection 1304
HAC 7th character A see Appendix B for HAC conditional logic

CC +7th **S73.005** **Unspecified dislocation of left hip**
CC Exclusion 7th character A see Appendix A PDX collection 1305
HAC 7th character A see Appendix B for HAC conditional logic

CC +7th **S73.006** **Unspecified dislocation of unspecified hip**
CC Exclusion 7th character A see Appendix A PDX collection 1306
HAC 7th character A see Appendix B for HAC conditional logic

\+ **S73.01** **Posterior subluxation and dislocation of hip**

CC +7th **S73.011** **Posterior subluxation of right hip**
CC Exclusion 7th character A see Appendix A PDX collection 1307
HAC 7th character A see Appendix B for HAC conditional logic

CC +7th **S73.012** **Posterior subluxation of left hip**
CC Exclusion 7th character A see Appendix A PDX collection 1308
HAC 7th character A see Appendix B for HAC conditional logic

CC +7th **S73.013** **Posterior subluxation of unspecified hip**
CC Exclusion 7th character A see Appendix A PDX collection 1309
HAC 7th character A see Appendix B for HAC conditional logic

CC +7th **S73.014** **Posterior dislocation of right hip**
CC Exclusion 7th character A see Appendix A PDX collection 1307
HAC 7th character A see Appendix B for HAC conditional logic

CC +7th **S73.015** **Posterior dislocation of left hip**
CC Exclusion 7th character A see Appendix A PDX collection 1308
HAC 7th character A see Appendix B for HAC conditional logic

CC +7th **S73.016** **Posterior dislocation of unspecified hip**
CC Exclusion 7th character A see Appendix A PDX collection 1309
HAC 7th character A see Appendix B for HAC conditional logic

+ S73.02 Obturator subluxation and dislocation of hip
CC +7th **S73.021** Obturator subluxation of right hip
CC Exclusion 7th character A see Appendix A
PDX collection 1310
HAC 7th character A see Appendix B for HAC conditional logic
CC +7th **S73.022** Obturator subluxation of left hip
CC Exclusion 7th character A see Appendix A
PDX collection 1311
HAC 7th character A see Appendix B for HAC conditional logic
CC +7th **S73.023** Obturator subluxation of unspecified hip
CC Exclusion 7th character A see Appendix A
PDX collection 1312
HAC 7th character A see Appendix B for HAC conditional logic
CC +7th **S73.024** Obturator dislocation of right hip
CC Exclusion 7th character A see Appendix A
PDX collection 1310
HAC 7th character A see Appendix B for HAC conditional logic
CC +7th **S73.025** Obturator dislocation of left hip
CC Exclusion 7th character A see Appendix A
PDX collection 1311
HAC 7th character A see Appendix B for HAC conditional logic
CC +7th **S73.026** Obturator dislocation of unspecified hip
CC Exclusion 7th character A see Appendix A
PDX collection 1312
HAC 7th character A see Appendix B for HAC conditional logic
+ S73.03 Other anterior subluxation and dislocation of hip
CC +7th **S73.031** Other anterior subluxation of right hip
CC Exclusion 7th character A see Appendix A
PDX collection 1313
HAC 7th character A see Appendix B for HAC conditional logic
CC +7th **S73.032** Other anterior subluxation of left hip
CC Exclusion 7th character A see Appendix A
PDX collection 1314
HAC 7th character A see Appendix B for HAC conditional logic
CC +7th **S73.033** Other anterior subluxation of unspecified hip
CC Exclusion 7th character A see Appendix A
PDX collection 1315
HAC 7th character A see Appendix B for HAC conditional logic
CC +7th **S73.034** Other anterior dislocation of right hip
CC Exclusion 7th character A see Appendix A
PDX collection 1313
HAC 7th character A see Appendix B for HAC conditional logic
CC +7th **S73.035** Other anterior dislocation of left hip
CC Exclusion 7th character A see Appendix A
PDX collection 1314
HAC 7th character A see Appendix B for HAC conditional logic
CC +7th **S73.036** Other anterior dislocation of unspecified hip
CC Exclusion 7th character A see Appendix A
PDX collection 1315
HAC 7th character A see Appendix B for HAC conditional logic
+ S73.04 Central subluxation and dislocation of hip
CC +7th **S73.041** Central subluxation of right hip
CC Exclusion 7th character A see Appendix A
PDX collection 1304
HAC 7th character A see Appendix B for HAC conditional logic
CC +7th **S73.042** Central subluxation of left hip
CC Exclusion 7th character A see Appendix A
PDX collection 1305
HAC 7th character A see Appendix B for HAC conditional logic
CC +7th **S73.043** Central subluxation of unspecified hip
CC Exclusion 7th character A see Appendix A
PDX collection 1306
HAC 7th character A see Appendix B for HAC conditional logic
CC +7th **S73.044** Central dislocation of right hip
CC Exclusion 7th character A see Appendix A
PDX collection 1304
HAC 7th character A see Appendix B for HAC conditional logic
CC +7th **S73.045** Central dislocation of left hip
CC Exclusion 7th character A see Appendix A
PDX collection 1305
HAC 7th character A see Appendix B for HAC conditional logic
CC +7th **S73.046** Central dislocation of unspecified hip
CC Exclusion 7th character A see Appendix A
PDX collection 1306
HAC 7th character A see Appendix B for HAC conditional logic
+ S73.1 Sprain of hip
+ S73.10 Unspecified sprain of hip
+7th S73.101 Unspecified sprain of right hip
+7th S73.102 Unspecified sprain of left hip
+7th S73.109 Unspecified sprain of unspecified hip
+ S73.11 Iliofemoral ligament sprain of hip
+7th S73.111 Iliofemoral ligament sprain of right hip
+7th S73.112 Iliofemoral ligament sprain of left hip
+7th S73.119 Iliofemoral ligament sprain of unspecified hip
+ S73.12 Ischiocapsular (ligament) sprain of hip
+7th S73.121 Ischiocapsular ligament sprain of right hip
+7th S73.122 Ischiocapsular ligament sprain of left hip
+7th S73.129 Ischiocapsular ligament sprain of unspecified hip
+ S73.19 Other sprain of hip
+7th S73.191 Other sprain of right hip
+7th S73.192 Other sprain of left hip
AHA CC: 4Q, 2014, 25
+7th S73.199 Other sprain of unspecified hip

S74 Injury of nerves at hip and thigh level

Code also any associated open wound (S71.-)
Excludes2: *injury of nerves at ankle and foot level (S94.-)*
injury of nerves at lower leg level (S84.-)

The appropriate 7th character is to be added to each code from category S74
A initial encounter
D subsequent encounter
S sequela

+ S74.0 Injury of sciatic nerve at hip and thigh level
X+7th S74.00 Injury of sciatic nerve at hip and thigh level, unspecified leg
X+7th S74.01 Injury of sciatic nerve at hip and thigh level, right leg
X+7th S74.02 Injury of sciatic nerve at hip and thigh level, left leg
+ S74.1 Injury of femoral nerve at hip and thigh level
X+7th S74.10 Injury of femoral nerve at hip and thigh level, unspecified leg
X+7th S74.11 Injury of femoral nerve at hip and thigh level, right leg
X+7th S74.12 Injury of femoral nerve at hip and thigh level, left leg
+ S74.2 Injury of cutaneous sensory nerve at hip and thigh level
X+7th S74.20 Injury of cutaneous sensory nerve at hip and thigh level, unspecified leg
X+7th S74.21 Injury of cutaneous sensory nerve at hip and high level, right leg
X+7th S74.22 Injury of cutaneous sensory nerve at hip and thigh level, left leg
+ S74.8 Injury of other nerves at hip and thigh level
+ S74.8X Injury of other nerves at hip and thigh level
+7th S74.8X1 Injury of other nerves at hip and thigh level, right leg
+7th S74.8X2 Injury of other nerves at hip and thigh level, left leg
+7th S74.8X9 Injury of other nerves at hip and thigh level, unspecified leg
+ S74.9 Injury of unspecified nerve at hip and thigh level
X+7th S74.90 Injury of unspecified nerve at hip and thigh level, unspecified leg
X+7th S74.91 Injury of unspecified nerve at hip and thigh level, right leg
X+7th S74.92 Injury of unspecified nerve at hip and thigh level, left leg

S75 Injury of blood vessels at hip and thigh level

Code also any associated open wound (S71.-)

Excludes2: *injury of blood vessels at lower leg level (S85.-)*
injury of popliteal artery (S85.0)

The appropriate 7th character is to be added to each code from category S75
A initial encounter
D subsequent encounter
S sequela

\+ **S75.0 Injury of femoral artery**

\+ **S75.00 Unspecified injury of femoral artery**

MCC +7th **S75.001 Unspecified injury of femoral artery, right leg**
MCC Exclusion 7th character A see Appendix A PDX collection 1316

MCC +7th **S75.002 Unspecified injury of femoral artery, left leg**
MCC Exclusion 7th character A see Appendix A PDX collection 1317

MCC +7th **S75.009 Unspecified injury of femoral artery, unspecified leg**
MCC Exclusion 7th character A see Appendix A PDX collection 1318

\+ **S75.01 Minor laceration of femoral artery**
Incomplete transection of femoral artery
Laceration of femoral artery NOS
Superficial laceration of femoral artery

MCC +7th **S75.011 Minor laceration of femoral artery, right leg**
MCC Exclusion 7th character A see Appendix A PDX collection 1316

MCC +7th **S75.012 Minor laceration of femoral artery, left leg**
MCC Exclusion 7th character A see Appendix A PDX collection 1317

MCC +7th **S75.019 Minor laceration of femoral artery, unspecified leg**
MCC Exclusion 7th character A see Appendix A PDX collection 1318

\+ **S75.02 Major laceration of femoral artery**
Complete transection of femoral artery
Traumatic rupture of femoral artery

MCC +7th **S75.021 Major laceration of femoral artery, right leg**
MCC Exclusion 7th character A see Appendix A PDX collection 1316

MCC +7th **S75.022 Major laceration of femoral artery, left leg**
MCC Exclusion 7th character A see Appendix A PDX collection 1317

MCC +7th **S75.029 Major laceration of femoral artery, unspecified leg**
MCC Exclusion 7th character A see Appendix A PDX collection 1318

\+ **S75.09 Other specified injury of femoral artery**

MCC +7th **S75.091 Other specified injury of femoral artery, right leg**
MCC Exclusion 7th character A see Appendix A PDX collection 1316

MCC +7th **S75.092 Other specified injury of femoral artery, left leg**
MCC Exclusion 7th character A see Appendix A PDX collection 1317

MCC +7th **S75.099 Other specified injury of femoral artery, unspecified leg**
MCC Exclusion 7th character A see Appendix A PDX collection 1318

\+ **S75.1 Injury of femoral vein at hip and thigh level**

\+ **S75.10 Unspecified injury of femoral vein at hip and thigh level**

MCC +7th **S75.101 Unspecified injury of femoral vein at hip and thigh level, right leg**
MCC Exclusion 7th character A see Appendix A PDX collection 1319

MCC +7th **S75.102 Unspecified injury of femoral vein at hip and thigh level, left leg**
MCC Exclusion 7th character A see Appendix A PDX collection 1320

MCC +7th **S75.109 Unspecified injury of femoral vein at hip and thigh level, unspecified leg**
MCC Exclusion 7th character A see Appendix A PDX collection 1321

\+ **S75.11 Minor laceration of femoral vein at hip and thigh level**
Incomplete transection of femoral vein at hip and thigh level
Laceration of femoral vein at hip and thigh level NOS
Superficial laceration of femoral vein at hip and thigh level

MCC +7th **S75.111 Minor laceration of femoral vein at hip and thigh level, right leg**
MCC Exclusion 7th character A see Appendix A PDX collection 1319

MCC +7th **S75.112 Minor laceration of femoral vein at hip and thigh level, left leg**
MCC Exclusion 7th character A see Appendix A PDX collection 1320

MCC +7th **S75.119 Minor laceration of femoral vein at hip and thigh level, unspecified leg**
MCC Exclusion 7th character A see Appendix A PDX collection 1321

\+ **S75.12 Major laceration of femoral vein at hip and thigh level**
Complete transection of femoral vein at hip and thigh level
Traumatic rupture of femoral vein at hip and thigh level

MCC +7th **S75.121 Major laceration of femoral vein at hip and thigh level, right leg**
MCC Exclusion 7th character A see Appendix A PDX collection 1319

MCC +7th **S75.122 Major laceration of femoral vein at hip and thigh level, left leg**
MCC Exclusion 7th character A see Appendix A PDX collection 1320

MCC +7th **S75.129 Major laceration of femoral vein at hip and thigh level, unspecified leg**
MCC Exclusion 7th character A see Appendix A PDX collection 1321

\+ **S75.19 Other specified injury of femoral vein at hip and thigh level**

MCC +7th **S75.191 Other specified injury of femoral vein at hip and thigh level, right leg**
MCC Exclusion 7th character A see Appendix A PDX collection 1319

MCC +7th **S75.192 Other specified injury of femoral vein at hip and thigh level, left leg**
MCC Exclusion 7th character A see Appendix A PDX collection 1320

MCC +7th **S75.199 Other specified injury of femoral vein at hip and thigh level, unspecified leg**
MCC Exclusion 7th character A see Appendix A PDX collection 1321

\+ **S75.2 Injury of greater saphenous vein at hip and thigh level**

Excludes1: *greater saphenous vein NOS (S85.3)*

\+ **S75.20 Unspecified injury of greater saphenous vein at hip and thigh level**

CC +7th **S75.201 Unspecified injury of greater saphenous vein at hip and thigh level, right leg**
CC Exclusion 7th character A see Appendix A PDX collection 1322

CC +7th **S75.202 Unspecified injury of greater saphenous vein at hip and thigh level, left leg**
CC Exclusion 7th character A see Appendix A PDX collection 1323

CC +7th **S75.209 Unspecified injury of greater saphenous vein at hip and thigh level, unspecified leg**
CC Exclusion 7th character A see Appendix A PDX collection 1324

\+ **S75.21 Minor laceration of greater saphenous vein at hip and thigh level**
Incomplete transection of greater saphenous vein at hip and thigh level
Laceration of greater saphenous vein at hip and thigh level NOS
Superficial laceration of greater saphenous vein at hip and thigh level

CC +7th **S75.211 Minor laceration of greater saphenous vein at hip and thigh level, right leg**
CC Exclusion 7th character A see Appendix A PDX collection 1322

CC +7th **S75.212 Minor laceration of greater saphenous vein at hip and thigh level, left leg**
CC Exclusion 7th character A see Appendix A PDX collection 1323

CC +7th **S75.219 Minor laceration of greater saphenous vein at hip and thigh level, unspecified leg**
CC Exclusion 7th character A see Appendix A
PDX collection 1324

\+ **S75.22 Major laceration of greater saphenous vein at hip and thigh level**
Complete transection of greater saphenous vein at hip and thigh level
Traumatic rupture of greater saphenous vein at hip and thigh level

CC +7th **S75.221 Major laceration of greater saphenous vein at hip and thigh level, right leg**
CC Exclusion 7th character A see Appendix A
PDX collection 1322

CC +7th **S75.222 Major laceration of greater saphenous vein at hip and thigh level, left leg**
CC Exclusion 7th character A see Appendix A
PDX collection 1323

CC +7th **S75.229 Major laceration of greater saphenous vein at hip and thigh level, unspecified leg**
CC Exclusion 7th character A see Appendix A
PDX collection 1324

\+ **S75.29 Other specified injury of greater saphenous vein at hip and thigh level**

CC +7th **S75.291 Other specified injury of greater saphenous vein at hip and thigh level, right leg**
CC Exclusion 7th character A see Appendix A
PDX collection 1322

CC +7th **S75.292 Other specified injury of greater saphenous vein at hip and thigh level, left leg**
CC Exclusion 7th character A see Appendix A
PDX collection 1323

CC +7th **S75.299 Other specified injury of greater saphenous vein at hip and thigh level, unspecified leg**
CC Exclusion 7th character A see Appendix A
PDX collection 1324

\+ **S75.8 Injury of other blood vessels at hip and thigh level**

\+ **S75.80 Unspecified injury of other blood vessels at hip and thigh level**

CC +7th **S75.801 Unspecified injury of other blood vessels at hip and thigh level, right leg**
CC Exclusion 7th character A see Appendix A
PDX collection 1325

CC +7th **S75.802 Unspecified injury of other blood vessels at hip and thigh level, left leg**
CC Exclusion 7th character A see Appendix A
PDX collection 1326

CC +7th **S75.809 Unspecified injury of other blood vessels at hip and thigh level, unspecified leg**
CC Exclusion 7th character A see Appendix A
PDX collection 1327

\+ **S75.81 Laceration of other blood vessels at hip and thigh level**

CC +7th **S75.811 Laceration of other blood vessels at hip and thigh level, right leg**
CC Exclusion 7th character A see Appendix A
PDX collection 1325

CC +7th **S75.812 Laceration of other blood vessels at hip and thigh level, left leg**
CC Exclusion 7th character A see Appendix A
PDX collection 1326

CC +7th **S75.819 Laceration of other blood vessels at hip and thigh level, unspecified leg**
CC Exclusion 7th character A see Appendix A
PDX collection 1327

\+ **S75.89 Other specified injury of other blood vessels at hip and thigh level**

CC +7th **S75.891 Other specified injury of other blood vessels at hip and thigh level, right leg**
CC Exclusion 7th character A see Appendix A
PDX collection 1325

CC +7th **S75.892 Other specified injury of other blood vessels at hip and thigh level, left leg**
CC Exclusion 7th character A see Appendix A
PDX collection 1326

CC +7th **S75.899 Other specified injury of other blood vessels at hip and thigh level, unspecified leg**
CC Exclusion 7th character A see Appendix A
PDX collection 1327

\+ **S75.9 Injury of unspecified blood vessel at hip and thigh level**

\+ **S75.90 Unspecified injury of unspecified blood vessel at hip and thigh level**

CC +7th **S75.901 Unspecified injury of unspecified blood vessel at hip and thigh level, right leg**
CC Exclusion 7th character A see Appendix A
PDX collection 1325

CC +7th **S75.902 Unspecified injury of unspecified blood vessel at hip and thigh level, left leg**
CC Exclusion 7th character A see Appendix A
PDX collection 1326

CC +7th **S75.909 Unspecified injury of unspecified blood vessel at hip and thigh level, unspecified leg**
CC Exclusion 7th character A see Appendix A
PDX collection 1327

\+ **S75.91 Laceration of unspecified blood vessel at hip and thigh level**

CC +7th **S75.911 Laceration of unspecified blood vessel at hip and thigh level, right leg**
CC Exclusion 7th character A see Appendix A
PDX collection 1325

CC +7th **S75.912 Laceration of unspecified blood vessel at hip and thigh level, left leg**
CC Exclusion 7th character A see Appendix A
PDX collection 1326

CC +7th **S75.919 Laceration of unspecified blood vessel at hip and thigh level, unspecified leg**
CC Exclusion 7th character A see Appendix A
PDX collection 1327

\+ **S75.99 Other specified injury of unspecified blood vessel at hip and thigh level**

CC +7th **S75.991 Other specified injury of unspecified blood vessel at hip and thigh level, right leg**
CC Exclusion 7th character A see Appendix A
PDX collection 1325

CC +7th **S75.992 Other specified injury of unspecified blood vessel at hip and thigh level, left leg**
CC Exclusion 7th character A see Appendix A
PDX collection 1326

CC +7th **S75.999 Other specified injury of unspecified blood vessel at hip and thigh level, unspecified leg**
CC Exclusion 7th character A see Appendix A
PDX collection 1327

S76 Injury of muscle, fascia and tendon at hip and thigh level

Code also any associated open wound (S71.-)

Excludes2: *injury of muscle, fascia and tendon at lower leg level (S86)*
sprain of joint and ligament of hip (S73.1)

The appropriate 7th character is to be added to each code from category S76
A initial encounter
D subsequent encounter
S sequela

\+ **S76.0 Injury of muscle, fascia and tendon of hip**

\+ **S76.00 Unspecified injury of muscle, fascia and tendon of hip**

+7th **S76.001 Unspecified injury of muscle, fascia and tendon of right hip**

+7th **S76.002 Unspecified injury of muscle, fascia and tendon of left hip**

+7th **S76.009 Unspecified injury of muscle, fascia and tendon of unspecified hip**

\+ **S76.01 Strain of muscle, fascia and tendon of hip**

+7th **S76.011 Strain of muscle, fascia and tendon of right hip**

+7th **S76.012 Strain of muscle, fascia and tendon of left hip**

+7th **S76.019 Strain of muscle, fascia and tendon of unspecified hip**

\+ **S76.02 Laceration of muscle, fascia and tendon of hip**

CC +7th **S76.021 Laceration of muscle, fascia and tendon of right hip**
CC Exclusion 7th character A see Appendix A
PDX collection 1328

CC +7th **S76.022 Laceration of muscle, fascia and tendon of left hip**
CC Exclusion 7th character A see Appendix A
PDX collection 1329

CC +7th **S76.029 Laceration of muscle, fascia and tendon of unspecified hip**
CC Exclusion 7th character A see Appendix A
PDX collection 1330

+ **S76.09** **Other specified injury of muscle, fascia and tendon of hip**
  - +7th **S76.091** **Other specified injury of muscle, fascia and tendon of right hip**
  - +7th **S76.092** **Other specified injury of muscle, fascia and tendon of left hip**
  - +7th **S76.099** **Other specified injury of muscle, fascia and tendon of unspecified hip**

+ **S76.1** **Injury of quadriceps muscle, fascia and tendon**
  Injury of patellar ligament (tendon)
+ **S76.10** **Unspecified injury of quadriceps muscle, fascia and tendon**
  - +7th **S76.101** **Unspecified injury of right quadriceps muscle, fascia and tendon**
  - +7th **S76.102** **Unspecified injury of left quadriceps muscle, fascia and tendon**
  - +7th **S76.109** **Unspecified injury of unspecified quadriceps muscle, fascia and tendon**
+ **S76.11** **Strain of quadriceps muscle, fascia and tendon**
  - +7th **S76.111** **Strain of right quadriceps muscle, fascia and tendon**
  - +7th **S76.112** **Strain of left quadriceps muscle, fascia and tendon**
  - +7th **S76.119** **Strain of unspecified quadriceps muscle, fascia and tendon**
+ **S76.12** **Laceration of quadriceps muscle, fascia and tendon**
  - CC +7th **S76.121** **Laceration of right quadriceps muscle, fascia and tendon**
    CC Exclusion 7th character A see Appendix A
    PDX collection 1328
  - CC +7th **S76.122** **Laceration of left quadriceps muscle, fascia and tendon**
    CC Exclusion 7th character A see Appendix A
    PDX collection 1329
  - CC +7th **S76.129** **Laceration of unspecified quadriceps muscle, fascia and tendon**
    CC Exclusion 7th character A see Appendix A
    PDX collection 1330
+ **S76.19** **Other specified injury of quadriceps muscle, fascia and tendon**
  - +7th **S76.191** **Other specified injury of right quadriceps muscle, fascia and tendon**
  - +7th **S76.192** **Other specified injury of left quadriceps muscle, fascia and tendon**
  - +7th **S76.199** **Other specified injury of unspecified quadriceps muscle, fascia and tendon**

+ **S76.2** **Injury of adductor muscle, fascia and tendon of thigh**
+ **S76.20** **Unspecified injury of adductor muscle, fascia and tendon of thigh**
  - +7th **S76.201** **Unspecified injury of adductor muscle, fascia and tendon of right thigh**
  - +7th **S76.202** **Unspecified injury of adductor muscle, fascia and tendon of left thigh**
  - +7th **S76.209** **Unspecified injury of adductor muscle, fascia and tendon of unspecified thigh**
+ **S76.21** **Strain of adductor muscle, fascia and tendon of thigh**
  - +7th **S76.211** **Strain of adductor muscle, fascia and tendon of right thigh**
  - +7th **S76.212** **Strain of adductor muscle, fascia and tendon of left thigh**
  - +7th **S76.219** **Strain of adductor muscle, fascia and tendon of unspecified thigh**
+ **S76.22** **Laceration of adductor muscle, fascia and tendon of thigh**
  - CC +7th **S76.221** **Laceration of adductor muscle, fascia and tendon of right thigh**
    CC Exclusion 7th character A see Appendix A
    PDX collection 1328
  - CC +7th **S76.222** **Laceration of adductor muscle, fascia and tendon of left thigh**
    CC Exclusion 7th character A see Appendix A
    PDX collection 1329
  - CC +7th **S76.229** **Laceration of adductor muscle, fascia and tendon of unspecified thigh**
    CC Exclusion 7th character A see Appendix A
    PDX collection 1330
+ **S76.29** **Other injury of adductor muscle, fascia and tendon of thigh**
  - +7th **S76.291** **Other injury of adductor muscle, fascia and tendon of right thigh**
  - +7th **S76.292** **Other injury of adductor muscle, fascia and tendon of left thigh**
  - +7th **S76.299** **Other injury of adductor muscle, fascia and tendon of unspecified thigh**

+ **S76.3** **Injury of muscle, fascia and tendon of the posterior muscle group at thigh level**
+ **S76.30** **Unspecified injury of muscle, fascia and tendon of the posterior muscle group at thigh level**
  - +7th **S76.301** **Unspecified injury of muscle, fascia and tendon of the posterior muscle group at thigh level, right thigh**
  - +7th **S76.302** **Unspecified injury of muscle, fascia and tendon of the posterior muscle group at thigh level, left thigh**
  - +7th **S76.309** **Unspecified injury of muscle, fascia and tendon of the posterior muscle group at thigh level, unspecified thigh**
+ **S76.31** **Strain of muscle, fascia and tendon of the posterior muscle group at thigh level**
  - +7th **S76.311** **Strain of muscle, fascia and tendon of the posterior muscle group at thigh level, right thigh**
  - +7th **S76.312** **Strain of muscle, fascia and tendon of the posterior muscle group at thigh level, left thigh**
  - +7th **S76.319** **Strain of muscle, fascia and tendon of the posterior muscle group at thigh level, unspecified thigh**
+ **S76.32** **Laceration of muscle, fascia and tendon of the posterior muscle group at thigh level**
  - CC +7th **S76.321** **Laceration of muscle, fascia and tendon of the posterior muscle group at thigh level, right thigh**
    CC Exclusion 7th character A see Appendix A
    PDX collection 1328
  - CC +7th **S76.322** **Laceration of muscle, fascia and tendon of the posterior muscle group at thigh level, left thigh**
    CC Exclusion 7th character A see Appendix A
    PDX collection 1329
  - CC +7th **S76.329** **Laceration of muscle, fascia and tendon of the posterior muscle group at thigh level, unspecified thigh**
    CC Exclusion 7th character A see Appendix A
    PDX collection 1330
+ **S76.39** **Other specified injury of muscle, fascia and tendon of the posterior muscle group at thigh level**
  - +7th **S76.391** **Other specified injury of muscle, fascia and tendon of the posterior muscle group at thigh level, right thigh**
  - +7th **S76.392** **Other specified injury of muscle, fascia and tendon of the posterior muscle group at thigh level, left thigh**
  - +7th **S76.399** **Other specified injury of muscle, fascia and tendon of the posterior muscle group at thigh level, unspecified thigh**

+ **S76.8** **Injury of other specified muscles, fascia and tendons at thigh level**
+ **S76.80** **Unspecified injury of other specified muscles, fascia and tendons at thigh level**
  - +7th **S76.801** **Unspecified injury of other specified muscles, fascia and tendons at thigh level, right thigh**
  - +7th **S76.802** **Unspecified injury of other specified muscles, fascia and tendons at thigh level, left thigh**
  - +7th **S76.809** **Unspecified injury of other specified muscles, fascia and tendons at thigh level, unspecified thigh**
+ **S76.81** **Strain of other specified muscles, fascia and tendon at thigh level**
  - +7th **S76.811** **Strain of other specified muscles, fascia and tendons at thigh level, right thigh**
  - +7th **S76.812** **Strain of other specified muscles, fascia and tendons at thigh level, left thigh**
  - +7th **S76.819** **Strain of other specified muscles, fascia and tendons at thigh level, unspecified thigh**

+ S76.82 Laceration of other specified muscles, fascia and tendons at thigh level
  - CC +7th S76.821 Laceration of other specified muscles, fascia and tendons at thigh level, right thigh
    CC Exclusion 7th character A see Appendix A PDX collection 1328
  - CC +7th S76.822 Laceration of other specified muscles, fascia and tendons at thigh level, left thigh
    CC Exclusion 7th character A see Appendix A PDX collection 1329
  - CC +7th S76.829 Laceration of other specified muscles, fascia and tendons at thigh level, unspecified thigh
    CC Exclusion 7th character A see Appendix A PDX collection 1330

+ S76.89 Other injury of other specified muscles, fascia and tendons at thigh level
  - +7th S76.891 Other injury of other specified muscles, fascia and tendons at thigh level, right thigh
  - +7th S76.892 Other injury of other specified muscles, fascia and tendons at thigh level, left thigh
  - +7th S76.899 Other injury of other specified muscles, fascia and tendons at thigh level, unspecified thigh

+ S76.9 Injury of unspecified muscles, fascia and tendons at thigh level

+ S76.90 Unspecified injury of unspecified muscles, fascia and tendons at thigh level
  - +7th S76.901 Unspecified injury of unspecified muscles, fascia and tendons at thigh level, right thigh
  - +7th S76.902 Unspecified injury of unspecified muscles, fascia and tendons at thigh level, left thigh
  - +7th S76.909 Unspecified injury of unspecified muscles, fascia and tendons at thigh level, unspecified thigh

+ S76.91 Strain of unspecified muscles, fascia and tendons at thigh level
  - +7th S76.911 Strain of unspecified muscles, fascia and tendons at thigh level, right thigh
  - +7th S76.912 Strain of unspecified muscles, fascia and tendons at thigh level, left thigh
  - +7th S76.919 Strain of unspecified muscles, fascia and tendons at thigh level, unspecified thigh

+ S76.92 Laceration of unspecified muscles, fascia and tendons at thigh level
  - CC +7th S76.921 Laceration of unspecified muscles, fascia and tendons at thigh level, right thigh
    CC Exclusion 7th character A see Appendix A PDX collection 1328
  - CC +7th S76.922 Laceration of unspecified muscles, fascia and tendons at thigh level, left thigh
    CC Exclusion 7th character A see Appendix A PDX collection 1329
  - CC +7th S76.929 Laceration of unspecified muscles, fascia and tendons at thigh level, unspecified thigh
    CC Exclusion 7th character A see Appendix A PDX collection 1330

+ S76.99 Other specified injury of unspecified muscles, fascia and tendons at thigh level
  - +7th S76.991 Other specified injury of unspecified muscles, fascia and tendons at thigh level, right thigh
  - +7th S76.992 Other specified injury of unspecified muscles, fascia and tendons at thigh level, left thigh
  - +7th S76.999 Other specified injury of unspecified muscles, fascia and tendons at thigh level, unspecified thigh

S77 Crushing injury of hip and thigh

Use additional code(s) for all associated injuries

Excludes2: *crushing injury of ankle and foot (S97.-)*
crushing injury of lower leg (S87.-)

> The appropriate 7th character is to be added to each code from category S77
> A initial encounter
> D subsequent encounter
> S sequela

+ S77.0 Crushing injury of hip
  - CC X+7th S77.00 Crushing injury of unspecified hip
    CC Exclusion 7th character A see Appendix A PDX collection 1331
    HAC 7th character A see Appendix B for HAC conditional logic
  - CC X+7th S77.01 Crushing injury of right hip
    CC Exclusion 7th character A see Appendix A PDX collection 1331
    HAC 7th character A see Appendix B for HAC conditional logic
  - CC X+7th S77.02 Crushing injury of left hip
    CC Exclusion 7th character A see Appendix A PDX collection 1331
    HAC 7th character A see Appendix B for HAC conditional logic

+ S77.1 Crushing injury of thigh
  - CC X+7th S77.10 Crushing injury of unspecified thigh
    CC Exclusion 7th character A see Appendix A PDX collection 1331
    HAC 7th character A see Appendix B for HAC conditional logic
  - CC X+7th S77.11 Crushing injury of right thigh
    CC Exclusion 7th character A see Appendix A PDX collection 1331
    HAC 7th character A see Appendix B for HAC conditional logic
  - CC X+7th S77.12 Crushing injury of left thigh
    CC Exclusion 7th character A see Appendix A PDX collection 1331
    HAC 7th character A see Appendix B for HAC conditional logic

+ S77.2 Crushing injury of hip with thigh
  - X+7th S77.20 Crushing injury of unspecified hip with thigh
  - X+7th S77.21 Crushing injury of right hip with thigh
  - X+7th S77.22 Crushing injury of left hip with thigh

S78 Traumatic amputation of hip and thigh

An amputation not identified as partial or complete should be coded to complete

Excludes1: *traumatic amputation of knee (S88.0-)*

> The appropriate 7th character is to be added to each code from category S78
> A initial encounter
> D subsequent encounter
> S sequela

+ S78.0 Traumatic amputation at hip joint

+ S78.01 Complete traumatic amputation at hip joint
  - CC +7th S78.011 Complete traumatic amputation at right hip joint
    CC Exclusion 7th character A see Appendix A PDX collection 1333
  - CC +7th S78.012 Complete traumatic amputation at left hip joint
    CC Exclusion 7th character A see Appendix A PDX collection 1334
  - CC +7th S78.019 Complete traumatic amputation at unspecified hip joint
    CC Exclusion 7th character A see Appendix A PDX collection 1335

+ S78.02 Partial traumatic amputation at hip joint
  - CC +7th S78.021 Partial traumatic amputation at right hip joint
    CC Exclusion 7th character A see Appendix A PDX collection 1333
  - CC +7th S78.022 Partial traumatic amputation at left hip joint
    CC Exclusion 7th character A see Appendix A PDX collection 1334
  - CC +7th S78.029 Partial traumatic amputation at unspecified hip joint
    CC Exclusion 7th character A see Appendix A PDX collection 1335

+ **S78.1 Traumatic amputation at level between hip and knee**
Excludes1: *traumatic amputation of knee (S88.0-)*

+ **S78.11 Complete traumatic amputation at level between hip and knee**

CC +7th **S78.111 Complete traumatic amputation at level between right hip and knee**
CC Exclusion 7th character A see Appendix A PDX collection 1333

CC +7th **S78.112 Complete traumatic amputation at level between left hip and knee**
CC Exclusion 7th character A see Appendix A PDX collection 1334

CC +7th **S78.119 Complete traumatic amputation at level between unspecified hip and knee**
CC Exclusion 7th character A see Appendix A PDX collection 1335

+ **S78.12 Partial traumatic amputation at level between hip and knee**

CC +7th **S78.121 Partial traumatic amputation at level between right hip and knee**
CC Exclusion 7th character A see Appendix A PDX collection 1333

CC +7th **S78.122 Partial traumatic amputation at level between left hip and knee**
CC Exclusion 7th character A see Appendix A PDX collection 1334

CC +7th **S78.129 Partial traumatic amputation at level between unspecified hip and knee**
CC Exclusion 7th character A see Appendix A PDX collection 1335

+ **S78.9 Traumatic amputation of hip and thigh, level unspecified**

+ **S78.91 Complete traumatic amputation of hip and thigh, level unspecified**

CC +7th **S78.911 Complete traumatic amputation of right hip and thigh, level unspecified**
CC Exclusion 7th character A see Appendix A PDX collection 1333

CC +7th **S78.912 Complete traumatic amputation of left hip and thigh, level unspecified**
CC Exclusion 7th character A see Appendix A PDX collection 1334

CC +7th **S78.919 Complete traumatic amputation of unspecified hip and thigh, level unspecified**
CC Exclusion 7th character A see Appendix A PDX collection 1335

+ **S78.92 Partial traumatic amputation of hip and thigh, level unspecified**

CC +7th **S78.921 Partial traumatic amputation of right hip and thigh, level unspecified**
CC Exclusion 7th character A see Appendix A PDX collection 1333

CC +7th **S78.922 Partial traumatic amputation of left hip and thigh, level unspecified**
CC Exclusion 7th character A see Appendix A PDX collection 1334

CC +7th **S78.929 Partial traumatic amputation of unspecified hip and thigh, level unspecified**
CC Exclusion 7th character A see Appendix A PDX collection 1335

S79 Other and unspecified injuries of hip and thigh

NOTE A fracture not indicated as open or closed should be coded to closed

The appropriate 7th character is to be added to each code from subcategories **S79.0** and **S79.1**
A initial encounter for closed fracture
D subsequent encounter for fracture with routine healing
G subsequent encounter for fracture with delayed healing
K subsequent encounter for fracture with nonunion
P subsequent encounter for fracture with malunion
S sequela

Review coding guideline C.19.c

+ **S79.0 Physeal fracture of upper end of femur**
Excludes1: *apophyseal fracture of upper end of femur (S72.13-)*
nontraumatic slipped upper femoral epiphysis (M93.0-)

+ **S79.00 Unspecified physeal fracture of upper end of femur**

CC MCC +7th **S79.001 Unspecified physeal fracture of upper end of right femur**
CC Exclusion 7th characters K & P see Appendix A PDX collection 0897
MCC Exclusion 7th character A see Appendix A PDX collection 1297
HAC 7th character A see Appendix B for HAC conditional logic

CC MCC +7th **S79.002 Unspecified physeal fracture of upper end of left femur**
CC Exclusion 7th characters K & P see Appendix A PDX collection 0897
MCC Exclusion 7th character A see Appendix A PDX collection 1299
HAC 7th character A see Appendix B for HAC conditional logic

CC MCC +7th **S79.009 Unspecified physeal fracture of upper end of unspecified femur**
CC Exclusion 7th characters K & P see Appendix A PDX collection 0897
MCC Exclusion 7th character A see Appendix A PDX collection 1298
HAC 7th character A see Appendix B for HAC conditional logic

+ **S79.01 Salter-Harris Type I physeal fracture of upper end of femur**
Acute on chronic slipped capital femoral epiphysis (traumatic)
Acute slipped capital femoral epiphysis (traumatic)
Capital femoral epiphyseal fracture
Excludes1: *chronic slipped upper femoral epiphysis (nontraumatic) (M93.02-)*

CC MCC +7th **S79.011 Salter-Harris Type I physeal fracture of upper end of right femur**
CC Exclusion 7th characters K & P see Appendix A PDX collection 0897
MCC Exclusion 7th character A see Appendix PDX collection 1297
HAC 7th character A see Appendix B for HAC conditional logic

CC MCC +7th **S79.012 Salter-Harris Type I physeal fracture of upper end of left femur**
CC Exclusion 7th characters K & P see Appendix A PDX collection 0897
MCC Exclusion 7th character A see Appendix PDX collection 1299
HAC 7th character A see Appendix B for HAC conditional logic

CC MCC +7th **S79.019 Salter-Harris Type I physeal fracture of upper end of unspecified femur**
CC Exclusion 7th characters K & P see Appendix A PDX collection 0897
MCC Exclusion 7th character A see Appendix PDX collection 1298
HAC 7th character A see Appendix B for HAC conditional logic

+ **S79.09 Other physeal fracture of upper end of femur**

CC MCC +7th **S79.091 Other physeal fracture of upper end of right femur**
CC Exclusion 7th characters K & P see Appendix A PDX collection 0897
MCC Exclusion 7th character A see Appendix PDX collection 1297
HAC 7th character A see Appendix B for HAC conditional logic

CC MCC +7th **S79.092 Other physeal fracture of upper end of left femur**
CC Exclusion 7th characters K & P see Appendix A PDX collection 0897
MCC Exclusion 7th character A see Appendix PDX collection 1299
HAC 7th character A see Appendix B for HAC conditional logic

CC MCC +7th **S79.099 Other physeal fracture of upper end of unspecified femur**
CC Exclusion 7th characters K & P see Appendix A PDX collection 0897
MCC Exclusion 7th character A see Appendix PDX collection 1298
HAC 7th character A see Appendix B for HAC conditional logic

\+ S79.1 **Physeal fracture of lower end of femur**

\+ S79.10 **Unspecified physeal fracture of lower end of femur**

CC +7th **S79.101** **Unspecified physeal fracture of lower end of right femur**
CC Exclusion 7th character A see Appendix A PDX collection 1300
CC Exclusion 7th characters K & P see Appendix A PDX collection 0897
HAC 7th character A see Appendix B for HAC conditional logic

CC +7th **S79.102** **Unspecified physeal fracture of lower end of left femur**
CC Exclusion 7th character A see Appendix A PDX collection 1302
CC Exclusion 7th characters K & P see Appendix A PDX collection 0897
HAC 7th character A see Appendix B for HAC conditional logic

CC +7th **S79.109** **Unspecified physeal fracture of lower end of unspecified femur**
CC Exclusion 7th character A see Appendix A PDX collection 1301
CC Exclusion 7th characters K & P see Appendix A PDX collection 0897
HAC 7th character A see Appendix B for HAC conditional logic

\+ S79.11 **Salter-Harris Type I physeal fracture of lower end of femur**

CC +7th **S79.111** **Salter-Harris Type I physeal fracture of lower end of right femur**
CC Exclusion 7th character A see Appendix A PDX collection 1300
CC Exclusion 7th characters K & P see Appendix A PDX collection 0897
HAC 7th character A see Appendix B for HAC conditional logic

CC +7th **S79.112** **Salter-Harris Type I physeal fracture of lower end of left femur**
CC Exclusion 7th character A see Appendix A PDX collection 1302
CC Exclusion 7th characters K & P see Appendix A PDX collection 0897
HAC 7th character A see Appendix B for HAC conditional logic

CC +7th **S79.119** **Salter-Harris Type I physeal fracture of lower end of unspecified femur**
CC Exclusion 7th character A see Appendix A PDX collection 1301
CC Exclusion 7th characters K & P see Appendix A PDX collection 0897
HAC 7th character A see Appendix B for HAC conditional logic

\+ S79.12 **Salter-Harris Type II physeal fracture of lower end of femur**

CC +7th **S79.121** **Salter-Harris Type II physeal fracture of lower end of right femur**
CC Exclusion 7th character A see Appendix A PDX collection 1300
CC Exclusion 7th characters K & P see Appendix A PDX collection 0897
HAC 7th character A see Appendix B for HAC conditional logic

CC +7th **S79.122** **Salter-Harris Type II physeal fracture of lower end of left femur**
CC Exclusion 7th character A see Appendix A PDX collection 1302
CC Exclusion 7th characters K & P see Appendix A PDX collection 0897
HAC 7th character A see Appendix B for HAC conditional logic

CC +7th **S79.129** **Salter-Harris Type II physeal fracture of lower end of unspecified femur**
CC Exclusion 7th character A see Appendix A PDX collection 1301
CC Exclusion 7th characters K & P see Appendix A PDX collection 0897
HAC 7th character A see Appendix B for HAC conditional logic

\+ S79.13 **Salter-Harris Type III physeal fracture of lower end of femur**

CC +7th **S79.131** **Salter-Harris Type III physeal fracture of lower end of right femur**
CC Exclusion 7th character A see Appendix A PDX collection 1300
CC Exclusion 7th characters K & P see Appendix A PDX collection 0897
HAC 7th character A see Appendix B for HAC conditional logic

CC +7th **S79.132** **Salter-Harris Type III physeal fracture of lower end of left femur**
CC Exclusion 7th character A see Appendix A PDX collection 1302
CC Exclusion 7th characters K & P see Appendix A PDX collection 0897
HAC 7th character A see Appendix B for HAC conditional logic

CC +7th **S79.139** **Salter-Harris Type III physeal fracture of lower end of unspecified femur**
CC Exclusion 7th character A see Appendix A PDX collection 1301
CC Exclusion 7th characters K & P see Appendix A PDX collection 0897
HAC 7th character A see Appendix B for HAC conditional logic

\+ S79.14 **Salter-Harris Type IV physeal fracture of lower end of femur**

CC +7th **S79.141** **Salter-Harris Type IV physeal fracture of lower end of right femur**
CC Exclusion 7th character A see Appendix A PDX collection 1300
CC Exclusion 7th characters K & P see Appendix A PDX collection 0897
HAC 7th character A see Appendix B for HAC conditional logic

CC +7th **S79.142** **Salter-Harris Type IV physeal fracture of lower end of left femur**
CC Exclusion 7th character A see Appendix A PDX collection 1302
CC Exclusion 7th characters K & P see Appendix A PDX collection 0897
HAC 7th character A see Appendix B for HAC conditional logic

CC +7th **S79.149** **Salter-Harris Type IV physeal fracture of lower end of unspecified femur**
CC Exclusion 7th character A see Appendix A PDX collection 1301
CC Exclusion 7th characters K & P see Appendix A PDX collection 0897
HAC 7th character A see Appendix B for HAC conditional logic

\+ S79.19 **Other physeal fracture of lower end of femur**

CC +7th **S79.191** **Other physeal fracture of lower end of right femur**
CC Exclusion 7th character A see Appendix A PDX collection 1300
CC Exclusion 7th characters K & P see Appendix A PDX collection 0897
HAC 7th character A see Appendix B for HAC conditional logic

CC +7th **S79.192** **Other physeal fracture of lower end of left femur**
CC Exclusion 7th character A see Appendix A PDX collection 1302
CC Exclusion 7th characters K & P see Appendix A PDX collection 0897
HAC 7th character A see Appendix B for HAC conditional logic

CC +7th **S79.199** **Other physeal fracture of lower end of unspecified femur**
CC Exclusion 7th character A see Appendix A PDX collection 1301
CC Exclusion 7th characters K & P see Appendix A PDX collection 0897
HAC 7th character A see Appendix B for HAC conditional logic

\+ S79.8 **Other specified injuries of hip and thigh**

The appropriate 7th character is to be added to each code in subcategory **S79.8**
A initial encounter
D subsequent encounter
S sequela

\+ S79.81 **Other specified injuries of hip**
+7th **S79.811** **Other specified injuries of right hip**
+7th **S79.812** **Other specified injuries of left hip**
+7th **S79.819** **Other specified injuries of unspecified hip**

\+ S79.82 **Other specified injuries of thigh**
+7th **S79.821** **Other specified injuries of right thigh**
+7th **S79.822** **Other specified injuries of left thigh**
+7th **S79.829** **Other specified injuries of unspecified thigh**

\+ **S79.9 Unspecified injury of hip and thigh**

The appropriate 7th character is to be added to each code in subcategory **S79.9**
A - initial encounter
D - subsequent encounter
S - sequela

\+ **S79.91 Unspecified injury of hip**
+7th **S79.911 Unspecified injury of right hip**
+7th **S79.912 Unspecified injury of left hip**
+7th **S79.919 Unspecified injury of unspecified hip**
\+ **S79.92 Unspecified injury of thigh**
+7th **S79.921 Unspecified injury of right thigh**
+7th **S79.922 Unspecified injury of left thigh**
+7th **S79.929 Unspecified injury of unspecified thigh**

Injuries to the knee and lower leg (S80-S89)

Excludes2: *burns and corrosions (T20-T32)*
frostbite (T33-T34)
injuries of ankle and foot, except fracture of ankle and malleolus (S90-S99)
insect bite or sting, venomous (T63.4)

S80 Superficial injury of knee and lower leg

Excludes2: *superficial injury of ankle and foot (S90.-)*

The appropriate 7th character is to be added to each code from category S80
A initial encounter
D subsequent encounter
S sequela

Knee Tendons and Ligaments

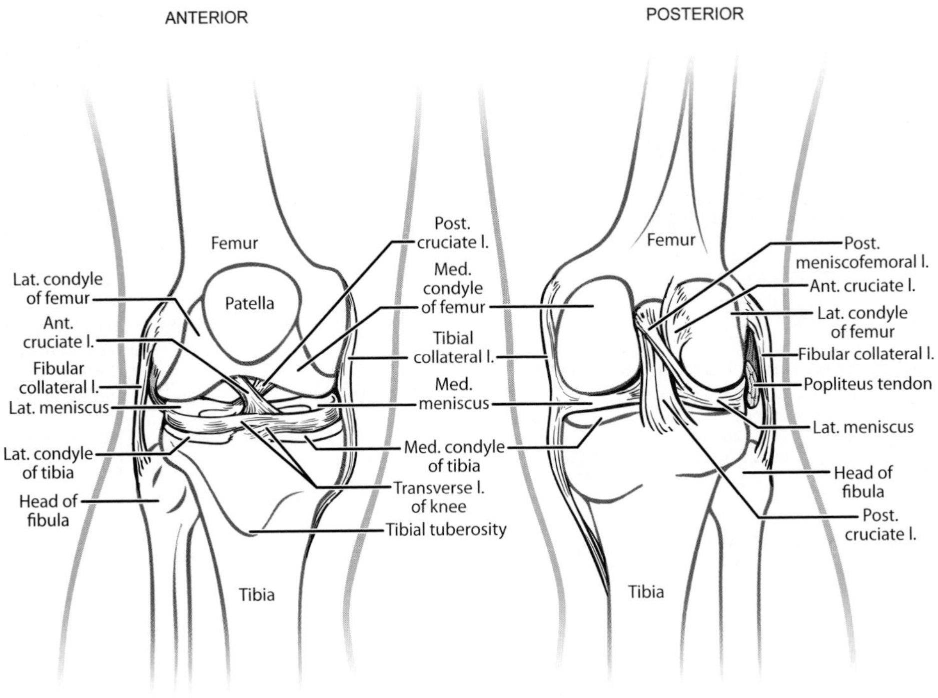

Bursa of the Knee

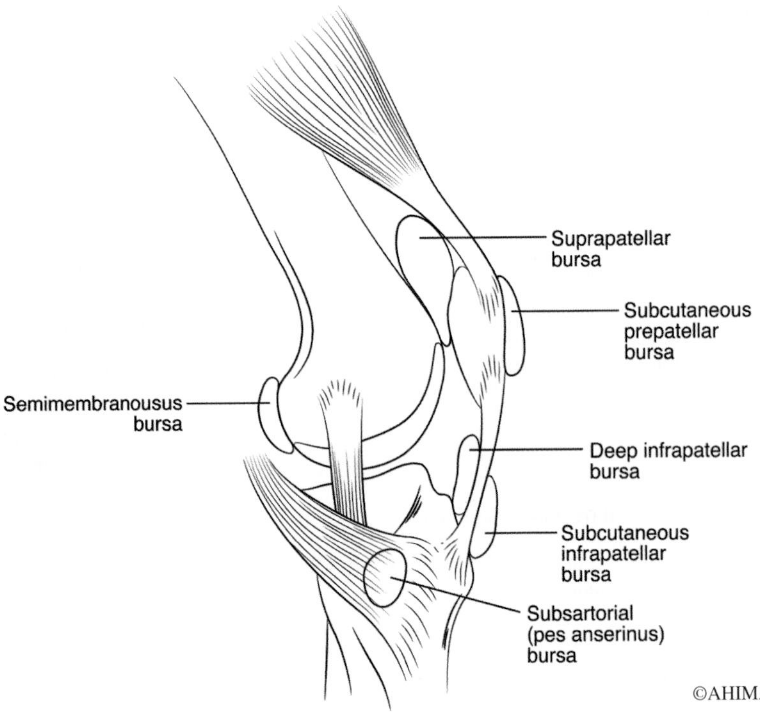

+ **S80.0 Contusion of knee**
X+7th **S80.00 Contusion of unspecified knee**
X+7th **S80.01 Contusion of right knee**
X+7th **S80.02 Contusion of left knee**
+ **S80.1 Contusion of lower leg**
X+7th **S80.10 Contusion of unspecified lower leg**
X+7th **S80.11 Contusion of right lower leg**
X+7th **S80.12 Contusion of left lower leg**
+ **S80.2 Other superficial injuries of knee**
+ **S80.21 Abrasion of knee**
+7th **S80.211 Abrasion, right knee**
+7th **S80.212 Abrasion, left knee**
+7th **S80.219 Abrasion, unspecified knee**
+ **S80.22 Blister (nonthermal) of knee**
+7th **S80.221 Blister (nonthermal), right knee**
+7th **S80.222 Blister (nonthermal), left knee**
+7th **S80.229 Blister (nonthermal), unspecified knee**
+ **S80.24 External constriction of knee**
+7th **S80.241 External constriction, right knee**
+7th **S80.242 External constriction, left knee**
+7th **S80.249 External constriction, unspecified knee**
+ **S80.25 Superficial foreign body of knee**
Splinter in the knee
+7th **S80.251 Superficial foreign body, right knee**
+7th **S80.252 Superficial foreign body, left knee**
+7th **S80.259 Superficial foreign body, unspecified knee**
+ **S80.26 Insect bite (nonvenomous) of knee**
+7th **S80.261 Insect bite (nonvenomous), right knee**
+7th **S80.262 Insect bite (nonvenomous), left knee**
+7th **S80.269 Insect bite (nonvenomous), unspecified knee**
+ **S80.27 Other superficial bite of knee**
Excludes1: *open bite of knee (S81.05-)*
+7th **S80.271 Other superficial bite of right knee**
+7th **S80.272 Other superficial bite of left knee**
+7th **S80.279 Other superficial bite of unspecified knee**
+ **S80.8 Other superficial injuries of lower leg**
+ **S80.81 Abrasion of lower leg**
+7th **S80.811 Abrasion, right lower leg**
+7th **S80.812 Abrasion, left lower leg**
+7th **S80.819 Abrasion, unspecified lower leg**
+ **S80.82 Blister (nonthermal) of lower leg**
+7th **S80.821 Blister (nonthermal), right lower leg**
+7th **S80.822 Blister (nonthermal), left lower leg**
+7th **S80.829 Blister (nonthermal), unspecified lower leg**
+ **S80.84 External constriction of lower leg**
+7th **S80.841 External constriction, right lower leg**
+7th **S80.842 External constriction, left lower leg**
+7th **S80.849 External constriction, unspecified lower leg**
+ **S80.85 Superficial foreign body of lower leg**
Splinter in the lower leg
+7th **S80.851 Superficial foreign body, right lower leg**
+7th **S80.852 Superficial foreign body, left lower leg**
+7th **S80.859 Superficial foreign body, unspecified lower leg**
+ **S80.86 Insect bite (nonvenomous) of lower leg**
+7th **S80.861 Insect bite (nonvenomous), right lower leg**
+7th **S80.862 Insect bite (nonvenomous), left lower leg**
+7th **S80.869 Insect bite (nonvenomous), unspecified lower leg**
+ **S80.87 Other superficial bite of lower leg**
Excludes1: *open bite of lower leg (S81.85-)*
+7th **S80.871 Other superficial bite, right lower leg**
+7th **S80.872 Other superficial bite, left lower leg**
+7th **S80.879 Other superficial bite, unspecified lower leg**
+ **S80.9 Unspecified superficial injury of knee and lower leg**
+ **S80.91 Unspecified superficial injury of knee**
+7th **S80.911 Unspecified superficial injury of right knee**
+7th **S80.912 Unspecified superficial injury of left knee**
+7th **S80.919 Unspecified superficial injury of unspecified knee**
+ **S80.92 Unspecified superficial injury of lower leg**
+7th **S80.921 Unspecified superficial injury of right lower leg**
+7th **S80.922 Unspecified superficial injury of left lower leg**
+7th **S80.929 Unspecified superficial injury of unspecified lower leg**

S81 **Open wound of knee and lower leg**

Code also any associated wound infection

Excludes1: *open fracture of knee and lower leg (S82.-)*
traumatic amputation of lower leg (S88.-)

Excludes2: *open wound of ankle and foot (S91.-)*

The appropriate 7th character is to be added to each code from category S81
A initial encounter
D subsequent encounter
S sequela

\+ **S81.0 Open wound of knee**
\+ **S81.00 Unspecified open wound of knee**
+7th **S81.001 Unspecified open wound, right knee**
+7th **S81.002 Unspecified open wound, left knee**
+7th **S81.009 Unspecified open wound, unspecified knee**
\+ **S81.01 Laceration without foreign body of knee**
+7th **S81.011 Laceration without foreign body, right knee**
+7th **S81.012 Laceration without foreign body, left knee**
+7th **S81.019 Laceration without foreign body, unspecified knee**
\+ **S81.02 Laceration with foreign body of knee**
+7th **S81.021 Laceration with foreign body, right knee**
+7th **S81.022 Laceration with foreign body, left knee**
+7th **S81.029 Laceration with foreign body, unspecified knee**
\+ **S81.03 Puncture wound without foreign body of knee**
+7th **S81.031 Puncture wound without foreign body, right knee**
+7th **S81.032 Puncture wound without foreign body, left knee**
+7th **S81.039 Puncture wound without foreign body, unspecified knee**
\+ **S81.04 Puncture wound with foreign body of knee**
+7th **S81.041 Puncture wound with foreign body, right knee**
+7th **S81.042 Puncture wound with foreign body, left knee**
+7th **S81.049 Puncture wound with foreign body, unspecified knee**
\+ **S81.05 Open bite of knee**
Bite of knee NOS
Excludes1: *superficial bite of knee (S80.27-)*
+7th **S81.051 Open bite, right knee**
+7th **S81.052 Open bite, left knee**
+7th **S81.059 Open bite, unspecified knee**
\+ **S81.8 Open wound of lower leg**
\+ **S81.80 Unspecified open wound of lower leg**
+7th **S81.801 Unspecified open wound, right lower leg**
+7th **S81.802 Unspecified open wound, left lower leg**
+7th **S81.809 Unspecified open wound, unspecified lower leg**
\+ **S81.81 Laceration without foreign body of lower leg**
+7th **S81.811 Laceration without foreign body, right lower leg**
+7th **S81.812 Laceration without foreign body, left lower leg**
+7th **S81.819 Laceration without foreign body, unspecified lower leg**
\+ **S81.82 Laceration with foreign body of lower leg**
+7th **S81.821 Laceration with foreign body, right lower leg**
+7th **S81.822 Laceration with foreign body, left lower leg**
+7th **S81.829 Laceration with foreign body, unspecified lower leg**
\+ **S81.83 Puncture wound without foreign body of lower leg**
+7th **S81.831 Puncture wound without foreign body, right lower leg**
+7th **S81.832 Puncture wound without foreign body, left lower leg**
+7th **S81.839 Puncture wound without foreign body, unspecified lower leg**
\+ **S81.84 Puncture wound with foreign body of lower leg**
+7th **S81.841 Puncture wound with foreign body, right lower leg**
AHA CC: 3Q, 2016, 24
+7th **S81.842 Puncture wound with foreign body, left lower leg**
+7th **S81.849 Puncture wound with foreign body, unspecified lower leg**
\+ **S81.85 Open bite of lower leg**
Bite of lower leg NOS
Excludes1: *superficial bite of lower leg (S80.86-, S80.87-)*
+7th **S81.851 Open bite, right lower leg**
+7th **S81.852 Open bite, left lower leg**
+7th **S81.859 Open bite, unspecified lower leg**

S82 **Fracture of lower leg, including ankle**

NOTE A fracture not indicated as displaced or nondisplaced should be coded to displaced
A fracture not indicated as open or closed should be coded to closed
The open fracture designations are based on the Gustilo open fracture classification

Includes: fracture of malleolus

Excludes1: *traumatic amputation of lower leg (S88.-)*

Excludes2: *fracture of foot, except ankle (S92.-)*
periprosthetic fracture of prosthetic implant of knee (M97.0-)

The appropriate 7th character is to be added to all codes from category S82
A initial encounter for closed fracture
B initial encounter for open fracture type I or II
initial encounter for open fracture NOS
C initial encounter for open fracture type IIIA, IIIB, or IIIC
D subsequent encounter for closed fracture with routine healing
E subsequent encounter for open fracture type I or II with routine healing
F subsequent encounter for open fracture type IIIA, IIIB, or IIIC with routine healing
G subsequent encounter for closed fracture with delayed healing
H subsequent encounter for open fracture type I or II with delayed healing
J subsequent encounter for open fracture type IIIA, IIIB, or IIIC with delayed healing
K subsequent encounter for closed fracture with nonunion
M subsequent encounter for open fracture type I or II with nonunion
N subsequent encounter for open fracture type IIIA, IIIB, or IIIC with nonunion
P subsequent encounter for closed fracture with malunion
Q subsequent encounter for open fracture type I or II with malunion
R subsequent encounter for open fracture type IIIA, IIIB, or IIIC with malunion
S sequela

Review coding guideline C.19.c

\+ **S82.0 Fracture of patella**
Knee cap
\+ **S82.00 Unspecified fracture of patella**
CC +7th **S82.001 Unspecified fracture of right patella**
CC Exclusion 7th character A see Appendix A PDX collection 1336
CC Exclusion 7th characters B & C see Appendix A PDX collection 1337
CC Exclusion 7th characters K - R see Appendix A PDX collection 0897
HAC 7th characters A - C see Appendix B for HAC conditional logic
CC +7th **S82.002 Unspecified fracture of left patella**
CC Exclusion 7th character A see Appendix A PDX collection 1338
CC Exclusion 7th characters B & C see Appendix A PDX collection 1337
CC Exclusion 7th characters K - R see Appendix A PDX collection 0897
HAC 7th characters A - C see Appendix B for HAC conditional logic
CC +7th **S82.009 Unspecified fracture of unspecified patella**
CC Exclusion 7th character A see Appendix A PDX collection 1339
CC Exclusion 7th characters B & C see Appendix A PDX collection 1337
CC Exclusion 7th characters K - R see Appendix A PDX collection 0897
HAC 7th characters A - C see Appendix B for HAC conditional logic

+ **S82.01 Osteochondral fracture of patella**

CC +7th **S82.011 Displaced osteochondral fracture of right patella**
CC Exclusion 7th character A see Appendix A PDX collection 1336
CC Exclusion 7th characters B & C see Appendix A PDX collection 1337
CC Exclusion 7th characters K - R see Appendix A PDX collection 0897
HAC 7th characters A - C see Appendix B for HAC conditional logic

CC +7th **S82.012 Displaced osteochondral fracture of left patella**
CC Exclusion 7th character A see Appendix A PDX collection 1338
CC Exclusion 7th characters B & C see Appendix A PDX collection 1337
CC Exclusion 7th characters K - R see Appendix A PDX collection 0897
HAC 7th characters A - C see Appendix B for HAC conditional logic

CC +7th **S82.013 Displaced osteochondral fracture of unspecified patella**
CC Exclusion 7th character A see Appendix A PDX collection 1339
CC Exclusion 7th characters B & C see Appendix A PDX collection 1337
CC Exclusion 7th characters K - R see Appendix A PDX collection 0897
HAC 7th characters A - C see Appendix B for HAC conditional logic

CC +7th **S82.014 Nondisplaced osteochondral fracture of right patella**
CC Exclusion 7th character A see Appendix A PDX collection 1336
CC Exclusion 7th characters B & C see Appendix A PDX collection 1337
CC Exclusion 7th characters K - R see Appendix A PDX collection 0897
HAC 7th characters A - C see Appendix B for HAC conditional logic

CC +7th **S82.015 Nondisplaced osteochondral fracture of left patella**
CC Exclusion 7th character A see Appendix A PDX collection 1338
CC Exclusion 7th characters B & C see Appendix A PDX collection 1337
CC Exclusion 7th characters K - R see Appendix A PDX collection 0897
HAC 7th characters A - C see Appendix B for HAC conditional logic

CC +7th **S82.016 Nondisplaced osteochondral fracture of unspecified patella**
CC Exclusion 7th character A see Appendix A PDX collection 1339
CC Exclusion 7th characters B & C see Appendix A PDX collection 1337
CC Exclusion 7th characters K - R see Appendix A PDX collection 0897
HAC 7th characters A - C see Appendix B for HAC conditional logic

+ **S82.02 Longitudinal fracture of patella**

CC +7th **S82.021 Displaced longitudinal fracture of right patella**
CC Exclusion 7th character A see Appendix A PDX collection 1336
CC Exclusion 7th characters B & C see Appendix A PDX collection 1337
CC Exclusion 7th characters K - R see Appendix A PDX collection 0897
HAC 7th characters A - C see Appendix B for HAC conditional logic

CC +7th **S82.022 Displaced longitudinal fracture of left patella**
CC Exclusion 7th character A see Appendix A PDX collection 1338
CC Exclusion 7th characters B & C see Appendix A PDX collection 1337
CC Exclusion 7th characters K - R see Appendix A PDX collection 0897
HAC 7th characters A - C see Appendix B for HAC conditional logic

CC +7th **S82.023 Displaced longitudinal fracture of unspecified patella**
CC Exclusion 7th character A see Appendix A PDX collection 1339
CC Exclusion 7th characters B & C see Appendix A PDX collection 1337
CC Exclusion 7th characters K - R see Appendix A PDX collection 0897
HAC 7th characters A - C see Appendix B for HAC conditional logic

CC +7th **S82.024 Nondisplaced longitudinal fracture of right patella**
CC Exclusion 7th character A see Appendix A PDX collection 1336
CC Exclusion 7th characters B & C see Appendix A PDX collection 1337
CC Exclusion 7th characters K - R see Appendix A PDX collection 0897
HAC 7th characters A - C see Appendix B for HAC conditional logic

CC +7th **S82.025 Nondisplaced longitudinal fracture of left patella**
CC Exclusion 7th character A see Appendix A PDX collection 1338
CC Exclusion 7th characters B & C see Appendix A PDX collection 1337
CC Exclusion 7th characters K - R see Appendix A PDX collection 0897
HAC 7th characters A - C see Appendix B for HAC conditional logic

CC +7th **S82.026 Nondisplaced longitudinal fracture of unspecified patella**
CC Exclusion 7th character A see Appendix A PDX collection 1339
CC Exclusion 7th characters B & C see Appendix A PDX collection 1337
CC Exclusion 7th characters K - R see Appendix A PDX collection 0897
HAC 7th characters A - C see Appendix B for HAC conditional logic

+ **S82.03 Transverse fracture of patella**

CC +7th **S82.031 Displaced transverse fracture of right patella**
CC Exclusion 7th character A see Appendix A PDX collection 1336
CC Exclusion 7th characters B & C see Appendix A PDX collection 1337
CC Exclusion 7th characters K - R see Appendix A PDX collection 0897
HAC 7th characters A - C see Appendix B for HAC conditional logic

CC +7th **S82.032 Displaced transverse fracture of left patella**
CC Exclusion 7th character A see Appendix A PDX collection 1338
CC Exclusion 7th characters B & C see Appendix A PDX collection 1337
CC Exclusion 7th characters K - R see Appendix A PDX collection 0897
HAC 7th characters A - C see Appendix B for HAC conditional logic

CC +7th **S82.033 Displaced transverse fracture of unspecified patella**
CC Exclusion 7th character A see Appendix A PDX collection 1339
CC Exclusion 7th characters B & C see Appendix A PDX collection 1337
CC Exclusion 7th characters K - R see Appendix A PDX collection 0897
HAC 7th characters A - C see Appendix B for HAC conditional logic

CC +7th **S82.034 Nondisplaced transverse fracture of right patella**
CC Exclusion 7th character A see Appendix A PDX collection 1336
CC Exclusion 7th characters B & C see Appendix A PDX collection 1337
CC Exclusion 7th characters K - R see Appendix A PDX collection 0897
HAC 7th characters A - C see Appendix B for HAC conditional logic

CC +7th **S82.035 Nondisplaced transverse fracture of left patella**
CC Exclusion 7th character A see Appendix A PDX collection 1338
CC Exclusion 7th characters B & C see Appendix A PDX collection 1337
CC Exclusion 7th characters K - R see Appendix A PDX collection 0897
HAC 7th characters A - C see Appendix B for HAC conditional logic

CC +7th **S82.036 Nondisplaced transverse fracture of unspecified patella**
CC Exclusion 7th character A see Appendix A PDX collection 1339
CC Exclusion 7th characters B & C see Appendix A PDX collection 1337
CC Exclusion 7th characters K - R see Appendix A PDX collection 0897
HAC 7th characters A - C see Appendix B for HAC conditional logic

\+ **S82.04 Comminuted fracture of patella**

CC +7th **S82.041 Displaced comminuted fracture of right patella**
CC Exclusion 7th character A see Appendix A PDX collection 1336
CC Exclusion 7th characters B & C see Appendix A PDX collection 1337
CC Exclusion 7th characters K - R see Appendix A PDX collection 0897
HAC 7th characters A - C see Appendix B for HAC conditional logic

CC +7th **S82.042 Displaced comminuted fracture of left patella**
CC Exclusion 7th character A see Appendix A PDX collection 1338
CC Exclusion 7th characters B & C see Appendix A PDX collection 1337
CC Exclusion 7th characters K - R see Appendix A PDX collection 0897
HAC 7th characters A - C see Appendix B for HAC conditional logic

CC +7th **S82.043 Displaced comminuted fracture of unspecified patella**
CC Exclusion 7th character A see Appendix A PDX collection 1339
CC Exclusion 7th characters B & C see Appendix A PDX collection 1337
CC Exclusion 7th characters K - R see Appendix A PDX collection 0897
HAC 7th characters A - C see Appendix B for HAC conditional logic

CC +7th **S82.044 Nondisplaced comminuted fracture of right patella**
CC Exclusion 7th character A see Appendix A PDX collection 1336
CC Exclusion 7th characters B & C see Appendix A PDX collection 1337
CC Exclusion 7th characters K - R see Appendix A PDX collection 0897
HAC 7th characters A - C see Appendix B for HAC conditional logic

CC +7th **S82.045 Nondisplaced comminuted fracture of left patella**
CC Exclusion 7th character A see Appendix A PDX collection 1338
CC Exclusion 7th characters B & C see Appendix A PDX collection 1337
CC Exclusion 7th characters K - R see Appendix A PDX collection 0897
HAC 7th characters A - C see Appendix B for HAC conditional logic

CC +7th **S82.046 Nondisplaced comminuted fracture of unspecified patella**
CC Exclusion 7th character A see Appendix A PDX collection 1339
CC Exclusion 7th characters B & C see Appendix A PDX collection 1337
CC Exclusion 7th characters K - R see Appendix A PDX collection 0897
HAC 7th characters A - C see Appendix B for HAC conditional logic

\+ **S82.09 Other fracture of patella**

CC +7th **S82.091 Other fracture of right patella**
CC Exclusion 7th character A see Appendix A PDX collection 1336
CC Exclusion 7th characters B & C see Appendix A PDX collection 1337
CC Exclusion 7th characters K - R see Appendix A PDX collection 0897
HAC 7th characters A - C see Appendix B for HAC conditional logic

CC +7th **S82.092 Other fracture of left patella**
CC Exclusion 7th character A see Appendix A PDX collection 1338
CC Exclusion 7th characters B & C see Appendix A PDX collection 1337
CC Exclusion 7th characters K - R see Appendix A PDX collection 0897
HAC 7th characters A - C see Appendix B for HAC conditional logic

CC +7th **S82.099 Other fracture of unspecified patella**
CC Exclusion 7th character A see Appendix A PDX collection 1339
CC Exclusion 7th characters B & C see Appendix A PDX collection 1337
CC Exclusion 7th characters K - R see Appendix A PDX collection 0897
HAC 7th characters A - C see Appendix B for HAC conditional logic

\+ **S82.1 Fracture of upper end of tibia**
Fracture of proximal end of tibia
Excludes2: *fracture of shaft of tibia (S82.2-)*
physeal fracture of upper end of tibia (S89.0-)

\+ **S82.10 Unspecified fracture of upper end of tibia**

CC MCC +7th **S82.101 Unspecified fracture of upper end of right tibia**
CC Exclusion 7th character A see Appendix A PDX collection 1340
CC Exclusion 7th characters K - R see Appendix A PDX collection 0897
MCC Exclusion 7th characters B & C see Appendix A PDX collection 1341
HAC 7th characters A - C see Appendix B for HAC conditional logic

CC MCC +7th **S82.102 Unspecified fracture of upper end of left tibia**
CC Exclusion 7th character A see Appendix A PDX collection 1342
CC Exclusion 7th characters K - R see Appendix A PDX collection 0897
MCC Exclusion 7th characters B & C see Appendix A PDX collection 1341
HAC 7th characters A - C see Appendix B for HAC conditional logic

CC MCC +7th **S82.109 Unspecified fracture of upper end of unspecified tibia**
CC Exclusion 7th character A see Appendix A PDX collection 1341
CC Exclusion 7th characters K - R see Appendix A PDX collection 0897
MCC Exclusion 7th characters B & C see Appendix A PDX collection 1341
HAC 7th characters A - C see Appendix B for HAC conditional logic

\+ **S82.11 Fracture of tibial spine**

CC MCC +7th **S82.111 Displaced fracture of right tibial spine**
CC Exclusion 7th character A see Appendix A PDX collection 1340
CC Exclusion 7th characters K - R see Appendix A PDX collection 0897
MCC Exclusion 7th characters B & C see Appendix A PDX collection 1341
HAC 7th characters A - C see Appendix B for HAC conditional logic

CC MCC +7th **S82.112 Displaced fracture of left tibial spine**
CC Exclusion 7th character A see Appendix A PDX collection 1342
CC Exclusion 7th characters K - R see Appendix A PDX collection 0897
MCC Exclusion 7th characters B & C see Appendix A PDX collection 1341
HAC 7th characters A - C see Appendix B for HAC conditional logic

CC MCC +7th **S82.113 Displaced fracture of unspecified tibial spine**
CC Exclusion 7th character A see Appendix A PDX collection 1341
CC Exclusion 7th characters K - R see Appendix A PDX collection 0897
MCC Exclusion 7th characters B & C see Appendix A PDX collection 1341
HAC 7th characters A - C see Appendix B for HAC conditional logic

CC MCC +7th **S82.114 Nondisplaced fracture of right tibial spine**
CC Exclusion 7th character A see Appendix A PDX collection 1340
CC Exclusion 7th characters K - R see Appendix A PDX collection 0897
MCC Exclusion 7th characters B & C see Appendix A PDX collection 1341
HAC 7th characters A - C see Appendix B for HAC conditional logic

CC MCC +7th **S82.115 Nondisplaced fracture of left tibial spine**
CC Exclusion 7th character A see Appendix A PDX collection 1342
CC Exclusion 7th characters K - R see Appendix A PDX collection 0897
MCC Exclusion 7th characters B & C see Appendix A PDX collection 1341
HAC 7th characters A - C see Appendix B for HAC conditional logic

CC MCC +7th **S82.116 Nondisplaced fracture of unspecified tibial spine**
CC Exclusion 7th character A see Appendix A PDX collection 1341
CC Exclusion 7th characters K - R see Appendix A PDX collection 0897
MCC Exclusion 7th characters B & C see Appendix A PDX collection 1341
HAC 7th characters A - C see Appendix B for HAC conditional logic

+ **S82.12 Fracture of lateral condyle of tibia**

CC MCC +7th **S82.121 Displaced fracture of lateral condyle of right tibia**
CC Exclusion 7th character A see Appendix A PDX collection 1340
CC Exclusion 7th characters K - R see Appendix A PDX collection 0897
MCC Exclusion 7th characters B & C see Appendix A PDX collection 1341
HAC 7th characters A - C see Appendix B for HAC conditional logic

CC MCC +7th **S82.122 Displaced fracture of lateral condyle of left tibia**
CC Exclusion 7th character A see Appendix A PDX collection 1342
CC Exclusion 7th characters K - R see Appendix A PDX collection 0897
MCC Exclusion 7th characters B & C see Appendix A PDX collection 1341
HAC 7th characters A - C see Appendix B for HAC conditional logic

CC MCC +7th **S82.123 Displaced fracture of lateral condyle of unspecified tibia**
CC Exclusion 7th character A see Appendix A PDX collection 1341
CC Exclusion 7th characters K - R see Appendix A PDX collection 0897
MCC Exclusion 7th characters B & C see Appendix A PDX collection 1341
HAC 7th characters A - C see Appendix B for HAC conditional logic

CC MCC +7th **S82.124 Nondisplaced fracture of lateral condyle of right tibia**
CC Exclusion 7th character A see Appendix A PDX collection 1340
CC Exclusion 7th characters K - R see Appendix A PDX collection 0897
MCC Exclusion 7th characters B & C see Appendix A PDX collection 1341
HAC 7th characters A - C see Appendix B for HAC conditional logic

CC MCC +7th **S82.125 Nondisplaced fracture of lateral condyle of left tibia**
CC Exclusion 7th character A see Appendix A PDX collection 1342
CC Exclusion 7th characters K - R see Appendix A PDX collection 0897
MCC Exclusion 7th characters B & C see Appendix A PDX collection 1341
HAC 7th characters A - C see Appendix B for HAC conditional logic

CC MCC +7th **S82.126 Nondisplaced fracture of lateral condyle of unspecified tibia**
CC Exclusion 7th character A see Appendix A PDX collection 1341
CC Exclusion 7th characters K - R see Appendix A PDX collection 0897
MCC Exclusion 7th characters B & C see Appendix A PDX collection 1341
HAC 7th characters A - C see Appendix B for HAC conditional logic

+ **S82.13 Fracture of medial condyle of tibia**

CC MCC +7th **S82.131 Displaced fracture of medial condyle of right tibia**
CC Exclusion 7th character A see Appendix A PDX collection 1340
CC Exclusion 7th characters K - R see Appendix A PDX collection 0897
MCC Exclusion 7th characters B & C see Appendix A PDX collection 1341
HAC 7th characters A - C see Appendix B for HAC conditional logic

CC MCC +7th **S82.132 Displaced fracture of medial condyle of left tibia**
CC Exclusion 7th character A see Appendix A PDX collection 1342
CC Exclusion 7th characters K - R see Appendix A PDX collection 0897
MCC Exclusion 7th characters B & C see Appendix A PDX collection 1341
HAC 7th characters A - C see Appendix B for HAC conditional logic

CC MCC +7th **S82.133 Displaced fracture of medial condyle of unspecified tibia**
CC Exclusion 7th character A see Appendix A PDX collection 1341
CC Exclusion 7th characters K - R see Appendix A PDX collection 0897
MCC Exclusion 7th characters B & C see Appendix A PDX collection 1341
HAC 7th characters A - C see Appendix B for HAC conditional logic

CC MCC +7th **S82.134 Nondisplaced fracture of medial condyle of right tibia**
CC Exclusion 7th character A see Appendix A PDX collection 1340
CC Exclusion 7th characters K - R see Appendix A PDX collection 0897
MCC Exclusion 7th characters B & C see Appendix A PDX collection 1341
HAC 7th characters A - C see Appendix B for HAC conditional logic

CC MCC +7th **S82.135 Nondisplaced fracture of medial condyle of left tibia**
CC Exclusion 7th character A see Appendix A PDX collection 1342
CC Exclusion 7th characters K - R see Appendix A PDX collection 0897
MCC Exclusion 7th characters B & C see Appendix A PDX collection 1341
HAC 7th characters A - C see Appendix B for HAC conditional logic

CC MCC +7th **S82.136 Nondisplaced fracture of medial condyle of unspecified tibia**
CC Exclusion 7th character A see Appendix A PDX collection 1341
CC Exclusion 7th characters K - R see Appendix A PDX collection 0897
MCC Exclusion 7th characters B & C see Appendix A PDX collection 1341
HAC 7th characters A - C see Appendix B for HAC conditional logic

+ **S82.14 Bicondylar fracture of tibia**
Fracture of tibial plateau NOS

CC MCC +7th **S82.141 Displaced bicondylar fracture of right tibia**
CC Exclusion 7th character A see Appendix A PDX collection 1340
CC Exclusion 7th characters K - R see Appendix A PDX collection 0897
MCC Exclusion 7th characters B & C see Appendix A PDX collection 1341
HAC 7th characters A - C see Appendix B for HAC conditional logic

CC MCC +7th **S82.142 Displaced bicondylar fracture of left tibia**
CC Exclusion 7th character A see Appendix A PDX collection 1342
CC Exclusion 7th characters K - R see Appendix A PDX collection 0897
MCC Exclusion 7th characters B & C see Appendix A PDX collection 1341
HAC 7th characters A - C see Appendix B for HAC conditional logic

CC MCC +7th **S82.143 Displaced bicondylar fracture of unspecified tibia**
CC Exclusion 7th character A see Appendix A PDX collection 1341
CC Exclusion 7th characters K - R see Appendix A PDX collection 0897
MCC Exclusion 7th characters B & C see Appendix A PDX collection 1341
HAC 7th characters A - C see Appendix B for HAC conditional logic

CC MCC +7th **S82.144 Nondisplaced bicondylar fracture of right tibia**
CC Exclusion 7th character A see Appendix A PDX collection 1340
CC Exclusion 7th characters K - R see Appendix A PDX collection 0897
MCC Exclusion 7th characters B & C see Appendix A PDX collection 1341
HAC 7th characters A - C see Appendix B for HAC conditional logic

CC MCC +7th **S82.145 Nondisplaced bicondylar fracture of left tibia**
CC Exclusion 7th character A see Appendix A PDX collection 1342
CC Exclusion 7th characters K - R see Appendix A PDX collection 0897
MCC Exclusion 7th characters B & C see Appendix A PDX collection 1341
HAC 7th characters A - C see Appendix B for HAC conditional logic

CC MCC +7th **S82.146 Nondisplaced bicondylar fracture of unspecified tibia**
CC Exclusion 7th character A see Appendix A PDX collection 1341
CC Exclusion 7th characters K - R see Appendix A PDX collection 0897
MCC Exclusion 7th characters B & C see Appendix A PDX collection 1341
HAC 7th characters A - C see Appendix B for HAC conditional logic

\+ **S82.15 Fracture of tibial tuberosity**

CC MCC +7th **S82.151 Displaced fracture of right tibial tuberosity**
CC Exclusion 7th character A see Appendix A PDX collection 1340
CC Exclusion 7th characters K - R see Appendix A PDX collection 0897
MCC Exclusion 7th characters B & C see Appendix A PDX collection 1341
HAC 7th characters A - C see Appendix B for HAC conditional logic

CC MCC +7th **S82.152 Displaced fracture of left tibial tuberosity**
CC Exclusion 7th character A see Appendix A PDX collection 1342
CC Exclusion 7th characters K - R see Appendix A PDX collection 0897
MCC Exclusion 7th characters B & C see Appendix A PDX collection 1341
HAC 7th characters A - C see Appendix B for HAC conditional logic

CC MCC +7th **S82.153 Displaced fracture of unspecified tibial tuberosity**
CC Exclusion 7th character A see Appendix A PDX collection 1341
CC Exclusion 7th characters K - R see Appendix A PDX collection 0897
MCC Exclusion 7th characters B & C see Appendix A PDX collection 1341
HAC 7th characters A - C see Appendix B for HAC conditional logic

CC MCC +7th **S82.154 Nondisplaced fracture of right tibial tuberosity**
CC Exclusion 7th character A see Appendix A PDX collection 1340
CC Exclusion 7th characters K - R see Appendix A PDX collection 0897
MCC Exclusion 7th characters B & C see Appendix A PDX collection 1341
HAC 7th characters A - C see Appendix B for HAC conditional logic

CC MCC +7th **S82.155 Nondisplaced fracture of left tibial tuberosity**
CC Exclusion 7th character A see Appendix A PDX collection 1342
CC Exclusion 7th characters K - R see Appendix A PDX collection 0897
MCC Exclusion 7th characters B & C see Appendix A PDX collection 1341
HAC 7th characters A - C see Appendix B for HAC conditional logic

CC MCC +7th **S82.156 Nondisplaced fracture of unspecified tibial tuberosity**
CC Exclusion 7th character A see Appendix A PDX collection 1341
CC Exclusion 7th characters K - R see Appendix A PDX collection 0897
MCC Exclusion 7th characters B & C see Appendix A PDX collection 1341
HAC 7th characters A - C see Appendix B for HAC conditional logic

\+ **S82.16 Torus fracture of upper end of tibia**

The appropriate 7th character is to be added to all codes in subcategory **S82.16**
A initial encounter for closed fracture
D subsequent encounter for fracture with routine healing
G subsequent encounter for fracture with delayed healing
K subsequent encounter for fracture with nonunion
P subsequent encounter for fracture with malunion
S sequela

CC +7th **S82.161 Torus fracture of upper end of right tibia**
CC Exclusion 7th character A see Appendix A PDX collection 1343
CC Exclusion 7th characters K & P see Appendix A PDX collection 0897
HAC 7th character A see Appendix B for HAC conditional logic

CC +7th **S82.162 Torus fracture of upper end of left tibia**
CC Exclusion 7th character A see Appendix A PDX collection 1344
CC Exclusion 7th characters K & P see Appendix A PDX collection 0897
HAC 7th character A see Appendix B for HAC conditional logic

CC +7th **S82.169 Torus fracture of upper end of unspecified tibia**
CC Exclusion 7th character A see Appendix A PDX collection 1345
CC Exclusion 7th characters K & P see Appendix A PDX collection 0897
HAC 7th character A see Appendix B for HAC conditional logic

\+ **S82.19 Other fracture of upper end of tibia**

CC MCC +7th **S82.191 Other fracture of upper end of right tibia**
CC Exclusion 7th character A see Appendix A PDX collection 1340
CC Exclusion 7th characters K - R see Appendix A PDX collection 0897
MCC Exclusion 7th characters B & C see Appendix A PDX collection 1341
HAC 7th characters A - C see Appendix B for HAC conditional logic

CC MCC +7th **S82.192 Other fracture of upper end of left tibia**
CC Exclusion 7th character A see Appendix A PDX collection 1342
CC Exclusion 7th characters K - R see Appendix A PDX collection 0897
MCC Exclusion 7th characters B & C see Appendix A PDX collection 1341
HAC 7th characters A - C see Appendix B for HAC conditional logic

CC MCC +7th **S82.199 Other fracture of upper end of unspecified tibia**
CC Exclusion 7th character A see Appendix A PDX collection 1341
CC Exclusion 7th characters K - R see Appendix A PDX collection 0897
MCC Exclusion 7th characters B & C see Appendix A PDX collection 1341
HAC 7th characters A - C see Appendix B for HAC conditional logic

+ **S82.2 Fracture of shaft of tibia**

+ **S82.20 Unspecified fracture of shaft of tibia**
Fracture of tibia NOS

CC MCC +7th **S82.201 Unspecified fracture of shaft of right tibia**
CC Exclusion 7th character A see Appendix A PDX collection 1346
CC Exclusion 7th characters K - R see Appendix A PDX collection 0897
MCC Exclusion 7th characters B & C see Appendix A PDX collection 1341
HAC 7th characters A - C see Appendix B for HAC conditional logic

CC MCC +7th **S82.202 Unspecified fracture of shaft of left tibia**
CC Exclusion 7th character A see Appendix A PDX collection 1342
CC Exclusion 7th characters K - R see Appendix A PDX collection 0897
MCC Exclusion 7th characters B & C see Appendix A PDX collection 1341
HAC 7th characters A - C see Appendix B for HAC conditional logic

CC MCC +7th **S82.209 Unspecified fracture of shaft of unspecified tibia**
CC Exclusion 7th character A see Appendix A PDX collection 1341
CC Exclusion 7th characters K - R see Appendix A PDX collection 0897
MCC Exclusion 7th characters B & C see Appendix A PDX collection 1341
HAC 7th characters A - C see Appendix B for HAC conditional logic

+ **S82.22 Transverse fracture of shaft of tibia**

CC MCC +7th **S82.221 Displaced transverse fracture of shaft of right tibia**
CC Exclusion 7th character A see Appendix A PDX collection 1340
CC Exclusion 7th characters K - R see Appendix A PDX collection 0897
MCC Exclusion 7th characters B & C see Appendix A PDX collection 1341
HAC 7th characters A - C see Appendix B for HAC conditional logic

CC MCC +7th **S82.222 Displaced transverse fracture of shaft of left tibia**
CC Exclusion 7th character A see Appendix A PDX collection 1342
CC Exclusion 7th characters K - R see Appendix A PDX collection 0897
MCC Exclusion 7th characters B & C see Appendix A PDX collection 1341
HAC 7th characters A - C see Appendix B for HAC conditional logic

CC MCC +7th **S82.223 Displaced transverse fracture of shaft of unspecified tibia**
CC Exclusion 7th character A see Appendix A PDX collection 1341
CC Exclusion 7th characters K - R see Appendix A PDX collection 0897
MCC Exclusion 7th characters B & C see Appendix A PDX collection 1341
HAC 7th characters A - C see Appendix B for HAC conditional logic

CC MCC +7th **S82.224 Nondisplaced transverse fracture of shaft of right tibia**
CC Exclusion 7th character A see Appendix A PDX collection 1340
CC Exclusion 7th characters K - R see Appendix A PDX collection 0897
MCC Exclusion 7th characters B & C see Appendix A PDX collection 1341
HAC 7th characters A - C see Appendix B for HAC conditional logic

CC MCC +7th **S82.225 Nondisplaced transverse fracture of shaft of left tibia**
CC Exclusion 7th character A see Appendix A PDX collection 1342
CC Exclusion 7th characters K - R see Appendix A PDX collection 0897
MCC Exclusion 7th characters B & C see Appendix A PDX collection 1341
HAC 7th characters A - C see Appendix B for HAC conditional logic

CC MCC +7th **S82.226 Nondisplaced transverse fracture of shaft of unspecified tibia**
CC Exclusion 7th character A see Appendix A PDX collection 1341
CC Exclusion 7th characters K - R see Appendix A PDX collection 0897
MCC Exclusion 7th characters B & C see Appendix A PDX collection 1341
HAC 7th characters A - C see Appendix B for HAC conditional logic

+ **S82.23 Oblique fracture of shaft of tibia**

CC MCC +7th **S82.231 Displaced oblique fracture of shaft of right tibia**
CC Exclusion 7th character A see Appendix A PDX collection 1340
CC Exclusion 7th characters K - R see Appendix A PDX collection 0897
MCC Exclusion 7th characters B & C see Appendix A PDX collection 1341
HAC 7th characters A - C see Appendix B for HAC conditional logic

CC MCC +7th **S82.232 Displaced oblique fracture of shaft of left tibia**
CC Exclusion 7th character A see Appendix A PDX collection 1342
CC Exclusion 7th characters K - R see Appendix A PDX collection 0897
MCC Exclusion 7th characters B & C see Appendix A PDX collection 1341
HAC 7th characters A - C see Appendix B for HAC conditional logic

CC MCC +7th **S82.233 Displaced oblique fracture of shaft of unspecified tibia**
CC Exclusion 7th character A see Appendix A PDX collection 1341
CC Exclusion 7th characters K - R see Appendix A PDX collection 0897
MCC Exclusion 7th characters B & C see Appendix A PDX collection 1341
HAC 7th characters A - C see Appendix B for HAC conditional logic

CC MCC +7th **S82.234 Nondisplaced oblique fracture of shaft of right tibia**
CC Exclusion 7th character A see Appendix A PDX collection 1340
CC Exclusion 7th characters K - R see Appendix A PDX collection 0897
MCC Exclusion 7th characters B & C see Appendix A PDX collection 1341
HAC 7th characters A - C see Appendix B for HAC conditional logic
AHA CC: 1Q, 2015, 3-21

CC MCC +7th **S82.235 Nondisplaced oblique fracture of shaft of left tibia**
CC Exclusion 7th character A see Appendix A PDX collection 1342
CC Exclusion 7th characters K - R see Appendix A PDX collection 0897
MCC Exclusion 7th characters B & C see Appendix A PDX collection 1341
HAC 7th characters A - C see Appendix B for HAC conditional logic

CC MCC +7th **S82.236 Nondisplaced oblique fracture of shaft of unspecified tibia**
CC Exclusion 7th character A see Appendix A PDX collection 1341
CC Exclusion 7th characters K - R see Appendix A PDX collection 0897
MCC Exclusion 7th characters B & C see Appendix A PDX collection 1341
HAC 7th characters A - C see Appendix B for HAC conditional logic

+ **S82.24 Spiral fracture of shaft of tibia**
Toddler fracture

CC MCC +7th **S82.241 Displaced spiral fracture of shaft of right tibia**
CC Exclusion 7th character A see Appendix A PDX collection 1340
CC Exclusion 7th characters K - R see Appendix A PDX collection 0897
MCC Exclusion 7th characters B & C see Appendix A PDX collection 1341
HAC 7th characters A - C see Appendix B for HAC conditional logic

CC MCC +7th **S82.242 Displaced spiral fracture of shaft of left tibia**
CC Exclusion 7th character A see Appendix A PDX collection 1342
CC Exclusion 7th characters K - R see Appendix A PDX collection 0897
MCC Exclusion 7th characters B & C see Appendix A PDX collection 1341
HAC 7th characters A - C see Appendix B for HAC conditional logic

CC MCC +7th **S82.243 Displaced spiral fracture of shaft of unspecified tibia**
CC Exclusion 7th character A see Appendix A PDX collection 1341
CC Exclusion 7th characters K - R see Appendix A PDX collection 0897
MCC Exclusion 7th characters B & C see Appendix A PDX collection 1341
HAC 7th characters A - C see Appendix B for HAC conditional logic

CC MCC +7th **S82.244 Nondisplaced spiral fracture of shaft of right tibia**
CC Exclusion 7th character A see Appendix A PDX collection 1340
CC Exclusion 7th characters K - R see Appendix A PDX collection 0897
MCC Exclusion 7th characters B & C see Appendix A PDX collection 1341
HAC 7th characters A - C see Appendix B for HAC conditional logic

CC MCC +7th **S82.245 Nondisplaced spiral fracture of shaft of left tibia**
CC Exclusion 7th character A see Appendix A PDX collection 1342
CC Exclusion 7th characters K - R see Appendix A PDX collection 0897
MCC Exclusion 7th characters B & C see Appendix A PDX collection 1341
HAC 7th characters A - C see Appendix B for HAC conditional logic

CC MCC +7th **S82.246 Nondisplaced spiral fracture of shaft of unspecified tibia**
CC Exclusion 7th character A see Appendix A PDX collection 1341
CC Exclusion 7th characters K - R see Appendix A PDX collection 0897
MCC Exclusion 7th characters B & C see Appendix A PDX collection 1341
HAC 7th characters A - C see Appendix B for HAC conditional logic

+ **S82.25 Comminuted fracture of shaft of tibia**

CC MCC +7th **S82.251 Displaced comminuted fracture of shaft of right tibia**
CC Exclusion 7th character A see Appendix A PDX collection 1340
CC Exclusion 7th characters K - R see Appendix A PDX collection 0897
MCC Exclusion 7th characters B & C see Appendix A PDX collection 1341
HAC 7th characters A - C see Appendix B for HAC conditional logic
AHA CC: 2Q, 2015, 6-7

CC MCC +7th **S82.252 Displaced comminuted fracture of shaft of left tibia**
CC Exclusion 7th character A see Appendix A PDX collection 1342
CC Exclusion 7th characters K - R see Appendix A PDX collection 0897
MCC Exclusion 7th characters B & C see Appendix A PDX collection 1341
HAC 7th characters A - C see Appendix B for HAC conditional logic

CC MCC +7th **S82.253 Displaced comminuted fracture of shaft of unspecified tibia**
CC Exclusion 7th character A see Appendix A PDX collection 1341
CC Exclusion 7th characters K - R see Appendix A PDX collection 0897
MCC Exclusion 7th characters B & C see Appendix A PDX collection 1341
HAC 7th characters A - C see Appendix B for HAC conditional logic

CC MCC +7th **S82.254 Nondisplaced comminuted fracture of shaft of right tibia**
CC Exclusion 7th character A see Appendix A PDX collection 1340
CC Exclusion 7th characters K - R see Appendix A PDX collection 0897
MCC Exclusion 7th characters B & C see Appendix A PDX collection 1341
HAC 7th characters A - C see Appendix B for HAC conditional logic

CC MCC +7th **S82.255 Nondisplaced comminuted fracture of shaft of left tibia**
CC Exclusion 7th character A see Appendix A PDX collection 1342
CC Exclusion 7th characters K - R see Appendix A PDX collection 0897
MCC Exclusion 7th characters B & C see Appendix A PDX collection 1341
HAC 7th characters A - C see Appendix B for HAC conditional logic

CC MCC +7th **S82.256 Nondisplaced comminuted fracture of shaft of unspecified tibia**
CC Exclusion 7th character A see Appendix A PDX collection 1341
CC Exclusion 7th characters K - R see Appendix A PDX collection 0897
MCC Exclusion 7th characters B & C see Appendix A PDX collection 1341
HAC 7th characters A - C see Appendix B for HAC conditional logic

+ **S82.26 Segmental fracture of shaft of tibia**

CC MCC +7th **S82.261 Displaced segmental fracture of shaft of right tibia**
CC Exclusion 7th character A see Appendix A PDX collection 1340
CC Exclusion 7th characters K - R see Appendix A PDX collection 0897
MCC Exclusion 7th characters B & C see Appendix A PDX collection 1341
HAC 7th characters A - C see Appendix B for HAC conditional logic

CC MCC +7th **S82.262 Displaced segmental fracture of shaft of left tibia**
CC Exclusion 7th character A see Appendix A PDX collection 1342
CC Exclusion 7th characters K - R see Appendix A PDX collection 0897
MCC Exclusion 7th characters B & C see Appendix A PDX collection 1341
HAC 7th characters A - C see Appendix B for HAC conditional logic

CC MCC +7th **S82.263 Displaced segmental fracture of shaft of unspecified tibia**
CC Exclusion 7th character A see Appendix A PDX collection 1341
CC Exclusion 7th characters K - R see Appendix A PDX collection 0897
MCC Exclusion 7th characters B & C see Appendix A PDX collection 1341
HAC 7th characters A - C see Appendix B for HAC conditional logic

CC MCC +7th **S82.264 Nondisplaced segmental fracture of shaft of right tibia**
CC Exclusion 7th character A see Appendix A PDX collection 1340
CC Exclusion 7th characters K - R see Appendix A PDX collection 0897
MCC Exclusion 7th characters B & C see Appendix A PDX collection 1341
HAC 7th characters A - C see Appendix B for HAC conditional logic

CC MCC +7th **S82.265 Nondisplaced segmental fracture of shaft of left tibia**
CC Exclusion 7th character A see Appendix A PDX collection 1342
CC Exclusion 7th characters K - R see Appendix A PDX collection 0897
MCC Exclusion 7th characters B & C see Appendix A PDX collection 1341
HAC 7th characters A - C see Appendix B for HAC conditional logic

CC MCC +7th **S82.266 Nondisplaced segmental fracture of shaft of unspecified tibia**
CC Exclusion 7th character A see Appendix A PDX collection 1341
CC Exclusion 7th characters K - R see Appendix A PDX collection 0897
MCC Exclusion 7th characters B & C see Appendix A PDX collection 1341
HAC 7th characters A - C see Appendix B for HAC conditional logic

\+ **S82.29 Other fracture of shaft of tibia**

CC MCC +7th **S82.291 Other fracture of shaft of right tibia**
CC Exclusion 7th character A see Appendix A PDX collection 1340
CC Exclusion 7th characters K - R see Appendix A PDX collection 0897
MCC Exclusion 7th characters B & C see Appendix A PDX collection 1341
HAC 7th characters A - C see Appendix B for HAC conditional logic

CC MCC +7th **S82.292 Other fracture of shaft of left tibia**
CC Exclusion 7th character A see Appendix A PDX collection 1342
CC Exclusion 7th characters K - R see Appendix A PDX collection 0897
MCC Exclusion 7th characters B & C see Appendix A PDX collection 1341
HAC 7th characters A - C see Appendix B for HAC conditional logic

CC MCC +7th **S82.299 Other fracture of shaft of unspecified tibia**
CC Exclusion 7th character A see Appendix A PDX collection 1341
CC Exclusion 7th characters K - R see Appendix A PDX collection 0897
MCC Exclusion 7th characters B & C see Appendix A PDX collection 1341
HAC 7th characters A - C see Appendix B for HAC conditional logic

\+ **S82.3 Fracture of lower end of tibia**
Excludes1: *bimalleolar fracture of lower leg (S82.84-)*
fracture of medial malleolus alone (S82.5-)
Maisonneuve's fracture (S82.86-)
pilon fracture of distal tibia (S82.87-)
trimalleolar fractures of lower leg (S82.85-)

\+ **S82.30 Unspecified fracture of lower end of tibia**

CC +7th **S82.301 Unspecified fracture of lower end of right tibia**
CC Exclusion 7th characters B & C see Appendix A PDX collection 1347
CC Exclusion 7th characters K - R see Appendix A PDX collection 0897
HAC 7th characters B & C see Appendix B for HAC conditional logic

CC +7th **S82.302 Unspecified fracture of lower end of left tibia**
CC Exclusion 7th characters B & C see Appendix A PDX collection 1347
CC Exclusion 7th characters K - R see Appendix A PDX collection 0897
HAC 7th characters B & C see Appendix B for HAC conditional logic

CC +7th **S82.309 Unspecified fracture of lower end of unspecified tibia**
CC Exclusion 7th characters B & C see Appendix A PDX collection 1347
CC Exclusion 7th characters K - R see Appendix A PDX collection 0897
HAC 7th characters B & C see Appendix B for HAC conditional logic

\+ **S82.31 Torus fracture of lower end of tibia**

The appropriate 7th character is to be added to all codes in subcategory **S82.31**
A initial encounter for closed fracture
D subsequent encounter for fracture with routine healing
G subsequent encounter for fracture with delayed healing
K subsequent encounter for fracture with nonunion
P subsequent encounter for fracture with malunion
S sequela

CC +7th **S82.311 Torus fracture of lower end of right tibia**
CC Exclusion 7th character A see Appendix A PDX collection 1343
CC Exclusion 7th characters K & P see Appendix A PDX collection 0897
HAC 7th character A see Appendix B for HAC conditional logic

CC +7th **S82.312 Torus fracture of lower end of left tibia**
CC Exclusion 7th character A see Appendix A PDX collection 1344
CC Exclusion 7th characters K & P see Appendix A PDX collection 0897
HAC 7th character A see Appendix B for HAC conditional logic

CC +7th **S82.319 Torus fracture of lower end of unspecified tibia**
CC Exclusion 7th character A see Appendix A PDX collection 1345
CC Exclusion 7th characters K & P see Appendix A PDX collection 0897
HAC 7th character A see Appendix B for HAC conditional logic

\+ **S82.39 Other fracture of lower end of tibia**

CC +7th **S82.391 Other fracture of lower end of right tibia**
CC Exclusion 7th characters B & C see Appendix A PDX collection 1347
CC Exclusion 7th characters K - R see Appendix A PDX collection 0897
HAC 7th characters B & C see Appendix B for HAC conditional logic

CC +7th **S82.392 Other fracture of lower end of left tibia**
CC Exclusion 7th characters B & C see Appendix A PDX collection 1347
CC Exclusion 7th characters K - R see Appendix A PDX collection 0897
HAC 7th characters B & C see Appendix B for HAC conditional logic
AHA CC: 1Q, 2015, 25

CC +7th **S82.399 Other fracture of lower end of unspecified tibia**
CC Exclusion 7th characters B & C see Appendix A PDX collection 1347
CC Exclusion 7th characters K - R see Appendix A PDX collection 0897
HAC 7th characters B & C see Appendix B for HAC conditional logic

\+ **S82.4 Fracture of shaft of fibula**
Excludes2: *fracture of lateral malleolus alone (S82.6-)*

\+ **S82.40 Unspecified fracture of shaft of fibula**

CC MCC +7th **S82.401 Unspecified fracture of shaft of right fibula**
CC Exclusion 7th characters K - R see Appendix A PDX collection 0897
MCC Exclusion 7th characters B & C see Appendix A PDX collection 1341
HAC 7th characters B & C see Appendix B for HAC conditional logic

CC MCC +7th **S82.402 Unspecified fracture of shaft of left fibula**
CC Exclusion 7th characters K - R see Appendix A PDX collection 0897
MCC Exclusion 7th characters B & C see Appendix A PDX collection 1341
HAC 7th characters B & C see Appendix B for HAC conditional logic

CC MCC +7th **S82.409 Unspecified fracture of shaft of unspecified fibula**
CC Exclusion 7th characters K - R see Appendix A PDX collection 0897
MCC Exclusion 7th characters B & C see Appendix A PDX collection 1341
HAC 7th characters B & C see Appendix B for HAC conditional logic

+ **S82.42 Transverse fracture of shaft of fibula**

CC MCC +7th **S82.421 Displaced transverse fracture of shaft of right fibula**
CC Exclusion 7th characters K - R see Appendix A PDX collection 0897
MCC Exclusion 7th characters B & C see Appendix A PDX collection 1341
HAC 7th characters B & C see Appendix B for HAC conditional logic

CC MCC +7th **S82.422 Displaced transverse fracture of shaft of left fibula**
CC Exclusion 7th characters K - R see Appendix A PDX collection 0897
MCC Exclusion 7th characters B & C see Appendix A PDX collection 1341
HAC 7th characters B & C see Appendix B for HAC conditional logic

CC MCC +7th **S82.423 Displaced transverse fracture of shaft of unspecified fibula**
CC Exclusion 7th characters K - R see Appendix A PDX collection 0897
MCC Exclusion 7th characters B & C see Appendix A PDX collection 1341
HAC 7th characters B & C see Appendix B for HAC conditional logic

CC MCC +7th **S82.424 Nondisplaced transverse fracture of shaft of right fibula**
CC Exclusion 7th characters K - R see Appendix A PDX collection 0897
MCC Exclusion 7th characters B & C see Appendix A PDX collection 1341
HAC 7th characters B & C see Appendix B for HAC conditional logic

CC MCC +7th **S82.425 Nondisplaced transverse fracture of shaft of left fibula**
CC Exclusion 7th characters K - R see Appendix A PDX collection 0897
MCC Exclusion 7th characters B & C see Appendix A PDX collection 1341
HAC 7th characters B & C see Appendix B for HAC conditional logic

CC MCC +7th **S82.426 Nondisplaced transverse fracture of shaft of unspecified fibula**
CC Exclusion 7th characters K - R see Appendix A PDX collection 0897
MCC Exclusion 7th characters B & C see Appendix A PDX collection 1341
HAC 7th characters B & C see Appendix B for HAC conditional logic

+ **S82.43 Oblique fracture of shaft of fibula**

CC MCC +7th **S82.431 Displaced oblique fracture of shaft of right fibula**
CC Exclusion 7th characters K - R see Appendix A PDX collection 0897
MCC Exclusion 7th characters B & C see Appendix A PDX collection 1341
HAC 7th characters B & C see Appendix B for HAC conditional logic

CC MCC +7th **S82.432 Displaced oblique fracture of shaft of left fibula**
CC Exclusion 7th characters K - R see Appendix A PDX collection 0897
MCC Exclusion 7th characters B & C see Appendix A PDX collection 1341
HAC 7th characters B & C see Appendix B for HAC conditional logic

CC MCC +7th **S82.433 Displaced oblique fracture of shaft of unspecified fibula**
CC Exclusion 7th characters K - R see Appendix A PDX collection 0897
MCC Exclusion 7th characters B & C see Appendix A PDX collection 1341
HAC 7th characters B & C see Appendix B for HAC conditional logic

CC MCC +7th **S82.434 Nondisplaced oblique fracture of shaft of right fibula**
CC Exclusion 7th characters K - R see Appendix A PDX collection 0897
MCC Exclusion 7th characters B & C see Appendix A PDX collection 1341
HAC 7th characters B & C see Appendix B for HAC conditional logic

CC MCC +7th **S82.435 Nondisplaced oblique fracture of shaft of left fibula**
CC Exclusion 7th characters K - R see Appendix A PDX collection 0897
MCC Exclusion 7th characters B & C see Appendix A PDX collection 1341
HAC 7th characters B & C see Appendix B for HAC conditional logic

CC MCC +7th **S82.436 Nondisplaced oblique fracture of shaft of unspecified fibula**
CC Exclusion 7th characters K - R see Appendix A PDX collection 0897
MCC Exclusion 7th characters B & C see Appendix A PDX collection 1341
HAC 7th characters B & C see Appendix B for HAC conditional logic

+ **S82.44 Spiral fracture of shaft of fibula**

CC MCC +7th **S82.441 Displaced spiral fracture of shaft of right fibula**
CC Exclusion 7th characters K - R see Appendix A PDX collection 0897
MCC Exclusion 7th characters B & C see Appendix A PDX collection 1341
HAC 7th characters B & C see Appendix B for HAC conditional logic

CC MCC +7th **S82.442 Displaced spiral fracture of shaft of left fibula**
CC Exclusion 7th characters K - R see Appendix A PDX collection 0897
MCC Exclusion 7th characters B & C see Appendix A PDX collection 1341
HAC 7th characters B & C see Appendix B for HAC conditional logic

CC MCC +7th **S82.443 Displaced spiral fracture of shaft of unspecified fibula**
CC Exclusion 7th characters K - R see Appendix A PDX collection 0897
MCC Exclusion 7th characters B & C see Appendix A PDX collection 1341
HAC 7th characters B & C see Appendix B for HAC conditional logic

CC MCC +7th **S82.444 Nondisplaced spiral fracture of shaft of right fibula**
CC Exclusion 7th characters K - R see Appendix A PDX collection 0897
MCC Exclusion 7th characters B & C see Appendix A PDX collection 1341
HAC 7th characters B & C see Appendix B for HAC conditional logic

CC MCC +7th **S82.445 Nondisplaced spiral fracture of shaft of left fibula**
CC Exclusion 7th characters K - R see Appendix A PDX collection 0897
MCC Exclusion 7th characters B & C see Appendix A PDX collection 1341
HAC 7th characters B & C see Appendix B for HAC conditional logic

CC MCC +7th **S82.446 Nondisplaced spiral fracture of shaft of unspecified fibula**
CC Exclusion 7th characters K - R see Appendix A PDX collection 0897
MCC Exclusion 7th characters B & C see Appendix A PDX collection 1341
HAC 7th characters B & C see Appendix B for HAC conditional logic

+ **S82.45 Comminuted fracture of shaft of fibula**

CC MCC +7th **S82.451 Displaced comminuted fracture of shaft of right fibula**
CC Exclusion 7th characters K - R see Appendix A PDX collection 0897
MCC Exclusion 7th characters B & C see Appendix A PDX collection 1341
HAC 7th characters B & C see Appendix B for HAC conditional logic

CC MCC +7th **S82.452 Displaced comminuted fracture of shaft of left fibula**
CC Exclusion 7th characters K - R see Appendix A PDX collection 0897
MCC Exclusion 7th characters B & C see Appendix A PDX collection 1341
HAC 7th characters B & C see Appendix B for HAC conditional logic

CC MCC +7th **S82.453 Displaced comminuted fracture of shaft of unspecified fibula**
CC Exclusion 7th characters K - R see Appendix A PDX collection 0897
MCC Exclusion 7th characters B & C see Appendix A PDX collection 1341
HAC 7th characters B & C see Appendix B for HAC conditional logic

CC MCC +7th **S82.454 Nondisplaced comminuted fracture of shaft of right fibula**
CC Exclusion 7th characters K - R see Appendix A PDX collection 0897
MCC Exclusion 7th characters B & C see Appendix A PDX collection 1341
HAC 7th characters B & C see Appendix B for HAC conditional logic

CC MCC +7th **S82.455 Nondisplaced comminuted fracture of shaft of left fibula**
CC Exclusion 7th characters K - R see Appendix A PDX collection 0897
MCC Exclusion 7th characters B & C see Appendix A PDX collection 1341
HAC 7th characters B & C see Appendix B for HAC conditional logic

CC MCC +7th **S82.456 Nondisplaced comminuted fracture of shaft of unspecified fibula**
CC Exclusion 7th characters K - R see Appendix A PDX collection 0897
MCC Exclusion 7th characters B & C see Appendix A PDX collection 1341
HAC 7th characters B & C see Appendix B for HAC conditional logic

\+ **S82.46 Segmental fracture of shaft of fibula**

CC MCC +7th **S82.461 Displaced segmental fracture of shaft of right fibula**
CC Exclusion 7th characters K - R see Appendix A PDX collection 0897
MCC Exclusion 7th characters B & C see Appendix A PDX collection 1341
HAC 7th characters B & C see Appendix B for HAC conditional logic

CC MCC +7th **S82.462 Displaced segmental fracture of shaft of left fibula**
CC Exclusion 7th characters K - R see Appendix A PDX collection 0897
MCC Exclusion 7th characters B & C see Appendix A PDX collection 1341
HAC 7th characters B & C see Appendix B for HAC conditional logic

CC MCC +7th **S82.463 Displaced segmental fracture of shaft of unspecified fibula**
CC Exclusion 7th characters K - R see Appendix A PDX collection 0897
MCC Exclusion 7th characters B & C see Appendix A PDX collection 1341
HAC 7th characters B & C see Appendix B for HAC conditional logic

CC MCC +7th **S82.464 Nondisplaced segmental fracture of shaft of right fibula**
CC Exclusion 7th characters K - R see Appendix A PDX collection 0897
MCC Exclusion 7th characters B & C see Appendix A PDX collection 1341
HAC 7th characters B & C see Appendix B for HAC conditional logic

CC MCC +7th **S82.465 Nondisplaced segmental fracture of shaft of left fibula**
CC Exclusion 7th characters K - R see Appendix A PDX collection 0897
MCC Exclusion 7th characters B & C see Appendix A PDX collection 1341
HAC 7th characters B & C see Appendix B for HAC conditional logic

CC MCC +7th **S82.466 Nondisplaced segmental fracture of shaft of unspecified fibula**
CC Exclusion 7th characters K - R see Appendix A PDX collection 0897
MCC Exclusion 7th characters B & C see Appendix A PDX collection 1341
HAC 7th characters B & C see Appendix B for HAC conditional logic

\+ **S82.49 Other fracture of shaft of fibula**

CC MCC +7th **S82.491 Other fracture of shaft of right fibula**
CC Exclusion 7th characters K - R see Appendix A PDX collection 0897
MCC Exclusion 7th characters B & C see Appendix A PDX collection 1341
HAC 7th characters B & C see Appendix B for HAC conditional logic

CC MCC +7th **S82.492 Other fracture of shaft of left fibula**
CC Exclusion 7th characters K - R see Appendix A PDX collection 0897
MCC Exclusion 7th characters B & C see Appendix A PDX collection 1341
HAC 7th characters B & C see Appendix B for HAC conditional logic

CC MCC +7th **S82.499 Other fracture of shaft of unspecified fibula**
CC Exclusion 7th characters K - R see Appendix A PDX collection 0897
MCC Exclusion 7th characters B & C see Appendix A PDX collection 1341
HAC 7th characters B & C see Appendix B for HAC conditional logic

\+ **S82.5 Fracture of medial malleolus**
Excludes1: *pilon fracture of distal tibia (S82.87-)*
Salter-Harris type III of lower end of tibia (S89.13-)
Salter-Harris type IV of lower end of tibia (S89.14-)

CC X+7th **S82.51 Displaced fracture of medial malleolus of right tibia**
CC Exclusion 7th characters B & C see Appendix A PDX collection 1347
CC Exclusion 7th characters K - R see Appendix A PDX collection 0897
HAC 7th characters B & C see Appendix B for HAC conditional logic

CC X+7th **S82.52 Displaced fracture of medial malleolus of left tibia**
CC Exclusion 7th characters B & C see Appendix A PDX collection 1347
CC Exclusion 7th characters K - R see Appendix A PDX collection 0897
HAC 7th characters B & C see Appendix B for HAC conditional logic

CC X+7th **S82.53 Displaced fracture of medial malleolus of unspecified tibia**
CC Exclusion 7th characters B & C see Appendix A PDX collection 1347
CC Exclusion 7th characters K - R see Appendix A PDX collection 0897
HAC 7th characters B & C see Appendix B for HAC conditional logic

CC X+7th **S82.54 Nondisplaced fracture of medial malleolus of right tibia**
CC Exclusion 7th characters B & C see Appendix A PDX collection 1347
CC Exclusion 7th characters K - R see Appendix A PDX collection 0897
HAC 7th characters B & C see Appendix B for HAC conditional logic

CC X+7th **S82.55 Nondisplaced fracture of medial malleolus of left tibia**
CC Exclusion 7th characters B & C see Appendix A PDX collection 1347
CC Exclusion 7th characters K - R see Appendix A PDX collection 0897
HAC 7th characters B & C see Appendix B for HAC conditional logic

CC X+7th **S82.56 Nondisplaced fracture of medial malleolus of unspecified tibia**
CC Exclusion 7th characters B & C see Appendix A PDX collection 1347
CC Exclusion 7th characters K - R see Appendix A PDX collection 0897
HAC 7th characters B & C see Appendix B for HAC conditional logic

\+ **S82.6 Fracture of lateral malleolus**
Excludes1: *pilon fracture of distal tibia (S82.87-)*

CC X+7th **S82.61 Displaced fracture of lateral malleolus of right fibula**
CC Exclusion 7th characters B & C see Appendix A PDX collection 1347
CC Exclusion 7th characters K - R see Appendix A PDX collection 0897
HAC 7th characters B & C see Appendix B for HAC conditional logic

CC X+7th **S82.62 Displaced fracture of lateral malleolus of left fibula**
CC Exclusion 7th characters B & C see Appendix A PDX collection 1347
CC Exclusion 7th characters K - R see Appendix A PDX collection 0897
HAC 7th characters B & C see Appendix B for HAC conditional logic

CC X+7th **S82.63 Displaced fracture of lateral malleolus of unspecified fibula**
CC Exclusion 7th characters B & C see Appendix A PDX collection 1347
CC Exclusion 7th characters K - R see Appendix A PDX collection 0897
HAC 7th characters B & C see Appendix B for HAC conditional logic

CC X+7th **S82.64 Nondisplaced fracture of lateral malleolus of right fibula**
CC Exclusion 7th characters B & C see Appendix A PDX collection 1347
CC Exclusion 7th characters K - R see Appendix A PDX collection 0897
HAC 7th characters B & C see Appendix B for HAC conditional logic

CC X+7th **S82.65 Nondisplaced fracture of lateral malleolus of left fibula**
CC Exclusion 7th characters B & C see Appendix A PDX collection 1347
CC Exclusion 7th characters K - R see Appendix A PDX collection 0897
HAC 7th characters B & C see Appendix B for HAC conditional logic

CC X+7th **S82.66 Nondisplaced fracture of lateral malleolus of unspecified fibula**
CC Exclusion 7th characters B & C see Appendix A PDX collection 1347
CC Exclusion 7th characters K - R see Appendix A PDX collection 0897
HAC 7th characters B & C see Appendix B for HAC conditional logic

+ **S82.8 Other fractures of lower leg**

+ **S82.81 Torus fracture of upper end of fibula**

The appropriate 7th character is to be added to all codes in subcategory **S82.81**
A initial encounter for closed fracture
D subsequent encounter for fracture with routine healing
G subsequent encounter for fracture with delayed healing
K subsequent encounter for fracture with nonunion
P subsequent encounter for fracture with malunion
S sequela

CC +7th **S82.811 Torus fracture of upper end of right fibula**
CC Exclusion 7th characters K & P see Appendix A PDX collection 0897

CC +7th **S82.812 Torus fracture of upper end of left fibula**
CC Exclusion 7th characters K & P see Appendix A PDX collection 0897

CC +7th **S82.819 Torus fracture of upper end of unspecified fibula**
CC Exclusion 7th characters K & P see Appendix A PDX collection 0897

+ **S82.82 Torus fracture of lower end of fibula**

The appropriate 7th character is to be added to all codes in subcategory **S82.82**
A initial encounter for closed fracture
D subsequent encounter for fracture with routine healing
G subsequent encounter for fracture with delayed healing
K subsequent encounter for fracture with nonunion
P subsequent encounter for fracture with malunion
S sequela

CC +7th **S82.821 Torus fracture of lower end of right fibula**
CC Exclusion 7th characters K & P see Appendix A PDX collection 0897

CC +7th **S82.822 Torus fracture of lower end of left fibula**
CC Exclusion 7th characters K & P see Appendix A PDX collection 0897

CC +7th **S82.829 Torus fracture of lower end of unspecified fibula**
CC Exclusion 7th characters K & P see Appendix A PDX collection 0897

+ **S82.83 Other fracture of upper and lower end of fibula**

CC MCC +7th **S82.831 Other fracture of upper and lower end of right fibula**
CC Exclusion 7th characters K - R see Appendix A PDX collection 0897
MCC Exclusion 7th characters B & C see Appendix A PDX collection 1341
HAC 7th characters B & C see Appendix B for HAC conditional logic

CC MCC +7th **S82.832 Other fracture of upper and lower end of left fibula**
CC Exclusion 7th characters K - R see Appendix A PDX collection 0897
MCC Exclusion 7th characters B & C see Appendix A PDX collection 1341
HAC 7th characters B & C see Appendix B for HAC conditional logic
AHA CC: 1Q, 2015, 25

CC MCC +7th **S82.839 Other fracture of upper and lower end of unspecified fibula**
CC Exclusion 7th characters K - R see Appendix A PDX collection 0897
MCC Exclusion 7th characters B & C see Appendix A PDX collection 1341
HAC 7th characters B & C see Appendix B for HAC conditional logic

+ **S82.84 Bimalleolar fracture of lower leg**

CC +7th **S82.841 Displaced bimalleolar fracture of right lower leg**
CC Exclusion 7th characters B & C see Appendix A PDX collection 1347
CC Exclusion 7th characters K - R see Appendix A PDX collection 0897
HAC 7th characters B & C see Appendix B for HAC conditional logic

CC +7th **S82.842 Displaced bimalleolar fracture of left lower leg**
CC Exclusion 7th characters B & C see Appendix A PDX collection 1347
CC Exclusion 7th characters K - R see Appendix A PDX collection 0897
HAC 7th characters B & C see Appendix B for HAC conditional logic

CC +7th **S82.843 Displaced bimalleolar fracture of unspecified lower leg**
CC Exclusion 7th characters B & C see Appendix A PDX collection 1347
CC Exclusion 7th characters K - R see Appendix A PDX collection 0897
HAC 7th characters B & C see Appendix B for HAC conditional logic

CC +7th **S82.844 Nondisplaced bimalleolar fracture of right lower leg**
CC Exclusion 7th characters B & C see Appendix A PDX collection 1347
CC Exclusion 7th characters K - R see Appendix A PDX collection 0897
HAC 7th characters B & C see Appendix B for HAC conditional logic

CC +7th **S82.845 Nondisplaced bimalleolar fracture of left lower leg**
CC Exclusion 7th characters B & C see Appendix A PDX collection 1347
CC Exclusion 7th characters K - R see Appendix A PDX collection 0897
HAC 7th characters B & C see Appendix B for HAC conditional logic

CC +7th **S82.846 Nondisplaced bimalleolar fracture of unspecified lower leg**
CC Exclusion 7th characters B & C see Appendix A PDX collection 1347
CC Exclusion 7th characters K - R see Appendix A PDX collection 0897
HAC 7th characters B & C see Appendix B for HAC conditional logic

+ **S82.85 Trimalleolar fracture of lower leg**

CC +7th **S82.851 Displaced trimalleolar fracture of right lower leg**
CC Exclusion 7th characters B & C see Appendix A PDX collection 1347
CC Exclusion 7th characters K - R see Appendix A PDX collection 0897
HAC 7th characters B & C see Appendix B for HAC conditional logic

CC +7th **S82.852 Displaced trimalleolar fracture of left lower leg**
CC Exclusion 7th characters B & C see Appendix A PDX collection 1347
CC Exclusion 7th characters K - R see Appendix A PDX collection 0897
HAC 7th characters B & C see Appendix B for HAC conditional logic

CC +7th **S82.853 Displaced trimalleolar fracture of unspecified lower leg**
CC Exclusion 7th characters B & C see Appendix A PDX collection 1347
CC Exclusion 7th characters K - R see Appendix A PDX collection 0897
HAC 7th characters B & C see Appendix B for HAC conditional logic

CC +7th **S82.854 Nondisplaced trimalleolar fracture of right lower leg**
CC Exclusion 7th characters B & C see Appendix A PDX collection 1347
CC Exclusion 7th characters K - R see Appendix A PDX collection 0897
HAC 7th characters B & C see Appendix B for HAC conditional logic

CC +7th **S82.855 Nondisplaced trimalleolar fracture of left lower leg**
CC Exclusion 7th characters B & C see Appendix A PDX collection 1347
CC Exclusion 7th characters K - R see Appendix A PDX collection 0897
HAC 7th characters B & C see Appendix B for HAC conditional logic

CC +7th **S82.856 Nondisplaced trimalleolar fracture of unspecified lower leg**
CC Exclusion 7th characters B & C see Appendix A PDX collection 1347
CC Exclusion 7th characters K - R see Appendix A PDX collection 0897
HAC 7th characters B & C see Appendix B for HAC conditional logic

\+ **S82.86 Maisonneuve's fracture**

CC MCC +7th **S82.861 Displaced Maisonneuve's fracture of right leg**
CC Exclusion 7th characters K - R see Appendix A PDX collection 0897
MCC Exclusion 7th characters B & C see Appendix A PDX collection 1341
HAC 7th characters B & C see Appendix B for HAC conditional logic

CC MCC +7th **S82.862 Displaced Maisonneuve's fracture of left leg**
CC Exclusion 7th characters K - R see Appendix A PDX collection 0897
MCC Exclusion 7th characters B & C see Appendix A PDX collection 1341
HAC 7th characters B & C see Appendix B for HAC conditional logic

CC MCC +7th **S82.863 Displaced Maisonneuve's fracture of unspecified leg**
CC Exclusion 7th characters K - R see Appendix A PDX collection 0897
MCC Exclusion 7th characters B & C see Appendix A PDX collection 1341
HAC 7th characters B & C see Appendix B for HAC conditional logic

CC MCC +7th **S82.864 Nondisplaced Maisonneuve's fracture of right leg**
CC Exclusion 7th characters K - R see Appendix A PDX collection 0897
MCC Exclusion 7th characters B & C see Appendix A PDX collection 1341
HAC 7th characters B & C see Appendix B for HAC conditional logic

CC MCC +7th **S82.865 Nondisplaced Maisonneuve's fracture of left leg**
CC Exclusion 7th characters K - R see Appendix A PDX collection 0897
MCC Exclusion 7th characters B & C see Appendix A PDX collection 1341
HAC 7th characters B & C see Appendix B for HAC conditional logic

CC MCC +7th **S82.866 Nondisplaced Maisonneuve's fracture of unspecified leg**
CC Exclusion 7th characters K - R see Appendix A PDX collection 0897
MCC Exclusion 7th characters B & C see Appendix A PDX collection 1341
HAC 7th characters B & C see Appendix B for HAC conditional logic

\+ **S82.87 Pilon fracture of tibia**

CC +7th **S82.871 Displaced pilon fracture of right tibia**
CC Exclusion 7th characters B & C see Appendix A PDX collection 1347
CC Exclusion 7th characters K - R see Appendix A PDX collection 0897
HAC 7th characters B & C see Appendix B for HAC conditional logic

CC +7th **S82.872 Displaced pilon fracture of left tibia**
CC Exclusion 7th characters B & C see Appendix A PDX collection 1347
CC Exclusion 7th characters K - R see Appendix A PDX collection 0897
HAC 7th characters B & C see Appendix B for HAC conditional logic

CC +7th **S82.873 Displaced pilon fracture of unspecified tibia**
CC Exclusion 7th characters B & C see Appendix A PDX collection 1347
CC Exclusion 7th characters K - R see Appendix A PDX collection 0897
HAC 7th characters B & C see Appendix B for HAC conditional logic

CC +7th **S82.874 Nondisplaced pilon fracture of right tibia**
CC Exclusion 7th characters B & C see Appendix A PDX collection 1347
CC Exclusion 7th characters K - R see Appendix A PDX collection 0897
HAC 7th characters B & C see Appendix B for HAC conditional logic

CC +7th **S82.875 Nondisplaced pilon fracture of left tibia**
CC Exclusion 7th characters B & C see Appendix A PDX collection 1347
CC Exclusion 7th characters K - R see Appendix A PDX collection 0897
HAC 7th characters B & C see Appendix B for HAC conditional logic

CC +7th **S82.876 Nondisplaced pilon fracture of unspecified tibia**
CC Exclusion 7th characters B & C see Appendix A PDX collection 1347
CC Exclusion 7th characters K - R see Appendix A PDX collection 0897
HAC 7th characters B & C see Appendix B for HAC conditional logic

\+ **S82.89 Other fractures of lower leg**
Fracture of ankle NOS

CC +7th **S82.891 Other fracture of right lower leg**
CC Exclusion 7th characters B & C see Appendix A PDX collection 1347
CC Exclusion 7th characters K - R see Appendix A PDX collection 0897
HAC 7th characters B & C see Appendix B for HAC conditional logic

CC +7th **S82.892 Other fracture of left lower leg**
CC Exclusion 7th characters B & C see Appendix A PDX collection 1347
CC Exclusion 7th characters K - R see Appendix A PDX collection 0897
HAC 7th characters B & C see Appendix B for HAC conditional logic

CC +7th **S82.899 Other fracture of unspecified lower leg**
CC Exclusion 7th characters B & C see Appendix A PDX collection 1347
CC Exclusion 7th characters K - R see Appendix A PDX collection 0897
HAC 7th characters B & C see Appendix B for HAC conditional logic

\+ **S82.9 Unspecified fracture of lower leg**

CC X+7th **S82.90 Unspecified fracture of unspecified lower leg**
CC Exclusion 7th characters B & C see Appendix A PDX collection 1348
CC Exclusion 7th characters K - R see Appendix A PDX collection 0897
HAC 7th characters B & C see Appendix B for HAC conditional logic

CC X+7th **S82.91 Unspecified fracture of right lower leg**
CC Exclusion 7th characters B & C see Appendix A PDX collection 1348
CC Exclusion 7th characters K - R see Appendix A PDX collection 0897
HAC 7th characters B & C see Appendix B for HAC conditional logic

CC X+7th **S82.92 Unspecified fracture of left lower leg**
CC Exclusion 7th characters B & C see Appendix A PDX collection 1348
CC Exclusion 7th characters K - R see Appendix A PDX collection 0897
HAC 7th characters B & C see Appendix B for HAC conditional logic

S83 Dislocation and sprain of joints and ligaments of knee

Includes: avulsion of joint or ligament of knee
laceration of cartilage, joint or ligament of knee
sprain of cartilage, joint or ligament of knee
traumatic hemarthrosis of joint or ligament of knee
traumatic rupture of joint or ligament of knee
traumatic subluxation of joint or ligament of knee
traumatic tear of joint or ligament of knee

Code also any associated open wound

Excludes1: *derangement of patella (M22.0-M22.3)*
injury of patellar ligament (tendon) (S76.1-)
internal derangement of knee (M23.-)
old dislocation of knee (M24.36)
pathological dislocation of knee (M24.36)
recurrent dislocation of knee (M22.0)

Excludes2: *strain of muscle, fascia and tendon of lower leg (S86.-)*

The appropriate 7th character is to be added to each code from category S83
A initial encounter
D subsequent encounter
S sequela

\+ **S83.0 Subluxation and dislocation of patella**
\+ **S83.00 Unspecified subluxation and dislocation of patella**
+7th **S83.001 Unspecified subluxation of right patella**
+7th **S83.002 Unspecified subluxation of left patella**
+7th **S83.003 Unspecified subluxation of unspecified patella**
+7th **S83.004 Unspecified dislocation of right patella**
+7th **S83.005 Unspecified dislocation of left patella**
+7th **S83.006 Unspecified dislocation of unspecified patella**
\+ **S83.01 Lateral subluxation and dislocation of patella**
+7th **S83.011 Lateral subluxation of right patella**
+7th **S83.012 Lateral subluxation of left patella**
+7th **S83.013 Lateral subluxation of unspecified patella**
+7th **S83.014 Lateral dislocation of right patella**
+7th **S83.015 Lateral dislocation of left patella**
+7th **S83.016 Lateral dislocation of unspecified patella**
\+ **S83.09 Other subluxation and dislocation of patella**
+7th **S83.091 Other subluxation of right patella**
+7th **S83.092 Other subluxation of left patella**
+7th **S83.093 Other subluxation of unspecified patella**
+7th **S83.094 Other dislocation of right patella**
+7th **S83.095 Other dislocation of left patella**
+7th **S83.096 Other dislocation of unspecified patella**
\+ **S83.1 Subluxation and dislocation of knee**
Excludes2: *instability of knee prosthesis (T84.022, T84.023)*
\+ **S83.10 Unspecified subluxation and dislocation of knee**
+7th **S83.101 Unspecified subluxation of right knee**
+7th **S83.102 Unspecified subluxation of left knee**
+7th **S83.103 Unspecified subluxation of unspecified knee**
+7th **S83.104 Unspecified dislocation of right knee**
+7th **S83.105 Unspecified dislocation of left knee**
+7th **S83.106 Unspecified dislocation of unspecified knee**
\+ **S83.11 Anterior subluxation and dislocation of proximal end of tibia**
Posterior subluxation and dislocation of distal end of femur
+7th **S83.111 Anterior subluxation of proximal end of tibia, right knee**
+7th **S83.112 Anterior subluxation of proximal end of tibia, left knee**
+7th **S83.113 Anterior subluxation of proximal end of tibia, unspecified knee**
+7th **S83.114 Anterior dislocation of proximal end of tibia, right knee**
+7th **S83.115 Anterior dislocation of proximal end of tibia, left knee**
+7th **S83.116 Anterior dislocation of proximal end of tibia, unspecified knee**
\+ **S83.12 Posterior subluxation and dislocation of proximal end of tibia**
Anterior dislocation of distal end of femur
+7th **S83.121 Posterior subluxation of proximal end of tibia, right knee**
+7th **S83.122 Posterior subluxation of proximal end of tibia, left knee**
+7th **S83.123 Posterior subluxation of proximal end of tibia, unspecified knee**
+7th **S83.124 Posterior dislocation of proximal end of tibia, right knee**
+7th **S83.125 Posterior dislocation of proximal end of tibia, left knee**
+7th **S83.126 Posterior dislocation of proximal end of tibia, unspecified knee**
\+ **S83.13 Medial subluxation and dislocation of proximal end of tibia**
+7th **S83.131 Medial subluxation of proximal end of tibia, right knee**
+7th **S83.132 Medial subluxation of proximal end of tibia, left knee**
+7th **S83.133 Medial subluxation of proximal end of tibia, unspecified knee**
+7th **S83.134 Medial dislocation of proximal end of tibia, right knee**
+7th **S83.135 Medial dislocation of proximal end of tibia, left knee**
+7th **S83.136 Medial dislocation of proximal end of tibi unspecified knee**
\+ **S83.14 Lateral subluxation and dislocation of proximal end of tibia**
+7th **S83.141 Lateral subluxation of proximal end of tibia, right knee**
+7th **S83.142 Lateral subluxation of proximal end of tibia, left knee**
+7th **S83.143 Lateral subluxation of proximal end of tibia, unspecified knee**
+7th **S83.144 Lateral dislocation of proximal end of tibia, right knee**
+7th **S83.145 Lateral dislocation of proximal end of tibia, left knee**
+7th **S83.146 Lateral dislocation of proximal end of tibia, unspecified knee**
\+ **S83.19 Other subluxation and dislocation of knee**
+7th **S83.191 Other subluxation of right knee**
+7th **S83.192 Other subluxation of left knee**
+7th **S83.193 Other subluxation of unspecified knee**
+7th **S83.194 Other dislocation of right knee**
+7th **S83.195 Other dislocation of left knee**
+7th **S83.196 Other dislocation of unspecified knee**
\+ **S83.2 Tear of meniscus, current injury**
Excludes1: *old bucket-handle tear (M23.2)*
\+ **S83.20 Tear of unspecified meniscus, current injury**
Tear of meniscus of knee NOS
+7th **S83.200 Bucket-handle tear of unspecified meniscus, current injury, right knee**
+7th **S83.201 Bucket-handle tear of unspecified meniscus, current injury, left knee**
+7th **S83.202 Bucket-handle tear of unspecified meniscus, current injury, unspecified knee**
+7th **S83.203 Other tear of unspecified meniscus, current injury, right knee**
+7th **S83.204 Other tear of unspecified meniscus, current injury, left knee**
+7th **S83.205 Other tear of unspecified meniscus, current injury, unspecified knee**
+7th **S83.206 Unspecified tear of unspecified meniscus, current injury, right knee**
+7th **S83.207 Unspecified tear of unspecified meniscus, current injury, left knee**
+7th **S83.209 Unspecified tear of unspecified meniscus, current injury, unspecified knee**

+ **S83.21 Bucket-handle tear of medial meniscus, current injury**
  - +7th **S83.211 Bucket-handle tear of medial meniscus, current injury, right knee**
  - +7th **S83.212 Bucket-handle tear of medial meniscus, current injury, left knee**
  - +7th **S83.219 Bucket-handle tear of medial meniscus, current injury, unspecified knee**
+ **S83.22 Peripheral tear of medial meniscus, current injury**
  - +7th **S83.221 Peripheral tear of medial meniscus, current injury, right knee**
  - +7th **S83.222 Peripheral tear of medial meniscus, current injury, left knee**
  - +7th **S83.229 Peripheral tear of medial meniscus, current injury, unspecified knee**
+ **S83.23 Complex tear of medial meniscus, current injury**
  - +7th **S83.231 Complex tear of medial meniscus, current injury, right knee**
  - +7th **S83.232 Complex tear of medial meniscus, current injury, left knee**
  - +7th **S83.239 Complex tear of medial meniscus, current injury, unspecified knee**
+ **S83.24 Other tear of medial meniscus, current injury**
  - +7th **S83.241 Other tear of medial meniscus, current injury, right knee**
  - +7th **S83.242 Other tear of medial meniscus, current injury, left knee**
  - +7th **S83.249 Other tear of medial meniscus, current injury, unspecified knee**
+ **S83.25 Bucket-handle tear of lateral meniscus, current injury**
  - +7th **S83.251 Bucket-handle tear of lateral meniscus, current injury, right knee**
  - +7th **S83.252 Bucket-handle tear of lateral meniscus, current injury, left knee**
  - +7th **S83.259 Bucket-handle tear of lateral meniscus, current injury, unspecified knee**
+ **S83.26 Peripheral tear of lateral meniscus, current injury**
  - +7th **S83.261 Peripheral tear of lateral meniscus, current injury, right knee**
  - +7th **S83.262 Peripheral tear of lateral meniscus, current injury, left knee**
  - +7th **S83.269 Peripheral tear of lateral meniscus, current injury, unspecified knee**
+ **S83.27 Complex tear of lateral meniscus, current injury**
  - +7th **S83.271 Complex tear of lateral meniscus, current injury, right knee**
  - +7th **S83.272 Complex tear of lateral meniscus, current injury, left knee**
  - +7th **S83.279 Complex tear of lateral meniscus, current injury, unspecified knee**
+ **S83.28 Other tear of lateral meniscus, current injury**
  - +7th **S83.281 Other tear of lateral meniscus, current injury, right knee**
  - +7th **S83.282 Other tear of lateral meniscus, current injury, left knee**
  - +7th **S83.289 Other tear of lateral meniscus, current injury, unspecified knee**

+ **S83.3 Tear of articular cartilage of knee, current**
  - X+7th **S83.30 Tear of articular cartilage of unspecified knee, current**
  - X+7th **S83.31 Tear of articular cartilage of right knee, current**
  - X+7th **S83.32 Tear of articular cartilage of left knee, current**

+ **S83.4 Sprain of collateral ligament of knee**
  + **S83.40 Sprain of unspecified collateral ligament of knee**
    - +7th **S83.401 Sprain of unspecified collateral ligament of right knee**
    - +7th **S83.402 Sprain of unspecified collateral ligament of left knee**
    - +7th **S83.409 Sprain of unspecified collateral ligament of unspecified knee**
  + **S83.41 Sprain of medial collateral ligament of knee**
    Sprain of tibial collateral ligament
    - +7th **S83.411 Sprain of medial collateral ligament of right knee**
    - +7th **S83.412 Sprain of medial collateral ligament of left knee**
    - +7th **S83.419 Sprain of medial collateral ligament of unspecified knee**
  + **S83.42 Sprain of lateral collateral ligament of knee**
    Sprain of fibular collateral ligament
    - +7th **S83.421 Sprain of lateral collateral ligament of right knee**
    - +7th **S83.422 Sprain of lateral collateral ligament of left knee**
    - +7th **S83.429 Sprain of lateral collateral ligament of unspecified knee**

+ **S83.5 Sprain of cruciate ligament of knee**
  + **S83.50 Sprain of unspecified cruciate ligament of knee**
    - +7th **S83.501 Sprain of unspecified cruciate ligament of right knee**
    - +7th **S83.502 Sprain of unspecified cruciate ligament of left knee**
    - +7th **S83.509 Sprain of unspecified cruciate ligament of unspecified knee**
  + **S83.51 Sprain of anterior cruciate ligament of knee**
    - +7th **S83.511 Sprain of anterior cruciate ligament of right knee**
      AHA CC: 2Q, 2016, 3-4
    - +7th **S83.512 Sprain of anterior cruciate ligament of left knee**
    - +7th **S83.519 Sprain of anterior cruciate ligament of unspecified knee**
  + **S83.52 Sprain of posterior cruciate ligament of knee**
    - +7th **S83.521 Sprain of posterior cruciate ligament of right knee**
    - +7th **S83.522 Sprain of posterior cruciate ligament of left knee**
    - +7th **S83.529 Sprain of posterior cruciate ligament of unspecified knee**

+ **S83.6 Sprain of the superior tibiofibular joint and ligament**
  - X+7th **S83.60 Sprain of the superior tibiofibular joint and ligament, unspecified knee**
  - X+7th **S83.61 Sprain of the superior tibiofibular joint and ligament, right knee**
  - X+7th **S83.62 Sprain of the superior tibiofibular joint and ligament, left knee**

+ **S83.8 Sprain of other specified parts of knee**
  + **S83.8X Sprain of other specified parts of knee**
    - +7th **S83.8X1 Sprain of other specified parts of right knee**
    - +7th **S83.8X2 Sprain of other specified parts of left knee**
    - +7th **S83.8X9 Sprain of other specified parts of unspecified knee**

+ **S83.9 Sprain of unspecified site of knee**
  - X+7th **S83.90 Sprain of unspecified site of unspecified knee**
  - X+7th **S83.91 Sprain of unspecified site of right knee**
  - X+7th **S83.92 Sprain of unspecified site of left knee**

S84 Injury of nerves at lower leg level

Code also any associated open wound (S81.-)

Excludes2: *injury of nerves at ankle and foot level (S94.-)*

The appropriate 7th character is to be added to each code from category S84
- A initial encounter
- D subsequent encounter
- S sequela

+ **S84.0 Injury of tibial nerve at lower leg level**
  - X+7th **S84.00 Injury of tibial nerve at lower leg level, unspecified leg**
  - X+7th **S84.01 Injury of tibial nerve at lower leg level, right leg**
  - X+7th **S84.02 Injury of tibial nerve at lower leg level, left leg**

+ **S84.1 Injury of peroneal nerve at lower leg level**
  - X+7th **S84.10 Injury of peroneal nerve at lower leg level, unspecified leg**
  - X+7th **S84.11 Injury of peroneal nerve at lower leg level, right leg**
  - X+7th **S84.12 Injury of peroneal nerve at lower leg level, left leg**

+ **S84.2 Injury of cutaneous sensory nerve at lower leg level**
  - X+7th **S84.20 Injury of cutaneous sensory nerve at lower leg level, unspecified leg**
  - X+7th **S84.21 Injury of cutaneous sensory nerve at lower leg level, right leg**
  - X+7th **S84.22 Injury of cutaneous sensory nerve at lower leg level, left leg**

+ **S84.8 Injury of other nerves at lower leg level**
  + **S84.80 Injury of other nerves at lower leg level**
    - +7th **S84.801 Injury of other nerves at lower leg level, right leg**
    - +7th **S84.802 Injury of other nerves at lower leg level, left leg**
    - +7th **S84.809 Injury of other nerves at lower leg level, unspecified leg**

+ **S84.9 Injury of unspecified nerve at lower leg level**
  - X+7th **S84.90 Injury of unspecified nerve at lower leg level, unspecified leg**
  - X+7th **S84.91 Injury of unspecified nerve at lower leg level, right leg**
  - X+7th **S84.92 Injury of unspecified nerve at lower leg level, left leg**

S85 Injury of blood vessels at lower leg level

Code also any associated open wound (S81.-)

Excludes2: *injury of blood vessels at ankle and foot level (S95.-)*

The appropriate 7th character is to be added to each code from category S85
A initial encounter
D subsequent encounter
S sequela

+ **S85.0 Injury of popliteal artery**
  + **S85.00 Unspecified injury of popliteal artery**
    - MCC +7th **S85.001 Unspecified injury of popliteal artery, right leg**
      MCC Exclusion 7th character A see Appendix A PDX collection 1349
    - MCC +7th **S85.002 Unspecified injury of popliteal artery, left leg**
      MCC Exclusion 7th character A see Appendix A PDX collection 1350
    - MCC +7th **S85.009 Unspecified injury of popliteal artery, unspecified leg**
      MCC Exclusion 7th character A see Appendix A PDX collection 1351
  + **S85.01 Laceration of popliteal artery**
    - MCC +7th **S85.011 Laceration of popliteal artery, right leg**
      MCC Exclusion 7th character A see Appendix A PDX collection 1349
    - MCC +7th **S85.012 Laceration of popliteal artery, left leg**
      MCC Exclusion 7th character A see Appendix A PDX collection 1350
    - MCC +7th **S85.019 Laceration of popliteal artery, unspecified leg**
      MCC Exclusion 7th character A see Appendix A PDX collection 1351
  + **S85.09 Other specified injury of popliteal artery**
    - MCC +7th **S85.091 Other specified injury of popliteal artery, right leg**
      MCC Exclusion 7th character A see Appendix A PDX collection 1349
    - MCC +7th **S85.092 Other specified injury of popliteal artery, left leg**
      MCC Exclusion 7th character A see Appendix A PDX collection 1350
    - MCC +7th **S85.099 Other specified injury of popliteal artery, unspecified leg**
      MCC Exclusion 7th character A see Appendix A PDX collection 1351
+ **S85.1 Injury of tibial artery**
  + **S85.10 Unspecified injury of unspecified tibial artery**
    Injury of tibial artery NOS
    - CC +7th **S85.101 Unspecified injury of unspecified tibial artery, right leg**
      CC Exclusion 7th character A see Appendix A PDX collection 1352
    - CC +7th **S85.102 Unspecified injury of unspecified tibial artery, left leg**
      CC Exclusion 7th character A see Appendix A PDX collection 1353
    - CC +7th **S85.109 Unspecified injury of unspecified tibial artery, unspecified leg**
      CC Exclusion 7th character A see Appendix A PDX collection 1354
  + **S85.11 Laceration of unspecified tibial artery**
    - CC +7th **S85.111 Laceration of unspecified tibial artery, right leg**
      CC Exclusion 7th character A see Appendix A PDX collection 1352
    - CC +7th **S85.112 Laceration of unspecified tibial artery, left leg**
      CC Exclusion 7th character A see Appendix A PDX collection 1353
    - CC +7th **S85.119 Laceration of unspecified tibial artery, unspecified leg**
      CC Exclusion 7th character A see Appendix A PDX collection 1354
  + **S85.12 Other specified injury of unspecified tibial artery**
    - CC +7th **S85.121 Other specified injury of unspecified tibial artery, right leg**
      CC Exclusion 7th character A see Appendix A PDX collection 1352
    - CC +7th **S85.122 Other specified injury of unspecified tibial artery, left leg**
      CC Exclusion 7th character A see Appendix A PDX collection 1353
    - CC +7th **S85.129 Other specified injury of unspecified tibial artery, unspecified leg**
      CC Exclusion 7th character A see Appendix A PDX collection 1354
  + **S85.13 Unspecified injury of anterior tibial artery**
    - CC +7th **S85.131 Unspecified injury of anterior tibial artery, right leg**
      CC Exclusion 7th character A see Appendix A PDX collection 1355
    - CC +7th **S85.132 Unspecified injury of anterior tibial artery, left leg**
      CC Exclusion 7th character A see Appendix A PDX collection 1356
    - CC +7th **S85.139 Unspecified injury of anterior tibial artery, unspecified leg**
      CC Exclusion 7th character A see Appendix A PDX collection 1357
  + **S85.14 Laceration of anterior tibial artery**
    - CC +7th **S85.141 Laceration of anterior tibial artery, right leg**
      CC Exclusion 7th character A see Appendix A PDX collection 1355
    - CC +7th **S85.142 Laceration of anterior tibial artery, left leg**
      CC Exclusion 7th character A see Appendix A PDX collection 1356
    - CC +7th **S85.149 Laceration of anterior tibial artery, unspecified leg**
      CC Exclusion 7th character A see Appendix A PDX collection 1357
  + **S85.15 Other specified injury of anterior tibial artery**
    - CC +7th **S85.151 Other specified injury of anterior tibial artery, right leg**
      CC Exclusion 7th character A see Appendix A PDX collection 1355
    - CC +7th **S85.152 Other specified injury of anterior tibial artery, left leg**
      CC Exclusion 7th character A see Appendix A PDX collection 1356
    - CC +7th **S85.159 Other specified injury of anterior tibial artery, unspecified leg**
      CC Exclusion 7th character A see Appendix A PDX collection 1357
  + **S85.16 Unspecified injury of posterior tibial artery**
    - CC +7th **S85.161 Unspecified injury of posterior tibial artery, right leg**
      CC Exclusion 7th character A see Appendix A PDX collection 1358
    - CC +7th **S85.162 Unspecified injury of posterior tibial artery, left leg**
      CC Exclusion 7th character A see Appendix A PDX collection 1359
    - CC +7th **S85.169 Unspecified injury of posterior tibial artery, unspecified leg**
      CC Exclusion 7th character A see Appendix A PDX collection 1360
  + **S85.17 Laceration of posterior tibial artery**
    - CC +7th **S85.171 Laceration of posterior tibial artery, right leg**
      CC Exclusion 7th character A see Appendix A PDX collection 1358
    - CC +7th **S85.172 Laceration of posterior tibial artery, left leg**
      CC Exclusion 7th character A see Appendix A PDX collection 1359
    - CC +7th **S85.179 Laceration of posterior tibial artery, unspecified leg**
      CC Exclusion 7th character A see Appendix A PDX collection 1360
  + **S85.18 Other specified injury of posterior tibial artery**
    - CC +7th **S85.181 Other specified injury of posterior tibial artery, right leg**
      CC Exclusion 7th character A see Appendix A PDX collection 1358
    - CC +7th **S85.182 Other specified injury of posterior tibial artery, left leg**
      CC Exclusion 7th character A see Appendix A PDX collection 1359

CC +7th **S85.189 Other specified injury of posterior tibial artery, unspecified leg**
CC Exclusion 7th character A see Appendix A
PDX collection 1360

\+ **S85.2 Injury of peroneal artery**

\+ **S85.20 Unspecified injury of peroneal artery**

CC +7th **S85.201 Unspecified injury of peroneal artery, right leg**
CC Exclusion 7th character A see Appendix A
PDX collection 1325

CC +7th **S85.202 Unspecified injury of peroneal artery, left leg**
CC Exclusion 7th character A see Appendix A
PDX collection 1326

CC +7th **S85.209 Unspecified injury of peroneal artery, unspecified leg**
CC Exclusion 7th character A see Appendix A
PDX collection 1327

\+ **S85.21 Laceration of peroneal artery**

CC +7th **S85.211 Laceration of peroneal artery, right leg**
CC Exclusion 7th character A see Appendix A
PDX collection 1325

CC +7th **S85.212 Laceration of peroneal artery, left leg**
CC Exclusion 7th character A see Appendix A
PDX collection 1326

CC +7th **S85.219 Laceration of peroneal artery, unspecified leg**
CC Exclusion 7th character A see Appendix A
PDX collection 1327

\+ **S85.29 Other specified injury of peroneal artery**

CC +7th **S85.291 Other specified injury of peroneal artery, right leg**
CC Exclusion 7th character A see Appendix A
PDX collection 1325

CC +7th **S85.292 Other specified injury of peroneal artery, left leg**
CC Exclusion 7th character A see Appendix A
PDX collection 1326

CC +7th **S85.299 Other specified injury of peroneal artery, unspecified leg**
CC Exclusion 7th character A see Appendix A
PDX collection 1327

\+ **S85.3 Injury of greater saphenous vein at lower leg level**
Injury of greater saphenous vein NOS
Injury of saphenous vein NOS

\+ **S85.30 Unspecified injury of greater saphenous vein at lower leg level**

CC +7th **S85.301 Unspecified injury of greater saphenous vein at lower leg level, right leg**
CC Exclusion 7th character A see Appendix A
PDX collection 1322

CC +7th **S85.302 Unspecified injury of greater saphenous vein at lower leg level, left leg**
CC Exclusion 7th character A see Appendix A
PDX collection 1323

CC +7th **S85.309 Unspecified injury of greater saphenous vein at lower leg level, unspecified leg**
CC Exclusion 7th character A see Appendix A
PDX collection 1324

\+ **S85.31 Laceration of greater saphenous vein at lower leg level**

CC +7th **S85.311 Laceration of greater saphenous vein at lower leg level, right leg**
CC Exclusion 7th character A see Appendix A
PDX collection 1322

CC +7th **S85.312 Laceration of greater saphenous vein at lower leg level, left leg**
CC Exclusion 7th character A see Appendix A
PDX collection 1323

CC +7th **S85.319 Laceration of greater saphenous vein at lower leg level, unspecified leg**
CC Exclusion 7th character A see Appendix A
PDX collection 1324

\+ **S85.39 Other specified injury of greater saphenous vein at lower leg level**

CC +7th **S85.391 Other specified injury of greater saphenous vein at lower leg level, right leg**
CC Exclusion 7th character A see Appendix A
PDX collection 1322

CC +7th **S85.392 Other specified injury of greater saphenous vein at lower leg level, left leg**
CC Exclusion 7th character A see Appendix A
PDX collection 1323

CC +7th **S85.399 Other specified injury of greater saphenous vein at lower leg level, unspecified leg**
CC Exclusion 7th character A see Appendix A
PDX collection 1324

\+ **S85.4 Injury of lesser saphenous vein at lower leg level**

\+ **S85.40 Unspecified injury of lesser saphenous vein at lower leg level**

CC +7th **S85.401 Unspecified injury of lesser saphenous vein at lower leg level, right leg**
CC Exclusion 7th character A see Appendix A
PDX collection 1322

CC +7th **S85.402 Unspecified injury of lesser saphenous vein at lower leg level, left leg**
CC Exclusion 7th character A see Appendix A
PDX collection 1323

CC +7th **S85.409 Unspecified injury of lesser saphenous vein at lower leg level, unspecified leg**
CC Exclusion 7th character A see Appendix A
PDX collection 1324

\+ **S85.41 Laceration of lesser saphenous vein at lower leg level**

CC +7th **S85.411 Laceration of lesser saphenous vein at lower leg level, right leg**
CC Exclusion 7th character A see Appendix A
PDX collection 1322

CC +7th **S85.412 Laceration of lesser saphenous vein at lower leg level, left leg**
CC Exclusion 7th character A see Appendix A
PDX collection 1323

CC +7th **S85.419 Laceration of lesser saphenous vein at lower leg level, unspecified leg**
CC Exclusion 7th character A see Appendix A
PDX collection 1324

\+ **S85.49 Other specified injury of lesser saphenous vein at lower leg level**

CC +7th **S85.491 Other specified injury of lesser saphenous vein at lower leg level, right leg**
CC Exclusion 7th character A see Appendix A
PDX collection 1322

CC +7th **S85.492 Other specified injury of lesser saphenous vein at lower leg level, left leg**
CC Exclusion 7th character A see Appendix A
PDX collection 1323

CC +7th **S85.499 Other specified injury of lesser saphenous vein at lower leg level, unspecified leg**
CC Exclusion 7th character A see Appendix A
PDX collection 1324

\+ **S85.5 Injury of popliteal vein**

\+ **S85.50 Unspecified injury of popliteal vein**

MCC +7th **S85.501 Unspecified injury of popliteal vein, right leg**
MCC Exclusion 7th character A see Appendix A
PDX collection 1361

MCC +7th **S85.502 Unspecified injury of popliteal vein, left leg**
MCC Exclusion 7th character A see Appendix A
PDX collection 1362

MCC +7th **S85.509 Unspecified injury of popliteal vein, unspecified leg**
MCC Exclusion 7th character A see Appendix A
PDX collection 1363

\+ **S85.51 Laceration of popliteal vein**

MCC +7th **S85.511 Laceration of popliteal vein, right leg**
MCC Exclusion 7th character A see Appendix A
PDX collection 1361

MCC +7th **S85.512 Laceration of popliteal vein, left leg**
MCC Exclusion 7th character A see Appendix A
PDX collection 1362

MCC +7th **S85.519 Laceration of popliteal vein, unspecified leg**
MCC Exclusion 7th character A see Appendix A
PDX collection 1363

\+ **S85.59 Other specified injury of popliteal vein**

MCC +7th **S85.591 Other specified injury of popliteal vein, right leg**
MCC Exclusion 7th character A see Appendix A
PDX collection 1361

MCC +7th **S85.592 Other specified injury of popliteal vein, left leg**
MCC Exclusion 7th character A see Appendix A
PDX collection 1362

MCC +7th **S85.599 Other specified injury of popliteal vein, unspecified leg**
MCC Exclusion 7th character A see Appendix A
PDX collection 1363

+ **S85.8 Injury of other blood vessels at lower leg level**
  + **S85.80 Unspecified injury of other blood vessels at lower leg level**
    - CC +7th **S85.801 Unspecified injury of other blood vessels at lower leg level, right leg**
      CC Exclusion 7th character A see Appendix A
      PDX collection 1325
    - CC +7th **S85.802 Unspecified injury of other blood vessels at lower leg level, left leg**
      CC Exclusion 7th character A see Appendix A
      PDX collection 1326
    - CC +7th **S85.809 Unspecified injury of other blood vessels at lower leg level, unspecified leg**
      CC Exclusion 7th character A see Appendix A
      PDX collection 1327
  + **S85.81 Laceration of other blood vessels at lower leg level**
    - CC +7th **S85.811 Laceration of other blood vessels at lower leg level, right leg**
      CC Exclusion 7th character A see Appendix A
      PDX collection 1325
    - CC +7th **S85.812 Laceration of other blood vessels at lower leg level, left leg**
      CC Exclusion 7th character A see Appendix A
      PDX collection 1326
    - CC +7th **S85.819 Laceration of other blood vessels at lower leg level, unspecified leg**
      CC Exclusion 7th character A see Appendix A
      PDX collection 1327
  + **S85.89 Other specified injury of other blood vessels at lower leg level**
    - CC +7th **S85.891 Other specified injury of other blood vessels at lower leg level, right leg**
      CC Exclusion 7th character A see Appendix A
      PDX collection 1325
    - CC +7th **S85.892 Other specified injury of other blood vessels at lower leg level, left leg**
      CC Exclusion 7th character A see Appendix A
      PDX collection 1326
    - CC +7th **S85.899 Other specified injury of other blood vessels at lower leg level, unspecified leg**
      CC Exclusion 7th character A see Appendix A
      PDX collection 1327

+ **S85.9 Injury of unspecified blood vessel at lower leg level**
  + **S85.90 Unspecified injury of unspecified blood vessel at lower leg level**
    - CC +7th **S85.901 Unspecified injury of unspecified blood vessel at lower leg level, right leg**
      CC Exclusion 7th character A see Appendix A
      PDX collection 1325
    - CC +7th **S85.902 Unspecified injury of unspecified blood vessel at lower leg level, left leg**
      CC Exclusion 7th character A see Appendix A
      PDX collection 1326
    - CC +7th **S85.909 Unspecified injury of unspecified blood vessel at lower leg level, unspecified leg**
      CC Exclusion 7th character A see Appendix A
      PDX collection 1327
  + **S85.91 Laceration of unspecified blood vessel at lower leg level**
    - CC +7th **S85.911 Laceration of unspecified blood vessel at lower leg level, right leg**
      CC Exclusion 7th character A see Appendix A
      PDX collection 1325
    - CC +7th **S85.912 Laceration of unspecified blood vessel at lower leg level, left leg**
      CC Exclusion 7th character A see Appendix A
      PDX collection 1326
    - CC +7th **S85.919 Laceration of unspecified blood vessel at lower leg level, unspecified leg**
      CC Exclusion 7th character A see Appendix A
      PDX collection 1327
  + **S85.99 Other specified injury of unspecified blood vessel at lower leg level**
    - CC +7th **S85.991 Other specified injury of unspecified blood vessel at lower leg level, right leg**
      CC Exclusion 7th character A see Appendix A
      PDX collection 1325
    - CC +7th **S85.992 Other specified injury of unspecified blood vessel at lower leg level, left leg**
      CC Exclusion 7th character A see Appendix A
      PDX collection 1326
    - CC +7th **S85.999 Other specified injury of unspecified blood vessel at lower leg level, unspecified leg**
      CC Exclusion 7th character A see Appendix A
      PDX collection 1327

S86 Injury of muscle, fascia and tendon at lower leg level

Code also any associated open wound (S81.-)

Excludes2: *injury of muscle, fascia and tendon at ankle (S96.-)*
injury of patellar ligament (tendon) (S76.1-)
sprain of joints and ligaments of knee (S83.-)

The appropriate 7th character is to be added to each code from category S86
A initial encounter
D subsequent encounter
S sequela

+ **S86.0 Injury of Achilles tendon**
  + **S86.00 Unspecified injury of Achilles tendon**
    - +7th **S86.001 Unspecified injury of right Achilles tendon**
    - +7th **S86.002 Unspecified injury of left Achilles tendon**
    - +7th **S86.009 Unspecified injury of unspecified Achilles tendon**
  + **S86.01 Strain of Achilles tendon**
    - +7th **S86.011 Strain of right Achilles tendon**
    - +7th **S86.012 Strain of left Achilles tendon**
    - +7th **S86.019 Strain of unspecified Achilles tendon**
  + **S86.02 Laceration of Achilles tendon**
    - CC +7th **S86.021 Laceration of right Achilles tendon**
      CC Exclusion 7th character A see Appendix A
      PDX collection 1364
    - CC +7th **S86.022 Laceration of left Achilles tendon**
      CC Exclusion 7th character A see Appendix A
      PDX collection 1365
    - CC +7th **S86.029 Laceration of unspecified Achilles tendon**
      CC Exclusion 7th character A see Appendix A
      PDX collection 1366
  + **S86.09 Other specified injury of Achilles tendon**
    - +7th **S86.091 Other specified injury of right Achilles tendon**
    - +7th **S86.092 Other specified injury of left Achilles tendon**
    - +7th **S86.099 Other specified injury of unspecified Achilles tendon**

+ **S86.1 Injury of other muscle(s) and tendon(s) of posterior muscle group at lower leg level**
  + **S86.10 Unspecified injury of other muscle(s) and tendon(s) of posterior muscle group at lower leg level**
    - +7th **S86.101 Unspecified injury of other muscle(s) and tendon(s) of posterior muscle group at lower leg level, right leg**
    - +7th **S86.102 Unspecified injury of other muscle(s) and tendon(s) of posterior muscle group at lower leg level, left leg**
    - +7th **S86.109 Unspecified injury of other muscle(s) and tendon(s) of posterior muscle group at lower leg level, unspecified leg**
  + **S86.11 Strain of other muscle(s) and tendon(s) of posterior muscle group at lower leg level**
    - +7th **S86.111 Strain of other muscle(s) and tendon(s) of posterior muscle group at lower leg level, right leg**
    - +7th **S86.112 Strain of other muscle(s) and tendon(s) of posterior muscle group at lower leg level, left leg**
    - +7th **S86.119 Strain of other muscle(s) and tendon(s) of posterior muscle group at lower leg level, unspecified leg**
  + **S86.12 Laceration of other muscle(s) and tendon(s) of posterior muscle group at lower leg level**
    - CC +7th **S86.121 Laceration of other muscle(s) and tendon(s) of posterior muscle group at lower leg level, right leg**
      CC Exclusion 7th character A see Appendix A
      PDX collection 1364
    - CC +7th **S86.122 Laceration of other muscle(s) and tendon(s) of posterior muscle group at lower leg level, left leg**
      CC Exclusion 7th character A see Appendix A
      PDX collection 1365
    - CC +7th **S86.129 Laceration of other muscle(s) and tendon(s) of posterior muscle group at lower leg level, unspecified leg**
      CC Exclusion 7th character A see Appendix A
      PDX collection 1366
  + **S86.19 Other injury of other muscle(s) and tendon(s) of posterior muscle group at lower leg level**

+7th S86.191 Other injury of other muscle(s) and tendon(s) of posterior muscle group at lower leg level, right leg
+7th S86.192 Other injury of other muscle(s) and tendon(s) of posterior muscle group at lower leg level, left leg
+7th S86.199 Other injury of other muscle(s) and tendon(s) of posterior muscle group at lower leg level, unspecified leg
+ S86.2 Injury of muscle(s) and tendon(s) of anterior muscle group at lower leg level
+ S86.20 Unspecified injury of muscle(s) and tendon(s) of anterior muscle group at lower leg level
+7th S86.201 Unspecified injury of muscle(s) and tendon(s) of anterior muscle group at lower leg level, right leg
+7th S86.202 Unspecified injury of muscle(s) and tendon(s) of anterior muscle group at lower leg level, left leg
+7th S86.209 Unspecified injury of muscle(s) and tendon(s) of anterior muscle group at lower leg level, unspecified leg
+ S86.21 Strain of muscle(s) and tendon(s) of anterior muscle group at lower leg level
+7th S86.211 Strain of muscle(s) and tendon(s) of anterior muscle group at lower leg level, right leg
+7th S86.212 Strain of muscle(s) and tendon(s) of anterior muscle group at lower leg level, left leg
+7th S86.219 Strain of muscle(s) and tendon(s) of anterior muscle group at lower leg level, unspecified leg
+ S86.22 Laceration of muscle(s) and tendon(s) of anterior muscle group at lower leg level
CC +7th S86.221 Laceration of muscle(s) and tendon(s) of anterior muscle group at lower leg level, right leg
CC Exclusion 7th character A see Appendix A PDX collection 1364
CC +7th S86.222 Laceration of muscle(s) and tendon(s) of anterior muscle group at lower leg level, left leg
CC Exclusion 7th character A see Appendix A PDX collection 1365
CC +7th S86.229 Laceration of muscle(s) and tendon(s) of anterior muscle group at lower leg level, unspecified leg
CC Exclusion 7th character A see Appendix A PDX collection 1366
+ S86.29 Other injury of muscle(s) and tendon(s) of anterior muscle group at lower leg level
+7th S86.291 Other injury of muscle(s) and tendon(s) of anterior muscle group at lower leg level, right leg
+7th S86.292 Other injury of muscle(s) and tendon(s) of anterior muscle group at lower leg level, left leg
+7th S86.299 Other injury of muscle(s) and tendon(s) of anterior muscle group at lower leg level, unspecified leg
+ S86.3 Injury of muscle(s) and tendon(s) of peroneal muscle group at lower leg level
+ S86.30 Unspecified injury of muscle(s) and tendon(s) of peroneal muscle group at lower leg level
+7th S86.301 Unspecified injury of muscle(s) and tendon(s) of peroneal muscle group at lower leg level, right leg
+7th S86.302 Unspecified injury of muscle(s) and tendon(s) of peroneal muscle group at lower leg level, left leg
+7th S86.309 Unspecified injury of muscle(s) and tendon(s) of peroneal muscle group at lower leg level, unspecified leg
+ S86.31 Strain of muscle(s) and tendon(s) of peroneal muscle group at lower leg level
+7th S86.311 Strain of muscle(s) and tendon(s) of peroneal muscle group at lower leg level, right leg
+7th S86.312 Strain of muscle(s) and tendon(s) of peroneal muscle group at lower leg level, left leg
+7th S86.319 Strain of muscle(s) and tendon(s) of peroneal muscle group at lower leg level, unspecified leg
+ S86.32 Laceration of muscle(s) and tendon(s) of peroneal muscle group at lower leg level
CC +7th S86.321 Laceration of muscle(s) and tendon(s) of peroneal muscle group at lower leg level, right leg
CC Exclusion 7th character A see Appendix A PDX collection 1364
CC +7th S86.322 Laceration of muscle(s) and tendon(s) of peroneal muscle group at lower leg level, left leg
CC Exclusion 7th character A see Appendix A PDX collection 1365
CC +7th S86.329 Laceration of muscle(s) and tendon(s) of peroneal muscle group at lower leg level, unspecified leg
CC Exclusion 7th character A see Appendix A PDX collection 1366
+ S86.39 Other injury of muscle(s) and tendon(s) of peroneal muscle group at lower leg level
+7th S86.391 Other injury of muscle(s) and tendon(s) of peroneal muscle group at lower leg level, right leg
+7th S86.392 Other injury of muscle(s) and tendon(s) of peroneal muscle group at lower leg level, left leg
+7th S86.399 Other injury of muscle(s) and tendon(s) of peroneal muscle group at lower leg level, unspecified leg
+ S86.8 Injury of other muscles and tendons at lower leg level
+ S86.80 Unspecified injury of other muscles and tendons at lower leg level
+ S86.801 Unspecified injury of other muscle(s) and tendon(s) at lower leg level, right leg
+ S86.802 Unspecified injury of other muscle(s) and tendon(s) at lower leg level, left leg
+ S86.809 Unspecified injury of other muscle(s) and tendon(s) at lower leg level, unspecified leg
+ S86.81 Strain of other muscles and tendons at lower leg level
+7th S86.811 Strain of other muscle(s) and tendon(s) at lower leg level, right leg
+7th S86.812 Strain of other muscle(s) and tendon(s) at lower leg level, left leg
+7th S86.819 Strain of other muscle(s) and tendon(s) at lower leg level, unspecified leg
+ S86.82 Laceration of other muscles and tendons at lower leg level
CC +7th S86.821 Laceration of other muscle(s) and tendon(s) at lower leg level, right leg
CC Exclusion 7th character A see Appendix A PDX collection 1364
CC +7th S86.822 Laceration of other muscle(s) and tendon(s) at lower leg level, left leg
CC Exclusion 7th character A see Appendix A PDX collection 1365
CC +7th S86.829 Laceration of other muscle(s) and tendon(s) at lower leg level, unspecified leg
CC Exclusion 7th character A see Appendix A PDX collection 1366
+ S86.89 Other injury of other muscles and tendons at lower leg level
+7th S86.891 Other injury of other muscle(s) and tendon(s) at lower leg level, right leg
+7th S86.892 Other injury of other muscle(s) and tendon(s) at lower leg level, left leg
+7th S86.899 Other injury of other muscle(s) and tendon(s) at lower leg level, unspecified leg
+ S86.9 Injury of unspecified muscle and tendon at lower leg level
+ S86.90 Unspecified injury of unspecified muscle and tendon at lower leg level
+7th S86.901 Unspecified injury of unspecified muscle(s) and tendon(s) at lower leg level, right leg
+7th S86.902 Unspecified injury of unspecified muscle(s) and tendon(s) at lower leg level, left leg

+7th **S86.909 Unspecified injury of unspecified muscle(s) and tendon(s) at lower leg level, unspecified leg**

+ **S86.91 Strain of unspecified muscle and tendon at lower leg level**

+7th **S86.911 Strain of unspecified muscle(s) and tendon(s) at lower leg level, right leg**

+7th **S86.912 Strain of unspecified muscle(s) and tendon(s) at lower leg level, left leg**

+7th **S86.919 Strain of unspecified muscle(s) and tendon(s) at lower leg level, unspecified leg**

+ **S86.92 Laceration of unspecified muscle and tendon at lower leg level**

CC +7th **S86.921 Laceration of unspecified muscle(s) and tendon(s) at lower leg level, right leg**
CC Exclusion 7th character A see Appendix A
PDX collection 1364

CC +7th **S86.922 Laceration of unspecified muscle(s) and tendon(s) at lower leg level, left leg**
CC Exclusion 7th character A see Appendix A
PDX collection 1365

CC +7th **S86.929 Laceration of unspecified muscle(s) and tendon(s) at lower leg level, unspecified leg**
CC Exclusion 7th character A see Appendix A
PDX collection 1366

+ **S86.99 Other injury of unspecified muscle and tendon at lower leg level**

+7th **S86.991 Other injury of unspecified muscle(s) and tendon(s) at lower leg level, right leg**

+7th **S86.992 Other injury of unspecified muscle(s) and tendon(s) at lower leg level, left leg**

+7th **S86.999 Other injury of unspecified muscle(s) and tendon(s) at lower leg level, unspecified leg**

S87 Crushing injury of lower leg

Use additional code(s) for all associated injuries

Excludes2: *crushing injury of ankle and foot (S97.-)*

The appropriate 7th character is to be added to each code from category S87
A initial encounter
D subsequent encounter
S sequela

+ **S87.0 Crushing injury of knee**

X+7th **S87.00 Crushing injury of unspecified knee**

X+7th **S87.01 Crushing injury of right knee**

X+7th **S87.02 Crushing injury of left knee**

+ **S87.8 Crushing injury of lower leg**

X+7th **S87.80 Crushing injury of unspecified lower leg**

X+7th **S87.81 Crushing injury of right lower leg**

X+7th **S87.82 Crushing injury of left lower leg**

S88 Traumatic amputation of lower leg

NOTE An amputation not identified as partial or complete should be coded to complete

Excludes1: *traumatic amputation of ankle and foot (S98.-)*

The appropriate 7th character is to be added to each code from category S88
A initial encounter
D subsequent encounter
S sequela

+ **S88.0 Traumatic amputation at knee level**

+ **S88.01 Complete traumatic amputation at knee level**

CC +7th **S88.011 Complete traumatic amputation at knee level, right lower leg**
CC Exclusion 7th character A see Appendix A
PDX collection 1333

CC +7th **S88.012 Complete traumatic amputation at knee level, left lower leg**
CC Exclusion 7th character A see Appendix A
PDX collection 1334

CC +7th **S88.019 Complete traumatic amputation at knee level, unspecified lower leg**
CC Exclusion 7th character A see Appendix A
PDX collection 1335

+ **S88.02 Partial traumatic amputation at knee level**

CC +7th **S88.021 Partial traumatic amputation at knee level, right lower leg**
CC Exclusion 7th character A see Appendix A
PDX collection 1333

CC +7th **S88.022 Partial traumatic amputation at knee level, left lower leg**
CC Exclusion 7th character A see Appendix A
PDX collection 1334

CC +7th **S88.029 Partial traumatic amputation at knee level, unspecified lower leg**
CC Exclusion 7th character A see Appendix A
PDX collection 1335

+ **S88.1 Traumatic amputation at level between knee and ankle**

+ **S88.11 Complete traumatic amputation at level between knee and ankle**

CC +7th **S88.111 Complete traumatic amputation at level between knee and ankle, right lower leg**
CC Exclusion 7th character A see Appendix A
PDX collection 1333

CC +7th **S88.112 Complete traumatic amputation at level between knee and ankle, left lower leg**
CC Exclusion 7th character A see Appendix A
PDX collection 1334

CC +7th **S88.119 Complete traumatic amputation at level between knee and ankle, unspecified lower leg**
CC Exclusion 7th character A see Appendix A
PDX collection 1335

+ **S88.12 Partial traumatic amputation at level between knee and ankle**

CC +7th **S88.121 Partial traumatic amputation at level between knee and ankle, right lower leg**
CC Exclusion 7th character A see Appendix A
PDX collection 1333

CC +7th **S88.122 Partial traumatic amputation at level between knee and ankle, left lower leg**
CC Exclusion 7th character A see Appendix A
PDX collection 1334

CC +7th **S88.129 Partial traumatic amputation at level between knee and ankle, unspecified lower leg**
CC Exclusion 7th character A see Appendix A
PDX collection 1335

+ **S88.9 Traumatic amputation of lower leg, level unspecified**

+ **S88.91 Complete traumatic amputation of lower leg, level unspecified**

CC +7th **S88.911 Complete traumatic amputation of right lower leg, level unspecified**
CC Exclusion 7th character A see Appendix A
PDX collection 1333

CC +7th **S88.912 Complete traumatic amputation of left lower leg, level unspecified**
CC Exclusion 7th character A see Appendix A
PDX collection 1334

CC +7th **S88.919 Complete traumatic amputation of unspecified lower leg, level unspecified**
CC Exclusion 7th character A see Appendix A
PDX collection 1335

+ **S88.92 Partial traumatic amputation of lower leg, level unspecified**

CC +7th **S88.921 Partial traumatic amputation of right lower leg, level unspecified**
CC Exclusion 7th character A see Appendix A
PDX collection 1333

CC +7th **S88.922 Partial traumatic amputation of left lower leg, level unspecified**
CC Exclusion 7th character A see Appendix A
PDX collection 1334

CC +7th **S88.929 Partial traumatic amputation of unspecified lower leg, level unspecified**
CC Exclusion 7th character A see Appendix A
PDX collection 1335

S89 Other and unspecified injuries of lower leg

NOTE A fracture not indicated as open or closed should be coded to closed

Excludes2: *other and unspecified injuries of ankle and foot (S99.-)*

The appropriate 7th character is to be added to each code from subcategories **S89.0, S89.1, S89.2,** and **S89.3**
A initial encounter for closed fracture
D subsequent encounter for fracture with routine healing
G subsequent encounter for fracture with delayed healing
K subsequent encounter for fracture with nonunion
P subsequent encounter for fracture with malunion
S sequela

Review coding guideline C.19.c

+ S89.0 Physeal fracture of upper end of tibia
+ S89.00 Unspecified physeal fracture of upper end of tibia
CC +7th S89.001 Unspecified physeal fracture of upper end of right tibia
CC Exclusion 7th character A see Appendix A PDX collection 1340
CC Exclusion 7th characters K & P see Appendix A PDX collection 0897
HAC 7th character A see Appendix B for HAC conditional logic
CC +7th S89.002 Unspecified physeal fracture of upper end of left tibia
CC Exclusion 7th character A see Appendix A PDX collection 1342
CC Exclusion 7th characters K & P see Appendix A PDX collection 0897
HAC 7th character A see Appendix B for HAC conditional logic
CC +7th S89.009 Unspecified physeal fracture of upper end of unspecified tibia
CC Exclusion 7th character A see Appendix A PDX collection 1341
CC Exclusion 7th characters K & P see Appendix A PDX collection 0897
HAC 7th character A see Appendix B for HAC conditional logic
+ S89.01 Salter-Harris Type I physeal fracture of upper end of tibia
CC +7th S89.011 Salter-Harris Type I physeal fracture of upper end of right tibia
CC Exclusion 7th character A see Appendix A PDX collection 1340
CC Exclusion 7th characters K & P see Appendix A PDX collection 0897
HAC 7th character A see Appendix B for HAC conditional logic
CC +7th S89.012 Salter-Harris Type I physeal fracture of upper end of left tibia
CC Exclusion 7th character A see Appendix A PDX collection 1342
CC Exclusion 7th characters K & P see Appendix A PDX collection 0897
HAC 7th character A see Appendix B for HAC conditional logic
CC +7th S89.019 Salter-Harris Type I physeal fracture of upper end of unspecified tibia
CC Exclusion 7th character A see Appendix A PDX collection 1341
CC Exclusion 7th characters K & P see Appendix A PDX collection 0897
HAC 7th character A see Appendix B for HAC conditional logic
+ S89.02 Salter-Harris Type II physeal fracture of upper end of tibia
CC +7th S89.021 Salter-Harris Type II physeal fracture of upper end of right tibia
CC Exclusion 7th character A see Appendix A PDX collection 1340
CC Exclusion 7th characters K & P see Appendix A PDX collection 0897
HAC 7th character A see Appendix B for HAC conditional logic
CC +7th S89.022 Salter-Harris Type II physeal fracture of upper end of left tibia
CC Exclusion 7th character A see Appendix A PDX collection 1342
CC Exclusion 7th characters K & P see Appendix A PDX collection 0897
HAC 7th character A see Appendix B for HAC conditional logic
CC +7th S89.029 Salter-Harris Type II physeal fracture of upper end of unspecified tibia
CC Exclusion 7th character A see Appendix A PDX collection 1341
CC Exclusion 7th characters K & P see Appendix A PDX collection 0897
HAC 7th character A see Appendix B for HAC conditional logic
+ S89.03 Salter-Harris Type III physeal fracture of upper end of tibia
CC +7th S89.031 Salter-Harris Type III physeal fracture of upper end of right tibia
CC Exclusion 7th character A see Appendix A PDX collection 1340
CC Exclusion 7th characters K & P see Appendix A PDX collection 0897
HAC 7th character A see Appendix B for HAC conditional logic
CC +7th S89.032 Salter-Harris Type III physeal fracture of upper end of left tibia
CC Exclusion 7th character A see Appendix A PDX collection 1342
CC Exclusion 7th characters K & P see Appendix A PDX collection 0897
HAC 7th character A see Appendix B for HAC conditional logic
CC +7th S89.039 Salter-Harris Type III physeal fracture of upper end of unspecified tibia
CC Exclusion 7th character A see Appendix A PDX collection 1341
CC Exclusion 7th characters K & P see Appendix A PDX collection 0897
HAC 7th character A see Appendix B for HAC conditional logic
+ S89.04 Salter-Harris Type IV physeal fracture of upper end of tibia
CC +7th S89.041 Salter-Harris Type IV physeal fracture of upper end of right tibia
CC Exclusion 7th character A see Appendix A PDX collection 1340
CC Exclusion 7th characters K & P see Appendix A PDX collection 0897
HAC 7th character A see Appendix B for HAC conditional logic
CC +7th S89.042 Salter-Harris Type IV physeal fracture of upper end of left tibia
CC Exclusion 7th character A see Appendix A PDX collection 1342
CC Exclusion 7th characters K & P see Appendix A PDX collection 0897
HAC 7th character A see Appendix B for HAC conditional logic
CC +7th S89.049 Salter-Harris Type IV physeal fracture of upper end of unspecified tibia
CC Exclusion 7th character A see Appendix A PDX collection 1341
CC Exclusion 7th characters K & P see Appendix A PDX collection 0897
HAC 7th character A see Appendix B for HAC conditional logic
+ S89.09 Other physeal fracture of upper end of tibia
CC +7th S89.091 Other physeal fracture of upper end of right tibia
CC Exclusion 7th character A see Appendix A PDX collection 1340
CC Exclusion 7th characters K & P see Appendix A PDX collection 0897
HAC 7th character A see Appendix B for HAC conditional logic
CC +7th S89.092 Other physeal fracture of upper end of left tibia
CC Exclusion 7th character A see Appendix A PDX collection 1342
CC Exclusion 7th characters K & P see Appendix A PDX collection 0897
HAC 7th character A see Appendix B for HAC conditional logic
CC +7th S89.099 Other physeal fracture of upper end of unspecified tibia
CC Exclusion 7th character A see Appendix A PDX collection 1341
CC Exclusion 7th characters K & P see Appendix A PDX collection 0897
HAC 7th character A see Appendix B for HAC conditional logic
+ S89.1 Physeal fracture of lower end of tibia
+ S89.10 Unspecified physeal fracture of lower end of tibia
CC +7th S89.101 Unspecified physeal fracture of lower end of right tibia
CC Exclusion 7th characters K & P see Appendix A PDX collection 0897

CC +7th **S89.102 Unspecified physeal fracture of lower end of left tibia**
CC Exclusion 7th characters K & P see Appendix A PDX collection 0897

CC +7th **S89.109 Unspecified physeal fracture of lower end of unspecified tibia**
CC Exclusion 7th characters K & P see Appendix A PDX collection 0897

\+ **S89.11 Salter-Harris Type I physeal fracture of lower end of tibia**

CC +7th **S89.111 Salter-Harris Type I physeal fracture of lower end of right tibia**
CC Exclusion 7th characters K & P see Appendix A PDX collection 0897

CC +7th **S89.112 Salter-Harris Type I physeal fracture of lower end of left tibia**
CC Exclusion 7th characters K & P see Appendix A PDX collection 0897

CC +7th **S89.119 Salter-Harris Type I physeal fracture of lower end of unspecified tibia**
CC Exclusion 7th characters K & P see Appendix A PDX collection 0897

\+ **S89.12 Salter-Harris Type II physeal fracture of lower end of tibia**

CC +7th **S89.121 Salter-Harris Type II physeal fracture of lower end of right tibia**
CC Exclusion 7th characters K & P see Appendix A PDX collection 0897

CC +7th **S89.122 Salter-Harris Type II physeal fracture of lower end of left tibia**
CC Exclusion 7th characters K & P see Appendix A PDX collection 0897

CC +7th **S89.129 Salter-Harris Type II physeal fracture of lower end of unspecified tibia**
CC Exclusion 7th characters K & P see Appendix A PDX collection 0897

\+ **S89.13 Salter-Harris Type III physeal fracture of lower end of tibia**
Excludes1: *fracture of medial malleolus (adult) (S82.5-)*

CC +7th **S89.131 Salter-Harris Type III physeal fracture of lower end of right tibia**
CC Exclusion 7th characters K & P see Appendix A PDX collection 0897

CC +7th **S89.132 Salter-Harris Type III physeal fracture of lower end of left tibia**
CC Exclusion 7th characters K & P see Appendix A PDX collection 0897

CC +7th **S89.139 Salter-Harris Type III physeal fracture of lower end of unspecified tibia**
CC Exclusion 7th characters K & P see Appendix A PDX collection 0897

\+ **S89.14 Salter-Harris Type IV physeal fracture of lower end of tibia**
Excludes1: *fracture of medial malleolus (adult) (S82.5-)*

CC +7th **S89.141 Salter-Harris Type IV physeal fracture of lower end of right tibia**
CC Exclusion 7th characters K & P see Appendix A PDX collection 0897

CC +7th **S89.142 Salter-Harris Type IV physeal fracture of lower end of left tibia**
CC Exclusion 7th characters K & P see Appendix A PDX collection 0897

CC +7th **S89.149 Salter-Harris Type IV physeal fracture of lower end of unspecified tibia**
CC Exclusion 7th characters K & P see Appendix A PDX collection 0897

\+ **S89.19 Other physeal fracture of lower end of tibia**

CC +7th **S89.191 Other physeal fracture of lower end of right tibia**
CC Exclusion 7th characters K & P see Appendix A PDX collection 0897

CC +7th **S89.192 Other physeal fracture of lower end of left tibia**
CC Exclusion 7th characters K & P see Appendix A PDX collection 0897

CC +7th **S89.199 Other physeal fracture of lower end of unspecified tibia**
CC Exclusion 7th characters K & P see Appendix A PDX collection 0897

\+ **S89.2 Physeal fracture of upper end of fibula**

\+ **S89.20 Unspecified physeal fracture of upper end of fibula**

CC +7th **S89.201 Unspecified physeal fracture of upper end of right fibula**
CC Exclusion 7th characters K & P see Appendix A PDX collection 0897

CC +7th **S89.202 Unspecified physeal fracture of upper end of left fibula**
CC Exclusion 7th characters K & P see Appendix A PDX collection 0897

CC +7th **S89.209 Unspecified physeal fracture of upper end of unspecified fibula**
CC Exclusion 7th characters K & P see Appendix A PDX collection 0897

\+ **S89.21 Salter-Harris Type I physeal fracture of upper end of fibula**

CC +7th **S89.211 Salter-Harris Type I physeal fracture of upper end of right fibula**
CC Exclusion 7th characters K & P see Appendix A PDX collection 0897

CC +7th **S89.212 Salter-Harris Type I physeal fracture of upper end of left fibula**
CC Exclusion 7th characters K & P see Appendix A PDX collection 0897

CC +7th **S89.219 Salter-Harris Type I physeal fracture of upper end of unspecified fibula**
CC Exclusion 7th characters K & P see Appendix A PDX collection 0897

\+ **S89.22 Salter-Harris Type II physeal fracture of upper end of fibula**

CC +7th **S89.221 Salter-Harris Type II physeal fracture of upper end of right fibula**
CC Exclusion 7th characters K & P see Appendix A PDX collection 0897

CC +7th **S89.222 Salter-Harris Type II physeal fracture of upper end of left fibula**
CC Exclusion 7th characters K & P see Appendix A PDX collection 0897

CC +7th **S89.229 Salter-Harris Type II physeal fracture of upper end of unspecified fibula**
CC Exclusion 7th characters K & P see Appendix A PDX collection 0897

\+ **S89.29 Other physeal fracture of upper end of fibula**

CC +7th **S89.291 Other physeal fracture of upper end of right fibula**
CC Exclusion 7th characters K & P see Appendix A PDX collection 0897

CC +7th **S89.292 Other physeal fracture of upper end of left fibula**
CC Exclusion 7th characters K & P see Appendix A PDX collection 0897

CC +7th **S89.299 Other physeal fracture of upper end of unspecified fibula**
CC Exclusion 7th characters K & P see Appendix A PDX collection 0897

\+ **S89.3 Physeal fracture of lower end of fibula**

\+ **S89.30 Unspecified physeal fracture of lower end of fibula**

CC +7th **S89.301 Unspecified physeal fracture of lower end of right fibula**
CC Exclusion 7th characters K & P see Appendix A PDX collection 0897

CC +7th **S89.302 Unspecified physeal fracture of lower end of left fibula**
CC Exclusion 7th characters K & P see Appendix A PDX collection 0897

CC +7th **S89.309 Unspecified physeal fracture of lower end of unspecified fibula**
CC Exclusion 7th characters K & P see Appendix A PDX collection 0897

\+ **S89.31 Salter-Harris Type I physeal fracture of lower end of fibula**

CC +7th **S89.311 Salter-Harris Type I physeal fracture of lower end of right fibula**
CC Exclusion 7th characters K & P see Appendix A PDX collection 0897

CC +7th **S89.312 Salter-Harris Type I physeal fracture of lower end of left fibula**
CC Exclusion 7th characters K & P see Appendix A PDX collection 0897

CC +7th **S89.319 Salter-Harris Type I physeal fracture of lower end of unspecified fibula**
CC Exclusion 7th characters K & P see Appendix A PDX collection 0897

+ **S89.32 Salter-Harris Type II physeal fracture of lower end of fibula**
  - CC +7th **S89.321 Salter-Harris Type II physeal fracture of lower end of right fibula**
    - CC Exclusion 7th characters K & P see Appendix A PDX collection 0897
  - CC +7th **S89.322 Salter-Harris Type II physeal fracture of lower end of left fibula**
    - CC Exclusion 7th characters K & P see Appendix A PDX collection 0897
  - CC +7th **S89.329 Salter-Harris Type II physeal fracture of lower end of unspecified fibula**
    - CC Exclusion 7th characters K & P see Appendix A PDX collection 0897
+ **S89.39 Other physeal fracture of lower end of fibula**
  - CC +7th **S89.391 Other physeal fracture of lower end of right fibula**
    - CC Exclusion 7th characters K & P see Appendix A PDX collection 0897
  - CC +7th **S89.392 Other physeal fracture of lower end of left fibula**
    - CC Exclusion 7th characters K & P see Appendix A PDX collection 0897
  - CC +7th **S89.399 Other physeal fracture of lower end of unspecified fibula**
    - CC Exclusion 7th characters K & P see Appendix A PDX collection 0897

+ **S89.8 Other specified injuries of lower leg**

> The appropriate 7th character is to be added to each code in subcategory **S89.8**
> A initial encounter
> D subsequent encounter
> S sequela

- X+7th **S89.80 Other specified injuries of unspecified lower leg**
- X+7th **S89.81 Other specified injuries of right lower leg**
- X+7th **S89.82 Other specified injuries of left lower leg**

+ **S89.9 Unspecified injury of lower leg**

> The appropriate 7th character is to be added to each code in subcategory **S89.9**
> A initial encounter
> D subsequent encounter
> S sequela

- X+7th **S89.90 Unspecified injury of unspecified lower leg**
- X+7th **S89.91 Unspecified injury of right lower leg**
- X+7th **S89.92 Unspecified injury of left lower leg**

Injuries to the ankle and foot (S90-S99)

Excludes2: *burns and corrosions (T20-T32)*
fracture of ankle and malleolus (S82.-)
frostbite (T33-T34)
insect bite or sting, venomous (T63.4)

S90 Superficial injury of ankle, foot and toes

> The appropriate 7th character is to be added to each code from category S90
> A initial encounter
> D subsequent encounter
> S sequela

+ **S90.0 Contusion of ankle**
  - X+7th **S90.00 Contusion of unspecified ankle**
  - X+7th **S90.01 Contusion of right ankle**
  - X+7th **S90.02 Contusion of left ankle**
+ **S90.1 Contusion of toe without damage to nail**
  + **S90.11 Contusion of great toe without damage to nail**
    - +7th **S90.111 Contusion of right great toe without damage to nail**
    - +7th **S90.112 Contusion of left great toe without damage to nail**
    - +7th **S90.119 Contusion of unspecified great toe without damage to nail**
  + **S90.12 Contusion of lesser toe without damage to nail**
    - +7th **S90.121 Contusion of right lesser toe(s) without damage to nail**
    - +7th **S90.122 Contusion of left lesser toe(s) without damage to nail**
    - +7th **S90.129 Contusion of unspecified lesser toe(s) without damage to nail**
      - Contusion of toe NOS
+ **S90.2 Contusion of toe with damage to nail**
  + **S90.21 Contusion of great toe with damage to nail**
    - +7th **S90.211 Contusion of right great toe with damage to nail**
    - +7th **S90.212 Contusion of left great toe with damage to nail**
    - +7th **S90.219 Contusion of unspecified great toe with damage to nail**
  + **S90.22 Contusion of lesser toe with damage to nail**
    - +7th **S90.221 Contusion of right lesser toe(s) with damage to nail**
    - +7th **S90.222 Contusion of left lesser toe(s) with damage to nail**
    - +7th **S90.229 Contusion of unspecified lesser toe(s) with damage to nail**
+ **S90.3 Contusion of foot**
  - **Excludes2:** *contusion of toes (S90.1-, S90.2-)*
  - X+7th **S90.30 Contusion of unspecified foot**
    - Contusion of foot NOS
  - X+7th **S90.31 Contusion of right foot**
  - X+7th **S90.32 Contusion of left foot**
+ **S90.4 Other superficial injuries of toe**
  + **S90.41 Abrasion of toe**
    - +7th **S90.411 Abrasion, right great toe**
    - +7th **S90.412 Abrasion, left great toe**
    - +7th **S90.413 Abrasion, unspecified great toe**
    - +7th **S90.414 Abrasion, right lesser toe(s)**
    - +7th **S90.415 Abrasion, left lesser toe(s)**
    - +7th **S90.416 Abrasion, unspecified lesser toe(s)**
  + **S90.42 Blister (nonthermal) of toe**
    - +7th **S90.421 Blister (nonthermal), right great toe**
    - +7th **S90.422 Blister (nonthermal), left great toe**
    - +7th **S90.423 Blister (nonthermal), unspecified great toe**
    - +7th **S90.424 Blister (nonthermal), right lesser toe(s)**
    - +7th **S90.425 Blister (nonthermal), left lesser toe(s)**
    - +7th **S90.426 Blister (nonthermal), unspecified lesser toe(s)**
  + **S90.44 External constriction of toe**
    - Hair tourniquet syndrome of toe
    - +7th **S90.441 External constriction, right great toe**
    - +7th **S90.442 External constriction, left great toe**
    - +7th **S90.443 External constriction, unspecified great toe**
    - +7th **S90.444 External constriction, right lesser toe(s)**
    - +7th **S90.445 External constriction, left lesser toe(s)**
    - +7th **S90.446 External constriction, unspecified lesser toe(s)**
  + **S90.45 Superficial foreign body of toe**
    - Splinter in the toe
    - +7th **S90.451 Superficial foreign body, right great toe**
    - +7th **S90.452 Superficial foreign body, left great toe**
    - +7th **S90.453 Superficial foreign body, unspecified great toe**
    - +7th **S90.454 Superficial foreign body, right lesser toe(s)**
    - +7th **S90.455 Superficial foreign body, left lesser toe(s)**
    - +7th **S90.456 Superficial foreign body, unspecified lesser toe(s)**
  + **S90.46 Insect bite (nonvenomous) of toe**
    - +7th **S90.461 Insect bite (nonvenomous), right great toe**
    - +7th **S90.462 Insect bite (nonvenomous), left great toe**
    - +7th **S90.463 Insect bite (nonvenomous), unspecified great toe**
    - +7th **S90.464 Insect bite (nonvenomous), right lesser toe(s)**
    - +7th **S90.465 Insect bite (nonvenomous), left lesser toe(s)**
    - +7th **S90.466 Insect bite (nonvenomous), unspecified lesser toe(s)**
  + **S90.47 Other superficial bite of toe**
    - **Excludes1:** *open bite of toe (S91.15-, S91.25-)*
    - +7th **S90.471 Other superficial bite of right great toe**
    - +7th **S90.472 Other superficial bite of left great toe**
    - +7th **S90.473 Other superficial bite of unspecified great toe**
    - +7th **S90.474 Other superficial bite of right lesser toe(s)**
    - +7th **S90.475 Other superficial bite of left lesser toe(s)**
    - +7th **S90.476 Other superficial bite of unspecified lesser toe(s)**
+ **S90.5 Other superficial injuries of ankle**
  + **S90.51 Abrasion of ankle**
    - +7th **S90.511 Abrasion, right ankle**
    - +7th **S90.512 Abrasion, left ankle**
    - +7th **S90.519 Abrasion, unspecified ankle**

Ankle

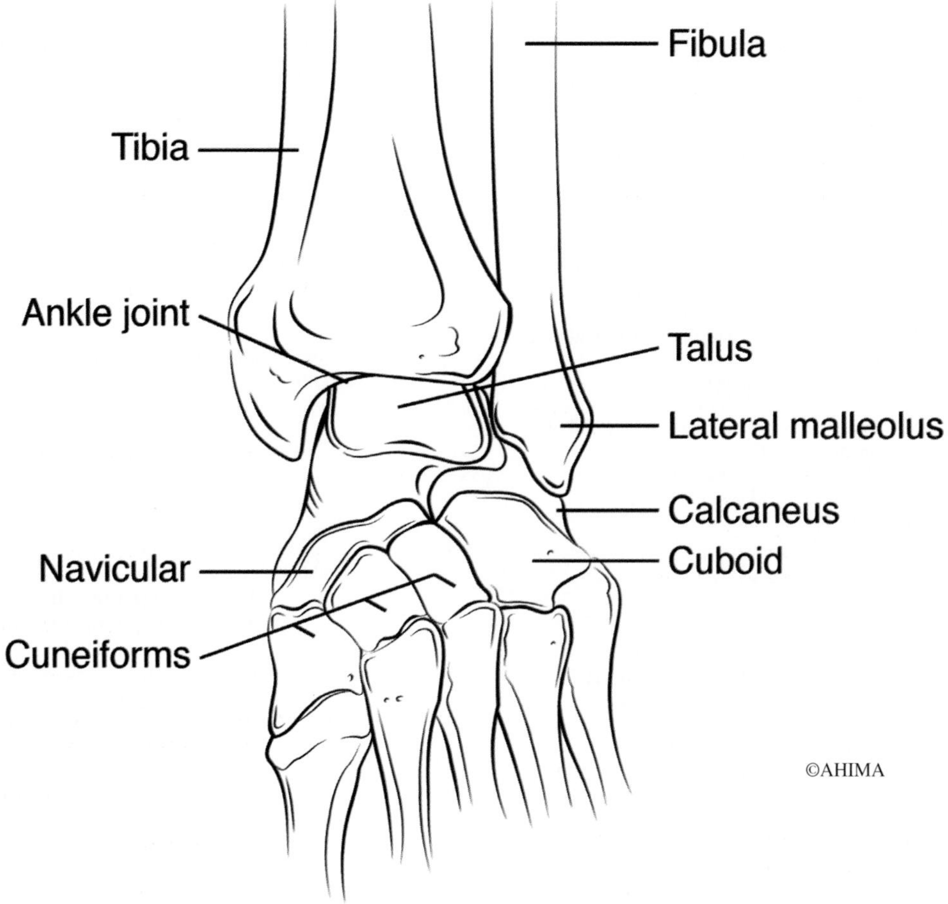
Fibula
Tibia
Ankle joint
Talus
Lateral malleolus
Calcaneus
Navicular
Cuboid
Cuneiforms
©AHIMA

Muscles of the Foot

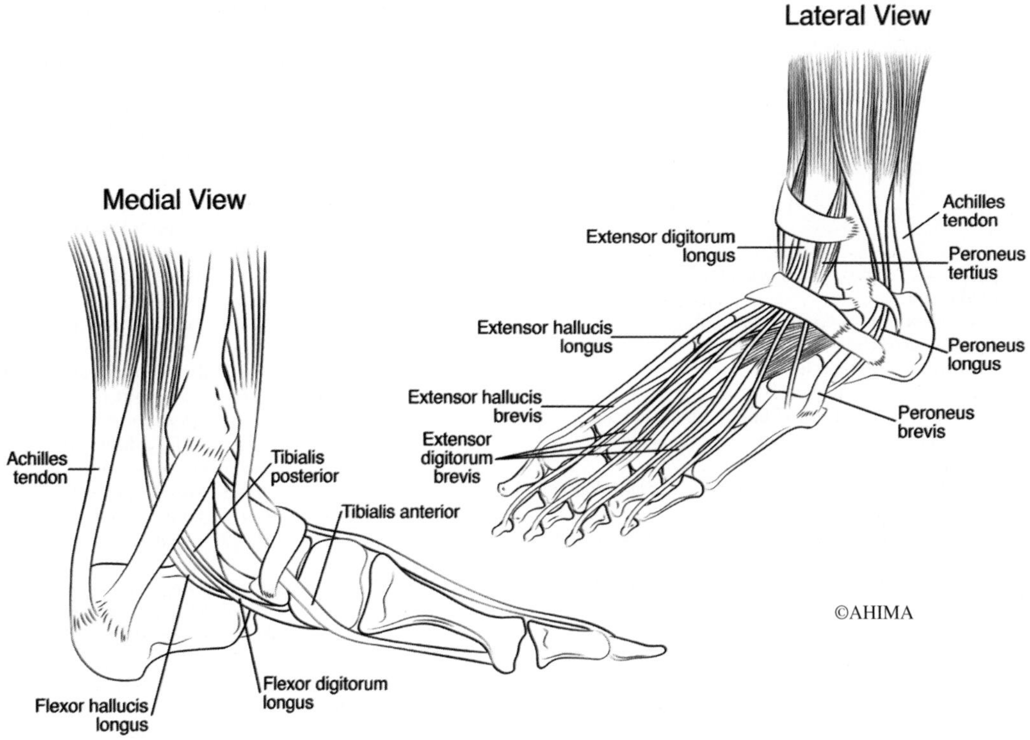
Lateral View
Achilles tendon
Extensor digitorum longus
Peroneus tertius
Extensor hallucis longus
Peroneus longus
Extensor hallucis brevis
Peroneus brevis
Extensor digitorum brevis
Medial View
Achilles tendon
Tibialis posterior
Tibialis anterior
Flexor hallucis longus
Flexor digitorum longus
©AHIMA

+ **S90.52 Blister (nonthermal) of ankle**
  - +7th **S90.521 Blister (nonthermal), right ankle**
  - +7th **S90.522 Blister (nonthermal), left ankle**
  - +7th **S90.529 Blister (nonthermal), unspecified ankle**
+ **S90.54 External constriction of ankle**
  - +7th **S90.541 External constriction, right ankle**
  - +7th **S90.542 External constriction, left ankle**
  - +7th **S90.549 External constriction, unspecified ankle**
+ **S90.55 Superficial foreign body of ankle**
  Splinter in the ankle
  - +7th **S90.551 Superficial foreign body, right ankle**
  - +7th **S90.552 Superficial foreign body, left ankle**
  - +7th **S90.559 Superficial foreign body, unspecified ankle**
+ **S90.56 Insect bite (nonvenomous) of ankle**
  - +7th **S90.561 Insect bite (nonvenomous), right ankle**
  - +7th **S90.562 Insect bite (nonvenomous), left ankle**
  - +7th **S90.569 Insect bite (nonvenomous), unspecified ankle**
+ **S90.57 Other superficial bite of ankle**
  Excludes1: *open bite of ankle (S91.05-)*
  - +7th **S90.571 Other superficial bite of ankle, right ankle**
  - +7th **S90.572 Other superficial bite of ankle, left ankle**
  - +7th **S90.579 Other superficial bite of ankle, unspecified ankle**

+ **S90.8 Other superficial injuries of foot**
+ **S90.81 Abrasion of foot**
  - +7th **S90.811 Abrasion, right foot**
  - +7th **S90.812 Abrasion, left foot**
  - +7th **S90.819 Abrasion, unspecified foot**
+ **S90.82 Blister (nonthermal) of foot**
  - +7th **S90.821 Blister (nonthermal), right foot**
  - +7th **S90.822 Blister (nonthermal), left foot**
  - +7th **S90.829 Blister (nonthermal), unspecified foot**
+ **S90.84 External constriction of foot**
  - +7th **S90.841 External constriction, right foot**
  - +7th **S90.842 External constriction, left foot**
  - +7th **S90.849 External constriction, unspecified foot**
+ **S90.85 Superficial foreign body of foot**
  Splinter in the foot
  - +7th **S90.851 Superficial foreign body, right foot**
  - +7th **S90.852 Superficial foreign body, left foot**
  - +7th **S90.859 Superficial foreign body, unspecified foot**
+ **S90.86 Insect bite (nonvenomous) of foot**
  - +7th **S90.861 Insect bite (nonvenomous), right foot**
  - +7th **S90.862 Insect bite (nonvenomous), left foot**
  - +7th **S90.869 Insect bite (nonvenomous), unspecified foot**
+ **S90.87 Other superficial bite of foot**
  Excludes1: *open bite of foot (S91.35-)*
  - +7th **S90.871 Other superficial bite of right foot**
  - +7th **S90.872 Other superficial bite of left foot**
  - +7th **S90.879 Other superficial bite of unspecified foot**

+ **S90.9 Unspecified superficial injury of ankle, foot and toe**
+ **S90.91 Unspecified superficial injury of ankle**
  - +7th **S90.911 Unspecified superficial injury of right ankle**
  - +7th **S90.912 Unspecified superficial injury of left ankle**
  - +7th **S90.919 Unspecified superficial injury of unspecified ankle**
+ **S90.92 Unspecified superficial injury of foot**
  - +7th **S90.921 Unspecified superficial injury of right foot**
  - +7th **S90.922 Unspecified superficial injury of left foot**
  - +7th **S90.929 Unspecified superficial injury of unspecified foot**
+ **S90.93 Unspecified superficial injury of toes**
  - +7th **S90.931 Unspecified superficial injury of right great toe**
  - +7th **S90.932 Unspecified superficial injury of left great toe**
  - +7th **S90.933 Unspecified superficial injury of unspecified great toe**
  - +7th **S90.934 Unspecified superficial injury of right lesser toe(s)**
  - +7th **S90.935 Unspecified superficial injury of left lesser toe(s)**
  - +7th **S90.936 Unspecified superficial injury of unspecified lesser toe(s)**

S91 Open wound of ankle, foot and toes

Code also any associated wound infection

Excludes1: *open fracture of ankle, foot and toes (S92.-with 7th character B)*
traumatic amputation of ankle and foot (S98.-)

The appropriate 7th character is to be added to each code from category S91
A initial encounter
D subsequent encounter
S sequela

+ **S91.0 Open wound of ankle**
+ **S91.00 Unspecified open wound of ankle**
  - +7th **S91.001 Unspecified open wound, right ankle**
  - +7th **S91.002 Unspecified open wound, left ankle**
  - +7th **S91.009 Unspecified open wound, unspecified ankle**
+ **S91.01 Laceration without foreign body of ankle**
  - +7th **S91.011 Laceration without foreign body, right ankle**
  - +7th **S91.012 Laceration without foreign body, left ankle**
  - +7th **S91.019 Laceration without foreign body, unspecified ankle**
+ **S91.02 Laceration with foreign body of ankle**
  - +7th **S91.021 Laceration with foreign body, right ankle**
  - +7th **S91.022 Laceration with foreign body, left ankle**
  - +7th **S91.029 Laceration with foreign body, unspecified ankle**
+ **S91.03 Puncture wound without foreign body of ankle**
  - +7th **S91.031 Puncture wound without foreign body, right ankle**
  - +7th **S91.032 Puncture wound without foreign body, left ankle**
  - +7th **S91.039 Puncture wound without foreign body, unspecified ankle**
+ **S91.04 Puncture wound with foreign body of ankle**
  - +7th **S91.041 Puncture wound with foreign body, right ankle**
  - +7th **S91.042 Puncture wound with foreign body, left ankle**
  - +7th **S91.049 Puncture wound with foreign body, unspecified ankle**
+ **S91.05 Open bite of ankle**
  Excludes1: *superficial bite of ankle (S90.56-, S90.57-)*
  - +7th **S91.051 Open bite, right ankle**
  - +7th **S91.052 Open bite, left ankle**
  - +7th **S91.059 Open bite, unspecified ankle**

+ **S91.1 Open wound of toe without damage to nail**
+ **S91.10 Unspecified open wound of toe without damage to nail**
  - +7th **S91.101 Unspecified open wound of right great toe without damage to nail**
  - +7th **S91.102 Unspecified open wound of left great toe without damage to nail**
  - +7th **S91.103 Unspecified open wound of unspecified great toe without damage to nail**
  - +7th **S91.104 Unspecified open wound of right lesser toe(s) without damage to nail**
  - +7th **S91.105 Unspecified open wound of left lesser toe(s) without damage to nail**
  - +7th **S91.106 Unspecified open wound of unspecified lesser toe(s) without damage to nail**
  - +7th **S91.109 Unspecified open wound of unspecified toe(s) without damage to nail**
+ **S91.11 Laceration without foreign body of toe without damage to nail**
  - +7th **S91.111 Laceration without foreign body of right great toe without damage to nail**
  - +7th **S91.112 Laceration without foreign body of left great toe without damage to nail**
  - +7th **S91.113 Laceration without foreign body of unspecified great toe without damage to nail**
  - +7th **S91.114 Laceration without foreign body of right lesser toe(s) without damage to nail**
  - +7th **S91.115 Laceration without foreign body of left lesser toe(s) without damage to nail**
  - +7th **S91.116 Laceration without foreign body of unspecified lesser toe(s) without damage to nail**
  - +7th **S91.119 Laceration without foreign body of unspecified toe without damage to nail**

+ **S91.12** **Laceration with foreign body of toe without damage to nail**
  - +7th **S91.121** **Laceration with foreign body of right great toe without damage to nail**
  - +7th **S91.122** **Laceration with foreign body of left great toe without damage to nail**
  - +7th **S91.123** **Laceration with foreign body of unspecified great toe without damage to nail**
  - +7th **S91.124** **Laceration with foreign body of right lesser toe(s) without damage to nail**
  - +7th **S91.125** **Laceration with foreign body of left lesser toe(s) without damage to nail**
  - +7th **S91.126** **Laceration with foreign body of unspecified lesser toe(s) without damage to nail**
  - +7th **S91.129** **Laceration with foreign body of unspecified toe(s) without damage to nail**

+ **S91.13** **Puncture wound without foreign body of toe without damage to nail**
  - +7th **S91.131** **Puncture wound without foreign body of right great toe without damage to nail**
  - +7th **S91.132** **Puncture wound without foreign body of left great toe without damage to nail**
  - +7th **S91.133** **Puncture wound without foreign body of unspecified great toe without damage to nail**
  - +7th **S91.134** **Puncture wound without foreign body of right lesser toe(s) without damage to nail**
  - +7th **S91.135** **Puncture wound without foreign body of left lesser toe(s) without damage to nail**
  - +7th **S91.136** **Puncture wound without foreign body of unspecified lesser toe(s) without damage to nail**
  - +7th **S91.139** **Puncture wound without foreign body of unspecified toe(s) without damage to nail**

+ **S91.14** **Puncture wound with foreign body of toe without damage to nail**
  - +7th **S91.141** **Puncture wound with foreign body of right great toe without damage to nail**
  - +7th **S91.142** **Puncture wound with foreign body of left great toe without damage to nail**
  - +7th **S91.143** **Puncture wound with foreign body of unspecified great toe without damage to nail**
  - +7th **S91.144** **Puncture wound with foreign body of right lesser toe(s) without damage to nail**
  - +7th **S91.145** **Puncture wound with foreign body of left lesser toe(s) without damage to nail**
  - +7th **S91.146** **Puncture wound with foreign body of unspecified lesser toe(s) without damage to nail**
  - +7th **S91.149** **Puncture wound with foreign body of unspecified toe(s) without damage to nail**

+ **S91.15** **Open bite of toe without damage to nail**
  Bite of toe NOS
  Excludes1: *superficial bite of toe (S90.46-, S90.47-)*
  - +7th **S91.151** **Open bite of right great toe without damage to nail**
  - +7th **S91.152** **Open bite of left great toe without damage to nail**
  - +7th **S91.153** **Open bite of unspecified great toe without damage to nail**
  - +7th **S91.154** **Open bite of right lesser toe(s) without damage to nail**
  - +7th **S91.155** **Open bite of left lesser toe(s) without damage to nail**
  - +7th **S91.156** **Open bite of unspecified lesser toe(s) without damage to nail**
  - +7th **S91.159** **Open bite of unspecified toe(s) without damage to nail**

+ **S91.2** **Open wound of toe with damage to nail**

+ **S91.20** **Unspecified open wound of toe with damage to nail**
  - +7th **S91.201** **Unspecified open wound of right great toe with damage to nail**
  - +7th **S91.202** **Unspecified open wound of left great toe with damage to nail**
  - +7th **S91.203** **Unspecified open wound of unspecified great toe with damage to nail**
  - +7th **S91.204** **Unspecified open wound of right lesser toe(s) with damage to nail**
  - +7th **S91.205** **Unspecified open wound of left lesser toe(with damage to nail**
  - +7th **S91.206** **Unspecified open wound of unspecified lesser toe(s) with damage to nail**
  - +7th **S91.209** **Unspecified open wound of unspecified toe(s) with damage to nail**

+ **S91.21** **Laceration without foreign body of toe with damag to nail**
  - +7th **S91.211** **Laceration without foreign body of right great toe with damage to nail**
  - +7th **S91.212** **Laceration without foreign body of left great toe with damage to nail**
  - +7th **S91.213** **Laceration without foreign body of unspecified great toe with damage to nail**
  - +7th **S91.214** **Laceration without foreign body of right lesser toe(s) with damage to nail**
  - +7th **S91.215** **Laceration without foreign body of left lesser toe(s) with damage to nail**
  - +7th **S91.216** **Laceration without foreign body of unspecified lesser toe(s) with damage to nail**
  - +7th **S91.219** **Laceration without foreign body of unspecified toe(s) with damage to nail**

+ **S91.22** **Laceration with foreign body of toe with damage to nail**
  - +7th **S91.221** **Laceration with foreign body of right gre toe with damage to nail**
  - +7th **S91.222** **Laceration with foreign body of left great toe with damage to nail**
  - +7th **S91.223** **Laceration with foreign body of unspecified great toe with damage to nail**
  - +7th **S91.224** **Laceration with foreign body of right less toe(s) with damage to nail**
  - +7th **S91.225** **Laceration with foreign body of left lesser toe(s) with damage to nail**
  - +7th **S91.226** **Laceration with foreign body of unspecified lesser toe(s) with damage to nail**
  - +7th **S91.229** **Laceration with foreign body of unspecified toe(s) with damage to nail**

+ **S91.23** **Puncture wound without foreign body of toe with damage to nail**
  - +7th **S91.231** **Puncture wound without foreign body of right great toe with damage to nail**
  - +7th **S91.232** **Puncture wound without foreign body of left great toe with damage to nail**
  - +7th **S91.233** **Puncture wound without foreign body of unspecified great toe with damage to nail**
  - +7th **S91.234** **Puncture wound without foreign body of right lesser toe(s) with damage to nail**
  - +7th **S91.235** **Puncture wound without foreign body of left lesser toe(s) with damage to nail**
  - +7th **S91.236** **Puncture wound without foreign body of unspecified lesser toe(s) with damage to nail**
  - +7th **S91.239** **Puncture wound without foreign body of unspecified toe(s) with damage to nail**

+ **S91.24** **Puncture wound with foreign body of toe with damage to nail**
  - +7th **S91.241** **Puncture wound with foreign body of rig great toe with damage to nail**
  - +7th **S91.242** **Puncture wound with foreign body of left great toe with damage to nail**
  - +7th **S91.243** **Puncture wound with foreign body of unspecified great toe with damage to nail**
  - +7th **S91.244** **Puncture wound with foreign body of rig lesser toe(s) with damage to nail**
  - +7th **S91.245** **Puncture wound with foreign body of left lesser toe(s) with damage to nail**
  - +7th **S91.246** **Puncture wound with foreign body of unspecified lesser toe(s) with damage to nail**
  - +7th **S91.249** **Puncture wound with foreign body of unspecified toe(s) with damage to nail**

+ **S91.25** **Open bite of toe with damage to nail**
  Bite of toe with damage to nail NOS
  Excludes1: *superficial bite of toe (S90.46-, S90.47-)*

+7th **S91.251 Open bite of right great toe with damage to nail**
+7th **S91.252 Open bite of left great toe with damage to nail**
+7th **S91.253 Open bite of unspecified great toe with damage to nail**
+7th **S91.254 Open bite of right lesser toe(s) with damage to nail**
+7th **S91.255 Open bite of left lesser toe(s) with damage to nail**
+7th **S91.256 Open bite of unspecified lesser toe(s) with damage to nail**
+7th **S91.259 Open bite of unspecified toe(s) with damage to nail**

\+ **S91.3 Open wound of foot**

\+ **S91.30 Unspecified open wound of foot**
+7th **S91.301 Unspecified open wound, right foot**
+7th **S91.302 Unspecified open wound, left foot**
+7th **S91.309 Unspecified open wound, unspecified foot**

\+ **S91.31 Laceration without foreign body of foot**
+7th **S91.311 Laceration without foreign body, right foot**
+7th **S91.312 Laceration without foreign body, left foot**
+7th **S91.319 Laceration without foreign body, unspecified foot**

\+ **S91.32 Laceration with foreign body of foot**
+7th **S91.321 Laceration with foreign body, right foot**
+7th **S91.322 Laceration with foreign body, left foot**
+7th **S91.329 Laceration with foreign body, unspecified foot**

\+ **S91.33 Puncture wound without foreign body of foot**
+7th **S91.331 Puncture wound without foreign body, right foot**
+7th **S91.332 Puncture wound without foreign body, left foot**
+7th **S91.339 Puncture wound without foreign body, unspecified foot**

\+ **S91.34 Puncture wound with foreign body of foot**
+7th **S91.341 Puncture wound with foreign body, right foot**
+7th **S91.342 Puncture wound with foreign body, left foot**
+7th **S91.349 Puncture wound with foreign body, unspecified foot**

\+ **S91.35 Open bite of foot**
Excludes1: *superficial bite of foot (S90.86-, S90.87-)*
+7th **S91.351 Open bite, right foot**
+7th **S91.352 Open bite, left foot**
+7th **S91.359 Open bite, unspecified foot**

S92 Fracture of foot and toe, except ankle

NOTE A fracture not indicated as displaced or nondisplaced should be coded to displaced
A fracture not indicated as open or closed should be coded to closed

Excludes1: *traumatic amputation of ankle and foot (S98.-)*
Excludes2: *fracture of ankle (S82.-)*
fracture of malleolus (S82.-)

The appropriate 7th character is to be added to each code from category S92
A initial encounter for closed fracture
B initial encounter for open fracture
D subsequent encounter for fracture with routine healing
G subsequent encounter for fracture with delayed healing
K subsequent encounter for fracture with nonunion
P subsequent encounter for fracture with malunion
S sequela

Review coding guideline C.19.c

\+ **S92.0 Fracture of calcaneus**
Heel bone
Os calcis
Excludes2: *Physeal fracture of calcaneus (S99.0-)*

\+ **S92.00 Unspecified fracture of calcaneus**

CC +7th **S92.001 Unspecified fracture of right calcaneus**
CC Exclusion 7th character B see Appendix A PDX collection 1367
CC Exclusion 7th characters K & P see Appendix A PDX collection 0897
HAC 7th character B see Appendix B for HAC conditional logic

CC +7th **S92.002 Unspecified fracture of left calcaneus**
CC Exclusion 7th character B see Appendix A PDX collection 1367
CC Exclusion 7th characters K & P see Appendix A PDX collection 0897
HAC 7th character B see Appendix B for HAC conditional logic

CC +7th **S92.009 Unspecified fracture of unspecified calcaneus**
CC Exclusion 7th character B see Appendix A PDX collection 1367
CC Exclusion 7th characters K & P see Appendix A PDX collection 0897
HAC 7th character B see Appendix B for HAC conditional logic

\+ **S92.01 Fracture of body of calcaneus**

CC +7th **S92.011 Displaced fracture of body of right calcaneus**
CC Exclusion 7th character B see Appendix A PDX collection 1367
CC Exclusion 7th characters K & P see Appendix A PDX collection 0897
HAC 7th character B see Appendix B for HAC conditional logic

CC +7th **S92.012 Displaced fracture of body of left calcaneus**
CC Exclusion 7th character B see Appendix A PDX collection 1367
CC Exclusion 7th characters K & P see Appendix A PDX collection 0897
HAC 7th character B see Appendix B for HAC conditional logic

CC +7th **S92.013 Displaced fracture of body of unspecified calcaneus**
CC Exclusion 7th character B see Appendix A PDX collection 1367
CC Exclusion 7th characters K & P see Appendix A PDX collection 0897
HAC 7th character B see Appendix B for HAC conditional logic

CC +7th **S92.014 Nondisplaced fracture of body of right calcaneus**
CC Exclusion 7th character B see Appendix A PDX collection 1367
CC Exclusion 7th characters K & P see Appendix A PDX collection 0897
HAC 7th character B see Appendix B for HAC conditional logic

CC +7th **S92.015 Nondisplaced fracture of body of left calcaneus**
CC Exclusion 7th character B see Appendix A PDX collection 1367
CC Exclusion 7th characters K & P see Appendix A PDX collection 0897
HAC 7th character B see Appendix B for HAC conditional logic

CC +7th **S92.016 Nondisplaced fracture of body of unspecified calcaneus**
CC Exclusion 7th character B see Appendix A PDX collection 1367
CC Exclusion 7th characters K & P see Appendix A PDX collection 0897
HAC 7th character B see Appendix B for HAC conditional logic

\+ **S92.02 Fracture of anterior process of calcaneus**

CC +7th **S92.021 Displaced fracture of anterior process of right calcaneus**
CC Exclusion 7th character B see Appendix A PDX collection 1367
CC Exclusion 7th characters K & P see Appendix A PDX collection 0897
HAC 7th character B see Appendix B for HAC conditional logic

CC +7th **S92.022 Displaced fracture of anterior process of left calcaneus**
CC Exclusion 7th character B see Appendix A PDX collection 1367
CC Exclusion 7th characters K & P see Appendix A PDX collection 0897
HAC 7th character B see Appendix B for HAC conditional logic

CC +7th **S92.023 Displaced fracture of anterior process of unspecified calcaneus**
CC Exclusion 7th character B see Appendix A PDX collection 1367
CC Exclusion 7th characters K & P see Appendix A PDX collection 0897
HAC 7th character B see Appendix B for HAC conditional logic

CC +7th **S92.024 Nondisplaced fracture of anterior process of right calcaneus**
CC Exclusion 7th character B see Appendix A PDX collection 1367
CC Exclusion 7th characters K & P see Appendix A PDX collection 0897
HAC 7th character B see Appendix B for HAC conditional logic

CC +7th **S92.025 Nondisplaced fracture of anterior process of left calcaneus**
CC Exclusion 7th character B see Appendix A PDX collection 1367
CC Exclusion 7th characters K & P see Appendix A PDX collection 0897
HAC 7th character B see Appendix B for HAC conditional logic

CC +7th **S92.026 Nondisplaced fracture of anterior process of unspecified calcaneus**
CC Exclusion 7th character B see Appendix A PDX collection 1367
CC Exclusion 7th characters K & P see Appendix A PDX collection 0897
HAC 7th character B see Appendix B for HAC conditional logic

\+ **S92.03 Avulsion fracture of tuberosity of calcaneus**

CC +7th **S92.031 Displaced avulsion fracture of tuberosity of right calcaneus**
CC Exclusion 7th character B see Appendix A PDX collection 1367
CC Exclusion 7th characters K & P see Appendix A PDX collection 0897
HAC 7th character B see Appendix B for HAC conditional logic

CC +7th **S92.032 Displaced avulsion fracture of tuberosity of left calcaneus**
CC Exclusion 7th character B see Appendix A PDX collection 1367
CC Exclusion 7th characters K & P see Appendix A PDX collection 0897
HAC 7th character B see Appendix B for HAC conditional logic

CC +7th **S92.033 Displaced avulsion fracture of tuberosity of unspecified calcaneus**
CC Exclusion 7th character B see Appendix A PDX collection 1367
CC Exclusion 7th characters K & P see Appendix A PDX collection 0897
HAC 7th character B see Appendix B for HAC conditional logic

CC +7th **S92.034 Nondisplaced avulsion fracture of tuberosity of right calcaneus**
CC Exclusion 7th character B see Appendix A PDX collection 1367
CC Exclusion 7th characters K & P see Appendix A PDX collection 0897
HAC 7th character B see Appendix B for HAC conditional logic

CC +7th **S92.035 Nondisplaced avulsion fracture of tuberosity of left calcaneus**
CC Exclusion 7th character B see Appendix A PDX collection 1367
CC Exclusion 7th characters K & P see Appendix A PDX collection 0897
HAC 7th character B see Appendix B for HAC conditional logic

CC +7th **S92.036 Nondisplaced avulsion fracture of tuberosity of unspecified calcaneus**
CC Exclusion 7th character B see Appendix A PDX collection 1367
CC Exclusion 7th characters K & P see Appendix A PDX collection 0897
HAC 7th character B see Appendix B for HAC conditional logic

\+ **S92.04 Other fracture of tuberosity of calcaneus**

CC +7th **S92.041 Displaced other fracture of tuberosity of right calcaneus**
CC Exclusion 7th character B see Appendix A PDX collection 1367
CC Exclusion 7th characters K & P see Appendix A PDX collection 0897
HAC 7th character B see Appendix B for HAC conditional logic

CC +7th **S92.042 Displaced other fracture of tuberosity of left calcaneus**
CC Exclusion 7th character B see Appendix A PDX collection 1367
CC Exclusion 7th characters K & P see Appendix A PDX collection 0897
HAC 7th character B see Appendix B for HAC conditional logic

CC +7th **S92.043 Displaced other fracture of tuberosity of unspecified calcaneus**
CC Exclusion 7th character B see Appendix A PDX collection 1367
CC Exclusion 7th characters K & P see Appendix A PDX collection 0897
HAC 7th character B see Appendix B for HAC conditional logic

CC +7th **S92.044 Nondisplaced other fracture of tuberosity of right calcaneus**
CC Exclusion 7th character B see Appendix A PDX collection 1367
CC Exclusion 7th characters K & P see Appendix A PDX collection 0897
HAC 7th character B see Appendix B for HAC conditional logic

CC +7th **S92.045 Nondisplaced other fracture of tuberosity of left calcaneus**
CC Exclusion 7th character B see Appendix A PDX collection 1367
CC Exclusion 7th characters K & P see Appendix A PDX collection 0897
HAC 7th character B see Appendix B for HAC conditional logic

CC +7th **S92.046 Nondisplaced other fracture of tuberosity of unspecified calcaneus**
CC Exclusion 7th character B see Appendix A PDX collection 1367
CC Exclusion 7th characters K & P see Appendix A PDX collection 0897
HAC 7th character B see Appendix B for HAC conditional logic

\+ **S92.05 Other extraarticular fracture of calcaneus**

CC +7th **S92.051 Displaced other extraarticular fracture of right calcaneus**
CC Exclusion 7th character B see Appendix A PDX collection 1367
CC Exclusion 7th characters K & P see Appendix A PDX collection 0897
HAC 7th character B see Appendix B for HAC conditional logic

CC +7th **S92.052 Displaced other extraarticular fracture of left calcaneus**
CC Exclusion 7th character B see Appendix A PDX collection 1367
CC Exclusion 7th characters K & P see Appendix A PDX collection 0897
HAC 7th character B see Appendix B for HAC conditional logic

CC +7th **S92.053 Displaced other extraarticular fracture of unspecified calcaneus**
CC Exclusion 7th character B see Appendix A PDX collection 1367
CC Exclusion 7th characters K & P see Appendix A PDX collection 0897
HAC 7th character B see Appendix B for HAC conditional logic

CC +7th **S92.054 Nondisplaced other extraarticular fracture of right calcaneus**
CC Exclusion 7th character B see Appendix A PDX collection 1367
CC Exclusion 7th characters K & P see Appendix A PDX collection 0897
HAC 7th character B see Appendix B for HAC conditional logic

CC +7th **S92.055** **Nondisplaced other extraarticular fracture of left calcaneus**
CC Exclusion 7th character B see Appendix A PDX collection 1367
CC Exclusion 7th characters K & P see Appendix A PDX collection 0897
HAC 7th character B see Appendix B for HAC conditional logic

CC +7th **S92.056** **Nondisplaced other extraarticular fracture of unspecified calcaneus**
CC Exclusion 7th character B see Appendix A PDX collection 1367
CC Exclusion 7th characters K & P see Appendix A PDX collection 0897
HAC 7th character B see Appendix B for HAC conditional logic

\+ **S92.06** **Intraarticular fracture of calcaneus**

CC +7th **S92.061** **Displaced intraarticular fracture of right calcaneus**
CC Exclusion 7th character B see Appendix A PDX collection 1367
CC Exclusion 7th characters K & P see Appendix A PDX collection 0897
HAC 7th character B see Appendix B for HAC conditional logic

CC +7th **S92.062** **Displaced intraarticular fracture of left calcaneus**
CC Exclusion 7th character B see Appendix A PDX collection 1367
CC Exclusion 7th characters K & P see Appendix A PDX collection 0897
HAC 7th character B see Appendix B for HAC conditional logic

CC +7th **S92.063** **Displaced intraarticular fracture of unspecified calcaneus**
CC Exclusion 7th character B see Appendix A PDX collection 1367
CC Exclusion 7th characters K & P see Appendix A PDX collection 0897
HAC 7th character B see Appendix B for HAC conditional logic

CC +7th **S92.064** **Nondisplaced intraarticular fracture of right calcaneus**
CC Exclusion 7th character B see Appendix A PDX collection 1367
CC Exclusion 7th characters K & P see Appendix A PDX collection 0897
HAC 7th character B see Appendix B for HAC conditional logic

CC +7th **S92.065** **Nondisplaced intraarticular fracture of left calcaneus**
CC Exclusion 7th character B see Appendix A PDX collection 1367
CC Exclusion 7th characters K & P see Appendix A PDX collection 0897
HAC 7th character B see Appendix B for HAC conditional logic

CC +7th **S92.066** **Nondisplaced intraarticular fracture of unspecified calcaneus**
CC Exclusion 7th character B see Appendix A PDX collection 1367
CC Exclusion 7th characters K & P see Appendix A PDX collection 0897
HAC 7th character B see Appendix B for HAC conditional logic

\+ **S92.1** **Fracture of talus**
Astragalus

\+ **S92.10** **Unspecified fracture of talus**

CC +7th **S92.101** **Unspecified fracture of right talus**
CC Exclusion 7th character B see Appendix A PDX collection 1368
CC Exclusion 7th characters K & P see Appendix A PDX collection 0897
HAC 7th character B see Appendix B for HAC conditional logic

CC +7th **S92.102** **Unspecified fracture of left talus**
CC Exclusion 7th character B see Appendix A PDX collection 1368
CC Exclusion 7th characters K & P see Appendix A PDX collection 0897
HAC 7th character B see Appendix B for HAC conditional logic

CC +7th **S92.109** **Unspecified fracture of unspecified talus**
CC Exclusion 7th character B see Appendix A PDX collection 1368
CC Exclusion 7th characters K & P see Appendix A PDX collection 0897
HAC 7th character B see Appendix B for HAC conditional logic

\+ **S92.11** **Fracture of neck of talus**

CC +7th **S92.111** **Displaced fracture of neck of right talus**
CC Exclusion 7th character B see Appendix A PDX collection 1368
CC Exclusion 7th characters K & P see Appendix A PDX collection 0897
HAC 7th character B see Appendix B for HAC conditional logic

CC +7th **S92.112** **Displaced fracture of neck of left talus**
CC Exclusion 7th character B see Appendix A PDX collection 1368
CC Exclusion 7th characters K & P see Appendix A PDX collection 0897

CC +7th **S92.113** **Displaced fracture of neck of unspecified talus**
CC Exclusion 7th character B see Appendix A PDX collection 1368
CC Exclusion 7th characters K & P see Appendix A PDX collection 0897
HAC 7th character B see Appendix B for HAC conditional logic

CC +7th **S92.114** **Nondisplaced fracture of neck of right talus**
CC Exclusion 7th character B see Appendix A PDX collection 1368
CC Exclusion 7th characters K & P see Appendix A PDX collection 0897
HAC 7th character B see Appendix B for HAC conditional logic

CC +7th **S92.115** **Nondisplaced fracture of neck of left talus**
CC Exclusion 7th character B see Appendix A PDX collection 1368
CC Exclusion 7th characters K & P see Appendix A PDX collection 0897
HAC 7th character B see Appendix B for HAC conditional logic

CC +7th **S92.116** **Nondisplaced fracture of neck of unspecified talus**
CC Exclusion 7th character B see Appendix A PDX collection 1368
CC Exclusion 7th characters K & P see Appendix A PDX collection 0897
HAC 7th character B see Appendix B for HAC conditional logic

\+ **S92.12** **Fracture of body of talus**

CC +7th **S92.121** **Displaced fracture of body of right talus**
CC Exclusion 7th character B see Appendix A PDX collection 1368
CC Exclusion 7th characters K & P see Appendix A PDX collection 0897
HAC 7th character B see Appendix B for HAC conditional logic

CC +7th **S92.122** **Displaced fracture of body of left talus**
CC Exclusion 7th character B see Appendix A PDX collection 1368
CC Exclusion 7th characters K & P see Appendix A PDX collection 0897
HAC 7th character B see Appendix B for HAC conditional logic

CC +7th **S92.123** **Displaced fracture of body of unspecified talus**
CC Exclusion 7th character B see Appendix A PDX collection 1368
CC Exclusion 7th characters K & P see Appendix A PDX collection 0897
HAC 7th character B see Appendix B for HAC conditional logic

CC +7th **S92.124** **Nondisplaced fracture of body of right talus**
CC Exclusion 7th character B see Appendix A PDX collection 1368
CC Exclusion 7th characters K & P see Appendix A PDX collection 0897
HAC 7th character B see Appendix B for HAC conditional logic

CC +7th **S92.125 Nondisplaced fracture of body of left talus**
CC Exclusion 7th character B see Appendix A PDX collection 1368
CC Exclusion 7th characters K & P see Appendix A PDX collection 0897
HAC 7th character B see Appendix B for HAC conditional logic

CC +7th **S92.126 Nondisplaced fracture of body of unspecified talus**
CC Exclusion 7th character B see Appendix A PDX collection 1368
CC Exclusion 7th characters K & P see Appendix A PDX collection 0897
HAC 7th character B see Appendix B for HAC conditional logic

\+ **S92.13 Fracture of posterior process of talus**

CC +7th **S92.131 Displaced fracture of posterior process of right talus**
CC Exclusion 7th character B see Appendix A PDX collection 1368
CC Exclusion 7th characters K & P see Appendix A PDX collection 0897
HAC 7th character B see Appendix B for HAC conditional logic

CC +7th **S92.132 Displaced fracture of posterior process of left talus**
CC Exclusion 7th character B see Appendix A PDX collection 1368
CC Exclusion 7th characters K & P see Appendix A PDX collection 0897
HAC 7th character B see Appendix B for HAC conditional logic

CC +7th **S92.133 Displaced fracture of posterior process of unspecified talus**
CC Exclusion 7th character B see Appendix A PDX collection 1368
CC Exclusion 7th characters K & P see Appendix A PDX collection 0897
HAC 7th character B see Appendix B for HAC conditional logic

CC +7th **S92.134 Nondisplaced fracture of posterior process of right talus**
CC Exclusion 7th character B see Appendix A PDX collection 1368
CC Exclusion 7th characters K & P see Appendix A PDX collection 0897
HAC 7th character B see Appendix B for HAC conditional logic

CC +7th **S92.135 Nondisplaced fracture of posterior process of left talus**
CC Exclusion 7th character B see Appendix A PDX collection 1368
CC Exclusion 7th characters K & P see Appendix A PDX collection 0897
HAC 7th character B see Appendix B for HAC conditional logic

CC +7th **S92.136 Nondisplaced fracture of posterior process of unspecified talus**
CC Exclusion 7th character B see Appendix A PDX collection 1368
CC Exclusion 7th characters K & P see Appendix A PDX collection 0897
HAC 7th character B see Appendix B for HAC conditional logic

\+ **S92.14 Dome fracture of talus**
Excludes1: *osteochondritis dissecans (M93.2)*

CC +7th **S92.141 Displaced dome fracture of right talus**
CC Exclusion 7th character B see Appendix A PDX collection 1368
CC Exclusion 7th characters K & P see Appendix A PDX collection 0897
HAC 7th character B see Appendix B for HAC conditional logic

CC +7th **S92.142 Displaced dome fracture of left talus**
CC Exclusion 7th character B see Appendix A PDX collection 1368
CC Exclusion 7th characters K & P see Appendix A PDX collection 0897
HAC 7th character B see Appendix B for HAC conditional logic

CC +7th **S92.143 Displaced dome fracture of unspecified talus**
CC Exclusion 7th character B see Appendix A PDX collection 1368
CC Exclusion 7th characters K & P see Appendix A PDX collection 0897
HAC 7th character B see Appendix B for HAC conditional logic

CC +7th **S92.144 Nondisplaced dome fracture of right talus**
CC Exclusion 7th character B see Appendix A PDX collection 1368
CC Exclusion 7th characters K & P see Appendix A PDX collection 0897
HAC 7th character B see Appendix B for HAC conditional logic

CC +7th **S92.145 Nondisplaced dome fracture of left talus**
CC Exclusion 7th character B see Appendix A PDX collection 1368
CC Exclusion 7th characters K & P see Appendix A PDX collection 0897
HAC 7th character B see Appendix B for HAC conditional logic

CC +7th **S92.146 Nondisplaced dome fracture of unspecified talus**
CC Exclusion 7th character B see Appendix A PDX collection 1368
CC Exclusion 7th characters K & P see Appendix A PDX collection 0897
HAC 7th character B see Appendix B for HAC conditional logic

\+ **S92.15 Avulsion fracture (chip fracture) of talus**

CC +7th **S92.151 Displaced avulsion fracture (chip fracture) of right talus**
CC Exclusion 7th character B see Appendix A PDX collection 1368
CC Exclusion 7th characters K & P see Appendix A PDX collection 0897
HAC 7th character B see Appendix B for HAC conditional logic

CC +7th **S92.152 Displaced avulsion fracture (chip fracture) of left talus**
CC Exclusion 7th character B see Appendix A PDX collection 1368
CC Exclusion 7th characters K & P see Appendix A PDX collection 0897
HAC 7th character B see Appendix B for HAC conditional logic

CC +7th **S92.153 Displaced avulsion fracture (chip fracture) of unspecified talus**
CC Exclusion 7th character B see Appendix A PDX collection 1368
CC Exclusion 7th characters K & P see Appendix A PDX collection 0897
HAC 7th character B see Appendix B for HAC conditional logic

CC +7th **S92.154 Nondisplaced avulsion fracture (chip fracture) of right talus**
CC Exclusion 7th character B see Appendix A PDX collection 1368
CC Exclusion 7th characters K & P see Appendix A PDX collection 0897
HAC 7th character B see Appendix B for HAC conditional logic

CC +7th **S92.155 Nondisplaced avulsion fracture (chip fracture) of left talus**
CC Exclusion 7th character B see Appendix A PDX collection 1368
CC Exclusion 7th characters K & P see Appendix A PDX collection 0897
HAC 7th character B see Appendix B for HAC conditional logic

CC +7th **S92.156 Nondisplaced avulsion fracture (chip fracture) of unspecified talus**
CC Exclusion 7th character B see Appendix A PDX collection 1368
CC Exclusion 7th characters K & P see Appendix A PDX collection 0897
HAC 7th character B see Appendix B for HAC conditional logic

+ S92.19 Other fracture of talus

CC +7th **S92.191** **Other fracture of right talus**
CC Exclusion 7th character B see Appendix A PDX collection 1368
CC Exclusion 7th characters K & P see Appendix A PDX collection 0897
HAC 7th character B see Appendix B for HAC conditional logic

CC +7th **S92.192** **Other fracture of left talus**
CC Exclusion 7th character B see Appendix A PDX collection 1368
CC Exclusion 7th characters K & P see Appendix A PDX collection 0897
HAC 7th character B see Appendix B for HAC conditional logic

CC +7th **S92.199** **Other fracture of unspecified talus**
CC Exclusion 7th character B see Appendix A PDX collection 1368
CC Exclusion 7th characters K & P see Appendix A PDX collection 0897
HAC 7th character B see Appendix B for HAC conditional logic

+ S92.2 Fracture of other and unspecified tarsal bone(s)

+ S92.20 Fracture of unspecified tarsal bone(s)

CC +7th **S92.201** **Fracture of unspecified tarsal bone(s) of right foot**
CC Exclusion 7th character B see Appendix A PDX collection 1369
CC Exclusion 7th characters K & P see Appendix A PDX collection 0897
HAC 7th character B see Appendix B for HAC conditional logic

CC +7th **S92.202** **Fracture of unspecified tarsal bone(s) of left foot**
CC Exclusion 7th character B see Appendix A PDX collection 1369
CC Exclusion 7th characters K & P see Appendix A PDX collection 0897
HAC 7th character B see Appendix B for HAC conditional logic

CC +7th **S92.209** **Fracture of unspecified tarsal bone(s) of unspecified foot**
CC Exclusion 7th character B see Appendix A PDX collection 1369
CC Exclusion 7th characters K & P see Appendix A PDX collection 0897
HAC 7th character B see Appendix B for HAC conditional logic

+ S92.21 Fracture of cuboid bone

CC +7th **S92.211** **Displaced fracture of cuboid bone of right foot**
CC Exclusion 7th character B see Appendix A PDX collection 1368
CC Exclusion 7th characters K & P see Appendix A PDX collection 0897
HAC 7th character B see Appendix B for HAC conditional logic

CC +7th **S92.212** **Displaced fracture of cuboid bone of left foot**
CC Exclusion 7th character B see Appendix A PDX collection 1368
CC Exclusion 7th characters K & P see Appendix A PDX collection 0897
HAC 7th character B see Appendix B for HAC conditional logic

CC +7th **S92.213** **Displaced fracture of cuboid bone of unspecified foot**
CC Exclusion 7th character B see Appendix A PDX collection 1368
CC Exclusion 7th characters K & P see Appendix A PDX collection 0897
HAC 7th character B see Appendix B for HAC conditional logic

CC +7th **S92.214** **Nondisplaced fracture of cuboid bone of right foot**
CC Exclusion 7th character B see Appendix A PDX collection 1368
CC Exclusion 7th characters K & P see Appendix A PDX collection 0897
HAC 7th character B see Appendix B for HAC conditional logic

CC +7th **S92.215** **Nondisplaced fracture of cuboid bone of left foot**
CC Exclusion 7th character B see Appendix A PDX collection 1368
CC Exclusion 7th characters K & P see Appendix A PDX collection 0897
HAC 7th character B see Appendix B for HAC conditional logic

CC +7th **S92.216** **Nondisplaced fracture of cuboid bone of unspecified foot**
CC Exclusion 7th character B see Appendix A PDX collection 1368
CC Exclusion 7th characters K & P see Appendix A PDX collection 0897
HAC 7th character B see Appendix B for HAC conditional logic

+ S92.22 Fracture of lateral cuneiform

CC +7th **S92.221** **Displaced fracture of lateral cuneiform of right foot**
CC Exclusion 7th character B see Appendix A PDX collection 1368
CC Exclusion 7th characters K & P see Appendix A PDX collection 0897
HAC 7th character B see Appendix B for HAC conditional logic

CC +7th **S92.222** **Displaced fracture of lateral cuneiform of left foot**
CC Exclusion 7th character B see Appendix A PDX collection 1368
CC Exclusion 7th characters K & P see Appendix A PDX collection 0897
HAC 7th character B see Appendix B for HAC conditional logic

CC +7th **S92.223** **Displaced fracture of lateral cuneiform of unspecified foot**
CC Exclusion 7th character B see Appendix A PDX collection 1368
CC Exclusion 7th characters K & P see Appendix A PDX collection 0897
HAC 7th character B see Appendix B for HAC conditional logic

CC +7th **S92.224** **Nondisplaced fracture of lateral cuneiform of right foot**
CC Exclusion 7th character B see Appendix A PDX collection 1368
CC Exclusion 7th characters K & P see Appendix A PDX collection 0897
HAC 7th character B see Appendix B for HAC conditional logic

CC +7th **S92.225** **Nondisplaced fracture of lateral cuneiform of left foot**
CC Exclusion 7th character B see Appendix A PDX collection 1368
CC Exclusion 7th characters K & P see Appendix A PDX collection 0897
HAC 7th character B see Appendix B for HAC conditional logic

CC +7th **S92.226** **Nondisplaced fracture of lateral cuneiform of unspecified foot**
CC Exclusion 7th character B see Appendix A PDX collection 1368
CC Exclusion 7th characters K & P see Appendix A PDX collection 0897
HAC 7th character B see Appendix B for HAC conditional logic

+ S92.23 Fracture of intermediate cuneiform

CC +7th **S92.231** **Displaced fracture of intermediate cuneiform of right foot**
CC Exclusion 7th character B see Appendix A PDX collection 1368
CC Exclusion 7th characters K & P see Appendix A PDX collection 0897
HAC 7th character B see Appendix B for HAC conditional logic

CC +7th **S92.232** **Displaced fracture of intermediate cuneiform of left foot**
CC Exclusion 7th character B see Appendix A PDX collection 1368
CC Exclusion 7th characters K & P see Appendix A PDX collection 0897
HAC 7th character B see Appendix B for HAC conditional logic

CC +7th **S92.233 Displaced fracture of intermediate cuneiform of unspecified foot**
CC Exclusion 7th character B see Appendix A PDX collection 1368
CC Exclusion 7th characters K & P see Appendix A PDX collection 0897
HAC 7th character B see Appendix B for HAC conditional logic

CC +7th **S92.234 Nondisplaced fracture of intermediate cuneiform of right foot**
CC Exclusion 7th character B see Appendix A PDX collection 1368
CC Exclusion 7th characters K & P see Appendix A PDX collection 0897
HAC 7th character B see Appendix B for HAC conditional logic

CC +7th **S92.235 Nondisplaced fracture of intermediate cuneiform of left foot**
CC Exclusion 7th character B see Appendix A PDX collection 1368
CC Exclusion 7th characters K & P see Appendix A PDX collection 0897
HAC 7th character B see Appendix B for HAC conditional logic

CC +7th **S92.236 Nondisplaced fracture of intermediate cuneiform of unspecified foot**
CC Exclusion 7th character B see Appendix A PDX collection 1368
CC Exclusion 7th characters K & P see Appendix A PDX collection 0897
HAC 7th character B see Appendix B for HAC conditional logic

\+ **S92.24 Fracture of medial cuneiform**

CC +7th **S92.241 Displaced fracture of medial cuneiform of right foot**
CC Exclusion 7th character B see Appendix A PDX collection 1368
CC Exclusion 7th characters K & P see Appendix A PDX collection 0897
HAC 7th character B see Appendix B for HAC conditional logic

CC +7th **S92.242 Displaced fracture of medial cuneiform of left foot**
CC Exclusion 7th character B see Appendix A PDX collection 1368
CC Exclusion 7th characters K & P see Appendix A PDX collection 0897
HAC 7th character B see Appendix B for HAC conditional logic

CC +7th **S92.243 Displaced fracture of medial cuneiform of unspecified foot**
CC Exclusion 7th character B see Appendix A PDX collection 1368
CC Exclusion 7th characters K & P see Appendix A PDX collection 0897
HAC 7th character B see Appendix B for HAC conditional logic

CC +7th **S92.244 Nondisplaced fracture of medial cuneiform of right foot**
CC Exclusion 7th character B see Appendix A PDX collection 1368
CC Exclusion 7th characters K & P see Appendix A PDX collection 0897
HAC 7th character B see Appendix B for HAC conditional logic

CC +7th **S92.245 Nondisplaced fracture of medial cuneiform of left foot**
CC Exclusion 7th character B see Appendix A PDX collection 1368
CC Exclusion 7th characters K & P see Appendix A PDX collection 0897
HAC 7th character B see Appendix B for HAC conditional logic

CC +7th **S92.246 Nondisplaced fracture of medial cuneiform of unspecified foot**
CC Exclusion 7th character B see Appendix A PDX collection 1368
CC Exclusion 7th characters K & P see Appendix A PDX collection 0897
HAC 7th character B see Appendix B for HAC conditional logic

\+ **S92.25 Fracture of navicular [scaphoid] of foot**

CC +7th **S92.251 Displaced fracture of navicular [scaphoid] of right foot**
CC Exclusion 7th character B see Appendix A PDX collection 1368
CC Exclusion 7th characters K & P see Appendix A PDX collection 0897
HAC 7th character B see Appendix B for HAC conditional logic

CC +7th **S92.252 Displaced fracture of navicular [scaphoid] of left foot**
CC Exclusion 7th character B see Appendix A PDX collection 1368
CC Exclusion 7th characters K & P see Appendix A PDX collection 0897
HAC 7th character B see Appendix B for HAC conditional logic

CC +7th **S92.253 Displaced fracture of navicular [scaphoid] of unspecified foot**
CC Exclusion 7th character B see Appendix A PDX collection 1368
CC Exclusion 7th characters K & P see Appendix A PDX collection 0897
HAC 7th character B see Appendix B for HAC conditional logic

CC +7th **S92.254 Nondisplaced fracture of navicular [scaphoid] of right foot**
CC Exclusion 7th character B see Appendix A PDX collection 1368
CC Exclusion 7th characters K & P see Appendix A PDX collection 0897
HAC 7th character B see Appendix B for HAC conditional logic

CC +7th **S92.255 Nondisplaced fracture of navicular [scaphoid] of left foot**
CC Exclusion 7th character B see Appendix A PDX collection 1368
CC Exclusion 7th characters K & P see Appendix A PDX collection 0897
HAC 7th character B see Appendix B for HAC conditional logic

CC +7th **S92.256 Nondisplaced fracture of navicular [scaphoid] of unspecified foot**
CC Exclusion 7th character B see Appendix A PDX collection 1368
CC Exclusion 7th characters K & P see Appendix A PDX collection 0897
HAC 7th character B see Appendix B for HAC conditional logic

\+ **S92.3 Fracture of metatarsal bone(s)**
Excludes2: *Physeal fracture of metatarsal (S99.1-)*

\+ **S92.30 Fracture of unspecified metatarsal bone(s)**

CC +7th **S92.301 Fracture of unspecified metatarsal bone(s right foot**
CC Exclusion 7th character B see Appendix A PDX collection 1368
CC Exclusion 7th characters K & P see Appendix A PDX collection 0897
HAC 7th character B see Appendix B for HAC conditional logic

CC +7th **S92.302 Fracture of unspecified metatarsal bone(s left foot**
CC Exclusion 7th character B see Appendix A PDX collection 1368
CC Exclusion 7th characters K & P see Appendix A PDX collection 0897
HAC 7th character B see Appendix B for HAC conditional logic

CC +7th **S92.309 Fracture of unspecified metatarsal bone(s unspecified foot**
CC Exclusion 7th character B see Appendix A PDX collection 1368
CC Exclusion 7th characters K & P see Appendix A PDX collection 0897

\+ **S92.31 Fracture of first metatarsal bone**

CC +7th **S92.311 Displaced fracture of first metatarsal bon right foot**
CC Exclusion 7th character B see Appendix A PDX collection 1368
CC Exclusion 7th characters K & P see Appendix A PDX collection 0897
HAC 7th character B see Appendix B for HAC conditional logic

CC +7th **S92.312 Displaced fracture of first metatarsal bone, left foot**
CC Exclusion 7th character B see Appendix A PDX collection 1368
CC Exclusion 7th characters K & P see Appendix A PDX collection 0897
HAC 7th character B see Appendix B for HAC conditional logic

CC +7th **S92.313 Displaced fracture of first metatarsal bone, unspecified foot**
CC Exclusion 7th character B see Appendix A PDX collection 1368
CC Exclusion 7th characters K & P see Appendix A PDX collection 0897
HAC 7th character B see Appendix B for HAC conditional logic

CC +7th **S92.314 Nondisplaced fracture of first metatarsal bone, right foot**
CC Exclusion 7th character B see Appendix A PDX collection 1368
CC Exclusion 7th characters K & P see Appendix A PDX collection 0897
HAC 7th character B see Appendix B for HAC conditional logic

CC +7th **S92.315 Nondisplaced fracture of first metatarsal bone, left foot**
CC Exclusion 7th character B see Appendix A PDX collection 1368
CC Exclusion 7th characters K & P see Appendix A PDX collection 0897
HAC 7th character B see Appendix B for HAC conditional logic

CC +7th **S92.316 Nondisplaced fracture of first metatarsal bone, unspecified foot**
CC Exclusion 7th character B see Appendix A PDX collection 1368
CC Exclusion 7th characters K & P see Appendix A PDX collection 0897
HAC 7th character B see Appendix B for HAC conditional logic

+ **S92.32 Fracture of second metatarsal bone**

CC +7th **S92.321 Displaced fracture of second metatarsal bone, right foot**
CC Exclusion 7th character B see Appendix A PDX collection 1368
CC Exclusion 7th characters K & P see Appendix A PDX collection 0897
HAC 7th character B see Appendix B for HAC conditional logic

CC +7th **S92.322 Displaced fracture of second metatarsal bone, left foot**
CC Exclusion 7th character B see Appendix A PDX collection 1368
CC Exclusion 7th characters K & P see Appendix A PDX collection 0897
HAC 7th character B see Appendix B for HAC conditional logic

CC +7th **S92.323 Displaced fracture of second metatarsal bone, unspecified foot**
CC Exclusion 7th character B see Appendix A PDX collection 1368
CC Exclusion 7th characters K & P see Appendix A PDX collection 0897
HAC 7th character B see Appendix B for HAC conditional logic

CC +7th **S92.324 Nondisplaced fracture of second metatarsal bone, right foot**
CC Exclusion 7th character B see Appendix A PDX collection 1368
CC Exclusion 7th characters K & P see Appendix A PDX collection 0897
HAC 7th character B see Appendix B for HAC conditional logic

CC +7th **S92.325 Nondisplaced fracture of second metatarsal bone, left foot**
CC Exclusion 7th character B see Appendix A PDX collection 1368
CC Exclusion 7th characters K & P see Appendix A PDX collection 0897
HAC 7th character B see Appendix B for HAC conditional logic

CC +7th **S92.326 Nondisplaced fracture of second metatarsal bone, unspecified foot**
CC Exclusion 7th character B see Appendix A PDX collection 1368
CC Exclusion 7th characters K & P see Appendix A PDX collection 0897
HAC 7th character B see Appendix B for HAC conditional logic

+ **S92.33 Fracture of third metatarsal bone**

CC +7th **S92.331 Displaced fracture of third metatarsal bone, right foot**
CC Exclusion 7th character B see Appendix A PDX collection 1368
CC Exclusion 7th characters K & P see Appendix A PDX collection 0897
HAC 7th character B see Appendix B for HAC conditional logic

CC +7th **S92.332 Displaced fracture of third metatarsal bone, left foot**
CC Exclusion 7th character B see Appendix A PDX collection 1368
CC Exclusion 7th characters K & P see Appendix A PDX collection 0897
HAC 7th character B see Appendix B for HAC conditional logic

CC +7th **S92.333 Displaced fracture of third metatarsal bone, unspecified foot**
CC Exclusion 7th character B see Appendix A PDX collection 1368
CC Exclusion 7th characters K & P see Appendix A PDX collection 0897
HAC 7th character B see Appendix B for HAC conditional logic

CC +7th **S92.334 Nondisplaced fracture of third metatarsal bone, right foot**
CC Exclusion 7th character B see Appendix A PDX collection 1368
CC Exclusion 7th characters K & P see Appendix A PDX collection 0897
HAC 7th character B see Appendix B for HAC conditional logic

CC +7th **S92.335 Nondisplaced fracture of third metatarsal bone, left foot**
CC Exclusion 7th character B see Appendix A PDX collection 1368
CC Exclusion 7th characters K & P see Appendix A PDX collection 0897
HAC 7th character B see Appendix B for HAC conditional logic

CC +7th **S92.336 Nondisplaced fracture of third metatarsal bone, unspecified foot**
CC Exclusion 7th character B see Appendix A PDX collection 1368
CC Exclusion 7th characters K & P see Appendix A PDX collection 0897
HAC 7th character B see Appendix B for HAC conditional logic

+ **S92.34 Fracture of fourth metatarsal bone**

CC +7th **S92.341 Displaced fracture of fourth metatarsal bone, right foot**
CC Exclusion 7th character B see Appendix A PDX collection 1368
CC Exclusion 7th characters K & P see Appendix A PDX collection 0897
HAC 7th character B see Appendix B for HAC conditional logic

CC +7th **S92.342 Displaced fracture of fourth metatarsal bone, left foot**
CC Exclusion 7th character B see Appendix A PDX collection 1368
CC Exclusion 7th characters K & P see Appendix A PDX collection 0897
HAC 7th character B see Appendix B for HAC conditional logic

CC +7th **S92.343 Displaced fracture of fourth metatarsal bone, unspecified foot**
CC Exclusion 7th character B see Appendix A PDX collection 1368
CC Exclusion 7th characters K & P see Appendix A PDX collection 0897
HAC 7th character B see Appendix B for HAC conditional logic

CC +7th **S92.344 Nondisplaced fracture of fourth metatarsal bone, right foot**
CC Exclusion 7th character B see Appendix A PDX collection 1368
CC Exclusion 7th characters K & P see Appendix A PDX collection 0897
HAC 7th character B see Appendix B for HAC conditional logic

CC +7th **S92.345 Nondisplaced fracture of fourth metatarsal bone, left foot**
CC Exclusion 7th character B see Appendix A PDX collection 1368
CC Exclusion 7th characters K & P see Appendix A PDX collection 0897
HAC 7th character B see Appendix B for HAC conditional logic

CC +7th **S92.346 Nondisplaced fracture of fourth metatarsal bone, unspecified foot**
CC Exclusion 7th character B see Appendix A PDX collection 1368
CC Exclusion 7th characters K & P see Appendix A PDX collection 0897
HAC 7th character B see Appendix B for HAC conditional logic

\+ **S92.35 Fracture of fifth metatarsal bone**

CC +7th **S92.351 Displaced fracture of fifth metatarsal bone, right foot**
CC Exclusion 7th character B see Appendix A PDX collection 1368
CC Exclusion 7th characters K & P see Appendix A PDX collection 0897
HAC 7th character B see Appendix B for HAC conditional logic

CC +7th **S92.352 Displaced fracture of fifth metatarsal bone, left foot**
CC Exclusion 7th character B see Appendix A PDX collection 1368
CC Exclusion 7th characters K & P see Appendix A PDX collection 0897
HAC 7th character B see Appendix B for HAC conditional logic

CC +7th **S92.353 Displaced fracture of fifth metatarsal bone, unspecified foot**
CC Exclusion 7th character B see Appendix A PDX collection 1368
CC Exclusion 7th characters K & P see Appendix A PDX collection 0897
HAC 7th character B see Appendix B for HAC conditional logic

CC +7th **S92.354 Nondisplaced fracture of fifth metatarsal bone, right foot**
CC Exclusion 7th character B see Appendix A PDX collection 1368
CC Exclusion 7th characters K & P see Appendix A PDX collection 0897
HAC 7th character B see Appendix B for HAC conditional logic

CC +7th **S92.355 Nondisplaced fracture of fifth metatarsal bone, left foot**
CC Exclusion 7th character B see Appendix A PDX collection 1368
CC Exclusion 7th characters K & P see Appendix A PDX collection 0897
HAC 7th character B see Appendix B for HAC conditional logic

CC +7th **S92.356 Nondisplaced fracture of fifth metatarsal bone, unspecified foot**
CC Exclusion 7th character B see Appendix A PDX collection 1368
CC Exclusion 7th characters K & P see Appendix A PDX collection 0897
HAC 7th character B see Appendix B for HAC conditional logic

\+ **S92.4 Fracture of great toe**
Excludes2: *Physeal fracture of phalanx of toe (S99.2-)*

\+ **S92.40 Unspecified fracture of great toe**

CC +7th **S92.401 Displaced unspecified fracture of right great toe**
CC Exclusion 7th characters K & P see Appendix A PDX collection 0897

CC +7th **S92.402 Displaced unspecified fracture of left great toe**
CC Exclusion 7th characters K & P see Appendix A PDX collection 0897

CC +7th **S92.403 Displaced unspecified fracture of unspecified great toe**
CC Exclusion 7th characters K & P see Appendix A PDX collection 0897

CC +7th **S92.404 Nondisplaced unspecified fracture of rig great toe**
CC Exclusion 7th characters K & P see Appendix A PDX collection 0897

CC +7th **S92.405 Nondisplaced unspecified fracture of left great toe**
CC Exclusion 7th characters K & P see Appendix A PDX collection 0897

CC +7th **S92.406 Nondisplaced unspecified fracture of unspecified great toe**
CC Exclusion 7th characters K & P see Appendix A PDX collection 0897

\+ **S92.41 Fracture of proximal phalanx of great toe**

CC +7th **S92.411 Displaced fracture of proximal phalanx right great toe**
CC Exclusion 7th characters K & P see Appendix A PDX collection 0897

CC +7th **S92.412 Displaced fracture of proximal phalanx left great toe**
CC Exclusion 7th characters K & P see Appendix A PDX collection 0897

CC +7th **S92.413 Displaced fracture of proximal phalanx unspecified great toe**
CC Exclusion 7th characters K & P see Appendix A PDX collection 0897

CC +7th **S92.414 Nondisplaced fracture of proximal phala of right great toe**
CC Exclusion 7th characters K & P see Appendix A PDX collection 0897

CC +7th **S92.415 Nondisplaced fracture of proximal phala of left great toe**
CC Exclusion 7th characters K & P see Appendix A PDX collection 0897

CC +7th **S92.416 Nondisplaced fracture of proximal phala of unspecified great toe**
CC Exclusion 7th characters K & P see Appendix A PDX collection 0897

\+ **S92.42 Fracture of distal phalanx of great toe**

CC +7th **S92.421 Displaced fracture of distal phalanx of right great toe**
CC Exclusion 7th characters K & P see Appendix A PDX collection 0897

CC +7th **S92.422 Displaced fracture of distal phalanx of l great toe**
CC Exclusion 7th characters K & P see Appendix A PDX collection 0897

CC +7th **S92.423 Displaced fracture of distal phalanx of unspecified great toe**
CC Exclusion 7th characters K & P see Appendix A PDX collection 0897

CC +7th **S92.424 Nondisplaced fracture of distal phalanx right great toe**
CC Exclusion 7th characters K & P see Appendix A PDX collection 0897

CC +7th **S92.425 Nondisplaced fracture of distal phalanx left great toe**
CC Exclusion 7th characters K & P see Appendix A PDX collection 0897

CC +7th **S92.426 Nondisplaced fracture of distal phalanx unspecified great toe**
CC Exclusion 7th characters K & P see Appendix A PDX collection 0897

\+ **S92.49 Other fracture of great toe**

CC +7th **S92.491 Other fracture of right great toe**
CC Exclusion 7th characters K & P see Appendix A PDX collection 0897

CC +7th **S92.492 Other fracture of left great toe**
CC Exclusion 7th characters K & P see Appendix A PDX collection 0897

CC +7th **S92.499 Other fracture of unspecified great toe**
CC Exclusion 7th characters K & P see Appendix A PDX collection 0897

\+ **S92.5 Fracture of lesser toe(s)**
Excludes2: *Physeal fracture of phalanx of toe (S99.2-)*

\+ **S92.50 Unspecified fracture of lesser toe(s)**

CC +7th **S92.501 Displaced unspecified fracture of right lesser toe(s)**
CC Exclusion 7th characters K & P see Appendix A PDX collection 0897

CC +7th **S92.502 Displaced unspecified fracture of left lesser toe(s)**
CC Exclusion 7th characters K & P see Appendix A PDX collection 0897

CC +7th **S92.503 Displaced unspecified fracture of unspecified lesser toe(s)**
CC Exclusion 7th characters K & P see Appendix A PDX collection 0897

CC +7th **S92.504 Nondisplaced unspecified fracture of right lesser toe(s)**
CC Exclusion 7th characters K & P see Appendix A PDX collection 0897

CC +7th **S92.505 Nondisplaced unspecified fracture of left lesser toe(s)**
CC Exclusion 7th characters K & P see Appendix A PDX collection 0897

CC +7th **S92.506 Nondisplaced unspecified fracture of unspecified lesser toe(s)**
CC Exclusion 7th characters K & P see Appendix A PDX collection 0897

\+ **S92.51 Fracture of proximal phalanx of lesser toe(s)**

CC +7th **S92.511 Displaced fracture of proximal phalanx of right lesser toe(s)**
CC Exclusion 7th characters K & P see Appendix A PDX collection 0897

CC +7th **S92.512 Displaced fracture of proximal phalanx of left lesser toe(s)**
CC Exclusion 7th characters K & P see Appendix A PDX collection 0897

CC +7th **S92.513 Displaced fracture of proximal phalanx of unspecified lesser toe(s)**
CC Exclusion 7th characters K & P see Appendix A PDX collection 0897

CC +7th **S92.514 Nondisplaced fracture of proximal phalanx of right lesser toe(s)**
CC Exclusion 7th characters K & P see Appendix A PDX collection 0897

CC +7th **S92.515 Nondisplaced fracture of proximal phalanx of left lesser toe(s)**
CC Exclusion 7th characters K & P see Appendix A PDX collection 0897

CC +7th **S92.516 Nondisplaced fracture of proximal phalanx of unspecified lesser toe(s)**
CC Exclusion 7th characters K & P see Appendix A PDX collection 0897

\+ **S92.52 Fracture of middle phalanx of lesser toe(s)**

CC +7th **S92.521 Displaced fracture of middle phalanx of right lesser toe(s)**
CC Exclusion 7th characters K & P see Appendix A PDX collection 0897

CC +7th **S92.522 Displaced fracture of middle phalanx of left lesser toe(s)**
CC Exclusion 7th characters K & P see Appendix A PDX collection 0897

CC +7th **S92.523 Displaced fracture of middle phalanx of unspecified lesser toe(s)**
CC Exclusion 7th characters K & P see Appendix A PDX collection 0897

CC +7th **S92.524 Nondisplaced fracture of middle phalanx of right lesser toe(s)**
CC Exclusion 7th characters K & P see Appendix A PDX collection 0897

CC +7th **S92.525 Nondisplaced fracture of middle phalanx of left lesser toe(s)**
CC Exclusion 7th characters K & P see Appendix A PDX collection 0897

CC +7th **S92.526 Nondisplaced fracture of middle phalanx of unspecified lesser toe(s)**
CC Exclusion 7th characters K & P see Appendix A PDX collection 0897

\+ **S92.53 Fracture of distal phalanx of lesser toe(s)**

CC +7th **S92.531 Displaced fracture of distal phalanx of right lesser toe(s)**
CC Exclusion 7th characters K & P see Appendix A PDX collection 0897

CC +7th **S92.532 Displaced fracture of distal phalanx of left lesser toe(s)**
CC Exclusion 7th characters K & P see Appendix A PDX collection 0897

CC +7th **S92.533 Displaced fracture of distal phalanx of unspecified lesser toe(s)**
CC Exclusion 7th characters K & P see Appendix A PDX collection 0897

CC +7th **S92.534 Nondisplaced fracture of distal phalanx of right lesser toe(s)**
CC Exclusion 7th characters K & P see Appendix A PDX collection 0897

CC +7th **S92.535 Nondisplaced fracture of distal phalanx of left lesser toe(s)**
CC Exclusion 7th characters K & P see Appendix A PDX collection 0897

CC +7th **S92.536 Nondisplaced fracture of distal phalanx of unspecified lesser toe(s)**
CC Exclusion 7th characters K & P see Appendix A PDX collection 0897

\+ **S92.59 Other fracture of lesser toe(s)**

CC +7th **S92.591 Other fracture of right lesser toe(s)**
CC Exclusion 7th characters K & P see Appendix A PDX collection 0897

CC +7th **S92.592 Other fracture of left lesser toe(s)**
CC Exclusion 7th characters K & P see Appendix A PDX collection 0897

CC +7th **S92.599 Other fracture of unspecified lesser toe(s)**
CC Exclusion 7th characters K & P see Appendix A PDX collection 0897
Add the following new codes after S92.599.

\+ **S92.8 Other fracture of foot, except ankle**

\+ **S92.81 Other fracture of foot**
Sesamoid fracture of foot
AHA CC: 4Q, 2016, 68

CC +7th **S92.811 Other fracture of right foot**
CC Exclusion 7th character B see Appendix A PDX collection 1369
CC Exclusion 7th characters K & P see Appendix A PDX collection 0897
HAC 7th character B see Appendix B for HAC conditional logic

CC +7th **S92.812 Other fracture of left foot**
CC Exclusion 7th character B see Appendix A PDX collection 1369
CC Exclusion 7th characters K & P see Appendix A PDX collection 0897
HAC 7th character B see Appendix B for HAC conditional logic

CC +7th **S92.819 Other fracture of unspecified foot**
CC Exclusion 7th character B see Appendix A PDX collection 1369
CC Exclusion 7th characters K & P see Appendix A PDX collection 0897
HAC 7th character B see Appendix B for HAC conditional logic

\+ **S92.9 Unspecified fracture of foot and toe**

\+ **S92.90 Unspecified fracture of foot**

CC +7th **S92.901 Unspecified fracture of right foot**
CC Exclusion 7th character B see Appendix A PDX collection 1369
CC Exclusion 7th characters K & P see Appendix A PDX collection 0897
HAC 7th character B see Appendix B for HAC conditional logic

CC +7th **S92.902 Unspecified fracture of left foot**
CC Exclusion 7th character B see Appendix A PDX collection 1369
CC Exclusion 7th characters K & P see Appendix A PDX collection 0897
HAC 7th character B see Appendix B for HAC conditional logic

CC +7th **S92.909 Unspecified fracture of unspecified foot**
CC Exclusion 7th character B see Appendix A PDX collection 1369
CC Exclusion 7th characters K & P see Appendix A PDX collection 0897
HAC 7th character B see Appendix B for HAC conditional logic

\+ **S92.91 Unspecified fracture of toe**

CC +7th **S92.911 Unspecified fracture of right toe(s)**
CC Exclusion 7th characters K & P see Appendix A PDX collection 0897

CC +7th **S92.912 Unspecified fracture of left toe(s)**
CC Exclusion 7th characters K & P see Appendix A PDX collection 0897

CC +7th **S92.919 Unspecified fracture of unspecified toe(s)**
CC Exclusion 7th characters K & P see Appendix A PDX collection 0897

S93 Dislocation and sprain of joints and ligaments at ankle, foot and toe level

Includes: avulsion of joint or ligament of ankle, foot and toe
laceration of cartilage, joint or ligament of ankle, foot and toe
sprain of cartilage, joint or ligament of ankle, foot and toe
traumatic hemarthrosis of joint or ligament of ankle, foot and toe
traumatic rupture of joint or ligament of ankle, foot and toe
traumatic subluxation of joint or ligament of ankle, foot and toe
traumatic tear of joint or ligament of ankle, foot and toe

Code also any associated open wound

Excludes2: *strain of muscle and tendon of ankle and foot (S96.-)*

The appropriate 7th character is to be added to each code from category S93
A initial encounter
D subsequent encounter
S sequela

+ **S93.0 Subluxation and dislocation of ankle joint**
  Subluxation and dislocation of astragalus
  Subluxation and dislocation of fibula, lower end
  Subluxation and dislocation of talus
  Subluxation and dislocation of tibia, lower end
  - X+7th **S93.01 Subluxation of right ankle joint**
  - X+7th **S93.02 Subluxation of left ankle joint**
  - X+7th **S93.03 Subluxation of unspecified ankle joint**
  - X+7th **S93.04 Dislocation of right ankle joint**
  - X+7th **S93.05 Dislocation of left ankle joint**
  - X+7th **S93.06 Dislocation of unspecified ankle joint**

+ **S93.1 Subluxation and dislocation of toe**
  + **S93.10 Unspecified subluxation and dislocation of toe**
    Dislocation of toe NOS
    Subluxation of toe NOS
    - +7th **S93.101 Unspecified subluxation of right toe(s)**
    - +7th **S93.102 Unspecified subluxation of left toe(s)**
    - +7th **S93.103 Unspecified subluxation of unspecified toe(s)**
    - +7th **S93.104 Unspecified dislocation of right toe(s)**
    - +7th **S93.105 Unspecified dislocation of left toe(s)**
    - +7th **S93.106 Unspecified dislocation of unspecified toe(s)**
  + **S93.11 Dislocation of interphalangeal joint**
    - +7th **S93.111 Dislocation of interphalangeal joint of right great toe**
    - +7th **S93.112 Dislocation of interphalangeal joint of left great toe**
    - +7th **S93.113 Dislocation of interphalangeal joint of unspecified great toe**
    - +7th **S93.114 Dislocation of interphalangeal joint of right lesser toe(s)**
    - +7th **S93.115 Dislocation of interphalangeal joint of left lesser toe(s)**
    - +7th **S93.116 Dislocation of interphalangeal joint of unspecified lesser toe(s)**
    - +7th **S93.119 Dislocation of interphalangeal joint of unspecified toe(s)**
  + **S93.12 Dislocation of metatarsophalangeal joint**
    - +7th **S93.121 Dislocation of metatarsophalangeal joint of right great toe**
    - +7th **S93.122 Dislocation of metatarsophalangeal joint of left great toe**
    - +7th **S93.123 Dislocation of metatarsophalangeal joint of unspecified great toe**
    - +7th **S93.124 Dislocation of metatarsophalangeal joint of right lesser toe(s)**
    - +7th **S93.125 Dislocation of metatarsophalangeal joint of left lesser toe(s)**
    - +7th **S93.126 Dislocation of metatarsophalangeal joint of unspecified lesser toe(s)**
    - +7th **S93.129 Dislocation of metatarsophalangeal joint of unspecified toe(s)**
  + **S93.13 Subluxation of interphalangeal joint**
    - +7th **S93.131 Subluxation of interphalangeal joint of right great toe**
    - +7th **S93.132 Subluxation of interphalangeal joint of left great toe**
    - +7th **S93.133 Subluxation of interphalangeal joint of unspecified great toe**
    - +7th **S93.134 Subluxation of interphalangeal joint of right lesser toe(s)**
    - +7th **S93.135 Subluxation of interphalangeal joint of left lesser toe(s)**
    - +7th **S93.136 Subluxation of interphalangeal joint of unspecified lesser toe(s)**
    - +7th **S93.139 Subluxation of interphalangeal joint of unspecified toe(s)**
  + **S93.14 Subluxation of metatarsophalangeal joint**
    - +7th **S93.141 Subluxation of metatarsophalangeal joint of right great toe**
    - +7th **S93.142 Subluxation of metatarsophalangeal joint of left great toe**
    - +7th **S93.143 Subluxation of metatarsophalangeal joint of unspecified great toe**
    - +7th **S93.144 Subluxation of metatarsophalangeal joint of right lesser toe(s)**
    - +7th **S93.145 Subluxation of metatarsophalangeal joint of left lesser toe(s)**
    - +7th **S93.146 Subluxation of metatarsophalangeal joint of unspecified lesser toe(s)**
    - +7th **S93.149 Subluxation of metatarsophalangeal joint of unspecified toe(s)**

+ **S93.3 Subluxation and dislocation of foot**
  Excludes2: *dislocation of toe (S93.1-)*
  + **S93.30 Unspecified subluxation and dislocation of foot**
    Dislocation of foot NOS
    Subluxation of foot NOS
    - +7th **S93.301 Unspecified subluxation of right foot**
    - +7th **S93.302 Unspecified subluxation of left foot**
    - +7th **S93.303 Unspecified subluxation of unspecified foot**
    - +7th **S93.304 Unspecified dislocation of right foot**
    - +7th **S93.305 Unspecified dislocation of left foot**
    - +7th **S93.306 Unspecified dislocation of unspecified foot**
  + **S93.31 Subluxation and dislocation of tarsal joint**
    - +7th **S93.311 Subluxation of tarsal joint of right foot**
    - +7th **S93.312 Subluxation of tarsal joint of left foot**
    - +7th **S93.313 Subluxation of tarsal joint of unspecified foot**
    - +7th **S93.314 Dislocation of tarsal joint of right foot**
    - +7th **S93.315 Dislocation of tarsal joint of left foot**
    - +7th **S93.316 Dislocation of tarsal joint of unspecified foot**
  + **S93.32 Subluxation and dislocation of tarsometatarsal joint**
    - +7th **S93.321 Subluxation of tarsometatarsal joint of right foot**
    - +7th **S93.322 Subluxation of tarsometatarsal joint of left foot**
    - +7th **S93.323 Subluxation of tarsometatarsal joint of unspecified foot**
    - +7th **S93.324 Dislocation of tarsometatarsal joint of right foot**
    - +7th **S93.325 Dislocation of tarsometatarsal joint of left foot**
    - +7th **S93.326 Dislocation of tarsometatarsal joint of unspecified foot**
  + **S93.33 Other subluxation and dislocation of foot**
    - +7th **S93.331 Other subluxation of right foot**
    - +7th **S93.332 Other subluxation of left foot**
    - +7th **S93.333 Other subluxation of unspecified foot**
    - +7th **S93.334 Other dislocation of right foot**
    - +7th **S93.335 Other dislocation of left foot**
    - +7th **S93.336 Other dislocation of unspecified foot**

+ **S93.4 Sprain of ankle**
  Excludes2: *injury of Achilles tendon (S86.0-)*
  + **S93.40 Sprain of unspecified ligament of ankle**
    Sprain of ankle NOS
    Sprained ankle NOS
    - +7th **S93.401 Sprain of unspecified ligament of right ankle**
    - +7th **S93.402 Sprain of unspecified ligament of left ankle**
    - +7th **S93.409 Sprain of unspecified ligament of unspecified ankle**
  + **S93.41 Sprain of calcaneofibular ligament**
    - +7th **S93.411 Sprain of calcaneofibular ligament of right ankle**
    - +7th **S93.412 Sprain of calcaneofibular ligament of left ankle**
    - +7th **S93.419 Sprain of calcaneofibular ligament of unspecified ankle**
  + **S93.42 Sprain of deltoid ligament**
    - +7th **S93.421 Sprain of deltoid ligament of right ankle**
    - +7th **S93.422 Sprain of deltoid ligament of left ankle**
    - +7th **S93.429 Sprain of deltoid ligament of unspecified ankle**

\+ **S93.43 Sprain of tibiofibular ligament**
+7th **S93.431 Sprain of tibiofibular ligament of right ankle**
+7th **S93.432 Sprain of tibiofibular ligament of left ankle**
+7th **S93.439 Sprain of tibiofibular ligament of unspecified ankle**
\+ **S93.49 Sprain of other ligament of ankle**
Sprain of internal collateral ligament
Sprain of talofibular ligament
+7th **S93.491 Sprain of other ligament of right ankle**
+7th **S93.492 Sprain of other ligament of left ankle**
+7th **S93.499 Sprain of other ligament of unspecified ankle**
\+ **S93.5 Sprain of toe**
\+ **S93.50 Unspecified sprain of toe**
+7th **S93.501 Unspecified sprain of right great toe**
+7th **S93.502 Unspecified sprain of left great toe**
+7th **S93.503 Unspecified sprain of unspecified great toe**
+7th **S93.504 Unspecified sprain of right lesser toe(s)**
+7th **S93.505 Unspecified sprain of left lesser toe(s)**
+7th **S93.506 Unspecified sprain of unspecified lesser toe(s)**
+7th **S93.509 Unspecified sprain of unspecified toe(s)**
\+ **S93.51 Sprain of interphalangeal joint of toe**
+7th **S93.511 Sprain of interphalangeal joint of right great toe**
+7th **S93.512 Sprain of interphalangeal joint of left great toe**
+7th **S93.513 Sprain of interphalangeal joint of unspecified great toe**
+7th **S93.514 Sprain of interphalangeal joint of right lesser toe(s)**
+7th **S93.515 Sprain of interphalangeal joint of left lesser toe(s)**
+7th **S93.516 Sprain of interphalangeal joint of unspecified lesser toe(s)**
+7th **S93.519 Sprain of interphalangeal joint of unspecified toe(s)**
\+ **S93.52 Sprain of metatarsophalangeal joint of toe**
+7th **S93.521 Sprain of metatarsophalangeal joint of right great toe**
+7th **S93.522 Sprain of metatarsophalangeal joint of left great toe**
+7th **S93.523 Sprain of metatarsophalangeal joint of unspecified great toe**
+7th **S93.524 Sprain of metatarsophalangeal joint of right lesser toe(s)**
+7th **S93.525 Sprain of metatarsophalangeal joint of left lesser toe(s)**
+7th **S93.526 Sprain of metatarsophalangeal joint of unspecified lesser toe(s)**
+7th **S93.529 Sprain of metatarsophalangeal joint of unspecified toe(s)**
\+ **S93.6 Sprain of foot**
Excludes2: *sprain of metatarsophalangeal joint of toe (S93.52-) sprain of toe (S93.5-)*
\+ **S93.60 Unspecified sprain of foot**
+7th **S93.601 Unspecified sprain of right foot**
+7th **S93.602 Unspecified sprain of left foot**
+7th **S93.609 Unspecified sprain of unspecified foot**
\+ **S93.61 Sprain of tarsal ligament of foot**
+7th **S93.611 Sprain of tarsal ligament of right foot**
+7th **S93.612 Sprain of tarsal ligament of left foot**
+7th **S93.619 Sprain of tarsal ligament of unspecified foot**
\+ **S93.62 Sprain of tarsometatarsal ligament of foot**
+7th **S93.621 Sprain of tarsometatarsal ligament of right foot**
+7th **S93.622 Sprain of tarsometatarsal ligament of left foot**
+7th **S93.629 Sprain of tarsometatarsal ligament of unspecified foot**
\+ **S93.69 Other sprain of foot**
+7th **S93.691 Other sprain of right foot**
+7th **S93.692 Other sprain of left foot**
+7th **S93.699 Other sprain of unspecified foot**

S94 Injury of nerves at ankle and foot level
Code also any associated open wound (S91.-)

The appropriate 7th character is to be added to each code from category S94
A initial encounter
D subsequent encounter
S sequela

\+ **S94.0 Injury of lateral plantar nerve**
X+7th **S94.00 Injury of lateral plantar nerve, unspecified leg**
X+7th **S94.01 Injury of lateral plantar nerve, right leg**
X+7th **S94.02 Injury of lateral plantar nerve, left leg**
\+ **S94.1 Injury of medial plantar nerve**
X+7th **S94.10 Injury of medial plantar nerve, unspecified leg**
X+7th **S94.11 Injury of medial plantar nerve, right leg**
X+7th **S94.12 Injury of medial plantar nerve, left leg**
\+ **S94.2 Injury of deep peroneal nerve at ankle and foot level**
Injury of terminal, lateral branch of deep peroneal nerve
X+7th **S94.20 Injury of deep peroneal nerve at ankle and foot level, unspecified leg**
X+7th **S94.21 Injury of deep peroneal nerve at ankle and foot level, right leg**
X+7th **S94.22 Injury of deep peroneal nerve at ankle and foot level, left leg**
\+ **S94.3 Injury of cutaneous sensory nerve at ankle and foot level**
X+7th **S94.30 Injury of cutaneous sensory nerve at ankle and foot level, unspecified leg**
X+7th **S94.31 Injury of cutaneous sensory nerve at ankle and foot level, right leg**
X+7th **S94.32 Injury of cutaneous sensory nerve at ankle and foot level, left leg**
\+ **S94.8 Injury of other nerves at ankle and foot level**
\+ **S94.8X Injury of other nerves at ankle and foot level**
+7th **S94.8X1 Injury of other nerves at ankle and foot level, right leg**
+7th **S94.8X2 Injury of other nerves at ankle and foot level, left leg**
+7th **S94.8X9 Injury of other nerves at ankle and foot level, unspecified leg**
\+ **S94.9 Injury of unspecified nerve at ankle and foot level**
X+7th **S94.90 Injury of unspecified nerve at ankle and foot level, unspecified leg**
X+7th **S94.91 Injury of unspecified nerve at ankle and foot level, right leg**
X+7th **S94.92 Injury of unspecified nerve at ankle and foot level, left leg**

S95 Injury of blood vessels at ankle and foot level
Code also any associated open wound (S91.-)
Excludes2: *injury of posterior tibial artery and vein (S85.1-, S85.8-)*

The appropriate 7th character is to be added to each code from category S95
A initial encounter
D subsequent encounter
S sequela

\+ **S95.0 Injury of dorsal artery of foot**
\+ **S95.00 Unspecified injury of dorsal artery of foot**
CC +7th **S95.001 Unspecified injury of dorsal artery of right foot**
CC Exclusion 7th character A see Appendix A PDX collection 1325
CC +7th **S95.002 Unspecified injury of dorsal artery of left foot**
CC Exclusion 7th character A see Appendix A PDX collection 1326
CC +7th **S95.009 Unspecified injury of dorsal artery of unspecified foot**
CC Exclusion 7th character A see Appendix A PDX collection 1327
\+ **S95.01 Laceration of dorsal artery of foot**
CC +7th **S95.011 Laceration of dorsal artery of right foot**
CC Exclusion 7th character A see Appendix A PDX collection 1325
CC +7th **S95.012 Laceration of dorsal artery of left foot**
CC Exclusion 7th character A see Appendix A PDX collection 1326
CC +7th **S95.019 Laceration of dorsal artery of unspecified foot**
CC Exclusion 7th character A see Appendix A PDX collection 1327

+ **S95.09 Other specified injury of dorsal artery of foot**
  - CC +7th **S95.091 Other specified injury of dorsal artery of right foot**
    CC Exclusion 7th character A see Appendix A PDX collection 1325
  - CC +7th **S95.092 Other specified injury of dorsal artery of left foot**
    CC Exclusion 7th character A see Appendix A PDX collection 1326
  - CC +7th **S95.099 Other specified injury of dorsal artery of unspecified foot**
    CC Exclusion 7th character A see Appendix A PDX collection 1327

+ **S95.1 Injury of plantar artery of foot**
+ **S95.10 Unspecified injury of plantar artery of foot**
  - CC +7th **S95.101 Unspecified injury of plantar artery of right foot**
    CC Exclusion 7th character A see Appendix A PDX collection 1370
  - CC +7th **S95.102 Unspecified injury of plantar artery of left foot**
    CC Exclusion 7th character A see Appendix A PDX collection 1371
  - CC +7th **S95.109 Unspecified injury of plantar artery of unspecified foot**
    CC Exclusion 7th character A see Appendix A PDX collection 1372
+ **S95.11 Laceration of plantar artery of foot**
  - CC +7th **S95.111 Laceration of plantar artery of right foot**
    CC Exclusion 7th character A see Appendix A PDX collection 1370
  - CC +7th **S95.112 Laceration of plantar artery of left foot**
    CC Exclusion 7th character A see Appendix A PDX collection 1371
  - CC +7th **S95.119 Laceration of plantar artery of unspecified foot**
    CC Exclusion 7th character A see Appendix A PDX collection 1372
+ **S95.19 Other specified injury of plantar artery of foot**
  - CC +7th **S95.191 Other specified injury of plantar artery of right foot**
    CC Exclusion 7th character A see Appendix A PDX collection 1370
  - CC +7th **S95.192 Other specified injury of plantar artery of left foot**
    CC Exclusion 7th character A see Appendix A PDX collection 1371
  - CC +7th **S95.199 Other specified injury of plantar artery of unspecified foot**
    CC Exclusion 7th character A see Appendix A PDX collection 1372

+ **S95.2 Injury of dorsal vein of foot**
+ **S95.20 Unspecified injury of dorsal vein of foot**
  - CC +7th **S95.201 Unspecified injury of dorsal vein of right foot**
    CC Exclusion 7th character A see Appendix A PDX collection 1325
  - CC +7th **S95.202 Unspecified injury of dorsal vein of left foot**
    CC Exclusion 7th character A see Appendix A PDX collection 1326
  - CC +7th **S95.209 Unspecified injury of dorsal vein of unspecified foot**
    CC Exclusion 7th character A see Appendix A PDX collection 1327
+ **S95.21 Laceration of dorsal vein of foot**
  - CC +7th **S95.211 Laceration of dorsal vein of right foot**
    CC Exclusion 7th character A see Appendix A PDX collection 1325
  - CC +7th **S95.212 Laceration of dorsal vein of left foot**
    CC Exclusion 7th character A see Appendix A PDX collection 1326
  - CC +7th **S95.219 Laceration of dorsal vein of unspecified foot**
    CC Exclusion 7th character A see Appendix A PDX collection 1327
+ **S95.29 Other specified injury of dorsal vein of foot**
  - CC +7th **S95.291 Other specified injury of dorsal vein of right foot**
    CC Exclusion 7th character A see Appendix A PDX collection 1325
  - CC +7th **S95.292 Other specified injury of dorsal vein of left foot**
    CC Exclusion 7th character A see Appendix A PDX collection 1326
  - CC +7th **S95.299 Other specified injury of dorsal vein of unspecified foot**
    CC Exclusion 7th character A see Appendix A PDX collection 1327

S95.8 Injury of other blood vessels at ankle and foot level
+ **S95.80 Unspecified injury of other blood vessels at ankle and foot level**
  - CC +7th **S95.801 Unspecified injury of other blood vessels at ankle and foot level, right leg**
    CC Exclusion 7th character A see Appendix A PDX collection 1325
  - CC +7th **S95.802 Unspecified injury of other blood vessels at ankle and foot level, left leg**
    CC Exclusion 7th character A see Appendix A PDX collection 1326
  - CC +7th **S95.809 Unspecified injury of other blood vessels at ankle and foot level, unspecified leg**
    CC Exclusion 7th character A see Appendix A PDX collection 1327
+ **S95.81 Laceration of other blood vessels at ankle and foot level**
  - CC +7th **S95.811 Laceration of other blood vessels at ankle and foot level, right leg**
    CC Exclusion 7th character A see Appendix A PDX collection 1325
  - CC +7th **S95.812 Laceration of other blood vessels at ankle and foot level, left leg**
    CC Exclusion 7th character A see Appendix A PDX collection 1326
  - CC +7th **S95.819 Laceration of other blood vessels at ankle and foot level, unspecified leg**
    CC Exclusion 7th character A see Appendix A PDX collection 1327
+ **S95.89 Other specified injury of other blood vessels at ankle and foot level**
  - CC +7th **S95.891 Other specified injury of other blood vessels at ankle and foot level, right leg**
    CC Exclusion 7th character A see Appendix A PDX collection 1325
  - CC +7th **S95.892 Other specified injury of other blood vessels at ankle and foot level, left leg**
    CC Exclusion 7th character A see Appendix A PDX collection 1326
  - CC +7th **S95.899 Other specified injury of other blood vessels at ankle and foot level, unspecified leg**
    CC Exclusion 7th character A see Appendix A PDX collection 1327

+ **S95.9 Injury of unspecified blood vessel at ankle and foot level**
+ **S95.90 Unspecified injury of unspecified blood vessel at ankle and foot level**
  - CC +7th **S95.901 Unspecified injury of unspecified blood vessel at ankle and foot level, right leg**
    CC Exclusion 7th character A see Appendix A PDX collection 1325
  - CC +7th **S95.902 Unspecified injury of unspecified blood vessel at ankle and foot level, left leg**
    CC Exclusion 7th character A see Appendix A PDX collection 1326
  - CC +7th **S95.909 Unspecified injury of unspecified blood vessel at ankle and foot level, unspecified leg**
    CC Exclusion 7th character A see Appendix A PDX collection 1327
+ **S95.91 Laceration of unspecified blood vessel at ankle and foot level**
  - CC +7th **S95.911 Laceration of unspecified blood vessel at ankle and foot level, right leg**
    CC Exclusion 7th character A see Appendix A PDX collection 1325
  - CC +7th **S95.912 Laceration of unspecified blood vessel at ankle and foot level, left leg**
    CC Exclusion 7th character A see Appendix A PDX collection 1326
  - CC +7th **S95.919 Laceration of unspecified blood vessel at ankle and foot level, unspecified leg**
    CC Exclusion 7th character A see Appendix A PDX collection 1327
+ **S95.99 Other specified injury of unspecified blood vessel at ankle and foot level**
  - CC +7th **S95.991 Other specified injury of unspecified blood vessel at ankle and foot level, right leg**
    CC Exclusion 7th character A see Appendix A PDX collection 1325

CC +7th **S95.992** **Other specified injury of unspecified blood vessel at ankle and foot level, left leg**
CC Exclusion 7th character A see Appendix A
PDX collection 1326

CC +7th **S95.999** **Other specified injury of unspecified blood vessel at ankle and foot level, unspecified leg**
CC Exclusion 7th character A see Appendix A
PDX collection 1327

S96 Injury of muscle and tendon at ankle and foot level

Code also any associated open wound (S91.-)

Excludes2: *injury of Achilles tendon (S86.0-)*
sprain of joints and ligaments of ankle and foot (S93.-)

The appropriate 7th character is to be added to each code from category S96
A initial encounter
D subsequent encounter
S sequela

\+ **S96.0** **Injury of muscle and tendon of long flexor muscle of toe at ankle and foot level**

\+ **S96.00** **Unspecified injury of muscle and tendon of long flexor muscle of toe at ankle and foot level**

+7th **S96.001** **Unspecified injury of muscle and tendon of long flexor muscle of toe at ankle and foot level, right foot**

+7th **S96.002** **Unspecified injury of muscle and tendon of long flexor muscle of toe at ankle and foot level, left foot**

+7th **S96.009** **Unspecified injury of muscle and tendon of long flexor muscle of toe at ankle and foot level, unspecified foot**

\+ **S96.01** **Strain of muscle and tendon of long flexor muscle of toe at ankle and foot level**

+7th **S96.011** **Strain of muscle and tendon of long flexor muscle of toe at ankle and foot level, right foot**

+7th **S96.012** **Strain of muscle and tendon of long flexor muscle of toe at ankle and foot level, left foot**

+7th **S96.019** **Strain of muscle and tendon of long flexor muscle of toe at ankle and foot level, unspecified foot**

\+ **S96.02** **Laceration of muscle and tendon of long flexor muscle of toe at ankle and foot level**

CC +7th **S96.021** **Laceration of muscle and tendon of long flexor muscle of toe at ankle and foot level, right foot**
CC Exclusion 7th character A see Appendix A
PDX collection 1364

CC +7th **S96.022** **Laceration of muscle and tendon of long flexor muscle of toe at ankle and foot level, left foot**
CC Exclusion 7th character A see Appendix A
PDX collection 1365

CC +7th **S96.029** **Laceration of muscle and tendon of long flexor muscle of toe at ankle and foot level, unspecified foot**
CC Exclusion 7th character A see Appendix A
PDX collection 1366

\+ **S96.09** **Other injury of muscle and tendon of long flexor muscle of toe at ankle and foot level**

+7th **S96.091** **Other injury of muscle and tendon of long flexor muscle of toe at ankle and foot level, right foot**

+7th **S96.092** **Other injury of muscle and tendon of long flexor muscle of toe at ankle and foot level, left foot**

+7th **S96.099** **Other injury of muscle and tendon of long flexor muscle of toe at ankle and foot level, unspecified foot**

\+ **S96.1** **Injury of muscle and tendon of long extensor muscle of toe at ankle and foot level**

\+ **S96.10** **Unspecified injury of muscle and tendon of long extensor muscle of toe at ankle and foot level**

+7th **S96.101** **Unspecified injury of muscle and tendon of long extensor muscle of toe at ankle and foot level, right foot**

+7th **S96.102** **Unspecified injury of muscle and tendon of long extensor muscle of toe at ankle and foot level, left foot**

+7th **S96.109** **Unspecified injury of muscle and tendon of long extensor muscle of toe at ankle and foot level, unspecified foot**

\+ **S96.11** **Strain of muscle and tendon of long extensor muscle of toe at ankle and foot level**

+7th **S96.111** **Strain of muscle and tendon of long extensor muscle of toe at ankle and foot level, right foot**

+7th **S96.112** **Strain of muscle and tendon of long extensor muscle of toe at ankle and foot level, left foot**

+7th **S96.119** **Strain of muscle and tendon of long extensor muscle of toe at ankle and foot level, unspecified foot**

\+ **S96.12** **Laceration of muscle and tendon of long extensor muscle of toe at ankle and foot level**

CC +7th **S96.121** **Laceration of muscle and tendon of long extensor muscle of toe at ankle and foot level, right foot**
CC Exclusion 7th character A see Appendix A
PDX collection 1364

CC +7th **S96.122** **Laceration of muscle and tendon of long extensor muscle of toe at ankle and foot level, left foot**
CC Exclusion 7th character A see Appendix A
PDX collection 1365

CC +7th **S96.129** **Laceration of muscle and tendon of long extensor muscle of toe at ankle and foot level, unspecified foot**
CC Exclusion 7th character A see Appendix A
PDX collection 1366

\+ **S96.19** **Other specified injury of muscle and tendon of long extensor muscle of toe at ankle and foot level**

+7th **S96.191** **Other specified injury of muscle and tendon of long extensor muscle of toe at ankle and foot level, right foot**

+7th **S96.192** **Other specified injury of muscle and tendon of long extensor muscle of toe at ankle and foot level, left foot**

+7th **S96.199** **Other specified injury of muscle and tendon of long extensor muscle of toe at ankle and foot level, unspecified foot**

\+ **S96.2** **Injury of intrinsic muscle and tendon at ankle and foot level**

\+ **S96.20** **Unspecified injury of intrinsic muscle and tendon at ankle and foot level**

+7th **S96.201** **Unspecified injury of intrinsic muscle and tendon at ankle and foot level, right foot**

+7th **S96.202** **Unspecified injury of intrinsic muscle and tendon at ankle and foot level, left foot**

+7th **S96.209** **Unspecified injury of intrinsic muscle and tendon at ankle and foot level, unspecified foot**

\+ **S96.21** **Strain of intrinsic muscle and tendon at ankle and foot level**

+7th **S96.211** **Strain of intrinsic muscle and tendon at ankle and foot level, right foot**

+7th **S96.212** **Strain of intrinsic muscle and tendon at ankle and foot level, left foot**

+7th **S96.219** **Strain of intrinsic muscle and tendon at ankle and foot level, unspecified foot**

\+ **S96.22** **Laceration of intrinsic muscle and tendon at ankle and foot level**

CC +7th **S96.221** **Laceration of intrinsic muscle and tendon at ankle and foot level, right foot**
CC Exclusion 7th character A see Appendix A
PDX collection 1364

CC +7th **S96.222** **Laceration of intrinsic muscle and tendon at ankle and foot level, left foot**
CC Exclusion 7th character A see Appendix A
PDX collection 1365

CC +7th **S96.229** **Laceration of intrinsic muscle and tendon at ankle and foot level, unspecified foot**
CC Exclusion 7th character A see Appendix A
PDX collection 1366

\+ **S96.29** **Other specified injury of intrinsic muscle and tendon at ankle and foot level**

+7th **S96.291** **Other specified injury of intrinsic muscle and tendon at ankle and foot level, right foot**

+7th **S96.292** **Other specified injury of intrinsic muscle and tendon at ankle and foot level, left foot**

+7th **S96.299** **Other specified injury of intrinsic muscle and tendon at ankle and foot level, unspecified foot**

+ **S96.8** **Injury of other specified muscles and tendons at ankle and foot level**

+ **S96.80** **Unspecified injury of other specified muscles and tendons at ankle and foot level**

+7th **S96.801** **Unspecified injury of other specified muscles and tendons at ankle and foot level, right foot**

+7th **S96.802** **Unspecified injury of other specified muscles and tendons at ankle and foot level, left foot**

+7th **S96.809** **Unspecified injury of other specified muscles and tendons at ankle and foot level, unspecified foot**

+ **S96.81** **Strain of other specified muscles and tendons at ankle and foot level**

+7th **S96.811** **Strain of other specified muscles and tendons at ankle and foot level, right foot**

+7th **S96.812** **Strain of other specified muscles and tendons at ankle and foot level, left foot**

+7th **S96.819** **Strain of other specified muscles and tendons at ankle and foot level, unspecified foot**

+ **S96.82** **Laceration of other specified muscles and tendons at ankle and foot level**

CC +7th **S96.821** **Laceration of other specified muscles and tendons at ankle and foot level, right foot**
CC Exclusion 7th character A see Appendix A
PDX collection 1364

CC +7th **S96.822** **Laceration of other specified muscles and tendons at ankle and foot level, left foot**
CC Exclusion 7th character A see Appendix A
PDX collection 1365

CC +7th **S96.829** **Laceration of other specified muscles and tendons at ankle and foot level, unspecified foot**
CC Exclusion 7th character A see Appendix A
PDX collection 1366

+ **S96.89** **Other specified injury of other specified muscles and tendons at ankle and foot level**

+7th **S96.891** **Other specified injury of other specified muscles and tendons at ankle and foot level, right foot**

+7th **S96.892** **Other specified injury of other specified muscles and tendons at ankle and foot level, left foot**

+7th **S96.899** **Other specified injury of other specified muscles and tendons at ankle and foot level, unspecified foot**

+ **S96.9** **Injury of unspecified muscle and tendon at ankle and foot level**

+ **S96.90** **Unspecified injury of unspecified muscle and tendon at ankle and foot level**

+7th **S96.901** **Unspecified injury of unspecified muscle and tendon at ankle and foot level, right foot**

+7th **S96.902** **Unspecified injury of unspecified muscle and tendon at ankle and foot level, left foot**

+7th **S96.909** **Unspecified injury of unspecified muscle and tendon at ankle and foot level, unspecified foot**

+ **S96.91** **Strain of unspecified muscle and tendon at ankle and foot level**

+7th **S96.911** **Strain of unspecified muscle and tendon at ankle and foot level, right foot**

+7th **S96.912** **Strain of unspecified muscle and tendon at ankle and foot level, left foot**

+7th **S96.919** **Strain of unspecified muscle and tendon at ankle and foot level, unspecified foot**

+ **S96.92** **Laceration of unspecified muscle and tendon at ankle and foot level**

CC +7th **S96.921** **Laceration of unspecified muscle and tendon at ankle and foot level, right foot**
CC Exclusion 7th character A see Appendix A
PDX collection 1364

CC +7th **S96.922** **Laceration of unspecified muscle and tendon at ankle and foot level, left foot**
CC Exclusion 7th character A see Appendix A
PDX collection 1365

CC +7th **S96.929** **Laceration of unspecified muscle and tendon at ankle and foot level, unspecifie foot**
CC Exclusion 7th character A see Appendix
PDX collection 1366

+ **S96.99** **Other specified injury of unspecified muscle and tendon at ankle and foot level**

+7th **S96.991** **Other specified injury of unspecified muscle and tendon at ankle and foot leve right foot**

+7th **S96.992** **Other specified injury of unspecified muscle and tendon at ankle and foot leve left foot**

+7th **S96.999** **Other specified injury of unspecified muscle and tendon at ankle and foot leve unspecified foot**

S97 Crushing injury of ankle and foot

Use additional code(s) for all associated injuries

The appropriate 7th character is to be added to each code from category S97
A initial encounter
D subsequent encounter
S sequela

+ **S97.0** **Crushing injury of ankle**

X+7th **S97.00** **Crushing injury of unspecified ankle**

X+7th **S97.01** **Crushing injury of right ankle**

X+7th **S97.02** **Crushing injury of left ankle**

+ **S97.1** **Crushing injury of toe**

+ **S97.10** **Crushing injury of unspecified toe(s)**

+7th **S97.101** **Crushing injury of unspecified right toe**

+7th **S97.102** **Crushing injury of unspecified left toe(s)**

+7th **S97.109** **Crushing injury of unspecified toe(s)**
Crushing injury of toe NOS

+ **S97.11** **Crushing injury of great toe**

+7th **S97.111** **Crushing injury of right great toe**

+7th **S97.112** **Crushing injury of left great toe**

+7th **S97.119** **Crushing injury of unspecified great toe**

+ **S97.12** **Crushing injury of lesser toe(s)**

+7th **S97.121** **Crushing injury of right lesser toe(s)**

+7th **S97.122** **Crushing injury of left lesser toe(s)**

+7th **S97.129** **Crushing injury of unspecified lesser toe**

+ **S97.8** **Crushing injury of foot**

X+7th **S97.80** **Crushing injury of unspecified foot**
Crushing injury of foot NOS

X+7th **S97.81** **Crushing injury of right foot**

X+7th **S97.82** **Crushing injury of left foot**

S98 Traumatic amputation of ankle and foot

NOTE An amputation not identified as partial or complete should be coded to complete

The appropriate 7th character is to be added to each code from category S98
A initial encounter
D subsequent encounter
S sequela

+ **S98.0** **Traumatic amputation of foot at ankle level**

+ **S98.01** **Complete traumatic amputation of foot at ankle le**

CC +7th **S98.011** **Complete traumatic amputation of righ foot at ankle level**
CC Exclusion 7th character A see Appendix
PDX collection 1333

CC +7th **S98.012** **Complete traumatic amputation of left at ankle level**
CC Exclusion 7th character A see Appendix
PDX collection 1334

CC +7th **S98.019** **Complete traumatic amputation of unspecified foot at ankle level**
CC Exclusion 7th character A see Appendix
PDX collection 1335

+ **S98.02** **Partial traumatic amputation of foot at ankle leve**

CC +7th **S98.021** **Partial traumatic amputation of right fo at ankle level**
CC Exclusion 7th character A see Appendix
PDX collection 1333

CC +7th **S98.022** **Partial traumatic amputation of left foo ankle level**
CC Exclusion 7th character A see Appendix
PDX collection 1334

CC +7th **S98.029** **Partial traumatic amputation of unspecified foot at ankle level**
CC Exclusion 7th character A see Appendix A PDX collection 1335

\+ **S98.1** **Traumatic amputation of one toe**

\+ **S98.11** **Complete traumatic amputation of great toe**

+7th **S98.111** **Complete traumatic amputation of right great toe**

+7th **S98.112** **Complete traumatic amputation of left great toe**

+7th **S98.119** **Complete traumatic amputation of unspecified great toe**

\+ **S98.12** **Partial traumatic amputation of great toe**

+7th **S98.121** **Partial traumatic amputation of right great toe**

+7th **S98.122** **Partial traumatic amputation of left great toe**

+7th **S98.129** **Partial traumatic amputation of unspecified great toe**

\+ **S98.13** **Complete traumatic amputation of one lesser toe**
Traumatic amputation of toe NOS

+7th **S98.131** **Complete traumatic amputation of one right lesser toe**

+7th **S98.132** **Complete traumatic amputation of one left lesser toe**

+7th **S98.139** **Complete traumatic amputation of one unspecified lesser toe**

\+ **S98.14** **Partial traumatic amputation of one lesser toe**

+7th **S98.141** **Partial traumatic amputation of one right lesser toe**

+7th **S98.142** **Partial traumatic amputation of one left lesser toe**

+7th **S98.149** **Partial traumatic amputation of one unspecified lesser toe**

\+ **S98.2** **Traumatic amputation of two or more lesser toes**

\+ **S98.21** **Complete traumatic amputation of two or more lesser toes**

+7th **S98.211** **Complete traumatic amputation of two or more right lesser toes**

+7th **S98.212** **Complete traumatic amputation of two or more left lesser toes**

+7th **S98.219** **Complete traumatic amputation of two or more unspecified lesser toes**

\+ **S98.22** **Partial traumatic amputation of two or more lesser toes**

+7th **S98.221** **Partial traumatic amputation of two or more right lesser toes**

+7th **S98.222** **Partial traumatic amputation of two or more left lesser toes**

+7th **S98.229** **Partial traumatic amputation of two or more unspecified lesser toes**

\+ **S98.3** **Traumatic amputation of midfoot**

\+ **S98.31** **Complete traumatic amputation of midfoot**

CC +7th **S98.311** **Complete traumatic amputation of right midfoot**
CC Exclusion 7th character A see Appendix A PDX collection 1333

CC +7th **S98.312** **Complete traumatic amputation of left midfoot**
CC Exclusion 7th character A see Appendix A PDX collection 1334

CC +7th **S98.319** **Complete traumatic amputation of unspecified midfoot**
CC Exclusion 7th character A see Appendix A PDX collection 1335

\+ **S98.32** **Partial traumatic amputation of midfoot**

CC +7th **S98.321** **Partial traumatic amputation of right midfoot**
CC Exclusion 7th character A see Appendix A PDX collection 1333

CC +7th **S98.322** **Partial traumatic amputation of left midfoot**
CC Exclusion 7th character A see Appendix A PDX collection 1334

CC +7th **S98.329** **Partial traumatic amputation of unspecified midfoot**
CC Exclusion 7th character A see Appendix A PDX collection 1335

\+ **S98.9** **Traumatic amputation of foot, level unspecified**

\+ **S98.91** **Complete traumatic amputation of foot, level unspecified**

CC +7th **S98.911** **Complete traumatic amputation of right foot, level unspecified**
CC Exclusion 7th character A see Appendix A PDX collection 1333

CC +7th **S98.912** **Complete traumatic amputation of left foot, level unspecified**
CC Exclusion 7th character A see Appendix A PDX collection 1334

CC +7th **S98.919** **Complete traumatic amputation of unspecified foot, level unspecified**
CC Exclusion 7th character A see Appendix A PDX collection 1335

\+ **S98.92** **Partial traumatic amputation of foot, level unspecified**

CC +7th **S98.921** **Partial traumatic amputation of right foot, level unspecified**
CC Exclusion 7th character A see Appendix A PDX collection 1333

CC +7th **S98.922** **Partial traumatic amputation of left foot, level unspecified**
CC Exclusion 7th character A see Appendix A PDX collection 1334

CC +7th **S98.929** **Partial traumatic amputation of unspecified foot, level unspecified**
CC Exclusion 7th character A see Appendix A PDX collection 1335

S99 Other and unspecified injuries of ankle and foot

\+ **S99.0** **Physeal fracture of calcaneus**
AHA CC: 4Q, 2016, 68-69

The appropriate 7th character is to be added to each code in subcategory **S99.0**

A initial encounter for closed fracture
B initial encounter for open fracture
D subsequent encounter for fracture with routine healing
G subsequent encounter for fracture with delayed healing
K subsequent encounter for fracture with nonunion
P subsequent encounter for fracture with malunion
S sequela

\+ **S99.00** **Unspecified physeal fracture of calcaneus**
Unspecified physeal fracture of calcaneus

+7th **S99.001** **Unspecified physeal fracture of right calcaneus**

+7th **S99.002** **Unspecified physeal fracture of left calcaneus**

+7th **S99.009** **Unspecified physeal fracture of unspecified calcaneus**

\+ **S99.01** **Salter-Harris Type I physeal fracture of calcaneus**

+7th **S99.011** **Salter-Harris Type I physeal fracture of right calcaneus**

+7th **S99.012** **Salter-Harris Type I physeal fracture of left calcaneus**

+7th **S99.019** **Salter-Harris Type I physeal fracture of unspecified calcaneus**

\+ **S99.02** **Salter-Harris Type II physeal fracture of calcaneus**

+7th **S99.021** **Salter-Harris Type II physeal fracture of right calcaneus**

+7th **S99.022** **Salter-Harris Type II physeal fracture of left calcaneus**

+7th **S99.029** **Salter-Harris Type II physeal fracture of unspecified calcaneus**

\+ **S99.03** **Salter-Harris Type III physeal fracture of calcaneus**

+7th **S99.031** **Salter-Harris Type III physeal fracture of right calcaneus**

+7th **S99.032** **Salter-Harris Type III physeal fracture of left calcaneus**

+7th **S99.039** **Salter-Harris Type III physeal fracture of unspecified calcaneus**

\+ **S99.04** **Salter-Harris Type IV physeal fracture of calcaneus**

+7th **S99.041** **Salter-Harris Type IV physeal fracture of right calcaneus**

+7th **S99.042** **Salter-Harris Type IV physeal fracture of left calcaneus**

+7th **S99.049** **Salter-Harris Type IV physeal fracture of unspecified calcaneus**

\+ **S99.09** **Other physeal fracture of calcaneus**

+7th **S99.091** **Other physeal fracture of right calcaneus**

+7th **S99.092** **Other physeal fracture of left calcaneus**

+7th **S99.099** **Other physeal fracture of unspecified calcaneus**

+ **S99.1 Physeal fracture of metatarsal**

The appropriate 7th character is to be added to each code in subcategory **S99.1**
A initial encounter for closed fracture
B initial encounter for open fracture
D subsequent encounter for fracture with routine healing
G subsequent encounter for fracture with delayed healing
K subsequent encounter for fracture with nonunion
P subsequent encounter for fracture with malunion
S sequela

+ **S99.10 Unspecified physeal fracture of metatarsal**
+7th **S99.101 Unspecified physeal fracture of right metatarsal**
+7th **S99.102 Unspecified physeal fracture of left metatarsal**
+7th **S99.109 Unspecified physeal fracture of unspecified metatarsal**
+ **S99.11 Salter-Harris Type I physeal fracture of metatarsal**
+7th **S99.111 Salter-Harris Type I physeal fracture of right metatarsal**
+7th **S99.112 Salter-Harris Type I physeal fracture of left metatarsal**
+7th **S99.119 Salter-Harris Type I physeal fracture of unspecified metatarsal**
+ **S99.12 Salter-Harris Type II physeal fracture of metatarsal**
+7th **S99.121 Salter-Harris Type II physeal fracture of right metatarsal**
+7th **S99.122 Salter-Harris Type II physeal fracture of left metatarsal**
+7th **S99.129 Salter-Harris Type II physeal fracture of unspecified metatarsal**
+ **S99.13 Salter-Harris Type III physeal fracture of metatarsal**
+7th **S99.131 Salter-Harris Type III physeal fracture of right metatarsal**
+7th **S99.132 Salter-Harris Type III physeal fracture of left metatarsal**
+7th **S99.139 Salter-Harris Type III physeal fracture of unspecified metatarsal**
+ **S99.14 Salter-Harris Type IV physeal fracture of metatarsal**
+7th **S99.141 Salter-Harris Type IV physeal fracture of right metatarsal**
+7th **S99.142 Salter-Harris Type IV physeal fracture of left metatarsal**
+7th **S99.149 Salter-Harris Type IV physeal fracture of unspecified metatarsal**
+ **S99.19 Other physeal fracture of metatarsal**
+7th **S99.191 Other physeal fracture of right metatarsal**
+7th **S99.192 Other physeal fracture of left metatarsal**
+7th **S99.199 Other physeal fracture of unspecified metatarsal**

+ **S99.2 Phseal fracture of phalanx of toe**

The appropriate 7th character is to be added to each code in subcategory **S99.2**
A initial encounter for closed fracture
B initial encounter for open fracture
D subsequent encounter for fracture with routine healing
G subsequent encounter for fracture with delayed healing
K subsequent encounter for fracture with nonunion
P subsequent encounter for fracture with malunion
S sequela

+ **S99.20 Unspecified physeal fracture of phalanx of toe**
+7th **S99.201 Unspecified physeal fracture of phalanx of right toe**
+7th **S99.202 Unspecified physeal fracture of phalanx of left toe**
+7th **S99.209 Unspecified physeal fracture of phalanx of unspecified toe**
+ **S99.21 Salter-Harris Type I physeal fracture of phalanx of toe**
+7th **S99.211 Salter-Harris Type I physeal fracture of phalanx of right toe**
+7th **S99.212 Salter-Harris Type I physeal fracture of phalanx of left toe**
+7th **S99.219 Salter-Harris Type I physeal fracture of phalanx of unspecified toe**
+ **S99.22 Salter-Harris Type II physeal fracture of phalanx of toe**
+7th **S99.221 Salter-Harris Type II physeal fracture of phalanx of right toe**
+7th **S99.222 Salter-Harris Type II physeal fracture of phalanx of left toe**
+7th **S99.229 Salter-Harris Type II physeal fracture of phalanx of unspecified toe**
+ **S99.23 Salter-Harris Type III physeal fracture of phalanx toe**
+7th **S99.231 Salter-Harris Type III physeal fracture o phalanx of right toe**
+7th **S99.232 Salter-Harris Type III physeal fracture o phalanx of left toe**
+7th **S99.239 Salter-Harris Type III physeal fracture o phalanx of unspecified toe**
+ **S99.24 Salter-Harris Type IV physeal fracture of phalanx toe**
+7th **S99.241 Salter-Harris Type IV physeal fracture o phalanx of right toe**
+7th **S99.242 Salter-Harris Type IV physeal fracture o phalanx of left toe**
+7th **S99.249 Salter-Harris Type IV physeal fracture o phalanx of unspecified toe**
+ **S99.29 Other physeal fracture of phalanx of toe**
+7th **S99.291 Other physeal fracture of phalanx of rig toe**
+7th **S99.292 Other physeal fracture of phalanx of left toe**
+7th **S99.299 Other physeal fracture of phalanx of unspecified toe**

+ **S99.8 Other specified injuries of ankle and foot**

The appropriate 7th character is to be added to each code from category **S99.8**
A initial encounter
D subsequent encounter
S sequela

+ **S99.81 Other specified injuries of ankle**
+7th **S99.811 Other specified injuries of right ankle**
+7th **S99.812 Other specified injuries of left ankle**
+7th **S99.819 Other specified injuries of unspecified ankle**
+ **S99.82 Other specified injuries of foot**
+7th **S99.821 Other specified injuries of right foot**
+7th **S99.822 Other specified injuries of left foot**
+7th **S99.829 Other specified injuries of unspecified fo**

+ **S99.9 Unspecified injury of ankle and foot**

The appropriate 7th character is to be added to each code from category **S99.9**
A initial encounter
D subsequent encounter
S sequela

+ **S99.91 Unspecified injury of ankle**
+7th **S99.911 Unspecified injury of right ankle**
+7th **S99.912 Unspecified injury of left ankle**
+7th **S99.919 Unspecified injury of unspecified ankle**
+ **S99.92 Unspecified injury of foot**
+7th **S99.921 Unspecified injury of right foot**
+7th **S99.922 Unspecified injury of left foot**
+7th **S99.929 Unspecified injury of unspecified foot**

INJURY, POISONING AND CERTAIN OTHER CONSEQUENCES OF EXTERNAL CAUSES (T07-T88)

Injuries involving multiple body regions (T07)

Excludes1: *burns and corrosions (T20-T32)*
frostbite (T33-T34)
insect bite or sting, venomous (T63.4)
sunburn (L55.-)

T07 Unspecified multiple injuries

The appropriate 7th character is to be added to each code from category T07
A initial encounter
D subsequent encounter
S sequela

Excludes1: *injury NOS (T14.90)*
Review coding guideline C.19.b

njury of unspecified body region (T14)

T14 Injury of unspecified body region

The appropriate 7th character is to be added to each code from category T14
A initial encounter
D subsequent encounter
S sequela

Excludes1: *multiple unspecified injuries (T07)*

T14.8 Other injury of unspecified body region
Abrasion NOS
Contusion NOS
Crush injury NOS
Fracture NOS
Skin injury NOS
Vascular injury NOS
Wound NOS

\+ **T14.9 Unspecified injury**
T14.90 Injury, unspecified
Injury NOS
T14.91 Suicide attempt
Attempted suicide NOS

;ffects of foreign body entering through natural orifice T15-T19)

xcludes2: *foreign body accidentally left in operation wound (T81.5-)*
foreign body in penetrating wound - See open wound by body region
residual foreign body in soft tissue (M79.5)
splinter, without open wound - See superficial injury by body region

T15 Foreign body on external eye

Excludes2: *foreign body in penetrating wound of orbit and eye ball (S05.4-, S05.5-)*
open wound of eyelid and periocular area (S01.1-)
retained foreign body in eyelid (H02.8-)
retained (old) foreign body in penetrating wound of orbit and eye ball (H05.5-, H44.6-, H44.7-)
superficial foreign body of eyelid and periocular area (S00.25-)

The appropriate 7th character is to be added to each code from category T15
A initial encounter
D subsequent encounter
S sequela

\+ **T15.0 Foreign body in cornea**
X+7th **T15.00 Foreign body in cornea, unspecified eye**
X+7th **T15.01 Foreign body in cornea, right eye**
X+7th **T15.02 Foreign body in cornea, left eye**
\+ **T15.1 Foreign body in conjunctival sac**
X+7th **T15.10 Foreign body in conjunctival sac, unspecified eye**
X+7th **T15.11 Foreign body in conjunctival sac, right eye**
X+7th **T15.12 Foreign body in conjunctival sac, left eye**
\+ **T15.8 Foreign body in other and multiple parts of external eye**
Foreign body in lacrimal punctum
X+7th **T15.80 Foreign body in other and multiple parts of external eye, unspecified eye**
X+7th **T15.81 Foreign body in other and multiple parts of external eye, right eye**
X+7th **T15.82 Foreign body in other and multiple parts of external eye, left eye**
\+ **T15.9 Foreign body on external eye, part unspecified**
X+7th **T15.90 Foreign body on external eye, part unspecified, unspecified eye**
X+7th **T15.91 Foreign body on external eye, part unspecified, right eye**
X+7th **T15.92 Foreign body on external eye, part unspecified, left eye**

T16 Foreign body in ear

Includes: foreign body in auditory canal

The appropriate 7th character is to be added to each code from category T16
A initial encounter
D subsequent encounter
S sequela

X+7th **T16.1 Foreign body in right ear**
X+7th **T16.2 Foreign body in left ear**
X+7th **T16.9 Foreign body in ear, unspecified ear**

T17 Foreign body in respiratory tract

The appropriate 7th character is to be added to each code from category T17
A initial encounter
D subsequent encounter
S sequela

X+7th **T17.0 Foreign body in nasal sinus**
X+7th **T17.1 Foreign body in nostril**
Foreign body in nose NOS
\+ **T17.2 Foreign body in pharynx**
Foreign body in nasopharynx
Foreign body in throat NOS
\+ **T17.20 Unspecified foreign body in pharynx**
+7th **T17.200 Unspecified foreign body in pharynx causing asphyxiation**
+7th **T17.208 Unspecified foreign body in pharynx causing other injury**
\+ **T17.21 Gastric contents in pharynx**
Aspiration of gastric contents into pharynx
Vomitus in pharynx
+7th **T17.210 Gastric contents in pharynx causing asphyxiation**
+7th **T17.218 Gastric contents in pharynx causing other injury**
\+ **T17.22 Food in pharynx**
Bones in pharynx
Seeds in pharynx
+7th **T17.220 Food in pharynx causing asphyxiation**
+7th **T17.228 Food in pharynx causing other injury**
\+ **T17.29 Other foreign object in pharynx**
+7th **T17.290 Other foreign object in pharynx causing asphyxiation**
+7th **T17.298 Other foreign object in pharynx causing other injury**
\+ **T17.3 Foreign body in larynx**
\+ **T17.30 Unspecified foreign body in larynx**
+7th **T17.300 Unspecified foreign body in larynx causing asphyxiation**
+7th **T17.308 Unspecified foreign body in larynx causing other injury**
\+ **T17.31 Gastric contents in larynx**
Aspiration of gastric contents into larynx
Vomitus in larynx
+7th **T17.310 Gastric contents in larynx causing asphyxiation**
+7th **T17.318 Gastric contents in larynx causing other injury**
\+ **T17.32 Food in larynx**
Bones in larynx
Seeds in larynx
+7th **T17.320 Food in larynx causing asphyxiation**
+7th **T17.328 Food in larynx causing other injury**
\+ **T17.39 Other foreign object in larynx**
+7th **T17.390 Other foreign object in larynx causing asphyxiation**
+7th **T17.398 Other foreign object in larynx causing other injury**
\+ **T17.4 Foreign body in trachea**
\+ **T17.40 Unspecified foreign body in trachea**
CC +7th **T17.400 Unspecified foreign body in trachea causing asphyxiation**
CC Exclusion 7th character A see Appendix A PDX collection 1373
CC +7th **T17.408 Unspecified foreign body in trachea causing other injury**
CC Exclusion 7th character A see Appendix A PDX collection 1373
\+ **T17.41 Gastric contents in trachea**
Aspiration of gastric contents into trachea
Vomitus in trachea
CC +7th **T17.410 Gastric contents in trachea causing asphyxiation**
CC Exclusion 7th character A see Appendix A PDX collection 1373
CC +7th **T17.418 Gastric contents in trachea causing other injury**
CC Exclusion 7th character A see Appendix A PDX collection 1373

+ **T17.42 Food in trachea**
  Bones in trachea
  Seeds in trachea
  CC +7th **T17.420 Food in trachea causing asphyxiation**
  CC Exclusion 7th character A see Appendix A
  PDX collection 1373
  CC +7th **T17.428 Food in trachea causing other injury**
  CC Exclusion 7th character A see Appendix A
  PDX collection 1373
+ **T17.49 Other foreign object in trachea**
  CC +7th **T17.490 Other foreign object in trachea causing asphyxiation**
  CC Exclusion 7th character A see Appendix A
  PDX collection 1373
  CC +7th **T17.498 Other foreign object in trachea causing other injury**
  CC Exclusion 7th character A see Appendix A
  PDX collection 1373

+ **T17.5 Foreign body in bronchus**
+ **T17.50 Unspecified foreign body in bronchus**
  CC +7th **T17.500 Unspecified foreign body in bronchus causing asphyxiation**
  CC Exclusion 7th character A see Appendix A
  PDX collection 1374
  CC +7th **T17.508 Unspecified foreign body in bronchus causing other injury**
  CC Exclusion 7th character A see Appendix A
  PDX collection 1374
+ **T17.51 Gastric contents in bronchus**
  Aspiration of gastric contents into bronchus
  Vomitus in bronchus
  CC +7th **T17.510 Gastric contents in bronchus causing asphyxiation**
  CC Exclusion 7th character A see Appendix A
  PDX collection 1374
  CC +7th **T17.518 Gastric contents in bronchus causing other injury**
  CC Exclusion 7th character A see Appendix A
  PDX collection 1374
+ **T17.52 Food in bronchus**
  Bones in bronchus
  Seeds in bronchus
  CC +7th **T17.520 Food in bronchus causing asphyxiation**
  CC Exclusion 7th character A see Appendix A
  PDX collection 1374
  CC +7th **T17.528 Food in bronchus causing other injury**
  CC Exclusion 7th character A see Appendix A
  PDX collection 1374
+ **T17.59 Other foreign object in bronchus**
  CC +7th **T17.590 Other foreign object in bronchus causing asphyxiation**
  CC Exclusion 7th character A see Appendix A
  PDX collection 1374
  CC +7th **T17.598 Other foreign object in bronchus causing other injury**
  CC Exclusion 7th character A see Appendix A
  PDX collection 1374

+ **T17.8 Foreign body in other parts of respiratory tract**
  Foreign body in bronchioles
  Foreign body in lung
+ **T17.80 Unspecified foreign body in other parts of respiratory tract**
  CC +7th **T17.800 Unspecified foreign body in other parts of respiratory tract causing asphyxiation**
  CC Exclusion 7th character A see Appendix A
  PDX collection 1374
  CC +7th **T17.808 Unspecified foreign body in other parts of respiratory tract causing other injury**
  CC Exclusion 7th character A see Appendix A
  PDX collection 1374
+ **T17.81 Gastric contents in other parts of respiratory tract**
  Aspiration of gastric contents into other parts of respiratory tract
  Vomitus in other parts of respiratory tract
  CC +7th **T17.810 Gastric contents in other parts of respiratory tract causing asphyxiation**
  CC Exclusion 7th character A see Appendix A
  PDX collection 1374
  CC +7th **T17.818 Gastric contents in other parts of respiratory tract causing other injury**
  CC Exclusion 7th character A see Appendix A
  PDX collection 1374
+ **T17.82 Food in other parts of respiratory tract**
  Bones in other parts of respiratory tract
  Seeds in other parts of respiratory tract
  CC +7th **T17.820 Food in other parts of respiratory tract causing asphyxiation**
  CC Exclusion 7th character A see Appendix A
  PDX collection 1374
  CC +7th **T17.828 Food in other parts of respiratory tract causing other injury**
  CC Exclusion 7th character A see Appendix A
  PDX collection 1374
+ **T17.89 Other foreign object in other parts of respiratory tract**
  CC +7th **T17.890 Other foreign object in other parts of respiratory tract causing asphyxiation**
  CC Exclusion 7th character A see Appendix A
  PDX collection 1374
  CC +7th **T17.898 Other foreign object in other parts of respiratory tract causing other injury**
  CC Exclusion 7th character A see Appendix A
  PDX collection 1374

T17.9 Foreign body in respiratory tract, part unspecified
+ **T17.90 Unspecified foreign body in respiratory tract, part unspecified**
  +7th **T17.900 Unspecified foreign body in respiratory tract, part unspecified causing asphyxiation**
  +7th **T17.908 Unspecified foreign body in respiratory tract, part unspecified causing other injury**
+ **T17.91 Gastric contents in respiratory tract, part unspecified**
  Aspiration of gastric contents into respiratory tract, part unspecified
  Vomitus in trachea respiratory tract, part unspecified
  +7th **T17.910 Gastric contents in respiratory tract, part unspecified causing asphyxiation**
  +7th **T17.918 Gastric contents in respiratory tract, part unspecified causing other injury**
+ **T17.92 Food in respiratory tract, part unspecified**
  Bones in respiratory tract, part unspecified
  Seeds in respiratory tract, part unspecified
  +7th **T17.920 Food in respiratory tract, part unspecified causing asphyxiation**
  +7th **T17.928 Food in respiratory tract, part unspecified causing other injury**
+ **T17.99 Other foreign object in respiratory tract, part unspecified**
  +7th **T17.990 Other foreign object in respiratory tract, part unspecified in causing asphyxiation**
  +7th **T17.998 Other foreign object in respiratory tract, part unspecified causing other injury**

T18 Foreign body in alimentary tract

Excludes2: *foreign body in pharynx (T17.2-)*

The appropriate 7th character is to be added to each code from category T18
A initial encounter
D subsequent encounter
S sequela

X+7th **T18.0 Foreign body in mouth**
+ **T18.1 Foreign body in esophagus**
  Excludes2: *foreign body in respiratory tract (T17.-)*
+ **T18.10 Unspecified foreign body in esophagus**
  +7th **T18.100 Unspecified foreign body in esophagus causing compression of trachea**
  Unspecified foreign body in esophagus causing obstruction of respiration
  +7th **T18.108 Unspecified foreign body in esophagus causing other injury**

+ **T18.11 Gastric contents in esophagus**
Vomitus in esophagus
+7th **T18.110 Gastric contents in esophagus causing compression of trachea**
Gastric contents in esophagus causing obstruction of respiration
+7th **T18.118 Gastric contents in esophagus causing other injury**
+ **T18.12 Food in esophagus**
Bones in esophagus
Seeds in esophagus
+7th **T18.120 Food in esophagus causing compression of trachea**
Food in esophagus causing obstruction of respiration
+7th **T18.128 Food in esophagus causing other injury**
+ **T18.19 Other foreign object in esophagus**
+7th **T18.190 Other foreign object in esophagus causing compression of trachea**
Other foreign body in esophagus causing obstruction of respiration
AHA CC: 1Q, 2015, 23-24
+7th **T18.198 Other foreign object in esophagus causing other injury**
AHA CC: 1Q, 2015, 23-24
X+7th **T18.2 Foreign body in stomach**
X+7th **T18.3 Foreign body in small intestine**
X+7th **T18.4 Foreign body in colon**
X+7th **T18.5 Foreign body in anus and rectum**
Foreign body in rectosigmoid (junction)
X+7th **T18.8 Foreign body in other parts of alimentary tract**
X+7th **T18.9 Foreign body of alimentary tract, part unspecified**
Foreign body in digestive system NOS
Swallowed foreign body NOS

T19 Foreign body in genitourinary tract

Excludes2: *complications due to implanted mesh (T83.7-)*
mechanical complications of contraceptive device (intrauterine) (vaginal) (T83.3-)
presence of contraceptive device (intrauterine) (vaginal) (Z97.5)

The appropriate 7th character is to be added to each code from category T19
A initial encounter
D subsequent encounter
S sequela

X+7th **T19.0 Foreign body in urethra**
X+7th **T19.1 Foreign body in bladder**
♀ X+7th **T19.2 Foreign body in vulva and vagina**
♀ X+7th **T19.3 Foreign body in uterus**
♂ X+7th **T19.4 Foreign body in penis**
X+7th **T19.8 Foreign body in other parts of genitourinary tract**
X+7th **T19.9 Foreign body in genitourinary tract, part unspecified**

BURNS AND CORROSIONS (T20-T32)

Includes: burns (thermal) from electrical heating appliances
burns (thermal) from electricity
burns (thermal) from flame
burns (thermal) from friction
burns (thermal) from hot air and hot gases
burns (thermal) from hot objects
burns (thermal) from lightning
burns (thermal) from radiation
chemical burn [corrosion] (external) (internal)
scalds

Excludes2: *erythema [dermatitis] ab igne (L59.0)*
radiation-related disorders of the skin and subcutaneous tissue (L55-L59)
sunburn (L55.-)

Burns and corrosions of external body surface, specified by site (T20-T25)

Includes: burns and corrosions of first degree [erythema]
burns and corrosions of second degree [blisters][epidermal loss]
burns and corrosions of third degree [deep necrosis of underlying tissue] [full- thickness skin loss]

Use additional code from category T31 or T32 to identify extent of body surface involved

Review coding guideline C.19.d

T20 Burn and corrosion of head, face, and neck

Excludes2: *burn and corrosion of ear drum (T28.41, T28.91)*
burn and corrosion of eye and adnexa (T26.-)
burn and corrosion of mouth and pharynx (T28.0)

The appropriate 7th character is to be added to each code from category T20
A initial encounter
D subsequent encounter
S sequela

+ **T20.0 Burn of unspecified degree of head, face, and neck**
Use additional external cause code to identify the source, place and intent of the burn (X00-X19, X75-X77, X96-X98, Y92)
X+7th **T20.00 Burn of unspecified degree of head, face, and neck, unspecified site**
+ **T20.01 Burn of unspecified degree of ear [any part, except ear drum]**
Excludes2: *burn of ear drum (T28.41-)*
+7th **T20.011 Burn of unspecified degree of right ear [any part, except ear drum]**
+7th **T20.012 Burn of unspecified degree of left ear [any part, except ear drum]**
+7th **T20.019 Burn of unspecified degree of unspecified ear [any part, except ear drum]**
X+7th **T20.02 Burn of unspecified degree of lip(s)**
X+7th **T20.03 Burn of unspecified degree of chin**
X+7th **T20.04 Burn of unspecified degree of nose (septum)**
X+7th **T20.05 Burn of unspecified degree of scalp [any part]**
X+7th **T20.06 Burn of unspecified degree of forehead and cheek**
X+7th **T20.07 Burn of unspecified degree of neck**
X+7th **T20.09 Burn of unspecified degree of multiple sites of head, face, and neck**
+ **T20.1 Burn of first degree of head, face, and neck**
Use additional external cause code to identify the source, place and intent of the burn (X00-X19, X75-X77, X96-X98, Y92)
X+7th **T20.10 Burn of first degree of head, face, and neck, unspecified site**
+ **T20.11 Burn of first degree of ear [any part, except ear drum]**
Excludes2: *burn of ear drum (T28.41-)*
+7th **T20.111 Burn of first degree of right ear [any part, except ear drum]**
+7th **T20.112 Burn of first degree of left ear [any part, except ear drum]**
+7th **T20.119 Burn of first degree of unspecified ear [any part, except ear drum]**
X+7th **T20.12 Burn of first degree of lip(s)**
X+7th **T20.13 Burn of first degree of chin**
X+7th **T20.14 Burn of first degree of nose (septum)**
X+7th **T20.15 Burn of first degree of scalp [any part]**
X+7th **T20.16 Burn of first degree of forehead and cheek**
X+7th **T20.17 Burn of first degree of neck**
X+7th **T20.19 Burn of first degree of multiple sites of head, face, and neck**
+ **T20.2 Burn of second degree of head, face, and neck**
Use additional external cause code to identify the source, place and intent of the burn (X00-X19, X75-X77, X96-X98, Y92)
X+7th **T20.20 Burn of second degree of head, face, and neck, unspecified site**
+ **T20.21 Burn of second degree of ear [any part, except ear drum]**
Excludes2: *burn of ear drum (T28.41-)*
+7th **T20.211 Burn of second degree of right ear [any part, except ear drum]**
+7th **T20.212 Burn of second degree of left ear [any part, except ear drum]**
+7th **T20.219 Burn of second degree of unspecified ear [any part, except ear drum]**
X+7th **T20.22 Burn of second degree of lip(s)**
X+7th **T20.23 Burn of second degree of chin**

X+7th **T20.24 Burn of second degree of nose (septum)**
X+7th **T20.25 Burn of second degree of scalp [any part]**
AHA CC: 1Q, 2015, 3-21
X+7th **T20.26 Burn of second degree of forehead and cheek**
X+7th **T20.27 Burn of second degree of neck**
X+7th **T20.29 Burn of second degree of multiple sites of head, face, and neck**

\+ **T20.3 Burn of third degree of head, face, and neck**
Use additional external cause code to identify the source, place and intent of the burn (X00-X19, X75-X77, X96-X98, Y92)

CC X+7th **T20.30 Burn of third degree of head, face, and neck, unspecified site**
CC Exclusion 7th character A see Appendix A PDX collection 1375
HAC 7th character A see Appendix B for HAC conditional logic

\+ **T20.31 Burn of third degree of ear [any part, except ear drum]**
Excludes2: *burn of ear drum (T28.41-)*

CC +7th **T20.311 Burn of third degree of right ear [any part, except ear drum]**
CC Exclusion 7th character A see Appendix A PDX collection 1376
HAC 7th character A see Appendix B for HAC conditional logic

CC +7th **T20.312 Burn of third degree of left ear [any part, except ear drum]**
CC Exclusion 7th character A see Appendix A PDX collection 1376
HAC 7th character A see Appendix B for HAC conditional logic
AHA CC: 1Q, 2015, 3-21

CC +7th **T20.319 Burn of third degree of unspecified ear [any part, except ear drum]**
CC Exclusion 7th character A see Appendix A PDX collection 1376
HAC 7th character A see Appendix B for HAC conditional logic

CC X+7th **T20.32 Burn of third degree of lip(s)**
CC Exclusion 7th character A see Appendix A PDX collection 1377
HAC 7th character A see Appendix B for HAC conditional logic

CC X+7th **T20.33 Burn of third degree of chin**
CC Exclusion 7th character A see Appendix A PDX collection 1378
HAC 7th character A see Appendix B for HAC conditional logic

CC X+7th **T20.34 Burn of third degree of nose (septum)**
CC Exclusion 7th character A see Appendix A PDX collection 1379
HAC 7th character A see Appendix B for HAC conditional logic

CC X+7th **T20.35 Burn of third degree of scalp [any part]**
CC Exclusion 7th character A see Appendix A PDX collection 1380
HAC 7th character A see Appendix B for HAC conditional logic

CC X+7th **T20.36 Burn of third degree of forehead and cheek**
CC Exclusion 7th character A see Appendix A PDX collection 1381
HAC 7th character A see Appendix B for HAC conditional logic

CC X+7th **T20.37 Burn of third degree of neck**
CC Exclusion 7th character A see Appendix A PDX collection 1382
HAC 7th character A see Appendix B for HAC conditional logic

CC X+7th **T20.39 Burn of third degree of multiple sites of head, face, and neck**
CC Exclusion 7th character A see Appendix A PDX collection 1383
HAC 7th character A see Appendix B for HAC conditional logic

\+ **T20.4 Corrosion of unspecified degree of head, face, and neck**
Code first (T51-T65) to identify chemical and intent external cause code to identify place (Y92)

X+7th **T20.40 Corrosion of unspecified degree of head, face, and neck, unspecified site**

\+ **T20.41 Corrosion of unspecified degree of ear [any part, except ear drum]**
Excludes2: *corrosion of ear drum (T28.91-)*

+7th **T20.411 Corrosion of unspecified degree of right ear [any part, except ear drum]**
+7th **T20.412 Corrosion of unspecified degree of left ear [any part, except ear drum]**
+7th **T20.419 Corrosion of unspecified degree of unspecified ear [any part, except ear drum]**

X+7th **T20.42 Corrosion of unspecified degree of lip(s)**
X+7th **T20.43 Corrosion of unspecified degree of chin**
X+7th **T20.44 Corrosion of unspecified degree of nose (septum)**
X+7th **T20.45 Corrosion of unspecified degree of scalp [any part]**
X+7th **T20.46 Corrosion of unspecified degree of forehead and cheek**
X+7th **T20.47 Corrosion of unspecified degree of neck**
X+7th **T20.49 Corrosion of unspecified degree of multiple sites of head, face, and neck**

\+ **T20.5 Corrosion of first degree of head, face, and neck**
Code first (T51-T65) to identify chemical and intent

Use additional external cause code to identify place (Y92)

X+7th **T20.50 Corrosion of first degree of head, face, and neck, unspecified site**

\+ **T20.51 Corrosion of first degree of ear [any part, except ear drum]**
Excludes2: *corrosion of ear drum (T28.91-)*

+7th **T20.511 Corrosion of first degree of right ear [any part, except ear drum]**
+7th **T20.512 Corrosion of first degree of left ear [any part, except ear drum]**
+7th **T20.519 Corrosion of first degree of unspecified ear [any part, except ear drum]**

X+7th **T20.52 Corrosion of first degree of lip(s)**
X+7th **T20.53 Corrosion of first degree of chin**
X+7th **T20.54 Corrosion of first degree of nose (septum)**
X+7th **T20.55 Corrosion of first degree of scalp [any part]**
X+7th **T20.56 Corrosion of first degree of forehead and cheek**
X+7th **T20.57 Corrosion of first degree of neck**
X+7th **T20.59 Corrosion of first degree of multiple sites of head, face, and neck**

\+ **T20.6 Corrosion of second degree of head, face, and neck**
Code first (T51-T65) to identify chemical and intent

Use additional external cause code to identify place (Y92)

X+7th **T20.60 Corrosion of second degree of head, face, and neck, unspecified site**

\+ **T20.61 Corrosion of second degree of ear [any part, except ear drum]**
Excludes2: *corrosion of ear drum (T28.91-)*

+7th **T20.611 Corrosion of second degree of right ear [any part, except ear drum]**
+7th **T20.612 Corrosion of second degree of left ear [any part, except ear drum]**
+7th **T20.619 Corrosion of second degree of unspecified ear [any part, except ear drum]**

X+7th **T20.62 Corrosion of second degree of lip(s)**
X+7th **T20.63 Corrosion of second degree of chin**
X+7th **T20.64 Corrosion of second degree of nose (septum)**
X+7th **T20.65 Corrosion of second degree of scalp [any part]**
X+7th **T20.66 Corrosion of second degree of forehead and cheek**
X+7th **T20.67 Corrosion of second degree of neck**
X+7th **T20.69 Corrosion of second degree of multiple sites of head, face, and neck**

\+ **T20.7 Corrosion of third degree of head, face, and neck**
Code first (T51-T65) to identify chemical and intent

Use additional external cause code to identify place (Y92)

CC X+7th **T20.70 Corrosion of third degree of head, face, and neck, unspecified site**
CC Exclusion 7th character A see Appendix A PDX collection 1375
HAC 7th character A see Appendix B for HAC conditional logic

\+ **T20.71 Corrosion of third degree of ear [any part, except ear drum]**
Excludes2: *corrosion of ear drum (T28.91-)*
CC +7th **T20.711 Corrosion of third degree of right ear [any part, except ear drum]**
CC Exclusion 7th character A see Appendix A PDX collection 1376
HAC 7th character A see Appendix B for HAC conditional logic
CC +7th **T20.712 Corrosion of third degree of left ear [any part, except ear drum]**
CC Exclusion 7th character A see Appendix A PDX collection 1376
HAC 7th character A see Appendix B for HAC conditional logic
CC +7th **T20.719 Corrosion of third degree of unspecified ear [any part, except ear drum]**
CC Exclusion 7th character A see Appendix A PDX collection 1376
HAC 7th character A see Appendix B for HAC conditional logic
CC X+7th **T20.72 Corrosion of third degree of lip(s)**
CC Exclusion 7th character A see Appendix A PDX collection 1377
HAC 7th character A see Appendix B for HAC conditional logic
CC X+7th **T20.73 Corrosion of third degree of chin**
CC Exclusion 7th character A see Appendix A PDX collection 1378
HAC 7th character A see Appendix B for HAC conditional logic
CC X+7th **T20.74 Corrosion of third degree of nose (septum)**
CC Exclusion 7th character A see Appendix A PDX collection 1379
HAC 7th character A see Appendix B for HAC conditional logic
CC X+7th **T20.75 Corrosion of third degree of scalp [any part]**
CC Exclusion 7th character A see Appendix A PDX collection 1380
HAC 7th character A see Appendix B for HAC conditional logic
CC X+7th **T20.76 Corrosion of third degree of forehead and cheek**
CC Exclusion 7th character A see Appendix A PDX collection 1381
HAC 7th character A see Appendix B for HAC conditional logic
CC X+7th **T20.77 Corrosion of third degree of neck**
CC Exclusion 7th character A see Appendix A PDX collection 1382
HAC 7th character A see Appendix B for HAC conditional logic
CC X+7th **T20.79 Corrosion of third degree of multiple sites of head, face, and neck**
CC Exclusion 7th character A see Appendix A PDX collection 1383
HAC 7th character A see Appendix B for HAC conditional logic

T21 Burn and corrosion of trunk

Includes: burns and corrosion of hip region
Excludes2: *burns and corrosion of axilla (T22.- with fifth character 4)*
burns and corrosion of scapular region (T22.- with fifth character 6)
burns and corrosion of shoulder (T22.- with fifth character 5)

The appropriate 7th character is to be added to each code from category T21
A initial encounter
D subsequent encounter
S sequela

\+ **T21.0 Burn of unspecified degree of trunk**
Use external cause code to identify the source, place and intent of the burn (X00-X19, X75-X77, X96-X98, Y92)
X+7th **T21.00 Burn of unspecified degree of trunk, unspecified site**
X+7th **T21.01 Burn of unspecified degree of chest wall**
Burn of of unspecified degree of breast
X+7th **T21.02 Burn of unspecified degree of abdominal wall**
Burn of unspecified degree of flank
Burn of unspecified degree of groin
X+7th **T21.03 Burn of unspecified degree of upper back**
Burn of unspecified degree of interscapular region
X+7th **T21.04 Burn of unspecified degree of lower back**
X+7th **T21.05 Burn of unspecified degree of buttock**
Burn of unspecified degree of anus
♂ X+7th **T21.06 Burn of unspecified degree of male genital region**
Burn of unspecified degree of penis
Burn of unspecified degree of scrotum
Burn of unspecified degree of testis
♀ X+7th **T21.07 Burn of unspecified degree of female genital region**
Burn of unspecified degree of labium (majus) (minus)
Burn of unspecified degree of perineum
Burn of unspecified degree of vulva
Excludes2: *burn of vagina (T28.3)*
X+7th **T21.09 Burn of unspecified degree of other site of trunk**
\+ **T21.1 Burn of first degree of trunk**
Use external cause code to identify the source, place and intent of the burn (X00-X19, X75-X77, X96-X98, Y92)
X+7th **T21.10 Burn of first degree of trunk, unspecified site**
X+7th **T21.11 Burn of first degree of chest wall**
Burn of first degree of breast
X+7th **T21.12 Burn of first degree of abdominal wall**
Burn of first degree of flank
Burn of first degree of groin
X+7th **T21.13 Burn of first degree of upper back**
Burn of first degree of interscapular region
X+7th **T21.14 Burn of first degree of lower back**
X+7th **T21.15 Burn of first degree of buttock**
Burn of first degree of anus
♂ X+7th **T21.16 Burn of first degree of male genital region**
Burn of first degree of penis
Burn of first degree of scrotum
Burn of first degree of testis
♀ X+7th **T21.17 Burn of first degree of female genital region**
Burn of first degree of labium (majus) (minus)
Burn of first degree of perineum
Burn of first degree of vulva
Excludes2: *burn of vagina (T28.3)*
X+7th **T21.19 Burn of first degree of other site of trunk**
\+ **T21.2 Burn of second degree of trunk**
Use external cause code to identify the source, place and intent of the burn (X00-X19, X75-X77, X96-X98, Y92)
X+7th **T21.20 Burn of second degree of trunk, unspecified site**
X+7th **T21.21 Burn of second degree of chest wall**
Burn of second degree of breast
X+7th **T21.22 Burn of second degree of abdominal wall**
Burn of second degree of flank
Burn of second degree of groin
X+7th **T21.23 Burn of second degree of upper back**
Burn of second degree of interscapular region
X+7th **T21.24 Burn of second degree of lower back**
X+7th **T21.25 Burn of second degree of buttock**
Burn of second degree of anus
♂ X+7th **T21.26 Burn of second degree of male genital region**
Burn of second degree of penis
Burn of second degree of scrotum
Burn of second degree of testis
♀ X+7th **T21.27 Burn of second degree of female genital region**
Burn of second degree of labium (majus) (minus)
Burn of second degree of perineum
Burn of second degree of vulva
Excludes2: *burn of vagina (T28.3)*
X+7th **T21.29 Burn of second degree of other site of trunk**
\+ **T21.3 Burn of third degree of trunk**
Use additional external cause code to identify the source, place and intent of the burn (X00-X19, X75-X77, X96-X98, Y92)
CC X+7th **T21.30 Burn of third degree of trunk, unspecified site**
CC Exclusion 7th character A see Appendix A PDX collection 1384
HAC 7th character A see Appendix B for HAC conditional logic
CC X+7th **T21.31 Burn of third degree of chest wall**
Burn of third degree of breast
CC Exclusion 7th character A see Appendix A PDX collection 1385
AHA CC: 2Q, 2016, 5-6
HAC 7th character A see Appendix B for HAC conditional logic
CC X+7th **T21.32 Burn of third degree of abdominal wall**
Burn of third degree of flank
Burn of third degree of groin
CC Exclusion 7th character A see Appendix A PDX collection 1386
HAC 7th character A see Appendix B for HAC conditional logic

CC X+7th **T21.33 Burn of third degree of upper back**
Burn of third degree of interscapular region
CC Exclusion 7th character A see Appendix A PDX collection 1387
HAC 7th character A see Appendix B for HAC conditional logic

CC X+7th **T21.34 Burn of third degree of lower back**
CC Exclusion 7th character A see Appendix A PDX collection 1387
HAC 7th character A see Appendix B for HAC conditional logic

CC X+7th **T21.35 Burn of third degree of buttock**
Burn of third degree of anus
CC Exclusion 7th character A see Appendix A PDX collection 1387
HAC 7th character A see Appendix B for HAC conditional logic

CC X+7th **T21.36 Burn of third degree of male genital region**
Burn of third degree of penis
Burn of third degree of scrotum
Burn of third degree of testis
CC Exclusion 7th character A see Appendix A PDX collection 1388
HAC 7th character A see Appendix B for HAC conditional logic

CC X+7th **T21.37 Burn of third degree of female genital region**
Burn of third degree of labium (majus) (minus)
Burn of third degree of perineum
Burn of third degree of vulva
Excludes2: *burn of vagina (T28.3)*
CC Exclusion 7th character A see Appendix A PDX collection 1388
HAC 7th character A see Appendix B for HAC conditional logic

CC X+7th **T21.39 Burn of third degree of other site of trunk**
CC Exclusion 7th character A see Appendix A PDX collection 1384
HAC 7th character A see Appendix B for HAC conditional logic

\+ **T21.4 Corrosion of unspecified degree of trunk**
Code first (T51-T65) to identify chemical and intent

Use additional external cause code to identify place (Y92)

X+7th **T21.40 Corrosion of unspecified degree of trunk, unspecified site**
X+7th **T21.41 Corrosion of unspecified degree of chest wall**
Corrosion of unspecified degree of breast
X+7th **T21.42 Corrosion of unspecified degree of abdominal wall**
Corrosion of unspecified degree of flank
Corrosion of unspecified degree of groin
X+7th **T21.43 Corrosion of unspecified degree of upper back**
Corrosion of unspecified degree of interscapular region
X+7th **T21.44 Corrosion of unspecified degree of lower back**
X+7th **T21.45 Corrosion of unspecified degree of buttock**
Corrosion of unspecified degree of anus
♂ X+7th **T21.46 Corrosion of unspecified degree of male genital region**
Corrosion of unspecified degree of penis
Corrosion of unspecified degree of scrotum
Corrosion of unspecified degree of testis
♀ X+7th **T21.47 Corrosion of unspecified degree of female genital region**
Corrosion of unspecified degree of labium (majus) (minus)
Corrosion of unspecified degree of perineum
Corrosion of unspecified degree of vulva
Excludes2: *corrosion of vagina (T28.8)*
X+7th **T21.49 Corrosion of unspecified degree of other site of trunk**

\+ **T21.5 Corrosion of first degree of trunk**
Code first (T51-T65) to identify chemical and intent

Use additional external cause code to identify place (Y92)

X+7th **T21.50 Corrosion of first degree of trunk, unspecified site**
X+7th **T21.51 Corrosion of first degree of chest wall**
Corrosion of first degree of breast
X+7th **T21.52 Corrosion of first degree of abdominal wall**
Corrosion of first degree of flank
Corrosion of first degree of groin
X+7th **T21.53 Corrosion of first degree of upper back**
Corrosion of first degree of interscapular region
X+7th **T21.54 Corrosion of first degree of lower back**
X+7th **T21.55 Corrosion of first degree of buttock**
Corrosion of first degree of anus
♂ X+7th **T21.56 Corrosion of first degree of male genital region**
Corrosion of first degree of penis
Corrosion of first degree of scrotum
Corrosion of first degree of testis
♀ X+7th **T21.57 Corrosion of first degree of female genital region**
Corrosion of first degree of labium (majus) (minus)
Corrosion of first degree of perineum
Corrosion of first degree of vulva
Excludes2: *corrosion of vagina (T28.8)*
X+7th **T21.59 Corrosion of first degree of other site of trunk**

\+ **T21.6 Corrosion of second degree of trunk**
Code first (T51-T65) to identify chemical and intent

Use additional external cause code to identify place (Y92)

X+7th **T21.60 Corrosion of second degree of trunk, unspecified site**
X+7th **T21.61 Corrosion of second degree of chest wall**
Corrosion of second degree of breast
X+7th **T21.62 Corrosion of second degree of abdominal wall**
Corrosion of second degree of flank
Corrosion of second degree of groin
X+7th **T21.63 Corrosion of second degree of upper back**
Corrosion of second degree of interscapular region
X+7th **T21.64 Corrosion of second degree of lower back**
X+7th **T21.65 Corrosion of second degree of buttock**
Corrosion of second degree of anus
♂ X+7th **T21.66 Corrosion of second degree of male genital region**
Corrosion of second degree of penis
Corrosion of second degree of scrotum
Corrosion of second degree of testis
♀ X+7th **T21.67 Corrosion of second degree of female genital region**
Corrosion of second degree of labium (majus) (minus)
Corrosion of second degree of perineum
Corrosion of second degree of vulva
Excludes2: *corrosion of vagina (T28.8)*
X+7th **T21.69 Corrosion of second degree of other site of trunk**

\+ **T21.7 Corrosion of third degree of trunk**
Code first (T51-T65) to identify chemical and intent

Use additional external cause code to identify place (Y92)

CC X+7th **T21.70 Corrosion of third degree of trunk, unspecified site**
CC Exclusion 7th character A see Appendix A PDX collection 1384
HAC 7th character A see Appendix B for HAC conditional logic

CC X+7th **T21.71 Corrosion of third degree of chest wall**
Corrosion of third degree of breast
CC Exclusion 7th character A see Appendix A PDX collection 1385
HAC 7th character A see Appendix B for HAC conditional logic

CC X+7th **T21.72 Corrosion of third degree of abdominal wall**
Corrosion of third degree of flank
Corrosion of third degree of groin
CC Exclusion 7th character A see Appendix A PDX collection 1386
HAC 7th character A see Appendix B for HAC conditional logic

CC X+7th **T21.73 Corrosion of third degree of upper back**
Corrosion of third degree of interscapular region
CC Exclusion 7th character A see Appendix A PDX collection 1387
HAC 7th character A see Appendix B for HAC conditional logic

CC X+7th **T21.74 Corrosion of third degree of lower back**
CC Exclusion 7th character A see Appendix A PDX collection 1387
HAC 7th character A see Appendix B for HAC conditional logic

CC X+7th **T21.75 Corrosion of third degree of buttock**
Corrosion of third degree of anus
CC Exclusion 7th character A see Appendix A PDX collection 1387
HAC 7th character A see Appendix B for HAC conditional logic

CC X+7th **T21.76 Corrosion of third degree of male genital region**
Corrosion of third degree of penis
Corrosion of third degree of scrotum
Corrosion of third degree of testis
CC Exclusion 7th character A see Appendix A PDX collection 1388
HAC 7th character A see Appendix B for HAC conditional logic

CC X+7th **T21.77 Corrosion of third degree of female genital region**
Corrosion of third degree of labium (majus) (minus)
Corrosion of third degree of perineum
Corrosion of third degree of vulva
Excludes2: *corrosion of vagina (T28.8)*
CC Exclusion 7th character A see Appendix A PDX collection 1388
HAC 7th character A see Appendix B for HAC conditional logic

CC X+7th **T21.79 Corrosion of third degree of other site of trunk**
CC Exclusion 7th character A see Appendix A PDX collection 1384
HAC 7th character A see Appendix B for HAC conditional logic

T22 Burn and corrosion of shoulder and upper limb, except wrist and hand

Excludes2: *burn and corrosion of interscapular region (T21.-)*
burn and corrosion of wrist and hand (T23.-)

The appropriate 7th character is to be added to each code from category T22
A initial encounter
D subsequent encounter
S sequela

+ **T22.0 Burn of unspecified degree of shoulder and upper limb, except wrist and hand**
Use additional external cause code to identify the source, place and intent of the burn (X00-X19, X75-X77, X96-X98, Y92)
X+7th **T22.00 Burn of unspecified degree of shoulder and upper limb, except wrist and hand, unspecified site**
+ **T22.01 Burn of unspecified degree of forearm**
+7th **T22.011 Burn of unspecified degree of right forearm**
+7th **T22.012 Burn of unspecified degree of left forearm**
+7th **T22.019 Burn of unspecified degree of unspecified forearm**
+ **T22.02 Burn of unspecified degree of elbow**
+7th **T22.021 Burn of unspecified degree of right elbow**
+7th **T22.022 Burn of unspecified degree of left elbow**
+7th **T22.029 Burn of unspecified degree of unspecified elbow**
+ **T22.03 Burn of unspecified degree of upper arm**
+7th **T22.031 Burn of unspecified degree of right upper arm**
+7th **T22.032 Burn of unspecified degree of left upper arm**
+7th **T22.039 Burn of unspecified degree of unspecified upper arm**
+ **T22.04 Burn of unspecified degree of axilla**
+7th **T22.041 Burn of unspecified degree of right axilla**
+7th **T22.042 Burn of unspecified degree of left axilla**
+7th **T22.049 Burn of unspecified degree of unspecified axilla**
+ **T22.05 Burn of unspecified degree of shoulder**
+7th **T22.051 Burn of unspecified degree of right shoulder**
+7th **T22.052 Burn of unspecified degree of left shoulder**
+7th **T22.059 Burn of unspecified degree of unspecified shoulder**
+ **T22.06 Burn of unspecified degree of scapular region**
+7th **T22.061 Burn of unspecified degree of right scapular region**
+7th **T22.062 Burn of unspecified degree of left scapular region**
+7th **T22.069 Burn of unspecified degree of unspecified scapular region**
+ **T22.09 Burn of unspecified degree of multiple sites of shoulder and upper limb, except wrist and hand**
+7th **T22.091 Burn of unspecified degree of multiple sites of right shoulder and upper limb, except wrist and hand**
+7th **T22.092 Burn of unspecified degree of multiple sites of left shoulder and upper limb, except wrist and hand**
+7th **T22.099 Burn of unspecified degree of multiple sites of unspecified shoulder and upper limb, except wrist and hand**

+ **T22.1 Burn of first degree of shoulder and upper limb, except wrist and hand**
Use additional external cause code to identify the source, place and intent of the burn (X00-X19, X75-X77, X96-X98, Y92)
X+7th **T22.10 Burn of first degree of shoulder and upper limb, except wrist and hand, unspecified site**
+ **T22.11 Burn of first degree of forearm**
+7th **T22.111 Burn of first degree of right forearm**
+7th **T22.112 Burn of first degree of left forearm**
+7th **T22.119 Burn of first degree of unspecified forearm**
+ **T22.12 Burn of first degree of elbow**
+7th **T22.121 Burn of first degree of right elbow**
+7th **T22.122 Burn of first degree of left elbow**
+7th **T22.129 Burn of first degree of unspecified elbow**
+ **T22.13 Burn of first degree of upper arm**
+7th **T22.131 Burn of first degree of right upper arm**
+7th **T22.132 Burn of first degree of left upper arm**
+7th **T22.139 Burn of first degree of unspecified upper arm**
+ **T22.14 Burn of first degree of axilla**
+7th **T22.141 Burn of first degree of right axilla**
+7th **T22.142 Burn of first degree of left axilla**
+7th **T22.149 Burn of first degree of unspecified axilla**
+ **T22.15 Burn of first degree of shoulder**
+7th **T22.151 Burn of first degree of right shoulder**
+7th **T22.152 Burn of first degree of left shoulder**
+7th **T22.159 Burn of first degree of unspecified shoulder**
+ **T22.16 Burn of first degree of scapular region**
+7th **T22.161 Burn of first degree of right scapular region**
+7th **T22.162 Burn of first degree of left scapular region**
+7th **T22.169 Burn of first degree of unspecified scapular region**
+ **T22.19 Burn of first degree of multiple sites of shoulder and upper limb, except wrist and hand**
+7th **T22.191 Burn of first degree of multiple sites of right shoulder and upper limb, except wrist and hand**
+7th **T22.192 Burn of first degree of multiple sites of left shoulder and upper limb, except wrist and hand**
+7th **T22.199 Burn of first degree of multiple sites of unspecified shoulder and upper limb, except wrist and hand**

+ **T22.2 Burn of second degree of shoulder and upper limb, except wrist and hand**
Use additional external cause code to identify the source, place and intent of the burn (X00-X19, X75-X77, X96-X98, Y92)
X+7th **T22.20 Burn of second degree of shoulder and upper limb, except wrist and hand, unspecified site**
+ **T22.21 Burn of second degree of forearm**
+7th **T22.211 Burn of second degree of right forearm**
+7th **T22.212 Burn of second degree of left forearm**
+7th **T22.219 Burn of second degree of unspecified forearm**
+ **T22.22 Burn of second degree of elbow**
+7th **T22.221 Burn of second degree of right elbow**
+7th **T22.222 Burn of second degree of left elbow**
+7th **T22.229 Burn of second degree of unspecified elbow**
+ **T22.23 Burn of second degree of upper arm**
+7th **T22.231 Burn of second degree of right upper arm**
+7th **T22.232 Burn of second degree of left upper arm**
+7th **T22.239 Burn of second degree of unspecified upper arm**
+ **T22.24 Burn of second degree of axilla**
+7th **T22.241 Burn of second degree of right axilla**
+7th **T22.242 Burn of second degree of left axilla**
+7th **T22.249 Burn of second degree of unspecified axilla**
+ **T22.25 Burn of second degree of shoulder**
+7th **T22.251 Burn of second degree of right shoulder**
+7th **T22.252 Burn of second degree of left shoulder**
+7th **T22.259 Burn of second degree of unspecified shoulder**
+ **T22.26 Burn of second degree of scapular region**
+7th **T22.261 Burn of second degree of right scapular region**
+7th **T22.262 Burn of second degree of left scapular region**
+7th **T22.269 Burn of second degree of unspecified scapular region**

+ **T22.29 Burn of second degree of multiple sites of shoulder and upper limb, except wrist and hand**
  - +7th **T22.291 Burn of second degree of multiple sites of right shoulder and upper limb, except wrist and hand**
  - +7th **T22.292 Burn of second degree of multiple sites of left shoulder and upper limb, except wrist and hand**
  - +7th **T22.299 Burn of second degree of multiple sites of unspecified shoulder and upper limb, except wrist and hand**

+ **T22.3 Burn of third degree of shoulder and upper limb, except wrist and hand**

Use additional external cause code to identify the source, place and intent of the burn (X00-X19, X75-X77, X96-X98, Y92)

CC X+7th **T22.30 Burn of third degree of shoulder and upper limb, except wrist and hand, unspecified site**
CC Exclusion 7th character A see Appendix A PDX collection 1389
HAC 7th character A see Appendix B for HAC conditional logic

+ **T22.31 Burn of third degree of forearm**

CC +7th **T22.311 Burn of third degree of right forearm**
CC Exclusion 7th character A see Appendix A PDX collection 1390
HAC 7th character A see Appendix B for HAC conditional logic

CC +7th **T22.312 Burn of third degree of left forearm**
CC Exclusion 7th character A see Appendix A PDX collection 1390
HAC 7th character A see Appendix B for HAC conditional logic

CC +7th **T22.319 Burn of third degree of unspecified forearm**
CC Exclusion 7th character A see Appendix A PDX collection 1390
HAC 7th character A see Appendix B for HAC conditional logic

+ **T22.32 Burn of third degree of elbow**

CC +7th **T22.321 Burn of third degree of right elbow**
CC Exclusion 7th character A see Appendix A PDX collection 1391
HAC 7th character A see Appendix B for HAC conditional logic

CC +7th **T22.322 Burn of third degree of left elbow**
CC Exclusion 7th character A see Appendix A PDX collection 1391
HAC 7th character A see Appendix B for HAC conditional logic

CC +7th **T22.329 Burn of third degree of unspecified elbow**
CC Exclusion 7th character A see Appendix A PDX collection 1391
HAC 7th character A see Appendix B for HAC conditional logic

+ **T22.33 Burn of third degree of upper arm**

CC +7th **T22.331 Burn of third degree of right upper arm**
CC Exclusion 7th character A see Appendix A PDX collection 1392
HAC 7th character A see Appendix B for HAC conditional logic

CC +7th **T22.332 Burn of third degree of left upper arm**
CC Exclusion 7th character A see Appendix A PDX collection 1392
HAC 7th character A see Appendix B for HAC conditional logic

CC +7th **T22.339 Burn of third degree of unspecified upper arm**
CC Exclusion 7th character A see Appendix A PDX collection 1392
HAC 7th character A see Appendix B for HAC conditional logic

+ **T22.34 Burn of third degree of axilla**

CC +7th **T22.341 Burn of third degree of right axilla**
CC Exclusion 7th character A see Appendix A PDX collection 1393
HAC 7th character A see Appendix B for HAC conditional logic

CC +7th **T22.342 Burn of third degree of left axilla**
CC Exclusion 7th character A see Appendix A PDX collection 1393
HAC 7th character A see Appendix B for HAC conditional logic

CC +7th **T22.349 Burn of third degree of unspecified axilla**
CC Exclusion 7th character A see Appendix A PDX collection 1393
HAC 7th character A see Appendix B for HAC conditional logic

+ **T22.35 Burn of third degree of shoulder**

CC +7th **T22.351 Burn of third degree of right shoulder**
CC Exclusion 7th character A see Appendix A PDX collection 1394
HAC 7th character A see Appendix B for HAC conditional logic

CC +7th **T22.352 Burn of third degree of left shoulder**
CC Exclusion 7th character A see Appendix A PDX collection 1394
HAC 7th character A see Appendix B for HAC conditional logic

CC +7th **T22.359 Burn of third degree of unspecified shoulder**
CC Exclusion 7th character A see Appendix A PDX collection 1394
HAC 7th character A see Appendix B for HAC conditional logic

+ **T22.36 Burn of third degree of scapular region**

CC +7th **T22.361 Burn of third degree of right scapular regi**
CC Exclusion 7th character A see Appendix A PDX collection 1395
HAC 7th character A see Appendix B for HAC conditional logic

CC +7th **T22.362 Burn of third degree of left scapular regi**
CC Exclusion 7th character A see Appendix A PDX collection 1395
HAC 7th character A see Appendix B for HAC conditional logic

CC +7th **T22.369 Burn of third degree of unspecified scapular region**
CC Exclusion 7th character A see Appendix A PDX collection 1395
HAC 7th character A see Appendix B for HAC conditional logic

+ **T22.39 Burn of third degree of multiple sites of shoulder and upper limb, except wrist and hand**

CC +7th **T22.391 Burn of third degree of multiple sites of right shoulder and upper limb, except wrist and hand**
CC Exclusion 7th character A see Appendix A PDX collection 1389
HAC 7th character A see Appendix B for HAC conditional logic

CC +7th **T22.392 Burn of third degree of multiple sites of l shoulder and upper limb, except wrist an hand**
CC Exclusion 7th character A see Appendix A PDX collection 1389
HAC 7th character A see Appendix B for HAC conditional logic

CC +7th **T22.399 Burn of third degree of multiple sites of unspecified shoulder and upper limb, except wrist and hand**
CC Exclusion 7th character A see Appendix A PDX collection 1389
HAC 7th character A see Appendix B for HAC conditional logic

+ **T22.4 Corrosion of unspecified degree of shoulder and upper limb, except wrist and hand**

Code first (T51-T65) to identify chemical and intent

Use additional external cause code to identify place (Y92)

X+7th **T22.40 Corrosion of unspecified degree of shoulder and upper limb, except wrist and hand, unspecified sit**

+ **T22.41 Corrosion of unspecified degree of forearm**
  - +7th **T22.411 Corrosion of unspecified degree of right forearm**
  - +7th **T22.412 Corrosion of unspecified degree of left forearm**
  - +7th **T22.419 Corrosion of unspecified degree of unspecified forearm**

+ **T22.42 Corrosion of unspecified degree of elbow**
  - +7th **T22.421 Corrosion of unspecified degree of right elbow**
  - +7th **T22.422 Corrosion of unspecified degree of left elbow**
  - +7th **T22.429 Corrosion of unspecified degree of unspecified elbow**

+ T22.43 Corrosion of unspecified degree of upper arm
 +7th T22.431 Corrosion of unspecified degree of right upper arm
 +7th T22.432 Corrosion of unspecified degree of left upper arm
 +7th T22.439 Corrosion of unspecified degree of unspecified upper arm
+ T22.44 Corrosion of unspecified degree of axilla
 +7th T22.441 Corrosion of unspecified degree of right axilla
 +7th T22.442 Corrosion of unspecified degree of left axilla
 +7th T22.449 Corrosion of unspecified degree of unspecified axilla
+ T22.45 Corrosion of unspecified degree of shoulder
 +7th T22.451 Corrosion of unspecified degree of right shoulder
 +7th T22.452 Corrosion of unspecified degree of left shoulder
 +7th T22.459 Corrosion of unspecified degree of unspecified shoulder
+ T22.46 Corrosion of unspecified degree of scapular region
 +7th T22.461 Corrosion of unspecified degree of right scapular region
 +7th T22.462 Corrosion of unspecified degree of left scapular region
 +7th T22.469 Corrosion of unspecified degree of unspecified scapular region
+ T22.49 Corrosion of unspecified degree of multiple sites of shoulder and upper limb, except wrist and hand
 +7th T22.491 Corrosion of unspecified degree of multiple sites of right shoulder and upper limb, except wrist and hand
 +7th T22.492 Corrosion of unspecified degree of multiple sites of left shoulder and upper limb, except wrist and hand
 +7th T22.499 Corrosion of unspecified degree of multiple sites of unspecified shoulder and upper limb, except wrist and hand
+ T22.5 Corrosion of first degree of shoulder and upper limb, except wrist and hand
 Code first (T51-T65) to identify chemical and intent

 Use additional external cause code to identify place (Y92)
X+7th T22.50 Corrosion of first degree of shoulder and upper limb, except wrist and hand unspecified site
+ T22.51 Corrosion of first degree of forearm
 +7th T22.511 Corrosion of first degree of right forearm
 +7th T22.512 Corrosion of first degree of left forearm
 +7th T22.519 Corrosion of first degree of unspecified forearm
+ T22.52 Corrosion of first degree of elbow
 +7th T22.521 Corrosion of first degree of right elbow
 +7th T22.522 Corrosion of first degree of left elbow
 +7th T22.529 Corrosion of first degree of unspecified elbow
+ T22.53 Corrosion of first degree of upper arm
 +7th T22.531 Corrosion of first degree of right upper arm
 +7th T22.532 Corrosion of first degree of left upper arm
 +7th T22.539 Corrosion of first degree of unspecified upper arm
+ T22.54 Corrosion of first degree of axilla
 +7th T22.541 Corrosion of first degree of right axilla
 +7th T22.542 Corrosion of first degree of left axilla
 +7th T22.549 Corrosion of first degree of unspecified axilla
+ T22.55 Corrosion of first degree of shoulder
 +7th T22.551 Corrosion of first degree of right shoulder
 +7th T22.552 Corrosion of first degree of left shoulder
 +7th T22.559 Corrosion of first degree of unspecified shoulder
+ T22.56 Corrosion of first degree of scapular region
 +7th T22.561 Corrosion of first degree of right scapular region
 +7th T22.562 Corrosion of first degree of left scapular region
 +7th T22.569 Corrosion of first degree of unspecified scapular region
+ T22.59 Corrosion of first degree of multiple sites of shoulder and upper limb, except wrist and hand
 +7th T22.591 Corrosion of first degree of multiple sites of right shoulder and upper limb, except wrist and hand
 +7th T22.592 Corrosion of first degree of multiple sites of left shoulder and upper limb, except wrist and hand
 +7th T22.599 Corrosion of first degree of multiple sites of unspecified shoulder and upper limb, except wrist and hand
+ T22.6 Corrosion of second degree of shoulder and upper limb, except wrist and hand
 Code first (T51-T65) to identify chemical and intent

 Use additional external cause code to identify place (Y92)
X+7th T22.60 Corrosion of second degree of shoulder and upper limb, except wrist and hand, unspecified site
+ T22.61 Corrosion of second degree of forearm
 +7th T22.611 Corrosion of second degree of right forearm
 +7th T22.612 Corrosion of second degree of left forearm
 +7th T22.619 Corrosion of second degree of unspecified forearm
+ T22.62 Corrosion of second degree of elbow
 +7th T22.621 Corrosion of second degree of right elbow
 +7th T22.622 Corrosion of second degree of left elbow
 +7th T22.629 Corrosion of second degree of unspecified elbow
+ T22.63 Corrosion of second degree of upper arm
 +7th T22.631 Corrosion of second degree of right upper arm
 +7th T22.632 Corrosion of second degree of left upper arm
 +7th T22.639 Corrosion of second degree of unspecified upper arm
+ T22.64 Corrosion of second degree of axilla
 +7th T22.641 Corrosion of second degree of right axilla
 +7th T22.642 Corrosion of second degree of left axilla
 +7th T22.649 Corrosion of second degree of unspecified axilla
+ T22.65 Corrosion of second degree of shoulder
 +7th T22.651 Corrosion of second degree of right shoulder
 +7th T22.652 Corrosion of second degree of left shoulder
 +7th T22.659 Corrosion of second degree of unspecified shoulder
+ T22.66 Corrosion of second degree of scapular region
 +7th T22.661 Corrosion of second degree of right scapular region
 +7th T22.662 Corrosion of second degree of left scapular region
 +7th T22.669 Corrosion of second degree of unspecified scapular region
+ T22.69 Corrosion of second degree of multiple sites of shoulder and upper limb, except wrist and hand
 +7th T22.691 Corrosion of second degree of multiple sites of right shoulder and upper limb, except wrist and hand
 +7th T22.692 Corrosion of second degree of multiple sites of left shoulder and upper limb, except wrist and hand
 +7th T22.699 Corrosion of second degree of multiple sites of unspecified shoulder and upper limb, except wrist and hand
+ T22.7 Corrosion of third degree of shoulder and upper limb, except wrist and hand
 Code first (T51-T65) to identify chemical and intent external cause code to identify place (Y92)
CC X+7th T22.70 Corrosion of third degree of shoulder and upper limb, except wrist and hand, unspecified site
 CC Exclusion 7th character A see Appendix A PDX collection 1389
 HAC 7th character A see Appendix B for HAC conditional logic
+ T22.71 Corrosion of third degree of forearm
 CC +7th T22.711 Corrosion of third degree of right forearm
 CC Exclusion 7th character A see Appendix A PDX collection 1390
 HAC 7th character A see Appendix B for HAC conditional logic

CC +7th **T22.712 Corrosion of third degree of left forearm**
CC Exclusion 7th character A see Appendix A
PDX collection 1390
HAC 7th character A see Appendix B for HAC conditional logic

CC +7th **T22.719 Corrosion of third degree of unspecified forearm**
CC Exclusion 7th character A see Appendix A
PDX collection 1390
HAC 7th character A see Appendix B for HAC conditional logic

+ **T22.72 Corrosion of third degree of elbow**

CC +7th **T22.721 Corrosion of third degree of right elbow**
CC Exclusion 7th character A see Appendix A
PDX collection 1391
HAC 7th character A see Appendix B for HAC conditional logic

CC +7th **T22.722 Corrosion of third degree of left elbow**
CC Exclusion 7th character A see Appendix A
PDX collection 1391
HAC 7th character A see Appendix B for HAC conditional logic

CC +7th **T22.729 Corrosion of third degree of unspecified elbow**
CC Exclusion 7th character A see Appendix A
PDX collection 1391
HAC 7th character A see Appendix B for HAC conditional logic

+ **T22.73 Corrosion of third degree of upper arm**

CC +7th **T22.731 Corrosion of third degree of right upper arm**
CC Exclusion 7th character A see Appendix A
PDX collection 1392
HAC 7th character A see Appendix B for HAC conditional logic

CC +7th **T22.732 Corrosion of third degree of left upper arm**
CC Exclusion 7th character A see Appendix A
PDX collection 1392
HAC 7th character A see Appendix B for HAC conditional logic

CC +7th **T22.739 Corrosion of third degree of unspecified upper arm**
CC Exclusion 7th character A see Appendix A
PDX collection 1392
HAC 7th character A see Appendix B for HAC conditional logic

+ **T22.74 Corrosion of third degree of axilla**

CC +7th **T22.741 Corrosion of third degree of right axilla**
CC Exclusion 7th character A see Appendix A
PDX collection 1393
HAC 7th character A see Appendix B for HAC conditional logic

CC +7th **T22.742 Corrosion of third degree of left axilla**
CC Exclusion 7th character A see Appendix A
PDX collection 1393
HAC 7th character A see Appendix B for HAC conditional logic

CC +7th **T22.749 Corrosion of third degree of unspecified axilla**
CC Exclusion 7th character A see Appendix A
PDX collection 1393
HAC 7th character A see Appendix B for HAC conditional logic

+ **T22.75 Corrosion of third degree of shoulder**

CC +7th **T22.751 Corrosion of third degree of right shoulder**
CC Exclusion 7th character A see Appendix A
PDX collection 1394
HAC 7th character A see Appendix B for HAC conditional logic

CC +7th **T22.752 Corrosion of third degree of left shoulder**
CC Exclusion 7th character A see Appendix A
PDX collection 1394
HAC 7th character A see Appendix B for HAC conditional logic

CC +7th **T22.759 Corrosion of third degree of unspecified shoulder**
CC Exclusion 7th character A see Appendix A
PDX collection 1394
HAC 7th character A see Appendix B for HAC conditional logic

+ **T22.76 Corrosion of third degree of scapular region**

CC +7th **T22.761 Corrosion of third degree of right scapula region**
CC Exclusion 7th character A see Appendix A
PDX collection 1395
HAC 7th character A see Appendix B for HAC conditional logic

CC +7th **T22.762 Corrosion of third degree of left scapular region**
CC Exclusion 7th character A see Appendix A
PDX collection 1395
HAC 7th character A see Appendix B for HAC conditional logic

CC +7th **T22.769 Corrosion of third degree of unspecified scapular region**
CC Exclusion 7th character A see Appendix A
PDX collection 1395
HAC 7th character A see Appendix B for HAC conditional logic

+ **T22.79 Corrosion of third degree of multiple sites of shoulder and upper limb, except wrist and hand**

CC +7th **T22.791 Corrosion of third degree of multiple site of right shoulder and upper limb, except wrist and hand**
CC Exclusion 7th character A see Appendix A
PDX collection 1389
HAC 7th character A see Appendix B for HAC conditional logic

CC +7th **T22.792 Corrosion of third degree of multiple site of left shoulder and upper limb, except wrist and hand**
CC Exclusion 7th character A see Appendix A
PDX collection 1389
HAC 7th character A see Appendix B for HAC conditional logic

CC +7th **T22.799 Corrosion of third degree of multiple site of unspecified shoulder and upper limb, except wrist and hand**
CC Exclusion 7th character A see Appendix A
PDX collection 1389
HAC 7th character A see Appendix B for HAC conditional logic

T23 Burn and corrosion of wrist and hand

The appropriate 7th character is to be added to each code from catego T23
A initial encounter
D subsequent encounter
S sequela

+ **T23.0 Burn of unspecified degree of wrist and hand**
Use additional external cause code to identify the source, plac and intent of the burn (X00-X19, X75-X77, X96-X98, Y92

+ **T23.00 Burn of unspecified degree of hand, unspecified sit**

+7th **T23.001 Burn of unspecified degree of right hand, unspecified site**

+7th **T23.002 Burn of unspecified degree of left hand, unspecified site**

+7th **T23.009 Burn of unspecified degree of unspecified hand, unspecified site**

+ **T23.01 Burn of unspecified degree of thumb (nail)**

+7th **T23.011 Burn of unspecified degree of right thum (nail)**

+7th **T23.012 Burn of unspecified degree of left thumb (nail)**

+7th **T23.019 Burn of unspecified degree of unspecified thumb (nail)**

+ **T23.02 Burn of unspecified degree of single finger (nail) except thumb**

+7th **T23.021 Burn of unspecified degree of single righ finger (nail) except thumb**

+7th **T23.022 Burn of unspecified degree of single left finger (nail) except thumb**

+7th **T23.029 Burn of unspecified degree of unspecifie single finger (nail) except thumb**

+ **T23.03 Burn of unspecified degree of multiple fingers (nail), not including thumb**
  - +7th **T23.031 Burn of unspecified degree of multiple right fingers (nail), not including thumb**
  - +7th **T23.032 Burn of unspecified degree of multiple left fingers (nail), not including thumb**
  - +7th **T23.039 Burn of unspecified degree of unspecified multiple fingers (nail), not including thumb**
+ **T23.04 Burn of unspecified degree of multiple fingers (nail), including thumb**
  - +7th **T23.041 Burn of unspecified degree of multiple right fingers (nail), including thumb**
  - +7th **T23.042 Burn of unspecified degree of multiple left fingers (nail), including thumb**
  - +7th **T23.049 Burn of unspecified degree of unspecified multiple fingers (nail), including thumb**
+ **T23.05 Burn of unspecified degree of palm**
  - +7th **T23.051 Burn of unspecified degree of right palm**
  - +7th **T23.052 Burn of unspecified degree of left palm**
  - +7th **T23.059 Burn of unspecified degree of unspecified palm**
+ **T23.06 Burn of unspecified degree of back of hand**
  - +7th **T23.061 Burn of unspecified degree of back of right hand**
  - +7th **T23.062 Burn of unspecified degree of back of left hand**
  - +7th **T23.069 Burn of unspecified degree of back of unspecified hand**
+ **T23.07 Burn of unspecified degree of wrist**
  - +7th **T23.071 Burn of unspecified degree of right wrist**
  - +7th **T23.072 Burn of unspecified degree of left wrist**
  - +7th **T23.079 Burn of unspecified degree of unspecified wrist**
+ **T23.09 Burn of unspecified degree of multiple sites of wrist and hand**
  - +7th **T23.091 Burn of unspecified degree of multiple sites of right wrist and hand**
  - +7th **T23.092 Burn of unspecified degree of multiple sites of left wrist and hand**
  - +7th **T23.099 Burn of unspecified degree of multiple sites of unspecified wrist and hand**

+ **T23.1 Burn of first degree of wrist and hand**

  Use additional external cause code to identify the source, place and intent of the burn (X00-X19, X75-X77, X96-X98, Y92)

+ **T23.10 Burn of first degree of hand, unspecified site**
  - +7th **T23.101 Burn of first degree of right hand, unspecified site**
  - +7th **T23.102 Burn of first degree of left hand, unspecified site**
  - +7th **T23.109 Burn of first degree of unspecified hand, unspecified site**
+ **T23.11 Burn of first degree of thumb (nail)**
  - +7th **T23.111 Burn of first degree of right thumb (nail)**
  - +7th **T23.112 Burn of first degree of left thumb (nail)**
  - +7th **T23.119 Burn of first degree of unspecified thumb (nail)**
+ **T23.12 Burn of first degree of single finger (nail) except thumb**
  - +7th **T23.121 Burn of first degree of single right finger (nail) except thumb**
  - +7th **T23.122 Burn of first degree of single left finger (nail) except thumb**
  - +7th **T23.129 Burn of first degree of unspecified single finger (nail) except thumb**
+ **T23.13 Burn of first degree of multiple fingers (nail), not including thumb**
  - +7th **T23.131 Burn of first degree of multiple right fingers (nail), not including thumb**
  - +7th **T23.132 Burn of first degree of multiple left fingers (nail), not including thumb**
  - +7th **T23.139 Burn of first degree of unspecified multiple fingers (nail), not including thumb**
+ **T23.14 Burn of first degree of multiple fingers (nail), including thumb**
  - +7th **T23.141 Burn of first degree of multiple right fingers (nail), including thumb**
  - +7th **T23.142 Burn of first degree of multiple left fingers (nail), including thumb**
  - +7th **T23.149 Burn of first degree of unspecified multiple fingers (nail), including thumb**
+ **T23.15 Burn of first degree of palm**
  - +7th **T23.151 Burn of first degree of right palm**
  - +7th **T23.152 Burn of first degree of left palm**
  - +7th **T23.159 Burn of first degree of unspecified palm**
+ **T23.16 Burn of first degree of back of hand**
  - +7th **T23.161 Burn of first degree of back of right hand**
  - +7th **T23.162 Burn of first degree of back of left hand**
  - +7th **T23.169 Burn of first degree of back of unspecified hand**
+ **T23.17 Burn of first degree of wrist**
  - +7th **T23.171 Burn of first degree of right wrist**
  - +7th **T23.172 Burn of first degree of left wrist**
  - +7th **T23.179 Burn of first degree of unspecified wrist**
+ **T23.19 Burn of first degree of multiple sites of wrist and hand**
  - +7th **T23.191 Burn of first degree of multiple sites of right wrist and hand**
  - +7th **T23.192 Burn of first degree of multiple sites of left wrist and hand**
  - +7th **T23.199 Burn of first degree of multiple sites of unspecified wrist and hand**

+ **T23.2 Burn of second degree of wrist and hand**

  Use additional external cause code to identify the source, place and intent of the burn (X00-X19, X75-X77, X96-X98, Y92)

+ **T23.20 Burn of second degree of hand, unspecified site**
  - +7th **T23.201 Burn of second degree of right hand, unspecified site**
  - +7th **T23.202 Burn of second degree of left hand, unspecified site**
  - +7th **T23.209 Burn of second degree of unspecified hand, unspecified site**
+ **T23.21 Burn of second degree of thumb (nail)**
  - +7th **T23.211 Burn of second degree of right thumb (nail)**
  - +7th **T23.212 Burn of second degree of left thumb (nail)**
  - +7th **T23.219 Burn of second degree of unspecified thumb (nail)**
+ **T23.22 Burn of second degree of single finger (nail) except thumb**
  - +7th **T23.221 Burn of second degree of single right finger (nail) except thumb**
  - +7th **T23.222 Burn of second degree of single left finger (nail) except thumb**
  - +7th **T23.229 Burn of second degree of unspecified single finger (nail) except thumb**
+ **T23.23 Burn of second degree of multiple fingers (nail), not including thumb**
  - +7th **T23.231 Burn of second degree of multiple right fingers (nail), not including thumb**
  - +7th **T23.232 Burn of second degree of multiple left fingers (nail), not including thumb**
  - +7th **T23.239 Burn of second degree of unspecified multiple fingers (nail), not including thumb**
+ **T23.24 Burn of second degree of multiple fingers (nail), including thumb**
  - +7th **T23.241 Burn of second degree of multiple right fingers (nail), including thumb**
  - +7th **T23.242 Burn of second degree of multiple left fingers (nail), including thumb**
  - +7th **T23.249 Burn of second degree of unspecified multiple fingers (nail), including thumb**
+ **T23.25 Burn of second degree of palm**
  - +7th **T23.251 Burn of second degree of right palm**
  - +7th **T23.252 Burn of second degree of left palm**
  - +7th **T23.259 Burn of second degree of unspecified palm**
+ **T23.26 Burn of second degree of back of hand**
  - +7th **T23.261 Burn of second degree of back of right hand**
  - +7th **T23.262 Burn of second degree of back of left hand**
  - +7th **T23.269 Burn of second degree of back of unspecified hand**
+ **T23.27 Burn of second degree of wrist**
  - +7th **T23.271 Burn of second degree of right wrist**
  - +7th **T23.272 Burn of second degree of left wrist**
  - +7th **T23.279 Burn of second degree of unspecified wrist**

+ **T23.29 Burn of second degree of multiple sites of wrist and hand**
  - +7th **T23.291 Burn of second degree of multiple sites of right wrist and hand**
  - +7th **T23.292 Burn of second degree of multiple sites of left wrist and hand**
  - +7th **T23.299 Burn of second degree of multiple sites of unspecified wrist and hand**

+ **T23.3 Burn of third degree of wrist and hand**
  Use additional external cause code to identify the source, place and intent of the burn (X00-X19, X75-X77, X96-X98, Y92)

+ **T23.30 Burn of third degree of hand, unspecified site**
  - CC +7th **T23.301 Burn of third degree of right hand, unspecified site**
    CC Exclusion 7th character A see Appendix A
    PDX collection 1396
    AHA CC: 1Q, 2015, 3-21
    HAC 7th character A see Appendix B for HAC conditional logic
  - CC +7th **T23.302 Burn of third degree of left hand, unspecified site**
    CC Exclusion 7th character A see Appendix A
    PDX collection 1396
    AHA CC: 2Q, 2016, 5
    HAC 7th character A see Appendix B for HAC conditional logic
  - CC +7th **T23.309 Burn of third degree of unspecified hand, unspecified site**
    CC Exclusion 7th character A see Appendix A
    PDX collection 1396
    HAC 7th character A see Appendix B for HAC conditional logic

+ **T23.31 Burn of third degree of thumb (nail)**
  - CC +7th **T23.311 Burn of third degree of right thumb (nail)**
    CC Exclusion 7th character A see Appendix A
    PDX collection 1397
    HAC 7th character A see Appendix B for HAC conditional logic
  - CC +7th **T23.312 Burn of third degree of left thumb (nail)**
    CC Exclusion 7th character A see Appendix A
    PDX collection 1397
    HAC 7th character A see Appendix B for HAC conditional logic
  - CC +7th **T23.319 Burn of third degree of unspecified thumb (nail)**
    CC Exclusion 7th character A see Appendix A
    PDX collection 1397
    HAC 7th character A see Appendix B for HAC conditional logic

+ **T23.32 Burn of third degree of single finger (nail) except thumb**
  - CC +7th **T23.321 Burn of third degree of single right finger (nail) except thumb**
    CC Exclusion 7th character A see Appendix A
    PDX collection 1398
    HAC 7th character A see Appendix B for HAC conditional logic
  - CC +7th **T23.322 Burn of third degree of single left finger (nail) except thumb**
    CC Exclusion 7th character A see Appendix A
    PDX collection 1398
    HAC 7th character A see Appendix B for HAC conditional logic
  - CC +7th **T23.329 Burn of third degree of unspecified single finger (nail) except thumb**
    CC Exclusion 7th character A see Appendix A
    PDX collection 1398
    HAC 7th character A see Appendix B for HAC conditional logic

+ **T23.33 Burn of third degree of multiple fingers (nail), not including thumb**
  - CC +7th **T23.331 Burn of third degree of multiple right fingers (nail), not including thumb**
    CC Exclusion 7th character A see Appendix A
    PDX collection 1399
    HAC 7th character A see Appendix B for HAC conditional logic
  - CC +7th **T23.332 Burn of third degree of multiple left fingers (nail), not including thumb**
    CC Exclusion 7th character A see Appendix A
    PDX collection 1399
    HAC 7th character A see Appendix B for HAC conditional logic
  - CC +7th **T23.339 Burn of third degree of unspecified multiple fingers (nail), not including thum**
    CC Exclusion 7th character A see Appendix A
    PDX collection 1399

+ **T23.34 Burn of third degree of multiple fingers (nail), including thumb**
  - CC +7th **T23.341 Burn of third degree of multiple right fingers (nail), including thumb**
    CC Exclusion 7th character A see Appendix A
    PDX collection 1400
    HAC 7th character A see Appendix B for HAC conditional logic
  - CC +7th **T23.342 Burn of third degree of multiple left finge (nail), including thumb**
    CC Exclusion 7th character A see Appendix A
    PDX collection 1400
    HAC 7th character A see Appendix B for HAC conditional logic
  - CC +7th **T23.349 Burn of third degree of unspecified multiple fingers (nail), including thumb**
    CC Exclusion 7th character A see Appendix A
    PDX collection 1400
    HAC 7th character A see Appendix B for HAC conditional logic

+ **T23.35 Burn of third degree of palm**
  - CC +7th **T23.351 Burn of third degree of right palm**
    CC Exclusion 7th character A see Appendix A
    PDX collection 1401
    HAC 7th character A see Appendix B for HAC conditional logic
  - CC +7th **T23.352 Burn of third degree of left palm**
    CC Exclusion 7th character A see Appendix A
    PDX collection 1401
    HAC 7th character A see Appendix B for HAC conditional logic
  - CC +7th **T23.359 Burn of third degree of unspecified palm**
    CC Exclusion 7th character A see Appendix A
    PDX collection 1401
    HAC 7th character A see Appendix B for HAC conditional logic

+ **T23.36 Burn of third degree of back of hand**
  - CC +7th **T23.361 Burn of third degree of back of right han**
    CC Exclusion 7th character A see Appendix
    PDX collection 1402
    HAC 7th character A see Appendix B for HAC conditional logic
  - CC +7th **T23.362 Burn of third degree of back of left hand**
    CC Exclusion 7th character A see Appendix
    PDX collection 1402
    HAC 7th character A see Appendix B for HAC conditional logic
  - CC +7th **T23.369 Burn of third degree of back of unspecifi hand**
    CC Exclusion 7th character A see Appendix
    PDX collection 1402
    HAC 7th character A see Appendix B for HAC conditional logic

+ **T23.37 Burn of third degree of wrist**
  - CC +7th **T23.371 Burn of third degree of right wrist**
    CC Exclusion 7th character A see Appendix
    PDX collection 1403
    HAC 7th character A see Appendix B for HA conditional logic
  - CC +7th **T23.372 Burn of third degree of left wrist**
    CC Exclusion 7th character A see Appendix
    PDX collection 1403
    HAC 7th character A see Appendix B for HA conditional logic
  - CC +7th **T23.379 Burn of third degree of unspecified wris**
    CC Exclusion 7th character A see Appendix
    PDX collection 1403
    HAC 7th character A see Appendix B for HA conditional logic

+ **T23.39 Burn of third degree of multiple sites of wrist and hand**
  - CC +7th **T23.391 Burn of third degree of multiple sites of right wrist and hand**
    CC Exclusion 7th character A see Appendix
    PDX collection 1396
    HAC 7th character A see Appendix B for HA conditional logic

CC +7th **T23.392 Burn of third degree of multiple sites of left wrist and hand**
CC Exclusion 7th character A see Appendix A PDX collection 1396
HAC 7th character A see Appendix B for HAC conditional logic

CC +7th **T23.399 Burn of third degree of multiple sites of unspecified wrist and hand**
CC Exclusion 7th character A see Appendix A PDX collection 1396
HAC 7th character A see Appendix B for HAC conditional logic

\+ **T23.4 Corrosion of unspecified degree of wrist and hand**
Code first (T51-T65) to identify chemical and intent

Use additional external cause code to identify place (Y92)

\+ **T23.40 Corrosion of unspecified degree of hand, unspecified site**
+7th **T23.401 Corrosion of unspecified degree of right hand, unspecified site**
+7th **T23.402 Corrosion of unspecified degree of left hand, unspecified site**
+7th **T23.409 Corrosion of unspecified degree of unspecified hand, unspecified site**

\+ **T23.41 Corrosion of unspecified degree of thumb (nail)**
+7th **T23.411 Corrosion of unspecified degree of right thumb (nail)**
+7th **T23.412 Corrosion of unspecified degree of left thumb (nail)**
+7th **T23.419 Corrosion of unspecified degree of unspecified thumb (nail)**

\+ **T23.42 Corrosion of unspecified degree of single finger (nail) except thumb**
+7th **T23.421 Corrosion of unspecified degree of single right finger (nail) except thumb**
+7th **T23.422 Corrosion of unspecified degree of single left finger (nail) except thumb**
+7th **T23.429 Corrosion of unspecified degree of unspecified single finger (nail) except thumb**

\+ **T23.43 Corrosion of unspecified degree of multiple fingers (nail), not including thumb**
+7th **T23.431 Corrosion of unspecified degree of multiple right fingers (nail), not including thumb**
+7th **T23.432 Corrosion of unspecified degree of multiple left fingers (nail), not including thumb**
+7th **T23.439 Corrosion of unspecified degree of unspecified multiple fingers (nail), not including thumb**

\+ **T23.44 Corrosion of unspecified degree of multiple fingers (nail), including thumb**
+7th **T23.441 Corrosion of unspecified degree of multiple right fingers (nail), including thumb**
+7th **T23.442 Corrosion of unspecified degree of multiple left fingers (nail), including thumb**
+7th **T23.449 Corrosion of unspecified degree of unspecified multiple fingers (nail), including thumb**

\+ **T23.45 Corrosion of unspecified degree of palm**
+7th **T23.451 Corrosion of unspecified degree of right palm**
+7th **T23.452 Corrosion of unspecified degree of left palm**
+7th **T23.459 Corrosion of unspecified degree of unspecified palm**

\+ **T23.46 Corrosion of unspecified degree of back of hand**
+7th **T23.461 Corrosion of unspecified degree of back of right hand**
+7th **T23.462 Corrosion of unspecified degree of back of left hand**
+7th **T23.469 Corrosion of unspecified degree of back of unspecified hand**

\+ **T23.47 Corrosion of unspecified degree of wrist**
+7th **T23.471 Corrosion of unspecified degree of right wrist**
+7th **T23.472 Corrosion of unspecified degree of left wrist**
+7th **T23.479 Corrosion of unspecified degree of unspecified wrist**

\+ **T23.49 Corrosion of unspecified degree of multiple sites of wrist and hand**
+7th **T23.491 Corrosion of unspecified degree of multiple sites of right wrist and hand**
+7th **T23.492 Corrosion of unspecified degree of multiple sites of left wrist and hand**
+7th **T23.499 Corrosion of unspecified degree of multiple sites of unspecified wrist and hand**

\+ **T23.5 Corrosion of first degree of wrist and hand**
Code first (T51-T65) to identify chemical and intent

Use additional external cause code to identify place (Y92)

\+ **T23.50 Corrosion of first degree of hand, unspecified site**
+7th **T23.501 Corrosion of first degree of right hand, unspecified site**
+7th **T23.502 Corrosion of first degree of left hand, unspecified site**
+7th **T23.509 Corrosion of first degree of unspecified hand, unspecified site**

\+ **T23.51 Corrosion of first degree of thumb (nail)**
+7th **T23.511 Corrosion of first degree of right thumb (nail)**
+7th **T23.512 Corrosion of first degree of left thumb (nail)**
+7th **T23.519 Corrosion of first degree of unspecified thumb (nail)**

\+ **T23.52 Corrosion of first degree of single finger (nail) except thumb**
+7th **T23.521 Corrosion of first degree of single right finger (nail) except thumb**
+7th **T23.522 Corrosion of first degree of single left finger (nail) except thumb**
+7th **T23.529 Corrosion of first degree of unspecified single finger (nail) except thumb**

\+ **T23.53 Corrosion of first degree of multiple fingers (nail), not including thumb**
+7th **T23.531 Corrosion of first degree of multiple right fingers (nail), not including thumb**
+7th **T23.532 Corrosion of first degree of multiple left fingers (nail), not including thumb**
+7th **T23.539 Corrosion of first degree of unspecified multiple fingers (nail), not including thumb**

\+ **T23.54 Corrosion of first degree of multiple fingers (nail), including thumb**
+7th **T23.541 Corrosion of first degree of multiple right fingers (nail), including thumb**
+7th **T23.542 Corrosion of first degree of multiple left fingers (nail), including thumb**
+7th **T23.549 Corrosion of first degree of unspecified multiple fingers (nail), including thumb**

\+ **T23.55 Corrosion of first degree of palm**
+7th **T23.551 Corrosion of first degree of right palm**
+7th **T23.552 Corrosion of first degree of left palm**
+7th **T23.559 Corrosion of first degree of unspecified palm**

\+ **T23.56 Corrosion of first degree of back of hand**
+7th **T23.561 Corrosion of first degree of back of right hand**
+7th **T23.562 Corrosion of first degree of back of left hand**
+7th **T23.569 Corrosion of first degree of back of unspecified hand**

\+ **T23.57 Corrosion of first degree of wrist**
+7th **T23.571 Corrosion of first degree of right wrist**
+7th **T23.572 Corrosion of first degree of left wrist**
+7th **T23.579 Corrosion of first degree of unspecified wrist**

\+ **T23.59 Corrosion of first degree of multiple sites of wrist and hand**
+7th **T23.591 Corrosion of first degree of multiple sites of right wrist and hand**
+7th **T23.592 Corrosion of first degree of multiple sites of left wrist and hand**
+7th **T23.599 Corrosion of first degree of multiple sites of unspecified wrist and hand**

+ **T23.6 Corrosion of second degree of wrist and hand**
  Code first (T51-T65) to identify chemical and intent
  Use additionalexternal cause code to identify place (Y92)
  + **T23.60 Corrosion of second degree of hand, unspecified site**
    +7th **T23.601 Corrosion of second degree of right hand, unspecified site**
    +7th **T23.602 Corrosion of second degree of left hand, unspecified site**
    +7th **T23.609 Corrosion of second degree of unspecified hand, unspecified site**
  + **T23.61 Corrosion of second degree of thumb (nail)**
    +7th **T23.611 Corrosion of second degree of right thumb (nail)**
    +7th **T23.612 Corrosion of second degree of left thumb (nail)**
    +7th **T23.619 Corrosion of second degree of unspecified thumb (nail)**
  + **T23.62 Corrosion of second degree of single finger (nail) except thumb**
    +7th **T23.621 Corrosion of second degree of single right finger (nail) except thumb**
    +7th **T23.622 Corrosion of second degree of single left finger (nail) except thumb**
    +7th **T23.629 Corrosion of second degree of unspecified single finger (nail) except thumb**
  + **T23.63 Corrosion of second degree of multiple fingers (nail), not including thumb**
    +7th **T23.631 Corrosion of second degree of multiple right fingers (nail), not including thumb**
    +7th **T23.632 Corrosion of second degree of multiple left fingers (nail), not including thumb**
    +7th **T23.639 Corrosion of second degree of unspecified multiple fingers (nail), not including thumb**
  + **T23.64 Corrosion of second degree of multiple fingers (nail), including thumb**
    +7th **T23.641 Corrosion of second degree of multiple right fingers (nail), including thumb**
    +7th **T23.642 Corrosion of second degree of multiple left fingers (nail), including thumb**
    +7th **T23.649 Corrosion of second degree of unspecified multiple fingers (nail), including thumb**
  + **T23.65 Corrosion of second degree of palm**
    +7th **T23.651 Corrosion of second degree of right palm**
    +7th **T23.652 Corrosion of second degree of left palm**
    +7th **T23.659 Corrosion of second degree of unspecified palm**
  + **T23.66 Corrosion of second degree of back of hand**
    +7th **T23.661 Corrosion of second degree back of right hand**
    +7th **T23.662 Corrosion of second degree back of left hand**
    +7th **T23.669 Corrosion of second degree back of unspecified hand**
  + **T23.67 Corrosion of second degree of wrist**
    +7th **T23.671 Corrosion of second degree of right wrist**
    +7th **T23.672 Corrosion of second degree of left wrist**
    +7th **T23.679 Corrosion of second degree of unspecified wrist**
  + **T23.69 Corrosion of second degree of multiple sites of wrist and hand**
    +7th **T23.691 Corrosion of second degree of multiple sites of right wrist and hand**
    +7th **T23.692 Corrosion of second degree of multiple sites of left wrist and hand**
    +7th **T23.699 Corrosion of second degree of multiple sites of unspecified wrist and hand**

+ **T23.7 Corrosion of third degree of wrist and hand**
  Code first (T51-T65) to identify chemical and intent
  Use additional external cause code to identify place (Y92)
  + **T23.70 Corrosion of third degree of hand, unspecified site**
    CC +7th **T23.701 Corrosion of third degree of right hand, unspecified site**
      CC Exclusion 7th character A see Appendix A PDX collection 1396
      HAC 7th character A see Appendix B for HAC conditional logic
    CC +7th **T23.702 Corrosion of third degree of left hand, unspecified site**
      CC Exclusion 7th character A see Appendix A PDX collection 1396
      HAC 7th character A see Appendix B for HAC conditional logic
    CC +7th **T23.709 Corrosion of third degree of unspecified hand, unspecified site**
      CC Exclusion 7th character A see Appendix A PDX collection 1396
      HAC 7th character A see Appendix B for HAC conditional logic
  + **T23.71 Corrosion of third degree of thumb (nail)**
    CC +7th **T23.711 Corrosion of third degree of right thumb (nail)**
      CC Exclusion 7th character A see Appendix A PDX collection 1397
      HAC 7th character A see Appendix B for HAC conditional logic
    CC +7th **T23.712 Corrosion of third degree of left thumb (nail)**
      CC Exclusion 7th character A see Appendix A PDX collection 1397
      HAC 7th character A see Appendix B for HAC conditional logic
    CC +7th **T23.719 Corrosion of third degree of unspecified thumb (nail)**
      CC Exclusion 7th character A see Appendix A PDX collection 1397
      HAC 7th character A see Appendix B for HAC conditional logic
  + **T23.72 Corrosion of third degree of single finger (nail) except thumb**
    CC +7th **T23.721 Corrosion of third degree of single right finger (nail) except thumb**
      CC Exclusion 7th character A see Appendix A PDX collection 1398
      HAC 7th character A see Appendix B for HAC conditional logic
    CC +7th **T23.722 Corrosion of third degree of single left finger (nail) except thumb**
      CC Exclusion 7th character A see Appendix A PDX collection 1398
      HAC 7th character A see Appendix B for HAC conditional logic
    CC +7th **T23.729 Corrosion of third degree of unspecified single finger (nail) except thumb**
      CC Exclusion 7th character A see Appendix A PDX collection 1398
      HAC 7th character A see Appendix B for HAC conditional logic
  + **T23.73 Corrosion of third degree of multiple fingers (nail), not including thumb**
    CC +7th **T23.731 Corrosion of third degree of multiple righ fingers (nail), not including thumb**
      CC Exclusion 7th character A see Appendix A PDX collection 1399
      HAC 7th character A see Appendix B for HAC conditional logic
    CC +7th **T23.732 Corrosion of third degree of multiple left fingers (nail), not including thumb**
      CC Exclusion 7th character A see Appendix A PDX collection 1399
      HAC 7th character A see Appendix B for HAC conditional logic
    CC +7th **T23.739 Corrosion of third degree of unspecified multiple fingers (nail), not including thum**
      CC Exclusion 7th character A see Appendix A PDX collection 1399
      HAC 7th character A see Appendix B for HAC conditional logic
  + **T23.74 Corrosion of third degree of multiple fingers (nail), including thumb**
    CC +7th **T23.741 Corrosion of third degree of multiple rigl fingers (nail), including thumb**
      CC Exclusion 7th character A see Appendix A PDX collection 1400
      HAC 7th character A see Appendix B for HAC conditional logic

CC +7th **T23.742** **Corrosion of third degree of multiple left fingers (nail), including thumb**
CC Exclusion 7th character A see Appendix A PDX collection 1400
HAC 7th character A see Appendix B for HAC conditional logic

CC +7th **T23.749** **Corrosion of third degree of unspecified multiple fingers (nail), including thumb**
CC Exclusion 7th character A see Appendix A PDX collection 1400
HAC 7th character A see Appendix B for HAC conditional logic

\+ **T23.75** **Corrosion of third degree of palm**

CC +7th **T23.751** **Corrosion of third degree of right palm**
CC Exclusion 7th character A see Appendix A PDX collection 1401
HAC 7th character A see Appendix B for HAC conditional logic

CC +7th **T23.752** **Corrosion of third degree of left palm**
CC Exclusion 7th character A see Appendix A PDX collection 1401
HAC 7th character A see Appendix B for HAC conditional logic

CC +7th **T23.759** **Corrosion of third degree of unspecified palm**
CC Exclusion 7th character A see Appendix A PDX collection 1401
HAC 7th character A see Appendix B for HAC conditional logic

\+ **T23.76** **Corrosion of third degree of back of hand**

CC +7th **T23.761** **Corrosion of third degree of back of right hand**
CC Exclusion 7th character A see Appendix A PDX collection 1402
HAC 7th character A see Appendix B for HAC conditional logic

CC +7th **T23.762** **Corrosion of third degree of back of left hand**
CC Exclusion 7th character A see Appendix A PDX collection 1402
HAC 7th character A see Appendix B for HAC conditional logic

CC +7th **T23.769** **Corrosion of third degree back of unspecified hand**
CC Exclusion 7th character A see Appendix A PDX collection 1402
HAC 7th character A see Appendix B for HAC conditional logic

\+ **T23.77** **Corrosion of third degree of wrist**

CC +7th **T23.771** **Corrosion of third degree of right wrist**
CC Exclusion 7th character A see Appendix A PDX collection 1403
HAC 7th character A see Appendix B for HAC conditional logic

CC +7th **T23.772** **Corrosion of third degree of left wrist**
CC Exclusion 7th character A see Appendix A PDX collection 1403
HAC 7th character A see Appendix B for HAC conditional logic

CC +7th **T23.779** **Corrosion of third degree of unspecified wrist**
CC Exclusion 7th character A see Appendix A PDX collection 1403
HAC 7th character A see Appendix B for HAC conditional logic

\+ **T23.79** **Corrosion of third degree of multiple sites of wrist and hand**

CC +7th **T23.791** **Corrosion of third degree of multiple sites of right wrist and hand**
CC Exclusion 7th character A see Appendix A PDX collection 1396
HAC 7th character A see Appendix B for HAC conditional logic

CC +7th **T23.792** **Corrosion of third degree of multiple sites of left wrist and hand**
CC Exclusion 7th character A see Appendix A PDX collection 1396
HAC 7th character A see Appendix B for HAC conditional logic

CC +7th **T23.799** **Corrosion of third degree of multiple sites of unspecified wrist and hand**
CC Exclusion 7th character A see Appendix A PDX collection 1396
HAC 7th character A see Appendix B for HAC conditional logic

T24 Burn and corrosion of lower limb, except ankle and foot

Excludes2: *burn and corrosion of ankle and foot (T25.-)*
burn and corrosion of hip region (T21.-)

The appropriate 7th character is to be added to each code from category T24
A initial encounter
D subsequent encounter
S sequela

\+ **T24.0** **Burn of unspecified degree of lower limb, except ankle and foot**
Use additional external cause code to identify the source, place and intent of the burn (X00-X19, X75-X77, X96-X98, Y92)

\+ **T24.00** **Burn of unspecified degree of unspecified site of lower limb, except ankle and foot**
+7th **T24.001** **Burn of unspecified degree of unspecified site of right lower limb, except ankle and foot**
+7th **T24.002** **Burn of unspecified degree of unspecified site of left lower limb, except ankle and foot**
+7th **T24.009** **Burn of unspecified degree of unspecified site of unspecified lower limb, except ankle and foot**

\+ **T24.01** **Burn of unspecified degree of thigh**
+7th **T24.011** **Burn of unspecified degree of right thigh**
+7th **T24.012** **Burn of unspecified degree of left thigh**
+7th **T24.019** **Burn of unspecified degree of unspecified thigh**

\+ **T24.02** **Burn of unspecified degree of knee**
+7th **T24.021** **Burn of unspecified degree of right knee**
+7th **T24.022** **Burn of unspecified degree of left knee**
+7th **T24.029** **Burn of unspecified degree of unspecified knee**

\+ **T24.03** **Burn of unspecified degree of lower leg**
+7th **T24.031** **Burn of unspecified degree of right lower leg**
+7th **T24.032** **Burn of unspecified degree of left lower leg**
+7th **T24.039** **Burn of unspecified degree of unspecified lower leg**

\+ **T24.09** **Burn of unspecified degree of multiple sites of lower limb, except ankle and foot**
+7th **T24.091** **Burn of unspecified degree of multiple sites of right lower limb, except ankle and foot**
+7th **T24.092** **Burn of unspecified degree of multiple sites of left lower limb, except ankle and foot**
+7th **T24.099** **Burn of unspecified degree of multiple sites of unspecified lower limb, except ankle and foot**

\+ **T24.1** **Burn of first degree of lower limb, except ankle and foot**
Use additional external cause code to identify the source, place and intent of the burn (X00-X19, X75-X77, X96-X98, Y92)

\+ **T24.10** **Burn of first degree of unspecified site of lower limb, except ankle and foot**
+7th **T24.101** **Burn of first degree of unspecified site of right lower limb, except ankle and foot**
+7th **T24.102** **Burn of first degree of unspecified site of left lower limb, except ankle and foot**
+7th **T24.109** **Burn of first degree of unspecified site of unspecified lower limb, except ankle and foot**

\+ **T24.11** **Burn of first degree of thigh**
+7th **T24.111** **Burn of first degree of right thigh**
+7th **T24.112** **Burn of first degree of left thigh**
+7th **T24.119** **Burn of first degree of unspecified thigh**

\+ **T24.12** **Burn of first degree of knee**
+7th **T24.121** **Burn of first degree of right knee**
+7th **T24.122** **Burn of first degree of left knee**
+7th **T24.129** **Burn of first degree of unspecified knee**

\+ **T24.13** **Burn of first degree of lower leg**
+7th **T24.131** **Burn of first degree of right lower leg**
+7th **T24.132** **Burn of first degree of left lower leg**
+7th **T24.139** **Burn of first degree of unspecified lower leg**

\+ **T24.19** **Burn of first degree of multiple sites of lower limb, except ankle and foot**
+7th **T24.191** **Burn of first degree of multiple sites of right lower limb, except ankle and foot**
+7th **T24.192** **Burn of first degree of multiple sites of left lower limb, except ankle and foot**
+7th **T24.199** **Burn of first degree of multiple sites of unspecified lower limb, except ankle and foot**

+ **T24.2 Burn of second degree of lower limb, except ankle and foot**
  Use additional external cause code to identify the source, place and intent of the burn (X00-X19, X75-X77, X96-X98, Y92)
  + **T24.20 Burn of second degree of unspecified site of lower limb, except ankle and foot**
    +7th **T24.201 Burn of second degree of unspecified site of right lower limb, except ankle and foot**
    +7th **T24.202 Burn of second degree of unspecified site of left lower limb, except ankle and foot**
    +7th **T24.209 Burn of second degree of unspecified site of unspecified lower limb, except ankle and foot**
  + **T24.21 Burn of second degree of thigh**
    +7th **T24.211 Burn of second degree of right thigh**
    +7th **T24.212 Burn of second degree of left thigh**
    +7th **T24.219 Burn of second degree of unspecified thigh**
  + **T24.22 Burn of second degree of knee**
    +7th **T24.221 Burn of second degree of right knee**
    +7th **T24.222 Burn of second degree of left knee**
    +7th **T24.229 Burn of second degree of unspecified knee**
  + **T24.23 Burn of second degree of lower leg**
    +7th **T24.231 Burn of second degree of right lower leg**
    +7th **T24.232 Burn of second degree of left lower leg**
    +7th **T24.239 Burn of second degree of unspecified lower leg**
  + **T24.29 Burn of second degree of multiple sites of lower limb, except ankle and foot**
    +7th **T24.291 Burn of second degree of multiple sites of right lower limb, except ankle and foot**
    +7th **T24.292 Burn of second degree of multiple sites of left lower limb, except ankle and foot**
    +7th **T24.299 Burn of second degree of multiple sites of unspecified lower limb, except ankle and foot**

+ **T24.3 Burn of third degree of lower limb, except ankle and foot**
  Use additional external cause code to identify the source, place and intent of the burn (X00-X19, X75-X77, X96-X98, Y92)
  + **T24.30 Burn of third degree of unspecified site of lower limb, except ankle and foot**
    CC +7th **T24.301 Burn of third degree of unspecified site of right lower limb, except ankle and foot**
      CC Exclusion 7th character A see Appendix A PDX collection 1404
      HAC 7th character A see Appendix B for HAC conditional logic
    CC +7th **T24.302 Burn of third degree of unspecified site of left lower limb, except ankle and foot**
      CC Exclusion 7th character A see Appendix A PDX collection 1404
      HAC 7th character A see Appendix B for HAC conditional logic
    CC +7th **T24.309 Burn of third degree of unspecified site of unspecified lower limb, except ankle and foot**
      CC Exclusion 7th character A see Appendix A PDX collection 1404
      HAC 7th character A see Appendix B for HAC conditional logic
  + **T24.31 Burn of third degree of thigh**
    CC +7th **T24.311 Burn of third degree of right thigh**
      CC Exclusion 7th character A see Appendix A PDX collection 1405
      HAC 7th character A see Appendix B for HAC conditional logic
    CC +7th **T24.312 Burn of third degree of left thigh**
      CC Exclusion 7th character A see Appendix A PDX collection 1405
      HAC 7th character A see Appendix B for HAC conditional logic
    CC +7th **T24.319 Burn of third degree of unspecified thigh**
      CC Exclusion 7th character A see Appendix A PDX collection 1405
      HAC 7th character A see Appendix B for HAC conditional logic
  + **T24.32 Burn of third degree of knee**
    CC +7th **T24.321 Burn of third degree of right knee**
      CC Exclusion 7th character A see Appendix A PDX collection 1406
      HAC 7th character A see Appendix B for HAC conditional logic
    CC +7th **T24.322 Burn of third degree of left knee**
      CC Exclusion 7th character A see Appendix A PDX collection 1406
      HAC 7th character A see Appendix B for HAC conditional logic
    CC +7th **T24.329 Burn of third degree of unspecified knee**
      CC Exclusion 7th character A see Appendix A PDX collection 1406
      HAC 7th character A see Appendix B for HAC conditional logic
  + **T24.33 Burn of third degree of lower leg**
    CC +7th **T24.331 Burn of third degree of right lower leg**
      CC Exclusion 7th character A see Appendix A PDX collection 1407
      HAC 7th character A see Appendix B for HAC conditional logic
    CC +7th **T24.332 Burn of third degree of left lower leg**
      CC Exclusion 7th character A see Appendix A PDX collection 1407
      HAC 7th character A see Appendix B for HAC conditional logic
    CC +7th **T24.339 Burn of third degree of unspecified lower leg**
      CC Exclusion 7th character A see Appendix A PDX collection 1407
      HAC 7th character A see Appendix B for HAC conditional logic
  + **T24.39 Burn of third degree of multiple sites of lower limb, except ankle and foot**
    CC +7th **T24.391 Burn of third degree of multiple sites of right lower limb, except ankle and foot**
      CC Exclusion 7th character A see Appendix A PDX collection 1404
      AHA CC: 2Q, 2016, 4
      HAC 7th character A see Appendix B for HAC conditional logic
    CC +7th **T24.392 Burn of third degree of multiple sites of left lower limb, except ankle and foot**
      CC Exclusion 7th character A see Appendix A PDX collection 1404
      AHA CC: 2Q, 2016, 4
      HAC 7th character A see Appendix B for HAC conditional logic
    CC +7th **T24.399 Burn of third degree of multiple sites of unspecified lower limb, except ankle and foot**
      CC Exclusion 7th character A see Appendix A PDX collection 1404
      HAC 7th character A see Appendix B for HAC conditional logic

+ **T24.4 Corrosion of unspecified degree of lower limb, except ankle and foot**
  Code first (T51-T65) to identify chemical and intent
  Use additional external cause code to identify place (Y92)
  + **T24.40 Corrosion of unspecified degree of unspecified site of lower limb, except ankle and foot**
    +7th **T24.401 Corrosion of unspecified degree of unspecified site of right lower limb, except ankle and foot**
    +7th **T24.402 Corrosion of unspecified degree of unspecified site of left lower limb, except ankle and foot**
    +7th **T24.409 Corrosion of unspecified degree of unspecified site of unspecified lower limb, except ankle and foot**
  + **T24.41 Corrosion of unspecified degree of thigh**
    +7th **T24.411 Corrosion of unspecified degree of right thigh**
    +7th **T24.412 Corrosion of unspecified degree of left thigh**
    +7th **T24.419 Corrosion of unspecified degree of unspecified thigh**
  + **T24.42 Corrosion of unspecified degree of knee**
    +7th **T24.421 Corrosion of unspecified degree of right knee**
    +7th **T24.422 Corrosion of unspecified degree of left knee**
    +7th **T24.429 Corrosion of unspecified degree of unspecified knee**

+ T24.43 Corrosion of unspecified degree of lower leg
  - +7th T24.431 Corrosion of unspecified degree of right lower leg
  - +7th T24.432 Corrosion of unspecified degree of left lower leg
  - +7th T24.439 Corrosion of unspecified degree of unspecified lower leg
+ T24.49 Corrosion of unspecified degree of multiple sites of lower limb, except ankle and foot
  - +7th T24.491 Corrosion of unspecified degree of multiple sites of right lower limb, except ankle and foot
  - +7th T24.492 Corrosion of unspecified degree of multiple sites of left lower limb, except ankle and foot
  - +7th T24.499 Corrosion of unspecified degree of multiple sites of unspecified lower limb, except ankle and foot

+ T24.5 Corrosion of first degree of lower limb, except ankle and foot

  Code first (T51-T65) to identify chemical and intent

  Use additional external cause code to identify place (Y92)

+ T24.50 Corrosion of first degree of unspecified site of lower limb, except ankle and foot
  - +7th T24.501 Corrosion of first degree of unspecified site of right lower limb, except ankle and foot
  - +7th T24.502 Corrosion of first degree of unspecified site of left lower limb, except ankle and foot
  - +7th T24.509 Corrosion of first degree of unspecified site of unspecified lower limb, except ankle and foot
+ T24.51 Corrosion of first degree of thigh
  - +7th T24.511 Corrosion of first degree of right thigh
  - +7th T24.512 Corrosion of first degree of left thigh
  - +7th T24.519 Corrosion of first degree of unspecified thigh
+ T24.52 Corrosion of first degree of knee
  - +7th T24.521 Corrosion of first degree of right knee
  - +7th T24.522 Corrosion of first degree of left knee
  - +7th T24.529 Corrosion of first degree of unspecified knee
+ T24.53 Corrosion of first degree of lower leg
  - +7th T24.531 Corrosion of first degree of right lower leg
  - +7th T24.532 Corrosion of first degree of left lower leg
  - +7th T24.539 Corrosion of first degree of unspecified lower leg
+ T24.59 Corrosion of first degree of multiple sites of lower limb, except ankle and foot
  - +7th T24.591 Corrosion of first degree of multiple sites of right lower limb, except ankle and foot
  - +7th T24.592 Corrosion of first degree of multiple sites of left lower limb, except ankle and foot
  - +7th T24.599 Corrosion of first degree of multiple sites of unspecified lower limb, except ankle and foot

+ T24.6 Corrosion of second degree of lower limb, except ankle and foot

  Code first (T51-T65) to identify chemical and intent

  Use additional external cause code to identify place (Y92)

+ T24.60 Corrosion of second degree of unspecified site of lower limb, except ankle and foot
  - +7th T24.601 Corrosion of second degree of unspecified site of right lower limb, except ankle and foot
  - +7th T24.602 Corrosion of second degree of unspecified site of left lower limb, except ankle and foot
  - +7th T24.609 Corrosion of second degree of unspecified site of unspecified lower limb, except ankle and foot
+ T24.61 Corrosion of second degree of thigh
  - +7th T24.611 Corrosion of second degree of right thigh
  - +7th T24.612 Corrosion of second degree of left thigh
  - +7th T24.619 Corrosion of second degree of unspecified thigh
+ T24.62 Corrosion of second degree of knee
  - +7th T24.621 Corrosion of second degree of right knee
  - +7th T24.622 Corrosion of second degree of left knee
  - +7th T24.629 Corrosion of second degree of unspecified knee
+ T24.63 Corrosion of second degree of lower leg
  - +7th T24.631 Corrosion of second degree of right lower leg
  - +7th T24.632 Corrosion of second degree of left lower leg
  - +7th T24.639 Corrosion of second degree of unspecified lower leg
+ T24.69 Corrosion of second degree of multiple sites of lower limb, except ankle and foot
  - +7th T24.691 Corrosion of second degree of multiple sites of right lower limb, except ankle and foot
  - +7th T24.692 Corrosion of second degree of multiple sites of left lower limb, except ankle and foot
  - +7th T24.699 Corrosion of second degree of multiple sites of unspecified lower limb, except ankle and foot

+ T24.7 Corrosion of third degree of lower limb, except ankle and foot

  Code first (T51-T65) to identify chemical and intent

  Use additional external cause code to identify place (Y92)

+ T24.70 Corrosion of third degree of unspecified site of lower limb, except ankle and foot
  - CC +7th T24.701 Corrosion of third degree of unspecified site of right lower limb, except ankle and foot
    CC Exclusion 7th character A see Appendix A PDX collection 1404
    HAC 7th character A see Appendix B for HAC conditional logic
  - CC +7th T24.702 Corrosion of third degree of unspecified site of left lower limb, except ankle and foot
    CC Exclusion 7th character A see Appendix A PDX collection 1404
    HAC 7th character A see Appendix B for HAC conditional logic
  - CC +7th T24.709 Corrosion of third degree of unspecified site of unspecified lower limb, except ankle and foot
    CC Exclusion 7th character A see Appendix A PDX collection 1404
    HAC 7th character A see Appendix B for HAC conditional logic
+ T24.71 Corrosion of third degree of thigh
  - CC +7th T24.711 Corrosion of third degree of right thigh
    CC Exclusion 7th character A see Appendix A PDX collection 1405
    HAC 7th character A see Appendix B for HAC conditional logic
  - CC +7th T24.712 Corrosion of third degree of left thigh
    CC Exclusion 7th character A see Appendix A PDX collection 1405
    HAC 7th character A see Appendix B for HAC conditional logic
  - CC +7th T24.719 Corrosion of third degree of unspecified thigh
    CC Exclusion 7th character A see Appendix A PDX collection 1405
    HAC 7th character A see Appendix B for HAC conditional logic
+ T24.72 Corrosion of third degree of knee
  - CC +7th T24.721 Corrosion of third degree of right knee
    CC Exclusion 7th character A see Appendix A PDX collection 1406
    HAC 7th character A see Appendix B for HAC conditional logic
  - CC +7th T24.722 Corrosion of third degree of left knee
    CC Exclusion 7th character A see Appendix A PDX collection 1406
    HAC 7th character A see Appendix B for HAC conditional logic
  - CC +7th T24.729 Corrosion of third degree of unspecified knee
    CC Exclusion 7th character A see Appendix A PDX collection 1406
    HAC 7th character A see Appendix B for HAC conditional logic

+ **T24.73 Corrosion of third degree of lower leg**
  - CC +7th **T24.731 Corrosion of third degree of right lower leg**
    CC Exclusion 7th character A see Appendix A PDX collection 1407
    HAC 7th character A see Appendix B for HAC conditional logic
  - CC +7th **T24.732 Corrosion of third degree of left lower leg**
    CC Exclusion 7th character A see Appendix A PDX collection 1407
    HAC 7th character A see Appendix B for HAC conditional logic
  - CC +7th **T24.739 Corrosion of third degree of unspecified lower leg**
    CC Exclusion 7th character A see Appendix A PDX collection 1407
    HAC 7th character A see Appendix B for HAC conditional logic

+ **T24.79 Corrosion of third degree of multiple sites of lower limb, except ankle and foot**
  - CC +7th **T24.791 Corrosion of third degree of multiple sites of right lower limb, except ankle and foot**
    CC Exclusion 7th character A see Appendix A PDX collection 1404
    HAC 7th character A see Appendix B for HAC conditional logic
  - CC +7th **T24.792 Corrosion of third degree of multiple sites of left lower limb, except ankle and foot**
    CC Exclusion 7th character A see Appendix A PDX collection 1404
    HAC 7th character A see Appendix B for HAC conditional logic
  - CC +7th **T24.799 Corrosion of third degree of multiple sites of unspecified lower limb, except ankle and foot**
    CC Exclusion 7th character A see Appendix A PDX collection 1404
    HAC 7th character A see Appendix B for HAC conditional logic

T25 Burn and corrosion of ankle and foot

The appropriate 7th character is to be added to each code from category T25
A initial encounter
D subsequent encounter
S sequela

+ **T25.0 Burn of unspecified degree of ankle and foot**
  Use additional external cause code to identify the source, place and intent of the burn (X00-X19, X75-X77, X96-X98, Y92)
  + **T25.01 Burn of unspecified degree of ankle**
    - +7th **T25.011 Burn of unspecified degree of right ankle**
    - +7th **T25.012 Burn of unspecified degree of left ankle**
    - +7th **T25.019 Burn of unspecified degree of unspecified ankle**
  + **T25.02 Burn of unspecified degree of foot**
    Excludes2: *burn of unspecified degree of toe(s) (nail) (T25.03-)*
    - +7th **T25.021 Burn of unspecified degree of right foot**
    - +7th **T25.022 Burn of unspecified degree of left foot**
    - +7th **T25.029 Burn of unspecified degree of unspecified foot**
  + **T25.03 Burn of unspecified degree of toe(s) (nail)**
    - +7th **T25.031 Burn of unspecified degree of right toe(s) (nail)**
    - +7th **T25.032 Burn of unspecified degree of left toe(s) (nail)**
    - +7th **T25.039 Burn of unspecified degree of unspecified toe(s) (nail)**
  + **T25.09 Burn of unspecified degree of multiple sites of ankle and foot**
    - +7th **T25.091 Burn of unspecified degree of multiple sites of right ankle and foot**
    - +7th **T25.092 Burn of unspecified degree of multiple sites of left ankle and foot**
    - +7th **T25.099 Burn of unspecified degree of multiple sites of unspecified ankle and foot**

+ **T25.1 Burn of first degree of ankle and foot**
  Use additional external cause code to identify the source, place and intent of the burn (X00-X19, X75-X77, X96-X98, Y92)
  + **T25.11 Burn of first degree of ankle**
    - +7th **T25.111 Burn of first degree of right ankle**
    - +7th **T25.112 Burn of first degree of left ankle**
    - +7th **T25.119 Burn of first degree of unspecified ankle**
  + **T25.12 Burn of first degree of foot**
    Excludes2: *burn of first degree of toe(s) (nail) (T25.13-)*
    - +7th **T25.121 Burn of first degree of right foot**
    - +7th **T25.122 Burn of first degree of left foot**
    - +7th **T25.129 Burn of first degree of unspecified foot**
  + **T25.13 Burn of first degree of toe(s) (nail)**
    - +7th **T25.131 Burn of first degree of right toe(s) (nail)**
    - +7th **T25.132 Burn of first degree of left toe(s) (nail)**
    - +7th **T25.139 Burn of first degree of unspecified toe(s) (nail)**
  + **T25.19 Burn of first degree of multiple sites of ankle and foot**
    - +7th **T25.191 Burn of first degree of multiple sites of right ankle and foot**
    - +7th **T25.192 Burn of first degree of multiple sites of left ankle and foot**
    - +7th **T25.199 Burn of first degree of multiple sites of unspecified ankle and foot**

+ **T25.2 Burn of second degree of ankle and foot**
  Use additional external cause code to identify the source, place and intent of the burn (X00-X19, X75-X77, X96-X98, Y92)
  + **T25.21 Burn of second degree of ankle**
    - +7th **T25.211 Burn of second degree of right ankle**
    - +7th **T25.212 Burn of second degree of left ankle**
    - +7th **T25.219 Burn of second degree of unspecified ankle**
  + **T25.22 Burn of second degree of foot**
    Excludes2: *burn of second degree of toe(s) (nail) (T25.23-)*
    - +7th **T25.221 Burn of second degree of right foot**
    - +7th **T25.222 Burn of second degree of left foot**
    - +7th **T25.229 Burn of second degree of unspecified foot**
  + **T25.23 Burn of second degree of toe(s) (nail)**
    - +7th **T25.231 Burn of second degree of right toe(s) (nail)**
    - +7th **T25.232 Burn of second degree of left toe(s) (nail)**
    - +7th **T25.239 Burn of second degree of unspecified toe(s) (nail)**
  + **T25.29 Burn of second degree of multiple sites of ankle and foot**
    - +7th **T25.291 Burn of second degree of multiple sites of right ankle and foot**
    - +7th **T25.292 Burn of second degree of multiple sites of left ankle and foot**
    - +7th **T25.299 Burn of second degree of multiple sites of unspecified ankle and foot**

+ **T25.3 Burn of third degree of ankle and foot**
  Use external cause code to identify the source, place and intent of the burn (X00-X19, X75-X77, X96-X98, Y92)
  + **T25.31 Burn of third degree of ankle**
    - CC +7th **T25.311 Burn of third degree of right ankle**
      CC Exclusion 7th character A see Appendix A PDX collection 1408
      HAC 7th character A see Appendix B for HAC conditional logic
    - CC +7th **T25.312 Burn of third degree of left ankle**
      CC Exclusion 7th character A see Appendix A PDX collection 1408
      HAC 7th character A see Appendix B for HAC conditional logic
    - CC +7th **T25.319 Burn of third degree of unspecified ankle**
      CC Exclusion 7th character A see Appendix A PDX collection 1408
      HAC 7th character A see Appendix B for HAC conditional logic
  + **T25.32 Burn of third degree of foot**
    Excludes2: *burn of third degree of toe(s) (nail) (T25.33-)*
    - CC +7th **T25.321 Burn of third degree of right foot**
      CC Exclusion 7th character A see Appendix A PDX collection 1409
      HAC 7th character A see Appendix B for HAC conditional logic

CC +7th **T25.322** **Burn of third degree of left foot**
CC Exclusion 7th character A see Appendix A PDX collection 1409
HAC 7th character A see Appendix B for HAC conditional logic

CC +7th **T25.329** **Burn of third degree of unspecified foot**
CC Exclusion 7th character A see Appendix A PDX collection 1409
HAC 7th character A see Appendix B for HAC conditional logic

+ **T25.33** **Burn of third degree of toe(s) (nail)**

CC +7th **T25.331** **Burn of third degree of right toe(s) (nail)**
CC Exclusion 7th character A see Appendix A PDX collection 1410
HAC 7th character A see Appendix B for HAC conditional logic

CC +7th **T25.332** **Burn of third degree of left toe(s) (nail)**
CC Exclusion 7th character A see Appendix A PDX collection 1410
HAC 7th character A see Appendix B for HAC conditional logic

CC +7th **T25.339** **Burn of third degree of unspecified toe(s) (nail)**
CC Exclusion 7th character A see Appendix A PDX collection 1410
HAC 7th character A see Appendix B for HAC conditional logic

+ **T25.39** **Burn of third degree of multiple sites of ankle and foot**

CC +7th **T25.391** **Burn of third degree of multiple sites of right ankle and foot**
CC Exclusion 7th character A see Appendix A PDX collection 1404
HAC 7th character A see Appendix B for HAC conditional logic

CC +7th **T25.392** **Burn of third degree of multiple sites of left ankle and foot**
CC Exclusion 7th character A see Appendix A PDX collection 1404
HAC 7th character A see Appendix B for HAC conditional logic

CC +7th **T25.399** **Burn of third degree of multiple sites of unspecified ankle and foot**
CC Exclusion 7th character A see Appendix A PDX collection 1404
HAC 7th character A see Appendix B for HAC conditional logic

+ **T25.4** **Corrosion of unspecified degree of ankle and foot**
Code first (T51-T65) to identify chemical and intent

Use additional external cause code to identify place (Y92)

+ **T25.41** **Corrosion of unspecified degree of ankle**
+7th **T25.411** **Corrosion of unspecified degree of right ankle**
+7th **T25.412** **Corrosion of unspecified degree of left ankle**
+7th **T25.419** **Corrosion of unspecified degree of unspecified ankle**

+ **T25.42** **Corrosion of unspecified degree of foot**
Excludes2: *corrosion of unspecified degree of toe(s) (nail) (T25.43-)*
+7th **T25.421** **Corrosion of unspecified degree of right foot**
+7th **T25.422** **Corrosion of unspecified degree of left foot**
+7th **T25.429** **Corrosion of unspecified degree of unspecified foot**

+ **T25.43** **Corrosion of unspecified degree of toe(s) (nail)**
+7th **T25.431** **Corrosion of unspecified degree of right toe(s) (nail)**
+7th **T25.432** **Corrosion of unspecified degree of left toe(s) (nail)**
+7th **T25.439** **Corrosion of unspecified degree of unspecified toe(s) (nail)**

+ **T25.49** **Corrosion of unspecified degree of multiple sites of ankle and foot**
+7th **T25.491** **Corrosion of unspecified degree of multiple sites of right ankle and foot**
+7th **T25.492** **Corrosion of unspecified degree of multiple sites of left ankle and foot**
+7th **T25.499** **Corrosion of unspecified degree of multiple sites of unspecified ankle and foot**

+ **T25.5** **Corrosion of first degree of ankle and foot**
Code first (T51-T65) to identify chemical and intent

Use additional external cause code to identify place (Y92)

+ **T25.51** **Corrosion of first degree of ankle**
+7th **T25.511** **Corrosion of first degree of right ankle**
+7th **T25.512** **Corrosion of first degree of left ankle**
+7th **T25.519** **Corrosion of first degree of unspecified ankle**

+ **T25.52** **Corrosion of first degree of foot**
Excludes2: *corrosion of first degree of toe(s) (nail) (T25.53-)*
+7th **T25.521** **Corrosion of first degree of right foot**
+7th **T25.522** **Corrosion of first degree of left foot**
+7th **T25.529** **Corrosion of first degree of unspecified foot**

+ **T25.53** **Corrosion of first degree of toe(s) (nail)**
+7th **T25.531** **Corrosion of first degree of right toe(s) (nail)**
+7th **T25.532** **Corrosion of first degree of left toe(s) (nail)**
+7th **T25.539** **Corrosion of first degree of unspecified toe(s) (nail)**

+ **T25.59** **Corrosion of first degree of multiple sites of ankle and foot**
+7th **T25.591** **Corrosion of first degree of multiple sites of right ankle and foot**
+7th **T25.592** **Corrosion of first degree of multiple sites of left ankle and foot**
+7th **T25.599** **Corrosion of first degree of multiple sites of unspecified ankle and foot**

+ **T25.6** **Corrosion of second degree of ankle and foot**
Code first (T51-T65) to identify chemical and intent

Use additional external cause code to identify place (Y92)

+ **T25.61** **Corrosion of second degree of ankle**
+7th **T25.611** **Corrosion of second degree of right ankle**
+7th **T25.612** **Corrosion of second degree of left ankle**
+7th **T25.619** **Corrosion of second degree of unspecified ankle**

+ **T25.62** **Corrosion of second degree of foot**
Excludes2: *corrosion of second degree of toe(s) (nail) (T25.63-)*
+7th **T25.621** **Corrosion of second degree of right foot**
+7th **T25.622** **Corrosion of second degree of left foot**
+7th **T25.629** **Corrosion of second degree of unspecified foot**

+ **T25.63** **Corrosion of second degree of toe(s) (nail)**
+7th **T25.631** **Corrosion of second degree of right toe(s) (nail)**
+7th **T25.632** **Corrosion of second degree of left toe(s) (nail)**
+7th **T25.639** **Corrosion of second degree of unspecified toe(s) (nail)**

+ **T25.69** **Corrosion of second degree of multiple sites of ankle and foot**
+7th **T25.691** **Corrosion of second degree of right ankle and foot**
+7th **T25.692** **Corrosion of second degree of left ankle and foot**
+7th **T25.699** **Corrosion of second degree of unspecified ankle and foot**

+ **T25.7** **Corrosion of third degree of ankle and foot**
Code first (T51-T65) to identify chemical and intent

Use additional external cause code to identify place (Y92)

+ **T25.71** **Corrosion of third degree of ankle**

CC +7th **T25.711** **Corrosion of third degree of right ankle**
CC Exclusion 7th character A see Appendix A PDX collection 1408
HAC 7th character A see Appendix B for HAC conditional logic

CC +7th **T25.712** **Corrosion of third degree of left ankle**
CC Exclusion 7th character A see Appendix A PDX collection 1408
HAC 7th character A see Appendix B for HAC conditional logic

CC +7th **T25.719** **Corrosion of third degree of unspecified ankle**
CC Exclusion 7th character A see Appendix A PDX collection 1408
HAC 7th character A see Appendix B for HAC conditional logic

+ **T25.72 Corrosion of third degree of foot**
Excludes2: corrosion of third degree of toe(s) (nail) (T25.73-)

CC +7th **T25.721 Corrosion of third degree of right foot**
CC Exclusion 7th character A see Appendix A PDX collection 1409
HAC 7th character A see Appendix B for HAC conditional logic

CC +7th **T25.722 Corrosion of third degree of left foot**
CC Exclusion 7th character A see Appendix A PDX collection 1409
HAC 7th character A see Appendix B for HAC conditional logic

CC +7th **T25.729 Corrosion of third degree of unspecified foot**
CC Exclusion 7th character A see Appendix A PDX collection 1409
HAC 7th character A see Appendix B for HAC conditional logic

+ **T25.73 Corrosion of third degree of toe(s) (nail)**

CC +7th **T25.731 Corrosion of third degree of right toe(s) (nail)**
CC Exclusion 7th character A see Appendix A PDX collection 1410
HAC 7th character A see Appendix B for HAC conditional logic

CC +7th **T25.732 Corrosion of third degree of left toe(s) (nail)**
CC Exclusion 7th character A see Appendix A PDX collection 1410
HAC 7th character A see Appendix B for HAC conditional logic

CC +7th **T25.739 Corrosion of third degree of unspecified toe(s) (nail)**
CC Exclusion 7th character A see Appendix A PDX collection 1410
HAC 7th character A see Appendix B for HAC conditional logic

+ **T25.79 Corrosion of third degree of multiple sites of ankle and foot**

CC +7th **T25.791 Corrosion of third degree of multiple sites of right ankle and foot**
CC Exclusion 7th character A see Appendix A PDX collection 1404
HAC 7th character A see Appendix B for HAC conditional logic

CC +7th **T25.792 Corrosion of third degree of multiple sites of left ankle and foot**
CC Exclusion 7th character A see Appendix A PDX collection 1404
HAC 7th character A see Appendix B for HAC conditional logic

CC +7th **T25.799 Corrosion of third degree of multiple sites of unspecified ankle and foot**
CC Exclusion 7th character A see Appendix A PDX collection 1404
HAC 7th character A see Appendix B for HAC conditional logic

Burns and corrosions confined to eye and internal organs (T26-T28)

Review coding guideline C.19.d

T26 Burn and corrosion confined to eye and adnexa

The appropriate 7th character is to be added to each code from category T26
A initial encounter
D subsequent encounter
S sequela

+ **T26.0 Burn of eyelid and periocular area**
Use additional external cause code to identify the source, place and intent of the burn (X00-X19, X75-X77, X96-X98, Y92)

X+7th **T26.00 Burn of unspecified eyelid and periocular area**
X+7th **T26.01 Burn of right eyelid and periocular area**
X+7th **T26.02 Burn of left eyelid and periocular area**

+ **T26.1 Burn of cornea and conjunctival sac**
Use additional external cause code to identify the source, place and intent of the burn (X00-X19, X75-X77, X96-X98, Y92)

X+7th **T26.10 Burn of cornea and conjunctival sac, unspecified eye**
X+7th **T26.11 Burn of cornea and conjunctival sac, right eye**
X+7th **T26.12 Burn of cornea and conjunctival sac, left eye**

+ **T26.2 Burn with resulting rupture and destruction of eyeball**
Use additional external cause code to identify the source, place and intent of the burn (X00-X19, X75-X77, X96-X98, Y92)

CC X+7th **T26.20 Burn with resulting rupture and destruction of unspecified eyeball**
No CC Exclusions
HAC 7th character A see Appendix B for HAC conditional logic

CC X+7th **T26.21 Burn with resulting rupture and destruction of right eyeball**
No CC Exclusions
HAC 7th character A see Appendix B for HAC conditional logic

CC X+7th **T26.22 Burn with resulting rupture and destruction of left eyeball**
No CC Exclusions
HAC 7th character A see Appendix B for HAC conditional logic

+ **T26.3 Burns of other specified parts of eye and adnexa**
Use additional external cause code to identify the source, place and intent of the burn (X00-X19, X75-X77, X96-X98, Y92)

X+7th **T26.30 Burns of other specified parts of unspecified eye and adnexa**
X+7th **T26.31 Burns of other specified parts of right eye and adnexa**
X+7th **T26.32 Burns of other specified parts of left eye and adnexa**

+ **T26.4 Burn of eye and adnexa, part unspecified**
Use additional external cause code to identify the source, place and intent of the burn (X00-X19, X75-X77, X96-X98, Y92)

X+7th **T26.40 Burn of unspecified eye and adnexa, part unspecified**
X+7th **T26.41 Burn of right eye and adnexa, part unspecified**
X+7th **T26.42 Burn of left eye and adnexa, part unspecified**

+ **T26.5 Corrosion of eyelid and periocular area**
Code first (T51-T65) to identify chemical and intent

Use additional external cause code to identify place (Y92)

X+7th **T26.50 Corrosion of unspecified eyelid and periocular area**
X+7th **T26.51 Corrosion of right eyelid and periocular area**
X+7th **T26.52 Corrosion of left eyelid and periocular area**

+ **T26.6 Corrosion of cornea and conjunctival sac**
Code first (T51-T65) to identify chemical and intent

Use additional external cause code to identify place (Y92)

X+7th **T26.60 Corrosion of cornea and conjunctival sac, unspecified eye**
X+7th **T26.61 Corrosion of cornea and conjunctival sac, right eye**
X+7th **T26.62 Corrosion of cornea and conjunctival sac, left eye**

+ **T26.7 Corrosion with resulting rupture and destruction of eyeball**
Code first (T51-T65) to identify chemical and intent

Use additional external cause code to identify place (Y92)

CC X+7th **T26.70 Corrosion with resulting rupture and destruction of unspecified eyeball**
No CC Exclusions
HAC 7th character A see Appendix B for HAC conditional logic

CC X+7th **T26.71 Corrosion with resulting rupture and destruction of right eyeball**
No CC Exclusions
HAC 7th character A see Appendix B for HAC conditional logic

CC X+7th **T26.72 Corrosion with resulting rupture and destruction of left eyeball**
No CC Exclusions
HAC 7th character A see Appendix B for HAC conditional logic

+ **T26.8 Corrosions of other specified parts of eye and adnexa**
Code first (T51-T65) to identify chemical and intent

Use add itional external cause code to identify place (Y92)

X+7th **T26.80 Corrosions of other specified parts of unspecified eye and adnexa**
X+7th **T26.81 Corrosions of other specified parts of right eye and adnexa**
X+7th **T26.82 Corrosions of other specified parts of left eye and adnexa**

+ T26.9 **Corrosion of eye and adnexa, part unspecified**
Code first (T51-T65) to identify chemical and intent

Use additional external cause code to identify place (Y92)

X+7th T26.90 **Corrosion of unspecified eye and adnexa, part unspecified**
X+7th T26.91 **Corrosion of right eye and adnexa, part unspecified**
X+7th T26.92 **Corrosion of left eye and adnexa, part unspecified**

T27 **Burn and corrosion of respiratory tract**

Use additional external cause code to identify the source and intent of the burn (X00-X19, X75-X77, X96-X98)

Use external cause code to identify place (Y92)

The appropriate 7th character is to be added to each code from category T27
A initial encounter
D subsequent encounter
S sequela

CC X+7th T27.0 **Burn of larynx and trachea**
CC Exclusion 7th character A see Appendix A PDX collection 1411
HAC 7th character A see Appendix B for HAC conditional logic

CC X+7th T27.1 **Burn involving larynx and trachea with lung**
CC Exclusion 7th character A see Appendix A PDX collection 1411
HAC 7th character A see Appendix B for HAC conditional logic

CC X+7th T27.2 **Burn of other parts of respiratory tract**
Burn of thoracic cavity
CC Exclusion 7th character A see Appendix A PDX collection 1411
HAC 7th character A see Appendix B for HAC conditional logic

CC X+7th T27.3 **Burn of respiratory tract, part unspecified**
CC Exclusion 7th character A see Appendix A PDX collection 1411
HAC 7th character A see Appendix B for HAC conditional logic

CC X+7th T27.4 **Corrosion of larynx and trachea**
Code first (T51-T65) to identify chemical and intent
CC Exclusion 7th character A see Appendix A PDX collection 1411
HAC 7th character A see Appendix B for HAC conditional logic

CC X+7th T27.5 **Corrosion involving larynx and trachea with lung**
CC Exclusion 7th character A see Appendix A PDX collection 1411
HAC 7th character A see Appendix B for HAC conditional logic

CC X+7th T27.6 **Corrosion of other parts of respiratory tract**
Code first (T51-T65) to identify chemical and intent
CC Exclusion 7th character A see Appendix A PDX collection 1411
HAC 7th character A see Appendix B for HAC conditional logic

CC X+7th T27.7 **Corrosion of respiratory tract, part unspecified**
Code first (T51-T65) to identify chemical and intent
CC Exclusion 7th character A see Appendix A PDX collection 1411
HAC 7th character A see Appendix B for HAC conditional logic

T28 **Burn and corrosion of other internal organs**

Use additional external cause code to identify the source and intent of the burn (X00-X19, X75-X77, X96-X98)

Use external cause code to identify place (Y92)

The appropriate 7th character is to be added to each code from category T28
A initial encounter
D subsequent encounter
S sequela

X+7th T28.0 **Burn of mouth and pharynx**

CC X+7th T28.1 **Burn of esophagus**
CC Exclusion 7th character A see Appendix A PDX collection 1412
HAC 7th character A see Appendix B for HAC conditional logic

CC X+7th T28.2 **Burn of other parts of alimentary tract**
CC Exclusion 7th character A see Appendix A PDX collection 1413
HAC 7th character A see Appendix B for HAC conditional logic

X+7th T28.3 **Burn of internal genitourinary organs**

+ T28.4 **Burns of other and unspecified internal organs**
Code first (T51-T65) to identify chemical and intent

X+7th T28.40 **Burn of unspecified internal organ**
+ T28.41 **Burn of ear drum**
+7th T28.411 **Burn of right ear drum**
+7th T28.412 **Burn of left ear drum**
+7th T28.419 **Burn of unspecified ear drum**
X+7th T28.49 **Burn of other internal organ**

X+7th T28.5 **Corrosion of mouth and pharynx**
Code first (T51-T65) to identify chemical and intent

CC X+7th T28.6 **Corrosion of esophagus**
Code first (T51-T65) to identify chemical and intent
CC Exclusion 7th character A see Appendix A PDX collection 1412
HAC 7th character A see Appendix B for HAC conditional logic

CC X+7th T28.7 **Corrosion of other parts of alimentary tract**
Code first (T51-T65) to identify chemical and intent
CC Exclusion 7th character A see Appendix A PDX collection 1413
HAC 7th character A see Appendix B for HAC conditional logic

X+7th T28.8 **Corrosion of internal genitourinary organs**
Code first (T51-T65) to identify chemical and intent

+ T28.9 **Corrosions of other and unspecified internal organs**
Code first (T51-T65) to identify chemical and intent

X+7th T28.90 **Corrosions of unspecified internal organs**
+ T28.91 **Corrosions of ear drum**
+7th T28.911 **Corrosions of right ear drum**
+7th T28.912 **Corrosions of left ear drum**
+7th T28.919 **Corrosions of unspecified ear drum**
X+7th T28.99 **Corrosions of other internal organs**

Burns and corrosions of multiple and unspecified body regions (T30-T32)

T30 **Burn and corrosion, body region unspecified**

Review coding guideline C.19.d.5

T30.0 **Burn of unspecified body region, unspecified degree**
This code is not for inpatient use. Code to specified site and degree of burns
Burn NOS
Multiple burns NOS

T30.4 **Corrosion of unspecified body region, unspecified degree**
This code is not for inpatient use. Code to specified site and degree of corrosion
Corrosion NOS
Multiple corrosion NOS

T31 **Burns classified according to extent of body surface involved**

NOTE This category is to be used as the primary code only when the site of the burn is unspecified. It should be used as a supplementary code with categories T20-T25 when the site is specified.

Review coding guideline C.19.d.6

T31.0 **Burns involving less than 10% of body surface**

+ T31.1 **Burns involving 10-19% of body surface**

CC T31.10 **Burns involving 10-19% of body surface with 0% to 9% third degree burns**
Burns involving 10-19% of body surface NOS
CC Exclusion see Appendix A PDX collection 1414
HAC see Appendix B for HAC conditional logic

CC T31.11 **Burns involving 10-19% of body surface with 10-19% third degree burns**
CC Exclusion see Appendix A PDX collection 1414
HAC see Appendix B for HAC conditional logic

+ T31.2 **Burns involving 20-29% of body surface**

CC T31.20 **Burns involving 20-29% of body surface with 0% to 9% third degree burns**
Burns involving 20-29% of body surface NOS
CC Exclusion see Appendix A PDX collection 1414
HAC see Appendix B for HAC conditional logic

MCC T31.21 **Burns involving 20-29% of body surface with 10-19% third degree burns**
MCC Exclusion see Appendix A PDX collection 1414
HAC see Appendix B for HAC conditional logic

MCC T31.22 **Burns involving 20-29% of body surface with 20-29% third degree burns**
MCC Exclusion see Appendix A PDX collection 1414
HAC see Appendix B for HAC conditional logic

+ T31.3 **Burns involving 30-39% of body surface**

CC T31.30 **Burns involving 30-39% of body surface with 0% to 9% third degree burns**
Burns involving 30-39% of body surface NOS
CC Exclusion see Appendix A PDX collection 1414
HAC see Appendix B for HAC conditional logic

MCC T31.31 **Burns involving 30-39% of body surface with 10-19% third degree burns**
MCC Exclusion see Appendix A PDX collection 1414
HAC see Appendix B for HAC conditional logic

MCC T31.32 **Burns involving 30-39% of body surface with 20-29% third degree burns**
MCC Exclusion see Appendix A PDX collection 1414
HAC see Appendix B for HAC conditional logic

MCC T31.33 **Burns involving 30-39% of body surface with 30-39% third degree burns**
MCC Exclusion see Appendix A PDX collection 1414
HAC see Appendix B for HAC conditional logic

+ **T31.4 Burns involving 40-49% of body surface**

CC **T31.40 Burns involving 40-49% of body surface with 0% to 9% third degree burns**
Burns involving 40-49% of body surface NOS
CC Exclusion see Appendix A PDX collection 1414
HAC see Appendix B for HAC conditional logic

MCC **T31.41 Burns involving 40-49% of body surface with 10-19% third degree burns**
MCC Exclusion see Appendix A PDX collection 1414
HAC see Appendix B for HAC conditional logic

MCC **T31.42 Burns involving 40-49% of body surface with 20-29% third degree burns**
MCC Exclusion see Appendix A PDX collection 1414
HAC see Appendix B for HAC conditional logic

MCC **T31.43 Burns involving 40-49% of body surface with 30-39% third degree burns**
MCC Exclusion see Appendix A PDX collection 1414
HAC see Appendix B for HAC conditional logic

MCC **T31.44 Burns involving 40-49% of body surface with 40-49% third degree burns**
MCC Exclusion see Appendix A PDX collection 1414
HAC see Appendix B for HAC conditional logic

+ **T31.5 Burns involving 50-59% of body surface**

CC **T31.50 Burns involving 50-59% of body surface with 0% to 9% third degree burns**
Burns involving 50-59% of body surface NOS
CC Exclusion see Appendix A PDX collection 1414
HAC see Appendix B for HAC conditional logic

MCC **T31.51 Burns involving 50-59% of body surface with 10-19% third degree burns**
MCC Exclusion see Appendix A PDX collection 1414
HAC see Appendix B for HAC conditional logic

MCC **T31.52 Burns involving 50-59% of body surface with 20-29% third degree burns**
MCC Exclusion see Appendix A PDX collection 1414
HAC see Appendix B for HAC conditional logic

MCC **T31.53 Burns involving 50-59% of body surface with 30-39% third degree burns**
MCC Exclusion see Appendix A PDX collection 1414
HAC see Appendix B for HAC conditional logic

MCC **T31.54 Burns involving 50-59% of body surface with 40-49% third degree burns**
MCC Exclusion see Appendix A PDX collection 1414
HAC see Appendix B for HAC conditional logic

MCC **T31.55 Burns involving 50-59% of body surface with 50-59% third degree burns**
MCC Exclusion see Appendix A PDX collection 1414
HAC see Appendix B for HAC conditional logic

+ **T31.6 Burns involving 60-69% of body surface**

CC **T31.60 Burns involving 60-69% of body surface with 0% to 9% third degree burns**
Burns involving 60-69% of body surface NOS
CC Exclusion see Appendix A PDX collection 1414
HAC see Appendix B for HAC conditional logic

MCC **T31.61 Burns involving 60-69% of body surface with 10-19% third degree burns**
MCC Exclusion see Appendix A PDX collection 1414
HAC see Appendix B for HAC conditional logic

MCC **T31.62 Burns involving 60-69% of body surface with 20-29% third degree burns**
MCC Exclusion see Appendix A PDX collection 1414
HAC see Appendix B for HAC conditional logic

MCC **T31.63 Burns involving 60-69% of body surface with 30-39% third degree burns**
MCC Exclusion see Appendix A PDX collection 1414
HAC see Appendix B for HAC conditional logic

MCC **T31.64 Burns involving 60-69% of body surface with 40-49% third degree burns**
MCC Exclusion see Appendix A PDX collection 1414
HAC see Appendix B for HAC conditional logic

MCC **T31.65 Burns involving 60-69% of body surface with 50-59% third degree burns**
MCC Exclusion see Appendix A PDX collection 1414
HAC see Appendix B for HAC conditional logic

MCC **T31.66 Burns involving 60-69% of body surface with 60-69% third degree burns**
MCC Exclusion see Appendix A PDX collection 1414
HAC see Appendix B for HAC conditional logic

+ **T31.7 Burns involving 70-79% of body surface**

CC **T31.70 Burns involving 70-79% of body surface with 0% to 9% third degree burns**
Burns involving 70-79% of body surface NOS
CC Exclusion see Appendix A PDX collection 1414
HAC see Appendix B for HAC conditional logic

MCC **T31.71 Burns involving 70-79% of body surface with 10-19% third degree burns**
MCC Exclusion see Appendix A PDX collection 1414
HAC see Appendix B for HAC conditional logic

MCC **T31.72 Burns involving 70-79% of body surface with 20-29% third degree burns**
MCC Exclusion see Appendix A PDX collection 1414
HAC see Appendix B for HAC conditional logic

MCC **T31.73** **Burns involving 70-79% of body surface with 30-39% third degree burns**
MCC Exclusion see Appendix A PDX collection 1414
HAC see Appendix B for HAC conditional logic

MCC **T31.74** **Burns involving 70-79% of body surface with 40-49% third degree burns**
MCC Exclusion see Appendix A PDX collection 1414
HAC see Appendix B for HAC conditional logic

MCC **T31.75** **Burns involving 70-79% of body surface with 50-59% third degree burns**
MCC Exclusion see Appendix A PDX collection 1414
HAC see Appendix B for HAC conditional logic

MCC **T31.76** **Burns involving 70-79% of body surface with 60-69% third degree burns**
MCC Exclusion see Appendix A PDX collection 1414
HAC see Appendix B for HAC conditional logic

MCC **T31.77** **Burns involving 70-79% of body surface with 70-79% third degree burns**
MCC Exclusion see Appendix A PDX collection 1414
HAC see Appendix B for HAC conditional logic

+ **T31.8** **Burns involving 80-89% of body surface**

CC **T31.80** **Burns involving 80-89% of body surface with 0% to 9% third degree burns**
Burns involving 80-89% of body surface NOS
CC Exclusion see Appendix A PDX collection 1414
HAC see Appendix B for HAC conditional logic

MCC **T31.81** **Burns involving 80-89% of body surface with 10-19% third degree burns**
MCC Exclusion see Appendix A PDX collection 1414
HAC see Appendix B for HAC conditional logic

MCC **T31.82** **Burns involving 80-89% of body surface with 20-29% third degree burns**
MCC Exclusion see Appendix A PDX collection 1414
HAC see Appendix B for HAC conditional logic

MCC **T31.83** **Burns involving 80-89% of body surface with 30-39% third degree burns**
MCC Exclusion see Appendix A PDX collection 1414
HAC see Appendix B for HAC conditional logic

MCC **T31.84** **Burns involving 80-89% of body surface with 40-49% third degree burns**
MCC Exclusion see Appendix A PDX collection 1414
HAC see Appendix B for HAC conditional logic

MCC **T31.85** **Burns involving 80-89% of body surface with 50-59% third degree burns**
MCC Exclusion see Appendix A PDX collection 1414
HAC see Appendix B for HAC conditional logic

MCC **T31.86** **Burns involving 80-89% of body surface with 60-69% third degree burns**
MCC Exclusion see Appendix A PDX collection 1414
HAC see Appendix B for HAC conditional logic

MCC **T31.87** **Burns involving 80-89% of body surface with 70-79% third degree burns**
MCC Exclusion see Appendix A PDX collection 1414
HAC see Appendix B for HAC conditional logic

MCC **T31.88** **Burns involving 80-89% of body surface with 80-89% third degree burns**
MCC Exclusion see Appendix A PDX collection 1414
HAC see Appendix B for HAC conditional logic

+ **T31.9** **Burns involving 90% or more of body surface**

CC **T31.90** **Burns involving 90% or more of body surface with 0% to 9% third degree burns**
Burns involving 90% or more of body surface NOS
CC Exclusion see Appendix A PDX collection 1414
HAC see Appendix B for HAC conditional logic

MCC **T31.91** **Burns involving 90% or more of body surface with 10-19% third degree burns**
MCC Exclusion see Appendix A PDX collection 1414
HAC see Appendix B for HAC conditional logic

MCC **T31.92** **Burns involving 90% or more of body surface with 20-29% third degree burns**
MCC Exclusion see Appendix A PDX collection 1414
HAC see Appendix B for HAC conditional logic

MCC **T31.93** **Burns involving 90% or more of body surface with 30-39% third degree burns**
MCC Exclusion see Appendix A PDX collection 1414
HAC see Appendix B for HAC conditional logic

MCC **T31.94** **Burns involving 90% or more of body surface with 40-49% third degree burns**
MCC Exclusion see Appendix A PDX collection 1414
HAC see Appendix B for HAC conditional logic

MCC **T31.95** **Burns involving 90% or more of body surface with 50-59% third degree burns**
MCC Exclusion see Appendix A PDX collection 1414
HAC see Appendix B for HAC conditional logic

MCC **T31.96** **Burns involving 90% or more of body surface with 60-69% third degree burns**
MCC Exclusion see Appendix A PDX collection 1414
HAC see Appendix B for HAC conditional logic

MCC **T31.97** **Burns involving 90% or more of body surface with 70-79% third degree burns**
MCC Exclusion see Appendix A PDX collection 1414
HAC see Appendix B for HAC conditional logic

MCC **T31.98** **Burns involving 90% or more of body surface with 80-89% third degree burns**
MCC Exclusion see Appendix A PDX collection 1414
HAC see Appendix B for HAC conditional logic

MCC **T31.99** **Burns involving 90% or more of body surface with 90% or more third degree burns**
MCC Exclusion see Appendix A PDX collection 1414
HAC see Appendix B for HAC conditional logic

T32 Corrosions classified according to extent of body surface involved

NOTE This category is to be used as the primary code only when the site of the corrosion is unspecified. It may be used as a supplementary code with categories T20-T25 when the site is specified.

Review coding guideline C.19.d.6

T32.0 **Corrosions involving less than 10% of body surface**

+ **T32.1** **Corrosions involving 10-19% of body surface**

CC **T32.10** **Corrosions involving 10-19% of body surface with 0% to 9% third degree corrosion**
Corrosions involving 10-19% of body surface NOS
CC Exclusion see Appendix A PDX collection 1414
HAC see Appendix B for HAC conditional logic

CC **T32.11** **Corrosions involving 10-19% of body surface with 10-19% third degree corrosion**
CC Exclusion see Appendix A PDX collection 1414
HAC see Appendix B for HAC conditional logic

+ **T32.2** **Corrosions involving 20-29% of body surface**

CC **T32.20** **Corrosions involving 20-29% of body surface with 0% to 9% third degree corrosion**
CC Exclusion see Appendix A PDX collection 1414
HAC see Appendix B for HAC conditional logic

MCC **T32.21** **Corrosions involving 20-29% of body surface with 10-19% third degree corrosion**
MCC Exclusion see Appendix A PDX collection 1414
HAC see Appendix B for HAC conditional logic

MCC **T32.22** **Corrosions involving 20-29% of body surface with 20-29% third degree corrosion**
MCC Exclusion see Appendix A PDX collection 1414
HAC see Appendix B for HAC conditional logic

+ **T32.3** **Corrosions involving 30-39% of body surface**

CC **T32.30** **Corrosions involving 30-39% of body surface with 0% to 9% third degree corrosion**
CC Exclusion see Appendix A PDX collection 1414
HAC see Appendix B for HAC conditional logic

MCC **T32.31** **Corrosions involving 30-39% of body surface with 10-19% third degree corrosion**
MCC Exclusion see Appendix A PDX collection 1414
HAC see Appendix B for HAC conditional logic

MCC **T32.32** **Corrosions involving 30-39% of body surface with 20-29% third degree corrosion**
MCC Exclusion see Appendix A PDX collection 1414
HAC see Appendix B for HAC conditional logic

MCC **T32.33** **Corrosions involving 30-39% of body surface with 30-39% third degree corrosion**
MCC Exclusion see Appendix A PDX collection 1414
HAC see Appendix B for HAC conditional logic

+ **T32.4** **Corrosions involving 40-49% of body surface**

CC **T32.40** **Corrosions involving 40-49% of body surface with 0% to 9% third degree corrosion**
CC Exclusion see Appendix A PDX collection 1414
HAC see Appendix B for HAC conditional logic

MCC **T32.41** **Corrosions involving 40-49% of body surface with 10-19% third degree corrosion**
MCC Exclusion see Appendix A PDX collection 1414
HAC see Appendix B for HAC conditional logic

MCC **T32.42** **Corrosions involving 40-49% of body surface with 20-29% third degree corrosion**
MCC Exclusion see Appendix A PDX collection 1414
HAC see Appendix B for HAC conditional logic

MCC **T32.43** Corrosions involving 40-49% of body surface with 30-39% third degree corrosion
MCC Exclusion see Appendix A PDX collection 1414
HAC see Appendix B for HAC conditional logic

MCC **T32.44** Corrosions involving 40-49% of body surface with 40-49% third degree corrosion
MCC Exclusion see Appendix A PDX collection 1414
HAC see Appendix B for HAC conditional logic

\+ T32.5 Corrosions involving 50-59% of body surface

CC T32.50 Corrosions involving 50-59% of body surface with 0% to 9% third degree corrosion
CC Exclusion see Appendix A PDX collection 1414
HAC see Appendix B for HAC conditional logic

MCC **T32.51** Corrosions involving 50-59% of body surface with 10-19% third degree corrosion
MCC Exclusion see Appendix A PDX collection 1414
HAC see Appendix B for HAC conditional logic

MCC **T32.52** Corrosions involving 50-59% of body surface with 20-29% third degree corrosion
MCC Exclusion see Appendix A PDX collection 1414
HAC see Appendix B for HAC conditional logic

MCC **T32.53** Corrosions involving 50-59% of body surface with 30-39% third degree corrosion
MCC Exclusion see Appendix A PDX collection 1414
HAC see Appendix B for HAC conditional logic

MCC **T32.54** Corrosions involving 50-59% of body surface with 40-49% third degree corrosion
MCC Exclusion see Appendix A PDX collection 1414
HAC see Appendix B for HAC conditional logic

MCC **T32.55** Corrosions involving 50-59% of body surface with 50-59% third degree corrosion
MCC Exclusion see Appendix A PDX collection 1414
HAC see Appendix B for HAC conditional logic

\+ T32.6 Corrosions involving 60-69% of body surface

CC T32.60 Corrosions involving 60-69% of body surface with 0% to 9% third degree corrosion
CC Exclusion see Appendix A PDX collection 1414
HAC see Appendix B for HAC conditional logic

MCC **T32.61** Corrosions involving 60-69% of body surface with 10-19% third degree corrosion
MCC Exclusion see Appendix A PDX collection 1414
HAC see Appendix B for HAC conditional logic

MCC **T32.62** Corrosions involving 60-69% of body surface with 20-29% third degree corrosion
MCC Exclusion see Appendix A PDX collection 1414
HAC see Appendix B for HAC conditional logic

MCC **T32.63** Corrosions involving 60-69% of body surface with 30-39% third degree corrosion
MCC Exclusion see Appendix A PDX collection 1414
HAC see Appendix B for HAC conditional logic

MCC **T32.64** Corrosions involving 60-69% of body surface with 40-49% third degree corrosion
MCC Exclusion see Appendix A PDX collection 1414
HAC see Appendix B for HAC conditional logic

MCC **T32.65** Corrosions involving 60-69% of body surface with 50-59% third degree corrosion
MCC Exclusion see Appendix A PDX collection 1414
HAC see Appendix B for HAC conditional logic

MCC **T32.66** Corrosions involving 60-69% of body surface with 60-69% third degree corrosion
MCC Exclusion see Appendix A PDX collection 1414
HAC see Appendix B for HAC conditional logic

\+ T32.7 Corrosions involving 70-79% of body surface

CC T32.70 Corrosions involving 70-79% of body surface with 0% to 9% third degree corrosion
CC Exclusion see Appendix A PDX collection 1414
HAC see Appendix B for HAC conditional logic

MCC **T32.71** Corrosions involving 70-79% of body surface with 10-19% third degree corrosion
MCC Exclusion see Appendix A PDX collection 1414
HAC see Appendix B for HAC conditional logic

MCC **T32.72** Corrosions involving 70-79% of body surface with 20-29% third degree corrosion
MCC Exclusion see Appendix A PDX collection 1414
HAC see Appendix B for HAC conditional logic

MCC **T32.73** Corrosions involving 70-79% of body surface with 30-39% third degree corrosion
MCC Exclusion see Appendix A PDX collection 1414
HAC see Appendix B for HAC conditional logic

MCC **T32.74** Corrosions involving 70-79% of body surface with 40-49% third degree corrosion
MCC Exclusion see Appendix A PDX collection 1414
HAC see Appendix B for HAC conditional logic

MCC **T32.75** Corrosions involving 70-79% of body surface with 50-59% third degree corrosion
MCC Exclusion see Appendix A PDX collection 1414
HAC see Appendix B for HAC conditional logic

MCC **T32.76** Corrosions involving 70-79% of body surface with 60-69% third degree corrosion
MCC Exclusion see Appendix A PDX collection 1414
HAC see Appendix B for HAC conditional logic

MCC **T32.77** Corrosions involving 70-79% of body surface with 70-79% third degree corrosion
MCC Exclusion see Appendix A PDX collection 1414
HAC see Appendix B for HAC conditional logic

\+ T32.8 Corrosions involving 80-89% of body surface

CC T32.80 Corrosions involving 80-89% of body surface with 0% to 9% third degree corrosion
CC Exclusion see Appendix A PDX collection 1414
HAC see Appendix B for HAC conditional logic

MCC **T32.81** Corrosions involving 80-89% of body surface with 10-19% third degree corrosion
MCC Exclusion see Appendix A PDX collection 1414
HAC see Appendix B for HAC conditional logic

MCC **T32.82** Corrosions involving 80-89% of body surface with 20-29% third degree corrosion
MCC Exclusion see Appendix A PDX collection 1414
HAC see Appendix B for HAC conditional logic

MCC **T32.83** Corrosions involving 80-89% of body surface with 30-39% third degree corrosion
MCC Exclusion see Appendix A PDX collection 1414
HAC see Appendix B for HAC conditional logic

MCC **T32.84** Corrosions involving 80-89% of body surface with 40-49% third degree corrosion
MCC Exclusion see Appendix A PDX collection 1414
HAC see Appendix B for HAC conditional logic

MCC **T32.85** Corrosions involving 80-89% of body surface with 50-59% third degree corrosion
MCC Exclusion see Appendix A PDX collection 1414
HAC see Appendix B for HAC conditional logic

MCC **T32.86** Corrosions involving 80-89% of body surface with 60-69% third degree corrosion
MCC Exclusion see Appendix A PDX collection 1414
HAC see Appendix B for HAC conditional logic

MCC **T32.87** Corrosions involving 80-89% of body surface with 70-79% third degree corrosion
MCC Exclusion see Appendix A PDX collection 1414
HAC see Appendix B for HAC conditional logic

MCC **T32.88** Corrosions involving 80-89% of body surface with 80-89% third degree corrosion
MCC Exclusion see Appendix A PDX collection 1414
HAC see Appendix B for HAC conditional logic

\+ T32.9 Corrosions involving 90% or more of body surface

CC T32.90 Corrosions involving 90% or more of body surface with 0% to 9% third degree corrosion
CC Exclusion see Appendix A PDX collection 1414
HAC see Appendix B for HAC conditional logic

MCC **T32.91** Corrosions involving 90% or more of body surface with 10-19% third degree corrosion
MCC Exclusion see Appendix A PDX collection 1414
HAC see Appendix B for HAC conditional logic

MCC **T32.92** Corrosions involving 90% or more of body surface with 20-29% third degree corrosion
MCC Exclusion see Appendix A PDX collection 1414
HAC see Appendix B for HAC conditional logic

MCC **T32.93** Corrosions involving 90% or more of body surface with 30-39% third degree corrosion
MCC Exclusion see Appendix A PDX collection 1414
HAC see Appendix B for HAC conditional logic

MCC **T32.94** Corrosions involving 90% or more of body surface with 40-49% third degree corrosion
MCC Exclusion see Appendix A PDX collection 1414
HAC see Appendix B for HAC conditional logic

MCC **T32.95** Corrosions involving 90% or more of body surface with 50-59% third degree corrosion
MCC Exclusion see Appendix A PDX collection 1414
HAC see Appendix B for HAC conditional logic

MCC **T32.96** **Corrosions involving 90% or more of body surface with 60-69% third degree corrosion**
MCC Exclusion see Appendix A PDX collection 1414
HAC see Appendix B for HAC conditional logic

MCC **T32.97** **Corrosions involving 90% or more of body surface with 70-79% third degree corrosion**
MCC Exclusion see Appendix A PDX collection 1414
HAC see Appendix B for HAC conditional logic

MCC **T32.98** **Corrosions involving 90% or more of body surface with 80-89% third degree corrosion**
MCC Exclusion see Appendix A PDX collection 1414
HAC see Appendix B for HAC conditional logic

MCC **T32.99** **Corrosions involving 90% or more of body surface with 90% or more third degree corrosion**
MCC Exclusion see Appendix A PDX collection 1414
HAC see Appendix B for HAC conditional logic

Frostbite (T33-T34)

Excludes2: *hypothermia and other effects of reduced temperature (T68, T69.-)*

T33 Superficial frostbite

Includes: frostbite with partial thickness skin loss

The appropriate 7th character is to be added to each code from category T33
A initial encounter
D subsequent encounter
S sequela

\+ **T33.0 Superficial frostbite of head**

\+ **T33.01 Superficial frostbite of ear**

CC +7th **T33.011 Superficial frostbite of right ear**
CC Exclusion 7th character A see Appendix A PDX collection 1415
HAC 7th character A see Appendix B for HAC conditional logic

CC +7th **T33.012 Superficial frostbite of left ear**
CC Exclusion 7th character A see Appendix A PDX collection 1415
HAC 7th character A see Appendix B for HAC conditional logic

CC +7th **T33.019 Superficial frostbite of unspecified ear**
CC Exclusion 7th character A see Appendix A PDX collection 1415
HAC 7th character A see Appendix B for HAC conditional logic

CC X+7th **T33.02 Superficial frostbite of nose**
CC Exclusion 7th character A see Appendix A PDX collection 1415
HAC 7th character A see Appendix B for HAC conditional logic

CC X+7th **T33.09 Superficial frostbite of other part of head**
CC Exclusion 7th character A see Appendix A PDX collection 1415
HAC 7th character A see Appendix B for HAC conditional logic

CC X+7th **T33.1 Superficial frostbite of neck**
CC Exclusion 7th character A see Appendix A PDX collection 1415
HAC 7th character A see Appendix B for HAC conditional logic

CC X+7th **T33.2 Superficial frostbite of thorax**
CC Exclusion 7th character A see Appendix A PDX collection 1416
HAC 7th character A see Appendix B for HAC conditional logic

CC X+7th **T33.3 Superficial frostbite of abdominal wall, lower back and pelvis**
CC Exclusion 7th character A see Appendix A PDX collection 1416
HAC 7th character A see Appendix B for HAC conditional logic

\+ **T33.4 Superficial frostbite of arm**
Excludes2: *superficial frostbite of wrist and hand (T33.5-)*

CC X+7th **T33.40 Superficial frostbite of unspecified arm**
CC Exclusion 7th character A see Appendix A PDX collection 1416
HAC 7th character A see Appendix B for HAC conditional logic

CC X+7th **T33.41 Superficial frostbite of right arm**
CC Exclusion 7th character A see Appendix A PDX collection 1416
HAC 7th character A see Appendix B for HAC conditional logic

CC X+7th **T33.42 Superficial frostbite of left arm**
CC Exclusion 7th character A see Appendix A PDX collection 1416
HAC 7th character A see Appendix B for HAC conditional logic

\+ **T33.5 Superficial frostbite of wrist, hand, and fingers**

\+ **T33.51 Superficial frostbite of wrist**

CC +7th **T33.511 Superficial frostbite of right wrist**
CC Exclusion 7th character A see Appendix A PDX collection 1417
HAC 7th character A see Appendix B for HAC conditional logic

CC +7th **T33.512 Superficial frostbite of left wrist**
CC Exclusion 7th character A see Appendix A PDX collection 1417
HAC 7th character A see Appendix B for HAC conditional logic

CC +7th **T33.519 Superficial frostbite of unspecified wrist**
CC Exclusion 7th character A see Appendix A PDX collection 1417
HAC 7th character A see Appendix B for HAC conditional logic

\+ **T33.52 Superficial frostbite of hand**
Excludes2: *superficial frostbite of fingers (T33.53-)*

CC +7th **T33.521 Superficial frostbite of right hand**
CC Exclusion 7th character A see Appendix A PDX collection 1417
HAC 7th character A see Appendix B for HAC conditional logic

CC +7th **T33.522 Superficial frostbite of left hand**
CC Exclusion 7th character A see Appendix A PDX collection 1417
HAC 7th character A see Appendix B for HAC conditional logic

CC +7th **T33.529 Superficial frostbite of unspecified hand**
CC Exclusion 7th character A see Appendix A PDX collection 1417
HAC 7th character A see Appendix B for HAC conditional logic

\+ **T33.53 Superficial frostbite of finger(s)**

CC +7th **T33.531 Superficial frostbite of right finger(s)**
CC Exclusion 7th character A see Appendix A PDX collection 1417
HAC 7th character A see Appendix B for HAC conditional logic

CC +7th **T33.532 Superficial frostbite of left finger(s)**
CC Exclusion 7th character A see Appendix A PDX collection 1417
HAC 7th character A see Appendix B for HAC conditional logic

CC +7th **T33.539 Superficial frostbite of unspecified finger(s)**
CC Exclusion 7th character A see Appendix A PDX collection 1417
HAC 7th character A see Appendix B for HAC conditional logic

\+ **T33.6 Superficial frostbite of hip and thigh**

CC X+7th **T33.60 Superficial frostbite of unspecified hip and thigh**
CC Exclusion 7th character A see Appendix A PDX collection 1416
HAC 7th character A see Appendix B for HAC conditional logic

CC X+7th **T33.61 Superficial frostbite of right hip and thigh**
CC Exclusion 7th character A see Appendix A PDX collection 1416
HAC 7th character A see Appendix B for HAC conditional logic

CC X+7th **T33.62 Superficial frostbite of left hip and thigh**
CC Exclusion 7th character A see Appendix A PDX collection 1416
HAC 7th character A see Appendix B for HAC conditional logic

\+ **T33.7 Superficial frostbite of knee and lower leg**
Excludes2: *superficial frostbite of ankle and foot (T33.8-)*

CC X+7th **T33.70 Superficial frostbite of unspecified knee and lower leg**
CC Exclusion 7th character A see Appendix A PDX collection 1416
HAC 7th character A see Appendix B for HAC conditional logic

CC X+7th **T33.71 Superficial frostbite of right knee and lower leg**
CC Exclusion 7th character A see Appendix A PDX collection 1416
HAC 7th character A see Appendix B for HAC conditional logic

CC X+7th **T33.72 Superficial frostbite of left knee and lower leg**
CC Exclusion 7th character A see Appendix A PDX collection 1416
HAC 7th character A see Appendix B for HAC conditional logic

+ **T33.8 Superficial frostbite of ankle, foot, and toe(s)**

+ **T33.81 Superficial frostbite of ankle**

CC +7th **T33.811 Superficial frostbite of right ankle**
CC Exclusion 7th character A see Appendix A PDX collection 1418
HAC 7th character A see Appendix B for HAC conditional logic

CC +7th **T33.812 Superficial frostbite of left ankle**
CC Exclusion 7th character A see Appendix A PDX collection 1418
HAC 7th character A see Appendix B for HAC conditional logic

CC +7th **T33.819 Superficial frostbite of unspecified ankle**
CC Exclusion 7th character A see Appendix A PDX collection 1418
HAC 7th character A see Appendix B for HAC conditional logic

+ **T33.82 Superficial frostbite of foot**

CC +7th **T33.821 Superficial frostbite of right foot**
CC Exclusion 7th character A see Appendix A PDX collection 1418
HAC 7th character A see Appendix B for HAC conditional logic

CC +7th **T33.822 Superficial frostbite of left foot**
CC Exclusion 7th character A see Appendix A PDX collection 1418
HAC 7th character A see Appendix B for HAC conditional logic

CC +7th **T33.829 Superficial frostbite of unspecified foot**
CC Exclusion 7th character A see Appendix A PDX collection 1418
HAC 7th character A see Appendix B for HAC conditional logic

+ **T33.83 Superficial frostbite of toe(s)**

CC +7th **T33.831 Superficial frostbite of right toe(s)**
CC Exclusion 7th character A see Appendix A PDX collection 1418
HAC 7th character A see Appendix B for HAC conditional logic

CC +7th **T33.832 Superficial frostbite of left toe(s)**
CC Exclusion 7th character A see Appendix A PDX collection 1418
HAC 7th character A see Appendix B for HAC conditional logic

CC +7th **T33.839 Superficial frostbite of unspecified toe(s)**
CC Exclusion 7th character A see Appendix A PDX collection 1418
HAC 7th character A see Appendix B for HAC conditional logic

+ **T33.9 Superficial frostbite of other and unspecified sites**

CC X+7th **T33.90 Superficial frostbite of unspecified sites**
Superficial frostbite NOS
CC Exclusion 7th character A see Appendix A PDX collection 1416
HAC 7th character A see Appendix B for HAC conditional logic

CC X+7th **T33.99 Superficial frostbite of other sites**
Superficial frostbite of leg NOS
Superficial frostbite of trunk NOS
CC Exclusion 7th character A see Appendix A PDX collection 1416
HAC 7th character A see Appendix B for HAC conditional logic

T34 Frostbite with tissue necrosis

The appropriate 7th character is to be added to each code from category T34
A initial encounter
D subsequent encounter
S sequela

+ **T34.0 Frostbite with tissue necrosis of head**

+ **T34.01 Frostbite with tissue necrosis of ear**

CC +7th **T34.011 Frostbite with tissue necrosis of right ear**
CC Exclusion 7th character A see Appendix A PDX collection 1415
HAC 7th character A see Appendix B for HAC conditional logic

CC +7th **T34.012 Frostbite with tissue necrosis of left ear**
CC Exclusion 7th character A see Appendix A PDX collection 1415
HAC 7th character A see Appendix B for HAC conditional logic

CC +7th **T34.019 Frostbite with tissue necrosis of unspecified ear**
CC Exclusion 7th character A see Appendix A PDX collection 1415
HAC 7th character A see Appendix B for HAC conditional logic

CC X+7th **T34.02 Frostbite with tissue necrosis of nose**
CC Exclusion 7th character A see Appendix A PDX collection 1415
HAC 7th character A see Appendix B for HAC conditional logic

CC X+7th **T34.09 Frostbite with tissue necrosis of other part of head**
CC Exclusion 7th character A see Appendix A PDX collection 1415
HAC 7th character A see Appendix B for HAC conditional logic

CC X+7th **T34.1 Frostbite with tissue necrosis of neck**
CC Exclusion 7th character A see Appendix A PDX collection 1415
HAC 7th character A see Appendix B for HAC conditional logic

CC X+7th **T34.2 Frostbite with tissue necrosis of thorax**
CC Exclusion 7th character A see Appendix A PDX collection 1416
HAC 7th character A see Appendix B for HAC conditional logic

CC X+7th **T34.3 Frostbite with tissue necrosis of abdominal wall, lower back and pelvis**
CC Exclusion 7th character A see Appendix A PDX collection 1416
HAC 7th character A see Appendix B for HAC conditional logic

+ **T34.4 Frostbite with tissue necrosis of arm**
Excludes2: *frostbite with tissue necrosis of wrist and hand (T34.5-)*

CC X+7th **T34.40 Frostbite with tissue necrosis of unspecified arm**
CC Exclusion 7th character A see Appendix A PDX collection 1416
HAC 7th character A see Appendix B for HAC conditional logic

CC X+7th **T34.41 Frostbite with tissue necrosis of right arm**
CC Exclusion 7th character A see Appendix A PDX collection 1416
HAC 7th character A see Appendix B for HAC conditional logic

CC X+7th **T34.42 Frostbite with tissue necrosis of left arm**
CC Exclusion 7th character A see Appendix A PDX collection 1416
HAC 7th character A see Appendix B for HAC conditional logic

+ **T34.5 Frostbite with tissue necrosis of wrist, hand, and finger(s)**

+ **T34.51 Frostbite with tissue necrosis of wrist**

CC +7th **T34.511 Frostbite with tissue necrosis of right wrist**
CC Exclusion 7th character A see Appendix A PDX collection 1417
HAC 7th character A see Appendix B for HAC conditional logic

CC +7th **T34.512 Frostbite with tissue necrosis of left wrist**
CC Exclusion 7th character A see Appendix A PDX collection 1417
HAC 7th character A see Appendix B for HAC conditional logic

CC +7th **T34.519 Frostbite with tissue necrosis of unspecified wrist**
CC Exclusion 7th character A see Appendix A PDX collection 1417
HAC 7th character A see Appendix B for HAC conditional logic

+ **T34.52 Frostbite with tissue necrosis of hand**
Excludes2: *frostbite with tissue necrosis of finger(s) (T34.53-)*

CC +7th **T34.521 Frostbite with tissue necrosis of right hand**
CC Exclusion 7th character A see Appendix A PDX collection 1417
HAC 7th character A see Appendix B for HAC conditional logic

CC +7th **T34.522 Frostbite with tissue necrosis of left hand**
CC Exclusion 7th character A see Appendix A PDX collection 1417
HAC 7th character A see Appendix B for HAC conditional logic

CC +7th **T34.529 Frostbite with tissue necrosis of unspecified hand**
CC Exclusion 7th character A see Appendix A PDX collection 1417
HAC 7th character A see Appendix B for HAC conditional logic

\+ **T34.53 Frostbite with tissue necrosis of finger(s)**

CC +7th **T34.531 Frostbite with tissue necrosis of right finger(s)**
CC Exclusion 7th character A see Appendix A PDX collection 1417
HAC 7th character A see Appendix B for HAC conditional logic

CC +7th **T34.532 Frostbite with tissue necrosis of left finger(s)**
CC Exclusion 7th character A see Appendix A PDX collection 1417
HAC 7th character A see Appendix B for HAC conditional logic

CC +7th **T34.539 Frostbite with tissue necrosis of unspecified finger(s)**
CC Exclusion 7th character A see Appendix A PDX collection 1417
HAC 7th character A see Appendix B for HAC conditional logic

\+ **T34.6 Frostbite with tissue necrosis of hip and thigh**

CC X+7th **T34.60 Frostbite with tissue necrosis of unspecified hip and thigh**
CC Exclusion 7th character A see Appendix A PDX collection 1416
HAC 7th character A see Appendix B for HAC conditional logic

CC X+7th **T34.61 Frostbite with tissue necrosis of right hip and thigh**
CC Exclusion 7th character A see Appendix A PDX collection 1416
HAC 7th character A see Appendix B for HAC conditional logic

CC X+7th **T34.62 Frostbite with tissue necrosis of left hip and thigh**
CC Exclusion 7th character A see Appendix A PDX collection 1416
HAC 7th character A see Appendix B for HAC conditional logic

\+ **T34.7 Frostbite with tissue necrosis of knee and lower leg**
Excludes2: *frostbite with tissue necrosis of ankle and foot (T34.8-)*

CC X+7th **T34.70 Frostbite with tissue necrosis of unspecified knee and lower leg**
CC Exclusion 7th character A see Appendix A PDX collection 1416
HAC 7th character A see Appendix B for HAC conditional logic

CC X+7th **T34.71 Frostbite with tissue necrosis of right knee and lower leg**
CC Exclusion 7th character A see Appendix A PDX collection 1416
HAC 7th character A see Appendix B for HAC conditional logic

CC X+7th **T34.72 Frostbite with tissue necrosis of left knee and lower leg**
CC Exclusion 7th character A see Appendix A PDX collection 1416
HAC 7th character A see Appendix B for HAC conditional logic

\+ **T34.8 Frostbite with tissue necrosis of ankle, foot, and toe(s)**

\+ **T34.81 Frostbite with tissue necrosis of ankle**

CC +7th **T34.811 Frostbite with tissue necrosis of right ankle**
CC Exclusion 7th character A see Appendix A PDX collection 1418
HAC 7th character A see Appendix B for HAC conditional logic

CC +7th **T34.812 Frostbite with tissue necrosis of left ankle**
CC Exclusion 7th character A see Appendix A PDX collection 1418
HAC 7th character A see Appendix B for HAC conditional logic

CC +7th **T34.819 Frostbite with tissue necrosis of unspecified ankle**
CC Exclusion 7th character A see Appendix A PDX collection 1418
HAC 7th character A see Appendix B for HAC conditional logic

\+ **T34.82 Frostbite with tissue necrosis of foot**

CC +7th **T34.821 Frostbite with tissue necrosis of right foot**
CC Exclusion 7th character A see Appendix A PDX collection 1418
HAC 7th character A see Appendix B for HAC conditional logic

CC +7th **T34.822 Frostbite with tissue necrosis of left foot**
CC Exclusion 7th character A see Appendix A PDX collection 1418
HAC 7th character A see Appendix B for HAC conditional logic

CC +7th **T34.829 Frostbite with tissue necrosis of unspecified foot**
CC Exclusion 7th character A see Appendix A PDX collection 1418
HAC 7th character A see Appendix B for HAC conditional logic

\+ **T34.83 Frostbite with tissue necrosis of toe(s)**

CC +7th **T34.831 Frostbite with tissue necrosis of right toe(s)**
CC Exclusion 7th character A see Appendix A PDX collection 1418
HAC 7th character A see Appendix B for HAC conditional logic

CC +7th **T34.832 Frostbite with tissue necrosis of left toe(s)**
CC Exclusion 7th character A see Appendix A PDX collection 1418
HAC 7th character A see Appendix B for HAC conditional logic

CC +7th **T34.839 Frostbite with tissue necrosis of unspecified toe(s)**
CC Exclusion 7th character A see Appendix A PDX collection 1418
HAC 7th character A see Appendix B for HAC conditional logic

\+ **T34.9 Frostbite with tissue necrosis of other and unspecified sites**

CC X+7th **T34.90 Frostbite with tissue necrosis of unspecified sites**
Frostbite with tissue necrosis NOS
CC Exclusion 7th character A see Appendix A PDX collection 1416
HAC 7th character A see Appendix B for HAC conditional logic

CC X+7th **T34.99 Frostbite with tissue necrosis of other sites**
Frostbite with tissue necrosis of leg NOS
Frostbite with tissue necrosis of trunk NOS
CC Exclusion 7th character A see Appendix A PDX collection 1416
HAC 7th character A see Appendix B for HAC conditional logic

Poisoning by, adverse effects of and underdosing of drugs, medicaments and biological substances (T36-T50)

Includes: adverse effect of correct substance properly administered
poisoning by overdose of substance
poisoning by wrong substance given or taken in error
underdosing by (inadvertently) (deliberately) taking less substance than prescribed or instructed

Code first: for adverse effects, the nature of the adverse effect, such as:
adverse effect NOS (T88.7)
aspirin gastritis (K29.-)
blood disorders (D56-D76)
contact dermatitis (L23-L25)
dermatitis due to substances taken internally (L27.-)
nephropathy (N14.0-N14.2)

NOTE The drug giving rise to the adverse effect should be identified by use of codes from categories T36-T50 with fifth or sixth character 5.

Use additional: code(s) to specify:
manifestations of poisoning
underdosing or failure in dosage during medical and surgical care (Y63.6, Y63.8-Y63.9)
underdosing of medication regimen (Z91.12-, Z91.13-)

Excludes1: *toxic reaction to local anesthesia in pregnancy (O29.3-)*

Excludes2: *abuse and dependence of psychoactive substances (F10-F19)*
abuse of non-dependence-producing substances (F55.-)
drug reaction and poisoning affecting newborn (P00-P96)
pathological drug intoxication (inebriation) (F10-F19)

Review coding guideline C.19.e

T36 Poisoning by, adverse effect of and underdosing of systemic antibiotics

Excludes1: *antineoplastic antibiotics (T45.1-)*
locally applied antibiotic NEC (T49.0)
topically used antibiotic for ear, nose and throat (T49.6)
topically used antibiotic for eye (T49.5)

The appropriate 7th character is to be added to each code from category T36
A initial encounter
D subsequent encounter
S sequela

+ **T36.0 Poisoning by, adverse effect of and underdosing of penicillins**
+ **T36.0X Poisoning by, adverse effect of and underdosing of penicillins**
+7th **T36.0X1 Poisoning by penicillins, accidental (unintentional)**
Poisoning by penicillins NOS
+7th **T36.0X2 Poisoning by penicillins, intentional self-harm**
+7th **T36.0X3 Poisoning by penicillins, assault**
+7th **T36.0X4 Poisoning by penicillins, undetermined**
+7th **T36.0X5 Adverse effect of penicillins**
+7th **T36.0X6 Underdosing of penicillins**
+ **T36.1 Poisoning by, adverse effect of and underdosing of cephalosporins and other beta-lactam antibiotics**
+ **T36.1X Poisoning by, adverse effect of and underdosing of cephalosporins and other beta-lactam antibiotics**
+7th **T36.1X1 Poisoning by cephalosporins and other beta-lactam antibiotics, accidental (unintentional)**
Poisoning by cephalosporins and other beta-lactam antibiotics NOS
+7th **T36.1X2 Poisoning by cephalosporins and other beta-lactam antibiotics, intentional self-harm**
+7th **T36.1X3 Poisoning by cephalosporins and other beta-lactam antibiotics, assault**
+7th **T36.1X4 Poisoning by cephalosporins and other beta-lactam antibiotics, undetermined**
+7th **T36.1X5 Adverse effect of cephalosporins and other beta-lactam antibiotics**
+7th **T36.1X6 Underdosing of cephalosporins and other beta-lactam antibiotics**
+ **T36.2 Poisoning by, adverse effect of and underdosing of chloramphenicol group**
+ **T36.2X Poisoning by, adverse effect of and underdosing of chloramphenicol group**
+7th **T36.2X1 Poisoning by chloramphenicol group, accidental (unintentional)**
Poisoning by chloramphenicol group NOS
+7th **T36.2X2 Poisoning by chloramphenicol group, intentional self-harm**
+7th **T36.2X3 Poisoning by chloramphenicol group, assault**
+7th **T36.2X4 Poisoning by chloramphenicol group, undetermined**
+7th **T36.2X5 Adverse effect of chloramphenicol group**
+7th **T36.2X6 Underdosing of chloramphenicol group**
+ **T36.3 Poisoning by, adverse effect of and underdosing of macrolides**
+ **T36.3X Poisoning by, adverse effect of and underdosing of macrolides**
+7th **T36.3X1 Poisoning by macrolides, accidental (unintentional)**
Poisoning by macrolides NOS
+7th **T36.3X2 Poisoning by macrolides, intentional self-harm**
+7th **T36.3X3 Poisoning by macrolides, assault**
+7th **T36.3X4 Poisoning by macrolides, undetermined**
+7th **T36.3X5 Adverse effect of macrolides**
+7th **T36.3X6 Underdosing of macrolides**
+ **T36.4 Poisoning by, adverse effect of and underdosing of tetracyclines**
+ **T36.4X Poisoning by, adverse effect of and underdosing of tetracyclines**
+7th **T36.4X1 Poisoning by tetracyclines, accidental (unintentional)**
Poisoning by tetracyclines NOS
+7th **T36.4X2 Poisoning by tetracyclines, intentional self-harm**
+7th **T36.4X3 Poisoning by tetracyclines, assault**
+7th **T36.4X4 Poisoning by tetracyclines, undetermined**
+7th **T36.4X5 Adverse effect of tetracyclines**
+7th **T36.4X6 Underdosing of tetracyclines**
+ **T36.5 Poisoning by, adverse effect of and underdosing of aminoglycosides**
Poisoning by, adverse effect of and underdosing of streptomyci
+ **T36.5X Poisoning by, adverse effect of and underdosing of aminoglycosides**
+7th **T36.5X1 Poisoning by aminoglycosides, accidental (unintentional)**
Poisoning by aminoglycosides NOS
+7th **T36.5X2 Poisoning by aminoglycosides, intentional self-harm**
+7th **T36.5X3 Poisoning by aminoglycosides, assault**
+7th **T36.5X4 Poisoning by aminoglycosides, undetermined**
+7th **T36.5X5 Adverse effect of aminoglycosides**
+7th **T36.5X6 Underdosing of aminoglycosides**
+ **T36.6 Poisoning by, adverse effect of and underdosing of rifampicins**
+ **T36.6X Poisoning by, adverse effect of and underdosing of rifampicins**
+7th **T36.6X1 Poisoning by rifampicins, accidental (unintentional)**
Poisoning by rifampicins NOS
+7th **T36.6X2 Poisoning by rifampicins, intentional self-harm**
+7th **T36.6X3 Poisoning by rifampicins, assault**
+7th **T36.6X4 Poisoning by rifampicins, undetermined**
+7th **T36.6X5 Adverse effect of rifampicins**
+7th **T36.6X6 Underdosing of rifampicins**
+ **T36.7 Poisoning by, adverse effect of and underdosing of antifungal antibiotics, systemically used**
+ **T36.7X Poisoning by, adverse effect of and underdosing of antifungal antibiotics, systemically used**
+7th **T36.7X1 Poisoning by antifungal antibiotics, systemically used, accidental (unintentional)**
Poisoning by antifungal antibiotics, systemically used NOS
+7th **T36.7X2 Poisoning by antifungal antibiotics, systemically used, intentional self-harm**
+7th **T36.7X3 Poisoning by antifungal antibiotics, systemically used, assault**
+7th **T36.7X4 Poisoning by antifungal antibiotics, systemically used, undetermined**
+7th **T36.7X5 Adverse effect of antifungal antibiotics, systemically used**
+7th **T36.7X6 Underdosing of antifungal antibiotics, systemically used**
+ **T36.8 Poisoning by, adverse effect of and underdosing of other systemic antibiotics**
+ **T36.8X Poisoning by, adverse effect of and underdosing of other systemic antibiotics**
+7th **T36.8X1 Poisoning by other systemic antibiotics, accidental (unintentional)**
Poisoning by other systemic antibiotics NO
+7th **T36.8X2 Poisoning by other systemic antibiotics, intentional self-harm**
+7th **T36.8X3 Poisoning by other systemic antibiotics, assault**
+7th **T36.8X4 Poisoning by other systemic antibiotics, undetermined**
+7th **T36.8X5 Adverse effect of other systemic antibiotic**
AHA CC: 1Q, 2017, 39
+7th **T36.8X6 Underdosing of other systemic antibiotics**
+ **T36.9 Poisoning by, adverse effect of and underdosing of unspecified systemic antibiotic**
X+7th **T36.91 Poisoning by unspecified systemic antibiotic, accidental (unintentional)**
Poisoning by systemic antibiotic NOS
X+7th **T36.92 Poisoning by unspecified systemic antibiotic, intentional self-harm**
X+7th **T36.93 Poisoning by unspecified systemic antibiotic, assault**

X+7th **T36.94 Poisoning by unspecified systemic antibiotic, undetermined**
X+7th **T36.95 Adverse effect of unspecified systemic antibiotic**
X+7th **T36.96 Underdosing of unspecified systemic antibiotic**

T37 Poisoning by, adverse effect of and underdosing of other systemic anti- infectives and antiparasitics

Excludes1: *anti-infectives topically used for ear, nose and throat (T49.6-)*
anti-infectives topically used for eye (T49.5-)
locally applied anti-infectives NEC (T49.0-)

The appropriate 7th character is to be added to each code from category T37
A initial encounter
D subsequent encounter
S sequela

+ **T37.0 Poisoning by, adverse effect of and underdosing of sulfonamides**
+ **T37.0X Poisoning by, adverse effect of and underdosing of sulfonamides**
+7th **T37.0X1 Poisoning by sulfonamides, accidental (unintentional)**
Poisoning by sulfonamides NOS
+7th **T37.0X2 Poisoning by sulfonamides, intentional self-harm**
+7th **T37.0X3 Poisoning by sulfonamides, assault**
+7th **T37.0X4 Poisoning by sulfonamides, undetermined**
+7th **T37.0X5 Adverse effect of sulfonamides**
+7th **T37.0X6 Underdosing of sulfonamides**
+ **T37.1 Poisoning by, adverse effect of and underdosing of antimycobacterial drugs**
Excludes1: *rifampicins (T36.6-)*
streptomycin (T36.5-)
+ **T37.1X Poisoning by, adverse effect of and underdosing of antimycobacterial drugs**
+7th **T37.1X1 Poisoning by antimycobacterial drugs, accidental (unintentional)**
Poisoning by antimycobacterial drugs NOS
+7th **T37.1X2 Poisoning by antimycobacterial drugs, intentional self-harm**
+7th **T37.1X3 Poisoning by antimycobacterial drugs, assault**
+7th **T37.1X4 Poisoning by antimycobacterial drugs, undetermined**
+7th **T37.1X5 Adverse effect of antimycobacterial drugs**
+7th **T37.1X6 Underdosing of antimycobacterial drugs**
+ **T37.2 Poisoning by, adverse effect of and underdosing of antimalarials and drugs acting on other blood protozoa**
Excludes1: *hydroxyquinoline derivatives (T37.8-)*
+ **T37.2X Poisoning by, adverse effect of and underdosing of antimalarials and drugs acting on other blood protozoa**
+7th **T37.2X1 Poisoning by antimalarials and drugs acting on other blood protozoa, accidental (unintentional)**
Poisoning by antimalarials and drugs acting on other blood protozoa NOS
+7th **T37.2X2 Poisoning by antimalarials and drugs acting on other blood protozoa, intentional self-harm**
+7th **T37.2X3 Poisoning by antimalarials and drugs acting on other blood protozoa, assault**
+7th **T37.2X4 Poisoning by antimalarials and drugs acting on other blood protozoa, undetermined**
+7th **T37.2X5 Adverse effect of antimalarials and drugs acting on other blood protozoa**
+7th **T37.2X6 Underdosing of antimalarials and drugs acting on other blood protozoa**
+ **T37.3 Poisoning by, adverse effect of and underdosing of other antiprotozoal drugs**
+ **T37.3X Poisoning by, adverse effect of and underdosing of other antiprotozoal drugs**
+7th **T37.3X1 Poisoning by other antiprotozoal drugs, accidental (unintentional)**
Poisoning by other antiprotozoal drugs NOS
+7th **T37.3X2 Poisoning by other antiprotozoal drugs, intentional self-harm**
+7th **T37.3X3 Poisoning by other antiprotozoal drugs, assault**
+7th **T37.3X4 Poisoning by other antiprotozoal drugs, undetermined**
+7th **T37.3X5 Adverse effect of other antiprotozoal drugs**
+7th **T37.3X6 Underdosing of other antiprotozoal drugs**
+ **T37.4 Poisoning by, adverse effect of and underdosing of anthelminthics**
+ **T37.4X Poisoning by, adverse effect of and underdosing of anthelminthics**
+7th **T37.4X1 Poisoning by anthelminthics, accidental (unintentional)**
Poisoning by anthelminthics NOS
+7th **T37.4X2 Poisoning by anthelminthics, intentional self-harm**
+7th **T37.4X3 Poisoning by anthelminthics, assault**
+7th **T37.4X4 Poisoning by anthelminthics, undetermined**
+7th **T37.4X5 Adverse effect of anthelminthics**
+7th **T37.4X6 Underdosing of anthelminthics**
+ **T37.5 Poisoning by, adverse effect of and underdosing of antiviral drugs**
Excludes1: *amantadine (T42.8-)*
cytarabine (T45.1-)
+ **T37.5X Poisoning by, adverse effect of and underdosing of antiviral drugs**
+7th **T37.5X1 Poisoning by antiviral drugs, accidental (unintentional)**
Poisoning by antiviral drugs NOS
+7th **T37.5X2 Poisoning by antiviral drugs, intentional self-harm**
+7th **T37.5X3 Poisoning by antiviral drugs, assault**
+7th **T37.5X4 Poisoning by antiviral drugs, undetermined**
+7th **T37.5X5 Adverse effect of antiviral drugs**
+7th **T37.5X6 Underdosing of antiviral drugs**
+ **T37.8 Poisoning by, adverse effect of and underdosing of other specified systemic anti-infectives and antiparasitics**
Poisoning by, adverse effect of and underdosing of hydroxyquinoline derivatives
Excludes1: *antimalarial drugs (T37.2-)*
+ **T37.8X Poisoning by, adverse effect of and underdosing of other specified systemic anti-infectives and antiparasitics**
+7th **T37.8X1 Poisoning by other specified systemic anti-infectives and antiparasitics, accidental (unintentional)**
Poisoning by other specified systemic anti-infectives and antiparasitics NOS
+7th **T37.8X2 Poisoning by other specified systemic anti-infectives and antiparasitics, intentional self-harm**
+7th **T37.8X3 Poisoning by other specified systemic anti-infectives and antiparasitics, assault**
+7th **T37.8X4 Poisoning by other specified systemic anti-infectives and antiparasitics, undetermined**
+7th **T37.8X5 Adverse effect of other specified systemic anti-infectives and antiparasitics**
+7th **T37.8X6 Underdosing of other specified systemic anti-infectives and antiparasitics**
+ **T37.9 Poisoning by, adverse effect of and underdosing of unspecified systemic anti-infective and antiparasitics**
X+7th **T37.91 Poisoning by unspecified systemic anti-infective and antiparasitics, accidental (unintentional)**
Poisoning by, adverse effect of and underdosing of systemic anti-infective and antiparasitics NOS
X+7th **T37.92 Poisoning by unspecified systemic anti-infective and antiparasitics, intentional self-harm**
X+7th **T37.93 Poisoning by unspecified systemic anti-infective and antiparasitics, assault**
X+7th **T37.94 Poisoning by unspecified systemic anti-infective and antiparasitics, undetermined**
X+7th **T37.95 Adverse effect of unspecified systemic anti-infective and antiparasitic**
X+7th **T37.96 Underdosing of unspecified systemic anti-infectives and antiparasitics**

T38 Poisoning by, adverse effect of and underdosing of hormones and their synthetic substitutes and antagonists, not elsewhere classified

Excludes1: *mineralocorticoids and their antagonists (T50.0-)*
oxytocic hormones (T48.0-)
parathyroid hormones and derivatives (T50.9-)

The appropriate 7th character is to be added to each code from category T38
A initial encounter
D subsequent encounter
S sequela

+ **T38.0 Poisoning by, adverse effect of and underdosing of glucocorticoids and synthetic analogues**
  Excludes1: *glucocorticoids, topically used (T49.-)*
  + **T38.0X Poisoning by, adverse effect of and underdosing of glucocorticoids and synthetic analogues**
    +7th **T38.0X1 Poisoning by glucocorticoids and synthetic analogues, accidental (unintentional)**
    Poisoning by glucocorticoids and synthetic analogues NOS
    +7th **T38.0X2 Poisoning by glucocorticoids and synthetic analogues, intentional self-harm**
    +7th **T38.0X3 Poisoning by glucocorticoids and synthetic analogues, assault**
    +7th **T38.0X4 Poisoning by glucocorticoids and synthetic analogues, undetermined**
    +7th **T38.0X5 Adverse effect of glucocorticoids and synthetic analogues**
    +7th **T38.0X6 Underdosing of glucocorticoids and synthetic analogues**

+ **T38.1 Poisoning by, adverse effect of and underdosing of thyroid hormones and substitutes**
  + **T38.1X Poisoning by, adverse effect of and underdosing of thyroid hormones and substitutes**
    +7th **T38.1X1 Poisoning by thyroid hormones and substitutes, accidental (unintentional)**
    Poisoning by thyroid hormones and substitutes NOS
    +7th **T38.1X2 Poisoning by thyroid hormones and substitutes, intentional self-harm**
    +7th **T38.1X3 Poisoning by thyroid hormones and substitutes, assault**
    +7th **T38.1X4 Poisoning by thyroid hormones and substitutes, undetermined**
    +7th **T38.1X5 Adverse effect of thyroid hormones and substitutes**
    +7th **T38.1X6 Underdosing of thyroid hormones and substitutes**

+ **T38.2 Poisoning by, adverse effect of and underdosing of antithyroid drugs**
  + **T38.2X Poisoning by, adverse effect of and underdosing of antithyroid drugs**
    +7th **T38.2X1 Poisoning by antithyroid drugs, accidental (unintentional)**
    Poisoning by antithyroid drugs NOS
    +7th **T38.2X2 Poisoning by antithyroid drugs, intentional self-harm**
    +7th **T38.2X3 Poisoning by antithyroid drugs, assault**
    +7th **T38.2X4 Poisoning by antithyroid drugs, undetermined**
    +7th **T38.2X5 Adverse effect of antithyroid drugs**
    +7th **T38.2X6 Underdosing of antithyroid drugs**

+ **T38.3 Poisoning by, adverse effect of and underdosing of insulin and oral hypoglycemic [antidiabetic] drugs**
  + **T38.3X Poisoning by, adverse effect of and underdosing of insulin and oral hypoglycemic [antidiabetic] drugs**
    +7th **T38.3X1 Poisoning by insulin and oral hypoglycemic [antidiabetic] drugs, accidental (unintentional)**
    Poisoning by insulin and oral hypoglycemic [antidiabetic] drugs NOS
    Review coding guideline C.4.a.5.b
    +7th **T38.3X2 Poisoning by insulin and oral hypoglycemic [antidiabetic] drugs, intentional self-harm**
    +7th **T38.3X3 Poisoning by insulin and oral hypoglycemic [antidiabetic] drugs, assault**
    +7th **T38.3X4 Poisoning by insulin and oral hypoglycemic [antidiabetic] drugs, undetermined**
    +7th **T38.3X5 Adverse effect of insulin and oral hypoglycemic [antidiabetic] drugs**
    +7th **T38.3X6 Underdosing of insulin and oral hypoglycemic [antidiabetic] drugs**
    Review coding guideline C.4.a.5.a

+ **T38.4 Poisoning by, adverse effect of and underdosing of oral contraceptives**
  Poisoning by, adverse effect of and underdosing of multiple- and single-ingredient oral contraceptive preparations
  + **T38.4X Poisoning by, adverse effect of and underdosing of oral contraceptives**
    +7th **T38.4X1 Poisoning by oral contraceptives, accidental (unintentional)**
    Poisoning by oral contraceptives NOS
    +7th **T38.4X2 Poisoning by oral contraceptives, intentional self-harm**
    +7th **T38.4X3 Poisoning by oral contraceptives, assault**
    +7th **T38.4X4 Poisoning by oral contraceptives, undetermined**
    +7th **T38.4X5 Adverse effect of oral contraceptives**
    +7th **T38.4X6 Underdosing of oral contraceptives**

+ **T38.5 Poisoning by, adverse effect of and underdosing of other estrogens and progestogens**
  Poisoning by, adverse effect of and underdosing of estrogens and progestogens mixtures and substitutes
  + **T38.5X Poisoning by, adverse effect of and underdosing of other estrogens and progestogens**
    +7th **T38.5X1 Poisoning by other estrogens and progestogens, accidental (unintentional)**
    Poisoning by other estrogens and progestogens NOS
    +7th **T38.5X2 Poisoning by other estrogens and progestogens, intentional self-harm**
    +7th **T38.5X3 Poisoning by other estrogens and progestogens, assault**
    +7th **T38.5X4 Poisoning by other estrogens and progestogens, undetermined**
    +7th **T38.5X5 Adverse effect of other estrogens and progestogens**
    +7th **T38.5X6 Underdosing of other estrogens and progestogens**

+ **T38.6 Poisoning by, adverse effect of and underdosing of antigonadotrophins, antiestrogens, antiandrogens, not elsewhere classified**
  Poisoning by, adverse effect of and underdosing of tamoxifen
  + **T38.6X Poisoning by, adverse effect of and underdosing of antigonadotrophins, antiestrogens, antiandrogens, not elsewhere classified**
    +7th **T38.6X1 Poisoning by antigonadotrophins, antiestrogens, antiandrogens, not elsewhere classified, accidental (unintentional)**
    Poisoning by antigonadotrophins, antiestrogens, antiandrogens, not elsewhere classified NOS
    +7th **T38.6X2 Poisoning by antigonadotrophins, antiestrogens, antiandrogens, not elsewhere classified, intentional self-harm**
    +7th **T38.6X3 Poisoning by antigonadotrophins, antiestrogens, antiandrogens, not elsewhere classified, assault**
    +7th **T38.6X4 Poisoning by antigonadotrophins, antiestrogens, antiandrogens, not elsewhere classified, undetermined**
    +7th **T38.6X5 Adverse effect of antigonadotrophins, antiestrogens, antiandrogens, not elsewhere classified**
    +7th **T38.6X6 Underdosing of antigonadotrophins, antiestrogens, antiandrogens, not elsewhere classified**

+ **T38.7 Poisoning by, adverse effect of and underdosing of androgens and anabolic congeners**
  + **T38.7X Poisoning by, adverse effect of and underdosing of androgens and anabolic congeners**
    +7th **T38.7X1 Poisoning by androgens and anabolic congeners, accidental (unintentional)**
    Poisoning by androgens and anabolic congeners NOS
    +7th **T38.7X2 Poisoning by androgens and anabolic congeners, intentional self-harm**

+7th T38.7X3 Poisoning by androgens and anabolic congeners, assault
+7th T38.7X4 Poisoning by androgens and anabolic congeners, undetermined
+7th T38.7X5 Adverse effect of androgens and anabolic congeners
+7th T38.7X6 Underdosing of androgens and anabolic congeners
+ T38.8 Poisoning by, adverse effect of and underdosing of other and unspecified hormones and synthetic substitutes
+ T38.80 Poisoning by, adverse effect of and underdosing of unspecified hormones and synthetic substitutes
+7th T38.801 Poisoning by unspecified hormones and synthetic substitutes, accidental (unintentional)
Poisoning by unspecified hormones and synthetic substitutes NOS
+7th T38.802 Poisoning by unspecified hormones and synthetic substitutes, intentional self-harm
+7th T38.803 Poisoning by unspecified hormones and synthetic substitutes, assault
+7th T38.804 Poisoning by unspecified hormones and synthetic substitutes, undetermined
+7th T38.805 Adverse effect of unspecified hormones and synthetic substitutes
+7th T38.806 Underdosing of unspecified hormones and synthetic substitutes
+ T38.81 Poisoning by, adverse effect of and underdosing of anterior pituitary [adenohypophyseal] hormones
+7th T38.811 Poisoning by anterior pituitary [adenohypophyseal] hormones, accidental (unintentional)
Poisoning by anterior pituitary [adenohypophyseal] hormones NOS
+7th T38.812 Poisoning by anterior pituitary [adenohypophyseal] hormones, intentional self-harm
+7th T38.813 Poisoning by anterior pituitary [adenohypophyseal] hormones, assault
+7th T38.814 Poisoning by anterior pituitary [adenohypophyseal] hormones, undetermined
+7th T38.815 Adverse effect of anterior pituitary [adenohypophyseal] hormones
+7th T38.816 Underdosing of anterior pituitary [adenohypophyseal] hormones
+ T38.89 Poisoning by, adverse effect of and underdosing of other hormones and synthetic substitutes
+7th T38.891 Poisoning by other hormones and synthetic substitutes, accidental (unintentional)
Poisoning by other hormones and synthetic substitutes NOS
+7th T38.892 Poisoning by other hormones and synthetic substitutes, intentional self-harm
+7th T38.893 Poisoning by other hormones and synthetic substitutes, assault
+7th T38.894 Poisoning by other hormones and synthetic substitutes, undetermined
+7th T38.895 Adverse effect of other hormones and synthetic substitutes
+7th T38.896 Underdosing of other hormones and synthetic substitutes
+ T38.9 Poisoning by, adverse effect of and underdosing of other and unspecified hormone antagonists
+ T38.90 Poisoning by, adverse effect of and underdosing of unspecified hormone antagonists
+7th T38.901 Poisoning by unspecified hormone antagonists, accidental (unintentional)
Poisoning by unspecified hormone antagonists NOS
+7th T38.902 Poisoning by unspecified hormone antagonists, intentional self-harm
+7th T38.903 Poisoning by unspecified hormone antagonists, assault
+7th T38.904 Poisoning by unspecified hormone antagonists, undetermined
+7th T38.905 Adverse effect of unspecified hormone antagonists
+7th T38.906 Underdosing of unspecified hormone antagonists
+ T38.99 Poisoning by, adverse effect of and underdosing of other hormone antagonists
+7th T38.991 Poisoning by other hormone antagonists, accidental (unintentional)
Poisoning by other hormone antagonists NOS
+7th T38.992 Poisoning by other hormone antagonists, intentional self-harm
+7th T38.993 Poisoning by other hormone antagonists, assault
+7th T38.994 Poisoning by other hormone antagonists, undetermined
+7th T38.995 Adverse effect of other hormone antagonists
+7th T38.996 Underdosing of other hormone antagonists

T39 Poisoning by, adverse effect of and underdosing of nonopioid analgesics, antipyretics and antirheumatics

The appropriate 7th character is to be added to each code from category T39
A initial encounter
D subsequent encounter
S sequela

+ T39.0 Poisoning by, adverse effect of and underdosing of salicylates
+ T39.01 Poisoning by, adverse effect of and underdosing of aspirin
Poisoning by, adverse effect of and underdosing of acetylsalicylic acid
+7th T39.011 Poisoning by aspirin, accidental (unintentional)
+7th T39.012 Poisoning by aspirin, intentional self-harm
+7th T39.013 Poisoning by aspirin, assault
+7th T39.014 Poisoning by aspirin, undetermined
+7th T39.015 Adverse effect of aspirin
AHA CC: 1Q, 2016, 15
+7th T39.016 Underdosing of aspirin
+ T39.09 Poisoning by, adverse effect of and underdosing of other salicylates
+7th T39.091 Poisoning by salicylates, accidental (unintentional)
Poisoning by salicylates NOS
+7th T39.092 Poisoning by salicylates, intentional self-harm
+7th T39.093 Poisoning by salicylates, assault
+7th T39.094 Poisoning by salicylates, undetermined
+7th T39.095 Adverse effect of salicylates
+7th T39.096 Underdosing of salicylates
+ T39.1 Poisoning by, adverse effect of and underdosing of 4-Aminophenol derivatives
+ T39.1X Poisoning by, adverse effect of and underdosing of 4-Aminophenol derivatives
+7th T39.1X1 Poisoning by 4-Aminophenol derivatives, accidental (unintentional)
Poisoning by 4-Aminophenol derivatives NOS
+7th T39.1X2 Poisoning by 4-Aminophenol derivatives, intentional self-harm
+7th T39.1X3 Poisoning by 4-Aminophenol derivatives, assault
+7th T39.1X4 Poisoning by 4-Aminophenol derivatives, undetermined
+7th T39.1X5 Adverse effect of 4-Aminophenol derivatives
+7th T39.1X6 Underdosing of 4-Aminophenol derivatives
+ T39.2 Poisoning by, adverse effect of and underdosing of pyrazolone derivatives
+ T39.2X Poisoning by, adverse effect of and underdosing of pyrazolone derivatives
+7th T39.2X1 Poisoning by pyrazolone derivatives, accidental (unintentional)
Poisoning by pyrazolone derivatives NOS
+7th T39.2X2 Poisoning by pyrazolone derivatives, intentional self-harm
+7th T39.2X3 Poisoning by pyrazolone derivatives, assault

+7th **T39.2X4 Poisoning by pyrazolone derivatives, undetermined**
+7th **T39.2X5 Adverse effect of pyrazolone derivatives**
+7th **T39.2X6 Underdosing of pyrazolone derivatives**

\+ **T39.3 Poisoning by, adverse effect of and underdosing of other nonsteroidal anti-inflammatory drugs [NSAID]**

\+ **T39.31 Poisoning by, adverse effect of and underdosing of propionic acid derivatives**
Poisoning by, adverse effect of and underdosing of fenoprofen
Poisoning by, adverse effect of and underdosing of flurbiprofen
Poisoning by, adverse effect of and underdosing of ibuprofen
Poisoning by, adverse effect of and underdosing of ketoprofen
Poisoning by, adverse effect of and underdosing of naproxen
Poisoning by, adverse effect of and underdosing of oxaprozin

+7th **T39.311 Poisoning by propionic acid derivatives, accidental (unintentional)**
+7th **T39.312 Poisoning by propionic acid derivatives, intentional self-harm**
+7th **T39.313 Poisoning by propionic acid derivatives, assault**
+7th **T39.314 Poisoning by propionic acid derivatives, undetermined**
+7th **T39.315 Adverse effect of propionic acid derivatives**
+7th **T39.316 Underdosing of propionic acid derivatives**

\+ **T39.39 Poisoning by, adverse effect of and underdosing of other nonsteroidal anti-inflammatory drugs [NSAID]**

+7th **T39.391 Poisoning by other nonsteroidal anti-inflammatory drugs [NSAID], accidental (unintentional)**
Poisoning by other nonsteroidal anti-inflammatory drugs NOS
+7th **T39.392 Poisoning by other nonsteroidal anti-inflammatory drugs [NSAID], intentional self-harm**
+7th **T39.393 Poisoning by other nonsteroidal anti-inflammatory drugs [NSAID], assault**
+7th **T39.394 Poisoning by other nonsteroidal anti-inflammatory drugs [NSAID], undetermined**
+7th **T39.395 Adverse effect of other nonsteroidal anti-inflammatory drugs [NSAID]**
+7th **T39.396 Underdosing of other nonsteroidal anti-inflammatory drugs [NSAID]**

\+ **T39.4 Poisoning by, adverse effect of and underdosing of antirheumatics, not elsewhere classified**
Excludes1: *poisoning by, adverse effect of and underdosing of glucocorticoids (T38.0-)*
poisoning by, adverse effect of and underdosing of salicylates (T39.0-)

\+ **T39.4X Poisoning by, adverse effect of and underdosing of antirheumatics, not elsewhere classified**

+7th **T39.4X1 Poisoning by antirheumatics, not elsewhere classified, accidental (unintentional)**
Poisoning by antirheumatics, not elsewhere classified NOS
+7th **T39.4X2 Poisoning by antirheumatics, not elsewhere classified, intentional self-harm**
+7th **T39.4X3 Poisoning by antirheumatics, not elsewhere classified, assault**
+7th **T39.4X4 Poisoning by antirheumatics, not elsewhere classified, undetermined**
+7th **T39.4X5 Adverse effect of antirheumatics, not elsewhere classified**
+7th **T39.4X6 Underdosing of antirheumatics, not elsewhere classified**

\+ **T39.8 Poisoning by, adverse effect of and underdosing of other nonopioid analgesics and antipyretics, not elsewhere classified**

\+ **T39.8X Poisoning by, adverse effect of and underdosing of other nonopioid analgesics and antipyretics, not elsewhere classified**

+7th **T39.8X1 Poisoning by other nonopioid analgesics and antipyretics, not elsewhere classified, accidental (unintentional)**
Poisoning by other nonopioid analgesics and antipyretics, not elsewhere classified NOS
+7th **T39.8X2 Poisoning by other nonopioid analgesics and antipyretics, not elsewhere classified, intentional self-harm**
+7th **T39.8X3 Poisoning by other nonopioid analgesics and antipyretics, not elsewhere classified, assault**
+7th **T39.8X4 Poisoning by other nonopioid analgesics and antipyretics, not elsewhere classified, undetermined**
+7th **T39.8X5 Adverse effect of other nonopioid analgesics and antipyretics, not elsewhere classified**
+7th **T39.8X6 Underdosing of other nonopioid analgesics and antipyretics, not elsewhere classified**

\+ **T39.9 Poisoning by, adverse effect of and underdosing of unspecified nonopioid analgesic, antipyretic and antirheumatic**

x+7th **T39.91 Poisoning by unspecified nonopioid analgesic, antipyretic and antirheumatic, accidental (unintentional)**
Poisoning by nonopioid analgesic, antipyretic and antirheumatic NOS
x+7th **T39.92 Poisoning by unspecified nonopioid analgesic, antipyretic and antirheumatic, intentional self-harm**
x+7th **T39.93 Poisoning by unspecified nonopioid analgesic, antipyretic and antirheumatic, assault**
x+7th **T39.94 Poisoning by unspecified nonopioid analgesic, antipyretic and antirheumatic, undetermined**
x+7th **T39.95 Adverse effect of unspecified nonopioid analgesic, antipyretic and antirheumatic**
x+7th **T39.96 Underdosing of unspecified nonopioid analgesic, antipyretic and antirheumatic**

T40 Poisoning by, adverse effect of and underdosing of narcotics and psychodysleptics [hallucinogens]

Excludes2: *drug dependence and related mental and behavioral disorders due to psychoactive substance use (F10.-F19.-)*

The appropriate 7th character is to be added to each code from category T40
A initial encounter
D subsequent encounter
S sequela

\+ **T40.0 Poisoning by, adverse effect of and underdosing of opium**

\+ **T40.0X Poisoning by, adverse effect of and underdosing of opium**

+7th **T40.0X1 Poisoning by opium, accidental (unintentional)**
Poisoning by opium NOS
+7th **T40.0X2 Poisoning by opium, intentional self-harm**
+7th **T40.0X3 Poisoning by opium, assault**
+7th **T40.0X4 Poisoning by opium, undetermined**
+7th **T40.0X5 Adverse effect of opium**
+7th **T40.0X6 Underdosing of opium**

\+ **T40.1 Poisoning by and adverse effect of heroin**

\+ **T40.1X Poisoning by and adverse effect of heroin**

+7th **T40.1X1 Poisoning by heroin, accidental (unintentional)**
Poisoning by heroin NOS
+7th **T40.1X2 Poisoning by heroin, intentional self-harm**
+7th **T40.1X3 Poisoning by heroin, assault**
+7th **T40.1X4 Poisoning by heroin, undetermined**

\+ **T40.2 Poisoning by, adverse effect of and underdosing of other opioids**

\+ **T40.2X Poisoning by, adverse effect of and underdosing of other opioids**

+7th **T40.2X1 Poisoning by other opioids, accidental (unintentional)**
Poisoning by other opioids NOS
+7th **T40.2X2 Poisoning by other opioids, intentional self-harm**
+7th **T40.2X3 Poisoning by other opioids, assault**
+7th **T40.2X4 Poisoning by other opioids, undetermined**

+7th T40.2X5 Adverse effect of other opioids
+7th T40.2X6 Underdosing of other opioids

+ T40.3 Poisoning by, adverse effect of and underdosing of methadone
+ T40.3X Poisoning by, adverse effect of and underdosing of methadone
+7th T40.3X1 Poisoning by methadone, accidental (unintentional)
Poisoning by methadone NOS
+7th T40.3X2 Poisoning by methadone, intentional self-harm
+7th T40.3X3 Poisoning by methadone, assault
+7th T40.3X4 Poisoning by methadone, undetermined
+7th T40.3X5 Adverse effect of methadone
+7th T40.3X6 Underdosing of methadone

+ T40.4 Poisoning by, adverse effect of and underdosing of other synthetic narcotics
+ T40.4X Poisoning by, adverse effect of and underdosing of other synthetic narcotics
+7th T40.4X1 Poisoning by other synthetic narcotics, accidental (unintentional)
Poisoning by other synthetic narcotics NOS
+7th T40.4X2 Poisoning by other synthetic narcotics, intentional self-harm
+7th T40.4X3 Poisoning by other synthetic narcotics, assault
+7th T40.4X4 Poisoning by other synthetic narcotics, undetermined
+7th T40.4X5 Adverse effect of other synthetic narcotics
+7th T40.4X6 Underdosing of other synthetic narcotics

+ T40.5 Poisoning by, adverse effect of and underdosing of cocaine
+ T40.5X Poisoning by, adverse effect of and underdosing of cocaine
+7th T40.5X1 Poisoning by cocaine, accidental (unintentional)
Poisoning by cocaine NOS
AHA CC: 2Q, 2016, 8-9
+7th T40.5X2 Poisoning by cocaine, intentional self-harm
+7th T40.5X3 Poisoning by cocaine, assault
+7th T40.5X4 Poisoning by cocaine, undetermined
+7th T40.5X5 Adverse effect of cocaine
+7th T40.5X6 Underdosing of cocaine

+ T40.6 Poisoning by, adverse effect of and underdosing of other and unspecified narcotics
+ T40.60 Poisoning by, adverse effect of and underdosing of unspecified narcotics
+7th T40.601 Poisoning by unspecified narcotics, accidental (unintentional)
Poisoning by narcotics NOS
+7th T40.602 Poisoning by unspecified narcotics, intentional self-harm
+7th T40.603 Poisoning by unspecified narcotics, assault
+7th T40.604 Poisoning by unspecified narcotics, undetermined
+7th T40.605 Adverse effect of unspecified narcotics
+7th T40.606 Underdosing of unspecified narcotics
+ T40.69 Poisoning by, adverse effect of and underdosing of other narcotics
+7th T40.691 Poisoning by other narcotics, accidental (unintentional)
Poisoning by other narcotics NOS
+7th T40.692 Poisoning by other narcotics, intentional self-harm
+7th T40.693 Poisoning by other narcotics, assault
+7th T40.694 Poisoning by other narcotics, undetermined
+7th T40.695 Adverse effect of other narcotics
+7th T40.696 Underdosing of other narcotics

+ T40.7 Poisoning by, adverse effect of and underdosing of cannabis (derivatives)
+ T40.7X Poisoning by, adverse effect of and underdosing of cannabis (derivatives)
+7th T40.7X1 Poisoning by cannabis (derivatives), accidental (unintentional)
Poisoning by cannabis NOS
+7th T40.7X2 Poisoning by cannabis (derivatives), intentional self-harm
+7th T40.7X3 Poisoning by cannabis (derivatives), assault
+7th T40.7X4 Poisoning by cannabis (derivatives), undetermined
+7th T40.7X5 Adverse effect of cannabis (derivatives)
+7th T40.7X6 Underdosing of cannabis (derivatives)

+ T40.8 Poisoning by and adverse effect of lysergide [LSD]
+ T40.8X Poisoning by and adverse effect of lysergide [LSD]
+7th T40.8X1 Poisoning by lysergide [LSD], accidental (unintentional)
Poisoning by lysergide [LSD]NOS
+7th T40.8X2 Poisoning by lysergide [LSD], intentional self-harm
+7th T40.8X3 Poisoning by lysergide [LSD], assault
+7th T40.8X4 Poisoning by lysergide [LSD], undetermined

+ T40.9 Poisoning by, adverse effect of and underdosing of other and unspecified psychodysleptics [hallucinogens]
+ T40.90 Poisoning by, adverse effect of and underdosing of unspecified psychodysleptics [hallucinogens]
+7th T40.901 Poisoning by unspecified psychodysleptics [hallucinogens], accidental (unintentional)
+7th T40.902 Poisoning by unspecified psychodysleptics [hallucinogens], intentional self-harm
+7th T40.903 Poisoning by unspecified psychodysleptics [hallucinogens], assault
+7th T40.904 Poisoning by unspecified psychodysleptics [hallucinogens], undetermined
+7th T40.905 Adverse effect of unspecified psychodysleptics [hallucinogens]
+7th T40.906 Underdosing of unspecified psychodysleptics
+ T40.99 Poisoning by, adverse effect of and underdosing of other psychodysleptics [hallucinogens]
+7th T40.991 Poisoning by other psychodysleptics [hallucinogens], accidental (unintentional)
Poisoning by other psychodysleptics [hallucinogens] NOS
+7th T40.992 Poisoning by other psychodysleptics [hallucinogens], intentional self-harm
+7th T40.993 Poisoning by other psychodysleptics [hallucinogens], assault
+7th T40.994 Poisoning by other psychodysleptics [hallucinogens], undetermined
+7th T40.995 Adverse effect of other psychodysleptics [hallucinogens]
+7th T40.996 Underdosing of other psychodysleptics

T41 Poisoning by, adverse effect of and underdosing of anesthetics and therapeutic gases

Excludes1: *benzodiazepines (T42.4-)*
cocaine (T40.5-)
complications of anesthesia during pregnancy (O29.-)
complications of anesthesia during labor and delivery (O74.-)
complications of anesthesia during the puerperium (O89.-)
opioids (T40.0-T40.2-)

The appropriate 7th character is to be added to each code from category T41
A initial encounter
D subsequent encounter
S sequela

+ T41.0 Poisoning by, adverse effect of and underdosing of inhaled anesthetics
Excludes1: *oxygen (T41.5-)*
+ T41.0X Poisoning by, adverse effect of and underdosing of inhaled anesthetics
+7th T41.0X1 Poisoning by inhaled anesthetics, accidental (unintentional)
Poisoning by inhaled anesthetics NOS
+7th T41.0X2 Poisoning by inhaled anesthetics, intentional self-harm
+7th T41.0X3 Poisoning by inhaled anesthetics, assault
+7th T41.0X4 Poisoning by inhaled anesthetics, undetermined
+7th T41.0X5 Adverse effect of inhaled anesthetics
+7th T41.0X6 Underdosing of inhaled anesthetics

+ T41.1 Poisoning by, adverse effect of and underdosing of intravenous anesthetics
Poisoning by, adverse effect of and underdosing of thiobarbiturates
+ T41.1X Poisoning by, adverse effect of and underdosing of intravenous anesthetics

+7th T41.1X1 Poisoning by intravenous anesthetics, accidental (unintentional)
Poisoning by intravenous anesthetics NOS
+7th T41.1X2 Poisoning by intravenous anesthetics, intentional self-harm
+7th T41.1X3 Poisoning by intravenous anesthetics, assault
+7th T41.1X4 Poisoning by intravenous anesthetics, undetermined
+7th T41.1X5 Adverse effect of intravenous anesthetics
+7th T41.1X6 Underdosing of intravenous anesthetics

+ T41.2 Poisoning by, adverse effect of and underdosing of other and unspecified general anesthetics
+ T41.20 Poisoning by, adverse effect of and underdosing of unspecified general anesthetics
+7th T41.201 Poisoning by unspecified general anesthetics, accidental (unintentional)
Poisoning by general anesthetics NOS
+7th T41.202 Poisoning by unspecified general anesthetics, intentional self-harm
+7th T41.203 Poisoning by unspecified general anesthetics, assault
+7th T41.204 Poisoning by unspecified general anesthetics, undetermined
+7th T41.205 Adverse effect of unspecified general anesthetics
AHA CC: 4Q, 2016, 72-73
+7th T41.206 Underdosing of unspecified general anesthetics
+ T41.29 Poisoning by, adverse effect of and underdosing of other general anesthetics
+7th T41.291 Poisoning by other general anesthetics, accidental (unintentional)
Poisoning by other general anesthetics NOS
+7th T41.292 Poisoning by other general anesthetics, intentional self-harm
+7th T41.293 Poisoning by other general anesthetics, assault
+7th T41.294 Poisoning by other general anesthetics, undetermined
+7th T41.295 Adverse effect of other general anesthetics
+7th T41.296 Underdosing of other general anesthetics

+ T41.3 Poisoning by, adverse effect of and underdosing of local anesthetics
Cocaine (topical)
Excludes2: *poisoning by cocaine used as a central nervous system stimulant (T40.5X1-T40.5X4)*
+ T41.3X Poisoning by, adverse effect of and underdosing of local anesthetics
+7th T41.3X1 Poisoning by local anesthetics, accidental (unintentional)
Poisoning by local anesthetics NOS
+7th T41.3X2 Poisoning by local anesthetics, intentional self-harm
+7th T41.3X3 Poisoning by local anesthetics, assault
+7th T41.3X4 Poisoning by local anesthetics, undetermined
+7th T41.3X5 Adverse effect of local anesthetics
+7th T41.3X6 Underdosing of local anesthetics

+ T41.4 Poisoning by, adverse effect of and underdosing of unspecified anesthetic
X+7th T41.41 Poisoning by unspecified anesthetic, accidental (unintentional)
Poisoning by anesthetic NOS
X+7th T41.42 Poisoning by unspecified anesthetic, intentional self-harm
X+7th T41.43 Poisoning by unspecified anesthetic, assault
X+7th T41.44 Poisoning by unspecified anesthetic, undetermined
X+7th T41.45 Adverse effect of unspecified anesthetic
X+7th T41.46 Underdosing of unspecified anesthetics

+ T41.5 Poisoning by, adverse effect of and underdosing of therapeutic gases
+ T41.5X Poisoning by, adverse effect of and underdosing of therapeutic gases
+7th T41.5X1 Poisoning by therapeutic gases, accidental (unintentional)
Poisoning by therapeutic gases NOS
+7th T41.5X2 Poisoning by therapeutic gases, intentional self-harm
+7th T41.5X3 Poisoning by therapeutic gases, assault
+7th T41.5X4 Poisoning by therapeutic gases, undetermined
+7th T41.5X5 Adverse effect of therapeutic gases
+7th T41.5X6 Underdosing of therapeutic gases

T42 Poisoning by, adverse effect of and underdosing of antiepileptic, sedative- hypnotic and antiparkinsonism drugs

Excludes2: *drug dependence and related mental and behavioral disorders due to psychoactive substance use (F10.--F19.-)*

The appropriate 7th character is to be added to each code from categor T42
A initial encounter
D subsequent encounter
S sequela

+ T42.0 Poisoning by, adverse effect of and underdosing of hydantoin derivatives
+ T42.0X Poisoning by, adverse effect of and underdosing of hydantoin derivatives
+7th T42.0X1 Poisoning by hydantoin derivatives, accidental (unintentional)
Poisoning by hydantoin derivatives NOS
+7th T42.0X2 Poisoning by hydantoin derivatives, intentional self-harm
+7th T42.0X3 Poisoning by hydantoin derivatives, assau
+7th T42.0X4 Poisoning by hydantoin derivatives, undetermined
+7th T42.0X5 Adverse effect of hydantoin derivatives
+7th T42.0X6 Underdosing of hydantoin derivatives

+ T42.1 Poisoning by, adverse effect of and underdosing of iminostilbenes
Poisoning by, adverse effect of and underdosing of carbamazepine
+ T42.1X Poisoning by, adverse effect of and underdosing of iminostilbenes
+7th T42.1X1 Poisoning by iminostilbenes, accidental (unintentional)
Poisoning by iminostilbenes NOS
+7th T42.1X2 Poisoning by iminostilbenes, intentional self-harm
+7th T42.1X3 Poisoning by iminostilbenes, assault
+7th T42.1X4 Poisoning by iminostilbenes, undetermine
+7th T42.1X5 Adverse effect of iminostilbenes
+7th T42.1X6 Underdosing of iminostilbenes

+ T42.2 Poisoning by, adverse effect of and underdosing of succinimides and oxazolidinediones
+ T42.2X Poisoning by, adverse effect of and underdosing of succinimides and oxazolidinediones
+7th T42.2X1 Poisoning by succinimides and oxazolidinediones, accidental (unintentional)
Poisoning by succinimides and oxazolidinediones NOS
+7th T42.2X2 Poisoning by succinimides and oxazolidinediones, intentional self-harm
+7th T42.2X3 Poisoning by succinimides and oxazolidinediones, assault
+7th T42.2X4 Poisoning by succinimides and oxazolidinediones, undetermined
+7th T42.2X5 Adverse effect of succinimides and oxazolidinediones
+7th T42.2X6 Underdosing of succinimides and oxazolidinediones

+ T42.3 Poisoning by, adverse effect of and underdosing of barbiturates
Excludes1: *poisoning by, adverse effect of and underdosing c thiobarbiturates (T41.1-)*
+ T42.3X Poisoning by, adverse effect of and underdosing of barbiturates
+7th T42.3X1 Poisoning by barbiturates, accidental (unintentional)
Poisoning by barbiturates NOS
+7th T42.3X2 Poisoning by barbiturates, intentional sel harm
+7th T42.3X3 Poisoning by barbiturates, assault
+7th T42.3X4 Poisoning by barbiturates, undetermined
+7th T42.3X5 Adverse effect of barbiturates
+7th T42.3X6 Underdosing of barbiturates

+ **T42.4 Poisoning by, adverse effect of and underdosing of benzodiazepines**

+ **T42.4X Poisoning by, adverse effect of and underdosing of benzodiazepines**

+7th **T42.4X1 Poisoning by benzodiazepines, accidental (unintentional)**
Poisoning by benzodiazepines NOS

+7th **T42.4X2 Poisoning by benzodiazepines, intentional self-harm**

+7th **T42.4X3 Poisoning by benzodiazepines, assault**

+7th **T42.4X4 Poisoning by benzodiazepines, undetermined**

+7th **T42.4X5 Adverse effect of benzodiazepines**

+7th **T42.4X6 Underdosing of benzodiazepines**

+ **T42.5 Poisoning by, adverse effect of and underdosing of mixed antiepileptics**

+ **T42.5X Poisoning by, adverse effect of and underdosing of antiepileptics**

+7th **T42.5X1 Poisoning by mixed antiepileptics, accidental (unintentional)**
Poisoning by mixed antiepileptics NOS

+7th **T42.5X2 Poisoning by mixed antiepileptics, intentional self-harm**

+7th **T42.5X3 Poisoning by mixed antiepileptics, assault**

+7th **T42.5X4 Poisoning by mixed antiepileptics, undetermined**

+7th **T42.5X5 Adverse effect of mixed antiepileptics**

+7th **T42.5X6 Underdosing of mixed antiepileptics**

+ **T42.6 Poisoning by, adverse effect of and underdosing of other antiepileptic and sedative-hypnotic drugs**
Poisoning by, adverse effect of and underdosing of methaqualone
Poisoning by, adverse effect of and underdosing of valproic acid
Excludes1: *poisoning by, adverse effect of and underdosing of carbamazepine (T42.1-)*

+ **T42.6X Poisoning by, adverse effect of and underdosing of other antiepileptic and sedative-hypnotic drugs**

+7th **T42.6X1 Poisoning by other antiepileptic and sedative-hypnotic drugs, accidental (unintentional)**
Poisoning by other antiepileptic and sedative-hypnotic drugs NOS

+7th **T42.6X2 Poisoning by other antiepileptic and sedative-hypnotic drugs, intentional self-harm**

+7th **T42.6X3 Poisoning by other antiepileptic and sedative-hypnotic drugs, assault**

+7th **T42.6X4 Poisoning by other antiepileptic and sedative-hypnotic drugs, undetermined**

+7th **T42.6X5 Adverse effect of other antiepileptic and sedative-hypnotic drugs**

+7th **T42.6X6 Underdosing of other antiepileptic and sedative-hypnotic drugs**

+ **T42.7 Poisoning by, adverse effect of and underdosing of unspecified antiepileptic and sedative-hypnotic drugs**

X+7th **T42.71 Poisoning by unspecified antiepileptic and sedative-hypnotic drugs, accidental (unintentional)**
Poisoning by antiepileptic and sedative-hypnotic drugs NOS

X+7th **T42.72 Poisoning by unspecified antiepileptic and sedative-hypnotic drugs, intentional self-harm**

X+7th **T42.73 Poisoning by unspecified antiepileptic and sedative-hypnotic drugs, assault**

X+7th **T42.74 Poisoning by unspecified antiepileptic and sedative-hypnotic drugs, undetermined**

X+7th **T42.75 Adverse effect of unspecified antiepileptic and sedative-hypnotic drugs**

X+7th **T42.76 Underdosing of unspecified antiepileptic and sedative-hypnotic drugs**

+ **T42.8 Poisoning by, adverse effect of and underdosing of antiparkinsonism drugs and other central muscle-tone depressants**
Poisoning by, adverse effect of and underdosing of amantadine

+ **T42.8X Poisoning by, adverse effect of and underdosing of antiparkinsonism drugs and other central muscle-tone depressants**

+7th **T42.8X1 Poisoning by antiparkinsonism drugs and other central muscle-tone depressants, accidental (unintentional)**
Poisoning by antiparkinsonism drugs and other central muscle-tone depressants NOS

+7th **T42.8X2 Poisoning by antiparkinsonism drugs and other central muscle-tone depressants, intentional self-harm**

+7th **T42.8X3 Poisoning by antiparkinsonism drugs and other central muscle-tone depressants, assault**

+7th **T42.8X4 Poisoning by antiparkinsonism drugs and other central muscle-tone depressants, undetermined**

+7th **T42.8X5 Adverse effect of antiparkinsonism drugs and other central muscle-tone depressants**

+7th **T42.8X6 Underdosing of antiparkinsonism drugs and other central muscle-tone depressants**

T43 Poisoning by, adverse effect of and underdosing of psychotropic drugs, not elsewhere classified

Excludes1: *appetite depressants (T50.5-)*
barbiturates (T42.3-)
benzodiazepines (T42.4-)
methaqualone (T42.6-)
psychodysleptics [hallucinogens] (T40.7-T40.9-)

Excludes2: *drug dependence and related mental and behavioral disorders due to psychoactive substance use (F10.- -F19.-)*

The appropriate 7th character is to be added to each code from category T43
A initial encounter
D subsequent encounter
S sequela

+ **T43.0 Poisoning by, adverse effect of and underdosing of tricyclic and tetracyclic antidepressants**

+ **T43.01 Poisoning by, adverse effect of and underdosing of tricyclic antidepressants**

+7th **T43.011 Poisoning by tricyclic antidepressants, accidental (unintentional)**
Poisoning by tricyclic antidepressants NOS

+7th **T43.012 Poisoning by tricyclic antidepressants, intentional self-harm**

+7th **T43.013 Poisoning by tricyclic antidepressants, assault**

+7th **T43.014 Poisoning by tricyclic antidepressants, undetermined**

+7th **T43.015 Adverse effect of tricyclic antidepressants**

+7th **T43.016 Underdosing of tricyclic antidepressants**

+ **T43.02 Poisoning by, adverse effect of and underdosing of tetracyclic antidepressants**

+7th **T43.021 Poisoning by tetracyclic antidepressants, accidental (unintentional)**
Poisoning by tetracyclic antidepressants NOS

+7th **T43.022 Poisoning by tetracyclic antidepressants, intentional self-harm**

+7th **T43.023 Poisoning by tetracyclic antidepressants, assault**

+7th **T43.024 Poisoning by tetracyclic antidepressants, undetermined**

+7th **T43.025 Adverse effect of tetracyclic antidepressants**

+7th **T43.026 Underdosing of tetracyclic antidepressants**

+ **T43.1 Poisoning by, adverse effect of and underdosing of monoamine-oxidase-inhibitor antidepressants**

+ **T43.1X Poisoning by, adverse effect of and underdosing of monoamine-oxidase-inhibitor antidepressants**

+7th **T43.1X1 Poisoning by monoamine-oxidase-inhibitor antidepressants, accidental (unintentional)**
Poisoning by monoamine-oxidase-inhibitor antidepressants NOS

+7th **T43.1X2 Poisoning by monoamine-oxidase-inhibitor antidepressants, intentional self-harm**

+7th **T43.1X3 Poisoning by monoamine-oxidase-inhibitor antidepressants, assault**

+7th **T43.1X4 Poisoning by monoamine-oxidase-inhibitor antidepressants, undetermined**

+7th **T43.1X5 Adverse effect of monoamine-oxidase-inhibitor antidepressants**

+7th **T43.1X6 Underdosing of monoamine-oxidase-inhibitor antidepressants**

+ **T43.2 Poisoning by, adverse effect of and underdosing of other and unspecified antidepressants**
  + **T43.20 Poisoning by, adverse effect of and underdosing of unspecified antidepressants**
    - +7th **T43.201 Poisoning by unspecified antidepressants, accidental (unintentional)**
      Poisoning by antidepressants NOS
    - +7th **T43.202 Poisoning by unspecified antidepressants, intentional self-harm**
    - +7th **T43.203 Poisoning by unspecified antidepressants, assault**
    - +7th **T43.204 Poisoning by unspecified antidepressants, undetermined**
    - +7th **T43.205 Adverse effect of unspecified antidepressants**
      Antidepressant discontinuation syndrome
    - +7th **T43.206 Underdosing of unspecified antidepressants**
  + **T43.21 Poisoning by, adverse effect of and underdosing of selective serotonin and norepinephrine reuptake inhibitors**
    Poisoning by, adverse effect of and underdosing of SSNRI antidepressants
    - +7th **T43.211 Poisoning by selective serotonin and norepinephrine reuptake inhibitors, accidental (unintentional)**
    - +7th **T43.212 Poisoning by selective serotonin and norepinephrine reuptake inhibitors, intentional self-harm**
    - +7th **T43.213 Poisoning by selective serotonin and norepinephrine reuptake inhibitors, assault**
    - +7th **T43.214 Poisoning by selective serotonin and norepinephrine reuptake inhibitors, undetermined**
    - +7th **T43.215 Adverse effect of selective serotonin and norepinephrine reuptake inhibitors**
    - +7th **T43.216 Underdosing of selective serotonin and norepinephrine reuptake inhibitors**
  + **T43.22 Poisoning by, adverse effect of and underdosing of selective serotonin reuptake inhibitors**
    Poisoning by, adverse effect of and underdosing of SSRI antidepressants
    - +7th **T43.221 Poisoning by selective serotonin reuptake inhibitors, accidental (unintentional)**
    - +7th **T43.222 Poisoning by selective serotonin reuptake inhibitors, intentional self-harm**
    - +7th **T43.223 Poisoning by selective serotonin reuptake inhibitors, assault**
    - +7th **T43.224 Poisoning by selective serotonin reuptake inhibitors, undetermined**
    - +7th **T43.225 Adverse effect of selective serotonin reuptake inhibitors**
    - +7th **T43.226 Underdosing of selective serotonin reuptake inhibitors**
  + **T43.29 Poisoning by, adverse effect of and underdosing of other antidepressants**
    - +7th **T43.291 Poisoning by other antidepressants, accidental (unintentional)**
      Poisoning by other antidepressants NOS
    - +7th **T43.292 Poisoning by other antidepressants, intentional self-harm**
    - +7th **T43.293 Poisoning by other antidepressants, assault**
    - +7th **T43.294 Poisoning by other antidepressants, undetermined**
    - +7th **T43.295 Adverse effect of other antidepressants**
    - +7th **T43.296 Underdosing of other antidepressants**
+ **T43.3 Poisoning by, adverse effect of and underdosing of phenothiazine antipsychotics and neuroleptics**
  + **T43.3X Poisoning by, adverse effect of and underdosing of phenothiazine antipsychotics and neuroleptics**
    - +7th **T43.3X1 Poisoning by phenothiazine antipsychotics and neuroleptics, accidental (unintentional)**
      Poisoning by phenothiazine antipsychotics and neuroleptics NOS
    - +7th **T43.3X2 Poisoning by phenothiazine antipsychotics and neuroleptics, intentional self-harm**
    - +7th **T43.3X3 Poisoning by phenothiazine antipsychotics and neuroleptics, assault**
    - +7th **T43.3X4 Poisoning by phenothiazine antipsychotics and neuroleptics, undetermined**
    - +7th **T43.3X5 Adverse effect of phenothiazine antipsychotics and neuroleptics**
    - +7th **T43.3X6 Underdosing of phenothiazine antipsychotics and neuroleptics**
+ **T43.4 Poisoning by, adverse effect of and underdosing of butyrophenone and thiothixene neuroleptics**
  + **T43.4X Poisoning by, adverse effect of and underdosing of butyrophenone and thiothixene neuroleptics**
    - +7th **T43.4X1 Poisoning by butyrophenone and thiothixene neuroleptics, accidental (unintentional)**
      Poisoning by butyrophenone and thiothixe neuroleptics NOS
    - +7th **T43.4X2 Poisoning by butyrophenone and thiothixene neuroleptics, intentional self-harm**
    - +7th **T43.4X3 Poisoning by butyrophenone and thiothixene neuroleptics, assault**
    - +7th **T43.4X4 Poisoning by butyrophenone and thiothixene neuroleptics, undetermined**
    - +7th **T43.4X5 Adverse effect of butyrophenone and thiothixene neuroleptics**
    - +7th **T43.4X6 Underdosing of butyrophenone and thiothixene neuroleptics**
+ **T43.5 Poisoning by, adverse effect of and underdosing of other and unspecified antipsychotics and neuroleptics**
  Excludes1: *poisoning by, adverse effect of and underdosing o rauwolfia (T46.5-)*
  + **T43.50 Poisoning by, adverse effect of and underdosing of unspecified antipsychotics and neuroleptics**
    - +7th **T43.501 Poisoning by unspecified antipsychotics and neuroleptics, accidental (unintention**
      Poisoning by antipsychotics and neuroleptics NOS
    - +7th **T43.502 Poisoning by unspecified antipsychotics and neuroleptics, intentional self-harm**
    - +7th **T43.503 Poisoning by unspecified antipsychotics and neuroleptics, assault**
    - +7th **T43.504 Poisoning by unspecified antipsychotics and neuroleptics, undetermined**
    - +7th **T43.505 Adverse effect of unspecified antipsychoti and neuroleptics**
    - +7th **T43.506 Underdosing of unspecified antipsychotic and neuroleptics**
  + **T43.59 Poisoning by, adverse effect of and underdosing of other antipsychotics and neuroleptics**
    - +7th **T43.591 Poisoning by other antipsychotics and neuroleptics, accidental (unintentional)**
      Poisoning by other antipsychotics and neuroleptics NOS
    - +7th **T43.592 Poisoning by other antipsychotics and neuroleptics, intentional self-harm**
      AHA CC: 1Q, 2017, 40
    - +7th **T43.593 Poisoning by other antipsychotics and neuroleptics, assault**
    - +7th **T43.594 Poisoning by other antipsychotics and neuroleptics, undetermined**
    - +7th **T43.595 Adverse effect of other antipsychotics an neuroleptics**
    - +7th **T43.596 Underdosing of other antipsychotics and neuroleptics**
+ **T43.6 Poisoning by, adverse effect of and underdosing of psychostimulants**
  Excludes1: *poisoning by, adverse effect of and underdosing o cocaine (T40.5-)*
  + **T43.60 Poisoning by, adverse effect of and underdosing of unspecified psychostimulant**
    - +7th **T43.601 Poisoning by unspecified psychostimulan accidental (unintentional)**
      Poisoning by psychostimulants NOS
    - +7th **T43.602 Poisoning by unspecified psychostimulan intentional self-harm**
    - +7th **T43.603 Poisoning by unspecified psychostimulan assault**
    - +7th **T43.604 Poisoning by unspecified psychostimulan undetermined**
    - +7th **T43.605 Adverse effect of unspecified psychostimulants**
    - +7th **T43.606 Underdosing of unspecified psychostimulants**

+ **T43.61 Poisoning by, adverse effect of and underdosing of caffeine**
- +7th **T43.611 Poisoning by caffeine, accidental (unintentional)**
  Poisoning by caffeine NOS
- +7th **T43.612 Poisoning by caffeine, intentional self-harm**
- +7th **T43.613 Poisoning by caffeine, assault**
- +7th **T43.614 Poisoning by caffeine, undetermined**
- +7th **T43.615 Adverse effect of caffeine**
- +7th **T43.616 Underdosing of caffeine**

+ **T43.62 Poisoning by, adverse effect of and underdosing of amphetamines**
  Poisoning by, adverse effect of and underdosing of methamphetamines
- +7th **T43.621 Poisoning by amphetamines, accidental (unintentional)**
  Poisoning by amphetamines NOS
- +7th **T43.622 Poisoning by amphetamines, intentional self-harm**
- +7th **T43.623 Poisoning by amphetamines, assault**
- +7th **T43.624 Poisoning by amphetamines, undetermined**
- +7th **T43.625 Adverse effect of amphetamines**
- +7th **T43.626 Underdosing of amphetamines**

+ **T43.63 Poisoning by, adverse effect of and underdosing of methylphenidate**
- +7th **T43.631 Poisoning by methylphenidate, accidental (unintentional)**
  Poisoning by methylphenidate NOS
- +7th **T43.632 Poisoning by methylphenidate, intentional self-harm**
- +7th **T43.633 Poisoning by methylphenidate, assault**
- +7th **T43.634 Poisoning by methylphenidate, undetermined**
- +7th **T43.635 Adverse effect of methylphenidate**
- +7th **T43.636 Underdosing of methylphenidate**

+ **T43.69 Poisoning by, adverse effect of and underdosing of other psychostimulants**
- +7th **T43.691 Poisoning by other psychostimulants, accidental (unintentional)**
  Poisoning by other psychostimulants NOS
- +7th **T43.692 Poisoning by other psychostimulants, intentional self-harm**
- +7th **T43.693 Poisoning by other psychostimulants, assault**
- +7th **T43.694 Poisoning by other psychostimulants, undetermined**
- +7th **T43.695 Adverse effect of other psychostimulants**
- +7th **T43.696 Underdosing of other psychostimulants**

+ **T43.8 Poisoning by, adverse effect of and underdosing of other psychotropic drugs**

+ **T43.8X Poisoning by, adverse effect of and underdosing of other psychotropic drugs**
- +7th **T43.8X1 Poisoning by other psychotropic drugs, accidental (unintentional)**
  Poisoning by other psychotropic drugs NOS
- +7th **T43.8X2 Poisoning by other psychotropic drugs, intentional self-harm**
- +7th **T43.8X3 Poisoning by other psychotropic drugs, assault**
- +7th **T43.8X4 Poisoning by other psychotropic drugs, undetermined**
- +7th **T43.8X5 Adverse effect of other psychotropic drugs**
- +7th **T43.8X6 Underdosing of other psychotropic drugs**

+ **T43.9 Poisoning by, adverse effect of and underdosing of unspecified psychotropic drug**
- X+7th **T43.91 Poisoning by unspecified psychotropic drug, accidental (unintentional)**
  Poisoning by psychotropic drug NOS
- X+7th **T43.92 Poisoning by unspecified psychotropic drug, intentional self-harm**
- X+7th **T43.93 Poisoning by unspecified psychotropic drug, assault**
- X+7th **T43.94 Poisoning by unspecified psychotropic drug, undetermined**
- X+7th **T43.95 Adverse effect of unspecified psychotropic drug**
- X+7th **T43.96 Underdosing of unspecified psychotropic drug**

T44 Poisoning by, adverse effect of and underdosing of drugs primarily affecting the autonomic nervous system

The appropriate 7th character is to be added to each code from category T44
A initial encounter
D subsequent encounter
S sequela

+ **T44.0 Poisoning by, adverse effect of and underdosing of anticholinesterase agents**

+ **T44.0X Poisoning by, adverse effect of and underdosing of anticholinesterase agents**
- +7th **T44.0X1 Poisoning by anticholinesterase agents, accidental (unintentional)**
  Poisoning by anticholinesterase agents NOS
- +7th **T44.0X2 Poisoning by anticholinesterase agents, intentional self-harm**
- +7th **T44.0X3 Poisoning by anticholinesterase agents, assault**
- +7th **T44.0X4 Poisoning by anticholinesterase agents, undetermined**
- +7th **T44.0X5 Adverse effect of anticholinesterase agents**
- +7th **T44.0X6 Underdosing of anticholinesterase agents**

+ **T44.1 Poisoning by, adverse effect of and underdosing of other parasympathomimetics [cholinergics]**

+ **T44.1X Poisoning by, adverse effect of and underdosing of other parasympathomimetics [cholinergics]**
- +7th **T44.1X1 Poisoning by other parasympathomimetics [cholinergics], accidental (unintentional)**
  Poisoning by other parasympathomimetics [cholinergics] NOS
- +7th **T44.1X2 Poisoning by other parasympathomimetics [cholinergics], intentional self-harm**
- +7th **T44.1X3 Poisoning by other parasympathomimetics [cholinergics], assault**
- +7th **T44.1X4 Poisoning by other parasympathomimetics [cholinergics], undetermined**
- +7th **T44.1X5 Adverse effect of other parasympathomimetics [cholinergics]**
- +7th **T44.1X6 Underdosing of other parasympathomimetics**

+ **T44.2 Poisoning by, adverse effect of and underdosing of ganglionic blocking drugs**

+ **T44.2X Poisoning by, adverse effect of and underdosing of ganglionic blocking drugs**
- +7th **T44.2X1 Poisoning by ganglionic blocking drugs, accidental (unintentional)**
  Poisoning by ganglionic blocking drugs NOS
- +7th **T44.2X2 Poisoning by ganglionic blocking drugs, intentional self-harm**
- +7th **T44.2X3 Poisoning by ganglionic blocking drugs, assault**
- +7th **T44.2X4 Poisoning by ganglionic blocking drugs, undetermined**
- +7th **T44.2X5 Adverse effect of ganglionic blocking drugs**
- +7th **T44.2X6 Underdosing of ganglionic blocking drugs**

+ **T44.3 Poisoning by, adverse effect of and underdosing of other parasympatholytics [anticholinergics and antimuscarinics] and spasmolytics**
  Poisoning by, adverse effect of and underdosing of papaverine

+ **T44.3X Poisoning by, adverse effect of and underdosing of other parasympatholytics [anticholinergics and antimuscarinics] and spasmolytics**
- +7th **T44.3X1 Poisoning by other parasympatholytics [anticholinergics and antimuscarinics] and spasmolytics, accidental (unintentional)**
  Poisoning by other parasympatholytics [anticholinergics and antimuscarinics] and spasmolytics NOS
- +7th **T44.3X2 Poisoning by other parasympatholytics [anticholinergics and antimuscarinics] and spasmolytics, intentional self-harm**
- +7th **T44.3X3 Poisoning by other parasympatholytics [anticholinergics and antimuscarinics] and spasmolytics, assault**
- +7th **T44.3X4 Poisoning by other parasympatholytics [anticholinergics and antimuscarinics] and spasmolytics, undetermined**

+7th **T44.3X5 Adverse effect of other parasympatholytics [anticholinergics and antimuscarinics] and spasmolytics**

+7th **T44.3X6 Underdosing of other parasympatholytics [anticholinergics and antimuscarinics] and spasmolytics**

+ **T44.4 Poisoning by, adverse effect of and underdosing of predominantly alpha-adrenoreceptor agonists**

Poisoning by, adverse effect of and underdosing of metaraminol

+ **T44.4X Poisoning by, adverse effect of and underdosing of predominantly alpha-adrenoreceptor agonists**

+7th **T44.4X1 Poisoning by predominantly alpha-adrenoreceptor agonists, accidental (unintentional)**

Poisoning by predominantly alpha-adrenoreceptor agonists NOS

+7th **T44.4X2 Poisoning by predominantly alpha-adrenoreceptor agonists, intentional self-harm**

+7th **T44.4X3 Poisoning by predominantly alpha-adrenoreceptor agonists, assault**

+7th **T44.4X4 Poisoning by predominantly alpha-adrenoreceptor agonists, undetermined**

+7th **T44.4X5 Adverse effect of predominantly alpha-adrenoreceptor agonists**

+7th **T44.4X6 Underdosing of predominantly alpha-adrenoreceptor agonists**

+ **T44.5 Poisoning by, adverse effect of and underdosing of predominantly beta-adrenoreceptor agonists**

Excludes1: *poisoning by, adverse effect of and underdosing of beta-adrenoreceptor agonists used in asthma therapy (T48.6-)*

+ **T44.5X Poisoning by, adverse effect of and underdosing of predominantly beta-adrenoreceptor agonists**

+7th **T44.5X1 Poisoning by predominantly beta-adrenoreceptor agonists, accidental (unintentional)**

Poisoning by predominantly beta-adrenoreceptor agonists NOS

+7th **T44.5X2 Poisoning by predominantly beta-adrenoreceptor agonists, intentional self-harm**

+7th **T44.5X3 Poisoning by predominantly beta-adrenoreceptor agonists, assault**

+7th **T44.5X4 Poisoning by predominantly beta-adrenoreceptor agonists, undetermined**

+7th **T44.5X5 Adverse effect of predominantly beta-adrenoreceptor agonists**

+7th **T44.5X6 Underdosing of predominantly beta-adrenoreceptor agonists**

+ **T44.6 Poisoning by, adverse effect of and underdosing of alpha-adrenoreceptor antagonists**

Excludes1: *poisoning by, adverse effect of and underdosing of ergot alkaloids (T48.0)*

+ **T44.6X Poisoning by, adverse effect of and underdosing of alpha-adrenoreceptor antagonists**

+7th **T44.6X1 Poisoning by alpha-adrenoreceptor antagonists, accidental (unintentional)**

Poisoning by alpha-adrenoreceptor antagonists NOS

+7th **T44.6X2 Poisoning by alpha-adrenoreceptor antagonists, intentional self-harm**

+7th **T44.6X3 Poisoning by alpha-adrenoreceptor antagonists, assault**

+7th **T44.6X4 Poisoning by alpha-adrenoreceptor antagonists, undetermined**

+7th **T44.6X5 Adverse effect of alpha-adrenoreceptor antagonists**

+7th **T44.6X6 Underdosing of alpha-adrenoreceptor antagonists**

+ **T44.7 Poisoning by, adverse effect of and underdosing of beta-adrenoreceptor antagonists**

+ **T44.7X Poisoning by, adverse effect of and underdosing of beta-adrenoreceptor antagonists**

+7th **T44.7X1 Poisoning by beta-adrenoreceptor antagonists, accidental (unintentional)**

Poisoning by beta-adrenoreceptor antagonists NOS

+7th **T44.7X2 Poisoning by beta-adrenoreceptor antagonists, intentional self-harm**

+7th **T44.7X3 Poisoning by beta-adrenoreceptor antagonists, assault**

+7th **T44.7X4 Poisoning by beta-adrenoreceptor antagonists, undetermined**

+7th **T44.7X5 Adverse effect of beta-adrenoreceptor antagonists**

+7th **T44.7X6 Underdosing of beta-adrenoreceptor antagonists**

+ **T44.8 Poisoning by, adverse effect of and underdosing of centrally-acting and adrenergic-neuron- blocking agents**

Excludes1: *poisoning by, adverse effect of and underdosing of clonidine (T46.5)*
poisoning by, adverse effect of and underdosing of guanethidine (T46.5)

+ **T44.8X Poisoning by, adverse effect of and underdosing of centrally-acting and adrenergic- neuron-blocking agents**

+7th **T44.8X1 Poisoning by centrally-acting and adrenergic-neuron-blocking agents, accidental (unintentional)**

Poisoning by centrally-acting and adrenergic-neuron-blocking agents NOS

+7th **T44.8X2 Poisoning by centrally-acting and adrenergic-neuron-blocking agents, intentional self-harm**

+7th **T44.8X3 Poisoning by centrally-acting and adrenergic-neuron-blocking agents, assau**

+7th **T44.8X4 Poisoning by centrally-acting and adrenergic-neuron-blocking agents, undetermined**

+7th **T44.8X5 Adverse effect of centrally-acting and adrenergic-neuron-blocking agents**

+7th **T44.8X6 Underdosing of centrally-acting and adrenergic-neuron-blocking agents**

+ **T44.9 Poisoning by, adverse effect of and underdosing of other and unspecified drugs primarily affecting the autonomic nervous system**

Poisoning by, adverse effect of and underdosing of drug stimulating both alpha and beta-adrenoreceptors

+ **T44.90 Poisoning by, adverse effect of and underdosing of unspecified drugs primarily affecting the autonomi nervous system**

+7th **T44.901 Poisoning by unspecified drugs primarily affecting the autonomic nervous system, accidental (unintentional)**

Poisoning by unspecified drugs primarily affecting the autonomic nervous system NOS

+7th **T44.902 Poisoning by unspecified drugs primarily affecting the autonomic nervous system, intentional self-harm**

+7th **T44.903 Poisoning by unspecified drugs primarily affecting the autonomic nervous system, assault**

+7th **T44.904 Poisoning by unspecified drugs primarily affecting the autonomic nervous system, undetermined**

+7th **T44.905 Adverse effect of unspecified drugs primarily affecting the autonomic nervou system**

+7th **T44.906 Underdosing of unspecified drugs primarily affecting the autonomic nervou system**

+ **T44.99 Poisoning by, adverse effect of and underdosing of other drugs primarily affecting the autonomic nervous system**

+7th **T44.991 Poisoning by other drug primarily affecting the autonomic nervous system, accidental (unintentional)**

Poisoning by other drugs primarily affectin the autonomic nervous system NOS

+7th **T44.992 Poisoning by other drug primarily affecting the autonomic nervous system, intentional self-harm**

+7th **T44.993 Poisoning by other drug primarily affecting the autonomic nervous system, assault**

+7th **T44.994 Poisoning by other drug primarily affecting the autonomic nervous system, undetermined**

+7th **T44.995 Adverse effect of other drug primarily affecting the autonomic nervous system**
+7th **T44.996 Underdosing of other drug primarily affecting the autonomic nervous system**

T45 Poisoning by, adverse effect of and underdosing of primarily systemic and hematological agents, not elsewhere classified

The appropriate 7th character is to be added to each code from category T45
A initial encounter
D subsequent encounter
S sequela

+ **T45.0 Poisoning by, adverse effect of and underdosing of antiallergic and antiemetic drugs**
Excludes1: *poisoning by, adverse effect of and underdosing of phenothiazine-based neuroleptics (T43.3)*
+ **T45.0X Poisoning by, adverse effect of and underdosing of antiallergic and antiemetic drugs**
+7th **T45.0X1 Poisoning by antiallergic and antiemetic drugs, accidental (unintentional)**
Poisoning by antiallergic and antiemetic drugs NOS
+7th **T45.0X2 Poisoning by antiallergic and antiemetic drugs, intentional self-harm**
+7th **T45.0X3 Poisoning by antiallergic and antiemetic drugs, assault**
+7th **T45.0X4 Poisoning by antiallergic and antiemetic drugs, undetermined**
+7th **T45.0X5 Adverse effect of antiallergic and antiemetic drugs**
+7th **T45.0X6 Underdosing of antiallergic and antiemetic drugs**

+ **T45.1 Poisoning by, adverse effect of and underdosing of antineoplastic and immunosuppressive drugs**
Excludes1: *poisoning by, adverse effect of and underdosing of tamoxifen (T38.6)*
+ **T45.1X Poisoning by, adverse effect of and underdosing of antineoplastic and immunosuppressive drugs**
+7th **T45.1X1 Poisoning by antineoplastic and immunosuppressive drugs, accidental (unintentional)**
Poisoning by antineoplastic and immunosuppressive drugs NOS
+7th **T45.1X2 Poisoning by antineoplastic and immunosuppressive drugs, intentional self-harm**
+7th **T45.1X3 Poisoning by antineoplastic and immunosuppressive drugs, assault**
+7th **T45.1X4 Poisoning by antineoplastic and immunosuppressive drugs, undetermined**
+7th **T45.1X5 Adverse effect of antineoplastic and immunosuppressive drugs**
Review coding guideline C.2.c.2
AHA CC: 4Q, 2014, 22-23
+7th **T45.1X6 Underdosing of antineoplastic and immunosuppressive drugs**

+ **T45.2 Poisoning by, adverse effect of and underdosing of vitamins**
Excludes2: *poisoning by, adverse effect of and underdosing of nicotinic acid (derivatives) (T46.7)*
poisoning by, adverse effect of and underdosing of iron (T45.4)
poisoning by, adverse effect of and underdosing of vitamin K (T45.7)
+ **T45.2X Poisoning by, adverse effect of and underdosing of vitamins**
+7th **T45.2X1 Poisoning by vitamins, accidental (unintentional)**
Poisoning by vitamins NOS
+7th **T45.2X2 Poisoning by vitamins, intentional self-harm**
+7th **T45.2X3 Poisoning by vitamins, assault**
+7th **T45.2X4 Poisoning by vitamins, undetermined**
+7th **T45.2X5 Adverse effect of vitamins**
+7th **T45.2X6 Underdosing of vitamins**
Excludes1: *vitamin deficiencies (E50-E56)*

+ **T45.3 Poisoning by, adverse effect of and underdosing of enzymes**
+ **T45.3X Poisoning by, adverse effect of and underdosing of enzymes**
+7th **T45.3X1 Poisoning by enzymes, accidental (unintentional)**
Poisoning by enzymes NOS
+7th **T45.3X2 Poisoning by enzymes, intentional self-harm**
+7th **T45.3X3 Poisoning by enzymes, assault**
+7th **T45.3X4 Poisoning by enzymes, undetermined**
+7th **T45.3X5 Adverse effect of enzymes**
+7th **T45.3X6 Underdosing of enzymes**

+ **T45.4 Poisoning by, adverse effect of and underdosing of iron and its compounds**
+ **T45.4X Poisoning by, adverse effect of and underdosing of iron and its compounds**
+7th **T45.4X1 Poisoning by iron and its compounds, accidental (unintentional)**
Poisoning by iron and its compounds NOS
+7th **T45.4X2 Poisoning by iron and its compounds, intentional self-harm**
+7th **T45.4X3 Poisoning by iron and its compounds, assault**
+7th **T45.4X4 Poisoning by iron and its compounds, undetermined**
+7th **T45.4X5 Adverse effect of iron and its compounds**
+7th **T45.4X6 Underdosing of iron and its compounds**
Excludes1: *iron deficiency (E61.1)*

+ **T45.5 Poisoning by, adverse effect of and underdosing of anticoagulants and antithrombotic drugs**
+ **T45.51 Poisoning by, adverse effect of and underdosing of anticoagulants**
+7th **T45.511 Poisoning by anticoagulants, accidental (unintentional)**
Poisoning by anticoagulants NOS
+7th **T45.512 Poisoning by anticoagulants, intentional self-harm**
+7th **T45.513 Poisoning by anticoagulants, assault**
+7th **T45.514 Poisoning by anticoagulants, undetermined**
+7th **T45.515 Adverse effect of anticoagulants**
AHA CC: 2Q, 2013, 34-35; 1Q, 2016, 14-15
+7th **T45.516 Underdosing of anticoagulants**
+ **T45.52 Poisoning by, adverse effect of and underdosing of antithrombotic drugs**
Poisoning by, adverse effect of and underdosing of antiplatelet drugs
Excludes2: *poisoning by, adverse effect of and underdosing of aspirin (T39.01-)*
poisoning by, adverse effect of and underdosing of acetylsalicylic acid (T39.01-)
+7th **T45.521 Poisoning by antithrombotic drugs, accidental (unintentional)**
Poisoning by antithrombotic drug NOS
+7th **T45.522 Poisoning by antithrombotic drugs, intentional self-harm**
+7th **T45.523 Poisoning by antithrombotic drugs, assault**
+7th **T45.524 Poisoning by antithrombotic drugs, undetermined**
+7th **T45.525 Adverse effect of antithrombotic drugs**
AHA CC: 1Q, 2016, 15
+7th **T45.526 Underdosing of antithrombotic drugs**

+ **T45.6 Poisoning by, adverse effect of and underdosing of fibrinolysis-affecting drugs**
+ **T45.60 Poisoning by, adverse effect of and underdosing of unspecified fibrinolysis-affecting drugs**
+7th **T45.601 Poisoning by unspecified fibrinolysis-affecting drugs, accidental (unintentional)**
Poisoning by fibrinolysis-affecting drug NOS
+7th **T45.602 Poisoning by unspecified fibrinolysis-affecting drugs, intentional self-harm**
+7th **T45.603 Poisoning by unspecified fibrinolysis-affecting drugs, assault**
+7th **T45.604 Poisoning by unspecified fibrinolysis-affecting drugs, undetermined**
+7th **T45.605 Adverse effect of unspecified fibrinolysis-affecting drugs**
+7th **T45.606 Underdosing of unspecified fibrinolysis-affecting drugs**
+ **T45.61 Poisoning by, adverse effect of and underdosing of thrombolytic drugs**
+7th **T45.611 Poisoning by thrombolytic drug, accidental (unintentional)**
Poisoning by thrombolytic drug NOS

+7th **T45.612 Poisoning by thrombolytic drug, intentional self-harm**
+7th **T45.613 Poisoning by thrombolytic drug, assault**
+7th **T45.614 Poisoning by thrombolytic drug, undetermined**
+7th **T45.615 Adverse effect of thrombolytic drugs**
AHA CC: 2Q, 2017, 9-10
+7th **T45.616 Underdosing of thrombolytic drugs**
+ **T45.62 Poisoning by, adverse effect of and underdosing of hemostatic drugs**
+7th **T45.621 Poisoning by hemostatic drug, accidental (unintentional)**
Poisoning by hemostatic drug NOS
+7th **T45.622 Poisoning by hemostatic drug, intentional self-harm**
+7th **T45.623 Poisoning by hemostatic drug, assault**
+7th **T45.624 Poisoning by hemostatic drug, undetermined**
+7th **T45.625 Adverse effect of hemostatic drug**
+7th **T45.626 Underdosing of hemostatic drugs**
+ **T45.69 Poisoning by, adverse effect of and underdosing of other fibrinolysis-affecting drugs**
+7th **T45.691 Poisoning by other fibrinolysis-affecting drugs, accidental (unintentional)**
Poisoning by other fibrinolysis-affecting drug NOS
+7th **T45.692 Poisoning by other fibrinolysis-affecting drugs, intentional self-harm**
+7th **T45.693 Poisoning by other fibrinolysis-affecting drugs, assault**
+7th **T45.694 Poisoning by other fibrinolysis-affecting drugs, undetermined**
+7th **T45.695 Adverse effect of other fibrinolysis-affecting drugs**
+7th **T45.696 Underdosing of other fibrinolysis-affecting drugs**
+ **T45.7 Poisoning by, adverse effect of and underdosing of anticoagulant antagonists, vitamin K and other coagulants**
+ **T45.7X Poisoning by, adverse effect of and underdosing of anticoagulant antagonists, vitamin K and other coagulants**
+7th **T45.7X1 Poisoning by anticoagulant antagonists, vitamin K and other coagulants, accidental (unintentional)**
Poisoning by anticoagulant antagonists, vitamin K and other coagulants NOS
+7th **T45.7X2 Poisoning by anticoagulant antagonists, vitamin K and other coagulants, intentional self-harm**
+7th **T45.7X3 Poisoning by anticoagulant antagonists, vitamin K and other coagulants, assault**
+7th **T45.7X4 Poisoning by anticoagulant antagonists, vitamin K and other coagulants, undetermined**
+7th **T45.7X5 Adverse effect of anticoagulant antagonists, vitamin K and other coagulants**
+7th **T45.7X6 Underdosing of anticoagulant antagonist, vitamin K and other coagulants**
Excludes1: *vitamin K deficiency (E56.1)*
+ **T45.8 Poisoning by, adverse effect of and underdosing of other primarily systemic and hematological agents**
Poisoning by, adverse effect of and underdosing of liver preparations and other antianemic agents
Poisoning by, adverse effect of and underdosing of natural blood and blood products
Poisoning by, adverse effect of and underdosing of plasma substitute
Excludes2: *poisoning by, adverse effect of and underdosing of immunoglobulin (T50.Z1)*
poisoning by, adverse effect of and underdosing of iron (T45.4)
transfusion reactions (T80.-)
+ **T45.8X Poisoning by, adverse effect of and underdosing of other primarily systemic and hematological agents**
+7th **T45.8X1 Poisoning by other primarily systemic and hematological agents, accidental (unintentional)**
Poisoning by other primarily systemic and hematological agents NOS
+7th **T45.8X2 Poisoning by other primarily systemic and hematological agents, intentional self-harm**
+7th **T45.8X3 Poisoning by other primarily systemic and hematological agents, assault**
+7th **T45.8X4 Poisoning by other primarily systemic and hematological agents, undetermined**
+7th **T45.8X5 Adverse effect of other primarily systemic and hematological agents**
AHA CC: 4Q, 2016, 41-42
+7th **T45.8X6 Underdosing of other primarily systemic and hematological agents**
+ **T45.9 Poisoning by, adverse effect of and underdosing of unspecified primarily systemic and hematological agent**
X+7th **T45.91 Poisoning by unspecified primarily systemic and hematological agent, accidental (unintentional)**
Poisoning by primarily systemic and hematological agent NOS
X+7th **T45.92 Poisoning by unspecified primarily systemic and hematological agent, intentional self-harm**
X+7th **T45.93 Poisoning by unspecified primarily systemic and hematological agent, assault**
X+7th **T45.94 Poisoning by unspecified primarily systemic and hematological agent, undetermined**
X+7th **T45.95 Adverse effect of unspecified primarily systemic and hematological agent**
X+7th **T45.96 Underdosing of unspecified primarily systemic and hematological agent**

T46 Poisoning by, adverse effect of and underdosing of agents primarily affecting the cardiovascular system

Excludes1: *poisoning by, adverse effect of and underdosing of metaraminol (T44.4)*

The appropriate 7th character is to be added to each code from category T46
A initial encounter
D subsequent encounter
S sequela

+ **T46.0 Poisoning by, adverse effect of and underdosing of cardiac-stimulant glycosides and drugs of similar action**
+ **T46.0X Poisoning by, adverse effect of and underdosing of cardiac-stimulant glycosides and drugs of similar action**
+7th **T46.0X1 Poisoning by cardiac-stimulant glycosides and drugs of similar action, accidental (unintentional)**
Poisoning by cardiac-stimulant glycosides and drugs of similar action NOS
+7th **T46.0X2 Poisoning by cardiac-stimulant glycosides and drugs of similar action, intentional self-harm**
+7th **T46.0X3 Poisoning by cardiac-stimulant glycosides and drugs of similar action, assault**
+7th **T46.0X4 Poisoning by cardiac-stimulant glycosides and drugs of similar action, undetermined**
+7th **T46.0X5 Adverse effect of cardiac-stimulant glycosides and drugs of similar action**
+7th **T46.0X6 Underdosing of cardiac-stimulant glycosides and drugs of similar action**
+ **T46.1 Poisoning by, adverse effect of and underdosing of calcium-channel blockers**
+ **T46.1X Poisoning by, adverse effect of and underdosing of calcium-channel blockers**
+7th **T46.1X1 Poisoning by calcium-channel blockers, accidental (unintentional)**
Poisoning by calcium-channel blockers NOS
+7th **T46.1X2 Poisoning by calcium-channel blockers, intentional self-harm**
+7th **T46.1X3 Poisoning by calcium-channel blockers, assault**
+7th **T46.1X4 Poisoning by calcium-channel blockers, undetermined**
+7th **T46.1X5 Adverse effect of calcium-channel blockers**
+7th **T46.1X6 Underdosing of calcium-channel blockers**
+ **T46.2 Poisoning by, adverse effect of and underdosing of other antidysrhythmic drugs, not elsewhere classified**
Excludes1: *poisoning by, adverse effect of and underdosing of beta-adrenoreceptor antagonists (T44.7-)*

+ **T46.2X Poisoning by, adverse effect of and underdosing of other antidysrhythmic drugs**
  - +7th **T46.2X1 Poisoning by other antidysrhythmic drugs, accidental (unintentional)**
    Poisoning by other antidysrhythmic drugs NOS
  - +7th **T46.2X2 Poisoning by other antidysrhythmic drugs, intentional self-harm**
  - +7th **T46.2X3 Poisoning by other antidysrhythmic drugs, assault**
  - +7th **T46.2X4 Poisoning by other antidysrhythmic drugs, undetermined**
  - +7th **T46.2X5 Adverse effect of other antidysrhythmic drugs**
  - +7th **T46.2X6 Underdosing of other antidysrhythmic drugs**

+ **T46.3 Poisoning by, adverse effect of and underdosing of coronary vasodilators**
  Poisoning by, adverse effect of and underdosing of dipyridamole
  Excludes1: *poisoning by, adverse effect of and underdosing of calcium-channel blockers (T46.1)*
+ **T46.3X Poisoning by, adverse effect of and underdosing of coronary vasodilators**
  - +7th **T46.3X1 Poisoning by coronary vasodilators, accidental (unintentional)**
    Poisoning by coronary vasodilators NOS
  - +7th **T46.3X2 Poisoning by coronary vasodilators, intentional self-harm**
  - +7th **T46.3X3 Poisoning by coronary vasodilators, assault**
  - +7th **T46.3X4 Poisoning by coronary vasodilators, undetermined**
  - +7th **T46.3X5 Adverse effect of coronary vasodilators**
  - +7th **T46.3X6 Underdosing of coronary vasodilators**

+ **T46.4 Poisoning by, adverse effect of and underdosing of angiotensin-converting-enzyme inhibitors**
+ **T46.4X Poisoning by, adverse effect of and underdosing of angiotensin-converting-enzyme inhibitors**
  - +7th **T46.4X1 Poisoning by angiotensin-converting-enzyme inhibitors, accidental (unintentional)**
    Poisoning by angiotensin-converting-enzyme inhibitors NOS
  - +7th **T46.4X2 Poisoning by angiotensin-converting-enzyme inhibitors, intentional self-harm**
  - +7th **T46.4X3 Poisoning by angiotensin-converting-enzyme inhibitors, assault**
  - +7th **T46.4X4 Poisoning by angiotensin-converting-enzyme inhibitors, undetermined**
  - +7th **T46.4X5 Adverse effect of angiotensin-converting-enzyme inhibitors**
  - +7th **T46.4X6 Underdosing of angiotensin-converting-enzyme inhibitors**

+ **T46.5 Poisoning by, adverse effect of and underdosing of other antihypertensive drugs**
  Excludes2: *poisoning by, adverse effect of and underdosing of beta-adrenoreceptor antagonists (T44.7)*
  poisoning by, adverse effect of and underdosing of calcium-channel blockers (T46.1)
  poisoning by, adverse effect of and underdosing of diuretics (T50.0-T50.2)
+ **T46.5X Poisoning by, adverse effect of and underdosing of other antihypertensive drugs**
  - +7th **T46.5X1 Poisoning by other antihypertensive drugs, accidental (unintentional)**
    Poisoning by other antihypertensive drugs NOS
  - +7th **T46.5X2 Poisoning by other antihypertensive drugs, intentional self-harm**
  - +7th **T46.5X3 Poisoning by other antihypertensive drugs, assault**
  - +7th **T46.5X4 Poisoning by other antihypertensive drugs, undetermined**
  - +7th **T46.5X5 Adverse effect of other antihypertensive drugs**
  - +7th **T46.5X6 Underdosing of other antihypertensive drugs**

+ **T46.6 Poisoning by, adverse effect of and underdosing of antihyperlipidemic and antiarteriosclerotic drugs**
+ **T46.6X Poisoning by, adverse effect of and underdosing of antihyperlipidemic and antiarteriosclerotic drugs**
  - +7th **T46.6X1 Poisoning by antihyperlipidemic and antiarteriosclerotic drugs, accidental (unintentional)**
    Poisoning by antihyperlipidemic and antiarteriosclerotic drugs NOS
  - +7th **T46.6X2 Poisoning by antihyperlipidemic and antiarteriosclerotic drugs, intentional self-harm**
  - +7th **T46.6X3 Poisoning by antihyperlipidemic and antiarteriosclerotic drugs, assault**
  - +7th **T46.6X4 Poisoning by antihyperlipidemic and antiarteriosclerotic drugs, undetermined**
  - +7th **T46.6X5 Adverse effect of antihyperlipidemic and antiarteriosclerotic drugs**
  - +7th **T46.6X6 Underdosing of antihyperlipidemic and antiarteriosclerotic drugs**

+ **T46.7 Poisoning by, adverse effect of and underdosing of peripheral vasodilators**
  Poisoning by, adverse effect of and underdosing of nicotinic acid (derivatives)
  Excludes1: *poisoning by, adverse effect of and underdosing of papaverine (T44.3)*
+ **T46.7X Poisoning by, adverse effect of and underdosing of peripheral vasodilators**
  - +7th **T46.7X1 Poisoning by peripheral vasodilators, accidental (unintentional)**
    Poisoning by peripheral vasodilators NOS
  - +7th **T46.7X2 Poisoning by peripheral vasodilators, intentional self-harm**
  - +7th **T46.7X3 Poisoning by peripheral vasodilators, assault**
  - +7th **T46.7X4 Poisoning by peripheral vasodilators, undetermined**
  - +7th **T46.7X5 Adverse effect of peripheral vasodilators**
  - +7th **T46.7X6 Underdosing of peripheral vasodilators**

+ **T46.8 Poisoning by, adverse effect of and underdosing of antivaricose drugs, including sclerosing agents**
+ **T46.8X Poisoning by, adverse effect of and underdosing of antivaricose drugs, including sclerosing agents**
  - +7th **T46.8X1 Poisoning by antivaricose drugs, including sclerosing agents, accidental (unintentional)**
    Poisoning by antivaricose drugs, including sclerosing agents NOS
  - +7th **T46.8X2 Poisoning by antivaricose drugs, including sclerosing agents, intentional self-harm**
  - +7th **T46.8X3 Poisoning by antivaricose drugs, including sclerosing agents, assault**
  - +7th **T46.8X4 Poisoning by antivaricose drugs, including sclerosing agents, undetermined**
  - +7th **T46.8X5 Adverse effect of antivaricose drugs, including sclerosing agents**
  - +7th **T46.8X6 Underdosing of antivaricose drugs, including sclerosing agents**

+ **T46.9 Poisoning by, adverse effect of and underdosing of other and unspecified agents primarily affecting the cardiovascular system**
+ **T46.90 Poisoning by, adverse effect of and underdosing of unspecified agents primarily affecting the cardiovascular system**
  - +7th **T46.901 Poisoning by unspecified agents primarily affecting the cardiovascular system, accidental (unintentional)**
  - +7th **T46.902 Poisoning by unspecified agents primarily affecting the cardiovascular system, intentional self-harm**
  - +7th **T46.903 Poisoning by unspecified agents primarily affecting the cardiovascular system, assault**
  - +7th **T46.904 Poisoning by unspecified agents primarily affecting the cardiovascular system, undetermined**
  - +7th **T46.905 Adverse effect of unspecified agents primarily affecting the cardiovascular system**
  - +7th **T46.906 Underdosing of unspecified agents primarily affecting the cardiovascular system**

+ **T46.99** **Poisoning by, adverse effect of and underdosing of other agents primarily affecting the cardiovascular system**
  - +7th **T46.991** **Poisoning by other agents primarily affecting the cardiovascular system, accidental (unintentional)**
  - +7th **T46.992** **Poisoning by other agents primarily affecting the cardiovascular system, intentional self-harm**
  - +7th **T46.993** **Poisoning by other agents primarily affecting the cardiovascular system, assault**
  - +7th **T46.994** **Poisoning by other agents primarily affecting the cardiovascular system, undetermined**
  - +7th **T46.995** **Adverse effect of other agents primarily affecting the cardiovascular system**
  - +7th **T46.996** **Underdosing of other agents primarily affecting the cardiovascular system**

T47 **Poisoning by, adverse effect of and underdosing of agents primarily affecting the gastrointestinal system**

The appropriate 7th character is to be added to each code from category T47
A initial encounter
D subsequent encounter
S sequela

+ **T47.0** **Poisoning by, adverse effect of and underdosing of histamine H2-receptor blockers**
  + **T47.0X** **Poisoning by, adverse effect of and underdosing of histamine H2-receptor blockers**
    - +7th **T47.0X1** **Poisoning by histamine H2-receptor blockers, accidental (unintentional)**
      Poisoning by histamine H2-receptor blockers NOS
    - +7th **T47.0X2** **Poisoning by histamine H2-receptor blockers, intentional self-harm**
    - +7th **T47.0X3** **Poisoning by histamine H2-receptor blockers, assault**
    - +7th **T47.0X4** **Poisoning by histamine H2-receptor blockers, undetermined**
    - +7th **T47.0X5** **Adverse effect of histamine H2-receptor blockers**
    - +7th **T47.0X6** **Underdosing of histamine H2-receptor blockers**
+ **T47.1** **Poisoning by, adverse effect of and underdosing of other antacids and anti-gastric-secretion drugs**
  + **T47.1X** **Poisoning by, adverse effect of and underdosing of other antacids and anti-gastric-secretion drugs**
    - +7th **T47.1X1** **Poisoning by other antacids and anti-gastric-secretion drugs, accidental (unintentional)**
      Poisoning by other antacids and anti-gastric-secretion drugs NOS
    - +7th **T47.1X2** **Poisoning by other antacids and anti-gastric-secretion drugs, intentional self-harm**
    - +7th **T47.1X3** **Poisoning by other antacids and anti-gastric-secretion drugs, assault**
    - +7th **T47.1X4** **Poisoning by other antacids and anti-gastric-secretion drugs, undetermined**
    - +7th **T47.1X5** **Adverse effect of other antacids and anti-gastric-secretion drugs**
    - +7th **T47.1X6** **Underdosing of other antacids and anti-gastric-secretion drugs**
+ **T47.2** **Poisoning by, adverse effect of and underdosing of stimulant laxatives**
  + **T47.2X** **Poisoning by, adverse effect of and underdosing of stimulant laxatives**
    - +7th **T47.2X1** **Poisoning by stimulant laxatives, accidental (unintentional)**
      Poisoning by stimulant laxatives NOS
    - +7th **T47.2X2** **Poisoning by stimulant laxatives, intentional self-harm**
    - +7th **T47.2X3** **Poisoning by stimulant laxatives, assault**
    - +7th **T47.2X4** **Poisoning by stimulant laxatives, undetermined**
    - +7th **T47.2X5** **Adverse effect of stimulant laxatives**
    - +7th **T47.2X6** **Underdosing of stimulant laxatives**
+ **T47.3** **Poisoning by, adverse effect of and underdosing of saline and osmotic laxatives**
  + **T47.3X** **Poisoning by and adverse effect of saline and osmoti laxatives**
    - +7th **T47.3X1** **Poisoning by saline and osmotic laxatives, accidental (unintentional)**
      Poisoning by saline and osmotic laxatives NOS
    - +7th **T47.3X2** **Poisoning by saline and osmotic laxatives, intentional self-harm**
    - +7th **T47.3X3** **Poisoning by saline and osmotic laxatives, assault**
    - +7th **T47.3X4** **Poisoning by saline and osmotic laxatives, undetermined**
    - +7th **T47.3X5** **Adverse effect of saline and osmotic laxatives**
    - +7th **T47.3X6** **Underdosing of saline and osmotic laxatives**
+ **T47.4** **Poisoning by, adverse effect of and underdosing of other laxatives**
  + **T47.4X** **Poisoning by, adverse effect of and underdosing of other laxatives**
    - +7th **T47.4X1** **Poisoning by other laxatives, accidental (unintentional)**
      Poisoning by other laxatives NOS
    - +7th **T47.4X2** **Poisoning by other laxatives, intentional self-harm**
    - +7th **T47.4X3** **Poisoning by other laxatives, assault**
    - +7th **T47.4X4** **Poisoning by other laxatives, undetermine**
    - +7th **T47.4X5** **Adverse effect of other l axatives**
    - +7th **T47.4X6** **Underdosing of other laxatives**
+ **T47.5** **Poisoning by, adverse effect of and underdosing of digestants**
  + **T47.5X** **Poisoning by, adverse effect of and underdosing of digestants**
    - +7th **T47.5X1** **Poisoning by digestants, accidental (unintentional)**
      Poisoning by digestants NOS
    - +7th **T47.5X2** **Poisoning by digestants, intentional self-harm**
    - +7th **T47.5X3** **Poisoning by digestants, assault**
    - +7th **T47.5X4** **Poisoning by digestants, undetermined**
    - +7th **T47.5X5** **Adverse effect of digestants**
    - +7th **T47.5X6** **Underdosing of digestants**
+ **T47.6** **Poisoning by, adverse effect of and underdosing of antidiarrheal drugs**
  Excludes2: *poisoning by, adverse effect of and underdosing of systemic antibiotics and other anti-infectives (T36-T37)*
  + **T47.6X** **Poisoning by, adverse effect of and underdosing of antidiarrheal drugs**
    - +7th **T47.6X1** **Poisoning by antidiarrheal drugs, accidental (unintentional)**
      Poisoning by antidiarrheal drugs NOS
    - +7th **T47.6X2** **Poisoning by antidiarrheal drugs, intentional self-harm**
    - +7th **T47.6X3** **Poisoning by antidiarrheal drugs, assault**
    - +7th **T47.6X4** **Poisoning by antidiarrheal drugs, undetermined**
    - +7th **T47.6X5** **Adverse effect of antidiarrheal drugs**
    - +7th **T47.6X6** **Underdosing of antidiarrheal drugs**
+ **T47.7** **Poisoning by, adverse effect of and underdosing of emetics**
  + **T47.7X** **Poisoning by, adverse effect of and underdosing of emetics**
    - +7th **T47.7X1** **Poisoning by emetics, accidental (unintentional)**
      Poisoning by emetics NOS
    - +7th **T47.7X2** **Poisoning by emetics, intentional self-harn**
    - +7th **T47.7X3** **Poisoning by emetics, assault**
    - +7th **T47.7X4** **Poisoning by emetics, undetermined**
    - +7th **T47.7X5** **Adverse effect of emetics**
    - +7th **T47.7X6** **Underdosing of emetics**
+ **T47.8** **Poisoning by, adverse effect of and underdosing of other agen primarily affecting gastrointestinal system**
  + **T47.8X** **Poisoning by, adverse effect of and underdosing of other agents primarily affecting gastrointestinal system**

+7th T47.8X1 **Poisoning by other agents primarily affecting gastrointestinal system, accidental (unintentional)**
Poisoning by other agents primarily affecting gastrointestinal system NOS
+7th T47.8X2 **Poisoning by other agents primarily affecting gastrointestinal system, intentional self-harm**
+7th T47.8X3 **Poisoning by other agents primarily affecting gastrointestinal system, assault**
+7th T47.8X4 **Poisoning by other agents primarily affecting gastrointestinal system, undetermined**
+7th T47.8X5 **Adverse effect of other agents primarily affecting gastrointestinal system**
+7th T47.8X6 **Underdosing of other agents primarily affecting gastrointestinal system**

+ T47.9 **Poisoning by, adverse effect of and underdosing of unspecified agents primarily affecting the gastrointestinal system**
X+7th T47.91 **Poisoning by unspecified agents primarily affecting the gastrointestinal system, accidental (unintentional)**
Poisoning by agents primarily affecting the gastrointestinal system NOS
X+7th T47.92 **Poisoning by unspecified agents primarily affecting the gastrointestinal system, intentional self-harm**
X+7th T47.93 **Poisoning by unspecified agents primarily affecting the gastrointestinal system, assault**
X+7th T47.94 **Poisoning by unspecified agents primarily affecting the gastrointestinal system, undetermined**
X+7th T47.95 **Adverse effect of unspecified agents primarily affecting the gastrointestinal system**
X+7th T47.96 **Underdosing of unspecified agents primarily affecting the gastrointestinal system**

T48 Poisoning by, adverse effect of and underdosing of agents primarily acting on smooth and skeletal muscles and the respiratory system

The appropriate 7th character is to be added to each code from category T48
A initial encounter
D subsequent encounter
S sequela

+ T48.0 **Poisoning by, adverse effect of and underdosing of oxytocic drugs**
Excludes1: *poisoning by, adverse effect of and underdosing of estrogens, progestogens and antagonists (T38.4-T38.6)*
+ T48.0X **Poisoning by, adverse effect of and underdosing of oxytocic drugs**
+7th T48.0X1 **Poisoning by oxytocic drugs, accidental (unintentional)**
Poisoning by oxytocic drugs NOS
+7th T48.0X2 **Poisoning by oxytocic drugs, intentional self-harm**
+7th T48.0X3 **Poisoning by oxytocic drugs, assault**
+7th T48.0X4 **Poisoning by oxytocic drugs, undetermined**
+7th T48.0X5 **Adverse effect of oxytocic drugs**
+7th T48.0X6 **Underdosing of oxytocic drugs**

+ T48.1 **Poisoning by, adverse effect of and underdosing of skeletal muscle relaxants [neuromuscular blocking agents]**
+ T48.1X **Poisoning by, adverse effect of and underdosing of skeletal muscle relaxants [neuromuscular blocking agents]**
+7th T48.1X1 **Poisoning by skeletal muscle relaxants [neuromuscular blocking agents], accidental (unintentional)**
Poisoning by skeletal muscle relaxants [neuromuscular blocking agents] NOS
+7th T48.1X2 **Poisoning by skeletal muscle relaxants [neuromuscular blocking agents], intentional self-harm**
+7th T48.1X3 **Poisoning by skeletal muscle relaxants [neuromuscular blocking agents], assault**
+7th T48.1X4 **Poisoning by skeletal muscle relaxants [neuromuscular blocking agents], undetermined**
+7th T48.1X5 **Adverse effect of skeletal muscle relaxants [neuromuscular blocking agents]**
+7th T48.1X6 **Underdosing of skeletal muscle relaxants [neuromuscular blocking agents]**

+ T48.2 **Poisoning by, adverse effect of and underdosing of other and unspecified drugs acting on muscles**
+ T48.20 **Poisoning by, adverse effect of and underdosing of unspecified drugs acting on muscles**
+7th T48.201 **Poisoning by unspecified drugs acting on muscles, accidental (unintentional)**
Poisoning by unspecified drugs acting on muscles NOS
+7th T48.202 **Poisoning by unspecified drugs acting on muscles, intentional self-harm**
+7th T48.203 **Poisoning by unspecified drugs acting on muscles, assault**
+7th T48.204 **Poisoning by unspecified drugs acting on muscles, undetermined**
+7th T48.205 **Adverse effect of unspecified drugs acting on muscles**
+7th T48.206 **Underdosing of unspecified drugs acting on muscles**
+ T48.29 **Poisoning by, adverse effect of and underdosing of other drugs acting on muscles**
+7th T48.291 **Poisoning by other drugs acting on muscles, accidental (unintentional)**
Poisoning by other drugs acting on muscles NOS
+7th T48.292 **Poisoning by other drugs acting on muscles, intentional self-harm**
+7th T48.293 **Poisoning by other drugs acting on muscles, assault**
+7th T48.294 **Poisoning by other drugs acting on muscles, undetermined**
+7th T48.295 **Adverse effect of other drugs acting on muscles**
+7th T48.296 **Underdosing of other drugs acting on muscles**

+ T48.3 **Poisoning by, adverse effect of and underdosing of antitussives**
+ T48.3X **Poisoning by, adverse effect of and underdosing of antitussives**
+7th T48.3X1 **Poisoning by antitussives, accidental (unintentional)**
Poisoning by antitussives NOS
+7th T48.3X2 **Poisoning by antitussives, intentional self-harm**
+7th T48.3X3 **Poisoning by antitussives, assault**
+7th T48.3X4 **Poisoning by antitussives, undetermined**
+7th T48.3X5 **Adverse effect of antitussives**
+7th T48.3X6 **Underdosing of antitussives**

+ T48.4 **Poisoning by, adverse effect of and underdosing of expectorants**
+ T48.4X **Poisoning by, adverse effect of and underdosing of expectorants**
+7th T48.4X1 **Poisoning by expectorants, accidental (unintentional)**
Poisoning by expectorants NOS
+7th T48.4X2 **Poisoning by expectorants, intentional self-harm**
+7th T48.4X3 **Poisoning by expectorants, assault**
+7th T48.4X4 **Poisoning by expectorants, undetermined**
+7th T48.4X5 **Adverse effect of expectorants**
+7th T48.4X6 **Underdosing of expectorants**

+ T48.5 **Poisoning by, adverse effect of and underdosing of other anti-common-cold drugs**
Poisoning by, adverse effect of and underdosing of decongestants
Excludes2: *poisoning by, adverse effect of and underdosing of antipyretics, NEC (T39.9-)*
poisoning by, adverse effect of and underdosing of non-steroidal antiinflammatory drugs (T39.3-)
poisoning by, adverse effect of and underdosing of salicylates (T39.0-)
+ T48.5X **Poisoning by, adverse effect of and underdosing of other anti-common-cold drugs**
+7th T48.5X1 **Poisoning by other anti-common-cold drugs, accidental (unintentional)**
Poisoning by other anti-common-cold drugs NOS
+7th T48.5X2 **Poisoning by other anti-common-cold drugs, intentional self-harm**

+7th **T48.5X3 Poisoning by other anti-common-cold drugs, assault**
+7th **T48.5X4 Poisoning by other anti-common-cold drugs, undetermined**
+7th **T48.5X5 Adverse effect of other anti-common-cold drugs**
+7th **T48.5X6 Underdosing of other anti-common-cold drugs**

+ **T48.6 Poisoning by, adverse effect of and underdosing of antiasthmatics, not elsewhere classified**
Poisoning by, adverse effect of and underdosing of beta-adrenoreceptor agonists used in asthma therapy
Excludes1: *poisoning by, adverse effect of and underdosing of beta-adrenoreceptor agonists not used in asthma therapy (T44.5)*
poisoning by, adverse effect of and underdosing of anterior pituitary [adenohypophyseal] hormones (T38.8)

+ **T48.6X Poisoning by, adverse effect of and underdosing of antiasthmatics**
+7th **T48.6X1 Poisoning by antiasthmatics, accidental (unintentional)**
Poisoning by antiasthmatics NOS
+7th **T48.6X2 Poisoning by antiasthmatics, intentional self-harm**
+7th **T48.6X3 Poisoning by antiasthmatics, assault**
+7th **T48.6X4 Poisoning by antiasthmatics, undetermined**
+7th **T48.6X5 Adverse effect of antiasthmatics**
+7th **T48.6X6 Underdosing of antiasthmatics**

+ **T48.9 Poisoning by, adverse effect of and underdosing of other and unspecified agents primarily acting on the respiratory system**
+ **T48.90 Poisoning by, adverse effect of and underdosing of unspecified agents primarily acting on the respiratory system**
+7th **T48.901 Poisoning by unspecified agents primarily acting on the respiratory system, accidental (unintentional)**
+7th **T48.902 Poisoning by unspecified agents primarily acting on the respiratory system, intentional self-harm**
+7th **T48.903 Poisoning by unspecified agents primarily acting on the respiratory system, assault**
+7th **T48.904 Poisoning by unspecified agents primarily acting on the respiratory system, undetermined**
+7th **T48.905 Adverse effect of unspecified agents primarily acting on the respiratory system**
+7th **T48.906 Underdosing of unspecified agents primarily acting on the respiratory system**
+ **T48.99 Poisoning by, adverse effect of and underdosing of other agents primarily acting on the respiratory system**
+7th **T48.991 Poisoning by other agents primarily acting on the respiratory system, accidental (unintentional)**
+7th **T48.992 Poisoning by other agents primarily acting on the respiratory system, intentional self-harm**
+7th **T48.993 Poisoning by other agents primarily acting on the respiratory system, assault**
+7th **T48.994 Poisoning by other agents primarily acting on the respiratory system, undetermined**
+7th **T48.995 Adverse effect of other agents primarily acting on the respiratory system**
+7th **T48.996 Underdosing of other agents primarily acting on the respiratory system**

T49 Poisoning by, adverse effect of and underdosing of topical agents primarily affecting skin and mucous membrane and by ophthalmological, otorhinorlaryngological and dental drugs
Includes: poisoning by, adverse effect of and underdosing of glucocorticoids, topically used

The appropriate 7th character is to be added to each code from category T49
A initial encounter
D subsequent encounter
S sequela

+ **T49.0 Poisoning by, adverse effect of and underdosing of local antifungal, anti-infective and anti-inflammatory drugs**
+ **T49.0X Poisoning by, adverse effect of and underdosing of local antifungal, anti-infective and anti-inflammatory drugs**
+7th **T49.0X1 Poisoning by local antifungal, anti-infective and anti-inflammatory drugs, accidental (unintentional)**
Poisoning by local antifungal, anti-infective and anti-inflammatory drugs NOS
+7th **T49.0X2 Poisoning by local antifungal, anti-infective and anti-inflammatory drugs, intentional self-harm**
+7th **T49.0X3 Poisoning by local antifungal, anti-infective and anti-inflammatory drugs, assault**
+7th **T49.0X4 Poisoning by local antifungal, anti-infective and anti-inflammatory drugs, undetermined**
+7th **T49.0X5 Adverse effect of local antifungal, anti-infective and anti-inflammatory drugs**
+7th **T49.0X6 Underdosing of local antifungal, anti-infective and anti-inflammatory drugs**

+ **T49.1 Poisoning by, adverse effect of and underdosing of antipruritics**
+ **T49.1X Poisoning by, adverse effect of and underdosing of antipruritics**
+7th **T49.1X1 Poisoning by antipruritics, accidental (unintentional)**
Poisoning by antipruritics NOS
+7th **T49.1X2 Poisoning by antipruritics, intentional self-harm**
+7th **T49.1X3 Poisoning by antipruritics, assault**
+7th **T49.1X4 Poisoning by antipruritics, undetermined**
+7th **T49.1X5 Adverse effect of antipruritics**
+7th **T49.1X6 Underdosing of antipruritics**

+ **T49.2 Poisoning by, adverse effect of and underdosing of local astringents and local detergents**
+ **T49.2X Poisoning by, adverse effect of and underdosing of local astringents and local detergents**
+7th **T49.2X1 Poisoning by local astringents and local detergents, accidental (unintentional)**
Poisoning by local astringents and local detergents NOS
+7th **T49.2X2 Poisoning by local astringents and local detergents, intentional self-harm**
+7th **T49.2X3 Poisoning by local astringents and local detergents, assault**
+7th **T49.2X4 Poisoning by local astringents and local detergents, undetermined**
+7th **T49.2X5 Adverse effect of local astringents and local detergents**
+7th **T49.2X6 Underdosing of local astringents and local detergents**

+ **T49.3 Poisoning by, adverse effect of and underdosing of emollients, demulcents and protectants**
+ **T49.3X Poisoning by, adverse effect of and underdosing of emollients, demulcents and protectants**
+7th **T49.3X1 Poisoning by emollients, demulcents and protectants, accidental (unintentional)**
Poisoning by emollients, demulcents and protectants NOS
+7th **T49.3X2 Poisoning by emollients, demulcents and protectants, intentional self-harm**
+7th **T49.3X3 Poisoning by emollients, demulcents and protectants, assault**
+7th **T49.3X4 Poisoning by emollients, demulcents and protectants, undetermined**
+7th **T49.3X5 Adverse effect of emollients, demulcents and protectants**
+7th **T49.3X6 Underdosing of emollients, demulcents and protectants**

+ **T49.4 Poisoning by, adverse effect of and underdosing of keratolytics, keratoplastics, and other hair treatment drugs and preparations**
+ **T49.4X Poisoning by, adverse effect of and underdosing of keratolytics, keratoplastics, and other hair treatment drugs and preparations**

+7th **T49.4X1 Poisoning by keratolytics, keratoplastics, and other hair treatment drugs and preparations, accidental (unintentional)**
Poisoning by keratolytics, keratoplastics, and other hair treatment drugs and preparations NOS
+7th **T49.4X2 Poisoning by keratolytics, keratoplastics, and other hair treatment drugs and preparations, intentional self-harm**
+7th **T49.4X3 Poisoning by keratolytics, keratoplastics, and other hair treatment drugs and preparations, assault**
+7th **T49.4X4 Poisoning by keratolytics, keratoplastics, and other hair treatment drugs and preparations, undetermined**
+7th **T49.4X5 Adverse effect of keratolytics, keratoplastics, and other hair treatment drugs and preparations**
+7th **T49.4X6 Underdosing of keratolytics, keratoplastics, and other hair treatment drugs and preparations**

\+ **T49.5 Poisoning by, adverse effect of and underdosing of ophthalmological drugs and preparations**
\+ **T49.5X Poisoning by, adverse effect of and underdosing of ophthalmological drugs and preparations**
+7th **T49.5X1 Poisoning by ophthalmological drugs and preparations, accidental (unintentional)**
Poisoning by ophthalmological drugs and preparations NOS
+7th **T49.5X2 Poisoning by ophthalmological drugs and preparations, intentional self-harm**
+7th **T49.5X3 Poisoning by ophthalmological drugs and preparations, assault**
+7th **T49.5X4 Poisoning by ophthalmological drugs and preparations, undetermined**
+7th **T49.5X5 Adverse effect of ophthalmological drugs and preparations**
+7th **T49.5X6 Underdosing of ophthalmological drugs and preparations**

\+ **T49.6 Poisoning by, adverse effect of and underdosing of otorhinolaryngological drugs and preparations**
\+ **T49.6X Poisoning by, adverse effect of and underdosing of otorhinolaryngological drugs and preparations**
+7th **T49.6X1 Poisoning by otorhinolaryngological drugs and preparations, accidental (unintentional)**
Poisoning by otorhinolaryngological drugs and preparations NOS
+7th **T49.6X2 Poisoning by otorhinolaryngological drugs and preparations, intentional self-harm**
+7th **T49.6X3 Poisoning by otorhinolaryngological drugs and preparations, assault**
+7th **T49.6X4 Poisoning by otorhinolaryngological drugs and preparations, undetermined**
+7th **T49.6X5 Adverse effect of otorhinolaryngological drugs and preparations**
+7th **T49.6X6 Underdosing of otorhinolaryngological drugs and preparations**

\+ **T49.7 Poisoning by, adverse effect of and underdosing of dental drugs, topically applied**
\+ **T49.7X Poisoning by, adverse effect of and underdosing of dental drugs, topically applied**
+7th **T49.7X1 Poisoning by dental drugs, topically applied, accidental (unintentional)**
Poisoning by dental drugs, topically applied NOS
+7th **T49.7X2 Poisoning by dental drugs, topically applied, intentional self-harm**
+7th **T49.7X3 Poisoning by dental drugs, topically applied, assault**
+7th **T49.7X4 Poisoning by dental drugs, topically applied, undetermined**
+7th **T49.7X5 Adverse effect of dental drugs, topically applied**
+7th **T49.7X6 Underdosing of dental drugs, topically applied**

\+ **T49.8 Poisoning by, adverse effect of and underdosing of other topical agents**
Poisoning by, adverse effect of and underdosing of spermicides
\+ **T49.8X Poisoning by, adverse effect of and underdosing of other topical agents**
+7th **T49.8X1 Poisoning by other topical agents, accidental (unintentional)**
Poisoning by other topical agents NOS
+7th **T49.8X2 Poisoning by other topical agents, intentional self-harm**
+7th **T49.8X3 Poisoning by other topical agents, assault**
+7th **T49.8X4 Poisoning by other topical agents, undetermined**
+7th **T49.8X5 Adverse effect of other topical agents**
+7th **T49.8X6 Underdosing of other topical agents**

\+ **T49.9 Poisoning by, adverse effect of and underdosing of unspecified topical agent**
X+7th **T49.91 Poisoning by unspecified topical agent, accidental (unintentional)**
X+7th **T49.92 Poisoning by unspecified topical agent, intentional self-harm**
X+7th **T49.93 Poisoning by unspecified topical agent, assault**
X+7th **T49.94 Poisoning by unspecified topical agent, undetermined**
X+7th **T49.95 Adverse effect of unspecified topical agent**
X+7th **T49.96 Underdosing of unspecified topical agent**

T50 Poisoning by, adverse effect of and underdosing of diuretics and other and unspecified drugs, medicaments and biological substances

The appropriate 7th character is to be added to each code from category T50
A initial encounter
D subsequent encounter
S sequela

\+ **T50.0 Poisoning by, adverse effect of and underdosing of mineralocorticoids and their antagonists**
\+ **T50.0X Poisoning by, adverse effect of and underdosing of mineralocorticoids and their antagonists**
+7th **T50.0X1 Poisoning by mineralocorticoids and their antagonists, accidental (unintentional)**
Poisoning by mineralocorticoids and their antagonists NOS
+7th **T50.0X2 Poisoning by mineralocorticoids and their antagonists, intentional self-harm**
+7th **T50.0X3 Poisoning by mineralocorticoids and their antagonists, assault**
+7th **T50.0X4 Poisoning by mineralocorticoids and their antagonists, undetermined**
+7th **T50.0X5 Adverse effect of mineralocorticoids and their antagonists**
+7th **T50.0X6 Underdosing of mineralocorticoids and their antagonists**

\+ **T50.1 Poisoning by, adverse effect of and underdosing of loop [high-ceiling] diuretics**
\+ **T50.1X Poisoning by, adverse effect of and underdosing of loop [high-ceiling] diuretics**
+7th **T50.1X1 Poisoning by loop [high-ceiling] diuretics, accidental (unintentional)**
Poisoning by loop [high-ceiling] diuretics NOS
+7th **T50.1X2 Poisoning by loop [high-ceiling] diuretics, intentional self-harm**
+7th **T50.1X3 Poisoning by loop [high-ceiling] diuretics, assault**
+7th **T50.1X4 Poisoning by loop [high-ceiling] diuretics, undetermined**
+7th **T50.1X5 Adverse effect of loop [high-ceiling] diuretics**
+7th **T50.1X6 Underdosing of loop [high-ceiling] diuretics**

\+ **T50.2 Poisoning by, adverse effect of and underdosing of carbonic-anhydrase inhibitors, benzothiadiazides and other diuretics**
Poisoning by, adverse effect of and underdosing of acetazolamide
\+ **T50.2X Poisoning by, adverse effect of and underdosing of carbonic-anhydrase inhibitors, benzothiadiazides and other diuretics**
+7th **T50.2X1 Poisoning by carbonic-anhydrase inhibitors, benzothiadiazides and other diuretics, accidental (unintentional)**
Poisoning by carbonic-anhydrase inhibitors, benzothiadiazides and other diuretics NOS

+7th **T50.2X2** **Poisoning by carbonic-anhydrase inhibitors, benzothiadiazides and other diuretics, intentional self-harm**
+7th **T50.2X3** **Poisoning by carbonic-anhydrase inhibitors, benzothiadiazides and other diuretics, assault**
+7th **T50.2X4** **Poisoning by carbonic-anhydrase inhibitors, benzothiadiazides and other diuretics, undetermined**
+7th **T50.2X5** **Adverse effect of carbonic-anhydrase inhibitors, benzothiadiazides and other diuretics**
+7th **T50.2X6** **Underdosing of carbonic-anhydrase inhibitors, benzothiadiazides and other diuretics**

+ **T50.3** **Poisoning by, adverse effect of and underdosing of electrolytic, caloric and water-balance agents**
Poisoning by, adverse effect of and underdosing of oral rehydration salts
+ **T50.3X** **Poisoning by, adverse effect of and underdosing of electrolytic, caloric and water-balance agents**
+7th **T50.3X1** **Poisoning by electrolytic, caloric and water-balance agents, accidental (unintentional)**
Poisoning by electrolytic, caloric and water-balance agents NOS
+7th **T50.3X2** **Poisoning by electrolytic, caloric and water-balance agents, intentional self-harm**
+7th **T50.3X3** **Poisoning by electrolytic, caloric and water-balance agents, assault**
+7th **T50.3X4** **Poisoning by electrolytic, caloric and water-balance agents, undetermined**
+7th **T50.3X5** **Adverse effect of electrolytic, caloric and water-balance agents**
+7th **T50.3X6** **Underdosing of electrolytic, caloric and water-balance agents**

+ **T50.4** **Poisoning by, adverse effect of and underdosing of drugs affecting uric acid metabolism**
+ **T50.4X** **Poisoning by, adverse effect of and underdosing of drugs affecting uric acid metabolism**
+7th **T50.4X1** **Poisoning by drugs affecting uric acid metabolism, accidental (unintentional)**
Poisoning by drugs affecting uric acid metabolism NOS
+7th **T50.4X2** **Poisoning by drugs affecting uric acid metabolism, intentional self-harm**
+7th **T50.4X3** **Poisoning by drugs affecting uric acid metabolism, assault**
+7th **T50.4X4** **Poisoning by drugs affecting uric acid metabolism, undetermined**
+7th **T50.4X5** **Adverse effect of drugs affecting uric acid metabolism**
+7th **T50.4X6** **Underdosing of drugs affecting uric acid metabolism**

+ **T50.5** **Poisoning by, adverse effect of and underdosing of appetite depressants**
+ **T50.5X** **Poisoning by, adverse effect of and underdosing of appetite depressants**
+7th **T50.5X1** **Poisoning by appetite depressants, accidental (unintentional)**
Poisoning by appetite depressants NOS
+7th **T50.5X2** **Poisoning by appetite depressants, intentional self-harm**
+7th **T50.5X3** **Poisoning by appetite depressants, assault**
+7th **T50.5X4** **Poisoning by appetite depressants, undetermined**
+7th **T50.5X5** **Adverse effect of appetite depressants**
+7th **T50.5X6** **Underdosing of appetite depressants**

+ **T50.6** **Poisoning by, adverse effect of and underdosing of antidotes and chelating agents**
Poisoning by, adverse effect of and underdosing of alcohol deterrents
+ **T50.6X** **Poisoning by, adverse effect of and underdosing of antidotes and chelating agents**
+7th **T50.6X1** **Poisoning by antidotes and chelatingagents, accidental (unintentional)**
Poisoning by antidotes and chelating agents NOS
+7th **T50.6X2** **Poisoning by antidotes and chelating agents, intentional self-harm**
+7th **T50.6X3** **Poisoning by antidotes and chelating agents, assault**
+7th **T50.6X4** **Poisoning by antidotes and chelating agents, undetermined**
+7th **T50.6X5** **Adverse effect of antidotes and chelating agents**
+7th **T50.6X6** **Underdosing of antidotes and chelating agents**

+ **T50.7** **Poisoning by, adverse effect of and underdosing of analeptics and opioid receptor antagonists**
+ **T50.7X** **Poisoning by, adverse effect of and underdosing of analeptics and opioid receptor antagonists**
+7th **T50.7X1** **Poisoning by analeptics and opioid receptor antagonists, accidental (unintentional)**
Poisoning by analeptics and opioid receptor antagonists NOS
+7th **T50.7X2** **Poisoning by analeptics and opioid receptor antagonists, intentional self-harm**
+7th **T50.7X3** **Poisoning by analeptics and opioid receptor antagonists, assault**
+7th **T50.7X4** **Poisoning by analeptics and opioid receptor antagonists, undetermined**
+7th **T50.7X5** **Adverse effect of analeptics and opioid receptor antagonists**
+7th **T50.7X6** **Underdosing of analeptics and opioid receptor antagonists**

+ **T50.8** **Poisoning by, adverse effect of and underdosing of diagnostic agents**
+ **T50.8X** **Poisoning by, adverse effect of and underdosing of diagnostic agents**
+7th **T50.8X1** **Poisoning by diagnostic agents, accidental (unintentional)**
Poisoning by diagnostic agents NOS
+7th **T50.8X2** **Poisoning by diagnostic agents, intentional self-harm**
+7th **T50.8X3** **Poisoning by diagnostic agents, assault**
+7th **T50.8X4** **Poisoning by diagnostic agents, undetermined**
+7th **T50.8X5** **Adverse effect of diagnostic agents**
+7th **T50.8X6** **Underdosing of diagnostic agents**

+ **T50.A** **Poisoning by, adverse effect of and underdosing of bacterial vaccines**
+ **T50.A1** **Poisoning by, adverse effect of and underdosing of pertussis vaccine, including combinations with a pertussis component**
+7th **T50.A11** **Poisoning by pertussis vaccine, including combinations with a pertussis component, accidental (unintentional)**
+7th **T50.A12** **Poisoning by pertussis vaccine, including combinations with a pertussis component, intentional self-harm**
+7th **T50.A13** **Poisoning by pertussis vaccine, including combinations with a pertussis component, assault**
+7th **T50.A14** **Poisoning by pertussis vaccine, including combinations with a pertussis component, undetermined**
+7th **T50.A15** **Adverse effect of pertussis vaccine, including combinations with a pertussis component**
+7th **T50.A16** **Underdosing of pertussis vaccine, including combinations with a pertussis component**
+ **T50.A2** **Poisoning by, adverse effect of and underdosing of mixed bacterial vaccines without a pertussis component**
+7th **T50.A21** **Poisoning by mixed bacterial vaccines without a pertussis component, accidental (unintentional)**
+7th **T50.A22** **Poisoning by mixed bacterial vaccines without a pertussis component, intentional self-harm**
+7th **T50.A23** **Poisoning by mixed bacterial vaccines without a pertussis component, assault**
+7th **T50.A24** **Poisoning by mixed bacterial vaccines without a pertussis component, undetermined**

+7th **T50.A25** Adverse effect of mixed bacterial vaccines without a pertussis component
+7th **T50.A26** Underdosing of mixed bacterial vaccines without a pertussis component
+ **T50.A9** Poisoning by, adverse effect of and underdosing of other bacterial vaccines
+7th **T50.A91** Poisoning by other bacterial vaccines, accidental (unintentional)
+7th **T50.A92** Poisoning by other bacterial vaccines, intentional self-harm
+7th **T50.A93** Poisoning by other bacterial vaccines, assault
+7th **T50.A94** Poisoning by other bacterial vaccines, undetermined
+7th **T50.A95** Adverse effect of other bacterial vaccines
+7th **T50.A96** Underdosing of other bacterial vaccines
+ **T50.B** Poisoning by, adverse effect of and underdosing of viral vaccines
+ **T50.B1** Poisoning by, adverse effect of and underdosing of smallpox vaccines
+7th **T50.B11** Poisoning by smallpox vaccines, accidental (unintentional)
+7th **T50.B12** Poisoning by smallpox vaccines, intentional self-harm
+7th **T50.B13** Poisoning by smallpox vaccines, assault
+7th **T50.B14** Poisoning by smallpox vaccines, undetermined
+7th **T50.B15** Adverse effect of smallpox vaccines
+7th **T50.B16** Underdosing of smallpox vaccines
+ **T50.B9** Poisoning by, adverse effect of and underdosing of other viral vaccines
+7th **T50.B91** Poisoning by other viral vaccines, accidental (unintentional)
+7th **T50.B92** Poisoning by other viral vaccines, intentional self-harm
+7th **T50.B93** Poisoning by other viral vaccines, assault
+7th **T50.B94** Poisoning by other viral vaccines, undetermined
+7th **T50.B95** Adverse effect of other viral vaccines
+7th **T50.B96** Underdosing of other viral vaccines
+ **T50.Z** Poisoning by, adverse effect of and underdosing of other vaccines and biological substances
+ **T50.Z1** Poisoning by, adverse effect of and underdosing of immunoglobulin
+7th **T50.Z11** Poisoning by immunoglobulin, accidental (unintentional)
+7th **T50.Z12** Poisoning by immunoglobulin, intentional self-harm
+7th **T50.Z13** Poisoning by immunoglobulin, assault
+7th **T50.Z14** Poisoning by immunoglobulin, undetermined
+7th **T50.Z15** Adverse effect of immunoglobulin
+7th **T50.Z16** Underdosing of immunoglobulin
+ **T50.Z9** Poisoning by, adverse effect of and underdosing of other vaccines and biological substances
+7th **T50.Z91** Poisoning by other vaccines and biological substances, accidental (unintentional)
+7th **T50.Z92** Poisoning by other vaccines and biological substances, intentional self-harm
+7th **T50.Z93** Poisoning by other vaccines and biological substances, assault
+7th **T50.Z94** Poisoning by other vaccines and biological substances, undetermined
+7th **T50.Z95** Adverse effect of other vaccines and biological substances
+7th **T50.Z96** Underdosing of other vaccines and biological substances
+ **T50.9** Poisoning by, adverse effect of and underdosing of other and unspecified drugs, medicaments and biological substances
+ **T50.90** Poisoning by, adverse effect of and underdosing of unspecified drugs, medicaments and biological substances
+7th **T50.901** Poisoning by unspecified drugs, medicaments and biological substances, accidental (unintentional)
AHA CC: 1Q, 2015, 3-21
+7th **T50.902** Poisoning by unspecified drugs, medicaments and biological substances, intentional self-harm
+7th **T50.903** Poisoning by unspecified drugs, medicaments and biological substances, assault
+7th **T50.904** Poisoning by unspecified drugs, medicaments and biological substances, undetermined
+7th **T50.905** Adverse effect of unspecified drugs, medicaments and biological substances
+7th **T50.906** Underdosing of unspecified drugs, medicaments and biological substances
+ **T50.99** Poisoning by, adverse effect of and underdosing of other drugs, medicaments and biological substances
+7th **T50.991** Poisoning by other drugs, medicaments and biological substances, accidental (unintentional)
+7th **T50.992** Poisoning by other drugs, medicaments and biological substances, intentional self-harm
+7th **T50.993** Poisoning by other drugs, medicaments and biological substances, assault
+7th **T50.994** Poisoning by other drugs, medicaments and biological substances, undetermined
+7th **T50.995** Adverse effect of other drugs, medicaments and biological substances
+7th **T50.996** Underdosing of other drugs, medicaments and biological substances

Toxic effects of substances chiefly nonmedicinal as to source (T51-T65)

NOTE When no intent is indicated code to accidental. Undetermined intent is only for use when there is specific documentation in the record that the intent of the toxic effect cannot be determined.

Use additional code(s):
for all associated manifestations of toxic effect, such as: respiratory conditions due to external agents (J60-J70)
personal history of foreign body fully removed (Z87.821)
to identify any retained foreign body, if applicable (Z18.-)

Excludes1: *contact with and (suspected) exposure to toxic substances (Z77.-)*

Review coding guideline C.19.e

T51 Toxic effect of alcohol

The appropriate 7th character is to be added to each code from category T51
A initial encounter
D subsequent encounter
S sequela

+ **T51.0** Toxic effect of ethanol
Toxic effect of ethyl alcohol
Excludes2: acute alcohol intoxication or 'hangover' effects
drunkenness (F10.129, F10.229, F10.929)
pathological (F10.129, F10.229, F10.929)
alcohol intoxication (F10.129, F10.229, F10.929)
+ **T51.0X** Toxic effect of ethanol
+7th **T51.0X1** Toxic effect of ethanol, accidental (unintentional)
Toxic effect of ethanol NOS
+7th **T51.0X2** Toxic effect of ethanol, intentional self-harm
+7th **T51.0X3** Toxic effect of ethanol, assault
+7th **T51.0X4** Toxic effect of ethanol, undetermined
+ **T51.1** Toxic effect of methanol
Toxic effect of methyl alcohol
+ **T51.1X** Toxic effect of methanol
+7th **T51.1X1** Toxic effect of methanol, accidental (unintentional)
Toxic effect of methanol NOS
+7th **T51.1X2** Toxic effect of methanol, intentional self-harm
+7th **T51.1X3** Toxic effect of methanol, assault
+7th **T51.1X4** Toxic effect of methanol, undetermined
+ **T51.2** Toxic effect of 2-Propanol
Toxic effect of isopropyl alcohol
+ **T51.2X** Toxic effect of 2-Propanol
+7th **T51.2X1** Toxic effect of 2-Propanol, accidental (unintentional)
Toxic effect of 2-Propanol NOS
+7th **T51.2X2** Toxic effect of 2-Propanol, intentional self-harm

+7th **T51.2X3 Toxic effect of 2-Propanol, assault**
+7th **T51.2X4 Toxic effect of 2-Propanol, undetermined**

+ **T51.3 Toxic effect of fusel oil**
Toxic effect of amyl alcohol
Toxic effect of butyl [1-butanol] alcohol
Toxic effect of propyl [1-propanol] alcohol
+ **T51.3X Toxic effect of fusel oil**
+7th **T51.3X1 Toxic effect of fusel oil, accidental (unintentional)**
Toxic effect of fusel oil NOS
+7th **T51.3X2 Toxic effect of fusel oil, intentional self-harm**
+7th **T51.3X3 Toxic effect of fusel oil, assault**
+7th **T51.3X4 Toxic effect of fusel oil, undetermined**

+ **T51.8 Toxic effect of other alcohols**
+ **T51.8X Toxic effect of other alcohols**
+7th **T51.8X1 Toxic effect of other alcohols, accidental (unintentional)**
Toxic effect of other alcohols NOS
+7th **T51.8X2 Toxic effect of other alcohols, intentional self-harm**
+7th **T51.8X3 Toxic effect of other alcohols, assault**
+7th **T51.8X4 Toxic effect of other alcohols, undetermined**

+ **T51.9 Toxic effect of unspecified alcohol**
X+7th **T51.91 Toxic effect of unspecified alcohol, accidental (unintentional)**
X+7th **T51.92 Toxic effect of unspecified alcohol, intentional self-harm**
X+7th **T51.93 Toxic effect of unspecified alcohol, assault**
X+7th **T51.94 Toxic effect of unspecified alcohol, undetermined**

T52 Toxic effect of organic solvents

Excludes1: *halogen derivatives of aliphatic and aromatic hydrocarbons (T53.-)*

The appropriate 7th character is to be added to each code from category T52
A initial encounter
D subsequent encounter
S sequela

+ **T52.0 Toxic effects of petroleum products**
Toxic effects of gasoline [petrol]
Toxic effects of kerosene [paraffin oil]
Toxic effects of paraffin wax
Toxic effects of ether petroleum
Toxic effects of naphtha petroleum
Toxic effects of spirit petroleum
+ **T52.0X Toxic effects of petroleum products**
+7th **T52.0X1 Toxic effect of petroleum products, accidental (unintentional)**
Toxic effects of petroleum products NOS
+7th **T52.0X2 Toxic effect of petroleum products, intentional self-harm**
+7th **T52.0X3 Toxic effect of petroleum products, assault**
+7th **T52.0X4 Toxic effect of petroleum products, undetermined**

+ **T52.1 Toxic effects of benzene**
Excludes1: homologues of benzene (T52.2)
nitroderivatives and aminoderivatives of benzene and its homologues (T65.3)
+ **T52.1X Toxic effects of benzene**
+7th **T52.1X1 Toxic effect of benzene, accidental (unintentional)**
Toxic effects of benzene NOS
+7th **T52.1X2 Toxic effect of benzene, intentional self-harm**
+7th **T52.1X3 Toxic effect of benzene, assault**
+7th **T52.1X4 Toxic effect of benzene, undetermined**

+ **T52.2 Toxic effects of homologues of benzene**
Toxic effects of toluene [methylbenzene]
Toxic effects of xylene [dimethylbenzene]
+ **T52.2X Toxic effects of homologues of benzene**
+7th **T52.2X1 Toxic effect of homologues of benzene, accidental (unintentional)**
Toxic effects of homologues of benzene NOS
+7th **T52.2X2 Toxic effect of homologues of benzene, intentional self-harm**
+7th **T52.2X3 Toxic effect of homologues of benzene, assault**
+7th **T52.2X4 Toxic effect of homologues of benzene, undetermined**

+ **T52.3 Toxic effects of glycols**
+ **T52.3X Toxic effects of glycols**
+7th **T52.3X1 Toxic effect of glycols, accidental (unintentional)**
Toxic effects of glycols NOS
+7th **T52.3X2 Toxic effect of glycols, intentional self-harm**
+7th **T52.3X3 Toxic effect of glycols, assault**
+7th **T52.3X4 Toxic effect of glycols, undetermined**

+ **T52.4 Toxic effects of ketones**
+ **T52.4X Toxic effects of ketones**
+7th **T52.4X1 Toxic effect of ketones, accidental (unintentional)**
Toxic effects of ketones NOS
+7th **T52.4X2 Toxic effect of ketones, intentional self-harm**
+7th **T52.4X3 Toxic effect of ketones, assault**
+7th **T52.4X4 Toxic effect of ketones, undetermined**

+ **T52.8 Toxic effects of other organic solvents**
+ **T52.8X Toxic effects of other organic solvents**
+7th **T52.8X1 Toxic effect of other organic solvents, accidental (unintentional)**
Toxic effects of other organic solvents NOS
+7th **T52.8X2 Toxic effect of other organic solvents, intentional self-harm**
+7th **T52.8X3 Toxic effect of other organic solvents, assault**
+7th **T52.8X4 Toxic effect of other organic solvents, undetermined**

+ **T52.9 Toxic effects of unspecified organic solvent**
X+7th **T52.91 Toxic effect of unspecified organic solvent, accidental (unintentional)**
X+7th **T52.92 Toxic effect of unspecified organic solvent, intentional self-harm**
X+7th **T52.93 Toxic effect of unspecified organic solvent, assault**
X+7th **T52.94 Toxic effect of unspecified organic solvent, undetermined**

T53 Toxic effect of halogen derivatives of aliphatic and aromatic hydrocarbons

The appropriate 7th character is to be added to each code from category T53
A initial encounter
D subsequent encounter
S sequela

+ **T53.0 Toxic effects of carbon tetrachloride**
Toxic effects of tetrachloromethane
+ **T53.0X Toxic effects of carbon tetrachloride**
+7th **T53.0X1 Toxic effect of carbon tetrachloride, accidental (unintentional)**
Toxic effects of carbon tetrachloride NOS
+7th **T53.0X2 Toxic effect of carbon tetrachloride, intentional self-harm**
+7th **T53.0X3 Toxic effect of carbon tetrachloride, assault**
+7th **T53.0X4 Toxic effect of carbon tetrachloride, undetermined**

+ **T53.1 Toxic effects of chloroform**
Toxic effects of trichloromethane
+ **T53.1X Toxic effects of chloroform**
+7th **T53.1X1 Toxic effect of chloroform, accidental (unintentional)**
Toxic effects of chloroform NOS
+7th **T53.1X2 Toxic effect of chloroform, intentional self-harm**
+7th **T53.1X3 Toxic effect of chloroform, assault**
+7th **T53.1X4 Toxic effect of chloroform, undetermined**

+ **T53.2 Toxic effects of trichloroethylene**
Toxic effects of trichloroethene
+ **T53.2X Toxic effects of trichloroethylene**
+7th **T53.2X1 Toxic effect of trichloroethylene, accidental (unintentional)**
Toxic effects of trichloroethylene NOS
+7th **T53.2X2 Toxic effect of trichloroethylene, intentional self-harm**
+7th **T53.2X3 Toxic effect of trichloroethylene, assault**
+7th **T53.2X4 Toxic effect of trichloroethylene, undetermined**

+ T53.3 **Toxic effects of tetrachloroethylene**

Toxic effects of perchloroethylene
Toxic effect of tetrachloroethene

+ T53.3X **Toxic effects of tetrachloroethylene**
  - +7th T53.3X1 **Toxic effect of tetrachloroethylene, accidental (unintentional)**
    Toxic effects of tetrachloroethylene NOS
  - +7th T53.3X2 **Toxic effect of tetrachloroethylene, intentional self-harm**
  - +7th T53.3X3 **Toxic effect of tetrachloroethylene, assault**
  - +7th T53.3X4 **Toxic effect of tetrachloroethylene, undetermined**

+ T53.4 **Toxic effects of dichloromethane**

Toxic effects of methylene chloride

+ T53.4X **Toxic effects of dichloromethane**
  - +7th T53.4X1 **Toxic effect of dichloromethane, accidental (unintentional)**
    Toxic effects of dichloromethane NOS
  - +7th T53.4X2 **Toxic effect of dichloromethane, intentional self-harm**
  - +7th T53.4X3 **Toxic effect of dichloromethane, assault**
  - +7th T53.4X4 **Toxic effect of dichloromethane, undetermined**

+ T53.5 **Toxic effects of chlorofluorocarbons**

+ T53.5X **Toxic effects of chlorofluorocarbons**
  - +7th T53.5X1 **Toxic effect of chlorofluorocarbons, accidental (unintentional)**
    Toxic effects of chlorofluorocarbons NOS
  - +7th T53.5X2 **Toxic effect of chlorofluorocarbons, intentional self-harm**
  - +7th T53.5X3 **Toxic effect of chlorofluorocarbons, assault**
  - +7th T53.5X4 **Toxic effect of chlorofluorocarbons, undetermined**

+ T53.6 **Toxic effects of other halogen derivatives of aliphatic hydrocarbons**

+ T53.6X **Toxic effects of other halogen derivatives of aliphatic hydrocarbons**
  - +7th T53.6X1 **Toxic effect of other halogen derivatives of aliphatic hydrocarbons, accidental (unintentional)**
    Toxic effects of other halogen derivatives of aliphatic hydrocarbons NOS
  - +7th T53.6X2 **Toxic effect of other halogen derivatives of aliphatic hydrocarbons, intentional self-harm**
  - +7th T53.6X3 **Toxic effect of other halogen derivatives of aliphatic hydrocarbons, assault**
  - +7th T53.6X4 **Toxic effect of other halogen derivatives of aliphatic hydrocarbons, undetermined**

+ T53.7 **Toxic effects of other halogen derivatives of aromatic hydrocarbons**

+ T53.7X **Toxic effects of other halogen derivatives of aromatic hydrocarbons**
  - +7th T53.7X1 **Toxic effect of other halogen derivatives of aromatic hydrocarbons, accidental (unintentional)**
    Toxic effects of other halogen derivatives of aromatic hydrocarbons NOS
  - +7th T53.7X2 **Toxic effect of other halogen derivatives of aromatic hydrocarbons, intentional self-harm**
  - +7th T53.7X3 **Toxic effect of other halogen derivatives of aromatic hydrocarbons, assault**
  - +7th T53.7X4 **Toxic effect of other halogen derivatives of aromatic hydrocarbons, undetermined**

+ T53.9 **Toxic effects of unspecified halogen derivatives of aliphatic and aromatic hydrocarbons**
  - X+7th T53.91 **Toxic effect of unspecified halogen derivatives of aliphatic and aromatic hydrocarbons, accidental (unintentional)**
  - X+7th T53.92 **Toxic effect of unspecified halogen derivatives of aliphatic and aromatic hydrocarbons, intentional self-harm**
  - X+7th T53.93 **Toxic effect of unspecified halogen derivatives of aliphatic and aromatic hydrocarbons, assault**
  - X+7th T53.94 **Toxic effect of unspecified halogen derivatives of aliphatic and aromatic hydrocarbons, undetermined**

T54 Toxic effect of corrosive substances

> The appropriate 7th character is to be added to each code from category T54
> A initial encounter
> D subsequent encounter
> S sequela

+ T54.0 **Toxic effects of phenol and phenol homologues**

+ T54.0X **Toxic effects of phenol and phenol homologues**
  - +7th T54.0X1 **Toxic effect of phenol and phenol homologues, accidental (unintentional)**
    Toxic effects of phenol and phenol homologues NOS
  - +7th T54.0X2 **Toxic effect of phenol and phenol homologues, intentional self-harm**
  - +7th T54.0X3 **Toxic effect of phenol and phenol homologues, assault**
  - +7th T54.0X4 **Toxic effect of phenol and phenol homologues, undetermined**

+ T54.1 **Toxic effects of other corrosive organic compounds**

+ T54.1X **Toxic effects of other corrosive organic compounds**
  - +7th T54.1X1 **Toxic effect of other corrosive organic compounds, accidental (unintentional)**
    Toxic effects of other corrosive organic compounds NOS
  - +7th T54.1X2 **Toxic effect of other corrosive organic compounds, intentional self-harm**
  - +7th T54.1X3 **Toxic effect of other corrosive organic compounds, assault**
  - +7th T54.1X4 **Toxic effect of other corrosive organic compounds, undetermined**

+ T54.2 **Toxic effects of corrosive acids and acid-like substances**

Toxic effects of hydrochloric acid
Toxic effects of sulfuric acid

+ T54.2X **Toxic effects of corrosive acids and acid-like substances**
  - +7th T54.2X1 **Toxic effect of corrosive acids and acid-like substances, accidental (unintentional)**
    Toxic effects of corrosive acids and acid-like substances NOS
  - +7th T54.2X2 **Toxic effect of corrosive acids and acid-like substances, intentional self-harm**
  - +7th T54.2X3 **Toxic effect of corrosive acids and acid-like substances, assault**
  - +7th T54.2X4 **Toxic effect of corrosive acids and acid-like substances, undetermined**

+ T54.3 **Toxic effects of corrosive alkalis and alkali-like substances**

Toxic effects of potassium hydroxide
Toxic effects of sodium hydroxide

+ T54.3X **Toxic effects of corrosive alkalis and alkali-like substances**
  - +7th T54.3X1 **Toxic effect of corrosive alkalis and alkali-like substances, accidental (unintentional)**
    Toxic effects of corrosive alkalis and alkali-like substances NOS
  - +7th T54.3X2 **Toxic effect of corrosive alkalis and alkali-like substances, intentional self-harm**
  - +7th T54.3X3 **Toxic effect of corrosive alkalis and alkali-like substances, assault**
  - +7th T54.3X4 **Toxic effect of corrosive alkalis and alkali-like substances, undetermined**

+ T54.9 **Toxic effects of unspecified corrosive substance**
  - X+7th T54.91 **Toxic effect of unspecified corrosive substance, accidental (unintentional)**
  - X+7th T54.92 **Toxic effect of unspecified corrosive substance, intentional self-harm**
  - X+7th T54.93 **Toxic effect of unspecified corrosive substance, assault**
  - X+7th T54.94 **Toxic effect of unspecified corrosive substance, undetermined**

T55 Toxic effect of soaps and detergents

> The appropriate 7th character is to be added to each code from category T55
> A initial encounter
> D subsequent encounter
> S sequela

+ T55.0 **Toxic effect of soaps**

+ T55.0X **Toxic effect of soaps**

+7th **T55.0X1 Toxic effect of soaps, accidental (unintentional)**
Toxic effect of soaps NOS
+7th **T55.0X2 Toxic effect of soaps, intentional self-harm**
+7th **T55.0X3 Toxic effect of soaps, assault**
+7th **T55.0X4 Toxic effect of soaps, undetermined**
+ **T55.1 Toxic effect of detergents**
+ **T55.1X Toxic effect of detergents**
+7th **T55.1X1 Toxic effect of detergents, accidental (unintentional)**
Toxic effect of detergents NOS
+7th **T55.1X2 Toxic effect of detergents, intentional self-harm**
+7th **T55.1X3 Toxic effect of detergents, assault**
+7th **T55.1X4 Toxic effect of detergents, undetermined**

T56 Toxic effect of metals

Includes: toxic effects of fumes and vapors of metals
toxic effects of metals from all sources, except medicinal substances
Use additional code to identify any retained metal foreign body, if applicable (Z18.0-, T18.1-)
Excludes1: *arsenic and its compounds (T57.0)*
manganese and its compounds (T57.2)

The appropriate 7th character is to be added to each code from category T56
A initial encounter
D subsequent encounter
S sequela

+ **T56.0 Toxic effects of lead and its compounds**
+ **T56.0X Toxic effects of lead and its compounds**
+7th **T56.0X1 Toxic effect of lead and its compounds, accidental (unintentional)**
Toxic effects of lead and its compounds NOS
+7th **T56.0X2 Toxic effect of lead and its compounds, intentional self-harm**
+7th **T56.0X3 Toxic effect of lead and its compounds, assault**
+7th **T56.0X4 Toxic effect of lead and its compounds, undetermined**
+ **T56.1 Toxic effects of mercury and its compounds**
+ **T56.1X Toxic effects of mercury and its compounds**
+7th **T56.1X1 Toxic effect of mercury and its compounds, accidental (unintentional)**
Toxic effects of mercury and its compounds NOS
+7th **T56.1X2 Toxic effect of mercury and its compounds, intentional self-harm**
+7th **T56.1X3 Toxic effect of mercury and its compounds, assault**
+7th **T56.1X4 Toxic effect of mercury and its compounds, undetermined**
+ **T56.2 Toxic effects of chromium and its compounds**
+ **T56.2X Toxic effects of chromium and its compounds**
+7th **T56.2X1 Toxic effect of chromium and its compounds, accidental (unintentional)**
Toxic effects of chromium and its compounds NOS
+7th **T56.2X2 Toxic effect of chromium and its compounds, intentional self-harm**
+7th **T56.2X3 Toxic effect of chromium and its compounds, assault**
+7th **T56.2X4 Toxic effect of chromium and its compounds, undetermined**
+ **T56.3 Toxic effects of cadmium and its compounds**
+ **T56.3X Toxic effects of cadmium and its compounds**
+7th **T56.3X1 Toxic effect of cadmium and its compounds, accidental (unintentional)**
Toxic effects of cadmium and its compounds NOS
+7th **T56.3X2 Toxic effect of cadmium and its compounds, intentional self-harm**
+7th **T56.3X3 Toxic effect of cadmium and its compounds, assault**
+7th **T56.3X4 Toxic effect of cadmium and its compounds, undetermined**
+ **T56.4 Toxic effects of copper and its compounds**
+ **T56.4X Toxic effects of copper and its compounds**
+7th **T56.4X1 Toxic effect of copper and its compounds, accidental (unintentional)**
Toxic effects of copper and its compounds NOS
+7th **T56.4X2 Toxic effect of copper and its compounds, intentional self-harm**
+7th **T56.4X3 Toxic effect of copper and its compounds, assault**
+7th **T56.4X4 Toxic effect of copper and its compounds, undetermined**
+ **T56.5 Toxic effects of zinc and its compounds**
+ **T56.5X Toxic effects of zinc and its compounds**
+7th **T56.5X1 Toxic effect of zinc and its compounds, accidental (unintentional)**
Toxic effects of zinc and its compounds NOS
+7th **T56.5X2 Toxic effect of zinc and its compounds, intentional self-harm**
+7th **T56.5X3 Toxic effect of zinc and its compounds, assault**
+7th **T56.5X4 Toxic effect of zinc and its compounds, undetermined**
+ **T56.6 Toxic effects of tin and its compounds**
+ **T56.6X Toxic effects of tin and its compounds**
+7th **T56.6X1 Toxic effect of tin and its compounds, accidental (unintentional)**
Toxic effects of tin and its compounds NOS
+7th **T56.6X2 Toxic effect of tin and its compounds, intentional self-harm**
+7th **T56.6X3 Toxic effect of tin and its compounds, assault**
+7th **T56.6X4 Toxic effect of tin and its compounds, undetermined**
+ **T56.7 Toxic effects of beryllium and its compounds**
+ **T56.7X Toxic effects of beryllium and its compounds**
+7th **T56.7X1 Toxic effect of beryllium and its compounds, accidental (unintentional)**
Toxic effects of beryllium and its compounds NOS
+7th **T56.7X2 Toxic effect of beryllium and its compounds, intentional self-harm**
+7th **T56.7X3 Toxic effect of beryllium and its compounds, assault**
+7th **T56.7X4 Toxic effect of beryllium and its compounds, undetermined**
+ **T56.8 Toxic effects of other metals**
+ **T56.81 Toxic effect of thallium**
+7th **T56.811 Toxic effect of thallium, accidental (unintentional)**
Toxic effect of thallium NOS
+7th **T56.812 Toxic effect of thallium, intentional self-harm**
+7th **T56.813 Toxic effect of thallium, assault**
+7th **T56.814 Toxic effect of thallium, undetermined**
+ **T56.89 Toxic effects of other metals**
+7th **T56.891 Toxic effect of other metals, accidental (unintentional)**
Toxic effects of other metals NOS
+7th **T56.892 Toxic effect of other metals, intentional self-harm**
+7th **T56.893 Toxic effect of other metals, assault**
+7th **T56.894 Toxic effect of other metals, undetermined**
+ **T56.9 Toxic effects of unspecified metal**
X+7th **T56.91 Toxic effect of unspecified metal, accidental (unintentional)**
X+7th **T56.92 Toxic effect of unspecified metal, intentional self-harm**
X+7th **T56.93 Toxic effect of unspecified metal, assault**
X+7th **T56.94 Toxic effect of unspecified metal, undetermined**

T57 Toxic effect of other inorganic substances

The appropriate 7th character is to be added to each code from category T57
A initial encounter
D subsequent encounter
S sequela

+ **T57.0 Toxic effect of arsenic and its compounds**
+ **T57.0X Toxic effect of arsenic and its compounds**

+7th **T57.0X1 Toxic effect of arsenic and its compounds, accidental (unintentional)**
Toxic effect of arsenic and its compounds NOS
+7th **T57.0X2 Toxic effect of arsenic and its compounds, intentional self-harm**
+7th **T57.0X3 Toxic effect of arsenic and its compounds, assault**
+7th **T57.0X4 Toxic effect of arsenic and its compounds, undetermined**

\+ **T57.1 Toxic effect of phosphorus and its compounds**
Excludes1: *organophosphate insecticides (T60.0)*
\+ **T57.1X Toxic effect of phosphorus and its compounds**
+7th **T57.1X1 Toxic effect of phosphorus and its compounds, accidental (unintentional)**
Toxic effect of phosphorus and its compounds NOS
+7th **T57.1X2 Toxic effect of phosphorus and its compounds, intentional self-harm**
+7th **T57.1X3 Toxic effect of phosphorus and its compounds, assault**
+7th **T57.1X4 Toxic effect of phosphorus and its compounds, undetermined**

\+ **T57.2 Toxic effect of manganese and its compounds**
\+ **T57.2X Toxic effect of manganese and its compounds**
+7th **T57.2X1 Toxic effect of manganese and its compounds, accidental (unintentional)**
Toxic effect of manganese and its compounds NOS
+7th **T57.2X2 Toxic effect of manganese and its compounds, intentional self-harm**
+7th **T57.2X3 Toxic effect of manganese and its compounds, assault**
+7th **T57.2X4 Toxic effect of manganese and its compounds, undetermined**

\+ **T57.3 Toxic effect of hydrogen cyanide**
\+ **T57.3X Toxic effect of hydrogen cyanide**
+7th **T57.3X1 Toxic effect of hydrogen cyanide, accidental (unintentional)**
Toxic effect of hydrogen cyanide NOS
+7th **T57.3X2 Toxic effect of hydrogen cyanide, intentional self-harm**
+7th **T57.3X3 Toxic effect of hydrogen cyanide, assault**
+7th **T57.3X4 Toxic effect of hydrogen cyanide, undetermined**

\+ **T57.8 Toxic effect of other specified inorganic substances**
\+ **T57.8X Toxic effect of other specified inorganic substances**
+7th **T57.8X1 Toxic effect of other specified inorganic substances, accidental (unintentional)**
Toxic effect of other specified inorganic substances NOS
+7th **T57.8X2 Toxic effect of other specified inorganic substances, intentional self-harm**
+7th **T57.8X3 Toxic effect of other specified inorganic substances, assault**
+7th **T57.8X4 Toxic effect of other specified inorganic substances, undetermined**

\+ **T57.9 Toxic effect of unspecified inorganic substance**
X+7th **T57.91 Toxic effect of unspecified inorganic substance, accidental (unintentional)**
X+7th **T57.92 Toxic effect of unspecified inorganic substance, intentional self-harm**
X+7th **T57.93 Toxic effect of unspecified inorganic substance, assault**
X+7th **T57.94 Toxic effect of unspecified inorganic substance, undetermined**

T58 Toxic effect of carbon monoxide

Includes: asphyxiation from carbon monoxide
toxic effect of carbon monoxide from all sources

The appropriate 7th character is to be added to each code from category T58
A initial encounter
D subsequent encounter
S sequela

\+ **T58.0 Toxic effect of carbon monoxide from motor vehicle exhaust**
Toxic effect of exhaust gas from gas engine
Toxic effect of exhaust gas from motor pump
X+7th **T58.01 Toxic effect of carbon monoxide from motor vehicle exhaust, accidental (unintentional)**
X+7th **T58.02 Toxic effect of carbon monoxide from motor vehicle exhaust, intentional self-harm**
X+7th **T58.03 Toxic effect of carbon monoxide from motor vehicle exhaust, assault**
X+7th **T58.04 Toxic effect of carbon monoxide from motor vehicle exhaust, undetermined**

\+ **T58.1 Toxic effect of carbon monoxide from utility gas**
Toxic effect of acetylene
Toxic effect of gas NOS used for lighting, heating, cooking
Toxic effect of water gas
X+7th **T58.11 Toxic effect of carbon monoxide from utility gas, accidental (unintentional)**
X+7th **T58.12 Toxic effect of carbon monoxide from utility gas, intentional self-harm**
X+7th **T58.13 Toxic effect of carbon monoxide from utility gas, assault**
X+7th **T58.14 Toxic effect of carbon monoxide from utility gas, undetermined**

\+ **T58.2 Toxic effect of carbon monoxide from incomplete combustion of other domestic fuels**
Toxic effect of carbon monoxide from incomplete combustion of coal, coke, kerosene, wood
\+ **T58.2X Toxic effect of carbon monoxide from incomplete combustion of other domestic fuels**
+7th **T58.2X1 Toxic effect of carbon monoxide from incomplete combustion of other domestic fuels, accidental (unintentional)**
+7th **T58.2X2 Toxic effect of carbon monoxide from incomplete combustion of other domestic fuels, intentional self-harm**
+7th **T58.2X3 Toxic effect of carbon monoxide from incomplete combustion of other domestic fuels, assault**
+7th **T58.2X4 Toxic effect of carbon monoxide from incomplete combustion of other domestic fuels, undetermined**

\+ **T58.8 Toxic effect of carbon monoxide from other source**
Toxic effect of carbon monoxide from blast furnace gas
Toxic effect of carbon monoxide from fuels in industrial use
Toxic effect of carbon monoxide from kiln vapor
\+ **T58.8X Toxic effect of carbon monoxide from other source**
+7th **T58.8X1 Toxic effect of carbon monoxide from other source, accidental (unintentional)**
+7th **T58.8X2 Toxic effect of carbon monoxide from other source, intentional self-harm**
+7th **T58.8X3 Toxic effect of carbon monoxide from other source, assault**
+7th **T58.8X4 Toxic effect of carbon monoxide from other source, undetermined**

\+ **T58.9 Toxic effect of carbon monoxide from unspecified source**
X+7th **T58.91 Toxic effect of carbon monoxide from unspecified source, accidental (unintentional)**
X+7th **T58.92 Toxic effect of carbon monoxide from unspecified source, intentional self-harm**
X+7th **T58.93 Toxic effect of carbon monoxide from unspecified source, assault**
X+7th **T58.94 Toxic effect of carbon monoxide from unspecified source, undetermined**

T59 Toxic effect of other gases, fumes and vapors

Includes: aerosol propellants
Excludes1: *chlorofluorocarbons (T53.5)*

The appropriate 7th character is to be added to each code from category T59
A initial encounter
D subsequent encounter
S sequela

\+ **T59.0 Toxic effect of nitrogen oxides**
\+ **T59.0X Toxic effect of nitrogen oxides**
+7th **T59.0X1 Toxic effect of nitrogen oxides, accidental (unintentional)**
Toxic effect of nitrogen oxides NOS
+7th **T59.0X2 Toxic effect of nitrogen oxides, intentional self-harm**
+7th **T59.0X3 Toxic effect of nitrogen oxides, assault**
+7th **T59.0X4 Toxic effect of nitrogen oxides, undetermined**

\+ **T59.1 Toxic effect of sulfur dioxide**
\+ **T59.1X Toxic effect of sulfur dioxide**

+7th **T59.1X1 Toxic effect of sulfur dioxide, accidental (unintentional)**
Toxic effect of sulfur dioxide NOS
+7th **T59.1X2 Toxic effect of sulfur dioxide, intentional self-harm**
+7th **T59.1X3 Toxic effect of sulfur dioxide, assault**
+7th **T59.1X4 Toxic effect of sulfur dioxide, undetermined**

+ **T59.2 Toxic effect of formaldehyde**
+ **T59.2X Toxic effect of formaldehyde**
+7th **T59.2X1 Toxic effect of formaldehyde, accidental (unintentional)**
Toxic effect of formaldehyde NOS
+7th **T59.2X2 Toxic effect of formaldehyde, intentional self-harm**
+7th **T59.2X3 Toxic effect of formaldehyde, assault**
+7th **T59.2X4 Toxic effect of formaldehyde, undetermined**

+ **T59.3 Toxic effect of lacrimogenic gas**
Toxic effect of tear gas
+ **T59.3X Toxic effect of lacrimogenic gas**
+7th **T59.3X1 Toxic effect of lacrimogenic gas, accidental (unintentional)**
Toxic effect of lacrimogenic gas NOS
+7th **T59.3X2 Toxic effect of lacrimogenic gas, intentional self-harm**
+7th **T59.3X3 Toxic effect of lacrimogenic gas, assault**
+7th **T59.3X4 Toxic effect of lacrimogenic gas, undetermined**

+ **T59.4 Toxic effect of chlorine gas**
+ **T59.4X Toxic effect of chlorine gas**
+7th **T59.4X1 Toxic effect of chlorine gas, accidental (unintentional)**
Toxic effect of chlorine gas NOS
+7th **T59.4X2 Toxic effect of chlorine gas, intentional self-harm**
+7th **T59.4X3 Toxic effect of chlorine gas, assault**
+7th **T59.4X4 Toxic effect of chlorine gas, undetermined**

+ **T59.5 Toxic effect of fluorine gas and hydrogen fluoride**
+ **T59.5X Toxic effect of fluorine gas and hydrogen fluoride**
+7th **T59.5X1 Toxic effect of fluorine gas and hydrogen fluoride, accidental (unintentional)**
Toxic effect of fluorine gas and hydrogen fluoride NOS
+7th **T59.5X2 Toxic effect of fluorine gas and hydrogen fluoride, intentional self-harm**
+7th **T59.5X3 Toxic effect of fluorine gas and hydrogen fluoride, assault**
+7th **T59.5X4 Toxic effect of fluorine gas and hydrogen fluoride, undetermined**

+ **T59.6 Toxic effect of hydrogen sulfide**
+ **T59.6X Toxic effect of hydrogen sulfide**
+7th **T59.6X1 Toxic effect of hydrogen sulfide, accidental (unintentional)**
Toxic effect of hydrogen sulfide NOS
+7th **T59.6X2 Toxic effect of hydrogen sulfide, intentional self-harm**
+7th **T59.6X3 Toxic effect of hydrogen sulfide, assault**
+7th **T59.6X4 Toxic effect of hydrogen sulfide, undetermined**

+ **T59.7 Toxic effect of carbon dioxide**
+ **T59.7X Toxic effect of carbon dioxide**
+7th **T59.7X1 Toxic effect of carbon dioxide, accidental (unintentional)**
Toxic effect of carbon dioxide NOS
+7th **T59.7X2 Toxic effect of carbon dioxide, intentional self-harm**
+7th **T59.7X3 Toxic effect of carbon dioxide, assault**
+7th **T59.7X4 Toxic effect of carbon dioxide, undetermined**

+ **T59.8 Toxic effect of other specified gases, fumes and vapors**
+ **T59.81 Toxic effect of smoke**
Smoke inhalation
Excludes2: *toxic effect of cigarette (tobacco) smoke (T65.22-)*
+7th **T59.811 Toxic effect of smoke, accidental (unintentional)**
Toxic effect of smoke NOS
+7th **T59.812 Toxic effect of smoke, intentional self-harm**
+7th **T59.813 Toxic effect of smoke, assault**
+7th **T59.814 Toxic effect of smoke, undetermined**
+ **T59.89 Toxic effect of other specified gases, fumes and vapors**
+7th **T59.891 Toxic effect of other specified gases, fumes and vapors, accidental (unintentional)**
+7th **T59.892 Toxic effect of other specified gases, fumes and vapors, intentional self-harm**
+7th **T59.893 Toxic effect of other specified gases, fumes and vapors, assault**
+7th **T59.894 Toxic effect of other specified gases, fumes and vapors, undetermined**

+ **T59.9 Toxic effect of unspecified gases, fumes and vapors**
X+7th **T59.91 Toxic effect of unspecified gases, fumes and vapors, accidental (unintentional)**
X+7th **T59.92 Toxic effect of unspecified gases, fumes and vapors, intentional self-harm**
X+7th **T59.93 Toxic effect of unspecified gases, fumes and vapors, assault**
X+7th **T59.94 Toxic effect of unspecified gases, fumes and vapors, undetermined**

T60 Toxic effect of pesticides

Includes: toxic effect of wood preservatives

The appropriate 7th character is to be added to each code from category T60
A initial encounter
D subsequent encounter
S sequela

+ **T60.0 Toxic effect of organophosphate and carbamate insecticides**
+ **T60.0X Toxic effect of organophosphate and carbamate insecticides**
+7th **T60.0X1 Toxic effect of organophosphate and carbamate insecticides, accidental (unintentional)**
Toxic effect of organophosphate and carbamate insecticides NOS
+7th **T60.0X2 Toxic effect of organophosphate and carbamate insecticides, intentional self-harm**
+7th **T60.0X3 Toxic effect of organophosphate and carbamate insecticides, assault**
+7th **T60.0X4 Toxic effect of organophosphate and carbamate insecticides, undetermined**

+ **T60.1 Toxic effect of halogenated insecticides**
Excludes1: *chlorinated hydrocarbon (T53.-)*
+ **T60.1X Toxic effect of halogenated insecticides**
+7th **T60.1X1 Toxic effect of halogenated insecticides, accidental (unintentional)**
Toxic effect of halogenated insecticides NOS
+7th **T60.1X2 Toxic effect of halogenated insecticides, intentional self-harm**
+7th **T60.1X3 Toxic effect of halogenated insecticides, assault**
+7th **T60.1X4 Toxic effect of halogenated insecticides, undetermined**

+ **T60.2 Toxic effect of other insecticides**
+ **T60.2X Toxic effect of other insecticides**
+7th **T60.2X1 Toxic effect of other insecticides, accidental (unintentional)**
Toxic effect of other insecticides NOS
+7th **T60.2X2 Toxic effect of other insecticides, intentional self-harm**
+7th **T60.2X3 Toxic effect of other insecticides, assault**
+7th **T60.2X4 Toxic effect of other insecticides, undetermined**

+ **T60.3 Toxic effect of herbicides and fungicides**
+ **T60.3X Toxic effect of herbicides and fungicides**
+7th **T60.3X1 Toxic effect of herbicides and fungicides, accidental (unintentional)**
Toxic effect of herbicides and fungicides NOS
+7th **T60.3X2 Toxic effect of herbicides and fungicides, intentional self-harm**
+7th **T60.3X3 Toxic effect of herbicides and fungicides, assault**
+7th **T60.3X4 Toxic effect of herbicides and fungicides, undetermined**

+ **T60.4 Toxic effect of rodenticides**
Excludes1: *strychnine and its salts (T65.1)*
thallium (T56.81-)
+ **T60.4X Toxic effect of rodenticides**
+7th **T60.4X1 Toxic effect of rodenticides, accidental (unintentional)**
Toxic effect of rodenticides NOS
+7th **T60.4X2 Toxic effect of rodenticides, intentional self-harm**
+7th **T60.4X3 Toxic effect of rodenticides, assault**
+7th **T60.4X4 Toxic effect of rodenticides, undetermined**
+ **T60.8 Toxic effect of other pesticides**
+ **T60.8X Toxic effect of other pesticides**
+7th **T60.8X1 Toxic effect of other pesticides, accidental (unintentional)**
Toxic effect of other pesticides NOS
+7th **T60.8X2 Toxic effect of other pesticides, intentional self-harm**
+7th **T60.8X3 Toxic effect of other pesticides, assault**
+7th **T60.8X4 Toxic effect of other pesticides, undetermined**
+ **T60.9 Toxic effect of unspecified pesticide**
X+7th **T60.91 Toxic effect of unspecified pesticide, accidental (unintentional)**
X+7th **T60.92 Toxic effect of unspecified pesticide, intentional self-harm**
X+7th **T60.93 Toxic effect of unspecified pesticide, assault**
X+7th **T60.94 Toxic effect of unspecified pesticide, undetermined**

T61 Toxic effect of noxious substances eaten as seafood

Excludes1: *allergic reaction to food, such as:*
anaphylactic reaction or shock due to adverse food reaction (T78.0-)
bacterial foodborne intoxications (A05.-)
dermatitis (L23.6, L25.4, L27.2)
food protein-induced enterocolitis syndrome (K52.21)
food protein-induced enteropathy (K52.22)
gastroenteritis (noninfective) (K52.29)
toxic effect of aflatoxin and other mycotoxins (T64)
toxic effect of cyanides (T65.0-)
toxic effect of harmful algae bloom (T65.82-)
toxic effect of hydrogen cyanide (T57.3-)
toxic effect of mercury (T56.1-)
toxic effect of red tide (T65.82-)

The appropriate 7th character is to be added to each code from category T61
A initial encounter
D subsequent encounter
S sequela

+ **T61.0 Ciguatera fish poisoning**
X+7th **T61.01 Ciguatera fish poisoning, accidental (unintentional)**
X+7th **T61.02 Ciguatera fish poisoning, intentional self-harm**
X+7th **T61.03 Ciguatera fish poisoning, assault**
X+7th **T61.04 Ciguatera fish poisoning, undetermined**
+ **T61.1 Scombroid fish poisoning**
Histamine-like syndrome
X+7th **T61.11 Scombroid fish poisoning, accidental (unintentional)**
X+7th **T61.12 Scombroid fish poisoning, intentional self-harm**
X+7th **T61.13 Scombroid fish poisoning, assault**
X+7th **T61.14 Scombroid fish poisoning, undetermined**
+ **T61.7 Other fish and shellfish poisoning**
+ **T61.77 Other fish poisoning**
+7th **T61.771 Other fish poisoning, accidental (unintentional)**
+7th **T61.772 Other fish poisoning, intentional self-harm**
+7th **T61.773 Other fish poisoning, assault**
+7th **T61.774 Other fish poisoning, undetermined**
+ **T61.78 Other shellfish poisoning**
+7th **T61.781 Other shellfish poisoning, accidental (unintentional)**
+7th **T61.782 Other shellfish poisoning, intentional self-harm**
+7th **T61.783 Other shellfish poisoning, assault**
+7th **T61.784 Other shellfish poisoning, undetermined**
+ **T61.8 Toxic effect of other seafood**
+ **T61.8X Toxic effect of other seafood**
+7th **T61.8X1 Toxic effect of other seafood, accidental (unintentional)**
+7th **T61.8X2 Toxic effect of other seafood, intentional self-harm**
+7th **T61.8X3 Toxic effect of other seafood, assault**
+7th **T61.8X4 Toxic effect of other seafood, undetermined**
+ **T61.9 Toxic effect of unspecified seafood**
X+7th **T61.91 Toxic effect of unspecified seafood, accidental (unintentional)**
X+7th **T61.92 Toxic effect of unspecified seafood, intentional self-harm**
X+7th **T61.93 Toxic effect of unspecified seafood, assault**
X+7th **T61.94 Toxic effect of unspecified seafood, undetermined**

T62 Toxic effect of other noxious substances eaten as food

Excludes1: *allergic reaction to food, such as:*
anaphylactic shock (reaction) due to adverse food reaction (T78.0-)
bacterial food borne intoxications (A05.-)
dermatitis (L23.6, L25.4, L27.2)
food protein-induced enterocolitis syndrome (K52.21)
food protein-induced enteropathy (K52.22)
gastroenteritis (noninfective) (K52.29)
toxic effect of aflatoxin and other mycotoxins (T64)
toxic effect of cyanides (T65.0-)
toxic effect of hydrogen cyanide (T57.3-)
toxic effect of mercury (T56.1-)

The appropriate 7th character is to be added to each code from category T62
A initial encounter
D subsequent encounter
S sequela

+ **T62.0 Toxic effect of ingested mushrooms**
+ **T62.0X Toxic effect of ingested mushrooms**
+7th **T62.0X1 Toxic effect of ingested mushrooms, accidental (unintentional)**
Toxic effect of ingested mushrooms NOS
+7th **T62.0X2 Toxic effect of ingested mushrooms, intentional self-harm**
+7th **T62.0X3 Toxic effect of ingested mushrooms, assault**
+7th **T62.0X4 Toxic effect of ingested mushrooms, undetermined**
+ **T62.1 Toxic effect of ingested berries**
+ **T62.1X Toxic effect of ingested berries**
+7th **T62.1X1 Toxic effect of ingested berries, accidental (unintentional)**
Toxic effect of ingested berries NOS
+7th **T62.1X2 Toxic effect of ingested berries, intentional self-harm**
+7th **T62.1X3 Toxic effect of ingested berries, assault**
+7th **T62.1X4 Toxic effect of ingested berries, undetermined**
+ **T62.2 Toxic effect of other ingested (parts of) plant(s)**
+ **T62.2X Toxic effect of other ingested (parts of) plant(s)**
+7th **T62.2X1 Toxic effect of other ingested (parts of) plant(s), accidental (unintentional)**
Toxic effect of other ingested (parts of) plant(s) NOS
+7th **T62.2X2 Toxic effect of other ingested (parts of) plant(s), intentional self-harm**
+7th **T62.2X3 Toxic effect of other ingested (parts of) plant(s), assault**
+7th **T62.2X4 Toxic effect of other ingested (parts of) plant(s), undetermined**
+ **T62.8 Toxic effect of other specified noxious substances eaten as food**
+ **T62.8X Toxic effect of other specified noxious substances eaten as food**
+7th **T62.8X1 Toxic effect of other specified noxious substances eaten as food, accidental (unintentional)**
Toxic effect of other specified noxious substances eaten as food NOS
+7th **T62.8X2 Toxic effect of other specified noxious substances eaten as food, intentional self-harm**
+7th **T62.8X3 Toxic effect of other specified noxious substances eaten as food, assault**
+7th **T62.8X4 Toxic effect of other specified noxious substances eaten as food, undetermined**
+ **T62.9 Toxic effect of unspecified noxious substance eaten as food**
X+7th **T62.91 Toxic effect of unspecified noxious substance eaten as food, accidental (unintentional)**
Toxic effect of unspecified noxious substance eaten as food NOS

X+7th **T62.92** **Toxic effect of unspecified noxious substance eaten as food, intentional self-harm**
X+7th **T62.93** **Toxic effect of unspecified noxious substance eaten as food, assault**
X+7th **T62.94** **Toxic effect of unspecified noxious substance eaten as food, undetermined**

T63 Toxic effect of contact with venomous animals and plants

Includes: bite or touch of venomous animal
pricked or stuck by thorn or leaf
Excludes2: *ingestion of toxic animal or plant (T61.-, T62.-)*

The appropriate 7th character is to be added to each code from category T63
A initial encounter
D subsequent encounter
S sequela

+ **T63.0 Toxic effect of snake venom**
+ **T63.00 Toxic effect of unspecified snake venom**
+7th **T63.001 Toxic effect of unspecified snake venom, accidental (unintentional)**
Toxic effect of unspecified snake venom NOS
+7th **T63.002 Toxic effect of unspecified snake venom, intentional self-harm**
+7th **T63.003 Toxic effect of unspecified snake venom, assault**
+7th **T63.004 Toxic effect of unspecified snake venom, undetermined**
+ **T63.01 Toxic effect of rattlesnake venom**
+7th **T63.011 Toxic effect of rattlesnake venom, accidental (unintentional)**
Toxic effect of rattlesnake venom NOS
+7th **T63.012 Toxic effect of rattlesnake venom, intentional self-harm**
+7th **T63.013 Toxic effect of rattlesnake venom, assault**
+7th **T63.014 Toxic effect of rattlesnake venom, undetermined**
+ **T63.02 Toxic effect of coral snake venom**
+7th **T63.021 Toxic effect of coral snake venom, accidental (unintentional)**
Toxic effect of coral snake venom NOS
+7th **T63.022 Toxic effect of coral snake venom, intentional self-harm**
+7th **T63.023 Toxic effect of coral snake venom, assault**
+7th **T63.024 Toxic effect of coral snake venom, undetermined**
+ **T63.03 Toxic effect of taipan venom**
+7th **T63.031 Toxic effect of taipan venom, accidental (unintentional)**
Toxic effect of taipan venom NOS
+7th **T63.032 Toxic effect of taipan venom, intentional self-harm**
+7th **T63.033 Toxic effect of taipan venom, assault**
+7th **T63.034 Toxic effect of taipan venom, undetermined**
+ **T63.04 Toxic effect of cobra venom**
+7th **T63.041 Toxic effect of cobra venom, accidental (unintentional)**
Toxic effect of cobra venom NOS
+7th **T63.042 Toxic effect of cobra venom, intentional self-harm**
+7th **T63.043 Toxic effect of cobra venom, assault**
+7th **T63.044 Toxic effect of cobra venom, undetermined**
+ **T63.06 Toxic effect of venom of other North and South American snake**
+7th **T63.061 Toxic effect of venom of other North and South American snake, accidental (unintentional)**
Toxic effect of venom of other North and South American snake NOS
+7th **T63.062 Toxic effect of venom of other North and South American snake, intentional self-harm**
+7th **T63.063 Toxic effect of venom of other North and South American snake, assault**
+7th **T63.064 Toxic effect of venom of other North and South American snake, undetermined**
+ **T63.07 Toxic effect of venom of other Australian snake**
+7th **T63.071 Toxic effect of venom of other Australian snake, accidental (unintentional)**
Toxic effect of venom of other Australian snake NOS
+7th **T63.072 Toxic effect of venom of other Australian snake, intentional self-harm**
+7th **T63.073 Toxic effect of venom of other Australian snake, assault**
+7th **T63.074 Toxic effect of venom of other Australian snake, undetermined**
+ **T63.08 Toxic effect of venom of other African and Asian snake**
+7th **T63.081 Toxic effect of venom of other African and Asian snake, accidental (unintentional)**
Toxic effect of venom of other African and Asian snake NOS
+7th **T63.082 Toxic effect of venom of other African and Asian snake, intentional self-harm**
+7th **T63.083 Toxic effect of venom of other African and Asian snake, assault**
+7th **T63.084 Toxic effect of venom of other African and Asian snake, undetermined**
+ **T63.09 Toxic effect of venom of other snake**
+7th **T63.091 Toxic effect of venom of other snake, accidental (unintentional)**
Toxic effect of venom of other snake NOS
+7th **T63.092 Toxic effect of venom of other snake, intentional self-harm**
+7th **T63.093 Toxic effect of venom of other snake, assault**
+7th **T63.094 Toxic effect of venom of other snake, undetermined**
+ **T63.1 Toxic effect of venom of other reptiles**
+ **T63.11 Toxic effect of venom of gila monster**
+7th **T63.111 Toxic effect of venom of gila monster, accidental (unintentional)**
Toxic effect of venom of gila monster NOS
+7th **T63.112 Toxic effect of venom of gila monster, intentional self-harm**
+7th **T63.113 Toxic effect of venom of gila monster, assault**
+7th **T63.114 Toxic effect of venom of gila monster, undetermined**
+ **T63.12 Toxic effect of venom of other venomous lizard**
+7th **T63.121 Toxic effect of venom of other venomous lizard, accidental (unintentional)**
Toxic effect of venom of other venomous lizard NOS
+7th **T63.122 Toxic effect of venom of other venomous lizard, intentional self-harm**
+7th **T63.123 Toxic effect of venom of other venomous lizard, assault**
+7th **T63.124 Toxic effect of venom of other venomous lizard, undetermined**
+ **T63.19 Toxic effect of venom of other reptiles**
+7th **T63.191 Toxic effect of venom of other reptiles, accidental (unintentional)**
Toxic effect of venom of other reptiles NO
+7th **T63.192 Toxic effect of venom of other reptiles, intentional self-harm**
+7th **T63.193 Toxic effect of venom of other reptiles, assault**
+7th **T63.194 Toxic effect of venom of other reptiles, undetermined**
+ **T63.2 Toxic effect of venom of scorpion**
+ **T63.2X Toxic effect of venom of scorpion**
+7th **T63.2X1 Toxic effect of venom of scorpion, accidental (unintentional)**
Toxic effect of venom of scorpion NOS
+7th **T63.2X2 Toxic effect of venom of scorpion, intentional self-harm**
+7th **T63.2X3 Toxic effect of venom of scorpion, assault**
+7th **T63.2X4 Toxic effect of venom of scorpion, undetermined**
+ **T63.3 Toxic effect of venom of spider**
+ **T63.30 Toxic effect of unspecified spider venom**
+7th **T63.301 Toxic effect of unspecified spider venom, accidental (unintentional)**
+7th **T63.302 Toxic effect of unspecified spider venom, intentional self-harm**
+7th **T63.303 Toxic effect of unspecified spider venom, assault**
+7th **T63.304 Toxic effect of unspecified spider venom, undetermined**
+ **T63.31 Toxic effect of venom of black widow spider**

+7th **T63.311** Toxic effect of venom of black widow spider, accidental (unintentional)
+7th **T63.312** Toxic effect of venom of black widow spider, intentional self-harm
+7th **T63.313** Toxic effect of venom of black widow spider, assault
+7th **T63.314** Toxic effect of venom of black widow spider, undetermined

\+ **T63.32** Toxic effect of venom of tarantula
+7th **T63.321** Toxic effect of venom of tarantula, accidental (unintentional)
+7th **T63.322** Toxic effect of venom of tarantula, intentional self-harm
+7th **T63.323** Toxic effect of venom of tarantula, assault
+7th **T63.324** Toxic effect of venom of tarantula, undetermined

\+ **T63.33** Toxic effect of venom of brown recluse spider
+7th **T63.331** Toxic effect of venom of brown recluse spider, accidental (unintentional)
+7th **T63.332** Toxic effect of venom of brown recluse spider, intentional self-harm
+7th **T63.333** Toxic effect of venom of brown recluse spider, assault
+7th **T63.334** Toxic effect of venom of brown recluse spider, undetermined

\+ **T63.39** Toxic effect of venom of other spider
+7th **T63.391** Toxic effect of venom of other spider, accidental (unintentional)
+7th **T63.392** Toxic effect of venom of other spider, intentional self-harm
+7th **T63.393** Toxic effect of venom of other spider, assault
+7th **T63.394** Toxic effect of venom of other spider, undetermined

\+ **T63.4** Toxic effect of venom of other arthropods

\+ **T63.41** Toxic effect of venom of centipedes and venomous millipedes
+7th **T63.411** Toxic effect of venom of centipedes and venomous millipedes, accidental (unintentional)
+7th **T63.412** Toxic effect of venom of centipedes and venomous millipedes, intentional self-harm
+7th **T63.413** Toxic effect of venom of centipedes and venomous millipedes, assault
+7th **T63.414** Toxic effect of venom of centipedes and venomous millipedes, undetermined

\+ **T63.42** Toxic effect of venom of ants
+7th **T63.421** Toxic effect of venom of ants, accidental (unintentional)
+7th **T63.422** Toxic effect of venom of ants, intentional self-harm
+7th **T63.423** Toxic effect of venom of ants, assault
+7th **T63.424** Toxic effect of venom of ants, undetermined

\+ **T63.43** Toxic effect of venom of caterpillars
+7th **T63.431** Toxic effect of venom of caterpillars, accidental (unintentional)
+7th **T63.432** Toxic effect of venom of caterpillars, intentional self-harm
+7th **T63.433** Toxic effect of venom of caterpillars, assault
+7th **T63.434** Toxic effect of venom of caterpillars, undetermined

\+ **T63.44** Toxic effect of venom of bees
+7th **T63.441** Toxic effect of venom of bees, accidental (unintentional)
+7th **T63.442** Toxic effect of venom of bees, intentional self-harm
+7th **T63.443** Toxic effect of venom of bees, assault
+7th **T63.444** Toxic effect of venom of bees, undetermined

\+ **T63.45** Toxic effect of venom of hornets
+7th **T63.451** Toxic effect of venom of hornets, accidental (unintentional)
+7th **T63.452** Toxic effect of venom of hornets, intentional self-harm
+7th **T63.453** Toxic effect of venom of hornets, assault
+7th **T63.454** Toxic effect of venom of hornets, undetermined

\+ **T63.46** Toxic effect of venom of wasps
Toxic effect of yellow jacket
+7th **T63.461** Toxic effect of venom of wasps, accidental (unintentional)
+7th **T63.462** Toxic effect of venom of wasps, intentional self-harm
+7th **T63.463** Toxic effect of venom of wasps, assault
+7th **T63.464** Toxic effect of venom of wasps, undetermined

\+ **T63.48** Toxic effect of venom of other arthropod
+7th **T63.481** Toxic effect of venom of other arthropod, accidental (unintentional)
+7th **T63.482** Toxic effect of venom of other arthropod, intentional self-harm
+7th **T63.483** Toxic effect of venom of other arthropod, assault
+7th **T63.484** Toxic effect of venom of other arthropod, undetermined

\+ **T63.5** Toxic effect of contact with venomous fish
Excludes2: *poisoning by ingestion of fish (T61.-)*

\+ **T63.51** Toxic effect of contact with stingray
+7th **T63.511** Toxic effect of contact with stingray, accidental (unintentional)
+7th **T63.512** Toxic effect of contact with stingray, intentional self-harm
+7th **T63.513** Toxic effect of contact with stingray, assault
+7th **T63.514** Toxic effect of contact with stingray, undetermined

\+ **T63.59** Toxic effect of contact with other venomous fish
+7th **T63.591** Toxic effect of contact with other venomous fish, accidental (unintentional)
+7th **T63.592** Toxic effect of contact with other venomous fish, intentional self-harm
+7th **T63.593** Toxic effect of contact with other venomous fish, assault
+7th **T63.594** Toxic effect of contact with other venomous fish, undetermined

\+ **T63.6** Toxic effect of contact with other venomous marine animals
Excludes1: *sea-snake venom (T63.09)*
Excludes2: *poisoning by ingestion of shellfish (T61.78-)*

\+ **T63.61** Toxic effect of contact with Portugese Man-o-war
Toxic effect of contact with bluebottle
+7th **T63.611** Toxic effect of contact with Portugese Man-o-war, accidental (unintentional)
+7th **T63.612** Toxic effect of contact with Portugese Man-o-war, intentional self-harm
+7th **T63.613** Toxic effect of contact with Portugese Man-o-war, assault
+7th **T63.614** Toxic effect of contact with Portugese Man-o-war, undetermined

\+ **T63.62** Toxic effect of contact with other jellyfish
+7th **T63.621** Toxic effect of contact with other jellyfish, accidental (unintentional)
+7th **T63.622** Toxic effect of contact with other jellyfish, intentional self-harm
+7th **T63.623** Toxic effect of contact with other jellyfish, assault
+7th **T63.624** Toxic effect of contact with other jellyfish, undetermined

\+ **T63.63** Toxic effect of contact with sea anemone
+7th **T63.631** Toxic effect of contact with sea anemone, accidental (unintentional)
+7th **T63.632** Toxic effect of contact with sea anemone, intentional self-harm
+7th **T63.633** Toxic effect of contact with sea anemone, assault
+7th **T63.634** Toxic effect of contact with sea anemone, undetermined

\+ **T63.69** Toxic effect of contact with other venomous marine animals
+7th **T63.691** Toxic effect of contact with other venomous marine animals, accidental (unintentional)
+7th **T63.692** Toxic effect of contact with other venomous marine animals, intentional self-harm
+7th **T63.693** Toxic effect of contact with other venomous marine animals, assault
+7th **T63.694** Toxic effect of contact with other venomous marine animals, undetermined

\+ **T63.7** Toxic effect of contact with venomous plant

\+ **T63.71** Toxic effect of contact with venomous marine plant
+7th **T63.711** Toxic effect of contact with venomous marine plant, accidental (unintentional)

+7th **T63.712** Toxic effect of contact with venomous marine plant, intentional self-harm
+7th **T63.713** Toxic effect of contact with venomous marine plant, assault
+7th **T63.714** Toxic effect of contact with venomous marine plant, undetermined
\+ **T63.79** Toxic effect of contact with other venomous plant
+7th **T63.791** Toxic effect of contact with other venomous plant, accidental (unintentional)
+7th **T63.792** Toxic effect of contact with other venomous plant, intentional self-harm
+7th **T63.793** Toxic effect of contact with other venomous plant, assault
+7th **T63.794** Toxic effect of contact with other venomous plant, undetermined
\+ **T63.8** Toxic effect of contact with other venomous animals
\+ **T63.81** Toxic effect of contact with venomous frog
Excludes1: *contact with nonvenomous frog (W62.0)*
+7th **T63.811** Toxic effect of contact with venomous frog, accidental (unintentional)
+7th **T63.812** Toxic effect of contact with venomous frog, intentional self-harm
+7th **T63.813** Toxic effect of contact with venomous frog, assault
+7th **T63.814** Toxic effect of contact with venomous frog, undetermined
\+ **T63.82** Toxic effect of contact with venomous toad
Excludes1: *contact with nonvenomous toad (W62.1)*
+7th **T63.821** Toxic effect of contact with venomous toad, accidental (unintentional)
+7th **T63.822** Toxic effect of contact with venomous toad, intentional self-harm
+7th **T63.823** Toxic effect of contact with venomous toad, assault
+7th **T63.824** Toxic effect of contact with venomous toad, undetermined
\+ **T63.83** Toxic effect of contact with other venomous amphibian
Excludes1: *contact with nonvenomous amphibian (W62.9)*
+7th **T63.831** Toxic effect of contact with other venomous amphibian, accidental (unintentional)
+7th **T63.832** Toxic effect of contact with other venomous amphibian, intentional self-harm
+7th **T63.833** Toxic effect of contact with other venomous amphibian, assault
+7th **T63.834** Toxic effect of contact with other venomous amphibian, undetermined
\+ **T63.89** Toxic effect of contact with other venomous animals
+7th **T63.891** Toxic effect of contact with other venomous animals, accidental (unintentional)
+7th **T63.892** Toxic effect of contact with other venomous animals, intentional self-harm
+7th **T63.893** Toxic effect of contact with other venomous animals, assault
+7th **T63.894** Toxic effect of contact with other venomous animals, undetermined
\+ **T63.9** Toxic effect of contact with unspecified venomous animal
X+7th **T63.91** Toxic effect of contact with unspecified venomous animal, accidental (unintentional)
X+7th **T63.92** Toxic effect of contact with unspecified venomous animal, intentional self-harm
X+7th **T63.93** Toxic effect of contact with unspecified venomous animal, assault
X+7th **T63.94** Toxic effect of contact with unspecified venomous animal, undetermined

T64 Toxic effect of aflatoxin and other mycotoxin food contaminants

The appropriate 7th character is to be added to each code from category T64
A initial encounter
D subsequent encounter
S sequela

\+ **T64.0** Toxic effect of aflatoxin
X+7th **T64.01** Toxic effect of aflatoxin, accidental (unintentional)
X+7th **T64.02** Toxic effect of aflatoxin, intentional self-harm
X+7th **T64.03** Toxic effect of aflatoxin, assault
X+7th **T64.04** Toxic effect of aflatoxin, undetermined
\+ **T64.8** Toxic effect of other mycotoxin food contaminants
X+7th **T64.81** Toxic effect of other mycotoxin food contaminants, accidental (unintentional)
X+7th **T64.82** Toxic effect of other mycotoxin food contaminants, intentional self-harm
X+7th **T64.83** Toxic effect of other mycotoxin food contaminants, assault
X+7th **T64.84** Toxic effect of other mycotoxin food contaminants, undetermined

T65 Toxic effect of other and unspecified substances

The appropriate 7th character is to be added to each code from category T65
A initial encounter
D subsequent encounter
S sequela

\+ **T65.0** Toxic effect of cyanides
Excludes1: *hydrogen cyanide (T57.3-)*
\+ **T65.0X** Toxic effect of cyanides
+7th **T65.0X1** Toxic effect of cyanides, accidental (unintentional)
Toxic effect of cyanides NOS
+7th **T65.0X2** Toxic effect of cyanides, intentional self-harm
+7th **T65.0X3** Toxic effect of cyanides, assault
+7th **T65.0X4** Toxic effect of cyanides, undetermined
\+ **T65.1** Toxic effect of strychnine and its salts
\+ **T65.1X** Toxic effect of strychnine and its salts
+7th **T65.1X1** Toxic effect of strychnine and its salts, accidental (unintentional)
Toxic effect of strychnine and its salts NOS
+7th **T65.1X2** Toxic effect of strychnine and its salts, intentional self-harm
+7th **T65.1X3** Toxic effect of strychnine and its salts, assault
+7th **T65.1X4** Toxic effect of strychnine and its salts, undetermined
\+ **T65.2** Toxic effect of tobacco and nicotine
Excludes2: *nicotine dependence (F17.-)*
\+ **T65.21** Toxic effect of chewing tobacco
+7th **T65.211** Toxic effect of chewing tobacco, accidental (unintentional)
Toxic effect of chewing tobacco NOS
+7th **T65.212** Toxic effect of chewing tobacco, intentional self-harm
+7th **T65.213** Toxic effect of chewing tobacco, assault
+7th **T65.214** Toxic effect of chewing tobacco, undetermined
\+ **T65.22** Toxic effect of tobacco cigarettes
Toxic effect of tobacco smoke
Use additional code for exposure to second hand tobacco smoke (Z57.31, Z77.22)
+7th **T65.221** Toxic effect of tobacco cigarettes, accidental (unintentional)
Toxic effect of tobacco cigarettes NOS
+7th **T65.222** Toxic effect of tobacco cigarettes, intentional self-harm
+7th **T65.223** Toxic effect of tobacco cigarettes, assault
+7th **T65.224** Toxic effect of tobacco cigarettes, undetermined
\+ **T65.29** Toxic effect of other tobacco and nicotine
+7th **T65.291** Toxic effect of other tobacco and nicotine, accidental (unintentional)
Toxic effect of other tobacco and nicotine NOS
+7th **T65.292** Toxic effect of other tobacco and nicotine, intentional self-harm
+7th **T65.293** Toxic effect of other tobacco and nicotine, assault
+7th **T65.294** Toxic effect of other tobacco and nicotine, undetermined
\+ **T65.3** Toxic effect of nitroderivatives and aminoderivatives of benzene and its homologues
Toxic effect of anilin [benzenamine]
Toxic effect of nitrobenzene
Toxic effect of trinitrotoluene
\+ **T65.3X** Toxic effect of nitroderivatives and aminoderivatives of benzene and its homologues

+7th T65.3X1 **Toxic effect of nitroderivatives and aminoderivatives of benzene and its homologues, accidental (unintentional)**
Toxic effect of nitroderivatives and aminoderivatives of benzene and its homologues NOS
+7th T65.3X2 **Toxic effect of nitroderivatives and aminoderivatives of benzene and its homologues, intentional self-harm**
+7th T65.3X3 **Toxic effect of nitroderivatives and aminoderivatives of benzene and its homologues, assault**
+7th T65.3X4 **Toxic effect of nitroderivatives and aminoderivatives of benzene and its homologues, undetermined**
+ T65.4 **Toxic effect of carbon disulfide**
+ T65.4X **Toxic effect of carbon disulfide**
+7th T65.4X1 **Toxic effect of carbon disulfide, accidental (unintentional)**
Toxic effect of carbon disulfide NOS
+7th T65.4X2 **Toxic effect of carbon disulfide, intentional self-harm**
+7th T65.4X3 **Toxic effect of carbon disulfide, assault**
+7th T65.4X4 **Toxic effect of carbon disulfide, undetermined**
+ T65.5 **Toxic effect of nitroglycerin and other nitric acids and esters**
Toxic effect of 1,2,3-Propanetriol trinitrate
+ T65.5X **Toxic effect of nitroglycerin and other nitric acids and esters**
+7th T65.5X1 **Toxic effect of nitroglycerin and other nitric acids and esters, accidental (unintentional)**
Toxic effect of nitroglycerin and other nitric acids and esters NOS
+7th T65.5X2 **Toxic effect of nitroglycerin and other nitric acids and esters, intentional self-harm**
+7th T65.5X3 **Toxic effect of nitroglycerin and other nitric acids and esters, assault**
+7th T65.5X4 **Toxic effect of nitroglycerin and other nitric acids and esters, undetermined**
+ T65.6 **Toxic effect of paints and dyes, not elsewhere classified**
+ T65.6X **Toxic effect of paints and dyes, not elsewhere classified**
+7th T65.6X1 **Toxic effect of paints and dyes, not elsewhere classified, accidental (unintentional)**
Toxic effect of paints and dyes NOS
+7th T65.6X2 **Toxic effect of paints and dyes, not elsewhere classified, intentional self-harm**
+7th T65.6X3 **Toxic effect of paints and dyes, not elsewhere classified, assault**
+7th T65.6X4 **Toxic effect of paints and dyes, not elsewhere classified, undetermined**
+ T65.8 **Toxic effect of other specified substances**
+ T65.81 **Toxic effect of latex**
+7th T65.811 **Toxic effect of latex, accidental (unintentional)**
Toxic effect of latex NOS
+7th T65.812 **Toxic effect of latex, intentional self-harm**
+7th T65.813 **Toxic effect of latex, assault**
+7th T65.814 **Toxic effect of latex, undetermined**
+ T65.82 **Toxic effect of harmful algae and algae toxins**
Toxic effect of (harmful) algae bloom NOS
Toxic effect of blue-green algae bloom
Toxic effect of brown tide
Toxic effect of cyanobacteria bloom
Toxic effect of Florida red tide
Toxic effect of pfiesteria piscicida
Toxic effect of red tide
+7th T65.821 **Toxic effect of harmful algae and algae toxins, accidental (unintentional)**
Toxic effect of harmful algae and algae toxins NOS
+7th T65.822 **Toxic effect of harmful algae and algae toxins, intentional self-harm**
+7th T65.823 **Toxic effect of harmful algae and algae toxins, assault**
+7th T65.824 **Toxic effect of harmful algae and algae toxins, undetermined**
+ T65.83 **Toxic effect of fiberglass**
+7th T65.831 **Toxic effect of fiberglass, accidental (unintentional)**
Toxic effect of fiberglass NOS
+7th T65.832 **Toxic effect of fiberglass, intentional self-harm**
+7th T65.833 **Toxic effect of fiberglass, assault**
+7th T65.834 **Toxic effect of fiberglass, undetermined**
+ T65.89 **Toxic effect of other specified substances**
+7th T65.891 **Toxic effect of other specified substances, accidental (unintentional)**
Toxic effect of other specified substances NOS
+7th T65.892 **Toxic effect of other specified substances, intentional self-harm**
+7th T65.893 **Toxic effect of other specified substances, assault**
+7th T65.894 **Toxic effect of other specified substances, undetermined**
+ T65.9 **Toxic effect of unspecified substance**
X+7th T65.91 **Toxic effect of unspecified substance, accidental (unintentional)**
Poisoning NOS
X+7th T65.92 **Toxic effect of unspecified substance, intentional self-harm**
X+7th T65.93 **Toxic effect of unspecified substance, assault**
X+7th T65.94 **Toxic effect of unspecified substance, undetermined**

Other and unspecified effects of external causes (T66-T78)

T66 Radiation sickness, unspecified
X+7th
Excludes1: *specified adverse effects of radiation, such as:*
burns (T20-T31)
leukemia (C91-C95)
radiation gastroenteritis and colitis (K52.0)
radiation pneumonitis (J70.0)
radiation related disorders of the skin and subcutaneous tissue (L55-L59)
sunburn (L55.-)

The appropriate 7th character is to be added to code T66
A initial encounter
D subsequent encounter
S sequela

T67 Effects of heat and light
Excludes1: *erythema [dermatitis] ab igne (L59.0)*
malignant hyperpyrexia due to anesthesia (T88.3)
radiation-related disorders of the skin and subcutaneous tissue (L55-L59)
Excludes2: *burns (T20-T31)*
sunburn (L55.-)
sweat disorder due to heat (L74-L75)

The appropriate 7th character is to be added to each code from category T67
A initial encounter
D subsequent encounter
S sequela

CC X+7th T67.0 **Heatstroke and sunstroke**
Heat apoplexy
Heat pyrexia
Siriasis
Thermoplegia
Use additional code(s) to identify any associated complications of heatstroke, such as:
coma and stupor (R40.-)
systemic inflammatory response syndrome (R65.1-)
CC Exclusion 7th character A see Appendix A PDX collection 1419
HAC 7th character A see Appendix B for HAC conditional logic
X+7th T67.1 **Heat syncope**
Heat collapse
X+7th T67.2 **Heat cramp**
X+7th T67.3 **Heat exhaustion, anhydrotic**
Heat prostration due to water depletion
Excludes1: *heat exhaustion due to salt depletion (T67.4)*
X+7th T67.4 **Heat exhaustion due to salt depletion**
Heat prostration due to salt (and water) depletion
X+7th T67.5 **Heat exhaustion, unspecified**
Heat prostration NOS
X+7th T67.6 **Heat fatigue, transient**

X+7th **T67.7 Heat edema**
X+7th **T67.8 Other effects of heat and light**
X+7th **T67.9 Effect of heat and light, unspecified**

T68 Hypothermia
X+7th
Accidental hypothermia
Hypothermia NOS
Use additional code to identify source of exposure:
Exposure to excessive cold of man-made origin (W93)
Exposure to excessive cold of natural origin (X31)
Excludes1: *hypothermia following anesthesia (T88.51)*
hypothermia not associated with low environmental temperature (R68.0)
hypothermia of newborn (P80.-)
Excludes2: *frostbite (T33-T34)*

The appropriate 7th character is to be added to code T68
A initial encounter
D subsequent encounter
S sequela

T69 Other effects of reduced temperature
Use additional code to identify source of exposure:
Exposure to excessive cold of man-made origin (W93)
Exposure to excessive cold of natural origin (X31)
Excludes2: *frostbite (T33-T34)*

The appropriate 7th character is to be added to each code from category T69
A initial encounter
D subsequent encounter
S sequela

\+ **T69.0 Immersion hand and foot**
\+ **T69.01 Immersion hand**
+7th **T69.011 Immersion hand, right hand**
+7th **T69.012 Immersion hand, left hand**
+7th **T69.019 Immersion hand, unspecified hand**
\+ **T69.02 Immersion foot**
Trench foot
CC +7th **T69.021 Immersion foot, right foot**
CC Exclusion 7th character A see Appendix A PDX collection 1420
HAC 7th character A see Appendix B for HAC conditional logic
CC +7th **T69.022 Immersion foot, left foot**
CC Exclusion 7th character A see Appendix A PDX collection 1420
HAC 7th character A see Appendix B for HAC conditional logic
CC +7th **T69.029 Immersion foot, unspecified foot**
CC Exclusion 7th character A see Appendix A PDX collection 1420
HAC 7th character A see Appendix B for HAC conditional logic
X+7th **T69.1 Chilblains**
X+7th **T69.8 Other specified effects of reduced temperature**
X+7th **T69.9 Effect of reduced temperature, unspecified**

T70 Effects of air pressure and water pressure

The appropriate 7th character is to be added to each code from category T70
A initial encounter
D subsequent encounter
S sequela

X+7th **T70.0 Otitic barotrauma**
Aero-otitis media
Effects of change in ambient atmospheric pressure or water pressure on ears
X+7th **T70.1 Sinus barotrauma**
Aerosinusitis
Effects of change in ambient atmospheric pressure on sinuses
\+ **T70.2 Other and unspecified effects of high altitude**
Excludes2: *polycythemia due to high altitude (D75.1)*
X+7th **T70.20 Unspecified effects of high altitude**
X+7th **T70.29 Other effects of high altitude**
Alpine sickness
Anoxia due to high altitude
Barotrauma NOS
Hypobaropathy
Mountain sickness
CC X+7th **T70.3 Caisson disease [decompression sickness]**
Compressed-air disease
Diver's palsy or paralysis
CC Exclusion 7th character A see Appendix A PDX collection 1421
HAC 7th character A see Appendix B for HAC conditional logic
X+7th **T70.4 Effects of high-pressure fluids**
Hydraulic jet injection (industrial)
Pneumatic jet injection (industrial)
Traumatic jet injection (industrial)
X+7th **T70.8 Other effects of air pressure and water pressure**
X+7th **T70.9 Effect of air pressure and water pressure, unspecified**

T71 Asphyxiation
Mechanical suffocation
Traumatic suffocation
Excludes1: *acute respiratory distress (syndrome) (J80)*
anoxia due to high altitude (T70.2)
asphyxia NOS (R09.01)
asphyxia from carbon monoxide (T58.-)
asphyxia from inhalation of food or foreign body (T17.-)
asphyxia from other gases, fumes and vapors (T59.-)
respiratory distress (syndrome) in newborn (P22.-)

The appropriate 7th character is to be added to each code from categor
T71
A initial encounter
D subsequent encounter
S sequela

\+ **T71.1 Asphyxiation due to mechanical threat to breathing**
Suffocation due to mechanical threat to breathing
\+ **T71.11 Asphyxiation due to smothering under pillow**
CC +7th **T71.111 Asphyxiation due to smothering under pillow, accidental**
Asphyxiation due to smothering under pillow NOS
CC Exclusion 7th character A see Appendix A PDX collection 1422
HAC 7th character A see Appendix B for HAC conditional logic
CC +7th **T71.112 Asphyxiation due to smothering under pillow, intentional self-harm**
CC Exclusion 7th character A see Appendix A PDX collection 1422
HAC 7th character A see Appendix B for HAC conditional logic
CC +7th **T71.113 Asphyxiation due to smothering under pillow, assault**
CC Exclusion 7th character A see Appendix A PDX collection 1422
HAC 7th character A see Appendix B for HAC conditional logic
CC +7th **T71.114 Asphyxiation due to smothering under pillow, undetermined**
CC Exclusion 7th character A see Appendix A PDX collection 1422
HAC 7th character A see Appendix B for HAC conditional logic
\+ **T71.12 Asphyxiation due to plastic bag**
CC +7th **T71.121 Asphyxiation due to plastic bag, accident**
Asphyxiation due to plastic bag NOS
CC Exclusion 7th character A see Appendix A PDX collection 1422
HAC 7th character A see Appendix B for HAC conditional logic
CC +7th **T71.122 Asphyxiation due to plastic bag, intention self-harm**
CC Exclusion 7th character A see Appendix A PDX collection 1422
HAC 7th character A see Appendix B for HAC conditional logic
CC +7th **T71.123 Asphyxiation due to plastic bag, assault**
CC Exclusion 7th character A see Appendix A PDX collection 1422
HAC 7th character A see Appendix B for HAC conditional logic
CC +7th **T71.124 Asphyxiation due to plastic bag, undetermined**
CC Exclusion 7th character A see Appendix A PDX collection 1422
HAC 7th character A see Appendix B for HAC conditional logic

+ **T71.13 Asphyxiation due to being trapped in bed linens**

CC +7th **T71.131 Asphyxiation due to being trapped in bed linens, accidental**
Asphyxiation due to being trapped in bed linens NOS
CC Exclusion 7th character A see Appendix A PDX collection 1422
HAC 7th character A see Appendix B for HAC conditional logic

CC +7th **T71.132 Asphyxiation due to being trapped in bed linens, intentional self-harm**
CC Exclusion 7th character A see Appendix A PDX collection 1422
HAC 7th character A see Appendix B for HAC conditional logic

CC +7th **T71.133 Asphyxiation due to being trapped in bed linens, assault**
CC Exclusion 7th character A see Appendix A PDX collection 1422
HAC 7th character A see Appendix B for HAC conditional logic

CC +7th **T71.134 Asphyxiation due to being trapped in bed linens, undetermined**
CC Exclusion 7th character A see Appendix A PDX collection 1422
HAC 7th character A see Appendix B for HAC conditional logic

+ **T71.14 Asphyxiation due to smothering under another person's body (in bed)**

CC +7th **T71.141 Asphyxiation due to smothering under another person's body (in bed), accidental**
Asphyxiation due to smothering under another person's body (in bed) NOS
CC Exclusion 7th character A see Appendix A PDX collection 1422
HAC 7th character A see Appendix B for HAC conditional logic

CC +7th **T71.143 Asphyxiation due to smothering under another person's body (in bed), assault**
CC Exclusion 7th character A see Appendix A PDX collection 1422
HAC 7th character A see Appendix B for HAC conditional logic

CC +7th **T71.144 Asphyxiation due to smothering under another person's body (in bed), undetermined**
CC Exclusion 7th character A see Appendix A PDX collection 1422
HAC 7th character A see Appendix B for HAC conditional logic

+ **T71.15 Asphyxiation due to smothering in furniture**

CC +7th **T71.151 Asphyxiation due to smothering in furniture, accidental**
Asphyxiation due to smothering in furniture NOS
CC Exclusion 7th character A see Appendix A PDX collection 1422
HAC 7th character A see Appendix B for HAC conditional logic

CC +7th **T71.152 Asphyxiation due to smothering in furniture, intentional self-harm**
CC Exclusion 7th character A see Appendix A PDX collection 1422
HAC 7th character A see Appendix B for HAC conditional logic

CC +7th **T71.153 Asphyxiation due to smothering in furniture, assault**
CC Exclusion 7th character A see Appendix A PDX collection 1422
HAC 7th character A see Appendix B for HAC conditional logic

CC +7th **T71.154 Asphyxiation due to smothering in furniture, undetermined**
CC Exclusion 7th character A see Appendix A PDX collection 1422
HAC 7th character A see Appendix B for HAC conditional logic

+ **T71.16 Asphyxiation due to hanging**
Hanging by window shade cord
Use additional code for any associated injuries, such as:
crushing injury of neck (S17.-)
fracture of cervical vertebrae (S12.0-S12.2-)
open wound of neck (S11.-)

CC +7th **T71.161 Asphyxiation due to hanging, accidental**
Asphyxiation due to hanging NOS
Hanging NOS
CC Exclusion 7th character A see Appendix A PDX collection 1422
HAC 7th character A see Appendix B for HAC conditional logic

CC +7th **T71.162 Asphyxiation due to hanging, intentional self-harm**
CC Exclusion 7th character A see Appendix A PDX collection 1422
HAC 7th character A see Appendix B for HAC conditional logic

CC +7th **T71.163 Asphyxiation due to hanging, assault**
CC Exclusion 7th character A see Appendix A PDX collection 1422
HAC 7th character A see Appendix B for HAC conditional logic

CC +7th **T71.164 Asphyxiation due to hanging, undetermined**
CC Exclusion 7th character A see Appendix A PDX collection 1422
HAC 7th character A see Appendix B for HAC conditional logic

+ **T71.19 Asphyxiation due to mechanical threat to breathing due to other causes**

CC +7th **T71.191 Asphyxiation due to mechanical threat to breathing due to other causes, accidental**
Asphyxiation due to other causes NOS
CC Exclusion 7th character A see Appendix A PDX collection 1422
AHA CC: 4Q, 2016, 74-76
HAC 7th character A see Appendix B for HAC conditional logic

CC +7th **T71.192 Asphyxiation due to mechanical threat to breathing due to other causes, intentional self-harm**
CC Exclusion 7th character A see Appendix A PDX collection 1422
HAC 7th character A see Appendix B for HAC conditional logic

CC +7th **T71.193 Asphyxiation due to mechanical threat to breathing due to other causes, assault**
CC Exclusion 7th character A see Appendix A PDX collection 1422
HAC 7th character A see Appendix B for HAC conditional logic

CC +7th **T71.194 Asphyxiation due to mechanical threat to breathing due to other causes, undetermined**
CC Exclusion 7th character A see Appendix A PDX collection 1422
HAC 7th character A see Appendix B for HAC conditional logic

+ **T71.2 Asphyxiation due to systemic oxygen deficiency due to low oxygen content in ambient air**
Suffocation due to systemic oxygen deficiency due to low oxygen content in ambient air

CC X+7th **T71.20 Asphyxiation due to systemic oxygen deficiency due to low oxygen content in ambient air due to unspecified cause**
CC Exclusion 7th character A see Appendix A PDX collection 1422
HAC 7th character A see Appendix B for HAC conditional logic

CC X+7th **T71.21 Asphyxiation due to cave-in or falling earth**
Use additional code for any associated cataclysm (X34-X38)
CC Exclusion 7th character A see Appendix A PDX collection 1422
HAC 7th character A see Appendix B for HAC conditional logic

+ **T71.22 Asphyxiation due to being trapped in a car trunk**

CC +7th **T71.221 Asphyxiation due to being trapped in a car trunk, accidental**
CC Exclusion 7th character A see Appendix A PDX collection 1422

CC +7th **T71.222 Asphyxiation due to being trapped in a car trunk, intentional self-harm**
CC Exclusion 7th character A see Appendix A PDX collection 1422

CC +7th **T71.223 Asphyxiation due to being trapped in a car trunk, assault**
CC Exclusion 7th character A see Appendix A PDX collection 1422

CC +7th **T71.224 Asphyxiation due to being trapped in a car trunk, undetermined**
CC Exclusion 7th character A see Appendix A PDX collection 1422

\+ **T71.23 Asphyxiation due to being trapped in a (discarded) refrigerator**

CC +7th **T71.231 Asphyxiation due to being trapped in a (discarded) refrigerator, accidental**
CC Exclusion 7th character A see Appendix A PDX collection 1422

CC +7th **T71.232 Asphyxiation due to being trapped in a (discarded) refrigerator, intentional self-harm**
CC Exclusion 7th character A see Appendix A PDX collection 1422

CC +7th **T71.233 Asphyxiation due to being trapped in a (discarded) refrigerator, assault**
CC Exclusion 7th character A see Appendix A PDX collection 1422

CC +7th **T71.234 Asphyxiation due to being trapped in a (discarded) refrigerator, undetermined**
CC Exclusion 7th character A see Appendix A PDX collection 1422

CC X+7th **T71.29 Asphyxiation due to being trapped in other low oxygen environment**
CC Exclusion 7th character A see Appendix A PDX collection 1422
HAC 7th character A see Appendix B for HAC conditional logic

CC X+7th **T71.9 Asphyxiation due to unspecified cause**
Suffocation (by strangulation) due to unspecified cause
Suffocation NOS
Systemic oxygen deficiency due to low oxygen content in ambient air due to unspecified cause
Systemic oxygen deficiency due to mechanical threat to breathing due to unspecified cause
Traumatic asphyxia NOS
CC Exclusion 7th character A see Appendix A PDX collection 1422
HAC 7th character A see Appendix B for HAC conditional logic

T73 Effects of other deprivation

The appropriate 7th character is to be added to each code from category T73
A initial encounter
D subsequent encounter
S sequela

X+7th **T73.0 Starvation**
Deprivation of food
X+7th **T73.1 Deprivation of water**
X+7th **T73.2 Exhaustion due to exposure**
X+7th **T73.3 Exhaustion due to excessive exertion**
Exhaustion due to overexertion
X+7th **T73.8 Other effects of deprivation**
X+7th **T73.9 Effect of deprivation, unspecified**

T74 Adult and child abuse, neglect and other maltreatment, confirmed

Use additional code, if applicable, to identify any associated current injury.

Use additional external cause code to identify perpetrator, if known (Y07.-)

Excludes1: *abuse and maltreatment in pregnancy (O9A.3-, O9A.4-, O9A.5-)*
adult and child maltreatment, suspected (T76.-)

The appropriate 7th character is to be added to each code from category T74
A initial encounter
D subsequent encounter
S sequela

Review coding guideline C.19.f

\+ **T74.0 Neglect or abandonment, confirmed**

● CC X+7th **T74.01 Adult neglect or abandonment, confirmed**
CC Exclusion 7th character A see Appendix A PDX collection 1423

● CC X+7th **T74.02 Child neglect or abandonment, confirmed**
CC Exclusion 7th character A see Appendix A PDX collection 1423

\+ **T74.1 Physical abuse, confirmed**
Excludes2: *sexual abuse (T74.2-)*

● CC X+7th **T74.11 Adult physical abuse, confirmed**
CC Exclusion 7th character A see Appendix A PDX collection 1423

● CC X+7th **T74.12 Child physical abuse, confirmed**
Excludes2: *shaken infant syndrome (T74.4)*
CC Exclusion 7th character A see Appendix A PDX collection 1423

\+ **T74.2 Sexual abuse, confirmed**
Rape, confirmed
Sexual assault, confirmed

● CC X+7th **T74.21 Adult sexual abuse, confirmed**
CC Exclusion 7th character A see Appendix A PDX collection 1423

● CC X+7th **T74.22 Child sexual abuse, confirmed**
CC Exclusion 7th character A see Appendix A PDX collection 1423

\+ **T74.3 Psychological abuse, confirmed**
CC Exclusion 7th character A see Appendix A PDX collection 1423

● X+7th **T74.31 Adult psychological abuse, confirmed**
CC Exclusion 7th character A see Appendix A PDX collection 1423

● CC X+7th **T74.32 Child psychological abuse, confirmed**
CC Exclusion 7th character A see Appendix A PDX collection 1423

● CC X+7th **T74.4 Shaken infant syndrome**
CC Exclusion 7th character A see Appendix A PDX collection 1423

\+ **T74.9 Unspecified maltreatment, confirmed**

● CC X+7th **T74.91 Unspecified adult maltreatment, confirmed**
CC Exclusion 7th character A see Appendix A PDX collection 1424

● CC X+7th **T74.92 Unspecified child maltreatment, confirmed**
CC Exclusion 7th character A see Appendix A PDX collection 1423

T75 Other and unspecified effects of other external causes

Excludes1: *adverse effects NEC (T78.-)*
Excludes2: *burns (electric) (T20-T31)*

The appropriate 7th character is to be added to each code from category T75
A initial encounter
D subsequent encounter
S sequela

\+ **T75.0 Effects of lightning**
Struck by lightning

X+7th **T75.00 Unspecified effects of lightning**
Struck by lightning NOS
X+7th **T75.01 Shock due to being struck by lightning**
X+7th **T75.09 Other effects of lightning**
Use additional code for other effects of lightning

CC X+7th **T75.1 Unspecified effects of drowning and nonfatal submersion**
Immersion
Excludes1: *specified effects of drowning- code to effects*
CC Exclusion 7th character A see Appendix A PDX collection 1425
HAC 7th character A see Appendix B for HAC conditional logic

\+ **T75.2 Effects of vibration**

X+7th **T75.20 Unspecified effects of vibration**
X+7th **T75.21 Pneumatic hammer syndrome**
X+7th **T75.22 Traumatic vasospastic syndrome**
X+7th **T75.23 Vertigo from infrasound**
Excludes1: *vertigo NOS (R42)*
X+7th **T75.29 Other effects of vibration**

X+7th **T75.3 Motion sickness**
Airsickness
Seasickness
Travel sickness
Use additional external cause code to identify vehicle or type motion (Y92.81-, Y93.5-)

X+7th **T75.4 Electrocution**
Shock from electric current
Shock from electroshock gun (taser)

\+ **T75.8 Other specified effects of external causes**

X+7th **T75.81 Effects of abnormal gravitation [G] forces**
X+7th **T75.82 Effects of weightlessness**
X+7th **T75.89 Other specified effects of external causes**

T76 Adult and child abuse, neglect and other maltreatment, suspected

Use additional code, if applicable, to identify any associated current injury

Excludes1: adult and child maltreatment, confirmed (T74.-)
suspected abuse and maltreatment in pregnancy (O9A.3-, O9A.4-, O9A.5-)
suspected adult physical abuse, ruled out (Z04.71)
suspected adult sexual abuse, ruled out (Z04.41)
suspected child physical abuse, ruled out (Z04.72)
suspected child sexual abuse, ruled out (Z04.42)

The appropriate 7th character is to be added to each code from category T76
A initial encounter
D subsequent encounter
S sequela

Review coding guideline C.19.f

\+ **T76.0 Neglect or abandonment, suspected**

● CC X+7th **T76.01 Adult neglect or abandonment, suspected**
CC Exclusion 7th character A see Appendix A PDX collection 1423

● CC X+7th **T76.02 Child neglect or abandonment, suspected**
CC Exclusion 7th character A see Appendix A PDX collection 1423

\+ **T76.1 Physical abuse, suspected**

● CC X+7th **T76.11 Adult physical abuse, suspected**
CC Exclusion 7th character A see Appendix A PDX collection 1423

● CC X+7th **T76.12 Child physical abuse, suspected**
CC Exclusion 7th character A see Appendix A PDX collection 1423

\+ **T76.2 Sexual abuse, suspected**
Rape, suspected
Excludes1: *alleged abuse, ruled out (Z04.7)*

● CC X+7th **T76.21 Adult sexual abuse, suspected**
CC Exclusion 7th character A see Appendix A PDX collection 1423

● CC X+7th **T76.22 Child sexual abuse, suspected**
CC Exclusion 7th character A see Appendix A PDX collection 1423

\+ **T76.3 Psychological abuse, suspected**

● X+7th **T76.31 Adult psychological abuse, suspected**

● CC X+7th **T76.32 Child psychological abuse, suspected**
CC Exclusion 7th character A see Appendix A PDX collection 1423

\+ **T76.9 Unspecified maltreatment, suspected**

● CC X+7th **T76.91 Unspecified adult maltreatment, suspected**
CC Exclusion 7th character A see Appendix A PDX collection 1424

● CC X+7th **T76.92 Unspecified child maltreatment, suspected**
CC Exclusion 7th character A see Appendix A PDX collection 1423

T78 Adverse effects, not elsewhere classified

Excludes2: *complications of surgical and medical care NEC (T80-T88)*

The appropriate 7th character is to be added to each code from category T78
A initial encounter
D subsequent encounter
S sequela

\+ **T78.0 Anaphylactic reaction due to food**
Anaphylactic reaction due to adverse food reaction
Anaphylactic shock or reaction due to nonpoisonous foods
Anaphylactoid reaction due to food

CC X+7th **T78.00 Anaphylactic reaction due to unspecified food**
CC Exclusion 7th character A see Appendix A PDX collection 1426

CC X+7th **T78.01 Anaphylactic reaction due to peanuts**
CC Exclusion 7th character A see Appendix A PDX collection 1426

CC X+7th **T78.02 Anaphylactic reaction due to shellfish (crustaceans)**
CC Exclusion 7th character A see Appendix A PDX collection 1426

CC X+7th **T78.03 Anaphylactic reaction due to other fish**
CC Exclusion 7th character A see Appendix A PDX collection 1426

CC X+7th **T78.04 Anaphylactic reaction due to fruits and vegetables**
CC Exclusion 7th character A see Appendix A PDX collection 1426

CC X+7th **T78.05 Anaphylactic reaction due to tree nuts and seeds**
Excludes2: *anaphylactic reaction due to peanuts (T78.01)*
CC Exclusion 7th character A see Appendix A PDX collection 1426

CC X+7th **T78.06 Anaphylactic reaction due to food additives**
CC Exclusion 7th character A see Appendix A PDX collection 1426

CC X+7th **T78.07 Anaphylactic reaction due to milk and dairy products**
CC Exclusion 7th character A see Appendix A PDX collection 1426

CC X+7th **T78.08 Anaphylactic reaction due to eggs**
CC Exclusion 7th character A see Appendix A PDX collection 1426

CC X+7th **T78.09 Anaphylactic reaction due to other food products**
CC Exclusion 7th character A see Appendix A PDX collection 1426

X+7th **T78.1 Other adverse food reactions, not elsewhere classified**
Use additional code to identify the type of reaction, if applicable
Excludes1: *anaphylactic reaction or shock due to adverse food reaction (T78.0-)*
anaphylactic reaction due to food (T78.0-)
bacterial food borne intoxications (A05.-)
Excludes2: *allergic and dietetic gastroenteritis and colitis (K52.29)*
allergic rhinitis due to food (J30.5)
dermatitis due to food in contact with skin (L23.6, L24.6, L25.4)
dermatitis due to ingested food (L27.2)
food protein-induced entercolitis syndrome (K52.21)
food protein-induced enteropathy (K52.22)

CC X+7th **T78.2 Anaphylactic shock, unspecified**
Allergic shock
Anaphylactic reaction
Anaphylaxis
Excludes1: *anaphylactic reaction or shock due to adverse effect of correct medicinal substance properly administered (T88.6)*
anaphylactic reaction or shock due to adverse food reaction (T78.0-)
anaphylactic reaction or shock due to serum (T80.5-)
CC Exclusion 7th character A see Appendix A PDX collection 1426

X+7th **T78.3 Angioneurotic edema**
Allergic angioedema
Giant urticaria
Quincke's edema
Excludes1: *serum urticaria (T80.6-)*
urticaria (L50.-)

\+ **T78.4 Other and unspecified allergy**
Excludes1: *specified types of allergic reaction such as:*
allergic diarrhea (K52.29)
allergic gastroenteritis and colitis (K52.29)
dermatitis (L23-L25, L27.-)
food protein-induced entercolitis syndrome (K52.21)
food protein-induced enteropathy (K52.22)
hay fever (J30.1)

X+7th **T78.40 Allergy, unspecified**
Allergic reaction NOS
Hypersensitivity NOS

X+7th **T78.41 Arthus phenomenon**
Arthus reaction

X+7th **T78.49 Other allergy**

X+7th **T78.8 Other adverse effects, not elsewhere classified**

Certain early complications of trauma (T79)

T79 Certain early complications of trauma, not elsewhere classified

Excludes2: *acute respiratory distress syndrome (J80)*
complications occurring during or following medical procedures (T80-T88)
complications of surgical and medical care NEC (T80-T88)
newborn respiratory distress syndrome (P22.0)

The appropriate 7th character is to be added to each code from category T79
A initial encounter
D subsequent encounter
S sequela

MCC X+7th **T79.0 Air embolism (traumatic)**

Excludes1: *air embolism complicating abortion or ectopic or molar pregnancy (O00-O07, O08.2)*
air embolism complicating pregnancy, childbirth and the puerperium (O88.0)
air embolism following infusion, transfusion, and therapeutic injection (T80.0)
air embolism following procedure NEC (T81.7-)

MCC Exclusion 7th character A see Appendix A PDX collection 1427

MCC X+7th **T79.1 Fat embolism (traumatic)**

Excludes1: *fat embolism complicating:*
abortion or ectopic or molar pregnancy (O00-O07, O08.2)
pregnancy, childbirth and the puerperium (O88.8)

MCC Exclusion 7th character A see Appendix A PDX collection 1428

CC X+7th **T79.2 Traumatic secondary and recurrent hemorrhage and seroma**

CC Exclusion 7th character A see Appendix A PDX collection 1429

MCC X+7th **T79.4 Traumatic shock**

Shock (immediate) (delayed) following injury

Excludes1: *anaphylactic shock due to adverse food reaction (T78.0-)*
anaphylactic shock due to correct medicinal substance properly administered (T88.6)
anaphylactic shock due to serum (T80.5-)
anaphylactic shock NOS (T78.2)
anesthetic shock (T88.2)
electric shock (T75.4)
nontraumatic shock NEC (R57.-)
obstetric shock (O75.1)
postprocedural shock (T81.1-)
septic shock (R65.21)
shock complicating abortion or ectopic or molar pregnancy (O00-O07, O08.3)
shock due to lightning (T75.01)
shock NOS (R57.9)

MCC Exclusion 7th character A see Appendix A PDX collection 1430

MCC X+7th **T79.5 Traumatic anuria**

Crush syndrome
Renal failure following crushing

MCC Exclusion 7th character A see Appendix A PDX collection 1431

X+7th **T79.6 Traumatic ischemia of muscle**

Traumatic rhabdomyolysis
Volkmann's ischemic contracture

Excludes2: *anterior tibial syndrome (M76.8)*
compartment syndrome (traumatic) (T79.A-)
nontraumatic ischemia of muscle (M62.2-)

CC X+7th **T79.7 Traumatic subcutaneous emphysema**

Excludes1: *emphysema NOS (J43)*
emphysema (subcutaneous) resulting from a procedure (T81.82)

CC Exclusion 7th character A see Appendix A PDX collection 1432

\+ **T79.A Traumatic compartment syndrome**

Excludes1: *fibromyalgia (M79.7)*
nontraumatic compartment syndrome (M79.A-)
traumatic ischemic infarction of muscle (T79.6)

CC X+7th **T79.A0 Compartment syndrome, unspecified**

Compartment syndrome NOS

CC Exclusion 7th character A see Appendix A PDX collection 0896

\+ **T79.A1 Traumatic compartment syndrome of upper extremity**

Traumatic compartment syndrome of shoulder, arm, forearm, wrist, hand, and fingers

CC +7th **T79.A11 Traumatic compartment syndrome of right upper extremity**

CC Exclusion 7th character A see Appendix A PDX collection 1433

CC +7th **T79.A12 Traumatic compartment syndrome of left upper extremity**

CC Exclusion 7th character A see Appendix A PDX collection 1433

CC +7th **T79.A19 Traumatic compartment syndrome of unspecified upper extremity**

CC Exclusion 7th character A see Appendix A PDX collection 1433

\+ **T79.A2 Traumatic compartment syndrome of lower extremity**

Traumatic compartment syndrome of hip, buttock, thigh, leg, foot, and toes

CC +7th **T79.A21 Traumatic compartment syndrome of right lower extremity**

CC Exclusion 7th character A see Appendix A PDX collection 1433

CC +7th **T79.A22 Traumatic compartment syndrome of left lower extremity**

CC Exclusion 7th character A see Appendix A PDX collection 1433

CC +7th **T79.A29 Traumatic compartment syndrome of unspecified lower extremity**

CC Exclusion 7th character A see Appendix A PDX collection 1433

CC X+7th **T79.A3 Traumatic compartment syndrome of abdomen**

CC Exclusion 7th character A see Appendix A PDX collection 1434

CC X+7th **T79.A9 Traumatic compartment syndrome of other sites**

CC Exclusion 7th character A see Appendix A PDX collection 0896

X+7th **T79.8 Other early complications of trauma**

X+7th **T79.9 Unspecified early complication of trauma**

Complications of surgical and medical care, not elsewhere classified (T80-T88)

Use additional code for adverse effect, if applicable, to identify drug (T36-T50 with fifth or sixth character 5)

Use additional code(s) to identify the specified condition resulting from the complication

Use additional code to identify devices involved and details of circumstances (Y62-Y82)

Excludes2: *any encounters with medical care for postprocedural conditions in which no complications are present, such as:*
artificial opening status (Z93.-)
closure of external stoma (Z43.-)
fitting and adjustment of external prosthetic device (Z44.-)
burns and corrosions from local applications and irradiation (T20-T32)
complications of surgical procedures during pregnancy, childbirth and the puerperium (O00-O9A)
mechanical complication of respirator [ventilator] (J95.850)
poisoning and toxic effects of drugs and chemicals (T36-T65 with fifth or sixth character 1-4 or 6)
postprocedural fever (R50.82)
specified complications classified elsewhere, such as:
cerebrospinal fluid leak from spinal puncture (G97.0)
colostomy malfunction (K94.0-)
disorders of fluid and electrolyte imbalance (E86-E87)
functional disturbances following cardiac surgery (I97.0-I97.1)
intraoperative and postprocedural complications of specified body systems (D78.-, E36.-, E89.-, G97.3-, G97.4, H59.3-, H59.-, H95.2-, H95.3, I97.4-, I97.5, J95.6-, J95.7, K91.6-, L76.-, M96.-, N99.-)
ostomy complications (J95.0-, K94.-, N99.5-)
postgastric surgery syndromes (K91.1)
postlaminectomy syndrome NEC (M96.1)
postmastectomy lymphedema syndrome (I97.2)
postsurgical blind-loop syndrome (K91.2)
ventilator associated pneumonia (J95.851)

T80 Complications following infusion, transfusion and therapeutic injection

Includes: complications following perfusion

Excludes2: *bone marrow transplant rejection (T86.01)*
febrile nonhemolytic transfusion reaction (R50.84)
fluid overload due to transfusion (E87.71)
posttransfusion purpura (D69.51)
transfusion associated circulatory overload (TACO) (E87.71)
transfusion (red blood cell) associated hemochromatosis (E83.111)
transfusion related acute lung injury (TRALI) (J95.84)

The appropriate 7th character is to be added to each code from category T80
A initial encounter
D subsequent encounter
S sequela

MCC X+7th **T80.0 Air embolism following infusion, transfusion and therapeutic injection**

MCC Exclusion 7th character A see Appendix A PDX collection 1

HAC 7th character A see Appendix B for HAC conditional logic

CC X+7th **T80.1 Vascular complications following infusion, transfusion and therapeutic injection**
Use additional code to identify the vascular complication
Excludes2: *extravasation of vesicant agent (T80.81-)*
infiltration of vesicant agent (T80.81-)
vascular complications specified as due to prosthetic devices, implants and grafts (T82.8-, T83.8-, T84.8-, T85.8-)
postprocedural vascular complications (T81.7-)
CC Exclusion 7th character A see Appendix A PDX collection 1436

\+ **T80.2 Infections following infusion, transfusion and therapeutic injection**
Use additional code to identify the specific infection, such as:
sepsis (A41.9)
Use additional code (R65.2-) to identify severe sepsis, if applicable
Excludes2: *infections specified as due to prosthetic devices, implants and grafts (T82.6-T82.7, T83.5-T83.6, T84.5-T84.7, T85.7)*
postprocedural infections (T81.4-)
Review coding guideline C.1.d.5

\+ **T80.21 Infection due to central venous catheter**
Infection due to pulmonary artery catheter (Swan-Ganz catheter)

CC +7th **T80.211 Bloodstream infection due to central venous catheter**
Catheter-related bloodstream infection (CRBSI) NOS
Central line-associated bloodstream infection (CLABSI)
Bloodstream infection due to Hickman catheter
Bloodstream infection due to peripherally inserted central catheter (PICC)
Bloodstream infection due to portacath (port-a-cath)
Bloodstream infection due to pulmonary artery catheter
Bloodstream infection due to triple lumen catheter
Bloodstream infection due to umbilical venous catheter
CC Exclusion 7th character A see Appendix A PDX collection 0948
HAC 7th character A see Appendix B for HAC conditional logic

CC +7th **T80.212 Local infection due to central venous catheter**
Exit or insertion site infection
Local infection due to Hickman catheter
Local infection due to peripherally inserted central catheter (PICC)
Local infection due to portacath (port-a-cath)
Local infection due to pulmonary artery catheter
Local infection due to triple lumen catheter
Local infection due to umbilical venous catheter
Port or reservoir infection
Tunnel infection
CC Exclusion 7th character A see Appendix A PDX collection 0948
HAC 7th character A see Appendix B for HAC conditional logic

CC +7th **T80.218 Other infection due to central venous catheter**
Other central line-associated infection
Other infection due to Hickman catheter
Other infection due to peripherally inserted central catheter (PICC)
Other infection due to portacath (port-a-cath)
Other infection due to pulmonary artery catheter
Other infection due to triple lumen catheter
Other infection due to umbilical venous catheter
CC Exclusion 7th character A see Appendix A PDX collection 0948
HAC 7th character A see Appendix B for HAC conditional logic

CC +7th **T80.219 Unspecified infection due to central venous catheter**
Central line-associated infection NOS
Unspecified infection due to Hickman catheter
Unspecified infection due to peripherally inserted central catheter (PICC)
Unspecified infection due to portacath (port-a-cath)
Unspecified infection due to pulmonary artery catheter
Unspecified infection due to triple lumen catheter
Unspecified infection due to umbilical venous catheter
CC Exclusion 7th character A see Appendix A PDX collection 0948
HAC 7th character A see Appendix B for HAC conditional logic

CC X+7th **T80.22 Acute infection following transfusion, infusion, or injection of blood and blood products**
CC Exclusion 7th character A see Appendix A PDX collection 0948

CC X+7th **T80.29 Infection following other infusion, transfusion and therapeutic injection**
CC Exclusion 7th character A see Appendix A PDX collection 0948

\+ **T80.3 ABO incompatibility reaction due to transfusion of blood or blood products**
Excludes1: *minor blood group antigens reactions (Duffy) (E) (K(ell)) (Kidd) (Lewis) (M) (N) (P) (S) (T80.A)*

CC X+7th **T80.30 ABO incompatibility reaction due to transfusion of blood or blood products, unspecified**
ABO incompatibility blood transfusion NOS
Reaction to ABO incompatibility from transfusion NOS
CC Exclusion 7th character A see Appendix A PDX collection 1437
HAC 7th character A see Appendix B for HAC conditional logic

\+ **T80.31 ABO incompatibility with hemolytic transfusion reaction**

CC +7th **T80.310 ABO incompatibility with acute hemolytic transfusion reaction**
ABO incompatibility with hemolytic transfusion reaction less than 24 hours after transfusion
Acute hemolytic transfusion reaction (AHTR) due to ABO incompatibility
CC Exclusion 7th character A see Appendix A PDX collection 1437
HAC 7th character A see Appendix B for HAC conditional logic

CC +7th **T80.311 ABO incompatibility with delayed hemolytic transfusion reaction**
ABO incompatibility with hemolytic transfusion reaction 24 hours or more after transfusion
Delayed hemolytic transfusion reaction (DHTR) due to ABO incompatibility
CC Exclusion 7th character A see Appendix A PDX collection 1437
HAC 7th character A see Appendix B for HAC conditional logic

CC +7th **T80.319 ABO incompatibility with hemolytic transfusion reaction, unspecified**
ABO incompatibility with hemolytic transfusion reaction at unspecified time after transfusion
Hemolytic transfusion reaction (HTR) due to ABO
incompatibility NOS
CC Exclusion 7th character A see Appendix A PDX collection 1437
HAC 7th character A see Appendix B for HAC conditional logic

CC X+7th **T80.39 Other ABO incompatibility reaction due to transfusion of blood or blood products**
Delayed serologic transfusion reaction (DSTR) from ABO incompatibility
Other ABO incompatible blood transfusion
Other reaction to ABO incompatible blood transfusion
CC Exclusion 7th character A see Appendix A PDX collection 1437
HAC 7th character A see Appendix B for HAC conditional logic

\+ **T80.4 Rh incompatibility reaction due to transfusion of blood or blood products**
Reaction due to incompatibility of Rh antigens (C) (c) (D) (E) (e)

CC X+7th **T80.40 Rh incompatibility reaction due to transfusion of blood or blood products, unspecified**
Reaction due to Rh factor in transfusion NOS
Rh incompatible blood transfusion NOS
CC Exclusion 7th character A see Appendix A PDX collection 1437

\+ **T80.41 Rh incompatibility with hemolytic transfusion reaction**

CC +7th **T80.410 Rh incompatibility with acute hemolytic transfusion reaction**
Acute hemolytic transfusion reaction (AHTR) due to Rh incompatibility
Rh incompatibility with hemolytic transfusion reaction less than 24 hours after transfusion
CC Exclusion 7th character A see Appendix A PDX collection 1437

CC +7th **T80.411 Rh incompatibility with delayed hemolytic transfusion reaction**
Delayed hemolytic transfusion reaction (DHTR) due to Rh incompatibility
Rh incompatibility with hemolytic transfusion reaction 24 hours or more after transfusion
CC Exclusion 7th character A see Appendix A PDX collection 1437

CC +7th **T80.419 Rh incompatibility with hemolytic transfusion reaction, unspecified**
Rh incompatibility with hemolytic transfusion reaction at unspecified time after transfusion
Hemolytic transfusion reaction (HTR) due to Rh incompatibility NOS
CC Exclusion 7th character A see Appendix A PDX collection 1437

CC X+7th **T80.49 Other Rh incompatibility reaction due to transfusion of blood or blood products**
Delayed serologic transfusion reaction (DSTR) from Rh incompatibility
Other reaction to Rh incompatible blood transfusion
CC Exclusion 7th character A see Appendix A PDX collection 1438

\+ **T80.A Non-ABO incompatibility reaction due to transfusion of blood or blood products**
Reaction due to incompatibility of minor antigens (Duffy) (Kell) (Kidd) (Lewis) (M) (N) (P) (S)

CC X+7th **T80.A0 Non-ABO incompatibility reaction due to transfusion of blood or blood products, unspecified**
Non-ABO antigen incompatibility reaction from transfusion NOS
CC Exclusion 7th character A see Appendix A PDX collection 1438

\+ **T80.A1 Non-ABO incompatibility with hemolytic transfusion reaction**

CC +7th **T80.A10 Non-ABO incompatibility with acute hemolytic transfusion reaction**
Acute hemolytic transfusion reaction (AHTR) due to non-ABO incompatibility
Non-ABO incompatibility with hemolytic transfusion reaction less than 24 hours after transfusion
CC Exclusion 7th character A see Appendix A PDX collection 1438

CC +7th **T80.A11 Non-ABO incompatibility with delayed hemolytic transfusion reaction**
Delayed hemolytic transfusion reaction (DHTR) due to non-ABO incompatibili
Non-ABO incompatibility with hemolytic transfusion reaction 24 or more hours after transfusion
CC Exclusion 7th character A see Appendix A PDX collection 1438

CC +7th **T80.A19 Non-ABO incompatibility with hemolytic transfusion reaction, unspecified**
Hemolytic transfusion reaction (HTR) due to non-ABO incompatibility NOS
Non-ABO incompatibility with hemolytic transfusion reaction at unspecified time after transfusion
CC Exclusion 7th character A see Appendix A PDX collection 1438

CC X+7th **T80.A9 Other non-ABO incompatibility reaction due to transfusion of blood or blood products**
Delayed serologic transfusion reaction (DSTR) from non-ABO incompatibility
Other reaction to non-ABO incompatible blood transfusion
CC Exclusion 7th character A see Appendix A PDX collection 1437

\+ **T80.5 Anaphylactic reaction due to serum**
Allergic shock due to serum
Anaphylactic shock due to serum
Anaphylactoid reaction due to serum
Anaphylaxis due to serum
Excludes1: *ABO incompatibility reaction due to transfusion blood or blood products (T80.3-)*
allergic reaction or shock NOS (T78.2)
anaphylactic reaction or shock NOS (T78.2)
anaphylactic reaction or shock due to adverse effect of correct medicinal substance properly administered (T88.6)
other serum reaction (T80.6-)

CC X+7th **T80.51 Anaphylactic reaction due to administration of blo and blood products**
CC Exclusion 7th character A see Appendix A PDX collection 1439

CC X+7th **T80.52 Anaphylactic reaction due to vaccination**
CC Exclusion 7th character A see Appendix A PDX collection 1439

CC X+7th **T80.59 Anaphylactic reaction due to other serum**
CC Exclusion 7th character A see Appendix A PDX collection 1439

\+ **T80.6 Other serum reactions**
Intoxication by serum
Protein sickness
Serum rash
Serum sickness
Serum urticaria
Excludes2: *serum hepatitis (B16-B19)*

CC X+7th **T80.61 Other serum reaction due to administration of blo and blood products**
CC Exclusion 7th character A see Appendix A PDX collection 1439

CC X+7th **T80.62 Other serum reaction due to vaccination**
CC Exclusion 7th character A see Appendix A PDX collection 1439

CC X+7th **T80.69 Other serum reaction due to other serum**
Code also, if applicable, arthropathy in hypersensitivity reactions classified elsewhere (M36.4)
CC Exclusion 7th character A see Appendix A PDX collection 1440

\+ **T80.8 Other complications following infusion, transfusion and therapeutic injection**

\+ **T80.81 Extravasation of vesicant agent**
Infiltration of vesicant agent

CC +7th **T80.810 Extravasation of vesicant antineoplastic chemotherapy**
Infiltration of vesicant antineoplastic chemotherapy
CC Exclusion 7th character A see Appendix PDX collection 1436

CC +7th **T80.818 Extravasation of other vesicant agent**
Infiltration of other vesicant agent
CC Exclusion 7th character A see Appendix PDX collection 1436

X+7th **T80.89 Other complications following infusion, transfusion and therapeutic injection**
Delayed serologic transfusion reaction (DSTR), unspecified incompatibility
Use additional code to identify graft-versus-host reaction, if applicable, (D89.81-)

+ **T80.9 Unspecified complication following infusion, transfusion and therapeutic injection**

X+7th **T80.90 Unspecified complication following infusion and therapeutic injection**

+ **T80.91 Hemolytic transfusion reaction, unspecified incompatibility**
Excludes1: *ABO incompatibility with hemolytic transfusion reaction (T80.31-)*
Non-ABO incompatibility with hemolytic transfusion reaction (T80.A1-)
Rh incompatibility with hemolytic transfusion reaction (T80.41-)

CC +7th **T80.910 Acute hemolytic transfusion reaction, unspecified incompatibility**
CC Exclusion 7th character A see Appendix A PDX collection 1437

CC +7th **T80.911 Delayed hemolytic transfusion reaction, unspecified incompatibility**
CC Exclusion 7th character A see Appendix A PDX collection 1437

CC +7th **T80.919 Hemolytic transfusion reaction, unspecified incompatibility, unspecified as acute or delayed**
Hemolytic transfusion reaction NOS
CC Exclusion 7th character A see Appendix A PDX collection 1437

X+7th **T80.92 Unspecified transfusion reaction**
Transfusion reaction NOS

T81 Complications of procedures, not elsewhere classified
Use additional code for adverse effect, if applicable, to identify drug (T36-T50 with fifth or sixth character 5)
Excludes2: *complications following immunization (T88.0-T88.1)*
complications following infusion, transfusion and therapeutic injection (T80.-)
complications of transplanted organs and tissue (T86.-)
specified complications classified elsewhere, such as:
complication of prosthetic devices, implants and grafts (T82-T85)
dermatitis due to drugs and medicaments (L23.3, L24.4, L25.1, L27.0-L27.1)
endosseous dental implant failure (M27.6-)
floppy iris syndrome (IFIS) (intraoperative) H21.81
intraoperative and postprocedural complications of specific body system (D78.-, E36.-, E89.-, G97.3-, G97.4, H59.3-, H59.-, H95.2-, H95.3, I97.4-, I97.5, J95, K91.-, L76.-, M96.-, N99.-)
ostomy complications (J95.0-, K94.-, N99.5-)
plateau iris syndrome (post-iridectomy) (postprocedural) (H21.82)
poisoning and toxic effects of drugs and chemicals (T36-T65 with fifth or sixth character 1-4 or 6)

The appropriate 7th character is to be added to each code from category T81
A initial encounter
D subsequent encounter
S sequela

+ **T81.1 Postprocedural shock**
Shock during or resulting from a procedure, not elsewhere classified
Excludes1: *anaphylactic shock NOS (T78.2)*
anaphylactic shock due to correct substance properly administered (T88.6)
anaphylactic shock due to serum (T80.5-)
anesthetic shock (T88.2)
electric shock (T75.4)
obstetric shock (O75.1)
septic shock (R65.21)
shock following abortion or ectopic or molar pregnancy (O00-O07, O08.3)
traumatic shock (T79.4)

CC X+7th **T81.10 Postprocedural shock unspecified**
Collapse NOS during or resulting from a procedure, not elsewhere classified
Postprocedural failure of peripheral circulation
Postprocedural shock NOS
CC Exclusion 7th character A see Appendix A PDX collection 1441

MCC X+7th **T81.11 Postprocedural cardiogenic shock**
MCC Exclusion 7th character A see Appendix A PDX collection 1441

MCC X+7th **T81.12 Postprocedural septic shock**
Postprocedural endotoxic shock resulting from a procedure, not elsewhere classified
Postprocedural gram-negative shock resulting from a procedure, not elsewhere classified
Code first underlying infection
Use additional code, to identify any associated acute organ dysfunction, if applicable
MCC Exclusion 7th character A see Appendix A PDX collection 1441
Review coding guideline C.1.d.2

MCC X+7th **T81.19 Other postprocedural shock**
Postprocedural hypovolemic shock
MCC Exclusion 7th character A see Appendix A PDX collection 1441

+ **T81.3 Disruption of wound, not elsewhere classified**
Disruption of any suture materials or other closure methods
Excludes1: *breakdown (mechanical) of permanent sutures (T85.612)*
displacement of permanent sutures (T85.622)
disruption of cesarean delivery wound (O90.0)
disruption of perineal obstetric wound (O90.1)
mechanical complication of permanent sutures NEC (T85.692)
AHA CC: 1Q, 2014, 23

CC X+7th **T81.30 Disruption of wound, unspecified**
Disruption of wound NOS
CC Exclusion 7th character A see Appendix A PDX collection 1442

CC X+7th **T81.31 Disruption of external operation (surgical) wound, not elsewhere classified**
Dehiscence of operation wound NOS
Disruption of operation wound NOS
Disruption or dehiscence of closure of cornea
Disruption or dehiscence of closure of mucosa
Disruption or dehiscence of closure of skin and subcutaneous tissue
Full-thickness skin disruption or dehiscence
Superficial disruption or dehiscence of operation wound
Excludes1: *dehiscence of amputation stump (T87.81)*
CC Exclusion 7th character A see Appendix A PDX collection 1442
AHA CC: 1Q, 2015, 3-21

CC X+7th **T81.32 Disruption of internal operation (surgical) wound, not elsewhere classified**
Deep disruption or dehiscence of operation wound NOS
Disruption or dehiscence of closure of internal organ or other internal tissue
Disruption or dehiscence of closure of muscle or muscle flap
Disruption or dehiscence of closure of ribs or rib cage
Disruption or dehiscence of closure of skull or craniotomy
Disruption or dehiscence of closure of sternum or sternotomy
Disruption or dehiscence of closure of tendon or ligament
Disruption or dehiscence of closure of superficial or muscular fascia
CC Exclusion 7th character A see Appendix A PDX collection 1442

CC X+7th **T81.33 Disruption of traumatic injury wound repair**
Disruption or dehiscence of closure of traumatic laceration (external) (internal)
CC Exclusion 7th character A see Appendix A PDX collection 1442

CC X+7th **T81.4 Infection following a procedure**
Intra-abdominal abscess following a procedure
Postprocedural infection, not elsewhere classified
Sepsis following a procedure
Stitch abscess following a procedure
Subphrenic abscess following a procedure
Wound abscess following a procedure
Use additional code to identify infection
Use additional code (R65.2-) to identify severe sepsis, if applicable
Excludes1: *obstetric surgical wound infection (O86.0)*
postprocedural fever NOS (R50.82)
postprocedural retroperitoneal abscess (K68.11)
Excludes2: *bleb associated endophthalmitis (H59.4-)*
infection due to infusion, transfusion and therapeutic injection (T80.2-)
infection due to prosthetic devices, implants and grafts (T82.6-T82.7, T83.5-T83.6, T84.5-T84.7, T85.7)
CC Exclusion 7th character A see Appendix A PDX collection 0805
HAC 7th character A see Appendix B for HAC conditional logic
AHA CC: 1Q, 2014, 23; 4Q, 2015, 37
Review coding guideline C.1.d.5

+ **T81.5 Complications of foreign body accidentally left in body following procedure**

+ **T81.50 Unspecified complication of foreign body accidentally left in body following procedure**

CC +7th **T81.500 Unspecified complication of foreign body accidentally left in body following surgical operation**
CC Exclusion 7th character A see Appendix A PDX collection 1443
HAC 7th character A see Appendix B for HAC conditional logic

CC +7th **T81.501 Unspecified complication of foreign body accidentally left in body following infusion or transfusion**
CC Exclusion 7th character A see Appendix A PDX collection 1443
HAC 7th character A see Appendix B for HAC conditional logic

CC +7th **T81.502 Unspecified complication of foreign body accidentally left in body following kidney dialysis**
CC Exclusion 7th character A see Appendix A PDX collection 1443
HAC 7th character A see Appendix B for HAC conditional logic

CC +7th **T81.503 Unspecified complication of foreign body accidentally left in body following injection or immunization**
CC Exclusion 7th character A see Appendix A PDX collection 1443
HAC 7th character A see Appendix B for HAC conditional logic

CC +7th **T81.504 Unspecified complication of foreign body accidentally left in body following endoscopic examination**
CC Exclusion 7th character A see Appendix A PDX collection 1443
HAC 7th character A see Appendix B for HAC conditional logic

CC +7th **T81.505 Unspecified complication of foreign body accidentally left in body following heart catheterization**
CC Exclusion 7th character A see Appendix A PDX collection 1443
HAC 7th character A see Appendix B for HAC conditional logic

CC +7th **T81.506 Unspecified complication of foreign body accidentally left in body following aspiration, puncture or other catheterization**
CC Exclusion 7th character A see Appendix A PDX collection 1443
HAC 7th character A see Appendix B for HAC conditional logic

CC +7th **T81.507 Unspecified complication of foreign body accidentally left in body following removal of catheter or packing**
CC Exclusion 7th character A see Appendix A PDX collection 1443
HAC 7th character A see Appendix B for HAC conditional logic

CC +7th **T81.508 Unspecified complication of foreign body accidentally left in body following other procedure**
CC Exclusion 7th character A see Appendix A PDX collection 1443
HAC 7th character A see Appendix B for HAC conditional logic

CC +7th **T81.509 Unspecified complication of foreign body accidentally left in body following unspecified procedure**
CC Exclusion 7th character A see Appendix A PDX collection 1443
HAC 7th character A see Appendix B for HAC conditional logic

+ **T81.51 Adhesions due to foreign body accidentally left in body following procedure**

CC +7th **T81.510 Adhesions due to foreign body accidentally left in body following surgical operation**
CC Exclusion 7th character A see Appendix A PDX collection 1443
HAC 7th character A see Appendix B for HAC conditional logic

CC +7th **T81.511 Adhesions due to foreign body accidentally left in body following infusion or transfusion**
CC Exclusion 7th character A see Appendix A PDX collection 1443
HAC 7th character A see Appendix B for HAC conditional logic

CC +7th **T81.512 Adhesions due to foreign body accidentally left in body following kidney dialysis**
CC Exclusion 7th character A see Appendix A PDX collection 1443
HAC 7th character A see Appendix B for HAC conditional logic

CC +7th **T81.513 Adhesions due to foreign body accidentally left in body following injection or immunization**
CC Exclusion 7th character A see Appendix A PDX collection 1443
HAC 7th character A see Appendix B for HAC conditional logic

CC +7th **T81.514 Adhesions due to foreign body accidentally left in body following endoscopic examination**
CC Exclusion 7th character A see Appendix A PDX collection 1443
HAC 7th character A see Appendix B for HAC conditional logic

CC +7th **T81.515 Adhesions due to foreign body accidentally left in body following heart catheterization**
CC Exclusion 7th character A see Appendix A PDX collection 1443
HAC 7th character A see Appendix B for HAC conditional logic

CC +7th **T81.516 Adhesions due to foreign body accidentally left in body following aspiration, puncture or other catheterization**
CC Exclusion 7th character A see Appendix A PDX collection 1443
HAC 7th character A see Appendix B for HAC conditional logic

CC +7th **T81.517 Adhesions due to foreign body accidentally left in body following removal of catheter or packing**
CC Exclusion 7th character A see Appendix A PDX collection 1443
HAC 7th character A see Appendix B for HAC conditional logic

CC +7th **T81.518 Adhesions due to foreign body accidentally left in body following other procedure**
CC Exclusion 7th character A see Appendix A PDX collection 1443
HAC 7th character A see Appendix B for HAC conditional logic

CC +7th **T81.519** **Adhesions due to foreign body accidentally left in body following unspecified procedure**
CC Exclusion 7th character A see Appendix A
PDX collection 1443
HAC 7th character A see Appendix B for HAC conditional logic

\+ **T81.52** **Obstruction due to foreign body accidentally left in body following procedure**

CC +7th **T81.520** **Obstruction due to foreign body accidentally left in body following surgical operation**
CC Exclusion 7th character A see Appendix A
PDX collection 1443
HAC 7th character A see Appendix B for HAC conditional logic

CC +7th **T81.521** **Obstruction due to foreign body accidentally left in body following infusion or transfusion**
CC Exclusion 7th character A see Appendix A
PDX collection 1443
HAC 7th character A see Appendix B for HAC conditional logic

CC +7th **T81.522** **Obstruction due to foreign body accidentally left in body following kidney dialysis**
CC Exclusion 7th character A see Appendix A
PDX collection 1443
HAC 7th character A see Appendix B for HAC conditional logic

CC +7th **T81.523** **Obstruction due to foreign body accidentally left in body following injection or immunization**
CC Exclusion 7th character A see Appendix A
PDX collection 1443
HAC 7th character A see Appendix B for HAC conditional logic

CC +7th **T81.524** **Obstruction due to foreign body accidentally left in body following endoscopic examination**
CC Exclusion 7th character A see Appendix A
PDX collection 1443
HAC 7th character A see Appendix B for HAC conditional logic

CC +7th **T81.525** **Obstruction due to foreign body accidentally left in body following heart catheterization**
CC Exclusion 7th character A see Appendix A
PDX collection 1443
HAC 7th character A see Appendix B for HAC conditional logic

CC +7th **T81.526** **Obstruction due to foreign body accidentally left in body following aspiration, puncture or other catheterization**
CC Exclusion 7th character A see Appendix A
PDX collection 1443
HAC 7th character A see Appendix B for HAC conditional logic

CC +7th **T81.527** **Obstruction due to foreign body accidentally left in body following removal of catheter or packing**
CC Exclusion 7th character A see Appendix A
PDX collection 1443
HAC 7th character A see Appendix B for HAC conditional logic

CC +7th **T81.528** **Obstruction due to foreign body accidentally left in body following other procedure**
CC Exclusion 7th character A see Appendix A
PDX collection 1443
HAC 7th character A see Appendix B for HAC conditional logic

CC +7th **T81.529** **Obstruction due to foreign body accidentally left in body following unspecified procedure**
CC Exclusion 7th character A see Appendix A
PDX collection 1443
HAC 7th character A see Appendix B for HAC conditional logic

\+ **T81.53** **Perforation due to foreign body accidentally left in body following procedure**

CC +7th **T81.530** **Perforation due to foreign body accidentally left in body following surgical operation**
CC Exclusion 7th character A see Appendix A
PDX collection 1443
HAC 7th character A see Appendix B for HAC conditional logic

CC +7th **T81.531** **Perforation due to foreign body accidentally left in body following infusion or transfusion**
CC Exclusion 7th character A see Appendix A
PDX collection 1443
HAC 7th character A see Appendix B for HAC conditional logic

+7th **T81.532** **Perforation due to foreign body accidentally left in body following kidney dialysis**
CC Exclusion 7th character A see Appendix A
PDX collection 1443
HAC 7th character A see Appendix B for HAC conditional logic

CC +7th **T81.533** **Perforation due to foreign body accidentally left in body following injection or immunization**
CC Exclusion 7th character A see Appendix A
PDX collection 1443
HAC 7th character A see Appendix B for HAC conditional logic

CC +7th **T81.534** **Perforation due to foreign body accidentally left in body following endoscopic examination**
CC Exclusion 7th character A see Appendix A
PDX collection 1443
HAC 7th character A see Appendix B for HAC conditional logic

CC +7th **T81.535** **Perforation due to foreign body accidentally left in body following heart catheterization**
CC Exclusion 7th character A see Appendix A
PDX collection 1443
HAC 7th character A see Appendix B for HAC conditional logic

CC +7th **T81.536** **Perforation due to foreign body accidentally left in body following aspiration, puncture or other catheterization**
CC Exclusion 7th character A see Appendix A
PDX collection 1443
HAC 7th character A see Appendix B for HAC conditional logic

CC +7th **T81.537** **Perforation due to foreign body accidentally left in body following removal of catheter or packing**
CC Exclusion 7th character A see Appendix A
PDX collection 1443
HAC 7th character A see Appendix B for HAC conditional logic

CC +7th **T81.538** **Perforation due to foreign body accidentally left in body following other procedure**
CC Exclusion 7th character A see Appendix A
PDX collection 1443
HAC 7th character A see Appendix B for HAC conditional logic

CC +7th **T81.539** **Perforation due to foreign body accidentally left in body following unspecified procedure**
CC Exclusion 7th character A see Appendix A
PDX collection 1443
HAC 7th character A see Appendix B for HAC conditional logic

\+ **T81.59** **Other complications of foreign body accidentally left in body following procedure**
Excludes2: *obstruction or perforation due to prosthetic devices and implants intentionally left in body (T82.0-T82.5, T83.0-T83.4, T83.7, T84.0-T84.4, T85.0-T85.6)*

CC +7th **T81.590 Other complications of foreign body accidentally left in body following surgical operation**
CC Exclusion 7th character A see Appendix A PDX collection 1443
HAC 7th character A see Appendix B for HAC conditional logic
AHA CC: 4Q, 2014, 24

CC +7th **T81.591 Other complications of foreign body accidentally left in body following infusion or transfusion**
CC Exclusion 7th character A see Appendix A PDX collection 1443
HAC 7th character A see Appendix B for HAC conditional logic

CC +7th **T81.592 Other complications of foreign body accidentally left in body following kidney dialysis**
CC Exclusion 7th character A see Appendix A PDX collection 1443
HAC 7th character A see Appendix B for HAC conditional logic

CC +7th **T81.593 Other complications of foreign body accidentally left in body following injection or immunization**
CC Exclusion 7th character A see Appendix A PDX collection 1443
HAC 7th character A see Appendix B for HAC conditional logic

CC +7th **T81.594 Other complications of foreign body accidentally left in body following endoscopic examination**
CC Exclusion 7th character A see Appendix A PDX collection 1443
HAC 7th character A see Appendix B for HAC conditional logic

CC +7th **T81.595 Other complications of foreign body accidentally left in body following heart catheterization**
CC Exclusion 7th character A see Appendix A PDX collection 1443
HAC 7th character A see Appendix B for HAC conditional logic

CC +7th **T81.596 Other complications of foreign body accidentally left in body following aspiration, puncture or other catheterization**
CC Exclusion 7th character A see Appendix A PDX collection 1443
HAC 7th character A see Appendix B for HAC conditional logic

CC +7th **T81.597 Other complications of foreign body accidentally left in body following removal of catheter or packing**
CC Exclusion 7th character A see Appendix A PDX collection 1443
HAC 7th character A see Appendix B for HAC conditional logic

CC +7th **T81.598 Other complications of foreign body accidentally left in body following other procedure**
CC Exclusion 7th character A see Appendix A PDX collection 1443
HAC 7th character A see Appendix B for HAC conditional logic

CC +7th **T81.599 Other complications of foreign body accidentally left in body following unspecified procedure**
CC Exclusion 7th character A see Appendix A PDX collection 1443
HAC 7th character A see Appendix B for HAC conditional logic

\+ **T81.6 Acute reaction to foreign substance accidentally left during a procedure**
Excludes2: *complications of foreign body accidentally left in body cavity or operation wound following procedure (T81.5-)*

CC X+7th **T81.60 Unspecified acute reaction to foreign substance accidentally left during a procedure**
CC Exclusion 7th character A see Appendix A PDX collection 1444
HAC 7th character A see Appendix B for HAC conditional logic

CC X+7th **T81.61 Aseptic peritonitis due to foreign substance accidentally left during a procedure**
Chemical peritonitis
CC Exclusion 7th character A see Appendix A PDX collection 1444
HAC 7th character A see Appendix B for HAC conditional logic

CC X+7th **T81.69 Other acute reaction to foreign substance accidentally left during a procedure**
CC Exclusion 7th character A see Appendix A PDX collection 1444
HAC 7th character A see Appendix B for HAC conditional logic

\+ **T81.7 Vascular complications following a procedure, not elsewhere classified**
Air embolism following procedure NEC
Phlebitis or thrombophlebitis resulting from a procedure
Excludes1: *embolism complicating abortion or ectopic or molar pregnancy (O00-O07, O08.2)*
embolism complicating pregnancy, childbirth and the puerperium (O88.-)
traumatic embolism (T79.0)
Excludes2: *embolism due to prosthetic devices, implants and grafts (T82.8-, T83.81, T84.8-, T85.81-)*
embolism following infusion, transfusion and therapeutic injection (T80.0)

\+ **T81.71 Complication of artery following a procedure, not elsewhere classified**

CC +7th **T81.710 Complication of mesenteric artery following a procedure, not elsewhere classified**
CC Exclusion 7th character A see Appendix A PDX collection 1445

CC +7th **T81.711 Complication of renal artery following a procedure, not elsewhere classified**
CC Exclusion 7th character A see Appendix A PDX collection 1445

CC +7th **T81.718 Complication of other artery following a procedure, not elsewhere classified**
CC Exclusion 7th character A see Appendix A PDX collection 1446

CC +7th **T81.719 Complication of unspecified artery following a procedure, not elsewhere classified**
CC Exclusion 7th character A see Appendix A PDX collection 1446

CC X+7th **T81.72 Complication of vein following a procedure, not elsewhere classified**
CC Exclusion 7th character A see Appendix A PDX collection 1446

\+ **T81.8 Other complications of procedures, not elsewhere classified**
Excludes2: *hypothermia following anesthesia (T88.51)*
malignant hyperpyrexia due to anesthesia (T88.3)

X+7th **T81.81 Complication of inhalation therapy**

X+7th **T81.82 Emphysema (subcutaneous) resulting from a procedure**

CC X+7th **T81.83 Persistent postprocedural fistula**
CC Exclusion 7th character A see Appendix A PDX collection 1447

X+7th **T81.89 Other complications of procedures, not elsewhere classified**
Use additional code to specify complication, such as: postprocedural delirium (F05)
AHA CC: 1Q, 2014, 23

X+7th **T81.9 Unspecified complication of procedure**

T82 Complications of cardiac and vascular prosthetic devices, implants and grafts
Excludes2: *failure and rejection of transplanted organs and tissue (T86.-)*

The appropriate 7th character is to be added to each code from category T82
A initial encounter
D subsequent encounter
S sequela

\+ **T82.0 Mechanical complication of heart valve prosthesis**
Mechanical complication of artificial heart valve
Excludes1: *mechanical complication of biological heart valve graft (T82.22-)*

CC X+7th **T82.01 Breakdown (mechanical) of heart valve prosthesis**
CC Exclusion 7th character A see Appendix A PDX collection 1448

CC X+7th **T82.02 Displacement of heart valve prosthesis**
Malposition of heart valve prosthesis
CC Exclusion 7th character A see Appendix A PDX collection 1448

CC X+7th **T82.03 Leakage of heart valve prosthesis**
CC Exclusion 7th character A see Appendix A PDX collection 1448

CC X+7th **T82.09 Other mechanical complication of heart valve prosthesis**
Obstruction (mechanical) of heart valve prosthesis
Perforation of heart valve prosthesis
Protrusion of heart valve prosthesis
CC Exclusion 7th character A see Appendix A PDX collection 1448

+ **T82.1 Mechanical complication of cardiac electronic device**

+ **T82.11 Breakdown (mechanical) of cardiac electronic device**

CC +7th **T82.110 Breakdown (mechanical) of cardiac electrode**
CC Exclusion 7th character A see Appendix A PDX collection 1449

CC +7th **T82.111 Breakdown (mechanical) of cardiac pulse generator (battery)**
CC Exclusion 7th character A see Appendix A PDX collection 1449

CC +7th **T82.118 Breakdown (mechanical) of other cardiac electronic device**
CC Exclusion 7th character A see Appendix A PDX collection 1449

CC +7th **T82.119 Breakdown (mechanical) of unspecified cardiac electronic device**
CC Exclusion 7th character A see Appendix A PDX collection 1449

+ **T82.12 Displacement of cardiac electronic device**
Malposition of cardiac electronic device

CC +7th **T82.120 Displacement of cardiac electrode**
CC Exclusion 7th character A see Appendix A PDX collection 1449

CC +7th **T82.121 Displacement of cardiac pulse generator (battery)**
CC Exclusion 7th character A see Appendix A PDX collection 1449

CC +7th **T82.128 Displacement of other cardiac electronic device**
CC Exclusion 7th character A see Appendix A PDX collection 1449

CC +7th **T82.129 Displacement of unspecified cardiac electronic device**
CC Exclusion 7th character A see Appendix A PDX collection 1449

+ **T82.19 Other mechanical complication of cardiac electronic device**
Leakage of cardiac electronic device
Obstruction of cardiac electronic device
Perforation of cardiac electronic device
Protrusion of cardiac electronic device

CC +7th **T82.190 Other mechanical complication of cardiac electrode**
CC Exclusion 7th character A see Appendix A PDX collection 1449

CC +7th **T82.191 Other mechanical complication of cardiac pulse generator (battery)**
CC Exclusion 7th character A see Appendix A PDX collection 1449

CC +7th **T82.198 Other mechanical complication of other cardiac electronic device**
CC Exclusion 7th character A see Appendix A PDX collection 1449

CC +7th **T82.199 Other mechanical complication of unspecified cardiac electronic device**
CC Exclusion 7th character A see Appendix A PDX collection 1449

+ **T82.2 Mechanical complication of coronary artery bypass graft and biological heart valve graft**
Excludes1: *mechanical complication of artificial heart valve prosthesis (T82.0-)*

+ **T82.21 Mechanical complication of coronary artery bypass graft**

CC +7th **T82.211 Breakdown (mechanical) of coronary artery bypass graft**
CC Exclusion 7th character A see Appendix A PDX collection 1450

CC +7th **T82.212 Displacement of coronary artery bypass graft**
Malposition of coronary artery bypass graft
CC Exclusion 7th character A see Appendix A PDX collection 1450

CC +7th **T82.213 Leakage of coronary artery bypass graft**
CC Exclusion 7th character A see Appendix A PDX collection 1450

CC +7th **T82.218 Other mechanical complication of coronary artery bypass graft**
Obstruction, mechanical of coronary artery bypass graft
Perforation of coronary artery bypass graft
Protrusion of coronary artery bypass graft
CC Exclusion 7th character A see Appendix A PDX collection 1450

+ **T82.22 Mechanical complication of biological heart valve graft**

CC +7th **T82.221 Breakdown (mechanical) of biological heart valve graft**
CC Exclusion 7th character A see Appendix A PDX collection 1451

CC +7th **T82.222 Displacement of biological heart valve graft**
Malposition of biological heart valve graft
CC Exclusion 7th character A see Appendix A PDX collection 1451

CC +7th **T82.223 Leakage of biological heart valve graft**
CC Exclusion 7th character A see Appendix A PDX collection 1451

CC +7th **T82.228 Other mechanical complication of biological heart valve graft**
Obstruction of biological heart valve graft
Perforation of biological heart valve graft
Protrusion of biological heart valve graft
CC Exclusion 7th character A see Appendix A PDX collection 1451

+ **T82.3 Mechanical complication of other vascular grafts**

+ **T82.31 Breakdown (mechanical) of other vascular grafts**

CC +7th **T82.310 Breakdown (mechanical) of aortic (bifurcation) graft (replacement)**
CC Exclusion 7th character A see Appendix A PDX collection 1452

CC +7th **T82.311 Breakdown (mechanical) of carotid arterial graft (bypass)**
CC Exclusion 7th character A see Appendix A PDX collection 1452

CC +7th **T82.312 Breakdown (mechanical) of femoral arterial graft (bypass)**
CC Exclusion 7th character A see Appendix A PDX collection 1452

CC +7th **T82.318 Breakdown (mechanical) of other vascular grafts**
CC Exclusion 7th character A see Appendix A PDX collection 1452

CC +7th **T82.319 Breakdown (mechanical) of unspecified vascular grafts**
CC Exclusion 7th character A see Appendix A PDX collection 1452

+ **T82.32 Displacement of other vascular grafts**
Malposition of other vascular grafts

CC +7th **T82.320 Displacement of aortic (bifurcation) graft (replacement)**
CC Exclusion 7th character A see Appendix A PDX collection 1452

CC +7th **T82.321 Displacement of carotid arterial graft (bypass)**
CC Exclusion 7th character A see Appendix A PDX collection 1452

CC +7th **T82.322 Displacement of femoral arterial graft (bypass)**
CC Exclusion 7th character A see Appendix A PDX collection 1452

CC +7th **T82.328 Displacement of other vascular grafts**
CC Exclusion 7th character A see Appendix A PDX collection 1452

CC +7th **T82.329 Displacement of unspecified vascular grafts**
CC Exclusion 7th character A see Appendix A
PDX collection 1452

+ **T82.33 Leakage of other vascular grafts**

CC +7th **T82.330 Leakage of aortic (bifurcation) graft (replacement)**
CC Exclusion 7th character A see Appendix A
PDX collection 1452

CC +7th **T82.331 Leakage of carotid arterial graft (bypass)**
CC Exclusion 7th character A see Appendix A
PDX collection 1452

CC +7th **T82.332 Leakage of femoral arterial graft (bypass)**
CC Exclusion 7th character A see Appendix A
PDX collection 1452

CC +7th **T82.338 Leakage of other vascular grafts**
CC Exclusion 7th character A see Appendix A
PDX collection 1452

CC +7th **T82.339 Leakage of unspecified vascular graft**
CC Exclusion 7th character A see Appendix A
PDX collection 1452

+ **T82.39 Other mechanical complication of other vascular grafts**
Obstruction (mechanical) of other vascular grafts
Perforation of other vascular grafts
Protrusion of other vascular grafts

CC +7th **T82.390 Other mechanical complication of aortic (bifurcation) graft (replacement)**
CC Exclusion 7th character A see Appendix A
PDX collection 1452

CC +7th **T82.391 Other mechanical complication of carotid arterial graft (bypass)**
CC Exclusion 7th character A see Appendix A
PDX collection 1452

CC +7th **T82.392 Other mechanical complication of femoral arterial graft (bypass)**
CC Exclusion 7th character A see Appendix A
PDX collection 1452

CC +7th **T82.398 Other mechanical complication of other vascular grafts**
CC Exclusion 7th character A see Appendix A
PDX collection 1452

CC +7th **T82.399 Other mechanical complication of unspecified vascular grafts**
CC Exclusion 7th character A see Appendix A
PDX collection 1452

+ **T82.4 Mechanical complication of vascular dialysis catheter**
Mechanical complication of hemodialysis catheter
Excludes1: *mechanical complication of intraperitoneal dialysis catheter (T85.62)*

CC X+7th **T82.41 Breakdown (mechanical) of vascular dialysis catheter**
CC Exclusion 7th character A see Appendix A PDX collection 1452

CC X+7th **T82.42 Displacement of vascular dialysis catheter**
Malposition of vascular dialysis catheter
CC Exclusion 7th character A see Appendix A PDX collection 1452

CC X+7th **T82.43 Leakage of vascular dialysis catheter**
CC Exclusion 7th character A see Appendix A PDX collection 1452

CC X+7th **T82.49 Other complication of vascular dialysis catheter**
Obstruction (mechanical) of vascular dialysis catheter
Perforation of vascular dialysis catheter
Protrusion of vascular dialysis catheter
CC Exclusion 7th character A see Appendix A PDX collection 1452

+ **T82.5 Mechanical complication of other cardiac and vascular devices and implants**
Excludes2: *mechanical complication of epidural and subdural infusion catheter (T85.61)*

+ **T82.51 Breakdown (mechanical) of other cardiac and vascular devices and implants**

CC +7th **T82.510 Breakdown (mechanical) of surgically created arteriovenous fistula**
CC Exclusion 7th character A see Appendix A
PDX collection 1452

CC +7th **T82.511 Breakdown (mechanical) of surgically created arteriovenous shunt**
CC Exclusion 7th character A see Appendix A
PDX collection 1452

CC +7th **T82.512 Breakdown (mechanical) of artificial heart**
CC Exclusion 7th character A see Appendix A
PDX collection 1452

CC +7th **T82.513 Breakdown (mechanical) of balloon (counterpulsation) device**
CC Exclusion 7th character A see Appendix A
PDX collection 1451

CC +7th **T82.514 Breakdown (mechanical) of infusion catheter**
CC Exclusion 7th character A see Appendix A
PDX collection 1452

CC +7th **T82.515 Breakdown (mechanical) of umbrella device**
CC Exclusion 7th character A see Appendix A
PDX collection 1452

CC +7th **T82.518 Breakdown (mechanical) of other cardiac and vascular devices and implants**
CC Exclusion 7th character A see Appendix A
PDX collection 1452

CC +7th **T82.519 Breakdown (mechanical) of unspecified cardiac and vascular devices and implants**
CC Exclusion 7th character A see Appendix A
PDX collection 1453

+ **T82.52 Displacement of other cardiac and vascular devices and implants**
Malposition of other cardiac and vascular devices and implants

CC +7th **T82.520 Displacement of surgically created arteriovenous fistula**
CC Exclusion 7th character A see Appendix A
PDX collection 1452

CC +7th **T82.521 Displacement of surgically created arteriovenous shunt**
CC Exclusion 7th character A see Appendix A
PDX collection 1452

CC +7th **T82.522 Displacement of artificial heart**
CC Exclusion 7th character A see Appendix A
PDX collection 1451

CC +7th **T82.523 Displacement of balloon (counterpulsation) device**
CC Exclusion 7th character A see Appendix A
PDX collection 1452

CC +7th **T82.524 Displacement of infusion catheter**
CC Exclusion 7th character A see Appendix A
PDX collection 1452

CC +7th **T82.525 Displacement of umbrella device**
CC Exclusion 7th character A see Appendix A
PDX collection 1452

CC +7th **T82.528 Displacement of other cardiac and vascular devices and implants**
CC Exclusion 7th character A see Appendix A
PDX collection 1452

CC +7th **T82.529 Displacement of unspecified cardiac and vascular devices and implants**
CC Exclusion 7th character A see Appendix A
PDX collection 1452

+ **T82.53 Leakage of other cardiac and vascular devices and implants**

CC +7th **T82.530 Leakage of surgically created arteriovenous fistula**
CC Exclusion 7th character A see Appendix A
PDX collection 1452

CC +7th **T82.531 Leakage of surgically created arteriovenous shunt**
CC Exclusion 7th character A see Appendix A
PDX collection 1452

CC +7th **T82.532 Leakage of artificial heart**
CC Exclusion 7th character A see Appendix A
PDX collection 1451

CC +7th **T82.533 Leakage of balloon (counterpulsation) device**
CC Exclusion 7th character A see Appendix A
PDX collection 1452

CC +7th **T82.534 Leakage of infusion catheter**
CC Exclusion 7th character A see Appendix A
PDX collection 1452

CC +7th **T82.535 Leakage of umbrella device**
CC Exclusion 7th character A see Appendix A
PDX collection 1452

CC +7th **T82.538 Leakage of other cardiac and vascular devices and implants**
CC Exclusion 7th character A see Appendix A
PDX collection 1452

CC +7th **T82.539 Leakage of unspecified cardiac and vascular devices and implants**
CC Exclusion 7th character A see Appendix A PDX collection 1453

\+ **T82.59 Other mechanical complication of other cardiac and vascular devices and implants**
Obstruction (mechanical) of other cardiac and vascular devices and implants
Perforation of other cardiac and vascular devices and implants
Protrusion of other cardiac and vascular devices and implants

CC +7th **T82.590 Other mechanical complication of surgically created arteriovenous fistula**
CC Exclusion 7th character A see Appendix A PDX collection 1452

CC +7th **T82.591 Other mechanical complication of surgically created arteriovenous shunt**
CC Exclusion 7th character A see Appendix A PDX collection 1452

CC +7th **T82.592 Other mechanical complication of artificial heart**
CC Exclusion 7th character A see Appendix A PDX collection 1451

CC +7th **T82.593 Other mechanical complication of balloon (counterpulsation) device**
CC Exclusion 7th character A see Appendix A PDX collection 1452

CC +7th **T82.594 Other mechanical complication of infusion catheter**
CC Exclusion 7th character A see Appendix A PDX collection 1451

CC +7th **T82.595 Other mechanical complication of umbrella device**
CC Exclusion 7th character A see Appendix A PDX collection 1452

CC +7th **T82.598 Other mechanical complication of other cardiac and vascular devices and implants**
CC Exclusion 7th character A see Appendix A PDX collection 1451

CC +7th **T82.599 Other mechanical complication of unspecified cardiac and vascular devices and implants**
CC Exclusion 7th character A see Appendix A PDX collection 1453

C X+7th **T82.6 Infection and inflammatory reaction due to cardiac valve prosthesis**
Use additional code to identify infection
CC Exclusion 7th character A see Appendix A PDX collection 1454
HAC 7th character A see Appendix B for HAC conditional logic

C X+7th **T82.7 Infection and inflammatory reaction due to other cardiac and vascular devices, implants and grafts**
Use additional code to identify infection
CC Exclusion 7th character A see Appendix A PDX collection 1454
HAC 7th character A see Appendix B for HAC conditional logic
AHA CC: 1Q, 2015, 3-21

\+ **T82.8 Other specified complications due to cardiac and vascular prosthetic devices, implants and grafts**

\+ **T82.81 Embolism due to cardiac and vascular prosthetic devices, implants and grafts**

CC +7th **T82.817 Embolism due to cardiac prosthetic devices, implants and grafts**
CC Exclusion 7th character A see Appendix A PDX collection 1455

CC +7th **T82.818 Embolism due to vascular prosthetic devices, implants and grafts**
CC Exclusion 7th character A see Appendix A PDX collection 1454

\+ **T82.82 Fibrosis due to cardiac and vascular prosthetic devices, implants and grafts**

CC +7th **T82.827 Fibrosis due to cardiac prosthetic devices, implants and grafts**
CC Exclusion 7th character A see Appendix A PDX collection 1455

CC +7th **T82.828 Fibrosis due to vascular prosthetic devices, implants and grafts**
CC Exclusion 7th character A see Appendix A PDX collection 1454

\+ **T82.83 Hemorrhage due to cardiac and vascular prosthetic devices, implants and grafts**

CC +7th **T82.837 Hemorrhage due to cardiac prosthetic devices, implants and grafts**
CC Exclusion 7th character A see Appendix A PDX collection 1455

CC +7th **T82.838 Hemorrhage due to vascular prosthetic devices, implants and grafts**
CC Exclusion 7th character A see Appendix A PDX collection 1454

\+ **T82.84 Pain due to cardiac and vascular prosthetic devices, implants and grafts**

CC +7th **T82.847 Pain due to cardiac prosthetic devices, implants and grafts**
CC Exclusion 7th character A see Appendix A PDX collection 1455

CC +7th **T82.848 Pain due to vascular prosthetic devices, implants and grafts**
CC Exclusion 7th character A see Appendix A PDX collection 1454

\+ **T82.85 Stenosis due to cardiac and vascular prosthetic devices, implants and grafts**

CC +7th **T82.855 Stenosis of coronary artery stent**
In-stent stenosis (restenosis) of coronary artery stent
Restenosis of coronary artery stent
CC Exclusion 7th character A see Appendix A PDX collection 1455
AHA CC: 4Q, 2016, 69

CC +7th **T82.856 Stenosis of peripheral vascular stent**
In-stent stenosis (restenosis) of peripheral vascular stent
Restenosis of peripheral vascular stent
CC Exclusion 7th character A see Appendix A PDX collection 1456
AHA CC: 4Q, 2016, 69

CC +7th **T82.857 Stenosis of other cardiac prosthetic devices, implants and grafts**
CC Exclusion 7th character A see Appendix A PDX collection 1455

CC +7th **T82.858 Stenosis of other vascular prosthetic devices, implants and grafts**
CC Exclusion 7th character A see Appendix A PDX collection 1454

\+ **T82.86 Thrombosis due to cardiac and vascular prosthetic devices, implants and grafts**

CC +7th **T82.867 Thrombosis due to cardiac prosthetic devices, implants and grafts**
CC Exclusion 7th character A see Appendix A PDX collection 1455

CC +7th **T82.868 Thrombosis due to vascular prosthetic devices, implants and grafts**
CC Exclusion 7th character A see Appendix A PDX collection 1454

\+ **T82.89 Other specified complication of cardiac and vascular prosthetic devices, implants and grafts**

CC +7th **T82.897 Other specified complication of cardiac prosthetic devices, implants and grafts**
CC Exclusion 7th character A see Appendix A PDX collection 1455

CC +7th **T82.898 Other specified complication of vascular prosthetic devices, implants and grafts**
CC Exclusion 7th character A see Appendix A PDX collection 1454

CC X+7th **T82.9 Unspecified complication of cardiac and vascular prosthetic device, implant and graft**
CC Exclusion 7th character A see Appendix A PDX collection 1455

T83 Complications of genitourinary prosthetic devices, implants and grafts

Excludes2: *failure and rejection of transplanted organs and tissue (T86.-)*
AHA CC: 4Q, 2016, 70-71

The appropriate 7th character is to be added to each code from category T83
A initial encounter
D subsequent encounter
S sequela

\+ **T83.0 Mechanical complication of urinary catheter**
Excludes2: *complications of stoma of urinary tract (N99.5-)*

\+ **T83.01 Breakdown (mechanical) of urinary catheter**

CC +7th **T83.010 Breakdown (mechanical) of cystostomy catheter**
CC Exclusion 7th character A see Appendix A PDX collection 1456

+7th **T83.011 Breakdown (mechanical) of indwelling urethral catheter**

+7th **T83.012 Breakdown (mechanical) of nephrostomy catheter**

+7th **T83.018 Breakdown (mechanical) of other urinary catheter**
Breakdown (mechanical) of Hopkins catheter
Breakdown (mechanical) of ileostomy catheter
Breakdown (mechanical) of urostomy catheter

+ **T83.02 Displacement of urinary catheter**
Malposition of urinary catheter

CC +7th **T83.020 Displacement of cystostomy catheter**
CC Exclusion 7th character A see Appendix A
PDX collection 1456

+7th **T83.021 Displacement of indwelling urethral catheter**

+7th **T83.022 Displacement of nephrostomy catheter**

+7th **T83.028 Displacement of other urinary catheter**
Displacement of Hopkins catheter
Displacement of ileostomy catheter
Displacement of urostomy catheter

+ **T83.03 Leakage of urinary catheter**

CC +7th **T83.030 Leakage of cystostomy catheter**
CC Exclusion 7th character A see Appendix A
PDX collection 1456

+7th **T83.031 Leakage of indwelling urethral catheter**

+7th **T83.032 Leakage of nephrostomy catheter**

+7th **T83.038 Leakage of other urinary catheter**
Leakage of Hopkins catheter
Leakage of ileostomy catheter
Leakage of urostomy catheter

+ **T83.09 Other mechanical complication of urinary catheter**
Obstruction (mechanical) of urinary catheter
Perforation of urinary catheter
Protrusion of urinary catheter

CC +7th **T83.090 Other mechanical complication of cystostomy catheter**
CC Exclusion 7th character A see Appendix A
PDX collection 1456

+7th **T83.091 Other mechanical complication of indwelling urethral catheter**

+7th **T83.092 Other mechanical complication of nephrostomy catheter**

+7th **T83.098 Other mechanical complication of other urinary catheter**
Other mechanical complication of Hopkins catheter
Other mechanical complication of ileostomy catheter
Other mechanical complication of urostomy catheter

+ **T83.1 Mechanical complication of other urinary devices and implants**

+ **T83.11 Breakdown (mechanical) of other urinary devices and implants**

CC +7th **T83.110 Breakdown (mechanical) of urinary electronic stimulator device**
Excludes2: *breakdown (mechanical) of electrode (lead) for sacral nerve neurostimulator (T85.111)*
breakdown (mechanical) of implanted electronic sacral neurostimulator, pulse generator or receiver (T85.113)
CC Exclusion 7th character A see Appendix A
PDX collection 1456

CC +7th **T83.111 Breakdown (mechanical) of implanted urinary sphincter**
CC Exclusion 7th character A see Appendix A
PDX collection 1456

CC +7th **T83.112 Breakdown (mechanical) of indwelling ureteral stent**
CC Exclusion 7th character A see Appendix A
PDX collection 1456

CC +7th **T83.113 Breakdown (mechanical) of other urinary stents**
Breakdown (mechanical) of ileal conduit stent
Breakdown (mechanical) of nephroureteral stent
CC Exclusion 7th character A see Appendix A
PDX collection 1456

CC +7th **T83.118 Breakdown (mechanical) of other urinary devices and implants**
CC Exclusion 7th character A see Appendix A
PDX collection 1456

+ **T83.12 Displacement of other urinary devices and implants**
Malposition of other urinary devices and implants

CC +7th **T83.120 Displacement of urinary electronic stimulator device**
Excludes2: *displacement of electrode (lead) for sacral nerve neurostimulator (T85.121)*
displacement of implanted electronic sacral neurostimulator, pulse generator or receiver (T85.123)
CC Exclusion 7th character A see Appendix A
PDX collection 1456

CC +7th **T83.121 Displacement of implanted urinary sphincter**
CC Exclusion 7th character A see Appendix A
PDX collection 1456

CC +7th **T83.122 Displacement of indwelling ureteral stent**
CC Exclusion 7th character A see Appendix A
PDX collection 1456

CC +7th **T83.123 Displacement of other urinary stents**
Displacement of ileal conduit stent
Displacement of nephroureteral stent
CC Exclusion 7th character A see Appendix A
PDX collection 1456

CC +7th **T83.128 Displacement of other urinary devices and implants**
CC Exclusion 7th character A see Appendix A
PDX collection 1456

+ **T83.19 Other mechanical complication of other urinary devices and implants**
Leakage of other urinary devices and implants
Obstruction (mechanical) of other urinary devices and implants
Perforation of other urinary devices and implants
Protrusion of other urinary devices and implants

CC +7th **T83.190 Other mechanical complication of urinary electronic stimulator device**
Excludes2: *other mechanical complication of electrode (lead) for sacral nerve neurostimulator (T85.191)*
other mechanical complication of implanted electronic sacral neurostimulator, pulse generator or receiver (T85.193)
CC Exclusion 7th character A see Appendix A
PDX collection 1456

CC +7th **T83.191 Other mechanical complication of implanted urinary sphincter**
CC Exclusion 7th character A see Appendix A
PDX collection 1456

CC +7th **T83.192 Other mechanical complication of indwelling ureteral stent**
CC Exclusion 7th character A see Appendix A
PDX collection 1456

CC +7th **T83.193 Other mechanical complication of other urinary stent**
Other mechanical complication of ileal conduit stent
Other mechanical complication of nephroureteral stent
CC Exclusion 7th character A see Appendix A
PDX collection 1456

CC +7th **T83.198 Other mechanical complication of other urinary devices and implants**
CC Exclusion 7th character A see Appendix A
PDX collection 1456

+ **T83.2 Mechanical complication of graft of urinary organ**

CC X+7th **T83.21 Breakdown (mechanical) of graft of urinary organ**
CC Exclusion 7th character A see Appendix A PDX collection 1456

CC X+7th **T83.22 Displacement of graft of urinary organ**
Malposition of graft of urinary organ
CC Exclusion 7th character A see Appendix A PDX collection 1456

CC X+7th **T83.23 Leakage of graft of urinary organ**
CC Exclusion 7th character A see Appendix A PDX collection 1456

CC X+7th **T83.24 Erosion of graft of urinary organ**
CC Exclusion 7th character A see Appendix A PDX collection 1456

CC X+7th **T83.25** **Exposure of graft of urinary organ**
CC Exclusion 7th character A see Appendix A PDX collection 1456

CC X+7th **T83.29** **Other mechanical complication of graft of urinary organ**
Obstruction (mechanical) of graft of urinary organ
Perforation of graft of urinary organ
Protrusion of graft of urinary organ
CC Exclusion 7th character A see Appendix A PDX collection 1456

\+ **T83.3** **Mechanical complication of intrauterine contraceptive device**

♀ X+7th **T83.31** **Breakdown (mechanical) of intrauterine contraceptive device**

♀ X+7th **T83.32** **Displacement of intrauterine contraceptive device**
Malposition of intrauterine contraceptive device
Missing string of intrauterine contraceptive device

♀ X+7th **T83.39** **Other mechanical complication of intrauterine contraceptive device**
Leakage of intrauterine contraceptive device
Obstruction (mechanical) of intrauterine contraceptive device
Perforation of intrauterine contraceptive device
Protrusion of intrauterine contraceptive device

\+ **T83.4** **Mechanical complication of other prosthetic devices, implants and grafts of genital tract**

\+ **T83.41** **Breakdown (mechanical) of other prosthetic devices, implants and grafts of genital tract**

♂ CC +7th **T83.410** **Breakdown (mechanical) of implanted penile prosthesis**
Breakdown (mechanical) of penile prosthesis cylinder
Breakdown (mechanical) of penile prosthesis pump
Breakdown (mechanical) of penile prosthesis reservoir
CC Exclusion 7th character A see Appendix A PDX collection 1456

CC +7th **T83.411** **Breakdown (mechanical) of implanted testicular prosthesis**
CC Exclusion 7th character A see Appendix A PDX collection 1456

CC +7th **T83.418** **Breakdown (mechanical) of other prosthetic devices, implants and grafts of genital tract**
CC Exclusion 7th character A see Appendix A PDX collection 1456

\+ **T83.42** **Displacement of other prosthetic devices, implants and grafts of genital tract**
Malposition of other prosthetic devices, implants and grafts of genital tract

♂ CC +7th **T83.420** **Displacement of implanted penile prosthesis**
Displacement of penile prosthesis cylinder
Displacement of penile prosthesis pump
Displacement of penile prosthesis reservoir
CC Exclusion 7th character A see Appendix A PDX collection 1456

CC +7th **T83.421** **Displacement of implanted testicular prosthesis**
CC Exclusion 7th character A see Appendix A PDX collection 1456

CC +7th **T83.428** **Displacement of other prosthetic devices, implants and grafts of genital tract**
CC Exclusion 7th character A see Appendix A PDX collection 1456

\+ **T83.49** **Other mechanical complication of other prosthetic devices, implants and grafts of genital tract**
Leakage of other prosthetic devices, implants and grafts of genital tract
Obstruction, mechanical of other prosthetic devices, implants and grafts of genital tract
Perforation of other prosthetic devices, implants and grafts of genital tract
Protrusion of other prosthetic devices, implants and grafts of genital tract

♂ CC +7th **T83.490** **Other mechanical complication of implanted penile prosthesis**
Other mechanical complication of penile prosthesis cylinder
Other mechanical complication of penile prosthesis pump
Other mechanical complication of penile prosthesis reservoir
CC Exclusion 7th character A see Appendix A PDX collection 1456

CC +7th **T83.491** **Other mechanical complication of implanted testicular prosthesis**
CC Exclusion 7th character A see Appendix A PDX collection 1456

CC +7th **T83.498** **Other mechanical complication of other prosthetic devices, implants and grafts of genital tract**
CC Exclusion 7th character A see Appendix A PDX collection 1456

\+ **T83.5** **Infection and inflammatory reaction due to prosthetic device, implant and graft in urinary system**
Use additional code to identify infection

\+ **T83.51** **Infection and inflammatory reaction due to urinary catheter**
Excludes2: *complications of stoma of urinary tract (N99.5-)*

CC +7th **T83.510** **Infection and inflammatory reaction due to cystostomy catheter**
CC Exclusion 7th character A see Appendix A PDX collection 1458

CC +7th **T83.511** **Infection and inflammatory reaction due to indwelling urethral catheter**
CC Exclusion 7th character A see Appendix A PDX collection 1457
HAC 7th character A see Appendix B for HAC conditional logic

CC +7th **T83.512** **Infection and inflammatory reaction due to nephrostomy catheter**
CC Exclusion 7th character A see Appendix A PDX collection 1458

CC +7th **T83.518** **Infection and inflammatory reaction due to other urinary catheter**
Infection and inflammatory reaction due to Hopkins catheter
Infection and inflammatory reaction due to ileostomy catheter
Infection and inflammatory reaction due to urostomy catheter
CC Exclusion 7th character A see Appendix A PDX collection 1458
HAC 7th character A see Appendix B for HAC conditional logic

\+ **T83.59** **Infection and inflammatory reaction due to prosthetic device, implant and graft in urinary system**

CC +7th **T83.590** **Infection and inflammatory reaction due to implanted urinary neurostimulation device**
Excludes2: *infection and inflammatory reaction due to electrode lead of sacral nerve neurostimulator (T85.732)*
infection and inflammatory reaction due to pulse generator or receiver of sacral nerve neurostimulator (T85.734)
CC Exclusion 7th character A see Appendix A PDX collection 1458

CC +7th **T83.591** **Infection and inflammatory reaction due to implanted urinary sphincter**
CC Exclusion 7th character A see Appendix A PDX collection 1458

CC +7th **T83.592** **Infection and inflammatory reaction due to indwelling ureteral stent**
CC Exclusion 7th character A see Appendix A PDX collection 1458

CC +7th **T83.593** **Infection and inflammatory reaction due to other urinary stents**
Infection and inflammatory reaction due to ileal conduit stents
Infection and inflammatory reaction due to nephroureteral stent
CC Exclusion 7th character A see Appendix A PDX collection 1458

CC +7th **T83.598 Infection and inflammatory reaction due to other prosthetic device, implant and graft in urinary system**
CC Exclusion 7th character A see Appendix A PDX collection 1458

+ **T83.6 Infection and inflammatory reaction due to prosthetic device, implant and graft in genital tract**
Use additional code to identify infection

CC X+7th **T83.61 Infection and inflammatory reaction due to implanted penile prosthesis**
Infection and inflammatory reaction due to penile prosthesis cylinder
Infection and inflammatory reaction due to penile prosthesis pump
Infection and inflammatory reaction due to penile prosthesis reservoir
CC Exclusion 7th character A see Appendix A PDX collection 1458

CC X+7th **T83.62 Infection and inflammatory reaction due to implanted testicular prosthesis**
CC Exclusion 7th character A see Appendix A PDX collection 1458

CC X+7th **T83.69 Infection and inflammatory reaction due to other prosthetic device, implant and graft in genital tract**
CC Exclusion 7th character A see Appendix A PDX collection 1458

+ **T83.7 Complications due to implanted mesh and other prosthetic materials**

+ **T83.71 Erosion of implanted mesh and other prosthetic materials to surrounding organ or tissue**

♀ +7th **T83.711 Erosion of implanted vaginal mesh to surrounding organ or tissue**
Erosion of implanted vaginal mesh into pelvic floor muscles

CC +7th **T83.712 Erosion of implanted urethral mesh to surrounding organ or tissue**
Erosion of implanted female urethral sling
Erosion of implanted male urethral sling
Erosion of implanted urethral mesh into pelvic floor muscles
CC Exclusion 7th character A see Appendix A PDX collection 1456

CC +7th **T83.713 Erosion of implanted urethral bulking agent to surrounding organ or tissue**
CC Exclusion 7th character A see Appendix A PDX collection 1456

CC +7th **T83.714 Erosion of implanted ureteral bulking agent to surrounding organ or tissue**
CC Exclusion 7th character A see Appendix A PDX collection 1456

CC +7th **T83.718 Erosion of other implanted mesh to organ or tissue**
CC Exclusion 7th character A see Appendix A PDX collection 1456

CC +7th **T83.719 Erosion of other prosthetic materials to surrounding organ or tissue**
CC Exclusion 7th character A see Appendix A PDX collection 1456

+ **T83.72 Exposure of implanted mesh and other prosthetic materials into surrounding organ or tissue**
Extrusion of implanted mesh

♀ +7th **T83.721 Exposure of implanted vaginal mesh into vagina**
Exposure of implanted vaginal mesh through vaginal wall

CC +7th **T83.722 Exposure of implanted urethral mesh into urethra**
Exposure of implanted female urethral sling
Exposure of implanted male urethral sling
Exposure of implanted urethral mesh through urethral wall
CC Exclusion 7th character A see Appendix A PDX collection 1456

CC +7th **T83.723 Exposure of implanted urethral bulking agent into urethra**
CC Exclusion 7th character A see Appendix A PDX collection 1456

CC +7th **T83.724 Exposure of implanted ureteral bulking agent into ureter**
CC Exclusion 7th character A see Appendix A PDX collection 1456

CC +7th **T83.728 Exposure of other implanted mesh into organ or tissue**
CC Exclusion 7th character A see Appendix A PDX collection 1456

CC +7th **T83.729 Exposure of other prosthetic materials into organ or tissue**
CC Exclusion 7th character A see Appendix A PDX collection 1456

CC X+7th **T83.79 Other specified complications due to other genitourinary prosthetic materials**
CC Exclusion 7th character A see Appendix A PDX collection 1456

+ **T83.8 Other specified complications of genitourinary prosthetic devices, implants and grafts**

CC X+7th **T83.81 Embolism due to genitourinary prosthetic devices, implants and grafts**
CC Exclusion 7th character A see Appendix A PDX collection 1458

CC X+7th **T83.82 Fibrosis due to genitourinary prosthetic devices, implants and grafts**
CC Exclusion 7th character A see Appendix A PDX collection 1458

CC X+7th **T83.83 Hemorrhage due to genitourinary prosthetic devices, implants and grafts**
CC Exclusion 7th character A see Appendix A PDX collection 1458

CC X+7th **T83.84 Pain due to genitourinary prosthetic devices, implants and grafts**
CC Exclusion 7th character A see Appendix A PDX collection 1458

CC X+7th **T83.85 Stenosis due to genitourinary prosthetic devices, implants and grafts**
CC Exclusion 7th character A see Appendix A PDX collection 1458

CC X+7th **T83.86 Thrombosis due to genitourinary prosthetic devices, implants and grafts**
CC Exclusion 7th character A see Appendix A PDX collection 1458

CC X+7th **T83.89 Other specified complication of genitourinary prosthetic devices, implants and grafts**
CC Exclusion 7th character A see Appendix A PDX collection 1458

CC X+7th **T83.9 Unspecified complication of genitourinary prosthetic device, implant and graft**
CC Exclusion 7th character A see Appendix A PDX collection 1458

T84 Complications of internal orthopedic prosthetic devices, implants and grafts

Excludes2: *failure and rejection of transplanted organs and tissues (T86.-)*
fracture of bone following insertion of orthopedic implant, joint prosthesis or bone plate (M96.6)

The appropriate 7th character is to be added to each code from category T84
A initial encounter
D subsequent encounter
S sequela

+ **T84.0 Mechanical complication of internal joint prosthesis**

+ **T84.01 Broken internal joint prosthesis**
Breakage (fracture) of prosthetic joint
Broken prosthetic joint implant
Excludes1: *periprosthetic joint implant fracture (M97.-)*

CC +7th **T84.010 Broken internal right hip prosthesis**
CC Exclusion 7th character A see Appendix A PDX collection 0911

CC +7th **T84.011 Broken internal left hip prosthesis**
CC Exclusion 7th character A see Appendix A PDX collection 0911

CC +7th **T84.012 Broken internal right knee prosthesis**
CC Exclusion 7th character A see Appendix A PDX collection 0911

CC +7th **T84.013 Broken internal left knee prosthesis**
CC Exclusion 7th character A see Appendix A PDX collection 0911

CC +7th **T84.018 Broken internal joint prosthesis, other site**
Use additional code to identify the joint (Z96.6-)
CC Exclusion 7th character A see Appendix A PDX collection 0911

CC +7th **T84.019 Broken internal joint prosthesis, unspecified site**
CC Exclusion 7th character A see Appendix A PDX collection 0911

+ T84.02 **Dislocation of internal joint prosthesis**
Instability of internal joint prosthesis
Subluxation of internal joint prosthesis

CC +7th **T84.020** **Dislocation of internal right hip prosthesis**
CC Exclusion 7th character A see Appendix A
PDX collection 0911

CC +7th **T84.021** **Dislocation of internal left hip prosthesis**
CC Exclusion 7th character A see Appendix A
PDX collection 0911

CC +7th **T84.022** **Instability of internal right knee prosthesis**
CC Exclusion 7th character A see Appendix A
PDX collection 0911

CC +7th **T84.023** **Instability of internal left knee prosthesis**
CC Exclusion 7th character A see Appendix A
PDX collection 0911

CC +7th **T84.028** **Dislocation of other internal joint prosthesis**
Use additional code to identify the joint (Z96.6-)
CC Exclusion 7th character A see Appendix A
PDX collection 0911

CC +7th **T84.029** **Dislocation of unspecified internal joint prosthesis**
CC Exclusion 7th character A see Appendix A
PDX collection 0911

+ T84.03 **Mechanical loosening of internal prosthetic joint**
Aseptic loosening of prosthetic joint

CC +7th **T84.030** **Mechanical loosening of internal right hip prosthetic joint**
CC Exclusion 7th character A see Appendix A
PDX collection 0911

CC +7th **T84.031** **Mechanical loosening of internal left hip prosthetic joint**
CC Exclusion 7th character A see Appendix A
PDX collection 0911

CC +7th **T84.032** **Mechanical loosening of internal right knee prosthetic joint**
CC Exclusion 7th character A see Appendix A
PDX collection 0911

CC +7th **T84.033** **Mechanical loosening of internal left knee prosthetic joint**
CC Exclusion 7th character A see Appendix A
PDX collection 0911

CC +7th **T84.038** **Mechanical loosening of other internal prosthetic joint**
Use additional code to identify the joint (Z96.6-)
CC Exclusion 7th character A see Appendix A
PDX collection 0911

CC +7th **T84.039** **Mechanical loosening of unspecified internal prosthetic joint**
CC Exclusion 7th character A see Appendix A
PDX collection 0911

+ T84.05 **Periprosthetic osteolysis of internal prosthetic joint**
Use additional code to identify major osseous defect, if applicable (M89.7-)
CC Exclusion 7th character A see Appendix A
PDX collection 0911

CC +7th **T84.050** **Periprosthetic osteolysis of internal prosthetic right hip joint**
CC Exclusion 7th character A see Appendix A
PDX collection 0911

CC +7th **T84.051** **Periprosthetic osteolysis of internal prosthetic left hip joint**
CC Exclusion 7th character A see Appendix A
PDX collection 0911

CC +7th **T84.052** **Periprosthetic osteolysis of internal prosthetic right knee joint**
CC Exclusion 7th character A see Appendix A
PDX collection 0911

CC +7th **T84.053** **Periprosthetic osteolysis of internal prosthetic left knee joint**
CC Exclusion 7th character A see Appendix A
PDX collection 0911

CC +7th **T84.058** **Periprosthetic osteolysis of other internal prosthetic joint**
Use additional code to identify the joint (Z96.6-)
CC Exclusion 7th character A see Appendix A
PDX collection 0911

CC +7th **T84.059** **Periprosthetic osteolysis of unspecified internal prosthetic joint**
CC Exclusion 7th character A see Appendix A
PDX collection 0911

+ T84.06 **Wear of articular bearing surface of internal prosthetic joint**

CC +7th **T84.060** **Wear of articular bearing surface of internal prosthetic right hip joint**
CC Exclusion 7th character A see Appendix A
PDX collection 0911

CC +7th **T84.061** **Wear of articular bearing surface of internal prosthetic left hip joint**
CC Exclusion 7th character A see Appendix A
PDX collection 0911

CC +7th **T84.062** **Wear of articular bearing surface of internal prosthetic right knee joint**
CC Exclusion 7th character A see Appendix A
PDX collection 0911

CC +7th **T84.063** **Wear of articular bearing surface of internal prosthetic left knee joint**
CC Exclusion 7th character A see Appendix A
PDX collection 0911

CC +7th **T84.068** **Wear of articular bearing surface of other internal prosthetic joint**
Use additional code to identify the joint (Z96.6-)
CC Exclusion 7th character A see Appendix A
PDX collection 0911

CC +7th **T84.069** **Wear of articular bearing surface of unspecified internal prosthetic joint**
CC Exclusion 7th character A see Appendix A
PDX collection 0911

+ T84.09 **Other mechanical complication of internal joint prosthesis**
Prosthetic joint implant failure NOS

CC +7th **T84.090** **Other mechanical complication of internal right hip prosthesis**
CC Exclusion 7th character A see Appendix A
PDX collection 0911

CC +7th **T84.091** **Other mechanical complication of internal left hip prosthesis**
CC Exclusion 7th character A see Appendix A
PDX collection 0911

CC +7th **T84.092** **Other mechanical complication of internal right knee prosthesis**
CC Exclusion 7th character A see Appendix A
PDX collection 0911

CC +7th **T84.093** **Other mechanical complication of internal left knee prosthesis**
CC Exclusion 7th character A see Appendix A
PDX collection 0911

CC +7th **T84.098** **Other mechanical complication of other internal joint prosthesis**
Use additional code to identify the joint (Z96.6-)
CC Exclusion 7th character A see Appendix A
PDX collection 0911

CC +7th **T84.099** **Other mechanical complication of unspecified internal joint prosthesis**
CC Exclusion 7th character A see Appendix A
PDX collection 0911

+ T84.1 **Mechanical complication of internal fixation device of bones of limb**
Excludes2: *mechanical complication of internal fixation device of bones of feet (T84.2-)*
mechanical complication of internal fixation device of bones of fingers (T84.2-)
mechanical complication of internal fixation device of bones of hands (T84.2-)
mechanical complication of internal fixation device of bones of toes (T84.2-)

+ T84.11 **Breakdown (mechanical) of internal fixation device of bones of limb**

CC +7th **T84.110** **Breakdown (mechanical) of internal fixation device of right humerus**
CC Exclusion 7th character A see Appendix A
PDX collection 0911

CC +7th **T84.111** **Breakdown (mechanical) of internal fixation device of left humerus**
CC Exclusion 7th character A see Appendix A
PDX collection 0911

CC +7th **T84.112** **Breakdown (mechanical) of internal fixation device of bone of right forearm**
CC Exclusion 7th character A see Appendix A
PDX collection 0911

CC +7th **T84.113** **Breakdown (mechanical) of internal fixation device of bone of left forearm**
CC Exclusion 7th character A see Appendix A
PDX collection 0911

CC +7th **T84.114** **Breakdown (mechanical) of internal fixation device of right femur**
CC Exclusion 7th character A see Appendix A
PDX collection 0911

CC +7th **T84.115** **Breakdown (mechanical) of internal fixation device of left femur**
CC Exclusion 7th character A see Appendix A
PDX collection 0911

CC +7th **T84.116** **Breakdown (mechanical) of internal fixation device of bone of right lower leg**
CC Exclusion 7th character A see Appendix A
PDX collection 0911

CC +7th **T84.117** **Breakdown (mechanical) of internal fixation device of bone of left lower leg**
CC Exclusion 7th character A see Appendix A
PDX collection 0911

CC +7th **T84.119** **Breakdown (mechanical) of internal fixation device of unspecified bone of limb**
CC Exclusion 7th character A see Appendix A
PDX collection 0911

\+ **T84.12** **Displacement of internal fixation device of bones of limb**
Malposition of internal fixation device of bones of limb

CC +7th **T84.120** **Displacement of internal fixation device of right humerus**
CC Exclusion 7th character A see Appendix A
PDX collection 0911

CC +7th **T84.121** **Displacement of internal fixation device of left humerus**
CC Exclusion 7th character A see Appendix A
PDX collection 0911

CC +7th **T84.122** **Displacement of internal fixation device of bone of right forearm**
CC Exclusion 7th character A see Appendix A
PDX collection 0911

CC +7th **T84.123** **Displacement of internal fixation device of bone of left forearm**
CC Exclusion 7th character A see Appendix A
PDX collection 0911

CC +7th **T84.124** **Displacement of internal fixation device of right femur**
CC Exclusion 7th character A see Appendix A
PDX collection 0911

CC +7th **T84.125** **Displacement of internal fixation device of left femur**
CC Exclusion 7th character A see Appendix A
PDX collection 0911

CC +7th **T84.126** **Displacement of internal fixation device of bone of right lower leg**
CC Exclusion 7th character A see Appendix A
PDX collection 0911

CC +7th **T84.127** **Displacement of internal fixation device of bone of left lower leg**
CC Exclusion 7th character A see Appendix A
PDX collection 0911

CC +7th **T84.129** **Displacement of internal fixation device of unspecified bone of limb**
CC Exclusion 7th character A see Appendix A
PDX collection 0911

\+ **T84.19** **Other mechanical complication of internal fixation device of bones of limb**
Obstruction (mechanical) of internal fixation device of bones of limb
Perforation of internal fixation device of bones of limb
Protrusion of internal fixation device of bones of limb

CC +7th **T84.190** **Other mechanical complication of internal fixation device of right humerus**
CC Exclusion 7th character A see Appendix A
PDX collection 0911

CC +7th **T84.191** **Other mechanical complication of internal fixation device of left humerus**
CC Exclusion 7th character A see Appendix A
PDX collection 0911

CC +7th **T84.192** **Other mechanical complication of internal fixation device of bone of right forearm**
CC Exclusion 7th character A see Appendix A
PDX collection 0911

CC +7th **T84.193** **Other mechanical complication of internal fixation device of bone of left forearm**
CC Exclusion 7th character A see Appendix A
PDX collection 0911

CC +7th **T84.194** **Other mechanical complication of internal fixation device of right femur**
CC Exclusion 7th character A see Appendix A
PDX collection 0911

CC +7th **T84.195** **Other mechanical complication of internal fixation device of left femur**
CC Exclusion 7th character A see Appendix A
PDX collection 0911

CC +7th **T84.196** **Other mechanical complication of internal fixation device of bone of right lower leg**
CC Exclusion 7th character A see Appendix A
PDX collection 0911

CC +7th **T84.197** **Other mechanical complication of internal fixation device of bone of left lower leg**
CC Exclusion 7th character A see Appendix A
PDX collection 0911

CC +7th **T84.199** **Other mechanical complication of internal fixation device of unspecified bone of limb**
CC Exclusion 7th character A see Appendix A
PDX collection 0911

\+ **T84.2** **Mechanical complication of internal fixation device of other bones**

\+ **T84.21** **Breakdown (mechanical) of internal fixation device of other bones**

CC +7th **T84.210** **Breakdown (mechanical) of internal fixation device of bones of hand and finger**
CC Exclusion 7th character A see Appendix A
PDX collection 0911

CC +7th **T84.213** **Breakdown (mechanical) of internal fixation device of bones of foot and toes**
CC Exclusion 7th character A see Appendix A
PDX collection 0911

CC +7th **T84.216** **Breakdown (mechanical) of internal fixation device of vertebrae**
CC Exclusion 7th character A see Appendix A
PDX collection 0911

CC +7th **T84.218** **Breakdown (mechanical) of internal fixation device of other bones**
CC Exclusion 7th character A see Appendix A
PDX collection 0911

\+ **T84.22** **Displacement of internal fixation device of other bones**
Malposition of internal fixation device of other bones

CC +7th **T84.220** **Displacement of internal fixation device of bones of hand and fingers**
CC Exclusion 7th character A see Appendix A
PDX collection 0911

CC +7th **T84.223** **Displacement of internal fixation device of bones of foot and toes**
CC Exclusion 7th character A see Appendix A
PDX collection 0911

CC +7th **T84.226** **Displacement of internal fixation device of vertebrae**
CC Exclusion 7th character A see Appendix A
PDX collection 0911

CC +7th **T84.228** **Displacement of internal fixation device of other bones**
CC Exclusion 7th character A see Appendix A
PDX collection 0911

\+ **T84.29** **Other mechanical complication of internal fixation device of other bones**
Obstruction (mechanical) of internal fixation device of other bones
Perforation of internal fixation device of other bones
Protrusion of internal fixation device of other bones

CC +7th **T84.290** **Other mechanical complication of internal fixation device of bones of hand and finger**
CC Exclusion 7th character A see Appendix A
PDX collection 0911

CC +7th **T84.293** **Other mechanical complication of internal fixation device of bones of foot and toes**
CC Exclusion 7th character A see Appendix A
PDX collection 0911

CC +7th **T84.296** **Other mechanical complication of internal fixation device of vertebrae**
CC Exclusion 7th character A see Appendix A PDX collection 0911

CC +7th **T84.298** **Other mechanical complication of internal fixation device of other bones**
CC Exclusion 7th character A see Appendix A PDX collection 0911

+ **T84.3** **Mechanical complication of other bone devices, implants and grafts**
Excludes2: *other complications of bone graft (T86.83-)*

+ **T84.31** **Breakdown (mechanical) of other bone devices, implants and grafts**

CC +7th **T84.310** **Breakdown (mechanical) of electronic bone stimulator**
CC Exclusion 7th character A see Appendix A PDX collection 0911

CC +7th **T84.318** **Breakdown (mechanical) of other bone devices, implants and grafts**
CC Exclusion 7th character A see Appendix A PDX collection 0911

+ **T84.32** **Displacement of other bone devices, implants and grafts**
Malposition of other bone devices, implants and grafts

CC +7th **T84.320** **Displacement of electronic bone stimulator**
CC Exclusion 7th character A see Appendix A PDX collection 0911

CC +7th **T84.328** **Displacement of other bone devices, implants and grafts**
CC Exclusion 7th character A see Appendix A PDX collection 0911
AHA CC: 4Q, 2014, 28-29

+ **T84.39** **Other mechanical complication of other bone devices, implants and grafts**
Obstruction (mechanical) of other bone devices, implants and grafts
Perforation of other bone devices, implants and grafts
Protrusion of other bone devices, implants and grafts

CC +7th **T84.390** **Other mechanical complication of electronic bone stimulator**
CC Exclusion 7th character A see Appendix A PDX collection 0911

CC +7th **T84.398** **Other mechanical complication of other bone devices, implants and grafts**
CC Exclusion 7th character A see Appendix A PDX collection 0911

+ **T84.4** **Mechanical complication of other internal orthopedic devices, implants and grafts**

+ **T84.41** **Breakdown (mechanical) of other internal orthopedic devices, implants and grafts**

CC +7th **T84.410** **Breakdown (mechanical) of muscle and tendon graft**
CC Exclusion 7th character A see Appendix A PDX collection 0911

CC +7th **T84.418** **Breakdown (mechanical) of other internal orthopedic devices, implants and grafts**
CC Exclusion 7th character A see Appendix A PDX collection 0911

+ **T84.42** **Displacement of other internal orthopedic devices, implants and grafts**
Malposition of other internal orthopedic devices, implants and grafts

CC +7th **T84.420** **Displacement of muscle and tendon graft**
CC Exclusion 7th character A see Appendix A PDX collection 0911

CC +7th **T84.428** **Displacement of other internal orthopedic devices, implants and grafts**
CC Exclusion 7th character A see Appendix A PDX collection 0911

+ **T84.49** **Other mechanical complication of other internal orthopedic devices, implants and grafts**
Mechanical complication of other internal orthopedic devices, implants and grafts NOS
Obstruction (mechanical) of other internal orthopedic devices, implants and grafts
Perforation of other internal orthopedic devices, implants and grafts
Protrusion of other internal orthopedic devices, implants and grafts

CC +7th **T84.490** **Other mechanical complication of muscle and tendon graft**
CC Exclusion 7th character A see Appendix A PDX collection 0911

CC +7th **T84.498** **Other mechanical complication of other internal orthopedic devices, implants and grafts**
CC Exclusion 7th character A see Appendix A PDX collection 0911

+ **T84.5** **Infection and inflammatory reaction due to internal joint prosthesis**
Use additional code to identify infection

CC X+7th **T84.50** **Infection and inflammatory reaction due to unspecified internal joint prosthesis**
CC Exclusion 7th character A see Appendix A PDX collection 1459

CC X+7th **T84.51** **Infection and inflammatory reaction due to internal right hip prosthesis**
CC Exclusion 7th character A see Appendix A PDX collection 1459
AHA CC: 4Q, 2015, 36

CC X+7th **T84.52** **Infection and inflammatory reaction due to internal left hip prosthesis**
CC Exclusion 7th character A see Appendix A PDX collection 1459
AHA CC: 1Q, 2015, 3-21

CC X+7th **T84.53** **Infection and inflammatory reaction due to internal right knee prosthesis**
CC Exclusion 7th character A see Appendix A PDX collection 1459

CC X+7th **T84.54** **Infection and inflammatory reaction due to internal left knee prosthesis**
CC Exclusion 7th character A see Appendix A PDX collection 1459

CC X+7th **T84.59** **Infection and inflammatory reaction due to other internal joint prosthesis**
CC Exclusion 7th character A see Appendix A PDX collection 1459

+ **T84.6** **Infection and inflammatory reaction due to internal fixation device**
Use additional code to identify infection

CC X+7th **T84.60** **Infection and inflammatory reaction due to internal fixation device of unspecified site**
CC Exclusion 7th character A see Appendix A PDX collection 1459
HAC 7th character A see Appendix B for HAC conditional logic

+ **T84.61** **Infection and inflammatory reaction due to internal fixation device of arm**

CC +7th **T84.610** **Infection and inflammatory reaction due to internal fixation device of right humerus**
CC Exclusion 7th character A see Appendix A PDX collection 1459
HAC 7th character A see Appendix B for HAC conditional logic

CC +7th **T84.611** **Infection and inflammatory reaction due to internal fixation device of left humerus**
CC Exclusion 7th character A see Appendix A PDX collection 1459
HAC 7th character A see Appendix B for HAC conditional logic

CC +7th **T84.612** **Infection and inflammatory reaction due to internal fixation device of right radius**
CC Exclusion 7th character A see Appendix A PDX collection 1459
HAC 7th character A see Appendix B for HAC conditional logic

CC +7th **T84.613** **Infection and inflammatory reaction due to internal fixation device of left radius**
CC Exclusion 7th character A see Appendix A PDX collection 1459
HAC 7th character A see Appendix B for HAC conditional logic

CC +7th **T84.614** **Infection and inflammatory reaction due to internal fixation device of right ulna**
CC Exclusion 7th character A see Appendix A PDX collection 1459
HAC 7th character A see Appendix B for HAC conditional logic

CC +7th **T84.615** **Infection and inflammatory reaction due to internal fixation device of left ulna**
CC Exclusion 7th character A see Appendix A PDX collection 1459
HAC 7th character A see Appendix B for HAC conditional logic

CC +7th **T84.619 Infection and inflammatory reaction due to internal fixation device of unspecified bone of arm**
CC Exclusion 7th character A see Appendix A PDX collection 1459
HAC 7th character A see Appendix B for HAC conditional logic

+ **T84.62 Infection and inflammatory reaction due to internal fixation device of leg**

CC +7th **T84.620 Infection and inflammatory reaction due to internal fixation device of right femur**
CC Exclusion 7th character A see Appendix A PDX collection 1459

CC +7th **T84.621 Infection and inflammatory reaction due to internal fixation device of left femur**
CC Exclusion 7th character A see Appendix A PDX collection 1459

CC +7th **T84.622 Infection and inflammatory reaction due to internal fixation device of right tibia**
CC Exclusion 7th character A see Appendix A PDX collection 1459

CC +7th **T84.623 Infection and inflammatory reaction due to internal fixation device of left tibia**
CC Exclusion 7th character A see Appendix A PDX collection 1459

CC +7th **T84.624 Infection and inflammatory reaction due to internal fixation device of right fibula**
CC Exclusion 7th character A see Appendix A PDX collection 1459

CC +7th **T84.625 Infection and inflammatory reaction due to internal fixation device of left fibula**
CC Exclusion 7th character A see Appendix A PDX collection 1459

CC +7th **T84.629 Infection and inflammatory reaction due to internal fixation device of unspecified bone of leg**
CC Exclusion 7th character A see Appendix A PDX collection 1459

CC X+7th **T84.63 Infection and inflammatory reaction due to internal fixation device of spine**
CC Exclusion 7th character A see Appendix A PDX collection 1459
HAC 7th character A see Appendix B for HAC conditional logic

CC X+7th **T84.69 Infection and inflammatory reaction due to internal fixation device of other site**
CC Exclusion 7th character A see Appendix A PDX collection 1459
HAC 7th character A see Appendix B for HAC conditional logic

CC X+7th **T84.7 Infection and inflammatory reaction due to other internal orthopedic prosthetic devices, implants and grafts**
Use additional code to identify infection
CC Exclusion 7th character A see Appendix A PDX collection 1459
HAC 7th character A see Appendix B for HAC conditional logic

+ **T84.8 Other specified complications of internal orthopedic prosthetic devices, implants and grafts**

CC X+7th **T84.81 Embolism due to internal orthopedic prosthetic devices, implants and grafts**
CC Exclusion 7th character A see Appendix A PDX collection 1459

CC X+7th **T84.82 Fibrosis due to internal orthopedic prosthetic devices, implants and grafts**
CC Exclusion 7th character A see Appendix A PDX collection 1459

CC X+7th **T84.83 Hemorrhage due to internal orthopedic prosthetic devices, implants and grafts**
CC Exclusion 7th character A see Appendix A PDX collection 1459

CC X+7th **T84.84 Pain due to internal orthopedic prosthetic devices, implants and grafts**
CC Exclusion 7th character A see Appendix A PDX collection 1459

CC X+7th **T84.85 Stenosis due to internal orthopedic prosthetic devices, implants and grafts**
CC Exclusion 7th character A see Appendix A PDX collection 1459

CC X+7th **T84.86 Thrombosis due to internal orthopedic prosthetic devices, implants and grafts**
CC Exclusion 7th character A see Appendix A PDX collection 1459

CC X+7th **T84.89 Other specified complication of internal orthopedic prosthetic devices, implants and grafts**
CC Exclusion 7th character A see Appendix A PDX collection 1459

CC X+7th **T84.9 Unspecified complication of internal orthopedic prosthetic device, implant and graft**
CC Exclusion 7th character A see Appendix A PDX collection 1459

T85 Complications of other internal prosthetic devices, implants and grafts

Excludes2: *failure and rejection of transplanted organs and tissue (T86.-)*

AHA CC: 4Q, 2016, 71-72

The appropriate 7th character is to be added to each code from category T85
A initial encounter
D subsequent encounter
S sequela

+ **T85.0 Mechanical complication of ventricular intracranial (communicating) shunt**

CC X+7th **T85.01 Breakdown (mechanical) of ventricular intracranial (communicating) shunt**
CC Exclusion 7th character A see Appendix A PDX collection 1460

CC X+7th **T85.02 Displacement of ventricular intracranial (communicating) shunt**
Malposition of ventricular intracranial (communicating) shunt
CC Exclusion 7th character A see Appendix A PDX collection 1460

CC X+7th **T85.03 Leakage of ventricular intracranial (communicating) shunt**
CC Exclusion 7th character A see Appendix A PDX collection 1460

CC X+7th **T85.09 Other mechanical complication of ventricular intracranial (communicating) shunt**
Obstruction (mechanical) of ventricular intracranial (communicating) shunt
Perforation of ventricular intracranial (communicating) shunt
Protrusion of ventricular intracranial (communicating) shunt
CC Exclusion 7th character A see Appendix A PDX collection 1460

+ **T85.1 Mechanical complication of implanted electronic stimulator of nervous system**

+ **T85.11 Breakdown (mechanical) of implanted electronic stimulator of nervous system**

CC +7th **T85.110 Breakdown (mechanical) of implanted electronic neurostimulator of brain electrode (lead)**
CC Exclusion 7th character A see Appendix A PDX collection 1460

CC +7th **T85.111 Breakdown (mechanical) of implanted electronic neurostimulator of peripheral nerve electrode (lead)**
Breakdown of electrode (lead) for cranial nerve neurostimulators
Breakdown of electrode (lead) for gastric neurostimulators
Breakdown of electrode (lead) for sacral nerve neurostimulators
Breakdown of electrode (lead) for vagal nerve neurostimulators
CC Exclusion 7th character A see Appendix A PDX collection 1460

CC +7th **T85.112 Breakdown (mechanical) of implanted electronic neurostimulator of spinal cord electrode (lead)**
CC Exclusion 7th character A see Appendix A PDX collection 1460

CC +7th **T85.113 Breakdown (mechanical) of implanted electronic neurostimulator, generator**
Breakdown (mechanical) of implanted electronic neurostimulator generator, brain, peripheral, gastric, spinal
Breakdown (mechanical) of implanted electronic sacral neurostimulator, pulse generator receiver
CC Exclusion 7th character A see Appendix A PDX collection 1460

CC +7th **T85.118 Breakdown (mechanical) of other implanted electronic stimulator of nervous system**
CC Exclusion 7th character A see Appendix A PDX collection 1460

+ **T85.12 Displacement of implanted electronic stimulator of nervous system**
Malposition of implanted electronic stimulator of nervous system

CC +7th **T85.120 Displacement of implanted electronic neurostimulator of brain electrode (lead)**
CC Exclusion 7th character A see Appendix A PDX collection 1460

CC +7th **T85.121 Displacement of implanted electronic neurostimulator of peripheral nerve electrode (lead)**
Displacement of electrode (lead) for cranial nerve neurostimulators
Displacement of electrode (lead) for gastric neurostimulators
Displacement of electrode (lead) for sacral nerve neurostimulators
Displacement of electrode (lead) for vagal nerve neurostimulators
CC Exclusion 7th character A see Appendix A PDX collection 1460

CC +7th **T85.122 Displacement of implanted electronic neurostimulator of spinal cord electrode (lead)**
CC Exclusion 7th character A see Appendix A PDX collection 1460

CC +7th **T85.123 Displacement of implanted electronic neurostimulator, generator**
Displacement of implanted electronic neurostimulator generator, brain, peripheral, gastric, spinal
Displacement of implanted electronic sacral neurostimulator, pulse generator receiver
CC Exclusion 7th character A see Appendix A PDX collection 1460

CC +7th **T85.128 Displacement of other implanted electronic stimulator of nervous system**
CC Exclusion 7th character A see Appendix A PDX collection 1460

+ **T85.19 Other mechanical complication of implanted electronic stimulator of nervous system**
Leakage of implanted electronic stimulator of nervous system
Obstruction (mechanical) of implanted electronic stimulator of nervous system
Perforation of implanted electronic stimulator of nervous system
Protrusion of implanted electronic stimulator of nervous system

CC +7th **T85.190 Other mechanical complication of implanted electronic neurostimulator of brain electrode (lead)**
CC Exclusion 7th character A see Appendix A PDX collection 1460

CC +7th **T85.191 Other mechanical complication of implanted electronic neurostimulator of peripheral nerve electrode (lead)**
Other mechanical complication of electrode (lead) for cranial nerve neurostimulators
Other mechanical complication of electrode (lead) for gastric neurostimulators
Other mechanical complication of electrode (lead) for sacral nerve neurostimulators
Other mechanical complication of electrode (lead) for vagal nerve neurostimulators
CC Exclusion 7th character A see Appendix A PDX collection 1460

CC +7th **T85.192 Other mechanical complication of implanted electronic neurostimulator of spinal cord electrode (lead)**
CC Exclusion 7th character A see Appendix A PDX collection 1460

CC +7th **T85.193 Other mechanical complication of implanted electronic neurostimulator, generator**
Other mechanical complication of implanted electronic neurostimulator generator, brain, peripheral, gastric, spinal
Other mechanical complication of implanted electronic sacral neurostimulator, pulse generator receiver
CC Exclusion 7th character A see Appendix A PDX collection 1460

CC +7th **T85.199 Other mechanical complication of other implanted electronic stimulator of nervous system**
CC Exclusion 7th character A see Appendix A PDX collection 1460

+ **T85.2 Mechanical complication of intraocular lens**

CC X+7th **T85.21 Breakdown (mechanical) of intraocular lens**
CC Exclusion 7th character A see Appendix A PDX collection 1461

CC X+7th **T85.22 Displacement of intraocular lens**
Malposition of intraocular lens
CC Exclusion 7th character A see Appendix A PDX collection 1461

CC X+7th **T85.29 Other mechanical complication of intraocular lens**
Obstruction (mechanical) of intraocular lens
Perforation of intraocular lens
Protrusion of intraocular lens
CC Exclusion 7th character A see Appendix A PDX collection 1461

+ **T85.3 Mechanical complication of other ocular prosthetic devices, implants and grafts**
Excludes2: *other complications of corneal graft (T86.84-)*

+ **T85.31 Breakdown (mechanical) of other ocular prosthetic devices, implants and grafts**

CC +7th **T85.310 Breakdown (mechanical) of prosthetic orbit of right eye**
CC Exclusion 7th character A see Appendix A PDX collection 1462

CC +7th **T85.311 Breakdown (mechanical) of prosthetic orbit of left eye**
CC Exclusion 7th character A see Appendix A PDX collection 1462

+7th **T85.318 Breakdown (mechanical) of other ocular prosthetic devices, implants and grafts**

+ **T85.32 Displacement of other ocular prosthetic devices, implants and grafts**
Malposition of other ocular prosthetic devices, implants and grafts

CC +7th **T85.320 Displacement of prosthetic orbit of right eye**
CC Exclusion 7th character A see Appendix A PDX collection 1462

CC +7th **T85.321 Displacement of prosthetic orbit of left eye**
CC Exclusion 7th character A see Appendix A PDX collection 1462

+7th **T85.328 Displacement of other ocular prosthetic devices, implants and grafts**

+ **T85.39 Other mechanical complication of other ocular prosthetic devices, implants and grafts**
Obstruction (mechanical) of other ocular prosthetic devices, implants and grafts
Perforation of other ocular prosthetic devices, implants and grafts
Protrusion of other ocular prosthetic devices, implants and grafts

CC +7th **T85.390 Other mechanical complication of prosthetic orbit of right eye**
CC Exclusion 7th character A see Appendix A PDX collection 1462

CC +7th **T85.391 Other mechanical complication of prosthetic orbit of left eye**
CC Exclusion 7th character A see Appendix A PDX collection 1462

+7th **T85.398 Other mechanical complication of other ocular prosthetic devices, implants and grafts**

+ **T85.4 Mechanical complication of breast prosthesis and implant**

CC X+7th **T85.41 Breakdown (mechanical) of breast prosthesis and implant**
CC Exclusion 7th character A see Appendix A PDX collection 1463

CC X+7th **T85.42 Displacement of breast prosthesis and implant**
Malposition of breast prosthesis and implant
CC Exclusion 7th character A see Appendix A PDX collection 1463

CC X+7th **T85.43 Leakage of breast prosthesis and implant**
CC Exclusion 7th character A see Appendix A PDX collection 1463

CC X+7th **T85.44 Capsular contracture of breast implant**
CC Exclusion 7th character A see Appendix A PDX collection 1463

CC X+7th **T85.49 Other mechanical complication of breast prosthesis and implant**
Obstruction (mechanical) of breast prosthesis and implant
Perforation of breast prosthesis and implant
Protrusion of breast prosthesis and implant
CC Exclusion 7th character A see Appendix A PDX collection 1463

+ **T85.5 Mechanical complication of gastrointestinal prosthetic devices, implants and grafts**

+ **T85.51 Breakdown (mechanical) of gastrointestinal prosthetic devices, implants and grafts**

CC +7th **T85.510 Breakdown (mechanical) of bile duct prosthesis**
CC Exclusion 7th character A see Appendix A PDX collection 1464

CC +7th **T85.511 Breakdown (mechanical) of esophageal anti-reflux device**
CC Exclusion 7th character A see Appendix A PDX collection 1464

CC +7th **T85.518 Breakdown (mechanical) of other gastrointestinal prosthetic devices, implants and grafts**
CC Exclusion 7th character A see Appendix A PDX collection 1464

+ **T85.52 Displacement of gastrointestinal prosthetic devices, implants and grafts**
Malposition of gastrointestinal prosthetic devices, implants and grafts

CC +7th **T85.520 Displacement of bile duct prosthesis**
CC Exclusion 7th character A see Appendix A PDX collection 1464

CC +7th **T85.521 Displacement of esophageal anti-reflux device**
CC Exclusion 7th character A see Appendix A PDX collection 1464

CC +7th **T85.528 Displacement of other gastrointestinal prosthetic devices, implants and grafts**
CC Exclusion 7th character A see Appendix A PDX collection 1464

+ **T85.59 Other mechanical complication of gastrointestinal prosthetic devices, implants and**
Obstruction, mechanical of gastrointestinal prosthetic devices, implants and grafts
Perforation of gastrointestinal prosthetic devices, implants and grafts
Protrusion of gastrointestinal prosthetic devices, implants and grafts

CC +7th **T85.590 Other mechanical complication of bile duct prosthesis**
CC Exclusion 7th character A see Appendix A PDX collection 1464

CC +7th **T85.591 Other mechanical complication of esophageal anti-reflux device**
CC Exclusion 7th character A see Appendix A PDX collection 1464

CC +7th **T85.598 Other mechanical complication of other gastrointestinal prosthetic devices, implants and grafts**
CC Exclusion 7th character A see Appendix A PDX collection 1464

+ **T85.6 Mechanical complication of other specified internal and external prosthetic devices, implants and grafts**
Review coding guidelines C.4.a.5.a and C.4.a.5.b

+ **T85.61 Breakdown (mechanical) of other specified internal prosthetic devices, implants and grafts**

CC +7th **T85.610 Breakdown (mechanical) of cranial or spinal infusion catheter**
Breakdown (mechanical) of epidural infusion catheter
Breakdown (mechanical) of intrathecal infusion catheter
Breakdown (mechanical) of subarachnoid infusion catheter
Breakdown (mechanical) of subdural infusion catheter
CC Exclusion 7th character A see Appendix A PDX collection 1465

CC +7th **T85.611 Breakdown (mechanical) of intraperitoneal dialysis catheter**
Excludes1: *mechanical complication of vascular dialysis catheter (T82.4-)*
CC Exclusion 7th character A see Appendix A PDX collection 1466

CC +7th **T85.612 Breakdown (mechanical) of permanent sutures**
Excludes1: *mechanical complication of permanent (wire) suture used in bone repair (T84.1-T84.2)*
CC Exclusion 7th character A see Appendix A PDX collection 1467

CC +7th **T85.613 Breakdown (mechanical) of artificial skin graft and decellularized allodermis**
Failure of artificial skin graft and decellularized allodermis
Non-adherence of artificial skin graft and decellularized allodermis
Poor incorporation of artificial skin graft and decellularized allodermis
Shearing of artificial skin graft and decellularized allodermis
CC Exclusion 7th character A see Appendix A PDX collection 1468

CC +7th **T85.614 Breakdown (mechanical) of insulin pump**
CC Exclusion 7th character A see Appendix A PDX collection 1469

CC +7th **T85.615 Breakdown (mechanical) of other nervous system device, implant or graft**
Breakdown (mechanical) of intrathecal infusion pump
CC Exclusion 7th character A see Appendix A PDX collection 1467

CC +7th **T85.618 Breakdown (mechanical) of other specified internal prosthetic devices, implants and grafts**
CC Exclusion 7th character A see Appendix A PDX collection 1467

+ **T85.62 Displacement of other specified internal prosthetic devices, implants and grafts**
Malposition of other specified internal prosthetic devices, implants and grafts

CC +7th **T85.620 Displacement of cranial or spinal infusion catheter**
Displacement of epidural infusion catheter
Displacement of intrathecal infusion catheter
Displacement of subarachnoid infusion catheter
Displacement of subdural infusion catheter
CC Exclusion 7th character A see Appendix A PDX collection 1465

CC +7th **T85.621 Displacement of intraperitoneal dialysis catheter**
Excludes1: *mechanical complication of vascular dialysis catheter (T82.4-)*
CC Exclusion 7th character A see Appendix A PDX collection 1466

CC +7th **T85.622 Displacement of permanent sutures**
Excludes1: *mechanical complication of permanent (wire) suture used in bone repair (T84.1-T84.2)*
CC Exclusion 7th character A see Appendix A PDX collection 1467

CC +7th **T85.623 Displacement of artificial skin graft and decellularized allodermis**
Dislodgement of artificial skin graft and decellularized allodermis
CC Exclusion 7th character A see Appendix A
PDX collection 1468

CC +7th **T85.624 Displacement of insulin pump**
CC Exclusion 7th character A see Appendix A
PDX collection 1469

CC +7th **T85.625 Displacement of other nervous system device, implant or graft**
Displacement of intrathecal infusion pump
CC Exclusion 7th character A see Appendix A
PDX collection 1467

CC +7th **T85.628 Displacement of other specified internal prosthetic devices, implants and grafts**
CC Exclusion 7th character A see Appendix A
PDX collection 1467
AHA CC: 1Q, 2015, 3-21

\+ **T85.63 Leakage of other specified internal prosthetic devices, implants and grafts**

CC +7th **T85.630 Leakage of cranial or spinal infusion catheter**
Leakage of epidural infusion catheter
Leakage of intrathecal infusion catheter
Leakage of subarachnoid infusion catheter
Leakage of subdural infusion catheter
CC Exclusion 7th character A see Appendix A
PDX collection 1465

CC +7th **T85.631 Leakage of intraperitoneal dialysis catheter**
Excludes1: *mechanical complication of vascular dialysis catheter (T82.4)*
CC Exclusion 7th character A see Appendix A
PDX collection 1466

CC +7th **T85.633 Leakage of insulin pump**
CC Exclusion 7th character A see Appendix A
PDX collection 1469

CC +7th **T85.635 Leakage of other nervous system device, implant or graft**
Leakage of intrathecal infusion pump
CC Exclusion 7th character A see Appendix A
PDX collection 1467

CC +7th **T85.638 Leakage of other specified internal prosthetic devices, implants and grafts**
CC Exclusion 7th character A see Appendix A
PDX collection 1467

\+ **T85.69 Other mechanical complication of other specified internal prosthetic devices, implants and grafts**
Obstruction, mechanical of other specified internal prosthetic devices, implants and grafts
Perforation of other specified internal prosthetic devices, implants and grafts
Protrusion of other specified internal prosthetic devices, implants and grafts

CC +7th **T85.690 Other mechanical complication of cranial or spinal infusion catheter**
Other mechanical complication of epidural infusion catheter
Other mechanical complication of intrathecal infusion catheter
Other mechanical complication of subarachnoid infusion catheter
Other mechanical complication of subdural infusion catheter
CC Exclusion 7th character A see Appendix A
PDX collection 1465

CC +7th **T85.691 Other mechanical complication of intraperitoneal dialysis catheter**
Excludes1: *mechanical complication of vascular dialysis catheter (T82.4)*
CC Exclusion 7th character A see Appendix A
PDX collection 1466

CC +7th **T85.692 Other mechanical complication of permanent sutures**
Excludes1: *mechanical complication of permanent(wire)sutureused in bone repair(T84.1-T84.2)*
CC Exclusion 7th character A see Appendix A
PDX collection 1467

CC +7th **T85.693 Other mechanical complication of artificial skin graft and decellularized allodermis**
CC Exclusion 7th character A see Appendix A
PDX collection 1468

CC +7th **T85.694 Other mechanical complication of insulin pump**
CC Exclusion 7th character A see Appendix A
PDX collection 1469

CC +7th **T85.695 Other mechanical complication of other nervous system device, implant or graft**
Other mechanical complication of intrathecal infusion pump
CC Exclusion 7th character A see Appendix A
PDX collection 1467

CC +7th **T85.698 Other mechanical complication of other specified internal prosthetic devices, implants and grafts**
Mechanical complication of nonabsorbable surgical material NOS
CC Exclusion 7th character A see Appendix A
PDX collection 1467

\+ **T85.7 Infection and inflammatory reaction due to other internal prosthetic devices, implants and grafts**
Use additional code to identify infection

CC X+7th **T85.71 Infection and inflammatory reaction due to peritoneal dialysis catheter**
CC Exclusion 7th character A see Appendix A PDX collection 1467

CC X+7th **T85.72 Infection and inflammatory reaction due to insulin pump**
CC Exclusion 7th character A see Appendix A PDX collection 1470

\+ **T85.73 Infection and inflammatory reaction due to nervous system devices, implants and graft**

CC +7th **T85.730 Infection and inflammatory reaction due to ventricular intracranial (communicating) shunt**
CC Exclusion 7th character A see Appendix A
PDX collection 1470

CC +7th **T85.731 Infection and inflammatory reaction due to implanted electronic neurostimulator of brain, electrode (lead)**
CC Exclusion 7th character A see Appendix A
PDX collection 1470

CC +7th **T85.732 Infection and inflammatory reaction due to implanted electronic neurostimulator of peripheral nerve, electrode (lead)**
Infection and inflammatory reaction due to electrode (lead) for cranial nerve neurostimulators
Infection and inflammatory reaction due to electrode (lead) for gastric neurostimulators
Infection and inflammatory reaction due to electrode (lead) for sacral nerve neurostimulators
Infection and inflammatory reaction due to electrode (lead) for vagal nerve neurostimulators
CC Exclusion 7th character A see Appendix A
PDX collection 1470

CC +7th **T85.733 Infection and inflammatory reaction due to implanted electronic neurostimulator of spinal cord, electrode (lead)**
CC Exclusion 7th character A see Appendix A
PDX collection 1470

CC +7th **T85.734 Infection and inflammatory reaction due to implanted electronic neurostimulator, generator**
Generator pocket infection
CC Exclusion 7th character A see Appendix A
PDX collection 1470

CC +7th **T85.735 Infection and inflammatory reaction due to cranial or spinal infusion catheter**
Infection and inflammatory reaction due to epidural catheter
Infection and inflammatory reaction due to intrathecal infsuion catheter
Infection and inflammatory reaction due to subarachnoid catheter
Infection and inflammatory reaction due to subdural catheter
CC Exclusion 7th character A see Appendix A PDX collection 1470

CC +7th **T85.738 Infection and inflammatory reaction due to other nervous system device, implant or graft**
Infection and inflammatory reaction due to intrathecal infusion pump
CC Exclusion 7th character A see Appendix A PDX collection 1470

CC X+7th **T85.79 Infection and inflammatory reaction due to other internal prosthetic devices, implants and grafts**
CC Exclusion 7th character A see Appendix A PDX collection 1470

+ **T85.8 Other specified complications of internal prosthetic devices, implants and grafts, not elsewhere classified**

+ **T85.81 Embolism due to internal prosthetic devices, implants and grafts, not elsewhere classified**

CC +7th **T85.810 Embolism due to nervous system prosthetic devices, implants and grafts**
CC Exclusion 7th characters A & D see Appendix A PDX collection 1470

+7th **T85.818 Embolism due to other internal prosthetic devices, implants and grafts**

+ **T85.82 Fibrosis due to internal prosthetic devices, implants and grafts, not elsewhere classified**

CC +7th **T85.820 Fibrosis due to nervous system prosthetic devices, implants and grafts**
CC Exclusion 7th characters A & D see Appendix A PDX collection 1470

+7th **T85.828 Fibrosis due to other internal prosthetic devices, implants and grafts**

+ **T85.83 Hemorrhage due to internal prosthetic devices, implants and grafts, not elsewhere classified**

CC +7th **T85.830 Hemorrhage due to nervous system prosthetic devices, implants and grafts**
CC Exclusion 7th characters A & D see Appendix A PDX collection 1470

+7th **T85.838 Hemorrhage due to other internal prosthetic devices, implants and grafts**

+ **T85.84 Pain due to internal prosthetic devices, implants and grafts, not elsewhere classified**

CC +7th **T85.840 Pain due to nervous system prosthetic devices, implants and grafts**
CC Exclusion 7th characters A & D see Appendix A PDX collection 1470

+7th **T85.848 Pain due to other internal prosthetic devices, implants and grafts**

+ **T85.85 Stenosis due to internal prosthetic devices, implants and grafts, not elsewhere classified**

CC +7th **T85.850 Stenosis due to nervous system prosthetic devices, implants and grafts**
CC Exclusion 7th characters A & D see Appendix A PDX collection 1470

+7th **T85.858 Stenosis due to other internal prosthetic devices, implants and grafts**

+ **T85.86 Thrombosis due to internal prosthetic devices, implants and grafts, not elsewhere classified**

CC +7th **T85.860 Thrombosis due to nervous system prosthetic devices, implants and grafts**
CC Exclusion 7th characters A & D see Appendix A PDX collection 1470

+7th **T85.868 Thrombosis due to other internal prosthetic devices, implants and grafts**

+ **T85.89 Other specified complication of internal prosthetic devices, implants and grafts, not elsewhere classified**
Erosion or breakdown of subcutaneous device pocket

CC +7th **T85.890 Other specified complication of nervous system prosthetic devices, implants and grafts**
CC Exclusion 7th characters A & D see Appendix A PDX collection 1470

+7th **T85.898 Other specified complication of other internal prosthetic devices, implants and grafts**

X+7th **T85.9 Unspecified complication of internal prosthetic device, implant and graft**
Complication of internal prosthetic device, implant and graft NOS

T86 Complications of transplanted organs and tissue

Use additional code to identify other transplant complications, such as:
graft-versus-host disease (D89.81-)
malignancy associated with organ transplant (C80.2)
post-transplant lymphoproliferative disorders (PTLD) (D47.Z1)
Review coding guideline C.2.r
Review coding guideline C.19.g.3

+ **T86.0 Complications of bone marrow transplant**

CC **T86.00 Unspecified complication of bone marrow transplant**
CC Exclusion see Appendix A PDX collection 0514

CC **T86.01 Bone marrow transplant rejection**
CC Exclusion see Appendix A PDX collection 0514

CC **T86.02 Bone marrow transplant failure**
CC Exclusion see Appendix A PDX collection 0514

CC **T86.03 Bone marrow transplant infection**
CC Exclusion see Appendix A PDX collection 0514

CC **T86.09 Other complications of bone marrow transplant**
CC Exclusion see Appendix A PDX collection 0514

+ **T86.1 Complications of kidney transplant**
Review coding guideline C.19.g.3.b

CC **T86.10 Unspecified complication of kidney transplant**
CC Exclusion see Appendix A PDX collection 1471

CC **T86.11 Kidney transplant rejection**
CC Exclusion see Appendix A PDX collection 1471

CC **T86.12 Kidney transplant failure**
CC Exclusion see Appendix A PDX collection 1471
AHA CC: 1Q, 2014, 24

CC **T86.13 Kidney transplant infection**
Use additional code to specify infection
CC Exclusion see Appendix A PDX collection 1471

CC **T86.19 Other complication of kidney transplant**
CC Exclusion see Appendix A PDX collection 1471

+ **T86.2 Complications of heart transplant**
Excludes1: *complication of:*
artificial heart device (T82.5)
heart-lung transplant (T86.3)

CC **T86.20 Unspecified complication of heart transplant**
CC Exclusion see Appendix A PDX collection 1472

CC **T86.21 Heart transplant rejection**
CC Exclusion see Appendix A PDX collection 1472

CC **T86.22 Heart transplant failure**
CC Exclusion see Appendix A PDX collection 1472

CC **T86.23 Heart transplant infection**
Use additional code to specify infection
CC Exclusion see Appendix A PDX collection 1472

+ **T86.29 Other complications of heart transplant**

CC **T86.290 Cardiac allograft vasculopathy**
Excludes1: *atherosclerosis of coronary arteries (I25.75-, I25.76-, I25.81-)*
CC Exclusion see Appendix A PDX collection 1472

CC **T86.298 Other complications of heart transplant**
CC Exclusion see Appendix A PDX collection 147

+ **T86.3 Complications of heart-lung transplant**

CC **T86.30 Unspecified complication of heart-lung transplant**
CC Exclusion see Appendix A PDX collection 1472

CC **T86.31 Heart-lung transplant rejection**
CC Exclusion see Appendix A PDX collection 1472

CC **T86.32 Heart-lung transplant failure**
CC Exclusion see Appendix A PDX collection 1472

CC **T86.33 Heart-lung transplant infection**
Use additional code to specify infection
CC Exclusion see Appendix A PDX collection 1472

CC **T86.39 Other complications of heart-lung transplant**
CC Exclusion see Appendix A PDX collection 1472

+ **T86.4 Complications of liver transplant**

CC **T86.40 Unspecified complication of liver transplant**
CC Exclusion see Appendix A PDX collection 1473

CC **T86.41 Liver transplant rejection**
CC Exclusion see Appendix A PDX collection 1473

CC **T86.42 Liver transplant failure**
CC Exclusion see Appendix A PDX collection 1473

CC **T86.43 Liver transplant infection**
Use additional code to identify infection, such as:
Cytomegalovirus (CMV) infection (B25.-)
CC Exclusion see Appendix A PDX collection 1473

CC T86.49 Other complications of liver transplant
CC Exclusion see Appendix A PDX collection 1473

CC T86.5 Complications of stem cell transplant
Complications from stem cells from peripheral blood
Complications from stem cells from umbilical cord
CC Exclusion see Appendix A PDX collection 1474

+ T86.8 Complications of other transplanted organs and tissues

+ T86.81 Complications of lung transplant
Excludes1: *complication of heart-lung transplant (T86.3-)*

CC T86.810 Lung transplant rejection
CC Exclusion see Appendix A PDX collection 1475

CC T86.811 Lung transplant failure
CC Exclusion see Appendix A PDX collection 1475

CC T86.812 Lung transplant infection
Use additional code to specify infection
CC Exclusion see Appendix A PDX collection 1475

CC T86.818 Other complications of lung transplant
CC Exclusion see Appendix A PDX collection 1475

CC T86.819 Unspecified complication of lung transplant
CC Exclusion see Appendix A PDX collection 1475

+ T86.82 Complications of skin graft (allograft) (autograft)
Excludes2: *complication of artificial skin graft (T85.693)*

CC T86.820 Skin graft (allograft) rejection
CC Exclusion see Appendix A PDX collection 1476

CC T86.821 Skin graft (allograft) (autograft) failure
CC Exclusion see Appendix A PDX collection 1476

CC T86.822 Skin graft (allograft) (autograft) infection
Use additional code to specify infection
CC Exclusion see Appendix A PDX collection 1476

CC T86.828 Other complications of skin graft (allograft) (autograft)
CC Exclusion see Appendix A PDX collection 1476

CC T86.829 Unspecified complication of skin graft (allograft) (autograft)
CC Exclusion see Appendix A PDX collection 1476

+ T86.83 Complications of bone graft
Excludes2: *mechanical complications of bone graft (T84.3-)*

CC T86.830 Bone graft rejection
CC Exclusion see Appendix A PDX collection 1477

CC T86.831 Bone graft failure
CC Exclusion see Appendix A PDX collection 1477

CC T86.832 Bone graft infection
Use additional code to specify infection
CC Exclusion see Appendix A PDX collection 1477

CC T86.838 Other complications of bone graft
CC Exclusion see Appendix A PDX collection 1477

CC T86.839 Unspecified complication of bone graft
CC Exclusion see Appendix A PDX collection 1477

+ T86.84 Complications of corneal transplant
Excludes2: *mechanical complications of corneal graft (T85.3-)*

CC T86.840 Corneal transplant rejection
CC Exclusion see Appendix A PDX collection 1478

CC T86.841 Corneal transplant failure
CC Exclusion see Appendix A PDX collection 1478

CC T86.842 Corneal transplant infection
Use additional code to specify infection
CC Exclusion see Appendix A PDX collection 1479

CC T86.848 Other complications of corneal transplant
CC Exclusion see Appendix A PDX collection 1479

CC T86.849 Unspecified complication of corneal transplant
CC Exclusion see Appendix A PDX collection 1479

+ T86.85 Complication of intestine transplant

CC T86.850 Intestine transplant rejection
CC Exclusion see Appendix A PDX collection 0495

CC T86.851 Intestine transplant failure
CC Exclusion see Appendix A PDX collection 0495

CC T86.852 Intestine transplant infection
Use additional code to specify infection
CC Exclusion see Appendix A PDX collection 0495

CC T86.858 Other complications of intestine transplant
CC Exclusion see Appendix A PDX collection 0495

CC T86.859 Unspecified complication of intestine transplant
CC Exclusion see Appendix A PDX collection 0495

+ T86.89 Complications of other transplanted tissue
Transplant failure or rejection of pancreas

CC T86.890 Other transplanted tissue rejection
CC Exclusion see Appendix A PDX collection 1480

CC T86.891 Other transplanted tissue failure
CC Exclusion see Appendix A PDX collection 1480

CC T86.892 Other transplanted tissue infection
Use additional code to specify infection
CC Exclusion see Appendix A PDX collection 1480

CC T86.898 Other complications of other transplanted tissue
CC Exclusion see Appendix A PDX collection 1480

CC T86.899 Unspecified complication of other transplanted tissue
CC Exclusion see Appendix A PDX collection 1480

+ T86.9 Complication of unspecified transplanted organ and tissue

CC T86.90 Unspecified complication of unspecified transplanted organ and tissue
CC Exclusion see Appendix A PDX collection 0495

CC T86.91 Unspecified transplanted organ and tissue rejection
CC Exclusion see Appendix A PDX collection 0495

CC T86.92 Unspecified transplanted organ and tissue failure
CC Exclusion see Appendix A PDX collection 0495

CC T86.93 Unspecified transplanted organ and tissue infection
Use additional code to specify infection
CC Exclusion see Appendix A PDX collection 0495

CC T86.99 Other complications of unspecified transplanted organ and tissue
CC Exclusion see Appendix A PDX collection 0495

T87 Complications peculiar to reattachment and amputation

+ T87.0 Complications of reattached (part of) upper extremity

+ T87.0X Complications of reattached (part of) upper extremity

CC T87.0X1 Complications of reattached (part of) right upper extremity
CC Exclusion see Appendix A PDX collection 1481

CC T87.0X2 Complications of reattached (part of) left upper extremity
CC Exclusion see Appendix A PDX collection 1481

CC T87.0X9 Complications of reattached (part of) unspecified upper extremity
CC Exclusion see Appendix A PDX collection 1481

+ T87.1 Complications of reattached (part of) lower extremity

+ T87.1X Complications of reattached (part of) lower extremity

CC T87.1X1 Complications of reattached (part of) right lower extremity
CC Exclusion see Appendix A PDX collection 1482

CC **T87.1X2 Complications of reattached (part of) left lower extremity**
CC Exclusion see Appendix A PDX collection 1482

CC **T87.1X9 Complications of reattached (part of) unspecified lower extremity**
CC Exclusion see Appendix A PDX collection 1482

CC **T87.2 Complications of other reattached body part**
CC Exclusion see Appendix A PDX collection 1483

+ **T87.3 Neuroma of amputation stump**

T87.30 Neuroma of amputation stump, unspecified extremity

T87.31 Neuroma of amputation stump, right upper extremity

T87.32 Neuroma of amputation stump, left upper extremity

T87.33 Neuroma of amputation stump, right lower extremity

T87.34 Neuroma of amputation stump, left lower extremity

+ **T87.4 Infection of amputation stump**

CC **T87.40 Infection of amputation stump, unspecified extremity**
CC Exclusion see Appendix A PDX collection 1484

CC **T87.41 Infection of amputation stump, right upper extremity**
CC Exclusion see Appendix A PDX collection 1484

CC **T87.42 Infection of amputation stump, left upper extremity**
CC Exclusion see Appendix A PDX collection 1484

CC **T87.43 Infection of amputation stump, right lower extremity**
CC Exclusion see Appendix A PDX collection 1484

CC **T87.44 Infection of amputation stump, left lower extremity**
CC Exclusion see Appendix A PDX collection 1484

+ **T87.5 Necrosis of amputation stump**

T87.50 Necrosis of amputation stump, unspecified extremity

T87.51 Necrosis of amputation stump, right upper extremity

T87.52 Necrosis of amputation stump, left upper extremity

T87.53 Necrosis of amputation stump, right lower extremity

T87.54 Necrosis of amputation stump, left lower extremity

+ **T87.8 Other complications of amputation stump**

T87.81 Dehiscence of amputation stump

T87.89 Other complications of amputation stump
Amputation stump contracture
Amputation stump contracture of next proximal joint
Amputation stump flexion
Amputation stump edema
Amputation stump hematoma
Excludes2: *phantom limb syndrome (G54.6-G54.7)*

T87.9 Unspecified complications of amputation stump

T88 Other complications of surgical and medical care, not elsewhere classified

Excludes2: *complication following infusion, transfusion and therapeutic injection (T80.-)*
complication following procedure NEC (T81.-)
complications of anesthesia in labor and delivery (O74.-)
complications of anesthesia in pregnancy (O29.-)
complications of anesthesia in puerperium (O89.-)
complications of devices, implants and grafts (T82-T85)
complications of obstetric surgery and procedure (O75.4)
dermatitis due to drugs and medicaments (L23.3, L24.4, L25.1, L27.0-L27.1)
poisoning and toxic effects of drugs and chemicals (T36-T65 with fifth or sixth character 1-4 or 6)
specified complications classified elsewhere

The appropriate 7th character is to be added to each code from category T88
A initial encounter
D subsequent encounter
S sequela

CC X+7th **T88.0 Infection following immunization**
Sepsis following immunization
CC Exclusion 7th character A see Appendix A PDX collection 0948
Review coding guideline C.1.d.5

CC X+7th **T88.1 Other complications following immunization, not elsewhere classified**
Generalized vaccinia
Rash following immunization
Excludes1: *vaccinia not from vaccine (B08.011)*
Excludes2: *anaphylactic shock due to serum (T80.5-)*
other serum reactions (T80.6-)
postimmunization arthropathy (M02.2)
postimmunization encephalitis (G04.02)
postimmunization fever (R50.83)
CC Exclusion 7th character A see Appendix A PDX collection 1485

CC X+7th **T88.2 Shock due to anesthesia**
Use additional code for adverse effect, if applicable, to identify drug (T41.- with fifth or sixth character 5)
Excludes1: *complications of anesthesia (in):*
labor and delivery (O74.-)
pregnancy (O29.-)
puerperium (O89.-)
postprocedural shock NOS (T81.1-)
CC Exclusion 7th character A see Appendix A PDX collection 1441

CC X+7th **T88.3 Malignant hyperthermia due to anesthesia**
Use additional code for adverse effect, if applicable, to identify drug (T41.- with fifth or sixth character 5)
CC Exclusion 7th character A see Appendix A PDX collection 1486

X+7th **T88.4 Failed or difficult intubation**

+ **T88.5 Other complications of anesthesia**
Use additional code for adverse effect, if applicable, to identify drug (T41.- with fifth or sixth character 5)
AHA CC: 4Q, 2016, 72-73

X+7th **T88.51 Hypothermia following anesthesia**

X+7th **T88.52 Failed moderate sedation during procedure**
Failed conscious sedation during procedure
Excludes2: *personal history of failed moderate sedation (Z92.83)*

X+7th **T88.53 Unintended awareness under general anesthesia during procedure**
Excludes2: *personal history of unintended awareness under general anesthesia (Z92.84)*
AHA CC: 4Q, 2016, 72-73

X+7th **T88.59 Other complications of anesthesia**

CC X+7th **T88.6 Anaphylactic reaction due to adverse effect of correct drug or medicament properly administered**
Anaphylactic shock due to adverse effect of correct drug or medicament properly administered
Anaphylactoid reaction NOS
Use additional code for adverse effect, if applicable, to identify drug (T36-T50 with fifth or sixth character 5)
Excludes1: *anaphylactic reaction due to serum (T80.5-)*
anaphylactic shock or reaction due to adverse food reaction (T78.0-)
CC Exclusion 7th character A see Appendix A PDX collection 1426

X+7th **T88.7 Unspecified adverse effect of drug or medicament**
Drug hypersensitivity NOS
Drug reaction NOS
Use additional code for adverse effect, if applicable, to identify drug (T36-T50 with fifth or sixth character 5)
Excludes1: *specified adverse effects of drugs and medicaments (A00-R94 and T80-T88.6, T88.8)*

X+7th **T88.8 Other specified complications of surgical and medical care, not elsewhere classified**
Use additional code to identify the complication

X+7th **T88.9 Complication of surgical and medical care, unspecified**

Chapter 20: External Causes of Morbidity (V00-Y99)

NOTE This chapter permits the classification of environmental events and circumstances as the cause of injury, and other adverse effects. Where a code from this section is applicable, it is intended that it shall be used secondary to a code from another chapter of the Classification indicating the nature of the condition. Most often, the condition will be classifiable to Chapter 19, Injury, poisoning and certain other consequences of external causes (S00-T88). Other conditions that may be stated to be due to external causes are classified in Chapters 1 to 18. For these conditions, codes from Chapter 20 should be used to provide additional information as to the cause of the condition.

AHA CC: 1Q, 2015, 3-21

This chapter contains the following category blocks:

V00-X58	Accidents
V00-V99	Transport accidents
V00-V09	Pedestrian injured in transport accident
V10-V19	Pedal cycle rider injured in transport accident
V20-V29	Motorcycle rider injured in transport accident
V30-V39	Occupant of three-wheeled motor vehicle injured in transport accident
V40-V49	Car occupant injured in transport accident
V50-V59	Occupant of pick-up truck or van injured in transport accident
V60-V69	Occupant of heavy transport vehicle injured in transport accident
V70-V79	Bus occupant injured in transport accident
V80-V89	Other land transport accidents
V90-V94	Water transport accidents
V95-V97	Air and space transport accidents
V98-V99	Other and unspecified transport accidents
W00-X58	Other external causes of accidental injury
W00-W19	Slipping, tripping, stumbling and falls
W20-W49	Exposure to inanimate mechanical forces
W50-W64	Exposure to animate mechanical forces
W65-W74	Accidental non-transport drowning and submersion
W85-W99	Exposure to electric current, radiation and extreme ambient air temperature and pressure
X00-X08	Exposure to smoke, fire and flames
X10-X19	Contact with heat and hot substances
X30-X39	Exposure to forces of nature
X52-X58	Accidental exposure to other specified factors
X71-X83	Intentional self-harm
X92-Y09	Assault
Y21-Y33	Event of undetermined intent
Y35-Y38	Legal intervention, operations of war, military operations, and terrorism
Y62-Y84	Complications of medical and surgical care
Y62-Y69	Misadventures to patients during surgical and medical care
Y70-Y82	Medical devices associated with adverse incidents in diagnostic and therapeutic use
Y83-Y84	Surgical and other medical procedures as the cause of abnormal reaction of the patient, or of later complication, without mention of misadventure at the time of the procedure
Y90-Y99	Supplementary factors related to causes of morbidity classified elsewhere

C. Chapter-Specific Coding Guidelines

In addition to general coding guidelines, there are guidelines for specific diagnoses and/or conditions in the classification. Unless otherwise indicated, these guidelines apply to all health care settings. Please refer to Section II for guidelines on the selection of principal diagnosis.

20. Chapter 20: External Causes of Morbidity (V00-Y99)

The external causes of morbidity codes should never be sequenced as the first-listed or principal diagnosis.

External cause codes are intended to provide data for injury research and evaluation of injury prevention strategies. These codes capture how the injury or health condition happened (cause), the intent (unintentional or accidental; or intentional, such as suicide or assault), the place where the event occurred the activity of the patient at the time of the event, and the person's status (e.g., civilian, military).

There is no national requirement for mandatory ICD-10-CM external cause code reporting. Unless a provider is subject to a state-based external cause code reporting mandate or these codes are required by a particular payer, reporting of ICD-10-CM codes in Chapter 20, External Causes of Morbidity, is not required. In the absence of a mandatory reporting requirement, providers are encouraged to voluntarily report external cause codes, as they provide valuable data for injury research and evaluation of injury prevention strategies.

a. General External Cause Coding Guidelines

1) Used with any code in the range of A00.0-T88.9, Z00-Z99

An external cause code may be used with any code in the range of A00.0-T88.9, Z00-Z99, classification that **represents** a health condition due to an external cause. Though they are most applicable to injuries, they are also valid for use with such things as infections or diseases due to an external source, and other health conditions, such as a heart attack that occurs during strenuous physical activity.

2) External cause code used for length of treatment

Assign the external cause code, with the appropriate 7th character (initial encounter, subsequent encounter or sequela) for each encounter for which the injury or condition is being treated.

Most categories in chapter 20 have a 7th character requirement for each applicable code. Most categories in this chapter have three 7th character values: A, initial encounter, D, subsequent encounter and S, sequela. While the patient may be seen by a new or different provider over the course of treatment for an injury or condition, assignment of the 7th character for external cause should match the 7th character of the code assigned for the associated injury or condition for the encounter.

3) Use the full range of external cause codes

Use the full range of external cause codes to completely describe the cause, the intent, the place of occurrence, and if applicable, the activity of the patient at the time of the event, and the patient's status, for all injuries, and other health conditions due to an external cause.

4) Assign as many external cause codes as necessary

Assign as many external cause codes as necessary to fully explain each cause. If only one external code can be recorded, assign the code most related to the principal diagnosis.

5) The selection of the appropriate external cause code

The selection of the appropriate external cause code is guided by the Alphabetic Index of External Causes and by Inclusion and Exclusion notes in the Tabular List.

6) External cause code can never be a principal diagnosis

An external cause code can never be a principal (first-listed) diagnosis.

7) Combination external cause codes

Certain of the external cause codes are combination codes that identify sequential events that result in an injury, such as a fall which results in striking against an object. The injury may be due to either event or both. The combination external cause code used should correspond to the sequence of events regardless of which caused the most serious injury.

8) No external cause code needed in certain circumstances

No external cause code from Chapter 20 is needed if the external cause and intent are included in a code from another chapter (e.g. T36.0X1-Poisoning by penicillins, accidental (unintentional)).

b. Place of Occurrence Guideline

Codes from category Y92, Place of occurrence of the external cause, are secondary codes for use after other external cause codes to identify the location of the patient at the time of injury or other condition.

Generally, a place of occurrent code is assigned only once, at the initial encounter for treatment. However, in the rare instance that a new injury occurs during hospitalization, an additional place of occurrence code may be assigned. No 7th characters are used for Y92.

Do not use place of occurrence code Y92.9 if the place is not stated or is not applicable.

c. Activity Code

Assign a code from category Y93, Activity code, to describe the activity of the patient at the time the injury or other health condition occurred.

An activity code is used only once, at the initial encounter for treatment. Only one code from Y93 should be recorded on a medical record.

The activity codes are not applicable to poisonings, adverse effects, misadventures or sequela.

Do not assign Y93.9, Unspecified activity, if the activity is not stated.

A code from category Y93 is appropriate for use with external cause and intent codes if identifying the activity provides additional information about the event.

d. Place of Occurrence, Activity, and Status Codes Used with other External Cause Code

When applicable, place of occurrence, activity, and external cause status codes are sequenced after the main external cause code(s). Regardless of the number of external cause codes assigned, there should be only one place of occurrence code, one activity code, and one external cause status code assigned to an encounter. However, in the rare instance that a new injury occurs during hospitalization, an additional place of occurrence code may be assigned.

e. If the Reporting Format Limits the Number of External Cause Codes

If the reporting format limits the number of external cause codes that can be used in reporting clinical data, report the code for the cause/intent most related to the principal diagnosis. If the format permits capture of additional external cause codes, the cause/intent, including medical misadventures, of the additional events should be reported rather than the codes for place, activity, or external status.

f. Multiple External Cause Coding Guidelines

More than one external cause code is required to fully describe the external cause of an illness or injury. The assignment of external cause codes should be sequenced in the following priority:

If two or more events cause separate injuries, an external cause code should be assigned for each cause. The first-listed external cause code will be selected in the following order:

External codes for child and adult abuse take priority over all other external cause codes.

See Section I.C.19., Child and Adult abuse guidelines.

External cause codes for terrorism events take priority over all other external cause codes except child and adult abuse.

External cause codes for cataclysmic events take priority over all other external cause codes except child and adult abuse and terrorism.

External cause codes for transport accidents take priority over all other external cause codes except cataclysmic events, child and adult abuse and terrorism.

Activity and external cause status codes are assigned following all causal (intent) external cause codes.

The first-listed external cause code should correspond to the cause of the most serious diagnosis due to an assault, accident, or self-harm, following the order of hierarchy listed above.

g. Child and Adult Abuse Guideline

Adult and child abuse, neglect and maltreatment are classified as assault. Any of the assault codes may be used to indicate the external cause of any injury resulting from the confirmed abuse.

For confirmed cases of abuse, neglect and maltreatment, when the perpetrator is known, a code from Y07, Perpetrator of maltreatment and neglect, should accompany any other assault codes.

See Section I.C.19. Adult and child abuse, neglect and other maltreatment

h. Unknown or Undetermined Intent Guideline

If the intent (accident, self-harm, assault) of the cause of an injury or other condition is unknown or unspecified, code the intent as accidental intent. All transport accident categories assume accidental intent.

1) Use of undetermined intent

External cause codes for events of undetermined intent are only for use if the documentation in the record specifies that the intent cannot be determined.

i. Sequelae (Late Effects) of External Cause Guidelines

1) Sequelae external cause codes

Sequela are reported using the external cause code with the 7th character "S" for sequela. These codes should be used with any report of a late effect or sequela resulting from a previous injury.

See Section I.B.10 Sequela (Late Effects)

2) Sequela external cause code with a related current injury

A sequela external cause code should never be used with a related current nature of injury code.

3) Use of sequela external cause codes for subsequent visits

Use a late effect external cause code for subsequent visits when a late effect of the initial injury is being treated. Do not use a late effect external cause code for subsequent visits for follow- up care (e.g., to assess healing, to receive rehabilitative therapy) of the injury when no late effect of the injury has been documented.

j. Terrorism Guidelines

1) Cause of injury identified by the Federal Government (FBI) as terrorism

When the cause of an injury is identified by the Federal Government (FBI) as terrorism, the first-listed external cause code should be a code from category Y38, Terrorism. The definition of terrorism employed by the FBI is found at the inclusion note at the beginning of category Y38. Use additional code for place of occurrence (Y92.-). More than one Y38 code may be assigned if the injury is the result of more than one mechanism of terrorism.

2) Cause of an injury is suspected to be the result of terrorism

When the cause of an injury is suspected to be the result of terrorism a code from category Y38 should not be assigned. Suspected cases should be classified as assault.

3) Code Y38.9, Terrorism, secondary effects

Assign code Y38.9, Terrorism, secondary effects, for conditions occurring subsequent to the terrorist event. This code should not be assigned for conditions that are due to the initial terrorist act.

It is acceptable to assign code Y38.9 with another code from Y38 if there is an injury due to the initial terrorist event and an injury that is a subsequent result of the terrorist event.

k. External cause status

A code from category Y99, External cause status, should be assigned whenever any other external cause code is assigned for an encounter, including an Activity code, except for the events noted below. Assign a code from category Y99, External cause status, to indicate the work status of the person at the time the event occurred. The status code indicates whether the event occurred during military activity, whether a non-military person was at work, whether an individual including a student or volunteer was involved in a non-work activity at the time of the causal event.

A code from Y99, External cause status, should be assigned, when applicable, with other external cause codes, such as transport accidents and falls. The external cause status codes are not applicable to poisonings, adverse effects, misadventures or late effects. Do not assign a code from category Y99 if no other external cause codes (cause, activity) are applicable for the encounter.

An external cause status code is used only once, at the initial encounter for treatment. Only one code from Y99 should be recorded on a medical record.

Do not assign code Y99.9, Unspecified external cause status, if the status is not stated.

Accidents (V00-X58)

Transport accidents (V00-V99)

NOTE This section is structured in 12 groups. Those relating to land transport accidents (V00-V89) reflect the victim's mode of transport and are subdivided to identify the victim's 'counterpart' or the type of event. The vehicle of which the injured person is an occupant is identified in the first two characters since it is seen as the most important factor to identify for prevention purposes. A transport accident is one in which the vehicle involved must be moving or running or in use for transport purposes at the time of the accident.

Use additional code to identify:
Airbag injury (W22.1)
Type of street or road (Y92.4-)
Use of cellular telephone and other electronic equipment at the time of the transport accident (Y93.C-)

Excludes1: *agricultural vehicles in stationary use or maintenance (W31.-)*
assault by crashing of motor vehicle (Y03.-)
automobile or motor cycle in stationary use or maintenance- code to type of accident
crashing of motor vehicle, undetermined intent (Y32)
intentional self-harm by crashing of motor vehicle (X82)

Excludes2: *transport accidents due to cataclysm (X34-X38)*

NOTE Definitions related to transport accidents:

(a) A transport accident (V00-V99) is any accident involving a device designed primarily for, or used at the time primarily for, conveying persons or goods from one place to another.

(b) A public highway [trafficway] or street is the entire width between property lines (or other boundary lines) of land open to the public as a matter of right or custom for purposes of moving persons or property from one place to another. A roadway is that part of the public highway designed, improved and customarily used for vehicular traffic.

(c) A traffic accident is any vehicle accident occurring on the public highway [i.e. originating on, terminating on, or involving a vehicle partially on the highway]. A vehicle accident is assumed to have occurred on the public highway unless another place is specified, except i the case of accidents involving only off-road motor vehicles, which are classified as nontraffic accidents unless the contrary is stated.

(d) A nontraffic accident is any vehicle accident that occurs entirely in any place other than a public highway.

(e) A pedestrian is any person involved in an accident who was not at the time of the accident riding in or on a motor vehicle, railway train, streetcar or animal-drawn or other vehicle, or on a pedal cycle or animal. This includes, a person changing a tire, working on a parked care, or a person on foot. It also includes the user of a pedestrian conveyance such as a babystroller, ice-skates, skis, sled, roller skates, a skateboard, nonmotorized or motorized wheelchair, motorized mobility scooter, or nonmotorized scooter.
(f) A driver is an occupant of a transport vehicle who is operating or intending to operate it.
(g) A passenger is any occupant of a transport vehicle other than the driver, except a person traveling on the outside of the vehicle.
(h) A person on the outside of a vehicle is any person being transported by a vehicle but not occupying the space normally reserved for the driver or passengers, or the space intended for the transport of property. This includes a person travailing on the bodywork, bumper, fender, roof, running board or step of a vehicle, as well as, hanging on the outside of the vehicle.
(i) A pedal cycle is any land transport vehicle operated solely by nonmotorized pedals including a bicycle or tricycle.
(j) A pedal cyclist is any person riding a pedal cycle or in a sidecar or trailer attached to a pedal cycle.
(k) A motorcycle is a two-wheeled motor vehicle with one or two riding saddles and sometimes with a third wheel for the support of a sidecar. The sidecar is considered part of the motorcycle. This includes a moped, motor scooter, or motorized bicycle.
(l) A motorcycle rider is any person riding a motorcycle or in a sidecar or trailer attached to the motorcycle.
(m) A three-wheeled motor vehicle is a motorized tricycle designed primarily for on-road use. This includes a motor-driven tricycle, a motorized rickshaw, or a three-wheeled motor car.
(n) A car [automobile] is a four-wheeled motor vehicle designed primarily for carrying up to 7 persons. A trailer being towed by the car is considered par of the car. It does not include a van or minivan - see definition (o)
(o) A pick-up truck or van is a four or six-wheeled motor vehicle designed for carrying passengers as well as property or cargo weighing less than the local limit for classification as a heavy goods vehicle, and not requiring a special driver's license. this includes a minivan and a sport-utility vehicle (SUV)
(p) A heavy transport vehicle is a motor vehicle designed primarily for carrying property, meeting local criteria for classification as a heavy goods vehicle in terms of weight and requiring a special driver's license.
(q) A bus (coach) is a motor vehicle designed or adapted primarily for carrying more than 10 passengers, and requiring a special driver's license.
(r) A railway train or railway vehicle is any device, with or without freight or passenger cars couple to it, designed for traffic on a railway track. This includes subterranean (subways) or elevated trains.
(s) A streetcar, is a device designed and used primarily for transporting passengers within a municipality, running on rails, usually subject to normal traffic control signals, and operated principally on a right-of-way that forms part of the roadway. This includes a tram or trolley that runs on rails. A trailer being towed by a streetcar is considered part of the streetcar.
(t) A special vehicle mainly used on industrial premises is a motor vehicle designed primarily for use within the building and premises of industrial or commercial establishments. This includes battery-powered airport passenger vehicles or baggage/mail trucks, forklifts, coal-cars in a coal min, logging cars and trucks used in mines or quarries.
(u) A special vehicle mainly used in agriculture is a motor vehicle designed specifically for use in farming and agriculture (horticulture), to work the land, tend and harvest crops and transport materials on the farm. This includes harvesters, farm machinery and tractor and trailers.
(v) A special construction vehicle is a motor vehicle designed specifically for use on construction and demolition sites. This includes bulldozers, diggers, earth levellers, dump trucks, backhoes, front-end loaders, pavers, and mechanical shovels.
(w) A special all-terrain vehicle is a motor vehicle of special design to enable it to negotiate over rough or soft terrain, snow or sand. Examples of special design are high construction, special wheels and tires, tracks, and support on a cushion of air. This includes snow mobiles, All terrain vehicles (ATV), and dune buggies. It does not include passenger vehicle designated as Sport Utility Vehicles (SUV).
(x) A water craft is any device designed for transporting passengers or goods on water. This includes motor or sail boats, ships, and hovercraft.
(y) An aircraft is any device for transporting passengers or goods in the air. This includes hot-air balloons, gliders, helicopters and airplanes.
(z) A military vehicle is any motorized vehicle operating on a public roadway owned by the military and being operated by a member of the military.

Pedestrian injured in transport accident (V00-V09)

Includes: person changing tire on transport vehicle
person examining engine of vehicle broken down in (on side of) road

Excludes1: *fall due to non-transport collision with other person (W03)*
pedestrian on foot falling (slipping) on ice and snow (W00.-)
struck or bumped by another person (W51)

V00 Pedestrian conveyance accident

Use additional place of occurrence and activity external cause codes, if known (Y92.-, Y93.-)

Excludes1: *collision with another person without fall (W51)*
fall due to person on foot colliding with another person on foot (W03)
fall from non-moving wheelchair, nonmotorized scooter and motorized mobility scooter without collision (W05.-)
pedestrian (conveyance) collision with other land transport vehicle (V01-V09)
pedestrian on foot falling (slipping) on ice and snow (W00.-)

The appropriate 7th character is to be added to each code from category V00
A initial encounter
D subsequent encounter
S sequela

\+ **V00.0 Pedestrian on foot injured in collision with pedestrian conveyance**
X+7th **V00.01 Pedestrian on foot injured in collision with roller-skater**
X+7th **V00.02 Pedestrian on foot injured in collision with skateboarder**
X+7th **V00.09 Pedestrian on foot injured in collision with other pedestrian conveyance**

\+ **V00.1 Rolling-type pedestrian conveyance accident**
Excludes1: *accident with babystroller (V00.82-)*
accident with wheelchair (powered) (V00.81-)
accident with motorized mobility scooter (V00.83-)

\+ **V00.11 In-line roller-skate accident**
+7th **V00.111 Fall from in-line roller-skates**
+7th **V00.112 In-line roller-skater colliding with stationary object**
+7th **V00.118 Other in-line roller-skate accident**
Excludes1: *roller-skater collision with other land transport vehicle (V01-V09 with 5th character 1)*

\+ **V00.12 Non-in- line roller-skate accident**
+7th **V00.121 Fall from non-in-line roller-skates**
+7th **V00.122 Non-in-line roller-skater colliding with stationary object**
+7th **V00.128 Other non-in-line roller-skating accident**
Excludes1: *roller-skater collision with other land transport vehicle (V01-V09 with 5th character 1)*

\+ **V00.13 Skateboard accident**
+7th **V00.131 Fall from skateboard**
+7th **V00.132 Skateboarder colliding with stationary object**
+7th **V00.138 Other skateboard accident**
Excludes1: *skateboarder collision with other land transport vehicle (V01-V09 with 5th character 2)*

\+ **V00.14 Scooter (nonmotorized) accident**
Excludes1: *motorscooter accident (V20-V29)*
+7th **V00.141 Fall from scooter (nonmotorized)**
+7th **V00.142 Scooter (nonmotorized) colliding with stationary object**
+7th **V00.148 Other scooter (nonmotorized) accident**
Excludes1: *scooter (nonmotorized) collision with other land transport vehicle (V01-V09 with fifth character 9)*

\+ **V00.15 Heelies accident**
Rolling shoe
Wheeled shoe
Wheelies accident
+7th **V00.151 Fall from heelies**

+7th **V00.152 Heelies colliding with stationary object**
+7th **V00.158 Other heelies accident**
+ **V00.18 Accident on other rolling-type pedestrian conveyance**
+7th **V00.181 Fall from other rolling-type pedestrian conveyance**
+7th **V00.182 Pedestrian on other rolling-type pedestrian conveyance colliding with stationary object**
+7th **V00.188 Other accident on other rolling-type pedestrian conveyance**
+ **V00.2 Gliding-type pedestrian conveyance accident**
+ **V00.21 Ice-skates accident**
+7th **V00.211 Fall from ice-skates**
+7th **V00.212 Ice-skater colliding with stationary object**
+7th **V00.218 Other ice-skates accident**
Excludes1: *ice-skater collision with other land transport vehicle (V01-V09 with 5th digit 9)*
+ **V00.22 Sled accident**
+7th **V00.221 Fall from sled**
+7th **V00.222 Sledder colliding with stationary object**
+7th **V00.228 Other sled accident**
Excludes1: *sled collision with other land transport vehicle (V01-V09 with 5th digit 9)*
+ **V00.28 Other gliding-type pedestrian conveyance accident**
+7th **V00.281 Fall from other gliding-type pedestrian conveyance**
+7th **V00.282 Pedestrian on other gliding-type pedestrian conveyance colliding with stationary object**
+7th **V00.288 Other accident on other gliding-type pedestrian conveyance**
Excludes1: *gliding-type pedestrian conveyance collision with other land transport vehicle (V01-V09 with 5th digit 9)*
+ **V00.3 Flat-bottomed pedestrian conveyance accident**
+ **V00.31 Snowboard accident**
+7th **V00.311 Fall from snowboard**
+7th **V00.312 Snowboarder colliding with stationary object**
+7th **V00.318 Other snowboard accident**
Excludes1: *snowboarder collision with other land transport vehicle (V01-V09 with 5th digit 9)*
+ **V00.32 Snow-ski accident**
+7th **V00.321 Fall from snow-skis**
AHA CC: 1Q, 2015, 3-21
+7th **V00.322 Snow-skier colliding with stationary object**
+7th **V00.328 Other snow-ski accident**
Excludes1: *snow-skier collision with other land transport vehicle (V01-V09 with 5th digit 9)*
+ **V00.38 Other flat-bottomed pedestrian conveyance accident**
+7th **V00.381 Fall from other flat-bottomed pedestrian conveyance**
+7th **V00.382 Pedestrian on other flat-bottomed pedestrian conveyance colliding with stationary object**
+7th **V00.388 Other accident on other flat-bottomed pedestrian conveyance**
+ **V00.8 Accident on other pedestrian conveyance**
+ **V00.81 Accident with wheelchair (powered)**
+7th **V00.811 Fall from moving wheelchair (powered)**
Excludes1: *fall from non-moving wheelchair (W05.0)*
+7th **V00.812 Wheelchair (powered) colliding with stationary object**
+7th **V00.818 Other accident with wheelchair (powered)**
+ **V00.82 Accident with babystroller**
+7th **V00.821 Fall from babystroller**
+7th **V00.822 Babystroller colliding with stationary object**
+7th **V00.828 Other accident with babystroller**
+ **V00.83 Accident with motorized mobility scooter**
+7th **V00.831 Fall from motorized mobility scooter**
Excludes1: *fall from non-moving motorized mobility scooter (W05.2)*
+7th **V00.832 Motorized mobility scooter colliding with stationary object**
+7th **V00.838 Other accident with motorized mobility scooter**
+ **V00.89 Accident on other pedestrian conveyance**
+7th **V00.891 Fall from other pedestrian conveyance**
+7th **V00.892 Pedestrian on other pedestrian conveyance colliding with stationary object**
+7th **V00.898 Other accident on other pedestrian conveyance**
Excludes1: *other pedestrian (conveyance) collision with other land transport vehicle (V01-V09 with 5th digit 9)*

V01 Pedestrian injured in collision with pedal cycle

The appropriate 7th character is to be added to each code from category V01
A initial encounter
D subsequent encounter
S sequela

+ **V01.0 Pedestrian injured in collision with pedal cycle in nontraffic accident**
X+7th **V01.00 Pedestrian on foot injured in collision with pedal cycle in nontraffic accident**
Pedestrian NOS injured in collision with pedal cycle in nontraffic accident
X+7th **V01.01 Pedestrian on roller-skates injured in collision with pedal cycle in nontraffic accident**
X+7th **V01.02 Pedestrian on skateboard injured in collision with pedal cycle in nontraffic accident**
X+7th **V01.09 Pedestrian with other conveyance injured in collision with pedal cycle in nontraffic accident**
Pedestrian with babystroller injured in collision with pedal cycle in nontraffic accident
Pedestrian on ice-skates injured in collision with pedal cycle in nontraffic accident
Pedestrian on nonmotorized scooter injured in collision with pedal cycle in nontraffic accident
Pedestrian on sled injured in collision with pedal cycle in nontraffic accident
Pedestrian on snowboard injured in collision with pedal cycle in nontraffic accident
Pedestrian on snow-skis injured in collision with pedal cycle in nontraffic accident
Pedestrian in wheelchair (powered) injured in collision with pedal cycle in nontraffic accident
Pedestrian in motorized mobility scooter injured in collision with pedal cycle in nontraffic accident
+ **V01.1 Pedestrian injured in collision with pedal cycle in traffic accident**
X+7th **V01.10 Pedestrian on foot injured in collision with pedal cycle in traffic accident**
Pedestrian NOS injured in collision with pedal cycle in traffic accident
X+7th **V01.11 Pedestrian on roller-skates injured in collision with pedal cycle in traffic accident**
X+7th **V01.12 Pedestrian on skateboard injured in collision with pedal cycle in traffic accident**
X+7th **V01.19 Pedestrian with other conveyance injured in collision with pedal cycle in traffic accident**
Pedestrian with babystroller injured in collision with pedal cycle in traffic accident
Pedestrian on ice-skates injured in collision with pedal cycle in traffic accident
Pedestrian on nonmotorized scooter injured in collision with pedal cycle in traffic accident
Pedestrian on sled injured in collision with pedal cycle in traffic accident
Pedestrian on snowboard injured in collision with pedal cycle in traffic accident
Pedestrian on snow-skis injured in collision with pedal cycle in traffic accident
Pedestrian in wheelchair (powered) injured in collision with pedal cycle in traffic accident
Pedestrian in motorized mobility scooter injured in collision with pedal cycle in traffic accident

+ **V01.9 Pedestrian injured in collision with pedal cycle, unspecified whether traffic or nontraffic accident**

X+7th **V01.90 Pedestrian on foot injured in collision with pedal cycle, unspecified whether traffic or nontraffic accident**

Pedestrian NOS injured in collision with pedal cycle, unspecified whether traffic or nontraffic accident

X+7th **V01.91 Pedestrian on roller-skates injured in collision with pedal cycle, unspecified whether traffic or nontraffic accident**

X+7th **V01.92 Pedestrian on skateboard injured in collision with pedal cycle, unspecified whether traffic or nontraffic accident**

X+7th **V01.99 Pedestrian with other conveyance injured in collision with pedal cycle, unspecified whether traffic or nontraffic accident**

Pedestrian with babystroller injured in collision with pedal cycle, unspecified whether traffic or nontraffic accident

Pedestrian on ice-skates injured in collision with pedal cycle unspecified, whether traffic or nontraffic accident

Pedestrian on nonmotorized scooter injured in collision with pedal cycle, unspecified whether traffic or nontraffic accident

Pedestrian on sled injured in collision with pedal cycle unspecified, whether traffic or nontraffic accident

Pedestrian on snowboard injured in collision with pedal cycle, unspecified whether traffic or nontraffic accident

Pedestrian on snow-skis injured in collision with pedal cycle, unspecified whether traffic or nontraffic accident

Pedestrian in wheelchair (powered) injured in collision with pedal cycle, unspecified whether traffic or nontraffic accident

Pedestrian in motorized mobility scooter injured in collision with pedal cycle, unspecified whether traffic or nontraffic accident

V02 Pedestrian injured in collision with two- or three-wheeled motor vehicle

The appropriate 7th character is to be added to each code from category V02
A initial encounter
D subsequent encounter
S sequela

+ **V02.0 Pedestrian injured in collision with two- or three-wheeled motor vehicle in nontraffic accident**

X+7th **V02.00 Pedestrian on foot injured in collision with two- or three-wheeled motor vehicle in nontraffic accident**

Pedestrian NOS injured in collision with two- or three-wheeled motor vehicle in nontraffic accident

X+7th **V02.01 Pedestrian on roller-skates injured in collision with two- or three-wheeled motor vehicle in nontraffic accident**

X+7th **V02.02 Pedestrian on skateboard injured in collision with two- or three-wheeled motor vehicle in nontraffic accident**

X+7th **V02.09 Pedestrian with other conveyance injured in collision with two- or three-wheeled motor vehicle in nontraffic accident**

Pedestrian with babystroller injured in collision with two- or three-wheeled motor vehicle in nontraffic accident

Pedestrian on ice-skates injured in collision with two- or three-wheeled motor vehicle in nontraffic accident

Pedestrian on nonmotorized scooter injured in collision with two- or three-wheeled motor vehicle in nontraffic accident

Pedestrian on sled injured in collision with two- or three-wheeled motor vehicle in nontraffic accident

Pedestrian on snowboard injured in collision with two- or three-wheeled motor vehicle in nontraffic accident

Pedestrian on snow-skis injured in collision with two- or three-wheeled motor vehicle in nontraffic accident

Pedestrian in wheelchair (powered) injured in collision with two- or three-wheeled motor vehicle in nontraffic accident

Pedestrian in motorized mobility scooter injured in collision with two- or three-wheeled motor vehicle in nontraffic accident

+ **V02.1 Pedestrian injured in collision with two- or three-wheeled motor vehicle in traffic accident**

X+7th **V02.10 Pedestrian on foot injured in collision with two- or three-wheeled motor vehicle in traffic accident**

Pedestrian NOS injured in collision with two- or three-wheeled motor vehicle in traffic accident

X+7th **V02.11 Pedestrian on roller-skates injured in collision with two- or three-wheeled motor vehicle in traffic accident**

X+7th **V02.12 Pedestrian on skateboard injured in collision with two- or three-wheeled motor vehicle in traffic accident**

V02.19 Pedestrian with other conveyance injured in collision with two- or three-wheeled motor vehicle in traffic accident

Pedestrian with babystroller injured in collision with two- or three-wheeled motor vehicle in traffic accident

Pedestrian on ice-skates injured in collision with two- or three-wheeled motor vehicle in traffic accident

Pedestrian on nonmotorized scooter injured in collision with two- or three-wheeled motor vehicle in traffic accident

Pedestrian on sled injured in collision with two- or three-wheeled motor vehicle in traffic accident

Pedestrian on snowboard injured in collision with two- or three-wheeled motor vehicle in traffic accident

Pedestrian on snow-skis injured in collision with two- or three-wheeled motor vehicle in traffic accident

Pedestrian in wheelchair (powered) injured in collision with two- or three-wheeled motor vehicle in traffic accident

Pedestrian in motorized mobility scooter injured in collision with two- or three-wheeled motor vehicle in traffic accident

+ **V02.9 Pedestrian injured in collision with two- or three-wheeled motor vehicle, unspecified whether traffic or nontraffic accident**

X+7th **V02.90 Pedestrian on foot injured in collision with two- or three-wheeled motor vehicle, unspecified whether traffic or nontraffic accident**

Pedestrian NOS injured in collision with two- or three-wheeled motor vehicle, unspecified whether traffic or nontraffic accident

X+7th **V02.91 Pedestrian on roller-skates injured in collision with two- or three-wheeled motor vehicle, unspecified whether traffic or nontraffic accident**

X+7th **V02.92 Pedestrian on skateboard injured in collision with two- or three-wheeled motor vehicle, unspecified whether traffic or nontraffic accident**

X+7th **V02.99 Pedestrian with other conveyance injured in collision with two- or three-wheeled motor vehicle, unspecified whether traffic or nontraffic accident**

Pedestrian with babystroller injured in collision with two- or three-wheeled motor vehicle, unspecified whether traffic or nontraffic accident

Pedestrian on ice-skates injured in collision with two- or three-wheeled motor vehicle, unspecified whether traffic or nontraffic accident

Pedestrian on nonmotorized scooter injured in collision with two- or three-wheeled motor vehicle, unspecified whether traffic or nontraffic accident

Pedestrian on sled injured in collision with two- or three-wheeled motor vehicle, unspecified whether traffic or nontraffic accident

Pedestrian on snowboard injured in collision with two- or three-wheeled motor vehicle, unspecified whether traffic or nontraffic accident

Pedestrian on snow-skis injured in collision with two- or three-wheeled motor vehicle, unspecified whether traffic or nontraffic accident

Pedestrian in wheelchair (powered) injured in collision with two- or three-wheeled motor vehicle, unspecified whether traffic or nontraffic accident

Pedestrian in motorized mobility scooter injured in collision with two- or three-wheeled motor vehicle, unspecified whether traffic or nontraffic accident

V03 Pedestrian injured in collision with car, pick-up truck or van

The appropriate 7th character is to be added to each code from category V03
- A initial encounter
- D subsequent encounter
- S sequela

\+ **V03.0 Pedestrian injured in collision with car, pick-up truck or van in nontraffic accident**

X+7th **V03.00 Pedestrian on foot injured in collision with car, pick-up truck or van in nontraffic accident**

Pedestrian NOS injured in collision with car, pick-up truck or van in nontraffic accident

X+7th **V03.01 Pedestrian on roller-skates injured in collision with car, pick-up truck or van in nontraffic accident**

X+7th **V03.02 Pedestrian on skateboard injured in collision with car, pick-up truck or van in nontraffic accident**

X+7th **V03.09 Pedestrian with other conveyance injured in collision with car, pick-up truck or van in nontraffic accident**

Pedestrian with babystroller injured in collision with car, pick-up truck or van in nontraffic accident

Pedestrian on ice-skates injured in collision with car, pick-up truck or van in nontraffic accident

Pedestrian on nonmotorized scooter injured in collision with car, pick-up truck or van in nontraffic accident

Pedestrian on sled injured in collision with car, pick-up truck or van in nontraffic accident

Pedestrian on snowboard injured in collision with car, pick-up truck or van in nontraffic accident

Pedestrian on snow-skis injured in collision with car, pick-up truck or van in nontraffic accident

Pedestrian in wheelchair (powered) injured in collision with car, pick-up truck or van in nontraffic accident

Pedestrian in motorized mobility scooter injured in collision with car, pick-up truck or van in nontraffic accident

\+ **V03.1 Pedestrian injured in collision with car, pick-up truck or van in traffic accident**

X+7th **V03.10 Pedestrian on foot injured in collision with car, pick-up truck or van in traffic accident**

Pedestrian NOS injured in collision with car, pick-up truck or van in traffic accident

X+7th **V03.11 Pedestrian on roller-skates injured in collision with car, pick-up truck or van in traffic accident**

X+7th **V03.12 Pedestrian on skateboard injured in collision with car, pick-up truck or van in traffic accident**

X+7th **V03.19 Pedestrian with other conveyance injured in collision with car, pick-up truck or van in traffic accident**

Pedestrian with babystroller injured in collision with car, pick-up truck or van in traffic accident

Pedestrian on ice-skates injured in collision with car, pick-up truck or van in traffic accident

Pedestrian on nonmotorized scooter injured in collision with car, pick-up truck or van in traffic accident

Pedestrian on sled injured in collision with car, pick-up truck or van in traffic accident

Pedestrian on snowboard injured in collision with car, pick-up truck or van in traffic accident

Pedestrian on snow-skis injured in collision with car, pick-up truck or van in traffic accident

Pedestrian in wheelchair (powered) injured in collision with car, pick-up truck or van in traffic accident

Pedestrian in motorized mobility scooter injured in collision with car, pick-up truck or van in traffic accident

\+ **V03.9 Pedestrian injured in collision with car, pick-up truck or van, unspecified whether traffic or nontraffic accident**

X+7th **V03.90 Pedestrian on foot injured in collision with car, pick-up truck or van, unspecified whether traffic or nontraffic accident**

Pedestrian NOS injured in collision with car, pick-up truck or van, unspecified whether traffic or nontraffic accident

X+7th **V03.91 Pedestrian on roller-skates injured in collision with car, pick-up truck or van, unspecified whether traffic or nontraffic accident**

X+7th **V03.92 Pedestrian on skateboard injured in collision with car, pick-up truck or van, unspecified whether traffic or nontraffic accident**

X+7th **V03.99 Pedestrian with other conveyance injured in collision with car, pick-up truck or van, unspecified whether traffic or nontraffic accident**

Pedestrian with babystroller injured in collision with car, pick-up truck or van, unspecified whether traffic or nontraffic accident

Pedestrian on ice-skates injured in collision with car, pick-up truck or van, unspecified whether traffic or nontraffic accident

Pedestrian on nonmotorized scooter injured in collision with car, pick-up truck or van, unspecified whether traffic or nontraffic accident

Pedestrian on sled injured in collision with car, pick-up truck or van in nontraffic accident

Pedestrian on snowboard injured in collision with car, pick-up truck or van, unspecified whether traffic or nontraffic accident

Pedestrian on snow-skis injured in collision with car, pick-up truck or van, unspecified whether traffic or nontraffic accident

Pedestrian in wheelchair (powered) injured in collision with car, pick-up truck or van, unspecified whether traffic or nontraffic accident

Pedestrian in motorized mobility scooter injured in collision with car, pick-up truck or van, unspecified whether traffic or nontraffic accident

V04 Pedestrian injured in collision with heavy transport vehicle or bus

Excludes1: *pedestrian injured in collision with military vehicle (V09.01, V09.21)*

The appropriate 7th character is to be added to each code from category V04
- A initial encounter
- D subsequent encounter
- S sequela

\+ **V04.0 Pedestrian injured in collision with heavy transport vehicle or bus in nontraffic accident**

X+7th **V04.00 Pedestrian on foot injured in collision with heavy transport vehicle or bus in nontraffic accident**

Pedestrian NOS injured in collision with heavy transport vehicle or bus in nontraffic accident

X+7th **V04.01 Pedestrian on roller-skates injured in collision with heavy transport vehicle or bus in nontraffic accident**

X+7th **V04.02 Pedestrian on skateboard injured in collision with heavy transport vehicle or bus in nontraffic accident**

X+7th **V04.09 Pedestrian with other conveyance injured in collision with heavy transport vehicle or bus in nontraffic accident**

Pedestrian with babystroller injured in collision with heavy transport vehicle or bus in nontraffic accident

Pedestrian on ice-skates injured in collision with heavy transport vehicle or bus in nontraffic accident

Pedestrian on nonmotorized scooter injured in collision with heavy transport vehicle or bus in nontraffic accident

Pedestrian on sled injured in collision with heavy transport vehicle or bus in nontraffic accident

Pedestrian on snowboard injured in collision with heavy transport vehicle or bus in nontraffic accident

Pedestrian on snow-skis injured in collision with heavy transport vehicle or bus in nontraffic accident

Pedestrian in wheelchair (powered) injured in collision with heavy transport vehicle or bus in nontraffic accident

Pedestrian in motorized mobility scooter injured in collision with heavy transport vehicle or bus in nontraffic accident

\+ **V04.1 Pedestrian injured in collision with heavy transport vehicle or bus in traffic accident**

X+7th **V04.10 Pedestrian on foot injured in collision with heavy transport vehicle or bus in traffic accident**

Pedestrian NOS injured in collision with heavy transport vehicle or bus in traffic accident

X+7th **V04.11 Pedestrian on roller-skates injured in collision with heavy transport vehicle or bus in traffic accident**

X+7th **V04.12 Pedestrian on skateboard injured in collision with heavy transport vehicle or bus in traffic accident**

X+7th **V04.19 Pedestrian with other conveyance injured in collision with heavy transport vehicle or bus in traffic accident**

Pedestrian with babystroller injured in collision with heavy transport vehicle or bus in traffic accident

Pedestrian on ice-skates injured in collision with heavy transport vehicle or bus in traffic accident

Pedestrian on nonmotorized scooter injured in collision with heavy transport vehicle or bus in traffic accident

Pedestrian on sled injured in collision with heavy transport vehicle or bus in traffic accident

Pedestrian on snowboard injured in collision with heavy transport vehicle or bus in traffic accident

Pedestrian on snow-skis injured in collision with heavy transport vehicle or bus in traffic accident

Pedestrian in wheelchair (powered) injured in collision with heavy transport vehicle or bus in traffic accident

Pedestrian in motorized mobility scooter injured in collision with heavy transport vehicle or bus in traffic accident

\+ **V04.9 Pedestrian injured in collision with heavy transport vehicle or bus, unspecified whether traffic or nontraffic accident**

X+7th **V04.90 Pedestrian on foot injured in collision with heavy transport vehicle or bus, unspecified whether traffic or nontraffic accident**

Pedestrian NOS injured in collision with heavy transport vehicle or bus, unspecified whether traffic or nontraffic accident

X+7th **V04.91 Pedestrian on roller-skates injured in collision with heavy transport vehicle or bus, unspecified whether traffic or nontraffic accident**

X+7th **V04.92 Pedestrian on skateboard injured in collision with heavy transport vehicle or bus, unspecified whether traffic or nontraffic accident**

X+7th **V04.99 Pedestrian with other conveyance injured in collision with heavy transport vehicle or bus, unspecified whether traffic or nontraffic accident**

Pedestrian with babystroller injured in collision with heavy transport vehicle or bus, unspecified whether traffic or nontraffic accident

Pedestrian on ice-skates injured in collision with heavy transport vehicle or bus, unspecified whether traffic or nontraffic accident

Pedestrian on nonmotorized scooter injured in collision with heavy transport vehicle or bus, unspecified whether traffic or nontraffic accident

Pedestrian on sled injured in collision with heavy transport vehicle or bus, unspecified whether traffic or nontraffic accident

Pedestrian on snowboard injured in collision with heavy transport vehicle or bus, unspecified whether traffic or nontraffic accident

Pedestrian on snow-skis injured in collision with heavy transport vehicle or bus, unspecified whether traffic or nontraffic accident

Pedestrian in wheelchair (powered) injured in collision with heavy transport vehicle or bus, unspecified whether traffic or nontraffic accident

Pedestrian in motorized mobility scooter injured in collision with heavy transport vehicle or bus, unspecified whether traffic or nontraffic accident

V05 Pedestrian injured in collision with railway train or railway vehicle

The appropriate 7th character is to be added to each code from category V05
A initial encounter
D subsequent encounter
S sequela

\+ **V05.0 Pedestrian injured in collision with railway train or railway vehicle in nontraffic accident**

X+7th **V05.00 Pedestrian on foot injured in collision with railway train or railway vehicle in nontraffic accident**

Pedestrian NOS injured in collision with railway train or railway vehicle in nontraffic accident

X+7th **V05.01 Pedestrian on roller-skates injured in collision with railway train or railway vehicle in nontraffic accident**

X+7th **V05.02 Pedestrian on skateboard injured in collision with railway train or railway vehicle in nontraffic accident**

X+7th **V05.09 Pedestrian with other conveyance injured in collision with railway train or railway vehicle in nontraffic accident**

Pedestrian with babystroller injured in collision with railway train or railway vehicle in nontraffic accident

Pedestrian on ice-skates injured in collision with railway train or railway vehicle in nontraffic accident

Pedestrian on nonmotorized scooter injured in collision with railway train or railway vehicle in nontraffic accident

Pedestrian on sled injured in collision with railway train or railway vehicle in nontraffic accident

Pedestrian on snowboard injured in collision with railway train or railway vehicle in nontraffic accident

Pedestrian on snow-skis injured in collision with railway train or railway vehicle in nontraffic accident

Pedestrian in wheelchair (powered) injured in collision with railway train or railway vehicle in nontraffic accident

Pedestrian in motorized mobility scooter injured in collision with railway train or railway vehicle in nontraffic accident

\+ **V05.1 Pedestrian injured in collision with railway train or railway vehicle in traffic accident**

X+7th **V05.10 Pedestrian on foot injured in collision with railway train or railway vehicle in traffic accident**

Pedestrian NOS injured in collision with railway train or railway vehicle in traffic accident

X+7th **V05.11 Pedestrian on roller-skates injured in collision with railway train or railway vehicle in traffic accident**

X+7th **V05.12 Pedestrian on skateboard injured in collision with railway train or railway vehicle in traffic accident**

X+7th **V05.19 Pedestrian with other conveyance injured in collision with railway train or railway vehicle in traffic accident**

Pedestrian with babystroller injured in collision with railway train or railway vehicle in traffic accident
Pedestrian on ice-skates injured in collision with railway train or railway vehicle in traffic accident
Pedestrian on nonmotorized scooter injured in collision with railway train or railway vehicle in traffic accident
Pedestrian on sled injured in collision with railway train or railway vehicle in traffic accident
Pedestrian on snowboard injured in collision with railway train or railway vehicle in traffic accident
Pedestrian on snow-skis injured in collision with railway train or railway vehicle in traffic accident
Pedestrian in wheelchair (powered) injured in collision with railway train or railway vehicle in traffic accident
Pedestrian in motorized mobility scooter injured in collision with railway train or railway vehicle in traffic accident

+ **V05.9 Pedestrian injured in collision with railway train or railway vehicle, unspecified whether traffic or nontraffic accident**

X+7th **V05.90 Pedestrian on foot injured in collision with railway train or railway vehicle, unspecified whether traffic or nontraffic accident**

Pedestrian NOS injured in collision with railway train or railway vehicle, unspecified whether traffic or nontraffic accident

X+7th **V05.91 Pedestrian on roller-skates injured in collision with railway train or railway vehicle, unspecified whether traffic or nontraffic accident**

X+7th **V05.92 Pedestrian on skateboard injured in collision with railway train or railway vehicle, unspecified whether traffic or nontraffic accident**

X+7th **V05.99 Pedestrian with other conveyance injured in collision with railway train or railway vehicle, unspecified whether traffic or nontraffic accident**

Pedestrian with babystroller injured in collision with railway train or railway vehicle, unspecified whether traffic or nontraffic
Pedestrian on ice-skates injured in collision with railway train or railway vehicle, unspecified whether traffic or nontraffic
Pedestrian on nonmotorized scooter injured in collision with railway train or railway vehicle, unspecified whether traffic or nontraffic
Pedestrian on sled injured in collision with railway train or railway vehicle, unspecified whether traffic or nontraffic
Pedestrian on snowboard injured in collision with railway train or railway vehicle, unspecified whether traffic or nontraffic
Pedestrian on snow-skis injured in collision with railway train or railway vehicle, unspecified whether traffic or nontraffic
Pedestrian in wheelchair (powered) injured in collision with railway train or railway vehicle, unspecified whether traffic or nontraffic
Pedestrian in motorized mobility scooter injured in collision with railway train or railway vehicle, unspecified whether traffic or nontraffic

V06 Pedestrian injured in collision with other nonmotor vehicle

Includes: collision with animal-drawn vehicle, animal being ridden, nonpowered streetcar

Excludes1: *pedestrian injured in collision with pedestrian conveyance (V00.0-)*

The appropriate 7th character is to be added to each code from category V06
A initial encounter
D subsequent encounter
S sequela

+ **V06.0 Pedestrian injured in collision with other nonmotor vehicle in nontraffic accident**

X+7th **V06.00 Pedestrian on foot injured in collision with other nonmotor vehicle in nontraffic accident**

Pedestrian NOS injured in collision with other nonmotor vehicle in nontraffic accident

X+7th **V06.01 Pedestrian on roller-skates injured in collision with other nonmotor vehicle in nontraffic accident**

X+7th **V06.02 Pedestrian on skateboard injured in collision with other nonmotor vehicle in nontraffic accident**

X+7th **V06.09 Pedestrian with other conveyance injured in collision with other nonmotor vehicle in nontraffic accident**

Pedestrian with babystroller injured in collision with other nonmotor vehicle in nontraffic accident
Pedestrian on ice-skates injured in collision with other nonmotor vehicle in nontraffic accident
Pedestrian on nonmotorized scooter injured in collision with other nonmotor vehicle in nontraffic accident
Pedestrian on sled injured in collision with other nonmotor vehicle in nontraffic accident
Pedestrian on snowboard injured in collision with other nonmotor vehicle in nontraffic accident
Pedestrian on snow-skis injured in collision with other nonmotor vehicle in nontraffic accident
Pedestrian in wheelchair (powered) injured in collision with other nonmotor vehicle in nontraffic accident
Pedestrian in motorized mobility scooter injured in collision with other nonmotor vehicle in nontraffic accident

+ **V06.1 Pedestrian injured in collision with other nonmotor vehicle in traffic accident**

X+7th **V06.10 Pedestrian on foot injured in collision with other nonmotor vehicle in traffic accident**

Pedestrian NOS injured in collision with other nonmotor vehicle in traffic accident

X+7th **V06.11 Pedestrian on roller-skates injured in collision with other nonmotor vehicle in traffic accident**

X+7th **V06.12 Pedestrian on skateboard injured in collision with other nonmotor vehicle in traffic accident**

X+7th **V06.19 Pedestrian with other conveyance injured in collision with other nonmotor vehicle in traffic accident**

Pedestrian with babystroller injured in collision with other nonmotor vehicle in nontraffic accident
Pedestrian on ice-skates injured in collision with other nonmotor vehicle in traffic accident
Pedestrian on nonmotorized scooter injured in collision with other nonmotor vehicle in traffic accident
Pedestrian on sled injured in collision with other nonmotor vehicle in traffic accident
Pedestrian on snowboard injured in collision with other nonmotor vehicle in traffic accident
Pedestrian on snow-skis injured in collision with other nonmotor vehicle in traffic accident
Pedestrian in wheelchair (powered) injured in collision with other nonmotor vehicle in traffic accident
Pedestrian in motorized mobility scooter injured in collision with other nonmotor vehicle in traffic accident

+ **V06.9 Pedestrian injured in collision with other nonmotor vehicle, unspecified whether traffic or nontraffic accident**

X+7th **V06.90 Pedestrian on foot injured in collision with other nonmotor vehicle, unspecified whether traffic or nontraffic accident**

Pedestrian NOS injured in collision with other nonmotor vehicle, unspecified whether traffic or nontraffic accident

X+7th **V06.91 Pedestrian on roller-skates injured in collision with other nonmotor vehicle, unspecified whether traffic or nontraffic accident**

X+7th **V06.92 Pedestrian on skateboard injured in collision with other nonmotor vehicle, unspecified whether traffic or nontraffic accident**

X+7th **V06.99 Pedestrian with other conveyance injured in collision with other nonmotor vehicle, unspecified whether traffic or nontraffic accident**
Pedestrian with babystroller injured in collision with other nonmotor vehicle, unspecified whether traffic or nontraffic accident
Pedestrian on ice-skates injured in collision with other nonmotor vehicle, unspecified whether traffic or nontraffic accident
Pedestrian on nonmotorized scooter injured in collision with other nonmotor vehicle, unspecified whether traffic or nontraffic accident
Pedestrian on sled injured in collision with other nonmotor vehicle, unspecified whether traffic or nontraffic accident
Pedestrian on snowboard injured in collision with other nonmotor vehicle, unspecified whether traffic or nontraffic accident
Pedestrian on snow-skis injured in collision with other nonmotor vehicle, unspecified whether traffic or nontraffic accident
Pedestrian in wheelchair (powered) injured in collision with other nonmotor vehicle, unspecified whether traffic or nontraffic accident
Pedestrian in motorized mobility scooter injured in collision with other nonmotor vehicle, unspecified whether traffic or nontraffic accident

V09 Pedestrian injured in other and unspecified transport accidents

The appropriate 7th character is to be added to each code from category V09
A initial encounter
D subsequent encounter
S sequela

\+ **V09.0 Pedestrian injured in nontraffic accident involving other and unspecified motor vehicles**
X+7th **V09.00 Pedestrian injured in nontraffic accident involving unspecified motor vehicles**
X+7th **V09.01 Pedestrian injured in nontraffic accident involving military vehicle**
X+7th **V09.09 Pedestrian injured in nontraffic accident involving other motor vehicles**
Pedestrian injured in nontraffic accident by special vehicle
X+7th **V09.1 Pedestrian injured in unspecified nontraffic accident**
\+ **V09.2 Pedestrian injured in traffic accident involving other and unspecified motor vehicles**
X+7th **V09.20 Pedestrian injured in traffic accident involving unspecified motor vehicles**
X+7th **V09.21 Pedestrian injured in traffic accident involving military vehicle**
X+7th **V09.29 Pedestrian injured in traffic accident involving other motor vehicles**
X+7th **V09.3 Pedestrian injured in unspecified traffic accident**
X+7th **V09.9 Pedestrian injured in unspecified transport accident**

edal cycle rider injured in transport accident (V10-V19)

cludes: any non-motorized vehicle, excluding an animal-drawn vehicle, or a sidecar or trailer attached to the pedal cycle
cludes2: *rupture of pedal cycle tire (W37.0)*

V10 Pedal cycle rider injured in collision with pedestrian or animal
Excludes1: *pedal cycle rider collision with animal-drawn vehicle or animal being ridden (V16.-)*

The appropriate 7th character is to be added to each code from category V10
A initial encounter
D subsequent encounter
S sequela

X+7th **V10.0 Pedal cycle driver injured in collision with pedestrian or animal in nontraffic accident**
X+7th **V10.1 Pedal cycle passenger injured in collision with pedestrian or animal in nontraffic accident**
X+7th **V10.2 Unspecified pedal cyclist injured in collision with pedestrian or animal in nontraffic accident**
X+7th **V10.3 Person boarding or alighting a pedal cycle injured in collision with pedestrian or animal**
X+7th **V10.4 Pedal cycle driver injured in collision with pedestrian or animal in traffic accident**
X+7th **V10.5 Pedal cycle passenger injured in collision with pedestrian or animal in traffic accident**
X+7th **V10.9 Unspecified pedal cyclist injured in collision with pedestrian or animal in traffic accident**

V11 Pedal cycle rider injured in collision with other pedal cycle

The appropriate 7th character is to be added to each code from category V11
A initial encounter
D subsequent encounter
S sequela

X+7th **V11.0 Pedal cycle driver injured in collision with other pedal cycle in nontraffic accident**
X+7th **V11.1 Pedal cycle passenger injured in collision with other pedal cycle in nontraffic accident**
X+7th **V11.2 Unspecified pedal cyclist injured in collision with other pedal cycle in nontraffic accident**
X+7th **V11.3 Person boarding or alighting a pedal cycle injured in collision with other pedal cycle**
X+7th **V11.4 Pedal cycle driver injured in collision with other pedal cycle in traffic accident**
X+7th **V11.5 Pedal cycle passenger injured in collision with other pedal cycle in traffic accident**
X+7th **V11.9 Unspecified pedal cyclist injured in collision with other pedal cycle in traffic accident**

V12 Pedal cycle rider injured in collision with two- or three-wheeled motor vehicle

The appropriate 7th character is to be added to each code from category V12
A initial encounter
D subsequent encounter
S sequela

X+7th **V12.0 Pedal cycle driver injured in collision with two- or three-wheeled motor vehicle in nontraffic accident**
X+7th **V12.1 Pedal cycle passenger injured in collision with two- or three-wheeled motor vehicle in nontraffic accident**
X+7th **V12.2 Unspecified pedal cyclist injured in collision with two- or three-wheeled motor vehicle in nontraffic accident**
X+7th **V12.3 Person boarding or alighting a pedal cycle injured in collision with two- or three-wheeled motor vehicle**
X+7th **V12.4 Pedal cycle driver injured in collision with two- or three-wheeled motor vehicle in traffic accident**
X+7th **V12.5 Pedal cycle passenger injured in collision with two- or three-wheeled motor vehicle in traffic accident**
X+7th **V12.9 Unspecified pedal cyclist injured in collision with two- or three-wheeled motor vehicle in traffic accident**

V13 Pedal cycle rider injured in collision with car, pick-up truck or van

The appropriate 7th character is to be added to each code from category V13
A initial encounter
D subsequent encounter
S sequela

X+7th **V13.0 Pedal cycle driver injured in collision with car, pick-up truck or van in nontraffic accident**
X+7th **V13.1 Pedal cycle passenger injured in collision with car, pick-up truck or van in nontraffic accident**
X+7th **V13.2 Unspecified pedal cyclist injured in collision with car, pick-up truck or van in nontraffic accident**
X+7th **V13.3 Person boarding or alighting a pedal cycle injured in collision with car, pick-up truck or van**
X+7th **V13.4 Pedal cycle driver injured in collision with car, pick-up truck or van in traffic accident**
X+7th **V13.5 Pedal cycle passenger injured in collision with car, pick-up truck or van in traffic accident**
X+7th **V13.9 Unspecified pedal cyclist injured in collision with car, pick-up truck or van in traffic accident**

V14 Pedal cycle rider injured in collision with heavy transport vehicle or bus
Excludes1: *pedal cycle rider injured in collision with military vehicle (V19.81)*

The appropriate 7th character is to be added to each code from category V14
A initial encounter
D subsequent encounter
S sequela

X+7th **V14.0 Pedal cycle driver injured in collision with heavy transport vehicle or bus in nontraffic accident**

X+7th **V14.1** **Pedal cycle passenger injured in collision with heavy transport vehicle or bus in nontraffic accident**

X+7th **V14.2** **Unspecified pedal cyclist injured in collision with heavy transport vehicle or bus in nontraffic accident**

X+7th **V14.3** **Person boarding or alighting a pedal cycle injured in collision with heavy transport vehicle or bus**

X+7th **V14.4** **Pedal cycle driver injured in collision with heavy transport vehicle or bus in traffic accident**

X+7th **V14.5** **Pedal cycle passenger injured in collision with heavy transport vehicle or bus in traffic accident**

X+7th **V14.9** **Unspecified pedal cyclist injured in collision with heavy transport vehicle or bus in traffic accident**

V15 **Pedal cycle rider injured in collision with railway train or railway vehicle**

The appropriate 7th character is to be added to each code from category V15
A initial encounter
D subsequent encounter
S sequela

X+7th **V15.0** **Pedal cycle driver injured in collision with railway train or railway vehicle in nontraffic accident**

X+7th **V15.1** **Pedal cycle passenger injured in collision with railway train or railway vehicle in nontraffic accident**

X+7th **V15.2** **Unspecified pedal cyclist injured in collision with railway train or railway vehicle in nontraffic accident**

X+7th **V15.3** **Person boarding or alighting a pedal cycle injured in collision with railway train or railway vehicle**

X+7th **V15.4** **Pedal cycle driver injured in collision with railway train or railway vehicle in traffic accident**

X+7th **V15.5** **Pedal cycle passenger injured in collision with railway train or railway vehicle in traffic accident**

X+7th **V15.9** **Unspecified pedal cyclist injured in collision with railway train or railway vehicle in traffic accident**

V16 **Pedal cycle rider injured in collision with other nonmotor vehicle**

Includes: collision with animal-drawn vehicle, animal being ridden, streetcar

The appropriate 7th character is to be added to each code from category V16
A initial encounter
D subsequent encounter
S sequela

X+7th **V16.0** **Pedal cycle driver injured in collision with other nonmotor vehicle in nontraffic accident**

X+7th **V16.1** **Pedal cycle passenger injured in collision with other nonmotor vehicle in nontraffic accident**

X+7th **V16.2** **Unspecified pedal cyclist injured in collision with other nonmotor vehicle in nontraffic accident**

X+7th **V16.3** **Person boarding or alighting a pedal cycle injured in collision with other nonmotor vehicle in nontraffic accident**

X+7th **V16.4** **Pedal cycle driver injured in collision with other nonmotor vehicle in traffic accident**

X+7th **V16.5** **Pedal cycle passenger injured in collision with other nonmotor vehicle in traffic accident**

X+7th **V16.9** **Unspecified pedal cyclist injured in collision with other nonmotor vehicle in traffic accident**

V17 **Pedal cycle rider injured in collision with fixed or stationary object**

The appropriate 7th character is to be added to each code from category V17
A initial encounter
D subsequent encounter
S sequela

X+7th **V17.0** **Pedal cycle driver injured in collision with fixed or stationary object in nontraffic accident**

X+7th **V17.1** **Pedal cycle passenger injured in collision with fixed or stationary object in nontraffic accident**

X+7th **V17.2** **Unspecified pedal cyclist injured in collision with fixed or stationary object in nontraffic accident**

X+7th **V17.3** **Person boarding or alighting a pedal cycle injured in collision with fixed or stationary object**

X+7th **V17.4** **Pedal cycle driver injured in collision with fixed or stationary object in traffic accident**

X+7th **V17.5** **Pedal cycle passenger injured in collision with fixed or stationary object in traffic accident**

X+7th **V17.9** **Unspecified pedal cyclist injured in collision with fixed or stationary object in traffic accident**

V18 **Pedal cycle rider injured in noncollision transport accident**

Includes: fall or thrown from pedal cycle (without antecedent collision)
overturning pedal cycle NOS
overturning pedal cycle without collision

The appropriate 7th character is to be added to each code from category V18
A initial encounter
D subsequent encounter
S sequela

X+7th **V18.0** **Pedal cycle driver injured in noncollision transport accident i nontraffic accident**

X+7th **V18.1** **Pedal cycle passenger injured in noncollision transport accident in nontraffic accident**

X+7th **V18.2** **Unspecified pedal cyclist injured in noncollision transport accident in nontraffic accident**

X+7th **V18.3** **Person boarding or alighting a pedal cycle injured in noncollision transport accident**

X+7th **V18.4** **Pedal cycle driver injured in noncollision transport accident i traffic accident**

X+7th **V18.5** **Pedal cycle passenger injured in noncollision transport accident in traffic accident**

X+7th **V18.9** **Unspecified pedal cyclist injured in noncollision transport accident in traffic accident**

V19 **Pedal cycle rider injured in other and unspecified transport accidents**

The appropriate 7th character is to be added to each code from categoı V19
A initial encounter
D subsequent encounter
S sequela

\+ **V19.0** **Pedal cycle driver injured in collision with other and unspecified motor vehicles in nontraffic accident**

X+7th **V19.00** **Pedal cycle driver injured in collision with unspecified motor vehicles in nontraffic accident**

X+7th **V19.09** **Pedal cycle driver injured in collision with other motor vehicles in nontraffic accident**

\+ **V19.1** **Pedal cycle passenger injured in collision with other and unspecified motor vehicles in nontraffic accident**

X+7th **V19.10** **Pedal cycle passenger injured in collision with unspecified motor vehicles in nontraffic accident**

X+7th **V19.19** **Pedal cycle passenger injured in collision with othe motor vehicles in nontraffic accident**

\+ **V19.2** **Unspecified pedal cyclist injured in collision with other and unspecified motor vehicles in nontraffic accident**

X+7th **V19.20** **Unspecified pedal cyclist injured in collision with unspecified motor vehicles in nontraffic accident**
Pedal cycle collision NOS, nontraffic

X+7th **V19.29** **Unspecified pedal cyclist injured in collision with other motor vehicles in nontraffic accident**

X+7th **V19.3** **Pedal cyclist (driver) (passenger) injured in unspecified nontraffic accident**
Pedal cycle accident NOS, nontraffic
Pedal cyclist injured in nontraffic accident NOS

\+ **V19.4** **Pedal cycle driver injured in collision with other and unspecified motor vehicles in traffic accident**

X+7th **V19.40** **Pedal cycle driver injured in collision with unspecified motor vehicles in traffic accident**

X+7th **V19.49** **Pedal cycle driver injured in collision with other motor vehicles in traffic accident**

\+ **V19.5** **Pedal cycle passenger injured in collision with other and unspecified motor vehicles in traffic accident**

X+7th **V19.50** **Pedal cycle passenger injured in collision with unspecified motor vehicles in traffic accident**

X+7th **V19.59** **Pedal cycle passenger injured in collision with othe motor vehicles in traffic accident**

\+ **V19.6** **Unspecified pedal cyclist injured in collision with other and unspecified motor vehicles in traffic accident**

X+7th **V19.60** **Unspecified pedal cyclist injured in collision with unspecified motor vehicles in traffic accident**
Pedal cycle collision NOS (traffic)

X+7th **V19.69** **Unspecified pedal cyclist injured in collision with other motor vehicles in traffic accident**

+ **V19.8 Pedal cyclist (driver) (passenger) injured in other specified transport accidents**

X+7th **V19.81 Pedal cyclist (driver) (passenger) injured in transport accident with military vehicle**

X+7th **V19.88 Pedal cyclist (driver) (passenger) injured in other specified transport accidents**

X+7th **V19.9 Pedal cyclist (driver) (passenger) injured in unspecified traffic accident**
Pedal cycle accident NOS

Motorcycle rider injured in transport accident (V20-V29)

Includes: moped
motorcycle with sidecar
motorized bicycle
motor scooter

Excludes1: *three-wheeled motor vehicle (V30-V39)*

V20 Motorcycle rider injured in collision with pedestrian or animal

Excludes1: *motorcycle rider collision with animal-drawn vehicle or animal being ridden (V26.-)*

The appropriate 7th character is to be added to each code from category V20
A initial encounter
D subsequent encounter
S sequela

X+7th **V20.0 Motorcycle driver injured in collision with pedestrian or animal in nontraffic accident**

X+7th **V20.1 Motorcycle passenger injured in collision with pedestrian or animal in nontraffic accident**

X+7th **V20.2 Unspecified motorcycle rider injured in collision with pedestrian or animal in nontraffic accident**

X+7th **V20.3 Person boarding or alighting a motorcycle injured in collision with pedestrian or animal**

X+7th **V20.4 Motorcycle driver injured in collision with pedestrian or animal in traffic accident**

X+7th **V20.5 Motorcycle passenger injured in collision with pedestrian or animal in traffic accident**

X+7th **V20.9 Unspecified motorcycle rider injured in collision with pedestrian or animal in traffic accident**

V21 Motorcycle rider injured in collision with pedal cycle

The appropriate 7th character is to be added to each code from category V21
A initial encounter
D subsequent encounter
S sequela

X+7th **V21.0 Motorcycle driver injured in collision with pedal cycle in nontraffic accident**

X+7th **V21.1 Motorcycle passenger injured in collision with pedal cycle in nontraffic accident**

X+7th **V21.2 Unspecified motorcycle rider injured in collision with pedal cycle in nontraffic accident**

X+7th **V21.3 Person boarding or alighting a motorcycle injured in collision with pedal cycle**

X+7th **V21.4 Motorcycle driver injured in collision with pedal cycle in traffic accident**

X+7th **V21.5 Motorcycle passenger injured in collision with pedal cycle in traffic accident**

X+7th **V21.9 Unspecified motorcycle rider injured in collision with pedal cycle in traffic accident**

V22 Motorcycle rider injured in collision with two- or three-wheeled motor vehicle

The appropriate 7th character is to be added to each code from category V22
A initial encounter
D subsequent encounter
S sequela

X+7th **V22.0 Motorcycle driver injured in collision with two- or three-wheeled motor vehicle in nontraffic accident**

X+7th **V22.1 Motorcycle passenger injured in collision with two- or three-wheeled motor vehicle in nontraffic accident**

X+7th **V22.2 Unspecified motorcycle rider injured in collision with two- or three-wheeled motor vehicle in nontraffic accident**

X+7th **V22.3 Person boarding or alighting a motorcycle injured in collision with two- or three-wheeled motor vehicle**

X+7th **V22.4 Motorcycle driver injured in collision with two- or three-wheeled motor vehicle in traffic accident**

X+7th **V22.5 Motorcycle passenger injured in collision with two- or three-wheeled motor vehicle in traffic accident**

X+7th **V22.9 Unspecified motorcycle rider injured in collision with two- or three-wheeled motor vehicle in traffic accident**

V23 Motorcycle rider injured in collision with car, pick-up truck or van

The appropriate 7th character is to be added to each code from category V23
A initial encounter
D subsequent encounter
S sequela

X+7th **V23.0 Motorcycle driver injured in collision with car, pick-up truck or van in nontraffic accident**

X+7th **V23.1 Motorcycle passenger injured in collision with car, pick-up truck or van in nontraffic accident**

X+7th **V23.2 Unspecified motorcycle rider injured in collision with car, pick-up truck or van in nontraffic accident**

X+7th **V23.3 Person boarding or alighting a motorcycle injured in collision with car, pick-up truck or van**

X+7th **V23.4 Motorcycle driver injured in collision with car, pick-up truck or van in traffic accident**

X+7th **V23.5 Motorcycle passenger injured in collision with car, pick-up truck or van in traffic accident**

X+7th **V23.9 Unspecified motorcycle rider injured in collision with car, pick-up truck or van in traffic accident**

V24 Motorcycle rider injured in collision with heavy transport vehicle or bus

Excludes1: *motorcycle rider injured in collision with military vehicle (V29.81)*

The appropriate 7th character is to be added to each code from category V24
A initial encounter
D subsequent encounter
S sequela

X+7th **V24.0 Motorcycle driver injured in collision with heavy transport vehicle or bus in nontraffic accident**

X+7th **V24.1 Motorcycle passenger injured in collision with heavy transport vehicle or bus in nontraffic accident**

X+7th **V24.2 Unspecified motorcycle rider injured in collision with heavy transport vehicle or bus in nontraffic accident**

X+7th **V24.3 Person boarding or alighting a motorcycle injured in collision with heavy transport vehicle or bus**

X+7th **V24.4 Motorcycle driver injured in collision with heavy transport vehicle or bus in traffic accident**

X+7th **V24.5 Motorcycle passenger injured in collision with heavy transport vehicle or bus in traffic accident**

X+7th **V24.9 Unspecified motorcycle rider injured in collision with heavy transport vehicle or bus in traffic accident**

V25 Motorcycle rider injured in collision with railway train or railway vehicle

The appropriate 7th character is to be added to each code from category V25
A initial encounter
D subsequent encounter
S sequela

X+7th **V25.0 Motorcycle driver injured in collision with railway train or railway vehicle in nontraffic accident**

X+7th **V25.1 Motorcycle passenger injured in collision with railway train or railway vehicle in nontraffic accident**

X+7th **V25.2 Unspecified motorcycle rider injured in collision with railway train or railway vehicle in nontraffic accident**

X+7th **V25.3 Person boarding or alighting a motorcycle injured in collision with railway train or railway vehicle**

X+7th **V25.4 Motorcycle driver injured in collision with railway train or railway vehicle in traffic accident**

X+7th **V25.5 Motorcycle passenger injured in collision with railway train or railway vehicle in traffic accident**

X+7th **V25.9 Unspecified motorcycle rider injured in collision with railway train or railway vehicle in traffic accident**

V26 Motorcycle rider injured in collision with other nonmotor vehicle

Includes: collision with animal-drawn vehicle, animal being ridden, streetcar

The appropriate 7th character is to be added to each code from category V26
A initial encounter
D subsequent encounter
S sequela

X+7th **V26.0 Motorcycle driver injured in collision with other nonmotor vehicle in nontraffic accident**
X+7th **V26.1 Motorcycle passenger injured in collision with other nonmotor vehicle in nontraffic accident**
X+7th **V26.2 Unspecified motorcycle rider injured in collision with other nonmotor vehicle in nontraffic accident**
X+7th **V26.3 Person boarding or alighting a motorcycle injured in collision with other nonmotor vehicle**
X+7th **V26.4 Motorcycle driver injured in collision with other nonmotor vehicle in traffic accident**
X+7th **V26.5 Motorcycle passenger injured in collision with other nonmotor vehicle in traffic accident**
X+7th **V26.9 Unspecified motorcycle rider injured in collision with other nonmotor vehicle in traffic accident**

V27 Motorcycle rider injured in collision with fixed or stationary object

The appropriate 7th character is to be added to each code from category V27
A initial encounter
D subsequent encounter
S sequela

X+7th **V27.0 Motorcycle driver injured in collision with fixed or stationary object in nontraffic accident**
X+7th **V27.1 Motorcycle passenger injured in collision with fixed or stationary object in nontraffic accident**
X+7th **V27.2 Unspecified motorcycle rider injured in collision with fixed or stationary object in nontraffic accident**
X+7th **V27.3 Person boarding or alighting a motorcycle injured in collision with fixed or stationary object**
X+7th **V27.4 Motorcycle driver injured in collision with fixed or stationary object in traffic accident**
X+7th **V27.5 Motorcycle passenger injured in collision with fixed or stationary object in traffic accident**
X+7th **V27.9 Unspecified motorcycle rider injured in collision with fixed or stationary object in traffic accident**

V28 Motorcycle rider injured in noncollision transport accident

Includes: fall or thrown from motorcycle (without antecedent collision)
overturning motorcycle NOS
overturning motorcycle without collision

The appropriate 7th character is to be added to each code from category V28
A initial encounter
D subsequent encounter
S sequela

X+7th **V28.0 Motorcycle driver injured in noncollision transport accident in nontraffic accident**
X+7th **V28.1 Motorcycle passenger injured in noncollision transport accident in nontraffic accident**
X+7th **V28.2 Unspecified motorcycle rider injured in noncollision transport accident in nontraffic accident**
X+7th **V28.3 Person boarding or alighting a motorcycle injured in noncollision transport accident**
X+7th **V28.4 Motorcycle driver injured in noncollision transport accident in traffic accident**
X+7th **V28.5 Motorcycle passenger injured in noncollision transport accident in traffic accident**
X+7th **V28.9 Unspecified motorcycle rider injured in noncollision transport accident in traffic accident**

V29 Motorcycle rider injured in other and unspecified transport accidents

The appropriate 7th character is to be added to each code from category V29
A initial encounter
D subsequent encounter
S sequela

+ **V29.0 Motorcycle driver injured in collision with other and unspecified motor vehicles in nontraffic accident**
X+7th **V29.00 Motorcycle driver injured in collision with unspecified motor vehicles in nontraffic accident**
X+7th **V29.09 Motorcycle driver injured in collision with other motor vehicles in nontraffic accident**
+ **V29.1 Motorcycle passenger injured in collision with other and unspecified motor vehicles in nontraffic accident**
X+7th **V29.10 Motorcycle passenger injured in collision with unspecified motor vehicles in nontraffic accident**
X+7th **V29.19 Motorcycle passenger injured in collision with other motor vehicles in nontraffic accident**
+ **V29.2 Unspecified motorcycle rider injured in collision with other and unspecified motor vehicles in nontraffic accident**
X+7th **V29.20 Unspecified motorcycle rider injured in collision with unspecified motor vehicles in nontraffic accident**
Motorcycle collision NOS, nontraffic
X+7th **V29.29 Unspecified motorcycle rider injured in collision with other motor vehicles in nontraffic accident**
X+7th **V29.3 Motorcycle rider (driver) (passenger) injured in unspecified nontraffic accident**
Motorcycle accident NOS, nontraffic
Motorcycle rider injured in nontraffic accident NOS
+ **V29.4 Motorcycle driver injured in collision with other and unspecified motor vehicles in traffic accident**
X+7th **V29.40 Motorcycle driver injured in collision with unspecified motor vehicles in traffic accident**
X+7th **V29.49 Motorcycle driver injured in collision with other motor vehicles in traffic accident**
+ **V29.5 Motorcycle passenger injured in collision with other and unspecified motor vehicles in traffic accident**
X+7th **V29.50 Motorcycle passenger injured in collision with unspecified motor vehicles in traffic accident**
X+7th **V29.59 Motorcycle passenger injured in collision with other motor vehicles in traffic accident**
+ **V29.6 Unspecified motorcycle rider injured in collision with other and unspecified motor vehicles in traffic accident**
X+7th **V29.60 Unspecified motorcycle rider injured in collision with unspecified motor vehicles in traffic accident**
Motorcycle collision NOS (traffic)
X+7th **V29.69 Unspecified motorcycle rider injured in collision with other motor vehicles in traffic accident**
+ **V29.8 Motorcycle rider (driver) (passenger) injured in other specified transport accidents**
X+7th **V29.81 Motorcycle rider (driver) (passenger) injured in transport accident with military vehicle**
X+7th **V29.88 Motorcycle rider (driver) (passenger) injured in other specified transport accidents**
X+7th **V29.9 Motorcycle rider (driver) (passenger) injured in unspecified traffic accident**
Motorcycle accident NOS

Occupant of three-wheeled motor vehicle injured in transport accident (V30-V39)

Includes: motorized tricycle
motorized rickshaw
three-wheeled motor car

Excludes1: *all-terrain vehicles (V86.-)*
motorcycle with sidecar (V20-V29)
vehicle designed primarily for off-road use (V86.-)

V30 Occupant of three-wheeled motor vehicle injured in collision with pedestrian or animal

Excludes1: *three-wheeled motor vehicle collision with animal-drawn vehicle or animal being ridden (V36.-)*

The appropriate 7th character is to be added to each code from category V30
A initial encounter
D subsequent encounter
S sequela

X+7th **V30.0 Driver of three-wheeled motor vehicle injured in collision with pedestrian or animal in nontraffic accident**
X+7th **V30.1 Passenger in three-wheeled motor vehicle injured in collision with pedestrian or animal in nontraffic accident**
X+7th **V30.2 Person on outside of three-wheeled motor vehicle injured in collision with pedestrian or animal in nontraffic accident**
X+7th **V30.3 Unspecified occupant of three-wheeled motor vehicle injured in collision with pedestrian or animal in nontraffic accident**
X+7th **V30.4 Person boarding or alighting a three-wheeled motor vehicle injured in collision with pedestrian or animal**
X+7th **V30.5 Driver of three-wheeled motor vehicle injured in collision with pedestrian or animal in traffic accident**

X+7th **V30.6 Passenger in three-wheeled motor vehicle injured in collision with pedestrian or animal in traffic accident**

X+7th **V30.7 Person on outside of three-wheeled motor vehicle injured in collision with pedestrian or animal in traffic accident**

X+7th **V30.9 Unspecified occupant of three-wheeled motor vehicle injured in collision with pedestrian or animal in traffic accident**

V31 Occupant of three-wheeled motor vehicle injured in collision with pedal cycle

The appropriate 7th character is to be added to each code from category V31
A initial encounter
D subsequent encounter
S sequela

X+7th **V31.0 Driver of three-wheeled motor vehicle injured in collision with pedal cycle in nontraffic accident**

X+7th **V31.1 Passenger in three-wheeled motor vehicle injured in collision with pedal cycle in nontraffic accident**

X+7th **V31.2 Person on outside of three-wheeled motor vehicle injured in collision with pedal cycle in nontraffic accident**

X+7th **V31.3 Unspecified occupant of three-wheeled motor vehicle injured in collision with pedal cycle in nontraffic accident**

X+7th **V31.4 Person boarding or alighting a three-wheeled motor vehicle injured in collision with pedal cycle**

X+7th **V31.5 Driver of three-wheeled motor vehicle injured in collision with pedal cycle in traffic accident**

X+7th **V31.6 Passenger in three-wheeled motor vehicle injured in collision with pedal cycle in traffic accident**

X+7th **V31.7 Person on outside of three-wheeled motor vehicle injured in collision with pedal cycle in traffic accident**

X+7th **V31.9 Unspecified occupant of three-wheeled motor vehicle injured in collision with pedal cycle in traffic accident**

V32 Occupant of three-wheeled motor vehicle injured in collision with two- or three-wheeled motor vehicle

The appropriate 7th character is to be added to each code from category V32
A initial encounter
D subsequent encounter
S sequela

X+7th **V32.0 Driver of three-wheeled motor vehicle injured in collision with two- or three-wheeled motor vehicle in nontraffic accident**

X+7th **V32.1 Passenger in three-wheeled motor vehicle injured in collision with two- or three-wheeled motor vehicle in nontraffic accident**

X+7th **V32.2 Person on outside of three-wheeled motor vehicle injured in collision with two- or three-wheeled motor vehicle in nontraffic accident**

X+7th **V32.3 Unspecified occupant of three-wheeled motor vehicle injured in collision with two- or three-wheeled motor vehicle in nontraffic accident**

X+7th **V32.4 Person boarding or alighting a three-wheeled motor vehicle injured in collision with two- or three-wheeled motor vehicle**

X+7th **V32.5 Driver of three-wheeled motor vehicle injured in collision with two- or three-wheeled motor vehicle in traffic accident**

X+7th **V32.6 Passenger in three-wheeled motor vehicle injured in collision with two- or three-wheeled motor vehicle in traffic accident**

X+7th **V32.7 Person on outside of three-wheeled motor vehicle injured in collision with two- or three-wheeled motor vehicle in traffic accident**

X+7th **V32.9 Unspecified occupant of three-wheeled motor vehicle injured in collision with two- or three-wheeled motor vehicle in traffic accident**

V33 Occupant of three-wheeled motor vehicle injured in collision with car, pick-up truck or van

The appropriate 7th character is to be added to each code from category V33
A initial encounter
D subsequent encounter
S sequela

X+7th **V33.0 Driver of three-wheeled motor vehicle injured in collision with car, pick-up truck or van in nontraffic accident**

X+7th **V33.1 Passenger in three-wheeled motor vehicle injured in collision with car, pick-up truck or van in nontraffic accident**

X+7th **V33.2 Person on outside of three-wheeled motor vehicle injured in collision with car, pick-up truck or van in nontraffic accident**

X+7th **V33.3 Unspecified occupant of three-wheeled motor vehicle injured in collision with car, pick-up truck or van in nontraffic accident**

X+7th **V33.4 Person boarding or alighting a three-wheeled motor vehicle injured in collision with car, pick-up truck or van**

X+7th **V33.5 Driver of three-wheeled motor vehicle injured in collision with car, pick-up truck or van in traffic accident**

X+7th **V33.6 Passenger in three-wheeled motor vehicle injured in collision with car, pick-up truck or van in traffic accident**

X+7th **V33.7 Person on outside of three-wheeled motor vehicle injured in collision with car, pick-up truck or van in traffic accident**

X+7th **V33.9 Unspecified occupant of three-wheeled motor vehicle injured in collision with car, pick-up truck or van in traffic accident**

V34 Occupant of three-wheeled motor vehicle injured in collision with heavy transport vehicle or bus

Excludes1: *occupant of three-wheeled motor vehicle injured in collision with military vehicle (V39.81)*

The appropriate 7th character is to be added to each code from category V34
A initial encounter
D subsequent encounter
S sequela

X+7th **V34.0 Driver of three-wheeled motor vehicle injured in collision with heavy transport vehicle or bus in nontraffic accident**

X+7th **V34.1 Passenger in three-wheeled motor vehicle injured in collision with heavy transport vehicle or bus in nontraffic accident**

X+7th **V34.2 Person on outside of three-wheeled motor vehicle injured in collision with heavy transport vehicle or bus in nontraffic accident**

X+7th **V34.3 Unspecified occupant of three-wheeled motor vehicle injured in collision with heavy transport vehicle or bus in nontraffic accident**

X+7th **V34.4 Person boarding or alighting a three-wheeled motor vehicle injured in collision with heavy transport vehicle or bus**

X+7th **V34.5 Driver of three-wheeled motor vehicle injured in collision with heavy transport vehicle or bus in traffic accident**

X+7th **V34.6 Passenger in three-wheeled motor vehicle injured in collision with heavy transport vehicle or bus in traffic accident**

X+7th **V34.7 Person on outside of three-wheeled motor vehicle injured in collision with heavy transport vehicle or bus in traffic accident**

X+7th **V34.9 Unspecified occupant of three-wheeled motor vehicle injured in collision with heavy transport vehicle or bus in traffic accident**

V35 Occupant of three-wheeled motor vehicle injured in collision with railway train or railway vehicle

The appropriate 7th character is to be added to each code from category V35
A initial encounter
D subsequent encounter
S sequela

X+7th **V35.0 Driver of three-wheeled motor vehicle injured in collision with railway train or railway vehicle in nontraffic accident**

X+7th **V35.1 Passenger in three-wheeled motor vehicle injured in collision with railway train or railway vehicle in nontraffic accident**

X+7th **V35.2 Person on outside of three-wheeled motor vehicle injured in collision with railway train or railway vehicle in nontraffic accident**

X+7th **V35.3 Unspecified occupant of three-wheeled motor vehicle injured in collision with railway train or railway vehicle in nontraffic accident**

X+7th **V35.4 Person boarding or alighting a three-wheeled motor vehicle injured in collision with railway train or railway vehicle**

X+7th **V35.5 Driver of three-wheeled motor vehicle injured in collision with railway train or railway vehicle in traffic accident**

X+7th **V35.6 Passenger in three-wheeled motor vehicle injured in collision with railway train or railway vehicle in traffic accident**

X+7th **V35.7 Person on outside of three-wheeled motor vehicle injured in collision with railway train or railway vehicle in traffic accident**

X+7th **V35.9 Unspecified occupant of three-wheeled motor vehicle injured in collision with railway train or railway vehicle in traffic accident**

V36 Occupant of three-wheeled motor vehicle injured in collision with other nonmotor vehicle

Includes: collision with animal-drawn vehicle, animal being ridden, streetcar

The appropriate 7th character is to be added to each code from category V36
A initial encounter
D subsequent encounter
S sequela

X+7th **V36.0 Driver of three-wheeled motor vehicle injured in collision with other nonmotor vehicle in nontraffic accident**

X+7th **V36.1 Passenger in three-wheeled motor vehicle injured in collision with other nonmotor vehicle in nontraffic accident**
X+7th **V36.2 Person on outside of three-wheeled motor vehicle injured in collision with other nonmotor vehicle in nontraffic accident**
X+7th **V36.3 Unspecified occupant of three-wheeled motor vehicle injured in collision with other nonmotor vehicle in nontraffic accident**
X+7th **V36.4 Person boarding or alighting a three-wheeled motor vehicle injured in collision with other nonmotor vehicle**
X+7th **V36.5 Driver of three-wheeled motor vehicle injured in collision with other nonmotor vehicle in traffic accident**
X+7th **V36.6 Passenger in three-wheeled motor vehicle injured in collision with other nonmotor vehicle in traffic accident**
X+7th **V36.7 Person on outside of three-wheeled motor vehicle injured in collision with other nonmotor vehicle in traffic accident**
X+7th **V36.9 Unspecified occupant of three-wheeled motor vehicle injured in collision with other nonmotor vehicle in traffic accident**

V37 Occupant of three-wheeled motor vehicle injured in collision with fixed or stationary object

The appropriate 7th character is to be added to each code from category V37
A initial encounter
D subsequent encounter
S sequela

X+7th **V37.0 Driver of three-wheeled motor vehicle injured in collision with fixed or stationary object in nontraffic accident**
X+7th **V37.1 Passenger in three-wheeled motor vehicle injured in collision with fixed or stationary object in nontraffic accident**
X+7th **V37.2 Person on outside of three-wheeled motor vehicle injured in collision with fixed or stationary object in nontraffic accident**
X+7th **V37.3 Unspecified occupant of three-wheeled motor vehicle injured in collision with fixed or stationary object in nontraffic accident**
X+7th **V37.4 Person boarding or alighting a three-wheeled motor vehicle injured in collision with fixed or stationary object**
X+7th **V37.5 Driver of three-wheeled motor vehicle injured in collision with fixed or stationary object in traffic accident**
X+7th **V37.6 Passenger in three-wheeled motor vehicle injured in collision with fixed or stationary object in traffic accident**
X+7th **V37.7 Person on outside of three-wheeled motor vehicle injured in collision with fixed or stationary object in traffic accident**
X+7th **V37.9 Unspecified occupant of three-wheeled motor vehicle injured in collision with fixed or stationary object in traffic accident**

V38 Occupant of three-wheeled motor vehicle injured in noncollision transport accident

Includes: fall or thrown from three-wheeled motor vehicle
overturning of three-wheeled motor vehicle NOS
overturning of three-wheeled motor vehicle without collision

The appropriate 7th character is to be added to each code from category V38
A initial encounter
D subsequent encounter
S sequela

X+7th **V38.0 Driver of three-wheeled motor vehicle injured in noncollision transport accident in nontraffic accident**
X+7th **V38.1 Passenger in three-wheeled motor vehicle injured in noncollision transport accident in nontraffic accident**
X+7th **V38.2 Person on outside of three-wheeled motor vehicle injured in noncollision transport accident in nontraffic accident**
X+7th **V38.3 Unspecified occupant of three-wheeled motor vehicle injured in noncollision transport accident in nontraffic accident**
X+7th **V38.4 Person boarding or alighting a three-wheeled motor vehicle injured in noncollision transport accident**
X+7th **V38.5 Driver of three-wheeled motor vehicle injured in noncollision transport accident in traffic accident**
X+7th **V38.6 Passenger in three-wheeled motor vehicle injured in noncollision transport accident in traffic accident**
X+7th **V38.7 Person on outside of three-wheeled motor vehicle injured in noncollision transport accident in traffic accident**
X+7th **V38.9 Unspecified occupant of three-wheeled motor vehicle injured in noncollision transport accident in traffic accident**

V39 Occupant of three-wheeled motor vehicle injured in other and unspecified transport accidents

The appropriate 7th character is to be added to each code from category V39
A initial encounter
D subsequent encounter
S sequela

\+ **V39.0 Driver of three-wheeled motor vehicle injured in collision with other and unspecified motor vehicles in nontraffic accident**
X+7th **V39.00 Driver of three-wheeled motor vehicle injured in collision with unspecified motor vehicles in nontraffic accident**
X+7th **V39.09 Driver of three-wheeled motor vehicle injured in collision with other motor vehicles in nontraffic accident**
\+ **V39.1 Passenger in three-wheeled motor vehicle injured in collision with other and unspecified motor vehicles in nontraffic accident**
X+7th **V39.10 Passenger in three-wheeled motor vehicle injured in collision with unspecified motor vehicles in nontraffic accident**
X+7th **V39.19 Passenger in three-wheeled motor vehicle injured in collision with other motor vehicles in nontraffic accident**
\+ **V39.2 Unspecified occupant of three-wheeled motor vehicle injured in collision with other and unspecified motor vehicles in nontraffic accident**
X+7th **V39.20 Unspecified occupant of three-wheeled motor vehicle injured in collision with unspecified motor vehicles in nontraffic accident**
Collision NOS involving three-wheeled motor vehicle, nontraffic
X+7th **V39.29 Unspecified occupant of three-wheeled motor vehicle injured in collision with other motor vehicles in nontraffic accident**
X+7th **V39.3 Occupant (driver) (passenger) of three-wheeled motor vehicle injured in unspecified nontraffic accident**
Accident NOS involving three-wheeled motor vehicle, nontraffic
Occupant of three-wheeled motor vehicle injured in nontraffic accident NOS
\+ **V39.4 Driver of three-wheeled motor vehicle injured in collision with other and unspecified motor vehicles in traffic accident**
X+7th **V39.40 Driver of three-wheeled motor vehicle injured in collision with unspecified motor vehicles in traffic accident**
X+7th **V39.49 Driver of three-wheeled motor vehicle injured in collision with other motor vehicles in traffic accident**
\+ **V39.5 Passenger in three-wheeled motor vehicle injured in collision with other and unspecified motor vehicles in traffic accident**
X+7th **V39.50 Passenger in three-wheeled motor vehicle injured in collision with unspecified motor vehicles in traffic accident**
X+7th **V39.59 Passenger in three-wheeled motor vehicle injured in collision with other motor vehicles in traffic accident**
\+ **V39.6 Unspecified occupant of three-wheeled motor vehicle injured in collision with other and unspecified motor vehicles in traffic accident**
X+7th **V39.60 Unspecified occupant of three-wheeled motor vehicle injured in collision with unspecified motor vehicles in traffic accident**
Collision NOS involving three-wheeled motor vehicle (traffic)
X+7th **V39.69 Unspecified occupant of three-wheeled motor vehicle injured in collision with other motor vehicles in traffic accident**
\+ **V39.8 Occupant (driver) (passenger) of three-wheeled motor vehicle injured in other specified transport accidents**
X+7th **V39.81 Occupant (driver) (passenger) of three-wheeled motor vehicle injured in transport accident with military vehicle**
X+7th **V39.89 Occupant (driver) (passenger) of three-wheeled motor vehicle injured in other specified transport accidents**
X+7th **V39.9 Occupant (driver) (passenger) of three-wheeled motor vehicle injured in unspecified traffic accident**
Accident NOS involving three-wheeled motor vehicle

Car occupant injured in transport accident (V40-V49)

Includes: a four-wheeled motor vehicle designed primarily for carrying passengers
automobile (pulling a trailer or camper)

Excludes1: *bus (V50-V59)*
minibus (V50-V59)
minivan (V50-V59)
motorcoach (V70-V79)
pick-up truck (V50-V59)
sport utility vehicle (SUV) (V50-V59)

V40 Car occupant injured in collision with pedestrian or animal

Excludes1: *car collision with animal-drawn vehicle or animal being ridden (V46.-)*

The appropriate 7th character is to be added to each code from category V40
A initial encounter
D subsequent encounter
S sequela

X+7th **V40.0 Car driver injured in collision with pedestrian or animal in nontraffic accident**
X+7th **V40.1 Car passenger injured in collision with pedestrian or animal in nontraffic accident**
X+7th **V40.2 Person on outside of car injured in collision with pedestrian or animal in nontraffic accident**
X+7th **V40.3 Unspecified car occupant injured in collision with pedestrian or animal in nontraffic accident**
X+7th **V40.4 Person boarding or alighting a car injured in collision with pedestrian or animal**
X+7th **V40.5 Car driver injured in collision with pedestrian or animal in traffic accident**
X+7th **V40.6 Car passenger injured in collision with pedestrian or animal in traffic accident**
X+7th **V40.7 Person on outside of car injured in collision with pedestrian or animal in traffic accident**
X+7th **V40.9 Unspecified car occupant injured in collision with pedestrian or animal in traffic accident**

V41 Car occupant injured in collision with pedal cycle

The appropriate 7th character is to be added to each code from category V41
A initial encounter
D subsequent encounter
S sequela

X+7th **V41.0 Car driver injured in collision with pedal cycle in nontraffic accident**
X+7th **V41.1 Car passenger injured in collision with pedal cycle in nontraffic accident**
X+7th **V41.2 Person on outside of car injured in collision with pedal cycle in nontraffic accident**
X+7th **V41.3 Unspecified car occupant injured in collision with pedal cycle in nontraffic accident**
X+7th **V41.4 Person boarding or alighting a car injured in collision with pedal cycle**
X+7th **V41.5 Car driver injured in collision with pedal cycle in traffic accident**
X+7th **V41.6 Car passenger injured in collision with pedal cycle in traffic accident**
X+7th **V41.7 Person on outside of car injured in collision with pedal cycle in traffic accident**
X+7th **V41.9 Unspecified car occupant injured in collision with pedal cycle in traffic accident**

V42 Car occupant injured in collision with two- or three-wheeled motor vehicle

The appropriate 7th character is to be added to each code from category V42
A initial encounter
D subsequent encounter
S sequela

X+7th **V42.0 Car driver injured in collision with two- or three-wheeled motor vehicle in nontraffic accident**
X+7th **V42.1 Car passenger injured in collision with two- or three-wheeled motor vehicle in nontraffic accident**
X+7th **V42.2 Person on outside of car injured in collision with two- or three-wheeled motor vehicle in nontraffic accident**
X+7th **V42.3 Unspecified car occupant injured in collision with two- or three-wheeled motor vehicle in nontraffic accident**
X+7th **V42.4 Person boarding or alighting a car injured in collision with two- or three-wheeled motor vehicle**
X+7th **V42.5 Car driver injured in collision with two- or three-wheeled motor vehicle in traffic accident**
X+7th **V42.6 Car passenger injured in collision with two- or three-wheeled motor vehicle in traffic accident**
X+7th **V42.7 Person on outside of car injured in collision with two- or three-wheeled motor vehicle in traffic accident**
X+7th **V42.9 Unspecified car occupant injured in collision with two- or three-wheeled motor vehicle in traffic accident**

V43 Car occupant injured in collision with car, pick-up truck or van

The appropriate 7th character is to be added to each code from category V43
A initial encounter
D subsequent encounter
S sequela

\+ **V43.0 Car driver injured in collision with car, pick-up truck or van in nontraffic accident**
X+7th **V43.01 Car driver injured in collision with sport utility vehicle in nontraffic accident**
X+7th **V43.02 Car driver injured in collision with other type car in nontraffic accident**
X+7th **V43.03 Car driver injured in collision with pick-up truck in nontraffic accident**
X+7th **V43.04 Car driver injured in collision with van in nontraffic accident**

\+ **V43.1 Car passenger injured in collision with car, pick-up truck or van in nontraffic accident**
X+7th **V43.11 Car passenger injured in collision with sport utility vehicle in nontraffic accident**
X+7th **V43.12 Car passenger injured in collision with other type car in nontraffic accident**
X+7th **V43.13 Car passenger injured in collision with pick-up in nontraffic accident**
X+7th **V43.14 Car passenger injured in collision with van in nontraffic accident**

\+ **V43.2 Person on outside of car injured in collision with car, pick-up truck or van in nontraffic accident**
X+7th **V43.21 Person on outside of car injured in collision with sport utility vehicle in nontraffic accident**
X+7th **V43.22 Person on outside of car injured in collision with other type car in nontraffic accident**
X+7th **V43.23 Person on outside of car injured in collision with pick-up truck in nontraffic accident**
X+7th **V43.24 Person on outside of car injured in collision with van in nontraffic accident**

\+ **V43.3 Unspecified car occupant injured in collision with car, pick-up truck or van in nontraffic accident**
X+7th **V43.31 Unspecified car occupant injured in collision with sport utility vehicle in nontraffic accident**
X+7th **V43.32 Unspecified car occupant injured in collision with other type car in nontraffic accident**
X+7th **V43.33 Unspecified car occupant injured in collision with pick-up truck in nontraffic accident**
X+7th **V43.34 Unspecified car occupant injured in collision with van in nontraffic accident**

\+ **V43.4 Person boarding or alighting a car injured in collision with car, pick-up truck or van**
X+7th **V43.41 Person boarding or alighting a car injured in collision with sport utility vehicle**
X+7th **V43.42 Person boarding or alighting a car injured in collision with other type car**
X+7th **V43.43 Person boarding or alighting a car injured in collision with pick-up truck**
X+7th **V43.44 Person boarding or alighting a car injured in collision with van**

\+ **V43.5 Car driver injured in collision with car, pick-up truck or van in traffic accident**
X+7th **V43.51 Car driver injured in collision with sport utility vehicle in traffic accident**
X+7th **V43.52 Car driver injured in collision with other type car in traffic accident**
X+7th **V43.53 Car driver injured in collision with pick-up truck in traffic accident**
X+7th **V43.54 Car driver injured in collision with van in traffic accident**

\+ **V43.6 Car passenger injured in collision with car, pick-up truck or van in traffic accident**
X+7th **V43.61 Car passenger injured in collision with sport utility vehicle in traffic accident**
AHA CC: 1Q, 2015, 3-21

X+7th **V43.62** **Car passenger injured in collision with other type car in traffic accident**
X+7th **V43.63** **Car passenger injured in collision with pick-up truck in traffic accident**
X+7th **V43.64** **Car passenger injured in collision with van in traffic accident**
\+ **V43.7** **Person on outside of car injured in collision with car, pick-up truck or van in traffic accident**
X+7th **V43.71** **Person on outside of car injured in collision with sport utility vehicle in traffic accident**
X+7th **V43.72** **Person on outside of car injured in collision with other type car in traffic accident**
X+7th **V43.73** **Person on outside of car injured in collision with pick-up truck in traffic accident**
X+7th **V43.74** **Person on outside of car injured in collision with van in traffic accident**
\+ **V43.9** **Unspecified car occupant injured in collision with car, pick-up truck or van in traffic accident**
X+7th **V43.91** **Unspecified car occupant injured in collision with sport utility vehicle in traffic accident**
X+7th **V43.92** **Unspecified car occupant injured in collision with other type car in traffic accident**
X+7th **V43.93** **Unspecified car occupant injured in collision with pick-up truck in traffic accident**
X+7th **V43.94** **Unspecified car occupant injured in collision with van in traffic accident**

V44 Car occupant injured in collision with heavy transport vehicle or bus

Excludes1: *car occupant injured in collision with military vehicle (V49.81)*

The appropriate 7th character is to be added to each code from category V44
A initial encounter
D subsequent encounter
S sequela

X+7th **V44.0** **Car driver injured in collision with heavy transport vehicle or bus in nontraffic accident**
X+7th **V44.1** **Car passenger injured in collision with heavy transport vehicle or bus in nontraffic accident**
X+7th **V44.2** **Person on outside of car injured in collision with heavy transport vehicle or bus in nontraffic accident**
X+7th **V44.3** **Unspecified car occupant injured in collision with heavy transport vehicle or bus in nontraffic accident**
X+7th **V44.4** **Person boarding or alighting a car injured in collision with heavy transport vehicle or bus**
X+7th **V44.5** **Car driver injured in collision with heavy transport vehicle or bus in traffic accident**
X+7th **V44.6** **Car passenger injured in collision with heavy transport vehicle or bus in traffic accident**
X+7th **V44.7** **Person on outside of car injured in collision with heavy transport vehicle or bus in traffic accident**
X+7th **V44.9** **Unspecified car occupant injured in collision with heavy transport vehicle or bus in traffic accident**

V45 Car occupant injured in collision with railway train or railway vehicle

The appropriate 7th character is to be added to each code from category V45
A initial encounter
D subsequent encounter
S sequela

X+7th **V45.0** **Car driver injured in collision with railway train or railway vehicle in nontraffic accident**
X+7th **V45.1** **Car passenger injured in collision with railway train or railway vehicle in nontraffic accident**
X+7th **V45.2** **Person on outside of car injured in collision with railway train or railway vehicle in nontraffic accident**
X+7th **V45.3** **Unspecified car occupant injured in collision with railway train or railway vehicle in nontraffic accident**
X+7th **V45.4** **Person boarding or alighting a car injured in collision with railway train or railway vehicle**
X+7th **V45.5** **Car driver injured in collision with railway train or railway vehicle in traffic accident**
X+7th **V45.6** **Car passenger injured in collision with railway train or railway vehicle in traffic accident**
X+7th **V45.7** **Person on outside of car injured in collision with railway train or railway vehicle in traffic accident**
X+7th **V45.9** **Unspecified car occupant injured in collision with railway train or railway vehicle in traffic accident**

V46 Car occupant injured in collision with other nonmotor vehicle

Includes: collision with animal-drawn vehicle, animal being ridden, streetcar

The appropriate 7th character is to be added to each code from category V46
A initial encounter
D subsequent encounter
S sequela

X+7th **V46.0** **Car driver injured in collision with other nonmotor vehicle in nontraffic accident**
X+7th **V46.1** **Car passenger injured in collision with other nonmotor vehicle in nontraffic accident**
X+7th **V46.2** **Person on outside of car injured in collision with other nonmotor vehicle in nontraffic accident**
X+7th **V46.3** **Unspecified car occupant injured in collision with other nonmotor vehicle in nontraffic accident**
X+7th **V46.4** **Person boarding or alighting a car injured in collision with other nonmotor vehicle**
X+7th **V46.5** **Car driver injured in collision with other nonmotor vehicle in traffic accident**
X+7th **V46.6** **Car passenger injured in collision with other nonmotor vehicle in traffic accident**
X+7th **V46.7** **Person on outside of car injured in collision with other nonmotor vehicle in traffic accident**
X+7th **V46.9** **Unspecified car occupant injured in collision with other nonmotor vehicle in traffic accident**

V47 Car occupant injured in collision with fixed or stationary object

AHA CC: 4Q, 2016, 73

The appropriate 7th character is to be added to each code from category V47
A initial encounter
D subsequent encounter
S sequela

X+7th **V47.0** **Car driver injured in collision with fixed or stationary object in nontraffic accident**
X+7th **V47.1** **Car passenger injured in collision with fixed or stationary object in nontraffic accident**
X+7th **V47.2** **Person on outside of car injured in collision with fixed or stationary object in nontraffic accident**
X+7th **V47.3** **Unspecified car occupant injured in collision with fixed or stationary object in nontraffic accident**
X+7th **V47.4** **Person boarding or alighting a car injured in collision with fixed or stationary object**
X+7th **V47.5** **Car driver injured in collision with fixed or stationary object in traffic accident**
X+7th **V47.6** **Car passenger injured in collision with fixed or stationary object in traffic accident**
X+7th **V47.7** **Person on outside of car injured in collision with fixed or stationary object in traffic accident**
X+7th **V47.9** **Unspecified car occupant injured in collision with fixed or stationary object in traffic accident**

V48 Car occupant injured in noncollision transport accident

Includes: overturning car NOS
overturning car without collision

The appropriate 7th character is to be added to each code from category V48
A initial encounter
D subsequent encounter
S sequela

X+7th **V48.0** **Car driver injured in noncollision transport accident in nontraffic accident**
X+7th **V48.1** **Car passenger injured in noncollision transport accident in nontraffic accident**
X+7th **V48.2** **Person on outside of car injured in noncollision transport accident in nontraffic accident**
X+7th **V48.3** **Unspecified car occupant injured in noncollision transport accident in nontraffic accident**
X+7th **V48.4** **Person boarding or alighting a car injured in noncollision transport accident**
X+7th **V48.5** **Car driver injured in noncollision transport accident in traffic accident**
X+7th **V48.6** **Car passenger injured in noncollision transport accident in traffic accident**
X+7th **V48.7** **Person on outside of car injured in noncollision transport accident in traffic accident**
X+7th **V48.9** **Unspecified car occupant injured in noncollision transport accident in traffic accident**

V49 Car occupant injured in other and unspecified transport accidents

The appropriate 7th character is to be added to each code from category V49
A initial encounter
D subsequent encounter
S sequela

+ **V49.0 Driver injured in collision with other and unspecified motor vehicles in nontraffic accident**
  - X+7th **V49.00 Driver injured in collision with unspecified motor vehicles in nontraffic accident**
  - X+7th **V49.09 Driver injured in collision with other motor vehicles in nontraffic accident**

+ **V49.1 Passenger injured in collision with other and unspecified motor vehicles in nontraffic accident**
  - X+7th **V49.10 Passenger injured in collision with unspecified motor vehicles in nontraffic accident**
  - X+7th **V49.19 Passenger injured in collision with other motor vehicles in nontraffic accident**

+ **V49.2 Unspecified car occupant injured in collision with other and unspecified motor vehicles in nontraffic accident**
  - X+7th **V49.20 Unspecified car occupant injured in collision with unspecified motor vehicles in nontraffic accident**
    Car collision NOS, nontraffic
  - X+7th **V49.29 Unspecified car occupant injured in collision with other motor vehicles in nontraffic accident**

X+7th **V49.3 Car occupant (driver) (passenger) injured in unspecified nontraffic accident**
Car accident NOS, nontraffic
Car occupant injured in nontraffic accident NOS

+ **V49.4 Driver injured in collision with other and unspecified motor vehicles in traffic accident**
  - X+7th **V49.40 Driver injured in collision with unspecified motor vehicles in traffic accident**
  - X+7th **V49.49 Driver injured in collision with other motor vehicles in traffic accident**

+ **V49.5 Passenger injured in collision with other and unspecified motor vehicles in traffic accident**
  - X+7th **V49.50 Passenger injured in collision with unspecified motor vehicles in traffic accident**
  - X+7th **V49.59 Passenger injured in collision with other motor vehicles in traffic accident**

+ **V49.6 Unspecified car occupant injured in collision with other and unspecified motor vehicles in traffic accident**
  - X+7th **V49.60 Unspecified car occupant injured in collision with unspecified motor vehicles in traffic accident**
    Car collision NOS (traffic)
  - X+7th **V49.69 Unspecified car occupant injured in collision with other motor vehicles in traffic accident**

+ **V49.8 Car occupant (driver) (passenger) injured in other specified transport accidents**
  - X+7th **V49.81 Car occupant (driver) (passenger) injured in transport accident with military vehicle**
  - X+7th **V49.88 Car occupant (driver) (passenger) injured in other specified transport accidents**

X+7th **V49.9 Car occupant (driver) (passenger) injured in unspecified traffic accident**
Car accident NOS
AHA CC: 1Q, 2015, 3-21

ccupant of pick-up truck or van injured in transport ccident (V50-V59)

cludes: a four or six wheel motor vehicle designed primarily for carrying passengers and property but weighing less than the local limit for classification as a heavy goods vehicle
minibus
minivan
sport utility vehicle (SUV)
truck
van

cludes1: *heavy transport vehicle (V60-V69)*

V50 Occupant of pick-up truck or van injured in collision with pedestrian or animal

Excludes1: *pick-up truck or van collision with animal-drawn vehicle or animal being ridden (V56.-)*

The appropriate 7th character is to be added to each code from category V50
A initial encounter
D subsequent encounter
S sequela

X+7th **V50.0 Driver of pick-up truck or van injured in collision with pedestrian or animal in nontraffic accident**
X+7th **V50.1 Passenger in pick-up truck or van injured in collision with pedestrian or animal in nontraffic accident**
X+7th **V50.2 Person on outside of pick-up truck or van injured in collision with pedestrian or animal in nontraffic accident**
X+7th **V50.3 Unspecified occupant of pick-up truck or van injured in collision with pedestrian or animal in nontraffic accident**
X+7th **V50.4 Person boarding or alighting a pick-up truck or van injured in collision with pedestrian or animal**
X+7th **V50.5 Driver of pick-up truck or van injured in collision with pedestrian or animal in traffic accident**
X+7th **V50.6 Passenger in pick-up truck or van injured in collision with pedestrian or animal in traffic accident**
X+7th **V50.7 Person on outside of pick-up truck or van injured in collision with pedestrian or animal in traffic accident**
X+7th **V50.9 Unspecified occupant of pick-up truck or van injured in collision with pedestrian or animal in traffic accident**

V51 Occupant of pick-up truck or van injured in collision with pedal cycle

The appropriate 7th character is to be added to each code from category V51
A initial encounter
D subsequent encounter
S sequela

X+7th **V51.0 Driver of pick-up truck or van injured in collision with pedal cycle in nontraffic accident**
X+7th **V51.1 Passenger in pick-up truck or van injured in collision with pedal cycle in nontraffic accident**
X+7th **V51.2 Person on outside of pick-up truck or van injured in collision with pedal cycle in nontraffic accident**
X+7th **V51.3 Unspecified occupant of pick-up truck or van injured in collision with pedal cycle in nontraffic accident**
X+7th **V51.4 Person boarding or alighting a pick-up truck or van injured in collision with pedal cycle**
X+7th **V51.5 Driver of pick-up truck or van injured in collision with pedal cycle in traffic accident**
X+7th **V51.6 Passenger in pick-up truck or van injured in collision with pedal cycle in traffic accident**
X+7th **V51.7 Person on outside of pick-up truck or van injured in collision with pedal cycle in traffic accident**
X+7th **V51.9 Unspecified occupant of pick-up truck or van injured in collision with pedal cycle in traffic accident**

V52 Occupant of pick-up truck or van injured in collision with two- or three-wheeled motor vehicle

The appropriate 7th character is to be added to each code from category V52
A initial encounter
D subsequent encounter
S sequela

X+7th **V52.0 Driver of pick-up truck or van injured in collision with two- or three-wheeled motor vehicle in nontraffic accident**
X+7th **V52.1 Passenger in pick-up truck or van injured in collision with two- or three-wheeled motor vehicle in nontraffic accident**
X+7th **V52.2 Person on outside of pick-up truck or van injured in collision with two- or three-wheeled motor vehicle in nontraffic accident**
X+7th **V52.3 Unspecified occupant of pick-up truck or van injured in collision with two- or three-wheeled motor vehicle in nontraffic accident**
X+7th **V52.4 Person boarding or alighting a pick-up truck or van injured in collision with two- or three-wheeled motor vehicle**
X+7th **V52.5 Driver of pick-up truck or van injured in collision with two- or three-wheeled motor vehicle in traffic accident**
X+7th **V52.6 Passenger in pick-up truck or van injured in collision with two- or three-wheeled motor vehicle in traffic accident**
X+7th **V52.7 Person on outside of pick-up truck or van injured in collision with two- or three-wheeled motor vehicle in traffic accident**
X+7th **V52.9 Unspecified occupant of pick-up truck or van injured in collision with two- or three-wheeled motor vehicle in traffic accident**

V53 Occupant of pick-up truck or van injured in collision with car, pick-up truck or van

The appropriate 7th character is to be added to each code from category V53
A initial encounter
D subsequent encounter
S sequela

X+7th **V53.0 Driver of pick-up truck or van injured in collision with car, pick-up truck or van in nontraffic accident**
X+7th **V53.1 Passenger in pick-up truck or van injured in collision with car, pick-up truck or van in nontraffic accident**
X+7th **V53.2 Person on outside of pick-up truck or van injured in collision with car, pick-up truck or van in nontraffic accident**
X+7th **V53.3 Unspecified occupant of pick-up truck or van injured in collision with car, pick-up truck or van in nontraffic accident**
X+7th **V53.4 Person boarding or alighting a pick-up truck or van injured in collision with car, pick-up truck or van**
X+7th **V53.5 Driver of pick-up truck or van injured in collision with car, pick-up truck or van in traffic accident**
X+7th **V53.6 Passenger in pick-up truck or van injured in collision with car, pick-up truck or van in traffic accident**
X+7th **V53.7 Person on outside of pick-up truck or van injured in collision with car, pick-up truck or van in traffic accident**
X+7th **V53.9 Unspecified occupant of pick-up truck or van injured in collision with car, pick-up truck or van in traffic accident**

V54 Occupant of pick-up truck or van injured in collision with heavy transport vehicle or bus

Excludes1: *occupant of pick-up truck or van injured in collision with military vehicle (V59.81)*

The appropriate 7th character is to be added to each code from category V54
A initial encounter
D subsequent encounter
S sequela

X+7th **V54.0 Driver of pick-up truck or van injured in collision with heavy transport vehicle or bus in nontraffic accident**
X+7th **V54.1 Passenger in pick-up truck or van injured in collision with heavy transport vehicle or bus in nontraffic accident**
X+7th **V54.2 Person on outside of pick-up truck or van injured in collision with heavy transport vehicle or bus in nontraffic accident**
X+7th **V54.3 Unspecified occupant of pick-up truck or van injured in collision with heavy transport vehicle or bus in nontraffic accident**
X+7th **V54.4 Person boarding or alighting a pick-up truck or van injured in collision with heavy transport vehicle or bus**
X+7th **V54.5 Driver of pick-up truck or van injured in collision with heavy transport vehicle or bus in traffic accident**
X+7th **V54.6 Passenger in pick-up truck or van injured in collision with heavy transport vehicle or bus in traffic accident**
X+7th **V54.7 Person on outside of pick-up truck or van injured in collision with heavy transport vehicle or bus in traffic accident**
X+7th **V54.9 Unspecified occupant of pick-up truck or van injured in collision with heavy transport vehicle or bus in traffic accident**

V55 Occupant of pick-up truck or van injured in collision with railway train or railway vehicle

The appropriate 7th character is to be added to each code from category V55
A initial encounter
D subsequent encounter
S sequela

X+7th **V55.0 Driver of pick-up truck or van injured in collision with railway train or railway vehicle in nontraffic accident**
X+7th **V55.1 Passenger in pick-up truck or van injured in collision with railway train or railway vehicle in nontraffic accident**
X+7th **V55.2 Person on outside of pick-up truck or van injured in collision with railway train or railway vehicle in nontraffic accident**
X+7th **V55.3 Unspecified occupant of pick-up truck or van injured in collision with railway train or railway vehicle in nontraffic accident**
X+7th **V55.4 Person boarding or alighting a pick-up truck or van injured in collision with railway train or railway vehicle**
X+7th **V55.5 Driver of pick-up truck or van injured in collision with railway train or railway vehicle in traffic accident**
X+7th **V55.6 Passenger in pick-up truck or van injured in collision with railway train or railway vehicle in traffic accident**
X+7th **V55.7 Person on outside of pick-up truck or van injured in collision with railway train or railway vehicle in traffic accident**
X+7th **V55.9 Unspecified occupant of pick-up truck or van injured in collision with railway train or railway vehicle in traffic accident**

V56 Occupant of pick-up truck or van injured in collision with other nonmotor vehicle

Includes: collision with animal-drawn vehicle, animal being ridden, streetcar

The appropriate 7th character is to be added to each code from category V56
A initial encounter
D subsequent encounter
S sequela

X+7th **V56.0 Driver of pick-up truck or van injured in collision with other nonmotor vehicle in nontraffic accident**
X+7th **V56.1 Passenger in pick-up truck or van injured in collision with other nonmotor vehicle in nontraffic accident**
X+7th **V56.2 Person on outside of pick-up truck or van injured in collision with other nonmotor vehicle in nontraffic accident**
X+7th **V56.3 Unspecified occupant of pick-up truck or van injured in collision with other nonmotor vehicle in nontraffic accident**
X+7th **V56.4 Person boarding or alighting a pick-up truck or van injured i collision with other nonmotor vehicle**
X+7th **V56.5 Driver of pick-up truck or van injured in collision with other nonmotor vehicle in traffic accident**
X+7th **V56.6 Passenger in pick-up truck or van injured in collision with other nonmotor vehicle in traffic accident**
X+7th **V56.7 Person on outside of pick-up truck or van injured in collision with other nonmotor vehicle in traffic accident**
X+7th **V56.9 Unspecified occupant of pick-up truck or van injured in collision with other nonmotor vehicle in traffic accident**

V57 Occupant of pick-up truck or van injured in collision with fixed or stationary object

The appropriate 7th character is to be added to each code from category V57
A initial encounter
D subsequent encounter
S sequela

X+7th **V57.0 Driver of pick-up truck or van injured in collision with fixed stationary object in nontraffic accident**
X+7th **V57.1 Passenger in pick-up truck or van injured in collision with fixed or stationary object in nontraffic accident**
X+7th **V57.2 Person on outside of pick-up truck or van injured in collision with fixed or stationary object in nontraffic accident**
X+7th **V57.3 Unspecified occupant of pick-up truck or van injured in collision with fixed or stationary object in nontraffic accident**
X+7th **V57.4 Person boarding or alighting a pick-up truck or van injured i collision with fixed or stationary object**
X+7th **V57.5 Driver of pick-up truck or van injured in collision with fixed stationary object in traffic accident**
X+7th **V57.6 Passenger in pick-up truck or van injured in collision with fixed or stationary object in traffic accident**
X+7th **V57.7 Person on outside of pick-up truck or van injured in collision with fixed or stationary object in traffic accident**
X+7th **V57.9 Unspecified occupant of pick-up truck or van injured in collision with fixed or stationary object in traffic accident**

V58 Occupant of pick-up truck or van injured in noncollision transport accident

Includes: overturning pick-up truck or van NOS
overturning pick-up truck or van without collision

The appropriate 7th character is to be added to each code from category V58
A initial encounter
D subsequent encounter
S sequela

X+7th **V58.0 Driver of pick-up truck or van injured in noncollision transport accident in nontraffic accident**
X+7th **V58.1 Passenger in pick-up truck or van injured in noncollision transport accident in nontraffic accident**
X+7th **V58.2 Person on outside of pick-up truck or van injured in noncollision transport accident in nontraffic accident**
X+7th **V58.3 Unspecified occupant of pick-up truck or van injured in noncollision transport accident in nontraffic accident**
X+7th **V58.4 Person boarding or alighting a pick-up truck or van injured i noncollision transport accident**

X+7th **V58.5 Driver of pick-up truck or van injured in noncollision transport accident in traffic accident**
X+7th **V58.6 Passenger in pick-up truck or van injured in noncollision transport accident in traffic accident**
X+7th **V58.7 Person on outside of pick-up truck or van injured in noncollision transport accident in traffic accident**
X+7th **V58.9 Unspecified occupant of pick-up truck or van injured in noncollision transport accident in traffic accident**

V59 Occupant of pick-up truck or van injured in other and unspecified transport accidents

The appropriate 7th character is to be added to each code from category V59
A initial encounter
D subsequent encounter
S sequela

\+ **V59.0 Driver of pick-up truck or van injured in collision with other and unspecified motor vehicles in nontraffic accident**
X+7th **V59.00 Driver of pick-up truck or van injured in collision with unspecified motor vehicles in nontraffic accident**
X+7th **V59.09 Driver of pick-up truck or van injured in collision with other motor vehicles in nontraffic accident**
\+ **V59.1 Passenger in pick-up truck or van injured in collision with other and unspecified motor vehicles in nontraffic accident**
X+7th **V59.10 Passenger in pick-up truck or van injured in collision with unspecified motor vehicles in nontraffic accident**
X+7th **V59.19 Passenger in pick-up truck or van injured in collision with other motor vehicles in nontraffic accident**
\+ **V59.2 Unspecified occupant of pick-up truck or van injured in collision with other and unspecified motor vehicles in nontraffic accident**
X+7th **V59.20 Unspecified occupant of pick-up truck or van injured in collision with unspecified motor vehicles in nontraffic accident**
Collision NOS involving pick-up truck or van, nontraffic
X+7th **V59.29 Unspecified occupant of pick-up truck or van injured in collision with other motor vehicles in nontraffic accident**
X+7th **V59.3 Occupant (driver) (passenger) of pick-up truck or van injured in unspecified nontraffic accident**
Accident NOS involving pick-up truck or van, nontraffic
Occupant of pick-up truck or van injured in nontraffic accident NOS
\+ **V59.4 Driver of pick-up truck or van injured in collision with other and unspecified motor vehicles in traffic accident**
X+7th **V59.40 Driver of pick-up truck or van injured in collision with unspecified motor vehicles in traffic accident**
X+7th **V59.49 Driver of pick-up truck or van injured in collision with other motor vehicles in traffic accident**
\+ **V59.5 Passenger in pick-up truck or van injured in collision with other and unspecified motor vehicles in traffic accident**
X+7th **V59.50 Passenger in pick-up truck or van injured in collision with unspecified motor vehicles in traffic accident**
X+7th **V59.59 Passenger in pick-up truck or van injured in collision with other motor vehicles in traffic accident**
\+ **V59.6 Unspecified occupant of pick-up truck or van injured in collision with other and unspecified motor vehicles in traffic accident**
X+7th **V59.60 Unspecified occupant of pick-up truck or van injured in collision with unspecified motor vehicles in traffic accident**
Collision NOS involving pick-up truck or van (traffic)
X+7th **V59.69 Unspecified occupant of pick-up truck or van injured in collision with other motor vehicles in traffic accident**
\+ **V59.8 Occupant (driver) (passenger) of pick-up truck or van injured in other specified transport accidents**
X+7th **V59.81 Occupant (driver) (passenger) of pick-up truck or van injured in transport accident with military vehicle**
X+7th **V59.88 Occupant (driver) (passenger) of pick-up truck or van injured in other specified transport accidents**
X+7th **V59.9 Occupant (driver) (passenger) of pick-up truck or van injured in unspecified traffic accident**
Accident NOS involving pick-up truck or van

Occupant of heavy transport vehicle injured in transport accident (V60-V69)

Includes: 18 wheeler
armored car
panel truck

Excludes1: *bus*
motorcoach

V60 Occupant of heavy transport vehicle injured in collision with pedestrian or animal

Excludes1: *heavy transport vehicle collision with animal-drawn vehicle or animal being ridden (V66.-)*

The appropriate 7th character is to be added to each code from category V60
A initial encounter
D subsequent encounter
S sequela

X+7th **V60.0 Driver of heavy transport vehicle injured in collision with pedestrian or animal in nontraffic accident**
X+7th **V60.1 Passenger in heavy transport vehicle injured in collision with pedestrian or animal in nontraffic accident**
X+7th **V60.2 Person on outside of heavy transport vehicle injured in collision with pedestrian or animal in nontraffic accident**
X+7th **V60.3 Unspecified occupant of heavy transport vehicle injured in collision with pedestrian or animal in nontraffic accident**
X+7th **V60.4 Person boarding or alighting a heavy transport vehicle injured in collision with pedestrian or animal**
X+7th **V60.5 Driver of heavy transport vehicle injured in collision with pedestrian or animal in traffic accident**
X+7th **V60.6 Passenger in heavy transport vehicle injured in collision with pedestrian or animal in traffic accident**
X+7th **V60.7 Person on outside of heavy transport vehicle injured in collision with pedestrian or animal in traffic accident**
X+7th **V60.9 Unspecified occupant of heavy transport vehicle injured in collision with pedestrian or animal in traffic accident**

V61 Occupant of heavy transport vehicle injured in collision with pedal cycle

The appropriate 7th character is to be added to each code from category V61
A initial encounter
D subsequent encounter
S sequela

X+7th **V61.0 Driver of heavy transport vehicle injured in collision with pedal cycle in nontraffic accident**
X+7th **V61.1 Passenger in heavy transport vehicle injured in collision with pedal cycle in nontraffic accident**
X+7th **V61.2 Person on outside of heavy transport vehicle injured in collision with pedal cycle in nontraffic accident**
X+7th **V61.3 Unspecified occupant of heavy transport vehicle injured in collision with pedal cycle in nontraffic accident**
X+7th **V61.4 Person boarding or alighting a heavy transport vehicle injured in collision with pedal cycle while boarding or alighting**
X+7th **V61.5 Driver of heavy transport vehicle injured in collision with pedal cycle in traffic accident**
X+7th **V61.6 Passenger in heavy transport vehicle injured in collision with pedal cycle in traffic accident**
X+7th **V61.7 Person on outside of heavy transport vehicle injured in collision with pedal cycle in traffic accident**
X+7th **V61.9 Unspecified occupant of heavy transport vehicle injured in collision with pedal cycle in traffic accident**

V62 Occupant of heavy transport vehicle injured in collision with two- or three-wheeled motor vehicle

The appropriate 7th character is to be added to each code from category V62
A initial encounter
D subsequent encounter
S sequela

X+7th **V62.0 Driver of heavy transport vehicle injured in collision with two- or three-wheeled motor vehicle in nontraffic accident**
X+7th **V62.1 Passenger in heavy transport vehicle injured in collision with two- or three-wheeled motor vehicle in nontraffic accident**
X+7th **V62.2 Person on outside of heavy transport vehicle injured in collision with two- or three-wheeled motor vehicle in nontraffic accident**
X+7th **V62.3 Unspecified occupant of heavy transport vehicle injured in collision with two- or three-wheeled motor vehicle in nontraffic accident**

X+7th **V62.4 Person boarding or alighting a heavy transport vehicle injured in collision with two- or three-wheeled motor vehicle**

X+7th **V62.5 Driver of heavy transport vehicle injured in collision with two- or three-wheeled motor vehicle in traffic accident**

X+7th **V62.6 Passenger in heavy transport vehicle injured in collision with two- or three-wheeled motor vehicle in traffic accident**

X+7th **V62.7 Person on outside of heavy transport vehicle injured in collision with two- or three-wheeled motor vehicle in traffic accident**

X+7th **V62.9 Unspecified occupant of heavy transport vehicle injured in collision with two- or three-wheeled motor vehicle in traffic accident**

V63 Occupant of heavy transport vehicle injured in collision with car, pick-up truck or van

The appropriate 7th character is to be added to each code from category V63
A initial encounter
D subsequent encounter
S sequela

X+7th **V63.0 Driver of heavy transport vehicle injured in collision with car, pick-up truck or van in nontraffic accident**

X+7th **V63.1 Passenger in heavy transport vehicle injured in collision with car, pick-up truck or van in nontraffic accident**

X+7th **V63.2 Person on outside of heavy transport vehicle injured in collision with car, pick-up truck or van in nontraffic accident**

X+7th **V63.3 Unspecified occupant of heavy transport vehicle injured in collision with car, pick-up truck or van in nontraffic accident**

X+7th **V63.4 Person boarding or alighting a heavy transport vehicle injured in collision with car, pick-up truck or van**

X+7th **V63.5 Driver of heavy transport vehicle injured in collision with car, pick-up truck or van in traffic accident**

X+7th **V63.6 Passenger in heavy transport vehicle injured in collision with car, pick-up truck or van in traffic accident**

X+7th **V63.7 Person on outside of heavy transport vehicle injured in collision with car, pick-up truck or van in traffic accident**

X+7th **V63.9 Unspecified occupant of heavy transport vehicle injured in collision with car, pick-up truck or van in traffic accident**

V64 Occupant of heavy transport vehicle injured in collision with heavy transport vehicle or bus

Excludes1: *occupant of heavy transport vehicle injured in collision with military vehicle (V69.81)*

The appropriate 7th character is to be added to each code from category V64
A initial encounter
D subsequent encounter
S sequela

X+7th **V64.0 Driver of heavy transport vehicle injured in collision with heavy transport vehicle or bus in nontraffic accident**

X+7th **V64.1 Passenger in heavy transport vehicle injured in collision with heavy transport vehicle or bus in nontraffic accident**

X+7th **V64.2 Person on outside of heavy transport vehicle injured in collision with heavy transport vehicle or bus in nontraffic accident**

X+7th **V64.3 Unspecified occupant of heavy transport vehicle injured in collision with heavy transport vehicle or bus in nontraffic accident**

X+7th **V64.4 Person boarding or alighting a heavy transport vehicle injured in collision with heavy transport vehicle or bus while boarding or alighting**

X+7th **V64.5 Driver of heavy transport vehicle injured in collision with heavy transport vehicle or bus in traffic accident**

X+7th **V64.6 Passenger in heavy transport vehicle injured in collision with heavy transport vehicle or bus in traffic accident**

X+7th **V64.7 Person on outside of heavy transport vehicle injured in collision with heavy transport vehicle or bus in traffic accident**

X+7th **V64.9 Unspecified occupant of heavy transport vehicle injured in collision with heavy transport vehicle or bus in traffic accident**

V65 Occupant of heavy transport vehicle injured in collision with railway train or railway vehicle

The appropriate 7th character is to be added to each code from category V65
A initial encounter
D subsequent encounter
S sequela

X+7th **V65.0 Driver of heavy transport vehicle injured in collision with railway train or railway vehicle in nontraffic accident**

X+7th **V65.1 Passenger in heavy transport vehicle injured in collision with railway train or railway vehicle in nontraffic accident**

X+7th **V65.2 Person on outside of heavy transport vehicle injured in collision with railway train or railway vehicle in nontraffic accident**

X+7th **V65.3 Unspecified occupant of heavy transport vehicle injured in collision with railway train or railway vehicle in nontraffic accident**

X+7th **V65.4 Person boarding or alighting a heavy transport vehicle injured in collision with railway train or railway vehicle**

X+7th **V65.5 Driver of heavy transport vehicle injured in collision with railway train or railway vehicle in traffic accident**

X+7th **V65.6 Passenger in heavy transport vehicle injured in collision with railway train or railway vehicle in traffic accident**

X+7th **V65.7 Person on outside of heavy transport vehicle injured in collision with railway train or railway vehicle in traffic accident**

X+7th **V65.9 Unspecified occupant of heavy transport vehicle injured in collision with railway train or railway vehicle in traffic accident**

V66 Occupant of heavy transport vehicle injured in collision with other nonmotor vehicle

Includes: collision with animal-drawn vehicle, animal being ridden, streetcar

The appropriate 7th character is to be added to each code from category V66
A initial encounter
D subsequent encounter
S sequela

X+7th **V66.0 Driver of heavy transport vehicle injured in collision with other nonmotor vehicle in nontraffic accident**

X+7th **V66.1 Passenger in heavy transport vehicle injured in collision with other nonmotor vehicle in nontraffic accident**

X+7th **V66.2 Person on outside of heavy transport vehicle injured in collision with other nonmotor vehicle in nontraffic accident**

X+7th **V66.3 Unspecified occupant of heavy transport vehicle injured in collision with other nonmotor vehicle in nontraffic accident**

X+7th **V66.4 Person boarding or alighting a heavy transport vehicle injured in collision with other nonmotor vehicle**

X+7th **V66.5 Driver of heavy transport vehicle injured in collision with other nonmotor vehicle in traffic accident**

X+7th **V66.6 Passenger in heavy transport vehicle injured in collision with other nonmotor vehicle in traffic accident**

X+7th **V66.7 Person on outside of heavy transport vehicle injured in collision with other nonmotor vehicle in traffic accident**

X+7th **V66.9 Unspecified occupant of heavy transport vehicle injured in collision with other nonmotor vehicle in traffic accident**

V67 Occupant of heavy transport vehicle injured in collision with fixed or stationary object

The appropriate 7th character is to be added to each code from category V67
A initial encounter
D subsequent encounter
S sequela

X+7th **V67.0 Driver of heavy transport vehicle injured in collision with fixed or stationary object in nontraffic accident**

X+7th **V67.1 Passenger in heavy transport vehicle injured in collision with fixed or stationary object in nontraffic accident**

X+7th **V67.2 Person on outside of heavy transport vehicle injured in collision with fixed or stationary object in nontraffic accident**

X+7th **V67.3 Unspecified occupant of heavy transport vehicle injured in collision with fixed or stationary object in nontraffic accident**

X+7th **V67.4 Person boarding or alighting a heavy transport vehicle injured in collision with fixed or stationary object**

X+7th **V67.5 Driver of heavy transport vehicle injured in collision with fixed or stationary object in traffic accident**

X+7th **V67.6 Passenger in heavy transport vehicle injured in collision with fixed or stationary object in traffic accident**

X+7th **V67.7 Person on outside of heavy transport vehicle injured in collision with fixed or stationary object in traffic accident**

X+7th **V67.9 Unspecified occupant of heavy transport vehicle injured in collision with fixed or stationary object in traffic accident**

V68 Occupant of heavy transport vehicle injured in noncollision transport accident

Includes: overturning heavy transport vehicle NOS
overturning heavy transport vehicle without collision

The appropriate 7th character is to be added to each code from category V68
A initial encounter
D subsequent encounter
S sequela

X+7th **V68.0 Driver of heavy transport vehicle injured in noncollision transport accident in nontraffic accident**
X+7th **V68.1 Passenger in heavy transport vehicle injured in noncollision transport accident in nontraffic accident**
X+7th **V68.2 Person on outside of heavy transport vehicle injured in noncollision transport accident in nontraffic accident**
X+7th **V68.3 Unspecified occupant of heavy transport vehicle injured in noncollision transport accident in nontraffic accident**
X+7th **V68.4 Person boarding or alighting a heavy transport vehicle injured in noncollision transport accident**
X+7th **V68.5 Driver of heavy transport vehicle injured in noncollision transport accident in traffic accident**
X+7th **V68.6 Passenger in heavy transport vehicle injured in noncollision transport accident in traffic accident**
X+7th **V68.7 Person on outside of heavy transport vehicle injured in noncollision transport accident in traffic accident**
X+7th **V68.9 Unspecified occupant of heavy transport vehicle injured in noncollision transport accident in traffic accident**

V69 Occupant of heavy transport vehicle injured in other and unspecified transport accidents

The appropriate 7th character is to be added to each code from category V69
A initial encounter
D subsequent encounter
S sequela

\+ **V69.0 Driver of heavy transport vehicle injured in collision with other and unspecified motor vehicles in nontraffic accident**
X+7th **V69.00 Driver of heavy transport vehicle injured in collision with unspecified motor vehicles in nontraffic accident**
X+7th **V69.09 Driver of heavy transport vehicle injured in collision with other motor vehicles in nontraffic accident**
\+ **V69.1 Passenger in heavy transport vehicle injured in collision with other and unspecified motor vehicles in nontraffic accident**
X+7th **V69.10 Passenger in heavy transport vehicle injured in collision with unspecified motor vehicles in nontraffic accident**
X+7th **V69.19 Passenger in heavy transport vehicle injured in collision with other motor vehicles in nontraffic accident**
\+ **V69.2 Unspecified occupant of heavy transport vehicle injured in collision with other and unspecified motor vehicles in nontraffic accident**
X+7th **V69.20 Unspecified occupant of heavy transport vehicle injured in collision with unspecified motor vehicles in nontraffic accident**
Collision NOS involving heavy transport vehicle, nontraffic
X+7th **V69.29 Unspecified occupant of heavy transport vehicle injured in collision with other motor vehicles in nontraffic accident**
X+7th **V69.3 Occupant (driver) (passenger) of heavy transport vehicle injured in unspecified nontraffic accident**
Accident NOS involving heavy transport vehicle, nontraffic
Occupant of heavy transport vehicle injured in nontraffic accident NOS
\+ **V69.4 Driver of heavy transport vehicle injured in collision with other and unspecified motor vehicles in traffic accident**
X+7th **V69.40 Driver of heavy transport vehicle injured in collision with unspecified motor vehicles in traffic accident**
X+7th **V69.49 Driver of heavy transport vehicle injured in collision with other motor vehicles in traffic accident**
\+ **V69.5 Passenger in heavy transport vehicle injured in collision with other and unspecified motor vehicles in traffic accident**
X+7th **V69.50 Passenger in heavy transport vehicle injured in collision with unspecified motor vehicles in traffic accident**
X+7th **V69.59 Passenger in heavy transport vehicle injured in collision with other motor vehicles in traffic accident**
\+ **V69.6 Unspecified occupant of heavy transport vehicle injured in collision with other and unspecified motor vehicles in traffic accident**
X+7th **V69.60 Unspecified occupant of heavy transport vehicle injured in collision with unspecified motor vehicles in traffic accident**
Collision NOS involving heavy transport vehicle (traffic)
X+7th **V69.69 Unspecified occupant of heavy transport vehicle injured in collision with other motor vehicles in traffic accident**
\+ **V69.8 Occupant (driver) (passenger) of heavy transport vehicle injured in other specified transport accidents**
X+7th **V69.81 Occupant (driver) (passenger) of heavy transport vehicle injured in transport accidents with military vehicle**
X+7th **V69.88 Occupant (driver) (passenger) of heavy transport vehicle injured in other specified transport accidents**
X+7th **V69.9 Occupant (driver) (passenger) of heavy transport vehicle injured in unspecified traffic accident**
Accident NOS involving heavy transport vehicle

Bus occupant injured in transport accident (V70-V79)

Includes: motorcoach

Excludes1: *minibus (V50-V59)*

V70 Bus occupant injured in collision with pedestrian or animal

The appropriate 7th character is to be added to each code from category V70
A initial encounter
D subsequent encounter
S sequela

Excludes1: *bus collision with animal-drawn vehicle or animal being ridden (V76.-)*

X+7th **V70.0 Driver of bus injured in collision with pedestrian or animal in nontraffic accident**
X+7th **V70.1 Passenger on bus injured in collision with pedestrian or animal in nontraffic accident**
X+7th **V70.2 Person on outside of bus injured in collision with pedestrian or animal in nontraffic accident**
X+7th **V70.3 Unspecified occupant of bus injured in collision with pedestrian or animal in nontraffic accident**
X+7th **V70.4 Person boarding or alighting from bus injured in collision with pedestrian or animal**
X+7th **V70.5 Driver of bus injured in collision with pedestrian or animal in traffic accident**
X+7th **V70.6 Passenger on bus injured in collision with pedestrian or animal in traffic accident**
X+7th **V70.7 Person on outside of bus injured in collision with pedestrian or animal in traffic accident**
X+7th **V70.9 Unspecified occupant of bus injured in collision with pedestrian or animal in traffic accident**

V71 Bus occupant injured in collision with pedal cycle

The appropriate 7th character is to be added to each code from category V71
A initial encounter
D subsequent encounter
S sequela

X+7th **V71.0 Driver of bus injured in collision with pedal cycle in nontraffic accident**
X+7th **V71.1 Passenger on bus injured in collision with pedal cycle in nontraffic accident**
X+7th **V71.2 Person on outside of bus injured in collision with pedal cycle in nontraffic accident**
X+7th **V71.3 Unspecified occupant of bus injured in collision with pedal cycle in nontraffic accident**
X+7th **V71.4 Person boarding or alighting from bus injured in collision with pedal cycle**
X+7th **V71.5 Driver of bus injured in collision with pedal cycle in traffic accident**
X+7th **V71.6 Passenger on bus injured in collision with pedal cycle in traffic accident**
X+7th **V71.7 Person on outside of bus injured in collision with pedal cycle in traffic accident**
X+7th **V71.9 Unspecified occupant of bus injured in collision with pedal cycle in traffic accident**

V72 Bus occupant injured in collision with two- or three-wheeled motor vehicle

The appropriate 7th character is to be added to each code from category V72
A initial encounter
D subsequent encounter
S sequela

X+7th **V72.0 Driver of bus injured in collision with two- or three-wheeled motor vehicle in nontraffic accident**
X+7th **V72.1 Passenger on bus injured in collision with two- or three-wheeled motor vehicle in nontraffic accident**
X+7th **V72.2 Person on outside of bus injured in collision with two- or three-wheeled motor vehicle in nontraffic accident**
X+7th **V72.3 Unspecified occupant of bus injured in collision with two- or three-wheeled motor vehicle in nontraffic accident**
X+7th **V72.4 Person boarding or alighting from bus injured in collision with two- or three-wheeled motor vehicle**
X+7th **V72.5 Driver of bus injured in collision with two- or three-wheeled motor vehicle in traffic accident**
X+7th **V72.6 Passenger on bus injured in collision with two- or three-wheeled motor vehicle in traffic accident**
X+7th **V72.7 Person on outside of bus injured in collision with two- or three-wheeled motor vehicle in traffic accident**
X+7th **V72.9 Unspecified occupant of bus injured in collision with two- or three-wheeled motor vehicle in traffic accident**

V73 Bus occupant injured in collision with car, pick-up truck or van

The appropriate 7th character is to be added to each code from category V73
A initial encounter
D subsequent encounter
S sequela

X+7th **V73.0 Driver of bus injured in collision with car, pick-up truck or van in nontraffic accident**
X+7th **V73.1 Passenger on bus injured in collision with car, pick-up truck or van in nontraffic accident**
X+7th **V73.2 Person on outside of bus injured in collision with car, pick-up truck or van in nontraffic accident**
X+7th **V73.3 Unspecified occupant of bus injured in collision with car, pick-up truck or van in nontraffic accident**
X+7th **V73.4 Person boarding or alighting from bus injured in collision with car, pick-up truck or van**
X+7th **V73.5 Driver of bus injured in collision with car, pick-up truck or van in traffic accident**
X+7th **V73.6 Passenger on bus injured in collision with car, pick-up truck or van in traffic accident**
X+7th **V73.7 Person on outside of bus injured in collision with car, pick-up truck or van in traffic accident**
X+7th **V73.9 Unspecified occupant of bus injured in collision with car, pick-up truck or van in traffic accident**

V74 Bus occupant injured in collision with heavy transport vehicle or bus

Excludes1: *bus occupant injured in collision with military vehicle (V79.81)*

The appropriate 7th character is to be added to each code from category V74
A initial encounter
D subsequent encounter
S sequela

X+7th **V74.0 Driver of bus injured in collision with heavy transport vehicle or bus in nontraffic accident**
X+7th **V74.1 Passenger on bus injured in collision with heavy transport vehicle or bus in nontraffic accident**
X+7th **V74.2 Person on outside of bus injured in collision with heavy transport vehicle or bus in nontraffic accident**
X+7th **V74.3 Unspecified occupant of bus injured in collision with heavy transport vehicle or bus in nontraffic accident**
X+7th **V74.4 Person boarding or alighting from bus injured in collision with heavy transport vehicle or bus**
X+7th **V74.5 Driver of bus injured in collision with heavy transport vehicle or bus in traffic accident**
X+7th **V74.6 Passenger on bus injured in collision with heavy transport vehicle or bus in traffic accident**
X+7th **V74.7 Person on outside of bus injured in collision with heavy transport vehicle or bus in traffic accident**
X+7th **V74.9 Unspecified occupant of bus injured in collision with heavy transport vehicle or bus in traffic accident**

V75 Bus occupant injured in collision with railway train or railway vehicle

The appropriate 7th character is to be added to each code from category V75
A initial encounter
D subsequent encounter
S sequela

X+7th **V75.0 Driver of bus injured in collision with railway train or railway vehicle in nontraffic accident**
X+7th **V75.1 Passenger on bus injured in collision with railway train or railway vehicle in nontraffic accident**
X+7th **V75.2 Person on outside of bus injured in collision with railway train or railway vehicle in nontraffic accident**
X+7th **V75.3 Unspecified occupant of bus injured in collision with railway train or railway vehicle in nontraffic accident**
X+7th **V75.4 Person boarding or alighting from bus injured in collision with railway train or railway vehicle**
X+7th **V75.5 Driver of bus injured in collision with railway train or railway vehicle in traffic accident**
X+7th **V75.6 Passenger on bus injured in collision with railway train or railway vehicle in traffic accident**
X+7th **V75.7 Person on outside of bus injured in collision with railway train or railway vehicle in traffic accident**
X+7th **V75.9 Unspecified occupant of bus injured in collision with railway train or railway vehicle in traffic accident**

V76 Bus occupant injured in collision with other nonmotor vehicle

Includes: collision with animal-drawn vehicle, animal being ridden, streetcar

The appropriate 7th character is to be added to each code from category V76
A initial encounter
D subsequent encounter
S sequela

X+7th **V76.0 Driver of bus injured in collision with other nonmotor vehicle in nontraffic accident**
X+7th **V76.1 Passenger on bus injured in collision with other nonmotor vehicle in nontraffic accident**
X+7th **V76.2 Person on outside of bus injured in collision with other nonmotor vehicle in nontraffic accident**
X+7th **V76.3 Unspecified occupant of bus injured in collision with other nonmotor vehicle in nontraffic accident**
X+7th **V76.4 Person boarding or alighting from bus injured in collision with other nonmotor vehicle**
X+7th **V76.5 Driver of bus injured in collision with other nonmotor vehicle in traffic accident**
X+7th **V76.6 Passenger on bus injured in collision with other nonmotor vehicle in traffic accident**
X+7th **V76.7 Person on outside of bus injured in collision with other nonmotor vehicle in traffic accident**
X+7th **V76.9 Unspecified occupant of bus injured in collision with other nonmotor vehicle in traffic accident**

V77 Bus occupant injured in collision with fixed or stationary object

The appropriate 7th character is to be added to each code from category V77
A initial encounter
D subsequent encounter
S sequela

X+7th **V77.0 Driver of bus injured in collision with fixed or stationary object in nontraffic accident**
X+7th **V77.1 Passenger on bus injured in collision with fixed or stationary object in nontraffic accident**
X+7th **V77.2 Person on outside of bus injured in collision with fixed or stationary object in nontraffic accident**
X+7th **V77.3 Unspecified occupant of bus injured in collision with fixed or stationary object in nontraffic accident**
X+7th **V77.4 Person boarding or alighting from bus injured in collision with fixed or stationary object**
X+7th **V77.5 Driver of bus injured in collision with fixed or stationary object in traffic accident**
X+7th **V77.6 Passenger on bus injured in collision with fixed or stationary object in traffic accident**
X+7th **V77.7 Person on outside of bus injured in collision with fixed or stationary object in traffic accident**
X+7th **V77.9 Unspecified occupant of bus injured in collision with fixed or stationary object in traffic accident**

V78 Bus occupant injured in noncollision transport accident

Includes: overturning bus NOS
overturning bus without collision

The appropriate 7th character is to be added to each code from category V78
A initial encounter
D subsequent encounter
S sequela

X+7th **V78.0 Driver of bus injured in noncollision transport accident in nontraffic accident**
X+7th **V78.1 Passenger on bus injured in noncollision transport accident in nontraffic accident**
X+7th **V78.2 Person on outside of bus injured in noncollision transport accident in nontraffic accident**
X+7th **V78.3 Unspecified occupant of bus injured in noncollision transport accident in nontraffic accident**
X+7th **V78.4 Person boarding or alighting from bus injured in noncollision transport accident**
X+7th **V78.5 Driver of bus injured in noncollision transport accident in traffic accident**
X+7th **V78.6 Passenger on bus injured in noncollision transport accident in traffic accident**
X+7th **V78.7 Person on outside of bus injured in noncollision transport accident in traffic accident**
X+7th **V78.9 Unspecified occupant of bus injured in noncollision transport accident in traffic accident**

V79 Bus occupant injured in other and unspecified transport accidents

The appropriate 7th character is to be added to each code from category V79
A initial encounter
D subsequent encounter
S sequela

\+ **V79.0 Driver of bus injured in collision with other and unspecified motor vehicles in nontraffic accident**
X+7th **V79.00 Driver of bus injured in collision with unspecified motor vehicles in nontraffic accident**
X+7th **V79.09 Driver of bus injured in collision with other motor vehicles in nontraffic accident**
\+ **V79.1 Passenger on bus injured in collision with other and unspecified motor vehicles in nontraffic accident**
X+7th **V79.10 Passenger on bus injured in collision with unspecified motor vehicles in nontraffic accident**
X+7th **V79.19 Passenger on bus injured in collision with other motor vehicles in nontraffic accident**
\+ **V79.2 Unspecified bus occupant injured in collision with other and unspecified motor vehicles in nontraffic accident**
X+7th **V79.20 Unspecified bus occupant injured in collision with unspecified motor vehicles in nontraffic accident**
Bus collision NOS, nontraffic
X+7th **V79.29 Unspecified bus occupant injured in collision with other motor vehicles in nontraffic accident**
X+7th **V79.3 Bus occupant (driver) (passenger) injured in unspecified nontraffic accident**
Bus accident NOS, nontraffic
Bus occupant injured in nontraffic accident NOS
\+ **V79.4 Driver of bus injured in collision with other and unspecified motor vehicles in traffic accident**
X+7th **V79.40 Driver of bus injured in collision with unspecified motor vehicles in traffic accident**
X+7th **V79.49 Driver of bus injured in collision with other motor vehicles in traffic accident**
\+ **V79.5 Passenger on bus injured in collision with other and unspecified motor vehicles in traffic accident**
X+7th **V79.50 Passenger on bus injured in collision with unspecified motor vehicles in traffic accident**
X+7th **V79.59 Passenger on bus injured in collision with other motor vehicles in traffic accident**
\+ **V79.6 Unspecified bus occupant injured in collision with other and unspecified motor vehicles in traffic accident**
X+7th **V79.60 Unspecified bus occupant injured in collision with unspecified motor vehicles in traffic accident**
Bus collision NOS (traffic)
X+7th **V79.69 Unspecified bus occupant injured in collision with other motor vehicles in traffic accident**
\+ **V79.8 Bus occupant (driver) (passenger) injured in other specified transport accidents**
X+7th **V79.81 Bus occupant (driver) (passenger) injured in transport accidents with military vehicle**
X+7th **V79.88 Bus occupant (driver) (passenger) injured in other specified transport accidents**
X+7th **V79.9 Bus occupant (driver) (passenger) injured in unspecified traffic accident**
Bus accident NOS

Other land transport accidents (V80-V89)

V80 Animal-rider or occupant of animal-drawn vehicle injured in transport accident

The appropriate 7th character is to be added to each code from category V80
A initial encounter
D subsequent encounter
S sequela

\+ **V80.0 Animal-rider or occupant of animal drawn vehicle injured by fall from or being thrown from animal or animal-drawn vehicle in noncollision accident**
\+ **V80.01 Animal-rider injured by fall from or being thrown from animal in noncollision accident**
+7th **V80.010 Animal-rider injured by fall from or being thrown from horse in noncollision accident**
+7th **V80.018 Animal-rider injured by fall from or being thrown from other animal in noncollision accident**
X+7th **V80.02 Occupant of animal-drawn vehicle injured by fall from or being thrown from animal-drawn vehicle in noncollision accident**
Overturning animal-drawn vehicle NOS
Overturning animal-drawn vehicle without collision
\+ **V80.1 Animal-rider or occupant of animal-drawn vehicle injured in collision with pedestrian or animal**
Excludes1: *animal-rider or animal-drawn vehicle collision with animal-drawn vehicle or animal being ridden (V80.7)*
X+7th **V80.11 Animal-rider injured in collision with pedestrian or animal**
X+7th **V80.12 Occupant of animal-drawn vehicle injured in collision with pedestrian or animal**
\+ **V80.2 Animal-rider or occupant of animal-drawn vehicle injured in collision with pedal cycle**
X+7th **V80.21 Animal-rider injured in collision with pedal cycle**
X+7th **V80.22 Occupant of animal-drawn vehicle injured in collision with pedal cycle**
\+ **V80.3 Animal-rider or occupant of animal-drawn vehicle injured in collision with two- or three-wheeled motor vehicle**
X+7th **V80.31 Animal-rider injured in collision with two- or three-wheeled motor vehicle**
X+7th **V80.32 Occupant of animal-drawn vehicle injured in collision with two- or three-wheeled motor vehicle**
\+ **V80.4 Animal-rider or occupant of animal-drawn vehicle injured in collision with car, pick-up truck, van, heavy transport vehicle or bus**
Excludes1: *animal-rider injured in collision with military vehicle (V80.910)*
occupant of animal-drawn vehicle injured in collision with military vehicle (V80.920)
X+7th **V80.41 Animal-rider injured in collision with car, pick-up truck, van, heavy transport vehicle or bus**
X+7th **V80.42 Occupant of animal-drawn vehicle injured in collision with car, pick-up truck, van, heavy transport vehicle or bus**
\+ **V80.5 Animal-rider or occupant of animal-drawn vehicle injured in collision with other specified motor vehicle**
X+7th **V80.51 Animal-rider injured in collision with other specified motor vehicle**
X+7th **V80.52 Occupant of animal-drawn vehicle injured in collision with other specified motor vehicle**
\+ **V80.6 Animal-rider or occupant of animal-drawn vehicle injured in collision with railway train or railway vehicle**
X+7th **V80.61 Animal-rider injured in collision with railway train or railway vehicle**
X+7th **V80.62 Occupant of animal-drawn vehicle injured in collision with railway train or railway vehicle**

+ **V80.7 Animal-rider or occupant of animal-drawn vehicle injured in collision with other nonmotor vehicles**
X+7th **V80.71 Animal-rider or occupant of animal-drawn vehicle injured in collision with animal being ridden**
X+7th **V80.710 Animal-rider injured in collision with other animal being ridden**
X+7th **V80.711 Occupant of animal-drawn vehicle injured in collision with animal being ridden**
X+7th **V80.72 Animal-rider or occupant of animal-drawn vehicle injured in collision with other animal-drawn vehicle**
X+7th **V80.720 Animal-rider injured in collision with animal-drawn vehicle**
X+7th **V80.721 Occupant of animal-drawn vehicle injured in collision with other animal-drawn vehicle**
+ **V80.73 Animal-rider or occupant of animal-drawn vehicle injured in collision with streetcar**
X+7th **V80.730 Animal-rider injured in collision with streetcar**
X+7th **V80.731 Occupant of animal-drawn vehicle injured in collision with streetcar**
X+7th **V80.79 Animal-rider or occupant of animal-drawn vehicle injured in collision with other nonmotor vehicles**
X+7th **V80.790 Animal-rider injured in collision with other nonmotor vehicles**
X+7th **V80.791 Occupant of animal-drawn vehicle injured in collision with other nonmotor vehicles**
+ **V80.8 Animal-rider or occupant of animal-drawn vehicle injured in collision with fixed or stationary object**
X+7th **V80.81 Animal-rider injured in collision with fixed or stationary object**
X+7th **V80.82 Occupant of animal-drawn vehicle injured in collision with fixed or stationary object**
+ **V80.9 Animal-rider or occupant of animal-drawn vehicle injured in other and unspecified transport accidents**
+ **V80.91 Animal-rider injured in other and unspecified transport accidents**
+7th **V80.910 Animal-rider injured in transport accident with military vehicle**
+7th **V80.918 Animal-rider injured in other transport accident**
+7th **V80.919 Animal-rider injured in unspecified transport accident**
Animal rider accident NOS
+ **V80.92 Occupant of animal-drawn vehicle injured in other and unspecified transport accidents**
+7th **V80.920 Occupant of animal-drawn vehicle injured in transport accident with military vehicle**
+7th **V80.928 Occupant of animal-drawn vehicle injured in other transport accident**
+7th **V80.929 Occupant of animal-drawn vehicle injured in unspecified transport accident**
Animal-drawn vehicle accident NOS

V81 Occupant of railway train or railway vehicle injured in transport accident

Includes: derailment of railway train or railway vehicle
person on outside of train
Excludes1: *streetcar (V82.-)*

The appropriate 7th character is to be added to each code from category V81
A initial encounter
D subsequent encounter
S sequela

X+7th **V81.0 Occupant of railway train or railway vehicle injured in collision with motor vehicle in nontraffic accident**
Excludes1: *Occupant of railway train or railway vehicle injured due to collision with military vehicle (V81.83)*
X+7th **V81.1 Occupant of railway train or railway vehicle injured in collision with motor vehicle in traffic accident**
Excludes1: *Occupant of railway train or railway vehicle injured due to collision with military vehicle (V81.83)*
X+7th **V81.2 Occupant of railway train or railway vehicle injured in collision with or hit by rolling stock**
X+7th **V81.3 Occupant of railway train or railway vehicle injured in collision with other object**
Railway collision NOS
X+7th **V81.4 Person injured while boarding or alighting from railway train or railway vehicle**
X+7th **V81.5 Occupant of railway train or railway vehicle injured by fall in railway train or railway vehicle**
X+7th **V81.6 Occupant of railway train or railway vehicle injured by fall from railway train or railway vehicle**
X+7th **V81.7 Occupant of railway train or railway vehicle injured in derailment without antecedent collision**
+ **V81.8 Occupant of railway train or railway vehicle injured in other specified railway accidents**
X+7th **V81.81 Occupant of railway train or railway vehicle injured due to explosion or fire on train**
X+7th **V81.82 Occupant of railway train or railway vehicle injured due to object falling onto train**
Occupant of railway train or railway vehicle injured due to falling earth onto train
Occupant of railway train or railway vehicle injured due to falling rocks onto train
Occupant of railway train or railway vehicle injured due to falling snow onto train
Occupant of railway train or railway vehicle injured due to falling trees onto train
X+7th **V81.83 Occupant of railway train or railway vehicle injured due to collision with military vehicle**
X+7th **V81.89 Occupant of railway train or railway vehicle injured due to other specified railway accident**
X+7th **V81.9 Occupant of railway train or railway vehicle injured in unspecified railway accident**
Railway accident NOS

V82 Occupant of powered streetcar injured in transport accident

Includes: interurban electric car
person on outside of streetcar
tram (car)
trolley (car)
Excludes1: *bus (V70-V79)*
motorcoach (V70-V79)
nonpowered streetcar (V76.-)
train (V81.-)

The appropriate 7th character is to be added to each code from category V82
A initial encounter
D subsequent encounter
S sequela

X+7th **V82.0 Occupant of streetcar injured in collision with motor vehicle in nontraffic accident**
X+7th **V82.1 Occupant of streetcar injured in collision with motor vehicle in traffic accident**
X+7th **V82.2 Occupant of streetcar injured in collision with or hit by rolling stock**
X+7th **V82.3 Occupant of streetcar injured in collision with other object**
Excludes1: *collision with animal-drawn vehicle or animal being ridden (V82.8)*
X+7th **V82.4 Person injured while boarding or alighting from streetcar**
X+7th **V82.5 Occupant of streetcar injured by fall in streetcar**
Excludes1: *fall in streetcar:*
while boarding or alighting (V82.4)
with antecedent collision (V82.0-V82.3)
X+7th **V82.6 Occupant of streetcar injured by fall from streetcar**
Excludes1: *fall from streetcar:*
while boarding or alighting (V82.4)
with antecedent collision (V82.0-V82.3)
X+7th **V82.7 Occupant of streetcar injured in derailment without antecedent collision**
Excludes1: *occupant of streetcar injured in derailment with antecedent collision (V82.0-V82.3)*
X+7th **V82.8 Occupant of streetcar injured in other specified transport accidents**
Streetcar collision with military vehicle
Streetcar collision with train or nonmotor vehicles
X+7th **V82.9 Occupant of streetcar injured in unspecified traffic accident**
Streetcar accident NOS

V83 Occupant of special vehicle mainly used on industrial premises injured in transport accident

Includes: battery-powered airport passenger vehicle
battery-powered truck (baggage) (mail)
coal-car in mine
forklift (truck)
logging car
self-propelled industrial truck
station baggage truck (powered)
tram, truck, or tub (powered) in mine or quarry

Excludes1: *special construction vehicles (V85.-)*
special industrial vehicle in stationary use or maintenance (W31.-)

The appropriate 7th character is to be added to each code from category V83
A initial encounter
D subsequent encounter
S sequela

X+7th **V83.0 Driver of special industrial vehicle injured in traffic accident**
X+7th **V83.1 Passenger of special industrial vehicle injured in traffic accident**
X+7th **V83.2 Person on outside of special industrial vehicle injured in traffic accident**
X+7th **V83.3 Unspecified occupant of special industrial vehicle injured in traffic accident**
X+7th **V83.4 Person injured while boarding or alighting from special industrial vehicle**
X+7th **V83.5 Driver of special industrial vehicle injured in nontraffic accident**
X+7th **V83.6 Passenger of special industrial vehicle injured in nontraffic accident**
X+7th **V83.7 Person on outside of special industrial vehicle injured in nontraffic accident**
X+7th **V83.9 Unspecified occupant of special industrial vehicle injured in nontraffic accident**
Special-industrial-vehicle accident NOS

V84 Occupant of special vehicle mainly used in agriculture injured in transport accident

Includes: self-propelled farm machinery
tractor (and trailer)

Excludes1: *animal-powered farm machinery accident (W30.8-)*
contact with combine harvester (W30.0)
special agricultural vehicle in stationary use or maintenance (W30.-)

The appropriate 7th character is to be added to each code from category V84
A initial encounter
D subsequent encounter
S sequela

X+7th **V84.0 Driver of special agricultural vehicle injured in traffic accident**
X+7th **V84.1 Passenger of special agricultural vehicle injured in traffic accident**
X+7th **V84.2 Person on outside of special agricultural vehicle injured in traffic accident**
X+7th **V84.3 Unspecified occupant of special agricultural vehicle injured in traffic accident**
X+7th **V84.4 Person injured while boarding or alighting from special agricultural vehicle**
X+7th **V84.5 Driver of special agricultural vehicle injured in nontraffic accident**
X+7th **V84.6 Passenger of special agricultural vehicle injured in nontraffic accident**
X+7th **V84.7 Person on outside of special agricultural vehicle injured in nontraffic accident**
X+7th **V84.9 Unspecified occupant of special agricultural vehicle injured in nontraffic accident**
Special-agricultural vehicle accident NOS

V85 Occupant of special construction vehicle injured in transport accident

Includes: bulldozer
digger
dump truck
earth-leveller
mechanical shovel
road-roller

Excludes1: *special industrial vehicle (V83.-)*
special construction vehicle in stationary use or maintenance (W31.-)

The appropriate 7th character is to be added to each code from category V85
A initial encounter
D subsequent encounter
S sequela

X+7th **V85.0 Driver of special construction vehicle injured in traffic accident**
X+7th **V85.1 Passenger of special construction vehicle injured in traffic accident**
X+7th **V85.2 Person on outside of special construction vehicle injured in traffic accident**
X+7th **V85.3 Unspecified occupant of special construction vehicle injured in traffic accident**
X+7th **V85.4 Person injured while boarding or alighting from special construction vehicle**
X+7th **V85.5 Driver of special construction vehicle injured in nontraffic accident**
X+7th **V85.6 Passenger of special construction vehicle injured in nontraffic accident**
X+7th **V85.7 Person on outside of special construction vehicle injured in nontraffic accident**
X+7th **V85.9 Unspecified occupant of special construction vehicle injured in nontraffic accident**
Special-construction-vehicle accident NOS

V86 Occupant of special all-terrain or other off-road motor vehicle, injured in transport accident

Excludes1: *special all-terrain vehicle in stationary use or maintenance (W31.-)*
sport-utility vehicle (V50-V59)
three-wheeled motor vehicle designed for on-road use (V30-V39)

The appropriate 7th character is to be added to each code from category V86
A initial encounter
D subsequent encounter
S sequela

\+ **V86.0 Driver of special all-terrain or other off-road motor vehicle injured in traffic accident**
+7th **V86.01 Driver of ambulance or fire engine injured in traffic accident**
+7th **V86.02 Driver of snowmobile injured in traffic accident**
+7th **V86.03 Driver of dune buggy injured in traffic accident**
+7th **V86.04 Driver of military vehicle injured in traffic accident**
+7th **V86.05 Driver of 3- or 4- wheeled all-terrain vehicle (ATV) injured in traffic accident**
+7th **V86.06 Driver of dirt bike or motor/cross bike injured in traffic accident**
+7th **V86.09 Driver of other special all-terrain or other off-road motor vehicle injured in traffic accident**
Driver of dirt bike injured in traffic accident
Driver of go cart injured in traffic accident
Driver of golf cart injured in traffic accident

\+ **V86.1 Passenger of special all-terrain or other off-road motor vehicle injured in traffic accident**
+7th **V86.11 Passenger of ambulance or fire engine injured in traffic accident**
+7th **V86.12 Passenger of snowmobile injured in traffic accident**
+7th **V86.13 Passenger of dune buggy injured in traffic accident**
+7th **V86.14 Passenger of military vehicle injured in traffic accident**
+7th **V86.15 Passenger of 3- or 4- wheeled all-terrain vehicle (ATV) injured in traffic accident**

+7th **V86.16** **Passenger of dirt bike or motor/cross bike injured in traffic accident**

+7th **V86.19** **Passenger of other special all-terrain or other off-road motor vehicle injured in traffic accident**
Passenger of dirt bike injured in traffic accident
Passenger of go cart injured in traffic accident
Passenger of golf cart injured in traffic accident

\+ **V86.2** **Person on outside of special all-terrain or other off-road motor vehicle injured in traffic accident**

+7th **V86.21** **Person on outside of ambulance or fire engine injured in traffic accident**

+7th **V86.22** **Person on outside of snowmobile injured in traffic accident**

+7th **V86.23** **Person on outside of dune buggy injured in traffic accident**

+7th **V86.24** **Person on outside of military vehicle injured in traffic accident**

+7th **V86.25** **Person on outside of 3- or 4- wheeled all-terrain vehicle (ATV) injured in traffic accident**

+7th **V86.26** **Person on outside of dirt bike or motor/cross bike injured in traffic accident**

+7th **V86.29** **Person on outside of other special all-terrain or other off-road motor vehicle injured in traffic accident**
Person on outside of dirt bike injured in traffic accident
Person on outside of go cart in traffic accident
Person on outside of golf cart injured in traffic accident

\+ **V86.3** **Unspecified occupant of special all-terrain or other off-road motor vehicle injured in traffic accident**

+7th **V86.31** **Unspecified occupant of ambulance or fire engine injured in traffic accident**

+7th **V86.32** **Unspecified occupant of snowmobile injured in traffic accident**

+7th **V86.33** **Unspecified occupant of dune buggy injured in traffic accident**

+7th **V86.34** **Unspecified occupant of military vehicle injured in traffic accident**

+7th **V86.35** **Unspecified occupant of 3- or 4- wheeled all-terrain vehicle (ATV) injured in traffic accident**

+7th **V86.36** **Unspecified occupant of dirt bike or motor/cross bike injured in traffic accident**

+7th **V86.39** **Unspecified occupant of other special all-terrain or other off-road motor vehicle injured in traffic accident**
Unspecified occupant of dirt bike injured in traffic accident
Unspecified occupant of go cart injured in traffic accident
Unspecified occupant of golf cart injured in traffic accident

\+ **V86.4** **Person injured while boarding or alighting from special all-terrain or other off-road motor vehicle**

+7th **V86.41** **Person injured while boarding or alighting from ambulance or fire engine**

+7th **V86.42** **Person injured while boarding or alighting from snowmobile**

+7th **V86.43** **Person injured while boarding or alighting from dune buggy**

+7th **V86.44** **Person injured while boarding or alighting from military vehicle**

+7th **V86.45** **Person injured while boarding or alighting from a 3- or 4- wheeled all-terrain vehicle (ATV)**

+7th **V86.46** **Person injured while boarding or alighting from a dirt bike or motor/cross bike**

+7th **V86.49** **Person injured while boarding or alighting from other special all-terrain or other off-road motor vehicle**
Person injured while boarding or alighting from dirt bike
Person injured while boarding or alighting from go cart
Person injured while boarding or alighting from golf cart

\+ **V86.5** **Driver of special all-terrain or other off-road motor vehicle injured in nontraffic accident**

+7th **V86.51** **Driver of ambulance or fire engine injured in nontraffic accident**

+7th **V86.52** **Driver of snowmobile injured in nontraffic accident**

+7th **V86.53** **Driver of dune buggy injured in nontraffic accident**

+7th **V86.54** **Driver of military vehicle injured in nontraffic accident**

+7th **V86.55** **Driver of 3- or 4- wheeled all-terrain vehicle (ATV) injured in nontraffic accident**

+7th **V86.56** **Driver of dirt bike or motor/cross bike injured in nontraffic accident, initial encounter**

+7th **V86.59** **Driver of other special all-terrain or other off-road motor vehicle injured in nontraffic accident**
Driver of dirt bike injured in nontraffic accident
Driver of go cart injured in nontraffic accident
Driver of golf cart injured in nontraffic accident

\+ **V86.6** **Passenger of special all-terrain or other off-road motor vehicle injured in nontraffic accident**

+7th **V86.61** **Passenger of ambulance or fire engine injured in nontraffic accident**

+7th **V86.62** **Passenger of snowmobile injured in nontraffic accident**

+7th **V86.63** **Passenger of dune buggy injured in nontraffic accident**

+7th **V86.64** **Passenger of military vehicle injured in nontraffic accident**

+7th **V86.65** **Passenger of 3- or 4- wheeled all-terrain vehicle (ATV) injured in nontraffic accident**

+7th **V86.66** **Passenger of dirt bike or motor/cross bike injured in nontraffic accident**

+7th **V86.69** **Passenger of other special all-terrain or other off-road motor vehicle injured in nontraffic accident**
Passenger of dirt bike injured in nontraffic accident
Passenger of go cart injured in nontraffic accident
Passenger of golf cart injured in nontraffic accident

\+ **V86.7** **Person on outside of special all-terrain or other off-road motor vehicle injured in nontraffic accident**

+7th **V86.71** **Person on outside of ambulance or fire engine injured in nontraffic accident**

+7th **V86.72** **Person on outside of snowmobile injured in nontraffic accident**

+7th **V86.73** **Person on outside of dune buggy injured in nontraffic accident**

+7th **V86.74** **Person on outside of military vehicle injured in nontraffic accident**

+7th **V86.75** **Person on outside of 3- or 4- wheeled all-terrain vehicle (ATV) injured in nontraffic accident**

+7th **V86.76** **Person on outside of dirt bike or motor/cross bike injured in nontraffic accident**

+7th **V86.79** **Person on outside of other special all-terrain or other off-road motor vehicles injured in nontraffic accident**
Person on outside of dirt bike injured in nontraffic accident
Person on outside of go cart injured in nontraffic accident
Person on outside of golf cart injured in nontraffic accident

\+ **V86.9** **Unspecified occupant of special all-terrain or other off-road motor vehicle injured in nontraffic accident**

+7th **V86.91** **Unspecified occupant of ambulance or fire engine injured in nontraffic accident**

+7th **V86.92** **Unspecified occupant of snowmobile injured in nontraffic accident**

+7th **V86.93** **Unspecified occupant of dune buggy injured in nontraffic accident**

+7th **V86.94** **Unspecified occupant of military vehicle injured in nontraffic accident**

+7th **V86.95** **Unspecified occupant of 3- or 4- wheeled all-terrain vehicle (ATV) injured in nontraffic accident**

+7th **V86.96** **Unspecified occupant of dirt bike or motor/cross bike injured in nontraffic accident**

+7th **V86.99** **Unspecified occupant of other special all-terrain or other off-road motor vehicle injured in nontraffic accident**
Off-road motor-vehicle accident NOS
Other motor-vehicle accident NOS
Unspecified occupant of go cart injured in nontraffic accident
Unspecified occupant of golf cart injured in nontraffic accident

V87 Traffic accident of specified type but victim's mode of transport unknown

Excludes1: *collision involving:*
pedal cycle (V10-V19)
pedestrian (V01-V09)

The appropriate 7th character is to be added to each code from category V87
A initial encounter
D subsequent encounter
S sequela

X+7th **V87.0 Person injured in collision between car and two- or three-wheeled powered vehicle (traffic)**
X+7th **V87.1 Person injured in collision between other motor vehicle and two- or three-wheeled motor vehicle (traffic)**
X+7th **V87.2 Person injured in collision between car and pick-up truck or van (traffic)**
X+7th **V87.3 Person injured in collision between car and bus (traffic)**
X+7th **V87.4 Person injured in collision between car and heavy transport vehicle (traffic)**
X+7th **V87.5 Person injured in collision between heavy transport vehicle and bus (traffic)**
X+7th **V87.6 Person injured in collision between railway train or railway vehicle and car (traffic)**
X+7th **V87.7 Person injured in collision between other specified motor vehicles (traffic)**
X+7th **V87.8 Person injured in other specified noncollision transport accidents involving motor vehicle (traffic)**
X+7th **V87.9 Person injured in other specified (collision) (noncollision) transport accidents involving nonmotor vehicle (traffic)**

V88 Nontraffic accident of specified type but victim's mode of transport unknown

Excludes1: *collision involving:*
pedal cycle (V10-V19)
pedestrian (V01-V09)

The appropriate 7th character is to be added to each code from category V88
A initial encounter
D subsequent encounter
S sequela

X+7th **V88.0 Person injured in collision between car and two- or three-wheeled motor vehicle, nontraffic**
X+7th **V88.1 Person injured in collision between other motor vehicle and two- or three-wheeled motor vehicle, nontraffic**
X+7th **V88.2 Person injured in collision between car and pick-up truck or van, nontraffic**
X+7th **V88.3 Person injured in collision between car and bus, nontraffic**
X+7th **V88.4 Person injured in collision between car and heavy transport vehicle, nontraffic**
X+7th **V88.5 Person injured in collision between heavy transport vehicle and bus, nontraffic**
X+7th **V88.6 Person injured in collision between railway train or railway vehicle and car, nontraffic**
X+7th **V88.7 Person injured in collision between other specified motor vehicle, nontraffic**
X+7th **V88.8 Person injured in other specified noncollision transport accidents involving motor vehicle, nontraffic**
X+7th **V88.9 Person injured in other specified (collision)(noncollision) transport accidents involving nonmotor vehicle, nontraffic**

V89 Motor- or nonmotor-vehicle accident, type of vehicle unspecified

The appropriate 7th character is to be added to each code from category V89
A initial encounter
D subsequent encounter
S sequela

X+7th **V89.0 Person injured in unspecified motor-vehicle accident, nontraffic**
Motor-vehicle accident NOS, nontraffic
X+7th **V89.1 Person injured in unspecified nonmotor-vehicle accident, nontraffic**
Nonmotor-vehicle accident NOS (nontraffic)
X+7th **V89.2 Person injured in unspecified motor-vehicle accident, traffic**
Motor-vehicle accident [MVA] NOS
Road (traffic) accident [RTA] NOS
X+7th **V89.3 Person injured in unspecified nonmotor-vehicle accident, traffic**
Nonmotor-vehicle traffic accident NOS
X+7th **V89.9 Person injured in unspecified vehicle accident**
Collision NOS

Water transport accidents (V90-V94)

V90 Drowning and submersion due to accident to watercraft

Excludes1: *civilian water transport accident involving military watercraft (V94.81-)*
fall into water not from watercraft (W16.-)
military watercraft accident in military or war operations (Y36.0-, Y37.0-)
water-transport-related drowning or submersion without accident to watercraft (V92.-)

The appropriate 7th character is to be added to each code from category V90
A initial encounter
D subsequent encounter
S sequela

\+ **V90.0 Drowning and submersion due to watercraft overturning**
X+7th **V90.00 Drowning and submersion due to merchant ship overturning**
X+7th **V90.01 Drowning and submersion due to passenger ship overturning**
Drowning and submersion due to Ferry-boat overturning
Drowning and submersion due to Liner overturning
X+7th **V90.02 Drowning and submersion due to fishing boat overturning**
X+7th **V90.03 Drowning and submersion due to other powered watercraft overturning**
Drowning and submersion due to Hovercraft (on open water) overturning
Drowning and submersion due to Jet ski overturning
X+7th **V90.04 Drowning and submersion due to sailboat overturning**
X+7th **V90.05 Drowning and submersion due to canoe or kayak overturning**
X+7th **V90.06 Drowning and submersion due to (nonpowered) inflatable craft overturning**
X+7th **V90.08 Drowning and submersion due to other unpowered watercraft overturning**
Drowning and submersion due to windsurfer overturning
X+7th **V90.09 Drowning and submersion due to unspecified watercraft overturning**
Drowning and submersion due to boat NOS overturning
Drowning and submersion due to ship NOS overturning
Drowning and submersion due to watercraft NOS overturning

\+ **V90.1 Drowning and submersion due to watercraft sinking**
X+7th **V90.10 Drowning and submersion due to merchant ship sinking**
X+7th **V90.11 Drowning and submersion due to passenger ship sinking**
Drowning and submersion due to Ferry-boat sinking
Drowning and submersion due to Liner sinking
X+7th **V90.12 Drowning and submersion due to fishing boat sinking**
X+7th **V90.13 Drowning and submersion due to other powered watercraft sinking**
Drowning and submersion due to Hovercraft (on open water) sinking
Drowning and submersion due to Jet ski sinking
X+7th **V90.14 Drowning and submersion due to sailboat sinking**
X+7th **V90.15 Drowning and submersion due to canoe or kayak sinking**
X+7th **V90.16 Drowning and submersion due to (nonpowered) inflatable craft sinking**
X+7th **V90.18 Drowning and submersion due to other unpowered watercraft sinking**
X+7th **V90.19 Drowning and submersion due to unspecified watercraft sinking**
Drowning and submersion due to boat NOS sinking
Drowning and submersion due to ship NOS sinking
Drowning and submersion due to watercraft NOS sinking

+ **V90.2 Drowning and submersion due to falling or jumping from burning watercraft**
  - X+7th **V90.20 Drowning and submersion due to falling or jumping from burning merchant ship**
  - X+7th **V90.21 Drowning and submersion due to falling or jumping from burning passenger ship**
    - Drowning and submersion due to falling or jumping from burning Ferry-boat
    - Drowning and submersion due to falling or jumping from burning Liner
  - X+7th **V90.22 Drowning and submersion due to falling or jumping from burning fishing boat**
  - X+7th **V90.23 Drowning and submersion due to falling or jumping from other burning powered watercraft**
    - Drowning and submersion due to falling and jumping from burning Hovercraft (on open water)
    - Drowning and submersion due to falling and jumping from burning Jet ski
  - X+7th **V90.24 Drowning and submersion due to falling or jumping from burning sailboat**
  - X+7th **V90.25 Drowning and submersion due to falling or jumping from burning canoe or kayak**
  - X+7th **V90.26 Drowning and submersion due to falling or jumping from burning (nonpowered) inflatable craft**
  - X+7th **V90.27 Drowning and submersion due to falling or jumping from burning water-skis**
  - X+7th **V90.28 Drowning and submersion due to falling or jumping from other burning unpowered watercraft**
    - Drowning and submersion due to falling and jumping from burning surf-board
    - Drowning and submersion due to falling and jumping from burning windsurfer
  - X+7th **V90.29 Drowning and submersion due to falling or jumping from unspecified burning watercraft**
    - Drowning and submersion due to falling or jumping from burning boat NOS
    - Drowning and submersion due to falling or jumping from burning ship NOS
    - Drowning and submersion due to falling or jumping from burning watercraft NOS

+ **V90.3 Drowning and submersion due to falling or jumping from crushed watercraft**
  - X+7th **V90.30 Drowning and submersion due to falling or jumping from crushed merchant ship**
  - X+7th **V90.31 Drowning and submersion due to falling or jumping from crushed passenger ship**
    - Drowning and submersion due to falling and jumping from crushed Ferry boat
    - Drowning and submersion due to falling and jumping from crushed Liner
  - X+7th **V90.32 Drowning and submersion due to falling or jumping from crushed fishing boat**
  - X+7th **V90.33 Drowning and submersion due to falling or jumping from other crushed powered watercraft**
    - Drowning and submersion due to falling and jumping from crushed Hovercraft
    - Drowning and submersion due to falling and jumping from crushed Jet ski
  - X+7th **V90.34 Drowning and submersion due to falling or jumping from crushed sailboat**
  - X+7th **V90.35 Drowning and submersion due to falling or jumping from crushed canoe or kayak**
  - X+7th **V90.36 Drowning and submersion due to falling or jumping from crushed (nonpowered) inflatable craft**
  - X+7th **V90.37 Drowning and submersion due to falling or jumping from crushed water-skis**
  - X+7th **V90.38 Drowning and submersion due to falling or jumping from other crushed unpowered watercraft**
    - Drowning and submersion due to falling and jumping from crushed surf-board
    - Drowning and submersion due to falling and jumping from crushed windsurfer
  - X+7th **V90.39 Drowning and submersion due to falling or jumping from crushed unspecified watercraft**
    - Drowning and submersion due to falling and jumping from crushed boat NOS
    - Drowning and submersion due to falling and jumping from crushed ship NOS
    - Drowning and submersion due to falling and jumping from crushed watercraft NOS

+ **V90.8 Drowning and submersion due to other accident to watercraft**
  - X+7th **V90.80 Drowning and submersion due to other accident to merchant ship**
  - X+7th **V90.81 Drowning and submersion due to other accident to passenger ship**
    - Drowning and submersion due to other accident to Ferry-boat
    - Drowning and submersion due to other accident to Liner
  - X+7th **V90.82 Drowning and submersion due to other accident to fishing boat**
  - X+7th **V90.83 Drowning and submersion due to other accident to other powered watercraft**
    - Drowning and submersion due to other accident to Hovercraft (on open water)
    - Drowning and submersion due to other accident to Jet ski
  - X+7th **V90.84 Drowning and submersion due to other accident to sailboat**
  - X+7th **V90.85 Drowning and submersion due to other accident to canoe or kayak**
  - X+7th **V90.86 Drowning and submersion due to other accident to (nonpowered) inflatable craft**
  - X+7th **V90.87 Drowning and submersion due to other accident to water-skis**
  - X+7th **V90.88 Drowning and submersion due to other accident to other unpowered watercraft**
    - Drowning and submersion due to other accident to surf-board
    - Drowning and submersion due to other accident to windsurfer
  - X+7th **V90.89 Drowning and submersion due to other accident to unspecified watercraft**
    - Drowning and submersion due to other accident to boat NOS
    - Drowning and submersion due to other accident to ship NOS
    - Drowning and submersion due to other accident to watercraft NOS

V91 Other injury due to accident to watercraft

Includes: any injury except drowning and submersion as a result of ar accident to watercraft

Excludes1: *civilian water transport accident involving military watercraft (V94.81-)*
military watercraft accident in military or war operations (Y36, Y37.-)

Excludes2: *drowning and submersion due to accident to watercraft (V90.-)*

The appropriate 7th character is to be added to each code from category V91
A initial encounter
D subsequent encounter
S sequela

+ **V91.0 Burn due to watercraft on fire**
  - ***Excludes1:*** *burn from localized fire or explosion on board shi without accident to watercraft (V93.-)*
  - X+7th **V91.00 Burn due to merchant ship on fire**
  - X+7th **V91.01 Burn due to passenger ship on fire**
    - Burn due to Ferry-boat on fire
    - Burn due to Liner on fire
  - X+7th **V91.02 Burn due to fishing boat on fire**
  - X+7th **V91.03 Burn due to other powered watercraft on fire**
    - Burn due to Hovercraft (on open water) on fire
    - Burn due to Jet ski on fire
  - X+7th **V91.04 Burn due to sailboat on fire**
  - X+7th **V91.05 Burn due to canoe or kayak on fire**
  - X+7th **V91.06 Burn due to (nonpowered) inflatable craft on fire**
  - X+7th **V91.07 Burn due to water-skis on fire**
  - X+7th **V91.08 Burn due to other unpowered watercraft on fire**
  - X+7th **V91.09 Burn due to unspecified watercraft on fire**
    - Burn due to boat NOS on fire
    - Burn due to ship NOS on fire
    - Burn due to watercraft NOS on fire

+ **V91.1 Crushed between watercraft and other watercraft or other object due to collision**

Crushed by lifeboat after abandoning ship in a collision

NOTE Select the specified type of watercraft that the victim was on at the time of the collision

X+7th **V91.10 Crushed between merchant ship and other watercraft or other object due to collision**

X+7th **V91.11 Crushed between passenger ship and other watercraft or other object due to collision**

Crushed between Ferry-boat and other watercraft or other object due to collision

Crushed between Liner and other watercraft or other object due to collision

X+7th **V91.12 Crushed between fishing boat and other watercraft or other object due to collision**

X+7th **V91.13 Crushed between other powered watercraft and other watercraft or other object due to collision**

Crushed between Hovercraft (on open water) and other watercraft or other object due to collision

Crushed between Jet ski and other watercraft or other object due to collision

X+7th **V91.14 Crushed between sailboat and other watercraft or other object due to collision**

X+7th **V91.15 Crushed between canoe or kayak and other watercraft or other object due to collision**

X+7th **V91.16 Crushed between (nonpowered) inflatable craft and other watercraft or other object due to collision**

X+7th **V91.18 Crushed between other unpowered watercraft and other watercraft or other object due to collision**

Crushed between surfboard and other watercraft or other object due to collision

Crushed between windsurfer and other watercraft or other object due to collision

X+7th **V91.19 Crushed between unspecified watercraft and other watercraft or other object due to collision**

Crushed between boat NOS and other watercraft or other object due to collision

Crushed between ship NOS and other watercraft or other object due to collision

Crushed between watercraft NOS and other watercraft or other object due to collision

+ **V91.2 Fall due to collision between watercraft and other watercraft or other object**

Fall while remaining on watercraft after collision

NOTE Select the specified type of watercraft that the victim was on at the time of the collision

Excludes1: *crushed between watercraft and other watercraft and other object due to collision (V91.1-)*
drowning and submersion due to falling from crushed watercraft (V90.3-)

X+7th **V91.20 Fall due to collision between merchant ship and other watercraft or other object**

X+7th **V91.21 Fall due to collision between passenger ship and other watercraft or other object**

Fall due to collision between Ferry-boat and other watercraft or other object

Fall due to collision between Liner and other watercraft or other object

X+7th **V91.22 Fall due to collision between fishing boat and other watercraft or other object**

X+7th **V91.23 Fall due to collision between other powered watercraft and other watercraft or other object**

Fall due to collision between Hovercraft (on open water) and other watercraft or other object

Fall due to collision between Jet ski and other watercraft or other object

X+7th **V91.24 Fall due to collision between sailboat and other watercraft or other object**

X+7th **V91.25 Fall due to collision between canoe or kayak and other watercraft or other object**

X+7th **V91.26 Fall due to collision between (nonpowered) inflatable craft and other watercraft or other object**

X+7th **V91.29 Fall due to collision between unspecified watercraft and other watercraft or other object**

Fall due to collision between boat NOS and other watercraft or other object

Fall due to collision between ship NOS and other watercraft or other object

Fall due to collision between watercraft NOS and other watercraft or other object

+ **V91.3 Hit or struck by falling object due to accident to watercraft**

Hit or struck by falling object (part of damaged watercraft or other object) after falling or jumping from damaged watercraft

Excludes2: *drowning or submersion due to fall or jumping from damaged watercraft (V90.2-, V90.3-)*

X+7th **V91.30 Hit or struck by falling object due to accident to merchant ship**

X+7th **V91.31 Hit or struck by falling object due to accident to passenger ship**

Hit or struck by falling object due to accident to Ferry-boat

Hit or struck by falling object due to accident to Liner

X+7th **V91.32 Hit or struck by falling object due to accident to fishing boat**

X+7th **V91.33 Hit or struck by falling object due to accident to other powered watercraft**

Hit or struck by falling object due to accident to Hovercraft (on open water)

Hit or struck by falling object due to accident to Jet ski

X+7th **V91.34 Hit or struck by falling object due to accident to sailboat**

X+7th **V91.35 Hit or struck by falling object due to accident to canoe or kayak**

X+7th **V91.36 Hit or struck by falling object due to accident to (nonpowered) inflatable craft**

X+7th **V91.37 Hit or struck by falling object due to accident to water-skis**

Hit by water-skis after jumping off of waterskis

X+7th **V91.38 Hit or struck by falling object due to accident to other unpowered watercraft**

Hit or struck by surf-board after falling off damaged surf-board

Hit or struck by object after falling off damaged windsurfer

X+7th **V91.39 Hit or struck by falling object due to accident to unspecified watercraft**

Hit or struck by falling object due to accident to boat NOS

Hit or struck by falling object due to accident to ship NOS

Hit or struck by falling object due to accident to watercraft NOS

+ **V91.8 Other injury due to other accident to watercraft**

X+7th **V91.80 Other injury due to other accident to merchant ship**

X+7th **V91.81 Other injury due to other accident to passenger ship**

Other injury due to other accident to Ferry-boat

Other injury due to other accident to Liner

X+7th **V91.82 Other injury due to other accident to fishing boat**

X+7th **V91.83 Other injury due to other accident to other powered watercraft**

Other injury due to other accident to Hovercraft (on open water)

Other injury due to other accident to Jet ski

X+7th **V91.84 Other injury due to other accident to sailboat**

X+7th **V91.85 Other injury due to other accident to canoe or kayak**

X+7th **V91.86 Other injury due to other accident to (nonpowered) inflatable craft**

X+7th **V91.87 Other injury due to other accident to water-skis**

X+7th **V91.88 Other injury due to other accident to other unpowered watercraft**

Other injury due to other accident to surf-board

Other injury due to other accident to windsurfer

X+7th **V91.89 Other injury due to other accident to unspecified watercraft**

Other injury due to other accident to boat NOS

Other injury due to other accident to ship NOS

Other injury due to other accident to watercraft NOS

V92 Drowning and submersion due to accident on board watercraft, without accident to watercraft

Excludes1: *civilian water transport accident involving military watercraft (V94.81-)*
drowning or submersion due to accident to watercraft (V90-V91)
drowning or submersion of diver who voluntarily jumps from boat not involved in an accident (W16.711, W16.721)
fall into water without watercraft (W16.-)
military watercraft accident in military or war operations (Y36, Y37)

The appropriate 7th character is to be added to each code from category V92
A initial encounter
D subsequent encounter
S sequela

+ **V92.0 Drowning and submersion due to fall off watercraft**
Drowning and submersion due to fall from gangplank of watercraft
Drowning and submersion due to fall overboard watercraft
Excludes2: *hitting head on object or bottom of body of water due to fall from watercraft (V94.0-)*

X+7th **V92.00 Drowning and submersion due to fall off merchant ship**

X+7th **V92.01 Drowning and submersion due to fall off passenger ship**
Drowning and submersion due to fall off Ferry-boat
Drowning and submersion due to fall off Liner

X+7th **V92.02 Drowning and submersion due to fall off fishing boat**

X+7th **V92.03 Drowning and submersion due to fall off other powered watercraft**
Drowning and submersion due to fall off Hovercraft (on open water)
Drowning and submersion due to fall off Jet ski

X+7th **V92.04 Drowning and submersion due to fall off sailboat**

X+7th **V92.05 Drowning and submersion due to fall off canoe or kayak**

X+7th **V92.06 Drowning and submersion due to fall off (nonpowered) inflatable craft**

X+7th **V92.07 Drowning and submersion due to fall off water-skis**
Excludes1: *drowning and submersion due to falling off burning water-skis (V90.27)*
drowning and submersion due to falling off crushed water-skis (V90.37)
hit by boat while water-skiing NOS (V94.X)

X+7th **V92.08 Drowning and submersion due to fall off other unpowered watercraft**
Drowning and submersion due to fall off surf-board
Drowning and submersion due to fall off windsurfer
Excludes1: *drowning and submersion due to fall off burningunpoweredwatercraft(V90.28)*
drowning and submersion due to fall off crushedunpoweredwatercraft(V90.38)
drowning and submersion due to fall off damaged unpowered watercraft (V90.88)
drowning and submersion due to rider of nonpowered watercraft being hit by other watercraft (V94.-)
other injury due to rider of nonpowered watercraftbeinghitbyotherwatercraft (V94.-)

X+7th **V92.09 Drowning and submersion due to fall off unspecified watercraft**
Drowning and submersion due to fall off boat NOS
Drowning and submersion due to fall off ship
Drowning and submersion due to fall off watercraft NOS

+ **V92.1 Drowning and submersion due to being thrown overboard by motion of watercraft**
Excludes1: *drowning and submersion due to fall off surf-board (V92.08)*
drowning and submersion due to fall off water-skis (V92.07)
drowning and submersion due to fall off windsurfer (V92.08)

X+7th **V92.10 Drowning and submersion due to being thrown overboard by motion of merchant ship**

X+7th **V92.11 Drowning and submersion due to being thrown overboard by motion of passenger ship**
Drowning and submersion due to being thrown overboard by motion of Ferry-boat
Drowning and submersion due to being thrown overboard by motion of Liner

X+7th **V92.12 Drowning and submersion due to being thrown overboard by motion of fishing boat**

X+7th **V92.13 Drowning and submersion due to being thrown overboard by motion of other powered watercraft**
Drowning and submersion due to being thrown overboard by motion of Hovercraft

X+7th **V92.14 Drowning and submersion due to being thrown overboard by motion of sailboat**

X+7th **V92.15 Drowning and submersion due to being thrown overboard by motion of canoe or kayak**

X+7th **V92.16 Drowning and submersion due to being thrown overboard by motion of (nonpowered) inflatable craft**

X+7th **V92.19 Drowning and submersion due to being thrown overboard by motion of unspecified watercraft**
Drowning and submersion due to being thrown overboard by motion of boat NOS
Drowning and submersion due to being thrown overboard by motion of ship NOS
Drowning and submersion due to being thrown overboard by motion of watercraft NOS

+ **V92.2 Drowning and submersion due to being washed overboard from watercraft**
Code first any associated cataclysm (X37.0-)

X+7th **V92.20 Drowning and submersion due to being washed overboard from merchant ship**

X+7th **V92.21 Drowning and submersion due to being washed overboard from passenger ship**
Drowning and submersion due to being washed overboard from Ferry-boat
Drowning and submersion due to being washed overboard from Liner

X+7th **V92.22 Drowning and submersion due to being washed overboard from fishing boat**

X+7th **V92.23 Drowning and submersion due to being washed overboard from other powered watercraft**
Drowning and submersion due to being washed overboard from Hovercraft (on open water)
Drowning and submersion due to being washed overboard from Jet ski

X+7th **V92.24 Drowning and submersion due to being washed overboard from sailboat**

X+7th **V92.25 Drowning and submersion due to being washed overboard from canoe or kayak**

X+7th **V92.26 Drowning and submersion due to being washed overboard from (nonpowered) inflatable craft**

X+7th **V92.27 Drowning and submersion due to being washed overboard from water-skis**
Excludes1: *drowning and submersion due to fall off water-skis (V92.07)*

X+7th **V92.28 Drowning and submersion due to being washed overboard from other unpowered watercraft**
Drowning and submersion due to being washed overboard from surf-board
Drowning and submersion due to being washed overboard from windsurfer

X+7th **V92.29 Drowning and submersion due to being washed overboard from unspecified watercraft**
Drowning and submersion due to being washed overboard from boat NOS
Drowning and submersion due to being washed overboard from ship NOS
Drowning and submersion due to being washed overboard from watercraft NOS

V93 Other injury due to accident on board watercraft, without accident to watercraft

Excludes1: *civilian water transport accident involving military watercraft (V94.81-)*
other injury due to accident to watercraft (V91.-)
military watercraft accident in military or war operations (Y36, Y37.-)

Excludes2: *drowning and submersion due to accident on board watercraft, without accident to watercraft (V92.-)*

The appropriate 7th character is to be added to each code from category V93
A initial encounter
D subsequent encounter
S sequela

\+ **V93.0 Burn due to localized fire on board watercraft**
Excludes1: *burn due to watercraft on fire (V91.0-)*
X+7th **V93.00 Burn due to localized fire on board merchant vessel**
X+7th **V93.01 Burn due to localized fire on board passenger vessel**
Burn due to localized fire on board Ferry-boat
Burn due to localized fire on board Liner
X+7th **V93.02 Burn due to localized fire on board fishing boat**
X+7th **V93.03 Burn due to localized fire on board other powered watercraft**
Burn due to localized fire on board Hovercraft
Burn due to localized fire on board Jet ski
X+7th **V93.04 Burn due to localized fire on board sailboat**
X+7th **V93.09 Burn due to localized fire on board unspecified watercraft**
Burn due to localized fire on board boat NOS
Burn due to localized fire on board ship NOS
Burn due to localized fire on board watercraft NOS

\+ **V93.1 Other burn on board watercraft**
Burn due to source other than fire on board watercraft
Excludes1: *burn due to watercraft on fire (V91.0-)*
X+7th **V93.10 Other burn on board merchant vessel**
X+7th **V93.11 Other burn on board passenger vessel**
Other burn on board Ferry-boat
Other burn on board Liner
X+7th **V93.12 Other burn on board fishing boat**
X+7th **V93.13 Other burn on board other powered watercraft**
Other burn on board Hovercraft
Other burn on board Jet ski
X+7th **V93.14 Other burn on board sailboat**
X+7th **V93.19 Other burn on board unspecified watercraft**
Other burn on board boat NOS
Other burn on board ship NOS
Other burn on board watercraft NOS

\+ **V93.2 Heat exposure on board watercraft**
Excludes1: *exposure to man-made heat not aboard watercraft (W92)*
exposure to natural heat while on board watercraft (X30)
exposure to sunlight while on board watercraft (X32)
Excludes2: *burn due to fire on board watercraft (V93.0-)*
X+7th **V93.20 Heat exposure on board merchant ship**
X+7th **V93.21 Heat exposure on board passenger ship**
Heat exposure on board Ferry-boat
Heat exposure on board Liner
X+7th **V93.22 Heat exposure on board fishing boat**
X+7th **V93.23 Heat exposure on board other powered watercraft**
Heat exposure on board hovercraft
X+7th **V93.24 Heat exposure on board sailboat**
X+7th **V93.29 Heat exposure on board unspecified watercraft**
Heat exposure on board boat NOS
Heat exposure on board ship NOS
Heat exposure on board watercraft NOS

\+ **V93.3 Fall on board watercraft**
Excludes1: *fall due to collision of watercraft (V91.2-)*
X+7th **V93.30 Fall on board merchant ship**
X+7th **V93.31 Fall on board passenger ship**
Fall on board Ferry-boat
Fall on board Liner
X+7th **V93.32 Fall on board fishing boat**
X+7th **V93.33 Fall on board other powered watercraft**
Fall on board Hovercraft (on open water)
Fall on board Jet ski
X+7th **V93.34 Fall on board sailboat**
X+7th **V93.35 Fall on board canoe or kayak**
X+7th **V93.36 Fall on board (nonpowered) inflatable craft**
X+7th **V93.38 Fall on board other unpowered watercraft**
X+7th **V93.39 Fall on board unspecified watercraft**
Fall on board boat NOS
Fall on board ship NOS
Fall on board watercraft NOS

\+ **V93.4 Struck by falling object on board watercraft**
Hit by falling object on board watercraft
Excludes1: *struck by falling object due to accident to watercraft (V91.3)*
X+7th **V93.40 Struck by falling object on merchant ship**
X+7th **V93.41 Struck by falling object on passenger ship**
Struck by falling object on Ferry-boat
Struck by falling object on Liner
X+7th **V93.42 Struck by falling object on fishing boat**
X+7th **V93.43 Struck by falling object on other powered watercraft**
Struck by falling object on Hovercraft
X+7th **V93.44 Struck by falling object on sailboat**
X+7th **V93.48 Struck by falling object on other unpowered watercraft**
X+7th **V93.49 Struck by falling object on unspecified watercraft**

\+ **V93.5 Explosion on board watercraft**
Boiler explosion on steamship
Excludes2: *fire on board watercraft (V93.0-)*
X+7th **V93.50 Explosion on board merchant ship**
X+7th **V93.51 Explosion on board passenger ship**
Explosion on board Ferry-boat
Explosion on board Liner
X+7th **V93.52 Explosion on board fishing boat**
X+7th **V93.53 Explosion on board other powered watercraft**
Explosion on board Hovercraft
Explosion on board Jet ski
X+7th **V93.54 Explosion on board sailboat**
X+7th **V93.59 Explosion on board unspecified watercraft**
Explosion on board boat NOS
Explosion on board ship NOS
Explosion on board watercraft NOS

\+ **V93.6 Machinery accident on board watercraft**
Excludes1: *machinery explosion on board watercraft (V93.4-)*
machinery fire on board watercraft (V93.0-)
X+7th **V93.60 Machinery accident on board merchant ship**
X+7th **V93.61 Machinery accident on board passenger ship**
Machinery accident on board Ferry-boat
Machinery accident on board Liner
X+7th **V93.62 Machinery accident on board fishing boat**
X+7th **V93.63 Machinery accident on board other powered watercraft**
Machinery accident on board Hovercraft
X+7th **V93.64 Machinery accident on board sailboat**
X+7th **V93.69 Machinery accident on board unspecified watercraft**
Machinery accident on board boat NOS
Machinery accident on board ship NOS
Machinery accident on board watercraft NOS

\+ **V93.8 Other injury due to other accident on board watercraft**
Accidental poisoning by gases or fumes on watercraft
X+7th **V93.80 Other injury due to other accident on board merchant ship**
X+7th **V93.81 Other injury due to other accident on board passenger ship**
Other injury due to other accident on board Ferry-boat
Other injury due to other accident on board Liner
X+7th **V93.82 Other injury due to other accident on board fishing boat**
X+7th **V93.83 Other injury due to other accident on board other powered watercraft**
Other injury due to other accident on board Hovercraft
Other injury due to other accident on board Jet ski
X+7th **V93.84 Other injury due to other accident on board sailboat**
X+7th **V93.85 Other injury due to other accident on board canoe or kayak**
X+7th **V93.86 Other injury due to other accident on board (nonpowered) inflatable craft**
X+7th **V93.87 Other injury due to other accident on board water-skis**
Hit or struck by object while waterskiing
X+7th **V93.88 Other injury due to other accident on board other unpowered watercraft**
Hit or struck by object while surfing
Hit or struck by object while on board windsurfer

X+7th **V93.89 Other injury due to other accident on board unspecified watercraft**
Other injury due to other accident on board boat NOS
Other injury due to other accident on board ship NOS
Other injury due to other accident on board watercraft NOS

V94 Other and unspecified water transport accidents

Excludes1: *military watercraft accidents in military or war operations (Y36, Y37)*

The appropriate 7th character is to be added to each code from category V94
A initial encounter
D subsequent encounter
S sequela

X+7th **V94.0 Hitting object or bottom of body of water due to fall from watercraft**
Excludes2: *drowning and submersion due to fall from watercraft (V92.0-)*

+ **V94.1 Bather struck by watercraft**
Swimmer hit by watercraft
X+7th **V94.11 Bather struck by powered watercraft**
X+7th **V94.12 Bather struck by nonpowered watercraft**

+ **V94.2 Rider of nonpowered watercraft struck by other watercraft**
X+7th **V94.21 Rider of nonpowered watercraft struck by other nonpowered watercraft**
Canoer hit by other nonpowered watercraft
Surfer hit by other nonpowered watercraft
Windsurfer hit by other nonpowered watercraft
X+7th **V94.22 Rider of nonpowered watercraft struck by powered watercraft**
Canoer hit by motorboat
Surfer hit by motorboat
Windsurfer hit by motorboat

+ **V94.3 Injury to rider of (inflatable) watercraft being pulled behind other watercraft**
X+7th **V94.31 Injury to rider of (inflatable) recreational watercraft being pulled behind other watercraft**
Injury to rider of inner-tube pulled behind motor boat
X+7th **V94.32 Injury to rider of non-recreational watercraft being pulled behind other watercraft**
Injury to occupant of dingy being pulled behind boat or ship
Injury to occupant of life-raft being pulled behind boat or ship

X+7th **V94.4 Injury to barefoot water-skier**
Injury to person being pulled behind boat or ship

+ **V94.8 Other water transport accident**
+ **V94.81 Water transport accident involving military watercraft**
+7th **V94.810 Civilian watercraft involved in water transport accident with military watercraft**
Passenger on civilian watercraft injured due to accident with military watercraft
+7th **V94.811 Civilian in water injured by military watercraft**
+7th **V94.818 Other water transport accident involving military watercraft**
X+7th **V94.89 Other water transport accident**

X+7th **V94.9 Unspecified water transport accident**
Water transport accident NOS

Air and space transport accidents (V95-V97)

Excludes1: *military aircraft accidents in military or war operations (Y36, Y37.-)*

V95 Accident to powered aircraft causing injury to occupant

The appropriate 7th character is to be added to each code from category V95
A initial encounter
D subsequent encounter
S sequela

+ **V95.0 Helicopter accident injuring occupant**
X+7th **V95.00 Unspecified helicopter accident injuring occupant**
X+7th **V95.01 Helicopter crash injuring occupant**
X+7th **V95.02 Forced landing of helicopter injuring occupant**
X+7th **V95.03 Helicopter collision injuring occupant**
Helicopter collision with any object, fixed, movable or moving
X+7th **V95.04 Helicopter fire injuring occupant**
X+7th **V95.05 Helicopter explosion injuring occupant**
X+7th **V95.09 Other helicopter accident injuring occupant**

+ **V95.1 Ultralight, microlight or powered-glider accident injuring occupant**
X+7th **V95.10 Unspecified ultralight, microlight or powered-glide accident injuring occupant**
X+7th **V95.11 Ultralight, microlight or powered-glider crash injuring occupant**
X+7th **V95.12 Forced landing of ultralight, microlight or powered glider injuring occupant**
X+7th **V95.13 Ultralight, microlight or powered-glider collision injuring occupant**
Ultralight, microlight or powered-glider collision wi any object, fixed, movable or moving
X+7th **V95.14 Ultralight, microlight or powered-glider fire injuri occupant**
X+7th **V95.15 Ultralight, microlight or powered-glider explosion injuring occupant**
X+7th **V95.19 Other ultralight, microlight or powered-glider accident injuring occupant**

+ **V95.2 Other private fixed-wing aircraft accident injuring occupant**
X+7th **V95.20 Unspecified accident to other private fixed-wing aircraft, injuring occupant**
X+7th **V95.21 Other private fixed-wing aircraft crash injuring occupant**
X+7th **V95.22 Forced landing of other private fixed-wing aircraft injuring occupant**
X+7th **V95.23 Other private fixed-wing aircraft collision injuring occupant**
Other private fixed-wing aircraft collision with any object, fixed, movable or moving
X+7th **V95.24 Other private fixed-wing aircraft fire injuring occupant**
X+7th **V95.25 Other private fixed-wing aircraft explosion injurin occupant**
X+7th **V95.29 Other accident to other private fixed-wing aircraft injuring occupant**

+ **V95.3 Commercial fixed-wing aircraft accident injuring occupant**
X+7th **V95.30 Unspecified accident to commercial fixed-wing aircraft injuring occupant**
X+7th **V95.31 Commercial fixed-wing aircraft crash injuring occupant**
X+7th **V95.32 Forced landing of commercial fixed-wing aircraft injuring occupant**
X+7th **V95.33 Commercial fixed-wing aircraft collision injuring occupant**
Commercial fixed-wing aircraft collision with any object, fixed, movable or moving
X+7th **V95.34 Commercial fixed-wing aircraft fire injuring occupant**
X+7th **V95.35 Commercial fixed-wing aircraft explosion injuring occupant**
X+7th **V95.39 Other accident to commercial fixed-wing aircraft injuring occupant**

+ **V95.4 Spacecraft accident injuring occupant**
X+7th **V95.40 Unspecified spacecraft accident injuring occupant**
X+7th **V95.41 Spacecraft crash injuring occupant**
X+7th **V95.42 Forced landing of spacecraft injuring occupant**
X+7th **V95.43 Spacecraft collision injuring occupant**
Spacecraft collision with any object, fixed, moveable or moving
X+7th **V95.44 Spacecraft fire injuring occupant**
X+7th **V95.45 Spacecraft explosion injuring occupant**
X+7th **V95.49 Other spacecraft accident injuring occupant**

X+7th **V95.8 Other powered aircraft accidents injuring occupant**

X+7th **V95.9 Unspecified aircraft accident injuring occupant**
Aircraft accident NOS
Air transport accident NOS

V96 Accident to nonpowered aircraft causing injury to occupant

The appropriate 7th character is to be added to each code from catego V96
A initial encounter
D subsequent encounter
S sequela

+ **V96.0 Balloon accident injuring occupant**
X+7th **V96.00 Unspecified balloon accident injuring occupant**
X+7th **V96.01 Balloon crash injuring occupant**
X+7th **V96.02 Forced landing of balloon injuring occupant**
X+7th **V96.03 Balloon collision injuring occupant**
Balloon collision with any object, fixed, moveable o moving

X+7th **V96.04 Balloon fire injuring occupant**
X+7th **V96.05 Balloon explosion injuring occupant**
X+7th **V96.09 Other balloon accident injuring occupant**
\+ **V96.1 Hang-glider accident injuring occupant**
X+7th **V96.10 Unspecified hang-glider accident injuring occupant**
X+7th **V96.11 Hang-glider crash injuring occupant**
X+7th **V96.12 Forced landing of hang-glider injuring occupant**
X+7th **V96.13 Hang-glider collision injuring occupant**
Hang-glider collision with any object, fixed, moveable or moving
X+7th **V96.14 Hang-glider fire injuring occupant**
X+7th **V96.15 Hang-glider explosion injuring occupant**
X+7th **V96.19 Other hang-glider accident injuring occupant**
\+ **V96.2 Glider (nonpowered) accident injuring occupant**
X+7th **V96.20 Unspecified glider (nonpowered) accident injuring occupant**
X+7th **V96.21 Glider (nonpowered) crash injuring occupant**
X+7th **V96.22 Forced landing of glider (nonpowered) injuring occupant**
X+7th **V96.23 Glider (nonpowered) collision injuring occupant**
Glider (nonpowered) collision with any object, fixed, moveable or moving
X+7th **V96.24 Glider (nonpowered) fire injuring occupant**
V96.25 Glider (nonpowered) explosion injuring occupant
X+7th **V96.29 Other glider (nonpowered) accident injuring occupant**
X+7th **V96.8 Other nonpowered-aircraft accidents injuring occupant**
Kite carrying a person accident injuring occupant
X+7th **V96.9 Unspecified nonpowered-aircraft accident injuring occupant**
Nonpowered-aircraft accident NOS

V97 Other specified air transport accidents

The appropriate 7th character is to be added to each code from category V97
A initial encounter
D subsequent encounter
S sequela

X+7th **V97.0 Occupant of aircraft injured in other specified air transport accidents**
Fall in, on or from aircraft in air transport accident
Excludes1: *accident while boarding or alighting aircraft (V97.1)*
X+7th **V97.1 Person injured while boarding or alighting from aircraft**
\+ **V97.2 Parachutist accident**
X+7th **V97.21 Parachutist entangled in object**
Parachutist landing in tree
X+7th **V97.22 Parachutist injured on landing**
X+7th **V97.29 Other parachutist accident**
\+ **V97.3 Person on ground injured in air transport accident**
X+7th **V97.31 Hit by object falling from aircraft**
Hit by crashing aircraft
Injured by aircraft hitting house
Injured by aircraft hitting car
X+7th **V97.32 Injured by rotating propeller**
X+7th **V97.33 Sucked into jet engine**
X+7th **V97.39 Other injury to person on ground due to air transport accident**
\+ **V97.8 Other air transport accidents, not elsewhere classified**
Excludes1: *aircraft accident NOS (V95.9)*
exposure to changes in air pressure during ascent or descent (W94.-)
\+ **V97.81 Air transport accident involving military aircraft**
+7th **V97.810 Civilian aircraft involved in air transport accident with military aircraft**
Passenger in civilian aircraft injured due to accident with military aircraft
+7th **V97.811 Civilian injured by military aircraft**
+7th **V97.818 Other air transport accident involving military aircraft**
X+7th **V97.89 Other air transport accidents, not elsewhere classified**
Injury from machinery on aircraft

Other and unspecified transport accidents (V98-V99)

Excludes1: *vehicle accident, type of vehicle unspecified (V89.-)*

V98 Other specified transport accidents

The appropriate 7th character is to be added to each code from category V98
A initial encounter
D subsequent encounter
S sequela

X+7th **V98.0 Accident to, on or involving cable-car, not on rails**
Caught or dragged by cable-car, not on rails
Fall or jump from cable-car, not on rails
Object thrown from or in cable-car, not on rails
X+7th **V98.1 Accident to, on or involving land-yacht**
X+7th **V98.2 Accident to, on or involving ice yacht**
X+7th **V98.3 Accident to, on or involving ski lift**
Accident to, on or involving ski chair-lift
Accident to, on or involving ski-lift with gondola
X+7th **V98.8 Other specified transport accidents**

V99 Unspecified transport accident
X+7th
The appropriate 7th character is to be added to code V99
A initial encounter
D subsequent encounter
S sequela

Other external causes of accidental injury (W00-X58)

Slipping, tripping, stumbling and falls (W00-W19)

Excludes1: *assault involving a fall (Y01-Y02)*
fall from animal (V80.-)
fall (in) (from) machinery (in operation) (W28-W31)
fall (in) (from) transport vehicle (V01-V99)
intentional self-harm involving a fall (X80-X81)

Excludes2: *at risk for fall (history of fall) (Z91.81)*
fall (in) (from) burning building (X00.-)
fall into fire (X00-X04, X08)

W00 Fall due to ice and snow

Includes: pedestrian on foot falling (slipping) on ice and snow
Excludes1: *fall on (from) ice and snow involving pedestrian conveyance (V00.-)*
fall from stairs and steps not due to ice and snow (W10.-)

The appropriate 7th character is to be added to each code from category W00
A initial encounter
D subsequent encounter
S sequela

X+7th **W00.0 Fall on same level due to ice and snow**
AHA CC: 2Q, 2016, 4-5
X+7th **W00.1 Fall from stairs and steps due to ice and snow**
X+7th **W00.2 Other fall from one level to another due to ice and snow**
X+7th **W00.9 Unspecified fall due to ice and snow**

W01 Fall on same level from slipping, tripping and stumbling

Includes: fall on moving sidewalk
Excludes1: *fall due to bumping (striking) against object (W18.0-)*
fall in shower or bathtub (W18.2-)
fall on same level NOS (W18.30)
fall on same level from slipping, tripping and stumbling due to ice or snow (W00.0)
fall off or from toilet (W18.1-)
slipping, tripping and stumbling NOS (W18.40)
slipping, tripping and stumbling without falling (W18.4-)

The appropriate 7th character is to be added to each code from category W01
A initial encounter
D subsequent encounter
S sequela

X+7th **W01.0 Fall on same level from slipping, tripping and stumbling without subsequent striking against object**
Falling over animal
\+ **W01.1 Fall on same level from slipping, tripping and stumbling with subsequent striking against object**
X+7th **W01.10 Fall on same level from slipping, tripping and stumbling with subsequent striking against unspecified object**

+ **W01.11 Fall on same level from slipping, tripping and stumbling with subsequent striking against sharp object**

+7th **W01.110 Fall on same level from slipping, tripping and stumbling with subsequent striking against sharp glass**

+7th **W01.111 Fall on same level from slipping, tripping and stumbling with subsequent striking against power tool or machine**

+7th **W01.118 Fall on same level from slipping, tripping and stumbling with subsequent striking against other sharp object**

+7th **W01.119 Fall on same level from slipping, tripping and stumbling with subsequent striking against unspecified sharp object**

+ **W01.19 Fall on same level from slipping, tripping and stumbling with subsequent striking against other object**

+7th **W01.190 Fall on same level from slipping, tripping and stumbling with subsequent striking against furniture**

+7th **W01.198 Fall on same level from slipping, tripping and stumbling with subsequent striking against other object**

W03 Other fall on same level due to collision with another person
X+7th

Fall due to non-transport collision with other person

Excludes1: *collision with another person without fall (W51)*
crushed or pushed by a crowd or human stampede (W52)
fall involving pedestrian conveyance (V00-V09)
fall due to ice or snow (W00)
fall on same level NOS (W18.30)

AHA CC: 4Q, 2012, 108; 1Q, 2015, 3-21

The appropriate 7th character is to be added to code W03
A initial encounter
D subsequent encounter
S sequela

W04 Fall while being carried or supported by other persons
X+7th

Accidentally dropped while being carried

The appropriate 7th character is to be added to code W04
A initial encounter
D subsequent encounter
S sequela

W05 Fall from non-movitng wheelchair, nonmotorized scooter and motorized mobility scooter

Excludes1: *fall from moving wheelchair (powered) (V00.811)*
fall from moving motorized mobility scooter (V00.831)
fall from nonmotorized scooter (V00.141)

The appropriate 7th character is to be added to each code from category W05
A initial encounter
D subsequent encounter
S sequela

X+7th **W05.0 Fall from non-moving wheelchair**
X+7th **W05.1 Fall from non-moving nonmotorized scooter**
X+7th **W05.2 Fall from non-moving motorized mobility scooter**

W06 Fall from bed
X+7th

The appropriate 7th character is to be added to code W06
A initial encounter
D subsequent encounter
S sequela

W07 Fall from chair
X+7th

The appropriate 7th character is to be added to code W07
A initial encounter
D subsequent encounter
S sequela

W08 Fall from other furniture
X+7th

The appropriate 7th character is to be added to code W08
A initial encounter
D subsequent encounter
S sequela

W09 Fall on and from playground equipment

Excludes1: *fall involving recreational machinery (W31)*

The appropriate 7th character is to be added to each code from category W09
A initial encounter
D subsequent encounter
S sequela

X+7th **W09.0 Fall on or from playground slide**
X+7th **W09.1 Fall from playground swing**
X+7th **W09.2 Fall on or from jungle gym**
X+7th **W09.8 Fall on or from other playground equipment**

W10 Fall on and from stairs and steps

Excludes1: *Fall from stairs and steps due to ice and snow (W00.1)*

The appropriate 7th character is to be added to each code from category W10
A initial encounter
D subsequent encounter
S sequela

X+7th **W10.0 Fall (on)(from) escalator**
X+7th **W10.1 Fall (on)(from) sidewalk curb**
X+7th **W10.2 Fall (on)(from) incline**
Fall (on) (from) ramp
X+7th **W10.8 Fall (on) (from) other stairs and steps**
X+7th **W10.9 Fall (on) (from) unspecified stairs and steps**

W11 Fall on and from ladder
X+7th

The appropriate 7th character is to be added to code W11
A initial encounter
D subsequent encounter
S sequela

W12 Fall on and from scaffolding
X+7th

The appropriate 7th character is to be added to code W12
A initial encounter
D subsequent encounter
S sequela

W13 Fall from, out of or through building or structure

The appropriate 7th character is to be added to each code from category W13
A initial encounter
D subsequent encounter
S sequela

X+7th **W13.0 Fall from, out of or through balcony**
Fall from, out of or through railing
X+7th **W13.1 Fall from, out of or through bridge**
X+7th **W13.2 Fall from, out of or through roof**
X+7th **W13.3 Fall through floor**
X+7th **W13.4 Fall from, out of or through window**
Excludes2: *fall with subsequent striking against sharp glass (W01.110)*
X+7th **W13.8 Fall from, out of or through other building or structure**
Fall from, out of or through viaduct
Fall from, out of or through wall
Fall from, out of or through flag-pole
X+7th **W13.9 Fall from, out of or through building, not otherwise specified**
Excludes1: *collapse of a building or structure (W20.-)*
fall or jump from burning building or structure (X00.-)

W14 Fall from tree
X+7th

The appropriate 7th character is to be added to code W14
A initial encounter
D subsequent encounter
S sequela

W15 Fall from cliff
X+7th

The appropriate 7th character is to be added to code W15
A initial encounter
D subsequent encounter
S sequela

W16 Fall, jump or diving into water

Excludes1: *accidental non-watercraft drowning and submersion not involving fall (W65-W74)*
effects of air pressure from diving (W94.-)
fall into water from watercraft (V90-V94)
hitting an object or against bottom when falling from watercraft (V94.0)

Excludes2: *striking or hitting diving board (W21.4)*

The appropriate 7th character is to be added to each code from category W16
A initial encounter
D subsequent encounter
S sequela

\+ **W16.0 Fall into swimming pool**
Fall into swimming pool NOS
Excludes1: *fall into empty swimming pool (W17.3)*

\+ **W16.01 Fall into swimming pool striking water surface**

+7th **W16.011 Fall into swimming pool striking water surface causing drowning and submersion**
Excludes1: *drowning and submersion while inswimmingpoolwithoutfall (W67)*

+7th **W16.012 Fall into swimming pool striking water surface causing other injury**

\+ **W16.02 Fall into swimming pool striking bottom**

+7th **W16.021 Fall into swimming pool striking bottom causing drowning and submersion**
Excludes1: *drowning and submersion while inswimmingpoolwithoutfall (W67)*

+7th **W16.022 Fall into swimming pool striking bottom causing other injury**

\+ **W16.03 Fall into swimming pool striking wall**

+7th **W16.031 Fall into swimming pool striking wall causing drowning and submersion**
Excludes1: *drowning and submersion while inswimmingpoolwithoutfall (W67)*

+7th **W16.032 Fall into swimming pool striking wall causing other injury**

\+ **W16.1 Fall into natural body of water**
Fall into lake
Fall into open sea
Fall into river
Fall into stream

\+ **W16.11 Fall into natural body of water striking water surface**

+7th **W16.111 Fall into natural body of water striking water surface causing drowning and submersion**
Excludes1: *drowning and submersion while in natural body of water without fall (W69)*

+7th **W16.112 Fall into natural body of water striking water surface causing other injury**

\+ **W16.12 Fall into natural body of water striking bottom**

+7th **W16.121 Fall into natural body of water striking bottom causing drowning and submersion**
Excludes1: *drowning and submersion while in natural body of water without fall (W69)*

+7th **W16.122 Fall into natural body of water striking bottom causing other injury**

\+ **W16.13 Fall into natural body of water striking side**

+7th **W16.131 Fall into natural body of water striking side causing drowning and submersion**
Excludes1: *drowning and submersion while in natural body of water without fall (W69)*

+7th **W16.132 Fall into natural body of water striking side causing other injury**

\+ **W16.2 Fall in (into) filled bathtub or bucket of water**

\+ **W16.21 Fall in (into) filled bathtub**
Excludes1: *fall into empty bathtub (W18.2)*

+7th **W16.211 Fall in (into) filled bathtub causing drowning and submersion**
Excludes1: *drowning and submersion while in filled bathtub without fall (W65)*

+7th **W16.212 Fall in (into) filled bathtub causing other injury**

\+ **W16.22 Fall in (into) bucket of water**

+7th **W16.221 Fall in (into) bucket of water causing drowning and submersion**

+7th **W16.222 Fall in (into) bucket of water causing other injury**

\+ **W16.3 Fall into other water**
Fall into fountain
Fall into reservoir

\+ **W16.31 Fall into other water striking water surface**

+7th **W16.311 Fall into other water striking water surface causing drowning and submersion**
Excludes1: *drowning and submersion while in other water without fall (W73)*

+7th **W16.312 Fall into other water striking water surface causing other injury**

\+ **W16.32 Fall into other water striking bottom**

+7th **W16.321 Fall into other water striking bottom causing drowning and submersion**
Excludes1: *drowning and submersion while in other water without fall (W73)*

+7th **W16.322 Fall into other water striking bottom causing other injury**

\+ **W16.33 Fall into other water striking wall**

+7th **W16.331 Fall into other water striking wall causing drowning and submersion**
Excludes1: *drowning and submersion while in other water without fall (W73)*

+7th **W16.332 Fall into other water striking wall causing other injury**

\+ **W16.4 Fall into unspecified water**

X+7th **W16.41 Fall into unspecified water causing drowning and submersion**

X+7th **W16.42 Fall into unspecified water causing other injury**

\+ **W16.5 Jumping or diving into swimming pool**

\+ **W16.51 Jumping or diving into swimming pool striking water surface**

+7th **W16.511 Jumping or diving into swimming pool striking water surface causing drowning and submersion**
Excludes1: *drowning and submersion while in swimming pool without jumping or diving (W67)*

+7th **W16.512 Jumping or diving into swimming pool striking water surface causing other injury**

\+ **W16.52 Jumping or diving into swimming pool striking bottom**

+7th **W16.521 Jumping or diving into swimming pool striking bottom causing drowning and submersion**
Excludes1: *drowning and submersion while in swimming pool without jumping or diving (W67)*

+7th **W16.522 Jumping or diving into swimming pool striking bottom causing other injury**

\+ **W16.53 Jumping or diving into swimming pool striking wall**

+7th **W16.531 Jumping or diving into swimming pool striking wall causing drowning and submersion**
Excludes1: *drowning and submersion while in swimming pool without jumping or diving (W67)*

+7th **W16.532 Jumping or diving into swimming pool striking wall causing other injury**

\+ **W16.6 Jumping or diving into natural body of water**
Jumping or diving into lake
Jumping or diving into open sea
Jumping or diving into river
Jumping or diving into stream

\+ **W16.61 Jumping or diving into natural body of water striking water surface**

+7th **W16.611 Jumping or diving into natural body of water striking water surface causing drowning and submersion**
Excludes1: *drowning and submersion while in natural body of water without jumping or diving (W69)*

+7th **W16.612 Jumping or diving into natural body of water striking water surface causing other injury**

+ **W16.62 Jumping or diving into natural body of water striking bottom**

+7th **W16.621 Jumping or diving into natural body of water striking bottom causing drowning and submersion**

Excludes1: *drowning and submersion while in natural body of water without jumping or diving (W69)*

+7th **W16.622 Jumping or diving into natural body of water striking bottom causing other injury**

+ **W16.7 Jumping or diving from boat**

Excludes1: *Fall from boat into water -see watercraft accident (V90-V94)*

+ **W16.71 Jumping or diving from boat striking water surface**

+7th **W16.711 Jumping or diving from boat striking water surface causing drowning and submersion**

+7th **W16.712 Jumping or diving from boat striking water surface causing other injury**

+ **W16.72 Jumping or diving from boat striking bottom**

+7th **W16.721 Jumping or diving from boat striking bottom causing drowning and submersion**

+7th **W16.722 Jumping or diving from boat striking bottom causing other injury**

+ **W16.8 Jumping or diving into other water**

Jumping or diving into fountain
Jumping or diving into reservoir

+ **W16.81 Jumping or diving into other water striking water surface**

+7th **W16.811 Jumping or diving into other water striking water surface causing drowning and submersion**

Excludes1: *drowning and submersion while in other water without jumping or diving (W73)*

+7th **W16.812 Jumping or diving into other water striking water surface causing other injury**

+ **W16.82 Jumping or diving into other water striking bottom**

+7th **W16.821 Jumping or diving into other water striking bottom causing drowning and submersion**

Excludes1: *drowning and submersion while in other water without jumping or diving (W73)*

+7th **W16.822 Jumping or diving into other water striking bottom causing other injury**

+ **W16.83 Jumping or diving into other water striking wall**

+7th **W16.831 Jumping or diving into other water striking wall causing drowning and submersion**

Excludes1: *drowning and submersion while in other water without jumping or diving (W73)*

+7th **W16.832 Jumping or diving into other water striking wall causing other injury**

+ **W16.9 Jumping or diving into unspecified water**

X+7th **W16.91 Jumping or diving into unspecified water causing drowning and submersion**

X+7th **W16.92 Jumping or diving into unspecified water causing other injury**

W17 Other fall from one level to another

The appropriate 7th character is to be added to each code from category W17
A initial encounter
D subsequent encounter
S sequela

X+7th **W17.0 Fall into well**

X+7th **W17.1 Fall into storm drain or manhole**

X+7th **W17.2 Fall into hole**

Fall into pit

X+7th **W17.3 Fall into empty swimming pool**

Excludes1: *fall into filled swimming pool (W16.0-)*

X+7th **W17.4 Fall from dock**

+ **W17.8 Other fall from one level to another**

X+7th **W17.81 Fall down embankment (hill)**

X+7th **W17.82 Fall from (out of) grocery cart**

Fall due to grocery cart tipping over

X+7th **W17.89 Other fall from one level to another**

Fall from cherry picker
Fall from lifting device
Fall from mobile elevated work platform [MEWP]
Fall from sky lift

AHA CC: 2Q, 2015, 6-7

W18 Other slipping, tripping and stumbling and falls

The appropriate 7th character is to be added to each code from category W18
A initial encounter
D subsequent encounter
S sequela

+ **W18.0 Fall due to bumping against object**

Striking against object with subsequent fall

Excludes1: *fall on same level due to slipping, tripping, or stumbling with subsequent striking against object (W01.1-)*

X+7th **W18.00 Striking against unspecified object with subsequent fall**

X+7th **W18.01 Striking against sports equipment with subsequent fall**

X+7th **W18.02 Striking against glass with subsequent fall**

X+7th **W18.09 Striking against other object with subsequent fall**

+ **W18.1 Fall from or off toilet**

X+7th **W18.11 Fall from or off toilet without subsequent striking against object**

Fall from (off) toilet NOS

X+7th **W18.12 Fall from or off toilet with subsequent striking against object**

X+7th **W18.2 Fall in (into) shower or empty bathtub**

Excludes1: *fall in full bathtub causing drowning or submersi (W16.21-)*

+ **W18.3 Other and unspecified fall on same level**

X+7th **W18.30 Fall on same level, unspecified**

X+7th **W18.31 Fall on same level due to stepping on an object**

Fall on same level due to stepping on an animal

Excludes1: *slipping, tripping and stumbling withou fall due to stepping on animal (W18.41)*

X+7th **W18.39 Other fall on same level**

+ **W18.4 Slipping, tripping and stumbling without falling**

Excludes1: *collision with another person without fall (W51)*

X+7th **W18.40 Slipping, tripping and stumbling without falling, unspecified**

X+7th **W18.41 Slipping, tripping and stumbling without falling d to stepping on object**

Slipping, tripping and stumbling without falling due stepping on animal

Excludes1: *slipping, tripping and stumbling with fa due to stepping on animal (W18.31)*

X+7th **W18.42 Slipping, tripping and stumbling without falling d to stepping into hole or opening**

X+7th **W18.43 Slipping, tripping and stumbling without falling d to stepping from one level to another**

X+7th **W18.49 Other slipping, tripping and stumbling without falling**

W19 Unspecified fall
X+7th

Accidental fall NOS

AHA CC: 4Q, 2012, 95-96

The appropriate 7th character is to be added to code W19
A initial encounter
D subsequent encounter
S sequela

xposure to inanimate mechanical forces (W20-W49)

cludes1: *assault (X92-Y09)*
contact or collision with animals or persons (W50-W64)
exposure to inanimate mechanical forces involving military or war operations (Y36.-, Y37.-)
intentional self-harm (X71-X83)

W20 Struck by thrown, projected or falling object

Code first any associated:
cataclysm (X34-X39)
lightning strike (T75.00)

Excludes1: *falling object in machinery accident (W24, W28-W31)*
falling object in transport accident (V01-V99)
object set in motion by explosion (W35-W40)
object set in motion by firearm (W32-W34)
struck by thrown sports equipment (W21.-)

The appropriate 7th character is to be added to each code from category W20
A initial encounter
D subsequent encounter
S sequela

X+7th **W20.0 Struck by falling object in cave-in**
Excludes2: *asphyxiation due to cave-in (T71.21)*
X+7th **W20.1 Struck by object due to collapse of building**
Excludes1: *struck by object due to collapse of burning building (X00.2, X02.2)*
X+7th **W20.8 Other cause of strike by thrown, projected or falling object**
Excludes1: *struck by thrown sports equipment (W21.-)*

W21 Striking against or struck by sports equipment

Excludes1: *assault with sports equipment (Y08.0-)*
striking against or struck by sports equipment with subsequent fall (W18.01)

The appropriate 7th character is to be added to each code from category W21
A initial encounter
D subsequent encounter
S sequela

\+ **W21.0 Struck by hit or thrown ball**
X+7th **W21.00 Struck by hit or thrown ball, unspecified type**
X+7th **W21.01 Struck by football**
X+7th **W21.02 Struck by soccer ball**
X+7th **W21.03 Struck by baseball**
X+7th **W21.04 Struck by golf ball**
X+7th **W21.05 Struck by basketball**
X+7th **W21.06 Struck by volleyball**
X+7th **W21.07 Struck by softball**
X+7th **W21.09 Struck by other hit or thrown ball**
\+ **W21.1 Struck by bat, racquet or club**
X+7th **W21.11 Struck by baseball bat**
X+7th **W21.12 Struck by tennis racquet**
X+7th **W21.13 Struck by golf club**
X+7th **W21.19 Struck by other bat, racquet or club**
\+ **W21.2 Struck by hockey stick or puck**
\+ **W21.21 Struck by hockey stick**
+7th **W21.210 Struck by ice hockey stick**
+7th **W21.211 Struck by field hockey stick**
\+ **W21.22 Struck by hockey puck**
X+7th **W21.220 Struck by ice hockey puck**
X+7th **W21.221 Struck by field hockey puck**
\+ **W21.3 Struck by sports foot wear**
X+7th **W21.31 Struck by shoe cleats**
Stepped on by shoe cleats
X+7th **W21.32 Struck by skate blades**
Skated over by skate blades
X+7th **W21.39 Struck by other sports foot wear**
X+7th **W21.4 Striking against diving board**
Use additional code for subsequent falling into water, if applicable (W16.-)

\+ **W21.8 Striking against or struck by other sports equipment**
X+7th **W21.81 Striking against or struck by football helmet**
X+7th **W21.89 Striking against or struck by other sports equipment**
X+7th **W21.9 Striking against or struck by unspecified sports equipment**

W22 Striking against or struck by other objects

Excludes1: *striking against or struck by object with subsequent fall (W18.09)*

The appropriate 7th character is to be added to each code from category W22
A initial encounter
D subsequent encounter
S sequela

\+ **W22.0 Striking against stationary object**
Excludes1: *striking against stationary sports equipment (W21.8)*
X+7th **W22.01 Walked into wall**
X+7th **W22.02 Walked into lamppost**
X+7th **W22.03 Walked into furniture**
\+ **W22.04 Striking against wall of swimming pool**
+7th **W22.041 Striking against wall of swimming pool causing drowning and submersion**
Excludes1: *drowning and submersion while swimming without striking against wall (W67)*
+7th **W22.042 Striking against wall of swimming pool causing other injury**
X+7th **W22.09 Striking against other stationary object**
\+ **W22.1 Striking against or struck by automobile airbag**
X+7th **W22.10 Striking against or struck by unspecified automobile airbag**
X+7th **W22.11 Striking against or struck by driver side automobile airbag**
X+7th **W22.12 Striking against or struck by front passenger side automobile airbag**
X+7th **W22.19 Striking against or struck by other automobile airbag**
X+7th **W22.8 Striking against or struck by other objects**
Striking against or struck by object NOS
Excludes1: *struck by thrown, projected or falling object (W20.-)*

W23 Caught, crushed, jammed or pinched in or between objects

Excludes1: *injury caused by cutting or piercing instruments (W25-W27)*
injury caused by firearms malfunction (W32.1, W33.1-, W34.1-)
injury caused by lifting and transmission devices (W24.-)
injury caused by machinery (W28-W31)
injury caused by nonpowered hand tools (W27.-)
injury caused by transport vehicle being used as a means of transportation (V01-V99)
injury caused by struck by thrown, projected or falling object (W20.-)

The appropriate 7th character is to be added to each code from category W23
A initial encounter
D subsequent encounter
S sequela

X+7th **W23.0 Caught, crushed, jammed, or pinched between moving objects**
X+7th **W23.1 Caught, crushed, jammed, or pinched between stationary objects**

W24 Contact with lifting and transmission devices, not elsewhere classified

Excludes1: *transport accidents (V01-V99)*

The appropriate 7th character is to be added to each code from category W24
A initial encounter
D subsequent encounter
S sequela

X+7th **W24.0 Contact with lifting devices, not elsewhere classified**
Contact with chain hoist
Contact with drive belt
Contact with pulley (block)
X+7th **W24.1 Contact with transmission devices, not elsewhere classified**
Contact with transmission belt or cable

W25 Contact with sharp glass
X+7th
Code first any associated:
injury due to flying glass from explosion or firearm discharge (W32-W40)
transport accident (V00-V99)
Excludes1: *fall on same level due to slipping, tripping and stumbling with subsequent striking against sharp glass (W01.10)*
striking against sharp glass with subsequent fall (W18.02)
Excludes2: *glass embedded in skin (W45)*

The appropriate 7th character is to be added to code W25
A initial encounter
D subsequent encounter
S sequela

W26 Contact with other sharp objects
Excludes2: *sharp object(s) embedded in skin (W45)*
AHA CC: 4Q, 2016, 73

The appropriate 7th character is to be added to each code from category W26
A initial encounter
D subsequent encounter
S sequela

X+7th **W26.0 Contact with knife**
Excludes1: *contact with electric knife (W29.1)*
X+7th **W26.1 Contact with sword or dagger**
X+7th **W26.2 Contact with edge of stiff paper**
Paper cut
X+7th **W26.8 Contact with other sharp object(s), not elsewhere classified**
Contact with tin can lid
X+7th **W26.9 Contact with unspecified sharp object(s)**

W27 Contact with nonpowered hand tool

The appropriate 7th character is to be added to each code from category W27
A initial encounter
D subsequent encounter
S sequela

X+7th **W27.0 Contact with workbench tool**
Contact with auger
Contact with axe
Contact with chisel
Contact with handsaw
Contact with screwdriver
X+7th **W27.1 Contact with garden tool**
Contact with hoe
Contact with nonpowered lawn mower
Contact with pitchfork
Contact with rake
X+7th **W27.2 Contact with scissors**
X+7th **W27.3 Contact with needle (sewing)**
Excludes1: *contact with hypodermic needle (W46.-)*
X+7th **W27.4 Contact with kitchen utensil**
Contact with fork
Contact with ice-pick
Contact with can-opener NOS
X+7th **W27.5 Contact with paper-cutter**
X+7th **W27.8 Contact with other nonpowered hand tool**
Contact with nonpowered sewing machine
Contact with shovel

W28 Contact with powered lawn mower
X+7th
Powered lawn mower (commercial) (residential)
Excludes1: *contact with nonpowered lawn mower (W27.1)*
Excludes2: *exposure to electric current (W86.-)*

The appropriate 7th character is to be added to code W28
A initial encounter
D subsequent encounter
S sequela

W29 Contact with other powered hand tools and household machinery
Excludes1: *contact with commercial machinery (W31.82)*
contact with hot household appliance (X15)
contact with nonpowered hand tool (W27.-)
exposure to electric current (W86)

The appropriate 7th character is to be added to each code from category W29
A initial encounter
D subsequent encounter
S sequela

X+7th **W29.0 Contact with powered kitchen appliance**
Contact with blender
Contact with can-opener
Contact with garbage disposal
Contact with mixer
X+7th **W29.1 Contact with electric knife**
X+7th **W29.2 Contact with other powered household machinery**
Contact with electric fan
Contact with powered dryer (clothes) (powered) (spin)
Contact with washing-machine
Contact with sewing machine
X+7th **W29.3 Contact with powered garden and outdoor hand tools and machinery**
Contact with chainsaw
Contact with edger
Contact with garden cultivator (tiller)
Contact with hedge trimmer
Contact with other powered garden tool
Excludes1: *contact with powered lawn mower (W28)*
X+7th **W29.4 Contact with nail gun**
X+7th **W29.8 Contact with other powered hand tools and household machinery**
Contact with do-it-yourself tool NOS

W30 Contact with agricultural machinery
Includes: animal-powered farm machine
Excludes1: *agricultural transport vehicle accident (V01-V99)*
explosion of grain store (W40.8)
exposure to electric current (W86.-)

The appropriate 7th character is to be added to each code from category W30
A initial encounter
D subsequent encounter
S sequela

X+7th **W30.0 Contact with combine harvester**
Contact with reaper
Contact with thresher
X+7th **W30.1 Contact with power take-off devices (PTO)**
X+7th **W30.2 Contact with hay derrick**
X+7th **W30.3 Contact with grain storage elevator**
Excludes1: *explosion of grain store (W40.8)*
\+ **W30.8 Contact with other specified agricultural machinery**
X+7th **W30.81 Contact with agricultural transport vehicle in stationary use**
Contact with agricultural transport vehicle under repair, not on public roadway
Excludes1: *agricultural transport vehicle accident (V01-V99)*
X+7th **W30.89 Contact with other specified agricultural machinery**
X+7th **W30.9 Contact with unspecified agricultural machinery**
Contact with farm machinery NOS

W31 Contact with other and unspecified machinery
Excludes1: *contact with agricultural machinery (W30.-)*
contact with machinery in transport under own power or being towed by a vehicle (V01-V99)
exposure to electric current (W86)

The appropriate 7th character is to be added to each code from category W31
A initial encounter
D subsequent encounter
S sequela

X+7th **W31.0 Contact with mining and earth-drilling machinery**
Contact with bore or drill (land) (seabed)
Contact with shaft hoist
Contact with shaft lift
Contact with undercutter

X+7th **W31.1 Contact with metalworking machines**
Contact with abrasive wheel
Contact with forging machine
Contact with lathe
Contact with mechanical shears
Contact with metal drilling machine
Contact with milling machine
Contact with power press
Contact with rolling-mill
Contact with metal sawing machine

X+7th **W31.2 Contact with powered woodworking and forming machines**
Contact with band saw
Contact with bench saw
Contact with circular saw
Contact with molding machine
Contact with overhead plane
Contact with powered saw
Contact with radial saw
Contact with sander
Excludes1: *nonpowered woodworking tools (W27.0)*

X+7th **W31.3 Contact with prime movers**
Contact with gas turbine
Contact with internal combustion engine
Contact with steam engine
Contact with water driven turbine

\+ **W31.8 Contact with other specified machinery**

X+7th **W31.81 Contact with recreational machinery**
Contact with roller coaster

X+7th **W31.82 Contact with other commercial machinery**
Contact with commercial electric fan
Contact with commercial kitchen appliances
Contact with commercial powered dryer (clothes) (powered) (spin)
Contact with commercial washing-machine
Contact with commercial sewing machine
Excludes1: *contact with household machinery (W29.-)*
contact with powered lawn mower (W28)

X+7th **W31.83 Contact with special construction vehicle in stationary use**
Contact with special construction vehicle under repair, not on public roadway
Excludes1: *special construction vehicle accident (V01-V99)*

X+7th **W31.89 Contact with other specified machinery**

X+7th **W31.9 Contact with unspecified machinery**
Contact with machinery NOS

W32 Accidental handgun discharge and malfunction

Includes: accidental discharge and malfunction of gun for single hand use
accidental discharge and malfunction of pistol
accidental discharge and malfunction of revolver
Handgun discharge and malfunction NOS

Excludes1: *accidental airgun discharge and malfunction (W34.010, W34.110)*
accidental BB gun discharge and malfunction (W34.010, W34.110)
accidental pellet gun discharge and malfunction (W34.010, W34.110)
accidental shotgun discharge and malfunction (W33.01, W33.11)
assault by handgun discharge (X93)
handgun discharge involving legal intervention (Y35.0-)
handgun discharge involving military or war operations (Y36.4-)
intentional self-harm by handgun discharge (X72)
Very pistol discharge and malfunction (W34.09, W34.19)

The appropriate 7th character is to be added to each code from category W32
A initial encounter
D subsequent encounter
S sequela

X+7th **W32.0 Accidental handgun discharge**

X+7th **W32.1 Accidental handgun malfunction**
Injury due to explosion of handgun (parts)
Injury due to malfunction of mechanism or component of handgun
Injury due to recoil of handgun
Powder burn from handgun

W33 Accidental rifle, shotgun and larger firearm discharge and malfunction

Includes: rifle, shotgun and larger firearm discharge and malfunction NOS

Excludes1: *accidental airgun discharge and malfunction (W34.010, W34.110)*
accidental BB gun discharge and malfunction (W34.010, W34.110)
accidental handgun discharge and malfunction (W32.-)
accidental pellet gun discharge and malfunction (W34.010, W34.110)
assault by rifle, shotgun and larger firearm discharge (X94)
firearm discharge involving legal intervention (Y35.0-)
firearm discharge involving military or war operations (Y36.4-)
intentional self-harm by rifle, shotgun and larger firearm discharge (X73)

The appropriate 7th character is to be added to each code from category W33
A initial encounter
D subsequent encounter
S sequela

\+ **W33.0 Accidental rifle, shotgun and larger firearm discharge**

X+7th **W33.00 Accidental discharge of unspecified larger firearm**
Discharge of unspecified larger firearm NOS

X+7th **W33.01 Accidental discharge of shotgun**
Discharge of shotgun NOS

X+7th **W33.02 Accidental discharge of hunting rifle**
Discharge of hunting rifle NOS

X+7th **W33.03 Accidental discharge of machine gun**
Discharge of machine gun NOS

X+7th **W33.09 Accidental discharge of other larger firearm**
Discharge of other larger firearm NOS

\+ **W33.1 Accidental rifle, shotgun and larger firearm malfunction**
Injury due to explosion of rifle, shotgun and larger firearm (parts)
Injury due to malfunction of mechanism or component of rifle, shotgun and larger firearm
Injury due to piercing, cutting, crushing or pinching due to (by) slide trigger mechanism, scope or other gun part
Injury due to recoil of rifle, shotgun and larger firearm
Powder burn from rifle, shotgun and larger firearm

X+7th **W33.10 Accidental malfunction of unspecified larger firearm**
Malfunction of unspecified larger firearm NOS

X+7th **W33.11 Accidental malfunction of shotgun**
Malfunction of shotgun NOS

X+7th **W33.12 Accidental malfunction of hunting rifle**
Malfunction of hunting rifle NOS

X+7th **W33.13 Accidental malfunction of machine gun**
Malfunction of machine gun NOS

X+7th **W33.19 Accidental malfunction of other larger firearm**
Malfunction of other larger firearm NOS

W34 Accidental discharge and malfunction from other and unspecified firearms and guns

The appropriate 7th character is to be added to each code from category W34
A initial encounter
D subsequent encounter
S sequela

\+ **W34.0 Accidental discharge from other and unspecified firearms and guns**

X+7th **W34.00 Accidental discharge from unspecified firearms or gun**
Discharge from firearm NOS
Gunshot wound NOS
Shot NOS
AHA CC: 1Q, 2015, 3-21

\+ **W34.01 Accidental discharge of gas, air or spring-operated guns**

+7th **W34.010 Accidental discharge of airgun**
Accidental discharge of BB gun
Accidental discharge of pellet gun

+7th **W34.011 Accidental discharge of paintball gun**
Accidental injury due to paintball discharge

+7th **W34.018 Accidental discharge of other gas, air or spring-operated gun**

X+7th **W34.09 Accidental discharge from other specified firearms**
Accidental discharge from Very pistol [flare]

+ **W34.1 Accidental malfunction from other and unspecified firearms and guns**
  - X+7th **W34.10 Accidental malfunction from unspecified firearms or gun**
    Firearm malfunction NOS
  - + **W34.11 Accidental malfunction of gas, air or spring-operated guns**
    - +7th **W34.110 Accidental malfunction of airgun**
      Accidental malfunction of BB gun
      Accidental malfunction of pellet gun
    - +7th **W34.111 Accidental malfunction of paintball gun**
      Accidental injury due to paintball gun malfunction
    - +7th **W34.118 Accidental malfunction of other gas, air or spring-operated gun**
  - X+7th **W34.19 Accidental malfunction from other specified firearms**
    Accidental malfunction from Very pistol [flare]

W35 Explosion and rupture of boiler
X+7th

Excludes1: *explosion and rupture of boiler on watercraft (V93.4)*

The appropriate 7th character is to be added to code W35
A initial encounter
D subsequent encounter
S sequela

W36 Explosion and rupture of gas cylinder

The appropriate 7th character is to be added to each code from category W36
A initial encounter
D subsequent encounter
S sequela

X+7th **W36.1 Explosion and rupture of aerosol can**
X+7th **W36.2 Explosion and rupture of air tank**
X+7th **W36.3 Explosion and rupture of pressurized-gas tank**
X+7th **W36.8 Explosion and rupture of other gas cylinder**
X+7th **W36.9 Explosion and rupture of unspecified gas cylinder**

W37 Explosion and rupture of pressurized tire, pipe or hose

The appropriate 7th character is to be added to each code from category W37
A initial encounter
D subsequent encounter
S sequela

X+7th **W37.0 Explosion of bicycle tire**
X+7th **W37.8 Explosion and rupture of other pressurized tire, pipe or hose**

W38 Explosion and rupture of other specified pressurized devices
X+7th

The appropriate 7th character is to be added to code W38
A initial encounter
D subsequent encounter
S sequela

W39 Discharge of firework
X+7th

The appropriate 7th character is to be added to code W39
A initial encounter
D subsequent encounter
S sequela

W40 Explosion of other materials

Excludes1: *assault by explosive material (X96)*
explosion involving legal intervention (Y35.1-)
explosion involving military or war operations (Y36.0-, Y36.2-)
intentional self-harm by explosive material (X75)

The appropriate 7th character is to be added to each code from category W40
A initial encounter
D subsequent encounter
S sequela

X+7th **W40.0 Explosion of blasting material**
Explosion of blasting cap
Explosion of detonator
Explosion of dynamite
Explosion of explosive (any) used in blasting operations

X+7th **W40.1 Explosion of explosive gases**
Explosion of acetylene
Explosion of butane
Explosion of coal gas
Explosion in mine NOS
Explosion of explosive gas
Explosion of fire damp
Explosion of gasoline fumes
Explosion of methane
Explosion of propane

X+7th **W40.8 Explosion of other specified explosive materials**
Explosion in dump NOS
Explosion in factory NOS
Explosion in grain store
Explosion in munitions
Excludes1: *explosion involving legal intervention (Y35.1-)*
explosion involving military or war operations (Y36.0-, Y36.2-)

X+7th **W40.9 Explosion of unspecified explosive materials**
Explosion NOS

W42 Exposure to noise

The appropriate 7th character is to be added to each code from category W42
A initial encounter
D subsequent encounter
S sequela

X+7th **W42.0 Exposure to supersonic waves**
X+7th **W42.9 Exposure to other noise**
Exposure to sound waves NOS

W45 Foreign body or object entering through skin

Includes: foreign body or object embedded in skin
nail embedded in skin
Excludes2: *contact with hand tools (nonpowered) (powered) (W27-W29)*
contact with other sharp object(s) (W26.-)
contact with sharp glass (W25.-)
struck by objects (W20-W22)

The appropriate 7th character is to be added to each code from category W45
A initial encounter
D subsequent encounter
S sequela

X+7th **W45.0 Nail entering through skin**
X+7th **W45.8 Other foreign body or object entering through skin**
Splinter in skin NOS

W46 Contact with hypodermic needle

The appropriate 7th character is to be added to each code from category W46
A initial encounter
D subsequent encounter
S sequela

X+7th **W46.0 Contact with hypodermic needle**
Hypodermic needle stick NOS
X+7th **W46.1 Contact with contaminated hypodermic needle**

W49 Exposure to other inanimate mechanical forces

Includes: exposure to abnormal gravitational [G] forces
exposure to inanimate mechanical forces NEC
Excludes1: *exposure to inanimate mechanical forces involving milit[...] or war operations (Y36.-, Y37.-)*

The appropriate 7th character is to be added to each code from category W49
A initial encounter
D subsequent encounter
S sequela

+ **W49.0 Item causing external constriction**
  - X+7th **W49.01 Hair causing external constriction**
  - X+7th **W49.02 String or thread causing external constriction**
  - X+7th **W49.03 Rubber band causing external constriction**
  - X+7th **W49.04 Ring or other jewelry causing external constrictio[...]**
  - X+7th **W49.09 Other specified item causing external constriction**

X+7th **W49.9 Exposure to other inanimate mechanical forces**

xposure to animate mechanical forces (W50-W64)

xcludes1: *Toxic effect of contact with venomous animals and plants (T63.-)*

W50 Accidental hit, strike, kick, twist, bite or scratch by another person

Includes: hit, strike, kick, twist, bite, or scratch by another person NOS

Excludes1: *assault by bodily force (Y04)*
struck by objects (W20-W22)

The appropriate 7th character is to be added to each code from category W50
A initial encounter
D subsequent encounter
S sequela

X+7th **W50.0 Accidental hit or strike by another person**
Hit or strike by another person NOS

X+7th **W50.1 Accidental kick by another person**
Kick by another person NOS

X+7th **W50.2 Accidental twist by another person**
Twist by another person NOS
AHA CC: 1Q, 2015, 3-21

X+7th **W50.3 Accidental bite by another person**
Human bite
Bite by another person NOS

X+7th **W50.4 Accidental scratch by another person**
Scratch by another person NOS

W51 Accidental striking against or bumped into by another person X+7th

Excludes1: *assault by striking against or bumping into by another person (Y04.2)*
fall due to collision with another person (W03)

The appropriate 7th character is to be added to code W51
A initial encounter
D subsequent encounter
S sequela

W52 Crushed, pushed or stepped on by crowd or human stampede X+7th

Crushed, pushed or stepped on by crowd or human stampede with or without fall

The appropriate 7th character is to be added to code W52
A initial encounter
D subsequent encounter
S sequela

+ **W53 Contact with rodent**

Includes: contact with saliva, feces or urine of rodent

The appropriate 7th character is to be added to each code from category W53
A initial encounter
D subsequent encounter
S sequela

+ **W53.0 Contact with mouse**
X+7th **W53.01 Bitten by mouse**
X+7th **W53.09 Other contact with mouse**

+ **W53.1 Contact with rat**
X+7th **W53.11 Bitten by rat**
X+7th **W53.19 Other contact with rat**

+ **W53.2 Contact with squirrel**
X+7th **W53.21 Bitten by squirrel**
X+7th **W53.29 Other contact with squirrel**

+ **W53.8 Contact with other rodent**
X+7th **W53.81 Bitten by other rodent**
X+7th **W53.89 Other contact with other rodent**

W54 Contact with dog

Includes: contact with saliva, feces or urine of dog

The appropriate 7th character is to be added to each code from category W54
A initial encounter
D subsequent encounter
S sequela

X+7th **W54.0 Bitten by dog**

X+7th **W54.1 Struck by dog**
Knocked over by dog

X+7th **W54.8 Other contact with dog**

W55 Contact with other mammals

Includes: contact with saliva, feces or urine of mammal

Excludes1: *animal being ridden- see transport accidents*
bitten or struck by dog (W54)
bitten or struck by rodent (W53.-)
contact with marine mammals (W56.-)

The appropriate 7th character is to be added to each code from category W55
A initial encounter
D subsequent encounter
S sequela

+ **W55.0 Contact with cat**
X+7th **W55.01 Bitten by cat**
X+7th **W55.03 Scratched by cat**
X+7th **W55.09 Other contact with cat**

+ **W55.1 Contact with horse**
X+7th **W55.11 Bitten by horse**
X+7th **W55.12 Struck by horse**
X+7th **W55.19 Other contact with horse**

+ **W55.2 Contact with cow**
Contact with bull
X+7th **W55.21 Bitten by cow**
X+7th **W55.22 Struck by cow**
Gored by bull
X+7th **W55.29 Other contact with cow**

+ **W55.3 Contact with other hoof stock**
Contact with goats
Contact with sheep
X+7th **W55.31 Bitten by other hoof stock**
X+7th **W55.32 Struck by other hoof stock**
Gored by goat
Gored by ram
X+7th **W55.39 Other contact with other hoof stock**

+ **W55.4 Contact with pig**
X+7th **W55.41 Bitten by pig**
X+7th **W55.42 Struck by pig**
X+7th **W55.49 Other contact with pig**

+ **W55.5 Contact with raccoon**
X+7th **W55.51 Bitten by raccoon**
X+7th **W55.52 Struck by raccoon**
X+7th **W55.59 Other contact with raccoon**

+ **W55.8 Contact with other mammals**
X+7th **W55.81 Bitten by other mammals**
X+7th **W55.82 Struck by other mammals**
X+7th **W55.89 Other contact with other mammals**

W56 Contact with nonvenomous marine animal

Excludes1: *contact with venomous marine animal (T63.-)*

The appropriate 7th character is to be added to each code from category W56
A initial encounter
D subsequent encounter
S sequela

+ **W56.0 Contact with dolphin**
X+7th **W56.01 Bitten by dolphin**
X+7th **W56.02 Struck by dolphin**
X+7th **W56.09 Other contact with dolphin**

+ **W56.1 Contact with sea lion**
X+7th **W56.11 Bitten by sea lion**
X+7th **W56.12 Struck by sea lion**
X+7th **W56.19 Other contact with sea lion**

+ **W56.2 Contact with orca**
Contact with killer whale
X+7th **W56.21 Bitten by orca**
X+7th **W56.22 Struck by orca**
X+7th **W56.29 Other contact with orca**

+ **W56.3 Contact with other marine mammals**
X+7th **W56.31 Bitten by other marine mammals**
X+7th **W56.32 Struck by other marine mammals**
X+7th **W56.39 Other contact with other marine mammals**

+ **W56.4 Contact with shark**
X+7th **W56.41 Bitten by shark**
X+7th **W56.42 Struck by shark**
X+7th **W56.49 Other contact with shark**

+ **W56.5 Contact with other fish**
X+7th **W56.51 Bitten by other fish**
X+7th **W56.52 Struck by other fish**
X+7th **W56.59 Other contact with other fish**

+ W56.8 Contact with other nonvenomous marine animals
  - X+7th W56.81 Bitten by other nonvenomous marine animals
  - X+7th W56.82 Struck by other nonvenomous marine animals
  - X+7th W56.89 Other contact with other nonvenomous marine animals

W57 Bitten or stung by nonvenomous insect and other nonvenomous arthropods X+7th

Excludes1: contact with venomous insects and arthropods (T63.2-, T63.3-, T63.4-)

The appropriate 7th character is to be added to code W57
A initial encounter
D subsequent encounter
S sequela

W58 Contact with crocodile or alligator

The appropriate 7th character is to be added to each code from category W58
A initial encounter
D subsequent encounter
S sequela

+ W58.0 Contact with alligator
  - X+7th W58.01 Bitten by alligator
  - X+7th W58.02 Struck by alligator
  - X+7th W58.03 Crushed by alligator
  - X+7th W58.09 Other contact with alligator
+ W58.1 Contact with crocodile
  - X+7th W58.11 Bitten by crocodile
  - X+7th W58.12 Struck by crocodile
  - X+7th W58.13 Crushed by crocodile
  - X+7th W58.19 Other contact with crocodile

W59 Contact with other nonvenomous reptiles

Excludes1: contact with venomous reptile (T63.0-, T63.1-)

The appropriate 7th character is to be added to each code from category W59
A initial encounter
D subsequent encounter
S sequela

+ W59.0 Contact with nonvenomous lizards
  - X+7th W59.01 Bitten by nonvenomous lizards
  - X+7th W59.02 Struck by nonvenomous lizards
  - X+7th W59.09 Other contact with nonvenomous lizards
    Exposure to nonvenomous lizards
+ W59.1 Contact with nonvenomous snakes
  - X+7th W59.11 Bitten by nonvenomous snake
  - X+7th W59.12 Struck by nonvenomous snake
  - X+7th W59.13 Crushed by nonvenomous snake
  - X+7th W59.19 Other contact with nonvenomous snake
+ W59.2 Contact with turtles
  Excludes1: contact with tortoises (W59.8-)
  - X+7th W59.21 Bitten by turtle
  - X+7th W59.22 Struck by turtle
  - X+7th W59.29 Other contact with turtle
    Exposure to turtles
+ W59.8 Contact with other nonvenomous reptiles
  - X+7th W59.81 Bitten by other nonvenomous reptiles
  - X+7th W59.82 Struck by other nonvenomous reptiles
  - X+7th W59.83 Crushed by other nonvenomous reptiles
  - X+7th W59.89 Other contact with other nonvenomous reptiles

W60 Contact with nonvenomous plant thorns and spines and sharp leaves X+7th

Excludes1: Contact with venomous plants (T63.7-)

The appropriate 7th character is to be added to code W60
A initial encounter
D subsequent encounter
S sequela

W61 Contact with birds (domestic) (wild)

Includes: contact with excreta of birds

The appropriate 7th character is to be added to each code from category W61
A initial encounter
D subsequent encounter
S sequela

+ W61.0 Contact with parrot
  - X+7th W61.01 Bitten by parrot
  - X+7th W61.02 Struck by parrot
  - X+7th W61.09 Other contact with parrot
    Exposure to parrots
+ W61.1 Contact with macaw
  - X+7th W61.11 Bitten by macaw
  - X+7th W61.12 Struck by macaw
  - X+7th W61.19 Other contact with macaw
    Exposure to macaws
+ W61.2 Contact with other psittacines
  - X+7th W61.21 Bitten by other psittacines
  - X+7th W61.22 Struck by other psittacines
  - X+7th W61.29 Other contact with other psittacines
    Exposure to other psittacines
+ W61.3 Contact with chicken
  - X+7th W61.32 Struck by chicken
  - X+7th W61.33 Pecked by chicken
  - X+7th W61.39 Other contact with chicken
    Exposure to chickens
+ W61.4 Contact with turkey
  - X+7th W61.42 Struck by turkey
  - X+7th W61.43 Pecked by turkey
  - X+7th W61.49 Other contact with turkey
+ W61.5 Contact with goose
  - X+7th W61.51 Bitten by goose
  - X+7th W61.52 Struck by goose
  - X+7th W61.59 Other contact with goose
+ W61.6 Contact with duck
  - X+7th W61.61 Bitten by duck
  - X+7th W61.62 Struck by duck
  - X+7th W61.69 Other contact with duck
+ W61.9 Contact with other birds
  - X+7th W61.91 Bitten by other birds
  - X+7th W61.92 Struck by other birds
  - X+7th W61.99 Other contact with other birds
    Contact with bird NOS

W62 Contact with nonvenomous amphibians

Excludes1: contact with venomous amphibians (T63.81-R63.83)

The appropriate 7th character is to be added to each code from category W62
A initial encounter
D subsequent encounter
S sequela

- X+7th W62.0 Contact with nonvenomous frogs
- X+7th W62.1 Contact with nonvenomous toads
- X+7th W62.9 Contact with other nonvenomous amphibians

W64 Exposure to other animate mechanical forces X+7th

Includes: exposure to nonvenomous animal NOS
Excludes1: contact with venomous animal (T63.-)

The appropriate 7th character is to be added to code W64
A initial encounter
D subsequent encounter
S sequela

Accidental non-transport drowning and submersion (W65-W74)

Excludes1: accidental drowning and submersion due to fall into water (W16.-)
accidental drowning and submersion due to water transport accident (V90.-, V92.-)

Excludes2: accidental drowning and submersion due to cataclysm (X34-X39)

W65 Accidental drowning and submersion while in bath-tub X+7th

Excludes1: accidental drowning and submersion due to fall in (into) bathtub (W16.211)

The appropriate 7th character is to be added to code W65
A initial encounter
D subsequent encounter
S sequela

W67 Accidental drowning and submersion while in swimming-pool X+7th

Excludes1: accidental drowning and submersion due to fall into swimming pool (W16.011, W16.021, W16.031)
accidental drowning and submersion due to striking into wall of swimming pool (W22.041)

The appropriate 7th character is to be added to code W67
A initial encounter
D subsequent encounter
S sequela

W69 Accidental drowning and submersion while in natural water
X+7th

Accidental drowning and submersion while in lake
Accidental drowning and submersion while in open sea
Accidental drowning and submersion while in river
Accidental drowning and submersion while in stream

Excludes1: *accidental drowning and submersion due to fall into natural body of water (W16.111, W16.121, W16.131)*

The appropriate 7th character is to be added to code W69
A initial encounter
D subsequent encounter
S sequela

W73 Other specified cause of accidental non-transport drowning and submersion
X+7th

Accidental drowning and submersion while in quenching tank
Accidental drowning and submersion while in reservoir

Excludes1: *accidental drowning and submersion due to fall into other water (W16.311, W16.321, W16.331)*

The appropriate 7th character is to be added to code W73
A initial encounter
D subsequent encounter
S sequela

W74 Unspecified cause of accidental drowning and submersion
X+7th

Drowning NOS

The appropriate 7th character is to be added to code W74
A initial encounter
D subsequent encounter
S sequela

xposure to electric current, radiation and extreme ambient r temperature and pressure (W85-W99)

cludes1: *exposure to:*
failure in dosage of radiation or temperature during surgical and medical care (Y63.2-Y63.5)
lightning (T75.0-)
natural cold (X31)
natural heat (X30)
natural radiation NOS (X39)
radiological procedure and radiotherapy (Y84.2)
sunlight (X32)

W85 Exposure to electric transmission lines
X+7th

Broken power line

The appropriate 7th character is to be added to code W85
A initial encounter
D subsequent encounter
S sequela

W86 Exposure to other specified electric current

The appropriate 7th character is to be added to each code from category W86
A initial encounter
D subsequent encounter
S sequela

X+7th **W86.0 Exposure to domestic wiring and appliances**
X+7th **W86.1 Exposure to industrial wiring, appliances and electrical machinery**
Exposure to conductors
Exposure to control apparatus
Exposure to electrical equipment and machinery
Exposure to transformers
X+7th **W86.8 Exposure to other electric current**
Exposure to wiring and appliances in or on farm (not farmhouse)
Exposure to wiring and appliances outdoors
Exposure to wiring and appliances in or on public building
Exposure to wiring and appliances in or on residential institutions
Exposure to wiring and appliances in or on schools

W88 Exposure to ionizing radiation

Excludes1: *exposure to sunlight (X32)*

The appropriate 7th character is to be added to each code from category W88
A initial encounter
D subsequent encounter
S sequela

X+7th **W88.0 Exposure to X-rays**
X+7th **W88.1 Exposure to radioactive isotopes**
X+7th **W88.8 Exposure to other ionizing radiation**

W89 Exposure to man-made visible and ultraviolet light

Includes: exposure to welding light (arc)
Excludes1: *exposure to sunlight (X32)*

The appropriate 7th character is to be added to each code from category W89
A initial encounter
D subsequent encounter
S sequela

X+7th **W89.0 Exposure to welding light (arc)**
X+7th **W89.1 Exposure to tanning bed**
X+7th **W89.8 Exposure to other man-made visible and ultraviolet light**
X+7th **W89.9 Exposure to unspecified man-made visible and ultraviolet light**

W90 Exposure to other nonionizing radiation

Excludes1: *exposure to sunlight (X32)*

The appropriate 7th character is to be added to each code from category W90
A initial encounter
D subsequent encounter
S sequela

X+7th **W90.0 Exposure to radiofrequency**
X+7th **W90.1 Exposure to infrared radiation**
X+7th **W90.2 Exposure to laser radiation**
X+7th **W90.8 Exposure to other nonionizing radiation**

W92 Exposure to excessive heat of man-made origin
X+7th

The appropriate 7th character is to be added to code W92
A initial encounter
D subsequent encounter
S sequela

W93 Exposure to excessive cold of man-made origin

The appropriate 7th character is to be added to each code from category W93
A initial encounter
D subsequent encounter
S sequela

\+ **W93.0 Contact with or inhalation of dry ice**
X+7th **W93.01 Contact with dry ice**
X+7th **W93.02 Inhalation of dry ice**
\+ **W93.1 Contact with or inhalation of liquid air**
X+7th **W93.11 Contact with liquid air**
Contact with liquid hydrogen
Contact with liquid nitrogen
X+7th **W93.12 Inhalation of liquid air**
Inhalation of liquid hydrogen
Inhalation of liquid nitrogen
X+7th **W93.2 Prolonged exposure in deep freeze unit or refrigerator**
X+7th **W93.8 Exposure to other excessive cold of man-made origin**

W94 Exposure to high and low air pressure and changes in air pressure

The appropriate 7th character is to be added to each code from category W94
A initial encounter
D subsequent encounter
S sequela

X+7th **W94.0 Exposure to prolonged high air pressure**
\+ **W94.1 Exposure to prolonged low air pressure**
X+7th **W94.11 Exposure to residence or prolonged visit at high altitude**
X+7th **W94.12 Exposure to other prolonged low air pressure**
\+ **W94.2 Exposure to rapid changes in air pressure during ascent**
X+7th **W94.21 Exposure to reduction in atmospheric pressure while surfacing from deep-water diving**
X+7th **W94.22 Exposure to reduction in atmospheric pressure while surfacing from underground**

X+7th **W94.23 Exposure to sudden change in air pressure in aircraft during ascent**
X+7th **W94.29 Exposure to other rapid changes in air pressure during ascent**
+ **W94.3 Exposure to rapid changes in air pressure during descent**
X+7th **W94.31 Exposure to sudden change in air pressure in aircraft during descent**
X+7th **W94.32 Exposure to high air pressure from rapid descent in water**
X+7th **W94.39 Exposure to other rapid changes in air pressure during descent**

W99 Exposure to other man-made environmental factors
X+7th
The appropriate 7th character is to be added to code W99
A initial encounter
D subsequent encounter
S sequela

Exposure to smoke, fire and flames (X00-X08)

Excludes1: *arson (X97)*

Excludes2: *explosions (W35-W40)*
lightning (T75.0-)
transport accident (V01-V99)

X00 Exposure to uncontrolled fire in building or structure

Includes: conflagration in building or structure
Code first any associated cataclysm
Excludes2: *Exposure to ignition or melting of nightwear (X05)*
Exposure to ignition or melting of other clothing and apparel (X06.-)
Exposure to other specified smoke, fire and flames (X08.-)

The appropriate 7th character is to be added to each code from category X00
A initial encounter
D subsequent encounter
S sequela

X+7th **X00.0 Exposure to flames in uncontrolled fire in building or structure**
AHA CC: 1Q, 2015, 3-21; 2Q, 2016, 5-6
X+7th **X00.1 Exposure to smoke in uncontrolled fire in building or structure**
X+7th **X00.2 Injury due to collapse of burning building or structure in uncontrolled fire**
Excludes1: *injury due to collapse of building not on fire (W20.1)*
X+7th **X00.3 Fall from burning building or structure in uncontrolled fire**
X+7th **X00.4 Hit by object from burning building or structure in uncontrolled fire**
X+7th **X00.5 Jump from burning building or structure in uncontrolled fire**
X+7th **X00.8 Other exposure to uncontrolled fire in building or structure**

X01 Exposure to uncontrolled fire, not in building or structure

Includes: exposure to forest fire

The appropriate 7th character is to be added to each code from category X01
A initial encounter
D subsequent encounter
S sequela

X+7th **X01.0 Exposure to flames in uncontrolled fire, not in building or structure**
X+7th **X01.1 Exposure to smoke in uncontrolled fire, not in building or structure**
X+7th **X01.3 Fall due to uncontrolled fire, not in building or structure**
X+7th **X01.4 Hit by object due to uncontrolled fire, not in building or structure**
X+7th **X01.8 Other exposure to uncontrolled fire, not in building or structure**

X02 Exposure to controlled fire in building or structure

Includes: exposure to fire in fireplace
exposure to fire in stove

The appropriate 7th character is to be added to each code from category X02
A initial encounter
D subsequent encounter
S sequela

X+7th **X02.0 Exposure to flames in controlled fire in building or structure**
X+7th **X02.1 Exposure to smoke in controlled fire in building or structure**
X+7th **X02.2 Injury due to collapse of burning building or structure in controlled fire**
Excludes1: *injury due to collapse of building not on fire (W20.*
X+7th **X02.3 Fall from burning building or structure in controlled fire**
X+7th **X02.4 Hit by object from burning building or structure in controlle fire**
X+7th **X02.5 Jump from burning building or structure in controlled fire**
X+7th **X02.8 Other exposure to controlled fire in building or structure**

X03 Exposure to controlled fire, not in building or structure

Includes: exposure to bon fire
exposure to camp-fire
exposure to trash fire

The appropriate 7th character is to be added to each code from category X03
A initial encounter
D subsequent encounter
S sequela

X+7th **X03.0 Exposure to flames in controlled fire, not in building or structure**
AHA CC: 1Q, 2015, 3-21
X+7th **X03.1 Exposure to smoke in controlled fire, not in building or structure**
X+7th **X03.3 Fall due to controlled fire, not in building or structure**
X+7th **X03.4 Hit by object due to controlled fire, not in building or structu**
X+7th **X03.8 Other exposure to controlled fire, not in building or structure**

X04 Exposure to ignition of highly flammable material
X+7th
Exposure to ignition of gasoline
Exposure to ignition of kerosene
Exposure to ignition of petrol
Excludes2: *exposure to ignition or melting of nightwear (X05)*
exposure to ignition or melting of other clothing and apparel (X06)
AHA CC: 2Q, 2016, 4

The appropriate 7th character is to be added to code X04
A initial encounter
D subsequent encounter
S sequela

X05 Exposure to ignition or melting of nightwear
X+7th
Excludes2: *exposure to uncontrolled fire in building or structure (X00*
exposure to uncontrolled fire, not in building or structure (X01.-)
exposure to controlled fire in building or structure (X02.-
exposure to controlled fire, not in building or structure (X03.-)
exposure to ignition of highly flammable materials (X04.-

The appropriate 7th character is to be added to code X05
A initial encounter
D subsequent encounter
S sequela

X06 Exposure to ignition or melting of other clothing and apparel

Excludes2: *exposure to uncontrolled fire in building or structure (X0*
exposure to uncontrolled fire, not in building or structure (X01.-)
exposure to controlled fire in building or structure (X02.-
exposure to controlled fire, not in building or structure (X0
exposure to ignition of highly flammable materials (X04.-

The appropriate 7th character is to be added to each code from category X06
A initial encounter
D subsequent encounter
S sequela

X+7th **X06.0 Exposure to ignition of plastic jewelry**
X+7th **X06.1 Exposure to melting of plastic jewelry**
X+7th **X06.2 Exposure to ignition of other clothing and apparel**
X+7th **X06.3 Exposure to melting of other clothing and apparel**

X08 Exposure to other specified smoke, fire and flames

The appropriate 7th character is to be added to each code from category X08
A initial encounter
D subsequent encounter
S sequela

+ **X08.0 Exposure to bed fire**
Exposure to mattress fire
X+7th **X08.00 Exposure to bed fire due to unspecified burning material**

X+7th **X08.01 Exposure to bed fire due to burning cigarette**
AHA CC: 1Q, 2015, 3-21
X+7th **X08.09 Exposure to bed fire due to other burning material**
+ **X08.1 Exposure to sofa fire**
X+7th **X08.10 Exposure to sofa fire due to unspecified burning material**
X+7th **X08.11 Exposure to sofa fire due to burning cigarette**
X+7th **X08.19 Exposure to sofa fire due to other burning material**
+ **X08.2 Exposure to other furniture fire**
X+7th **X08.20 Exposure to other furniture fire due to unspecified burning material**
X+7th **X08.21 Exposure to other furniture fire due to burning cigarette**
X+7th **X08.29 Exposure to other furniture fire due to other burning material**
X+7th **X08.8 Exposure to other specified smoke, fire and flames**

Contact with heat and hot substances (X10-X19)

Excludes1: *exposure to excessive natural heat (X30)*
exposure to fire and flames (X00-X08)

X10 Contact with hot drinks, food, fats and cooking oils

The appropriate 7th character is to be added to each code from category X10
A initial encounter
D subsequent encounter
S sequela

X+7th **X10.0 Contact with hot drinks**
X+7th **X10.1 Contact with hot food**
X+7th **X10.2 Contact with fats and cooking oils**

X11 Contact with hot tap-water

Includes: contact with boiling tap-water
contact with boiling water NOS
Excludes1: *contact with water heated on stove (X12)*

The appropriate 7th character is to be added to each code from category X11
A initial encounter
D subsequent encounter
S sequela

X+7th **X11.0 Contact with hot water in bath or tub**
Excludes1: *contact with running hot water in bath or tub (X11.1)*
X+7th **X11.1 Contact with running hot water**
Contact with hot water running out of hose
Contact with hot water running out of tap
X+7th **X11.8 Contact with other hot tap-water**
Contact with hot water in bucket
Contact with hot tap-water NOS

X12 Contact with other hot fluids
X+7th
Contact with water heated on stove
Excludes1: *hot (liquid) metals (X18)*

The appropriate 7th character is to be added to code X12
A initial encounter
D subsequent encounter
S sequela

X13 Contact with steam and other hot vapors

The appropriate 7th character is to be added to each code from category X13
A initial encounter
D subsequent encounter
S sequela

X+7th **X13.0 Inhalation of steam and other hot vapors**
X+7th **X13.1 Other contact with steam and other hot vapors**

X14 Contact with hot air and other hot gases

The appropriate 7th character is to be added to each code from category X14
A initial encounter
D subsequent encounter
S sequela

X+7th **X14.0 Inhalation of hot air and gases**
X+7th **X14.1 Other contact with hot air and other hot gases**

X15 Contact with hot household appliances

Excludes1: *contact with heating appliances (X16)*
contact with powered household appliances (W29.-)
exposure to controlled fire in building or structure due to household appliance (X02.8)
exposure to household appliances electrical current (W86.0)

The appropriate 7th character is to be added to each code from category X15
A initial encounter
D subsequent encounter
S sequela

X+7th **X15.0 Contact with hot stove (kitchen)**
X+7th **X15.1 Contact with hot toaster**
X+7th **X15.2 Contact with hotplate**
X+7th **X15.3 Contact with hot saucepan or skillet**
X+7th **X15.8 Contact with other hot household appliances**
Contact with cooker
Contact with kettle
Contact with light bulbs

X16 Contact with hot heating appliances, radiators and pipes
X+7th
Excludes1: *contact with powered appliances (W29.-)*
exposure to controlled fire in building or structure due to appliance (X02.8)
exposure to industrial appliances electrical current (W86.1)

The appropriate 7th character is to be added to code X16
A initial encounter
D subsequent encounter
S sequela

X17 Contact with hot engines, machinery and tools
X+7th
Excludes1: *contact with hot heating appliances, radiators and pipes (X16)*
contact with hot household appliances (X15)

The appropriate 7th character is to be added to code X17
A initial encounter
D subsequent encounter
S sequela

X18 Contact with other hot metals
X+7th
Contact with liquid metal

The appropriate 7th character is to be added to code X18
A initial encounter
D subsequent encounter
S sequela

X19 Contact with other heat and hot substances
X+7th
Excludes1: *objects that are not normally hot, e.g., an object made hot by a house fire (X00-X08)*

The appropriate 7th character is to be added to code X19
A initial encounter
D subsequent encounter
S sequela

Exposure to forces of nature (X30-X39)

X30 Exposure to excessive natural heat
X+7th
Exposure to excessive heat as the cause of sunstroke
Exposure to heat NOS
Excludes1: *excessive heat of man-made origin (W92)*
exposure to man-made radiation (W89)
exposure to sunlight (X32)
exposure to tanning bed (W89)

The appropriate 7th character is to be added to code X30
A initial encounter
D subsequent encounter
S sequela

X31 Exposure to excessive natural cold
X+7th
Excessive cold as the cause of chilblains NOS
Excessive cold as the cause of immersion foot or hand
Exposure to cold NOS
Exposure to weather conditions
Excludes1: *cold of man-made origin (W93.-)*
contact with or inhalation of dry ice (W93.-)
contact with or inhalation of liquefied gas (W93.-)

The appropriate 7th character is to be added to code X31
A initial encounter
D subsequent encounter
S sequela

X32 Exposure to sunlight
X+7th
Excludes1: *man-made radiation (tanning bed) (W89)*
Excludes2: *radiation-related disorders of the skin and subcutaneous tissue (L55-L59)*

The appropriate 7th character is to be added to code X32
A initial encounter
D subsequent encounter
S sequela

X34 Earthquake
X+7th
Excludes2: *tidal wave (tsunami) due to earthquake (X37.41)*

The appropriate 7th character is to be added to code X34
A initial encounter
D subsequent encounter
S sequela

X35 Volcanic eruption
X+7th
Excludes2: *tidal wave (tsunami) due to volcanic eruption (X37.41)*

The appropriate 7th character is to be added to code X35
A initial encounter
D subsequent encounter
S sequela

X36 Avalanche, landslide and other earth movements
X+7th
Includes: victim of mudslide of cataclysmic nature
Excludes1: *earthquake (X34)*
Excludes2: *transport accident involving collision with avalanche or landslide not in motion (V01-V99)*

The appropriate 7th character is to be added to each code from category X36
A initial encounter
D subsequent encounter
S sequela

X36.0 Collapse of dam or man-made structure causing earth movement
X36.1 Avalanche, landslide, or mudslide

X37 Cataclysmic storm

The appropriate 7th character is to be added to each code from category X37
A initial encounter
D subsequent encounter
S sequela

X+7th **X37.0 Hurricane**
Storm surge
Typhoon
X+7th **X37.1 Tornado**
Cyclone
Twister
X+7th **X37.2 Blizzard (snow)(ice)**
X+7th **X37.3 Dust storm**
\+ **X37.4 Tidalwave**
X+7th **X37.41 Tidal wave due to earthquake or volcanic eruption**
Tidal wave NOS
Tsunami
X+7th **X37.42 Tidal wave due to storm**
X+7th **X37.43 Tidal wave due to landslide**
X+7th **X37.8 Other cataclysmic storms**
Cloudburst
Torrential rain
Excludes2: *flood (X38)*
X+7th **X37.9 Unspecified cataclysmic storm**
Storm NOS
Excludes1: *collapse of dam or man-made structure causing earth movement (X39.0)*

X38 Flood
X+7th
Flood arising from remote storm
Flood of cataclysmic nature arising from melting snow
Flood resulting directly from storm
Excludes1: *collapse of dam or man-made structure causing earth movement (X39.0)*
tidal wave NOS (X37.41)
tidal wave caused by storm (X37.2)

The appropriate 7th character is to be added to code X38
A initial encounter
D subsequent encounter
S sequela

X39 Exposure to other forces of nature

The appropriate 7th character is to be added to each code from category X39
A initial encounter
D subsequent encounter
S sequela

\+ **X39.0 Exposure to natural radiation**
Excludes1: *contact with and (suspected) exposure to radon and other naturally occuring radiation (Z77.123)*
exposure to man-made radiation (W88-W90)
exposure to sunlight (X32)
X+7th **X39.01 Exposure to radon**
X+7th **X39.08 Exposure to other natural radiation**
X+7th **X39.8 Other exposure to forces of nature**

Overexertion and strenuous or repetitive movements (X50)

X50 Overexertion and strenuous or repetitive movements
AHA CC: 4Q, 2016, 73-74

The appropriate 7th character is to be added to each code from category X50
A initial encounter
D subsequent encounter
S sequela

X+7th **X50.0 Overexertion from strenuous movement or load**
Lifting heavy objects
Lifting weights
X+7th **X50.1 Overexertion from prolonged static or awkward postures**
Prolonged bending
Prolonged kneeling
Prolonged reaching
Prolonged sitting
Prolonged standing
Prolonged twisting
Static bending
Static kneeling
Static reaching
Static sitting
Static standing
Static twisting
X+7th **X50.3 Overexertion from repetitive movements**
Use of hand as hammer.
Excludes2: Overuse from prolonged static or awkward postures (X50.1)
X+7th **X50.9 Other and unspecified overexertion or strenuous movements or postures**
Contact pressure
Contact stress

Accidental exposure to other specified factors (X52-X58)

X52 Prolonged stay in weightless environment
X+7th
Weightlessness in spacecraft (simulator)

The appropriate 7th character is to be added to code X52
A initial encounter
D subsequent encounter
S sequela

X58 Exposure to other specified factors
X+7th
Accident NOS
Exposure NOS

The appropriate 7th character is to be added to code X58
A initial encounter
D subsequent encounter
S sequela

Intentional self-harm (X71-X83)

Purposely self-inflicted injury
Suicide (attempted)

X71 Intentional self-harm by drowning and submersion

The appropriate 7th character is to be added to each code from category X71
A initial encounter
D subsequent encounter
S sequela

X+7th **X71.0 Intentional self-harm by drowning and submersion while in bathtub**
X+7th **X71.1 Intentional self-harm by drowning and submersion while in swimming pool**
X+7th **X71.2 Intentional self-harm by drowning and submersion after jump into swimming pool**
X+7th **X71.3 Intentional self-harm by drowning and submersion in natural water**
X+7th **X71.8 Other intentional self-harm by drowning and submersion**
X+7th **X71.9 Intentional self-harm by drowning and submersion, unspecified**

X72 Intentional self-harm by handgun discharge
X+7th

Intentional self-harm by gun for single hand use
Intentional self-harm by pistol
Intentional self-harm by revolver
Excludes1: *Very pistol (X74.8)*

The appropriate 7th character is to be added to code X72
A initial encounter
D subsequent encounter
S sequela

X73 Intentional self-harm by rifle, shotgun and larger firearm discharge
X+7th

Excludes1: *airgun (X74.01)*

The appropriate 7th character is to be added to each code from category X73
A initial encounter
D subsequent encounter
S sequela

X+7th **X73.0 Intentional self-harm by shotgun discharge**
X+7th **X73.1 Intentional self-harm by hunting rifle discharge**
X+7th **X73.2 Intentional self-harm by machine gun discharge**
X+7th **X73.8 Intentional self-harm by other larger firearm discharge**
X+7th **X73.9 Intentional self-harm by unspecified larger firearm discharge**

X74 Intentional self-harm by other and unspecified firearm and gun discharge

The appropriate 7th character is to be added to each code from category X74
A initial encounter
D subsequent encounter
S sequela

\+ **X74.0 Intentional self-harm by gas, air or spring-operated guns**
X+7th **X74.01 Intentional self-harm by airgun**
Intentional self-harm by BB gun discharge
Intentional self-harm by pellet gun discharge
X+7th **X74.02 Intentional self-harm by paintball gun**
X+7th **X74.09 Intentional self-harm by other gas, air or spring-operated gun**
X+7th **X74.8 Intentional self-harm by other firearm discharge**
Intentional self-harm by Very pistol [flare] discharge
X+7th **X74.9 Intentional self-harm by unspecified firearm discharge**

X75 Intentional self-harm by explosive material
X+7th

The appropriate 7th character is to be added to code X75
A initial encounter
D subsequent encounter
S sequela

X76 Intentional self-harm by smoke, fire and flames
X+7th

The appropriate 7th character is to be added to code X76
A initial encounter
D subsequent encounter
S sequela

X77 Intentional self-harm by steam, hot vapors and hot objects

The appropriate 7th character is to be added to each code from category X77
A initial encounter
D subsequent encounter
S sequela

X+7th **X77.0 Intentional self-harm by steam or hot vapors**
X+7th **X77.1 Intentional self-harm by hot tap water**
X+7th **X77.2 Intentional self-harm by other hot fluids**
X+7th **X77.3 Intentional self-harm by hot household appliances**
X+7th **X77.8 Intentional self-harm by other hot objects**
X+7th **X77.9 Intentional self-harm by unspecified hot objects**

X78 Intentional self-harm by sharp object

The appropriate 7th character is to be added to each code from category X78
A initial encounter
D subsequent encounter
S sequela

X+7th **X78.0 Intentional self-harm by sharp glass**
X+7th **X78.1 Intentional self-harm by knife**
X+7th **X78.2 Intentional self-harm by sword or dagger**
X+7th **X78.8 Intentional self-harm by other sharp object**
X+7th **X78.9 Intentional self-harm by unspecified sharp object**

X79 Intentional self-harm by blunt object
X+7th

The appropriate 7th character is to be added to code X79
A initial encounter
D subsequent encounter
S sequela

X80 Intentional self-harm by jumping from a high place
X+7th

Intentional fall from one level to another

The appropriate 7th character is to be added to code X80
A initial encounter
D subsequent encounter
S sequela

X81 Intentional self-harm by jumping or lying in front of moving object

The appropriate 7th character is to be added to each code from category X81
A initial encounter
D subsequent encounter
S sequela

X+7th **X81.0 Intentional self-harm by jumping or lying in front of motor vehicle**
X+7th **X81.1 Intentional self-harm by jumping or lying in front of (subway) train**
X+7th **X81.8 Intentional self-harm by jumping or lying in front of other moving object**

X82 Intentional self-harm by crashing of motor vehicle

The appropriate 7th character is to be added to each code from category X82
A initial encounter
D subsequent encounter
S sequela

X+7th **X82.0 Intentional collision of motor vehicle with other motor vehicle**
X+7th **X82.1 Intentional collision of motor vehicle with train**
X+7th **X82.2 Intentional collision of motor vehicle with tree**
X+7th **X82.8 Other intentional self-harm by crashing of motor vehicle**

X83 Intentional self-harm by other specified means

Excludes1: *intentional self-harm by poisoning or contact with toxic substance- See Table of Drugs and Chemicals*

The appropriate 7th character is to be added to each code from category X83
A initial encounter
D subsequent encounter
S sequela

X+7th **X83.0 Intentional self-harm by crashing of aircraft**
X+7th **X83.1 Intentional self-harm by electrocution**
X+7th **X83.2 Intentional self-harm by exposure to extremes of cold**
X+7th **X83.8 Intentional self-harm by other specified means**

Assault (X92-Y09)

Includes: homicide
injuries inflicted by another person with intent to injure or kill, by any means

Excludes1: *injuries due to legal intervention (Y35.-)*
injuries due to operations of war (Y36.-)
injuries due to terrorism (Y38.-)

Review coding guideline C.19.f

X92 Assault by drowning and submersion

The appropriate 7th character is to be added to each code from category X92
A initial encounter
D subsequent encounter
S sequela

X+7th **X92.0 Assault by drowning and submersion while in bathtub**
X+7th **X92.1 Assault by drowning and submersion while in swimming pool**
X+7th **X92.2 Assault by drowning and submersion after push into swimming pool**
X+7th **X92.3 Assault by drowning and submersion in natural water**
X+7th **X92.8 Other assault by drowning and submersion**
X+7th **X92.9 Assault by drowning and submersion, unspecified**

X93 Assault by handgun discharge
X+7th
Assault by discharge of gun for single hand use
Assault by discharge of pistol
Assault by discharge of revolver
Excludes1: *Very pistol (X95.8)*

The appropriate 7th character is to be added to code X93
A initial encounter
D subsequent encounter
S sequela

X94 Assault by rifle, shotgun and larger firearm discharge

Excludes1: *airgun (X95.01)*

The appropriate 7th character is to be added to each code from category X94
A initial encounter
D subsequent encounter
S sequela

X+7th **X94.0 Assault by shotgun**
X+7th **X94.1 Assault by hunting rifle**
X+7th **X94.2 Assault by machine gun**
X+7th **X94.8 Assault by other larger firearm discharge**
X+7th **X94.9 Assault by unspecified larger firearm discharge**

X95 Assault by other and unspecified firearm and gun discharge

The appropriate 7th character is to be added to each code from category X95
A initial encounter
D subsequent encounter
S sequela

\+ **X95.0 Assault by gas, air or spring-operated guns**
X+7th **X95.01 Assault by airgun discharge**
Assault by BB gun discharge
Assault by pellet gun discharge
X+7th **X95.02 Assault by paintball gun discharge**
X+7th **X95.09 Assault by other gas, air or spring-operated gun**
X+7th **X95.8 Assault by other firearm discharge**
Assault by very pistol [flare] discharge
X+7th **X95.9 Assault by unspecified firearm discharge**
AHA CC: 3Q, 2016, 24

X96 Assault by explosive material

Excludes1: *incendiary device (X97)*
terrorism involving explosive material (Y38.2-)

The appropriate 7th character is to be added to each code from category X96
A initial encounter
D subsequent encounter
S sequela

X+7th **X96.0 Assault by antipersonnel bomb**
Excludes1: *antipersonnel bomb use in military or war (Y36.2-)*
X+7th **X96.1 Assault by gasoline bomb**
X+7th **X96.2 Assault by letter bomb**
X+7th **X96.3 Assault by fertilizer bomb**
X+7th **X96.4 Assault by pipe bomb**
X+7th **X96.8 Assault by other specified explosive**
X+7th **X96.9 Assault by unspecified explosive**

X97 Assault by smoke, fire and flames
X+7th
Assault by arson
Assault by cigarettes
Assault by incendiary device

The appropriate 7th character is to be added to code X97
A initial encounter
D subsequent encounter
S sequela

X98 Assault by steam, hot vapors and hot objects

The appropriate 7th character is to be added to each code from category X98
A initial encounter
D subsequent encounter
S sequela

X+7th **X98.0 Assault by steam or hot vapors**
X+7th **X98.1 Assault by hot tap water**
X+7th **X98.2 Assault by hot fluids**
X+7th **X98.3 Assault by hot household appliances**
X+7th **X98.8 Assault by other hot objects**
X+7th **X98.9 Assault by unspecified hot objects**

X99 Assault by sharp object

Excludes1: *assault by strike by sports equipment (Y08.0-)*

The appropriate 7th character is to be added to each code from category X99
A initial encounter
D subsequent encounter
S sequela

X+7th **X99.0 Assault by sharp glass**
X+7th **X99.1 Assault by knife**
X+7th **X99.2 Assault by sword or dagger**
X+7th **X99.8 Assault by other sharp object**
X+7th **X99.9 Assault by unspecified sharp object**
Assault by stabbing NOS

Y00 Assault by blunt object
X+7th
Excludes1: *assault by strike by sports equipment (Y08.0-)*

The appropriate 7th character is to be added to code Y00
A initial encounter
D subsequent encounter
S sequela

Y01 Assault by pushing from high place
X+7th
The appropriate 7th character is to be added to code Y01
A initial encounter
D subsequent encounter
S sequela

Y02 Assault by pushing or placing victim in front of moving object

The appropriate 7th character is to be added to each code from category Y02
A initial encounter
D subsequent encounter
S sequela

X+7th **Y02.0 Assault by pushing or placing victim in front of motor vehicl**
X+7th **Y02.1 Assault by pushing or placing victim in front of (subway) tra**
X+7th **Y02.8 Assault by pushing or placing victim in front of other movin object**

Y03 Assault by crashing of motor vehicle

The appropriate 7th character is to be added to each code from catego Y03
A initial encounter
D subsequent encounter
S sequela

X+7th **Y03.0 Assault by being hit or run over by motor vehicle**
X+7th **Y03.8 Other assault by crashing of motor vehicle**

Y04 Assault by bodily force

Excludes1: *assault by:*
submersion (X92.-)
use of weapon (X93-X95, X99, Y00)

The appropriate 7th character is to be added to each code from category Y04
A initial encounter
D subsequent encounter
S sequela

X+7th **Y04.0 Assault by unarmed brawl or fight**

X+7th **Y04.1 Assault by human bite**
X+7th **Y04.2 Assault by strike against or bumped into by another person**
X+7th **Y04.8 Assault by other bodily force**
Assault by bodily force NOS

Y07 Perpetrator of assault, maltreatment and neglect

NOTE Codes from this category are for use only in cases of confirmed abuse (T74.-)
Selection of the correct perpetrator code is based on the relationship between the perpetrator and the victim

Includes: perpetrator of abandonment
perpetrator of emotional neglect
perpetrator of mental cruelty
perpetrator of physical abuse
perpetrator of physical neglect
perpetrator of sexual abuse
perpetrator of torture

Review coding guideline C.20.g

\+ **Y07.0 Spouse or partner, perpetrator of maltreatment and neglect**
Spouse or partner, perpetrator of maltreatment and neglect against spouse or partner
Y07.01 Husband, perpetrator of maltreatment and neglect
Y07.02 Wife, perpetrator of maltreatment and neglect
Y07.03 Male partner, perpetrator of maltreatment and neglect
Y07.04 Female partner, perpetrator of maltreatment and neglect

\+ **Y07.1 Parent (adoptive) (biological), perpetrator of maltreatment and neglect**
Y07.11 Biological father, perpetrator of maltreatment and neglect
Y07.12 Biological mother, perpetrator of maltreatment and neglect
Y07.13 Adoptive father, perpetrator of maltreatment and neglect
Y07.14 Adoptive mother, perpetrator of maltreatment and neglect

\+ **Y07.4 Other family member, perpetrator of maltreatment and neglect**
\+ **Y07.41 Sibling, perpetrator of maltreatment and neglect**
Excludes1: *stepsibling, perpetrator of maltreatment and neglect (Y07.435, Y07.436)*
Y07.410 Brother, perpetrator of maltreatment and neglect
Y07.411 Sister, perpetrator of maltreatment and neglect
\+ **Y07.42 Foster parent, perpetrator of maltreatment and neglect**
Y07.420 Foster father, perpetrator of maltreatment and neglect
Y07.421 Foster mother, perpetrator of maltreatment and neglect
\+ **Y07.43 Stepparent or stepsibling, perpetrator of maltreatment and neglect**
Y07.430 Stepfather, perpetrator of maltreatment and neglect
Y07.432 Male friend of parent (co-residing in household), perpetrator of maltreatment and neglect
Y07.433 Stepmother, perpetrator of maltreatment and neglect
Y07.434 Female friend of parent (co-residing in household), perpetrator of maltreatment and neglect
Y07.435 Stepbrother, perpetrator or maltreatment and neglect
Y07.436 Stepsister, perpetrator of maltreatment and neglect
\+ **Y07.49 Other family member, perpetrator of maltreatment and neglect**
Y07.490 Male cousin, perpetrator of maltreatment and neglect
Y07.491 Female cousin, perpetrator of maltreatment and neglect
Y07.499 Other family member, perpetrator of maltreatment and neglect

\+ **Y07.5 Non-family member, perpetrator of maltreatment and neglect**
Y07.50 Unspecified non-family member, perpetrator of maltreatment and neglect
\+ **Y07.51 Daycare provider, perpetrator of maltreatment and neglect**
Y07.510 At-home childcare provider, perpetrator of maltreatment and neglect
Y07.511 Daycare center childcare provider, perpetrator of maltreatment and neglect
Y07.512 At-home adultcare provider, perpetrator of maltreatment and neglect
Y07.513 Adultcare center provider, perpetrator of maltreatment and neglect
Y07.519 Unspecified daycare provider, perpetrator of maltreatment and neglect
\+ **Y07.52 Healthcare provider, perpetrator of maltreatment and neglect**
Y07.521 Mental health provider, perpetrator of maltreatment and neglect
Y07.528 Other therapist or healthcare provider, perpetrator of maltreatment and neglect
Nurse perpetrator of maltreatment and neglect
Occupational therapist perpetrator of maltreatment and neglect
Physical therapist perpetrator of maltreatment and neglect
Speech therapist perpetrator of maltreatment and neglect
Y07.529 Unspecified healthcare provider, perpetrator of maltreatment and neglect
Y07.53 Teacher or instructor, perpetrator of maltreatment and neglect
Coach, perpetrator of maltreatment and neglect
Y07.59 Other non-family member, perpetrator of maltreatment and neglect
Y07.9 Unspecified perpetrator of maltreatment and neglect

Y08 Assault by other specified means

The appropriate 7th character is to be added to each code from category Y08
A initial encounter
D subsequent encounter
S sequela

\+ **Y08.0 Assault by strike by sport equipment**
X+7th **Y08.01 Assault by strike by hockey stick**
X+7th **Y08.02 Assault by strike by baseball bat**
X+7th **Y08.09 Assault by strike by other specified type of sport equipment**
\+ **Y08.8 Assault by other specified means**
X+7th **Y08.81 Assault by crashing of aircraft**
X+7th **Y08.89 Assault by other specified means**

Y09 Assault by unspecified means

Assassination (attempted) NOS
Homicide (attempted) NOS
Manslaughter (attempted) NOS
Murder (attempted) NOS
Valid 3-character code, no further characters required

Event of undetermined intent (Y21-Y33)

Undetermined intent is only for use when there is specific documentation in the record that the intent of the injury cannot be determined. If no such documentation is present, code to accidental (unintentional)

Y21 Drowning and submersion, undetermined intent

The appropriate 7th character is to be added to each code from category Y21
A initial encounter
D subsequent encounter
S sequela

X+7th **Y21.0 Drowning and submersion while in bathtub, undetermined intent**
X+7th **Y21.1 Drowning and submersion after fall into bathtub, undetermined intent**
X+7th **Y21.2 Drowning and submersion while in swimming pool, undetermined intent**
X+7th **Y21.3 Drowning and submersion after fall into swimming pool, undetermined intent**
X+7th **Y21.4 Drowning and submersion in natural water, undetermined intent**
X+7th **Y21.8 Other drowning and submersion, undetermined intent**
X+7th **Y21.9 Unspecified drowning and submersion, undetermined intent**

X+7th **Y22 Handgun discharge, undetermined intent**

Discharge of gun for single hand use, undetermined intent
Discharge of pistol, undetermined intent
Discharge of revolver, undetermined intent
Excludes2: *very pistol (Y24.8)*

The appropriate 7th character is to be added to code Y22
A initial encounter
D subsequent encounter
S sequela

Y23 Rifle, shotgun and larger firearm discharge, undetermined intent

Excludes2: *airgun (Y24.0)*

The appropriate 7th character is to be added to each code from category Y23
A initial encounter
D subsequent encounter
S sequela

X+7th **Y23.0 Shotgun discharge, undetermined intent**
X+7th **Y23.1 Hunting rifle discharge, undetermined intent**
X+7th **Y23.2 Military firearm discharge, undetermined intent**
X+7th **Y23.3 Machine gun discharge, undetermined intent**
X+7th **Y23.8 Other larger firearm discharge, undetermined intent**
X+7th **Y23.9 Unspecified larger firearm discharge, undetermined intent**

Y24 Other and unspecified firearm discharge, undetermined intent

The appropriate 7th character is to be added to each code from category Y24
A initial encounter
D subsequent encounter
S sequela

X+7th **Y24.0 Airgun discharge, undetermined intent**
BB gun discharge, undetermined intent
Pellet gun discharge, undetermined intent
X+7th **Y24.8 Other firearm discharge, undetermined intent**
Paintball gun discharge, undetermined intent
Very pistol [flare] discharge, undetermined intent
X+7th **Y24.9 Unspecified firearm discharge, undetermined intent**

Y25 Contact with explosive material, undetermined intent
X+7th
The appropriate 7th character is to be added to code Y25
A initial encounter
D subsequent encounter
S sequela

Y26 Exposure to smoke, fire and flames, undetermined intent
X+7th
The appropriate 7th character is to be added to code Y26
A initial encounter
D subsequent encounter
S sequela

Y27 Contact with steam, hot vapors and hot objects, undetermined intent

The appropriate 7th character is to be added to each code from category Y27
A initial encounter
D subsequent encounter
S sequela

X+7th **Y27.0 Contact with steam and hot vapors, undetermined intent**
X+7th **Y27.1 Contact with hot tap water, undetermined intent**
X+7th **Y27.2 Contact with hot fluids, undetermined intent**
X+7th **Y27.3 Contact with hot household appliance, undetermined intent**
X+7th **Y27.8 Contact with other hot objects, undetermined intent**
X+7th **Y27.9 Contact with unspecified hot objects, undetermined intent**

Y28 Contact with sharp object, undetermined intent

The appropriate 7th character is to be added to each code from category Y28
A initial encounter
D subsequent encounter
S sequela

X+7th **Y28.0 Contact with sharp glass, undetermined intent**
X+7th **Y28.1 Contact with knife, undetermined intent**
X+7th **Y28.2 Contact with sword or dagger, undetermined intent**
X+7th **Y28.8 Contact with other sharp object, undetermined intent**
X+7th **Y28.9 Contact with unspecified sharp object, undetermined intent**

Y29 Contact with blunt object, undetermined intent
X+7th
The appropriate 7th character is to be added to code Y29
A initial encounter
D subsequent encounter
S sequela

Y30 Falling, jumping or pushed from a high place, undetermined intent
X+7th
Victim falling from one level to another, undetermined intent

The appropriate 7th character is to be added to code Y30
A initial encounter
D subsequent encounter
S sequela

Y31 Falling, lying or running before or into moving object, undetermined intent
X+7th

The appropriate 7th character is to be added to code Y31
A initial encounter
D subsequent encounter
S sequela

Y32 Crashing of motor vehicle, undetermined intent
X+7th
The appropriate 7th character is to be added to code Y32
A initial encounter
D subsequent encounter
S sequela

Y33 Other specified events, undetermined intent
X+7th
The appropriate 7th character is to be added to code Y33
A initial encounter
D subsequent encounter
S sequela

Legal intervention, operations of war, military operations, and terrorism (Y35-Y38)

Y35 Legal intervention

Includes: any injury sustained as a result of an encounter with any law enforcement official, serving in any capacity at the time of the encounter, whether on-duty or off-duty. Includes: a injury to law enforcement official, suspect and bystander

The appropriate 7th character is to be added to each code from category Y35
A initial encounter
D subsequent encounter
S sequela

\+ **Y35.0 Legal intervention involving firearm discharge**
\+ **Y35.00 Legal intervention involving unspecified firearm discharge**
Legal intervention involving gunshot wound
Legal intervention involving shot NOS
+7th **Y35.001 Legal intervention involving unspecified firearm discharge, law enforcement official injured**
+7th **Y35.002 Legal intervention involving unspecified firearm discharge, bystander injured**
+7th **Y35.003 Legal intervention involving unspecified firearm discharge, suspect injured**
\+ **Y35.01 Legal intervention involving injury by machine gun**
+7th **Y35.011 Legal intervention involving injury by machine gun, law enforcement official injured**
+7th **Y35.012 Legal intervention involving injury by machine gun, bystander injured**
+7th **Y35.013 Legal intervention involving injury by machine gun, suspect injured**
\+ **Y35.02 Legal intervention involving injury by handgun**
+7th **Y35.021 Legal intervention involving injury by handgun, law enforcement official injured**
+7th **Y35.022 Legal intervention involving injury by handgun, bystander injured**
+7th **Y35.023 Legal intervention involving injury by handgun, suspect injured**
\+ **Y35.03 Legal intervention involving injury by rifle pellet**
+7th **Y35.031 Legal intervention involving injury by rifle pellet, law enforcement official injured**
+7th **Y35.032 Legal intervention involving injury by rifle pellet, bystander injured**
+7th **Y35.033 Legal intervention involving injury by rifle pellet, suspect injured**
\+ **Y35.04 Legal intervention involving injury by rubber bullet**
+7th **Y35.041 Legal intervention involving injury by rubber bullet, law enforcement official injured**

+7th **Y35.042** **Legal intervention involving injury by rubber bullet, bystander injured**
+7th **Y35.043** **Legal intervention involving injury by rubber bullet, suspect injured**
\+ **Y35.09** **Legal intervention involving other firearm discharge**
+7th **Y35.091** **Legal intervention involving other firearm discharge, law enforcement official injured**
+7th **Y35.092** **Legal intervention involving other firearm discharge, bystander injured**
+7th **Y35.093** **Legal intervention involving other firearm discharge, suspect injured**
\+ **Y35.1** **Legal intervention involving explosives**
\+ **Y35.10** **Legal intervention involving unspecified explosives**
+7th **Y35.101** **Legal intervention involving unspecified explosives, law enforcement official injured**
+7th **Y35.102** **Legal intervention involving unspecified explosives, bystander injured**
+7th **Y35.103** **Legal intervention involving unspecified explosives, suspect injured**
\+ **Y35.11** **Legal intervention involving injury by dynamite**
+7th **Y35.111** **Legal intervention involving injury by dynamite, law enforcement official injured**
+7th **Y35.112** **Legal intervention involving injury by dynamite, bystander injured**
+7th **Y35.113** **Legal intervention involving injury by dynamite, suspect injured**
\+ **Y35.12** **Legal intervention involving injury by explosive shell**
+7th **Y35.121** **Legal intervention involving injury by explosive shell, law enforcement official injured**
+7th **Y35.122** **Legal intervention involving injury by explosive shell, bystander injured**
+7th **Y35.123** **Legal intervention involving injury by explosive shell, suspect injured**
\+ **Y35.19** **Legal intervention involving other explosives**
Legal intervention involving injury by grenade
Legal intervention involving injury by mortar bomb
+7th **Y35.191** **Legal intervention involving other explosives, law enforcement official injured**
+7th **Y35.192** **Legal intervention involving other explosives, bystander injured**
+7th **Y35.193** **Legal intervention involving other explosives, suspect injured**
\+ **Y35.2** **Legal intervention involving gas**
Legal intervention involving asphyxiation by gas
Legal intervention involving poisoning by gas
\+ **Y35.20** **Legal intervention involving unspecified gas**
+7th **Y35.201** **Legal intervention involving unspecified gas, law enforcement official injured**
+7th **Y35.202** **Legal intervention involving unspecified gas, bystander injured**
+7th **Y35.203** **Legal intervention involving unspecified gas, suspect injured**
\+ **Y35.21** **Legal intervention involving injury by tear gas**
+7th **Y35.211** **Legal intervention involving injury by tear gas, law enforcement official injured**
+7th **Y35.212** **Legal intervention involving injury by tear gas, bystander injured**
+7th **Y35.213** **Legal intervention involving injury by tear gas, suspect injured**
\+ **Y35.29** **Legal intervention involving other gas**
+7th **Y35.291** **Legal intervention involving other gas, law enforcement official injured**
+7th **Y35.292** **Legal intervention involving other gas, bystander injured**
+7th **Y35.293** **Legal intervention involving other gas, suspect injured**
\+ **Y35.3** **Legal intervention involving blunt objects**
Legal intervention involving being hit or struck by blunt object
\+ **Y35.30** **Legal intervention involving unspecified blunt objects**
+7th **Y35.301** **Legal intervention involving unspecified blunt objects, law enforcement official injured**
+7th **Y35.302** **Legal intervention involving unspecified blunt objects, bystander injured**
+7th **Y35.303** **Legal intervention involving unspecified blunt objects, suspect injured**
\+ **Y35.31** **Legal intervention involving baton**
+7th **Y35.311** **Legal intervention involving baton, law enforcement official injured**
+7th **Y35.312** **Legal intervention involving baton, bystander injured**
+7th **Y35.313** **Legal intervention involving baton, suspect injured**
\+ **Y35.39** **Legal intervention involving other blunt objects**
+7th **Y35.391** **Legal intervention involving other blunt objects, law enforcement official injured**
+7th **Y35.392** **Legal intervention involving other blunt objects, bystander injured**
+7th **Y35.393** **Legal intervention involving other blunt objects, suspect injured**
\+ **Y35.4** **Legal intervention involving sharp objects**
Legal intervention involving being cut by sharp objects
Legal intervention involving being stabbed by sharp objects
\+ **Y35.40** **Legal intervention involving unspecified sharp objects**
+7th **Y35.401** **Legal intervention involving unspecified sharp objects, law enforcement official injured**
+7th **Y35.402** **Legal intervention involving unspecified sharp objects, bystander injured**
+7th **Y35.403** **Legal intervention involving unspecified sharp objects, suspect injured**
\+ **Y35.41** **Legal intervention involving bayonet**
+7th **Y35.411** **Legal intervention involving bayonet, law enforcement official injured**
+7th **Y35.412** **Legal intervention involving bayonet, bystander injured**
+7th **Y35.413** **Legal intervention involving bayonet, suspect injured**
\+ **Y35.49** **Legal intervention involving other sharp objects**
+7th **Y35.491** **Legal intervention involving other sharp objects, law enforcement official injured**
+7th **Y35.492** **Legal intervention involving other sharp objects, bystander injured**
+7th **Y35.493** **Legal intervention involving other sharp objects, suspect injured**
\+ **Y35.8** **Legal intervention involving other specified means**
\+ **Y35.81** **Legal intervention involving manhandling**
+7th **Y35.811** **Legal intervention involving manhandling, law enforcement official injured**
+7th **Y35.812** **Legal intervention involving manhandling, bystander injured**
+7th **Y35.813** **Legal intervention involving manhandling, suspect injured**
\+ **Y35.89** **Legal intervention involving other specified means**
+7th **Y35.891** **Legal intervention involving other specified means, law enforcement official injured**
+7th **Y35.892** **Legal intervention involving other specified means, bystanderinjured**
+7th **Y35.893** **Legal intervention involving other specified means, suspect injured**
\+ **Y35.9** **Legal intervention, means unspecified**
X+7th **Y35.91** **Legal intervention, means unspecified, law enforcement official injured**
X+7th **Y35.92** **Legal intervention, means unspecified, bystander injured**
X+7th **Y35.93** **Legal intervention, means unspecified, suspect injured**

Y36 Operations of war

Includes: injuries to military personnel and civilians caused by war, civil insurrection, and peacekeeping missions

Excludes1: *injury to military personnel occurring during peacetime military operations (Y37.-)*

military vehicles involved in transport accidents with non-military vehicle during peacetime (V09.01, V09.21, V19.81, V29.81, V39.81, V49.81, V59.81, V69.81, V79.81)

AHA CC: 3Q, 2014, 4-5

The appropriate 7th character is to be added to each code from category Y36
A initial encounter
D subsequent encounter
S sequela

+ **Y36.0 War operations involving explosion of marine weapons**
+ **Y36.00 War operations involving explosion of unspecified marine weapon**
War operations involving underwater blast NOS
+7th **Y36.000 War operations involving explosion of unspecified marine weapon, military personnel**
+7th **Y36.001 War operations involving explosion of unspecified marine weapon, civilian**
+ **Y36.01 War operations involving explosion of depth-charge**
+7th **Y36.010 War operations involving explosion of depth-charge, military personnel**
+7th **Y36.011 War operations involving explosion of depth-charge, civilian**
+ **Y36.02 War operations involving explosion of marine mine**
War operations involving explosion of marine mine, at sea or in harbor
+7th **Y36.020 War operations involving explosion of marine mine, military personnel**
+7th **Y36.021 War operations involving explosion of marine mine, civilian**
+ **Y36.03 War operations involving explosion of sea-based artillery shell**
+7th **Y36.030 War operations involving explosion of sea-based artillery shell, military personnel**
+7th **Y36.031 War operations involving explosion of sea-based artillery shell, civilian**
+ **Y36.04 War operations involving explosion of torpedo**
+7th **Y36.040 War operations involving explosion of torpedo, military personnel**
+7th **Y36.041 War operations involving explosion of torpedo, civilian**
+ **Y36.05 War operations involving accidental detonation of onboard marine weapons**
+7th **Y36.050 War operations involving accidental detonation of onboard marine weapons, military personnel**
+7th **Y36.051 War operations involving accidental detonation of onboard marine weapons, civilian**
+ **Y36.09 War operations involving explosion of other marine weapons**
+7th **Y36.090 War operations involving explosion of other marine weapons, military personnel**
+7th **Y36.091 War operations involving explosion of other marine weapons, civilian**
+ **Y36.1 War operations involving destruction of aircraft**
+ **Y36.10 War operations involving unspecified destruction of aircraft**
+7th **Y36.100 War operations involving unspecified destruction of aircraft, military personnel**
+7th **Y36.101 War operations involving unspecified destruction of aircraft, civilian**
+ **Y36.11 War operations involving destruction of aircraft due to enemy fire or explosives**
War operations involving destruction of aircraft due to air to air missile
War operations involving destruction of aircraft due to explosive placed on aircraft
War operations involving destruction of aircraft due to rocket propelled grenade [RPG]
War operations involving destruction of aircraft due to small arms fire
War operations involving destruction of aircraft due to surface to air missile
+7th **Y36.110 War operations involving destruction of aircraft due to enemy fire or explosives, military personnel**
+7th **Y36.111 War operations involving destruction of aircraft due to enemy fire or explosives, civilian**
+ **Y36.12 War operations involving destruction of aircraft due to collision with other aircraft**
+7th **Y36.120 War operations involving destruction of aircraft due to collision with other aircraft military personnel**
+7th **Y36.121 War operations involving destruction of aircraft due to collision with other aircraft civilian**
+ **Y36.13 War operations involving destruction of aircraft due to onboard fire**
+7th **Y36.130 War operations involving destruction of aircraft due to onboard fire, military personnel**
+7th **Y36.131 War operations involving destruction of aircraft due to onboard fire, civilian**
+ **Y36.14 War operations involving destruction of aircraft due to accidental detonation of onboard munitions and explosives**
+7th **Y36.140 War operations involving destruction of aircraft due to accidental detonation of onboard munitions and explosives, militar personnel**
+7th **Y36.141 War operations involving destruction of aircraft due to accidental detonation of onboard munitions and explosives, civilian**
+ **Y36.19 War operations involving other destruction of aircra**
+7th **Y36.190 War operations involving other destructio of aircraft, military personnel**
+7th **Y36.191 War operations involving other destructio of aircraft, civilian**
+ **Y36.2 War operations involving other explosions and fragments**

Excludes1: *war operations involving explosion of aircraft (Y36.1-)*
war operations involving explosion of marine weapons (Y36.0-)
war operations involving explosion of nuclear weapons (Y36.5-)
war operations involving explosion occurring afte cessation of hostilities (Y36.8-)

+ **Y36.20 War operations involving unspecified explosion and fragments**
War operations involving air blast NOS
War operations involving blast NOS
War operations involving blast fragments NOS
War operations involving blast wave NOS
War operations involving blast wind NOS
War operations involving explosion NOS
War operations involving explosion of bomb NOS
+7th **Y36.200 War operations involving unspecified explosion and fragments, military personnel**
+7th **Y36.201 War operations involving unspecified explosion and fragments, civilian**
+ **Y36.21 War operations involving explosion of aerial bomb**
+7th **Y36.210 War operations involving explosion of aerial bomb, military personnel**
+7th **Y36.211 War operations involving explosion of aerial bomb, civilian**
+ **Y36.22 War operations involving explosion of guided missi**
+7th **Y36.220 War operations involving explosion of guided missile, military personnel**
+7th **Y36.221 War operations involving explosion of guided missile, civilian**
+ **Y36.23 War operations involving explosion of improvised explosive device [IED]**
War operations involving explosion of person-borne improvised explosive device [IED]
War operations involving explosion of vehicle-borne improvised explosive device [IED]
War operations involving explosion of roadside improvised explosive device [IED]

+7th **Y36.230 War operations involving explosion of improvised explosive device [IED], military personnel**
+7th **Y36.231 War operations involving explosion of improvised explosive device [IED], civilian**
+ **Y36.24 War operations involving explosion due to accidental detonation and discharge of own munitions or munitions launch device**
+7th **Y36.240 War operations involving explosion due to accidental detonation and discharge of own munitions or munitions launch device, military personnel**
+7th **Y36.241 War operations involving explosion due to accidental detonation and discharge of own munitions or munitions launch device, civilian**
+ **Y36.25 War operations involving fragments from munitions**
+7th **Y36.250 War operations involving fragments from munitions, military personnel**
+7th **Y36.251 War operations involving fragments from munitions, civilian**
+ **Y36.26 War operations involving fragments of improvised explosive device [IED]**
War operations involving fragments of person-borne improvised explosive device [IED]
War operations involving fragments of vehicle-borne improvised explosive device [IED]
War operations involving fragments of roadside improvised explosive device [IED]
+7th **Y36.260 War operations involving fragments of improvised explosive device [IED], military personnel**
+7th **Y36.261 War operations involving fragments of improvised explosive device [IED], civilian**
+ **Y36.27 War operations involving fragments from weapons**
+7th **Y36.270 War operations involving fragments from weapons, military personnel**
+7th **Y36.271 War operations involving fragments from weapons, civilian**
+ **Y36.29 War operations involving other explosions and fragments**
War operations involving explosion of grenade
War operations involving explosions of land mine
War operations involving shrapnel NOS
+7th **Y36.290 War operations involving other explosions and fragments, military personnel**
+7th **Y36.291 War operations involving other explosions and fragments, civilian**
+ **Y36.3 War operations involving fires, conflagrations and hot substances**
War operations involving smoke, fumes, and heat from fires, conflagrations and hot substances
Excludes1: *war operations involving fires and conflagrations aboard military aircraft (Y36.1-)*
war operations involving fires and conflagrations aboard military watercraft (Y36.0-)
war operations involving fires and conflagrations caused indirectly by conventional weapons (Y36.2-)
war operations involving fires and thermal effects of nuclear weapons (Y36.53-)
+ **Y36.30 War operations involving unspecified fire, conflagration and hot substance**
+7th **Y36.300 War operations involving unspecified fire, conflagration and hot substance, military personnel**
+7th **Y36.301 War operations involving unspecified fire, conflagration and hot substance, civilian**
+ **Y36.31 War operations involving gasoline bomb**
War operations involving incendiary bomb
War operations involving petrol bomb
+7th **Y36.310 War operations involving gasoline bomb, military personnel**
+7th **Y36.311 War operations involving gasoline bomb, civilian**
+ **Y36.32 War operations involving incendiary bullet**
+7th **Y36.320 War operations involving incendiary bullet, military personnel**
+7th **Y36.321 War operations involving incendiary bullet, civilian**
+ **Y36.33 War operations involving flamethrower**
+7th **Y36.330 War operations involving flamethrower, military personnel**
+7th **Y36.331 War operations involving flamethrower, civilian**
+ **Y36.39 War operations involving other fires, conflagrations and hot substances**
+7th **Y36.390 War operations involving other fires, conflagrations and hot substances, military personnel**
+7th **Y36.391 War operations involving other fires, conflagrations and hot substances, civilian**
+ **Y36.4 War operations involving firearm discharge and other forms of conventional warfare**
+ **Y36.41 War operations involving rubber bullets**
+7th **Y36.410 War operations involving rubber bullets, military personnel**
+7th **Y36.411 War operations involving rubber bullets, civilian**
+ **Y36.42 War operations involving firearms pellets**
+7th **Y36.420 War operations involving firearms pellets, military personnel**
+7th **Y36.421 War operations involving firearms pellets, civilian**
+ **Y36.43 War operations involving other firearms discharge**
War operations involving bullets NOS
Excludes1: *war operations involving munitions fragments (Y36.25-)*
war operations involving incendiary bullets (Y36.32-)
+7th **Y36.430 War operations involving other firearms discharge, military personnel**
+7th **Y36.431 War operations involving other firearms discharge, civilian**
+ **Y36.44 War operations involving unarmed hand to hand combat**
Excludes1: *war operations involving combat using blunt or piercing object (Y36.45-)*
war operations involving intentional restriction of air and airway (Y36.46-)
war operations involving unintentional restriction of air and airway (Y36.47-)
+7th **Y36.440 War operations involving unarmed hand to hand combat, military personnel**
+7th **Y36.441 War operations involving unarmed hand to hand combat, civilian**
+ **Y36.45 War operations involving combat using blunt or piercing object**
+7th **Y36.450 War operations involving combat using blunt or piercing object, military personnel**
+7th **Y36.451 War operations involving combat using blunt or piercing object, civilian**
+ **Y36.46 War operations involving intentional restriction of air and airway**
+7th **Y36.460 War operations involving intentional restriction of air and airway, military personnel**
+7th **Y36.461 War operations involving intentional restriction of air and airway, civilian**
+ **Y36.47 War operations involving unintentional restriction of air and airway**
+7th **Y36.470 War operations involving unintentional restriction of air and airway, military personnel**
+7th **Y36.471 War operations involving unintentional restriction of air and airway, civilian**
+ **Y36.49 War operations involving other forms of conventional warfare**
+7th **Y36.490 War operations involving other forms of conventional warfare, military personnel**
+7th **Y36.491 War operations involving other forms of conventional warfare, civilian**
+ **Y36.5 War operations involving nuclear weapons**
War operations involving dirty bomb NOS
+ **Y36.50 War operations involving unspecified effect of nuclear weapon**
+7th **Y36.500 War operations involving unspecified effect of nuclear weapon, military personnel**
+7th **Y36.501 War operations involving unspecified effect of nuclear weapon, civilian**

+ **Y36.51 War operations involving direct blast effect of nuclear weapon**
  War operations involving blast pressure of nuclear weapon
  - +7th **Y36.510 War operations involving direct blast effect of nuclear weapon, military personnel**
  - +7th **Y36.511 War operations involving direct blast effect of nuclear weapon, civilian**

+ **Y36.52 War operations involving indirect blast effect of nuclear weapon**
  War operations involving being thrown by blast of nuclear weapon
  War operations involving being struck or crushed by blast debris of nuclear weapon
  - +7th **Y36.520 War operations involving indirect blast effect of nuclear weapon, military personnel**
  - +7th **Y36.521 War operations involving indirect blast effect of nuclear weapon, civilian**

+ **Y36.53 War operations involving thermal radiation effect of nuclear weapon**
  War operations involving direct heat from nuclear weapon
  War operation involving fireball effects from nuclear weapon
  - +7th **Y36.530 War operations involving thermal radiation effect of nuclear weapon, military personnel**
  - +7th **Y36.531 War operations involving thermal radiation effect of nuclear weapon, civilian**

+ **Y36.54 War operation involving nuclear radiation effects of nuclear weapon**
  War operation involving acute radiation exposure from nuclear weapon
  War operation involving exposure to immediate ionizing radiation from nuclear weapon
  War operation involving fallout exposure from nuclear weapon
  War operation involving secondary effects of nuclear weapons
  - +7th **Y36.540 War operation involving nuclear radiation effects of nuclear weapon, military personnel**
  - +7th **Y36.541 War operation involving nuclear radiation effects of nuclear weapon, civilian**

+ **Y36.59 War operation involving other effects of nuclear weapons**
  - +7th **Y36.590 War operation involving other effects of nuclear weapons, military personnel**
  - +7th **Y36.591 War operation involving other effects of nuclear weapons, civilian**

+ **Y36.6 War operations involving biological weapons**
  + **Y36.6X War operations involving biological weapons**
    - +7th **Y36.6X0 War operations involving biological weapons, military personnel**
    - +7th **Y36.6X1 War operations involving biological weapons, civilian**

+ **Y36.7 War operations involving chemical weapons and other forms of unconventional warfare**
  Excludes1: *war operations involving incendiary devices (Y36.3-, Y36.5-)*
  + **Y36.7X War operations involving chemical weapons and other forms of unconventional warfare**
    - +7th **Y36.7X0 War operations involving chemical weapons and other forms of unconventional warfare, military personnel**
    - +7th **Y36.7X1 War operations involving chemical weapons and other forms of unconventional warfare, civilian**

+ **Y36.8 War operations occurring after cessation of hostilities**
  War operations classifiable to categories Y36.0-Y36.8 but occurring after cessation of hostilities
  + **Y36.81 Explosion of mine placed during war operations but exploding after cessation of hostilities**
    - +7th **Y36.810 Explosion of mine placed during war operations but exploding after cessation of hostilities, military personnel**
    - +7th **Y36.811 Explosion of mine placed during war operations but exploding after cessation of hostilities, civilian**
  + **Y36.82 Explosion of bomb placed during war operations but exploding after cessation of hostilities**
    - +7th **Y36.820 Explosion of bomb placed during war operations but exploding after cessation of hostilities, military personnel**
    - +7th **Y36.821 Explosion of bomb placed during war operations but exploding after cessation of hostilities, civilian**
  + **Y36.88 Other war operations occurring after cessation of hostilities**
    - +7th **Y36.880 Other war operations occurring after cessation of hostilities, military personnel**
    - +7th **Y36.881 Other war operations occurring after cessation of hostilities, civilian**
  + **Y36.89 Unspecified war operations occurring after cessation of hostilities**
    - +7th **Y36.890 Unspecified war operations occurring after cessation of hostilities, military personnel**
    - +7th **Y36.891 Unspecified war operations occurring after cessation of hostilities, civilian**

+ **Y36.9 Other and unspecified war operations**
  - X+7th **Y36.90 War operations, unspecified**
  - X+7th **Y36.91 War operations involving unspecified weapon of mass destruction [WMD]**
  - X+7th **Y36.92 War operations involving friendly fire**

Y37 Military operations

Includes: injuries to military personnel and civilians occurring during peacetime on military property and during routine military exercises and operations

Excludes1: *military aircraft involved in aircraft accident with civilian aircraft (V97.81-)*
military vehicles involved in transport accident with civilian vehicle (V09.01, V09.21, V19.81, V29.81, V39.81, V49.81, V59.81, V69.81, V79.81)
military watercraft involved in water transport accident with civilian watercraft (V94.81-)
war operations (Y36.-)

The appropriate 7th character is to be added to each code from category Y37
A initial encounter
D subsequent encounter
S sequela

+ **Y37.0 Military operations involving explosion of marine weapons**
  + **Y37.00 Military operations involving explosion of unspecified marine weapon**
    Military operations involving underwater blast NOS
    - +7th **Y37.000 Military operations involving explosion of unspecified marine weapon, military personnel**
    - +7th **Y37.001 Military operations involving explosion of unspecified marine weapon, civilian**
  + **Y37.01 Military operations involving explosion of depth-charge**
    - +7th **Y37.010 Military operations involving explosion of depth-charge, military personnel**
    - +7th **Y37.011 Military operations involving explosion of depth-charge, civilian**
  + **Y37.02 Military operations involving explosion of marine mine**
    Military operations involving explosion of marine mine, at sea or in harbor
    - +7th **Y37.020 Military operations involving explosion of marine mine, military personnel**
    - +7th **Y37.021 Military operations involving explosion of marine mine, civilian**
  + **Y37.03 Military operations involving explosion of sea-based artillery shell**
    - +7th **Y37.030 Military operations involving explosion of sea-based artillery shell, military personnel**
    - +7th **Y37.031 Military operations involving explosion of sea-based artillery shell, civilian**
  + **Y37.04 Military operations involving explosion of torpedo**
    - +7th **Y37.040 Military operations involving explosion of torpedo, military personnel**
    - +7th **Y37.041 Military operations involving explosion of torpedo, civilian**

+ **Y37.05 Military operations involving accidental detonation of onboard marine weapons**
  - +7th **Y37.050 Military operations involving accidental detonation of onboard marine weapons, military personnel**
  - +7th **Y37.051 Military operations involving accidental detonation of onboard marine weapons, civilian**

+ **Y37.09 Military operations involving explosion of other marine weapons**
  - +7th **Y37.090 Military operations involving explosion of other marine weapons, military personnel**
  - +7th **Y37.091 Military operations involving explosion of other marine weapons, civilian**

+ **Y37.1 Military operations involving destruction of aircraft**

+ **Y37.10 Military operations involving unspecified destruction of aircraft**
  - +7th **Y37.100 Military operations involving unspecified destruction of aircraft, military personnel**
  - +7th **Y37.101 Military operations involving unspecified destruction of aircraft, civilian**

+ **Y37.11 Military operations involving destruction of aircraft due to enemy fire or explosives**

  Military operations involving destruction of aircraft due to air to air missile
  Military operations involving destruction of aircraft due to explosive placed on aircraft
  Military operations involving destruction of aircraft due to rocket propelled grenade [RPG]
  Military operations involving destruction of aircraft due to small arms fire
  Military operations involving destruction of aircraft due to surface to air missile
  - +7th **Y37.110 Military operations involving destruction of aircraft due to enemy fire or explosives, military personnel**
  - +7th **Y37.111 Military operations involving destruction of aircraft due to enemy fire or explosives, civilian**

+ **Y37.12 Military operations involving destruction of aircraft due to collision with other aircraft**
  - +7th **Y37.120 Military operations involving destruction of aircraft due to collision with other aircraft, military personnel**
  - +7th **Y37.121 Military operations involving destruction of aircraft due to collision with other aircraft, civilian**

+ **Y37.13 Military operations involving destruction of aircraft due to onboard fire**
  - +7th **Y37.130 Military operations involving destruction of aircraft due to onboard fire, military personnel**
  - +7th **Y37.131 Military operations involving destruction of aircraft due to onboard fire, civilian**

+ **Y37.14 Military operations involving destruction of aircraft due to accidental detonation of onboard munitions and explosives**
  - +7th **Y37.140 Military operations involving destruction of aircraft due to accidental detonation of onboard munitions and explosives, military personnel**
  - +7th **Y37.141 Military operations involving destruction of aircraft due to accidental detonation of onboard munitions and explosives, civilian**

+ **Y37.19 Military operations involving other destruction of aircraft**
  - +7th **Y37.190 Military operations involving other destruction of aircraft, military personnel**
  - +7th **Y37.191 Military operations involving other destruction of aircraft, civilian**

+ **Y37.2 Military operations involving other explosions and fragments**

  Excludes1: *military operations involving explosion of aircraft (Y37.1-)*
  military operations involving explosion of marine weapons (Y37.0-)
  military operations involving explosion of nuclear weapons (Y37.5-)

+ **Y37.20 Military operations involving unspecified explosion and fragments**

  Military operations involving air blast NOS
  Military operations involving blast NOS
  Military operations involving blast fragments NOS
  Military operations involving blast wave NOS
  Military operations involving blast wind NOS
  Military operations involving explosion NOS
  Military operations involving explosion of bomb NOS
  - +7th **Y37.200 Military operations involving unspecified explosion and fragments, military personnel**
  - +7th **Y37.201 Military operations involving unspecified explosion and fragments, civilian**

+ **Y37.21 Military operations involving explosion of aerial bomb**
  - +7th **Y37.210 Military operations involving explosion of aerial bomb, military personnel**
  - +7th **Y37.211 Military operations involving explosion of aerial bomb, civilian**

+ **Y37.22 Military operations involving explosion of guided missile**
  - +7th **Y37.220 Military operations involving explosion of guided missile, military personnel**
  - +7th **Y37.221 Military operations involving explosion of guided missile, civilian**

+ **Y37.23 Military operations involving explosion of improvised explosive device [IED]**

  Military operations involving explosion of person-borne improvised explosive device [IED]
  Military operations involving explosion of vehicle-borne improvised explosive device [IED]
  Military operations involving explosion of roadside improvised explosive device [IED]
  - +7th **Y37.230 Military operations involving explosion of improvised explosive device [IED], military personnel**
  - +7th **Y37.231 Military operations involving explosion of improvised explosive device [IED], civilian**

+ **Y37.24 Military operations involving explosion due to accidental detonation and discharge of own munitions or munitions launch device**
  - +7th **Y37.240 Military operations involving explosion due to accidental detonation and discharge of own munitions or munitions launch device, military personnel**
  - +7th **Y37.241 Military operations involving explosion due to accidental detonation and discharge of own munitions or munitions launch device, civilian**

+ **Y37.25 Military operations involving fragments from munitions**
  - +7th **Y37.250 Military operations involving fragments from munitions, military personnel**
  - +7th **Y37.251 Military operations involving fragments from munitions, civilian**

+ **Y37.26 Military operations involving fragments of improvised explosive device [IED]**

  Military operations involving fragments of person-borne improvised explosive device [IED]
  Military operations involving fragments of vehicle-borne improvised explosive device [IED]
  Military operations involving fragments of roadside improvised explosive device [IED]
  - +7th **Y37.260 Military operations involving fragments of improvised explosive device [IED], military personnel**
  - +7th **Y37.261 Military operations involving fragments of improvised explosive device [IED], civilian**

+ **Y37.27 Military operations involving fragments from weapons**
  - +7th **Y37.270 Military operations involving fragments from weapons, military personnel**
  - +7th **Y37.271 Military operations involving fragments from weapons, civilian**

+ **Y37.29 Military operations involving other explosions and fragments**

  Military operations involving explosion of grenade
  Military operations involving explosions of land mine
  Military operations involving shrapnel NOS
  - +7th **Y37.290 Military operations involving other explosions and fragments, military personnel**

+7th **Y37.291 Military operations involving other explosions and fragments,civilian**

\+ **Y37.3 Military operations involving fires, conflagrations and hot substances**

Military operations involving smoke, fumes, and heat from fires, conflagrations and hot substances

Excludes1: *military operations involving fires and conflagrations aboard military aircraft (Y37.1-)*
military operations involving fires and conflagrations aboard military watercraft (Y37.0-)
military operations involving fires and conflagrations caused indirectly by conventional weapons (Y37.2-)
military operations involving fires and thermal effects of nuclear weapons (Y36.53-)

\+ **Y37.30 Military operations involving unspecified fire, conflagration and hot substance**

+7th **Y37.300 Military operations involving unspecified fire, conflagration and hot substance, military personnel**

+7th **Y37.301 Military operations involving unspecified fire, conflagration and hot substance, civilian**

\+ **Y37.31 Military operations involving gasoline bomb**

Military operations involving incendiary bomb
Military operations involving petrol bomb

+7th **Y37.310 Military operations involving gasoline bomb, military personnel**

+7th **Y37.311 Military operations involving gasoline bomb, civilian**

\+ **Y37.32 Military operations involving incendiary bullet**

+7th **Y37.320 Military operations involving incendiary bullet, military personnel**

+7th **Y37.321 Military operations involving incendiary bullet, civilian**

\+ **Y37.33 Military operations involving flamethrower**

+7th **Y37.330 Military operations involving flamethrower, military personnel**

+7th **Y37.331 Military operations involving flamethrower, civilian**

\+ **Y37.39 Military operations involving other fires, conflagrations and hot substances**

+7th **Y37.390 Military operations involving other fires, conflagrations and hot substances, military personnel**

+7th **Y37.391 Military operations involving other fires, conflagrations and hot substances, civilian**

\+ **Y37.4 Military operations involving firearm discharge and other forms of conventional warfare**

\+ **Y37.41 Military operations involving rubber bullets**

+7th **Y37.410 Military operations involving rubber bullets, military personnel**

+7th **Y37.411 Military operations involving rubber bullets, civilian**

\+ **Y37.42 Military operations involving firearms pellets**

+7th **Y37.420 Military operations involving firearms pellets, military personnel**

+7th **Y37.421 Military operations involving firearms pellets, civilian**

\+ **Y37.43 Military operations involving other firearms discharge**

Military operations involving bullets NOS

Excludes1: *military operations involving munitions fragments (Y37.25-)*
military operations involving incendiary bullets (Y37.32-)

+7th **Y37.430 Military operations involving other firearms discharge, military personnel**

+7th **Y37.431 Military operations involving other firearms discharge, civilian**

\+ **Y37.44 Military operations involving unarmed hand to hand combat**

Excludes1: *military operations involving combat using blunt or piercing object (Y37.45-)*
military operations involving intentional restriction of air and airway (Y37.46-)
military operations involving unintentional restriction of air and airway (Y37.47-)

+7th **Y37.440 Military operations involving unarmed hand to hand combat, military personnel**

+7th **Y37.441 Military operations involving unarmed hand to hand combat, civilian**

\+ **Y37.45 Military operations involving combat using blunt or piercing object**

+7th **Y37.450 Military operations involving combat using blunt or piercing object, military personnel**

+7th **Y37.451 Military operations involving combat using blunt or piercing object, civilian**

\+ **Y37.46 Military operations involving intentional restriction of air and airway**

+7th **Y37.460 Military operations involving intentional restriction of air and airway, military personnel**

+7th **Y37.461 Military operations involving intentional restriction of air and airway, civilian**

\+ **Y37.47 Military operations involving unintentional restriction of air and airway**

+7th **Y37.470 Military operations involving unintentional restriction of air and airway, military personnel**

+7th **Y37.471 Military operations involving unintentional restriction of air and airway, civilian**

\+ **Y37.49 Military operations involving other forms of conventional warfare**

+7th **Y37.490 Military operations involving other forms of conventional warfare, military personnel**

+7th **Y37.491 Military operations involving other forms of conventional warfare, civilian**

\+ **Y37.5 Military operations involving nuclear weapons**

Military operation involving dirty bomb NOS

\+ **Y37.50 Military operations involving unspecified effect of nuclear weapon**

+7th **Y37.500 Military operations involving unspecified effect of nuclear weapon, military personnel**

+7th **Y37.501 Military operations involving unspecified effect of nuclear weapon, civilian**

\+ **Y37.51 Military operations involving direct blast effect of nuclear weapon**

Military operations involving blast pressure of nuclear weapon

+7th **Y37.510 Military operations involving direct blast effect of nuclear weapon, military personnel**

+7th **Y37.511 Military operations involving direct blast effect of nuclear weapon, civilian**

\+ **Y37.52 Military operations involving indirect blast effect of nuclear weapon**

Military operations involving being thrown by blast of nuclear weapon
Military operations involving being struck or crushed by blast debris of nuclear weapon

+7th **Y37.520 Military operations involving indirect blast effect of nuclear weapon, military personnel**

+7th **Y37.521 Military operations involving indirect blast effect of nuclear weapon, civilian**

\+ **Y37.53 Military operations involving thermal radiation effect of nuclear weapon**

Military operations involving direct heat from nuclear weapon
Military operation involving fireball effects from nuclear weapon

+7th **Y37.530 Military operations involving thermal radiation effect of nuclear weapon, military personnel**

+7th **Y37.531 Military operations involving thermal radiation effect of nuclear weapon, civilian**

\+ **Y37.54 Military operation involving nuclear radiation effects of nuclear weapon**

Military operation involving acute radiation exposure from nuclear weapon
Military operation involving exposure to immediate ionizing radiation from nuclear weapon
Military operation involving fallout exposure from nuclear weapon
Military operation involving secondary effects of nuclear weapons

+7th **Y37.540 Military operation involving nuclear radiation effects of nuclear weapon, military personnel**

+7th **Y37.541 Military operation involving nuclear radiation effects of nuclear weapon, civilian**

+ **Y37.59 Military operation involving other effects of nuclear weapons**

+7th **Y37.590 Military operation involving other effects of nuclear weapons, military personnel**

+7th **Y37.591 Military operation involving other effects of nuclear weapons, civilian**

+ **Y37.6 Military operations involving biological weapons**

+ **Y37.6X Military operations involving biological weapons**

+7th **Y37.6X0 Military operations involving biological weapons, military personnel**

+7th **Y37.6X1 Military operations involving biological weapons, civilian**

+ **Y37.7 Military operations involving chemical weapons and other forms of unconventional warfare**

Excludes1: *military operations involving incendiary devices (Y36.3-, Y36.5-)*

+ **Y37.7X Military operations involving chemical weapons and other forms of unconventional warfare**

+7th **Y37.7X0 Military operations involving chemical weapons and other forms of unconventional warfare, military personnel**

+7th **Y37.7X1 Military operations involving chemical weapons and other forms of unconventional warfare, civilian**

+ **Y37.9 Other and unspecified military operations**

X+7th **Y37.90 Military operations, unspecified**

X+7th **Y37.91 Military operations involving unspecified weapon of mass destruction [WMD]**

X+7th **Y37.92 Military operations involving friendly fire**

Y38 Terrorism

These codes are for use to identify injuries resulting from the unlawful use of force or violence against persons or property to intimidate or coerce a Government, the civilian population, or any segment thereof, in furtherance of political or social objective

Use additional code for place of occurrence (Y92.-)

The appropriate 7th character is to be added to each code from category Y38
A initial encounter
D subsequent encounter
S sequela

Review coding guideline C.20.j

+ **Y38.0 Terrorism involving explosion of marine weapons**

Terrorism involving depth-charge
Terrorism involving marine mine
Terrorism involving mine NOS, at sea or in harbor
Terrorism involving sea-based artillery shell
Terrorism involving torpedo
Terrorism involving underwater blast

+ **Y38.0X Terrorism involving explosion of marine weapons**

+7th **Y38.0X1 Terrorism involving explosion of marine weapons, public safety official injured**

+7th **Y38.0X2 Terrorism involving explosion of marine weapons, civilian injured**

+7th **Y38.0X3 Terrorism involving explosion of marine weapons, terrorist injured**

+ **Y38.1 Terrorism involving destruction of aircraft**

Terrorism involving aircraft burned
Terrorism involving aircraft exploded
Terrorism involving aircraft being shot down
Terrorism involving aircraft used as a weapon

+ **Y38.1X Terrorism involving destruction of aircraft**

+7th **Y38.1X1 Terrorism involving destruction of aircraft, public safety official injured**

+7th **Y38.1X2 Terrorism involving destruction of aircraft, civilian injured**

+7th **Y38.1X3 Terrorism involving destruction of aircraft, terrorist injured**

+ **Y38.2 Terrorism involving other explosions and fragments**

Terrorism involving antipersonnel (fragments) bomb
Terrorism involving blast NOS
Terrorism involving explosion NOS
Terrorism involving explosion of breech block
Terrorism involving explosion of cannon block
Terrorism involving explosion (fragments) of artillery shell
Terrorism involving explosion (fragments) of bomb
Terrorism involving explosion (fragments) of grenade
Terrorism involving explosion (fragments) of guided missile
Terrorism involving explosion (fragments) of land mine
Terrorism involving explosion of mortar bomb
Terrorism involving explosion of munitions
Terrorism involving explosion (fragments) of rocket
Terrorism involving explosion (fragments) of shell
Terrorism involving shrapnel
Terrorism involving mine NOS, on land

Excludes1: *terrorism involving explosion of nuclear weapon (Y38.5)*
terrorism involving suicide bomber (Y38.81)

+ **Y38.2X Terrorism involving other explosions and fragments**

+7th **Y38.2X1 Terrorism involving other explosions and fragments, public safety official injured**

+7th **Y38.2X2 Terrorism involving other explosions and fragments, civilian injured**

+7th **Y38.2X3 Terrorism involving other explosions and fragments, terrorist injured**

+ **Y38.3 Terrorism involving fires, conflagration and hot substances**

Terrorism involving conflagration NOS
Terrorism involving fire NOS
Terrorism involving petrol bomb

Excludes1: *terrorism involving fire or heat of nuclear weapon (Y38.5)*

+ **Y38.3X Terrorism involving fires, conflagration and hot substances**

+7th **Y38.3X1 Terrorism involving fires, conflagration and hot substances, public safety official injured**

+7th **Y38.3X2 Terrorism involving fires, conflagration and hot substances, civilian injured**

+7th **Y38.3X3 Terrorism involving fires, conflagration and hot substances, terrorist injured**

+ **Y38.4 Terrorism involving firearms**

Terrorism involving carbine bullet
Terrorism involving machine gun bullet
Terrorism involving pellets (shotgun)
Terrorism involving pistol bullet
Terrorism involving rifle bullet
Terrorism involving rubber (rifle) bullet

+ **Y38.4X Terrorism involving firearms**

+7th **Y38.4X1 Terrorism involving firearms, public safety official injured**

+7th **Y38.4X2 Terrorism involving firearms, civilian injured**

+7th **Y38.4X3 Terrorism involving firearms, terrorist injured**

+ **Y38.5 Terrorism involving nuclear weapons**

Terrorism involving blast effects of nuclear weapon
Terrorism involving exposure to ionizing radiation from nuclear weapon
Terrorism involving fireball effect of nuclear weapon
Terrorism involving heat from nuclear weapon

+ **Y38.5X Terrorism involving nuclear weapons**

+7th **Y38.5X1 Terrorism involving nuclear weapons, public safety official injured**

+7th **Y38.5X2 Terrorism involving nuclear weapons, civilian injured**

+7th **Y38.5X3 Terrorism involving nuclear weapons, terrorist injured**

+ **Y38.6 Terrorism involving biological weapons**

Terrorism involving anthrax
Terrorism involving cholera
Terrorism involving smallpox

+ **Y38.6X Terrorism involving biological weapons**

+7th **Y38.6X1 Terrorism involving biological weapons, public safety official injured**

+7th **Y38.6X2 Terrorism involving biological weapons, civilian injured**

+7th **Y38.6X3 Terrorism involving biological weapons, terrorist injured**

+ Y38.7 **Terrorism involving chemical weapons**
  Terrorism involving gases, fumes, chemicals
  Terrorism involving hydrogen cyanide
  Terrorism involving phosgene
  Terrorism involving sarin
  + Y38.7X **Terrorism involving chemical weapons**
    +7th Y38.7X1 **Terrorism involving chemical weapons, public safety official injured**
    +7th Y38.7X2 **Terrorism involving chemical weapons, civilian injured**
    +7th Y38.7X3 **Terrorism involving chemical weapons, terrorist injured**
+ Y38.8 **Terrorism involving other and unspecified means**
  X+7th Y38.80 **Terrorism involving unspecified means**
    Terrorism NOS
  + Y38.81 **Terrorism involving suicide bomber**
    +7th Y38.811 **Terrorism involving suicide bomber, public safety official injured**
    +7th Y38.812 **Terrorism involving suicide bomber, civilian injured**
  + Y38.89 **Terrorism involving other means**
    Terrorism involving drowning and submersion
    Terrorism involving lasers
    Terrorism involving piercing or stabbing instruments
    +7th Y38.891 **Terrorism involving other means, public safety official injured**
    +7th Y38.892 **Terrorism involving other means, civilian injured**
    +7th Y38.893 **Terrorism involving other means, terrorist injured**
+ Y38.9 **Terrorism, secondary effects**
  NOTE This code is for use to identify conditions occurring subsequent to a terrorist attack not those that are due to the initial terrorist attack
  + Y38.9X **Terrorism, secondary effects**
    +7th Y38.9X1 **Terrorism, secondary effects, public safety official injured**
    +7th Y38.9X2 **Terrorism, secondary effects, civilian injured**

Complications of medical and surgical care (Y62-Y84)

Includes: complications of medical devices surgical and medical procedures as the cause of abnormal reaction of the patient, or of later complication, without mention of misadventure at the time of the procedure

Misadventures to patients during surgical and medical care (Y62-Y69)

Excludes1: *surgical and medical procedures as the cause of abnormal reaction of the patient, without mention of misadventure at the time of the procedure (Y83-Y84)*

Excludes2: *breakdown or malfunctioning of medical device (during procedure) (after implantation) (ongoing use) (Y70-Y82)*

Y62 Failure of sterile precautions during surgical and medical care

Y62.0 Failure of sterile precautions during surgical operation
Y62.1 Failure of sterile precautions during infusion or transfusion
Y62.2 Failure of sterile precautions during kidney dialysis and other perfusion
Y62.3 Failure of sterile precautions during injection or immunization
Y62.4 Failure of sterile precautions during endoscopic examination
Y62.5 Failure of sterile precautions during heart catheterization
Y62.6 Failure of sterile precautions during aspiration, puncture and other catheterization
Y62.8 Failure of sterile precautions during other surgical and medical care
Y62.9 Failure of sterile precautions during unspecified surgical and medical care

Y63 Failure in dosage during surgical and medical care

Excludes2: *accidental overdose of drug or wrong drug given in error (T36-T50)*

Y63.0 Excessive amount of blood or other fluid given during transfusion or infusion
Y63.1 Incorrect dilution of fluid used during infusion
Y63.2 Overdose of radiation given during therapy
Y63.3 Inadvertent exposure of patient to radiation during medical care
Y63.4 Failure in dosage in electroshock or insulin-shock therapy
Y63.5 Inappropriate temperature in local application and packing
Y63.6 Underdosing and nonadministration of necessary drug, medicament or biological substance
Review coding guideline C.19.e.5.c
Y63.8 Failure in dosage during other surgical and medical care
Review coding guideline C.19.e.5.c
Y63.9 Failure in dosage during unspecified surgical and medical ca
Review coding guideline C.19.e.5.c

Y64 Contaminated medical or biological substances

Y64.0 Contaminated medical or biological substance, transfused or infused
Y64.1 Contaminated medical or biological substance, injected or used for immunization
Y64.8 Contaminated medical or biological substance administered other means
Y64.9 Contaminated medical or biological substance administered unspecified means
Administered contaminated medical or biological substance NC

Y65 Other misadventures during surgical and medical care

Y65.0 Mismatched blood in transfusion
Y65.1 Wrong fluid used in infusion
Y65.2 Failure in suture or ligature during surgical operation
Y65.3 Endotracheal tube wrongly placed during anesthetic procedu
Y65.4 Failure to introduce or to remove other tube or instrument
+ **Y65.5 Performance of wrong procedure (operation)**
  Y65.51 Performance of wrong procedure (operation) on correct patient
    Wrong device implanted into correct surgical site
    Excludes1: *performance of correct procedure (operation) on wrong side or body part (Y65.53)*
  Y65.52 Performance of procedure (operation) on patient n scheduled for surgery
    Performance of procedure (operation) intended for another patient
    Performance of procedure (operation) on wrong patie
  Y65.53 Performance of correct procedure (operation) on wrong side or body part
    Performance of correct procedure (operation) on wrong side
    Performance of correct procedure (operation) on wrong site
Y65.8 Other specified misadventures during surgical and medical ca

Y66 Nonadministration of surgical and medical care

Premature cessation of surgical and medical care
Excludes1: *DNR status (Z66)*
palliative care (Z51.5)
Valid 3-character code, no further characters required

Y69 Unspecified misadventure during surgical and medical care

Valid 3-character code, no further characters required

Medical devices associated with adverse incidents in diagnost and therapeutic use (Y70-Y82)

Includes: breakdown or malfunction of medical devices (during use) (after implantation) (ongoing use)

Excludes2: *breakdown or malfunctioning of medical device (after implantation) (during procedure) (ongoing use) (Y70-Y82)*
later complications following use of medical devices without breakdown or malfunctioning of device (Y83-Y84)
misadventure to patients during surgical and medical care, classifiable to (Y62-Y69)
surgical and other medical procedures as the cause of abnormal reaction of the patient, or of later complication, without mention misadventure at the time of the procedure (Y83-Y84)

Y70 Anesthesiology devices associated with adverse incidents

Y70.0 Diagnostic and monitoring anesthesiology devices associated with adverse incidents
Y70.1 Therapeutic (nonsurgical) and rehabilitative anesthesiology devices associated with adverse incidents
Y70.2 Prosthetic and other implants, materials and accessory anesthesiology devices associated with adverse incidents
Y70.3 Surgical instruments, materials and anesthesiology devices (including sutures) associated with adverse incidents
Y70.8 Miscellaneous anesthesiology devices associated with advers incidents, not elsewhere classified

Y71 Cardiovascular devices associated with adverse incidents

Y71.0 Diagnostic and monitoring cardiovascular devices associated with adverse incidents
Y71.1 Therapeutic (nonsurgical) and rehabilitative cardiovascular devices associated with adverse incidents

Y71.2 Prosthetic and other implants, materials and accessory cardiovascular devices associated with adverse incidents
Y71.3 Surgical instruments, materials and cardiovascular devices (including sutures) associated with adverse incidents
Y71.8 Miscellaneous cardiovascular devices associated with adverse incidents, not elsewhere classified

Y72 Otorhinolaryngological devices associated with adverse incidents
Y72.0 Diagnostic and monitoring otorhinolaryngological devices associated with adverse incidents
Y72.1 Therapeutic (nonsurgical) and rehabilitative otorhinolaryngological devices associated with adverse incidents
Y72.2 Prosthetic and other implants, materials and accessory otorhinolaryngological devices associated with adverse incidents
Y72.3 Surgical instruments, materials and otorhinolaryngological devices (including sutures) associated with adverse incidents
Y72.8 Miscellaneous otorhinolaryngological devices associated with adverse incidents, not elsewhere classified

Y73 Gastroenterology and urology devices associated with adverse incidents
Y73.0 Diagnostic and monitoring gastroenterology and urology devices associated with adverse incidents
Y73.1 Therapeutic (nonsurgical) and rehabilitative gastroenterology and urology devices associated with adverse incidents
Y73.2 Prosthetic and other implants, materials and accessory gastroenterology and urology devices associated with adverse incidents
Y73.3 Surgical instruments, materials and gastroenterology and urology devices (including sutures) associated with adverse incidents
Y73.8 Miscellaneous gastroenterology and urology devices associated with adverse incidents, not elsewhere classified

Y74 General hospital and personal-use devices associated with adverse incidents
Y74.0 Diagnostic and monitoring general hospital and personal-use devices associated with adverse incidents
Y74.1 Therapeutic (nonsurgical) and rehabilitative general hospital and personal-use devices associated with adverse incidents
Y74.2 Prosthetic and other implants, materials and accessory general hospital and personal-use devices associated with adverse incidents
Y74.3 Surgical instruments, materials and general hospital and personal-use devices (including sutures) associated with adverse incidents
Y74.8 Miscellaneous general hospital and personal-use devices associated with adverse incidents, not elsewhere classified

Y75 Neurological devices associated with adverse incidents
Y75.0 Diagnostic and monitoring neurological devices associated with adverse incidents
Y75.1 Therapeutic (nonsurgical) and rehabilitative neurological devices associated with adverse incidents
Y75.2 Prosthetic and other implants, materials and neurological devices associated with adverse incidents
Y75.3 Surgical instruments, materials and neurological devices (including sutures) associated with adverse incidents
Y75.8 Miscellaneous neurological devices associated with adverse incidents, not elsewhere classified

Y76 Obstetric and gynecological devices associated with adverse incidents
♀ Y76.0 Diagnostic and monitoring obstetric and gynecological devices associated with adverse incidents
♀ Y76.1 Therapeutic (nonsurgical) and rehabilitative obstetric and gynecological devices associated with adverse incidents
♀ Y76.2 Prosthetic and other implants, materials and accessory obstetric and gynecological devices associated with adverse incidents
♀ Y76.3 Surgical instruments, materials and obstetric and gynecological devices (including sutures) associated with adverse incidents
♀ Y76.8 Miscellaneous obstetric and gynecological devices associated with adverse incidents, not elsewhere classified

Y77 Ophthalmic devices associated with adverse incidents
Y77.0 Diagnostic and monitoring ophthalmic devices associated with adverse incidents
Y77.1 Therapeutic (nonsurgical) and rehabilitative ophthalmic devices associated with adverse incidents
Y77.2 Prosthetic and other implants, materials and accessory ophthalmic devices associated with adverse incidents
Y77.3 Surgical instruments, materials and ophthalmic devices (including sutures) associated with adverse incidents
Y77.8 Miscellaneous ophthalmic devices associated with adverse incidents, not elsewhere classified

Y78 Radiological devices associated with adverse incidents
Y78.0 Diagnostic and monitoring radiological devices associated with adverse incidents
Y78.1 Therapeutic (nonsurgical) and rehabilitative radiological devices associated with adverse incidents
Y78.2 Prosthetic and other implants, materials and accessory radiological devices associated with adverse incidents
Y78.3 Surgical instruments, materials and radiological devices (including sutures) associated with adverse incidents
Y78.8 Miscellaneous radiological devices associated with adverse incidents, not elsewhere classified

Y79 Orthopedic devices associated with adverse incidents
Y79.0 Diagnostic and monitoring orthopedic devices associated with adverse incidents
Y79.1 Therapeutic (nonsurgical) and rehabilitative orthopedic devices associated with adverse incidents
Y79.2 Prosthetic and other implants, materials and accessory orthopedic devices associated with adverse incidents
Y79.3 Surgical instruments, materials and orthopedic devices (including sutures) associated with adverse incidents
Y79.8 Miscellaneous orthopedic devices associated with adverse incidents, not elsewhere classified

Y80 Physical medicine devices associated with adverse incidents
Y80.0 Diagnostic and monitoring physical medicine devices associated with adverse incidents
Y80.1 Therapeutic (nonsurgical) and rehabilitative physical medicine devices associated with adverse incidents
Y80.2 Prosthetic and other implants, materials and accessory physical medicine devices associated with adverse incidents
Y80.3 Surgical instruments, materials and physical medicine devices (including sutures) associated with adverse incidents
Y80.8 Miscellaneous physical medicine devices associated with adverse incidents, not elsewhere classified

Y81 General- and plastic-surgery devices associated with adverse incidents
Y81.0 Diagnostic and monitoring general- and plastic-surgery devices associated with adverse incidents
Y81.1 Therapeutic (nonsurgical) and rehabilitative general- and plastic-surgery devices associated with adverse incidents
Y81.2 Prosthetic and other implants, materials and accessory general- and plastic-surgery devices associated with adverse incidents
Y81.3 Surgical instruments, materials and general- and plastic-surgery devices (including sutures) associated with adverse incidents
Y81.8 Miscellaneous general- and plastic-surgery devices associated with adverse incidents, not elsewhere classified

Y82 Other and unspecified medical devices associated with adverse incidents
Y82.8 Other medical devices associated with adverse incidents
Y82.9 Unspecified medical devices associated with adverse incidents

Surgical and other medical procedures as the cause of abnormal reaction of the patient, or of later complication, without mention of misadventure at the time of the procedure (Y83-Y84)

Excludes1: *misadventures to patients during surgical and medical care, classifiable to (Y62-Y69)*

Excludes2: *breakdown or malfunctioning of medical device (after implantation) (during procedure) (ongoing use) (Y70-Y82)*

Y83 Surgical operation and other surgical procedures as the cause of abnormal reaction of the patient, or of later complication, without mention of misadventure at the time of the procedure
Y83.0 Surgical operation with transplant of whole organ as the cause of abnormal reaction of the patient, or of later complication, without mention of misadventure at the time of the procedure
Y83.1 Surgical operation with implant of artificial internal device as the cause of abnormal reaction of the patient, or of later complication, without mention of misadventure at the time of the procedure

Y83.2 Surgical operation with anastomosis, bypass or graft as the cause of abnormal reaction of the patient, or of later complication, without mention of misadventure at the time of the procedure

Y83.3 Surgical operation with formation of external stoma as the cause of abnormal reaction of the patient, or of later complication, without mention of misadventure at the time of the procedure

Y83.4 Other reconstructive surgery as the cause of abnormal reaction of the patient, or of later complication, without mention of misadventure at the time of the procedure

Y83.5 Amputation of limb(s) as the cause of abnormal reaction of the patient, or of later complication, without mention of misadventure at the time of the procedure

Y83.6 Removal of other organ (partial) (total) as the cause of abnormal reaction of the patient, or of later complication, without mention of misadventure at the time of the procedure

Y83.8 Other surgical procedures as the cause of abnormal reaction of the patient, or of later complication, without mention of misadventure at the time of the procedure

Y83.9 Surgical procedure, unspecified as the cause of abnormal reaction of the patient, or of later complication, without mention of misadventure at the time of the procedure

Y84 Other medical procedures as the cause of abnormal reaction of the patient, or of later complication, without mention of misadventure at the time of the procedure

Y84.0 Cardiac catheterization as the cause of abnormal reaction of the patient, or of later complication, without mention of misadventure at the time of the procedure

Y84.1 Kidney dialysis as the cause of abnormal reaction of the patient, or of later complication, without mention of misadventure at the time of the procedure

Y84.2 Radiological procedure and radiotherapy as the cause of abnormal reaction of the patient, or of later complication, without mention of misadventure at the time of the procedure

Review coding guideline C.2.c.2

Y84.3 Shock therapy as the cause of abnormal reaction of the patient, or of later complication, without mention of misadventure at the time of the procedure

Y84.4 Aspiration of fluid as the cause of abnormal reaction of the patient, or of later complication, without mention of misadventure at the time of the procedure

Y84.5 Insertion of gastric or duodenal sound as the cause of abnormal reaction of the patient, or of later complication, without mention of misadventure at the time of the procedure

Y84.6 Urinary catheterization as the cause of abnormal reaction of the patient, or of later complication, without mention of misadventure at the time of the procedure

Y84.7 Blood-sampling as the cause of abnormal reaction of the patient, or of later complication, without mention of misadventure at the time of the procedure

Y84.8 Other medical procedures as the cause of abnormal reaction of the patient, or of later complication, without mention of misadventure at the time of the procedure

AHA CC: 4Q, 2014, 24

Y84.9 Medical procedure, unspecified as the cause of abnormal reaction of the patient, or of later complication, without mention of misadventure at the time of the procedure

Supplementary factors related to causes of morbidity classified elsewhere (Y90-Y99)

NOTE These categories may be used to provide supplementary information concerning causes of morbidity. They are not to be used for single-condition coding.

Y90 Evidence of alcohol involvement determined by blood alcohol level

Code first any associated alcohol related disorders (F10)

Y90.0 Blood alcohol level of less than 20 mg/100 ml
Y90.1 Blood alcohol level of 20-39 mg/100 ml
Y90.2 Blood alcohol level of 40-59 mg/100 ml
Y90.3 Blood alcohol level of 60-79 mg/100 ml
Y90.4 Blood alcohol level of 80-99 mg/100 ml
Y90.5 Blood alcohol level of 100-119 mg/100 ml
Y90.6 Blood alcohol level of 120-199 mg/100 ml
Y90.7 Blood alcohol level of 200-239 mg/100 ml
Y90.8 Blood alcohol level of 240 mg/100 ml or more
Y90.9 Presence of alcohol in blood, level not specified

Y92 Place of occurrence of the external cause

The following category is for use, when relevant, to identify the place of occurrence of the external cause. Use in conjunction with an activity code.

Place of occurrence should be recorded only at the initial encounter for treatment

Review coding guideline C.20.b

\+ Y92.0 Non-institutional (private) residence as the place of occurrence of the external cause

Excludes1: *abandoned or derelict house (Y92.89)*
home under construction but not yet occupied (Y92.6-)
institutional place of residence (Y92.1-)

\+ Y92.00 Unspecified non-institutional (private) residence as the place of occurrence of the external cause

Y92.000 Kitchen of unspecified non-institutional (private) residence as the place of occurrence of the external cause

Y92.001 Dining room of unspecified non-institutional (private) residence as the place of occurrence of the external cause

Y92.002 Bathroom of unspecified non-institutional (private) residence single-family (private) house as the place of occurrence of the external cause

Y92.003 Bedroom of unspecified non-institutional (private) residence as the place of occurrence of the external cause

Y92.007 Garden or yard of unspecified non-institutional (private) residence as the place of occurrence of the external cause

Y92.008 Other place in unspecified non-institutional (private) residence as the place of occurrence of the external cause

Y92.009 Unspecified place in unspecified non-institutional (private) residence as the place of occurrence of the external cause

Home (NOS) as the place of occurrence of the external cause

\+ Y92.01 Single-family non-institutional (private) house as the place of occurrence of the external cause

Farmhouse as the place of occurrence of the external cause

Excludes1: *barn (Y92.71)*
chicken coop or hen house (Y92.72)
farm field (Y92.73)
orchard (Y92.74)
single family mobile home or trailer (Y92.02-)
slaughter house (Y92.86)

Y92.010 Kitchen of single-family (private) house as the place of occurrence of the external cause

Y92.011 Dining room of single-family (private) house as the place of occurrence of the external cause

Y92.012 Bathroom of single-family (private) house as the place of occurrence of the external cause

Y92.013 Bedroom of single-family (private) house as the place of occurrence of the external cause

Y92.014 Private driveway to single-family (private house as the place of occurrence of the external cause

Y92.015 Private garage of single-family (private) house as the place of occurrence of the external cause

Y92.016 Swimming-pool in single-family (private) house or garden as the place of occurrenc of the external cause

Y92.017 Garden or yard in single-family (private) house as the place of occurrence of the external cause

Y92.018 Other place in single-family (private) hou as the place of occurrence of the external cause

Y92.019 Unspecified place in single-family (privat house as the place of occurrence of the external cause

+ **Y92.02 Mobile home as the place of occurrence of the external cause**
  - **Y92.020 Kitchen in mobile home as the place of occurrence of the external cause**
  - **Y92.021 Dining room in mobile home as the place of occurrence of the external cause**
  - **Y92.022 Bathroom in mobile home as the place of occurrence of the external cause**
  - **Y92.023 Bedroom in mobile home as the place of occurrence of the external cause**
  - **Y92.024 Driveway of mobile home as the place of occurrence of the external cause**
  - **Y92.025 Garage of mobile home as the place of occurrence of the external cause**
  - **Y92.026 Swimming-pool of mobile home as the place of occurrence of the external cause**
  - **Y92.027 Garden or yard of mobile home as the place of occurrence of the external cause**
  - **Y92.028 Other place in mobile home as the place of occurrence of the external cause**
  - **Y92.029 Unspecified place in mobile home as the place of occurrence of the external cause**

+ **Y92.03 Apartment as the place of occurrence of the external cause**

  Condominium as the place of occurrence of the external cause

  Co-op apartment as the place of occurrence of the external cause
  - **Y92.030 Kitchen in apartment as the place of occurrence of the external cause**
  - **Y92.031 Bathroom in apartment as the place of occurrence of the external cause**
  - **Y92.032 Bedroom in apartment as the place of occurrence of the external cause**
  - **Y92.038 Other place in apartment as the place of occurrence of the external cause**
  - **Y92.039 Unspecified place in apartment as the place of occurrence of the external cause**

+ **Y92.04 Boarding-house as the place of occurrence of the external cause**
  - **Y92.040 Kitchen in boarding-house as the place of occurrence of the external cause**
  - **Y92.041 Bathroom in boarding-house as the place of occurrence of the external cause**
  - **Y92.042 Bedroom in boarding-house as the place of occurrence of the external cause**
  - **Y92.043 Driveway of boarding-house as the place of occurrence of the external cause**
  - **Y92.044 Garage of boarding-house as the place of occurrence of the external cause**
  - **Y92.045 Swimming-pool of boarding-house as the place of occurrence of the external cause**
  - **Y92.046 Garden or yard of boarding-house as the place of occurrence of the external cause**
  - **Y92.048 Other place in boarding-house as the place of occurrence of the external cause**
  - **Y92.049 Unspecified place in boarding-house as the place of occurrence of the external cause**

+ **Y92.09 Other non-institutional residence as the place of occurrence of the external cause**
  - **Y92.090 Kitchen in other non-institutional residence as the place of occurrence of the external cause**
  - **Y92.091 Bathroom in other non-institutional residence as the place of occurrence of the external cause**
  - **Y92.092 Bedroom in other non-institutional residence as the place of occurrence of the external cause**
  - **Y92.093 Driveway of other non-institutional residence as the place of occurrence of the external cause**
  - **Y92.094 Garage of other non-institutional residence as the place of occurrence of the external cause**
  - **Y92.095 Swimming-pool of other non-institutional residence as the place of occurrence of the external cause**
  - **Y92.096 Garden or yard of other non-institutional residence as the place of occurrence of the external cause**
  - **Y92.098 Other place in other non-institutional residence as the place of occurrence of the external cause**

    AHA CC: 2Q, 2017, 10-11
  - **Y92.099 Unspecified place in other non-institutional residence as the place of occurrence of the external cause**

+ **Y92.1 Institutional (nonprivate) residence as the place of occurrence of the external cause**
  - **Y92.10 Unspecified residential institution as the place of occurrence of the external cause**

+ **Y92.11 Children's home and orphanage as the place of occurrence of the external cause**
  - **Y92.110 Kitchen in children's home and orphanage as the place of occurrence of the external cause**
  - **Y92.111 Bathroom in children's home and orphanage as the place of occurrence of the external cause**
  - **Y92.112 Bedroom in children's home and orphanage as the place of occurrence of the external cause**
  - **Y92.113 Driveway of children's home and orphanage as the place of occurrence of the external cause**
  - **Y92.114 Garage of children's home and orphanage as the place of occurrence of the external cause**
  - **Y92.115 Swimming-pool of children's home and orphanage as the place of occurrence of the external cause**
  - **Y92.116 Garden or yard of children's home and orphanage as the place of occurrence of the external cause**
  - **Y92.118 Other place in children's home and orphanage as the place of occurrence of the external cause**
  - **Y92.119 Unspecified place in children's home and orphanage as the place of occurrence of the external cause**

+ **Y92.12 Nursing home as the place of occurrence of the external cause**

  Home for the sick as the place of occurrence of the external cause

  Hospice as the place of occurrence of the external cause
  - **Y92.120 Kitchen in nursing home as the place of occurrence of the external cause**
  - **Y92.121 Bathroom in nursing home as the place of occurrence of the external cause**
  - **Y92.122 Bedroom in nursing home as the place of occurrence of the external cause**
  - **Y92.123 Driveway of nursing home as the place of occurrence of the external cause**
  - **Y92.124 Garage of nursing home as the place of occurrence of the external cause**
  - **Y92.125 Swimming-pool of nursing home as the place of occurrence of the external cause**
  - **Y92.126 Garden or yard of nursing home as the place of occurrence of the external cause**
  - **Y92.128 Other place in nursing home as the place of occurrence of the external cause**
  - **Y92.129 Unspecified place in nursing home as the place of occurrence of the external cause**

+ **Y92.13 Military base as the place of occurrence of the external cause**

  Excludes1: *military training grounds (Y92.83)*
  - **Y92.130 Kitchen on military base as the place of occurrence of the external cause**
  - **Y92.131 Mess hall on military base as the place of occurrence of the external cause**
  - **Y92.133 Barracks on military base as the place of occurrence of the external cause**
  - **Y92.135 Garage on military base as the place of occurrence of the external cause**
  - **Y92.136 Swimming-pool on military base as the place of occurrence of the external cause**

Y92.137 **Garden or yard on military base as the place of occurrence of the external cause**
Y92.138 **Other place on military base as the place of occurrence of the external cause**
Y92.139 **Unspecified place military base as the place of occurrence of the external cause**

+ **Y92.14 Prison as the place of occurrence of the external cause**
Y92.140 **Kitchen in prison as the place of occurrence of the external cause**
Y92.141 **Dining room in prison as the place of occurrence of the external cause**
Y92.142 **Bathroom in prison as the place of occurrence of the external cause**
Y92.143 **Cell of prison as the place of occurrence of the external cause**
Y92.146 **Swimming-pool of prison as the place of occurrence of the external cause**
Y92.147 **Courtyard of prison as the place of occurrence of the external cause**
Y92.148 **Other place in prison as the place of occurrence of the external cause**
Y92.149 **Unspecified place in prison as the place of occurrence of the external cause**

+ **Y92.15 Reform school as the place of occurrence of the external cause**
Y92.150 **Kitchen in reform school as the place of occurrence of the external cause**
Y92.151 **Dining room in reform school as the place of occurrence of the external cause**
Y92.152 **Bathroom in reform school as the place of occurrence of the external cause**
Y92.153 **Bedroom in reform school as the place of occurrence of the external cause**
Y92.154 **Driveway of reform school as the place of occurrence of the external cause**
Y92.155 **Garage of reform school as the place of occurrence of the external cause**
Y92.156 **Swimming-pool of reform school as the place of occurrence of the external cause**
Y92.157 **Garden or yard of reform school as the place of occurrence of the external cause**
Y92.158 **Other place in reform school as the place of occurrence of the external cause**
Y92.159 **Unspecified place in reform school as the place of occurrence of the external cause**

+ **Y92.16 School dormitory as the place of occurrence of the external cause**
Excludes1: *reform school as the place of occurrence of the external cause (Y92.15-)*
school buildings and grounds as the place of occurrence of the external cause (Y92.2-)
school sports and athletic areas as the place of occurrence of the external cause (Y92.3-)
Y92.160 **Kitchen in school dormitory as the place of occurrence of the external cause**
Y92.161 **Dining room in school dormitory as the place of occurrence of the external cause**
Y92.162 **Bathroom in school dormitory as the place of occurrence of the external cause**
Y92.163 **Bedroom in school dormitory as the place of occurrence of the external cause**
Y92.168 **Other place in school dormitory as the place of occurrence of the external cause**
Y92.169 **Unspecified place in school dormitory as the place of occurrence of the external cause**

+ **Y92.19 Other specified residential institution as the place of occurrence of the external cause**
Y92.190 **Kitchen in other specified residential institution as the place of occurrence of the external cause**
Y92.191 **Dining room in other specified residential institution as the place of occurrence of the external cause**
Y92.192 **Bathroom in other specified residential institution as the place of occurrence of the external cause**
Y92.193 **Bedroom in other specified residential institution as the place of occurrence of the external cause**
Y92.194 **Driveway of other specified residential institution as the place of occurrence of the external cause**
Y92.195 **Garage of other specified residential institution as the place of occurrence of the external cause**
Y92.196 **Pool of other specified residential institution as the place of occurrence of the external cause**
Y92.197 **Garden or yard of other specified residential institution as the place of occurrence of the external cause**
Y92.198 **Other place in other specified residential institution as the place of occurrence of the external cause**
Y92.199 **Unspecified place in other specified residential institution as the place of occurrence of the external cause**

+ **Y92.2 School, other institution and public administrative area as the place of occurrence of the external cause**
Building and adjacent grounds used by the general public or by a particular group of the public
Excludes1: *building under construction as the place of occurrence of the external cause (Y92.6)*
residential institution as the place of occurrence of the external cause (Y92.1)
school dormitory as the place of occurrence of the external cause (Y92.16-)
sports and athletics area of schools as the place of occurrence of the external cause (Y92.3-)

+ **Y92.21 School (private) (public) (state) as the place of occurrence of the external cause**
Y92.210 **Daycare center as the place of occurrence of the external cause**
Y92.211 **Elementary school as the place of occurrence of the external cause**
Kindergarten as the place of occurrence of the external cause
Y92.212 **Middle school as the place of occurrence of the external cause**
Y92.213 **High school as the place of occurrence of the external cause**
AHA CC: 4Q, 2012, 108
Y92.214 **College as the place of occurrence of the external cause**
University as the place of occurrence of the external cause
Y92.215 **Trade school as the place of occurrence of the external cause**
Y92.218 **Other school as the place of occurrence of the external cause**
Y92.219 **Unspecified school as the place of occurrence of the external cause**

+ **Y92.22 Religious institution as the place of occurrence of the external cause**
Church as the place of occurrence of the external cause
Mosque as the place of occurrence of the external cause
Synagogue as the place of occurrence of the external cause

+ **Y92.23 Hospital as the place of occurrence of the external cause**
Excludes1: *ambulatory (outpatient) health services establishments (Y92.53-)*
home for the sick as the place of occurrence of the external cause (Y92.12-)
hospice as the place of occurrence of the external cause (Y92.12-)
nursing home as the place of occurrence of the external cause (Y92.12-)
Y92.230 **Patient room in hospital as the place of occurrence of the external cause**
Y92.231 **Patient bathroom in hospital as the place of occurrence of the external cause**
Y92.232 **Corridor of hospital as the place of occurrence of the external cause**

Y92.233 **Cafeteria of hospital as the place of occurrence of the external cause**

Y92.234 **Operating room of hospital as the place of occurrence of the external cause**

Y92.238 **Other place in hospital as the place of occurrence of the external cause**

Y92.239 **Unspecified place in hospital as the place of occurrence of the external cause**

+ Y92.24 **Public administrative building as the place of occurrence of the external cause**

Y92.240 **Courthouse as the place of occurrence of the external cause**

Y92.241 **Library as the place of occurrence of the external cause**

Y92.242 **Post office as the place of occurrence of the external cause**

Y92.243 **City hall as the place of occurrence of the external cause**

Y92.248 **Other public administrative building as the place of occurrence of the external cause**

+ Y92.25 **Cultural building as the place of occurrence of the external cause**

Y92.250 **Art Gallery as the place of occurrence of the external cause**

Y92.251 **Museum as the place of occurrence of the external cause**

Y92.252 **Music hall as the place of occurrence of the external cause**

Y92.253 **Opera house as the place of occurrence of the external cause**

Y92.254 **Theater (live) as the place of occurrence of the external cause**

Y92.258 **Other cultural public building as the place of occurrence of the external cause**

Y92.26 **Movie house or cinema as the place of occurrence of the external cause**

Y92.29 **Other specified public building as the place of occurrence of the external cause**

Assembly hall as the place of occurrence of the external cause

Clubhouse as the place of occurrence of the external cause

+ Y92.3 **Sports and athletics area as the place of occurrence of the external cause**

+ Y92.31 **Athletic court as the place of occurrence of the external cause**

Excludes1: *tennis court in private home or garden (Y92.09)*

Y92.310 **Basketball court as the place of occurrence of the external cause**

Y92.311 **Squash court as the place of occurrence of the external cause**

Y92.312 **Tennis court as the place of occurrence of the external cause**

Y92.318 **Other athletic court as the place of occurrence of the external cause**

+ Y92.32 **Athletic field as the place of occurrence of the external cause**

Y92.320 **Baseball field as the place of occurrence of the external cause**

Y92.321 **Football field as the place of occurrence of the external cause**

Y92.322 **Soccer field as the place of occurrence of the external cause**

Y92.328 **Other athletic field as the place of occurrence of the external cause**

Cricket field as the place of occurrence of the external cause

Hockey field as the place of occurrence of the external cause

+ Y92.33 **Skating rink as the place of occurrence of the external cause**

Y92.330 **Ice skating rink (indoor) (outdoor) as the place of occurrence of the external cause**

Y92.331 **Roller skating rink as the place of occurrence of the external cause**

Y92.34 **Swimming pool (public) as the place of occurrence of the external cause**

Excludes1: *swimming pool in private home or garden (Y92.016)*

Y92.39 **Other specified sports and athletic area as the place of occurrence of the external cause**

Golf-course as the place of occurrence of the external cause

Gymnasium as the place of occurrence of the external cause

Riding-school as the place of occurrence of the external cause

Stadium as the place of occurrence of the external cause

+ Y92.4 **Street, highway and other paved roadways as the place of occurrence of the external cause**

Excludes1: *private driveway of residence (Y92.014, Y92.024, Y92.043, Y92.093, Y92.113, Y92.123, Y92.154, Y92.194)*

+ Y92.41 **Street and highway as the place of occurrence of the external cause**

Y92.410 **Unspecified street and highway as the place of occurrence of the external cause**

Road NOS as the place of occurrence of the external cause

Y92.411 **Interstate highway as the place of occurrence of the external cause**

Freeway as the place of occurrence of the external cause

Motorway as the place of occurrence of the external cause

Y92.412 **Parkway as the place of occurrence of the external cause**

Y92.413 **State road as the place of occurrence of the external cause**

Y92.414 **Local residential or business street as the place of occurrence of the external cause**

Y92.415 **Exit ramp or entrance ramp of street or highway as the place of occurrence of the external cause**

+ Y92.48 **Other paved roadways as the place of occurrence of the external cause**

Y92.480 **Sidewalk as the place of occurrence of the external cause**

Y92.481 **Parking lot as the place of occurrence of the external cause**

Y92.482 **Bike path as the place of occurrence of the external cause**

Y92.488 **Other paved roadways as the place of occurrence of the external cause**

+ Y92.5 **Trade and service area as the place of occurrence of the external cause**

Excludes1: *garage in private home (Y92.015)*
schools and other public administration buildings (Y92.2-)

+ Y92.51 **Private commercial establishments as the place of occurrence of the external cause**

Y92.510 **Bank as the place of occurrence of the external cause**

Y92.511 **Restaurant or café as the place of occurrence of the external cause**

Y92.512 **Supermarket, store or market as the place of occurrence of the external cause**

Y92.513 **Shop (commercial) as the place of occurrence of the external cause**

+ Y92.52 **Service areas as the place of occurrence of the external cause**

Y92.520 **Airport as the place of occurrence of the external cause**

Y92.521 **Bus station as the place of occurrence of the external cause**

Y92.522 **Railway station as the place of occurrence of the external cause**

Y92.523 **Highway rest stop as the place of occurrence of the external cause**

Y92.524 **Gas station as the place of occurrence of the external cause**

Petroleum station as the place of occurrence of the external cause

Service station as the place of occurrence of the external cause

+ **Y92.53 Ambulatory health services establishments as the place of occurrence of the external cause**
  - **Y92.530 Ambulatory surgery center as the place of occurrence of the external cause**
    - Outpatient surgery center, including that connected with a hospital as the place of occurrence of the external cause
    - Same day surgery center, including that connected with a hospital as the place of occurrence of the external cause
  - **Y92.531 Health care provider office as the place of occurrence of the external cause**
    - Physician office as the place of occurrence of the external cause
  - **Y92.532 Urgent care center as the place of occurrence of the external cause**
  - **Y92.538 Other ambulatory health services establishments as the place of occurrence of the external cause**

Y92.59 Other trade areas as the place of occurrence of the external cause
- Office building as the place of occurrence of the external cause
- Casino as the place of occurrence of the external cause
- Garage (commercial) as the place of occurrence of the external cause
- Hotel as the place of occurrence of the external cause
- Radio or television station as the place of occurrence of the external cause
- Shopping mall as the place of occurrence of the external cause
- Warehouse as the place of occurrence of the external cause

+ **Y92.6 Industrial and construction area as the place of occurrence of the external cause**
  - **Y92.61 Building [any] under construction as the place of occurrence of the external cause**
  - **Y92.62 Dock or shipyard as the place of occurrence of the external cause**
    - Dockyard as the place of occurrence of the external cause
    - Dry dock as the place of occurrence of the external cause
    - Shipyard as the place of occurrence of the external cause
  - **Y92.63 Factory as the place of occurrence of the external cause**
    - Factory building as the place of occurrence of the external cause
    - Factory premises as the place of occurrence of the external cause
    - Industrial yard as the place of occurrence of the external cause
  - **Y92.64 Mine or pit as the place of occurrence of the external cause**
    - Mine as the place of occurrence of the external cause
  - **Y92.65 Oil rig as the place of occurrence of the external cause**
    - Pit (coal) (gravel) (sand) as the place of occurrence of the external cause
  - **Y92.69 Other specified industrial and construction area as the place of occurrence of the external cause**
    - Gasworks as the place of occurrence of the external cause
    - Power-station (coal) (nuclear) (oil) as the place of occurrence of the external cause
    - Tunnel under construction as the place of occurrence of the external cause
    - Workshop as the place of occurrence of the external cause

+ **Y92.7 Farm as the place of occurrence of the external cause**
  - Ranch as the place of occurrence of the external cause
  - ***Excludes1:*** *farmhouse and home premises of farm (Y92.01-)*
  - **Y92.71 Barn as the place of occurrence of the external cause**
  - **Y92.72 Chicken coop as the place of occurrence of the external cause**
    - Hen house as the place of occurrence of the external cause
  - **Y92.73 Farm field as the place of occurrence of the external cause**
  - **Y92.74 Orchard as the place of occurrence of the external cause**
  - **Y92.79 Other farm location as the place of occurrence of the external cause**

+ **Y92.8 Other places as the place of occurrence of the external cause**
  + **Y92.81 Transport vehicle as the place of occurrence of the external cause**
    - ***Excludes1:*** *transport accidents (V00-V99)*
    - **Y92.810 Car as the place of occurrence of the external cause**
    - **Y92.811 Bus as the place of occurrence of the external cause**
    - **Y92.812 Truck as the place of occurrence of the external cause**
    - **Y92.813 Airplane as the place of occurrence of the external cause**
    - **Y92.814 Boat as the place of occurrence of the external cause**
    - **Y92.815 Train as the place of occurrence of the external cause**
    - **Y92.816 Subway car as the place of occurrence of the external cause**
    - **Y92.818 Other transport vehicle as the place of occurrence of the external cause**
  + **Y92.82 Wilderness area**
    - **Y92.820 Desert as the place of occurrence of the external cause**
    - **Y92.821 Forest as the place of occurrence of the external cause**
    - **Y92.828 Other wilderness area as the place of occurrence of the external cause**
      - Swamp as the place of occurrence of the external cause
      - Mountain as the place of occurrence of the external cause
      - Marsh as the place of occurrence of the external cause
      - Prairie as the place of occurrence of the external cause
  + **Y92.83 Recreation area as the place of occurrence of the external cause**
    - **Y92.830 Public park as the place of occurrence of the external cause**
    - **Y92.831 Amusement park as the place of occurrence of the external cause**
    - **Y92.832 Beach as the place of occurrence of the external cause**
      - Seashore as the place of occurrence of the external cause
    - **Y92.833 Campsite as the place of occurrence of the external cause**
    - **Y92.834 Zoological garden (Zoo) as the place of occurrence of the external cause**
    - **Y92.838 Other recreation area as the place of occurrence of the external cause**
  - **Y92.84 Military training ground as the place of occurrence of the external cause**
  - **Y92.85 Railroad track as the place of occurrence of the external cause**
  - **Y92.86 Slaughter house as the place of occurrence of the external cause**
  - **Y92.89 Other specified places as the place of occurrence of the external cause**
    - Derelict house as the place of occurrence of the external cause

Y92.9 Unspecified place or not applicable

Y93 Activity codes

NOTE Category Y93 is provided for use to indicate the activity of the person seeking healthcare for an injury or health condition, such as a heart attack while shoveling snow, which resulted from, or was contributed to, by the activity. These codes are appropriate for use for both acute injuries, such as those from chapter 19, and conditions that are due to the long-term, cumulative effects of an activity, such as those from chapter 13. They are also appropriate for use with external cause codes for cause and intent if identifying the activity provides additional information on the event. These codes should be used in conjunction with codes for external cause status (Y99) and place of occurrence (Y92).

This section contains the following broad activity categories:

Y93.0 Activities involving walking and running
Y93.1 Activities involving water and water craft
Y93.2 Activities involving ice and snow
Y93.3 Activities involving climbing, rappelling, and jumping off
Y93.4 Activities involving dancing and other rhythmic movement
Y93.5 Activities involving other sports and athletics played individually
Y93.6 Activities involving other sports and athletics played as a team or group
Y93.7 Activities involving other specified sports and athletics
Y93.A Activities involving other cardiorespiratory exercise
Y93.B Activities involving other muscle strengthening exercises
Y93.C Activities involving computer technology and electronic devices
Y93.D Activities involving arts and handcrafts
Y93.E Activities involving personal hygiene and interior property and clothing maintenance
Y93.F Activities involving caregiving
Y93.G Activities involving food preparation, cooking and grilling
Y93.H Activities involving exterior property and land maintenance, building and construction
Y93.I Activities involving roller coasters and other types of external motion
Y93.J Activities involving playing musical instrument
Y93.K Activities involving animal care
Y93.8 Activities, other specified
Y93.9 Activity, unspecified

Review coding guideline C.20.c

+ **Y93.0 Activities involving walking and running**
Excludes1: *activity, walking an animal (Y93.K1)*
activity, walking or running on a treadmill (Y93.A1)
Y93.01 Activity, walking, marching and hiking
Activity, walking, marching and hiking on level or elevated terrain
Excludes1: *activity, mountain climbing (Y93.31)*
Y93.02 Activity, running

+ **Y93.1 Activities involving water and water craft**
Excludes1: *activities involving ice (Y93.2-)*
Y93.11 Activity, swimming
Y93.12 Activity, springboard and platform diving
Y93.13 Activity, water polo
Y93.14 Activity, water aerobics and water exercise
Y93.15 Activity, underwater diving and snorkeling
Activity, SCUBA diving
Y93.16 Activity, rowing, canoeing, kayaking, rafting and tubing
Activity, canoeing, kayaking, rafting and tubing in calm and turbulent water
Y93.17 Activity, water skiing and wake boarding
Y93.18 Activity, surfing, windsurfing and boogie boarding
Activity, water sliding
Y93.19 Activity, other involving water and watercraft
Activity involving water NOS
Activity, parasailing
Activity, water survival training and testing

+ **Y93.2 Activities involving ice and snow**
Excludes1: *activity, shoveling ice and snow (Y93.H1)*
Y93.21 Activity, ice skating
Activity, figure skating (singles) (pairs)
Activity, ice dancing
Excludes1: *activity, ice hockey (Y93.22)*
Y93.22 Activity, ice hockey
Y93.23 Activity, snow (alpine) (downhill) skiing, snow boarding, sledding, tobogganing and snow tubing
Excludes1: *activity, cross country skiing (Y93.24)*
Y93.24 Activity, cross country skiing
Activity, nordic skiing
Y93.29 Activity, other involving ice and snow
Activity involving ice and snow NOS

+ **Y93.3 Activities involving climbing, rappelling and jumping off**
Excludes1: *activity, hiking on level or elevated terrain (Y93.01)*
activity, jumping rope (Y93.56)
activity, trampoline jumping (Y93.44)
Y93.31 Activity, mountain climbing, rock climbing and wall climbing
Y93.32 Activity, rappelling
Y93.33 Activity, BASE jumping
Activity, Building, Antenna, Span, Earth jumping
Y93.34 Activity, bungee jumping
Y93.35 Activity, hang gliding
Y93.39 Activity, other involving climbing, rappelling and jumping off

+ **Y93.4 Activities involving dancing and other rhythmic movement**
Excludes1: *activity, martial arts (Y93.75)*
Y93.41 Activity, dancing
AHA CC: 4Q, 2012, 108
Y93.42 Activity, yoga
Y93.43 Activity, gymnastics
Activity, rhythmic gymnastics
Excludes1: *activity, trampolining (Y93.44)*
Y93.44 Activity, trampolining
Y93.45 Activity, cheerleading
Y93.49 Activity, other involving dancing and other rhythmic movements

+ **Y93.5 Activities involving other sports and athletics played individually**
Excludes1: *activity, dancing (Y93.41)*
activity, gymnastic (Y93.43)
activity, trampolining (Y93.44)
activity, yoga (Y93.42)
Y93.51 Activity, roller skating (inline) and skateboarding
Y93.52 Activity, horseback riding
Y93.53 Activity, golf
Y93.54 Activity, bowling
Y93.55 Activity, bike riding
Y93.56 Activity, jumping rope
Y93.57 Activity, non-running track and field events
Excludes1: *activity, running (any form) (Y93.02)*
Y93.59 Activity, other involving other sports and athletics played individually
Excludes1: *activities involving climbing, rappelling, and jumping (Y93.3-)*
activities involving ice and snow (Y93.2-)
activities involving walking and running (Y93.0-)
activities involving water and watercraft (Y93.1-)

+ **Y93.6 Activities involving other sports and athletics played as a team or group**
Excludes1: *activity, ice hockey (Y93.22)*
activity, water polo (Y93.13)
Y93.61 Activity, american tackle football
Activity, football NOS
Y93.62 Activity, american flag or touch football
Y93.63 Activity, rugby
Y93.64 Activity, baseball
Activity, softball
Y93.65 Activity, lacrosse and field hockey
AHA CC: 1Q, 2015, 3-21
Y93.66 Activity, soccer
Y93.67 Activity, basketball
Y93.68 Activity, volleyball (beach) (court)
Y93.6A Activity, physical games generally associated with school recess, summer camp and children
Activity, capture the flag
Activity, dodge ball
Activity, four square
Activity, kickball
Y93.69 Activity, other involving other sports and athletics played as a team or group
Activity, cricket

+ **Y93.7 Activities involving other specified sports and athletics**
Y93.71 Activity, boxing
Y93.72 Activity, wrestling
Y93.73 Activity, racquet and hand sports
Activity, handball
Activity, racquetball
Activity, squash
Activity, tennis

Y93.74 **Activity, frisbee**
Activity, ultimate frisbee
Y93.75 **Activity, martial arts**
Activity, combatives
Y93.79 **Activity, other specified sports and athletics**
Excludes1: *sports and athletics activities specified in categories Y93.0-Y93.6*

+ **Y93.A Activities involving other cardiorespiratory exercise**
Activities involving physical training
Y93.A1 **Activity, exercise machines primarily for cardiorespiratory conditioning**
Activity, elliptical and stepper machines
Activity, stationary bike
Activity, treadmill
Y93.A2 **Activity, calisthenics**
Activity, jumping jacks
Activity, warm up and cool down
Y93.A3 **Activity, aerobic and step exercise**
Y93.A4 **Activity, circuit training**
Y93.A5 **Activity, obstacle course**
Activity, challenge course
Activity, confidence course
Y93.A6 **Activity, grass drills**
Activity, guerilla drills
Y93.A9 **Activity, other involving cardiorespiratory exercise**
Excludes1: *activities involving cardiorespiratory exercise specified in categories Y93.0-Y93.7*

+ **Y93.B Activities involving other muscle strengthening exercises**
Y93.B1 **Activity, exercise machines primarily for muscle strengthening**
Y93.B2 **Activity, push-ups, pull-ups, sit-ups**
Y93.B3 **Activity, free weights**
Activity, barbells
Activity, dumbbells
Y93.B4 **Activity, pilates**
Y93.B9 **Activity, other involving muscle strengthening exercises**
Excludes1: *activities involving muscle strengthening specified in categories Y93.0-Y93.A*

+ **Y93.C Activities involving computer technology and electronic devices**
Excludes1: *activity, electronic musical keyboard or instruments (Y93.J-)*
Y93.C1 **Activity, computer keyboarding**
Activity, electronic game playing using keyboard or other stationary device
Y93.C2 **Activity, hand held interactive electronic device**
Activity, cellular telephone and communication device
Activity, electronic game playing using interactive device
Excludes1: *activity, electronic game playing using keyboard or other stationary device (Y93.C1)*
Y93.C9 **Activity, other involving computer technology and electronic devices**

+ **Y93.D Activities involving arts and handcrafts**
Excludes1: *activities involving playing musical instrument (Y93.J-)*
Y93.D1 **Activity, knitting and crocheting**
Y93.D2 **Activity, sewing**
Y93.D3 **Activity, furniture building and finishing**
Activity, furniture repair
Y93.D9 **Activity, other involving arts and handcrafts**

+ **Y93.E Activities involving personal hygiene and interior property and clothing maintenance**
Excludes1: *activities involving cooking and grilling (Y93.G-)*
activities involving exterior property and land maintenance, building and construction (Y93.H-)
activities involving caregiving (Y93.F-)
activity, dishwashing (Y93.G1)
activity, food preparation (Y93.G1)
activity, gardening (Y93.H2)
Y93.E1 **Activity, personal bathing and showering**
Y93.E2 **Activity, laundry**
Y93.E3 **Activity, vacuuming**
Y93.E4 **Activity, ironing**
Y93.E5 **Activity, floor mopping and cleaning**
Y93.E6 **Activity, residential relocation**
Activity, packing up and unpacking involved in moving to a new residence
Y93.E8 **Activity, other personal hygiene**
Y93.E9 **Activity, other interior property and clothing maintenance**

+ **Y93.F Activities involving caregiving**
Activity involving the provider of caregiving
Y93.F1 **Activity, caregiving, bathing**
Y93.F2 **Activity, caregiving, lifting**
AHA CC: 4Q, 2016, 73-74
Y93.F9 **Activity, other caregiving**

+ **Y93.G Activities involving food preparation, cooking and grilling**
Y93.G1 **Activity, food preparation and clean up**
Activity, dishwashing
Y93.G2 **Activity, grilling and smoking food**
Y93.G3 **Activity, cooking and baking**
Activity, use of stove, oven and microwave oven
Y93.G9 **Activity, other involving cooking and grilling**

+ **Y93.H Activities involving exterior property and land maintenance, building and construction**
Y93.H1 **Activity, digging, shoveling and raking**
Activity, dirt digging
Activity, raking leaves
Activity, snow shoveling
Y93.H2 **Activity, gardening and landscaping**
Activity, pruning, trimming shrubs, weeding
Y93.H3 **Activity, building and construction**
Y93.H9 **Activity, other involving exterior property and land maintenance, building and construction**

+ **Y93.I Activities involving roller coasters and other types of external motion**
Y93.I1 **Activity, roller coaster riding**
Y93.I9 **Activity, other involving external motion**

+ **Y93.J Activities involving playing musical instrument**
Activity involving playing electric musical instrument
Y93.J1 **Activity, piano playing**
Activity, musical keyboard (electronic) playing
Y93.J2 **Activity, drum and other percussion instrument playing**
Y93.J3 **Activity, string instrument playing**
Y93.J4 **Activity, winds and brass instrument playing**

+ **Y93.K Activities involving animal care**
Excludes1: *activity, horseback riding (Y93.52)*
Y93.K1 **Activity, walking an animal**
Y93.K2 **Activity, milking an animal**
Y93.K3 **Activity, grooming and shearing an animal**
Y93.K9 **Activity, other involving animal care**

+ **Y93.8 Activities, other specified**
Y93.81 **Activity, refereeing a sports activity**
Y93.82 **Activity, spectator at an event**
Y93.83 **Activity, rough housing and horseplay**
AHA CC: 1Q, 2015, 3-21
Y93.84 **Activity, sleeping**
Y93.85 **Activity, choking game**
Activity, blackout game
Activity, fainting game
Activity, pass out game
AHA CC: 4Q, 2016, 74-76
Y93.89 **Activity, other specified**

Y93.9 Activity, unspecified

Y95 Nosocomial condition
Valid 3-character code, no further characters required
AHA CC: 4Q, 2013, 119

Y99 External cause status

NOTE A single code from category Y99 should be used in conjunction with the external cause code(s) assigned to a record to indicate the status of the person at the time the event occurred.

Review coding guideline C.20.k

Y99.0 Civilian activity done for income or pay

Civilian activity done for financial or other compensation

Excludes1: *military activity (Y99.1)*
volunteer activity (Y99.2)

AHA CC: 4Q, 2016, 73-74

Y99.1 Military activity

Excludes1: *activity of off duty military personnel (Y99.8)*

Y99.2 Volunteer activity

Excludes1: *activity of child or other family member assisting in compensated work of other family member (Y99.8)*

Y99.8 Other external cause status

Activity NEC
Activity of child or other family member assisting in compensated work of other family member
Hobby not done for income
Leisure activity
Off-duty activity of military personnel
Recreation or sport not for income or while a student
Student activity

Excludes1: *civilian activity done for income or compensation (Y99.0)*
military activity (Y99.1)

AHA CC: 4Q, 2012, 108

Y99.9 Unspecified external cause status

Chapter 21: Factors Influencing Health Status and Contact with Health Services (Z00-Z99)

NOTE Z codes represent reasons for encounters. A corresponding procedure code must accompany a Z code if a procedure is performed. Categories Z00-Z99 are provided for occasions when circumstances other than a disease, injury or external cause classifiable to categories A00-Y89 are recorded as 'diagnoses' or 'problems'. This can arise in two main ways:
(a) When a person who may or may not be sick encounters the health services for some specific purpose, such as to receive limited care or service for a current condition, to donate an organ or tissue, to receive prophylactic vaccination (immunization), or to discuss a problem which is in itself not a disease or injury.
(b) When some circumstance or problem is present which influences the person's health status but is not in itself a current illness or injury.

This chapter contains the following category blocks:

Z00-Z13	Persons encountering health services for examinations
Z14-Z15	Genetic carrier and genetic susceptibility to disease
Z16	Resistance to antimicrobial drugs
Z17	Estrogen receptor status
Z18	Retained foreign body fragments
Z20-Z29	Persons with potential health hazards related to communicable diseases
Z30-Z39	Persons encountering health services in circumstances related to reproduction
Z40-Z53	Encounters for other specific health care
Z55-Z65	Persons with potential health hazards related to socioeconomic and psychosocial circumstances
Z66	Do not resuscitate status
Z67	Blood type
Z68	Body mass index (BMI)
Z69-Z76	Persons encountering health services in other circumstances
Z77-Z99	Persons with potential health hazards related to family and personal history and certain conditions influencing health status

C. Chapter-Specific Coding Guidelines

In addition to general coding guidelines, there are guidelines for specific diagnoses and/or conditions in the classification. Unless otherwise indicated, these guidelines apply to all health care settings. Please refer to Section II for guidelines on the selection of principal diagnosis.

21. Chapter 21: Factors Influencing Health Status and Contact with Health Services (Z00-Z99)

NOTE The chapter specific guidelines provide additional information about the use of Z codes for specified encounters.

a. Use of Z codes in any healthcare setting

Z codes are for use in any healthcare setting. Z codes may be used as either a first-listed (principal diagnosis code in the inpatient setting) or secondary code, depending on the circumstances of the encounter. Certain Z codes may only be used as first-listed or principal diagnosis.

b. Z Codes indicate a reason for an encounter

Z codes are not procedure codes. A corresponding procedure code must accompany a Z code to describe any procedure performed.

c. Categories of Z Codes

1) Contact/Exposure

Category Z20 indicates contact with, and suspected exposure to, communicable diseases. These codes are for patients who do not show any sign or symptom of a disease but are suspected to have been exposed to it by close personal contact with an infected individual or are in an area where a disease is epidemic.

Category Z77, Other contact with and (suspected) exposures hazardous to health, indicates contact with and suspected exposures hazardous to health.

Contact/exposure codes may be used as a first-listed code to explain an encounter for testing, or, more commonly, as a secondary code to identify a potential risk.

2) Inoculations and vaccinations

Code Z23 is for encounters for inoculations and vaccinations. It indicates that a patient is being seen to receive a prophylactic inoculation against a disease. Procedure codes are required to identify the actual administration of the injection and the type(s) of immunizations given. Code Z23 may be used as a secondary code if the inoculation is given as a routine part of preventive health care, such as a well-baby visit.

3) Status

Status codes indicate that a patient is either a carrier of a disease or has the sequelae or residual of a past disease or condition. This includes such things as the presence of prosthetic or mechanical devices resulting from past treatment. A status code is informative, because the status may affect the course of treatment and its outcome. A status code is distinct from a history code. The history code indicates that the patient no longer has the condition.

A status code should not be used with a diagnosis code from one of the body system chapters, if the diagnosis code includes the information provided by the status code. For example, code Z94.1, Heart transplant status, should not be used with a code from subcategory T86.2, Complications of heart transplant. The status code does not provide additional information. The complication code indicates that the patient is a heart transplant patient.

For encounters for weaning from a mechanical ventilator, assign a code from subcategory J96.1, Chronic respiratory failure, followed by code Z99.11, Dependence on respirator [ventilator] status.

The status Z codes/categories are:

Z14 Genetic carrier
Genetic carrier status indicates that a person carries a gene associated with a particular disease, which may be passed to offspring who may develop that disease. The person does not have the disease and is not at risk of developing the disease.

Z15 Genetic susceptibility to disease
Genetic susceptibility indicates that a person has a gene that increases the risk of that person developing the disease.

Codes from category Z15 should not be used as principal or first listed codes. If the patient has the condition to which he/she is susceptible, and that condition is the reason for the encounter, the code for the current condition should be sequenced first. If the patient is being seen for follow-up after completed treatment for this condition, and the condition no longer exists, a follow-up code should be sequenced first, followed by the appropriate personal history and genetic susceptibility codes. If the purpose of the encounter is genetic counseling associated with procreative management, code Z31.5, Encounter for genetic counseling, should be assigned as the first-listed code, followed by a code from category Z15. Additional codes should be assigned for any applicable family or personal history.

Z16 Resistance to antimicrobial drugs
This code indicates that a patient has a condition that is resistant to antimicrobial drug treatment. Sequence the infection code first.

Z17 Estrogen receptor status

Z18 Retained foreign body fragments

Z19 Hormone sensitivity malignancy status

Z21 Asymptomatic HIV infection status
This code indicates that a patient has tested positive for HIV but has manifested no signs or symptoms of the disease.

Z22 Carrier of infectious disease
Carrier status indicates that a person harbors the specific organisms of a disease without manifest symptoms and is capable of transmitting the infection.

Z28.3 Underimmunization status

Z33.1 Pregnant state, incidental
This code is a secondary code only for use when the pregnancy is in no way complicating the reason for visit. Otherwise, a code from the obstetric chapter is required.

Z66 Do not resuscitate
This code may be used when it is documented by the provider that a patient is on do not resuscitate status at any time during the stay.

Z67 Blood type

Z68 Body mass index (BMI)
As with all other secondary diagnosis codes, the BMI codes should only be assigned when they meet the definition of a reportable diagnosis (see Section III, Reporting Additional Diagnoses).

Z74.01 Bed confinement status

Z76.82 Awaiting organ transplant status

Z78 Other specified health status
Code Z78.1, Physical restraint status, may be used when it is documented by the provider that a patient has been put in restraints during the current encounter. Please note that this code should not be reported when it is documented by the provider that a patient is temporarily restrained during a procedure.

Z79 Long-term (current) drug therapy
Codes from this category indicate a patient's continuous use of a prescribed drug (including such things as aspirin therapy) for the long-term treatment of a condition or for prophylactic use. It is not for use for patients who have addictions to drugs. This subcategory is not for use of medications for detoxification or maintenance programs to prevent withdrawal symptoms in patients with drug dependence (e.g., methadone maintenance for opiate dependence). Assign the appropriate code for the drug dependence instead.

Assign a code from Z79 if the patient is receiving a medication for an extended period as a prophylactic measure (such as for the prevention of deep vein thrombosis) or as treatment of a chronic condition (such as arthritis) or a disease requiring a lengthy course of treatment (such as cancer). Do not assign a code from category Z79 for medication being administered for a brief period of time to treat an acute illness or injury (such as a course of antibiotics to treat acute bronchitis).

Z88 Allergy status to drugs, medicaments and biological substances
Except: Z88.9, Allergy status to unspecified drugs, medicaments and biological substances status

Z89 Acquired absence of limb

Z90 Acquired absence of organs, not elsewhere classified

Z91.0- Allergy status, other than to drugs and biological substances

Z92.82 Status post administration of tPA (rtPA) in a different facility within the last 24 hours prior to admission to a current facility

Assign code Z92.82, Status post administration of tPA (rtPA) in a different facility within the last 24 hours prior to admission to current facility, as a secondary diagnosis when a patient is received by transfer into a facility and documentation indicates they were administered tissue plasminogen activator (tPA) within the last 24 hours prior to admission to the current facility.

This guideline applies even if the patient is still receiving the tPA at the time they are received into the current facility.

The appropriate code for the condition for which the tPA was administered (such as cerebrovascular disease or myocardial infarction) should be assigned first.

Code Z92.82 is only applicable to the receiving facility record and not to the transferring facility record.

Z93 Artificial opening status

Z94 Transplanted organ and tissue status

Z95 Presence of cardiac and vascular implants and grafts

Z96 Presence of other functional implants

Z97 Presence of other devices

Z98 Other postprocedural states
Assign code Z98.85, Transplanted organ removal status, to indicate that a transplanted organ has been previously removed. This code should not be assigned for the encounter in which the transplanted organ is removed. The complication necessitating removal of the transplant organ should be assigned for that encounter.
See section I.C19. for information on the coding of organ transplant complications.

Z99 Dependence on enabling machines and devices, not elsewhere classified

NOTE Categories Z89-Z90 and Z93-Z99 are for use only if there are no complications or malfunctions of the organ or tissue replaced, the amputation site or the equipment on which the patient is dependent.

4) History (of)

There are two types of history Z codes, personal and family. Personal history codes explain a patient's past medical condition that no longer exists and is not receiving any treatment, but that has the potential for recurrence, and therefore may require continued monitoring.

Family history codes are for use when a patient has a family member(s) who has had a particular disease that causes the patient to be at higher risk of also contracting the disease.

Personal history codes may be used in conjunction with follow- up codes and family history codes may be used in conjunction with screening codes to explain the need for a test or procedure. History codes are also acceptable on any medical record regardless of the reason for visit. A history of an illness, even if no longer present, is important information that may alter the type of treatment ordered.

The history Z code categories are:

Z80 Family history of primary malignant neoplasm

Z81 Family history of mental and behavioral disorders

Z82 Family history of certain disabilities and chronic diseases (leading to disablement)

Z83 Family history of other specific disorders

Z84 Family history of other conditions

Z85 Personal history of malignant neoplasm

Z86 Personal history of certain other diseases

Z87 Personal history of other diseases and conditions

Z91.4- Personal history of psychological trauma, not elsewhere classified

Z91.5 Personal history of self-harm

Z91.81 History of falling

Z91.82 Personal history of military deployment

Z92 Personal history of medical treatment
Except: Z92.0, Personal history of contraception Except: Z92.82, Status post administration of tPA (rtPA) in a different facility within the last 24 hours prior to admission to a current facility

5) Screening

Screening is the testing for disease or disease precursors in seemingly well individuals so that early detection and treatment can be provided for those who test positive for the disease (e.g., screening mammogram).

The testing of a person to rule out or confirm a suspected diagnosis because the patient has some sign or symptom is a diagnostic examination, not a screening. In these cases, the sign or symptom is used to explain the reason for the test.

A screening code may be a first-listed code if the reason for the visit is specifically the screening exam. It may also be used as an additional code if the screening is done during an office visit for other health problems. A screening code is not necessary if the screening is inherent to a routine examination, such as a pap smear done during a routine pelvic examination.

Should a condition be discovered during the screening then the code for the condition may be assigned as an additional diagnosis.

The Z code indicates that a screening exam is planned. A procedure code is required to confirm that the screening was performed.

The screening Z codes/categories:

Z11 Encounter for screening for infectious and parasitic diseases

Z12 Encounter for screening for malignant neoplasms

Z13 Encounter for screening for other diseases and disorders
Except: Z13.9, Encounter for screening, unspecified

Z36 Encounter for antenatal screening for mother

6) Observation

There are three observation Z code categories. They are for use in very limited circumstances when a person is being observed for a suspected condition that is ruled out. The observation codes are not for use if an injury or illness or any signs or symptoms related to the suspected condition are present. In such cases the diagnosis/symptom code is used with the corresponding external cause code.

The observation codes are to be used as principal diagnosis only. The only exception to this is when the principal diagnosis is required to be a code from category Z38, Liveborn infants according to place of birth and type of delivery. Then a code form category Z05, Encounter for observation and evaluation of newborn for suspected diseases and conditions ruled out, is sequenced after the Z38 code. Additional codes may be used in addition to the observation code but only if they are unrelated to the suspected condition being observed.

Codes from subcategory Z03.7, Encounter for suspected maternal and fetal conditions ruled out, may either be used as a first-listed or as an additional code assignment depending on the case. They are for use in very limited circumstances on a maternal record when an encounter is for a suspected maternal or fetal condition that is ruled out during that encounter (for example, a maternal or fetal condition may be suspected due to an abnormal test result). These codes should not be used when the condition is confirmed. In those cases, the confirmed condition should be coded. In addition, these codes are not for use if an illness or any signs or symptoms related to the suspected condition or problem are present. In such cases the diagnosis/symptom code is used.

Additional codes may be used in addition to the code from subcategory Z03.7, but only if they are unrelated to the suspected condition being evaluated.

Codes from subcategory Z03.7 may not be used for encounters for antenatal screening of mother. *See Section I.C.21. Screening.*

For encounters for suspected fetal condition that are inconclusive following testing and evaluation, assign the appropriate code from category O35, O36, O40 or O41.

The observation Z code categories:

Z03 Encounter for medical observation for suspected diseases and conditions ruled out

Z04 Encounter for examination and observation for other reasons
Except: Z04.9, Encounter for examination and observation for unspecified reason

Z05 Encounter for observation and evaluation of newborn for suspected diseases and conditions ruled out

7) Aftercare

Aftercare visit codes cover situations when the initial treatment of a disease has been performed and the patient requires continued care during the healing or recovery phase, or for the long-term consequences of the disease. The aftercare Z code should not be used if treatment is directed at a current, acute disease. The diagnosis code is to be used in these cases. Exceptions to this rule are codes Z51.0, Encounter for antineoplastic radiation therapy, and codes from subcategory Z51.1, Encounter for antineoplastic chemotherapy and immunotherapy. These codes are to be first-listed, followed by the diagnosis code when a patient's encounter is solely to receive radiation therapy, chemotherapy, or immunotherapy for the treatment of a neoplasm. If the reason for the encounter is more than one type of antineoplastic therapy, code Z51.0 and a code from subcategory Z51.1 may be assigned together, in which case one of these codes would be reported as a secondary diagnosis.

The aftercare Z codes should also not be used for aftercare for injuries. For aftercare of an injury, assign the acute injury code with the appropriate 7th character (for subsequent encounter).

The aftercare codes are generally first-listed to explain the specific reason for the encounter. An aftercare code may be used as an additional code when some type of aftercare is provided in addition to the reason for admission and no diagnosis code is applicable. An example of this would be the closure of a colostomy during an encounter for treatment of another condition.

Aftercare codes should be used in conjunction with other aftercare codes or diagnosis codes to provide better detail on the specifics of an aftercare encounter visit, unless otherwise directed by the classification. Should a patient receive multiple types of antineoplastic therapy during the same encounter, code Z51.0, Encounter for antineoplastic radiation therapy, and codes from subcategory Z51.1, Encounter for antineoplastic chemotherapy and immunotherapy, may be used together on a record. The sequencing of multiple aftercare codes depends on the circumstances of the encounter.

Certain aftercare Z code categories need a secondary diagnosis code to describe the resolving condition or sequelae. For others, the condition is included in the code title.

Additional Z code aftercare category terms include fitting and adjustment, and attention to artificial openings.

Status Z codes may be used with aftercare Z codes to indicate the nature of the aftercare. For example code Z95.1, Presence of aortocoronary bypass graft, may be used with code Z48.812, Encounter for surgical aftercare following surgery on the circulatory system, to indicate the surgery for which the aftercare is being performed. A status code should not be used when the aftercare code indicates the type of status, such as using Z43.0, Encounter for attention to tracheostomy, with Z93.0, Tracheostomy status.

The aftercare Z category/codes:

Z42	Encounter for plastic and reconstructive surgery following medical procedure or healed injury
Z43	Encounter for attention to artificial openings
Z44	Encounter for fitting and adjustment of external prosthetic device
Z45	Encounter for adjustment and management of implanted device
Z46	Encounter for fitting and adjustment of other devices
Z47	Orthopedic aftercare
Z48	Encounter for other postprocedural aftercare
Z49	Encounter for care involving renal dialysis
Z51	Encounter for other aftercare and medical care

8) Follow-up

The follow-up codes are used to explain continuing surveillance following completed treatment of a disease, condition, or injury. They imply that the condition has been fully treated and no longer exists. They should not be confused with aftercare codes, or injury codes with a 7th character for subsequent encounter, that explain ongoing care of a healing condition or its sequelae. Follow-up codes may be used in conjunction with history codes to provide the full picture of the healed condition and its treatment. The follow-up code is sequenced first, followed by the history code.

A follow-up code may be used to explain multiple visits. Should a condition be found to have recurred on the follow-up visit, then the diagnosis code for the condition should be assigned in place of the follow-up code.

The follow-up Z code categories:

Z08	Encounter for follow-up examination after completed treatment for malignant neoplasm
Z09	Encounter for follow-up examination after completed treatment for conditions other than malignant neoplasm
Z39	Encounter for maternal postpartum care and examination

9) Donor

Codes in category Z52, Donors of organs and tissues, are used for living individuals who are donating blood or other body tissue. These codes are only for individuals donating for others, not for self-donations. They are not used to identify cadaveric donations.

10) Counseling

Counseling Z codes are used when a patient or family member receives assistance in the aftermath of an illness or injury, or when support is required in coping with family or social problems.

The counseling Z codes/categories:

Z30.0-	Encounter for general counseling and advice on contraceptio
Z31.5	Encounter for **procreative** genetic counseling
Z31.6-	Encounter for general counseling and advice on procreation
Z32.2	Encounter for childbirth instruction
Z32.3	Encounter for childcare instruction
Z69	Encounter for mental health services for victim and perpetrato of abuse
Z70	Counseling related to sexual attitude, behavior and orientation
Z71	Persons encountering health services for other counseling an medical advice, not elsewhere classified
Z76.81	Expectant mother prebirth pediatrician visit

11) Encounters for Obstetrical and Reproductive Services

See Section I.C.15. Pregnancy, Childbirth, and the Puerperium, for furthe instruction on the use of these codes.

Z codes for pregnancy are for use in those circumstances when none of th problems or complications included in the codes from the Obstetrics chapte exist (a routine prenatal visit or postpartum care). Codes in category Z34 Encounter for supervision of normal pregnancy, are always first-listed an are not to be used with any other code from the OB chapter.

Codes in category Z3A, Weeks of gestation, may be assigned to provid additional information about the pregnancy. Category Z3A codes should no be assigned for pregnancies with abortive outcomes (categories O00-O08 elective termination of pregnancy (code **Z33.2**), nor for postpartu conditions, as category Z3A is not applicable to these conditions. Th date of the admission should be used to determine weeks of gestation fo inpatient admissions that encompass more than one gestational week.

The outcome of delivery, category Z37, should be included on all materna delivery records. It is always a secondary code. Codes in category Z3 should not be used on the newborn record.

Z codes for family planning (contraceptive) or procreative manageme and counseling should be included on an obstetric record either during th pregnancy or the postpartum stage, if applicable.

Z codes/categories for obstetrical and reproductive services:

Z30	Encounter for contraceptive management
Z31	Encounter for procreative management
Z32.2	Encounter for childbirth instruction
Z32.3	Encounter for childcare instruction
Z33	Pregnant state
Z34	Encounter for supervision of normal pregnancy
Z36	Encounter for antenatal screening of mother
Z3A	Weeks of gestation
Z37	Outcome of delivery
Z39	Encounter for maternal postpartum care and examination
Z76.81	Expectant mother prebirth pediatrician visit

12) Newborns and Infants

See Section I.C.16. Newborn (Perinatal) Guidelines, for further instructio on the use of these codes.

Newborn Z codes/categories:

Z76.1	Encounter for health supervision and care of foundling
Z00.1-	Encounter for routine child health examination
Z38	Liveborn infants according to place of birth and type c delivery

13) Routine and administrative examinations

The Z codes allow for the description of encounters for routine examinations such as, a general check-up, or, examinations for administrative purposes such as, a pre-employment physical. The codes are not to be used if th examination is for diagnosis of a suspected condition or for treatme purposes. In such cases the diagnosis code is used. During a routine exam should a diagnosis or condition be discovered, it should be coded as a additional code. Pre-existing and chronic conditions and history code may also be included as additional codes as long as the examination is fc administrative purposes and not focused on any particular condition.

Some of the codes for routine health examinations distinguish betwee "with" and "without" abnormal findings. Code assignment depends on th information that is known at the time the encounter is being coded. Fo example, if no abnormal findings were found during the examination, bu the encounter is being coded before test results are back, it is acceptable t assign the code for "without abnormal findings." When assigning a cod for "with abnormal findings," additional code(s) should be assigned t identify the specific abnormal finding(s).

Pre-operative examination and pre-procedural laboratory examination Z codes are for use only in those situations when a patient is being cleare for a procedure or surgery and no treatment is given.

The Z codes/categories for routine and administrative examinations:

Z00 Encounter for general examination without complaint, suspected or reported diagnosis
Z01 Encounter for other special examination without complaint, suspected or reported diagnosis
Z02 Encounter for administrative examination Except: Z02.9, Encounter for administrative examinations, unspecified
Z32.0- Encounter for pregnancy test

14) **Miscellaneous Z codes**

The miscellaneous Z codes capture a number of other health care encounters that do not fall into one of the other categories. Certain of these codes identify the reason for the encounter; others are for use as additional codes that provide useful information on circumstances that may affect a patient's care and treatment.

Prophylactic Organ Removal

For encounters specifically for prophylactic removal of an organ (such as prophylactic removal of breasts due to a genetic susceptibility to cancer or a family history of cancer), the principal or first-listed code should be a code from category Z40, Encounter for prophylactic surgery, followed by the appropriate codes to identify the associated risk factor (such as genetic susceptibility or family history).

If the patient has a malignancy of one site and is having prophylactic removal at another site to prevent either a new primary malignancy or metastatic disease, a code for the malignancy should also be assigned in addition to a code from subcategory Z40.0, Encounter for prophylactic surgery for risk factors related to malignant neoplasms. A Z40.0 code should not be assigned if the patient is having organ removal for treatment of a malignancy, such as the removal of the testes for the treatment of prostate cancer.

Miscellaneous Z codes/categories:

Z28 Immunization not carried out
Except: Z28.3, Underimmunization status
Z29 Encounter for other prophylactic measures
Z40 Encounter for prophylactic surgery
Z41 Encounter for procedures for purposes other than remedying health state
Except: Z41.9, Encounter for procedure for purposes other than remedying health state, unspecified
Z53 Persons encountering health services for specific procedures and treatment, not carried out
Z55 Problems related to education and literacy
Z56 Problems related to employment and unemployment
Z57 Occupational exposure to risk factors
Z58 Problems related to physical environment
Z59 Problems related to housing and economic circumstances
Z60 Problems related to social environment
Z62 Problems related to upbringing
Z63 Other problems related to primary support group, including family circumstances
Z64 Problems related to certain psychosocial circumstances
Z65 Problems related to other psychosocial circumstances
Z72 Problems related to lifestyle
Note: These codes should be assigned only when the documentation specifies that the patient has an associated problem.
Z73 Problems related to life management difficulty
Z74 Problems related to care provider dependency
Except: Z74.01, Bed confinement status
Z75 Problems related to medical facilities and other health care
Z76.0 Encounter for issue of repeat prescription
Z76.3 Healthy person accompanying sick person
Z76.4 Other boarder to healthcare facility
Z76.5 Malingerer [conscious simulation]
Z91.1- Patient's noncompliance with medical treatment and regimen
Z91.83 Wandering in diseases classified elsewhere
Z91.84- Oral health risk factors
Z91.89 Other specified personal risk factors, not elsewhere classified

15) **Nonspecific Z codes**

Certain Z codes are so non-specific, or potentially redundant with other codes in the classification, that there can be little justification for their use in the inpatient setting. Their use in the outpatient setting should be limited to those instances when there is no further documentation to permit more precise coding. Otherwise, any sign or symptom or any other reason for visit that is captured in another code should be used.

Nonspecific Z codes/categories:

Z02.9 Encounter for administrative examinations, unspecified
Z04.9 Encounter for examination and observation for unspecified reason
Z13.9 Encounter for screening, unspecified
Z41.9 Encounter for procedure for purposes other than remedying health state, unspecified
Z52.9 Donor of unspecified organ or tissue
Z86.59 Personal history of other mental and behavioral disorders
Z88.9 Allergy status to unspecified drugs, medicaments and biological substances status
Z92.0 Personal history of contraception

16) **Z Codes That May Only be Principal/First-Listed Diagnosis**

The following Z codes/categories may only be reported as the principal/first-listed diagnosis, except when there are multiple encounters on the same day and the medical records for the encounters are combined:

Z00 Encounter for general examination without complaint, suspected or reported diagnosis
Except: Z00.6
Z01 Encounter for other special examination without complaint, suspected or reported diagnosis
Z02 Encounter for administrative examination
Z03 Encounter for medical observation for suspected diseases and conditions ruled out
Z04 Encounter for examination and observation for other reasons
Z33.2 Encounter for elective termination of pregnancy
Z31.81 Encounter for male factor infertility in female patient
Z31.83 Encounter for assisted reproductive fertility procedure cycle
Z31.84 Encounter for fertility preservation procedure
Z34 Encounter for supervision of normal pregnancy
Z39 Encounter for maternal postpartum care and examination
Z38 Liveborn infants according to place of birth and type of delivery
Z40 Encounter for prophylactic surgery
Z42 Encounter for plastic and reconstructive surgery following medical procedure or healed injury
Z51.0 Encounter for antineoplastic radiation therapy
Z51.1- Encounter for antineoplastic chemotherapy and immunotherapy
Z52 Donors of organs and tissues
Except: Z52.9, Donor of unspecified organ or tissue
Z76.1 Encounter for health supervision and care of foundling
Z76.2 Encounter for health supervision and care of other healthy infant and child
Z99.12 Encounter for respirator [ventilator] dependence during power failure

Persons encountering health services for examinations (Z00-Z13)

NOTE Nonspecific abnormal findings disclosed at the time of these examinations are classified to categories R70-R94.

Excludes1: *examinations related to pregnancy and reproduction (Z30-Z36, Z39.-)*

Z00 Encounter for general examination without complaint, suspected or reported diagnosis

Excludes1: *encounter for examination for administrative purposes (Z02.-)*

Excludes2: *encounter for pre-procedural examinations (Z01.81-)*
special screening examinations (Z11-Z13)

Review coding guidelines C.21.c.13 and C.21.c.16

+ **Z00.0 Encounter for general adult medical examination**

Encounter for adult periodic examination (annual) (physical) and any associated laboratory and radiologic examinations

Excludes1: *encounter for examination of sign or symptom- code to sign or symptom*
general health check-up of infant or child (Z00.12.-)

• **Z00.00 Encounter for general adult medical examination without abnormal findings**

Encounter for adult health check-up NOS

AHA CC: 1Q, 2016, 36-37

• **Z00.01 Encounter for general adult medical examination with abnormal findings**

Use additional code to identify abnormal findings

AHA CC: 1Q, 2016, 35-36

+ **Z00.1 Encounter for newborn, infant and child health examinations**

Review coding guideline C.21.c.12

+ **Z00.11 Newborn health examination**

Health check for child under 29 days old

Use additional code to identify any abnormal findings

Excludes1: *health check for child over 28 days old (Z00.12-)*

• **Z00.110 Health examination for newborn under 8 days old**

Health check for newborn under 8 days old

• **Z00.111 Health examination for newborn 8 to 28 days old**

Health check for newborn 8 to 28 days old
Newborn weight check

+ Z00.12 **Encounter for routine child health examination**
Encounter for development testing of infant or child
Health check (routine) for child over 28 days old
Excludes1: *health check for child under 29 days old (Z00.11-)*
health supervision of foundling or other healthy infant or child (Z76.1-Z76.2)
newborn health examination (Z00.11-)
• **Z00.121 Encounter for routine child health examination with abnormal findings**
Use additional code to identify abnormal findings
AHA CC: 1Q, 2016, 34-35
• **Z00.129 Encounter for routine child health examination without abnormal findings**
Encounter for routine child health examination NOS
AHA CC: 1Q, 2016, 34-35
• **Z00.2 Encounter for examination for period of rapid growth in childhood**
• **Z00.3 Encounter for examination for adolescent development state**
Encounter for puberty development state
Z00.5 Encounter for examination of potential donor of organ and tissue
Z00.6 Encounter for examination for normal comparison and control in clinical research program
Examination of participant or control in clinical research program
+ Z00.7 **Encounter for examination for period of delayed growth in childhood**
• **Z00.70 Encounter for examination for period of delayed growth in childhood without abnormal findings**
• **Z00.71 Encounter for examination for period of delayed growth in childhood with abnormal findings**
Use additional code to identify abnormal findings
Z00.8 Encounter for other general examination
Encounter for health examination in population surveys

Z01 Encounter for other special examination without complaint, suspected or reported diagnosis
Includes: routine examination of specific system
NOTE Codes from category Z01 represent the reason for the encounter. A separate procedure code is required to identify any examinations or procedures performed
Excludes1: *encounter for examination for administrative purposes (Z02.-)*
encounter for examination for suspected conditions, proven not to exist (Z03.-)
encounter for laboratory and radiologic examinations as a component of general medical examinations (Z00.0-)
encounter for laboratory, radiologic and imaging examinations for sign(s) and symptom(s) - code to the sign(s) or symptom(s)
Excludes2: *screening examinations (Z11-Z13)*
Review coding guidelines C.21.c.13 and C.21.c.16
+ Z01.0 **Encounter for examination of eyes and vision**
Excludes1: *examination for driving license (Z02.4)*
Z01.00 Encounter for examination of eyes and vision without abnormal findings
Encounter for examination of eyes and vision NOS
Z01.01 Encounter for examination of eyes and vision with abnormal findings
Use additional code to identify abnormal findings
AHA CC: 4Q, 2016, 21
+ Z01.1 **Encounter for examination of ears and hearing**
Z01.10 Encounter for examination of ears and hearing without abnormal findings
Encounter for examination of ears and hearing NOS
AHA CC: 4Q, 2016, 21
+ Z01.11 **Encounter for examination of ears and hearing with abnormal findings**
Z01.110 Encounter for hearing examination following failed hearing screening
AHA CC: 3Q, 2016, 18-19
Z01.118 Encounter for examination of ears and hearing with other abnormal findings
Use additional code to identify abnormal findings
AHA CC: 3Q, 2016, 17
Z01.12 Encounter for hearing conservation and treatment
+ Z01.2 **Encounter for dental examination and cleaning**
Z01.20 Encounter for dental examination and cleaning without abnormal findings
Encounter for dental examination and cleaning NOS
Z01.21 Encounter for dental examination and cleaning with abnormal findings
Use additional code to identify abnormal findings
+ Z01.3 **Encounter for examination of blood pressure**
Z01.30 Encounter for examination of blood pressure without abnormal findings
Encounter for examination of blood pressure NOS
Z01.31 Encounter for examination of blood pressure with abnormal findings
Use additional code to identify abnormal findings
+ Z01.4 **Encounter for gynecological examination**
Excludes2: *pregnancy examination or test (Z32.0-)*
routine examination for contraceptive maintenance (Z30.4-)
+ Z01.41 **Encounter for routine gynecological examination**
Encounter for general gynecological examination with or without cervical smear
Encounter for gynecological examination (general) (routine) NOS
Encounter for pelvic examination (annual) (periodic)
Use additional code:
for screening for human papillomavirus, if applicable, (Z11.51)
for screening vaginal pap smear, if applicable (Z12.72)
to identify acquired absence of uterus, if applicable (Z90.71-)
Excludes1: *gynecologic examination status-post hysterectomy for malignant condition (Z08)*
screening cervical pap smear not a part of a routine gynecological examination (Z12.4)
♀ **Z01.411 Encounter for gynecological examination (general) (routine) with abnormal findings**
Use additional code to identify abnormal findings.
♀ **Z01.419 Encounter for gynecological examination (general) (routine) without abnormal findings**
♀ **Z01.42 Encounter for cervical smear to confirm findings of recent normal smear following initial abnormal smear**
+ Z01.8 **Encounter for other specified special examinations**
+ Z01.81 **Encounter for preprocedural examinations**
Encounter for preoperative examinations
Encounter for radiological and imaging examinations as part of preprocedural examination
Z01.810 Encounter for preprocedural cardiovascular examination
Z01.811 Encounter for preprocedural respiratory examination
Z01.812 Encounter for preprocedural laboratory examination
Blood and urine tests prior to treatment or procedure
Z01.818 Encounter for other preprocedural examination
Encounter for preprocedural examination NOS
Encounter for examinations prior to antineoplastic chemotherapy
Z01.82 Encounter for allergy testing
Excludes1: *encounter for antibody response examination (Z01.84)*
Z01.83 Encounter for blood typing
Encounter for Rh typing
Z01.84 Encounter for antibody response examination
Encounter for immunity status testing
Excludes1: *encounter for allergy testing (Z01.82)*
Z01.89 Encounter for other specified special examinations

Z02 Encounter for administrative examination
Review coding guidelines C.21.c.13 and C.21.c.16
Z02.0 Encounter for examination for admission to educational institution
Encounter for examination for admission to preschool (education)
Encounter for examination for re-admission to school following illness or medical treatment
Z02.1 Encounter for pre-employment examination
Z02.2 Encounter for examination for admission to residential institution
Excludes1: *examination for admission to prison (Z02.89)*
Z02.3 Encounter for examination for recruitment to armed forces
Z02.4 Encounter for examination for driving license

Z02.5 **Encounter for examination for participation in sport**
Excludes1: *blood-alcohol and blood-drug test (Z02.83)*
Z02.6 **Encounter for examination for insurance purposes**
+ **Z02.7** **Encounter for issue of medical certificate**
Excludes1: *encounter for general medical examination (Z00-Z01, Z02.0-Z02.6, Z02.8-Z02.9,)*
Z02.71 **Encounter for disability determination**
Encounter for issue of medical certificate of incapacity
Encounter for issue of medical certificate of invalidity
Z02.79 **Encounter for issue of other medical certificate**
+ **Z02.8** **Encounter for other administrative examinations**
Z02.81 **Encounter for paternity testing**
Z02.82 **Encounter for adoption services**
Z02.83 **Encounter for blood-alcohol and blood-drug test**
Use additional code for findings of alcohol or drugs in blood (R78.-)
Z02.89 **Encounter for other administrative examinations**
Encounter for examination for admission to prison
Encounter for examination for admission to summer camp
Encounter for immigration examination
Encounter for naturalization examination
Encounter for premarital examination
Excludes1: *health supervision of foundling or other healthy infant or child (Z76.1-Z76.2)*
Z02.9 **Encounter for administrative examinations, unspecified**

Z03 **Encounter for medical observation for suspected diseases and conditions ruled out**

This category is to be used when a person without a diagnosis is suspected of having an abnormal condition, without signs or symptoms, which requires study, but after examination and observation, is ruled out. This category is also for use for administrative and legal observation status.
Excludes1: *contact with and (suspected) exposures hazardous to health (Z77.-)*
encounter for observation and evaluation of newborn for suspected diseases and conditions, ruled out (Z05.0-)
person with feared complaint in whom no diagnosis is made (Z71.1)
signs or symptoms under study- code to signs or symptoms
Review coding guidelines C.21.c.6 and C.21.c.16
Z03.6 **Encounter for observation for suspected toxic effect from ingested substance ruled out**
Encounter for observation for suspected adverse effect from drug
Encounter for observation for suspected poisoning
+ **Z03.7** **Encounter for suspected maternal and fetal conditions ruled out**
Encounter for suspected maternal and fetal conditions not found
Excludes1: *known or suspected fetal anomalies affecting management of mother, not ruled out (O26.-, O35.-, O36.-, O40.-, O41.-)*
● ♀ **Z03.71** **Encounter for suspected problem with amniotic cavity and membrane ruled out**
Encounter for suspected oligohydramnios ruled out
Encounter for suspected polyhydramnios ruled out
● ♀ **Z03.72** **Encounter for suspected placental problem ruled out**
● ♀ **Z03.73** **Encounter for suspected fetal anomaly ruled out**
AHA CC: 4Q, 2016, 4-7
● ♀ **Z03.74** **Encounter for suspected problem with fetal growth ruled out**
● ♀ **Z03.75** **Encounter for suspected cervical shortening ruled out**
● ♀ **Z03.79** **Encounter for other suspected maternal and fetal conditions ruled out**
AHA CC: 4Q, 2016, 4-7
+ **Z03.8** **Encounter for observation for other suspected diseases and conditions ruled out**
Z03.81 **Encounter for observation for suspected exposure to biological agents ruled out**
Z03.810 **Encounter for observation for suspected exposure to anthrax ruled out**
Z03.818 **Encounter for observation for suspected exposure to other biological agents ruled out**
Z03.89 **Encounter for observation for other suspected diseases and conditions ruled out**

Z04 **Encounter for examination and observation for other reasons**

Includes: encounter for examination for medicolegal reasons
This category is to be used when a person without a diagnosis is suspected of having an abnormal condition, without signs or symptoms, which requires study, but after examination and observation, is ruled-out. This category is also for use for administrative and legal observation status.
Review coding guidelines C.21.c.6 and C.21.c.16
Z04.1 **Encounter for examination and observation following transport accident**
Excludes1: *encounter for examination and observation following work accident (Z04.2)*
Z04.2 **Encounter for examination and observation following work accident**
Z04.3 **Encounter for examination and observation following other accident**
+ **Z04.4** **Encounter for examination and observation following alleged rape**
Encounter for examination and observation of victim following alleged rape
Encounter for examination and observation of victim following alleged sexual abuse
● **Z04.41** **Encounter for examination and observation following alleged adult rape**
Suspected adult rape, ruled out
Suspected adult sexual abuse, ruled out
Review coding guideline C.19.f
● **Z04.42** **Encounter for examination and observation following alleged child rape**
Suspected child rape, ruled out
Suspected child sexual abuse, ruled out
Review coding guideline C.19.f
Z04.6 **Encounter for general psychiatric examination, requested by authority**
+ **Z04.7** **Encounter for examination and observation following alleged physical abuse**
● **Z04.71** **Encounter for examination and observation following alleged adult physical abuse**
Suspected adult physical abuse, ruled out
Excludes1: *confirmed case of adult physical abuse (T74.-)*
encounter for examination and observation following alleged adult sexual abuse (Z04.41)
suspected case of adult physical abuse, not ruled out (T76.-)
Review coding guideline C.19.f
● **Z04.72** **Encounter for examination and observation following alleged child physical abuse**
Suspected child physical abuse, ruled out
Excludes1: *confirmed case of child physical abuse (T74.-)*
encounter for examination and observation following alleged child sexual abuse (Z04.42)
suspected case of child physical abuse, not ruled out (T76.-)
Review coding guideline C.19.f
Z04.8 **Encounter for examination and observation for other specified reasons**
Encounter for examination and observation for request for expert evidence
Z04.9 **Encounter for examination and observation for unspecified reason**
Encounter for observation NOS

Z05 **Encounter for observation and evaluation of newborn for suspected diseases and conditions ruled out**

NOTE This category is to be used for newborns, within the neonatal period (the first 28 days of life), who are suspected of having an abnormal condition, but without signs or symptoms, and which, after examination and observation, is ruled out.
Review coding guideline C.16.b
Review coding guideline C.21.c.6
AHA CC: 4Q, 2016, 77
Z05.0 **Observation and evaluation of newborn for suspected cardiac condition ruled out**
Z05.1 **Observation and evaluation of newborn for suspected infectious condition ruled out**

Z05.2 Observation and evaluation of newborn for suspected neurological condition ruled out

Z05.3 Observation and evaluation of newborn for suspected respiratory condition ruled out

+ **Z05.4 Observation and evaluation of newborn for suspected genetic, metabolic or immunologic condition ruled out**

Z05.41 Observation and evaluation of newborn for suspected genetic condition ruled out

AHA CC: 4Q, 2016, 54-55

Z05.42 Observation and evaluation of newborn for suspected metabolic condition ruled out

Z05.43 Observation and evaluation of newborn for suspected immunologic condition ruled out

Z05.5 Observation and evaluation of newborn for suspected gastrointestinal condition ruled out

Z05.6 Observation and evaluation of newborn for suspected genitourinary condition ruled out

+ **Z05.7 Observation and evaluation of newborn for suspected skin, subcutaneous, musculoskeletal and connective tissue condition ruled out**

Z05.71 Observation and evaluation of newborn for suspected skin and subcutaneous tissue condition ruled out

Z05.72 Observation and evaluation of newborn for suspected musculoskeletal condition ruled out

Z05.73 Observation and evaluation of newborn for suspected connective tissue condition ruled out

Z05.8 Observation and evaluation of newborn for other specified suspected condition ruled out

Z05.9 Observation and evaluation of newborn for unspecified suspected condition ruled out

Z08 Encounter for follow-up examination after completed treatment for malignant neoplasm

Medical surveillance following completed treatment

Use additional code to identify any acquired absence of organs (Z90.-)

Use additional code to identify the personal history of malignant neoplasm (Z85.-)

Excludes1: *aftercare following medical care (Z43-Z49, Z51)*

Review coding guideline C.21.c.8

Valid 3-character code, no further characters required

Z09 Encounter for follow-up examination after completed treatment for conditions other than malignant neoplasm

Medical surveillance following completed treatment

Use additional code to identify any applicable history of disease code (Z86.-, Z87.-)

Excludes1: *aftercare following medical care (Z43-Z49, Z51)*
surveillance of contraception (Z30.4-)
surveillance of prosthetic and other medical devices (Z44-Z46)

Review coding guideline C.21.c.8

AHA CC: 1Q, 2017, 9

Valid 3-character code, no further characters required

Z11 Encounter for screening for infectious and parasitic diseases

Screening is the testing for disease or disease precursors in asymptomatic individuals so that early detection and treatment can be provided for those who test positive for the disease.

Excludes1: *encounter for diagnostic examination-code to sign or symptom*

Review coding guideline C.21.c.5

Z11.0 Encounter for screening for intestinal infectious diseases

Z11.1 Encounter for screening for respiratory tuberculosis

Z11.2 Encounter for screening for other bacterial diseases

Z11.3 Encounter for screening for infections with a predominantly sexual mode of transmission

Excludes2: *encounter for screening for human immunodeficiency virus [HIV] (Z11.4)*
encounter for screening for human papillomavirus (Z11.51)

Z11.4 Encounter for screening for human immunodeficiency virus [HIV]

Review coding guideline C.1.a.2.h

+ **Z11.5 Encounter for screening for other viral diseases**

Excludes2: *encounter for screening for viral intestinal disease (Z11.0)*

Z11.51 Encounter for screening for human papillomavirus (HPV)

Z11.59 Encounter for screening for other viral diseases

Z11.6 Encounter for screening for other protozoal diseases and helminthiases

Excludes2: *encounter for screening for protozoal intestinal disease (Z11.0)*

Z11.8 Encounter for screening for other infectious and parasitic diseases

Encounter for screening for chlamydia

Encounter for screening for rickettsial

Encounter for screening for spirochetal

Encounter for screening for mycoses

Z11.9 Encounter for screening for infectious and parasitic diseases, unspecified

Z12 Encounter for screening for malignant neoplasms

Screening is the testing for disease or disease precursors in asymptomatic individuals so that early detection and treatment can be provided for those who test positive for the disease.

Use additional code to identify any family history of malignant neoplasm (Z80.-)

Excludes1: *encounter for diagnostic examination-code to sign or symptom*

Review coding guideline C.21.c.5

Z12.0 Encounter for screening for malignant neoplasm of stomach

+ **Z12.1 Encounter for screening for malignant neoplasm of intestinal tract**

Z12.10 Encounter for screening for malignant neoplasm of intestinal tract, unspecified

Z12.11 Encounter for screening for malignant neoplasm of colon

Encounter for screening colonoscopy NOS

AHA CC: 1Q, 2017, 8-9

Z12.12 Encounter for screening for malignant neoplasm of rectum

Z12.13 Encounter for screening for malignant neoplasm of small intestine

Z12.2 Encounter for screening for malignant neoplasm of respiratory organs

+ **Z12.3 Encounter for screening for malignant neoplasm of breast**

Z12.31 Encounter for screening mammogram for malignant neoplasm of breast

Excludes1: *inconclusive mammogram (R92.2)*

AHA CC: 1Q, 2015, 24

Z12.39 Encounter for other screening for malignant neoplasm of breast

♀ **Z12.4 Encounter for screening for malignant neoplasm of cervix**

Encounter for screening pap smear for malignant neoplasm of cervix

Excludes1: *when screening is part of general gynecological examination (Z01.4-)*

Excludes2: *encounter for screening for human papillomavirus (Z11.51)*

♂ **Z12.5 Encounter for screening for malignant neoplasm of prostate**

Z12.6 Encounter for screening for malignant neoplasm of bladder

+ **Z12.7 Encounter for screening for malignant neoplasm of other genitourinary organs**

♂ **Z12.71 Encounter for screening for malignant neoplasm of testis**

♀ **Z12.72 Encounter for screening for malignant neoplasm of vagina**

Vaginal pap smear status-post hysterectomy for non-malignant condition

Use additional code to identify acquired absence of uterus (Z90.71-)

Excludes1: *vaginal pap smear status-post hysterectomy for malignant conditions (Z08)*

♀ **Z12.73 Encounter for screening for malignant neoplasm of ovary**

Z12.79 Encounter for screening for malignant neoplasm of other genitourinary organs

+ **Z12.8 Encounter for screening for malignant neoplasm of other sites**

Z12.81 Encounter for screening for malignant neoplasm of oral cavity

Z12.82 Encounter for screening for malignant neoplasm of nervous system

Z12.83 Encounter for screening for malignant neoplasm of skin

Z12.89 Encounter for screening for malignant neoplasm of other sites

Z12.9 Encounter for screening for malignant neoplasm, site unspecified

Z13 Encounter for screening for other diseases and disorders

Screening is the testing for disease or disease precursors in asymptomatic individuals so that early detection and treatment can be provided for those who test positive for the disease.

Excludes1: *encounter for diagnostic examination-code to sign or symptom*

Review coding guideline C.21.c.5

Z13.0 Encounter for screening for diseases of the blood and blood-forming organs and certain disorders involving the immune mechanism

Z13.1 Encounter for screening for diabetes mellitus

+ **Z13.2 Encounter for screening for nutritional, metabolic and other endocrine disorders**

Z13.21 Encounter for screening for nutritional disorder

+ **Z13.22 Encounter for screening for metabolic disorder**

Z13.220 Encounter for screening for lipoid disorders

Encounter for screening for cholesterol level

Encounter for screening for hypercholesterolemia

Encounter for screening for hyperlipidemia

Z13.228 Encounter for screening for other metabolic disorders

Z13.29 Encounter for screening for other suspected endocrine disorder

Excludes1: *encounter for screening for diabetes mellitus (Z13.1)*

• **Z13.4 Encounter for screening for certain developmental disorders in childhood**

Encounter for screening for developmental handicaps in early childhood

Excludes1: *routine development testing of infant or child (Z00.1-)*

Z13.5 Encounter for screening for eye and ear disorders

Excludes2: *encounter for general hearing examination (Z01.1-)*
encounter for general vision examination (Z01.0-)

AHA CC: 3Q, 2016, 17

Z13.6 Encounter for screening for cardiovascular disorders

+ **Z13.7 Encounter for screening for genetic and chromosomal anomalies**

Excludes1: *genetic testing for procreative management (Z31.4-)*

Z13.71 Encounter for nonprocreative screening for genetic disease carrier status

Z13.79 Encounter for other screening for genetic and chromosomal anomalies

+ **Z13.8 Encounter for screening for other specified diseases and disorders**

Excludes2: *screening for malignant neoplasms (Z12.-)*

+ **Z13.81 Encounter for screening for digestive system disorders**

Z13.810 Encounter for screening for upper gastrointestinal disorder

Z13.811 Encounter for screening for lower gastrointestinal disorder

Excludes1: *encounter for screening for intestinal infectious disease (Z11.0)*

Z13.818 Encounter for screening for other digestive system disorders

+ **Z13.82 Encounter for screening for musculoskeletal disorder**

Z13.820 Encounter for screening for osteoporosis

Z13.828 Encounter for screening for other musculoskeletal disorder

Z13.83 Encounter for screening for respiratory disorder NEC

Excludes1: *encounter for screening for respiratory tuberculosis (Z11.1)*

Z13.84 Encounter for screening for dental disorders

+ **Z13.85 Encounter for screening for nervous system disorders**

Z13.850 Encounter for screening for traumatic brain injury

Z13.858 Encounter for screening for other nervous system disorders

Z13.88 Encounter for screening for disorder due to exposure to contaminants

Excludes1: *those exposed to contaminants without suspected disorders (Z57.-, Z77.-)*

Z13.89 Encounter for screening for other disorder

Encounter for screening for genitourinary disorders

Z13.9 Encounter for screening, unspecified

Genetic carrier and genetic susceptibility to disease (Z14-Z15)

Z14 Genetic carrier

Review coding guideline C.21.c.3

+ **Z14.0 Hemophilia A carrier**

Z14.01 Asymptomatic hemophilia A carrier

Z14.02 Symptomatic hemophilia A carrier

Z14.1 Cystic fibrosis carrier

Z14.8 Genetic carrier of other disease

Z15 Genetic susceptibility to disease

Includes: confirmed abnormal gene

Use additional code, if applicable, for any associated family history of the disease (Z80-Z84)

Excludes1: *chromosomal anomalies (Q90-Q99)*

Review coding guideline C.21.c.3

+ **Z15.0 Genetic susceptibility to malignant neoplasm**

Code first , if applicable, any current malignant neoplasm (C00-C75, C81-C96)

Use additional code, if applicable, for any personal history of malignant neoplasm (Z85.-)

Z15.01 Genetic susceptibility to malignant neoplasm of breast

♀ **Z15.02 Genetic susceptibility to malignant neoplasm of ovary**

♂ **Z15.03 Genetic susceptibility to malignant neoplasm of prostate**

♀ **Z15.04 Genetic susceptibility to malignant neoplasm of endometrium**

Z15.09 Genetic susceptibility to other malignant neoplasm

+ **Z15.8 Genetic susceptibility to other disease**

Z15.81 Genetic susceptibility to multiple endocrine neoplasia [MEN]

Excludes1: *multiple endocrine neoplasia [MEN] syndromes (E31.2-)*

Z15.89 Genetic susceptibility to other disease

Resistance to antimicrobial drugs (Z16)

Z16 Resistance to antimicrobial drugs

NOTE The codes in this category are provided for use as additional codes to identify the resistance and non-responsiveness of a condition to antimicrobial drugs.

Code first the infection

Excludes1: *Methicillin resistant Staphylococcus aureus infection (A49.02)*
Methicillin resistant Staphylococcus aureus pneumonia (J15.212)
Sepsis due to Methicillin resistant Staphylococcus aureus (A41.02)

Review coding guideline C.1.c

Review coding guideline C.21.c.3

+ **Z16.1 Resistance to beta lactam antibiotics**

Z16.10 Resistance to unspecified beta lactam antibiotics

Z16.11 Resistance to penicillins

Resistance to amoxicillin

Resistance to ampicillin

Review coding guidelines C.1.e.1.a and C.1.e.1.b

Z16.12 Extended spectrum beta lactamase (ESBL) resistance

Excludes2: *Methicillin resistant Staphylococcus aureus infection in diseases classified elsewhere (B95.62)*

Z16.19 Resistance to other specified beta lactam antibiotics

Resistance to cephalosporins

+ **Z16.2 Resistance to other antibiotics**

Z16.20 Resistance to unspecified antibiotic

Resistance to antibiotics NOS

Z16.21 Resistance to vancomycin

Z16.22 Resistance to vancomycin related antibiotics

Z16.23 Resistance to quinolones and fluoroquinolones

Z16.24 Resistance to multiple antibiotics

Z16.29 Resistance to other single specified antibiotic

Resistance to aminoglycosides

Resistance to macrolides

Resistance to sulfonamides

Resistance to tetracyclines

+ **Z16.3 Resistance to other antimicrobial drugs**

Excludes1: *resistance to antibiotics (Z16.1-, Z16.2-)*

Z16.30 Resistance to unspecified antimicrobial drugs

Drug resistance NOS

Z16.31 Resistance to antiparasitic drug(s)

Resistance to quinine and related compounds

Z16.32 **Resistance to antifungal drug(s)**
Z16.33 **Resistance to antiviral drug(s)**
\+ **Z16.34** **Resistance to antimycobacterial drug(s)**
Resistance to tuberculostatics
Z16.341 **Resistance to single antimycobacterial drug**
Resistance to antimycobacterial drug NOS
Z16.342 **Resistance to multiple antimycobacterial drugs**
Z16.35 **Resistance to multiple antimicrobial drugs**
Excludes1: *Resistance to multiple antibiotics only (Z16.24)*
Z16.39 **Resistance to other specified antimicrobial drug**

Estrogen receptor status (Z17)

Z17 Estrogen receptor status
Code first malignant neoplasm of breast (C50.-)
Review coding guideline C.21.c.3
Z17.0 **Estrogen receptor positive status [ER+]**
Z17.1 **Estrogen receptor negative status [ER-]**

Retained foreign body fragments (Z18)

Z18 Retained foreign body fragments
Includes: embedded fragment (status)
embedded splinter (status)
retained foreign body status
Excludes1: *artificial joint prosthesis status (Z96.6-)*
foreign body accidentally left during a procedure (T81.5-)
foreign body entering through orifice (T15-T19)
in situ cardiac device (Z95.-)
organ or tissue replaced by means other than transplant (Z96.-, Z97.-)
organ or tissue replaced by transplant (Z94.-)
personal history of retained foreign body fully removed (Z87.821)
superficial foreign body (non-embedded splinter) - code to superficial foreign body, by site
Review coding guideline C.21.c.3
\+ **Z18.0** **Retained radioactive fragments**
Z18.01 **Retained depleted uranium fragments**
Z18.09 **Other retained radioactive fragments**
Other retained depleted isotope fragments
Retained nontherapeutic radioactive fragments
\+ **Z18.1** **Retained metal fragments**
Excludes1: *retained radioactive metal fragments (Z18.01-Z18.09)*
Z18.10 **Retained metal fragments, unspecified**
Retained metal fragment NOS
Z18.11 **Retained magnetic metal fragments**
Z18.12 **Retained nonmagnetic metal fragments**
Z18.2 **Retained plastic fragments**
Acrylics fragments
Diethylhexylphthalates fragments
Isocyanate fragments
\+ **Z18.3** **Retained organic fragments**
Z18.31 **Retained animal quills or spines**
Z18.32 **Retained tooth**
Z18.33 **Retained wood fragments**
Z18.39 **Other retained organic fragments**
\+ **Z18.8** **Other specified retained foreign body**
Z18.81 **Retained glass fragments**
Z18.83 **Retained stone or crystalline fragments**
Retained concrete or cement fragments
Z18.89 **Other specified retained foreign body fragments**
AHA CC: 3Q, 2016, 24
Z18.9 **Retained foreign body fragments, unspecified material**

Hormone sensitivity malignancy status (Z19)

Z19 Hormone sensitivity malignancy status
Code first malignant neoplasm - see Table of Neoplasms, by site, malignant
Review coding guideline C.21.c.3
AHA CC: 4Q, 2016, 76
Z19.1 **Hormone sensitive malignancy status**
Z19.2 **Hormone resistant malignancy status**
Castrate resistant prostate malignancy status

Persons with potential health hazards related to communicable diseases (Z20-Z29)

Z20 Contact with and (suspected) exposure to communicable diseases
Excludes1: *carrier of infectious disease (Z22.-)*
diagnosed current infectious or parasitic disease -see Alphabetic Index
Excludes2: *personal history of infectious and parasitic diseases (Z86.1-)*
Review coding guideline C.21.c.1
\+ **Z20.0** **Contact with and (suspected) exposure to intestinal infectious diseases**
Z20.01 **Contact with and (suspected) exposure to intestinal infectious diseases due to Escherichia coli (E. coli)**
Z20.09 **Contact with and (suspected) exposure to other intestinal infectious diseases**
Z20.1 **Contact with and (suspected) exposure to tuberculosis**
Z20.2 **Contact with and (suspected) exposure to infections with a predominantly sexual mode of transmission**
Z20.3 **Contact with and (suspected) exposure to rabies**
Z20.4 **Contact with and (suspected) exposure to rubella**
Z20.5 **Contact with and (suspected) exposure to viral hepatitis**
Z20.6 **Contact with and (suspected) exposure to human immunodeficiency virus [HIV]**
Excludes1: *asymptomatic human immunodeficiency virus [HIV] HIV infection status (Z21)*
Z20.7 **Contact with and (suspected) exposure to pediculosis, acariasis and other infestations**
\+ **Z20.8** **Contact with and (suspected) exposure to other communicable diseases**
\+ **Z20.81** **Contact with and (suspected) exposure to other bacterial communicable diseases**
Z20.810 **Contact with and (suspected) exposure to anthrax**
Z20.811 **Contact with and (suspected) exposure to meningococcus**
Z20.818 **Contact with and (suspected) exposure to other bacterial communicable diseases**
\+ **Z20.82** **Contact with and (suspected) exposure to other viral communicable diseases**
Z20.820 **Contact with and (suspected) exposure to varicella**
Z20.828 **Contact with and (suspected) exposure to other viral communicable diseases**
AHA CC: 4Q, 2016, 4-7
Z20.89 **Contact with and (suspected) exposure to other communicable diseases**
Z20.9 **Contact with and (suspected) exposure to unspecified communicable disease**

Z21 Asymptomatic human immunodeficiency virus [HIV] infection status
HIV positive NOS
Code first Human immunodeficiency virus [HIV] disease complicating pregnancy, childbirth and the puerperium, if applicable (O98.7-)
Excludes1: *acquired immunodeficiency syndrome (B20)*
contact with human immunodeficiency virus [HIV] (Z20.6)
exposure to human immunodeficiency virus [HIV] (Z20.6)
human immunodeficiency virus [HIV] disease (B20)
inconclusive laboratory evidence of human immunodeficiency virus [HIV] (R75)
Review coding guidelines C.1.a.2.d, C.1.a.2.f and C.1.a.2.g
Review coding guideline C.15.f
Review coding guideline C.21.c.3
Valid 3-character code, no further characters required

Z22 Carrier of infectious disease
Includes: colonization status
suspected carrier
Excludes2: *carrier of viral hepatitis (B18.-)*
Review coding guideline C.21.c.3
Z22.0 **Carrier of typhoid**
Z22.1 **Carrier of other intestinal infectious diseases**
Z22.2 **Carrier of diphtheria**
\+ **Z22.3** **Carrier of other specified bacterial diseases**
Z22.31 **Carrier of bacterial disease due to meningococci**
\+ **Z22.32** **Carrier of bacterial disease due to staphylococci**
Z22.321 **Carrier or suspected carrier of Methicillin susceptible Staphylococcus aureus**
MSSA colonization
Review coding guidelines C.1.e.1.c and C.1.e.1.d

Z22.322 **Carrier or suspected carrier of Methicillin resistant Staphylococcus aureus**
MRSA colonization
Review coding guidelines C.1.e.1.c and C.1.e.1.d

+ Z22.33 **Carrier of bacterial disease due to streptococci**
Z22.330 **Carrier of Group B streptococcus**
Excludes1: *carrier of streptococcus group B (GBS) complicating pregnancy, childbirth and the puerperium (O99.82-)*
Z22.338 **Carrier of other streptococcus**
Z22.39 **Carrier of other specified bacterial diseases**
Z22.4 **Carrier of infections with a predominantly sexual mode of transmission**
Z22.6 **Carrier of human T-lymphotropic virus type-1 [HTLV-1] infection**
Z22.8 **Carrier of other infectious diseases**
Z22.9 **Carrier of infectious disease, unspecified**

Z23 **Encounter for immunization**
Code first any routine childhood examination
NOTE Procedure codes are required to identify the types of immunizations given
Review coding guideline C.21.c.2
Valid 3-character code, no further characters required

Z28 **Immunization not carried out and underimmunization status**
Includes: vaccination not carried out
+ Z28.0 **Immunization not carried out because of contraindication**
Z28.01 **Immunization not carried out because of acute illness of patient**
Z28.02 **Immunization not carried out because of chronic illness or condition of patient**
Z28.03 **Immunization not carried out because of immune compromised state of patient**
Z28.04 **Immunization not carried out because of patient allergy to vaccine or component**
Z28.09 **Immunization not carried out because of other contraindication**
Z28.1 **Immunization not carried out because of patient decision for reasons of belief or group pressure**
Immunization not carried out because of religious belief
+ Z28.2 **Immunization not carried out because of patient decision for other and unspecified reason**
Z28.20 **Immunization not carried out because of patient decision for unspecified reason**
Z28.21 **Immunization not carried out because of patient refusal**
Z28.29 **Immunization not carried out because of patient decision for other reason**
Z28.3 **Underimmunization status**
Delinquent immunization status
Lapsed immunization schedule status
Review coding guideline C.21.c.3
+ Z28.8 **Immunization not carried out for other reason**
Z28.81 **Immunization not carried out due to patient having had the disease**
Z28.82 **Immunization not carried out because of caregiver refusal**
Immunization not carried out because of guardian refusal
Immunization not carried out because of parent refusal
Excludes1: *immunization not carried out because of caregiver refusal because of religious belief (Z28.1)*
Z28.89 **Immunization not carried out for other reason**
Z28.9 **Immunization not carried out for unspecified reason**

Z29 **Encounter for other prophylactic measures**
Excludes1: *desensitization to allergens (Z51.6)*
prophylactic surgery (Z40.-)
Review coding guideline C.21.c.14
AHA CC: 4Q, 2016, 78-79
+ Z29.1 **Encounter for prophylactic immunotherapy**
Encounter for administration of immunoglobulin
Z29.11 **Encounter for prophylactic immunotherapy for respiratory syncytial virus (RSV)**
Z29.12 **Encounter for prophylactic antivenin**
Z29.13 **Encounter for prophylactic Rho(D) immune globulin**
Z29.14 **Encounter for prophylactic rabies immune globin**
Z29.3 **Encounter for prophylactic fluoride administration**
Z29.8 **Encounter for other specified prophylactic measures**
Z29.9 **Encounter for prophylactic measures, unspecified**

Persons encountering health services in circumstances related to reproduction (Z30-Z39)

Z30 **Encounter for contraceptive management**
Review coding guideline C.21.c.11
AHA CC: 4Q, 2016, 78
+ Z30.0 **Encounter for general counseling and advice on contraception**
Review coding guideline C.21.c.10
+ Z30.01 **Encounter for initial prescription of contraceptives**
Excludes1: *encounter for surveillance of contraceptives (Z30.4-)*
♀ Z30.011 **Encounter for initial prescription of contraceptive pills**
♀ Z30.012 **Encounter for prescription of emergency contraception**
Encounter for postcoital contraception
♀ Z30.013 **Encounter for initial prescription of injectable contraceptive**
♀ Z30.014 **Encounter for initial prescription of intrauterine contraceptive device**
Excludes1: *encounter for insertion of intrauterine contraceptive device (Z30.430, Z30.432)*
Z30.015 **Encounter for initial prescription of vaginal ring hormonal contraceptive**
Z30.016 **Encounter for initial prescription of transdermal patch hormonal contraceptive device**
Z30.017 **Encounter for initial prescription of implantable subdermal contraceptive**
♀ Z30.018 **Encounter for initial prescription of other contraceptives**
Encounter for initial prescription of barrier contraception
Encounter for initial prescription of diaphragm
♀ Z30.019 **Encounter for initial prescription of contraceptives, unspecified**
Z30.02 **Counseling and instruction in natural family planning to avoid pregnancy**
Z30.09 **Encounter for other general counseling and advice on contraception**
Encounter for family planning advice NOS
Z30.2 **Encounter for sterilization**
+ Z30.4 **Encounter for surveillance of contraceptives**
Z30.40 **Encounter for surveillance of contraceptives, unspecified**
♀ Z30.41 **Encounter for surveillance of contraceptive pills**
Encounter for repeat prescription for contraceptive pill
♀ Z30.42 **Encounter for surveillance of injectable contraceptive**
+ Z30.43 **Encounter for surveillance of intrauterine contraceptive device**
♀ Z30.430 **Encounter for insertion of intrauterine contraceptive device**
♀ Z30.431 **Encounter for routine checking of intrauterine contraceptive device**
♀ Z30.432 **Encounter for removal of intrauterine contraceptive device**
♀ Z30.433 **Encounter for removal and reinsertion of intrauterine contraceptive device**
Encounter for replacement of intrauterine contraceptive device
♀ Z30.44 **Encounter for surveillance of vaginal ring hormonal contraceptive device**
♀ Z30.45 **Encounter for surveillance of transdermal patch hormonal contraceptive device**
♀ Z30.46 **Encounter for surveillance of implantable subdermal contraceptive**
Encounter for checking, reinsertion or removal of implantable subdermal contraceptive
♀ Z30.49 **Encounter for surveillance of other contraceptives**
Encounter for surveillance of barrier contraception
Encounter for surveillance of diaphragm
Z30.8 **Encounter for other contraceptive management**
Encounter for postvasectomy sperm count
Encounter for routine examination for contraceptive maintenance
Excludes1: *sperm count following sterilization reversal (Z31.42)*
sperm count for fertility testing (Z31.41)
Z30.9 **Encounter for contraceptive management, unspecified**

Z31 Encounter for procreative management

Excludes1: *complications associated with artificial fertilization (N98.-)*
female infertility (N97.-)
male infertility (N46.-)
Review coding guideline C.21.c.11

Z31.0 Encounter for reversal of previous sterilization

+ **Z31.4 Encounter for procreative investigation and testing**
Excludes1: *postvasectomy sperm count (Z30.8)*

Z31.41 Encounter for fertility testing
Encounter for fallopian tube patency testing
Encounter for sperm count for fertility testing

Z31.42 Aftercare following sterilization reversal
Sperm count following sterilization reversal

+ **Z31.43 Encounter for genetic testing of female for procreative management**
Use additional code for recurrent pregnancy loss, if applicable (N96, O26.2-)
Excludes1: *nonprocreative genetic testing (Z13.7-)*

♀ **Z31.430 Encounter of female for testing for genetic disease carrier status for procreative management**

♀ **Z31.438 Encounter for other genetic testing of female for procreative management**

+ **Z31.44 Encounter for genetic testing of male for procreative management**
Excludes1: *nonprocreative genetic testing (Z13.7-)*

♂ **Z31.440 Encounter of male for testing for genetic disease carrier status for procreative management**

• ♂ **Z31.441 Encounter for testing of male partner of patient with recurrent pregnancy loss**

• ♂ **Z31.448 Encounter for other genetic testing of male for procreative management**

Z31.49 Encounter for other procreative investigation and testing

Z31.5 Encounter for procreative genetic counseling
Review coding guideline C.21.c.10

+ **Z31.6 Encounter for general counseling and advice on procreation**
Review coding guideline C.21.c.10

Z31.61 Procreative counseling and advice using natural family planning

Z31.62 Encounter for fertility preservation counseling
Encounter for fertility preservation counseling prior to cancer therapy
Encounter for fertility preservation counseling prior to surgical removal of gonads

Z31.69 Encounter for other general counseling and advice on procreation

Z31.7 Encounter for procreative management and counseling for gestational carrier
Excludes1: *pregnant state, gestational carrier (Z33.3)*
AHA CC: 4Q, 2016, 78

+ **Z31.8 Encounter for other procreative management**

♀ **Z31.81 Encounter for male factor infertility in female patient**
Review coding guideline C.21.c.16

♀ **Z31.82 Encounter for Rh incompatibility status**
Review coding guideline C.21.c.16
AHA CC: 4Q, 2014, 17

♀ **Z31.83 Encounter for assisted reproductive fertility procedure cycle**
Patient undergoing in vitro fertilization cycle
Use additional code to identify the type of infertility
Excludes1: *pre-cycle diagnosis and testing - code to reason for encounter*
Review coding guideline C.21.c.16

Z31.84 Encounter for fertility preservation procedure
Encounter for fertility preservation procedure prior to cancer therapy
Encounter for fertility preservation procedure prior to surgical removal of gonads
Review coding guideline C.21.c.16

Z31.89 Encounter for other procreative management

Z31.9 Encounter for procreative management, unspecified

Z32 Encounter for pregnancy test and childbirth and childcare instruction

+ **Z32.0 Encounter for pregnancy test**
Review coding guideline C.21.c.13

♀ **Z32.00 Encounter for pregnancy test, result unknown**
Encounter for pregnancy test NOS

• ♀ **Z32.01 Encounter for pregnancy test, result positive**

♀ **Z32.02 Encounter for pregnancy test, result negative**

Z32.2 Encounter for childbirth instruction
Review coding guidelines C.21.c.10 and C.21.c.11

Z32.3 Encounter for childcare instruction
Encounter for prenatal or postpartum childcare instruction
Review coding guidelines C.21.c.10 and C.21.c.11

Z33 Pregnant state
Review coding guideline C.21.c.11
AHA CC: 4Q, 2016, 78

• ♀ **Z33.1 Pregnant state, incidental**
Pregnant state NOS
Excludes1: *complications of pregnancy (O00-O9A)*
pregnant state, gestational carrier (Z33.3)
Review coding guideline C.15.a.1
Review coding guidelines C.21.c.3

• ♀ **Z33.2 Encounter for elective termination of pregnancy**
Excludes1: *early fetal death with retention of dead fetus (O02.1)*
late fetal death (O36.4)
spontaneous abortion (O03)
Review coding guidelines C.15.q.1 and C.15.q.2
Review coding guidelines C.21.c.16

• ♀ **Z33.3 Pregnant state, gestational carrier**
Excludes1: *encounter for procreative management and counseling for gestational carrier (Z31.7)*

Z34 Encounter for supervision of normal pregnancy

Excludes1: *any complication of pregnancy (O00-O9A)*
encounter for pregnancy test (Z32.0-)
encounter for supervision of high risk pregnancy (O09.-)
Review coding guideline C.15.b.1
Review coding guidelines C.21.c.11 and C.21.c.16
AHA CC: 4Q, 2016, 4-7

+ **Z34.0 Encounter for supervision of normal first pregnancy**

• ♀ **Z34.00 Encounter for supervision of normal first pregnancy, unspecified trimester**

• ♀ **Z34.01 Encounter for supervision of normal first pregnancy, first trimester**

• ♀ **Z34.02 Encounter for supervision of normal first pregnancy, second trimester**

• ♀ **Z34.03 Encounter for supervision of normal first pregnancy, third trimester**

+ **Z34.8 Encounter for supervision of other normal pregnancy**

• ♀ **Z34.80 Encounter for supervision of other normal pregnancy, unspecified trimester**

• ♀ **Z34.81 Encounter for supervision of other normal pregnancy, first trimester**

• ♀ **Z34.82 Encounter for supervision of other normal pregnancy, second trimester**

• ♀ **Z34.83 Encounter for supervision of other normal pregnancy, third trimester**
AHA CC: 4Q, 2014, 17

+ **Z34.9 Encounter for supervision of normal pregnancy, unspecified**

• ♀ **Z34.90 Encounter for supervision of normal pregnancy, unspecified, unspecified trimester**

• ♀ **Z34.91 Encounter for supervision of normal pregnancy, unspecified, first trimester**

• ♀ **Z34.92 Encounter for supervision of normal pregnancy, unspecified, second trimester**

• ♀ **Z34.93 Encounter for supervision of normal pregnancy, unspecified, third trimester**

Z36 Encounter for antenatal screening of mother

Includes: Encounter for placental sample (taken vaginally)
Screening is the testing for disease or disease precursors in asymptomatic individuals so that early detection and treatment can be provided for those who test positive for the disease.
Excludes1: *diagnostic examination- code to sign or symptom*
encounter for suspected maternal and fetal conditions ruled out (Z03.7-)
suspected fetal condition affecting management of pregnancy - code to condition in Chapter 15
Excludes2: *abnormal findings on antenatal screening of mother (O28.-)*
genetic counseling and testing (Z31.43-, Z31.5)
routine prenatal care (Z34)
Review coding guidelines C.21.c.5 and C.21.c.11

• ♀ **Z36.0 Encounter for antenatal screening for chromosomal anomalies**

• ♀ **Z36.1 Encounter for antenatal screening for raised alphafetoprotein level**
Encounter for antenatal screening for elevated maternal serum alphafetoprotein level

• ♀ **Z36.2 Encounter for other antenatal screening follow-up**
Non-visualized anatomy on a previous scan

- • ♀ Z36.3 **Encounter for antenatal screening for malformations**
  Screening for suspected anomaly
- • ♀ Z36.4 **Encounter for antenatal screening for fetal growth retardation**
  Intrauterine growth restriction (IUGR)/small-for-dates
- • ♀ Z36.5 **Encounter for antenatal screening for isoimmunization**
- + Z36.8 **Encounter for other antenatal screening**
  - • ♀ Z36.81 **Encounter for antenatal screening for hydrops fetails**
  - • ♀ Z36.82 **Encounter for antenatal screening fornuchal translucency**
  - • ♀ Z36.83 **Encounter for antenatal screening for congenital cardiac abnormalities**
  - • ♀ Z36.84 **Encounter for antenatal screening for fetal lung maturity**
  - • ♀ Z36.85 **Encounter for antenatal screening for Streptococcus B**
  - • ♀ Z36.86 **Encounter for antenatal screening for for cervical length**
    Screening for risk of pre-term labor
  - • ♀ Z36.87 **Encounter for antenatal screening for uncertain dates**
  - • ♀ Z36.88 **Encounter for antenatal screening for fetal macrosomia**
    Screening for large-for-dates
  - • ♀ Z36.89 **Encounter for other specified antenatal screening**
  - • ♀ Z36.8A **Encounter for antenatal screening for other genetic defects**
- • ♀ Z36.9 **Encounter for antenatal screening, unspecified**

Z3A Weeks of gestation

NOTE Codes from category Z3A are for use, only on the maternal record, to indicate the weeks of gestation of the pregnancy, if known.

Code first complications of pregnancy, childbirth and the puerperium (O09-O9A)

Review coding guideline C.21.c.11

- + Z3A.0 **Weeks of gestation of pregnancy, unspecified or less than 10 weeks**
  - • ♀ Z3A.00 **Weeks of gestation of pregnancy not specified**
  - • ♀ Z3A.01 **Less than 8 weeks gestation of pregnancy**
  - • ♀ Z3A.08 **8 weeks gestation of pregnancy**
  - • ♀ Z3A.09 **9 weeks gestation of pregnancy**
- + Z3A.1 **Weeks of gestation of pregnancy, weeks 10-19**
  - • ♀ Z3A.10 **10 weeks gestation of pregnancy**
  - • ♀ Z3A.11 **11 weeks gestation of pregnancy**
  - • ♀ Z3A.12 **12 weeks gestation of pregnancy**
  - • ♀ Z3A.13 **13 weeks gestation of pregnancy**
  - • ♀ Z3A.14 **14 weeks gestation of pregnancy**
  - • ♀ Z3A.15 **15 weeks gestation of pregnancy**
  - • ♀ Z3A.16 **16 weeks gestation of pregnancy**
    AHA CC: 4Q, 2016, 4-7
  - • ♀ Z3A.17 **17 weeks gestation of pregnancy**
  - • ♀ Z3A.18 **18 weeks gestation of pregnancy**
  - • ♀ Z3A.19 **19 weeks gestation of pregnancy**
- + Z3A.2 **Weeks of gestation of pregnancy, weeks 20-29**
  - • ♀ Z3A.20 **20 weeks gestation of pregnancy**
    AHA CC: 4Q, 2016, 4-7
  - • ♀ Z3A.21 **21 weeks gestation of pregnancy**
  - • ♀ Z3A.22 **22 weeks gestation of pregnancy**
    AHA CC: 4Q, 2016, 4-7
  - • ♀ Z3A.23 **23 weeks gestation of pregnancy**
  - • ♀ Z3A.24 **24 weeks gestation of pregnancy**
  - • ♀ Z3A.25 **25 weeks gestation of pregnancy**
  - • ♀ Z3A.26 **26 weeks gestation of pregnancy**
  - • ♀ Z3A.27 **27 weeks gestation of pregnancy**
  - • ♀ Z3A.28 **28 weeks gestation of pregnancy**
  - • ♀ Z3A.29 **29 weeks gestation of pregnancy**
- + Z3A.3 **Weeks of gestation of pregnancy, weeks 30-39**
  - • ♀ Z3A.30 **30 weeks gestation of pregnancy**
  - • ♀ Z3A.31 **31 weeks gestation of pregnancy**
  - • ♀ Z3A.32 **32 weeks gestation of pregnancy**
    AHA CC: 4Q, 2016, 4-7
  - • ♀ Z3A.33 **33 weeks gestation of pregnancy**
  - • ♀ Z3A.34 **34 weeks gestation of pregnancy**
  - • ♀ Z3A.35 **35 weeks gestation of pregnancy**
  - • ♀ Z3A.36 **36 weeks gestation of pregnancy**
  - • ♀ Z3A.37 **37 weeks gestation of pregnancy**
  - • ♀ Z3A.38 **38 weeks gestation of pregnancy**
    AHA CC: 2Q, 2016, 34
  - • ♀ Z3A.39 **39 weeks gestation of pregnancy**
- + Z3A.4 **Weeks of gestation of pregnancy, weeks 40 or greater**
  - • ♀ Z3A.40 **40 weeks gestation of pregnancy**
    AHA CC: 2Q, 2014, 9
  - • ♀ Z3A.41 **41 weeks gestation of pregnancy**
  - • ♀ Z3A.42 **42 weeks gestation of pregnancy**
    AHA CC: 4Q, 2014, 23
  - • ♀ Z3A.49 **Greater than 42 weeks gestation of pregnancy**

Z37 Outcome of delivery

This category is intended for use as an additional code to identify the outcome of delivery on the mother's record. It is not for use on the newborn record.

Excludes1: *stillbirth (P95)*

Review coding guidelines C.15.b.5
Review coding guidelines C.15.n.3 and C.15.q.1
Review coding guidelines C.21.c.11

- • ♀ Z37.0 **Single live birth**
  AHA CC: 2Q, 2014, 9; 4Q, 2014, 17-18; 2Q, 2016, 34
- • ♀ Z37.1 **Single stillbirth**
- • ♀ Z37.2 **Twins, both liveborn**
- • ♀ Z37.3 **Twins, one liveborn and one stillborn**
- • ♀ Z37.4 **Twins, both stillborn**
- + Z37.5 **Other multiple births, all liveborn**
  - • ♀ Z37.50 **Multiple births, unspecified, all liveborn**
  - • ♀ Z37.51 **Triplets, all liveborn**
  - • ♀ Z37.52 **Quadruplets, all liveborn**
  - • ♀ Z37.53 **Quintuplets, all liveborn**
  - • ♀ Z37.54 **Sextuplets, all liveborn**
  - • ♀ Z37.59 **Other multiple births, all liveborn**
- + Z37.6 **Other multiple births, some liveborn**
  - • ♀ Z37.60 **Multiple births, unspecified, some liveborn**
  - • ♀ Z37.61 **Triplets, some liveborn**
  - • ♀ Z37.62 **Quadruplets, some liveborn**
  - • ♀ Z37.63 **Quintuplets, some liveborn**
  - • ♀ Z37.64 **Sextuplets, some liveborn**
  - • ♀ Z37.69 **Other multiple births, some liveborn**
- • ♀ Z37.7 **Other multiple births, all stillborn**
- • ♀ Z37.9 **Outcome of delivery, unspecified**
  Multiple birth NOS
  Single birth NOS

Z38 Liveborn infants according to place of birth and type of delivery

This category is for use as the principal code on the initial record of a newborn baby. It is to be used for the initial birth record only. It is not to be used on the mother's record.

Review coding guideline C.16.a.2
Review coding guideline C.17
Review coding guidelines C.21.c.6, C.21.c.12 and C.21.c.16
AHA CC: 2Q, 2015, 15; 4Q, 2016, 4-7, 54-55

- + Z38.0 **Single liveborn infant, born in hospital**
  Single liveborn infant, born in birthing center or other health care facility
  AHA CC: 2Q, 2017, 5-7
  - • Z38.00 **Single liveborn infant, delivered vaginally**
  - • Z38.01 **Single liveborn infant, delivered by cesarean**
    AHA CC: 3Q, 2016, 18
- • Z38.1 **Single liveborn infant, born outside hospital**
- • Z38.2 **Single liveborn infant, unspecified as to place of birth**
  Single liveborn infant NOS
- + Z38.3 **Twin liveborn infant, born in hospital**
  - • Z38.30 **Twin liveborn infant, delivered vaginally**
  - • Z38.31 **Twin liveborn infant, delivered by cesarean**
- • Z38.4 **Twin liveborn infant, born outside hospital**
- • Z38.5 **Twin liveborn infant, unspecified as to place of birth**
- + Z38.6 **Other multiple liveborn infant, born in hospital**
  - • Z38.61 **Triplet liveborn infant, delivered vaginally**
  - • Z38.62 **Triplet liveborn infant, delivered by cesarean**
  - • Z38.63 **Quadruplet liveborn infant, delivered vaginally**
  - • Z38.64 **Quadruplet liveborn infant, delivered by cesarean**
  - • Z38.65 **Quintuplet liveborn infant, delivered vaginally**
  - • Z38.66 **Quintuplet liveborn infant, delivered by cesarean**
  - • Z38.68 **Other multiple liveborn infant, delivered vaginally**
  - • Z38.69 **Other multiple liveborn infant, delivered by cesarean**
- • Z38.7 **Other multiple liveborn infant, born outside hospital**
- • Z38.8 **Other multiple liveborn infant, unspecified as to place of birth**

Z39 Encounter for maternal postpartum care and examination

Review coding guidelines C.21.c.8, C.21.c.11 and C.21.c.16

- • ♀ Z39.0 **Encounter for care and examination of mother immediately after delivery**
  Care and observation in uncomplicated cases when the delivery occurs outside a healthcare facility
  Excludes1: *care for postpartum complication- see Alphabetic index*
  Review coding guideline C.15.o.4

• ♀ **Z39.1** **Encounter for care and examination of lactating mother**
Encounter for supervision of lactation
Excludes1: *disorders of lactation (O92.-)*

• ♀ **Z39.2** **Encounter for routine postpartum follow-up**

Encounters for other specific health care (Z40-Z53)

Categories Z40-Z53 are intended for use to indicate a reason for care. They may be used for patients who have already been treated for a disease or injury, but who are receiving aftercare or prophylactic care, or care to consolidate the treatment, or to deal with a residual state

Excludes2: *follow-up examination for medical surveillance after treatment (Z08-Z09)*

Z40 Encounter for prophylactic surgery

Excludes1: *organ donations (Z52.-)*
therapeutic organ removal-code to condition
Review coding guideline C.21.c.14 and C21.c.16

+ **Z40.0** **Encounter for prophylactic surgery for risk factors related to malignant neoplasms**
Admission for prophylactic organ removal
Use additional code to identify risk factor
Z40.00 **Encounter for prophylactic removal of unspecified organ**
Z40.01 **Encounter for prophylactic removal of breast**
♀ **Z40.02** **Encounter for prophylactic removal of ovary(s)**
Encounter for prophylactic removal of ovary(s) and fallopian tube(s)
♀ **Z40.03** **Encounter for prophylactic removal of fallopian tube(s)**
Z40.09 **Encounter for prophylactic removal of other organ**

Z40.8 **Encounter for other prophylactic surgery**
Z40.9 **Encounter for prophylactic surgery, unspecified**

Z41 Encounter for procedures for purposes other than remedying health state

Z41.1 **Encounter for cosmetic surgery**
Encounter for cosmetic breast implant
Encounter for cosmetic procedure
Excludes1: *encounter for plastic and reconstructive surgery following medical procedure or healed injury (Z42.-)*
encounter for post-mastectomy breast implantation (Z42.1)

♂ **Z41.2** **Encounter for routine and ritual male circumcision**
Z41.3 **Encounter for ear piercing**
Z41.8 **Encounter for other procedures for purposes other than remedying health state**
Z41.9 **Encounter for procedure for purposes other than remedying health state, unspecified**

Z42 Encounter for plastic and reconstructive surgery following medical procedure or healed injury

Excludes1: *encounter for cosmetic plastic surgery (Z41.1)*
encounter for plastic surgery for treatment of current injury - code to relevent injury
Review coding guidelines C.21.c.7 and C.21.c.16

• **Z42.1** **Encounter for breast reconstruction following mastectomy**
Excludes1: *deformity and disproportion of reconstructed breast (N65.1-)*

Z42.8 **Encounter for other plastic and reconstructive surgery following medical procedure or healed injury**
AHA CC: 1Q, 2017, 42-43

Z43 Encounter for attention to artificial openings

Includes: closure of artificial openings
passage of sounds or bougies through artificial openings
reforming artificial openings
removal of catheter from artificial openings
toilet or cleansing of artificial openings
Excludes1: *complications of external stoma (J95.0-, K94.-, N99.5-)*
Excludes2: *fitting and adjustment of prosthetic and other devices (Z44-Z46)*
Review coding guideline C.21.c.7

Z43.0 **Encounter for attention to tracheostomy**
CC **Z43.1** **Encounter for attention to gastrostomy**
CC Exclusion see Appendix A PDX collection 1487
Excludes2: *artificial opening status only, without need for care (Z93.-)*
Z43.2 **Encounter for attention to ileostomy**
AHA CC: 3Q, 2016, 5
Z43.3 **Encounter for attention to colostomy**
Z43.4 **Encounter for attention to other artificial openings of digestive tract**
Z43.5 **Encounter for attention to cystostomy**
Z43.6 **Encounter for attention to other artificial openings of urinary tract**
Encounter for attention to nephrostomy
Encounter for attention to ureterostomy
Encounter for attention to urethrostomy
Z43.7 **Encounter for attention to artificial vagina**
Z43.8 **Encounter for attention to other artificial openings**
Z43.9 **Encounter for attention to unspecified artificial opening**

Z44 Encounter for fitting and adjustment of external prosthetic device

Includes: removal or replacement of external prosthetic device
Excludes1: *malfunction or other complications of device - see Alphabetical Index*
presence of prosthetic device (Z97.-)
Review coding guideline C.21.c.7

+ **Z44.0** **Encounter for fitting and adjustment of artificial arm**
+ **Z44.00** **Encounter for fitting and adjustment of unspecified artificial arm**
Z44.001 **Encounter for fitting and adjustment of unspecified right artificial arm**
Z44.002 **Encounter for fitting and adjustment of unspecified left artificial arm**
Z44.009 **Encounter for fitting and adjustment of unspecified artificial arm, unspecified arm**
+ **Z44.01** **Encounter for fitting and adjustment of complete artificial arm**
Z44.011 **Encounter for fitting and adjustment of complete right artificial arm**
Z44.012 **Encounter for fitting and adjustment of complete left artificial arm**
Z44.019 **Encounter for fitting and adjustment of complete artificial arm, unspecified arm**
+ **Z44.02** **Encounter for fitting and adjustment of partial artificial arm**
Z44.021 **Encounter for fitting and adjustment of partial artificial right arm**
Z44.022 **Encounter for fitting and adjustment of partial artificial left arm**
Z44.029 **Encounter for fitting and adjustment of partial artificial arm, unspecified arm**

+ **Z44.1** **Encounter for fitting and adjustment of artificial leg**
+ **Z44.10** **Encounter for fitting and adjustment of unspecified artificial leg**
Z44.101 **Encounter for fitting and adjustment of unspecified right artificial leg**
Z44.102 **Encounter for fitting and adjustment of unspecified left artificial leg**
Z44.109 **Encounter for fitting and adjustment of unspecified artificial leg, unspecified leg**
+ **Z44.11** **Encounter for fitting and adjustment of complete artificial leg**
Z44.111 **Encounter for fitting and adjustment of complete right artificial leg**
Z44.112 **Encounter for fitting and adjustment of complete left artificial leg**
Z44.119 **Encounter for fitting and adjustment of complete artificial leg, unspecified leg**
+ **Z44.12** **Encounter for fitting and adjustment of partial artificial leg**
Z44.121 **Encounter for fitting and adjustment of partial artificial right leg**
Z44.122 **Encounter for fitting and adjustment of partial artificial left leg**
Z44.129 **Encounter for fitting and adjustment of partial artificial leg, unspecified leg**

+ **Z44.2** **Encounter for fitting and adjustment of artificial eye**
Excludes1: *mechanical complication of ocular prosthesis (T85.3)*
Z44.20 **Encounter for fitting and adjustment of artificial eye unspecified**
Z44.21 **Encounter for fitting and adjustment of artificial right eye**
Z44.22 **Encounter for fitting and adjustment of artificial left eye**

+ **Z44.3 Encounter for fitting and adjustment of external breast prosthesis**

Excludes1: *complications of breast implant (T85.4-)*
encounter for adjustment or removal of breast implant (Z45.81-)
encounter for initial breast implant insertion for cosmetic breast augmentation (Z41.1)
encounter for breast reconstruction following mastectomy (Z42.1)

Z44.30 Encounter for fitting and adjustment of external breast prosthesis, unspecified breast

Z44.31 Encounter for fitting and adjustment of external right breast prosthesis

Z44.32 Encounter for fitting and adjustment of external left breast prosthesis

Z44.8 Encounter for fitting and adjustment of other external prosthetic devices

Z44.9 Encounter for fitting and adjustment of unspecified external prosthetic device

Z45 Encounter for adjustment and management of implanted device

Includes: removal or replacement of implanted device
Excludes1: *malfunction or other complications of device - see Alphabetical Index*
Excludes2: *encounter for fitting and adjustment of non-implanted device (Z46.-)*
Review coding guideline C.21.c.7

+ **Z45.0 Encounter for adjustment and management of cardiac device**

+ **Z45.01 Encounter for adjustment and management of cardiac pacemaker**

Encounter for adjustment and management of cardiac resynchronization therapy pacemaker (CRT-P)
Excludes1: *encounter for adjustment and management of automatic implantable cardiac defibrillator with synchronous cardiac pacemaker (Z45.02)*

Z45.010 Encounter for checking and testing of cardiac pacemaker pulse generator [battery]

Encounter for replacing cardiac pacemaker pulse generator [battery]

Z45.018 Encounter for adjustment and management of other part of cardiac pacemaker

Excludes2: *presence of prosthetic and other devices (Z95-Z97)*

Z45.02 Encounter for adjustment and management of automatic implantable cardiac defibrillator

Encounter for adjustment and management of automatic implantable cardiac defibrillator with synchronous cardiac pacemaker
Encounter for adjustment and management of cardiac resynchronization therapy defibrillator (CRT-D)

Z45.09 Encounter for adjustment and management of other cardiac device

Z45.1 Encounter for adjustment and management of infusion pump

Z45.2 Encounter for adjustment and management of vascular access device

Encounter for adjustment and management of vascular catheters
Excludes1: *encounter for adjustment and management of renal dialysis catheter (Z49.01)*

+ **Z45.3 Encounter for adjustment and management of implanted devices of the special senses**

Z45.31 Encounter for adjustment and management of implanted visual substitution device

+ **Z45.32 Encounter for adjustment and management of implanted hearing device**

Excludes1: *Encounter for fitting and adjustment of hearing aide (Z46.1)*

Z45.320 Encounter for adjustment and management of bone conduction device

Z45.321 Encounter for adjustment and management of cochlear device

Z45.328 Encounter for adjustment and management of other implanted hearing device

+ **Z45.4 Encounter for adjustment and management of implanted nervous system device**

Z45.41 Encounter for adjustment and management of cerebrospinal fluid drainage device

Encounter for adjustment and management of cerebral ventricular (communicating) shunt

Z45.42 Encounter for adjustment and management of neuropacemaker (brain) (peripheral nerve) (spinal cord)

Z45.49 Encounter for adjustment and management of other implanted nervous system device

AHA CC: 3Q, 2014, 19-20

+ **Z45.8 Encounter for adjustment and management of other implanted devices**

+ **Z45.81 Encounter for adjustment or removal of breast implant**

Encounter for elective implant exchange (different material) (different size)
Encounter removal of tissue expander without synchronous insertion of permanent implant
Excludes1: *complications of breast implant (T85.4-)*
encounter for initial breast implant insertion for cosmetic breast augmentation (Z41.1)
encounter for breast reconstruction following mastectomy (Z42.1)

Z45.811 Encounter for adjustment or removal of right breast implant

Z45.812 Encounter for adjustment or removal of left breast implant

Z45.819 Encounter for adjustment or removal of unspecified breast implant

Z45.82 Encounter for adjustment or removal of myringotomy device (stent) (tube)

Z45.89 Encounter for adjustment and management of other implanted devices

AHA CC: 4Q, 2014, 26-28

Z45.9 Encounter for adjustment and management of unspecified implanted device

Z46 Encounter for fitting and adjustment of other devices

Includes: removal or replacement of other device
Excludes1: *malfunction or other complications of device - see Alphabetical Index*
Excludes2: *encounter for fitting and management of implanted devices (Z45.-)*
issue of repeat prescription only (Z76.0)
presence of prosthetic and other devices (Z95-Z97)
Review coding guideline C.21.c.7

Z46.0 Encounter for fitting and adjustment of spectacles and contact lenses

Z46.1 Encounter for fitting and adjustment of hearing aid

Excludes1: *encounter for adjustment and management of implanted hearing device (Z45.32-)*

Z46.2 Encounter for fitting and adjustment of other devices related to nervous system and special senses

Excludes2: *encounter for adjustment and management of implanted nervous system device (Z45.4-)*
encounter for adjustment and management of implanted visual substitution device (Z45.31)

Z46.3 Encounter for fitting and adjustment of dental prosthetic device

Encounter for fitting and adjustment of dentures

Z46.4 Encounter for fitting and adjustment of orthodontic device

+ **Z46.5 Encounter for fitting and adjustment of other gastrointestinal appliance and device**

Excludes1: *encounter for attention to artificial openings of digestive tract (Z43.1-Z43.4)*

Z46.51 Encounter for fitting and adjustment of gastric lap band

Z46.59 Encounter for fitting and adjustment of other gastrointestinal appliance and device

Z46.6 Encounter for fitting and adjustment of urinary device

Excludes2: *attention to artificial openings of urinary tract (Z43.5, Z43.6)*

+ **Z46.8 Encounter for fitting and adjustment of other specified devices**

Z46.81 Encounter for fitting and adjustment of insulin pump

Encounter for insulin pump titration
Encounter for insulin pump instruction and training

Z46.82 Encounter for fitting and adjustment of non-vascular catheter

Z46.89 Encounter for fitting and adjustment of other specified devices

Encounter for fitting and adjustment of wheelchair

Z46.9 Encounter for fitting and adjustment of unspecified device

Z47 Orthopedic aftercare

Excludes1: *aftercare for healing fracture-code to fracture with 7th character D*

Review coding guideline C.21.c.7

Z47.1 Aftercare following joint replacement surgery

Use additional code to identify the joint (Z96.6-)

Z47.2 Encounter for removal of internal fixation device

Excludes1: *encounter for adjustment of internal fixation device for fracture treatment- code to fracture with appropriate 7th character*
encounter for removal of external fixation device- code to fracture with 7th character D
infection or inflammatory reaction to internal fixation device (T84.6-)
mechanical complication of internal fixation device (T84.1-)

+ Z47.3 Aftercare following explantation of joint prosthesis

Aftercare following explantation of joint prosthesis, staged procedure
Encounter for joint prosthesis insertion following prior explantation of joint prosthesis

Z47.31 Aftercare following explantation of shoulder joint prosthesis

Excludes1: *acquired absence of shoulder joint following prior explantation of shoulder joint prosthesis (Z89.23-)*
shoulder joint prosthesis explantation status (Z89.23-)

Z47.32 Aftercare following explantation of hip joint prosthesis

Excludes1: *acquired absence of hip joint following prior explantation of hip joint prosthesis (Z89.62-)*
hip joint prosthesis explantation status (Z89.62-)

AHA CC: 1Q, 2015, 16-17

Z47.33 Aftercare following explantation of knee joint prosthesis

Excludes1: *acquired absence of knee joint following prior explantation of knee prosthesis (Z89.52-*
knee joint prosthesis explantation status (Z89.52-)

+ Z47.8 Encounter for other orthopedic aftercare

Z47.81 Encounter for orthopedic aftercare following surgical amputation

Use additional code to identify the limb amputated (Z89.-)

Z47.82 Encounter for orthopedic aftercare following scoliosis surgery

Z47.89 Encounter for other orthopedic aftercare

Z48 Encounter for other postprocedural aftercare

Excludes1: *encounter for aftercare following injury - code to Injury, by site, with appropriate 7th character for subsequent encounter*
encounter for follow-up examination after completed treatment (Z08-Z09)

Excludes2: *encounter for attention to artificial openings (Z43.-)*
encounter for fitting and adjustment of prosthetic and other devices (Z44-Z46)

Review coding guideline C.21.c.7

+ Z48.0 Encounter for attention to dressings, sutures and drains

Excludes1: *encounter for planned postprocedural wound closure (Z48.1)*

Z48.00 Encounter for change or removal of nonsurgical wound dressing

Encounter for change or removal of wound dressing NOS

Z48.01 Encounter for change or removal of surgical wound dressing

AHA CC: 4Q, 2015, 38

Z48.02 Encounter for removal of sutures

Encounter for removal of staples

Z48.03 Encounter for change or removal of drains

Z48.1 Encounter for planned postprocedural wound closure

Excludes1: *encounter for attention to dressings and sutures (Z48.0-)*

+ Z48.2 Encounter for aftercare following organ transplant

CC **Z48.21 Encounter for aftercare following heart transplant**

CC Exclusion see Appendix A PDX collection 1488

CC **Z48.22 Encounter for aftercare following kidney transplant**

CC Exclusion see Appendix A PDX collection 1489

CC **Z48.23 Encounter for aftercare following liver transplant**

CC Exclusion see Appendix A PDX collection 1490

CC **Z48.24 Encounter for aftercare following lung transplant**

CC Exclusion see Appendix A PDX collection 1491

+ Z48.28 Encounter for aftercare following multiple organ transplant

CC **Z48.280 Encounter for aftercare following heart-lung transplant**

CC Exclusion see Appendix A PDX collection 1488

Z48.288 Encounter for aftercare following multiple organ transplant

+ Z48.29 Encounter for aftercare following other organ transplant

CC **Z48.290 Encounter for aftercare following bone marrow transplant**

CC Exclusion see Appendix A PDX collection 1492

Z48.298 Encounter for aftercare following other organ transplant

Z48.3 Aftercare following surgery for neoplasm

Use additional code to identify the neoplasm

+ Z48.8 Encounter for other specified postprocedural aftercare

+ Z48.81 Encounter for surgical aftercare following surgery on specified body systems

These codes identify the body system requiring aftercare. They are for use in conjunction with other aftercare codes to fully explain the aftercare encounter. The condition treated should also be coded if still present.

Excludes1: *aftercare for injury- code the injury with 7th character D*
aftercare following surgery for neoplasm (Z48.3)

Excludes2: *aftercare following organ transplant (Z48.2-)*
orthopedic aftercare (Z47.-)

Z48.810 Encounter for surgical aftercare following surgery on the sense organs

Z48.811 Encounter for surgical aftercare following surgery on the nervous system

Excludes2: *encounter for surgical aftercare following surgery on the sense organs (Z48.810)*

Z48.812 Encounter for surgical aftercare following surgery on the circulatory system

AHA CC: 4Q, 2012, 96-97

Z48.813 Encounter for surgical aftercare following surgery on the respiratory system

Z48.814 Encounter for surgical aftercare following surgery on the teeth or oral cavity

Z48.815 Encounter for surgical aftercare following surgery on the digestive system

AHA CC: 4Q, 2015, 38

Z48.816 Encounter for surgical aftercare following surgery on the genitourinary system

Excludes1: *encounter for aftercare following sterilization reversal (Z31.42)*

Z48.817 Encounter for surgical aftercare following surgery on the skin and subcutaneous tissue

Z48.89 Encounter for other specified surgical aftercare

Z49 Encounter for5 care involving renal dialysis

Code also associated end stage renal disease (N18.6)

Review coding guideline C.21.c.7

+ Z49.0 Preparatory care for renal dialysis

Encounter for dialysis instruction and training

Z49.01 Encounter for fitting and adjustment of extracorporeal dialysis catheter

Removal or replacement of renal dialysis catheter
Toilet or cleansing of renal dialysis catheter

Z49.02 Encounter for fitting and adjustment of peritoneal dialysis catheter

+ Z49.3 Encounter for adequacy testing for dialysis

Z49.31 Encounter for adequacy testing for hemodialysis

Z49.32 Encounter for adequacy testing for peritoneal dialysis

Encounter for peritoneal equilibration test

Z51 **Encounter for other aftercare and medical care**

Code also condition requiring care

Excludes1: *follow-up examination after treatment (Z08-Z09)*

Review coding guidelines C.2.a, C.2.e.2 and C.2.e.3

Review coding guideline C.21.c.7

Z51.0 **Encounter for antineoplastic radiation therapy**

Review coding guidelines C.21.c.7 and C.21.c.16

+ Z51.1 **Encounter for antineoplastic chemotherapy and immunotherapy**

Excludes2: *encounter for chemotherapy and immunotherapy for nonneoplastic condition - code to condition*

Review coding guidelines C.21.c.7 and C21.c.16

Z51.11 **Encounter for antineoplastic chemotherapy**

AHA CC: 3Q, 2015, 19-20

Z51.12 **Encounter for antineoplastic immunotherapy**

Z51.5 **Encounter for palliative care**

AHA CC: 1Q, 2017, 48-49

Z51.6 **Encounter for desensitization to allergens**

AHA CC: 4Q, 2016, 77

+ Z51.8 **Encounter for other specified aftercare**

Excludes1: *holiday relief care (Z75.5)*

Z51.81 **Encounter for therapeutic drug level monitoring**

Code also any long-term (current) drug therapy (Z79.-)

Excludes1: *encounter for blood-drug test for administrative or medicolegal reasons (Z02.83)*

Z51.89 **Encounter for other specified aftercare**

AHA CC: 4Q, 2012, 96-97

NOTE Z51.89 is an acceptable PDX when reported with a secondary diagnosis.

Z52 **Donors of organs and tissues**

Includes: autologous and other living donors

Excludes1: *cadaveric donor - omit code*
examination of potential donor (Z00.5)

Review coding guidelines C.21.c.9 and C.21.c.16

+ Z52.0 **Blood donor**

+ Z52.00 **Unspecified blood donor**

Z52.000 **Unspecified donor, whole blood**

Z52.001 **Unspecified donor, stem cells**

Z52.008 **Unspecified donor, other blood**

+ Z52.01 **Autologous blood donor**

Z52.010 **Autologous donor, whole blood**

Z52.011 **Autologous donor, stem cells**

Z52.018 **Autologous donor, other blood**

+ Z52.09 **Other blood donor**

Volunteer donor

Z52.090 **Other blood donor, whole blood**

Z52.091 **Other blood donor, stem cells**

Z52.098 **Other blood donor, other blood**

+ Z52.1 **Skin donor**

Z52.10 **Skin donor, unspecified**

Z52.11 **Skin donor, autologous**

Z52.19 **Skin donor, other**

+ Z52.2 **Bone donor**

Z52.20 **Bone donor, unspecified**

Z52.21 **Bone donor, autologous**

Z52.29 **Bone donor, other**

Z52.3 **Bone marrow donor**

Z52.4 **Kidney donor**

Z52.5 **Cornea donor**

Z52.6 **Liver donor**

+ Z52.8 **Donor of other specified organs or tissues**

+ Z52.81 **Egg (Oocyte) donor**

♀ Z52.810 **Egg (Oocyte) donor under age 35, anonymous recipient**

Egg donor under age 35 NOS

♀ Z52.811 **Egg (Oocyte) donor under age 35, designated recipient**

♀ Z52.812 **Egg (Oocyte) donor age 35 and over, anonymous recipient**

Egg donor age 35 and over NOS

♀ Z52.813 **Egg (Oocyte) donor age 35 and over, designated recipient**

♀ Z52.819 **Egg (Oocyte) donor, unspecified**

Z52.89 **Donor of other specified organs or tissues**

Z52.9 **Donor of unspecified organ or tissue**

Donor NOS

Z53 **Persons encountering health services for specific procedures and treatment, not carried out**

+ Z53.0 **Procedure and treatment not carried out because of contraindication**

Z53.01 **Procedure and treatment not carried out due to patient smoking**

Z53.09 **Procedure and treatment not carried out because of other contraindication**

Z53.1 **Procedure and treatment not carried out because of patient's decision for reasons of belief and group pressure**

+ Z53.2 **Procedure and treatment not carried out because of patient's decision for other and unspecified reasons**

Z53.20 **Procedure and treatment not carried out because of patient's decision for unspecified reasons**

Z53.21 **Procedure and treatment not carried out due to patient leaving prior to being seen by health care provider**

Z53.29 **Procedure and treatment not carried out because of patient's decision for other reasons**

+ Z53.3 **Procedure converted to open procedure**

AHA CC: 4Q, 2016, 79

Z53.31 **Laparoscopic surgical procedure converted to open procedure**

AHA CC: 4Q, 2016, 100-101

Z53.32 **Thoracoscopic surgical procedure converted to open procedure**

Z53.33 **Arthroscopic surgical procedure converted to open procedure**

Z53.39 **Other specified procedure converted to open procedure**

Z53.8 **Procedure and treatment not carried out for other reasons**

Z53.9 **Procedure and treatment not carried out, unspecified reason**

Persons with potential health hazards related to socioeconomic and psychosocial circumstances (Z55-Z65)

Z55 **Problems related to education and literacy**

Excludes1: *disorders of psychological development (F80-F89)*

Z55.0 **Illiteracy and low-level literacy**

Z55.1 **Schooling unavailable and unattainable**

Z55.2 **Failed school examinations**

Z55.3 **Underachievement in school**

Z55.4 **Educational maladjustment and discord with teachers and classmates**

Z55.8 **Other problems related to education and literacy**

Problems related to inadequate teaching

Z55.9 **Problems related to education and literacy, unspecified**

Academic problems NOS

Z56 **Problems related to employment and unemployment**

Excludes2: *occupational exposure to risk factors (Z57.-)*
problems related to housing and economic circumstances (Z59.-)

Z56.0 **Unemployment, unspecified**

• Z56.1 **Change of job**

Z56.2 **Threat of job loss**

Z56.3 **Stressful work schedule**

Z56.4 **Discord with boss and workmates**

Z56.5 **Uncongenial work environment**

Difficult conditions at work

Z56.6 **Other physical and mental strain related to work**

+ Z56.8 **Other problems related to employment**

Z56.81 **Sexual harassment on the job**

Z56.82 **Military deployment status**

Individual (civilian or military) currently deployed in theater or in support of military war, peacekeeping and humanitarian operations

Z56.89 **Other problems related to employment**

Z56.9 **Unspecified problems related to employment**

Occupational problems NOS

Z57 **Occupational exposure to risk factors**

Z57.0 **Occupational exposure to noise**

Z57.1 **Occupational exposure to radiation**

Z57.2 **Occupational exposure to dust**

+ Z57.3 **Occupational exposure to other air contaminants**

Z57.31 **Occupational exposure to environmental tobacco smoke**

Excludes2: *exposure to environmental tobacco smoke (Z77.22)*

Z57.39 **Occupational exposure to other air contaminants**

Z57.4 Occupational exposure to toxic agents in agriculture
Occupational exposure to solids, liquids, gases or vapors in agriculture
Z57.5 Occupational exposure to toxic agents in other industries
Occupational exposure to solids, liquids, gases or vapors in other industries
Z57.6 Occupational exposure to extreme temperature
Z57.7 Occupational exposure to vibration
Z57.8 Occupational exposure to other risk factors
Z57.9 Occupational exposure to unspecified risk factor

Z59 Problems related to housing and economic circumstances

Excludes2: *problems related to upbringing (Z62.-)*
Z59.0 Homelessness
Z59.1 Inadequate housing
Lack of heating
Restriction of space
Technical defects in home preventing adequate care
Unsatisfactory surroundings
Excludes1: *problems related to the natural and physical environment (Z77.1-)*
Z59.2 Discord with neighbors, lodgers and landlord
Z59.3 Problems related to living in residential institution
Boarding-school resident
Excludes1: *institutional upbringing (Z62.2)*
Z59.4 Lack of adequate food and safe drinking water
Inadequate drinking water supply
Excludes1: *effects of hunger (T73.0)*
inappropriate diet or eating habits (Z72.4)
malnutrition (E40-E46)
Z59.5 Extreme poverty
Z59.6 Low income
Z59.7 Insufficient social insurance and welfare support
Z59.8 Other problems related to housing and economic circumstances
Foreclosure on loan
Isolated dwelling
Problems with creditors
Z59.9 Problem related to housing and economic circumstances, unspecified

Z60 Problems related to social environment

Z60.0 Problems of adjustment to life-cycle transitions
Empty nest syndrome
Phase of life problem
Problem with adjustment to retirement [pension]
Z60.2 Problems related to living alone
Z60.3 Acculturation difficulty
Problem with migration
Problem with social transplantation
Z60.4 Social exclusion and rejection
Exclusion and rejection on the basis of personal characteristics, such as unusual physical appearance, illness or behavior.
Excludes1: *target of adverse discrimination such as for racial or religious reasons (Z60.5)*
Z60.5 Target of (perceived) adverse discrimination and persecution
Excludes1: *social exclusion and rejection (Z60.4)*
Z60.8 Other problems related to social environment
Z60.9 Problem related to social environment, unspecified

Z62 Problems related to upbringing

Includes: current and past negative life events in childhood
current and past problems of a child related to upbringing
Excludes2: *maltreatment syndrome (T74.-)*
problems related to housing and economic circumstances (Z59.-)
Z62.0 Inadequate parental supervision and control
Z62.1 Parental overprotection
+ **Z62.2 Upbringing away from parents**
Excludes1: *problems with boarding school (Z59.3)*
• **Z62.21 Child in welfare custody**
Child in care of non-parental family member
Child in foster care
Excludes2: *problem for parent due to child in welfare custody (Z63.5)*
Z62.22 Institutional upbringing
Child living in orphanage or group home
Z62.29 Other upbringing away from parents
• **Z62.3 Hostility towards and scapegoating of child**
Z62.6 Inappropriate (excessive) parental pressure
+ **Z62.8 Other specified problems related to upbringing**
+ **Z62.81 Personal history of abuse in childhood**
Z62.810 Personal history of physical and sexual abuse in childhood
Excludes1: *current child physical abuse (T74.12, T76.12)*
current child sexual abuse (T74.22, T76.22)
Z62.811 Personal history of psychological abuse in childhood
Excludes1: *current child psychological abuse (T74.32, T76.32)*
Z62.812 Personal history of neglect in childhood
Excludes1: *current child neglect (T74.02, T76.02)*
Z62.819 Personal history of unspecified abuse in childhood
Excludes1: *current child abuse NOS (T74.92, T76.92)*
+ **Z62.82 Parent-child conflict**
Z62.820 Parent-biological child conflict
Parent-child problem NOS
Z62.821 Parent-adopted child conflict
Z62.822 Parent-foster child conflict
+ **Z62.89 Other specified problems related to upbringing**
Z62.890 Parent-child estrangement NEC
Z62.891 Sibling rivalry
Z62.898 Other specified problems related to upbringing
Z62.9 Problem related to upbringing, unspecified

Z63 Other problems related to primary support group, including family circumstances

Excludes2: *maltreatment syndrome (T74.-, T76)*
parent-child problems (Z62.-)
problems related to negative life events in childhood (Z62.-
problems related to upbringing (Z62.-)
Z63.0 Problems in relationship with spouse or partner
Relationship distress with spouse or intimate partner
Excludes1: *counseling for spousal or partner abuse problems (Z69.1)*
counseling related to sexual attitude, behavior, and orientation (Z70.-)
Z63.1 Problems in relationship with in-laws
+ **Z63.3 Absence of family member**
Excludes1: *absence of family member due to disappearance and death (Z63.4)*
absence of family member due to separation and divorce (Z63.5)
Z63.31 Absence of family member due to military deployment
Individual or family affected by other family member being on military deployment
Excludes1: *family disruption due to return of family member from military deployment (Z63.71)*
Z63.32 Other absence of family member
Z63.4 Disappearance and death of family member
Assumed death of family member
Bereavement
AHA CC: 1Q, 2014, 25
Z63.5 Disruption of family by separation and divorce
Marital estrangement
Z63.6 Dependent relative needing care at home
+ **Z63.7 Other stressful life events affecting family and household**
Z63.71 Stress on family due to return of family member from military deployment
Individual or family affected by family member having returned from military deployment (current or past conflict)
Z63.72 Alcoholism and drug addiction in family
Z63.79 Other stressful life events affecting family and household
Anxiety (normal) about sick person in family
Health problems within family
Ill or disturbed family member
Isolated family

Z63.8 **Other specified problems related to primary support group**
Family discord NOS
Family estrangement NOS
High expressed emotional level within family
Inadequate family support NOS
Inadequate or distorted communication within family
Z63.9 **Problem related to primary support group, unspecified**
Relationship disorder NOS

Z64 Problems related to certain psychosocial circumstances
♀ Z64.0 **Problems related to unwanted pregnancy**
♀ Z64.1 **Problems related to multiparity**
Z64.4 **Discord with counselors**
Discord with probation officer
Discord with social worker

Z65 Problems related to other psychosocial circumstances
Z65.0 **Conviction in civil and criminal proceedings without imprisonment**
Z65.1 **Imprisonment and other incarceration**
Z65.2 **Problems related to release from prison**
Z65.3 **Problems related to other legal circumstances**
Arrest
Child custody or support proceedings
Litigation
Prosecution
Z65.4 **Victim of crime and terrorism**
Victim of torture
• Z65.5 **Exposure to disaster, war and other hostilities**
Excludes1: *target of perceived discrimination or persecution (Z60.5)*
Z65.8 **Other specified problems related to psychosocial circumstances**
Religious or spiritual problem
Z65.9 **Problem related to unspecified psychosocial circumstances**

Do not resuscitate status (Z66)

Z66 Do not resuscitate
DNR status
Review coding guideline C.21.c.3
Valid 3-character code, no further characters required

Blood type (Z67)

Z67 Blood type
Review coding guideline C.21.c.3
AHA CC: 3Q, 2015, 40
+ Z67.1 **Type A blood**
Z67.10 **Type A blood, Rh positive**
Z67.11 **Type A blood, Rh negative**
+ Z67.2 **Type B blood**
Z67.20 **Type B blood, Rh positive**
Z67.21 **Type B blood, Rh negative**
+ Z67.3 **Type AB blood**
Z67.30 **Type AB blood, Rh positive**
Z67.31 **Type AB blood, Rh negative**
+ Z67.4 **Type O blood**
Z67.40 **Type O blood, Rh positive**
Z67.41 **Type O blood, Rh negative**
+ Z67.9 **Unspecified blood type**
Z67.90 **Unspecified blood type, Rh positive**
Z67.91 **Unspecified blood type, Rh negative**

Body mass index [BMI] (Z68)

Z68 Body mass index [BMI]
Kilograms per meters squared
NOTE BMI adult codes are for use for persons 21 years of age or older
BMI pediatric codes are for use for persons 2-20 years of age. These percentiles are based on the growth charts published by the Centers for Disease Control and Prevention (CDC)
Review coding guideline C.21.c.3
• CC Z68.1 **Body mass index (BMI) 19.9 or less, adult**
CC Exclusion see Appendix A PDX collection 1493
AHA CC: 1Q, 2017, 39
+ Z68.2 **Body mass index (BMI) 20-29, adult**
• Z68.20 **Body mass index (BMI) 20.0-20.9, adult**
• Z68.21 **Body mass index (BMI) 21.0-21.9, adult**
• Z68.22 **Body mass index (BMI) 22.0-22.9, adult**
• Z68.23 **Body mass index (BMI) 23.0-23.9, adult**
• Z68.24 **Body mass index (BMI) 24.0-24.9, adult**
• Z68.25 **Body mass index (BMI) 25.0-25.9, adult**
• Z68.26 **Body mass index (BMI) 26.0-26.9, adult**
• Z68.27 **Body mass index (BMI) 27.0-27.9, adult**
• Z68.28 **Body mass index (BMI) 28.0-28.9, adult**
• Z68.29 **Body mass index (BMI) 29.0-29.9, adult**
+ Z68.3 **Body mass index (BMI) 30-39, adult**
• Z68.30 **Body mass index (BMI) 30.0-30.9, adult**
• Z68.31 **Body mass index (BMI) 31.0-31.9, adult**
• Z68.32 **Body mass index (BMI) 32.0-32.9, adult**
• Z68.33 **Body mass index (BMI) 33.0-33.9, adult**
• Z68.34 **Body mass index (BMI) 34.0-34.9, adult**
• Z68.35 **Body mass index (BMI) 35.0-35.9, adult**
• Z68.36 **Body mass index (BMI) 36.0-36.9, adult**
• Z68.37 **Body mass index (BMI) 37.0-37.9, adult**
• Z68.38 **Body mass index (BMI) 38.0-38.9, adult**
• Z68.39 **Body mass index (BMI) 39.0-39.9, adult**
+ Z68.4 **Body mass index (BMI) 40 or greater, adult**
• CC Z68.41 **Body mass index (BMI) 40.0-44.9, adult**
CC Exclusion see Appendix A PDX collection 1494
• CC Z68.42 **Body mass index (BMI) 45.0-49.9, adult**
CC Exclusion see Appendix A PDX collection 1494
• CC Z68.43 **Body mass index (BMI) 50-59.9 , adult**
CC Exclusion see Appendix A PDX collection 1494
• CC Z68.44 **Body mass index (BMI) 60.0-69.9, adult**
CC Exclusion see Appendix A PDX collection 1494
• CC Z68.45 **Body mass index (BMI) 70 or greater, adult**
CC Exclusion see Appendix A PDX collection 1494
+ Z68.5 **Body mass index (BMI) pediatric**
Z68.51 **Body mass index (BMI) pediatric, less than 5th percentile for age**
Z68.52 **Body mass index (BMI) pediatric, 5th percentile to less than 85th percentile for age**
Z68.53 **Body mass index (BMI) pediatric, 85th percentile to less than 95th percentile for age**
Z68.54 **Body mass index (BMI) pediatric, greater than or equal to 95th percentile for age**

Persons encountering health services in other circumstances (Z69-Z76)

Z69 Encounter for mental health services for victim and perpetrator of abuse
Includes: counseling for victims and perpetrators of abuse
Review coding guideline C.21.c.10
+ Z69.0 **Encounter for mental health services for child abuse problems**
+ Z69.01 **Encounter for mental health services for parental child abuse**
• Z69.010 **Encounter for mental health services for victim of parental child abuse**
Encounter for mental health services for victim of child abuse by parent
Encounter for mental health services for victim of child neglect by parent
Encounter for mental health services for victim of child psychological abuse by parent
Encounter for mental health services for victim of child sexual abuse by parent
Z69.011 **Encounter for mental health services for perpetrator of parental child abuse**
Encounter for mental health services for perpetrator of parental child neglect
Encounter for mental health services for perpetrator of parental child psychological abuse
Encounter for mental health services for perpetrator of parental child sexual abuse
Excludes1: *encounter for mental health services for non-parental child abuse (Z69.02-)*
+ Z69.02 **Encounter for mental health services for non-parental child abuse**
• Z69.020 **Encounter for mental health services for victim of non-parental child abuse**
Encounter for mental health services for victim of non-parental child neglect
Encounter for mental health services for victim of non-parental child psychological abuse
Encounter for mental health services for victim of non-parental child sexual abuse

Z69.021 Encounter for mental health services for perpetrator of non-parental child abuse
Encounter for mental health services for perpetrator of non-parental child neglect
Encounter for mental health services for perpetrator of non-parental child psychological abuse
Encounter for mental health services for perpetrator of non-parental child sexual abuse

+ **Z69.1 Encounter for mental health services for spousal or partner abuse problems**

Z69.11 Encounter for mental health services for victim of spousal or partner abuse
Encounter for mental health services for victim of spouse or partner neglect
Encounter for mental health services for victim of spouse or partner psychological abuse
Encounter for mental health services for victim of spouse or partner violence, physical

Z69.12 Encounter for mental health services for perpetrator of spousal or partner abuse
Encounter for mental health services for perpetrator of spouse or partner neglect
Encounter for mental health services for perpetrator of spouse or partner psychological abuse
Encounter for mental health services for perpetrator of spouse or partner violence, physical

+ **Z69.8 Encounter for mental health services for victim or perpetrator of other abuse**

Z69.81 Encounter for mental health services for victim of other abuse
Encounter for mental health services for perpetrator of non-spousal adult abuse
Encounter for mental health services for victim of non-spousal adult abuse
Encounter for mental health services for victim of spouse or partner violence, sexual
Encounter for rape victim counseling

Z69.82 Encounter for mental health services for perpetrator of other abuse

Z70 Counseling related to sexual attitude, behavior and orientation

Includes: encounter for mental health services for sexual attitude, behavior and orientation
Excludes2: *contraceptive or procreative counseling (Z30-Z31)*
Review coding guideline C.21.c.10

Z70.0 Counseling related to sexual attitude

Z70.1 Counseling related to patient's sexual behavior and orientation
Patient concerned regarding impotence
Patient concerned regarding non-responsiveness
Patient concerned regarding promiscuity
Patient concerned regarding sexual orientation

Z70.2 Counseling related to sexual behavior and orientation of third party
Advice sought regarding sexual behavior and orientation of child
Advice sought regarding sexual behavior and orientation of partner
Advice sought regarding sexual behavior and orientation of spouse

Z70.3 Counseling related to combined concerns regarding sexual attitude, behavior and orientation

Z70.8 Other sex counseling
Encounter for sex education

Z70.9 Sex counseling, unspecified

Z71 Persons encountering health services for other counseling and medical advice, not elsewhere classified

Excludes2: *contraceptive or procreation counseling (Z30-Z31)*
sex counseling (Z70.-)
Review coding guideline C.21.c.10

Z71.0 Person encountering health services to consult on behalf of another person
Person encountering health services to seek advice or treatment for non-attending third party
Excludes2: *anxiety (normal) about sick person in family (Z63.7)*
expectant (adoptive) parent(s) pre-birth pediatrician visit (Z76.81)

Z71.1 Person with feared health complaint in whom no diagnosis is made
Person encountering health services with feared condition which was not demonstrated
Person encountering health services in which problem was normal state
'Worried well'
Excludes1: *medical observation for suspected diseases and conditions proven not to exist (Z03.-)*
AHA CC: 4Q, 2016, 4-7

Z71.2 Person consulting for explanation of examination or test findings

Z71.3 Dietary counseling and surveillance
Use additional code for any associated underlying medical condition

Use additional code to identify body mass index (BMI), if known (Z68.-)

+ **Z71.4 Alcohol abuse counseling and surveillance**
Use additional code for alcohol abuse or dependence (F10.-)

Z71.41 Alcohol abuse counseling and surveillance of alcoholic

Z71.42 Counseling for family member of alcoholic
Counseling for significant other, partner, or friend of alcoholic

+ **Z71.5 Drug abuse counseling and surveillance**
Use additional code for drug abuse or dependence (F11-F16, F18-F19)

Z71.51 Drug abuse counseling and surveillance of drug abuser

Z71.52 Counseling for family member of drug abuser
Counseling for significant other, partner, or friend of drug abuser

Z71.6 Tobacco abuse counseling
Use additional code for nicotine dependence (F17.-)

Z71.7 Human immunodeficiency virus [HIV] counseling
Review coding guideline C.1.a.2.h

+ **Z71.8 Other specified counseling**
Excludes2: *counseling for contraception (Z30.0-)*

Z71.81 Spiritual or religious counseling

Z71.82 Exercise counseling

Z71.83 Encounter for nonprocreative genetic counseling
Exludes1: *counseling for procreative genetics (Z31.5)*
counseling for procreative management (Z31.6)

Z71.89 Other specified counseling

Z71.9 Counseling, unspecified
Encounter for medical advice NOS

Z72 Problems related to lifestyle

Excludes2: *problems related to life-management difficulty (Z73.-)*
problems related to socioeconomic and psychosocial circumstances (Z55-Z65)
Review coding guideline C.21.c.14

Z72.0 Tobacco use
Tobacco use NOS
Excludes1: *history of tobacco dependence (Z87.891)*
nicotine dependence (F17.2-)
tobacco dependence (F17.2-)
tobacco use during pregnancy (O99.33-)
Review coding guideline C.15.l.2

Z72.3 Lack of physical exercise

Z72.4 Inappropriate diet and eating habits
Excludes1: *behavioral eating disorders of infancy or childhood (F98.2-F98.3)*
eating disorders (F50.-)
lack of adequate food (Z59.4)
malnutrition and other nutritional deficiencies (E40-E64)

+ **Z72.5 High risk sexual behavior**
Promiscuity
Excludes1: *paraphilias (F65)*

Z72.51 High risk heterosexual behavior

Z72.52 High risk homosexual behavior

Z72.53 High risk bisexual behavior

Z72.6 Gambling and betting
Excludes1: *compulsive or pathological gambling (F63.0)*

+ **Z72.8 Other problems related to lifestyle**

+ **Z72.81 Antisocial behavior**
Excludes1: *conduct disorders (F91.-)*

• **Z72.810 Child and adolescent antisocial behavior**
Antisocial behavior (child) (adolescent) without manifest psychiatric disorder
Delinquency NOS
Group delinquency
Offenses in the context of gang membership
Stealing in company with others
Truancy from school

• **Z72.811 Adult antisocial behavior**
Adult antisocial behavior without manifest psychiatric disorder

+ **Z72.82 Problems related to sleep**

Z72.820 Sleep deprivation
Lack of adequate sleep
Excludes1: *insomnia (G47.0-)*

Z72.821 Inadequate sleep hygiene
Bad sleep habits
Irregular sleep habits
Unhealthy sleep wake schedule
Excludes1: *insomnia (F51.0-, G47.0-)*

Z72.89 Other problems related to lifestyle
Self-damaging behavior

Z72.9 Problem related to lifestyle, unspecified

Z73 Problems related to life management difficulty

Excludes2: *problems related to socioeconomic and psychosocial circumstances (Z55-Z65)*

Z73.0 Burn-out
Z73.1 Type A behavior pattern
Z73.2 Lack of relaxation and leisure
Z73.3 Stress, not elsewhere classified
Physical and mental strain NOS
Excludes1: *stress related to employment or unemployment (Z56.-)*
Z73.4 Inadequate social skills, not elsewhere classified
Z73.5 Social role conflict, not elsewhere classified
Z73.6 Limitation of activities due to disability
Excludes1: *care-provider dependency (Z74.-)*

+ **Z73.8 Other problems related to life management difficulty**

+ **Z73.81 Behavioral insomnia of childhood**

• **Z73.810 Behavioral insomnia of childhood, sleep-onset association type**
• **Z73.811 Behavioral insomnia of childhood, limit setting type**
• **Z73.812 Behavioral insomnia of childhood, combined type**
• **Z73.819 Behavioral insomnia of childhood, unspecified type**

Z73.82 Dual sensory impairment
Z73.89 Other problems related to life management difficulty

Z73.9 Problem related to life management difficulty, unspecified

Z74 Problems related to care provider dependency

Excludes2: *dependence on enabling machines or devices NEC (Z99.-)*

+ **Z74.0 Reduced mobility**

Z74.01 Bed confinement status
Bedridden
Review coding guideline C.21.c.3

Z74.09 Other reduced mobility
Chairridden
Reduced mobility NOS
Excludes2: *wheelchair dependence (Z99.3)*

Z74.1 Need for assistance with personal care
Z74.2 Need for assistance at home and no other household member able to render care
Z74.3 Need for continuous supervision
Z74.8 Other problems related to care provider dependency
Z74.9 Problem related to care provider dependency, unspecified

Z75 Problems related to medical facilities and other health care

Z75.0 Medical services not available in home
Excludes1: *no other household member able to render care (Z74.2)*
Z75.1 Person awaiting admission to adequate facility elsewhere
Z75.2 Other waiting period for investigation and treatment
Z75.3 Unavailability and inaccessibility of health-care facilities
Excludes1: *bed unavailable (Z75.1)*
Z75.4 Unavailability and inaccessibility of other helping agencies
Z75.5 Holiday relief care
Z75.8 Other problems related to medical facilities and other health care
Z75.9 Unspecified problem related to medical facilities and other health care

Z76 Persons encountering health services in other circumstances

Z76.0 Encounter for issue of repeat prescription
Encounter for issue of repeat prescription for appliance
Encounter for issue of repeat prescription for medicaments
Encounter for issue of repeat prescription for spectacles
Excludes2: *issue of medical certificate (Z02.7)*
repeat prescription for contraceptive (Z30.4-)

Z76.1 Encounter for health supervision and care of foundling
Review coding guidelines C.21.c.12 and C.21.c.16

• **Z76.2 Encounter for health supervision and care of other healthy infant and child**
Encounter for medical or nursing care or supervision of healthy infant under circumstances such as adverse socioeconomic conditions at home
Encounter for medical or nursing care or supervision of healthy infant under circumstances such as awaiting foster or adoptive placement
Encounter for medical or nursing care or supervision of healthy infant under circumstances such as maternal illness
Encounter for medical or nursing care or supervision of healthy infant under circumstances such as number of children at home preventing or interfering with normal care
Review coding guideline C.21.c.16

Z76.3 Healthy person accompanying sick person
Z76.4 Other boarder to healthcare facility
Excludes1: *homelessness (Z59.0)*
Z76.5 Malingerer [conscious simulation]
Person feigning illness (with obvious motivation)
Excludes1: *factitious disorder (F68.1-)*
peregrinating patient (F68.1-)

+ **Z76.8 Persons encountering health services in other specified circumstances**

Z76.81 Expectant parent(s) prebirth pediatrician visit
Pre-adoption pediatrician visit for adoptive parent(s)
Review coding guideline C.21.c.10

Z76.82 Awaiting organ transplant status
Patient waiting for organ availability
Review coding guideline C.21.c.3

Z76.89 Persons encountering health services in other specified circumstances
Persons encountering health services NOS
AHA CC: 2Q, 2014, 10

Persons with potential health hazards related to family and personal history and certain conditions influencing health status (Z77-Z99)

Code also any follow-up examination (Z08-Z09)

Z77 Other contact with and (suspected) exposures hazardous to health

Includes: contact with and (suspected) exposures to potential hazards to health

Excludes2: *contact with and (suspected) exposure to communicable diseases (Z20.-)*
exposure to (parental) (environmental) tobacco smoke in the perinatal period (P96.81)
newborn affected by noxious substances transmitted via placenta or breast milk (P04.-)
occupational exposure to risk factors (Z57.-)
retained foreign body (Z18.-)
retained foreign body fully removed (Z87.821)
toxic effects of substances chiefly nonmedicinal as to source (T51-T65)

Review coding guideline C.21.c.1

+ **Z77.0 Contact with and (suspected) exposure to hazardous, chiefly nonmedicinal, chemicals**

+ **Z77.01 Contact with and (suspected) exposure to hazardous metals**

Z77.010 Contact with and (suspected) exposure to arsenic
Z77.011 Contact with and (suspected) exposure to lead
Z77.012 Contact with and (suspected) exposure to uranium
Excludes1: *retained depleted uranium fragments (Z18.01)*

Z77.018 Contact with and (suspected) exposure to other hazardous metals
Contact with and (suspected) exposure to chromium compounds
Contact with and (suspected) exposure to nickel dust

+ **Z77.02 Contact with and (suspected) exposure to hazardous aromatic compounds**
Z77.020 Contact with and (suspected) exposure to aromatic amines
Z77.021 Contact with and (suspected) exposure to benzene
Z77.028 Contact with and (suspected) exposure to other hazardous aromatic compounds
Aromatic dyes NOS
Polycyclic aromatic hydrocarbons

+ **Z77.09 Contact with and (suspected) exposure to other hazardous, chiefly nonmedicinal, chemicals**
Z77.090 Contact with and (suspected) exposure to asbestos
Z77.098 Contact with and (suspected) exposure to other hazardous, chiefly nonmedicinal, chemicals
Dyes NOS

+ **Z77.1 Contact with and (suspected) exposure to environmental pollution and hazards in the physical environment**
+ **Z77.11 Contact with and (suspected) exposure to environmental pollution**
Z77.110 Contact with and (suspected) exposure to air pollution
Z77.111 Contact with and (suspected) exposure to water pollution
Z77.112 Contact with and (suspected) exposure to soil pollution
Z77.118 Contact with and (suspected) exposure to other environmental pollution

+ **Z77.12 Contact with and (suspected) exposure to hazards in the physical environment**
Z77.120 Contact with and (suspected) exposure to mold (toxic)
Z77.121 Contact with and (suspected) exposure to harmful algae and algae toxins
Contact with and (suspected) exposure to (harmful) algae bloom NOS
Contact with and (suspected) exposure to blue-green algae bloom
Contact with and (suspected) exposure to brown tide
Contact with and (suspected) exposure to cyanobacteria bloom
Contact with and (suspected) exposure to Florida red tide
Contact with and (suspected) exposure to pfiesteria piscicida
Contact with and (suspected) exposure to red tide
Z77.122 Contact with and (suspected) exposure to noise
Z77.123 Contact with and (suspected) exposure to radon and other naturally occuring radiation
Excludes2: *radiation exposure as the cause of a confirmed condition (W88-W90, X39.0-)*
radiation sickness NOS (T66)
Z77.128 Contact with and (suspected) exposure to other hazards in the physical environment

+ **Z77.2 Contact with and (suspected) exposure to other hazardous substances**
Z77.21 Contact with and (suspected) exposure to potentially hazardous body fluids
Z77.22 Contact with and (suspected) exposure to environmental tobacco smoke (acute) (chronic)
Exposure to second hand tobacco smoke (acute) (chronic)
Passive smoking (acute) (chronic)
Excludes1: *nicotine dependence (F17.-)*
tobacco use (Z72.0)
Excludes2: *occupational exposure to environmental tobacco smoke (Z57.31)*

Z77.29 Contact with and (suspected) exposure to other hazardous substances
AHA CC: 2Q, 2016, 34

Z77.9 Other contact with and (suspected) exposures hazardous to health

Z78 Other specified health status

Excludes2: *asymptomatic human immunodeficiency virus [HIV] infection status (Z21)*
postprocedural status (Z93-Z99)
sex reassignment status (Z87.890)
Review coding guideline C.21.c.3

• ♀ **Z78.0 Asymptomatic menopausal state**
Menopausal state NOS
Postmenopausal status NOS
Excludes2: *symptomatic menopausal state (N95.1)*

Z78.1 Physical restraint status
Excludes1: *physical restraint due to a procedure - omit code*

Z78.9 Other specified health status

Z79 Long term (current) drug therapy

Includes: long term (current) drug use for prophylactic purposes
Code also any therapeutic drug level monitoring (Z51.81)
Excludes2: *drug abuse and dependence (F11-F19)*
drug use complicating pregnancy, childbirth, and the puerperium (O99.32-)
long term (current) use of oral antidiabetic drugs (Z79.84)
long term (current) use of oral hypoglycemic drugs (Z79.84)
Review coding guideline C.21.c.3

+ **Z79.0 Long term (current) use of anticoagulants and antithrombotics/antiplatelets**
Excludes2: *long term (current) use of aspirin (Z79.82)*
Z79.01 Long term (current) use of anticoagulants
Z79.02 Long term (current) use of antithrombotics/ antiplatelets

Z79.1 Long term (current) use of non-steroidal anti-inflammatories (NSAID)
Excludes2: *long term (current) use of aspirin (Z79.82)*

Z79.2 Long term (current) use of antibiotics

Z79.3 Long term (current) use of hormonal contraceptives
Long term (current) use of birth control pill or patch

Z79.4 Long term (current) use of insulin
Review coding guidelines C.4.a.3 and C.4.a.6
Review coding guidelines C.15.h and C.15.i

+ **Z79.5 Long term (current) use of steroids**
Z79.51 Long term (current) use of inhaled steroids
Z79.52 Long term (current) use of systemic steroids

+ **Z79.8 Other long term (current) drug therapy**
+ **Z79.81 Long term (current) use of agents affecting estrogen receptors and estrogen levels**
Code first if applicable:
malignant neoplasm of breast (C50.-)
malignant neoplasm of prostate (C61)

Use additional code, if applicable, to identify:
estrogen receptor positive status (Z17.0)
family history of breast cancer (Z80.3)
genetic susceptibility to malignant neoplasm (cancer) (Z15.0-)
personal history of breast cancer (Z85.3)
personal history of prostate cancer (Z85.46)
postmenopausal status (Z78.0)
Excludes1: *hormone replacement therapy (Z79.890)*

Z79.810 Long term (current) use of selective estrogen receptor modulators (SERMs)
Long term (current) use of raloxifene (Evista)
Long term (current) use of tamoxifen (Nolvadex)
Long term (current) use of toremifene (Fareston)

Z79.811 Long term (current) use of aromatase inhibitors
Long term (current) use of anastrozole (Arimidex)
Long term (current) use of exemestane (Aromasin)
Long term (current) use of letrozole (Femara)

Z79.818 **Long term (current) use of other agents affecting estrogen receptors and estrogen levels**
Long term (current) use of estrogen receptor downregulators
Long term (current) use of fulvestrant (Faslodex)
Long term (current) use of gonadotropin-releasing hormone (GnRH) agonist
Long term (current) use of goserelin acetate (Zoladex)
Long term (current) use of leuprolide acetate (leuprorelin) (Lupron)
Long term (current) use of megestrol acetate (Megace)

Z79.82 **Long term (current) use of aspirin**

Z79.83 **Long term (current) use of bisphosphonates**
AHA CC: 4Q, 2016, 21

Z79.84 **Long term (current) use of oral hypoglycemic drugs**
Long term (current) use of oral antidiabetic drugs
Excludes2: *long term (current) use of insulin (Z79.4)*
Review coding guidelines C.4.a.e and C.4.a.6
Review coding guidelines C.15.h and C.15.i
AHA CC: 4Q, 2016, 76

\+ Z79.89 **Other long term (current) drug therapy**

Z79.890 **Hormone replacement therapy**

Z79.891 **Long term (current) use of opiate analgesic**
Long term (current) use of methadone for pain management
Excludes1: *methodone use NOS (F11.9-)*
use of methodone for treatment of heroin addiction (F11.2-)

Z79.899 **Other long term (current) drug therapy**
AHA CC: 3Q, 2015, 21-22; 4Q, 2015, 34

Z80 **Family history of primary malignant neoplasm**
Review coding guideline C.21.c.4

Z80.0 **Family history of malignant neoplasm of digestive organs**
Conditions classifiable to C15-C26

Z80.1 **Family history of malignant neoplasm of trachea, bronchus and lung**
Conditions classifiable to C33-C34

Z80.2 **Family history of malignant neoplasm of other respiratory and intrathoracic organs**
Conditions classifiable to C30-C32, C37-C39

Z80.3 **Family history of malignant neoplasm of breast**
Conditions classifiable to C50.-

\+ Z80.4 **Family history of malignant neoplasm of genital organs**
Conditions classifiable to C51-C63

Z80.41 **Family history of malignant neoplasm of ovary**

Z80.42 **Family history of malignant neoplasm of prostate**

Z80.43 **Family history of malignant neoplasm of testis**

Z80.49 **Family history of malignant neoplasm of other genital organs**

\+ Z80.5 **Family history of malignant neoplasm of urinary tract**
Conditions classifiable to C64-C68

Z80.51 **Family history of malignant neoplasm of kidney**

Z80.52 **Family history of malignant neoplasm of bladder**

Z80.59 **Family history of malignant neoplasm of other urinary tract organ**

Z80.6 **Family history of leukemia**
Conditions classifiable to C91-C95

Z80.7 **Family history of other malignant neoplasms of lymphoid, hematopoietic and related tissues**
Conditions classifiable to C81-C90, C96.-

Z80.8 **Family history of malignant neoplasm of other organs or systems**
Conditions classifiable to C00-C14, C40-C49, C69-C79

Z80.9 **Family history of malignant neoplasm, unspecified**
Conditions classifiable to C80.1

Z81 **Family history of mental and behavioral disorders**
Review coding guideline C.21.c.4

Z81.0 **Family history of intellectual disabilities**
Conditions classifiable to F70-F79

Z81.1 **Family history of alcohol abuse and dependence**
Conditions classifiable to F10.-

Z81.2 **Family history of tobacco abuse and dependence**
Conditions classifiable to F17.-

Z81.3 **Family history of other psychoactive substance abuse and dependence**
Conditions classifiable to F11-F16, F18-F19

Z81.4 **Family history of other substance abuse and dependence**
Conditions classifiable to F55

Z81.8 **Family history of other mental and behavioral disorders**
Conditions classifiable elsewhere in F01-F99

Z82 **Family history of certain disabilities and chronic diseases (leading to disablement)**
Review coding guideline C.21.c.4

Z82.0 **Family history of epilepsy and other diseases of the nervous system**
Conditions classifiable to G00-G99

Z82.1 **Family history of blindness and visual loss**
Conditions classifiable to H54.-

Z82.2 **Family history of deafness and hearing loss**
Conditions classifiable to H90-H91

Z82.3 **Family history of stroke**
Conditions classifiable to I60-I64

\+ Z82.4 **Family history of ischemic heart disease and other diseases of the circulatory system**
Conditions classifiable to I00-I52, I65-I99

Z82.41 **Family history of sudden cardiac death**

Z82.49 **Family history of ischemic heart disease and other diseases of the circulatory system**

Z82.5 **Family history of asthma and other chronic lower respiratory diseases**
Conditions classifiable to J40-J47
Excludes2: *family history of other diseases of the respiratory system (Z83.6)*

\+ Z82.6 **Family history of arthritis and other diseases of the musculoskeletal system and connective tissue**
Conditions classifiable to M00-M99

Z82.61 **Family history of arthritis**

Z82.62 **Family history of osteoporosis**

Z82.69 **Family history of other diseases of the musculoskeletal system and connective tissue**

\+ Z82.7 **Family history of congenital malformations, deformations and chromosomal abnormalities**
Conditions classifiable to Q00-Q99

Z82.71 **Family history of polycystic kidney**

Z82.79 **Family history of other congenital malformations, deformations and chromosomal abnormalities**

Z82.8 **Family history of other disabilities and chronic diseases leading to disablement, not elsewhere classified**

Z83 **Family history of other specific disorders**
Excludes2: *contact with and (suspected) exposure to communicable disease in the family (Z20.-)*
Review coding guideline C.21.c.4

Z83.0 **Family history of human immunodeficiency virus [HIV] disease**
Conditions classifiable to B20

Z83.1 **Family history of other infectious and parasitic diseases**
Conditions classifiable to A00-B19, B25-B94, B99

Z83.2 **Family history of diseases of the blood and blood-forming organs and certain disorders involving the immune mechanism**
Conditions classifiable to D50-D89

Z83.3 **Family history of diabetes mellitus**
Conditions classifiable to E08-E13

\+ Z83.4 **Family history of other endocrine, nutritional and metabolic diseases**
Conditions classifiable to E00-E07, E15-E88

Z83.41 **Family history of multiple endocrine neoplasia [MEN] syndrome**

Z83.42 **Family history of familial hypercholesterolemia**
AHA CC: 4Q, 2016, 77

Z83.49 **Family history of other endocrine, nutritional and metabolic diseases**

\+ Z83.5 **Family history of eye and ear disorders**

\+ Z83.51 **Family history of eye disorders**
Conditions classifiable to H00-H53, H55-H59
Excludes2: *family history of blindness and visual loss (Z82.1)*

Z83.511 **Family history of glaucoma**

Z83.518 **Family history of other specified eye disorder**

Z83.52 **Family history of ear disorders**
Conditions classifiable to H60-H83, H92-H95
Excludes2: *family history of deafness and hearing loss (Z82.2)*

Z83.6 Family history of other diseases of the respiratory system
Conditions classifiable to J00-J39, J60-J99
Excludes2: *family history of asthma and other chronic lower respiratory diseases (Z82.5)*

+ **Z83.7 Family history of diseases of the digestive system**
Conditions classifiable to K00-K93

Z83.71 Family history of colonic polyps
Excludes2: *family history of malignant neoplasm of digestive organs (Z80.0)*

Z83.79 Family history of other diseases of the digestive system

Z84 Family history of other conditions

Review coding guideline C.21.c.4

Z84.0 Family history of diseases of the skin and subcutaneous tissue
Conditions classifiable to L00-L99

Z84.1 Family history of disorders of kidney and ureter
Conditions classifiable to N00-N29

Z84.2 Family history of other diseases of the genitourinary system
Conditions classifiable to N30-N99

Z84.3 Family history of consanguinity

+ **Z84.8 Family history of other specified conditions**

Z84.81 Family history of carrier of genetic disease

Z84.82 Family history of sudden infant death syndrome
Family history of SIDS
AHA CC: 4Q, 2016, 77

Z84.89 Family history of other specified conditions

Z85 Personal history of malignant neoplasm

Code first any follow-up examination after treatment of malignant neoplasm (Z08)

Use additional code to identify:
alcohol use and dependence (F10.-)
exposure to environmental tobacco smoke (Z77.22)
history of tobacco dependence (Z87.891)
occupational exposure to environmental tobacco smoke (Z57.31)
tobacco dependence (F17.-)
tobacco use (Z72.0)

Excludes2: *personal history of benign neoplasm (Z86.01-)*
personal history of carcinoma-in-situ (Z86.00-)

Review coding guidelines C.2.d and C.2.m
Review coding guideline C.21.c.4

+ **Z85.0 Personal history of malignant neoplasm of digestive organs**

Z85.00 Personal history of malignant neoplasm of unspecified digestive organ

Z85.01 Personal history of malignant neoplasm of esophagus
Conditions classifiable to C15

+ **Z85.02 Personal history of malignant neoplasm of stomach**

Z85.020 Personal history of malignant carcinoid tumor of stomach
Conditions classifiable to C7A.092

Z85.028 Personal history of other malignant neoplasm of stomach
Conditions classifiable to C16

+ **Z85.03 Personal history of malignant neoplasm of large intestine**

Z85.030 Personal history of malignant carcinoid tumor of large intestine
Conditions classifiable to C7A.022-C7A.025, C7A.029

Z85.038 Personal history of other malignant neoplasm of large intestine
Conditions classifiable to C18

+ **Z85.04 Personal history of malignant neoplasm of rectum, rectosigmoid junction, and anus**

Z85.040 Personal history of malignant carcinoid tumor of rectum
Conditions classifiable to C7A.026

Z85.048 Personal history of other malignant neoplasm of rectum, rectosigmoid junction, and anus
Conditions classifiable to C19-C21

Z85.05 Personal history of malignant neoplasm of liver
Conditions classifiable to C22

+ **Z85.06 Personal history of malignant neoplasm of small intestine**

Z85.060 Personal history of malignant carcinoid tumor of small intestine
Conditions classifiable to C7A.01-

Z85.068 Personal history of other malignant neoplasm of small intestine
Conditions classifiable to C17

Z85.07 Personal history of malignant neoplasm of pancreas
Conditions classifiable to C25

Z85.09 Personal history of malignant neoplasm of other digestive organs

+ **Z85.1 Personal history of malignant neoplasm of trachea, bronchus and lung**

+ **Z85.11 Personal history of malignant neoplasm of bronchus and lung**

Z85.110 Personal history of malignant carcinoid tumor of bronchus and lung
Conditions classifiable to C7A.090

Z85.118 Personal history of other malignant neoplasm of bronchus and lung
Conditions classifiable to C34

Z85.12 Personal history of malignant neoplasm of trachea
Conditions classifiable to C33

+ **Z85.2 Personal history of malignant neoplasm of other respiratory and intrathoracic organs**

Z85.20 Personal history of malignant neoplasm of unspecified respiratory organ

Z85.21 Personal history of malignant neoplasm of larynx
Conditions classifiable to C32

Z85.22 Personal history of malignant neoplasm of nasal cavities, middle ear, and accessory sinuses
Conditions classifiable to C30-C31

+ **Z85.23 Personal history of malignant neoplasm of thymus**

Z85.230 Personal history of malignant carcinoid tumor of thymus
Conditions classifiable to C7A.091

Z85.238 Personal history of other malignant neoplasm of thymus
Conditions classifiable to C37

Z85.29 Personal history of malignant neoplasm of other respiratory and intrathoracic organs

Z85.3 Personal history of malignant neoplasm of breast
Conditions classifiable to C50.-

+ **Z85.4 Personal history of malignant neoplasm of genital organs**
Conditions classifiable to C51-C63

♀ **Z85.40 Personal history of malignant neoplasm of unspecified female genital organ**

♀ **Z85.41 Personal history of malignant neoplasm of cervix uteri**

♀ **Z85.42 Personal history of malignant neoplasm of other parts of uterus**

♀ **Z85.43 Personal history of malignant neoplasm of ovary**

♀ **Z85.44 Personal history of malignant neoplasm of other female genital organs**

♂ **Z85.45 Personal history of malignant neoplasm of unspecified male genital organ**

♂ **Z85.46 Personal history of malignant neoplasm of prostate**

♂ **Z85.47 Personal history of malignant neoplasm of testis**

♂ **Z85.48 Personal history of malignant neoplasm of epididymis**

♂ **Z85.49 Personal history of malignant neoplasm of other male genital organs**

+ **Z85.5 Personal history of malignant neoplasm of urinary tract**
Conditions classifiable to C64-C68

Z85.50 Personal history of malignant neoplasm of unspecified urinary tract organ

Z85.51 Personal history of malignant neoplasm of bladder

+ **Z85.52 Personal history of malignant neoplasm of kidney**
Excludes1: *personal history of malignant neoplasm of renal pelvis (Z85.53)*

Z85.520 Personal history of malignant carcinoid tumor of kidney
Conditions classifiable to C7A.093

Z85.528 Personal history of other malignant neoplasm of kidney
Conditions classifiable to C64

Z85.53 Personal history of malignant neoplasm of renal pelvis

Z85.54 Personal history of malignant neoplasm of ureter

Z85.59 Personal history of malignant neoplasm of other urinary tract organ

Z85.6 Personal history of leukemia
Conditions classifiable to C91-C95
Excludes1: *leukemia in remission C91.0-C95.9 with 5th character 1*
Review coding guideline C.2.n

+ Z85.7 **Personal history of other malignant neoplasms of lymphoid, hematopoietic and related tissues**
  - **Z85.71 Personal history of Hodgkin lymphoma**
    Conditions classifiable to C81
  - **Z85.72 Personal history of non-Hodgkin lymphomas**
    Conditions classifiable to C82-C85
  - **Z85.79 Personal history of other malignant neoplasms of lymphoid, hematopoietic and related tissues**
    Conditions classifiable to C88-C90, C96
    Excludes1: *multiple myeloma in remission (C90.01)*
    plasma cell leukemia in remission (C90.11)
    plasmacytoma in remission (C90.21)
    Review coding guideline C.2.n

+ Z85.8 **Personal history of malignant neoplasms of other organs and systems**
  Conditions classifiable to C00-C14, C40-C49, C69-C75, C7A.098, C76-C79
  - + Z85.81 **Personal history of malignant neoplasm of lip, oral cavity, and pharynx**
    - **Z85.810 Personal history of malignant neoplasm of tongue**
    - **Z85.818 Personal history of malignant neoplasm of other sites of lip, oral cavity, and pharynx**
    - **Z85.819 Personal history of malignant neoplasm of unspecified site of lip, oral cavity, and pharynx**
  - + Z85.82 **Personal history of malignant neoplasm of skin**
    - **Z85.820 Personal history of malignant melanoma of skin**
      Conditions classifiable to C43
    - **Z85.821 Personal history of Merkel cell carcinoma**
      Conditions classifiable to C4A
    - **Z85.828 Personal history of other malignant neoplasm of skin**
      Conditions classifiable to C44
  - + Z85.83 **Personal history of malignant neoplasm of bone and soft tissue**
    - **Z85.830 Personal history of malignant neoplasm of bone**
    - **Z85.831 Personal history of malignant neoplasm of soft tissue**
      Excludes2: *personal history of malignant neoplasm of skin (Z85.82-)*
  - + Z85.84 **Personal history of malignant neoplasm of eye and nervous tissue**
    - **Z85.840 Personal history of malignant neoplasm of eye**
    - **Z85.841 Personal history of malignant neoplasm of brain**
    - **Z85.848 Personal history of malignant neoplasm of other parts of nervous tissue**
  - + Z85.85 **Personal history of malignant neoplasm of endocrine glands**
    - **Z85.850 Personal history of malignant neoplasm of thyroid**
    - **Z85.858 Personal history of malignant neoplasm of other endocrine glands**
  - **Z85.89 Personal history of malignant neoplasm of other organs and systems**

Z85.9 Personal history of malignant neoplasm, unspecified
Conditions classifiable to C7A.00, C80.1

Z86 Personal history of certain other diseases

Code first any follow-up examination after treatment (Z09)
Review coding guideline C.21.c.4

+ Z86.0 **Personal history of in-situ and benign neoplasms and neoplasms of uncertain behavior**
  Excludes2: *personal history of malignant neoplasms (Z85.-)*
  - + Z86.00 **Personal history of in-situ neoplasm**
    Conditions classifiable to D00-D09
    - **Z86.000 Personal history of in-situ neoplasm of breast**
    - ♀ **Z86.001 Personal history of in-situ neoplasm of cervix uteri**
      Personal history of cervical intraepithelial neoplasia III [CINIII]
    - **Z86.008 Personal history of in-situ neoplasm of other site**
      Personal history of vaginal intraepithelial neoplasia III [VAINIII]
      Personal history of vulvar intraepithelial neoplasia III [VINIII]
  - + Z86.01 **Personal history of benign neoplasm**
    - **Z86.010 Personal history of colonic polyps**
      AHA CC: 1Q, 2017, 9
    - **Z86.011 Personal history of benign neoplasm of the brain**
    - **Z86.012 Personal history of benign carcinoid tumor**
    - **Z86.018 Personal history of other benign neoplasm**
  - **Z86.03 Personal history of neoplasm of uncertain behavior**

+ Z86.1 **Personal history of infectious and parasitic diseases**
  Conditions classifiable to A00-B89, B99
  Excludes1: *personal history of infectious diseases specific to a body system*
  sequelae of infectious and parasitic diseases (B90-B94)
  AHA CC: 4Q, 2016, 4-7
  - **Z86.11 Personal history of tuberculosis**
  - **Z86.12 Personal history of poliomyelitis**
  - **Z86.13 Personal history of malaria**
  - **Z86.14 Personal history of Methicillin resistant Staphylococcus aureus infection**
    Personal history of MRSA infection
  - **Z86.19 Personal history of other infectious and parasitic diseases**

Z86.2 Personal history of diseases of the blood and blood-forming organs and certain disorders involving the immune mechanism
Conditions classifiable to D50-D89

+ Z86.3 **Personal history of endocrine, nutritional and metabolic diseases**
  Conditions classifiable to E00-E88
  - **Z86.31 Personal history of diabetic foot ulcer**
    Excludes2: *current diabetic foot ulcer (E08.621, E09.621, E10.621, E11.621, E13.621)*
  - ♀ **Z86.32 Personal history of gestational diabetes**
    Personal history of conditions classifiable to O24.4-
    Excludes1: *gestational diabetes mellitus in current pregnancy (O24.4-)*
  - **Z86.39 Personal history of other endocrine, nutritional and metabolic disease**

+ Z86.5 **Personal history of mental and behavioral disorders**
  Conditions classifiable to F40-F59
  - • **Z86.51 Personal history of combat and operational stress reaction**
  - **Z86.59 Personal history of other mental and behavioral disorders**

+ Z86.6 **Personal history of diseases of the nervous system and sense organs**
  Conditions classifiable to G00-G99, H00-H95
  - **Z86.61 Personal history of infections of the central nervous system**
    Personal history of encephalitis
    Personal history of meningitis
  - **Z86.69 Personal history of other diseases of the nervous system and sense organs**
    AHA CC: 4Q, 2016, 21

+ Z86.7 **Personal history of diseases of the circulatory system**
  Conditions classifiable to I00-I99
  Excludes2: *old myocardial infarction (I25.2)*
  personal history of anaphylactic shock (Z87.892)
  postmyocardial infarction syndrome (I24.1)
  - + Z86.71 **Personal history of venous thrombosis and embolism**
    - **Z86.711 Personal history of pulmonary embolism**
    - **Z86.718 Personal history of other venous thrombosis and embolism**
  - **Z86.72 Personal history of thrombophlebitis**
  - **Z86.73 Personal history of transient ischemic attack (TIA), and cerebral infarction without residual deficits**
    Personal history of prolonged reversible ischemic neurological deficit (PRIND)
    Personal history of stroke NOS without residual deficits
    Excludes1: *personal history of traumatic brain injury (Z87.820)*
    sequelae of cerebrovascular disease (I69.-)
    Review coding guideline C.9.d.3

Z86.74 **Personal history of sudden cardiac arrest**
Personal history of sudden cardiac death successfully resuscitated
Z86.79 **Personal history of other diseases of the circulatory system**

Z87 **Personal history of other diseases and conditions**
Code first any follow-up examination after treatment (Z09)
Review coding guideline C.21.c.4
+ **Z87.0** **Personal history of diseases of the respiratory system**
Conditions classifiable to J00-J99
Z87.01 **Personal history of pneumonia (recurrent)**
Z87.09 **Personal history of other diseases of the respiratory system**
+ **Z87.1** **Personal history of diseases of the digestive system**
Conditions classifiable to K00-K93
Z87.11 **Personal history of peptic ulcer disease**
Z87.19 **Personal history of other diseases of the digestive system**
AHA CC: 1Q, 2017, 14-15
Z87.2 **Personal history of diseases of the skin and subcutaneous tissue**
Conditions classifiable to L00-L99
Excludes2: *personal history of diabetic foot ulcer (Z86.31)*
+ **Z87.3** **Personal history of diseases of the musculoskeletal system and connective tissue**
Conditions classifiable to M00-M99
Excludes2: *personal history of (healed) traumatic fracture (Z87.81)*
+ **Z87.31** **Personal history of (healed) nontraumatic fracture**
Z87.310 **Personal history of (healed) osteoporosis fracture**
Personal history of (healed) fragility fracture
Personal history of (healed) collapsed vertebra due to osteoporosis
Review coding guideline C.13.d.1
Z87.311 **Personal history of (healed) other pathological fracture**
Personal history of (healed) collapsed vertebra NOS
Excludes2: *personal history of osteoporosis fracture (Z87.310)*
Z87.312 **Personal history of (healed) stress fracture**
Personal history of (healed) fatigue fracture
Z87.39 **Personal history of other diseases of the musculoskeletal system and connective tissue**
+ **Z87.4** **Personal history of diseases of genitourinary system**
Conditions classifiable to N00-N99
+ **Z87.41** **Personal history of dysplasia of the female genital tract**
Excludes1: *personal history of malignant neoplasm of female genital tract (Z85.40-Z85.44)*
personal history of intraepithelial neoplasia III of female genital tract (Z86.001, Z86.008)
♀ **Z87.410** **Personal history of cervical dysplasia**
♀ **Z87.411** **Personal history of vaginal dysplasia**
♀ **Z87.412** **Personal history of vulvar dysplasia**
♀ **Z87.42** **Personal history of other diseases of the female genital tract**
+ **Z87.43** **Personal history of diseases of male genital organs**
♂ **Z87.430** **Personal history of prostatic dysplasia**
Excludes1: *personal history of malignant neoplasm of prostate (Z85.46)*
♂ **Z87.438** **Personal history of other diseases of male genital organs**
+ **Z87.44** **Personal history of diseases of urinary system**
Excludes1: *personal history of malignant neoplasm of cervix uteri (Z85.41)*
Z87.440 **Personal history of urinary (tract) infections**
Z87.441 **Personal history of nephrotic syndrome**
Z87.442 **Personal history of urinary calculi**
Personal history of kidney stones
Z87.448 **Personal history of other diseases of urinary system**
+ **Z87.5** **Personal history of complications of pregnancy, childbirth and the puerperium**
Conditions classifiable to O00-O9A
Excludes2: *recurrent pregnancy loss (N96)*
♀ **Z87.51** **Personal history of pre-term labor**
Excludes1: *current pregnancy with history of pre-term labor (O09.21-)*
♀ **Z87.59** **Personal history of other complications of pregnancy, childbirth and the puerperium**
Personal history of trophoblastic disease
+ **Z87.7** **Personal history of (corrected) congenital malformations**
Conditions classifiable to Q00-Q89 that have been repaired or corrected
Excludes1: *congenital malformations that have been partially corrected or repair but which still require medical treatment - code to condition*
Excludes2: *other postprocedural states (Z98.-)*
personal history of medical treatment (Z92.-)
presence of cardiac and vascular implants and grafts (Z95.-)
presence of other devices (Z97.-)
presence of other functional implants (Z96.-)
transplanted organ and tissue status (Z94.-)
+ **Z87.71** **Personal history of (corrected) congenital malformations of genitourinary system**
♂ **Z87.710** **Personal history of (corrected) hypospadias**
Z87.718 **Personal history of other specified (corrected) congenital malformations of genitourinary system**
+ **Z87.72** **Personal history of (corrected) congenital malformations of nervous system and sense organs**
Z87.720 **Personal history of (corrected) congenital malformations of eye**
Z87.721 **Personal history of (corrected) congenital malformations of ear**
Z87.728 **Personal history of other specified (corrected) congenital malformations of nervous system and sense organs**
+ **Z87.73** **Personal history of (corrected) congenital malformations of digestive system**
Z87.730 **Personal history of (corrected) cleft lip and palate**
Z87.738 **Personal history of other specified (corrected) congenital malformations of digestive system**
Z87.74 **Personal history of (corrected) congenital malformations of heart and circulatory system**
Z87.75 **Personal history of (corrected) congenital malformations of respiratory system**
Z87.76 **Personal history of (corrected) congenital malformations of integument, limbs and musculoskeletal system**
+ **Z87.79** **Personal history of other (corrected) congenital malformations**
Z87.790 **Personal history of (corrected) congenital malformations of face and neck**
Z87.798 **Personal history of other (corrected) congenital malformations**
+ **Z87.8** **Personal history of other specified conditions**
Excludes2: *personal history of self harm (Z91.5)*
Z87.81 **Personal history of (healed) traumatic fracture**
Excludes2: *personal history of (healed) nontraumatic fracture (Z87.31-)*
+ **Z87.82** **Personal history of other (healed) physical injury and trauma**
Conditions classifiable to S00-T88, except traumatic fractures
Z87.820 **Personal history of traumatic brain injury**
Excludes1: *personal history of transient ischemic attack (TIA), and cerebral infarction without residual deficits (Z86.73)*
Z87.821 **Personal history of retained foreign body fully removed**
Z87.828 **Personal history of other (healed) physical injury and trauma**
+ **Z87.89** **Personal history of other specified conditions**
Z87.890 **Personal history of sex reassignment**
Z87.891 **Personal history of nicotine dependence**
Excludes1: *current nicotine dependence (F17.2-)*
AHA CC: 2Q, 2017, 26-28

Z87.892 **Personal history of anaphylaxis**
Code also allergy status such as:
allergy status to drugs, medicaments and biological substances (Z88.-)
allergy status, other than to drugs and biological substances (Z91.0-)

Z87.898 **Personal history of other specified conditions**
AHA CC: 1Q, 2013, 21

Z88 Allergy status to drugs, medicaments and biological substances

Excludes2: *Allergy status, other than to drugs and biological substances (Z91.0-)*
Review coding guideline C.21.c.3

Z88.0 **Allergy status to penicillin**
Z88.1 **Allergy status to other antibiotic agents status**
Z88.2 **Allergy status to sulfonamides status**
AHA CC: 3Q, 2015, 23
Z88.3 **Allergy status to other anti-infective agents status**
Z88.4 **Allergy status to anesthetic agent status**
Z88.5 **Allergy status to narcotic agent status**
Z88.6 **Allergy status to analgesic agent status**
Z88.7 **Allergy status to serum and vaccine status**
Z88.8 **Allergy status to other drugs, medicaments and biological substances status**
Z88.9 **Allergy status to unspecified drugs, medicaments and biological substances status**

Z89 Acquired absence of limb

Includes: amputation status
postprocedural loss of limb
post-traumatic loss of limb
Excludes1: *acquired deformities of limbs (M20-M21)*
congenital absence of limbs (Q71-Q73)
Review coding guideline C.21.c.3

+ Z89.0 **Acquired absence of thumb and other finger(s)**
  + Z89.01 **Acquired absence of thumb**
    Z89.011 **Acquired absence of right thumb**
    Z89.012 **Acquired absence of left thumb**
    Z89.019 **Acquired absence of unspecified thumb**
  + Z89.02 **Acquired absence of other finger(s)**
    Excludes2: *acquired absence of thumb (Z89.01-)*
    Z89.021 **Acquired absence of right finger(s)**
    Z89.022 **Acquired absence of left finger(s)**
    Z89.029 **Acquired absence of unspecified finger(s)**
+ Z89.1 **Acquired absence of hand and wrist**
  + Z89.11 **Acquired absence of hand**
    Z89.111 **Acquired absence of right hand**
    Z89.112 **Acquired absence of left hand**
    Z89.119 **Acquired absence of unspecified hand**
  + Z89.12 **Acquired absence of wrist**
    Disarticulation at wrist
    Z89.121 **Acquired absence of right wrist**
    Z89.122 **Acquired absence of left wrist**
    Z89.129 **Acquired absence of unspecified wrist**
+ Z89.2 **Acquired absence of upper limb above wrist**
  + Z89.20 **Acquired absence of upper limb, unspecified level**
    Z89.201 **Acquired absence of right upper limb, unspecified level**
    Z89.202 **Acquired absence of left upper limb, unspecified level**
    Z89.209 **Acquired absence of unspecified upper limb, unspecified level**
    Acquired absence of arm NOS
  + Z89.21 **Acquired absence of upper limb below elbow**
    Z89.211 **Acquired absence of right upper limb below elbow**
    Z89.212 **Acquired absence of left upper limb below elbow**
    Z89.219 **Acquired absence of unspecified upper limb below elbow**
  + Z89.22 **Acquired absence of upper limb above elbow**
    Disarticulation at elbow
    Z89.221 **Acquired absence of right upper limb above elbow**
    Z89.222 **Acquired absence of left upper limb above elbow**
    Z89.229 **Acquired absence of unspecified upper limb above elbow**
  + Z89.23 **Acquired absence of shoulder**
    Acquired absence of shoulder joint following explantation of shoulder joint prosthesis, with or without presence of antibiotic-impregnated cement spacer
    Z89.231 **Acquired absence of right shoulder**
    Z89.232 **Acquired absence of left shoulder**
    Z89.239 **Acquired absence of unspecified shoulder**
+ Z89.4 **Acquired absence of toe(s), foot, and ankle**
  + Z89.41 **Acquired absence of great toe**
    Z89.411 **Acquired absence of right great toe**
    Z89.412 **Acquired absence of left great toe**
    Z89.419 **Acquired absence of unspecified great toe**
  + Z89.42 **Acquired absence of other toe(s)**
    Excludes2: *acquired absence of great toe (Z89.41-)*
    Z89.421 **Acquired absence of other right toe(s)**
    Z89.422 **Acquired absence of other left toe(s)**
    Z89.429 **Acquired absence of other toe(s), unspecified side**
  + Z89.43 **Acquired absence of foot**
    Z89.431 **Acquired absence of right foot**
    Z89.432 **Acquired absence of left foot**
    Z89.439 **Acquired absence of unspecified foot**
  + Z89.44 **Acquired absence of ankle**
    Disarticulation of ankle
    Z89.441 **Acquired absence of right ankle**
    Z89.442 **Acquired absence of left ankle**
    Z89.449 **Acquired absence of unspecified ankle**
+ Z89.5 **Acquired absence of leg below knee**
  + Z89.51 **Acquired absence of leg below knee**
    Z89.511 **Acquired absence of right leg below knee**
    Z89.512 **Acquired absence of left leg below knee**
    Z89.519 **Acquired absence of unspecified leg below knee**
  + Z89.52 **Acquired absence of knee**
    Acquired absence of knee joint following explantation of knee joint prosthesis, with or without presence of antibiotic-impregnated cement spacer
    Z89.521 **Acquired absence of right knee**
    Z89.522 **Acquired absence of left knee**
    Z89.529 **Acquired absence of unspecified knee**
+ Z89.6 **Acquired absence of leg above knee**
  + Z89.61 **Acquired absence of leg above knee**
    Acquired absence of leg NOS
    Disarticulation at knee
    Z89.611 **Acquired absence of right leg above knee**
    Z89.612 **Acquired absence of left leg above knee**
    Z89.619 **Acquired absence of unspecified leg above knee**
  + Z89.62 **Acquired absence of hip**
    Acquired absence of hip joint following explantation of hip joint prosthesis, with or without presence of antibiotic-impregnated cement spacer
    Disarticulation at hip
    Z89.621 **Acquired absence of right hip joint**
    Z89.622 **Acquired absence of left hip joint**
    Z89.629 **Acquired absence of unspecified hip joint**
Z89.9 **Acquired absence of limb, unspecified**

Z90 Acquired absence of organs, not elsewhere classified

Includes: postprocedural or post-traumatic loss of body part NEC
Excludes1: *congenital absence - see Alphabetical Index*
Excludes2: *postprocedural absence of endocrine glands (E89.-)*
Review coding guideline C.21.c.3

+ Z90.0 **Acquired absence of part of head and neck**
  Z90.01 **Acquired absence of eye**
  Z90.02 **Acquired absence of larynx**
  Z90.09 **Acquired absence of other part of head and neck**
  Acquired absence of nose
  Excludes2: *teeth (K08.1)*
+ Z90.1 **Acquired absence of breast and nipple**
  Z90.10 **Acquired absence of unspecified breast and nipple**
  Z90.11 **Acquired absence of right breast and nipple**
  Z90.12 **Acquired absence of left breast and nipple**
  Z90.13 **Acquired absence of bilateral breasts and nipples**
Z90.2 **Acquired absence of lung [part of]**
Z90.3 **Acquired absence of stomach [part of]**
+ Z90.4 **Acquired absence of other specified parts of digestive tract**
  + Z90.41 **Acquired absence of pancreas**
    Code also exocrine pancreatic insufficiency (K86.81)

    Use additional code to identify any associated:
    insulin use (Z79.4)
    diabetes mellitus, postpancreatectomy (E13.-)
    Review coding guideline C.4.a.6.b.i

Z90.410 Acquired total absence of pancreas
Acquired absence of pancreas NOS
Z90.411 Acquired partial absence of pancreas
Z90.49 Acquired absence of other specified parts of digestive tract
Z90.5 Acquired absence of kidney
Z90.6 Acquired absence of other parts of urinary tract
Acquired absence of bladder
+ Z90.7 Acquired absence of genital organ(s)
Excludes1: *personal history of sex reassignment (Z87.890)*
Excludes2: *female genital mutilation status (N90.81-)*
+ Z90.71 Acquired absence of cervix and uterus
♀ **Z90.710 Acquired absence of both cervix and uterus**
Acquired absence of uterus NOS
Status post total hysterectomy
♀ **Z90.711 Acquired absence of uterus with remaining cervical stump**
Status post partial hysterectomy with remaining cervical stump
♀ **Z90.712 Acquired absence of cervix with remaining uterus**
+ Z90.72 Acquired absence of ovaries
♀ **Z90.721 Acquired absence of ovaries, unilateral**
♀ **Z90.722 Acquired absence of ovaries, bilateral**
Z90.79 Acquired absence of other genital organ(s)
+ Z90.8 Acquired absence of other organs
Z90.81 Acquired absence of spleen
Z90.89 Acquired absence of other organs

Z91 Personal risk factors, not elsewhere classified

Excludes2: *contact with and (suspected) exposures hazardous to health (Z77.-)*
exposure to pollution and other problems related to physical environment (Z77.1-)
female genital mutilation status (N90.81-)
personal history of physical injury and trauma (Z87.81, Z87.82-)
occupational exposure to risk factors (Z57.-)

+ Z91.0 Allergy status, other than to drugs and biological substances
Excludes2: *Allergy status to drugs, medicaments, and biological substances (Z88.-)*
Review coding guideline C.21.c.3
+ Z91.01 Food allergy status
Excludes2: *food additives allergy status (Z91.02)*
Z91.010 Allergy to peanuts
Z91.011 Allergy to milk products
Excludes1: *lactose intolerance (E73.-)*
Z91.012 Allergy to eggs
Z91.013 Allergy to seafood
Allergy to shellfish
Allergy to octopus or squid ink
Z91.018 Allergy to other foods
Allergy to nuts other than peanuts
Z91.02 Food additives allergy status
+ Z91.03 Insect allergy status
Z91.030 Bee allergy status
Z91.038 Other insect allergy status
+ Z91.04 Nonmedicinal substance allergy status
Z91.040 Latex allergy status
Latex sensitivity status
Z91.041 Radiographic dye allergy status
Allergy status to contrast media used for diagnostic X-ray procedure
Z91.048 Other nonmedicinal substance allergy status
Z91.09 Other allergy status, other than to drugs and biological substances
+ Z91.1 Patient's noncompliance with medical treatment and regimen
Z91.11 Patient's noncompliance with dietary regimen
+ Z91.12 Patient's intentional underdosing of medication regimen
Code first underdosing of medication (T36-T50) with fifth or sixth character 6
Excludes1: *adverse effect of prescribed drug taken as directed- code to adverse effect*
poisoning (overdose) -code to poisoning
Review coding guideline C.19.e.5.c
Z91.120 Patient's intentional underdosing of medication regimen due to financial hardship
Z91.128 Patient's intentional underdosing of medication regimen for other reason
+ Z91.13 Patient's unintentional underdosing of medication regimen
Code first underdosing of medication (T36-T50) with fifth or sixth character 6
Excludes1: *adverse effect of prescribed drug taken as directed- code to adverse effect*
poisoning (overdose) -code to poisoning
Review coding guideline C.19.e.5.c
Z91.130 Patient's unintentional underdosing of medication regimen due to age-related debility
Z91.138 Patient's unintentional underdosing of medication regimen for other reason
Z91.14 Patient's other noncompliance with medication regimen
Patient's underdosing of medication NOS
Z91.15 Patient's noncompliance with renal dialysis
Z91.19 Patient's noncompliance with other medical treatment and regimen
Nonadherence to medical treatment
+ Z91.4 Personal history of psychological trauma, not elsewhere classified
Review coding guideline C.21.c.4
+ Z91.41 Personal history of adult abuse
Excludes2: *personal history of abuse in childhood (Z62.81-)*
• **Z91.410 Personal history of adult physical and sexual abuse**
Excludes1: *current adult physical abuse (T74.11, T76.11)*
current adult sexual abuse (T74.21-T76.11)
• **Z91.411 Personal history of adult psychological abuse**
• **Z91.412 Personal history of adult neglect**
Excludes1: *current adult neglect (T74.01, T76.01)*
• **Z91.419 Personal history of unspecified adult abuse**
Z91.49 Other personal history of psychological trauma, not elsewhere classified
Z91.5 Personal history of self-harm
Personal history of parasuicide
Personal history of self-poisoning
Personal history of suicide attempt
Review coding guideline C.21.c.4
+ Z91.8 Other specified personal risk factors, not elsewhere classified
Review coding guideline C.21.c.4
Z91.81 History of falling
At risk for falling
Review coding guideline C.18.d and C21.c.4
• **Z91.82 Personal history of military deployment**
Individual (civilian or military) with past history of military war, peacekeeping and humanitarian deployment (current or past conflict)
Returned from military deployment
Review coding guideline C.21.c.4
Z91.83 Wandering in diseases classified elsewhere
Code first underlying disorder such as:
Alzheimer's disease (G30.-)
autism or pervasive developmental disorder (F84.-)
intellectual disabilities (F70-F79)
unspecified dementia with behavioral disturbance (F03.9-)
+ Z91.84 Oral health risk factors
Review coding guideline C.21.c.14
Z91.841 Risk for dental caries, low
Z91.842 Risk for dental caries, moderate
Z91.843 Risk for dental caries, high
Z91.849 Unspecified risk for dental caries
Z91.89 Other specified personal risk factors, not elsewhere classified
AHA CC: 1Q, 2017, 45-46

Z92 Personal history of medical treatment

Excludes2: *postprocedural states (Z98.-)*
Review coding guideline C.21.c.4
Z92.0 Personal history of contraception
Excludes1: *counseling or management of current contraceptive practices (Z30.-)*
long term (current) use of contraception (Z79.3)
presence of (intrauterine) contraceptive device (Z97.5)

+ Z92.2 **Personal history of drug therapy**
Excludes2: *long term (current) drug therapy (Z79.-)*
Z92.21 **Personal history of antineoplastic chemotherapy**
Z92.22 **Personal history of monoclonal drug therapy**
Z92.23 **Personal history of estrogen therapy**
+ Z92.24 **Personal history of steroid therapy**
Z92.240 **Personal history of inhaled steroid therapy**
Z92.241 **Personal history of systemic steroid therapy**
Personal history of steroid therapy NOS
Z92.25 **Personal history of immunosupression therapy**
Excludes2: *personal history of steroid therapy (Z92.24)*
Z92.29 **Personal history of other drug therapy**
Z92.3 **Personal history of irradiation**
Personal history of exposure to therapeutic radiation
Excludes1: *exposure to radiation in the physical environment (Z77.12)*
occupational exposure to radiation (Z57.1)
+ Z92.8 **Personal history of other medical treatment**
Z92.81 **Personal history of extracorporeal membrane oxygenation (ECMO)**
Z92.82 **Status post administration of tPA (rtPA) in a different facility within the last 24 hours prior to admission to current facility**
Code first condition requiring tPA administration, such as:
acute cerebral infarction (I63.-)
acute myocardial infarction (I21.-, I22.-)
AHA CC: 4Q, 2013, 124
Review coding guideline C.21.c.3
Z92.83 **Personal history of failed moderate sedation**
Personal history of failed conscious sedation
Excludes2: *failed moderate sedation during procedure (T88.52)*
Z92.84 **Personal history of unintended awareness under general anesthesia**
Excludes2: *unintended awareness under general anesthesia during procedure (T88.53)*
AHA CC: 4Q, 2016, 72-73, 77
Z92.89 **Personal history of other medical treatment**

Z93 Artificial opening status

Excludes1: *artificial openings requiring attention or management (Z43.-)*
complications of external stoma (J95.0-, K94.-, N99.5-)
Review coding guideline C.21.c.3
Z93.0 **Tracheostomy status**
AHA CC: 4Q, 2013, 129
Z93.1 **Gastrostomy status**
Z93.2 **Ileostomy status**
Z93.3 **Colostomy status**
Z93.4 **Other artificial openings of gastrointestinal tract status**
+ Z93.5 **Cystostomy status**
Z93.50 **Unspecified cystostomy status**
Z93.51 **Cutaneous-vesicostomy status**
Z93.52 **Appendico-vesicostomy status**
Z93.59 **Other cystostomy status**
Z93.6 **Other artificial openings of urinary tract status**
Nephrostomy status
Ureterostomy status
Urethrostomy status
Z93.8 **Other artificial opening status**
Z93.9 **Artificial opening status, unspecified**

Z94 Transplanted organ and tissue status

Includes: organ or tissue replaced by heterogenous or homogenous transplant
Excludes1: *complications of transplanted organ or tissue - see Alphabetical Index*
Excludes2: *presence of vascular grafts (Z95.-)*
Review coding guideline C.21.c.3
CC Z94.0 **Kidney transplant status**
CC Exclusion see Appendix A PDX collection 1489
Review coding guideline C.14.a.2
CC Z94.1 **Heart transplant status**
Excludes1: *artificial heart status (Z95.812)*
heart-valve replacement status (Z95.2-Z95.4)
CC Exclusion see Appendix A PDX collection 1488
CC Z94.2 **Lung transplant status**
CC Exclusion see Appendix A PDX collection 1491
CC Z94.3 **Heart and lungs transplant status**
CC Exclusion see Appendix A PDX collection 1488
CC Z94.4 **Liver transplant status**
CC Exclusion see Appendix A PDX collection 1490
Z94.5 **Skin transplant status**
Autogenous skin transplant status
Z94.6 **Bone transplant status**
Z94.7 **Corneal transplant status**
+ Z94.8 **Other transplanted organ and tissue status**
CC Z94.81 **Bone marrow transplant status**
CC Exclusion see Appendix A PDX collection 1492
CC Z94.82 **Intestine transplant status**
CC Exclusion see Appendix A PDX collection 1495
CC Z94.83 **Pancreas transplant status**
CC Exclusion see Appendix A PDX collection 1496
CC Z94.84 **Stem cells transplant status**
CC Exclusion see Appendix A PDX collection 1497
Z94.89 **Other transplanted organ and tissue status**
Z94.9 **Transplanted organ and tissue status, unspecified**

Z95 Presence of cardiac and vascular implants and grafts

Excludes2: *complications of cardiac and vascular devices, implants and grafts (T82.-)*
Review coding guideline C.21.c.3
Z95.0 **Presence of cardiac pacemaker**
Presence of cardiac resynchronization therapy (CRT-P) pacemaker
Excludes1: *adjustment or management of cardiac device (Z45.0-)*
adjustment or management of cardiac pacemaker (Z45.0)
presence of automatic (implantable) cardiac defibrillator with synchronous cardiac pacemaker (Z95.810)
Z95.1 **Presence of aortocoronary bypass graft**
Presence of coronary artery bypass graft
Z95.2 **Presence of prosthetic heart valve**
Presence of heart valve NOS
Z95.3 **Presence of xenogenic heart valve**
Z95.4 **Presence of other heart-valve replacement**
Z95.5 **Presence of coronary angioplasty implant and graft**
Excludes1: *coronary angioplasty status without implant and graft (Z98.61)*
+ Z95.8 **Presence of other cardiac and vascular implants and grafts**
+ Z95.81 **Presence of other cardiac implants and grafts**
Z95.810 **Presence of automatic (implantable) cardiac defibrillator**
Presence of automatic (implantable) cardiac defibrillator with synchronous cardiac pacemaker
Presence of cardiac resynchronization therapy defibrillator (CRT-D)
Present of cardioverter-defribrillator (ICD)
CC Z95.811 **Presence of heart assist device**
CC Exclusion see Appendix A PDX collection 1498
CC Z95.812 **Presence of fully implantable artificial heart**
CC Exclusion see Appendix A PDX collection 1498
Z95.818 **Presence of other cardiac implants and grafts**
+ Z95.82 **Presence of other vascular implants and grafts**
Z95.820 **Peripheral vascular angioplasty status with implants and grafts**
Excludes1: *peripheral vascular angioplasty without implant and graft (Z98.62)*
Z95.828 **Presence of other vascular implants and grafts**
Presence of intravascular prosthesis NEC
Z95.9 **Presence of cardiac and vascular implant and graft, unspecified**

Z96 Presence of other functional implants

Excludes2: *complications of internal prosthetic devices, implants and grafts (T82-T85)*
fitting and adjustment of prosthetic and other devices (Z44-Z46)
Review coding guideline C.21.c.3

Z96.0 **Presence of urogenital implants**
Z96.1 **Presence of intraocular lens**
Presence of pseudophakia
+ **Z96.2** **Presence of otological and audiological implants**
Z96.20 **Presence of otological and audiological implant, unspecified**
Z96.21 **Cochlear implant status**
Z96.22 **Myringotomy tube(s) status**
Z96.29 **Presence of other otological and audiological implants**
Presence of bone-conduction hearing device
Presence of eustachian tube stent
Stapes replacement
Z96.3 **Presence of artificial larynx**
+ **Z96.4** **Presence of endocrine implants**
Z96.41 **Presence of insulin pump (external) (internal)**
Z96.49 **Presence of other endocrine implants**
Z96.5 **Presence of tooth-root and mandibular implants**
+ **Z96.6** **Presence of orthopedic joint implants**
Z96.60 **Presence of unspecified orthopedic joint implant**
+ **Z96.61** **Presence of artificial shoulder joint**
Z96.611 **Presence of right artificial shoulder joint**
Z96.612 **Presence of left artificial shoulder joint**
Z96.619 **Presence of unspecified artificial shoulder joint**
+ **Z96.62** **Presence of artificial elbow joint**
Z96.621 **Presence of right artificial elbow joint**
Z96.622 **Presence of left artificial elbow joint**
Z96.629 **Presence of unspecified artificial elbow joint**
+ **Z96.63** **Presence of artificial wrist joint**
Z96.631 **Presence of right artificial wrist joint**
Z96.632 **Presence of left artificial wrist joint**
Z96.639 **Presence of unspecified artificial wrist joint**
+ **Z96.64** **Presence of artificial hip joint**
Hip-joint replacement (partial) (total)
Z96.641 **Presence of right artificial hip joint**
AHA CC: 3Q, 2016, 16-17
Z96.642 **Presence of left artificial hip joint**
AHA CC: 1Q, 2015, 16-17
Z96.643 **Presence of artificial hip joint, bilateral**
Z96.649 **Presence of unspecified artificial hip joint**
+ **Z96.65** **Presence of artificial knee joint**
Z96.651 **Presence of right artificial knee joint**
Z96.652 **Presence of left artificial knee joint**
Z96.653 **Presence of artificial knee joint, bilateral**
Z96.659 **Presence of unspecified artificial knee joint**
+ **Z96.66** **Presence of artificial ankle joint**
Z96.661 **Presence of right artificial ankle joint**
Z96.662 **Presence of left artificial ankle joint**
Z96.669 **Presence of unspecified artificial ankle joint**
+ **Z96.69** **Presence of other orthopedic joint implants**
Z96.691 **Finger-joint replacement of right hand**
Z96.692 **Finger-joint replacement of left hand**
Z96.693 **Finger-joint replacement, bilateral**
Z96.698 **Presence of other orthopedic joint implants**
Z96.7 **Presence of other bone and tendon implants**
Presence of skull plate
+ **Z96.8** **Presence of other specified functional implants**
Z96.81 **Presence of artificial skin**
Z96.89 **Presence of other specified functional implants**
Z96.9 **Presence of functional implant, unspecified**

Z97 Presence of other devices

Excludes1: *complications of internal prosthetic devices, implants and grafts (T82-T85)*
fitting and adjustment of prosthetic and other devices (Z44-Z46)
Excludes2: *presence of cerebrospinal fluid drainage device (Z98.2)*
Review coding guideline C.21.c.3
Z97.0 **Presence of artificial eye**
+ **Z97.1** **Presence of artificial limb (complete) (partial)**
Z97.10 **Presence of artificial limb (complete) (partial), unspecified**
Z97.11 **Presence of artificial right arm (complete) (partial)**
Z97.12 **Presence of artificial left arm (complete) (partial)**
Z97.13 **Presence of artificial right leg (complete) (partial)**
Z97.14 **Presence of artificial left leg (complete) (partial)**
Z97.15 **Presence of artificial arms, bilateral (complete) (partial)**
Z97.16 **Presence of artificial legs, bilateral (complete) (partial)**
Z97.2 **Presence of dental prosthetic device (complete) (partial)**
Presence of dentures (complete) (partial)
Z97.3 **Presence of spectacles and contact lenses**
Z97.4 **Presence of external hearing-aid**
♀ **Z97.5** **Presence of (intrauterine) contraceptive device**
Excludes1: *checking, reinsertion or removal of implantable subdermal contraceptive (Z30.46)*
checking, reinsertion or removal of intrauterine contraceptive device (Z30.43-)
Z97.8 **Presence of other specified devices**

Z98 Other postprocedural states

Excludes2: *aftercare (Z43-Z49, Z51)*
follow-up medical care (Z08-Z09)
postprocedural complication - see Alphabetical Index
Review coding guideline C.21.c.3
Z98.0 **Intestinal bypass and anastomosis status**
Excludes2: *bariatric surgery status (Z98.84)*
gastric bypass status (Z98.84)
obesity surgery status (Z98.84)
Z98.1 **Arthrodesis status**
Z98.2 **Presence of cerebrospinal fluid drainage device**
Presence of CSF shunt
Z98.3 **Post therapeutic collapse of lung status**
Code first underlying disease
+ **Z98.4** **Cataract extraction status**
Use additional code to identify intraocular lens implant status (Z96.1)
Excludes1: *aphakia (H27.0)*
Z98.41 **Cataract extraction status, right eye**
Z98.42 **Cataract extraction status, left eye**
Z98.49 **Cataract extraction status, unspecified eye**
+ **Z98.5** **Sterilization status**
Excludes1: *female infertility (N97.-)*
male infertility (N46.-)
♀ **Z98.51** **Tubal ligation status**
● ♂ **Z98.52** **Vasectomy status**
+ **Z98.6** **Angioplasty status**
Z98.61 **Coronary angioplasty status**
Excludes1: *coronary angioplasty status with implant and graft (Z95.5)*
Z98.62 **Peripheral vascular angioplasty status**
Excludes1: *peripheral vascular angioplasty status with implant and graft (Z95.820)*
+ **Z98.8** **Other specified postprocedural states**
AHA CC: 4Q, 2016, 76
+ **Z98.81** **Dental procedure status**
Z98.810 **Dental sealant status**
Z98.811 **Dental restoration status**
Dental crown status
Dental fillings status
Z98.818 **Other dental procedure status**
Z98.82 **Breast implant status**
Excludes1: *breast implant removal status (Z98.86)*
Z98.83 **Filtering (vitreous) bleb after glaucoma surgery status**
Excludes1: *Inflammation (infection) of postprocedural bleb (H59.4-)*
Z98.84 **Bariatric surgery status**
Gastric banding status
Gastric bypass status for obesity
Obesity surgery status
Excludes1: *bariatric surgery status complicating pregnancy, childbirth, or the puerperium (O99.84)*
Excludes2: *intestinal bypass and anastomosis status (Z98.0)*
Z98.85 **Transplanted organ removal status**
Transplanted organ previously removed due to complication, failure, rejection or infection
Excludes1: *encounter for removal of transplanted organ -code to complication of transplanted organ (T86.-)*
Z98.86 **Personal history of breast implant removal**
+ **Z98.87** **Personal history of in utero procedure**

♀ **Z98.870 Personal history of in utero procedure during pregnancy**
Excludes2: *complications from in utero procedure for current pregnancy (O35.7)*
supervision of current pregnancy with history of in utero procedure during previous pregnancy (O09.82-)

Z98.871 Personal history of in utero procedure while a fetus

\+ **Z98.89 Other specified postprocedural states**

Z98.890 Other specified postprocedural states
Personal history of surgery, note elsewhere classified

Z98.891 History of uterine scar from previous surgery
Excludes1: *Maternal care due to uterine scar from previous surgery (O34.2-)*
AHA CC: 4Q, 2016, 51-52

Z99 Dependence on enabling machines and devices, not elsewhere classified
Excludes1: *cardiac pacemaker status (Z95.0)*
Review coding guideline C.21.c.3

Z99.0 Dependence on aspirator

\+ **Z99.1 Dependence on respirator**
Dependence on ventilator

CC **Z99.11 Dependence on respirator [ventilator] status**
CC Exclusion see Appendix A PDX collection 0759
AHA CC: 1Q, 2015, 21

CC **Z99.12 Encounter for respirator [ventilator] dependence during power failure**
Excludes1: *mechanical complication of respirator [ventilator] (J95.850)*
CC Exclusion see Appendix A PDX collection 0759
Review coding guideline C.21.c.16

Z99.2 Dependence on renal dialysis
Hemodialysis status
Peritoneal dialysis status
Presence of arteriovenous shunt for dialysis
Renal dialysis status NOS
Excludes1: *encounter for fitting and adjustment of dialysis catheter (Z49.0-)*
Excludes2: *noncompliance with renal dialysis (Z91.15)*

Z99.3 Dependence on wheelchair
Wheelchair confinement status
Code first cause of dependence, such as:
muscular dystrophy (G71.0)
obesity (E66.-)

\+ **Z99.8 Dependence on other enabling machines and devices**

Z99.81 Dependence on supplemental oxygen
Dependence on long-term oxygen
AHA CC: 4Q, 2013, 129

Z99.89 Dependence on other enabling machines and devices
Dependence on machine or device NOS

Appendix A: CC/MCC Exclusion Lists

Appendix A is provided online in an format suitable for spreadsheet and/or database use. Go to http://ahimapress.org/Casto5894, click the "Onlin Resources" link, and enter case-sensitive password AHIMA6uJ8f2017 to download the files.

Appendix B: Hospital-Acquired Conditions (HAC) List

Appendix B is provided online in an format suitable for spreadsheet and/or database use. Go to http://ahimapress.org/Casto5894, click the "Onlin Resources" link, and enter case-sensitive password AHIMA6uJ8f2017 to download the files.

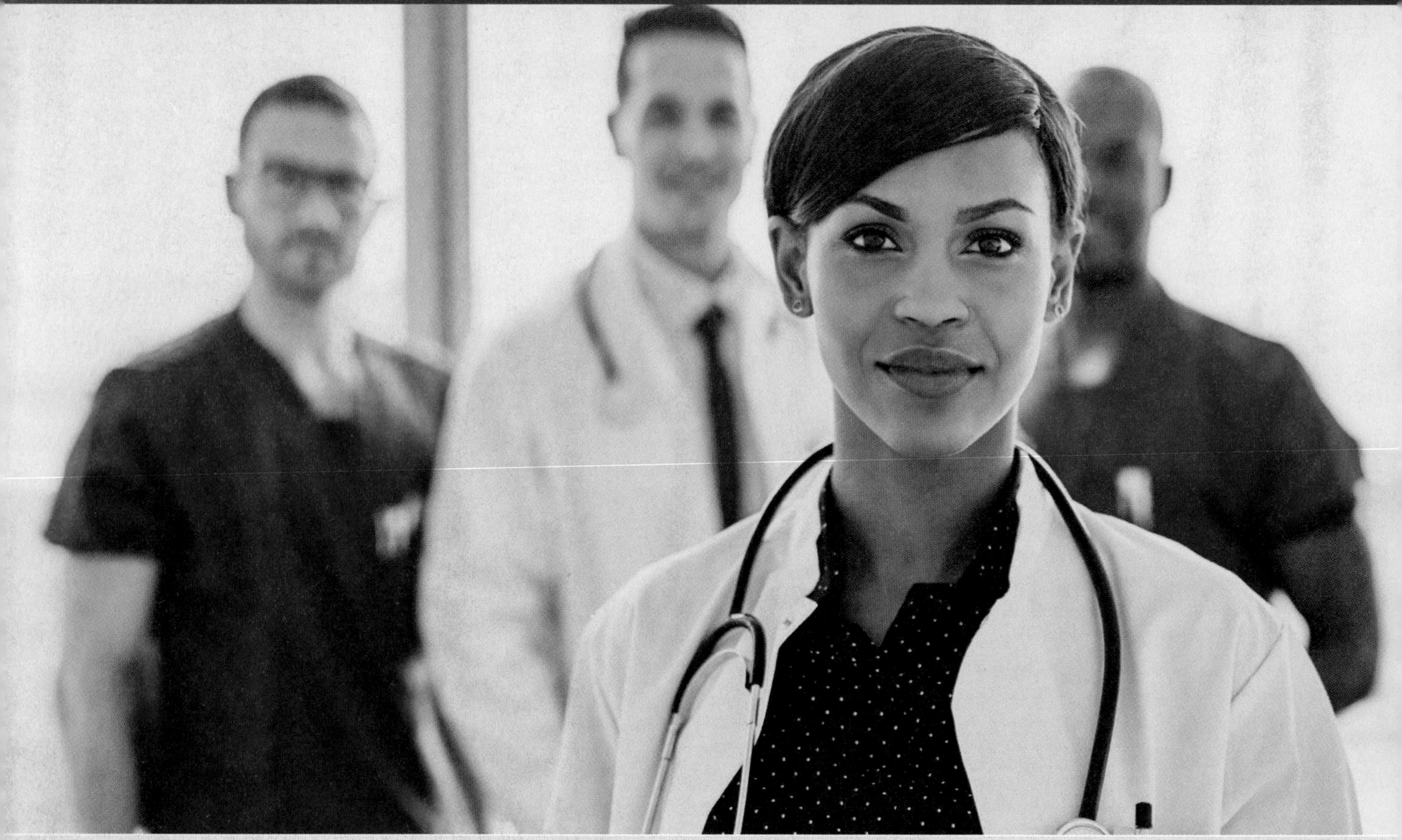